Mandell, Douglas, and Bennett's

PRINCIPLES AND PRACTICE OF
Infectious Diseases

VOLUME 1

Mandell, Douglas, and Bennett's

PRINCIPLES AND PRACTICE OF Infectious Diseases

Fifth Edition

Edited by

Gerald L. Mandell, M.D.
Professor of Medicine
Owen R. Cheatham Professor of the Sciences
Chief, Division of Infectious Diseases
University of Virginia Health Sciences Center
Charlottesville, Virginia

John E. Bennett, M.D.
Head, Clinical Mycology Section
Laboratory of Clinical Investigation
National Institute of Allergy and Infectious Diseases
National Institutes of Health
Bethesda, Maryland

Raphael Dolin, M.D.
Dean for Clinical Programs
Maxwell Finland Professor of Medicine
Harvard Medical School
Boston, Massachusetts

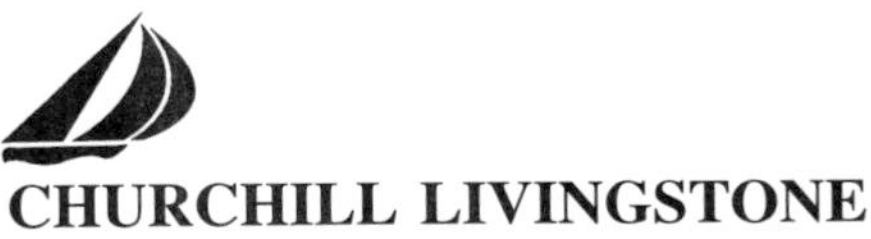

CHURCHILL LIVINGSTONE
A Harcourt Health Sciences Company
Philadelphia London Toronto Montreal Sydney Tokyo Edinburgh

CHURCHILL LIVINGSTONE
A Harcourt Health Sciences Company

The Curtis Center
Independence Square West
Philadelphia, Pennsylvania 19106

Library of Congress Cataloging-in-Publication Data

Mandell, Douglas, and Bennett's principles and practice of infectious diseases / edited by Gerald L. Mandell, John E. Bennett, Raphael Dolin.—5th ed.

p. cm.

Includes bibliographical references and index.

ISBN 0–443–07593–X

1. Communicable diseases. I. Mandell, Gerald L. II. Douglas, R. Gordon (Robert Gordon). III. Bennett, John E. (John Eugene). IV. Dolin, Raphael. V. Title: Principles and practice of infectious diseases. [DNLM: 1. Communicable Diseases. WC 100 M2713 2000]

RC111.P78 2000 616.9—dc21

DNLM/DLC 99-16736

ISBN 0–443–07593–X (set)
ISBN 0–443–07983–8 (Vol. 1)
ISBN 0–443–07524–7 (Vol. 2)

MANDELL, DOUGLAS, AND BENNETT'S PRINCIPLES AND PRACTICE OF INFECTIOUS DISEASES

Printed in the United States of America.

Last digit is the print number: 9 8 7 6 5 4 3 2 1

Contributors

N. Franklin Adkinson, Jr., M.D.
Professor of Medicine, Johns Hopkins University School of Medicine; Co-Director, Division of Allergy and Clinical Immunology, Johns Hopkins Asthma and Allergy Center, Baltimore, Maryland
β-Lactam Allergy

David M. Allen, M.D., FAMS
Adjunct Assistant Professor of Medicine, Weill Medical College of Cornell University, New York, New York; Partner and Attending Physician, ID Associates, Dallas, Texas
Acinetobacter *Species*

Harvey J. Alter, M.D.
Clinical Professor of Medicine, Georgetown University School of Medicine, Washington, DC; Chief, Infectious Diseases Section, and Associate Director, Research Department of Transfusion Medicine, Warren G. Magnuson Clinical Center, National Institutes of Health, Bethesda, Maryland
Hepatitis G Virus and TT Virus

Guy W. Amsden, Pharm.D.
Adjunct Assistant Professor, Department of Pharmacology, Columbia University College of Physicians and Surgeons, New York; Adjunct Assistant Professor, Department of Pharmacy Practice, Albany College of Pharmacy, Union University, Albany; Clinical Pharmacy Specialist and Research Scientist, Clinical Pharmacology Research Center, Bassett Healthcare, Cooperstown, New York
Pharmacokinetics and Pharmacodynamics of Anti-infective Agents; Tables of Antimicrobial Agent Pharmacology

Elias Anaissie, M.D.
Professor of Medicine and Director of Clinical Affairs, Myeloma and Transplantation Research Center, University of Arkansas Medical Sciences, Little Rock, Arkansas
Stenotrophomonas maltophilia *and* Burkholderia cepacia

Suresh J. Antony, M.D., FACP, FRCP
Assistant Professor, Texas Tech University Health Sciences Center School of Medicine; Infectious Disease Consultant, Texas Oncology Physician Associates, El Paso, Texas
Streptococcus intermedius *Group*

Michael A. Apicella, M.D.
Professor and Head, Department of Microbiology, University of Iowa College of Medicine, Iowa City, Iowa
Neisseria meningitidis

Gordon L. Archer, M.D.
Professor of Medicine and Microbiology/Immunology; Chairman, Division of Infectious Diseases, Department of Medicine, Virginia Commonwealth University School of Medicine, Richmond, Virginia
Staphylococcus epidermidis *and Other Coagulase-Negative Staphylococci*

David A. Ashford, D.V.M., M.P.H., D.Sc.
Medical Epidemiologist, Meningitis and Special Pathogens Branch, Division of Bacterial and Mycotic Diseases, Center for Infectious Diseases, Centers for Disease Control and Prevention, Atlanta, Georgia
Leptospira *Species (Leptospirosis)*

Carol J. Baker, M.D.
Professor and Head, Section of Infectious Diseases, Department of Pediatrics, and Professor, Department of Microbiology and Immunology, Baylor College of Medicine; Attending Physician, Texas Children's Hospital, Houston, Texas
Streptococcus agalactiae *(Group B Streptococcus)*

Ronald C. Ballard, Ph.D., M.I.Biol.
Associate Professor, Department of Clinical Microbiology and Infectious Diseases, School of Pathology, University of the Witwatersrand and South African Institute for Medical Research, Johannesburg, South Africa
Calymmatobacterium granulomatis *(Donovanosis, Granuloma Inguinale)*

Charles H. Ballow, M.S., Pharm.D.
Clinical Associate Professor, School of Pharmacy, State University of New York at Buffalo; Director, Antiinfectives Research, The Clinical Pharmacokinetics Laboratory, Kaleida Health/Millard Fillmore Hospital, Buffalo, New York
Pharmacokinetics and Pharmacodynamics of Anti-infective Agents

Kenneth J. Bart, M.D.
Dean, San Diego State University School of Public Health, San Diego, California
Immunization

Byron E. Batteiger, M.D.
Professor of Medicine and Microbiology and Immunology, Indiana University School of Medicine, Indianapolis, Indiana
Chlamydia trachomatis *(Trachoma, Perinatal Infections, Lymphogranuloma Venereum, and Other Genital Infections); Introduction to Chlamydial Diseases*

Stephen G. Baum, M.D.
Professor of Medicine and Microbiology and Immunology, Albert Einstein College of Medicine of Yeshiva University, Bronx; Chairman, Department of Medicine, Beth Israel Medical Center, New York, New York
Adenovirus; Introduction to Mycoplasma *Diseases; Mumps Virus;* Mycoplasma pneumoniae *and Atypical Pneumonia*

Arnold S. Bayer, M.D.
Professor of Medicine, University of California, Los Angeles, UCLA School of Medicine, Los Angeles; Associate Chief, Adult Infectious Diseases, Harbor–UCLA Medical Center, Torrance, California
Endocarditis and Intravascular Infections

John E. Bennett, M.D.
Head, Clinical Mycology Section, Laboratory of Clinical Investigation, National Institute of Allergy and Infectious Diseases, National Institutes of Health, Bethesda, Maryland
Antifungal Agents; Introduction to Mycoses; Miscellaneous Fungi and Prototheca

Joseph S. Bertino, Jr., Pharm.D.
Associate Professor of Clinical Pharmacology (in Medicine), Columbia University College of Physicians and Surgeons, New York; Co-Director, Clinical Pharmacology Research Center, Bassett Healthcare, Cooperstown, New York
Pharmacokinetics and Pharmacodynamics of Anti-infective Agents

Alan L. Bisno, M.D.
Professor and Vice-Chairman, Department of Medicine, University of Miami School of Medicine; Chief, Medical Service, Veterans Affairs Medical Center, Miami, Florida
Classification of Streptococci; Nonsuppurative Poststreptococcal Sequelae: Rheumatic Fever and Glomerulonephritis; Pharyngitis; Streptococcus pyogenes *(Including Streptococcal Toxic Shock Syndrome and Necrotizing Fasciitis)*

Martin J. Blaser, M.D.
Addison B. Scoville Professor of Medicine and Professor of Microbiology and Immunology, and Director, Division of Infectious Diseases, Vanderbilt University School of Medicine; Staff Physician, Veterans Affairs Medical Center, Nashville, Tennessee
Campylobacter jejuni *and Related Species;* Helicobacter pylori *and Related Organisms*

Thomas P. Bleck, M.D.
Louise Nerancy Professor of Neurology and Professor of Neurological Surgery and Internal Medicine, University of Virginia School of Medicine; Director, Neuroscience Intensive Care Unit, University of Virginia Hospital, Charlottesville, Virginia
Approach to the Patient with Central Nervous System Infection; Clostridium botulinum *(Botulism);* Clostridium tetani *(Tetanus); Epidural Abscess; Rabies Virus; Subdural Empyema; Suppurative Intracranial Phlebitis*

David A. Bobak, M.D.
Associate Professor of Medicine and Microbiology, University of Virginia School of Medicine; Director, Traveler's Clinic, and Attending Physician, University of Virginia Health Sciences Center, Charlottesville, Virginia
Nausea, Vomiting, and Noninflammatory Diarrhea

William Bonnez, M.D.
Associate Professor of Medicine, University of Rochester School of Medicine and Dentistry; Attending Physician, Department of Medicine, Strong Memorial Hospital, Rochester, New York
Papillomaviruses

R.C. Boucher, M.D.
Professor of Medicine, University of North Carolina at Chapel Hill School of Medicine; Director, Division of Pulmonary/Critical Care Medicine, and Director, Cystic Fibrosis/Pulmonary Research and Treatment Center, UNC Hospitals, Chapel Hill, North Carolina
Cystic Fibrosis

Barry D. Brause, M.D.
Clinical Professor of Medicine, Weill Medical College of Cornell University; Attending Physician, New York Presbyterian Hospital–Cornell Campus, and Hospital for Special Surgery, New York, New York
Infections with Prostheses in Bones and Joints

Arthur E. Brown, M.D.
Professor of Clinical Medicine and Pediatrics, Weill Medical College of Cornell University; Attending Physician, Infectious Disease Service, Memorial Sloan-Kettering Cancer Center; Attending Physician, New York Presbyterian Hospital–Cornell Campus; and Visiting Associate Physician, The Rockefeller University Hospital, New York, New York
Other Corynebacteria and Rhodococcus

Barbara A. Brown, M.S., MT, ASCP, SM
Senior Research Scientist and Supervisor, Mycobacteria/Nocardia Laboratory; Study Coordinator, Mycobacterial Clinical Trials, University of Texas Health Center, Tyler, Texas
Infections Due to Nontuberculous Mycobacteria

Eric J. Brown, M.D.
Professor, Program in Microbial Pathogenesis and Host Defense, University of California, San Francisco, School of Medicine, San Francisco, California
Cell-Mediated Immunity in Host Defense against Infectious Diseases

Kevin E. Brown, M.D.
Visiting Scientist, Hematology Branch, National Heart, Lung and Blood Institute, National Institutes of Health, Bethesda, Maryland
Parvovirus B19

Patricia D. Brown, M.D.
Assistant Professor of Medicine, Department of Internal Medicine, Division of Infectious Diseases, Wayne State University School of Medicine, Detroit, Michigan
Infections in Injection Drug Users

Ralph T. Bryan, M.D.
Clinical Associate Professor of Medicine, University of New Mexico School of Medicine, Albuquerque, New Mexico; Medical Epidemiologist, National Center for Infectious Diseases, Centers for Disease Control and Prevention, Atlanta, Georgia
Microsporidia

Richard E. Bryant, M.D.
Professor of Medicine (Emeritus), Department of Medicine, Infectious Diseases Division, Oregon Health Sciences University School of Medicine, Portland, Oregon
Pleural Effusion and Empyema

James E. Burns, M.D., M.B.A.
Attending Physician, University of Virginia Health System, Department of Pediatrics, Division of Infectious Diseases, Charlottesville, Virginia
Epiglottitis

Larry M. Bush, M.D., FACP
Chief of Staff and Chairman, Infectious Diseases, JFK Medical Center, West Palm Beach, Florida; formerly Assistant Clinical Professor of Medicine, Medical College of Pennsylvania (now MCP–Hahnemann School of Medicine), Philadelphia, Pennsylvania
Peritonitis and Other Intra-abdominal Infections

Thomas Butler, M.D.
Professor of Internal Medicine, Texas Tech University Health Sciences Center School of Medicine; Chief of Infectious Diseases, Department of Internal Medicine, University Medical Center, Lubbock, Texas
Yersinia *Species, Including Plague*

Jason Calhoun, M.D., FACS
Professor and Chair, Department of Orthopedics and Rehabilitation, University of Texas Medical Branch, University of Texas Medical School at Galveston, Galveston, Texas
Osteomyelitis

Ellis S. Caplan, M.D.
Associate Professor of Medicine, Program in Traumatology, University of Maryland School of Medicine; Chief, Section of Infectious Diseases, R. A. Cowley Shock Trauma Center, Baltimore, Maryland
Hyperbaric Oxygen; Multiple Trauma

Charles C. J. Carpenter, M.D.
Professor of Medicine, Brown University School of Medicine, Providence, Rhode Island
Other Pathogenic Vibrios

Mary T. Caserta, M.D.
Assistant Professor of Pediatrics, University of Rochester School of Medicine and Dentistry; Attending Physician, Department of Pediatrics, Strong Memorial Hospital, Rochester, New York
Acute Laryngitis

Richard E. Chaisson, M.D.
Professor of Medicine, Epidemiology, and International Health, Johns Hopkins University School of Medicine, Baltimore, Maryland
Gastrointestinal and Hepatobiliary Manifestations of Human Immunodeficiency Virus Infection; General Clinical Manifestations of Human Immunodeficiency Virus Infection (Including Oral, Cutaneous, Renal, Ocular, and Cardiac Diseases)

Henry F. Chambers, M.D.
Professor of Medicine, University of California, San Francisco, School of Medicine; Chief, Infectious Diseases, San Francisco General Hospital, San Francisco, California
Other β-Lactam Antibiotics; Penicillins

Stanley W. Chapman, M.D.
Professor of Medicine and Associate Professor of Microbiology, University of Mississippi School of Medicine; Director, Division of Infectious Diseases, University of Mississippi Medical Center, Jackson, Mississippi
Blastomyces dermatitidis

Linda A. Chiarello, R.N., M.S.
Hospital Infections Program, National Center for Infectious Diseases, Centers for Disease Control and Prevention, Atlanta, Georgia
Human Immunodeficiency Virus in Health Care Settings

Anthony W. Chow, M.D., FRCPC, FACP
Professor of Medicine and Director, MD/PhD Program, Faculty of Medicine and Graduate Studies, University of British Columbia; Consultant, Division of Infectious Diseases, Department of Medicine, Vancouver Hospital and Health Sciences Centre, Vancouver, British Columbia, Canada
Infections of the Oral Cavity, Neck, and Head

Jeffrey D. Chulay, M.D., DTM&H
Principal Clinical Program Head, HIV and Opportunistic Infections Clinical Development, Glaxo Wellcome Inc., Research Triangle Park, North Carolina
Treponema *Species (Yaws, Pinta, Bejel)*

Claudia Cicala, Ph.D.
Staff Scientist, National Institute of Allergy and Infectious Diseases, National Institutes of Health, Bethesda, Maryland
The Immunology of Human Immunodeficiency Virus Infection

H. Fred Clark, D.V.M., Ph.D.
Research Professor of Pediatrics, University of Pennsylvania School of Medicine, Philadelphia, Pennsylvania
Rotavirus

Rebecca A. Clark, M.D., Ph.D.
Associate Professor of Medicine, Tulane University School of Medicine; HIV Division Director, HIV Outpatient Program, Tulane University Hospital, New Orleans, Louisiana
Human Immunodeficiency Virus Infection in Women

Robert A. Clark, M.D.
Professor and Chairman, Department of Medicine, and Dan F. Parman Distinguished Chair in Medicine, University of Texas Medical School at San Antonio; Attending Physician, South Texas Veterans Health System and University Hospital, San Antonio, Texas
Granulocytic Phagocytes

Myron S. Cohen, M.D.
Professor of Medicine and Microbiology and Epidemiology, University of North Carolina at Chapel Hill School of Medicine; Chief, Division of Infectious Diseases, and Director, UNC Center for Infectious Diseases, Chapel Hill, North Carolina
The Acutely Ill Patient with Fever and Rash

Oren Cohen, M.D.
Assistant Director for Medical Affairs, National Institute of Allergy and Infectious Diseases, National Institutes of Health, Bethesda, Maryland
The Immunology of Human Immunodeficiency Virus Infection

Susan E. Cohn, M.D., M.P.H.
Associate Professor of Medicine, University of Rochester School of Medicine and Dentistry, Rochester, New York
Human Immunodeficiency Virus Infection in Women

Lawrence Corey, M.D.
Professor of Laboratory Medicine and Medicine, University of Washington School of Medicine; Head, Virology Division, University of Washington Medical Center, and Head, Program in Infectious Diseases, Fred Hutchinson Cancer Research Center, Seattle, Washington
Herpes Simplex Virus

J. Thomas Cross, Jr., M.D., M.P.H.
Associate Professor, Department of Internal Medicine, Division of Infectious Diseases, and Department of Pediatrics, Louisiana State University School of Medicine in Shreveport, Shreveport, Louisiana
Francisella tularensis *(Tularemia)*

Kent B. Crossley, M.D.
Professor of Medicine, University of Minnesota Medical School–Minneapolis; Chief, Education Service, Minneapolis Veterans Affairs Medical Center, Minneapolis, Minnesota
Infections in the Elderly

Clyde S. Crumpacker, M.D.
Professor of Medicine, Harvard Medical School; Attending Physician, Infectious Diseases Division, Beth Israel Deaconess Medical Center, Boston, Massachusetts
Cytomegalovirus

James W. Curran, M.D., M.P.H.
Professor of Epidemiology and Dean, Rollins School of Public Health of Emory University, Atlanta, Georgia
Epidemiology and Prevention of Acquired Immunodeficiency Syndrome and Human Immunodeficiency Virus Infection

Rabih O. Darouiche, M.D.
Associate Professor, Departments of Physical Medicine and Rehabilitation and Medicine, and Director, Center for Prostheses Infection, Baylor College of Medicine; Staff Physician, Spinal Cord Injury and Medical Services, Infectious Disease Section, Veterans Affairs Medical Center, Houston, Texas
Infections in Patients with Spinal Cord Injuries

George S. Deepe, Jr., M.D.
Morgan Professor of Medicine, University of Cincinnati College of Medicine; Chief, Division of Infectious Diseases, University Hospital, Cincinnati, Ohio
Histoplasma capsulatum

Carlos Del Rio, M.D.
Associate Professor of Medicine (Infectious Diseases), Emory University School of Medicine, and Adjunct Associate Professor of International Health, Rollins School of Public Health of Emory University; Associate Director of Clinical Activities, Grady Memorial Hospital and the Ponce de Leon Center, Atlanta, Georgia
Epidemiology and Prevention of Acquired Immunodeficiency Syndrome and Human Immunodeficiency Virus Infection; Other Gram-Negative Bacilli

Lisa M. Demeter, M.D.
Assistant Professor of Medicine and Microbiology and Immunology, University of Rochester School of Medicine and Dentistry, Rochester, New York
Detection of Human Immunodeficiency Virus Infection; JC, BK, and Other Polyomaviruses; Progressive Multifocal Leukoencephalopathy

David W. Denning, M.B.B.S., FRCP, FRCPath
Senior Lecturer in Medicine (Infectious Diseases), University of Manchester; Consultant in Infectious Diseases, North Manchester General and Hope Hospitals, Manchester, England
Aspergillus *species*

Peter Densen, M.D.
Professor of Internal Medicine and Associate Dean, University of Iowa College of Medicine, Iowa City, Iowa
Complement

Ben E. De Pauw, M.D., Ph.D.
Professor of Medicine for Supportive Care, Catholic University; Head, Blood Transfusion Service and Clinical Department of Hematology, University Hospital St. Radboud, Nijmegen, The Netherlands
Infections in the Immunocompromised Host: General Principles; Infections in Patients with Acute Leukemia and Lymphoma

Terence S. Dermody, M.D.
Associate Professor of Pediatrics and Microbiology and Immunology and Director, Elizabeth B. Lamb Center for Pediatric Research, Vanderbilt University School of Medicine, Nashville, Tennessee
Introduction to Viruses and Viral Diseases

Richard D. Diamond, M.D.
Professor of Medicine and Research and Professor of Biochemistry, Boston University School of Medicine; Attending Physician, Section of Infectious Diseases, Boston Medical Center, Boston, Massachusetts
Cryptococcus neoformans

William E. Dismukes, M.D.
Professor and Vice-Chairman, Department of Medicine, and Director, Division of Infectious Diseases, University of Alabama School of Medicine; Director, Internal Medicine Residency Training Program, University of Alabama at Birmingham Medical Center, Birmingham, Alabama
Chronic Pneumonia

Raphael Dolin, M.D.
Professor of Medicine and Dean for Clinical Programs, Harvard Medical School, Boston, Massachusetts
Astroviruses, Toroviruses, and Picobirnaviruses; Norwalk Virus and Other Caliciviruses; Vaccines for Human Immunodeficiency Virus Infection

J. Peter Donnelly, B.Sc., Ph.D.
Microbiologist, Division of Hematology, University Hospital, Nijmegen, The Netherlands
Infections in the Immunocompromised Host: General Principles

Gerald R. Donowitz, M.D.
Professor of Medicine, University of Virginia School of Medicine; Attending Physician, Department of Internal Medicine, Division of Infectious Diseases, University of Virginia Health Sciences Center, Charlottesville, Virginia
Acute Pneumonia; Oxazolidinones

J. Stephen Dumler, M.D.
Associate Professor, Departments of Pathology and Molecular Microbiology and Immunology, and Cellular and Molecular Medicine, Johns Hopkins University School of Medicine and School of Hygiene and Public Health; Director, Division of Medical Microbiology, Department of Pathology, Johns Hopkins Hospital, Baltimore, Maryland
Ehrlichia chaffeensis *(Human Monocytotropic Ehrlichiosis),* Ehrlichia phagocytophila *(Human Granulocytotropic Ehrlichiosis), and Other Ehrlichiae;* Rickettsia typhi *(Murine Typhus)*

J. Stephen Dummer, M.D.
Professor of Medicine, Vanderbilt University School of Medicine; Director, Transplant Infectious Diseases, The Transplant Center, Vanderbilt University Hospital, Nashville, Tennessee
Infections in Solid Organ Transplant Recipients; Risk Factors and Approaches to Infections in Transplant Recipients

Herbert L. DuPont, M.D.
H. Irving Schweppe, Jr., M.D. Chair in Internal Medicine, Baylor College of Medicine, and Mary W. Kelsey Professor, University of Texas Medical School at Houston; Chief, Internal Medicine Service, St. Luke's Episcopal Hospital, Houston, Texas
Shigella *Species (Bacillary Dysentery)*

David T. Durack, M.B., D.Phil., FRCP, FRACP, FACP
Consulting Professor of Medicine, Duke University School of Medicine, Durham, North Carolina; Worldwide Medical Director, Becton Dickinson Microbiology Systems, Sparks, Maryland
Fever of Unknown Origin; Prophylaxis of Infective Endocarditis

Michael B. Edmond, M.D., M.P.H.
Associate Professor and Associate Chair for Education, Department of Internal Medicine, Virginia Commonwealth University School of Medicine; Hospital Epidemiologist, Medical College of Virginia Hospitals, Richmond, Virginia
Isolation; Organization for Infection Control

John E. Edwards, Jr., M.D.
Professor of Medicine, University of California, Los Angeles, UCLA School of Medicine, Los Angeles; Chief, Division of Infectious Diseases, Harbor/UCLA Medical Center, Torrance, California
Candida *Species*

Morven S. Edwards, M.D.
Professor of Pediatrics, Baylor College of Medicine; Attending Physician, Texas Children's Hospital, Houston, Texas
Streptococcus agalactiae *(Group B Streptococcus)*

Barry I. Eisenstein, M.D.
Professor of Medicine, Harvard Medical School; Vice President, Office of Science and Technology, Beth Israel Deaconess Medical Center, Boston, Massachusetts
Enterobacteriaceae; Introduction to Bacterial Diseases

Jerrold J. Ellner, M.D.
Professor of Medicine, Case Western Reserve University School of Medicine; Executive Vice Chair, Department of Medicine, University Hospitals of Cleveland, Cleveland, Ohio
Chronic Meningitis; Mycobacterium avium *Complex*

Suzanne U. Emerson, Ph.D.
Head, Molecular Hepatitis Section, Laboratory of Infectious Diseases, National Institute of Allergy and Infectious Diseases, National Institutes of Health, Bethesda, Maryland
Hepatitis E Virus

N. Cary Engleberg, M.D.
Professor and Chief, Division of Infectious Diseases, Department of Internal Medicine, University of Michigan Medical School, Ann Arbor, Michigan
Chronic Fatigue Syndrome

Lawrence M. Fagan, M.D., Ph.D.
Co-Director, Medical Informatics Training Program, and Associate Director for External Affairs, Stanford Medical Informatics, Stanford University School of Medicine, Stanford, California
The Infectious Diseases Physician and the Internet

Stanley Falkow, Ph.D.
Professor of Microbiology and Immunology, Stanford University School of Medicine, Stanford, California
A Molecular Perspective of Microbial Pathogenicity

Judith Falloon, M.D.
Senior Investigator, National Institute of Allergy and Infectious Diseases, National Institutes of Health, Bethesda, Maryland
Pulmonary Manifestations of Human Immunodeficiency Virus Infection

Barry M. Farr, M.D., M.Sc.
Professor of Medicine, Division of Epidemiology, University of Virginia School of Medicine, Charlottesville, Virginia
Rifamycins

W. Edmund Farrar, M.D.
Professor Emeritus of Medicine, Medical University of South Carolina College of Medicine, Charleston, South Carolina
Erysipelothrix rhusiopathiae

Anthony S. Fauci, M.D.
Director, National Institute of Allergy and Infectious Diseases, National Institutes of Health, Bethesda, Maryland
The Immunology of Human Immunodeficiency Virus Infection

Daniel P. Fedorko, Ph.D.
Senior Staff Microbiologist, Department of Clinical Pathology, Warren G. Magnuson Clinical Center, National Institutes of Health, Bethesda, Maryland
The Clinician and the Microbiology Laboratory

Stephen M. Feinstone, M.D.
Chief, Laboratory of Hepatitis Viruses, Center for Biologic Evaluation and Research, Food and Drug Administration, Bethesda, Maryland
Acute Viral Hepatitis; Hepatitis A Virus

Robert Fekety, M.D.
Professor Emeritus of Internal Medicine, University of Michigan Medical School; Attending Physician, Division of Infectious Diseases, Department of Internal Medicine, University of Michigan Health System, Ann Arbor, Michigan
Vancomycin, Teicoplanin, and the Streptogramins: Quinupristin and Dalfopristin

Jo-David Fine, M.D.
Professor of Dermatology and Clinical Professor of Epidemiology, University of North Carolina at Chapel Hill School of Medicine; Attending Physician, UNC Hospitals; Principal Investigator and Head, National Epidermolysis Bullosa Registry, Chapel Hill, North Carolina
The Acutely Ill Patient with Fever and Rash

Steven M. Fine, M.D., Ph.D.
Senior Instructor in Medicine, Infectious Diseases Unit, University of Rochester School of Medicine and Dentistry; Attending Physician, Strong Memorial Hospital, Rochester, New York
Vesicular Stomatitis and Related Viruses

Sydney M. Finegold, M.D.
Professor of Medicine and Microbiology and Immunology, University of California, Los Angeles, UCLA School of Medicine; Staff Physician, Infectious Diseases Section, Veterans Affairs Medical Center West Los Angeles, Los Angeles, California
Anaerobic Bacteria: General Concepts; Lung Abscess; Metronidazole

Anthony E. Fiore, M.D.
Medical Epidemiologist, Division of Viral and Rickettsial Diseases, National Center for Infectious Diseases, Centers for Disease Control and Prevention, Atlanta, Georgia
Multiple Trauma

Neil O. Fishman, M.D.
Assistant Professor of Medicine, University of Pennsylvania School of Medicine; Director, Antimicrobial Management Program, University of Pennsylvania Health System, Philadelphia, Pennsylvania
Antimicrobial Management and Cost Containment

Michael O. Frank, M.D.
Associate Professor of Medicine, Division of Infectious Diseases, Medical College of Wisconsin, Milwaukee, Wisconsin
Immunomodulators

John Galgiani, M.D.
Professor of Medicine and Director, Valley Fever Center for Excellence, University of Arizona; Program Director, Infectious Diseases, Veterans Affairs Medical Center, Tucson, Arizona
Coccidioides immitis

Joel E. Gallant, M.D., M.P.H.
Associate Professor of Medicine, Division of Infectious Diseases, Johns Hopkins University School of Medicine; Director, Moore HIV Clinic, Johns Hopkins Hospital, Baltimore, Maryland
Global Perspectives on Human Immunodeficiency Virus Infection and Acquired Immunodeficiency Syndrome

John I. Gallin, M.D.
Director, Warren G. Magnuson Clinical Center, and Chief, Laboratory of Host Defenses, National Institute of Allergy and Infectious Diseases, National Institutes of Health, Bethesda, Maryland
Evaluation of the Patient with Suspected Immunodeficiency

Robert C. Gallo, M.D.
Institute of Human Virology, University of Maryland School of Medicine, Baltimore, Maryland
Human Immunodeficiency Viruses

Robert H. Gelber, M.D.
Clinical Professor of Medicine and Dermatology, University of California, San Francisco, School of Medicine; Attending Physician, San Francisco General Hospital, San Francisco, California
Mycobacterium leprae *(Leprosy, Hansen's Disease)*

Jeffrey A. Gelfand, M.D.
Professor of Medicine and Dean for Research, Tufts University School of Medicine; Senior Vice President, Research and Technology, New England Medical Center, Boston, Massachusetts
Babesia

Julie Louise Gerberding, M.D., M.P.H.
Hospital Infections Program, National Center for Infectious Diseases, Centers for Disease Control and Prevention, Atlanta, Georgia
Human Immunodeficiency Virus in Health Care Settings

Anne A. Gershon, M.D.
Professor of Pediatrics and Director, Pediatric Infectious Diseases, Columbia University College of Physicians and Surgeons, New York, New York
Measles Virus (Rubeola); Rubella Virus (German Measles)

David N. Gilbert, M.D.
Professor of Medicine, Oregon Health Sciences University School of Medicine; Director, Medical Education and Earle A. Chiles Research Institute, Providence Portland Medical Center, Portland, Oregon
Aminoglycosides

Vee J. Gill, Ph.D.
Special Expert, Microbiology, Microbiology Service, Department of Clinical Pathology, Warren G. Magnuson Clinical Center, National Institutes of Health, Bethesda, Maryland
Capnocytophaga; *The Clinician and the Microbiology Laboratory*

P. H. Gilligan, Ph.D.
Professor, Departments of Microbiology and Immunology and Pathology and Laboratory Medicine, University of North Carolina at Chapel Hill School of Medicine; Director, Clinical Microbiology/Immunology Laboratory, UNC Hospitals, Chapel Hill, North Carolina
Cystic Fibrosis

Howard S. Gold, M.D.
Instructor, Harvard Medical School; Attending Physician, Division of Infectious Diseases, Department of Medicine, Beth Israel Deaconess Medical Center, Boston, Massachusetts
Introduction to Bacterial Diseases

Ellie J. C. Goldstein, M.D.
Clinical Professor of Medicine, University of California, Los Angeles, UCLA School of Medicine, Los Angeles; Director, R. M. Alden Research Laboratory, Santa Monica–UCLA Medical Center; Private Practice, Santa Monica, California
Bites

Linnie M. Golightly, M.D.
Assistant Professor of Medicine, Division of International Medicine and Infectious Diseases, Weill Medical College of Cornell University; Assistant Attending Physician, New York Presbyterian Hospital–Cornell Campus, New York, New York
Borrelia *Species (Relapsing Fever)*

Eduardo Gotuzzo, M.D.
Professor, Universidad Peruana Cayetano Heredia; Head, Infectious Disease Department, Hospital Nacional Cayetano Heredia, Lima, Peru
Vibrio cholerae

Paul S. Graman, M.D.
Associate Professor of Medicine, University of Rochester School of Medicine and Dentistry; Attending Physician, and Clinical Director, Infectious Diseases Unit, Strong Memorial Hospital, Rochester, New York
Esophagitis

J. Thomas Grayston, M.D.
Professor, Department of Epidemiology, School of Public Health and Community Medicine, University of Washington, Seattle, Washington
Chlamydia pneumoniae

John E. Greenlee, M.D.
Professor and Vice-Chair, Department of Neurology, University of Utah School of Medicine; Chief, Neurology Service, Veterans Affairs Medical Center, Salt Lake City, Utah
Approach to the Patient with Central Nervous System Infection; Epidural Abscess; Subdural Empyema; Suppurative Intracranial Phlebitis

Diane E. Griffin, M.D., Ph.D.
Professor and Chair, Department of Molecular Microbiology and Immunology, Johns Hopkins University School of Hygiene and Public Health, and Professor of Medicine and Neurology, Johns Hopkins University School of Medicine, Baltimore, Maryland
Encephalitis, Myelitis, and Neuritis

Barbara M. Gripshover, M.D.
Assistant Professor of Medicine, Case Western Reserve University School of Medicine; Medical Director, John T. Carey Special Immunology Unit, University Hospitals of Cleveland, Cleveland, Ohio
Chronic Meningitis

David I. Grove, M.D.
Clinical Professor, Departments of Medicine and Microbiology, University of Adelaide; Director, Departments of Clinical Microbiology and Infectious Diseases, The Queen Elizabeth Hospital, Adelaide, South Australia, Australia
Tissue Nematodes (Trichinosis, Dracunculiasis, Filariasis)

Richard L. Guerrant, M.D.
Thomas H. Hunter Professor of International Medicine, Department of Medicine, University of Virginia School of Medicine; Chief, Division of Geographic and International Medicine, and Director, Office of International Health, University of Virginia Hospital, Charlottesville, Virginia
Enteric Fever and Other Causes of Abdominal Symptoms with Fever; Inflammatory Enteritides; Nausea, Vomiting, and Noninflammatory Diarrhea; Principles and Syndromes of Enteric Infection; Tropical Sprue/Enteropathy

Ian D. Gust, M.D.
Professor, Monash University Faculty of Medicine, Chadstone; Professional Associate, University of Melbourne Faculty of Medicine, Dentistry and Health Sciences, Parkville; Director, Research and Development, CSL Limited, Parkville, Victoria, Australia
Hepatitis A Virus

Jack M. Gwaltney, Jr., M.D.
Wade Hampton Frost Professor of Internal Medicine, Department of Medicine, University of Virginia School of Medicine; Head, Division of Epidemiology and Virology, and Director, Center for the Prevention of Disease and Injury, University of Virginia Health Sciences Center, Charlottesville, Virginia
Acute Bronchitis; The Common Cold; Pharyngitis; Rhinovirus; Sinusitis

David W. Haas, M.D.
Associate Professor of Medicine, Vanderbilt University School of Medicine; Director, Clinical Infectious Diseases Services, Vanderbilt University Medical Center, Nashville, Tennessee
Mycobacterium tuberculosis

Caroline Breese Hall, M.D.
Professor of Pediatrics and Medicine in Infectious Diseases, University of Rochester School of Medicine and Dentistry, Rochester, New York
Acute Laryngotracheobronchitis (Croup); Bronchiolitis; Respiratory Syncytial Virus

W. Lee Hand, M.D.
Professor and Assistant Dean for Research, Department of Internal Medicine, Texas Tech University Health Sciences Center School of Medicine, El Paso, Texas
Haemophilus *Species (Including Chancroid)*

H. Hunter Handsfield, M.D.
Professor of Medicine, University of Washington School of Medicine; Director, STD Control Program, Public Health–Seattle and King County, Seattle, Washington
Neisseria gonorrhoeae

George J. Hanna, M.D.
Research Fellow in Medicine, Harvard Medical School; Clinical and Research Fellow in Medicine, Massachusetts General Hospital, Boston, Massachusetts
Antiretroviral Therapy of Human Immunodeficiency Virus Infection

Barry J. Hartman, M.D.
Clinical Professor of Medicine, Weill Medical College of Cornell University; Attending Physician, New York Presbyterian Hospital–Cornell Campus, New York, New York
Acinetobacter *Species*

M. Shahbaz Hasan, M.B.B.S.
Assistant Professor, Department of Internal Medicine, University of Texas Southwestern Medical Center at Dallas Southwestern Medical School; Staff Physician, Dallas Veterans Affairs Medical Center, Dallas, Texas
Infectious Arthritis

Diane V. Havlir, M.D.
Associate Professor, Division of Infectious Disease, Department of Medicine, University of California, San Diego, School of Medicine, La Jolla, California
Mycobacterium avium *Complex*

Roderick J. Hay, D.M., FRCP, FRCPath
Mary Dunhill Professor of Cutaneous Medicine, St. John's Institute of Dermatology, Guys, King's and St. Thomas School of Medicine (KCL), London, England
Dermatophytosis and Other Superficial Mycoses

Frederick G. Hayden, M.D.
Stuart S. Richardson Professor of Clinical Virology and Professor of Internal Medicine and Pathology, University of Virginia School of Medicine; Associate Director, Clinical Microbiology Laboratory, University of Virginia Health Sciences Center, Charlottesville, Virginia
Antiviral Drugs (Other Than Antiretrovirals)

Craig W. Hedberg, Ph.D.
Acute Disease Epidemiology Section, Minnesota Department of Health, Minneapolis, Minnesota
Epidemiologic Principles

Frederick P. Heinzel, M.D.
Associate Professor, Department of Medicine, Division of Geographic Medicine, Case Western Reserve University School of Medicine; Staff Physician, Veterans Affairs Medical Center, Cleveland, Ohio
Antibodies

David K. Henderson, M.D.
Deputy Director, Warren G. Magnuson Clinical Center, National Institutes of Health, Bethesda, Maryland
Infections Due to Percutaneous Intravascular Devices; Nosocomial Herpesvirus Infections

J. Owen Hendley, M.D.
Professor of Pediatrics, University of Virginia School of Medicine; Attending Physician, Department of Pediatrics, Division of Pediatric Infectious Diseases, University of Virginia Health System, Charlottesville, Virginia
Epiglottitis

Erik L. Hewlett, M.D.
Professor of Medicine and Pharmacology and Associate Dean for Research, University of Virginia School of Medicine, Charlottesville, Virginia
Bordetella *Species; Toxins*

Adrian V. S. Hill, D.Phil., D.M.
Professor of Human Genetics, University of Oxford; Noffield Department of Medicine, John Radcliffe Hospital, Oxford, England
Human Genetics and Infection

David R. Hill, M.D.
Associate Professor, Department of Medicine, Division of Infectious Diseases, University of Connecticut School of Medicine; Director, International Travelers' Medical Service, University of Connecticut Health Center, Farmington, Connecticut
Giardia lamblia

Alan R. Hinman, M.D., M.P.H.
Senior Consultant for Public Health Programs, Task Force for Child Survival and Development, Decatur, Georgia
Immunization

Martin S. Hirsch, M.D.
Professor of Medicine, Harvard Medical School; Director, AIDS Clinical Research, Massachusetts General Hospital, Boston, Massachusetts
Antiretroviral Therapy of Human Immunodeficiency Virus Infection

Monto Ho, M.D.
Professor of Medicine and Microbiology and Pathology, Emeritus, Graduate School of Public Health and School of Medicine, University of Pittsburgh, Pittsburgh, Pennsylvania
Infections in Solid Organ Transplant Recipients; Risk Factors and Approaches to Infections in Transplant Recipients

Steven M. Holland, M.D.
Investigator and Head, Immunopathogenesis Unit, Clinical Pathophysiology Section, Laboratory of Host Defenses, National Institute of Allergy and Infectious Diseases, National Institutes of Health, Bethesda, Maryland
Evaluation of the Patient with Suspected Immunodeficiency

Robert G. Holloway, Jr., M.D., M.P.H.
Assistant Professor of Neurology and Community and Preventive Medicine, University of Rochester School of Medicine and Dentistry, Rochester, New York
Neurologic Manifestations of Human Immunodeficiency Virus Infection

David C. Hooper, M.D.
Associate Professor of Medicine, Harvard Medical School; Fellowship Program Director, Infectious Disease Division, and Associate Chief, Infection Control Unit, Massachusetts General Hospital, Boston, Massachusetts
Quinolones; Urinary Tract Agents: Nitrofurantoin and Methenamine

David L. Hoover, M.D.
Associate Professor, Department of Medicine, Uniformed Services University of the Health Sciences, F. Edward Hébert School of Medicine, Bethesda, Maryland; Department of Bacterial Diseases, Walter Reed Army Institute of Research, Washington, D.C.
Innate (General or Nonspecific) Host Defense Mechanisms

Duane R. Hospenthal, M.D., Ph.D.
Assistant Chief, Infectious Disease Service (MCHK-DMI), Tripler Army Medical Center, Honolulu, Hawaii
Miscellaneous Fungi and Prototheca

James M. Hughes, M.D.
Clinical Associate Professor of Medicine, Division of Infectious Diseases, Department of Medicine, Emory University School of Medicine, and Adjunct Professor, Department of Epidemiology, Rollins School of Public Health of Emory University; Director, National Center for Infectious Diseases, Centers for Disease Control and Prevention, Atlanta, Georgia
Foodborne Disease; New and Emerging Infectious Diseases

Jainulabdeen J. Ifthikharuddin, M.D., MRCP(UK), MRCPath
Senior Instructor, University of Rochester School of Medicine and Dentistry; Attending Physician, Strong Memorial Hospital, Rochester, New York
Human T-Cell Lymphotropic Virus Types I and II

Jonathan R. Iredell, M.B.B.S., Ph.D., FRACP, FRCPA
Senior Lecturer, Faculty of Medicine, University of Sydney; Staff Specialist, Centre for Infectious Diseases and Microbiology, Westmead Hospital, Westmead, New South Wales, Australia
Nocardia *Species*

Lisa A. Jackson, M.D., M.P.H.
Assistant Professor, Department of Epidemiology, School of Public Health and Community Medicine, University of Washington; Assistant Investigator, Center for Health Studies, Group Health Cooperative, Seattle, Washington
Chlamydia pneumoniae

Selma M. B. Jeronimo, M.D., Ph.D.
Professor of Biochemistry, Universidade Federal do Rio Grande do Norte, Natal, Rio Grande do Norte, Brazil
Leishmania *Species: Visceral (Kala-Azar), Cutaneous, and Mucosal Leishmaniasis*

Caroline C. Johnson, M.D.
Associate Professor of Medicine, MCP–Hahnemann School of Medicine; Medical Director, Acute Communicable Disease Control Program, Philadelphia Department of Public Health, Philadelphia, Pennsylvania
Viridans Streptococci and Groups C and G Streptococci

Raymond M. Johnson, M.D., Ph.D.
Howard Hughes Postdoctoral Fellow, Department of Infectious Diseases, Washington University School of Medicine, St. Louis, Missouri
Cell-Mediated Immunity in Host Defense against Infectious Diseases

Warren D. Johnson, Jr., M.D.
B. H. Kean Professor of Tropical Medicine and Professor of Medicine, Weill Medical College of Cornell University; Attending Physician and Medical Director, International Health Care Service, and Chief, Division of International Medicine and Infectious Diseases, New York Presbyterian Hospital–Cornell Campus, New York, New York
Borrelia *Species (Relapsing Fever)*

Robert B. Jones, M.D., Ph.D.
Professor of Medicine and Microbiology and Immunology, Indiana University School of Medicine, Indianapolis, Indiana
Chlamydia trachomatis *(Trachoma, Perinatal Infections, Lymphogranuloma Venereum, and Other Genital Infections); Introduction to Chlamydial Diseases*

Manjari Joshi, M.D.
R. A. Cowley Shock Trauma Center, University of Maryland Medical System, Baltimore, Maryland
Multiple Trauma

Allen B. Kaiser, M.D.
Professor and Vice-Chairman, Department of Medicine, Vanderbilt University School of Medicine, Nashville, Tennessee
Postoperative Infections and Antimicrobial Prophylaxis

Adolf W. Karchmer, M.D.
Professor of Medicine, Harvard Medical School; Chief, Division of Infectious Diseases, Beth Israel Deaconess Medical Center, Boston, Massachusetts
Cephalosporins; Infections of Prosthetic Valves and Intravascular Devices

Hiroshi Kawai, M.D.
Department of Internal Medicine, University of Kanazawa School of Medicine, Kanazawa, Japan
Acute Viral Hepatitis

Donald Kaye, M.D.
Professor of Medicine, MCP–Hahnemann School of Medicine, Philadelphia, Pennsylvania
Urinary Tract Infections

Michael C. Keefer, M.D.
Associate Professor of Medicine, University of Rochester School of Medicine and Dentistry, Rochester, New York
Vaccines for Human Immunodeficiency Virus-1 Infection

Douglas S. Kernodle, M.D.
Associate Professor, Department of Medicine, Vanderbilt University School of Medicine; Chief, Infectious Diseases Section, Veterans Affairs Medical Center, Nashville, Tennessee
Postoperative Infections and Antimicrobial Prophylaxis

Jay S. Keystone, M.D., M.Sc.(CTM), FRCPC
Professor of Medicine, University of Toronto Faculty of Medicine; Staff Physician, Centre for Travel and Tropical Medicine, Toronto General Hospital, Toronto, Ontario, Canada
Isospora belli, Sarcocystis *Species,* Blastocystis hominis, *and* Cyclospora

Karl D. Kieburtz, M.D., M.P.H.
Associate Professor of Neurology and Community and Preventive Medicine, University of Rochester School of Medicine and Dentistry, Rochester, New York
Neurologic Manifestations of Human Immunodeficiency Virus Infection

Charles H. King, M.D.
Associate Professor of Medicine and International Health, Case Western Reserve University School of Medicine; Attending Physician, University Hospitals, Cleveland, Ohio
Cestodes (Tapeworms)

Louis V. Kirchhoff, M.D., M.P.H.
Professor, Department of Internal Medicine, University of Iowa College of Medicine; Staff Physician, Medical Service, Department of Veterans Affairs Medical Center, Iowa City, Iowa
Agents of African Trypanosomiasis (Sleeping Sickness); Trypanosoma *Species (American Trypanosomiasis, Chagas' Disease): Biology of Trypanosomes*

Jerome O. Klein, M.D.
Professor of Pediatrics, Boston University School of Medicine; Vice-Chairman for Academic Affairs, Boston Medical Center, Boston, Massachusetts
Otitis Externa, Otitis Media, and Mastoiditis

M. R. Knowles, M.D.
Professor of Medicine, University of North Carolina at Chapel Hill School of Medicine; Associate Director, Division of Pulmonary Critical Care Medicine, and Director, Adult Cystic Fibrosis Center, UNC Hospitals, Chapel Hill, North Carolina
Cystic Fibrosis

Phyllis Kozarsky, M.D.
Associate Professor of Medicine, Emory University School of Medicine; Chief of Infectious Diseases, Emory Crawford Long Hospital, Atlanta, Georgia
Isospora belli, Sarcocystis *Species,* Blastocystis hominis, *and* Cyclospora

John N. Krieger, M.D.
Professor of Urology, University of Washington School of Medicine; Chief of Urology, Veterans Affairs Puget Sound Health Care System, and Attending Surgeon, University of Washington Medical Center and Harborview Medical Center, Seattle, Washington
Prostatitis, Epididymitis, and Orchitis

Donald J. Krogstad, M.D.
Henderson Professor and Chair, Department of Tropical Medicine, Tulane University School of Public Health and Tropical Medicine, New Orleans, Louisiana
Plasmodium *Species (Malaria)*

Joshua Lederberg, Ph.D., M.D.(Hic.)
Professor, The Rockefeller University, New York, New York
Biological Warfare and Bioterrorism

James W. Leduc, Ph.D.
Associate Director for Global Health, National Center for Infectious Diseases, Centers for Disease Control and Prevention, Atlanta, Georgia
Global Epidemiology of Infectious Diseases

Stanley M. Lemon, M.D.
Professor and Chairman, Department of Microbiology and Immunology, University of Texas Medical Branch University of Texas Medical School of Galveston, Galveston, Texas
Hepatitis C

Donald P. Levine, M.D.
Professor of Medicine, Department of Medicine, Division of Infectious Diseases, Wayne State University School of Medicine; Vice-Chief of Medicine and Section Head, Infectious Diseases, Detroit Receiving Hospital, Detroit, Michigan
Infections in Injection Drug Users

Matthew E. Levison, M.D.
Professor of Medicine and Public Health, MCP–Hahnemann School of Medicine; Chief, Division of Infectious Diseases, Hahnemann University Hospital, Philadelphia, Pennsylvania
Peritonitis and Other Intra-abdominal Infections

Daniel P. Lew, M.D.
Professor of Medicine, Geneva University Medical School; Chief, Infectious Diseases Division, Geneva University Hospital, Geneva, Switzerland
Bacillus anthracis *(Anthrax)*

Aldo A. M. Lima, M.D., Ph.D.
Professor of Medicine, Federal University of Ceará, Fortaleza, Brazil
Inflammatory Enteritides

Nathan Litman, M.D.
Professor of Pediatrics, Albert Einstein College of Medicine of Yeshiva University; Chief, Pediatric Service, Montefiore Medical Center, Bronx, New York
Mumps Virus

Bennett Lorber, M.D., D.Sc. (Hon.)
Thomas M. Durant Professor of Medicine and Professor of Microbiology and Immunology, Temple University School of Medicine; Chief, Section of Infectious Diseases, Temple University Hospital, Philadelphia, Pennsylvania
Bacteroides, Prevotella, Porphyromonas, *and* Fusobacterium *Species (and Other Medically Important Anaerobic Gram-Negative Bacilli); Gas Gangrene and Other* Clostridium*-Associated Diseases;* Listeria monocytogenes

Larry I. Lutwick, M.D.
Professor of Medicine, State University of New York Health Science Center at Brooklyn College of Medicine; Director, Infectious Diseases, Veterans Affairs New York Harbor Health Care System, Brooklyn Campus, Brooklyn, New York
Infections in Asplenic Patients

Rob Roy MacGregor, M.D.
Professor of Medicine, Department of Medicine, Division of Infectious Diseases, University of Pennsylvania School of Medicine; Attending Physician, Hospital of the University of Pennsylvania, and Acting Chief, Infectious Disease Division, Philadelphia Veterans Affairs Medical Center, Philadelphia, Pennsylvania
Corynebacterium diphtheriae

Philip A. Mackowiak, M.D.
Professor and Vice Chairman, Department of Medicine, University of Maryland School of Medicine; Chief, Medical Care Clinical Center, Veterans Affairs Maryland Health Care System, Baltimore, Maryland
Fever of Unknown Origin; Temperature Regulation and Pathogenesis of Fever

Antone A. Madeiros, M.D.
Professor of Medicine, Brown University School of Medicine; Director, Division of Infectious Diseases, Miriam Hospital, and Medical Director, Clinical Microbiology Laboratory, Lifespan Academic Medical Center, Providence, Rhode Island
Mechanisms of Bacterial Antibiotic Resistance

Jon T. Mader, M.D.
Professor, Department of Internal Medicine, Division of Infectious Diseases, University of Texas Medical Branch University of Texas Medical School at Galveston, Galveston, Texas
Osteomyelitis

El Sheikh Mahgoub, M.D., Ph.D., FRCPath
Professor of Medical Microbiology, Faculty of Medicine, University of Science and Technology, Jordan; Formerly Regional Adviser, Research Promotion and Strategy Coordination, World Health Organization, Eastern Mediterranean Region, Alexandria, Egypt
Agents of Mycetoma

Adel A. F. Mahmoud, M.D., Ph.D.
Formerly Professor and Chairman of Medicine, Case Western Reserve University School of Medicine, and Physician-in-Chief, University Hospitals, Cleveland, Ohio; President, Merck Vaccines, Merck & Co., Inc., Whitehouse Station, New Jersey
Intestinal Nematodes (Roundworms); Introduction to Helminth Infections; Trematodes (Schistosomiasis) and Other Flukes

Gerald L. Mandell, M.D.
Professor of Medicine and Owen R. Cheatham Professor of the Sciences, University of Virginia School of Medicine; Chief, Division of Infectious Diseases, University of Virginia Health Sciences Center, Charlottesville, Virginia
Acute Pneumonia; Immunomodulators

Lionel A. Mandell, M.D.
Professor of Medicine, McMaster Medical Unit, Henderson General Hospital, Hamilton, Ontario, Canada
Fusidic Acid

Barbara J. Mann, Ph.D.
Assistant Professor of Research, Department of Internal Medicine, Division of Infectious Diseases, University of Virginia School of Medicine, Charlottesville, Virginia
Microbial Adherence

Lewis Markoff, M.D.
Chief, Laboratory of Vector-Borne Virus Diseases, Division of Viral Products, Center for Biologic Evaluation and Research, Food and Drug Administration, Bethesda, Maryland
Alphaviruses

Thomas J. Marrie, M.D., FRCPC
Professor and Chair, Department of Medicine, University of Alberta Faculty of Medicine; Site Chief, Medicine, University of Alberta Hospital, Edmonton, Alberta, Canada
Coxiella burnetii *(Q Fever)*

Thomas Marth, M.D.
Professor of Internal Medicine II, Saarland University, Homburg, Germany
Whipple's Disease

Ellen M. Mascini, M.D., Ph.D.
Senior Fellow in Medical Microbiology, Eijkman-Winkler Institute for Microbiology, Infectious Diseases, and Inflammation, University Medical Centre, Utrecht, The Netherlands
Anaerobic Cocci; Anaerobic Gram-Positive Nonsporulating Bacilli

Henry Masur, M.D.
Chief, Critical Care Medicine Department, Clinical Center, National Institutes of Health, Bethesda, Maryland
Management of Opportunistic Infections Associated with Human Immunodeficiency Virus Infection

Michael Eric Mathieu, M.D.
Clinical Instructor in Dermatology, Dermatology Department, University of Virginia School of Medicine; Associate, Dermatology PLC of Charlottesville, Charlottesville, Virginia
Introduction to Ectoparasitic Diseases; Lice (Pediculosis); Mites (Including Chiggers); Myiasis; Scabies; Ticks (Including Tick Paralysis)

Kenneth H. Mayer, M.D.
Professor of Medicine and Community Health, Brown University School of Medicine, Providence, Rhode Island; Chief, Infectious Disease Service, Memorial Hospital of Rhode Island, Pawtucket, Rhode Island, and Medical Research Director, Fenway Community Health Center, Boston, Massachusetts
Mechanisms of Bacterial Antibiotic Resistance; Sulfonamides and Trimethoprim

John T. McBride, M.D.
Professor of Pediatrics, Northeast Ohio Universities College of Medicine, Rootstown; Vice-Chair, Department of Pediatrics, Children's Hospital Medical Center of Akron, Akron, Ohio
Acute Laryngotracheitis (Croup); Bronchiolitis

Carol A. McCarthy, M.D.
Associate Professor of Pediatrics, University of Vermont College of Medicine, Burlington, Vermont; Director, Pediatric Infectious Disease, Maine Medical Center, Portland, Maine
Respiratory Syncytial Virus

William M. McCormack, M.D.
Professor of Medicine and Obstetrics and Gynecology, State University of New York Health Science Center at Brooklyn College of Medicine, Brooklyn, New York
Urethritis

Joseph E. McDade, Ph.D.
Deputy Director, National Center for Infectious Diseases, Centers for Disease Control and Prevention, Atlanta, Georgia
New and Emerging Infectious Diseases

Kenneth McIntosh, M.D.
Professor of Pediatrics, Harvard Medical School; Chief, Division of Infectious Diseases, Children's Hospital, Boston, Massachusetts
Coronaviruses

Philip B. Mead, M.D.
Professor and Chair, Department of Obstetrics and Gynecology, University of Vermont College of Medicine; Obstetrician and Gynecologist-in-Chief, Fletcher Allen Health Care, Burlington, Vermont
Infections of the Female Pelvis

Michael H. Merson, M.D.
Professor and Dean of Public Health, and Chairman, Department of Epidemiology and Public Health, Yale University School of Medicine, New Haven, Connecticut
Global Perspectives on Human Immunodeficiency Virus Infection and Acquired Immunodeficiency Syndrome

Françoise Meunier, M.D., Ph.D.
Director, Central Office—Data Center, and Chairman, Invasive Fungal Infections Cooperative Group, European Organization for Research and Treatment of Cancer, Brussels, Belgium
Infections in Patients with Acute Leukemia and Lymphoma

Samuel I. Miller, M.D.
Professor of Medicine and Microbiology, Department of Medicine, Division of Allergy and Infectious Diseases, University of Washington School of Medicine, Seattle, Washington
Salmonella *Species, Including* Salmonella typhi

David H. Mitchell, M.B.B.S., M.Med.Sci.(Epi.)
Clinical Lecturer, Department of Infectious Disease, University of Sydney, Sydney; Staff Specialist, Centre for Infectious Diseases and Microbiology, Institute of Clinical Pathology and Medical Research, Westmead Hospital, Westmead, New South Wales, Australia
Nocardia *Species*

John F. Modlin, M.D.
Professor of Pediatrics and Medicine and Acting Chair, Department of Pediatrics, Dartmouth Medical School, Hanover; Attending Physician, Infectious Disease Section, Dartmouth–Hitchcock Medical Center, Lebanon, New Hampshire
Coxsackieviruses, Echoviruses, and Newer Enteroviruses; Introduction to Picornaviridae; Poliovirus

Robert C. Moellering, Jr., M.S., M.D., D.Sc.(hon)
Herrman L. Blumgart Professor of Medicine, Harvard Medical School; Physician-in-Chief and Chairman, Department of Medicine, and Chief Executive Officer, Harvard Medical Faculty Physicians, Beth Israel Deaconess Medical Center, Boston, Massachusetts
Enterococcus *Species,* Streptococcus bovis, *and* Leuconostoc *Species; Principles of Anti-infective Therapy*

Jose G. Montoya, M.D.
Assistant Professor of Medicine, Division of Infectious Diseases and Geographic Medicine, Stanford University School of Medicine, Stanford, California
Toxoplasma gondii

Kristine A. Moore, M.D., M.P.H.
Medical Director, Infection Control Advisory Network, Inc., Eden Prairie, Minnesota
Epidemiologic Principles

J. Glenn Morris, Jr., M.D., M.P.H.T.M.
Professor of Medicine, Epidemiology and Preventive Medicine, and Microbiology and Immunology, University of Maryland School of Medicine, Baltimore, Maryland
Human Illness Associated with Harmful Algal Blooms

E. Richard Moxon M.A., M.B., B.Chir.
Professor and Head, Department of Paediatrics, University of Oxford, and Head, Molecular Infectious Diseases Group, University of Oxford Institute of Molecular Medicine, John Radcliffe Hospital, Oxford, England
Haemophilus influenzae

Robert R. Muder, M.D.
Associate Professor of Medicine, University of Pittsburgh School of Medicine; Hospital Epidemiologist, Veterans Affairs Pittsburgh Healthcare System, Pittsburgh, Pennsylvania
Other Legionella *Species*

Jean Marie Mulinde, M.D.
Assistant Professor of Medicine, Program in Traumatology, University of Maryland School of Medicine; Attending Physician, Section of Infectious Diseases, R. A. Cowley Shock Trauma Center, Baltimore, Maryland
Hyperbaric Oxygen

Timothy F. Murphy, M.D.
Professor of Medicine and Microbiology, State University of New York at Buffalo School of Medicine and Biomedical Sciences; Chief, Division of Infectious Diseases, Veterans Affairs Medical Center, Buffalo, New York
Haemophilus influenzae; Moraxella (Branhamella) catarrhalis *and Other Gram-Negative Cocci*

Daniel M. Musher, M.D.
Professor of Medicine and Microbiology and Immunology, Baylor College of Medicine; Chief, Infectious Diseases Section, Veterans Affairs Medical Center, Houston, Texas
Streptococcus pneumoniae

Theodore E. Nash, M.D.
Senior Scientist, Laboratory of Parasitic Diseases, National Institute of Allergy and Infectious Diseases, National Institutes of Health, Bethesda, Maryland
Visceral Larva Migrans and Other Unusual Helminth Infections

William M. Nauseef, M.D.
Professor, Department of Internal Medicine, Inflammation Program, University of Iowa College of Medicine; Attending Physician, Veterans Affairs Medical Center, Iowa City, Iowa
Granulocytic Phagocytes

John M. Neff, M.D.
Professor of Pediatrics, University of Washington School of Medicine; Director, Center for Children with Special Needs and Chronic Health Conditions, Children's Hospital and Regional Medical Center, Seattle, Washington
Introduction to Poxviridae; Parapoxviruses, Molluscum Contagiosum, and Tanapox Viruses; Vaccinia *Virus (Cowpox); Variola (Smallpox) and Monkeypox Viruses*

Marguerite A. Neill, M.D.
Associate Professor, Department of Medicine, Division of Infectious Diseases, Brown University School of Medicine, Providence; Attending Physician, Division of Infectious Diseases, Memorial Hospital of Rhode Island, Pawtucket, Rhode Island
Other Pathogenic Vibrios

Terrence P. O'Brien, M.D.
Assistant Professor, Wilmer Eye Institute, Johns Hopkins Hospital, Baltimore, Maryland
Conjunctivitis; Endophthalmitis; Keratitis; Periocular Infections

Paul A. Offit, M.D.
Henle Professor of Immunologic and Infectious Diseases, University of Pennsylvania School of Medicine; Chief, Section of Infectious Diseases, Children's Hospital of Philadelphia, Philadelphia, Pennsylvania
Rotavirus

Pablo C. Okhuysen, M.D.
Associate Professor of Medicine, Division of Infectious Diseases, University of Texas Medical School at Houston; Assistant Professor of Biological Sciences, University of Texas–Houston School of Public Health, Houston, Texas
Sporothrix schenckii

Steven M. Opal, M.D.
Professor of Medicine, Brown University School of Medicine, Providence; Director, Infection Control Service, Memorial Hospital of Rhode Island, Pawtucket, Rhode Island
Mechanisms of Bacterial Antibiotic Resistance

Walter A. Orenstein, M.D.
Director, National Immunization Program, Centers for Disease Control and Prevention, and Assistant Surgeon General, U.S. Public Health Service, Atlanta, Georgia
Immunization

Michael T. Osterholm, Ph.D., M.P.H.
Chairman and Chief Executive Officer, Infection Control Advisory Network, Inc., Eden Prairie, Minnesota
Epidemiologic Principles

Stephen M. Ostroff, M.D.
Associate Director for Epidemiologic Science, National Center for Infectious Diseases, Centers for Disease Control and Prevention, Atlanta, Georgia
Global Epidemiology of Infectious Diseases

Michael N. Oxman, M.D.
Professor of Medicine and Pathology, University of California, San Diego, School of Medicine, La Jolla; Staff Physician, Infectious Diseases Section, Veterans Affairs San Diego Healthcare System, San Diego, California
Myocarditis and Pericarditis

Richard D. Pearson, M.D.
Professor, Department of Medicine, Division of Geographic and International Medicine, and Department of Pathology, University of Virginia School of Medicine, Charlottesville, Virginia
Agents Active Against Parasites and Pneumocystis carinii; *Enteric Fever and Other Causes of Abdominal Symptoms with Fever;* Leishmania *Species: Visceral (Kala-Azar), Cutaneous, and Mucosal Leishmaniasis*

David A. Pegues, M.D.
Assistant Clinical Professor, Department of Medicine, University of California, Los Angeles, UCLA School of Medicine; Hospital Epidemiologist and Attending Physician, Division of Infectious Diseases, UCLA Center for Health Sciences, Los Angeles, California
Salmonella *Species, Including* Salmonelli typhi

Robert L. Penn, M.D.
Professor, Department of Medicine, Louisiana State University School of Medicine in Shreveport; Chief, Infectious Diseases Section, Louisiana State University Hospital–Shreveport, Shreveport, Louisiana
Francisella tularensis *(Tularemia)*

Bradley A. Perkins, M.D.
Centers for Disease Control and Prevention, Atlanta, Georgia
Leptospira *Species (Leptospirosis)*

C. J. Peters, M.D.
Adjunct Professor, Department of Microbiology and Immunology, Emory University School of Medicine; Chief, Special Pathogens Branch, Centers for Disease Control and Prevention, Atlanta, Georgia
California Encephalitis, Hantavirus Pulmonary Syndrome, and Bunyaviridae Hemorrhagic Fevers; Lymphocytic Choriomeningitis Virus, Lassa Virus, and the South American Hemorrhagic Fevers; Marburg and Ebola Virus Hemorrhagic Fevers

Phillip K. Peterson, M.D.
Professor of Medicine, University of Minnesota Medical School; Director, Infectious Diseases Division, Department of Medicine, Hennepin County Medical Center, Minneapolis, Minnesota
Infections in the Elderly

William A. Petri, Jr., M.D., Ph.D.
Professor, Department of Internal Medicine, Division of Infectious Diseases, and Departments of Microbiology and Pathology, University of Virginia School of Medicine; Attending Physician and Associate Director of Clinical Microbiology, University of Virginia Hospital, Charlottesville, Virginia
Free-Living Amebas; Microbial Adherence

Peter Piot, M.D., Ph.D.
Executive Director, Joint United Nations Programme on HIV/AIDS, Geneva, Switzerland
Global Perspectives on Human Immunodeficiency Virus Infection and Acquired Immunodeficiency Syndrome

Philip A. Pizzo, M.D.
Thomas Morgan Rotch Professor and Chair, Department of Pediatrics, Harvard Medical School; Physician-in-Chief and Chair, Department of Medicine, Children's Hospital, Boston, Massachusetts
Empirical Therapy and Prevention of Infection in the Immunocompromised Host

Matthew Pollack, M.D.
Professor of Medicine, F. Edward Hébert School of Medicine, Uniformed Services University of the Health Sciences; Attending Staff Physician Internal Medicine, Infectious Diseases, National Naval Medical Center, Bethesda, Maryland
Pseudomonas aeruginosa

Debra Poutsiaka, M.D., Ph.D.
Assistant Professor of Medicine, Tufts University School of Medicine; Assistant Physician, Division of Geographic Medicine and Infectious Diseases, Department of Medicine, New England Medical Center, Boston, Massachusetts
Babesia

Robert H. Purcell, M.D.
Head, Hepatitis Viruses Section, Laboratory of Infectious Diseases, National Institute of Allergy and Infectious Diseases, National Institutes of Health, Bethesda, Maryland
Hepatitis E Virus

Anastacio de Queiroz Sousa, M.D.
Professor of Medicine, Department of Tropical Medicine, Universidade Federal do Ceará, Fortaleza; Secretary of Health, Ceará, Brazil
Leishmania *Species: Visceral (Kala-Azar), Cutaneous, and Mucosal Leishmaniasis*

Ronald P. Rabinowitz, M.D.
Assistant Professor, Department of Medicine, Division of Infectious Diseases, University of Maryland School of Medicine, Baltimore, Maryland
Multiple Trauma

Didier Raoult
Rickettsia Unit, Bacteriology-Serology-Virology Laboratory, Groupe Hospitalier de la Timone; Director, National Rickettsia Reference Center, Marseilles, France
Rickettsia rickettsii *and Other Spotted Fever Group Rickettsiae (Rocky Mountain Spotted Fever and Other Spotted Fevers)*

Jonathan I. Ravdin, M.D.
Nesbitt Professor and Chairman, Department of Medicine, University of Minnesota Medical School–Minneapolis; Chief of Medicine, Fairview–University Medical Center, Minneapolis, Minnesota
Entamoeba histolytica *(Amebiasis); Introduction to Protozoal Diseases*

Thomas H. Rea, M.D.
Emeritus Professor of Medicine (Dermatology), University of Southern California, Attending Physician, Los Angeles County/USC Medical Center, Los Angeles, California
Mycobacterium leprae *(Leprosy, Hansen's Disease)*

Annette C. Reboli, M.D.
Associate Professor of Medicine, University of Medicine and Dentistry of New Jersey Robert Wood Johnson Medical School at Camden; Hospital Epidemiologist, Cooper Hospital/University Medical Center, Camden, New Jersey
Erysipelothrix rhusiopathiae

Richard C. Reichman, M.D.
Professor of Medicine and Microbiology and Immunology, University of Rochester School of Medicine and Dentistry; Head, Infectious Diseases Unit, Strong Memorial Hospital, Rochester, New York
Detection of Human Immunodeficiency Virus Infection; Papillomaviruses

Michael F. Rein, M.D.
Professor, Department of Medicine, Division of Infectious Diseases, University of Virginia School of Medicine; Medical Director, Sexually Transmitted Disease Clinic, Thomas Jefferson District Health Department, Charlottesville, Virginia
Genital Skin and Mucous Membrane Lesions; Trichomonas vaginalis; *Urethritis; Vulvovaginitis and Cervicitis*

Marvin S. Reitz, Jr., Ph.D.
University of Maryland School of Medicine; Institute of Human Virology, Baltimore, Maryland
Human Immunodeficiency Viruses

David A. Relman, M.D.
Assistant Professor of Medicine and Microbiology and Immunology, Stanford University School of Medicine, Stanford; Staff Physician, Veterans Affairs Palo Alto Health Care System, Palo Alto, California
A Molecular Perspective of Microbial Pathogenicity

Jack S. Remington, M.D.
Professor, Department of Medicine, Division of Infectious Diseases and Geographic Medicine, Stanford University School of Medicine, Stanford; Marcus A. Krupp Research Chair and Chairman, Department of Immunology and Infectious Diseases, Research Institute, Palo Alto Medical Foundation, Palo Alto, California
Toxoplasma gondii

Angela Restrepo, Ph.D.
Senior Researcher and Scientific Director, Corporación para Investigaciones Biologicas (CIB), Medellin, Colombia
Paracoccidioides brasiliensis

John H. Rex, M.D.
Associate Professor of Medicine, University of Texas Medical School at Houston; Medical Director for Epidemiology, Hermann Hospital, Houston, Texas
Sporothrix schenckii

Herbert Y. Reynolds, M.D.
Professor and Chairman, Department of Medicine, Pennsylvania State University College of Medicine; Chief, Medical Clinical Operations, South Central Region, and Associate Director, Division of Medicine, Penn State Geisinger Health System, Hershey, Pennsylvania
Chronic Bronchitis and Acute Infectious Exacerbations

William S. Robinson, M.D.
Division of Infectious Diseases, Stanford University School of Medicine, Palo Alto, California
Hepatitis B Virus and Hepatitis D Virus

Joseph D. Rosenblatt, M.D.
Professor of Medicine and Microbiology and Immunology, University of Rochester School of Medicine and Dentistry; University of Rochester Cancer Center, Rochester, New York
Human T-Cell Lymphotropic Virus Types I and II

Mark E. Rupp, M.D.
Associate Professor, Department of Internal Medicine, University of Nebraska College of Medicine; Medical Director, Department of Healthcare Epidemiology, Nebraska Health System, Omaha, Nebraska
Meidastinitis

Charles E. Rupprecht, V.M.D., Ph.D.
Division of Viral and Rickettsial Diseases, Centers for Disease Control and Prevention, Atlanta, Georgia
Rabies Virus

Thomas A. Russo, M.D.
Assistant Professor, Department of Medicine, Division of Infectious Diseases, State University of New York at Buffalo School of Medicine and Biomedical Sciences; Staff Physician, Veterans Affairs Medical Center and Erie County Medical Center, Buffalo, New York
Agents of Actinomycosis

Alfred J. Saah, M.D., M.P.H.
Associate Director, Clinical Research, Infectious Diseases, Merck Research Laboratories, West Point, Pennsylvania
Introduction to Rickettsioses and Ehrlichioses; Orientia tsutsugamushi *(Scrub Typhus);* Rickettsia akari *(Rickettsialpox);* Rickettsia prowazekii *(Epidemic or Louse-Borne Typhus)*

Christopher J. Salmon, M.D.
Chest Radiologist, Scottsdale Medical Imaging, Ltd., Scottsdale, Arizona
Pleural Effusion and Empyema

Frank T. Saulsbury, M.D.
Professor of Pediatrics and Head, Division of Immunology and Rheumatology, Department of Pediatrics, University of Virginia School of Medicine, Charlottesville, Virginia
Kawasaki Syndrome

Maria C. Savoia, M.D.
Professor of Clinical Medicine and Associate Dean for Curriculum and Student Affairs, University of California, San Diego, School of Medicine, San Diego, California
Myocarditis and Pericarditis

W. Michael Scheld, M.D.
Professor of Medicine (Infectious Disease) and Neurosurgery, University of Virginia School of Medicine, Charlottesville, Virginia
Acute Meningitis; Brain Abscess; Endocarditis and Intravascular Infections

David Schlossberg, M.D.
Professor of Medicine, Jefferson Medical College of Thomas Jefferson University; Director, Department of Medicine, and Head, Infectious Disease Section, Episcopal Hospital, Philadelphia, Pennsylvania
Chlamydia psittaci *(Psittacosis)*

Robert T. Schooley, M.D.
Tim Gill Professor of Medicine, University of Colorado School of Medicine; Head, Division of Infectious Diseases, University of Colorado Health Sciences Center, Denver, Colorado
Epstein-Barr Virus (Infectious Mononucleosis)

David A. Schwartz, M.D.
Associate Professor of Pathology and Medicine, Emory University School of Medicine; Department of Pathology, Grady Memorial Hospital, Atlanta, Georgia
Microsporidia

Carlos Seas, M.D.
Assistant Professor of Medicine, Universidad Peruana Cayetano Heredia; Attending Physician, Hospital Nacional Cayetano Heredia, Lima, Peru
Vibrio cholerae

Kent A. Sepkowitz, M.D.
Associate Professor of Medicine, Weill Medical College of Cornell University; Associate Chairman, Clinical Affairs, Memorial Sloan-Kettering Cancer Center, New York, New York
Nosocomial Hepatitis and Other Infections Transmitted by Blood and Blood Products

Thomas A. Shaw-Stiffel, M.D.C.M., M.M.M.
Associate Professor of Medicine, University of Rochester School of Medicine and Dentistry; Director of Hepatology, Konar Center for Digestive and Liver Diseases, University of Rochester Medical Center, Rochester, New York
Chronic Hepatitis

Edward H. Shortliffe, M.D., Ph.D.
Professor, Departments of Medicine and Computer Science; Director, Medical Informatics Training Program; and Associate Dean for Information Resources and Technology, Stanford University School of Medicine; Attending Physician, UCSF Stanford Health Care System, Stanford, California
The Infectious Diseases Physician and the Internet

Upinder Singh, M.D.
Fellow, Department of Microbiology, Stanford University School of Medicine, Stanford, California
Free-Living Amebas

Leonard N. Slater, M.D.
Professor, Department of Medicine, University of Oklahoma College of Medicine; Vice-Chief, Infectious Diseases Section, Department of Medicine, University of Oklahoma Health Sciences Center; Attending Physician, University Hospital, Veterans Affairs Medical Center, and Presbyterian Hospital, Oklahoma City, Oklahoma
Bartonella *Species, Including Cat-Scratch Disease*

James W. Smith, M.D.
Professor, Department of Internal Medicine, University of Texas Southwestern Medical Center at Dallas Southwestern Medical School; Staff Physician, Infectious Diseases Section, Dallas Veterans Affairs Medical Center, Dallas, Texas
Infectious Arthritis

Jack D. Sobel, M.D.
Professor of Medicine, Wayne State University School of Medicine; Chief, Division of Infectious Diseases, Detroit Medical Center, Detroit, Michigan
Urinary Tract Infections

Tania C. Sorrell, M.D., FRACP
Professor of Clinical Infectious Diseases, Faculty of Medicine, University of Sydney, Sydney; Director, Centre for Infectious Diseases and Microbiology, Westmead Hospital, Westmead, New South Wales, Australia
Nocardia *Species*

P. Frederick Sparling, M.D.
J. Herbert Bate Professor of Medicine and Professor of Microbiology and Immunology, University of North Carolina at Chapel Hill School of Medicine, Chapel Hill, North Carolina
Neisseria gonorrhoeae

Carol A. Spiegel, Ph.D.
Associate Professor, Department of Pathology and Laboratory Medicine, University of Wisconsin Medical School; Director, Clinical Microbiology, University of Wisconsin Hospital and Clinics, Madison, Wisconsin
Gardnerella vaginalis *and* Mobiluncus *Species*

Harold C. Standiford, M.D.
Professor of Medicine, University of Maryland School of Medicine; Deputy Director, Medical Care Center, Veterans Affairs Maryland Health Care System, Baltimore, Maryland
Tetracyclines and Chloramphenicol

Allen C. Steere, M.D.
Zucker Professor of Medicine, Tufts University School of Medicine; Chief, Rheumatology/Immunology, New England Medical Center, Boston, Massachusetts
Borrelia burgdorferi *(Lyme Disease, Lyme Borreliosis)*

Neal H. Steigbigel, M.D.
Professor of Medicine, Albert Einstein College of Medicine of Yeshiva University; Head, Division of Infectious Diseases, Montefiore Medical Center, Bronx, New York
Macrolides and Clindamycin

James P. Steinberg, M.D.
Associate Professor, Department of Medicine, Division of Infectious Diseases, Emory University School of Medicine; Associate Chief of Medicine and Hospital Epidemiologist, Crawford W. Long Memorial Hospital, Atlanta, Georgia
Other Gram-Negative Bacilli

Theodore S. Steiner, M.D.
Assistant Professor, Department of Medicine, Division of Geographic and International Medicine, University of Virginia School of Medicine, Charlottesville, Virginia
Principles and Syndromes of Enteric Infection

Timothy R. Sterling, M.D.
Assistant Professor of Medicine and Epidemiology, Johns Hopkins University School of Medicine; Medical Director, Baltimore City Health Department TB Clinic, Baltimore, Maryland
General Clinical Manifestations of Human Immunodeficiency Virus Infection (Including Oral, Cutaneous, Renal, Ocular, and Cardiac Diseases)

David A. Stevens, M.D.
Professor, Department of Medicine, Stanford University School of Medicine, Stanford; Chief, Division of Infectious Diseases, Department of Medicine, Santa Clara Valley Medical Center; Principal Investigator, Infectious Diseases Research Laboratory, California Institute for Medical Research, San Jose, California
Antifungal Agents

Dennis L. Stevens, Ph.D., M.D.
Professor, Department of Medicine, University of Washington School of Medicine, Seattle, Washington; Chief, Infectious Disease Section, Veterans Affairs Medical Center, Boise, Idaho
Streptococcus pyogenes *(Including Streptococcal Toxic Shock Syndrome and Necrotizing Fasciitis)*

Charles W. Stratton, M.D.
Vanderbilt University School of Medicine, Nashville, Tennessee
Streptococcus intermedius *Group*

Stephen E. Straus, M.D.
Chief, Laboratory of Clinical Investigation, National Institute of Allergy and Infectious Diseases, National Institutes of Health, Bethesda, Maryland
Herpes B Virus; Human Herpesvirus Type 8 (Kaposi's Sarcoma–Associated Herpesvirus); Human Herpesvirus Types 6 and 7; Introduction to Herpesviridae

Larry J. Strausbaugh, M.D.
Professor of Medicine, Oregon Health Sciences University School of Medicine; Hospital Epidemiologist and Staff Physician, Veterans Affairs Medical Center, Portland, Oregon
Nosocomial Respiratory Infections

Howard Z. Streicher, M.D.
National Institutes of Health; Warren G. Magnuson Clinical Center, Bethesda, Maryland
Human Immunodeficiency Viruses

Alan M. Sugar, M.D.
Professor of Medicine, Boston University School of Medicine, Boston; Director HIV/AIDS Program, Cape Cod Hospital, Hyannis, Massachusetts
Agents of Mucormycosis and Related Species

Mark S. Sulkowski, M.D.
Assistant Professor, Department of Medicine, Division of Infectious Diseases, Johns Hopkins University School of Medicine, Baltimore, Maryland
Gastrointestinal and Hepatobiliary Manifestations of Human Immunodeficiency Virus Infection

Morton N. Swartz, M.D.
Professor of Medicine, Harvard Medical School; Chief, Jackson Firm Medical Service and Infectious Disease Unit, Massachusetts General Hospital, Boston, Massachusetts
Cellulitis and Subcutaneous Tissue Infections; Lymphadenitis and Lymphangitis; Myositis

David L. Swerdlow, M.D.
Medical Epidemiologist, Foodborne and Diarrheal Diseases Branch, National Center for Infectious Diseases, Centers for Disease Control and Prevention, Atlanta, Georgia
Foodborne Disease

Jordan W. Tappero, M.D., M.P.H.
Chief, Epidemiology Section, Division of Bacterial and Mycotic Diseases, National Center for Infectious Diseases, Centers for Disease Control and Prevention, Atlanta, Georgia
Leptospira *Species (Leptospirosis)*

Robert V. Tauxe, M.D., M.P.H.
Chief, Foodborne and Diarrheal Diseases Branch, Division of Bacterial and Mycotic Diseases, National Center for Infectious Diseases, Centers for Disease Control and Prevention, Atlanta, Georgia
Foodborne Disease

David Taylor-Robinson, M.D., MRCP, FRCPath
Emeritus Professor of Genitourinary Microbiology and Medicine, Department of Genitourinary Medicine and Communicable Diseases, Imperial College School of Medicine; St. Mary's Hospital, London, England
Ureaplasma urealyticum, Mycoplasma hominis, *and* Mycoplasma genitalium

Nathan M. Thielman, M.D., M.P.H.
Assistant Professor, Department of Medicine, Division of Infectious Diseases, Medical University of South Carolina, Charleston, South Carolina
Antibiotic-Associated Colitis

David L. Thomas, M.D., M.P.H.
Associate Professor of Medicine and Epidemiology, Johns Hopkins University School of Medicine, Baltimore, Maryland
Hepatitis C

Alan D. Tice, M.D.
Clinical Associate Professor, University of Washington School of Medicine, Seattle; Partner, Infections Limited, Tacoma, Washington
Outpatient Intravenous Antibiotic Therapy

Edmund C. Tramont, M.D.
Professor of Medicine (Infectious Diseases), University of Maryland School of Medicine; Associate Director, Institute of Human Virology, University of Maryland Biotechnology Institute, Baltimore, Maryland
Innate (General or Nonspecific) Host Defense Mechanisms; Treponema pallidum *(Syphilis)*

John J. Treanor, M.D.
Associate Professor, Department of Medicine, Division of Infectious Diseases, University of Rochester School of Medicine and Dentistry, Rochester, New York
Astroviruses, Toroviruses, and Picobirnaviruses; Influenza Virus; Norwalk Virus and Other Caliciviruses

Phoebe R. Trubowitz, M.D.
Clinical Fellow, Department of Medicine, Division of Hematology/Oncology, University of California, San Francisco, School of Medicine, San Francisco, California
Malignancies in Human Immunodeficiency Virus Infection

Theodore F. Tsai, M.D., M.P.H.
Director, Clinical Research, Wyeth Lederle Vaccines, Pearl River, New York
Coltiviruses (Colorado Tick Fever); Flaviviruses (Yellow Fever, Dengue, Dengue Hemorrhagic Fever, Japanese Encephalitis, St. Louis Encephalitis, Tick-Borne Encephalitis); Orthoreoviruses and Orbiviruses

Carmelita U. Tuazon, M.D., M.P.H.
Professor of Medicine, George Washington University School of Medicine and Health Sciences; Attending Physician, George Washington University Hospital, Washington, D.C.
Other Bacillus *Species*

Allan R. Tunkel, M.D., Ph.D.
Professor of Medicine and Associate Chair for Education, Department of Medicine, MCP–Hahnemann University; Director, Internal Medicine Residency Program, Hahnemann University Hospital, Philadelphia, Pennsylvania
Acute Meningitis; Brain Abscess; Topical Antibacterials; Viridans Streptococci and Groups C and G Streptococci

Kenneth L. Tyler, M.D.
Professor and Vice-Chairman, Department of Neurology, and Professor, Departments of Medicine and Microbiology and Immunology, University of Colorado School of Medicine; Chief, Neurology Service, Denver Veterans Affairs Medical Center, Denver, Colorado
Introduction to Viruses and Viral Diseases; Prions and Prion Diseases of the Central Nervous System (Transmissible Neurodegenerative Diseases)

Beth L. P. Ungar, M.D.
Clinical Associate Professor of Medicine, Georgetown University School of Medicine, Washington, D.C.
Cryptosporidium

Mauro Vaccarezza, M.D.
Visiting Fellow, National Institute of Allergy and Infectious Diseases, National Institutes of Health, Bethesda, Maryland
The Immunology of Human Immunodeficiency Virus Infection

Jo-Anne Van Burik, M.D.
Assistant Professor, Department of Medicine, Division of Infectious Diseases, University of Minnesota Medical School–Minneapolis, Minneapolis, Minnesota
Infections in Recipients of Blood and Marrow Transplantation

Ivo van de Rijn, Ph.D.
Professor, Department of Microbiology and Immunology, and Associate Professor, Department of Internal Medicine, Bowman Gray School of Medicine of Wake Forest University, Winston-Salem, North Carolina
Classification of Streptococci

Shahe Vartivarian, M.D.
Private Practice, Metropolitan Infectious Disease Associates, Houston, Texas
Stenotrophomonas maltophilia *and* Burkholderia cepacia

Jan Verhoef, M.D., Ph.D.
Professor of Medical Microbiology, University of Utrecht; Director, Eijkman-Winkler Institute for Microbiology, Infectious Diseases, and Inflammation, University Medical Centre, Utrecht, The Netherlands
Anaerobic Cocci; Anaerobic Gram-Negative Nonsporulating Bacilli

Paul A. Volberding, M.D.
Professor of Medicine, University of California, San Francisco, School of Medicine; Director, AIDS Program, San Francisco General Hospital, San Francisco, California
Malignancies in Human Immunodeficiency Virus Infection

Kenneth F. Wagner, D.O.
Associate Professor, Department of Medicine, Uniformed Services University of the Health Sciences, F. Edward Hébert School of Medicine; Attending Physician and Infectious Diseases Consultant, Department of Internal Medicine, National Naval Medical Center, Bethesda, Maryland
Agents of Chromomycosis

Francis A. Waldvogel, M.D.
Professor of Medicine, University of Geneva Medical School; Chairman, Department of Internal Medicine, University Hospital, Geneva, Switzerland
Staphylococcus aureus

David H. Walker, M.D.
Chair, Department of Pathology, University of Texas Medical Branch, Galveston, Texas
Ehrlichia chaffeensis *(Human Monocytotropic Ehrlichiosis),* Ehrlichia phagocytophila *(Human Granulocytotropic Ehrlichiosis) and Other Ehrlichiae;* Rickettsia rickettsii *and Other Spotted Fever Group Rickettsiae (Rocky Mountain Spotted Fever and Other Spotted Fevers);* Rickettsia typhi *(Murine Typhus)*

Richard J. Wallace, Jr., M.D.
Professor, Department of Medicine and Professor and Chairman, Department of Microbiology; Chief, Infectious Diseases, University of Texas Health Center, Tyler, Texas
Antimycobacterial Agents; Infections Due to Nontuberculous Mycobacteria

Peter D. Walzer, M.D.
Professor of Medicine, University of Cincinnati College of Medicine; Associate Chief of Staff for Research, Veterans Affairs Medical Center, Cincinnati, Ohio
Pneumocystis carinii

Christine A. Wanke, M.D.
Associate Professor of Community Health and Medicine, Tufts University School of Medicine; Staff Physician, Division of Infectious Diseases, New England Medical Center, Boston, Massachusetts
Tropical Sprue/Enteropathy

John W. Warren, M.D.
Professor and Head, Division of Infectious Diseases, Department of Medicine, University of Maryland School of Medicine, Baltimore, Maryland
Nosocomial Urinary Tract Infections

Ronald G. Washburn, M.D.
Associate Professor of Medicine, University of Nevada School of Medicine; Chief, Infectious Diseases, Veterans Affairs Medical Center, Reno, Nevada
Spirillum minus *(Rat-Bite Fever);* Streptobacillus moniliformis *(Rat-Bite Fever)*

David J. Weber, M.D.
Associate Professor of Medicine, Pediatrics, and Epidemiology and Assistant Dean, University of North Carolina at Chapel Hill School of Medicine; Associate Chief of Staff, UNC Hospitals, Chapel Hill, North Carolina
The Acutely Ill Patient with Fever and Rash

Rainer Weber, M.D.
Assistant Professor (Infectious Diseases), University of Zurich; Acting Head, Division of Infectious Diseases and Hospital Epidemiology, Department of Internal Medicine, University Hospital, Zurich, Switzerland
Microsporidia

Arnold N. Weinberg, M.D.
Professor of Medicine, Harvard Medical School, Boston; Attending Physician, Massachusetts General Hospital, Boston, and Medical Director, Massachusetts Institute of Technology, Cambridge, Massachusetts
Zoonoses

Geoffrey A. Weinberg, M.D.
Associate Professor, Department of Pediatrics, Division of Infectious Diseases, University of Rochester School of Medicine and Dentistry; Director, Pediatric HIV Program, Children's Hospital at Strong, Strong Memorial Hospital, Rochester, New York
Pediatric Human Immunodeficiency Virus Infection

Daniel Weisdorf, M.D.
Professor of Medicine, Department of Medicine, Division of Hematology, Oncology, and Transplantation, University of Minnesota Medical School–Minneapolis; Director, Adult Blood and Marrow Transplant Program, University of Minnesota Hospital and Clinic, Minneapolis, Minnesota
Infections in Recipients of Blood and Marrow Transplantation

Michael E. Weiss, M.D.
Clinical Associate Professor, Department of Medicine, Division of Allergy, University of Washington School of Medicine, Seattle, Washington
β-Lactam Allergy

David F. Welch, Ph.D.
Clinical Associate Professor of Pathology, University of Texas Southwestern Medical Center at Dallas Southwestern Medical School; Director, Clinical Microbiology Laboratories, Laboratory Corporation of America, Dallas, Texas
Bartonella *Species, Including Cat-Scratch Disease*

Richard P. Wenzel, M.D., M.Sc.
William Branch Porter Professor and Chair, Department of Internal Medicine, Virginia Commonwealth University School of Medicine, Richmond, Virginia
Health Care Reform and the Specialist in Infectious Diseases; Isolation; Organization for Infection Control; Disinfection, Sterilization, and Control of Hospital Waste

Melinda Wharton, M.D.
National Immunization Program, Centers for Disease Control and Prevention, Atlanta, Georgia
Immunization

Richard J. Whitley, M.D.
Professor of Pediatrics, Microbiology, and Medicine, University of Alabama School of Medicine, Birmingham, Alabama
Varicella-Zoster Virus

Barbara Braunstein Wilson, M.D.
Associate Professor, Department of Dermatology, University of Virginia School of Medicine; Attending Physician, University of Virginia Hospitals, Charlottesville, Virginia
Introduction to Ectoparasitic Diseases; Lice (Pediculosis); Mites (Including Chiggers); Myiasis; Scabies; Ticks (Including Tick Paralysis)

Brian Wispelwey, M.D.
Associate Professor, Department of Medicine, University of Virginia School of Medicine, Charlottesville, Virginia
Brain Abscess

Frank G. Witebsky, M.D.
Acting Chief, Microbiology Service, Clinical Pathology Department, Warren G. Magnuson Clinical Center, National Institutes of Health, Bethesda, Maryland
The Clinician and the Microbiology Laboratory

Martin S. Wolfe, M.D., D.C.M.T., FACP
Clinical Professor of Medicine, Georgetown University School of Medicine, and George Washington University School of Medicine and Health Sciences; Director, Traveler's Medical Service of Washington, D.C., Washington, D.C.
Protection of Travelers

Peter F. Wright, M.D.
Professor of Pediatrics, Microbiology and Immunology, and Pathology, and Director, Division of Infectious Disease, Vanderbilt University School of Medicine; Staff Physician, Department of Pediatrics, and Director, Clinical Diagnostic Virology Laboratory, Vanderbilt University Hospital, Nashville, Tennessee
Parainfluenza Viruses

Edward J. Young, M.D., M.S.
Professor of Medicine and Microbiology and Immunology, Baylor College of Medicine; Staff Physician, Veterans Affairs Medical Center, Houston, Texas
Brucella *Species*

Lowell S. Young, M.D.
Clinical Professor of Medicine, University of California, San Francisco, School of Medicine; Director, Kuzell Institute for Arthritis and Infectious Diseases, California Pacific Medical Center, San Francisco, California
Sepsis Syndrome

Victor L. Yu, M.D.
Professor of Medicine, University of Pittsburgh School of Medicine; Chief, Infectious Disease Section, Veterans Affairs Medical Center, Pittsburgh, Pennsylvania
The Infectious Diseases Physician and the Internet; Legionella pneumophila *(Legionnaires' Disease)*

Roger W. Yurt, M.D.
Johnson and Johnson Distinguished Professor and Vice-Chairman, Department of Surgery, Weill Medical College of Cornell University; Director, The Burn Center, New York Presbyterian Hospital–Cornell Campus, New York, New York
Burns

Mussaret Zaidi, M.D.
Associate Researcher, Department of Investigation, Hospital General O'Horán, Merida, Yucatan, Mexico
Disinfection, Sterilization, and Control of Hospital Waste

Dori F. Zaleznik, M.D.
Assistant Professor of Medicine, Harvard Medical School; Staff Physician, Beth Israel Deaconess Medical Center, Boston, Massachusetts
Enterobacteriaceae

Stephen H. Zinner, M.D.
Charles S. Davidson Professor of Medicine, Harvard Medical School, Boston; Chair, Department of Medicine, Mount Auburn Hospital, Cambridge, Massachusetts
Sulfonamides and Trimethoprim

John J. Zurlo, M.D.
Associate Professor, Department of Medicine, Section of Infectious Diseases and Epidemiology, Pennsylvania State University College of Medicine, Hershey, Pennsylvania
Pasteurella *Species*

Preface to the Fifth Edition

Infectious diseases remain the number one killer of human beings in the world as we approach the new millennium. Our knowledge of the role of infectious agents in malignancies, heart disease, rheumatic disease, gastrointestinal disease, and other "idiopathic" diseases continues to grow and expand. Preventive options and therapeutic strategies are changing rapidly, with the development of new vaccines, new antimicrobial agents, and innovative immunotherapies.

Our goal was to make this the most complete, authoritative, and up-to-date reference book in the world, and we believe that we and the contributing authors have succeeded.

In this, the fifth edition, we have added new chapters (e.g., Human genetics and infection; Global Epidemiology; New and Emerging Infectious Diseases; Hyperbaric oxygen; Oxazolidinones; Antimicrobial agent utilization and cost control; Home intravenous therapy; Human herpesvirus 8; Microbial warfare and terrorism; Health care reform and the ID specialist; The ID physician and the internet). The AIDS/HIV section has been completely rewritten and expanded. All chapters have been revised or rewritten, and new authors have been selected for many chapters. We are grateful to our authors and are in awe of their dedication and expertise.

Marc Strauss at Churchill Livingstone has been our advocate for excellence, and we thank him for that. Once again, Judith, Shirley, and Kelly get our thanks for putting up with distracted, overworked, and sometimes cranky husbands during the 2 years that it took to complete this latest and best edition.

Gerald L. Mandell, M.D.
John E. Bennett, M.D.
Raphael Dolin, M.D.

Preface to the First Edition

Infectious diseases traverse the usual boundaries established by medical specialists. All organ systems may be involved, and all physicians caring for patients may have to deal with infected patients. The format of this book was chosen with the intent that it would contain the necessary information to aid the practitioner in the understanding, diagnosis, and treatment of infectious diseases. Thus, internists, family or general practitioners, pediatricians, surgeons, obstetrician-gynecologists, urologists, residents and fellows in training, medical students, hospital infection control personnel, and clinical microbiologists should find the book a valuable reference.

In planning this book the editors considered several different patterns of organization. The system adopted allows the reader to approach an infected patient three different ways: (a) by major clinical syndrome, (b) by specific etiologic organisms, and (c) by host characteristics for patients who are compromised.

Principles and Practice of Infectious Diseases consists of four major parts. The book may be perused as whole, or individual chapters may be examined when the reader is concerned with a specific problem. Part I covers the basic principles necessary for a clear understanding of the concepts of diagnosis and management of infectious disease. Chapters dealing with microbial virulence factors, host defense mechanisms, the epidemiology of infectious diseases, and the clinician and microbiology laboratory are included. In addition, there is a comprehensive discussion of anti-infective chemotherapy.

Part II considers major clinical syndromes. The syndromes are described, followed by a discussion of the potential etiologic agents, evaluation of differential diagnostic possibilities, and an outline of presumptive therapy. All major infectious diseases are discussed in this part of the book.

Part III describes all important pathogenic microbes for man and the diseases they cause. The pathogen is classified and described, the epidemiology is discussed, clinical manifestations are listed, and specific information on therapy and prevention is presented. The most comprehensive discussion of a disease entity can be found by reading about both the etiologic agent and the clinical syndrome. Thus, a comprehensive treatment of pneumococcal pneumonia could be found in reading the appropriate sections of the chapters on acute pneumonia and *Streptococcus pneumoniae*. We attempted to make the chapters dealing with etiologic agents and those dealing with syndromes complete. Therefore some repetition was unavoidable.

The final section, Part IV, covers special problems in infectious diseases including nosocomial infections, infections in impaired hosts, immunizations, and protection of travelers.

The editors are grateful to our expert contributors. These physicians are the world's leaders in their fields, and they diligently prepared carefully written, well-referenced "state of the art" chapters. Our secretaries were skillful and meticulous in their attention to the complexities of assembling *Principles and Practice of Infectious Diseases*. John de Carville, executive editor of John Wiley & Sons, encouraged, cajoled, and advised us from the formative steps all the way through to completion. Lastly, and perhaps most important, we are grateful to our wives and children for putting up with interminable editorial work and meetings.

Gerald L. Mandell, M.D.

R. Gordon Douglas, Jr., M.D.

John E. Bennett, M.D.

NOTICE

Contents

DNA VIRUSES

Poxviridae

Herpesviridae

Adenoviridae

Papovaviridae

Hepadnaviridae

Parvoviridae

RNA VIRUSES

Reoviridae

Togaviridae

Flaviviruses

Coronaviridae

Paramyxoviridae

PART I

Basic Principles in the Diagnosis and Management of Infectious Diseases

SECTION A
MICROBIAL VIRULENCE FACTORS

Chapter 1

A Molecular Perspective of Microbial Pathogenicity

DAVID A. RELMAN
STANLEY FALKOW

The study of microbial pathogenicity at the molecular level has altered our view of host-parasite relationships dramatically and has forced the redefinition of some commonly used terms. *Infection, infectious disease,* and *virulence* have been defined and used in numerous and sometimes misleading ways. The essential feature of most infections, however, is the successful multiplication of a microbe on or within a host. This process is often of benefit to both participants. Thus, after birth, human exposure to myriad microorganisms leads to the establishment of protective microbial flora, stimulates the immune system, and, in addition, provides small amounts of human accessory growth factors. The human participants in these infections are most often asymptomatic or exhibit subclinical signs but are generally better off for their encounter with the infecting organism or organisms. It is probably fair to say that such is the usual outcome of most infections.

The term *infectious disease* applies when signs and symptoms result from infection and its associated damage or altered physiology. A *pathogen* is usually defined as any microorganism that has the capacity to cause disease. Yet not all pathogens have an equal probability of causing disease in the same host population. *Virulence* provides a quantitative measure of pathogenicity, or the likelihood of causing disease. For example, encapsulated pneumococci are more virulent than nonencapsulated pneumococci, and *Escherichia coli* strains that express Shiga-like toxins are more virulent than those that do not express these toxins. *Virulence factors* refer to the properties (i.e., gene products) that enable a microorganism to establish itself on or within a host of a particular species and enhance its potential to cause disease.

It is useful to distinguish "principal" pathogens, which *regularly* cause disease in some proportion of susceptible individuals with apparently *intact* defense systems, from other potentially pathogenic microorganisms. Certain microorganisms with potential for causing disease do not meet this definition. *Pseudomonas aeruginosa* is a good example. This microorganism does not usually cause disease in people with intact host defense systems, yet it can clearly cause devastating disease in many hospitalized and immunocompromised patients. Most microorganisms with a capacity for sustained multiplication in humans cause disease more readily in individuals with underlying chronic disease or in those who are otherwise compromised. The common term *opportunist* suits this category of pathogen well. One could extend this argument to say that for most organisms classified as principal pathogens, for example, *Staphylococcus aureus* and the pneumococcus, some impairment or local breakdown in normal host defense mechanisms must occur for these bacteria to cause disease. However, it seems clear that the capacity of certain microorganisms to cause disease in seemingly uncompromised human hosts on a regular basis reflects some fundamental difference in their virulence capabilities from those of opportunists or nonpathogens.

THE ATTRIBUTES OF MICROBIAL PATHOGENS

To be successful, a pathogen must find an appropriate host niche and multiply there. Disease is arguably only an inadvertent outcome of microbial multiplication. To cause infection, a microorganism must possess an interactive group of complementary genetic properties, sometimes coregulated, that promote its interaction with a particular host. For a given microorganism, these genetic traits define unique attributes that enable it to follow a common sequence of steps used by organisms that are successful in establishing infection or subsequent disease.[1, 2] These traits are reflected as phenotypes for which one or more genes and their gene products may be responsible. Elegant molecular techniques permit the identification, isolation, and characterization of many of these genes and their products. In complementary fashion, complete genome sequences provide important clues and insight into the potential of a microorganism for causing disease and facilitate genetic approaches.[3] Precise manipulation of the pathogen's genome has led to determination of the roles for some of these putative virulence factors.

An initial step required of a pathogen is for it to gain access to the host in sufficient numbers. Such access requires that the microorganism not only make contact with an appropriate surface but also then reach its unique niche or microenvironment on or within the host. This requirement is not trivial. Some pathogens must survive for varying periods in the external environment. Others have evolved an effective and suitable means of transmission. To accomplish this goal, the infecting microbe may make use of motility, chemotactic properties, and adhesive structures, or adhesins, that mediate binding to specific eukaryotic cell receptors (see Chapter 2).[4, 5] Preexisting microorganisms, the normal flora, provide competition against establishment of the newcomer; in addition, the latter must adapt, at least temporarily, to the particular nutrient environment in which it now finds itself.

Normal host defense mechanisms pose the next and most difficult set of obstacles to the arriving pathogen. For any set of specific host defenses, an individual pathogen may have devised a unique and distinctive counterstrategy. Some of the best known mechanisms for countering host defenses include the use of an antiphagocytic capsule and the elaboration of toxins and microbial enzymes that act on host immune cells and destroy anatomic barriers. In addition, microorganisms may use subtle mechanisms to avoid or even subvert host defenses, including immunoglobulin-specific protease, iron sequestration mechanisms, or coating themselves with host proteins to confuse the immune surveillance system. Examples of these mechanisms include the production of IgA_1 protease by *Haemophilus influenzae,* the use of receptors for iron-saturated human transferrin and lactoferrin by *Neisseria gonorrhoeae,* and the coating of *Treponema pallidum* with human soluble fibronectin. Antigenic variation and intracellular invasion are other common strategies used by successful pathogens to avoid immune detection.

The ability to multiply is a characteristic of all living organisms. Whether the pathogen's niche in the relevant host be intracellular or extracellular, mucosal or submucosal, within the blood stream or within a privileged anatomic site, the pathogen will have evolved a distinct set of biochemical tactics to achieve this goal. The success of a pathogen, indeed, of any microorganism, is measured by the degree to which it can multiply on reaching its specific niche and secure its potential transmission to a new susceptible host.

Thus, the outcome of the events just described is determined by the degree to which the pathogen has perpetuated itself and by the nature of the relationship it has established with its host. The result may be altered host physiology, tissue damage, and even clinical manifestations of disease. Disease is simply a byproduct of the method and site chosen by pathogens for replication and persistence; disease per se is not a measure of success. Death of the host is a rare event and one that must be viewed as most often detrimental to both parties involved! The more usual outcome is sufficient multiplication of the pathogen to ensure its establishment within the host (transient or long-term colonization) or its successful transmission to a new susceptible host.

Why do some pathogens cause disease more readily than others do? The strategy used for multiplication on or within the host often defines fundamental differences between pathogens that commonly cause disease and those that do not. An organism that can reach and multiply in privileged anatomic sites away from the competitive environment of skin and mucosal surfaces is more likely to disrupt homeostasis in the host and cause disease than is one that chooses a different strategy. If a microorganism has evolved a means to nullify or destroy phagocytic cells to multiply successfully, it is more likely a disease-causing pathogen. Commensal organisms are content to multiply just enough, in the midst of competing microflora, to persist but not damage the host's self-preserving homeostatic mechanisms. It is important to emphasize that a microorganism exceptionally equipped to cause infection may be an unexceptional pathogen and only infrequently, if ever, cause clinically manifested disease.

Why are some organisms such as *P. aeruginosa* only opportunists despite their impressive array of virulence factors? An organism has no presupposition about the state of the host defenses when it encounters a human host. For opportunistic pathogens, that state is the main determinant of whether disease will be the outcome of their interaction with the host. This pattern of infection reflects the fact that these organisms may lack an effective means to overcome normal host defense mechanisms. Opportunists may be very adept at establishing an infection, but because of their preferred growth locale (e.g., the mucosal surface) and preferred growth conditions (e.g., a microaerophilic environment), they may have limited growth opportunities outside their restricted niche in an unimpaired individual. As a result, disease may be only a rare consequence of the host-microbe encounter.

Pathogens were once viewed as organisms, largely unadapted to their hosts, that elaborated potent toxins or other powerful aggressive factors that caused the signs and symptoms of disease. The current view is that a microbial pathogen is a highly adapted organism that follows a strategy for survival requiring multiplication on or within another living organism. Occasionally, this survival strategy produces overt damage to the host. Of course, some infectious diseases occur predominantly in dramatic epidemic form, which argues against the evolution of a balanced host-parasite relationship; however, in many such epidemics, mitigating circumstances involving herd immunity and other underlying social, economic, and political issues impinge on this relationship. Furthermore, some of the most serious infectious diseases occur when humans are infected by microorganisms that prefer and are better adapted to another mammalian host.

THE CLONAL NATURE OF BACTERIAL PATHOGENS

Pathogenicity is not a microbial trait that has appeared by chance. Instead, particular microbial strains and species have evolved to carry very specific arrays of virulence-associated genes. By examining the genetic organization of pathogens, opportunists, and nonpathogenic bacteria, one can begin to understand the origins of pathogenicity.

Techniques used in the study of genetic relatedness include primary protein or nucleic acid sequence comparisons and DNA hybridization methods. Some genetic sequences, such as those of the small- and large-subunit ribosomal RNAs, have been used as reliable evolutionary clocks.[6] Comparative analysis of these sequences allows one to infer phylogenetic relationships among all known cellular life. Multilocus enzyme electrophoresis is a method by which chromosomal structure or genotype is deduced from the electrophoretic mobility variations in a number of common metabolic enzymes.[7] The increasing ease with which primary genomic sequence information can be acquired, differences quantified, and these data shared has led to more precise methods of strain characterization such as multilocus sequence typing.[8] These approaches avoid comparisons of phenotypes (i.e., gross observable characteristics of a microbe, which can be unreliable). When these techniques are used, a consistent finding emerges concerning the population structure of microorganisms: most natural populations of microorganisms consist of a number of discrete clonal lineages.[9]

The finding of a clonal population structure implies that the rates of recombination of chromosomal genes between different strains of the same species and between different bacterial species are very low. Clonal organization has been substantiated by the concordance between evolutionary trees derived from unrelated chromosomal sequences. At first view, this pattern may seem somewhat unexpected because well-established, naturally occurring mechanisms are in place for horizontal genetic exchange between and within species, including transformation, transduction, and conjugation. However, bacteria are haploid creatures. If horizontal transfer of genetic material and subsequent recombination were frequent occurrences, one would expect to see homogenization of bacterial species and little specialization. In fact, the opposite is true. Bacterial species have remained discrete and distinct taxonomic entities[10] because the bacterial chromosome is a highly integrated and coadapted entity that has resisted rearrangement. Nonetheless, global analysis of bacterial chromosomes reveals chimeric features, with evidence of exogenously acquired segments (approximately 18% of the *E. coli* genome) and subsequent amelioration of base composition and codon usage over millions of years.[11]

Analysis of natural populations of microorganisms with pathogenic potential has revealed the prominent representation of a relatively few clones. In fact, most cases of serious disease may be caused by a small proportion of the total number of extant clones that constitute a pathogenic bacterial species. Indeed, in some extreme cases, all members of a species such as *Shigella sonnei* or *Bordetella pertussis* belong to the same clonal type or small group of closely related types. Although it is true of most that have been studied, not all pathogenic bacterial species reveal this pattern of clonal organization. Two notable exceptions are *N. gonorrhoeae* and *P. aeruginosa,* which appear to use chromosomal recombination to increase their genetic diversity. The genetic variability among gonococcal isolates from discrete geographic locations suggests that this organism is essentially sexual. *Neisseria meningitidis* also demonstrates random chromosomal rearrangement; however, because single clones disseminate rapidly during an epidemic, the population structure of this species may falsely appear to be clonal.[12] *Salmonella* population analysis also suggests that serovars that are most adapted to a specific host species are less genetically diverse than those that infect a wider range of hosts.

Clonal analysis has generated other important conclusions concerning the evolution of bacterial species and pathogenic strains in particular. Study of *E. coli* populations in the human intestinal tract indicates that only a small number of clonal lineages persist while numerous unrelated cell lines appear and disappear.[9] *E. coli* urinary tract pathogens causing symptomatic disease in humans are even less genetically diverse than *E. coli* strains found in the intestinal flora or those that cause asymptomatic urinary tract colonization. The nonrandom association of particular versions of different genes within a distinct clone has led to speculation that this species has evolved, not by means of accumulated random recombinational events, but by "random sampling" of clonal populations from the environment with periodic selection and extinction.[11] The evolution of pathogenicity is revealed in part by examination of chromosomal structure and organization.

HORIZONTAL EXCHANGE OF VIRULENCE-ASSOCIATED GENES

Study of natural populations of bacteria suggests that the genetic potential for pathogenicity within a bacterial species has arisen among a small number of unrelated clones through means that do not compromise the genetic individuality of the organism or its unique place in nature but nonetheless in a fashion that provides the microbe with genetic and biochemical flexibility for a competitive environment. How might this adaptation have happened? The answer can be approached from two different temporal perspectives: events that take place over months to years and changes that are defined over millions of years (see the next section).

A number of separate observations indicate that microbes frequently carry virulence-associated genes on mobile genetic elements.[1] Bacteriophages and extrachromosomal elements such as bacterial plasmids are supplements to the bacterial genome that allow a microbe to maintain the integrity of its chromosome and still increase its genetic diversity.[13] Some of these mobile elements are able to enter a wide variety of host organisms and may facilitate the transfer of genes that have been selected for their ability to function in diverse genetic backgrounds.[14] These genetic exchanges are observed over the course of infection within a single host or within a population of microorganisms over the course of months to years. Clinicians are painfully aware that genes encoding antibiotic resistance are efficiently disseminated among different microbial species in nature by such means. The presence of virulence factors in pathogenic bacteria is also associated with the presence of plasmids,[15] transposons, and bacteriophages[13] to a striking degree, both in gram-positive and in gram-negative species (Table 1–1). For example, cholera toxin is encoded by a vibriophage that is found integrated within the *Vibrio cholerae* chromosome.[16] Expression of the fimbrial receptor for this phage is regulated by the same *V. cholerae* protein, ToxR, that controls expression of the cholera toxin genes (see later). Some transmissible elements such as bacteriophages prefer specific chromosomal sites for integration, for example, tRNA genes.[13] This specificity may explain the chromosomal distribution of some virulence genes.

Some bacteria readily exchange random fragments of their chromosome with other members of their species through a process known as *transformation.* For some of these species such as *N. gonorrhoeae,* transformation in nature may provide an additional means of acquiring genes that are advantageous to their growth in the host.

Plasmids, transposons, and phages provide bacteria with the potential for relatively rapid adaptation to an unfavorable, changing, or new environment. Although these mobile genetic elements are often dispensable to the host bacterium, they are typically conserved over substantial periods within diverse cell lineages.[17] This situation is hardly surprising if the mobile element enables the organism to successfully multiply in a host. Often, the mobile element carries multiple virulence-associated genes as a coadapted block, accompanied by a separate self-regulatory system.

GENOMICS AND THE EVOLUTION OF PATHOGENICITY

Comparisons of pathogenic and nonpathogenic representatives of a single genus or species usually demonstrate the nonpathogens to be totally devoid of genetic sequences encoding the pathogenic trait or traits. Inactive mutational variants or portions of virulence-associated genes infrequently occur in nonpathogenic strains of the same species. Not uncommonly, virulence-specific sequences are bounded by repeated DNA segments, some of which represent known insertion elements, which suggests that these virulence genes were once associated with a mobile genetic element or that these genes formerly occupied another chromosomal locale in either the same species or another microorganism altogether. Acquisition of an adhesin, toxin, or serum resistance factor might lead a previously nonpathogenic organism to cause disease in a host that had previously been nonsusceptible.

This concept has been supported by the discovery of "pathogenicity islands."[18, 19] The latter are 35- to 200-kilobase segments of chromosomal DNA flanked by insertion or repeat elements, with a nucleotide composition quite unlike the surrounding bacterial genome. Pathogenicity islands contain clusters of virulence-associated genes that encode specialized secretion systems, secreted effector molecules, adhesins, and regulatory proteins. *Salmonella typhimurium* is believed to have begun evolving as a pathogen approximately 130 million years ago through the sequential acquisition of at least two pathogenicity islands, one of which mediates internalization within host cells and the other, survival and replication within an intracellular vacuole.[20] The apparent genetic instability of some chromosomal regions, such as the *Helicobacter pylori cag* island, can give rise to an assortment of strains with differing virulence capabilities.

Full genome sequencing offers a more complete picture of microbial virulence-associated gene organization. The first complete genome sequence for a free-living organism, *H. influenzae,* was described in 1995.[21] Since then, more than 20 full microbial genome sequences have been completed and released to public databases. These sequences range in size and complexity from the minimal 0.58–mega–base pair (Mbp) genome of *Mycoplasma genitalium* with

TABLE 1–1 Examples of Plasmid- and Phage-Encoded Virulence Determinants

Organism	Virulence Factor	Biologic Function
Plasmid encoded		
Enterotoxigenic *Escherichia coli*	Heat-labile, heat-stable enterotoxins	Activation of adenylate/guanylate cyclase in the small bowel, which leads to diarrhea
	CFA/I and CFA/II	Adherence/colonization factors
Extraintestinal *E. coli*	Hemolysin	Cytotoxin
Shigella spp. and enteroinvasive *E. coli*	Gene products involved in invasion	Induces internalization by intestinal epithelial cells
Yersinia spp.	Adherence factors and gene products involved in invasion	Attachment/invasion
Bacillus anthracis	Edema factor, lethal factor, and protective antigen	Edema factor has adenylate cyclase activity
Staphylococcus aureus	Exfoliative toxin	Causes toxic epidermal necrolysis
Clostridium tetani	Tetanus neurotoxin	Blocks the release of inhibitory neurotransmitter, which leads to muscle spasms
Phage encoded		
Corynebacterium diphtheriae	Diphtheria toxin	Inhibition of eukaryotic protein synthesis
Streptococcus pyogenes	Erythrogenic toxin	Rash of scarlet fever
Clostridium botulinum	Neurotoxin	Blocks synaptic acetylcholine release, which leads to flaccid paralysis
Enterohemorrhagic *E. coli*	Shiga-like toxin	Inhibition of eukaryotic protein synthesis
Vibrio cholerae	Cholera toxin	Stimulates adenylate cyclase in host cells

Data from Elwell LP, Shipley PL. Plasmid-mediated factors associated with virulence of bacteria to animals. Annu Rev Microbiol. 1980;34:465–496; and Cheetham BR, Katz ME. A role for bacteriophages in the evolution and transfer of bacterial virulence determinants. Mol Microbiol. 1995;18:201–208.

its 470 putative protein-encoding open reading frames to the 1.66-, 4.4-, and 4.6-Mbp genomes of *H. pylori, Mycobacterium tuberculosis,* and *E. coli* (see http://www.tigr.org/tdb/mdb/mdb.html). Despite the obvious value of a primary genomic blueprint, it is increasingly clear that genetic, genomic, and epidemiologic approaches provide complementary advantages. Each contributes to the search for new chromosomal determinants of virulence. For example, epidemiologic findings in an outbreak of watery diarrhea in Minnesota led to the characterization of a novel *E. coli* strain with genomic features of both enteroaggregative and enteropathogenic strains.[22]

REGULATION OF BACTERIAL PATHOGENICITY

All bacteria respond to environmental changes with metabolic alterations. A successful host-parasite relationship demands that a pathogen sense its local host environment and distinguish between conditions favorable to rapid growth and those inhospitable and requiring an adaptive or protective response. Consequently, regulating the expression of virulence factors is an additional, yet essential complication of a pathogenic microbe's life.[23] The host presents an array of conditions strikingly distinct from those of the outside environment, conditions that are not easily reproduced in the laboratory. In fact, laboratory culture conditions bias our understanding of microbial adaptation to natural environments. This bias is reflected in the concept of a "viable but nonculturable state" for bacteria in their natural external environment.[24] *V. cholerae,* for example, is thought to persist in this state in brackish estuaries and other saline aquatic environments, sometimes associated with the chitinous exoskeleton of various marine organisms.[25, 26] Transition from this milieu to the contrasting environment of the human small intestinal lumen must be accompanied by substantial genetic regulatory events. The equally dramatic transition for *Borrelia burgdorferi* and *Yersinia pestis* from arthropod vector to human host is accompanied by significant changes in gene expression.[27] This adaptation has practical relevance: the recently approved vaccine against Lyme disease consists of an immunogenic outer surface protein, OspA, that is expressed by the bacterium while in the tick gut, turned off on entry into humans, and then expressed again during late disease. After attachment of an infected tick and initiation of a blood meal, anti-OspA antibodies enter the tick gut and mediate killing of *B. burgdorferi.*

Changes in temperature, ionic conditions, oxygen concentration, pH, and calcium, iron, and other metal concentrations that might appear more subtle also exert profound effects on the expression of virulence determinants.[28] The environmental regulatory signals that prepare the microbe for its transition from an extracellular to an intracellular state may include some of these parameters. For example, iron is a critical component of many cell metabolic processes; therefore, it is not surprising that animals rely on high-affinity iron binding and storage proteins to deprive microorganisms from access to this nutrient, especially at the mucosal surface. In turn, most pathogens sense iron availability and induce or repress various iron acquisition systems accordingly.[29]

Reversible regulation of the expression of virulence genes by temperature is a feature common to many pathogens, including enteropathogenic and uropathogenic *E. coli* (K-88 and K-99 fimbriae, pyelonephritis-associated pilus fimbriae, and K-1 capsular antigen), *Shigella* spp. (invasiveness and Shiga toxin), and *Yersinia* spp. (virulence-associated determinants, including a low-calcium response and outer-membrane proteins). Changes in DNA topology, mRNA conformation, and in the case of the heat shock response, protein stability mediate thermal regulation of these diverse virulence determinants.[30]

The number of well-characterized virulence regulatory systems is rapidly increasing. At the same time, relatively little is known about both the specific environmental signals to which these systems respond and the exact role of these responses in the course of human infection. One common mechanism for bacterial transduction of environmental signals involves a two-component regulatory system that acts on gene expression, usually at the transcriptional level.[31, 32] Such systems make use of similar pairs of proteins; one protein of the pair spans the cytoplasmic membrane, contains a transmitter domain, and may act as a sensor of environmental stimuli, whereas the other is a cytoplasmic protein ("response regulator") with a receiver domain and regulates responsive genes or proteins. Sensor proteins are often kinases that phosphorylate themselves at a conserved histidine residue. These high-energy intermediates then transfer their phosphate groups to a conserved aspartate residue within the receiver domain of the response regulator proteins. Competing dephosphorylases determine an overall phosphorylation state of these response regulators and hence their level of activity. Many of these regulators are DNA-binding proteins that regulate transcription of multiple gene targets. Systems of this type control, for example, the permeability properties of the *E. coli* cell envelope in response to osmotic stimuli (EnvZ/OmpR), motor control involved in *E. coli* chemotaxis (CheA/CheY, CheB), the switch from vegetative growth to sporulation by *Bacillus subtilis* (KinA/SpoOF, SpoOA), and even the ability of the soil bacterium *Agrobacterium tumefaciens* to induce tumors in susceptible plant cells in response to phenols found within plant wound exudates (VirA/VirG). *V. cholerae* ToxR and the BvgAS proteins of *B. pertussis* share several features common to these systems, but they also retain significant differences (discussed later).

The coordinated control of pathogenicity incorporates the important concept of a *regulon.* A regulon is a group of operons or individual genes controlled by a common regulator, usually a protein activator or repressor. This regulator may, in some cases, be the second component of a two-component system as described earlier. A regulon provides a means by which many genes can respond in concert to a particular stimulus. At other times the same genes may respond independently to other signals. Global regulatory networks are a common feature of microbial virulence, as well as basic microbial physiology (Table 1–2). The apparent complexity of virulence regulation in a single microbial pathogen is magnified by the coexistence of multiple interacting ("cross-talking") systems and by regulons within regulons. *E. coli,* for example, expresses more than 20 two-component systems, whereas *H. pylori* encodes 5. Perhaps the more restricted number and type of microenvironments occupied by the latter organism reduce the number of cues that it must recognize. Given the limited sensitivity of in vitro models, it appears that some, but not all regulatory systems are essential for virulence.

B. pertussis synthesizes a group of surface-associated or extracellular products that are responsible for the pathologic and clinical findings of pertussis. These products include pertussis toxin, filamentous hemagglutinin, adenylate cyclase, dermonecrotic toxin, fimbrial protein, and pertactin. Coordinate expression of these and other virulence factors is orchestrated by the two encoded products of the chromosomal *bvgAS* locus.[33, 34] *Trans*-activation and *trans*-repression are features of the Bvg regulon in which at least 20 unlinked chromosomal *bvg*-activated genes are expressed and a group of other *bvg*-repressed genes silenced, or vice versa, depending on the nature of the immediate environment (Fig. 1–1).

BvgS is a member of the histidine kinase sensor class of bacterial regulatory proteins, but unlike most other members of this class, it also contains a receiver communication module and a regulatory carboxyl-terminal domain (see Fig. 1–1). BvgS spans the cytoplasmic membrane and may exist as a multimer.[35] A periplasmic domain responds to temperature and ionic conditions, thereby modulating BvgS activity. At 37°C, BvgS autophosphorylates its transmitter domain, and an ensuing cascade of phosphotransfer events results in phosphorylation of the receiver domain of BvgA, a member of the class of bacterial protein response regulators.[36] BvgA then binds to a DNA recognition sequence located upstream of the *bvgAS* operon itself, the filamentous hemagglutinin structural gene, and other *bvg*-regulated loci and promotes transcription of these genes.[37] Gene repression by *bvg* also occurs at the level of transcription and is mediated by a *bvg*-activated *trans*-acting regulator protein, BvgR, encoded by a locus adjacent to *bvgAS*[38] (see Fig. 1–1). Regulatory

TABLE 1-2 Examples of Bacterial Virulence Regulatory Systems

Organism	Regulatory Gene(s)	Environmental Stimuli	Regulated Functions
Escherichia coli	*drdX*	Temperature	Pyelonephritis-associated pili
	fur	Iron concentration	Shiga-like toxin, siderophores
Bordetella pertussis	*bvgAS*	Temperature, ionic conditions, nicotinic acid	Pertussis toxin, filamentous hemagglutinin, adenylate cyclase, others
Vibrio cholerae	*toxR*	Temperature, osmolarity, pH, amino acids	Cholera toxin, pili, outer-membrane proteins
Yersinia spp.	*lcr* loci	Temperature, calcium	Secretion of effector proteins
	virF	Temperature	Adherence, invasiveness
Shigella spp.	*virR*	Temperature	Invasiveness
Salmonella typhimurium	*pag* genes	pH	Virulence, macrophage survival
Staphylococcus aureus	*agr* genes	Cell density	α-, β-Hemolysins; toxic shock syndrome toxin 1, protein A

Data from Miller JF, Mekalanos JJ, Falkow S. Coordinate regulation and sensory transduction in the control of bacterial virulence. Science. 1989;243:916–922; and Mekalanos JJ. Environmental signals controlling the expression of virulence determinants in bacteria. J Bacteriol. 1992;174:1–7.

cascades allow signal amplification and the possibility of sequential temporal gene expression. For example, with removal of downmodulating conditions, *bvgAS* autoactivation and expression of the crucial adherence factors filamentous hemagglutinin and fimbrial protein precede expression of the other *bvg*-activated genes.[39] With this type of regulatory system, *B. pertussis* can adapt in a measured fashion to the diverse local conditions within the human upper respiratory tract, its natural site of infection.[40] In addition, *bvg*-repressed genes are critical for survival of the related pathogen *Bordetella bronchiseptica* outside its animal hosts and may be detrimental during infection[41]; the role of *bvg*-repressed *B. pertussis* genes remains to be clarified.[42]

Regulation of the expression of virulence determinants by *V. cholerae* also illustrates the use of a global regulatory protein that in this case serves a dual function. The *toxR* gene product is a transmembrane, DNA-binding protein that activates transcription of the genes encoding cholera toxin, pilus colonization factor, and specific outer-membrane proteins.[43] The ToxR protein is thought to sense a variety of environmental regulatory signals, including osmolarity, amino acid concentration, temperature, and pH.[44] ToxR directs expression of these genes indirectly by activating transcription of ToxT, a member of the AraC family of transcriptional regulators.[40, 45] At the level of amino acid sequence, the ToxR protein contains features of both sensor and regulator proteins from the two-component sensory transduction system. The combination of these features into one protein may lead to increased specificity of action.

Quorum sensing is a means by which bacteria keep track of their cell density and regulate their behavior accordingly. Gram-negative organisms secrete and respond to acylated homoserine lactones as a means of cell-cell communication. Production of light by marine vibrios and tissue-degrading enzymes by *P. aeruginosa* is activated by these autoinducing compounds when they reach sufficient concentration.[46] Gram-positive organisms such as *S. aureus* use peptide autoinducers and repressors to sense cell density and regulate toxin expression; these secreted factors might serve as targets for novel immunoprophylactic approaches.[47]

Some microbial pathogens (e.g., *N. gonorrhoeae, Borrelia recurrentis,* and *Trypanosoma brucei*) periodically vary prominent antigenic components of their surface and, by so doing, may avoid the host immune response. Antigenic variations in *S. typhimurium* and *N. gonorrhoeae* provide examples of alternative molecular mechanisms (i.e., DNA rearrangements) that mediate regulation of the expression of virulence factors. *S. typhimurium* varies an immunodominant antigen by alternating between the expression of two different flagellin genes, H1 and H2. The mechanism for this form of variation has been well characterized: inversion of a 995-bp chromosomal DNA sequence orients a promoter such that transcription of the H2 flagellin gene occurs together with that of a gene encoding a *trans*-acting repressor of the H1 gene.[48] The opposite orientation allows relief of H1 gene repression and prevents transcription of H2. Inversion is catalyzed by the *hin* gene product. It promotes site-specific recombination between the 14-bp inverted repeats that flank the invertible segment. In this manner, *S. typhimurium* avoids the host antibody response directed against it.

Pili are essential for virulence of the gonococcus in the human host, probably as a result of their role in adherence to the mucosal target surface.[49] They also elicit a specific local and systemic host antibody response.[50] Intermittent production of pili, as well as variation in the antigenic type of pilus, may be strategies used by the gonococcus to avoid the host immune response. The molecular mechanisms behind these strategies are complex. In general terms, phase and antigenic variation results from DNA rearrangements that move pilin-related sequences scattered around the gonococcal chromosome (in silent *pilS* loci) to the expression site (*pilE* locus).[51] Numerous different pilus types may be expressed by derivatives of a single *N. gonorrhoeae* strain. Gene conversion and other recombination mechanisms may be involved. Among other microbial pathogens, DNA rearrangements account for the antigenic variation of variant surface glycoproteins of *T. brucei*[52] and the antigenic variation of variable major proteins in *Borrelia* spp.[53] A DNA rearrangement is also associated with the expression of type I pili in *E. coli.*

Proper presentation of certain virulence-associated gene products on the microbial surface is now recognized to be as important to pathogenicity as the initial expression of these genes. Presentation entails export pathways, association with other periplasmic or surface factors, and sometimes macromolecular assembly at the surface and is also subject to regulation. Among bacterial pathogens, shared homology is apparent among families of proteins involved in these processes. One family consists of proteins that are known as *chaperones* and *ushers,* concepts first proposed in a model for the assembly of uroepithelium-adherent *E. coli* P pili.[54] Periplasmic chaperones such as PapD escort protein subunits from the cytoplasmic to the outer membrane and assist in their proper folding. Outer-membrane ushers such as PapC target these complexes to a surface assembly site. Folding, transport, and assembly enable a microorganism to present a specific array of surface molecules necessary for eukaryotic cell tropism, intoxication, or entry.[5] A precise configuration of microbial surface molecules might be viewed as an "attack complex," with properties not found in any of the individual components.

MICROBIAL PATHOGENS AS INTRACELLULAR PARASITES

Despite their capacity for an extracellular existence, a wide variety of bacterial and protozoal pathogens have evolved the means to enter, survive, and multiply within host eukaryotic cells. By so doing, a microorganism avoids host immune defenses and gains access to what are otherwise restricted nutrients.[55] These advantages impose a strong selective evolutionary pressure that is dramatically reflected in the refined strategies developed by microbial pathogens for life

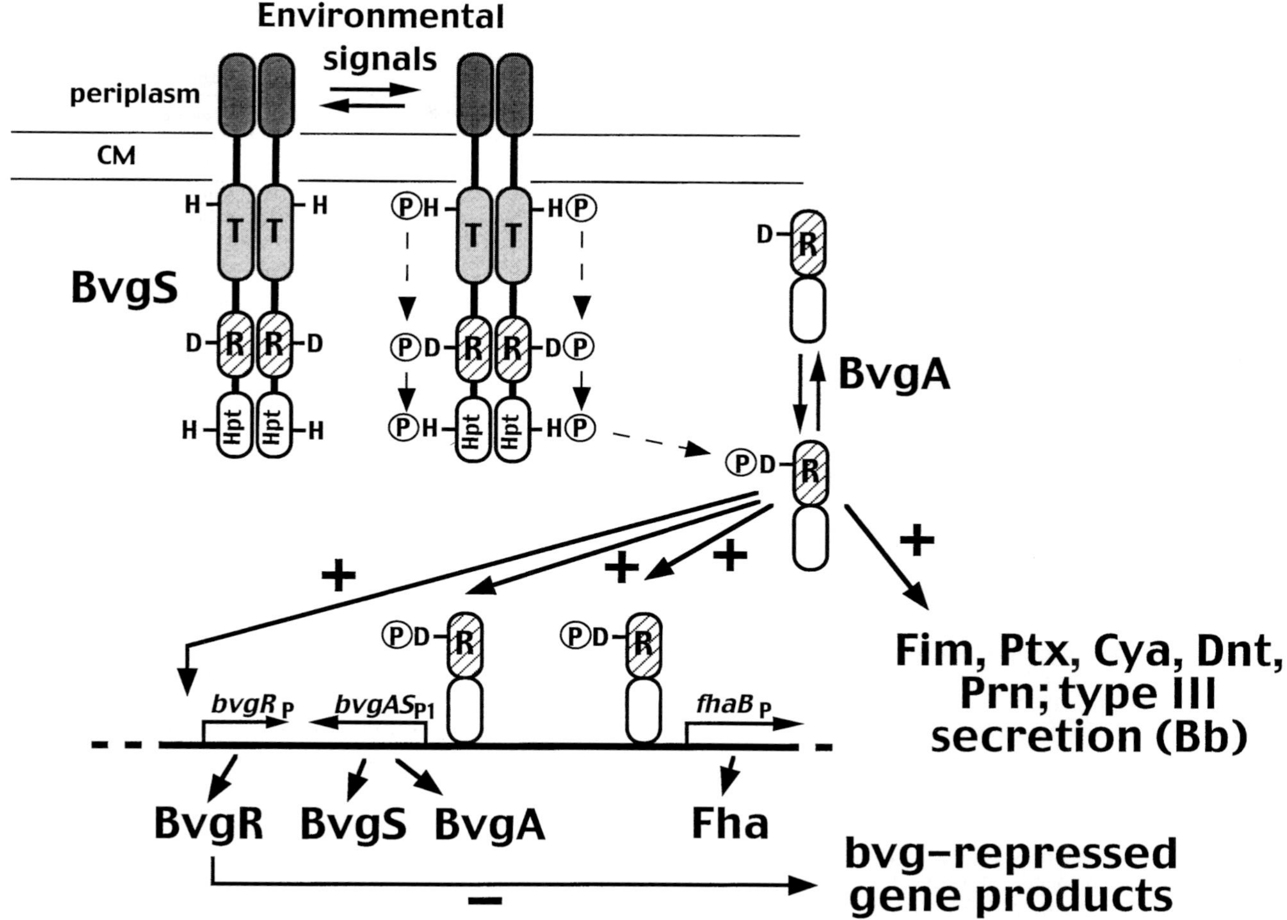

FIGURE 1–1. Schematic model of the *Bordetella pertussis* Bvg regulatory system, by which a variety of virulence-associated genes are coordinately expressed or repressed in response to specific environmental signals (see text). This type of "two-component" regulatory system is found in a number of other microbial pathogens. *Abbreviations:* Bb, *Bordetella bronchiseptica*; CM, bacterial cytoplasmic membrane; Cya, adenylate cyclase; D, aspartic acid; Dnt, dermonecrotic toxin; Fha, filamentous hemagglutinin; Fim, fimbrial protein; H, histidine; Hpt, histidine phosphotransfer domain; P, phosphorylated residue; P subscript, transcriptional promoter; Prn, pertactin; Ptx, pertussis toxin; R, receiver protein domain; T, transmitter protein domain; + and −, positive and negative regulatory signals, respectively.

within a host cell. These strategies include molecular mimicry, coercion, and intimate adaption to eukaryotic cellular processes. Collaborative efforts of molecular microbiologists and cell biologists have begun to reveal some of the details of these strategies.[56] Some common themes are described in this section and the next.

To a large degree, the mechanisms used by a microorganism to adhere to a eukaryotic cell dictate whether and how it enters the cell and its subsequent intracellular fate. Most, if not all intracellular pathogens have multiple means for attachment to a eukaryotic cell surface; the particular combination of microbial attachment factors and cognate host receptors favors selection of one of several entry pathways and predetermines basic features of the intracellular vacuole. However, in a general sense, it is unclear to what extent microbial pathogens accept preprogrammed pathways dictated by phagocytic (e.g., complement and Fc receptors) and nonphagocytic receptors and to what extent they may be able to modify these pathways. *Toxoplasma gondii* invades and replicates within all types of nucleated mammalian cells. After entry and through unidentified receptors, *T. gondii* resides within a parasitophorous vacuole that is permanently incapable of fusion with other intracellular organelles, including lysosomes. Parasite survival within this vacuole depends on the accompanying lack of acidification, exclusion of lysosomal contents, and specific mechanisms for nutrient acquisition and environmental sensing.[57] However, when this organism is directed to enter eukaryotic cells by means of an alternative pathway (i.e., mediated by receptors for the constant region of immunoglobulin G, Fc), this vacuole fusion block is overcome.[58] Presumably, parasite-directed modifications of the surrounding vacuolar membrane and exclusion of certain host proteins during the earliest stages of entry help create conditions necessary for growth and development of the pathogen.

Some pathogenic microorganisms seem to regulate when and where they enter host cells by using preexistent host signaling pathways.[59] Among the receptors that recognize pathogens and mediate entry are integrins (*Yersinia* spp.), the cadherins (*Listeria monocytogenes*),[60] dystroglycans (arenaviruses and possibly *Mycobacterium leprae*),[61, 62] growth factor receptors (*S. typhimurium*), and the cystic fibrosis transmembrane conductance regulator (CFTR) (*Salmonella typhi*). In some of these cases, the pathogen(s) do not depend on only one receptor family for cellular entry. In addition, cell or organ tropism may be determined by recognition of different members of the same family. *S. typhi* is recognized by wild-type CFTR and translocates across the intestinal mucosa as a consequence of binding; however, mutant alleles of CFTR associated with cystic fibrosis are impaired in recognition of this pathogen and may confer some resistance in the host to typhoid fever.[63]

Signaling events at the surface of the host cell, between pathogens of the same type, and between pathogen and host cell indicate a complex, highly evolved process of coadaptation and cooptation.[46, 56] Many of these signals induce rearrangement of host cell cytoskeleton to the advantage of the pathogen. In a particularly dramatic example, enteropathogenic *E. coli* induces the effacement of normal epithelial cell surface architecture and the formation of a specialized structure containing reorganized actin that protrudes from the host cell surface and is called a "pedestal" or pseudopod[64] (Fig. 1–2). Pedestals facilitate intimate attachment but not entry of enteropathogenic *E. coli* to the host cell; attachment is mediated by the bacterial adhesin intimin and a receptor, Tir, that is secreted by enteropathogenic *E. coli* into the host cell and then localized to the host cell membrane at the apical surface of the pedestal.[65] These events require a specialized secretion system (see later) that delivers not only Tir but effector proteins that direct host cell phosphorylation of Tir and stimulate other signaling pathways. All these factors are encoded by genes found within a pathogenicity island known as the locus for enterocyte effacement; this chromosomal island is also found in some strains of Shiga toxin–producing *E. coli.* Tir from Shiga toxin–producing *E. coli* is immunogenic in humans and exhibits sequence and antigenic diversity among different isolates.[66]

Other forms of cytoskeletal rearrangements are essential to the process by which *Salmonella, Shigella,* and other intracellular pathogens enter host cells. *Salmonella* induces "ruffling" of the host cell membrane, which then engulfs the bacterium and leads to internalization via macropinocytosis. This response by nonphagocytic cells is similar to that provoked by growth factors. *Salmonella* Sip proteins and the related *Shigella* Ipa proteins are secreted into host cells after surface contact and are each necessary for the cytoskeletal responses of the host cell and for pathogen entry.

Microbial pathogens that have adapted to an intracellular environment possess diverse and specific strategies for survival and replication. Some pathogens remain within a vacuole (e.g., *Toxoplasma, Salmonella*), and some lyse the initial phagosomal membrane and replicate within the host cell cytoplasm (*Shigella, Listeria, Trypanosoma,* some *Rickettsia* species). Maintenance of specific and favorable vacuolar conditions may entail inhibition of phagolysosomal fusion and acidification (*Toxoplasma*), association of eukaryotic organelles with bacteria-containing vacuoles (*Legionella, Salmonella*), and regulation of pH (*Salmonella*). Some of the details of the molecular mechanisms behind these phenomena are now available. For example, the *Legionella pneumophila* DotA protein plays a major role in the inhibition of phagolysosomal fusion, as well as recruitment of vesicles, mitochondria, and ribosomes to the bacterial phagosome.[67] Furthermore, *S. typhimurium* delays and attenuates macrophage phagosomal acidification, during which various regulons (e.g., the PhoP/PhoQ two-component system) mediate bacterial adaptation to a radically changing environment.[68] Some of these regulated *Salmonella* gene products, such as PhoP-activated PagC, are essential for survival within macrophages and recognize pH as a transcriptional signal.

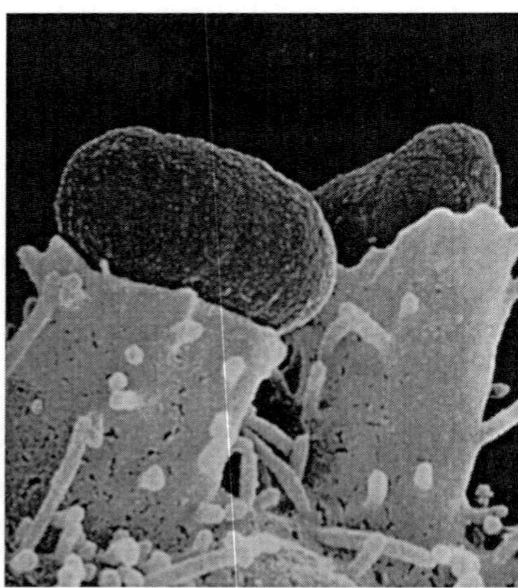

FIGURE 1–2. Scanning electron micrograph depicting pseudopod or "pedestal" formation by enteropathogenic *Escherichia coli* (EPEC) as it interacts with the surface of an epithelial cell. This form of intimate adherence requires a bacterial adhesin, intimin; a receptor of bacterial origin, Tir, that is injected into the host cell; and a series of EPEC-initiated signaling events. Disruption of normal absorptive function results in diarrhea. Other bacterial pathogens are also capable of inducing pedestal formation on intestinal epithelial cells. (From Rosenshine I, Ruschkowski S, Stein M, et al. A pathogenic bacterium triggers epithelial signals to form a functional bacterial receptor that mediates actin pseudopod formation. EMBO J. 1996;15:2613–2624. Courtesy of BB Finlay.)

Early escape from the vacuole is essential for the growth and virulence of some intracellular pathogens. *L. monocytogenes* relies on several molecules for lysis of the early phagosome, including a pore-forming hemolysin (listeriolysin O) and two forms of phospholipase C.[69] Once in the cytoplasm, *Listeria* replicates and induces its own movement through a remarkable process of host cell actin polymerization and formation of microfilaments within a comet-like tail. *Shigella* also lyses the phagosomal vacuole and induces the formation of similar structures for the purpose of intracytoplasmic movement and cell-cell spread. In both cases, bacterial factors involved in actin polymerization have been identified.[70, 71] In the same way that microbial pathogens fare differently in their interactions with phagocytic cells, the outcome of intracellular parasitism for the host cell also varies considerably, depending on the specific host cell and pathogen involved.

SUBVERSION OF HOST CELLULAR PROCESSES AND IMMUNE DEFENSES

Pathogens can be distinguished from commensal microorganisms by their ability to subvert host cellular processes for their own advantage.[56, 72] Enhanced adherence or internalization of the pathogen, inhibition of host cell antimicrobial activity, altered inflammatory responses, enhanced multiplication, and death are potential outcomes for the host cell and goals for the pathogen. As mentioned earlier, one common mechanism by which bacterial pathogens alter or subvert the host cell involves a specialized secretion system, the type III or contact-dependent secretion pathway.[73] Type III secretion systems from diverse bacterial pathogens share structural and functional features that suggest an evolutionary relationship with the bacterial flagellar apparatus. These systems are encoded by blocks of genes that are usually located within pathogenicity islands. Using a supramolecular structure that spans the entire cell wall and resembles a hypodermic syringe,[74] pathogens secrete effector molecules directly across host cell membranes. Whereas *Salmonella* and *Shigella* use type III secretion systems (SPI-1 and invasion plasmid systems, respectively) to mediate entry into host cells, *Salmonella* relies on a second type III system (SPI-2) for successful replication within an intracellular vacuole; this second system is expressed only when the organism occupies this privileged niche.

Type III secreted effector molecules mediate diverse tasks. *Salmonella* SopE is secreted by the SPI-1 system and binds directly to members of the Rho small-molecular-weight guanosine triphosphatase protein family in the host cell cytoplasm; this action activates membrane ruffling.[75] SopE also stimulates mitogen-activated protein kinases and, thus, NFκB and AP-1–mediated nuclear transcriptional responses. The *Yersinia* YopH effector protein is a potent protein tyrosine phosphatase,[76] virulence factor, and antiphagocytic factor. YopJ induces apoptosis in activated macrophages, suppresses tumor necrosis factor-α production, and is critical for *Yersinia* translocation from Peyer's patches to lymphoid tissue and replication in the spleen.[77, 78] A number of pathogens, including *Shigella,* are capable of inducing apoptosis in selected host cells, although each accomplishes this outcome through different mechanisms.[79, 80]

Manipulation of host cell fate and orchestrated choreography of inflammatory responses are recurrent themes in the strategies of microbial pathogens. Because they establish dependent relationships with host cells, viruses often manipulate host cells in dramatic fashion. Human papillomaviruses and other animal viruses induce expansion of their preferred host niche by interfering with critical cell-cycle controls.[81] In an interesting analogy, *Rickettsia rickettsii* blocks a host cell apoptosis defensive strategy to prolong the life of the infected cell, facilitate rickettsial replication, and then spread to other host cells.[82] Molluscum contagiosum virus protects its host cell from oxidative or ultraviolet-induced damage by expressing a glutathione peroxidase–like selenoprotein that acts as a scavenger of toxic oxygen metabolites.[83] Other opportunistic strategies of viral pathogens include suppression of viral antigen presentation by host cells and interference with host cytokine, complement, and interferon activities.[84–86] Bacteria also modulate local cytokine networks.[87]

IDENTIFICATION AND CHARACTERIZATION OF VIRULENCE GENES

Characterization of microbial pathogenicity at the molecular level begins with the identification of a virulence-associated phenotype. Such identification may come from clinical observation, epidemiologic investigation, or the use of a model system that reliably reproduces the microbial phenotype in a manner similar to that seen in natural infection. Traditionally, a virulent strain was compared with a naturally occurring avirulent variant. Such variants, however, may have complex genotypic alterations involving multiple genetic loci. Comparison of strains of naturally occurring virulent and nonvirulent organisms may be even more confounding now that we understand that they may represent entirely different clones.

Analysis using mutant strains with an identical genetic background is a more desirable approach to the definition of virulence phenotypes. The goal is to define a single, well-defined genetic lesion that alters a recognizable phenotype and then test the effect of this alteration on the pathogenicity or virulence of the organism in an appropriate model system. The use of insertional elements (e.g., antibiotic-resistant transposons) as mutational agents is an attractive means of accomplishing this aim. Transposons are pieces of DNA that are able to translocate from one genomic site to another. Insertion into a gene usually disrupts its function. Transposons have the advantage of marking the mutagenized genetic locus with a new selectable phenotype, typically antibiotic resistance, but the disadvantage of possible pleiotropic effects on cotranscribed genes or on overall microbial fitness. The development of broad–host range plasmid vectors carrying well-defined transposons has extended this method of analysis to a number of pathogenic species for which a method of genetic manipulation was not previously available. Once a gene is identified, more precise characterization of the gene product usually follows. By using transposable elements with unique genetic tags, negative selection can be applied to a pool of random mutants in a relevant model of pathogenesis. This approach, known as *signature-tagged mutagenesis,* has identified a number of genes in gram-negative and gram-positive bacteria that are essential for virulence.[88, 89]

Genes of interest are usually isolated by screening a "library" of overlapping pieces of a fragmented microbial genome that have been inserted into an appropriate plasmid or bacteriophage vector, which is then introduced into a carrier microorganism. Although *E. coli* K-12 has traditionally served as the carrier, other organisms may be far more useful than *E. coli* if they are easily manipulated genetically and more closely related to the pathogen of interest, for example, use of *B. subtilis* or even *Listeria innocua* to study *L. monocytogenes.* In some instances, only a few hundred carrier organisms bearing such recombinant molecules need to be examined to screen effectively an entire, average-sized bacterial genome. Typical strategies for screening a genomic library may or may not depend on expression of the cloned gene of interest by the carrier organisms. Tools for screening include DNA fragments or oligonucleotides as hybridization probes and antisera for expressed gene products. In some cases, a recombinant host expressing the cloned gene will display a corresponding phenotype that can be exploited for screening purposes: expression of the cloned *inv* locus from *Yersinia pseudotuberculosis* confers on the *E. coli* host an ability to invade certain types of cultured eukaryotic cells in vitro.[90] The carrier organisms bearing the recombinant clones, once intracellular, are uniquely resistant to the killing effect of gentamicin, which acts only on extracellular bacteria.

A number of powerful methods have been developed for the identification of virulence-associated genes based on the recognition that they are regulated by the transitions between external and internal host and cellular environments.[3] For example, one can select for mutations that cause a defect in the intracellular growth of certain bacterial pathogens by studying auxotrophic strains that die upon replication in conditions that mimic those found within the host cell. One then imposes a requirement upon a pool of mutagenized auxotrophs that they survive serial passage within host cells under these limiting conditions. This method was the one that first revealed the *Legionella dotA* gene (see earlier).[67] Two more recently devised approaches allow one to select for genes and promoters that are preferentially expressed by a microbial pathogen within a host cell or within a host organ. These approaches rely on specially designed vectors into which a complete library of chromosomal genes are cloned such that when the promoters for these genes are activated they turn on the expression of factors that can be easily selected, either by expression of antibiotics, by complementation of an engineered growth-attenuating mutation in the pathogen, or by expression of a fluorescent protein. The application of *in vivo expression technology* to *V. cholerae* and *S. typhimurium* has clarified the conditions encountered by pathogens in vivo, as well as their regulatory responses.[91, 92] By using a technique termed *differential fluorescence induction,* one identifies promoters that are selectively induced within host cells or tissues by fusing random fragments of a pathogen's genome to the gene encoding green fluorescent protein and then applying fluorescence-activated flow cytometry to a pool of recombinant organisms bearing these reporter gene fusions.[93] As an example, differential fluorescence induction has revealed the differential expression of the *Salmonella* SPI-2 pathogenicity island within the phagosomal vacuole.

Broad-based, nonselective approaches for screening an entire genome and its complement of expressed genes are now quite feasible with subtractive hybridization, full genome sequences, and DNA microarray technology. Methods based on subtractive hybridization techniques facilitate the detection of subtle differences between two populations of DNA or RNA. These differences can be amplified by polymerase chain reaction (PCR).[94] An approach of this type was used to identify differences in genomic content among a group of *H. pylori* strains.[95] DNA microarrays are high-density grids of probes displayed on a solid surface; tens of thousands of probes can be arrayed in an area of 1 cm^2. Hybridization of fluorescently tagged target RNA or DNA is detected and quantified by scanning the array with a laser. Although this technology is quite new, it already promises to yield important insight into pathogen biology. For example, by displaying probes for every gene of a given pathogen on a microarray and hybridizing labeled cDNA one can obtain a complete gene expression profile for the pathogen under any desired condition.[96] With these approaches, genes and their products are incriminated by their relationship with a disease-associated process. Final proof, however, that a gene is associated with pathogenicity requires that certain criteria be met (see the next section).

ASSOCIATION OF GENES WITH VIRULENCE: PROOF BY A MOLECULAR FORM OF KOCH'S POSTULATES

Technical advances have brought about a proliferation of reports describing genes thought to be involved in microbial pathogenicity.

These advances have dramatized the need for defined criteria by which genes may be assigned a role in pathogenesis. In a manner analogous to Koch's original postulates, these criteria must include return of the putative causal agent (the cloned virulence-associated gene mutated or intact) to the host of origin. Unless one can demonstrate an effect on pathogenicity by this kind of controlled genetic manipulation, causality with respect to virulence has not been proved. Just as the original Henle-Koch postulates have provided a reference point for later revised criteria of microbial causality,[97] the criteria to be outlined in this section best serve as guidelines, in this case for an experimental approach to the molecular genetic basis of pathogenicity.

A molecular form of Koch's postulates[98] can be stated as follows: (1) the phenotype or property under investigation should be associated significantly more often with pathogenic members of a genus or pathogenic strains of a species than with nonpathogenic members or strains. (2) Specific inactivation of the gene or genes associated with the suspected virulence trait should lead to a measurable decrease in virulence. If inactivation of the gene has taken place in a cloned copy carried by a recombinant host, this mutated gene must be exchanged for the wild-type copy of the gene in the host of origin; the latter must suffer a loss of virulence after the exchange. (3) Restoration of full pathogenicity should accompany replacement of the mutated version of the gene with the wild-type version in the strain of origin.

Technical limitations often face investigators who wish to apply these postulates to an organism poorly characterized from a genetic standpoint. The ability to exchange alleles in the organism under investigation is crucial because it allows a virulence-associated gene to be studied in an isogenic background. Cloned genes carried into the strain of origin on plasmid vectors are exchanged for the analogous chromosomal version of the same genes by means of homologous recombination, an enzyme-catalyzed process by which a segment of DNA replaces an equivalent segment elsewhere that has identical or nearly identical nucleotide sequences. A suicide plasmid cloning vector can be used for this purpose; these vectors are plasmids that can be manipulated in *E. coli,* for example, but are unable to replicate in the organism under investigation. When conjugation is performed in the presence of an antibiotic that selects for the presence of the suicide plasmid, the plasmid becomes recombined into the recipient organism's chromosome because of homology with the cloned gene copy in the plasmid. Subsequent antibiotic selection against the presence of the suicide plasmid allows detection of a second recombinational event that results in excision of the plasmid and replacement of the original chromosomal gene copy with that carried by the plasmid. In this way, chromosomal virulence genes can be modified in a directed fashion.

Another difficulty in the application of a molecular form of Koch's postulates is similar to a problem that faced Koch in his own day: finding an appropriate animal model system. This problem limits the study of microbial pathogenesis as much as any other. It does little good to return a carefully constructed virulence gene mutation to the original strain if its effect on a particular virulence phenotype cannot be evaluated. A model must duplicate relevant pathology commonly observed in the normal host. The animal host must become consistently infected by using a natural route. Clearly, a model of this sort does not exist for many pathogens. At the same time, it should be remembered that exposure to a known human pathogen does not uniformly lead to disease in all humans.

The postulates just outlined are meant to provide principles by which one may study the genes and gene products associated with microbial pathogenesis. This kind of approach can also be used to analyze the internal structure of these genes and the corresponding functional domains of the encoded proteins.

MOLECULAR MICROBIOLOGY AT THE BEDSIDE: PATHOGEN DETECTION AND DISCOVERY

As mechanisms of microbial pathogenicity, acquisition of virulence, and drug resistance are revealed, pathogen detection, strain identification, and pathogen discovery assume increasing importance in the practice of clinical infectious diseases.[99] It is already apparent that studies of microbial pathogenicity at the molecular level have made substantial contributions to our understanding of the epidemiology, clinical manifestations, diagnosis, treatment, and immunoprophylaxis of infectious diseases. Even the fundamental issue of disease causation and the possible role of microorganisms in chronic diseases of uncertain etiology must be reexamined in light of newer experimental methods and insight.[100, 101]

Infectious disease epidemiology hinges on a clear definition of the clinical problem under study and, moreover, precise identification of the etiologic agent. Molecular techniques provide for the sensitive and specific detection of putative pathogens and supply a means for establishing relationships among multiple isolates of the same species. As a result, seemingly unrelated cases occurring during an outbreak have been connected; similarly, geographically or temporally distinct outbreaks have been linked to the same pathogenic clone. Molecular techniques have been used in other epidemiologic investigations to study transmission mechanisms and the role of avirulent microbial variants in the spread of disease.

Several methods are available with which to define clonal relationships among pathogens in an epidemiologic investigation of disease outbreaks, including restriction endonuclease genomic fingerprinting, pulsed-field gel electrophoresis, plasmid analysis, randomly amplified polymorphic DNA analysis, and primary sequence-based methods such as multilocus sequence typing.[8, 102–106] Molecular strain typing data sometimes provide the only clue that a group of cases are related, that is, that an outbreak of disease has occurred.[107] Morphologic and metabolic features often fail to indicate the important genetic diversity found within strains; for example, sequence-based typing of *Cryptosporidium parvum* distinguishes animal- from human-adapted isolates, and *Plasmodium falciparum* isolates can be traced geographically.[108, 109]

One of the most exciting and profound technical advances in the past 15 years has been the development of nucleic acid amplification techniques and their application to the study of microbial pathogenesis and the diagnosis of infectious diseases. PCR, originally described by Saiki and colleagues,[110] is currently the most widely used of these techniques.[111] With this technique it is possible to detect the presence of a single target DNA or RNA sequence in a sample of 10^5 cells. This degree of sensitivity is far greater than that achieved by Southern hybridization with a specific DNA probe. Specific PCR assays and DNA probes are now available for a long and rapidly growing list of microbial pathogens.[104, 111] The more informative of these assays target microbial genetic sequences that encode specific virulence determinants or antimicrobial-resistance factors. Probes linked to nonradioactive detection systems are readily applied to field investigations and are widely used in laboratory diagnosis, both with cultivated microbial pathogens and directly with clinical samples. On the other hand, the extraordinary sensitivity of PCR and potential problems with cross-contamination have thus far restricted its use to reference and research laboratories. Suboptimal sample preparation methods and the PCR inhibitors found in many types of clinical specimens pose additional challenges. Other nucleic acid and probe amplification methods include self-sustaining sequence replication, strand displacement amplification, ligase chain reaction, and Q replicase–based probe amplification.[111]

Southern hybridization–DNA probe technology has been applied widely to infectious disease outbreak investigations and field surveillance. Fingerprint patterns have been used to type strains, track isolates, and incriminate particular strains in multiple cases of disease.[112] PCR- and microarray-based methods may eventually supplant Southern hybridization techniques in many of these sorts of investigations. For example, a variety of arthropod-borne microbial pathogens (such as *Y. pestis, R. rickettsii, Babesia microti,* and some arboviruses) are readily detected in their natural vectors with PCR. *B. burgdorferi* sequences have been amplified from archival tick samples and used to clarify the geographic and temporal origins of Lyme disease in the United States.[113]

Current methods for the identification of microbial pathogens rely heavily on cultivation or propagation in the laboratory. Molecular pathogen discovery methods provide alternative approaches and have spawned new searches for microorganisms that might play important causal roles in a wide variety of poorly explained acute and chronic diseases.[99, 101] The principle behind these methods is reliance on molecular signatures to identify or classify a previously unrecognized pathogen; the most commonly used signature is the genomic sequence, but other small molecules may prove useful. One of these methods targets highly conserved regions of ribosomal DNA sequences by amplifying them directly from digested, infected human tissue.[114] Reliable evolutionary relationships of a putative organism can then be established from these amplified ribosomal DNA sequences. A number of organisms resistant to cultivation or propagation have now been identified with non–culture-based methods.[99, 114–118] Some of these methods originated in earlier efforts to understand better the diversity of microorganisms in the external environment.[119, 120] With the discovery of novel bacterial kingdoms in soil, thermal springs, lakes, and oceans, questions might be raised about our understanding of diversity within the commensal microbial communities that populate the skin and mucosal surfaces of the human body. With the detection of microbial sequences by highly sensitive methods, new challenges are also posed for clarifying the role of the inferred putative organisms in disease causation.[100, 121]

The application of molecular techniques and theory to infectious disease therapeutics and prophylaxis has yet to be fully realized. As virulence factors for essential steps in pathogenesis are identified in individual pathogens, it should be possible to interfere with their function. As they become better characterized, manipulation of global virulence regulatory systems may have therapeutic value. New acellular or recombinant live-attenuated vaccines have already resulted from the identification of immunoprotective antigens through molecular approaches. The current Lyme disease vaccine is an example. Another is an acellular pertussis vaccine based on engineered inactivation of the amino acid residues that are crucial for adenosine diphosphate–ribosyltransferase activity of the pertussis toxin S1 subunit.[122] The increasing availability of microbial full genome sequences will accelerate these efforts.[123] The result should be a more informed and effective approach to the detection, treatment, and prevention of infectious diseases.

REFERENCES

1. Finlay BB, Falkow S. Common themes in microbial pathogenicity revisited. Microbiol Mol Biol Rev. 1997;61:136–169.
2. Falkow S. The microbe's view of infection (Editorial). Ann Intern Med. 1998;129:247–248.
3. Strauss EJ, Falkow S. Microbial pathogenesis: Genomics and beyond. Science. 1997;276:707–712.
4. Jones GW, Isaacson RE. Proteinaceous bacterial adhesins and their receptors. CRC Crit Rev Microbiol. 1983;10:229–260.
5. Hultgren SJ, Abraham S, Caparon M, et al. Pilus and nonpilus bacterial adhesins: Assembly and function in cell recognition. Cell. 1993;73:887–901.
6. Woese CR. Bacterial evolution. Microbiol Rev. 1987;51:221–271.
7. Selander RK, Caugant DA, Ochman H, et al. Methods of multilocus enzyme electrophoresis for bacterial population genetics and systematics. Appl Environ Microbiol. 1986;51:873–884.
8. Maiden MC, Bygraves JA, Feil E, et al. Multilocus sequence typing: A portable approach to the identification of clones within populations of pathogenic microorganisms. Proc Natl Acad Sci U S A. 1998;95:3140–3145.
9. Whittam TS. Genetic variation and evolutionary processes in natural populations of *Escherichia coli.* In: Neidhardt FC, ed. *Escherichia coli* and *Salmonella typhimurium.* 2nd ed. Washington, DC: American Society for Microbiology; 1996:2708–2720.
10. Falkow S. The evolution of pathogenicity in *Escherichia, Shigella,* and *Salmonella.* In: Neidhardt FC, ed. *Escherichia coli* and *Salmonella typhimurium.* 2nd ed. Washington, DC: American Society for Microbiology; 1996:2723–2729.
11. Lawrence JG, Ochman H. Molecular archaeology of the *Escherichia coli* genome. Proc Natl Acad Sci U S A. 1998;95:9413–9417.
12. Maynard Smith J, Smith NH, O'Rourke M, Spratt BG. How clonal are bacteria? Proc Natl Acad Sci U S A. 1993;90:4384–4388.
13. Cheetham BF, Katz ME. A role for bacteriophages in the evolution and transfer of bacterial virulence determinants. Mol Microbiol. 1995;18:201–208.
14. Campbell A. Evolutionary significance of accessory DNA elements in bacteria. Annu Rev Microbiol. 1981;35:55–83.
15. Elwell LP, Shipley PL. Plasmid-mediated factors associated with virulence of bacteria to animals. Annu Rev Microbiol. 1980;34:465–496.
16. Waldor MK, Mekalanos JJ. Lysogenic conversion by a filamentous phage encoding cholera toxin. Science. 1996;272:1910–1914.
17. Mercer AA, Morelli G, Heuzenroeder M, et al. Conservation of plasmids among *Escherichia coli* K1 isolates of diverse origins. Infect Immun. 1984;46:649–657.
18. Groisman EA, Ochman H. Pathogenicity islands: Bacterial evolution in quantum leaps. Cell. 1996;87:791–794.
19. Hacker J, Blum-Oehler G, Muhldorfer I, Tschape H. Pathogenicity islands of virulent bacteria: Structure, function and impact on microbial evolution. Mol Microbiol. 1997;23:1089–1097.
20. Groisman EA, Ochman H. How *Salmonella* became a pathogen. Trends Microbiol. 1997;5:343–349.
21. Fleischmann RD, Adams MD, White O, et al. Whole-genome random sequencing and assembly of *Haemophilus influenzae* Rd. Science. 1995;269:496–512.
22. Hedberg CW, Savarino SJ, Besser JM et al. An outbreak of foodborne illness caused by *Escherichia coli* O39:NM, an agent not fitting into the existing scheme for classifying diarrheogenic *E. coli.* J Infect Dis. 1997;176:1625–1628.
23. Guiney DG. Regulation of bacterial virulence gene expression by the host environment. J Clin Invest. 1997;99:565–569.
24. Roszak DB, Colwell RR. Survival strategies of bacteria in the natural environment. Microbiol Rev. 1987;51:365–379.
25. Huq A, Small EB, West PA, et al. Ecological relationships between *Vibrio cholerae* and planktonic crustacean copepods. Appl Environ Microbiol. 1983;45:275–283.
26. Perez-Rosas N, Hazen TC. In situ survival of *Vibrio cholerae* and *Escherichia coli* in tropical coral reefs. Appl Environ Microbiol. 1988;54:1–9.
27. deSilva AM, Fikrig E. Arthropod- and host-specific gene expression by *Borrelia burgdorferi.* J Clin Invest. 1997;99:377–379.
28. Mekalanos JJ. Environmental signals controlling the expression of virulence determinants in bacteria. J Bacteriol. 1992;174:1–7.
29. Crosa JH. Signal transduction and transcriptional and posttranscriptional control of iron-regulated genes in bacteria. Microbiol Mol Biol Rev. 1997;61:319–336.
30. Hurme R, Rhen M. Temperature sensing in bacterial gene regulation—what it all boils down to. Mol Microbiol. 1998;30:1–6.
31. Stock JB, Stock AM, Mottonen JM. Signal transduction in bacteria. Nature. 1990;344:395–400.
32. Parkinson JS. Signal transduction schemes of bacteria. Cell. 1993;73:857–871.
33. Weiss AA, Falkow S. Genetic analysis of phase change in *Bordetella pertussis.* Infect Immun. 1984;43:263–269.
34. Arico B, Miller JF, Roy C, et al. Sequences required for expression of *Bordetella pertussis* virulence factors share homology with prokaryotic signal transduction proteins. Proc Natl Acad Sci U S A. 1989;86:6671–6675.
35. Stibitz S, Yang MS. Subcellular localization and immunological detection of proteins encoded by the *vir* locus of *Bordetella pertussis.* J Bacteriol. 1991;173:4288–4296.
36. Uhl MA, Miller JF. Integration of multiple domains in a two-component sensor protein: The *Bordetella pertussis* BvgAS phosphorelay. EMBO J. 1996;15:1028–1036.
37. Akerley BJ, Miller JF. Understanding signal transduction during bacterial infection. Trends Microbiol. 1996;4:141–146.
38. Merkel TJ, Barros C, Stibitz S. Characterization of the *bvgR* locus of *Bordetella pertussis.* J Bacteriol. 1998;180:1682–1690.
39. Scarlato V, Arico B, Prugnola A, Rappuoli R. Sequential activation and environmental regulation of virulence genes in *Bordetella pertussis.* EMBO J. 1991;10:3971–3975.
40. Cotter PA, Miller JF. In vivo and ex vivo regulation of bacterial virulence gene expression. Curr Opin Microbiol. 1998;1:17–26.
41. Akerley BJ, Cotter PA, Miller JF. Ectopic expression of the flagellar regulon alters development of the *Bordetella*-host interaction. Cell. 1995;80:611–620.
42. Merkel TJ, Stibitz S, Keith JM, et al. Contribution of regulation by the *bvg* locus to respiratory infection of mice by *Bordetella pertussis.* Infect Immun. 1998;66:4367–4373.
43. Miller VL, Taylor RK, Mekalanos JJ. Cholera toxin transcriptional activator *toxR* is a transmembrane DNA binding protein. Cell. 1987;48:271–279.
44. Miller VL, Mekalanos JJ. A novel suicide vector and its use in construction of insertion mutations: Osmoregulation of outer membrane proteins and virulence determinants in *Vibrio cholerae* requires *toxR.* J Bacteriol. 1988;170:2575–2583.
45. DiRita VJ, Parsot C, Jander G, et al. Regulatory cascade controls virulence in *Vibrio cholerae.* Proc Natl Acad Sci U S A. 1991;88:5403–5407.
46. Fuqua C, Greenberg EP. Self perception in bacteria: Quorum sensing with acylated homoserine lactones. Curr Opin Microbiol. 1998;1:183–189.
47. Balaban N, Goldkorn T, Nhan RT, et al. Autoinducer of virulence as a target for vaccine and therapy against *Staphylococcus aureus.* Science. 1998;280:438–440.
48. Simon M, Zieg J, Silverman M, et al. Phase variation: Evolution of a controlling element. Science. 1980;209:1370–1374.
49. McGee ZA, Johnson AP, Taylor-Robinson D. Pathogenic mechanisms of *Neisseria gonorrhoeae:* Observations on damage to human fallopian tubes in organ culture by gonococci of colony type 1 or type 4. J Infect Dis. 1981;143:413–422.

50. McChesney D, Tramont EC, Boslego JW, et al. Genital antibody response to a parenteral gonococcal pilus vaccine. Infect Immun. 1982;36:1006–1012.
51. Seifert HS, So M. Genetic mechanisms of bacterial antigenic variation. Microbiol Rev. 1988;52:327–336.
52. Borst P. Discontinuous transcription and antigenic variation in trypanosomes. Annu Rev Biochem. 1986;55:701–732.
53. Meier JT, Simon MI, Barbour AG. Antigenic variation is associated with DNA rearrangements in a relapsing fever borrelia. Cell. 1985;41:403–409.
54. Jones CH, Jacob-Dubuisson F, Dodson K, et al. Adhesin presentation in bacteria requires molecular chaperones and ushers. Infect Immun. 1992;60:4445–4451.
55. Falkow S. Bacterial entry into eukaryotic cells. Cell. 1991;65:1099–1102.
56. Finlay BB, Cossart P. Exploitation of mammalian host cell functions by bacterial pathogens. Science. 1997;276:718–725.
57. Joiner KA, Dubremetz JF. *Toxoplasma gondii:* A protozoan for the nineties. Infect Immun. 1993;61:1169–1172.
58. Joiner KA, Fuhrman SA, Miettinen HM, et al. *Toxoplasma gondii:* Fusion competence of parasitophorous vacuoles in Fc receptor–transfected fibroblasts. Science. 1990;249:641–646.
59. Bliska JB, Galan JE, Falkow S. Signal transduction in the mammalian cell during bacterial attachment and entry. Cell. 1993;73:903–920.
60. Mengaud J, Ohayon H, Guonon P, et al. E-cadherin is the receptor for internalin, a surface protein required for entry of *L. monocytogenes* into epithelial cells. Cell. 1996;84:923–932.
61. Cao W, Henry MD, Borrow P, et al. Identification of alpha-dystroglycan as a receptor for lymphocytic choriomeningitis virus and Lassa fever virus. Science. 1998;282:2079–2081.
62. Rambukkana A, Yamada H, Zanazzi G, et al. Role of alpha-dystroglycan as a Schwann cell receptor for *Mycobacterium leprae.* Science. 1998;282:2076–2079.
63. Pier GB, Grout M, Zaidi T, et al. *Salmonella typhi* uses CFTR to enter intestinal epithelial cells. Nature. 1998;393:79–82.
64. Rosenshine I, Ruschkowski S, Stein M, et al. A pathogenic bacterium triggers epithelial signals to form a functional bacterial receptor that mediates actin pseudopod formation. EMBO J. 1996;15:2613–2624.
65. Kenny B, DeVinney R, et al. Enteropathogenic *E. coli* (EPEC) transfers its receptor for intimate adherence into mammalian cells. Cell. 1997;91:511–520.
66. Paton AW, Manning PA, Woodrow MC, Paton JC. Translocated intimin receptors (Tir) of Shiga-toxigenic *Escherichia coli* isolates belonging to serogroups O26, O111, and O157 react with sera from patients with hemolytic-uremic syndrome and exhibit marked sequence heterogeneity. Infect Immun. 1998;66:5580–5586.
67. Roy CR, Berger KH, Isberg RR. *Legionella pneumophila* DotA protein is required for early phagosome trafficking decisions that occur within minutes of bacterial uptake. Mol Microbiol. 1998;28:663–674.
68. Alpuche-Aranda CM, Swanson JA, Loomis WP, Miller SI. *Salmonella typhimurium* activates virulence gene transcription within acidified macrophage lysosomes. Proc Natl Acad Sci U S A. 1992;89:10079–10083.
69. Cossart P, Lecuit M. Interactions of *Listeria monocytogenes* with mammalian cells during entry and actin-based movement: Bacterial factors, cellular ligands and signaling. EMBO J. 1998;17:3797–3806.
70. Goldberg MB, Barzu O, Parsot C, Sansonetti PJ. Unipolar localization and ATPase activity of IcsA, a *Shigella flexneri* protein involved in intracellular movement. J Bacteriol. 1993;175:2189–2196.
71. Kocks C, Gouin E, Tabouret M, et al. *L. monocytogenes*–induced actin assembly requires the *actA* gene product, a surface protein. Cell. 1992;68:521–531.
72. Galan JE. Interactions of *Salmonella* with host cells: Encounters of the closest kind. Proc Natl Acad Sci U S A. 1998;95:14006–14008.
73. Hueck CJ. Type III protein secretion systems in bacterial pathogens of animals and plants. Microbiol Mol Biol Rev. 1998;62:379–433.
74. Kubori T, Matsushima Y, Nakamura D, et al. Supramolecular structure of the *Salmonella typhimurium* type III protein secretion system. Science. 1998;280:602–605.
75. Hardt WD, Chen LM, Schuebel KE, et al. *S. typhimurium* encodes an activator of Rho GTPases that induces membrane ruffling and nuclear responses in host cells. Cell. 1998;93:815–826.
76. Clemens JC, Guan K, Bliska JB, et al. Microbial pathogenesis and tyrosine dephosphorylation: Surprising bedfellows. Mol Microbiol. 1991;5:2617–2620.
77. Monack DM, Mecsas J, Bouley D, Falkow S. *Yersinia*-induced apoptosis in vivo aids in the establishment of a systemic infection of mice. J Exp Med. 1998;188:2127–2137.
78. Schesser K, Spiik AK, Dukuzumuremyi JM, et al. The *yopJ* locus is required for *Yersinia*-mediated inhibition of NF-kappaB activation and cytokine expression: YopJ contains a eukaryotic SH2-like domain that is essential for its repressive activity. Mol Microbiol. 1998;28:1067–1079.
79. Zychlinsky A, Prevost MC, Sansonetti PJ. *Shigella flexneri* induces apoptosis in infected macrophages. Nature. 1992;358:167–169.
80. Zychlinsky A, Sansonetti P. Perspectives series: Host/pathogen interactions. Apoptosis in bacterial pathogenesis. J Clin Invest. 1997;100:493–495.
81. Galloway DA, McDougall JK. The disruption of cell cycle checkpoints by papillomavirus oncoproteins contributes to anogenital neoplasia. Semin Cancer Biol. 1996;7:309–315.
82. Clifton DR, Goss RA, Sahni SK, et al. NF-kappa B–dependent inhibition of apoptosis is essential for host cell survival during *Rickettsia rickettsii* infection. Proc Natl Acad Sci U S A. 1998;95:4646–4651.
83. Shisler JL, Senkevich TG, Berry MJ, Moss B. Ultraviolet-induced cell death blocked by a selenoprotein from a human dermatotropic poxvirus. Science. 1998;279:102–105.
84. Marrack P, Kappler J. Subversion of the immune system by pathogens. Cell. 1994;76:323–332.
85. Smith GL. Virus strategies for evasion of the host response to infection. Trends Microbiol. 1994;2:81–88.
86. McFadden G. Even viruses can learn to cope with stress. Science. 1998;279:40–41.
87. Wilson M, Seymour R, Henderson B, et al. Bacterial perturbation of cytokine networks. Infect Immun. 1998;66:2401–2409.
88. Hensel M, Shea JE, Gleeson C, et al. Simultaneous identification of bacterial virulence genes by negative selection. Science. 1995;269:400–403.
89. Mei JM, Nourbakhsh F, Ford CW, Holden DW. Identification of *Staphylococcus aureus* virulence genes in a murine model of bacteraemia using signature-tagged mutagenesis. Mol Microbiol. 1997;26:399–407.
90. Isberg RR, Falkow S. A single genetic locus encoded by *Yersinia pseudotuberculosis* permits invasion of cultured animal cells by *Escherichia coli* K-12. Nature. 1985;317:262–264.
91. Mahan MJ, Slauch JM, Mekalanos JJ. Selection of bacterial virulence genes that are specifically induced in host tissues. Science. 1993;259:686–688.
92. Heithoff DM, Conner CP, Hanna PC, et al. Bacterial infection as assessed by in vivo gene expression. Proc Natl Acad Sci U S A. 1997;94:934–939.
93. Valdivia RH, Falkow S. Fluorescence-based isolation of bacterial genes expressed within host cells. Science. 1997;277:2007–2011.
94. Lisitsyn N, Lisitsyn N, Wigler M. Cloning the differences between two complex genomes. Science. 1993;259:946–951.
95. Akopyants NS, Fradkov A, Diatchenko L, et al. PCR-based subtractive hybridization and differences in gene content among strains of *Helicobacter pylori.* Proc Natl Acad Sci U S A. 1998;95:13108–13113.
96. deSaizieu A, Certa U, Warrington J, et al. Bacterial transcript imaging by hybridization of total RNA to oligonucleotide arrays. Nat Biotechnol. 1998;16:45–48.
97. Evans AS. Causation and disease: The Henle-Koch postulates revisited. Yale J Biol Med. 1976;49:175–195.
98. Falkow S. Molecular Koch's postulates applied to microbial pathogenicity. Rev Infect Dis. 1988;10(Suppl):S274–S276.
99. Relman DA. Detection and identification of previously unrecognized microbial pathogens. Emerg Infect Dis. 1998;4:382–389.
100. Fredricks DN, Relman DA. Sequence-based identification of microbial pathogens: A reconsideration of Koch's postulates. Clin Microbiol Rev. 1996;9:18–33.
101. Fredricks DN, Relman DA. Infectious agents and the etiology of chronic idiopathic diseases. Curr Clin Top Infect Dis. 1998;18:180–200.
102. Welsh J, McClelland M. Fingerprinting genomes using PCR with arbitrary primers. Nucleic Acids Res. 1990;18:7213–7218.
103. Naber SP. Molecular pathology—diagnosis of infectious disease. N Engl J Med. 1994;331:1212–1215.
104. Ieven M, Goossens H. Relevance of nucleic acid amplification techniques for diagnosis of respiratory tract infections in the clinical laboratory. Clin Microbiol Rev. 1997;10:242–256.
105. Tang YW, Procop GW, Persing DH. Molecular diagnostics of infectious diseases. Clin Chem. 1997;43:2021–2038.
106. Lipuma JJ. Molecular tools for epidemiologic study of infectious diseases. Pediatr Infect Dis J. 1998;17:667–675.
107. Bender JB, Hedberg CW, Besser JM, et al. Surveillance by molecular subtype for *Escherichia coli* O157:H7 infections in Minnesota by molecular subtyping. N Engl J Med. 1997;337:388–394.
108. Awad-El-Kariem FM, Robinson HA, Petry F, et al. Differentiation between human and animal isolates of *Cryptosporidium parvum* using molecular and biological markers. Parasitol Res. 1998;84:297–301.
109. Robson KJ, Dolo A, Hackford IR, et al. Natural polymorphism in the thrombospondin-related adhesive protein of *Plasmodium falciparum.* Am J Trop Med Hyg. 1998;58:81–89.
110. Saiki RK, Gelfand DH, Stoffel S, et al. Primer-directed enzymatic amplification of DNA with a thermostable DNA polymerase. Science. 1988;239:487–491.
111. Persing DH, Smith TF, Tenover FC, White TJ, eds. Diagnostic Molecular Microbiology: Principles and Applications. Washington, DC: American Society for Microbiology; 1993.
112. Behr MA, Warren SA, Salamon H, et al. Transmission of *Mycobacterium tuberculosis* from patients smear-negative for acid-fast bacilli. Lancet. 1999; 353:444–449.
113. Persing DH, Telford SR III, Rys PN, et al. Detection of *Borrelia burgdorferi* DNA in museum specimens of *Ixodes dammini* ticks. Science. 1990;249:1420–1423.
114. Relman DA, Loutit JS, Schmidt TM, et al. The agent of bacillary angiomatosis: An approach to the identification of uncultured pathogens. N Engl J Med. 1990;323:1573–1580.
115. Wilson KH, Blitchington R, Frothingham R, et al. Phylogeny of the Whipple's-disease–associated bacterium. Lancet. 1991;338:474–475.
116. Relman DA, Schmidt TM, MacDermott RP, et al. Identification of the uncultured bacillus of Whipple's disease. N Engl J Med. 1992;327:293–301.
117. Chang Y, Cesarman E, Pessin MS, et al. Identification of herpesvirus-like DNA sequences in AIDS-associated Kaposi's sarcoma. Science. 1994;266:1865–1869.
118. Santamaria FM, Fajardo LF, Sogin ML, et al. Lethal infection by a previously unrecognised metazoan parasite. Lancet. 1996;347:1797–1801.
119. Pace NR. A molecular view of microbial diversity and the biosphere. Science. 1997;276:734–740.

120. Hugenholtz P, Goebel BM, Pace MR. Impact of culture-independent studies on the emerging phylogenetic view of bacterial diversity. J Bacteriol. 1998;180:4765–4774.
121. Relman DA. The search for unrecognized pathogens. Science. 1999;284:1308–1310.
122. Pizza M, Covacci A, Bartoloni A, et al. Mutants of pertussis toxin suitable for vaccine development. Science. 1989;246:497–500.
123. Moxon ER. Applications of molecular microbiology to vaccinology. Lancet. 1997;350:1240–1244.

Chapter 2

Microbial Adherence

WILLIAM A. PETRI, JR.
BARBARA J. MANN

Adherence is the initial interaction of a pathogenic microorganism with its host. Adherence is the route to cellular invasion by intracellular parasites and the first step in host cell killing and toxin delivery by microbial pathogens. Adhesins are microbial molecules that mediate adherence or binding of microbes to the host (Fig. 2–1). Receptors are the host molecules or ligands that microbial adhesins bind to initiate adherence. A single adhesin may have more than one receptor, and a single receptor may be recognized by many different adhesins.

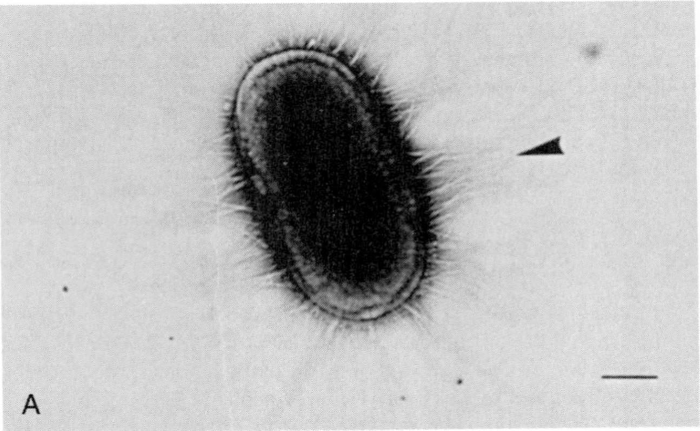

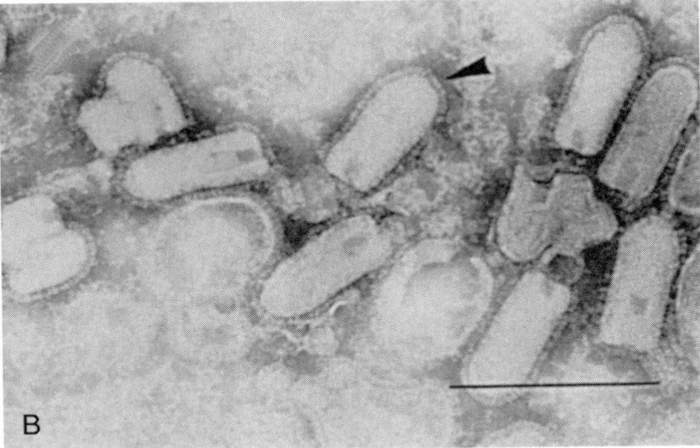

FIGURE 2–1. Vesicular stomatitis virus and *Escherichia coli* adhesins. Electron micrographs of *E. coli* expressing P fimbriae *(arrowhead) (A)* and vesicular stomatitis virus, demonstrating the spikelike protrusions *(arrowhead)* of the viral adherence glycoprotein *(B)*. Bar = 0.25 μm. (*A* from Klemm P. Fimbrial adhesins of *Escherichia coli*. Rev Infect Dis. 1985;7:321–340.)

EXPERIMENTAL IDENTIFICATION OF AN ADHESIN

Understanding a microbe's adherence mechanism begins with the development of an adherence assay (Table 2–1). Care must be taken that the assay is designed to measure adherence and not motility or invasion. Experiments to measure adherence are often performed at 4°C, a temperature at which motility and invasion are inhibited. Juxtaposition of microbe and target cell can be accomplished by centrifugation, so motility of the microbe is not required for adherence to take place. Bacterial adherence to cells may also be distinguished from invasion by adding aminoglycosides to the medium after adherence has occurred. Only extracellular bacteria should be killed because aminoglycosides do not penetrate into cells in sufficient quantities to kill intracellular bacteria. Other approaches include mild fixation of target cells to prevent intracellular invasion.

A physiologically relevant substrate can also be an important component of an adherence assay. Receptors for some microorganisms such as influenza or *Entamoeba histolytica* are ubiquitous, so little, if any species or tissue restriction to adherence in vitro is noted. However, the adherence of many microorganisms such as polioviruses and rhinoviruses is species specific and, in the case of pathogens such as Epstein-Barr virus (EBV) and the human immunodeficiency virus (HIV), is species and cell type specific. An adherence assay that measures hepatitis B virus binding to human hepatocytes is more likely to yield information relevant to pathogenesis than one measuring binding to mouse fibroblasts, for example.

Adherence can often be measured visually. The influenza virus adhesin is named *hemagglutinin* (HA) because of the initial observation that purified influenza virions agglutinate erythrocytes. Cell rosetting assays performed with larger microorganisms are a modification of these hemagglutination assays. Radioactive labeling of the microbe is often used as a means to measure adherence to cells. Care must be taken that the labeling procedure does not kill or significantly alter the microbe; a good test is to show that binding of the radiolabeled microorganism can be inhibited by excess unlabeled microorganism. Likewise, binding of soluble receptors such as extracellular matrix components to microorganisms is performed by radiolabeling the receptors, with "specific" binding defined as the amount of radiolabeled receptor bound that is inhibited by excess cold receptor.

Once an assay has been developed to measure the adherence of a pathogen to a cell or substrate, steps can be taken to identify the microbial components participating in adherence. Because the binding of many microbes to host tissues is mediated by microbial lectins, an initial approach is to test whether adherence can be blocked with simple sugars or complex oligosaccharides. Definition of the carbohydrate specificity of adherence can lead to identification of the responsible adhesin via carbohydrate affinity chromatography. Another common approach is to screen monoclonal antibodies produced against the microorganism for their ability to block adherence; inhibitory monoclonal antibodies can be used to identify and purify the putative adhesin.

Antibody inhibition of adherence is most convincing if performed

TABLE 2–1 Approaches to the Identification of Adhesins of Pathogenic Microorganisms

Develop an assay that measures adherence to a physiologically relevant substrate.
Inhibit adherence with simple sugars or Fab fragments of monoclonal antibodies directed against the microorganism.
Demonstrate receptor binding activity of the purified putative adhesin and show that excess adhesin blocks adherence of intact organsisms.
Mutate the adhesin gene and demonstrate a change in the adhesive phenotype of the organism.

TABLE 2–2 Approaches to the Identification of Host Cell Receptors for Pathogenic Microorganisms

Transfer DNA from a permissive to a nonpermissive cell; identify the transfected DNA that confers permissiveness. This technique exploits the fact that many microorganisms have restricted host ranges (e.g., rhinovirus infects only human and chimpanzee cells) and tissue tropism (e.g., HIV and CD4 cells, Epstein-Barr virus, and B cells)
Produce monoclonal antibodies against host cell surface antigens; screen the antibody for inhibition of binding or infection. Characterize the antigen recognized by the monoclonal antibody.
Identify lectin (carbohydrate recognition) activity of the microorganism's adhesin by blocking adherence, infectivity, or both of the permissive cell with simple or complex carbohydrates (e.g., sialic acid and influenza hemagglutinin; HIV and galactosylcerebroside).
Affinity-purify the host cell receptor by using microbial adhesin (rarely successful because of the generally low affinity of the adhesin for the solubilized receptor).

TABLE 2–4 Classes of Microbial Adhesins for Host Cell Receptors

Lectins: Sialic acid binding (hemagglutinin envelope glycoproteins of orthomyxoviruses), galactose binding (*Entamoeba histolytica* adherence lectin), galactosylcerebroside binding (HIV gp120/gp41), *trans*-sialidase (*Trypanosoma cruzi*)
Fimbria (pili): Filamentous bacterial adhesins of *Escherichia coli* (P, S, type 1, K-88, K-99, CFA-1), *Neisseria gonorrhoeae* (type 4), *Salmonella* (type 1), *Vibrio cholerae* (Tcp)
Nonfimbrial bacterial adhesins: Yersinia (Inv and Ail proteins), *Bordetella pertussis* (pertactin), *Mycoplasma pneumoniae* (P1 cytoadhesin), *Treponema pallidum* (fibronectin-binding protein)
Lipid: Streptococcus pyogenes (lipoteichoic acid), *Leishmania* (lipophosphoglycan)
Glycosaminoglycan: Chlamydia trachomatis (heparin sulfate–like glycosaminoglycan)
Viral capsid proteins: Rhinovirus (VP1/VP3); aphthovirus (VP1)
Mechanical: Giardia lamblia (gripping disk)

with Fab fragments of antibody, which reduces the likelihood of nonspecific effects of the antibodies from agglutination, steric hindrance, or cross-linking on the microbial surface, or performed with monoclonal antibodies, where epitope-specific inhibition of adherence can be demonstrated (monoclonal antibody to some but not all epitopes on an adhesin blocks its adhesive function, thereby making nonspecific effects of the monoclonal antibody less likely). The purified putative adhesin should be demonstrated to bind to the microbe's receptor, and excess adhesin should be able to inhibit adherence of the intact microbe competitively by preventing binding to the host receptor.

EXPERIMENTAL IDENTIFICATION OF A HOST RECEPTOR

Identification of the receptor for an adhesin is important to understanding the interactions of microbial pathogens with their hosts (Table 2–2). In several pathogens the species specificity, or tissue or cell tropism, of a microorganism can be explained by the presence or absence of a receptor for the microbial adhesin. Examples include the B-lymphocyte CR2 receptor for EBV,[1] the T-cell CD4 receptor for HIV,[2, 3] and the aminopeptidase N receptor for the pig coronavirus TGEV.[4, 5] Species specificity of adherence of microbial pathogens has also been demonstrated for poliovirus[6, 7] and the major group of rhinoviruses,[8–10] where viral receptors are present on human but not murine cells (Tables 2–3 and 2–4).

Species or tissue specificity for receptors for microbial adhesins suggests an obvious approach to their identification: transfection of DNA from a receptor-positive to a receptor-negative cell line, followed by identification and sequencing of the DNA segment that confers receptor positivity. This approach has been successfully used to identify intercellular adhesion molecule 1 (ICAM-1) as the human receptor for the major group of rhinoviruses[9, 10] and to identify the poliovirus receptor, a member of the immunoglobulin gene superfamily.[6, 7] The advantage of this approach to receptor identification is that the receptor is cloned and sequenced at the same time that it is identified.

When a restricted host range or tissue tropism cannot be exploited, monoclonal antibodies produced against the host cell have been used to identify the receptor. Monoclonal antibodies that block adherence to or infection of host cells were used to identify ICAM-1 as the receptor for the major group of rhinoviruses,[8] CD4 as the HIV receptor,[2, 3] aminopeptidase N as the TGEV coronavirus receptor,[4, 5] and VLA-2 as the receptor for echovirus-1.[11]

If the microbial adhesin is a lectin, the carbohydrate structure recognized by the adhesin on host cells can be determined by the effect of different oligosaccharides on inhibition of adherence. In this manner, the detailed structure of the sialic acid–containing oligosaccharide recognized by influenza virus HA has been determined.[12]

If the adhesin itself is purified, it can be used to affinity-purify its receptor from the host cell. This approach is not likely to be successful if the interaction of adhesin with receptor is of low affinity, which may be a particular problem when adhesin and receptor have been solubilized in purification. However, this approach successfully identified CR2 as the receptor for EBV.

CENTRAL CONCEPTS IN THE INTERACTIONS OF ADHESINS AND RECEPTORS

Many adhesins require post-translational processing, especially proteolytic fragmentation, to manifest full biologic activity (Table 2–5). The membrane fusion activity of HA, which is required for viral infectivity, requires processing by a host protease of the intact hemagglutinin (HA_0) into HA_1 and HA_2. This proteolytic fragmentation exposes a highly conserved hydrophobic sequence at the amino terminus of HA_2 that, at acidic pH, is involved in viral entry into the cell by fusion of the viral membrane to the endocytic vacuole cell membrane[12] (Fig. 2–2). Similar processing events are required for the gp160 adhesin of HIV to have functional cell fusion activity, as will be described later. The requirement for host proteases to activate the fusion activity of adhesins may partly explain the tissue tropism of microbial pathogens inasmuch as the proteases required to activate the adhesins may be present only in certain tissues.

A second important concept is the "canyon hypothesis," in which

TABLE 2–3 Classes of Host Cell Receptors for Microbial Adhesins

Sugars: Sialic acid (orthomyxoviruses and paramyxoviruses, polyomaviruses), galactose (*Entamoeba histolytica*), galactosylcerebroside (HIV)
Immunoglobulin superfamily: ICAM-1 (rhinoviruses, major group), CD4 (HIV), polioviruses receptor (polio)
Growth factors or growth factor receptors: ECF receptors (vaccinia), erythropoietin receptor (Friend leukemia virus), interleukin-6 (hepatitis B virus)
Integrins: VLA-2 (echovirus)
Extracellular matrix components: Laminin (*toxoplasma gondii*), fibronectin (streptococci)
Transport proteins: Basic amino acid and phosphate transporter (certain retroviruses)
Complement receptors: CR2 (Epstein-Barr virus)
Antibody-dependent or complement-dependent enhancement of adherence: Antibody-coated dengue virus entry into macrophages via Fcγ1 and IgA-coated Epstein-Barr virus entry via IgA receptor; HIV antibody-dependent enhancement via CR2

Abbreviations: EGF, Epidermal growth factor; ICAM-1, intercellular adhesion molecule 1.

TABLE 2–5 Key Concepts in Microbial Adhesin–Host Cell Receptor Interactions

Proteolytic processing of the adhesin is often required for the full biologic activity of the adhesin to be manifested.
Canyon hypothesis postulates that active sites of adhesins for receptor interaction will reside in antibody-inaccessible pockets in the adhesin.
Activity of adhesins may be conformationally controlled, especially in the case of adhesins that also function as fusion proteins.
Multiple receptors may bind to the same adhesin.
Anti-adhesin antibodies may enhance infection by altering adhesin-receptor interactions

the active site of the adhesin may be inaccessible to antibody because of its location in a "canyon" or depression in the molecule. This location shields the receptor site from antibody and enables the microbe to conserve the amino acids required for formation of the binding site in the face of antibody-driven variation in the rest of the adhesin sequence. For example, the sialic acid–binding site of influenza HA is formed by the highly conserved amino acids Tyr98, Trp153, His183, Glu190, and Leu194, which are found in an antibody-inaccessible depression at the distal end of the HA; the surface-exposed residues, however, are subject to antigenic variation.[12] In a similar manner, the binding site on the major group of rhinoviruses for the ICAM-1 receptor is located in a canyon formed by the capsid proteins that is only partially accessible to antibody[13] (Fig. 2–3).

Human adhesins such as LFA-1, CR3, and integrins require activation in addition to cell surface expression to mediate adherence,[14, 15] and microbial adhesins also exist in active and inactive states. One example is the galactose-specific adhesin of *E. histolytica*: antibodies against different epitopes on this adhesin either enhance or inhibit the galactose-binding activity of the adhesin, presumably by altering conformations from inactive to active configurations (see later).

Conformational changes in adhesin may also activate other functions of the adhesin, such as the fusion activities of enveloped virus glycoproteins. Some viral adherence glycoproteins, upon binding to a receptor or upon exposure to low pH in endosomes, undergo conformational changes that expose the hydrophobic fusion domains of the envelope glycoproteins.[16, 17]

Single adhesins can have multiple receptors. For example, gp120/41 of HIV binds to CD4 on T cells and to galactosylcerebroside on $CD4^-$ neural cell lines and interacts with membrane-bound chemokine receptors (see later) before initiation of viral–host cell membrane fusion.

The immune response to an adhesin, in particular, antiadhesin

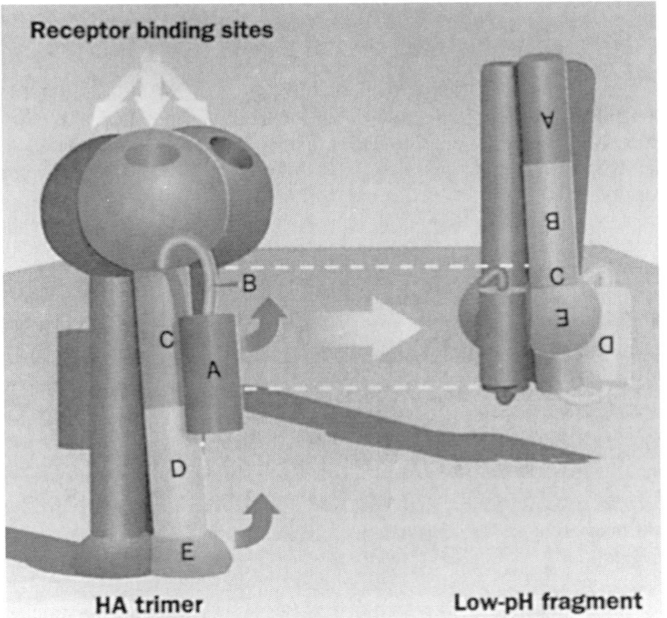

FIGURE 2–2. Schematic representation of the conformation of the influenza hemagglutinin molecule at neutral and acidic pH. The HA trimer is shown protruding from a plane representing the surface of the viral membrane. The main structural units of the low pH structure (from about residues 40 to 155 of the HA_2 chain) are labeled A to E from the N-terminal end. The fusion peptide, N-terminal to unit A, would protrude well above the heads bearing the receptor binding sites, ideally placed to engage the membrane of the target cell. (Reprinted by permission from Stuart D. Virus structure: Docking mission accomplished. Nature. 1994;371:19–20, Macmillan Magazines Ltd.)

antibodies, may enhance adherence, infectivity, or both by facilitating alternative routes of adherence and invasion. Examples of this phenomenon can be found in infections with HIV, *E. histolytica,* dengue virus, and EBV. Enhancement of adherence and infection of Fc receptor–positive monocytes and macrophages by subneutralizing antibodies has been demonstrated for some flaviviruses, including dengue. However, the importance of antibody-dependent enhancement in the pathogenesis of dengue hemorrhagic fever remains controversial.[18] EBV entry into a human epithelial cell line was promoted by polymeric IgA specific for EBV. The virus entered the cells via secretory component–mediated transport when bound to IgA instead of the usual route of entry via the CR2 receptor in B cells and other epithelial cell lines.[19]

The species, tissue, and cell tropism of a microbe is often determined by adhesin-receptor interactions. Examples include EBV and the CR2 receptor on B cells, poliovirus and the poliovirus receptor of human cells, and rhinoviruses and the human ICAM-1 receptor.

SPECIFIC ADHERENCE MECHANISMS AND THEIR ROLES IN PATHOGENESIS

HIV gp120/160

The development of an immune response to the gp120/41 adhesin of HIV to block adherence and invasion by the virus has been an important approach to the development of HIV vaccines, as discussed in Chapter 117.[20, 21] Infection of cells with HIV and other enveloped viruses requires fusion of the viral and cell membranes. The fusion event releases the viral nucleocapsid into the cell cytoplasm and thereby initiates the process of viral infection and replication.[22] This fusion event can occur at the cell surface between the plasma membrane and the viral membrane, as it does for paramyxoviruses, or it can occur between the endosome and viral membranes after phagocytosis of the virus, as in influenza virus infection. The adherence and fusion events are generally mediated by the same viral glycoprotein. In the case of HIV, it appears that the fusion event occurs at the plasma membrane because neutralization of acidic endosomes with weak bases does not interfere with viral entry and mutation of CD4 to a glycolipid-anchored form that is endocytosed poorly also has no effect on HIV entry.[23, 24]

The HIV cell surface glycoprotein is synthesized as a 160-kD glycoprotein. Proteolytic cleavage of gp160 to gp120 and gp41 at a site containing several basic amino acids (arginine and lysine) is required for activation of the glycoprotein and production of infectious virions. Cleavage of gp160 is thought to occur in the trans-Golgi compartment and has been shown in vitro to be mediated by the endoproteinase furin, which cleaves at the consensus sequence Arg-X-Lys/Arg-Arg.[25] Furin also activates the HA protein of the fowl plague influenza virus. In fact, the cleavage sites of the fusion proteins for orthomyxoviruses, paramyxoviruses, and retroviruses are all remarkably conserved. Inhibition of gp160 cleavage with peptide moieties containing the furin consensus sequence or by the ionophore monensin blocks HIV glycoprotein-induced syncytia formation and results in the production of virions with greatly reduced infectivity.[25] Mutation of the carboxyl-terminal amino acid 518 of gp120 from arginine to threonine abolishes both gp160 cleavage and syncytia formation.[26]

Cleavage of gp160 results in the production of gp41 and gp120 and activates the fusion ability of the viral glycoprotein. gp41 contains the transmembrane carboxyl terminus of gp160; gp120 remains attached to the virion via noncovalent interactions with gp41. The amino terminus created on gp41 by cleavage of gp160 is hydrophobic and contains the Phe-X-Gly sequence present in the amino termini of the activated fusion proteins of the paramyxoviruses. Mutations in gp160 that affect fusion activity map to the amino terminus of gp41. Thus, the requirement for cleavage of gp160 to gp41 and gp120 is in large part necessary to expose the fusion domain of gp41 for the virion to enter the cell via viral–cell plasma membrane fusion.[23–26]

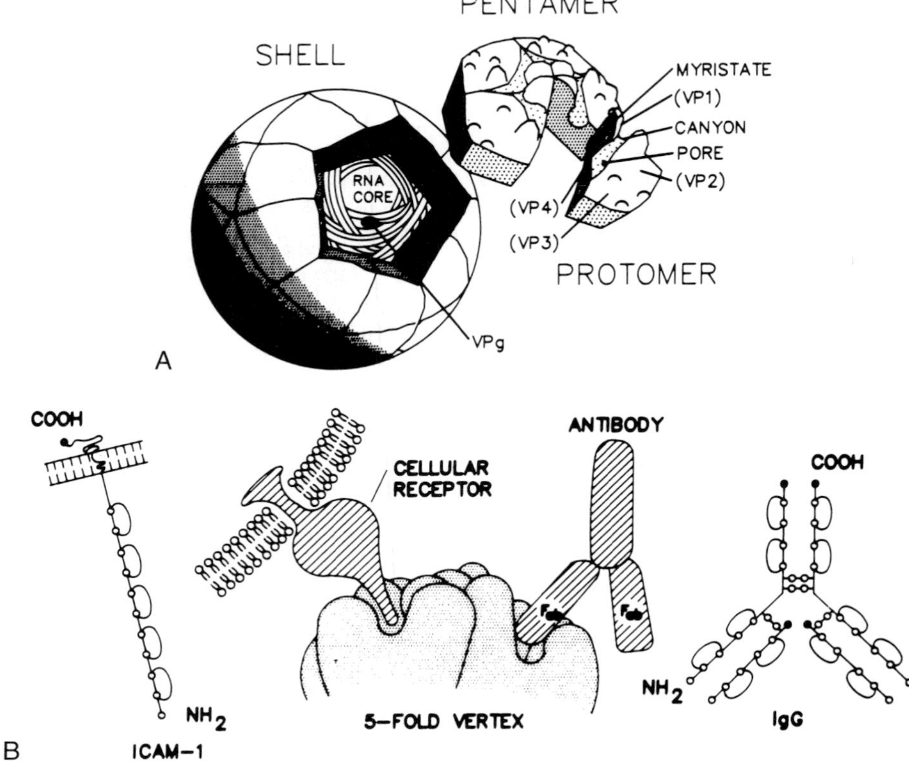

FIGURE 2–3. Key features in the adherence function of a typical picornavirus. *A,* Exploded diagram showing location of canyon in the middle of the center of the viral capsid protein VP4 pentamer. *B,* Binding of cellular receptor to the floor of the canyon. Note that the binding site of the ICAM-1 molecule, identified as ICAM-1 for major group rhinoviruses, has a diameter roughly half that of an IgG antibody molecule. (From Rueckert RR. Picornaviridae and their replication. In: Fields BN, Knipe DM, Howley PM, eds. Fields Virology. 3rd ed. Philadelphia: Lippincott-Raven; 1996:623.)

Binding of HIV to CD4 and galactosylcerebroside is mediated by gp120.[2, 3, 27, 28] Galactosylcerebroside apparently acts as a receptor for gp120 on neural cells that lack CD4 but are infected by HIV. Binding of CD4 by gp120 is a high-affinity interaction and results in the exposure of cryptic epitopes on gp120 and gp41 and shedding of gp120 from the virion, which indicates that CD4 binding has resulted in a conformational change in the virion glycoproteins.[29] Binding of HIV to CD4 is insufficient for the fusion of viral and cell membranes because cell surface expression of CD4 in murine cells enabled HIV to bind to, but not infect the cells.[30] The requirement for something in addition to CD4 to allow entry of HIV led to the recent discovery of chemokine coreceptors for HIV. Macrophage-tropic strains of HIV invade after interaction with the CCR5 chemokine receptor; T-cell–tropic strains require the CXCR4 chemokine receptor.[28, 29] CCR5 and CXCR4 consist of seven transmembrane domain G-coupled receptors for chemokines, a group of chemoattractant polypeptides involved in inflammation and infection. Additional chemokine receptors may also serve as HIV coreceptors or even as primary receptors. Interaction of HIV gp120 with the coreceptor is thought to permit interaction of the fusion domain of gp41 with the host cell (Fig. 2–4). Interestingly, a deletion mutation in CCR5 is associated with resistance to HIV infection in whites.[29]

Cell tropism (T4 cells versus macrophages) of HIV-1 is determined in large part by the interaction of the third variable (V3) loop of gp120 with the macrophage coreceptor CCR5 or the T-cell coreceptor CXCR4. Production of a chimeric gp120 containing the V3 loop of the macrophage-tropic BaL isolate of HIV-1 conferred macrophage tropism on the human T-cell leukemia/lymphoma virus IIIB, which is normally a T-cell–tropic virus. The sensitivity of HIV isolates to inhibition by soluble CD4 is also determined by the sequence in the V3 loop.[31–34] Amino acid substitutions in the V3 loop block cell fusion and infectivity without affecting gp160 processing to gp120/gp41 or CD4 binding.[35] Evidence has demonstrated interaction of the V3 loop of gp120 with distinct membrane-bound serine proteinases from T-cell and promonocytic cell lines. These membrane-bound proteinases cleave gp120 at the V3 loop only upon prolonged (several hours) incubation in vitro, so it is not clear whether the proteinase functions solely as a second receptor for gp120 or protease-mediated cleavage of gp120 at the V3 loop is required for virus–cell membrane fusion[36] (see Fig. 2–4).

Enhancement of HIV infection of cells has also been observed in the presence of anti-gp120/gp41 antibodies. Most of the antibodies enhancing HIV infection have been mapped to the V3 loop; enhancement of infection appears to occur when anti–V3 loop antibodies derived from infection or immunization with gp120 from one strain cross react with, but do not neutralize the V3 region of another strain. Apparently, V3 hypervariable loops from one isolate may elicit antibodies enhancing infection by another HIV isolate.[37] Antibody-mediated enhancement of HIV infection may be independent of complement or may be mediated by complement and the CR2 receptor; antibodies to the CR2 receptor blocked enhanced infectivity in one experimental system.[38]

Entamoeba histolytica Galactose Adhesin

E. histolytica trophozoites adhere to human colonic mucins and mammalian cells in culture via a surface lectin or adhesin that preferentially recognizes galactose in a β1–4 linkage to *N*-acetylglucosamine[39–41] (Fig. 2–5). Colonic mucins, by binding to and neutralizing the galactose-specific lectin, may serve as receptors for amebic colonization and also provide a nonimmune defense against amebic invasion by preventing adherence and contact-dependent killing of intestinal epithelial cells.

Contact-dependent killing of host cells requires the activity of the galactose adhesin. Blockade of the galactose adhesin in vitro with colonic mucins or galactose prevents amebic contact-dependent cytolysis of immune effector cells, including human macrophages and neutrophils.[39, 40, 42, 43] The ability of antiadhesin monoclonal antibody to block cytolysis after adherence has occurred suggests that the adhesin either signals the initiation of cytolysis or directly participates in the cytolytic event.[44, 45]

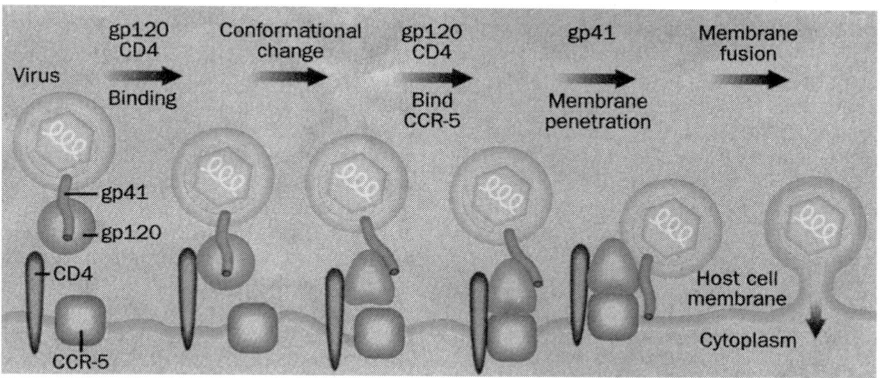

FIGURE 2–4. Adherence and fusion mechanisms of HIV gp120/gp41. After gp120 binds to CD4, a conformational change in gp120 ensues, allowing it to bind to a second receptor, CCR5. This change allows the amino terminus of gp41 to insert into the membrane of the CD4 cell and causes the membrane of the virus and cell to fuse. Membrane fusion thus allows the contents of the virus to enter the cell. (From Wain-Hobson S. One on one meets two. Nature. 1996;384:117–118.)

The role of the galactose lectin in adherence has been demonstrated in several ways. Inhibition of lectin activity with galactose or antilectin antibodies completely inhibited adherence to human colonic mucin glycoproteins and Chinese hamster ovary (CHO) cells.[39, 40] The adhesin, purified by galactose-affinity chromatography, was shown to bind to CHO cells in a galactose-specific manner and thereby competitively inhibit amebic adherence to CHO cells.[41, 46]

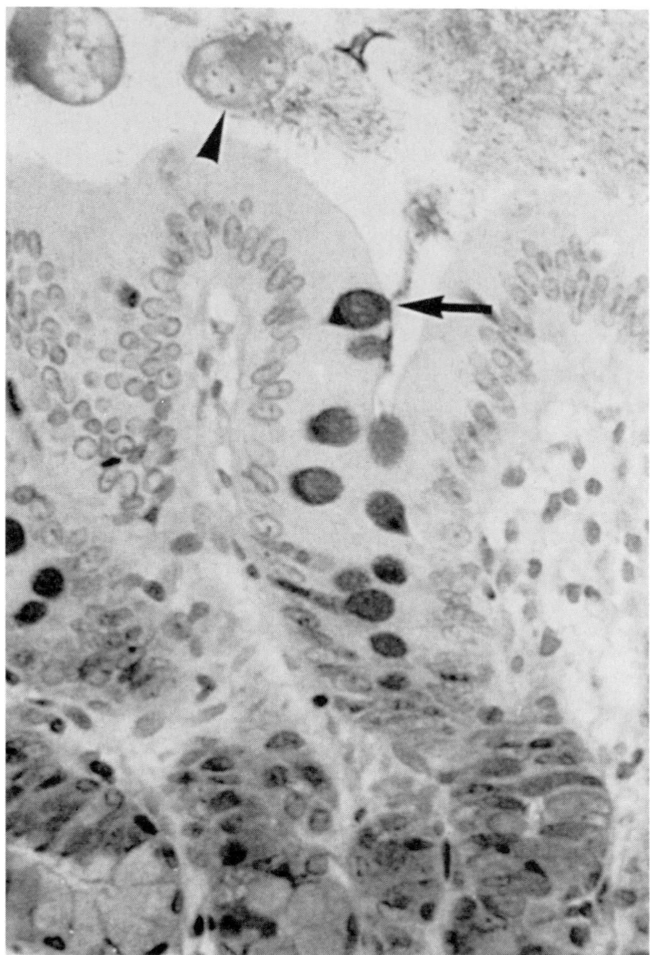

FIGURE 2–5. *Entamoeba histolytica* trophozoites *(arrowhead)* adhering to colonic mucins in rat colon. Note the goblet cell with apical protrusion *(arrow)* in the interglandular epithelium. Bar = 0.06 mm. (HRE, ×312.) (From Petri WA Jr. Invasive amebiasis and the galactose lectin of *Entamoeba histolytica.* ASM News. 1991;57:299–306.)

CHO cells deficient in terminal *N*-acetyl-lactosamine (galactose β_{1-4} glucosamine) residues on their glycoproteins and glycolipids were resistant to amebic adherence and killing.[47, 48]

The galactose lectin may resemble other eukaryotic adhesins such as LFA-1 and CR3 in requiring activation in addition to surface expression to mediate adherence. Monoclonal antibodies that bound to epitopes 1 and 2 on the 170-kD subunit increased the galactose-binding activity of the lectin, apparently by inducing a change to the active configuration of the lectin. Activation of the extracellular lectin is mediated by inside-out signaling via its cytoplasmic tail.[49] Activation and deactivation of the adhesin may explain the observed ability of amebas both to attach to and to detach from galactose-containing substrates. In addition, antiadhesin antibody responses may not necessarily be protective and, if adherence enhancing, could instead facilitate *E. histolytica* colonization and invasion. It is interesting in this light that only the adherence-enhancing epitopes 1 and 2 are conserved in both pathogenic *E. histolytica*[50] and nonpathogenic *Entamoeba dispar.* Protection from invasive infection with *E. histolytica* is associated with the production of antibodies against the adhesin's carbohydrate binding domain.[51]

The galactose-specific adhesin appears to function not only in adherence and host cell killing but also in evasion of the complement system of defense. Monoclonal antibodies against epitopes 6 and 7 on the 170-kD subunit increased *E. histolytica* lysis by human sera. These antiadhesin monoclonal antibodies and their Fab fragments also inhibited amebic resistance to lysis by the purified human complement components C5b–C9, which form the membrane attack complex. The 170-kD subunit has limited sequence identity with CD59 (a human inhibitor of the C5b–C9 membrane attack complex) near the region where monoclonal antibodies to epitopes 6 and 7 bind and anti-CD59 antibodies cross react with the adhesin. The purified adhesin conferred C5b–C9 resistance when reconstituted into C5b–C9–sensitive amebas, which is a direct demonstration of its C5b–C9–inhibitory activity.[52]

Escherichia coli P Fimbriae

Bacteria have specific organelles called *fimbriae* or *pili* that mediate attachment to host tissues. Fimbriae are proteinaceous, 2- to 7-nm rodlike structures that are peritrichously arranged on the surface in numbers from 100 to 1000 per cell[53, 54] (see Fig. 2–1). They are easily distinguishable from flagella, which are about 20 nm in diameter.[55] Some fimbriae are associated with certain sites of infection. One example is P or Pap (*p*ili *a*ssociated with *p*yelonephritis) fimbriae on uropathogenic *E. coli.* The presence of P fimbriae has been clearly established as a virulence factor that promotes urinary tract colonization and invasion. Over 95% of *E. coli* isolates from children and 50 to 90% from adults with pyelonephritis express P fimibriae.[56–59]

P fimbriae have been shown to bind specifically to uroepithelial cells and P blood group antigens on human erythrocytes. The receptors for P fimbriae on these cells are globo series glycolipids con-

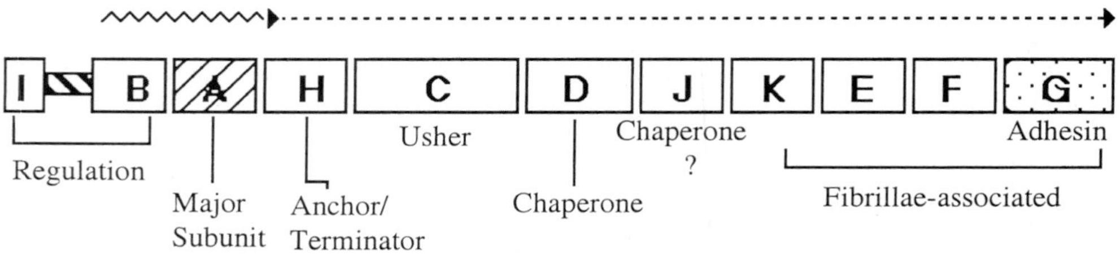

I B A H C D J K E F G

Regulation · Major Subunit · Anchor/ Terminator · Usher · Chaperone · Chaperone ? · Adhesin · Fibrillae-associated

FIGURE 2–6. Organization of the genes of the *pap* operon. Proposed functions for each gene are listed. The hatched bar represents the operator-promoter region of the DNA that binds the regulatory proteins described in text. The *wavy line* represents mRNA transcripts. Most transcripts terminate after *papA*. The *dotted line* indicates that transcription continues through to *papG*, but at a lower level owing to differential mRNA stability, processing, and partial termination or attenuation.

taining the disaccharide α-D-galactopyranosyl-(1,4)-β-D-galactopyranose (Gal-Gal).[60, 61] Gal-Gal, which is the minimal receptor moiety, can inhibit hemagglutination[62] and block the attachment of P fimbriated bacteria to uroepithelial cells.[63]

Women with recurrent infections are two to three times more likely to be nonsecretors of P blood group substance. Uroepithelial cells from nonsecretors show more adherence of P fimbriated bacteria than do cells from secretors.[64] It has been speculated that Gal-Gal receptors on nonsecretor cells may be more accessible because of the lack of fucosyltransferase-mediated synthesis of A, B, and H antigens and that the presence of these histo–blood group antigens on secretor cells may block or modify the essential Gal-Gal receptors.[60] Other investigators have reported the isolation of unique globo series glycolipids from nonsecretor uroepithelial cells but not from secretor cells.[65] These results raise the possibility that the increased risk of urinary tract infections in nonsecretors may be due to the presence of a unique receptor for P fimbriated bacteria on their uroepithelial cells.

P fimbriae biosynthesis, assembly, and regulation are encoded by the *pap* gene operon found on the *E. coli* chromosome[66, 67] (Fig. 2–6). In *E. coli,* many genes with related functions are often organized in operons. In the *pap* operon, a regulatory protein and RNA polymerase bind to DNA at specific sites called *operator* and *promoter* sites, respectively, located just upstream of the structural genes. As RNA transcription proceeds, a single polycistronic mRNA transcript is made that encodes all the structural genes. This type of system allows for coordinated expression and regulation of all the genes that are essential for fimbriae production.

The functional roles of the genes in the *pap* operon have been elucidated by analyzing mutations in each individual gene.[66, 67] *papI* and *papB* encode positive regulatory proteins necessary for expression of the structural genes. *papA* codes for the major fimbrial subunit that polymerizes to form the fimbrial rod. *papH* mutants have unusually long fimbriae, and it has been proposed that PapH functions as an anchor or terminator of fimbrial polymerization. Mutations in *papC, papD, papK,* or *papJ* fail to express fimbriae on the bacterial surface, thus indicating a role for these genes in surface assembly. The PapC protein is found in the outer membrane and functions as a molecular usher that helps translocate fimbrial subunits across the outer membrane. PapC also functions as an assembly center for fimbrial polymerization. PapD acts as a "chaperone" in fimbrial assembly. Chaperones stabilize other proteins by maintaining a protein in a non-native conformation that will allow the protein to be secreted across the cytoplasmic membrane or to assemble at the proper time or location. A mutation in *papD* results in rapid degradation of the other major and minor fimbrial subunits and has been isolated as complexes with PapG and PapE. PapJ may also function as a chaperone.

PapK, PapE, PapF, and PapG are all associated with the fibrillar tip.[68, 69] A model for fimbrial organization and structure is depicted in Figure 2–7. PapE forms the fibrillar shaft, and PapK is thought to terminate the fibrillar shaft and create a binding site for PapA subunits. PapF functions as an adapter for the attachment of PapG to the tip of the fibrillae. PapG has been identified as the actual Gal-Gal binding subunit by complementation studies and has been shown to localize to the tip of the fimbriae by immune electron microscopy.[69, 70]

The three classes or alleles of PapG each have a different binding specificity for Gal-Gal globo series glycolipids and contribute to tissue tropism.[71] Class II PapG is most the most common allele in isolates from acute pyelonephritis and first-time cystitis patients. Class II binds to the Gal-Gal globoside GbO_4, which predominates in the upper urinary tract of humans.[72] The saccharides flanking GbO_4 have also been shown to be important for recognition, thus lending further specificity to the interaction.[73] The class III adhesin is frequently found on human cystitis isolates and rarely on pyelonephritic isolates. Class III adhesin recognizes GbO_5, or Forssman's antigen, and globoA. Isolates with class III adhesin also frequently occur in secretor-positive individuals who carry globoA on their uroepithelial cells.[74]

P fimbriae undergo a type of phase variation in which an individ-

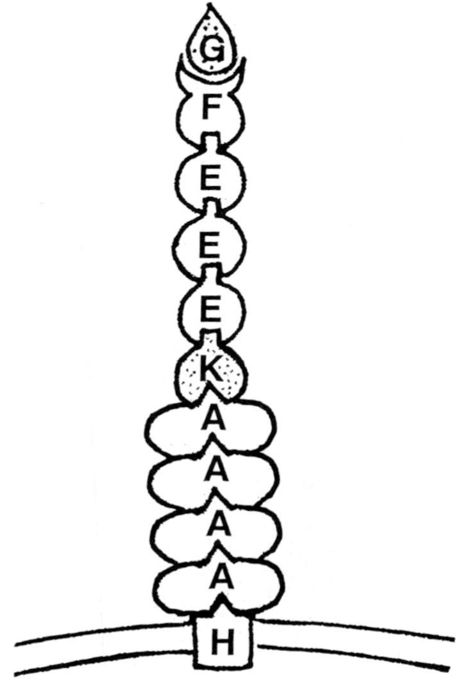

FIGURE 2–7. Model for the organization of P fimbriae subunits. Subunits *PapG, F, E* and *K* constitute the fibrillar tip. The fimbrial rod is composed of *papA* and anchored in the membrane by *papH.* See text for details. Subunits are not drawn to scale.

ual bacterium can turn on or off expression of the fimbrial genes. Consequently, within a clonal population not all bacteria containing the P fimbrial genes will be expressing P fimbriae on their surface. The ability to control the expression of P fimbriae may be advantageous to the bacteria by enabling detachment and migration to different sites or by providing a mechanism of antigenic variation to avoid recognition by the immune system.[75]

Fimbriae are logical targets for antimicrobial therapy and vaccine development. Purified fimbriae have served as effective, well-established vaccines for veterinary use for several years. One of the first effective fimbrial vaccines was based on K-88 antigen, or fimbriae found on *E. coli* strains that cause diarrheal disease in pigs.[76]

Purified P fimbriae have been tested as protective antigens in several animal models. Protection against pyelonephritis in monkeys has been achieved by immunization with purified P fimbriae. Protection was shown to correlate with a high titer of anti–P fimbrial antibodies.[77] Another study reports that PapG-mediated protection is dependent on the presence of a specific cognate receptor.[78] Primates immunized with P fimbriated *E. coli* bearing the class II PapG adhesin were protected against challenge. Immunization with strains of bacteria expressing P fimbriae that lacked PapG or carried a class III PapG allele (whose receptor is not present in the primate bladder) did not result in protective immunity even though these strains produced bladder infections similar to those produced by the wild type. Interestingly, animals immunized with bacteria expressing class II PapG were protected against challenge with either the mutant or the class III–bearing bacteria, which suggests that the PapG-receptor complex may have signaling functions that are important for the development of a protective immune response. The application of DNA recombinant technology to express specific protective epitopes may increase the effectiveness of fimbrial vaccines. However, the antigenic variation of P fimbriae and perhaps the requirement for the appropriate host ligand receptor will have to be considered in development of a broadly effective vaccine.

MICROBIAL BIOFILMS

Many of the studies of bacterial adherence have been done on free-floating "planktonic" bacteria growing in culture. In nature, however, many bacteria exist in a complex community-like structure known as a biofilm. Biofilms are matrix-enclosed bacterial populations that adhere to a surface, interface, or each other.[79] Bacteria form microcolonies with conelike and mushroom-shaped morphologies (Fig. 2–8). Water-filled channels surround the microcolonies and function somewhat like a primitive circulatory system allowing access to nutrients, elimination of wastes, and interbacterial communication. Biofilms are responsible for such things as dental plaque, fouling of storage tanks, and clogging of water pipes. Biofilms have become of interest to the medical community because of their formation on synthetic medical implants, including intravascular catheters, artificial valves, pacemakers, orthopedic devices, and contact lenses.[80] Biofilms are an area of increasing medical concern because one of the properties of biofilms is an increased resistance to antibiotics. Bacterial biofilms have been reported to be 500 times more resistant to antibiotics than planktonic cells are.[79] The mechanism for resistance is not well understood, but some studies suggest that the exopolysaccharide matrix, or "slime," that surrounds the cells may create an exclusion barrier to antimicrobials or more directly complex with these agents to inactive them.[81]

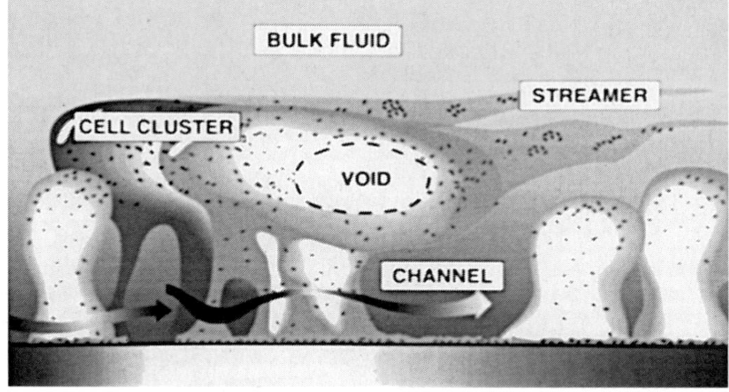

FIGURE 2–8. Conceptual model of biofilm architecture. At the microscopic level biofilms are heterogeneous in structure. Commonly seen characteristics include cell clusters and void spaces, water channels, and a variety of "slime structures," including "streamers" affected by flow in the fluid surrounding the biofilm. (From the Center for Biofilm Engineering, Montana State University-Bozeman, illustrator Peg Dirckx.)

Biofilm is formed in two phases. The first phase is an initial, reversible adherence to a surface. Several factors are thought to contribute to this initial adherence, including surface hydrophobicity, proteinaceous adhesins, and capsular polysaccharides. The second phase involves intercellular adhesion, which results in microcolony formation and the complex biofilm architecture.

The molecular mechanisms of biofilm formation are beginning to be dissected by identifying biofilm formation mutants. *Pseudomonas aeruginosa* forms biofilms in storage tanks and in the lungs of patients with cystic fibrosis. *Pseudomonas* bacteria with a mutation in the gene *lasI,* which is involved in generation of the quorum-sensing molecule acetylated homoserine lactone, have been shown to be defective in biofilm formation.[82] Quorum sensors are signaling molecules secreted by bacteria in proportion to the density of the bacteria.[83] They control a variety of activities, including exoenzyme synthesis, virulence factors, and bioluminescence. Mutant *lasI* bacteria are able to attach to a surface and multiply, but they fail to form channels and create the complex biofilm architecture. These experiments indicate that cell-cell communication is an important aspect of biofilm formation.

Another example of a biofilm former of medical importance is *Staphylococcus epidermidis.* This bacterium is a common component of the normal microflora; however, it is also one of the major culprits in biofilm formation on synthetic medical implants.[84] Several cell surface proteins have been identified that contribute to the ability of *S. epidermidis* to initially adhere to plastic surfaces.[85] Fimbrial-like adhesins, SSP-1 and SSP-2, have been described that contribute to adherence to plastic.[86] In addition, a protein with 61% identity to *Staphylococcus aureus* autolysin, AltE, has been identified by mutational analysis to be deficient in the initial attachment step of biofilm formation.[80] AltE in *S. aureus* is a protein that is involved in cell wall hydrolytic activities. Involvement in biofilm formation would represent a newly identified function for this autolysin.

After initial adherence to the surface, bacteria multiply and form microcolonies and higher-ordered structures, which requires intercellular adherence. In *S. epidermidis,* a unique polysaccharide intercellular adhesin molecule has been identified that mediates intercellular adherence. *S. epidermidis* polysaccharide intercellular adhesin is a linear polymer of β1, 6-linked 2-deoxy-2-aminoglucopyranosyl residues. Approximately 85% of the residues are *N*-acetylated.[87] This molecule is somewhat reminiscent of chitin or cellulose; however, the use of a β1,6 linkage rather than a β1,4, which is found in chitin or cellulose, predicts a less compact and more flexible structure. The unbranched structure may provide long-range contacts and interactions between the cell wall or lectin-like proteins on the surface of cells. An operon consisting of three genes, *icaA, icaB,* and *icaC,* has been identified that is essential for polysaccharide intercellular adhesin synthesis and biofilm formation.[80] Elucidation of the molecular mechanisms of biofilm formation should identify new targets for chemotherapy and provide new approaches to controlling the formation of biofilms.

REFERENCES

1. Fingeroth JD, Weiss JJ, Tedder TF, et al. Epstein-Barr virus receptor of human B lymphocytes is the C3d receptor CR2. Proc Natl Acad Sci U S A. 1984;81:4510–4514.

2. Dagleish AG, Beverley PCL, Clapham PR, et al. The CD4 (T4) antigen is an essential component of the receptor for the AIDS retrovirus. Nature. 1984;312:763–767.
3. Klatzmann D, Champagne E, Chamaret S, et al. T lymphocyte T4 molecule behaves as the receptor for human retrovirus LAV. Nature. 1984;312:767–768.
4. Delmas B, Gelfi J, L'Haridon R, et al. Aminopeptidase N is a major receptor for the enteropathogenic coronavirus TGEV. Nature. 1992;357:417–420.
5. Yeager CL, Ashmun RA, Williams RK, et al. Human aminopeptidase N is a receptor for human coronavirus 229E. Nature. 1992;357:420–422.
6. Mendelsohn CL, Wimmer E, Racaniello VR. Cellular receptor for poliovirus: Molecular cloning, nucleotide sequence, and expression of a new member of the immunoglobulin superfamily. Cell. 1989;56:855–865.
7. Koike S, Horie H, Ise I, et al. The poliovirus receptor protein is produced both as membrane-bound and secreted forms. EMBO J. 1990;9:3217–3224.
8. Tomassini JE, Colonno RJ. Isolation of a receptor protein involved in attachment of human rhinoviruses. J Virol. 1986;58:290–295.
9. Greve JM, Davis G, Meyer AM, et al. The major human rhinovirus receptor is ICAM-1. Cell. 1989;56:839–847.
10. Staunton DE, Merluzzi VJ, Rothlein R, et al. A cell adhesion molecule, ICAM-1, is the major surface receptor for rhinoviruses. Cell. 1989;56:849–853.
11. Bergelson JM, Shepley MP, Chan BMC, et al. Identification of the integrin VLA-2 as a receptor for echovirus 1. Science. 1992;255:1718–1720.
12. Wiley DC, Skehel JJ. The structure and function of the hemagglutinin membrane glycoprotein of influenza virus. Annu Rev Biochem. 1989;56:365.
13. Rossman MG, Arnold E, Erickson JW, et al. The structure of a human common cold virus (rhinovirus 14) and its functional relations to other picornaviruses. Nature. 1985;317:145–153.
14. Altieri DC, Edginton TS. A monoclonal antibody reacting with distinct adhesion molecules defines a transition in the functional state of the receptor CD11b/CD18 (Mac-1). J Immunol. 1988;141:2656.
15. Dustin ML, Springer TA. T cell receptor cross-linking transiently stimulates adhesiveness through LFA-1. Nature. 1989;341:619.
16. Flynn DC, Meyer WJ, MacKenzie JM Jr, et al. A conformational change in Sindbis virus glycoprotein E1 and E2 is detected at the plasma membrane as a consequence of early virus-cell interaction. J Virol. 1990;64:3643–3653.
17. Wahlberg JM, Garoff H. Membrane fusion process of Semliki forest virus I: Low pH–induced rearrangement in spike protein quaternary structure precedes virus penetration into cells. J Cell Biol. 1992;116:339–348.
18. Halstead SB. Pathogenesis of dengue: Challenges to molecular biology. Science. 1988;239:476–481.
19. Sixbey JW, Yao QY. Immunoglobulin A induced shift of Epstein-Barr virus tissue tropism. Science. 1992;255:1578–1580.
20. Emini EA, Schleif WA, Nunberg JH, et al. Prevention of HIV-1 infection in chimpanzees by gp120 V3 domain–specific monoclonal antibody. Nature. 1992;355:728–730.
21. Hu SL, Abrams K, Barber GN, et al. Protection of macaques against SIV infection by subunit vaccines of SIV envelope glycoprotein gp160. Science. 1992;255:456–459.
22. White J, Kielian M, Helenius A. Membrane fusion proteins of enveloped animal viruses. Q Rev Biophys. 1983;16:151–195.
23. Nara PL, Garrity RR, Goudsmit J. Neutralization of HIV-1: A paradox of humoral proportions. FASEB J. 1991;5:2437–2455.
24. Wain-Hobson S. One on one meets two. Nature. 1996;384:117–118.
25. Hallenberger S, Bosch V, Angliker H, et al. Inhibition of furin-mediated cleavage activation of HIV-1 glycoprotein gp160. Nature. 1992;360:358–361.
26. Freed EO, Myers DJ, Risser R. Mutational analysis of the cleavage sequence of the human immunodeficiency virus type 1 envelope glycoprotein precursor gp160. J Virol. 1989;63:4670–4675.
27. Harouse JM, Bhat S, Spitalnik SL, et al. Inhibition of entry of HIV-1 in neural cells by antibodies against galactosyl ceramide. Science. 1991;253:320–323.
28. Feng Y, Broder CC, Kennedy PE, Berger EA. HIV-1 entry co-factor: Functional cDNA cloning of a seven-transmembrane G protein–coupled receptor. Science. 1996;272:872–877.
29. Fauci AS. Host factors and the pathogenesis of HIV-induced disease. Nature. 1996;384:529–534.
30. Maddon PJ, Dalgleish AG, McDougal JS, et al. The T4 gene encodes the AIDS virus receptor and is expressed in the immune system and brain. Cell. 1986;47:333.
31. Safrit JT, Fung MSC, Andrews CA, et al. hu-PBL-SCID mice can be protected from HIV-1 infection by passive transfer of monoclonal antibody to the principal neutralizing determinant of envelope gp120. AIDS. 1993;7:15–21.
32. Hwang SS, Boyle TJ, Lyerly HK, et al. Identification of the envelope V3 loop as the primary determinant of cell tropism in HIV-1. Science. 1991;253:71–74.
33. Hwang SS, Boyle TJ, Lyerly HK, et al. Identification of the envelope V3 loop as the major determinant of CD4 neutralization sensitivity of HIV-1. Science. 1992;257:535–537.
34. Shioda T, Levy JA, Cheng-Mayer C. Macrophage and T cell tropisms of HIV-1 are determined by specific regions of the envelope gp120 gene. Nature. 1991;349:167–169.
35. Page KA, Stearns SM, Littman DR. Analysis of mutations in the V3 domain of gp160 that affect fusion and infectivity. J Virol. 1992;66:524–533.
36. Avril LE, Martino-Ferrer MD, Barin F, et al. Interaction between a membrane-associated serine proteinase of U-937 monocytes and peptides from the V3 loop of the human immunodeficiency virus type 1 gp 120 envelope glycoprotein. FEBS Lett. 1993;317:167–172.
37. Jiang S, Lin K, Neurath AR. Enhancement of human immunodeficiency virus type 1 infection by antisera to peptides from the envelope glycoproteins gp120/gp41. J Exp Med. 1991;174:1557–1563.
38. Tremblay M, Meloche S, Sekaly RP, et al. Complement receptor 2 mediates enhancement of human immunodeficiency virus 1 infection in Epstein-Barr virus carrying B cells. J Exp Med. 1990;171:1791–1796.
39. Ravdin JI, Guerrant RL. Role of adherence in cytopathic mechanisms of *Entamoeba histolytica*. Study with mammalian tissue culture cells and human erythrocytes. J Clin Invest. 1981;68:1305–1313.
40. Chadee K, Petri WA Jr, Innes DJ, et al. Rat and human colonic mucins bind to and inhibit the adherence lectin of *Entamoeba histolytica.* J Clin Invest. 1987;80:1245–1254.
41. Saffer LD, Petri WA Jr. *Entamoeba histolytica:* Recognition of α- and β-galactose by the 260 kDa adherence lectin. Exp Parasitol. 1991;72:106–108.
42. Guerrant RL, Brush J, Ravdin JI, et al. Interaction between *Entamoeba histolytica* and human polymorphonuclear neutrophils. J Infect Dis. 1981;143:83–93.
43. Chadee K, Meerovitch E. *Entamoeba histolytica:* Early progressive pathology in the cecum of the gerbil *(Meriones unguiculatus)*. Am J Trop Med Hyg. 1985;34:283–291.
44. Ravdin JI, Croft BY, Guerrant RL. Cytopathogenic mechanisms of *Entamoeba histolytica.* J Exp Med. 1980;152:377–390.
45. Saffer LD, Petri WA Jr. Role of the galactose lectin of *Entamoeba histolytica* in adherence-dependent killing of mammalian cells. Infect Immun. 1991;59:4681–4683.
46. Petri WA Jr, Smith RD, Schlesinger PH, et al. Isolation of the galactose binding lectin of *Entamoeba histolytica.* J Clin Invest. 1987;80:1238–1244.
47. Li E, Becker A, Stanley SL. Chinese hamster ovary cells deficient in *N*-acetylglucosaminyltransferase I activity are resistant to *Entamoeba histolytica*–mediated cytotoxicity. Infect Immun. 1989;57:8–12.
48. Ravdin JI, Stanley P, Murphy CF, et al. Characterization of cell surface carbohydrate receptors for *Entamoeba histolytica* adherence lectin. Infect Immun. 1989;57:2179–2186.
49. Vines RR, Ramakrishnan G, Rogers JB, et al. Regulation of adherence and virulence by the *Entamoeba histolytica* lectin cytoplasmic domain, which contains a β2 integrin regulatory motif disrupts adherence and virulence. Mol Biol Cell. 1998;9:2069–2079.
50. Petri WA Jr, Jackson TFHG, Gathiram V, et al. Pathogenic and nonpathogenic strains of *Entamoeba histolytica* can be differentiated by monoclonal antibodies to the galactose-specific adherence lectin. Infect Immun. 1990;58:1802–1806.
51. Dodson JM, Lenkowski PW Jr, Eubanks AC, et al. Role of the *Entamoeba histolytica* adhesin carbohydrate recognition domain in infection and immunity. J Infect Dis. 1999;179:460–466.
52. Braga LL, Ninomiya H, McCoy JJ, et al. Inhibition of the complement membrane attack complex by the galactose-specific adhesin of *Entamoeba histolytica.* J Clin Invest. 1992;90:1131–1137.
53. Brinton CC Jr. The structure, function, synthesis and genetic control of bacterial pili and a molecular model for DNA and RNA transport in gram negative bacteria. Trans N Y Acad Sci. 1965;27:1003–1054.
54. Houwink AL, van Itersen W. Electron microscopic observations on bacterial cytology. II. A study on flagellation. Biochim Biophys Acta. 1950;5:10–44.
55. Silverman M, Simon MI. Bacterial flagella. Annu Rev Microbiol. 1977;31:397–419.
56. Kallenius G, Svenson SB, Hultberg H, et al. Occurrence of P fimbriated *Escherichia coli* in urinary tract infection. Lancet. 1981;2:1369–1372.
57. Latham RH, Stamm WE. Role of fimbriated *Escherichia coli* in urinary tract infections in adult women: Correlation with localization studies. J Infect Dis. 1984;149:835–840.
58. Svanborg-Eden C, Eriksson B, Hanson LA, et al. Adhesion to normal human uroepithelial cells of *Escherichia coli* from children with various forms of urinary tract infection. J Pediatr. 1978;93:398–403.
59. O'Hanley P, Low D, Romero I, et al. Gal-gal binding and hemolysin phenotypes and genotypes associated with uropathogenic *Escherichia coli.* N Engl J Med. 1985;313:414–420.
60. Kallenius G, Mollby R, Svenson SB, et al. The p^k antigen as receptor for the haemagglutinin of pyelonephritic *Escherichia coli* strains. FEMS Microbiol Lett. 1980;7:297–302.
61. Leffler H, Svanborg-Eden C. Chemical identification of glycosphingolipid receptor for *Escherichia coli* attaching to human urinary tract epithelial cells and agglutinating human erythrocytes. FEMS Microbiol Lett. 1980;8:127–134.
62. O'Hanley P, Lark D, Normark S, et al. Mannose-sensitive and gal-gal binding pili of *Escherichia coli* from recombinant strains. J Exp Med. 1983;158:1713–1719.
63. Svanborg-Eden C, Freter R, Hagberg L, et al. Inhibition of experimental ascending urinary tract infection by an epithelial cell-surface receptor analogue. Nature. 1982;298:560–562.
64. Lomberg H, Cedergren B, Leffler H, et al. Influence of blood group antigen on the availability of receptors for attachment of uropathogenic *Escherichia coli.* Infect Immun. 1986;51:919–926.
65. Stapleton A, Nudelman E, Clasuen H, et al. Binding of uropathogenic *Escherichia coli* R45 to glycolipids extracted from vaginal epithelial cells is dependent on histo–blood group secretor status. J Clin Invest. 1992;90:965–972.
66. Hultgren SJ, Normark S. Chaperone-assisted assembly and molecular architecture of adhesive pili. Annu Rev Microbiol. 1991;45:383–415.
67. Tennent JM, Hultgren S, Marklund B, et al. Genetics of adhesin expression in *Escherichia coli.* In: Iglewski BH, Clark VL, eds. The Bacteria. v. II. New York: Academic Press; 1990:79–110.
68. Kuehn MJ, Heuser J, Normark S, et al. P pili in uropathogenic *E. coli* are composite fibres with distinct fibrillar adhesive tips. Nature. 1992;356:252–255.

69. Lindberg F, Lund B, Johansson L, et al. Localization of the receptor-binding protein adhesin at the tip of the bacterial pilus. Nature. 1987;328:84–87.
70. Lund B, Lindberg F, Marklund BI, et al. The PapG protein is the α-D-galactopyranosyl-(1-4)-β-D-galactopyranose–binding adhesin of uropathogenic *Escherichia coli.* Proc Natl Acad Sci U S A. 1987;84:5898–5902.
71. Stromberg N, Nyholm P-G, Pashcer I, et al. Saccharide orientation at the cell surface affects glycolipid receptor function. Proc Natl Acad Sci U S A. 1991;88:9340–9344.
72. Johanson I-M, Plos K, Marklund BI, et al. *Pap, papG* and *prsG* DNA sequences in *Escherichia coli* from the fecal flora and the urinary tract. Microb Pathog. 1993;15:121–129.
73. Striker R, Nilsson U, Stonecipher A, et al. Structural requirements for the glycolipid receptor of humna uropathogenic *Escherichia coli.* Mol Microbiol. 1995;16:1021–1029.
74. Lindstedt R, Larson G, Falk P, et al. The receptor repertoire defines the host range for attaching *Escherichia coli* strains that recognize globo-A. Infect Immun. 1991;59:1086–1092.
75. van der Woude M, Braaten B, Low D. Epigenetic phase variation of the *pap* operon in *Escherichia coli.* Trends Microbiol. 1996;4:5–9
76. Greenwood PE, Clark SJ, Cahill AD, et al. Development and protective efficacy of a recombinant-DNA derived fimbrial vaccine against enterotoxic colibacillosis in neonatal piglets. Vaccine. 1988;6:389–392.
77. Roberts J, Hardaway K, Kaack B, et al. Prevention of pyelonephritis by immunization with P-fimbriae. J Urol. 1984;131:602–607.
78. Soderhill M, Normark S, Ishikawa K, et al. Induction of protective immunity after *Escherichia coli* bladder infection in primates. J Clin Invest. 1997;100:364–372.
79. Costerton JW, Lewandowski Z, Caldwell DE, et al. Microbial biofilms. Annu Rev Microbiol. 1995;49:711–745.
80. Heilmann C, Schweitzer O, Gerke C, et al. Molecular basis of intercellular adhesion in the biofilm-forming *Staphylococcus epidermidis.* Mol Microbiol. 1996;20:1083–1091.
81. Gander S. Bacterial biofilms: Resistance to antimicrobial agents. J Antimicrob Chemother. 1996;37:1047–1050.
82. Davies DG, Parsek MR, Pearson JP et al. The involvement of cell-to-cell signals in the development of a bacterial biofilm. Science. 1998;280:295–298.
83. Latifi A, Winson MK, Foglino M, et al. Multiple homologues of LuxR and LuxI control expression of virulence determinants and secondary metabolites through quorum sensing in *Pseudomonas aeruginosa* PAO1. Mol Microbiol. 1995;17:333–343.
84. Christensen GD, Baldassarri L, Simpson WA. Colonization of medical devices by coagulase-negative staphylococci. In: Bisno AL, Waldvogel FA, eds. Infections Associated with Indwelling Medical Devices. Washington DC: ASM Press; 1994:45–78.
85. Heilmann C, Hussain M, Peters G, et al. Evidence for autolysin-mediated primary attachment of *Staphylococcus epidermidis* to a polystyrene surface. Mol Microbiol. 1997;24:1013–1024.
86. Veenstra GJC, Cremers FFM, van Dijk H, et al. Ultrastructural organization and regulation of a bio-material adhesin of *Staphylococcus epidermidis.* J Bacteriol. 1996;178:797–803.
87. Mack D, Werner F, Krokotsch A, et al. The intercellular adhesin involved in biofilm accumulation of *Staphylococcus epidermidis* is a linear β-1-,6–linked glucosaminoglycan: Purification and structural analysis. J Bacteriol. 1996;178:175–183.

Chapter 3

Toxins

ERIK L. HEWLETT

CLASSIFICATION OF TOXINS

Toxins such as tetanus toxin and diphtheria toxin were among the first bacterial virulence factors identified and isolated, which led to the belief that all microorganisms elicit their adverse effects on hosts by elaboration of toxins. It is now clear, however, that the pathogenic process is complex and represents a well-orchestrated sequence of events in which many microbial components play a part, even for diseases that are classically considered to be primarily toxin mediated. These diverse microbial products allow the pathogen access to the appropriate site in the host, provide a means for environmental signals to be transmitted to the bacterium to indicate that the conditions are right for expression of toxins and other virulence determinants, and protect the microbe against clearance by host defenses. The development of microbial pathogenesis as a distinct discipline and the availability of bacterial genome sequences have facilitated the identification of additional virulence factors involved in the activities required for production of infection and disease (see Chapter 1).[1–3] In addition, the distinction between toxins and other virulence factors, such as exoenzymes, that affect tissue permeability or clotting, is increasingly blurred. Some molecules of this type, such as exoenzymes with no known extracellular function, are now recognized to be "injected" into host cells from cell-bound bacteria possessing a novel secretory apparatus called the type III secretion pathway.[4, 5]

This chapter is focused on the structure, mechanisms of action, and consequences to the host of molecules that fit the classic definition of "toxin." This word is derived from the Greek *toxikon,* or "bow poison," and refers to the poisonous material placed on arrows by Greek warriors. The implication of this choice of terms is that the bacterium produces a molecule that it "releases" to affect host cells at a distance. The term was first used by Roux and Yersin to describe a factor released into the culture medium by *Corynebacterium diphtheriae* that caused the death of recipient animals.[6]

Subsequently, many toxins have been identified, and confusion has arisen concerning the terminology used to describe and classify different toxins. Exotoxin was originally used to refer to toxins produced by and released from gram-positive bacteria during growth, whereas endotoxin was used for the intracellular and cell-associated toxic components of gram-negative organisms, including the lipopolysaccharide component that now bears the name endotoxin. Because gram-negative bacteria are now recognized to elaborate classic protein toxins, it seems prudent that the term *exotoxin* be used for bacterial products that are protein in nature, are released from the bacterium during exponential growth, and are toxic for target cells or experimental animals. This definition excludes protein toxins that are intracellular in location and released only after lysis of the bacterial cell (intracellular or cell-associated toxins). In addition, gram-negative bacterial lipopolysaccharide and bacterial virulence factors that may be involved in attachment, local or systemic dissemination, and acquisition of nutrients but possess no capacity for direct toxicity to the host are also classified separately. The biologic effects of endotoxin from gram-negative organisms are addressed in Chapter 63.

Many of the molecules fitting the definition of "toxin" are enzymes with very specific intracellular targets within host cells, and a general structural model to which a number of these exotoxins conform has been elaborated. According to the A-B model described by Gill and colleagues, each of these toxins is composed of a binding (B) domain, component, or subunit and an enzymatic (A) domain/subunit that is responsible for the toxic effect once inside the cell.[7] Isolated A subunits are enzymatically active but lack binding and cell entry capability and thus have no biologic activity (the ability to intoxicate intact cells). Isolated B subunits may bind to target cells and even block the action of holotoxin, but they are, in many instances, nontoxic and biologically inactive. Recently, however, an increasing number of exceptions to this principle have been discovered. First, isolated B subunits from several toxins such as pertussis toxin and cholera toxin elicit biologic effects simply by interacting with their receptors on the surface of target cells.[8, 9] This phenomenon appears to arise when the molecule to which the toxin binds is a receptor for some hormone or other endogenous signaling agent and is usurped by the toxin for binding and cell entry. Specific examples of B subunit activities are noted in the discussion of toxins to which this concept is relevant.

Other criteria by which toxins may be classified are (1) their cellular or tissue target of action (i.e., enterotoxins, neurotoxins, leukotoxins); (2) their mechanisms of action (proteolytic toxins, adenosine diphosphate [ADP]-ribosylating toxins, adenylate cyclase toxins; Table 3–1); (3) their intracellular targets (small-molecular-weight G proteins such as Rho or trimeric G proteins such as G_s or G_i); (4) their major biologic effects (dermonecrotic toxin, edema-

TABLE 3–1 Representative Bacterial Toxins with Enzymatic Mechanisms

Toxin Type	Toxin	Organism	Molecular Mechanism and Biologic Effect
Adenylate cyclase toxins	Adenylate cyclase toxin	*Bordetella* species	Activation by calmodulin results in the production of cAMP in the host cell and cAMP-mediated effects, depending on the cell type
	Edema factor (plus protective antigen)	*Bacillus anthracis*	Same as adenylate cyclase toxin
	Adenylate cyclase	*Pseudomonas aeruginosa*	Introduced into the host cell by type III secretion; activation by calmodulin results in the production of cAMP in the host cell and cAMP-mediated effects, depending on the cell type
ADP-ribosylating toxins	Cholera toxin	*Vibrio cholerae*	ADP-ribosylation of $G_{s\alpha}$ activates host cell adenylate cyclase and increases cAMP-level and cAMP-elicited fluid secretion
	Heat-labile toxin	*Escherichia coli*	Same as cholera toxin
	Diphtheria toxin	*Corynebacterium diphtheriae*	ADP-ribosylation of EF-2 inhibits protein synthesis and causes cell death
	Exotoxin A	*Pseudomonas aeruginosa*	Same as diphtheria toxin
	Pertussis toxin	*Bordetella pertussis*	ADP-ribosylation of several heterotrimeric G proteins results in blockade of signal transduction mediated by those proteins
	C2 toxin	*Clostridium botulinum*	ADP-ribosylation of actin results in inhibition of polymerization and causes cell rounding
	C3 ADP-ribosyltransferase	*Clostridium botulinum*	ADP-ribosylation of Rho A, B, or C causes their inactivation and cytopathic changes in target cells
Deamidating toxins	Cytotoxic necrotizing factor (CNF1, CNF2)	*Escherichia coli*	Deamidation of Rho inhibits its GTPase activity and results in constitutive activation and an increase in actin stress fibers and focal adhesion
	Dermonecrotic toxin	*Bordetella pertussis*	Probably the same as cytotoxic necrotizing factor
Glucosylating toxins	Toxins A and B	*Clostridium difficile*	Monoglucosylation of Rho proteins (Rho, Rac, CDC42) causes their inactivation and subsequent cytopathic changes in target cells and cytokine release
Metalloprotease toxins	*B. fragilis* enterotoxin	*Bacillus fragilis*	Cleavage of E-cadherin (zonula adherens protein) allows disruption of the tight intestinal junction and consequently F-actin rearrangement and fluid secretion
	Botulinum neurotoxins	*Clostridium botulinum*	Cleavage of secretory complex proteins (SNAP-25, serotypes A, E; synaptobrevin, serotypes B, D, F, G; syntaxin, serotype C1) blocks ACh secretion and causes flaccid paralysis
	Tetanus neurotoxin	*Clostridium tetani*	Cleavage of the secretory complex protein synaptobrevin/VAMP blocks neurotransmitter secretion and causes spastic paralysis
	Lethal factor (plus protective antigen)	*Bacillus anthracis*	Cleavage of MAPKK and probably other cytoplasmic protein substrates and stimulation of cytokine release result in death of the host animal
RNA glycosidase toxins	Shiga toxin	*Shigella dysenteriae*	Single-site depurination of ribosomal RNA causes inhibition of protein synthesis and cell death
	Shiga-like toxin	*Escherichia coli*	Same as Shiga toxin

Abbreviations: ACh, Acetylcholine; ADP, adenosine diphosphate; cAMP, cyclic adenosine monophosphate; EF-2, elongation factor-2; GTPase, guanosine triphosphatase.

producing toxin, hemolytic toxin, lymphocytosis-promoting toxin); or (5) the organisms that produce them (pertussis toxin, cholera toxin). Quite clearly, the difficulties associated with describing and classifying these bacterial products reflect limitations in knowledge of their production, target cell interaction, mechanism of action, and clinical significance. The use of powerful investigative techniques provided by genomic and proteomic analyses in combination with cellular and molecular biology has resulted in a dramatic increase in the quantity and quality of information on bacterial toxins. These recent developments include the discovery of new toxins, determination of the amino acid sequence and crystal structure of many toxins, recognition of molecular mechanisms of action, and identification of family relationships among apparently disparate molecules.

CONTROL OF SYNTHESIS AND RELEASE OF TOXINS

Molecular biologic approaches have revealed an unanticipated level of complexity in the regulation of microbial virulence, including toxin production and secretion.[1, 10–13] Synthesis of many bacterial toxins and other virulence factors is tightly controlled by regulatory systems that are responsive to environmental conditions (see Chapter 1). For example, the production of diphtheria toxin is virtually eliminated by the presence of iron in the medium, virulence gene expression in *Yersinia* is repressed by calcium, and the expression of cholera toxin and associated virulence factors is controlled by environmental osmolarity.[14–16] In many cases, two-component, environmental-sensing systems are responsible for coordinated control of the expression of a group of toxins and virulence factors in a regulon and allow for their concurrent production during a particular phase of infection.[17–19] Recently, several genetic selection systems have been developed to allow detection of bacterial genes activated in vivo, thus providing powerful tools for evaluating putative virulence genes.[20–23] In *Bordetella pertussis,* induction of the synthesis of different virulence components is staggered such that attachment factors are initially produced to establish the infection and toxins are synthesized and later released to protect against the host response and promote survival.[18]

In addition to the regulatory elements within a given toxin operon, one or more structural genes may encode the toxin and other genes for proteins involved in activation and export of the toxin after synthesis.[10, 24] Furthermore, the regulatory and structural genes may be chromosomal in location, as is the case for cholera toxin, or plasmid encoded, as is the case for the family of immunologically and functionally homologous heat-labile toxins of *Escherichia coli.*[25] The structural gene for diphtheria toxin is located on a bacteriophage, but the inhibition of toxin synthesis by excess iron is mediated through a metalloregulatory protein, DtxR, that is encoded on the bacterial chromosome.[26, 27] The structural gene for tetanus toxin is now known to be located on a large (75 kilobase) plasmid.[28] The pertussis toxin gene is chromosomal and present in three *Bordetella* species, but it is expressed only in *B. pertussis* because of mutations in the promoter region of the gene in *Bordetella parapertussis* and *Bordetella bronchiseptica.*[29, 30] Finally, the gene for staphylococcal enterotoxin may be either chromosomal or plasmid in location, but its production is regulated by genes on a plasmid.[31]

The processes by which large protein molecules such as toxins are exported from the bacterial cell have been further elucidated by analysis of toxin operons.[32–34] The mechanisms involved have been thoroughly discussed in recent reviews, and it has been shown that not only do bacteria have specialized pathways for toxin export, but structures known to be involved in other functions such as conjugation may also be usurped for secretion.[13] Many of the classic exotoxins are synthesized with an NH-terminal signal or leader sequence consisting of a few (1 to 3) charged amino acids and a stretch (14 to 20) of hydrophobic amino acids. The signal sequence may bind and be inserted into the cytoplasmic membrane during translation such that the polypeptide is secreted while being synthesized. The signal peptide is then cleaved, which leaves the intact toxin molecule free in the periplasm. Alternatively, the protein may be synthesized intracytoplasmically. Subsequent binding via the leader sequence to the cytoplasmic membrane may cause a conformational change allowing the protein to traverse the membrane with or without the help of pores or transport molecules. Frequently, chaperone proteins are required to guide this process. As is the case with many toxins, the synthesis and release of *E. coli* hemolysin, *B. pertussis* adenylate cyclase toxin, and pertussis toxin clearly entail a process requiring the products of multiple genes involved in processing and transport.[24, 35, 36] Some multicomponent toxins such as cholera toxin have their subunits secreted separately; they are then assembled in the periplasmic space with the assistance of disulfide isomerase–like enzymes.[37, 38]

Discovery and characterization of the type III secretion pathway have revealed an alternative mechanism for bacterial virulence factors to be delivered to target cells.[4, 5, 39, 40] Numerous proteins produced by *Yersinia* species gain access to host cells by injection across the cytoplasmic membrane when *Yersinia* organisms are adherent.[41, 42] Some of these bacterial products have until now been orphans in that they are found in the culture medium and have enzymatic activities that can affect the function of target cells when they are introduced through permeabilized membranes. By virtue of containing no B subunit for binding to the cell surface, however, they have no apparent means for cell entry. For example, several products of *Pseudomonas,* including exoenzyme S, are responsible for covalent modification of vimentin, small molecular weight G proteins, and other substrates by transfer of ADP-ribose moiety to a specific amino acid on the target protein. These, and a recently discovered adenylate cyclase, are now recognized to be injected into the host cell from adherent bacteria via the type III secretion pathway.[43–45] The results of virulence factors on the target cell are comparable to intoxication by the classic process of binding and internalization described in the next section. The type III secretion apparatus that is responsible for this delivery mechanism has been visualized by microscopy and bears a remarkable resemblance to a hypodermic needle.[46]

ATTACHMENT AND ENTRY OF TOXINS

Some toxins such as the hemolytic phospholipases are bacterial exoenzymes that appear to interact with the external surface of host cell membranes to catalyze their specific reactions and elicit their specific toxic effects without cell entry.[47] A number of toxins, however, act on intracellular substrates and thus require cell entry to be effective. Most of them conform to the A-B model described earlier and have binding components that interact with specific receptors on target cells, such as the sialoganglioside GM_1 for cholera toxin, GT_1 for tetanus toxin, and probably GD_{1b} for botulinum toxin.[7, 48] The relatively wide distribution of GM_1 ganglioside among cell types accounts for the apparent lack of selectivity of cholera toxin in vitro. The specificity of the effect of cholera toxin during infection (secretory diarrhea), however, is due to localization of the organisms and the toxin to the intestinal tract. Pertussis toxin has been shown to interact with sialic acid–containing glycoproteins,[8, 49–52] and most cells are sensitive to intoxication by pertussis toxin. Cumulative data, however, reveal that the various sensitive cell types often do not contain the same receptors, which suggests that a common carbohydrate motif (presumably containing sialic acid) is present on different proteins.[52] Diphtheria toxin and *Pseudomonas* exotoxin A catalyze the identical reaction intracellularly and are both distributed systemically during infection, yet the resultant disease processes are quite distinct. The differences between the two appear to reside, at least in part, at the level of target cell specificities, with diphtheria toxin binding to an epidermal growth factor precursor molecule and exotoxin A to the α_2-macroglobulin/low-density lipoprotein receptor.[53–55]

Several different mechanisms can be used by the A subunits of A/B toxins to enter the target cell. In each case, however, a large protein molecule must insert into or cross the lipid bilayer.[7, 56–58] This activity is reflected in the ability of a number of intact A/B toxins or their B subunits to insert into artificial lipid bilayers and create ion-permeable pathways.[59–61] In some cases such as diphtheria toxin, binding to a surface receptor, uptake into an endocytotic vesicle, and acidification of that vesicle appear to result in a conformational change that enables a part of the toxin molecule to traverse the membrane.[62] The final step in diphtheria toxin translocation is energy requiring and dependent on membrane potential and a proton gradient.[63] *Pseudomonas* exotoxin A appears to be internalized somewhat differently, with endocytosis into coated pits and routing to the trans-Golgi compartment, where proteolytic activation occurs before entry into the cytosol.[64] The entry of pertussis toxin to reach its G protein substrates is now known to involve membrane vesicle trafficking, which can be disrupted by blockers of acidification and microtubule function.[65, 66]

Toxins with identical enzymatic mechanisms may enter cells by completely separate and distinct pathways. Adenylate cyclase toxins from *B. pertussis* and *Bacillus anthracis* both catalyze the production of cyclic adenosine monophosphate (cAMP) from host intracellular adenosine triphosphate stores.[67–69] Anthrax toxin (edema factor plus protective antigen) enters by receptor-mediated endocytosis, whereas pertussis adenylate cyclase toxin traverses the cell membrane directly from the environment through a process that appears to include the membrane potential as a driving force.[67, 70, 71] For many toxins such as tetanus and botulinum toxins, entry and trafficking are critical events in production of the specific clinical syndrome.[72] Putative ganglioside receptors have been identified, but the mechanisms for entry and differential intracellular distribution remain a mystery.

MECHANISM OF TOXIN ACTION AND ROLE IN CLINICAL DISEASE

As noted earlier, bacterial toxins do not operate in isolation to cause disease. With the exception of preformed toxins responsible for foodborne illnesses, toxins are produced by organisms during the course of local or systemic infection of the host, and a complex array of virulence factors is generally involved. In the following sections, several toxins are described along with their mechanisms of action, when known, and their apparent roles in the clinical disease with which they are associated. This list is by no means complete, but rather provides only some examples of major toxins that are well studied and for which information is more complete. Important toxins that contribute substantially to infectious diseases and are not mentioned here are discussed in the chapters corresponding to the specific organisms or the resultant disease.

Diphtheria Toxin

One of the most extensively studied of all bacterial toxins is that produced by bacteriophage-infected *C. diphtheriae*.[62] Diphtheria toxin, the prototype ADP-ribosylating toxin, inhibits protein synthesis in target cells by catalyzing the transfer of ADP-ribose from nicotinamide adenine dinucleotide to a novel amino acid (diphthamide) on elongation factor-2, a host protein required for translocation of ribosomal mRNA. Without doubt, other products of *C. diphtheriae* are involved in establishment of the infection and production and dissemination of the toxin. Nevertheless, the widespread control of clinical diphtheria with the use of diphtheria toxoid attests to the dominant role of this toxin both in the local infection and in the systemic toxicity, morbidity, and mortality of this disease. Diphtheria toxin has been crystallized and the structure of nucleotide-bound and free forms resolved, and thus its functional domains can be modeled.[73, 74] The receptor for diphtheria toxin on eukaryotic cells has been identified as the extracellular domain of a heparin-binding, epidermal growth factor–like precursor molecule that also has transmembrane and cytosolic domains.[54, 75] Structural studies have continued with crystallization of the toxin–extracellular domain complex.[76] An additional host cell component that may interact with the receptor has been identified by Iwamoto and colleagues.[77] Bound diphtheria toxin enters the cell by receptor-mediated endocytosis, with A subunit being released into the cytosol.

As noted in Table 3–1, exotoxin A of *Pseudomonas aeruginosa* catalyzes an identical reaction to that of diphtheria toxin but is associated with disease processes that are clearly distinct from those of diphtheria. The cellular receptor for exotoxin A has been identified as the α_2-macroglobulin/low-density lipoprotein receptor.[53] It is likely that the distinct differences between diphtheria and infection with an exotoxin A–producing *P. aeruginosa* are due to different receptors with different cellular distributions and to the fact that exotoxin A is only one of a number of virulence factors involved in *Pseudmonas*-induced disease whereas diphtheria toxin is the major determinant in clinical diphtheria.[78, 79]

Clostridial Neurotoxins

Advances in knowledge of the mechanisms of action of the neurotoxins produced by *Clostridium tetani* and *Clostridium botulinum* have revealed how they cause their respective neurologic diseases and have validated their use as important research probes for cell secretory processes, even beyond the nervous system.[72, 80–83] These molecules are metalloproteases that have as their targets several different proteins of the secretory complex required for fusion of neurotransmitter-containing vesicles with the presynaptic membrane.[72, 81] The truly remarkable aspect of these observations is that the serologically distinct botulinum toxins, some of which elicit slightly different clinical manifestations, act on several different proteins in this secretory apparatus.[82]

Tetanus Toxin

In contrast to diphtheria, immunization with tetanus toxoid has no effect on the establishment of infection with *C. tetani.* However, the resultant antibody response totally prevents the disease process of clinical tetanus, a direct consequence of the action of tetanus toxin (tetanospasmin). Tetanus toxin exhibits striking selectivity for neural tissue and is believed to be taken up at myoneural junctions for retrograde axonal transport within alpha motor neurons after binding to a receptor, which may be the gangliosides GT_1 or GD_{1b}.[84] The toxin ultimately crosses the synapses in a retrograde direction by an unknown mechanism to reach the axons of inhibitory γ-aminobutyric acid neurons in the spinal cord. It is the toxin-induced inhibition of neurotransmitter release, specifically in the inhibitory neuron, that results in the spasms characteristic of the disease. However, at high local concentrations, tetanus toxin can cause inhibition of acetylcholine release at the myoneural junction and flaccid paralysis similar to that elicited by botulinum toxin.[85]

Tetanus toxin is a zinc-dependent metalloprotease that appears to act by selective cleavage of a protein component of synaptic vesicles, synaptobrevin II.[72, 80, 81] Toxicity can be prevented by metalloprotease inhibitors such as the angiotensin-converting enzyme inhibitor captopril, which raises the possibility of specific therapeutic intervention that has not been available heretofore.

Botulinum Toxin

Botulinum toxin is among the most potent toxins known, with a lethal dose (toxin type A) of approximately 1 ng/kg.[86] Botulinum toxin consists of a family of seven immunologically distinct molecules, most of which cause flaccid paralysis by inhibiting myoneural junction acetylcholine release.[87] The mechanism of this neurotoxic activity is the same as that of tetanus toxin, namely, proteolytic cleavage of proteins involved in vesicle secretion. Interestingly, however, some of the substrates and sites of cleavage are not only different from those of tetanus toxin but also differ among the serotypes of botulinum toxin[82] (see Table 3–1).

The classic features of clinical botulism result from the ingestion of preformed toxin in improperly prepared foods, but a subacute intoxication can occur in infants (infant botulism) and adults harboring *C. botulinum* in their gastrointestinal tracts.[88–90] In most cases, the low-level toxin absorption results in listlessness and hypotonia, but the course can be fulminant and infant botulism has been proposed as a cause of sudden infant death syndrome.[91] The ability of botulinum toxin to block muscle contraction at the myoneural junction has led to its use therapeutically in disorders such as blepharospasm, spastic torticollis, and strabismus.[89, 92]

Many strains of *C. botulinum* types C and D also produce a different molecule, C2 toxin, that ADP-ribosylates actin; this action inhibits the polymerization of actin, affects the shape of target cells, and results in enterotoxin activity in vivo.[93, 94] C2 toxin is now known to represent a family of clostridial ADP-ribosylating toxins that modify actin.

Enterotoxins

The list of bacterial proteins with enterotoxic activities continues to grow, and the heterogeneous molecules included in this group have been discussed extensively in reviews.[95, 96] These diverse molecules elicit enterotoxic activity by a variety of mechanisms, including some that remain poorly understood.[95–97] In this section, several representative examples will be described briefly, and additional information about individual enterotoxins can be obtained from the appropriate chapter on the enterotoxin-producing organism.

Cholera Toxin

The classic enterotoxin, that produced by *Vibrio cholerae,* is believed to be responsible for the voluminous watery diarrhea characteristic of clinical cholera.[98] Cholera toxin activates adenylate cyclase of the intestinal epithelial cell by ADP-ribosylation of the B subunit of the stimulatory G protein G_1.[99] Although the resultant elevation in mucosal cell cAMP levels does produce chloride and isotonic intestinal fluid secretion,[100, 101] it is increasingly likely that additional bacterial components and additional regulatory pathways with other mediators are involved.[95, 102–104] Prostaglandin, platelet-activating factor, and perhaps 5-hydroxytryptamine have been implicated as potential intermediates in or synergistic components for cholera toxin action.[102, 103, 105] Furthermore, an intestinal secretory response in volunteers challenged with strains of *V. cholerae* in which the cholera toxin gene had been deleted or disrupted suggested a role for other factors.[106] Subsequent studies have identified accessory cholera enterotoxin, zonula occludens toxin, and most recently, an RTX-like molecule in the armamentarium of *V. cholerae.*[95, 105, 107] The relative roles, if any, of these molecules in diarrhea caused by cholera remain to be determined.

In addition to its well-known action as an enterotoxin, cholera toxin is also recognized as an adjuvant for preparations of antigens with which it is administered.[95, 108–110] Despite extensive investigation, however, the mechanism of this adjuvant effect and the requirement for holotoxin possessing ADP-ribosyltransferase activity remain controversial.[109, 110] Probably the most appropriate resolution of the data at present is the conclusion that the B subunit of cholera toxin does have a modest adjuvant effect but that the enzymatically intact holotoxin is more potent.[109]

Escherichia coli *Heat-Labile Toxin*

The heat-labile toxins produced by *E. coli* share their molecular mechanism of action with cholera toxin but are divided into two categories, LT-I and LT-II, which are distinguished immunologically. LT-I toxins are closely related to cholera toxin and have no major structural or functional differences.[111] Organisms producing this toxin infect primarily humans, but the disease is generally milder than that of cholera for reasons that are not well understood. The LT-II heat-labile toxins are associated with diarrheal disease in animals and have an immunologically distinct B subunit and different receptor.[112]

Escherichia coli *Heat-Stable Toxin*

E. coli organisms can produce toxins other than the heat-labile toxin discussed in the previous section. Heat-stable toxin, known as STa or ST-I, is synthesized as a peptide of 72 amino acids and is cleaved to an active species of 18 or 19 amino acids.[113] It causes diarrhea by binding to and activating endogenous particulate guanylate cyclase, thus eliciting cyclic guanosine monophosphate (cGMP) production.[114–117] Unlike cholera toxin and *E. coli* heat-labile toxin, heat-stable toxin exhibits striking target cell specificity with little activity in extraintestinal tissues, except when the cells have been transfected with the gene for particulate guanylate cyclase.[118] The endogenous ligand for this receptor, called guanylin, has been identified in extracts of rat jejunum and shown to stimulate cGMP production and chloride secretion in intestinal cells.[119] Recent studies have revealed that phosphorylation of the heat-stable toxin receptor/guanylate cyclase by protein kinase C produces a synergistic activation when heat-stable toxin is added.[120]

Enteropathogenic *E. coli* elicit activation of protein kinase C and an enhanced sensitivity to heat-stable toxin in cells to which they adhere, and that combination may be responsible for the diarrhea occurring in patients infected with those organisms.[121] Other bacterial species such as *Yersinia enterocolitica,* non-01 *V. cholerae,* and *Citrobacter freundii* also produce toxins related to heat-stable toxin, but their role in diarrheal illnesses is unclear.[122]

Clostridium difficile *Toxins A and B*

Clostridium difficile, a causative agent of antibiotic-associated pseudomembranous colitis, produces two large protein toxins, toxin A (308 kD) and toxin B (270 kD).[123] Toxin A is classified as an enterotoxin and toxin B as a cytotoxin based on their activities when administered separately, but both have cytotoxic effects, as reflected by cytoskeletal disruption in treated cells. Toxin A appears to be more important in clinical pseudomembranous colitis because of its ability to elicit inflammatory responses by induction of cytokine release.[124] The inflammation and cytokines may be responsible for the decreases in monolayer resistance observed after treatment with toxin A, but it does not alone produce an increase in short-circuit current.[125] The in vivo secretory effects elicited by toxin A apparently involve other mediators because they can be blocked by inhibitors of phospholipase A_2 and platelet-activating factor.[126] Toxin A (and probably toxin B) acts by glucosylation of Rho, which disrupts its ability to promote actin polymerization, thus adding another toxin to the growing list of bacterial products that target Rho.[93]

Bacteroides fragilis *Enterotoxin*

Diarrhea-associated strains of *B. fragilis* produce a 20-kD protein that causes a decrease in monolayer resistance and disruption of the morphology of human intestinal epithelial cells.[127] This toxin elicits fluid secretion in vivo and alters actin cytoskeleton structure in vitro.[128, 129] These effects appear to be the result of a newly described mechanism, namely, proteolytic cleavage of the zonula adherens protein E-cadherin causing loosening of the tight junction and perhaps signaling some other intracellular events.[130]

Toxins of *Bordetella pertussis*

B. pertussis, the causative agent of whooping cough, produces several toxins that have striking effects in experimental systems and are hypothesized to be major contributors to the pathogenesis of the clinical illness.[131] Pertussis toxin, also known as lymphocytosis-promoting factor, histamine-sensitizing factor, or islet-activating protein, is expressed only by *B. pertussis,* although a transcriptionally silent copy of the gene is present in *B. parapertussis* and *B. bronchiseptica.*[30] Pertussis toxin acts by ADP-ribosylation of several members of the family of guanine nucleotide–binding (G) proteins involved in signal transduction.[132] The result of this covalent modification is inhibition of G protein function and, consequently, interruption of the signal from a variety of receptors to effector systems, such as inhibition of adenylate cyclase, activation of phospholipases, and modulation of ion channels. Although pertussis toxin is clearly a virulence factor for *B. pertussis* and a protective antigen present in all acellular pertussis vaccines licensed to date, its target tissue and role in clinical pertussis remain unclear.[131, 133] Unlike tetanus and diphtheria, however, the clinical manifestations of pertussis cannot be mimicked by experimental administration of pertussis toxin. This conclusion is illustrated by a study in which pertussis toxin (1 μg/kg intravenously) was given to human volunteers who neither got whooping cough nor suffered adverse effects.[134]

Bordetella species also produce other toxins that are significant virulence factors, including adenylate cyclase toxin and tracheal cytotoxin. Adenylate cyclase toxin enters host cells and catalyzes the production of supraphysiologic levels of cAMP, which impair the normal activities of neutrophils and other immune effector cells and may produce fluid and mucous secretion in the respiratory tract.[131, 135, 136] Tracheal cytotoxin is a disaccharide-tetrapeptide that is derived from the bacterial peptidoglycan.[137] It is cytotoxic to respiratory epithelial cells, apparently by eliciting interleukin-1 release and nitric oxide production.[138–140]

An additional toxin from *Bordetella* species, dermonecrotic toxin, has not been clearly implicated in the pathogenesis of pertussis but appears to have a mechanism of action like that of the recently studied cytotoxic necrotizing factor from invasive strains of *E. coli.*[141–144] As its name implies, dermonecrotic toxin causes dermonecrosis when injected into the skin of suckling mice. It has significant sequence homology with cytotoxic necrotizing factor, and both toxins alter the cytoskeleton of affected cells, with enhanced actin stress fiber assembly and focal adhesions. These effects are now known to be the result of constitutive activation of Rho by deamidation of glutamine 63 and abolition of its intrinsic guanosinetriphosphatase activity.[145, 146] This action represents yet another molecular basis for toxin alteration of this critical signaling protein.[93]

Anthrax Toxins

B. anthracis produces three toxin components that are novel in their interaction with cells.[68] None of the three components—edema factor, lethal factor, or protective antigen—has toxin activity alone. Protective antigen is the binding moiety that interacts with target cells to promote the entry of edema factor or lethal factor. Protective antigen binds to a glycoprotein receptor on target cells and is cleaved by a host protease that is furin or furin-like.[147] This process results in the release of a 20-kD fragment and activates the remaining portion of protective antigen to allow edema factor or lethal factor binding. The complex is internalized by receptor-mediated endocytosis.[148] Protective antigen has been shown to produce a heptamer that inserts into the target cell membrane to form an ion-permeable pore.[61, 149] This structure is hypothesized to be involved in the delivery of edema factor or lethal factor to the cell interior, but no direct data support that concept. When edema factor enters the cytosol, it is activated by calmodulin to produce supraphysiologic levels of cAMP.[68] Lethal factor is a zinc-dependent protease that has been demonstrated to cleave the N-terminus of the mitogen-activated protein kinase kinases Mek1 and Mek2 and results in their inactivation.[150, 151] Although it remains to be determined whether these substrates are responsible for the rapidly lethal effects of this toxin complex, these data provide convincing evidence of protease activity in vivo. Protective antigen and lethal factor together also elicit mediator (interleukin-1 and others) release by a process that may or may not be related to mitogen-activated protein kinase kinase proteolysis.[152]

Shiga and Shiga-like Toxins

Shiga toxin is the prototype of a family of toxins produced by *Shigella dysenteriae* (Shiga toxin), *E. coli, C. freundii,* and other organisms (Shiga-like toxins SLT-I and SLT-II, previously known as Vero toxins).[153, 154] SLT-I molecules react with antiserum to Shiga toxin, whereas SLT-II molecules do not despite possessing a common mechanism of action. The members of this family conform to the A/B model with a subunit structure similar to that of cholera toxin (A-5B).[155] The binding pentamer interacts with the glycolipid globotriaosylceramide, and the toxin is internalized via receptor-mediated endocytosis through clathrin-coated pits and eventually traffics to the trans-Golgi apparatus.[57, 153] Within the cytoplasm, the A subunit causes inhibition of protein synthesis by enzymatic inactivation of the 28S RNA within the 60S ribosomal subunit.[156] This inactivation occurs by enzymatic removal of adenine from a specific adenosine residue, which is the same process catalyzed by the plant toxin ricin.

Despite the cytotoxicity elicited in vitro, the role of these toxins in shigellosis and diarrhea associated with infection by Shiga-like toxin–positive, enterohemorrhagic *E. coli* and others remains controversial.[95, 153] Shiga toxin, especially in combination with lipopolysaccharide, causes damage to vascular endothelial cells in a fashion that may explain the hemolytic-uremic syndrome known to be associated with infection by *S. dysenteriae* and enterohemorrhagic *E. coli.*[157, 158] In this setting, lipopolysaccharide increases expression of the globotriaosylceramide receptor on vascular endothelial cells in a process involving tumor necrosis factor and interleukin-1.[159] Cell damage also appears to depend on endothelial cell production of procoagulant and arachidonic acid metabolites.[160] Even the enterotoxin activity (intestinal fluid accumulation) may represent toxin effects on the villus cells and on the vasculature of the intestinal mucosa.

Pyrogenic Exotoxins

The pyrogenic exotoxins compose a growing family of molecules that are responsible for a systemic syndrome manifested by fever, shock, and profound immunomodulation.[161, 162] Included in this group are toxic shock syndrome toxins, staphylococcal enterotoxins and exfoliative toxins, and pyrogenic exotoxins from *Streptococcus pyogenes* and group B, C, F, and G streptococci.[161] In addition to their recognized roles in toxic shock syndrome, scarlet fever, and other streptococcal diseases, evidence now implicates toxic shock syndrome toxin–producing and exfoliative toxin–secreting *Staphylococcus aureus* in Kawasaki syndrome.[163, 164] These proteins share the ability to stimulate T-cell proliferation by interaction with the class II major histocompatibility complex on antigen-presenting cells and specific V_β chains of the T-cell receptor and are thereby designated superantigens.[165] The important feature of this interaction is the resultant production of cytokines such as interleukin-1, tumor necrosis factor, macrophage migration inhibition factor, and other monokines and lymphokines, which appear to be the principal mediators of the disease processes associated with these toxins. The crystal structures have been solved for at least some of these superantigens, which allows for closer examination of their interaction with the T-cell receptor complex, in addition to permitting mutational analysis.[166–168]

At this time, it is not clear whether superantigen activity is the sole mechanism of these illnesses or whether other actions of the toxins may contribute. Staphylococcal enterotoxins elicit emesis in experimental animals, but this activity may occur with other superantigens with different potencies.[161] In addition, toxic shock syndrome toxin 1 has been shown to be cytotoxic for aortic endothelial cells in vitro, a setting in which cytokines should not be present.[169] Thus, it is possible that the various clinical syndromes produced by the organisms that make these toxins reflect the activities of numerous bacterial components directly on host cells, as well as the effects of massive mediator release via their function as superantigens.

Other Toxins

The list of toxins discussed in the preceding sections is by no means inclusive. It is merely exemplary of the many different toxin molecules that have been implicated in clinical diseases in humans. Many other toxins have been the subject of basic investigations concerning structure and molecular mechanisms of action, with little knowledge of their contribution to clinical disease. These other toxins include pore-forming toxins and cytotoxins. For example, a large number of toxins have the ability to lyse erythrocytes and are thus defined as "hemolysins." They act by a variety of mechanisms, including phospholipase C activity, and result in membrane damage from the cell exterior and pore formation leading to osmotic lysis. Some of these hemolysins also have leukotoxic activity and have been found, on the basis of amino acid sequence, to contain a glycine-rich repeat region and thus belong to a family of toxins termed RTX (for *r*epea*t* in to*x*in).[170] These and other classes of toxins are discussed in several books devoted to toxins and pathogenesis.[171–172a]

THERAPEUTIC USES OF BACTERIAL TOXINS

In light of the remarkable specificity of the enzymatically based cytotoxicities of many bacterial toxins, it was logical that these natural products be considered for use as antitumor agents.[173–176] Several bacterial toxins such as diphtheria toxin, A subunit, and *Pseudomonas* exotoxin A have been combined genetically or chemically to ligands that can target the toxic moiety selectively to the malignant cell.[177] For example, interleukin-2 has been used as the binding domain for the A subunit of diphtheria toxin in a fusion protein for treatment of interleukin-2 receptor–positive lymphoma and Sézary syndrome.[178] This construct has reached the point of phase III trials with some success and little toxicity.

As described earlier, botulinum neurotoxin type A has been developed as a therapeutic reagent for the treatment of neuromuscular disorders that involve uncontrolled muscle contractions. For example, injection of nanogram quantities of type A botulinum neurotoxin into involved muscles has been effective in blepharospasm and torticollis[92] and most recently has been used for cosmetic purposes in the elimination of wrinkles. Despite the carefully controlled conditions under which this dangerous toxin is used, systemic toxicity has occurred in some cases.[89]

In addition to these special applications of toxins, other uses are being developed for the future. Insertion of foreign epitopes into toxins that enter the cytoplasm of host cells provides a mechanism for delivering those antigens to the major histocompatibility complex class I pathway. This concept has been used with several toxins, including adenylate cyclase toxins from *B. pertussis* and *B. anthracis.*[179–181]

REFERENCES

1. Strauss EJ, Falkow S. Microbial pathogenesis: Genomics and beyond. Science. 1997;276:707–712.
2. Falkow S. Invasion and intracellular sorting of bacteria: Searching for bacterial

genes expressed during host/pathogen interactions. J Clin Invest. 1997;100:239–243.
3. Finlay BB, Cossart P. Exploitation of mammalian host cell functions by bacterial pathogens. Science. 1997;276:718–725.
4. Lee CA. Type III secretion systems: Machines to deliver bacterial proteins into eukaryotic cells? Trends Microbiol. 1997;5:148–156.
5. Hueck CJ. Type III protein secretion systems in bacterial pathogens of animals and plants. Microbiol Mol Biol Rev. 1998;62:379–433.
6. Roux E, Yersin A. Contribution a l'etude de la diphtherie. Ann Inst Pasteur. 1888;2:629–661.
7. Gill DM. Seven toxic peptides that cross cell membranes. In: Jeljaszewicz J, Wadstrom T, eds. Bacterial Toxins and Cell Membranes. New York: Academic; 1978:291–332.
8. Wong WS, Rosoff PM. Pharmacology of pertussis toxin B-oligomer. Can J Physiol Pharmacol. 1996;74:559–564.
9. Masco D, Van de Walle M, Spiegel S. Interaction of ganglioside GM_1 with the B subunit of cholera toxin modulates growth and differentiation of neuroblastoma N18 cells. J Neurosci. 1991;11:2443–2452.
10. DiRita VJ, Mekalanos JJ. Genetic regulation of bacterial virulence. Annu Rev Genet. 1989;23:455–482.
11. Kaper JB, McDaniel TK, Jarvis KG, Gomez-Duarte O. Genetics of virulence of enteropathogenic *E. coli.* Adv Exp Med Biol. 1997;412:279–287.
12. Sandkvist M, Michel LO, Hough LP, et al. General secretion pathway *(eps)* genes required for toxin secretion and outer membrane biogenesis in *Vibrio cholerae.* J Bacteriol. 1997;179:6994–7003.
13. Winans SC, Burns DL, Christie PJ. Adaptation of a conjugal transfer system for the export of pathogenic macromolecules. Trends Microbiol. 1996;4:64–68.
14. Pappenheimer AM Jr. Diphtheria toxin. Annu Rev Biochem. 1977;46:69–94.
15. Straley SC, Plano GV, Skrzypek E, et al. Regulation by Ca^{2+} in the *Yersinia* low Ca^{2+} response. Mol Microbiol. 1993;8:1005–1010.
16. Miller VL, Taylor RK, Mekalanos JJ. Cholera toxin transcriptional activator toxR is a transmembrane DNA binding protein. Cell. 1987;48:271–279.
17. Miller JF, Johnson SA, Black WJ, et al. Constitutive sensory transduction mutations in the *Bordetella pertussis bvgS* gene. J Bacteriol. 1992;174:970–979.
18. Scarlato V, Arico B, Domenighini M, Rappuoli R. Environmental regulation of virulence factors in *Bordetella* species. Bioessays. 1993;15:99–104.
19. Merkel TJ, Stibitz S, Keith JM, et al. Contribution of regulation by the *bvg* locus to respiratory infection of mice by *Bordetella pertussis.* Infect Immun. 1998;66:4367–4373.
20. Mahan MJ, Slauch JM, Mekalanos JJ. Selection of bacterial virulence genes that are specifically induced in host tissues. Science. 1993;259:686–688.
21. Akerley BJ, Rubin EJ, Camilli A, et al. Systematic identification of essential genes by *in vitro* mariner mutagenesis. Proc Natl Acad Sci U S A. 1998;95:8927–8932.
22. Chiang SL, Mekalanos JJ. Use of signature-tagged transposon mutagenesis to identify *Vibrio cholerae* genes critical for colonization. Mol Microbiol. 1998;27:797–805.
23. Camilli A, Mekalanos JJ. Use of recombinase gene fusions to identify *Vibrio cholerae* genes induced during infection. Mol Microbiol. 1995;18:671–683.
24. Welch RA. Pore-forming cytolysins of gram-negative bacteria. Mol Microbiol. 1991;5:521–528.
25. Betley MJ, Miller VL, Mekalanos JJ. Genetics of bacterial enterotoxins. Annu Rev Microbiol. 1986;40:577–605.
26. Pohl E, Holmes RK, Hol WG. Motion of the DNA-binding domain with respect to the core of the diphtheria toxin repressor (DtxR) revealed in the crystal structures of apo- and holo-DtxR. J Biol Chem. 1998;273:22420–22427.
27. White A, Ding X, vanderSpek JC, et al. Structure of the metal-ion–activated diphtheria toxin repressor/tox operator complex. Nature. 1998;394:502–506.
28. Finn CWJ, Silver RP, Habig WH, et al. The structural gene for tetanus neurotoxin is on a plasmid. Science. 1984;224:881–884.
29. Locht C, Keith JM. Pertussis toxin gene: Nucleotide sequence and genetic organization. Science. 1986;232:1258–1264.
30. Arico B, Rappuoli R. *Bordetella parapertussis* and *Bordetella bronchiseptica* contain transcriptionally silent pertussis toxin genes. J Bacteriol. 1987;169:2847–2853.
31. Dyer DW, Iandolo JJ. Plasmid-chromosomal transition of genes important in staphylococcal enterotoxin B expression. Infect Immun. 1981;33:450–458.
32. Russel M. Macromolecular assembly and secretion across the bacterial cell envelope: Type II protein secretion systems. J Mol Biol. 1998;279:485–499.
33. Pugsley AP, Francetic O, Possot OM, et al. Recent progress and future directions in studies of the main terminal branch of the general secretory pathway in gram-negative bacteria—a review. Gene. 1997;192:13–19.
34. Hardie KR, Seydel A, Guilvout I, Pugsley AP. The secretin-specific, chaperone-like protein of the general secretory pathway: Separation of proteolytic protection and piloting functions. Mol Microbiol. 1996;22:967–976.
35. Bellalou J, Ladant D, Sakamoto H. Synthesis and secretion of *Bordetella pertussis* adenylate cyclase as a 200-kilodalton protein. Infect Immun. 1990;58:1195–1200.
36. Weiss AA, Johnson FD, Burns DL. Molecular characterization of an operon required for pertussis toxin secretion. Proc Natl Acad Sci U S A. 1993;90:2970–2974.
37. Yu J, McLaughlin S, Freedman RB, Hirst TR. Cloning and active site mutagenesis of *Vibrio cholerae* DsbA, a periplasmic enzyme that catalyzes disulfide bond formation. J Biol Chem. 1993;268:4326–4330.
38. Connell TD, Metzger DJ, Wang M, et al. Initial studies of the structural signal for extracellular transport of cholera toxin and other proteins recognized by *Vibrio cholerae.* Infect Immun. 1995;63:4091–4098.
39. Mecsas JJ, Strauss EJ. Molecular mechanisms of bacterial virulence: Type III secretion and pathogenicity islands. Emerg Infect Dis. 1996;2:270–288.
40. Shea JE, Hensel M, Gleeson C, Holden DW. Identification of a virulence locus encoding a second type III secretion system in *Salmonella typhimurium.* Proc Natl Acad Sci U S A. 1996;93:2593–2597.
41. Mecsas J, Raupach B, Falkow S. The *Yersinia* Yops inhibit invasion of *Listeria, Shigella* and *Edwardsiella* but not *Salmonella* into epithelial cells. Mol Microbiol. 1998;28:1269–1281.
42. Cornelis GR. The *Yersinia* Yop virulon, a bacterial system to subvert cells of the primary host defense. Folia Microbiol. 1998;43:253–261.
43. Yahr TL, Goranson J, Frank DW. Exoenzyme S of *Pseudomonas aeruginosa* is secreted by a type III pathway. Mol Microbiol. 1996;22:991–1003.
44. Frithz-Lindsten E, Du Y, Rosqvist R, Forsberg A. Intracellular targeting of exoenzyme S of *Pseudomonas aeruginosa* via type III–dependent translocation induces phagocytosis resistance, cytotoxicity and disruption of actin microfilaments. Mol Microbiol. 1997;25:1125–1139.
45. Knight DA, Barbieri JT. Ecto-ADP-ribosyltransferase activity of *Pseudomonas aeruginosa* exoenzyme S. Infect Immun. 1997;65:3304–3309.
46. Kubori T, Matsushima Y, Nakamura D, et al. Supramolecular structure of the *Salmonella typhimurium* type III protein secretion system. Science. 1998;280:602–605.
47. Mollby R, Jeljaszewicz J, Wadstrom T, eds. Bacterial Phospholipases. New York: Academic; 1978:367–424.
48. Eidels L, Proia RL, Hart DA. Membrane receptors for bacterial toxins. Microbiol Rev. 1983;47:596–620.
49. Brennan MJ, David JL, Kenimer JG, Manclark CR. Lectin-like binding of pertussis toxin to a 165-kilodalton Chinese hamster ovary cell glycoprotein. J Biol Chem. 1988;263:4895–4899.
50. Saukkonen K, Burnette WN, Mar VL, et al. Pertussis toxin has eukaryotic-like carbohydrate recognition domains. Proc Natl Acad Sci U S A. 1992;89:118–122.
51. Clark CG, Armstrong GD. Lymphocyte receptors for pertussis toxin. Infect Immun. 1990;58:3840–3846.
52. Sindt K, Redpath G, Hewlett E, et al. Pertussis toxin activates platelets through an interaction with platelet glycoprotein 1b. Infect Immun. 1994;62:3108–3114.
53. Kounnas MZ, Morris RE, Thompson MR, et al. The α_2-macroglobulin receptor/low density lipoprotein receptor–related protein binds and internalizes *Pseudomonas* exotoxin A. J Biol Chem. 1992;267:12420–12423.
54. Naglich JG, Metherall JE, Russell DW, Eidels L. Expression cloning of a diphtheria toxin receptor: Identity with a heparin-binding EGF-like growth factor precursor. Cell. 1992;69:1051–1061.
55. Middlebrook JL, Dorland RB. Response of cultured mammalian cells to the exotoxins of *Pseudomonas aeruginosa* and *Corynebacterium diphtheriae:* Differential cytotoxicity. Can J Microbiol. 1977;23:183–189.
56. Saelinger CB. Toxin structure and function. In: Saelinger CB, ed. Trafficking of Bacterial Toxins. Boca Raton, Fla: CRC; 1990:2–13.
57. Sandvig K, Garred O, van Deurs B. Intracellular transport and processing of protein toxins produced by enteric bacteria. Adv Exp Med Biol. 1997;412:225–232.
58. Cabiaux V, Wolff C, Ruysschaert JM. Interaction with a lipid membrane: A key step in bacterial toxins virulence. Int J Biol Macromol. 1997;21:285–298.
59. Kagan BL, Reich KA, Collier RJ. Orientation of the diphtheria toxin channel in lipid bilayers. Biophys J. 1984;45:102–104.
60. Finkelstein A. Channels formed in phospholipid bilayer membranes by diphtheria, tetanus, botulinum and anthrax toxin. J Physiol (Paris). 1990;84:188–190.
61. Benson EL, Huynh PD, Finkelstein A, Collier RJ. Identification of residues lining the anthrax protective antigen channel. Biochemistry. 1998;37:3941–3948.
62. Collier RJ. ADP-ribosylating toxins and G proteins. In: Moss J, Vaughan M, eds. Diphtheria Toxin: Structure and Function of a Cytocidal Protein. Washington, DC: American Society for Microbiology; 1990:3–19.
63. Hudson TH, Scharff J, Kimak MAG, Neville DM Jr. Energy requirements for diphtheria toxin translocation are coupled to the maintenance of a plasma membrane potential and a proton gradient. J Biol Chem. 1988;263:4773–4781.
64. Morris RE. Interaction between *Pseudomonas* exotoxin A and mouse LM fibroblast cells. In: Saelinger CB, ed. Trafficking of Bacterial Toxins. Boca Raton, Fla: CRC Press; 1990:50–70.
65. Xu Y, Barbieri JT. Pertussis toxin–catalyzed ADP-ribosylation of Gi-2 and Gi-3 in CHO cells is modulated by inhibitors of intracellular trafficking. Infect Immun. 1996;64:593–599.
66. Xu Y, Barbieri JT. Pertussis toxin–mediated ADP-ribosylation of target proteins in Chinese hamster ovary cells involves a vesicle trafficking mechanism. Infect Immun. 1995;63:825–832.
67. Gordon VM, Young WW Jr, Lechler SM, et al. Adenylate cyclase toxins from *Bacillus anthracis* and *Bordetella pertussis.* Different processes for interaction with and entry into target cells. J Biol Chem. 1989;264:14792–14796.
68. Leppla SH. Anthrax toxin edema factor: A bacterial adenylate cyclase that increases cyclic AMP concentrations in eukaryotic cells. Proc Natl Acad Sci U S A. 1982;79:3162–3166.
69. Hewlett, EL, Gordon VM. Adenylate cyclase toxin of *Bordetella pertussis.* In: Wardlaw AC, Parton R, eds. Pathogenesis and Immunity in Pertussis. New York: John Wiley & Sons; 1988:193–209.
70. Otero AS, Yi XB, Gray MC, et al. Membrane depolarization prevents cell invasion by *Bordetella pertussis* adenylate cyclase toxin. J Biol Chem. 1995;270:9695–9697.
71. Karimova G, Fayolle C, Gmira S, et al. Charge-dependent translocation of *Bordetella pertussis* adenylate cyclase toxin into eukaryotic cells: Implication for the *in vivo* delivery of CD8+ T cell epitopes into antigen-presenting cells. Proc Natl Acad Sci U S A. 1998;95:12532–12537.

72. Schiavo G, Rossetto O, Tonello F, Montecucco C. Intracellular targets and metalloprotease activity of tetanus and botulism neurotoxins. Curr Top Microbiol Immunol. 1995;195:257–274.
73. Choe S, Bennett MJ, Fujii G, et al. The crystal structure of diphtheria toxin. Nature. 1992;357:216–222.
74. Bell CE, Eisenberg D. Crystal structure of nucleotide-free diphtheria toxin. Biochemistry. 1997;36:481–488.
75. Cha JH, Brooke JS, Eidels L. Toxin binding site of the diphtheria toxin receptor: Loss and gain of diphtheria toxin binding of monkey and mouse heparin-binding, epidermal growth factor–like growth factor precursors by reciprocal site-directed mutagenesis. Mol Microbiol. 1998;29:1275–1284.
76. Louie GV, Yang W, Bowman ME, Choe S. Crystal structure of the complex of diphtheria toxin with an extracellular fragment of its receptor. Mol Cell. 1997;1:67–78.
77. Iwamoto R, Senoh H, Okada Y, et al. An antibody that inhibits the binding of diphtheria toxin to cells revealed the association of a 27-kDa membrane protein with the diphtheria toxin receptor. J Biol Chem. 1991;266:20463–20469.
78. Pollack M, Young LS. Protective activity of antibodies to exotoxin A and lipopolysaccharide at the onset of *Pseudomonas aeruginosa* septicemia in man. J Clin Invest. 1979;63:276–286.
79. Tang HB, DiMango E, Bryan R, et al. Contribution of specific *Pseudomonas aeruginosa* virulence factors to pathogenesis of pneumonia in a neonatal mouse model of infection. Infect Immun. 1996;64:37–43.
80. Schiavo G, Benfenati F, Poulain B, et al. Tetanus and botulinum-B neurotoxins block neurotransmitter release by proteolytic cleavage of synaptobrevin. Nature. 1992;359:832–835.
81. Schiavo G, Rossetto O, Benfenati F, et al. Tetanus and botulinum neurotoxins are zinc proteases specific for components of the neuroexocytosis apparatus. Ann N Y Acad Sci. 1994;710:65–75.
82. Niemann H, Blasi J, Jahn R. Clostridial neurotoxins: New tools for dissecting exocytosis. Trends Cell Biol. 1994;4:179–185.
83. Nemoz-Gaillard E, Bosshard A, Regazzi R, et al. Expression of SNARE proteins in enteroendocrine cell lines and functional role of tetanus toxin–sensitive proteins in cholecystokinin release. FEBS Lett. 1998;425:66–70.
84. Van Heyningen S. Tetanus role. In: Dorner F, Drews J, eds. Pharmacology of Bacterial Toxins. Oxford: Pergamon; 1986:549–570.
85. Habermann E, Dreyer F, Bigalke H. Tetanus toxin blocks the neuromuscular transmission *in vitro* like botulinum A toxin. Naunyn Schmiedebergs Arch Pharmacol. 1980;311:33–40.
86. Gill DM. Bacterial toxins: A table of lethal amounts. Microbiol Rev. 1982;46:86–94.
87. Simpson LL. Clostridial and related protein toxins: A short overview. In: Witholt B, Alouf JE, eds. Bacterial Protein Toxins. Stuttgart, Germany: Gustav Fischer Verlag; 1992:20–30.
88. Shapiro RL, Hatheway C, Swerdlow DL. Botulism in the United States: A clinical and epidemiologic review. Ann Intern Med. 1998;129:221–228.
89. Cherington M. Clinical spectrum of botulism. Muscle Nerve. 1998;21:701–710.
90. Glatman-Freedman A. Infant botulism. Pediatr Rev 1996;17(5):185–186.
91. Arnon SS. Infant botulism. Annu Rev Med. 1980;31:541–560.
92. Denislic M, Pirtosek Z, Vodusek DB, et al. Botulinum toxin in the treatment of neurological disorders. Ann N Y Acad Sci. 1994;710:76–87.
93. Aktories K. Bacterial toxins that target Rho proteins. J Clin Invest. 1997;99:827–829.
94. Boquet P, Munro P, Fiorentini C, Just I. Toxins from anaerobic bacteria: Specificity and molecular mechanisms of action. Curr Opin Microbiol. 1998;1:66–74.
95. Sears CL, Kaper JB. Enteric bacterial toxins: Mechanisms of action and linkage to intestinal secretion. Microbiol Rev. 1996;60:167–215.
96. Ishibashi Y, Arai T. Specific inhibition of phagosome-lysosome fusion in murine macrophages mediated by *Salmonella typhimurium* infection. FEMS Microbiol Immunol. 1990;2:35–43.
97. Popoff MR. Interactions between bacterial toxins and intestinal cells. Toxicon. 1998;36:665–685.
98. Kaper JB, Morris JGJ, Levine MM. Cholera [published erratum appears in Clin Microbiol Rev 1995 Apr;8(2):316]. Clin Microbiol Rev. 1995;8:48–86.
99. Moss J, Vaughan M. Mechanism of action of choleragen and *E. coli* heat-labile enterotoxin: Activation of adenylate cyclase by ADP-ribosylation. Mol Cell Biochem. 1981;37:75–90.
100. Field M. Intestinal electrolyte secretion. History of a paradigm. Arch Surg. 1993;128:273–278.
101. Field M, Fromm D, Al-Awqati Q, Greenough WB. Effect of cholera enterotoxin on ion transport across isolated ileal mucosa. J Clin Invest. 1972;51:796–804.
102. Thielman NM, Marcinkiewicz M, Sarosiek J, et al. Role of platelet-activating factor in Chinese hamster ovary cell responses to cholera toxin. J Clin Invest. 1997;99:1999–2004.
103. Turvill JL, Mourad FH, Farthing MJ. Crucial role for 5-HT in cholera toxin but not *Escherichia coli* heat-labile enterotoxin-intestinal secretion in rats. Gastroenterology. 1998;115:883–890.
104. Lundgren O. 5-Hydroxytryptamine, enterotoxins, and intestinal fluid secretion. Gastroenterology. 1998;115:1009–1012.
105. Smith PL, Blumberg JB, Stoff JS, Field M. Antisecretory effects of indomethacin on rabbit ileal mucosa *in vitro*. Gastroenterology. 1981;80:356–365.
106. Levine MM, Kaper JB. Live oral vaccines against cholera: An update. Vaccine. 1993;11:207–212.
107. Baudry B, Fasano A, Ketley J, Kaper JB. Cloning of a gene *(zot)* encoding a new toxin produced by *Vibrio cholerae*. Infect Immun. 1992;60:428–434.
108. Pierce NF, Cray WCJ, Sacci JBJ. Oral immunization of dogs with purified cholera toxin, crude cholera toxin, or B subunit: Evidence for synergistic protection by antitoxic and antibacterial mechanisms. Infect Immun. 1982;37:687–694.
109. Lycke N. The mechanism of cholera toxin adjuvanticity. Res Immunol. 1997;148:504–520.
110. Yamamoto S, Takeda Y, Yamamoto M, et al. Mutants in the ADP-ribosyltransferase cleft of cholera toxin lack diarrheagenicity but retain adjuvanticity. J Exp Med. 1997;185:1203–1210.
111. Spangler BD. Structure and function of cholera toxin and the related *Escherichia coli* heat-labile enterotoxin. Microbiol Rev. 1992;56:622–647.
112. Pickett CL, Twiddy EM, Coker C, Holmes RK. Cloning, nucleotide sequence, and hybridization studies of the type IIb heat-labile enterotoxin gene of *Escherichia coli*. J Bacteriol. 1989;171:4945–4952.
113. Rasheed JK, Guzman-Verduzco LM, Kupersztoch YM. Two precursors of the heat-stable enterotoxin of *Escherichia coli:* Evidence of extracellular processing. Mol Microbiol. 1990;4:265–273.
114. Field M, Graf LHJ, Laird WJ, Smith PL. Heat-stable enterotoxin of *Escherichia coli:* In vitro effects on guanylate cyclase activity, cyclic GMP concentration, and ion transport in small intestine. Proc Natl Acad Sci U S A. 1978;75:2800–2804.
115. Hughes JM, Murad F, Chang B, Guerrant RL. Role of cyclic GMP in the action of heat-stable enterotoxin of *Escherichia coli*. Nature. 1978;271:755–756.
116. Schulz S, Green CK, Yuen PS, Garbers DL. Guanylyl cyclase is a heat-stable enterotoxin receptor. Cell. 1990;63:941–948.
117. Guerrant RL, Hughes JM, Chang B, et al. Activation of intestinal guanylate cyclase by heat-stable enterotoxin of *Escherichia coli:* Studies of tissue specificity, potential receptors, and intermediates. J Infect Dis. 1980;142:220–228.
118. de Sauvage FJ, Camerato TR, Goeddel DV. Primary structure and functional expression of the human receptor for *Escherichia coli* heat-stable enterotoxin. J Biol Chem. 1991;266:17912–17918.
119. Forte LR, Eber SL, Turner JT, et al. Guanylin stimulation of Cl^- secretion in human intestinal T84 cells via cyclic guanosine monophosphate. J Clin Invest. 1993;91:2423–2428.
120. Crane JK, Shanks KL. Phosphorylation and activation of the intestinal guanylyl cyclase receptor for *Escherichia coli* heat-stable toxin by protein kinase C. Mol Cell Biochem. 1996;165:111–120.
121. Crane JK, Oh JS. Activation of host cell protein kinase C by enteropathogenic *Escherichia coli*. Infect Immun. 1997;65:3277–3285.
122. Guarino A, Capano G, Malamisura B, et al. Production of *Escherichia coli* STa-like heat-stable enterotoxin by *Citrobacter freundii* isolated from humans. J Clin Microbiol. 1987;25:110–114.
123. Wren BW. Molecular characterisation of *Clostridium difficile* toxins A and B. Rev Med Microbiol. 1992;3:21–27.
124. Rocha MFG, Maia MET, Bezerra LRPS, et al. *Clostridium difficile* toxin A induces the release of neutrophil chemotactic factors from rat peritoneal macrophages: Role of interleukin-1β, tumor necrosis factor alpha, and leukotrienes. Infect Immun. 1997;65:2740–2746.
125. Hecht G, Pothoulakis C, LaMont JT, Madara JL. *Clostridium diffcle* toxin A perturbs cytoskeletal structure and tight junction permeability of cultured human intestinal epithelial monolayers. J Clin Invest. 1988;82:1516–1524.
126. Fonteles M, Fang G, Thielman NM, et al. Role of platelet activating factor in the inflammatory and secretory effects of *Clostridium difficile* toxin A. J Lipid Mediat Cell Signal. 1995;11:133–143.
127. Chambers FG, Koshy SS, Saidi RF, et al. *Bacteroides fragilis* toxin exhibits polar activity on monolayers of human intestinal epithelial cells (T84 cells) *in vitro*. Infect Immun. 1997;65:3561–3570.
128. Obiso RJ Jr, Lyerly DM, Van Tassell RL, Wilkins TD. Proteolytic activity of the *Bacteroides fragilis* enterotoxin causes fluid secretion and intestinal damage in vivo. Infect Immun. 1995;63:3820–3826.
129. Saidi RF, Jaeger K, Montrose MH, et al. *Bacteroides fragilis* toxin rearranges the actin cytoskeleton of HT29/C1 cells without direct proteolysis of actin or decrease in F-actin content. Cell Motil Cytoskeleton. 1997;37:159–165.
130. Wu S, Lim KC, Huang J, et al. *Bacteroides fragilis* enterotoxin cleaves the zonula adherens protein, E-cadherin. Proc Natl Acad Sci U S A. 1998;95:14979–14984.
131. Hewlett EL. Pertussis: Current concepts of pathogenesis and prevention. Pediatr Infect Dis J. 1997;16(Suppl):S78–S84.
132. Ui M. Pertussis toxin as a valuable probe for G-protein involvement in signal transduction. In: Moss J, Vaughan M, eds. ADP-Ribosylating Toxins and G Proteins. Washington, DC: American Society for Microbiology; 1990:45–78.
133. Hewlett EL, Cherry JD. New and improved vaccines against pertussis. In: Cobon GS, Kaper JB, Woodrow GC, et al, eds. New Generation Vaccines. 2nd ed. New York: Marcel Dekker; 1997:387–416.
134. Toyota T, Kai Y, Kakizaki M, et al. Effects of islet-activating protein (IAP) on blood glucose and plasma insulin in healthy volunteers (phase 1 studies). Tohoku J Exp Med. 1980;130:105–116.
135. Confer DL, Eaton JW. Phagocyte impotence caused by an invasive bacterial adenylate cyclase. Science. 1982;217:948–950.
136. Hewlett EL, Maloney NJ. Adenylyl cyclase toxin from *Bordetella pertussis*. In: Iglewski B, Moss J, Tu AT, et al, eds. Handbook of Natural Toxins, v. 8. Microbial Toxins. New York: Marcel Dekker; 1994:425–439.
137. Cookson BT, Cho HL, Herwaldt LA, Goldman WE. Biological activities and chemical composition of purified tracheal cytotoxin of *Bordetella pertussis*. Infect Immun. 1989;57:2223–2229.
138. Luker KE, Tyler AN, Marshall GR, Goldman WE. Tracheal cytotoxin structural requirements for respiratory epithelial damage in pertussis. Mol Microbiol. 1995;16:733–743.

139. Flak TA, Goldman WE. Autotoxicity of nitric oxide in airway disease. Am J Respir Crit Care Med. 1996;154(Suppl):S202–S206.
140. Heiss LN, Flak TA, Lancaster JRJ, et al. Nitric oxide mediates *Bordetella pertussis* tracheal cytotoxin damage to the respiratory epithelium. Infect Agents Dis. 1993;2:173–177.
141. Lacerda HM, Pullinger GD, Lax AJ, Rozengurt E. Cytotoxic necrotizing factor 1 from *Escherichia coli* and dermonecrotic toxin from *Bordetella bronchiseptica* induce p21[rho]-dependent tyrosine phosphorylation of focal adhesion kinase and paxillin in Swiss 3T3 cells. J Biol Chem. 1997;272:9587–9596.
142. Oswald E, Sugai M, Labigne A, et al. Cytotoxic necrotizing factor type 2 produced by virulent *Escherichia coli* modifies the small GTP-binding proteins Rho involved in assembly of actin stress fibers. Proc Natl Acad Sci U S A. 1994;91:3814–3818.
143. Horiguchi Y, Senda T, Sugimoto N, et al. *Bordetella bronchiseptica* dermonecrotizing toxin stimulates assembly of actin stress fibers and focal adhesions by modifying the small GTP-binding protein rho. J Cell Sci. 1995;108:3243–3251.
144. Boquet P. Cytotoxic necrotizing factor 1 from *Escherichia coli:* A toxin with a new intracellular activity for eukaryotic cells. Folia Microbiol. 1998;43:285–289.
145. Schmidt G, Sehr P, Wilm M, et al. Gln 63 of Rho is deamidated by *Escherichia coli* cytotoxic necrotizing factor-1. Nature. 1997;387:725–729.
146. Flatau G, Lemichez E, Gauthier M, et al. Toxin-induced activation of the G protein p21 Rho by deamidation of glutamine. Nature. 1997;387:729–733.
147. Gordon VM, Klimpel KR, Arora N, et al. Proteolytic activation of bacterial toxins by eukaryotic cells is performed by furin and by additional cellular proteases. Infect Immun. 1995;63:82–87.
148. Gordon VM, Leppla SH, Hewlett EL. Inhibitors of receptor-mediated endocytosis block the entry of *Bacillus anthracis* adenylate cyclase toxin but not that of *Bordetella pertussis* adenylate cyclase toxin. Infect Immun. 1988;56:1066–1069.
149. Petosa C, Collier RJ, Klimpel KR, et al. Crystal structure of the anthrax toxin protective antigen. Nature. 1997;385:833–838.
150. Duesbery NS, Webb CP, Leppla SH, et al. Proteolytic inactivation of MAP-kinase-kinase by anthrax lethal factor. Science. 1998;280:734–737.
151. Vitale G, Pellizzari R, Recchi C, et al. Anthrax lethal factor cleaves the N-terminus of MAPKKs and induces tyrosine/threonine phosphorylation of MAPKs in cultured macrophages. Biochem Biophys Res Commun. 1998;248:706–711.
152. Hanna PC, Acosta D, Collier RJ. On the role of macrophages in anthrax. Proc Natl Acad Sci U S A. 1993;90:10198–10201.
153. O'Brien AD, Tesh VL, Donohue-Rolfe A, et al. Shiga toxin: Biochemistry, genetics, mode of action, and role in pathogenesis. Curr Top Microbiol Immunol. 1992;180:65–94.
154. Schmidt H, Montag M, Bockemuhl J, et al. Shiga-like toxin II–related cytotoxins in *Citrobacter freundii* strains from humans and beef samples. Infect Immun. 1993;61:534–543.
155. Stein PE, Boodhoo A, Tyrrell GJ, et al. Crystal structure of the cell-binding B oligomer of verotoxin-1 from *E. coli.* Nature. 1992;355:748–750.
156. Obrig TG, Moran TP, Colinas RJ. Ribonuclease activity associated with the 60S ribosome-inactivating proteins ricin A, phytolaccin and Shiga toxin. Biochem Biophys Res Commun. 1985;130:879–884.
157. Louise CB, Obrig TG. Shiga toxin–associated hemolytic uremic syndrome: Combined cytotoxic effects of Shiga toxin and lipopolysaccharide (endotoxin) on human vascular endothelial cells *in vitro.* Infect Immun. 1992;60:1536–1543.
158. Kaplan BS. Shiga toxin–induced tubular injury in hemolytic uremic syndrome (Editorial). Kidney Int. 1998;54:648–649.
159. Louise CB, Tran MC, Obrig TG. Sensitization of human umbilical vein endothelial cells to Shiga toxin: Involvement of protein kinase C and NF-kappaB. Infect Immun. 1997;65:3337–3344.
160. Adler S, Bollu R. Glomerular endothelial cell injury mediated by Shinga-like toxin-1. Kidney Blood Press Res. 1998;21:13–21.
161. Bohach GA, Stauffacher CV, Ohlendorf DH, et al. The staphylococcal and streptococcal pyrogenic toxin family. Adv Exp Med Biol. 1996;391:131–154.
162. Rago JV, Schlievert PM. Mechanisms of pathogenesis of staphylococcal and streptococcal superantigens. Curr Top Microbiol Immunol. 1998;225:81–97.
163. Leung DY, Meissner C, Fulton D, Schlievert PM. The potential role of bacterial superantigens in the pathogenesis of Kawasaki syndrome. J Clin Immunol. 1995;15(Suppl):S11–S17.
164. Leung DY, Sullivan KE, Brown-Whitehorn TF, et al. Association of toxic shock syndrome toxin–secreting and exfoliative toxin–secreting *Staphylococcus aureus* with Kawasaki syndrome complicated by coronary artery disease. Pediatr Res. 1997;42:268–272.
165. Marrack P, Kappler J. The staphylococcal enterotoxins and their relatives. Science. 1990;248:705–711.
166. Leder L, Llera A, Lavoie PM, et al. A mutational analysis of the binding of staphylococcal enterotoxins B and C3 to the T cell receptor beta chain and major histocompatibility complex class II. J Exp Med. 1998;187:823–833.
167. Bohach GA. Staphylococcal enterotoxins B and C. Structural requirements for superantigenic and enterotoxigenic activities. Prep Biochem Biotechnol. 1997;27:79–110.
168. Schlievert PM, Bohach GA, Ohlendorf DH, et al. Molecular structure of staphylococcus and streptococcus superantigens [published erratum appears in J Clin Immunol 1996 Mar;16(2):126]. J Clin Immunol. 1995;15(Suppl):S4–S10.
169. Lee PK, Vercellotti GM, Deringer JR, Schlievert PM. Effects of staphylococcal toxic shock syndrome toxin 1 on aortic endothelial cells. J Infect Dis. 1991;164:711–719.
170. Phylogenetic analyses of the RTX toxin family. In: Welch RA. Roth JA, eds. Virulence Mechanisms of Bacterial Pathogens. 2nd ed. Washington, DC: American Society for Microbiology; 1995:195–206.
171. Rappuoli R, Montecucco C, eds. Guidebook to Protein Toxins and Their Use in Cell Biology. New York: Oxord; 1997:1.
172. Alouf JE, Freer JH, eds. Bacterial Protein Toxins. Handbook of Experimental Pharmacology. Kent: Academic Press; 1999. In press.
172a. Alouf JE, Freer JH, eds. The Comprehensive Sourcebook of Bacterial Protein Toxins. 2nd ed. Kent: Academic Press; 1999.
173. Saleh MN, LeMaistre CF, Kuzel TM, et al. Antitumor activity of DAB389IL-2 fusion toxin in mycosis fungoides. J Am Acad Dermatol. 1998;39:63–73.
174. Klimka A, Barth S, Drillich S, et al. A deletion mutant of *Pseudomonas* exotoxin-A fused to recombinant human interleukin-9 (rhIL-9-ETA′) shows specific cytotoxicity against IL-9-receptor–expressing cell lines. Cytokines Mol Ther. 1996;2:139–146.
175. Nechushtan A, Yarkoni S, Marianovsky I, Lorberboum-Galski H. Adenocarcinoma cells are targeted by the new GnRH-PE66 chimeric toxin through specific gonadotropin-releasing hormone binding sites. J Biol Chem. 1997;272:11597–11603.
176. Gu L, Zhou M, Jurickova I, et al. Expression of interleukin-6 receptors by pediatric acute lymphoblastic leukemia cells with the t(4;11) translocation: A possible target for therapy with recombinant IL6-*Pseudomonas* exotoxin. Leukemia. 1997;11:1779–1786.
177. FitzGerald D, Pastan I, Robertus J, et al, eds. Current Topics in Microbiology and Immunology. Berlin: Springer-Verlag; 1998.
178. Foss FM, Saleh MN, Krueger JG, et al. Diphtheria toxin fusion proteins. Curr Top Microbiol Immunol. 1998;234:63–81.
179. Goletz TJ, Klimpel KR, Leppla SH, et al. Delivery of antigens to the MHC class I pathway using bacterial toxins. Hum Immunol. 1997;54:129–136.
180. Fayolle C, Sebo P, Ladant D, et al. In vivo induction of CTL responses by recombinant adenylate cyclase of *Bordetella pertussis* carrying viral CD8+ T cell epitopes. J Immunol. 1996;156:4697–4706.
181. Ballard JD, Collier RJ, Starnbach MN. Anthrax toxin as a molecular tool for stimulation of cytotoxic T lymphocytes: Disulfide-linked epitopes, multiple injections, and role of CD4(+) cells. Infect Immun. 1998;66:4696–4699.

SECTION B

HOST DEFENSE MECHANISMS

Chapter 4

Innate (General or Nonspecific) Host Defense Mechanisms

EDMUND C. TRAMONT
DAVID L. HOOVER

Innate (general or nonspecific) host defense mechanisms represent a formidable array of host resistance factors that interfere with and provide the initial defense against microbes. The protective effects are a result of innate steady-state resistance caused by physical barriers (e.g., intact skin, mucous membranes, mucus, cilia, peristalsis, resident microflora, lysozyme, complement) and a consequence of the presence or invasion of any foregin substance that results in the activation of a multitude of cellular and soluble factors (e.g., cytokines/chemokines, natural killer (NK) cells) and leads to the release or production of acute phase reactants (acute phase proteins) that promote phagocytosis and stimulate complementary cytokines/chemokines.

Innate nonspecific host defense mechanisms represent an effective, broad–based surveillance program that serves as a transitional defense system holding a foreign invader at bay while setting the stage for the host to develop specific adaptive immunity. These mechanisms provide a critical first encounter against any microorganism. Because of their general nature, the innate nonspecific host defense mechanisms are difficult to quantify, and because they are so efficient they are often taken for granted (Tables 4–1 and 4–2). Taken as a whole, the effect of this first line of defense is impressive; taken individually, each mechanism or factor is less dramatic than are the adaptive specific humoral and cellular immune responses, such as antibodies and cytotoxic lymphocytes, that arise from clonal expansion of lymphocytes to confer resistance to specific infectious agents.

NORMAL INDIGENOUS MICROBIAL FLORA

With the exception of a preformed toxin or other microbial by-product, a microorganism must gain access into or onto the host to develop a particular relationship with that host. This host-parasite relationship may be symbiotic, commensal, or parasitic, depending on the particular situation that is encountered. For example, *Escherichia coli* is usually a commensal organism in the gastrointestinal tract, but it is almost always a parasite (pathogen) in the lung. Certain organisms behave in a predictable fashion. For example, in humans, the rabies virus is always considered a pathogen, whereas lactobacilli are seldom considered pathogens. From the point of view of the microorganism, the better adapted it becomes to exist in a symbiotic or commensal relationship with its host, the better its own chances for survival.

The normal commensal flora constitute a critical ecosystem that plays an important role in protecting the host from microbial invasion by "pathogenic" organisms.[1] Its protective mechanisms include the following: (1) competition for the same nutrients (interference); (2) competition for the same receptors on host cells (tropism); (3) production of secreted products such as bacteriocins (antibiotics) that are toxic to other organisms, usually of the same species; (4) production of volatile fatty acids or other metabolites that are toxic to competing microbes; (5) continual stimulation of the immune system to maintain low but constant levels of class II histocompatibility (HLA-DR) molecule expression on macrophages and other antigen-presenting cells; and (6) stimulation of cross-protective immune factors such as "natural" antibodies (see later discussion).

The ultimate effect of the first three protective mechanisms is to limit the quantity or dominance of any one species. For example, broad-spectrum antibiotic therapy decreases the total numbers of bacteria in the gut. This results in an increased proportion of normally commensal fungal species and resistant bacterial strains. When the antibiotic therapy is stopped, a natural rebound results and the gut is repopulated, but to the advantage of the faster-growing aerobic Enterobacteriaceae over the slower-replicating anaerobes, thereby increasing the probability of gram-negative bacteremia.

The microbial flora harbored by the host can be divided into two groups: (1) normal resident flora that is regularly found and, if perturbed, promptly reestablishes itself and (2) a transient microbial flora that may colonize the host for periods ranging from hours to weeks but does not permanently establish itself.

Certain organisms characteristically colonize certain body sites (tropism). This is taken into consideration when deciding whether a particular organism is behaving in a pathogenic fashion. Bacteria and fungi make up the great majority of commensal and symbiotic organisms. Protozoa are less ubiquitous, almost always reside in the gastrointestinal tract, and are more prevalent in developing countries. Mycoplasmas and viruses are much less prevalent members of the host commensal flora.

The species that make up the normal commensal flora are influenced by environmental factors such as diet, sanitary conditions, air pollution, and hygienic habits.[2] For example, lactobacilli are common intestinal commensals whenever dairy products make up a significant proportion of the dietary intake; protozoa are common intestinal inhabitants of those persons living where sanitation is poor; and a patient with underlying chronic bronchitis is more likely than others to harbor *Haemophilus influenzae* in the tracheobronchial tree.

The normal commensal flora may also be influenced by hormones. Premenarchal and postmenopausal vaginal flora differ significantly from that present during the childbearing period.

The normal commensal flora is also influenced by genetically

TABLE 4–1 Factors Contributing to Host Nonspecific Resistance to Infection

Normal indigenous microflora
Genetic factors
Natural antibodies
Morphologic integrity
Normal excretory secretions and flow
Phagocytosis
Natural killer cells
Nutrition
Non–antigen-specific immune response
Fibronectin
Hormonal factors
Natural anticoagulants
$\gamma\delta$ T cells

TABLE 4–2 Comparison of Innate and Acquired Immunity

Parameter	Innate (Nonspecific)	Acquired (Specific)
Availability	Rapid	Delayed
Dependency on T or B cells	No	Yes
Exhibits memory	No	Yes
Components	Physical barriers Soluble factors Normal flora	Lymphocytes Macrophages

determined host cell receptors to which microorganisms attach and which determine or select the microbes that adhere to the host's cells.

An important beneficial effect of the normal flora on the immune system is to keep it "primed" and therefore more rapid and efficient in its response to invading microorganisms. Antigens are normally presented to the immune system in an ordered and specified way. For example, T cells recognize antigens only after they are displayed on the surface of a macrophage (or other antigen-presenting cell) in physical association with a DR molecule. Normally, 75 to 85% of circulating monocytes in adults maintain relatively high levels of DR molecule expression. DR expression is much lower on monocytes of human newborns, neonatal mice, and germ-free animals. The constant stimulation by the host's indigenous microbial flora maintains the relatively high level of DR molecule expression on macrophages, and perhaps other antigen-presenting cells, which serves to keep the immune system primed. This modulation results, at least in part, from low-level production of interferon-γ (INF-γ), interleukin-4 (IL-4), and other cytokines and chemokines by activated T cells (see "Cytokines") (Table 4–3) and endothelial cells.

In contrast to these benefits, detrimental consequences of colonization with indigenous flora include the stimulation of nonfunctional blocking antibodies, cross-reactive responses to host tissues, inappropriate T-cell responses,[2a] and chronic low-grade inflammation.[2b, 2c]

TISSUE TROPISMS AND HEREDITARY FACTORS

Population studies have shown that susceptibility to and mortality from an infection are significantly influenced by heredity; for example, if a child's parent died from an infectious disease such as pneumonia, then the child has a significantly increased chance of dying from an infection[3] (Fig. 4–1). This susceptibility is at least in part a consequence of the presence of receptors on cells that serve as anchor sites to permit the attachment of a particular genus, species, or strain of microorganism. The attachment of a microorganism to a receptor depends on the presence of a complementary ligand or adhesin on that microorganism (see Chapter 2).

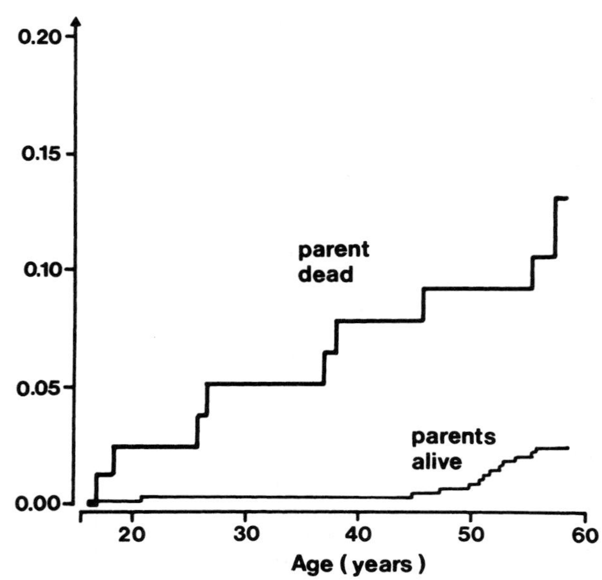

FIGURE 4–1. Probability of dying from an infection before a given age for adoptees with at least one biologic parent who died before the age of 50 (parent dead) of an infection versus adoptees whose biologic parents were alive at that age (parents alive).

TABLE 4–3 Cytokines and Chemokines in Innate Immunity

Class	Examples	Main Cell Source	Action
Proinflammatory cytokines	IL-1β	M, T	Increases selectins, acute phase proteins, IL-1, IL-1Ra, IL-2R and IL-2, IL-6, CSFs, chemokines, prostaglandins; causes fever
	TNF-α	M, T	Increases selectins, IL-1, IL-1Ra, IL-2R and IL-2, IL-6, IL-12, IFN-γ, CSFs, chemokines, prostaglandins; causes fever
	IL-12, IL-18	M, D M, Ep	Increases IL-12, IFN-γ in NK and T; decreases IL-10
Anti-inflammatory cytokines	IL-1Ra	M	Inhibits IL-1
	IL-10	M, L	Inhibits IL-1, TNF-α, IL-12, increases NK cytotoxicity, decreases M microbicidal activity, decreases MHC
	IL-6 and other gp130 cytokines	M, F	Increases acute phase proteins, ACTH, B-cell differentiation, NK cytotoxicity, decreases IL-1, TNF-α; induces fever
	IFN-α/β	Many	Antiviral activity, increases NK cytotoxicity, IL-1Ra, TNFR(II), IL-1R, decreases IL-1, TNF-α
Chemokines	IL-8, other CXC family	M, En, P, many others	Chemotaxis of M, D, NK, T, and especially P
	MCPs, MIPs, other CC family	M, En, many others	M, D, T, E, Ba
	Eotaxins	M, En, many others	E, Ba, D
Activating cytokines	IFN-γ	NK, T	Increases M and NK microbicidal activity, lowers threshold for granule exocytosis by P and LPS triggering of M, drives T (especially Th1) response, increases MHC expression
	GM-CSF	T, NK, activated M	Increases M and P microbicidal activity and myelopoiesis

Abbreviations: ACTH, Adrenocorticotropic hormone; Ba, basophil; CSFs, colony-stimulating factors; D, dendritic cell; E, eosinophil; En, endothelial cell; Ep, epithelial cell; F, = fibroblast; GM-CSF, granulocyte-macrophage colony-stimulating factor; IFN, interferon; IL, interleukin; L, lymphocyte; LPS, lipopolysaccharide; M, monocyte-macrophage; MCP, monocyte chemotactic proteins; MHC, major histocompatibility complex; MIP, macrophage inflammatory protein; NK, NK cell; P, polymorphonuclear leukocyte; T, T cell; TNF, tumor necrosis factor.

The ligand and the receptor vary independently as to their specificity: a receptor may bind to one or many different organisms (ligands), a ligand to one or many different receptors. Most organisms preferentially colonize certain cells (tissues) and spare others. This phenomenon, referred to as *cellular tropism* or *tissue tropism*, is a critical determinant of host–microorganism relationships. For example, influenza virus and mycoplasmas preferentially adhere to respiratory epithelial cells, *E. coli* and *Vibrio cholerae* to intestinal cells, and *Streptococcus mutans* to tooth enamel. Gram-positive organisms more readily attach to heart valves than do gram-negative organisms. *Treponema pallidum*, on the other hand, binds to many different tissue receptors, and untreated syphilis may affect any organ. An example of cellular tropism is the monotropic human immunodeficiency virus (HIV-1), which requires the presence of the chemokine receptor CCR5 (in conjunction with the CD_4 molecule) to infect a cell.

Receptors on host cells may change. For example, there is evidence to suggest that a viral illness can affect tissue tropisms of the oropharynx to allow easier colonization by gram-negative organisms.[4] Also, urinary epithelial cells from persons with recurrent urinary tract infections support the attachment of urinary pathogens more than do urinary epithelial cells obtained from persons not prone to develop these infections.[5] As the genetics and cellular characteristics of tissue tropisms become better known, they will offer a new paradigm for the development of treatment modalities and vaccines.

Ligands on microorganisms may also change. One of the oldest known examples is trypanosomiasis (see Chapter 266). More recently, the switch by HIV-1 from a monotropic or nonsyncytial-inducing (NSI) phenotype to a T-cell or syncytial inducing (SI) phenotype has been related to disease progression.

Infections represent one of the strongest selection pressures in human evolution (see Chapter 5). Tuberculosis, measles, and smallpox, for example, had devastating effects on native populations of North America. Conversely, the sickle cell trait has a protective effect against falciparum malaria, and the trait benefits inhabitants of areas where this disease is endemic. It has been shown that persons homozygous for a mutation in the gene that codes for the CCR5 chemokine receptor (*Δ32CCR5*) are resistant to contracting HIV-1 through sexual contact.[6] Persons of Western European descent, especially persons from the British Isles, are more likely to carry this deletion than are Africans and Asians, who almost never do.[7] Also, persons heterozygous for the *Δ32CCR5* deletion or other chemokine deletions progress to AIDS at a slower rate.[8] Susceptibility to tuberculosis has been linked to variations in the *NRAMP1* gene, an HLA-DQ allele, and IL-12 deficiency.[9, 10, 10a] Susceptibility to pneumococcal disease has been linked to defective production of antibody to the pneumococcal capsule,[11] and the congenital absence of a terminal component of complement predisposes to repeated episodes of disseminated neisserial infections (see Chapter 266).

Other known linkages include HLA-B27 and reactive arthropathy (Reiter syndrome), HLA-DR4 and chronic Lyme arthritis, and the predisposition of persons with blood group O to cholera, which is presumably linked to the expression of glycosphingolipids in the small bowel mucosa. There is also evidence of HLA-linked relationships for tuberculoid leprosy, acute glomerulonephritis, paralytic poliomyelitis, and responsiveness to antigenic stimuli. The list is destined to grow.

NATURAL ANTIBODIES

Natural antibodies is the term used to designate antibodies that are specific to a microbe found in healthy people without a previous history of infection with the microbe. These antibodies are of great importance to the immune defense against many bacteria, especially encapsulated bacteria such as *Neisseria meningitidis* and *H. influenzae* type b.

Some of these antibodies are thought to be stimulated as a result of colonization of the oropharynx, gut, or other sites by organisms sharing cross-reactive (cross-protective) antigens. Other antibodies apparently develop independently of antigen stimulation; are "polyreactive" (e.g., react individually with related epitopes); are found in serum and in secretions; and have been observed in newborns, in nude mice, and in germ-free animals.[12] However, these antibodies are not always beneficial. For example, specific serum immunoglobulin A (IgA) antibodies to *N. meningitidis* may predispose an otherwise immune person to become susceptible by preferentially attaching to the organism, thus blocking the beneficial bactericidal effect of protective IgG and IgM antibodies.[13] The blood group antibodies are a consequence of colonization of the gut by microorganisms bearing cross-reactive antigens.

NATURAL BARRIERS TO THE ENTRY OF MICROORGANISMS INTO THE BODY

The morphologic integrity of body surfaces is an important and effective first line of defense.

Skin and Mucous Membranes

The intact skin forms an effective mechanical barrier to invasion by microorganisms. Because very few organisms have the innate ability to penetrate the skin, they must gain access by some physical means such as an arthropod vector, trauma, surgical incision, or intravenous catheter.

The specific antimicrobial properties of skin have not been exhaustively studied. However, the relative dryness or desiccating effect of skin, its mild acidity (acid mantle, pH 5 to 6), and the normal skin flora act in concert to form an effective prohibitive environment. Inflamed skin is more permeable to water and therefore is more hospitable to colonization. It has been speculated that oily skin may retard evaporation of water, resulting in increased numbers of colonizing organisms. The acidity of the skin results from the breakdown of lipids into fatty acids. Sebum contains few esterified fatty acids, but the normal skin flora partially hydrolyzes the triglycerides, thereby liberating fatty acids. Desquamation of skin scales also aids in the elimination of microorganisms.

Because of the inherent moisture with which they are associated, mucous membranes support a broad spectrum and large number of microorganisms. However, body secretions, including cerebral spinal fluid, are endowed with unique antimicrobial properties. For example, cervical mucus, prostatic fluid, and tears have been shown to be toxic to a variety of microorganisms. Two of the more potent antimicrobial substances are lysozyme and *N*-acetyl muramyl-L-alanine amidase (NAMLAA). Both substances are particularly effective against gram-positive bacteria because they hydrolyze the amino acid backbone of peptidoglycan.[14] Other inhibitory substances include the broad family of small cationic antimicrobial peptides or defensins.[14a, 14b]

Local secretions also contain immunoglobulins, principally IgG and secretory IgA, which act primarily to agglutinate microorganisms or competitively block the attachment of organisms to receptors on host cells, or both.

More secretory IgA than total IgG is produced. The immunoglobulin is made relatively resistant to proteolysis by complexing with secretory piece and protein Fv.[15] There is also evidence that mucosal IgA is able to bind intracellular pathogens or products as it is transported to the cell surface before complexing to secretory piece.[16]

Mucosal secretions also contain significant amounts of iron-binding proteins. The importance of iron for microorganisms is well recognized, and all fluids that are potentially exposed to microbes are enriched with iron-binding proteins that act to keep this important factor from the microorganisms. In contrast, microorganisms that routinely colonize skin and mucosal surfaces have evolved mechanisms to acquire iron.[17, 17a]

Respiratory Tract

The respiratory tract has formidable antimicrobial defense mechanisms.[18, 19] First, inhaled particles must survive and penetrate the aerodynamic filtration system of the upper airway and tracheobronchial tree. The airflow in these areas is turbulent, causing large particles to affect the mucosal surfaces. Humidification also causes hygroscopic organisms to increase in size, thereby aiding trapping.

Once a particle is deposited, the mucociliary blanket transports the invading offender away from the lung. Coughing aids this expulsion. This system is amazingly efficient: 90% of deposited material is cleared in less than 1 hour. In addition, the bronchial secretions contain various antimicrobial substances such as lysozyme, NAMLAA, and the β-defensin hBD-1, hBD-2.[20]

After a particle reaches the alveoli, physical expulsion becomes much less effective, and the alveolar macrophages and tissue histiocytes play a more prominent role in protecting the host. These phagocytes are assisted in their defense by the collectin surfactants SP-A and SP-D, which bind to and opsonize diverse organisms, including gram-negative bacteria, fungi, and *Pneumocystis carinii*.[21]

Like all defense mechanisms, these nonspecific mechanisms can be overcome by the introduction of large numbers of invading organisms (e.g., contaminated respirator), particularly if the host is exposed for an extended period. Furthermore, their effectiveness is decreased by air pollutants (e.g., cigarette smoke), mechanical respirators, tracheostomy, concomitant infection, and allergenic agents.

Intestinal Tract

The acid pH of the stomach, the antibacterial effect of the various pancreatic enzymes, and bile and intestinal secretions are effective antimicrobial factors. Paneth cells of the small intestine, located in the crypts of Lieberkühn, secrete defensins hD-5 and hD-6, lysozyme, and type II phospholipase A.[22]

Peristalsis and the normal loss of epithelial cells also act to purge the intestinal tract of harmful microorganisms. Alteration of these parameters can lead to increased susceptibility of the host to infection. For example, *Salmonella* and *Mycobacterium tuberculosis* infections are more common in achlorhydric patients, and slowing peristalsis with belladonna or opium alkaloids prolongs symptomatic shigellosis.

Normal bowel flora competition for nutrients (10^{12} organisms per gram of feces) plays an extremely important protective role. Altering this flora with broad-spectrum antibiotics can lead to overgrowth of inherently pathogenic organisms (e.g., *Salmonella typhimurium*) or suprainfection with ordinarily commensal organisms (e.g., *Candida albicans*). Nevertheless, the interfering competitive capacity of the normal flora can be overcome by the introduction of large numbers of virulent organisms. For example, the probability of development of salmonellosis is directly related to the number of *Salmonella* organisms ingested.

Genitourinary Tract

Urine is normally sterile. The factors that contribute to the ability of the urinary tract to resist infection are complex. Urine is bactericidal for some strains of bacteria, mostly because of its pH, although factors such as hypertonicity, urea, and other solutes play a role. Tamm-Horsfall protein is a glycoprotein produced by the kidneys and excreted in large amounts in urine (approximately 50 mg/liter). Because certain bacteria avidly bind to it, the protein acts as a natural host defense mechanism against colonization and subsequent infection by preventing these bacteria from gaining a foothold in the urinary tract.[23]

The lower urinary tract is flushed with urine four to eight times each day, eliminating potential pathogenic organisms unless they are capable of firmly attaching to epithelial cells of the urinary tract (e.g., *Neisseria gonorrhoeae*, certain strains of *E. coli*). The length of the male urethra (20 cm in the adult) also provides passive protection, and bacteria seldom gain access to the bladder in men unless introduced by instrumentation. The female urethra is much shorter (5 cm in the adult) and is more readily traversed by microorganisms, which may be one reason why urinary tract infections are 14 times more common in women than in men.

The hypotonic state of the kidney medulla presents an unfavorable milieu for most microorganisms. This natural barrier is most often breached by increased glucose levels secondary to hyperglycemia, which accounts for the increased incidence of pyelonephritis in diabetic patients.

The vagina has a unique mechanism of protection. Under hormonal influence, especially that of estrogens, the vaginal epithelium contains increased amounts of glycogen that *Döderlein's bacilli* and other commensals metabolize into lactic acid. *Döderlein's bacilli* is an all-encompassing term used to describe acidogenic gram-positive rods, especially lactobacilli, residing in the vagina. Normal vaginal secretions contain up to 10^8 such bacteria per milliliter. They establish an acid environment that is unfavorable to most pathogenic microorganisms. The vaginal secretions of women with nonspecific vaginitis or vaginosis, a perturbation of the normally protective vaginal ecosystem, are characterized by an elevated pH.

The Eye

Constant bathing of the eye by tears is an effective means of protection. Foreign substances are continually diluted and washed away via the tear ducts into the nasal cavity. Tears also contain large amounts of lysozyme and other antimicrobial substances.

STEADY-STATE COMPONENTS OF NONSPECIFIC IMMUNITY

After microbes breach the integumentary barriers, they encounter additional innate host defenses mediated by soluble factors and cells. The level and localization of these humoral and cellular components are regulated primarily by cytokines and chemokines.

Complement

Complement refers to a group of 20 or more serum proteins that interact in an orderly fashion that is referred to as the *complement cascade*. Complement can be activated by specific antibody or by the acute phase reactant, C-reactive protein (classic pathway); by the surface components of microorganisms (alternative pathway); and by the collectin mannose-binding protein via interaction with the cell surface receptors C1R and C1S.[21, 24, 25]

Complement activation can lead to microbial lysis, but it also plays important roles in phagocytosis, cytokine/chemokine production, and attraction of leukocytes to infected sites. The lytic action of complement is very effective: the overwhelming majority of intestinal bacteria are susceptible to complement-mediated lysis. In contrast, strains of enteric bacteria that cause invasive disease typically resist complement-mediated serum bactericidal activity. Most complement components are synthesized by macrophages, with increased production in response to infection (see Chapter 7).

Fibronectin

Fibronectin is a high-molecular-weight glycoprotein found in plasma and on cell surfaces that plays a central role in cell-cell adhesion, cell–basement membrane adhesion, clot stabilization, fibroblast migration, and macrophage function. As with all aspects of the host-parasite relationship, a yin-yang phenomenon occurs: fibronectin covers the receptors of surface cells and thereby blocks the attachment of many organisms, such as *Pseudomonas aeruginosa*, but it enhances the binding of other organisms, such as *Staphylococcus aureus*, to host cells.[26]

Phagocytosis

Microorganisms that enter the lymphatics, lung, or blood stream are engulfed and killed by a variety of phagocytic cells. Polymorphonuclear leukocytes and monocytes, which circulate in blood and migrate through the tissues, are attracted to sites of inflammation primarily through the action of chemokines. Opsonin-independent phagocytosis by polymorphonuclear leukocytes (PMNs) is related to the contact angle between the microorganism and the surface on which it rests. As a consequence of this physical relationship, phagocytosis is most efficient when organisms are trapped in small tissue spaces (e.g., alveoli) than when they reside on smooth, open surfaces (e.g., synovium).[27]

Mononuclear phagocytes in blood, lymph nodes, spleen, liver, bone marrow, and lung constitute the reticuloendothelial system. These cells recognize microbes, particulate matter, and damaged or senescent host cells by "pattern recognition receptors" on the macrophage surface. The scavenger receptor family (SRAI and SRAII, MACRO, CD36, CD68, and CLA-1)[28] and the mannose receptor[29] detect phospholipid- and mannose-containing structures, respectively. These structures are frequently present on microbes but are not present on normal host cells. Integrins, notably CD11b/CD18, CD11c/CD18, α_V/β_1, and α_V/β_3, indirectly recognize particulate targets by binding soluble host constituents, including activated complement components, vitronectin, and fibronectin. These soluble molecules interact with fragments of damaged cells, collagen debris, altered platelets, and microbes to enhance their clearance by macrophages.[29, 30] Recognition of collectins (mannose-binding protein, complement component C1q, and the surfactant SP-A) by macrophage receptor C1qRp also enhances phagocytosis of microorganisms coated with these ligands.[31] In addition, CD14 recognizes lipid A from gram-negative bacteria and lipoteichoic acid from gram-positive bacteria. Binding of lipid A to CD14 is facilitated by its attachment to lipopolysaccharide (LPS)–binding protein (LBP). When these receptors are engaged, macrophages are programmed to remove the recognized complexed particles from circulation.

Under resting or steady-state conditions, macrophages and monocytes kill ingested microorganisms by the generation of toxic oxygen metabolites such as hydrogen peroxide and superoxide, the acidification of phagosomal vacuoles, the deposition of acid hydrolases and other lysosomal enzymes into phagolysosomes, and the production of a variety of granule-associated antimicrobial molecules, including neutrophil peptides 1 through 4, lysozyme, elastase, antileukoproteases, azurocidin, cathepsin G, and bactericidal/permeability-increasing protein (BPI).[32–34] These molecules are also released into the plasma and other bodily fluids during inflammation.[35] Their microbicidal capability, however, is relatively limited compared with that of PMNs and activated macrophages stimulated initially by the acute phase reactants (proteins) and later by an adaptive immune response.

Persons whose spleens have been surgically removed or functionally impaired dramatically demonstrate the importance of the reticuloendothelial system: when encapsulated bacteria such as pneumococci are poorly filtered from the blood, they can more easily overwhelm the host to replicate freely in the blood (see Chapter 307).

ACUTE PHASE RESPONSE

When an invader sufficiently perturbs the baseline defensive capabilities of humoral components and phagocytes, a generalized, coordinated, but nonspecific reaction termed the *acute phase response*[35a] ensues. This response augments or depresses the concentration and function of humoral defensive components collectively referred to as *acute phase proteins*, including C-reactive protein, LBP,[36] serum amyloid A, haptoglobin, ceruloplasmin, fibrinogen, α_1-acid glycoprotein, complement components C3, C4, C9, Factor B, C1 inhibitor, and C4b binding protein, transferrin, procalcitonin, prealbumin, and natural anti-coagulants such as protein C, protein S, antithrombin plasminogen, tissue plasminogen activator, urokinase, vitronectin, plasminogen-activator inhibitor 1, α_1-protease inhibitor, α_1-antichymotrypsin, pancreatic secretory trypsin inhibitor, Interleukin-1-receptor antagonist, GCSF, fibronectin, ferritin, angiotensinogen, alpha-fetoprotein, thyroxine-binding globulin, and factor XII.[37] These omnipresent proteins increase the number and function of phagocytic cells, facilitate delivery of humoral and cellular components to sites of inflammation, and direct the pattern of antigen-specific immune responses. The acute phase response is mediated by gamma-delta ($\gamma\delta$) T cells,[37a] reactions of preexisting humoral defenses, and by de novo production of active regulatory molecules (e.g., cytokines/chemokines, prostaglandins and other eicosanoids, hormones) by phagocytes, lymphocytes, and endothelial cells.

Cytokines

Engagement of many of the pattern recognition receptors that lead to microbial clearance, with the general exception of the scavenger receptors[38] also leads to the production of cytokines and chemokines by mononuclear phagocytes and dendritic cells. Other important regulators of the acute phase response include NK cells, $\gamma\delta$-T cells, and endothelial cells. Epithelial cells may also contribute, particularly at the initiation of infection. The intricacy, pleomorphism, and redundancy of the cytokine network have become increasingly apparent (see Chapter 9). Most cytokines are secreted by more than one cell type and most cells that secrete one cytokine secrete many (Fig. 4–2; Table 4–3). In addition, cytokines may enhance or diminish the release of themselves, other cytokines, or other components of the regulatory network.

Mononuclear phagocytes, the most broadly reactive cells of this group, are important producers of the proinflammatory cytokines IL-1β, tumor necrosis factor-α (TNF-α), IL-12,[39] and IL-18,[40] which profoundly affect the inflammatory response and provide priming signals for induction of adaptive immunity. They also make INF-α and INF-β, important nonspecific antiviral molecules and enhancers of T-cell–mediated immune responses. Macrophages also produce prostaglandins and other arachidonic acid metabolites that play a prominent role in inflammation and generally provide feedback inhibition on proinflammatory cytokine release.

Macrophage production of IL-10 and IL-6,[41] also inhibits proinflammatory cytokine production. LPS-induced release of IL-1 receptor antagonist and soluble TNF and IL-1 receptors leads to further modulation of cytokine binding and agonistic activity.[42] Transforming growth factor-β, a product of many cell types including macrophages and platelets, also inhibits PMN and macrophage antimicrobial activity.[43]

Endothelial cells also secrete IL-1, TNF-α, and IL-6, particularly in response to TNF-α, IL-1, and gram-negative bacterial LPS. In addition, they produce large amounts of IL-8, the primary chemokine mediator of PMN localization.[6, 44]

NK cells recognize and destroy virus-infected cells in response to INF-α/β and are further activated for cytotoxicity by IL-10, IL-12, IL-18, and INF-γ. NK cells are the major source of INF-γ in the innate immune response, before specifically sensitized T cells are produced.[45] This cytokine mediates macrophage microbicidal activity, primes PMNs for granule exocytosis and superoxide production, and enhances T-cell–mediated immune responses, especially type 1 (Th1) responses. Another source of INF-γ is $\gamma\delta$-T cells, which recognize peptide and non-peptide antigens of intracellular organisms like *Listeria* and mycobacteria[46] and initiate responses faster than α/β-T cells do. Cytokines not only have direct effects on cells and modulate each other's production but also induce release of adrenocorticotropic hormone, endorphins, prolactin, neurotransmitters, and growth hor-

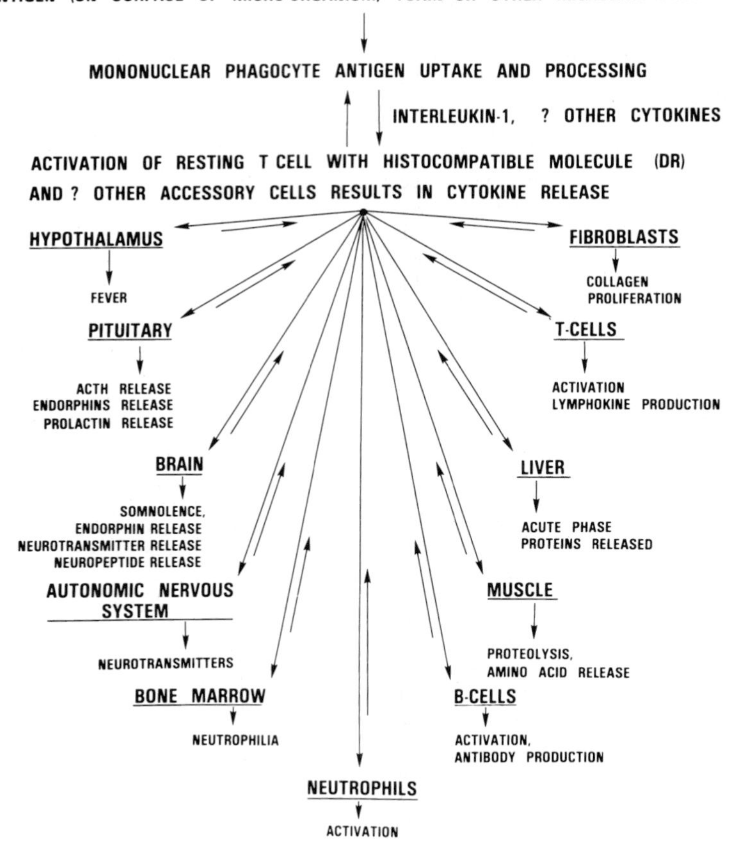

FIGURE 4–2. The cytokine cascade.

mone, which further regulate nonspecific and specific immune responses.[47]

Metabolic Changes. Fever is the most obvious clinical sign of the acute phase response, but the febrile and the acute phase response appear to be regulated independently. Numerous cytokines, notably IL-1, TNF-α, IL-6, and INF-γ, increase prostaglandin production by cells in or near the hypothalamic thermoregulatory center. These prostaglandins raise the temperature setpoint and result in fever. The beneficial versus detrimental effects of fever have long been debated.[48] The consistent expression of fever in response to moderate to severe infection, however, suggests that it plays a beneficial role in resistance to microbial attack (see Chapter 43).

A number of other metabolic changes reflect mobilization of the host's resources for defense. These include increased production of thyroid-stimulating hormone, vasopressin, insulin, and glucagon. Profound catabolism of muscle protein also occurs as amino acids are used for synthesis of defensive cells and proteins and resting muscle metabolic activity or shivering increases to raise body temperature.

Soluble Defensive Molecules. Serum complement components, fibronectin, mannose-binding protein, haptoglobin, amyloid A protein, C-reactive protein, LBP, a number of glycoproteins, and certain protease inhibitors including α_1-antitrypsin and β_2-macroglobulin, also increase as a consequence of infection. LBP mediates binding of LPS to monocytes and macrophages via a specific cell receptor (CD14) and increases sensitivity of cells to LPS stimulation.[49] Increased hepatic synthesis of many of these defensive proteins occurs primarily under the influence of IL-1β and the IL-6 cytokine family members at the expense of serum albumin synthesis, as host metabolism shifts from homeostasis to defense.[50, 51]

A decrease in serum iron has long been recognized as a component of the acute phase response. Many microorganisms must scavenge iron from their environment for optimal growth. Transferrin, an iron-binding protein secreted by hepatocytes under the influence of IL-6, complexes with free iron and limits its availability to microorganisms. Macrophages internalize iron-transferrin complexes, retain the iron, and recycle transferrin, further reducing the availability of both free and total serum iron to any potential invader.[52]

Increased Phagocyte Number and Function. Numbers and functions of phagocytes also increase as an immediate consequence of infection (see Chapter 8). Production of IL-1, TNF-α, IL-3, and stem cell factor by macrophages or lymphocytes (or both) enhances replication of bone marrow stem cells. Replication and differentiation of bone marrow cells toward mature phagocytes are further augmented by granulocyte-macrophage colony-stimulating factor (GM-CSF) and granulocyte colony-stimulating factor (G-CSF).[53]

In addition to providing increased numbers of phagocytes available for defense, cytokines play an important role in enhancing microbicidal activity. TNF-α, IL-1, GM-CSF, INF-γ, and IL-2, alone or in various combinations, lead to increased destruction of microbes through increased production of toxic oxygen products and release of granule-bound antimicrobial molecules. TNF-α and IL-1 also promote expression of complement receptor 3 (CR3), the receptor of iC3b, and thereby enhance ingestion of organisms opsonized by complement.

Inflammation. As part of the acute phase response, phagocyte and soluble antimicrobial substances are directed to sites of microbial invasion. Cytokines, especially TNF-α and IL-1, increase expression of adhesion molecules on endothelial cells, PMNs, NK cells, and monocytes. Production of chemokines by endothelial cells, monocytes, and PMNs in response to other cytokines or microbial products further modulates expression of adhesion molecules and provides chemotactic signals that promote emigration of leukocytes from the blood to the inflammatory site.

Two main families of chemokines direct leukocyte migration.[6, 44, 44a] Members of the CXC family, whose first two cysteines are separated by a single amino acid, stimulate chemotaxis of PMNs, eosinophils, monocytes, dendritic cells, NK cells, and T lymphocytes. Members of the CC family, whose first two cysteines adjoin each other, stimulate all these leukocytes except PMNs, which do not express receptors for CC chemokines. More than 40 chemokines, 8 receptors for CC chemokines, and 5 receptors for CXC chemokines have been described so far. Chemokines upregulate adhesion molecules, stimulate leukocyte migration, and lower the threshold for cell activation.

Although the interactions of chemokines on target cell populations are extraordinarily complex, IL-8 and eotaxin are, respectively, the predominant chemokine modulators of PMN and eosinophil migration. Resting T cells express few chemokine receptors, but these are strongly upregulated by IL-2 in conjunction with stimulation via the antigen receptor. Therefore, the most vigorous immigration of T cells to inflammatory sites occurs in conjunction with acquired immunity rather than during the innate response.

Chemotaxis and release of granule contents in response to complement components (e.g., C5a) or microbial products (e.g., LPS, formylmethionine-leucine-phenylalanine) are also enhanced by INF-γ. These granule contents increase vascular permeability. Other, noncytokine products of macrophages, such as the arachidonic acid products, prostaglandins, and leukotrienes, also increase vascular permeability and cause vasodilatation. As a consequence of these activities, local extravasation of soluble defensive components and plasma and further immigration of phagocytes occur. Kinins generated as a consequence of activation of the coagulation cascade contribute to vasodilatation and stimulate pain-sensitive neuronal endings. Thus, the classic hallmarks of inflammation (swelling, warmth, redness, pain) appear. As more complement components, fibronectin, PMNs, and macrophages accumulate at the inflammatory site, they release more cytokines, chemokines, and other reactants that promote further chemotaxis, inflammation, and enhanced microbicidal activity.

A number of other phenomena, of uncertain consequence, also occur as part of the acute phase reaction. Zinc levels decrease. This metal, which has no known tissue stores, enhances lymphocyte responsiveness, aids wound healing, and participates in protein synthesis.[54] Zinc plays a crucial role in regulation of DNA transcription and RNA translation. Its decrease in infection may reflect its increased use by actively metabolizing cells.

Ceruloplasmin, a superoxide-scavenging, copper-binding protein synthesized by hepatocytes, also increases during the acute phase response under the influence of IL-6. The consequences of this increase on the host response are not known.

INITIATION AND BIASING OF SPECIFIC IMMUNITY

The acute phase response not only provides substantial antimicrobial activity but also sets the stage for the development of specific, adaptive immunity.[37a] In their initial response to microbial invaders, mononuclear phagocytes play a pivotal role in this process by secreting powerful regulatory cytokines, IL-10, IL-12, and IL-18.[39, 40] IL-12 and IL-18 cooperatively promote secretion of INF-γ by NK cells, driving specific immunity toward Th1 T-cell responses, which are characterized by high levels of INF-γ production, development of delayed-type hypersensitivity, and defense against intracellular microbes. Monocytes also produce IL-10, which inhibits IL-12 production, stimulates B-cell proliferation and immunoglobulin synthesis, and drives specific immunity toward Th2 responses, which are characterized by high levels of IL-4 production and synthesis of antibody, particularly IgE. Type 2 (Th2) responses are important for the defense against some viruses, encapsulated bacteria, and large extracellular eukaryotes, especially worms. In addition, IL-10 and IL-18 enhance NK cells and IL-10 enhances CD8 T-cell–mediated cytotoxicity, which protects against viruses.[55]

IMPAIRMENT AND EXAGGERATION OF INNATE (NONSPECIFIC) IMMUNITY

Impaired natural immunity, most conveniently detected by testing for cutaneous delayed hypersensitivity, can occur as a consequence of numerous illnesses. In the United States, end-stage cancer, renal disease, end-stage HIV infection (AIDS), liver disease, and alcoholism are the most common underlying illnesses resulting in diminished cellular immune responsiveness. Worldwide, malnutrition is the leading cause of increased susceptibility to and severity of several infections. These include life-threatening bacterial infections of the middle ear, pervasive dental caries, HIV, and common childhood infections, especially measles.[55, 56]

Nutrition

It is well established that persons with malnutrition, whether preexisting (protein-energy malnutrition) or disease-induced (cytokine-induced malnutrition), have more severe infections. Vitamin A in particular plays a central role.[56, 57] Cellular immune dysfunction is disproportionately affected, and nutritional support has a demonstrable beneficial effect on outcome.[58] For example, before the advent of antibiotics, tuberculosis was often successfully treated by nutrition-based therapies that in some patients included consumption of 20 to 30 eggs per day.

Aging

Although the data regarding the effects of aging on immunity and infection are confusing and sometimes conflicting, this process has an impact on the immune system that can best be summarized as immunosenescence. Superimposed and interrelated with this generalized impairment are social isolation and age-related decrements in organ structure and function. Regardless of the setting, there is a higher incidence in elderly persons of pneumonias (2-fold), cholecystitis (2- to 8-fold), appendicitis (15- to 20-fold), diverticulitis, bacteremia (3-fold), asymptomatic bacteriuria, urinary tract infections (5- to 10-fold), reactivation of varicella-zoster virus and tuberculosis (10-fold), bacterial meningitis (3-fold), and even bacterial endocarditis (2- to 3-fold). The greatest impact of aging is on cell-mediated immunity; there is a lesser but substantial impact on humoral immunity.[59]

Stress

A growing body of evidence has demonstrated an inverse relation between stress and immune function; the end result is an increased susceptibility to infection.[60]

Hormones

Increased production of adrenocorticotropic hormone occurs during the acute phase response and appears to augment the host's survival potential. The depressive effect of excess corticosteroids on inflammation is well known and probably represents an important feedback mechanism to modulate an inflammatory response.

Estrogen affects the lining of the vagina, resulting in increased nonspecific resistance. T-cell function is blunted during pregnancy, which may account for the severity of certain infections, such as those caused by poliomyelitis virus, *Coccidioides immitis*, group A β-hemolytic streptococci, influenza virus, and *N. gonorrhoeae*, particularly in the third trimester.[61]

Dysregulation

The initial nonspecific response is usually effective in controlling microbial invasion. With overwhelming infection and release of large amounts of microbial products, however, the failure of feedback control may lead to the catastrophic syndrome of septic shock. In addition, if infections are not controlled and become chronic, some acute derangements (e.g., decreased serum albumin, iron sequestration, muscle wasting) persist and become profound.

REFERENCES

1. Mackowiak PA. The normal microbial flora. N Engl J Med. 1982;307:83–86.
2. Moore WEC, Burmeister JA, Brooke CW, et al. Investigation of the influences on puberty, genetics and environment on the composition of subgingival peridontal flora. Infect Immun. 1993;61:2891–2898.
2a. Looney RJ, Falsey D, Campbell D, et al. Role of cytomegalovirus in the T cell changes seen in elderly individuals. Clin Immunol. 1999;90:213–219.
2b. Wilson M, Seymour R, Hendeerson B. Bacterial perturbation of cytokine networks. Infect Immun. 1998;66:2401–2409.
2c. Mattila KJ, Valtonen VV, Nieminen MS. Role of infection as a risk factor for atherosclerosis, myocardial infarction and stroke. Clin Infect Dis. 1998;26:719–734.
3. Sorensen TIA, Neilson GG, Anderson PK, et al. Genetic and environmental influences on premature death in adult adoptees. N Engl J Med. 1988;318:727–732.
4. Ramirez-Ronda CH, Fuxench-Lopez Z, Nevarez M. Increased pharyngeal bacterial colonization during viral illness. Arch Intern Med. 1981;141:1599.
5. Svanburg-Eden C, Jodal V. Attachment of *E. coli* to urinary sediment epithelial cells from urinary tract infection prone healthy children. Infect Immun. 1979;26:837.
6. Luster AD. Chemokines: Chemotactic cytokines that mediate inflammation. N Engl J Med. 1998;338:436–445.
7. Samson M, Libert F, Doranz BJ, et al. Resistance to HIV-1 infection in caucasian individuals bearing mutant alleles of the CCR-5 chemokine receptor gene. Nature. 1996;382:722–725.
8. Stewart G. Chemokine genes: Beating the odds. Nat Med. 1998;4:275–277.
9. Bellamy R, Ruwenda C, Corrah T, et al. Variations in the NRAMP1 gene and susceptibility to tuberculosis in West Africans. N Engl J Med. 1998;338:640–643.
10. Goldfeld AE, Delgado JO, Thim S, et al. Association of an HLA-DQ allele with clinical tuberculosis. JAMA. 1998;279:226–228.
10a. Altare F, Durandy A, Lammas D, et al. Impairment of mycobacterial immunity in human interleukin-12 receptor deficiency. Science. 1998;280:1432–1438.
11. Ekdahl K, Braconier HJ, Svanborg C. Impaired antibody response to pneumococcal capsular polysaccharide and phosphorylcholine in adult patients with a history of bacteremic pneumococcal infection. Clin Infect Dis. 1997;25:654–660.
12. Quinn CP, Bernemen A, Pires R, et al. Natural polyreactive secretory immunoglobulin A autoantibodies as a possible barrier to infection in humans. Infect Immun. 1997;65:3997–4004.
13. Griffiss JM. Bactericidal activity by IgA of lytic antibody in human convalescent sera. J Immunol. 1975;114:1779.
14. Hoijer MA, deGroot R, Lieshout L. Differences in *N*-acetylmurmyl-t-alanineamidase and lysozyme in serum and cerebrospinal fluid of patients with bacterial memingitis. J Infect Dis. 1998;177:102–106.
14a. Krisanaprakornkit S, Weinberg A, Perez CN, et al. Expression of the peptide antibiotic human β-defensin 1 in cultured gingival epithelial cells and gingival tissue. Infect Immun. 1988;66:4222–4228.
14b. Bals R, Wang X, Wu Z, et al. Human beta-defensin-2 is a salt-sensitive peptide antibiotic expressed in human lung. J Clin Invest. 1998;102(5):874–880.
15. Bauvet JP, Pries R, Isaki S, et al. Non-immune macromolecular complexes of Ig in the human gut lumen. J Immun. 1993;151:2562–2571.
16. Mazamec MB, Kaetzel CS, Lamm LE. Intracellular neutralization of virus by immunoglobulin A antibodies. Proc Natl Acad Sci U S A. 1992;89:6901–6905.
17. Weinberg ED. Iron withholdings: A defense against infection and neoplasia. Physiol Rev. 1984;64:65–102.
17a. Hill PJ, Cockayne A, Landers P, et al. SirR, a novel iron-dependent repressor in *Staphylococcus epidermidis*. Infect Immun. 1998;66:4123–4129.
18. Tsai H, Raj PA, Bobek LA. Candidacidal activity of recombinant human salivary histadine-5 and varients. Infect Immun. 1996;64:5000–5007.
19. Green GM. In defense of the lung. Am Rev Respir Dis. 1970;102:691.
20. Zhao C, Wang I, Lehrer RI. Widespread expression of beta-defensin hBD-1 in human secretory glands and epithelial cells. FEBS Lett. 1996;396:319–322.
21. Epstein J, Eichbaum Q, Sheriff S, et al. The collectins in innate immunity. Curr Opin Immunol. 1996;8:29–35.
22. Ouellette AJ, Selsted ME. Paneth cell defensins: Endogenous peptide components of intestinal host defense. FASEB J. 1996;10:1280–1289.
23. Israde V, Darabi A, McCracken GH. The role of bacterial virulence factors and Tamm-Horsfall protein in the pathogenesis of *E. coli* urinary tract infections in infants. Am J Dis Child. 1987;147:1230–1234.
24. Wolbink GJ, Bossink AW, Groeneveld AB, et al. Complement activation in patients with sepsis is in part medicated by C-reactive protein. J Infect Dis. 1998;177:81–87.
25. Szalai AJ, Arawal A, Greenhough TJ, et al. C-reactive protein: Structural biology, gene expression, and host defense function. Immunol Res. 1997;16:127–126.
26. Vandaux P, Didier P, Haeberli A, et al. Fibronectin is more active than fibrin or fibrinogen in promoting *S. aureus* adherence to inserted intravascular catheters. J Infect Dis. 1993;167:633–641.
27. Van Oss CJ, Gillman CF. Phagocytosis as a surface phenomenon: I. Contact angles and phagocytosis of nonopsonized bacteria. J Reticuloendothel Soc. 1972;12:283.
28. Yamada Y, Doi T, Hamakubo T, et al. Scavenger receptor family proteins: Roles for atherosclerosis, host defense and disorders of the central nervous system. Cell Mol Life Sci. 1998;54(7):628–640.
29. Ofek I, Goldhar J, Keisari Y, et al. Nonopsonic phagocytosis of microorganisms. Annu Rev Microbiol. 1995;49:239–276.
30. Hayashi T, Rao SP, Catanzaro A. Binding of the 68-kilodalton protein of *Mycobacterium avium* to alpha (v) beta3 on human monocyte-derived macrophages enhances complement receptor type 3 expression. Infect Immun. 1997;65:1211–1216.
31. Nepomuceno RR, Tenner AJ. C1qRP, the C1q receptor that enhances phagocytosis, is detected specifically in human cells of myeloid lineage, endothelial cells, and platelets. J Immunol. 1998;160:1929–1935.
32. Yagisawa M, Yuo A, Yonemaru M, et al. Superoxide release and NADPH oxidase components in mature human phagocytes: Correlation between functional capacity and amount of functional proteins. Biochem Biophys Res Commun. 1996;228:510–516.
33. Tomee JF, Hiemstra PS, Heinzel WR, et al. Antileukoprotease: An endogenous protein in the innate mucosal defense against fungi. J Infect Dis. 1997;176:740–747.
34. Vaara M. Agents that increase the permeability of the outer membrane. Microbiol Rev. 1992;56:395–411.
35. Ihi T, Nakazato M, Mukae H, et al. Elevated concentrations of human neutrophil peptides in plasma, blood, and body fluids from patients with infections [see comments]. Clin Infect Dis. 1997;25:1134–1140.
35a. Gabay C, Kushner I. Acute-phase proteins and other systemic responses to inflammation. N Engl J Med. 1999;340:448–454.
36. Dentener MA, Francot GJ, Hiemstra PS, et al. Bactericidal/permeability-increasing protein release in whole blood ex vivo: Strong induction by lipopolysaccharide and tumor necrosis factor-alpha. J Infect Dis. 1997;175:108–117.
37. Smith OP, White B, Vaughan D, et al. Use of protein C concentrate, heparin, and haemodiafiltration in meningococcus induced purpura fulminans. Lancet. 1997;350:1590–1593.
37a. Mak TW, Ferrick DA. The γδ T-cell bridge: Linking innate and acquired immunity. Nat Med. 1998;4:764–765.
38. Haworth R, Platt N, Keshav S, et al. The macrophage scavenger receptor type A is expressed by activated macrophages and protects the host against lethal endotoxic shock. J Exp. Med 1997;186:1431–1439.
39. Trinchieri G. Cytokines acting on or secreted by macrophages during intracelluar infection (IL-10, IL-12, INF-gamma). Curr Opin Immunol. 1997;9:17–23.
40. Kohno K, Kurimoto M. Interleukin 18, a cytokine which resembles IL-1 sructurally and IL-12 functionally but exerts its effect independently of both. Clin Immunol Immunopathol. 1998;86:11–15.
41. Dinarello CA. Interleukin-1, interleukin-1 receptors and interleukin-1 receptor antagonist. Int Rev Immunol. 1998;16:457–499.
42. Dinarello CA. Biologic basis for interleukin-1 in disease. Blood. 1996;87:2095–2147.
43. Letterio JJ, Roberts AB. TGF-beta: A critical modulator of immune cell function. Clin Immunol Immunopathol. 1997;84:244–250.
44. Baggiolini M, Dewald B, Moser B. Human chemokines: An update. Annu Rev Immunol. 1997;15:675–705.
44a. Baggiolini M. Chemokines and leukocyte traffic. Nature. 1998;392(6676):565–568.
45. Timonen T. Natural killer cells: Endothelial interactions, migration, and target cell recognition. J Leukoc Biol. 1997;62:693–701.
46. Boismenu R, Havran WL. Gammadelta T cells in host defense and epithelial cell biology. Clin Immunol Immunopathol. 1998;86:121–133.
47. Sullivan GW, Mandell GL. The role of cytokines in infection. Curr Opin Infect Dis. 1991;4:344–349.
48. Mackowiak PA, Bartlett JG, Borden EC, et al. Concepts of fever: Recent advances and lingering dogma. Clin Infect Dis. 1997;25:119–138.
49. Wright SD, Ramos RA, Tobias PT, et al. CD14, a receptor for complexes of lipopolysaccharide (LPS) and LPS binding protein. Science. 1990;249:1431–1433.
50. Taga T, Kishimoto T. Gp130 and the intrerleukin-6 family of cytokines. Annu Rev Immunol. 1997;15:797–819.
51. Moshage H. Cytokines and the hepatic acute phase response. J Pathol. 1997;181:257–266.
52. Ward CG. Influence of iron on infection. Am J Surg. 1986;151:291–295.
53. Opdenakker G, Fibbe WE, Van Damme J. The molecular basis of leukocytosis. Immunol Today. 1998;19:182–189.
54. Keen CL, Gershwin ME. Zinc deficiency and immune function. Annu Rev Nutr. 1990;10:415–431.
55. Carson WE, Lindemann MJ, Baiocchi R, et al. The functional characterization of interleukin-10 receptor expression on human natural killer cells. Blood. 1995;85:3577–3585.
56. Corman LC. The relationship between nutrition, infection, and immunity. Med Clin North Am. 1985;69:519–531.
57. Semba RD, Graham NM, Caiaffa WT, et al. Increased mortality associated with vitamin A deficiency during human immunodeficiency virus type 1 infection. Arch Intern Med. 1993;153:2149–2154.
58. Souba WW. Nutritional support. N Engl J Med. 1997;336:41–48.
59. Yoshikawa TT. Perspective: Aging and infectious diseases—past, present, and future. J Infect Dis. 1997;176:1053–1057.
60. Peterson PK, Chao CC, Molitor T, et al. Stress and pathogenesis of infectious disease. Rev Infect Dis. 1991;13:710–720.
61. Weinberg ED. Pregnancy-associated depression of cell-mediated immunity. Rev Infect Dis. 1984;6:814–831.

Chapter 5

Human Genetics and Infection

ADRIAN V. S. Hill

The course of infectious diseases caused by many microorganisms is influenced substantially by genetic variation in the host. Such interactions have been well studied in human infectious diseases, in which the pathogens and the host genome are well characterized. In recent years the methodology and techniques available for analyzing human genetic variation have advanced rapidly, leading to the identification of a large number of genes associated with altered susceptibility to infectious pathogens. However, it is likely that those characterized so far represent only a small fraction of the relevant genes. Indeed, susceptibility to most infectious diseases in humans is likely to be highly polygenic, and the identification of susceptibility and resistance genes is providing new insights into disease pathogenesis and resistance mechanisms. Conversely, it appears increasingly likely that a substantial proportion of the functional variation in the human genome has evolved to facilitate defense against infectious pathogens, which points to the observed polygenic variation in susceptibility among individuals and human populations.

MAGNITUDE OF THE HOST GENETIC EFFECT

Various types of evidence demonstrate a significant role for host genetics in variable susceptibility to infectious disease. For some infections such as leprosy, disease is noted to cluster in families,[1] but it is often difficult to assess the relative importance of proximity to an index case and shared genes. Nonetheless, the increased risk of disease in a sibling compared with the general population risk is a useful index of the extent of the genetic component in a multifactorial disease[2] and appears to be on the order of 1.5 to 5 for several infectious diseases.

Apparent interpopulation and racial differences in susceptibility have also been noted.[3,4] Particularly striking have been the apparent increased susceptibility to viral infections and tuberculosis noted in some previously unexposed populations.[5] After some decades of exposure to tuberculosis, rates of disease in the Qu'Appelle tribe in Saskatchewan dropped 50-fold.[6] The use of malaria therapy for syphilis in nonimmune individuals[7] and the accidental vaccination of some children with *Mycobacterium tuberculosis* rather than Calmette-Guérin bacillus in Lubeck, Germany, provided direct evidence of variable susceptibility to these pathogens.

In addition to observational data, studies of adoptees and twins have provided more direct quantification of the importance of host genetics in susceptibility to infectious disease. In a study of more than 900 Scandinavian adoptees, early death of a biologic but not an adoptive parent from an infectious disease was associated with an almost sixfold increase in risk for an infectious cause of death in the adoptee, evidence that is consistent with a substantial role for host genetics.[8] Also, several studies of twins have found higher concordance rates among monozygotic than among dizygotic twin pairs, who share, respectively, 100% and, on average, 50% of their genes. The diseases studied include tuberculosis, poliomyelitis, leprosy, persistent hepatitis B virus infection, *Helicobacter pylori* infection, and malaria (Table 5–1).[9–14] In general, it has been easier to demonstrate a significant role for host genetic factors in infections in which only a proportion of those infected develop disease, in chronic rather than acute infections, and in the severity of infectious disease rather than the susceptibility to infection per se.[15]

Approaches

Several different and usually complementary approaches have been taken in identifying genes involved in susceptibility to infectious diseases. By far the most widely adopted strategy has been the assessment of candidate genes in case-control studies. Here the frequencies of variants of a gene with a suspected role in resistance are compared in individuals who have and who do not have the disease. In general, large sample sizes are necessary, particularly for rare alleles or multiallelic genes, and such candidate genes have come from a variety of sources. A particular geographic distribution of certain hemoglobin variants suggested that they might play a role in malaria resistance. A few genes have been identified by mapping susceptibility genes in different strains of mice, leading to assessment of their human homologues. A much larger number of candidate genes have been suggested by studies of the susceptibility of various gene knockout mice to infectious pathogens. Finally, genes known to play roles in immune or innate resistance to infection, such as human leukocyte antigen (HLA) and mannose-binding lectin variants, have been assessed based on their known function.

A different approach is to search for genetic linkage to, rather than association with, an infectious disease in family studies. Identification of a chromosomal region genetically linked to susceptibility indicates that there is a susceptibility gene in that region.[2] The advantage of this approach is that unknown genes may be mapped and identified without prior information on their function. Although the statistical power of this approach is more limited than that of case-control studies, it does allow a comprehensive screen of the whole genome to be undertaken for major susceptibility genes. A similar approach in mice has led to the mapping of numerous susceptibility genes, and a few of these, such as the macrophage gene *Nramp1*, have then been identified.[16] The human homologue in this case, NRAMP1, has been found to affect susceptibility to tuberculosis,[17] but the human homologue of other murine susceptibility genes, such as the *MX* influenza resistance gene,[18] may be functionally invariant in humans.

SPECIFIC SUSCEPTIBILITY AND RESISTANCE GENES (Tables 5–2 to 5–4)

Blood Groups

ABO blood groups have been investigated in large numbers of infectious diseases, but the results of many early studies were inconsistent and may have suffered from poor matching of cases and controls. An association of blood group O with increased severity of cholera symptoms has been found consistently in several studies.[19,20] Blood group O has been associated repeatedly with peptic ulceration, which in turn is associated with *H. pylori* infection. A possible mechanism for this association was suggested by the finding that fucosylation of the Leb receptor for *H. pylori* in the gastric mucosa, found in individuals with A or B blood groups, impaired binding of the bacteria.[21] However, *H. pylori* infection is not clearly influenced by ABO blood group type.[22] The ability to secrete blood group substances into saliva and at other mucosal surfaces is determined genetically. Most individuals are secretors, but about 20% of most populations are nonsecretors owing to a mutation in the fucosyla-

TABLE 5–1 Twin Studies of Infectious Diseases

Disease	Population	Reference*
Tuberculosis	Germany	128
	United States	129
	United States	130
	United Kingdom	9
Poliomyelitis	United States	10
Chest infection	United Kingdom	131
Leprosy	India	11
Hepatitis B	Taiwan	12
Helicobacter pylori	Sweden	13
Malaria	Gambia	14

*All showed significantly higher concordances in monozygotic than in dizygotic twin pairs.

TABLE 5–2 Some Susceptibility and Resistance Genes Implicated in Parasitic Diseases

Gene	Variant	Disease	Effect
Beta-globin	Sickle, thalassemias	Malaria (Pf)	Resistance
Alpha-globin	Thalassemias	Malaria (Pf)	Resistance
Erythrocyte band 3	27 bp deletion	Malaria (Pf, Pv)	Resistance
Duffy chemokine receptor	Promoter variant	Malaria (Pv)	Resistance
G6PD	Deficiency variants	Malaria (Pf)	Resistance
HLA-B	HLA-B53	Malaria (Pf)	Resistance
HLA-DR	HLA-DRB1*1302	Malaria (Pf)	Resistance
ICAM-1	Kilifi variant	Malaria (Pf)	Susceptibility
Tumor necrosis factor	Promoter-308	Malaria (Pf)	Susceptibility
Tumor necrosis factor	Promoter-308	Leishmaniasis	Susceptibility

Abbreviations: Pf, *Plasmodium falciparum;* Pv, *Plasmodium vivax.*

TABLE 5–4 Some Susceptibility and Resistance Genes Implicated in Viral Diseases

Gene	Variant	Disease	Effect
CCR5	32 bp deletion	HIV infection/progression	Resistance
CCR2	Codon 64	HIV progression	Resistance
SDF-1	3′ UTR variant	HIV progression	Resistance
HLA-DR	HLA-DRB1*1302	HBV persistence	Resistance
HLA-DR	HLA-DRB1*11	HCV persistence	Resistance
PRP	Codon 129	Creutzfeldt-Jakob disease	Susceptibility

Abbreviations: HBV, Hepatitis B virus; HCV, hepatitis C virus; HIV, human immunodeficiency virus.

transferase-2 gene.[23] In relatively small studies, nonsecretion has been suggested to be associated with susceptibility to some bacterial and fungal infections and with resistance to certain common viral infections.[24, 25] The most convincing association is between nonsecretor status and susceptibility to recurrent urinary tract infection,[26] and a possible mechanism for this has been proposed.[27]

The most striking blood group association is that relating the Duffy blood group and susceptibility to *Plasmodium vivax* malaria. This parasite uses the Duffy blood group antigen as the receptor to invade erythrocytes.[28] The Duffy blood group antigen is a promiscuous chemokine receptor. Most sub-Saharan Africans are Duffy blood group negative owing to homozygosity for a mutation in the promoter of this gene. They are thus completely resistant to *P. vivax* infections. Interestingly, such individuals express the Duffy antigen on some other tissues because the promoter mutation, which is in the recognition site for an erythroid-specific enhancer, is tissue specific.[29] It is unclear whether the Duffy negative genotype prevented *P. vivax* from ever entering Africa or whether an earlier more virulent form of this parasitic infection might have selected this variant in Africa.

Hemoglobin Gene Variants

Based on the distribution of thalassemia in the Mediterranean, Haldane proposed that certain hemoglobin gene variants might have reached high frequencies in malarious regions by providing resistance to this disease.[30] The protective efficacy of sickle hemoglobin in heterozygotes against *Plasmodium falciparum* malaria was discovered a few years later.[31] The greatest protection is afforded against death and severe, life-threatening malaria, somewhat less protection is offered against uncomplicated disease, and the least protection is present against becoming infected. This pattern of greater protection against disease than infection appears to be present for many infectious disease–resistant genes. The α and β thalassemias are extremely common disorders of hemoglobin synthesis that lead to unbalanced globin chain production.[32] More than 200 different mutations of the α and β globin genes have been identified as the cause of thalassemia, and the mild forms of thalassemia are among the most prevalent single gene disorders.[33] Both α and β thalassaemias have been shown to afford some protection against *P. falciparum* malaria, in keeping with their geographic distribution.[34–37] Although the geographic distribution of hemoglobins C and E suggest that they may also protect against malaria, this protection has not been demonstrated. However, hemoglobin E behaves as a mild form of β-thalassemia, suggesting that it is probably weakly protective.

The mechanism of protection afforded by these hemoglobinopathies remains unclear. Several differences observed in vitro with variant compared with normal red blood cells have been proposed as the relevant mechanism. Initially, it was suggested that increased sickling of parasitized erythrocytes from heterozygotes in vivo might be protective.[38] It was subsequently found that at low oxygen tensions both parasite invasion and growth in HbAS erythrocytes were reduced.[39, 40] Infants with major hemoglobinopathies also have a slower rate of decline of fetal hemoglobin—hemoglobin F—which has been found to impair parasite growth.[41] However, it is unclear whether these in vitro findings are applicable in vivo. Furthermore, in the case of erythrocytes from individuals with mild forms of thalassemia, it has usually not been possible to identify any decreased invasion or growth of parasites in vitro. However, other mechanisms such as decreased rosetting of parasitized cells,[42] decreased expression of a major parasite neoantigen on the erythrocyte surface,[43] and increased reticuloendothelial clearance in thalassemia may be relevant. Finally, there is some limited evidence that altered immune responses in individuals with globin gene variants may play a part in their resistance to malaria.[44, 45]

Glucose-6-Phosphate Dehydrogenase Deficiency

Erythrocyte glucose-6-phosphate dehydrogenase (G6PD) deficiency is found at high frequencies in many tropical and subtropical populations. This is an X-linked genetic disorder that is associated with red blood cell destruction under certain conditions.[46] A variety of drugs, some infections, and ingestion of fava beans can trigger acute hemolysis, and male G6PD-deficient infants may have neonatal jaundice. More than 100 different mutations of G6PD have been described using molecular analysis, and a small group of uncommon variants is associated with chronic hemolytic anemia in the absence of any environmental agents. The majority of G6PD variants are associated with lesser degrees of enzyme deficiency and are found at higher frequencies. As for the hemoglobinopathies, the geographic distribution of G6PD deficiency in the "malaria belt" suggests its

TABLE 5–3 Some Susceptibility and Resistance Genes Implicated in Bacterial Diseases

Gene	Variant	Disease	Effect
HLA-DR	HLA-DR2	Tuberculosis	Susceptibility
NRAMP1	5′ and 3′ variants	Tuberculosis	Susceptibility
Vitamin D receptor	3′ variant	Tuberculosis	Resistance
HLA-DR	HLA-DR2	Leprosy	Susceptibility
TNF	Promoter-308	Lepromatous leprosy	Susceptibility
ABO	Blood group O	Cholera	Susceptibility
FUT2	Nonsecretors	Urinary tract infection	Susceptibility
MBL	Coding variants	Pneumococcus	Susceptibility
γ-Interferon receptor	Various mutations	Disseminated bacille Calmette-Guérin	Susceptibility

selective advantage.[6] In several locations, populations with a history of malaria exposure had a significantly higher frequency of G6PD deficiency than related populations not exposed to malarial selection. As with the hemoglobinopathies, a variety of molecular mutations are associated with this enzyme deficiency. In Africa G6PD A- is the common variant; in the Mediterranean basin it is G6PD-Med, and in Asia and Melanesia several different G6PD variant are found.[47] In some studies, malaria parasite densities and counts were found to be lower in enzyme-deficient females and sometimes in males.[48] However, more recent studies of severe malaria in both East and West Africa have shown that both heterozygous females and hemizygous males are significantly protected.[49] This is in keeping with in vitro studies showing impaired *P. falciparum* growth in G6PD-deficient red blood cells.[50] In contrast to its protective effects against malaria, G6PD deficiency has been associated with more severe forms of Rocky Mountain and Mediterranean spotted fevers.[51, 52]

Human Leukocyte Antigens

The pivotal position of HLAs in the initiation and regulation of immune responses, together with their well-documented polymorphism, has led to numerous studies of their influence on infectious disease susceptibility. The first evidence of HLA effects came from studies of the mycobacterial diseases leprosy and tuberculosis.[53] HLA-DR2, the class II HLA, was found to be both associated with and genetically linked to susceptibility to tuberculoid leprosy in India.[54, 55] Although initially it appeared that HLA might predominantly influence leprosy type, most studies now indicate that HLA-DR2 in Asian populations predisposes to the development of leprosy per se.[56, 57] In several Asian populations, but not in other continents, the same HLA type has been associated with susceptibility to tuberculosis.[58–60] The mechanism of these susceptibility associations remains unclear, but it has been speculated that HLA-DR2 may influence the type of immune response that develops, leading to stronger humoral but weaker protective cellular responses to mycobacterial antigens.

Studies of malaria susceptibility in African children identified protective associations between particular HLA types and infectious disease. In a large Gambian study, the HLA class I antigen HLA-B53 (now denoted B*5301) was associated with resistance to severe malaria.[61] This HLA type is particularly common in Africans, possibly as a result of natural selection by malaria. Cytotoxic T lymphocytes restricted by this HLA class I molecule recognize a peptide epitope from the liver stage of the malaria parasite's life cycle and may mediate this protective association.[62] In the same study, an HLA class II molecule, HLA-DRB1*1302, a subtype of HLA-DR13 in the older nomenclature, was also associated with resistance to a form of severe malaria, presumably indicating a protective action of $CD4^+$ T cells restricted by this HLA-DR molecule.[61] Thus, both HLA class I and II alleles influence malaria susceptibility in Africa, but it is likely that the particular alleles showing associations differ among populations, and there is some evidence that this is so.[63] Such interpopulation heterogeneity can result from many causes, but a prominent one in malaria is likely to be the marked polymorphism of immunodominant malaria antigens. Indeed, HLA has also been found to influence the strain of malaria parasite associated with clinical malaria, and complex interactions among parasite strains may lead to further variability in HLA associations.[64] It seems likely that the predominant immune protective mechanisms against malaria may vary geographically with transmission patterns.

In West Africa the HLA class II type implicated in malaria resistance, HLA-DRB1*1302, has also been associated with clearance of hepatitis B virus infection.[65] In European populations, HLA-DR11 has been associated with resistance to persistent hepatitis C virus infection.[66] Strong evidence of HLA associations with disease manifestations has also been presented for human papillomavirus infection.[67, 68] Numerous studies of HLA and human immunodeficiency virus (HIV) infection have been undertaken that mainly have assessed the influence of HLA type on the rate of disease progression after infection. Although there are marked differences among studies, some of the alleles in question have been associated with susceptibility or resistance in more than one population. HLA-B35 and the HLA-A1-B8-DR3 haplotype have been associated with more rapid disease progression,[69, 70] and HLA-B27 and HLA-B57 may be associated with a slower rate.[71] Particular combinations of HLA class I and II alleles and variants of the transporter associated with antigen processing (TAP) genes have also been implicated.[72] Although all of these alllelic associations are relatively weak, the finding of genetic linkage of the major histocompatibility complex to rate of CD4 T-cell decline provided strong support for the relevance of polymorphism as a whole in this gene cluster.[73] Part of the difficulty in assessing individual reports is the small sample size of most studies (usually fewer than 200 individuals in each group). Further heterogeneity among studies may be attributed to polymorphism in HIV because variation in viral epitopes for HLA molecules is well described both among and within individuals.

The accumulating evidence that particular HLA types are associated with altered susceptibility to infectious disease supports the view that the remarkable diversity of HLA types has been generated and maintained through natural selection by infectious pathogens. The relatively modest magnitude of the reported associations, compared with some HLA associations with autoimmune disease, is in keeping with this possibility. Small selective effects can over time markedly change allele frequencies. The observation that cellular immune responses are restricted by HLA molecules suggests an attractive mechanism whereby heterozygosity for HLA type might be evolutionarily advantageous.[74] Heterozygotes should be able to recognize more peptide epitopes in a foreign pathogen than homozygotes to permit a more protective immune response. However, a protective effect of heterozygosity has to date been observed only in relation to HLA class II antigens and clearance of hepatitis B virus.[75] Another feature of HLA associations with infectious disease is that associations often vary geographically. In some cases this may result from geographic strain variation in the infectious pathogen, and an HLA association with the strain of parasite causing infection has been reported in malaria.[64] More detailed analysis of the mechanisms of identified associations should explain further this population diversity and provide insights into immune mechanisms of protection and pathogenesis.

Cytokine Genes

Increasing understanding of the pleiotropic regulatory role of various cytokines in immune defense has led to analysis of the role of cytokine genes in several infectious diseases. Studies of the tumor necrosis factor (TNF) gene, located in the class III region of the major histocompatibility complex, have been most rewarding. Several point mutations are found in the promoter of this gene, which may affect the level of TNF production. A variant at position −308 has been associated with susceptibility to cerebral malaria in Africa,[76] mucocutaneous leishmaniasis in South America,[77] and lepromatous leprosy in India.[78] Interestingly, serum levels of TNF have been found to be elevated in all of these conditions, and the genetic associations suggest that the elevated TNF levels play a pathogenic role. Interestingly, these genetic associations were identified before there was any in vitro evidence that the promoter variant is associated with increased levels of TNF gene expression.[79] Associations have also been described with susceptibility to trachoma[80] and persistent hepatitis B virus infection. Other TNF promoter variants may also be associated with altered susceptibility to infectious diseases.[81] These associations with the TNF gene have supported attempts to modulate the severity of diseases such as cerebral malaria using a variety of anti-TNF reagents. Studies of the families of children with meningococcal disease found that individuals from families with low TNF and high interleukin (IL)-10 production in response to endotoxin stimulation in vitro had much higher mortality rates in meningococcal disease,[82] suggesting a protective role for a proinflammatory cytokine profile.

To date, searches for infectious disease associations with other cytokine genes have been less fruitful. However, a susceptibility gene for worm burden in schistosomiasis has been mapped to a region of the long arm of chromosome 5 that encodes a large number of cytokine genes, and it has been suggested that one of these may be causative.[83] Also, rare defects in the genes for the interferon-γ receptor-1 and the IL-12 receptor β_2 chain result in marked susceptibility to some nontuberculous mycobacteria.[84–87]

Chemokine Receptors

The relatively recent discovery that certain chemokine receptors act as coreceptors for the invasion of macrophages and lymphocytes by HIVs has led to numerous studies of these genes and variable susceptibility to HIV infection and disease progression to acquired immunodeficiency syndrome (AIDS). A 32-base pair deletion in the CCR5 chemokine receptor is found at allele frequencies of up to .10 in Europeans and derived populations[88] but is rare or absent in other populations.[89] CCR5 is the coreceptor for macrophage-tropic strains of HIV-1 involved in viral transmission. Heterozygotes for the 32-base pair deletion progress more slowly once infected but are not at reduced risk for HIV infection.[90] In contrast, homozygotes for this variant have very substantial resistance to HIV infection, and only a few infected homozygotes have been identified. Another rarer variant of this gene has been associated with resistance to infection,[91] and promoter variants may also be functionally relevant. An amino acid change in the linked CCR2 gene is also associated with slower disease progression to AIDS,[92] but this association might be secondary to linkage disequilibrium with variants of the CCR5 gene. Lymphotropic HIV viruses, which appear later in the course of infection, use the CXCR4 rather than the CCR5 receptor. The natural ligand for the CXCR4 receptor is stromal-derived factor 1 (SDF-1), and variation in the 3′-untranslated region of this gene has also been associated with altered rates of disease progression to AIDS.[93] The protective effects of these genetic variants underpin current attempts to develop pharmaceutic agents that will block interaction of HIV with these coreceptors.

Mannose-Binding Lectin

Mannose-binding lectin (MBL, previously termed *mannose-binding protein*) is a serum protein that plays a role in innate immunity. It is a collagenous lectin with two roles in host defense.[94] It binds to sugars, particularly *N*-acetylglucosamine and mannose, on the surface of microorganisms and facilitates their opsonization by macrophages. It also activates complement by means of two MBL-associated serine proteases. Perhaps surprisingly, inactivating mutations of this gene are very common in most populations. Single amino acid changes are found at codon 52, 54, or 57, each of which leads to a substantial reduction in MBL concentration in heterozygotes. Homozygotes or compound heterozygotes for these variants have absent or extremely low MBL levels in serum. Variation in the promoter of the gene also has measurable but less marked effects on MBL levels.[95] It was originally suggested that MBL might play a key role in immune defense in late infancy after maternal antibodies had waned and before acquired immunity had been well developed. However, this has not been demonstrated. Case reports and small-scale studies suggested that MBP deficiency might predispose to a variety of infectious diseases,[96] but initial studies of individual diseases— meningococcal disease, malaria, tuberculosis, and persistent hepatitis B virus infection—failed to show clear associations.[97, 98] However, homozygotes for MBL codon changes may be susceptible to invasive disease caused by encapsulated bacteria, particularly pneumococci (Roy et al., unpublished manuscript).

Natural Resistance–Associated Macrophage Protein 1

The relevance of natural resistance–associated macrophage protein 1 (NRAMP1) to tuberculosis susceptibility was discovered by an unusual route. In studies of various mouse strains, susceptibility to species of *Salmonella, Leishmania,* and some mycobacteria was found to be influenced by a single major gene that was mapped and identified by positional cloning.[16] The human homologue of this murine gene Nramp1 is termed NRAMP1. Several sequence changes in NRAMP1 have been associated with susceptibility to severe pulmonary tuberculosis in West Africa.[17] It is more likely that this gene affects susceptibility to clinical tuberculosis than susceptibility to infection. The function of the NRAMP1 gene product is unclear, but it is present only in macrophages on the membrane of the phagolysosome in which *M. tuberculosis* grows.[99] NRAMP1 is homologous to the recently described NRAMP2 gene, which encodes a divalent ion transporter,[100] and the former may influence intraphagosomal iron concentrations and thus mycobacterial multiplication.

Other Genes

Studies of twins have indicated that most of the genetic component of variation in cellular and humoral immune responses to some common infectious pathogens maps to genes outside of the major histocompatibility complex.[101] These genes are likely to be numerous and to affect susceptibility to several infectious diseases, but they have not been identified. One candidate for this type of role is the vitamin D receptor. The active form of vitamin D, vitamin D_3, has immunoregulatory functions as well as an important role in calcium metabolism.[102] The vitamin D receptor is expressed in macrophages and activated lymphocytes, and the presence of vitamin D_3 leads to increased macrophage activation and a shift in the cytokine secretion profile of lymphocytes to a more TH2-like pattern.[103] Variation in the vitamin D receptor has been associated with resistance to tuberculosis and persistent hepatitis B virus infection and appears to influence the type of leprosy developed, possibly by affecting the polarization of CD4 T cell responses.[104, 105] As with the vitamin D receptor association with osteoporosis,[106] gene-environment interactions are likely to be important, so that some population differences in the magnitude of such genetic associations are to be expected.

Other genes have been implicated in resistance to malaria. Melanesian carriers of a 27-base pair deletion in the erythrocyte band 3 gene appear to be very strongly protected from *P. falciparum,*[107] maintaining the deletion at frequencies of up to 0.35 even though homozygous fetuses do not survive gestation.[108] Malaria parasites vary in their capacity to form rosettes with uninfected erythrocytes and to sequester in capillary beds, and both of these phenotypes have been implicated in increased malaria severity.[109, 110] Evidence has been provided that a polymorphic host receptor involved in parasite sequestration—intercellular adhesion molecule-1—may influence susceptibility to cerebral malaria.[111] Furthermore, the polymorphic complement receptor, CD35 or CR1, has been found to play a role in rosetting of parasitized erythrocytes.[112] Thus, such host receptors that interact with the surface of the parasitized erythrocyte may add to the list of malaria resistance genes.

Small studies of the FcγRII immunoglobulin receptor CD32 have been undertaken in recurrent bacterial respiratory infection and in systemic meningococcal infection.[113, 114] The results of these studies suggested that alleles encoding histidine at amino acid position 132, which are associated with greater opsonic activity, may be less frequent in the disease group. However, larger studies are required.

Creutzfeld-Jakob disease is caused by infection with prions, proteinaceous particles that appear to lack all nucleic acid. Rare familial forms of the disease have been related to variation in the host human prion protein (PRP) gene.[115, 116] In both French and U.S. patients iatrogenically infected with the Creutzfeld-Jakob disease agent, a marked effect of a very common variation in PRP genotype on susceptibility to disease was observed.[117, 118] Homozygotes for either of the amino acids, methionine or valine, commonly found at position 129, were markedly more susceptible to disease than heterozygotes. In patients in the United Kingdom with new-variant Creutzfeld-Jakob disease, presumably related to infection with the prion that causes bovine spongiform encephalopathy in cattle, only methionine homozygotes have been found among cases.[117]

Cystic fibrosis is the commonest life-threatening autosomal recessive disorder in populations of European origin. Causative mutations in the cystic fibrosis transmembrane conductance regulator (CFTR) are found at frequencies of up to 0.04 in these populations. It is likely, but probably not essential,[119] that some selective advantage has contributed to the high frequencies of mutations in this gene.[120] Studies in a mouse model of cystic fibrosis led to the suggestion that cholera may have been the selective agent.[121] However, more recent studies have provided stronger support for selection by typhoid rather than by cholera.[122, 123] The CFTR molecule was found to be the receptor used by *Salmonella typhi* to enter human intestinal epithelial cells.[122] As yet there are no data on CFTR variation and susceptibility to typhoid in humans.

EVOLUTIONARY PERSPECTIVE

From an overview of the information currently available, it seems likely that susceptibility to most infectious diseases will prove to be highly polygenic. The contrary view, that there may be major single genes determining susceptibility to many infectious diseases, is supported only by complex segregation analysis[124] and may be incorrect.[125] The existence of multiple genes affecting susceptibility to some and perhaps all infectious diseases probably reflects the major role that infectious pathogens have played in shaping variation in the human genome through natural selection. Genes playing a role in host defense against infectious pathogens appear to evolve at a higher rate than any other class of genes. Natural selection for resistance to infectious pathogens may also explain why the observed effects of most individual genes are relatively modest in magnitude. In the absence of a counterbalancing selective force, alleles that markedly increased or decreased risk of a major infectious disease would be eliminated quickly or selected to very high frequency, eliminating polymorphism. Such polygenic susceptibility has also been found in extensive analyses of the genetic basis of susceptibility to autoimmune diseases in both humans and mice.[126]

Given the pressure for fixation of selectively advantageous variants, one of the major questions in evolutionary biology has related to the mechanisms maintaining substantial genetic diversity in populations. Some aspects of this question are particularly well addressed in human populations where the host genome and the infectious pathogens have been characterized in most detail. Heterozygote advantage is an attractive mechanism by which two alleles may be maintained in a population and is classically exemplified by the sickle hemoglobin polymorphism and resistance to malaria. However, this appears to be a relatively unusual means of maintaining genetic diversity, and other mechanisms such as frequency-dependent selection and fluctuations in selection may be more generally important. Another factor is likely to be variation in the genome of infectious pathogens. Increasing attention is being paid to specific interactions between variants of the host and the parasite. Particular HLA types have been associated with disease caused by specific serotypes of human papillomavirus,[67] and HLA type may also influence the strain of *P. falciparum* that causes malaria.[64] Furthermore, immunologic mechanisms have been identified that may underlie interactions among competing strains of microorganisms.[64] There may be exquisite specificity in some of these host-parasite interactions, leading to co-evolution of genetic variation in the host and pathogen. Thus, individual susceptibility to disease will be the result of a variety of genetic factors in both host and pathogen tempered by the constellation of environmental variables. This dynamic evolutionary perspective suggests that the genes affecting susceptibility to an infectious disease may show significant interpopulation heterogeneity due to geographic variation in the pathogen genome and in the frequencies of interacting genes in the host and to local variation in the environment, a prediction well supported by available data on malaria susceptibility.

APPLICATIONS

It is unlikely that most of the genetic components to any infectious disease can be accounted for by the polymorphisms and associations identified to date. There are several potential advantages to applying the power of modern molecular genetics to understand genetic susceptibility more fully. An obvious application is in risk prediction. This might influence behavior, the use of prophylactic antimicrobials, or immunizations and travel patterns. It is likely that in future it will be possible to offer a genetic profiling test to estimate individual susceptibility to particular pathogens.

Another application is in the understanding of particular pathways used in host resistance to infectious disease. For example, the HLA-B53 association with resistance to malaria[61] supported a protective role for $CD8^+$ T cells in this disease, encouraging efforts to develop vaccines that elicit this immune response.[127] The association of mannose-binding ligand deficiency with susceptibility to pneumococcal invasive disease has supported a role for this molecule in innate immunity to this bacterium.

A third application will be the identification of molecules and pathways that are targets for pharmacologic intervention. The demonstration of the almost complete resistance to HIV infection of homozygotes for a deletion in the CCR5 gene has underpinned attempts to develop pharmacologic blockers of this viral coreceptor. The NRAMP1 gene product may also turn out to be amenable to specific pharmacologic interventions. New techniques of genome-wide analysis offer the prospect of many new target molecules discovered through linkage analysis and positional cloning. The expected very large number of infectious disease resistance genes and the increasing power of methods to identify these suggest that there will be much to learn.

REFERENCES

1. Fine PE. Immunogenetics of susceptibility to leprosy, tuberculosis, and leishmaniasis. An epidemiological perspective. Int J Lepr Other Mycobact Dis. 1981;49(4):437–454.
2. Weeks DE, Lathrop GM. Polygenic disease: Methods for mapping complex disease traits. Trends Genet. 1995;11(12):513–519.
3. Modiano D, Petrarca V, Sirima BS, et al. Different response to *Plasmodium falciparum* malaria in west African sympatric ethnic groups. Proc Natl Acad Sci U S A. 1996;93(23):13206–13211.
4. Stead WW, Senner JW, Reddick WT, Lofgren JP. Racial differences in susceptibility to infection by *Mycobacterium tuberculosis*. N Engl J Med. 1990;322(7):422–427.
5. Black FL. Why did they die? Science. 1992;258(5089):1739–1740.
6. Motulsky AG. Metabolic polymorphisms and the role of infectious diseases in human evolution. Hum Biol. 1960;32:28–62.
7. James SP, Nicol WD, Shute PG. A study of induced malignant tertian malaria. Proc Soc Med. 1932;25:1153–1186.
8. Sorensen TI, Nielsen GG, Andersen PK, Teasdale TW. Genetic and environmental influences on premature death in adult adoptees. N Engl J Med. 1988;318(12):727–732.
9. Comstock GW. Tuberculosis in twins: A re-analysis of the Prophit survey. Am Rev Respir Dis. 1978;117(4):621–624.
10. Herndon CN, Jennings RG. A twin-family study of susceptibility to poliomyelitis. Am J Hum Genet. 1951;3:17–46.
11. Chakravarti MR, Vogel F. A Twin Study on Leprosy. Vol. I: Topics in Human Genetics. Stuttgart: Thieme; 1973.
12. Lin TM, Chen CJ, Wu MM, et al. Hepatitis B virus markers in Chinese twins. Anticancer Res. 1989;9(3):737–741.
13. Malaty HM, Engstrand L, Pedersen NL, Graham DY. *Helicobacter pylori* infection: Genetic and environmental influences. A study of twins. Ann Intern Med. 1994;120(12):982–986.
14. Jepson AP, Banya WA, Sisay-Joof F, et al. Genetic regulation of fever in *Plasmodium falciparum* malaria in Gambian twin children. J Infect Dis. 1995;172(1):316–319.
15. Jepson A. Twin studies for the analysis of heritability of infectious diseases. Res Infect Dis. 1998. In press.

16. Vidal SM, Malo D, Vogan K, et al. Natural resistance to infection with intracellular parasites: Isolation of a candidate for Bcg. Cell. 1993;73(3):469–485.
17. Bellamy R, Ruwende C, Corrah T, et al. Variations in the *NRAMP1* gene and susceptibility to tuberculosis in West Africans. N Engl J Med. 1998;338(10):640–644.
18. Staeheli P, Grob R, Meier E, et al. Influenza virus–susceptible mice carry Mx genes with a large deletion or a nonsense mutation. Mol Cell Biol. 1988;8(10):4518–4523.
19. Levine MM, Nalin DR, Rennels MB, et al. Genetic susceptibility to cholera. Ann Hum Biol. 1979;6(4):369–374.
20. Glass RI, Holmgren J, Haley CE, et al. Predisposition for cholera of individuals with O blood group. Possible evolutionary significance. Am J Epidemiol. 1985;121(6):791–796.
21. Boren T, Falk P, Roth KA, et al. Attachment of *Helicobacter pylori* to human gastric epithelium mediated by blood group antigens. Science. 1993;262(5141): 1892–1895.
22. Umlauft F, Keeffe EB, Offner F, et al. *Helicobacter pylori* infection and blood group antigens: Lack of clinical association. Am J Gastroenterol. 1996;91(10):2135–2138.
23. Kelly RJ, Rouquier S, Giorgi D, et al. Sequence and expression of a candidate for the human secretor blood group alpha(1,2)fucosyltransferase gene (FUT2). Homozygosity for an enzyme-inactivating nonsense mutation commonly correlates with the non-secretor phenotype. J Biol Chem. 1995;270(9):4640–4649.
24. Blackwell CC, Jonsdottir K, Hanson M, et al. Non-secretion of ABO antigens predisposing to infection by *Neisseria meningitidis* and *Streptococcus pneumoniae*. Lancet. 1986;2(8501):284–285.
25. Raza MW, Blackwell CC, Molyneaux P, et al. Association between secretor status and respiratory viral illness. BMJ. 1991;303(6806):815–818.
26. Sheinfeld J, Schaeffer AJ, Cordon-Cardo C, et al. Association of the Lewis blood-group phenotype with recurrent urinary tract infections in women. N Engl J Med. 1989;320(12):773–777.
27. Stapleton A, Nudelman E, Clausen H, et al. Binding of uropathogenic *Escherichia coli* R45 to glycolipids extracted from vaginal epithelial cells is dependent on histo-blood group secretor status. J Clin Invest. 1992;90(3):965–972.
28. Miller LH, Mason SJ, Clyde DF, McGinniss MH. The resistance factor to *Plasmodium vivax* in blacks. The Duffy-blood-group genotype, FyFy. N Engl J Med. 1976;295(6):302–304.
29. Tournamille C, Colin Y, Cartron JP, Le Van Kim C. Disruption of a GATA motif in the Duffy gene promoter abolishes erythroid gene expression in Duffy-negative individuals. Nat Genet. 1995;10(2):224–228.
30. Haldane JBS. Disease and evolution. La Ricercha scientifica. 1949;19(Suppl):68–76.
31. Allison AC. Protection afforded by sickle-cell trait against subtertian malarial infection. BMJ. 1954;1:290–294.
32. Weatherall DJ, Clegg JB, Higgs DR, Wood WG. The hemoglobinopathies. In: Scriver CR, Beaudet AL, Sly WS, Valle D, eds. The Metabolic and Molecular Basis of Inherited Disease. 7th ed. New York: McGraw-Hill; 1995:3417–3484.
33. Weatherall DJ, Clegg JB. Thalassemia—a global public health problem. Nat Med. 1996;2(8):847–849.
34. Flint J, Hill AVS, Bowden DK, et al. High frequencies of alpha-thalassaemia are the result of natural selection by malaria. Nature. 1986;321(6072):744–750.
35. Hill AVS, Bowden DK, DF OS, et al. Beta thalassemia in Melanesia: Association with malaria and characterization of a common variant (IVS-1 nt 5 G——C). Blood. 1988;72(1):9–14.
36. Allen SJ, O'Donnell A, Alexander ND, et al. Alpha+-Thalassemia protects children against disease caused by other infections as well as malaria. Proc Natl Acad Sci U S A. 1997;94(26):14736–14741.
37. Willcox M, Bjorkman A, Brohult J, et al. A case-control study in northern Liberia of *Plasmodium falciparum* malaria in haemoglobin S and beta-thalassaemia traits. Ann Trop Med Parasitol. 1983;77(3):239–246.
38. Luzzatto L, Nwachuku Jarrett ES, Reddy S. Increased sickling of parasitised erythrocytes as mechanism of resistance against malaria in the sickle-cell trait. Lancet. 1970;1(642):319–321.
39. Pasvol G, Weatherall DJ, Wilson RJ. Cellular mechanism for the protective effect of haemoglobin S against *P. falciparum* malaria. Nature. 1978;274(5672):701–703.
40. Friedman MJ. Oxidant damage mediates variant red cell resistance to malaria. Nature. 1979;280(5719):245–247.
41. Pasvol G, Weatherall DJ, Wilson RJ, et al. Fetal haemoglobin and malaria. Lancet. 1976;1(7972):1269–1272.
42. Carlson J, Nash GB, Gabutti V, et al. Natural protection against severe *Plasmodium falciparum* malaria due to impaired rosette formation. Blood. 1994;84(11):3909–3914.
43. Luzzi GA, Merry AH, Newbold CI, et al. Surface antigen expression on *Plasmodium falciparum*–infected erythrocytes is modified in alpha- and beta-thalassemia. J Exp Med. 1991;173(4):785–791.
44. Abu-Zeid YA, Theander TG, Abdulhadi NH, et al. Modulation of the cellular immune response during *Plasmodium falciparum* infections in sickle cell trait individuals. Clin Exp Immunol. 1992;88(1):112–118.
45. Williams TN, Maitland K, Bennett S, et al. High incidence of malaria in alpha-thalassaemic children. Nature. 1996;383(6600):522–525.
46. Motulsky AG, Stamatoyannopoulos G. Clinical implications of glucose-6-phosphate dehydrogenase deficiency. Ann Intern Med. 1966;65(6):1329–1334.
47. Vulliamy T, Beutler E, Luzzatto L. Variants of glucose-6-phosphate dehydrogenase are due to missense mutations spread throughout the coding region of the gene. Hum Mutat. 1993;2(3):159–167.
48. Bienzle U, Ayeni O, Lucas AO, Luzzatto L. Glucose-6-phosphate dehydrogenase and malaria. Greater resistance of females heterozygous for enzyme deficiency and of males with non-deficient variant. Lancet. 1972;1(742):107–110.
49. Ruwende C, Khoo SC, Snow RW, et al. Natural selection of hemi- and heterozygotes for G6PD deficiency in Africa by resistance to severe malaria. Nature. 1995;376(6537):246–249.
50. Roth EF, Jr., Raventos-Suarez C, Rinaldi A, Nagel RL. Glucose-6-phosphate dehydrogenase deficiency inhibits in vitro growth of *Plasmodium falciparum*. Proc Natl Acad Sci U S A. 1983;80(1):298–299.
51. Walker DH, Hawkins HK, Hudson P. Fulminant Rocky Mountain spotted fever. Its pathologic characteristics associated with glucose-6-phosphate dehydrogenase deficiency. Arch Pathol Lab Med. 1983;107(3):121–125.
52. Raoult D, Zuchelli P, Weiller PJ, et al. Incidence, clinical observations and risk factors in the severe form of Mediterranean spotted fever among patients admitted to hospital in Marseilles 1983–1984. J Infect. 1986;12(2):111–116.
53. de Vries RR, Fat RF, Nijenhuis LE, van Rood JJ. HLA-linked genetic control of host response to *Mycobacterium leprae*. Lancet. 1976;2(7999):1328–1330.
54. de Vries RR, Mehra NK, Vaidya MC, et al. HLA-linked control of susceptibility to tuberculoid leprosy and association with HLA-DR types. Tissue Antigens. 1980;16(4):294–304.
55. Singh SP, Mehra NK, Dingley HB, et al. Human leukocyte antigen (HLA)-linked control of susceptibility to pulmonary tuberculosis and association with HLA-DR types. J Infect Dis. 1983;148(4):676–681.
56. Todd JR, West BC, McDonald JC. Human leukocyte antigen and leprosy: Study in northern Louisiana and review. Rev Infect Dis. 1990;12(1):63–74.
57. Rani R, Fernandez Vina MA, Zaheer SA, et al. Study of HLA class II alleles by PCR oligotyping in leprosy patients from north India. Tissue Antigens. 1993;42(3):133–137.
58. Brahmajothi V, Pitchappan RM, Kakkanaiah VN, et al. Association of pulmonary tuberculosis and HLA in south India. Tubercle. 1991;72(2):123–132.
59. Bothamley GH, Beck JS, Schreuder GM, et al. Association of tuberculosis and *M. tuberculosis*–specific antibody levels with HLA. J Infect Dis. 1989;159(3):549–555.
60. Khomenko AG, Litvinov VI, Chukanova VP, Pospelov LE. Tuberculosis in patients with various HLA phenotypes. Tubercle. 1990;71(3):187–192.
61. Hill AVS, Allsopp CE, Kwiatkowski D, et al. Common west African HLA antigens are associated with protection from severe malaria. Nature. 1991;352(6336):595–600.
62. Hill AVS, Elvin J, Willis AC, et al. Molecular analysis of the association of HLA-B53 and resistance to severe malaria. Nature. 1992;360(6403):434–439.
63. Hill AVS, Yates SN, Allsopp CE, et al. Human leukocyte antigens and natural selection by malaria. Philos Trans R Soc Lond B Biol Sci. 1994;346:379–385.
64. Gilbert SC, Plebanski M, Gupta S, et al. Association of malaria parasite population structure, HLA, and immunological antagonism. Science. 1998;279(5354):1173–1177.
65. Thursz MR, Kwiatkowski D, Allsopp CE, et al. Association between an MHC class II allele and clearance of hepatitis B virus in the Gambia. N Engl J Med. 1995;332(16):1065–1069.
66. Zavaglia C, Bortolon C, Ferrioli G, et al. HLA typing in chronic type B, D and C hepatitis. J Hepatol. 1996;24(6):658–665.
67. Apple RJ, Erlich HA, Klitz W, et al. HLA DR-DQ associations with cervical carcinoma show papillomavirus-type specificity. Nat Genet. 1994;6(2):157–162.
68. Wank R, Thomssen C. High risk of squamous cell carcinoma of the cervix for women with HLA-DQw3. Nature. 1991;352(6337):723–725.
69. Scorza Smeraldi R, Fabio G, Lazzarin A, et al. HLA-associated susceptibility to acquired immunodeficiency syndrome in Italian patients with human-immunodeficiency-virus infection. Lancet. 1986;2(8517):1187–1189.
70. Kaslow RA, Duquesnoy R, VanRaden M, et al. A1, Cw7, B8, DR3 HLA antigen combination associated with rapid decline of T-helper lymphocytes in HIV-1 infection. A report from the Multicenter AIDS Cohort Study. Lancet. 1990;335(8695):927–930.
71. McNeil AJ, Yap PL, Gore SM, et al. Association of HLA types A1-B8-DR3 and B27 with rapid and slow progression of HIV disease. QJM. 1996;89(3):177–185.
72. Kaslow RA, Carrington M, Apple R, et al. Influence of combinations of major histocompatibility genes on the course of HIV-1 infection. Nat Med. 1996;2(4):405–411.
73. Kroner BL, Goedert JJ, Blattner WA, et al. Concordance of human leukocyte antigen haplotype-sharing, CD4 decline and AIDS in hemophilic siblings. Multicenter Hemophilia Cohort and Hemophilia Growth and Development Studies. AIDS. 1995;9(3):275–280.
74. Doherty PC, Zinkernagel RM. A biological role for the major histocompatibility antigens. Lancet. 1975;1(7922):1406–1409.
75. Thursz MR, Kwiatkowski D, Torok ME, et al. Association of hepatitis B surface antigen carriage with severe malaria in Gambian children. Nat Med. 1995;1(4):374–375.
76. McGuire W, Hill AVS, Allsopp CE, et al. Variation in the TNF-alpha promoter region associated with susceptibility to cerebral malaria. Nature. 1994;371(6497):508–510.
77. Cabrera M, Shaw M-A, Sharples C, et al. Polymorphism in tumor necrosis factor genes associated with mucocutaneous leishmaniasis. J Exp Med. 1995;182:1259–1264.
78. Roy S, McGuire W, Mascie-Taylor CG, et al. Tumor necrosis factor promoter polymorphism and susceptibility to lepromatous leprosy. J Infect Dis. 1997;176(2):530–532.
79. Wilson AG, Symons JA, McDowell TL, et al. Effects of a polymorphism in the

human tumor necrosis factor alpha promoter on transcriptional activation. Proc Natl Acad Sci U S A. 1997;94(7):3195–3199.
80. Conway DJ, Holland MJ, Bailey RL, et al. Scarring trachoma is associated with polymorphism in the tumor necrosis factor alpha (TNF-alpha) gene promoter and with elevated TNF-alpha levels in tear fluid. Infect Immun. 1997;65(3):1003–1006.
81. Hohler T, Kruger A, Gerken G, et al. A tumor necrosis factor-alpha (TNF-alpha) promoter polymorphism is associated with chronic hepatitis B infection. Clin Exp Immunol. 1998;111(3):579–582.
82. Westendorp RG, Langermans JA, Huizinga TW, et al. Genetic influence on cytokine production and fatal meningococcal disease. Lancet. 1997;349(9046):170–173.
83. Marquet S, Abel L, Hillaire D, et al. Genetic localization of a locus controlling the intensity of infection by *Schistosoma mansoni* on chromosome 5q31–q33. Nat Genet. 1996;14(2):181–184.
84. Newport MJ, Huxley CM, Huston S, et al. A mutation in the interferon-gamma–receptor gene and susceptibility to mycobacterial infection. N Engl J Med. 1996;335(26):1941–1949.
85. Jouanguy E, Altare F, Lamhamedi S, et al. Interferon-gamma–receptor deficiency in an infant with fatal bacille Calmette-Guérin infection. N Engl J Med. 1996;335(26):1956–1961.
86. Altare F, Durandy A, Lammas D, et al. Impairment of mycobacterial immunity in human interleukin-12–receptor deficiency. Science. 1998;280(5368):1432–1435.
87. Jong R, Altare F, Haagen IA, et al. Severe mycobacterial and salmonella infections in interleukin-12 receptor–deficient patients. Science. 1998;280(5368):1435–1438.
88. Liu R, Paxton WA, Choe S, et al. Homozygous defect in HIV-1 coreceptor accounts for resistance of some multiply-exposed individuals to HIV-1 infection. Cell. 1996;86(3):367–377.
89. Martinson JJ, Chapman NH, Rees DC, et al. Global distribution of the CCR5 gene 32-basepair deletion. Nat Genet. 1997;16(1):100–103.
90. Dean M, Carrington M, Winkler C, et al. Genetic restriction of HIV-1 infection and progression to AIDS by a deletion allele of the CKR5 structural gene. Hemophilia Growth and Development Study, Multicenter AIDS Cohort Study, Multicenter Hemophilia Cohort Study, San Francisco City Cohort, ALIVE Study. Science. 1996;273(5283):1856–1862.
91. Quillent C, Oberlin E, Braun J, et al. HIV-1-resistance phenotype conferred by combination of two separate inherited mutations of CCR5 gene. Lancet. 1998;351(9095):14–18.
92. Smith MW, Dean M, Carrington M, et al. Contrasting genetic influence of CCR2 and CCR5 variants on HIV-1 infection and disease progression. Hemophilia Growth and Development Study (HGDS), Multicenter AIDS Cohort Study (MACS), Multicenter Hemophilia Cohort Study (MHCS), San Francisco City Cohort (SFCC), ALIVE Study. Science. 1997;277(5328):959–965.
93. Winkler C, Modi W, Smith MW, et al. Genetic restriction of AIDS pathogenesis by an SDF-1 chemokine gene variant. ALIVE Study, Hemophilia Growth and Development Study (HGDS), Multicenter AIDS Cohort Study (MACS), Multicenter Hemophilia Cohort Study (MHCS), San Francisco City Cohort (SFCC). Science. 1998;279(5349):389–393.
94. Turner MW. Mannose-binding lectin: The pluripotent molecule of the innate immune system. Immunol Today. 1996;17(11):532–540.
95. Madsen HO, Garred P, Thiel S, et al. Interplay between promoter and structural gene variants control basal serum level of mannan-binding protein. J Immunol. 1995;155(6):3013–3020.
96. Summerfield JA, Ryder S, Sumiya M, et al. Mannose binding protein gene mutations associated with unusual and severe infections in adults. Lancet. 1995;345(8954):886–889.
97. Garred P, Michaelsen TE, Bjune G, et al. A low serum concentration of mannan-binding protein is not associated with serogroup B or C meningococcal disease. Scand J Immunol. 1993;37(4):468–470.
98. Bellamy R, Ruwende C, McAdam KP, et al. Mannose binding protein deficiency is not associated with malaria, hepatitis B carriage nor tuberculosis in Africans. QJM. 1998;91(1):13–18.
99. Gruenheid S, Pinner E, Desjardins M, Gros P. Natural resistance to infection with intracellular pathogens: The Nramp1 protein is recruited to the membrane of the phagosome. J Exp Med. 1997;185(4):717–730.
100. Gunshin H, Mackenzie B, Berger UV, et al. Cloning and characterization of a mammalian proton–coupled metal-ion transporter. Nature. 1997;388(6641):482–488.
101. Jepson A, Banya W, Sisay-Joof F, et al. Quantification of the relative contribution of major histocompatibility complex (MHC) and non-MHC genes to human immune responses to foreign antigens. Infect Immun. 1997;65(3):872–876.
102. Tsoukas CD, Provvedini DM, Manolagas SC. 1,25-dihydroxyvitamin D_3: A novel immunoregulatory hormone. Science. 1984;224(4656):1438–1440.
103. D'Ambrosio D, Cippitelli M, Cocciolo MG, et al. Inhibition of IL-12 production by 1,25-dihydroxyvitamin D_3. Involvement of NF-kappaB downregulation in transcriptional repression of the p40 gene. J Clin Invest. 1998;101(1):252–262.
104. Bellamy R, Ruwende C, et al. Association of vitamin D receptor polymorphism with susceptibility to tuberculosis and persistent hepatitis B virus infection. Submitted for publication.
105. Roy S, Frosham A, Saha B, et al. Association of vitamin D receptor variation with leprosy type. J Infect Dis. 1999;179:187–191.
106. Morrison NA, Qi JC, Tokita A, et al. Prediction of bone density from vitamin D receptor alleles. Nature. 1994;367(6460):284–287.
107. Genton B, al-Yaman F, Mgone CS, et al. Ovalocytosis and cerebral malaria. Nature. 1995;378(6557):564–565.
108. Mgone CS, Koki G, Paniu MM, et al. Occurrence of the erythrocyte band 3 (AE1) gene deletion in relation to malaria endemicity in Papua New Guinea. Trans R Soc Trop Med Hyg. 1996;90(3):228–231.
109. Carlson J, Helmby H, Hill AVS, et al. Human cerebral malaria: Association with erythrocyte rosetting and lack of anti-rosetting antibodies. Lancet. 1990;336(8729):1457–1460.
110. Marsh K, Snow RW. Host-parasite interaction and morbidity in malaria endemic areas. Philos Trans R Soc Lond B Biol Sci. 1997;352(1359):1385–1394.
111. Fernandez-Reyes D, Craig AG, Kyes SA, et al. A high frequency African coding polymorphism in the N-terminal domain of ICAM-1 predisposing to cerebral malaria in Kenya. Hum Mol Genet. 1997;6(8):1357–1360.
112. Rowe JA, Moulds JM, Newbold CI, Miller LH. *P. falciparum* rosetting mediated by a parasite-variant erythrocyte membrane protein and complement-receptor 1. Nature. 1997;388(6639):292–295.
113. Bredius RG, Derkx BH, Fijen CA, et al. Fc gamma receptor IIa (CD32) polymorphism in fulminant meningococcal septic shock in children. J Infect Dis. 1994;170(4):848–853.
114. Sanders LA, van de Winkel JG, Rijkers GT, et al. Fc gamma receptor IIa (CD32) heterogeneity in patients with recurrent bacterial respiratory tract infections. J Infect Dis. 1994;170(4):854–861.
115. Goldfarb LG, Brown P, Haltia M, et al. Creutzfeldt-Jakob disease cosegregates with the codon 178Asn PRNP mutation in families of European origin. Ann Neurol. 1992;31(3):274–281.
116. Chen SG, Parchi P, Brown P, et al. Allelic origin of the abnormal prion protein isoform in familial prion diseases. Nat Med. 1997;3(9):1009–1015.
117. Deslys J-P, Jaeglyy A, d'Aignaux JH, et al. Genotype at codon 129 and susceptibility to Creutzfeldt-Jacob disease. Lancet. 1998;351:1251.
118. Brown P, Cervenakova L, Goldfarb LG, et al. Iatrogenic Creutzfeldt-Jakob disease: An example of the interplay between ancient genes and modern medicine. Neurology. 1994;44(2):291–293.
119. Thompson EA, Neel JV. Allelic disequilibrium and allele frequency distribution as a function of social and demographic history. Am J Hum Genet. 1997;60(1):197–204.
120. Bertranpetit J, Calafell F. Genetic and geographical variability in cystic fibrosis: Evolutionary considerations. Ciba Found Symp. 1996;197:97–114.
121. Gabriel SE, Brigman KN, Koller BH, et al. Cystic fibrosis heterozygote resistance to cholera toxin in the cystic fibrosis mouse model. Science. 1994;266(5182):107–109.
122. Pier GB, Grout M, Zaidi T, et al. *Salmonella typhi* uses CFTR to enter intenstinal epithelial cells. Nature. 1998;393:79–82.
123. Cuthbert AW, Halstead J, Ratcliff R, et al. The genetic advantage hypothesis in cystic fibrosis heterozygotes: A murine study. J Physiol (Lond). 1995;482(Pt 2):449–454.
124. Abel L, Demenais F. Detection of major genes for susceptibility to leprosy and its subtypes in a Caribbean island: Desirade Island. Am J Hum Genet. 1988;42(2):256–266.
125. McGuffin P, Huckle P. Simulation of Mendelism revisited: The recessive gene for attending medical school. Am J Hum Genet. 1990;46(5):994–999.
126. Vyse TJ, Todd JA. Genetic analysis of autoimmune disease. Cell. 1996;85(3):311–318.
127. Lalvani A, Aidoo M, Allsopp CE, et al. An HLA-based approach to the design of a CTL-inducing vaccine against *Plasmodium falciparum*. Res Immunol. 1994;145(6):461–468.
128. Diehl K, Von Verscheur O. Der Erbeinfluss bei den Tuberkulose. Jena: Gustav Fischer; 1936.
129. Kallmann FJ, Reisner D. Twin studies on the significance of genetic factors in tuberculosis. Am Rev Tuberc. 1942;47:549–574.
130. Harvald B, Hauge M. Hereditary factors elucidated by twin studies. In: Neel JV, Shaw MW, Schull WJ, eds. Genetics and Epidemiology of Chronic Diseases. Washington, DC: U.S. Department of Health, Public Health Service; 1965:61–76.
131. Marshall AG, Hutchinson EO, Honisett J. Heredity in common diseases: A retrospective survey of twins in a hospital population. BMJ. 1962;1:1–6.

Chapter 6

Antibodies

FREDERICK P. HEINZEL

Antibodies are complex glycoprotein immunoglobulins that individually bind with high affinity and exquisite specificity to peptides, proteins, polysaccharides, glycolipids, and related biologic molecules. Once bound to their specific molecular target, or *antigen*, antibodies may elicit cellular and molecular responses important in the mediation of antimicrobial immunity. Along with the complement system, antibodies are major effectors of humoral immunity, and

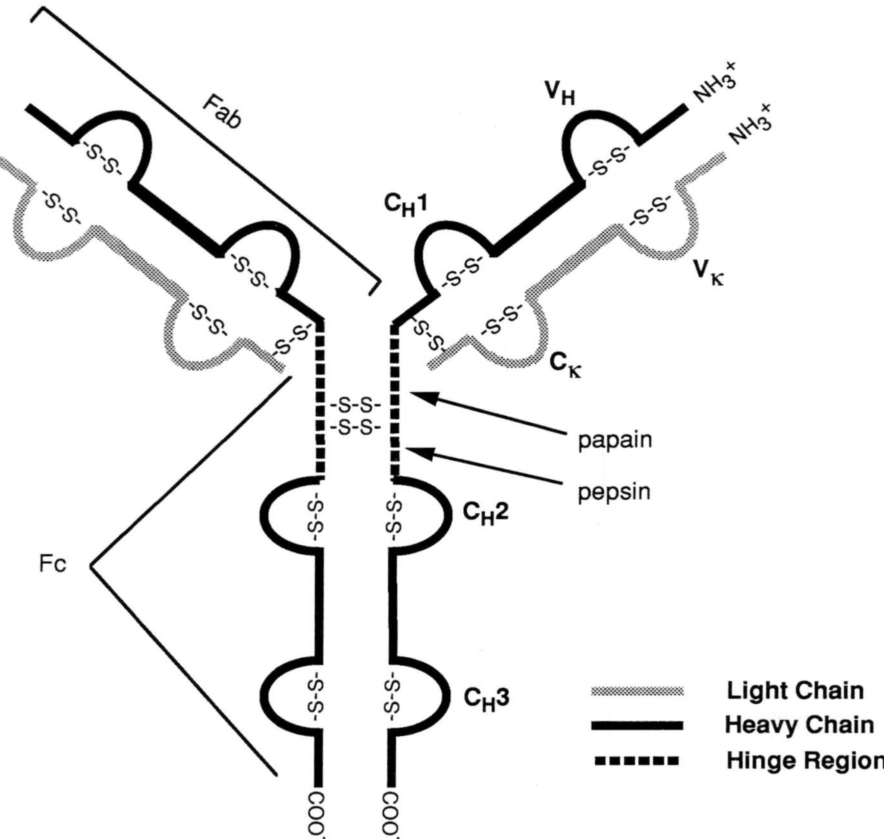

FIGURE 6–1. Schematic illustration demonstrating the structure of an IgG molecule. Two γ heavy chains and two κ light chains (shown as black or gray lines) are linked together by disulfide bonds (-S-S-). Individual domains are designated as V_H and V_κ for variable domains, and C_H 1–3 and C_κ for the three constant domains of the heavy chain and one constant domain of the light chain. The antigen-binding site is defined by the combination of V_H and V_κ sequences and is contained within the *Fab* fragment released on digestion by papain (indicated by the *arrow*). Also shown is the Fc portion of the molecule involved in activation of both the complement cascade and leukocyte Fc receptors. The heavy chain hinge region is shown as *cross-hatched line.* IgE and IgM each contain an additional C_H4 domain.

their presence in the circulation or on mucosal surfaces defines acquired resistance against many infectious agents. Two critical functions are encoded within the structure of the immunoglobulin molecule. The amino-terminal end of the molecule contains highly variable (V region) peptide sequences that uniquely define the antigen recognition site of the antibody and that collectively represent a repertoire of up to 10^8 possible amino acid sequences with distinct antigen-binding specificities. The relatively conserved carboxyl-terminal portion of the molecule falls into one of nine functionally distinct structural classes and subclasses that define the *isotype* of the immunoglobulin: IgD, IgM, IgG_1 through IgG_4, IgA_1, IgA_2, or IgE. In particular, the class-specific structure of the immunoglobulin determines the efficiency with which it activates complement and leukocyte responses and how it is distributed among different anatomic compartments.

Antibodies are produced by B lymphocytes (or B cells) that express surface-bound immunoglobulins of a single specificity. When these antigen receptors encounter the appropriate ligand, in the context of necessary coactivating signals, the B cells proliferate and begin to secrete soluble antibodies directed against the target molecule. B cells additionally function as antigen-presenting cells that can assist in T-lymphocyte–mediated immune responses (further defined in Chapter 9). These antibody responses are essential for the cure and prevention of many bacterial and viral infections. However, antibodies also contribute to the immunopathology of infectious diseases when they manifest as immune complexes or autoantibodies. Inherited or acquired defects in any of these B-lymphocyte functions can be associated with clinically significant immunodeficiencies that predispose to frequent severe infections as a result of antibody underproduction. The significant benefit for such patients that follows transfusion with immunoglobulin preparations further illustrates the clinical importance of the antibody system.

IMMUNOGLOBULINS

Structure and Chemistry

All classes of immunoglobulin have the same basic molecular structure, consisting of two identical peptide heterodimers linked by disulfide bonds. Each heterodimer consists of a *heavy chain* and a *light chain,* also joined by disulfide bridges (Fig. 6–1). Each chain is further subdivided into two to five structurally related peptide *domains* of approximately 110 amino acids, each domain containing one intrachain disulfide bond. The domain closest to the amino terminus on both heavy and light chains consists of conserved framework sequences interspersed with three hypervariable regions, stretches of 10 to 12 amino acid residues with markedly variant sequences. Light- and heavy-chain variable domains (V_L and V_H, respectively) jointly form a quaternary structure that defines the antigen-binding site of the fully assembled antibody.[1] Since the basic immunoglobulin molecule is composed of two heterodimers (each with one heavy and one light chain), antibodies are bivalent for antigen binding.

In addition to the one variable domain, heavy chains possess a *constant region* composed of three to four constant domains (C_H1, C_H2, C_H3, and C_H4). Within the constant region are peptide segments that determine the ability of the intact antibody to mediate important biologic functions after antigen binding.[2] Each heavy-chain constant region is the product of distinct genes that define the class of immunoglobulin produced and that are identified by Greek letters (i.e., δ, μ, γ, α, and ϵ). The number and location of inter–heavy-chain disulfide bridges vary among the different immunoglobulin classes. However, disulfide linkages between heavy chains at the C_H1 site on IgG or at the C_H2 site on IgM define a region with varying degrees of molecular flexibility called the immunoglobulin *hinge.* This structure determines rotation and flexion, or the variable reach of the antigen-binding regions around the heavy-chain stem. Immunoglobulin isotypes differ markedly in hinge region length and flexibility, and this characteristic may correlate with their disparate abilities to activate effector functions.[3]

Enzymatic cleavage of immunoglobulins has provided insights into the functional organization of the immunoglobulin molecule. Papain cleaves immunoglobulins proximal to the inter–heavy-chain disulfide bond or bonds, generating three fragments. Two, referred to as *Fab* fragments, are identical, bind to antigen, but cannot activate complement or leukocyte Fc receptors (see Fig. 6–1). The third, crystallizable (or *Fc)* fragment does not bind antigen but retains the ability to activate effector functions. Fab fragments are heterodimers composed of intact light chains covalently joined via disulfide bond to the variable (V_H) and first constant (C_H1) domains of the adjacent heavy chain. Each Fab fragment contains one antigen-binding site for a single antigenic determinant. The portion of the antigen recognized by the Fab fragment is referred to as the antigenic *epitope;* the complementary structure of the Fab binding site is called the antibody *paratope.* Structural analysis of Fab-antigen complexes have revealed much about the mechanism by which antibody noncovalently binds antigen. Both heavy and light chains generate a polypeptide pocket bounded by V_H and V_L hypervariable loops, into which the antigenic epitope fits by virtue of complementary molecular charge, size, and conformation.[4, 5] Approximately six complementarity-defining residues interact with the antigen. Rather than being a strictly "lock and key" fit, conformational changes may sometimes occur during binding to provide an "induced fit."[4] The enzyme pepsin cleaves immunoglobulins on the carboxyl-terminal side of the inter–heavy-chain disulfide bridge to generate a single large $F(ab')_2$ fragment consisting of two Fab fragments linked together by their heavy chains. As with monovalent Fab fragments, $F(ab')_2$ molecules also bind antigens with affinities similar to those of the parent molecule but lack the constant region domains required for activation of effector functions.

The Fc portion release by enzymatic cleavage is a homodimer composed of disulfide-linked heavy chains, truncated to include only the two to three domains closest to the carboxyl terminus of the protein (see Fig. 6–1). It is this region of the molecule that interacts with C1q to activate the complement system or binds to defined immunoglobulin receptors on the surface of immune effector cells (referred to as Fc receptors). Amino acid sequences within the IgG C_H2 and C_H3 domains define the C1q and Fc receptor-binding sites; immunoglobulin isotypes that are poor activators of these effector systems do not possess these sequences or contain steric impediments that block access to these sites.[6, 7] Membrane-spanning domains may be added to the carboxyl terminus of the heavy chain by alternative splicing of precursor RNA; this provides a mechanism for producing immunoglobulin that is either anchored to the surface of the B cell to act as an antigen receptor or released as a soluble antibody.[8] IgM and IgA molecules also contain additional carboxyl-terminal sequences that are recognition sites for J-chain cross-linking and polymerization (see next section).

Immunoglobulin Classes

Five immunoglobulin classes have been identified; they are defined by their heavy-chain composition and share the basic structure discussed in the previous section.[3, 5–12] Molecular differences include disparities in size, charge, and association into antibody multimers (Table 6–1). IgG and IgA classes are further divided into subclasses that are derived from distinct heavy-chain genes. Each heavy-chain gene product gives rise to a different immunoglobulin isotype. Allelic differences within each heavy-chain locus also result in serologically recognizable *allotypes.* There are two classes of light chains, the κ and λ proteins, which are encoded by a single Cκ locus and four distinct Cλ genes. Only a single class of light chain is expressed during the life span of each B-cell clone. Although all the heavy-chain classes can associate with either κ or λ peptides, the ratio of actual usage of κ to λ is about 7:3.

Immunoglobulin M. IgM is present in the serum as a 950-kD pentameric immunoglobulin. IgM can also be expressed as a transmembrane monomer on the surface of B cells, where it functions as an antigen receptor capable of transducing activating signals when bound to antigen. The IgM heavy chain consists of four constant domains, and the C_H4 domain at the carboxyl terminus contains an 18-amino-acid extension required for polymerization. Each IgM member of the pentamer is covalently linked to the others, either by direct intermolecular disulfide bonds or by indirect attachments through a 15-kD polypeptide called the J chain (Fig. 6–2).[13] The J

TABLE 6–1 Selected Molecular and Functional Properties of Human Immunoglobulins

Property	IgG	IgA	IgM	IgD	IgE
Basic structure	Monomer	Monomer/dimer	Pentamer	Monomer	Monomer
Molecular weight	150,000	160,000/400,000	900,000	180,000	190,000
Molecular formula	γ_2L_2	α_2L_2, $(\alpha_2L_2)_2$, secretory component, J chain	$(\mu_2L_2)_5J$	δ_2L_2	ϵ_2L_2
Mean serum concentration and range (mg/dl)	989 (600–1600)	200 (60–330)	120 (45–150)	Trace	Trace
	IgG_1 670–1050 IgG_2 250–420 IgG_3 54–100 IgG_4 38–67				
Serum $T_{1/2}$ (d)	23	6	5	3	2
Complement activation					
Classic pathway (C1q binding)	+ +	0	+ + + +	0	0
Alternative pathway	+	+	+	+	+
Opsonic activity (FcR binding)	+ + + +	+ +	0	0	0
Reaginic activity	0	0	0	0	+ + + +
Functions as antigen receptor on B-cell surface		+	+	+ + + +	+ + + +

Abbreviations: L, Light chain (either κ or γ); 0, no activity; + to + + + +, increasing activity.
Adapted from Stites DP, Stobo JD, Wells JV, eds. Basic and Clinical Immunology. 7th ed. Los Altos, Calif: Appleton & Lange; 1991, with permission.

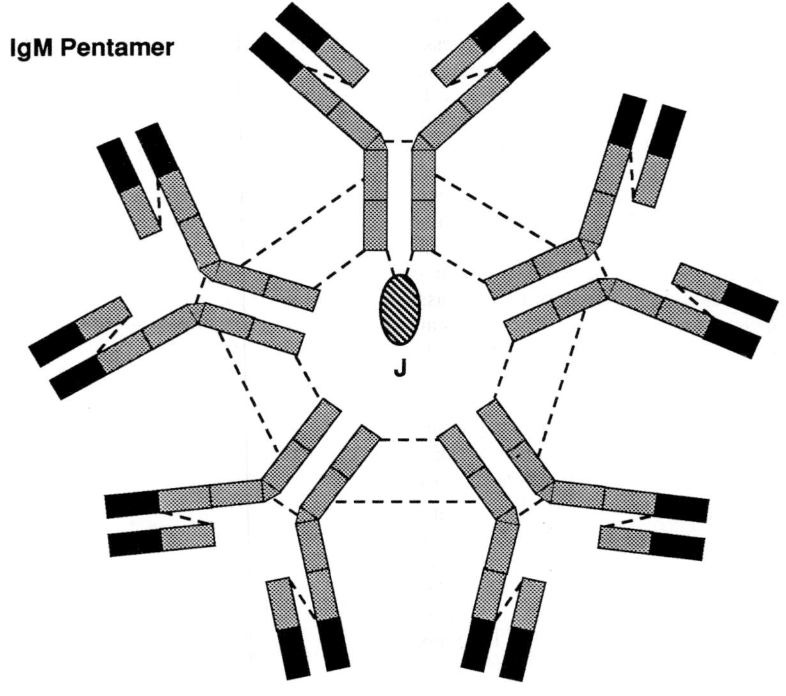

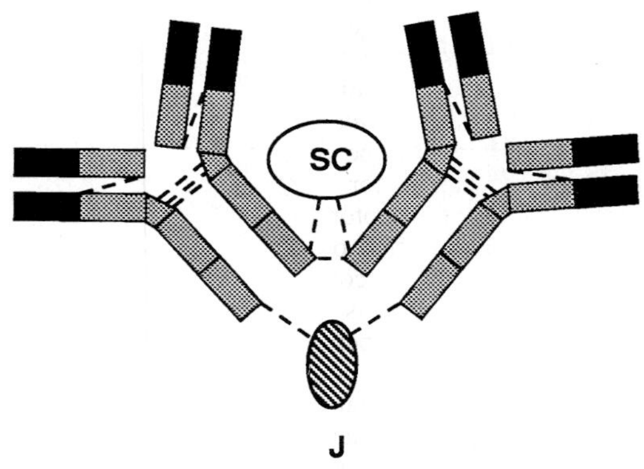

FIGURE 6–2. Schematic illustration of the molecular structure of an IgM pentamer and an IgA dimer. Individual immunoglobulins are joined to each other through intermolecular disulfide bonds, as shown by *dashed lines.* Similar disulfide linkages attach the J chain (J) or the secretory component (SC) to the antibody multimers. Constant domains are shown in gray and variable domains in black.

chain is cosynthesized by the IgM-secreting B cell and is necessary for IgM polymerization, a process catalyzed by a sulfhydryl oxidase on the surface of these cells.[14]

IgM is the first class of immunoglobulin synthesized by infants and is also the first isotype to appear after an immune response to new antigen.[15] Although the affinity of each IgM monomer for antigen is usually less than that of IgG, the pentameric structure of IgM may compensate for this deficiency by increasing the total number of antigen-antibody interactions. Pentavalent binding also assists in complement activation and in the aggregation of antigen or microbes. These virtues of the IgM molecule make it an important first response to microbial infection until IgG molecules, with higher affinity and more specialized function, can be generated.

IgM usually constitutes only 10% of serum immunoglobulins. Much of the circulating IgM consists of low-affinity antibody against common environmental determinants, including phosphocholine, dextrans, and other polysaccharide determinants, which may include blood type–specific isohemagglutinin antibodies.[16] Although some of these antibodies may be generated in response to cross-reactive environmental antigens, others may be natural antibodies produced without prior antigenic stimulation (see "B1 Cells and Natural Antibodies").

Immunoglobulin D. IgD is a 175-kD protein produced as a monomer. The greater size of the IgD molecule compared with IgG reflects the possession of an especially long hinge region. IgD is not abundant in the serum, comprising less than 0.2% of serum immunoglobulins. Instead, most of the IgD synthesized is expressed as surface-bound antigen receptor on B cells. Membrane IgD can be anchored to the cell surface either by a hydrophobic transmembrane peptide domain or by a glycosophosphoinositol linkage synthesized after peptide translation.[17]

Immunoglobulin G. IgG is the most abundant immunoglobulin in the serum of normal adults, providing 75% of the total immunoglobulin mass, and is more broadly distributed through tissues than are other isotypes. IgG crosses the placenta and provides much of the maternal antibody present during the first 6 months of life. IgG is also prevalent in the lower respiratory tract and appears at mucosal sites during exudative responses.[18] The four subclasses of IgG are each encoded by a different Cγ heavy-chain gene consisting of three

C_H domains. The different IgG isotypes vary in abundance ($IgG_1 > IgG_2 > IgG_3 > IgG_4$) and possess distinct functional capabilities. IgG_3 and IgG_1 both fix complement well, although several IgG molecules are required to provide the multivalent binding required for activation of C1q. IgG_1 and IgG_3, but not IgG_2 and IgG_4, can bind and activate leukocyte Fc receptors for IgG. Despite the relative inability of IgG_2 to activate Fc receptor–mediated functions, IgG_2 may activate complement if it is bound on microbial surfaces in high concentration.[19] In adults, IgG_2 is the predominant isotype generated with specificity for dense polysaccharide determinants on encapsulated bacteria.[20] Genetic or cellular deficiencies leading to defective IgG_2 production are sometimes associated with an increased frequency and severity of infections caused by *Streptococcus pneumoniae* or *Haemophilus influenzae*.[21, 22] IgG_4 is the least abundant isotype in the serum and has the least functional capability. Specifically, the short, inflexible hinge region of IgG_4 may result in steric hindrance by the Fab arms of the complement-fixing motif in C_H2.[7] IgG_4 is often produced in concert with IgE, leading to speculation that IgG_4 can block IgE interactions with antigen and the IgE Fc receptor.[23]

Immunoglobulin A. IgA is present as either a 160-kD monomer or a 400-kD dimer, with heavy chains provided by either the IgA_1 or IgA_2 genes.[24–26] Each heavy chain consists of three constant domains; the C_H3 domain contains the peptide sequence necessary for polymerization via J chain (see Fig. 6–2). Although IgA comprises only about 15% of total serum immunoglobulins, its serum half-life is shorter than that of IgG, and IgA production actually exceeds that of IgG (66 versus 30 mg/kg/day).[27] Generally, IgA_1 is produced in the bone marrow and provides most of the IgA present in the serum, 80% of which is monomeric. In contrast, both IgA_1 and IgA_2 are produced in the gut-associated lymphoid tissue as homodimeric molecules that can be secreted onto the mucosal surfaces.[28] Some IgA is polymerized beyond the dimer stage.

Transport of dimeric IgA from the intestinal submucosa to the lumen of the gut is mediated by a unique receptor-linked mechanism. A 100-kD peptide, called the *secretory component,* is expressed as an integral membrane protein on the basolateral surface of epithelial cells and serves as a receptor for dimeric IgA.[27, 29] Engagement of the secretory component receptor by IgA induces endocytosis, transcytosolic transport, and release of the immunoglobulin from the apical cellular surface into the mucosal lumen. During this process, the secretory component receptor is cleaved, and the IgA retains a piece of this covalently linked peptide. IgM can be transported similarly and constitutes a minor population of secretory antibodies.[25, 30] Secretory component–mediated IgA transport was identified as the cause of a shift in the cellular tropism of Epstein-Barr virus from B lymphocytes to the nasopharyngeal epithelium after coating of the virus with IgA.[31] IgA bound to antigen can also be transported through epithelial tissues by secretory component, and this may be a mechanism for disposal of submucosal antigen and viral particles.[32]

Secretory IgA is the predominant immunoglobulin present in the gastrointestinal fluids, nasal secretions, saliva, tears, and other mucous secretions of the body, where it provides an important host defense against infection entering via enteric or respiratory routes.[24] Colostrum is an especially abundant source of IgA, and the passive contribution of this maternal antibody to breast-fed infants may be responsible for their lower incidence of infection compared with formula-fed children.[33] Although secretory IgA does not activate complement well (nor are complement proteins abundant on mucosal surfaces), IgA can neutralize toxin activity and disrupt adherence of pathogens to mucosal cellular receptors. Passive protection mediated by IgA has been described in models of viral, bacterial, and protozoan infection.[34–37] Fc receptors capable of initiating phagocytosis of IgA-coated microorganisms have been recognized on neutrophils and monocytes derived from the pulmonary mucosa.[38] This suggests a broader role for mucosal IgA in mediating opsonophagocytosis. Although IgA is resistant to digestion by gastrointestinal proteases, some bacteria have evolved IgA-specific proteases that may confer a survival advantage to the pathogen.[39]

Another important function of IgA may be to mask commonly encountered dietary or environmental peptides and thereby avoid undesirable inflammatory responses mediated by T-cell responses or by other antibody isotypes. The relative inability of IgA to activate proinflammatory effector mechanisms would allow these antigens to be sequestered without deleterious consequences.[40] This form of "antigenic exclusion" of dietary proteins may account for the increased frequency of autoimmune or allergic diseases in patients with IgA deficiencies.[41, 42]

Immunoglobulin E. IgE is a 190-kD immunoglobulin composed of γ heavy chains containing four constant domains. Although present in low abundance in the serum, IgE can be expressed on the cell surface of mast cells and basophils through noncovalent binding to high-affinity IgE Fc receptors.[43] Immediate-type hypersensitivity, or *reaginic*, responses are triggered when cytophilic IgE encounters antigen and activates cellular degranulation and the synthesis of eicosanoid and peptide mediators of hypersensitivity (see "Immunoglobulin E Fc Receptors"). These potentially deleterious reactions presumably serve some host defense role that remains poorly defined. The expulsion of gastrointestinal nematodes mediated by the peristaltic and exudative effects of mast cell degranulation has been suggested as one protective role for IgE. Consistent with this, increased IgE serum levels and tissue mastocytosis develop during intestinal infection with worms.[44, 45] Epidemiologic evidence has also pointed to a direct correlation between increased IgE levels and decreased reinfection rates with *Schistosoma haematobium*.[46] Parasite burdens are similarly increased in IgE-deficient mice infected with *Schistosoma mansoni*.[47] The protective effects of IgE in this disease may be mediated in part by IgE-directed antibody-dependent cellular cytotoxicity (ADCC).[48] Putative effector cells in this response include monocytes, eosinophils, and platelets bearing the low-affinity IgE Fc receptor (FcεRII). The importance of IgE in recovery from intestinal helminthic infection is less clear, although mast cells and basophils bearing high-affinity IgE receptors are required for cure of these infections.[49]

Distribution and Catabolism of Antibodies

Concentrations of different immunoglobulin isotypes in the serum reflect disparate rates of synthesis and catabolism unique to each class of antibody (see Table 6–1). Human immunoglobulins are synthesized at estimated rates of 66, 30, and 2 mg/kg/day for IgA, IgG, and IgM, respectively; IgE and IgD are produced at even lower rates. Owing to differing rates of catabolism, immunoglobulin half-lives do not correlate strictly with these rates of synthesis; half-lives for IgG, IgA, IgM, IgE, and IgD are 21, 6, 5, 3, and 3 days, respectively.[50] Diseases that affect catabolic or synthetic rates of these proteins can sometimes lead to detectable immunoglobulin deficiencies (see "Immunoglobulin and Antibody Deficiency States"). The catabolic rate of IgG is directly proportional to its concentration within the serum, and possession of an intact Fc portion is required to prevent IgG degradation in vivo. These observations may reflect the function of saturable type I major histocompatibility complex (MHC I)–like Fc receptors (FcRn) that bind and transport to the cell surface IgG pinocytosed into the endosomal system and otherwise fated for catabolic degradation.[51]

IgG and IgA are the immunoglobulins that are most widely distributed throughout the different anatomic compartments. Only 50% of total IgG and IgA are present in the circulation, whereas 75% of IgM and IgD remain serum associated. IgG is the only class of immunoglobulin capable of crossing placental barriers, and therefore IgG molecules provide many of the maternal antibodies present during neonatal life. This represents active, transcytosolic transport of IgG bound by the same "neonatal" Fc receptor (FcRn) that is responsible for preventing IgG degradation in both children and adults.[52] Although IgA is the major immunoglobulin present at mucosal sites, IgG is actually present in greater concentrations in the

TABLE 6–2 Immunoglobulin Fc Receptors: Distribution and Function

Type	Cellular Distribution	Function
IgG Fc receptors (all bind IgG_1, IgG_3 > IgG_2, IgG_4)		
FcγRI (high-affinity), CD64	Monocytes, activated neutrophils	ADCC, phagocytosis, cell degranulation
FcγRII (low-affinity), CD32	Monocytes, neutrophils, eosinophils, B lymphocytes, platelets	Endocytosis of immune complexes, ADCC, phagocytosis, cell degranulation, superoxide anion generation; the B-cell isoform inhibits immunoglobulin production
FcγRIII (low-affinity), CD16	Macrophages, neutrophils, natural killer cells	Phagocytosis, removal of immune complexes, ADCC, cytokine generation
Other (class MHC I–like molecules)		
Neonatal Fc receptor (FcRn)	Placental tissues, intestinal epithelium, endothelium	Binds monomeric IgG in acidified endosomes, transcytosolic transport; responsible for IgG transplacental transport and uptake of IgG from maternal milk; rescues circulating IgG from catabolic degradation
IgE Fc receptors		
FcεRI (high-affinity)	Mast cells, basophils	Degranulation, leukotriene production, cytokine production
FcεRII (low-affinity) CD23	Eosinophils, T and B lymphocytes, macrophages, platelets	Antigen uptake, phagocytosis, ADCC
IgA Fc receptors		
FcαR	Macrophages, granulocytes	Phagocytosis, superoxide anion production

Abbreviations: ADCC, Antibody-dependent cellular cytotoxicity; Ig, immunoglobulin; MHC, major histocompatibility complex.

lower respiratory tract and, in the presence of IgA deficiency, secretory IgM may replace IgA on mucosal surfaces.[18, 30]

Immunoglobulin Fc Receptor

Cellular Fc receptors are transmembrane protein complexes that bind to the Fc portion of immunoglobulin and activate cell-specific functions (Table 6–2).[53] Fc receptors are specific for individual immunoglobulin classes; those that bind to IgA, IgE, and IgG are designated FcαR, FcεR, and FcγR, respectively. Most receptor subunits responsible for recognition and binding of different immunoglobulin Fc regions are members of a single gene family with highly conserved extracellular binding domains and richly diverse cytoplasmic sequences producing a wide variety of cellular functions.[54, 55] Accessory molecules necessary for receptor complex assembly and signal transduction are often shared between different Fc receptors. In contrast, the low-affinity receptor for IgE (FcεRII) is genetically distinct, being related to animal lectin receptors.[56] The FcRn, which binds IgG under acidic conditions, is a member of the MHC I molecular family. Whatever their specificity, Fc receptors mediate similar types of cell responses, including degranulation, phagocytosis, uptake of immune complexes, cytokine generation, and synthesis of eicosanoid and amine inflammatory mediators. However, the variety of Fc receptors expressed suggests a degree of specialization providing for distinct antibody-mediated effector responses in different cells.

Immunoglobulin G Fc Receptors. IgG_1 and IgG_3 induce phagocytosis of coated particles by neutrophils, monocytes, and macrophages by interacting either as monomers with high-affinity FcγRI receptors or as multivalent complexes with low-affinity FcγRII and FcγRIII receptors.[54, 55] IgG_2 and IgG_4 do not participate significantly in FcγR engagement. Phagocytosis mediated by FcγR triggers important microbicidal responses in granulocytes and macrophages, including activation of the oxidative burst[57] and generation of proinflammatory monokines.[58] Although FcγRII is also present on B lymphocytes, the cytoplasmic portion of this receptor is truncated and cannot mediate phagocytosis.[55] The B-cell receptor isoform may instead inhibit cellular responses when engaged by immune complexes, presumably providing a form of feedback inhibition during states of antibody excess.[59] Transmembrane FcγRIII on natural killer cells and macrophages can trigger ADCC; cross-linking of FcγRIII on natural killer cells additionally elicits production of interferon-γ, which may assist in control of infection.[60, 61] Granulocyte FcγRIII is attached to the cell surface by phosphoinositolglycan anchors. Because this mode of attachment may disrupt the usual mechanisms for signal transduction, the function of this receptor is not well understood.[62]

Immunoglobulin E Fc Receptors. The high-affinity receptor for IgE (FcεRI) is expressed on mast cells and basophils.[43] As with other FC receptors, FcεRI is a transmembrane protein multimer consisting of an IgE-binding ε-chain associated with other accessory molecules essential for assembly and signal transduction.[63] Because of the high affinity for its ligand, receptors capture and retain functional monomeric IgE on the cell surface. When this cytophilic IgE is cross-linked by antigen, the activated mast cells discharge granule contents containing preformed vasoactive amine and eicosanoid mediators that mediate the clinical manifestations of urticaria, anaphylaxis, and asthma (i.e., reaginic responses). They also release cytokines, such as interleukin-4 (IL-4), IL-3, IL-5, and granulocyte-macrophage colony-stimulating factor, that may influence T-cell and B-cell responses developing at the time of mast cell activation.[64] Mast cells and basophils have been identified as essential for control of intestinal worm infection.[49]

The low-affinity IgE receptor (FcεRII) is expressed on IL-4–stimulated B cells and many other leukocytic cells. Binding of IgE-antigen complexes to the receptor results in endocytosis and may lead to antigen processing with presentation of peptides to T cells.[65] FcεRII is also expressed on macrophages, platelets, and eosinophils and can trigger phagocytosis, degranulation, and ADCC. This response has been suggested to protect against reinfection by *S. haematobium.*[48]

Immunoglobulin A Fc Receptor. Part of the protective effect of IgA at mucosal surfaces may be mediated by enhanced phagocytosis of IgA-coated microbial pathogens. Mucosal macrophages and granulocytes, particularly in the lung, express a receptor for monomeric and dimeric IgA that was cloned and identified as a relative of IgG Fc receptors.[66] Engagement of this receptor triggers both phagocytosis and generation of superoxide.[67]

ANTIMICROBIAL FUNCTIONS OF ANTIBODIES

Complement Activation

The classic pathway of complement is activated when multiple sites on the hexameric C1q initiator molecule are engaged by the Fc regions of IgG and IgM. Defined peptide sequences within the C_H2 domains of IgG_1 and IgG_3 or the C_H3 domain of IgM are required for this noncovalent association.[2] Aggregation of IgG on a microbial surface is a prerequisite for complement fixation by this pathway, because immobilized IgG binds C1q with an affinity 10,000 times greater than that of soluble IgG.[68] Although pentameric IgM more readily activates complement when present at lower densities than does monomeric IgG, binding of IgM to substrate also is required for complement activation. This apparently reflects structural changes in the Fc region that interact with C1q, thereby preventing inappropriate activation by soluble antibody.[69] IgG_2 is less capable of C1q binding, although it may be effective when presented in high local concentrations, as would be expected when it binds to densely clustered polysaccharide determinants on encapsulated bacteria.[19] In contrast, IgG_4, IgE, and IgA do not have significant C1q-binding activities.

Activation of complement on bacterial cell surfaces mediates both lytic and opsonizing activities important in the resolution of infection.[70] Opsonizing antibodies of this sort have been identified during infection with pneumococcus, *Streptococcus pyogenes, H. influenzae,* and *Staphylococcus aureus.*[71–74] Further discussion of the complement cascade and the role of complement products in inflammation is given in Chapter 7. Although the alternative pathway of complement activation is typically defined by its antibody-independent nature, aggregates of immunoglobulin may facilitate the generation of C3 convertase by providing a favorable glycosylated substrate.[75, 76]

Phagocytosis

All three classes of IgG Fc receptors can efficiently mediate phagocytosis of antibody-coated particles by neutrophils, macrophages, and monocytes.[57, 77, 78] This process is generally limited to organisms coated with IgG_1 or IgG_3, or both, although IgA opsonizes microbes for ingestion via FcγR-mediated uptake by mucosal phagocytes.[67] Although Fc receptor interactions alone are sufficient to mediate phagocytosis, in most cases efficient ingestion of encapsulated bacteria requires coating with both antibody and complement.[74, 79] The respective roles of Fc receptors and complement receptors in opsonophagocytosis are addressed in Chapters 7 and 8. Cross-linking of FcγR and FcαR may also trigger an oxidative burst and the release of proinflammatory mediators, such as IL-1, tumor necrosis factor, and eicosanoids, as part of a coordinated microbicidal response. Mice that are deficient in Fc receptors for IgG have enhanced susceptibility to infection with *Cryptococcus neoformans.*[80]

Antibody-Dependent Cellular Cytotoxicity

Engagement of Fc receptors on leukocytes can induce contact-dependent killing of antibody-coated microbes or parasitized host cells.[81] Antibody provides both the target specificity and the activating stimulus for these responses. Natural killer cells expressing the low-affinity FcγRIII receptor therefore can lyse cells infected with virus when they express viral antigens on their surface.[82] When the density of bound antibody is sufficient to cross-link the Fc receptor, degranulation occurs with release of cytolytic perforin molecules and synthesis of cytotoxic cytokines, such as interferon-γ and tumor necrosis factor.[83] ADCC is also mediated by the FcγRII receptor on macrophages and neutrophils.[84] IgE-coated parasites can be targeted and killed in vitro by FcєRII-bearing eosinophils that release toxic molecules, such as major basic protein, onto the parasite surface in response to receptor cross-linking.[48]

Neutralization of Microbial Toxins

The ability of antibodies to neutralize disease-causing microbial toxins was among the earliest recognized forms of protective immunity and led directly to the clinical use of horse antiserum to treat diphtheria.[85] Neutralization presumably reflects steric disruption of toxin uptake and action through specific cellular receptors (see Chapter 1). The role of passive and active immunization in the prevention of toxin-mediated diseases such as tetanus,[86] botulism,[87] and pertussis[88] are further discussed in the appropriate chapters of this text.

The use of antibodies against bacterial endotoxin as therapy for gram-negative septic shock has been aggressively pursued since the observations that serotype-specific anti-endotoxin antibodies detoxify this normally proinflammatory substance and markedly reduce lethality in animal models.[89] However, protection is not extended to other serogroups, the great number of which have confounded the formulation of broadly reactive immunoglobulins. Despite the successful use of polyclonal antisera against the invariant core region of *Escherichia coli* J5 lipopolysaccharide in the prevention of bacteremic death,[90] two different monoclonal antibody preparations failed to show consistent benefit.[91, 92] However, IgM natural antibodies directed to lipopolysaccharide are necessary for innate resistance to endotoxic shock in animal models, suggesting that any beneficial effect of anti-J5 treatment may have been obscured by the activity of these endogenous anti-endotoxin antibodies.[93]

Neutralization of Viruses

Antibodies of the IgG, IgM, or IgA class inhibit the ability of extracellular viruses to infect host cells.[94, 95] This is best illustrated by the neutralizing antibody response to influenza, in which cellular adhesion, membrane fusion, and uncoating after entry are all inhibited by immunoglobulin A present on the mucosal surface.[96] Antibodies directed to determinants remote from the viral binding site may prevent infection by disrupting important molecular conformations or altering essential charge characteristics of the pathogen. A single antibody may thus neutralize infectivity despite the presence of as many as 60 separate binding sites on picornaviruses.[97] Antibodies can also coat and inactivate viral ribonucleoproteins required for transcription of viral genes.[98] The protective role of neutralizing antibodies in infections caused by viruses, especially hepatitis, polio, and rabies viruses, are reviewed in their respective chapters and Chapter 312 of this book.

Antibody responses are less effective against viruses sequestered within the cellular cytoplasm, and cell-mediated immunity plays the dominant role in recovery from these infections. However, antibodies recognizing cell-associated viral antigen may direct ADCC responses involved in viral clearance.[82] Furthermore, in epithelial cells possessing the polymeric IgA receptor, antibody may inhibit intracellular virus replication when virus and immunoglobulin are colocalized within the cytoplasm during IgA transport.[99, 100] This may constitute an important barrier defense against viral pathogens that initiate infection within the mucosal tissues.

Antiadhesion Antibodies

Adherence to epithelium is often a necessary prelude to tissue invasion or local proliferation of pathogenic microbes. Antibodies generated against microbial ligands for host cells [101] disrupt adherence and thereby abort infection.[26, 102] The protective effects of IgA in this regard have been demonstrated in experimental models of *Campylobacter* and *Shigella flexneri* infection.[37]

Agglutination

Polyvalent immunoglobulins have the ability to cross-link microbes or microbial antigens extensively. These IgM, IgG, or IgA antigenic complexes can then effect removal of the offending substance when complement is activated by classic or alternative pathways. Agglutination of microbes by IgA may assist in mucociliary clearance of the resulting particulate material within the respiratory tract.

IMMUNOPATHOLOGY CAUSED BY ANTIBODIES

Hypergammaglobulinemia

Chronic infection and inflammation can be associated with exaggerated antibody responses and abnormally high serum levels of immunoglobulin. This is commonly observed during infective endocarditis, secondary syphilis, infectious mononucleosis, the acquired immunodeficiency syndrome (AIDS), parasitic infection, and cystic fibrosis.[103–105] Polyclonal responses are thought to represent "bystander" activation of B cells producing antibody specificities unrelated to the infecting agent. Because Epstein-Barr viruses transiently infect and activate B cells, a variety of irrelevant antibody responses may occur during infectious mononucleosis as a result of polyclonal stimulation. These are frequently observed as antibody responses to nuclear antigens, leukocytes, and ampicillin.[106] Otherwise, polyclonal gammopathies resulting from infection usually are not linked to any definable pathology unless they are accompanied by formation of immune complexes or cryoglobulins. One exception to this rule is the presence of hyperimmunoglobulinemia D in the inherited periodic fever syndrome, a chronic inflammatory disease that may be mediated by IgD overproduction.[107]

Immune Complexes

Under favorable stoichiometric conditions, antigen and antibody form immune complexes that may damage tissues as a secondary consequence of an infectious disease. Damage is mediated through activation of leukocyte Fc receptors, causing release of proteases and production of reactive oxygen intermediates. Local complement activation by immune complexes further contributes to pathology.[108] The classic manifestation of immune complex-related pathology is seen in the immune glomerulopathies resulting from infection with hepatitis B, hepatitis C, and *S. pyogenes.*[109] Any chronic antigenemia from a microbial source, such as occurs during endocarditis or ventriculoatrial shunt infection ("shunt nephritis"), may lead to these complications.[110] Normal mechanisms for clearance of these immune complexes include removal by low-affinity Fc receptors on phagocytic cells and, via complement activation, by complement receptors on erythrocytes. Complement proteins may also help to solubilize aggregated IgG by disrupting noncovalent attractions between IgG Fc regions.[111]

Rheumatoid Factor

Rheumatoid factors (RF) are IgM or IgG antibodies that are directed specifically against autologous IgG.[16, 112] Although originally characterized as a pathologic concomitant of rheumatoid arthritis, IgM RF is a natural antibody produced by expression of germline sequences that encode RF specificity.[113, 114] Perhaps because of their low affinity for antigen, RF-positive B cells are not normally deleted during early development. In fact, B cells bearing surface antibody with this specificity are abundant in healthy persons, especially within the CD5-positive B cell population. This conservation suggests that RF+ B cells and their immunoglobulin products serve an important immunologic or host defense role. In this regard, it has been speculated that RF enhances opsonization of pathogens when IgG reactive with microbes is insufficiently concentrated on the target or of the wrong IgG subclass to permit efficient complement activation.[16] The normally weak affinity of natural RF for soluble IgG is overcome when the IgG is immobilized on solid surfaces, permitting multivalent binding. RF may similarly accelerate the clearance of immune complexes containing IgG-coated antigen. RF+ B cells may mediate important accessory cell functions by efficiently capturing IgG complexed to antigen, thus amplifying T-cell activation in response to low levels of antigen.[16, 115] RF responses become pathogenic when the autoantibody response increases in titer, the RF isotype switches to IgG, and higher-affinity RF variants appear as a result of somatic mutation or altered germline sequence usage.[114]

Cryoglobulinemia

Type II or mixed cryoglobulinemia is a vasculitis associated with purpura, arthralgias, and glomerulonephritis caused by cryoprecipitable immune complexes generated in the presence of IgM RF and increased serum levels of polyclonal IgG. Infection with hepatitis C or hepatitis B virus is frequently associated with this syndrome.[116, 117]

Autoantibodies

The formation of antibodies against host tissue determinants occurs frequently during infectious diseases. Most commonly, this represents the stimulation of RF or other low-affinity IgM molecules with broad reactivity toward polysaccharide and phospholipid determinants. These may be sufficiently predictable to permit indirect serodiagnosis of infection, as illustrated by the cold hemagglutinin response associated with *Mycoplasma* infections. Similarly, antibodies that are cross-reactive with cardiolipin are generated during syphilis. Cross-reactivity between microbes and humans may also reflect similarities in peptide sequence—so-called molecular mimicry.[118] For instance, autoimmunity against neural tissue during Chagas' disease has been linked to a cross-reactive 12-amino-acid antigenic peptide common to both *Trypanosoma cruzi* and mammalian neurons.[119] Highly conserved sequences within the heat shock proteins of humans and various microbial pathogens similarly induce autoimmune responses that may manifest as rheumatologic disease.[120] Cross-reactive epitopes shared by the M protein of *S. pyogenes* and proteins within the myocardial sarcolemma may contribute to the pathogenesis of rheumatic heart disease.[121]

CELLULAR MECHANISMS IN ANTIBODY PRODUCTION

Acquired antibody responses are defined by the appearance of protective or diagnostic antibodies after antigenic exposure. These are distinguished from *natural antibodies,* which are usually IgM molecules with polyreactive specificities spontaneously produced in the absence of antigenic stimulus. Natural antibodies are discussed in more detail in the context of the $CD5^+$ B-cell subset responsible for their production. Antibodies produced during the *primary antibody response* that occurs after an encounter with a new antigen are typically of the IgM isotype, appear 5 to 10 days after antigenic exposure, and express relatively low affinities for antigen. *Secondary antibody responses* result in the more rapid appearance (within 1 to 3 days) of antibodies that are more abundant and that are more likely to consist of IgG, IgA, or IgE. During the secondary response, the affinity of the antibody is also increased for its respective antigen, a process referred to as *affinity maturation.* The more rapid onset and greater amplitude of the secondary antibody response reflects the increased number of antigen-specific B cells generated previously during the primary response. Such *memory cells* also are more likely to produce mature antibody isotypes, and this process of *isotypic switching* is closely controlled by T cells and their cytokine products. Secondary antibody responses to protein antigens are quantitatively and qualitatively distinct from those elicited by polymeric polysaccharide antigens. This reflects different T-cell–dependent and –independent mechanisms of B-cell activation, as discussed in more detail in a later section.

The ability to produce antibodies against a broad range of exogenous antigens introduced by infection or immunization, while minimizing wasteful or autoreactive immune reactions, testifies to the complex and highly regulated biology of the B cell. The discussion that follows highlights important functions of B cells with regard to antibody production and immunologic specialization.

Generation of Antigen-Binding Diversity

The immunoglobulin antigen-binding repertoire is created during early B-lymphocyte development through the linear assembly of DNA segments derived from large families of related but sequence-disparate variable-region genes.[122–124] An estimated 10^8 possible antigen-binding specificities (idiotypes) result from this process. Similar mechanisms generate diversity in T-cell receptor genes. Although

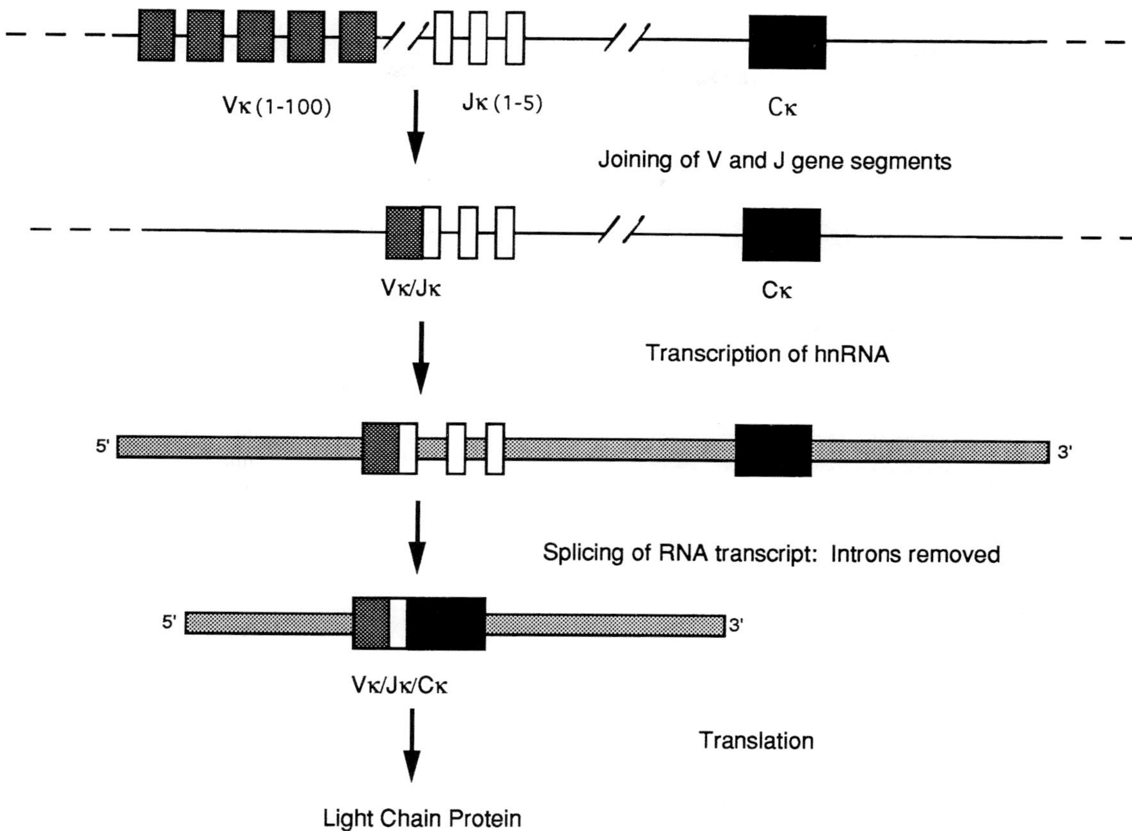

FIGURE 6–3. Illustration of events involved in the generation of antigen-binding diversity within the κ light chain gene complex. Recombination results in one of nearly a hundred Vκ gene segments being brought into proximity with one of the indicated Jκ segments through deletion of the intervening chromosomal DNA. Continuity with the rest of the chromosome is indicated by the *dashed lines* at either end of the gene complex. Transcription of the recombined gene complex leads to heterogeneous nuclear RNA (hnRNA) containing introns and irrelevant exons that are subsequently deleted during RNA processing to produce the mature messenger RNA.

heavy-chain genes rearrange first during B-cell ontogeny, the light-chain complexes are of simpler design and are discussed first here.

Gene complexes encoding the constant- and variable-region genes of the κ light chain are located on chromosome 2, and the genes for λ constant and variable regions are on chromosome 22. The variable-region sequence of each light-chain gene represents the fusion of one of almost 200 separate variable-segment genes with one of 5 to 10 short joining (J)–segment genes (Fig. 6–3). Although these gene segments are separated by as many as 1 million base pairs, the loci are juxtaposed when the intervening DNA is deleted by recombinase activity.[125] The mechanisms by which RAG1 and RAG2 gene products accomplish this process have been elucidated.[126] The κ light-chain complex contains one Cκ gene adjacent to the site of Vκ-Jκ joining, so that a single recombination forms a linear array of genes that can be transcribed to generate mature light-chain mRNA. The λ complex is differently constructed, having six or more Cλ genes, each adjacent to a distinct Jλ gene segment. Excision of intervening DNA associates one of several hundred Vλ sequences with any one of these Jλ-Cλ pairs to produce a complete transcriptional unit. In either case, diversity of the light-chain variable region is generated through the great number of possible V and J joinings. The relative inaccuracy of the joining process contributes an additional source of diversity by introducing one or two randomly selected amino acids at the VJ splice site. Only one successful variable-region rearrangement is allowed per cell; the first rearranged gene product suppresses recombination at the other three light-chain loci so that each mature B cell expresses only a single light-chain isotype (κ or λ).

The genes of the heavy-chain complex on chromosome 14 form a variable-region sequence in a similar fashion (Fig. 6–4). About 500 V_H genes and 4 J_H segments are available for fusion, providing 2000 possible VJ combinations. In addition, there are 10 or more short, diversity-generating (D_H) segment genes available for insertion between the V and J segments during assembly of the variable region, increasing the number of possible variable-region gene combinations to 20,000. One or two amino acid codons, called N sequences, are added to the VDJ splice sites by the enzyme terminal deoxynucleotidyltransferase.[127] In contrast to the light-chain genetic structure, each successfully rearranged VDJ gene can be expressed in conjunction with any of nine heavy-chain constant-region genes that, when translated, define the isotype of the final immunoglobulin. Furthermore, the heavy-chain variable region can later be spliced in front of another heavy-chain constant-region locus, causing an isotypic switch. These C_H genes are arranged in linear fashion near to the VDJ recombination site in the following order: Cμ, Cδ, Cγ3, Cγl, Cα1, Cγ2, Cγ4, Cε, and Cα2. At first, transcription initiated within the VDJ assembly extends only through the two proximal C_H genes, creating a polycistronic message that can be selectively spliced to produce either μ or δ heavy chains without further rearrangement of DNA. Heavy-chain switching can occur under the control of extrinsic immunologic signals, whereby antigen-binding specificity is maintained but antibody class is altered. Isotypic

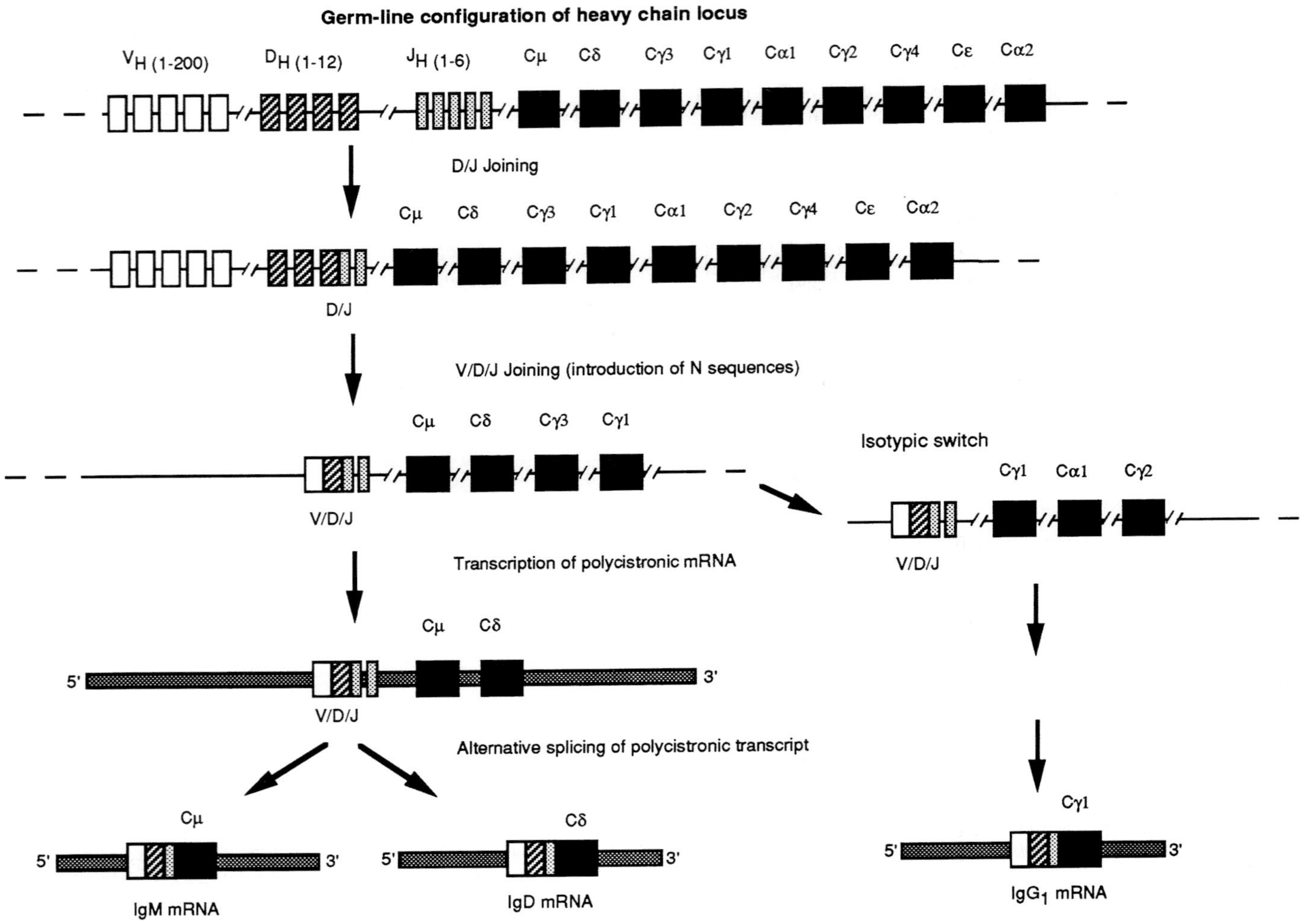

FIGURE 6–4. Illustration of events involved in the generation of antigen-binding diversity within the heavy chain complex and in the formation of different mature heavy chain isotypes. In the first recombination, one D_H gene segment is linked to a J_H segment (designated as D/J) through deletion of intervening chromosomal DNA. A second recombination adds one of nearly 200 V_H segments to the nascent variable region gene (V/D/J). At this time, junctional diversity is created through inexact joining of these segments and through addition of N-sequence amino acid codons. Transcription through the V/D/J gene and through the adjacent μ and δ heavy chain constant genes generates a polycistronic nuclear RNA (hnRNA) that can be spliced to provide mature mRNA encoding either IgM or IgD. Other types of alternative splicing may lead to the deletion or addition of a region within the tail of the heavy chain that determines whether the final immunoglobulin product is expressed on the surface of the B cell or is released as soluble antibody (not shown). Alternatively, deletion of intervening DNA can lead to the association and expression of the unaltered variable region sequences with a distal heavy chain gene.

switching is accomplished through the excision of intervening DNA and juxtaposition of the intact variable-region sequence and a new distal C_H gene. Excision occurs at defined "switch" regions and is preceded by the appearance of a long RNA molecule spanning the future deletion site. This transcript is not translated and has been proposed to function as a template to guide the excisional and splicing process.[128]

Because C_H genes proximal to the new splice site are deleted from the genome, isotypic switches to IgG, IgE, or IgA phenotype are irreversible. Therefore, the order of C_H genes in the genome crudely approximates the order of appearance of isotypes during advanced B-cell differentiation, IgM and IgD being the first immunoglobulins produced and IgG, IgE, or IgA appearing during later differentiation. The antigen-binding specificity is preserved during isotypic switches, because the heavy- and light-chain variable regions are not affected by this process. The switch to IgE and IgG_4 production or to IgA expression in response to appropriate regulatory signals has been well studied, and it is apparent now that each switch occurs as a single excisional deletion of intervening C_H genes and not in multiple, transient recombinations.[129] The control of immunoglobulin isotype switching by T cells and T-cell–derived cytokines is further discussed in a later section. Whatever the isotype, heavy-chain genes can generate either membrane-bound or soluble immunoglobulins, depending on the inclusion or deletion of two exons encoding a 40-amino-acid hydrophobic transmembrane domain.

In summary, antigen-binding diversity is generated through the *recombination* of V, D, and J sequences, through *junctional diversity* introduced by the inexact joining of these segments and the addition of N sequences, and through the *quaternary association* of both V_H and V_L into a complete antigen-binding site during immunoglobulin assembly. A fourth nonrecombinatorial mechanism further increases idiotype diversity after primary exposure to antigen. Specifically, comparisons of immunoglobulin gene sequences before and after secondary or tertiary antigenic challenges demonstrate increasing numbers of single-base mutations in the hypervariable regions of light and heavy chains.[125, 130] These mutations are restricted to specific areas within the hypervariable regions and are usually point mutations. It is thought that this process of *somatic mutation* underlies the phenomenon of affinity maturation, in which repeated antigenic challenges result in production of antibodies with incrementally increased affinity for the eliciting epitope. The selection of antibody-producing cells expressing increased antigenic affinity is discussed later as part of the cell biology of B lymphocytes.

Surface Molecules of the B Cell

Mature B lymphocytes are defined by their expression of surface immunoglobulin. Initially B cells are surface IgM and IgD positive, but with isotypic switching IgG, IgA, and IgE can be expressed as well. Further differentiation into antibody-secreting plasma cells results in the loss of surface immunoglobulin expression. Other molecules expressed on the B-cell surface have defined functions in B-cell activation and differentiation (Table 6–3) but are too numerous for all but the most important to be reviewed here (see Banchereau and Rousset[131] for complete review).

The B-Cell Receptor

Complex surface immunoglobulin functions as the antigen receptor of the B cell, defining the antigenic specificity of the cells but also providing the trigger for internalization of antigen into the MHC II processing pathway and for cellular activation.[131–133] Signals for antigen internalization are provided by specific functional motifs in the cytoplasmic tail of the immunoglobulin molecule.[134] In contrast, B-cell activation requires interactions between surface immunoglobulin and accessory molecules, providing an analogy with the multimeric T-cell receptor complex (Fig. 6–5).[135] The nonimmunoglobulin transmembrane proteins (Igα and Igβ) form a disulfide-linked heterodimer noncovalently associated with surface immunoglobulin. Cross-linking of surface immunoglobulin by polymeric antigens causes conformational changes that activate SRC-family tyrosine kinases (Fyn, Lyn, and Blk) through signals delivered by the cytoplasmic domains of Igα and Igβ.[136] Other transmembrane molecules associated noncovalently with the B-cell receptor complex decrease the threshold for B-cell activation. The most important of these is CD21, the complement receptor 2 (CR2) molecule that binds C3d complement proteins attached to microorganisms or antigens.[137] Cross-linking of the CD21 antigen, the closely associated CD19 transmembrane signal transduction protein, and the B-cell antigen receptor increases the immunogenicity of an antigen between 1000- and 10,000-fold. This increases B-cell responsiveness to monomeric protein antigens that would not activate the B cell through cross-linking of the antigen receptor alone. Because complement can be directly activated through the alternative pathway by microbial antigens, CD21 can assist B-cell function in the absence of a prior antibody response and is therefore an important bridge between innate and acquired immunity. Activation of the B-cell receptor complex by antigen and these accessory molecules results in a cascading phosphorylation of transmembrane and cytoplasmic proteins and calcium fluxes that leads to the transcription of cellular genes required for cell division, differentiation, and antibody production. The very complex cell biology of B-cell activation has been reviewed extensively elsewhere.[138]

Recognition of antigen alone is rarely sufficient for the full or sustained expression of B-cell function. Depending on the nature of the eliciting antigen, B cells may require further signals provided by physical interaction with activated T-helper cells—so-called *T-cell–dependent B-cell activation.* This requires that the B-cell function as an antigen-presenting cell by internalizing and processing antigen to be provided as peptides complexed on MHC II for recognition by the appropriate T-cell partner.[139] The joint recognition of different epitopes of the same antigen by B cells and T cells constitutes the phenomenon previously identified as hapten-carrier cooperation.[140] The B-cell receptor generally binds to native, unprocessed protein determinants, whereas the T-cell receptor is limited to the recognition of linear peptide determinants previously processed by the B cell. A very different type of B-cell activation takes place in response to highly polymerized antigens, characteristically bacterial polysaccharides, which cause extensive cross-linking of the B-cell receptor complex and generate activation signals of sufficient intensity to drive B-cell proliferation and antibody production in the absence of cognate T-cell interactions. This is referred to as *T-cell–independent B-cell activation.*

TABLE 6–3 Important B-Cell Surface Molecules

Molecules	Function
IgM, IgD	Antigen-specific receptor on B-cells; triggers cell activation and endocytosis of bound antigen
Igα, Igβ	Accessory molecules of the B-cell receptor complex; associates with IgM and IgD and transduces activating signals via cytoplasmic domains
B7 molecules (CD86, CD80)	Marker of activated B cells; induced by cross-linking of surface immunoglobulin or MHC II; adhesion receptor for T-cell CD28; provides critical costimulus for T-cell activation
CD5	Ligand for CD72; expressed by the B1 subset of B cells; may modulate activation signals
CD19	Associates with surface immunoglobulin and CD21; lowers threshold for activation during Ig cross-linking
CD21 (CR2)	Binds the C3d fragment(s) of C3 and activates CD19
CD22	Transmembrane molecule with tyrosine kinase activity; involved in signal transduction; adhesion receptor for T-cell CD45RO and other uncharacterized ligands
CD40	Receptor for T-cell help, activated by binding to CD40 ligand expressed on T cells; transduces signals necessary for growth and differentiation of activated B cells; X-linked CD40 ligand deficiency causes the hyper-IgM syndrome
CD45	Protein phosphatase required for activation; expressed throughout B-cell ontogeny
CD72	Ligand for CD5 expressed on T cells and the B1 subset of B cells
Fc receptors	See Table 6–2
MHC II	Involved in presentation of antigenic peptides to complementary T-cell receptor heterodimer
Cytokine receptors	Transduce signals required for proliferation, activation, and differentiation

Abbreviations: Ig, Immunoglobulin; MHC, major histocompatibility complex.

T-Cell–Dependent B-Cell Activation

Both the B-cell receptor and its bound ligand are internalized and delivered to a protease-rich lysosomal compartment where antigen is processed into component peptides that are complexed with nascent MHC II molecules.[141] B cells constitutively express large amounts of MHC II on their surface in support of their accessory cell functions. In contrast to other antigen-presenting cells (e.g., macrophages, dendritic cells) that process antigens from proteins obtained by bulk endocytosis, the high affinity of B-cell antigen receptors for their ligand means that B cells can activate T cells when specific antigen is present in concentrations almost 10,000-fold less than that required for macrophage antigen-presenting cell function.[142] This ability to present antigens efficiently during secondary immune responses is markedly increased when the previous encounter has increased the available number of antigen-specific B cells in the lymphoid tissues.

The formation of a T- and B-cell cognate pair is a highly orchestrated event that depends on multiple noncovalent interactions between complementary adhesion molecules expressed on the surface of each cell.[139] Many of these molecules also transduce functionally important signals through their cytoplasmic domain or through associated transmembrane molecules. This results in a bidirectional, antigen-specific activation of the engaged lymphocytes during the transient intercellular adhesion process. Antigen specificity is provided by the recognition of MHC II—peptide complexes by the appropriate T-cell receptors. The usually weak interactions involved in the coupling of MHC II, peptide, and T-cell receptors are stabilized by

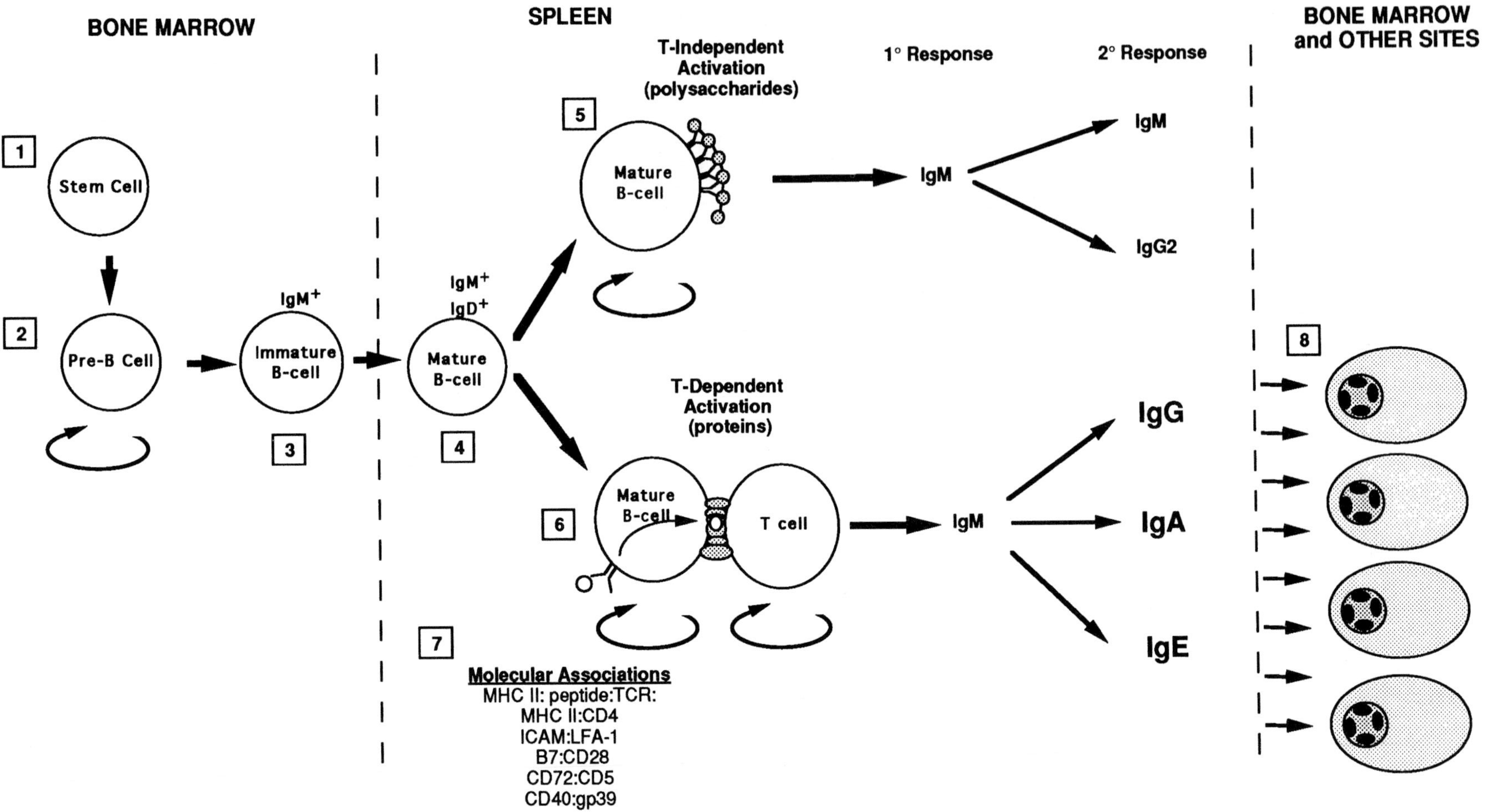

FIGURE 6–5. Important stages in the development of B cells from primitive bone marrow stem cells to antibody-secreting plasma cells. *(1)* Antigen-independent proliferation of bone marrow stem cells leads to large numbers of pre-B cells. Proliferative stages are indicated by the semicircular arrow. *(2)* Recombination of heavy and light chain gene complexes occurs during the pre-B cell stage and generates the antigen-binding diversity of the future B-cell repertoire. *(3)* Approximately 10% of cells achieve a functional recombination and thereupon express surface IgM. These surface IgM–positive cells are defined as immature B cells until they are capable of activation by antigen exposure. At this stage autoreactive B cells are removed by programmed cell death (apoptosis) should they recognize a self-antigen. *(4)* Survivors of this process of negative selection evolve into mature B cells (surface IgM- and IgD-positive cells) that can be activated to proliferate and produce antibodies following recognition of their respective antigen. Activation by two distinct pathways is shown at this stage. *(5)* In the T-cell–independent pathway, B cells are activated when surface immunoglobulins are extensively cross-linked by polymeric antigens—such as the repetitive carbohydrate structure of bacterial polysaccharides, leading to antigen-specific B-cell proliferation and IgM production during the primary antibody response (1° response). T-cell–independent activation results in poor memory cell formation; therefore the amount of antibody produced during the secondary response (2° response) is low. Little differentiation of isotype occurs, the secondary response is composed largely of IgM with some production of IgG (often IgG-2). *(6)* In the T-cell–dependent pathway, specific immunoglobulin receptors identify and internalize low concentrations of monomeric antigens that are processed and incorporated as peptide fragments bound to surface MHC II. T cells recognize and bind to the MHC II-peptide complex, thereby activating multiple intercellular molecular interactions as listed *(7)*. This results in mutual activation of T and B cells. Activated B cells proliferate and produce IgM as part of the primary antibody response. Compared with T-cell–independent responses, T-cell–dependent responses result in more efficient memory cell formation and a consequently larger secondary antibody response (indicated by the larger type). Affinity maturation of antibody takes place in the germinal center at this time. Isotypic switching results in the appearance of IgG, IgA, and IgE isotypes during the secondary response. The type of immunoglobulin made is controlled by T cells through their ligation of B-cell CD40 and through the generation of soluble cytokines such as IL-4, which promotes IgE formation, and IL-5/TGF-β, which induce IgA production. *(8)* With repeated stimulation, short-lived plasma cells producing large amounts of antibody production appear in the bone marrow and in other tissues.

specific and inducible interactions between CD4, CD28, CD5, and LFA-1 on T cells and their complementary B-cell ligands MHC II, B7, CD72, and intracellular adhesion molecule (ICAM).[143, 144] This process is reviewed in detail in Chapter 9. Some of these receptor-ligand pairings generate signals important in B-cell function. Specifically, binding of B-cell CD40 to the CD40 ligand on activated T cells is essential for continued B-cell proliferation and viability after activation by antigen.[145] Because signals provided by CD40 ligation are necessary for B-cell differentiation into IgG-, IgA-, and IgE-producing cells, disabling mutations within the gene for CD40 ligand cause a severe immunodeficiency characterized by deficient production of these isotypes. Instead, antibody responses are dominated by IgM and are inadequate to defend against bacterial and viral pathogens.[146] The hyper-IgM immunodeficiency syndrome is discussed later (see "Immunoglobulin and Antibody Deficiency States"). Similarly, patients who lack β_2 integrins (the leukocyte adhesion deficiency syndrome) are less able to generate antibodies against protein antigens, but their production of antipolysaccharide antibodies is unimpaired.[147]

T-Cell–Independent B-Cell Activation

Certain polymeric antigens, especially bacterial polysaccharides containing repetitive carbohydrate determinants, can activate B cells without requiring cognate signals from T cells.[148] The polymeric structure of these antigens suggests that extensive cross-linking of surface immunoglobulin is an important feature of T-independent responses. Antibody responses generated by T-independent activation are distinct from those induced by T-cell–dependent B-cell activation, and this has important clinical ramifications. First, immunoglobulin isotypes produced in response to antigens causing T-independent antigens, typified by *S. pneumoniae* and *H. influenzae* polysaccharide vaccines, consist largely of IgM and IgG_2.[20] Second, memory cell formation is inefficient during T-cell–independent B-cell activation, and repeated antigenic challenges with T-independent antigens generate low-level antibody responses compared with T-dependent antigens. This poses a practical problem for vaccine design when the immunogen is a bacterial polysaccharide that elicits only low titers of antibody that may be nonprotective. Coupling of the desired determinants with a protein antigen can convert a T-independent response into a T-cell–driven immune reaction and result in strong IgG recall responses. This is well illustrated by the greater vaccine efficacy of *H. influenzae* type b capsular polysaccharide antigen when it is coupled with diphtheria or tetanus toxoid.[149]

B-Cell Ontogeny and Differentiation

Almost 1 billion B cells are produced in the adult bone marrow daily. These arise continuously from stem cells and proceed through a series of highly programmed maturational stages before emerging into the peripheral lymphoid system as fully competent B cells defined by their expression of surface immunoglobulin.[150] After initial differentiation into spontaneously proliferating, surface immunoglobulin–negative B-cell precursors (referred to as *pre-B cells*), the future antigenic specificity of these cells is generated by immunoglobulin gene rearrangements that, if successful, lead to the synthesis of a μ heavy chain and a λ or κ light chain, as previously discussed. Gene rearrangement occurs first in the heavy-chain gene complex, starting in one parental chromosome and progressing to the other if the first does not provide a functional rearrangement. Cytoplasmic μ heavy chain appears when this process is complete and is expressed on the cell surface bound to surrogate light chains not used in mature B cells.[151] One of the four λ or κ light-chain gene complexes is next to rearrange, with sequential activation of the remaining gene complexes if the initial rearrangements are dysfunctional. Owing to frame shift errors and mutations during VJ or VDJ joining, a great majority of immunoglobulin gene rearrangements are nonfunctional. Almost 90% of pre-B cells encounter such difficulty and are removed through a process of programmed cell death or apoptosis.[152] B cells then express IgM on the surface of the B cell. Only one functional light-chain or heavy-chain rearrangement is observed per cell, because production of intact immunoglobulin suppresses further gene recombination. The process of suppression, by an immunoglobulin chain, of activation of the analogous gene locus on the other parental chromosome is termed *allelic exclusion.* Concurrent suppression of κ-chain rearrangement by successful λ-chain recombination (or vice versa) is referred to as *isotypic exclusion.*

Antigen-independent proliferation ceases with attainment of the B-cell phenotype. During a brief *immature B-cell stage,* the newly emerged IgM-positive B cells are subjected to a process of negative selection to remove or suppress autoreactive specificities. Exposure to self-antigen within the bone marrow or in the periphery removes nascent self-reactive clones. Apparently surface immunoglobulin–mediated signals are transiently programmed to induce cell death by apoptosis, whereas failure to detect self-antigen during this critical period allows further maturation into an antigen-responsive or *mature* B cell.[151, 153] Intermediate degrees of self-reactivity may instead result in *tolerance,* in which the autoreactive B-cell clone does not die but is rendered unresponsive to future activating stimuli.[154] However, the mere presence of tolerized B-cell specificities in the body introduces the potential for future autoimmune responses.[151, 155]

Whereas immature B cells express only surface IgM, mature B cells surviving negative selection are positive for both surface IgM and surface IgD. The reason for maintaining two different isotypes of B-cell receptor is not well defined. Signaling through either IgM or IgD receptors does not provide for distinct tolerizing or activating responses,[156] and IgD-deficient mice suffer only a delay in the onset of affinity maturation after B-cell activation.[157] These mature B cells leave the bone marrow and next appear in the periarteriolar sheath of the spleen and peripheral lymph node tissues. When activated by exposure to antigen, through mechanisms described previously, the B cells are triggered to proliferate and differentiate into antibody-secreting and/or memory cells. The proliferative phase that follows primary or secondary sensitization by antigen is associated with a translocation of the activated B cell from the periarteriolar sheath into the germinal center, where the cells enlarge into "centroblasts" as defined by morphologic criteria. Affinity maturation occurs during this phase, reflecting a process of somatic hypermutation within the hypervariable regions of the immunoglobulin and subsequent selection by antigen-expressing follicular dendritic cells.[158] Mutations resulting in high-affinity or kinetically favorable receptor-antigen interactions are preserved for further clonal amplification, whereas low-affinity somatic mutants are removed by apoptotic death.[159] Responses engendered by a single antigen may result in the occupation of each germinal center by only a few amplified clones derived from a single antigen-response precursor cell.[160] Alternatively, reexpression of *RAG* recombinase genes in germinal-center B cells may provide a mechanism for rescuing autoreactive cells through the provision of a new immunoglobulin specificity.[161] Follicular dendritic cells are critically involved in this selection process through their presentation to B cells of antigenic complexes. These antigens are displayed on the cell surface of the follicular dendritic cell for prolonged periods and are capable of supporting B-cell proliferation and affinity maturation long after circulating antigen has disappeared.[162]

B-Cell Differentiation

After primary antigenic exposure, the activated B cells may undergo isotypic switching, wherein the expressed immunoglobulin isotype is changed to IgG, IgA, or IgE with preserved variable regions and antigenic specificity.[129] Although the bulk of B cells previously exposed to antigen and capable of priming the secondary response (memory B cells) remain surface IgM positive, they are capable of rapid production of IgG isotype after restimulation.[163] This process of isotypic switching is regulated by exposure to T-cell cytokines and T-cell cognate interactions. Heavy-chain switching to produce IgE requires that the responding B cells receive differentiating stimuli provided by the T-cell lymphokine IL-4 and engagement of the B-cell CD40 molecule by its respective T-cell ligand.[145] Similarly, CD40 ligation in the presence of transforming growth factor-β and IL-5 results in switching to the IgA isotype. A variety of cytokine combinations promote IgG production. The expression of IgG, IgA, and IgE by B cells tends to reflect the dominant cytokine milieu provided by antigen-responsive CD4-positive T cells. As discussed in greater detail in the chapter on T-cell immunity, this may explain the propensity for B cells to evolve into IgA-secreting cells within the gut-associated lymphatics, where the local T-cell environment is strongly biased in favor of T-helper type 2 cytokine responses that would support IgA isotypic switches.

With continued stimulation, some B cells leave the lymphoid tissues and evolve into surface immunoglobulin–negative, nonproliferating plasma cells that are characterized by markedly expanded endoplasmic reticulum and Golgi structures committed to the sole function of producing large quantities of antibody.[131] Plasma cells are present mostly in the bone marrow and in the lamina propria of the gut and are an important source of circulating IgG and IgA. Infiltration of nonlymphoid tissues by plasma cells may characterize many chronic infectious diseases associated with hypergammaglobulinemia.

B1 Cells and Natural Antibodies

A small subpopulation of functionally distinct B lymphocytes express the CD5 surface protein and spontaneously produce IgM with unusual polyreactive specificities to both endogenous and exogenous forms of phosphocholine, DNA, and polysaccharide antigen. The unique polyspecificity of these "natural" antibodies is determined by the expression of certain, unmutated germline V-region gene sequences. $CD5^+$ B1 cells are distributed within peritoneal and other serosal cavities, but are rare within lymphoid tissues, where the more numerous CD5− B2 cells reside.[164, 165] B1 cells replicate autonomously at these sites, may arise from distinct precursor cells, and probably constitute a separate lymphocyte lineage altogether. Natural antibodies are normally present in serum and provide a type of clinically significant, "innate" humoral immunity against infectious agents, tumors, and endotoxins that bear oligosaccharide determinants included within the cross-reactive specificity repertoire of these immunoglobulins.[93, 166, 167] Natural antibodies also demonstrate autoreactive idiotypes, such as low-affinity RF, that may serve special roles in enhancing antigen presentation and contributing to nonspecific innate immunity (see previous discussion of RF). Natural antibodies with specificity to DNA may be beneficial if they block the many proinflammatory effects of bacterial DNA that have been described.[168]

Regulation of B-Cell Activity

A variety of regulatory mechanisms have evolved to avoid development of autoreactive B cells and to select simultaneously for high-affinity antibodies directed against foreign antigens. As discussed, the antibody repertoire is actively shaped at different points in the life span of B cells. Negative selection during the immature B-cell stage removes autoreactive specificities through programmed cell death. B-cell tolerance to less intensely activating self-epitopes occurs both in the bone marrow and in the peripheral tissues and provides another layer of control over potentially autodestructive specificities. During the secondary response, both positive and negative selection results in the emergence of a few high-affinity B-cell clones within the germinal center. In addition, suppressor CD8+ T cells may inhibit antibody production in response to some antigens, although the mechanisms involved are not well understood.[169] Antibody overproduction may be regulated as well, either by feedback inhibition through downregulatory B-cell Fc receptors or via anti-idiotypic antibody networks in which inhibitory antibodies are generated against the overexpressed idiotype.[170]

IMMUNOGLOBULIN AND ANTIBODY DEFICIENCY STATES

These immunodeficiencies embrace a wide range of genetic and acquired disorders characterized at the extremes by the absence of circulating antibodies, which results in repeated, potentially fatal infections, or by the selective loss of a single class or subclass, which may be wholly asymptomatic. Several of the more significant humoral immunodeficiencies are single-gene defects within the X chromosome and therefore are diseases of young boys.[171] Because severe forms of antibody deficiency can be effectively treated with intravenous immunoglobulins (IVIGs), children or adults presenting with unusually frequent bacterial infections should be evaluated for immunoglobulin deficiencies. Delayed diagnosis is associated with worsened prognosis.[172]

The severe manifestations of agammaglobulinemia are most obviously related to the loss of IgG- and IgM-mediated serum opsonic, lytic, and neutralizing activities that critically defend against infection with encapsulated bacteria and many types of virus. The cause of susceptibility to infection in partial immunoglobulin deficiencies, such as IgG subclass disorders, may be driven as much by dysfunctional primary antibody responses as by quantitative changes in serum immunoglobulin levels. This can be measured in the patient's inability to generate antibody against defined bacterial polysaccharide or protein antigens. Several genetic diseases result in combined humoral and cellular immune deficiencies[173]; these are discussed in further depth in Chapter 9. Immunoglobulin deficiencies or functional abnormalities may be secondary manifestations of preexisting diseases that alter production or clearance of antibody. In these cases, the underlying disease may separately contribute to the enhanced susceptibility to infection.

Common Clinical Features of Antibody Deficiencies

The most severe antibody deficiencies, such as X-linked agammaglobulinemia (XLA), common variable immunodeficiency (CVI), and X-linked hyper-IgM syndrome, usually manifest in children or young adults as recurrent infections involving many different organ systems.[172–176] Unusually severe or recurrent pulmonary infections with *S. pneumoniae, H. influenzae, Mycoplasma* spp., and meningococci are especially characteristic. The persistent or repetitive nature of the infections can lead to chronic morbidity from bronchiectasis and related pulmonary disease. Chronic sinusitis and otitis are also frequent problems. Gastrointestinal infections are increased in severity and incidence and are caused by common pathogens, such as *Salmonella, Shigella, Campylobacter,* and rotavirus.[172, 177] Intestinal giardiasis may be prolonged in patients with hypogammaglobulinemia, reflecting a key role for secretory antibody in the control of this parasite.[178] Chronic giardiasis can result in prolonged malabsorption associated with nodular submucosal hyperplasia of lymphoid tissues in the small intestine.[176] In addition, gluten-sensitive enteropathies and Crohn's disease are suspected to be more common in these patients.[172, 179]

Rheumatologic disease occurs in about 10 to 30% of patients with humoral immunodeficiency.[180] This includes septic arthritis caused by the usual bacterial agents but also embraces joint infections caused by *Mycoplasma* and *Ureaplasma* spp. that may pose unusual diagnostic and therapeutic problems. *Mycoplasma* spp. are associated with a destructive arthritis with a subacute onset in these patients that is usually, but not always, associated with intra-articular purulence.[172, 175, 181] Diagnosis requires specialized culture procedures adapted for *Mycoplasma,* and empiric therapy with doxycycline should be considered whenever these patients develop arthritis that is culture negative by conventional microbiologic techniques. Rheumatoid-like, polyarticular synovitis also occurs in the absence of a definable infectious cause. Infusion with IVIGs may lead to clinical improvement. A syndrome that closely resembles polymyositis or dermatomyositis is caused by enteroviral infection of the skeletal muscle.[182] Finally, the incidence of autoimmune disorders, such as systemic lupus erythematosus, Sjögren's syndrome, and autoimmune hematologic disorders, is increased to as much as 20% in patients with CVI or IgA deficiency. These complications are notably lacking in patients with XLA.[175, 183]

Other unique infectious disease manifestations of hypogammaglobulinemia are noteworthy. Enterovirus can cause chronic meningitis that is often fatal despite the institution of combined intrathecal and IVIG therapies.[172, 175, 184] Although the humoral immune deficiencies do not generally predispose to fungal or parasitic infections, the occurrence of *Pneumocystis carinii* pneumonia in several agammaglobulinemic patients has been described.[185] This may reflect the frequent occurrence of neutropenia in these disorders[186] or relate to defects in T-cell function resulting from disrupted intracellular signaling between B cells and T cells.[146] Similarly, viral infections normally controlled by cell-mediated immunity (e.g., herpes simplex) can become recurrent or severe in these patients.[187]

Other immunologic functions unrelated to control of infection are affected by the loss of immunoglobulins. Serum and mucosal IgA is thought to play an important role in sequestering frequently encountered antigens derived from the diet or from the environment. Failure to mask these potential allergens may result in undesirable IgE-mediated responses. Indeed, a high rate of atopic disorders is observed in patients with isolated IgA deficiency.

Diagnosis of Antibody Deficiencies

Although frequent infections can also result from complement deficiencies, cystic fibrosis, dysmotile cilia syndrome, and AIDS, the availability of accurate laboratory assays of serum IgM, IgG, and IgA levels or of IgG subclass concentrations makes the diagnosis of immunoglobulin deficiency relatively straightforward.[188] Inherited immunodeficiencies can also be diagnosed by genetic analysis.[189] The biggest pitfall in the diagnosis of agammaglobulinemia is usually a failure to suspect the disorder. However, the clinician should be aware of important caveats in the interpretation of serum immunoglobulin levels.[173] The laboratory threshold defining the lower limits of normal are based on statistical, not functional, criteria. Therefore, most patients with low levels of immunoglobulin (5% of the population by definition) are not truly immunodeficient. A more useful rule of thumb is that susceptibility to recurrent infections more typically occurs in patients with levels of IgG that are 50% or less of the lower limit of normal—typically less than 200 mg/dl. Those antibody deficiencies most likely to require IVIG result in no detectable IgM or IgG in the serum. Additionally, normal immunoglobulin levels vary with age, and the laboratory should provide appropriate age-adjusted normal levels on request.

Low levels of immunoglobulin do not always correlate with patients' ability to generate specific antibody responses against new antigens.[173] In fact, most patients with demonstrably low IgG subclass levels have clinically adequate antibody responses to defined antigens. In situations in which a strong history of recurrent infection is associated with isolated subclass deficiencies or modestly depressed immunoglobulin levels, a useful functional test of humoral adequacy is to evaluate antibody responses to tetanus toxoid, pneumococcal vaccine, *H. influenzae* type b toxoid conjugate vaccine, or hepatitis B vaccine. Enzyme-linked immunosorbent assay (ELISA) determinations of these antibodies are available through commercial laboratories. A relatively normal antibody response either before or after immunization implies functional normalcy and argues strongly against a need for immunoglobulin replacement therapy. Similar tests may also be useful in the evaluation of diseases associated with dysfunctional antibody responses and only modestly abnormal immunoglobulin levels, including ataxia telangiectasia, and Wiskott-Aldrich syndrome.[190]

When diagnostic ambiguity exists or when resources are easily available, circulating B-lymphocyte numbers can be quantitated using fluorescent monoclonal antibodies and fluorescence-activated flow cytometry. XLA, but not CVI, is associated with an absence of peripheral B cells.[173, 188] Measurement of in vitro immunoglobulin production in response to B-cell mitogens is a research tool in selected institutions. The coordinated use of these tests in conjunction with assays of complement, phagocytes, T-lymphocyte function, and ciliary function, as well as tests for cystic fibrosis and AIDS, are described in further detail in Chapter 10.

Treatment of Immunoglobulin G Deficiency

The goals of therapy in patients with IgG deficiency are threefold: to treat acute infection effectively, to prevent repeated infections through infusion of IVIG, and to prevent or treat pulmonary disease resulting from repeated pneumonias and bronchitis.[173, 191] Because agammaglobulinemia leads to a failure of serum opsonization, acute infections require aggressive therapy with antibiotics. Antimicrobials should be given intravenously and for longer periods than is the usual practice. Empiric therapy should always include antibiotics active against typical encapsulated bacterial pathogens, notably *S. pneumoniae* and *H. influenzae.* Because infection may consume the small amounts of serum immunoglobulin available, IVIG administration during acute infection is probably indicated if serum immunoglobulin levels are considered subtherapeutic.

Prophylaxis against infection is based on the administration of preparations of human immunoglobulins specially formulated for intravenous delivery.[191–193] Historically, IgG replacement was subcutaneous because older methods of immune globulin preparation contained aggregated IgG that was toxic when given parenterally. Immunoglobulin preparations specifically formulated for intravenous injection are now available and can be administered in quantities sufficient to normalize serum IgG levels. These preparations are 95 to 99% IgG, with trace quantities of IgA, IgM, IgD, and IgE; the half-life of the delivered IgG is variable, but the average is about 20 days.[191] The efficacy of IVIG in improving symptoms and preventing infection among patients with severe hypogammaglobulinemia has been well documented. The average patient with complete immunoglobulin deficiency may require doses of 100 to 400 mg/kg delivered every 3 to 4 weeks to achieve protection. A comparative study showed that higher-dose regimens resulted in decreased incidence of pneumonia and meningitis and fewer days in the hospital; such regimens may prevent long-term sequelae, such as bronchiectasis or other chronic pulmonary disease.[194] Monitoring of trough immunoglobulin levels may assist in defining the optimal time between doses, because IgG clearance varies considerably among patients. It has been recommended that trough levels be maintained at 400 to 500 mg/dl during therapy for humoral immunodeficiencies.[191] The efficacy of therapy can be followed also by obtaining yearly pulmonary function tests and through the maintenance of patient diaries to document frequency of infections. Subcutaneous infusion of IVIG is a potentially cost-effective method of administration that achieves serum levels of IgG comparable to those generated by intravenous infusion.[195]

IVIG is typically well tolerated, although rate-related side effects are common. About 3 to 12% of patients experience fever, chills, headache, myalgia, and nausea with infusion. When symptoms are severe enough, the rate of infusion should be slowed (to 0.01 ml/kg/minute) and the patient should be pretreated with acetaminophen, antihistamines, and hydrocortisone to reduce these side effects.[191, 193] Tolerance to these effects develops after several doses, and the rate of infusion can be increased to minimize inconvenience. Home administration of IVIG has been advocated as a convenient and cost-conserving measure,[196] but the potential for complications needs to be considered.[191] Special precautions are necessary when treating isolated IgA deficiency with IVIG, because anti-IgE antibodies may develop against the exogenous IgA contained in the infusate and cause anaphylactic reactions.[197] The process used to prepare human immunoglobulins for infusion inactivates most viral pathogens, and the human immunodeficiency virus (HIV) has not been reported to be transferred by IVIG.[191] However, hepatitis C virus contaminating several lots of infusate caused an outbreak of non-A, non-B hepatitis before screening could be instituted to remove this infectious threat.[198]

Treatment of the chronic pulmonary disease resulting from repeated infection is also required, because structural lesions within the lung further predispose to infection and cor pulmonale. Pulmonary disease is an important cause of death in patients with agammaglobulinemia. Postural drainage or other physiotherapy may be required to clear pooled respiratory secretions. The role of prophylactic antibiotics or antibiotic "cleanouts" akin to those used in patients with lung disease resulting from cystic fibrosis has not been studied in cases of humoral immunodeficiency.

The ultimate treatment for genetic humoral immunodeficiencies is to provide the affected patient with normal bone marrow stem cells. This can be achieved through bone marrow transplantation in cases of severe combined immunodeficiency, XLA, or Wiskott-Aldrich syndrome, although the risks of allogeneic transplantation in the absence of suitable related donors may contraindicate this approach. Identification of the genetic lesions responsible for XLA and X-linked hyper-IgM syndrome has given rise to interest in adoptive gene therapy.[199]

Primary Disorders: Pure Antibody Deficiency

X-Linked Agammaglobulinemia. Originally described by Bruton[200] in 1952, XLA was the first immunodeficiency disorder to be identified. The disorder was recently mapped to a previously uncharacterized protein-tyrosine kinase that contained inactivating mutations in all the affected subjects studied.[201] The XLA genotype in male patients results in abortive B-cell development at the pre-B-cell stage. An autosomal recessive form of agammaglobulinemia is caused by genetic defects in the μ heavy-chain gene.[202] As a consequence, B cells and plasma cells are markedly diminished (<1% of normal) in blood, lymph nodes, and bone marrow.[203] IgG, IgM, and IgA are reduced to undetectable or extremely low levels in the serum. Affected infants are usually asymptomatic until 5 to 6 months of age, at which time maternal antibodies are reduced to levels ineffective against infection. The hypogammaglobulinemia then usually manifests as recurrent middle ear, sinopulmonary, and gastrointestinal tract infections with or without complicating bacteremia, meningitis, and cellulitis.[203] Less commonly, recurrent infections are clinically unappreciated until progressive pulmonary disease and bronchiectasis are identified. The presence of pulmonary disease at the time of diagnosis is considered a poor prognostic factor because mortality, usually in the second or third decade of life, is caused by progressive respiratory failure. Vaccination with inactivated antigen is usually futile, and live virus vaccinations are strictly contraindicated because of the risk of opportunistic infection. Poliomyelitis caused by vaccine strain virus has occurred in several patients with agammaglobulinemia.[173]

Diagnosis rests on the characteristic family history of severe illnesses in a young boy and failure to detect IgM, IgG, and IgA in the serum. IgG concentrations in particular are usually less than 100 mg/dl, a level below which antibody-dependent serum opsonization is severely affected. When appropriate laboratory resources are available, the absence of B cells in the peripheral blood and lymphatic tissues can be documented.[204] Antibody deficiency can also be identified by the absence of IgM isohemagglutinins against ABO blood group incompatibilities and an inability to generate antibodies against vaccine antigens after routine immunization. Although rarely indicated for diagnosis of XLA, biopsy specimens from appropriate tissues demonstrate a complete absence of plasma cells in the germinal centers of lymph nodes and in the lamina propria of the gut. Cellular immunity is completely intact. Many patients may have an associated cyclic or transient neutropenia that further aggravates their predisposition to infection. Related syndromes include XLA with isolated growth hormone deficiency and autosomal recessive hypogammaglobulinemia.[205]

Transient Hypogammaglobulinemia of Infancy. Transient hypogammaglobulinemia of infancy represents a delay in production of endogenous IgM and IgG, which leads to an exaggerated form of the normal reduction in serum IgG levels that occurs at 5 to 6 months.[206] Serum IgG concentrations may drop to as low as 350 mg/dl, and the infant may be subject to the same type of infections as children with XLA. In contrast to those with XLA, these infants are able to generate normal antibody responses to diphtheria, tetanus, and pertussis vaccines.[207] Because of their transient immunodeficiency, these children should not be immunized with live virus vaccine until recovery of serum immunoglobulins is established. Treatment with IVIG is only rarely required for severe infections, and infusion of immunoglobulin can be detrimental if it suppresses production of endogenous immunoglobulins.

Common Variable Immunodeficiency. The CVI antibody deficiencies are a heterogeneous group of disorders that have in common a late onset (15 to 25 years of age), hypogammaglobulinemia, and recurrent bacterial infections.[174, 208, 209] Because disease becomes manifest in adulthood, this disorder is often referred to as "acquired" hypogammaglobulinemia, although the familial occurrence suggests a genetic cause. The possession of rare alleles of complement genes within the MHC III complex on chromosome 6 is strongly associated with the development of CVI or IgA deficiency, or both.[210] The estimated prevalence of CVI is between 1 in 50,000 and 1 in 200,000 in the general population.[174]

The underlying cause of CVI-related antibody deficiency remains poorly defined. Early B-cell maturation is intact, and normal numbers of B cells are evident in the circulation and in lymph nodes, although their ability to secrete antibody is clearly lacking.[211] Although a defect intrinsic to the B cell may be present, half of these patients manifest T-cell dysfunction that is measurable by reduced production of IL-2 and other lymphokines.[183, 212] A separate T-cell defect would also explain the increased risk of neoplasm and autoimmunity encountered in these patients. As described previously, genetic linkages to the MHC III complex and the intrafamilial concurrence of both CVI and IgA deficiency suggest that these two disorders may be mechanistically related. Some patients with IgA deficiency later develop CVI.[210]

CVI is distinct in its manifestation, compared with XLA.[208] While IgG concentrations are invariably lower than 250 mg/dl in symptomatic patients, with comparable decreases in the levels of other immunoglobulins, this pattern is less pronounced or consistent when compared with that of patients with XLA. Mature B cells expressing surface immunoglobulin are apparent in near-normal numbers in the circulation. CVI affects men and women equally, and the infections are often less severe than those seen in patients with XLA. Some patients may merely experience an increased number or severity of sinopulmonary infections. Patients are predisposed to sprue-like malabsorption or regional enteritis, and autoimmune illnesses develop in up to a quarter of them. In contrast to XLA, generalized lymphoid hyperplasia with or without splenomegaly is a common finding, and a subset of CVI patients with lymphadenopathy develop systemic granulomatous disease, $CD4^+$ lymphopenia, and high levels of circulating tumor necrosis factor-α.[213, 214] This illness may resemble sarcoid, and the differential diagnosis of sarcoid and sarcoid-like granulomatous responses in CVI has been reviewed.[215] Patients with CVI are highly predisposed to malignancy and have an estimated 57-fold increased risk of gastric cancer and a 438-fold increased risk for development of lymphomas later in life.[174, 216]

The treatment of patients with the acquired form is similar to that of those with XLA and relies on the use of aggressive antibiotic therapy for acute infection combined with monthly infusions of IVIG to prevent future infections. Affected patients may require therapy for associated autoimmune disorders, and screening for malignancies should be regularly pursued. Treatments with polyethylene glycol–conjugated IL-2 have enhanced in vitro B-cell function and stabilized serum IgG levels but are available only on an experimental basis at present.[217]

X-Linked Hyper-IgM Syndrome. Affected male patients have increased serum IgM levels and diminished or absent IgG levels and experience recurrent pyogenic infections.[218, 219] This humoral immunodeficiency is also uniquely associated with an increased incidence of *Pneumocystis* pneumonia. Although initial B-cell maturation is intact, appropriate activating stimuli do not result in differentiation into IgG- or IgA-producing cells. Consequently, there is a characteristic increase in serum IgM concentrations in association with low-to-absent levels of IgA and IgG and a paucity of circulating B cells expressing IgG or IgA. Families with X-linked hyper-IgM syndrome express a variety of mutations in a gene on the X chromosome that encodes the CD40 ligand (CD154) responsible for costimulation of B-cell function.[146] Engagement of CD40 is also a prerequisite for the appearance of IgG- and IgA-producing cells, providing a satisfactory explanation for the clinical pattern of B-cell dysfunction seen in these patients.[131, 145] Supportive treatment with IVIG is similar to that for the other hypogammaglobulinemic disorders outlined previously. As in CVI, lymphoid hyperplasia is characteristic and may result in diagnostic misdirection.

Selective Immunoglobulin A Deficiency. Selective IgA deficiency is the most common disorder of antibody production, with an incidence of about 1 in 300 to 600 in the normal population.[42, 220] Whereas the majority of people with IgA deficiency are clinically normal, it is clear that this defect predisposes to a variety of diseases similar to those seen in patients with CVI, including recurrent sinopulmonary infections, atopy, gastrointestinal tract disease, autoimmune disorders (e.g., systemic lupus erythematosus, rheumatoid arthritis, pernicious anemia), and malignancy (diffuse histiocytic lymphoma or gastrointestinal carcinoma). These clinical manifestations are probably caused by the absence of protective IgA on mucosal surfaces[26] and the loss of serum IgA blocking antibody directed against environmental antigens. Affected patients have markedly reduced levels of IgA in both serum (<50 mg/dl) and secretions, generally without abnormalities within the other major immunoglobulin classes. Usually both IgA subclasses are affected, although selected deficiencies in IgA_2 have been described.[221] Some patients with IgA deficiency have decreased levels of IgG subclasses, notably IgG_2 and IgG_4, with or without an absence of serum IgE.

The variability in the predisposition of IgA-deficient persons to infection is largely unexplained; it has been speculated that associated IgG_2 subclass deficiencies account for such susceptibility.[21] However, cases of combined IgA-IgG_2 deficiency caused by deletions of heavy-chain genes have been identified by screening of blood donors without a history of increased susceptibility to infection.[222, 223] Secretory IgM directed against microbial antigens is present in greater concentrations in these subjects and may provide adequate compensation for deficient dimeric IgA at mucosal sites.[30] There is little evidence that IVIG therapy is required in patients with IgA deficiency. Patients may require frequent follow-up for the management of atopic or autoimmune disease and are at increased risk of malignancy. Some IgA-deficient patients go on to develop CVI.

Allergies in these patients are often directed against common dietary antigens, such as bovine albumin contained in milk products.[224] As a consequence, patients who are totally IgA deficient are at risk for development of IgE-mediated anaphylactic reactions directed against exogenous IgA neoantigens.[197] When identified, these subjects should not receive immunoglobulin preparations containing IgA and should receive only extensively washed red cell transfusions.

Immunoglobulin G Subclass Deficiency. Isolated deficiency of IgG_1 is rare. Because this subtype accounts for approximately 70% of the IgG class, its deficiency results in recognizable reductions in total IgG levels.[225] The clinical presentation with increased bacterial infections is very much like that of patients with hypogammaglobulinemia. Replacement immune globulin therapy is usually effective in reducing the incidence of infections.

IgG_2 subclass deficiencies have been identified and are usually combined with parallel decreases in IgG_4, IgE, and IgA. Total IgG is often in the normal range, reflecting the small contribution of IgG_2 to total IgG concentration. A subset of these patients may be at risk for recurrent bacterial infections.[21, 22] However, most patients with IgG_2 deficiency do not have an increased susceptibility to infectious disease.[226] It is likely that the predisposition to pulmonary infection instead reflects functional defects in the ability to generate specific anticapsular antibodies by a subset of patients with subclass deficiency.[227, 228] Because most patients with IgG subclass deficiency are not at risk for infection, IVIG therapy should be reserved for those who have clear-cut evidence of increased susceptibility to infectious diseases and who have demonstrated an inability to respond to capsular polysaccharide vaccines.

Combined T-Cell and Antibody Deficiencies

Severe Combined Immunodeficiency Disorders. These are a heterogeneous group of primary immunodeficiency disorders in which both antibody production and cellular immunity are impaired, usually because of a failure to generate mature B cells and T cells.[173, 176, 189] These infants (1 per 100,000 live births) are subject to a complex variety of infectious diseases and rarely survive past their second year of life without aggressive medical therapy. The various causes of this immunodeficiency are discussed in greater detail in Chapters 9 and 10. Because of extremely low immunoglobulin levels, these patients are at increased risk for bacterial pneumonia, otitis, and septicemia. However, the clinical picture is dominated mostly by opportunistic infections resulting from deficient cellular immunity. Treatment consists of bone marrow transplantation or enzyme replacement (when the deficiency is caused by loss of adenosine deaminase).

Wiskott-Aldrich Syndrome. Wiskott-Aldrich syndrome is a rare X-linked recessive disorder characterized by a triad of thrombocytopenia, severe eczematoid dermatitis, and deficient T-cell– and B-cell–mediated immune responses.[229] Young boys with this genotype usually present at a very early age with gastrointestinal bleeding or severe eczema. The immunodeficiency is associated not only with an increased risk of infection but also with an approximately 10% lifetime risk of cancer.[230] Because of the great risk of premature death from bleeding, sepsis, or malignancy in these young patients, bone marrow transplantation is often considered as a curative measure. The syndrome is probably caused by mutations in a gene encoding the Wiskott-Aldrich syndrome protein (or WASp), a functionally complex protein that links signal transduction to cytoskeletal and proliferative responses.[231] Although affected patients have normal numbers of B and T cells, IgM and IgG levels are low, IgE and IgA levels are high, and de novo synthesis of antibodies to T-independent antigens (e.g., bacterial polysaccharides) are subnormal.[232] Not surprisingly, severe infections with pneumococci and *H. influenzae* are common and may necessitate frequent antibiotic and IVIG prophylaxis.[229]

Ataxia-Telangiectasia. Ataxia-telangiectasia is a rare genetic disorder associated with heterogeneous defects in immunoglobulin levels and antigen-specific B-cell and T-cell responses.[233] The clinical picture is dominated by the progressive and disabling neurologic manifestations of the syndrome. Ocular telangiectases are also present in almost all affected persons. Markedly perturbed DNA repair mechanisms are characteristic of ataxia-telangiectasia syndrome and the

ATM gene mutated in this disease encodes a protein kinase required for activation of protective cellular responses to ionizing radiation.[234] Chromosomal damage near the T-cell receptor and immunoglobulin genes have been suggested as reasons for the observed defects in immunity. Because immunoglobulin levels are not usually critically diminished, the use of IVIG should be restricted to patients with recurring infection who are unable to generate antibodies against *H. influenzae* type b toxoid conjugate or other childhood vaccines.[176, 191]

Secondary Antibody Deficiencies

Malignancy. Chronic lymphocytic leukemia and multiple myeloma are commonly associated with clinically significant antibody deficiency.[235, 236] The cause of the hypogammaglobulinemia is uncertain, but low levels of IgG and decreased antipneumococcal antibody titers in these patients are correlated with more frequent infectious morbidity. Patients with chronic lymphocytic leukemia may benefit from regular administration of IVIG,[237] although the cost-effectiveness of this approach has been questioned.[238] Antibody dyscrasias, such as multiple myeloma and Waldenström's macroglobulinemia, are also associated with suppressed antibody responses by nonmalignant B cells.[239] This is related both to decreased numbers of normal B cells and to functional disorders that might be caused by triggering of immune feedback mechanisms in response to monoclonal hypergammaglobulinemia.[240] Increased catabolism of immunoglobulins as a result of saturation of MHC I–like Fc receptors by excess circulating antibody may also contribute to decreased levels of nonmalignant types of IgG. A biphasic susceptibility to infections with encapsulated and gram-negative bacteria is evident in these patients.[241, 242] Immunoglobulin supplementation protects against life-threatening infections in plateau-phase myeloma and is especially recommended for patients who cannot generate IgG antibody responses to pneumococcal vaccination.[243] Thymoma and rare lymphomas are associated with profound deficiencies in one or more classes of immunoglobulins.[244, 245]

Protein Wasting States. Immunoglobulin catabolism is increased in some patients with severe burns, protein-losing enteropathies, or the nephrotic syndrome. Immunoglobulins can be lost excessively in burned tissues,[246] whereas gastrointestinal or urinary tract losses of IgG are responsible for hypogammaglobulinemia in the other disorders. Treatment of the primary disease process brings about a reversal of these conditions.

Splenectomy and Sickle Cell Anemia. The spleen serves multiple host defense functions.[247] It acts as a phagocytic filter that nonspecifically removes circulating antigenic complexes, microbes, and parasitized erythrocytes. The spleen is especially efficient at removing poorly opsonized pathogens.[248] Antigen-presenting cells within the spleen are available for processing the captured antigens and presenting them to T cells contained in this organ. The spleen is also an important site of IgM production and memory B-cell differentiation during primary humoral responses.[249] Consequently, removal of the spleen by surgery or by disease results in a heightened predisposition to sepsis syndrome caused by pneumococci, other streptococci, *H. influenzae,* meningococci, and a variety of other encapsulated bacteria, such as *Capnocytophaga canimorsus* (DF-2 bacillus).[250, 251] Splenic hypofunction also predisposes to severe infection with intraerythrocytic parasites such as *Babesia microti.* Splenectomy during childhood is most associated with enhanced susceptibility to infection, although adult splenectomy is also associated with increased infection rates. The immune defect is probably related to decreased phagocytic removal of poorly opsonized bacteria from the blood stream.[248, 252]

Although the titer of antibody produced in response to pneumococcal vaccine is less than that of eusplenic patients, the protective efficacy can be as high as 85%.[253] Because antipneumococcal antibody responses decline over 2 to 5 years in asplenic hosts, revaccination 2 years after primary immunization has become accepted practice.[254, 255] *H. influenzae* type b conjugate vaccine administered to children undergoing splenectomy generates antibody responses deemed adequate for prophylaxis against infection.[256] Therefore, vaccination of asplenic patients with *H. influenzae* type b conjugate and pneumococcal vaccines is strongly recommended. Although these patients are also at risk for meningococcemia and respond well to meningococcal vaccine, the currently available preparations do not provide protection against the group B serotype common in the United States.[257] Daily oral penicillin or amoxicillin for life is still considered a mainstay therapy to prevent infection in the splenectomized child or adult.[258, 259] In contrast to trauma-related splenectomy, splenic removal during staging of Hodgkin's disease results in a substantial, although transient, loss of pneumococcal vaccine responses. This may be mediated by the lymphoma, by cytotoxic therapy, or by lymphoid irradiation.[260] Because antibody responses to polysaccharide vaccines are relatively intact before splenectomy, vaccination is recommended 2 weeks before the spleen is scheduled to be removed. Responses to polysaccharide-conjugate and polysaccharide vaccines return to normal 2 years after completion of therapy for Hodgkin's disease.[261]

Patients with sickle cell disease are functionally asplenic after infarction of that organ and have a 30- to 100-fold increased incidence of pneumococcal, *Haemophilus,* and meningococcal infections, including both pneumonia and septicemia.[262, 263] The increased susceptibility to infection in these patients has been variously ascribed to the loss of splenic clearance mechanisms, to poor anticapsular antibody responses, and to deficient serum opsonizing activity. In contrast to splenectomy, sickle cell disease is more clearly associated with a deficient response to available pneumococcal vaccines.[263] However, *H. influenzae* type b polysaccharide–tetanus protein conjugate vaccine stimulates antibody levels comparable to those in normal children.[264] Antibiotic prophylaxis and aggressive vaccination are advised to prevent infection with pneumococcus or *H. influenzae* in young patients with sickle cell disease.[263, 265]

Bone Marrow Transplantation. The preparative regimen used before bone marrow transplantation effectively removes bone marrow precursor B cells and memory B-cell populations in the lymphoid organs. Despite the prolonged half-life of serum immunoglobulin, the long time required for full engraftment of donor bone marrow usually results in a dramatic decrease in serum immunoglobulin levels, with a subsequent slow return to normal over 4 to 12 months.[266] In some respects this process recapitulates the transient hypogammaglobulinemia of infancy in that IgM recovery precedes that of IgG and IgA. During the posttransplantation recovery period, some patients are functionally antibody deficient in the face of bacterial and viral infections. In this regard, combinations of IVIG and ganciclovir appear to prevent cytomegalovirus infection in cytomegalovirus-seropositive patients.[267] Although the ability of IVIG to reduce bacterial infections significantly in these patients remains controversial, IVIG has been recommended as a general antimicrobial prophylaxis for the first 3 months after transplantation.[268] IVIG is also used after allogeneic transplantation as immunomodulatory therapy to prevent acute graft-versus-host disease and interstitial pneumonitis.[269] Because immunologic memory is lost, bone marrow transplantation patients should be revaccinated against tetanus, pertussis, pneumococcus, and *Haemophilus influenzae* type b 1 to 2 years after successful engraftment.[270] Alternatively, vaccination of the donor several weeks before marrow harvest may adoptively transfer protective antibody responses to the recipient.[271, 272]

HIV-Related Antibody Deficiency. Infection with HIV is associated with aberrant immunoglobulin production and B-cell function. Although adult patients may have normal to increased immunoglobulin levels, their ability to generate or maintain specific antibody responses to bacterial antigens is severely impaired even before $CD4^+$ T-lymphocyte counts begin to decline. This condition commonly manifests as poor antibody responses to polysaccharide and protein vaccines[273, 274] and an increasing inability to seroconvert during primary infections. Children typically have a much more severe humoral deficiency, probably because they have not formed sufficient memory B cells before CD4+ T-helper cell functions are lost. Both children and adults have markedly increased rates of pneumococcal and *H. influenzae* pneumonia and bacteremia.[275] Although immunization with pneumococcal vaccine does not reliably provoke strong antibody responses in AIDS patients, *H. influenzae* capsular antigens linked to diphtheria toxoid are markedly more effective than capsular polysaccharide alone in inducing adequate humoral responses.[276] Therefore, HIV-positive patients should receive pneumococcal, *H. influenzae*–toxoid conjugate and influenza vaccines as early as possible in the course of disease. Therapy with IVIG has been demonstrated to reduce the incidence of bacterial infections in HIV-infected children with CD4+ T-cell counts higher than 200 cells/mm^3 and may be indicated for severe repeated bacterial infections.[237, 277] There were no differences in the rates of other opportunistic infections.

In contrast, production of IgE may be increased during HIV infection. This increase is associated with a greater frequency (30 to 68%) of allergic rhinitis and sinusitis, leading to frequent bacterial sinusitis as a complication. Patients in the later stages of disease develop new allergies documentable by skin testing and maintain serum levels of IgE that are three to five times higher than normal values.[278] This spontaneous shift in immunoglobulin isotype may reflect alterations in the balance of T-helper types 1 and 2 CD4+ activities during the evolution of AIDS.

REFERENCES

1. Capra JD, Kehoe JM. Hypervariable regions, idiotypy, and the antibody-combining site. Adv Immunol. 1975;20:1–33.
2. Burton DR, Woof JM. Human antibody effector function. Adv Immunol. 1992;51:1–84.
3. Nezlin R. Internal movements in immunoglobulin molecules. Adv Immunol. 1990;48:1–40.
4. Rini J, Schulze-Gahmen U, Wilson IA. Structural evidence for an induced fit as a mechanism for antibody-antigen recognition. Science. 1992;255:959–965.
5. Davies DR, Cohen GH. Interactions of protein antigens with antibodies. Proc Natl Acad Sci U S A. 1996;93:7–12.
6. Canfield SM, Morrison SL. The binding affinity of human IgG for its high affinity Fc receptor is determined by multiple amino acids in the C_H2 domain and is modulated by the hinge region. J Exp Med. 1991;173:1483–1491.
7. Tao MH, Canfield SM, Morrison SL. The differential ability of human IgG1 and IgG4 to activate complement is determined by the COOH-terminal sequence of the C_H2 domain. J Exp Med. 1991;173:1025–1028.
8. Kehry M. The immunoglobulin μ chains of membrane-bound and secreted IgM molecules differ in their C-terminal segments. Cell. 1980;21:393.
9. Natvig J, Kunkel H. Immunoglobulins: Classes, subclasses, genetic variants, and idiotypes. Adv Immunol. 1973;16:1–26.
10. Goodman JW. Immunoglobulin structure and function. In: Stites D, Terr AI, eds. Basic and Clinical Immunology. 7th ed. San Mateo, Calif: Appleton & Lange, 1991;109–121.
11. Porter RR. Structural studies of immunoglobulins. Science. 1973;180:713–716.
12. Spiegelberg HL. Biological activities of immunoglobulins of different classes and subclasses. Adv Immunol. 1974;19:259–294.
13. Koshland ME. The coming of age of the immunoglobulin J chain. Annu Rev Immunol. 1985;3:425–453.
14. Roth RA, Koshland ME. Identification of a lymphocyte enzyme that catalyzes pentamer immunoglobulin M assembly. J Biol Chem. 1981;256:4633–4639.
15. Buckley RH, Dees SC, O'Fallon WM. Serum immunoglobulins: I. Levels in normal children and in uncomplicated childhood allergy. Pediatrics. 1968;41:600–611.
16. Carson DA, Chen PP, Kipps TJ. New roles for rheumatoid factor. J Clin Invest. 1991;87:379–383.
17. Wienands J, Reth M. Glycosyl-phosphatidylinositol linkage as a mechanism for cell-surface expression of immunoglobulin D. Nature. 1992;356:246–249.
18. Reynolds HY. Immunoglobulin G and its function in the human respiratory tract. Mayo Clin Proc. 1988;63:161–174.
19. Michaelsen TE, Garred P, Aase A. Human IgG subclass pattern of inducing complement-mediated cytolysis depends on antigen concentration and to a lesser extent on epitope patchiness, antibody affinity and complement concentration. Eur J Immunol. 1991;21:11–16.
20. Siber GR, Schur PH, Aisenberg AC, et al. Correlation between serum IgG2 concentrations and the antibody response to bacterial polysaccharide antigens. N Engl J Med. 1980;303:178–181.
21. Oxelius VA, Laurell AB, Lindquist B, et al. IgG subclasses in selective IgA deficiency: Importance of IgG2-IgA deficiency. N Engl J Med. 1981;304:1476–1477.
22. Bjorkander J, Bake B, Oxelius V, et al. Impaired lung function in patients with IgA deficiency and low levels of IgG2 or IgG3. N Engl J Med. 1985;313:720–724.
23. Stanworth DR, Smith AK. Inhibition of reagin-mediated PCA reactions in baboons by the human IgG4 sub-class. Clin Allergy. 1973;3:37–41.
24. Underdown B, Schiff M. Immunoglobulin A: Strategic defense initiative at the mucosal surface. Annu Rev Immunol. 1986;4:389–417.
25. Tomsai TB, Plaut AG. Humoral aspects of mucosal immunity. In: Gallin J, Fauci A, eds. Advances in Host Defense Mechanisms. New York: Raven; 1985:31–62.
26. Childers NK, Bruce MG, McGhee JR. Molecular mechanisms of immunoglobulin A defense. Annu Rev Microbiol. 1989;43:503–536.
27. Mestecky J, McGhee JR. Immunoglobulin A (IgA): Molecular and cellular interaction involved in IgA biosynthesis and immune response. Adv Immunol. 1987;40:153–189.
28. Lamm ME. Cellular aspects of immunoglobulin A. Adv Immunol. 1976;22:223–290.
29. Mostov KE, Deitcher DL. Polymeric immunoglobulin receptor expressed in MDCK cells transcytoses IgA. Cell. 1986;46:613–621.
30. Mellander L, Bjorkander J, Carlsson B, et al. Secretory antibodies in IgA-deficient and immunosuppressed individuals. J Clin Immunol. 1986;6:284–290.
31. Sixbey JW, Yao QY. Immunoglobulin A-induced shift of Epstein-Barr virus tissue tropism. Science. 1992;255:1578–1580.
32. Kaetzel CS, Robinson JK, Chintalacharuvu KR, et al. The polymeric immunoglobulin receptor (secretory component) mediates transport of immune complexes across epithelial cells: A local defense function for IgA. Proc Natl Acad Sci U S A. 1991;88:8796–8800.
33. Welsh JK, May JT. Antiinfective properties of breast milk. J Pediatr. 1979;94:1–9.
34. Ogra PL, Karzon DT, Righthand F, et al. Immunoglobulin response in serum and secretions after immunization with live and inactivated poliovaccine and natural infection. N Engl J Med. 1968;279:894–902.
35. Heyworth MF. Immunology of *Giardia* and *Cryptosporidium* infections. J Infect Dis. 1992;166:465–472.
36. Bessen D, Fischetti VA. Passive acquired mucosal immunity to group A streptococci by secretory immunoglobulin A. J Exp Med. 1988;167:1945–1950.
37. Phalipon A, Kaufmann M, Michetti P, et al. Monoclonal immunoglobulin A antibody directed against serotype-specific epitope of *Shigella flexneri* lipopolysaccharide protects against murine experimental shigellosis. J Exp Med. 1995;182:769–778.
38. Hostoffer RW, Krukovets I, Berger M. Increased FcαR expression and IgA-mediated function on neutrophils induced by chemoattractants. J Immunol. 1993;150:4532–4540.
39. Kilian M, Mestecky J, Russell MW. Defense mechanisms involving Fc-dependent functions of immunoglobulin A and their subversion by bacterial immunoglobulin A proteases. Microbiol Rev. 1988;52:296–303.
40. Stokes CR, Soothill JF, Turner MW. Immune exclusion is a function of IgA. Nature. 1975;255:745–746.
41. Walker W, Isselbacher KJ, Block K. Intestinal uptake of macromolecules: Effect of oral immunization. Science. 1972;177:608–610.
42. Burks A, Steele RW. Selective IgA deficiency. Ann Allergy. 1986;57:3–8.
43. Metzger H, Alcaraz G, Hohman R, et al. The receptor with high affinity for immunoglobulin E. Annu Rev Immunol. 1986;4:419–470.
44. Jarrett EE, Miller H. Production and activities of IgE in helminth infection. Prog Allergy. 1982;31:178–184.
45. Miller H. The protective mucosal response against gastrointestinal nematodes in ruminants and laboratory animals. Vet Immunol Immunopathol. 1984;6:167–174.
46. Hagan P, Blumenthal U, Dunn D, et al. Human IgE, IgG4 and resistance to reinfection with *Schistosoma haematobium*. Nature. 1991;349:243–246.
47. King CL, Xianli J, Malhotra I, et al. Mice with a targeted deletion of the IgE gene have increased worm burdens and reduced granulomatous inflammation following primary infection with *Schistosoma mansoni*. J Immunol. 1997;158:294–300.
48. Capron A, Dessaint JP. Immunologic aspects of schistosomiasis. Annu Rev Med. 1992;43:209–218.
49. Lantz CS, Boesiger J, Song CH, et al. Role for interleukin-3 in mast-cell and basophil development and in immunity to parasites. Nature. 1998;392:90–93.
50. Zuckier LS, Rodriguez LD, Scharff MD. Immunological and pharmacological concepts of monoclonal antibodies. Semin Nucl Med. 1989;19:166–186.
51. Liu Z, Roopenian DC, Zhou X, et al. β2-Microglobulin–deficient mice are resistant to bullous pemphigoid. J Exp Med. 1997;186:777–783.
52. Ravetch J, Margulies DH. New tricks for old molecules. Nature. 1994;372:323–324.
53. Fridman WH. Fc receptors and immunoglobulin binding factors. FASEB J. 1991;5:2684–2690.
54. Ravetch JV, Kinet JP. Fc receptors. Annu Rev Immunol. 1991;9:457–492.
55. Daeron M. Fc receptor biology. Annu Rev Immunol. 1997;15:203–234.
56. Conrad DH. FcεRII/CD23: The low affinity receptor for IgE. Annu Rev Immunol. 1990;8:623–645.
57. Huizinga T, van Kemenade F, Koenderman L, et al. The 40-kDa Fcγ receptor (FcγRII) on human neutrophils is essential for the IgG-induced respiratory burst and IgG-induced phagocytosis. J Immunol. 1989;142:2365–2369.
58. Debets JM, Van der Linden CJ, Dieteren IEM, et al. Fc-receptor cross-linking induces rapid secretion of tumor necrosis factor (cachectin) by human peripheral blood monocytes. J Immunol. 1988;141:1197–1201.
59. Bich-Thuy LT, Revillard JP. Selective suppression of human B lymphocyte differ-

entiation into IgG-producing cells by soluble Fc receptors. J Immunol. 1982;129:150–159.
60. Azzoni L, Kamoun M, Salcedo TW, et al. Stimulation of FcγRIIIA results in phospholipase C-γ1 tyrosine phosphorylation and p56[lck] activation. J Exp Med. 1992;176:1745–1750.
61. Cassatella M, Anegon I, Cuturi MC, et al. FcγR (CD16) interaction with ligand induces Ca^{2+} mobilization and phosphoinositide turnover in human natural killer cells: Role in transcription and expression of lymphokine genes. J Exp Med. 1989;169:549–567.
62. Hibbs ML, Selvaraj P, Carpen O, et al. Mechanisms for regulating expression of membrane isoforms of FcγRIII (CD16). Science. 1989;246:1608–1611.
63. Blank U, Ra C, Miller L, et al. Complete structure and expression in transfected cells of high affinity IgE receptor. Nature. 1989;337:187–189.
64. Paul WE, Seder RA, Plaut M. Lymphokine and cytokine production by FcεRI+ cells. Adv Immunol. 1993;53:1–29.
65. Kehry MR, Yamashita LC. Role of the low-affinity Fcε receptor in B-lymphocyte antigen presentation. Res Immunol. 1990;141:77–81.
66. Maliszewski CR, March CJ, Schoenborn MA, et al. Expression cloning of a human Fc receptor for IgA. J Exp Med. 1990;172:1665–1672.
67. Shen L, Lasser R, Fanger MW. My43, a monoclonal antibody that reacts with human myeloid cells, inhibits monocyte IgA binding and triggers function. J Immunol. 1989;143:4117–4121.
68. Burton DR. Immunoglobulin G: Functional sites. Mol Immunol. 1985;22:161–206.
69. Borsos T, Rapp HJ. Complement fixation on cell surfaces by 19S and 7S antibodies. Science. 1965;150:505–506.
70. Frank M, Joiner K, Hammer C. The function of antibody and complement in the lysis of bacteria. Rev Infect Dis. 1987;9:S537–S545.
71. Giebink GS, Verhoef J, Peterson P. Opsonic requirements for phagocytosis of *Streptococcus pneumoniae* types VI, XVIII, XXIII, and XXV. Infect Immunol. 1977;18:291–297.
72. Anderson P, Johnston R. Human serum activities against *Haemophilus influenzae*, type B. J Clin Invest. 1972;51:31–38.
73. Peterson P, Wilkinson B, Kim Y, et al. The key role of peptidoglycan in the opsonization of *Staphylococcus aureus*. J Clin Invest. 1978;61:597–609.
74. Horowitz MA. Phagocytosis of microorganisms. Rev Infect Dis. 1982;4:104–118.
75. Schneiderman RD, Lint TL, Knight KL. Activation of the alternative pathway of complement by 12 different rabbit-mouse chimeric transfectoma IgA isotypes. J Immunol. 1990;145:233–237.
76. Pfaffenbach G, Lamm ME, Gigli I. Activation of the guinea pig alternative complement pathway by mouse IgA immune complexes. J Exp Med. 1982;155:231–247.
77. Fanger MW, Erbe DV. Fc gamma receptors in cancer and infectious disease. Immunol Res. 1992;11:203–216.
78. Anderson CL, Shen L, Eicher DM. Phagocytosis mediated by three distinct Fcγ receptor classes on human leukocytes. J Exp Med. 1990;171:1333–1345.
79. Johnston R, Anderson P, Rosen F, et al. Characterization of human antibody to polyribose phosphate, the capsular antigen of *Haemophilus influenzae* type B. Clin Immunol Immunopathol. 1973;1:234–240.
80. Yuan RR, Clynes R, Oh J, et al. Antibody-mediated modulation of *Cryptococcus neoformans* infection is dependent on distinct Fc receptor functions and IgG subclass. J Exp Med. 1998;187:641–648.
81. Clark RA, Klebanoff SJ. Studies on the mechanism of antibody-dependent polymorphonuclear leukocyte-mediated cytotoxicity. J Immunol. 1977;119:1413–1418.
82. Sissons J, Oldstone M. Killing of virus infected cells by cytotoxic lymphocytes. J Infect Dis. 1980;142:114–119.
83. Trinchieri G. Biology of natural killer cells. Adv Immunol. 1989;47:187–376.
84. Fanger MW, Shen, L, Graziano, RF, et al. Cytotoxicity mediated by human Fc receptors for IgG. Immunol Today. 1989;10:92–99.
85. Ehrlich P. Die Wertbemessung des Diphtherieheilserums und deren theoretische Grundlagen. Klin Jahrbuch. 1897;6:299–312.
86. Blake PA, Feldman RA, Buchanan TM, et al. Serologic therapy of tetanus in the United States, 1965–1971. JAMA. 1976;235:42–44.
87. Metzer JF, Lewis GE. Human-derived immune globulins for the treatment of botulism. Rev Infect Dis. 1979;1:689–694.
88. English PC. Diphtheria and theories of infectious disease: Centennial appreciation of the critical role of diphtheria in the history of medicine. Pediatrics. 1985;71:1–9.
89. Johns M, Skehill A, McCabe WR. Immunization with rough mutants of *Salmonella minnesota*: IV. Protection by antisera to O and rough antigens of endotoxin. J Infect Dis. 1983;147:57–63.
90. Ziegler E, McCutchan J, Fierer J, et al. Treatment of gram-negative bacteremia and shock with human antiserum to a mutant *Escherichia coli*. N Engl J Med. 1982;307:1225–1230.
91. Ziegler E, Fisher C, Sprung C, et al. Treatment of gram-negative bacteremia and septic shock with HA-1A human monoclonal antibody against endotoxin: A randomized, double-blind, placebo-controlled trial. N Engl J Med. 1991;324:429–436.
92. Greenman R, Schein R, Martin M, et al. A controlled clinical trial of E5 murine monoclonal IgM antibody to endotoxin in the treatment of gram-negative sepsis. JAMA. 1991;266:1097–1102.
93. Reid RR, Prodeus AP, Khan W, et al. Endotoxin shock in antibody-deficient mice: Unraveling the role of natural antibody and complement in the clearance of lipopolysaccharide. J Immunol. 1997;159:970–975.
94. Mandel B. Neutralization of animal viruses. Adv Virus Res. 1974;23:205–269.
95. Dimmock NJ. Mechanisms of neutralization of animal viruses. J Gen Virol. 1984;65:1015–1022.
96. Taylor HP, Dimmock NJ. Mechanism of neutralization of influenza virus by secretory IgA is different from that of monomeric IgA or IgG. J Exp Med. 1985;161:198–209.
97. Rossman MG. Neutralization of small RNA viruses by antibodies and antiviral agents. FASEB J. 1989;3:2335–2343.
98. Armstrong SJ, Dimmock NJ. Neutralization of influenza virus by low concentrations of hemagglutinin-specific polymeric immunoglobulin A inhibits viral fusion activity, but activation of the ribonucleoprotein is also inhibited. J Virol. 1992;66:3823–3832.
99. Mazanec MB, Kaetzel CS, Lamm ME, et al. Intracellular neutralization of virus by immunoglobulin A antibodies. Proc Natl Acad Sci U S A. 1992;89:6901–6905.
100. Burns JW, Siadat-Pajouh M, Krishnaney AA, et al. Protective effect of rotavirus VP6-specific IgA monoclonal antibodies that lack neutralizing activity. Science. 1996;272:104–107.
101. Finlay BB, Falkow S. Common themes in microbial pathogenicity. Microbiol Rev. 1989;53:210–230.
102. Williams RC, Gibbons RJ. Inhibition of bacterial adherence by secretory immunoglobulin A: A mechanism of antigen disposal. Science. 1972;177:697–699.
103. Moss RB. Hypergammaglobulinemia in cystic fibrosis. Chest. 1987;91:523–526.
104. Phair J, Clarke J. Immunology of infective endocarditis. Prog Cardiovasc Dis. 1979;22:137–144.
105. Kobayakawa T, Louis J, Izui S, et al. Autoimmune response to DNA, red blood cells and thymocyte antigens in association with polyclonal antibody synthesis during experimental African trypanosomiasis. J Immunol. 1979;122:296–301.
106. Carter RL. Antibody formation in infectious mononucleosis: II. Other 19S antibodies and false positive serology. Br J Haematol. 1966;12:268–272.
107. Drenth JPH, Haagsma CJ, van der Meer JWM. Hyperimmunoglobulinemia D and periodic fever syndrome: The clinical spectrum in a series of 50 patients. Medicine (Baltimore). 1994;73:133–144.
108. Hoiby N, During G, Schiotz K. The role of immune complexes in the pathogenesis of bacterial infections. Annu Rev Microbiol. 1986;40:29–53.
109. Couser WG. Mechanisms of glomerular injury in immune-complex disease. Kidney Int. 1985;28:569–583.
110. Stickler GB, Shin M, Burke E. Diffuse glomerulonephritis associated with infected ventriculoatrial shunt. N Engl J Med. 1968;279:1077–1082.
111. Schifferli J, Ng YC, Peters DK. The role of complement and its receptor in the elimination of immune complexes. N Engl J Med. 1986;315:488–495.
112. Carson DA, Chen PP, Fox RI, et al. Rheumatoid factor and immune networks. Annu Rev Immunol. 1987;5:109–126.
113. Radoux V, Chen PP, Sorge JA, et al. A conserved human germline V gene directly encodes rheumatoid factor light chains. J Exp Med. 1986;164:2119–2124.
114. Pascual V, Randen I, Thompson K, et al. The complete nucleotide sequences of the heavy chain variable regions of six monospecific rheumatoid factors derived from Epstein-Barr virus-transformed B cells isolated from the synovial tissue of patients with rheumatoid arthritis. J Clin Invest. 1990;86:1320–1328.
115. Roosnek E, Lanzavecchia A. Efficient and selective presentation of antigen-antibody complexes by rheumatoid factor B cells. J Exp Med. 1991;173:487–489.
116. Agnello V, Chung RT, Kaplan LM. A role for hepatitis C virus infection in type II cryoglobulinemia. N Engl J Med. 1992;327:1490–1495.
117. Misiani R, Bellavita P, Fenili D, et al. Hepatitis C virus infection in patients with essential mixed cryoglobulinemia. Ann Intern Med. 1992;117:573–577.
118. Fritzler MJ, Salazar M. Diversity and origin of rheumatologic autoantibodies. Clin Microbiol Rev. 1991;4:256–269.
119. Van Voorhis WC, Schlekewy L, Trong HL. Molecular mimicry by *Trypanosoma cruzi*: The Fl-160 epitope that mimics mammalian nerve can be mapped to a 12-amino acid peptide. Proc Natl Acad Sci U S A. 1991;88:5993–5997.
120. Cohen IR, Young DB. Autoimmunity, microbial immunity and the immunological homunculus. Immunol Today. 1991;12:105–107.
121. Dale JB, Beachey EH. Epitopes of streptococcal M proteins shared with cardiac myosins. J Exp Med. 1985;162:583–591.
122. Tonegawa S. Somatic generation of antibody diversity. Nature. 1983;302:575–581.
123. Alt FW, Blackwell TK, Yancopoulos G. Development of the primary antibody repertoire. Science. 1987;238:1079–1087.
124. Yancopoulos GD, Alt FW. Regulation of the assembly and expression of variable-region genes. Annu Rev Immunol. 1986;4:339–368.
125. Schatz DG, Oettinger MA, Schlissel MS. V(D)J recombination: Molecular biology and regulation. Annu Rev Immunol. 1992;10:359–383.
126. Ramsden DA, Paull TT, Gellert M. Cell-free V(D)J recombination. Nature. 1997;388:488–491.
127. Landau NR, Schatz DG, Rosa M, et al. Increased frequency of N-regional insertion in a murine pre-B-cell line infected with a terminal deoxynucleotidyl transferase retroviral expression vector. Mol Cell Biol. 1987;7:3237–3243.
128. Harriman W, Volk H, Defranoux N, et al. Immunoglobulin class switch recombination. Annu Rev Immunol. 1993;11:361–384.
129. Coffman RL, Lebman DA, Rothman P. Mechanism and regulation of immunoglobulin isotype switching. Adv Immunol. 1993;54:229–270.
130. French DL, Laskov R, Scharff M. The role of somatic hypermutation in the generation of antibody diversity. Science. 1989;244:1152–1157.
131. Banchereau J, Rousset F. Human B lymphocytes: Phenotype, proliferation, and differentiation. Adv Immunol. 1992;52:125–251.
132. Clark EA, Lane PJ. Regulation of human B-cell activation and adhesion. Annu Rev Immunol. 1991;9:97–127.
133. Reth M. Antigen receptors on B lymphocytes. Annu Rev Immunol. 1992;10:97–121.

134. Tarlinton D. Antigen presentation by memory B cells: The sting is in the tail. Science. 1997;276:374–375.
135. Malissen B, Schmitt-Verhulst AM. Transmembrane signalling through the T cell receptor-CD3 complex. Curr Opin Immunol. 1993;5:324–333.
136. Clark M, Campbell K, Kazlauskas A, et al. The B cell antigen receptor complex: Association of Ig-α and Ig-β with distinct cytoplasmic effectors. Science. 1992;258:123–126.
137. Dempsey PW, Allison MED, Akkaraju S, et al. C3d of complement as a molecular adjuvant: Bridging innate and acquired immunity. Science. 1996;271:348–350.
138. Reth M, Wienands J. Initiation and processing of signals from the B cell antigen receptor. Annu Rev Immunol. 1997;15:453–479.
139. Parker DC. T cell-dependent B cell activation. Annu Rev Immunol. 1993;11:331–360.
140. Mitchinson NA. The carrier effect in the secondary response to hapten-carrier conjugates: II. Cellular cooperation. Eur J Immunol. 1971;1:18–26.
141. Germain RN, Margulies DH. The biochemistry and cell biology of antigen processing and presentation. Annu Rev Immunol. 1993;11:403–450.
142. Chestnut RW, Grey HM. Antigen presentation by B cells and its significance in T-B interactions. Adv Immunol. 1986;39:51–95.
143. Van de Velde H, von Hoegen I, Luo W, et al. The B-cell surface protein CD72/Lyb-2 is the ligand for CD5. Nature. 1991;351:662–665.
144. Linsley PS, Ledbetter JA. The role of the CD28 receptor during T cell responses to antigen. Annu Rev Immunol. 1993;11:191–212.
145. Banchereau J, Rousset F. Growing human B lymphocytes in the CD40 system. Nature. 1991;353:678–679.
146. Aruffo A, Farrington, M, Hollenbaugh D, et al. The CD40 ligand, gp39, is defective in activated T cells from patients with X-linked hyper-IgM syndrome. Cell. 1993;72:291–300.
147. Fischer A, Durandy A, Sterkers G. Role of the LFA-1 molecule in cellular interactions required for antibody production in humans. J Immunol. 1986;136:3198–3203.
148. Mond JJ, Lees A, Snapper CM. T cell-independent antigens type 2. Annu Rev Immunol. 1995;13:655–692.
149. Santosham M, Wolff M, Reid R, et al. The efficacy in Navajo infants of a conjugate vaccine consisting of *Haemophilus influenzae* type b polysaccharide and *Neisseria meningitidis* outer-membrane protein complex. N Engl J Med. 1991;324:1767–1772.
150. Cooper MD. B lymphocytes: Normal development and function. N Engl J Med. 1987;317:1452–1456.
151. Rajewsky K. Clonal selection and learning in the antibody system. Nature. 1996;381:751–757.
152. Motyka B, Reynolds JD. Apoptosis is associated with the extensive B cell death in the sheep ileal Peyer's patch and the chicken bursa of Fabricius: A possible role in B cell selection. Eur J Immunol. 1991;21:1951–1958.
153. Cohen J, Duke RC, Fadoik VA, et al. Apoptosis and programmed cell death in immunity. Annu Rev Immunol. 1992;10:267–294.
154. Goodnow CC. B-cell tolerance. Curr Opin Immunol. 1992;4:703–710.
155. Goodnow CC, Brink R, Adams E. Breakdown of self-tolerance in anergic B lymphocytes. Nature. 1991;352:532–536.
156. Brink R, Goodnow CC, Crosbie J, et al. Immunoglobulin M and D antigen receptors are both capable of mediating B lymphocyte activation, deletion, or anergy after interaction with specific antigen. J Exp Med. 1992;176:991–1005.
157. Roes J, Rajewsky K. Immunoglobulin D (IgD)-deficient mice reveal an auxiliary receptor function for IgD in antigen-mediated recruitment of B cells. J Exp Med. 1993;177:43–55.
158. Liu YJ. Sites of B lymphocyte selection, activation and tolerance in spleen. J Exp Med. 1997;186:625–629.
159. Foote J, Milstein C. Kinetic maturation of an immune response. Nature. 1991;352:530–532.
160. Jacob J, Kelsoe G, Rajewsky K, et al. Intraclonal generation of antibody mutants in germinal centers. Nature. 1991;354:389–392.
161. Liu YJ. Reuse of B lymphocytes in germinal centers. Science. 1997;278:238–239.
162. Schriever F, Nadler LM. The central role of follicular dendritic cells in lymphoid tissue. Adv Immunol. 1992;51:243–284.
163. Gray D. Immunological memory. Annu Rev Immunol. 1993;11:49–77.
164. Kearney JF. $CD5^+$ B-cell networks. Curr Opin Immunol. 1993;5:223–226.
165. Kantor AB, Herzenberg LA. Origin of murine B cell lineages. Annu Rev Immunol. 1993;11:501–538.
166. Briles DE, Nahm M, Schroer K, et al. Antiphosphorylcholine antibodies found in normal mouse serum are protective against intravenous infections with type 3 *S. pneumoniae*. J Exp Med. 1981;153:694–705.
167. Goni F, Frangione B. Amino acid sequence of the Fv region of a human monoclonal IgM (protein WEA) with antibody activity against 3,4-pyruvylated galactose in *Klebsiella* polysaccharides K30 and K33. Proc Natl Acad Sci U S A. 1983;80:4837–4841.
168. Pisetsky DS. DNA and the immune system. Ann Intern Med. 1997;126:169–171.
169. Murphy DB. T cell mediated immunosuppression. Curr Opin Immunol. 1993;5:411–417.
170. Nisonoff A. Idiotypes: Concepts and applications. J Immunol. 1991;147:2429–2438.
171. Conley ME. Molecular approaches to analysis of X-linked immunodeficiencies. Annu Rev Immunol. 1992;10:215–238.
172. Hermaszewski RA, Webster AD. Primary hypogammaglobulinaemia: A survey of clinical manifestations and complications. QJM. 1993;86:31–42.
173. Buckley RH. Immunodeficiency diseases. JAMA. 1992;268:2797–2806.
174. Sneller MC, Strober W, Eisenstein E, et al. New insights into common variable immundeficiency. Ann Intern Med. 1993;118:720–730.
175. Spickett GP, Misbah SA, Chapel HM. Primary antibody deficiency in adults. Lancet. 1991;337:281–284.
176. Rosen FS, Cooper MD, Wedgwood RJ. The primary immunodeficiencies. N Engl J Med. 1995;333:431–440.
177. Saulsbury FT, Winkelstein JA, Yolken RH. Chronic rotavirus infection in immunodeficiency. J Pediatr. 1980;97:61–65.
178. Roberts-Thomson IC. Genetic studies of human and murine giardiasis. Clin Infect Dis. 1993;16(Suppl 2):S98–S104.
179. Abramowsky CR, Sorensen RU. Regional enteritis-like enteropathy in a patient with agammaglobulinemia: Histologic and immunocytologic studies. Hum Pathol. 1988;19:483–490.
180. Lee AH, Levinson AI, Schumacher HR. Hypogammaglobulinemia and rheumatic disease. Semin Arthritis Rheum. 1993;22:252–264.
181. Forgacs P, Kundsin RB, Margles SW, et al. A case of *Ureaplasma urealyticum* septic arthritis in a patient with hypogammaglobulinemia. Clin Infect Dis. 1993;16:293–294.
182. Crennan JM, Van Scoy RE, McKenna CH, et al. Echovirus polymyositits in patients with hypogammaglobulinemia: Failure of high-dose intravenous gammaglobulin therapy and review of the literature. Am J Med. 1986;81:35–42.
183. Sneller MC, Strober W. Abnormalities of lymphokine gene expression in patients with common variable immunodeficiency. J Immunol. 1990;144:3762–3769.
184. McKinney RE, Katz SE, Wilfert CM. Chronic enteroviral meningoencephalitis in agammaglobulinemic patients. Rev Infect Dis. 1987;9:334–356.
185. Saulsbury FT, Bernstein MT, Winkelstein JA. *Pneumocystis carinii* pneumonia as the presenting infection in congenital hypogammaglobulinemia. J Pediatr. 1979;95:559–561.
186. Webster A, Platts-Mills T, Jannossy G, et al. Autoimmune blood dyscrasias in five patients with hypogammaglobulinemia: Response of neutropenia to vincristine. J Clin Immunol. 1981;1:113–118.
187. Straus SE, Seidlin M, Takiff H, et al. Oral acyclovir to suppress recurring herpes simplex virus infections in immunodeficient patients. Ann Intern Med. 1984;100:522–524.
188. Lopez M, Fleisher T, deShazo RD. Use and interpretation of diagnostic immunologic laboratory tests. JAMA. 1992;268:2970–2990.
189. Weinberg KI, Kohn DB. Gene therapy for congenital immunodeficiency diseases. Immunol Allergy Clin North Am. 1996;16:453–476.
190. Gross S, Blaiss MS, Herrod HG. Role of immunoglobulin subclasses and specific antibody determinations in the evaluation of recurrent infection in children. J Pediatr. 1992;121:516–522.
191. Buckley RH, Schiff RI. The use of intravenous immune globulin in immunodeficiency diseases. N Engl J Med. 1991;325:110–117.
192. Stiehm ER, Ashida E, Kim KS, et al. Intravenous immunoglobulins as therapeutic agents. Ann Intern Med. 1987;107:367–382.
193. Berkman SA, Lee ML, Gale RP. Clinical uses of intravenous immunogloblulins. Ann Intern Med. 1990;112:278–292.
194. Liese JG, Wintergerst U, Tympner KD, et al. High- vs low-dose immunoglobulin therapy in the long-term treatment of X-linked agammaglobulinemia. Am J Dis Child. 1992;146:335–339.
195. Gardulf A, Andersen V, Bjorkander J, et al. Subcutaneous immunoglobulin replacement in patients with primary antibody deficiencies: Safety and costs. Lancet. 1995;345:365–369.
196. Kobayashi RH, Dobayashi AD, Lee N, et al. Home self-administration of intravenous immunoglobulin therapy in children. Pediatrics. 1990;85:705–709.
197. Burks AW, Sampson HA, Buckley RH. Anaphylactic reactions after gamma globulin administration in patients with hypogammaglobulinemia: Detection of IgE antibodies to IgA. N Engl J Med. 1986;314:560–564.
198. Bjoro K, Froland SS, Yun Z, et al. Hepatitis C infection in patients with primary hypogammaglobulinemia after treatment with contaminated immune globulin. N Engl J Med. 1994;331:1607–1611.
199. Cournoyer D, Caskey CT. Gene therapy of the immune system. Annu Rev Immunol. 1993;11:297–329.
200. Bruton OC. Agammaglobulinemia. Pediatrics. 1952;9:722–728.
201. Vetrie D, Vorechovsky I, Sideras P, et al. The gene involved in X-linked agammaglobulinaemia is a member of the *src* family of protein-tyrosine kinases. Nature. 1993;361:226–233.
202. Yel L, Minegishi Y, Coustan-Smith E, et al. Mutations in the mu heavy-chain gene in patients with agammaglobulinemia. N Engl J Med. 1996;335:1486–1493.
203. Lederman HM, Winkelstein JA. X-linked agammaglobulinemia: An analysis of 96 patients. Medicine (Baltimore). 1985;64:145–156.
204. Pezacalsakak G, Lim J, Good R. B lymphocytes in primary and secondary deficiencies of humoral immunity. Birth Defects. 1975;11:33–38.
205. Fleisher T, White R, Broder S, et al. X-linked hypogammaglobulinemia and isolated growth hormone deficiency. N Engl J Med. 1980;302:1492–1534.
206. Tiller TL, Buckley R. Transient hypogammaglobulinemia of infancy: Review of the literature, clinical and immunologic features of 11 new cases, and long-term follow up. J Pediatr. 1978;92:347–353.
207. McGready SJ. Transient hypogammaglobulinemia of infancy: Need to reconsider name and definition. J Pediatr. 1987;110:47–50.
208. Hermans P, Diaz-Buxo J, Stobo J. Idiopathic late onset immunoglobulin deficiency: Clinical observations in 50 patients. Am J Med. 1976;61:221–232.
209. Sicherer SH, Winkelstein JA. Primary immunodeficiency diseases in adults. JAMA. 1998;279:58–61.
210. Volanakis J, Zhu Z, Schaffer F, et al. Major histocompatibility complex III genes

and susceptibility to immunoglobulin A deficiency and common variable immunodeficiency. J Clin Invest. 1992;89:1914–1922.
211. Spickett GP, Webster A, Farrant J. Cellular abnormalities in common variable immunodeficiency. Immunodeficiency Rev. 1990;2:199–219.
212. Eisenstein EM, Jaffe J, Sneller MC, et al. Impaired and intact differentiation pathways in CD4 lymphocytes of patients with common variable immunodeficiency. J Allergy Clin Immunol. 1992;89:167.
213. Spickett GP, Zhang JG, Green T, et al. Granulomatous disease in common variable immunodeficiency: Effect on immunoglobulin replacement therapy and response to steroids and splenectomy. J Clin Pathol. 1996;49:431–434.
214. Aukrust P, Lien E, Kristoffersen AK, et al. Persistent activation of the tumor necrosis factor system in a subgroup of patients with common variable immunodeficiency: Possible immunologic and clinical consequences. Blood. 1996;87:674–681.
215. Fasano MB, Sullivan KE, Sarpong SB, et al. Sarcoidosis and common variable immunodeficiency: Report of 8 cases and review of the literature. Medicine (Baltimore). 1996;75:251–261.
216. Kinlen LJ, Webster A, Bird A, et al. Prospective study of cancer in patients with hypogammaglobulinaemia. Lancet. 1985;1:263–265.
217. Cunningham-Rundles C, Kazbay K, Hassett J, et al. Enhanced humoral immunity in common variable immunodeficiency after long-term treatment with polyethylene glycol-conjugated interleukin-2. N Engl J Med. 1994;331:918–921.
218. Levitt D, Haber P, Rich K, et al. Hyper IgM immunodeficiency. J Clin Invest. 1983;72:1650–1657.
219. Geha RS, Hyslop N, Alami S, et al. Hyper immunoglobulin M immunodeficiency (dysgammaglobulinemia). J Clin Invest. 1979;64:385–391.
220. Ammann AJ, Hong R. Selective IgA deficiency: Presentation of 30 cases and a review of the literature. Medicine (Baltimore). 1971;50:223–236.
221. Van Loghem E, Zegers BJM, Bast EJEG, et al. Selective deficiency of immunoglobulin A2. J Clin Invest. 1983;72:1918–1923.
222. Migane N, Oliviero S, DeLange G, et al. Multiple-gene deletions within the human immunoglobulin heavy chain cluster. Proc Natl Acad Sci U S A. 1984;81:5811–5815.
223. Carbonara A, Demarchi M. Genetics and techniques: Ig isotype deficiency caused by gene deletions. Monogr Allergy. 1986;20:13–17.
224. Cunningham-Rundles C, Brandeis W, Good R, et al. Milk precipitins, circulating immune complexes and IgA deficiency. Proc Natl Acad Sci U S A. 1978;75:3387–3392.
225. Schur P, Borel H, Gelfand G, et al. Selective gamma-G globulin deficiencies in patients with recurrent pyogenic infections. N Engl J Med. 1970;283:631–635.
226. Lefranc MP, Hammarstrom L, Smith C. Gene deletions in the human immunoglobulin heavy chain constant region locus: Molecular and immunological analysis. Immunol Rev. 1991;2:265–281.
227. Umetsu DT, Ambrosino DM, Geha RS. Children with selective IgG subclass deficiency and recurrent sinopulmonary infection: Impaired response to bacterial capsular polysaccharide antigens. Mongr Allergy. 1986;20:57–61.
228. Insel RA, Anderson PW. Response to oligosaccharide-protein conjugate vaccine against *Haemophilus influenzae* b in two patients with IgG2 deficiency unresponsive to capsular polysaccharide vaccine. N Engl J Med. 1986;315:499–503.
229. Standen GR. Wiskott-Aldrich syndrome: A multidisciplinary disease. J Clin Pathol. 1991;44:979–982.
230. Perry GS, Spector B, Schuman L, et al. The Wiskott-Alrich syndrome in the United States and Canada (1892–1979). J Pediatr. 1980;97:72–78.
231. Derry JM, Ochs HD, Francke U. Isolation of a novel gene mutated in Wiskott-Aldrich syndrome. Cell. 1994;78:635–644.
232. Spitler LE, Levein AS, Stites DP, et al. The Wiskott-Aldrich syndrome: Immunologic studies in nine patients and selected family members. Cell Immunol. 1975;19:201–218.
233. Woods CG, Taylor AM. Ataxia telangiectasia in the British Isles: The clinical and laboratory features of 70 affected individuals. QJM. 1992;82:169–179.
234. Baskaran R, Wood LD, Whitaker LL, et al. Ataxia telangiectasia mutant protein activates c-Abl tyrosine kinase in response to ionizing radiation. Science. 1997;387:516–523.
235. Ultmann J, Winthrop F, Osserman E, et al. The clinical implications of hypogammaglobulinemia in patients with chronic lymphocytic leukemia and lymphocytic lymphosarcoma. Ann Intern Med. 1959;51:501–516.
236. Chapel HM, Bunch C. Mechanisms of infection in chronic lymphocytic leukemia. Semin Hematol. 1987;24:291–296.
237. Cooperative Group for the Study of Immunoglobulin in Chronic Lymphocytic Leukemia. Intravenous immunoglobulin for the prevention of infection in chronic lymphocytic leukemia: A randomized, controlled clinical trial. N Engl J Med. 1988;319:902–907.
238. Weeks JC, Tierney MR, Weinstein MC. Cost effectiveness of prophylactic intravenous immune globulin in chronic lymphocytic leukemia. N Engl J Med. 1991;325:81–86.
239. Birgens H, Esperson F, Hertz J, et al. Antibody response to pneumococcal vaccination in patients with myelomatosis. Scand J Haematol. 1982;30:324–330.
240. Pilarksi LM, Andrews E, Mant MJ, et al. Humoral immune deficiency in multiple myeloma patients due to compromised B cell function. J Clin Immunol. 1986;6:491–501.
241. Meyers BR, Hirschman SZ, Axelrod J. Current patterns of infection in multiple myeloma. Am J Med. 1972;52:87–92.
242. Savage DG, Lindenbaum J, Garrett T. Biphasic pattern of bacterial infection in multiple myeloma. Ann Intern Med. 1982;96:47–50.
243. Chapel HM, Lee M, Hargreaves R, et al. Randomised trial of intravenous immunoglobulin as prophylaxis against infection in plateau-phase multiple myeloma. Lancet. 1994;343:1059–1063.
244. Miller DG. Patterns of immunologic deficiency in lymphomas and leukemias. Ann Intern Med. 1972;57:703–706.
245. Weitzman SA, Aisenberg AC, Siber GR. Impaired humoral immunity in treated Hodgkin's disease. N Engl J Med. 1977;297:245–248.
246. Hansbrough J, Miller L, Field T, et al. High dose intravenous immunoglobulin therapy in burn patients: Pharmacokinetics and effects on microbial opsonization and phagocytosis. Pediatr Infect Dis J. 1988;7:S49–S56.
247. Bohnsack JF, Brown EJ. The role of the spleen in resistance to infection. Annu Rev Med. 1986;37:49–59.
248. Hosea S, Brown E, Hamburger M, et al. Opsonic requirements for intravascular clearance after splenectomy. N Engl J Med. 1981;304:245–250.
249. Lockwood CM. Immunological functions of the spleen. Clin Haematol. 1983;12:449–465.
250. Brigden ML. Overwhelming postsplenectomy infections still a problem. West J Med. 1992;157:440–443.
251. Styrt B. Infection associated with asplenia: Risks, mechanisms, and prevention. Am J Med. 1990;88(5N):33N–42N.
252. Brown E, Hosea SW, Frank MM. The role of the spleen in experimental pneumococcal bacteremia. J Clin Invest. 1981;67:975–982.
253. Bolan G, Broome CV, Facklam RR, et al. Pneumococcal vaccine efficacy in selected populations int he United States. Ann Intern Med. 1986;104:1–6.
254. Konradsen HB, Pedersen F, Henrichsen J. Pneumococcal revaccination of splenectomized children. Pediatr Infect Dis J. 1990;9:258–263.
255. Grimfors G, Soderqvist M, Holm G, et al. A longitudinal study of class and subclass antibody responses to pneumococcal vaccination in splenectomized individuals with special reference to patients with Hodgkin's disease. Eur J Haematol. 1990;45:101–108.
256. Ambrosino D, Lee M, Chen D, et al. Response to *Haemophilus influenzae* type B conjugate vaccine in children undergoing splenectomy. J Pediatr Surg. 1992;27:1045–1047.
257. Ruben F, Hankins WA, Zeigler Z, et al. Antibody response to meningococcal polysaccharide vaccine in adults without a spleen. Am J Med. 1984;76:115–121.
258. Murdoch IA, Dos Anjos R. Continued need for pneumococcal prophylaxis after splenectomy. Arch Dis Child. 1990;65:1268–1269.
259. Working Party of the British Committee for Standards in Haematology Clincal Hematology Task Force. Guidelines for the prevention and treatment of infection in patients with an absent or dysfunctional spleen. BMJ. 1996;312:430–434.
260. Siber GR, Goman C, Martin P, et al. Antibody response to pretreatment immunization and post treatment boosting with bacterial polysaccharide vaccines in patients with Hodgkin's disease. Ann Intern Med. 1986;104:467–475.
261. Molrine DC, George S, Tarbell N, et al. Antibody responses to polysaccharide and polysaccharide-conjugate vaccines after treatment of Hodgkin disease. Ann Intern Med. 1995;123:828–834.
262. Wong WY, Overturf GD, Powars DR. Infection caused by *Streptococcus pneumoniae* in children with sickle cell disease: Epidemiology, immunologic mechanisms, prophylaxis and vaccination. Clin Infect Dis. 1992;14:1124–1136.
263. Wong WY, Powars DR, Chan L, et al. Polysaccharide encapsulated bacterial infection in sickle cell anemia: A thirty year epidemiologic experience. Am J Hematol. 1992;39:176–182.
264. Kaplan SL, Duckett T, Mahoney DH, et al. Immunogenicity of *Haemophilus influenzae* type b polysaccharide-tetanus protein conjugate vaccine in children with sickle hemoglobinopathy or malignancies, and after systemic *Haemophilus influenzae* type b infection. J Pediatr. 1992;120:367–370.
265. Gaston MH, Verter JI, Woods G, et al. Prophylaxis with oral penicillin in children with sickle cell anemia: A randomized trial. N Engl J Med. 1986;314:1593–1599.
266. Witherspoon RP, Storb R, Ochs HD. Recovery of antibody production in human allogeneic marrow graft recipients: Influence of time posttransplantation, the presence or absence of chronic graft-versus-host disease and antithymocyte globulin treatment. Blood. 1981;58:360–368.
267. Morgan M, Gale RP, Winston D. Intravenous immunoglobulin in bone marrow transplantation. Cancer. 1991;68(Suppl 6):1451–1453.
268. Wolff S, Fay JW, Herzig R, et al. High-dose weekly intravenous immunoglobulin to prevent infections in patients undergoing autologous bone marrow transplantation or severe myelosuppressive therapy. Ann Intern Med. 1993;118:937–942.
269. Sacher RA. Intravenous gammaglobulin therapy: Current role in bone marrow transplant, malignancy, and autoimmune hematologic disorders. Semin Hematol. 1992;29(Suppl 2):1–5.
270. Henning KJ, White MH, Sepkowitz KA, et al. A national survey of immunization practices following allogeneic bone marrow transplantation. JAMA. 1997;277:1148–1151.
271. Brugger SA, Oesterreicher C, Hofmann H, et al. Hepatitis B virus clearance by transplantation of bone marrow from hepatitis B immunised donor (Letter) (see comments). Lancet. 1997;349:996–997.
272. Molrine DC, Guinan EC, Antin JH, et al. Donor immunization with *Haemophilus influenzae* type b (HIB)-conjugate vaccine in allogeneic bone marrow transplantation. Blood. 1996;87:3012–3018.
273. Huang KL, Ruben FL, Rinaldo CR, et al. Antibody response after influenza and pneumococcal immunization in HIV-infected homosexual men. JAMA. 1987;257:2047–2050.
274. Collier AC, Corey L, Murphy VL, et al. Antibody to human immunodeficiency virus (HIV) and suboptimal response to hepatitis B vaccination. Ann Intern Med. 1988;109:101–105.
275. Janoff EN, Breiman RF, Daley CL, et al. Pneumococcal disease during HIV

infection: Epidemiologic, clinical and immunologic perspectives. Ann Intern Med. 1992;117:314–324.
276. Steinhoff MC, Auerbach BS, Nelson KE, et al. Antibody responses to *Haemophilus influenzae* type b vaccines in men with human immunodeficiency virus infection. N Engl J Med 1991;325:1837–1842.
277. Mofenson L, Moye J, Bethel J, et al. Prophylactic intravenous immunoglobulin in HIV-infected children with CD4+ counts of 0.20 × 10⁹/L or more: Effect on viral, opportunistic and bacterial infections. JAMA. 1992;268:483–488.
278. Small C, Kaufman A, Armenaka M, et al. Sinusitis and atopy in human immunodeficiency virus infection. J Infect Dis. 1993;167:283–290.
279. Stites DP, Stobo JD, Wells JV, eds. Basic and Clinical Immunology. 7th ed. Los Altos, Calif: Appleton & Lange; 1991.

Chapter 7

Complement

PETER DENSEN

Functional activity attributable to the complement system was first described in the period between 1888 and 1894.[1] Experiments at that time demonstrated that fresh serum contained a heat-labile bactericidal factor termed *alexin.* Subsequently it was shown that a heat-stable factor present in convalescent serum also contributed to bactericidal activity. At the turn of the century Paul Erlich employed the terms *complement* to describe the heat-labile factor and *ambocepto* (antibody) to describe the heat-stable factor. With the 20th century came the recognition that complement was composed of more than one component. However, it was not until 1941 that Louis Pillemer was able to separate functionally distinct components of the classical pathway from various serum fractions. In the early 1950s, Pillemer and coworkers also described and characterized an antibody-independent mechanism for complement activation that they termed the *properdin pathway.*[1–3] However, the protein purification techniques of the time were unable to provide complement components of sufficient purity to convince others of the existence of this pathway. With the 1960s and 1970s came the development of a mathematical model capable of describing the sequential activation of complement as well as new techniques for the purification of the individual complement components. The latter development led to rediscovery of Pillemer's work, characterization of these proteins, and delineation of mechanisms controlling their activity. The 1980s brought the recognition that the complement system consists not only of plasma proteins but also of membrane proteins that protect host cells from the detrimental effects of complement activation. This led to the appreciation that the complement cascade is intended to function at the interface between the fluid phase and the cell surface. Finally, the late-century outburst of advances in molecular biology has led to cloning and structural characterization of all the complement proteins and an understanding of the molecular basis for their deficiency states.

The complement system comprises more than 30 proteins (Table 7–1). Their activation results in sequential triggering of the various proteins and in this regard exhibits many similarities to the clotting cascade. The beneficial effects of complement activation for the host include development of an inflammatory response and elimination of microbial pathogens and immune complexes (Fig. 7–1).

The antibody and complement systems are grouped together be-

TABLE 7–1 Complement Plasma Proteins

Component	Approximate Serum Concentration (μg/ml)	Molecular Weight	Chain Structure*	Number of Genetic Loci	Chromosomal Assignment†
Classical pathway					
C1q	70	410,000	(A, B, C) × 6	3 (A, B, C)	1p
C1r	34	170,000	Dimer of two identical chains	1	12p
C1s	31	85,000	Dimer of two identical chains	1	12p
C4	600	206,000	β–α–γ	2 (C4A, C4B)	6p
C2	25	117,000	One chain	1	6p
Alternative pathway					
D (adipsin)	1	24,000	One chain	1	ND
C3	1300	195,000	β–α	1	19q
B	200	95,000	One chain	1	6p
Membrane attack complex					
C5	80	180,000	β–α	1	9q
C6	60	128,000	One chain	1	5p
C7	55	97,000	One chain	1	5p
C8	65	150,000	Three nonidentical chains α- - -γ, β	3 (A, B, G)	α, β 1p γ 9q
C9	60	79,000	One chain	1	5p
Control proteins					
Positive regulation					
Properdin	25	220,000	Cyclic polymers of a single 57-kD chain	1	Xp
Negative regulation					
C1 INH	200	105,000	One chain	1	11q
C4b BP	250	550,000	Seven identical chains	1	1q
Factor H	500	150,000	One chain	1	1q
Factor I	34	90,000	β–γ	1	4q
Anaphylatoxin inactivator (carboxypeptidase N)	35	310,000	Dimer of two nonidentical chains (H, L) × 2	ND	ND
S protein (vitronectin)	350	80,000	1 chain	1	ND
SP-40,40 (clusterin)	50	80,000	α–β	1	8p

*For multichain components, parentheses indicate subunit structure; commas indicate noncovalent linkage of chains arising from separate genes; solid lines indicate covalent linkage of chains arising from posttranslational cleavage of a proenzyme molecule, chains being listed in order beginning at the amino terminus of the proenzyme molecule; dashed line indicates covalent linkage of chains arising from separate genes.

†p indicates the short arm and q the long arm of the chromosome.

Abbreviations: BP, Binding protein; C1-INH, C1 inhibitor; H, heavy chain; L, light chain; ND, not determined.

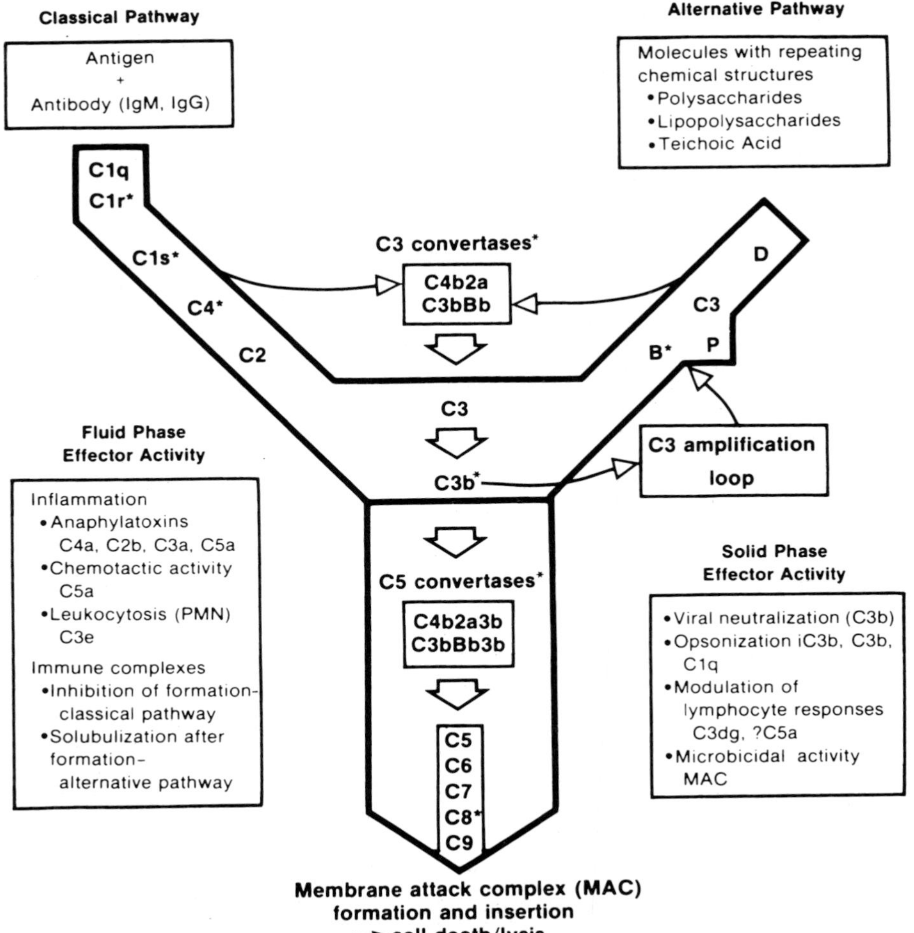

FIGURE 7–1. The complement cascade. Within each pathway, the components are arranged in order of their activation and aligned opposite their functional and structural analogue in the opposite pathway. Asterisks indicate sites of downregulation of complement activity (see Table 7–2).

cause of their historical and functional association and because they are soluble serum proteins.[4] However, antibody-mediated events are characterized by a high degree of specificity dictated by a given antibody for a given antigenic epitope. Consequently, after initial exposure to antigen there is a significant delay while protective antibody is synthesized to influence the course of the disease. In contrast, the complement system is activated by a wide variety of chemically diverse substances even in the absence of antibody. Consequently, the multiplicity of its physiologic effects is felt early in the course of infection. In many instances antibody and complement are synergistic in providing effective host defense. The presence of specific antibody leads to more rapid and efficient complement activation and serves to direct complement deposition to appropriate sites on the surface of invading pathogens. Opsonization of infectious agents with both antibody and complement leads to more efficient ingestion and killing of these microbes than does opsonization with either substance alone. Similarly, the presence of receptors on lymphocytes for immunoglobulin and complement suggests a cooperative role for these substances in both the affector and effector pathways of the immune response. "In such a way a highly specific response mediated by the tertiary structure of an antibody molecule can be coupled with the more general cellular or humoral responses of the phagocytic and complement system to eradicate attacking organisms."[4]

COMPLEMENT SYNTHESIS, CATABOLISM, AND DISTRIBUTION

Studies using cultured hepatocytes coupled with an examination of complement component polymorphisms in patients before and after orthotopic liver transplantation have established the liver as the major site of synthesis for most complement components.[5–7] The fractional catabolic rate for several complement components ranges from 1 to 60% per hour, indicating that they are among the most rapidly metabolized of all plasma proteins. The catabolic rates of these proteins are independent of their serum concentrations, whereas synthetic rates correlate with these levels, indicating that the rate of synthesis is the major determinant of plasma concentration.[8]

The concentrations of individual complement components fluctuate over time. In part this fluctuation reflects the fact that many of these proteins are acute phase reactants, the synthesis of which can be modulated twofold to fivefold by a variety of immune mediators, including interleukin-1 (IL-1), IL-6, tumor necrosis factor (TNF), interferon-γ, and endotoxin.[9, 10] In most cases, enhanced synthesis is mediated at the transcriptional level.

A variety of other cells also synthesize and secrete a number of complement proteins. Most notable among these are monocytes and macrophages, but microglia, astrocytes, fibroblasts, endothelial cells, and adipocytes are also important sites of local complement production.[11] Complement synthesis by monocytes can be modulated by interferon-γ, endotoxin,[12, 13] IL-1, and TNF. Local synthesis is an important aspect of complement-mediated host defense, as evidenced by the observation that monocytes and macrophages can synthesize sufficient amounts of complement to promote opsonization, ingestion, and killing of bacteria.[14]

In healthy persons the majority of complement is found in plasma. Concentrations of complement proteins in normal mucosal secretions are approximately 5 to 10% of serum levels and in normal spinal fluid even lower, perhaps 1% or less. In the presence of local inflammation, complement concentrations in mucosal secretions and in cerebrospinal fluid increase, most likely as a result of altered vascular permeability barriers but also as a consequence of enhanced synthesis and secretion by local mononuclear cells.

Serum complement activity is reduced in preterm infants in proportion to the magnitude of their immaturity.[15] In contrast, complement levels in healthy full-term infants range from 60 to 100% of those in healthy adults. Despite these almost normal levels, defective complement activation via either the classical or the alternative pathway has been noted in as many as 40% of such infants.[16–18]

COMPLEMENT ACTIVATION

Generation of the Classical Pathway C3 Convertase

Activation of the classical pathway most commonly occurs as a consequence of antigen-antibody recognition. Only immunoglobulin M (IgM) and certain IgG subclasses (IgG_3 > IgG_1 > IgG_2) are capable of initiating complement activation.[19] The third constant domain (C_H3) of the heavy chain of IgM, especially glycosylation at Asn 402, and the C_H2 and C_H3 regions of IgG play particularly important roles in the association of C1 with antibody.[20, 21] Amino acid sequence differences in the C_H2 region may account for the different complement-activating potentials among the IgG subclasses.[22]

C1 is a trimolecular complex containing one molecule of C1q and two molecules each of C1r and C1s. C1q consists of a central core with six radiating, collagen-like fibrillar strands that terminate in globular heads, which contain the antibody-binding sites.[19, 23] In the case of IgM, functionally important C1q binding occurs after the change in configuration that accompanies binding of a single IgM molecule to multiple sites on the target particle. In contrast, for IgG, functionally effective C1q binding requires that two IgG molecules be crosslinked via the globular heads on C1q. This topographic stipulation dictates that many IgG molecules be bound to a target particle to ensure sufficient density for doublet formation. At a functional level this requirement means that complement activation by IgG is less efficient than that by IgM, because the latter requires only that a single molecule be bound in the correct configuration.[19, 23]

Although antibody-antigen interactions are the most common means of initiating classic pathway activation, this pathway can also be activated directly via certain lectins. These lectins, including mannose-binding protein (MBP), pulmonary surfactant proteins, and bovine conglutin, are structurally homologous with C1q in that they possess collagen-like and globular domains. Like C1q, these molecules can bind directly to anionic structures such as lipid A ketodeoxyoctonate complexes on the surface of rough gram-negative bacteria. Under physiologic conditions, MBP complexes preferentially interact with other proteases, termed MBP-associated serum proteases (MASPs), to form a complex capable of cleaving C4 and C2 and eliciting the full range of classical pathway mediated activities.[24–29]

C1 binding by antibody results in a change in the structural configuration of the C1q molecule so that the C1r and C1s tetramer contained within the cagelike structure formed by the radiating pods of C1q becomes autocatalytically active. This structural alteration may involve the release of C1 inhibitor, which binds reversibly to proenzyme C1. C1r and C1s are structurally related molecules consisting of a head bearing the serine esterase enzymatic site and a tail bearing the binding site. The subunits are aligned linearly so that the central portion of the tetramer is formed by two C1r subunits linked through their catalytic domains. Each C1r molecule is joined to a C1s molecule via the binding sites in the tail regions of the respective subunits. This linear arrangement allows the tetramer to assume a figure-eight configuration so that all four catalytic domains are in close proximity. In this configuration, each C1r molecule is believed to activate the other C1r molecule, which in turn activates C1s.[19, 30, 31]

Expression of enzymatic activity by C1r and C1s represents the initial activation and amplification step in the classical pathway. Many molecules of substrate are cleaved by a given enzyme complex, resulting in the fixation of subsequent complement components in the cascade in close proximity to the antibody-binding site on the surface of the target particle. Therefore, antibody serves not only to activate complement in a kinetically efficient manner but also to direct complement deposition to specific sites on the target surface.

Activated C1s cleaves a 9-kD fragment, C4a, from the amino terminus of the α-chain of C4. This results in exposure of an internal thioester bond linking the SH group of a cysteine residue with the terminal carboxyl group of glutamic acid. This bond is subject to nucleophilic attack by hydroxyl or amino groups, leading to the formation of covalent ester or amide linkages.[32–34] Through this reaction and the analogous one involving C3 (Fig. 7–2), the complement system acquires a chemically stable association with the target surface. Because of gene duplication there are two slightly different C4 genes, C4A and C4B. The product of the C4A gene preferentially forms amide bonds with target surfaces and is hemolytically less active than the product of the C4B gene, which preferentially forms ester bonds.[35–37] Consequently, C4A binds more effectively to proteins (e.g., antigen-antibody complexes) than does C4B.[36, 38, 39] The molecular basis for this difference in binding efficiency appears to be the presence of an aspartic acid residue in the C4A molecule and a histidine residue in the C4B molecule at a site distant from the thioester in the primary structure of C4. The tertiary configuration of the molecule probably brings these charged amino acids into close proximity with the thioester so that they influence the nucleophilic attack on the thioester bond by amino or hydroxyl groups on the target surface. The difference in reactivity of the C4A and C4B molecules may play a role in determining the clinical picture observed in patients with inherited deficiencies of these respective genes.[38, 39]

Activated C1s also cleaves C2 to produce a small fragment, C2b, which is released into the environment, and a larger fragment, C2a, which binds to C4b on the surface of the target particle. This complex, C4b2a, is the classical pathway C3 convertase (see Fig. 7–1). It is inherently labile, but after its dissociation C4b can bind newly generated C2a derived from further cleavage of C2 by C1s.[19, 33]

Generation of the Alternative-Pathway C3 Convertase

Activation of complement by the alternative pathway displays several unique features. First, antibody is not required, although it can facilitate the activation process. Second, activation proceeds both in the fluid phase and on cell surfaces. Fluid-phase activation occurs continuously at a low rate that is tightly controlled by plasma regulatory proteins. Spillover from the fluid phase results in complement deposition on cells of the host as well as on intruding microorganisms. Therefore, host cells must possess a mechanism to limit the effects of complement fixation (i.e., they are "nonactivators"), whereas intruding microorganisms must provide a surface that allows complement activation to proceed further (i.e., they are "activators").[33, 40, 41] Third, a component of the activation process, C3b, is also a product of the reaction, so that a positive-feedback loop is generated that amplifies the activation process. Consequently, C3b deposition resulting from C3 cleavage by either the alternative- or the classical pathway C3 convertase can initiate the alternative-pathway amplification loop (see Fig. 7–1).[33, 40, 41] The time required

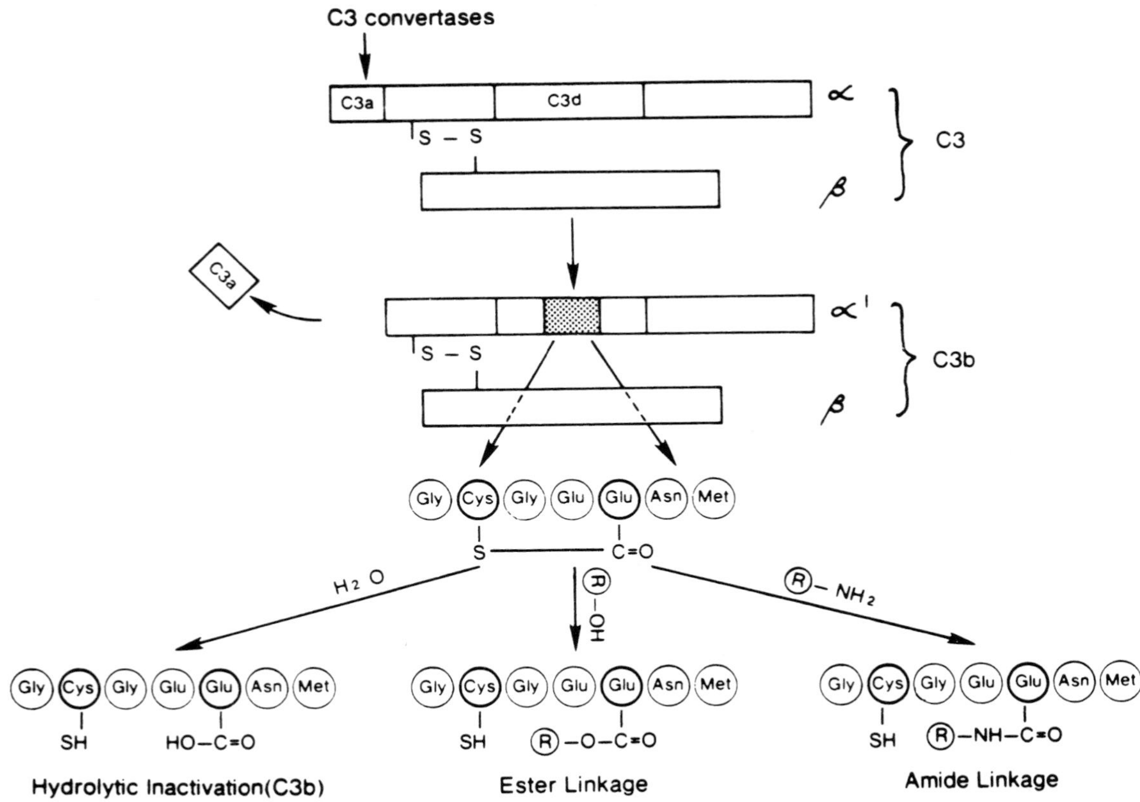

FIGURE 7–2. C3 activation and fate of the internal thiolester bond. During activation, C3a is released from the amino terminus of the α-chain of C3. The exposed internal thiolester bond becomes accessible to nucleophilic attack and can react with water or available hydroxyl or amine groups on cell surfaces. Analogous reactions occur with C4. Together these reactions involving C3 and C4 are responsible for covalently linking complement deposition to the cell surface. (From Gordon DL, Hostetter MK. Complement and host defense against microorganisms. Pathology. 1986;18:365–375.)

until amplification occurs makes complement activation via the alternative pathway three to five times less efficient kinetically than activation via the classic pathway on the same target.[42] This delay in activation is characteristic for a given target and differs among different target particles.[41, 42] Fourth, in contrast to the classical pathway, in which antibody directs covalent C4b binding in clusters about the antibody-binding site, covalent C3b binding mediated by the alternative pathway occurs randomly over the surface of the target particle.[40, 41] The random nature of this process contributes in part to the delay in complement activation via this pathway.

C3 is the critical reactant of the alternative pathway. It is structurally and functionally analogous to C4 (see Fig. 7–2) and contains the same internal thioester bond within its α-chain. This internal thioester bond undergoes spontaneous low-rate hydrolysis to form C3(H_2O), as shown in Figure 7–2. For a brief moment before its inactivation by the control proteins factors H and I, C3(H_2O) can form a complex with factor B. Once bound to C3, factor B can be cleaved by factor D, the rate-limiting enzyme in the alternative pathway, to yield C3(H_2O)Bb—the fluid phase C3 convertase. C3(H_2O)Bb reacts with intact C3 to cleave a 9-kD peptide fragment, C3a, from the amino terminus of the α-chain.[40, 41] Analogous to the situation with C4, this process results in exposure of the internal thioester in the α-chain. The resulting metastable C3b can form covalent ester or amide linkages with appropriate chemical constituents on the surface of nearby cells. Surface-bound C3b can bind additional factor B, which in turn can be cleaved by factor D to produce C3bBb. This complex is the alternative-pathway C3 convertase, which is capable of cleaving additional C3, thereby initiating the amplification phase of the alternative pathway. Like its classical pathway analogue, this convertase is inherently labile and has a half-life of approximately 90 seconds. Properdin binding to C3bBb stabilizes the complex and prolongs its half-life by 5- to 10-fold,[44, 45] thereby providing reaction conditions sufficient for further C3 cleavage and signaling the initiation of the amplification phase of alternative-pathway activation.

From these considerations it is apparent that any substance that stabilizes the alternative-pathway convertase will also promote C3 consumption. This situation arises in patients who develop autoantibodies to C3bBb that stabilize the convertase.[46] In addition, cobra venom contains a C3b-like factor that forms an extremely stable complex with factor B; this complex functions as a C3 convertase except that it is resistant to the action of the control proteins. Therefore, the addition of cobra venom factor to serum leads to the dramatic consumption of C3.[41, 47–49] Infusion of this factor can be used in experimental animals to delineate the role of the complement cascade in host defense or other disease processes.

Although antibody is not required for activation of the alternative pathway, it acts synergistically with properdin to facilitate the activation process.[50, 51] Facilitation depends on the Fab portion of the antibody molecule rather than the Fc fragment responsible for classical pathway activation.[51–55] Not all antibodies can enhance activation. For example, guinea pig IgG_1 but not IgG_2 can augment alternative-pathway activation.[56] The molecular basis for facilitation is uncertain but probably requires carbohydrate moieties present on IgG.[57] Antibody deposited on target surfaces can serve as a potential binding site for the covalent linkage of C3.[52] Moreover, the alternative-pathway C3 convertase C3bBb that is formed on IgG is relatively resistant to the action of the regulatory proteins.[58, 59] This property may contribute to the ability of antibody to facilitate alternative-pathway activation.

C3—The Linchpin of the Complement System

The critical importance of C3 in the complement cascade is evident from its position at the convergence of the classical and alternative pathways, its role in activating and amplifying alternative-pathway activation, the multitude of functional activities associated with its various cleavage products, the fact that it is a major point of regulation of complement activity (see Fig. 7–1), and the fact that its concentration in plasma (1.6 mg/ml) exceeds by 2- to 10-fold the concentration of all other complement components (see Table 7–1).[60] The α-chain of C3b is subject to proteolytic cleavage by factor I to yield C3bi and by less well-defined proteases to C3dg and C3d. Each of these progressively smaller C3 fragments remains linked to the cell surface via the original covalent bond, and each can react with specific receptors on phagocytic and lymphocytic cells. However, only C3b can perpetuate complement activation. C3b binding to the C3 convertases generates new complexes, C4bC2aC3b and C3bBbC3b, the C5 convertases, which are responsible for cleaving C5 and initiating assembly of the membrane attack complex (MAC).

Assembly of the Membrane Attack Complex

C5 is the structural homologue of C4 and C3 except that its α-chain does not contain an internal thioester bond. Instead, the amino acids cysteine and glutamine, which form the internal thioester in C4 and C3, have been replaced by serine and alanine.[61, 62] Analogous to C4 and C3, activation of C5 proceeds via cleavage of an 11.2-kD fragment, C5a, from the amino terminus of its α-chain. The resulting C5b binds noncovalently to the surface of the target particle.[63] The remaining terminal complement components, C6, C7, C8β, C8α-γ, and C9, share a high level of structural organization at both the DNA and protein levels.[64–66] Unlike the early components of the classical and alternative pathways, these proteins lack enzymatic activity but as a group are characterized by their amphipathic properties. They circulate in plasma in hydrophilic form, undergoing hydrophobic transformation on binding to the nascent MAC.[63] Assembly of the MAC begins when C5b binds to hydrophobic sites on the cell surface and expresses a metastable binding site for C6. Both C6 and C7 bind to the α-chains of C5b through binding domains in their carboxyl termini to form a stable trimolecular complex, C5b–7.[63] Subsequently, C8 binds to C5b via a site on its β-chain.[67, 68] In the final step, C8 initiates polymerization of C9 through a binding site on C8α-γ.[69] A current model of this process suggests that the function of C5b–8 is to create a discontinuity in the membrane lipid bilayer, thereby establishing an environment for the stepwise unfolding, insertion, and polymerization of monomeric C9.[70] In its completely assembled state the MAC consists of a single molecule each of C5b, C6, C7, and C8 and multiple (1 to 18) molecules of C9.[63]

Fully inserted and polymerized C9 has a tubular shape and the properties of an integral membrane protein.[63, 70] It is responsible for the characteristic electron microscopic appearance of the membrane holes that appear during effective complement activation. The inner aspect of this tubular structure is hydrophilic and allows the passage of water and ions, whereas the outer surface of the structure is hydrophobic and causes varying degrees of membrane disorganization during insertion.[63, 70] Both of these effects are thought to contribute to the microbicidal and cytolytic properties of the MAC.

REGULATION OF COMPLEMENT ACTIVATION

A major feature of the complement cascade is the controlled production of an inflammatory reaction sufficient to enhance host defense and the immune response yet not strong enough to lead to host injury. Upregulation of this process is achieved by the inherent property of enzymes to turn over multiple substrate molecules rapidly and by stabilization of enzyme complexes (e.g., by properdin). Downregulation is achieved in a temporal fashion by the short half-lives of the enzymatic complexes and the anaphylatoxins and in a spatial manner by direction of complement activation to the target surface (e.g., by antibody). Modulation of the potential injurious effects of indiscriminant complement activation is achieved by specific regulatory proteins acting at three major levels: activation (C1), effector initiation (C3), and cytolysis (MAC). Unique disease entities resulting from a deficiency of these control proteins are testimony to the importance of complement regulation.

Regulation of C1 Activation

As described previously, C1 esterase inhibitor (C1-INH) binds reversibly to pro-C1, thereby preventing its spontaneous activation.[23] Binding of C1q to antibody subverts this control by causing dissociation of C1-INH from pro-C1 and allowing autocatalytic cleavage to proceed. At some point after C1 activation, C1-INH binds to the active sites on C1r and C1s, inactivating their catalytic function and dissociating them from C1q. C1-INH neither prevents nor inhibits initial activation; rather, its role is to prevent amplification of fluid-phase C1 activation and to limit excessive activation on the target cell. Complete C1 inactivation requires the binding of four molecules of C1-INH, one per catalytic site. In contrast to its binding to pro-C1, C1-INH binding to C1r and C1s is irreversible and thereby prevents cleavage of C4 and controls the initial amplification step of classical pathway activation.[23, 71]

Regulation of the C3 Convertases

As indicated in Figure 7–1, the classical and alternative-pathway C3 convertases are functionally analogous molecules. Control of their activity occurs via three basic mechanisms using functionally identical or shared regulator proteins (Table 7–2).[33, 41, 42, 46] First, both convertases are inherently labile and undergo spontaneous decay, with the loss of C2a or Bb from their respective complexes. Second, the rate of spontaneous decay can be accelerated by regulatory proteins. These proteins compete with C2a and Bb for binding sites on C4b and C3b, thereby inhibiting new convertase formation and enhancing the rate of dissociation of already formed convertases. Third, functionally active C3b and C4b can be cleaved by factor I, thereby eliminating the ability of these molecules to reform their respective C3 convertases.[46, 72, 73]

Several additional points have emerged from the many studies on C3 convertase regulation. First, control of C3 convertase activity is expressed both in the fluid phase and on host cell surfaces. Despite similarity in function, the proteins responsible for this regulation are distinct. Serum proteins (C4b binding protein [C4b BP], factor H) primarily serve to control activation in the fluid phase, whereas membrane-bound proteins (complement receptor 1 [CR1], membrane cofactor protein [MCP], decay-accelerating factor [DAF]) primarily serve to control complement activation on cell surfaces. Second, control proteins serve to accelerate the decay of the C3 convertases (decay factors, DAF) or to promote factor I–mediated cleavage of C3b or C4b (cofactor activity, MCP), or both (CR1, C4b BP, factor H). Third, C4b BP and factor H, unlike their membrane-bound counterparts, exhibit specificity for the classical and alternative pathway C3 convertases, respectively.[72–74]

The combined actions of these membrane-bound and serum proteins serve to confine the spread of complement activation and, by inactivating cell-bound C4 and C3, to protect host cells. They thereby serve to distinguish self from nonself with respect to the deleterious effects of complement activation.[75]

Regulation of the Membrane Attack Complex

Assembly of the MAC is controlled in two ways: by proteins that bind to the C5b–7 complex and by those that inhibit C9 incorporation and polymerization within the MAC. Nascent C5b–7 molecules have the potential to insert into any cell membrane and are not restricted

TABLE 7–2 Plasma and Membrane Proteins That Regulate or Mediate Complement Activity

Location, Protein	Specificity	Function
Plasma		
C1-INH	C1r, C1s	Binds to and inactivates C1r and C1s in the C1 complex
C4b BP	C4b	Inhibits assembly and accelerates decay of C4b2a; cofactor for C4b cleavage by factor I
Factor H	C3b	Inhibits assembly and accelerates decay of C3bBb; cofactor for C3b cleavage by factor I
Factor I	C4b, C3b	Proteolytic inactivation of C4b and C3b
Properdin	C3bBb	Stabilizes alternative pathway C3 convertase
S protein (vitronectin), SP-40,40 (clusterin)	C5b–7	Binds fluid-phase C5b–7; prevents attachment of C5b–7 and C5b–9 to membranes
Carboxypeptidase N	C4a, C3a, C5a	Inactivates these anaphylatoxins by removal of carboxyl-terminal arginine
Cell membranes		
CR1 (CD35)	C3b, C4b, C3bi	Inhibits assembly and accelerates decay of C3 convertases
Membrane cofactor protein (CD46)	C3b, C4b	Cofactor for cleavage of C4b/C3b by factor I
Decay-accelerating factor (CD55)	C4b2a, C3bBb	Promotes decay of alternative pathway C3 convertase
CR1 (CD35)	C3b, C4b, iC3b	Binds immune complexes to erythrocytes; phagocytosis
CR2 (CD21)	C3d, C3dg	Phagocytosis
	C3bi, C3b	Modulates B-cell responses; Epstein-Barr virus receptor
CR3 (CD11b/CD18)	C3bi	Phagocytosis
CR4 (CD11c/CD18)	C3dg, C3d	Phagocytosis
CD59	C8 in C5b–8	Binds to C8; inhibits polymerization of C9
C3a/C4aR	C3a, C4a	Vasodilation
C5aR	C5a, C5a des Arg	Chemotaxis
C1qR	C1q	Phagocytosis

Abbreviation: CR, Complement receptor.

to the surface on which complement is activated. By binding to this trimolecular complex, S protein (vitronectin) and clusterin abrogate its ability to insert into cell membranes and consequently its hemolytic potential. Both proteins, by binding to C8, C9, or both, can also inhibit the incorporation of these components into the nascent MAC, but they act much more potently at the level of C5b–7. Clusterin concentrations in seminal plasma are high, suggesting a role for this protein in protecting sperm from immune-mediated cytolysis.[72]

Although several proteins inhibit C9 incorporation and polymerization within the MAC, by far the most potent is CD59. CD59 is very widely distributed. Its presence as a membrane protein probably accounts for homologous restriction,[76] a phenomenon whereby cells are not lysed by complement from the same species but can be (though are not always) lysed by complement from a different species. Although it is clear that CD59 binds to C9, the site of binding and the mechanism by which it prevents C9 incorporation and polymerization within the MAC are unclear.[72]

Nucleated eukaryotic cells are resistant to complement-mediated cytolysis even in the face of a nonhomologous complement source. Resistance is associated with the capacity of the cell to maintain high synthetic rates of membrane lipids and the ability to shed MAC from the cell surface.[77–79] Insertion of the MAC in eukaryotic cell membranes is accompanied by a rapid influx of calcium, generation of multiple signals, and stimulation of arachidonic acid metabolism.[80–82] These events probably promote normal physiologic functions and contribute to host cell injury.

Basis for Discriminating between Host and Microbial Cell Surfaces

The capacity of C4 and C3 to form covalent bonds with reactive groups on cell surfaces, thereby establishing the nidus for C3 convertase formation, is inherently incapable of distinguishing between host and microbial cells. Consequently, for the beneficial effects of complement activation to be expressed as an effective host defense mechanism, additional factors must allow discrimination between self and nonself.[75] These factors must inhibit activation of complement amplification on host cells ("nonactivators") yet permit amplification on the surface of microbial organisms ("activators"). One element of this discriminatory process is the presence of the complement regulatory proteins in the membranes of host cells but not on the cells of microbial organisms.[75] The other important determinant of complement activation is the chemical composition of the cell surface. Because covalent bond formation is nondiscriminatory, the basis for discrimination must lie in the capacity for chemical differences to affect the outcome of the competition between factor B and factor H for the binding site on C3b, which in turn determines C3 convertase formation or decay and whether a particular cell surface will activate the alternative pathway. For example, C3b bound to the surface of a nonactivating particle binds factor H with about 100-fold greater affinity than C3b bound to an activator particle. Consequently, factor B binding and subsequent amplification of complement activation is favored on the latter particle.[33, 41, 42, 46]

Chemical constituents that influence the competition between factor B and factor H for C3b include sialic acid and sulfated acid mucopolysaccharides (e.g., heparin sulfate). These molecules, present on most human cells, act through an anion binding site on factor H to enhance its affinity for C3b, thereby contributing to the nonactivator status of host cells.[83–86] From the standpoint of infectious diseases, sialic acid is also a prominent chemical constituent of the capsular polysaccharides present on type 3 group B streptococci, K1 *Escherichia coli,* and groups B and C meningococci.[46] Consequently, the capsules of these organisms are nonactivators of the alternative pathway and, because sialic acid is a constituent of host cells, constitute a poor stimulus for antibody production. In this context it is noteworthy that K1 *E. coli,* group B streptococci, and group B meningococci are prominent causes of neonatal and infant sepsis and meningitis. The frequent absence in these patients of specific antibody to activate the classic pathway, coupled with bacterial sialic acid–mediated inhibition of alternative-pathway activity, may provide the ideal clinical setting for infection with these organisms.

Chemical constituents other than sialic acid must also affect the outcome of the competition between factors B and H for C3b. For example, sheep and human erythrocytes contain an extensive amount of sialic acid on their surface and are normally nonactivators of the alternative pathway.[84–87] Enzymatic removal of sialic acid from these cells converts sheep but not human erythrocytes into activating particles. Moreover, the chemical introduction of lipopolysaccharide molecules capable of activating the alternative pathway into the membrane of sheep erythrocytes converts them from a nonactivating to activating particles despite the presence of sialic acid.[87]

In summary, the C3 convertases represent the major site of both complement amplification and complement regulation. The membranes of host cells contain specific proteins that act to downregulate the C3 convertases and other chemical constituents that enhance the affinity of fluid-phase factor H for surface-bound C3b and promote its regulatory activity. In contrast, most microbial surfaces lack specific factors capable of downregulating complement activation and possess a chemical composition that decreases the affinity of factor H for cell-bound C3b. Therefore, factor B binding to C3b and alternative-pathway activation and amplification are favored on most microbial surfaces.

COMPLEMENT RECEPTORS

Complement receptors have been described primarily on peripheral blood cells, including erythrocytes, neutrophils, monocytes, B and T lymphocytes, and platelets. They fall into two broad categories: those that bind complement components deposited on cell surfaces so that the component serves as a bifunctional ligand linking the target cell to the receptor and those that bind diffusible complement fragments released during activation of the complement cascade. The latter are responsible for many of the manifestations of the inflammatory response.

The former category of receptors includes C1qR, CR1, CR2, CR3, and CR4. The C1qR is a carbohydrate-rich protein expressed on phagocytic cells and lymphocytes that modulates phagocytosis, cytokine release, cytotoxicity, and interactions with endothelial cells. Functional ligands in addition to C1q that are recognized by C1qR include MBP, surfactant protein A, and conglutinin, all of which exhibit structural homology with C1q.[24]

Receptors for the cleavage products of C3 and C4 (CR1, CR2, CR3, and CR4) have been studied more extensively. Although they recognize closely related ligands, each of these receptors is structurally distinct and exhibits a unique pattern of distribution on peripheral blood cells.[88, 89] A portion of these receptors is linked to the cellular cytoskeleton, an association that is probably important in signal transduction.[90]

CR1, the C3b/C4b receptor, is present on erythrocytes, neutrophils, monocytes, B cells, subpopulations of T cells, follicular dendritic cells, and glomerular podocytes. There are four polymorphic variants that vary in size (190 to 280 kD) and in the number of C3b/C4b-binding sites.[91] The number of CR1 molecules per cell is genetically determined but varies with cell type and disease activity. CR1 mediates immune complex binding and clearance, promotes ingestion of C3b/C4b-bearing particles, modulates certain lymphocyte functions,[88, 89] and carries certain blood group antigens.[92]

CR3 and CR4 are members of the integrin family of heterodimeric proteins.[93] They recognize C3bi as their major binding ligand. However, CR3 also binds to C3b and C3dg and bears a lectin-like domain that recognizes specific carbohydrates on microbial surfaces.[94] The three-amino-acid sequence arginine-glycine-aspartic acid (Arg-Gly-Asp), which is present in C3 and other ligands, represents an important binding motif for CR3.[94–96] Together CR3 and CR4, particularly the former, recognize the various combinations of C3b, C3bi, and C3dg present on the surface of microbial cells and play a major role in their elimination by phagocytic cells.[97] In addition, CR3 plays an important role in the adherence-related functions of neutrophils (see Chapter 8).

CR2 is present on B lymphocytes and follicular dendritic cells and serves to recognize C3dg. The association of CR2 and CD19 in the B-cell membrane constitutes an important mechanism for B-cell activation.[98] CR2 acts to localize C3dg-bearing particles or immune complexes to lymphocyte-rich areas in the spleen and lymph nodes, thereby driving antigen activation of these cells.

Receptors for complement-derived mediators of the inflammatory response, including C4a, C3a, and C5a, have also been described. Of these, the high-affinity C5a receptor has been best studied. It is present on neutrophils and monocytes, and its perturbation causes directed migration (chemotaxis) of these cells in the direction of increasing C5a concentration. Experimental evidence has confirmed the presence of receptors for C3a on B lymphocytes, guinea pig ileum, vascular endothelium, and mast cells.[99]

FAMILIES OF COMPLEMENT PROTEINS

The preceding material and the representation of the complement cascade presented in Figure 7–1 emphasize features shared by both pathways with respect to their activation and regulation. It is apparent from these similarities that a number of complement components belong to several different protein families. These include the serine protease family (C1r, C1s, C2, factor D, factor B, and factor I); disulfide-linked, multichained molecules with homology to an ancestral protein that contained an internal thioester bond (C4, C3, and C5); proteins that are the products of class 3 major histocompatibility complex (MHC) genes located on chromosome 6 (C2, factor B, C4A, and C4B); proteins that bind C3 and C4 fragments and belong to a closely clustered supergene family located on the long arm of chromosome 1 (C4b BP, factor H, DAF, MCP, CR1, and CR2); and proteins sharing homology with the low-density lipoprotein (LDL) receptors (C6, C7, C8α, C8β, and C9).[100]

Among these families, interest has focused on those components that are the products of the class III MHC genes, the regulatory protein supergene family on chromosome 1, and the proteins with homology to the LDL receptor. MHC III genes are located between the class I and class II loci on the short arm of chromosome 6.[101] The genetic material in this region appears to have undergone two duplication events, resulting on the one hand in the structurally and functionally related proteins C2 and factor B and on the other in the C4 and 21-hydroxylase A and B variants.[100–102] Recombinant events in this region of the chromosome tend to be suppressed, thereby leading to the usual inheritance of the entire region intact from each parent.[103] The polymorphic variants of the complement components encoded by these genes in a given individual are referred to as *complotypes*.[104] The association of specific complotypes with specific products of the MHC I and II genes probably contributes to the association of specific complotypes with certain disease states (e.g., systemic lupus erythematosus [SLE]).[105]

Proteins encoded by the complement regulatory protein loci on the long arm of chromosome 1 share a common structural organization with each other, with other complement components that bind to C3 and C4 (e.g., C2, factor B), and with some other complement and noncomplement proteins that do not bind these two components.[106, 107] These molecules contain a structural motif called complement control protein repeats (CCPRs). CCPRs are tandem repeats of approximately 60 amino acids that share a conserved consensus sequence in which paired cysteine residues are linked to form a double loop structure that constitutes a binding domain. The number of repeats varies considerably among the proteins: MCP and DAF contain 4, CR2 has 16, factor H has 20, CR1 has 30, and C4b BP has 59. Two to four CCPRs are required to form a complete binding site.[107, 108]

The LDL receptor–related complement proteins are cysteine-rich molecules. Each molecule (except C8α) contains an even number of cysteine residues, which are clustered at the amino and carboxyl ends of the protein and participate in disulfide bond formation. Those clustered at the amino terminus of the molecule share homology with the LDL receptor, whereas those at the carboxyl terminus share homology with epidermal growth factor. The large number of disulfide bonds in these molecules is thought to convey a tertiary structure that facilitates the hydrophilic-hydrophobic transition that occurs on their interaction with lipid membranes during the assembly of the MAC.[64, 65]

COMPLEMENT-MEDIATED FUNCTIONS

Complement plays a major role in initiating the inflammatory response, clearing immune complexes, modulating immunoglobulin production, opsonizing microbial pathogens, and killing certain gram-negative bacteria (see Fig. 7–1). Small, diffusible peptide fragments released from C4, C3, C5, and probably C2 during their activation help to modulate the inflammatory response.[99] Collectively,

C4a, C3a, and C5a are referred to as *anaphylatoxins*, and together they stimulate histamine release from mast cells (C3a), promote vascular dilation (C3a, C4a), increase endothelial permeability (C3a), and stimulate neutrophil responses (C5a). In addition to these proinflammatory activities, C3a also acts via its receptor on B cells to downregulate cytokine synthesis and antibody production.[109] Carboxypeptidase N–mediated removal of the carboxyl-terminal arginine from the anaphylatoxins abrogates their functional activity by preventing their interaction with specific receptors.[99] In the case of C5a des Arg (the inactivated form of C5a), chemotactic activity is restored by association with vitamin D–binding protein.[110, 111] The activity of this complex is inhibited by free Bb, which is found in the sera of some patients with SLE.[112]

The incorporation of complement in immune complexes enhances their clearance and helps to minimize their potential for causing tissue damage.[113, 114] This process includes inhibition of immune complex precipitation, solubilization of immune complexes, and clearance of C3b-bearing immune complexes via the CR1 receptor. Under conditions of antibody excess or antibody-antigen equivalence, the probability that both antigen-binding sites on a single antibody will bind to epitopes on a single antigen and the probability that multiple antibody molecules will bind to a given molecule of antigen are increased. This situation provides an opportunity for antibody-antibody interactions via their Fc fragments, a condition that leads to immune complex precipitation.[113] C1q binding inhibits these Fc-Fc interactions and leads to complement activation with covalent binding of C3b to the immune complex. Subsequent recruitment of the alternative pathway via the C3b amplification loop promotes further C3b deposition within the immune complex lattice, thereby reducing the forces holding the lattice together and causing separation (solubilization) of smaller complexes from the lattice network. Thus the classical pathway functions to inhibit immune complex precipitation, whereas the alternative pathway promotes solubilization of the immune complex.[113, 114] In the context of disease pathogenesis, however, it is important to stress that complement is 10 times more efficient in inhibiting immune complex precipitation than in solubilizing precipitated complexes.

Immune complexes bearing C3b are bound to cells bearing C3b receptors (CR1). The number of these receptors per cell varies from a low of 950 for erythrocytes to a high of 57,000 for neutrophils.[115] However, because there are 1000 times more erythrocytes than leukocytes, 95% of the total CR1 receptors in the peripheral circulation are located on erythrocytes. Consequently, immune complexes bearing C3b are 500 to 1000 times more likely to be cleared from the circulation by erythrocytes than by leukocytes.[115] These complexes are removed along with the CR1 from the erythrocyte during passage through the liver and, to a lesser extent, through the spleen. This extraction probably involves CR1 on fixed macrophages lining the sinusoids of these organs.[116]

Substantial data indicate that C3 modulates the immune response.[117] This evidence includes (1) the absolute requirement for C3 in antigen localization within splenic germinal centers; (2) the presence of complement receptors, especially CR2, on B and T lymphocytes, follicular dendritic cells, and other antigen-presenting cells; (3) impaired antibody responses in animals or humans lacking one of the complement components (C1, C2, C4, C3) required for classical pathway C3 convertase formation and restoration of the immune response by replacement of the missing component; and (4) the association of these deficiencies in humans with significantly depressed concentrations of IgG_4 and IgG_2.[32, 117–121] In general, these studies demonstrate that soluble C3 fragments (especially C3a) inhibit immune responses, whereas C3 fragments (especially C3d) covalently linked to target particles enhance these responses. In particular, ligation of C3d to its receptor, CR2, leads to its association with CD19 in the B-cell membrane, thereby constituting an important signal for the activation of these cells[98] and reducing the antigen concentration necessary for their activation.[119] In addition to enhancing responses to primary antigenic exposure, C3 fragments facilitate isotype switching and anamnestic responses after secondary antigenic exposure.[117] An intriguing observation in this regard is the apparent inverse correlation between the extent of C3b degradation on a given pneumococcal polysaccharide and the ability of that polysaccharide to elicit an immune response when administered as part of the polyvalent vaccine.[122] In summary, although an absolute complement requirement does not exist for the generation of the humoral immune response, C3 facilitates antigen localization and presentation, acts as an immune adjuvant to reduce the amount of antigen required to evoke an optimal immune response, and participates both directly in the activation of B cells and indirectly by promoting cytokine synthesis.

Cell-bound fragments of C3, particularly C3b and C3bi, serve as bifunctional ligands linking target particles with cells bearing receptors for these fragments. In the case of bacteria, opsonization with C3b or C3bi, especially in conjunction with IgG, promotes ingestion of the organism and triggers the microbicidal mechanisms of phagocytic cells (see Chapter 8). Ingestion appears to be more efficient when the organism is opsonized with C3bi than with C3b.[123, 124] A small fragment, C3e, derived from the α-chain of C3, promotes the development of leukocytosis. This observation may help explain the failure of some C3-deficient patients to develop leukocytosis in response to infection.[33]

The complete activation of the complement cascade, with assembly of the MAC and its effective insertion into cell membranes, results in the death and eventual lysis of the cell. Death and lysis are independent events, and in the case of prokaryotes evidence suggests that a metabolic response is required by the organism before the lethal effects of the MAC can be expressed.[125] For some organisms, the assembly of the MAC through C8 is sufficient for killing[126]; however, in all cases the incorporation of C9 accelerates this process. Complement-mediated virucidal activity has also been well described and in some cases seems to require deposition of only the early components of the classical pathway.[127]

MICROBIAL INTERACTIONS WITH THE COMPLEMENT SYSTEM

The demonstration by Roantree and Rantz[128] that gram-negative bacteria isolated from blood were almost always resistant to complement-mediated killing whereas two thirds of those isolated from mucosal surfaces were serum sensitive was one of the first to suggest an important clinical role for complement in host defense. This suggestion was borne out by subsequent studies of complement-deficient persons (see later discussion) and by the elucidation of the strategies and extent to which microorganisms go to escape host defense mechanisms. In the case of complement, these strategies parallel those employed by host cells to circumvent injury during the inflammatory response. That is, they are focused on decreasing complement activation, accelerating convertase decay, and inhibiting the formation or insertion of the MAC.[129, 130] In many instances, the microbial proteins responsible for these effects share molecular, structural, immunologic, and functional homology with their human counterparts.

Elegant experiments correlating virulence with lipopolysaccharide composition and complement activation in three isogenic *Salmonella typhimurium* variants demonstrated the importance to bacteria of limiting complement deposition on their surface. These variants differ only in the chemical structure of their lipopolysaccharide side chains, yet their abilities to activate complement via the alternative pathway differ substantially, varying inversely with their relative in vivo virulence. The greatest rate of C3 consumption and extent of C3b deposition are initiated by the least virulent strains. Although the chemical structure of the lipopolysaccharide O antigen clearly determines the magnitude of C3b deposition, it has no effect on the subsequent cleavage and breakdown of the bound C3b. Rather, the effect of O-antigen structure is expressed at the level of alternative-pathway amplification, as manifested in the greater affinity of factor

B for C3b on the surface of the least virulent compared with the most virulent strains. In contrast, the affinity of factor H for C3b is the same on all strains.[131–136]

In addition to these effects, the long lipopolysaccharide O-antigen side chains on gram-negative bacilli restrict complement activation to sites distant from the outer membrane and hinder access of C5b–9 complexes to it. The failure of these complexes to localize to hydrophobic domains in the outer membrane results in their shedding and the survival of the organism and contributes to their serum resistance.[129, 137]

Gram-negative bacteria possessing truncated lipopolysaccharide molecules (e.g., *Haemophilus influenzae,* meningococci, gonococci) are not innately resistant to the bactericidal effects of the complement system but do require antibody for effective sensitization and complement deposition. The absence of bactericidal antibody renders these organisms serum resistant and contributes to the greater frequency of *H. influenzae* and meningococcal disease during the first several years of life.

Gonococci isolated from patients with disseminated gonococcal infection are resistant to the bactericidal activity of normal human serum.[138] The serum resistance of these strains is multifactorial. In the absence of bactericidal antibody, the MAC is assembled on the organism surface but fails to insert properly into the outer membrane.[139, 140] MAC insertion and killing occur normally in the presence of antilipopolysaccharide IgG found in the convalescent serum of some patients with this infection.[141, 142] However, some sera also contain IgG specific for gonococcal outer membrane protein 3.[143, 144] This antibody competes with bactericidal antibody for binding sites on the surface of the organism, thereby blocking its bactericidal effect. Although the blocking antibody promotes complement deposition on the organism, it apparently does so at sites that do not lead to the killing of the organism.[145] Blocking antibody also appears to account for the resistance of meningococci to killing by the serum of some adults who acquire this infection.[146, 147] These findings illustrate the influence of the composition of the outer membrane of gram-negative bacteria in determining sensitivity to complement-mediated killing and the importance to the host of specific antibody in overcoming the resistance of these organisms to killing.[148]

Other organisms owe their serum resistance to functional homologues of CD59, the protein that interferes with MAC assembly on host cell membranes. For example, the galactose-specific adhesin of *Entamoeba histolytica* not only functions in this manner but also shares DNA sequence homology and antigenic cross-reactivity with CD59.[149] Plasmids in *Salmonella typhimurium* and *Yersinia enterocolitica* contain the *rck* and *Ail* genes, respectively, which encode products of a family of virulence-associated outer membrane proteins. By preventing C9 polymerization, these proteins mediate serum resistance and therefore function similarly to CD59.[150, 151]

To date, molecules analogous to the complement regulatory proteins that accelerate the decay of the C3 convertases have not been identified in bacteria, although they are well described in multicellular parasites and viruses. The striking metamorphosis that protozoans undergo during transformation from insect- to human-infective forms is accompanied by the acquisition of resistance to complement-dependent killing. This phenomenon has been studied most extensively in *Trypanosoma cruzi,* for which surface proteins, gp72 and gp160, have been identified that block the assembly and promote the decay of the alternative-pathway C3 convertase.[129, 130, 152] These proteins function in a manner identical to human CR1 and DAF (see Table 7–2). In the case of gp160, structural homology to DAF appears to underlie functional homology.

The increasing availability of DNA sequence data banks and investigations into molecular pathogenesis have served to focus attention on virus-complement interactions and the mechanisms by which these organisms elude complement-mediated attack. Studies of the human immunodeficiency virus (HIV) are particularly illustrative. During viral replication, the virus is assembled and released from the infected cell by budding—a process that incorporates host cell membrane proteins into the viral envelope. Host cell DAF and CD59 incorporated into the viral envelope in this manner function efficiently to limit amplified complement deposition on HIV and its subsequent lysis. In addition, the HIV-specific envelope proteins gp120 and gp41 both contain factor H binding domains, which in the case of the latter protein demonstrate significant homology with C3. Factor H passively absorbed from serum and secretions serves to further limit complement deposition on the virus.[153, 154]

Appropriation of complement regulatory proteins is a strategy also employed by group A streptococci. Streptococcal M protein contains repetitive domains, known as C repeats, that promote binding of proteins that control C3 convertase activity—C4b BP, factor H, and MCP. In this manner, M protein not only limits complement deposition on the streptococcal surface but also promotes adhesion to the surface of keratinocytes in the skin.[155]

A variation on this theme occurs in serum-sensitive gonococci isolated from patients with symptomatic local genital disease. These organisms possess a sialyl transferase but lack the ability to synthesize cytidine monophospho-*N*-acetyl neuraminic acid (CMP-NANA). Consequently, they are incapable of endogenous sialylation of their lipopolysaccharide; rather, they appropriate host CMP-NANA for this purpose. Exogenous sialylation confers serum resistance to these gonococci by reducing the binding of bactericidal antibody.[156] It also reduces phagocytic uptake and may alter C3 cleavage and intracellular survival. *T. cruzi* accomplishes the same effect via a *trans*-sialidase that removes terminal sialic acid residues from host glycoconjugates and transfers them to acceptor molecules on the parasite surface.[152]

Other organisms employ different but related strategies. The envelope of type 1 herpes simplex virus contains a virus-specific protein, gC-1, that interferes with properdin-dependent stabilization of the alternative-pathway C3 convertase, thereby limiting complement-mediated effects. Deletion mutants lacking gC-1 are exquisitely sensitive to complement-mediated lysis. Natural mutants have not been isolated with any frequency in surveys of clinical specimens, attesting to the importance of this protein and perhaps this mechanism in the pathogenesis of infection. Vaccinia virus bears a C4b BP structural and functional homologue that accelerates the decay of the classical pathway convertase.[130, 154, 157, 158]

Capsular polysaccharides are another example of microbial surface structures that modulate the effect of complement deposition on the organism and its interaction with the host. In the absence of specific antibody, these polysaccharides—especially those on serogroup B and Y meningococci and type III group B streptococci, which contain sialic acid—are poor activators of complement. The capsule, by masking C3 deposited on subcapsular structures, serves to block its interaction with appropriate complement receptors on phagocytic cells. These effects account in large measure for the antiphagocytic property of these structures. In addition, capsular polysaccharides and outer membrane blebs are shed during organism growth and complement attack. Shedding serves to abort complement attack at the organism surface and may act to decoy complement activation away from the intact organism.[129] The ability of capsular-specific antibody to reverse these effects is testimony to the importance of antibody in redirecting complement deposition to a relevant site on the surface of the organism.[159]

There has been growing appreciation of the number of intracellular pathogens that use complement receptors to gain entry into cells.[108] Entry in this fashion varies as to whether it initiates an appropriate signal transduction response and whether it is sufficient to establish effective intracellular infection. For example, gp350 on Epstein-Barr virus serves as a ligand for CR2 to initiate viral entry into B cells. The resulting cellular transformation probably contributes to the polyclonal gammopathy observed early in infectious mononucleosis.[160–162] In addition to its factor H binding domain, HIV gp120 contains several C3b binding regions. Cells harboring latent HIV can be activated by the uptake of additional HIV or other particles via CR3. Interactions via this receptor can induce the NFκB cellular transcription factor, which in turn binds to promoter regions in the virus to stimulate generation of progeny virus. *Leishmania* species, *Legionella pneumophila,* and various *Mycobacteria* and *Babesia* spp. also use CR1 and CR3, alone or in combination, to gain intracellular access. However, the effects of these modes of entry on cellular activation and organism replication have not been well elucidated.

COMPLEMENT DEFICIENCY STATES

Frequency

Complement deficiency states can be either acquired or inherited. Acquired deficiency states can occur acutely, as part of an abrupt insult such as infection, or in conjunction with chronic rheumatologic or autoimmune diseases. The frequency of inherited complement deficiencies in the general population is about 0.03%. Because these states are rare, the utility of screening tests is greatest in populations that contain the clinical correlates of abnormal complement inheritance—that is, persons with rheumatologic diseases or recurrent bacterial infections.[163, 164] The frequency of complement deficiencies reported among persons with these disorders is affected by both methodological and biologic factors.[165] The most important methodological variables are the sample size and degree of ascertainment. The most important biologic considerations are the ethnic makeup of the population and the incidence of the target disease in that population.

One such study, employing immunologic and functional assays, detected a single individual with homozygous C2 deficiency among 545 patients with rheumatologic disease.[166] This frequency (0.2%) is approximately 10-fold greater than that in the general population. Studies in which DNA typing techniques were applied have found the frequency of homozygous C2 deficiency in whites with SLE to be about 1.7%.[167, 168] These studies provide clear support for the association of complement deficiency states with certain rheumatologic disorders, in particular, SLE.[169]

Reports of an association between systemic meningococcal and gonococcal infections and inherited deficiency of C5, C6, C7, or C8 have led to several studies of the frequency of such deficiencies among patients with these infections. These studies have found from as few as 0 of 47 (<2%) to as many as 8 of 16 (50%) complement-deficient individuals presenting with a first episode of documented meningococcal disease.[164, 165] Analysis of these studies reveals an inverse relation between the prevalence of complement deficiency in persons with meningococcal disease and the incidence of the disease in the general population (Fig. 7–3). This suggests that the overall prevalence of complement deficiencies is relatively constant (0.03 to 0.11%) but that, among populations in which the level of protective antibody is low and meningococcal disease is epidemic, more normal than complement-deficient persons will be infected because there are significantly more of the former than the latter. As the level of immunity in the population increases, the incidence of meningococcal disease falls. However, because the prevalence of complement deficiency in the general population is relatively stable, the frequency of these states among persons with meningococcal disease increases—that is, complement deficiency becomes a proportionately greater determinant of the risk of infection.[165] Therefore, the best estimate of inherited complement deficiency states among patients with endemic neisserial disease is about 5 to 10%, although the likelihood of a complement deficiency is increased dramatically (31%) among patients who have had more than one episode of meningococcal infection.

Although the number of infections caused *by Streptococcus pneumoniae* and *H. influenzae* appears to be increased in patients with complement deficiencies, the prevalence of complement deficiency among persons with systemic infections caused by these organisms does not appear to be markedly different from that in the population at large.[170] The basis for this apparent paradox, especially for *H. influenzae,* which share many features with meningococci, is unknown.

Classical Pathway Deficiencies

The association of immune disorders, in particular SLE, with complement deficiency states is most evident in persons lacking C1, C4, C2, or C3 (Table 7–3). This association exhibits a striking decreasing frequency among these deficiencies: 87%, 75%, 33%, and 16% for C1q, C1, C4, C2, and C3 deficiencies, respectively. This hierarchical relationship is also evident in the severity of SLE and in the frequency and type of autoantibodies present in the sera of these patients. SLE is severe in patients with C1q, C1r, C1s, or C4 deficiency. In these persons, central nervous system disease and

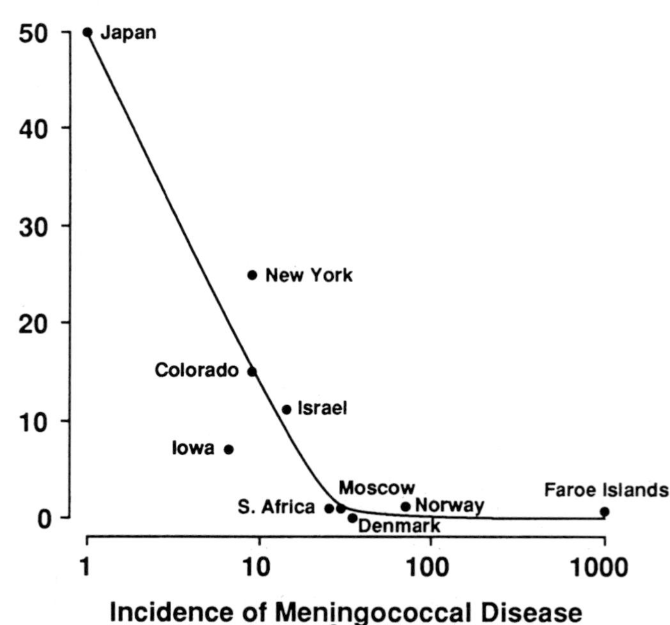

FIGURE 7–3. Relationship between the prevalence of complement deficiency and the incidence of meningococcal disease. (From Figueroa JE, Densen P. Infectious diseases associated with complement deficiencies. Clin Microbiol Rev. 1991;4:359–395.)

TABLE 7–3 Complement Deficiency States

Component	No. of Reported Patients	Mode of Inheritance	Functional Defects	Disease Associations
Classical pathway				
C1qrs	31	ACD	Impaired IC handling, delayed C′ activation, impaired immune response	CVD, 48%; infection (encaps bact), 22%; both, 18%; healthy, 12%
C4	21	ACD		
C2	109	ACD		
Alternative pathway				
D	3	ACD	Impaired C′ activation in absence of specific antibody	Infection (meningococcal), 74%; healthy, 26%
P	70	XL		
Junction of classical and alternative pathways				
C3	19	ACD	Impaired IC handling, opson/phag; granulocytosis, CTX, immune response and absent SBA	CVD, 79%; recurrent infection (encaps bact), 71%
Terminal components				
C5	27	ACD	Impaired CTX; absent SBA	Infection (*Neisseria,* primarily meningococcal), 58%; CVD, 4%
C6	77	ACD	Absent SBA	Both, 1%
C7	73	ACD		Healthy, 25%
C8	73	ACD		
C9	165	ACD	Impaired SBA	Healthy, 91%; infection, 9%
Plasma proteins regulating C′ activation				
C1-INH	Many	AD Acq	Uncontrolled generation of an inflammatory mediator on C′ activation	Hereditary angioedema
H	13	ACD	Uncontrolled AP activation → low C3	CVD, 40%; CVD plus infection (encaps bact), 40%; healthy, 20%
I	14	ACD	Uncontrolled AP activation → low C3	Infection (encaps bact), 100%
Membrane proteins regulating C′ activation				
Decay-accelerating factor	Many	Acq	Impaired regulation of C3b and C8 deposited on host RBC; PMN, platelets → cell lysis	Paroxysmal nocturnal hemoglobinuria
Homologous restriction factor				
CD59				
CR3	>20	ACD	Impaired PMN adhesive functions (i.e., margination), CTX, C3bi-mediated opson/phag	Infection (*Staphylococcus aureus, Pseudomonas* spp.), 100%
Autoantibodies				
C3 nephritic factors	>59	Acq	Stabilize AP, convertase → low C3	MPGN, 41%; PLD, 25%; infection (encaps bact), 16%; MPGN plus PLD, 10%; PLD plus infection, 5%; MPGN plus PLD plus infection, 3%; MPGN plus infection, 2%
C4 nephritic factor		Acq	Stabilize CP, C3 convertase → low C3	Glomerulonephritis, 50%; CVD, 50%

Abbreviations: ACD, Autosomal codominant; Acq, acquired; AD, autosomal dominant; AP, alternative pathway; C′, complement; CP, classical pathway; CTX, chemotaxis; CVD, collagen vascular disease; encaps bact, encapsulated bacteria; IC, immune complex, MPGN, membranoproliferative glomerulonephritis; PLD, partial lipodystrophy; PMN, polymorphonuclear neutrophil; RBC, red blood cells; SBA, serum bactericidal activity; XL, X-linked.
Data from refs. 163 and 164.

glomerulonephritis are common and disease manifests at a median age of 7 years.[171, 172] In persons with C2 deficiency, the severity of SLE appears to be similar to that in the general population, whereas in C3-deficient persons it may be less severe.[169, 173]

Uncertainty exists as to whether these complement deficiencies constitute a risk factor for SLE in both the homozygous and heterozygous conditions or in just the former states. Earlier studies employing immunologic and functional assays suggested an association in both homozygous and heterozygous deficient persons. More recent studies employing DNA typing techniques strongly suggest that, at least in C1q and C2 deficiency, the association exists only for the homozygous state.[167, 168] The situation in partial C4 deficiency is complicated by two factors: the existence of two C4 genes and the association of the null genes with an extended haplotype associated with a number of autoimmune diseases.

The existence of two separate C4 genes, C4A and C4B, dictates that complete C4 deficiency (i.e., the absence of the products of all four C4 genetic loci) is extremely rare. Conversely, heterozygous C4 deficiency is very common, occurring in approximately 25% of the general population.[174]

As a result of linkage disequilibrium, the C2 and C4 null genes occur predominantly as part of distinct extended haplotypes. These haplotypes include MHC I, MHC II, complement, and TNF genes, each of which are candidate disease susceptibility genes. The specific haplotype associated with C2 deficiency, DR2, C4A4, C4B4, BFS, C2Q0, B18, A25, DQB1*0201, DQA1*0501, DRB1*0103, C4B1, C4AQ0, BfS, TNFA*1, TNFB*2, B8, A1, occurs in about 93% of affected persons.[175] For C4 deficiency, this haplotype is HLA-A1, B8, DRB1*0103, DQA1*0501, DQB1*0201, Bf*s, C2*C, C4AQ0, C4B1, TNFA*1, TNFB*2.[176, 177] Multivariate analysis of DR and C4 gene types has confirmed an independent contribution of the C4AQ0 and the DR antigens to the development of SLE. The C4B null gene (C4BQ0) was not associated with SLE.[178] The chemical preference of the internal thioester in C4A to form amide bonds and to react with immune complexes may contribute to the effect of the C4A null gene on the development of SLE.[36, 38, 39]

The pathophysiologic basis for the association between these complement deficiencies and SLE is incompletely understood. Both the impaired handling of immune complexes that is a direct consequence of these deficiencies and the tight genetic linkage of the C2 and C4 loci to the MHC I and MHC II genes, perhaps by modulation of antigen presentation and autoantibody formation, probably contribute to disease pathogenesis.[171, 177, 179–180] However, impaired immune complex clearance unquestionably exerts a greater impact, because this association is apparent for all four of these complement deficiencies, especially C1q, whereas only C4 and C2 are MHC linked. Additional support for this conclusion stems from the occurrence of SLE in some patients with acquired hypocomplementemia.

Of these, C1 inhibitor deficiency is especially interesting, because the absence of this regulatory protein is associated with uncontrolled consumption of the classical pathway complement components, which is particularly severe and prolonged in a small number of patients. It appears that it is these patients who are at risk for development of SLE.[171]

The role of the early components of the classical pathway in inhibiting immune complex precipitation has been documented by in vitro experiments using sera from patients with deficiencies of these components.[181, 182] Studies in both deficient and hypocomplementemic subjects confirmed a striking impairment in the in vivo clearance of immune complexes by the liver and spleen, which was corrected by the replacement of the missing component or components.[171] Moreover, abnormal humoral immune system regulation and the presence of autoantibodies, including rheumatoid factors, have been demonstrated in C2- and C4-deficient guinea pigs[183] and, more recently, in C1q knockout mice.[184]

The low frequency of infection (20%) in persons with a deficiency of C1, C4, or C2, compared with other component deficiencies (see Table 7–3), has been attributed to the presence of an intact alternative pathway in these patients. Bacterial infection, when it occurs, is usually caused by encapsulated bacteria, especially *S. pneumoniae,* and may be recurrent. The most common sites of infection are the sinopulmonary tree, meninges, and blood.[163, 164]

Alternative-Pathway Deficiencies

Inherited deficiencies of the components of the alternative pathway are less common than those of other complement proteins. To date, no individuals with homozygous factor B deficiency have been identified (see Table 7–3). In the presence of specific antibody persons with alternative-pathway defects activate the classical pathway normally, but in the absence of specific antibody a defect in alternative-pathway activation leads to a profound abnormality in complement activation and serum bactericidal activity. Infection in such persons may therefore be expected to have dire consequences, a prediction borne out in patients with properdin deficiency (Table 7–4). However, this prediction is not borne out in factor B knockout mice. These mice breed, develop, and survive normally when reared in conventional housing. They also demonstrate normal lymphoid maturation and antibody production and are no more susceptible to endotoxin challenge than control mice.[185, 186] Resolution of this apparent discrepancy awaits identification of humans with this deficiency.

Properdin deficiency is an X-linked trait that predisposes three quarters of affected persons to meningococcal infections. These infections are frequently characterized by a fulminant course and high mortality rate, and, consequently, recurrent infections are uncommon.[187, 188] Three properdin-deficient variants have been described: type 1, characterized by extremely low concentrations (<0.1 μg/ml) of properdin and absent properdin function[187, 188]; type 2, characterized by a low concentration (~2 μg/ml) of antigenically detectable but functionally altered properdin; and type 3, characterized by a normal concentration (~25 μg/ml) of antigenically detectable properdin but absent function.[189, 190]

C3 Deficiency

C3 deficiency is uncommon (see Table 7–3). As expected from its position and function as the linchpin of the complement cascade, virtually all persons with this defect are seriously ill.[163, 164] Approximately three quarters develop SLE or a related rheumatologic syndrome. Moreover, the inability to use either the classical or the alternative pathway results in a multitude of severe defects in host defense, including impairments in opsonization, immune response, neutrophil chemotaxis, and the ability to generate serum bactericidal activity. Consequently, severe and recurrent pneumococcal, *H. influenzae,* and meningococcal infections involving the sinopulmonary tree, meninges, and blood stream are common, occurring in about 70% of such patients.[163, 164]

A comparable clinical picture is observed in persons with an inherited deficiency of either factor H or factor I and in those who develop autoantibody to C3 (C3 nephritic factor).[163, 164] The similar clinical picture results from uncontrolled alternative-pathway activation and resultant low levels of C3 (<10%) in serum. Recurrent infection and collagen vascular disorders occur less commonly in patients with C3 nephritic factor, presumably because of the somewhat higher levels of C3 in these patients.

Patients with autoantibody to C3 have increased incidences of membranoproliferative glomerulonephritis and partial lipodystrophy (see Table 7–3).[191, 192] The identity of complement factor D and adipsin, a secretory product of adipocytes that is deficient in several animal models of obesity, has been established.[193, 194] This finding has led to the recognition that adipose tissue is a significant site of synthesis for all of the alternative-pathway components.[195] Moreover, it has been shown that C3a stimulates glucose uptake by adipocytes and increases the activity of diacyltransferase. Impairment of these actions, coupled with C3 nephritic factor–dependent adipocyte lysis, suggests potential mechanisms for the association of this antibody with partial lipodystrophy.[196]

Late Complement Component Deficiencies

Persons with a deficiency of one of the terminal complement components exhibit a striking susceptibility to systemic neisserial infections, especially meningococcal disease. Despite the chemotactic defect associated with C5 deficiency, the clinical manifestations of meningococcal disease in persons with this defect and in those with other terminal component deficiencies are remarkably similar.[165]

TABLE 7–4 Comparison of Meningococcal Disease in Normal and Late Complement Component– and Properdin-Deficient Patients

Characteristics	Normal	Deficient in C5, C6, C7, or C8	Deficient in C9	Properdin Deficient*
No. of homozygotes	—	250	165	54–70
No. with meningococcal disease	—	146	15	25–37
Frequency of infection (%)	0.0072	58	9.1	46–53
Median age at first episode (y)	3	17	16	14–11.5
Recurrence rate (%)	0.34	44	0	2–1.4
Relapse rate (%)	0.6	7.9	0	0
Mortality per 100 episodes (%)	19	1.5	0	12–51.4
Infecting serogroup				
No. of isolates	3184	67	2	16
B (%)	50	19.4	50	18.7
Y (%)	4.4	32.8	0	37.5

*Where a range is given the first number refers to documented cases and the second number refers to documented plus probable and possible cases.

From Densen P. Human complement deficiency states and infection. In: Whaley K, Loos M, Weiler JM, eds. Complement in Health and Disease. Dordrecht, The Netherlands: Kluwer Academic Publishers; 1993:173–197, with permission.

Therefore, the basis for the association of meningococcal disease in these persons appears to be their inability to assemble the MAC and express complement-dependent bactericidal activity.

This conclusion is supported by detailed population-based epidemiologic studies demonstrating an approximate 5000-fold increase in risk of meningococcal disease in C7-deficient compared with complement-sufficient Japanese patients. In contrast, C9-deficient Japanese patients experienced an approximate 700-fold increase in risk.[197] The increased risk of meningococcal disease in persons deficient in C5, C6, C7, or C8, compared with those deficient in C9, is consistent with in vitro studies demonstrating that C9-deficient sera can kill meningococci, albeit at a slower rate.[126] This dose-response relation, coupled with the fact that the structural genes encoding these proteins are located on multiple chromosomes, provides strong evidence for a cause-and-effect relationship between the absence of complement-dependent bactericidal activity and the increased susceptibility of these persons to meningococcal disease.

Molecular Basis for Inherited Complement Deficiencies

As with most other inherited conditions, the basis for complement deficiency states exhibits substantial heterogeneity, especially among persons representing different ethnic or racial ancestries. Within a defined ethnic or racial population, the probability that a single molecular defect will predominate is substantially increased. A corollary of this principle is that the same deficiency occurring among persons of different backgrounds is likely to exhibit molecular heterogeneity. The latter generalization is useful in selecting patients whose deficiencies, when characterized at the molecular level, are likely to yield new information. Future studies may focus on the possible association of various component polymorphisms with different disease states.

Classical Pathway Deficiencies. C1q is the product of three separate genes (A, B, and C; see Table 7–1). Mutations in each of these genes have been associated with C1q deficiency. A predominant mutation has not yet emerged from the few patients whose defect has been characterized, nor is there any apparent difference in the clinical picture among persons with these various defects.[198]

C2 deficiency is probably the most common of all the complement deficiencies. It occurs predominantly in white persons of northern European extraction and is inherited in association with a distinct haplotype. The molecular basis for this defect in 93% of cases is a 28-bp gene deletion that causes skipping of exon 6 during mRNA splicing. Exon skipping in turn results in the generation of a premature stop codon and synthesis of a nonfunctional protein.[199, 200]

The predominant molecular basis for C4A and C4B deficiencies involves large deletions encompassing both the respective C4 and associated 21-hydroxylase genes.[176] A 2-bp insertion in exon 29 of the C4A gene has been reported in association with the haplotype HLA-B60 DR6.[201]

Alternative Pathway Deficiencies. Factor H deficiency has been characterized in a single individual who was found to be a compound heterozygote. Both mutations were single-base-pair substitutions that led to the replacement of cysteine residues by an arginine and a tyrosine thereby disrupting disulfide pairing within the short consensus repeat modules. These effects resulted in a failure to secrete the altered factor H.[202]

The molecular basis for factor I deficiency has been established in two kindred. Three of the four null alleles were identical and led to the substitution of a leucine for a histidine. The altered protein was secreted in vitro, but no factor I was detected in the patients' sera, suggesting that the secreted molecules were catabolized extracellularly.[203]

As noted previously, three phenotypic forms of properdin deficiency have been described based on the concentration and residual function of properdin in patient sera. The molecular basis of this deficiency has been delineated in four families with type 1 deficiency (no detectable properdin), two with type 2 deficiency (low levels of functional properdin), and one with type 3 deficiency (normal levels of a dysfunctional molecule) and has proved to be highly heterogeneous.[204] Type 1 deficiency stems from different mutations, all of which result in premature stop codon formation and the production of truncated proteins, which are presumably neither functional nor secreted.[205] Type 2 deficiency arises from separate mutations that lead to amino acid substitutions that could affect molecular charge. The altered molecules are secreted normally but appear to have an accelerated rate of extracellular catabolism.[205] Type 3 deficiency results from an amino acid substitution that does not affect the secretion of the molecule or its extracellular catabolism. Instead, folding of the molecule appears to be altered and to lead indirectly to a decreased affinity of properdin for C3b.[206]

C3 Deficiency. Primary C3 deficiency is uncommon; when recognized, it has occurred in ethnically diverse populations. The molecular basis for this deficiency has been characterized in four patients and has revealed two different splicing defects, a substantial deletion and a single-base-pair change leading to a defect in C3 secretion.[207]

Late Complement Component Deficiencies. The basis for C5 deficiency is molecularly heterogeneous, with multiple but different defects in whites and African Americans. All of the African American patients were compound heterozygotes and possessed nonsense mutations in exons 1 and 36.[208]

Several distinct types of C6 deficiency have been described, including complete deficiency and two different subtotal deficiencies, one of which occurs in association with subtotal C7 deficiency. Worldwide, complete C6 deficiency is molecularly diffuse. This deficiency is particularly common among native Africans from the Western Cape in South Africa. Three separate single-base-pair deletions have been described in this population. Of these, the 879delG is most common. Together with an 1195delG null allele, it accounts for a characteristic set of C6/C7 DNA haplotypes. The 1195delG and 1936delG alleles have also been reported in African Americans.[209, 210] Isolated subtotal C6 deficiency is caused by an abnormal 5′ splice donor site in intron 15, which results in the reduced secretion of a C6 molecule that is 13.5% shorter than normal but retains functional activity.[211]

A missense mutation in exon 9 appears to account for most of the cases of C7 deficiency among Israeli families of Moroccan Sephardic Jewish descent.[212] In contrast, deletion of exons 7 and 8 appears to be the predominant cause of this deficiency among the Irish population.[213]

The structural genes for C6 and C7 are tightly linked on chromosome 5 (see Table 7–1). Combined subtotal C6/C7 deficiency (SD) states represents novel combinations of the C6 SD allele with a C7 SD allele and various C6 and C7 null alleles. These partial deficiencies typically come to clinical attention when some initiating event generates production of the C5b6 complex, which in turn converts a partial deficiency to a total one. Persons in whom the two SD alleles are shared in combination with a C6 null allele are functionally C6 SD. Their serum contains a near-normal concentration of C7 despite the presence of the C7 SD allele, because the markedly reduced C6 activity is insufficient to lead to consumption of the existing C7. Complement consumption converts the subtotal state to complete C6 deficiency. In contrast, persons in whom the C6 SD allele is paired with two different C7 SD alleles are functionally C7 deficient despite the expression, albeit reduced, of functional C7, because the C5b6 complex consumes the C7.[214, 215]

Three genes (see Table 7–1) encode the C8 molecule, but defects have been reported only in the A and B genes. C8β deficiency occurs predominantly in white persons, especially those of Russian descent. About 85% of the C8β null alleles described to date have been caused by a C→T transition in exon 9, and 95% of all the C8β null alleles characterized to date have been caused by C→T transitions. It is unclear why C→T transitions should be such a common underlying mechanism for this deficiency.[216] A splicing defect in the C8A gene that results in a 10-bp insertion in the associated RNA has been described as the basis for C8α deficiency in several African Americans with C8α-γ deficiency.[217] In contrast, a point mutation disrupting the universally conserved 5′ splice site sequence at the boundary between the second exon and intron appears common in the Japanese.[217a]

C9 deficiency is particularly common in the Japanese population. To date the molecular basis for this deficiency has not been described in that population. Its basis among white populations is molecularly diverse.[218, 219]

Meningococcal Infection in Complement Deficiency States

Meningococcal disease is the single most common infection sustained by persons with complement deficiency, accounting for 75 to 85% of etiologically identified infections.[163, 164] Although meningococcal disease has been reported in persons with a deficiency of any of the plasma complement proteins, it is most common in those with a deficiency of properdin, C5, C6, C7, or C8, of whom 50 to 60% experience at least one episode during their lifetime. This striking association confirms the importance of the complement system in host defense against meningococci.

Meningococcal disease in patients with these complement deficiencies exhibits several unique features that help to distinguish it from that in complement-sufficient persons (see Table 7–4). These features provide important clinical clues that should suggest to the clinician the underlying presence of a deficiency and the need to screen for a complement deficiency state. These features are unlikely to result solely from ascertainment bias for the following reasons. First, they have been confirmed in multiple studies in varied populations around the world. Second, each feature has been borne out by investigations of complement-deficient families after exclusion of the proband from the analysis. Third, at least in the case of the late complement component deficiencies, family studies have failed to reveal undiagnosed infections or unexplained or premature deaths.

Data compiled from the literature and from a detailed population-based study suggest that these complement deficiency states increase the risk of meningococcal disease by 5000- to 10,000-fold. In the general population the median age at onset of meningococcal infection is 3 years and 56% of the infections occur before 5 years of age; in contrast, the median age of first infection in complement-deficient patients is 17 years and only 10% of the infections occur before 5 years. Therefore, most deficient persons pass through the age of life when the deficiency might be expected to increase maximally their susceptibility to meningococcal disease without evidence of that susceptibility. The basis for this observation is unknown, but it suggests that unidentified factors may modulate the susceptibility of deficient persons to infection later in life.

Meningococcal disease in complement-deficient patients is caused by uncommon serogroups—particularly groups Y, W135, and X—more often than in persons without complement deficiencies.[163, 164, 220] Conversely, the prevalence of these deficiencies is increased among patients with meningococcal disease caused by these serogroups.[221] The physiologic basis for this observation is not known with certainty, but factors that may be important include (1) the critical requirement for anticapsular antibody for prevention of disease in deficient compared with normal persons; (2) better elimination of group B isolates by phagocytic cells in the absence of capsular antibody[222]; and (3) the propensity for uncommon meningococcal serogroup organisms to cause disease in older persons.[223] Nevertheless, meningococci and gonococci isolated from complement-deficient patients with systemic neisserial infection do not differ significantly in their biologic properties from the same organisms isolated from complement-sufficient patients.[224] Therefore, the absence of complement-dependent bactericidal activity does not automatically provide access to the blood stream by less virulent, serum-sensitive organisms.

Recurrent meningococcal disease, defined as a new infection occurring more than 1 month after a previous episode, occurs in about 40 to 45% of persons deficient in C5, C6, C7, or C8. This recurrence rate is approximately 100 to 150 times greater than that in the general population. Results of statistical analysis of the number of patients with a specified number of episodes of meningococcal disease are consistent with the interpretation that the risk of meningococcal disease in complement-deficient persons is independent of prior infection.[164] That is, prior disease does not reduce the risk of subsequent meningococcal infection in these patients. In that study, the estimated probability of each infection was 0.39.[164] A similar analysis, using a slightly different statistical approach, arrived at an identical conclusion and produced an estimated probability of infection of 0.6.[225, 226] The latter analysis also demonstrated that the interval between infections (4 to 5 years) did not differ, again suggesting that prior disease does not reduce the risk of subsequent meningococcal infection. The explanation for the failure of prior infection to reduce the risk of subsequent episodes of meningococcal disease in these complement-deficient persons appears to lie in their critical dependence on capsular antibodies for protection and the fact that infection constitutes a relatively poor stimulus for production of these antibodies. These antibodies are highly efficient in promoting opsonophagocytic elimination of meningococci. In contrast, antibodies to subcapsular antigens, although bactericidal and protective in the normal host, are poor opsonins and afford little protection in complement-deficient patients who lack the effector proteins necessary for the expression of bactericidal activity.[227]

Relapse of meningococcal disease, defined as infection with the same serogroup occurring less than 1 month after the initial infection, occurs in 7.6% of the patients deficient in C5 through C8 with meningococcal disease reported in the literature. This frequency is approximately 10 times greater than that in the general population and suggests that meningococci may be sequestered intracellularly, where they are relatively protected from antibiotics.[164]

One of the most striking aspects of meningococcal disease in persons with late complement component deficiencies is that, despite a several-thousand-fold increase in the risk of infection, they experience a 5- to 10-fold reduction in the chance of dying from the disease, compared with normal persons.[164] Therefore, the same defect that predisposes to infection appears to provide protection from the lethal consequences of the disease. This remarkable observation suggests that the host's exuberant response to the organism is as much responsible for the clinical manifestations and outcome as is the organism itself. This deduction is supported by the report of Brandtzaeg and colleagues[228] of a close correlation between the extent of complement activation and mortality in meningococcal disease and suggests that the latter is in part dependent on the assembly of the MAC.

The basis for the lower mortality from meningococcal disease in persons deficient in late complement components is unknown, but variables that may be relevant include milder disease,[225] the possibility that fewer organisms are required to initiate infection, an ability to tolerate better a given endotoxin load,[229] and less host cell injury.

The possibility that fewer organisms may be required to establish systemic meningococcal disease in deficient than in normal persons is attractive, but data addressing this point are conspicuously absent in the literature. Such an affect would account for the increased number of infections and also for the milder disease and the decreased case fatality rate, since mortality is directly related to the number of organisms in the blood stream.[230, 231] A reduction in the organism load might translate into a lower concentration of circulating endotoxin and less systemic inflammation. Alternatively, because insertion of the MAC into the outer membrane of gram-negative organisms results in the release of free endotoxin, the inability of persons with late complement component deficiencies to assemble the MAC may be associated with a reduction in the quantity of circulating endotoxin for a given load of organisms. This reduction in turn might lessen ongoing complement activation and decrease secretion of various cytokines linked to the development of septic shock in meningococcal disease.[228, 232–236] Finally, insertion of the MAC into host cell membranes might occur in vivo as a consequence of exuberant complement activation in the vicinity of innocent bystander cells or as a consequence of endotoxin binding to these cells and subsequent complement activation on their surfaces. For example, MAC insertion activates leukocytes, stimulating release of a plethora of potentially noxious mediators[237–239] and increased expression of procoagulant molecules on endothelial cells.[240] Interruption of these processes in the patient with a late complement component deficiency would result in an improved ability to tolerate a given load of organisms and endotoxin.

Attention has been drawn to functional differences among the various polymorphic forms of the FcγRIIa receptor on phagocytic cells and the possible linkage of a poor IgG_2 binding allotype to meningococcal disease in the general population.[241] Characterization of these polymorphisms in patients with late complement component deficiency revealed a significant association of the FcγRIIa allotype with infection, whereas neutrophils from persons with LCCD without infection were more likely to bear FcγRIIIb and to phagocytose and kill meningococci effectively. These observations suggest a possible explanation for the fact that not all patients with late complement component deficiency become infected with meningococci.[242–244]

Other Complement Deficiency States

Hereditary Angioedema—C1 Inhibitor Deficiency. Persons lacking C1-INH present with a distinctive clinical picture historically referred to as hereditary angioneurotic edema (HANE or HAE).[245] The hereditary form of this disease was recognized more than 100 years ago, and an acquired variant was identified as a distinct entity more recently. HAE is an autosomal dominant disorder, but about 20% of newly identified patients lack a positive family history and reflect spontaneous mutations. Type 1 HAE accounts for 75 to 85% of cases and is characterized by the presence of low (5 to 30%) levels of normal C1-INH protein arising from the intact allele. Type 2 HAE is characterized by the presence of normal to increased levels of antigenic C1-INH, representing a mixture of functional and dysfunctional gene products.[71, 245–247]

The acquired forms of this disorder (AAE) are considerably less common. Historically, two variants have been recognized: one occurs in association with B-lymphocyte disorders and the other because of the presence of an autoantibody to C1-INH. However, studies suggest that this distinction may be inaccurate and that autoantibodies account for both types of AAE. Antibody binding does not interfere with cleavage of C1-INH by C1s but rather prevents the formation of a covalent linkage between the enzyme and the cleaved inhibitor. This alteration effectively converts C1-INH from an inhibitor to a substrate and permits C1s action to continue unchecked. In turn, this leads to complement consumption in the fluid phase and associated low levels of C1s, C1r, C4, and C2 that are the hallmark of the disease.[247–249]

Because the hereditary form of this disorder is inherited as an autosomal dominant trait, the serum from all of these patients contains some normally functioning C1-INH.[71] In contrast, persons with the acquired variants have markedly reduced or absent functional C1-INH activity in their serum. As a consequence of this basic difference, the serum from patients with the hereditary form of this disorder contains normal amounts of C1 and C1q but reduced levels of C4 and C2, whereas serum from those with the acquired variants contains strikingly reduced amounts of C1, C1q, C4, and C2.[71, 245, 246]

The health of patients with this disorder is punctuated by attacks of nonpitting, nonpruritic, and nonpainful edema of the extremities, face, or larynx. Angioedema of the larynx is the most severe complication of the disorder and is a common cause of death in these patients. The gastrointestinal tract may also be affected, and such attacks manifest as episodes of acute, crampy abdominal pain frequently associated with nausea, vomiting, and occasionally diarrhea. In the inherited form of the disorder, attacks generally begin in childhood, increase in frequency and worsen in severity during adolescence, increase during menstruation, are markedly reduced during pregnancy, and diminish gradually in the fifth and sixth decades of life. A typical attack lasts 2 to 3 days. Acute, life-threatening attacks should be treated with C1-INH concentrate. Administration of impeded androgens to increase the biosynthesis of C1-INH has been employed successfully for chronic management of the hereditary form of the disease.[71, 245]

The mechanism whereby C1-INH deficiency produces the clinical syndrome of angioedema is incompletely understood. Evidence exists to support a role for both complement-derived and contact system mediators. Intradermal injection of activated C1s leads to nonpainful, nonpruritic swelling in both humans and guinea pigs. This response does not occur if activated C1 is injected into C2-deficient humans or guinea pigs but is observed after injection into C3-deficient patients.[250] These data provide support for a C2-derived anaphylatoxin in the clinical picture of angioedema. However, in addition to its role as the sole inhibitor of C1 esterase, C1-INH is also an important inhibitor, if not the major inhibitor, of factor XII and kallikrein in the contact system. Plasma from patients with HAE exhibits an impaired ability to inactivate these mediators. Detailed studies of a particular family with dysfunctional C1-INH demonstrated that the molecule was defective in its ability to inhibit C1r and C1s but retained full ability to complex and inhibit kallikrein and factor XIIa. None of the 10 family members whose sera possessed this dysfunctional C1-INH had ever experienced an attack of angioedema.[251] These data support an important role of the contact system in the clinical picture of HAE. Together these separate lines of inquiry suggest that symptoms probably result from the interaction of several factors within these cascade systems.[71, 252]

As expected from the different C1-INH protein phenotypes, the genetic basis for HAE is heterogeneous. A substantial proportion of the type I HAE defects are associated with mutations within short interspersed nucleotide elements called *Alu* clusters. These mutations cause a variety of rearrangements leading to deletions or duplications within the gene, impaired transcription, and reduced levels of specific mRNA and plasma concentrations of C1-INH. In contrast, type II HAE, which is generally associated with normal concentrations of a dysfunctional protein, is typically caused by point mutations. These mutations usually affect the arginine at the reactive center of the molecule or amino acids in its immediate vicinity. Occasionally mutations affect C1-INH glycosylation. In all instances the mutation leads to the synthesis of a protein with an altered ability to react with its substrates. The resulting altered catabolism is responsible for the normal or elevated concentration of plasma C1-INH.[253–255]

Paroxysmal Nocturnal Hemoglobinuria. Paroxysmal nocturnal hemoglobinuria (PNH) is an uncommon syndrome that typically occurs in adults in their thirties to fifties. Classically, affected persons present with bouts of intravascular hemolysis that are worse at night and last for several days to weeks. The events precipitating hemolysis are usually inapparent. The basis for the increased hemolysis at night is unclear but may relate to a lower pH in the small vessels of the peripheral venous circulation. In contrast, the more common presentation, occurring in about half of the patients, is one of chronic hemolysis. Patients may have back pain, cramping abdominal pain, and headaches. Although the major clinical features of the disease relate to intravascular hemolysis, the full syndrome includes a propensity to venous thrombosis and diminished hematopoiesis. The thrombosis is unusual in that it typically involves major intra-abdominal and hepatic veins and is often precipitated by surgery.[256–258]

The basic problem in patients with PNH is an increased susceptibility of their erythrocytes to hemolysis. The peripheral blood of these patients contains varying proportions of three populations of erythrocytes. PNH type 1 cells are normal, whereas type 2 and type 3 PNH cells exhibit, respectively, 3- to 6-fold and 15- to 25-fold increased sensitivity to complement-mediated lysis. The severity of the clinical picture correlates best with the proportion of type 3 cells present in the peripheral circulation.[259]

PNH cells lack more than 20 different surface proteins. The presence of these molecules in normal amounts on endothelial cells in persons with PNH supports the clonal origin of this disorder within bone marrow precursor cells. The feature shared by these proteins is their linkage to the cell membrane through a carboxyl-terminal glycosylphosphatidylinositol (GPI) anchor.[260] Two of these proteins are the complement regulatory proteins DAF and CD59.[261, 262] However, persons with an inherited defect affecting expression of only DAF on their erythrocyte membranes do not exhibit the PNH phenotype, whereas those lacking solely CD59 do manifest this phenotype.[263, 264] Therefore the absence of the CD59 molecule directly accounts for the increased susceptibility of PNH cells to intravascular hemolysis.

In the absence of CD59, many MACs are inserted in the platelet membrane, cause vesiculation, and provide sites to generate prothrombinase with resultant thrombin formation. These alterations may contribute to the susceptibility of patients with PNH to thrombosis. In addition, the absence of the GPI-linked urokinase receptor from PNH cells may render clots more resistant to dissolution, although neither of these abnormalities explains the propensity for intra-abdominal thrombus formation. Similarly, the absence of the GPI-linked FcγRIII receptor from phagocytic cells may contribute to the slightly increased susceptibility of these patients to infection. Studies concerning the diminished hematopoiesis that occurs in patients with PNH suggest that PNH cells do not possess a proliferative advantage within the marrow. However, in an abnormal marrow in which normal cells are at a survival disadvantage, PNH cells appear to be resistant to abnormal influences and emerge as the predominant cell type. The absence of a GPI-linked receptor (e.g., for a growth factor) has been postulated as the basis for this effect. Whether the factors that contribute to the development of an abnormal marrow environment are the same as those giving rise to the somatic mutation responsible for PNH is unknown.[257, 258, 260, 265]

PNH arises as a result of a defect in the first step of the synthesis of the GPI anchor responsible for linking the missing surface proteins to the cell membrane. This step is catalyzed by an enzyme that transfers activated *N*-acetyl glucose to the phosphatidylinositol acceptor.[266] This enzyme is the presumed product of the *PIGA* gene, and multiple mutations in this gene have been reported in association with PNH. Unlike most defects affecting synthetic pathways, these genetic abnormalities are expressed in dominant fashion in progeny cells. This unusual event arises because the *PIGA* gene is located on the X chromosome and the somatic mutations in this gene arise after inactivation of one of the X chromosomes.[258, 260]

COMPLEMENT IN DISEASE STATES

The increasing availability of knockout mice coupled with modern molecular techniques is leading to a progressively sophisticated understanding of the role of complement in different types of inflammation and in the pathogenesis of tissue injury and repair. Mediators released during complement activation may play a role in the development of symptoms or in the outcome of these disorders. Evidence supporting this suggestion includes the fact that the extent of complement activation often parallels disease activity, the occurrence of complement deposition at the site of tissue injury, and the demonstration that in animal models of these disorders specific manipulation of complement activation modulates the course of disease. The role of complement has been studied most extensively in infectious diseases, rheumatologic disorders, and glomerulonephritis that are characterized by obvious inflammation. However, it has become increasingly clear that complement activation and mediator generation play important roles in such diverse entities as atherosclerosis,[267] restenosis, postperfusion injury,[268] demyelination disorders,[269–271] a variety of dermatoses,[272] and hyperacute graft rejection in xenogeneic transplantation.[273, 274] Damage in these disorders is complement dependent. It can be prevented by complement depletion or infusion of proteins that regulate complement activation such as soluble CR1 and CD46[275–277] or, in the case of xenotransplantation, by the development of transgenic animals whose organs express the genes for human complement regulatory molecules.[278]

Infectious Diseases

Complement activation during infections is particularly impressive in diseases like dengue fever, bacterial endocarditis, and bacteremia, in which the organisms or their products react with antibodies to form circulating immune complexes and initiate complement consumption. It is especially striking in meningococcal disease and other forms of gram-negative sepsis and septic shock. Studies have convincingly demonstrated a protective role for complement in endotoxin shock. Genetically engineered C3- and C4-deficient mice did not clear endotoxin as efficiently, had higher levels of TNF and IL-1, and had much higher mortality rates than wild-type mice. C1-INH and fibrinogen levels were also lower in the deficient mice. Reconstitution of the deficient mice with C1-INH significantly reduced mortality and restored fibrinogen concentrations to normal despite the persistent deficiency of C3 or C4. Together these findings indicate that endotoxin-containing immune complexes initiate complement consumption via the classic pathway and that the failure to incorporate C3 into the immune complexes leads to deficient endotoxin clearance, ongoing complement consumption, and C1-INH depletion. The absence of C1-INH permits contact system activation, as manifested by fibrinogen consumption (a potential counterpart of disseminated intravascular coagulopathy in humans). The fact that C1-INH replacement protected the deficient animals and restored fibrinogen levels to normal strongly implicates the direct involvement of the contact system in endotoxin shock and death.[279] Subsequent experiments demonstrated that the immune complexes initiating this sequence of events were composed of IgM natural antibody with specificity for the endotoxin O antigen.[280] In this respect these results are reminiscent of those implicating natural antibody and complement consumption via the classical pathway in reperfusion injury.[268]

Additional studies suggest that other complement components also modulate the interaction of the host with endotoxin. Circulating C5a has been associated with the development of the acute respiratory distress syndrome in humans[281, 282] and in a monkey model of gram-negative shock.[283] In the monkey model, mortality could be prevented and morbidity attenuated by the administration of antibody to C5a.[283] The observation that persons with inherited C5, C6, C7, or C8 deficiency have a 6000-fold greater frequency of meningococcal disease but 10-fold less mortality than do those with a normal complement system (see Table 7–4) suggests that MAC assembly may increase mortality in the sufficient host, perhaps by facilitating greater release of endotoxin from the bacteria or through an action on host cells (see previous discussion).[163]

Complement, in conjunction with the reticuloendothelial system, plays a critical role in the removal of encapsulated bacteria from the blood stream.[284] Delineation of the contribution of these variables to the clearance process has been accomplished in an animal model of pneumococcal bacteremia and has demonstrated that the more virulent the organism, the greater the role of the spleen in performing this clearance function.[285, 286] Complement depletion led to a significant decrease in the number of pneumococci needed to kill 50% of the animals, demonstrating an important role for complement in the clearance function. In addition, clearance of pneumococci was similar in healthy and in C4-deficient animals, indicating that complement activation and fixation to the bacteria via the alternative pathway were particularly relevant in this process. Moreover, the presence of immune antibody shifted the burden of clearance from the spleen to the liver, and this effect was absolutely dependent on a functional alternative complement pathway.[287]

An increased susceptibility to infection is observed both in persons undergoing splenectomy and in those with intact but nonfunctioning spleens (e.g., patients with sickle cell anemia).[288, 289] The incidence of infection varies from a low of approximately 1% in persons undergoing incidental splenectomy to a high of approximately 25% in those undergoing splenectomy as treatment for thalassemia.[289] The mortality rate in these patients varies between 40 and 80%, depending on the underlying condition prompting splenectomy. A wide variety of organisms have been reported to cause overwhelming sepsis in splenectomized patients, but the pneumococcus accounts for 50 to 70% of such infections, with the bulk of the remainder being accounted for by the meningococcus, *H. influenzae,* and, to a lesser extent, *E. coli.*[288] The typical presentation of such patients is that of septic shock, disseminated intravascular coagulopathy, and the adult respiratory distress syndrome occurring in the absence of a primary site of infection.[290]

Rheumatologic Disorders

Substantial clinical and experimental evidence links complement deficiency syndromes and complement activation to a variety of rheumatologic diseases, most notably SLE.[291] Additional support for this relation is the finding that pharmacologic agents (e.g., hydralazine, isoniazid) associated with the drug-induced form of SLE inactivate C4 by nucleophilic attack on its internal thioester and formation of amide bonds.[292] Evidence that complement activation may be associated with the manifestations of the disease and with tissue injury includes the demonstration of C3 and immune complex deposition at the dermal-epidermal junction in cutaneous lesions from patients with either SLE or discoid lupus erythematosus. Similar immunohistochemical alterations have been demonstrated in biopsy specimens of healthy skin from the same patients. However, the finding of MAC in areas of affected but not unaffected skin from these patients strengthens the hypothesis that complement activation may partly mediate tissue injury in these disorders.[272]

In addition to these effects, sera from about 40% of patients with SLE contain an inhibitor of C5a-derived chemotactic activity.[293–295] Its presence correlates with disease activity and the resultant chemotactic defect with the enhanced susceptibility of these patients to infection. The inhibitor has been identified as the Bb fragment of factor B, and it exerts its effect by blocking the interaction of C5a des Arg with its cochemotaxin in serum.[112] The presence of free Bb in the serum of these patients reflects alternative-pathway activation and substantiates the utility of complement component quantitation in assessing disease activity.

Incorporation of C3 into immune complexes promotes their binding to C3b receptors (CR1) on erythrocytes. Erythrocyte CR1 are removed along with immune complexes during passage through the liver and spleen. The number of erythrocyte CR1 molecules is reduced in persons with disorders such as SLE that are characterized by circulating immune complexes.[296] The degree of CR1 reduction correlates well with disease activity and with the extent of complement activation. The decrease in CR1, coupled with the inability of circulating erythrocytes to resynthesize them, further exacerbates the defect in immune complex clearance, thereby promoting their deposition in the tissues, with resultant damage to the host. The number of erythrocyte CR1 molecules returns to the genetically prescribed level on control of disease activity and replenishment of the circulating erythrocyte pool.

Renal Disorders

Complement deposition in renal diseases that are associated with immune disorders is related to the deposition of immune complexes within the kidney,[297–303] whereas complement deposition in the absence of immune complexes is postulated to occur by activation of the alternative pathway.[304] In a rat model of chronic tubulointerstitial disease, loss of renal mass and function was correlated with increased ammonia production and systemic acidosis. Under these conditions, peritubular deposition of C3 and the MAC was readily demonstrated. However, deposition of these components and evidence of tubulointerstitial inflammation were markedly decreased in diseased animals treated with sodium bicarbonate. These and other results suggest that ammonia attacks the C3 internal thioester to form amidated C3. Amidated C3 serves to activate the alternative complement pathway in the fluid phase, leads to C3 and C5b–9 deposition in the tissue, and elicits an inflammatory response and tissue injury.[304, 305] The resulting intrarenal complement depletion may also contribute to the development of chronic bacterial pyelonephritis.[306]

Local ammonia production may also play a role in complement deposition in ischemic tissue. The mechanisms of ammonia formation in such tissues involve the release of adenosine from affected cells and its deamination to ammonia by the adenosine deamidase present in circulating erthyrocytes.[307, 308]

Experiments using C6-sufficient and -deficient rabbits and the infusion of C8-deficient serum into rats have clearly demonstrated that the development of proteinuria in membranous glomerulonephritis depends on the assembly and deposition of a complete MAC on the glomerular epithelial cells.[299, 302] A substantial portion of this injury results from MAC-mediated stimulation of prostaglandin and thromboxane synthesis, because development of proteinuria could be inhibited by treatment with indomethacin, an inhibitor of cyclooxygenase.[309]

Many patients with chronic renal disease ultimately require hemodialysis. Exposure of plasma to first-use filter membranes during dialysis results in complement activation.[310] Anaphylatoxins released during this process (e.g., C5a) have been associated in a concentration-dependent and temporal fashion with the onset of respiratory distress in some dialysis patients.[282, 310, 311] This association is believed to relate in part to C5a-dependent neutrophil aggregation and stimulation and the formation of microemboli and their deposition in the lung[282] (see Chapter 8).

EVALUATION AND TREATMENT OF COMPLEMENT DISORDERS

Evaluation

Evaluation of the complement system is indicated when the diagnosis of a complement deficiency state is being considered or when specific measures of complement proteins are being used to assess disease activity or response to therapy. As pointed out previously, several clinical clues should lead the clinician to suspect a complement deficiency state.[163, 164] Foremost among these is a medical or family history of recurrent systemic infection caused by encapsulated bacteria, especially meningococci. A family history of fulminant meningococcal disease occurring in males in skipped generations should suggest the possibility of X-linked properdin deficiency. Meningococcal disease occurring in persons older than 10 years of age, especially when caused by non–group B meningococci, warrants evaluation of the complement system, because 5 to 10% of these patients have a complement deficiency state, even in the absence of recurrent disease. Likewise, a history of SLE in family members or the occurrence of atypical features of SLE should also suggest the need to evaluate the complement system. Specific syndromes, including partial lipodystrophy, angioedema, and PNH, are other indications for the specific measurement of complement function or related activities.

Because any of a number of specific complement deficiencies can produce one of the typical clinical syndromes associated with these disorders, it is important to use a test that measures the function of the entire complement cascade during the initial evaluation of such patients. The most common of these tests is the CH_{50}, which measures the function of the classical and terminal complement pathways. When defects in the alternative pathway are being considered, an analogous test evaluating alternative-pathway function should be requested. Many hospital laboratories do not perform the latter test, so it may be necessary to contact a research or commercial laboratory with specific expertise in this area. A negative or extremely low result in either of these two assays warrants further diagnostic evaluation. The combined results of the tests of classical and alternative-pathway functions should suggest which additional tests need to be performed. If both the classical and alternative-pathway CH_{50} values are extremely low, the defect must lie in one of the components shared by both pathways: C3 through C9 (see Fig. 7–1). If the alternative pathway is normal but the classical pathway is not, the deficient component must be C1, C2, or C4. Conversely, a normal classical but a defective alternative pathway suggests a defect in factor D, factor B, or properdin. The diagnosis of these specific defects can frequently be accomplished by the use of immunochemical methods to demonstrate an absence of the relevant antigen. However, several complement deficiency states involve absent function in the presence of normal amounts of antigenic protein. Hence, confirmation of the diagnosis of a specific component deficiency should be documented by specific functional assays for the protein under consideration and by demonstration that replacement of the missing component restores both specific and total complement activity. Such assays usually require the expertise of a complement laboratory.

Treatment

There are two aspects of the treatment of complement deficiency states: replacement of the missing protein and prevention of infection. Although advances in knowledge of the molecular basis of the various complement deficiency states may provide an alternative means of therapy in the future, replacement of a deficient component at the present time usually requires the infusion of fresh-frozen plasma. This approach has been successfully employed in therapy for acute attacks of angioedema,[71, 245] in restoring C3 levels toward normal in patients with C3 deficiency, and in the treatment of a C2-deficient patient with SLE unresponsive to conventional therapy.[312, 313] This approach has several drawbacks. First, the half-life of most complement proteins in vivo is short,[8] although a notable exception occurs in patients with low C3 levels caused by factor I deficiency. In these patients, replacement therapy restores factor I activity, thereby markedly reducing the accelerated breakdown of C3 that is observed in this disorder.[314] Second, replacement of a genetically absent protein may stimulate the production of antibody to the missing component, thereby limiting the value of subsequent therapy. This consideration is of limited concern in persons with autosomally inherited disorders such as hereditary angioedema whose serum contains some normal protein or in persons with other complement deficiency disorders characterized by the presence of antigenically normal amounts of a dysfunctional protein. Third, the relative infrequency of infection in most of these patients must be balanced against the potential risk of acquisition of a variety of blood-borne infections during plasma infusion, especially since alternative modes of therapy are available. Whether the acute infusion of fresh-frozen plasma might be beneficial in the treatment of life-threatening infections,[315] especially in properdin-deficient patients, remains untested. The use of impeded androgens to enhance the in vivo biosynthesis of C1-INH provides a long-term alternative approach to replacement of this protein.[71, 245, 316]

Prevention of infection in complement-deficient patients is best achieved through vaccination. All deficient persons should be vaccinated with the tetravalent meningococcal vaccine. Those with classical pathway deficiencies should also receive the polyvalent pneumococcal and conjugated *H. influenzae* vaccines. Given the low cost and high potential benefit of these vaccines, all three vaccines should probably be administered to any individual with complement deficiency. Conjugate vaccines, such as that for *H. influenzae*, that initiate a T-cell–dependent response appear to stimulate the production of higher antibody concentrations and longer persistence of the antibody. The T-cell dependence of this vaccine may help to circumvent the qualitative defect in antibody production observed in these patients.[118]

Successful vaccination leads to the production of anticapsular antibodies that promote utilization of the classical pathway in patients with an alternative-pathway defect and facilitate alternative-pathway utilization in patients lacking one of the classical pathway components.[50, 188] In such patients, these antibodies may promote bactericidal activity as well as microbial elimination by enhancing opsonophagocytosis.

Neither clinical nor in vitro studies have explored the potential for vaccination to help protect C3-deficient persons from infection. The theoretical basis for this approach lies in the ability of antibody alone to facilitate phagocytic elimination of organisms, albeit at a reduced rate of killing. This property is most relevant to the clearance of organisms from the blood stream via the reticuloendothelial system, in which the structural architecture and lining of the sinusoids with tissue macrophages contribute greatly to surface phagocytosis.[284, 285] In view of the suboptimal response to protein and polysaccharide antigens in C1-, C2-, C4-, and C3-deficient humans and animals, documentation of the patient's response to vaccination with these antigens seems prudent.

Although anticapsular antibody cannot enhance serum bactericidal activity in persons with a deficiency of one of the terminal complement proteins, it promotes opsonization and killing of these organisms by phagocytic cells.[222] In vitro studies of prevaccination and postvaccination sera have documented the ability of these patients to respond to the tetravalent meningococcal vaccine and for that response to facilitate phagocytic killing of the corresponding meningococci.[227, 317, 318] In addition, clinical investigations have documented that vaccination reduces the frequency of infection from 0.15 to 0.04 episodes per year and prolongs the interval between infections from 3.6 to more than 6 years.[319, 320] These studies, like those in other groups of complement-deficient individuals, attest to the utility of vaccination as an immunologic means to circumvent the major clinical manifestations of these deficiencies.

An alternative strategy for the prevention of meningococcal disease is the use of prophylactic antibiotics.[321] This approach significantly reduces the frequency of infection in C6-deficient persons and has its greatest use in populations in whom group B disease is highly prevalent.[322] It is unclear whether prophylaxis should be lifelong or whether the development of antibiotic resistance will limit the efficacy of this approach.

REFERENCES

1. Ross GD. Introduction and history of complement research. In: Ross GD, ed. Immunobiology of the Complement System. Orlando, Fla: Academic Press; 1986:1–20.
2. Ratnoff WD. A war with the molecules: Louis Pillemer and the history of properdin. Perspect Biol Med. 1980;23:638–657.
3. Lepow IH. Louis Pillemer, properdin, and scientific controversy. J Immunol. 1980;125:471–478.
4. Root RK, Ryan JL. Humoral immunity and complement. In: Mandell GL, Douglas RG Jr, Bennett JE, eds. Principles and Practice of Infectious Diseases. 2nd ed. New York: Churchill Livingstone; 1985;31–56.
5. Morris KM, Aden DP, Knowles BB, et al. Complement biosynthesis by the human hepatoma-derived cell line HepG2. J Clin Invest. 1982;70:906–913.
6. Perlmutter DH, Colten HR. Molecular immunobiology of complement biosynthesis: A model of single-cell control of effector–inhibitor balance. Annu Rev Immunol. 1986;4:231–251.
7. Alper CA, Raum D, Awdeh ZL, et al. Studies of hepatic synthesis in vivo of plasma proteins, including orosomucoid, transferrin, α_1-antitrypsin, C8, and factor B. Clin Immunol Immunopathol. 1980;16:84–89.
8. Ruddy S, Carpenter CB, Chin KW, et al. Human complement metabolism: An analysis of 144 studies. Medicine (Baltimore). 1975;54:165–178.
9. Mier JW, Dinarello CA, Atkins MB, et al. Regulation of hepatic acute phase protein synthesis by products of interleukin 2 (IL-2)-stimulated human peripheral blood mononuclear cells. J Immunol. 1987;139:1268–1272.
10. Baumann H, Richards C, Gauldie J. Interaction among hepatocyte-stimulating factors, interleukin 1, and glucocorticoids for regulation of acute phase plasma proteins in human hepatoma (HepG2) cells. J Immunol. 1987;139:4122–4128.
11. Morgan BP, Gasque P. Extrahepatic complement biosynthesis: Where, when and why? Clin Exp Immunol. 1997;107:1–7.

12. Strunk RC, Cole FS, Perlmutter DH, et al. γ-Interferon increases expression of class III complement genes C2 and factor B in human monocytes and in murine fibroblasts transfected with human C2 and factor B genes. J Biol Chem. 1985;260:15280–15285.
13. Strunk RC, Whitehead AS, Cole FS. Pretranslational regulation of the synthesis of the third component of complement in human mononuclear phagocytes by the lipid A portion of lipopolysaccharide. J Clin Invest. 1985;76:985–990.
14. Hetland G, Eskeland T. Formation of the functional alternative pathway of complement by human monocytes in vitro as demonstrated by phagocytosis of agarose beads. Scand J Immunol. 1986;23:301–308.
15. Notarangelo LD, Chirico G, Chaira A, et al. Activity of classical and alternative pathways of complement in preterm and small for gestational age infants. Pediatr Res. 1984;18:281–285.
16. Johnston RB Jr, Altenburger KM, Atkinson AW Jr, et al. Complement in the newborn infant. Pediatrics. 1979;64(Suppl):781–786.
17. Mills EL, Björksten B, Quie PG. Deficient alternative complement pathway activity in newborn sera. Pediatr Res. 1979;13:1341–1344.
18. Edwards MS, Buffone GJ, Fuselier PA, et al. Deficient classical complement pathway activity in newborn sera. Pediatr Res. 1983;17:685–688.
19. Lachmann PJ, Hughes-Jones NC. Initiation of complement activation. Springer Semin Immunopathol. 1984;7:143–162.
20. Muraoka S, Shulman MJ. Structural requirements for IgM assembly and cytolytic activity: Effects of mutations in the oligosaccharide acceptor site at Asn402. J Immunol. 1989;142:695–701.
21. Wright JF, Shulman MJ, Isenman DE, et al. C1 binding by mouse IgM. The effect of abnormal glycosylation at position 402 resulting from a serine to asparagine exchange at residue 406 of the μ-chain. J Biol Chem. 1990;265:10506–10513.
22. Tao M-H, Canfield SM, Morrison SL. The differential ability of human IgG1 and IgG4 to activate complement is determined by the COOH-terminal sequence of the C_H2 domain. J Exp Med. 1991;173:1025–1028.
23. Cooper NR. The classical complement pathway: Activation and regulation of the first complement component. Adv Immunol. 1985;37:151–216.
24. Malhotra R, Sim RB, Reid KBM. Interaction of C1q, and other proteins containing collagen-like domains, with the C1q receptor. Biochem Soc Trans. 1990;18:1145–1148.
25. Acton S, Resnick D, Freeman M, et al. The collagenous domains of macrophage scavenger receptors and complement component C1q mediate their similar, but not identical, binding specificities for polyanionic ligands. J Biol Chem. 1993;268:3530–3537.
26. Whaley K, Schwaeble W. Complement and complement deficiencies. Semin Liver Dis 1997;17:297–310.
27. Schweinie JE, Ezekowitz RAB, Tenner AJ, et al. Human mannose-binding protein activates the alternative complement pathway and enhances serum bactericidal activity on a mannose-rich isolate of *Salmonella.* J Clin Invest. 1989;84:1821–1829.
28. Lu J, Thiel S, Wiedemann H, et al. Binding of the pentamer/hexamer forms of mannan-binding protein to zymosan activates the proenzyme $C1r_2C1s_2$ complex, of the classical pathway of complement, without involvement of C1q. J Immunol. 1990;144:2287–2294.
29. Matsushita M, Fujita T. Activation of the classical complement pathway by mannose-binding protein in association with a novel C1s-like serine protease. J Exp Med. 1992;176:1497–1502.
30. Arlaud GJ, Colomb MG, Gagnon J. A functional model of the human C1 complex. Immunol Today. 1987;8:106–111.
31. Schumaker VN, Zavodszky P, Poon RH. Activation of the first component of complement. Annu Rev Immunol. 1987;5:21–42.
32. Fearon DT. Complement. J Allergy Clin Immunol. 1983;71:520–529.
33. Müller-Eberhard HJ. Molecular organization and function of the complement system. Annu Rev Biochem. 1988;57:321–347.
34. Isenman DE, Young JR. The molecular basis for the difference in immune hemolysis activity of the Chido and Rodgers isotypes of human complement component C4. J Immunol. 1984;132:3019–3027.
35. Law SKA, Dodds AW, Porter RR. A comparison of the properties of two classes, C4A and C4B, of the human complement component C4. EMBO J. 1984;3:1819–1823.
36. Dodds AW, Law SK, Porter RR. The origin of the very variable haemolytic activities of the common human complement component C4 allotypes including C4–A6. EMBO J. 1985;4:2239–2244.
37. Schifferli JA, Steiger G, Paccaud J-P, et al. Difference in the biological properties of the two forms of the fourth component of human complement (C4). Clin Exp Immunol. 1986;63:473–477.
38. Schifferli JA, Hauptmann G, Paccaud J-P. Complement-mediated adherence of immune complexes to human erythrocytes. FEBS Lett. 1987;213:415–418.
39. Naama JK, Niven IP, Zoma A, et al. Complement, antigen–antibody complexes and immune complex disease. J Clin Lab Immunol. 1985;17:59–67.
40. Pangburn MK, Müller-Eberhard HJ. The alternative pathway of complement. Springer Semin Immunopathol. 1984;7:163–192.
41. Pangburn MK. The alternative pathway. In: Ross GD, ed. Immunobiology of the Complement System. Orlando, Fla: Academic Press; 1986:45–62.
42. Densen P, McRill C, Ross SC. The contribution of the alternative and classical complement pathways to gonococcal killing and C3 fixation. In: Poolman JT, Zanen HC, Meyer TF, et al, eds. Gonococci and Meningococci. Dordrecht: Kluwer Academic Publishers; 1988;693–697.
43. Gordon DL, Hostetter MK. Complement and host defense against microorganisms. Pathology. 1986;18:365–375.
44. Fearon DT, Austen KF. Properdin: Initiation of alternative complement pathway. Immunology. 1975;72:3220–3224.
45. Fearon DT, Austen KF. Properdin: Binding to C3b and stabilization of the C3b-dependent C3 convertase. J Exp Med. 1975;142:856–863.
46. Fearon DT, Austen KF. The alternative pathway of complement: A system for host resistance to microbial infection. N Engl J Med. 1980;303:259–263.
47. Hunsicker LG, Ruddy S, Austen KF. Alternate complement pathway: Factors involved in cobra venom factor (CoVF) activation of the third component of complement (C3). J Immunol. 1973;110:128–138.
48. Müller-Eberhard HJ, Schreiber RD. Molecular biology and chemistry of the alternative pathway of complement. Adv Immunol. 1980;29:1–53.
49. Vogel C-W, Smith CA, Müller-Eberhard HJ. Cobra venom factor: Structural homology with the third component of human complement. J Immunol. 1984;133:3235–3241.
50. Söderstöm C, Braconier JH, Danielssen D, et al. Bactericidal activity for *Neisseria meningitidis* in properdin-deficient sera. J Infect Dis. 1987;156:107–112.
51. Schenkein HA, Ruddy S. The role of immunoglobulins in alternative complement pathway activation by zymosan: II. The effect of IgG on the kinetics of the alternative pathway. J Immunol. 1981;126:11–15.
52. Ratnoff WD, Fearon DT, Austen KF. The role of antibody in the activation of the alternative complement pathway. Springer Semin Immunopathol. 1983;6:361–371.
53. Winkelstein JA, Shin HS. The role of immunoglobulin in the interaction of pneumococci and the properdin pathway: Evidence for its specificity and lack of requirement for the Fc portion of the molecule. J Immunol. 1974;112:1635–1642.
54. Nelson B, Ruddy S. Enhancing role of IgG in lysis of rabbit erythrocytes by the alternative pathway of human complement. J Immunol. 1979;122:1994–1999.
55. Schenkein HA, Ruddy S. The role of immunoglobulins in alternative complement pathway activation by zymosan: I. Human IgG with specificity for zymosan enhances alternative pathway activation by zymosan. J Immunol. 1981;126:7–10.
56. Nicholson-Weller A, Daha MR, Austen KF. Different functions for specific guinea pig IgG1 and IgG2 in the lysis of sheep erythrocytes by C4-deficient guinea pig serum. J Immunol. 1981;126:1800–1804.
57. Capel PJA, Groeneboer O, Grosveld G, et al. The binding of activated C3 to polysaccharides and immunoglobulins. J Immunol. 1978;121:2566–2572.
58. Fries LF, Gaither TA, Hammer CH, et al. C3b covalently bound to IgG demonstrates a reduced rate of inactivation by factors H and I. J Exp Med. 1984;160:1640–1655.
59. Joiner KA, Fries LF, Schmetz MA, et al. IgG bearing covalently bound C3b has enhanced bactericidal activity for *Escherichia coli* O111. J Exp Med. 1985;162:877–889.
60. Lambris JD, Müller-Eberhard HJ. The multifunctional role of C3: Structural analysis of its interactions with physiological ligands. Mol Immunol. 1986;23:1237–1242.
61. Wetsel RA, Lemons RS, Le Beau MM, et al. Molecular analysis of human complement component C5: Localization of the structural gene to chromosome 9. Biochemistry. 1988;27:1474–1482.
62. Lundwall AB, Wetsel RA, Kristenson T, et al. Isolation and sequence analysis of a cDNA clone encoding the fifth complement component. J Biol Chem. 1985;260:2108–2112.
63. Müller-Eberhard HJ. The membrane attack complex of complement. Annu Rev Immunol. 1986;4:503–528.
64. Stanley K, Luzio P. A family of killer proteins. Nature. 1988;334:475–476.
65. Tschopp J, Mollnes T-E. Antigenic crossreactivity of the α subunit of complement component C8 with the cysteine-rich domain shared by complement component C9 and low density lipoprotein receptor. Proc Natl Acad Sci U S A. 1986;83:4223–4227.
66. Haefliger J-A, Tschopp J, Nardelli D, et al. Complementary DNA cloning of complement C8β and its sequence homology to C9. Biochemistry. 1987;26:3551–3556.
67. Monahan JB, Sodetz JM. Binding of the eighth component of human complement to the soluble cytolytic complex is mediated by its β subunit. J Biol Chem. 1980;255:10579–10582.
68. Stewart JL, Kolb WP, Sodetz JM. Evidence that C5b recognizes and mediates C8 incorporation into the cytolytic complex of complement. J Immunol. 1987;139:1960–1964.
69. Stewart JL, Sodetz JM. Analysis of the specific association of the eighth and ninth components of human complement: identification of a direct role for the α subunit of C8. Biochemistry. 1985;24:4598–4602.
70. Stanley KK, Page M, Campbell AK, et al. A mechanism for the insertion of complement component C9 into target membranes. Mol Immunol. 1986;23:451–458.
71. Davis AE III. C1 inhibitor and hereditary angioneurotic edema. Annu Rev Immunol. 1988;6:595–628.
72. Liszewski MK, Farries TC, Lublin DM, et al. Control of the complement system. Adv Immunol. 1996;61:201—283.
73. Holers VM, Cole JL, Lublin DM, et al. Human C3b- and C4b-regulatory proteins: A new multi-gene family. Immunol Today. 1985;6:188–192.
74. Davies A. Policing the membrane: Cell surface proteins which regulate complement. Res Immunol. 1997;147:82—87.
75. Atkinson JP, Farries T. Separation of self from non-self in the complement system. Immunol Today. 1987;8:212–215.
76. Rollins SA, Zhao J, Ninomiya H, et al. Inhibition of homologous complement by CD59 is mediated by a species-selective recognition conferred through binding to C8 within C5b-8 or C9 within C5b-9. J Immunol. 1991;146:2345–2351.
77. Carney DF, Koski CL, Shin ML. Elimination of terminal complement intermediates

from the plasma membrane of nucleated cells: The rate of disappearance differs for cells carrying C5b-7 or C5b-8 or a mixture of C5b-8 with a limited number of C5b-9. J Immunol. 1985;134:1804–1809.
78. Ramm LE, Whitlow MB, Koski CL, et al. Elimination of complement channels from the plasma membranes of U937, a nucleated mammalian cell line: Temperature dependence of the elimination rate. J Immunol. 1983;131:1411–1415.
79. Schlager SI, Ohanian SH, Borsos T. Correlations between the ability of tumor cells to resist humoral immune attack and their ability to synthesize lipid. J Immunol. 1978;120:463–471.
80. Imagawa DK, Osifchin NE, Paznekas WA, et al. Consequences of cell membrane attack by complement: Release of arachidonate and formation of inflammatory derivatives. Proc Natl Acad Sci U S A. 1983;80:6647–6651.
81. Betz M, Hansch GM. Release of arachidonic acid: A new function of the late complement components. Immunobiology. 1984;166:473–483.
82. Carney DF, Lang TJ, Shin ML. Multiple signal messengers generated by terminal complement complexes and their role in terminal complement complex elimination. J Immunol. 1990;145:623–629.
83. Gordon DL, Kaufman RM, Blackmore TK, et al. Identification of complement regulatory domains in human factor H. J Immunol. 1995;155:348–356.
84. Fearon DT, Austen KF. Activation of the alternative complement pathway with rabbit erythrocytes by circumvention of the regulatory action of endogenous control proteins. J Exp Med. 1977;146:22–33.
85. Fearon DT. Regulation by membrane sialic acid of β1H-dependent decay-dissociation of amplification C3 convertase of the alternative complement pathway. Proc Natl Acad Sci U S A. 1978;75:1971–1975.
86. Kazatchkine MD, Fearon DT, Austen KF. Human alternative complement pathway: Membrane-associated sialic acid regulates the competition between B and β1H for cell-bound C3b. J Immunol. 1979;122:75–81.
87. Pangburn MK, Morrison DC, Schreiber RD, et al. Activation of the alternative complement pathway: Recognition of surface structures on activators by bound C3b. J Immunol. 1980;124:977–982.
88. Ross GD, Medof ME. Membrane complement receptors specific for bound fragments of C3. Adv Immunol. 1985;37:217–267.
89. Wilson JG, Andriopoulos NA, Fearon DT. CR1 and the cell membrane proteins that bind C3 and C4: A basic and clinical review. Immunol Res. 1987;6:192–209.
90. Jack RM, Ezzell RM, Hartwig J, et al. Differential interaction of the C3b/C4b receptor and MHC class I with the cytoskeleton of human neutrophils. J Immunol. 1986;137:3996–4003.
91. Krych M, Hourcade D, Atkinson JP. Sites within the complement C3b/C4b receptor important for the specificity of ligand binding. Proc Natl Acad Sci U S A. 1991;88:4353–4357.
92. Moulds JM, Nickells MW, Moulds JJ, et al. The C3b/C4b receptor is recognized by the Knops, McCoy, Swain-Langley, and York blood group antisera. J Exp Med. 1991;173:1159–1163.
93. Hynes RO. Integrins: A family of cell surface receptors. Cell. 1987;48:549–554.
94. Wright SD, Levin SM, Jong MTC, et al. CR3 (CD11b/CD18) expresses one binding site for Arg-Gly-Asp-containing peptides and a second site for bacterial lipopolysaccharide. J Exp Med. 1989;169:175–183.
95. Wright SD, Reddy A, Jong MTC, et al. C3bi receptor (complement receptor type 3) recognizes a region of complement protein C3 containing the sequence Arg-Gly-Asp. Proc Natl Acad Sci U S A. 1987;84:1965–1968.
96. Ruoslahti E, Pierschbacher MD. Arg-Gly-Asp: A versatile cell recognition signal. Cell. 1986;44:517–518.
97. Myones BL, Dalzell JG, Hogg N, et al. Neutrophil and monocyte cell surface p150,95 has iC3b-receptor (CR4) activity resembling CR3. J Clin Invest. 1988;81:64–51.
98. Matsumoto AK, Kopicky-Burd J, Carter RH, et al. Intersection of the complement and immune systems: A signal transduction complex of the B lymphocyte–containing complement receptor type 2 and CD19. J Exp Med. 1991;173:55–64.
99. Hugli TE. Biological activities of fragments derived from human complement components. Prog Immunol. 1983:419–426.
100. Perlmutter DH, Colten HR. Complement molecular genetics. In: Gallin JI, Goldstein IM, Snyderman R, eds. Inflammation: Basic Principles and Clinical Correlates. New York: Raven; 1988:75–88.
101. Campbell RD. The molecular genetics and polymorphism of C2 and factor B. Br Med Bull. 1987;43:37–49.
102. Campbell RD, Law SKA, Reid KBM, et al. Structure, organization, and regulation of the complement genes. Annu Rev Immunol. 1988;6:161–195.
103. Awdeh ZL, Raum D, Yunis EJ, et al. Extended HLA/complement allele haplotypes: Evidence for T/t-like complex in man. Proc Natl Acad Sci U S A. 1983;80:259–263.
104. Alper CA, Raum D, Karp S, et al. Serum complement "supergenes" of the major histocompatibility complex in man (complotypes). Vox Sang. 1983;45:62–67.
105. Porter RR. Complement polymorphism, the major histocompatibility complex and associated diseases: A speculation. Mol Biol Med. 1983;1:161–168.
106. Kristensen T, D'Eustachio P, Ogata RT, et al. The superfamily of C3b/C4b-binding proteins. FASEB J. 1987;46:2463–2469.
107. Reid KBM, Bentley DR, Campbell RD, et al. Complement system proteins which interact with C3b or C4b: A superfamily of structurally related proteins. Immunol Today. 1986;7:230–234.
108. Seya T. Human regulator of complement activation (RCA) gene family proteins and their relationship to microbial infection. Microbiol Immunol. 1995;39:295–305.
109. Fischer WH, Hugli TE. Regulation of B cell functions by C3a and C3a^{desArg}: Suppression of TNF-α, IL-6, and the polyclonal immune response. J Immunol 1997;159:4279–4286.
110. Perez HD, Kelly E, Chenoweth D, et al. Identification of the C5a des Arg cochemotaxin: Homology with vitamin D–binding protein (group-specific component globulin). J Clin Invest. 1988;82:360–363.
111. Kew RR, Webster RO. Ge-globulin (vitamin D–binding protein) enhances the neutrophil chemotactic activity of C5a and C5a des Arg. J Clin Invest. 1988;82:364–369.
112. Perez HD, Hooper C, Volanakis J, et al. Specific inhibitor of complement (C5)–derived chemotactic activity in systemic lupus erythematosus related antigenically to the Bb fragment of human factor B. J Immunol. 1987;139:484–489.
113. Miller GW, Nusenzweig V. A new complement function: Solubilization of antigen–antibody aggregates. Proc Natl Acad Sci U S A. 1975;72:418–422.
114. Schifferli JA, Ng YC, Peters DK. The role of complement and its receptor in the elimination of immune complexes. N Engl J Med. 1986;315:488–495.
115. Siegel I, Liu TL, Gleicher N. The red-cell immune system. Lancet. 1981;2:556–559.
116. Cornacoff JB, Hebert LA, Smead WL, et al. Primate erythrocyte-immune complex-clearing mechanism. J Clin Invest. 1983;71:236–247.
117. Erdei A, Fust G, Gergely J. The role of C3 in the immune response. Immunol Today. 1991;12:332–337.
118. Papamichail M, Gutierrez C, Embling P, et al. Complement dependence of localisation of aggregated IgG in germinal centres. Scand J Immunol. 1975;4:343–347.
119. Bird P, Lachmann PJ. The regulation of IgG subclass production in man: Low serum IgG4 in inherited deficiencies of the classical pathway of C3 activation. J Immunol. 1988;18:1217–1222.
120. Dempsey PW, Allison MED, Akkaraju S, et al. C3d of complement as a molecular adjuvant: Bridging innate and acquired immunity. Science. 1996;271:348–350.
121. Böttger EC, Bitter-Suermann D. Complement and the regulation of humoral immune responses. Immunol Today. 1987;8:261–264.
122. Hostetter MK. Serotypic variations among virulent pneumococci in deposition and degradation of covalently bound C3b: Implications for phagocytosis and antibody production. J Infect Dis. 1986;153:682–693.
123. Gordon DL, Hostetter MK. Complement and host defense against micro-organisms. Pathology. 1986;18:365–375.
124. Hostetter MK, Krueger RA, Schmeling DJ. The biochemistry of opsonization: Central role of the reactive thiolester of the third component of complement. J Infect Dis. 1984;150:653–661.
125. Taylor PW. Bactericidal and bacteriolytic activity of serum against gram-negative bacteria. Microbiol Rev. 1983;47:46–83.
126. Harriman GR, Esser AF, Podack ER, et al. The role of C9 in complement-mediated killing of *Neisseria*. J Immunol. 1981;127:2386–2390.
127. Cooper NR, Nemerow GR. Complement-dependent mechanisms of virus neutralization. In: Ross GD, ed. Immunobiology of the Complement System. Orlando, Fla: Academic Press; 1986:139–162.
128. Roantree RJ, Rantz LA. A study of the relationship of the normal bactericidal activity of human serum to bacterial infection. J Clin Invest. 1960;39:72–81.
129. Joiner K. Complement evasion by bacteria and parasites. Annu Rev Microbiol. 1988;42:201–230.
130. Cooper NR. Complement evasion strategies of microorganisms. Immunol Today. 1991;12:327–332.
131. Leive LL, Jimenez-Lucho VE. Lipopolysaccharide O-antigen structure controls alternative pathway activation of complement: Effects on phagocytosis and virulence of *Salmonella*. In: Leive L, ed. Microbiology. Washington, DC: American Society for Microbiology; 1986:14–17.
132. Liang-Takasaki C-J, Mäkelä PH, Leive L. Phagocytosis of bacteria by macrophages: Changing the carbohydrate of lipopolysaccharide alters interaction with complement and macrophages. J Immunol. 1982;128:1229–1235.
133. Liang-Takasaki C-J, Saxén H, Mäkelä PH, et al. Complement activation by polysaccharide of lipopolysaccharide: An important virulence determinant of *Salmonella*. Infect Immun. 1983;41:563–569.
134. Grossman N, Leive L. Complement activation via the alternative pathway by purified *Salmonella* lipopolysaccharide is affected by its structure but not its O-antigen length. J Immunol. 1984;132:376–385.
135. Grossman N, Joiner KA, Frank MM, et al. C3b binding, but not its breakdown, is affected by the structure of the O-antigen polysaccharide in lipopolysaccharide from *Salmonella*. J Immunol. 1986;136:2208–2215.
136. Jimenez-Lucho VE, Joiner KA, Foulds J, et al. C3b generation is affected by the structure of the O-antigen polysaccharide in lipopolysaccharide from *Salmonella*. J Immunol. 1987;139:1253–1259.
137. Joiner KA, Grossman N, Schmetz M, et al. C3 binds preferentially to long-chain lipopolysaccharide during alternative pathway activation by *Salmonella montevideo*. J Immunol. 1986;136:710–715.
138. Schoolnik GK, Buchman TM, Holmes KK. Gonococci causing disseminated gonococcal infection are resistant to the bactericidal action of normal human sera. J Clin Invest. 1976;58:1163–1173.
139. Joiner KA, Warren KA, Brown EJ, et al. Studies on the mechanism of bacterial resistance to complement-mediated killing: IV. C5b-9 forms high molecular weight complexes with bacterial outer membrane constituents on serum-resistant but not on serum-sensitive *Neisseria gonorrhoeae*. J Immunol. 1983;131:1443–1451.
140. Harriman GR, Podack ER, Braude AI, et al. Activation of complement by serum-resistant *Neisseria gonorrhoeae*. J Exp Med. 1982;156:1235–1249.
141. Rice PA, Kasper DL. Characterization of gonococcal antigens responsible for induction of bactericidal antibody in disseminated infection. J Clin Invest. 1977;60:1149–1158.
142. Densen P, Gulati S, Rice PA. Specificity of antibodies against *Neisseria gonor-*

rhoeae that stimulate neutrophil chemotaxis: Role of antibodies directed against lipooligosaccharides. J Clin Invest. 1987;80:78–87.
143. Rice PA, Kasper KL. Characterization of serum resistance of *Neisseria gonorrhoeae* that disseminate: Roles of blocking antibody and gonococcal outer membrane proteins. J Clin Invest. 1982;70:157–167.
144. Rice PA, Vayo HE, Tam MR, et al. Immunoglobulin G antibodies directed against protein III block killing of serum-resistant *Neisseria gonorrhoeae* by immune serum. J Exp Med. 1986;164:1735–1748.
145. Joiner KA, Scales R, Warren KA, et al. Mechanism of action of blocking immunoglobulin G for *Neisseria gonorrhoeae*. J Clin Invest. 1985;76:1765–1772.
146. Griffiss MJ, Bertram MA. Immunoepidemiology of meningococcal disease in military recruits: II. Blocking of serum bactericidal activity by circulating IgA early in the course of invasive disease. J Infect Dis. 1977;136:733–739.
147. Griffiss JM. Epidemic meningococcal disease: Synthesis of a hypothetical immunoepidemiologic model. Rev Infect Dis. 1982;4:159–172.
148. Frank MM, Joiner K, Hammer C. The function of antibody and complement in the lysis of bacteria. Rev Infect Dis. 1987;9(Suppl 5):537–545.
149. Braga LL, Ninomiya H, McCoy JJ, et al. Inhibition of the complement membrane attack complex by the galactose-specific adhesin of *Entamoeba histolytica*. J Clin Invest. 1992;90:1131–1137.
150. Heffernan EJ, Reed S, Hackett J, et al. Mechanism of resistance to complement-mediated killing of bacteria encoded by the *Salmonella typhimurium* virulence plasmid gene *rck*. J Clin Invest. 1992;90:953–964.
151. Bliska JB, Falkow S. Bacterial resistance to complement killing mediated by the Ail protein of *Yersinia enterocolitica*. Proc Natl Acad Sci U S A. 1992;89:3561–3565.
152. Hall BF, Joiner KA. Developmentally regulated virulence factors of *Trypanosoma cruzi* and their relationship to evasion of host defences. J Eukaryot Microbiol. 1993;40:207–213.
153. Stoiber H, Clivio A, Dierich MP. Role of complement in HIV infection. Ann Rev Immunol. 1997;15:649–674.
154. Lachmann PJ, Davies A. Complement and immunity to viruses. Immunol Rev. 1997;159:69–77.
155. Thern A, Stenberg L, Dahlbäck B, et al. Ig-binding surface proteins of *Streptococcus pyogenes* also bind human C4b-binding protein (C4BP), a regulatory component of the complement system. J Immunol. 1995;154:375–386.
156. Smith H, Cole JA, Parsons NJ. The sialylation of gonococcal lipopolysaccharide by host factors: A major impact on pathogenicity. FEMS Microbiol Lett. 1992;100:287–292.
157. Kotwal GJ, Moss B. Vaccinia virus encodes a secretory polypeptide structurally related to complement control proteins. Nature. 1988;335:176–178.
158. Kotwal GJ, Isaacs SN, McKenzie R, et al. Inhibition of the complement cascade by the major secretory protein of vaccinia virus. Science. 1990;250:827–830.
159. Brown EJ. Interaction of gram-positive microorganisms with complement. Curr Top Microbiol Immunol. 1985;121:159–197.
160. Cooper NR, Moore MD, Nemerow GR. Immunobiology of CR2, the B lymphocyte receptor for Epstein-Barr virus and the C3d complement fragment. Annu Rev Immunol. 1988;6:85–113.
161. Fingeroth JD, Weis JJ, Tedder TF, et al. Epstein-Barr virus receptor of human B lymphocytes is the C3d receptor CR2. Proc Natl Acad Sci U S A. 1984;81:4510–4514.
162. Montefiori DC, Stewart K, Ahearn JM, et al. Complement-mediated binding of naturally glycosylated and glycosylation-modified human immunodeficency virus type 1 to human CR2 (CD21). J Virol. 1993;67:2699–2706.
163. Ross SC, Densen P. Complement deficiency states and infection: Epidemiology, pathogenesis and consequences of neisserial and other infections in an immune deficiency. Medicine (Baltimore). 1984;63:243–273.
164. Figueroa JE, Densen P. Infectious diseases associated with complement deficiencies. Clin Microbiol Rev. 1991;4:359–395.
165. Densen P. Human complement deficiency states and infection. In: Whaley K, Loos M, Weiler JM, eds. Complement in Health and Disease. Dordrecht, The Netherlands: Kluwer Academic Publishers; 1993:173–197.
166. Glass D, Raum D, Gibson D, et al. Inherited deficiency of the second component of complement. J Clin Invest. 1976;58:853–861.
167. Truedsson L, Sturfelt G, Nived O. Prevalence of the type I complement C2 deficiency gene in Swedish systemic lupus erythematosus patients. Lupus 1993;2:325–327.
168. Sullivan KE, Petri MA, Schmeckpeper BJ, et al. Prevalence of a mutation causing C2 deficiency in systemic lupus erythematosus. J Rheumatol. 1994;21:1128–1133.
169. Agnello V. Lupus diseases associated with hereditary and acquired deficiencies of complement. Springer Semin Immunopathol. 1986;9:161–178.
170. Ekdahl K, Truedsson L, Sjöholm AG, et al. Complement analysis in adult patients with a history of bacteremic pneumococcal infections or recurrent pneumonia. Scand J Infect Dis. 1995;27:111–117.
171. Davies KA, Schifferli JA, Walport MJ. Complement deficiency and immune complex disease. Springer Semin Immunopathol. 1994;15:397–416.
172. Bowness P, Davies KA, Norsworthy PJ, et al. Hereditary C1q deficiency and systemic lupus erythematosus. QJM. 1994;87:455–464.
173. Provost TT, Arnett FC, Reichlin M. Homozygous C2 deficiency, lupus erythematosus, and anti-Ro (SSA) antibodies. Arthritis Rheum. 1983;26:1279–1282.
174. Hauptmann G, Goetz J, Uring-Lambert B, et al. Component deficiencies: 2. The fourth component. Prog Allergy. 1986;39:1232–1249.
175. Awdeh ZL, Raum DD, Glass D, et al. Complement-human histocompatibility antigen haplotypes in C2 deficiency. J Clin Invest. 1981;67:581–583.
176. Kemp ME, Atkinson JP, Skanes VM, et al. Deletion of C4A genes in patients with systemic lupus erythematosus. Arthritis Rheum. 1987;30:1015–1022.
177. Walport MJ, Davies KA, Morley BJ, et al. Complement deficiency and autoimmunity. Ann N Y Acad Sci. 1997;815:267–281.
178. Howard PF, Hochberg MC, Bias WB, et al. Relationship between C4 null genes, HLA-D region antigens, and genetic susceptibility to systemic lupus erythematosus in Caucasian and Black Americans. Am J Med. 1986;81:187–193.
179. Davis AE III. The efficiency of complement activation in MHC-linked diseases. Immunol Today. 1983;4:250–252.
180. Walport MJ, Davies KA. Complement and immune complexes. Res Immunol. 1996;147:103–109.
181. Schifferli JA, Peters DK. Complement, the immune-complex lattice, and the pathophysiology of complement-deficiency syndromes. Lancet. 1983;2:957–959.
182. Schifferli JA, Steiger G, Hauptmann G, et al. Formation of soluble immune complexes by complement in sera of patients with various hypocomplementemic states. J Clin Invest. 1985;76:2127–2133.
183. Böttger EC, Hoffmann T, Hadding U, et al. Guinea pigs with inherited deficiencies of complement components C2 or C4 have characteristics of immune complex disease. J Clin Invest. 1986;78:689–695.
184. Würzner R, Dierich MP. Complement in human disease. Immunol Today. 1997;18:460–463.
185. Matsumoto M, Fukuda W, Circolo A, et al. Abrogation of the alternative complement pathway by targeted deletion of murine factor B. Proc Natl Acad Sci U S A. 1997;94:8720–8725.
186. Pekna M, Hietala MA, Landin A, et al. Mice deficient for the complement factor B develop and reproduce normally. Scand J Immunol. 1998;47:375–380.
187. Sjöholm AG, Braconier J-H, Söderström C. Properdin deficiency in a family with fulminant meningococcal infections. Clin Exp Immunol. 1982;50:291–297.
188. Densen P, Weiler JM, Griffiss JM, et al. Familial properdin deficiency and fatal meningococcemia: Correction of the bactericidal defect by vaccination. N Engl J Med. 1987;316:922–926.
189. Sjöholm AG, Söderström C, Nilsson L-A. A second variant of properdin deficiency: The detection of properdin at low concentration in affected males. Complement. 1988;5:130–140.
190. Sjöholm AG, Kuijper EJ, Tijssen CC, et al. Dysfunctional properdin in a Dutch family with meningococcal disease. N Engl J Med. 1988;319:33–37.
191. Sissons JGP, West RJ, Fallow J, et al. The complement abnormalities of lipodystrophy. N Engl J Med. 1976;294:461–465.
192. Ipp MM, Minta JO, Gelfand EW. Disorders of the complement system in lipodystrophy. Clin Immunol Immunopathol. 1977;7:281–287.
193. Rosen BS, Cook KS, Yaglom J, et al. Adipsin and complement factor D activity: An immune-related defect in obesity. Science. 1989;244:1483–1487.
194. White RT, Damm D, Hancock N, et al. Human adipsin is identical to complement factor D and is expressed at high levels in adipose tissue. J Biol Chem. 1992;267:9210–9213.
195. Choy LN, Rosen BS, Spiegelman BM. Adipsin and an endogenous pathway of complement from adipose cells. J Biol Chem. 1992;267:12736–12741.
196. Mathieson PW, Wurzner R, Oliveira DBG, et al. Complement-mediated adipocyte lysis by nephritic factor sera. J Exp Med. 1993;177:1827–1831.
197. Nagata M, Hara T, Aoki T, et al. Inherited deficiency of ninth component of complement: An increased risk of meningococcal meningitis. J Pediatr. 1989;114:260–264.
198. Slingsby JH, Norsworthy P, Pearce G, et al. Homozygous hereditary C1q deficiency and systemic lupus erythematosus: A new family and the molecular basis of C1q deficiency in three families. Arthritis Rheum. 1996;39:663–670.
199. Johnson C, Densen P, Cole FS, et al. Molecular heterogeneity of human C2 deficiency. N Engl J Med. 1992;326:871–874.
200. Johnson CA, Densen P, Hurford R, et al. Type I human complement C2 deficiency: A 28-base pair gene deletion causes skipping of exon 6 during RNA splicing. J Biol Chem. 1992;267:9347–9353.
201. Barba G, Rittner C, Schneider PM. Genetic basis of human complement C4a deficiency. J Clin Invest. 1993;91:1681–1686.
202. Ault BH, Schmidt BZ, Fowler NL, et al. Human factor H deficiency: Mutations in framework cysteine residues and block in H protein secretion and intracellular catabolism. J Biol Chem. 1997;272:25168–25175.
203. Vyse TJ, Morley BJ, Bartók I, et al. The molecular basis of hereditary complement factor I deficiency. J Clin Invest. 1996;97:925–933.
204. Truedsson L, Westberg J, Fredrikson GN, et al. Human properdin deficiency has a heterogeneous genetic background. Immunopharmacology. 1997;38:203–206.
205. Westberg J, Fredrikson GN, Truedsson L, et al. Sequence-based analysis of properdin deficiency: Identification of point mutations in two phenotypic forms of an X-linked immunodeficiency. Genomics. 1995;29:1–8.
206. Fredrikson GN, Westberg J, Kuijper EJ, et al. Molecular characterization of properdin deficiency type III: Dysfunction produced by a single point mutation in exon 9 of the structural gene causing a tyrosine to aspartic acid interchange. J Immunol. 1996;157:3666–3671.
207. Singer L, Colten HR, Wetsel RA. Complement C3 deficiency: Human, animal and experimental models. Pathobiology. 1994;62:14–28.
208. Wang X, Fleischer DT, Whitehead WT, et al. Inherited human complement C5 deficiency: Nonsense mutations in exons 1 (Gln1 to Stop) and 36 (Arg1458 to Stop) and compound heterozygosity in three African-American families. J Immunol. 1995;154:5464–5471.
209. Hobart MJ, Fernie BA, Fijen KA, et al. The molecular bases of C6 deficiency in the Western Cape, South Africa. Hum Genet. 1998;103:506–512.
210. Nishizaka H, Horiuchi T, Zhu ZB, et al. Molecular bases for inherited human

complement component C6 deficiency in two unrelated individuals. J Immunol. 1996;156:2309–2315.
211. Würzner R, Hobart MJ, Fernie BA, et al. Molecular basis of subtotal complement C6 deficiency: A carboxy-terminally truncated but functionally active C6. J Clin Invest. 1995;95:1877–1883.
212. Fernie BA, Orren A, Sheehan G, et al. Molecular bases of C7 deficiency: Three different defects. J Immunol. 1997;159:1019–1026.
213. O'Hara AM, Moran AP, Fernie BA, et al. Molecular bases of deficiency of the seventh complement component, deletion of exons 7 and 8. Royal Academy of Medicine in Ireland, Biomedical Sciences Section. 1998. Abstract accepted for publication.
214. Fernie BA, Würzner R, Orren A, et al. Molecular bases of combined subtotal deficiencies of C6 and C7: Their effects in combination with other C6 and C7 deficiencies. J Immunol. 1996;157:3648–3657.
215. Würzner R, Platonov AE, Beloborodov VB, et al. How partial C7 deficiency with chronic and recurrent bacterial infections can mimic total C7 deficiency: Temporary restoration of host C7 levels following plasma transfusion. Immunology. 1996;88:407–411.
216. Saucedo L, Ackermann L, Platonov AE, et al. Delineation of additional genetic bases for C8β deficiency: Prevalence of null alleles and predominance of C→T transition in their genesis. J Immunol. 1995;155:5022–5028.
217. Densen P, Ackermann L, Saucedo L, et al. The genetic basis for human C8-α-γ deficiency (Abstract). XVI International Complement Workshop, Boston, Mass, USA, 1996.
217a. Kojima T, Horiuchi T, Nishizacki H, et al. Genetic basis of human complement C8α-γ deficiency. J Immunol. 1998;161:3762–3766.
218. Witzel-Schlömp K, Späth PJ, Hobart MJ, et al. The human complement C9 gene: Identification of two mutations causing deficiency and revision of the gene structure. J Immunol. 1997;158:5043–5049.
219. Witzel-Schlömp K, Hobart MJ, Fernie BA, et al. Heterogeneity in the genetic basis of human complement C9 deficiency. Immunogenetics. 1998;48:144–147.
220. Fijen CAP, Kuijper EJ, Tjia HG, et al. Complement deficiency predisposes for meningitis due to nongroupable meningococci and *Neisseria*-related bacteria. Clin Infect Dis. 1994;18:780–784.
221. Fijen CA, Kuijper EJ, Hannema AJ, et al. Complement deficiencies in patients over ten years old with meningococcal disease due to uncommon serogroups. Lancet. 1989;2:585–588.
222. Ross SC, Rosenthal PJ, Berberich HM, et al. Killing of *Neisseria meningitidis* by human neutrophils: Implications for normal and complement-deficient individuals. J Infect Dis. 1987;155:1266–1275.
223. Anonymous. Analysis of endemic meningococcal disease by serogroup and evaluation of chemoprophylaxis. J Infect Dis. 1976;134:201–204.
224. Ross SC, Berberich HM, Densen P. Natural serum bactericidal activity against *Neisseria meningitidis* isolates from disseminated infections in normal and complement-deficient hosts. J Infect Dis. 1985;152:1332–1335.
225. Beloborodov VB, Platonov AE. Meningococcal disease in the USSR in patients with deficiencies in late complement components. In: Achtman M, Kohl P, Marchal C, et al. Neisseriae 1990. Berlin: Walter de Gruyter; 1991:659–663.
226. Platonov AE, Beloborodov VB, Vershinina IV. Meningococcal disease in patients with late complement deficiency: Studies in the U.S.S.R. Medicine (Baltimore). 1993;72:374–392.
227. Andreoni J, Käyhty H, Densen P. Vaccination and the role of capsular polysaccharide antibody in prevention of recurrent meningococcal disease in late complement component-deficient individuals. J Infect Dis. 1993;168:227–231.
228. Brandtzaeg P, Mollnes TE, Kierulf P. Complement activation and endotoxin levels in systemic meningococcal disease. J Infect Dis. 1989;160:58–65.
229. Brown DL, Lachmann PJ. The behaviour of complement and platelets in lethal endotoxin shock in rabbits. Int Arch Allergy Immunol. 1973;45:193–205.
230. Zwahlen A, Waldvogel FA. Magnitude of bacteremia and complement activation during *Neisseria meningitidis* infection: Study of two co-primary cases with different clinical presentations. Eur J Clin Microbiol. 1984;3:439–441.
231. Sullivan TD, LaScolea LJ Jr. *Neisseria meningitidis* bacteremia in children: Quantitation of bacteremia and spontaneous clinical recovery without antibiotic therapy. Pediatrics. 1987;80:63–67.
232. Brandtzaeg P, Kierulf P, Gaustad P, et al. Plasma endotoxin as a predictor of multiple organ failure and death in systemic meningococcal disease. J Infect Dis. 1989;159:195–204.
233. Waage A, Brandtzaeg P, Halstensen A, et al. The complex pattern of cytokines in serum from patients with meningococcal septic shock: Association between interleukin 6, interleukin 1, and fatal outcome. J Exp Med. 1989;169:333–338.
234. Girardin E, Grau GE, Dayer JM, et al. Tumor necrosis factor and interleukin-1 in the serum of children with severe infectious purpura. N Engl J Med. 1988;319:397–400.
235. Waage A, Halstensen A, Espevik T. Association between tumour necrosis factor in serum and fatal outcome in patients with meningococcal disease. Lancet. 1987;1:355–357.
236. Waage A, Halstensen A, Shalaby R, et al. Local production of tumor necrosis factor α, interleukin 1, and interleukin 6 in meningococcal meningitis: Relation to the inflammatory response. J Exp Med. 1989;170:1859–1867.
237. Morgan BP. Mechanisms of tissue damage by the membrane attack complex of complement. Complement Inflamm. 1989;6:104–111.
238. Sims PJ, Wiedmer T. The response of human platelets to activated components of the complement system. Immunol Today. 1991;12:338–342.
239. Platonov AE, Gracheva AM. Effects of lipopolysaccharide from *N. meningitidis* on human granulocyte lysis and chemiluminescence. In: Achtman M, Kohl P, Marchal C, et al, eds. Neisseriae 1990. Berlin: Walter de Gruyter; 1991:627–631.
240. Hamilton KK, Hattori R, Esmon CT, et al. Complement proteins C5b–9 induce vesiculation of the endothelial plasma membrane and expose catalytic surface for assembly of the prothrombinase enzyme complex. J Biol Chem. 1990;265:3809–3814.
241. Bredius RGM, Derkx BHF, Fijen CAP, et al. Fc receptor IIa (CD32) polymorphism in fulminant meningococcal septic shock in children. J Infect Dis. 1994:170:848–853.
242. Fijen CAP, Bredius RGM, Kuijper EJ. Polymorphism of IgG Fc receptors in meningococcal disease (Letter). Ann Intern Med. 1993;119:636.
243. Fijen CAP, et al. Complement deficiency and the role of Fc receptors, properdin and C3 in phagocytosis of meningococci. In: Fijen CAP, ed. Meningococcal disease and complement deficiencies in the Netherlands. Amsterdam: University of Amsterdam; 1995;157–175.
244. Platonov AE, Kuijper EJ, Vershinina IV, et al. Meningococcal disease and polymorphism of FcγRIIa (CD32) in late complement component-deficient individuals. Clin Exp Immunol. 1998;111:97–101.
245. Frank MM, Gelfand JA, Atkinson JP. Hereditary angioedema: The clinical syndrome and its management. Ann Intern Med. 1976;84:580–593.
246. Frank MM. C1 esterase inhibitor: Clinical clues to the pathophysiology of angioedema. J Allergy Clin Immunol. 1986;78:848–850.
247. Cicardi M, Agostoni A. Hereditary angioedema. N Engl J Med. 1996;334:1666–1667.
248. Whaley K, Sim RB, He S. Autoimmune C1-inhibitor deficiency. Clin Exp Immunol. 1996;106:423–426.
249. Cicardi M, Beretta A, Colombo M, et al. Relevance of lymphoproliferative disorders and of anti-C1-inhibitor autoantibodies in acquired angioedema. Clin Exp Immunol. 1996;106:475–480.
250. Strang CJ, Auerbach HS, Rosen FS. C1s-induced vascular permeability in C2-deficient guinea pigs. J Immunol. 1986;137:631–635.
251. Zahedi R, Bissler JJ, Davis AE, et al. Unique C1 inhibitor dysfunction in a kindred without angioedema: II. Identification of an Ala[443]Val substitution and functional analysis of the recombinant mutant protein. J Clin Invest. 1995;95:1299–1305.
252. Zahedi R, Wisnieski J, Davis AE. Role of the P2 residue of complement 1 inhibitor (Ala[443]) in determination of target protease specificity: Inhibition of complement and contact system proteases. J Immunol. 1997;159:983–988.
253. Davis AE. C1 inhibitor: Functional analysis of naturally-occurring mutant proteins. In: Church FC, Cunningham DD, Ginsburg D, et al. eds. Chemistry and Biology of Serpins. New York: Plenum; 1997:185–194.
254. Agostini A, Cicardi M. Herediatry and acquired C1-inhibitor deficiency: Biological and clinical characteristics in 235 patients. Medicine (Baltimore). 1992;71:206–215.
255. Donaldson VH, Bissler JJ. C1 inhibitors and their genes: An update. J Lab Clin Med. 1993;119:330–333.
256. Rosse WF, Parker CJ. Paroxysmal nocturnal haemoglobinuria. Clin Haematol. 1985;14:105–125.
257. Rosse WF. Hematopoiesis and the defect in paroxysmal nocturnal hemoglobinuria (Editorial). J Clin Invest. 1997;100:953–954.
258. Luzzatto L, Bessler M, Rotoli B. Somatic mutations in paroxysmal nocturnal hemoglobinuria: A blessing in disguise? Cell. 1997;88:1–4.
259. Rosse WF. The control of complement activation by the blood cells in paroxysmal nocturnal hemoglobinuria. Blood. 1986;67:268–269.
260. Rosse WF, Ware RE. The molecular basis of paroxysmal nocturnal hemoglobinuria. Blood. 1995;86:3277–3286.
261. Nicholson-Weller A, March JP, Rosenfeld SI, et al. Affected erythrocytes of patients with paroxysmal nocturnal hemoglobinuria are deficient in the complement regulatory protein, decay accelerating factor. Proc Natl Acad Sci U S A. 1983;80:5066–5070.
262. Holguin MH, Fredrick LR, Bernshaw NJ, et al. Isolation and characterization of a membrane protein from normal human erythrocytes that inhibits reactive lysis of the erythrocytes of paroxysmal nocturnal hemoglobinuria. J Clin Invest. 1989;84:7–17.
263. Holguin MH, Wilcox LA, Bernshaw NJ, et al. Relationship between the membrane inhibitor of reactive lysis and the erythrocyte phenotypes of paroxysmal nocturnal hemoglobinuria. J Clin Invest. 1989;84:1387–1394.
264. Yamashina M, Ueda E, Kinoshita T, et al. Inherited complete deficiency of 20-kilodalton homologous restriction factor (CD59) as a cause of paroxysmal nocturnal hemoglobinuria. N Engl J Med. 1990;323:1184–1189.
265. Devetten MP, Liu JM, Ling V, et al. Paroxysmal nocturnal hemoglobinuria: New insights from murine Pig-a-deficient hematopoiesis. Proc Assoc Am Physicians. 1997;109:99–110.
266. Armstrong C, Schubert J, Ueda E, et al. Affected paroxysmal nocturnal hemoglobinuria T lymphocytes harbor a common defect in assembly of *N*-acetyl-D-glucosamine inositol phospholipid corresponding to that in class A thy-1-murine lymphoma mutants. J Biol Chem. 1992;267:25347–25351.
267. Torzewski J, Bowyer DE, Waltenberger J, et al. Processes in atherogenesis: Complement activation. Atherosclerosis. 1997;132:131–138.
268. Weiser MR, Williams JP, Moore FD, et al. Reperfusion injury of ischemic skeletal muscle is mediated by natural antibody and complement. J Exp Med. 1996;183:2343–2348.
269. Koski CL, Sanders ME, Swoveland PT, et al. Activation of terminal components of complement in patients with Guillain-Barré syndrome and other demyelinating neuropathies. J Clin Invest. 1987;80:1492–1497.
270. Cammer W, Brosnan CF, Basile C, et al. Complement potentiates the degradation

of myelin proteins by plasmin: Implications for a mechanism of inflammatory demyelination. Brain Res. 1986;364:91–101.
271. Mollnes TE, Vandvik B, Lea T, et al. Intrathecal complement activation in neurological diseases evaluated by analysis of the terminal complement complex. J Neurol Sci. 1987;78:17–28.
272. Biesecker G, Lavin L, Ziskind M, et al. Cutaneous localization of the membrane attack complex in discoid and systemic lupus erythematosus. N Engl J Med. 1982;306:264–270.
273. Platt JL, Vercellotti GM, Dalmasso AP, et al. Transplantation of discordant xenografts: A review of progress. Immunol Today. 1990;11:450–455.
274. Dalmasso AP, Vercellotti GM, Fischel RJ, et al. Mechanism of complement activation in the hyperacute rejection of porcine organs transplanted into primate recipients. Am J Pathol. 1992;140:1157–1166.
275. Xia W, Fearon DT, Kirkman RL. Effect of repetitive doses of soluble human complement receptor type 1 on survival of discordant cardiac xenografts. Transplant Proc. 1993;25:410–411.
276. Loveland BE, Johnstone RW, Russell SM, et al. CD46 (MCP) confers protection from lysis by xenogeneic antibodies. Transplant Proc. 1993;25:396–397.
277. Weisman HF, Bartow T, Leppo MK, et al. Soluble human complement receptor type 1: In vivo inhibitor of complement suppressing post-ischemic myocardial inflammation and necrosis. Science. 1990;249:146–151.
278. White DJG, Yannoutsos N. Production of pigs transgenic for human DAF to overcome complement-mediated hyperacute xenograft rejection in man. Res Immunol. 1996;147:88–94.
279. Fischer MB, Prodeus AP, Nicholson-Weller A, et al. Increased susceptibility to endotoxin shock in complement C3- and C4-deficient mice is corrected by C1 inhibitor replacement. J Immunol. 1997;159:976–982.
280. Reid RR, Prodeus AP, Khan W, et al. Endotoxin shock in antibody-deficient mice. J Immunol. 1997;159:970–975.
281. Weaver LJ, Craddock PR, Jacob HS. Association of complement activation and elevated plasma-C5a with adult respiratory distress syndrome: Pathophysiological relevance and possible prognostic value. Lancet. 1980;1:947–949.
282. Jacob HS, Craddock PR, Hammerschmidt DE, et al. Complement-induced granulocyte aggregation: An unsuspected mechanism of disease. N Engl J Med. 1980;302:789–794.
283. Stevens JH, O'Hanley P, Shapiro JM, et al. Effect of anti-C5a antibodies on the adult respiratory distress syndrome in septic primates. J Clin Invest. 1986;77:1812–1816.
284. Hosea SW, Brown EJ, Frank MM. The critical role of complement in experimental pneumococcal sepsis. J Infect Dis. 1980;142:903–909.
285. Brown EJ, Hosea SW, Frank MM. The role of the spleen in experimental pneumococcal bacteremia. J Clin Invest. 1981;67:975–982.
286. Bohnsack JF, Brown EJ. The role of the spleen in resistance to infection. Annu Rev. Med. 1986;37:49–59.
287. Brown EJ, Hosea SW, Frank MM. The role of antibody and complement in the reticuloendothelial clearance of pneumococci from the bloodstream. Rev Infect Dis. 1985;5(Suppl):797–805.
288. Singer DB. Postsplenectomy sepsis. Perspect Pediatr Pathol. 1973;1:285–311.
289. Winkelstein JA, Drachman RH. Deficiency of pneumococcal serum opsonizing activity in sickle-cell disease. N Engl J Med. 1968;279:459–466.
290. Bisno AL, Freeman JC. The syndrome of asplenia, pneumococcal sepsis, and disseminated intravascular coagulation. Ann Intern Med. 1970;72:389–393.
291. Atkinson JP. Complement activation and complement receptors in systemic lupus erythematosus. Springer Semin Immunopathol. 1986;9:179–194.
292. Sim E, Gill EW, Sim RB. Drugs that induce systemic lupus erythematosus inhibit complement component C4. Lancet. 1984;2:422–424.
293. Clark RA, Kimball HR, Decker JL. Neutrophil chemotaxis in systemic lupus erythematosus. Ann Rheum Dis. 1974;33:167–172.
294. Perez HD, Lipton M, Goldstein IM. A specific inhibitor of complement (C5)–derived chemotactic activity in serum from patients with systemic lupus erythematosus. J Clin Invest. 1978;62:29–38.
295. Perez HD, Goldstein IM. Polymorphonuclear leukocyte chemotaxis in systemic lupus erythematosus. J Rheumatol. 1987;14:53–58.
296. Ross GD, Yount WJ, Walport MJ, et al. Disease-associated loss of erythrocyte complement receptors (CR1, C3b receptors) in patients with systemic lupus erythematosus and other diseases involving autoantibodies and/or complement activation. J Immunol. 1985;135:2005–2014.
297. Biesecker G, Katz S, Koffler D. Renal localization of the membrane attack complex in systemic lupus erythematosus nephritis. J Exp Med. 1981;151:1790–1791.
298. Falk RJ, Dalmasso AP, Kim Y, et al. Neoantigen of the polymerized ninth component of complement: Characterization of a monoclonal antibody and immunohistochemical localization in renal disease. J Clin Invest. 1983;72:560–573.
299. Groggel GC, Adler S, Rennke HG, et al. Role of the terminal complement pathway in experimental membranous nephropathy in the rabbit. J Clin Invest. 1983;72:1948–1957.
300. Adler S, Baker PJ, Pritzl P, et al. Detection of terminal complement components in experimental immune glomerular injury. Kidney Int. 1984;26:830–837.
301. Cybulsky AV, Rennke HG, Feintzeig ID, et al. Complement-induced glomerular epithelial cell injury: Role of the membrane attack complex in rat membranous nephropathy. J Clin Invest. 1986;77:1096–1107.
302. Cybulsky AV, Quigg RJ, Salant DJ. The membrane attack complex in complement-mediated glomerular epithelial cell injury: Formation and stability of C5b-9 and C5b-7 in rat membranous nephropathy. J Immunol. 1986;137:1511–1516.
303. Rus HG, Niculescu F, Nanulescu M, et al. Immunohistochemical detection of the terminal C5b-9 complement complex in children with glomerular diseases. Clin Exp Immunol. 1986;65:66–72.
304. Nath KA, Hostetter MK, Hostetter TH. Pathophysiology of chronic tubulointerstitial disease in rats: Interactions of dietary acid load, ammonia, and complement component C3. J Clin Invest. 1985;76:667–675.
305. Gordon DL, Krueger RA, Quie PG, et al. Amidation of C3 at the thiolester site: Stimulation of chemiluminescence and phagocytosis by a new inflammatory mediator. J Immunol. 1985;134:3339–3345.
306. Beeson PB, Rowley D. The anticomplementary effect of kidney tissue: Its association with ammonia production. J Exp Med. 1959;110:685–698.
307. Hostetter MK, Gordon DL. Biochemistry of C3 and related thiolester proteins in infection and inflammation. Rev Infect Dis. 1987;9:97–109.
308. Rubio R, Berne RM, Katori M. Release of adenosine in reactive hyperemia of the dog. Am J Physiol. 1969;216:56–62.
309. Cybulsky AV, Lieberthal W, Quigg RJ, et al. A role for thromboxane in complement-mediated glomerular injury. Am J Pathol. 1987;128:45–51.
310. Hakim RM, Breillatt J, Lazarus MJ, et al. Complement activation and hypersensitivity reactions to dialysis membranes. N Engl J Med. 1984;311:878–882.
311. Craddock PR. Complement and granulocyte activation and deactivation during hemodialysis. In: Lysaght MJ, Gurland JG, eds. Plasma Separation and Plasma Fractionation. Basel: S Karger AG; 1983:14–21.
312. Steinsson K, Erlendsson K, Valdimarsson H. Successful treatment with plasma infusions in a patient with deficiency of the second component of complement and systemic lupus erythematosus: Clinical experience over a 45 month period. Arthritis Rheum. 1989;32:906.
313. Erlendsson K, Traustadóttir K, Freysdóttir J, et al. Reciprocal changes in complement activity and immune-complex levels during plasma infusion in a C2-deficient SLE patient. Lupus. 1993;2:161–165.
314. Barrett DJ, Boyle MDP. Restoration of complement function in vivo by plasma infusion in factor I (C3b inactivator) deficiency. J Pediatr. 1984;104:76–81.
315. Rao CP, Minta JO, Laski B, et al. Inherited C8β subunit deficiency in a patient with recurrent meningococcal infections: In vivo functional kinetic analysis of C8. Clin Exp Immunol. 1985;60:183–190.
316. Pitts JS, Donaldson VH, Forristal J, et al. Remissions induced in hereditary angioneurotic edema with an attenuated androgen (danazol): Correlation between concentrations of C1-inhibitor and the fourth and second components of complement. J Lab Clin Med. 1978;92:501–507.
317. Platonov AE, Beloborodov VB, Pavlova LI, et al. Vaccination of patients deficient in a late complement component with tetravalent meningococcal capsular polysaccharide vaccine. Clin Exp Immunol. 1995;100:32–39.
318. Biselli R, Casapollo I, D'Amelio R, et al. Antibody response to meningococcal polysaccharides A and C in patients with complement defects. Scand J Immunol. 1993;37:644–650.
319. Fijen CAP, Kuijper EJ, van Leeuwen Y, et al. Antibody response of complement deficient patients to tetravalent meningococcal polysaccharide vaccine (Abstract). Proceedings of the Ninth International Pathogenic Neisseria Conference, Winchester, England, September 26–30, 1994:440.
320. Platonov AE, Vershinina IV, Dankert J, et al. Long-term follow-up of late complement component deficient patients vaccinated with meningococcal polysaccharide vaccine: Antibody persistence and efficacy of vaccination (Abstract). Abstracts of the Tenth International Pathogenic Neisseria Conference, Baltimore, Maryland, September 8–13, 1996:235.
321. Densen P, Brown EJ, O'Neill GJ. Inherited deficiency of C8 in a patient with recurrent meningococcal infections: Further evidence for a dysfunctional C8 molecule and nonlinkage to the HLA system. J Clin Immunol. 1983;3:90–99.
322. Potter PC, Frasch CE, van der Sande WJ, et al. Prophylaxis against *Neisseria meningitidis* infections and antibody responses in patients with deficiency of the sixth component of complement. J Infect Dis. 1990;161:932–937.

Chapter 8

Granulocytic Phagocytes

WILLIAM M. NAUSEEF
ROBERT A. CLARK

In general, vertebrates possess two fundamental mechanisms to respond to infection, the innate and the acquired immune systems. *Innate (natural) immunity* is the ability to respond immediately to an infectious challenge, regardless of previous exposure of the host to the invading agent. This type of immunity represents mechanisms encoded in germline genes. Elements of the innate system include phagocytic cells, namely polymorphonuclear leukocytes (PMNs) and mononuclear phagocytes, and the complement cascade of circulating soluble proteins. This relatively nonspecific "pattern recognition" system has functional analogues in the immune systems of a wide variety of multicellular organisms, including plants and insects. As such, this evolutionarily ancient system represents a rapid and sensitive surveillance mechanism of host defense when the organism is challenged with an invading microorganism previously "unseen" by the host's immune system.

In contrast, *acquired (adaptive) immunity* is the product of somatic gene rearrangement and has remarkable capacity to recognize and respond to a wide diversity of structures and to discriminate precisely among them. Lymphocytes (both B and T cells) and antibodies represent the cellular and circulating protein elements, respectively, of adaptive immunity. In contrast to the innate system, adaptive immunity is restricted to vertebrates and represents a precisely tuned means by which host cells define specifically the nature of the invading pathogen or tumor cell. Such precision, however, requires time for antigens to be processed and specific antibodies to be generated. Therefore, the adaptive system is slower to respond to new challenges than is the innate system, although the latter lacks specificity.

Vertebrate immunity represents an integration of these two complex and regulated mechanisms of host defense.[1, 2] Granulocytes, the most numerous leukocytes in the peripheral circulation, include neutrophils, eosinophils, and basophils. Structurally these cells share a multilobed nucleus and the presence of numerous membrane-bound, characteristically staining cytoplasmic granules, but functionally they differ significantly.

NEUTROPHILS

Development

Neutrophils arise from pluripotent stem cells located in the bone marrow. The processes of proliferation and differentiation are precisely orchestrated by the coordinated activity of colony-stimulating factors (CSF) for myeloid cells.[3, 4] These molecules influence the survival and direct the maturation and proliferation of myeloid cells. Each factor is named for the colony produced under its influence: GM-CSF, for granulocytes and macrophages; G-CSF, for granulocytes; M-CSF, for monocytes and macrophages; and multi-CSF (or interleukin-3 [IL-3]), for a variety of colonies including neutrophils, macrophages, eosinophils, megakaryocytes, and erythroid cells. Although lineage-specific cytokines mediate acquisition of granulocytic features, precise details of their regulation are not understood.[5–7] In addition cytokines, including GM-CSF and G-CSF, may enhance function and prolong neutrophil survival by delaying the apoptosis these cells usually undergo.[8]

Granulocyte development in the bone marrow can be divided into a mitotic phase and a nonmitotic phase, each lasting approximately 1 week. During the mitotic phase, cells mature sequentially from myeloblasts into promyelocytes and myelocytes.[9] Maturation is associated with the appearance of the cytoplasmic granules characteristic of neutrophils, basophils, and eosinophils. The nonmitotic phase of development includes metamyelocytes, band (or immature) neutrophils, and mature neutrophils.

Coincident with the morphologic changes, the cells acquire the specific surface markers and functional properties of more mature cells.[10] For example, Fc receptors appear as the cells develop into promyelocytes, cells become competent for phagocytosis in the early myelocyte stage, and complement receptors appear in the late myelocyte and metamyelocyte stages. Oxygen-dependent microbicidal activity appears in the early metamyelocyte stage, and cells in the late metamyelocyte–band stage demonstrate increased adhesiveness, cell motility, and chemotactic responses.[10] In addition, coordinated expression of genes encoding the granule proteins is synchronized with early stages of myeloid development, and normal granulocytic differentiation is intimately linked with expression of proteins localized in specific granules.[11] Although they are incompletely understood at this time, the hematopoietic growth factors direct myeloid differentiation by modulating transcription factors that regulate genes responsible for a specific myeloid phenotype.[7, 11]

Morphologic and Structural Characteristics

The earliest histochemical studies of neutrophils classified the membrane-bound intracellular granules by their staining characteristics. Two populations of granules were distinguished based on staining with azure A: the positively-staining azurophilic granules and the unstained specific granules. Sophisticated subcellular fractionation and analysis of neutrophil organelles have refined significantly our appreciation of the complexity and heterogeneity of neutrophil granules.[12] In addition to insights into the biologic roles of the various proteins in the matrix of the granules, studies have identified functionally important proteins within the membranes of particular granule subsets.

At a first approximation, neutrophil granules can be categorized based on peroxidase staining. The peroxidase-positive granules are also known as *primary granules*, because they arise first in granulopoiesis, and as *azurophilic granules*, based on histochemical staining.[13] Azurophilic granules contain myeloperoxidase (MPO)[14]; a variety of proteolytic enzymes, including cathepsins, proteinase-3,[15] and elastase[16]; and the antimicrobial defensins[17] and bactericidal permeability-increasing protein (BPI)[18] (Table 8–1). Because of the acid hydrolase activity of the azurophilic granule contents, this compartment has been considered lysosomal in nature. However azurophilic granules lack lysosome-associated membrane protein, an identifying marker for lysosomes. Moreover proteins such as MPO[19] and the defensins[20] do not segregate into the azurophilic granule by means of the mannose-6-phosphate receptor, a targeting system characteristic of lysosomal proteins. Taken together, these observations suggest that the azurophilic granule may be a specialized organelle that is distinctly different from conventional primary lysosomes.

Based in large part on studies by Borregaard and colleagues,[12, 21] the peroxidase-negative granules can be categorized as *specific granules, gelatinase granules,* and *secretory vesicles*. The contents of the specific and gelatinase granules overlap to a significant extent[22] (see Table 8–1) but differ from those of azurophilic granules and secretory

TABLE 8–1 Characteristics of Neutrophil Granules

Characteristics	Primary (Azurophil)	Specific (Secondary)
Contents	Acid hydrolases	Lactoferrin
	β-Glucuronidase	Lysozyme
	α-Mannosidase	Vitamin B_{12}-binding protein
	Arylsulfatase	Collagenase (?)
	5′-Nucleotidase	Monocyte chemotactic factor
	Acid protease (cathepsin)	C3 and C5 cleaving proteases
	Neutral proteases	Membrane-bound receptors
	Cathepsin G	CR3
	Elastase	CR4
	Collagenase (?)	C5a
	Myeloperoxidase	FMLP
	Cationic proteins	Laminin
	Defensins	Membrane-bound components of NADPH oxidase system
	Lysozyme	Cytochrome-b_{558}
	Acid mucopolysaccharide	
pH optimum	5.5–6.5	7.0–7.5
Degranulation	Degranulation delayed >50% into phagosome	Degranulates first >90% Exocytosis
Function	Microbial killing Digestion	Inflammatory process

Abbreviations: FMLP, Formylmethyl-leucyl-phenylaline; NADPH, nicotinamide adenine dinucleotide phosphate.

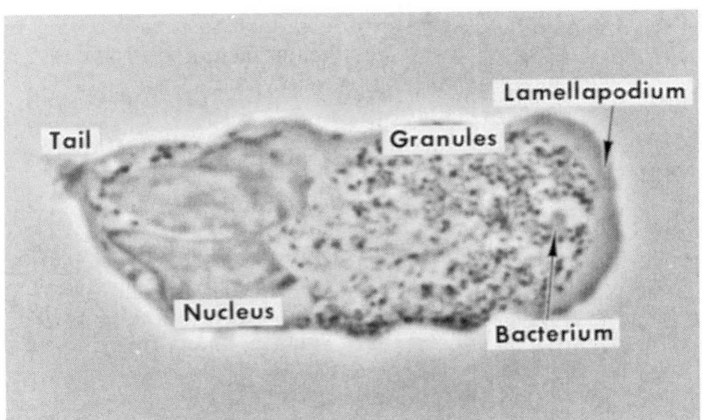

FIGURE 8–1. Phase-contrast photomicrograph of a human neutrophil.

vesicles. More striking, however, is the distribution of functionally important plasma membrane proteins in the membranes of peroxidase-negative granules.[23] These membranes contain cytochrome-b_{558},[24, 25] an essential component of the nicotinamide adenine dinucleotide phosphate (NADPH)–dependent oxidase (discussed later); receptors for chemotactic peptides[26, 27]; extracellular matrix proteins[28]; cytokines[29]; opsonins[30]; and adhesion proteins.[27, 31, 32] They therefore represent an intracellular reservoir of functionally important membrane proteins that can be quickly recruited to the cell surface during neutrophil activation. The presence of such compartments is ideally suited to the central role of neutrophils as the major circulating cell in the innate immune system; a reservoir of readily accessible functional proteins allows a rapid response without the delays that would be incurred by requirements for new protein synthesis. The functional consequences of this compartmentalization of proteins in the matrix and in the membrane of granules is discussed later.

During maturation, the nucleus becomes segmented and the cytoskeletal elements, microfilaments and microtubules, appear in the cytoplasm. A meshwork of microfilaments makes up the clear cortical veil that surrounds the cell and forms the lamellipodium of an advancing cell (Fig. 8–1). These structures are polymers of actin, a protein representing 5 to 10% of the total cellular protein. Actin, together with a number of other interacting proteins, constitutes the contractile machinery of the cell that generates locomotion.[33] Actin monomers (G-actin), in the presence of actin-binding protein, polymerize to form cross-linked actin filaments (F-actin). Regulation of the length of the filaments and the degree of cross-linking provides for the physicochemical dynamics of actin flux between the gel and sol states. Filament length is controlled by several different proteins. Profilin serves to sequester G-actin and may provide a mechanism for rapid transport of actin to sites of polymerization. Acumentin, by initiating multiple sites of filament formation (nucleation) and preferentially inhibiting actin monomer exchange from the "slow-growing" end of elongating filaments, maintains actin in short filaments. Gelsolin, a calcium-modulated protein that initiates filament nucleation, binds to the "fast-growing" end of the filaments and can split preformed actin filaments. In the presence of adenosine triphosphate (ATP), myosin repetitively dissociates and binds to cross-linked actin. Myosin binding changes the cross-linking angle between actin filaments from 90 to 45 degrees, which results in movement of the filaments. In this way myosin serves to harness the changes in the physicochemical state of actin so as to give directionality to cell movement. Changes in calcium concentration that occur with membrane perturbation, directly and in concert with calmodulin, exert control over the contractile process by regulating myosin kinase and gelsolin. As a result, intracellular calcium gradients provide for an increase in polymerized actin in regions of high calcium concentration.

Actin filaments are associated with the cytoskeleton or with the plasma membrane via membrane skeletal proteins.[34] Stimulation of the cell with chemotactic factors causes an abrupt increase in the amount of actin associated with the cytoskeleton[35] and a shift in microfilament organization from a parallel strand to a cross-hatched meshwork most evident at the leading edge of the directionally polarized cell.[36]

Microtubules are hollow structures composed of dimers of tubulin. In contrast to the role of microfilaments in directed locomotion and changes in cell shape, microtubules appear to be necessary for the initial orientation of the cell in a chemotactic gradient and for the spatial organization of structures within the cell during locomotion. They also may be involved in vesicle transport, degranulation, and the regulation of cell surface microviscosity during phagocytosis.[37]

Mature neutrophils (Figs. 8–1 and 8–2) are characterized by a paucity of ribosomal material and mitochondria, in keeping with the low levels of synthetic processes in these cells. However, neutrophils actively synthesize a selective group of proteins, including major histocompatibility complex (MHC) class I molecules,[38] complement receptors,[39] IL-8,[40] tumor necrosis factor-α (TNF-α), G-CSF, M-CSF, IL-1, IL-6, and interferon-α (IFN-α).[41] Glycogen granules fill the cytoplasm and serve as a source of energy for neutrophil function.

Receptors with specificity for a number of humoral substances, including immunoglobulin G (IgG),[42] IgA, the complement fragments C3b and iC3b,[43] and several chemotactic factors (most notably the formyl peptide receptor family[44]) have been identified and characterized both functionally and structurally.[45–49] These receptors are homogeneously distributed over the surface of the resting cell but undergo an asymmetric clustering at the front of the cell when it becomes polarized in response to a chemotactic stimulus. The distribution of receptors with different ligand specificities can be independently regulated even though stimulation via these receptors may result in similar functional effects.[50] Moreover, the various neutrophil functional responses exhibit differential requirements for receptor occupancy. For example, maximal degranulation requires brief receptor occupancy, whereas sustained oxidative responses depend on continuous ligand binding to the receptor.[51]

Neutrophil Kinetics

The daily production of mature PMNs in a healthy adult is on the order of 10^{11} cells. During acute infection or other inflammatory stresses, neutrophils are mobilized from the marrow reserve, which contains up to 10 times the normal daily neutrophil requirement. In the face of a persistent stimulus this reserve may be depleted, but

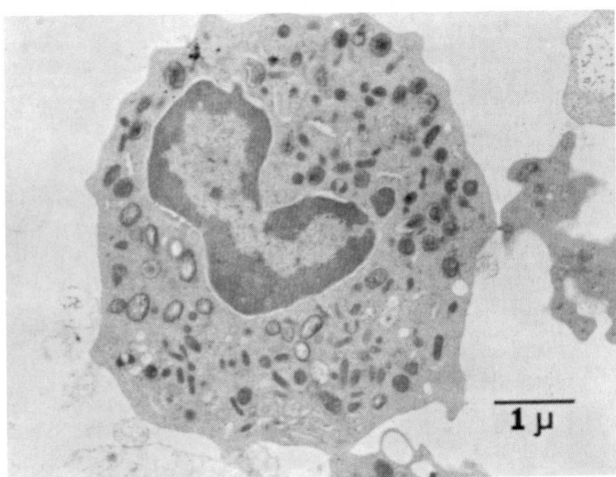

FIGURE 8–2. Electron micrograph of a human neutrophil. Note the granules *(large oval structures)*, glycogen particles *(small dark particles)*, but few other visible organelles.

only if there is nutritional deficiency or other disorder (e.g., ethanol abuse) that compromises mechanisms for augmenting delivery to meet demands. Increased stem cell input, increased mitoses during the mitotic stage of development, use of a store of cells whose maturation had been inhibited (so-called hiatal cells), and shortening of the maturation time within the marrow may all occur.[52] Multiplication and differentiation of stem cells is stimulated by the CSFs produced by peripheral blood monocytes, tissue macrophages, and stimulated lymphocytes.[52, 53]

Approximately 5% (about 4×10^8 cells per kilogram of body weight) of the total granulocyte pool is located in two compartments of similar size, the intravascular circulating cells and the marginating cells. A dynamic equilibrium exists between these two compartments, as cells exhibit transient endothelial interactions (margination) and then resume rapid flow, reflecting the balance between intercellular adherence and shear forces. The intravascular half-life of these cells is 6 to 8 hours, whereas their persistence in extravascular sites ranges from a few hours to several days. Granulocytosis, the hallmark of acute inflammation, is a consequence of certain physiologic and pharmacologic stimuli that typically alter the distribution of neutrophils among the various granulocyte pools rather than increase cell production. For example, the acute administration of corticosteroids or endotoxin, perhaps mimicking pathophysiologic events that occur in severe infection, promotes granulocyte release from the marrow reserve. Chronic steroid administration produces granulocytosis primarily by decreasing neutrophil adherence and shifting cells from the marginating to the circulating pool. Similarly, exercise, stress, epinephrine, hypoxia, aspirin, and alcohol cause granulocytosis by mobilizing marginating cells.

Recruitment to the Inflammatory Site

Circulating neutrophils are functionally heterogeneous, and the majority (80%) have the capacity to form IgG rosettes.[54] Because release from the bone marrow is not synchronized, this heterogeneity probably reflects maturational differences within a single cell line, although its biologic significance is uncertain. Differences in the distributions of these cells may contribute to the development of "impaired" neutrophil function in certain disease states. In contrast, tissue neutrophils are homogeneous, and more than 96% are capable of IgG rosette formation.[54] They contain fewer lysosomal granules and more glycogen than do their circulating counterparts, because anaerobic glycolysis provides the energy for cell movement through the tissues.[55]

To combat invading microorganisms, neutrophils must emigrate from the circulation and into the extravascular tissue space. Extravascular recruitment of neutrophils represents the summation of coordinated interactions of cells, specific receptors, and soluble mediators. The process involves at least four discrete steps: rolling adhesion, integrin activation, firm adhesion, and transmigration[56, 57] (Fig. 8–3).

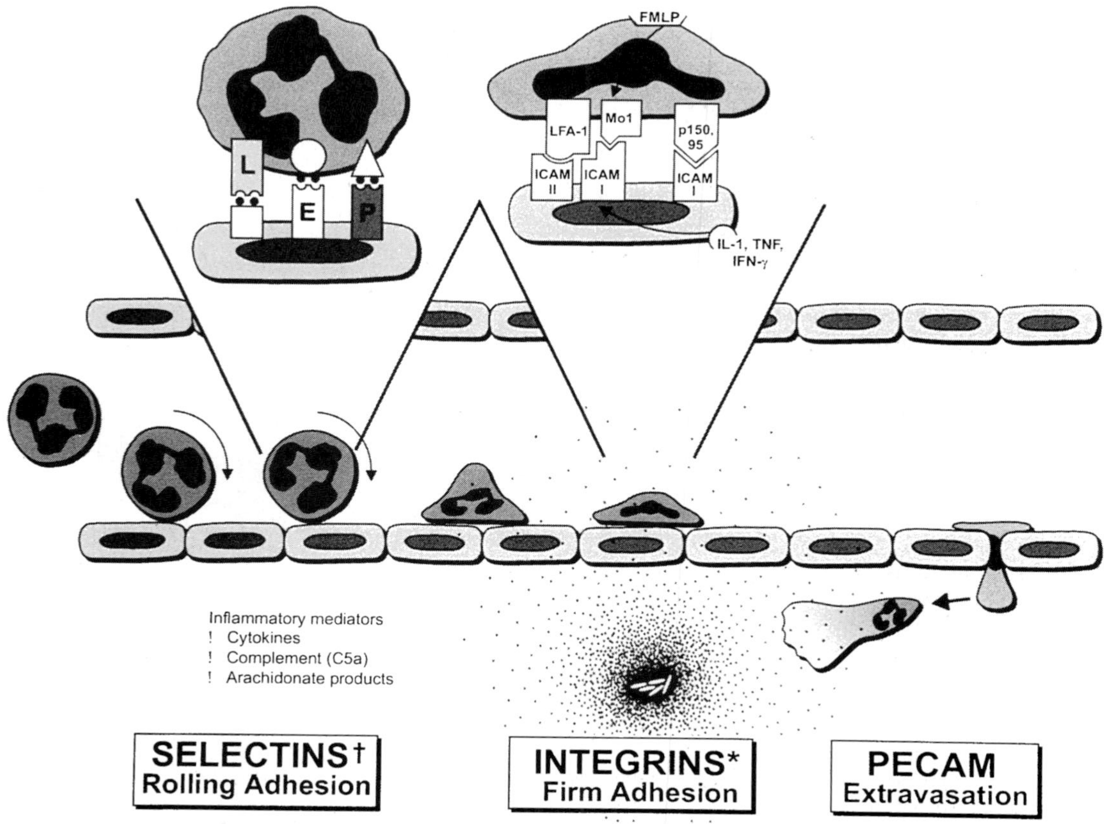

FIGURE 8–3. Steps in the emigration of neutrophils from the vascular space. Neutrophils are depicted entering the marginating pool in a postcapillary venule. Initial adhesion is mediated by neutrophil (L) and endothelial (E, P) selectins and by their respective carbohydrate ligands on the opposing cell surface. Blood flow shear forces propel the lightly adherent neutrophils forward with a rolling or tumbling motion. Inflammatory mediators diffusing into the blood stream from sites of microbial invasion in the tissues bind to specific receptors and upregulate the functional expression of β_2-integrins (LFA-1; Mo-1; p150,95) on neutrophils as well as intercellular adhesion molecules (ICAM) on endothelial cells. These alterations promote a change in neutrophil shape and the firm adhesion of these cells to the vessel wall. Platelet-endothelial cell adhesion molecules (PECAM) localized to interendothelial cell junctions interact with PECAM on the neutrophil surface to permit neutrophil migration between endothelial cells. Once in the tissues, the polarized neutrophils move up the mediator concentration gradient to reach the site of microbial invasion. Type 2 leukocyte adhesion deficiency (†) is caused by the absence on neutrophil glycoproteins of the primary carbohydrate ligand (small dots in diagram), sLe^x, for E-selectin. Type 1 leukocyte adhesion deficiency (*) is caused by the lack of β_2-integrin expression on the neutrophil surface.

In turn these events are mediated by four classes of adhesion proteins: selectins, integrins, immunoglobulin-like proteins, and mucin-like selectin ligands. In addition to neutrophils and endothelial cells, platelets figure prominently in the initiation of the inflammatory response, colocalizing with neutrophils and participating in P-selectin–dependent leukocyte binding.[58, 59] Taken together, the cooperation of several cell types and their secreted products culminates in events necessary to recruit circulating neutrophils to the site of inflammation, and the activation of autocrine and paracrine feedback loops modulates the extent of the host response.[60]

Through a process of repetitive ligand-receptor binding and release, marginating granulocytes become lightly adherent to endothelial cells and, under the influence of the physiologic shear forces of blood flow, tumble or roll slowly along the vessel wall (see Fig. 8–3). The molecules mediating rolling adhesion are called *selectins* "to highlight the amino terminal lectin domain and to indicate [their] selective function and cellular expression."[56] These molecules are homologous to C-type lectins and therefore require calcium for expression of binding activity. Individual members of this family are named for the cell type on which they were originally identified (E, endothelia; L, lymphocytes; P, platelets). Although attention has focused on binding to sialylated Lewis X and A (sLe^X, sLe^A) glycoproteins, selectins also interact with sulfated and phosphorylated polysaccharides such as heparin and mannose-6-phosphate. Individual selectins exhibit different but overlapping binding specificities, the bases for which largely remain to be determined.[61–63]

The presence of unique selectins on endothelial cells and neutrophils means that rolling adhesion can be modulated bidirectionally. For example, L-selectin is constitutively expressed on neutrophils and appears to be shed after cell activation. In contrast, little or no E-selectin is present on resting endothelial cells, either in vitro or in vivo. Stimulation of these cells leads to inducible and transient E-selectin expression, which peaks about 4 hours after stimulation and dissipates over 24 hours.[56]

When neutrophils tumbling along the venule wall encounter inflammatory mediators and stimulated endothelial cells, adhesion between the two cell types rapidly shifts to a high-affinity state. This second step in transendothelial migration reflects activation of β_2 integrins. The β_2 or leukocyte integrins are members of a large family of heterodimeric molecules that mediate cell-cell and cell-matrix interactions.[64] This family is subdivided on the basis of eight different β-chains, any one of which can associate with multiple α-chains to form a unique α β pair. Both the α- and β-chains are transmembrane molecules with short cytoplasmic tails and large extracellular globular heads that interact to form the ligand-binding site. The three neutrophil integrins have a common 95-kD β-chain, which is identical to CD18, and distinct α-chains. These molecular complexes are also referred to as leukocyte function-associated antigen-1 or LFA-1 ($\alpha_L\beta_2$, CD11a/CD18), Mo-1 or Mac-1 ($\alpha_M\beta_2$, CD11b/CD18), and p150,95 ($\alpha_X\beta_2$, CD11c/CD18).[65] Mo-1 and p150,95 also function as receptors (CR3 and CR4, respectively) for the opsonic C3 fragments iC3b and C3d. Endothelial counterreceptors for the β_2 integrins include intercellular adhesion molecule-1 (ICAM-1) and ICAM-2. LFA-1 binds to both ICAM-1 and ICAM-2, whereas Mo-1 and p150,95 bind only to ICAM-1 but at different sites from that for LFA-1. An additional LFA-1 counterreceptor, ICAM-3, is not present on endothelium but is expressed on all hematopoietic cells, where it may be involved in leukocyte-leukocyte interactions.[66, 67] In addition to the β_2 integrins, PMNs possess on their surface the leukocyte response integrin,[68] which, together with integrin-associated protein, modulates cellular responses, particularly those induced by extracellular matrix proteins.[69–71] Although the precise details of the interactions of these various proteins are unknown, their importance is inferred from the observation that mice deficient in integrin-associated protein are unable to mount an inflammatory response after intraperitoneal challenge.[72]

Integrin function requires calcium, a specific membrane environment, and appropriate stimuli such as chemoattractant peptides.[65] These stimuli appear to modulate integrin binding affinity by altering the interaction of the intracytoplasmic tails with each other and with the cytoskeleton. Integrin activation results in increased number and avidity of β_2 integrins as well as clustering of receptors and cytoskeletal rearrangement. Neutrophils change from spherical granulocytes with relatively little surface area involved in cell-cell contact to flattened cells with a broad surface area for cellular interactions (see Fig. 8–3). Blood flow shear forces are no longer able to propel them forward along the vessel wall. This firm adhesion, the third step in transmigration, is mediated through interactions between β_2 integrins on neutrophils and ICAM-1 and -2 on endothelial cells.[73]

ICAM-2 is constitutively expressed on endothelial cells and therefore may provide the initial endothelial ligand underlying the rapid development of firm adhesion. In contrast, ICAM-1, like E-selectin, undergoes marked upregulation when endothelium is exposed to IL-1 or TNF. It differs from E-selectin in that low-level expression is present on unstimulated cells, peak expression occurs over 12 to 24 hours and is sustained, and expression is also induced by IFN-γ.[56] The ability of corticosteroids to inhibit E-selectin and ICAM-1 upregulation in the face of endotoxin, a potent stimulus for their expression, attests to the feasibility of anti-inflammatory strategies directed at adhesion molecules.

Endothelial cells play an active role in upregulating adherence events. For example, stimulated endothelial cells secrete IL-8, which both attracts and directly activates neutrophils, and upregulates expression of platelet-activating factor, which can engage its receptor on neutrophils.[56] Transmigration, the final step in neutrophil emigration into tissue (see Fig. 8–3), involves at least two specific proteins, platelet-endothelial cell adhesion molecule (PECAM or CD31) and integrin-associated protein (IAP or CD47). Both proteins are localized at the intercellular junctions between endothelial cells, and antibodies to each block transmigration.[73] Current dogma dictates that transmigration occurs between endothelial cells, perhaps by neutrophil-dependent transient disorganization of adherens junctions at cell-cell interfaces,[74] although one study indicates that neutrophil extravasation may also occur by transcellular pathways.[75]

Although this paradigm applies to neutrophil extravasation, transmigration of neutrophils across epithelial barriers, which is necessary in infections involving the gastrointestinal, genitourinary, and respiratory tracts, deviates significantly from this theme. Major insights into the mechanisms of neutrophil interaction with polarized epithelial cells have derived from studies with human cell lines such as T84 and HT29.[76] Neutrophils can bind to either surface of these cells, and transmigration can occur in either direction. Binding to the basolateral surface of T84 cells is mediated by neutrophil β_2 integrins and an unidentified counterligand on the epithelial cell that is neither ICAM-1 nor a known selectin. In contrast, neutrophil binding to the apical surface of intestinal epithelial cells is dependent on ICAM-1.[76–78] Basolateral-to-apical migration of neutrophils across T84 cells requires expression of CD47,[79, 80] but the determinants of apical-to-basolateral migration have not been identified. Evidence suggests that the mechanism for transmigration in each direction is distinct, because immunomodulators such as lipoxin A4[81] and IFN-γ[82] stimulate movement toward the basolateral surface but inhibit luminal migration. Eventual characterization of regulated neutrophil movement across epithelium will provide important insights into the pathogenesis of infectious diseases at such epithelial surfaces.

Neutrophil extravasation and migration through tissue is the consequence of a carefully regulated process involving the sequential release and compartmentalization of a wide variety of inflammatory mediators. Early (0 to 5 hours) neutrophil influx into an area of induced injury appears predominantly to reflect the effects of IFN-γ, C5a, and leukotriene B_4. IL-8 and IL-6 appear in a second wave of mediator activity (at 5 to 24 hours) and IL-1α, GM-CSF, and TNF-α in a third wave of activity (8 to 24 hours), whereas concentrations of IL-1, IL-2, and IL-4 remain unchanged. C5a, leukotriene B_4, and IL-8 are potent neutrophil chemoattractants, as are hydroxyeicosatetraenoic acids (HETE) and microbial oligopeptides analogous to *N*-formyl-methionyl-leucyl-phenylalanine (FMLP).

Among the soluble mediators that can recruit leukocytes, the chemokines represent a diverse and biologically important class of proteins. Chemokines are a family of structurally related, pluripotent proteins that trigger leukocyte activation,[83–85] including adherence, chemotaxis, degranulation, and priming of the neutrophil oxidase; participate in angiogenesis; and figure prominently in host response to infection with human immunodeficiency virus (HIV).[86] Chemokines are classified into two major families, CXC and CC, distinguished by the presence or absence of an amino acid between the first two cysteines in the protein. All chemokines targeted for neutrophils are in the CXC family, the most important of which is IL-8. Secreted by leukocytes, platelets, fibroblasts, epithelial cells, and activated endothelium, IL-8 triggers the full range of cellular responses in neutrophils. IL-8 activation of neutrophils is mediated by engagement of one of two G-protein–coupled membrane receptors that specifically recognize the chemokine.[87]

Of importance from the point of view of pathogenesis of infection, several organisms have mimicked chemokine receptors as a means by which to enter cells. For example, US28, a gene product of human cytomegalovirus,[44] and ECRF3, a protein of the herpesvirus of Saimiri,[88] represent virally encoded proteins with significant structural homology to chemokine receptors. In addition, HIV enters target cells by utilizing CD4 and specific chemokine receptors.[89, 90] Moreover, genetic polymorphisms in certain of these chemokine receptors have significant effects on susceptibility to or rate of progression of HIV-1 infection.[91] It is clear that chemokines and their receptors have a pivotal place in the inflammatory response and in the pathogenesis of certain infectious diseases.[92]

Chemotactic stimuli bind to high-affinity receptors on the leukocyte surface. Receptors for IL-8, FMLP, and C5a are members of a large family of proteins characterized by an external ligand-binding domain, seven membrane-spanning segments, and cytoplasmic regions that couple to G proteins.[44] In the presence of chemoattractant gradients across the cell as small as 0.1 to 1.0% (e.g., as the attractant diffuses from a focus of infection), ligand-linked receptors distribute asymmetrically and trigger the directed movement (chemotaxis) and net accumulation of neutrophils at sites of increasing concentrations of attractant (Fig. 8–4). How the chemoattractant signal is transduced to cell movement is not precisely understood, but calcium fluxes, actin, and a number of actin-binding and regulatory proteins of the cytoskeleton are centrally involved,[93] as are leukocyte adherence molecules and the extracellular matrix. The binding of chemoattractants to their receptors also initiates elements of the microbicidal response, namely, degranulation and the respiratory burst, although these responses generally require higher concentrations of the stimulus than does chemotaxis. For this reason, activation of these distal events may be delayed until the cell is in close proximity to the infected tissue site.

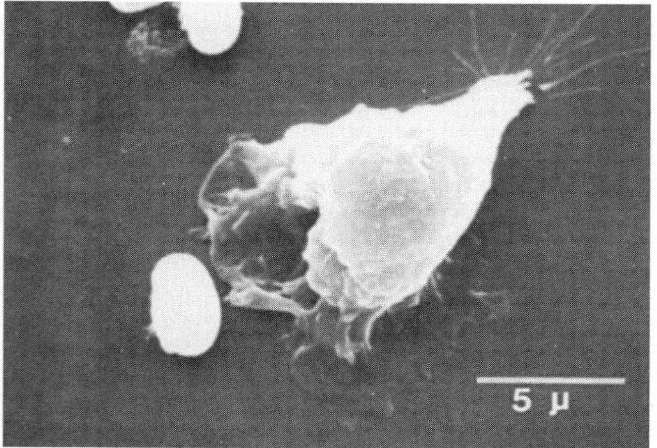

FIGURE 8–4. Scanning electron micrograph of a neutrophil extending a pseudopod toward *Candida albicans.*

Phagocytosis

Phagocytosis is the intracellular uptake of particles greater than 0.5 mm by a mechanism independent of clathrin but dependent on the polymerization of actin. After attachment to the cell surface, the phagocytic particle is internalized, with subsequent phagosome maturation (described later) and eventual delivery to and fusion with the lysosome to form a phagolysosome.[94] Neutrophils may ingest some microorganisms in the absence of serum factors by a process known as lectinophagocytosis,[95] wherein surface proteins on one or both cells recognize specific carbohydrates on the other cell. However, most bacteria must be opsonized for attachment to and ingestion by neutrophils to occur efficiently.[96]

Specific IgG and complement are the major opsonic factors promoting recognition and ingestion of most microorganisms by neutrophils. Antibody promotes phagocytic uptake by neutralizing antiphagocytic molecules on the bacterial surface (e.g., capsular polysaccharide), efficiently activating the classic pathway of complement and promoting deposition of opsonic fragments of C3 on the bacterial surface, physically linking the organism to the neutrophils and engaging the IgG receptor in the neutrophil membrane.[97, 98] Activation of complement via either the alternative or the classic pathway leads to C3b and iC3b deposition on the microbial surface (see Chapter 7), and C1q deposition enhances Fc receptor-dependent ingestion.[99] Opsonization directly alters the organism by making the relatively hydrophilic microbial surface more hydrophobic and therefore more readily ingested.[100]

Distinct receptors for IgG (FcγRI through RIII), but not other immunoglobulins, and for C3b (CR1) and iC3b (CR3) are present in the neutrophil membrane.[42, 43] In addition to its iC3b-binding site, CR3 also bears a carbohydrate recognition domain that may play a role in lectinophagocytosis. Data suggest that Fcγ receptors mediate phagocytosis via calcium-dependent pathways, whereas CR1 and CR3 use calcium-independent pathways.[98, 101] FcγRII and RIII are low- to moderate-affinity receptors that are constitutively expressed, whereas the high-affinity FcγRI is present only after cell stimulation (e.g., by IFN-γ).[102] Intracellular pools of Fc receptors have not been identified, but reserves have been described for both CR1 and CR3.[43] These receptor pools are rapidly mobilized to the surface after stimulation of the cell by a variety of inflammatory mediators.

Binding of either IgG or C3 increases the rate of phagocytosis of appropriately sensitized erythrocytes. However, Fc receptor–dependent interactions with this target initiate microfilament polymerization and ingestion only in unprimed cells.[103, 104] In contrast, complement deposition alone is sufficient to promote ingestion of a number of bacteria, a finding that emphasizes the heterogeneity among opsonic requirements for different particles. In most cases phagocytosis is most efficient when organisms are coated with both IgG and C3, thereby allowing cooperative interaction of the two types of receptors.

Ingestion is the result of the sequential interaction between opsonic ligands distributed over the particle surface and their receptors on the phagocyte membrane.[105] The sequential interaction of these opsonic ligands with their receptors in the phagocytic membrane initiates polymerization of actin microfilaments in the cytoplasm underlying the site of particle attachment and results in circumferential flow of the cell membrane about the opsonized particle and its enclosure within a phagosome[106, 107] (Figs. 8–4 and 8–5).

Increased attention has been paid to the important phagocytic role played by receptors that do not bind to opsonins, especially in soft tissues where neutrophil function is most critical. Receptors for fibronectin and laminin, proteins that constitute part of the extracellular matrix secreted by endothelial cells, recognize the Arg-Gly-Asp

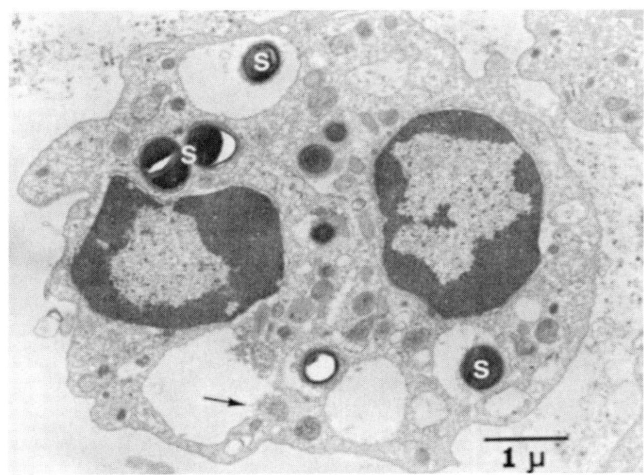

FIGURE 8–5. Electron micrograph of a neutrophil that has ingested *Staphylococcus aureus* (S). Bacteria are in phagocytic vacuoles formed by invagination of external cell membrane. Degranulation into a phagocytic vacuole can be seen at the lower left *(arrow)*.

(RGD) amino acid sequence in these extracellular matrix proteins.[108] Although these proteins in solution fail to promote ingestion of target particles, neutrophils adherent to surfaces coated with proteins containing this sequence display enhanced capacity to ingest C3-coated particles when stimulated with a variety of chemotactic factors. This enhancement requires neutrophil adherence to the matrix protein but not interaction of the matrix protein with the target particles or an increase in FcγR or C3 receptor number. Hence, these proteins are not opsonins but rather enhance phagocytosis by converting C3 receptors from a binding mode to one mediating ingestion. Studies have assigned an important role for the vitronectin receptor ($\alpha_V\beta_3$) in modulating phagocytosis via the $\alpha_5\beta_1$ receptor on mononuclear phagocytes.[109] Such findings reinforce the notion that migrating phagocytes modulate their phagocytic capacity according to the tissue context in which they function.

Postphagocytic Events

Once internalization has begun, actin polymerization in the cytoplasm immediately adjacent to the nascent phagosome occurs and actin-binding proteins are recruited to the periphagosomal space.[94] In an orderly fashion, cytosolic proteins associate with and disassociate from the phagosome sequentially, with eventual fusion of the phagosome with the neutrophil granules. In the mature phagosome, optimal microbicidal activity represents the coordinated generation of oxygen-derived species by activation of the NADPH-dependent oxidase and release of granule components. As discussed later, the successful survival of several intracellular pathogens reflects their ability to elude or undermine events critical for normal phagosomal maturation and complete recruitment of the elements essential for microbicidal action.

Oxidative Burst. The oxidative or respiratory burst is mediated by a multicomponent system present as an enzymatically active complex in the plasma membrane and phagosomal membrane of stimulated neutrophils.[110, 111] Such enzymatic activity is not detected in resting, nonstimulated neutrophils. A similar, if not identical, enzyme system is found in stimulated eosinophils, monocytes, and macrophages. The respiratory burst enzyme transports electrons from cytosolic NADPH to molecular oxygen to generate superoxide anion ($O_2^{\cdot-}$), the one-electron reduction product of oxygen, as the immediate product:

$$2O_2 + NADPH \rightarrow 2O_2^{\cdot-} + H^+ + NADP^+$$

Important features of the oxidase include the 1:1 stoichiometry between oxygen consumption and superoxide formation, the two-electron oxidation of the pyridine nucleotide compared with the one-electron reduction of oxygen, the formation of protons, and the generation of $NADP^+$, which must be reduced back to NADPH to sustain the reaction.

Most of the superoxide formed readily undergoes dismutation to hydrogen peroxide and oxygen:

$$2O_2^{\cdot-} + 2H^+ \rightarrow H_2O_2 + O_2$$

This reaction occurs spontaneously with rapid kinetics at acidic pH, where a significant portion of the superoxide exists in its protonated form, the perhydroxy radical ($HO_2^{\cdot}$). This is a result of the very high rate constant for the reaction between $O_2^{\cdot-}$ and $HO_2^{\cdot}$. In the acidic environment of the phagocytic vacuole, superoxide is converted quantitatively to hydrogen peroxide. Because 1 mole of oxygen is regenerated for each mole of hydrogen peroxide formed, there is a net 1:1 stoichiometry between oxygen consumption and hydrogen peroxide formation, but a 2:1 relation between $O_2^{\cdot-}$ and H_2O_2.

Detoxification of $O_2^{\cdot-}$ and H_2O_2 is carried out by cellular enzyme systems. At neutral pH, superoxide dismutase markedly accelerates the dismutation reaction. H_2O_2 is metabolized either by catalase or through the glutathione system. Catalase converts H_2O_2 directly to water and oxygen, whereas glutathione peroxidase utilizes reduced glutathione (GSH) to reduce H_2O_2 to water. NADPH provides the reducing equivalents for the glutathione reductase–catalyzed regeneration of GSH from glutathione (GSSG). NADPH levels must be maintained in order to support both the superoxide-forming oxidase and the glutathione cycle. The reduced pyridine nucleotide is regenerated by the activity of the hexose monophosphate shunt, which is enhanced 15- to 30-fold during phagocytosis.[112]

The dormant respiratory burst oxidase of the resting neutrophil is activated as the cell is stimulated (e.g., during phagocytosis). The lag period between stimulus exposure and expression of NADPH oxidase activity varies from 10 or 20 seconds to 1 or 2 minutes, depending on the stimulus. It appears that the lag time reflects the period required for assembly of the multiple components of the oxidase at the cytoplasmic face of the plasma membrane or phagocytic vacuole membrane. On the basis of studies in both intact neutrophils and in vitro cell-free systems, the components of the NADPH oxidase comprise integral membrane proteins as well as soluble cytosolic proteins[111, 113] (Fig. 8–6).

Within the membrane is cytochrome-b_{558}, so designated because of a characteristic 558-nm peak in its redox difference spectrum.[114–122] It is a heterodimer composed of large and small subunits, gp91*phox* and p22*phox* (*phox* stands for *ph*agocyte *ox*idase), respectively, which are firmly but noncovalently associated. This protein has two different types of redox centers, a flavin adenine dinucleotide (FAD) domain and two (or possibly more) heme prosthetic groups.[123–125] There is evidence that cytochrome-b_{558} is the sole catalytic subunit of the oxidase, although this is not yet unequivocally established. According to this view the substrate, NADPH, binds to a domain within the flavoprotein portion of the molecule and is oxidized by the transfer of two electrons to FAD. Then follow two single-electron reductions of the heme groups ($Fe^{3+} \rightarrow Fe^{2+}$). The very low midpoint potential of the reduced hemes allows them to react directly with molecular oxygen, reoxidizing the iron moieties and forming two molecules of superoxide, $O_2^{\cdot-}$.

Although cytochrome-b_{558} appears to mediate the catalytic functions of the respiratory burst oxidase, other proteins are required for enzyme activation and activity. Two necessary proteins, p47*phox* and p67*phox*, are present in neutrophil cytosol,[126–130] existing, at least in part, as a complex with one another.[111, 112, 131] The primary structure of p47*phox* includes a very cationic carboxyl-terminal domain containing several serine residues that serve as substrates for phosphorylation by several kinases including protein kinase C (PKC) or related enzymes.[129] In the stimulated neutrophil, some sites on p47*phox*

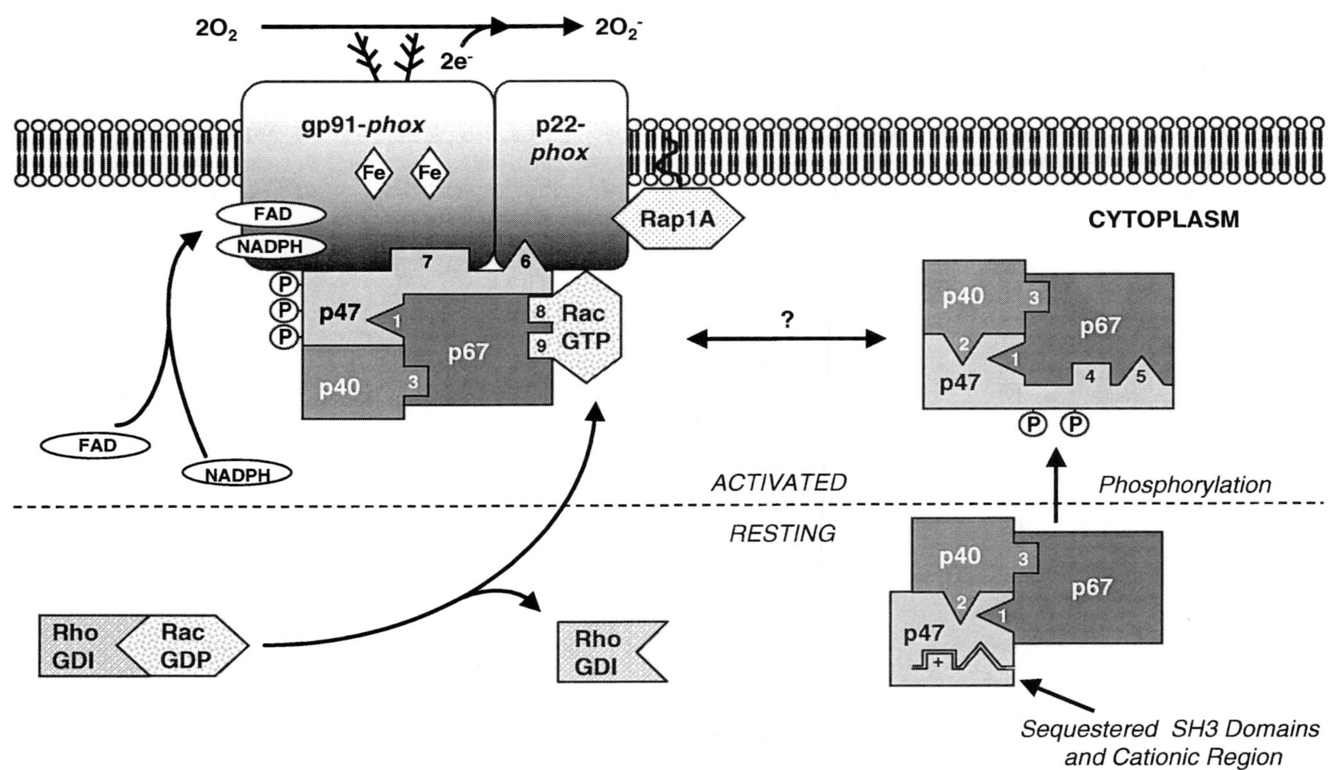

FIGURE 8–6. Model of the agonist-dependent assembly of the neutrophil respiratory burst oxidase. Numbers 1–7 represent associations mediated by interactions between SH3 domains and proline-rich regions *(triangular shapes)* or by other protein-protein binding motifs *(square shapes).* (Modified from DeLeo FR, Quinn MT. Assembly of the phagocyte NADPH oxidase: Molecular interactions of oxidase proteins. J Leukoc Biol. 1996; 60:677–691.)

are phosphorylated and the partially phosphorylated protein then translocates to the plasma membrane, where additional sites are phosphorylated.[132–136] There is also evidence for phosphorylation-independent determinants of p47*phox* translocation.[137]

The functioning oxidase assembles at the plasma membrane, and cytochrome-b_{558} appears to be the membrane docking site for p47*phox*.[113] Specific sites of gp91*phox* and p22*phox* have been implicated as mediating interactions with the cytosolic components.[138–141] Neutrophil stimulation also results in membrane translocation of p67*phox*, probably as a result of its association with p47*phox*; p67*phox* fails to translocate in the absence of p47*phox*, although p47*phox* is competent for translocation by itself.[135]

Both p47*phox* and p67*phox* contain two copies of a 50-amino-acid domain related to a region of the SRC oncoprotein designated SH3 (*src* homology region 3).[128, 130] Proline-rich motifs similar to those that bind to SH3 domains in other proteins[142, 143] are present in p47*phox*, p67*phox*, and p22*phox*. In general, SH3 domains are thought to mediate binding to cytoskeletal and membrane elements. Both SH3 and proline-rich segments of the oxidase proteins are involved in the protein-protein interactions required for oxidase activation and function.[144, 145] The net effect of phosphorylation and translocation of cytosolic components is the assembly on the membrane of the active oxidase complex, composed of the cytochrome-b_{558} subunits, p47*phox*, p67*phox*, and perhaps other constituents including RAC2 and p40*phox*.

In cell-free model systems, requirements for additional proteins have been demonstrated. In keeping with the enhancement of oxidase activation in these systems by guanoside triphosphate (GTP) or nonhydrolyzable GTP analogues,[99, 115, 116] the low-molecular-weight GTP-binding proteins RAC1 or RAC2, depending on species and type of phagocytic cell,[146–152] have been implicated as essential elements of the oxidase. The RAC proteins are isolated together with another protein, *rho*GDI (the guanoside diphosphatase dissociation inhibitor of p21*rho*), which may also be involved in the oxidase system. Modification of the carboxyl terminus of *RAC* by isoprenylation with a 20-carbon (geranylgeranyl) fatty acid and carboxymethylation promotes association with *rho*GDI and with membranes and is required for optimal activity.[153, 154] During neutrophil stimulation, RAC translocates to the plasma membrane but in a fashion independent of the redistribution of p47*phox* and p67*phox*.[155–157] Another small GTP-binding protein, RAP1A, is closely associated with cytochrome-b_{558}, but whether it is involved in NADPH oxidase assembly or function is unknown.[158–160] An additional oxidase-related cytosolic protein, p40*phox*, exhibits homology to p47*phox*,[161–163] including the presence of an SH3 domain, and may serve as a negative regulator of enzyme activation.[164]

The active respiratory burst oxidase is topographically oriented in the membrane to promote the delivery of toxic products of oxygen reduction to the ingested microorganism. The binding site for NADPH is on the cytoplasmic face of the membrane, whereas the reaction product superoxide is formed at the vacuolar side. Oxidase activation on the external plasma membrane results in extracellular release of superoxide, a process important in the oxidative attack on attached but uningested organisms (e.g., protozoa) and on adjacent host cells. Despite indirect evidence that reactive products of the oxidase inactivate the enzyme,[165] the precise mechanisms by which oxidase activity is regulated and terminated are unknown.

Degranulation. In parallel with activation of the oxidative burst, stimulated neutrophils undergo exocytosis and release their granule contents.[166] This process is remarkably selective in its regulation of distinct granule subpopulations for fusion with different membranes. For example, fusion of granule membranes with the phagosome, with subsequent exocytosis into the phagolysosome, involves different fusogenic proteins and different granule populations than does extracellular release of granule contents.[166] Most extensively studied have been the differential calcium requirements for exocytosis of neutrophil granules.[167, 168] In addition, the release of given granule populations depends on the specific stimulus and the particular opsonin used.[169]

Stimulated exocytosis requires cytoskeletal rearrangement[170, 171] with redistribution of actin-binding proteins such as myristoylated alanine-rich C-kinase substrates (MARCKS).[172, 173] Fusogenic proteins on the granules, including annexins,[174] syntaxin 4, vesicle-associated membrane protein-2 (VAMP-2), and other cytosolic soluble *N*-ethylmaleimide-sensitive attachment proteins (SNAPs),[175, 176] mediate association at the target membranes with specific receptors, including various target SNAP receptors (t-SNAREs).[176, 177] Lipid modification probably contributes critically to fusion of the granule membrane with the plasma or phagosomal membrane, and such remodeling depends on the redistribution and activation of cytosolic phospholipases.[178, 179] The intraphagosomal pH must be modified for optimal activation of some of the granule contents. To that end, activation recruits to the phagosomal membrane Na^+/H^+ exchangers, Na^+,K^+-ATPases, and vacuolar-type proton ATPases from membrane-bound granule intracellularly.[180, 181]

As discussed previously, the granules of neutrophils differ not only in the luminal contents but also in the proteins inserted in their membranes. Azurophilic granules fuse predominantly with the phagosome, thereby delivering to the ingested organism microbicidal and hydrolytic proteins at high concentration. On the other hand, specific granules and secretory vesicles fuse preferentially with the plasma membrane, releasing contents extracellularly and bringing to the cell surface a variety of functionally important membrane proteins, including integrins, cytochrome-b_{558}, and receptors for chemotactic agents and opsonins. Taken together, the process of degranulation affords concurrent recruitment of critical membrane proteins (e.g., cytochrome-b_{558}) to the cell surface, release of essential elements of the oxygen-dependent microbicidal system (e.g., MPO), and discharge of proteins that possess direct antimicrobial activity (e.g., defensins, BPI).

Signal Transduction

Exposure of the neutrophil to various stimuli is linked to functional responses through receptor-dependent generation of intracellular second messengers.[182] Binding of a specific ligand to a receptor on the neutrophil surface initiates a cascade of reactions at the membrane level and in the cytoplasm. A key initial feature is the activation of a phospholipase that cleaves specific membrane phospholipids to generate active products. Phospholipase C is a prototype in neutrophils and a wide variety of other cells. The link between an occupied receptor and the phospholipase is provided by a G protein. Dissociation of the active γ-subunit, the GTP-binding component, leads to activation of the phospholipase. In the case of phospholipase Cγ, phosphatidylinositol 4,5-bisphosphate is then cleaved to form inositol 1,4,5-trisphosphate (IP_3) and diacylglycerol (DAG).[183] The water-soluble IP_3 diffuses into the cytoplasm, where it binds to high-affinity receptors in the membranes of intracellular Ca^{2+} storage organelles. The IP_3 receptor functions as a ligand-gated Ca^{2+} channel, permitting rapid release into the cytosol of a large amount of Ca^{2+} from high-capacity, low-affinity Ca^{2+} storage proteins.[184] The resulting initial spike in cytoplasmic Ca^{2+} concentration is then supplemented by an influx of Ca^{2+} through plasma membrane channels. These channels appear to be opened by a signal generated via emptying of the intracellular Ca^{2+} stores or possibly by products of IP_3 metabolism, including 1,3,4,5-tetraphosphate (IP_4).[185] In any case, the net effect is an increase in cytosolic Ca^{2+} from baseline levels of less than 100 nmol/liter to micromolar concentrations.

Ca^{2+} has many targets, including cytoskeletal proteins and a number of enzymatic systems such as the Ca^{2+}-dependent PKC. Also converging at this point is the second product of phospholipase Cγ action, DAG, which remains membrane associated and promotes the membrane translocation and activation of PKC. Thus, both IP_3 and DAG participate in PKC activation. PKC then phosphorylates a variety of regulatory proteins whose functional properties are altered by this covalent modification.

In addition to the phospholipase C pathway, mechanisms of neutrophil signal transduction involving phospholipases D and A_2 appear to be operative under certain conditions.[186, 187] Phospholipase D cleaves phosphatidylcholine to form phosphatidic acid, which may trigger distal activation pathways either directly or via its conversion by a phosphohydrolase enzyme to DAG, which in turn activates PKC. Phospholipase A_2 acts on phospholipids or phosphatidic acid to form lysophospholipds or lysophosphatidic acid, respectively, plus free arachidonic acid. Both the lyso compounds and arachidonate may go on to signal cellular activation.

Studies have examined the role of tyrosine phosphorylation and involvement of the mitogen-activated protein kinase pathways in neutrophil activation.[188, 189] Data implicate direct or indirect tyrosine phosphorylation–dependent events in a wide variety of neutrophil responses, including microbicidal activity,[190] adherence,[191] spreading,[192] β_2-integrin activation,[193] phagocytosis,[194] immune complex[195] or GM-CSF[196] activation, stimulation of the oxidase,[197] acute changes in cell volume,[198] and interactions between neutrophils and endothelium.[199] Understanding how various signaling pathways are integrated into the precise and regulated responses of activated neutrophils will provide important insights into new therapeutic interventions to modulate clinical inflammatory diseases.

Priming of Neutrophil Responses

Concentrations of mediators that are too low to stimulate neutrophils directly nevertheless prepare the cell for an enhanced response to a second, unrelated stimulus, in a phenomenon known as *priming*.[200] A broad array of inflammatory mediators, including chemotactic factors, endotoxin, cytokines, and certain lipids, can prime the neutrophil, and the primed state exists with respect to each of the major aspects of neutrophil function. This state of enhanced responsiveness persists for an extended period (longer than 20 minutes) in relation to the response elicited by direct stimulation of the cell, and it is reversible. Although the molecular basis for priming of neutrophils is not understood, one study of the effects of endotoxin on neutrophil oxidase activity suggests that partial assembly of the oxidase at the plasma membrane may be responsible in part for the altered activation state of the cell.[201]

Microbicidal Mechanisms

As described previously, the postphagocytic events deliver the products of degranulation and the respiratory burst to the phagocytic vacuole, a closed space in which an ingested microbe is exposed to high concentrations of toxic substances while the exposure of the phagocyte and other cells to these potentially injurious agents is limited (see Fig. 8–5).

Oxygen-dependent bactericidal mechanisms can be divided into MPO-dependent and MPO-independent reactions. The essential requirements for the MPO-mediated bactericidal mechanisms, as first described by Klebanoff, are MPO (released from the primary granule), hydrogen peroxide (generated by the respiratory burst), and a halide ion. In addition, the low pH present in the phagocytic vacuole enhances MPO activity. Hydrogen peroxide by itself has bactericidal properties, but in the presence of MPO the potency of this system for bacteria is enhanced 50-fold. The halide used in the MPO–hydrogen peroxide reaction also affects potency, the effect of iodide being greater than that of bromide, which is greater than that of chloride. However, on the basis of concentration, chloride appears to be the physiologic cofactor for this reaction in the cell.[202]

Hypochlorous acid, formed by the neutrophil when chloride is the relevant halide, is a potent oxidizing and microbicidal agent.[203, 204] Other agents, including chlorine gas, chlorinated sterols, tyrosyl radicals, and nitric oxide–derived reactants, are generated by neutrophils in an MPO-dependent fashion.[205–209] The precise event responsible for the microbicidal activity of this system is incompletely characterized. Candidate sites in bacteria include components of the electron transport chain, iron-sulfur centers, penicillin-binding proteins, and sites in bacterial membranes that are necessary for initiation of chromosomal replication.[210–215] Oxidation of some of these molecules may lead to the release of free iron, which can then participate in the formation of the highly reactive hydroxyl radical.[216] In addition to these effects, the MPO–hydrogen peroxide–halide system promotes the formation of singlet oxygen, decarboxylation of amino acids to form toxic aldehydes, and generation of chloramines,[217] agents that may contribute to neutrophil microbicidal activity.[218] Studies have implicated the MPO–hydrogen peroxide–halide system in the oxidation of lipids and possibly in atherogenesis, extending the biologic importance of this system beyond its microbicidal activity.[219–221]

Metabolites of oxygen for which a role in neutrophil bactericidal activity has been suggested include hydrogen peroxide, superoxide, singlet oxygen, and hydroxyl radical. The facts that catalase, which destroys hydrogen peroxide, protects bacteria from the bactericidal effects of neutrophils[222] and that the bactericidal activity of MPO-deficient neutrophils remains high are strong pieces of evidence supporting a direct germicidal effect of hydrogen peroxide. Superoxide, by itself, is thought to play little role in the killing of microorganisms, because bacteria incubated in a cell-free, superoxide-generating system survive normally. However, under appropriate conditions superoxide can react with other products of oxygen to generate hydroxyl radical and singlet oxygen. The bactericidal effect of these oxygen-derived free radicals may result from the initiation of a chain of oxidizing events in the bacterial cell wall.[218] Hydroxyl radical is a potent bactericidal agent that can be formed by the direct reaction of superoxide with hydrogen peroxide, a reaction that occurs too slowly to be of biologic importance but can be catalyzed by ferric salts.[223]

Sensitive analytical systems indicate that activated neutrophils can produce hydroxyl radical by two different mechanisms. One of these mechanisms depends on the catalytic activity of MPO,[224] and the other requires participation of transition metals in the Haber-Weiss reaction.[225] The relative contribution of each mechanism to the overall production of hydroxyl radical in vivo depends on the availability of exogenous transition metals, usually iron. In the presence of supplemental iron, hydroxyl radical generation occurs through the Haber-Weiss reaction. However, in vivo lactoferrin and transferrin bind iron in a form that cannot catalyze this reaction. Therefore, under most physiologic conditions, the small amount of hydroxyl radical generated by stimulated neutrophils is derived from the MPO-dependent pathway.

Underemphasized in the past has been the importance of oxygen-independent antimicrobial systems in overall innate immunity and neutrophil-dependent host defense.[226, 227] The importance of these mechanisms in neutrophils is clearly demonstrated by the ability of these cells to kill some organisms under anaerobic conditions.[228] Substances contributing to oxygen-independent microbicidal activity include acid, defensins, BPI, lactoferrin, lysozyme, and a variety of cationic proteins. In human neutrophils, the pH in the phagosome decreases to about 6.0.[229] Although pneumococci are readily killed by the effect of acid alone, most bacteria are little affected by the acid environment. The main effect of the low pH in the phagocytic vacuole is to potentiate the microbicidal and degradative activity of the granule enzymes.

Defensins are potent antimicrobial peptides in the primary granules of neutrophils[230, 231] and in epithelial cells of the gut and the genitourinary tract.[232–234] Defensins and closely related proteins are widely distributed in nature (e.g., the hemolymph of insects[235]) and probably represent an ancient mechanism for host defense. In general, defensins are small (3 to 4 kD), are rich in arginine, and contain a characteristic disulfide motif. Elegant studies have defined many of the physical properties of purified defensins[236–238] and may provide insight into their mechanism of action. The spectrum of organisms against which defensins are active is extremely broad and includes gram-positive and gram-negative bacteria, fungi, and enveloped viruses.

BPI is a 59-kD protein located in the primary granule of neutrophils. Its antimicrobial activity resides in a 25-kD amino-terminal fragment.[239–240] In addition, BPI binds to lipopolysaccharide[241] and blocks the release of TNF elicited by bacteria,[242] properties that portend a potential clinical use of recombinant BPI, or a fragment thereof, in the treatment or prevention of lipopolysaccharide-dependent sequelae of acute bacterial infection. Clinical trials with recombinant amino-terminal BPI have demonstrated efficacy in ameliorating morbidity and mortality in disseminated meningococcal disease in children.[243]

Lactoferrin is an iron-binding protein found in secretions bathing mucosal membranes and in the specific granules of neutrophils.[244] The bacteriostatic effect of lactoferrin reflects its ability to deprive bacteria of the iron required for growth, an effect eliminated by saturation of both iron-binding sites.[244] Lactoferrin plays a role in the alteration of the physicochemical properties of the neutrophil membrane that occurs during degranulation,[245] in the modulation of hydroxyl radical production,[223] in the regulation of granulopoiesis,[246] and in the modulation of complement function.[247]

Lysozyme, found mainly in the specific granules but also present in the primary granules, hydrolyzes the glycoside bond between *N*-acetylmuramic acid and *N*-acetylglucosamine, a component of the peptidoglycan in bacterial cell walls. Although the bactericidal properties of lysozyme reflect this activity, peptide substitutions on the *N*-acetylmuramic acid residue in most bacteria make this bond inaccessible to lysozyme, thereby limiting its bacteriolytic properties. However, in the context of the complex environment of an inflammatory reaction, a bacterial cell wall already damaged by complement or granule proteins may allow access of lysozyme to its site of action.

Additional cationic proteins isolated from neutrophil primary granules[226, 239] demonstrate preferential activity against specific bacterial species. These proteins include a 37-kD cationic antimicrobial protein, the activity of which is favored by the intraphagosomal acid pH[248, 249]; p15s[250]; azuricidin[251]; indolicin[252]; and cathelicidins.[253] Understanding of the principles of antimicrobial activity of these proteins is incomplete at this time. In some cases it involves temperature-independent binding to the organism via ionic interactions followed by temperature-dependent insertion into the outer membrane via hydrophobic interactions.[239] These sequential events result in increased permeability of the bacterial outer membrane and the subsequent death of the organism.

Microbial Defenses against Phagocytes

Ongoing investigation in microbial pathogenesis reflects the scientific advances in molecular microbiology and eukaryotic cell biology. It is clear that pathogens have evolved molecular strategies for neutralizing one or more of the discrete steps in normal host defense.[254, 255] To that end, the invading microorganism may exploit aspects of normal mammalian cell biology, including adhesive properties, signal transduction pathways, cytoskeletal rearrangements, and vacuolar trafficking. In some cases these properties are manifest only when microbes are in the appropriate host, demonstrating the exquisitely precise manner in which the invading microorganism has adapted to the context of the mammalian host.[256, 257]

In some cases bacteria adhere to surface proteins on target phagocytes, as with certain *Neisseria* and CD66 on the neutrophil surface.[258] In other situations, bacterial proteins secreted into target cells may modify the host cell response, as is the case with the Yop proteins of *Yersinia*. Once secreted into the host cell, the various members of the Yop family of proteins impair phagocytosis, induce apoptosis, paralyze cellular actin, and, in the case of the tyrosine phosphatase YopH, block Fc receptor–mediated activation of the respiratory burst oxidase.[259–261] In other settings, multiple mammalian cell types are targeted. For example, a glycoprotein of Ebola virus, in its secreted form, engages the neutrophil Fc receptor and inhibits cell activation and, in its transmembrane form, interacts with endothelial cells. In this way the virus simultaneously inhibits the neutrophil-dependent early inflammatory response and induces endothelial cell damage, the clinical hallmark of Ebola virus infection.[262]

Even within the phagocyte microbes have devised ways to subvert or avoid host defenses and survive. For example, within mononuclear phagocytes, mycobacteria block the fusion of lysosomes with phagosomes and inhibit recruitment of the endosomal vacuolar proton ATPase that mediates phagosomal acidification.[263] The aberrant compartmentalization of mycobacteria depends on the viability of the organism,[264] assigning the organism an active role in the subversion of fusion, and results in the avoidance by the organism of the microbicidal and hydrolytic contents of the phagocyte's lysosomes. In an analogous fashion, *Chlamydia* remain in an intracellular vacuole dissociated from the endosomal pathway of the host cell.[265] On the other hand, in the case of intraphagocytic *Leishmania* species, the phagosomes acquire markers from the lysosomal compartment and the intraphagolysosomal pH is appropriately acidic, although organisms survive.[266, 267] Other organisms escape the vacuole and invade the cytoplasm of the host cell, targeting a variety of host proteins or organellar systems.[268] Even with the limited details available, it is clear that there is as broad a range of microbial tactics for pathogenesis as there are host cell targets.

DEFECTS IN NEUTROPHIL FUNCTION

Defects in neutrophil function can result from decreased numbers of mature neutrophils or abnormalities in chemotaxis, ingestion, or bactericidal mechanisms.[269] Table 8–2 summarizes these defects. Infections resulting from quantitative or qualitative defects in neutrophil function share a tendency to be prolonged, to respond slowly to antibiotics, and to be recurrent. Staphylococci, gram-negative organisms, and fungi are the usual organisms responsible for these infections. Patients with defective serum opsonic activity frequently are infected by encapsulated bacteria.

Qualitative defects may be intrinsic or extrinsic to the neutrophil. In general, the intrinsic defects of qualitative neutrophil function are more severe than are the extrinsic defects. Chemotactic defects are frequently expressed as cutaneous infections with associated adenitis. Unlike quantitative defects or defects in phagocytosis or intracellular killing, they rarely result in bacteremia or metastatic spread of infection. This is probably because, although neutrophil accumulation is delayed, phagocytosis and bactericidal activity often proceed normally once neutrophils encounter the microorganism.

TABLE 8–2 Defects in Neutrophil Function

- Neutropenia
  - Acquired
    - Drug-induced
    - Autoimmune
    - Cancer-related
  - Hereditary
    - Infantile genetic agranulocytosis
    - Familial neutropenia
    - Cyclic neutropenia
- Qualitative defects
  - Adhesion defects
    - Leukocyte adhesion deficiency
      - Type 1, integrin deficiency
      - Type 2, E-selectin ligand deficiency
  - Chemotactic defects
    - Humoral
      - Complement deficiency
      - Inhibitors
      - Immune complexes
      - Hyperimmunoglobulinemia E (Job's) syndrome
    - Cellular
      - Chédiak-Higashi syndrome
      - Hypophosphatemia
      - Lazy leukocyte syndrome
  - Opsonic defects
    - Complement deficiency
    - Antibody deficiency
  - Defects in intracellular killing
    - Abnormal respiratory burst
      - Chronic granulomatous disease
      - Glucose-6-phosphate dehydrogenase deficiency
    - Granule abnormalities
      - Myeloperoxidase deficiency
      - Specific granule deficiency
      - Chédiak-Higashi syndrome

Neutropenia

The most common granulocyte defect encountered is the absolute reduction of circulating neutrophils. The lower limit of normal for circulating neutrophils is 1500 to 2000 cells/mm^3. The risk of acquiring an infection increases progressively with both the duration and the magnitude of the granulocytopenia below 1500 cells/mm^3. Below 500 cells/mm^3, there is a dramatic increase in the incidence of infection.[270]

The acquired neutropenias are most often related to drug therapy and may be a predictable result of therapy or an idiosyncratic reaction. The former are frequently encountered during chemotherapy for various neoplastic and immunologic disorders. Neutropenia caused by an idiosyncratic drug reaction is observed with phenothiazines, sulfonamides, penicillins, cephalosporins, and vancomycin. Chloramphenicol can cause both a predictable and an idiosyncratic neutropenia. The latter is rare, but when it occurs is frequently fatal. Increased granulocyte destruction may occur as a result of splenic sequestration, which may be immunologically mediated by antibody[271] or secondary to any of the causes of hypersplenism. Splenectomy may be beneficial in restoring neutrophil counts toward normal.

The availability of recombinant CSF has afforded clinicians a therapeutic option for treatment of acquired cytopenias.[4, 270] Most clinical experience has been with G-CSF and GM-CSF, primarily for treatment of the granulocytopenia associated with cancer chemotherapy and bone marrow transplantation. These agents have been used to stimulate hematopoiesis in myelodysplastic syndromes, aplastic anemia, and cytopenias resulting from chemotherapy. Likewise, GM-CSF has been used to overcome HIV-mediated leukopenias[272] and, in some cases, to permit use of myelosuppressive antiviral agents. Not only is the number of circulating cells increased, but the biologic function and bactericidal activity of the recruited cells are normal.[273] However, current data do not support the use of these agents as an adjunct to antibiotics in infected patients with normal neutrophil production.

Hereditary neutropenia is observed either as a solitary defect or in association with other defects. The neutropenia can be severe as in infantile genetic agranulocytosis, moderate as in familial (benign) neutropenia, or cyclic. Infantile genetic agranulocytosis (Kostmann's syndrome) is an autosomal recessive disorder characterized by granulocyte maturation arrest and severe infection with death in infancy. Progenitor cells from some patients with Kostmann's syndrome are hyporesponsive to G-CSF and, in some cases, have a somatic point mutation in the gene encoding the G-CSF receptor.[274, 275] Some hereditary neutropenias are accompanied by an apparent compensatory monocytosis. Cyclic neutropenia is a rare autosomal dominant defect of myelopoiesis that is characterized by the periodic disappearance of neutrophils and other blood elements from the circulation. Early granulocyte precursors are present in the marrow during the neutropenia, which suggests a transient maturation arrest. The duration of neutropenia ranges from 5 to 8 days, followed by a 2- to 5-week period with normal numbers of circulating neutrophils. In a given patient, the periodic oscillations are highly predictable. During the neutropenic state, the patient experiences aphthous stomatitis, fever, malaise, and cutaneous infections. The disease is usually recognized during childhood, and there is no amelioration with age. Treatment with either recombinant G-CSF[276] or alternate-day prednisolone[277] attenuates the oscillations in neutrophil maturation.

Leukocyte Adhesion Deficiency Syndromes

The hallmark of the leukocyte adhesion deficiency (LAD) syndromes is severe, prolonged, and recurrent infection in the face of a marked granulocytosis. Cell counts are often 2 to 20 times higher than normal even in the absence of infection. Despite this impressive granulocytosis, pus formation (the accumulation of neutrophils in tissues) is poor, and patients develop "cold" abscesses. This abnormality reflects impaired adhesion of affected cells within the vasculature and their inability to emigrate into the tissue. Two types of LAD have been described: LAD-1,[278] in which integrin expression is abnormal, and LAD-2,[279] in which expression of the primary selectin ligand sLe^x on granulocytes is essentially absent (see Fig. 8–3). In vivo, cells from persons with type 1 deficiency display normal rolling adhesion but are unable to adhere firmly to the venule walls or to emigrate from the vasculature.[280] In contrast, cells from those with type 2 deficiency fail to adhere to stimulated venules exposed to normal shear forces, and they do not exhibit rolling adhesion. Because integrin function is intact, these cells can adhere to the vessel wall and can emigrate into the tissues if shear forces are absent.

LAD-1 results from mutations in the gene encoding the β_2-integrin subunit CD18 and is inherited in an autosomal recessive manner. There is frequently a history of consanguinity, and both severe and moderate phenotypes are recognized. Patients with this syndrome typically present with prolonged and/or recurrent staphylococcal and *Pseudomonas* infections beginning in infancy, often in the perinatal period. Patients with the severe phenotype exhibit poor wound healing. As a consequence, they often have delayed separation of the umbilical cord and may develop omphalitis. Infections involving the soft tissues, mucosal surfaces, and the intestinal tract are common. Cutaneous infections frequently become necrotic. Initially these lesions may resemble ecthyma gangrenosum, whereas later they may assume a pyoderma gangrenosum appearance. Affected persons who survive infancy universally develop acute gingivitis with eruption of primary dentition. The gingivitis persists and results in progressive gingival hypertrophy and alveolar bone loss. Although survival into adulthood is well described, particularly in patients with the moderate phenotype, 41% of affected individuals die before the age of 2 years.[278, 281]

Evaluation of neutrophil function demonstrates impaired adherence to artificial substrates, impaired chemotaxis in vivo and in vitro, and impaired respiratory burst in response to the ingestion of particles coated with iC3b but not IgG.[269, 278] Affected neutrophils exhibit an above- or below-normal burst in oxidative metabolism after stimulation with soluble stimuli, depending on which stimulus is used and the nature of the association between its receptor and the cytoskeleton.[282]

Leukocytes from patients with the severe phenotypic expression of LAD-1 bear less than 0.3% of the normal quantity of all three β_2 integrins, whereas moderately affected patients have 2.5 to 6% of the integrin expression of healthy people.[281] In affected individuals, the surface expression of both the α- and β-chains is abnormal. However, the α-chain is present in normal amounts within the cell. The predominant basis for this syndrome is abnormal β-chain synthesis and the requirement for intracellular assembly of the αβ-heterodimer for transport of the molecular complex to the cell surface.[283] Molecular analysis has demonstrated a spectrum of β-gene mutations that cause abnormalities ranging from failure to produce mRNA in some persons with the severe disease phenotype, to production of an abnormally sized precursor β-protein, to absence of any readily apparent defect.[284]

LAD-2 is an autosomal recessive disorder that has been described in two unrelated Arab families. In addition to the infectious complications seen in patients with LAD-1, these persons have a distinct facial appearance, short stature, microcephaly, mental retardation,[279] and the rare Bombay blood phenotype (hh). They develop recurrent bacterial infections, primarily pneumonia, beginning early in life. Periodontal infections, otitis media, and focal cellulitis have also been reported, but infection caused by a predominant organism has not been striking.[285] The two patients described with LAD-2 lack fucosylated glycoconjugates, and their underlying defect appears to be defective GDP-fucose biosynthesis.[286] Despite the generalized nature of the defect, endothelial cells from LAD-2 patients support neutrophil rolling in vitro, demonstrating that the fucose is not essential for function of L-selectin ligands on vascular endothelium.[286]

In vivo assessment of neutrophil function reveals a marked impairment of both random motility and directed migration. Oxidative response to a particulate stimulus is within the normal range, although lower than that from simultaneously evaluated normal cells. Phorbol myristate acetate, a soluble stimulus, also evokes a normal although somewhat greater than average oxidative response from these cells. Lymphocyte number, subset distribution, and mitogenic responses are normal, as is natural killer cell activity.[279]

Chemotactic Defects

Extrinsic Abnormalities

Neutrophil chemotactic defects resulting from extrinsic factors may be caused by abnormalities involving the complement cascade. These include genetic deficiencies (C3, C5) and decreased synthesis (cirrhosis, kwashiorkor, premature birth), hypercatabolism, and increased loss (severe burns) of serum proteins. Some investigators have noted a depression in neutrophil chemotactic responses in patients with diabetes mellitus that is independent of serum osmolality. The defect is mild and is most readily demonstrated in juvenile-onset diabetics. Chemotactic responsiveness of diabetic neutrophils can be restored in vitro by incubation with insulin.[287]

Chemotactic inhibitors may express their effect directly or indirectly by neutralizing the chemotactic effect of complement. Polymeric IgA is cytophilic for neutrophils and can markedly depress chemotaxis.[288] Defective chemotaxis has been described in a number of diseases characterized by circulating immune complexes, including rheumatoid arthritis, systemic lupus erythematosus, and subacute bacterial endocarditis. The sera from about 40% of patients with systemic lupus erythematosus contain an inhibitor that is specific for C5-derived chemotactic activity but does not interfere with the expression of other C5-mediated functions. Its presence correlates with disease activity and the resultant chemotactic defect with the enhanced susceptibility of these patients to infection.[289] The inhibitor has been identified as the Bb fragment of complement factor B, and it exerts its effect by inhibiting the interaction of C5a des Arg with cochemotaxin in serum.[290]

A chemotactic defect has been described in patients with juvenile periodontitis, a familial disorder characterized by periodontitis occurring in the absence of severe dental disease. Serum from some of these patients contains an inhibitor of chemotaxis, and the resultant defect in chemotaxis has been postulated to play a role in the pathogenesis of this disease.[291] In addition, neutrophils from some of these patients bear fewer chemotactic receptors than do cells from unaffected persons, and an apparent structural abnormality of certain isoforms of the formyl peptide chemoattractant receptor has been reported.[292, 293] Of particular note in this regard is the report of an acquired neutrophil chemotactic defect in two adults with gingival infection caused by *Capnocytophaga* (*Bacteroides ochraceus*). Eradication of infection resulted in a return to normal of neutrophil function. Sonicates of *Capnocytophaga* and filtrates of broth in which the organism had been grown inhibited the chemotactic response of normal neutrophils. These findings suggest that the chemotactic defect associated with some forms of periodontal disease may be caused by the presence of bacterial products in the circulation.[294]

Chemotactic inhibitors whose mode of action appears to be the inactivation of chemotactic substances have been described in Hodgkin's disease, sarcoidosis, leprosy, and cirrhosis. These inhibitors are usually present in low concentration in normal serum and affect chemotaxis only when present in high concentrations. Recurrent skin infections and abnormal neutrophil chemotaxis have also been associated with an IgG antineutrophil antibody.[295]

Intrinsic Abnormalities

Chédiak-Higashi Syndrome. Chédiak-Higashi syndrome (CHS) is a rare autosomal recessive trait caused by mutations of the *LYST* gene at chromosome 1q42-43.[296] The disease affects lysosomes in melanocytes, Schwann cells, renal tubular cells, thyroid cells, and all types of leukocytes (Fig. 8–7). The giant and dysmorphic lysosomes account for the physical findings of partial oculocutaneous albinism, rotatory nystagmus, peripheral neuropathy, and recurrent infections. Laboratory abnormalities include anemia, leukopenia, thrombocytopenia, and evidence of intramedullary destruction of blood elements with secondary elevations in serum lysozyme and deficiencies in iron and folate concentrations. In some patients there is an unpredictable transformation of the disease to a lymphoma-like accelerated phase with associated hepatosplenomegaly, lymphadenopathy, and lymphocytic infiltration of organs. Both T-cell– and natural killer cell–mediated cytotoxicity are depressed, and studies have identified defective MHC class II peptide loading and antigen presentation in cells derived from patients with this CHS.[297]

Neutrophils from patients with the CHS exhibit a defective chemotactic response[298] and, although ingestion occurs normally, many bacteria exhibit prolonged intracellular survival. Bacterial killing rates are most abnormal during the first 20 minutes of contact in vitro but approach normal levels at 2 hours, reflecting the delayed release of lysosomal enzymes within phagocytic vacuoles. Because the metabolic burst is normal,[299] the intracellular killing defect appears to result primarily from delayed degranulation into the phagosome.

Although infections are common in patients with this syndrome, significant morbidity also results from the progressive peripheral neuropathy caused by axonal dysfunction.[300] The primary cellular defect in CHS is the function of a lysosomal trafficking regulator, the product of the *LYST* gene,[301, 302] which is essential for normal vesicle sorting in the endosomal pathway.

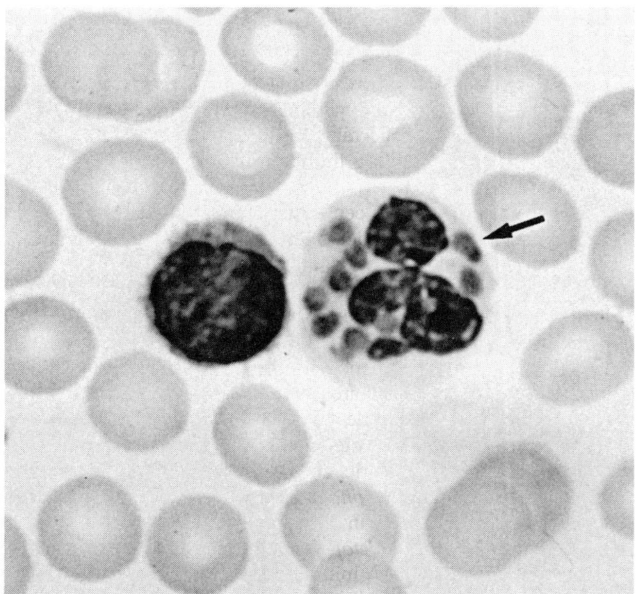

FIGURE 8–7. Neutrophil and lymphocyte from a patient with Chédiak-Higashi syndrome. Note the large abnormal granules *(arrow).*

Current management of patients with CHS is limited to prophylactic use of antibiotics such as trimethoprim-sulfamethoxazole and supportive care. Bone marrow transplantation is effective therapy for the chronic progressive symptoms and the accelerated phase of the disease but has no impact on the peripheral neuropathy.[303]

Hyperimmunoglobulinemia E with Impaired Chemotaxis (Job's Syndrome). Job's syndrome, as originally described, is an affliction of fair-skinned, red-haired women that is characterized by eczema, recurrent "cold" staphylococcal skin abscesses, sinusitis, and otitis media.[304] However, the disorder also occurs in blacks and in men.[305] Many of the patients have coarse facial features and a broad nasal bridge. In addition to cutaneous staphylococcal infection, recurrent pneumonia and mucocutaneous candidiasis are common. Patients may have mild eosinophilia, and the neutrophils of most patients exhibit a chemotactic abnormality, although this feature is variable. The chemotactic defect appears to correlate best with the severity of the eczema, and patients have been reported in whom a chemotactic defect could be demonstrated only during relapses of their dermatitis. Mononuclear cells from these patients but not from persons with or without atopy spontaneously produce a factor that inhibits the chemotactic responses of normal neutrophils and monocytes.[306] All patients have markedly elevated (more than 10 times normal) serum levels of IgE because of a decreased fractional catabolic rate of this immunoglobulin.[307] Antistaphylococcal and anti-*Candida* IgE antibodies have been demonstrated in sera from patients with Job's syndrome but not from healthy people, patients with hyperimmunoglobulinemia E caused by atopic disease or parasitic infection, or patients with chronic staphylococcal infections. Antistaphylococcal antibody of the IgM class is also elevated in the sera from these patients, whereas specific IgA is low and the IgG level no different from that in healthy people. Infection is inversely related to the concentrations of specific IgE, IgA, and IgM, suggesting that these antibodies normally exert a protective rather than a permissive effect against staphylococci.[308] It therefore appears that Job's syndrome does not represent an intrinsic defect of neutrophil function but rather is the result of aberrant immune regulation.

A well-controlled clinical trial established that levamisole, which had been reported to improve neutrophil function in patients with Job's syndrome, failed to reduce and was actually associated with an increase in the number of infections.[309] Therefore, management should be directed toward early detection of infection, prolonged treatment with antibiotics, and early surgical drainage of "cold" abscesses.[305]

Other Disorders. A mild and variable chemotactic defect has been described in patients with Kartagener's (immotile cilia) syndrome, in which there is an abnormality in the linkage between microtubules and cilia.[310] An acquired but reversible defect in neutrophil function has been documented with severe hypophosphatemia (less than 1 mg/dl) caused by phosphate-free hyperalimentation. The defect in these cells is thought to result from an inability to generate ATP from anaerobic glycolysis.[311]

Abnormal Phagocytosis

Defective opsonization occurs with inherited or acquired deficiencies of the early complement components (especially C3) or immunoglobulin. Similar derangements accompany the paraproteinemias and a number of other neoplastic and non-neoplastic disorders characterized by hypoglobulinemia or hypocomplementemia. Patients with these types of opsonic disorders frequently have recurrent infections with encapsulated bacteria, particularly pneumococci and *Haemophilus influenzae.* Infection with these organisms in the splenectomized person can manifest as fulminant bacteremia or meningitis accompanied by disseminated intravascular coagulation.[312]

In 1968, Miller and colleagues[313] reported that sera from 5 to 7% of the population were defective in opsonizing baker's yeast. A number of these individuals suffered recurrent upper respiratory tract infections, and some had diarrhea with associated failure to thrive. The basis for this defect remained obscure until Turner and coworkers[314] discovered that the concentration of mannan-binding protein (MBP) was low in affected subjects. MBP acts to enhance complement activation and deposition on mannose-rich surfaces.[315, 316] The usual molecular basis for this defect is a point mutation resulting in the replacement in exon 1 of a glycine residue with aspartic acid, a change postulated to interfere with MBP triple helix formation, with consequent retention of the protein and intracellular degradation.[317]

Defects in Intracellular Killing

Impaired neutrophil intracellular microbicidal activity may be a consequence of either an abnormal respiratory burst oxidase or the failure to deliver active granule enzymes. Those diseases in which microbicidal defects have been well characterized represent inherited disorders.[318, 319] Although functional decreases in microbial killing have been described in patients with certain acquired inflammatory, metabolic, and malignant diseases, these observations have been neither widely confirmed nor characterized at a biochemical level.

Abnormal Respiratory Burst

Chronic Granulomatous Disease. Patients with the hereditary disorder known as chronic granulomatous disease (CGD) characteristically experience recurrent and often severe pyogenic infections, a granulomatous tissue response, and impaired phagocyte microbicidal activity due to the absence of respiratory burst oxidase activity.[320–323] Although initially described as an X-linked disorder, with males affected and mothers and sisters serving as heterozygous carriers, CGD can be transmitted with the inheritance pattern of either an autosomal or an X-linked disease, depending on the molecular defect.[323] The remarkable insights into the components and regulation of the NADPH-dependent oxidase made possible by the development of the broken cell assay[324, 325] also provided investigators with a means by which to classify the various forms of CGD (Table 8–3).

The membrane component of the NADPH oxidase is the heterodimeric cytochrome-b_{558}. The gene for the large subunit (gp91*phox*) is located on the X chromosome and is the site of mutation in all patients with X-linked CGD.[115, 326–328] Rarely (in less than 5% of CGD patients), mutations occur in the gene for the small subunit (p22*phox*), which is on chromosome 16. In most cases deletion or frameshift mutations result in a failure to synthesize the affected subunit of the cytochrome. When one subunit is absent neither is inserted into the membrane, and the characteristic heme spectrum featuring a 558-nm peak is not present.[329] In rare kindreds single point mutations result in synthesis of nonfunctional flavocytochrome,[330] especially when defects are present in critical functional domains such as the binding site for NADPH or flavin. Mutations also include alterations in the site on the cytochrome for docking p47*phox*, leaving affected cells unable to assemble a functional oxidase.[331]

In most patients with autosomally inherited CGD, the neutrophils lack the cytosolic oxidase component p47*phox*.[321, 332] Mutations in the p47*phox* gene account for approximately one third of all cases of CGD. Unlike the cytochrome-*b* mutations, which comprise many different lesions, most examples of p47*phox* deficiency[111, 333, 334] are caused by a two-base deletion at an exon splice site that results in a frameshift and early termination of translation. Most of the patients studied to date appear to be homozygous for this deletion, although examples have been described of patients who are compound heterozygotes for this mutation and either a single-base frameshift deletion at another site or missense mutations.[111, 334] The high prevalence of this deletion of guanine and thymine, also present in a homologous pseudogene on chromosome 7, may reflect recombination of normal and pseudogene sequences.[335] Mutations in the gene for p67*phox* are less common, accounting for perhaps 5% of CGD cases.[332] The p67*phox* protein is usually absent, and several specific mutations have been defined.[323, 336] In one kindred, a p67*phox* allele with a triplet nucleotide deletion resulted in an in-frame loss of a lysine residue that was shown in vitro to disrupt p67*phox*-RAC1 binding.[337]

In all thoroughly characterized cases to date, the CGD phenotype is explained by a defect in a gene for one of the four peptide oxidase components—the two cytochrome-*b* subunits and the cytosolic proteins p47*phox* and p67*phox*. These findings underscore the critical roles that each of these proteins plays in oxidase function. Although other components could be involved in oxidase activation or function, and in fact the GTP-binding protein RAC2 is required in cell-free systems, their genetic deficiency as a cause of CGD, if it exists, is rare. In spite of genetic heterogeneity, the biochemical phenotype common to all forms of CGD is the failure of phagocytic cells to generate a respiratory burst in response to any phagocytic or soluble stimulus. Because no oxygen-derived microbicidal agents (e.g., superoxide, hydrogen peroxide, hydroxyl radical, hypochlorous acid) are formed, there is a severe defect in intracellular killing of phagocytized microorganisms. Catalase-negative organisms such as the streptococci are killed normally, because microbial hydrogen peroxide accumulates within the phagocytic vacuole and essentially reconstitutes the defective MPO–hydrogen peroxide–halide system. The preservation of microbicidal activity of CGD cells against catalase-negative microorganisms translates into an absence of major clinical infections caused by these species in patients with CGD.

In general the clinical manifestations of the different genetic forms of CGD are quite similar, notwithstanding some evidence for a more severe course in X-linked compared with autosomally inherited disease. Infectious complications often begin in infancy and recur throughout childhood and adolescence. In those patients who survive into adulthood, there may be a lessening of clinical severity. Occasionally, there is a relatively mild clinical course during childhood, and some patients may not come to medical attention until they are adolescents or even adults.[338, 339] Infections may involve virtually any organ system, but the most common manifestations are suppurative lymphadenitis, subcutaneous abscesses, pneumonia, lung abscess, liver abscess, and osteomyelitis. Stomatitis, blepharitis, and pyogenic

TABLE 8–3 Genetic Types of Chronic Granulomatous Disease (CGD)

Defective Component	Relative Frequency (%)*	Gene Locus	Mutations	Biochemical Features	
				Membranes	Cytosol
gp91*phox*	55–60	Xp21.1	Large deletions, deletion/frameshift, missense	Cytochrome *b* absent in most, but present in missense mutations	Normal
p22*phox*	<5	16q24	Deletion/frameshift missense	Same as for gp91*phox*	Normal
p47*phox*	30–35	7q11.23	Deletion/frameshift missense	Normal	p47*phox* absent
p67*phox*	<5	1q25	Unknown	Normal	p67*phox* absent

*Percent of all CGD patients.[260, 261]

dermatitis frequently are recurring problems. The most characteristic pathogens are *Staphylococcus aureus, Serratia marcescens, Pseudomonas cepacia,* and *Aspergillus* spp., although a wide variety of other catalase-positive bacteria and fungi may cause disease as well. Although one study of morbidity and mortality of a p47*phox* knockout mouse infected with various strains of *Aspergillus nidulans* suggests that the presence of catalase may not represent a significant virulence factor for successful fungal infection of hosts with impaired oxidase function,[340] the observations were predictable, given the failure of *Aspergillus* to generate hydrogen peroxide. The presence of catalase represents a determinant of an organism's virulence in patients with CGD only when the pathogen has the potential to generate hydrogen peroxide. *Serratia marcescens* osteomyelitis is particularly suggestive of the diagnosis of CGD.

Infections can follow an acute course, but more often there is a subacute or chronic progression with poor wound healing, a mixed acute and chronic inflammatory response, and granuloma formation. The basis for the granulomatous inflammation is not clear, but it is thought to relate to the persistence of viable intracellular microorganisms. In certain tissue sites obstructive lesions may develop, as in xanthogranulomatous urinary tract disease[341] or granulomatous bowel involvement that resembles Crohn's disease.[342] Perirectal involvement with fissures or inflammatory masses is a rather common manifestation. The physical examination often shows dermatitis, lymphadenitis, enlargement of liver and spleen, and retardation of normal rates of growth and development. Routine laboratory studies may indicate anemia of inflammation, leukocytosis to a moderate level (generally less than 15,000 to 20,000 cells/mm^3), hyperglobulinemia, and an elevated erythrocyte sedimentation rate. Pathologic examination of infected tissues usually demonstrates inflammatory masses with granulomas that may progress to areas of frank necrosis, sometimes with well-defined abscesses. Lipid-filled histiocytes are found in liver, spleen, lymph nodes, gut, and other tissues of some CGD patients.

The diagnosis of CGD can be made with assays for any of the products of the neutrophil respiratory burst. The most useful method is the nitroblue tetrazolium (NBT) slide test. Neutrophils adherent to a microscope coverslip are stimulated in the presence of NBT, a soluble yellow dye that is reduced by superoxide to formazan, an insoluble precipitate that stains the cells dark blue or black. In normal control subjects, essentially 100% of the neutrophils stain with NBT. In contrast, neutrophils from CGD patients are uniformly NBT negative, whereas female carriers of X-linked CGD exhibit a mixture of NBT-positive and NBT-negative cells owing to the expression of only one of the X chromosomes in any somatic female cell (lyonization). Although the average distribution of the two cell types is 50:50, skewing toward a higher proportion of either defective (CGD) or normal cells occurs. Most female carriers of CGD maintain good health and normal host defenses, but some develop either a cutaneous syndrome similar to discoid lupus or systemic lupus erythematosus.[343] Clinical manifestations in carriers are more likely when lyonization is skewed toward predominantly CGD-like neutrophils.

The management of patients with CGD is based largely on the early recognition and aggressive treatment of infections. Specific microbiologic diagnosis should be established whenever possible and, if necessary, empiric therapy should be directed against the pathogens characteristically encountered in such patients (i.e., *S. aureus*, certain gram-negative bacilli). Surgical incision and drainage are often required, although the surgeon may encounter an inflammatory granulomatous mass rather than a discrete abscess. Obstructive lesions are occasionally responsive to steroids, which when used in a limited fashion do not increase substantially the risk of secondary infection. Because the utility of granulocyte transfusions has not been established, they are not generally recommended, although their use in severe infections unresponsive to standard treatment may be worth considering. Prophylactic use of antimicrobial agents is of well-established benefit in patients with CGD,[344] and trimethoprim-sulfamethoxazole is generally preferred. In patients who experience morbidity from infections despite prophylactic antibiotics, the use of recombinant IFN-γ should be considered. This agent, given in a dose of 50 μg/m^2 three times weekly by the subcutaneous route, reduced by 72% the incidence of serious infections, regardless of the genetic form of the disease and with relatively few side effects. Notwithstanding the reported effects of IFN-γ on oxidative metabolism and microbicidal activity of CGD phagocytes,[345–347] the mechanism of action in patients is not clear.[348] In a rare kindred with a defect in the regulatory domain of the gp91*phox* subunit of cytochrome-b_{558}, the cytokine appears to upregulate gene expression and restore cytochrome synthesis and function to normal,[349] although clearly this is not the mechanism of action in most patients.

Long-term reconstitution of normal phagocyte function in patients with CGD might be achieved by bone marrow transplantation.[350] However, the morbidity and mortality of this mode of treatment are high, and results in a few CGD patients have been variable. Gene transfer may ultimately prove to be the preferred means of definitive treatment. In vitro reconstitution of oxidase function in CGD cells has been achieved in several systems, including peripheral blood CD34$^+$ progenitor cells from subjects with p47*phox* or p67*phox* deficiency.[351, 352] Very promising is the report of studies by Malech in which five patients with p47*phox* deficiency achieved extended, albeit low-level, reconstitution of oxidase function in vivo.[353] Better targeting vectors and specialized conditioning regimens for patients offer the promise of a durable correction of oxidase dysfunction by genetic therapy in the future.[354] The prognosis in CGD patients has improved considerably over the last 20 years, based on increased recognition, aggressive treatment of infections, and prophylactic approaches to preventing infectious complications.

Glucose-6-Phosphate Dehydrogenase Deficiency. Although erythrocyte and leukocyte glucose-6-phosphate dehydrogenase (G6PD) are products of the same gene, the common form of G6PD deficiency that manifests as a hemolytic anemia in African Americans is not associated with neutrophil dysfunction. This discrepancy reflects the fact that this deficiency is caused by an unstable enzyme, the activity of which diminishes over a period that exceeds the life expectancy of the neutrophil. Neutrophil dysfunction does occur in rare cases of G6PD deficiency in whites who are missing or have less than 5% of the normal levels of G6PD. Neutrophil function is abnormal in this disorder because, in the absence of G6PD, glucose cannot be metabolized via the hexose monophosphate shunt and, as a consequence, NADPH cannot be regenerated from NADP to support oxidase activity. Aside from the presence of a hemolytic anemia, the clinical, laboratory, and genetic (X-linked) presentation is very similar to that of CGD. The NBT test is abnormal, as are other parameters of the respiratory burst. The failure of methylene blue to stimulate hexose monophosphate shunt activity and the low level of G6PD distinguish this defect from CGD.[355]

Myeloperoxidase Deficiency

Once thought to be a rare disorder, neutrophil MPO deficiency is now recognized as the most common of all neutrophil functional disorders, with a frequency of 1 per 2000 to 4000 people for whom leukocyte counts are performed. This discrepancy is explained by the facts that the overwhelming majority of such persons are healthy and that detection of this condition has been greatly facilitated by the widespread use of flow cytometry techniques that use peroxidase staining for leukocyte differential counts.[356] Eosinophil peroxidase is normal in this disorder. An autosomal recessive manner of inheritance has been reported, but the inheritance pattern is much more complex, probably reflecting the heterogeneity of the responsible genotypes.[357] Of all the patients recognized with this disorder, only six have had serious infections. Systemic candidiasis occurred in four of these patients, three of whom also had diabetes mellitus.[318, 319, 358]

Because the cell is devoid of MPO-dependent but not other

oxidative killing mechanisms, there is delayed but not absent intracellular killing in MPO-deficient neutrophils. Delayed killing is more pronounced for fungi than for bacteria,[359] which suggests an explanation for the clinical findings in this disorder. Chemotaxis, phagocytosis, and degranulation are normal, but the respiratory burst is enhanced. The supranormal oxidative metabolism may be caused by absent MPO-dependent inactivation of the oxidase system[165] and may help explain the lack of clinical expression of this defect in most patients.

Normal MPO is the product of a single gene on chromosome 17. Post-translational processing of a glycosylated (89-kD) primary gene product results in a mature molecule containing heavy (59-kD) α-chain and light (13.5-kD) β-chains.[319, 360–364] The current structural model suggests that the chain content of mature MPO is an $\alpha_2\beta_2$ molecule and that processing and lysosomal targeting are independent of the mannose-6-phosphate receptor system.[360, 365] Most patients with MPO deficiency have a defect in post-translational processing such that their neutrophils have immunochemical evidence of an MPO precursor but no mature protein.[366, 367] However, one report described a patient with a pretranslational defect causing MPO deficiency,[368] highlighting the heterogeneity of the molecular defects causing this disorder. To date, three mutations in the coding sequence of MPO have been identified in persons with inherited deficiency,[367, 369, 370] but it is probable that many different mutations underlie this common disorder.[357, 371]

MPO deficiency has also been recognized as an acquired defect accompanying some myeloproliferative disorders, particularly acute myelogenous leukemia. In the leukemic but not the preleukemic state, this deficiency is associated with an increased risk of infection.[372] However, large population studies suggest that MPO deficiency may predispose to infection and certain forms of malignant disease.[373, 374]

Specific Granule Deficiency

The absence of specific granules has been recognized in five patients with recurrent infection.[375] The peripheral leukocyte count in such patients is normal when they are uninfected, and the diagnosis is established by the apparent absence of intracellular granules on routine Wright's stain (primary granules do not take up Wright's stain). Close examination reveals a bilobed nuclear morphology with nuclear blocks and clefts. In addition, eosinophils are affected in this disorder.[376] Specific granule contents (e.g., lactoferrin, vitamin B_{12}-binding protein) are absent, as is membrane alkaline phosphatase.[375] Unexpectedly, the neutrophils of affected patients are almost completely devoid of defensins, proteins that normally constitute one third of the azurophilic granule contents.[377] Only myeloid cells are affected, because the lactoferrin content of nasal secretions and tears is normal.[378] Because of this observation and the fact that the affected genes are not located on the same chromosome but are expressed during a specific period of myeloid development, it is likely that specifc granule deficiency represents a disorder of myeloid differentiation. Elegant ongoing studies in the laboratory of Berliner[11] promise to provide important insights into normal myeloid development and the mechanisms important to coordinated regulation of the genes encoding the various granule proteins.

Therapy for Neutrophil Defects

Antimicrobial Therapy. The recurrent and severe infections that occur in many patients with abnormal neutrophil function have made the administration of prophylactic antibiotics common despite concerns about colonization and infection with resistant microorganisms. The low prevalence of these disorders has made controlled trials of prophylactic antibiotics almost impossible. Nonetheless, the broad antimicrobial spectrum of trimethoprim-sulfamethoxazole against both gram-positive and gram-negative bacteria, coupled with its penetration and concentration within neutrophils, probably explains its apparent effectiveness in reducing infections in patients with CGD.[379] Prophylactic antibiotic therapy in patients with CGD has been associated with an increase in the average infection-free interval from 9.6 to 40 months.[344] The effect of antibiotics on intracellular killing mechanisms received attention with the demonstration that staphylococci exposed to sublethal concentrations of cell wall–active antibiotics for a short time were more readily killed by neutrophils than were staphylococci grown in the absence of antibiotics. Improved killing resulted from an enhancement in nonoxidative bactericidal mechanisms and was both organism and antibiotic specific.[380] The significance of these findings for patient management is unknown.

Granulocyte Transfusions. Granulocyte transfusions have been used therapeutically in febrile granulocytopenic patients. Theoretically, to achieve a blood neutrophil count of 1000 cells/mm^3 after transfusion, approximately 1×10^{10} neutrophils (all the neutrophils in 2 to 3 liters of blood) are required for the average adult per day. However, many patients show no significant rise in the peripheral leukocyte count after transfusion of this number of cells.[381] Two basic methods of procurement have been devised: centrifugation and filtration leukapheresis. The former method uses differences in density among blood cells to achieve separation. Filtration makes use of the ability of neutrophils to adhere to nylon wool to achieve separation from other cells. Cells obtained by both procedures are functional both in vitro and in vivo, but those obtained by filtration leukapheresis exhibit cytoplasmic vacuolization and surface distortion as well as a loss of granule contents and reduced bactericidal capacity.[381, 382] In addition, up to 75% of the recipients of cells obtained by leukapheresis have transfusion reactions, predominantly fever and chills, compared with 15% of the recipients of cells obtained by centrifugation.[383] Despite these differences, administration of cells obtained by either method to granulocytopenic patients with infection has been beneficial in some but not all controlled trials.[384, 385] Granulocytopenic patients with proven bacterial infection who received daily granulocyte transfusions for the duration of their infection survived longer than did infected nontransfused control patients. Both groups received therapy appropriate for their infection.[383, 386] Leukocyte transfusions have also been therapeutically successful when administered to a limited number of patients with neutrophil bactericidal defects and progressive infection. By using a positive NBT test as a marker, delivery to and persistence of transfused normal leukocytes at the site of infection was documented in a patient with CGD.[387]

Although leukocyte transfusion may be beneficial for certain infected granulocytopenic patients, associated complications have limited their use. These complications include (1) transfusion-associated cytomegalovirus infection, (2) allosensitization to human leukocyte antigens, (3) difficulties in locating adequate numbers of suitable donors, (4) risks to the donor, (5) high cost of the procedure, and (6) an increased incidence of acute pulmonary reactions when transfusions are given in conjunction with amphotericin B administration.[388, 389] This reaction most commonly occurs when amphotericin B treatment is initiated simultaneously with or after transfusion and is characterized by the acute onset of respiratory decompensation, pulmonary infiltrates, and intra-alveolar hemorrhage.[389]

A potentially serious complication of red cell or white cell transfusions in patients with CGD may occur because of abnormalities of the Kell antigen system and the Kell-related antigen K_x. This antigen is present on the surface of red and white blood cells from healthy people and from patients with autosomally transmitted CGD. K_x is absent from the neutrophils of most patients with the X-linked form of the disease because of the close linkage of the CGD and X_k genes on the X chromosome.[390–392] In addition, some patients with X-linked CGD exhibit the rare McLeod phenotype, in which K_x and the standard Kell antigens are absent from erythrocytes and leukocytes and a mild hemolytic anemia occurs. Failure to recognize this antigenic abnormality can result in severe transfusion reactions.[393] As a consequence of these complicating aspects, leukocyte transfusion seems best reserved for the patient with severe granulocytopenia or functionally defective neutrophils who has a serious bacterial or fungal infection that has not responded to appropriate antimicrobial therapy. Donors should preferably be seronegative for cytomegalovirus.

Bone Marrow Transplantation. Several patients, one with LAD and three with CGD,[394] have undergone successful bone marrow engraftment with subsequent clinical improvement. Two of the patients with CGD ultimately rejected their transplant but continued to enjoy clinical improvement. This result illustrates the difficulty in meaningfully evaluating this procedure in these types of patients. Moreover, given the increased infection-free interval and survival rates observed with the use of prophylactic antibiotics and IFN-γ in patients with CGD,[344] it seems reasonable to reserve such aggressive therapy for unusual situations.

Evaluating Phagocyte Function

The most important step in the evaluation of possible abnormalities of neutrophil function is to obtain a good clinical history and a leukocyte count with a stained blood smear. Serum immunoglobulin and complement levels should be determined. An NBT test, requiring only a drop or two of blood, is simple and can be performed quickly. Further evaluation depends on the results of these simple screening tests (Table 8–4) (see Chapter 10).

EOSINOPHILS

Eosinophils are bone marrow–derived, tissue-based granulocytes located subjacent to the skin and mucosal lining of the respiratory and gastrointestinal tracts.[395, 396] In these locations they play a role in host defense against helminthic infection; hypersensitivity diseases, especially bronchial asthma; and certain dermatologic conditions. In general, eosinophils have a functional repertoire similar to that of neutrophils,[395, 397] although there are several significant differences in the activities of these two phagocytic granulocytes.

Eosinophils develop from marrow stem cells over a 5- to 6-day period.[398] Eosinophilopoiesis in humans appears to be uniquely dependent on IL-5, with IL-3 and GM-CSF also contributing to a lesser degree. IL-5 concentrations correlate with the appearance and magnitude of eosinophilia in vivo.[399] Eosinophil maturation is accompanied by the appearance of three characteristic granule populations: primary, secondary, and small granules (Fig. 8–8). Primary granules are electron dense and appear during the promyelocyte stage of development. Secondary granules are distinguished by their larger size, an electron-dense crystalloid core containing major basic protein (MBP), and an electron-lucent matrix containing eosinophil cationic protein, eosinophil-derived neurotoxin, and eosinophil peroxidase. Small granules contain acid phosphatase and arylsulfatase B. Mature eosinophils also possess secretory IgA receptors as well as low-affinity IgG (FcγRII) and IgE receptors. Receptors for complement (CRI, CR3, ClqR, C5a), cytokines (IL-5, IL-3, GM-CSF, IFN-γ,

TABLE 8–4 Evaluation of Neutrophil Function[413, 414]

Leukocyte and differential count
Adherence
Migration to site
Chemotaxis
Phagocytosis and bactericidal activity[415]
Postphagocytic activity
Oxygen consumption
Hexose monophosphate shunt
Iodination
Nitroblue tetrazolium[416, 417]
Degranulation
Chemiluminescence[418]

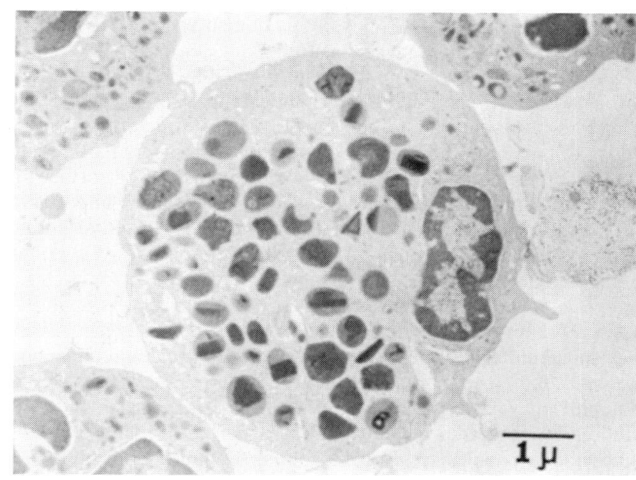

FIGURE 8–8. Electron micrograph of a human eosinophil. Note the prominent granules with crystalloid cores.

TNF), platelet-activating factor, and leukotriene B_4 have also been reported.[400] The number and functional competence of these receptors are presumably regulated in a manner analogous to that documented for neutrophils.

Circulating eosinophils can be separated into two populations based on their buoyant density. Most of the eosinophils in normal persons are characterized as dense or normodense. Hypodense eosinophils are cells that have been activated: they express a greater number of functionally competent receptors, exhibit a higher resting level of oxidative metabolism, and predominate in the blood and tissues of persons with eosinophilia.

The intravascular half-life of eosinophils is about 2 hours. Eosinophil migration involves different adhesion molecules than does neutrophil transmigration.[401, 402] In addition to the β2 integrins also expressed by neutrophils, eosinophils express $\alpha_4\beta_1$, $\alpha_4\beta_7$, and $\alpha_6\beta_1$[403] integrins and display a form of P-selectin glycoprotein ligand 1 (PSGL-1) that binds more avidly to endothelial P-selectin than does the form expressed by neutrophils.[404–406] That eosinophil transmigration is normal in LAD-1 provides evidence that β2 integrins are not required for this process. Association with endothelium appears to be mediated by IL-5–dependent upregulation of $\alpha_4\beta_1$ on eosinophils and its counterreceptor, vascular cell adhesion molecule-1, on endothelial cells.[407]

In murine models of helminthic infection, the major source of IL-5 is the T-helper cell subset, Th2. The outcome of the infection appears to depend on whether Th1 or Th2 cell responses predominate and on the identity of the parasites. Because IL-5 is intimately involved in eosinophil production, activation, and transmigration in humans, its modulation is an attractive therapeutic strategy for affecting this type of eosinophil-dependent event.[399]

Substantial evidence supports a role for eosinophils in immunity to helminthic parasites, as demonstrated by the greater worm burden and tissue damage in animals treated with antieosinophil serum and by the finding that the transfer of passive immunity requires the presence of these cells. This conclusion is buttressed by the demonstration of eosinophils on and around degenerating parasites in vivo and by the ability of eosinophils to kill these organisms in vitro.[408, 409]

Killing of parasites is related to exocytosis of eosinophil granule contents onto the parasite surface while it is in close apposition to the eosinophils.[410, 411] The eosinophil peroxidase–hydrogen peroxide–halide oxidation system plays a minor role in antihelminthic activity. Rather, the cationic granule proteins are responsible for the bulk of this activity. On a molar, basis eosinophil cationic protein exerts a more potent antihelminthic effect than does MBP, but the greater quantity of the latter in the eosinophil makes its contribution more significant. The effect of these proteins is also specific for different stages in the life cycle of the parasite.

Recognition that eosinophil granules contain a number of substances capable of inactivating the chemical mediators of anaphylaxis has led to the suggestion that the eosinophil may modulate the severity of type I hypersensitivity reactions.[412] In this scenario, stimulation of basophils and mast cells by the interaction of surface IgE with specific antigen results in the release of substances important in type I hypersensitivity reactions. These include vasoactive amines, slow-reacting substances of anaphylaxis (leukotrienes C, D, and E), platelet-activating factor, and eosinophil chemotactic factor of anaphylaxis (ECF-A). Histamine and ECF-A attract eosinophils to the site of antigen reaction with basophils and mast cells. ECF-A can also stimulate eosinophil degranulation, as can immune complexes that the eosinophil phagocytizes. Histaminase secreted by the eosinophil may inactivate local histamine, and further histamine secretion by basophils may be inhibited by a substance present in eosinophils. Arylsulfatase and phospholipase present in the smaller eosinophil granules are capable of inactivating leukotrienes C, D, and E and platelet-activating factor. Therefore, eosinophils may modulate immediate hypersensitivity reactions by inhibiting the release of mediators of the type I reaction as well as by destroying mediators that have already been released.[412]

The association of eosinophilia of several weeks' duration with the development of endocardial lesions and the isolation of an eosinophil-derived neurotoxin capable of reproducing the neurologic picture observed in patients with cerebrospinal fluid eosinophilia strongly support a role for the eosinophil in the pathogenesis of tissue injury in certain disorders, most prominent of which is bronchial asthma. Substantial evidence indicates that eosinophil MBP is an important mediator of tissue injury. For example, increased quantities of MBP are detectable in the bronchial washings from patients with asthma but not from those with other pulmonary disorders. Nanomolar concentrations of MBP but not other cationic proteins cause exfoliation of epithelial cells, impaired ciliary function, net chloride secretion, and bronchial hyperreactivity. Immunofluorescent staining of bronchial epithelium in autopsy specimens from patients who died from asthma revealed extensive deposition of MBP in the peribronchial areas and overlying regions of bronchial epithelial denudation. These findings were not observed in autopsy material obtained from patients whose deaths were related to other pulmonary diseases. The importance of epithelial denudation lies in the resultant enhanced responsiveness of the underlying bronchial smooth muscle to contractile agonists, including acetylcholine and histamine, as well as leukotriene C_4 produced by eosinophils.[400]

REFERENCES

1. Carroll MC, Prodeus AP. Linkages of innate and acquired immunity. Curr Opin Immunol. 1998;10:36–40.
2. Medzhitov R, Janeway CA Jr. An ancient system of host defense. Curr Opin Immunol. 1998;10:12–15.
3. Broxmeyer HE, Mantel CR, Aronica SM. Biology and mechanisms of action of synergistically stimulated myeloid progenitor cell proliferation and suppression by chemokines. Stem Cells. 1974;15:67–77.
4. Nemuaitis J. A comparative review of colony-stimulating factors. Drugs. 1997;54:709–729.
5. Kehrl JH. Hematopoietic lineage commitment: Role of transcription factors. Stem Cells. 1995;13:223–241.
6. Metcalf D. Hematopoietic regulation: Redundancy or subtlety? Blood. 1993;82:3515–3523.
7. Tenen DG, Hromas R, Licht JD, et al. Transcription factors, normal myeloid development, and leukemia. Blood. 1997;90:489–519.
8. Colotta F, Re F, Polentarutti N, et al. Modulation of granulocyte survival and programmed cell death by cytokines and bacterial products. Blood. 1992; 80:2012–2020.
9. Bainton DF. Differentiation of human neutrophilic granulocytes: Normal and abnormal. Prog Clin Biol Res. 1977;13:1.
10. Glasser L, Fiederlein RL. Functional differentiation of normal human neutrophils. Blood. 1987;69:937–944.
11. Sigurdsson F, Khanna-Gupta A, Lawson N, et al. Control of late neutrophil-specific gene expression: Insights into regulation of myeloid differentiation. Semin Hematol. 1990;34:303–310.
12. Borregaard N, Cowland JB. Granules of the human neutrophilic polymorphonuclear leukocyte. Blood. 1997;89:3503–3521.
13. Bainton DF, Farquhar MG. Origin of granules in polymorphonuclear leukocytes. J Cell Biol. 1966;28:277.
14. Cramer E, Pryzwansky KB, Villeval J-C, et al. Ultrastructural localization of lactoferrin and myeloperoxidase in human neutrophils by immunogold. Blood. 1985;65:423–432.
15. Csernok E, Ludemann J, Gross WL, et al. Ultrastructural localization of proteinase 3, the target antigen of anti-cytoplasmic antibodies circulating in Wegener's granulomatosis. Am J Pathol. 1990;137:1113–1120.
16. Ohlsson K, Olsson I. The neutral proteases of human granulocytes: Isolation and partial characterization of granulocyte elastase. Eur J Biochem. 1974;42:519–527.
17. Rice WG, Ganz T, Kinkade JM, et al. Defensin-rich dense granules of human neutrophils. Blood. 1987;70:757–765.
18. Weiss J, Olsson I. Cellular and subcellular localization of the bactericidal/permeability-increasing protein of neutrophils. Blood. 1987;69:652–659.
19. Nauseef WM, McCormick S, Yi H. Roles of heme insertion and the mannose-6-phosphate receptor in processing of the human myeloid lysosomal enzyme, myeloperoxidase. Blood. 1992;80:2622–2633.
20. Valore EV, Ganz T. Posttranslational processing of defensin precursors in immature human myeloid cells. Blood. 1992;79:1538–1544.
21. Sengelov H, Nielsen MH, Borregaard N. Separation of human neutrophil plasma membrane from intracellular vesicles containing alkaline phosphatase and NADPH oxidase activity by free flow electrophoresis. J Biol Chem. 1992;267:14912–14917.
22. Kjeldsen L, Bainton DF, Sengelov H, et al. Structural and functional heterogeneity among peroxidase-negative granules in human neutrophils: Identification of a distinct gelatinase-containing granule subset by combined immunocytochemistry and subcellular fractionation. Blood. 1993;82:3183–3191.
23. Borregaard N, Kjeldsen L, Lollike K. Granules and vesicles of human neutrophils: The role of endomembranes as source of plasma membrane proteins. Eur J Haematol. 1993;51:318–322.
24. Calafat J, Kuijpers TW, Janssen H, et al. Evidence for small intracellular vesicles in human blood phagocytes containing cytochrome b558 and the adhesion molecule CD11b/CD18. Blood. 1993;81:3122–3129.
25. Borregaard N, Heiple JM, Simons ER, et al. Subcellular localization of the b-cytochrome component of the human neutrophil microbicidal oxidase: translocation during activation. J Cell Biol. 1983;97:52–61.
26. Sengelov H, Boulay F, Kjeldsen L, et al. Subcellular localization and translocation of the receptor for *N*-formylmethionyl-leucyl-phenylalanine in human neutrophils. Biochem J. 1994;299:473–479.
27. English D, Graves V. Simultaneous mobilization of Mac-1 (CD11b/CD18) and formyl peptide chemoattractant receptors in human neutrophils. Blood. 1992;80:776–787.
28. Singer II, Scott S, Kawka DW, et al. Adhesomes: Specific granules containing receptors for laminin, C3bi/fibrinogen, fibronectin, and vitronectin in human polymorphonuclear leukocytes and monocytes. J Cell Biol. 1989;109:3169–3182.
29. Porteu F, Nathan CF. Mobilizable intracellular pool of p55 (type I) tumor necrosis factor receptors in human neutrophils. J Leukoc Biol. 1992;52:122–124.
30. Sengelov H, Kjeldsen L, Kroeze W, et al. Secretory vesicles are the intracellular reservoir of complement receptor 1 in human neutrophils. J Immunol. 1994;153:804–810.
31. Borregaard N, Kjeldsen L, Sengelov H, et al. Changes in subcellular localization and surface expression of L-selectin, alkaline phosphatase, and Mac-1 in human neutrophils during stimulation with inflammatory mediators. J Leukocyte Biol. 1994;56:80–87.
32. Sengelov H, Kjeldsen L, Diamond MS, et al. Subcellular localization and dynamics of Mac-1 ($\alpha_m\beta_2$) in human neutrophils. J Clin Invest. 1993;92:1467–1476.
33. Stossel TP. On the crawling of animal cells. Science. 1993;260:1086–1094.
34. Pestonjamasp K, Amieva MR, Strassel CP, et al. Moesin, ezrin, and p205 are actin-binding proteins associated with neutrophil plasma membranes. Mol Biol Cell. 1995;6:247–259.
35. White JR, Naccache PH, Sha'afi RI. Stimulation by chemotactic factor of actin association with the cytoskeleton in rabbit neutrophils. J Biol Chem. 1983; 258:14041–14047.
36. Ryder MI, Weinreb RN, Niederman R. The organization of actin filaments in human polymorphonuclear leukocytes. Anat Rec. 1984;209:7–20.
37. Berlin RD, Fera JP. Changes in membrane microviscosity associated with phagocytosis: Effects of colchicine. Proc Natl Acad Sci U S A. 1977;74:1072.
38. Neuman E, Huleatt JW, Vargas H, et al. Regulation of MHC class I synthesis and expression by human neutrophils. J Immunol. 1992;148:3520–3527.
39. Neuman E, Huleatt JW, Jack RM. Granulocyte-macrophage colony-stimulating factor increases synthesis and expression of CR1 and CR3 by human peripheral blood neutrophils. J Immunol. 1990;145:3325–3332.
40. Cassatella MA, Bazzoni F, Ceska M, et al. IL-8 production by human polymorphonuclear leukocytes: The chemoattractant formyl-methionyl-leucyl-phenylalanine induces the gene expression and release of IL-8 through a pertussis toxin-sensitive pathway. J Immunol. 1992;148:3216–3220.
41. Jack RM, Fearon DT. Selective synthesis of mRNA and proteins by human peripheral blood neutrophils. J Immunol. 1988;140:4286–4293.
42. McKenzie SE, Schreiber AD. Fc gamma receptors in phagocytes. Curr Opin Hematol. 1998;5:16–21.
43. Sengelov H. Complement receptors in neutrophils. Crit Rev Immunol. 1995;15:107–131.

44. Murphy PM. The molecular biology of leukocyte chemoattractant receptors. Annu Rev Immunol. 1994;12:593–633.
45. Messner RP, Jelinek J. Receptors for human gamma-globulin on human neutrophils. J Clin Invest. 1970;49:2165.
46. Lay WH, Nussenzweig V. Receptors for complement on leukocytes. J Exp Med. 1968;129:991.
47. Williams LT, Snyderman R, Pike MC, et al. Specific receptor sites for chemotactic peptides on human polymorphonuclear leukocytes. Proc Natl Acad Sci U S A. 1977;74:1204.
48. Chenoweth DE, Hughli TE. Demonstration of specific C5a receptor on intact human polymorphonuclear leukocytes. Proc Natl Acad Sci U S A. 1978;75:3943.
49. Daeron M. Fc receptor biology. Ann Rev Immunol. 1997;15:203–234.
50. Bender JG, Van Epps DE, Chenoweth DE. Independent regulation of human neutrophil chemotactic receptors after activation. J Immunol. 1987;139:3028–3033.
51. Korchak HM, Wildenfeld C, Rich AM, et al. Stimulus response coupling in the human neutrophil. J Biol Chem. 1984;259:7439–7445.
52. Walker RI, Willemze R. Neutrophil kinetics and regulation of granulopoiesis. Rev Infect Dis. 1980;2:282–292.
53. Sachs L. The molecular control of blood cell development. Science. 1987;238:1374–1379.
54. Gallin JI. Human neutrophil heterogeneity exists, but is it meaningful? Blood. 1984;63:977–983.
55. Robinson JM, Karnovsky ML, Karnovsky MJ. Glycogen accumulation in polymorphonuclear leukocytes, and other intracellular alterations that occur during inflammation. J Cell Biol. 1982;95:933.
56. Bevilacqua MP. Endothelial-leukocyte adhesion molecules. Annu Rev Immunol. 1993;11:767–804.
57. Springer TA. Traffic signals for lymphocyte recirculation and leukocyte emigration: The multistep paradigm. Cell. 1994;76:301–314.
58. Frenette PS, Moyna C, Hartwell DW, et al. Platelet-endothelial interactions in inflamed mesenteric venules. Blood. 1998;91:1318–1324.
59. Yeaman, MR, Bayer AS, Koo S-P, et al. Platelet microbicidal proteins and neutrophil defensin disrupt the *Staphylococcus aureus* cytoplasmic membrane by distinct mechanisms of action. J Clin Invest. 1998;101:178–187.
60. Celi A, Lorenzet R, Furie B, et al. Platelet-leukocyte-endothelial cell interaction on the blood vessel wall. Semin Hematol. 1997;34:327–335.
61. Fuhlbrigge RC, Alon R, Puri KD, et al. Sialylated, fucosylated ligands for L-selectin expressed on leukocytes mediate tethering and rolling adhesions in physiologic flow conditions. J Cell Biol. 1997;135:837–848.
62. Nelson RM, Venot A, Bevilacqua MP, et al. Carbohydrate-protein interactions in vascular biology. Annu Rev Cell Dev Biol. 1995;11:601–631.
63. Kansas GS. Selectins and their ligands: Current concepts and controversies. Blood. 1996;88:3259–3287.
64. Gahmberg CG, Tovanen M, Kotovuori P. Leukocyte adhesion: Structure and function of human leukocyte 2 integrins and their cellular ligands. Eur J Biochem. 1997;245:215–232.
65. Smyth SS, Joneckis CC, Parise LV. Regulation of vascular integrins. Blood. 1993;81:2827–2843.
66. De Fougerolles AR, Klickstein LB, Springer TA. Cloning and expression of intercellular adhesion molecule 3 reveals strong homology to the immunoglobulin family counter-receptors for lymphocyte function-associated antigen 1. J Exp Med. 1993;177:1187–1192.
67. De Fougerolles AR, Diamond MS, Springer TA. Heterogenous glucosylation of ICAM-3 and lack of interaction with Mac-1 and p150,95. Eur J Immunol. 1995;25:1008–1012.
68. Gresham HD, Goodwin JL, Allen PM, et al. A novel member of the integrin receptor family mediates Arg-Gly-Asp-stimulated neutrophil phagocytosis. J Cell Biol. 1989;108:1935–1943.
69. Gresham HD, Graham IL, Griffin GL, et al. Domain-specific interactions between entactin and neutrophil integrins. J Biol Chem. 1996;271:30587–30594.
70. Lindberg FP, Gresham HD, Reinhold MI, et al. Integrin-associated protein immunoglobulin domain is necessary for efficient vitronectin bead binding. J Cell Biol. 1996;134:1313–1322.
71. Zhou M, Brown EJ. Leukocyte response integrin and integrin-associated protein act as a signal transduction unit in generation of a phagocyte respiratory burst. J Exp Med. 1993;178:1165–1174.
72. Nitsch M, Gabrijelcic D, Tschesche H. Separation of granule subpopulations in human polymorphonuclear leukocytes. Biol Chem Hoppe-Seyler. 1990;371:611–615.
73. Brown E. Neutrophil adhesion and the therapy of inflammation. Semin Hematol. 1997;34:319–326.
74. Del Maschio A, Zanetti A, Corada M, et al. Polymorphonuclear leukocyte adhesion triggers the disorganization of endothelial cell-to-cell adherens junctions. J Cell Biol. 1996;135:497–510.
75. Feng D, Nagy JA, Pyne K, et al. Neutrophils emigrate from venules by a transendothelial cell pathway in response to FMLP. J Exp Med. 1998;187:903–915.
76. Parkos CA, Colgan SP, Madara JL. Interactions of neutrophils with epithelial cells: Lessons from the intestine. J Am Soc Nephrol. 1994;5:138–152.
77. Huang GT, Eckmann L, Savidge TC, et al. Infection of human intestinal epithelial cells with invasive bacteria upregulates apical intercellular adhesion molecule-1 (ICAM-1) expression and neutrophil adhesion. J Clin Invest. 1996;98:572–583.
78. Parkos CA, Colgan SP, Bacarra AE, et al. Intestinal epithelia (T84) possess basolateral ligands for CD11b/CD18-mediated neutrophil adherence. Am J Physiol. 1995;268:C472–C479.
79. Parkos CA, Colgan SP, Liang TW, et al. CD47 mediates post-adhesive events required for neutrophil migration across polarized intestinal epithelia. J Cell Biol. 1996;132:437–450.
80. Lindberg FP, Bullard DC, Caver DE, et al. Decreased resistance to bacterial infection and granulocyte defects in IAP-deficient mice. Science. 1996;274:795–798.
81. Colgan SP, Serhan CN, Parkos CA, et al. Lipoxin A4 modulates transmigration of human neutrophils across intestinal epithelial monolayers. J Clin Invest. 1993;92:75–82.
82. Colgan SP, Parkos CA, Delp C, et al. Neutrophil migration across cultured intestinal epithelial monolayers is modulated by epithelial exposure to IFN-gamma in a highly polarized fashion. J Cell Biol. 1993;120:785–798.
83. Baggiolini M. Chemokines and leukocyte traffic. Nature. 1998;392:565–568.
84. Camussi G, Turello E, Tetta C, et al. Tumor necrosis factor induces contraction of mesangial cells and alters their cytoskeletons. Kidney Int. 1990;38:795–802.
85. Murphy PM. Neutrophil receptors for interleukin-8 and related CXC chemokines. Semin Hematol. 1997;34:311–318.
86. Adams DH, Lloyd AR. Chemokines: Leucocyte recruitment and activation cytokines. Lancet. 1997;349:490–495.
87. Baggiolini M, Dewald B, Moser B. Interleukin-8 and related chemotactic chemokines: CXC and CC chemokines. Adv Immunol. 1994;55:97–179.
88. Ahuja SK, Murphy PM. Molecular piracy of mammalian interleukin-8 receptor type B by Herpesvirus saimiri. J Biol Chem. 1993;268:20961–20964.
89. Dragic T, Litwin V, Allaway GP, et al. HIV-1 entry into CD4+ cells is mediated by the chemokine receptor CC-CKR-5. Nature. 1996;381:667–673.
90. Deng HK, Liu R, Ellemeirer W, et al. Identification of a major co-receptor for primary isolates of HIV. Nature. 1996;381:661–666.
91. Mummidi S, Gonzalez E, Ahuja SS, et al. Genealogy of the CCR5 locus and chemokine system gene variants associated with altered rates of HIV-1 disease progression. Nat Med. 1998;4:786–793.
92. Roger M. Influence of host genes on HIV-1 disease progression. FASEB J. 1998;12:625–632.
93. Hallett MB. Controlling the molecular motor of neutrophil chemotaxis. Bioessays. 1997;19:615–621.
94. Allen L-AH, Aderem A. Mechanisms of phagocytosis. Curr Opin Immunol. 1996;8:36–40.
95. Gordon LI, Douglas SD, Kay NE, et al. Modulation of neutrophil function by lysozyme. J Clin Invest. 1979;64:226.
96. Brown EJ. Phagocytosis. Bioessays. 1995;17:109–117.
97. Greenberg S. Signal transduction of phagocytosis. Trends Cell Biol. 1995;5:93–99.
98. Greenberg S, Chang P, Wang D, et al. Clustered syk tyrosine kinase domains trigger phagocytosis. Proc Natl Acad Sci U S A. 1996;93:1103–1107.
99. Bobak DA, Gaither TA, Frank MM, et al. Modulation of FcR function by complement: Subcomponent Clq enhances the phagocytosis of IgG-opsonized targets by human monocytes and culture-derived macrophages. J Immunol. 1987;138:1150–1156.
100. van Oss CJ. Phagocytosis as a surface phenomenon. Annu Rev Microbiol. 1978;32:19.
101. Lew DP, Andersson T, Hed J, et al. Ca^{2+}-dependent and Ca^{2+}-independent phagocytosis in human neutrophils. Nature. 1985;315:509–511.
102. Petroni KC, Shen L, Guyre PM. Modulation of human polymorphonuclear leukocyte IgG Fc receptors and Fc receptor-mediated functions by IFN-γ and glucocorticoids. J Immunol. 1988;140:3467–3472.
103. Lawrence WD, Packman CH, Rowe JM, et al. Attachment of particle bound IgG and complement to human neutrophils. Blood. 1981;58:772.
104. Newman S, Johnston RB Jr. Role of binding through C3b and IgG in polymorphonuclear neutrophil function: Studies with trypsin generated C3b. J Immunol. 1979;123:1839.
105. Swanson JA, Baer SC. Phagocytosis by zippers and triggers. Trends Cell Biol. 1995;5:89–93.
106. Griffin FM, Griffin JH, Leider JE, et al. Studies on the mechanism of phagocytosis: I. Requirements for circumferential attachment of particle bound ligands to specific receptors on the macrophage plasma membrane. J Exp Med. 1975;142:1263.
107. Griffin FM, Griffin JA, Silverstein SC. Studies on the mechanism of phagocytosis: II. The interaction of macrophages with anti-immunoglobulin IgG-coated bone marrow derived lymphocytes. J Exp Med. 1976;144:788.
108. Ruoslahti E, Pierschbacher MD. Arg-Gly-Asp: A versatile cell recognition signal. Cell. 1986;44:517–518.
109. Blystone SD, Graham IL, Lindberg FP, et al. Integrin $\alpha5\beta1$ differentially regulates adhesion and phagocytic functions of the fibronectin receptor, $\alpha5\beta1$. J Cell Biol. 1994;127:1129–1137.
110. Henderson LM, Chappel JB. NADPH oxidase of neutrophils. Biochim Biophys Acta. 1996;1273:87–107.
111. Heyworth PG, Peveri P, Curnutte JT: Cytosolic components of NADPH oxidase: Identity, function, and role in regulation of oxidase activity. In: Cochrane CG, Gimbrone MA, eds. Cellular and Molecular Mechanisms of Inflammation. New York: Academic Press; 1992:43–81.
112. Eggleston LV, Krebs AA. Regulation of the pentose phosphate cycle. Biochem J. 1974;138:424.
113. DeLeo FR, Quinn MT. Assembly of the phagocyte NADPH oxidase: Molecular interactions of oxidase proteins. J Leukoc Biol. 1996;60:677–691.
114. Segal AW. Absence of both cytochrome b-245 subunits from neutrophils in X-linked chronic granulomatous disease. Nature. 1987;326:88–91.
115. Teahan C, Rowe P, Parker P, et al. The X-linked chronic granulomatous disease gene codes for the b-chain of cytochrome b-245. Nature. 1987;327:720–721.

116. Segal AW, Jones OTG. Novel cytochrome b system in phagocytic vacuoles of human granulocytes. Nature. 1978;276:515–517.
117. Segal AW, Jones OTG, Webster D, et al. Absence of a newly described cytochrome b from neutrophils of patients with chronic granulomatous disease. Lancet. 1978;2:446–449.
118. Segal AW, Cross AR, Garcia RC, et al. Absence of cytochrome b-245 in chronic granulomatous disease: A multicenter European evaluation of its incidence and relevance. N Engl J Med. 1983;308:245–251.
119. Borregaard N, Simons ER, Clark RA. Involvement of cytochrome b-245 in the respiratory burst of human neutrophils. Infect Immun. 1982;38:1301–1303.
120. Gabig TG, Schervish EW, Santinga JT. Functional relationship of the cytochrome b to the superoxide-generating oxidase of human neutrophils. J Biol Chem. 1982;257:4114–4119.
121. Parkos CA, Allen RA, Cochrane CG, et al. Purified cytochrome b from human granulocyte plasma membrane is comprised of two polypeptides with relative molecular weights of 91,000 and 22,000. J Clin Invest. 1987;80:732–742.
122. Dinauer MC, Orkin SH, Brown R, et al. The glycoprotein encoded by the X-linked chronic granulomatous disease locus is a component of the neutrophil cytochrome b complex. Nature. 1987;327:717–720.
123. Quinn MT, Mullen ML, Jesaitis AJ. Human neutrophil cytochrome b contains multiple hemes: Evidence for heme associated with both subunits. J Biol Chem. 1992;267:7303–7309.
124. Rotrosen D, Yeung CL, Leto TL, et al. Cytochrome b_{558}: The flavin-binding component of the phagocyte NADPH oxidase. Science. 1992;256:1459–1462.
125. Segal AW, West I, Wientjes F, et al. Cytochrome b_{-245} is a flavocytochrome containing FAD and the NADPH-binding site of the microbicidal oxidase of phagocytes. Biochem J. 1992;284:781–788.
126. Volpp BD, Nauseef WM, Clark RA. Two cytosolic neutrophil oxidase components absent in autosomal chronic granulomatous disease. Science. 1988;242:1295–1297.
127. Nunoi H, Rotrosen D, Gallin JI, et al. Two forms of autosomal chronic granulomatous disease lack distinct neutrophil cytosol factors. Science. 1988;242:1298–1301.
128. Volpp BD, Nauseef WM, Donelson JE, et al. Cloning of the cDNA and functional expression of the 47 kilodalton cytosolic component of the human neutrophil respiratory burst oxidase. Proc Natl Acad Sci U S A. 1989;86:7195–7199.
129. Lomax KJ, Leto TL, Nunoi H, et al. Recombinant 47-kilodalton cytosol factor restores NADPH oxidase in chronic granulomatous disease. Science. 1989;245:409–412.
130. Leto TL, Lomax KJ, Volpp BD, et al. Cloning of a 67-kD neutrophil oxidase factor with similarity to a noncatalytic region of $p60^{c\text{-}src}$. Science. 1990;248:727–730.
131. Park J-W, Ma M, Ruedi JM, et al. The cytosolic components of the respiratory burst oxidase exist as a M_r (approx.) 240,00 complex that acquires a membrane-binding site during activation of the oxidase in a cell-free system. J Biol Chem. 1992;267:17327–17332.
132. Heyworth PG, Shrimpton CF, Segal AW. Localization of the 47 kDa phosphoprotein involved in the respiratory-burst NADPH oxidase of phagocytic cells. Biochem J. 1989;260:243–248.
133. Rotrosen D, Leto TL. Phosphorylation of neutrophil 47-kDa cytosolic oxidase factor: Translocation to membrane is associated with distinct phosphorylation events. J Biol Chem. 1990;265:19910–19915.
134. Clark RA, Volpp BD, Leidal KG, et al. Two cytosolic components of the human neutrophil respiratory burst oxidase translocate to the plasma membrane during cell activation. J Clin Invest. 1990;85:714–721.
135. Heyworth PG, Curnutte JT, Nauseef WM, et al. Neutrophil nicotinamide adenine dinucleotide phosphate oxidase assembly: Translocation of *p47-phox* and *p67-phox* requires interaction between *p47-phox* and cytochrome b_{558}. J Clin Invest. 1991;87:352–356.
136. Nauseef WM, Volpp BD, McCormick S, et al. Assembly of the neutrophil respiratory burst oxidase: Protein kinase C promotes cytoskeletal and membrane association of cytosolic oxidase components. J Biol Chem. 1991:266:5911–5917.
137. Nauseef WM, McCormick S, Renee J, et al. Functional domain in an arginine-rich carboxyl-terminal region of p47phox. J Biol Chem. 1993:268:23646–23651.
138. Rotrosen D, Kleinberg ME, Nunoi H, et al. Evidence for a functional cytoplasmic domain of phagocyte oxidase cytochrome b558. J Biol Chem. 1990:265:8745–8750.
139. Kleinberg ME, Mital D, Rotrosen D, et al. Characterization of a phagocyte cytochrome b_{558} 91-kilodalton subunit functional domain: Identification of peptide sequence and amino acids essential for activity. Biochemistry. 1992:31:2686–2690.
140. Schoedon G, Schneemann M, Walter R, et al. Nitric oxide and infection: Another view. Clin Infect Dis. 1995;21(Suppl 2):S152–S157.
141. DeLeo FR, Yu L, Burritt JB, et al. Mapping sites of interaction of p47-phox and flavocytochrome *b* with random-sequence peptide phage display libraries. Proc Natl Acad Sci U S A. 1995;92:7110–7114.
142. Ren R, Mayer BJ, Cicchetti P, et al. Identification of a ten-amino acid proline-rich SH3 binding site. Science. 1993;259:1157–1161.
143. Pawson T, Schlessinger J. SH2 and SH3 domains. Curr Biol. 1993;3:434–442.
144. McPhail LC. SH3-dependent assembly of the phagocyte NADPH oxidase. J Exp Med. 1994;180:2011–2015.
145. Leto TL, Adams AG, de Mendez I. Assembly of the phagocyte NADPH oxidase: Binding of Src homology 3 domains to proline-rich targets. Proc Natl Acad Sci U S A. 1994;91:10650–10654.
146. Seifert R, Schultz G. Fatty-acid-induced activation of NADPH oxidase in plasma membranes of human neutrophils depends on neutrophil cytosol and is potentiated by stable guanine nucleotides. Eur J Biochem. 1987;162:563–569.
147. Gabig TG, English D, Akard LP, et al. Regulation of neutrophil NADPH oxidase activation in a cell-free system by guanine nucleotides and fluoride. J Biol Chem. 1987;262:1685–1690.
148. Abo A, Pick E, Hall A, et al. Activation of the NADPH oxidase involves the small GTP-binding protein $p21^{rac1}$. Nature. 1991;353:668–670.
149. Abo A, Pick E. Purification and characterization of a third cytosolic component of the superoxide-generating NADPH oxidase of macrophages. J Biol Chem. 1991;266:23577–23585.
150. Knaus UG. Heyworth PG, Evans T, et al. Regulation of phagocyte oxygen radical production by the GTP-binding protein Rac 2. Science. 1991;254:1512–1515.
151. Knaus UG, Heyworth PG, Kinsella BT, et al. Purification and characterization of Rac 2: A cytosolic GTP-binding protein that regulates human neutrophil NADPH oxidase. J Biol Chem. 1992;267:23575–23582.
152. Kwong CH, Malech HL, Rotrosen D, et al. Regulation of the human neutrophil NADPH oxidase by *rho-* related G-proteins. Biochemistry. 1993;32:5711–5717.
153. Philips MR, Pillinger MH, Staud R, et al. Carboxyl methylation of Ras-related proteins during signal transduction in neutrophils. Science. 1993;259:977–980.
154. Ando S, Kaibuchi K, Sasaki T, et al. Post-translational processing of *rac* p21s is important both for their interaction with the GDP/GTP exchange proteins and for their activation of NADPH oxidase. J Biol Chem. 1992;267:25709–25713.
155. Quinn MT, Evans T, Loetterle LR, et al. Translocation of Rac correlates with NADPH oxidase activation: Evidence for equimolar translocation of oxidase components. J Biol Chem. 1993;268:20983–20987.
156. Abo A, Webb MR, Grogan A, et al. Activation of NADPH oxidase involves the dissociation of $p21^{rac}$ from its inhibitory GDP/GTP exchange protein (rhoGDI) followed by its translocation to the plasma membrane. Biochem J. 1994;298:585–591.
157. Heyworth PG, Bohl BP, Bokoch GM, et al. Rac translocates independently of the neutrophil NADPH oxidase components $p47^{phox}$ and $p67^{phox}$: Evidence for its interaction with flavocytochrome b_{558}. J Biol Chem. 1994;269:30749–30752.
158. Quinn MT, Parkos CA, Walker L, et al. Association of a Ras-related protein with cytochrome b of human neutrophils. Nature. 1989;342:198–200.
159. Bokoch GM, Quilliam LA, Bohl BP, et al. Inhibition of RaplA binding to cytochrome b_{558} of NADPH oxidase by phosphorylation of RaplA. Science. 1991;254:1794–1796.
160. Quinn MT, Mullen ML, Jesaitis AJ, et al. Subcellular distribution of the Rap 1A protein in human neutrophils: Colocalization and cotranslocation with cytochrome b_{559}. Blood. 1992;79:1563–1573.
161. Tsunawaki S, Mizunari H, Nagata M, et al. A novel cytosolic component, $p40^{phox}$, of respiratory burst oxidase associates with $p67^{phox}$ and is absent in patients with chronic granulomatous disease who lack $p67^{phox}$. Biochem Biophys Res Commun. 1994;199:1378–1387.
162. Wientjes FB, Hsuan JJ, Totty NF, et al. p40phox, a third cytosolic component of the activation complex of the NADPH oxidase to contain src homology 3 domains. Biochem J. 1993;296:557–561.
163. Wientjes FB, Panayotou G, Reeves E, et al. Interactions between cytosolic components of the NADPH oxidase: $p40^{phox}$ interacts with both $p67^{phox}$ and $p47^{phox}$. Biochem J. 1996;317:919–924.
164. Sathyamoorthy M, de Mendez I, Adams AG, et al. $p40^{phox}$ down-regulates NADPH oxidase activity through interactions with its SH3 domain. J Biol Chem. 1997;272:9141–9146.
165. Jandl RC, Andre-Schwartz J, Borges-Dubois L, et al. Termination of the respiratory burst in human neutrophils. J Clin Invest. 1978;61:1176.
166. Tapper H. The secretion of preformed granules by macrophages and neutrophils. J Leukoc Biol. 1996;59:613–622.
167. Nüsse O, Serrander L, Lew DP, et al. KH. Ca^{++}-induced exocytosis in individual human neutrophils: High- and low-affinity granule populations and submaximal responses. EMBO J. 1998;17:1279–1288.
168. Nüsse O, Serrander L, Foyouzi-Youssefi R, et al. Store-operated Ca^{++} influx and stimulation of exocytosis in HL-60 granulocytes. J Biol Chem. 1997;272:28360–28363.
169. Tapper H, Grinstein S. Fc receptor-triggered insertion of secretory granules into the plasma membrane of human neutrophils: Selective retrieval during phagocytosis. J Immunol. 1997;159:409–418.
170. Aunis D, Bader M-F. The cytoskeleton as a barrier to exocytosis in secretory cells. J Exp Biol. 1988;139:253–266.
171. Boyles J, Bainton DF. Changes in plasma-membrane-associated filaments during endocytosis and exocytosis in polymorphonuclear leukocytes. Cell. 1981;24:905–914.
172. Allen L-AH, Aderem A. Protein kinase C regulates MARCKS cycling between the plasma membrane and lysosomes in fibroblasts. EMBO J. 1995;14:1109–1120.
173. Allen L-AH, Aderem A. A role for MARCKS, the isozyme of protein kinase C and myosin I in zymosan phagocytosis by macrophages. J Exp Med. 1995;182:829–840.
174. Rosales JL, Ernst JD. Calcium-dependent neutrophil secretion: Characterization and regulation by annexins. J Immunol. 1997;159:6195–6202.
175. Whiteheart SW, Kubalek EW. SNAPs and NSF: General members of the fusion apparatus. Trends Cell Biol. 1995;5:64–68.
176. Brumell JH, Volchuk A, Sengelov H, et al. Subcellular distribution of docking/fusion proteins in neutrophils, secretory cells with multiple exocytic compartments. J Immunol. 1995;155:5750–5759.
177. Hackam DJ, Rotstein OD, Bennett MK, et al. Characterization and subcellular localization of target membrane soluble NSF attachment protein receptors (t-SNAREs) in macrophages: Syntaxins 2, 3, and 4 are present on phagosomal membranes. J Immunol. 1996;156:4377–4383.
178. Blackwood RA, Smolen JE, Tranoue A, et al. Phospholipase D activity facilitates

Ca^{++}-induced aggregation and fusion of complex liposomes. Am J Physiol. 1997;242:C1285.
179. Hessler RJ, Blackwood RA, Brock TG, et al. Identification of glyceraldehyde-3-phosphate dehydrogenase as a Ca^{++}-dependent fusogen in human neutophil cytosol. J Leukoc Biol. 1998;63:331–336.
180. Hackam DJ, Rotstein OD, Zheng WJ, et al. Regulation of phagosomal acidification. Differential targeting of Na^+/H^+ exchangers, Na^+K^+-ATPases, and vacuolar-type H^+-ATPases. J Biol Chem. 1997;272:29810–29820.
181. Nanda A, Brumell JH, Nordström T, et al. Activation of proton pumping in human neutrophils occurs by exocytosis of vesicles bearing vacuolar-type H^+-ATPases. J Biol Chem. 1996;271:15963–15970.
182. Bokoch GM. Chemoattractant signaling and leukocyte activation. Blood. 1995; 86:1649–1660.
183. Berridge MJ. Inositol trisphosphate and calcium signalling. Nature. 1993;361:315–325.
184. Mikoshiba K. Inositol 1,4,5-trisphosphate receptor. Trends Pharmacol Sci. 1993;14:86–89.
185. Putney JW Jr, Bird GSJ. The signal for capacitative calcium entry. Cell. 1993:75:199–201.
186. Dana R, Malech HL, Levy R. The requirement for phospholipase A_2 for activation of the assembled NADPH oxidase in human neutrophils. Biochem J. 1994;297:217–223.
187. Exton JH. New developments in phospholipase D. J Biol Chem. 1997;272:15579–15582.
188. Nahas N, Molski TFP, Fernandez GA, et al. Tyrosine phosphorylation and activation of a new mitogen-activated protein (MAP)-kinase cascade in human neutrophils stimulated with various agonists. Biochem J. 1996;318:247–253.
189. Brummel JH, Grinstein S. Serine/threonine kinase activation in human neutrophils: Relationship to tyrosine phosphorylation. Am J Physiol. 1994;267:C1574–C1581.
190. Downey GP, Butler JR, Tapper H, et al. Importance of MEK in neutrophil microbicidal responsiveness. J Immunol. 1998;160:434–443.
191. Fuortes M, Jin W-W, Nathan C. Adhesion-dependent protein tyrosine phosphorylation in neutrophils treated with tumor necrosis factor. J Cell Biol. 1993;120:777–784.
192. Fernandez R, Suchard SJ. Syk activation is required for spreading and H_2O_2 release in adherent neutrophils. J Immunol. 1998;160:5154–5162.
193. Berton G, Fumagalli L, Laudanna C, et al. β2 Integrin-dependent protein tyrosine phosphorylation and activation of the FGR protein tyrosine kinase in human neutrophils. J Cell Biol. 1994;126:1111–1121.
194. Greenberg S, Chang P, Silverstein SC. Tyrosine phosphorylation is required for Fc receptor-mediated phagocytosis in mouse macrophages. J Exp Med. 1993;177:529–534.
195. Dusi S, Donimi M, Della-Bianca V, et al. In human neutrophils the binding of immunocomplexes induces the tyrosine phosphorylation of Fc gamma RII but this phosphorylation is not an essential signal for Fc-mediated phagocytosis. Biochem Biophys Res Commun. 1994;201:30–37.
196. Al-Shami A, Bourgoin SG, Naccache PH. Granulocyte-macrophage colony-stimulating factor-activated signaling pathways in human neutrophils: 1. Tyrosine phosphorylation-dependent stimulation of phosphotidylinositol 3-kinase and inhibition by phorbol esters. Blood. 1997;89:1035–1044.
197. Fialkow L, Chan CK, Grinstein S, et al. Regulation of tyrosine phosphorylation in neutrophils by the NADPH oxidase: Role of reactive oxygen intermediates. J Biol Chem. 1993;268:17131–17137.
198. Krump E, Nikitas K, Grinstein S. Induction of tyrosine phosphorylation and NA^+/H^+ exchanger activation during shrinkage of human neutrophils. J Biol Chem. 1997;272:17303–17311.
199. Hidari KI, Weyrich AS, Zimmerman GA, et al. Engagement of P-selectin glycoprotein ligand-1 enhances tyrosine phosphorylation and activates integrin-activated protein kinase in human neutrophils. J Biol Chem. 1997;272:28750–28756.
200. Bender JG, McPhail LC, Van Epps DE. Exposure of human neutrophils to chemotactic factors potentiates activation of the respiratory burst enzyme. J Immunol. 1983:130:2316–2323.
201. DeLeo FR, Renee J, McCormick S, et al. Neutrophils exposed to bacterial lipopolysaccharide up-regulate NADPH oxidase assembly. J Clin Invest. 1998;101:455–463.
202. Klebanoff SJ. Myeloperoxidase: Occurrence and biological function. In: Everse J, Everse K, Grisham M, eds. Peroxidases in Chemistry and Biology. Boca Raton, Fla: CRC Press; 1991:1–36.
203. Klebanoff SJ. Antimicrobial mechanisms in neutrophilic PMN leukocytes. Semin Hematol. 1975;12:117.
204. Hurst JK. Myeloperoxidase: Active site structure and catalytic mechanisms. In: Everse J, Everse KE, Grisham MB, eds. Peroxidases in Chemistry and Biology. Boca Raton, Fla: CRC Press; 1991:37–62.
205. Jiang Q, Griffin DA, Barofsky DF, et al. Intraphagosomal chlorination dynamics and yields determinded using unique fluorescent bacterial mimics. Chem Res Toxicol. 1997;10:1080–1089.
206. Hazen SL, Hsu FF, Mueller DM, et al. Human neutrophils employ chlorine gas as an oxidant during phagocytosis. J Clin Invest. 1996;98:1283–1289.
207. Hazen SL, Hsu FF, Duffin K, et al. Molecular chlorine generated by the myeloperoxidase-hydrogen peroxide-chloride system of phagocytes converts low density lipoprotein cholesterol into a family of chlorinated sterols. J Biol Chem. 1996;271:23080–23088.
208. Jacob JS, Cistola DP, Hsu FF, et al. Human phagocytes employ the myeloperoxidase-hydrogen peroxide system to synthesize dityrosine, trityrosine, pulcherosine, and isodityrosine by a tyrosyl radical-dependent pathway. J Biol Chem. 1996;271:19950–19956.
209. Eiserich JP, Hristova M, Cross CE, et al. Formation of nitric oxide-derived inflammatory oxidants by myeloperoxidase in neutrophils. Nature. 1998;391:393–397.
210. Rosen H, Michel BR, VanDevanter DR at al. Differential effects of myeloperoxidase-derived oxidants on *Escherichia coli* DNA replication. Infect Immun. 1998;66:2655–2659.
211. Rakita RM, Michel BR, Rosen H. Differential inactivation of *Escherichia coli* membrane dehydrogenases by a myeloperoxidase-mediated antimicrobial system. Biochemistry. 1990:29:1075–1080.
212. Rosen H, Orman J, Rakita RM, et al. Loss of DNA-membrane interactions and cessation of DNA synthesis in myeloperoxidase-treated *Escherichia coli*. Proc Natl Acad Sci U S A. 1990;87:10048–10052.
213. Rakita RM, Rosen H. Penicillin-binding protein inactivation by human neutrophil myeloperoxidase. J Clin Invest. 1991;88:750–754.
214. Rakita RM, Michel BR, Rosen H. Myeloperoxidase-mediated inhibition of microbial respiration: Damage to *Escherichia coli* ubiquinol oxidase. Biochemistry. 1989:28:3031–3036.
215. Hurst JK, Barrette WC Jr, Michel BR, et al. Hypochlorous acid and myeloperoxidase-catalyzed oxidation of iron-sulfur clusters in bacterial respiratory dehydrogenases. Eur J Biochem. 1991;202:1275–1282.
216. Rosen H, Klebanoff SJ. Oxidation of microbial iron-sulfur centers by the myeloperoxidase-H_2O_2-halide antimicrobial system. Infect Immun. 1985;47:613–618.
217. Thomas EL, Jefferson MM, Grisham MB. Myeloperoxidase-catalyzed incorporation of amines into proteins: Role of hypochlorous acid and dichloramines. Biochemistry. 1982;24:6299–6308.
218. Klebanoff SJ. Oxygen-dependent cytotoxic mechanisms of phagocytes. Adv Host Defense Mech. 1982;1:111.
219. Berliner JA, Heinecke JW. The role of oxidized lipoproteins in atherogenesis. Free Radic Biol Med. 1996;20:707–727.
220. Hazen SL, Heinecke JW. 3-Chlorotyrosine, a specific marker of myeloperoxidase-catalyzed oxidation, is markedly elevated in low density lipoprotein isolated from human atherosclerotic intima. J Clin Invest. 1997;99:2075–2081.
221. Daugherty A, Dunn JL, Rateri DL, et al. Myeloperoxidase, a catalyst for lipoprotein oxidation, is expressed in human atherosclerotic lesions. J Clin Invest. 1994;94:437–444.
222. Mandell GL. Catalase, superoxide dismutase, and virulence of *S. aureus*. J Clin Invest. 1975:55:561.
223. Cohen MS, Britigan BE, Hassett DJ, et al. Phagocytes, O_2 reduction, and hydroxyl radical. Rev Infect Dis. 1988;10:1088.
224. Ramos CL, Pou S, Britigan BE, et al. Spin trapping evidence for myeloperoxidase-dependent hydroxyl radical formation by human neutrophils and monocytes. J Biol Chem. 1992;267:8307–8312.
225. Pou S, Cohen MS, Britigan BE, et al. Spin trapping and human neutrophils: Limits of detection of hydroxyl radical. J Biol Chem. 1989;264:12299–12302.
226. Levy O. Antibiotic proteins of polymorphonuclear leukocytes. Eur J Haematol. 1996;56:263–277.
227. Ganz T, Weiss J. Antimicrobial peptides of phagocytes and epithelia. Semin Hematol. 1997;34:343–354.
228. Mandell GL. Bactericidal activity of aerobic and anaerobic polymorphonuclear neutrophils. Infect Immun. 1974;9:337.
229. Mandell GL. Intraphagosomal pH of human polymorphonuclear neutrophils. Proc Soc Exp Biol Med. 1970;134:447.
230. Lehrer RI, Ganz T, Selsted ME. Defensins: Endogenous antibiotic peptides of animal cells. Cell. 1991;64:229–230.
231. Lehrer RI, Lichtenstein AK, Ganz T. Defensins: Antimicrobial and cytotoxic peptides of mammalian cells. Annu Rev Immunol. 1993;11:105–128.
232. Ouellette AJ, Miller SI, Henschen AH, et al. Purification and primary structure of murine cryptdin-l, a Paneth cell defensin. FEBS Lett. 1992;304:146–148.
233. Selsted ME, Miller SI, Henschan AH, et al. Enteric defensins: Antibiotic peptide components of intestinal host defense. J Cell Biol. 1992;118:929–936.
234. Valore EV, Park CH, Quayle AJ, et al. Human β-defensin-1: An antimicrobial peptide of urogenital tissues. J Clin Invest. 1998;101:1633–1642.
235. Hoffmann JA, Hetru C. Insect defensins: Inducible antibacterial peptides. Immunol Today. 1992;13:411–415.
236. Hill CP, Yee J, Selsted ME, et al. Crystal structure of defensin HNP-3, an amphiphilic dimer: Mechanisms of membrane permeabilization. Science. 1991;251:1481–1485.
237. Zhang X-L, Selsted ME, Pardi A. NMR studies of defensin antimicrobial peptides: 1. Resonance assignment and secondary structure determination of rabbit NP-2 and human HNP-1. Biochemistry. 1992;31:11348–11356.
238. Pardi A, Zhang X-L, Selsted ME, et al. NMR studies of defensin antimicrobial peptides: 2. Three-dimensional structures of rabbit NP-2 and human HNP-I. Biochemistry. 1992;31:11357–11364.
239. Elsbach P, Weiss J. Oxygen-independent bactericidal systems of polymorphonuclear leukocytes. In: Weissmann G, ed. Advances in Inflammation Research, v. 2. New York: Raven; 1981:95.
240. Ooi CE, Weiss J, Elsbach P, et al. A 25-kD NH2-terminal fragment carries all the antibacterial activities of the human neutrophil 60-kD bactericidal/permeability-increasing protein. J Biol Chem. 1987;262:14891.
241. Tobias PS, Soldau K, Iovine NM, et al. Lipopolysaccharide (LPS)–binding proteins BPI and LBP form different types of complexes with LPS. J Biol Chem. 1997;272:18682–18685.
242. Weiss J, Elsbach P, Shu C, et al. Human bactericidal/permeability-increasing

protein and a recombinant NH-terminal fragment cause killing of serum-resistant gram-negative bacteria in whole blood and inhibit tumor necrosis factor release induced by the bacteria. J Clin Invest. 1992;90:1122–1130.
243. Giroir BP, Quint PA, Barton P, et al. Preliminary evaluation of recombinant amino-terminal fragment of human bactericidal/permeability-increasing protein in children with severe meningococcal sepsis. Lancet. 1997;350:1439–1443.
244. Oram JD, Reiter B. Inhibition of bacteria by lactoferrin and other iron-chelating agents. Biochim Biophys Acta. 1968;170:351.
245. Boxer LA, Coates TD, Haak RA, et al. Lactoferrin deficiency associated with altered granulocyte function. N Engl J Med. 1982;387:404.
246. Broxmeyer HE, Smithyman A, Eger RR, et al. Identification of lactoferrin as the granulocyte-derived inhibitor of colony-stimulating activity production. J Exp Med. 1978;148:1052.
247. Kijlstra A, Jeurissen HM. Modulation of classical C3 convertase of complement by tear lactoferrin. Immunology. 1982;47:263.
248. Shafer WM, Martin LE, Spitznagel JK. Cationic antimicrobial proteins isolated from human neutrophil granulocytes in the presence of diisopropyl flurophosphate. Infect Immun. 1984;45:29.
249. Shafer WM, Martin LE, Spitznagel JK. Late intraphagosomal hydrogen ion concentration favors the in vitro antimicrobial capacity of a 37-kilodalton cationic granule protein of human neutrophil granulocytes. Infect Immun. 1986;53:651.
250. Levy O, Weiss J, Zarember K, et al. Antibacterial 15-kDa protein isoforms (p15s) are members of a novel family of leukocyte proteins. J Biol Chem. 1993;268:6058–6063.
251. Campanelli D, Detmers PA, Nathan CF, et al. Azurocidin and a homologous serine protease from neutrophils: Differential antimicrobial and proteolytic properties. J Clin Invest. 1990;85:904–915.
252. Selsted ME, Novotny MJ, Morris WL, et al. Indolicidin, a novel bactericidal tridecapeptide amide from neutrophils. J Biol Chem. 1992;267:4292–4295.
253. Zanetti M, Gennaro R, Romeo D. Cathelicidins: A novel protein family with a common proregion and a variable C-terminal antimicrobial domain. FEBS Lett. 1996;374:1–5.
254. Finlay BB, Cossart P. Exploitation of mammalian host cell functions by bacterial pathogens. Science. 1997;276:718–725.
255. Theriot JA. The cell biology of infection by intracellular bacterial pathogens. Annu Rev Cell Dev Biol. 1995;11:213–239.
256. Vlavidia RH, Falkow S. Probing bacterial gene expression within host cells. Trends Microbiol. 1997;5:360–363.
257. Guiney DG. Regulation of bacterial virulence gene expression by the host environment. J Clin Invest. 1998;99:565–569.
258. Virgi M, Makepeace K, Ferguson DJ, et al. Carcinoembryonic antigens (CD66) on epithelial cells and neutrophils and receptor for Opa proteins of pathogenic neisseriae. Mol Microbiol. 1996;22:941–950.
259. Monack DM, Mecsas J, Ghori J, et al. Yersinia signals macrophages to undergo apoptosis and YopJ is necessary for this cell death. Proc Natl Acad Sci U S A. 1997;94:10385–10390.
260. Ginsel LA, Onderwater JJM, Fransen JAM, et al. Localization of the low-M_r subunit of cytochrome b_{558} in human blood phagocytes by immunoelectron microscopy. Blood. 1990;76:2105–2116.
261. Sory MP, Boland A, Lambermont I, et al. Identification of the YopE and YopH domains required for secretion and internalization into the cytosol of macrophages, using cyaA gene fusion approach. Proc Natl Acad Sci U S A. 1995;92:11198–12002.
262. Yang Z, Delgado R, Xu L, et al. Distinct cellular interactions of secreted and transmembrane ebola virus glycoproteins. Science. 1998;279:1034–1037.
263. Sturgill-Koszycki S, Schlesinger PH, Chakraborty P, et al. Lack of acidification in *Mycobacterium* phagosomes produced by exclusion of the vesicular proton-ATPase. Science. 1994;263:678–681.
264. Barker LP, George KM, Falkow S, et al. Differential trafficking of live and dead *Mycobacterium marinum* organisms in macrophages. Infect Immun. 1997;65:1504.
265. Hackstadt T, Scidmore MA, Rockey DD. Lipid metabolism in *Chlamydia trachomatis*–infected cells: Directed trafficking of Golgi-derived sphingolipids to the chlamydial inclusion. Proc Natl Acad Sci U S A. 1995;92:4877–4881.
266. Russell DG, Xu S, Chakraborty P. Intracellular trafficking and the parisitophorous vacuole of *Leishmania mexicana*–infected macrophages. J Cell Sci. 1992;103:1193–1210.
267. Antoine JC, Prina E, Jovanne C, et al. Parasitophorous vacuoles of *Leishmania amazonensis*–infected macrophages maintain an acidic pH. Infect Immun. 1990;58:779–787.
268. Garcia-del Portillo F, Finlay BB. The varied lifestyles of intracellular pathogens within eukaryotic vacuolar compartments. Trends Microbiol. 1995;3:373–380.
269. Malech HL, Gallin JI. Neutrophils in human diseases. N Engl J Med. 1987;317:687.
270. Bodey GP, Buckley M, Sathe YS, et al. Quantitative relationship between circulating leukocytes and infection in patients with acute leukemia. Ann Intern Med. 1966;64:328.
271. Dale DC. Immune and idiopathic neutropenia. Curr Opin Hematol. 1998;5:33–36.
272. Scadden DT. The clinical applications of colony-stimulating factors in acquired immunodeficiency syndrome. Semin Hematol. 1992;29(Suppl 3):33–57.
273. Allen RC, Stevens PR, Price TH, et al. In vivo effects of recombinant human granulocyte colony-stimulating factor on neutrophil oxidative functions in normal human volunteers. J Infect Dis. 1997;175:1184–1192.
274. Dong F, Hoefsloot LH, Schelen AM, et al. Identification of a nonsense mutation in the granulocyte-colony-stimulating factor receptor in severe congenital neutropenia. Proc Natl Acad Sci U S A. 1994;91:4480–4484.
275. Avalos BR. The granulocyte colony-stimulating factor receptor and its role in disorders of granulopoiesis. Leuk Lymphoma. 1998;28:265–273.
276. Hammond WP, Price TH, Souza LM, et al. Treatment of cyclic neutropenia with granulocyte colony-stimulating factor. N Engl J Med. 1989;320:1306–1311.
277. Wright DG, Fauci AS, Dale DC, et al. Correction of human cyclic neutropenia with prednisolone. N Engl J Med. 1978;298:295.
278. Anderson DC, Springer TA. Leukocyte adhesion deficiency: An inherited defect in the Mac-l, LFA-1, and p150,95 glycoproteins. Annu Rev Med. 1987;38:1975–1994.
279. Etzioni A, Frydman M, Pollack S, et al. Recurrent severe infections caused by a novel leukocyte adhesion deficiency. N Engl J Med. 1992;327:1789–1792.
280. von Andrian UH, Berger EM, Ramezani L, et al. In vivo behavior of neutrophils from two patients with distinct inherited leukocyte adhesion deficiency syndromes. J Clin Invest. 1993;91:2893–2897.
281. Anderson DC, Schmalsteig FC, Finegold MJ, et al. The severe and moderate phenotypes of heritable Mac-l, LFA-I deficiency: Their quantitative definition and relation to leukocyte dysfunction and clinical features. J Infect Dis. 1985;152:668.
282. Nauseef WM, de Alarcon P, Bale JF, et al. Aberrant activation and regulation of the oxidative burst in neutrophils with Mo-1 glycoprotein deficiency. J Immunol. 1986;137:636.
283. Springer TA, Thompson WS, Miller LJ, et al. Inherited deficiency of the Mac-l, LFA-1, p150,95 glycoprotein family and its molecular basis. J Exp Med. 1984;160:1901.
284. Kishimoto TK, Hollander N, Roberts TM, et al. Heterogeneous mutations in the 13 subunit common to the LFA-1, Mac-l, and p150,95 glycoproteins cause leukocyte adhesion deficiency. Cell. 1987;50:193.
285. Frydman M, Etzioni A, Eidlitz-Markus T, et al. Rambam-Hasharon syndrome of psychomotor retardation, short stature, defective neutrophil motility, and Bombay phenotype. Am J Med Genet. 1992;44:297–302.
286. Karsan A, Cornejo CJ, Winn RK, et al. Leukocyte adhesion deficiency type II is a generalized defect of de novo GDP-fucose biosynthesis. J Clin Invest. 1998;101:2438–2445.
287. Gallin JI. Abnormal phagocyte chemotaxis: Pathophysiology, clinical manifestations, and management of patients. Rev Infect Dis. 1981;3:1196.
288. Van Epps DE, Williams RC. Suppression of leukocyte chemotaxis by human IgA myeloma components. J Exp Med. 1976;144:1227.
289. Perez HD, Lipton M, Goldstein IM. A specific inhibitor of complement (C5)-derived chemotactic activity in serum from patients with systemic lupus erythematosus. J Clin Invest. 1978;62:29.
290. Perez HD, Hooper C, Volanakis J, et al. Specific inhibitor of complement derived chemotactic activity in systemic lupus erythematosus related antigenically to the Bb fragment of human factor B. J Immunol. 1987;139:484.
291. Clark RA, Page RC, Wilde G. Defective neutrophil chemotaxis in juvenile periodontis. Infect Immun. 1977;18:694.
292. Van Dyke TE. Role of the neutrophil in oral disease: Receptor deficiency in leukocytes from patients with juvenile periodontitis. Rev Infect Dis. 1985;7:419.
293. Perez HD, Kelly E, Elfman F, et al. Defective polymorphonuclear leukocyte formyl peptide receptor(s) in juvenile periodontitis. J Clin Invest. 1991;87:971–976.
294. Shurin SB, Socransky SS, Sweeney E, et al. A neutrophil disorder induced by capnocytophaga: A dental micro-organism. N Engl J Med. 1979;301:849.
295. Kramer N, Perez HD, Goldstein IM. An immunoglobulin (IgG) inhibitor of polymorphonuclear leukocyte motility in a patient with recurrent infection. N Engl J Med. 1980;303:1253.
296. Barrat FJ, Auloge L, Pastural E, et al. Genetic and physical mapping of the Chédiak-Higashi syndrome on chromosome 1q42-43. Am J Hum Genet. 1996;59:625–632.
297. Faigle W, Raposo G, Tenza D, et al. Deficient peptide loading and MHC class II endosomal sorting in a human genetic immunodeficiency disease: the Chédiak-Higashi syndrome. J Cell Biol. 1998;141:1121–1134.
298. Clark RA, Kimball HR. Defective granulocyte chemotaxis in the Chédiak-Higashi syndrome. J Clin Invest. 1971;50:2645.
299. Root RK, Rosenthal AS, Balestra DJ. Abnormal bactericidal, metabolic, and lysosomal functions of Chédiak-Higashi syndrome leukocytes. J Clin Invest. 1972;51:649.
300. Spritz RA. Genetic defects in Chédiak-Higashi syndrome and the beige mouse. J Clin Immunol. 1998;18:97–105.
301. Barbosa MDFS, Nguyen QA, Tchernev VT, et al. Identification of the homologous beige and Chédiak-Higashi syndrome genes. Nature. 1996;382:262–265.
302. Nagle DL, Karim MA, Woolf EA, et al. Identification and mutation analysis of the complete gene for Chédiak-Higashi syndrome. Nat Genet. 1996;14:307–311.
303. Haddad E, Le Deist F, Blanche S, et al. Treatment of Chédiak-Higashi syndrome by allogenic bone marrow transplantation: Report of 10 cases. Blood. 1995;85:3328–3333.
304. Davis SD, Schaller J, Wedgwood RJ. Job's syndrome: Recurrent "cold" staphylococcal abscesses. Lancet. 1966;1:1013.
305. Donabedian H, Gallin JI. The hyperimmunoglobulinemia E recurrent-infection (Job's) syndrome. Medicine (Baltimore). 1983;62:195.
306. Donabedian H, Gallin JI. Mononuclear cells from patients with the hyperimmunoglobulinemia E recurrent infection syndrome produce an inhibitor of leukocyte chemotaxis. J Clin Invest. 1982;69:1155.
307. Dreskin SC, Goldsmith PK, Strober W, et al. Metabolism of immunoglobulin E in patients with markedly elevated serum immunoglobulin E levels. J Clin Invest. 1987;79:1764.
308. Dreskin SC, Goldsmith PK, Gallin JI. Immunoglobulins in the hyperimmunoglobulin E and recurrent infection (Job's) syndrome. J Clin Invest. 1985;75:26.
309. Donabedian H, Alling DW, Gallin JI. Levamisole is inferior to placebo in the

hyperimmunoglobulin E recurrent-infection (Job's) syndrome. N Engl J Med. 1982;307:290.

310. Ottonello L, Daprio P, Pastorino G, et al. Neutrophil dysfunction and increased susceptibility to infection. Eur J Clin Invest. 1998;19:434.
311. Craddock PR, Yawata P, Van Santen L, et al. Acquired phagocyte dysfunction: A complication of the hypophosphatemia of parenteral hyperalimentation. N Engl J Med. 1974;290:1403.
312. Bisno AL, Freeman JC. The syndrome of asplenia, pneumococcal sepsis, and disseminated intravascular coagulation. Ann Intern Med. 1970;72:389.
313. Miller ME, Seals J, Kaye R, et al. A familial, plasma associated defect of phagocytosis: A new cause of recurrent bacterial infections. Lancet. 1968;2:60–63.
314. Super M, Thiel S, Lu J, et al. Association of low levels of mannan-binding protein with a common defect of opsonisation. Lancet. 1989;1236–1239.
315. Turner MW, Seymour ND, Kazatchkine MD, et al. Suboptimal C3b/C3bi deposition and defective yeast opsonization: I. Evidence for the absence of essential cofactor activity. Clin Exp Immunol. 1985;62:427–434.
316. Super M, Levinsky RJ, Turner MW. The level of mannan-binding protein regulates the binding of complement-derived opsonins to mannan and zymosan at low serum concentrations. Clin Exp Immunol. 1990;79:144–150.
317. Garred P, Thiel S, Madsen HO, et al. Gene frequency and partial protein characterization of an allelic variant of mannan binding protein associated with low serum concentrations. Clin Exp Immunol. 1992;90:517–521.
318. Malech HL, Nauseef WM. Primary inherited defects in neutrophil function: Etiology and treatment. Semin Hematol. 1997;34:279–290.
319. Forehand JR, Nauseef WM, Curnutte JT, et al. Inherited disorders of phagocyte killing. In: Scriver CR, Beaudet AL, Sly WS, et al, eds. The Metabolic and Molecular Bases of Inherited Disease. 7th ed. New York: McGraw-Hill; 1995;3995–4026.
320. Curnutte JT. Chronic granulomatous disease: The solving of a clinical riddle at the molecular level. Clin Immunol Immunopathol. 1993;67:S2–S15.
321. Casimir C, Chetty M, Bohler M-C, et al. Identification of the defective NADPH-oxidase component in chronic granulomatous disease: A study of 57 European families. Eur J Clin Invest. 1992;22:403–406.
322. Dinauer MC, Orkin SH. Chronic granulomatous disease. Annu Rev Med. 1992;43:117–124.
323. Meischl C, Roos D. The molecular basis for chronic granulomatous disease. Springer Semin Immunopathol. 1998;19:417–434.
324. Bromberg Y, Pick E. Activation of NADPH-dependent superoxide production in a cell-free system by sodium dodecyl sulfate. J Biol Chem. 1985;260:13539–13545.
325. Heyneman RA, Vercauteren RE. Activation of a NADPH-dependent oxidase from horse polymorphonuclear leukocytes in a cell-free system. J Leukocyte Biol. 1984;36:751–759.
326. Royer-Pokora B, Kunkel LM, Monaco AP, et al. Cloning the gene for an inherited human disorder—chronic granulomatous disease—on the basis of its chromosomal location. Nature. 1986;322:32–38.
327. Rae J, Newburger PE, Dinauer MC, et al. X-linked chronic granulomatous disease: Mutations in the CYBB gene encoding the gp91-*phox* component of the respiratory burst oxidase. Am J Hum Genet. 1998;62:1320–1331.
328. Heyworth PG, Curnutte JT, Noack D, et al. Hematologically important mutations: X-linked chronic granulomatous disease, an update. Blood Cells Mol Dis. 1997;23:443–450.
329. Parkos CA, Dinauer MC, Jesaitis AJ, et al. Absence of both the 91 kD and 22 kD subunits of human neutrophil cytochrome b in two genetic forms of chronic granulomatous disease. Blood. 1989;73:1416–1420.
330. Dinauer MC, Curnutte JT, Rosen H, et al. A missense mutation in the cytochrome b heavy chain in cytochrome-positive X-linked chronic granulomatous disease. J Clin Invest. 1989;84:2012–2016.
331. Dinauer MC, Pierce EA; Erickson RW, et al. Point mutation in the cytoplasmic domain of the neutrophil *p22-phox* cytochrome b subunit is associated with a nonfunctional NADPH oxidase and chronic granulomatous disease. Proc Natl Acad Sci U S A. 1991;88:11231–11235.
332. Clark RA, Malech HL, Gallin JI, et al. Genetic variants of chronic granulomatous disease: Prevalence of deficiencies of two cytosolic components of the NADPH oxidase system. N Engl J Med. 1989;321:647–652.
333. Casimir CM, Bu-Ghanim HN, Rodaway ARF, et al. Autosomal recessive chronic granulomatous disease caused by deletion at a dinucleotide repeat. Proc Natl Acad Sci U S A. 1991;88:2753–2757.
334. Volpp BD, Lin Y. In vitro molecular reconstitution of the respiratory burst in B lymphoblasts from *p47-phox-deficient* chronic granulomatous disease. J Clin Invest. 1993;91:201–207.
335. Gorlach A, Lee PL, Roesler J, et al. A p47-*phox* pseudogene carries the most common mutation causing p47-*phox*-deficient chronic granulomatous disease. J Clin Invest. 1997;100:1907–1918.
336. Bonnizzato A, Russo MP, Donini M, et al. Identification of a double mutation (D160V-K161E) in the p67*phox* gene of a chronic granulomatous disease patient. Biochem Biophys Res Commun. 1997;231:861–863.
337. Leusen JHW, De Klein A, Hilarius PM, et al. Disturbed interaction of p21-*rac* with mutated p67-*phox* causes chronic granulomatous disease. J Exp Med. 1996;184:1243–1249.
338. Clark RA, Klebanoff SJ. Chronic granulomatous disease: Studies of a family with impaired neutrophil chemotactic, metabolic and bactericidal function. Am J Med. 1978;65:941–948.
339. Schapiro BL, Newburger PE, Klempner MS, et al. Chronic granulomatous disease presenting in a 69-year-old man. N Engl J Med. 1991;325:1786–1790.
340. Chang YC, Segal BH, Holland SM, et al. Virulence of catalase-deficient *Aspergillus nidulans* in p47$^{phox-/-}$ mice. J Clin Invest. 1998;101:1843–1850.
341. Aliabadi H, Gonzalez R, Quie PG. Urinary tract disorders in patients with chronic granulomatous disease. N Engl J Med. 1989;321:706–708.
342. Ament ME, Ochs HD. Gastrointestinal manifestations of chronic granulomatous disease. N Engl J Med. 1973;288:382–387.
343. Sillevis Smitt JH, Weening RS, Krieg SR, et al. Discoid lupus erythematosus-like lesions in carriers of X-linked chronic granulomatous disease. Br J Dermatol. 1990;122:643–650.
344. Gallin JI, Buescher ES, Seligmann BE, et al. Recent advances in chronic granulomatous disease. Ann Intern Med. 1983;99:657–674.
345. Sechler JMG, Malech HL, White CJ, et al. Recombinant human interferon-reconstitutes defective phagocyte function in patients with chronic granulomatous disease of childhood. Proc Natl Acad Sci U S A. 1988;85:4874–4878.
346. Ezekowitz RAB, Orkin SH, Newburger PE. Recombinant interferon gamma augments phagocyte superoxide production and X-chronic granulomatous disease gene expression in X-linked variant chronic granulomatous disease. J Clin Invest. 1987;80:1009–1016.
347. Ezekowitz RAB, Dinauer MC, Jaffee HS, et al. Partial correction of the phagocyte defect in patients with X-linked chronic granulomatous disease by subcutaneous interferon gamma. N Engl J Med. 1988;319:146–151.
348. Woodman RC, Erickson RW, Rae J, et al. Prolonged recombinant interferon-gamma therapy in chronic granulomatous disease: Evidence against enhanced neutrophil oxidase activity. Blood. 1992;79:1558–1562.
349. Newburger PE, Ezekowitz RAB. Cellular and molecular effects of recombinant interferon gamma in chronic granulomatous disease. Hematol Oncol Clin North Am. 1988;2:267–276.
350. Calvino MC, Maldonado MS, Otheo E, et al. Bone marrow transplantation in chronic granulomatous disease. Eur J Pediatr. 1996;155:877–879.
351. Sekhsaria S, Gallin JI, Linton GF, et al. Peripheral blood progenitors as a target for genetic correction of p47^{phox}-deficient chronic granulomatous disease. Proc Natl Acad Sci U S A. 1993;90:7446–7450.
352. Weil WM, Linton GF, Whiting-Theobald N, et al. Genetic correction of p67^{phox} deficient chronic granulomatous disease using peripheral blood progenitor cells as a target for retrovirus mediated gene transfer. Blood. 1997;89:1754–1761.
353. Malech HL, Maples PB, Whiting-Theobald N, et al. Prolonged production of NADPH oxidase-corrected granulocytes after gene therapy of chronic granulomatous disease. Proc Natl Acad Sci U S A. 1997;94:12133–12138.
354. Malech HL, Bauer TR Jr, Hickstein DD. Prospects for gene therapy for neutrophil defects. Semin Hematol. 1997;34:355–361.
355. Babior GL, Crowley CA. Chronic granulomatous disease and other disorders of killing by phagocytes. In: Steinbury JB, Wyngaarden JB, Frederickson DS, et al, eds. The Metabolic Basis of Inherited Disease. 5th ed. New York: McGraw-Hill; 1983;1969.
356. Parry MF, Root RK, Metcalf JA, et al. Myeloperoxidase deficiency: Prevalance and clinical significance. Ann Intern Med. 1981;95:293.
357. Nauseef WM, Cogley M, Bock S, et al. Pattern of inheritance in hereditary myeloperoxidase deficiency associated with the R569W missense mutation. J Leukoc Biol. 1998;63:264–269.
358. Nauseef WM, Olsson I, Strömberg-Arnljots K. Biosynthesis and processing of myeloperoxidase—a marker for myeloid differentiation. Eur J Haematol. 1988;40:97–110.
359. Lehrer RJ, Cline MJ. Leukocyte myeloperoxidase deficiency and disseminated candidiasis: The role of myeloperoxidase in resistance to candida infection. J Clin Invest. 1969;48:1478.
360. Koeffler HP, Ranyard J, Pertcheck M. Myeloperoxidase: Its structure and expression during myeloid differentiation. Blood. 1985;65:484.
361. Nauseef WM. Insights into myeloperoxidase biosynthesis gained from cases of inherited deficiency. J Mol Med. 1998;76:661–668.
362. Gullberg U, Andersson E, Garwicz D, et al. Biosynthesis, processing and sorting of neutrophil proteins: Insight into neutrophil granule development. Eur J Haematol. 1997;58:137–153.
363. Nauseef WM. Myeloperoxidase biosynthesis by a human promyelocytic leukemia cell line: Insight into myeloperoxidase deficiency. Blood. 1986;67:865–872.
364. Nauseef WM. Posttranslational processing of a human myeloid lysosomal protein, myeloperoxidase. Blood. 1987;70:1143–1150.
365. Nauseef WM, McCormick S, Yi H. Roles of heme insertion and the mannose-6-phosphate receptor in processing of the human myeloid lysosomal enzyme, myeloperoxidase. Blood. 1992;80:2622–2633.
366. Nauseef WM, Root RK, Malech HL. Biochemical and immunologic analysis of hereditary myeloperoxidase deficiency. J Clin Invest. 1983;71:1297.
367. Nauseef WM, Brigham S, Cogley M. Hereditary myeloperoxidase deficiency due to a missense mutation of arginine to tryptophan. J Biol Chem. 1994;369:1212–1216.
368. Tobler A, Selsted ME, Miller CW, et al. Evidence for a pretranslational defect in hereditary and acquired myeloperoxidase deficiency. Blood. 1989;73:1980–1986.
369. DeLeo FR, Goedken M, McCormick SJ, et al. A novel form of hereditary myeloperoxidase deficiency linked to endoplasmic reticulum/proteasome degradation. J Clin Invest. 1998;101:2900–2909.
370. Romano M, Dri P, Dadalt L, et al. Biochemical and molecular characterization of hereditary myeloperoxidase deficiency. Blood. 1997;90:4126–4134.
371. Petrides PE. Molecular genetics of peroxidase deficiency. J Mol Med. 1998;76:688–698.
372. Nauseef WM. Myeloperoxidase deficiency. Hematol Oncol Clin North Am. 1988;2:135.
373. Lanza F. Pathology of myeloperoxidase deficiency. J Mol Med. 1998;76:676–681.

374. Kutter, D. Recent developments in myeloperoxidase deficiency. J Mol Med. 1998;76:669–675.
375. Gallin JI. Neutrophil specific granule deficiency. Annu Rev Med. 1985;36:263.
376. Rosenberg HF, Gallin JI. Neutrophil-specific granule deficiency includes eosinophils. Blood. 1993;82:268–273.
377. Ganz T, Metcalf JA, Gallin JI, et al. Microbicidal/cytotoxic proteins of neutrophils are deficient in two disorders: Chédiak-Higashi syndrome and "specific" granule deficiency. J Clin Invest. 1988:82:552–556.
378. Lomax KJ, Gallin JI, Rotrosen D, et al. Selective defect in myeloid cell lactoferrin gene expression in neutrophil specific granule deficiency. J Clin Invest. 1989;83:514–519.
379. Gmumder RK, Seger RA. Chronic granulomatous disease: Mode of action of sulfamethoxazole/trimethoprim. Pediatr Res. 1981;15:1533.
380. Yourtee EL, Root RK. Antibiotic-neutrophil interactions in microbial killing. Adv Host Defense Mech. 1982;1:187.
381. Herzig GP, Graw RG. Granulocyte transfusion for bacterial infections. Prog Hematol. 1975;9:207.
382. Klock JC, Bainton DF. Degranulation and abnormal bactericidal function of granulocytes procured by reversible adhesion to nylon wool. Blood. 1976;48:149.
383. Herzig RH, Herzig GP, Grano RG, et al. Successful granulocyte transfusion therapy for gram-negative septicemia. N Engl J Med. 1977;296:701.
384. Strauss RG, Connett JE, Gale RP, et al. A controlled trial of prophylactic granulocyte transfusions during initial induction chemotherapy for acute myelogenous leukemia. N Engl J Med. 1981:305:597.
385. Winston DJ, Winston GH, Gale RP. Therapeutic granulocyte transfusions for documented infections. Ann Intern Med. 1982:97:509.
386. Alavi JB, Root RK, Djerassi I, et al. A randomized clinical trial of granulocyte transfusions for infections in acute leukemia. N Engl J Med. 1977:296:706.
387. Buescher ES, Gallin JI. Leukocyte transfusion in chronic granulomatous disease. N Engl J Med. 1982;307:800.
388. Young LS. Prophylactic granulocytes in the neutropenic host. Ann Intern Med. 1982;96:240.
389. Wright DG, Robichaud KJ, Pizzo PA, et al. Lethal pulmonary reactions associated with the combined use of amphotericin B and leukocyte transfusions. N Engl J Med. 1981;304:1185.
390. Marsh WL, Oyen R, Nichols ME. K_x antigen, the McLeod phenotype, and chronic granulomatous disease: Further studies. Vox Sang. 1976;31:356.
391. Densen P, Wilkinson-Kroovand S, Mandell GL, et al. K_x: Its relationship to chronic granulomatous disease and genetic linkage with Xg. Blood. 1981;58:34.
392. Frey D, Machler M, Seger R, et al. Gene deletion in a patient with chronic granulomatous disease and McLeod syndrome: Fine mapping of the Xk gene locus. Blood. 1988;71:252.
393. Giblett ER, Klebanoff SJ, Pincus SH, et al. Kell phenotypes in chronic granulomatous disease: A potential transfusion hazard. Lancet. 1971;1:1235.
394. van der Meer JWM, van den Broek PJ. Present status of the management of patients with defective phagocyte function. Rev Infect Dis. 1984;6:107.
395. Weller PF. Human eosinophils. J Allergy Clin Immunol. 1997;100:283–287.
396. Hirai K, Miyamasu M, Takaishi T, et al. Regulation of the function of eosinophils and basophils. Crit Rev Immunol. 1997;17:325–352.
397. Boyce JA. The pathology of eosinophilic inflammation. Allergy Asthma Proc. 1997;18:293–300.
398. Spry CJE. Mechanisms of eosinophilia: V. Kinetics of normal and accelerated eosinopoiesis. Cell Tissue Kinet. 1971:4:351.
399. Sanderson CJ. Interleukin-5, eosinophils, and disease. Blood. 1992:79:3101–3109.
400. Gleich GJ, Adolphson CR, Leiferman KM. The biology of eosinophilic leukocyte. Annu Rev Med. 1993:44:85–101.
401. Kitayama J, Mackay CR, Ponath PD, et al. The C-C chemokine receptor CCR3 participates in stimulation of eosinophil arrest on inflammatory endothelium in shear flow. J Clin Invest. 1998;101:2017–2024.
402. Henderson WR Jr, Chi EY, Albert RK, et al. Blockade of CD49d ($\alpha_4$integrin) on intrapulmonary but not circulating leukocytes inhibits airway inflammation and hyperresponsiveness in a mouse model of asthma. J Clin Invest. 1997;100:3083–3092.
403. Sriramarao P, Von Andrian UH, Butcher EC, et al. L-Selectin and very late antigen-4 integrin promote eosinophil rolling at physiological shear rates in vivo. J Immunol. 1994;153:4238–4246.
404. Henriques GMO, Miotla JM, Cordeiro RSB, et al. Selectins mediate eosinophil recruitment in vivo: A comparison with their role in neutrophil influx. Blood. 1996;87:5297–5304.
405. Nourshargh S. Mechanisms of neutrophil and eosinophil accumulation in vivo. Am Rev Respir Dis. 1993;148:S60–S64.
406. Wardlaw AJ, Walsh GM, Symon FA. Adhesion interactions involved in eosinophil migration through vascular endothelium. Ann N Y Acad Sci. 1996;796:124–137.
407. Dobrina A, Menegazzi R, Carlos TM, et al. Mechanisms of eosinophil adherence to cultured vascular endothelial cells: Eosinophils bind to the cytokine-induced endothelial ligand vascular cell adhesion molecule-1 via the very late activation antigen-4 integrin receptor. J Clin Invest. 1991;88:20–26.
408. David JR, Vadas MA, Butterworth AE, et al. Enhanced helminthotoxic capacity of eosinophils from patients with eosinophilia. N Engl J Med. 1980;303:1147.
409. Mahmoud AAF, Warren KS, Peters PA. A role for the eosinophil in acquired resistance to *Schistosoma mansoni* infection as determined by antieosinophil serum. J Exp Med. 1975;142:805.
410. McLaren DJ, MacKenzie CD, Ramalho-Pinto FJ. Ultrastructural observations on the in vitro interaction between rat eosinophils and some parasitic helminths (*Schistosoma mansoni, Trichinella spiralis* and *Nippostrongylus brasiliensis).* Clin Exp Immunol. 1977;30:105.
411. Densen P, Mahmoud AAF, Sullivan J, et al. Demonstration of eosinophil degranulation on the surface of opsonized schistosomules by phase-contrast cinemicrography. Infect Immun. 1978;22:282.
412. Weller PF, Goetzl EJ. The human eosinophil: Roles in host defense and tissue injury. Am J Pathol. 1980;100:790.
413. Metcalf JA, Gallin JI, Nauseef WM, et al. Laboratory of Neutrophil Function. New York: Raven; 1985.
414. Carulli G. Applications of flow cytometry in the study of human neutrophil biology and pathology. Hematopathol Mol Hematol. 1996;10:39–61.
415. Rest RF. Measurement of human neutrophil respiratory burst activity during phagocytosis of bacteria. Meth Enzymol. 1994;236:119–136.
416. Ochs HD, Igo RP. The nitroblue tetrazolium slide test: A simple screening method for detecting chronic granulomatous disease and female carriers. J Pediatr. 1973;83:77–82.
417. Baehner RL, Nathan DG. Quantitative nitroblue tetrazolium dye test in chronic granulomatous disease. N Engl J Med. 1968;278:971.
418. Allen RC. Phagocytic leukocyte oxygenation activities and chemiluminescence: A kinetic approach to analysis. Methods Enzymol. 1986;133:449–493.

Chapter 9

Cell-Mediated Immunity in Host Defense against Infectious Diseases

RAYMOND M. JOHNSON
ERIC J. BROWN

All organisms have evolved systems for self-defense against pathogens. Bacteria have unique restriction enzyme systems that cleave invading foreign DNA from bacteriophages. In simple metazoans, discrimination between self and nonself is based on molecular pattern recognition and is relatively nonspecific. Invertebrates depend on serum components and phagocytic cells for protection from invading pathogens. Vertebrates have retained the nonspecific defenses in the form of complement, natural killer (NK) cells, and phagocytic leukocytes. These relatively primitive defenses constitute *innate immunity.* In addition to the innate defenses conserved through evolution, mammals have developed a more sophisticated defense system that is capable of identifying and remembering specific pathogens. This defense system, termed *adaptive immunity*, consists of B and T lymphocytes expressing unique receptors that recognize invading pathogens. This more sophisticated defense system evolved in concert with the innate defense system and is intimately enmeshed with it. The combined innate and adaptive immune defenses allow mammals to defend themselves from a plethora of pathogens ranging from microscopic subcellular viruses to macroscopic multicellular nematodes.

Survival of the mammalian host depends on eliminating or at least controlling all pathogens that successfully penetrate the keratinized epithelium of the skin and epithelial tight junctions of the mucosa. Free-living pathogens, including most bacteria, nematodes, flukes, and cestodes, are susceptible to the innate defenses mediated by complement and granulocytes. Adaptive immunity in these infections plays a supportive role, largely through enhancement of innate defenses by the production of pathogen-specific antibodies. Antibodies enhance complement- and granulocyte-mediated killing of invading free-living pathogens. This branch of adaptive immunity is referred to as *humoral immunity.*

We thank Michael B. Brenner, Jerrold J. Ellner, Richard M. Locksley, Juneann W. Murphy, Marion G. Peters, and Arthur Weiss for contributing figures to this project.

A subset of pathogens, including viruses, some bacteria, some protozoans, and some fungi, has evolved to exploit a unique niche within the host, the host cell cytoplasm and intracellular spaces. This group of pathogens effectively evades most of the innate defenses. Complement and granulocytes are unable to kill pathogens that reside within host cells. Pathogen-specific antibodies can do little to enhance the innate defenses in this setting. NK cells have some ability to detect abnormal cells, but their mechanism for recognition is inefficient and often specifically compromised by the invading pathogen. It is for these intracellular pathogens that the adaptive immune system is critical for host survival.

All host cells have a surveillance system that monitors the intracellular compartments. T lymphocytes armed with a unique antigen receptor called the T-cell receptor (TCR) patrol the circulatory system and soft tissues looking for "nonself" presented by this universal surveillance system. T-lymphocyte surveillance is specifically recruited to areas of inflammation caused by pathogenic microbes and the innate defense system. When cells are identified that harbor "nonself" within their cytoplasm, they are lysed by T lymphocytes, thereby exposing the pathogen to antibodies, complement, and granulocytes capable of eliminating it or at least controlling it by the process of granuloma formation. This branch of the adaptive defense system is referred to as *cellular immunity*. In patients with compromised cellular immunity caused by use of immunosuppressive drugs, hematologic malignancies, chemotherapy, congenital abnormalities, or human immunodeficiency virus (HIV) infection, intracellular pathogens become particularly important infectious agents.

ANTIGEN RECOGNITION

The critical initial event in the cellular immune response to an invading pathogen is the recognition of a foreign molecule (antigen) by the TCR. Classically, this event requires a complex interplay between T lymphocytes and antigen-presenting cells (APCs). Most antigens can be recognized by T lymphocytes only when they are dissociated from the invading pathogen, degraded, and complexed with major histocompatibility complex (MHC) glycoproteins on the surface of an APC. In addition to the direct interaction between the TCR and the antigen-MHC complex, further T lymphocyte–APC interactions mediated by accessory molecules are required for optimal T-lymphocyte activation and expansion. The early portion of this chapter outlines the mechanics of cellular immunity as they are understood today. The chapter finishes by integrating clinical infectious disease practice with cellular immunology theory.

MAJOR HISTOCOMPATIBILITY ANTIGENS

The MHC is a family of glycoprotein heterodimers on APCs that is responsible for presenting foreign macromolecules to the TCR. In humans, the MHC genes are referred to as the human leukocyte antigen (HLA) complex and are found on two separate chromosomes. The classic HLA members HLA-A, -B, -C, -D and the nonclassic members HLA-E, -F, and -G are found on chromosome 6. A second family of nonclassic HLA glycoprotein loci, CD1A through CD1E, is found on chromosome 1. MHC-related genes that act as immunoglobulin G (IgG) Fc receptors or that have no characterized or immunologically related functions have been identified but go beyond the scope of this chapter.[1, 2] The murine MHC loci are referred to as the H-2 complex and are found on chromosome 17. The mouse CD1 genes, CD1D1 and CD1D2 (also known as CD1.1 and CD1.2), are located on chromosome 3.

MHC molecules present foreign antigens to T lymphocytes for the purpose of initiating and propagating a cellular immune response. The MHC molecules and types of antigen presentation can be divided into MHC class II, classic MHC class I (class Ia), nonclassic MHC class I (class Ib), and a miscellaneous category for MHC-related molecules such as heat shock proteins (HSPs) that are genetically and functionally related to MHC molecules. Antigen presentation to T lymphocytes occurs through polymorphic and nonpolymorphic MHC molecules. The nonpolymorphic MHC molecules (MHC Ib), present a limited number of foreign macromolecules unique to invading pathogens (danger signals), such as bacterial glycolipids and formylated peptides. In contrast, polymorphic MHC molecules have evolved to present a broad array of antigenic peptides so as to recognize the universe of potential pathogens. The human MHC complex contains six highly polymorphic loci (three MHC II loci and three MHC Ia loci). The high degree of polymorphism in these loci within the population means that most persons are heterozygous (i.e., they carry two nonidentical alleles) for several loci. This maximizes the number of foreign peptides that can be presented to T lymphocytes in any individual host. Antigen presentation by MHC II and MHC Ia molecules are the most thoroughly studied and understood (Figs. 9–1 and 9–2). Because MHC II antigen presentation is critical to the initiation of cellular immune responses, it is discussed first.

Class II

MHC II molecules are heterodimers consisting of an α-chain and a β-chain. Both chains are type I membrane proteins and are members of the immunoglobulin superfamily. Each chain of the heterodimer has two immunoglobulin domains in the extracellular portion of the molecule. The genes for the two chains are tightly linked in three loci designated DP, DR, and DQ in humans (I-A and I-E in mice). The class II region is highly polymorphic in all vertebrates. As of 1997 there were 62 DPβ, 8 DPα, 25 DQβ, 16 DQα, and 122 DRβ alleles.[3] An interesting exception to this high degree of polymorphism is DRα, which is monomorphic. The noncovalently linked 34-kD α- and 29-kD β-chains of MHC II are expressed constitutively on B cells, dendritic cells, macrophages, and thymic epithelial cells and can be induced by interferon gamma (IFN-γ) on others, including endothelial cells, epithelial cells, neurons, glial cells, and fibroblasts.[4–6]

MHC II molecules present peptides derived from exogenous foreign antigens to T lymphocytes. Antigen processing and presentation by the MHC II pathway occurs in an endocytic compartment specialized to degrade macromolecules or pathogens that enter the cell through pinocytosis or receptor-mediated endocytosis. Peptides generated in this compartment are loaded onto resident MHC II molecules for presentation to T lymphocytes. As a general rule, antigens presented by MHC II molecules are extracellular in origin and were not originally synthesized in the host cell cytoplasm.

MHC II αβ heterodimers present unfolded polypeptides ranging from 12 to 25 amino acids in length to the TCR at the surface of the APC.[7] The α_1 and β_1 domains of the αβ heterodimer form a peptide-binding groove or pocket with distinct characteristics and requirements. MHC II polymorphisms are concentrated in the α_1 and β_1 domains. The class II heterodimer peptide pocket is open-ended and can tolerate peptide residues extending beyond the 10- to 12-amino-acid capacity of the peptide-binding groove.[8–14] However, amino acids lying outside the peptide-binding groove do not seem to contribute to T-cell recognition. These amino acids may be removed by exopeptidase activity after the peptide-MHC complex has reached the cell surface without affecting T-cell responses. Although many different peptides are capable of interacting with a particular MHC allele, there is specificity to this interaction. The specificity is determined by the amino acid composition of the peptide-binding groove. The high degree of polymorphism in this region of MHC II molecules increases the diversity of peptides that can be presented as antigens by the population as a whole.

Peptide loading of MHC II molecules occurs predominately in a specialized endocytic compartment called MIIC.[15–19] Newly synthesized class II αβ heterodimers associate with a third peptide, called the *invariant chain*, in the endoplasmic reticulum (ER). The invariant chain serves three functions in MHC II processing. First, association with the invariant chain stabilizes the MHC II heterodimer. Second,

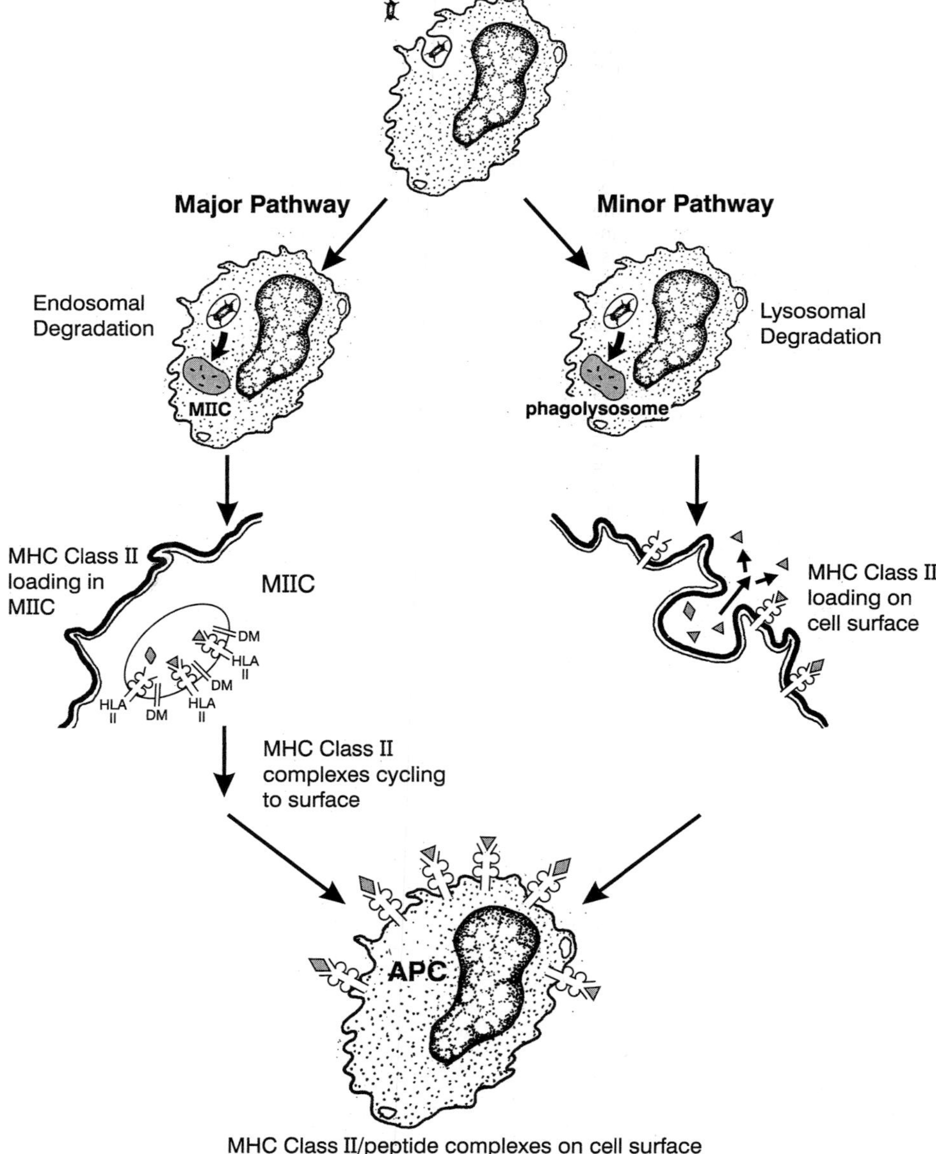

FIGURE 9–1. Pathways for processing and presentation of exogenous antigens by major histocompatibility complex (MHC) class II. The major pathway for MHC class II antigen presentation involves antigen proteolysis in intracellular acidic vacuolar compartments, followed by peptide loading in the MIIC and trafficking of the peptide-loaded MHC molecules to the cell surface, where they can interact with antigen-specific T cells. A minor pathway for class II antigen presentation involves release of antigenic peptides into the extracellular milieu, where they can compete for binding to class II molecules already at the cell surface. The minor pathway for presentation of endogenous antigens by MHC class II is not shown.

a portion of the invariant chain polypeptide, called the class II-associated invariant chain peptide (CLIP), prevents loading of peptide fragments in the ER by occupying the MHC II αβ peptide-binding groove. Third, it functions as a chaperone, guiding newly synthesized MHC II heterodimers from the ER to the MIIC endosomal compartment.[20] In this compartment, exogenous proteins or intact pathogens taken in by pinocytosis or receptor-mediated endocytosis are subjected to low pH, reduction, and proteolysis.[21] Efficient MHC II antigen processing requires an acidic environment and can be blocked by chloroquine, a weak base that prevents acidification of endosomes and the MIIC.[7] Peptides generated in the MIIC are exchanged for the CLIP peptide of the invariant chain. Displacement of the CLIP peptide and loading of exogenous peptides onto MHC II heterodimers is catalyzed by a class II–like molecule called HLA-DM (H2-M in mice).[22, 23] HLA-DM is a heterodimer encoded within the MHC complex near DP, and its synthesis, like that of the MHC II molecules, is stimulated by IFN-γ. Unlike DP, DQ, and DR, HLA-DM is found only in the MIIC.[24] In addition to catalyzing the displacement of the invariant-chain peptide CLIP from MHC II, the HLA-DM molecule is thought to hold MHC II complexes in the MIIC until they are loaded with peptides that form stable complexes.[25]

Loss of invariant chain or HLA-DM (H2-M) function compromises antigen presentation by the MHC II pathway. In the absence of invariant chain, class II heterodimers are retained in the ER and are not efficiently loaded with foreign peptides.[26, 27] Mice deficient in H2-M have normal cell-surface levels of stable class II heterodimers, but the majority of these complexes have CLIP rather than exogenous peptides in the peptide-binding grooves.[28] These mice are unable to present exogenous whole-protein antigens to antigen-specific T cells.[29] Some class II–restricted exogenous antigens are still presented in invariant chain and H2-M knockout mice, suggesting that peptide loading of MHC II αβ heterodimers may occur at a low level by alternative pathways.[30, 31] These pathways may involve regurgitation of peptides after lysosomal degradation and subsequent exchange of those peptides with MHC II–peptide complexes at the cell surface. There is evidence that proteolysis of MHC II–bound peptides continues on the cell surface after the MHC II–peptide complexes leave the endosomal compartment, suggesting that peptide–MHC II complexes exist in a dynamic state at the cell surface.[32]

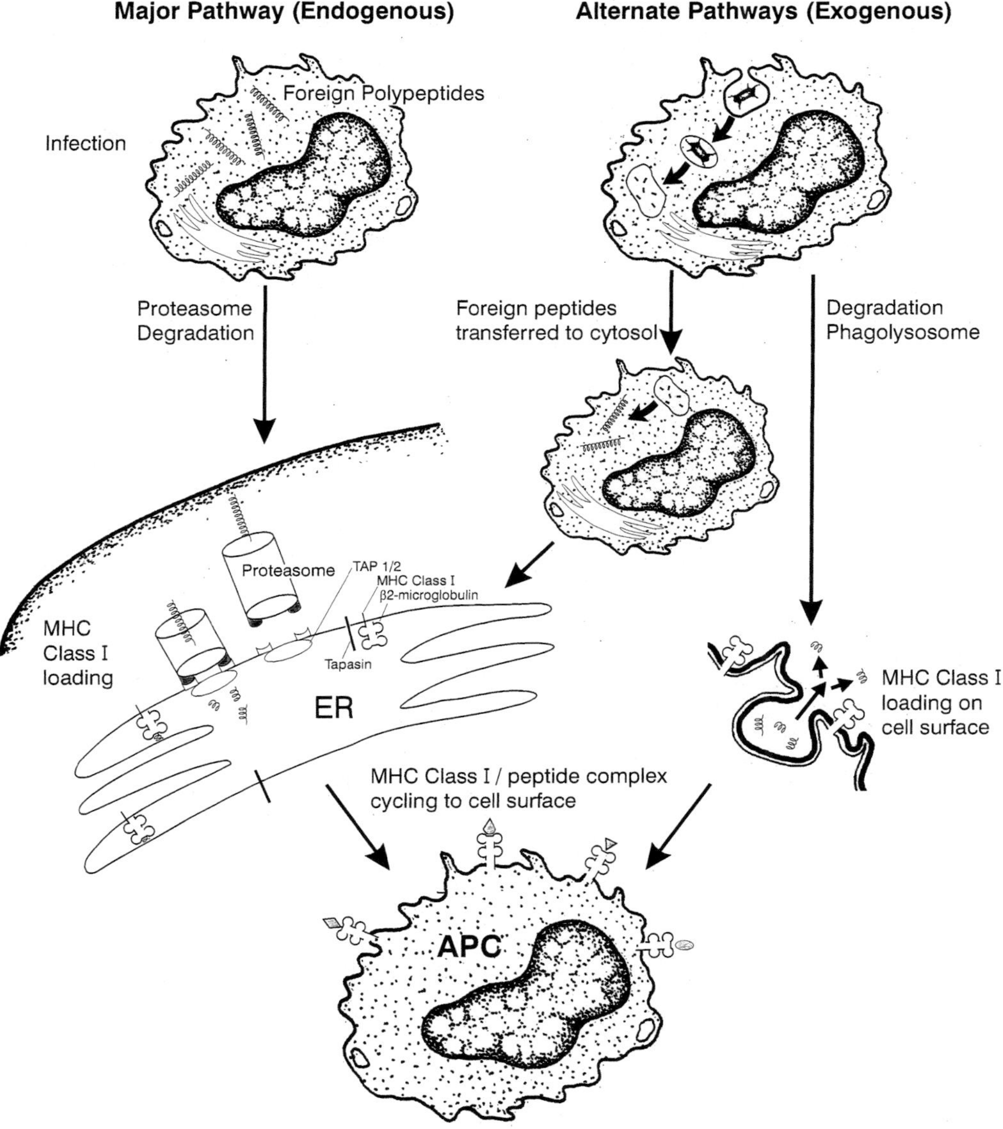

FIGURE 9–2. Pathways for processing and presentation of antigens by major histocompatibility complex (MHC) class I. The major pathway for MHC class I antigen presentation involves proteolysis of endogenous antigens by proteasome complexes in the cytosol, with class I peptide loading in the endoplasmic reticulum (ER). Peptide-bound complexes then traffic to the plasma membrane, where they can interact with antigen-specific T cells. One pathway for MHC class I presentation of proteins in phagocytic vacuoles involves direct transport of these proteins into the host cell cytoplasm, where they can intersect the major pathway. A second pathway involves antigen proteolysis in the phagolysosome, followed by release of peptides into the extracellular milieu, where they can compete for binding to class I molecules already at the cell surface.

Exogenous antigens reach the MIIC via pinocytosis or, more efficiently, via receptor-mediated endocytosis. Receptors known to mediate endocytosis and antigen presentation by MHC II include the B cell antigen receptors (IgG and IgE), complement receptors, and lectins (DEC205 and mannose receptors). For both soluble and particulate antigens, antigen receptor–mediated endocytosis in B cells increases the efficiency of MHC II antigen presentation by 1000 to 10,000 times.[33, 34] In the Langerhans cell, MHC II antigen presentation is enhanced by cell-surface IgE.[35] Similar enhancement of MHC II antigen presentation is seen with receptor-mediated endocytosis by members of the mannose receptor family.[36–40]

Although exogenous antigens are the principal source of peptides presented by MHC II αβ heterodimers, there are many examples of endogenous antigens (alloantigens, viral antigens, and genetically engineered proteins) that can be presented by MHC II molecules. The route of antigen processing for these peptides is less well understood than the model outlined for exogenous antigens.[41–46] Further clarification of this enigmatic pathway and its physiologic role is needed.

Pathogens have evolved mechanisms for interfering with MHC II antigen processing and presentation (Table 9–1).

Class Ia

Like the αβ heterodimer of MHC II, MHC I molecules are heterodimers containing four immunoglobulin domains. For MHC I, however, three immunoglobulin domains are encoded by the α-chain, while the fourth is supplied by a noncovalently-associated, non-MHC–encoded, nontransmembrane glycoprotein called β_2-microglobulin. Humans have three HLA class Ia genes, designated HLA-A, -B, and -C, with molecular weights of about 45 kD. (In mice, H-2K and H-2D are found in all strains, and an additional class I locus, H-2L, is present in some strains.) Like MHC II genes, the class Ia genes are highly polymorphic. Fifty-nine HLA-A, 126 HLA-B, and 36 HLA-C alleles are known.[3] MHC I molecules are more broadly expressed than MHC II molecules, and they are present at some level in virtually all cells in the body except mature erythro-

TABLE 9–1 Mechanisms of Pathogen Interference with Major Histocompatibility Class II Antigen Presentation

Pathogen	Mechanism	Reference
HCMV	Blocks IFN-γ–induced upregulation of MHC II molecules	459
MCMV	Blocks IFN-γ–induced upregulation of MHC II molecules	460
Listeria	Listeriolysin O mediated alteration of MHC II/peptide complex resulting in antigen-specific T lymphocyte anergy	461
Leishmania	Interferes with MHC II peptide loading by sequestering MHC II molecules in the parasitophorous vacuole	462

Abbreviations: HCMV, Human cytomegalovirus; IFN, interferon; MCMV, murine cytomegalovirus; MHC, major histocompatibility complex.

cytes. As with MHC II, MHC I gene expression is upregulated by IFN-γ.

The peptide-binding groove for MHC Ia molecules is formed by the α_1 and α_2 domains of the MHC molecule. As with MHC II, the peptide-binding groove is the most polymorphic region of the molecule. The MHC Ia peptide-binding groove has more rigid requirements for peptide length and sequence (anchor residues) than does that of MHC II. Typically, the MHC I–presented peptides are 8 to 11 residues in length. The peptides are secured within the peptide-binding groove by conserved anchor residues.[47–49]

β_2-microglobulin is a secreted 12-kD glycoprotein encoded by a locus outside of the MHC on chromosome 15 in humans (chromosome 2 in mice). It is noncovalently associated with the MHC Ia glycoprotein and serves to stabilize the conformation of the class Ia heterodimer, allowing peptide loading and transport to the APC cell surface.[50, 51] It does not contribute directly to the peptide-binding groove. Nonetheless, β_2-microglobulin is critical to MHC I presentation, because knockout mice deficient in β_2-microglobulin lack all cell-surface MHC I molecules.[51]

Antigen processing and loading of MHC I molecules differs considerably from the pathway described for MHC II presentation. Whereas MHC II processing and presentation is geared toward exogenous antigens, MHC I loci are dedicated to presentation of endogenous antigens. Endogenous antigens are those antigens that are synthesized by host cell ribosomes (e.g., from invading viruses) or are present in the cytoplasm after synthesis by other intracellular pathogens. Antigens present in the cytoplasm are degraded into peptides by an organelle known as the proteasome complex. Proteasomes are cylindrical organelles composed of 14 to 17 subunits. The active site for polypeptide cleavage lies within the hollow cylinder. Proteasomes provide the broad biologic function of degrading effete proteins and proteins meant to have transient effects, such as cell cycle proteins, transcription factors, and signal transduction pathway components. These proteins are marked for destruction by modification with ubiquitin. The proteasome also serves to recycle both ubiquinated and nonubiquinated proteins that have been denatured, oxidized, or incorrectly folded de novo.[52, 53] In performing these housekeeping functions, the proteasome is associated with a 19S regulatory unit that includes receptor activity for ubiquitin-conjugated proteins. Consistent with these functions, proteasomes are found in both the cytoplasm and the nucleus.[54]

In addition to the basic housekeeping functions just outlined, the proteasome complex plays a critical role in the generation of MHC Ia–restricted peptides. In professional APCs and in most cells stimulated with IFN-γ, the proteasome exchanges its 19S regulatory complex for an 11S regulatory complex (PA28) and incorporates new elements, including the low-molecular-mass polypeptides (LMPs) LMP-2 and LMP-7 and multicatalytic endopeptidase complex-like 1 (MECL1).[55, 56] LMP-2 and LMP-7 are encoded within the MHC locus on chromosome 6; MECL1 and PA28 are not. With the exchange of regulatory subunits, the proteasome complex optimizes its production of peptides suitable for transport by TAP (*t*ransporter associated with *a*ntigen *p*rocessing) and complexing with MHC Ia heterodimers.[57–59] It is strongly suspected that this change in regulatory complexes influences the association of the proteasome complex with the smooth ER and, either directly or indirectly, with TAP. Though it varies by cell type, approximately 10 to 15% of the total pool of proteasomes is localized to the ER.

MHC Ia chains are cotranslationally inserted into the ER, where they rapidly associate with a calcium-binding chaperone, calnexin, and then with β_2-microglobulin via conserved sequences on the α_3 domain, displacing calnexin in favor of calreticulin in the human system (the sequence of events is slightly different in mice).[60] This complex then docks with TAP via an intermediary protein, tapasin. TAP is an ER-resident integral membrane heterodimer, composed of two polypeptides called TAP1 and TAP2, that transports proteasome-generated peptides from the cytosol into the ER for loading onto MHC I heterodimers. The TAP genes are encoded within the MHC. Peptide transport is an active process driven by adenosine triphosphate hydrolysis. TAP preferentially transports short peptides of 8 to 12 amino acids, but it can transport longer peptides with decreased efficiency. Peptide binding to TAP is highly promiscuous; that is, it is minimally affected by the actual sequence of the polypeptide.[61]

Binding of an 8- to 11-amino-acid peptide to the class I heterodimer releases it from the TAP-tapasin-calreticulin complex. The peptide-containing MHC I complex then proceeds through the ER and Golgi complex to the cell surface for presentation of the bound peptide to CD8$^+$ T lymphocytes.[62, 63] Mutation of either TAP or tapasin greatly reduces cell-surface expression of MHC I–peptide complexes and therefore class Ia–restricted antigen presentation.[64–66]

The model of MHC Ia antigen presentation derived from these data explains degradation and peptide loading of cytosol-resident proteins but does not readily explain the presentation of peptides derived from integral membrane proteins or from secreted proteins that do not normally reside in the cytoplasm. Possible mechanisms for class I presentation of such epitopes include inefficient translation blockade by signal sequences on cytosolic ribosomes, resulting in peptide-chain synthesis in the cytosol, and initiation of translation from alternative initiation codons (removing the signal sequence) with subsequent synthesis and degradation in the cytosol.[67, 68] An additional mechanism for antigen processing has been identified for both integral membrane proteins and proteins resident in the ER lumen. These proteins can be transported into the cytoplasm,[69, 70] the likely retrograde transporter for this pathway being Sec61 complex.[71–73] Analysis of integral membrane glycoprotein epitopes demonstrated that degradation and TAP-mediated loading of MHC I heterodimers occurs after the nascent protein has been posttranslationally modified (glycosylated) in the ER.[74] This newly appreciated mechanism of antigen processing ensures that all endogenously synthesized peptides are subject to MHC I–mediated immunosurveillance.

The majority of MHC I–bound peptides generated from endogenous proteins are proteasome and TAP dependent. However, there are examples of TAP- and proteasome-independent epitopes. Most of these epitopes are generated from proteins that have signal sequences that deliver the proteins into the ER lumen (bypassing the requirement for TAP), with subsequent proteolytic generation of the peptide epitope and class I loading occurring in the ER, Golgi complex, or distal vesicle compartment.[75–79] Some of the relevant proteases are probably signal peptidases,[80] but these proteases alone cannot account for all MHC-associated TAP-independent peptides. Most details of this secondary pathway for endogenous epitope processing and loading remain to be characterized.

In some circumstances, exogenous antigen can be taken up by APCs and presented to MHC Ia–restricted CD8$^+$ cytotoxic T lymphocytes (CTLs or Tc cells). Exogenous antigens are typically poor immunogens for generation of MHC I–restricted Tc responses, but they reproducibly generate MHC II–restricted CD4$^+$ T-helper (Th) lymphocyte responses[81] (see later discussion). However, particulate exogenous antigens can gain access to the MHC I antigen presentation pathway. Exogenous antigens contained within bacteria and apoptotic cells can be presented by MHC I molecules. Bacterial cytosolic, periplasmic, and outer membrane proteins all can be presented to T lymphocytes via MHC I. This pathway of class Ia–restricted antigen processing and presentation requires phagocytosis but does not require new synthesis and trafficking of MHC I heterodimers. Therefore it uses already-formed MHC I molecules and is presumably TAP independent. MHC I–restricted epitopes presented in this manner appear to arise from regurgitation of peptides after endosomal or lysosomal degradation of bacteria or bacterial products, with subsequent binding of the peptides to cell-surface MHC I molecules.[82–86] This pathway of antigen presentation may increase the total number of antigenic epitopes recognized during an immune response. However, regurgitation of peptides that are subsequently loaded onto preexisting cell-surface MHC I molecules may result in T cell–mediated killing of uninfected bystander cells. This pathway may be responsible for the detrimental immunopathology seen in some infections.

The second pathway identified for exogenous MHC I–restricted antigen processing and presentation depends on TAP and requires direct transfer of bacterial peptides from phagosomes to the cytosol in the APCs.[87, 88] The mechanism for transfer of peptides from phagosome to cytosol may be similar to the Sec61-dependent pathway for MHC I–mediated presentation of endogenous antigens previously described. This pathway of antigen presentation has been demonstrated in vivo.[89]

Pathogens have evolved multiple mechanisms for interfering with MHC I antigen presentation (Table 9–2).

Class Ib

Class Ib nonclassic MHC molecules are similar to MHC Ia molecules in that they associate with β_2-microglobulin to form a functional unit. They differ considerably in the nature of the processed antigens that they are capable of presenting, their tissue distribution, and the degree of polymorphism in the population. The oligomorphic (nonclassic) MHC genes are subdivided into two distinct subclasses based on the degree of homology and physical relation to the MHC loci. HLA-E, -F, and -G genes (probably orthologous to the Q, T, and M genes in mice) are adjacent to the classic MHC genes on chromosome 6 in humans (chromosome 17 in mice) and have considerable homology to the class I genes HLA-A, -B, and -C (H2-K, -D, -L in mice).

The second subset of nonclassic MHC I genes are the CD1 genes (same terminology in mice). These genes have no significant homology to classic MHC I genes in the α_1 domain, significant homology in the α_2 domain, and a small amount of homology in the α_3 domain. CD1 genes have only 3 of 10 residues conserved in the class I α_3 domain known to interact with CD8. The CD1 genes are located on chromosome 1 in humans (chromosome 3 in mice).[90]

TABLE 9–2 Mechanisms of Pathogen Interference with Major Histocompatibility Complex Class I Antigen Presentation

Pathogen	Mechanism	Reference
Adenovirus	E3/19K sequesters HLA class I molecules in the ER	463
EBV	EBNA-1 contains a repeat structure that interferes with its proteolysis	464, 465
HSV	ICP47 inhibits the TAP transporter	466
CMV	US3 sequesters HLA class I molecules in the ER	467
	US2 & US11 dislocate HLA class I molecules into the cytosol where they are degraded by the proteosome complex	71, 468
	US6 inhibits translocation by TAP	469, 470
	Pp65 interferes with cytosolic proteolysis of CMV polypeptides	471
	UL18, an MHC 1 viral homologue, protects the virus from NK cell–mediated cytoxicity expected from viral-induced downregulation of MHC I molecules	472
	gp40 sequesters murine class I molecules in the Golgi	473
	M144, an MHC I viral homologue, protects the virus from NK cell–mediated cytotoxicity expected from viral-induced downregulation of MHC I molecules	474

Abbreviations: CMV, Cytomegalovirus; EBNA, Epstein-Barr virus–associated nuclear antigen; EBV, Epstein-Barr virus; ER, endoplasmic reticulum; HLA, human leukocyte antigen; HSV, herpes simplex virus; MHC, major histocompatibility complex; NK, natural killer; TAP, transporter associated with antigen processing.

HLA-E, -F, and -G and Murine Q, T, and M

The current understanding of HLA-E, -F, and -G in the cellular immune response is fairly limited. There are few alleles of these genes known in the human population.[91] Like the other MHC genes, these genes appear to be upregulated by IFN-γ.[92] Data exist to show that both HLA-E and HLA-G can bind peptides in a manner similar to classic MHC I genes, with apparent preferences for nonomers[93, 94] and dependence on the TAP transporter.[95, 96]

In vitro and in vivo cell-surface expression of HLA-E and -F has been difficult to demonstrate. Transcripts for HLA-E are present in multiple tissues, whereas HLA-F transcription is restricted to skin, T lymphocytes, B lymphocytes, and fetal liver.[97] To date no direct data exist for either HLA-E or HLA-F presentation of an antigen to T lymphocytes in vivo, or for any other biologic functions. In contrast, HLA-G is expressed on fetal cytotrophoblast populations at the fetomaternal interface, and its expression protects fetal tissue from NK cell–mediated cytolysis by engaging an NK-cell inhibitory receptor[98, 99] (see later discussion).

The murine Q (Qa-2), T (Qa-1), and M nonclassic genes may provide insight into roles for human HLA-E, HLA-F, or other yet unappreciated nonclassic MHC Ib molecules. Unlike the human HLA-E and HLA-F genes, these loci have been shown to present antigens in mice. These genes associate with β_2-microglobulin in the ER and apparently are loaded and cycled to the cell surface in a pathway very similar to that for MHC Ia molecules. Mutations in the TAP transport system decrease cell-surface expression of Q and M genes, implying that TAP-derived peptides are loaded into the $\alpha_1\alpha_2$ peptide-binding pocket, stabilizing these nonclassic MHC complexes and allowing them to exit from the ER.[64, 100, 101] Cell-surface expression of H2-T (Qa-1) molecules is unaffected in TAP-deficient cells, and it appears that H2-T molecules can be expressed on the cell surface without bound peptide.[102, 103] However, presentation of peptide antigens by H2-T still requires a functional TAP1/TAP2 transporter.[104]

H2-T molecules present *Listeria* antigens, suggesting a role in host defense.[105, 106] H2-T also can present signal peptides to alloreactive T cells.[104] This MHC molecule is capable of presenting a peptide derived from the influenza HA glycoprotein to naive T lymphocytes, but the significance of this fact for host defense is unclear, because that same epitope is not generated within influenza-infected cells and H2-T–restricted T cells have not been described in natural influenza infection.[107]

H2-Q (Qa-2) molecules have been shown to bind peptides,[108–110] but no physiologically relevant peptide has yet been shown to be presented by Qa-2. Qa-2 has been implicated in murine resistance to *Taenia crassiceps*, an animal model for cysticercosis, although the nature of the T-lymphocyte response has not been determined.[111] Qa-2 does not bind to T-cell CD8[112] and is the only MHC I or II molecule that is linked to the plasma membrane by a glycan phosphoinositol anchor rather by than a transmembrane domain.[113]

The most interesting of the murine nonclassic loci is H2-M3. This molecule presents formylated peptides from many different bacterial antigens to CD8$^+$ Tc cells. Teleologically such capability would have appeal as a mechanism for identifying invading bacteria, because only eubacteria, mitochondria, and chloroplasts generate formylated peptides. The presence of formylated peptides within the body (other than in the lumen of the gastrointestinal tract) would almost always represent a danger signal. Generation of H2-M3–restricted CD8$^+$ T cells can be demonstrated during the in vivo response to *Listeria monocytogenes* infection, and adoptive transfer of such T lymphocytes is protective against infection.[114, 115] Data suggest that H2-M3 can present these antigens by both TAP-dependent and TAP-independent pathways, because TAP-deficient bone marrow macrophages can present formylated peptides to an H2-M3–restricted T-cell clone, although not as efficiently as wild-type macrophages can.[116] The dual presentation pathway is consistent with both the intracellular location and the particulate nature of *L. monocytogenes*. In addition to the biologic data, the crystal structure of H2-M3 complexed with a formylated peptide has been solved.[117] It shows an overall structure similar to that of other MHC I heterodimer–peptide complexes, with the principal difference being the position of the N-terminal peptide amino acid within the peptide-binding groove. Murine H2-M3 shares some peptide-binding groove structural similarities with the human HLA-E molecule, but to date no presentation of formylated peptides has been documented in humans.

CD1 Family

The CD1 family of nonclassic MHC I molecules is less closely related to HLA-A, -B, and -C than are HLA-E, -F, and -G. It is estimated that HLA class I, class II, and CD1 genes first appeared at about the same time in phylogeny.[90, 118, 119] Consistent with this more distant evolutionary divergence is the presence of the CD1 gene locus on chromosome 1 (chromosome 3 in mice) rather than on chromosome 6 (chromosome 17 in mice), the site for all other HLA loci. Humans have five CD1 loci, designated CD1A, CD1B, CD1C, CD1D, and CD1E, and mice have two loci, CD1D1 and CD1D2 (also known as CD1.1 and CD1.2). The tissue distribution and cytokine regulation profile of CD1 genes is different from that of the other MHC I and II genes. CD1A, CD1B, and CD1C are expressed on thymocytes, B lymphocytes, and monocyte/macrophage/dendritic cell lineages. CD1D (murine CD1D1) is also expressed on nonhematopoietic cells, especially epithelial cells of the gastrointestinal tract.[90, 120–123] Expression of human CD1A, CD1B, and CD1C on monocytes is upregulated maximally by interleukin-4 (IL-4) and granulocyte-macrophage colony-stimulating factor (GM-CSF), or by IL-4 and IL-3, and is antagonized by IL-1[124] and apparently by IFN-γ.[90] In contrast, CD1D on epithelial cells is modestly upregulated by IFN-γ and unaffected by IL-4.[125] To date no protein products have been identified for the human CD1E or murine CD1D2 genes.

In 1992 Porcelli and colleagues[126] showed that $CD4^-8^-$ αβ TCR^+ T cells from the peripheral blood of a normal donor recognized a mycobacterial antigen in the context of CD1B. Presentation of this antigen was not affected by mutation of the TAP1/TAP2 transporter but was affected by pretreatment of monocytes with chloroquine. Subsequent work showed that these T cells recognized a mycolic acid as antigen.[127] Further characterization of the mycobacterial lipid antigens has shown that phosphoglycolipids lipoarabinomannan, lipomannan, glucose monomycolate, and phosphatidylinositol mannosides can be presented by CD1B and CD1C to $CD4^-8^-$ αβ TCR^+ T cells (antigen presentation by CD1A has not been documented). Presentation of mycobacterial lipid antigens to T lymphocytes is independent of the TAP transporter and HLA-DM molecules that play critical roles in MHC I and II antigen presentation, respectively. T-cell recognition of lipid antigens can be blocked by antibodies to CD1 molecules, by prefixing of monocyte APCs, or by pretreatment of monocyte APCs with chloroquine.[126, 128–130] Mycobacterial lipid antigen presentation by CD1 molecules shares many features of the MHC II antigen presentation pathway, including requirements for active endosomal trafficking and acidification of endosomal vesicles.[131] CD1D1 in the murine system has been shown to present glycosylceramides, lipids found in some bacterial cell walls, to $CD4^-8^-$ αβ TCR^+ T cells.[132, 133] Therefore, the role of the CD1 loci in cellular immunity appears to be presentation of bacterial glycolipids rather than peptides to CD4 − 8 − αβ TCR^+ T lymphocytes.

CD1 molecules, unlike HLA-A through HLA-G, localize to the MIIC compartments that are the sites of MHC II peptide loading. CD1 heavy chains are cotranslationally inserted into the ER, where they initially complex with the ER chaperone, calnexin. In the absence of β_2-microglobulin, the CD1 heavy chain remains confined to the ER. Association of the heavy chain with β_2-microglobulin allows CD1 to exit the ER.[134] Unlike classic MHC I molecules, CD1 heterodimers are stable in the absence of bound antigen.[135, 136] From the ER, CD1 heterodimers move out to the cell surface. CD1 on the cell surface is rapidly internalized via clathrin-coated pits and subsequently localized to MIIC compartments.[137] CD1 localization to MIIC is required for loading of lipid antigen onto CD1 molecules.[138] Acidification of the MIIC compartment is also required, as with MHC II peptide loading.[131]

The data outlined, in conjunction with the crystal structure of CD1D, support the following model. CD1 molecules present glycolipids by sequestering their paired hydrophobic tails in deep hydrophobic pockets within the antigen-binding groove.[139] Once loaded, the CD1 heterodimer recycles to the cell surface to present the lipid antigen to T lymphocytes. The TCR sees a contour formed by the $\alpha_1\alpha_2$ domains of the CD1 heavy chain and the hydrophilic portion of the complexed lipid antigen. The affinity and fine specificity of this interaction may mirror that seen with MHC Ia–restricted peptide antigens.[129, 132] T-cell recognition of the MHC-lipid complex results in T-cell activation, cytokine production, and cytolysis, just as occurs with recognition of peptide antigens complexed to classic MHC molecules.

All lipid-specific T-cell populations described to date have had a $CD4^-8^-$ αβ TCR^+ natural killer cell receptor $(NKR)^+$ phenotype,[128, 132] consistent with a subset of T lymphocytes known as natural T cells (discussed later). Evidence for the importance of CD1 to this T-cell subset is the dramatic loss of natural T cells in CD1D1 knockout mice.[140] No studies have been published on the susceptibility of CD1D1 knockout mice to mycobacterial infection. Data for CD1 interaction with CD8 or CD4 is equivocal[135, 141] and is unlikely to be important, because the majority of responding T cells lack both CD4 and CD8.

Heat Shock Proteins

HSPs, like MHC I and II molecules, are members of the immunoglobulin superfamily. Like MHC molecules, HSPs bind peptides. DNA and amino acid comparisons show significant evolutionary relationships between these molecules, including domains involved in peptide binding.[142] A relatively small but growing body of literature suggests that HSPs such as glucose regulated protein 94 (GRP94)/gp96 and HSP70 can selectively and efficiently deliver exogenous peptides to the MHC I antigen presentation pathway.

The first evidence that HSPs may play a role in antigen processing and presentation came from the field of tumor immunology. Immunization of mice with gp96 purified from a chemically induced syngeneic tumor protected the mice from subsequent tumor challenge. The protective effect was mediated by $CD8^+$ T lymphocytes and depended on the peptides associated with gp96 rather than gp96 itself.[143, 144] Similar antitumor effects have been obtained by immunization with HSP70.[145] In vitro loading of peptides onto HSPs requires heating of the complex, with 60°C optimal. Several different viral peptides that are recognized by virus-specific T cells can bind to gp96, and peritoneal macrophages primed with in vitro generated gp96–vesicular stomatitis virus (VSV) peptide complexes can present relevant peptide to VSV-specific T cells.[146] Finally, the K^b-restricted immunodominant peptide (RGYVYQGL) of VSV can be recovered from gp96 complexes isolated from VSV-infected cells.[147]

It is not clear how HSP-peptide complexes interact with the MHC I antigen presentation pathway. For endogenous proteins, the gp96-peptide delivery system may provide a mechanism for MHC I surveillance of the ER lumen (this function also is provided independently of HSPs by Sec61). It has been proposed that gp96 directly participates in TAP1/TAP2-mediated loading of peptides onto MHC I heterodimers or that it loads peptides onto MHC I independent of TAP1/TAP2, or both.[148, 149]

The discovery of HSPs as natural adjuvants for generation of $CD8^+$ T cells via presentation of peptide antigens is exciting because current immunization protocols with soluble antigens (especially peptides) rarely generate significant $CD8^+$ T cell responses. Nonetheless, the general applicability and overall contribution of this novel pathway for MHC I antigen presentation remain to be established.

ANTIGEN-PRESENTING CELLS

APCs play a critical role in the immune response and probably strongly influence the character of the response. An extensive review of APCs goes beyond the scope of this chapter, but a brief overview is necessary to appreciate the mechanics of the cellular immune response. APCs can be divided into two basic types, professional APCs and nonprofessional APCs. *Professional APCs* are hematopoietic in origin and include macrophages, monocytes, dendritic cells, and B lymphocytes. These cells are considered "professional" because they have the ability to express MHC II molecules and have specific mechanisms of phagocytosis and receptor-mediated uptake of soluble antigens that facilitate processing of MHC II–restricted epitopes. As discussed later, this function is critical for the activation of Th cells to produce cytokines that control both B-lymphocyte and Tc responses to infection. In addition to their ability to process and present antigen in the context of MHC II, professional APCs have important accessory molecules necessary for optimal T-cell activation, including CD58, intercellular adhesion molecule-3 (ICAM-3), B7-1 and B7-2. These accessory molecules are critical to activation of naive lymphocytes during primary immune responses.

Nonprofessional APCs include essentially all of the cell types not previously mentioned. They typically lack MHC II cell-surface expression, although many express class II molecules on exposure to IFN-γ. Nonprofessional APCs with MHC II expression induced by IFN-γ can present exogenous antigen to $CD4^+$ T lymphocytes.[150–153] However, when naive T lymphocytes (i.e., those that have never been exposed to their specific peptide antigen) interact with nonprofessional APC MHC II–peptide complexes, a hyporesponsive state rather than activation occurs.[154] Studies in murine models suggest that the array of MHC II epitopes generated by nonprofessional APC processing of exogenous antigens is much more limited than that seen with professional APCs.[155] Differences between professional and nonprofessional APCs have also been described for MHC I antigen processing and presentation.[156] Nonprofessional APCs typically lack many of the classic accessory molecules used by T lymphocytes to interact with professional APCs. Table 9–3 summarizes classic and nonclassic accessory molecules, their ligands, and cell expression.

Dendritic cells are the critical APCs in the early activation of the cellular immune response, because they are the only APCs that can efficiently activate naive T lymphocytes.[157] The prototypic immune response to an infection begins with general inflammation and necrosis caused by the invading pathogen and the innate defenses, including neutrophils, tissue macrophages, NK cells, and nonlymphoid cytokine production. Local dendritic cells take up antigen by phagocytosis, become activated, and increase expression of cell-surface MHC II complexes and accessory molecules. Activated dendritic cells migrate to the local lymph nodes and activate T cells bearing appropriate receptors. In secondary (recall) immune responses, both B cells and dendritic cells have important roles as APCs, as do inflammatory macrophages in the affected tissues.

T LYMPHOCYTES

The T-Cell Receptor

The principal effector cells in the adaptive response to infection are B and T lymphocytes that recognize pathogens by means of antigen-specific cell-surface receptors. B cells and the antibodies they produce in response to antigenic challenge are generally referred to as the humoral immune response. T-lymphocyte responses to antigenic challenges are called the cellular immune response. T lymphocytes can be categorized and functionally divided by the type of antigen receptor (TCR) used and a small number of unique accessory markers on their cell surfaces.

The primary event in initiation of an antigen-specific cellular

TABLE 9–3 T-Lymphocyte Accessory Molecules

Accessory Molecule	Ligand	Ligand Presence on APC*		Reference
		Professional	Nonprofessional	
Classic				
CD28	B7-1	+	−	475, 476
	B7-2	+	−	
CTLA-4	B7-1	+	−	475, 476
	B7-2	+	−	475, 476
CD2	CD58	+	+	477
LFA-1 (CD11a/CD18)	ICAM-1	+	+/−	478
	ICAM-2	+	−	478
	ICAM-3	+	−	479, 480
CD5	CD72	+	−	481, 482
	CD5L	+	−	483
CD27	CD70	+	−	484–486
CD40 ligand	CD40	+	−	487
FAS ligand	Fas	+	+	488
Nonclassic				
$\alpha_V\beta_3$	Arg-Gly-Asp–containing proteins	−	+	489
$\alpha_4\beta_1$ (VLA-4)	fibronectin, VCAM-1	−	+	489
$\alpha_5\beta_1$ (VLA-5)	fibronectin	−	+	489
$\alpha_6\beta_1$ (VLA-6)	laminin	−	+	489
CD44	hyaluronic acid	−	+	490, 491
Thy 1	?	?	+	492
CD7	?	+	?	493, 494
Ly-6C	?	?	+	492
?	CD59	+	+	495
Heat-stable antigen	?	+	?	496

*Professional APCs include dendritic cells, macrophage/monocytes, and B cells. Nonprofessional APCs for purposes of this table are all nonhematopoietic cells with the exception of endothelial cells.
Abbreviations: APC, Antigen-presenting cell; CTLA, cytotoxic T-lymphocyte–associated protein; ICAM, intercellular adhesion molecule; LFA, lymphocyte function antigen; VCAM, vascular cell adhesion molecule; VLA, very late antigen; +, present; −, absent; +/−, present on a small subset; ?, unknown.

immune response is the recognition of a peptide or glycolipid bound to an MHC molecule on the surface of an APC by an appropriate T lymphocyte. Antigen recognition is mediated by the TCR. There are two distinct families of TCRs. The prototypic TCR is composed of a TCR α-chain and a TCR β-chain, and the T lymphocytes bearing this receptor are called αβ T lymphocytes. The second type of TCR is composed of an analogous heterodimer containing distinct gene products, the γ-chain and the δ-chain, and the T lymphocytes bearing this receptor are called γδ T lymphocytes. The αβ and γδ heterodimers function as the antigen recognition units of the TCR. Each heterodimer associates with several additional plasma membrane proteins that transduce signals into the cell cytoplasm on engagement of the TCR. These proteins are called the CD3 complex and consist of one γ-chain (different from the TCR γ-chain), one δ-chain (different from the TCR δ-chain), two ϵ-chains, and a disulfide-linked ζ-dimer. The antigen recognition chains and the CD3 complex together are called the TCR complex. All components of the TCR complex except ζ are members of the immunoglobulin superfamily (Fig. 9–3).

αβ T-Cell Receptor–Positive T Lymphocytes

The TCR α- and β-chains are analogous to the immunoglobulin chains that make up B cell antigen receptor. Each chain has a variable region used for antigen recognition, a constant region, and a transmembrane portion with a short cytoplasmic tail. In humans, the α-chain has a mass of 40 to 57 kD and the β-chain has a mass of 40 to 44 kD. The TCR αβ heterodimer is disulfide linked. The variable domains of α- and β-chains together determine the antigen specificity of the TCR. Generation of a diverse repertoire of αβ TCRs occurs through somatic recombination, in a process similar to that responsible for immunoglobulin diversity. Functional α-chains are assembled by gene recombination that links one of 70 to 80 unique variable gene segments (V) to one of 61 unique joining segments (J) and a single constant region (C) of the α-chain; this is known as VJ rearrangement (Fig. 9–4*A*). β-Chain assembly is more complex due to incorporation of an additional gene segment known as D (diversity). In addition, the entire D-J-C region is duplicated so that a single V exon (chosen from 52 possible ones) can recombine with either $D\beta_1$ or $D\beta_2$. Following $D\beta_1$ are six potential J-chain exons and a single constant-region exon, $C\beta_1$; following $D\beta_2$ are seven potential J-chain exons and a distinct constant-region exon, $C\beta_2$ (see Fig. 9–4*B*). Diversity in the TCR repertoire is generated by the combinatorial possibilities of the V-J (α-chain) or V-D-J (β-chain) segments assembled to form each TCR chain. Additional coding variability between the V-D and D-J coding regions is generated by the addition of non-germline–encoded nucleotides at the V-J, V-D, and D-J junctions by terminal deoxynucleotidyl transferase during somatic recombination. The random pairing of Vα- and Vβ-chains in the αβ heterodimer imparts another degree of combinatorial diversity to the TCR repertoire. Total calculated diversity for the αβ TCR is approximately 10^{12} to 10^{15} unique receptors, theoretically enough to provide immunity against all potential pathogens.

T-Cell Recognition of the Peptide-Major Histocompatibility Complex

The αβ component of the TCR complex recognizes an epitope comprised of amino acids from both the antigenic peptide and the MHC molecule. Crystal structures of αβ TCRs interacting with MHC-antigen complexes show that the TCR recognizes a contour formed by antigenic peptides and the $\alpha_1\beta_1$ (class II) or $\alpha_1\alpha_2$ (class I) domains of MHC molecules.[13, 158–160] TCR α- and β-chains both contribute directly to antigen recognition.

The contribution of the MHC molecule to the antigenic structure recognized by the TCR accounts for the phenomenon of MHC restriction. The amino acid sequence of the MHC molecule affects T-cell recognition of the foreign peptide because the TCR makes extensive contact with the MHC molecule in addition to the peptide. A T cell that recognizes a foreign peptide associated with one MHC molecule cannot recognize the same peptide associated with another MHC molecule. The MHC not only presents peptides to the TCR but limits peptide recognition to certain TCRs. T-cell recognition of antigenic peptides is therefore constrained by the ability of the host MHC molecules to bind and present peptides. Several antigenic

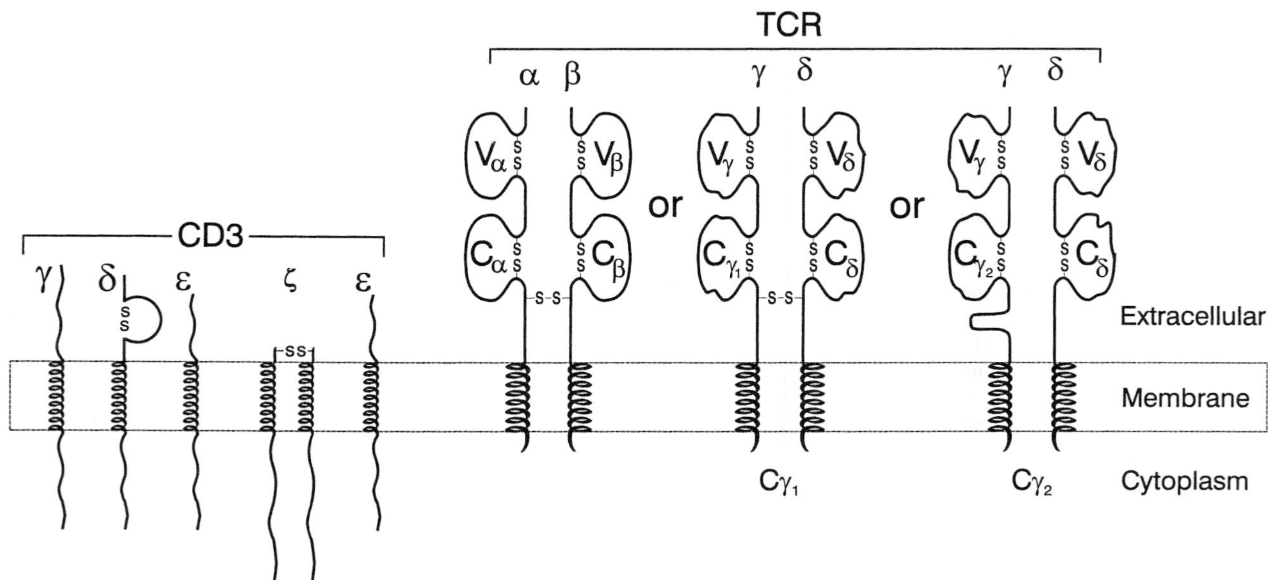

FIGURE 9–3. T-lymphocyte antigen receptor structures and the associated CD3 complex. The T-lymphocyte antigen receptor (T-cell receptor, TCR) is expressed on all T lymphocytes. It is a heterodimer consisting of an α and a β chain (αβ TCR) or of a γ and a δ chain (γδ TCR). All αβ TCRs are disulfide linked; γδ TCRs may be either disulfide linked ($\gamma_1\delta$) or not ($\gamma_2\delta$). Each T cell expresses only one of these forms of TCR, and all copies of the TCR on a single cell are identical. Each TCR is noncovalently associated with a CD3 complex, composed of γ, δ, ϵ, and ζ chains, which is responsible for signaling after TCR engagement by ligand. (Adapted from Weiss A. Structure and function of the T cell antigen receptor. J Clin Invest. 1990;86:1015–1022, by copyright permission of the American Society for Clinical Investigation; and Brenner MB, Strominger JL, Krangel MS. The gamma delta T cell receptor. Adv Immunol. 1988;43:133–192.)

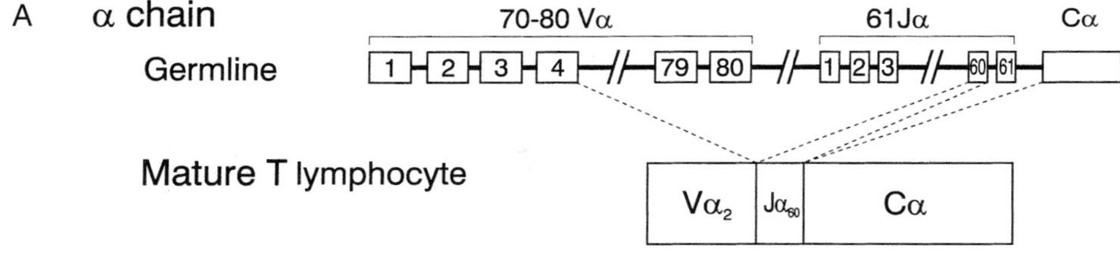

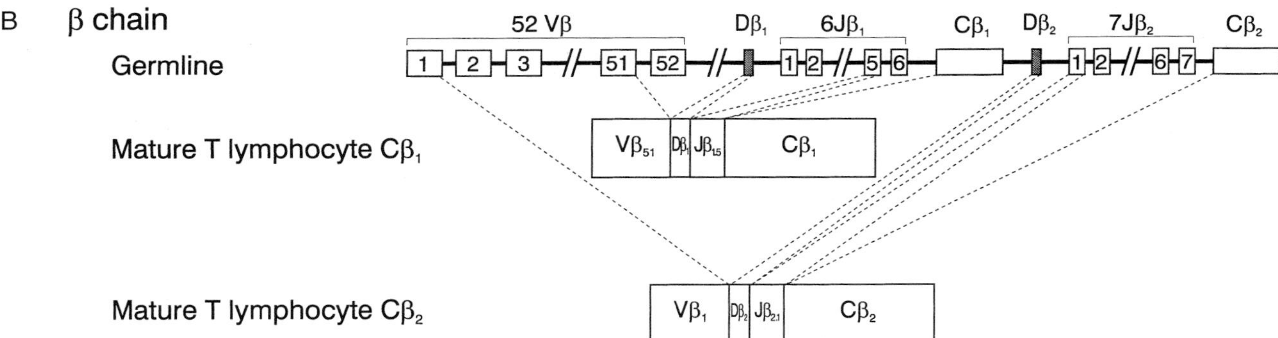

FIGURE 9–4. Somatic recombination in the T-cell receptor (TCR) α and β genes. *A*, Germline and mature T lymphocyte forms of the TCR α chain. The somatic rearrangement depicted results in a $V\alpha_4J\alpha_{60}C\alpha$ TCR α chain. *B*, Germline and mature T-lymphocyte forms of the TCR β chain. Somatic rearrangements depicted generate β chains that use different Cβ exons. For the purpose of illustration, the $C\beta_1$ TCR β chain depicted is $V\beta_{51}D\beta_1J\beta_{1.5}C\beta_1$, and the $C\beta_2$ chain is $V\beta_1D\beta_2J\beta_{2.1}C\beta_2$.

peptides have been analyzed in detail for how they interact with MHC and the TCR complex. In general, only a few amino acids are critical to anchor the peptide into the MHC molecule, and a separate subset of two or three amino acids is required for recognition by the TCR. By systematic alteration of the amino acids that contact the TCR, it is possible to generate peptides with high affinity for MHC but none for the TCR. Theoretically, these peptides could block immune responses to the original antigenic peptide by simple competition. More interesting are peptides that retain affinity for MHC molecules and have a diminished affinity for the TCR. These peptides, called altered peptide ligands, can induce a specific state of unresponsiveness to the original immunizing antigens (i.e., anergy). Generation of altered peptide ligands may be an important mechanism by which viruses such as HIV and hepatitis B limit the immune response during chronic infection.[161–163]

There seems to be equivalent specificity in TCR recognition of bacterial glycolipid antigens presented by CD1 molecules, although this phenomenon is less well studied. Fine specificity in lipid antigen recognition by the TCR was demonstrated for a T-cell line derived from a patient with leprosy that recognized lipoarabinomannan derived from *Mycobacterium leprae* but not *Mycobacterium tuberculosis*.[130]

CD4 and CD8 Coreceptors

Most αβ T lymphocytes express either CD4 or CD8 as a coreceptor. Expression of CD4 or CD8 as the coreceptor correlates closely with the role of the T lymphocyte in the adaptive immune response. Those αβ TCR^+ T cells expressing CD4 are commonly referred to as Th cells, and those expressing CD8 are known as Tc cells. Th cells recognize foreign peptides associated with MHC II and produce cytokines that "help" antibody production, Tc activation and expansion, and NK cell activation and expansion. Tc cells kill infected or neoplastic cells presenting a foreign peptide associated with MHC I.

In most circumstances, αβ TCR–mediated recognition of MHC-peptide complexes on APC surfaces is not sufficient for a productive interaction between T lymphocytes and APCs. Activation of most αβ T lymphocytes requires additional signals provided by CD4 or CD8. CD4 expressed on Th cells binds to monomorphic sequences on MHC II; CD8 expressed on Tc cells recognizes monomorphic sequences on MHC Ia. Therefore, one important role for CD4 and CD8 is to enhance the T-cell interaction with the MHC complex on the APC. Because these coreceptors are required for T-lymphocyte activation, $CD4^+$ Th cells can be activated by only peptides bound to MHC II, and $CD8^+$ Tc cells can be activated only by peptides bound to MHC Ia.

Both CD4 and CD8 are type I membrane proteins and members of the immunoglobulin superfamily. CD4 is expressed as a monomer on the surface of Th cells. The cytoplasmic tail of CD4 associates with the SRC-family tyrosine kinase p56/59 lymphocyte-specific protein tyrosine kinase (LCK), which plays a critical role in TCR signal transduction. CD8 is expressed on the cell surface of Tc cells as a disulfide-linked dimer. In the peripheral blood, most Tc cells have a dimer composed of closely related CD8 α- and β-chains. Tc cells associated with mucosal lymphoid tissues commonly express a CD8αα homodimer. The CD8αα homodimer is a marker for extrathymic T-cell development (see later discussion). As with CD4, the CD8 α-chain cytoplasmic tail associates with LCK, but with a lower affinity. It is possible that the CD8 β-chain cytoplasmic tail increases the affinity of the heterodimer for LCK, compared with the homodimer.[164] Therefore, a second important role for CD4 and CD8 is to augment tryosine kinase–mediated signaling after recognition of an appropriate MHC peptide complex.

γδ T-Cell Receptor–Positive T Lymphocytes

The γδ T lymphocytes use an alternate TCR heterodimer for antigen recognition, called the γδ TCR. In the human, the δ-chain gene is nested within the coding sequences for the α-chain locus on chromosome 14, and the γ-chain gene is independently located on chromosome 7. The γδ receptor shares many features with the αβ TCR. The γ-chain, like the α-chain, is assembled by somatic recombination of variable gene segments with joining segments (VJ rearrangement). However, the γ-chain has a much more limited potential repertoire than the TCR α-chain does. In humans, there are six to eight functional γ variable gene segments, five joining gene segments, and two different constant gene segments, $C\gamma_1$ and $C\gamma_2$ (Fig. 9–5*A*). $C\gamma_1$ has the cysteine required for disulfide linkage of the TCR heterodimer, but $C\gamma_2$ does not. Consistent with the amino acid sequence, $C\gamma_1$ γδ TCRs are disulfide linked (similar to αβ TCRs), but $C\gamma_2$ γδ TCRs are not (see Fig. 9–3). The murine γ-chain locus has a more complex organization, with three different γ constant gene segments. Significant variability in the coding sequence at the V-J junction occurs because of imprecise recombination and the activity of terminal nucleotidyl transferase.

The δ-chain is encoded by a locus nested within the α-chain locus of the αβ TCR. The actual number of variable gene segments used by the δ-chain has not been precisely determined and is complicated by δ-chain use of upstream Vα gene segments. There are three δ diversity exons, four δ joining exons, and a single δ constant exon located before the first Jα exon (see Fig. 9–5*B*).[165] Therefore, any rearrangement of the TCR α locus splices out the entire δ locus. The δ-chains can incorporate one or two diversity gene segments into the final gene product. Junctional diversity resulting from imprecise recombination and the activity of terminal nucleotidyl transferase exists at the V-D, D-D, and D-J junctions. The tremendous number of potential non-germline coding sequences in the δ-chain makes it the most diverse of all the TCR chains.[166, 167] Overall diversity of the γδ TCR repertoire is the product of the relatively limited diversity of the γ-chain and the tremendous diversity of the δ-chain. The diversity of the γδ TCR repertoire probably approaches or exceeds that of the αβ TCR repertoire.[168]

Human γδ TCR lymphocytes represent about 1 to 15% of the circulating T-lymphocyte pool in normal persons.[169] Eighty percent of γδ TCR lymphocytes in the peripheral circulation are $CD4^-8^-$, and 20% are weakly $CD8^+$. $CD4^+$ γδ T cells are extremely rare. Human γδ TCR^+ lymphocytes have tissue-specific biases in Vγ and Vδ usage.[170, 171] This phenomenon is even more pronounced in mice.[172] In addition to the lymphoid compartments (blood, lymph nodes, thymus, and spleen), γδ T cells are found in significant numbers in the gut, epidermis, and reproductive tract of adult animals. Initial population of the nonlymphoid compartments occurs early in embryonic development (day 14 to 18 of gestation in mice) by lymphocytes with relatively invariant γδ TCRs (limited junctional diversity and chain usage); γδ T lymphocytes that mature later in life have much more diverse TCR γ- and δ-chains.[173]

Antigen recognition by γδ TCR appears to be independent of antigen-processing pathways and MHC restriction elements, as might

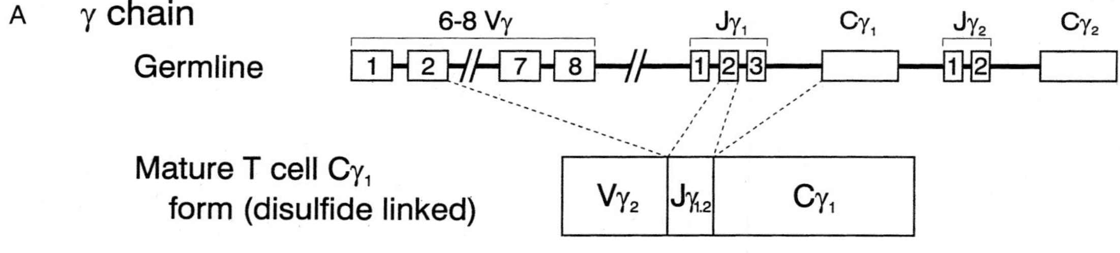

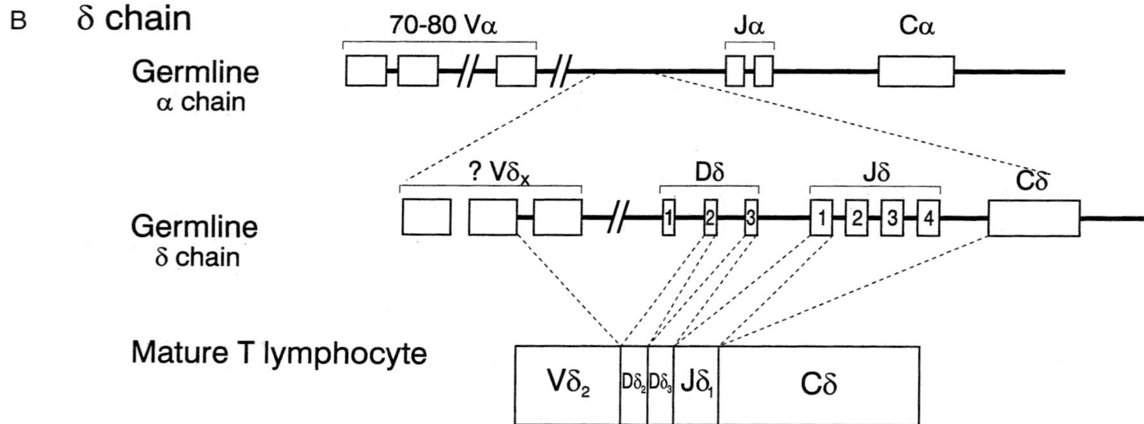

FIGURE 9–5. Somatic recombination in the T-cell receptor (TCR) γ and δ genes. *A*, Germline and mature T lymphocyte forms of the TCR γ chain. The somatic rearrangement depicted results in a $V\gamma_2J\gamma_{1.2}C\gamma_1$ TCR γ chain. Use of a $C\gamma_1$ constant exon results in a γδ TCR that is disulfide-linked. *B*, Germline and mature T lymphocyte forms of the TCR δ chain. The TCR δ chain coding sequences are nested within the TCR α chain locus between the α chain variable exons and the α chain joining exons. The somatic rearrangement depicted results in a $V\delta_2D\delta_2D\delta_3J\delta_1C\delta$ TCR δ chain. This particular rearrangement incorporates two D exons. Pairing of the γ and δ chains in this figure reconstitutes a γδ TCR from a *Mycobacterium tuberculosis*–reactive γδ T-cell clone isolated from the pleural fluid of a patient with tuberculous pleuritis. (From Ohmen JD, Barnes PF, Uyemura K, et al. The T cell receptors of human gamma delta T cells reactive to *Mycobacterium tuberculosis* are encoded by specific V genes but diverse V-J junctions. J Immunol. 1991;147:3353–3359.)

be expected with a CD4⁻8⁻ phenotype. The γδ TCR⁺ T lymphocytes recognize conformational epitopes of polypeptides and possibly carbohydrates in a manner similar to antibodies. In fact, sequence analysis of the antigen recognition sites suggests that the γδ TCR is more closely related to the B-cell immunoglobulin antigen receptor than to the αβ TCR.[174] Murine alloreactive γδ T cells specific for H2-T molecules and I-E^k do not require any antigen processing and can recognize their epitopes across species barriers, including recognition of recombinant molecules produced by *Drosophila* cell lines that synthesize MHC complexes devoid of peptides.[172] In addition, a herpes simplex virus (HSV)–specific γδ T-cell clone derived from an infected mouse recognizes HSV glycoprotein I in a manner independent of MHC and TAP. The γδ TCR recognizes the native conformation of the HSV glycoprotein in the absence of any processing.[175, 176] Numbers and distribution of γδ T cells are not affected by deficiencies of β_2-microglobulin or TAP that are known to have a dramatic impact on CD8⁺ αβ TCR⁺ T cells,[177, 178] by CD1 knockout known to decrease natural T-cell numbers,[140] or by invariant-chain or H2-M knockouts that decrease the number and function of CD4⁺ T lymphocytes.[26, 42]

T-Lymphocyte Maturation in the Thymus

The process of T-cell development and selection of T lymphocytes that express specific TCR rearrangements takes place in the thymus. Somatic recombination in γ, δ, α, β, and TCR loci also occurs within the thymus.[179] The process of lymphocyte development is complex, and a thorough review is beyond the scope of this chapter. In brief, T-lymphocyte precursors travel from the bone marrow to the thymus. On entering the thymus, these cells are TCR⁻, CD8⁻, and CD4⁻. Initial TCR rearrangements occur in the γ-chain and δ-chain loci. Successful rearrangement results in a CD4⁻8⁻ γδ T lymphocyte. The γδ T lymphocytes then undergo a poorly understood process of negative selection that eliminates autoreactive T cells before migration into the periphery. However, some γδ T cells appear to develop outside the thymus. In transgenic γδ TCR mouse models, thymic depletion of autoreactive γδ T lymphocytes applies only to lymphocytes that normally reside in the spleen and peripheral lymph nodes (systemic immune system). Autoreactive γδ T lymphocytes are not depleted in the intraepithelial lymphocyte (IEL) compartment, although their numbers do fade with time.[180, 181] γδ T-lymphocyte IELs are found in normal numbers in athymic mice.

In the thymus, failure to productively rearrange a γδ TCR allows developmental progression through the αβ TCR pathway. The initial event in the αβ pathway is rearrangement of the TCR β-chain. Precursor αβ T lymphocytes express this β-chain with a monomorphic α-chain surrogate called the pre-Tα, the CD3 complex, and CD25 (IL-2 receptor α-chain). After a period of expansion, CD25 expression decreases, both CD4 and CD8 are expressed, and the precursor αβ T lymphocytes begin to rearrange and express the TCR α-chain. Subsequently, either CD4 or CD8 coreceptor expression is lost. Once the αβ T-lymphocyte precursors have successfully rearranged to produce unique αβ TCRs, they undergo a selection process based on the affinity of the unique TCRs for MHC molecules loaded with self-peptides. TCRs that do not have any affinity for the available HLA elements (different for every individual) receive no signal and die. TCRs that have too high an affinity for the available self-peptide–loaded HLA elements (autoreactive) are overactivated and die (negative selection). TCRs that have the appropriate affinity for the available HLA-peptide complexes complete the maturation process (positive selection) and leave the thymus for the periphery as CD4⁺8⁻ or CD4⁻8⁺ αβ T lymphocytes.[182, 183] Both positive and negative selection depend on appropriate tyrosine kinase signaling through antigen-engaged TCRs.[184] Only about 10% of the T-lymphocyte precursors circulating through the thymus ever make it out into the periphery as functional T cells.[185]

T-Cell Activation

The process of T-cell activation is central to the development of antigen-specific peripheral T cells for host defense. When a T lymphocyte bearing an appropriate TCR recognizes MHC-bound peptide, signal transduction to the cell cytoplasm begins. T-lymphocyte activation is initiated by a tyrosine kinase cascade induced by the clustering of TCR complexes. The signaling occurs through the CD3 complex associated with the antigen-specific TCR. The first kinases activated are two members of the SRC kinase family, LCK and FYN. Although FYN associates directly with the TCR complex, LCK is associated with the CD4 or CD8 molecule and is brought into proximity to the TCR when both the TCR and the coreceptor molecule interact with the MHC-peptide complex. These kinases phosphorylate particular tyrosines in the cytoplasmic tails of the ε- and ζ-chains of the CD3 complex. The phosphorylated tyrosines then act as docking sites for the next kinases in the cascade, known as ζ-associated protein-70 (ZAP70) and SYK. Absence of ZAP70 leads to severe immunodeficiency in humans and mice; absence of spleen tyrosine kinase (SYK) is lethal because of its broader biologic role.[186]

In general, activation of αβ Th lymphocytes requires additional signals beyond TCR recognition of the MHC-peptide complex and the CD4 coreceptor. Molecules that mediate these additional cell-cell interactions to enhance T-cell proliferation are called costimulatory molecules (Fig. 9–6). One of the best understood Th costimulatory molecules is CD28, which interacts with two different ligands on APCs, termed B7-1 and B7-2.[187] Expression of these ligands is restricted to professional APCs such as macrophages, dendritic cells, and B cells. Without this additional signal interaction, engagement of the TCR by the MHC-peptide complex results in a hyporesponsive state called anergy, in which the Th lymphocyte is refractory to new

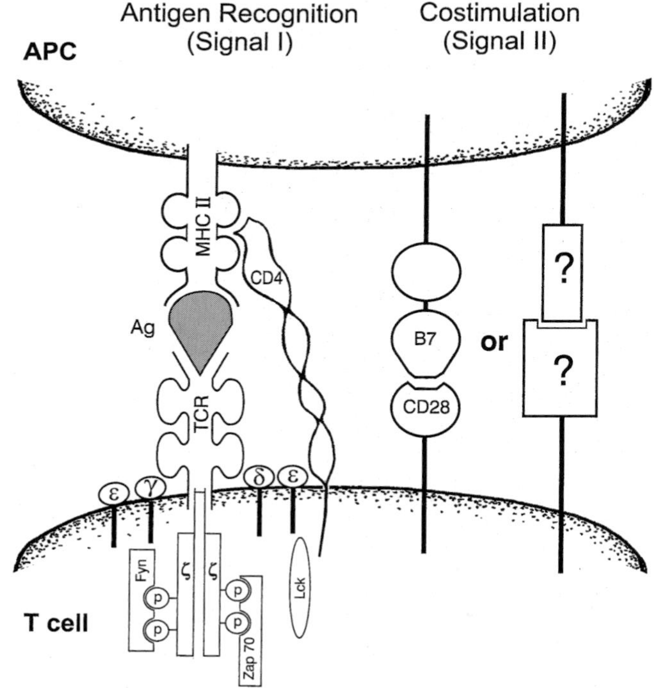

FIGURE 9–6. T-cell activation. T-cell activation requires two signals. The first signal is generated via the T-cell receptor complex and involves the phosphorylation of the CD3 complex and recruitment of src kinases that are associated with the CD4 or CD8 coreceptors. The second signal is commonly referred to as *costimulation*. In most Th lymphocytes this signal is delivered by CD28 interaction with its ligands B7-1 and B7-2 (also known as CD80 and CD86). In some Th and most Tc that are CD28⁻, the mediator(s) of signal II are less clear.

stimuli through the TCR.[188] The molecular mechanism for CD28 costimulation is not well understood, and there is no consensus about the signal transduction events that occur when CD28 binds to its counterreceptors on APCs. CD28 ligation does activate a lipid kinase, phosphatidylinositol 3-kinase, but whether this is important in its costimulatory activity is controversial.[189–191] CD28 may also activate a tyrosine kinase called interleukin-2 inducible T cell kinase (ITK),[192] but its role in costimulation also is uncertain.[193] There is evidence that, together with CD3 signals, CD28 can activate the *c*-JUN amino-terminal kinase (JNK), which is an important event in the activation of gene transcription in response to cell activation.[194] Despite these uncertainties, it is clear that CD28 is a major costimulatory molecule, because in mice that are deficient in CD28 important Th-mediated functions such as B-cell expansion, immunoglobulin class switching, and immunoglobulin production are deficient.[195] The interactions of CD28 with B7-1 and B7-2 are opposed by another T-cell surface molecule, cytotoxic T-lymphocyte–associated protein 4 (CTLA-4), which recognizes the same APC ligands. CTLA-4 interaction with these ligands is not costimulatory and may even inhibit T-cell activation.[196] CTLA-4 is not expressed until late in an immune response and therefore is thought to be part of the gene program for resolution of an inflammatory response. Soluble CTLA-4 has been used to treat chronic inflammatory diseases in several animal models and perhaps has potential as a therapeutic agent in human chronic inflammatory diseases.[197–199]

The role of CD28 in activation of T cells other than CD4$^+$ Th cells is less certain. In humans, approximately 10% of circulating CD8$^+$ T lymphocytes express CD28. Activation of Tc cells for cytolysis and lymphokine secretion is often by nonprofessional APCs. Nonprofessional APCs lack many of the classic accessory molecules used by T cells to interact with professional APCs. An alternate set of accessory molecules may be important for interactions with nonprofessional APCs (see Table 9–3).

T-CELL SUBSETS

Cytotoxic T Lymphocytes

The αβ TCR$^+$ T lymphocytes are functionally divided into Th and Tc cells based on the expression of CD4 or CD8, respectively. CD8$^+$ T cells recognize their antigenic peptides in the context of MHC I molecules and are called cytotoxic because their primary role and effector function is to kill infected or neoplastic cells. This effector function can be mediated by one of several basic mechanisms, all of which are usually active in concert. Activation of Tc lymphocytes upregulates FAS ligand (FASL) on their surfaces. Interaction of T-lymphocyte FASL with FAS (CD95) on the target cell results in programmed cell death (apoptosis) of the target cell. The death cascade involves activation of catabolic proteases (caspases), loss of mitochondrial integrity leading to loss of adenosine triphosphate, and finally activation of endonucleases that cleave nuclear DNA.[200] The second mechanism is a complement-like activity mediated by a Tc granule protein called perforin. Perforin has significant homology to the terminal component of complement (C9) and, like complement, is able to form a physical pore in planar lipid bilayers. This activity alone is sufficient to lyse non-nucleated targets, but many nucleated cells can survive an isolated perforin "hit." Perforin's role is to augment apoptosis by facilitating delivery of effector proteases called granzymes through the membrane channels it creates.[201, 202] Granzymes, like perforin, are stored in secretory granules in the Tc cell cytoplasm. Finally, CD8$^+$ Tc cells release the cytokines lymphotoxin-α (LT-α) and tumor necrosis factor-α (TNF-α), which can induce apoptosis in some cell types.

Classically, CD8$^+$ T cells play an important role in the control of viral infections by lysing infected cells. This is especially important for viruses that replicate by noncytolytic pathways.[203, 204] In addition, CD8$^+$ T lymphocytes play an important role in the control of many nonviral intracellular pathogens, including bacteria, fungi, and protozoa.[205, 206]

Activated Tc cells typically secrete a limited number of cytokines (IL-3, LT-α, and IFN-γ) on activation; unlike Th cells, they do not cooperate directly with B cells to generate antibody responses, although there may be some exceptions.[207]

T-Helper Lymphocytes

CD4$^+$ Th lymphocytes are MHC II restricted in their recognition of peptide antigens. Th-cell recognition of APCs bearing appropriate MHC II peptide complexes generally results in lymphokine release as the principal effector function. Helper cells are so named because they orchestrate (help) both Tc and B-cell responses. At the earliest stage of the adaptive immune response, a professional APC (most likely a dendritic cell) presents peptides derived from an invading pathogen (e.g., virus, bacteria, fungus, protozoan) in the context of MHC II molecules to antigen-specific CD4$^+$ T lymphocytes. Help for Tc responses is provided by release of IL-2, IFN-γ, and LT-α; Th-secreted IL-4, IL-5, IL-6, and IL-13 provide help for B-cell responses. This help is especially critical for activation and expansion of naive B and T lymphocytes.

CD4$^+$ T lymphocytes also have cytolytic machinery (perforin and FASL) and can mediate cytolysis, although this process is rarely as robust as that seen with CD8$^+$ T lymphocytes.[208, 209] It is not clear how CD4$^+$ T lymphocytes "decide" whether to release cytokines only or to release cytokines and deliver a lethal hit when they are activated by APCs bearing appropriate antigens. Perforin-dependent killing of infected or neoplastic targets by CD4$^+$ T lymphocytes may actually be controlled by CD8$^+$ T lymphocytes. Naive CD4$^+$ T cells stimulated by alloantigen in the absence of CD8$^+$ T cells and NK cells develop FASL and perforin-mediated cytotoxicity, whereas co-activation of CD4$^+$ and CD8$^+$ T lymphocytes results in CD4$^+$ T cells that can use only FASL for cytolysis. Regulation by CD8$^+$ T lymphocytes requires close proximity to the CD4$^+$ cells, suggesting that cell-cell contact, a low-abundance soluble mediator present in high concentration at the cell-cell interface, or a short-lived soluble mediator is responsible for the regulatory effect. These experiments suggest that CD4-mediated cytolysis is activated under circumstances in which there is little or no CD8$^+$ T-lymphocyte activation.[210]

The T-Helper 1/T-Helper 2 Paradigm

During the course of an immune response, Th cells can develop a bias in cytokine production that preferentially expands and activates either Tc or B lymphocytes. Th cells that secrete IL-2, LT-α, and IFN-γ to assist Tc responses are further classified as Th1 cells, whereas those that secrete IL-4, IL-5, IL-6, and IL-13 are referred to as Th2 cells. Since the late 1980s immunologists have attempted to categorize the cytokine profiles associated with infectious diseases according to the Th1/Th2 paradigm.

The paradigm was based initially on analyses of lymphokine profiles of CD4$^+$ T-cell clones. Mosmann and colleagues[211] found that activated murine CD4$^+$ T-cell clones made either IL-2 and IFN-γ, or IL-4 and IL-13, but not both IFN-γ and IL-4. Since this initial study, the model has been further refined. Th1 lymphocytes produce IL-2, IFN-γ, and LT-α on activation. These cytokines promote activation of Tc, NK, and macrophage cells and B-lymphocyte production of IgG_{2a}. Th2 lymphocytes secrete IL-4, IL-5, IL-6, and IL-13, which promote isotype switching to IgG_1 and IgE antibodies during development of an antibody response. Unlike Th1-secreted cytokines, these Th2 cytokines do not promote cell-mediated immunity. IL-3, IL-10, TNF-α, transforming growth factor (TGF)-β, and GM-CSF are secreted on activation of both Th1 and Th2 cells. Often, at the initiation of an immune response, Th lymphocytes make complex assortments of lymphokines that do not fit either a Th1 or a Th2 pattern; these are classified as Th0 cells.

The Th1/Th2 paradigm has been strengthened by in vitro and in vivo data showing antagonism between Th1 and Th2 lymphokines.

IL-4 promotes Th2 development and antagonizes Th1 development, whereas IFN-γ and IL-12 promote Th1 development and antagonize Th2 development.[212] In vivo, similar synergy and antagonism have been demonstrated in infectious diseases. In some instances, Th polarization has profound effects on the outcome of the infection.

The importance of Th1 versus Th2 polarization is best illustrated by immune responses to the intracellular pathogen *Leishmania major.* Balb/c mice show an increased susceptibility to chronic infection with this organism. The phenotype correlates with preferential production of IL-4 rather than IFN-γ by $CD4^+$ lymphocytes from infected mice, indicating a predominance of Th2 cells in the response to infection. Interventions that blunt the IL-4 response, including administration of anti-IL-4 antibodies or administration of exogenous IL-12 at the time of infection, increase the resistance of Balb/c mice to leishmaniasis. This alteration in susceptibility correlates with a switch from production of Th2 cytokines to Th1 cytokines.[213] A similar correlation of resistance with a Th1 cytokine profile is seen in infections by other intracellular pathogens, including *L. monocytogenes* and several mycobacteria.[205] Conversely, polarization toward development of Th2 cells and their associated cytokines has been associated with resistance to large extracellular pathogens such as nematodes and cestodes.[206, 214–216] In contrast to the situation with intracellular pathogens, interventions that blunt the IL-4 response, such as administration of exogenous IL-12 or IFN-γ, exacerbate parasitic infections.[217–219] These data suggest a dichotomy in T-lymphocyte responses, with Th1 responses leading to effective protection from intracellular pathogens and Th2 responses important in protection against extracellular parasitic infections. Consistent with the role of Th2 lymphocytes in defending against parasitic infections is the importance of the Th2 cytokines IL-4 and IL-5 in IgE production and eosinophil biology.[220, 221]

The current model for Th1/Th2 polarization in immune responses is diagrammed in Figure 9–7. An invading pathogen causes local inflammation and recruitment of the innate defense system. Macrophages and dendritic cells engulf either the whole living invading pathogen directly or pathogen debris resulting from the local inflammatory response and become activated to make IL-12, TNF-α, and other cytokines. Other innate effector cells also produce cytokines at this stage of the immune response. NK cells secrete IFN-γ, and natural T cells (discussed later) make IL-4. In the draining lymph node, naive antigen-specific $CD4^+$ Th0 T cells interact with dendritic cells bearing pathogen antigens in the context of MHC II. Based on the relative balance of pro-Th1 cytokines (IL-12, IFN-γ) versus pro-Th2 cytokines (IL-4, IL-10), Th0 $CD4^+$ T cells differentiate into either Th1 or Th2 cells. Once polarization has occurred, it is self-reinforcing, because IFN-γ suppresses Th2 development and, conversely, IL-4 and IL-10 suppress Th1 development. In this model, the polarity "decision" made by Th cells is made early in the immune response, based on the balance of pro-Th1 and pro-Th2 cytokines generated by effector cells of the innate immune response.[222]

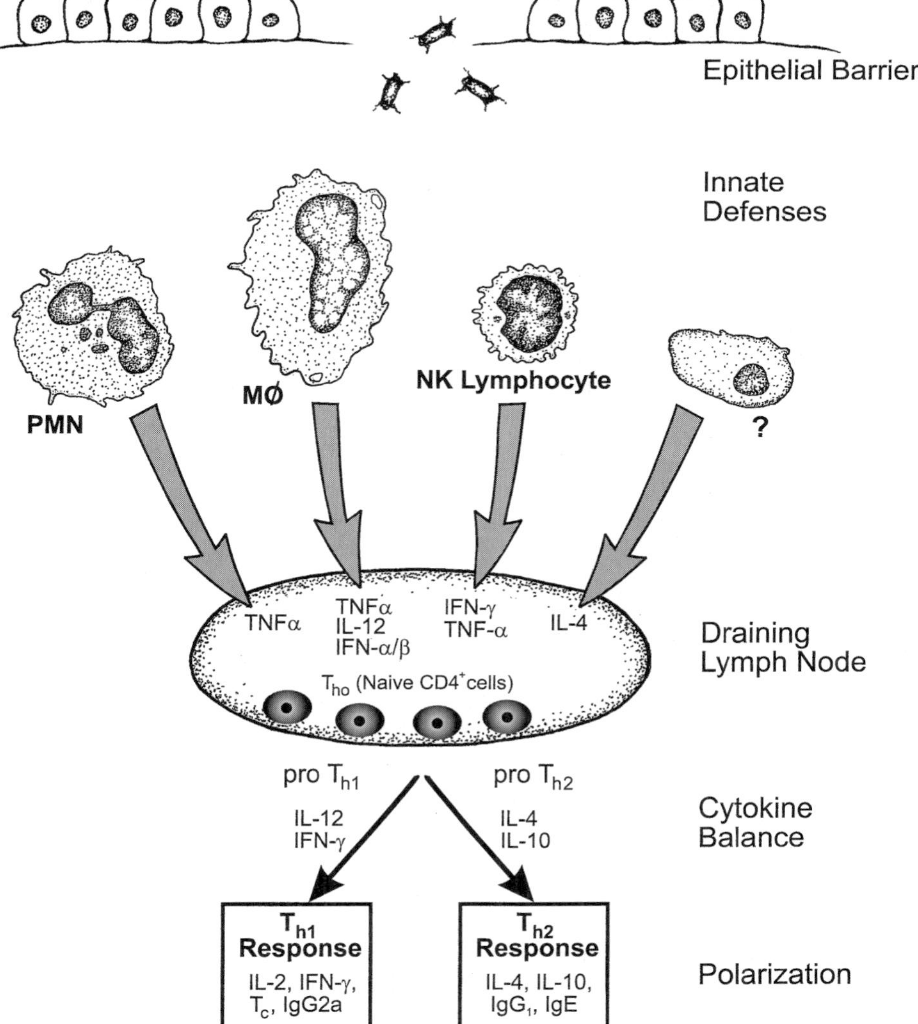

FIGURE 9–7. The Th1/Th2 paradigm. An invading microbe penetrates an epithelial barrier, triggering activation of the resident innate defenses. Antigens from the invading pathogen and cytokines produced by the innate defenses feed into the local draining lymph node via the afferent lymphatics. The relative abundance of pro-Th1 cytokines (IL-12 and IFN-γ) *versus* pro-Th2 cytokines (IL-4 and IL-10) influences naive antigen-stimulated $CD4^+$ T lymphocytes (Th0) to differentiate into either Th1 cells or Th2 cells.

The Th1/Th2 paradigm is important because it provides a framework within which to organize the complex and dynamic cytokine responses to infection. It is supported by elegant animal models and in vitro experiments. However, a decade of dedicated research in this field has stretched the paradigm. Experimental data inconsistent with the model have prompted some dissent.[223, 224] First, mice that naturally develop Th1-type responses to infections can be forced to shift to Th2 responses, but they do not maintain a Th2 response unless the external influences are maintained. C3H mice naturally develop a Th1-type response to infection with *L. major*. Treatment of these mice with antibodies against IL-12 or IFN-γ during infection results in a Th2-type response and persistent infection. The susceptible Th2 phenotype reverts to a resistant phenotype once the anti-IL-12 or anti-IFN-γ antibody treatment is stopped.[225] Second, the Th1/Th2 polarization correlation with resistance and susceptibility established for *L. major* has no predictive value for *Leishmania donovani* infections.[226, 227] IL-4–deficient mice are actually more susceptible to *L. donovani* infection than normal littermates.[228] Third, it has been difficult to identify the early effector cell that secretes IL-4 during the innate immune response to induce Th2 polarization. Natural T cells were an attractive candidate, but CD1 knockout mice deficient in this cell population have normal IgE class switching (a surrogate marker of Th2 function), and normal Th2 polarization occurs in β_2-microglobulin knockout mice also deficient in natural T cells.[229, 230] Finally, the Th1/Th2 paradigm is most clearly applicable to chronic infections, and it is therefore tempting to infer that Th1 and Th2 polarization represent extremes on a dynamic continuum rather than a categorical response to infection.

A modified version of the Th1/Th2 paradigm is presented in Figure 9–8. Pathogen invasion triggers local inflammation; its characteristics are determined by the cell types infected and the configuration of the innate immune response in the involved tissue. Antigen presentation by dendritic cells in the draining lymph nodes activates naive CD4$^+$ T cells to a Th0 phenotype, and they produce IL-2, IL-4, and IFN-γ. These lymphokines trigger an initial expansion of B cells, CD8$^+$ T cells, and NK cells and the activation of macrophages. The Th0 profile of lymphokines is consistent with general activation of all branches of the immune response. If the cytokine-stimulated CD8$^+$ T cells find infected cells bearing MHC I epitopes, they become activated and expand further, producing more IFN-γ. Most MHC I presentation requires that pathogen proteins be present in the host cytoplasm for proteolytic processing by proteasomes and loading onto MHC I heterodimers via the TAP1/TAP2 transporter. This is most likely to occur with intracellular pathogens. If class I–restricted antigens are present, CD8$^+$ Tc–generated IFN-γ can influence the evolving Th0 response toward Th1. On the other hand, if the CD8$^+$ T lymphocytes find few MHC I epitopes, then no significant activation or expansion of CD8$^+$ T lymphocytes occurs, B cells play a more prominent role in the immune response, and the evolving Th0 response shifts toward Th2.[231] In extracellular infections (e.g., with helminths), few MHC I epitopes are likely to be generated, leading to a diminished role for CD8$^+$ T cells and the development of a Th2-type response.

The critical step in this model is the generation of MHC I–restricted antigenic peptides by the proteasome complex in the infected cell cytoplasm, and a critical question is whether potential antigens of the pathogen are available to the proteasome in any infected cell. This alternative model can accommodate the inconsistencies in Th1/Th2 polarization seen within *Leishmania* strains or described in other infections.[232] Different strains may have different MHC I epitopes or a different intracellular biology, affecting processing and presentation of cytosolic antigens. Consistent with this model is the role that has been recognized for CD8$^+$ T cells in controlling nonviral intracellular pathogens,[205, 233] including *Leishmania*.[234] CD8$^+$ T cells are responsible for resolution of *Leishmania* infections in Balb/c mice manipulated to acquire a resistant phenotype.[235, 236] A direct role for CD8$^+$ T cells in determining Th1 versus Th2 polarization through IFN-γ production has been demonstrated in a murine model of respiratory syncytial virus infection.[237] Finally, classic Th1/Th2 polarization is seen in chronic infections, and polarization to Th1 or Th2 phenotypes typically requires 2 to 3 weeks in most experimental systems. In viral or acute intracellular bacterial infections, antigen-specific CD8$^+$ T cells are detectable as early as day 3 and usually peak within 1 week; this time course of the CD8$^+$ T-cell responses to infection is compatible with a role in regulation of Th1/Th2 polarization. Still, the modified Th1/Th2 paradigm cannot directly account for some observed phenomena, such as resistance to *Leishmania* infection in β_2-microglobulin–deficient mice.[238] It is likely that multiple overlapping host defense mechanisms contribute to susceptibility and resistance and the associated Th cytokine patterns.

In humans, immune responses to several chronic infections appear to polarize along Th1/Th2 lines.[239] One human pathogen to which the Th1/Th2 paradigm has been applied is *M. leprae*. Lepromatous leprosy (poorly controlled disease with high organism burden) is associated with Th2-type polarization, whereas tuberculoid leprosy (controlled infection with few organisms) is associated with a Th1-type response.[240] T cells isolated from tuberculoid leprosy lesions produce IFN-γ,[241, 242] and lepromatous leprosy lesions yield CD8$^+$ T cells that make IL-4.[242] Other studies report T-lymphocyte production of both IL-4 and IFN-γ (Th0) regardless of disease status.[243, 244] It is difficult to use the standard Th1/Th2 paradigm exclusively to understand the immune response to leprosy because Tc cells are a source of IL-4 in this disease and because γδ T lymphocytes are likely to have an important role in host protection from mycobacterial infections (see later discussion). Nonetheless, the role of IL-12 and IFN-γ in protection from mycobacteria (and salmonella) in humans is clear. Patients deficient in receptors for either of these lymphokines are vulnerable to severe infections by these intracellular pathogens.[245–249]

Progression of HIV infection has been reported to correlate with a shift from Th1 toward Th2 cytokine profiles,[250] but this view is controversial.[251] Interpretation of these data is complicated because of the destruction of CD4$^+$ cells by the virus and because CD8$^+$ Tc lymphocytes probably play a prominent role in preventing disease progression.[252–254]

A clinically useful way to analyze the host response to mycobacterial and other intracellular pathogen infections is to ask whether there has been adequate activation of macrophages and dendritic cells. In lepromatous leprosy, the tissue macrophage organism burden is very high, suggesting a profound inability to kill the intracellular pathogen. Similar findings are present in disseminated tuberculosis and in *Histoplasma* and *Leishmania* infections. This failure of macrophage activation presents a potential opportunity to intervene with immunomodulatory therapy. Likely candidates for intervention are the lymphokines that directly or indirectly affect cytocidal activity and antigen presentation, which are the Th1-like cytokines including IFN-γ, GM-CSF, macrophage colony-stimulating factor (M-CSF), TNF-α, and IL-1β. IL-12, alone or in combination with IL-2, increases IFN-γ and may also have other effects on cytokine dynamics.[255] Toxicity limits the clinical potential for some cytokines such as TNF-α and IL-1β.[256, 257] IL-12 administration appears to be associated with toxicity as well, because preliminary studies with IL-12 as a cancer therapy adjuvant showed IL-12–related mortality,[258] and phase I trials with IL-12 in HIV patients showed acute decreases in lymphocyte counts lasting about 1 week after the initial dose.[259] The mechanisms for these cytokine toxicities are not understood.

In contrast, IFN-γ is been less toxic and has been used successfully to treat refractory disseminated mycobacterial infections in both compromised and noncompromised hosts.[260–263] Use of IFN-γ or perhaps other cytokines in combination with directed antimicrobial therapy (if available) would be expected to give the greatest benefit. In animal models antimicrobial therapy can shift immune responses toward Th1-type lymphokines, and the same phenomenon (reversal reaction) is seen in patients with borderline leprosy treated with antibiotics.[264] As characterization of the immune deficiencies in com-

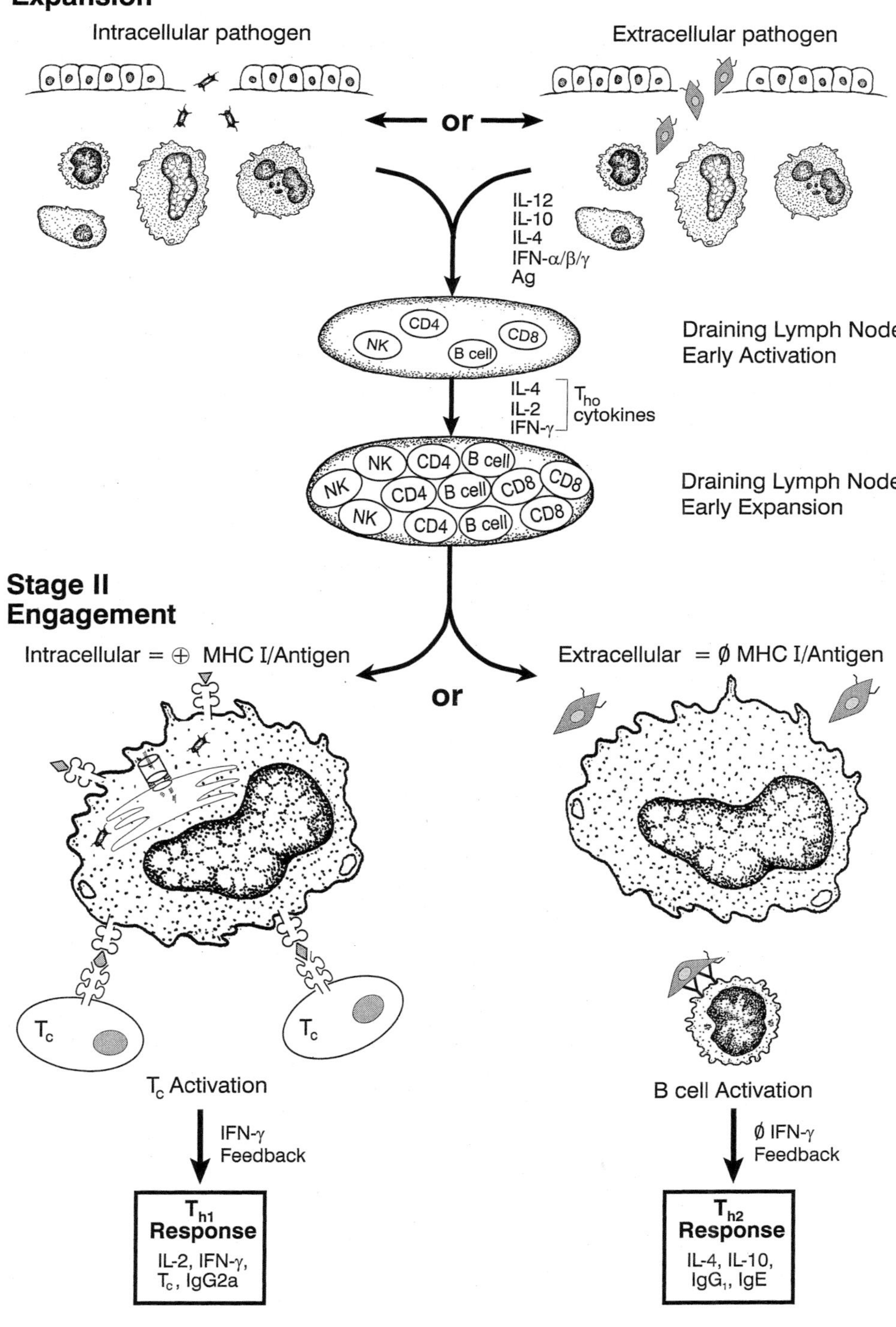

FIGURE 9–8. The modified Th1/Th2 paradigm. An invading microbe penetrates an epithelial barrier triggering activation of the resident innate defenses. Antigens from the invading pathogen and cytokines produced by the innate defenses feed into the local draining lymph node via afferent lymphatics. Activated naive $CD4^+$ T lymphocytes (Th0) drive an initial expansion of T cells, NK cells, and B cells, as well as activation of macrophages. Th1 versus Th2 polarization is determined by relative contributions of $CD8^+$ T lymphocytes versus B lymphocytes in the evolving adaptive immune response.

promised hosts becomes more complete, rational intervention with cytokines will become increasingly possible.

Intervention with cytokines with Th2 profiles would be most logical for parasitic infections. To date there are no examples for this type of clinical intervention. There are few clinical infectious disease processes in which an excessive Th1-type response causes significant morbidity and mortality. Th2 cytokines are also attractive immunomodulators for disease processes believed to be autoimmune in nature, such as rheumatoid arthritis and systemic lupus erythematosus.[265, 266] A complete review of lymphokines goes beyond the scope of this chapter (see Chapter 37). Table 9–4 presents a simplified listing of important cytokines and their functions in host defense and immunity.

Natural T Lymphocytes

An additional subset of αβ TCR^+ lymphocytes exists that expresses NK cell surface markers.[267] These T lymphocytes are typically $CD4^-$

TABLE 9–4 Cytokines

Cytokine	Principal Cell Source	Major Biologic Effects
Interleukin-1	Many cell types; mononuclear phagocytes are a major source	Fever acute phase response, corticotropin release
Interleukin-1 receptor antagonist	Mononuclear phagocytes contain secreted form	Antagonizes IL-1 by competing for IL-1R
Interleukin-2	T lymphocytes	Major mediator of T-cell proliferation; cofactor for B-cell proliferation and Ig production
Interleukin-3	T cells, mast cells	Promotes proliferation of pluripotent stem cells; growth factor for natural T cells
Interleukin-4	T cells, mast cells, basophils	Promotes proliferation of B and T cells; facilitates IgG_1 and IgE synthesis; inhibits macrophage activation; antagonizes Th1 development
Interleukin-5	T cells, mast cells	Promotes antibody production especially IgM, IgA, and IgE; eosinophil expansion and activation; expansion of T cell independent B cells; critical for protective immunity in some parasite infections
Interleukin-6	Many cell types; mononuclear phagocytes are a major source; T cells and endothelial cells	Mediates the acute phase response; enhances B-cell proliferation and Ig production; cofactor for T-cell proliferation
Interleukin-7	Bone marrow stromal cells	Major role in NK cell homeostasis; growth factor for B-cell development and thymocyte growth; cofactor for T-cell growth and macrophage activation
Interleukin-8 and the CXC chemokines	Many cell types; mononuclear phagocytes are a major source; endothelial cells, epithelial cells, T cells	Neutrophil chemoattractants
CC chemokines	Many cell types; mononuclear phagocytes are a major source; endothelial cells, epithelial cells, T cells	Lymphocyte and monocyte chemoattractants; eosinophil and basophil chemoattractants and activators
C chemokine lymphotactin	T cells, NK cells, mast cells	Lymphocyte chemoattractant
Interleukin-9	CD4+ lymphocytes	Cofactor for some CD4+ T cell clones; mast cell growth factor
Interleukin-10	Mononuclear phagocytes, CD4+ T cells, B cells, keratinocytes	Inhibits cytokine synthesis by macrophages, T cells, NK cells; downregulates MCH class II on macrophages; antagonizes Th1 development; enhances B-cell growth and antibody production; cofactor for mast cell growth
Interleukin-11	Bone marrow stromal cells	Mediates acute phase protein synthesis; enhances B-cell growth and differentiation to plasma cells
Interleukin-12	Mononuclear cells, B cells	Induces IFN-γ in T cells and NK cells; enhances T cell and NK cell cytotoxicity; growth factor for activated T cells; major cytokine for Th1 development
Interleukin-13	T lymphocytes	B-cell proliferation and immunoglobulin production; enhances IgE and IgG isotype switching; downregulates expression of macrophage inflammatory cytokines
Interleukin-14	B and T lymphocytes	Proliferation of activated B cells
Interleukin-15	Bone marrow stroma, gut/skin epithelium, macrophages	Major mediator of proliferation and homeostasis in extrathymic T-lymphocyte development; growth factor for αβ & γδ IEL and NK cells
Interleukin-16	Many cell types: T lymphocytes, B lymphocytes, eosinophils, epithelial cells, mast cells	Chemoattractant for T cells, monocytes, and eosinophils; growth factor for CD4+ lymphocytes
Interleukin-17	T lymphocytes	Induces stromal cells to produce IL-6, IL-8, G-CSF; complex effects on macrophage cytokine production
Interleukin-18	Macrophages, keratinocytes	Augments T-lymphocyte production of IFN-γ and TNF-α; related to IL-1 but uses a different receptor
Interferon-α	Mononuclear phagocytes, lymphocytes	Interferes with RNA virus replication; downregulates IL-12 production by macrophages; induces expansion of memory T lymphocytes early in inflammatory events; increases MHC I
Interferon-β	Fibroblasts, epithelial cells	Interferes with RNA virus replication; increases MHC I
Interferon-γ	T cells, NK cells	Increases expression of MHC I and II; activates macrophages enhancing cytocidal activity; major cytokine in Th1, development; antagonizes Th2 development
TNF-α	Mononuclear phagocytes, T cells, NK cells, mast cells, eosinophils	Fever; enhances leukocyte endothelial interactions; cofactor for B- and T-lymphocyte proliferation; direct cytotoxicity for some cell types
Lymphotoxin-α (LT-α)	T lymphocytes	Similar to TNF, but generally released in lesser quantity; developmental role in peripheral lymph nodes, spleen, and Peyer's patches
Lymphotoxin-β (LT-β)	T lymphocytes	Similar to LT-α; developmental role in peripheral lymph nodes and Peyer's patches
TGF-β	T lymphocytes, mononuclear phagocytes	Pleiotropic effects; on balance an anti-inflammatory cytokine; plays an important role in oral tolerance
GM-CSF	T cells, endothelial cells, mononuclear phagocytes, fibroblasts, mast cells	Growth of granulocyte macrophage precursors; enhances macrophage and granulocyte function
M-CSF	Monocytes, endothelial cells, fibroblasts	Growth of mononuclear phagocytes; enhances macrophage function
G-CSF	Mononuclear phagocytes, epithelial cells, fibroblasts	Promotes granulocyte production; enhances granulocyte function

Abbreviations: CSF, Colony-stimulating factor; G, granulocyte; GM, granulocyte-macrophage; IEL, intraepithelial lymphocyte; IFN, interferon; Ig, immunoglobulin; IL, interleukin; M, macrophage; MHC, major histocompatibility complex; NK, natural killer; TGF, transforming growth factor; TNF, tumor necrosis factor.
Adapted from Locksley RM, Wilson CB. Cell-mediated immunity and its role in host defense. In: Mandell GL, Bennett JE, Dolin R, eds. Principles and Practice of Infectious Diseases. 4th ed. New York: Churchill Livingstone; 1995.

and $CD8^-$, although a small subpopulation can be $CD4^+8^-$. This unique subset of T lymphocytes is called NK^+ T cells or *natural T cells*. Natural T cells are typically less than 1% of the peripheral T-cell pool, but in some normal persons they can be almost 10% of peripheral T cells.[268] In patients with autoimmune diseases, this subset can represent up to 50% of circulating T lymphocytes.[269, 270] Natural T cells are especially prominent in liver and bone marrow.[271] In addition to their unique cell-surface phenotype, these T lymphocytes also have unique growth characteristics. Unlike typical $CD4^+8^-$ or $CD4^-8^+$ αβ TCR^+ T cells or γδ T cells, natural T cells can utilize IL-3 as a growth factor.[272, 273] Despite carrying NK-cell receptors, this population of T lymphocytes displays little NK-like cytotoxicity.[274, 275]

Natural T lymphocytes are restricted in the composition and diversity of their TCRs. Unlike Tc and Th cells, natural T cells have an invariant TCR α-chain, $V\alpha_{24}$-J_Q in humans ($V\alpha_{14}$-J_{128} in mice).[276] In addition, the β-chain of the TCR seems skewed toward $V\beta_{11}$ ($V\beta_8$, $V\beta_7$, $V\beta_2$ in mice).[276, 277] There is junctional diversity (non-germline–encoded nucleotides) in the β-chain V-D and D-J junctions.[278, 279] Natural T cell development occurs predominantly in extrathymic compartments[280, 281] but also in the thymus.[271, 282] Normal development of natural T cells is critically dependent on CD1 antigen presentation both in the periphery and in the thymus[140] and therefore is independent of TAP. Indirect evidence suggests that H2-T molecules may influence natural T cell development,[283] although their role is not critical.[284]

The role of natural T cells in the cellular immune response is a matter of debate. It is possible that natural T cells are the source of IL-4 early in infections that polarize toward Th2 responses,[285] although this concept remains controversial.[229, 230] A role for natural T cells in host defense against free-living bacteria seems to be well supported. CD1 molecules present bacterial glycolipids to natural T cells, and this process presumably has a role in the activation of phagocytes, B cells, and other elements of humoral host defense. A natural T cell clone specific for *Escherichia coli* presented by peripheral blood monocytes has been isolated from a normal subject.[268] Localization of these T lymphocytes in the liver (the critical bacterial filter of the portal circulation) is consistent with the hypothesis that they play an important role in initial responses to bacterial infections.

γδ T-Lymphocyte Effector Functions

The γδ T-lymphocyte functions are not as well studied as those of αβ T cells, but these cells seem most similar to Tc cells in their cytolytic functions and lymphokine profiles. Cytolysis by γδ T lymphocytes can be mediated by either a perforin[286] or an FASL pathway.[287] Although lymphokine profiles of γδ T lymphocytes have not been exhaustively studied, lectin-stimulated murine γδ T cells secrete predominantly IFN-γ and TNF-α. In some animal models other cytokines may predominate[288, 289]; no data are available that specifically address this issue in human γδ T lymphocytes.

Nonpeptide molecules have been found to activate a subset of γδ T lymphocytes to proliferate and to lyse NK cell targets.[290] $V\gamma_2V\delta_2$ TCR (also known as $V\gamma_9V\delta_2$ TCR) γδ T cells are stimulated by a myriad of alkyl phosphate molecules of both natural and synthetic origin. These compounds have low molecular weights (100 to 600 Da) and represent precursors for synthesis of vitamins, lipids, and sterols. A mycobacterial product, isopentenyl pyrophosphate, also stimulates this γδ T-cell subset. Because this compound is synthesized by many bacteria, it is possible that these γδ T lymphocytes are an important part of antibacterial host defense. These small molecules can activate in vitro propagated γδ TCR clones directly, in the absence of exogenous APCs.[291–294] In contrast, activation of primary peripheral blood γδ lymphocytes requires both IL-2 and APCs in addition to alkyl phosphate antigens.[295] The potential role of these compounds as γδ TCR ligands is exciting but unsettled because of their extremely small size and the wide-ranging cross-reactivity among tested natural and synthetic alkyl phosphate compounds. These issues raise questions about the mechanism by which they activate γδ T cells. Understanding of this novel mechanism of T-cell activation will be greatly advanced by definitive data regarding the nature of the interaction of these compounds with the $V\gamma_2V\delta_2$ TCR.

The role of γδ T cells in controlling mycobacterial infections has received considerable clinical and experimental attention. $V\gamma_2V\delta_2$ TCR+ T lymphocytes are the predominant γδ T-cell subset in human peripheral blood. This γδ subset contains the γδ T lymphocytes reactive with mycobacteria.[296, 297] This same subset of γδ T lymphocytes is preferentially expanded by mycobacterial alkyl phosphates. These observations have led to speculation that the human γδ T-cell repertoire is skewed by interactions with mycobacterial pathogens, and that these T lymphocytes may play an important role in the control of mycobacterial diseases.

Data collected from patients with mycobacterial infections have neither confirmed nor refuted this hypothesis because they have not given a clear picture of γδ T-cell function in these diseases. In some studies mycobacteria-infected patients have elevated numbers of γδ T lymphocytes,[298–300] and in others they do not.[301–303] Patients with uncontrolled tuberculosis infection (pneumonia or miliary disease) have decreased γδ T-cell function (and numbers) locally and systemically, as measured by γδ TCR^+ T-lymphocyte responsiveness to *M. tuberculosis* in vitro.[303–305] *M. leprae* skin testing (lepromin reaction) shows an increased number of γδ T lymphocytes at the injection site in patients with the tuberculoid form of the disease,[306] whereas absence of *M. leprae* responsive γδ T lymphocytes is a hallmark of lepromatous leprosy.[303] Murine models using αβ TCR–deficient mice or γδ TCR–deficient mice support a role for γδ T lymphocytes in controlling *M. tuberculosis*, especially in the early stages of infection; γδ knockout mice have significantly higher mycobacterial organism burdens in liver, spleen, and lung after intravenous infection with a low inoculum and increased mortality at a higher inoculum.[307] Aerosol challenge with *M. tuberculosis* revealed an exacerbation in pulmonary lesions in γδ knockout mice, without a dramatic increase in bacterial growth compared with normal littermates; survival of aerosol-infected knockout animals compared with controls was not addressed.[308] Many studies of resistance to infection in γδ knockout mice have been done with intraperitoneal or intravenous challenges, but the localization of γδ T cells in epithelial tissues suggests that they may have a more prominent role in these sites. It is not clear that γδ T lymphocytes play any role in systemic immunity that is not also performed by the more abundant αβ T lymphocytes. More interesting would be infectious challenges at mucosal surfaces in the lungs, gastrointestinal tract, and reproductive tissues, where γδ T lymphocytes may play a unique role in controlling infections (see later discussion).

The γδ T-cell response to HSV infection is a good model for examining γδ T-lymphocyte function in adaptive immunity because mouse and human data are available. Knockout mice deficient in either αβ TCR or γδ TCR lymphocytes survive and clear HSV-1 footpad infections. Depletion of both αβ and γδ subsets results in failure to clear the infection, with death in most mice within 2 months, demonstrating that either the αβ or the γδ T-lymphocyte subset is sufficient to control HSV infection. In a second model, ocular infection of αβ TCR knockout mice causes significant morbidity but no mortality. If αβ T lymphocyte–deficient mice are depleted of γδ TCR^+ lymphocytes with the use of a monoclonal antibody, then 100% of the mice die within 40 days of HSV-1 encephalitis, again demonstrating a significant role for γδ T lymphocytes in controlling infection. γδ TCR^+ T lymphocytes specific for HSV-1 glycoprotein I can be isolated from αβ TCR knockout mice. The γδ T lymphocytes in these populations are polyclonal (i.e., use different γδ TCRs) and recognize unprocessed glycoprotein I as antigen.[309]

In humans, HSV-specific γδ TCR^+ T lymphocytes can reproducibly be found in the peripheral blood of HSV-seropositive but not -seronegative individuals. In many persons, γδ TCR^+ T lymphocytes represent the predominant HSV-specific cytolytic T-cell population

TABLE 9–5 Role of γδ T Lymphocytes in Infection

Pathogen	Species	Result	References
Viruses			
Coxsackievirus	Murine	Coxsackievirus-specific myocarditis associated with γδ T-lymphocyte subset; adoptive transfer of γδ T cells resulted in viral-specific myocarditis	497
Epstein-Barr virus	Human	γδ T lymphocytes expand during acute mononucleosis	498
Herpes simplex virus	(See text)		
Influenza virus	Murine	γδ T-lymphocyte mediated protection from lethal influenza infection; γδ T lymphocyte recognition of viral hemaglutinin as antigen	499
Papilloma virus	Bovine	γδ T lymphocytes localize in regressing papilloma lesions	500
Sendai virus	Murine	γδ T cell expansion early in pulmonary infection; Sendai virus–specific γδ T-cell recognition of infected macrophages	501
Bacteria			
Francisella tularensis	Murine	No significant role of γδ T lymphocytes	502
Listeria monocytogenes	Murine	Increased number of bacteria recovered early in infection from γδ T cell–depleted mice	503
	Murine	Mice deficient in αβ and γδ T cells were more susceptible to *Listeria* infection than mice deficient only in αβ T cells; direct role of γδ T cells demonstrated	504
	Human	In vivo γδ T-lymphocyte expansion to *Listeria* infection; *Listeria*-specific in vitro activation of peripheral blood γδ T cells but not αβ T cells taken from healthy donors	505
Mycobacteria	(See text)		
Salmonella	Murine	γδ T cell–depleted mice are more susceptible to oral infection	506
	Human	In vivo γδ T-lymphocyte expansion to *Salmonella* infection; *Salmonella*-specific activation of γδ T cells from infected patients but not controls in vitro	507
Protozoa			
Cryptosporidium	Murine	Increased shedding of organism in young γδ T-cell knockout mice compared with controls	508
Eimeria vermiformis	Murine	γδ T-cell knockout mice had increased mucosal damage without increased shedding of pathogen; postulated role in controlling αβ T lymphocyte–mediated inflammation	509
Plasmodium yoelii	Murine	Adoptive transfer of γδ T cells inhibited the liver stage of the parasite life cycle	510
Toxoplasma gondii	Murine	Adoptive transfer of γδ T cells prolonged survival; γδ T cells lysed infected macrophages	511
Trypanosoma cruzi	Murine	γδ T cells contributed to cytopathology but not control of infection	512

grown out in vitro.[310–312] These HSV-specific γδ TCR$^+$ lymphocytes are MHC unrestricted and use $V\gamma_2V\delta_2$ TCR receptors.

γδ T lymphocytes have been shown to have NK cell–like cytolytic activities.[313–315] Studies reveal that approximately 85% of human peripheral blood γδ T lymphocytes express one or more members of the NK cell receptors (CD94, NKR-P1, or p58; see next section).[313]

In addition to viral and mycobacterial infections, γδ T lymphocytes have been shown to play a role in other bacterial and protozoan infections, as outlined in Table 9–5. Few studies have addressed the role of γδ T lymphocytes in fungal infections.[316]

The simplest explanation of γδ T-cell function that encompasses all the available data would be that γδ T cells have roles in both the innate and adaptive immune responses: their function in the adaptive immune response depends on recognition of native antigen on infected cells through the TCR, whereas their innate function resembles NK-cell recognition of "missing self."

NATURAL KILLER CELLS

NK cells are a unique subset of host defense cells comprising approximately 10 to 15% of peripheral blood lymphocytes.[317, 318] They have the general appearance of large granular lymphocytes, carry macrophage and T-cell markers, use T-cell growth factors, secrete T cell–like cytokines, kill targets using perforin- and FASL-mediated pathways, but do not express a TCR or CD3 complex. NK cells and T lymphocytes arise from the same progenitor cell during differentiation.[319]

Long-standing confusion over how NK cells recognize their targets has been significantly reduced over the past several years. NK cells detect the absence of appropriate levels of MHC I on their cellular targets; this is commonly referred to as "missing self" recognition.[320] Decreased levels of cell-surface MHC I molecules are commonly found on infected cells and tumors and therefore provide a general marker for abnormal cells.[321]

NK cells depend on inhibitory receptor interaction with MHC I to prevent them from killing indiscriminately, whereas Tc cells depend on an activating signal produced by TCR interaction with peptide–MHC I complexes to induce them to kill specifically. NK-cell inhibitory receptors belong to one of two distinct families, the C-type lectin and immunoglobulin superfamilies. The C-type lectin receptors are disulfide-linked heterodimers of NK-specific genes (NKGs) NKG2A, NKG2B, NKG2C, NKG2D, or NKG2E paired with CD94. Immunoglobulin superfamily receptors, known as "killer inhibitory receptors (KIRs)," function as monomers or homodimers. Members of both receptor families have been shown to recognize specific MHC I molecules. Both killer inhibitory receptors and C-type lectin class I receptors have cytoplasmic tails containing immunoreceptor tyrosine inhibitory motifs (ITIMs), which are key to the specific repression of NK activation by class I molecules. On receptor ligation, ITIMs are phosphorylated on tyrosine and recruit phosphatases that act to dephosphorylate specific proteins and inositol phospholipids, leading to inhibition of activation pathways and prevention of cytolysis.[322, 323] Engagement of inhibitory receptors by MHC I is consistent with active suppression of NK function by recognition of self. However, some NK receptors from both inhibitory receptor families have identical extracellular ligand-binding domains but lack ITIM motifs in their cytoplasmic domains and actually deliver activating rather than deactivating signals on receptor ligation.[324–326] Currently, it is not clear how these molecules fit into the overall regulation of NK cells.[327, 328] A consequence of "missing self" activation of NK cells is that normal cells can be lysed by NK cells in vitro in the presence of antibodies against either the inhibitory NK receptors or MHC I molecules.

NK-cell detection of "missing self" leads to cytolysis and cytokine release.[322] NK cells express perforin, granzymes, and FASL, and NK cell–mediated cytolysis is mechanistically similar to that mediated by T lymphocytes.[329–331] NK cells also express CD16, a low-affinity IgG receptor (FcγRIII), and can mediate antibody-dependent cell-mediated cytotoxicity (ADCC). The presence of pathogen-specific antibody has been shown to be critical in some settings for NK-cell function.[332] Cytokines secreted by NK cells are similar to those produced by CD8$^+$ Tc cells. The principal NK-cell cytokines are IL-3, IFN-γ, TNF-α, LT-α, M-CSF, and GM-CSF, though additional cytokines have been reported.[333]

NK cells provide some degree of protection against viral, bacterial, and protozoan infections.[334] The role of NK cells in fungal infection in vivo has not been extensively investigated, but adoptive transfer experiments and genetic experiments have demonstrated a role for NK cells in control of *Cryptococcus neoformans* in a murine model.[335, 336]

Most of the NK-cell protective effect seen in animal models of infection can be reproduced or replaced by exogenous IFN-γ administration. For this reason, the role of NK cells in protection against intracellular bacteria (and probably against protozoans) is thought to be secretion of IFN-γ, which activates macrophage cytocidal activities.[337] In viral infections, the mechanism of NK protection probably involves NK cell–mediated cytolysis in addition to secretion of IFN-γ. Severe combined immunodeficient (SCID) mice are an important animal model for studying NK-cell effects. These mice lack functional B and T lymphocytes but have normal NK cells. Although NK cells can be shown in animal models to provide some degree of protection from infection, animals that are dependent solely on NK cells for protection rarely clear infections.[338] Patients deficient in NK-cell activity are predisposed to chronic bacterial infections (otitis, bronchiectasis) and severe manifestations of HSV, varicella-zoster virus (VZV), cytomegalovirus (HCMV), and acute Epstein-Barr virus mononucleosis.[339, 340] Consistent with an adjunctive role for NK cells in the immune response, these patients with decreased NK function appear to have a more severe clinical course but ultimately do clear their infections rather than developing chronic disease.

NK cells are typically considered part of the innate defense system because their activation to lyse infected targets does not require recognition of specific pathogen antigens, because they are functional without prior exposure to specific pathogens, and because they have no demonstrable memory. However, the functional distinction between NK cells and T lymphocytes has become more blurred since the realization that some αβ TCR^+ T lymphocytes (natural T cells and some $CD8^+$ αβ T cells) and γδ TCR^+ T lymphocytes express classic C-type lectin NK receptors. In addition, these T-cell subsets are capable of typical NK-like activities.[317, 341–345] It is now clear that inhibitory receptors containing ITIM motifs are not NK-specific and are more generally expressed than initially thought.[346] These inhibitory receptors may have a general role in growth regulation in many cell types. Like NK receptors, the inhibitory receptors have counterparts with identical extracellular domains that lack cytoplasmic ITIM sequences. Several members of this expanding family are expressed on other cells of the immune system, including $CD4^+$ T cells, B cells, and macrophages.[347–350] The role of these newly discovered inhibitory receptors in immunobiology remains to be clarified.

NEW ASPECTS OF CELL-MEDIATED IMMUNITY

Major Histocompatibility Complex–Independent T-Cell Antimicrobial Activity

One special problem for the immune system is the killing of large invading pathogens (eukaryotic pathogens). Frequently these pathogens are multicelluar, too large to be effectively engulfed by professional phagocytes, or resistant to phagocytosis because of capsular polysaccharides or other protective features. This class of pathogens includes fungi, protozoans, flukes, cestodes, and nematodes. T-cell deficiencies can predispose the host to severe infections with these pathogens.[351] One explanation for this phenomenon may be that cytokine deficiencies related to T-lymphocyte dysfunction decrease the recruitment or activation of eosinophils that are prominent cells in the host response to multicellular pathogens. However, not all of the infections with "big" pathogens are associated with significant eosinophilia, nor are eosinophils implicated in all big pathogen infections.[352, 353] An alternative, but not mutually exclusive, explanation for the increased susceptibility of patients with immune defects to these infections is that T lymphocytes and NK cells may have a role in direct killing of invading pathogens.

Human T lymphocytes and NK cells have an innate ability to bind to and kill eukaryotic and possibly even some prokaryotic pathogens.[354] This effector function is MHC independent, because no APC is present or required. The electron micrograph in Figure 9–9 shows human T lymphocytes interacting with *C. neoformans,* and Figure 9–10 is a phase contrast photomicrograph of human T lymphocytes interacting with *Schistosoma mansoni.* Both figures demonstrate T-lymphocyte adherence to pathogens and a T cell–associated cytopathic effect. NK cells and T lymphocytes isolated from the peripheral blood of normal human donors can directly inhibit growth of *C. neoformans* in vitro.[355] Experiments using IL-2–treated peripheral blood cells have demonstrated that both the $CD4^+$ and $CD8^+$ T lymphocyte subsets mediate the inhibitory effect.[356, 357] In mice, prior immunization enhances the T lymphocyte–mediated inhibition of cryptococcus growth.[358, 359] Activated human T lymphocytes also have been shown to have direct antimicrobial activity against *Entamoeba histolytica*[360] and *S. mansoni.*[361] T lymphocytes from mice immunized with fixed *Nocardia asteroides* have direct antimicrobial activity against this prokaryotic pathogen.[362]

For both eukaryotic and prokaryotic pathogens, many important features of this immune mechanism remain to be elucidated, including the mechanism of the antimicrobial effect. The question of γδ versus αβ T lymphocyte contribution to this type of immunity has not been addressed directly. It is tempting to speculate that IELs may play some role in this defense system, because they reside at portals of entry in a heightened state of activation. Better understanding of these phenomena may reveal an unanticipated role for T cells in innate host defense.

Role of Mast Cells in Bacterial Host Defense

Although not typically considered in the same company as NK cells, neutrophils, macrophages, and dendritic cells, tissue mast cells play an important role as an early component of host defense. Mice deficient in mast cells are markedly susceptible to experimental bacterial infections.[363] Mast cells are the only cell type shown to store presynthesized TNF-α in secretory granules.[364–366] They are also the only nonlymphoid cell type capable of IL-4 production.[367] Mast cells can sense invading bacteria either through direct binding of bacteria[368] or indirectly through receptors for C3a and C5a, products of bacterial activation of complement. Either mechanism can lead to mast cell degranulation and release of TNF-α. TNF-α induces inflammation by directing synthesis of proinflammatory molecules on overlying endothelium and by acting as a chemoattractant for polymorphonuclear lymphocytes. IL-4 is a potent B-cell growth factor and an important contributor to Th2 development. Presumably the role for mast cells in host defense involves their early activation and recruitment of these effector cells to sites of infection.

THE MUCOSAL IMMUNE SYSTEM

The mucosal immune system (mucosal-associated lymphoid tissue, or MALT) is a unique branch of adaptive immunity. These lymphocytes reside preferentially within the mucosa and are specialized to function within that environment. The number of T lymphocytes localized to the MALT is approximately equal to the number of T lymphocytes residing in the remaining lymphoid tissues (systemic immune system).[369] Three functional compartments can be identified within mucosal tissues of the gut, which is the best characterized of the mucosal immune sites (Fig. 9–11). The first is the intraepithelial compartment (IELs). These lymphocytes are directly incorporated into the epithelial cell layer. The second is the lamina propria (lamina propria lymphocytes, or LPLs) immediately below the mucosal epithelium, separated only by the basal lamina. The third compartment is the Peyer's patches, which are loosely organized lymphoid tissue centered below specialized epithelial cells that sample the antigenic milieu of the gut lumen. The IEL and LPL compartments differ mainly in the relative abundance of γδ T cells and B cells. γδ T lymphocytes are found predominately among the IEL, whereas B lymphocytes are localized to the LPL compartment; αβ TCR^+ lymphocytes are found in both compartments. B lymphocytes that reside

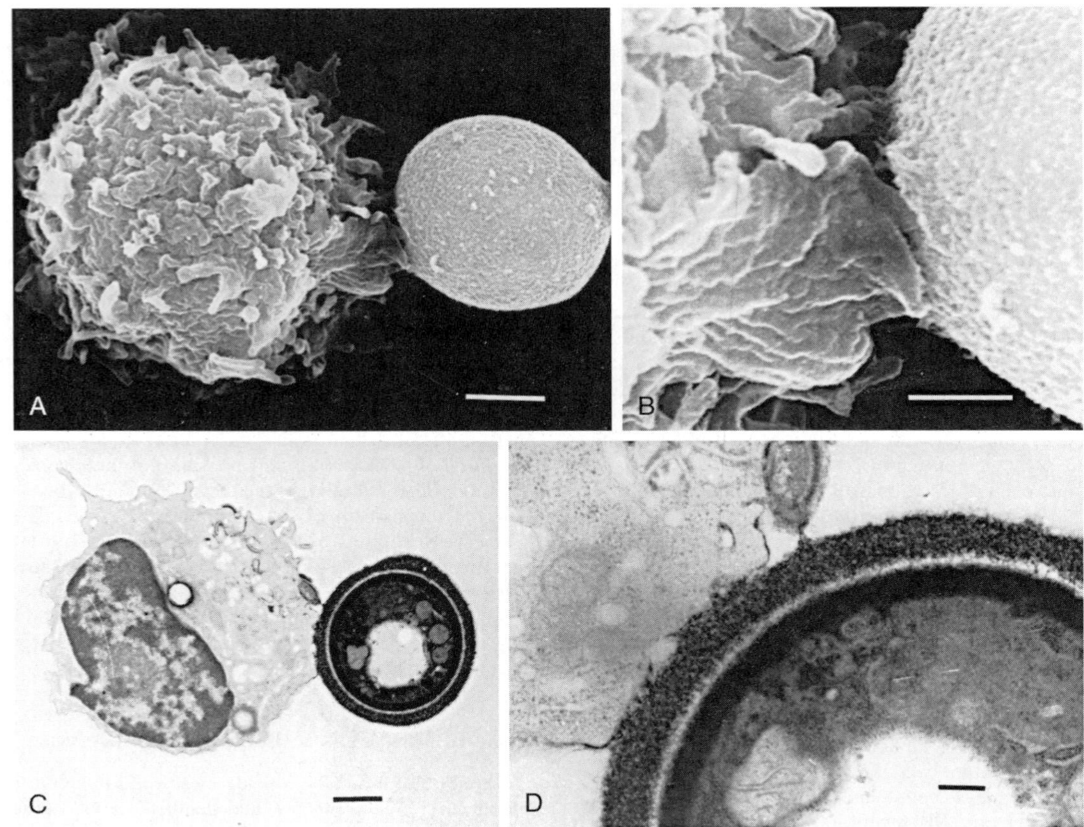

FIGURE 9–9. Direct antimicrobial activity of T lymphocytes. Scanning and transmission electron micrograph demonstrating binding of human T cells (left side of photomicrographs) to *Cryptococcus neoformans*. *A,* Scanning electron micrograph; *B,* higher magnification of the cell-cell contact area in *A*; *C,* transmission electron micrograph of a thin section through a T cell–*C. neoformans* conjugate; and *D,* higher magnification of the contact area in *C.* Scale bars = *A,* 1.2 μm; *B,* 0.45 μm; *C,* 1.0 μm; *D,* 0.1 μm. (From Levitz SM, Mathews HL, Murphy JW. Direct antimicrobial activity of T cells. Immunol Today. 1995;16:387–391, with permission from Elsevier Science.)

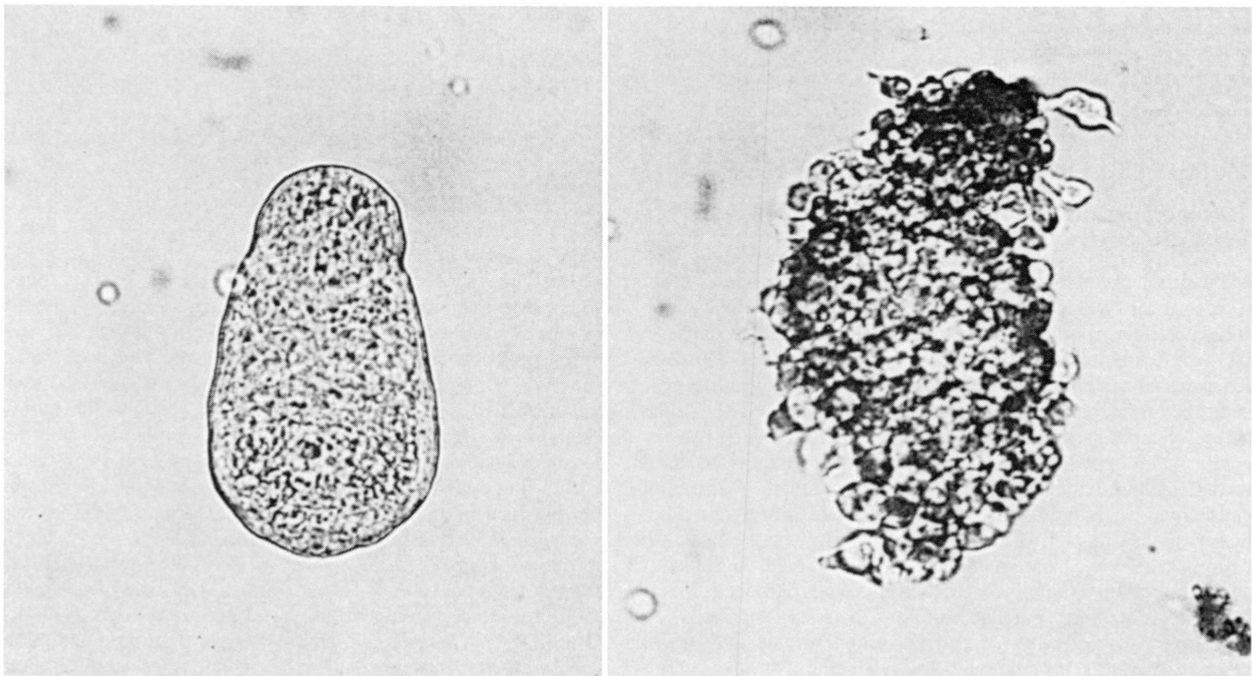

FIGURE 9–10. Direct T-cell cytotoxicity for invading pathogens. Morphologic appearance of shistosomula exposed to unstimulated and PHA-stimulated lymphocytes for 24 hours. *Left panel,* Shistosomula cultured with unstimulated T cells. The organism was viable, impermeable to dye, and motile. Few T cells adhere to the microbe. *Right panel,* Shistosomula cultured with PHA-stimulated T cells. The organism appeared disrupted, granular, permeable to dye, and encased by T cells (× 400). (From Ellner JJ, Olds GR, Lee CW, et al. Destruction of the multicellular parasite *Schistosoma mansoni* by T lymphocytes. J Clin Invest. 1982;70:369–378, with permission from The Rockefeller University Press.)

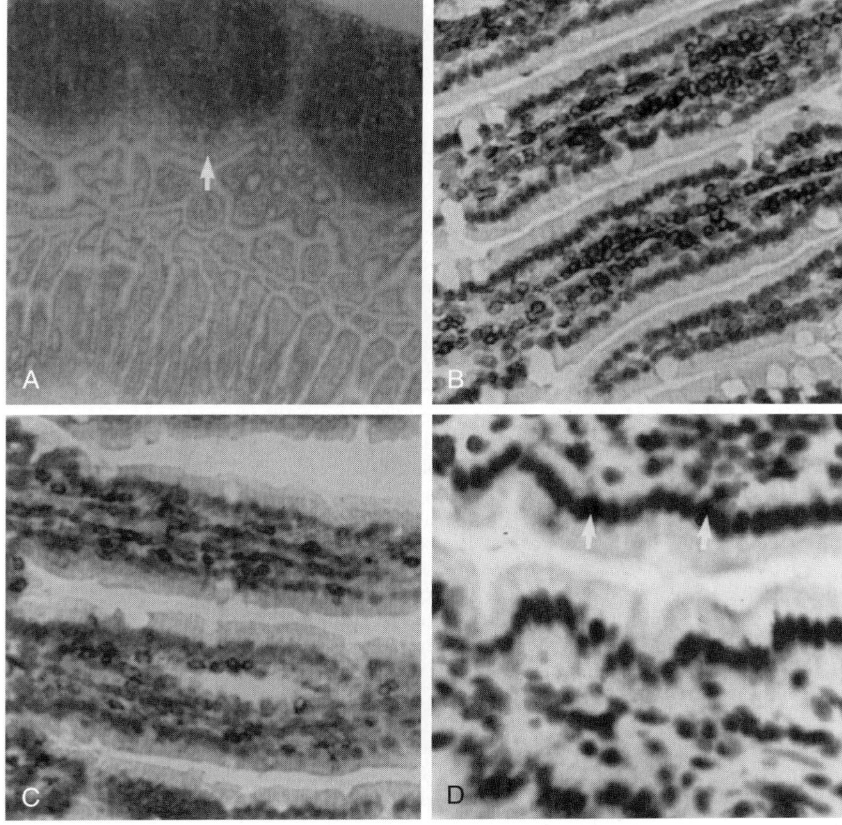

FIGURE 9–11. Morphology of the human gut-associated lymphoid tissues. *A,* Peyer's patches located in the small bowel. Arrow points to one of three Peyer's patches in the section. *B,* Staining of B lymphocytes showing their restriction to the lamina propria. *C,* Staining of CD8+ T lymphocytes showing their presence in both the LPL and IEL compartments. *D,* Staining of γδ T lymphocytes showing their presence in the IEL compartment. Arrows point to two examples of γδ IELs, clearly within the epithelial layer. (Figure provided by Marion G. Peters, MD.)

in the mucosa have unique properties. The most notable is the production of IgA, an immunoglobulin that is secreted across the epithelial surface to the external environment by a specialized transport system. These antibodies play an important role in preventing pathogenic microbes from adhering to host epithelial cells and in neutralizing bacterial toxins.[370]

Peyer's patches are lymphoid structures found within the gastrointestinal tract that serve roughly the same function in the MALT as lymph nodes do in the systemic immune system. This loosely organized lymphoid tissue is centered under unique epithelial patches that contain M cells. M cells are morphologically distinct epithelial cells specialized for efficient transcytosis of antigens from the gut lumen to the underlying macrophages and lymphocytes assembled in the Peyer's patches. In mice, M cells are clustered and the associated Peyer's patches are quite large. In humans, the M cells are more dispersed and the lymphoid tissue is less organized. Similar structures are formed in bronchi, tonsils, and the appendix. Antigen presentation within Peyer's patches is thought to occur by mechanisms analogous to antigen presentation in the systemic immune system. Th and Tc cells activated by antigen within Peyer's patches recirculate through the blood and populate all areas of MALT throughout the body, but they only inefficiently populate the systemic immune system.

Intraepithelial Lymphocytes

IELs have cell-surface phenotypes and TCR repertoires distinct from those found on the peripheral T lymphocytes of the systemic immune system. Approximately 60% of IELs express a CD8αα homodimer rather than the CD8αβ heterodimer seen on peripheral T lymphocytes, and, of these, up to half also express CD4. $CD4^+8^+$ T cells are never seen among peripheral T lymphocytes. Both CD8αβ and CD8αα IEL T lymphocytes exist in a heightened activation state and may not require costimulation for full activation.[371–373] αβ TCR^+ IELs express TCR Vβ gene segments that are not used by peripheral αβ T lymphocytes,[374] including autoreactive TCRs specifically depleted in the thymus.[375] This lack of thymic negative selection suggests that these cells mature in extrathymic sites. In addition, evidence from immune reconstitution experiments in mice supports thymus-independent development of some mucosal lymphocyte subsets. Intestinal cryopatches in athymic nude mice containing predominately $Thy1^+CD3^-4^-8^-$ cells are able to reconstitute the IEL compartment of irradiated SCID mice.[376] Active transcription of the RAG1/RAG2 recombinase responsible for TCR rearrangement has been documented in the MALT in normal mice.[377, 378] Transcription of these genes is tightly linked to TCR gene rearrangement and is not seen in mature lymphocytes, again supporting extrathymic T-lymphocyte maturation of some mucosal T cells. Nonetheless, some IELs in normal mice are thymus derived. Congenitally athymic nude mice that have essentially no T lymphocytes within the systemic immune system have reduced numbers of all IEL T-lymphocyte subsets. γδ TCR^+ IELs are reduced about 3-fold, αβ TCR^+ $CD8\alpha\alpha^+$ IELs about 30-fold, and αβ TCR^+ $CD8\alpha\beta^+$ IELs roughly 3- to 75-fold (variable from mouse to mouse).[371, 379–382] Peyer's patch T lymphocytes and LPLs appear to be thymus derived, similar to T lymphocytes of the systemic immune system. Memory T lymphocytes reside within the lamina propria and Peyer's patches.[383, 384] During the acute immune response to infection in the gastrointestinal tract, $CD8\alpha\beta^+$ T lymphocytes from the systemic immune system readily enter the LPL and IEL compartments.[385–387]

β_2-microglobulin–deficient mice lack MHC Ia and Ib and, as a result, αβ TCR^+ $CD8\alpha\beta^+$ IELs are absent. The presence of αβ TCR^+ $CD8\alpha\alpha^+$ IELs in β_2-microglobulin–deficient mice[177, 388] suggests that this mucosal-specific CD8αα subset is not entirely MHC I dependent. Similarly, MHC II restriction of αβ TCR^+ $CD4^+8^-$ and $CD4^+8\alpha\alpha^+$ T lymphocytes is doubtful. MHC II–deficient mice lack peripheral CD4+ T lymphocytes, but the CD4+ IEL compartment is unaffected.[389] Therefore, the nature of antigen recognition and MHC restriction by αβ TCR+ IEL subsets remains an open question.

Mucosa-Associated Lymphoid Tissue in Immunity to Infection

Antigen-specific cytolytic IELs develop during viral and bacterial enteritis. Mice infected intraduodenally with reovirus develop Tc cells within the IEL compartment that are antigen specific and MHC I restricted by day 6 of infection.[390] Microbial colonization of previously germ-free mice is associated with expansion of both αβ and γδ IEL subsets and probably represents intraepithelial or at least intramucosal expansion of these cells in response to bacterial colonization of the intestine.[391] In β_2-microglobulin–deficient mice, *L. monocytogenes* enteritis causes antigen-specific activation of both αβ TCR+ CD4−8αα+ and γδ TCR+ T lymphocytes in the IEL compartment.[392] Ideally, vaccination protocols would generate a durable mucosal immune response in addition to a systemic immune response. The portal of entry for almost all infectious agents is a mucosal or epithelial surface (oropharynyx, lungs, gastrointestinal tract, genitourinary tract, and skin). Lymphocytes activated in mucosal tissue recirculate to those tissues and participate in local immunity. Mucosally administered vaccines in current use are the Sabin oral polio vaccine and the oral *Salmonella typhi* vaccine (Vivotif). A live, attenuated, orally administered rotavirus vaccine has been approved for use, and a live, nasally administered flu vaccine has been shown to be effective.[393]

Animal models of HSV and HIV demonstrate the potential of mucosal vaccination for preventing disease. In one model, mice were immunized either systemically (intraperitoneally) or mucosally (intranasally) with an adenovirus engineered to express HSV type II glycoprotein B. Follow-up testing at 18 months showed preservation of antigen-specific Tc lymphocytes only at the site of original immunization. Mice immunized systemically had detectable Tc activity in the spleen but not in the MALT, whereas the reverse was true for intranasally immunized mice. This pattern of site-specific durable immunity had significant practical consequences, because intranasally immunized mice were better protected from both morbidity and mortality after lethal intravaginal challenge with HSV-2 than were naive or intraperitoneally immunized mice.[394, 395]

Rectal immunization of mice with an HIV polydeterminant peptide (including a gp160 peptide) and cholera toxin adjuvant generated antigen-specific Tc in the spleen, lamina propria, and Peyer's patches, whereas subcutaneous immunization generated antigen-specific Tc only in the spleen. Intrarectal immunization conferred significant protection from intrarectal viral infection with a recombinant vaccinia virus expressing HIV gp160. Rectally immunized animals showed a 4.5-log decrease in virus recovered from local tissues 6 days after infectious challenge.[396]

In summary, MALT consists of a resident population of T lymphocytes of αβ and γδ lineages that develop by mechanisms distinct from the those of the mature T lymphocytes of the systemic immune system. During immune responses, conventional thymus-dependent peripheral T lymphocytes enter the mucosal compartment and contribute to host defense. Dynamic changes within the resident IELs and LPLs also occur in response to infection. Resolution of infection is associated with generation of memory T lymphocytes that reside within the MALT. The mucosal immune system apparently can maintain its own pool of memory T lymphocytes, at least to some degree independent of systemic immunity. Generation of these T cells depends on the route of immunization or on the original site of infection. Their activity is critical to local immunity during rechallenge with infectious agents at mucosal portals of entry. Evolution of this field of cellular immunology will probably have a significant impact on how vaccines are administered in the coming years. Advances in this area may be critical to the development of an HIV vaccine, because HIV is an infection for which rapid control of the virus at the portal of entry may determine the efficacy of vaccination.

TRANSENDOTHELIAL MIGRATION

A fundamental mechanism in immune surveillance is the ability of T cells to migrate through lymph nodes throughout the body as scouts for potential foreign antigens. Antigens from invading pathogens can arrive in local lymph nodes either by direct passage of soluble molecules through lymph or because of the movement of antigen-bearing dendritic cells to lymph nodes draining areas of infection. T-cell recirculation through lymph nodes involves passage through the specialized endothelium in the blood vessels of lymph nodes, known as high endothelial venules (HEV). The key events in lymphocyte recirculation involve specific cell-cell interactions between circulating lymphocytes and HEVs. The molecules that mediate this recognition are called adhesion molecules; they are related to the molecules that mediate cell-cell interactions critical to the development of inflammation and an immune response at a site of infection.

Adhesion Molecules

The important adhesion molecules involved in cell-cell recognition in transendothelial migration are listed in Table 9–6. These molecules mostly fall into four molecular families. The first family is the selectins, a specialized group of cell-surface carbohydrate-binding molecules. These molecules all demonstrate Ca^{2+}-dependent recognition of their ligands, which are sialic acid– and fucose-containing carbohydrate epitopes called sialyl Lewis X. All circulating leukocytes express one member of this carbohydrate-binding family, called L-selectin. L-selectin is shed from the surface of leukocytes when they are activated by a mechanism involving the activation of a Zn^{2+}-dependent protease. Endothelial cells express two other members of this family, called P-selectin and E-selectin. These molecules are expressed constitutively in some microvascular beds. Their expression is markedly enhanced by proinflammatory cytokines such as IL-1, IFN-γ, and TNF-α and also can be stimulated by direct interaction of bacterial lipopolysaccharide with endothelium. Because leukocytes express carbohydrate ligands for these selectins, the effect of their increased expression on endothelium is enhanced interaction between leukocytes and endothelium.

The second family of adhesion molecules is the integrins. Integrins are heterodimers of type I membrane proteins involved in a variety of cell adhesion phenomena on virtually all cells in the body. They act as sites for plasma membrane anchoring of the component of the cytoskeleton known as microfilaments. As a result, interaction of integrins with their ligands leads to changes in cell shape and motility. In addition, integrin ligation enhances cell responses to growth factors and can lead directly to the induction of transcription of genes involved in the inflammatory response, such as extracellular matrix–degrading enzymes. Leukocytes express some integrins (mainly those that are involved in recognition of extracellular matrix components) that are also expressed by other cells. However, leukocytes also uniquely express some integrins involved in interaction with endothelium and in activation at sites of adhesion. These leukocyte-specific integrins include $\alpha_4\beta_1$ (very late antigen-4, or VLA-4), and the CD18 (β_2) integrin family that includes $\alpha_L\beta_2$ (lymphocyte function antigen-1, LFA-1 or CD11a), $\alpha_M\beta_2$ (Mac-1 or CD11b), $\alpha_X\beta_2$ (p150,95 or CD11c), and $\alpha_D\beta_2$. The $\alpha_M\beta_2$ and $\alpha_X\beta_2$ integrins are expressed primarily on myeloid cells, whereas $\alpha_L\beta_2$ is present on all leukocytes. The $\alpha_M\beta_2$ integrin also is expressed on NK cells, where its ligation can amplify cytolytic activity.

A special property of leukocyte integrins that is essential to their function in surveillance against infection is that they have regulatable affinity for their ligands. In circulating, unactivated leukocytes, leukocyte integrins mediate adhesion to ligand-coated surfaces very

TABLE 9–6 Leukocyte Adhesion Molecules Involved in Leukocyte Recirculation and Migration to Sites of Inflammation

Leukocyte Receptor	Leukocyte Expression	Counter-receptor	Function
L-selectin	All	Glycam-1, PSGL-1, MadCAM-1, others	Rolling on endothelium
$\alpha_L\beta_2$	All	ICAM-1, ICAM-2, ICAM-3	Stable adhesion to endothelium; leukocyte aggregation; FGR activation
$\alpha_M\beta_2$	Myeloid cells; NK cells	ICAM-1, fibrinogen, factor X, others	Stable adhesion; migration; membrane receptor complex formation
$\alpha_X\beta_2$	Myeloid cells	Fibrinogen	Stable adhesion; monocyte transendothelial migration
$\alpha_d\beta_2$	Myeloid cells; NK cells; lymphocyte subpopulation	ICAM-3	?
$\alpha_4\beta_1$	All	VCAM-1, fibronectin	Rolling and firm adhesion
$\alpha_4\beta_7$	Lymphocyte subset	MadCAM-1	Rolling and firm adhesion
$\alpha_E\beta_7$	Lymphocyte subset	E-cadherin	?
$\alpha_V\beta_3$	Myeloid cells and lymphocyte subset	Arg-Gly-Asp–containing proteins; ?PECAM-1	Modulation of migration[513]
PSGL-1	All	P-selectin; E-selectin; L-selectin	Rolling
ESL	PMN	E-selectin	Rolling
CD44	All	Hyaluronate	?

Abbreviations: CAM, Cell adhesion molecule (I, intercellular; PE, platelet/endothelial; V, vascular); ESL, E-selectin ligand; NK, natural killer; PMN, polymorphonuclear neutrophil leukocyte; PSGL, P-selectin glycoprotein ligand.

poorly. Many molecules found at sites of inflammation, including bacterial products such as lipopolysaccharide or formylated peptides, cytokines such as TNF-α, arachidonic acid metabolites such as leukotriene B_4, and peptide fragments of complement activation such as C5a, induce activation of the high-affinity state of leukocyte integrins, a process that requires specific signal transduction. Very important among these leukocyte activators are chemokines, which are discussed in more detail later.

The third group of adhesion molecules involved in cell homing is the immunoglobulin superfamily, the same structural family containing the molecules involved in T-cell interaction with APCs. The immunoglobulin superfamily members involved in interaction with endothelial cells are endothelial ligands for the leukocyte-specific integrins (see Table 9–6). One of these molecules, ICAM-2, is expressed constitutively on many endothelial cells. Two others, ICAM-1 and vascular cell adhesion molecule-1 (VCAM-1), are expressed on venules overlying inflammatory sites; their transcription is regulated by proinflammatory cytokines. A final immunoglobulin family member, mucosal addressin cell adhesion molecule-1 (MadCAM-1), is expressed only on mucosal endothelium and is important for homing of mucosal lymphocytes to the gut (see later discussion).[397, 398]

Mucins are heavily *o*-glycosylated ligands for the selectins that are present on endothelium and leukocytes. Several mucin ligands for selectins have now been characterized.[399, 400] It is clear that, although the sialyl Lewis X antigen is required for selectin recognition, there are characteristics of the protein backbone that are also required and that confer specificity on the ligand for interaction with a specific selectin. For example, a very unusual tyrosine sulfation occurs on the ligand for P-selectin called P-*s*electin glycoprotein ligand-1 (PSGL-1); without this modification, the ligand interacts with P-selectin very inefficiently.[401]

Finally, the heparin sulfate proteoglycan CD44 has been shown to have a role in lymphocyte homing to lymph nodes.[402, 403] CD44 is a transmembrane glycoprotein that has homology to cartilage link protein and, perhaps paradoxically, not only is decorated with heparan sulfates but recognizes them as ligands. Although blockade of CD44 with monoclonal antibodies blocks efficient lymph node homing, the mechanism of this effect is unclear.

Homing and recirculation of lymphocytes to tissue-specific environments is mediated by specific receptors on distinct T-lymphocyte subsets. Localization of T cells to Peyer's patches is mediated by $\alpha_4\beta_7$, L-selectin, and LFA-1[404–406]; to skin by a modified form of PSGL-1 called cutaneous lymphocyte antigen (CLA)[407–409]; and to peripheral nodes by L-selectin and $\alpha_4\beta_1$.[410–413] Localization of both αβ TCR$^+$ and γδ TCR$^+$ T lymphocytes to the IEL compartment correlates strongly with lymphocyte cell-surface expression of $\alpha_E\beta_7$.[414] Selective expression of these receptors by T-lymphocyte subsets based on the tissue type in which they were originally localized or activated presumably is responsible for the observed phenomenon of differential lymphocyte homing.[400] Of special interest is the discovery that P- and E-selectin can mediate the accumulation of Th1 but not Th2 lymphocytes at sites of inflammation.[415]

After circulating lymphocytes enter a lymph node expressing the correct "addressin" (a ligand for one of the lymphocyte's adhesion molecules), they begin to interact with the endothelium, usually by rolling along the endothelial surface. In peripheral lymph nodes, L-selectin ligands (mucins) are the most important addressins. In the absence of L-selectin, there is a major defect in the ability of lymphocytes to enter lymph nodes.[416] Different addressins are characteristic of normal peripheral nodes, Peyer's patches, skin, and lymph nodes draining sites of inflammation.

After initial L-selectin–mediated interaction, lymphocytes exit through the HEV into the lymph node only if they are stimulated by a chemotactic cytokine (chemokine). Chemokines are a large family of structurally related 10-kD secreted ligands that can be subdivided into families on the basis of the spacing of characteristic cysteine residues. Chemokines are recognized by cell-surface molecules on the lymphocytes that are members of the large family of seven-transmembrane, trimeric guanosine triphosphatase–associated receptors.[417] Much of the specificity of leukocyte responses to distinct inflammatory or immune stimuli is thought to reside in the nature of the chemokines produced at the site of infection, because each leukocyte subset has a distinct pattern of chemokine receptors. There are many different chemokines that can be chemotactic for lymphocytes. The most important chemokine in peripheral lymph nodes is 6-C-kine (also known as SLC), recognized by the lymphocyte receptor CCR7.[418–420] The presence of this receptor on naive and memory T cells means that both will be induced to migrate through the HEV into the lymph nodes, where they can potentially be exposed to antigens. These antigen-exposed cells can migrate to the site of infection through efferent lymphatics. If not exposed to relevant antigen on APCs in the lymph node, T cells exit into the lymph to migrate through tissue and eventually return to the blood via the thoracic duct.

As might be surmised from the fact that immune responses in the MALT develop so separately from the systemic immune system, the addressin for Peyer's patches is distinct from that for the peripheral nodes. It is a molecule called MadCAM-1. MadCAM-1 has immunoglobulin domains as well as a mucin domain and therefore can interact with both L-selectin and the integrin $\alpha_4\beta_7$ that is expressed almost exclusively on mucosal lymphocytes. Both L-selectin and $\alpha_4\beta_7$ can mediate lymphocyte rolling on MadCAM-expressing endothelium, so there are two mechanisms for the initial interaction of appropriate lymphocytes with the HEV of Peyer's patches.[421, 422] An additional integrin, called $\alpha_E\beta_7$, is closely related to $\alpha_4\beta_7$ and is expressed on LPLs and IELs. Mice deficient in β_7 integrins ($\alpha_4\beta_7$ and $\alpha_E\beta_7$) fail to populate the gut-associated lymphoid tissue (LPL and IEL), suggesting that these integrins are important for lymphocyte homing to this compartment.[423] Moreover, $\alpha_E\beta_7$-deficient lymphocytes fail to populate the IEL and LPL compartments normally. Although $\alpha_E\beta_7$ binds the epithelium-specific cell-cell adhesion molecule called E-cadherin,[424] it is not clear whether this is a relevant integrin ligand in lymphocyte homing to the mucosa. Because lamina propria does not express E-cadherin, there must be an additional ligand for $\alpha_E\beta_7$ to explain why it is required for homing of LPLs.

Recruitment of Leukocytes to Sites of Inflammation

The migration of leukocytes to sites of infection is absolutely required for successful host defense against invading pathogens. Studies have now elucidated many of the molecular interactions that mediate this critical event. The current paradigm is that leukocyte recognition of endothelium overlying a site of inflammation or infection and subsequent migration through the endothelium occurs in four steps, analogous to transendothelial migration in lymphocyte recirculation. In the first step, selectins and selectin ligands expressed by endothelium at a site of inflammation interact with mucins and L-selectin constitutively expressed by the leukocytes. Selectin-mucin binding, which is very rapid but has low affinity, leads in combination with the shear stress from blood flow to leukocyte rolling over the site of inflammation. This, in turn, dramatically slows leukocyte passage through the blood vessel, giving the cell time to sample the environment for activating stimuli, especially chemokines. If the rolling leukocyte has a receptor for a chemokine expressed at the site of inflammation, signal transduction from the chemokine receptor (step 2) occurs. This leads to activation of the leukocyte integrins to an adherent state, resulting in tight adhesion between the leukocyte and the endothelial cells if the latter express the appropriate integrin ligand (step 3). This tight adhesion is resistant to even high shear forces. Activated integrins also are required for the final step, transendothelial migration. This step is the least understood in the process, and it is not yet certain whether leukocytes always migrate through interendothelial junctions or sometimes move directly through endothelial cells.[425] Antibodies to two members of the immunoglobulin superfamily (platelet/endothelial cell adhesion molecule-1 [PECAM-1, also known as CD31] and integrin-associated protein [IAP, also known as CD47]) block transendothelial migration at a step after integrin activation.[426] However, because IAP and PECAM-1 are on both leukocytes and endothelial cells, the mechanism of antibody blockade is not clear.

OPPORTUNISTIC INFECTIONS IN PATIENTS WITH COMPROMISED CELLULAR IMMUNITY

Patients with compromised cellular immunity are especially susceptible to viruses, intracellular bacteria, and intracellular eukaryotic pathogens (protozoa and fungi) (Table 9–7). T cell–mediated immunity is critical for controlling many viral infections, and one of the consequences of dysfunctional cellular immunity is increased susceptibility to viral infections. The role of cellular immunity in protecting the host from nonviral intracellular pathogens also is well established. Tc-mediated killing of cells infected by many intracellular pathogens, including *Listeria*, *Mycobacterium*, *Leishmania*, and *Toxoplasma,* has been demonstrated.[427–434] In addition, IFN-γ released by activated T lymphocytes plays an important role in host defense by activating macrophages and NK cells.

Intracellular pathogens have a unique relationship with the infected host cell. In viral infections, all viral polypeptides are synthesized on host cell ribosomes in the cytosol and are therefore susceptible to proteasome-mediated degradation and loading onto MHC I molecules for antigen presentation. Intracellular bacterial, fungal, and protozoan pathogens have larger genomes and more complex arrays of polypeptides than viruses do, but they do not necessarily produce more MHC I–bound peptides. These pathogens synthesize polypeptides on their own ribosomes in their own cytosol. The only antigens available to the host cell proteasome–MHC I presentation pathway are those that are transported into the host cell cytoplasm. Some pathogens, including *Leishmania*, *Mycobacterium*, and *Legionella,* never truly enter the cytosol but live in specialized intracellular vacuoles called phagosomes. For these organisms, it is not clear whether and how pathogen antigens enter the cytosol of an infected host cell. The intraphagosomal location of these pathogens is likely to limit antigen presentation via MHC I molecules. This may in turn limit IFN-γ production for macrophage activation. If the intracellular pathogen also is resistant to the killing mechanisms of activated macrophages such as nitric oxide and superoxide, most of the host effector mechanisms for pathogen control have been evaded. This is the case for many successful intracellular pathogens. In this circumstance, active immunity is required for control of the infecting organism, either through granuloma formation or through cytokine suppression of intracellular growth. This control depends on an ongoing immune response and, as immunity wanes due to disease, age, or iatrogenic intervention, the pathogen recrudesces to cause disease. Infections acquired in the distant past (e.g., toxoplasmosis, tuberculosis, histoplasmosis) can cause serious infections in patients with compromised cellular immunity because an ongoing, active immune response is required to keep these organisms in check. Newly acquired infections with these organisms in the setting of cellular immune defects are an even greater problem, because the immune response required to control infection never develops.

Another important consequence of this complex host-pathogen interaction is the potential for pathologic Tc activation and tissue destruction without control of infection. Tc epitopes generated by the exogenous MHC I pathway (endosomal degradation) do not necessarily match the antigen epitopes generated endogenously in the infected cell (proteasome degradation). If there is a complete mismatch, then exogenous antigen presentation by the MHC I pathway can result in lysis of bystander cells rather than infected cells. This scenario may explain the phenomenon of disease exacerbation caused by immunization, as seen in animal models of *Leishmania* and other intracellular pathogens.[238, 435, 436] It may be clinically important that vaccine epitopes match endogenously generated epitopes in infected cells so as to avoid vaccine-associated immunopathology. This consideration is unique to intracellular pathogens that bring

TABLE 9–7 Important Intracellular Pathogens in Compromised Patients*

Viruses
Severe disease: RSV, adenovirus, parainfluenza, HCMV, HSV, VZV, HHV-6, HHV-7, JC virus, parvovirus B19
Chronic disease: Molluscum contagiosum, human papilloma virus
Bacteria
Listeria monocytogenes
Legionella pneumophila
Mycobacterium tuberculosis
Mycobacterium avium complex
Nocardia species
Rhodococcus equi
Salmonella species
Shigella species
Fungi
Histoplasma capsulatum
Pencillium marneffei
Protozoa
Cryptosporidium parvum
Leishmania species
Microsporidia species
Toxoplasma gondii

*Only microbes with documented intracellular lifestyles are included in the table.
Abbreviations: HCMV, Human cytomegalovirus; HHV, human herpesvirus; HSV, herpes simplex virus; RSV, respiratory syncytial virus; VZV, varicella-zoster virus.

with them their own protein synthesis machinery and exist within cells in highly specialized compartments.

Clinical Considerations

Three types of patients with compromised cellular immunity are commonly encountered in the clinic, and their cases highlight important aspects of cellular immunology theory. The first group of patients have had their immune systems ablated and then reconstituted from exogenous sources; this group is represented by patients undergoing bone marrow transplantation (see Chapter 303). During induction therapy, these patients have their entire innate and adaptive immune system ablated. They lose all memory B and T cells and are left with serum antibody as their only remnant of immunologic memory. In the best case, the bone marrow recipient is reconstituted with a matched, related donor. These patients are roughly in the same position as a newborn infant who has some pathogen-specific antibodies but a naive cellular immune compartment. However, adult bone marrow recipients are further compromised by a senile, mostly involuted thymus. The consequence is a lifelong diminished ability to generate immune responses to new antigens. With matched, unrelated donors and incomplete matches, cellular immunity is more severely compromised. The patient's adaptive immune system is replaced by a foreign immune system. Theoretically, the new donor T-lymphocyte precursors should be able to go through thymic maturation and development of peripheral tolerance normally. However, clinical experience suggests that thymic and peripheral tolerance mechanisms are dysfunctional, because patients who receive T cell–depleted CD34$^+$ pluripotent stem cells still get graft-versus-host disease.[437] The reasons for failure of peripheral tolerance and thymic negative selection are probably multifactoral and include thymic dysfunction as well as the profound inflammatory state associated with transplant conditioning.[438] Marked involvement of the skin and gut in graft-versus-host disease suggests that failure of tolerance in the mucosal and epithelial compartments may be a dominant problem. The net result of this situation is disruption of regulation of the adaptive immune response, a requirement for increased pharmacologic immunosuppression, and severely compromised cell-mediated immunity. In the early posttransplantation period, bone marrow recipients are markedly susceptible to all intracellular pathogens, including severe infections with endogenous latent viruses such as HCMV, HSV, and VZV. In addition, they are susceptible to fatal infections with relatively common endemic viruses, including respiratory syncytial virus, parainfluenza, and adenovirus.[439–442] Other viruses that cause increased morbidity include human herpesvirus-6 and -7.[443–445] Because of the complete ablation of preexisting memory T cells, reactivations of viral infections are clinically as severe as primary infections. In contrast to primary infections in immunocompetent persons, no immune response supervenes to limit tissue damage. Intracellular bacterial infections are also severe when they occur in this patient population.[446]

HIV-infected patients constitute the second group of commonly encountered patients with compromised cellular immunity (see Chapter 107). In these patients, the cellular immune response gradually fades over time. Decline in immune status parallels the decline in the CD4$^+$ T cell compartment. Loss of these Th cells leads to failure of optimal activation of Tc and other effector cells in response to infection. At a CD4$^+$ T-lymphocyte count of 200 cells/mm^3 a significant subset of patients no longer has effective cellular immunity against *Pneumocystis carinii,* and after a further decline to 50 cells/mm^3 a significant number of patients no longer have effective immunity to *Mycobacterium avium* complex or HCMV. As disease progresses, HIV-infected patients have significant problems with HSV, VZV, and HCMV. Chronic viral infections relatively unique to HIV patients include JC virus (manifesting as progressive multifocal leukoencephalopathy), pox viruses causing chronic molluscum contagiosum, and high rates of Epstein-Barr virus–related central nervous system lymphoma and non-Hodgkin's lymphoma.[447] HIV-infected patients are susceptible to intracellular bacteria including *M. tuberculosis*, *M. avium* complex, *Nocardia*, *Rhodococcus*, *Salmonella*, and *Legionella*. They are also susceptible to intracellular fungi such as *Histoplasma capsulatum* and *Penicillium marneffei*, and intracellular protozoans such as *Toxoplasma*, *Cryptosporidium*, *Microsporidia*, and *Leishmania*. The enhanced susceptibility to each of these agents undoubtedly arises from loss of CD4$^+$ T lymphocytes necessary for host defense as a consequence of infection by HIV. Aggressive intervention with highly active antiretroviral therapy can halt the decline of the cellular immune system, and in patients receiving effective therapy immune reconstitution has been demonstrated.[448, 449] One of the major issues in care of persons with HIV infection is determining how much immune reconstitution is enough for the purpose of discontinuing primary and secondary prophylaxis for opportunistic infections.

The third clinical setting in which unique problems arise from compromised cellular immunity is with patients who have received solid organ transplants (see Chapter 304). In this circumstance, the patient has an intact adaptive and innate immune system that is intentionally compromised by pharmacologic interventions to prevent its optimal activity, which would include rejection of the transplanted organ. A fascinating immunologic scenario exists within the transplanted organ itself, because solid organ transplants have HLA mismatches between donor and recipient. The recipient's cellular immune compartment consists of T lymphocytes that are educated in the patient's thymus to recognize antigenic peptides in the context of self-HLA. During T-cell ontogeny, T cells with TCRs that have too high or too low an affinity for self-HLA are deleted. However, the HLA molecules on the cells of the transplanted organ are distinct from those of the recipient. This has two consequences. The first and most obvious is that there has been no deletion of T cells that bear TCRs with high affinity for the HLA molecules of the transplanted organ. These are the T cells that cause rejection. The second, more subtle, consequence is the absence of prior positive thymic selection for T cells bearing TCR molecules that can interact in a productive fashion with the foreign HLA molecules in antigen presentation. Recipients of solid organ transplants therefore are uniquely susceptible to severe and potentially fatal viral infections focused in the transplanted organ. Adenoviruses in particular have been associated with isolated hepatitis in liver transplants. This viral infection occurs within the first 3 months after transplantation and results in significant graft failure and mortality in affected patients. In the pediatric transplantation population, isolated adenovirus hepatitis occurs in about 3% of patients.[450] Adenovirus hepatitis also is seen in adult liver transplantation patients but is much less common.[451] Especially severe or fatal respiratory viral infections involving respiratory syncytial virus, parainfluenza virus, and adenoviruses have been reported with lung transplantation.[452, 453] Cardiac transplantation can be complicated by isolated viral myocarditis caused by HCMV or parvovirus B19.[454–456] The unusual predilection of the viruses for transplanted organs probably reflects the dysfunctional relation between the recipient's T lymphocytes and the donor-organ HLA, as well as iatrogenic pharmacologic immunosuppression. Transplantation patients to greater or lesser degrees are susceptible to systemic infections with intracellular bacteria, fungi, and protozoans, depending on the level of immunosuppression required to prevent graft rejection. Current pharmacologic interventions to suppress transplant rejection are global in effect. Anti-thymocyte globulin and OKT3 deplete T lymphocytes directly. Glucocorticoids antagonize both T-lymphocyte and APC functions.[457] Azathioprine, methotrexate, and mycophenolate mofetil block lymphocyte proliferation through the use of DNA precursor poisons. FK506 and cyclosporine inhibit calcineurin/nuclear factor of activated T cells (NF-ATc) signaling generated by engagement of the TCR receptor, resulting in loss of several lymphokines including IL-2, IL-3, IL-4, and GM-CSF and accessory or effector molecules including CD40 ligand (CD40L) and FASL.[458] Rapamycin/sirolimus interferes with signal transduction via the IL-2 receptor. Current research in transplant immunosuppression is directed toward finding interventions with more precise and limited disruption of the immune defenses and greater preservation of global immune function.

There are a number of inborn abnormalities that affect various aspects of the cellular immune response. These patients present a complex set of problems including variable degrees of susceptibility to viruses and intracellular pathogens (see Chapters 10 and 298).

CONCLUSIONS

Cellular immunity contributes to host defense through two basic mechanisms. First, it enhances the innate defense systems. Cellular immune mechanisms produce cytokines that recruit and activate appropriate subsets of myeloid effector cells and stimulate the production of pathogen-specific antibodies that enhance the killing of pathogens by the innate defenses. Second, components of the cellular immune system patrol the body searching for intracellular pathogens that escape the innate immune defenses. The mechanism for detecting the presence of intracellular pathogens within host cells depends on the interaction of TCRs with MHC molecules that have bound peptides (or glycolipids) from foreign antigens. A better understanding of how pathogens interact with this unique surveillance system can lead to a more prominent role for immunotherapeutics in the treatment of clinical infectious diseases.

REFERENCES

1. Hashimoto K, Hirai M, Kurosawa Y. A gene outside the human MHC related to classical HLA class I genes. Science. 1995;269:693–695.
2. Lundin LG. Evolution of the vertebrate genome as reflected in paralogous chromosomal regions in man and the house mouse. Genomics. 1993;16:1–19.
3. Janeway CA Jr, Travers P. Immunobiology: The Immune System in Health and Disease. 2nd ed. New York: Garland Publishing; 1996.
4. Wong GH, Bartlett PF, Clark-Lewis I, et al. Inducible expression of H-2 and Ia antigens on brain cells. Nature. 1984;310:688–691.
5. Momburg F, Koch N, Moller P, et al. Differential expression of Ia and Ia-associated invariant chain in mouse tissues after in vivo treatment with IFN-gamma. J Immunol. 1986;136:940–948.
6. Muhlethaler-Mottet A, Otten LA, Steimle V, et al. Expression of MHC class II molecules in different cellular and functional compartments is controlled by differential usage of multiple promoters of the transactivator CIITA. EMBO J. 1997;16:2851–2860.
7. Unanue ER. The 1995 Albert Lasker Medical Research Award: The concept of antigen processing and presentation. JAMA. 1995;274:1071–1073.
8. Rudensky AY, Preston-Hurlburt P, Hong SC, et al. Sequence analysis of peptides bound to MHC class II molecules. Nature. 1991;353:622–627.
9. Hunt DF, Michel H, Dickinson TA, et al. Peptides presented to the immune system by the murine class II major histocompatibility complex molecule I-Ad. Science. 1992;256:1817–1820.
10. Chicz RM, Urban RG, Gorga JC, et al. Specificity and promiscuity among naturally processed peptides bound to HLA-DR alleles. J Exp Med. 1993;178:27–47.
11. Brown JH, Jardetzky TS, Gorga JC, et al. Three-dimensional structure of the human class II histocompatibility antigen HLA-DR1 (See comments). Nature. 1993;364:33–39.
12. Jardetzky TS, Brown JH, Gorga JC, et al. Three-dimensional structure of a human class II histocompatibility molecule complexed with superantigen. Nature. 1994;368:711–718.
13. Stern LJ, Brown JH, Jardetzky TS, et al. Crystal structure of the human class II MHC protein HLA-DR1 complexed with an influenza virus peptide. Nature. 1994;368:215–221.
14. Falk K, Rotzschke O, Stevanovic S, et al. Pool sequencing of natural HLA-DR, DQ, and DP ligands reveals detailed peptide motifs, constraints of processing, and general rules. Immunogenetics. 1994;39:230–242.
15. Peters PJ, Neefjes JJ, Oorschot V, et al. Segregation of MHC class II molecules from MHC class I molecules in the Golgi complex for transport to lysosomal compartments (See comments). Nature. 1991;349:669–676.
16. Amigorena S, Drake JR, Webster P, et al. Transient accumulation of new class II MHC molecules in a novel endocytic compartment in B lymphocytes (See comments). Nature. 1994;369:113–120.
17. Tulp A, Verwoerd D, Dobberstein B, et al. Isolation and characterization of the intracellular MHC class II compartment (See comments). Nature. 1994;369:120–126.
18. West MA, Lucocq JM, Watts C. Antigen processing and class II MHC peptide-loading compartments in human B-lymphoblastoid cells (See comments). Nature. 1994;369:147–151.
19. Peters PJ, Raposo G, Neefjes JJ, et al. Major histocompatibility complex class II compartments in human B lymphoblastoid cells are distinct from early endosomes. J Exp Med. 1995;182:325–334.
20. Germain RN. Binding domain regulation of MHC class II molecule assembly, trafficking, fate, and function. Semin Immunol. 1995;7:361–372.
21. Chapman HA. Endosomal proteolysis and MHC class II function. Curr Opin Immunol. 1998;10:93–102.
22. Sherman MA, Weber DA, Jensen PE. DM enhances peptide binding to class II MHC by release of invariant chain-derived peptide. Immunity. 1995;3:197–205.
23. Weber DA, Evavold BD, Jensen PE. Enhanced dissociation of HLA-DR-bound peptides in the presence of HLA-DM (See comments). Science. 1996;274:618–620.
24. Sanderson F, Kleijmeer MJ, Kelly A, et al. Accumulation of HLA-DM, a regulator of antigen presentation, in MHC class II compartments. Science. 1994;266:1566–1569.
25. Kropshofer H, Hammerling GJ, Vogt AB. How HLA-DM edits the MHC class II peptide repertoire: Survival of the fittest? Immunol Today. 1997;18:77–82.
26. Viville S, Neefjes J, Lotteau V, et al. Mice lacking the MHC class II-associated invariant chain. Cell. 1993;72:635–648.
27. Ceman S, Sant AJ. The function of invariant chain in class II-restricted antigen presentation. Semin Immunol. 1995;7:373–387.
28. Fung-Leung WP, Surh CD, Liljedahl M, et al. Antigen presentation and T cell development in H2-M-deficient mice. Science. 1996;271:1278–1281.
29. Miyazaki T, Wolf P, Tourne S, et al. Mice lacking H2-M complexes, enigmatic elements of the MHC class II peptide-loading pathway. Cell. 1996;84:531–541.
30. Escola JM, Grivel JC, Chavrier P, et al. Different endocytic compartments are involved in the tight association of class II molecules with processed hen egg lysozyme and ribonuclease A in B cells. J Cell Sci. 1995;108:2337–2345.
31. Nadimi F, Moreno J, Momburg F, et al. Antigen presentation of hen egg-white lysozyme but not of ribonuclease A is augmented by the major histocompatibility complex class II-associated invariant chain. Eur J Immunol. 1991;21:1255–1263.
32. Larsen SL, Pedersen LO, Buus S, et al. T cell responses affected by aminopeptidase N (CD13)-mediated trimming of major histocompatibility complex class II-bound peptides [published erratum appears in J Exp Med 1996;184:2073]. J Exp Med. 1996;184:183–189.
33. Lanzavecchia A. Receptor-mediated antigen uptake and its effect on antigen presentation to class II-restricted T lymphocytes. Annu Rev Immunol. 1990;8:773–793.
34. Vidard L, Kovacsovics-Bankowski M, Kraeft SK, et al. Analysis of MHC class II presentation of particulate antigens of B lymphocytes. J Immunol. 1996;156:2809–2818.
35. Mudde GC, Van Reijsen FC, Boland GJ, et al. Allergen presentation by epidermal Langerhans' cells from patients with atopic dermatitis is mediated by IgE. Immunology. 1990;69:335–341.
36. Parra-Lopez CA, Lindner R, Vidavsky I, et al. Presentation on class II MHC molecules of endogenous lysozyme targeted to the endocytic pathway. J Immunol. 1997;158:2670–2679.
37. Tan MC, Mommaas AM, Drijfhout JW, et al. Mannose receptor mediated uptake of antigens strongly enhances HLA-class II restricted antigen presentation by cultured dendritic cells. Adv Exp Med Biol. 1997;417:171–174.
38. Engering AJ, Cella M, Fluitsma DM, et al. Mannose receptor mediated antigen uptake and presentation in human dendritic cells. Adv Exp Med Biol. 1997;417:183–187.
39. Jiang W, Swiggard WJ, Heufler C, et al. The receptor DEC-205 expressed by dendritic cells and thymic epithelial cells is involved in antigen processing. Nature. 1995;375:151–155.
40. Stahl PD, Ezekowitz RA. The mannose receptor is a pattern recognition receptor involved in host defense. Curr Opin Immunol. 1998;10:50–55.
41. Nuchtern JG, Biddison WE, Klausner RD. Class II MHC molecules can use the endogenous pathway of antigen presentation. Nature. 1990;343:74–76.
42. Battegay M, Bachmann MF, Burhkart C, et al. Antiviral immune responses of mice lacking MHC class II or its associated invariant chain. Cell Immunol. 1996;167:115–121.
43. Malnati MS, Marti M, LaVaute T, et al. Processing pathways for presentation of cytosolic antigen to MHC class II-restricted T cells. Nature. 1992;357:702–704.
44. Loss GEJ, Elias CG, Fields PE, et al. Major histocompatibility complex class II-restricted presentation of an internally synthesized antigen displays cell-type variability and segregates from the exogenous class II and endogenous class I presentation pathways. J Exp Med. 1993;178:73–85.
45. Stebbins CC, Loss GEJ, Elias CG, et al. The requirement for DM in class II-restricted antigen presentation and SDS-stable dimer formation is allele and species dependent. J Exp Med. 1995;181:223–234.
46. Bodmer H, Viville S, Benoist C, et al. Diversity of endogenous epitopes bound to MHC class II molecules limited by invariant chain. Science. 1994;263:1284–1286.
47. Rammensee HG. Chemistry of peptides associated with MHC class I and class II molecules. Curr Opin Immunol. 1995;7:85–96.
48. Rammensee HG, Friede T, Stevanoviic S. MHC ligands and peptide motifs: First listing. Immunogenetics. 1995;41:178–228.
49. Batalia MA, Collins EJ. Peptide binding by class I and class II MHC molecules. Biopolymers. 1997;43:281–302.
50. Heemels MT, Ploegh H. Generation, translocation, and presentation of MHC class I-restricted peptides. Annu Rev Biochem. 1995;64:463–491.
51. Glas R, Ohlen C, Hoglund P, et al. The CD8+ T cell repertoire in beta 2-microglobulin-deficient mice is biased towards reactivity against self-major histocompatibility class I. J Exp Med. 1994;179:661–672.
52. Coux O, Tanaka K, Goldberg AL. Structure and functions of the 20S and 26S proteasomes. Annu Rev Biochem. 1996;65:801–847.

53. Hughes EA, Hammond C, Cresswell P. Misfolded major histocompatibility complex class I heavy chains are translocated into the cytoplasm and degraded by the proteasome. Proc Natl Acad Sci U S A. 1997;94:1896–1901.
54. Rivett AJ. Intracellular distribution of proteasomes. Curr Opin Immunol. 1998;10:110–114.
55. Aki M, Shimbara N, Takashina M, et al. Interferon-gamma induces different subunit organizations and functional diversity of proteasomes. J Biochem (Tokyo). 1994;115:257–269.
56. Groettrup M, Soza A, Kuckelkorn U, et al. Peptide antigen production by the proteasome: Complexity provides efficiency. Immunol Today. 1996;17:429–435.
57. Niedermann G, Grimm R, Geier E, et al. Potential immunocompetence of proteolytic fragments produced by proteasomes before evolution of the vertebrate immune system. J Exp Med. 1997;186:209–220.
58. Kuckelkorn U, Frentzel S, Kraft R, et al. Incorporation of major histocompatibility complex-encoded subunits LMP2 and LMP7 changes the quality of the 20S proteasome polypeptide processing products independent of interferon-gamma. Eur J Immunol. 1995;25:2605–2611.
59. Groettrup M, Ruppert T, Kuehn L, et al. The interferon-gamma-inducible 11 S regulator (PA28) and the LMP2/LMP7 subunits govern the peptide production by the 20S proteasome in vitro. J Biol Chem. 1995;270:23808–23815.
60. Elliott T. How does TAP associate with MHC class I molecules? Immunol Today. 1997;18:375–379.
61. Androlewicz MJ, Cresswell P. How selective is the transporter associated with antigen processing? Immunity. 1996;5:1–5.
62. Suh WK, Cohen-Doyle MF, Fruh K, et al. Interaction of MHC class I molecules with the transporter associated with antigen processing. Science. 1994;264:1322–1326.
63. Ortmann B, Androlewicz MJ, Cresswell P. MHC class I/beta 2-microglobulin complexes associate with TAP transporters before peptide binding. Nature. 1994;368:864–867.
64. Attaya M, Jameson S, Martinez CK, et al. Ham-2 corrects the class I antigen-processing defect in RMA-S cells. Nature. 1992;355:647–649.
65. Spies T, DeMars R. Restored expression of major histocompatibility class I molecules by gene transfer of a putative peptide transporter. Nature. 1991;351:323–324.
66. Sadasivan B, Lehner PJ, Ortmann B, et al. Roles for calreticulin and a novel glycoprotein, tapasin, in the interaction of MHC class I molecules with TAP. Immunity. 1996;5:103–114.
67. Yewdell JW, Bennink JR. Cell biology of antigen processing and presentation to major histocompatibility complex class I molecule-restricted T lymphocytes. Adv Immunol. 1992;52:1–123.
68. Ferris RL, Buck C, Hammond SA, et al. Class I-restricted presentation of an HIV-1 gp41 epitope containing an N-linked glycosylation site: Implications for the mechanism of processing of viral envelope proteins. J Immunol. 1996;156:834–840.
69. Jensen TJ, Loo MA, Pind S, et al. Multiple proteolytic systems, including the proteasome, contribute to CFTR processing. Cell. 1995;83:129–135.
70. Ward CL, Omura S, Kopito RR. Degradation of CFTR by the ubiquitin-proteasome pathway. Cell. 1995;83:121–127.
71. Wiertz EJ, Tortorella D, Bogyo M, et al. Sec61-mediated transfer of a membrane protein from the endoplasmic reticulum to the proteasome for destruction (See comments). Nature. 1996;384:432–438.
72. Kopito RR. ER quality control: The cytoplasmic connection. Cell. 1997;88:427–430.
73. Brodsky JL, Mccracken AA. ERr-associated and proteasome-mediated protein degradation: How two topologically restricted events came together. Trends Cell Biol. 1997;7:151–156.
74. Mosse CA, Meadows L, Luckey CJ, et al. The class I antigen-processing pathway for the membrane protein tyrosinase involves translation in the endoplasmic reticulum and processing in the cytosol. J Exp Med. 1998;187:37–48.
75. Henderson RA, Michel H, Sakaguchi K, et al. HLA-A2.1-associated peptides from a mutant cell line: A second pathway of antigen presentation. Science. 1992;255:1264–1266.
76. Wei ML, Cresswell P. HLA-A2 molecules in an antigen-processing mutant cell contain signal sequence-derived peptides (See comments). Nature. 1992;356:443–446.
77. Hammond SA, Bollinger RC, Tobery TW, et al. Transporter-independent processing of HIV-1 envelope protein for recognition by CD8+ T cells. Nature. 1993;364:158–161.
78. Lee SP, Thomas WA, Blake NW, et al. Transporter (TAP)-independent processing of a multiple membrane-spanning protein, the Epstein-Barr virus latent membrane protein 2. Eur J Immunol. 1996;26:1875–1883.
79. Snyder HL, Bacik I, Bennink JR, et al. Two novel routes of transporter associated with antigen processing (TAP)-independent major histocompatibility complex class I antigen processing. J Exp Med. 1997;186:1087–1098.
80. Hughes EA, Ortmann B, Surman M, et al. The protease inhibitor, *N*-acetyl-L-leucyl-L-leucyl-leucyl-L-norleucinal, decreases the pool of major histocompatibility complex class I-binding peptides and inhibits peptide trimming in the endoplasmic reticulum. J Exp Med. 1996;183:1569–1578.
81. Braciale TJ, Morrison LA, Sweetser MT, et al. Antigen presentation pathways to class I and class II MHC-restricted T lymphocytes. Immunol Rev. 1987;98:95–114.
82. Harding CV, Song R. Phagocytic processing of exogenous particulate antigens by macrophages for presentation by class I MHC molecules. J Immunol. 1994;153:4925–4933.
83. Pfeifer JD, Wick MJ, Roberts RL, et al. Phagocytic processing of bacterial antigens for class I MHC presentation to T cells. Nature. 1993;361:359–362.
84. Liu T, Zhou X, Orvell C, et al. Heat-inactivated Sendai virus can enter multiple MHC class I processing pathways and generate cytotoxic T lymphocyte responses in vivo. J Immunol. 1995;154:3147–3155.
85. Schirmbeck R, Melber K, Reimann J. Hepatitis B virus small surface antigen particles are processed in a novel endosomal pathway for major histocompatibility complex class I-restricted epitope presentation. Eur J Immunol. 1995;25:1063–1070.
86. Schirmbeck R, Bohm W, Melber K, et al. Processing of exogenous heat-aggregated (denatured) and particulate (native) hepatitis B surface antigen for class I-restricted epitope presentation. J Immunol. 1995;155:4676–4684.
87. Kovacsovics-Bankowski M, Clark K, Benacerraf B, et al KL. Efficient major histocompatibility complex class I presentation of exogenous antigen upon phagocytosis by macrophages. Proc Natl Acad Sci U S A. 1993;90:4942–4946.
88. Kovacsovics-Bankowski M, Rock KL. A phagosome-to-cytosol pathway for exogenous antigens presented on MHC class I molecules. Science. 1995;267:243–246.
89. Huang AY, Bruce AT, Pardoll DM, Levitsky HI. In vivo cross-priming of MHC class I-restricted antigens requires the TAP transporter. Immunity. 1996;4:349–355.
90. Porcelli SA. The CD1 family: A third lineage of antigen-presenting molecules. Adv Immunol. 1995;59:1–98.
91. Le Bouteiller P, Lenfant F. Antigen-presenting function(s) of the non-classical HLA-E, -F and -G class I molecules: The beginning of a story. Res Immunol. 1996;147:301–313.
92. Gustafson KS, Ginder GD. Interferon-gamma induction of the human leukocyte antigen-E gene is mediated through binding of a complex containing STAT1alpha to a distinct interferon-gamma-responsive element. J Biol Chem. 1996;271:20035–20046.
93. Braud V, Jones EY, McMichael A. The human major histocompatibility complex class Ib molecule HLA-E binds signal sequence-derived peptides with primary anchor residues at positions 2 and 9. Eur J Immunol. 1997;27:1164–1169.
94. Diehl M, Munz C, Keilholz W, et al. Nonclassical HLA-G molecules are classical peptide presenters. Curr Biol. 1996;6:305–314.
95. Ulbrecht M, Modrow S, Srivastava R, et al. Interaction of HLA-E with peptides and the peptide transporter in vitro: Implications for its function in antigen presentation. J Immunol. 1998;160:4375–4385.
96. Lee N, Malacko AR, Ishitani A, et al. The membrane-bound and soluble forms of HLA-G bind identical sets of endogenous peptides but differ with respect to TAP association. Immunity. 1995;3:591–600.
97. Le Bouteiller P. HLA class I chromosomal region, genes, and products: Facts and questions. Crit Rev Immunol. 1994;14:89–129.
98. Rouas-Freiss N, Goncalves RM, Menier C, et al. Direct evidence to support the role of HLA-G in protecting the fetus from maternal uterine natural killer cytolysis. Proc Natl Acad Sci U S A. 1997;94:11520–11525.
99. Perez-Villar JJ, Melero I, Navarro F, et al. The CD94/NKG2-A inhibitory receptor complex is involved in natural killer cell-mediated recognition of cells expressing HLA-G1. J Immunol. 1997;158:5736–5743.
100. Hermel E, Grigorenko E, Lindahl KF. Expression of medial class I histocompatibility antigens on RMA-S mutant cells. Int Immunol. 1991;3:407–412.
101. Shawar SM, Rodgers JR, Cook RG, et al. Specialized function of the nonclassical MHC class I molecule Hmt: A specific receptor for N-formylated peptides. Immunol Res. 1991;10:365–375.
102. Holcombe HR, Castano AR, Cheroutre H, et al. Nonclassical behavior of the thymus leukemia antigen: Peptide transporter-independent expression of a nonclassical class I molecule. J Exp Med. 1995;181:1433–1443.
103. Rodgers JR, Mehta V, Cook RG. Surface expression of beta 2-microglobulin-associated thymus-leukemia antigen is independent of TAP2. Eur J Immunol. 1995;25:1001–1007.
104. Aldrich CJ, DeCloux A, Woods AS, et al. Identification of a Tap-dependent leader peptide recognized by alloreactive T cells specific for a class Ib antigen. Cell. 1994;79:649–658.
105. Bouwer HG, Lindahl KF, Baldridge JR, et al. An H2-T MHC class Ib molecule presents *Listeria monocytogenes*-derived antigen to immune CD8+ cytotoxic T cells. J Immunol. 1994;152:5352–5360.
106. Bouwer HG, Seaman MS, Forman J, et al. MHC class Ib-restricted cells contribute to antilisterial immunity: Evidence for Qa-1b as a key restricting element for *Listeria*-specific CTLs. J Immunol. 1997;159:2795–2801.
107. Milligan GN, Flaherty L, Braciale VL, et al. Nonconventional (TL-encoded) major histocompatibility complex molecules present processed viral antigen to cytotoxic T lymphocytes. J Exp Med. 1991;174:133–138.
108. Joyce S, Tabaczewski P, Angeletti RH, et al. A nonpolymorphic major histocompatibility complex class Ib molecule binds a large array of diverse self-peptides. J Exp Med. 1994;179:579–588.
109. Rotzschke O, Falk K, Stevanovic S, et al. Qa-2 molecules are peptide receptors of higher stringency than ordinary class I molecules. Nature. 1993;361:642–644.
110. Tabaczewski P, Chiang E, Henson M, et al. Alternative peptide binding motifs of Qa-2 class Ib molecules define rules for binding of self and nonself peptides. J Immunol. 1997;159:2771–2781.
111. Fragoso G, Lamoyi E, Mellor A, et al. Increased resistance to *Taenia crassiceps* murine cysticercosis in Qa-2 transgenic mice. Infect Immun. 1998;66:760–764.
112. Aldrich CJ, Lowen LC, Mann D, et al. The Q7 alpha 3 domain alters T cell recognition of class I antigens. J Immunol. 1991;146:3082–3090.
113. Tabaczewski P, Stroynowski I. Expression of secreted and glycosylphosphatidylinositol-bound Qa-2 molecules is dependent on functional TAP-2 peptide transporter. J Immunol. 1994;152:5268–5274.
114. Kurlander RJ, Shawar SM, Brown ML, et al. Specialized role for a murine class I-b MHC molecule in prokaryotic host defenses. Science. 1992;257:678–679.

115. Pamer EG, Wang CR, Flaherty L, et al. H-2M3 presents a *Listeria monocytogenes* peptide to cytotoxic T lymphocytes. Cell. 1992;70:215–223.
116. Lenz LL, Dere B, Bevan MJ. Identification of an H2-M3-restricted *Listeria* epitope: Implications for antigen presentation by M3. Immunity. 1996;5:63–72.
117. Wang CR, Castano AR, Peterson PA, et al. Nonclassical binding of formylated peptide in crystal structure of the MHC class Ib molecule H2-M3. Cell. 1995;82:655–664.
118. Calabi F, Jarvis JM, Martin L, et al. Two classes of CD1 genes. Eur J Immunol. 1989;19:285–292.
119. Beckman EM, Brenner MB. MHC class I-like, class II-like and CD1 molecules: Distinct roles in immunity. Immunol Today. 1995;16:349–352.
120. Small TN, Knowles RW, Keever C, et al. M241 (CD1) expression on B lymphocytes. J Immunol. 1987;138:2864–2868.
121. Bleicher PA, Balk SP, Hagen SJ, et al. Expression of murine CD1 on gastrointestinal epithelium. Science. 1990;250:679–682.
122. Canchis PW, Bhan AK, Landau SB, et al. Tissue distribution of the non-polymorphic major histocompatibility complex class I-like molecule, CD1d. Immunology. 1993;80:561–565.
123. Blumberg RS, Terhorst C, Bleicher P, et al. Expression of a nonpolymorphic MHC class I-like molecule, CD1D, by human intestinal epithelial cells. J Immunol. 1991;147:2518–2524.
124. Thomssen H, Kahan M, Londei M. IL-3 in combination with IL-4, induces the expression of functional CD1 molecules on monocytes. Cytokine. 1996;8:476–481.
125. Colgan SP, Morales VM, Madara JL, et al. IFN-gamma modulates CD1d surface expression on intestinal epithelia. Am J Physiol. 1996;271:t-83.
126. Porcelli S, Morita CT, Brenner MB. CD1b restricts the response of human CD4−8− T lymphocytes to a microbial antigen. Nature. 1992;360:593–597.
127. Beckman EM, Porcelli SA, Morita CT, et al. Recognition of a lipid antigen by CD1-restricted alpha beta+ T cells (See comments). Nature. 1994;372:691–694.
128. Beckman EM, Melian A, Behar SM, et al. CD1c restricts responses of mycobacteria-specific T cells: Evidence for antigen presentation by a second member of the human CD1 family. J Immunol. 1996;157:2795–2803.
129. Moody DB, Reinhold BB, Guy MR, et al. Structural requirements for glycolipid antigen recognition by CD1b-restricted T cells. Science. 1997;278:283–286.
130. Sieling PA, Chatterjee D, Porcelli SA, et al. CD1-restricted T cell recognition of microbial lipoglycan antigens (See comments). Science. 1995;269:227–230.
131. Ernst WA, Maher J, Cho S, et al. Molecular interaction of CD1b with lipoglycan antigens. Immunity. 1998;8:331–340.
132. Kawano T, Cui J, Koezuka Y, et al. CD1d-restricted and TCR-mediated activation of valpha14 NKT cells by glycosylceramides. Science. 1997;278:1626–1629.
133. Kawasaki S, Moriguchi R, Sekiya K, et al. The cell envelope structure of the lipopolysaccharide-lacking gram-negative bacterium *Sphingomonas paucimobilis*. J Bacteriol. 1994;176:284–290.
134. Sugita M, Porcelli SA, Brenner MB. Assembly and retention of CD1b heavy chains in the endoplasmic reticulum. J Immunol. 1997;159:2358–2365.
135. Teitell M, Holcombe HR, Brossay L, et al. Nonclassical behavior of the mouse CD1 class I-like molecule. J Immunol. 1997;158:2143–2149.
136. Brutkiewicz RR, Bennink JR, Yewdell JW, et al. TAP-independent, beta 2-microglobulin-dependent surface expression of functional mouse CD1.1. J Exp Med. 1995;182:1913–1919.
137. Sugita M, Jackman RM, van Donselaar E, et al. Cytoplasmic tail-dependent localization of CD1b antigen-presenting molecules to MIICs. Science. 1996;273:349–352.
138. Jackman RM, Stenger S, Lee A, et al. The tyrosine-containing cytoplasmic tail of CD1b is essential for its efficient presentation of bacterial lipid antigens. Immunity. 1998;8:341–351.
139. Zeng Z, Castano AR, Segelke BW, et al. Crystal structure of mouse CD1: An MHC-like fold with a large hydrophobic binding groove (See comments). Science. 1997;277:339–345.
140. Mendiratta SK, Martin WD, Hong S, et al. CD1d1 mutant mice are deficient in natural T cells that promptly produce IL-4. Immunity. 1997;6:469–477.
141. Calabi F, Milstein C. A novel family of human major histocompatibility complex-related genes not mapping to chromosome 6. Nature. 1986;323:540–543.
142. Rippmann F, Taylor WR, Rothbard JB, et al. A hypothetical model for the peptide binding domain of hsp70 based on the peptide binding domain of HLA. EMBO J. 1991;10:1053–1059.
143. Srivastava PK. Peptide-binding heat shock proteins in the endoplasmic reticulum: Role in immune response to cancer and in antigen presentation. Adv Cancer Res. 1993;62:153–177.
144. Udono H, Levey DL, Srivastava PK. Cellular requirements for tumor-specific immunity elicited by heat shock proteins: Tumor rejection antigen gp96 primes CD8+ T cells in vivo. Proc Natl Acad Sci U S A. 1994;91:3077–3081.
145. Udono H, Srivastava PK. Heat shock protein 70-associated peptides elicit specific cancer immunity. J Exp Med. 1993;178:1391–1396.
146. Blachere NE, Li Z, Chandawarkar RY, et al. Heat shock protein-peptide complexes, reconstituted in vitro, elicit peptide-specific cytotoxic T lymphocyte response and tumor immunity. J Exp Med. 1997;186:1315–1322.
147. Nieland TJ, Tan MC, Monne-van MM, et al. Isolation of an immunodominant viral peptide that is endogenously bound to the stress protein GP96/GRP94. Proc Natl Acad Sci U S A. 1996;93:6135–6139.
148. Li Z, Srivastava PK. Tumor rejection antigen gp96/grp94 is an ATPase: Implications for protein folding and antigen presentation. EMBO J. 1993;12:3143–3151.
149. Arnold D, Wahl C, Faath S, et al. Influences of transporter associated with antigen processing (TAP) on the repertoire of peptides associated with the endoplasmic reticulum-resident stress protein gp96. J Exp Med. 1997;186:461–466.
150. Vidal K, Grosjean I, Kaiserlian D. Antigen presentation by a mouse duodenal epithelial cell line (MODE-K). Adv Exp Med Biol. 1995;371A:225–228.
151. Bland PW, Warren LG. Antigen presentation by epithelial cells of the rat small intestine. I: Kinetics, antigen specificity and blocking by anti-Ia antisera. Immunology. 1986;58:1–7.
152. Mayer L, Shlien R. Evidence for function of Ia molecules on gut epithelial cells in man. J Exp Med. 1987;166:1471–1483.
153. Kaiserlian D, Vidal K, Revillard JP. Murine enterocytes can present soluble antigen to specific class II-restricted CD4+ T cells. Eur J Immunol. 1989;19:1513–1516.
154. Marelli-Berg FM, Hargreaves RE, Carmichael P, et al. Major histocompatibility complex class II-expressing endothelial cells induce allospecific nonresponsiveness in naive T cells. J Exp Med. 1996;183:1603–1612.
155. Housseau F, Rouas-Freiss N, Roy M, et al. Antigen-presenting function of murine gonadal epithelial cell lines. Cell Immunol. 1997;177:93–101.
156. Butz EA, Bevan MJ. Differential presentation of the same MHC class I epitopes by fibroblasts and dendritic cells. J Immunol. 1998;160:2139–2144.
157. Steinman RM. The dendritic cell system and its role in immunogenicity. Annu Rev Immunol. 1991;9:271–296.
158. Garcia KC, Degano M, Stanfield RL, et al. An alphabeta T cell receptor structure at 2.5 Å and its orientation in the TCR-MHC complex (See comments). Science. 1996;274:209–219.
159. Garboczi DN, Ghosh P, Utz U, et al. Structure of the complex between human T-cell receptor, viral peptide and HLA-A2 [Comment]. Nature. 1996;384:134–141.
160. Wilson IA, Garcia KC. T-cell receptor structure and TCR complexes [published erratum appears in Curr Opin Struct Biol 1998;8:124–125]. Curr Opin Struct Biol. 1997;7:839–848.
161. Bertoletti A, Sette A, Chisari FV, et al. Natural variants of cytotoxic epitopes are T-cell receptor antagonists for antiviral cytotoxic T cells (See comments). Nature. 1994;369:407–410.
162. Burroughs NJ, Rand DA. Dynamics of T-cell antagonism: Enhanced viral diversity and survival. Proc R Soc Lond B Biol Sci. 1998;265:529–535.
163. Diepolder HM, Jung MC, Wierenga E, et al. Anergic TH1 clones specific for hepatitis B virus (HBV) core peptides are inhibitory to other HBV core-specific CD4+ T cells in vitro. J Virol. 1996;70:7540–7548.
164. Irie HY, Ravichandran KS, Burakoff SJ. CD8 beta chain influences CD8 alpha chain-associated Lck kinase activity. J Exp Med. 1995;181:1267–1273.
165. Genevee C, Chung V, Diu A, et al. TCR gene segments from at least one third of V alpha subfamilies rearrange at the delta locus. Mol Immunol. 1994;31:109–115.
166. Brenner MB, Strominger JL, Krangel MS. The gamma delta T cell receptor. Adv Immunol. 1988;43:133–192.
167. Arden B, Clark SP, Kabelitz D, et al. Human T-cell receptor variable gene segment families. Immunogenetics. 1995;42:455–500.
168. Davis MM, Bjorkman PJ. T-cell antigen receptor genes and T-cell recognition [published erratum appears in Nature 1988;335:744]. Nature. 1988;334:395–402.
169. Jitsukawa S, Faure F, Lipinski M, et al. A novel subset of human lymphocytes with a T cell receptor-gamma complex. J Exp Med. 1987;166:1192–1197.
170. Groh V, Porcelli S, Fabbi M, et al. Human lymphocytes bearing T cell receptor gamma/delta are phenotypically diverse and evenly distributed throughout the lymphoid system. J Exp Med. 1989;169:1277–1294.
171. Chowers Y, Holtmeier W, Harwood J, et al. The V delta 1 T cell receptor repertoire in human small intestine and colon. J Exp Med. 1994;180:183–190.
172. Bluestone JA, Khattri R, Sciammas R, et al. TCR gamma delta cells: A specialized T-cell subset in the immune system. Annu Rev Cell Dev Biol. 1995;11:307–353.
173. Allison JP, Havran WL. The immunobiology of T cells with invariant gamma delta antigen receptors. Annu Rev Immunol. 1991;9:679–705.
174. Rock EP, Sibbald PR, Davis MM, et al. CDR3 length in antigen-specific immune receptors. J Exp Med. 1994;179:323–328.
175. Johnson RM, Lancki DW, Sperling AI, et al. A murine CD4−, CD8− T cell receptor-gamma delta T lymphocyte clone specific for herpes simplex virus glycoprotein I. J Immunol. 1992;148:983–988.
176. Sciammas R, Johnson RM, Sperling AI, et al. Unique antigen recognition by a herpesvirus-specific TCR-gamma delta cell. J Immunol. 1994;152:5392–5397.
177. Correa I, Bix M, Liao NS, et al. Most gamma delta T cells develop normally in beta 2-microglobulin-deficient mice. Proc Natl Acad Sci U S A. 1992;89:653–657.
178. de la Salle H, Hanau D, Fricker D, et al. Homozygous human TAP peptide transporter mutation in HLA class I deficiency [published erratum appears in Science 1994;266:1464]. Science. 1994;265:237–241.
179. Godfrey DI, Zlotnik A. Control points in early T-cell development. Immunol Today. 1993;14:547–553.
180. Dent AL, Matis LA, Hooshmand F, et al. Self-reactive gamma delta T cells are eliminated in the thymus. Nature. 1990;343:714–719.
181. Barrett TA, Delvy ML, Kennedy DM, et al. Mechanism of self-tolerance of gamma/delta T cells in epithelial tissue. J Exp Med. 1992;175:65–70.
182. Nossal GJ. Negative selection of lymphocytes. Cell. 1994;76:229–239.
183. Jameson SC, Hogquist KA, Bevan MJ. Positive selection of thymocytes. Annu Rev Immunol. 1995;13:93–126.
184. Molina TJ, Kishihara K, Siderovski DP, et al. Profound block in thymocyte development in mice lacking p56lck (See comments). Nature. 1992;357:161–164.
185. Surh CD, Sprent J. T-cell apoptosis detected in situ during positive and negative selection in the thymus (See comments). Nature. 1994;372:100–103.
186. Cheng AM, Rowley B, Pao W, et al. Syk tyrosine kinase required for mouse viability and B-cell development. Nature. 1995;378:303–306.
187. June CH, Bluestone JA, Nadler LM, et al. The B7 and CD28 receptor families. Immunol Today. 1994;15:321–331.
188. Schwartz RH. T cell clonal anergy. Curr Opin Immunol. 1997;9:351–357.

189. Ni HT, Deeths MJ, Mescher MF. Phosphatidylinositol 3 kinase activity is not essential for B7-1-mediated costimulation of proliferation or development of cytotoxicity in murine T cells. J Immunol. 1996;157:2243–2246.
190. Truitt KE, Nagel T, Suen LF, et al. Structural requirements for CD28-mediated costimulation of IL-2 production in Jurkat T cells. J Immunol. 1996;156:4539–4541.
191. Cai YC, Cefai D, Schneider H, et al. Selective CD28pYMNM mutations implicate phosphatidylinositol 3-kinase in CD86-CD28-mediated costimulation. Immunity. 1995;3:417–426.
192. August A, Gibson S, Kawakami Y, et al. CD28 is associated with and induces the immediate tyrosine phosphorylation and activation of the Tec family kinase ITK/EMT in the human Jurkat leukemic T-cell line. Proc Natl Acad Sci U S A. 1994;91:9347–9351.
193. Liao XC, Fournier S, Killeen N, et al. Itk negatively regulates induction of T cell proliferation by CD28 costimulation. J Exp Med. 1997;186:221–228.
194. Su B, Jacinto E, Hibi M, et al. JNK is involved in signal integration during costimulation of T lymphocytes. Cell. 1994;77:727–736.
195. Shahinian A, Pfeffer K, Lee KP, et al. Differential T cell costimulatory requirements in CD28-deficient mice. Science. 1993;261:609–612.
196. Thompson CB, Allison JP. The emerging role of CTLA-4 as an immune attenuator. Immunity. 1997;7:445–450.
197. Finck BK, Linsley PS, Wofsy D. Treatment of murine lupus with CTLA4Ig. Science. 1994;265:1225–1227.
198. Padrid PA, Mathur M, Li X, et al. CTLA4Ig inhibits airway eosinophilia and hyperresponsiveness by regulating the development of Th1/Th2 subsets in a murine model of asthma. Am J Respir Cell Mol Biol. 1998;18:453–462.
199. Kirk AD, Harlan DM, Armstrong NN, et al. CTLA4-Ig and anti-CD40 ligand prevent renal allograft rejection in primates. Proc Natl Acad Sci U S A. 1997;94:8789–8794.
200. Penninger JM, Kroemer G. Molecular and cellular mechanisms of T lymphocyte apoptosis. Adv Immunol. 1998;68:51–144.
201. Liu CC, Walsh CM, Young JD. Perforin: Structure and function. Immunol Today. 1995;16:194–201.
202. Pham CT, Ley TJ. The role of granzyme B cluster proteases in cell-mediated cytotoxicity. Semin Immunol. 1997;9:127–133.
203. Doherty PC. Cytotoxic T cell effector and memory function in viral immunity. Curr Top Microbiol Immunol. 1996;206:1–14.
204. Kagi D, Seiler P, Pavlovic J, et al. The roles of perforin- and Fas-dependent cytotoxicity in protection against cytopathic and noncytopathic viruses. Eur J Immunol. 1995;25:3256–3262.
205. Kaufmann SH. Immunity to intracellular bacteria. Annu Rev Immunol. 1993; 11:129–163.
206. Sher A, Coffman RL. Regulation of immunity to parasites by T cells and T cell-derived cytokines. Annu Rev Immunol. 1992;10:385–409.
207. Cronin DC, Stack R, Fitch FW. IL-4-producing CD8+ T cell clones can provide B cell help. J Immunol. 1995;154:3118–3127.
208. Lancki DW, Fitch FW. Cytolytic T lymphocytes: An overview of their characteristics. Biotherapy. 1992;5:71–81.
209. Lancki DW, Hsieh CS, Fitch FW. Mechanisms of lysis by cytotoxic T lymphocyte clones: Lytic activity and gene expression in cloned antigen-specific CD4+ and CD8+ T lymphocytes. J Immunol. 1991;146:3242–3249.
210. Williams NS, Engelhard VH. Perforin-dependent cytotoxic activity and lymphokine secretion by CD4+ T cells are regulated by CD8+ T cells. J Immunol. 1997;159:2091–2099.
211. Mosmann TR, Cherwinski H, Bond MW, et al. Two types of murine helper T cell clone: I. Definition according to profiles of lymphokine activities and secreted proteins. J Immunol. 1986;136:2348–2357.
212. Fitch FW, McKisic MD, Lancki DW, et al. Differential regulation of murine T lymphocyte subsets. Annu Rev Immunol. 1993;11:29–48.
213. Reiner SL, Locksley RM. The regulation of immunity to *Leishmania major*. Annu Rev Immunol. 1995;13:151–177.
214. Else KJ, Grencis RK. Cellular immune responses to the murine nematode parasite *Trichuris muris*: I. Differential cytokine production during acute or chronic infection. Immunology. 1991;72:508–513.
215. Else KJ, Hultner L, Grencis RK. Cellular immune responses to the murine nematode parasite *Trichuris muris*: II. Differential induction of TH-cell subsets in resistant versus susceptible mice. Immunology. 1992;75:232–237.
216. Else KJ, Finkelman FD, Maliszewski CR, et al. Cytokine-mediated regulation of chronic intestinal helminth infection. J Exp Med. 1994;179:347–351.
217. Rotman HL, Schnyder-Candrian S, Scott P, et al. IL-12 eliminates the Th-2 dependent protective immune response of mice to larval *Strongyloides stercoralis*. Parasite Immunol. 1997;19:29–39.
218. Bancroft AJ, Else KJ, Sypek JP, et al. Interleukin-12 promotes a chronic intestinal nematode infection. Eur J Immunol. 1997;27:866–870.
219. Urban JFJ, Madden KB, Cheever AW, et al. IFN inhibits inflammatory responses and protective immunity in mice infected with the nematode parasite, *Nippostrongylus brasiliensis*. J Immunol. 1993;151:7086–7094.
220. Dent LA, Strath M, Mellor AL, et al. Eosinophilia in transgenic mice expressing interleukin 5. J Exp Med. 1990;172:1425–1431.
221. Tominaga A, Takaki S, Koyama N, et al. Transgenic mice expressing a B cell growth and differentiation factor gene (interleukin 5) develop eosinophilia and autoantibody production. J Exp Med. 1991;173:429–437.
222. Abbas AK, Murphy KM, Sher A. Functional diversity of helper T lymphocytes. Nature. 1996;383:787–793.
223. Kelso A. Th1 and Th2 subsets: Paradigms lost? Immunol Today. 1995;16:374–379.
224. Allen JE, Maizels RM. Th1-Th2: Reliable paradigm or dangerous dogma? (See comments). Immunol Today. 1997;18:387–392.
225. Hondowicz BD, Scharton-Kersten TM, Jones DE, et al. *Leishmania major*-infected C3H mice treated with anti-IL-12 mAb develop but do not maintain a Th2 response. J Immunol. 1997;159:5024–5031.
226. Kaye PM, Curry AJ, Blackwell JM. Differential production of Th1- and Th2-derived cytokines does not determine the genetically controlled or vaccine-induced rate of cure in murine visceral leishmaniasis. J Immunol. 1991;146:2763–2770.
227. Miralles GD, Stoeckle MY, McDermott DF, et al. Th1 and Th2 cell-associated cytokines in experimental visceral leishmaniasis. Infect Immun. 1994;62:1058–1063.
228. Satoskar A, Bluethmann H, Alexander J. Disruption of the murine interleukin-4 gene inhibits disease progression during *Leishmania mexicana* infection but does not increase control of *Leishmania donovani* infection. Infect Immun. 1995;63:4894–4899.
229. Brown DR, Fowell DJ, Corry DB, et al. Beta 2-microglobulin-dependent NK1.1+ T cells are not essential for T helper cell 2 immune responses. J Exp Med. 1996;184:1295–1304.
230. Zhang Y, Rogers KH, Lewis DB. Beta 2-microglobulin-dependent T cells are dispensable for allergen-induced T helper 2 responses. J Exp Med. 1996;184:1507–1512.
231. Macaulay AE, DeKruyff RH, Goodnow CC, et al. Antigen-specific B cells preferentially induce CD4+ T cells to produce IL-4. J Immunol. 1997;158:4171–4179.
232. Mencacci A, Del Sero G, Cenci E, et al. Endogenous interleukin 4 is required for development of protective CD4+ T helper type 1 cell responses to *Candida albicans*. J Exp Med. 1998;187:307–317.
233. Bhardwaj V, Kanagawa O, Swanson PE, et al. Chronic *Listeria* infection in SCID mice: Requirements for the carrier state and the dual role of T cells in transferring protection or suppression. J Immunol. 1998;160:376–384.
234. Muller I. Role of T cell subsets during the recall of immunologic memory to *Leishmania major*. Eur J Immunol. 1992;22:3063–3069.
235. Hill JO, Awwad M, North RJ. Elimination of CD4+ suppressor T cells from susceptible BALB/c mice releases CD8+ T lymphocytes to mediate protective immunity against *Leishmania*. J Exp Med. 1989;169:1819–1827.
236. Muller I, Pedrazzini T, Kropf P, et al. Establishment of resistance to *Leishmania major* infection in susceptible BALB/c mice requires parasite-specific CD8+ T cells. Int Immunol. 1991;3:587–597.
237. Hussell T, Baldwin CJ, O'Garra A, et al. CD8+ T cells control Th2-driven pathology during pulmonary respiratory syncytial virus infection. Eur J Immunol. 1997;27:3341–3349.
238. Wang ZE, Reiner SL, Hatam F, et al. Targeted activation of CD8 cells and infection of beta 2-microglobulin-deficient mice fail to confirm a primary protective role for CD8 cells in experimental leishmaniasis. J Immunol. 1993;151:2077–2086.
239. Romagnani S. Lymphokine production by human T cells in disease states. Annu Rev Immunol. 1994;12:227–257.
240. Yamamura M, Uyemura K, Deans RJ, et al. Defining protective responses to pathogens: Cytokine profiles in leprosy lesions [published erratum appears in Science 1992;255:12]. Science. 1991;254:277–279.
241. Haanen JB, de Waal M, Res PC, et al. Selection of a human T helper type 1-like T cell subset by mycobacteria. J Exp Med. 1991;174:583–592.
242. Salgame P, Abrams JS, Clayberger C, et al. Differing lymphokine profiles of functional subsets of human CD4 and CD8 T cell clones. Science. 1991;254:279–282.
243. Howe RC, Wondimu A, Demissee A, et al. Functional heterogeneity among CD4+ T-cell clones from blood and skin lesions of leprosy patients: Identification of T-cell clones distinct from Th0, Th1 and Th2. Immunology. 1995;84:585–594.
244. Misra N, Murtaza A, Walker B, et al. Cytokine profile of circulating T cells of leprosy patients reflects both indiscriminate and polarized T-helper subsets: T-helper phenotype is stable and uninfluenced by related antigens of *Mycobacterium leprae*. Immunology. 1995;86:97–103.
245. Altare F, Durandy A, Lammas D, et al. Impairment of mycobacterial immunity in human interleukin-12 receptor deficiency. Science. 1998;280:1432–1435.
246. de Jong R, Altare F, Haagen IA, et al. Severe mycobacterial and *Salmonella* infections in interleukin-12 receptor-deficient patients. Science. 1998;280:1435–1438.
247. Newport MJ, Huxley CM, Huston S, et al. A mutation in the interferon-gamma-receptor gene and susceptibility to mycobacterial infection. N Engl J Med. 1996;335:1941–1949.
248. Jouanguy E, Altare F, Lamhamedi S, et al. Interferon-gamma-receptor deficiency in an infant with fatal bacille Calmette-Guérin infection. N Engl J Med. 1996;335:1956–1961.
249. Pierre-Audigier C, Jouanguy E, Lamhamedi S, et al. Fatal disseminated *Mycobacterium smegmatis* infection in a child with inherited interferon gamma receptor deficiency. Clin Infect Dis. 1997;24:982–984.
250. Clerici M, Shearer GM. The Th1-Th2 hypothesis of HIV infection: New insights. Immunol Today. 1994;15:575–581.
251. Graziosi C, Pantaleo G, Gantt KR, et al. Lack of evidence for the dichotomy of TH1 and TH2 predominance in HIV-infected individuals (See comments). Science. 1994;265:248–252.
252. Ogg GS, Jin X, Bonhoeffer S, et al. Quantitation of HIV-1-specific cytotoxic T lymphocytes and plasma load of viral RNA. Science. 1998;279:2103–2106.
253. Borrow P, Lewicki H, Wei X, et al. Antiviral pressure exerted by HIV-1-specific cytotoxic T lymphocytes (CTLs) during primary infection demonstrated by rapid selection of CTL escape virus (See comments). Nat Med. 1997;3:205–211.
254. Goulder PJ, Phillips RE, Colbert RA, et al. Late escape from an immunodominant

cytotoxic T-lymphocyte response associated with progression to AIDS. Nat Med. 1997;3:212–217.
255. de Jong R, Janson AA, Faber WR, et al. IL-2 and IL-12 act in synergy to overcome antigen-specific T cell unresponsiveness in mycobacterial disease. J Immunol. 1997;159:786–793.
256. Waage A, Espevik T. Interleukin 1 potentiates the lethal effect of tumor necrosis factor alpha/cachectin in mice. J Exp Med. 1988;167:1987–1992.
257. Okusawa S, Gelfand JA, Ikejima T, et al. Interleukin 1 induces a shock-like state in rabbits: Synergism with tumor necrosis factor and the effect of cyclooxygenase inhibition. J Clin Invest. 1988;81:1162–1172.
258. Cohen J. IL-12 deaths: Explanation and a puzzle (News). Science. 1995;270:908.
259. Kohl S, Sigaroudinia M, Charlebois ED, et al. Interleukin-12 administered in vivo decreases human NK cell cytotoxicity and antibody-dependent cellular cytotoxicity to human immunodeficiency virus-infected cells. J Infect Dis. 1996;174:1105–1108.
260. Holland SM, Eisenstein EM, Kuhns DB, et al. Treatment of refractory disseminated nontuberculous mycobacterial infection with interferon gamma: A preliminary report. N Engl J Med. 1994;330:1348–1355.
261. Raad I, Hachem R, Leeds N, et al. Use of adjunctive treatment with interferon-gamma in an immunocompromised patient who had refractory multidrug-resistant tuberculosis of the brain. Clin Infect Dis. 1996;22:572–574.
262. Condos R, Rom WN, Schluger NW. Treatment of multidrug-resistant pulmonary tuberculosis with interferon-gamma via aerosol (See comments). Lancet. 1997;349:1513–1515.
263. Levin M, Newport MJ, D'Souza S, et al. Familial disseminated atypical mycobacterial infection in childhood: A human mycobacterial susceptibility gene? (See comments). Lancet. 1995;345:79–83.
264. Verhagen CE, Wierenga EA, Buffing AA, et al. Reversal reaction in borderline leprosy is associated with a polarized shift to type 1-like *Mycobacterium leprae* T cell reactivity in lesional skin: A follow-up study. J Immunol. 1997;159:4474–4483.
265. Jorgensen C, Apparailly F, Couret I, et al. Interleukin-4 and interleukin-10 are chondroprotective and decrease mononuclear cell recruitment in human rheumatoid synovium in vivo. Immunology. 1998;93:518–523.
266. van Roon JA, van Roy JL, Gmelig-Meyling FH, et al. Prevention and reversal of cartilage degradation in rheumatoid arthritis by interleukin-10 and interleukin-4. Arthritis Rheum. 1996;39:829–835.
267. Lanier LL, Chang C, Phillips JH. Human NKR-P1A: A disulfide-linked homodimer of the C-type lectin superfamily expressed by a subset of NK and T lymphocytes. J Immunol. 1994;153:2417–2428.
268. Dellabona P, Casorati G, Friedli B, et al. In vivo persistence of expanded clones specific for bacterial antigens within the human T cell receptor alpha/beta CD4−8− subset. J Exp Med. 1993;177:1763–1771.
269. Wirt DP, Brooks EG, Vaidya S, et al. Novel T-lymphocyte population in combined immunodeficiency with features of graft-versus-host disease (See comments). N Engl J Med. 1989;321:370–374.
270. Shivakumar S, Tsokos GC, Datta SK. T cell receptor alpha/beta expressing double-negative (CD4−/CD8−) and CD4+ T helper cells in humans augment the production of pathogenic anti-DNA autoantibodies associated with lupus nephritis. J Immunol. 1989;143:103–112.
271. Bendelac A, Killeen N, Littman DR, et al. A subset of CD4+ thymocytes selected by MHC class I molecules. Science. 1994;263:1774–1778.
272. Londei M, Verhoef A, De Berardinis P, et al. Definition of a population of CD4−8− T cells that express the alpha beta T-cell receptor and respond to interleukins 2, 3, and 4. Proc Natl Acad Sci U S A. 1989;86:8502–8506.
273. Kubota H, Okazaki H, Onuma M, et al. CD3+4−8− alpha beta T cell population with biased T cell receptor V gene usage: Presence in bone marrow and possible involvement of IL-3 for their extrathymic development. J Immunol. 1992;149:1143–1150.
274. Ballas ZK, Rasmussen W. NK1.1+ thymocytes: Adult murine CD4−, CD8− thymocytes contain an NK1.1+, CD3+, CD5hi, CD44hi, TCR-V beta 8+ subset. J Immunol. 1990;145:1039–1045.
275. Bendelac A, Rivera MN, Park SH, et al. Mouse CD1-specific NK1 T cells: Development, specificity, and function. Annu Rev Immunol. 1997;15:535–562.
276. Lantz O, Bendelac A. An invariant T cell receptor alpha chain is used by a unique subset of major histocompatibility complex class I-specific CD4+ and CD4−8− T cells in mice and humans. J Exp Med. 1994;180:1097–1106.
277. Arase H, Arase N, Ogasawara K, et al. An NK1.1+ CD4+8− single-positive thymocyte subpopulation that expresses a highly skewed T-cell antigen receptor V beta family. Proc Natl Acad Sci U S A. 1992;89:6506–6510.
278. Porcelli S, Yockey CE, Brenner MB, et al. Analysis of T cell antigen receptor (TCR) expression by human peripheral blood CD4−8− alpha/beta T cells demonstrates preferential use of several V beta genes and an invariant TCR alpha chain. J Exp Med. 1993;178:1–16.
279. Vicari AP, Zlotnik A. Mouse NK1.1+ T cells: A new family of T cells. Immunol Today. 1996;17:71–76.
280. Makino Y, Yamagata N, Sasho T, et al. Extrathymic development of V alpha 14-positive T cells. J Exp Med. 1993;177:1399–1408.
281. Makino Y, Kanno R, Koseki H, et al. Development of Valpha4+ NK T cells in the early stages of embryogenesis. Proc Natl Acad Sci U S A. 1996;93:6516–6520.
282. Bendelac A. Positive selection of mouse NK1+ T cells by CD1-expressing cortical thymocytes. J Exp Med. 1995;182:2091–2096.
283. Joyce S, Negishi I, Boesteanu A, et al. Expansion of natural (NK1+) T cells that express alpha beta T cell receptors in transporters associated with antigen presentation-1 null and thymus leukemia antigen positive mice. J Exp Med. 1996;184:1579–1584.
284. Bendelac A, Lantz O, Quimby ME, et al. CD1 recognition by mouse NK1+ T lymphocytes. Science. 1995;268:863–865.
285. Yoshimoto T, Paul WE. CD4pos, NK1.1pos T cells promptly produce interleukin 4 in response to in vivo challenge with anti-CD3. J Exp Med. 1994;179:1285–1295.
286. Boullier S, Dadaglio G, Lafeuillade A, et al. V delta 1 T cells expanded in the blood throughout HIV infection display a cytotoxic activity and are primed for TNF-alpha and IFN-gamma production but are not selected in lymph nodes. J Immunol. 1997;159:3629–3637.
287. Lin T, Brunner T, Tietz B, et al. Fas ligand-mediated killing by intestinal intraepithelial lymphocytes: Participation in intestinal graft-versus-host disease. J Clin Invest. 1998;101:570–577.
288. Duhindan N, Farley AJ, Humphreys S, et al. Patterns of lymphokine secretion amongst mouse gamma delta T cell clones. Eur J Immunol. 1997;27:1704–1712.
289. Ferrick DA, Schrenzel MD, Mulvania T, et al. Differential production of interferon-gamma and interleukin-4 in response to Th1- and Th2-stimulating pathogens by gamma delta T cells in vivo. Nature. 1995;373:255–257.
290. Tanaka Y, Sano S, Nieves E, et al. Nonpeptide ligands for human gamma delta T cells. Proc Natl Acad Sci U S A. 1994;91:8175–8179.
291. Tanaka Y, Morita CT, Nieves E, et al. Natural and synthetic non-peptide antigens recognized by human gamma delta T cells. Nature. 1995;375:155–158.
292. Poquet Y, Constant P, Halary F, et al. A novel nucleotide-containing antigen for human blood gamma delta T lymphocytes. Eur J Immunol. 1996;26:2344–2349.
293. Constant P, Davodeau F, Peyrat MA, et al. Stimulation of human gamma delta T cells by nonpeptidic mycobacterial ligands. Science. 1994;264:267–270.
294. De Libero G. Sentinel function of broadly reactive human gamma delta T cells. Immunol Today. 1997;18:22–26.
295. Wesch D, Marx S, Kabelitz D. Comparative analysis of alpha beta and gamma delta T cell activation by *Mycobacterium tuberculosis* and isopentenyl pyrophosphate. Eur J Immunol. 1997;27:952–956.
296. De Libero G, Casorati G, Giachino C, et al. Selection by two powerful antigens may account for the presence of the major population of human peripheral gamma/delta T cells. J Exp Med. 1991;173:1311–1322.
297. Parker CM, Groh V, Band H, et al. Evidence for extrathymic changes in the T cell receptor gamma/delta repertoire. J Exp Med. 1990;171:1597–1612.
298. Ito M, Kojiro N, Ikeda T, et al. Increased proportions of peripheral blood gamma delta T cells in patients with pulmonary tuberculosis. Chest. 1992;102:195–197.
299. Balbi B, Valle MT, Oddera S, et al. T-lymphocytes with gamma delta+ V delta 2+ antigen receptors are present in increased proportions in a fraction of patients with tuberculosis or with sarcoidosis. Am Rev Respir Dis. 1993;148:t–90.
300. Ueta C, Tsuyuguchi I, Kawasumi H, et al. Increase of gamma/delta T cells in hospital workers who are in close contact with tuberculosis patients. Infect Immun. 1994;62:5434–5441.
301. Tazi A, Bouchonnet F, Valeyre D, et al. Characterization of gamma/delta T-lymphocytes in the peripheral blood of patients with active tuberculosis: A comparison with normal subjects and patients with sarcoidosis. Am Rev Respir Dis. 1992;146:t–21.
302. Tazi A, Fajac I, Soler P, et al. Gamma/delta T-lymphocytes are not increased in number in granulomatous lesions of patients with tuberculosis or sarcoidosis. Am Rev Respir Dis. 1991;144:1373–1375.
303. Barnes PF, Grisso CL, Abrams JS, et al. Gamma delta T lymphocytes in human tuberculosis. J Infect Dis. 1992;165:506–512.
304. Li B, Rossman MD, Imir T, et al. Disease-specific changes in gammadelta T cell repertoire and function in patients with pulmonary tuberculosis. J Immunol. 1996;157:4222–4229.
305. Boom WH. The role of T-cell subsets in *Mycobacterium tuberculosis* infection. Infect Agents Dis. 1996;5:73–81.
306. Modlin RL, Pirmez C, Hofman FM, et al. Lymphocytes bearing antigen-specific gamma delta T-cell receptors accumulate in human infectious disease lesions. Nature. 1989;339:544–548.
307. Ladel CH, Blum C, Dreher A, et al. Protective role of gamma/delta T cells and alpha/beta T cells in tuberculosis [published erratum appears in Eur J Immunol 1995;25:3525]. Eur J Immunol. 1995;25:2877–2881.
308. D'Souza CD, Cooper AM, Frank AA, et al. An anti-inflammatory role for gamma delta T lymphocytes in acquired immunity to *Mycobacterium tuberculosis*. J Immunol. 1997;158:1217–1221.
309. Sciammas R, Kodukula P, Tang Q, et al. T cell receptor-gamma/delta cells protect mice from herpes simplex virus type 1-induced lethal encephalitis. J Exp Med. 1997;185:1969–1975.
310. Maccario R, Comoli P, Percivalle E, et al. Herpes simplex virus-specific human cytotoxic T-cell colonies expressing either gamma delta or alpha beta T-cell receptor: Role of accessory molecules on HLA-unrestricted killing of virus-infected targets. Immunology. 1995;85:49–56.
311. Maccario R, Revello MG, Comoli P, et al. HLA-unrestricted killing of HSV-1-infected mononuclear cells: Involvement of either gamma/delta+ or alpha/beta+ human cytotoxic T lymphocytes. J Immunol. 1993;150:1437–1445.
312. Bukowski JF, Morita CT, Brenner MB. Recognition and destruction of virus-infected cells by human gamma delta CTL. J Immunol. 1994;153:5133–5140.
313. Battistini L, Borsellino G, Sawicki G, et al. Phenotypic and cytokine analysis of human peripheral blood gamma delta T cells expressing NK cell receptors. J Immunol. 1997;159:3723–3730.
314. Sturm E, Braakman E, Fisch P, et al. Human V gamma 9-V delta 2 T cell receptor-gamma delta lymphocytes show specificity to Daudi Burkitt's lymphoma cells. J Immunol. 1990;145:3202–3208.
315. Hacker G, Kromer S, Falk M, et al. V delta 1+ subset of human gamma delta T

cells responds to ligands expressed by EBV-infected Burkitt lymphoma cells and transformed B lymphocytes. J Immunol. 1992;149:3984–3089.
316. Munk ME, Teixeira HC, Kuner A, et al. Human alpha beta and gamma delta T cells from unexposed individuals respond to protein antigens of the yeast form of *Paracoccidioides brasiliensis*. Int Immunol. 1994;6:1717–1725.
317. Lanier LL, Le AM, Civin CI, et al. The relationship of CD16 (Leu-11) and Leu-19 (NKH-1) antigen expression on human peripheral blood NK cells and cytotoxic T lymphocytes. J Immunol. 1986;136:4480–4486.
318. Nagler A, Lanier LL, Cwirla S, et al. Comparative studies of human FcRIII-positive and negative natural killer cells. J Immunol. 1989;143:3183–3191.
319. Spits H, Lanier LL, Phillips JH. Development of human T and natural killer cells. Blood. 1995;85:2654–2670.
320. Karre K, Ljunggren HG, Piontek G, et al. Selective rejection of H-2-deficient lymphoma variants suggests alternative immune defence strategy. Nature. 1986;319:675–678.
321. Maudsley DJ, Pound JD. Modulation of MHC antigen expression by viruses and oncogenes. Immunol Today. 1991;12:429–431.
322. Burshtyn DN, Long EO. Regulation through inhibitory receptors: Lessons from natural killer cells (Review). Trends Cell Biol. 1997;7:473–479.
323. Yokoyama WM. What goes up must come down: The emerging spectrum of inhibitory receptors (Comment). J Exp Med. 1997;186:1803–1808.
324. Moretta A, Sivori S, Vitale M, et al. Existence of both inhibitory (p58) and activatory (p50) receptors for HLA-C molecules in human natural killer cells. J Exp Med. 1995;182:875–884.
325. Mandelboim O, Davis DM, Reyburn HT, et al. Enhancement of class II-restricted T cell responses by costimulatory NK receptors for class I MHC proteins. Science. 1996;274:2097–2100.
326. Mason LH, Anderson SK, Yokoyama WM, et al. The Ly-49D receptor activates murine natural killer cells. J Exp Med. 1996;184:2119–2128.
327. Colonna M. Immunology. Unmasking the killer's accomplice (News; comment). Nature. 1998;391:642–643.
328. Lanier LL, Corliss BC, Wu J, et al. Immunoreceptor DAP12 bearing a tyrosine-based activation motif is involved in activating NK cells (See comments). Nature. 1998;391:703–707.
329. Kagi D, Ledermann B, Burki K, et al. Cytotoxicity mediated by T cells and natural killer cells is greatly impaired in perforin-deficient mice (See comments). Nature. 1994;369:31–37.
330. Shresta S, Heusel JW, Macivor DM, et al. Granzyme B plays a critical role in cytotoxic lymphocyte-induced apoptosis. Immunol Rev. 1995;146:211–221.
331. Nakazawa T, Agematsu K, Yabuhara A. Later development of Fas ligand-mediated cytotoxicity as compared with granule-mediated cytotoxicity during the maturation of natural killer cells. Immunology. 1997;92:180–187.
332. Kohl S, West MS, Prober CG, et al. Neonatal antibody-dependent cellular cytotoxic antibody levels are associated with the clinical presentation of neonatal herpes simplex virus infection. J Infect Dis. 1989;160:770–776.
333. Robertson MJ, Ritz J. Biology and clinical relevance of human natural killer cells. Blood. 1990;76:2421–2438.
334. Bancroft GJ. The role of natural killer cells in innate resistance to infection. Curr Opin Immunol. 1993;5:503–510.
335. Hidore MR, Murphy JW. Correlation of natural killer cell activity and clearance of *Cryptococcus neoformans* from mice after adoptive transfer of splenic nylon wool-nonadherent cells. Infect Immun. 1986;51:547–555.
336. Murphy JW. Natural killer cell-mediated resistance in cryptococcosis. In: Herberman RB, ed. NK cells and other natural effector cells. New York: Academic Press; 1982;1503–1507.
337. Tripp CS, Gately MK, Hakimi J, et al. Neutralization of IL-12 decreases resistance to Listeria in SCID and C.B-17 mice: Reversal by IFN-gamma. J Immunol. 1994;152:1883–1887.
338. Welsh RM, Brubaker JO, Vargas-Cortes M, et al. Natural killer (NK) cell response to virus infections in mice with severe combined immunodeficiency: The stimulation of NK cells and the NK cell-dependent control of virus infections occur independently of T and B cell function. J Exp Med. 1991;173:1053–1063.
339. Fleisher G, Starr S, Koven N, et al. A non-X-linked syndrome with susceptibility to severe Epstein-Barr virus infections. J Pediatr. 1982;100:727–730.
340. Biron CA, Byron KS, Sullivan JL. Severe herpesvirus infections in an adolescent without natural killer cells (See comments). N Engl J Med. 1989;320:1731–1735.
341. Halary F, Peyrat MA, Champagne E, et al. Control of self-reactive cytotoxic T lymphocytes expressing gamma delta T cell receptors by natural killer inhibitory receptors. Eur J Immunol. 1997;27:2812–2821.
342. Eichelberger M, Doherty PC. Gamma delta T cells from influenza-infected mice develop a natural killer cell phenotype following culture. Cell Immunol. 1994;159:94–102.
343. Schmidt RE, Murray C, Daley JF, et al. A subset of natural killer cells in peripheral blood displays a mature T cell phenotype. J Exp Med. 1986;164:351–356.
344. Acha-Orbea H, Groscurth P, Lang R, et al. Characterization of cloned cytotoxic lymphocytes with NK-like activity. J Immunol. 1983;130:2952–2959.
345. Lanier LL, Le AM, Ding A, et al. Expression of Leu-19 (NKH-1) antigen on IL 2-dependent cytotoxic and non-cytotoxic T cell lines. J Immunol. 1987;138:2019–2023.
346. Kharitonenkov A, Chen Z, Sures I, et al. A family of proteins that inhibit signalling through tyrosine kinase receptors. Nature. 1997;386:181–186.
347. Meyaard L, Adema GJ, Chang C, et al. LAIR-1, a novel inhibitory receptor expressed on human mononuclear leukocytes. Immunity. 1997;7:283–290.
348. Cosman D, Fanger N, Borges L, et al. A novel immunoglobulin superfamily receptor for cellular and viral MHC class I molecules. Immunity. 1997;7:273–282.
349. Samaridis J, Colonna M. Cloning of novel immunoglobulin superfamily receptors expressed on human myeloid and lymphoid cells: Structural evidence for new stimulatory and inhibitory pathways. Eur J Immunol. 1997;27:660–665.
350. Cella M, Dohring C, Samaridis J, et al. A novel inhibitory receptor (ILT3) expressed on monocytes, macrophages, and dendritic cells involved in antigen processing. J Exp Med. 1997;185:1743–1751.
351. Palau LA, Pankey GA. Strongyloides hyperinfection in a renal transplant recipient receiving cyclosporine: Possible *Strongyloides stercoralis* transmission by kidney transplant. Am J Trop Med Hyg. 1997;57:413–415.
352. Yoshida T, Ikuta K, Sugaya H, et al. Defective B-1 cell development and impaired immunity against *Angiostrongylus cantonensis* in IL-5R alpha-deficient mice. Immunity. 1996;4:483–494.
353. Kopf M, Brombacher F, Hodgkin PD, et al. IL-5-deficient mice have a developmental defect in CD5+ B-1 cells and lack eosinophilia but have normal antibody and cytotoxic T cell responses. Immunity. 1996;4:15–24.
354. Levitz SM, Mathews HL, Murphy JW. Direct antimicrobial activity of T cells. Immunol Today. 1995;16:387–391.
355. Murphy JW, Hidore MR, Wong SC. Direct interactions of human lymphocytes with the yeast-like organism, *Cryptococcus neoformans*. J Clin Invest. 1993;91:1553–1566.
356. Levitz SM, Dupont MP. Phenotypic and functional characterization of human lymphocytes activated by interleukin-2 to directly inhibit growth of *Cryptococcus neoformans* in vitro. J Clin Invest. 1993;91:1490–1498.
357. Levitz SM, Dupont MP, Smail EH. Direct activity of human T lymphocytes and natural killer cells against *Cryptococcus neoformans*. Infect Immun. 1994;62:194–202.
358. Fung PY, Murphy JW. In vitro interactions of immune lymphocytes and *Cryptococcus neoformans*. Infect Immun. 1982;36:1128–1138.
359. Muth SM, Murphy JW. Direct anticryptococcal activity of lymphocytes from *Cryptococcus neoformans*-immunized mice. Infect Immun. 1995;63:1637–1644.
360. Salata RA, Cox JG, Ravdin JI. The interaction of human T-lymphocytes and *Entamoeba histolytica*: Killing of virulent amoebae by lectin-dependent lymphocytes. Parasite Immunol. 1987;9:249–261.
361. Ellner JJ, Olds GR, Lee CW, et al. Destruction of the multicellular parasite *Schistosoma mansoni* by T lymphocytes. J Clin Invest. 1982;70:369–378.
362. Deem RL, Doughty FA, Beaman BL. Immunologically specific direct T lymphocyte-mediated killing of *Nocardia asteroides*. J Immunol. 1983;130:2401–2406.
363. Malaviya R, Ikeda T, Ross E, et al. Mast cell modulation of neutrophil influx and bacterial clearance at sites of infection through TNF-alpha (See comments). Nature. 1996;381:77–80.
364. Dvorak AM. New aspects of mast cell biology. Int Arch Allergy Immunol. 1997;114:1–9.
365. Abraham SN, Thankavel K, Malaviya R. Mast cells as modulators of host defense in the lung. Front Biosci. 1997;2:d78–d87.
366. Walsh LJ, Trinchieri G, Waldorf HA, et al. Human dermal mast cells contain and release tumor necrosis factor alpha, which induces endothelial leukocyte adhesion molecule 1. Proc Natl Acad Sci U S A. 1991;88:4220–4224.
367. Bradding P, Feather IH, Howarth PH, et al. Interleukin 4 is localized to and released by human mast cells. J Exp Med. 1992;176:1381–1386.
368. Malaviya R, Ross E, Jakschik BA, Abraham SN. Mast cell degranulation induced by type 1 fimbriated *Escherichia coli* in mice. J Clin Invest. 1994;93:1645–1653.
369. Guy-Grand D, Vassalli P. Gut intraepithelial T lymphocytes. Curr Opin Immunol. 1993;5:247–252.
370. Lamm ME. Interaction of antigens and antibodies at mucosal surfaces. Annu Rev Microbiol. 1997;51:311–340.
371. Emoto M, Emoto Y, Kaufmann SH. Development of CD8 alpha/beta + TCR alpha beta intestinal intraepithelial lymphocytes in athymic nu/nu mice and participation in regional immune responses. Immunology. 1996;88:531–536.
372. Lundqvist C, Melgar S, Yeung MM, et al. Intraepithelial lymphocytes in human gut have lytic potential and a cytokine profile that suggest T helper 1 and cytotoxic functions. J Immunol. 1996;157:1926–1934.
373. Goodman T, Lefrancois L. Expression of the gamma-delta T-cell receptor on intestinal CD8+ intraepithelial lymphocytes. Nature. 1988;333:855–858.
374. Rocha B, Vassalli P, Guy-Grand D. The V beta repertoire of mouse gut homodimeric alpha CD8+ intraepithelial T cell receptor alpha/beta + lymphocytes reveals a major extrathymic pathway of T cell differentiation. J Exp Med. 1991;173:483–486.
375. Kappler JW, Staerz U, White J, et al. Self-tolerance eliminates T cells specific for Mls-modified products of the major histocompatibility complex. Nature. 1988;332:35–40.
376. Saito H, Kanamori Y, Takemori T, et al. Generation of intestinal T cells from progenitors residing in gut cryptopatches (See comments). Science. 1998;280:275–278.
377. Guy-Grand D, Vanden Broecke C, Briottet C, et al. Different expression of the recombination activity gene RAG-1 in various populations of thymocytes, peripheral T cells and gut thymus-independent intraepithelial lymphocytes suggests two pathways of T cell receptor rearrangement. Eur J Immunol. 1992;22:505–510.
378. Sim GK, Rajaserkar R, Dessing M, et al. Homing and in situ differentiation of resident pulmonary lymphocytes. Int Immunol. 1994;6:1287–1295.
379. Bandeira A, Itohara S, Bonneville M, et al. Extrathymic origin of intestinal intraepithelial lymphocytes bearing T-cell antigen receptor gamma delta. Proc Natl Acad Sci U S A. 1991;88:43–47.
380. Wang J, Klein JR. Thymus-neuroendocrine interactions in extrathymic T cell development. Science. 1994;265:1860–1862.
381. Guy-Grand D, Cerf-Bensussan N, Malissen B, et al. Two gut intraepithelial CD8+

lymphocyte populations with different T cell receptors: A role for the gut epithelium in T cell differentiation. J Exp Med. 1991;173:471–481.
382. Ota Y, Kobata T, Seki M, et al. Extrathymic origin of V gamma 1/V delta 6 T cells in the skin. Eur J Immunol. 1992;22:595–598.
383. Offit PA, Dudzik KI. Rotavirus-specific cytotoxic T lymphocytes appear at the intestinal mucosal surface after rotavirus infection. J Virol. 1989;63:3507–3512.
384. Farstad IN, Halstensen TS, Kvale D, et al. Topographic distribution of homing receptors on B and T cells in human gut-associated lymphoid tissue: Relation of L-selectin and integrin alpha 4 beta 7 to naive and memory phenotypes. Am J Pathol. 1997;150:187–199.
385. Kim SK, Reed DS, Heath WR, et al. Activation and migration of CD8 T cells in the intestinal mucosa. J Immunol. 1997;159:4295–4306.
386. Poussier P, Julius M. T-cell development and selection in the intestinal epithelium. Semin Immunol. 1995;7:321–334.
387. Lefrancois L, Fuller B, Huleatt JW, et al. On the front lines: Intraepithelial lymphocytes as primary effectors of intestinal immunity. Springer Semin Immunopathol. 1997;18:463–475.
388. Neuhaus O, Emoto M, Blum C, et al. Control of thymus-independent intestinal intraepithelial lymphocytes by beta 2-microglobulin. Eur J Immunol. 1995;25:2332–2339.
389. Poussier P, Julius M. Thymus independent T cell development and selection in the intestinal epithelium. Annu Rev Immunol. 1994;12:521–553.
390. London SD, Cebra JJ, Rubin DH. Intraepithelial lymphocytes contain virus-specific, MHC-restricted cytotoxic cell precursors after gut mucosal immunization with reovirus serotype 1/Lang. Reg Immunol. 1989;2:98–102.
391. Imaoka A, Matsumoto S, Setoyama H, et al. Proliferative recruitment of intestinal intraepithelial lymphocytes after microbial colonization of germ-free mice. Eur J Immunol. 1996;26:945–948.
392. Emoto M, Neuhaus O, Emoto Y, et al. Influence of beta 2-microglobulin expression on gamma interferon secretion and target cell lysis by intraepithelial lymphocytes during intestinal *Listeria monocytogenes* infection. Infect Immun. 1996;64:569–575.
393. Belshe RB, Mendelman PM, Treanor J, et al. The efficacy of live attenuated, cold-adapted, trivalent, intranasal influenzavirus vaccine in children (See comments). N Engl J Med. 1998;338:1405–1412.
394. Gallichan WS, Rosenthal KL. Long-lived cytotoxic T lymphocyte memory in mucosal tissues after mucosal but not systemic immunization. J Exp Med. 1996;184:1879–1890.
395. Rosenthal KL, Gallichan WS. Challenges for vaccination against sexually-transmitted diseases: Induction and long-term maintenance of mucosal immune responses in the female genital tract. Semin Immunol. 1997;9:303–314.
396. Belyakov IM, Derby MA, Ahlers JD, et al. Mucosal immunization with HIV-1 peptide vaccine induces mucosal and systemic cytotoxic T lymphocytes and protective immunity in mice against intrarectal recombinant HIV-vaccinia challenge. Proc Natl Acad Sci U S A. 1998;95:1709–1714.
397. Shaw SK, Brenner MB. The beta 7 integrins in mucosal homing and retention. Semin Immunol. 1995;7:335–342.
398. Rott LS, Briskin MJ, Andrew DP, et al. A fundamental subdivision of circulating lymphocytes defined by adhesion to mucosal addressin cell adhesion molecule-1: Comparison with vascular cell adhesion molecule-1 and correlation with beta 7 integrins and memory differentiation. J Immunol. 1996;156:3727–3736.
399. Lasky LA. Selectin-carbohydrate interactions and the initiation of the inflammatory response. Annu Rev Biochem. 1995;64:113–139.
400. Springer TA. Traffic signals for lymphocyte recirculation and leukocyte emigration: The multistep paradigm. Cell. 1994;76:301–314.
401. Liu W, Ramachandran V, Kang J, et al. Identification of N-terminal residues on P-selectin glycoprotein ligand-1 required for binding to P-selectin. J Biol Chem. 1998;273:7078–7087.
402. Herrlich P, Zoller M, Pals ST, et al. CD44 splice variants: Metastases meet lymphocytes. Immunol Today. 1993;14:395–399.
403. Kraal G, Mebius RE. High endothelial venules: Lymphocyte traffic control and controlled traffic. Adv Immunol. 1997;65:347–395.
404. Berlin C, Berg EL, Briskin MJ, et al. Alpha 4 beta 7 integrin mediates lymphocyte binding to the mucosal vascular addressin MAdCAM-1. Cell. 1993;74:185–195.
405. Erle DJ, Briskin MJ, Butcher EC, et al. Expression and function of the MAdCAM-1 receptor, integrin alpha 4 beta 7, on human leukocytes. J Immunol. 1994;153:517–528.
406. Hamann A, Andrew DP, Jablonski-Westrich D, et al. Role of alpha 4-integrins in lymphocyte homing to mucosal tissues in vivo. J Immunol. 1994;152:3282–3293.
407. Berg EL, Yoshino T, Rott LS, et al. The cutaneous lymphocyte antigen is a skin lymphocyte homing receptor for the vascular lectin endothelial cell-leukocyte adhesion molecule 1. J Exp Med. 1991;174:1461–1466.
408. Picker LJ, Kishimoto TK, Smith CW, et al. ELAM-1 is an adhesion molecule for skin-homing T cells (See comments). Nature. 1991;349:796–799.
409. Fuhlbrigge RC, Kieffer JD, Armerding D, et al. Cutaneous lymphocyte antigen is a specialized form of PSGL-1 expressed on skin-homing T cells. Nature. 1997;389:978–981.
410. Camerini D, James SP, Stamenkovic I, et al. Leu-8/TQ1 is the human equivalent of the Mel-14 lymph node homing receptor. Nature. 1989;342:78–82.
411. Kishimoto TK, Jutila MA, Butcher EC. Identification of a human peripheral lymph node homing receptor: A rapidly down-regulated adhesion molecule. Proc Natl Acad Sci U S A. 1990;87:2244–2248.
412. Kansas GS. Structure and function of L-selectin. APMIS. 1992;100:287–293.
413. Picker LJ. Control of lymphocyte homing. Curr Opin Immunol. 1994;6:394–406.
414. Kilshaw PJ, Karecla P. Structure and function of the mucosal T-cell integrin alpha E beta 7. Biochem Soc Trans. 1997;25:433–439.
415. Austrup F, Vestweber D, Borges E, et al. P- and E-selectin mediate recruitment of T-helper-1 but not T-helper-2 cells into inflamed tissues. Nature. 1997;385:81–83.
416. Arbones ML, Ord DC, Ley K, et al. Lymphocyte homing and leukocyte rolling and migration are impaired in L-selectin-deficient mice. Immunity. 1994;1:247–260.
417. Ye RD, Boulay F. Structure and function of leukocyte chemoattractant receptors. Adv Pharmacol. 1997;39:221–289.
418. Campbell JJ, Hedrick J, Zlotnik A, et al. Chemokines and the arrest of lymphocytes rolling under flow conditions. Science. 1998;279:381–384.
419. Campbell JJ, Bowman EP, Murphy K, et al. 6-C-kine (SLC), a lymphocyte adhesion-triggering chemokine expressed by high endothelium, is an agonist for the MIP-3beta receptor CCR7. J Cell Biol. 1998;141:1053–1059.
420. Gunn MD, Tangemann K, Tam C, et al. A chemokine expressed in lymphoid high endothelial venules promotes the adhesion and chemotaxis of naive T lymphocytes. Proc Natl Acad Sci U S A. 1998;95:258–263.
421. Berg EL, McEvoy LM, Berlin C, et al. L-selectin-mediated lymphocyte rolling on MAdCAM-1 (See comments). Nature. 1993;366:695–698.
422. Berlin C, Bargatze RF, Campbell JJ, et al. Alpha 4 integrins mediate lymphocyte attachment and rolling under physiologic flow. Cell. 1995;80:413–422.
423. Wagner N, Lohler J, Kunkel EJ, et al. Critical role for beta7 integrins in formation of the gut-associated lymphoid tissue. Nature. 1996;382:366–370.
424. Cepek KL, Shaw SK, Parker CM, et al. Adhesion between epithelial cells and T lymphocytes mediated by E-cadherin and the alpha E beta 7 integrin. Nature. 1994;372:190–193.
425. Feng D, Nagy JA, Pyne K, et al. Neutrophils emigrate from venules by a transendothelial cell pathway in response to FMLP. J Exp Med. 1998;187:903–915.
426. Brown EJ. Adhesive interactions in the immune system. Trends Cell Biol. 1997;7:289–295.
427. Kaufmann SH, Rodewald HR, Hug E, et al. Cloned *Listeria monocytogenes* specific non-MHC-restricted Lyt-2+ T cells with cytolytic and protective activity. J Immunol. 1988;140:3173–3179.
428. Kaufmann SH, Hug E, De Libero G. *Listeria monocytogenes*-reactive T lymphocyte clones with cytolytic activity against infected target cells. J Exp Med. 1986;164:363–368.
429. De Libero G, Kaufmann SH. Antigen-specific Lyt-2+ cytolytic T lymphocytes from mice infected with the intracellular bacterium *Listeria monocytogenes*. J Immunol. 1986;137:2688–2694.
430. De Libero G, Flesch I, Kaufmann SH. Mycobacteria-reactive Lyt-2+ T cell lines. Eur J Immunol. 1988;18:59–66.
431. Stenger S, Mazzaccaro RJ, Uyemura K, et al. Differential effects of cytolytic T cell subsets on intracellular infection. Science. 1997;276:1684–1687.
432. Kima PE, Ruddle NH, McMahon-Pratt D. Presentation via the class I pathway by *Leishmania amazonensis*-infected macrophages of an endogenous leishmanial antigen to CD8+ T cells. J Immunol. 1997;159:1828–1834.
433. Hakim FT, Gazzinelli RT, Denkers E, et al. CD8+ T cells from mice vaccinated against *Toxoplasma gondii* are cytotoxic for parasite-infected or antigen-pulsed host cells. J Immunol. 1991;147:2310–2316.
434. Subauste CS, Koniaris AH, Remington JS. Murine CD8+ cytotoxic T lymphocytes lyse *Toxoplasma gondii*-infected cells. J Immunol. 1991;147:3955–3959.
435. Frankenburg S, Axelrod O, Kutner S, et al. Effective immunization of mice against cutaneous leishmaniasis using an intrinsically adjuvanted synthetic lipopeptide vaccine. Vaccine. 1996;14:923–929.
436. Petri WAJ, Ravdin JI. Protection of gerbils from amebic liver abscess by immunization with the galactose-specific adherence lectin of *Entamoeba histolytica*. Infect Immun. 1991;59:97–101.
437. Link H, Arseniev L, Bahre O, et al. Transplantation of allogeneic CD34+ blood cells. Blood. 1996;87:4903–4909.
438. Ehl S, Hombach J, Aichele P, et al. Viral and bacterial infections interfere with peripheral tolerance induction and activate CD8+ T cells to cause immunopathology. J Exp Med. 1998;187:763–774.
439. Hertz MI, Englund JA, Snover D, et al. Respiratory syncytial virus-induced acute lung injury in adult patients with bone marrow transplants: A clinical approach and review of the literature. Medicine (Baltimore). 1989;68:269–281.
440. Harrington RD, Hooton TM, Hackman RC, et al. An outbreak of respiratory syncytial virus in a bone marrow transplant center. J Infect Dis. 1992;165:987–993.
441. Lewis VA, Champlin R, Englund J, et al. Respiratory disease due to parainfluenza virus in adult bone marrow transplant recipients. Clin Infect Dis. 1996;23:1033–1037.
442. Blanke C, Clark C, Broun ER, et al. Evolving pathogens in allogeneic bone marrow transplantation: Increased fatal adenoviral infections. Am J Med. 1995;99:326–328.
443. Chan PK, Peiris JS, Yuen KY, et al. Human herpesvirus-6 and human herpesvirus-7 infections in bone marrow transplant recipients. J Med Virol. 1997;53:295–305.
444. Knox KK, Carrigan DR. Chronic myelosuppression associated with persistent bone marrow infection due to human herpesvirus 6 in a bone marrow transplant recipient. Clin Infect Dis. 1996;22:174–175.
445. Mookerjee BP, Vogelsang G. Human herpes virus-6 encephalitis after bone marrow transplantation: Successful treatment with ganciclovir. Bone Marrow Transplant. 1997;20:905–906.
446. Kugler JW, Armitage JO, Helms CM, et al. Nosocomial Legionnaires' disease: Occurrence in recipients of bone marrow transplants. Am J Med. 1983;74:281–288.
447. Moses A, Nelson J, Bagby GCJ. The influence of human immunodeficiency virus-1 on hematopoiesis. Blood. 1998;91:1479–1495.
448. Gorochov G, Neumann AU, Kereveur A, et al. Perturbation of CD4+ and CD8+

T-cell repertoires during progression to AIDS and regulation of the CD4+ repertoire during antiviral therapy (See comments). Nat Med. 1998;4:215–221.
449. Komanduri KV, Viswanathan MN, Wieder ED, et al. Restoration of cytomegalovirus-specific CD4+ T-lymphocyte responses after ganciclovir and highly active antiretroviral therapy in individuals infected with HIV-1. Nat Med. 1998;4:953–956.
450. Michaels MG, Green M, Wald ER, et al. Adenovirus infection in pediatric liver transplant recipients. J Infect Dis. 1992;165:170–174.
451. McGrath D, Falagas ME, Freeman R, et al. Adenovirus infection in adult orthotopic liver transplant recipients: Incidence and clinical significance. J Infect Dis. 1998;177:459–462.
452. Wendt CH, Fox JM, Hertz MI. Paramyxovirus infection in lung transplant recipients. J Heart Lung Transplant. 1995;14:479–485.
453. Simsir A, Greenebaum E, Nuovo G, et al. Late fatal adenovirus pneumonitis in a lung transplant recipient. Transplantation. 1998;65:592–594.
454. Millett R, Tomita T, Marshall HE, et al. Cytomegalovirus endomyocarditis in a transplanted heart: A case report with in situ hybridization. Arch Pathol Lab Med. 1991;115:511–515.
455. Gonwa TA, Capehart JE, Pilcher JW, et al. Cytomegalovirus myocarditis as a cause of cardiac dysfunction in a heart transplant recipient. Transplantation. 1989;47:197–199.
456. Schowengerdt KO, Ni J, Denfield SW, et al. Association of parvovirus B19 genome in children with myocarditis and cardiac allograft rejection: Diagnosis using the polymerase chain reaction. Circulation. 1997;96:3549–3554.
457. Didonato JA, Saatcioglu F, Karin M. Molecular mechanisms of immunosuppression and anti-inflammatory activities by glucocorticoids. Am J Respir Crit Care Med. 1996;154:t-5.
458. Ruhlmann A, Nordheim A. Effects of the immunosuppressive drugs CsA and FK506 on intracellular signalling and gene regulation. Immunobiology. 1997;198:192–206.
459. Miller DM, Rahill BM, Boss JM, et al. Human cytomegalovirus inhibits major histocompatibility complex class II expression by disruption of the Jak/Stat pathway. J Exp Med. 1998;187:675–683.
460. Heise MT, Connick M, Virgin HW. Murine cytomegalovirus inhibits interferon gamma-induced antigen presentation to CD4 T cells by macrophages via regulation of expression of major histocompatibility complex class II-associated genes. J Exp Med. 1998;187:1037–1046.
461. Darji A, Stockinger B, Wehland J, et al. Antigen-specific T cell receptor antagonism by antigen-presenting cells treated with the hemolysis of *Listeria monocytogenes*: A novel type of immune escape. Eur J Immunol. 1997;27:1696–1703.
462. Ojcius DM, Gachelin G, Dautry-Varsat A. Presentation of antigens derived from microorganisms residing in host-cell vacuoles. Trends Microbiol. 1996;4:53–59.
463. Paabo S, Severinsson L, Andersson M, et al. Adenovirus proteins and MHC expression. Adv Cancer Res. 1989;52:151–163.
464. Levitskaya J, Sharipo A, Leonchiks A, et al. Inhibition of ubiquitin/proteasome-dependent protein degradation by the Gly-Ala repeat domain of the Epstein-Barr virus nuclear antigen 1. Proc Natl Acad Sci U S A. 1997;94:12616–12621.
465. Sharipo A, Imreh M, Leonchiks A, et al. A minimal glycine-alanine repeat prevents the interaction of ubiquitinated I kappaB alpha with the proteasome: A new mechanism for selective inhibition of proteolysis (See comments). Nat Med. 1998;4:939–944.
466. York IA, Roop C, Andrews DW, et al. A cytosolic herpes simplex virus protein inhibits antigen presentation to CD8+ T lymphocytes. Cell. 1994;77:525–535.
467. Jones TR, Wiertz EJ, Sun L, et al. Human cytomegalovirus US3 impairs transport and maturation of major histocompatibility complex class I heavy chains. Proc Natl Acad Sci U S A. 1996;93:11327–11333.
468. Wiertz EJ, Jones TR, Sun L, et al. The human cytomegalovirus US11 gene product dislocates MHC class I heavy chains from the endoplasmic reticulum to the cytosol. Cell. 1996;84:769–779.
469. Ahn K, Gruhler A, Galocha B, et al. The ER-luminal domain of the HCMV glycoprotein US6 inhibits peptide translocation by TAP. Immunity. 1997;6:613–621.
470. Lehner PJ, Karttunen JT, Wilkinson GW, et al. The human cytomegalovirus US6 glycoprotein inhibits transporter associated with antigen processing-dependent peptide translocation. Proc Natl Acad Sci U S A. 1997;94:6904–6909.
471. Gilbert MJ, Riddell SR, Plachter B, et al. Cytomeglovirus selectively blocks antigen processing and presentation of its immediate-early gene product. Nature. 1996;383:720–722.
472. Reyburn HT, Mandelboim O, Vales-Gomez M, et al. The class I MHC homologue of human cytomegalovirus inhibits attack by natural killer cells (See comments). Nature. 1997;386:514–517.
473. Ziegler H, Thale R, Lucin P, et al. A mouse cytomegalovirus glycoprotein retains MHC class I complexes in the ERGIC/cis-Golgi compartments. Immunity. 1997;6:57–66.
474. Farrell HE, Vally H, Lynch DM, et al. Inhibition of natural killer cells by a cytomegalovirus MHC class I homologue in vivo (See comments). Nature. 1997;386:510–514.
475. Bluestone JA. New perspectives of CD28-B7-mediated T cell costimulation. Immunity. 1995;2:555–559.
476. Boise LH, Noel PJ, Thompson CB. CD28 and apoptosis. Curr Opin Immunol. 1995;7:620–625.
477. Bierer BE, Barbosa J, Herrmann S, et al. Interaction of CD2 with its ligand, LFA-3, in human T cell proliferation. J Immunol. 1988;140:3358–3363.
478. Springer TA. Adhesion receptors of the immune system. Nature. 1990;346:425–434.
479. Green JM, Thompson CB. Homotypic interactions mediated through LFA-1/ICAM-3 decrease the prolifertive response of activated T cells. Cell Immunol. 1996;171:126–131.
480. Teunissen MB, Koomen CW, Bos JD. Intercellular adhesion molecule-3 (CD50) on human epidermal Langerhans cells participates in T-cell activation. J Invest Dermatol. 1995;104:995–998.
481. Van dV, von HI, Luo W, et al. The B-cell surface protein CD72/Lyb-2 is the ligand for CD5 (See comments). Nature. 1991;351:662–665.
482. Luo W, Van de Velde H, von Hoegen I, et al. Ly-1 (CD5), a membrane glycoprotein of mouse T lymphocytes and a subset of B cells, is a natural ligand of the B cell surface protein Lyb-2 (CD72). J Immunol. 1992;148:1630–1634.
483. Biancone L, Bowen MA, Lim A, et al. Identification of a novel inducible cell-surface ligand of CD5 on activated lymphocytes. J Exp Med. 1996;184:811–819.
484. Tesselaar K, Gravestein LA, van Schijndel GM, et al. Characterization of murine CD70, the ligand of the TNF receptor family member CD27. J Immunol. 1997;159:4959–4965.
485. Bowman MR, Crimmins MA, Yetz-Aldape J, et al. The cloning of CD70 and its identification as the ligand for CD27. J Immunol. 1994;152:1756–1761.
486. Kobata T, Agematsu K, Kameoka J, et al. CD27 is a signal-transducing molecule involved in CD45RA+ naive T cell costimulation. J Immunol. 1994;153:5422–5432.
487. Borrow P, Tishon A, Lee S, et al. CD40L-deficient mice show deficits in antiviral immunity and have an impaired memory CD8+ CTL response. J Exp Med. 1996;183:2129–2142.
488. Suzuki I, Fink PJ. Maximal proliferation of cytotoxic T lymphocytes requires reverse signaling through Fas ligand. J Exp Med. 1998;187:123–128.
489. Shimizu Y, van Seventer GA, Horgan KJ, Shaw S. Costimulation of proliferative responses of resting CD4+ T cells by the interaction of VLA-4 and VLA-5 with fibronectin or VLA-6 with laminin. J Immunol. 1990;145:59–67.
490. Bourguignon LY, Lokeshwar VB, Chen X, et al. Hyaluronic acid-induced lymphocyte signal transduction and HA receptor (GP85/CD44)-cytoskeleton interaction. J Immunol. 1993;151:6634–6644.
491. Galandrini R, Galluzzo E, Albi N, et al. Hyaluronate is costimulatory for human T cell effector functions and binds to CD44 on activated T cells. J Immunol. 1994;153:21–31.
492. Johnson R, Lancki DW, Fitch FW. Accessory molecules involved in antigen-mediated cytolysis and lymphokine production by cytotoxic T lymphocyte subsets: I. Identification of functions for the T cell surface molecules Ly-6C and Thy-1. J Immunol. 1993;151:2986–2999.
493. Lazarovits AI, Karsh J. A monoclonal antibody, 7G5 (CD7), induces modulation of Tp40 and inhibits proliferation in the allogeneic and autologous mixed lymphocyte reactions. Transplant Proc. 1988;20:1253–1257.
494. Lee DM, Staats HF, Sundy JS, et al. Immunologic characterization of CD7-deficient mice. J Immunol. 1998;160:5749–5756.
495. Liversidge J, Dawson R, Hoey S, et al. CD59 and CD48 expressed by rat retinal pigment epithelial cells are major ligands for the CD2-mediated alternative pathway of T cell activation. J Immunol. 1996;156:3696–3703.
496. Liu Y, Jones B, Aruffo A, et al. Heat-stable antigen is a costimulatory molecule for CD4 T cell growth. J Exp Med. 1992;175:437–445.
497. Huber SA, Moraska A, Choate M. T cells expressing the gamma delta T-cell receptor potentiate coxsackievirus B3-induced myocarditis. J Virol. 1992;66:6541–6546.
498. De Paoli P, Gennari D, Martelli P, et al. Gamma delta T cell receptor-bearing lymphocytes during Epstein-Barr virus infection. J Infect Dis. 1990;161:1013–1016.
499. Hoq MM, Suzutani T, Toyoda T, et al. Role of gamma delta TCR+ lymphocytes in the augmented resistance of trehalose 6,6′-dimycolate-treated mice to influenza virus infection. J Gen Virol. 1997;78:1597–1603.
500. Knowles G, O'Neil BW, Campo MS. Phenotypical characterization of lymphocytes infiltrating regressing papillomas. J Virol. 1996;70:8451–8458.
501. Ogasawara T, Emoto M, Kiyotani K, et al. Sendai virus pneumonia: Evidence for the early recruitment of gamma delta T cells during the disease course. J Virol. 1994;68:4022–4027.
502. Yee D, Rhinehart-Jones TR, Elkins KL. Loss of either CD4+ or CD8+ T cells does not affect the magnitude of protective immunity to an intracellular pathogen, *Francisella tularensis* strain LVS. J Immunol. 1996;157:5042–5048.
503. Hiromatsu K, Yoshikai Y, Matsuzaki G, et al. A protective role of gamma/delta T cells in primary infection with *Listeria monocytogenes* in mice. J Exp Med. 1992;175:49–56.
504. Mombaerts P, Arnoldi J, Russ F, et al. Different roles of alpha beta and gamma delta T cells in immunity against an intracellular bacterial pathogen. Nature. 1993;365:53–56.
505. Jouen-Beades F, Paris E, Dieulois C, et al. In vivo and in vitro activation and expansion of gammadelta T cells during *Listeria monocytogenes* infection in humans. Infect Immun. 1997;65:4267–4272.
506. Mixter PF, Camerini V, Stone BJ, et al. Mouse T lymphocytes that express a gamma delta T-cell antigen receptor contribute to resistance to *Salmonella* infection in vivo. Infect Immun. 1994;62:4618–4621.
507. Hara T, Mizuno Y, Takaki K, et al. Predominant activation and expansion of V gamma 9-bearing gamma delta T cells in vivo as well as in vitro in *Salmonella* infection. J Clin Invest. 1992;90:204–210.
508. Waters WR, Harp JA. *Cryptosporidium parvum* infection in T-cell receptor (TCR)-alpha- and TCR-delta-deficient mice. Infect Immun. 1996;64:1854–1857.
509. Roberts SJ, Smith AL, West AB, et al. T-cell alpha beta + and gamma delta + deficient mice display abnormal but distinct phenotypes toward a natural, wide-

spread infection of the intestinal epithelium. Proc Natl Acad Sci U S A. 1996;93:11774–11779.
510. Tsuji M, Mombaerts P, Lefrancois L, et al. Gamma delta T cells contribute to immunity against the liver stages of malaria in alpha beta T-cell-deficient mice. Proc Natl Acad Sci U S A. 1994;91:345–349.
511. Kasper LH, Matsuura T, Fonseka S, et al. Induction of gammadelta T cells during acute murine infection with *Toxoplasma gondii*. J Immunol. 1996;157:5521–5527.
512. Santos LE, Minoprio P. Chagas' disease is attenuated in mice lacking gamma delta T cells. Infect Immun. 1996;64:215–221.
513. Piali L, Hammel P, Uherek C, et al. CD31/PECAM-1 is a ligand for alpha v beta 3 integrin involved in adhesion of leukocytes to endothelium. J Cell Biol. 1995;130:451–460.

Chapter 10

Evaluation of the Patient with Suspected Immunodeficiency

STEVEN M. HOLLAND
JOHN I. GALLIN

The most common causes of immunodeficiency are iatrogenic and a result of the widespread use of therapies that modulate the immune system either by design or incidentally. With the expanding recognition, characterization, and in an increasing number of cases, correction of immune abnormalities, making the correct diagnosis is no longer of only academic interest. Identification and cloning of disease-related genes have now made precise antenatal diagnosis and genetic counseling a reality. The promise of the emerging field of gene transfer technology makes a sensible, problem-oriented approach to the patient in whom these issues are raised essential. Following are some general principles involved in the consideration of whether a patient may have an immunodeficiency and how to proceed with a diagnostic evaluation before or as an adjunct to referral or discussion with a specialist.

THE INDEX OF SUSPICION

Concern about the immune status of a patient is usually raised on the basis of the frequency or severity of infections or the finding of an unusual infectious agent. Table 10–1 lists some infectious organisms and the affected limb of host defense implied by their isolation. Obviously, not every isolation of a herpesvirus or *Staphylococcus* implies an immunodeficiency in a specific patient. However, in the setting of abnormally frequent infections or failure to thrive, isolation of these organisms from patient samples should make one consider possible underlying diagnoses. In contrast, isolation of *Pneumocystis carinii, Burkholderia (Pseudomonas) cepacia, Aspergillus,* or *Nocardia* from a patient without a known immunodeficiency is sufficient grounds for pursuing the probability of an underlying defect.

Recurrent hematogenous neisserial infections indicate deficiencies in the late components of complement.[1] *P. carinii* pneumonia indicates T-cell abnormalities.[2] *B. cepacia* bacteremia strongly suggests chronic granulomatous disease.[3] Some specific immunodeficiencies are listed in Table 10–2, along with the gene defect, if known, and some pertinent findings. Recognition and appreciation of the genetic basis of these disorders have been critical to the development of therapy for them and are fundamental to the curative approaches that are now being implemented.

INITIAL EVALUATION

The screening approach to a patient with suspected immunodeficiency is listed in Table 10–3. Careful attention to historical detail is critical. Age of onset of the illness is helpful; Job's syndrome often has an onset within the first days to weeks of life, whereas antibody deficiency states appear only after several months of life when maternal immunoglobulin levels have fallen.[59] Failure to thrive and diarrhea are important points in favor of a substantial problem but are not specific in terms of etiology. Birth history should include the condition and time of separation of the umbilical stump because stump separation is abnormally delayed in leukocyte adhesion deficiency (LAD).[45] The past medical history should note the administration of vaccines, especially for measles, mumps, rubella and for Calmette-Guérin bacillus, difficulties with which are suggestive of dysfunctional T-cell or monocyte immunity. A dental history can be quite informative because patients with abnormalities of phagocytic defense often have gingivitis with periodontal disease[63] and patients with Job's syndrome have severely delayed exfoliation of the primary teeth.[60] Specific questioning regarding parental consanguinity is critical.

Physical examination can yield findings diagnostic or highly suggestive of lesions in specific arms of the immune system. Facial anomalies, including hypertelorism, a shortened philtrum, and downslanting palpebral fissures, are encountered in DiGeorge syndrome,[2] whereas characteristic facies with a broad nose and a triangular mandible are seen in the syndrome of extremely elevated IgE and recurrent infections (Job's syndrome).[60, 61] Hair with a silvery sheen and irregular melanin production is seen in Chédiak-Higashi syndrome.[42] In general, poor dentition, gingivitis, aphthous ulcers, and tooth loss are seen in phagocytic defects such as chronic granulomatous disease (CGD) and LAD,[63] whereas retained primary teeth are encountered in Job's syndrome.[60] Cutaneous signs of immune defects include telangiectases over the bulbar conjunctivae and skin in ataxia-telangiectasia, severe eczema that accompanies Job's syndrome, or the dystrophic scarring seen in LAD.

The initial laboratory examination should consist of a complete blood count with differential, platelet count, examination of the peripheral blood smear, and erythrocyte sedimentation rate. Chédiak-Higashi syndrome and neutrophil-specific granule deficiency can be detected on peripheral smear, whereas Kostmann's syndrome (congenital agranulocytosis) and Wiskott-Aldrich syndrome can be excluded by normal neutrophil or platelet counts, respectively. An immunoglobulin profile with total IgA, IgM, and IgG levels will help detect cases of IgA deficiency, as well as hypogammaglobulinemia. In cases in which eczema is a prominent feature or Job's syndrome is suspected, measurement of IgE levels is indicated. A functional challenge of the humoral immune system, such as preimmunization and postimmunization antibody levels, may be informative. Testing of total hemolytic complement (CH_{50}) gives a quick assessment of the functional integrity of the classic component of the complement cascade from C1 through the membrane attack complex (C5–C9). Plain radiographs of the chest can demonstrate pulmonary scarring, pneumatoceles, and destruction, often encountered in phagocyte defects and Job's syndrome. Scoliosis, osteoporosis, rib and long bone fractures, and their sequelae are frequently seen in Job's syndrome.[60, 61]

LYMPHOCYTE IMMUNE DEFECTS

T Cells and Cell-Mediated Immunity

The initial manifestation of congenital T-cell defects usually, but not always, occurs within the first few months of life and includes severe mucocutaneous candidiasis, recurrent, persistent respiratory infections, diarrhea, and failure to thrive. A broad spectrum of onset and severity is seen. Reticular dysgenesis occurs within the first weeks of life and is characterized by pancytopenia, infection, and early demise.[16, 17] The lymphocyte enzymopathies (adenosine deaminase deficiency and purine nucleoside phosphorylase deficiency) tend to occur after several months of life when lymphocyte counts begin to fall because of accumulation of the toxic metabolites deoxyadeno-

TABLE 10–1 Selected Disease-Associated Pathogens

Pathogen	History	Host Defense Affected	Clinical Examples
Pneumocystis carinii, Cryptococcus neoformans, herpesviruses	Disseminated infections, opportunistic infections, persistent viral infections	T cells	Severe combined immunodeficiency, acquired immunodeficiency syndrome
Haemophilus influenzae, Streptococcus pneumoniae, Giardia lamblia, Campylobacter spp., enteroviruses	Recurrent respiratory infections with encapsulated organisms, chronic diarrhea, aseptic meningitis	B cells	Common variable immunodeficiency, X-linked agammaglobulinemia
Staphylococcus aureus, Burkholderia cepacia, Serratia marcescens, Aspergillus spp., *Nocardia* spp.	Gingivitis, apthous ulcers, recurrent pyogenic infections, delayed umbilical stump separation	Phagocytes	Chronic granulomatous disease, Chédiak-Higashi syndrome, leukocyte adhesion deficiency[67]
Neisseria spp.	Recurrent bacteremia, recurrent meningitis	Complement	Late complement component deficiency
S. aureus, H. influenzae, S. pneumoniae, Candida albicans	Eczema, kyphoscoliosis, bony deformities and fractures, pulmonary and cutaneous infections, mucocutaneous candidiasis	T cells, phagocytes	Hyperimmunoglobulin E and recurrent infections (Job's syndrome)
Calmette-Guérin bacillus, nontuberculous mycobacteria, *Salmonella*	Disseminated infections	Monocytes	Interferon-γ receptor defects, IL-12 receptor defects, IL-12 p40 defects

sine triphosphate and deoxyguanosine triphosphate, respectively.[6, 9] The occurrence of *P. carinii* pneumonia, disseminated Calmette-Guérin bacillus infection after vaccination, persistent poliovirus infection after oral polio vaccination, or persistent respiratory virus infection should initiate consideration of a defect in lymphocyte function.[4] Graft-versus-host disease, either acquired from in utero transfer of maternal lymphocytes or through transfusion of unirradiated blood, may be the underlying cause of cutaneous eruptions, transaminase elevations, or malabsorption and diarrhea and is a strong indicator of defective T-cell immunity.[4]

In many forms of T-cell abnormality, B-cell function is also compromised, and both cell-mediated and humoral deficiencies occur, a state referred to as severe combined immunodeficiency.[4] This syndrome tends to be recognized after maternal antibody levels wane and recurrent bacterial infections begin. The finding of low immunoglobulin levels in association with marked lymphopenia in the appropriate setting should lead to the consideration of severe combined immunodeficiency.[2]

The most direct and simplest assessment of T-cell immune status is the determination of lymphocyte number, which is obtained in the screening differential count. Circulating lymphocyte numbers range from about 7000 cells/μl in infants to 4000 cells/μl in children and about 2000 cells/μl in adolescents and adults through old age.[64] Of these lymphocytes, roughly half are T cells, with the remainder split between B cells and natural killer cells. Severe quantitative abnormalities of lymphocytes are relatively uncommon; low absolute lymphocyte numbers are encountered in the great majority of cases of severe combined immunodeficiency, as well as in several other congenital immunodeficiencies (see Table 10–2). Acquired immunodeficiency syndrome (AIDS), high plasma corticosteroid levels (iatrogenic or endogenous), obstructed lymphatic circulation (e.g., intestinal lymphangiectasia), severe systemic illness (e.g., carcinomatosis, miliary tuberculosis), systemic lupus erythematosus, sarcoid, cytotoxic or immunosuppressive therapy, and severe right-sided congestive heart failure can also cause lymphocytopenia.

T-lymphocyte function is initially and most easily assayed in vivo by testing of type IV cell-mediated immunity, or delayed-type hypersensitivity (DTH) (Table 10–4). DTH is elicited by the intradermal injection of an antigen to which the patient has been exposed. Antigen-specific CD4$^+$ T cells are recruited; in turn, these T cells recruit macrophages with resulting interstitial fibrin deposition and induration. Erythema and edema are seen early after the injection but are not indicative of DTH. Frank induration is best appreciated between 24 and 48 hours and then gradually falls off. Effective DTH is indicated by induration. In the screening evaluation for immune defects it is important to consider the patient's antigenic experience, such as immunizations, previous infections, and regional exposure in the selection of antigens. It is critical to test several different antigens simultaneously for the determination of T-cell responsiveness, such as mumps, *Candida*, *Trichophyton*, streptococcal antigens, and tetanus. The demonstration of intact DTH confirms the presence of functional CD4$^+$ T cells and excludes most of the congenital defects in cell-mediated immunity. Importantly, DTH can be preserved until relatively late into human immunodeficiency virus (HIV) infection. Therefore, the presence of DTH should not be considered evidence against HIV infection per se. Selective anergy to the antigens of the offending organism has been observed in active visceral leishmaniasis and lepromatous leprosy. These specific defects have reversed after successful treatment of the underlying infection.[65] Complete anergy to a battery of antigens is a relatively nonspecific finding in terms of etiology insofar as the differential diagnosis includes all the entities that cause lymphopenia. However, anergy makes further evaluation of the cell-mediated immune system reasonable.

Fluorescence-activated cell sorting (FACS) analysis now allows rapid enumeration and characterization of lymphocyte, monocyte, and neutrophil subsets.[66] Access to FACS analysis is widely available. Lymphocyte subset determination, specifically for CD4$^+$ T cells, is standard in the management of HIV infection to provide guideposts for initiation of antiviral and prophylactic therapy. With the recent identification and cloning of certain immunodeficiency-related genes, FACS is able to confirm or exclude specific diagnoses.

Evaluation of T-cell function in vitro requires laboratory personnel skilled in the isolation, preparation, and stimulation of peripheral blood mononuclear cells. Stimulation is typically done on unseparated peripheral blood mononuclear cells and therefore represents the product of both lymphocyte and monocyte contributions. Proliferation is usually measured as ^{3}H-thymidine incorporation into the DNA of dividing lymphocytes after stimulation with cell membrane binding lectins (phytohemagglutinin, concanavalin A, pokeweed mitogen), direct stimulants of cellular signaling pathways that bypass the need for membrane components (phorbol myristate acetate and calcium ionophore), antigens (purified protein derivative, *Candida*, tetanus), cytokines (interleukin-2 [IL-2]), or allogeneic cells (mixed lymphocyte reaction).[66] Significantly low proliferation in vitro can result from absent cell surface receptors such as the CD3 complex,[67] antigen-specific anergy as in leishmaniasis,[65] IL-2 deficiencies,[13–15] or major histocompatibility complex abnormalities.[11] Two important CD4$^+$ T-cell subsets are distinguished. Th1 cells produce interferon-γ and IL-2 and are the predominant cells in the DTH response. Th2 cells produce IL-4, IL-5, and IL-10 and can regulate the differentiation of B cells and eosinophils. Both of these cell types regulate each other and therefore open new areas for the likely discovery of immune defects and new therapeutic manipulations of their relationship.[68] Cytokine levels in the supernatants of stimulated and unstimulated cells can be readily determined and may demonstrate states of either deficiency[13–15] or excess.

DiGeorge syndrome is caused by anomalous development of the third and fourth pharyngeal pouches with agenesis of the thymus and parathyroids and subsequent immunodeficiency and hypocalcemia. Neonatal tetany is an expected manifestation.[18] The defect in DiGeorge syndrome is due to interstitial deletions in chromosome 21, but specific genes have not yet been identified. Ataxia-telangiectasia is associated with low IgA and low CD3$^+$ and CD4$^+$ T-cell levels,

TABLE 10–2 Congenital Immunodeficiencies

Clinical Disease	Affected Gene Product*	Chromosomal Location	Inheritance	Functional Defect	Important Findings
T cells					
SCID[4]					
X-linked SCID[5]	Interleukin-2 receptor α-chain	Xq13-21.1	X	T-cell proliferation, antibody production	Lymphopenia, hypogammaglobulinemia
Adenosine deaminase deficiency[6–8]	Adenosine deaminase	20q13-ter	AR	T-cell functions, antibody production	Absent adenosine deaminase activity, lymphopenia, hypogammaglobulinemia
Purine nucleoside phosphorylase deficiency[7, 9, 10]	Purine nucleoside phosphorylase	14q13.1	AR	T-cell functions	Absent purine nucleoside phosphorylase activity, low CD3$^+$ cells, increased natural killer cells, low uric acid
Defective MHC molecules[11, 12]	RF-X	19q13	AR	Cell-mediated immunity	B cells normal, Ig normal or low, absent MHC molecules
IL-2 deficiency[13–15]	Nuclear factor–activated T cells	?	AR	Cell-mediated immunity, antibody production	Lymphopenia, hypogammaglobulinemia
Reticular dysgenesis[16, 17]	?	?	AR	Pancytopenia	Pancytopenia
DiGeorge syndrome[18, 18a]	ufd1?	22q11.21–q11.23	AD	Anomalous development of the 3rd and 4th pharyngeal pouches	Thymic aplasia, parathyroid aplasia, cardiac anomalies, abnormal facies
Ataxia-telangiectasia[19–21]	?	11q22.3	AR	DNA repair, T cells	Low IgA, low CD3$^+$ and CD4$^+$ cells
Wiskott-Aldrich syndrome[22–24]	WASP	Xq11-11.3	X	T cells and platelets	Thrombocytopenia, low IgM, high IgA
B cells					
X-linked agammaglobulinemia[25, 26]	B-cell progenitor kinase	Xq22	X	B cells	Very low antibody levels
X-linked immunodeficiency with hyper-IgM syndrome[27, 28]	CD40 ligand (gp39)	Xq26	X	B cells	High IgM, low IgG, IgA
X-linked lymphoproliferative syndrome (Duncan's syndrome)[29–31]	SLAM	Xq25	X	Epstein-Barr virus response	Low antibody to Epstein-Barr nuclear antigen
Common variable immunodeficiency[32]	?	?	?	Antibody synthesis	Low IgG, poor antibody response, low IgA common
IgA deficiency[32]	IgA	?6p21.3	AR	IgA	Associated with other immunodeficiencies
Phagocytes					
CGD					
X-linked CGD[33–36]	gp91^{phox}	Xp21.1	X	Bacterial and fungal killing defective in all forms of CGD	Infections with catalase-positive microbes, granulomas, and absent NBT reduction and superoxide generation in 60% of CGD
Autosomal recessive CGD[37–40]	p22^{phox}	16q24	AR		5% of CGD
	p47^{phox}	77q11.23	AR		30% of CGD
	p67^{phox}	1q25	AR		5% of CGD
Cyclic neutropenia[41]	?G-CSF	?5q	AR	Neutropenia	Cyclic hematopoiesis, cycle about 21 d
Chédiak-Higashi syndrome[42–44]	*Lyst*, lysosomal transport protein	1q43	AR	Chemotactic defect, neutropenia	Giant granules in neutrophils, oculocutaneous albinism
Leukocyte adhesion deficiency type 1[45–47]	CD18	21q22.3	AR	Absent integrins	Chronic leukocytosis, delayed umbilical cord separation, recurrent infections
Leukocyte adhesion deficiency type 2[48]	Sialyl-Lewis X	?19q	AR	E-selectin ligand, ?fucose metabolism	Short stature, mental retardation
Neutrophil-specific granule deficiency[49–51a]	C/EBPϵ	14q11.2	AR	Neutrophil granule products	Absent neutrophil-specific granules, absent defensins
Myeloperoxidase deficiency[52]	Myeloperoxidase	17q21-q23	AR	Conversion of superoxide to hydrogen peroxide	Absent myeloperoxidase, usually unassociated with infections
Interferon-γ receptor 1 deficiency[53–55]	IFN γR1	6q23-q24	AR, AD	Absence of interferon-γ binding	Recurrent nontuberculous mycobacterial and salmonella infections
Interferon-γ receptor 2 deficiency[56]	IFN γR2	21q22.1-q22.2	AR	Absence of interferon-γ signaling	Recurrent nontuberculous mycobacterial and salmonella infections
Interleukin-12 receptor β1 deficiency[57, 58]	IL-12RB1	19p13.1	AR	Absence of IL-12 signaling	Recurrent nontuberculous mycobacterial and salmonella infections
Hyper-IgE and recurrent infection syndrome (Job's syndrome)[59–62]	?	4q	AD	Intermittently poor chemotaxis, ?CD8$^+$ T-cell dysfunction	Extremely high IgE, eczema; facial, dental, and bony abnormalities; pneumatocele formation
Interleukin-12 p40 deficiency	IL-12 p40	5q31–q33	AR	Absence of IL-12	Recurrent nontuberculous mycobacterial and *Salmonella* infections

TABLE 10–2 Congenital Immunodeficiencies *Continued*

Clinical Disease	Affected Gene Product*	Chromosomal Location	Inheritance	Functional Defect	Important Findings
Complement					
Classic pathway					
		1p			
		12p13			
C1q deficiency[1]	C1q	12p13	AR		
C1r deficiency	C1r	6p21.3	AR		
C1s deficiency	C1s	19p13.2-p	AR		
C2 deficiency	C2	13.11	AR		Low CH_{50} is seen with all forms of classic complement component deficiency. Individual components are very low or absent. Autoimmune disease common in early component deficiencies (C1–C4). Bacteremia and meningitis are common in all types of complement deficiency
C3 deficiency	C3	6p21.3	AR		
C4A deficiency	C4A	6p21.3	AR		
C4B deficiency	C4B	9q22-q34	AR		
C5 deficiency	C5	5	AR		
C6 deficiency	C6	1p22	AR	Antibody-dependent complement lysis is depressed in all forms of classic complement component deficiencies	
C7 deficiency	C7	1p36.2-p2	AR		
C8 deficiency	C8	2.1	AR		
C9 deficiency	C9	5p14-p12	AR		
Alternative pathway				Antibody-independent complement lysis is depressed in alternative complement component deficiencies	More severe susceptibility to infection than with classic component deficiencies
Properdin deficiency	Properdin	Xp21-p11	X		
Factor H deficiency	Factor H	1q32	AR		
Factor I deficiency	Factor I	4q25	AR		

*The affected gene product is not always the gene in which the lesion has occurred. The genetic lesion may disable a regulatory gene required for expression or function of the affected gene product.
Abbreviations: AD, Autosomal dominant; AR, autosomal recessive; CGD, chronic granulomatous disease; CH_{50}, total hemolytic complement; G-CSF, granulocyte colony-stimulating factor; MHC, major histocompatibility complex; NBT, nitroblue tetrazolium; SCID, severe combined immunodeficiency; WASP, Wiskott-Aldrich syndrome protein; X, X-linked inheritance.

progressive ataxia, and oculocutaneous telangiectases. These patients usually experience recurrent bacterial respiratory infections and are at increased risk of malignancy because of abnormalities in DNA repair.[2, 19] Wiskott-Aldrich syndrome is characterized by eczema, thrombocytopenia, and recurrent opportunistic infections.[22] Recently, the gene product defective in Wiskott-Aldrich syndrome was identified as Wiskott-Aldrich syndrome protein *(WASP)*.[23, 24]

B Cells and Humoral Immunity

Almost 50 years have elapsed since the first description of an immunodeficiency syndrome, X-linked agammaglobulinemia, by Colonel Bruton.[69] The clinical features of immunoglobulin defects are distinct from those of T-cell or combined defects. The age of onset for congenital deficiencies is between 6 months and 2 years, and the initial infections are predominantly with encapsulated bacteria. The thymus gland is present and apparently normal in X-linked agammaglobulinemia, but peripheral lymphoid tissues such as tonsils and lymph nodes are essentially absent.[70] B cells and plasma cells in the circulation and the periphery are rare despite normal numbers of pre-B cells in the bone marrow. These patients have elevated T-cell numbers, normal T-cell subsets, and intact T-cell functions. Although they have significant problems with bacterial infections, patients with X-linked agammaglobulinemia also have severe difficulty with persistent, disseminated echovirus infections, especially in the central nervous system. Immunoglobulin G, A, and M levels are extremely low, as are those of isohemagglutinins. No antibody to either new or previously administered antigens is detectable. In contrast, patients with hyperimmunoglobulin M, an X-linked immunodeficiency caused by a deficiency of CD40 ligand (CD40L or CD154), may have preserved lymphoid tissue mass, hepatosplenomegaly, normal

TABLE 10–3 Screening Evaluations for Immune Defects

- History
  - Medications and treatments
  - Relatedness of parents, umbilical stump separation, age of onset, dental history
  - Frequency, severity, distribution, type of infections
  - Vaccination history, especially live vaccines
  - Causative infectious agents
- Physical examination
  - Weight and height
  - Hair: sheen, pigmentation
  - Abdomen: organomegaly
  - Skin: dystrophic scars, telangiectases, eczema
  - Oropharynx: thrush, ulcers, gingivitis, secondary tooth eruption
  - Facies: hypertelorism, eye slant, shortened philtrum
  - Skeleton: kyphoscoliosis, fractures
- Routine laboratory tests
  - Complete blood count
    - Differential: lymphopenia, neutropenia, eosinophilia
    - Peripheral smear: giant granules, specific (secondary) granules
    - Platelet count: thrombocytopenia
    - Erythrocyte sedimentation rate: usually elevated in infection
  - Chemistries
    - Serum calcium
    - Serum uric acid
    - Liver function tests
  - Immunoglobulins
    - IgA, IgM, IgG, IgE
    - Isohemagglutinins
    - Antibody titers (tetanus, pneumococcus, etc.)
  - Complement
    - Total hemolytic complement (CH_{50})
- Radiographs
  - Plain chest films: kyphoscoliosis, pneumatoceles, scarring

TABLE 10–4 Directed Tests of Immune Function

- T cells
  - Fluorescence-activated cell sorting
  - Delayed-type hypersensitivity: mumps, *Candida*, tetanus, *Trichophyton*
  - Lymphocyte enzymes (adenosine deaminase and purine nucleoside phosphorylase)
  - Cytokine production and response
  - In vitro proliferation: stimulation with antigen, lectin, antibody, allogeneic cells, phosphokinase C stimulants, and calcium ionophores
- B cells
  - Fluorescence-activated cell sorting
  - Antigen challenge, recall or new
  - In vitro antibody production
- Phagocytes
  - Fluorescence activated cell sorting
  - Nitroblue tetrazolium reduction, dihydrorhodamine oxidation
  - Superoxide generation, hydrogen peroxide generation
  - Adherence
  - Staphylococcicidal activity
  - Chemotaxis
  - Phagocytosis
- Complement
  - Assay of individual complement components, functional or quantitative

numbers of B cells and T cells, and variable neutropenia. Autoimmune phenomena such as Coombs-positive hemolytic anemia and thrombocytopenia are common. IgM is often elevated, and IgG and IgA are usually quite low; isohemagglutinins may be elevated.[70] The X-linked lymphoproliferative disorder Duncan's syndrome occurs in males only after infection with Epstein-Barr virus and results in a full-blown immunodeficiency syndrome that can be fatal.[29] The gene has recently been cloned and identified as *SLAM*, a critical T-cell signaling molecule.[71]

The initial test for the integrity of the humoral arm of immunity is a determination of levels of isohemagglutinins (see later) and levels of IgG, IgA, and IgM. Normal immunoglobulin levels are relatively low in infancy and childhood and increase with age. If immunoglobulin levels are appropriate, X-linked agammaglobulinemia can be excluded. Low immunoglobulin levels may be seen in the first year of life in the transient hypogammaglobulinemia of infancy.[2, 70] However, these infants usually have detectable isohemagglutinins and can mount antibody responses to new antigenic challenges. Despite family histories notable for relatives with immunodeficiencies, patients with transient hypogammaglobulinemia of infancy tend to normalize their immunoglobulin levels over the first 2 years of life. The finding of depressed levels of immunoglobulin, especially in an adult with recurrent bacterial sinopulmonary infections, raises the possibility of common variable immunodeficiency.[32] Common variable immunodeficiency is a heterogeneous group of diseases that share the features of hypogammaglobulinemia and an increased susceptibility to chronic enteric infections with *Giardia lamblia, Campylobacter,* and disseminated echovirus infections, in addition to sinopulmonary bacterial infections. Patients with common variable immunodeficiency often have low isohemagglutinin levels and abnormal DTH and fail to make antibody to new antigens. IgG subclass analysis may show selective defects in IgG_1 and IgG_3 or IgG_2 and IgG_4, in addition to defects in IgA.[32]

Isohemagglutinins are IgM antibodies directed against blood group A and B antigens, which occur in all healthy people except those with blood group AB. By the age of 3 years, 98% of patients with blood groups A, B, or O have isohemagglutinins with a titer of at least 1:16.[32] Isohemagglutinin levels are determined in blood banks as a prerequisite to transfusion. Challenge with antigen is probably the simplest and most effective method for determining the functional integrity of the humoral immune system. Use of a recall antigen allows for testing of anamnestic responses. Novel antigens such as bacteriophage ΦX174 or keyhole limpet hemocyanin make possible the testing of antibody responses during immunoglobulin administration. Pneumococcal vaccination examines the response to polysaccharide antigen, whereas tetanus challenge is more specific for peptide responses. Serum titers should be checked before and 2 weeks after immunization.

PHAGOCYTE IMMUNE DEFECTS: NEUTROPHILS

The clinical findings of patients with neutrophil disorders often share common features: gingivitis, periodontal disease, and oral ulceration.[63] Cutaneous infections with *Staphylococcus aureus* are recurrent and can be severe. In neutrophil disorders characterized by inadequate inflammation (neutropenia, LAD, Chédiak-Higashi syndrome, neutrophil-specific granule deficiency), infections can extend locally and subcutaneously with little reaction until marked destruction has taken place. Visceral and especially sinopulmonary involvement is a feature that helps distinguish neutrophil defects from other syndromes in the differential diagnosis. Hepatic abscess is a frequent manifestation of CGD and is most often due to *S. aureus,* an organism rarely encountered at that anatomic site in patients with normal neutrophils.

Neutropenia

A neutrophil count below 500 cells/μl carries a profound risk of bacterial and fungal infection.[72] Although this principle was first extensively documented and is still most frequently displayed in cancer and leukemia patients undergoing combination chemotherapy, its importance has been confirmed in patients with genetic disorders that affect neutrophil number. Cyclic neutropenia or cyclic hematopoiesis is a rare disease occurring in autosomal dominant, spontaneous, and acquired forms that is characterized by regular 21-day oscillations in the levels of blood neutrophils, monocytes, eosinophils, lymphocytes, platelets, and reticulocytes.[41] The defect is at the level of the hematopoietic stem cell and is associated with abnormal colony-stimulating factor responses in bone marrow precursor cells. It is postulated that cyclic neutropenia may represent dysregulated feedback from the circulating cell pool to the marrow. Patients are usually first seen in childhood and have recurrent episodes of fever, malaise, mucosal ulcers, and occasionally, life-threatening infections associated with periods of profound neutropenia (<200/μl).[41] Adult-onset cases have been described with an associated clonal proliferation of large granular lymphocytes ($CD8^+/CD57^+$) as well. Neutrophil number is transiently impaired, but function is normal. The diagnosis is suspected in children with recurrent stomatitis, gingivitis, cutaneous infections, lymphadenopathy, and fever. The diagnosis can only be established after repeated white blood cell counts with differentials at least three times per week for at least 6 weeks. In congenital agranulocytosis (Kostmann's syndrome[73]), neutrophil counts are consistently low from birth and show no periodicity. Both syndromes are successfully treated with recombinant granulocyte colony-stimulating factor.

Chédiak-Higashi Syndrome

Chédiak-Higashi syndrome is a rare autosomal recessive disorder caused by defects in the lysosomal transport protein (*Lyst*).[43, 44] It is characterized by recurrent bacterial infections, partial oculocutaneous albinism, photophobia, nystagmus, and peripheral neuropathy.[42] Many patients die in childhood from infection. An aggressive "lymphoproliferative" phase with diffuse organ infiltration and death develops in about half of the patients who survive into adolescence. Several patients have lived into adulthood, at which time an aggressive, severe, debilitating peripheral neuropathy is a common feature.[42] Pathologically, giant abnormal granules are found in neutrophils, melanocytes, hair, Schwann cells, the central nervous system, peripheral ganglia, capillary epithelium, renal tubular epithelium, erythroid precursors, fibroblasts, and other granule-containing cells.[42] In neutrophils, the granules are formed mainly by fusion of azurophilic or primary granules to each other and to a lesser extent by fusion to specific or secondary granules.[74]

Features of Chédiak-Higashi syndrome include central and peripheral nervous system involvement with peripheral neuropathy, myopathy, autonomic dysfunction, and leptomeningeal involvement.[42] Lymphohistiocytic infiltration of axons and myelin sheaths occurs in patients with peripheral neuropathy and in ganglia in patients with autonomic neuropathy. Melanin granules seen in the neurons of the substantia nigra are large, irregular, and clumped. These aggregates of melanosomes seem to increase in size and number with age. Low intelligence has been noted in some series.[42] The diagnosis of Chédiak-Higashi syndrome is easily made by inspection of the peripheral smear for giant lysosomes or microscopic examination of hair for characteristic melanin clumps.

Leukocyte Adhesion Deficiency

Leukocyte adhesion to endothelium and other leukocytes is mediated by several sets of molecules, among which are the integrins and the selectins. It is now recognized that defects in either of these two intercellular adhesion pathways can lead to overlapping clinical phenotypes. LAD type 1 is a rare autosomal recessive disorder involving one set of the leukocyte integrins, the molecules required for leukocyte adherence to endothelium, other leukocytes, and bacteria.[45, 75]

Deficiency of the integrin component CD18 leads to a corresponding deficiency of the complexes LFA-1, Mac-1, and p150,95 and resulting abnormalities of cellular adhesion. These abnormalities are predictable from the basic defect. The absence of a marginated pool of neutrophils leads to chronic leukocytosis, whereas the poor inflammatory response leads to recurrent infections.

LAD-1 falls into two broad categories, severe and moderate, depending on the degree of CD18 deficiency.[45] Patients with severe deficiency (<0.5%) of normal protein expression are characterized by delayed umbilical stump separation, umbilical stump infection, persistent leukocytosis in the absence of active infection (>15,000/μl), and severe destructive periodontitis with associated loss of dentition and alveolar bone. Recurrent infections of the skin, upper and lower airways, bowel, and perirectal area and septicemia are common and usually due to *S. aureus* or gram-negative rods, most notably *Pseudomonas* spp. Infections tend to be necrotizing and may progress to ulceration but demonstrate an almost complete absence of neutrophil invasion on histopathologic analysis. Patients with a moderate form of the disease (3 to 30% of normal expression) tend to have normal umbilical stump separation, have LAD diagnosed later in life, and less commonly have life-threatening infections. Leukocytosis is still the rule, as is delayed wound healing and periodontal disease. Although patients with a moderate form of the disease are less ill and tend to live past childhood, deaths from infection have been reported in young adults.[45]

Laboratory findings in general reflect the clinical differences between severe and moderate phenotypes of the disease, with the severe form showing more profound deficiencies than the moderate form. Abnormalities include grossly defective granulocyte and mononuclear cell mobilization into Rebuck skin windows in vivo and diminished neutrophil migration in response to the bacterial chemoattractant f-Met-Leu-Phe in vitro despite normal numbers of receptors.[45] These laboratory abnormalities are demonstrated in vivo in histologic sections of infected tissues, which show the presence of some mononuclear cells but very low numbers of neutrophils. Patient granulocyte adherence to glass, plastic, nylon wool, and other LAD granulocytes is greatly reduced and not stimulated by exposure to f-Met-Leu-Phe or phorbol myristate acetate. The absence of CD18 leads to the absence of Mac-1 and the iC3b receptor CR3. Therefore, complement-mediated phagocytosis is severely impaired whereas IgG-mediated phagocytosis is normal. Although viral infections are not usually special problems in LAD, antibody-dependent cellular cytotoxicity by patient cells is also diminished. Oxidative metabolism in response to phorbol myristate acetate or calcium ionophore is normal in patient granulocytes as measured by nitroblue tetrazolium reduction or chemiluminescence. Neutrophil primary and secondary granule release in response to phorbol myristate acetate or chemoattractants is normal in LAD cells, whereas the response after zymosan particle ingestion is depressed.

The diagnosis is established by eliciting a thorough history, with special attention directed to evidence of depressed inflammation in the neonatal period, delayed umbilical stump separation, and recurrent infections. A dental history is helpful inasmuch as most of these patients have severe problems with gingivitis, periodontal disease, tooth loss, and alveolar bone erosion. Wounds often heal abnormally, with dystrophic, paper-thin scars remaining. The diagnosis is confirmed by FACS, which shows reduction or absence of the components of the leukocyte adhesion molecules CD18, CD11a, CD11b, and CD11c.

In LAD-2, neutrophil adherence to endothelial cells is defective because of absence of the sialyl-Lewis X antigen on the neutrophil surface, which is the binding site for E-selectin.[48, 76, 77] The patients reported are the products of consanguineous marriages. They have had neutrophilia, recurrent pulmonary, periodontal, and cutaneous infections, abnormal chemotaxis, mental retardation, short stature, distinctive facies, and the Bombay (hh) blood phenotype. The underlying defect is probably autosomal recessive and appears to involve fucose metabolism.[48]

Neutrophil-Specific Granule Deficiency

Neutrophil-specific (secondary) granule deficiency is a rare (five cases reported), heterogeneous disease characterized by a profound reduction or absence of neutrophil-specific granules and their contents.[49] Associated abnormalities in the few patients reported include bilobed or trilobed neutrophil nuclei, absence of some neutrophil primary (azurophil) granule proteins, mononuclear eosinophils without eosinophil granules, and dysfunction of platelet α-granules. The neutrophil-specific granule protein lactoferrin has been shown to be diminished or absent in these patients' neutrophils, and the defective production of lactoferrin is relatively tissue specific, with normal production by lacrimal glands but no production in neutrophils or eosinophils.[49, 50, 78] Sibling deaths at early ages, consanguineous marriages in the parents of patients, and occurrence of the syndrome in females lead to the assumption of an autosomal recessive pattern of inheritance for neutrophil-specific granule deficiency. The development of a mouse model that displays clinical features of neutrophil-specific granule deficiency by deletion of the gene *C/EBPε*, a regulator of myeloid development, focused attention on this regulatory gene family in this disease.[51] One case of specific granule deficiency due to human mutation of c/EBPε has been confirmed.

Myeloperoxidase Deficiency

Myeloperoxidase (MPO; also called *verdoperoxidase*), the heme binding protein that makes pus green, catalyzes the conversion of hydrogen peroxide to hypochlorous acid (bleach). MPO deficiency, the most common neutrophil disorder, affects about 1 in 2000 persons but is quite silent in most cases. Neutrophil function is affected by MPO deficiency in a variety of ways. The respiratory burst in MPO-deficient neutrophils is prolonged, and as a result, exaggerated amounts of hydrogen peroxide are produced.[52] The increased hydrogen peroxide production probably compensates functionally for the defect in hypochlorous acid production. Phagocytosis is normal to increased in MPO-deficient neutrophils, whereas bactericidal activity is somewhat slower than normal. Killing of *Aspergillus* conidia by MPO-deficient neutrophils is retarded, whereas the combination of MPO-deficient neutrophils with CGD neutrophils (see the next section), which are unable to generate hydrogen peroxide but do produce MPO, results in normal killing of *Aspergillus* conidia.[79] Pathologic sequelae of MPO deficiency are only brought out in the presence of other impairments of host defense such as diabetes mellitus. A very few MPO-deficient diabetic patients have had severe yeast infections.

Chronic Granulomatous Disease

CGD is a genetically heterogeneous group of disorders of phagocytic cell oxidative metabolism characterized by recurrent life-threatening infections with bacteria and fungi and dysregulated granuloma formation.[33] The estimated frequency is 1 in 250,000 persons. CGD is caused by a defect in reduced nicotinamide-adenine dinucleotide phosphate oxidase, which is responsible for the respiratory burst and the generation of hydrogen peroxide. Clinically, CGD is quite variable; the time of onset occurs from infancy to late adulthood, with CGD diagnosed in most patients while toddlers and young children. However, CGD is diagnosed in a significant number of patients later in life.[33, 80] Children with CGD tend to be short and small for their age but eventually achieve the height predicted by their parents' height.[81]

Pulmonary, cutaneous, lymphatic, and hepatic infections are frequent. Osteomyelitis, perianal abscess, and gingivitis are also common.[80] The microbiology of infections associated with CGD is remarkable for its relative specificity: *S. aureus*, *B. cepacia*, *Serratia marcescens*, *Nocardia* spp., and *Aspergillus* spp. account for the overwhelming majority of infections. As in other neutrophil abnormalities, the most common offender in CGD is *S. aureus*. Whereas the typical case of liver abscess in an immunologically normal patient involves enteric organisms and is liquid and easily drainable, the liver abscesses encountered in patients with CGD are dense, caseous, and staphylococcal. In the absence of antibiotic prophylaxis, lung, skin, and bone infections are usually staphylococcal. However, *Aspergillus* spp. and some of the rarer fungi such as *Exophiala dermatitidis*[82] and *Paecilomyces* spp.[83] are encountered in CGD. Infections with *Nocardia* spp., *Chromobacterium violaceum, S. marcescens,* and *B. cepacia* are seen frequently in patients with CGD and should suggest the diagnosis.[3, 80, 84] Bony involvement can occur by direct extension in the case of *Aspergillus* or hematogeneously as in the case of *Staphylococcus* and *Nocardia*.[85] Infection with *Aspergillus nidulans* is especially aggressive and requires more intensive therapy than do infections with *Aspergillus fumigatus*.[86] The advent of antibiotic prophylaxis has altered the frequency of infections in CGD and reduced the frequency of staphylococcal infections in particular.[3, 81] The rate of fungal infections in CGD is lower than that for bacterial infections and has apparently not changed in the setting of prophylactic antibiotics.[87]

The granulomas that occur in CGD are presumed to originate from an inflammatory response to infectious or irritative foci (e.g., sutures) that fails to eradicate the infection or irritation. This persistent inflammatory reaction leads to exuberant and often obstructive granulomatous lesions. The gastrointestinal and genitourinary tracts are frequently involved by granulomatous lesions in CGD, sometimes as the site of the initial complaint, sometimes asymptomatically. Ament and Ochs[88] noted frequent malabsorption, intrinsic factor–unresponsive vitamin B_{12} deficiency, abundant lipid-pigmented histiocytes in small bowel biopsy specimens, and pigmented histiocytes and granulomas in rectal biopsy material. These findings were present in both autosomal and X-linked patients. Esophageal, jejunal, ileal, cecal, rectal, and perirectal involvement with granulomas, often mimicking Crohn's disease, has been described. Gastric outlet obstruction is an especially common manifestation and may be the initial feature of CGD. In a comprehensive review of genitourinary manifestations, Walther and colleagues[89] found that 38% of patients with CGD had some kind of urologic event, including bladder granulomas, ureteral obstruction, and urinary tract infection.

The diagnosis of CGD is made by assay of superoxide or hydrogen peroxide production, such as nitroblue tetrazolium reduction, chemiluminescence, or dihydrorhodamine oxidation. Mothers of boys with the X-linked form of CGD are obligate carriers of a defective X chromosome. Therefore, by lyonization, a certain proportion of the mother's cells will fail to reduce nitroblue tetrazolium and thus give a characteristic mosaic pattern. By performing a nitroblue tetrazolium or dihydrorhodamine test on the mother's blood, one can determine the broad lines of inheritance of CGD in a given male.

An important adjunct to therapy is interferon-γ, a cytokine with neutrophil and monocyte-macrophage stimulating properties that has reduced the frequency and severity of infections in patients with CGD.[90] Although granulocyte transfusions supply only a small portion of the body's normal neutrophil output in a day, we believe that they may be effective in helping to clear severe infections. Transfused granulocytes produce superoxide, which can be used by the intact MPO system in CGD neutrophils and thereby bypass the biochemical defect.[91] The granulomatous complications of CGD pose a special problem in management. Although these patients are already somewhat immunocompromised, the judicious use of corticosteroids in conjunction with antibiotics has been successful in opening and maintaining the patency of hollow visci in patients with CGD.[92]

PHAGOCYTE AND LYMPHOCYTE DEFECTS AFFECTING MONONUCLEAR CELLS

Although tuberculosis is highly virulent in humans and infects more than one third of the globe's population, infections with nontuberculous mycobacteria are much less common, and when these infections are disseminated, they bespeak substantial immunocompromise. If HIV infection and iatrogenic causes are excluded, one is left with patients with intrinsic immune defects, some of which have recently been characterized at a genetic level.

Interferon-γ is an absolutely critical cytokine in the control of mycobacteria.[93] It is produced by lymphocytes and acts through its cognate receptor on monocyte-macrophages to facilitate the killing of intracellular parasites such as mycobacteria. Therefore, it is expected and observed that severe, disseminated infections with nontuberculous mycobacteria such as *Mycobacterium avium* complex develop in humans with defects in either the ligand binding (interferon-γ receptor 1) or the signal transducing (interferon-γ receptor 2) chains of the interferon-γ receptor.[53–56] These infections often have their onset in childhood, and if Calmette-Guérin bacillus is given to these infants, it often disseminates. These patients characteristically fail to form granulomas and have very high mortality from their *M. avium* complex infections. They are also susceptible to recurrent disseminated infections with the intracellular pathogen *Salmonella*. One kindred has been identified in which a partial defect in interferon-γ receptor 1 resulted in an intermediate phenotype in which the children had severe mycobacterial infections but were able to be cured with standard antibiotics and retained the ability to form granulomas.[94] The diagnosis of complete interferon-γ receptor 1 deficiency is most easily accomplished by examination of the cell surface for interferon-γ receptor 1 expression by flow cytometry. However, demonstration of protein-positive interferon-γ receptor 1 deficiency or interferon-γ receptor 2 deficiency must still be performed by functional and molecular assays.

IL-12 is a monocyte-macrophage product that acts on lymphocytes to drive the production of interferon-γ. As expected, in the absence of IL-12 signal transduction as a result of defects in the IL-12 receptor or the absence of IL-12p40, disseminated infections with nontuberculous mycobacteria and *Salmonella* occur.[57, 58] However, because patients with IL-12 receptor defects have some residual interferon-γ production, granuloma formation is preserved and these patients tend to be less severely affected than those with complete interferon-γ receptor defects. Treatment of IL-12 receptor–deficient patients with disseminated mycobacterial infections can be greatly aided by the use of interferon-γ. The diagnosis of IL-12 receptor deficiency currently requires functional or molecular assays.

Hyperimmunoglobulin E–Recurrent Infection Syndrome (Job's Syndrome)

Job's syndrome is a rare disorder characterized by recurrent infections, typically of the lower respiratory system and skin, eczema, extremely elevated levels of IgE, and eosinophilia. Most patients have facial abnormalities, including ocular hypertelorism, a prominent, protruding, triangular mandible, and a broad, somewhat bulbous nose.[59–62] Failure of primary teeth to exfoliate is common and results in a frequent need for dental extractions to allow eruption of normal secondary teeth.[60] Moderate scoliosis develops in most patients. Many also have abnormalities of bone formation and metabolism, which may result in fractures.[95, 96] Craniosynostosis has been reported in several patients.[60–62] Job's syndrome appears to occur spontaneously in all racial and ethnic groups and seems to be transmitted as an autosomal dominant trait with variable penetrance.[59, 60]

Patients are usually noted within the first days to months of life to have severe eczema, mucocutaneous candidiasis, and cutaneous, sinus, or pulmonary infections predominantly with *S. aureus* or *Haemophilus influenzae*. Pneumatoceles are often noted by adolescence, and these in turn provide a hospitable site for subsequent infections with *Aspergillus* and *P. aeruginosa*. Otitis media and externa are relatively common, as are intertriginous infections and breast abscesses. Infections occur less frequently in bones and joints and very infrequently in the liver, kidneys, and gastrointestinal tract. Documented sepsis is rare. Deep tissue infections are frequently extensions of paronychia or apical abscesses. Recurrent "cold" abscesses of the skin are commonly due to staphylococci. The lack of robust inflammation is a manifestation of the impaired inflammatory response in these patients insofar as substantial infection may elicit only modest reaction and is often unassociated with a sense of illness on the part of the patient. Pathogens that have been recovered from patients with Job's syndrome include *S. aureus, H. influenzae, Aspergillus* spp., *P. aeruginosa, Streptococcus pneumoniae,* group A streptococci, *Cryptococcus neoformans,* and *Candida albicans.*[59–62]

The syndrome is defined by marked elevations of IgE (>2000 IU/ml), with levels of more than 50,000 IU/ml reported.[59–61] Levels may start out elevated in cord blood and then climb through infancy and childhood.[97] In addition, levels may decline into the normal range over time.[60] Therefore, although a high IgE level is part of the diagnostic criteria for Job's syndrome, authentic cases do at times lack this particular feature. Catabolism of IgE is abnormally reduced in both Job's syndrome and atopic dermatitis, thus further contributing to the elevated levels of IgE seen in these syndromes.[98] A high proportion of the IgE in Job's syndrome binds to *S. aureus* and *C. albicans.*[99] That this finding is specific was shown by the absence of binding to *Escherichia coli* and *S. pneumoniae.* The lack of similar binding activity in other patients frequently infected with *S. aureus* indicates that this abnormality is host, and not organism driven. The presence of elevated anti–*S. aureus* IgE is specific for Job's syndrome and has helped in the discrimination of this syndrome from severe atopic dermatitis with high IgE levels.[99] White blood cell counts are typically normal but have been reported to range from 1700 to 60,000/μl.[59–61] Chronic leukopenia with borderline neutropenia has been observed in several patients.[61] Mild to moderate eosinophilia is the rule, although exceptions do occur.[60] No correlation between IgE levels and the degree of eosinophilia or clinical disease has been made.[60, 61] Chemotaxis is abnormal in this syndrome, at least some of the time in most of the patients.[61] However, until the disease gene is found and its functions clearly defined, clinical criteria are the basis for making the diagnosis of hyperimmunoglobulin E–recurrent infection syndrome: extremely elevated IgE, eczema, and recurrent sinopulmonary infections. The added findings of failure of primary dental exfoliation, recurrent skin abscesses, scoliosis, characteristic facies, and a positive family history are helpful.[60]

Complement-Mediated Immunity

Deficiencies in complement components are clinically manifested as recurrent systemic bacterial infections. Bacteremia and meningitis are common in all the complement deficiencies.[1] Pneumonia is common in the early classic pathway (C1, C4, C2) and alternative pathway (factors I and H, properdin, C3) defects. Late-component defects (C5–C9) are associated with recurrent *Neisseria* bacteremia and meningitis. Surprisingly, the bacteremias associated with late-component defects occur at a much later age (average, 17 years) than does meningococcal bacteremia in the healthy population. Although these patients also have much higher rates of relapse and reinfection than healthy people do, their mortality from the infection is lower than normal. Patients with deficiencies of the early components of complement, C1, C4, C2, and C3, tend to have considerably higher rates of collagen-vascular disease such as systemic and discoid lupus erythematosus than do either healthy populations or patients with late-component defects.

Except for properdin deficiency, which is X-linked, complement deficiency states are inherited as autosomal recessive disorders. Heterozygotes have 50% of normal levels whereas homozygous defective persons tend to have very low levels, if any, of the affected component. Screening for the presence of complement deficiencies is best accomplished by use of the test for total hemolytic complement (CH_{50} assay). This test examines the integrity of the classic pathway of the complement system by determining the ability of complement in patient serum to lyse antibody-coated sheep erythrocytes in vitro. Cell lysis leads to the release of hemoglobin, which can be determined spectrophotometrically. Specific classic complement component defects can be detected by a modified CH_{50} assay that uses purified proteins and selectively omits the one to be assayed so that patient serum must supply the missing factor.[66] Direct determinations of immunologically reactive protein, including members of the alternative pathway, can be performed with enzyme-linked immunosorbent assays or diffusion assays. These types of direct assay systems do not offer functional data but can help quantify apparent functional defects.

Acquired Immune Deficiencies

The most common forms of immunodeficiency encountered are acquired after birth and are not clearly traceable to an immune genetic basis. Like other immunodeficiencies, they are best approached by a thorough history and physical examination to search for associated findings and to guide diagnostic testing. Special attention to the infecting organisms can point to underlying abnormalities in host defense. AIDS[100] is caused by HIV, which induces progressive $CD4^+$ T-cell depletion. A recently described syndrome that is manifested, like AIDS, by opportunistic infections but is unassociated with HIV infection is idiopathic $CD4^+$ lymphopenia.[101] The diagnosis is made by excluding all other known causes of immunodeficiency, including HIV, and determining that the $CD4^+$ T-cell count is 300/μl or less. Certain malignancies, particularly hematopoietic and lymphoid malignancies, result in immune dysfunction by causing a deficiency in immune effector cells or dysregulation of such activities as antibody synthesis and are associated with severe or opportunistic infections. Drug therapy can be complicated by rare or idiosyncratic reactions such as aplastic anemia with chloramphenicol or drug-induced neutropenia.[102] Iron overload and chelation therapy with deferoxamine provide a hospitable environment for certain bacteria, notably *Yersinia enterocolitica.*[103–105] Splenectomy, especially post-traumatic splenectomy, predisposes to overwhelming infection with encapsulated organisms such as *S. pneumoniae* and *Capnocytophaga canimorsus* (DF-2) and parasites such as *Babesia microti* and *Plasmodium* spp.[106] Severe thermal injury is associated with selective degranulation of neutrophil-specific granules, decreased chemotaxis, and profound susceptibility to infection.[107]

REFERENCES

1. Ross SC, Denson P. Complement deficiency states and infection: Epidemiology, pathogenesis and consequences of neisserial and other infections in an immune deficiency. Medicine (Baltimore). 1984;63:243–273.
2. Buckley RH. Immunodeficiency diseases. JAMA. 1992;268:2797–2806.
3. O'Neil KM, Herman JH, Modlin JF, et al. *Pseudomonas cepacia:* An emerging pathogen in chronic granulomatous disease. J Pediatr. 1986;108:940–942.
4. Fisher A. Severe combined immunodeficiencies. Immunodefic Rev. 1992;3:83–100.
5. Noguchi M, Yi H, Rosenblatt HM, et al. Interleukin-2 receptor gamma chain mutation results in X-linked severe combined immunodeficiency in humans. Cell. 1993;73:147–158.
6. Hirschhorn R. Adenosine deaminase deficiency. Immunodefic Rev. 1990;2: 175–198.
7. Markert ML, Hershfield MS, Schiff RI, Buckley R. Adenosine deaminase and purine nucleoside phosphorylase deficiencies: Evaluation of therapeutic interventions in eight patients. J Clin Immunol. 1987;7:389–399.
8. Parkman R, Gelfand EW, Rosen FS, et al. Severe combined immunodeficiency and adenosine deaminase deficiency. N Engl J Med. 1975;292:714–719.
9. Markert ML. Purine nucleoside phosphorylase deficiency. Immunodefic Rev. 1991;3:45–81.
10. Rich KC, Mejias E, Fox IH. Purine nucleoside phosphorylase deficiency: Improved metabolic and immunologic function with erythrocyte transfusions. N Engl J Med. 1980;303:973–977.
11. Griscelli C, Lisowska-Grospierre B, Mach B. Combined immunodeficiency with defective expression in MHC class II genes. Immunodefic Rev. 1989;1:135–153.
12. de Preval C, Lisowska-Grospierre B, Loche M, et al. A trans-acting class II regulatory gene unlinked to the MHC controls expression of HLA class II genes. Nature. 1985;318:291–293.
13. Pahwa R, Chatila T, Pahwa S, et al. Recombinant interleukin 2 therapy in severe combined immunodeficiency disease. Proc Natl Acad Sci U S A. 1989;86:5069–5073.
14. Weinberg K, Parkman R. Severe combined immunodeficiency due to a specific defect in the production of interleukin 2. N Engl J Med. 1990;322:1718–1723.
15. Chatila T, Castigli E, Pahwa R, et al. Primary combined immunodeficiency resulting from defective transcription of multiple T-cell lymphokine genes. Proc Natl Acad Sci U S A. 1990;87:10033–10037.

16. Ownby DR, Pizzo SV, Blackmon L, et al. Severe combined immunodeficiency with leukopenia (reticular dysgenesis) in siblings: Immunologic and histopathologic findings. J Pediatr. 1976;89:382–387.
17. Roper M, Parmley RT, Crist WM, et al. Severe congenital leukopenia (reticular dysgenesis): Immunologic and morphologic characterizations of leukocytes. Am J Dis Child. 1985;139:832–835.
18. Muller W, Peter HH, Wilken M, et al. The DiGeorge syndrome: I. Clinical evaluation and course of partial and complete forms of the syndrome. Eur J Pediatr. 1988;147:496–502.
18a. Yamagishi H, Garg V, Matsuoka R, et al. A molecular pathway revealing a genetic basis for human cardiac and craniofacial defects. Science. 1999;283:1158–1161.
19. Gatti RA, Boder E, Vinters HV, et al. Ataxia-telangiectasia: An interdisciplinary approach to pathogenesis. Medicine (Baltimore). 1991;70:99–117.
20. McFarlin DE, Strober W, Waldmann TA. Ataxia-telangiectasia. Medicine (Baltimore). 1972;51:281–314.
21. Gatti RA, Berkel I, Boder E, et al. Localization of an ataxia-telangiectasia gene to chromosome 11q22–23. Nature. 1988;336:577–580.
22. Aldrich RA, Steinberg AG, Campbell DC. Pedigree demonstrating a sex-linked recessive condition characterized by draining ears, eczematoid dermatitis, and bloody diarrhea. Pediatrics. 1954;13:133–139.
23. Derry JM, Ochs HD, Francke U. Isolation of a novel gene mutated in Wiskott-Aldrich syndrome. Cell. 1994;78:635–644.
24. Symons M, Derry JM, Karlak B, et al. Wiskott-Aldrich syndrome protein, a novel effector for the GTPase CDC42Hs, is implicated in actin polymerization. Cell. 1996;84:723–734.
25. Tsukada S, Saffran DC, Rawlings DJ, et al. Deficient expression of a B cell cytoplasmic tyrosine kinase in human X-linked agammaglobulinemia. Cell. 1993;72:279–290.
26. Vetrie D, Vorechovsky I, Sideras P, et al. The gene involved in X-linked agammaglobulinaemia is a member of the *src* family of protein-tyrosine kinases. Nature. 1993;361:226–233.
27. Allen RC, Armitage RJ, Conley ME, et al. CD40 ligand gene defects responsible for X-linked hyper-IgM syndrome. Science. 1993;259:990–993.
28. Aruffo A, Farrington M, Hollenbaugh D, et al. The CD40 ligand, gp39, is defective in activated T cells from patients with X-linked hyper-IgM syndrome. Cell. 1993;72:291–300.
29. Sullivan JL, Woda BA. X-linked lymphoproliferative syndrome. Immunodefic Rev. 1989;1:325–347.
30. Sullivan JL, Byron KS, Brewster FE, et al. X-linked lymphoproliferative syndrome: Natural history of the immunodeficiency. J Clin Invest. 1983;71:1765–1778.
31. Grierson H, Purtilo DT. Epstein-Barr virus infections in males with the X-linked lymphoproliferative syndrome. Ann Intern Med. 1987;106:538–545.
32. Sneller MC, Strober W, Eisenstein E, et al. New insights into common variable immunodeficiency. Ann Intern Med. 1993;118:720–730.
33. Gallin JI, Malech HL. Update on chronic granulomatous disease of childhood: Immunotherapy and potential for gene therapy. JAMA. 1990;263:1533–1537.
34. Royer-Pokora B, Kunkel LM, Monaco P, et al. Cloning the gene for an inherited human disorder—chronic granulomatous disease—on the basis of its chromosomal location. Nature. 1986;322:32–38.
35. Bolsher BGJM, deBoer M, de Klein A, et al. Point mutations in the B-subunit of cytochrome b558 leading to X-linked chronic granulomatous disease. Blood. 1991;77:2482–2487.
36. Shapiro BL, Newburger PE, Klempner MS, et al. Chronic granulomatous disease presenting in a 69-year-old man. N Engl J Med. 1991;325:1786–1790.
37. Dinauer MC, Pierce EA, Bruns GA, et al. Human neutrophil cytochrome b light chain (p22-phox). Gene structure, chromosomal location, and mutations in cytochrome negative autosomal recessive chronic granulomatous disease. J Clin Invest. 1990;86:1729–1737.
38. Clark RC, Malech HL, Gallin JI, et al. Genetic variants of chronic granulomatous disease: Prevalence of deficiencies of two cytosolic components of the NADPH oxidase system. N Engl J Med. 1989;321:647–652.
39. Casimir CM, Bu-Ganim HN, Rodaway ARF, et al. Autosomal recessive chronic granulomatous disease caused by deletion at a dinucleotide repeat. Proc Natl Acad Sci U S A. 1991;88:2753–2757.
40. Kenney RT, Malech HL, Leto TL. Structural characterization of the $p67^{phox}$ gene (Abstract). Clin Res. 1992;40:261.
41. Wright DG, Dale DC, Fauci AS, et al. Human cyclic neutropenia: Clinical review and long term follow up of patients. Medicine (Baltimore). 1981;60:1–13.
42. Blume RS, Wolff SM. The Chédiak-Higashi syndrome: Studies in four patients and a review of the literature. Medicine (Baltimore). 1972;51:247–280.
43. Barbosa MD, Nguyen QA, Tchernev VT, et al. Identification of the homologous beige and Chédiak-Higashi syndrome genes. Nature. 1996;382:262–265.
44. Nagle DL, Karim MA, Woolf EA, et al. Identification and mutation analysis of the complete gene for Chédiak-Higashi syndrome. Nat Genet. 1996;14:307–311.
45. Anderson DC, Schmalsteig FC, Finegold MJ, et al. The severe and moderate phenotypes of heritable Mac-1, LFA-1 deficiency: Their quantitative definition and relation to leukocyte dysfunction and clinical features. J Infect Dis. 1985;152: 668–689.
46. Kishimoto TK, Hollander N, Roberts TM, et al. Heterogeneous mutations in the β subunit common to the LFA-1, Mac-1, and P150,95 glycoproteins cause leukocyte adhesion deficiency. Cell. 1987;50:193–202.
47. Corbi AL, Larson RS, Kishimoto TK, et al. Chromosomal location of the genes encoding the leukocyte adhesion receptors LFA-1, Mac-1, and P150,95: Identification of a gene cluster involved in cell adhesion. J Exp Med. 1988;167:1597–1607.
48. Etzioni A, Frydman M, Pollack S, et al. Brief report: Recurrent severe infections caused by a novel leukocyte adhesion deficiency. N Engl J Med. 1992;327:1789–1792.
49. Gallin JI, Fletcher MP, Seligmann BE, et al. Human neutrophil specific granule deficiency: A model to assess the role of the neutrophil specific granules in the evolution of the inflammatory response. Blood. 1982;59:1317–1329.
50. Lomax KJ, Gallin JI, Rotrosen D, et al. Selective defect in myeloid cell lactoferrin gene expression in neutrophil specific granule deficiency. J Clin Invest. 1989;83:514–519.
51. Yamanaka R, Barlow C, Lekstrom-Himes J, et al. Impaired granulopoiesis, myelodysplasia, and early lethality in CCAAT/enhancer binding protein epsilon-deficient mice. Proc Natl Acad Sci U S A. 1997;94:13187–13192.
51a. Lekstrom-Himes J, Dorman SE, Kapar P, et al. Neutrophil-specific granule deficiency results from a novel mutation with loss of function of the transcription factor CCAAT/enhancer binding protein ϵ. J Emp Med. 1999;189:1842–1852.
52. Nauseef WM. Myeloperoxidase deficiency. Hematol Oncol Clin North Am. 1988;2:135–158.
53. Newport MJ, Huxley CM, Huston S, et al. A mutation in the interferon-gamma-receptor gene and susceptibility to mycobacterial infection. N Engl J Med. 1996;335:1941–1949.
54. Jouanguy E, Altare F, Lamhamedi S, et al. Interferon-gamma-receptor deficiency in an infant with fatal bacille Calmette-Guérin infection. N Engl J Med. 1996;335:1956–1961.
55. Holland SM, Dorman SE, Kwon A, et al. Abnormal regulation of interferon-gamma, interleukin-12, and tumor necrosis factor-alpha, in human interferon-gamma receptor 1 deficiency. J Infect Dis. 1998;178:1095–1104.
56. Dorman SE, Holland SM. Mutation in the signal-transducing chain of the interferon-gamma receptor and susceptibility to mycobacterial infection. J Clin Invest. 1998;101:2364–2369.
57. de Jong R, Altare F, Haagen IA, et al. Severe mycobacterial and *Salmonella* infections in interleukin-12 receptor–deficient patients. Science. 1998;280:1435–1438.
58. Altare F, Durandy A, Lammas D, et al. Impairment of mycobacterial immunity in human interleukin-12 receptor deficiency. Science. 1998;280:1432–1435.
58a. Altare F, Lammas D, Revy P, et al. Inherited interleukin 12 deficiency in a child with bacille Calmette-Guérin and *Salmonella* enteritidis disseminated infection. J Clin Invest. 1998;102:2035–2040.
59. Buckley RH, Becker WG. Abnormalities in the regulation of human IgE synthesis. Immunol Rev. 1978;41:288–314.
60. Grimbacher B, Holland SM, Gallin JI, et al. Hyper IgE syndrome with recurrent infections—an autosomal dominant multisystem disorder. N Engl J Med. 1999;340:692–702.
61. Donabedian H, Gallin JI. The hyperimmunoglobulin E recurrent infection (Job's) syndrome: A review of the NIH experience and the literature. Medicine (Baltimore). 1983;62:195–208.
62. Geha RS, Leung DYM. Hyper immunoglobulin E syndrome. Immunodefic Rev. 1989;1:155–172.
63. Charon JA, Mergenhagen SE, Gallin JI. Gingivitis and oral ulceration in patients with neutrophil dysfunction. J Oral Pathol. 1985;14:150–155.
64. Williams WJ, Nelson DA, Morris MW. Examination of the blood. In: Williams WA, Beutler E, Erslev AJ, et al, eds. Hematology. 4th ed. New York: McGraw-Hill; 1990:9–24.
65. Carvalho EM, Bacellaro O, Barral A, et al. Antigen specific immunosuppression in visceral leishmaniasis is cell mediated. J Clin Invest. 1989;83:860–864.
66. Lopez M, Fleisher T, deShazo RD. Use and interpretation of diagnostic immunologic laboratory tests. JAMA. 1992;268:2970–2990.
67. Alarcon B, Regueiro JR, Arnaiz-Villena A, et al. Familial defect in the surface expression of the T cell receptor–CD3 complex. N Engl J Med. 1988;319:1203–1208.
68. Mossmann TR, Moore KW. The role of IL10 in cross regulation of Th1 and Th2 responses. Immunol Today. 1991;12:48–53.
69. Bruton OC. Agammaglobulinemia. Pediatrics. 1952;9:722–728.
70. Waldmann TA. Immunodeficiency diseases: Primary and acquired. In: Samter M, ed. Immunological Diseases. 4th ed. New York: Little Brown; 1988:411–465.
71. Coffey AJ, Brooksbank RA, Brandau O, et al. Host response to EBV infection in X-linked lymphoproliferative disease results from mutations in an SH2-domain encoding gene. Nature Genet. 1998;20:129–135.
72. Bodey GP, Buckley M, Sathe YS, et al. Quantitative relationships between circulating leukocytes and infection in patients with acute leukemia. Ann Intern Med. 1966;64:328–340.
73. Bonilla MA, Gillio AP, Ruggiero M, et al. Effects of recombinant human granulocyte colony-stimulating factor on neutropenia in patients with congenital agranulocytosis. N Engl J Med. 1989;320:1574–1580.
74. Rausch PG, Pryzwansky KB, Spitznagel JK. Immunocytochemical identification of azurophilic and specific granule markers in the giant granules of Chédiak-Higashi neutrophils. N Engl J Med. 1978;298:693–698.
75. Kishimoto TK, Larson RS, Corbi AL, et al. The leukocyte integrins. Adv Immunol. 1989;46:149–182.
76. Springer TA. Adhesion receptors of the immune system. Nature. 1990;346: 425–434.
77. Butcher EC. Leukocyte–endothelial cell recognition: 3 (or more) steps to specificity and diversity. Cell. 1991;67:1033–1036.
78. Rosenberg HF, Gallin JI. Neutrophil specific granule deficiency includes eosinophils. Blood. 1993;82:268–273.
79. Rex JH, Bennett JE, Gallin JI, et al. Normal and deficient neutrophils can cooperate to damage *Aspergillus fumigatus* hyphae. J Infect Dis. 1990;162:523–528.

80. Muoy R, Fisher A, Vilmer E, et al. Incidence, severity and prevention of infections in chronic granulomatous disease. J Pediatr. 1989;114:555–560.
81. Buescher ES, Gallin JI. Stature and weight in chronic granulomatous disease. J Pediatr. 1984;104:911–913.
82. Kenney RT, Kwon-Chung KJ, Waytes AT, et al. Successful treatment of systemic *Exophiala dermatitidis* infection in a patient with chronic granulomatous disease. Clin Infect Dis. 1992;1:235–242.
83. Williamson PR, Kwon-Chung KJ, Gallin JI. Successful treatment of *Paecilomyces varioti* infection in a patient with chronic granulomatous disease and a review of *Paecilomyces* species infections. Clin Infect Dis. 1992;5:1023–1026.
84. Gallin JI, Buescher ES, Seligmann BE, et al. Recent advances in chronic granulomatous disease. Ann Intern Med. 1983;99:657–674.
85. Sponseller PD, Malech HL, McCarthy EF, et al. Skeletal involvement in chronic granulomatous disease of childhood. J Bone Joint Surg Am. 1991;73:37–51.
86. Segal BH, DeCarlo ES, Kwon-Chung KJ, et al. *Aspergillus nidulans* infection in chronic granulomatous disease. Medicine (Baltimore). 1998;77:345–354.
87. Margolis DM, Melnick DA, Alling DW, et al. Trimethoprim-sulfamethoxazole prophylaxis in the management of chronic granulomatous disease. J Infect Dis. 1990;162:723–726.
88. Ament ME, Ochs HD. Gastrointestinal manifestations of chronic granulomatous disease. N Engl J Med. 1973;288:382–387.
89. Walther MM, Malech H, Berman A, et al. The urologic manifestations of chronic granulomatous disease. J Urol. 1992;147:1314–1318.
90. International Chronic Granulomatous Disease Cooperative Study. A controlled trial of interferon gamma to prevent infection in chronic granulomatous disease. N Engl J Med. 1991;324:509–516.
91. Buescher ES, Gallin JI. Leukocyte transfusions in chronic granulomatous disease: Persistence of transfused leukocytes in sputum. N Engl J Med. 1982;307:800–803.
92. Chin TW, Steihm ER, Falloon J, et al. Corticosteroids in treatment of obstructive lesions of chronic granulomatous disease. J Pediatr. 1987;111:349–352.
93. Holland SM. Host defense against nontuberculous mycobacterial infections. Semin Respir Infect. 1996;11:217–230.
94. Jouanguy E, Lamhamedi-Cherradi S, Altare F, et al. Partial interferon gamma receptor 1 deficiency in a child with tuberculoid bacillus Calmette-Guérin infection and a sibling with clinical tuberculosis. J Clin Invest. 1997;100:2658–2664.
95. Lallemand D, Kalifa G, Buriot D, et al. Constitutional bone anomalies in congenital immune deficiencies. Ann Radiol. 1978;22:108–118.
96. Leung DYM, Key L, Steinberg JJ, et al. Increased in vitro bone resorption by monocytes in the hyperimmunoglobulin E syndrome. J Immunol. 1988;140:84–88.
97. Dreskin SC, Gallin JI. Evolution of the hyper immunoglobulin E and infection (HIE, Job's) syndrome in a young girl. J Allergy Clin Immunol. 1987;80:746–751.
98. Dreskin SC, Goldsmith PK, Strober W, et al. Metabolism of immunoglobulin E in patients with markedly elevated serum immunoglobulin E levels. J Clin Invest. 1987;79:1764–1772.
99. Berger M, Kirkpatrick CH, Goldsmith PK, et al. IgE antibodies to *Staphylococcus aureus* and *Candida albicans* in patients with the syndrome of hyperimmunoglobulin E and recurrent infections. J Immunol. 1980;125:2437–2443.
100. Pantaleo G, Graziosi C, Fauci AS. The immunopathogenesis of human immunodeficiency virus infection. N Engl J Med. 1993;328:327–335.
101. Smith DK, Neal JJ, Holmberg SD, Centers for Disease Control Idiopathic CD4+ T-Lymphocytopenia Task Force. Unexplained opportunistic infections and CD4+ T-lymphocytopenia without HIV infection—an investigation of cases in the United States. N Engl J Med. 1993;328:373–379.
102. Singh N, Yu VL, Mielles LA, et al. Beta-lactam antibiotic induced leukopenia in severe hepatic dysfunction: Risk factors and implications for dosing in patients with liver disease. Am J Med. 1993;94:251–256.
103. Leighton PM, MacSween HM. *Yersinia* hepatic abscesses subsequent to long term iron therapy. JAMA. 1987;257:964–965.
104. Gallant T, Freedman MH, Vellend H, et al. *Yersinia* sepsis in patients with iron overload treated with desferrioxamine (Letter). N Engl J Med. 1986;314:1643.
105. Mofenson HC, Caraccio TR, Sharieff N. Iron sepsis: *Yersinia enterocolitica* septicemia possibly caused by an overdose of iron (Letter). N Engl J Med. 1987;316:1092–1093.
106. Case 29-1986: DF-2 sepsis in a splenectomized patient. N Engl J Med. 1986;315:241–249.
107. Davis JM, Dineen P, Galin JI. Neutrophil degranulation and abnormal chemotaxis after thermal injury. J Immunol. 1990;124:1467–1471.

SECTION C

EPIDEMIOLOGY OF INFECTIOUS DISEASES

Chapter 11

Epidemiologic Principles

MICHAEL T. OSTERHOLM
CRAIG W. HEDBERG
KRISTINE A. MOORE

EPIDEMIOLOGIC STUDY METHODS

Epidemiology is the study of the distribution of health-related conditions or events and factors associated with the occurrence of these conditions or events in defined populations. The science of epidemiology was originally derived from the study of epidemics and has now been broadened to encompass all phenomena related to health in populations.[1] Simply stated, epidemiology involves the careful description of events within populations and the comparison of rates at which these events occur between groups within those populations. Similar concepts and methods of epidemiology apply to both infectious and noninfectious diseases.[2] The strength and adaptability of epidemiologic methods come from their underlying simplicity. For example, John Snow's application of epidemiologic study methods resulted in the classic investigation of the Broad Street pump outbreak of cholera in London in 1851. His work was based on a careful description of his observations and his quantitative approach in analyzing the occurrence of cholera among the citizens of London. The influence of his work led to legislation mandating that all the water companies in London filter their water. Of note, it was not until 1883 that Robert Koch discovered *Vibrio cholerae*.[3]

Goals of Epidemiologic Analysis

As applied to infectious diseases, at least 10 primary goals of epidemiologic analysis can be listed: (1) describe patterns of infection and disease occurrence in populations; (2) identify outbreaks or unusual rates of disease occurrence; (3) facilitate laboratory-based efforts to identify infectious agents; (4) describe the occurrence of asymptomatic infection and the spectrum of disease associated with specific agents; (5) provide population-based descriptions of clinical illness to improve the specificity of diagnosis for individual diseases; (6) assist in the understanding of disease pathogenesis; (7) identify and characterize factors in the chain of infection that contribute to agent transmission and the development of disease; (8) develop and evaluate treatment protocols through clinical trials; (9) develop and evaluate primary, secondary, and tertiary prevention and control measures for individuals; and (10) describe and assess the use of prevention measures on a community-wide basis. These comprehensive goals far exceed the often considered goal of epidemiologic analysis to investigate and control epidemics or outbreaks.

These goals can be illustrated by a historical review of the unfolding of the human immunodeficiency virus (HIV) epidemic. After the acquired immunodeficiency syndrome (AIDS) was initially described in 1981, a national epidemiologic surveillance case definition was developed. Subsequent disease surveillance was initiated to characterize the cases by standard measures of time, place, and person and to identify population groups at risk. Based on these efforts, an infectious etiology was hypothesized early in the epidemic, before the first laboratory evidence of an etiologic agent was presented. Combined clinical, epidemiologic, and laboratory studies led to identification of HIV as the cause of AIDS and to the development of sensitive and specific serologic tests for infection. This progress in turn led to studies that characterized the spectrum of illness associated with HIV infection. Epidemiologic studies of persons infected with HIV (with or without AIDS) have characterized the routes of HIV transmission, have shown that the occurrence of other sexually transmitted diseases can increase the risk of HIV transmission, and have demonstrated that HIV infection can enhance the transmission of other agents such as *Mycobacterium tuberculosis*. Clinical trials have been conducted (or are ongoing) to assess the efficacy of certain antiretroviral agents and, more recently, HIV vaccines. Multiple other trials have also been conducted to assess the efficacy of a range of antimicrobial agents aimed at preventing a variety of opportunistic infections. Finally, community-based programs developed on the basis of epidemiologic data have been developed to promote behavior change aimed at reducing the risk of HIV transmission. Epidemiologic methods have also been applied to the evaluation of these community-based programs. These examples illustrate the broad role that epidemiologic methods have played in understanding and controlling the HIV epidemic.

Defining Infections, Diseases, and Populations

An essential aspect of any epidemiologic study is careful definition of the infection, disease, condition, or factor that is being studied. The ability to detect meaningful and valid statistical associations between health status and risk factors is frequently dependent on the precision and reliability with which the study variables can be defined. For example, the occurrence of toxic shock syndrome in menstruating women was initially associated with the use of a single brand of tampons.[4] However, that brand had a disproportionately increased share of the high-absorbency tampon sales when compared with all other brands. Another epidemiologic study that controlled for the absorbency of tampons demonstrated that the use of all tampon brands was associated with toxic shock syndrome.[5]

Specificity and sensitivity are concepts that are frequently used in reference to laboratory test performance, particularly tests that are used for screening purposes.[1] However, in the epidemiologic study of infectious diseases, it is important to also apply the concepts of specificity and sensitivity more broadly in terms of diagnosis of infection and disease. For example, the diagnosis of smallpox infection and disease was both highly specific and sensitive. Few other diseases could be confused with smallpox (i.e., the diagnosis was specific), and clinical disease developed in most people who became infected with smallpox virus (i.e., the diagnosis was sensitive). These qualities, in addition to the fact that humans were the only important reservoir for the smallpox virus and highly immunogenic vaccines had been developed, led to the successful eradication of smallpox.[6] In contrast, the diagnosis of infection and disease with diarrheogenic *Escherichia coli* is neither specific nor sensitive because *E. coli* may have an array of virulence factors that can result in disease and yet are not detected by standard biochemical tests.[7] Without a specific and sensitive case definition based on microbial testing of stool, efforts are severely hampered to provide an accurate description of the epidemiology of this disease in the community.

Some clinical conditions or syndromes may be caused by more than one etiologic agent (e.g., meningitis or hemolytic-uremic syndrome). In such situations, for epidemiologic methods to be successful, the case definition needs to be kept as specific as possible. Conversely, some agents may lead to a broad spectrum of clinical illnesses. Depending on the goals of a particular study, investigators may choose a case definition that casts a wide net or may choose a more narrow case definition. The type of definition can have a substantial impact on study results and should be carefully considered before a specific study is undertaken.

Epidemiologic studies may be designed to evaluate outcome variables other than infection or disease occurrence. In these situations, how the outcome variables are defined and measured can affect interpretation of the results and the validity of the conclusions. For example, in the development of recombinant vaccines for hepatitis B virus, two vaccine formulations that differed primarily in the amount of hepatitis B surface antigen (HBsAg) in each dose were evaluated. Although higher antibody titers developed in subjects who were administered vaccine with 20 μg HBsAg per dose than in those who were provided vaccine with 10 μg HBsAg per dose, sufficient levels of antibody to be considered protective against infection developed in similar proportions of both groups. Based on similar qualitative responses in clinical trials, both vaccines were licensed by the Food and Drug Administration. However, among Minnesota hospital employees, those who received vaccine with 20 μg HBsAg per dose were more likely than persons given the other vaccine to have detectable antibody when tested within 6 months after completing the three-dose series.[8] The results of this investigation suggested that sociodemographic factors of the population studied, such as age, gender, weight, and smoking, affected the outcome of vaccination programs.

Establishing specific enrollment criteria for cases of infection or disease in epidemiologic studies is critical to obtaining valid and biologically meaningful results. For example, large multistate outbreaks of *E. coli* O157-H7 have been documented with increasing frequency. However, without molecular subtyping of *E. coli* O157-H7 strains, population-based surveillance is limited in its ability to detect and determine when an unexpected number or temporal clustering of cases actually documents a common vehicle-associated outbreak. In Minnesota during 1994 and 1995, of 317 reported cases of *E. coli* O157-H7 infection and for which isolates were available for pulsed-field gel electrophoresis (PFGE), 143 distinct PFGE patterns were identified.[9] Ten outbreaks of *E. coli* O157-H7 were identified during that time; these accounted for only 56 (18%) of the cases. Most cases represented sporadic infections not related to a single food vehicle.

A similar issue regarding the definition of cases and the population in which they occur confronts public health officials when they must consider intervention activities because of a possible outbreak of some selected infectious disease. It is common practice to define outbreaks as the occurrence of cases of disease at a frequency greater than expected.[1] When an outbreak occurs, it is necessary to define the population at risk (i.e., the denominator) if an accurate measure of the rate of disease is to be calculated. For example, it is not unusual to recognize a cluster of cases of *Neisseria meningitidis* disease in the community. Because outbreaks of invasive *N. meningitidis* disease are known to occur in closed populations, such as persons living in dormitories and barracks, and because a vaccine and antibiotic chemoprophylaxis are available to prevent or control these outbreaks, the occurrence of multiple cases of meningococcal disease inevitably prompts a rapid public health assessment. Cases of meningococcal disease tend to occur during well-described seasonal peak periods, so it is possible that a cluster of unrelated cases may occur in a defined population. The need for public health intervention is quite different for a cluster of cases related to a single outbreak-associated strain versus a cluster of cases in which each is caused by a different group or strain of *N. meningitidis*. However, in many situations, strains are not available for further subtyping because laboratory capacity to distinguish strains is limited.

A companion problem to defining the cases is the definition of the population at risk. To determine whether cases of disease are occurring at a frequency greater than expected, it is necessary to consider baseline incidence rates of disease. For example, in the United States, *N. meningitidis* invasive disease occurs at a rate of approximately 1 to 2 cases per 100,000 persons per year.[10] However, many of these cases occur seasonally (i.e., in the winter months) and among young children. Thus, expected temporal clustering in the winter months could make a short-term observed rate of occurrence appear excessive when compared with the annual rate of disease. A similar issue is the fact that cases often occur in one or more identified populations (i.e., school, workplace, church group) that are of limited size; therefore, rate comparisons may be meaningless. For example, 1 case of meningococcal disease in a school of 1000 students could be represented as a rate of 100 per 100,000 persons per year. Although this figure is 50 times the expected annual population rate, it cannot reasonably be interpreted as defining an outbreak. Thus, timely decisions regarding major community-based interventions after the observation of a cluster of meningococcal cases will often be made without adequate information regarding the status of a possible outbreak. Similar situations also occur with other pathogens.

Two common measures of the occurrence of disease in populations are incidence and prevalence.[1] *Incidence* represents the occurrence of new cases of infection or disease per unit of population per time period. It is common to express incidence rates in terms of person-years of exposure. *Prevalence* describes the number of current cases of disease per population unit at the time of observation. The relationship between incidence and prevalence depends on the duration of infection or disease. For example, the incidence of measles over the period of a year is always greater than its prevalence at a given point because the disease has a very short duration. In contrast, the prevalence of HIV infection is always greater than its incidence because the infection is chronic and infected persons may live for years after the initial infection.

Biology and Statistics

The results of epidemiologic studies to compare the risk of infection or disease and the presence or absence of specific risk factors are presented in terms of relative risk and odds ratios. *Relative risk* is the ratio of the rate of illness or infection among persons who were exposed and the rate of illness or infection in persons who were not exposed (Fig. 11–1). Relative risks may also be called rate ratios and are the products of cohort studies. In case-control studies, *odds ratios* are determined and approximate the relative risk. Odds ratios provide a valid estimate of the relative risk under conditions that prevail in most case-control studies: the cases of disease are newly diagnosed, prevalent cases are not included in the control group, and the selection of cases and controls is not based on exposure status.[11]

An increased relative risk or odds ratio (i.e., >1.0) for an exposure variable indicates that the exposure is related to an increased risk of disease. Similarly, a decreased relative risk or odds ratio (i.e., <1.0) indicates that the exposure variable is related to a decreased risk of disease. For example, the consumption of undercooked eggs has been associated with an increased risk of *Salmonella enteritidis* infection in outbreak settings and for sporadic *S. enteritidis* infections in the community.[12] Although relative risks and odds ratios do provide a measure of the risk of disease associated with a specific factor, they do not directly describe how much disease in the community can be attributed to that factor. Rather, the *attributable risk* or *fraction* considers both the relative risk for an exposure variable and the proportion of the population exposed to that variable. In Minnesota, persons who consumed undercooked eggs had approximately a four times greater risk of *S. enteritidis* infection than did those who did not eat undercooked eggs. Based on an estimate for the frequency of eating undercooked eggs among the general population, investigators estimated that 37% of sporadic *S. enteritidis* infections in Minnesota adults could be attributed to the consumption of undercooked

	Disease present	Disease absent
Exposure present	a	b
Exposure absent	c	d

A The relative risk is calculated as: $\frac{[a/(a+b)]}{[c/(c+d)]}$

The odds ratio is calculated as: $\frac{ad}{bc}$

B Calculation of population-attributable risk percent:

$$\frac{\text{(Prevalence of exposure)(relative risk-1)}}{1 + [\text{(Prevalence of exposure)(relative risk-1)}]} \times 100$$

FIGURE 11–1. The calculation of and relationship among relative risks, odds ratios, and attributable risks. *A,* The calculation of relative risks and odds ratios from a two-by-two table. The odds ratio provides a valid estimate of the relative risk under conditions that prevail in most case-control studies, including that the cases of disease are newly diagnosed, that prevalent cases are not included in the control group, and that the selection of cases and controls is not based on exposure status. *B,* The calculation of population-attributable risk percent. In a case-control study, attributable risk can be estimated from the prevalence of exposure among controls (b/b+d) and the odds ratio. The validity of this approach is limited by how representative controls are of the population and how well the odds ratio estimates the relative risk. (*A* from St Louis ME, Morse DL, Potter ME, et al. The emergence of grade A eggs as major source of *Salmonella enteritidis* infections. New implications of the control of salmonellosis. JAMA. 1988;259:2103–2107.)

eggs.[13] Thus, both relative risk and attributable risk are important measures for describing the epidemiology of infectious diseases and determining public health priorities.

In the process of studying the epidemiology of infectious diseases, many factors are evaluated to determine their relationship or association with a specific disease. Statistical associations, both positive and negative, may represent a true causal relationship, a confounding relationship with another factor, or a chance occurrence. When more than one factor is statistically associated with infection or disease status in univariate, or single-variable, analyses, the relationship between individual factors and infection or disease status can be evaluated by multivariate regression analysis.[14] These procedures allow the investigator to simultaneously control for a combination of factors in the analysis and to determine whether any of the risk factors are associated with infection or disease status independently of other factors. Another critical way of distinguishing between causation, confounding, and chance is by assessing the biologic plausibility of the association. An unexpected statistical association found in conjunction with an epidemiologic study may result in a new understanding of how agent transmission or disease occurs. The temptation to stretch the plausibility of biology to provide meaning to statistical results is a constant danger. However, such results may be a useful guide to evaluate new hypotheses in future studies.

Furthermore, "statistically significant results" may be unimportant from a disease control or a practical perspective. Statistical significance, which has historically been considered to be an event that happens less than once every 20 times by chance alone (i.e., $p < .05$), is a combination of both the sample size and the strength or degree of the association. Studies with a large number of persons enrolled can produce statistically significant results of weak associations (i.e., relative risks or odds ratios greater than 1 but less than 2), whereas studies with a limited number of persons enrolled may not be able to produce statistically significant results even with moderately strong or increased associations (i.e., relative risks or odds ratios greater than 5).

Determining Epidemiologic Methods Appropriate to the Study Setting

The clinical trial is cited as the gold standard of epidemiologic research. However, many epidemiologic studies cannot take place under such rigorously controlled conditions. Taking advantage of opportunities to study diseases in clinical and community settings is one of the strengths of epidemiology. In the setting of a clinical practice, epidemiology may involve studying a series of patients, participating in multicenter trials, or being a reporting source for cases of disease to public health officials. This last aspect of epidemiologic study may be a legal obligation, but it should also be viewed as an opportunity for all practicing clinicians to participate in the practice of community-based epidemiology. Academic-based research centers are often settings for clinical trials, studies requiring newly developed laboratory methods, or studies derived from referrals to clinical specialty groups. Public health departments typically do not have direct access to or contact with patients for clinical trials, but they are responsible for surveillance of reportable diseases and the investigation of outbreaks. Each of these settings provides opportunities for epidemiologic studies that have made major contributions to the understanding, prevention, and control of infectious diseases.

Several major constraints are confronted in the design of epidemiologic studies of infectious diseases. Time is frequently a problem in the investigation of outbreaks. The need to quickly design and conduct outbreak investigations necessarily limits the investigator's ability to fully explore the outbreak setting and can result in the loss of information. In any study involving the retrospective collection of data, information may be lost because of difficulty in recalling exposure or in verifying information about the exposure.

For many infectious diseases, it may also be difficult to identify sufficient numbers of cases in clinical settings to conduct meaningful epidemiologic studies. In such situations, multisite collaborative projects are often needed. For example, a Centers for Disease Control and Prevention (CDC) work group on prevention of invasive group A streptococcal disease among household contacts concluded in 1995 that the data available from a single study conducted in Ontario, Canada, were inadequate to recommend chemoprophylaxis to household contacts.[15, 16] Although the Canadian study suggested an increased risk of invasive disease among household contacts, this assessment was based on only four subsequent cases in households. Based on the recommendations of the work group, a multisite study coordinated by CDC was initiated in several states or areas with active surveillance of invasive group A streptococcal disease.

Types of Epidemiologic Studies

Several schemes can be used to classify or define types of epidemiologic studies (Table 11–1). Studies can be classified as *descriptive* or

TABLE 11–1 Classification Schemes for Epidemiologic Studies

	Observational	Experimental
Descriptive	Surveillance	
	Case series	
Analytic	Outbreak investigations	Clinical trials
	Cross-sectional surveys	Community interventions
	Seroprevalence surveys	
	Case-control studies	
	Cohort studies	
	Seroincidence studies	

analytic and *observational* or *experimental*. A descriptive study is designed to describe only the existing distribution of case characteristics without regard to causal or other hypotheses.[17] For example, the results of community-based surveillance for *Campylobacter* infection may include a summary of all cases reported in a given year by the date of onset, county of residence, age, sex, and race. An analytic study is one designed to examine associations, particularly hypothesized causal relationships.[17] A case-control study could be designed to examine whether consumption of hot dogs is a risk factor for cases of invasive listeriosis infections identified through surveillance activities. In addition to case-control studies, cohort studies, clinical trials, and cross-sectional surveys are common types of analytic studies. In practice, most epidemiologic studies involve both descriptive and analytic elements.

A more relevant distinction can be made between observational and experimental studies. Observational studies are conducted in natural settings where changes in one characteristic are studied in relation to others without the intervention of the investigator.[18] Observational studies represent the bulk of epidemiologic research because they focus on events, exposures, and diseases occurring in the population during the course of routine living conditions. In contrast, experimental studies are ones in which the study conditions are under the direct control of the investigator.[18] Such studies may include randomization of subjects to treatment or placebo groups and blinding of subject and investigator to placement status. Clinical trials are the prototypic experimental study. On a broader scale, community intervention trials can also be conducted.

Observational Studies

Disease Surveillance

Disease surveillance is an ongoing process that involves the systematic collection, analysis, and distribution of information regarding the occurrence of diseases in defined populations.[19] Surveillance can be conducted in the community and in institutional settings, where it may form the basis for an infection-control program. For most infectious diseases, community-based surveillance is the domain of public health departments at the local or state level. All jurisdictions require licensed physicians to report the occurrence of selected diseases to the health department.[20] Typically, such diseases include sexually transmitted diseases, vaccine-preventable diseases, bloodborne pathogens, tuberculosis, certain invasive bacterial diseases, and enteric infections caused by *Salmonella, Shigella,* and *Campylobacter.* In addition to categoric reporting, most states require reporting of disease outbreaks, regardless of the cause, and have some provision to solicit reports of new and emerging diseases. In some situations, syndromal surveillance may be appropriate, as opposed to surveillance based on isolation of a specific infectious agent. Surveillance of influenza-like illness in sentinel physician practices, nursing homes, or schools is a way to monitor influenza activity each influenza season. Surveillance for chronic liver disease may be a way to measure the burden of disease caused by hepatitis C in the United States.[21] Surveillance for unexplained deaths from possible infectious causes with characterization of such deaths based on the clinical syndrome at the initial evaluation is a way to monitor the emergence of potential new infectious disease threats.[22] Finally, syndromal surveillance may be useful when setting up early warning systems for the detection of bioterrorist events.

During the last 10 years, surveillance for certain pathogens has evolved to include surveillance for antimicrobial resistance. Surveillance for drug-resistant tuberculosis is now essentially routine in all jurisdictions.[23] The emergence of multidrug-resistant *Salmonella typhimurium* DT104 in the United States was recently detected through national surveillance to monitor resistant enteric infections.[24] Several state health departments now monitor the occurrence of drug-resistant pneumococcal infections in their jurisdictions, and national data have been developed as well.[25] The importance of surveillance for drug-resistant infections will continue to grow in the 21st century, and data collected through public health surveillance can be extremely useful to clinical care providers.

Surveillance can be conducted in an active or passive manner. *Active surveillance* involves a regular, systematic effort to contact reporting sources or to review records within an institution to ascertain information on the occurrence of newly diagnosed diseases or infections. An example of an active surveillance system for foodborne illnesses is the Foodborne Diseases Active Surveillance Network (FoodNet), which operates as part of CDC's Emerging Infections Program.[26] Active laboratory-based surveillance for confirmed cases of *Campylobacter, Cryptosporidium, Cyclospora, E. coli* O157-H7, *Listeria, Salmonella, Shigella,* and *Vibrio* was initiated in five Emerging Infections Program sites in 1996 and expanded to eight sites in 1999. Each clinical laboratory in the surveillance catchment areas is contacted weekly or monthly to ensure that all confirmed infections under surveillance have been reported. *Passive surveillance* relies on the individual clinician or laboratory to initiate the report.

Two key qualities of community-based surveillance for infectious diseases that must be considered when interpreting surveillance data are representativeness and timeliness. These qualities will vary by disease and depend on multiple factors. The first factor of importance is that the patient must seek medical attention. It is not common for persons with mild or limited illnesses to seek medical attention. Second, the physician must seek laboratory testing of appropriate clinical specimens to confirm the diagnosis. Third, the laboratory must have the capability to identify the agent. Fourth, the physician and laboratory must report the clinical and laboratory findings to public health officials in a timely manner. Fifth, the availability of molecular subtyping techniques such as PFGE and the ability to electronically compare PFGE patterns through the national computer network PulseNet can greatly increase both the sensitivity and the specificity of pathogen-specific surveillance. Even in states where laboratory-based infectious disease reporting is required, there may be confusion between the physician and laboratory officials over who has responsibility for reporting. Finally, public health agencies must have the resources to conduct timely and routine follow-up of such reports to ascertain basic case demographic and other relevant data. Failure at any step of this process will result in loss of information to the community-based surveillance system.

The efficiency of community-based surveillance systems varies greatly, depending on the disease and how the diagnosis is made and the resources targeted toward the surveillance effort.[19] Diseases that require a diagnosis based on clinical findings, such as Lyme disease, present difficulties because many patients may not be seen when the typical clinical manifestations of the disease are present and laboratory testing is not adequate to establish the diagnosis. In contrast, the diagnosis of measles can be confirmed by specific serologic testing regardless of whether the physician sees the patient when the pathognomonic clinical features of the disease are present. Surveillance for invasive bacterial diseases such as those caused by *Haemophilus influenzae* type B and *N. meningitidis* is facilitated by the need for medical treatment because of the relative severity of the disease and the laboratory-supported diagnosis. For diseases such as these, active case ascertainment can greatly enhance the effectiveness of surveillance activities. However, active surveillance requires the commitment of personnel and other resources that are limited for many reportable diseases. Typically, active surveillance may be conducted for a limited period when complete data are most critical. Examples include the characterization of emerging diseases such as AIDS or special surveillance projects aimed at assessing an intervention, such as evaluating the efficacy of *H. influenzae* type B vaccine in a defined population.[27]

Most infectious disease surveillance conducted by public health departments in the United States is passive in that it relies on the physician or the laboratory to initiate the report. Passive surveillance systems are subject to selection bias because disease reports are likely to come from a nonrepresentative sample of practicing physicians who may report specific diseases because of personal interest.[19] In addition, some data (i.e., age and gender versus clinical and pathologic information) may be more readily reported because of ease of ascertainment.[19]

Active surveillance is relatively more common in the hospital setting. For example, surveillance of nosocomial infections is an important hospital infection-control activity.[28] This highly specialized surveillance system has the operational advantage of a defined population, routine clinical observation of the patient population, and direct access to the laboratory. Hospital-based surveillance has been a primary epidemiologic tool in the study of drug-resistant organisms.[29]

Case Series

A common type of descriptive study that is conducted in clinical settings is the case series. A case series describes the clinical features of a disease and the demographic profiles and other interesting features of patients with the disease. They are typically the domain of practicing clinicians and serve as a way of communicating significant clinical observations. For example, in one Australian hospital, *Campylobacter upsaliensis* was isolated from the stool of 20 HIV-infected patients with diarrhea. In 13 patients, no other enteric pathogen was isolated. These findings suggest that *C. upsaliensis* was the cause of their prolonged diarrhea of mild to moderate severity.[30] Similar case series presaged the identification of *Cryptosporidium* and *Cyclospora* as important pathogens of immunocompetent persons.

Case-Control Studies

In case-control studies, persons with infection or disease are compared with controls (i.e., persons without the infection or disease under study) with respect to prior exposures likely to be related to agent transmission.[1] Case-control studies by nature are retrospective because the outcome (i.e., case status) is known at the outset of the study. Case-control studies are the most widely conducted type of epidemiologic study because they are relatively cheap, powerful, and adaptable to many settings.[14] For example, in a nationwide outbreak of *S. enteritidis* infection, the results of a case-control study identified the ice cream made by a large national producer as the source of the outbreak 10 days before *S. enteritidis* could be isolated from samples of the implicated ice cream.[31] When *S. enteritidis* was isolated from the ice cream, it was shown to be present at levels of less than one to six organisms per half-cup serving, levels that rendered microbiologic surveillance of ice cream insensitive. Furthermore, the case-control study identified contamination of pasteurized ice cream premix during transport in tanker trailers that had previously carried nonpasteurized liquid eggs, even though regulatory officials were not able to isolate *S. enteritidis* from any environmental samples.

The primary considerations in designing case-control studies are defining cases, establishing enrollment criteria, identifying suitable controls, and developing interview or other data collection processes that do not systematically result in different standards of data collection for cases versus controls. In the community setting it is customary to select controls from the same area of residence as the cases. It is desirable for controls to resemble cases with respect to variables that are not being studied. Controls may also be matched by age, gender, or any other factor that the investigator wishes to consider. For example, in studying risk factors for toxic shock syndrome in menstruating women, it was important to select or match controls based on gender. The use of male controls could have produced spurious associations between illness and any menses-related event. However, overmatching, such as requiring controls to have the same birthday as the case, may make it difficult to identify and recruit controls. Also, once a variable is used as a matching criterion, it is no longer available for evaluation. Thus, in the studies of toxic shock syndrome in menstruating women, requiring controls to use the same catemenial products (i.e., tampons) as the cases would have eliminated the possibility of studying this factor. In hospital settings, controls are frequently selected from patients with unrelated diagnoses who might otherwise be comparable to the cases.

Analysis of case-control studies involves comparing exposure differences between cases and controls. Such comparison allows for associations between exposure and disease to be studied even when the disease is a rare outcome of the exposure. For example, a case-control study of Guillain-Barré syndrome demonstrated an association between *Campylobacter* infection and Guillain-Barré syndrome.[32] This association could not have been easily evaluated in a prospective cohort study because of the population size necessary to identify a similar number of Guillain-Barré syndrome cases. The power of the case-control methodology comes from the fact that although illnesses may be uncommon outcomes of a given exposure, the common history of exposure among cases may stand in stark contrast to the exposure history of controls.

Cohort Studies

In cohort studies, the development of infection or disease is observed in groups who are either exposed or not exposed to the previously defined risk factors.[1] Cohort studies are traditionally considered prospective studies. However, this nomenclature is misleading because in reality, cohort studies can be prospective or retrospective, depending on how the exposed and comparison groups were identified and monitored. Cohort studies provide the advantage of a direct measurement of illness rates by exposure status, which allows direct measurement of relative risk. Furthermore, when conducted prospectively, cohort studies allow the investigator better control over data collection and identification of potential confounding variables. The use of cohort studies is limited to groups in which exposures can be defined and measured.

Cohort studies of homosexual men have helped evaluate risk factors for transmission of HIV, hepatitis B virus, and hepatitis C virus.[33, 34] These studies are also examples of *seroincidence surveys,* in which the appearance of antibody to an agent in the second of two sequentially collected specimens indicates infection with that agent somewhere between the two times of collection.[35] Seroincidence surveys allow the investigator to (1) define total infection rates, (2) relate infection rates to prior antibody levels, and (3) identify risk factors for infection.[35] Prospective cohort studies are limited because of the enrollment size and observation period requirements for diseases of low incidence. Retrospective cohort studies in which previous exposures can be identified offer the advantage of not requiring additional observation periods. However, they may be limited by the recall of study subjects or the adequacy of available medical records.

Cross-sectional Surveys

Cross-sectional surveys provide a point-in-time assessment of the population or study group. These surveys may be conducted to determine the prevalence of a disease in the community, but a more common use is to establish the prevalence of risk factors or serologic markers of infection.[11] For example, a cross-sectional survey of patients attending a sexually transmitted disease clinic demonstrated that hepatitis C virus infection occurred infrequently; however, patients with a history of intravenous drug use had a significantly higher rate of serologic markers for hepatitis C virus infection.[36]

An important type of cross-sectional survey is the *seroprevalence survey.* Serologic prevalence data reflect total infection rates and thus represent both clinical and subclinical (or asymptomatic) infections. Seroprevalence surveys can therefore provide information on patterns of infection or immunity to agents that could not be obtained by ordinary surveillance methods based on the reporting of clinical cases.[35] For example, the federally funded survey of newborn infants for antibody to HIV conducted by state and local health departments provided population-based HIV infection rates for childbearing women throughout the United States in the early 1990s.[37]

Outbreak Investigations

A final category of observational study that integrates multiple epidemiologic methods is the outbreak investigation. A special feature of outbreak investigations is that they are frequently conducted with a sense of urgency because of the ongoing occurrence of cases, the need to rapidly implement control measures, or intense public and media interest in the outbreak. Investigations of the first documented outbreak of legionnaires' disease and the 1993 outbreak of hantavirus-associated respiratory illness in the southwestern United States were lead stories for national news media. Standard methods for conducting outbreak investigations have been published.[18]

Specific surveillance systems have been established for outbreaks of foodborne and waterborne diseases, influenza, and a range of infections in institutional settings. At the local or state level, outbreaks may be reported because a physician or the public is aware of the health department's existence and desires some intervention. Once an outbreak has been recognized, it is necessary to determine the extent of the outbreak in terms of person, place, and time. For example, the nationwide outbreak associated with Schwan's ice cream initially appeared as an increased occurrence of cases in southeastern Minnesota.[31] These cases served to index the larger outbreak occurring throughout the distribution area for the implicated product. Similarly, the increased occurrence of *Salmonella agona* infection in several states during April and May 1998 led to the identification of a nationwide outbreak associated with toasted oats cereal, a previously unrecognized vehicle for salmonellosis. Molecular subtyping by PFGE was critical to identify the outbreak-associated strain of *S. agona,* exclude sporadic *S. agona* infections identified through surveillance, and provide for a specific case definition for use in the case-control study that implicated the cereal.[38]

Molecular subtyping by PFGE and comparison of subtype patterns through PulseNet facilitated identification of a multistate outbreak of listeriosis that occurred from August to December 1998.[39] The outbreak was associated with the consumption of hot dogs and luncheon meat manufactured at a single plant. Although subtype results allowed the identification of cases with a high degree of specificity, preliminary results of epidemiologic investigations that identified the likely source did not lead to appropriate public health interventions, and product recall and public notification were delayed until after the outbreak strain of *Listeria monocytogenes* was isolated from the implicated hot dogs.

The second major category of foodborne outbreaks consists of those that are recognized because of the occurrence of a similar illness among persons with a common exposure, such as eating at a restaurant or attending a banquet. Although many of these outbreaks may seem to be self-limited events unique to the establishment, they may serve to index much larger outbreaks. They also provide opportunities to identify emerging foodborne pathogens. For example, in both 1996 and 1997 the nationwide outbreaks of cyclosporiasis associated with raspberries imported from Guatemala were manifested as a large series of otherwise unrelated outbreaks associated with restaurants, banquets, and parties.[40, 41] It was only through collective investigation and tracing the product back from these individual events that the nature of the outbreak was recognized. Similarly, the investigation of an outbreak of gastrointestinal illness with clinical and epidemiologic features of enterotoxigenic *E. coli* at a restaurant led to the identification of a novel strain of atypical enteropathogenic *E. coli.*[7] Nationwide surveillance efforts conducted by individual states, coordinated by CDC, and facilitated by activities such as FoodNet and PulseNet offer great promise to enhance our understanding of foodborne diseases in the coming years.

Experimental Studies

Clinical Trials

Clinical trials are research activities that involve the administration of a treatment or prevention regimen to humans to evaluate its safety and efficacy.[1] In general, these trials involve a comparison of clinical outcomes in patients receiving treatment with the outcomes of a comparable control group. Most clinical trials of interest in infectious disease epidemiology involve trials of antimicrobial agents and vaccines. An early forerunner to the modern clinical trial was a U.S.-based smallpox trial conducted in 1800.[42] During the 1950s, several multicenter trials were developed to evaluate chemotherapy in the treatment of tuberculosis.[43] In 1953, the U.S. poliomyelitis vaccine trials were conducted in collaboration with the U.S. Public Health Service and state health departments.[44]

Many considerations are necessary when designing a clinical trial. First, should the trial be conducted at all? Is enough known about the safety and biologic activity of the treatment or vaccine to allow it to be administered to patients? This consideration requires some knowledge of the immunogenicity of candidate vaccines or the in vitro activity of an antibiotic against specific pathogens. Second, would patients be harmed by withholding either the treatment or vaccine? These issues have gained particular attention regarding trials of drugs for the treatment of HIV infection. Concern expressed by AIDS activists and some clinicians about withholding potentially life-extending treatments has forced the Food and Drug Administration to sanction the use of a secondary and less rigorous treatment and evaluation protocol in designated AIDS clinics.[45] More recently, concern has been expressed regarding the enrollment of individuals at risk for HIV infection in HIV vaccine trials. The need to maintain behavior-related education intervention for participants in the trials reduces the likelihood of demonstrating vaccine efficacy because of the lack of new infections among placebo recipients; however, to not provide such education would be unethical.

Other considerations include the specification of both test and control treatments, an outcome measure for evaluating the treatments, a bias-free method for assigning patients to treatment groups, and calculation of the necessary sample size.[46] Sample size calculations are affected by the number of treatment groups to be studied, the desired significance level for rejecting the null hypothesis, the statistical power to detect a difference, and the desired detectable treatment difference.

Community Intervention Trials

Community intervention trials are related to the clinical trial but are carried out on a larger scale. In these experiments, large groups or communities are selected to receive a therapeutic or preventive regimen.[46] For example, the efficacy of normal human immune globulin prophylaxis to control hepatitis A outbreaks in child care facilities was demonstrated in a community trial in Phoenix.[47] Community trials are particularly well suited to broad-based interventions such as changing physician antibiotic prescribing practices through the promotion of judicious antibiotic use.[48]

THE HOST-AGENT RELATIONSHIP

Although advances in medical science have made us less vulnerable to some infectious disease epidemics and pandemics, they continue to occur as they have throughout human history. As recently as the late 1960s, it was suggested by leading medical authorities in this country, including the Surgeon General, that it was time "to close the book on infectious diseases."[49] However, infectious diseases remain the leading cause of death worldwide. The world's human and animal populations continue to struggle against an increasingly recognized number of viral, bacterial, protozoal, helminthic, and fungal agents.

For the study of infectious disease epidemiology, it is important to consider both infection and disease, for these may be different. *Infection* results from an encounter with a potentially pathogenic agent with a susceptible human host in conjunction with a suitable portal of entry. The source of most human infections lies outside the individual human host; thus, exposure to the environment or other infected hosts is a key factor. *Disease* is one of the possible outcomes of infection, and its development is related to factors of both the host and the agent.

Whereas the clinician is primarily concerned with disease, the epidemiologist is interested in both infection and disease. Because infection without disease occurs frequently for many agents, a study of only clinical illness may provide a misleading understanding of the epidemiology of a specific infectious disease in the community. For example, adults infected with the hepatitis A virus (HAV) frequently experience clinical hepatitis, whereas infants and toddlers with HAV infection are usually asymptomatic.[50] Thus, to determine the incidence of hepatitis A associated with child care facilities and subsequent transmission to family members and child care providers, investigators need to determine both the diagnosis of asymptomatic HAV infection and the level of HAV-related disease.

If the balance between agent and host favors the agent, infection (and in some instances disease) will occur. This relationship between the agent, the route or mechanism of transmission, and the host is referred to as the *chain of infection.* Control and prevention of infection depend on sufficient understanding of the dynamics of these interrelating factors.

Frequently, characteristics of the agent or host are seen as independent factors. However, it is necessary to consider both the host and the agent together in any discussion of the relationship resulting in infection and disease. For example, smallpox was a disease of dramatic human suffering; historically, it has been one of the most feared of all infectious diseases. Yet, the ability of the smallpox virus (variola virus) to infect and cause disease only in humans and subhuman primates was an important consideration in approaches to control and prevention (i.e., vaccination of the human population).[51] Consideration of the smallpox virus as highly virulent must be tempered by the fact that inoculation studies of this virus into many animal species did not result in infection. In contrast, most *Salmonella* serotypes may cause mild to severe infections in humans and a variety of animal species. A notable exception is *Salmonella typhi,* which causes infections only in humans. Thus, any description of the characteristics for either the agent or the host must be understood in the context of their interrelationship.

AGENT

Any agent or microorganism is of epidemiologic importance if it can be transmitted through the environment, causes infection in a host (either human or animal), and produces clinical disease. These agents, regardless of their classification as bacterial, viral, protozoal, helminthic, or fungal, are considered the first necessary component of the chain of infection. Three characteristics of agents must be considered in terms of their epidemiologic importance[52]: (1) those characteristics of agents that are involved in their spread or transport through the environment, (2) the agent characteristics that are involved in the production of infection, and (3) those characteristics that are involved in the production of disease.

The characteristics of agents involved in spread through the environment vary with the method of transmission. However, regardless of the method of transmission, it is necessary for a minimum number of organisms to survive transport through the environment to reach and enter a susceptible host. For agents that are transmitted by direct person-to-person contact, their ability to survive stressful environmental conditions (such as changes in temperature, humidity, or pH) tends to be minimal. In contrast, agents that are capable of actual multiplication within the environment (i.e., in food products, water, soil, and plants) have a unique advantage for survival. Some agents such as *Legionella pneumophila* or *Bacillus anthracis* do not necessarily multiply within the environment; however, they can survive for months in relatively hostile conditions, including distilled water or soil.[53, 54] For those agents for which humans are the only known reservoir, the longer the time between the likelihood of contact between two susceptible hosts, the greater the resistance that the agent must have to environmental conditions such as heat, drying, ultraviolet light, or dilution by airflow. Finally, some agents have the capacity to infect a nonhuman host such as animals, birds, or an insect vector. Such nonhuman hosts may play an important role in maintenance of the agent in the environment.

The ability of an agent to cause infection or disease has to be considered in the context of host characteristics. For example, an agent is considered to *colonize* a host when its presence in that host does not cause a specific immune response or infection. However, should the relationship between the agent and the host change, such as the introduction of *E. coli* from the gastrointestinal tract into the blood stream, infection can result. These types of infection are known as *endogenous.* If the agent is transported from an external source to the host (*exogenous infection*) and the balance between the agent and host favors the agent, infection usually develops.

Several aspects of the agent-host relationship can be related to the agent. Other aspects must be considered only in the context of both agent and host characteristics. For example, *infectiousness* is a characteristic of an agent that is concerned with the relative ease with which it is transmitted to other hosts. A droplet-spread infection, such as a respiratory virus, tends to be more infectious than an infection transmitted by direct contact, such as a sexually transmitted disease. Characteristics of the portals of exit and entry are thus determinants of infectiousness, as is the agent's ability to survive away from the host. Some factors that are often ascribed to an agent are actually the result of both agent and host characteristics. These factors include infectivity, pathogenicity, virulence, and antigenicity or immunogenicity.

Infectivity is typically defined as the characteristic of the infectious agent that embodies its capability to enter, survive, and multiply in the host. A measure of infectivity is the *secondary attack rate.* Infectivity is often expressed as the number infected divided by the number susceptible and exposed. A population with an increased number of individuals with compromised specific or nonspecific immune responses may result in a higher proportion of exposed individuals actually becoming infected. For example, individuals who have decreased gastric acidity because of antacid use are at a higher risk for the development of salmonellosis at a lower infectious dose than are those with normal gastric pH.[55]

Pathogenicity is the property of an agent that determines the extent to which overt disease is produced in an infected population.[1] The pathogenicity of an agent is measured by the ratio of the number of persons in whom clinical disease develops to the number of infections. Again, pathogenicity is frequently considered a sole property of the agent; however, host characteristics play an important role in defining pathogenicity. For example, as noted earlier, the ratio of disease to total infections related to HAV varies widely by host age.[50] In general, those agents with the highest levels of pathogenicity possess characteristics that protect them against nonspecific host defenses. In addition, they may elaborate a number of enzymes or toxins or induce host-mediated disease associated with the immune response to the infection.

The *gradient of infection,* or *biologic gradient,* is the range of manifestations of illness in the host as a result of infection with an agent. It extends from death at one extreme to inapparent or subclinical illness at the other. In this regard, *virulence* is frequently used as a quantitative expression of the disease-producing potential of a pathogenic agent. It is defined as the ratio of the number of cases of serious or disability-producing infections among the total number of people infected.[1] When death is the only criterion in determining severity, it is referred to as the *case-fatality rate.*

From an epidemiologic perspective, the virulence of an organism must be viewed in light of the host. For example, the clinical outcome of hepatitis B infection ranging from limited, subclinical infection to the development of acute fulminant hepatitis is related to immune-mediated disease and important genetic factors of the host.[56] Similarly, the severity of tuberculosis is increased among African Americans with host characteristics similar to those of cases in other races.[57] The development of drug resistance among organisms (regardless of the mechanism) is an important consideration related to virulence. Infection that is caused by agents sensitive to a variety of antimicrobial drugs is less likely to cause serious disease if treated in a timely and appropriate manner than is infection caused by a highly resistant organism. With rapidly increasing drug resistance among all groups of infectious agents, this virulence characteristic will become even more important in the future.[58, 59]

Finally, the last characteristic usually ascribed to an agent is *antigenicity* or *immunogenicity.* It is defined as the ability of an agent to produce a systemic or local immunologic reaction in the host.[1] However, this characteristic must also be considered in the context of both agent and host. The antigenicity of an agent is important from a clinical perspective because it is a primary determinant in the host's ability to mount an initial immune response to infection, thus affecting both pathogenicity and virulence. It also determines the host's development of long-term immunity to a specific agent. Thus, it is a critical factor in the assessment and development of vaccines for human and animal use.

In general, the host immune system includes all physiologic mechanisms with the capacity to recognize materials foreign to itself and to neutralize, eliminate, or metabolize them with or without injury to its own tissues.[60] The immune response may be classified into two categories: specific and nonspecific. Specific immune responses depend on exposure to a foreign configuration, including infectious agents and the subsequent recognition of and reaction to that agent. An example of this type of response is the development of both humoral and cell-mediated immunity related to a specific agent.[61] A nonspecific response occurs after initial and subsequent exposure to a foreign antigen, and although selective in differentiating "self" from "nonself," it is not dependent on selective recognition. A number of factors modify the host immune mechanisms, including genetic, age, metabolic, environmental, anatomic, physiologic, and microbial factors.

An example of the complex nature of the interaction between an agent and host can be demonstrated by the relationship between *H. influenzae* type b and the age of the host. Children younger than 2 years do not mount an effective immune response to agents with capsular polysaccharide (i.e., *H. influenzae* type b, *N. meningitidis, Streptococcus pneumoniae*).[62] Polysaccharide antigens are T-cell–independent antigens, in contrast to protein antigens, which induce a T-cell effect. T-cell–independent antigens are poorly handled by children younger than 2 years because of the lack of maturation of their immune system. Thus, efforts were undertaken to develop vaccines for *H. influenzae* in younger children. This approach required that the *H. influenzae* type b polysaccharide be conjugated to various carrier proteins.[27, 62] This combination of polysaccharide and protein has resulted in vaccines with enhanced immunogenicity by inducing a T-cell response in infants. Use of the second-generation *H. influenzae* conjugate vaccines in infants in the United States has resulted in a dramatic decrease in the occurrence of invasive *H. influenzae* type b disease in children in that age group.[63] Similar efforts are under way to develop conjugated polysaccharide vaccines for *N. meningitidis* and *S. pneumoniae.* Because the use of vaccines has proved to be one of the most cost-effective methods of preventing infectious diseases, the need to understand antigenicity in terms of both the agent and host is a high priority.

HOST

As noted in the previous section regarding agent, the characteristics of the host also play an important role in the eventual outcome of an agent-host interaction. Host factors that influence exposure, infection, and disease are summarized in Table 11–2. Factors can be classified into two categories: those that influence exposure and those that influence the likelihood of infection and the occurrence and severity of disease.

All the factors that influence human exposure to an infectious agent depend on contact with sources of infection within the environment or the promotion of person-to-person transmission.[52] The importance of the factors that influence exposure tend to change by host age, culture, geographic residence, season, and family status.

TABLE 11–2 Host Factors That Influence Exposure, Infection, and Disease

Factors that influence exposure
Animal exposure, including pets
Behavioral factors related to age, drug usage, alcohol consumption
Blood or blood product receipt
Child daycare attendance
Closed living quarters: military barracks, dormitories, homeless shelters, facilities for the elderly and mentally handicapped, prisons
Food and water consumption
Familial exposure
Gender
Hospitalization or outpatient medical care
Hygienic practices, including toilet training and hand washing
Occupation
Recreational activities, including sports and recreational injecting drug use
Sexual activity: heterosexual and homosexual, type and number of partners
School attendance
Socioeconomic status
Travel, especially to developing countries
Vector exposure
Factors that influence infection and the occurrence and severity of disease
Age at the time of infection
Alcoholism
Anatomic defect
Antibiotic resistance (agent)
Antibiotic use (host)
Coexisting noninfectious diseases, especially chronic
Coexisting infections
Dosage: amount and virulence of the organism to which the host is exposed
Duration of exposure to the organism
Entry portal of the organism and presence of trauma at the site of implantation
Gender
Genetic makeup, especially influences on the immune response
Immune state at the time of infection, including immunization status
Immunodeficiency (specific or nonspecific): natural, drug induced, or viral (HIV)
Mechanism of disease production: inflammatory, immunopathologic, or toxic
Nutritional status
Receptors for organism on cells needed for attachment or entry of the organism

Adopted from Evans AS, Brachman PS. Bacterial Infections of Humans; Epidemiology and Control. 3rd ed. New York: Plenum; 1998.

Although most of the factors that influence infection and the occurrence and severity of disease are related to the host, the characteristics of both the agent and host, as described by pathogenicity, virulence, and antigenicity, are important. Also, the agent infectious dose, mechanisms of disease production, antibiotic resistance of the infecting agent, and portal of entry contribute to infection and disease status.[52] For most infections, two host factors play a key role in determining the likelihood of clinical illness and the severity of that illness: the immune status of the host and the age at the time of infection. The highest levels of pathogenicity and virulence associated with the agent-host relationship tends to occur very early in life, when immune disease mechanisms are immature, or at an old age, when they may be deteriorating. Finally, genetic factors tend to influence both susceptibility and disease outcome, although they are primarily related to the host immune response to infection.

ROUTES OF TRANSMISSION

Transmission of infectious agents is defined as any mechanism by which an infectious agent is spread through the environment or to another person.[1, 64] These mechanisms can be classified as either direct or indirect.

Of the three different modes of direct agent transmission, the most common mode is associated with direct and immediate transfer of an infectious agent to a receptive portal of entry through which the human infection is established. This type of direct contact transmission occurs in association with touching, kissing, or sexual intercourse or by the direct projection (droplet spread) of droplet spray from an infected host onto the conjunctiva or the mucous membranes of the nose or mouth. Typically, droplet spread is limited to a distance of approximately 1 m. The second type of direct transmission occurs when host susceptible tissue is exposed to the agent, such as by the bite of a rabid animal or when it comes in contact with soil or decaying matter in which the agent usually leads a saprophytic existence (e.g., systemic mycosis). Finally, transplacental transmission is another form of direct transmission.

The three primary mechanisms of indirect agent transmission are vehicle-borne, vector-borne, and airborne. Vehicle-borne transmission occurs when any material serves as an intermediate means by which an infectious agent is transported or introduced into the susceptible host through a suitable portal of entry. These materials may include water; food; biologic products such as blood, serum, plasma, tissues, and organs; and objects (fomites) such as toys, soiled clothing, bedding, or surgical instruments. It is not necessary that the agent multiply or develop in or on the vehicle before it is transmitted.

The second method of indirect transmission is vector-borne. The two different types of vector-borne transmission are mechanical and biologic. Mechanical transmission occurs when an insect carries an infectious agent through the soiling of its feet or proboscis or through carriage in its gastrointestinal tract. Mechanical transmission does not require multiplication or development of the organism. In contrast, biologic vector-borne transmission occurs when propagation (multiplication), cyclic development, or a combination of these events (cyclopropagative) is required before the arthropod can transmit the infected form of the agent to humans.

The third type of indirect transmission is airborne and involves the dissemination of aerosols with infectious agents to a suitable portal of entry in a host, usually the respiratory tract. These aerosols are suspensions of particles in the air that consist partially or wholly of infectious agents. The particles are in the range of 1 to 5 μm. (Note that airborne transmission does not include droplets and other large particles that promptly settle out. As noted earlier, these agents are included under direct transmission.) Some infections transmitted by the airborne route may be carried great distances from their sources, as documented by outbreaks of measles, legionnaires' disease, and anthrax.[65, 66] For this reason, there is particular concern that agents such as anthrax will be used as weapons of mass destruction in a civilian bioterrorism event.[67]

DISEASE PREVENTION AND CONTROL

Individual, Institutional, Community, and Globally Based Strategies

Disease prevention and control activities for infectious agents occur at four levels. The first level is targeted to the individual and is predominantly the domain of the clinician. A variety of prevention activities can be targeted to individuals through their primary care provider. Use of chemoprophylaxis to prevent surgical wound infections is an example of a control measure targeted to the individual. The second level is that of the institution, which is predominantly the domain of the infection-control practitioner or the school health official. This level includes health care facilities, nursing homes, other residential facilities, and schools. Programs to prevent the spread of blood-borne pathogens or tuberculosis to health care workers in hospitals are examples of control strategies targeted at the institutional level. The third level is targeted to the community in general and is predominantly the domain of public health agencies (at the local, state, and national levels). Removal of a contaminated food product from the market is an example of a control measure targeted to the community. Finally, the fourth level is related to global strategies. For a number of important pathogens, it has become clear that global control strategies are critical to have an impact on disease occurrence within the United States. The growing proportion of tuberculosis cases among refugees and immigrants to the United States and ongoing episodes of importation of measles from abroad are two examples pertinent to U.S. disease control in the late 1990s and early 21st century.

Although some control measures are specific to these different levels, a substantial amount of overlap can also occur. For example, immunization programs operate at all four levels. Clinicians play an important role in the health maintenance of their individual patients by providing immunizations against a variety of pathogens. Immunization programs are also an important activity at the institutional level, such as routine annual immunization against influenza in nursing homes and immunization of health care workers against hepatitis B virus. Public health agencies monitor vaccination levels in the community and provide vaccination clinics open to the public. Finally, ensuring that foreign travelers from countries with selected endemic vaccine-preventable diseases are adequately vaccinated before travel is a critical control measure for the prevention of diseases such as measles.

When assessing or developing disease prevention and control activities targeted to infectious diseases, the weakest link in the chain of infection (agent, transmission, host) also needs to be considered for each specific pathogen. In some situations, control of the agent in a specific reservoir may be the best way to reduce disease occurrence. Chlorination of water is an example of destroying an agent in its reservoir or eliminating a possible mode of transmission.

Strategies aimed at the level of transmission need to be tailored to the type of transmission involved. For example, the use of condoms in the prevention of sexually transmitted diseases is a control strategy targeted at preventing contact transmission. Transmission through common vehicles frequently involves food and water and may also involve other vehicles such as blood in the case of transfusions. Irradiation of food and screening blood for infectious agents are control activities targeted to a common vehicle. An example of a control activity targeted to airborne transmission is use of respirators to prevent transmission of tuberculosis in the health care setting. Finally, control of vector-borne transmission can be targeted toward destroying the vector or toward the use of protective clothing and repellents.

In some instances, the best mechanism to prevent disease occurrence is through modification of the host, such as developing or boosting immunity through active or passive immunization. Other examples of control activities targeted to the host include improving nutritional status or providing chemoprophylaxis against a variety of agents.

Assessment of Risk, Feasibility, Cost, and Effectiveness

When disease prevention and control strategies are being developed, several issues need to be considered, including risk, feasibility, cost, and effectiveness. Risk can be defined by the potential for exposure. Epidemiologic studies or analysis of surveillance data can serve to define persons or populations at risk and can also quantify risk within different populations. At the individual level, risk can be evaluated by assessing host characteristics, such as the need for prophylaxis against *Pneumocystis carinii* pneumonia for persons with HIV infection and T-cell depletion.[68] An example of evaluating risk at the institutional level is assessing occupational exposure to infectious agents such as blood-borne pathogens. At the community level, groups at risk for a variety of conditions can be defined by demographic features (such as age, race, country of origin, socioeconomic status, and geographic location). For example, persons born outside the United States are at increased risk for infectious diseases such as tuberculosis or of being chronic carriers of infections such as hepatitis B. Screening programs targeted to these populations with subsequent interventions (such as isoniazid prophylaxis for persons with *M. tuberculosis* infection or immunization of susceptible household contacts of hepatitis B virus carriers) can serve as important community-based strategies to prevent infectious disease occurrence.[69, 70] Another example of defining risk at the community level is assessing behavior that increases the risk for specific diseases, such as injecting drug use as a risk behavior for acquiring HIV or hepatitis C virus infection. Education and drug treatment programs targeted to this population can serve as an important disease prevention and control strategy.

In developing control programs, the feasibility of a strategy also needs to be assessed. Feasibility is dependent on the sociodemographic factors of the population involved. For example, high immunization rates can clearly prevent the occurrence of infectious diseases. In the United States, immunizations should be readily available; however, in the late 1980s, numerous large outbreaks of measles occurred in U.S. inner-city populations because of low immunization rates.[71] A variety of sociodemographic factors contributed to these low rates, such as inadequate access to medical care and other barriers to immunization. Until such barriers are removed and control strategies are developed to specifically target such populations, adequate control of vaccine-preventable diseases in the United States cannot be accomplished.[72]

Cost and the availability of resources also need to be considered when developing control strategies. Adequate water treatment facilities and distribution systems in developing countries would do much to eliminate the spread of cholera. However, in many countries, resources to build and develop such facilities are not available. Consequently, control strategies need to be focused on simpler, less expensive methods such as boiling water or improving water storage in the home.

Finally, control strategies need to be evaluated for their effectiveness. For example, the effectiveness of the control strategy is a critical issue in evaluating ways to curb the HIV epidemic in the absence of vaccination. Evaluation of HIV prevention educational programs or HIV counseling and testing programs is essential in assessing the effectiveness of currently available strategies. Cost-effectiveness models are often used in making recommendations for population-based vaccination programs.[73, 74]

Primary, Secondary, or Tertiary Prevention

Prevention strategies for infectious diseases can be characterized by using the traditional concepts of primary, secondary, or tertiary prevention.[1] *Primary prevention* can be defined as the prevention of infection by personal and community-wide efforts. *Secondary prevention* includes measures available to individuals and the population for detection of early infection and effective intervention. *Tertiary prevention* consists of measures available to reduce or eliminate the long-term impairment and disabilities caused by infectious diseases.

Primary Prevention

A key example of primary prevention is immunoprophylaxis, which can be active or passive. Active immunoprophylaxis involves the administration of all or part of a microorganism (live or inactivated) or a product of that microorganism (such as a toxoid) to alter the host by stimulating an immunologic response aimed at protecting against infection. Live vaccines are often more immunogenic than inactivated vaccines and may require fewer booster doses. Live-attenuated vaccines contain weakened or avirulent viruses or bacteria. They are generally contraindicated in immunocompromised persons. Examples of live-attenuated vaccines include vaccines against measles, mumps, rubella, and yellow fever; oral polio vaccine; oral typhoid vaccine; and Calmette-Guérin bacillus vaccine.[64] Examples of vaccines created from inactivated organisms include inactivated polio vaccine and vaccines against anthrax, influenza, hepatitis B, cholera, pertussis, and rabies.[64] Examples of polysaccharide vaccines include pneumococcal and meningococcal vaccines; *H. influenzae* type b conjugate vaccine is a polysaccharide-protein conjugate.[64] Examples of toxoid vaccines include tetanus, diphtheria, and botulinal toxoids.[64]

Currently, at least four types of active immunization programs are being conducted. The first is routine childhood immunization. Current practices include routine childhood immunization against measles, mumps, rubella, tetanus, diphtheria, pertussis, *H. influenzae* type b, and hepatitis B.[75] In many parts of the world, Calmette-Guérin bacillus vaccine is also given routinely in early childhood. Recently, childhood vaccines have become available to prevent infections caused by HAV, rotavirus, and varicella-zoster virus. As the routine childhood immunization schedule becomes increasingly complex, new methods of vaccine delivery need to be developed. Of particular interest is the development of new multiple-antigen vaccines to simplify the routine schedule and maximize efficiency of vaccine delivery. The goals of routine childhood immunization are twofold: first, to protect the individual and, second, to provide herd immunity, which can be effective in controlling certain diseases at the population level (such as measles, mumps, rubella, and *H. influenzae*.[76] Ongoing adequate surveillance for these diseases is essential to monitor the effectiveness of population-based immunization programs so that strategies can be adapted as needed. The expansion of measles immunization to a two-dose schedule in the United States in 1989 is an example of using surveillance data to revise immunization practices.[77]

A second type of immunization program is travel-related immunization. Examples include the administration of typhoid, yellow fever, Japanese encephalitis, and meningococcal vaccines for travel to areas endemic for these conditions. The third type of program is immunization of selected at-risk populations. For example, influenza vaccine is currently recommended in the United States annually for persons older than 65 years, residents of nursing homes, adults with certain chronic diseases, and children who are receiving long-term aspirin therapy and may be at risk for Reye's syndrome. Pneumococcal vaccine is also recommended for selected high-risk populations, including persons older than 65 years, persons with certain chronic diseases, and persons with certain immunosuppressive conditions. In outbreak settings, community-wide vaccination may be used to protect those at risk of exposure, such as during community outbreaks of serogroup C meningococcal disease.[78]

The final type of immunization program is based on occupational exposure. Recommendations for the immunization of health care workers have been made because of their special risk of exposure to a variety of vaccine-preventable diseases. Examples include immunization of laboratory workers against anthrax, rabies, and botulism in settings in which these organisms are handled and immunization of health care workers against measles and hepatitis B based on exposure to blood-borne pathogens.[79]

In 1998, the first Lyme disease vaccine was licensed in the United States. This vaccine represents a "hybrid" pattern of use; one target group for vaccination includes persons who work outdoors in areas endemic for Lyme disease. However, the larger target group comprises persons who live in endemic areas or who travel to these areas to pursue outdoor recreational activities. The probable protective effect of Lyme disease vaccine is based on inactivation of *Borrelia burgdorferi* in the tick midgut after exposure to antibodies ingested during feeding.[80] Thus, long-term protection depends on maintaining an adequate level of circulating antibodies to *B. burgdorferi.* Preliminary results from vaccine trials and our experience with hepatitis B vaccine suggest that persons older than 60 years may be less likely to acquire or maintain protective antibody levels.[8, 80]

Active immunization is also used in certain postexposure situations, including immunization after exposure to *N. meningitidis,* hepatitis B virus, measles, pertussis, and rabies. Some of these vaccines are given in conjunction with various types of immunoglobulin in the postexposure setting.

Passive immunization involves the administration of preformed antibodies, often to specific agents, after exposure. The broadest form of passive immunization is the use of normal human immune globulin (also referred to as gamma globulin). It is most often used after exposure to HAV and may be effective if given within 14 days after exposure.[70] Normal human immune globulin is also recommended before travel to countries endemic for hepatitis A. It may also be effective in reducing clinical disease in persons exposed to measles if provided within 6 days after exposure.[77] For persons with hypogammaglobulinemia or agammaglobulinemia, it may be given as IgG replacement therapy. Multiple specific types of immune globulin are also used in postexposure settings to prevent infection. Examples include immune globulin specific to hepatitis B virus, cytomegalovirus, rabies, varicella-zoster virus, and tetanus.

A second type of primary prevention is antimicrobial prophylaxis, often referred to as chemoprophylaxis. Use of effective chemoprophylaxis requires that the infectious agent be susceptible to the antimicrobial used. As a primary prevention strategy, it may be used before or after exposure to prevent infection. Examples of chemoprophylaxis in the postexposure setting include exposure to pertussis (e.g., erythromycin), *N. meningitidis* (e.g., rifampin), influenza A virus (e.g., amantadine or rimantadine), and HIV (e.g., zidovudine). Use of antiretroviral drugs by HIV-infected pregnant women has been shown to substantially reduce the risk of perinatal HIV infection.[81] Prophylaxis against surgical wound infections with broad-spectrum coverage before surgery and prophylaxis of neonates against ophthalmia neonatorum are examples of chemoprophylaxis used in the hospital setting. In such situations, chemoprophylaxis is used because a likelihood of exposure to pathogenic organisms is present, even though exposure is not clearly documented. Chemoprophylaxis is also used in anticipation of exposure during travel (such as prevention of malaria through the use of chloroquine or mefloquine), or antimicrobials against enteric pathogens can be used to prevent traveler's diarrhea.

In addition to immunoprophylaxis and chemoprophylaxis, other important primary prevention activities are aimed at the individual, institutional and community levels. Examples have been discussed in earlier sections of this chapter.

Secondary Prevention

Secondary prevention activities traditionally entail chemoprophylaxis and involve the identification of early or asymptomatic infection with subsequent treatment so that such infections are eradicated and sequelae are prevented. Although most secondary prevention programs involve intervention at the individual level through the use of chemoprophylaxis, such programs often operate within the context of a population-based or institutional-based screening effort. Routine screening programs for sexually transmitted diseases such as *Chlamydia* infection are examples of secondary prevention strategies.[82, 83] Contact investigations for partners of persons with sexually transmitted diseases are also part of a secondary prevention strategy focused on those at highest risk of infection (i.e., those with known exposure).[82] Another example of a secondary prevention program using chemoprophylaxis is screening of high-risk populations for tuberculosis infection and subsequent therapy with an antimicrobial such as isoniazid to prevent active disease.

Although most secondary prevention strategies involve chemoprophylaxis (and rarely, immunoprophylaxis), the concept can be broadened to other prevention efforts aimed at intervention and correction of a recognized specific health hazard. Most such efforts occur at the community level. Examples of community-based secondary prevention efforts include the early identification of contaminated products through outbreak investigations and subsequent removal of such products from the market to prevent additional illnesses and restore "the community's health." A boil-water order for a waterborne disease outbreak of cryptosporidiosis is another example of a secondary prevention strategy aimed at correcting an existing community-wide problem.

Tertiary Prevention

Tertiary prevention efforts are measures to eliminate long-term impairment and disabilities from an existing condition. Because most infectious diseases are treatable, tertiary prevention activities are less common than those found with chronic diseases such as hypertension, diabetes, and coronary artery disease. However, this concept is still applicable to the control of infectious diseases inasmuch as some viral infections are chronic and cannot be eradicated. Current treatment of HIV infection, including prophylaxis against other opportunistic agents, is an example of a tertiary prevention activity.

REFERENCES

1. Last JM, ed. A Dictionary of Epidemiology, 2nd ed. New York: Oxford; 1988.
2. Barrett-Connor E. Infectious and chronic disease epidemiology: Separate and unequal? Am J Epidemiol. 1979;109:245–249.
3. Snow J. On the Mode of Communication of Cholera. London: 1855. Reprinted in Frost WH, ed. Snow on Cholera. New York: Commonwealth Fund; 1936.
4. Centers for Disease Control. Follow-up on toxic shock syndrome. MMWR Morb Mortal Wkly Rep. 1980;29:297–299.
5. Osterholm MT, Davis JP, Gibson RW, et al. Tri-state toxic-shock syndrome study. I. Epidemiologic findings. J Infect Dis. 1982;145:431–440.
6. World Health Organization. Global eradication of smallpox. Bull World Health Organ. 1980;58:161–163.
7. Hedberg CW, Savarino SJ, Besser JM, et al. An outbreak of foodborne illness caused by *Escherichia coli* O39:NM, an agent not fitting into the existing scheme for classifying diarrheogenic *E. coli.* J Infect Dis. 1997;176:1625–1628.
8. Wood RC, MacDonald KL, White KE, et al. Risk factors for lack of detectable antibody following hepatitis B vaccination of Minnesota health care workers. JAMA. 1993;270:2935–2939.
9. Bender JB, Hedberg CW, Besser JM, et al. Surveillance for *Escherichia coli* O157:H7 infections in Minnesota by molecular subtyping. N Engl J Med. 1997;337:388–394.
10. Centers for Disease Control and Prevention. Summary of notifiable diseases, United States, 1992. MMWR Morb Mortal Wkly Rep. 1992;41(55):41.
11. Hennekens CH, Burning JE. Epidemiology in Medicine. Boston: Little, Brown; 1987.
12. St Louis ME, Morse DL, Potter ME, et al. The emergence of grade A eggs as a major source of *Salmonella enteritidis* infections. New implications of the control of salmonellosis. JAMA. 1988;259:2103–2107.
13. Hedberg CW, David MJ, White KE, et al. Role of egg consumption in sporadic *Salmonella enteritidis* and *Salmonella typhimurium* infections in Minnesota. J Infect Dis. 1993;167:107–111.
14. Schlesselman JJ, Stolley PD. Case-Control Studies. Design, Conduct, Analysis. New York: Oxford; 1982.
15. The Working Group on Prevention of Invasive Group A Streptococcal Infections. Prevention of invasive group A streptococcal disease among household contacts of case-patients: Is prophylaxis warranted? JAMA. 1998;279:1206–1210.
16. Davies HD, McGeer A, Schwartz B, et al. A prospective, population-based study of invasive group A streptococcal infections, including toxic shock syndrome and the risk of secondary invasive disease. N Engl J Med. 1996;335:547–554.
17. Lilienfeld AM, Lilienfeld DE. Foundations of Epidemiology. 2nd ed. New York: Oxford; 1980.
18. Kelsey JL, Thompson WD, Evans AS. Methods in Observational Epidemiology, v. 10. Monographs in Epidemiology and Biostatistics. New York: Oxford; 1986.
19. Thacker SB, Berkelman RL. Public health surveillance in the United States. Epidemiol Rev. 1988;10:164–190.
20. Chorba TL, Berkelman RL, Saffor SK, et al. Mandatory reporting of infectious diseases by clinicians. JAMA. 1989;262:3018–3026.
21. Centers for Disease Control and Prevention. Recommendations for prevention and control of hepatitis C virus (HCV) infection and HCV-related chronic disease. MMWR Morb Mortal Wkly Rep. 1998;47(RR-19):1–39.
22. Perkins BA, Flood JM, Danila R, et al. Unexplained deaths due to possibly infectious causes in the United States: Defining the problem and designing surveillance and laboratory approaches. Emerg Infect Dis. 1996;2:47–53.
23. Moore M, Onorato IM, McCray E, et al. Trends in drug-resistant tuberculosis in the United States, 1993–1996. JAMA. 1997;278:833–837.
24. Glynn MK, Bopp C, Dewitt W, et al. Emergence of multidrug-resistant *Salmonella enterica* serotype *typhimurium* DT104 infections in the United States. N Engl J Med. 1998;338:1333–1338.
25. Breiman RF, Butler JC, Tenover FC, et al. Emergence of drug-resistant pneumococcal infections in the United States. JAMA. 1994;271:1831–1835.
26. Centers for Disease Control and Prevention. The Foodborne Diseases Active Surveillance Network, 1996. MMWR Morb Mortal Wkly Rep. 1997;46:258–261.
27. Osterholm MT, Rambeck JH, White KE, et al. Lack of efficacy of *Haemophilus* b polysaccharide vaccine in Minnesota. JAMA. 1988;260:1423–1428.
28. Centers for Disease Control and Prevention. Public health: Surveillance, prevention and control of nosocomial infections. MMWR Morb Mortal Wkly Rep. 1992;41:783–787.
29. Williams REO. Changing perspectives in hospital infection. In: Proceedings of the International Conference on Nosocomial Infections. Atlanta: Centers for Disease Control; 1970:1–10.
30. Jenkin GA, Tee W. *Campylobacter upsaliensis*–associated diarrhea in human immunodeficiency virus–infected patients. Clin Infect Dis. 1998;27:816–821.

31. Hennessey TW, Hedberg CW, Slutsker L, et al. A national outbreak of *Salmonella enteritidis* infections from ice cream. N Engl J Med. 1996;334:1281–1286.
32. Mishu B, Blaser MJ. Role of infection due to *Campylobacter jejuni* in the initiation of Guillain-Barré syndrome. Clin Infect Dis. 1993;17:104–108.
33. Moss AR, Osmond D, Bacchetti P, et al. Risk factors for AIDS and HIV seropositivity in homosexual men. Am J Epidemiol. 1987;125:1035–1047.
34. Osmond DH, Charlebois E, Sheppard HW, et al. Comparison of risk factors for hepatitis C and hepatitis B infection in homosexual men. J Infect Dis. 1993;167:66–71.
35. Evans AS, ed. Viral Infections of Humans. Epidemiology and Control. 2nd ed. New York: Plenum; 1982.
36. Weinstock HS, Bolar G, Reingold AL, Polish LB. Hepatitis C virus infection among patients attending a clinic for sexually transmitted diseases. JAMA. 1993;269:392–394.
37. Gwinn M, Pappaioanou M, George JR, et al. Prevalence of HIV infection in childbearing women in the United States. Surveillance using newborn blood samples. JAMA. 1991;265:1704–1708.
38. Centers for Disease Control and Prevention. Multistate outbreak of *Salmonella* serotype *agona* infections linked to toasted oats cereal—United States, April–May 1998. MMWR Morb Mortal Wkly Rep. 1998;47:402–464.
39. Centers for Disease Control and Prevention. Multistate outbreak of listeriosis—United States, 1998. MMWR Morb Mortal Wkly Rep. 1998;47:1085–1086.
40. Herwaldt BL, Ackers ML. An outbreak in 1996 of cyclosporiasis associated with imported raspberries. The Cyclospora Working Group. N Engl J Med. 1997;336:1548–1556.
41. Herwaldt BL, Beach MJ. The return of *Cyclospora* in 1997: Another outbreak of cyclosporiasis in North America associated with imported raspberries. The Cyclospora Working Group. An Intern Med. 1999;130:210–220.
42. Waterhouse B. A Prospect for Exterminating the Smallpox. Cambridge, England: Cambridge; 1800.
43. Tucker WB. The evolution of the cooperative studies in the chemotherapy of tuberculosis of the Veteran's Administration and Armed Forces of the USA: An account of the evolving education of the physician in clinical pharmacology. Adv Tuber Res. 1960;10:1–68.
44. Francis T, Karns RF, Voight RB, et al. An evaluation of the 1954 poliomyelitis vaccine trial: Summary report. Am J Public Health. 1955;45(Suppl):S1–S51.
45. Austin SC, Stolley PD, Lasky T. The history of malariotherapy for neurosyphilis. Modern parallels. JAMA. 1992;268:516–519.
46. Meinert CL. Clinical Trials. Design, Conduct and Analysis, v. 8. Monographs in Epidemiology and Biostatistics. New York: Oxford; 1986.
47. Hadler SC, Erben JJ, Matthews D, et al. Effect of immunoglobulin on hepatitis A in day-care centers. JAMA. 1983;249:48–53.
48. Schwartz B. Preventing the spread of antimicrobial resistance among bacterial respiratory pathogens in industrialized countries: The case for judicious antimicrobial use. Clin Infect Dis. 1999;28:211–213.
49. Berkelman RL, Hughes JM. The conquest of infectious diseases: Who are we kidding? Ann Intern Med. 1993;119:426–428.
50. Hadler SC, Webster HM, Erben JJ, et al. Hepatitis A in day care centers—a community-wide assessment. N Engl J Med. 1980;302:1222–1227.
51. Benenson AS. Smallpox. In: Evans AS, ed. Viral Infections of Humans: Epidemiology and Control. New York: Plenum; 1982:541–568.
52. Evans AS, Brachman PS, eds. Bacterial Infections of Humans: Epidemiology and Control. 3rd ed. New York: Plenum; 1998.
53. Fox M, Kaufmann AF, Zendel SA, et al. Anthrax in Louisiana, 1971: Epizootiologic study. J Am Vet Med Assoc. 1973;163:446–451.
54. Skaliy P, McEachern HV. Survival of the legionnaires' disease bacterium in water. Ann Intern Med. 1979;90:577–580.
55. Black PH, Kunz LJ, Swartz MN. Salmonellosis—a review of some unusual aspects. N Engl J Med. 1960;262:811–816, 846–870, 921–927.
56. Lau JYN, Wright TL. Molecular virology and pathogenesis of hepatitis B. Lancet. 1993;342:1335–1339.
57. Stead WW, Senner JW, Reddick WT, Lofgren JP. Racial differences in susceptibility to infection by *Mycobacterium tuberculosis.* N Engl J Med. 1990;322:422–427.
58. Cohen ML. Epidemiology of drug resistance: Implications for a post-antimicrobial era. Science. 1992;257:1050–1055.
59. Levy SB. Confronting multidrug resistance: A role for each of us. JAMA. 1993;269:1840–1842.
60. Bellanti JA. Immunology II. Philadelphia: WB Saunders; 1978.
61. Nossal GJV. Current concepts: Immunology: The basic components of the immune system. N Engl J Med. 1987;316:1320–1325.
62. Granoff DM, Munson RS Jr. Prospects for prevention of *Haemophilus influenzae* type b disease by immunization. J Infect Dis. 1986;153:448–461.
63. Murphy TV, White KE, Pastor P, et al. Declining incidence of *Haemophilus influenzae* type b since introduction of vaccination. JAMA. 1993;269:246–248.
64. Benenson AS, ed. Control of Communicable Diseases in Man, 16th ed. Washington, DC: American Public Health Association; 1995.
65. Ehresmann KR, Hedberg CW, Grimm MB, et al. An outbreak of measles at an international sporting event with airborne transmission in a domed stadium. J Infect Dis. 1995;171:679–683.
66. Meselson M, Guillemin J, Hugh-Jones M, et al. The Sverdlovsk anthrax outbreak of 1979. Science. 1994;266:1202–1208.
67. Inglesby TV, Henderson DA, Bartlett JG, et al. Anthrax: Civilian medical and public health management following use of a biological weapon. JAMA. 1999;281:1735–1745.
68. Centers for Disease Control. Recommendations for prophylaxis against *Pneumocystis carinii* pneumonia for adults and adolescents infected with human immunodeficiency virus. MMWR Morb Mortal Wkly Rep. 1992;41(RR-4):1–11.
69. American Thoracic Society. Control of tuberculosis in the United States. Am Rev Respir Dis. 1992;146:1623–1633.
70. Centers for Disease Control. Protection against viral hepatitis: Recommendations of the Immunization Practices Advisory Committee. MMWR Morb Mortal Wkly Rep. 1990;39(RR-2):1–26.
71. The National Vaccine Advisory Committee. The measles epidemic: The problems, barriers, and recommendations. JAMA. 1991;266:1547–1552.
72. Shalala DE. Giving pediatric immunizations the priority they deserve. JAMA. 1993;269:1844–1845.
73. Tucker AW, Haddix AC, Bresee JS, et al. Cost-effectiveness analysis of a rotavirus immunization program for the United States. JAMA. 1998;279:1371–1376.
74. Sisk JE, Moskowitz AJ, Whang W, et al. Cost-effectiveness of vaccination against pneumococcal bacteremia among elderly people. JAMA. 1997;278:1333–1339.
75. Peter G, Lepow ML, McCracken GH Jr, Phillips CF, eds. Report of the Committee of Infectious Diseases, 22nd ed. Elk Grove Village, Ill: American Academy of Pediatrics; 1991.
76. Fine PE. Herd immunity: History, theory, practice. Epidemiol Rev. 1993;15:265–302.
77. Centers for Disease Control. Measles prevention: Recommendations of the Immunization Practices Advisory Committee. MMWR Morb Mortal Wkly Rep. 1989;38(S-9):1–13.
78. Centers for Disease Control and Prevention. Control and prevention of meningococcal disease and control and prevention of serogroup C meningococcal disease: Evaluation and management of suspected outbreaks: Recommendations of the Advisory Committee on Immunization Practices (ACIP). MMWR Morb Mortal Wkly Rep. 1997;46(RR-5):1–21.
79. Centers for Disease Control and Prevention. Immunization of health-care workers: Recommendations of the Advisory Committee on Immunization Practices (ACIP) and the Hospital Infection Control Practices Advisory Committee (HICPAC). MMWR Morb Mortal Wkly Rep. 1997;46(RR-18):1–42.
80. Wormser GP, Nowakowski J, Nadelman RB, et al. Efficacy of an OSPA vaccine preparation for prevention of Lyme disease in New York State. Infection. 1998;26:208–212.
81. Centers for Disease Control and Prevention. Public health services task force recommendations for the use of antiretroviral drugs in pregnant women infected with HIV-1 for maternal health and for reducing perinatal HIV-1 transmission in the United States. MMWR Morb Mortal Wkly Rep. 1998;47(RR-2):1–30.
82. Centers for Disease Control. 1993 sexually transmitted diseases treatment guidelines. MMWR Morb Mortal Wkly Rep. 1993;42(RR-14):1–102.
83. Centers for Disease Control and Prevention. Recommendations for the prevention and management of *Chlamydia trachomatis* infections, 1993. MMWR Morb Mortal Wkly Rep. 1993;42(RR-12):1–39.

Chapter 12

Global Epidemiology of Infectious Diseases

STEPHEN M. OSTROFF
JAMES W. LEDUC

One of the most striking achievements of medical science during the 20th century has been the remarkable gains in human life expectancy. In the United States, the average child born at the turn of the century could expect to live for less than 50 years.[1] A similar child born at the close of the century could expect to live for 77 years, and this figure continues to rise.[2] Parallel increases have occurred in most other developed countries, where average life expectancy now approaches or has reached 80 years in many locations.[3] On a global basis, human life expectancy has risen from 48 years in 1955 to 66 years in 1997, a rise of 38% in less than half a century.[3]

These gains in life expectancy have many causes, but one of the major contributors has been reduced morbidity and mortality from infectious diseases. Although the reasons for the declining impact of infectious diseases are themselves multifactorial, three major achievements can be cited. The first factor is improved sanitation and hygienic measures, including safer food from better processing and refrigeration, availability of safe drinking water, and improved waste management and disposal. The second factor is the development and mass delivery of effective vaccines, notably those used to prevent previously common childhood illnesses such as poliomyelitis and measles. The third factor is the discovery and production of safe and effective antimicrobial agents, beginning with the sulfa drugs and penicillins in the 1930s and 1940s.

Trends in tuberculosis in the United States serve to illustrate the changes in infectious disease mortality during the 20th century. In 1900, this disease was the leading cause of death in the United States, accounting for 1 in every 8.8 deaths.[4] In contrast, by 1995 it accounted for only 1341 deaths in the United States, or 1 in every 1726 deaths that occurred.[2, 5] The successful campaign for smallpox eradication, which was completed in 1977, is probably the best demonstration of the present ability to control and prevent infectious diseases worldwide.[6] An attempt to replicate this effort through the global campaign for poliomyelitis eradication has already been successful in the Western Hemisphere, as certified by the World Health Organization (WHO) in 1994.[7]

Despite these successes, infectious diseases remain one of the most significant health problems faced by humans. On a global basis, they remain the leading categorical cause of death. According to WHO statistics, one of every three deaths around the world in 1997 resulted from an infectious or parasitic disease.[3] As impressive as this statistic appears, it actually underestimates the true burden of death from infectious diseases, because many deaths with infectious causes are not included by WHO under the category of infectious and parasitic diseases. Examples are deaths from cancers caused by infection (e.g., hepatocellular carcinoma and cirrhosis from hepatitis B, cervical cancer from human papillomavirus infection, stomach cancer from *Helicobacter pylori* infection), cardiovascular deaths resulting from poststreptococcal rheumatic heart disease, and maternal deaths caused by puerperal sepsis.

The health gains from improved control and prevention of infectious diseases have not been equitably distributed between the developed and developing regions of the world. Approximately 95% of deaths from infectious diseases occur in developing countries, where 43% of deaths are caused by infections, compared with 1% in developed countries.[3] This disparity is clearly illustrated by the marked differences in life expectancy between persons in less developed countries (e.g., 38 years in Sierra Leone, 41 years in Malawi) and those in more developed countries (e.g., 80 years in Japan, 79 years in Switzerland).[3] Many of the infectious diseases responsible for the high mortality in developing countries affect young children disproportionately, further magnifying their societal impact. As a result, this category is among the greatest contributors to disability-adjusted life years around the world.[8]

The developed countries of the world have not escaped the fluctuations of infectious diseases. Declines in infectious disease mortality have slowed, and in some locations deaths from infections are increasing. This is primarily a result of the impact that the human immunodeficiency virus/acquired immunodeficiency syndrome (HIV/AIDS) epidemic has had in many developed countries. Even though it was recognized only in the early 1980s, by 1994 AIDS had became the leading cause of death among men between 25 and 44 years of age in the United States.[9] During this same period (1980 to 1992), overall infectious disease mortality in the United States rose by 58%.[10] Even when AIDS-associated deaths were removed from the mortality data analysis, infectious disease mortality still rose by 22%. Most of this increase occurred among older Americans for reasons that are not entirely understood but may be reflective of increasing longevity and improved ability to manage chronic diseases.

The leading global causes of infectious disease mortality are listed in Table 12–1. This chapter examines the epidemiology of these diseases and syndromes and the etiologic agents responsible for them. Many of these diseases and agents are discussed in greater detail elsewhere in this book. Because of their potential to affect global patterns of morbidity and mortality (as has been the case with HIV/AIDS), infectious diseases that are emerging or reemerging during the 1990s are mentioned here when appropriate.

TABLE 12–1 Global Mortality from Selected Infectious and Parasitic Diseases and Syndromes (1997 Estimates)

Disease	No. of Deaths	Percentage of All Deaths*
Acute lower respiratory infections	3,745,000	7.2
Tuberculosis	2,910,000	5.6
Diarrheal disease	2,455,000	4.7
HIV/AIDS	2,300,000	4.4
Malaria	1,5–2,700,000	2.9–5.2
Measles	960,000	1.8
Hepatitis B	605,000	1.2
Pertussis	410,000	0.8
Neonatal tetanus	275,000	0.5
Dengue fever	140,000	0.3

Abbreviations: AIDS, Acquired immunodeficiency syndrome; HIV, human immunodeficiency virus.
*Based on 52.2 million estimated deaths.
From World Health Organization. The World Health Report, 1998. Geneva: World Health Organization; 1998.

ACUTE RESPIRATORY INFECTIONS

Acute respiratory infections constitute the leading cause of mortality from infectious and parasitic diseases in the world. Each year almost 4 million persons die from respiratory tract infections.[3] This category includes infections of both the upper and lower respiratory tract, including acute pharyngitis, epiglottitis, bronchitis, and pneumonia. Although infection in any of these locations can produce severe illness (e.g., poststreptococcal rheumatic fever, streptococcal toxic shock syndrome), most deaths result from lower respiratory tract infections, particularly pneumonia in children younger than 5 years of age. In this age group, excluding measles and pertussis, more than 90% of deaths from acute respiratory infections are caused by pneumonia.[11] Significant influenza- and pneumonia-associated mortality also occurs in persons older than 65 years of age and in persons with chronic underlying pulmonary disease. In the United States, influenza and pneumonia are the leading causes of infectious disease–related mortality and are the sixth and seventh leading overall causes of death.[2] Pneumonia is also a significant nosocomial problem; it is the second most common infectious complication of hospitalization and the infectious complication most often leading to a fatal outcome.[12, 13]

Infants and young children (<5 years) throughout the world have been estimated to experience between 3 and 11 episodes of acute respiratory tract infection per year, with the highest incidence rates in the first year of life.[14–23] Studies examining the frequency of respiratory tract infections in children suggest that the incidence has remained stable over time and is similar among children in developed and developing countries and among those residing in temperate and tropical climates.[14–23] Despite these similarities, children in developing countries are at far greater risk of a fatal outcome from respiratory tract infections than those in developed countries. Estimates indicate that the risk is more than 30 times higher among such children, and therefore more than 95% of childhood deaths from respiratory tract infections occur in the less developed parts of the world.[11, 14]

Regardless of geographic location, the agents most commonly responsible for acute respiratory tract infections in children are viruses.[11] Respiratory syncytial virus, parainfluenza, adenovirus, and influenza are the viruses most frequently linked to childhood respiratory tract infections.[11] These agents most commonly produce self-limited illness, but they can be an important cause of pneumonia and death; this is especially true for respiratory syncytial virus.[24] Bacterial agents play a major role in acute lower respiratory tract infections and are considered the major reason for high mortality rates among children with pneumonia in the developing world. In this setting, lung puncture studies of children with clinically and radiologically diagnosed pneumonia have consistently demonstrated *Streptococcus pneumoniae*, *Haemophilus influenzae*, and *Staphylococcus aureus* to be the three most commonly isolated bacterial agents.[25] Analysis of nine lung puncture studies of children with pneumonia showed that the proportion of specimens yielding a bacterial pathogen was 63% (range, 21 to 78%).[25] The number of children enrolled in these studies ranged from 18 to 233. Among specimens that were positive for bacterial growth, 38% yielded *S. pneumoniae* (range, 18 to 83%), 37% yielded *H. influenzae* (range, 13 to 85%), and 23% yielded *S. aureus* (range, 0 to 37%). Observed differences among the studies, which were conducted at different times over a period of four decades, may reflect varying study designs, sampling methods, diagnostic criteria, or culture techniques. In a study of bacteremia among children with pneumonia in Pakistan, 36% of 601 blood cultures were positive for bacteria.[26] The most commonly isolated organisms were *S. pneumoniae* (50%) and *H. influenzae* (46%); only one specimen was positive for *S. aureus*. Other blood culture surveys from children with pneumonia have also found a higher proportion of pneumococci than of *H. influenzae* or *S. aureus*.[27, 28] The roles of other bacterial agents known to be major causes of pneumonia in adults in developed countries (e.g., *Chlamydia pneumoniae, Mycoplasma pneumoniae*) have not been well defined as causes of childhood pneumonia in the developing world.

A number of factors have been proposed to explain the increased likelihood that an episode of acute respiratory tract infection will be complicated by pneumonia and the high mortality rate from respiratory tract infections among children in developing countries. Factors associated with the host and the environment are both considered to be important. Low birth weight resulting from prematurity and intrauterine growth retardation[29] and malnutrition[30–32] are host risk factors that have been strongly associated with both an increased risk of pneumonia and fatal outcome from respiratory tract infection; breast-feeding has been shown to be protective.[33] Vitamin A deficiency has been identified as a risk factor for pneumonia in children.[34] However, a placebo-controlled study in Haiti suggested an increased risk of symptoms of respiratory tract infection after routine vitamin A supplementation.[35] Environmental determinants linked to childhood respiratory tract infections and pneumonia include household crowding,[18] smoking within the household,[36, 37] attendance in childcare settings,[36, 38] and environmental pollution,[39–41] particularly use of biomass smoke-producing fuels in the household, although the results of studies in the latter case have not been consistent. It is also possible that such environmental risks simply represent markers for other, undefined factors.

Approaches to control and prevention of childhood pneumonia, particularly in developing countries, are problematic because of difficulties making a definitive diagnosis and determining an etiologic agent. The WHO has devised a simple algorithm that uses detection of fast breathing, chest indrawing, and indicators of severe disease to identify children with pneumonia and those cases that require hospitalization.[42] This algorithm has a high sensitivity for childhood pneumonia but lower specificity and predictive values.[43–45] This design ensures that the children most likely to have pneumonia will receive treatment, specifically inexpensive antimicrobial therapy directed against *S. pneumoniae* and *H. influenzae*. Proper implementation of the WHO strategy has been shown to reduce mortality from childhood pneumonia by 28 to 55%.[46, 47] However, in addition to the need for trained first-line health workers, the success of this strategy depends on knowledge of the patterns of antimicrobial resistance for these two organisms.

Antimicrobial resistance among *S. pneumoniae*, first described in the 1960s in Australia, has now been reported throughout the world.[48] In many geographic areas, the frequency of resistance among pneumococci has risen rapidly during the 1990s.[49–51] The clinical significance of intermediate levels of resistance to penicillin among persons with pneumonia is questionable.[52, 53] There have been reports of high-level resistance being associated with treatment failure,[54] but even this finding has been inconsistent,[52] and prospective studies are difficult to perform because of delays in laboratory confirmation of resistance patterns. In the United States during the 1980s, only 1 (0.02%) of 5459 isolates of pneumococci from normally sterile sites exhibited high-level penicillin resistance.[55] By 1994, this proportion had increased to 3.2%,[56] and in some locations 7% of sterile site isolates were found to have high-level resistance to penicillin.[57] Similar problems exist in other locations in both developed and developing regions of the world. Data from Europe indicate that penicillin nonsusceptibility (intermediate and high-level resistance) has varied from 45% in Spain to 3% in Great Britain.[58] In one Hong Kong hospital, penicillin nonsusceptibility increased from 6.6% to 55.8% of isolates in only 2 years.[59] In Mexico City, 22% of pneumococcal isolates from children with invasive disease were found to have high-level resistance.[60] In other locations, low frequencies of penicillin resistance were found. In one survey in Ethiopia, no penicillin-resistant strains were identified.[61] *H. influenzae* isolates from children with pneumonia have also variably exhibited antimicrobial resistance.[62–64] As demonstrated in these examples, resistance patterns are highly variable, possibly reflecting different patterns of antimicrobial use and other, undefined factors. Local patterns of resistance must be understood for proper selection of therapy.

It is also important to define the serotype distribution among disease-causing *S. pneumoniae* and *H. influenzae* in order to define the potential utility of vaccines as a preventative strategy for childhood pneumonia and development of antimicrobial resistance. Between 34 and 94% of *H. influenzae* isolated from cultures taken from children with pneumonia were found to be non–type B, and a significant proportion were nontypable, suggesting a limited role for *H. influenzae* type B vaccine to prevent childhood pneumonia.[11] Currently available polyvalent polysaccharide pneumococcal vaccines are poorly immunogenic in children younger than 2 years old, the age group at highest risk of pneumonia-related mortality. However, it is important to define pneumococcal serotype distributions, which are known to vary geographically and temporally,[65] to aid in the formulation of conjugated pneumococcal vaccines that are under development, because the number of serotypes that can be included in these vaccines is lower than in the current 23-valent polysaccharide vaccine.[66, 67]

DIARRHEAL DISEASE

Diarrheal disease is the other non–disease-specific category of infectious diseases listed among the leading causes of death in the world. It accounted for slightly fewer than 2.5 million deaths in 1997.[3] Diarrheal disease affects all geographic locations and age groups, but, as with the pattern of mortality from acute respiratory tract infections, the greatest burden of severe illness and death falls on infants and young children in developing nations. Estimates indicate that more than 80% of all diarrheal disease deaths occur among children younger than 5 years of age in developing countries.[3] Diarrheal disease is among the leading causes of morbidity, with 4 billion acute episodes estimated to occur on an annual basis, and up to 10% of these resulting in persistent illness (>2 weeks).[68] Nonfatal diarrheal disease is also more common in the developing parts of the world than in developed areas. Studies among children in these settings have found a range of 1 to 10 episodes of diarrhea per year, with most finding 3 to 5 episodes per year.[68–72] In comparison, children in the developed parts of North America typically experience one to two diarrheal episodes annually.[68]

There are three principal ways in which the pathogens that produce diarrhea are transmitted. These are foodborne transmission, waterborne transmission, and person-to-person transmission. Although it has been difficult to perform systematic studies demonstrating the relative importance of these transmission patterns in different settings, they are likely to vary in importance between developed and developing countries. The pathogens that cause diarrheal illness also differ in their modes of transmission. For example, nontyphoidal

Salmonella species are principally transmitted through food, *Shigella* species are mainly transmitted in person-to-person fashion, and *Cryptosporidium parvum* is principally waterborne. Determining the patterns of pathogen distribution can provide a surrogate marker for the importance of different modes of transmission in a given location.

However, the causes of diarrheal disease do not remain static over time, even in a single location. Fluctuations may result from the introduction of a new organism, recognition of a new agent, or changing levels of sanitation. Such was the case when classic cholera was reintroduced into Latin America. Human illness from cholera had not been recognized in South America during the 20th century, but in January 1991, cases were identified in coastal Peru.[73] Within weeks, thousands of cases were occurring, and cholera quickly became the most commonly diagnosed cause of diarrheal illness in many parts of Peru.[74–76] Over the next 3 years, the disease spread throughout mainland South and Central America, significantly altering the distribution patterns of etiologic agents of diarrheal disease.[75] The international movement of foods can also alter the spectrum of diarrheal pathogens. In 1996, thousands of cases of cyclosporiasis, caused by the parasitic agent *Cyclospora cayetanensis,* occurred in the United States and Canada among persons who consumed fresh raspberries imported from Guatemala.[77] Before this episode, only small numbers of persons with cyclosporiasis had been recognized in North America, and these cases were mainly associated with travel to developing countries.[78]

Vibrio cholerae O139 is an example of a newly recognized pathogen that has had a significant impact on the distribution of agents producing diarrheal disease. This organism was first detected in South Asia in 1992, and it quickly spread to many regions of India and Bangladesh.[79–81] Studies conducted in Bangladesh suggested that shortly after its introduction *V. cholerae* O139 became the most common agent linked to cholera in that country, although this shift does not appear to have been sustained.[82] *Escherichia coli* O157:H7 is a newly recognized pathogen that has affected pathogen distribution patterns in the developed parts of the world.[83] First observed in the United States in 1982, in many locations in North America this foodborne agent rapidly became recognized as the most common cause of bloody diarrhea.[84] It has since become the fourth most commonly isolated bacterial agent of diarrheal disease in the United States.[84] Shigellosis is an example of a disease with rapid emergence in areas with disrupted sanitation. Along with cholera, it has been a common problem in areas with social disruption as a result of war, especially when large numbers of refugees have lacked access to water and sanitary services.[85–87]

Because the pathogens responsible for diarrheal disease vary over time even in the same location, longitudinal studies are important to define the etiology of diarrheal disease. Data from studies of the causes of acute diarrheal illness among young children in developing countries suggest that the most common etiologic agents are rotavirus, enterotoxigenic *E. coli*, and *Shigella* species.[68] Their relative importance is difficult to determine because findings have varied depending on the population studied, the types of specimens collected, which pathogens were tested for, and which detection methods were used. Rotavirus infects all age groups, but most cases involving severe illness and hospitalization occur in children younger than 2 years of age, in whom it often produces dehydrating diarrhea.[88–90] Infants are vulnerable to the complications of diarrhea, particularly dehydration, and rotavirus has been estimated to cause up to 30% of acute diarrheal deaths.[89] Two studies in the developing world found this agent in less than 20% of acute diarrheal episodes in children younger than 5 years of age.[91, 92] In these same studies, pathogenic forms of *E. coli* were found in less than 15% of episodes, and *Shigella* species accounted for between 6% and 13% of episodes. Because bacterial dysentery produced by *Shigella* species is severe and can be accompanied by the complication of hemolytic-uremic syndrome in children infected with *Shigella dysenteriae* type 1, the impact of shigellosis as a cause of diarrheal morbidity and mortality in developing countries is substantial.[93, 94] Other agents that are increasingly appreciated as important causes of diarrheal disease among children in developing countries are *Campylobacter jejuni/coli* and *Campylobacter parvum*, although these agents have not been as well studied.[95–98]

Rotavirus is also an important cause of childhood diarrhea and hospitalization in developed countries, with four out of five children in the United States experiencing this infection by the age of 5 years and an estimated 55,000 annual hospitalizations.[89] In the early 1990s, it was estimated that 5.2 per 1000 children younger than 5 years of age in England and Wales were hospitalized with rotavirus-associated illness during a 1-year period.[99] Among both children and adults in developed countries, viral agents, particularly small round structured viruses, including Norwalk-like agents, are among the most common causes of diarrhea.[100, 101] Systematic studies in the United States indicate that, among the bacterial diarrhea pathogens, *C. jejuni/coli* is the most common agent, followed by nontyphoidal *Salmonella* species, *Shigella*, and *E. coli* O157:H7.[84] Although this distribution is similar in other developed countries, serotypes other than O157:H7 can be the predominant form of Shiga-toxin producing *E. coli* in other locations.[102, 103] These findings suggest that foodborne sources are an important cause of diarrheal disease in the developed world, because all but *Shigella* species are transmitted principally from foods. Notifiable disease data demonstrate trends in the occurrence of these pathogens but severely underestimate their incidence. As an example, 45,970 cases of salmonellosis were reported in the United States in 1995, but calculations suggest that almost 2 million cases of this infection occur each year.[104, 105] The role of waterborne parasites, particularly *C. parvum*, is underappreciated in developed countries.[106]

Antimicrobial resistance has developed among many of the major diarrheal bacterial pathogens. In sub-Saharan Africa, *S. dysenteriae* has become resistant to multiple drugs, with strains that are resistant to all commonly available antimicrobial agents except the fluoroquinolones.[86] These multiple-drug–resistant strains have caused major disease outbreaks with high mortality in refugee settings.[86] In the United States, sequential surveys have documented increasing levels of resistance among *Salmonella* isolates from humans. In 1979–1980, a total of 17% of *Salmonella* isolates were found to exhibit antimicrobial resistance.[107] By 1989–1990, this proportion had risen to 31%, with 25% of strains demonstrating multiple-drug resistance.[108] In a 1997 national survey that used different methodology, a total of 34% of *Salmonella* strains were drug resistant, including 27% that were resistant to multiple drugs.[109] *Salmonella typhimurium* DT104 was first recognized in Great Britain in 1984 and is now the second most commonly isolated *Salmonella* subtype from humans in that country.[110] It was first recognized in the United States in 1985; although it did not appear to have become widespread until the late 1990s, it is now thought to produce more than 25% of all *S. typhimurium* infections.[111] This organism is invariably resistant to five antimicrobial agents, and 14% of isolates from Great Britain have also exhibited resistance to fluoroquinolone drugs.[112] Fluoroquinolone resistance among *C. jejuni/coli* strains causing human disease also appears to be increasing.[113] The use of antimicrobial agents as growth promoters in animals is thought to contribute to the rising levels of resistance among foodborne zoonotic pathogens, but other factors are also likely to be responsible.

The global patterns of diarrheal disease are constantly evolving. Vaccines have been licensed or are under development to prevent illness from rotavirus infection and enterotoxigenic *E. coli*.[114, 115] These vaccines have the potential to decrease the burden of diarrheal disease in the developing world. Food production practices are changing, with greater volumes of fresh fruits and vegetables grown in the developing world for export to developed countries. This practice has resulted in the transfer of agents such as *C. cayetanensis* and *V. cholerae* on exported products, a process that is likely to continue.[77, 116] Changes in food distribution practices increase the potential for widespread, multinational disease outbreaks.[117] Climate change, which has been reported to affect the spread of cholera; the increasing populations of immunocompromised persons, who have a different spectrum of pathogens responsible for diarrheal illness; and increasing global travel all can affect future trends in diarrheal disease in ways that may be difficult to predict.

SPECIFIC DISEASES

The eight other leading causes of global infectious disease mortality are specific etiologic agents that are described in greater depth elsewhere in this book. This section discusses factors that are relevant to their global epidemiology.

Tuberculosis

Mycobacterium tuberculosis is responsible for more deaths around the world than any other infectious agent, accounting for almost 3 million deaths annually.[3] These fatalities are mostly from a pool of more than 7 million new cases of tuberculosis per year and a prevalence of almost 16 million persons with active tuberculosis, half of whom have significant disability as a result of their disease.[3, 118] The global epidemiologic patterns of tuberculosis have changed as a result of the AIDS epidemic and development and spread of multiple-drug–resistant strains of *M. tuberculosis*.[119] New strategies to control tuberculosis, especially directly observed therapy, raise the potential to affect tuberculosis epidemiology in a positive way.[120]

In the developed countries of the world, illness and death from tuberculosis declined dramatically throughout much of the 20th century. These declines predated the availability of antituberculosis drugs, beginning in the 1940s with streptomycin, and probably were a result of improved living conditions and decreasing opportunity for exposure.[121] Antituberculosis therapy increased the slope of the decline, which in the United States averaged 6% per year until the mid-1980s to a nadir of 22,201 new cases in 1985.[104, 122] Tuberculosis incidence then began to increase, primarily because of the dismantling of the tuberculosis control infrastructure, the impact of HIV infection, and multiple-drug resistance of *M. tuberculosis*. By 1992, the annual number of new cases in the United States had increased by 20% to 26,673 persons.[104] Similar trends were observed in western European countries (Spain, 28% increase between 1990 and 1992; Italy, 27% increase between 1988 and 1992; Netherlands, 19% increase between 1987 and 1992).[123] Implementation of directly observed therapy has substantially increased therapeutic compliance and reduced the occurrence of disease transmission. By 1997, the number of new cases of tuberculosis reached a new low of 19,855 persons in the United States.[124] During this period, the epidemiologic patterns of tuberculosis were also in transition. Between 1986 and 1993, the number of new cases in the United States that occurred in persons born outside of the country increased from 22% to 30%; by 1997, this proportion had increased to 40%.[124, 125]

In the developing world, the tuberculosis situation is very different. In many locations, one third or more of the population is infected with tuberculosis (compared with 6% in the United States), and incidence rates of newly diagnosed tuberculosis are higher than 300 cases per 100,000 population in parts of Africa.[123, 126] HIV infection is known to be the strongest risk factor for the progression of tuberculosis infection to active disease. In non–HIV-infected persons infected with tuberculosis, the cumulative lifetime risk of active disease ranges between 5% and 10%.[122] In contrast, HIV-infected persons have a 10% annual risk of progression to active tuberculosis.[127] In areas of the world with rapid escalation of HIV prevalence, the impact on the occurrence of active tuberculosis has been dramatic. One study of data from sub-Saharan Africa demonstrated that tuberculosis rates were declining by 1.6% per year before 1985 but since then have increased by 7.7% annually.[128] In one city in Thailand, the proportion of tuberculosis patients who were HIV positive increased from 1.5% to 45.5% in only 4 years.[129] Estimates suggest that there are more than 5 million persons co-infected with tuberculosis and HIV in the developing world, largely in sub-Saharan Africa (3.8 million persons) and Asia (1.15 million persons).[118, 119, 127] Because HIV infection rates are rising rapidly in some areas of Asia, these numbers are likely to be underestimates today. Tuberculosis rates are also rapidly rising in areas of the former Soviet Union. Between 1990–1991 and 1993, the notification rate in Russia increased from 34 to 42.9 cases per 100,000 population.[130] In some populations in Russia, the rate of active disease is estimated to be as high as 10%. Because HIV infection is not currently widespread in this region, other explanations, including deterioration in the public health infrastructure and economic disruption, have been suggested to account for the increases in tuberculosis.[130]

Molecular subtyping of *M. tuberculosis* isolates using restriction fragment length polymorphisms (RFLPs) has contributed to the understanding of patterns of tuberculosis transmission.[131] Studies in hospital and community settings in developed countries have shown surprisingly consistent findings. A representative sample of these studies is shown in Table 12–2.[132–137] The ratio of individual RFLP patterns to enrolled patients was 0.66:1 (range, 0.59:1 to 0.8:1), with one "cluster" of patterns for every 10.4 persons enrolled (range, 8.7 to 13.8 persons). A cluster was defined as at least two matching RFLP patterns during the study period. Despite different settings and enrollment methods, these studies concluded that between 29% and 40% of all newly diagnosed cases of tuberculosis were caused by recent transmission. These figures are higher than had previously been suspected for locations thought to have effective control programs. They can be used as baselines to monitor the impact of improved tuberculosis control. Studies conducted in developing countries have shown less diversity of RFLP patterns than in developed countries.[138, 139] Although this suggests higher levels of recent transmission, selection bias in the specimens that were tested could also explain some of these findings. Other studies in developing countries have found transmission patterns similar to those in developed countries.[140, 141]

Drug resistance in tuberculosis, particularly resistance to the first-line bactericidal agents isoniazid and rifampin, has become a major

TABLE 12–2 Findings of Selected Epidemiologic Studies of Molecular Subtyping of *Mycobacterium tuberculosis* Isolates Using Restriction Fragment Length Polymorphisms (RFLP)

Study Location and Time Frame (Reference)	Study Type	No. of Patients or Isolates	RFLP Patterns*		Clusters†		Percent Recent‡
			No.	Ratio	No. (Range)	Ratio	
San Francisco 1991–1992[132]	PB	473	324	0.7:1	44 (2–30)	10.8:1	40
New York City 1991[133]	PB	429	252	0.6:1	31 (2–17)	13.8:1	37
Arkansas 1992–1993[136]	PB	235	148	0.6:1	24 (2–7)	9.8:1	33
Amsterdam 1992–1995[134]	PB	459	298	0.6:1	53 (2–29)	8.7:1	35
Seville 1993–1995[135]	H	175	128	0.7:1	19 (2–8)	9.2:1	38
Prague 1995[137]	PB	75	60	0.8:1	7 (2–6)	10.7:1	29

*Number of RFLP patterns per patient/isolate.
†Number of patients/isolates per cluster.
‡Percent of infections thought to result from recent tuberculosis transmission based on the number of clusters and number of isolates per cluster.
Abbreviations: H, Hospital based; PB, population based.

concern throughout the world.[142–144] The Global Tuberculosis Program of the WHO has summarized published data on patterns of drug resistance.[145] The findings of this survey for primary drug resistance (resistance in cases of newly diagnosed tuberculosis) are shown in Figure 12–1. These findings require cautious interpretation because the individual studies used different methodologies and were variably representative of the population in the study area. In general, levels of acquired drug resistance (resistance in cases of previously diagnosed and treated disease) were higher than those of primary drug resistance. The rates of primary multiple-drug–resistant tuberculosis (resistance to at least isoniazid and rifampin) around the world ranged from 0 to 11% (median, 0.5%), but high rates of acquired multiple-drug–resistant disease were found in several areas (Nepal, 48%; Gujarat, India, 33%; New York City, 30%). However, the levels of drug resistance in New York City have declined, a finding that probably reflects strengthened control programs and wider use of directly observed therapy.[146] Between 1991 and 1994, overall isoniazid resistance decreased from 26% to 18%, multiple-drug resistance decreased from 19% to 13%, and any drug resistance in newly diagnosed disease decreased from 22% to 13%. Because drug resistance increases the likelihood of a poor therapeutic outcome and increases the potential for ongoing transmission,[147] these improvements have had a great impact on overall disease incidence in New York, which declined by 50% from 4574 new cases in 1992 to 2265 cases in 1997.[124]

Malaria

Malaria is a disease that was considered a target for eradication as recently as the 1960s.[148] However, today malaria is one of the most common causes of global mortality, accounting for an estimated 1.5 to 2.7 million deaths and up to 500 million new cases per year.[3, 149] Although the other diseases and syndromes discussed in this chapter occur throughout the world, malaria is a mosquito-borne disease with transmission occurring mainly in tropical areas, amplifying its impact on mortality and morbidity in these regions.[149–152] Malaria can be transmitted outside of its usual range when the parasite is introduced into local mosquito populations via international commerce or travel.[153] However, in more recent episodes transmission has not been sustained even in locations that were formerly endemic for malaria.

Four species of *Plasmodium* are capable of producing malaria in humans: *P. falciparum*, *P. vivax*, *P. malariae*, and *P. ovale*. All are transmitted to humans by *Anopheles* species mosquitoes. The first two species cause most cases of human malaria. Although vivax malaria occurs more frequently than falciparum malaria, the latter is considered the greater public health concern because of its more severe clinical manifestations and association with mortality. According to WHO data from 1994, a total of 100 countries reported varying degrees of indigenous malaria transmission, with infection by *P. falciparum* (in addition to other species) reported in 92 countries and 8 reporting only *P. vivax* transmission.[150] *P. falciparum* causes more than 90% of all the malaria infections in sub-Saharan Africa and Haiti and more than two thirds of infections in Southeast Asia. *P. vivax* infections predominate in Central America, most malarious areas of South America, and the Indian subcontinent but are rare in Africa owing to genetic factors that inhibit red blood cell invasion by the parasite.[154] Vivax malaria has also become a problem in some areas of the former Soviet Union, including the Caucasus region and the central Asian republics.[152, 155, 156] *P. ovale* infection is limited to small foci in sub-Saharan Africa and Papua New Guinea, whereas *P. malariae* occurs in low frequencies in many of the areas with endemic malaria transmission.

As a result of eradication efforts during the 1950s and 1960s, which largely consisted of vector control and chemotherapy, malaria incidence fell, particularly in temperate zones and some island nations, and the disease was eliminated in Europe, the Asian former Soviet Union, the United States, and most of the Caribbean.[157] On cessation of eradication efforts, the disease rebounded in frequency

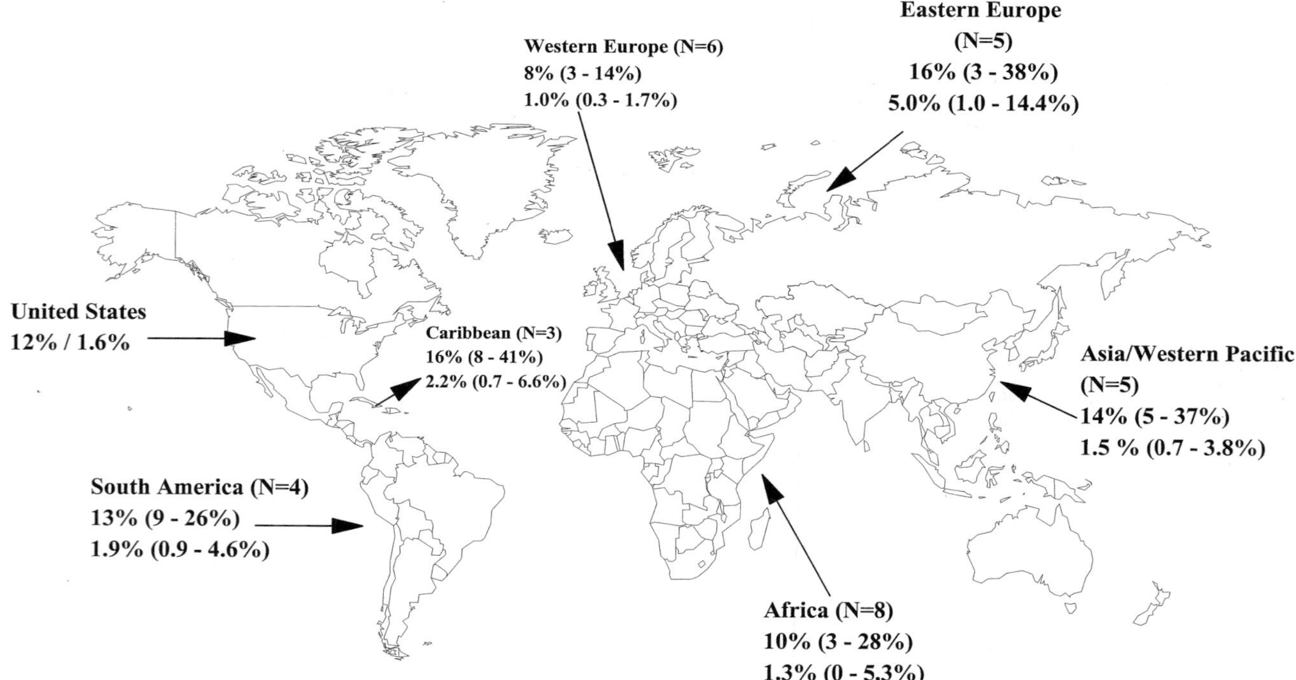

FIGURE 12–1. Patterns of primary drug resistance among *Mycobacterium tuberculosis* isolates by geographic region. N equals the number of countries with data per region. The first value for each region represents the percent of isolates with any primary drug resistance and the lowest and highest percentage among the countries in that region. The second value is the percent of isolates with primary multidrug resistance (resistance to at least isoniazid and rifampicin) and the range among the countries in that region. (Figure adapted from data published in Pablos-Mendez A, Raviglione MC, Laszlo A, et al. Global surveillance for antituberculous-drug resistance, 1994–1997. N Engl J Med. 1998; 338:1641–1649.)

and geographic extent.[157] According to WHO, during the 10 years between 1985 and 1994 the number of reported cases almost doubled, from slightly more than 18 million to almost 35 million.[150] Most of the increase occurred in Africa, which reported 27 million (77%) of these cases. These numbers, which reflect only reported cases and represent less than 10% of the estimated global burden of 300 to 500 million cases, have fluctuated on an annual basis owing to variable disease surveillance and reporting. It is estimated that the most intense malaria transmission occurs in sub-Saharan Africa, where more than 90% of malaria deaths occur. These deaths, caused by *P. falciparum*, occur mostly among children younger than 5 years of age; significant morbidity and mortality also occurs among pregnant women, especially during the first pregnancy.[158, 159] These patterns reflect the role of partial immunity, which develops from repeated exposure to the parasite in areas of intense disease transmission.[160, 161] In areas of less intense or intermittent malaria exposure partial immunity either does not develop or is not sustained, and all age groups can be affected by the disease. Areas with less intense transmission also have a higher potential for malaria outbreaks, as has been the case in highland areas of eastern Africa.[162]

The reemergence of malaria has several explanations. The expansion of human populations in tropical locations is one factor; ineffective or absent vector control programs is another.[157] Climate change may also play a role.[163] However, the evolution of drug resistance, particularly among *P. falciparum* parasites, is probably the most critical problem in malaria treatment and control.[157, 164, 165] Chloroquine was extensively used for treatment and mass prophylaxis during the malaria eradication campaigns, and by the early 1960s resistance was recognized in both South America and Thailand.[166] It took almost 2 decades for chloroquine-resistant strains to reach eastern Africa, but once they appeared in 1978 they spread steadily to all areas of the continent.[167] At present, chloroquine-resistant *P. falciparum* has been recognized in all parts of the world where the parasite occurs except for small foci in Egypt and Central America.[150] *P. falciparum* resistance has developed similarly with other antimalarial agents, including pyrimethamine, quinine, sulfadoxine-pyrimethamine (Fansidar), mefloquine, and more recently introduced agents such as halofantrine.[168] Resistance to these agents has risen rapidly after their introduction, particularly in locations in Southeast Asia, where multiple-drug–resistant strains of *P. falciparum* are present with few therapeutic options.[169] Because resistance patterns are highly variable, information on local patterns of resistance is vital. Despite the high levels of chloroquine resistance in Africa, the drug remains widely used, both because of its antipyretic effect and because of the lack of inexpensive, readily available alternatives.[150] Chloroquine resistance is a more recent phenomenon among *P. vivax* species, being first documented in 1989 in Papua New Guinea.[170] Even where it occurs the prevalence is low, and the drug has remained the therapeutic agent of choice for this pathogen. Chloroquine-resistant *P. vivax* is currently most common in Southeast Asia and in South America. Because the malaria parasite has consistently demonstrated its ability to develop drug resistance, and the vector to develop insecticide resistance,[171] other strategies will be necessary to control this disease. Insecticide-impregnated bed nets have been shown to reduce the incidence of malaria in areas of intense transmission when used appropriately.[172] The WHO has developed algorithms for malaria that seek to ensure children with the disease are treated while minimizing inappropriate antimalarial chemotherapy.[173] Although efforts to develop antimalarial vaccines have been disappointing, renewed interest has now been expressed.[174, 175]

As a result of international travel, commerce, and migration, malaria infection has remained a problem in most developed countries even though sustained indigenous transmission no longer occurs. In the United States, between 1000 and 1500 cases have been reported annually.[104] Approximately half of these cases occur in U.S. citizens who have traveled abroad, and the remainder are in persons from areas with malaria transmission who are visiting the United States.[176] During 1993–1994, infections caused by *P. vivax* were slightly more common (49%) than those caused by *P. falciparum* (37%). The most common source countries for *P. vivax* diagnosed among civilians in the United States are India, Honduras, and Guatemala; for *P. falciparum* the most common sources are Nigeria, Ghana, and India.[176, 177] Information collected from ill persons suggests that many cases occur among foreign-borne persons residing in the United States during a visit to their country of origin. In such persons, existing immunity may have waned since they relocated to the United States.

Measles, Neonatal Tetanus, Pertussis, and Hepatitis B

Although each of these diseases has different global epidemiologic features, they are considered together because all use vaccines as a primary prevention strategy. For tetanus, the first effective toxoids became available in the 1930s; vaccines for pertussis were developed in the 1940s; for measles, an effective live-attenuated vaccine became available in the 1960s; and the serum-derived vaccine for hepatitis B became available in the 1980s. These vaccines have had a marked impact on the distribution of disease where they have been effectively used. In the United States, during the decade in which measles vaccination became routine, measles incidence declined 10-fold, from 441,703 cases in 1960 to 47,351 cases in 1970.[104] It reached a record low of 138 cases in the United States in 1997.[178] Despite the availability of vaccines, however, these diseases remain among the leading global causes of death. This suggests that the benefits of the vaccines have not yet reached all parts of the world even though global mortality from these diseases has been declining.

Measles. In the prevaccine era, almost 2.5 million children died from measles annually. This figure has been reduced to less than 1 million children through vaccination programs, with almost all of these deaths occurring in the developing countries of the world, particularly countries in Africa, which account for 50% of measles deaths.[179] It has been estimated that more than 90% of the susceptible population must be adequately immunized against measles to interrupt transmission of this highly contagious virus, although outbreaks have been seen even with high levels of population immunity.[180] At present, the estimated global coverage of measles vaccine in children older than 1 year of age is 81%.[181] In some areas, higher levels have not been attained because of inadequate vaccination programs. There are 19 countries in which measles vaccine coverage is less than 50%, and 16 of these countries are in Africa.[179] In many developing countries, measles vaccine is administered to children at 9 months of age, when the immune response is not as vigorous as in older children.[182] This policy does protect younger children from measles infection, but it creates lower population immunity, forming a cohort for ongoing transmission of disease unless a second dose of vaccine is given later in life. This phenomenon in part explains the outbreaks of measles in older age cohorts in Brazil in 1997.[179] Despite these problems, substantial progress has been made in reducing measles incidence and complications. In 1994, the Pan American Health Organization targeted measles for hemispheric elimination by the year 2000,[183] and other experts have considered measles a global disease eradication target.[182]

Neonatal tetanus. Neonatal tetanus elimination was endorsed by the World Health Assembly in 1989, and progress has been made in controlling this disease.[184] As recently as 1994, almost 500,000 cases were estimated to occur in the developing countries of the world; this number is now lower than 300,000 cases as a result of improved vaccination programs.[185] However, neonatal tetanus is estimated to cause 23 to 73% of neonatal deaths in developing countries.[186] Efforts to control this disease concentrate on ensuring that women of childbearing age have received at least two doses of tetanus toxoid and ensuring that delivery and cord-handling practices are sanitary.[186] In Egypt, adoption of such practices resulted in an 85% decrease in reported cases of neonatal tetanus[187]; improvements have also been seen in other locations.[188] However, even among women attending prenatal clinics in developing countries, many fail to received tetanus immunization.[189] In 39% of countries surveyed, fewer than 75% of prenatal attendees received the vaccine.

Pertussis. Pertussis remains a problem throughout the world, although most fatalities from this disease occur among infants in developing countries who are too young to have received a full series of vaccinations.[190] The organism is highly contagious, and, as with measles, high levels of population immunity (>90%) must be achieved to interrupt transmission.[190] The critical role of adolescents and adults with inadequate or waning immunity in the epidemiology of pertussis, particularly as reservoirs for transmission to young children, has now been appreciated.[191, 192] Studies have suggested that up to 26% of episodes of acute cough illness of at least 7 days' duration in adults may represent pertussis infection.[193, 194] With the availability of acellular pertussis vaccines, the possibility of booster doses in adults to reduce the burden of disease in both children and adults has been raised.[194–196]

Hepatitis B. The global epidemiology of hepatitis B differs from that of the other vaccine-preventable diseases. This infection occurs throughout the world and causes substantial morbidity and mortality in both developed and developing countries, although its epidemiologic features are different in the two settings. In developing countries, most hepatitis B transmission occurs during the perinatal period and in early childhood (≤5 years), when the risk of chronic infection and subsequent hepatocellular carcinoma is highest.[197–202] The prevalence of chronic infection varies in these countries, but it is highest (>8%) in Southeast Asia, China, the Pacific Island nations, and Africa. Intermediate levels of infection (2 to 7%) are seen in parts of the former Soviet Union, South Asia, Central America, and the northern zones of South America, and developed countries generally have a prevalence of less than 2%.[197–201, 203] Among the estimated 350 million hepatitis B carriers, more than 75% are thought to reside in the western Pacific and Southeast Asia.[197]

In developed countries such as the United States, where perinatal transmission is low, the major risk factors for hepatitis B transmission include injection drug use and sexual transmission (both heterosexual and homosexual); household contact and transmission in the health care setting account for less than 5% of cases.[204] Because of these risk factors, most hepatitis B transmission occurs in teenagers and adults, when the risk of chronic infection is lower (<10%). Mortality from hepatitis B results from the sequelae of chronic infection, which include both hepatocellular carcinoma and cirrhosis. In India, hepatitis B is linked to 60% of cases of hepatocellular carcinoma and 80% of cases of cirrhosis of the liver.[200] In 1992, the World Health Assembly endorsed the concept of universal infant immunization for hepatitis B.[205] Infant immunization has been shown to reduce the prevalence of chronic infection by 80 to 90% and has been shown to reduce the frequency of hepatocellular carcinoma in Taiwanese children by 50%.[206–208] However, in most parts of the developing world, hepatitis B vaccination has not yet been incorporated into routine vaccination activities.

Human Immunodeficiency Virus

HIV infection represents the most significant emerging infectious disease of the late 20th century throughout the world. In the United States, HIV became the most common cause of death among persons between the ages of 25 to 44 years in slightly more than a decade, and it has resulted in devastating epidemics in Africa and, more recently, in Asia.[209, 210] Since its recognition in 1981, HIV-related AIDS has become one of the leading causes of death worldwide, and the Joint United Nations Programme on HIV/AIDS estimated that more than 30 million persons were infected with HIV by the end of 1997.[3]

HIV has also had a profound impact on the epidemiologic patterns of many of the diseases and syndromes discussed in this chapter. As examples, invasive pneumococcal disease is more than 100 times more prevalent among HIV-infected persons than in the rest of the population,[211] and *Pneumocystis carinii* is the most common cause of pneumonia in persons with HIV infection.[212] Cryptosporidiosis, microsporidiosis, and salmonellosis are among the diarrheal diseases whose epidemiology was altered by AIDS, and HIV is known to be the most powerful risk factor for progression of tuberculosis infection to active disease.[106, 127, 213, 214] In the United States, 95% of all cases of cryptosporidiosis occur in HIV-infected persons, as do 85% of cases of *Pneumocystis* pneumonia and 24% of cases of active tuberculosis.[215] Although associations between malaria and HIV were identified early in the epidemic, this relation was found to result from the frequent transfusions required by persons with malaria-associated anemia.[216]

Among other opportunistic pathogens, HIV has had a major impact on toxoplasmosis (increasing the death rate 86 times over baseline) and on nontuberculous mycobacterial infections (increasing the mortality rate 19 times over baseline).[215] In Southeast Asia, the fungus *Penicillium marneffei* was a rare cause of infection before HIV infection became common in locations such as Thailand.[217]

Dengue Fever

Since the mid-1950s, the frequency of dengue fever and its more severe complication, dengue hemorrhagic fever (DHF), has been on the increase in tropical regions of the world, and 80 to 100 million cases are estimated to occur annually.[218, 219] Dengue is a mosquito-borne virus disease caused by any of four antigenically distinct viruses (DEN-1, -2, -3, and -4). There is no durable cross-protection among the four viruses; therefore, a single person can experience four different episodes of dengue infection. Primary dengue infections most often lead to a self-limited febrile syndrome, sometimes accompanied by rash and severe joint and muscle pain.[219–221] Secondary infections can manifest similarly, but DHF is more commonly encountered among patients experiencing a secondary infection.[222, 223] DHF is a life-threatening condition characterized by capillary permeability that may lead to hypovolemic shock and death if not managed appropriately. In endemic areas, most deaths from dengue infection occur in children younger than 15 years of age.[219]

The mosquito *Aedes aegypti* is the primary vector of all four dengue viruses. Historically, this mosquito was found in Africa, but it spread throughout the tropical regions of the world during the 19th and 20th centuries as a result of international shipping. *A. aegypti* is well adapted to the urban environment, feeding almost exclusively on humans and breeding in containers found in cities, suburbs, and villages where water is stored or allowed to accumulate (e.g., discarded cans, bottles, plastic containers, and tires). As human urban populations have increased in the developing world, so too have the populations of *A. aegypti*, leading to enhanced dengue transmission and outbreaks. These outbreaks first occurred on a periodic basis and were caused by single serotypes, but they have now evolved into outbreaks characterized by multiple serotypes concurrently transmitted.[218, 224] This pattern was first observed in Southeast Asia beginning in the 1950s and has now evolved so that all four dengue viruses are in constant circulation. Because multiple infections raise the risk of DHF, the incidence of this complication has also increased, as has the mortality rate, especially in children.[218] Dengue infection is now the 10th leading cause of death throughout the world, responsible for almost 150,000 fatalities annually.[3]

The Pan American Health Organization mounted a hemispheric eradication campaign against *A. aegypti* in the 1960s and succeeded in eliminating the species from most of Central and South America. The campaign was abandoned, however, and today the vector has been reestablished in virtually all major cities of the region.[218, 225, 226] The patterns of dengue transmission in this area have become similar to those in Southeast Asia, and DHF has also become more common.

Epidemics of dengue fever are now routinely seen in Venezuela, Colombia, Brazil, and other locations in Latin America and the Caribbean.[218, 227] Today approximately 40% of the world's population live in areas at risk for dengue and DHF, and as urban centers continue to expand and international travel increases, the importance of dengue will continue to rise. There is no effective therapy for dengue infection, and treatment is symptomatic.[219] Vaccines are under development but are not currently available.[228] Prevention of infection through vector control is effective but is expensive and difficult to sustain.[229] Education of health care providers on appropriate management of patients with DHF has been shown to be effective in reducing mortality rates.

CONCLUSION

There are many other infectious diseases that cause significant global morbidity and mortality. Examples include infectious agents linked to malignancies (*H. pylori*, human papillomavirus, human herpesvirus 8); hepatitis C, which is estimated to affect almost 200 million persons around the world and is associated with cirrhosis and hepatocellular carcinoma; tropical parasitic diseases such as African trypanosomiasis and leishmaniasis; rabies; and meningococcal disease. The Global Burden of Disease Study supported by the WHO and the World Bank suggests that the impact of infectious diseases on mortality will decline in the coming decades as the socioeconomic status of the world's population continues to improve.[230] As the epidemiology of the current leading infectious causes of mortality demonstrates, most of these diseases affect the developing countries of the world disproportionately and can be influenced by social and economic upheavals. Infectious diseases can be highly volatile, and previous predictions of their decline and demise have not been borne out. The HIV/AIDS epidemic alone has had a significant impact on global patterns of morbidity and mortality. Although the predictions in the Global Burden of Disease Study for sustained reductions in infectious disease mortality may be realized, past experience suggests that they should be viewed with caution.

REFERENCES

1. United States Bureau of the Census. United States Life Tables 1890, 1901, 1910, and 1901–1910. Washington, DC: US Government Printing Office; 1921.
2. United States Department of Health and Human Services. Health, United States, 1998. Washington, DC: U.S. Government Printing Office; 1998.
3. World Health Organization. The World Health Report, 1998. Geneva: World Health Organization; 1998.
4. Linder FE, Grove RD. Vital Statistics Rates in the United States, 1900–1940. Washington, DC: U.S. Government Printing Office; 1947.
5. Centers for Disease Control and Prevention. Report on Tuberculosis in the United States, 1996. Washington, DC: U.S. Government Printing Office; 1997.
6. Centers for Disease Control and Prevention. Smallpox surveillance—worldwide, 1978. MMWR Morb Mortal Wkly Rep. 1997;46:991–994.
7. de Quadros CA, Hersh BS, Olive JM, et al. Eradication of wild poliovirus from the Americas: Acute flaccid paralysis surveillance, 1988–1995. J Infect Dis. 1997;175:S37–S42.
8. Murray CJ, Lopez AD. Global mortality, disability, and the contribution of risk factors: Global Burden of Disease Study. Lancet. 1997;349:1436–1442.
9. Centers for Disease Control and Prevention. Update: Trends in AIDS incidence, deaths, and prevalence—United States, 1996. MMWR Morb Mortal Wkly Rep. 1997;46:165–173.
10. Pinner RW, Teutsch SM, Simonsen L, et al. Trends in infectious disease mortality in the United States. JAMA. 1996;275:189–193.
11. Berman S. Epidemiology of acute respiratory infections in children of developing countries. Rev Infect Dis. 1991;13:S454–S462.
12. Craven DE, Steger KA. Hospital-acquired pneumonia: Perspectives for the health-care epidemiologist. Infect Control Hosp Epidemiol. 1997;18:783–795.
13. Greenaway CA, Embil J, Orr PH, et al. Nosocomial pneumonia on general medical and surgical wards in a tertiary-care hospital. Infect Control Hosp Epidemiol. 1997;18:749–756.
14. Graham NMH. The epidemiology of acute respiratory infections in children and adults: A global perspective. Epidemiol Rev. 1990;12:149–178.
15. Vathanophas K, Sangchai R, Raktham S, et al. A community-based study of acute respiratory tract infection in Thai children. Rev Infect Dis. 1990;12:S957–S965.
16. Borrero I, Fajardo L, Bedoya A, et al. Acute respiratory tract infections among a cohort of children from Cali, Colombia. Rev Infect Dis. 1990;12:S950–S956.
17. Tupasi TE, de Leon LE, Lupisan S, et al. Patterns of acute respiratory tract infection in children: A longitudinal study in a depressed community in Metro Manila. Rev Infect Dis. 1990;12:S940–S949.
18. Selwyn BJ. The epidemiology of acute respiratory tract infection in young children: Comparison of findings from several developing countries. Coordinated Data Group of BOSTID Researchers. Rev Infect Dis. 1990;12:S870–S888.
19. Zaman K, Baqui AH, Yunus M, et al. Acute respiratory infections in children: A community-based longitudinal study in rural Bangladesh. J Trop Pediatr. 1997;43:133–137.
20. Singh MP, Nayar S. Magnitude of acute respiratory infections in under five children. J Commun Dis. 1996;28:273–278.
21. Fagbule D, Parakoyi DB, Spiegel R. Acute respiratory infections in Nigerian children: Prospective cohort study of incidence and case management. J Trop Pediatr. 1994;40:279–284.
22. Hortal M, Contera M, Mogdasy C, et al. Acute respiratory infections in children from a deprived urban population from Uruguay. Rev Inst Med Trop Sao Paulo. 1994;36:51–57.
23. Monto AS, Sullivan KM. Acute respiratory illness in the community: Frequency of illness and the agents involved. Epidemiol Infect. 1993;110:145–160.
24. Ruuskanen O, Ogra PL. Respiratory syncytial virus. Curr Prob Pediatr. 1993;23:50–79.
25. Shann F. Etiology of severe pneumonia in children in developing countries. Pediatr Infect Dis. 1986;5:247–252.
26. Mastro TD, Nomani NK, Ishaq Z, et al. Use of nasopharyngeal isolates of *Streptococcus pneumoniae* and *Haemophilus influenzae* from children in Pakistan for surveillance for antimicrobial resistance. Pediatr Infect Dis J. 1993;12:824–830.
27. John TJ, Cherian T, Steinhoff MC, et al. Etiology of acute respiratory infections in children in tropical southern India. Rev Infect Dis. 1991;13:S463–S469.
28. Ostroff SM, Harrison LH, Khallaf N, et al. Resistance patterns of *Streptococcus pneumoniae* and *Haemophilus influenzae* isolates recovered in Egypt from children with pneumonia. Clin Infect Dis. 1996;23:1069–1074.
29. Datta N, Kumar V, Kumar L, et al. Application of case management to the control of acute respiratory infections in low-birth-weight infants: A feasibility study. Bull World Health Organ. 1987;65:77–82.
30. Tupasi TE, Velmonte MA, Sanvictores MEG, et al. Determinants of morbidity and mortality due to acute respiratory infections: Implications for intervention. J Infect Dis. 1988;157:615–623.
31. Keusch GT. Nutritional effects on response of children in developing countries to respiratory tract pathogens: Implications for vaccine development. Rev Infect Dis. 1991;13:S486–S491.
32. Victora CG, Smith PG, Barros FC, et al. Risk factors for deaths due to respiratory infections among Brazilian infants. Int J Epidemiol. 1989;18:918–925.
33. Watkins CJ, Leeder SR, Corkhill RT. The relationship between breast and bottle feeding and respiratory illness in the first year of life. J Epidemiol Community Health. 1979;33:180–182.
34. Sommer A, Katz J, Tarwotjo I. Increased risk of respiratory disease and diarrhea in children with preexisting mild vitamin A deficiency. Am J Clin Nutr. 1984;40:1090–1095.
35. Stansfield SK, Pierre-Louis M, Lerebours G, et al. Vitamin A supplementation and increased prevalence of childhood diarrhoea and acute respiratory infections. Lancet. 1993;342:578–582.
36. Forastiere F, Corbo GM, Michelozzi P, et al. Effects of environment and passive smoking on the respiratory health of children. Int J Epidemiol. 1992;21:66–73.
37. Holberg CJ, Wright AL, Martinez FD, et al. Child day care, smoking by caregivers, and lower respiratory tract illness in the first 3 years of life. Pediatrics. 1993;91:885–892.
38. Woodward A, Douglas RM, Graham NMH, et al. Acute respiratory illness in Adelaide children: The influence of child care. Med J Aust. 1991;154:805–808.
39. Frampton MW, Samet JM, Utell MJ. Environmental factors and atmospheric pollutants. Semin Respir Infect. 1991;6:185–193.
40. Armstrong JRM, Campbell H. Indoor air pollution and lower respiratory tract infections in young Gambian children. Int J Epidemiol. 1991;20:424–429.
41. Anonymous. Indoor air pollution and acute respiratory infections in children. Lancet. 1992;339:396–398.
42. Programme for the Control of Acute Respiratory Infections. Acute Respiratory Infections in Children: Case Management in Small Hospitals in Developing Countries. WHO/ARI/90.5. Geneva: World Health Organization, 1990.
43. Harari M, Shann F, Spooner V, et al. Clinical signs of pneumonia in children. Lancet. 1991;338:928–930.
44. Cherian T, John TJ, Simoes E, et al. Evaluation of simple clinical signs for the diagnosis of acute lower respiratory tract infections. Lancet. 1988;2;125–128.
45. Campbell H, Byass P, Lamont AC, et al. Assessment of clinical criteria for identification of severe acute lower respiratory tract infections in children. Lancet. 1989;1:297–299.
46. Pandey MR, Daulaire NMP, Starbuck ES, et al. Reduction in total under-five mortality in western Nepal through community-based antimicrobial treatment of pneumonia. Lancet. 1991;338:993–997.
47. Khan AJ, Khan JA, Akbar M, et al. Acute respiratory infections in children: A case management intervention in Abbottabad District, Pakistan. Bull World Health Organ. 1990;68:577–585.
48. Campbell GD Jr, Silberman R. Drug-resistant *Streptococcus pneumoniae*. Clin Infect Dis. 1998;26:1188–1195.
49. Appelbaum PC. Antimicrobial resistance in *Streptococcus pneumoniae*: An overview. Clin Infect Dis. 1992;15:77–83.

50. Breiman RF, Butler JC, Tenover FC, et al. Emergence of drug-resistant pneumococcal infections in the United States. JAMA. 1994;271:1831–1835.
51. Lonks JR, Medeiros AA. The growing threat of antibiotic-resistant *Streptococcus pneumoniae*. Med Clin North Am. 1995;79:523–535.
52. Palleres R, Liñares J, Vadillo M, et al. Resistance to penicillin and cephalosporin and mortality from severe pneumococcal pneumonia in Barcelona, Spain. N Engl J Med. 1995;333:474–480.
53. Friedland IR. Comparison of response to antimicrobial therapy of penicillin-resistant and penicillin-susceptible pneumococcal disease. Pediatr Infect Dis J. 1995;14:885–890.
54. Friedland IR, McCracken GH Jr. Management of infections caused by antibiotic-resistant *Streptococcus pneumoniae*. N Engl J Med. 1994;331:377–382.
55. Spika JS, Facklam RR, Plikaytis BD, et al. Antimicrobial resistance of *Streptococcus pneumoniae* in the United States 1979–1987. J Infect Dis. 1991;163:1273–1278.
56. Butler JC, Hofmann J, Cetron MS, et al. The continued emergence of drug-resistant *Streptococcus pneumoniae* in the United States: An update from the Centers for Disease Control and Prevention's Pneumococcal Sentinel Surveillance System. J Infect Dis. 1996;174:986–993.
57. Hofmann J, Cetron MS, Farley MM, et al. The prevalence of drug-resistant *Streptococcus pneumoniae* in Atlanta. N Engl J Med. 1995;333:481–486.
58. Pradier C, Dunais B, Carsenti-Etesse H, et al. Pneumococcal resistance patterns in Europe. Eur J Clin Microbiol Infect Dis. 1997;16:644–647.
59. Lyon DJ, Scheel O, Fung KS, et al. Rapid emergence of penicillin-resistant pneumococci in Hong Kong. Scand J Infect Dis. 1996;28:375–376.
60. Echaniz-Aviles G, Velazquez-Meza ME, Carnalla-Barajas MN, et al. Antimicrobial susceptibilities and capsular types of invasive *Streptococcus pneumoniae* isolated in children in Mexico City. Microb Drug Resist. 1997;3:153–157.
61. Ringertz S, Muhe L, Krantz I, et al. Prevalence of potential respiratory disease bacteria in children in Ethiopia: Antimicrobial susceptibility of the pathogens and use of antibiotics among the children. Acta Paediatr. 1993;82:843–848.
62. Scriver SR, Walmsley SL, Kau CL, et al. Determination of antimicrobial susceptibilities of Canadian isolates of *Haemophilus influenzae* and characterization of their beta-lactamases. Antimicrob Agents Chemother. 1994;38:1678–1680.
63. Bijlmer HA, van Alphen L, Greenwood BM, et al. Antibiotic susceptibility of invasive and non-invasive isolates of *Haemophilus influenzae* from the Gambia, West Africa. J Antimicrob Chemother. 1994;34:275–280.
64. Hussey G, Hitchcock J, Hanslo D, et al. Serotypes and antimicrobial susceptibility of *Haemophilus influenzae*. J Antimicrob Chemother. 1994;34:1031–1036.
65. Sniadack DH, Schwartz B, Lipman H, et al. Potential interventions for the prevention of childhood pneumonia: Geographic and temporal differences in serotype and serogroup distribution of sterile site pneumococcal isolates from children. Implications for vaccine strategies. Pediatr Infect Dis J. 1995;14:503–510.
66. Dagan R, Muallem M, Melamed R, et al. Reduction of pneumococcal nasopharyngeal carriage in early infancy after immunization with tetravalent pneumococcal vaccines conjugated to either tetanus toxoid or diphtheria toxoid. Pediatr Infect Dis J. 1997;16:1060–1064.
67. Rennels MB, Edwards KM, Keyserling HL, et al. Safety and immunogenecity of heptavalent pneumococcal vaccine conjugated to CRM197 in United States infants. Pediatrics. 1998;101:604–611.
68. DuPont HL. Diarrheal diseases in the developing world. Infect Dis Clin North Am. 1995;2:313–324.
69. Muhe L, Byass P, Friej L, et al. A one-year community study of under-fives in rural Ethiopia: Patterns of morbidity and mortality. Public Health. 1995;109:99–109.
70. Gupta DN, Sircar BK, Sengupta PG, et al. Epidemiological and clinical profiles of acute invasive diarrhoea with special reference to mucoid episodes: A rural community-based longitudinal study. Trans R Soc Trop Med Hyg. 1997;90:544–547.
71. Jousilahti P, Madkour SM, Lambrechts T, et al. Diarrhoeal disease morbidity and home treatment practices in Egypt. Public Health. 1997;111:5–10.
72. Mirza NM, Caulfield LE, Black RE, et al. Risk factors for diarrheal duration. Am J Epidemiol. 1997;146:776–785.
73. Gotuzzo E, Cieza J, Estremadoyro L, et al. Cholera: Lessons from the epidemic in Peru. Infect Dis Clin North Am. 1994;8:183–205.
74. Ries AA, Vugia DJ, Beingolea L, et al. Cholera in Piura, Peru: A modern urban epidemic. J Infect Dis. 1992;166:1429–1433.
75. Begue RE, Castellares G, Hayashi KE, et al. Diarrheal disease in Peru after the introduction of cholera. Am J Trop Med Hyg. 1994;51:585–589.
76. Vugia DJ, Rodriguez M, Vargas R, et al. Epidemic cholera in Trujillo, Peru 1992: Utility of a clinical case definition and shift in *Vibrio cholerae* O1 serotype. Am J Trop Med Hyg. 1994;50:566–569.
77. Herwaldt BL, Ackers ML, Cyclospora Working Group. An outbreak in 1996 of cyclosporiasis associated with imported raspberries. N Engl J Med. 1997;336:1548–1556.
78. Soave R. *Cyclospora*: An overview. Clin Infect Dis. 1996;23:429–437.
79. Nair GB, Ramamurthy T, Bhattacharya SK, et al. Spread of *Vibrio cholerae* O139 Bengal in India. J Infect Dis. 1994;169:1029–1034.
80. Siddique AK, Zaman K, Akram K, et al. Emergence of a new epidemic strain of *Vibrio cholerae* in Bangladesh: An epidemiological study. Trop Geogr Med. 1994;46:147–150.
81. Large epidemic of cholera-like disease in Bangladesh caused by *Vibrio cholerae* O139 synonym Bengal. Lancet. 1993;342:387–390.
82. Mahalanabis D, Faruque AS, Albert MJ, et al. An epidemic of cholera due to *Vibrio cholerae* O139 in Dhaka, Bangladesh: Clinical and epidemiological features. Epidemiol Infect. 1994;112:463–471.
83. Armstrong GL, Hollingsworth J, Morris JG Jr. Emerging foodborne pathogens: *Escherichia coli* O157:H7 as a model of entry of a new pathogen into the food supply of the developed world. Epidemiol Rev. 1996;18:29–51.
84. Slutsker L, Ries AA, Greene KD, et al. *Escherichia coli* O157:H7 diarrhea in the United States: Clinical and epidemiologic features. Ann Intern Med. 1997;126:505–513.
85. Hatch DL, Waldman RJ, Lungu GW, et al. Epidemic cholera during refugee resettlement in Malawi. Int J Epidemiol. 1994;23:1292–1299.
86. Engels D, Madaras T, Nyandwi S, et al. Epidemic dysentery caused by *Shigella dysenteriae* type 1: A sentinel site surveillance of antimicrobial resistance patterns in Burundi. Bull World Health Organ. 1995;73:787–791.
87. Shears P. Shigella infections. Ann Trop Med Parasitol. 1996;90:105–114.
88. Bishop RF. Natural history of human rotavirus infection. Arch Virol Suppl. 1996;12:119–128.
89. Glass RI, Kilgore PE, Holman RC, et al. The epidemiology of rotavirus diarrhea in the United States: Surveillance and estimates of disease burden. J Infect Dis. 1996:174:S5–S11.
90. Unicomb LE, Kilgore PE, Faruque SG, et al. Anticipating rotavirus vaccines: Hospital-based surveillance for rotavirus diarrhea and estimates of disease burden in Bangladesh. Pediatr Infect Dis J. 1997;16:947–951.
91. Suwatano O. Acute diarrhea in under five-year-old children admitted to King Mongkut Prachomklao Hospital, Phetchaburi province. J Med Assoc Thai. 1997;80:26–33.
92. Saida SM, Iijima Y, Sang WK, et al. Epidemiological study on infectious diarrheal diseases in children in a coastal rural area of Kenya. Microbiol Immunol. 1997;41:773–778.
93. Townes JM, Quick R, Gonzales OY, et al. Etiology of bloody diarrhea in Bolivian children: Implications for empiric therapy. J Infect Dis. 1997;175:1527–1530.
94. Bhimma R, Rollins NC, Coovadia HM, et al. Post-dysenteric hemolytic uremic syndrome in children during an epidemic of *Shigella* dysentery in Kwazulu/Natal. Pediatr Nephrol. 1997;11:560–564.
95. Lindblood GB, Ahren C, Changalucha J, et al. *Campylobacter jejuni/coli* and enterotoxigenic *Escherichia coli* (ETEC) in faeces from children and adults in Tanzania. Scand J Infect Dis. 1995;27:589–593.
96. Blaser MJ. Epidemiologic and clinical features of *Campylobacter jejuni* infections. J Infect Dis. 1997;176:S103–S105.
97. Bhattacharya MK, Teka T, Faruque AS, et al. *Cryptosporidium* infection in children in urban Bangladesh. J Trop Pediatr. 1997;43:282–286.
98. Agnew DG, Lima AA, Newman RD, et al. Cryptosporidiosis in northeastern Brazilian children: Association with increased diarrhea morbidity. J Infect Dis. 1998;177:754–760.
99. Ryan MJ, Ramsay M, Brown D, et al. Hospital admissions attributable to rotavirus infection in England and Wales. J Infect Dis. 1996;174:S12–S18.
100. Blacklow NR, Greenberg HB. Viral gastroenteritis. N Engl J Med. 1991;325:252–264.
101. Kapikian AZ. Overview of viral gastroenteritis. Arch Virol Suppl. 1996;12:7–19.
102. Goldwater PN, Bettelheim KA. The role of enterohemorrhagic *Escherichia coli* serotypes other than O157:H7 as causes of disease. Commun Dis Intell. 1995;19:2–4.
103. Huppertz HI, Busch D, Schmidt H, et al. Diarrhea in young children associated with *Escherichia coli* non-O157 organisms that produce Shiga-like toxin. J Pediatr. 1996;128:341–346.
104. Centers for Disease Control and Prevention. Summary of notifiable diseases—United States, 1995. MMWR Morb Mortal Wkly Rep. 1995;44:1–87.
105. Chalker RB, Blaser MJ. A review of human salmonellosis: III. Magnitude of *Salmonella* infection in the United States. Rev Infect Dis. 1988;10:111–124.
106. Meinhardt PL, Casemore DP, Miller KB. Epidemiologic aspects of human cryptosporidiosis and the role of waterborne transmission. Epidemiol Rev. 1996;18:118–136.
107. Riley LW, Cohen ML, Seals JE, et al. Importance of host factors in human salmonellosis caused by multiresistant strains of *Salmonella*. J Infect Dis. 1984;149:878–883.
108. Lee LA, Puhr ND, Maloney EK, et al. Increase in antimicrobial-resistant *Salmonella* infections in the United States, 1989–1990. J Infect Dis. 1994;170:128–134.
109. National Antimicrobial Resistance Monitoring System: 1997 Annual Report. Atlanta: Centers for Disease Control and Prevention; 1998.
110. Threlfall EJ, Frost JA, Ward LR, et al. Increasing spectrum of resistance in multiresistant *Salmonella typhimurium*. Lancet. 1996;347:1053–1054.
111. Glynn MK, Bopp C, Dewitt W, et al. Emergence of multidrug-resistant *Salmonella enterica* serotype Typhimurium DT104 infections in the United States. N Engl J Med. 1998;338:1333–1338.
112. Threlfall EJ, Ward LR, Rowe B. Increasing incidence of resistance to trimethoprim and ciprofloxacin in epidemic *Salmonella typhimurium* DT104 in England and Wales. Eurosurveillance. 1997;2:81–84.
113. Piddock LJ. Quinolone resistance and *Campylobacter* spp. J Antimicrob Chemother. 1995;36:891–898.
114. Perez-Schael I, Guntinas MJ, Perez M, et al. Efficacy of the rhesus rotavirus-based quadrivalent vaccine in infants and young children in Venezuela. N Engl J Med. 1997;337:1181–1187.
115. Savarino SJ, Brown FM, Hall E, et al. Safety and immunogenicity of an oral, killed enterotoxigenic *Escherichia coli*-cholera toxin B subunit vaccine in Egyptian adults. J Infect Dis. 1998;177:796–799.
116. Taylor JL, Tuttle J, Pramukul T, et al. An outbreak of cholera in Maryland associated with imported commercial frozen fresh coconut milk. J Infect Dis. 1993;167:1330–1335.
117. Threlfall EJ, Hampton MD, Ward LR, et al. Application of pulsed-field gel electro-

phoresis to an international outbreak of *Salmonella agona*. Emerg Infect Dis. 1996;2:130–132.
118. Dolin PJ, Raviglione MC, Kochi A. Global tuberculosis incidence and mortality during 1990–2000. Bull World Health Organ. 1994;72:213–220.
119. Raviglione MC, Snider DE, Kochi A. Global epidemiology of tuberculosis: Morbidity and mortality of a worldwide epidemic. JAMA. 1995;273:220–226.
120. Kochi A. Tuberculosis control: Is DOTS the health breakthrough of the 1990s? World Health Forum. 1997;18:225–232.
121. Wilson LG. The historical decline of tuberculosis in Europe and America: Its causes and significance. J Hist Med Allied Sci. 1990;45:366–396.
122. Rieder HL, Cauthen GM, Comstock GW, et al. Epidemiology of tuberculosis in the United States. Epidemiol Rev. 1989;11:79–98.
123. World Health Organization. TB, A Global Health Emergency: WHO Report on the TB Epidemic. WHO/TB/94.177. Geneva: World Health Organization; 1994.
124. Centers for Disease Control and Prevention. Tuberculosis morbidity—United States, 1997. MMWR Morb Mortal Wkly Rep. 1998;47:253–257.
125. McKenna MT, McCray E, Onorato I. The epidemiology of tuberculosis among foreign-born persons in the United States, 1986 to 1993. N Engl J Med. 1995;332:1071–1076.
126. Kochi A. The global tuberculosis situation and the new control strategy of the World Health Organization. Tubercle. 1991;72:1–6.
127. Shafer RW, Edlin BR. Tuberculosis in patients with human immunodeficiency virus: Perspective on the past decade. Clin Infect Dis. 1996;22:683–704.
128. Cantwell MF, Binkin NJ. Tuberculosis in sub-Saharan Africa: A regional assessment of the impact of the human immunodeficiency virus and National Tuberculosis Control Program quality. Tuber Lung Dis. 1996;77:220–225.
129. Yanai H, Uthaivoravit W, Panich V, et al. Rapid increase in HIV-related tuberculosis, Chiang Rai, Thailand, 1990–1994. AIDS. 1996;10:527–531.
130. Drobniewski F, Tayler E, Ignatenko N, et al. Tuberculosis in Siberia: 1. An epidemiological and microbiological assessment. Tuber Lung Dis. 1996;77:199–206.
131. Van Embden JD, Cave MD, Crawford JT, et al. Strain identification of *Mycobacterium tuberculosis* by DNA fingerprinting: Recommendations for a standardized methodology. J Clin Microbiol. 1993;31:406–409.
132. Small PM, Hopewell PC, Singh SP, et al. The epidemiology of tuberculosis in San Francisco: A population-based study using conventional and molecular methods. N Engl J Med. 1994;330:1703–1709.
133. Frieden TR, Woodley CL, Crawford JT, et al. The molecular epidemiology of tuberculosis in New York City: The importance of nosocomial transmission and laboratory error. Tuber Lung Dis. 1996;77:407–413.
134. van Deutekom H, Gerritsen JJ, van Soolingen D, et al. A molecular epidemiologic approach to studying the transmission of tuberculosis in Amsterdam. Clin Infect Dis. 1997;25:1071–1077.
135. Safi H, Aznar J, Palomares JC. Molecular epidemiology of *Mycobacterium tuberculosis* strains isolated during a 3-year period (1993 to 1995) in Seville, Spain. J Clin Microbiol. 1997;35:2472–2476.
136. Braden CR, Templeton GL, Cave MD, et al. Interpretation of restriction fragment length polymorphism analysis of *Mycobacterium tuberculosis* isolates from a state with a large rural population. J Infect Dis. 1997;175:1446–1452.
137. Kubin M, Riley LW, Havelkova M, et al. Molecular epidemiology of tuberculosis in Prague: Analysis by restriction fragment length polymorphism. Int J Infect Dis. 1998;2:155–158.
138. van Soolingen D, Hermans PW, de Haas PE, et al. Occurrence and stability of insertion sequences in *Mycobacterium tuberculosis* complex strains: Evaluation of an insertion sequence-dependent DNA polymorphism as a tool in the epidemiology of tuberculosis. J Clin Microbiol. 1991;29:2578–2586.
139. van Soolingen D, Qian L, de Haas PE, et al. Predominance of a single genotype of *Mycobacterium tuberculosis* in countries of east Asia. J Clin Microbiol. 1995;33:3234–3238.
140. Wilkinson D, Pillay M, Crump J, et al. Molecular epidemiology and transmission dynamics of *Mycobacterium tuberculosis* in rural Africa. Trop Med Int Health. 1997;2:747–753.
141. Yang ZH, Mtoni I, Chonde M, et al. DNA fingerprinting and phenotyping of *Mycobacterium tuberculosis* isolates from human immunodeficiency virus (HIV)-seropositive and HIV-seronegative patients in Tanzania. J Clin Microbiol. 1995;33:1064–1069.
142. Parsons LM, Driscoll JR, Taber HW, et al. Drug resistance in tuberculosis. Infect Dis Clin North Am. 1997;11:905–928.
143. Bradford WZ, Daley CL. Multiple drug-resistant tuberculosis. Infect Dis Clin North Am. 1998;12:157–172.
144. Snider DE Jr, Castro KG. The global threat of drug-resistant tuberculosis. N Engl J Med. 1998;338:1689–1690.
145. Pablos-Mendez A, Raviglione MC, Laszlo A, et al. Global surveillance for antituberculosis-drug resistance, 1994–1997. N Engl J Med. 1998;338:1641–1649.
146. Fujiwara PI, Cook SV, Rutherford CM, et al. A continuing survey of drug-resistant tuberculosis, New York City, April 1994. Arch Intern Med. 1997;157:531–536.
147. Goble M, Iseman MD, Madsen LA, et al. Treatment of 171 patients with pulmonary tuberculosis resistant to isoniazid and rifampin. N Engl J Med. 1993;328:527–532.
148. Pampana EJ. A Textbook of Malaria Eradication. London: Oxford University Press; 1963.
149. Olliaro P, Cattani J, Wirth D. Malaria, the submerged disease. JAMA. 1996;275:230–233.
150. World Health Organization. World malaria situation in 1994: Part I. Wkly Epidemiol Rec. 1997;72:269–274.
151. World Health Organization. World malaria situation in 1994: Part II. Wkly Epidemiol Rec. 1997;72:277–283.
152. World Health Organization. World malaria situation in 1994: Part III. Wkly Epidemiol Rec. 1997;72:285–290.
153. Zucker JR. Changing patterns of autochthonous malaria transmission in the United States: A review of recent outbreaks. Emerg Infect Dis. 1996;2:37–43.
154. Miller LH, McAuliffe FM, Mason SJ. Erythrocyte receptors for malaria merozoites. Am J Trop Med Hyg. 1977;26:204–208.
155. Centers for Disease Control and Prevention. Epidemic malaria—Tadjikistan, 1995. MMWR Morb Mortal Wkly Rep. 1996;45:513–516.
156. Centers for Disease Control and Prevention. Epidemic malaria transmission—Armenia, 1997. MMWR Morb Mortal Wkly Rep. 1998;47:526–528.
157. Krogstad DJ. Malaria as a reemerging disease. Epidemiol Rev. 1996;18:77–89.
158. Silver HM. Malarial infection during pregnancy. Infect Dis Clin North Am. 1997:11:99–107.
159. Steele RW. Malaria in children. Adv Pediatr Infect Dis. 1996;12:325–349.
160. Marsh K, Snow RW. Host-parasite interaction and morbidity in malaria endemic areas. Philos Trans R Soc Lond B Biol Sci. 1997;352:1385–1394.
161. Warsame M, Wernsdorfer WH, Perlmann H, et al. A malariometric survey in a rural community in the Muheza district, Tanzania: Age profiles in the development of humoral immune responses. Acta Trop. 1997;68:239–253.
162. Lindsay SW, Martens WJ. Malaria in the African highlands: Past, present and future. Bull World Health Organ. 1998;76:33–45.
163. Bourma MJ, Dye C. Cycles of malaria associated with El Nino in Venezuela. JAMA. 1997;278:1772–1774.
164. Wernsdorfer WH. The development and spread of drug-resistant malaria. Parasitol Today. 1991;7:297–303.
165. White NJ. Antimalarial drug resistance: The pace quickens. J Antimicrob Chemother. 1992;30:571–585.
166. Moore DV, Lanier JE. Observations on two *Plasmodium falciparum* infections with abnormal response to chloroquine. Am J Trop Med Hyg. 1961;10:5–9.
167. Campbell CC, Chin W, Collins WE, et al. Chloroquine-resistant *Plasmodium falciparum* from East Africa: Cultivation and drug sensitivity of the Tanzanian I/CDC strain from an American tourist. Lancet. 1979;2:1151–1154.
168. Barat LM, Bloland PB. Drug resistance among malaria and other parasites. Infect Dis Clin North Am. 1997;11:969–987.
169. Wongsrichanalai C, Webster HK, Wimonwattrawatee T, et al. Emergence of multidrug-resistant *Plasmodium falciparum* in Thailand: In vitro tracking. Am J Trop Med Hyg. 1992;47:112–116.
170. Rieckmann KH, Davis DR, Hutton DC. *Plasmodium vivax* resistance to chloroquine? Lancet. 1989;2:1183–1184.
171. Roberts DR, Andre RG. Insecticide resistance issues in vector-borne disease control. Am J Trop Med Hyg. 1994;50(6 Suppl):21–34.
172. D'Alessandro U, Olaleye BO, McGuire W, et al. Mortality and morbidity from malaria in Gambian children after introduction of an impregnated bednet programme. Lancet. 1995;345:479–483.
173. World Health Organization. Integrated management of the sick child. Bull World Health Organ. 1995;73:735–740.
174. D'Alessandro U, Leach A, Drakeley CJ, et al. Efficacy trial of malaria vaccine Spf66 in Gambian infants. Lancet. 1995;346:462–467.
175. Stoute JA, Slaoui M, Heppner G, et al. A preliminary evaluation of a recombinant circumsporozoite protein vaccine against *Plasmodium falciparum* malaria. N Engl J Med. 1997;336:86–91.
176. Centers for Disease Control and Prevention. Malaria surveillance—United States, 1993. MMWR Morb Mortal Wkly Rep. 1997;46:27–47.
177. Ostroff SM, Kozarsky P. Emerging infectious diseases and travel medicine. Infect Dis Clin North Am. 1998;12:231–241.
178. Centers for Disease Control and Prevention. Measles—United States, 1997. MMWR Morb Mortal Wkly Rep. 1998;47:273–276.
179. Centers for Disease Control and Prevention. Advances in global measles control and elimination: Summary of the 1997 international meeting. MMWR Morb Mortal Wkly Rep. 1998;47(RR-11):1–23.
180. Gustafson TL, Lievens AW, Brunell PA, et al. Measles outbreak in a fully immunized secondary school population. N Engl J Med. 1987;316:771–774.
181. Centers for Disease Control and Prevention. Progress toward global measles control and elimination, 1990–1996. MMWR Morb Mortal Wkly Rep. 1997;46:893–897.
182. Centers for Disease Control and Prevention. Measles eradication: Recommendations from a meeting cosponsored by the World Health Organization, the Pan American Health Organization, and CDC. MMWR Morb Mortal Wkly Rep. 1997;46(RR-11):1–21.
183. de Quadros CA, Olive JM, Hersh BS, et al. Measles elimination in the Americas. JAMA. 1996;275:224–229.
184. Centers for Disease Control and Prevention. Progress toward the global elimination of neonatal tetanus, 1989–1993. MMWR Morb Mortal Wkly Rep. 1994;43:885–887,893–894.
185. Thayaparan B, Nicoll A. Prevention and control of tetanus in childhood. Curr Opin Pediatr. 1998;10:4–8.
186. Gupta SD, Keyl PM. Effectiveness of prenatal tetanus toxoid immunization against neonatal tetanus in a rural area of India. Pediatr Infect Dis J. 1998;17:316–321.
187. Centers for Disease Control and Prevention. Progress towards elimination of neonatal tetanus—Egypt, 1988–1994. MMWR Morb Mortal Wkly Rep. 1996;45:89–92.
188. Chongsuvivatwong V, Bujakorn L, Kanpoy V, et al. Control of neonatal tetanus in Southern Thailand. Int J Epidemiol. 1993;22:931–935.

189. Buekens P, Tsui A, Kotelchuck M, Degraft-Johnson J. Tetanus immunization and prenatal care in developing countries. Int J Gynecol Obstet. 1995;48:91–94.
190. Ivanoff B, Robertson SE. Pertussis: A worldwide problem. Dev Biol Stand. 1997;89:3–13.
191. Miller E, Gay NJ. Epidemiological determinants of pertussis. Dev Biol Stand. 1997;89:15–23.
192. Deville JG, Cherry JD, Christenson PD, et al. Frequency of unrecognized *Bordetella pertussis* infections in adults. Clin Infect Dis. 1995;21:639–642.
193. Mink CM, Cherry JD, Christenson PD, et al. A search for *Bordetella pertussis* infection in university students. Clin Infect Dis. 1992;14:464–471.
194. Nennig ME, Shinefield H, Edwards KM, et al. Prevalence and incidence of adult pertussis in an urban population. JAMA. 1996;275:1672–1674.
195. Cherry JD. The role of *Bordetella pertussis* infections in adults in the epidemiology of pertussis. Dev Biol Standard. 1997;89:181–186.
196. He Q, Mertsola J. Epidemiology and prevention of pertussis. Curr Opin Pediatr. 1997;9:14–18.
197. Gust ID. Epidemiology of hepatitis B infection in the Western Pacific and South East Asia. Gut. 1996;38(Suppl 2):S18–S23.
198. Toukan AU. Hepatitis B in the Middle East: Aspects of epidemiology and liver disease after infection. Gut. 1996;38(Suppl 2):S2–S4.
199. Lansang MA. Epidemiology and control of hepatitis B infection: A perspective from the Philippines, Asia. Gut. 1996;38(Suppl 2):S43–S47.
200. Tandon BN, Acharya SK, Tandon A. Epidemiology of hepatitis B virus infection in India. Gut. 1996;38(Suppl 2):S56–S59.
201. Torres JR. Hepatitis B and hepatitis delta virus infection in South America. Gut. 1996;38(Suppl 2):S48–S55.
202. Edmunds WJ, Medley GF, Nokes DJ, et al. Epidemiological patterns of hepatitis B virus (HBV) in highly endemic areas. Epidemiol Infect. 1996;117:313–325.
203. Maynard JE, Kane MA, Hadler SC. Global control of hepatitis B through vaccination: Role of hepatitis B vaccine in the Expanded Programme on Immunization. Rev Infect Dis. 1989;11:S574–S578.
204. Alter MJ, Hadler SC, Margolis HS, et al. The changing epidemiology of hepatitis B in the United States: Need for alternative vaccination strategies. JAMA. 1990;263:1218–1222.
205. World Health Assembly. Immunization and vaccine quality. Document WHA 45.17. Geneva: 54th World Health Assembly; 1992.
206. Mahoney FJ, Woodruff BA, Erben JJ, et al. Effect of hepatitis B vaccination program on the prevalence of hepatitis B virus infection. J Infect Dis. 1993;167:203–207.
207. Chen HL, Chang MH, Hsu HY, et al. Seroepidemiology of hepatitis B virus infection in children: Ten years of mass vaccination in Taiwan. JAMA. 1996;276:906–908.
208. Chang MH, Chen CJ, Lai MS, et al. Universal hepatitis B vaccination in Taiwan and the incidence of hepatocellular carcinoma in children. N Engl J Med. 1997;337:1855–1859.
209. Centers for Disease Control and Prevention. Trends in AIDS incidence, death, and prevalence—United States, 1996. MMWR Morb Mortal Wkly Rep. 1997;46:165–173.
210. Mann JM, Tarantola D, eds. AIDS in the World, v. 2. Oxford: Oxford University Press; 1996.
211. Schuchat A, Broome CV, Hightower A, et al. Use of surveillance for invasive pneumococcal disease to estimate the size of the immunosuppressed HIV-infected population. JAMA. 1991;265:3275–3279.
212. Cohn SE, Klein JD, Weinstein RA, et al. Geographic variation in the management and outcome of patients with AIDS-related *Pneumocystis carinii*. J Acquir Immune Defic Syndr Hum Retrovirol. 1996;13:408–415.
213. Didier E. Microsporidiosis. Clin Infect Dis. 1998;27:1–8.
214. Gruenewald R, Blum S, Chan J. Relationship between human immunodeficiency virus infection and salmonellosis in 20- to 59-year old residents of New York City. Clin Infect Dis. 1994;18:358–363.
215. Selik RM, Karon JM, Ward JW. Effect of the human immunodeficiency virus epidemic on mortality from opportunistic infections in the United States in 1993. J Infect Dis. 1997;176:632–636.
216. Greenberg AE, Nguyen-Dinh P, Mann JM, et al. The association between malaria, blood transfusions, and HIV seropositivity in a pediatric population in Kinshasa, Zaire. JAMA. 1988;259:545–549.
217. Vanittanakom N, Sirisanthana T. *Penicillium marneffei* infection in patients infected with human immunodeficiency virus. Curr Top Med Mycol. 1997;8:35–42.
218. Penheiro FP, Corber SJ. Global situation of dengue and dengue haemorrhagic fever, and its emergence in the Americas. World Health Stat Q. 1997;50:161–169.
219. Kautner I, Robinson MJ, Kuhnle U. Dengue virus infection: Epidemiology, pathogenesis, clinical presentation, diagnosis, and prevention. J Pediatr. 1997;131:516–524.
220. Hayes EB, Gubler DJ. Dengue and dengue hemorrhagic fever. Pediatr Infect Dis J. 1992;11:311–317.
221. Kalayanarooj S, Vaughn DW, Nimmannitya S, et al. Early clinical and laboratory indicators of acute dengue illness. J Infect Dis. 1997;176:313–321.
222. Halstead SB. Pathogenesis of dengue: Challenge to molecular biology. Science. 1988;239:476–481.
223. Thein S, Aung MM, Shwe TN, et al. Risk factors in dengue shock syndrome. Am J Trop Med Hyg. 1997;56:566–572.
224. Richards AL, Bagus R, Baso SM, et al. The first reported outbreak of dengue hemorrhagic fever in Irian Jaya, Indonesia. Am J Trop Med Hyg. 1997;57:49–55.
225. Pan American Health Organization. Re-emergence of dengue in the Americas. Epidemiol Bull. 1997;18:1–6.
226. Brandling-Bennett AD, Penheiro F. Infectious diseases in Latin America and the Caribbean: Are they really emerging and increasing? Emerg Infect Dis. 1996;2:59–61.
227. Kouri G, Guzman MG, Valdes L, et al. Reemergence of dengue in Cuba: A 1997 epidemic in Santiago de Cuba. Emerg Infect Dis. 1998;4:89–92.
228. Vaughn DW, Hoke CH Jr, Yoksan S, et al. Testing of a dengue 2 live-attenuated vaccine (strain 16681 PDK 53) in ten American volunteers. Vaccine. 1996:14:329–336.
229. Gubler DJ. *Aedes aegypti* and *Aedes aegypti*-borne disease control in the 1990s: Top down or bottom up. Am J Trop Med Hyg. 1989;40:571–578.
230. Murray CJ, Lopez AD. Alternative projections of mortality and disability by cause, 1990–2020: Global Burden of Disease Study. Lancet. 1997;349:1498–1504.

Chapter 13

New and Emerging Infectious Diseases

JOSEPH E. McDADE
JAMES M. HUGHES

Infectious diseases have been a scourge since the dawn of civilization. Over the centuries, epidemics of cholera, plague, typhus, smallpox, and other infectious diseases periodically swept across different populations and shaped the course of history. Global spread of infectious diseases began in the 16th century when Spanish explorers reportedly brought smallpox to the New World and returned with syphilis.[1, 2] Major epidemics of infectious diseases have continued to the present day. For example, the great influenza pandemic of 1918 killed an estimated 25 million people worldwide; influenza pandemics occurred again in 1957 and 1968, with substantial morbidity and mortality. The recent emergence of influenza associated with a new strain of avian origin in Hong Kong illustrates the continuing threat of pandemic disease.[3]

During the 1960s and early 1970s, buoyed by success of vaccination programs and the ready availability of antibiotics, many scientists and public health officials concluded that the world was witnessing "the virtual elimination of the infectious disease as a significant factor in social life."[2] Unfortunately, this optimism was short-lived. Between 1980 and 1992, the mortality rate for infectious diseases, excluding acquired immunodeficiency syndrome (AIDS), increased by 22%. The rate of death from septicemia increased by 83%, and the rate of death from respiratory tract infections increased by 20%.[4] In 1990, diphtheria reemerged in the newly independent states of the former Soviet Union; by 1996, 125,000 cases and 4000 deaths had been reported.[5] In 1991, epidemic cholera reappeared in South America after a lengthy absence; more than 1 million cases occurred in Central and South America during the ensuing 3 years.[6] Pertussis reemerged in the Netherlands during the 1990s, despite ongoing immunization programs.[7]

Worldwide, infectious diseases remain the leading cause of death (Fig. 13–1); estimates of direct and indirect costs of infectious diseases exceed $120 billion annually.[8, 9] Major epidemics can be devastating to national economies, particularly those of developing nations. For example, an outbreak of plague in India in 1994 cost the country an estimated $1 billion to $2 billion in commerce, and in 1991, the cholera epidemic in Peru resulted in an estimated loss of $700 million in tourism and trade.

New infectious diseases and etiologic agents continue to be discovered with surprising frequency. Table 13–1 lists many of the important infectious diseases and pathogens identified since 1973. In some instances, infectious agents have been identified as the cause

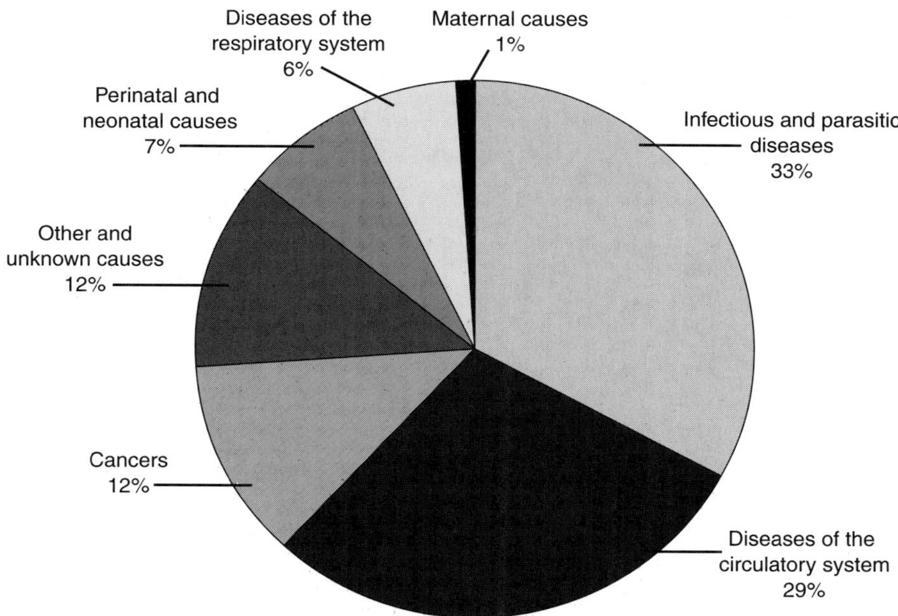

FIGURE 13–1. Distribution of global causes of death, 1997. (Data from the World Health Report 1998. Geneva: World Health Organization; 1998.)

of previously known diseases or syndromes (e.g., rotavirus as a cause of infantile diarrhea and parvovirus B19 as the etiologic agent of fifth disease). However, in other cases, diseases or etiologic agents have been newly identified (e.g., human immunodeficiency virus [HIV]/AIDS, hantavirus pulmonary syndrome, and hepatitis C virus infection). Increasingly, infectious agents also have been associated with chronic disease and neoplasia (Table 13–2).

The increasing prevalence of antimicrobial resistance complicates already serious infectious disease problems. Multiple-drug–resistant *Mycobacterium tuberculosis, Streptococcus pneumoniae, Staphylococcus aureus*, and *Neisseria gonorrhoeae* are just a few of the many pathogens that present significant treatment challenges.[40] Chloroquine-resistant malaria has become widespread, and multiple-drug–resistant malaria continues to increase (Fig. 13–2).

TABLE 13–1 Major Etiologic Agents and Infectious Diseases Identified since 1973

Year	Agent	Disease
1973	Rotavirus	Major cause of infantile diarrhea worldwide
1975	Parvovirus B19	Fifth disease; aplastic crisis in chronic hemolytic anemia
1976	*Cryptosporidium parvum*	Acute enterocolitis
1977	Ebola virus	Ebola hemorrhagic fever
1977	*Legionella pneumophila*	Legionnaires' disease
1977	Hantavirus	Hemorrhagic fever with renal syndrome (HFRS)
1977	*Campylobacter* sp.	Enteric pathogens distributed globally
1980	Human T-cell lymphotropic virus-1 (HTLV-1)	T-cell lymphoma-leukemia
1981	Toxin-producing strains of *Staphylococcus*	Toxic shock syndrome associated with tampon usage
1982	*Escherichia coli* O157 : H7	Hemorrhagic colitis; hemolytic uremic syndrome
1982	HTLV-II	Hairy cell leukemia
1982	*Borrelia burgdorferi*	Lyme disease
1983	Human immunodeficiency virus (HIV)	Acquired immunodeficiency syndrome
1983	*Helicobacter pylori*	Gastric ulcers
1986	*Cyclospora cayetanensis*	Persistent diarrhea
1988	Human herpesvirus-6 (HHV-6)	Roseola subitum
1988	Hepatitis E virus	Parenterally transmitted non-A, non-B hepatitis
1989	*Ehrlichia chaffeensis*	Human ehrlichiosis
1989	Hepatitis C	Parenterally transmitted non-A, non-B hepatitis
1991	Guanarito virus	Venezuelan hemorrhagic fever
1992	*Vibrio cholerae* O139	New strain associated with epidemic cholera
1992	*Bartonella* (= *Rochalimaea*) *henselae*	Cat-scratch disease; bacillary angiomatosis
1993	Sin Nombre virus	Hantavirus pulmonary syndrome
1994	Equine morbillivirus	Human pneumonia and encephalitis
1994	Sabia virus	Brazilian hemorrhagic fever
1995	Human herpesvirus-8 (HHV-8)	Associated with Kaposi's sarcoma in patients who have acquired immunodeficiency syndrome

Adapted from Satcher D. Emerging infections: Getting ahead of the curve. Emerg Infect Dis. 1995;1:1–6.

TABLE 13-2 Some Infectious Agents Tentatively Associated with Chronic Disease and Neoplasia

Disease	Agent	References
Coronary artery disease and stroke	*Chlamydia pneumoniae*	10–12
Deafness, hearing loss	Lassa fever virus	13
Gastric and duodenal ulcer	*Helicobacter pylori*	14
Infertility	*Chlamydia trachomatis*	15
Cryoglobulinemia, mixed leukocytoclastic vasculitis	Hepatitis C virus	16, 17
Cervical carcinoma	Human papillomavirus	18, 19
Gastric cancer	*H. pylori*	14, 20
Hepatocellular carcinoma	Hepatitis B and C viruses	21, 22
Kaposi's sarcoma	Human herpesvirus 8 (HHV-8)	23
Non-Hodgkin's lymphoma	Hepatitis C virus	24, 25
Lyme arthritis	*Borrelia burgdorferi*	26
Polyarthritis	Hepatitis C virus, human T-cell lymphotropic virus-1, and arthropod-borne viruses	27–29
Reactive arthritis	*Campylobacter jejuni, C. trachomatis, Salmonella, Shigella* spp., *Yersinia* spp.	30–32
Cranial neuropathies	*B. burgdorferi,* herpes simplex virus-1, varicella-zoster virus	33, 34
Guillain-Barré syndrome	*Campylobacter jejuni*	35, 36
Verruga peruana	*Bartonella bacilliformis*	37
Chorioretinitis and/or uveitis	*Toxoplasma gondii*	38, 39

IDENTIFYING ROOT CAUSES

In 1991, the Institute of Medicine (IOM) of the U.S. National Academy of Sciences convened a multidisciplinary committee to study issues related to infectious disease emergence. The report defined the issue as "new, re-emerging, or drug-resistant infections whose incidence in humans has increased within the past two decades or whose incidence threatens to increase in the near future." Their report, issued in 1992,[41] identified six factors underlying infectious disease emergence: (1) changes in human demographics and behavior, (2) the impact of new technologies and industries, (3) economic development and changes in land use, (4) increased international travel and commerce, (5) microbial adaptation and change, and (6) the breakdown of public health measures.

Many examples can illustrate how these factors contribute to the emergence of infectious diseases. Among many demographic changes, increased urbanization puts millions of people at risk for infection. At the beginning of the 19th century, less than 2% of the world's population lived in cities. By the year 2000, approximately 50% of the population will live in urban settings, and an estimated 25 cities will have populations exceeding 11 million people.[41] In developing countries, increased urbanization is all too frequently accompanied by overcrowding, inadequate sanitation and hygiene, insufficient supplies of clean drinking water, and malnutrition—factors that contribute to the emergence of infectious diseases. In industrialized nations, more young children attend daycare centers, where they are at increased risk for hepatitis A infection and respiratory illness and middle ear infections, which are often caused by drug-resistant organisms.[42] At the same time, the populations of industrialized nations are aging, and these older citizens are more susceptible to influenza, pneumonia, and other infections.[43]

Technological and industrial changes can also contribute to the emergence of infectious diseases. For example, contaminated water in cooling towers of air conditioning systems and in produce-misting devices in supermarkets has caused outbreaks of legionnaires' disease.[44, 45] Large-scale processing and distribution of apple juice in the Pacific Northwest resulted in widespread infection with *Escherichia coli* O157:H7; some patients with this infection developed hemolytic uremic syndrome.[46] Each year in the United States, an estimated 2 million persons acquire infections in hospitals, often in association with invasive medical procedures.[9]

Changes in land use in the northeastern United States were mainly responsible for the emergence of Lyme disease. Beginning in the early part of the 19th century, former farms reforested; this change allowed indigenous deer populations to expand, which then brought ticks that are vectors for Lyme disease *(Ixodes scapularis)* into proximity with residents in suburban communities.[41] Hantaviruses evidently have circulated harmlessly among rodent populations in certain areas of the world for thousands of years. However, recently, as forests are being cleared for economic development in South America, contact between rodents and humans has increased and has caused many fatal human infections.[47]

With modern transportation, a person infected with a disease can travel to any country in the world in 24 to 36 hours and can introduce the infection to an immunologically naive and unsuspecting population. Increasingly, imported foods constitute much of the diet of people in industrialized nations and may also contribute to the emergence of infectious diseases. For example, in 1996, large outbreaks of *Cyclospora* infection in the United States and Canada were associated with contaminated raspberries that had been imported from Guatemala.[48]

The 20th century has produced tremendous improvements in hygiene and sanitation and major scientific advances that have reduced the incidence of many infectious diseases in certain areas of the world. However, at the same time, the enormous increase in the human population, coupled with social, economic, and technological change, has provided continuing and even increased opportunities for contact between humans and infectious microorganisms.

The rapid generation time and mutation rate of microorganisms provide them with an incredible ability to adapt to changing ecologic conditions. The development of antimicrobial resistance is a good example of this. Penicillin was introduced in the 1940s; initially, it was uniformly effective for treating many diseases, especially pneumococcal pneumonia. Fifty years later, resistance to penicillin and its derivatives is commonplace. Previously susceptible bacteria, of human or animal origin, become resistant to antimicrobial compounds by spontaneous or induced genetic mutation or by acquiring resistance genes from related species. In some instances, resistance genes may originate in benign microorganisms, such as commensal species inhabiting the large intestine. For example, tetracycline-resistant genes in *S. pneumoniae* and *N. gonorrhoeae* are thought to have originated in *Enterococcus* species.[49] Newly resistant strains are then selected by use of antibiotics in humans and animals. Eventually, resistant microorganisms become widely disseminated, either by person-to-person spread or via contaminated food or water.[50] Development of antimicrobial resistance is notorious in populations following indiscriminate use of antibiotics. The recent emergence of multiple-drug–resistant *Salmonella typhimurium* DT 104 in England and Wales, at the same time that trimethoprim and enrofloxacin became widely used in cattle, is noteworthy.[51]

Continued erosion of the public health infrastructure also contributes to the emergence of infectious diseases. For example, the enormous outbreak of cryptosporidiosis in the greater Milwaukee area in 1993, where an estimated 400,000 people developed prolonged diarrheal illness, was traced to inadequately treated drinking water from a municipal system.[52] Ironically, that same year, in 12 of

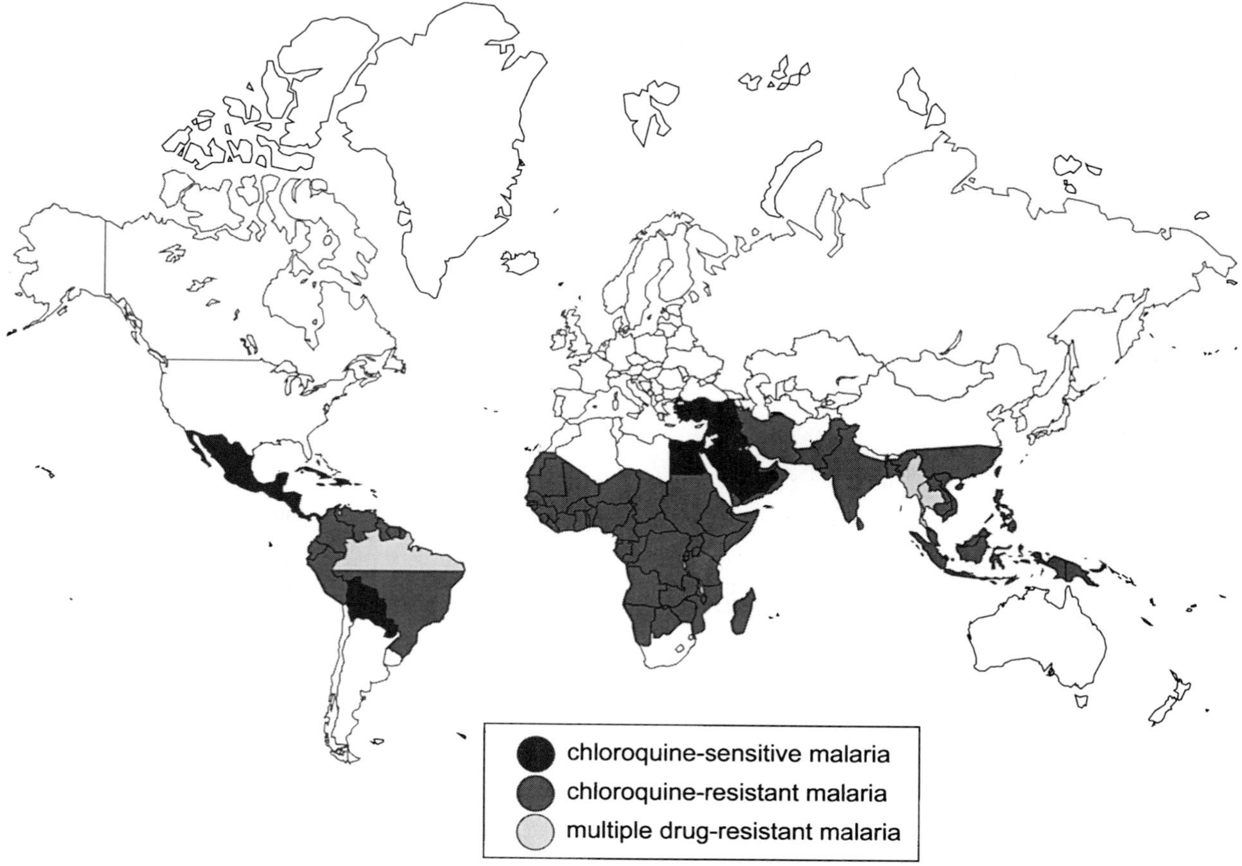

FIGURE 13–2. Distribution of malaria and drug-resistant *Plasmodium falciparum,* 1995. (Data from the Centers for Disease Control and Prevention, Atlanta, Ga.)

50 states, no personnel were assigned to conduct surveillance for waterborne or foodborne diseases.[53]

Events in Hong Kong during the winter of 1997–1998 illustrate the continuing threat of pandemic influenza. Eighteen previously healthy residents of Hong Kong became infected with an avian influenza strain (H5N1) for the first time in medical history; six (33%) of the cases were fatal.[3] Epidemiologic investigations found that most persons became infected by direct contact with infected poultry, but, in some instances, person-to-person transmission could not be ruled out. The outbreak was interrupted when more than 1 million chickens in the local marketplace were killed and the area was sanitized. In addition, patients were isolated while in the hospital to prevent the spread of infection. Had the H5N1 virus acquired the capability for efficient, person-to-person transmission, a worldwide pandemic could have resulted because the human population has acquired no underlying immunity from earlier exposure to the H5 subtype. Development of an appropriate influenza vaccine would then become an important public health priority.

In sum, microorganisms have survived ecologic change for millions of years because of their rapid rate of replication, mutation, and genetic recombination and exchange, and they will continue to do so as global ecology changes. Bacteria appeared on earth millions of years before humans and other mammals. Initially they grew in soil and water; as unicellular and multicellular plant and animal life evolved, bacteria established commensal or parasitic relationships with these new life forms. When humans and other mammals began to dominate the global ecosystem, bacteria exploited this ecologic niche. Pathogenicity was not necessarily a prerequisite for their continued survival. Instead, development of their ability to infect humans was merely a manifestation of their ability to exploit a nutritionally rich food source. Although humans are now the reservoir for many bacterial pathogens, some evidence of ancestral associations remains. For example, although humans are the principal reservoir for the cholera bacillus *(Vibrio cholerae), V. cholerae* also proliferate in association with copepods and other zooplankton in estuaries and brackish water in warm climates.[54]

INTERNATIONAL ASPECTS

All countries should have an interest in addressing these problems internationally. A Working Group on Emerging and Reemerging Infections under the auspices of the Committee on International Science, Engineering, and Technology (CISET) of the National Science and Technology Council developed 19 recommendations.[55] Six of the recommendations with highest priority address the need to establish global surveillance and response systems for infectious diseases, to enhance domestic infectious disease surveillance, to strengthen response capacity through collaboration with the private sector, to assist other countries in strengthening their national infectious disease systems, to establish the authority of U.S. agencies to make the most effective use of their resources, and to establish an interagency task force to facilitate the implementation of these recommendations.

The CISET report served as the basis for the Presidential Decision Directive (NSTC-7) from President Bill Clinton that Vice President Albert Gore announced in June 1996.[56] The directive contains six policy goals consistent with the CISET Work Group recommendations, including the need to strengthen domestic infectious disease surveillance and response systems; to establish a global infectious disease surveillance and response system; to strengthen research; to ensure the availability of drugs, vaccines, and diagnostic tests; to expand the missions and establish the authority of agencies of the U.S. government to contribute to worldwide networks; and to increase public awareness of these problems.

In 1995, the World Health Organization (WHO) created a new division of Emerging and Other Communicable Diseases Surveillance and Control.[57] The WHO has developed an emerging infections plan with goals similar to those of the Centers for Disease Control and Prevention plan. Some WHO regional offices have developed plans and are in the process of creating inventories of institutions in their regions that have the capacity to address many of these issues.

STRATEGIES FOR PREVENTION

It should be evident that, despite earlier predictions of a world free of infectious disease, the struggle for survival between humans and microorganisms will continue indefinitely, and new etiologic agents and infectious diseases will continue to emerge. The IOM Report on Emerging Infections recommended that several measures be implemented to improve preparedness against new and emerging infections. The recommendations were directed primarily to public health service agencies, such as the Centers for Disease Control and Prevention, the National Institutes of Health, and the Food and Drug Administration. The IOM Report emphasized the need for restoring essential public health infrastructure through improved surveillance, training, and research. However, improvements in these areas cannot be effected without active participation by the private sector.

Surveillance is the foundation of all public health programs.[58] Development of effective surveillance systems requires the combined expertise of clinicians, epidemiologists, laboratory technicians, and information systems specialists, among others. Because laboratory testing is necessary to confirm clinical diagnoses, collection and testing of appropriate clinical specimens is an essential component of the process. Prompt reporting of notifiable diseases to public health authorities is also critical.

Timely and accurate surveillance data have many useful applications. For example, surveillance can quantify the burden of infectious diseases in a given population and detect disease emergence and reemergence. In addition, surveillance for antibiotic resistance of locally circulating strains can help ensure prompt and cost-effective therapy for infections, thus minimizing the risk of development of resistance. Surveillance can also identify cases of a given illness, particularly newly discovered diseases, for detailed epidemiologic investigation to determine reservoirs of infectious microorganisms, their mode of transmission, and risk factors for infection.

Population-based surveillance data are essential for establishing national health goals and initiating intervention programs. Surveillance also allows the effectiveness of prevention programs to be evaluated. Occasionally, initial awareness and investigation of unusual events or clusters of cases may identify large outbreaks of disease. For example, unprecedented sales of loperamide, reported to public health officials by pharmacists, and high rates of absenteeism among students, school teachers, and hospital employees were the first signs of the outbreak of *Cryptosporidium* infection in the greater Milwaukee area.[52] Prompt reporting of undiagnosed cases of pneumonia by alert physicians and pathologists led ultimately to the discoveries of legionnaires' disease and Hantavirus pulmonary syndrome.[59, 60]

Clinical laboratories should submit representative isolates of microorganisms to state public health laboratories for follow-up testing for epidemiologic purposes. State public health laboratories subtype isolates of certain microorganisms, for example, enteric bacteria, to determine whether ill persons in a given population have been infected with the same or with different strains.[61] Identification of the same strain from multiple patients suggests a common source outbreak, and in some instances, a continuing epidemic. For example, in 1997 the Colorado Department of Health determined that 13 of 15 isolates from patients with *E. coli* O157:H7 infections were indistinguishable when analyzed by pulsed field gel electrophoresis. A follow-up epidemiologic investigation identified contaminated hamburger as the source of infection.[62] More than 24 million pounds of frozen hamburger patties from implicated lots were subsequently withdrawn from the market to prevent additional cases. The outbreak would not have been detected without collaboration among health care providers, clinical microbiology laboratories, state health departments, and other public health agencies and use of the molecular fingerprinting technique.

FUTURE CHALLENGES

Future challenges certainly include antimicrobial-resistant infections, the threat of another influenza pandemic, and the likelihood of increasing problems with dengue hemorrhagic fever and the risk of urban yellow fever in the Western Hemisphere. The global HIV epidemic will put large numbers of people at risk for currently recognized and new opportunistic infections.[43] The roles of hepatitis B and C viruses in chronic liver disease and hepatocellular carcinoma, of human papillomaviruses in cervical cancer, and of *Helicobacter pylori* infection in peptic ulcer disease and gastric cancer are now well established. Additional chronic diseases are likely to be found to have an infectious etiology.

Nobel laureate Joshua Lederberg has stressed the fact that emerging infectious diseases pose a threat to national security (see Chapter 313).[63] Recent experiences with terrorist incidents involving the chemical nerve agent sarin in Tokyo and explosive devices in New York City, Oklahoma City, and Atlanta provide grim reminders of the impact of terrorist activities. In contrast to incidents associated with toxic chemicals and explosive devices, an episode involving a biologic agent would occur following an incubation period, by which time exposed individuals would be dispersed geographically. Such an epidemic would require detection through infectious disease surveillance.

The need for partnerships is a recurrent theme in discussions of approaches to addressing emerging infectious diseases. Local, state, and territorial health departments, federal agencies, health care providers, microbiologists, pathologists, professional societies, the pharmaceutical industry, academic institutions, and the WHO and its regional offices all have critically important roles to play.

REFERENCES

1. McNeill WH. Plagues and Peoples. Garden City, NY: Anchor Press, Doubleday; 1976.
2. Burnet M, White DO. Natural History of Infectious Disease. London: Cambridge University Press; 1972.
3. Centers for Disease Control and Prevention. Update: Isolation of avian influenza A (H5N1) viruses from humans—Hong Kong, 1997–1998. MMWR Morb Mortal Wkly Rep. 1998;46:1245–1247.
4. Pinner RW, Teutsch SM, Simonsen L, et al. Trends in infectious disease mortality in the United States. JAMA. 1996;275:189–193.
5. Vitek CR, Wharton M. Diphtheria in the former Soviet Union: Re-emergence of a pandemic disease. Emerg Infect Dis. 1998;4:539–550.
6. Centers for Disease Control and Prevention. Update: *Vibrio cholerae* O1—Western hemisphere, 1991–1994 and *V. cholerae* O139—Asia, 1994. MMWR Morb Mortal Wkly Rep. 1994;44:215–219.
7. de Melker HE, Conyn-van Spaendonck MAE, Rumke HC, et al. Pertussis in the Netherlands: An outbreak despite high levels of immunization with whole-cell vaccine. Emerg Infect Dis. 1997;3:175–178.
8. Centers for Disease Control and Prevention. Addressing emerging infectious disease threats: A prevention strategy for the United States. Atlanta: Centers for Disease Control and Prevention; 1994.
9. National Institute for Allergy and Infectious Disease. Report of the Task Force on Microbiology and Infectious Disease. NIH Publication No. 2-3320. Bethesda, Md: National Institutes of Health; 1992.
10. Matilla KJ, Valtonen VV, Nieminen MS, et al. Role of infection as a risk factor for atherosclerosis, myocardial infarction, and stroke. Clin Infect Dis. 1998:26:719–734.
11. Danesh J, Collins R, Peto R. Chronic infections and coronary heart disease: Is there a link? Lancet. 1997;350:430–436.

12. Cook PJ, Honeybourne D, Lip GYH, et al. *Chlamydia pneumoniae* antibody titers are significantly associated with acute stroke and transient cerebral ischemia. Stroke. 1998;29:404–410.
13. Cummins D, McCormick JB, Bennett D, et al. Acute sensorineural deafness in Lassa fever. JAMA. 1990;264:2093–2096.
14. Dunn BE, Cohen H, Blaser MJ. *Helicobacter pylori*. Clin Microbiol Rev. 1997;10:720–741.
15. Peeling RW, Kimani J, Plummer F, et al. Antibody to chlamydial hsp60 predicts an increased risk for chlamydial pelvic inflammatory disease. J Infect Dis. 1997;175:1153–1158.
16. Agnello V. Hepatitis C virus infection and type II cryoglobulinemia: An immunological perspective. Hepatology. 1997;26:1375–1379.
17. Agnello V, Abel G. Localization of hepatitis C virus in cutaneous vasculitic lesions in patients with type II cryoglobulinemia. Arthritis Rheum. 1997;40:2007–2015.
18. Meschede W, Zumbach K, Braspenning J, et al. Antibodies against early proteins of human papillomavirus as diagnostic markers for invasive cervical cancer. J Clin Microbiol. 1998;36:475–480.
19. Munoz N, Bosch FA. The causal link between HPV and cervical cancer and its implications for prevention of cervical cancer. Bull Pan Am Health Organ. 1996;30:362–377.
20. Cheli R, Crespi M, Testino G, et al. Gastric cancer and *Helicobacter pylori*: Biologic and epidemiologic considerations. J Clin Gastroenterol. 1998;26:3–6.
21. Di Bisceglie AM. Hepatitis C and hepatocellular carcinoma. Hepatology. 1997;26(Suppl 1):34S–38S.
22. Montesano R, Hainaut P, Wild CP. Hepatocellular carcinoma: From gene to public health. J Natl Cancer Inst. 1997;89:1844–1851.
23. Moore PS, Chang Y. Kaposi's sarcoma (KS), KS-associated herpesvirus, and the criteria for causality in the age of molecular biology. Am J Epidemiol. 1998;147:217–221.
24. Kashyap A, Nademanee A, Molina A. Hepatitis C and B-cell lymphoma. Ann Intern Med. 1998;128:695.
25. Zuckerman E, Zuckerman T, Levine AM, et al. Hepatitis C virus infection in patients with B-cell non-Hodgkin lymphoma. Ann Intern Med. 1997;127:423–438.
26. Steere AC. Diagnosis and treatment of Lyme arthritis. Med Clin North Am. 1997;81:179–194.
27. Willson RA. Extrahepatic manifestations of chronic viral hepatitis. Am J Gastroenterol. 1997;92:4–17.
28. Nishioka K, Sumida T, Hasunuma T. Human T lymphotropic virus type I in arthropathy and autoimmune disorders. Arthritis Rheum. 1996;39:1410–1418.
29. Mackenzie JS, Smith DW. Mosquito-borne viruses and epidemic polyarthritis. Med J Aust. 1996;164:90–93.
30. Toivanen A, Toivanen P. Reactive arthritis. Curr Opin Rheumatol. 1997;9:321–327.
31. van der Heijden IM, Res PCM, Wilbrink B, et al. *Yersinia enterocolitica*: A cause of chronic polyarthritis. Clin Infect Dis. 1997;25:831–837.
32. Bremell T, Bjelle A, Svedham A. Rheumatic symptoms following an outbreak of *Campylobacter* enteritis: A five year follow-up. Ann Rheum Dis. 1995;50:934–938.
33. Belman AL, Reynolds L, Preston T, et al. Cerebrospinal fluid findings in children with Lyme disease–associated facial nerve palsy. Arch Pediatr Adolesc Med. 1997;151:1224–1228.
34. Murakami S, Mizobuchi M, Nakashiro Y, et al. Bell palsy and herpes simplex virus: Identification of viral DNA in endoneurial fluid and muscle. Ann Intern Med. 1996;124:27–30.
35. Allos BM. Association between *Campylobacter* infection and Guillain-Barré syndrome. J Infect Dis. 1997;176(Suppl 2):S125–S128.
36. Blaser MJ. Epidemiologic and clinical features of *Campylobacter jejuni* infections. J Infect Dis. 1997;176(Suppl 2):S103–S105.
37. Amano Y, Rumbea J, Knobloch J, et al. Bartonellosis in Ecuador: Serosurvey and current status of cutaneous verrucous disease. Am J Trop Med Hyg. 1997;57:174–179.
38. Ronday MJ, Stilma JS, Barbe RF, et al. Aetiology of uveitis in Sierra Leone, West Africa. Br J Ophthalmol. 1996;80:956–961.
39. Montoya JG, Remington JS. Toxoplasmic chorioretinitis in the setting of acute acquired toxoplasmosis. Clin Infect Dis. 1996;23:277–282.
40. Tenover FC, Hughes JM. The challenge of emerging infectious diseases. JAMA. 1996;275:300–304.
41. Institute of Medicine. Emerging infections: Microbial threats to health in the United States. Washington, DC: National Academy Press; 1992.
42. Schappert SM. Office visits for otitis media: United States, 1975–90. Advance Data from Vital and Health Statistics, No. 214. Hyattsville, Md: National Center for Health Statistics; 1992.
43. Kaplan JE, Hanson D, Jones J, et al. Opportunistic infections (OIs) as emerging infectious diseases: Challenges posed by OIs in the 1990s and beyond. In: Scheld WM, Craig WA, Hughes JM, eds. Emerging Infections 2. Washington, DC: ASM Press; 1998:257–272.
44. Dondero TJ Jr, Rendtorff RC, Mallison GF, et al. An outbreak of legionnaires' disease associated with a contaminated air conditioning cooling tower. N Engl J Med. 1980;302:365–370.
45. Mahoney FJ, Hoge CW, Farley TA, et al. Community-wide outbreak of legionnaires' disease associated with a grocery store mist machine. J Infect Dis. 1992;165:736–739.
46. Centers for Disease Control and Prevention. Outbreak of *Escherichia coli* O157:H7 infections associated with drinking unpasteurized commercial apple juice—British Columbia, California, Colorado, and Washington, October 1996. MMWR Morb Mortal Wkly Rep. 1996;45:975.
47. Parisi MN, Enria DA, Pina NC, et al. Detección retrospectiva de infecciones clínicas por hantavirus en la Argentina. Medicina (Buenos Aires). 1996;56:1–13.
48. Herwaldt B, Ackers ML, and the Cyclospora Working Group. An outbreak in 1996 of cyclosporiasis associated with imported raspberries. N Engl J Med. 1997;336:1548–1556.
49. Ferber D. New hunt for the roots of resistance. Science. 1998;280:27.
50. Tenover FC, McGowan JE Jr. Reasons for the emergence of antibiotic resistance. Am J Med Sci. 1996 311:9–16.
51. Threlfall EJ, Ward LR, Rowe B. Increased incidence of resistance of trimethoprim and ciprofloxacin in epidemic *Salmonella typhimurium* DT 104 in England and Wales. Eurosurveillance. 1997;2:81–84.
52. MacKenzie WR, Hoxie NJ, Proctor MS, et al. A massive outbreak in Milwaukee of *Cryptosporidium* infection transmitted through the public water supply. N Engl J Med. 331:161–167.
53. Osterholm MT, Birkhead GS, Meriwether RA. Impediments to public health surveillance in the 1990s: The lack of resources and the need for priorities. Public Health Manage Pract. 1996;2:11–15.
54. Colwell RR. Global climate and infectious disease: The cholera paradigm. Science. 1996;274:2025–2031.
55. Committee on International Science, Engineering, and Technology (CISET). Report of the NSTC CISET Working Group on Emerging and Reemerging Infectious Diseases. Washington, DC: National Science and Technology Council; 1995.
56. Gore A. Emerging infections threaten national and global security. ASM News. 1996 62:448–449.
57. LeDuc J. World Health Organization strategy for emerging infectious diseases. JAMA. 1996;275:318–320.
58. Berkelman RL, Stroup DF, Buehler JW. Public health surveillance. In: Detels R, Holland WW, McEwan J, et al, eds. Oxford Textbook of Public Health. 3rd ed. New York: Oxford University Press; 1997:735–750.
59. Fraser DW, Tsai TF, Orenstein W, et al. Legionnaires' disease. 1. Description of an epidemic. N Engl J Med. 1977;297:1189–1197.
60. Nichol ST, Spiropoulou CF, Morzunov S, et al. Genetic identification of a hantavirus associated with an outbreak of acute respiratory illness. Science. 1993;262:914–917.
61. Stephenson J. New approaches for detecting and curtailing foodborne microbial infections. JAMA. 1997;277:1337, 1339–1340.
62. Centers for Disease Control and Prevention. *Escherichia coli* O157:H7 infections associated with eating a nationally distributed commercial brand of frozen ground beef patties and burgers—Colorado, 1997. MMWR Morb Mortal Wkly Rep. 1997;46:777–778.
63. Lederberg J. Infectious diseases—a threat to global health and security. JAMA. 1996;276:417–419.

SECTION D

Chapter 14

The Clinician and the Microbiology Laboratory

VEE J. GILL
DANIEL P. FEDORKO
FRANK G. WITEBSKY

The clinician and the microbiology laboratory are partners in determining the etiology of infections, and as part of this process, it is essential that they actively communicate with each other. To attain an optimal working relationship between the laboratory and the infectious disease consultant, the following expectations regarding the laboratory's and the clinician's responsibilities should be recognized and addressed.

The laboratory must ensure that its operation meets all regulatory requirements (Clinical Laboratory Improvement Amendments of 1988 [CLIA]), including initial verification and ongoing validation of procedures that are used by the laboratory.[2] It should have a responsible program of quality control, as well as quality assurance benchmarks by which it can gauge its performance. Minimizing costs is essential but must be done without significantly compromising the quality of results. As part of an ongoing process, the laboratory director should be looking for state-of-the-art methodology that improves performance but is also relevant to the specific hospital population.[3] Through the hospital informational network, the laboratory should provide clinicians with easy access to specific guidelines for optimal collection and transport of specimens, as well as guidelines for common laboratory policies, for example, policies limiting the number of specimens per day or per week. These policies should be included on the ordering screens, which should also display practical information about specific tests, such as what pathogens are screened for when a routine bacterial stool culture is ordered. Reporting urgent and significant results is mandatory, such as reporting positive blood cultures, but provision of preliminary or interim "significant" reports should also be available to aid in patient management. It has become a more common practice for laboratories to include information on the culture report to help in the interpretation of results, particularly results that are unusual, for example, providing a brief description about an unusual bacterium. Critical to optimal functioning of a laboratory are its interactions with other hospital personnel, including patient care staff, hospital infection control officers, and pharmacists, in addition to the infectious disease specialists with whom the laboratory should be interacting on a daily basis. Establishing good notification and informational guidelines with each of these groups is important for maintaining effective hospital infection control and to deter the emergence of resistant organisms by the indiscriminate or inappropriate use of antibiotics.[4] If possible, laboratories with sufficient personnel and financial resources should also provide molecular-based typing of organisms because this service can have a significant impact on patient care.[5] By quickly defining potential outbreaks, particularly those with antibiotic-resistant organisms, control measures to prevent spread can be promptly instituted.

The responsibilities of the clinician, particularly the infectious disease specialist, include a substantive understanding of the laboratory's policies and methods used for commonly ordered cultures so that the infectious disease specialist can provide meaningful feedback to the patient's primary physician, who may be awaiting the test results. The laboratory expects that the infectious disease specialist will recommend the best specimen type and request the most appropriate test from the laboratory's menu and will contact the laboratory if further information or clarification is needed. The clinician should also alert the laboratory when looking for a particular organism that may be unusual or one that may require a special setup (e.g., *Corynebacterium diphtheriae, Bartonella* spp.) or when a potentially hazardous organism is expected (e.g., *Francisella tularensis,* multidrug-resistant *Mycobacterium tuberculosis, Coccidioides immitis*). On a similar note, discussion with the laboratory would be beneficial to explain out-of-the-ordinary situations in which deviation from normal laboratory policy would best serve the patient's interests (e.g., extended incubation, additional antibiotic susceptibility tests). In the care of immunocompromised patients or difficult diagnostic problems, numerous cultures or tests are often requested on a specimen for which there may be inadequate quantity; the clinician should prioritize the test requests for the laboratory based on the highest clinical suspicions because the laboratory cannot objectively assess test prioritization. The infectious disease specialist should bring to laboratory management's attention policies or procedures that, from experience, are recurrent problems for which solutions should be sought.

Both the microbiology laboratory and the infectious disease specialist need to regularly update their knowledge of organism nomenclature, which seems to be constantly changing. It is as difficult for laboratorians as it is for physicians to stay current with taxonomic changes and the discovery of new organisms. The laboratory must change and add names in a timely, yet appropriate fashion, and the infectious disease specialist must be aware of the significant changes or additions and be ready to discuss them with primary patient care physicians. Much of the taxonomic reorganization now under way is driven by our increased capability to group organisms because of molecular relatedness shown either by DNA hybridization or by specific gene sequencing analyses, such as 16S ribosomal DNA.[6] These analyses will lead us to taxonomic schemes that are more objective and, one hopes, more accurate in portraying the phylogenetic relationships of organisms.

Figure 14–1 is a general scheme of the types of methods used for the diagnosis of infectious agents. The specific methods and the relative usefulness of the tests will vary according to the microorganism being sought. In the following section we will summarize guidelines for specimen selection, collection, and transport and then briefly describe the detection and identification methods currently available. Recent advances in the use of molecular techniques to aid in the laboratory diagnosis of infectious diseases have added another dimension to the traditional stain, culture, and serology repertoire of the microbiology laboratory. Although such testing is currently limited in its availability and proven utility, molecular testing by the clinical laboratory has started and is likely to play an increasingly prominent role.

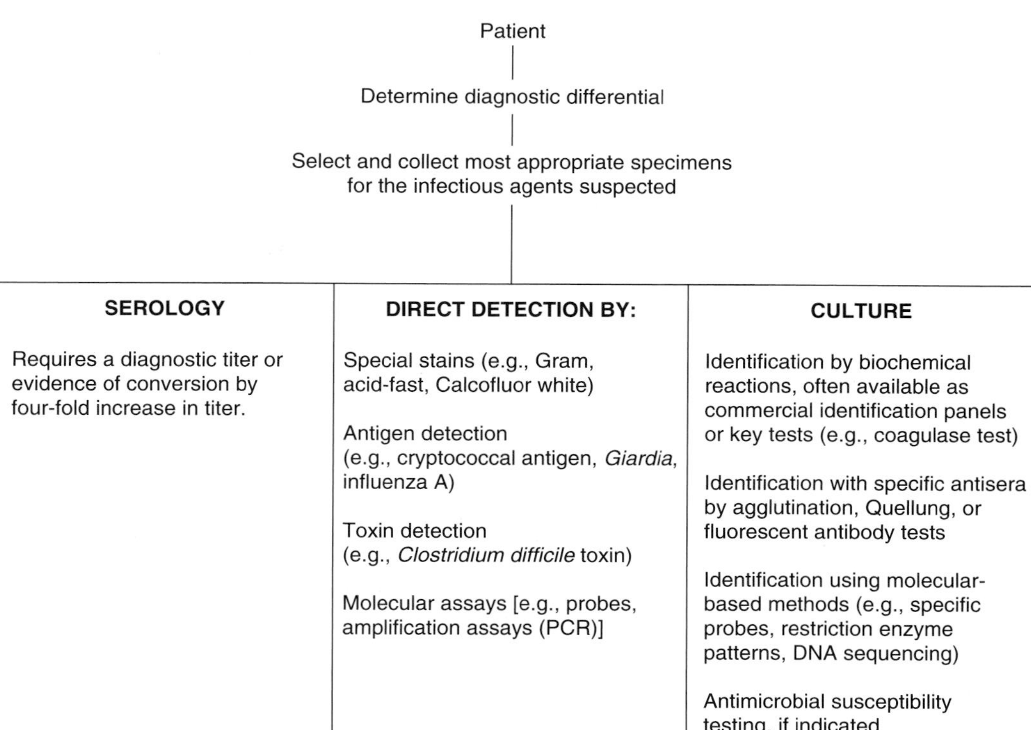

FIGURE 14–1. Methodologies used in the diagnosis of infectious agents.

SPECIMEN SELECTION, COLLECTION, AND PROCESSING

Submission of the best specimen type for a particular test or to recover a specific microorganism is of paramount importance for a successful outcome.[7, 8] It is obvious, however, that such a specimen, if placed in the wrong container, obtained incorrectly, or left undelivered for a prolonged period, will result in less reliable, if not falsely negative results. For many specimen types, the laboratory must also do some preliminary processing steps for the specimen to be suitable for culture or specific testing. Like the need for knowledgeable specimen selection and appropriate collection and transport, attention to recommended processing guidelines is critical for optimal testing.

General Criteria for Specimen Selection

Selection of the type of specimen to send for testing depends on multiple factors. Although it seems intuitively obvious that the best specimen is one that probably contains the infecting organism, a direct correlation is not always found between the apparently infected site and the success of detection. Specimen selection must also be based on the known characteristics of certain infectious processes or infectious agents. For example, pneumonia caused by *Legionella pneumophila* is only poorly diagnosed from expectorated sputum, whereas urine from the patient might yield a positive *Legionella* urinary antigen test. If, however, the patient is infected with *Legionella* spp. other than *L. pneumophila* serotype 1, the optimal specimen for diagnosis would be either bronchoalveolar lavage or lung biopsy because the urinary antigen test only detects serotype 1. Thus, selection of the most appropriate specimen must be done with knowledge of the relative yields of different specimens for different organisms for different tests. Here again, the laboratorian and the infectious diseases specialist must work to educate and provide physicians with this information. Selection of the best array of tests for specific types of infections or for specific microorganisms is not always obvious. In addition, patient tolerance of diagnostic procedures may limit the ability to obtain the most definitive specimen type.

General Criteria for Specimen Collection and Transport

Proper specimen collection should ideally start with collection performed before the administration of chemotherapeutic agents (antibiotic, antiviral, antifungal, etc.) to avoid possibly decreasing the recovery of microorganisms. Collection must then proceed with care to prevent contamination of the specimen with normal flora that may be encountered during the collection process, although such contamination may sometimes be unavoidable.

As part of the collection process, it is important to obtain amounts of material that are adequate for the tests needed. This information needs to be relayed by the infectious disease specialist to the individual obtaining the specimen, often a surgeon, dermatologist, or other specialist, who may not be aware of all the tests that will be ordered. Too often, laboratories are hampered by inadequate amounts of sterile body fluids, such as cerebrospinal fluid (CSF) or pleural fluid, that must be cultured or directly tested for multiple agents. This shortage of material is particularly significant when an invasive procedure is used to obtain the specimen because the procedure is unlikely to be repeated in the event of insufficient quantities. Even material taken with a swab must be examined to determine adequacy of the sampled material for the various tests that are to be requested. In general, swab cultures should be reserved for superficial skin lesions or throat swabs. It may be necessary to obtain two sets of swabs if multiple test requests will be made, particularly if both direct smears and cultures are intended. When a collection of fluid or pus is to be sampled, aspirated material is preferable to the use of swabs. A particularly important culture type that is dependent on adequate volume for maximal sensitivity is the blood culture. Although a sufficient volume of blood may be difficult to obtain from some patients, good effort should be made to obtain the recommended amount of blood to increase the likelihood of successful culture.

Complete instructions should be provided to those who will be collecting specimens that require special handling. Common questions, including what to put the biopsy in for transport to the laboratory, how to culture for anaerobes, how to collect and transport material for direct tests such as a fluorescent antibody test on skin lesions for varicella-zoster virus (VZV), what to use for *Chlamydia* cultures, and so forth, should be anticipated. Providing answers to these and similar questions could prevent discarding of specimens because of improper collection or having valuable specimens placed in bacteriostatic saline or formalin. All this information should be readily available and easily accessible to physicians and nurses through the hospital or laboratory computer system or in a widely distributed laboratory guide.

Transport of specimens to the microbiology laboratory must be done in a timely fashion and is particularly important in the handling of urgent requests. The laboratory should determine in what manner and how often specimens should be delivered and should periodically monitor this process to make sure that delivery to the laboratory is occurring as expected. Specimens should not be allowed to sit for hours; even if the specimen may remain perfectly suitable for culture, such as urine in buffered tubes, the delay in transport results in later processing and a shorter "overnight" incubation period. For some lengthy tests that may take 4 to 6 hours for completion such as certain immunoassays, late arrival may mean postponing performance of the test until the following day. Laboratories often have daily cutoff times for certain tests to complete the test on the same day as receipt of the specimen.

Table 14–1 summarizes generally accepted guidelines for specimen collection and transport of common specimen types. Although different laboratories have policies that are similar to one another, little absolute uniformity in the practice of microbiology is seen from laboratory to laboratory, so the clinician must be sure to understand the guidelines for a specific laboratory. Not all situations can be covered under general guidelines. For these instances, the physician should contact the laboratory to discuss the best procedures to ensure optimal handling of the specimen. For more extensive guidelines or recommendations that are beyond the scope of this chapter, numerous sources are available.[9–12]

SPECIFIC GUIDELINES AND RECOMMENDATIONS FOR MAJOR CATEGORIES OF INFECTION

This section summarizes pertinent laboratory information, predominantly for bacterial infections. Viral, fungal, and mycobacterial infections are only briefly mentioned here but are covered more specifically in separate sections to follow. Likewise, common parasitic test requests are included here, but more extensive discussion can be found in the relevant parasitology chapters.

Respiratory Tract Infections

Laboratories typically subdivide respiratory specimens into two major categories, upper respiratory and lower respiratory. Common upper respiratory specimens are throat swabs, nasopharyngeal swabs or washes, and mouth or oral cavity swabs or scrapings. Sinus aspiration and culture for otitis media are submitted only occasionally for specific problematic cases because empirical therapy without culture is generally effective.

From throat swabs, laboratories look for the presence or absence of group A streptococci (*Streptococcus pyogenes*) only unless specifically requested to look for other agents. Although it is recognized that group C and G β-hemolytic streptococci may also cause pharyngitis, the lack of proven rheumatic fever sequelae, as well as only rare reports of associated post-streptococcal glomerulonephritis, has deterred laboratories from screening for and reporting these isolates. Rapid antigen tests for detection of group A *streptococci* are used by some laboratories and physicians' offices because they give rapid results that if positive, can justify the initiation of antibiotic therapy. Although highly specific, rapid antigen tests are hampered by their lack of sensitivity for detecting very low numbers of organisms, and because the quality of the specimen depends on the effectiveness of the sampling process, very low numbers of organisms may still be significant. For that reason, it is recommended that all negative rapid direct tests be followed by a traditional culture for group A *streptococci.* Antibiotic susceptibility testing is not done on *S. pyogenes* because all isolates remain universally susceptible to penicillin.

To look for other agents of pharyngitis such as *Neisseria gonorrhoeae,* the laboratory must be notified because cultures for agents other than *S. pyogenes* are not routinely done. Throat swabs or nasopharyngeal specimens may also be submitted when diphtheria is suspected, but special smears and isolation media are used for culturing of *C. diphtheriae.* For *Bordetella pertussis* culture, either nasopharyngeal swabs or aspirates are recommended rather than throat swabs or "cough plates." Dacron or calcium alginate swabs should be used, and because special media are required for optimal growth of *Bordetella,* the laboratory should be notified in advance.[13]

Lower respiratory tract infections, primarily pneumonia, are most often initially cultured from expectorated sputa or tracheal aspirates because these specimens can be obtained with minimal patient discomfort. More aggressive culturing is attained by way of sputum induction for patients producing only scant sputum or by bronchoscopic procedures, including bronchial washes, bronchial brushes, transbronchial biopsies, and bronchoalveolar lavage.[14] In select situations, lung biopsies are performed, particularly when less invasive specimens have yielded no diagnosis. Although sputa and tracheal aspirates are readily obtained, the significance of the potential pathogens that are isolated is sometimes difficult to assess. Also important is that expectorated sputum is insensitive for the detection of *Legionella* or *Pneumocystis.* To eliminate unnecessary as well as potentially misleading culture results, laboratories use microscopy screening guidelines to reject sputum specimens that are poor in quality. Rejection is usually based on the observation of many squamous epithelial cells, which generally correlates with significant oropharyngeal contamination. The presence of polymorphonuclear leukocytes usually indicates good specimen quality, but this criterion should not be required in a granulocytopenic patient. Although sputa should be screened when submitted for routine bacterial culture, analogous rejection criteria have not been validated for fungal and mycobacterial cultures.

Lower respiratory specimens obtained by bronchoscopic procedures or by lung biopsy should always be regarded as important specimens requiring prompt laboratory attention. Diagnoses obtained by the use of bronchoalveolar lavage and transbronchial biopsy have significantly decreased the need for open lung biopsies. The range of microorganisms that cause lower respiratory tract infections is broad, and selection of appropriate tests relies on whether the infection is thought to be community acquired or nosocomial in origin and on other relevant clinical information, including the type of infiltrate, the immunologic status and underlying disease of the patient, history of exposure to known pathogens, travel or occupational exposure, and so on.[15] Table 14–2 summarizes the microorganisms that often enter into the differential diagnosis and the types of tests that can be used to establish an infectious etiology.[16] To help determine the significance of potential pathogens that could instead be mere colonizers, some laboratories use a quantitative procedure with suggested significance cutoffs to analyze the culture results from bronchoalveolar lavage fluids.[17] The specifics of the guidelines used by a laboratory should be known to the infectious disease consultant and the appropriateness of the interpretation assessed in light of the type of patient and clinical concerns.

Because the diagnosis of pneumonia in an immunocompromised host has become a more frequent and often urgent problem, laboratories have made significant strides in establishing some of these

TABLE 14–1 Collection and Transport* Guidelines for Commonly Submitted Specimens†

Specimen	Collection Guidelines	Other Comments
Abscess	Aspirate of pus or fluid in anaerobic transport vial is preferred. Swabs usually have insufficient material for Gram stain and culture. Specify location of abscess for optimal plating. Aspirate is appropriate for routine, anaerobic, fungal, and mycobacterial culture	Specimen sent immediately in syringe is also acceptable, but without a needle attached. Provide additional pertinent information, e.g., cat bite, needle aspirate of liver
Biopsies	Keep specimen moist and transport rapidly to lab. Do not use bacteriostatic saline or formalin. Biopsies are suitable specimens for routine, fungal, mycobacterial, viral, and anaerobic cultures, depending on the site of biopsy	Always specify the type of tissue and indicate the specific pathogen sought if other than routine bacteria, e.g., *Nocardia, Bartonella, Histoplasma*
Blood	Prepare site with 70% alcohol, then with tincture of iodine or an iodophor. Cleanse top of culture bottles/tubes with 70% alcohol; do not change needles to inoculate	All blood cultures should be transported ASAP to start incubation or processing. (Differing skin preparation methods have been proposed; follow specific hospital recommendations)
Routine bacteria	20–30 ml in adults, 1–3 ml in children is the *minimum* amount for each episode; peripheral draws are preferred. 3 culture sets/d maximum	Do not use smaller blood volumes in pediatric bottles for **adults** because culture sensitivity will be decreased. SPS may inhibit some organisms (see text)
Anaerobes	If anaerobic bottle is not part of lab's routine culture set, contact lab for instructions	
Bartonella	10 ml in lysis-centrifugation tube is preferred method. Bottle systems may be much slower; contact lab	
Brucella	Routine broth culture systems, biphasic systems, and lysis-centrifugation are used; contact lab	
Leptospira	1–3 drops of fresh or SPS blood are needed to inoculate special media; collect within first week of illness	Contact lab in advance
Fungi	Use routine blood culture system for *Candida,* 10 ml in lysis-centrifugation tube, or 3–5 ml in fungal blood culture bottle or biphasic systems	Specify if culture for *Malassezia* is needed
Mycobacteria	10 ml in lysis-centrifugation tube; amount of blood or lysed sediment needed for bottle systems for mycobacteria depends on system used	
Malaria or *Babesia*	Prepare thick and thin smears from fingerstick or EDTA blood; examine multiple specimens over 48–72 h	Transport for smear preparation ASAP
Trypanosomes	Prepare multiple thick and thin smears from fingerstick or EDTA blood during febrile episodes. Culture is possible, but not generally available	Transport for wet mount or smear preparation ASAP
Microfilariae	Obtain blood according to observed periodicity; concentration techniques such as thick smears can be used; contact lab	Transport for smear preparation ASAP
Bone marrow	Obtain 1–2 ml of marrow for diagnosis of histoplasmosis, miliary tuberculosis, brucellosis, *Salmonella typhi.* Also good for diagnosis of leishmaniasis	Aspirating more than 2 ml will dilute marrow with peripheral blood
Catheter		
Intravenous	Remove aseptically, cut at least a 2-inch segment from tip, and place segment in sterile container	Transport ASAP to prevent drying out
Foley	Not acceptable for culture	
Drainage	Not recommended for culture; needle aspirate of fluid or abscess preferred	Drainage tubes may be superficially contaminated and make interpretation difficult
Eye (lid, conjunctiva, corneal scrapings)	Bacterial, fungal, chlamydial, mycobacterial, or viral cultures may be requested from these sites	Notify lab if looking for *Acanthamoeba* or microsporidia
Fluids (body fluids other than blood, urine)		
Pleural, peritoneal, synovial, cardiac, etc.	Send at least 2–5 ml for bacteria, >10 ml for fungi and/or mycobacteria. Use anaerobic transport media if indicated. Viral etiology may be considered for pericardial fluids	Excess peritoneal fluid inoculated into blood culture bottles may increase sensitivity of culture for routine bacteria. Send ASAP
CSF	1–2 ml for bacteria, viruses; 5–10 ml for mycobacteria, fungi	Send immediately. Alert lab if anaerobic culture is indicated because anaerobes may not be detected by the lab's routine culture; also alert lab for diagnosis of primary amebic meningoencephalitis
Genital tract (commonly submitted specimens)		
Cervical, urethral, vaginal, or penile ulcer or discharge	Use transport media/containers appropriate for organisms sought (*Neisseria gonorrhoeae, Chlamydia, Ureaplasma,* etc.)	Transport quickly. Lab may want specimen planted directly; swabs or plates need to be transported to the lab ASAP
	Follow lab guidelines for syphilis, soft chancre, herpes, yeast, *Trichomonas, Gardnerella, N. gonorrhoeae*	Check with lab to determine which tests are available because some of these organisms are difficult to detect by culture. Anaerobic cultures are not performed
Respiratory, upper		
Nose	Anterior nares swabs usually submitted only for detection of staphylococcal or streptococcal carriers	Use bacterial transport media; specify organism, e.g., rule out MRSA
Nasopharynx	Nasopharyngeal specimen appropriate for *Bordetella pertussis, Corynebacterium diphtheriae, N. gonorrhoeoe, Neisseria meningitidis.* Alert laboratory before sending	Cough plates for pertussis are not recommended; use calcium alginate swabs and plate directly or send to lab ASAP
Oral cavity	Swabs or scrapings taken from oral lesions	
Bacteria	Not usually cultured, but direct smears may be used to demonstrate fusospirochetal disease	
Fungi	Gram stain, Calcofluor white stain, or KOH preparation can be used for direct detection of yeast. Culture not generally done unless identification or susceptibilities of yeast are wanted	Follow lab guidelines for submission of samples for direct smears
Sinus aspirate	Submit in anaerobic transport if anaerobes are suspected. Bacterial and fungal smears and cultures may be indicated	
Throat	Swab areas of purulence or ulceration. Notify lab if looking for organism other than group A streptococci	Use transport media. Be sure to specify when looking for diphtheria or pertussis
Respiratory, lower		
All specimens of lower respiratory secretions	Specimens should be refrigerated if transport will be delayed to prevent overgrowth with commensals. See below for specific guidelines	For multiple test requests, be sure that specimen volume is adequate

Table continued on following page

TABLE 14–1 Collection and Transport* Guidelines for Commonly Submitted Specimens† *Continued*

Specimen	Collection Guidelines	Other Comments
Sputum		
Bacteria	Sputa are screened for acceptability by absence or low numbers of squamous epithelial cells in the presence of neutrophils. Not suitable for anaerobic culture. Not recommended for *Legionella* culture	Expectorated sputa may not be best specimen for diagnosis of bacterial pneumonia. Lavage or biopsy material is more definitive. Concomitant blood cultures are recommended
Mycobacteria	First, early morning specimen is preferred, not pooled. Should not be screened for adequacy. Send 3 consecutive first morning specimens for optimal diagnosis	
Fungi	Should not be screened for adequacy. Send 3 consecutive first morning specimens for optimal diagnosis. **Induced** sputum recommended for *Pneumocystis*	If known, specify particular agent of concern, e.g., *Cryptococcus, Histoplasma, Nocardia,* etc. Isolation of *Candida* spp. from sputum is not diagnostic of *Candida* pneumonia
Parasites	Acceptable for parasite detection, e.g., *Stronglyoides, Ascaris* larvae	
Sputum, induced	Induction with nebulized saline is used primarily to obtain specimens suitable for either mycobacterial or *Pneumocystis* diagnosis	Quantity of specimen is generally limited (<2 ml), so tests requested should be prioritized. Substantial contamination with oral flora makes this specimen unsuitable for culture of routine bacteria
Tracheal aspirate	Acceptable for same tests as sputum; not screened for acceptability like sputa	Significance of potential pathogens such as gram-negative rods cannot be determined because of rapid, heavy colonization of these sites with such organisms
Transtracheal aspirate	Acceptable for same tests as sputum; this procedure bypasses the oral cavity, so anaerobic cultures are also acceptable	This procedure is only infrequently performed
Bronchial wash/brush	These specimens are not usually screened for acceptability like sputa	For detection of all pathogens, bronchoalveolar lavage (see below) is considered better than bronchial wash
Bacteria	Suitable for culture of common bacterial pathogens, but only sheathed brush specimens are acceptable for anaerobic cultures	Specimens are contaminated with oral flora, so assessment of the significance of routine bacteria is still problematic
Legionella	Process ASAP for *Legionella* because saline may be deterimental	
Mycobacteria	Preferable to expectorated sputum	
Fungi	Preferable to expectorated sputum. Also acceptable for detection of *Pneumocystis*	Growth of *Candida* and other opportunistic fungi does not necessarily predict significance
Parasites	Suitable for detection of *Stronglyloides,* cryptosporidia, microsporidia, *Toxoplasma*	
Bronchoalveolar lavage	Can be used for same tests as bronchial wash/brush. Particularly better than bronchial wash for *Pneumocystis*	Although properly obtained lavage fluid has minimal contamination with oral flora, significance of *Candida,* molds, and opportunistic bacteria may still be unclear. Some labs use quantitation of bacteria to help assess significance
Skin scrapings for dermatophytes	Scrape skin at active edge of lesion; avoid blood. Place in sterile Petri dish	
Skin lesion	Specimen taken from advancing edge is recommended. Biopsy may be more definitive than swabs of lesion. Appropriate for routine, fungal, and mycobacterial culture and for *Leishmania* by smear or culture	Transport swabs in transport media to prevent drying out. Specifying species of fungus or *Mycobacterium* sought is helpful
Rectal swabs (see "Stool")	Only rarely acceptable when looking for diarrheal pathogens. Send fresh stool instead (see stool guidelines below)	Occasionally an infant or very ill patient with diarrhea may necessitate use of a rectal swab
	Avoid fecal material on anal swabs for *N. gonorrhoeae* culture	
	Perianal samples used for detection of pinworm	For pinworm, use a clear plastic tape preparation or Swube device
Stool		
Bacteria	Send up to 3 specimens (1/d). Notify lab if *Vibrio, Yersinia, Aeromonas,* or enterohermorrhagic *Escherichia coli* is being sought. Transport immediately or hold in refrigerator (less desirable)	Be aware of what pathogens are "routinely" screened for by lab, in particular, *Campylobacter.* Stool from patients in hospital for >3 d is not accepted by some laboratories
Ova and parasites	Transport fresh specimen to lab quickly. Preservatives for transport may be supplied by labs. Three specimens on 3 separate days are sufficient for screening	Alert lab when specific pathogens are suspected, e.g., *Strongyloides,* cryptosporidia, microsporidia, *Isospora. Giardia* enzyme immunoassays may need to be specifically requested
Clostridium difficile toxin	No more than 1 per day or 3 specimens for initial screening is acceptable. Deliver ASAP or else refrigerate or freeze specimen. Isolation of organism is not generally done. Assays are usually for toxin	Find out what kind of assay is used, turnaround time, sensitivity, and specificity of assay
Urine	Keep refrigerated and transport to lab promptly or submit in urine tube with preservative	Proper instruction for midstream collection should be routinely provided. Straight catheter collection provides specimen with less or no external contamination
Bacteria	Most commonly clean voided. Only suprapubic aspirate is acceptable for anaerobic culture	*Candida* spp. will also be detected by routine bacterial cultures
Leptospira	Culture within 2 h or neutralize to pH 7.0; collect **after** first week of illness	Contact lab in advance
N. gonorrhoeae	LCR amplification assay for urine; can detect *Chlamydia* also	
Chlamydia	Urine is acceptable specimen for amplification assays, e.g., PCR, LCR, TMA. LCR can be used for simultaneous detection of *N. gonorrhoeae*	
Mycobacteria	Send >20 ml, use first morning urine	**Do not send** 24-h specimens
Fungi	Send >20 ml, specify fungus being sought	Check with lab on policy for *Candida* culture
Schistosoma haematobium	Collect mid-day urine, particularly urine containing mucus and blood	
Trichomonas	Collect first-voided urine and transport quickly. **Do not refrigerate**	For males, prostatic massage may increase detection
Wound (see "Abscess," "Skin lesion")	Decontaminate open lesion first. Aspirate if possible; if swabs must be used, be sure that quantity is sufficient for stains and cultures. Open superficial wounds are not suitable for anaerobic culturing. Identify type/location of wound	Transport in anaerobic transport media ASAP if anaerobes suspected. Use transport media for all swabs

*It is assumed that appropriate transport media will be provided and used.
†Recommendations for viruses presented separately.
Abbreviations: ASAP, As soon as possible; CSF, cerebrospinal fluid; EDTA, ethylenediaminetetraacetic acid; LCR, ligase chain reaction; MRSA, methicillin-resistant *Staphylococcus aureus*; PCR, polymerase chain reaction; SPS, sodium polyanethole sulfonate anticoagulant; TMA, transcription-mediated amplification.

TABLE 14–2 Diagnosis of Lower Respiratory Tract Pathogens

Organism	Acceptable Specimens	Tests Available	Comments
Common bacteria*	S, B, L	Gram stain, culture	1–5 d for isolation and identification
Legionella	B, L	FA	Poor test, not recommended
		Culture	Requires special media, incubation for 10–12 d
	Urine	Antigen assay	EIA for *L. pneumophila* serotype 1 only
Mycobacteria	S, IS, B, L	Acid-fast stains	Fluorochrome stains preferred
		Nucleic acid amplification	Approved for specimens smear positive for *M. tuberculosis*
		Culture	Rapid methods preferred, e.g., radiometric, newer automated systems; 4–6-wk incubation is standard
Nocardia	S, IS, B, L	Modified acid-fast stain	Include positive and negative controls when staining
		Culture	Incubate up to 4 wk
Fungi	S, IS, B, L	Calcofluor white stain	Superior to unstained wet mounts
		Culture	Specify if *Histoplasma* or *Coccidioides* is suspected. Incubate 6 wk
	Serum and CSF	Cryptococcal antigen	By latex agglutination or EIA
	Serum and urine	*Histoplasma* antigen	Not generally offered
Pneumocystis	IS, B, L	*Pneumocystis* stains (nonculturable agent)	FA, Giemsa, toluidine blue O, silver stains, etc.
Mycoplasma pneumoniae	S, NP, B, L	No direct stains	
		Culture	Not done routinely, 7–10 d. Species identification needed
	Serum	Serology (CF)	4–9-wk conversion time
		Cold agglutinins	CA titers are nonspecific
Chlamydia pneumoniae	NP, ?B, ?L	No direct stains	
		Culture	Fastidious, difficult to grow; not readily available
	Serum	Serology, CF	Cross reacts within the genus, 4–6-wk conversion time
		Serology, microimmunofluorescence	Not widely available
Viruses	NP, B, L	FA, EIAs	Available only for certain viruses
		Culture	Rapid shell vials, hold 2–5 d
			Standard tubes, hold 4–6 wk

*Common bacteria, including staphylococci, streptococci, *Enterobacteriaceae, Pseudomonas,* etc.
Abbreviations: B, Bronchial washes, brushings, biopsies, bronchoalveolar lavage fluid; CA, cold agglutinins; CF, complement fixation; EIA, enzyme immunoassay; FA, fluorescent antibody; IS, induced sputum; L, lung biopsy; NP, nasopharyngeal suction or swab; S, sputum, tracheal aspirates.

diagnoses more expeditiously than in the past. The diagnosis of *Pneumocystis* pneumonia can be made from either induced sputum or bronchoalveolar lavage fluid with stains that can be done within a few hours.[18, 19] Microbiology laboratories should make an effort to provide this service because in many situations they can provide results sooner than the cytopathology laboratory and these results may have a significant impact on patient management. Improved fungal stains with Calcofluor white rather than the traditional wet mount have greatly improved direct detection of fungi. Likewise, the use of fluorochrome smears for acid-fast bacilli rather than the older Ziehl-Neelsen or Kinyoun stains has improved the sensitivity of direct detection of mycobacteria. Radiometric culture methods, as well as other new culture systems for mycobacteria, have reduced time to detection; other advances in mycobacteriology will be discussed later in this chapter. Despite these improvements, more sensitive and specific methods are still needed for detection of *Legionella, Chlamydia, Mycoplasma,* and fungi, particularly *Histoplasma* and *Cryptococcus* in lower respiratory specimens. For these and other organisms, molecular amplification assays may be the best direction for improving our diagnostic capabilities.[20, 21]

Blood Stream Infections

Blood cultures are considered one of the most significant specimen types that the microbiology laboratory processes. Every laboratory has strict notification policies to ensure that positive blood cultures are promptly reported to the physician. The latest generation of automated blood culture systems now provides us with the capability of "continuous monitoring,"[22] which generally means that a growth reading is automatically done every 10 to 20 minutes throughout the day to detect positive cultures as quickly as possible. With these new systems, monitoring does not require entry into the bottles, so contamination rates remain low. Nonbottle systems such as the lysis-centrifugation system (Isolator) are also used in some hospitals for either routine bacteria, fungi, mycobacteria, or fastidious organisms such as *Bartonella* or *Brucella.* Although lysis-centrifugation offers advantages such as colony counts and isolated colonies for rapid identification, it remains a fairly labor-intensive method that has higher rates of contamination than bottle systems do and is therefore not widely used by laboratories with heavy workloads or few technical staff members.

For most common, nonfastidious pathogens, the type of blood culture system used is probably not as significant a factor in the reliable detection of septicemia as other important considerations. Two recent reviews of blood cultures discuss this subject in detail.[22, 23] Optimal blood culturing starts with proper skin preparation for venipuncture: the skin surface is first cleansed with 70% alcohol, followed by tincture of iodine (1 minute) or povidone iodine (2 minutes). The septum of the culture bottle or tube need only be wiped with 70% alcohol and the blood immediately injected without changing the needle. Blood cultures should be transported to the laboratory promptly so that processing and incubation can be started without delay. The volume of blood cultured and the number of sets drawn are particularly important factors that determine the success of detection. Often, the number of organisms per milliliter of blood is low, or circulation of organisms may be intermittent, so the current recommendations for adults are to draw at least two separate blood cultures totaling 30 to 40 ml of blood. Separate venipunctures should be performed to help interpret cultures that contain skin flora such as *Staphylococcus epidermidis* and *Corynebacterium* species. In cases of fever of unknown origin, subsequent sets at later times in the day may be indicated. For children, the maximum amount of blood that can be taken will depend on the weight and clinical status of the child; usually 1 to 3 ml may be obtained from a child younger than 6 years, whereas neonates may only be able to afford 0.5 to 1 ml. When the volume drawn is 2 ml or less, pediatric blood culture systems should be used to achieve the optimal blood-to-broth dilution ratio. The use of pediatric systems for adult patients or older children results in less blood cultured and should be discouraged except in most unusual circumstances because smaller volumes significantly compromise the effectiveness of blood cultures. For both children and adults, blood cultures should be obtained before the start of antibiotic therapy to prevent inhibition of organism growth.

In recent years, many bacteremias have been associated with the increased use of catheters for intravenous access, including long-term percutaneous catheters and subcutaneous implanted devices and short-term catheters used for a variety of limited vascular access needs. Hospitals in which the use of indwelling intravenous lines is commonplace have had an increase in organisms such as coagulase-negative staphylococci, corynebacteria, *Bacillus,* yeast, and even a variety of uncommon, but opportunistic gram-negative rods. Microbiologists have long recommended that blood for cultures not be drawn through catheters because a positive culture may not represent true septicemia but rather colonization or localized infection of the catheter. Laboratories most often do semiquantitative catheter tip cultures according to the guidelines of Maki and colleagues[24] to help determine the likelihood of catheter-related infection. Despite laboratory recommendations to not draw blood for cultures through intravenous catheters, the ease of drawing blood for cultures through these catheters, especially with little discomfort to the patient, has made this practice common. In addition, physicians may have clinically significant concerns about keeping the catheter in place and treating with antibiotics without removal of the catheter. For these reasons, the use of catheter-drawn blood for culture has and continues to increase in comparison to peripherally drawn blood to diagnose catheter-related infection. For laboratories using quantitative blood culture systems (e.g., Isolator), a substantially higher colony count from catheter-drawn blood versus peripheral blood cultures is commonly used to identify a catheter-related focus for the bacteremia.

Standard blood culture protocols usually provide for one aerobic and one anaerobic bottle for each blood culture set. Examination of the utility and cost-effectiveness of routinely including an anaerobic bottle for all blood cultures has led to the suggestion that anaerobic blood cultures be done only by specific request and that the second bottle instead be an additional aerobic bottle.[25] Such practice would increase the overall sensitivity of the culture for aerobic and facultatively anaerobic bacteria and fungi. However, unanticipated sepsis with anaerobes would place patients at high risk for serious, potentially life-threatening infection.[26] At present, each hospital should determine the combination of bottles that would be most desirable for its patient population.[23] In addition to an aerobic/anaerobic or aerobic/aerobic two-bottle set, the use of resin-containing bottles, different broth media, or fungal broth media can be considered.

Blood cultures are usually incubated for 5 to 7 days except for specific situations, for example, when fastidious organisms are anticipated such as *Brucella* and *Bartonella* or in cases of suspected subacute bacterial endocarditis or prolonged fever of unknown origin. Laboratory policies on extended incubation (e.g., from 2 to 4 weeks) vary according to the type of blood culture system used. For some bottle systems, weekly subcultures, acridine orange staining, or both are recommended to reliably detect organisms such as *Brucella, Bartonella, Campylobacter,* or *Helicobacter.* Organisms such as *N. gonorrhoeae, Neisseria meningitidis, Gardnerella vaginalis, Streptobacillus moniliformis,* and *Peptostreptococcus anaerobius* may be inhibited by the anticoagulant used in most blood culture systems, sodium polyanethole sulfonate, so culture for these agents requires media without this anticoagulant. Optimal methods should be used whenever possible for the growth of *Brucella, Bartonella, Campylobacter, Helicobacter, Abiotrophia, Legionella, Nocardia,* and *Malassezia.* Table 14–3 provides a general overview of the usefulness of specific blood culture methods for various organisms. Further discussion of blood cultures for mycobacteria, fungi, and viruses will be covered later in this chapter.

Intravenous Catheter Tip Cultures. As mentioned earlier, semiquantitative culture of catheter tips obtained by rolling the tip across a blood-agar plate is the method used most commonly. A breakpoint of 15 or more colonies suggests that these organisms are indicative of catheter infection,[24] although other investigators suggest that lower breakpoints such as 5 or more colonies more accurately identify infection.[27] Other methods include simple qualitative cultures done by incubating the tip immersed in broth, by culture of sonicates of segments or tips, or by intraluminal flushing of the catheter tip with broth to culture the inside of the catheter segment. Quantitative culture performed by flushing, sonicating, and/or vortexing the catheter segment and then preparing and plating a set of dilutions for colony counts is more labor intensive but may be a more accurate predictor of catheter-related sepsis.[28]

Central Nervous System Infections

CSF is another type of specimen that requires immediate processing, as well as prompt reporting of results of Gram stain or other direct tests such as cryptococcal antigen assays or acid-fast stains. These specimens must be transported to the laboratory quickly because fastidious organisms such as *N. meningitidis* may become nonviable if the specimen is allowed to sit at room temperature or in a refrigerator. Because multiple tubes are sent for microbiologic, hematologic, and chemistry analyses, it is important to use the most turbid specimen for microbiology and also allocate enough fluid to adequately cover the culture requests. Gram stain and routine culture may require only 1 to 2 ml of CSF; however, if fungal or mycobacterial infection is suspected, larger volumes of CSF, preferably more than 2 ml for each test, will increase the likelihood of successful culture.

Gram stains should be done on all spinal fluids either by using a concentrated sediment smear prepared by centrifugation or by using a cytocentrifuge.[29] Because the number of organisms present may be low yet the nature of the organisms seen on direct Gram stain could be of immediate critical assistance in starting optimal antibiotic coverage, it is particularly important that these stains be done on well-concentrated smears and results reported to the physician immediately. If properly done and read by someone with microscopic expertise, the direct Gram stain can provide a preliminary answer in 60 to 80% of untreated cases and is most sensitive for *Haemophilus influenzae* and less sensitive for *N. meningitidis* and *Streptococcus pneumoniae.*

Bacterial antigen tests for *S. pneumoniae, H. influenzae, N. meningitidis,* group B streptococci *(Streptococcus agalactiae),* and *Escherichia coli* K1 are offered by some laboratories, although their overall cost-effectiveness has become even more questionable because of the dramatic reduction of *H. influenzae* meningitis since the introduction of *H. influenzae* type b vaccine. Laboratories need to determine the real benefit, if any, of maintaining these tests in their hospital setting. In the absence of seeing organisms on the Gram stain, initiation of antibiotic therapy based on the most appropriate empirical coverage rather than in response to antigen testing may be considered a safer course of action when dealing with life-threatening situations. Culture yields the definitive diagnosis and should determine whether modification of empirical coverage is warranted. Bacterial antigen testing results should not be relied on to modify initial treatment decisions. Antigen testing for *Cryptococcus neoformans,* however, is both a sensitive and specific way of establishing the diagnosis of cryptococcal meningitis. Such testing can be done either by latex agglutination assays or by enzyme immunoassays (EIAs) and has replaced the India ink wet preparation as the direct test of choice.

Most bacteria causing acute meningitis grow well on chocolate agar, unless they have been partially treated by antibiotic intervention. This medium allows for good growth of the primary pathogens, including *E. coli* and group B streptococci in neonates and infants; *Listeria* in neonates, infants, immunosuppressed patients, and the elderly; *H. influenzae* predominantly in children; *N. meningitidis* either in children or in adults; and *S. pneumoniae* in children, adults, and the elderly. As previously mentioned, since the introduction of *H. influenzae* type b vaccine, a notable drop has occurred in meningitis caused by this organism, so *S. pneumoniae, N. meningitidis,* and *Listeria monocytogenes* are currently the most common agents of bacterial meningitis.[30] *C. neoformans,* particularly of concern in

TABLE 14–3 Special Blood Culture Methods

Organism	Method	Comments
Abiotrophia	LC	Primary blood plates must contain pyridoxal
	Bottle systems	Subculture either to blood agar with pyridoxal or place staphylococcal streak for satelliting growth
Bartonella	LC	More sensitive and faster than bottle systems. Use fresh blood agar; incubate 12–14 d
Brucella	LC (5–10% CO_2)	LC may be most sensitive with earliest detection (3–5 d)
	Biphasic systems (5–10% CO_2)	Regularly flood agar with broth phase
	Bottle systems (5–10% CO_2)	Do weekly blind subcultures. No growth in anaerobic bottles
Campylobacter and *Helicobacter*	Bottle systems	Stain with acridine orange; may have minimal growth indices, slow growth
	LC	Blood plates must be incubated in reduced O_2 atmosphere
Legionella	LC	Plate LC concentrate onto BCYE plates
	Bottle systems	May have negative growth indices; subculture on BCYE
Leptospira	Fletcher's semisolid or EMJH medium	Only during 1st week of illness; incubate in dark, in air, 28°C–29°C, 4–6 wk. Use darkfield or phase-contrast microscopy
Nocardia	LC or bottle systems	Extend incubation of primary blood-agar plates or bottles

*Blood cultures for mycobacteria and fungi are discussed in subsequent sections.
Abbreviations: BCYE, Buffered charcoal-yeast extract; EMJH, Elinghausen, McCullough, Johnson, and Harris medium for leptospires; LC, lysis-centrifugation.

immunocompromised patients, also grows well on chocolate or blood-agar plates, and colonies can be detected within a few days. Detection of mycobacteria and viruses from central nervous system specimens is discussed later in this chapter. Spinal fluid specimens are not generally cultured for anaerobic bacteria unless specifically requested.

Sterile Body Fluid Infections Other than Blood, Urine, and Cerebrospinal Fluid (Peritoneal Fluid/Dialysate; Pleural, Synovial, Pericardial Fluids)

Normally sterile body fluids are usually concentrated by either centrifugation or filtration if the volume of specimen is sufficient because the number of organisms may be low. To improve culture sensitivity, culturing larger volumes of fluid in blood culture bottles has been recommended, particularly for peritoneal and dialysate fluids.[31] This concept may be expanded to improve the recovery of organisms from all types of sterile fluid because some automated blood culture systems have been approved for use with these specimens. Although the use of blood culture bottles that are read by automated instrumentation streamlines work for laboratories, undiluted specimen should also be sent along with the bottles whenever possible so that direct Gram stains can be made and agar media inoculated. The type of organisms seen on direct Gram stain of the fluid can give initial guidance regarding antibiotic coverage, whereas the ability to work with isolated colonies from agar plates will provide more rapid organism identification and susceptibility testing than could be done with growth only in broth media. Direct plating of the fluids is also helpful to detect mixed infections, whereas growth in broth may initially reveal only the most rapidly growing organism. Unlike the narrow spectrum of organisms isolated from CSF, other body fluids can be infected with a wide range of bacteria, fungi, mycobacteria, and viruses. When fluid is limited in quantity, the clinician must prioritize and select the most appropriate array of tests to request. Although any growth from these fluids must be considered significant and reported immediately, clinical judgment is required to assess real significance because contamination during collection and processing of the specimen occasionally occurs.

Urinary Tract Infections

Urine cultures, primarily clean-voided midstream urine samples, remain one of the microbiology laboratory's largest-volume test. The accuracy and therefore the utility of the culture results, however, are dependent on how well the specimen is collected and how promptly it arrives at the laboratory. Specific detailed instructions should be given to each patient at the time of urine collection to minimize contamination of the specimen with genital bacteria. Laboratories should ensure that specimen delivery occur within 2 hours of collection or, if not possible, that either refrigeration be available until pickup or urine transport tubes containing preservatives be supplied. Laboratories will not culture Foley catheter tips. Suprapubic aspirates, done primarily in infants or other patients in whom assessment of clean-voided urine is difficult, should be clearly labeled as such so that all growth is identified and reported. This recommendation also holds for specimens obtained at cystoscopy or by other invasive procedures. Anaerobic cultures are not performed unless specifically requested, and these cultures must be done on suprapubic aspirated urine.

Rapid screening techniques for urinary tract infection include direct Gram stains, as well as a variety of commercially available products, including dipstick methods, bioluminescence, and filtration devices.[32] A Gram stain is prepared by placing a drop of well-mixed, uncentrifuged urine onto a slide, air-drying, and then staining. The slide is read with the oil immersion lens, and 1 or more organisms per oil immersion field is equivalent to 10^5 or more colony-forming units per milliliter. If the Gram stain is read by a well-trained microscopist, correlation of stain with culture results should be quite good for colony counts of 10^5 or greater. The presence of mixed bacterial types or a moderate amount of squamous epithelial cells usually indicates contamination with normal genital flora. Also, direct Gram stains cannot be used to detect situations in which 10^4 colony-forming units per milliliter or less might be considered significant. Use of the other rapid screening methods may provide for some efficiency if the method has a high negative predictive value and will be used to screen out specimens that would be culture negative. If detection of lower colony counts (10^4 to 10^5) will be desired, however, care should be taken to make sure that these specimens will not be eliminated through the screening procedure. In addition, the reliability of the screening system should be determined, particularly for patients who are neutropenic.

The most common urinary tract pathogens are fortunately easy to grow and grow quickly. These organisms include *Escherichia, Klebsiella, Enterobacter, Proteus, Pseudomonas, Enterococcus,* and *Staphylococcus* ssp. Contaminants that are generally disregarded include lactobacilli, diphtheroids, nonenterococcal α-hemolytic streptococci, and coagulase-negative staphylococci other than *Staphylococcus saprophyticus*. In some patient populations, high colony counts of *S. epidermidis* may also be considered significant. Yeast, particularly *Candida* species, may be isolated from routine midstream urine cultures, often in quantities deemed significant for bacteria. Determination of true urinary tract infection with yeast, however, may require more invasively obtained specimens because either heavy genital colonization, long-term urinary catheterization, or both may make this distinction difficult. The value of colony counts for predicting true yeast urinary infection has not been well documented or substantiated, particularly in recent years.

Urine specimens are also used for the detection of other fungi, mycobacteria, *Leptospira,* viruses, and *Chlamydia.* For these organisms, further discussion will be found later in this chapter, as well as in the specific chapters related to these organisms. For fungi and mycobacteria, first morning specimens are recommended.

Gastrointestinal Infections

Gastritis

The discovery of *Helicobacter pylori* and its association with gastritis has resulted in the need for diagnostic verification of the presence or absence of this organism.[33] Detection of serum antibody to *H. pylori* is widely used to provide evidence of past or recent infection. The urea breath test is another noninvasive test procedure that can be used. Culture of this organism requires gastric tissue that must be inoculated onto enriched media under microaerophilic conditions; growth is generally not visible before 3 days of incubation. Growth of the organism may be desired when treatment failure is thought to be related to antibiotic resistance, which requires in vitro antibiotic susceptibility testing for confirmation. Gastric tissue can also be used to demonstrate the organism by Gram stain or histologically with special stains or to perform rapid presumptive tests to detect the hydrolysis of urea caused by *H. pylori.* These rapid tests generally rely on an obvious color (pH) change caused by the presence of a potent urease when a specimen such as gastric biopsy tissue is inoculated into the test.

Diarrheal Disease

Acute diarrhea can have a wide variety of etiologies, including bacteria, viruses, and parasites. Stool specimens are preferred to rectal swabs and should be transported to the laboratory quickly. New recommendations to minimize unnecessary stool cultures advise laboratories to not accept routine bacterial stool cultures on patients who have been hospitalized for 3 days or longer.[34] Most laboratories also have guidelines limiting specimen submissions to one per day and no more than three specimens (on successive days) for initial screening of acute gastroenteritis.

The spectrum of bacterial diarrheal pathogens is relatively well defined, and all laboratories have a "routine" setup to look for the common agents, which should include *Campylobacter, Salmonella,* and *Shigella* at a minimum. The presence of white blood cells suggests invasive infection with *Campylobacter, Shigella,* or enteroinvasive *E. coli,* so direct Gram stains are sometimes requested to look for leukocytes. Enrichment broths to detect small numbers of organisms may or may not be performed, depending on each hospital's experience regarding their overall utility. When stool specimens are submitted for bacterial culture, it is important to know which organisms are routinely cultured for and which ones must be specifically requested because of variation from laboratory to laboratory.

Although enterohemorrhagic *E. coli* (also referred to as Shiga-like toxin– or Vero toxin–producing *E. coli,* including O157-H7) is a significant pathogen, recovery of this organism, even with selective media, is usually low unless dealing with an outbreak situation or with bloody stool specimens. For this reason, many laboratories have decided to screen for enterohemorrhagic *E. coli* only when specifically requested. All laboratories should have this capability because serious infections such as hemolytic-uremic syndrome and severe hemorrhagic colitis can be caused by enterohemorrhagic *E. coli.* Newer, commercially available enzyme-linked immunosorbent assays (ELISAs) and latex agglutination assays that can be used directly on stool specimens or on culture isolates are currently undergoing evaluation and development; these assays may provide simple, acceptable tests for the future. Other known pathogens, particularly the various types of diarrhea-producing *E. coli, Vibrio* spp. (*Vibrio cholerae* and halophilic vibrios), *Yersinia,* and *Aeromonas* spp., may also need to be specifically requested because they may not be detected by the laboratory's routine screening procedure. Additional specific selective media would need to be included for optimal sensitivity. Table 14–4 shows the selective media commonly used for bacterial enteric pathogens and the additional media for specific pathogens.

For *Clostridium difficile,* toxin detection rather than organism culture is recommended because nontoxigenic strains may be cultured from asymptomatic carriers. When culture is needed for epidemiologic or comparative study purposes, selective media (see Table 14–4) incubated anaerobically are required. Toxin assays vary in their sensitivity and specificity, with the labor-intensive, time-consuming tissue culture assay being the most specific. An early rapid latex agglutination assay and the early EIAs proved to be insufficiently sensitive and specific, but the newer-generation EIAs are beginning to approach the tissue culture assay in acceptable performance. These simpler, rapid assays can have a more immediate impact on patient care decisions because they can be done in a matter of hours rather than days. In the evaluation of new methods such as EIAs, however, difficulty is always encountered in establishing what constitutes a "true" positive because even the tissue culture assay may not be an adequately sensitive standard.

Parasitic etiologies have also become more commonplace in the past few years, particularly with the greater recognition of cryptosporidial infection. Fresh specimens are important, and if delay is expected, the specimen should be placed in an appropriate fixative generally supplied by the laboratory. When looking for *Cryptosporidium, Cyclospora,* or microsporidia, the request must be specified because special techniques are needed to detect these organisms. Detection of *Giardia* infection has been improved with the development of immunoassays.[35] As suggested for the submission of stool for routine cultures, it is similarly recommended that stool for parasitic evaluation be limited to the first 3 days of hospitalization.[36]

Genital Infections, Including Sexually Transmitted Diseases

The genital tract normally contains many organisms that reside as colonizing flora, including coagulase-negative staphylococci, lactobacilli, corynebacteria, streptococci, anaerobes, and yeast. On occasion, because of host factors, genital tract infection may be caused by members of this endogenous population, for example, by *G. vaginalis* or *S. agalactiae.* In addition, specific pathogens, particularly those

TABLE 14–4 Selective Media for Enteric Pathogens

Pathogen	Common Media/Methods Used
Salmonella and *Shigella*	Primary plates (1) MacConkey or eosin–methylene blue (2) Hektoen or xylose-lysine-desoxycholate Optional: *Salmonella-Shigella* agar, gram-negative or selenite enrichment broths
Campylobacter jejuni/coli	*Campylobacter*-selective agars incubated at 42°C under microaerophilic conditions, e.g., cefoperazone-vancomycin agar, Campy-BAP, Skirrow agar
	By special request
Aeromonas	Cefsulodin-irgasan-novobiocin agar incubated at 37°C, or screen colonies from blood agar for positive oxidase reaction
Clostridium difficile	Cycloserine cefoxitin egg yolk fructose agar incubated anaerobically. Toxin assay usually performed rather than culture
Escherichia coli, enterohemorrhagic (Vero or shiga toxin producers, including O157-H7)	MacConkey-sorbitol agar; used in conjunction with specific antisera
Vibrio	Thiosulfate-citrate-bile salts sucrose agar or screen colonies from blood agar for positive oxidase reaction
Yersinia	Cefsulodin-irgasan-novobiocin agar incubated at room temperature

involved in sexually transmitted diseases, must be considered when determining infectious etiologies. Commonly submitted specimens include vaginal or penile discharge, genital ulcers, and urethral, cervical, and anorectal swabs. Genital infections can be caused by many different bacteria, including actinomycetes, *Haemophilus* spp., *Staphylococcus aureus,* Enterobacteriaceae, *N. gonorrhoeae,* group A and group B streptococci, and anaerobes, to name a few. In addition to bacteria, *Ureaplasma urealyticum, Chlamydia trachomatis, Trichomonas,* and viruses may need to be included in the infectious differential. Certain pathogens are known to be associated with specific types of genital infections, so the physician will base the selection of culture requests on the type or location of infection.

Vaginitis with accompanying discharge can be caused by *Trichomonas vaginalis, Candida,* or bacteria, as in the case of bacterial vaginosis. *T. vaginalis* is often diagnosed microscopically in wet mounts of vaginal secretions, although culture of this organism has been shown to be more sensitive. More recently, monoclonal fluorescent antibody stains have become available; they are more costly than the traditional wet mounts but may increase the sensitivity of detection over wet mounts. Vaginal candidiasis is most frequently diagnosed by direct smears that show many budding yeast and pseudohyphae. Although culture of *Candida* can be accomplished rapidly and easily, because many asymptomatic women harbor *Candida* spp., growth of *Candida* is not necessarily diagnostic of candidal infection. The etiology of nonspecific vaginitis or bacterial vaginosis is controversial, with organisms such as *G. vaginalis, Mobiluncus, Mycoplasma hominis,* and anaerobic gram-negative rods thought to play a role, most likely through coinfection or overgrowth with these organisms. The diagnosis of bacterial vaginosis is not based on bacterial culture because growing plus identifying these presumed pathogens is difficult, slow, and therefore costly. Gram stain of vaginal secretions is used to suggest bacterial vaginosis when evidence of *Gardnerella* is detected by the presence of "clue cells" or a prevalence of delicate gram-negative and gram-variable curved or fusiform bacteria, along with a reduction or absence of typical lactobacillary forms. The watery character of the discharge, a pH greater than 4.5, and the characteristic fishy amine odor are also used to support this diagnosis.[37]

N. gonorrhoeae is a major pathogen in genital infections such as cervicitis, salpingitis, urethritis, and epididymitis. Because this organism is delicate, specimens should be sent in appropriate transport media, should be transported promptly, and should never be refrigerated. The specimen type will depend on the site of infection, but anorectal or oropharyngeal specimens may also be sent with a specific request to look for *N. gonorrhoeae.* Gram stain and culture still remain the mainstay of diagnosis, although newer nonculture methods, particularly DNA hybridization (probe) assays, are being increasingly used because of their relative speed and reasonable accuracy.[38] Isolation of *N. gonorrhoeae* would still be needed if antibiotic susceptibility testing is required. The direct Gram stain is the most rapid and inexpensive way of making an accurate presumptive diagnosis of gonococcal infection in symptomatic men. The sensitivity and specificity of urethral smears in these instances, when read by trained microscopists, are as high as 95%. This sensitivity decreases when looking at urethral specimens from asymptomatic men, although the specificity remains good. Gram stains of cervical discharge are thought to be less reliable because of the presence of other organisms, which can make interpretation error prone; these stains are done by some laboratories but may be discouraged by others because of concerns of accuracy.

Infections caused by *N. gonorrhoeae* and *C. trachomatis* are often clinically difficult to distinguish and coinfection is relatively common, so diagnostic testing should include methods that will detect both agents. Although cell culture methods and rapid shell vial cultures are available for the growth of *C. trachomatis,* they are done only by a limited number of laboratories because of the technical demands of these cultures. In place of cultures, laboratories welcomed the use of direct immunofluorescence using specific monoclonal antibodies or a commercially available EIA as the preferred diagnostic test. More recently, as for the diagnosis of *N. gonorrhoeae,* the commercial development of specific DNA probes has further advanced sensitive and specific detection of *C. trachomatis* in urethral and endocervical specimens, with the added advantage of using the same swab specimens to detect both organisms. New alternative molecular methods rely on nucleic acid amplification techniques (polymerase chain reaction [PCR], ligase chain reaction, and transcription-mediated amplification), which have also been designed to detect both organisms. Amplification methods can be used on urine samples with excellent sensitivity, which is a decided benefit. The increased sensitivity of these assays is attractive, although the increased cost of amplification tests must also be factored in.[39]

Other pathogens causing genital infections include *Treponema pallidum, Haemophilus ducreyi, Ureaplasma,* and herpes simplex virus (HSV). For diagnostic consideration of these and other organisms, which are beyond the scope of this section, consult the relevant chapters devoted to these organisms.

Skin, Skeletal, and Soft Tissue Infections

These infections most frequently involve bacteria and less commonly mycobacteria and fungi. Specimens sent to the laboratory include tissue biopsies, aspirates or swabs of abscesses, wound swabs, material obtained by surgical débridement, and drainage samples. The usefulness of these cultures may be limited by the character of the lesion being cultured because lesions connecting with skin, mucosal surfaces, or gastrointestinal contents will be encumbered by the presence of indigenous microflora. For meaningful culture results, laboratories prefer surgically obtained tissue samples, aspirates of closed abscesses, and an aliquot of pus or fluid rather than swab samples. When anaerobic bacteria are expected, the specimen should be inoculated into an anaerobic transport container and delivered promptly. Swabs of superficial skin ulcers, from the skin surface of a sinus tract, or from open abscesses commonly yield a host of mixed bacterial flora and often do not reflect the organisms of true infectious significance. For these infections, every effort should be made to sample from the deeper aspects of the lesion, with careful avoidance of the contaminated tissue surface to obtain the best possible specimen.

Wound infections and abscesses are caused by many organisms, including routine bacteria, anaerobic bacteria, mycobacteria, and fungi. A long listing of these organisms is not particularly helpful, but it is important for the clinician and the laboratory to recognize that certain organisms are often associated with particular types of wounds or abscesses. An infected animal bite may yield organisms such as *Pasteurella multocida* or *Capnocytophaga cynodegmi*; a post-traumatic hand infection may yield *S. aureus, Mycobacterium marinum,* or *Sporothrix schenckii,* depending on the source of trauma; and a postoperative wound infection might yield *Pseudomonas* or *Acinetobacter* spp., among others. Laboratory guidelines include media and methods suitable for the isolation of most rapidly growing bacteria. Fungal, mycobacterial, and anaerobic cultures must be specifically requested if these organisms are suspected. When looking for fastidious organisms such as *Francisella, Brucella,* or *Bartonella,* the laboratory should be notified so that cultures can be set up appropriately and held for prolonged incubation as needed. Providing the laboratory with the location or type of wound, abscess, or tissue is often useful because it may hasten the recognition of specific pathogens known to be associated with the type of infection (e.g., cat bite, brain abscess).

Whenever an ample amount of specimen is available, a direct Gram stain should be performed to give some preliminary indication of the infecting organism(s). In some instances, if antibiotic therapy has been initiated, direct smear may be the only available guide to the etiology because growth may be inhibited. On tissue specimens, impression smears made by gently pressing a freshly cut surface of the tissue onto a slide should be examined in place of or in addition to ground tissue smears. Impression smears are easier to read and interpret than those made from material that has been ground or macerated. In addition to Gram stains, Calcofluor white stains for fungi and acid-fast stains for mycobacteria can also be done on impression smears. Direct Gram stains are of significant value not only for providing the physician with preliminary information about the type of organism(s) present but also as a guide for the microbiologist examining the culture. The presence of many epithelial cells, for example, indicates skin contamination, whereas observation of many polymorphonuclear leukocytes would suggest a good-quality specimen. The types of organisms seen should be correlated with culture results because such correlation may sometimes help in recognizing organisms that do not grow well under routine aerobic culture conditions. For example, seeing faintly staining gram-negative rods that do not grow on routine aerobic plates should suggest the possibility of an anaerobic organism such as *Bacteroides.*

In some hospital settings, quantitative wound or tissue biopsy cultures have been used to help predict the likelihood of wound sepsis and also for the performance of skin grafts. Quantitative culture requires weighing and careful preparation of the specimen for serial dilutions to determine whether the colony count is greater than 10^5 colony-forming units per gram of tissue. Such colony counts are correlated with a greater likelihood of infection associated with wound closure. Direct Gram smears of known quantities of specimen can also be used to give an immediate assessment of organism load. Because quantitative cultures are time consuming and labor intensive, not all laboratories will have procedures in place to perform these assays; the availability of quantitative wound cultures should be checked by consulting with the laboratory before ordering.

DETECTION AND IDENTIFICATION METHODS

As was shown in Figure 14–1, microorganisms can be identified in patient materials either by direct detection, commonly accomplished by special stains, or by culture methods that rely on growth of the organisms. In this section, routine bacterial detection and identification will be discussed, with only superficial mention of methods used for mycobacteria, fungi, and viruses, each of which will be discussed in greater detail in later sections of this chapter. Parasitology methods, covered only briefly here, are covered more extensively in a separate chapter.

Direct Detection of Microorganisms in Patient Specimens

Microscopic Observation

Table 14–5 shows the most common stains used directly on patient specimens and the types of organisms that they detect. The Gram stain is a simple, yet reliable stain that can provide preliminary important information on whether a bacterial infection is being caused by a gram-negative or gram-positive organism and whether it is a rod or a coccus. When read by an individual with microscopy expertise, the Gram stain provides an indication about the quality of the specimen and, in addition to routine bacteria, may also reveal yeast, molds, and occasionally parasites, mycobacteria, and *Nocardia.* As with all other direct stains, detection sensitivity is limited by the amount of material that can be reviewed on a slide, and if the number of organisms is low, they may fail to be seen.

Although the Gram stain provides a category of organism as a preliminary guide, it is a nonspecific stain. Specific stains using antiserum conjugated to a fluorescent label are not used widely for direct detection of bacteria in patient specimens. At present, fluorescent antibody stains for *Legionella* and *B. pertussis* are the only ones that are still offered by some laboratories. Both of these commercially available stains are not considered to be effective for direct detection because the *Legionella* direct fluorescent antibody (DFA) stain has low sensitivity and *B. pertussis* DFA has low specificity. The results of DFA staining should be used with caution because

TABLE 14–5 Commonly Used Direct Stains for Microorganisms

Type of Stain	Comments
Gram stain	Determines gram-positive versus gram-negative bacteria and provides general morphology (rods or cocci); also stains yeast. Filamentous fungi stain poorly; *Nocardia* and mycobacteria stain variably, often with a beaded appearance
Acridine orange	Useful for viewing bacteria that are difficult to see on Gram stain, particularly in blood culture bottles (*Campylobacter, Helicobacter,* anaerobes, etc.). Requires a fluorescent microscope
Mycobacterial stains	Ziehl-Neelsen and Kinyoun stains are carbolfuchsin-based stains widely used for mycobacteria. Fluorochrome stains using auramine and rhodamine dyes that bind to cell wall mycolic acids are more sensitive and easier to screen.
Nocardial stains	Often referred to as modified acid-fast stains, these have weaker or shorter decolorization steps than do traditional acid-fast bacillus stains to demonstrate the acid-fastness of *Nocardia.* Can also be used for *Cryptosporidium, Cyclospora,* and *Isospora.*
Calcofluor white	Whitening agent that binds to cellulose and chitin and is useful for staining fungi. Yeast and molds fluoresce brightly, which makes this a more sensitive stain than traditional wet mounts, but it requires a fluorescent microscope
Fluorescent antibody stains	Use monoclonal or polyclonal antibodies against specific organisms. The assays can be either direct or indirect fluorescent antibody stains, but most commonly use fluorescein isothiocyanate as the fluorochrome

false positives may occur from cross-reactivity with other organisms and false negatives may occur from poor quality of the antiserum or too few organisms. Fluorescent antibody stains are always subject to technical concerns, primarily in reading and interpretation, which should only be done by trained individuals. DFA stains have been used successfully for other organisms, including *Chlamydia,* some viruses, and some parasites (see the specific chapters). Although fluorescent antibody stains are not used for the detection of common molds or yeast, the diagnosis of *Pneumocystis carinii* can be made by using monoclonal fluorescent antibodies specific for this organism, either on bronchoscopic specimens or on saline-induced sputa.

Wet mounts have traditionally been used to look for fungi and parasites. The addition of potassium hydroxide to a wet preparation helps clarify the background of tissue cells, mucus, or proteinaceous materials and allows for better visualization of yeast or hyphal structures. In recent years, many laboratories have adopted the use of a Calcofluor white stain. Although this stain requires a fluorescent microscope with a specific set of excitation and barrier filters for use with Calcofluor, the benefit of this stain is that it provides a more sensitive direct stain for fungi, which fluoresce brightly and are much easier to distinguish than in an unstained wet mount. Another type of wet mount, the India ink preparation, has been used to identify encapsulated *C. neoformans,* particularly in CSF. This stain has been replaced in most laboratories by either a latex agglutination test or an EIA for cryptococcal antigen, both of which have greater sensitivity than India ink does.

In addition to a monoclonal fluorescent antibody stain, *Pneumocystis* can also be rapidly diagnosed in the microbiology laboratory by staining with Giemsa or toluidine blue O, and the organism may also be seen on certain preparations of Calcofluor white. Other important microscopic stains include the traditional acid-fast stain and fluorochrome stains for mycobacteria, as well as the modified acid-fast or *Nocardia* stains for *Nocardia* spp. These stains will be discussed in later sections of this chapter.

Antigen Detection by Agglutination or Enzyme Immunoassays

Direct testing of patient specimens with simplified antigen assays has become more commonplace and has been developed for a variety of microorganisms. These types of tests are usually simple and rapid for laboratories to perform, and if reasonably sensitive and specific, such tests are adopted fairly rapidly into laboratory routine. Table 14–6 shows some of the assays that are currently being used regularly. Antigenic assays for *C. difficile* are different from the usual assays for bacteria in that most assays for *C. difficile* are based on detection of the toxin rather than the organism. On request, the laboratory should be able to supply the performance characteristics of the assays that they use so that an educated assessment of the meaning of a positive or negative test can be made. The sensitivities and specificities of different commercial products may vary, even when testing for the same organism.

Molecular-Based Assays

Development of molecular assays for the direct detection of microorganisms has been an actively growing specialty (see the review by Baselki[40]). The first commercially offered assays were based on hybridization with DNA probe technology to detect specific ribosomal RNA (Gen-Probe system), which gives the system a built-in amplification factor. This system currently uses acridinium ester–labeled, single-stranded DNA probes to detect complementary ribosomal RNA sequences of the target organism; this reaction is measured by chemiluminescence read on a luminometer. This method is used as a direct test only for a few bacteria, mainly *N. gonorrhoeae* and *C. trachomatis,* but it is more widely used for culture confirmation of an organism (dimorphic fungi and mycobacterial species) once growth is available.

Amplification techniques such as those using PCR or ligase chain reaction should provide increased sensitivity because of the extensive amplification of target nucleic acid that is achievable. Commercial amplification systems for the clinical laboratory that have been approved by the Food and Drug Administration are now becoming available, although in-house development of PCR technology has been under way for years. PCR assays developed in-house, as well as prospective commercial amplification systems under development, have been tested in many university- or research-affiliated institutions to validate the performance of these assays. Results from these investigations have been most encouraging and suggest that molecular diagnostics will usefully expand the ability of laboratories to detect organisms present in very low quantities, those that are difficult or slow to grow, and agents that are yet "undiscovered." The potential power of these tools is substantial, and simplification of technology will eventually make molecular methods more within the realm of possibility for the average clinical laboratory. At present, however, the spectrum of validated assays is limited, and performance of these assays is technically complex and requires well-trained and knowledgeable personnel. The experience of laboratories offering molecular amplification assays has highlighted the potential problems that both the physician and the microbiologist need to be aware of. The first critical issue is that of false-positive reactions because of amplicon (PCR product) contamination of the work area. False positives can lead to serious consequences in patient care, so laboratories must be particularly diligent about avoiding amplicon carryover. Control over this contamination can be exerted by allocating separate work areas, pipettes, and reagents for the various components of the assay, as well as by using methods designed to inactivate the product from further amplification (uridine triphosphate/uracil-*N*-glycosylase system[41] or postamplification sterilization with isopsoralen). A second source of error is false-negative results resulting from the inhibitors of the PCR reaction present in the patient's specimen. Although most assays include positive controls containing known target, as well as external amplification controls to detect inhibition as part of their quality control process, the best index of inhibition uses internal controls that mimic the target primers. Use of the internal controls included in the test reaction mixture gives the most accurate assessment of inhibition.[42, 43] In addition to these important technical considerations, clinical assessment of amplification assays has yet to be accomplished for most microorganisms. For agents that are considered infectious and needing treatment or intervention regardless of the quantity or source or regardless of the medical status of the host, a positive amplification result may be interpreted in the same manner as a positive culture or other currently accepted measure of diagnosis (DFA, EIA for antigen, etc.). For most other agents, however, amplification baseline information needs to be accumulated for various patient populations and correlated not only with traditional detection methods but also with utility for patient care purposes. Because it is likely that some PCR assays will be much more sensitive than the current traditional test for a particular organism, a higher rate of detection of "asymptomatic carriers" may occur, so the threshold for infection when using amplification techniques would be different from an assessment based on culture positivity. At this stage of molecular diagnostics in microbiology, it is prudent for the infectious disease specialist and the laboratory to be critical in their acceptance and interpretation of results. The transition from research-based testing to clinical laboratory routine testing is under way, and some of these questions and problem areas will be alleviated because the validation required by CLIA regulations must be provided by either the commercial vendors or those offering tests developed in-house.

TABLE 14–6 Direct Antigen Detection Tests by Agglutination Assays or by Enzyme Immunoassays

Latex Agglutination	Enzyme Immunoassays
Bacterial antigens (used primarily for CSF specimens):	Bacterial antigens
Group B *streptococci*	Group A *streptococci*
Haemophilus influenzae type B	*Legionella pneumophila* serotype 1
Streptococcus pneumoniae	Bacterial toxins
Neisseria meningitidis	*Clostridium difficile*
Fungal antigen	Shiga-like toxins of *Escherichia coli*
Cryptococcus neoformans	Fungal antigen
	Cryptococcus neoformans
	Parasitic antigens
	Giardia lamblia
	Cryptosporidium parvum
	Entamoeba dispar/histolytica
	Viral antigens
	Adenovirus 40/41
	Herpes simplex
	Influenza A
	Respiratory syncytial virus
	Rotavirus
	Chlamydial antigen
	Chlamydia trachomatis

Detection by Culture

Much of diagnostic bacteriology has long relied on the growth of organisms on appropriate culture media and identification based on biochemical characteristics. Many clinical microbiology textbooks and reference manuals are available to help a laboratory determine the "standard" culture setups for various organisms.[6, 10, 30] Culture and identification methods for the subspecialties of mycology, mycobacteriology, and virology are discussed in later sections of this chapter, and here we will focus mainly on culture of routine bacteria.

For common specimen types, laboratories use enriched all-purpose media such as blood or chocolate agars, which grow most of the ordinary bacterial pathogens. For specimens that might contain mixed microbial flora, additional plates such as MacConkey or eosin–methylene blue agar for gram-negative bacteria and phenylethyl alcohol agar for gram-positive bacteria would also be inoculated. Laboratories also use a broth medium into which a larger aliquot of specimen can be inoculated to detect small numbers of organisms. Table 14–7 provides examples of the types of media recommended for various specimen types, and Table 14–8 lists the organisms for which special enriched or selective media are required for optimal recovery. In addition to the selection of appropriate media, use of

TABLE 14–7 Commonly Used Bacteriologic Media

Medium	Description
Blood agar (5% sheep blood, SBA)	SBA is the most commonly used all-purpose medium. It grows most bacteria, fungi, and some mycobacteria but will not grow *Haemophilus, Legionella, Francisella,* or other very fastidious organisms. It is used to determine α- or β-hemolysis
Chocolate agar	Chocolate is another all-purpose medium that supports the growth of most bacteria, including *Haemophilus,* and provides better growth than SBA for fastidious organisms such as pathogenic *Neisseria*
Eosin–methylene blue agar (EMB), MacConkey agar (Mac)	EMB and Mac inhibit the growth of most gram-positive organisms and allow the growth of a wide variety of gram-negative rods. Both media have sugars and dyes that yield differential characteristics (e.g., lactose positive or negative). One of these plates is included in the primary setup of most non–sterile specimens (sputa, wounds, abscesses, etc.)
Phenylethyl alcohol agar (PEA), colistin–nalidixic acid agar (CNA)	These agars, primarily PEA, are used to inhibit the growth of gram-negative organisms and thereby permit isolation of gram-positive organisms. One of these plates is included in the primary setup of most nonsterile specimens
Broth media, e.g., thioglycollate, brain-heart infusion, trypticase soy, or fastidious broth	Broth media are frequently used in addition to agar plates so that a larger aliquot of specimen can be cultured. Ideally, the broth should support the growth of all types of organisms, including relatively fastidious bacteria. Unless specifically requested, however, the broth is not included for recovery of anaerobes

the optimal atmosphere (aerobic, aerobic with CO_2, microaerophilic, anaerobic) and temperature (25°C, 37°C, 42°C) is important.

Identification by Biochemical Methods

Once colony growth is evident on the agar media, Gram-stain morphology and characteristics such as colony size, color, shape, and the presence or absence of hemolytic activity are used by the microbiologist to select the appropriate identification procedure. An experienced microbiologist will often be able to provide reliable preliminary information on a culture from these early characteristics. For most common bacterial pathogens, identification can be done fairly simply and rapidly because of the availability of rapid key tests, as well as miniaturized identification panels. For example, an opaque white, gray, or light yellow colony that on Gram stain appears as gram-positive cocci predominantly in clusters will be tested promptly with a latex agglutination reagent for coagulase/protein A detection to determine whether it is *S. aureus* or a coagulase-negative *Staphylococcus* species. Specific laboratory procedures for identification of organisms are not uniform from laboratory to laboratory because of the multiple choices of commercial products available for identification of each bacterial species. Table 14–9 summarizes tests that are commonly used, along with colony and Gram-stain morphology, to identify certain species of bacteria.

Various identification schemes and flow charts for the major groups of bacteria are available in diagnostic microbiology and infectious diseases textbooks. These schemes are particularly useful for subdividing bacteria on the basis of key reactions so that the user can narrow the spectrum of possibilities down to a smaller subset of organisms. With some bacteria, identification to the species level can be relatively simple (e.g., *S. aureus, Pseudomonas aeruginosa*), whereas with others, identification to the species level may require many biochemical reactions (e.g., *Neisseria lactamica, Haemophilus paraphrophilus*). Figures 14–2 to 14–5 are schematic diagrams to help differentiate the most common bacteria encountered in clinical material.

Gram-Positive Cocci

Gram-positive cocci (Fig. 14–2) can be subdivided into several important categories. Aerobic or facultatively anaerobic gram-positive cocci are regarded as streptococcal-like by virtue of a negative catalase reaction and the appearance of cocci in pairs and chains in broth media or regarded as staphylococcal-like by virtue of a positive catalase reaction and microscopic morphology showing cocci in groups, clusters, or tetrads. In recent years, additional genera and species of gram-positive cocci have become clinically significant and have complicated earlier simplified schemes. These cocci include *Leuconostoc, Pediococcus, Aerococcus, Stomatococcus, Alloiococcus, Gemella,* and others, and although they are encountered as true pathogens on occasion, most of them still occur only infrequently. Anaerobic cocci can have either clusters or chains as their microscopic morphology; nomenclature and identification for this group can be found in the chapter devoted to anaerobic cocci.

The catalase test that distinguishes catalase-producing organisms

TABLE 14–8 Special Media Used for Specific Pathogens*

Organism	Medium	Comments
Bacteroides species	Kanamycin-vancomycin laked blood agar	Inhibits the growth of most gram-positive organisms. Selective for *Prevotella* and *Bacteroides* spp.
Bacteroides fragilis group	*Bacteroides* bile-esculin (with gentamicin and bile)	Positive esculin reaction gives rapid presumptive evidence of *B. fragilis* group; also selects *Bilophila* spp.
Bordetella pertussis	Bordet-Gengou agar plus methicillin or cephalexin Regan-Lowe cephalexin agar Horse blood–charcoal agar	Nasopharyngeal swabs rather than cough plates are recommended. *B. pertussis* will also grow on BCYE
Burkholderia cepacia	PC agar	Highly selective for *B. cepacia*; particularly useful for sputum cultures from patients with cystic fibrosis
Corynebacterium diphtheriae	Tinsdale agar Cystine-tellurite blood agar Löffler's slant	Brown halo around colonies on Tinsdale agar is presumptive for *C. diphtheriae.* Use Löffler's for "Chinese letter" forms
Francisella tularensis	Blood- or chocolate-cystine agar	*Francisella* will also grow on most chocolate and Thayer-Martin agars, as well as on BCYE agar
Legionella	BCYE agar	BCYE formula that includes antibiotics can be used to inhibit the growth of other organisms
Leptospira	Fletcher's or Stuart's medium with rabbit serum or *Leptospira* medium with BSA–Tween 80	Incubate cultures in the dark at 28°C–30°C for up to 6 wk and examine by darkfield microscopy
Neisseria gonorrhoeae, meningitidis	Modified Thayer-Martin agar New York City agar	Both media inhibit the growth of other bacteria and yeast

*Not including gastrointestinal pathogens (see Table 14–4).
Abbreviations: BSA, Bovine serum albumin; BCYE, buffered charcoal-yeast extract; PC, *Pseudomonas cepacia.*

TABLE 14–9 Common Biochemical Reactions Used to Identify Bacteria

Biochemical Test	Primary Use of Test
ALA test (δ-aminolevulinic acid)	Rapid presumptive differentiation of *Haemophilus influenzae* from *Haemophilus parainfluenzae* isolated from upper respiratory specimens
Bacitracin (A) disk (0.04 unit bacitracin)	For presumptive identification of group A β-hemolytic steptococci, which are all sensitive to low concentrations of bacitracin
Bile solubility	For rapid differentiation of pneumococci (which are bile soluble) from other α-hemolytic streptococci
Catalase	An important characteristic that defines significant major groups of bacteria, e.g., staphylococci (catalase positive), streptococci (catalase negative)
Coagulase	A positive coagulase test is the key criterion for identification of *Staphylococcus aureus*
Hippurate hydrolysis	A positive test is used for presumptive identification of group B streptococci and also for *Campylobacter jejuni*
Indole	A rapid test is used for presumptive identification of *Escherichia coli* from urine specimens, but indole production is also used for the identification of many different gram-negative rods
Optochin (Ethylhydrocupreine hydrochloride)	Susceptibility to optochin is presumptive identification of *Streptococcus pneumoniae*
Oxidase	This key reaction helps differentiate gram-negative rods; e.g., Enterobacteriaceae are oxidase negative, whereas *Pseudomonas* spp. are oxidase positive
PYR hydrolysis (L-pyrrolidonyl-β-naphthylamide)	Used primarily for gram-positive cocci in chains; a positive test suggests *Streptococcus pyogenes, Enterococcus* spp., or *Abiotrophia* spp.
X and V factor requirements	Factor requirements are used to help identify different species of *Haemophilus*; *H. influenzae* requires both X and V for growth, whereas *H. parainfluenzae* requires only V factor

such as *Staphylococcus* and *Micrococcus* from non–catalase producers such as *Streptococcus* and *Enterococcus* is performed by placing a drop of hydrogen peroxide onto colonies of the organism grown on a non–blood-containing medium. The presence of catalase results in the evolution of O_2 bubbles from H_2O_2. Micrococci are most definitively differentiated from staphylococci by their lack of fermentative capability, although this test is not routinely used. Instead, if *Micrococcus* is suspected, susceptibility to a bacitracin A disk is a simpler method of making this distinction. For gram-positive cocci that appear staphylococcal by colony morphology and color, a rapid test to separate coagulase-positive from coagulase-negative staphylococci is done. Methods include a standard tube coagulase test to look for fibrin clot formation in plasma, a slide coagulase test that requires a subsequent tube coagulase test for all negative reactions, or a more rapid latex agglutination test that detects both clumping factor and protein A. Latex agglutination tests take only a few minutes to perform, and unlike the slide coagulase test, negative reactions do not have to be repeated with a tube coagulase test. The reliability of these tests is high, although both false-positive and false-negative reactions occur. Some have reported that particular latex agglutination tests may not be reliable for the detection of methicillin-resistant *S. aureus,* although this experience does not appear to be generalized. Because the various commercial products vary in their performance, it is important to know the characteristics of the particular assay used. Newer products have increased sensitivity in an attempt to decrease false-negative reactions, but increased sensitivity may result in a higher false-positive rate. In most laboratories, an organism yielding a positive coagulase or latex agglutination test would be identified as *S. aureus,* whereas those that are negative would be classified as "coagulase-negative staphylococci." Because many species of coagulase-negative staphylococci are known, species determinations are not routinely done for all isolates. Some laboratories identify species of coagulase-negative staphylococci from cases of significant bacteremia or other significant infections, as well as from urine cultures with high colony counts. The latter identification commonly entails the use of resistance to novobiocin to detect *S. saprophyticus,* a known urinary tract pathogen predominantly in young women. Species identification may be obtained from commercially available staphylococcal identification panels. Such identification is reasonably reliable, particularly for the most common species, *S. epidermidis.* The accuracy of an identification panel depends on the completeness of the repository of organisms used to maintain the database from which the identification is made. More recently described organisms such as *Staphylococcus lugdunensis* and *Staphylococcus schleiferi* are missing from some commercial panel databases and thus either will not be identified or will be identified incorrectly as a different species.

In addition to *Staphylococcus* and *Micrococcus,* other gram-positive cocci that are arranged in tetrads or clusters and have become of more interest of late include *Pediococcus, Aerococcus, Gemella, Helcococcus, Stomatococcus,* and *Alloiococcus.* These genera consist of aerobic or facultatively anaerobic cocci that are assumed to reside as normal human flora, so recognition of these organisms will occur only when they are isolated from a critical site such as blood and are assumed to be a pathogen. Of these genera, *Pediococcus* is the only one that is usually vancomycin resistant and may be readily suspected by virtue of this feature. *Stomatococcus* has been isolated more frequently in blood cultures in association with intravenous line sepsis and may initially look like other coagulase-negative staphylococci until its colonies become adherent, gummy, and difficult to pick from the agar surface. Key features of these gram-positive cocci are shown in Figure 14–2. Laboratories do not have a lot of experience with these species because except for *Stomatococcus,* they are not encountered frequently.

Identification of streptococci and enterococci initially relies on the type of hemolysis observed on blood agar, as well as colony size and morphology. For β-hemolytic streptococci, it is now possible to rapidly test for group A *streptococci* (*S. pyogenes*) by using either this species' ability to hydrolyze L-pyrrolidonyl-β-naphthylamide (positive PYR test) or the presence of group A antigen as done by latex agglutination with specific antisera. Both of these tests take under 30 minutes to perform and can thus be done the same day that colonies are observed, whereas the traditional method using susceptibility to low-content bacitracin disks (A disk) requires overnight incubation and may yield false-positive reactions because of bacitracin-susceptible strains of group C and G β-hemolytic streptococci. β-Hemolytic streptococci from throat cultures are usually identified as group A or not group A. When β-hemolytic streptococci are isolated from other significant sources such as blood, group identification can be easily accomplished by latex agglutination, which is available for groups A, B, C, F, and G. Commercial panels for identification of streptococcal species identify the β-hemolytic species, but the accuracy of identification by these panels must be established before accepting these identifications. Group B *Streptococcus* (*S. agalactiae*) is an important pathogen that in the past was identified either by its ability to hydrolyze hippurate or by a positive CAMP (Christie, Atkins, and Munch-Petersen) test to demonstrate synergistic hemolysis with *S. aureus.* These tests may still be done in hospitals that frequently see group B streptococci because they are both inexpensive and reliably accurate.

The extent of identification of *Enterococcus* spp. is dependent on individual laboratory policies. A key reaction that rapidly suggests a presumptive identification as *Enterococcus* is a positive PYR test, as just described for *S. pyogenes.* For a nonhemolytic or α-hemolytic streptococcal organism, a positive PYR test is presumptive evidence of *Enterococcus.* For a β-hemolytic streptococcus that is PYR positive, the isolate is most likely *S. pyogenes,* for although β-hemolytic enterococci also exist, they are uncommon. Significant enterococcal isolates from blood and other sterile fluid sites are almost always identified to the species level, as are strains that are vancomycin resistant. Urinary or wound isolates, however, are often identified as *Enterococcus* without further species identification. Species of enterococci can be identified with commercially available panels,

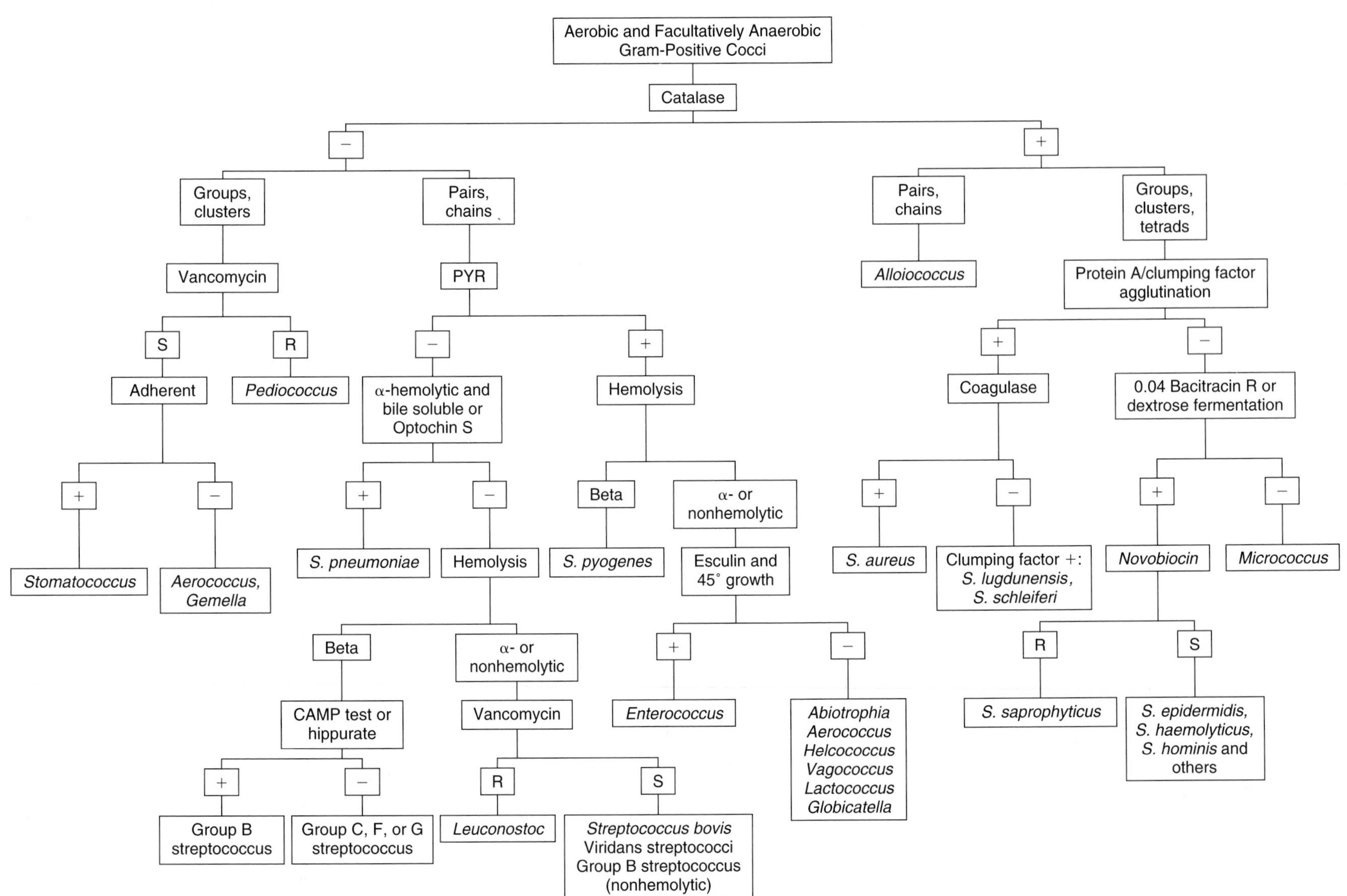

FIGURE 14–2. Schematic outline for the identification of aerobic and facultatively anaerobic gram-positive cocci.

and species identification has become of more interest and concern because of the emergence of vancomycin-resistant strains. *Enterococcus faecalis* is the most common species of *Enterococcus* encountered, although antibiotic-resistant strains of *Enterococcus faecium* are being seen with increasing frequency. Even though identification of *E. faecalis* by these panels is reasonably accurate, identification of *E. faecium* may be less reliable if *Enterococcus gallinarum* or *Enterococcus casseliflavus* is not included in the panel's database. Lack of inclusion of these species in the database requires that extra tests be set up, such as motility or detection of yellow pigment, to correctly identify the species.[44]

S. pneumoniae produces α-hemolytic colonies that have either a coin- or "checker"-shaped flat colony or a wet mucoid colony appearance. Rapid presumptive identification is made by placing a drop of desoxycholate onto the colonies and watching for disappearance of the colonies (bile solubility) or by latex agglutination with polyvalent (omni) pneumococcal antiserum. Presumptive identification of pneumococci can also be based on susceptibility to optochin (ethylhydrocupreine hydrochloride), which differentiates *S. pneumoniae* from other α-hemolytic streptococci, although this test requires overnight incubation. Rapid identification of pneumococcal infections has become more clinically significant because of the increased number of penicillin-intermediate and penicillin-resistant strains.

α-Hemolytic and nonhemolytic streptococci that are nongroupable and are not pneumococci or enterococci are commonly found as human oral or gastrointestinal flora. These organisms have been called "viridans" or "green" streptococci and are not generally identified unless clearly significant, as in cases of bacteremia in an immunocompromised host or subacute bacterial endocarditis. These species of streptococci are difficult to identify accurately, although some commercial identification panels attempt to do so. Recent modifications in taxonomy have simplified the grouping of these organisms so that they can be identified as related subgroups rather than species, e.g., *Streptococcus mitis* group or *Streptococcus sanguis* group. Although these streptococci used to be uniformly susceptible to penicillin, the emergence of intermediate as well as outright resistance has been seen, so in vitro susceptibility testing is warranted in serious infections.[45] Similar in morphology to α-hemolytic streptococci is the genus *Abiotrophia,* members of which were formerly called nutritionally deficient streptococci or "satelliting" streptococci. Members of this genus are recognized by their inability to grow on blood or chocolate agar unless the agar has been supplemented with pyridoxal, although they will grow in broth-based blood cultures (but fail to grow upon subculture onto unsupplemented agar). These organisms are also PYR positive like enterococci and *S. pyogenes,* but the PYR reactions are delayed and weak.

Other more recently described species that appear as gram-positive cocci or coccobacilli in chains belong to the genera *Leuconostoc, Lactococcus,* and *Globicatella.* Of these, *Leuconostoc* is notable because of its inherent vancomycin resistance. It is often initially thought to be a streptococcus until antibiotic susceptibility testing reveals the isolate to be vancomycin resistant. Additional tests needed to firmly identify the isolate as *Leuconostoc* include a negative leucine aminopeptidase reaction with a positive test for gas formation in MRS broth (deMan, Rogosa, and Sharpe broth). *Lactococcus* and *Globicatella* are unusual isolates that may be difficult to recognize and identify unless more extensive biochemical reactions are evaluated.

Gram-Positive Rods

The spectrum of clinically important gram-positive rods (Fig. 14–3) is quite diverse and has been succinctly summarized by Berkowitz.[46]

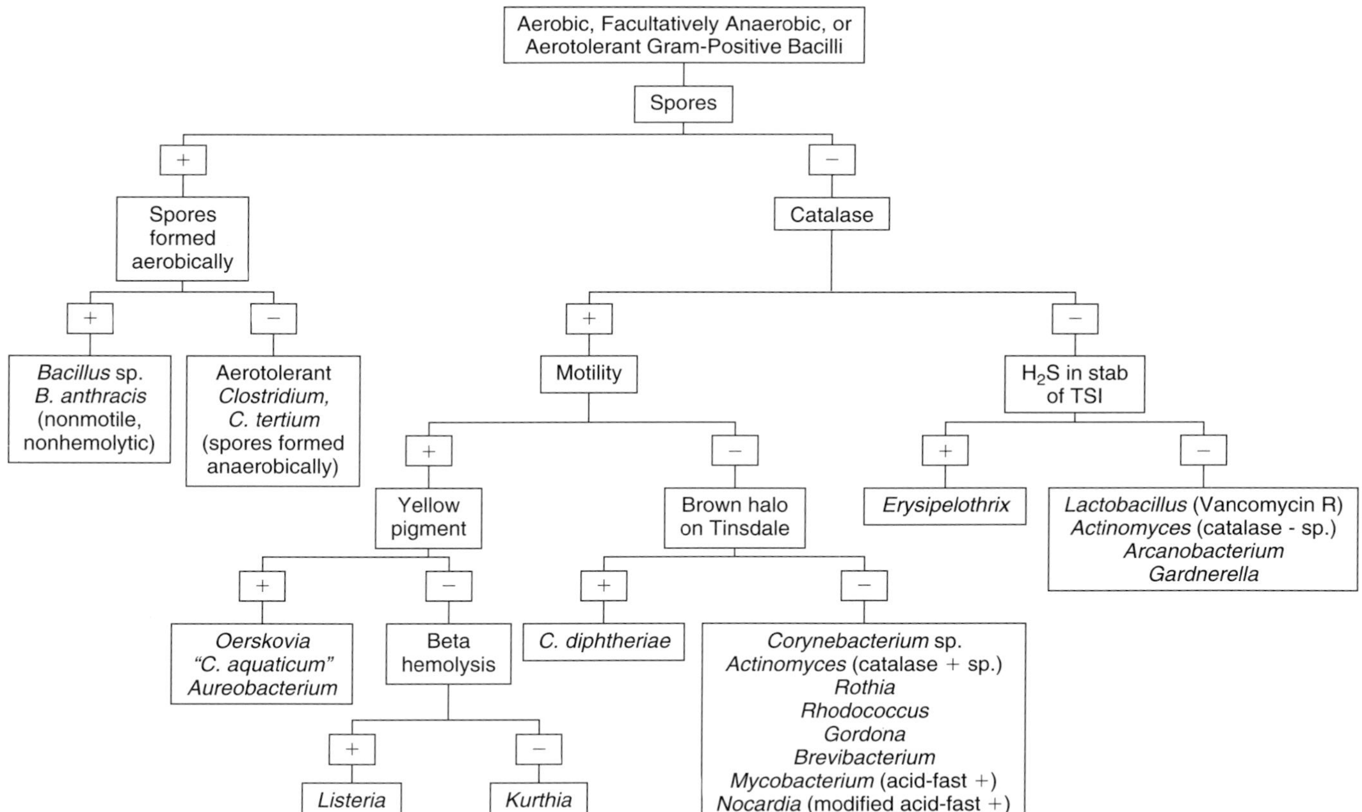

FIGURE 14–3. Schematic outline for the identification of aerobic, facultatively anaerobic, or aerotolerant gram-positive bacilli.

In this section only the aerobic and facultatively anaerobic gram-positive rods will be discussed; mycobacteria and *Nocardia* are covered later in this chapter. As can be seen from Figure 14–3, the first major distinction made in this group of bacteria is whether they are capable of forming spores. Demonstration of spores in an organism growing aerobically is considered presumptive identification of *Bacillus* spp. Although aerotolerant clostridial species such as *Clostridium tertium* exist, these organisms do not sporulate under aerobic conditions. Identification of the different species of *Bacillus* is labor intensive and time consuming because of the lack of commercially available identification panels for *Bacillus*. The need for such identification is minimal because most isolates of *Bacillus* are laboratory contaminants. On occasion, *Bacillus* causes bacteremia in an immunocompromised host, usually associated with intravenous catheters and most commonly with strains of *Bacillus subtilis, Bacillus cereus,* and *Bacillus licheniformis*. Isolation of *Bacillus anthracis* in the United States occurs only occasionally, yet because of its potential use as an agent of biologic warfare, infectious disease physicians and microbiologists must remain aware of how to best isolate and identify this organism,[47] which is described in depth in a separate chapter.

Non–spore-forming gram-positive rods can be preliminarily identified by a few key characteristics, including the type of hemolysis, catalase production, and motility. In addition, colony morphology and Gram-stain morphology are critically linked to the microbiologist's pathway of identification. Major pathogens that must be promptly recognized for optimal patient management include *L. monocytogenes, C. diphtheriae, Erysipelothrix rhusiopathiae, Actinomyces* spp., *Rhodococcus equi,* and *Corynebacterium jeikeium*. As can be seen from Figure 14–2, many other species of gram-positive rods exist than can be isolated, either as normal flora or at other times as opportunistic pathogens. Two recent reviews of *Corynebacterium* spp. and coryneform bacteria provide extensive, detailed information on this group of organisms.[48–50]

L. monocytogenes is vigorously catalase positive and should be recognized by its β-hemolytic colonies and its characteristic "tumbling" motility as observed by hanging drop, or "umbrella," motility at 25°C in semisolid motility medium. Other catalase-positive, motile, aerobic gram-positive rods such as *Oerskovia* or *Corynebacterium aquaticum* are not β-hemolytic. Confirmation of *Listeria* can be achieved by additional biochemical reactions or by using certain commercially available biochemical panels, for which such identification is usually highly reliable.

Except for *C. diphtheriae, Corynebacterium* species, including *C. jeikeium,* are commonly found on skin or mucosal surfaces. *C. diphtheriae* isolation and identification require prior notification of the laboratory because specific media and toxigenicity studies are needed for successful culturing and identification. The other corynebacteria and similar organisms that are catalase positive, nonmotile, and nonhemolytic are difficult for laboratories to identify to the species level. Although some panels are available for corynebacteria identification, they are not in widespread use. Identification of *C. jeikeium* relies on colony and Gram-stain morphology, although organisms such as *Corynebacterium urealyticum, Corynebacterium* Centers for Disease Control and Prevention (CDC) group G2, and *Corynebacterium minutissimum* may appear similar. Antibiotic-resistance profiles are used by many laboratories to confirm the identification of *C. jeikeium,* but it should be noted that *C. urealyticum* and CDC group G2 can also be resistant to multiple antibiotics.

R. equi, formerly *Corynebacterium equi,* can be a cause of serious, life-threatening pneumonia in patients with acquired immunodeficiency syndrome (AIDS). Like the corynebacteria, *R. equi* is nonmotile and catalase positive but can be distinguished by the mucoid, pink colony that it produces. Although it has been noted to be weakly acid fast, this characteristic should not be used as a preliminary screening test for this organism because it is frequently very difficult to demonstrate. Other species of *Rhodococcus* may be variously pigmented and nonmucoid but have not been reported to cause fulminant pneumonia.

Clinically important catalase-negative aerobic gram-positive rods are generally nonmotile. Important pathogens include *E. rhusiopathiae, Actinomyces* spp., and occasionally *Lactobacillus* spp. Both *E. rhusiopathiae* and *Lactobacillus* spp. have strains that may show in vitro vancomycin resistance. The production of H_2S in a triple sugar iron agar slant is a reaction that provides presumptive evidence of *Erysipelothrix*. This organism would also be suspected if isolated from a skin lesion in a person with a history suggestive of fish handling or, on occasion, when isolated from a blood culture from a patient with subacute bacterial endocarditis. Confirmation of identification as *E. rhusiopathiae* requires additional biochemical reactions. Vancomycin-resistant lactobacilli should be differentiated from vancomycin-resistant *Leuconostoc* species, which may be coccobacillary and thus mistakenly thought to be a gram-positive rod like *Lactobacillus*.

Identification of the various *Actinomyces* species is not simple, although anaerobic identification panels are currently available that attempt to do species identification. *Actinomyces* is suspected by the observation of short branching forms; frequently they appear diphtheroidal on solid media, but more definitively branching when grown in thioglycollate broth. Although the primary pathogens *Actinomyces israelii* and *Actinomyces naeslundii* are catalase negative, *Actinomyces viscosus, Actinomyces naeslundii* genomospecies II, and *Actinomyces neuii* are catalase positive. *A. israelii* usually requires anaerobic conditions for initial growth, whereas *A. naeslundii, A. viscosus,* and *Actinomyces odontolyticus* may also initiate growth in an aerobic environment supplemented with CO_2.

Gram-Negative Cocci

Aerobic gram-negative cocci (Fig. 14–4) belong to the genus *Neisseria* and do not produce coccobacillary forms. *Moraxella* and *Acinetobacter* are classified as gram-negative rods, although both genera are sometimes observed to appear as gram-negative cocci and thus need distinction from *Neisseria. Moraxella catarrhalis,* formerly named *Neisseria catarrhalis* and *Branhamella catarrhalis,* has microscopic morphology similar to that of *Neisseria*: it occurs as diplococci with flattened adjacent edges and, upon division, forms packets of four cocci rather than chains of coccobacilli like other *Moraxella* and *Acinetobacter* species. *M. catarrhalis* can be quickly identified, however, by either of two biochemical tests for which it is positive and *Neisseria* is negative, DNAse production or butyrate esterase production. *Neisseria* spp. are oxidase positive, which readily distinguishes them from *Acinetobacter* spp., which are oxidase negative.

Traditional identification of *Neisseria* species relies on the pattern of acid production from four sugars, glucose, maltose, lactose, and sucrose, as well as the ability of the organism to grow on nutrient agar and to grow at room temperature (see Fig. 14–3). These features, along with colony color and morphology, will guide species identification. Various kits for the identification of *Neisseria* species are available; some rely on sugar patterns, but more recently developed tests use detection of specific enzymes. The chapter on *Neisseria* covers isolation and identification in greater detail.

Aerobic and Facultatively Anaerobic Gram-Negative Rods

Gram-negative rods are usually grouped into four major categories for identification purposes: (1) aerobic and facultatively anaerobic, (2) nonfermentative, (3) fastidious, and (4) strictly anaerobic gram-negative rods (Fig. 14–5). Commercial companies have focused a lot of effort on accurate and timely identification of gram-negative rods because they constitute a large and important segment of clinically significant isolates. Although most of these identification products are good and have been in use for many years, some are better than

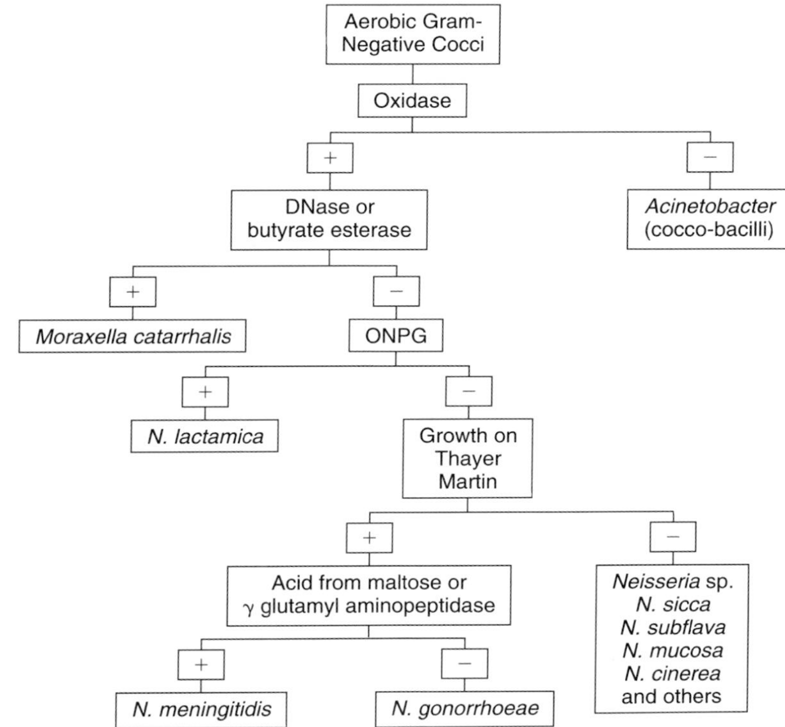

FIGURE 14–4. Schematic outline for the identification of aerobic gram-negative cocci.

others, and some are better for certain groups of gram-negative rods but do more poorly for others. To remain current, companies must regularly update their systems to keep up with name changes, as well as to add new organisms. As a consequence of delays in updating, microbial identification panel names will often lag behind accepted taxonomic changes.

The aerobic and facultatively anaerobic group, which includes members of the *Enterobacteriaceae* and *Vibrionaceae* (including *Vibrio, Aeromonas,* and *Plesiomonas*), is the most easily identified group, with many different commercial panels doing accurate identifications within 4 to 6 hours or overnight. *Vibrionaceae* can be quickly distinguished from the *Enterobacteriaceae* by their strong oxidase reaction. All these organisms generally grow luxuriantly after overnight incubation and grow well on MacConkey agar. When screening stool cultures for enteric pathogens, most laboratories use a two-tube screen (triple sugar iron agar/urea or lysine-iron agar/urea) to select those isolates most suggestive of being *Salmonella* or *Shigella* for further full biochemical profile.

The nonfermentative gram-negative rods include many important pathogens such as *Pseudomonas, Burkholderia, Acinetobacter,* and *Stenotrophomonas.*[51] The accuracy of different commercial panels to identify these genera to the species level varies with both the panel and the specific organism. Organisms that have fairly distinctive biochemical properties are usually readily identified correctly, for example, *P. aeruginosa, Acinetobacter baumanii,* or *Stenotrophomonas maltophilia.* When the nonfermentative gram-negative rod is biochemically inert or has few characteristics useful for differentiation, identification panels may yield incorrect or ambiguous results, often necessitating extra tests to make a definitive identification, for example, with different species of *Moraxella* or *Alcaligenes.*

Fastidious gram-negative rods include a very wide range of organisms.[51] Early descriptions of members of this group, primarily described because of their role in causing endocarditis, delineated them by the acronym HACEK, which refers to the first letter of each of the following genera: *Haemophilus aphrophilus, Actinobacillus actinomycetemcomitans, Cardiobacterium hominis, Eikenella corrodens,* and *Kingella kingae.* For purposes of discussion here, the fastidious group includes these organisms, as well as the host of other gram-negative rods that either grow slowly or need enriched or special media for cultivation. This group thus contains very significant pathogens, including *Haemophilus, Brucella, Francisella, Legionella, B. pertussis, Campylobacter, Capnocytophaga, Helicobacter, Pasteurella,* and *Bartonella.* Extensive discussions of these pathogens will be presented in chapters to follow. Identification of most of these organisms is often a challenge for the laboratory inasmuch as many are not identified with simple, commercially available panels. For most of these organisms, the laboratory must be notified in advance to optimize isolation by including specific media, temperature, or growth conditions or extending incubation times. Organisms such as *Brucella* and *Francisella* are laboratory hazards once they start to grow and need to be handled with caution. For a few of these fastidious species, simple tests are available to aid in identification. X factor (hemin) and V factor (nicotinamide adenine dinucleotide [NAD]) requirements or the ALA test (δ-aminolevulinic acid) are used to identify the common species of *Haemophilus.* For a delicate, curved organism growing well at 42°C from a stool culture, a positive hippurate hydrolysis reaction is regarded as sufficient to identify the organism as *Campylobacter jejuni,* whereas a similarly curved gram-negative rod that is strongly urease positive and isolated from a gastric biopsy specimen is likely to be *H. pylori.* A faintly staining slender gram-negative rod that only grows on charcoal-yeast extract agar is presumptively identified as *Legionella,* an identification that is usually confirmed by specific fluorescent antisera. *P. multocida* is one of the few organisms in the fastidious group that can be identified by using commercially available panels designed for fermentative gram-negative rods.

Anaerobic gram-negative rods will not be discussed here, except to note that systems for identification of the common species of *Bacteroides* and *Fusobacterium* are available and can provide genus or species identification promptly.

Identification Using Specific Antisera

In addition to biochemical methods of identification, laboratories also use antisera for culture confirmation of certain organisms. Ag-

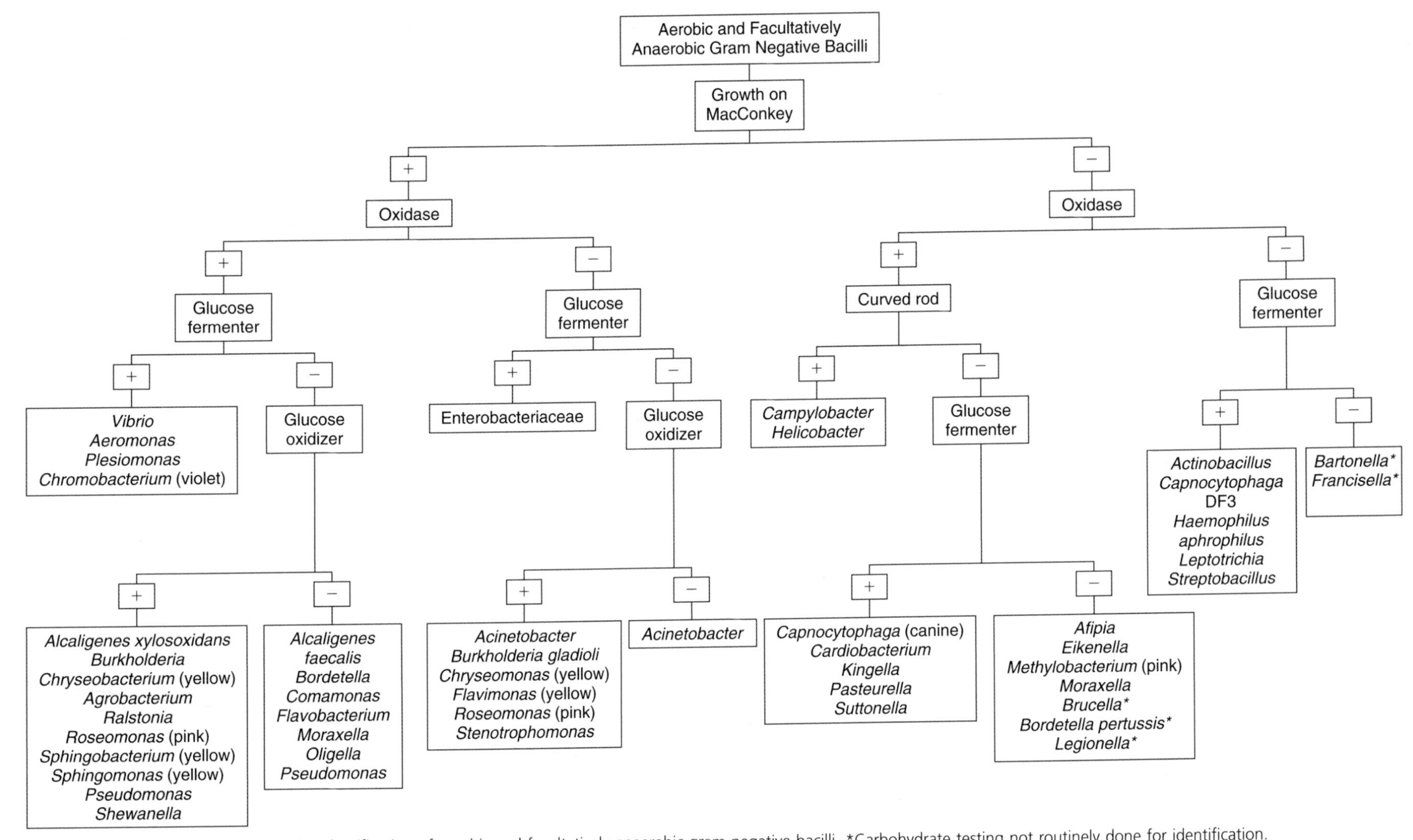

FIGURE 14–5. Schematic outline for the identification of aerobic and facultatively anaerobic gram-negative bacilli. *Carbohydrate testing not routinely done for identification.

glutination using whole-organism suspensions or latex agglutination using antibody bound to latex beads is technically simple to perform and takes a few minutes to complete. Agglutination and latex agglutination tests are used on colony growth by some laboratories to identify *S. pneumoniae,* groups of β-hemolytic streptococci, serotypes of *H. influenzae,* serogroups of *N. meningitidis, E. coli* 0157, and serogroups of *Salmonella* and *Shigella.* Detection of specific antigens by fluorescent antibody staining can also be used to identify colonies of *B. pertussis, S. pyogenes,* and the species and serotypes of *Legionella,* although lack of specificity of some antisera can lead to misidentification. The quellung reaction, which relies on the ability of specific antisera to interact with capsular polysaccharides of *S. pneumoniae,* can be used to confirm the identification as well as determine the serotype of these organisms, although this reaction is not routinely needed.

Identification Using Molecular Techniques

Chemiluminescent probes are available and can be used to identify colonies or broth cultures of dimorphic fungi and several important species of mycobacteria with a high degree of sensitivity and specificity. For these organisms, probe identification yields results much more rapidly than seen with traditional biochemical methods. The timeliness and accuracy of these procedures have been a major advance in mycology and mycobacteriology diagnostic testing, and although similar probes have been developed for other bacteria, their current usefulness lies mainly for dimorphic fungi and mycobacteria. Analysis of organisms based on nucleic acid sequencing of ribosomal RNA genes is currently being used taxonomically to help classify organisms more definitively. As more organisms become sequenced, however, this valuable repository of data sequences will provide us with another mechanism of identifying unknown or unusual organisms more quickly and accurately. Such identification based on 16S ribosomal RNA sequencing is already available through commercial and research laboratories.

ANTIMICROBIAL SUSCEPTIBILITY TESTING

Susceptibility testing of a presumed pathogen is indicated when its response to antimicrobial agents is not predictable from its identification.[52, 53] Unfortunately, with the continuing increase and dissemination of resistance mechanisms in bacteria, more and more species require at least some form of susceptibility testing. To ensure both clinical relevance and interlaboratory comparability of results, much effort has been devoted to the standardization of susceptibility testing. The basic problem is to demonstrate that in vitro growth inhibition of an infecting organism by a specific agent correlates with clinical response to that agent. The National Committee for Clinical Laboratory Standards (NCCLS) has published several standards pertaining to various aspects of bacterial susceptibility testing; many of these standards are updated regularly.[52–57] Because these documents reflect consensus statements by a committee of experts, laboratories cannot readily deviate from NCCLS recommendations without excellent data to justify their procedures. The CLIA amendments have also imposed stringent validation requirements on laboratories performing procedures developed in-house, further encouraging the use of standardized procedures for which proficiency testing is available.[1] Unfortunately, as both the number of organisms requiring testing and the number of antimicrobial agents available have increased, the NCCLS recommendations have become increasingly complex, with more and more organism- and drug-specific variables needing to be taken into account when obtaining and reporting susceptibility test results. Each new edition of an NCCLS susceptibility testing document must be carefully reviewed to ensure that the laboratory has incorporated the latest changes into its testing methodology.

Nearly all the more common and nonfastidious organisms can be tested and the results reported by using NCCLS criteria. The NCCLS also provides recommendations regarding the selection of antimicrobial agents to be tested against specific organisms; the committee has grouped those agents recommended for routine testing and those suggested for testing only under certain circumstances, such as the presence of a resistant strain in the institution in question. Another distinction, in terms of both antimicrobial selection and breakpoint criteria, depends on whether one is dealing with a urinary tract infection or some other infection (generally presumed to be systemic).

For less common or more fastidious organisms, as well as for nonstandard organism/drug combinations, the NCCLS guidelines are less complete. This shortcoming may be partly a consequence of the NCCLS requirement that in order to consider an organism susceptible to an agent, adequate data should be available to substantiate clinical responsiveness to that agent at species-specific (or group-specific) minimal inhibitory concentrations (MICs). Many organism/antibiotic combinations have inadequate clinical response data to help define sensitive and resistant MIC breakpoints. The consequent lack of interpretive criteria results in some vexing problems for both the laboratory and the clinician. For example, interpretive guidelines are not provided for organisms such as *Bacillus, Corynebacterium* and noncholera *Vibrio* or for many fastidious or unusual species (*Eikenella, Campylobacter, Capnocytophaga, H. pylori, Leuconostoc,* etc.). Many of these organisms may cause significant infections, and in the past laboratories used more "generally applicable" breakpoints, usually based on known achievable serum levels and the clinical response of other organisms with similar MICs, to help guide the clinician. Currently, to follow NCCLS recommendations, laboratories are more limited in what they can report because the guidelines specify the organism as well as the antimicrobial agents that can be reported. This lack of breakpoint criteria for a variety of organisms or organism/antibiotic combinations becomes particularly problematic for organisms that are resistant to many different antibiotics, in which case the laboratory would like to test and report agents that may not be recommended by the NCCLS for that specific organism. For organisms not included in the NCCLS standards, "consultation with an infectious disease specialist is recommended for guidance in determining the need for susceptibility testing and in the interpretation of results."[55]

The results obtained by any form of in vitro antibiotic testing depend not only on the particular antibiotic and organism but also on a host of other performance variables as well, including the organism inoculum concentration, the medium used, and the time, atmosphere, and temperature of incubation. The NCCLS documents provide detailed instructions for dealing with all the variables involved in susceptibility testing, including specific procedural modifications that may have to be made for specific organism-antimicrobial combinations.

Most bacterial species or groups of species have a susceptibility pattern characteristic for the species or group. Whenever an unusual susceptibility pattern for a particular species is obtained, it is worth checking to be sure that the susceptibility test was set up and interpreted correctly, that a pure culture was used, and that identification of the organism is correct.

Terminology

Susceptibility testing for most bacteria is performed either by a disk diffusion procedure or by a procedure (usually broth microdilution) that will provide an MIC. A relatively new procedure (Etest, from AB Biodisk) using a strip impregnated with a gradient of antimicrobial agent also provides an MIC. With the disk diffusion procedure, only a qualitative result (sensitive, intermediate, or resistant) is usually reported, whereas with MIC testing, both a quantitative result (the MIC) and a qualitative result (which "interprets" the MIC) may be reported. The MIC is the lowest concentration of a specific antimicrobial agent that inhibits the test organism. MICs can also be determined by an agar dilution procedure in which dilutions of antimicrobial agents are incorporated into an agar-based medium rather than dissolved in broth. Similarly, the *minimal bactericidal concentration* (MBC) (also known as the minimal lethal concentration) is the lowest concentration of a specific antimicrobial agent that kills the test organism. All these minimal concentrations have units of weight or mass divided by volume—usually they are given in micrograms per milliliter. A *serum bactericidal titration or test,* sometimes also called a Schlichter test, is a measure of the extent to which a patient's body fluid (usually serum) can be diluted and still exert bactericidal activity against an infecting organism isolated from the patient. The result is reported as a titer or ratio and therefore has no units.[58] An *antimicrobial level* is the amount of a specific drug in a patient's body fluid; the result is generally expressed in micrograms per milliliter.

Traditional quantitative susceptibility testing has used twofold dilution steps for the antimicrobial agent because such a dilution sequence is easy to perform. Increasingly, however, commercially prepared microdilution trays are used that do not contain an entire sequence of dilutions, only the most clinically relevant concentrations. This elimination of certain dilutions has consequences for the meaning of quantitative results. For example, if in a twofold dilution series of 2, 4, and 8 μg/ml the 4-μg/ml dilution were omitted, an organism with an actual MIC between 2 and 4 μg/ml would be reported as having an MIC of 8 μg/ml rather than the 4-μg/ml value that would be reported if the full twofold dilution series were used.

The following definitions of susceptible, intermediate, and resistant are presented in one of the NCCLS documents[55]:

1. Susceptible. The "susceptible" category implies that an infection due to the strain may be appropriately treated with the dosage of antimicrobial agent recommended for that type of infection and infecting species, unless otherwise contraindicated.
2. Intermediate. The "intermediate" category includes isolates with antimicrobial agent MICs that approach usually attainable blood and tissue levels and for which response rates may be lower than for susceptible isolates. The intermediate category implies clinical applicability in body sites where the drugs are physiologically concentrated (e.g., quinolones and β-lactams in urine) or when a high dosage of drug can be used (e.g., β-lactams). The intermediate category also includes a "buffer zone" that should prevent small, uncontrolled technical factors from causing major discrepancies in interpretations, especially for drugs with narrow pharmacotoxicity margins.
3. Resistant. Resistant strains are not inhibited by the usually achievable systemic concentrations of the agent with normal dosage schedules and/or fall in the range in which specific microbial resistance mechanisms are likely (e.g., β-lactamases) and clinical efficacy has not been reliable in treatment studies.

Specific Susceptibility Testing Procedures

Disk Diffusion Susceptibility Testing

Disk diffusion susceptibility testing,[52] still frequently referred to as the Kirby-Bauer procedure, should be used for rapidly growing organisms only. A disk containing a certain amount of antibiotic is placed on an agar plate immediately after it has been inoculated with the test organism. After incubation for 16 to 18 hours, the diameter of the zone of inhibition around the disk is measured. Interpretation of the organism as sensitive, intermediate, or resistant to the antibiotic depends on the zone diameter criteria for the particular organism-antibiotic combination. For example, for one of the *Enterobacteriaceae,* a zone diameter around an ampicillin disk of 17 mm or greater is considered susceptible, whereas for a *Staphylococcus* species, the zone diameter for ampicillin must be 29 mm or larger to be considered susceptible.

Zone diameter interpretive breakpoints are based on the inverse correlation of zone diameter with MIC; that is, the larger the zone diameter, the lower the MIC. The NCCLS lists the MIC correlates of its disk diffusion breakpoints in its tables. For example, the MIC equivalent to the zone diameter breakpoint for susceptibility to ampicillin for the *Enterobacteriaceae* is 8 μg/ml or less; for staphylococci, it is 0.25 μg/ml or less. However, with disk diffusion testing it is standard practice not to report an MIC, only an interpretive category.

Minimal Inhibitory Concentration Testing

MIC testing[53] is most often done by a broth microdilution technique on commercially available trays, which may also contain biochemical reactions used for organism identification. MIC testing may also be performed by broth macrodilution, by agar dilution, and by Etest.[59] All three dilution procedures involve the incorporation of known concentrations of antimicrobial agents into either broth or agar and then checking for the presence or absence of organism growth after a suitable incubation period, generally 16 to 18 hours. Broth macrodilution testing is very labor intensive and is rarely performed in a diagnostic laboratory. Agar dilution testing is cost-effective if a large number of isolates are tested at the same time; with this procedure, many different organisms can be tested simultaneously on each plate. The Etest is a relatively new procedure that uses a strip impregnated with a gradient of antimicrobial agent; after inoculation of a plate with an organism, the strip is applied to the plate. After incubation the plate is examined for growth; if the organism is susceptible to the antimicrobial agent, an oval of growth inhibition is produced that is widest at the end of the strip with the highest drug concentration. The MIC of the drug for the organism is read off the strip at the point at which the oval of inhibition intersects the strip.

Testing for Bactericidal Activity

The NCCLS published a tentative guideline for the determination of MBCs and other related bactericidal tests in 1992, but no approved standard has yet been published. The determination of bactericidal activity[57] is technically difficult. Given the lack of a fully standardized, approved methodology, the technical complexity and labor intensiveness of the procedure, the need to validate a procedure for CLIA purposes before reporting patient results, and the uncertain clinical relevance, very few laboratories offer such testing on a routine, nonresearch basis. As the NCCLS document itself states, "The determination of the MBC . . . is so subject to methodologic variables that the clinical relevance of MBCs is nearly impossible to assess."

Serum Bactericidal Test

The NCCLS published a tentative guideline in 1992 pertaining to the serum bactericidal test,[58] but as with the guideline pertaining to the measurement of bactericidal activity, no approved standard has been published, and the test is rarely available in routine diagnostic laboratories. The clinical relevance of the test remains uncertain. Use of the serum bactericidal test may even be contraindicated because it may stimulate an attempt to achieve an arbitrary bactericidal titer through modification of a treatment regimen that is in fact already adequate.[60]

Synergy Testing

Because no standardized methodology for synergy testing exists, this procedure remains essentially a research tool. However, a standardized method is available for predicting synergism between aminoglycosides and cell wall–active agents against enterococci (see later under susceptibility testing problems with enterococci).

Special Susceptibility Testing Problems

Staphylococci

All species of staphylococci that are oxacillin (or methicillin) resistant should be considered resistant to all β-lactam antibiotics, including imipenem, regardless of the actual in vitro result.[55] For either MIC or disk testing of staphylococcal susceptibility to oxacillin, a full 24 hours of incubation at 35°C are required to maximize the likelihood of detection of resistance; for coagulase-negative staphylococci, disk test results appear to correlate better with the presence or absence of the *mecA* gene than do microdilution results using current NCCLS breakpoints.[55, 61] An agar screening test using Mueller-Hinton agar with 4% NaCl and 6 μg/ml of oxacillin is quite reliable for detecting oxacillin-resistant *S. aureus* after 24 hours of incubation; 48 hours may be required for coagulase-negative staphylococci, but even with such extended incubation, a few oxacillin-resistant organisms may be missed.[55, 62]

Streptococcus pneumoniae

If a disk diffusion procedure is used to screen isolates for susceptibility to penicillin and related agents, an oxacillin disk is used. However, no result for oxacillin itself should be reported. If the zone around the oxacillin disk is 20 mm or larger, the isolate should be reported as susceptible to penicillin. If the zone is 19 mm or smaller, MIC testing with penicillin and either cefotaxime or ceftriaxone should be done because isolates with such a zone size may prove to be either susceptible, intermediate, or resistant to penicillin by MIC testing.[55]

Enterococci

Several issues pertain to susceptibility testing of enterococci:

1. Test results for the following agents should not be reported because the agents have not been found to be clinically effective: cephalosporins, clindamycin, trimethoprim/sulfamethoxazole, and (at usual testing levels) aminoglycosides.[55]
2. Testing at high levels for gentamicin (500 μg/ml) and streptomycin (1000 or 2000 μg/ml, depending on methodology) susceptibility is useful for the purpose of predicting synergy with cell wall–active agents. For gentamicin, 24 hours of incubation are required; for streptomycin, 48 hours are required unless the isolate is already resistant at 24 hours. An isolate susceptible to either agent at these high levels should exhibit a synergistic response to that agent plus a cell wall–active antimicrobial such as ampicillin.
3. Vancomycin resistance may be detected by using a screening procedure involving growth on brain-heart infusion agar containing 6 μg/ml of vancomycin.[55] A full 24 hours of incubation are required. The MIC of organisms that grow on the screening medium or that are determined to be vancomycin resistant by a breakpoint method can be more precisely determined to distinguish those with lower-level intrinsic *vanC*-mediated resistance from those with acquired, usually higher-level *vanA*- or *vanB*-mediated resistance.[55] A fourth resistance gene, *vanD,* has also been described.[63] The resistance classes can most reliably be distinguished by gene-based methods.[64] Also, it is important to be aware that automated identification systems may not be able to distinguish species with low-level resistance such as *Enterococcus casseliflavus* and *Enterococcus gallinarum* from *E. faecium.*[44]

Anaerobes

Anaerobes require susceptibility testing procedures different from those for organisms that can be grown aerobically, and the NCCLS has a separate standard pertaining to susceptibility testing of anaerobes.[56] That document and the relevant chapters in this text can be consulted for a discussion of the circumstances under which anaerobic susceptibility testing may be warranted.

Extended-Spectrum β-Lactamase Detection

Extended-spectrum β-lactamase (ESBL)-producing strains of *E. coli* and *Klebsiella* species are of increasing concern and may be difficult to detect in the laboratory. The NCCLS recommends that isolates of these species with MICs of 2 μg/ml or greater for cefpodoxime, ceftazidime, or aztreonam be considered possible ESBL producers.[55] Because ESBLs are inhibited by clavulanic acid, the MICs to these agents should decrease when testing is done with any of these agents along with clavulanic acid.[55] Initially, such organisms may appear to be susceptible to both cefoxitin and imipenem in vitro. However, cefoxitin is not recommended for treatment of infections caused by ESBL producers because resistance may develop during treatment; imipenem, on the other hand, has been found to be an effective agent.[65] The most sensitive single method for detecting ESBL production at present is susceptibility testing with cefpodoxime using an MIC breakpoint of 2 μg/ml or greater or a disk breakpoint of 22 mm or less as an indicator of possible ESBL production.[55, 65, 66] Both the Etest and double-disk potentiation methods are also available for further characterization of ESBL producers. In these assays, an ESBL producer is detected by virtue of its enhanced sensitivity to a test antibiotic such as ceftazidime in the presence of a β-lactamase inhibitor such as clavulanate. Although both procedures have been reported to perform well, at least the Etest does not detect all ESBL producers.[65–67]

Molecular Methods of Susceptibility Determination

The genetic basis for specific antimicrobial resistance in some organisms is now known, and it is possible to use molecular methods to reliably detect these resistance determinants. A well-studied example concerns the *mecA* gene for oxacillin resistance in staphylococci. A number of studies have examined the correlation between presence of the *mecA* gene and results with various susceptibility testing procedures. For *S. aureus,* current breakpoints used in both MIC and disk testing correlate well with presence of the *mecA* gene.[61] However, for coagulase-negative staphylococci, although the current disk breakpoint seems to have been clinically satisfactory, the current NCCLS MIC breakpoint fails to detect nearly 16% of *mecA*-containing organisms.[61] It would be interesting to know what percentage of the coagulase-negative staphylococcal isolates not determined to be oxacillin resistant by current NCCLS MIC criteria came from patients who had failed treatment with oxacillin or a related agent, but this information is not available. Some *S. aureus* strains lacking the *mecA* gene may be at least borderline oxacillin resistant on the basis of either β-lactamase production or modification of normal penicillin binding proteins.[68] Unfortunately, the absence of a gene or gene mutation known to confer resistance to an antimicrobial agent does not mean that an organism is susceptible to the agent because other mechanisms of resistance might be present. Also, molecular procedures for resistance determination are presently labor intensive, time consuming, and costly. Thus, because molecular methods are unable to determine susceptibility (as opposed to resistance) to specific agents, phenotypic procedures for susceptibility testing will continue to be required for the foreseeable future.

MYCOBACTERIA

Mycobacteria are aerobic, nonmotile, rod-shaped bacteria that are acid fast, that is, once stained with certain dyes, they resist decolorization with acid alcohol as a consequence of their cell wall structure.

Safety Issues

If bleach (5% sodium hypochlorite) is used to inactivate mycobacteria that may be present in a patient specimen, smears for the direct detection of mycobacteria can be prepared without special containment facilities. Processing of specimens, including digestion, decontamination, and planting, requires a biosafety level 2 facility and an appropriate biologic safety cabinet. Manipulation of cultures of *M. tuberculosis* requires a biosafety level 3 facility, including a room with unidirectional airflow that is entered through a series of two separate doors.[69]

Specimen Collection and Transport

Specimens for smear and culture for mycobacteria should be collected and transported in closed, leakproof, sterile containers. Containers contaminated with specimen on the outside are not acceptable because of the hazard posed to personnel. Gastric aspirates require pH neutralization soon after collection to ensure the viability of any mycobacteria that may be present; arrangements should be made in advance with the laboratory to ensure optimal specimen handling. Biopsies are preferable to swab specimens of tissue lesions for the isolation of mycobacteria. No special procedures are usually necessary for the collection and transport of sterile fluids, urine, and stool. However, organism concentrations in sterile fluids may be low, so a minimum of several milliliters (at least 10 ml if possible) should be obtained whenever mycobacterial infection is a serious consideration.[70] Blood may be collected for mycobacterial culture in a blood collection tube containing anticoagulant, collected in a lysis-centrifugation tube, or inoculated directly into a special bottle for mycobacterial blood culture, depending on laboratory protocol. Twenty-four-hour collections of sputum and urine are unacceptable because of the likelihood of bacterial overgrowth. For sputum and urine, it is recommended that at least three first morning specimens be obtained, with volumes of 5 to 10 ml for sputum and at least 40 ml for urine.[70]

Direct Organism Detection

Mycobacteria may be detected directly in patient specimens by visualization of stained organisms or by detection of specific mycobacterial nucleic acids or other cellular constituents.

The Gram stain is insensitive for the detection of mycobacteria. If visible at all, mycobacteria may appear as finely beaded gram-positive rods with only the beads visible (gram-positive) and the rest of the organism appearing gram-negative, or they may appear as negative images (rodlike clefts) in the specimen. Specific mycobacterial stains are based on the ability of mycobacteria to retain certain dyes after washing with an acid-alcohol decolorizer (hence "acid fast"), unlike other bacteria. The Ziehl-Neelsen and Kinyoun stains are both carbolfuchsin based and stain mycobacteria red. The Ziehl-Neelsen stain requires a heating step and has been largely replaced by the Kinyoun stain, which is a "cold" acid-fast stain. The auramine O and auramine-rhodamine stains use fluorescent compounds; although fluorescence microscopy is required to visualize the mycobacteria, the stains do not involve the use of an antibody but are based on the acid-fast properties of mycobacteria. Fluorescent stains are more sensitive for the detection of mycobacteria, particularly in direct specimens, because the organisms stain brightly and can be clearly distinguished from background material. In addition, because slides stained with a fluorescent dye can be examined reliably with an objective lens of lower magnification (25×) than the oil immersion lens (100×) required for carbolfuchsin-stained smears, reading of slides can be done faster. Rapidly growing mycobacteria may be less avidly acid fast than slow growers and may be more readily visualized with a modified acid-fast stain that uses a weaker decolorizing step than does a regular carbolfuchsin stain.[70] Some species of mycobacteria differ from others in the length, width, or arrangement of individual cells. *Mycobacterium kansasii,* for example, tends to be long and broad, sometimes with a banded rather than a beaded appearance, whereas *Mycobacterium avium* complex may appear coccobacillary, especially on a smear from a liquid medium. Cells of *M. tuberculosis* often group together in "cords" composed of long strands of organisms with their long axes parallel. However, the microscopic appearance of individual cells and groups of cells should at best be considered only suggestive of a certain species or group of species.

Amplification of mycobacterial nucleic acids can be used for the direct detection of mycobacteria in clinical material. Two commercially available procedures for the detection of organisms in the *M. tuberculosis* complex, the Gen-Probe MTD and the Roche Amplicor, have been approved by the Food and Drug Administration. Other procedures are under development.[71] The Gen-Probe and Roche procedures are approved only for use with smear-positive respiratory specimens, for which they have a sensitivity of better than 95% and a specificity approaching 100%.[72] Their sensitivity for smear-negative specimens has shown considerable variation in different studies and populations; overall it appears to be approximately 70%.[72]

Although direct detection of both mycobacterial antigens and tuberculostearic acid may have some utility for the diagnosis of tuberculosis, particularly tuberculous meningitis, such testing is not generally available.[73, 74] Nucleic acid amplification may be more sensitive than tuberculostearic acid detection for the diagnosis of both pulmonary and meningeal tuberculosis.[75, 76]

Specimen Processing and Planting

Specimens such as sputum, urine, and stool, which can be expected to contain considerable normal microbial flora, must be digested and decontaminated to prevent overgrowth of any mycobacteria present. These processing steps are inevitably somewhat toxic to mycobacteria, and a balance must be struck to minimize the loss of mycobacteria while simultaneously maximizing the elimination of as many other microorganisms as possible.[77] Concentration of the specimen occurs as part of the digestion and decontamination procedures, and smears of a specimen are prepared from such concentrates. The most commonly used digestion and decontamination procedure entails the use of a mixture of *N*-acetyl-L-cysteine and NaOH, although other procedures are occasionally used, such as the oxalic acid procedure for specimens heavily contaminated with *P. aeruginosa*.[77, 78] Normally sterile fluids such as CSF may be concentrated for smear preparation and planting but need not be subjected to digestion and decontamination. Biopsies obtained from normally sterile sites need to be ground before planting but do not require digestion and decontamination. Blood processed by a lysis-centrifugation method can be planted onto solid media, from which quantitation of growth (organisms per milliliter) in the blood can be determined. Currently, two types of mycobacterial blood culture bottles are available for direct inoculation, BACTEC 13A and BACTEC MYCO/F LYTIC (both from Becton Dickinson), and other systems are being developed, but quantitation cannot be obtained with liquid culture media.

It is recommended that a liquid in addition to a solid medium be used for planting specimens whenever practicable because the newer liquid media may enhance both the sensitivity of culture and the rapidity of organism detection.[70, 79] Most studies have shown improved mycobacterial isolation rates when both solid and liquid media are used. The benefit of using two different types of medium may derive from the preference of some mycobacterial isolates for one type of medium over another or simply from the increased sensitivity obtained by culturing a larger volume of specimen. Use of a liquid medium often results in the isolation of *M. tuberculosis* within 2 weeks and isolation of other slowly growing mycobacteria in even less time.[70] Consequently, when one of these liquid media has been used, one cannot assume that an organism detected after about a week of incubation is necessarily a rapid grower in the traditional sense. Solid media used for the initial isolation of mycobacteria are either egg based, such as Lowenstein-Jensen medium, or agar based, such as Middlebrook 7H11 medium. Antimicrobial agents may be added to solid media to help prevent overgrowth of contaminants; for example, Gruft is an egg-based medium containing penicillin and nalidixic acid, whereas Mitchison's or selective 7H11 medium is an agar-based medium containing polymixin B, amphotericin B, carbenicillin, and trimethoprim. Many of the liquid-based systems use an instrument for automated detection of organism growth, and at least two nonautomated systems are also available (Septi-Chek AFB System and Mycobacteria Growth Indicator Tube, both from Becton-Dickinson). Detection is based on such features as liberation of radiolabeled carbon dioxide from a ^{14}C-labeled substrate (BACTEC 460, Becton Dickinson), nonradiolabeled carbon dioxide production (MB/BacT, Organon-Teknika), oxygen consumption with activation of a fluorescent compound (BACTEC 9000MB and Mycobacteria Growth Indicator Tube, Becton-Dickinson) or change in vial gas pressure as a result of organism metabolism (ESP MYCO System, Accumed International).[78] Liquid media inoculated with specimens requiring digestion and decontamination are supplemented with an antimicrobial mixture as a further aid in suppressing bacterial overgrowth; an example is the PANTA (polymixin B, amphotericin B, nalidixic acid, trimethoprim, and azlocillin) added to BACTEC medium. Mycobacterial cultures are generally incubated at 36°C ± 1°C in an atmosphere of approximately 8% CO_2, the optimum conditions for isolation of *M. tuberculosis.* However, several species of pathogenic mycobacteria have different growth requirements or preferences that may have to be satisfied to ensure their isolation (Table 14–10). To optimize conditions for possible mycobacterial pathogens, some decisions need to be made regarding the initial handling of each specimen. Given the preference of several skin and subcutaneous pathogens (including *Mycobacterium haemophilum, M. marinum, Mycobacterium ulcerans,* and rapid growers) to grow at 30°C, at least a portion of all skin biopsies submitted for mycobacterial culture should be incubated at approximately 30°C.[78] It is also important that the clinician notify the laboratory if a pathogen with specific growth requirements, such as *M. haemophilum,* is suspected so that optimal culturing procedures can be used. *Mycobacterium paratuberculosis,* reported from some patients with Crohn's disease and the etiologic agent of Johne's disease in ruminants, cannot be isolated in the routine diagnostic laboratory.[80]

Significance of Isolation of Mycobacteria from Clinical Specimens

Isolation of certain species of mycobacteria, such as *M. avium* complex or a rapidly growing mycobacterium, may represent colonization or specimen contamination rather than active disease, but the potential significance of repeated isolation of the same species from the same source requires careful evaluation.[81] Most isolates of *Mycobacterium gordonae,* a water organism, are regarded as contaminants; only rarely is it a proven pathogen.[82–85] Unfortunately, the specimen processing steps required for mycobacterial culture make transfer of a mycobacterium from one specimen to another a rare, but real possibility. Therefore, the significance even of the isolation of *M. tuberculosis* from a solitary smear-negative specimen, especially in the absence of consistent histopathology or a highly consistent clinical picture, requires careful consideration.[86] A useful summary of recommendations for the diagnosis and treatment of disease caused by nontuberculous mycobacteria is provided by the American Thoracic Society.[81]

TABLE 14–10 Pathogenic Mycobacteria with Unusual Growth Requirements or Preferences

Mycobacterium bovis
- Growth said to be enhanced by 0.4% pyruvate, but apparently supplementation is not needed with the newer media

Mycobacterium haemophilum
- Requires ferric ion (provided as ferric ammonium citrate, hemin, or blood)
- Requires approximately 30°C for initial growth

Mycobacterium genavense
- Grows best in BACTEC media
- May grow on solid media supplemented with mycobactin J after prolonged incubation

Mycobacterium marinum
- May require approximately 30°C for initial growth

Mycobacterium paratuberculosis
- May require many months to grow
- Cultivation is not feasible in the diagnostic laboratory

Mycobacterium ulcerans
- May require approximately 30°C for initial growth
- Requires prolonged (up to 3 mo) incubation for detection

Mycobacterium xenopi
- Grows best at 42°C but will grow, at least slowly, at 36°C

Rapidly growing mycobacteria
- Often grow best at approximately 30°C, but often grow well at 36°C

Mycobacterial Identification

Traditional Categories and Methods

A mycobacterial species is placed into one of several categories, depending on its growth rate and its pigment production in relation to light stimulation. Rapid growers take less than 7 days for growth on subculture to a solid medium from a dilute suspension; however, they generally also take less than 7 days to grow on solid or in liquid medium on initial isolation. Slowly growing mycobacteria are further divided into photochromogens, scotochromogens, and nonphotochromogens, depending on their ability to produce pigment and the relationship of pigment production to light stimulation. Photochromogens produce pigment after light stimulation, but not when grown continuously in the dark. Scotochromogens produce pigment when grown in the dark, as well as after light exposure. Nonphotochromogens do not produce pigment even after light stimulation. However, not all isolates of some species will fall into the same categories. For example, most isolates of *M. avium* complex are nonphotochromogenic, but some are scotochromogenic; many isolates of *M. marinum* (a photochromogen) grow rapidly, and isolates of *Mycobacterium szulgai* are usually photochromogenic at 25°C but scotochromogenic at 36°C. These three categories (photochromogen, scotochromogen, and nonphotochromogen) correspond to the Runyoun groups I, II, and III, respectively, which along with group IV (rapid growers), were initially established for the categorization of mycobacteria other than *M. tuberculosis.* The Runyoun numerical group designations are rarely used today. *M. tuberculosis* complex, although by definition not a member of any of the Runyoun groups, is in fact a nonphotochromogen. In addition to the features of growth rate and pigment production, traditional identification of mycobacterial species is based on colony morphology and a variety of biochemical reactions.[78, 87] *M. tuberculosis,* for example, in addition to producing rough, buff colonies (which are considered nonpigmented), also produces niacin, reduces nitrate, and hydrolyzes urea. By conventional biochemical methods, *M. avium* is essentially indistinguishable from *Mycobacterium intracellulare*; serologic techniques (not generally available) may help distinguish between the two species, but the distinction is best made by newer procedures such as cell wall or nucleic acid–based analysis.

Rapid Methods

Three major categories of methods are available for the rapid identification of mycobacteria.

Nucleic Acid–Based Methods. Commercially available probes (AccuProbe [Gen-Probe]) are available for identification of *M. avium* complex, *M. gordonae, M. kansasii,* and *M. tuberculosis* complex. These chemiluminescent compound–labeled probes are DNA probes for ribosomal RNA; they can be used only with organisms grown in culture, not directly on patient specimens. Each is a single, separate probe, except for the *M. avium* complex probe, which is a mixture of three separate probes, one for each recognized member of the complex (Table 14–11). The procedure can be performed within a matter of hours from the time of organism isolation.[78] The sensitivity

TABLE 14–11 Mycobacteria Isolated from Clinical Specimens*

Nonphotochromogens	Scotochromogens
M. avium complex	*M. flavescens*
M. avium	*M. gordonae*
M. intracellulare	*M. interjectum*†
"X-cluster"	*M. lentiflavum*
M. branderi†	*M. scrofulaceum*
M. celatum†	*M. szulgai*
M. conspicuum†	Rapid growers
M. gastri‡	*M. aurum*†
M. genavense†	*M. chelonae* group
M. haemophilum	*M. abscessus*
M. heidelbergense†	*M. chelonae*
M. malmoense	*M. mucogenicum*
M. paratuberculosis	*M. fortuitum* group
M. shimoidei	*M. fortuitum*
M. terrae complex	*M. fortuitum*, third biovar
M. nonchromogenicum	*M. peregrinum*
M. terrae‡	*M. hassicacum*†
M. triplex†	*M. margeritense*†
M. triviale‡	*M. neoaurum*
M. tuberculosis complex§	*M. novocastrense*†
M. africanum	*M. phlei*
M. bovis	*M. smegmatis*
M. tuberculosis	*M. thermoresistible*
M. ulcerans	*M. vaccae*
M. xenopi	
Photochromogens	
M. asiaticum	
M. intermedium†	
M. kansasii	
M. marinum	
M. simiae	

*Includes most species of mycobacteria reported from clinical specimens; does not include *M. leprae*, which cannot be grown in vitro.

†Species newly described since 1990 (exclusive of organisms in *M. chelonae* and *M. fortuitum* groups).

‡May never be a pathogen.[102]

§Also includes *M. microti*, usually an animal pathogen and only recently implicated as a human pathogen.

of the procedure derives in part from the multiple copies of ribosomal RNA that exist in each bacterial cell, as opposed to a single copy of bacterial DNA. Laboratories not doing further testing of isolates of the *M. avium* complex and the *M. tuberculosis* complex should make it clear that their identifications have not gone beyond the level of the complex (e.g., they should report "*M. tuberculosis* complex," not "*M. tuberculosis,*" unless additional appropriate testing such as niacin and nitrate reactions has been done). Other nucleic acid–based methods for identification of mycobacterial species include amplification of a species-specific portion of the genome or amplification of a portion of the genome common to all mycobacteria, followed by the use of species-specific probes, by restriction fragment length polymorphism analysis, or by sequencing of the amplified material.[71] These latter techniques are not widely available.

Analysis of Cellular Constituents. Gas-liquid chromatography and high-performance liquid chromatography allow rapid identification of many species of mycobacteria via analysis of short- and long-chain fatty acids, respectively.[88] Because of the equipment and expertise required, these chromatographic identification procedures are available primarily in larger, specialized laboratories.

NAP Test. The NAP test, based on the inhibition of growth of members of the *M. tuberculosis* complex by *p*-nitro-α-acetylamino-β-hydroxypropiophenone (NAP), can be used with the BACTEC system and provides presumptive identification as *M. tuberculosis* complex or not *M. tuberculosis* complex in 5 days with a high degree of reliability. Occasional isolates of nontuberculous mycobacteria may have their growth delayed in the presence of NAP.[87]

Mycobacteria Isolated in the Clinical Laboratory

Table 14–11 lists most of the mycobacterial species that have been reported to date from clinical specimens, with each species placed in the category to which it is usually assigned.[87, 89–96] Of the slow growers, many are rarely isolated or newly described species, some of which can be identified at present only by the use of molecular methods. Unfortunately, some recent reports of unusual pathogens provide little, if any, data to substantiate identification of the species stated to be the infecting agent. Determination of the clinical significance of some of these species must await further resolution of their frequency of isolation, spectrum of illness, and therapeutic responsiveness. Within the group of rapid growers, certain organisms recently considered to be subspecies or biovariants are now regarded as separate species. With continuing use of molecular techniques, particularly sequencing of amplified portions of the bacterial genome, it can be anticipated that the description of new mycobacterial species will continue for some time.

Susceptibility Testing

In the United States, susceptibility testing of *M. tuberculosis* complex is done either by the proportion method using Middlebrook 7H10 agar or in BACTEC liquid medium. It is currently recommended that all initial isolates of *M. tuberculosis* complex be tested, as well as isolates from patients who are still culture positive after 3 months of therapy or who are clinically failing to respond. The use of liquid medium is recommended for testing the five primary antituberculous drugs because results are usually available within a week, as opposed to the 3 weeks required with solid medium. In the proportion method, an isolate is considered resistant to a specific concentration of antimicrobial if the number of colonies growing on the corresponding drug-containing quadrant of the plate is greater than 1% of the number of colonies on a drug-free quadrant. Ethambutol, isoniazid, pyrazinamide, rifampin, and streptomycin can be tested in the BACTEC system. Testing using the liquid medium has been standardized to be in accordance with results using the solid medium. It is considered most important to test the "critical concentration" of each drug, or the concentration that inhibits most cells in a fully sensitive strain.[77] These concentrations differ somewhat for solid and liquid media (e.g., the critical concentrations for isoniazid in 7H10 agar and BACTEC medium are 0.2 and 0.1 μg/ml, respectively). The NCCLS has published a tentative standard for susceptibility testing of *M. tuberculosis*; no standardized methodology exists for the susceptibility testing of other slowly growing mycobacteria.[97] Although procedures have been published for susceptibility testing of other slowly growing mycobacteria such as *M. avium* complex, the clinical relevance of such testing is controversial.[81, 98] Rapidly growing mycobacteria do not generally respond to the agents used for the treatment of tuberculosis. The NCCLS is developing a modification of the broth microdilution procedure used for bacterial susceptibility testing for use with rapid growers; the principal modifications will probably include an inoculum matching a 1 McFarland standard, temperature of incubation of 30°C, and incubation for 3 to 5 days.[99]

Epidemiology

Molecular fingerprinting can now be performed by a few laboratories to determine the relatedness of different isolates of *M. tuberculosis*. The method most widely used is based on the insertion sequence IS*6110*, which is found in 5 to 20 copies scattered in different locations in the chromosome in different strains. The DNA fragments produced by a specific endonuclease (which cleaves at only one site in each insertion sequence) are separated by gel electrophoresis. A probe is then used to detect the fragments containing the larger portion of the cleaved insertion sequence, and fragment patterns obtained from different isolates are compared to determine relatedness.[100] The procedure has been used for such purposes as investigating episodes of possible laboratory cross-contamination, tracing sources of infection in outbreak situations, determining whether a second episode of disease is due to a previously isolated strain or to a newly infecting strain, and determining whether an infection is caused by more than one strain of organism.[101] Other techniques are available when the IS*6110*-based technique is not practicable, such as for isolates with too few copies of the insertion sequence. Pulsed-field gel electrophoresis and randomly amplified polymorphic DNA PCR have been used for evaluation of the strain relatedness of rapid growers.[103]

Recommended Procedures and Target Times for Results for the Mycobacteriology Laboratory

To help control the resurgence of tuberculosis in the United States and deal with the increase in isolation of drug-resistant *M. tuberculosis,* the recommendations summarized in Table 14–12 have been made regarding diagnostic mycobacteriology laboratory procedures.[79]

AEROBIC ACTINOMYCETES

The aerobic actinomycetes are branching, gram-positive rods that grow best (or in many cases only) under aerobic conditions. They are similar in certain respects to both corynebacteria and mycobacteria, which are sometimes also included with the aerobic actinomycetes.[104] The taxonomy of this group is under active revision, and considerable nomenclatural change is occurring. Despite possible phylogenetic relationship to the aerobic actinomycetes, the morphologically similar anaerobic actinomycetes (including the genus *Actinomyces*), which have a preference or requirement for anaerobic growth conditions, are included with gram-positive anaerobic bacteria. Genera of aerobic actinomycetes that contain species pathogenic for humans include *Actinomadura, Dermatophilus, Gordona, Rhodococcus, Nocardia, Nocardiopsis, Oerskovia, Rothia, Streptomyces,* and *Tsukamurella.*[105] Organisms in the genera *Gordona, Nocardia, Rhodococcus,* and *Tsukamurella* are usually modified acid fast positive; of these, only isolates of *Nocardia* regularly produce an aerial mycelium.[105] Although true bacteria and not molds, these organisms have traditionally been identified in the mycology section of the laboratory, perhaps because they somewhat resemble molds both in their relatively slow growth rate and in their tendency to form long, branched structures reminiscent of hyphae. Because these organisms are widespread in the environment, colonization and specimen contamination can occur. Single colonies of *Streptomyces,* especially from nonsterile sites and from nonmycetomatous lesions, are very likely to represent contamination. However, most aerobic actinomycetes are very uncommon as laboratory contaminants, and their isolation should not be too quickly dismissed as insignificant.

TABLE 14–12 Recommended Procedures for the Diagnostic Mycobacteriology Laboratory

Recommended Procedure	Time for Recommended Procedures	Time for Conventional Procedures
Fluorochrome stain	Within 24 h of specimen receipt	Within 24 h of specimen receipt
Liquid medium for culture	Growth of *M. tuberculosis* within approximately 2 wk	Growth detected at approximately 3–6 wk
Rapid method for identification of *M. tuberculosis*	Within 24 h (by probes or chromatography) or 5 d (NAP) of organism isolation	Requires 3–6 wk after organism isolation and adequate organism growth
Susceptibility testing of *M. tuberculosis* in a liquid medium	Results available approximately 1 wk after organism isolation	Results available 3 wk after organism isolation and adequate organism growth

Abbreviation: NAP, *p*-nitro-α-acetylamino-β-hydroxypropiophenol.
Data from Della-Latta P, Weitzman I. Mycobacteriology. In: Isenberg HD, ed. Essential Procedures for Clinical Microbiology. Washington, DC: American Society for Microbiology; 1998:169–203; and Tenover FC, Crawford JT, Huebner RE, et al. The resurgence of tuberculosis: Is your laboratory ready? J Clin Microbiol. 1993;31:767–770.

Specimen Collection and Transport

Collection and transport procedures suitable for bacterial and fungal cultures are also adequate for the aerobic actinomycetes, but refrigeration of specimens should be avoided because some *Nocardia* strains lose viability at low temperatures.[104] If infection with an organism in this group is strongly suspected, alerting the laboratory is advisable because special staining and planting procedures are useful to enhance the likelihood of detecting the organism. Because these organisms may cause deep-seated infections such as brain abscess, biopsy may be necessary for isolation. These organisms are not considered a safety hazard in the laboratory.

Direct Organism Detection

In some infections caused by these organisms such as mycetoma, the organisms may grow in dense masses visible macroscopically as "grains" in purulent material. Detection of these "grains" may greatly facilitate isolation of the etiologic agent; hence, the laboratory should be notified in advance when such an infection is suspected.[105] The only generally available means of direct detection of these organisms in patient specimens is by staining. On Gram stain, many of these organisms appear as long, branching, somewhat beaded gram-positive rods. *Nocardia* tends to be especially thin and long and may appear to be composed mainly of tiny noncontiguous gram-positive beads. Organisms in other genera such as *Streptomyces* (and the anaerobic actinomycetes) tend to appear wider and more avidly gram-positive, but a definite genus assignment of any organism other than *Dermatophilus* cannot be made with certainty on the basis of organism morphology alone. *Nocardia* may also be "gram-invisible," and a modified acid-fast smear should always be requested if *Nocardia* infection is suspected. *Gordona* and *Rhodococcus* spp. may be unbranched, much shorter than *Nocardia,* and overall more coryneform in appearance. *Dermatophilus congolensis,* the only species in the genus, produces branching filaments with divisions occurring both parallel and perpendicular to the long axis of the filament. In Gram-stained material, the organism may appear too darkly stained for adequate visualization of structural detail, and some other stain such as a Giemsa stain may be necessary.[105] The modified acid-fast stain for aerobic actinomycetes is similar to the Kinyoun stain for mycobacteria but differs particularly in that a weaker decolorizing solution, a shorter time period, or both are used for decolorization. The stain requires some expertise for performance and interpretation and should always be done with appropriate positive and negative controls. *Nocardia* spp. are weakly acid fast in that they retain carbolfuchsin only if a weak decolorization procedure is performed; they are not acid fast with the decolorizing procedure used for mycobacteria. In addition to being weakly acid fast, they also tend to be only partially acid fast, particularly when stained from culture, which means that often only a small proportion of the cells retain the carbolfuchsin dye.

Specimen Processing and Planting

No special specimen processing is required for isolation of the aerobic actinomycetes, which will grow on many different types of media. However, they may not survive the specimen processing used to eliminate bacterial flora from specimens for mycobacterial culture. Because they may be present in low numbers and are relatively slowly growing, isolation of aerobic actinomycetes may be enhanced by using media containing antimicrobial agents to suppress the normal flora. A medium that has been found to be particularly useful for the isolation of *Nocardia* is buffered charcoal-yeast extract agar with antibiotics.[106] Cultures for *Nocardia* should be held for up to 3 weeks.[105]

Aerobic Actinomycete Identification

Colonies of *Nocardia* typically have a powdery, whitish surface because of the production of aerial mycelium and a tan to orange reverse surface. When stained from colonies, the organism often breaks up into coccobacillary fragments, with long, branching forms much less conspicuous than in direct patient material. Organisms stained from culture may be less acid fast than in stains prepared from the original specimen.

Nocardia asteroides has been determined to contain a number of different subgroups, at least three of which are now considered to be separate species: *N. asteroides* in the strict sense, *Nocardia farcinica,* and *Nocardia nova.* All three species together may be referred to as the *N. asteroides* complex. However, because even *N. asteroides* in the strict sense may be a set of several different species, some refer to this more restricted group itself as the *N. asteroides* complex. Other potentially pathogenic species of *Nocardia* include *Nocardia brasiliensis, Nocardia otitidiscaviarum* (formerly called *N. caviae*), and *Nocardia transvalensis. Nocardia pseudobrasiliensis* is a newly described pathogen that may be difficult to separate from *N. brasiliensis.*[107] Conventional identification procedures for *Nocardia* spp. as performed in most laboratories involve only a small number of biochemical tests, and these tests are insufficient to distinguish among members of the *N. asteroides* complex. Differences in the results of testing for susceptibility to certain antimicrobial agents may help distinguish among some of these species.[104, 105, 108]

Colonies of *R. equi,* which is the principal pathogen in the genus *Rhodococcus,* are generally somewhat mucoid and acquire a pink color after 4 days of incubation; the organism has been isolated from a variety of sites, including the respiratory tract and blood.[105, 109]

Amplification by PCR of a portion of the genome, followed by restriction fragment length polymorphism analysis, may prove to be the most rapid and reliable way for accurately identifying aerobic actinomycetes, but these techniques are not yet widely available.[110] Other procedures such as cell wall analysis are useful for identifying these organisms, but they are also available only in some reference laboratories. Thus, for accurate identification of many of these organisms, referral to a specialized laboratory is necessary.

Susceptibility Testing

Several different procedures have been proposed for susceptibility testing of *Nocardia,* but no standardized method yet exists.[111] Different investigators have used different susceptibility testing procedures, so caution should be used when comparing published results. Better correlation of in vitro and in vivo results are needed, but such correlations are difficult to perform in the absence of a standardized susceptibility testing methodology. For example, although some isolates of *N. otitidiscaviarum* have been found to be resistant to sulfonamides in vitro, the clinical relevance of this finding is unclear because of conflicting reports in the literature regarding the responsiveness of *N. otitidiscaviarum* infections to sulfonamides.[104, 112, 113] Reports of sulfonamide treatment failures in *Nocardia* infections have also appeared despite in vitro susceptibility.[114] At least one report suggests the development of sulfonamide resistance during treatment.[112] See the chapter on *Nocardia* infections in this text for a discussion of treatment options.

Epidemiology

Because infection with aerobic actinomycetes generally occurs on a sporadic basis, epidemiologic investigations are only rarely needed. To document that a pseudo-outbreak was the result of specimen cross-contamination with a single strain of *N. asteroides,* both pulsed-field gel electrophoresis and randomly amplified polymorphic DNA analysis have been used successfully.[115]

FUNGI

Like plants and animals, fungi are eukaryotic, a characteristic that distinguishes these three groups from bacteria. Fungi are now placed in their own separate kingdom. Thousands of species have been described, approximately 150 of which have been reported to be at least occasional human pathogens, with additional ones appearing in the literature regularly.[116, 117] The genus *Pneumocystis,* formerly considered to be a parasite, is now thought to be a fungus, although the human pathogen *P. carinii* remains for all practical purposes uncultivatable in vitro.[118] Other pathogens presumed to be fungi that have not yet been cultured in vitro include *Loboa loboi* and *Rhinosporidium seeberi.*[116] Organisms recovered from patients with hepatosplenic candidiasis, although often readily visible microscopically, are frequently uncultivatable in vitro.[119] The genus *Prototheca* is thought to be an achlorophyllous alga; organisms in this genus can be pathogenic and are usually included in discussions of fungi because they grow well on fungal media.[116]

Terminology

The diagnostic mycology laboratory uses terminology that although of little taxonomic significance, is useful in terms of assessing both clinical relevance and identification possibilities.[116, 117, 120, 121] *Yeasts* are organisms that grow as relatively smooth, creamy colonies, whereas *molds* produce fuzzy colonies because of the production of aerial hyphae. Some organisms may initially produce yeastlike colonies that become more moldlike with continued incubation. Microscopically, yeasts appear as round or oval cells that reproduce by budding. Many yeasts, such as most species of *Candida,* also produce hyphal structures. Hyphae are morphologically subdivided into pseudohyphae and true hyphae. *Pseudohyphae* resemble chains of sausages in that the hyphae tend to be constricted at the septa and each cell originates as a bud. The cell at the tip tends to be small and rounded, and a septum is often found at each branch point. In contrast, *true hyphae* tend to have straighter, parallel walls without constrictions at the septa and usually without a septum at the branch point. True hyphae may be either *septate* or *aseptate.* True hyphae that are septate suggest organisms such as *Aspergillus, Fusarium,* and *Pseudallescheria.* True aseptate hyphae may be broad and have a ribbon-like appearance; their presence suggests one of the zygomycetes (aseptate molds) such as *Rhizomucor.* Brown pigment in hyphae suggests that the organism is a *dermatiaceous* (black) mold; *hyaline* molds do not produce pigmented hyphae. These simplified distinctions are not absolute. Thus, some *Candida* species can form true hyphae, and the "aseptate" molds may have an occasional septum. *Dermatophytes* and *dimorphic* molds are considered separate categories of mold distinct from the other hyaline septate molds. The likelihood that an organism may be a dermatophyte is usually suggested by the specimen source (e.g., skin, hair, nails). Dimorphic molds have a nonmold form when growing in the patient but grow as a mold in the laboratory at 30°C. Table 14–13 summarizes some of the more significant and more commonly isolated genera and species according to the categories frequently used in the diagnostic laboratory. Of the clinically significant dimorphic molds, *Blastomyces dermatitidis, Histoplasma capsulatum, Paracoccidioides brasiliensis, Penicillium marneffei,* and *S. schenckii* grow as yeasts in the patient and at 37°C; *Coccidioides immitis* grows as thick-walled spherules in the patient and requires a special medium not widely available to be grown in this form in vitro.

Many molds have a morphologic form resulting from sexual reproduction that differs from the form resulting from asexual reproduction. The form resulting from sexual reproduction is known as the *teleomorph,* or perfect state; the form resulting from asexual reproduction is known as the *anamorph,* or imperfect state. Traditionally, each form has been given a different scientific name; for example, the sexual form of *H. capsulatum* is named *Ajellomyces capsulatum,* and the sexual form of *Scedosporium apiospermum* is named *Pseudallescheria boydii.*

TABLE 14–13 Laboratory Categorization of Selected Clinically Significant and/or Commonly Isolated Fungi

	Molds				
	Dematiaceous	*Hyaline Septate*			*Hyaline Aseptate*
Yeasts		*Dermatophyte*	*Dimorphic*	*Other*	
Candida *Cryptococcus* *Blastoschizomyces* *Malassezia* *Saccharomyces* *Rhodotorula* *Trichosporon*	*Alternaria* *Bipolaris* *Cladosporium* *Curvularia* *Exophiala* *Exserohilum* *Phialophora* *Xylohypha*	*Epidermophyton* *Microsporum* *Trichophyton*	*Blastomyces dermatitidis* *Coccidioides immitis* *Histoplasma capsulatum* *Paracoccidioides brasiliensis* *Penicillium marneffei* *Sporothrix schenckii*	*Aspergillus* *Fusarium* *Paecilomyces* *Penicillium* *Pseudallescheria*	*Cunninghamella* *Mucor* *Rhizomucor* *Rhizopus*

Adapted from Koneman EW, Roberts GD. Practical Laboratory Mycology. 3rd ed. Baltimore: Williams & Wilkins; 1985.

Safety Issues

Virtually all molds release their reproductive structures (conidia or spores) into the air, and for many fungal pathogens the respiratory tract is the initial portal of entry. Thus, it is not surprising that certain species, particularly *C. immitis* and *H. capsulatum,* can be significant laboratory hazards. Containment facilities (biosafety level 2 for specimen handling and initial isolation, biosafety level 3 for further culture workup) are needed for processing specimens and working with cultures of these organisms.[117, 122] Because infectious spores are not present in patient specimens such as sputa or biopsies, these specimens are not considered hazardous by the aerosol route, but of course they would be infectious by accidental inoculation.

Specimen Collection and Transport

The procedures used for the collection of specimens for bacterial culture will suffice for fungal culture. However, it is important to be sure that an adequate volume of specimen has been collected, as for example, in the case of CSF (up to 5 ml or even 30 ml for chronic meningitis) and urine (up to 200 ml).[116] Twenty-four-hour collections of urine or sputa are not suitable for fungal culture because of bacterial overgrowth; first morning specimens are considered optimal. Aspirated material can be transported to the laboratory in an anaerobic transport vial; as long as the specimen is received and processed promptly by the laboratory, there appears to be little loss of fungal viability.[123] Blood culture performed by lysis-centrifugation has been found to be the most sensitive procedure for the isolation of *H. capsulatum* from blood.[123] BACTEC 13A bottles designed for mycobacterial culture will also recover this organism from blood, although it is not known whether they are as sensitive for this purpose as lysis-centrifugation is.[124] Commercially available broth and biphasic systems have been shown to be quite sensitive for the isolation of other fungi from blood, particularly *Candida.* Terminal subculturing may be needed to optimize isolation of *C. neoformans* from at least some broth systems.[123] Certain specimen types are more useful than others for the detection of particular pathogens—these issues are dealt with in the chapters pertaining to specific organisms.

Direct Organism Detection

Fungi are detected in clinical specimens either by direct visualization of the organisms themselves or by detection of antigens produced by the organism. Fungi may be visualized histopathologically or cytologically by a variety of special stains such as the methenamine silver, periodic acid–Schiff, or Papanicolaou stains. In the microbiology laboratory, fungi are usually visualized directly by a Gram stain, a KOH (wet) mount, or a Calcofluor white stain.[123] With a Gram stain, yeast cells and pseudohyphae of *Candida* species usually stain uniformly throughout as gram-positive, whereas the cells of *C. neoformans* may be unevenly speckled with crystal violet and may be surrounded by an orange halo that is presumably capsular material. The true hyphae of organisms such as *Aspergillus* species are either gram-negative, visible as unstained negative images, or surprisingly, Gram-stain invisible. Although KOH wet mounts allow visualization of most fungi, organisms may actually be quite difficult to discern because they do not stand out prominently from the background; in addition, tissue components such as blood vessels can be mistaken for fungal elements, so considerable care and expertise are required for reading such preparations. In the Calcofluor white stain, a fluorescent compound binds to certain cell wall polysaccharides found in all fungi; organisms stained by this dye can be readily visualized with a fluorescence microscope.[116, 123] In the microbiology laboratory, *P. carinii* can be visualized by a Calcofluor white, toluidine blue O, Giemsa, or monoclonal antibody stain.[118, 123] The Calcofluor white and toluidine blue O stains (as well as the methenamine silver stain) only stain the cyst wall; a drawback of these stains is that they also stain yeast cells, which can be morphologically similar to *Pneumocystis* cysts. The Giemsa stain allows visualization of intracystic structures and trophozoites, but the cyst wall appears only as a negative image. Monoclonal antibody stains allow the visualization of both cysts and trophozoites of *P. carinii,* but even with these stains, some expertise is required to recognize the various forms of the organism and to distinguish them from staining artifacts. The Giemsa stain is also useful for detecting *H. capsulatum* within macrophages.[123]

Antigen detection for *C. neoformans* and for *H. capsulatum* has been demonstrated to be of sufficient sensitivity to have considerable diagnostic utility; antigen detection for other fungi is not yet of sufficient sensitivity to be widely used for diagnostic purposes.[123, 125] The capsular polysaccharide antigen of *C. neoformans* may be detected by either latex agglutination or EIA techniques. These tests can be performed on both CSF and serum. Detection of cryptococcal antigen has been demonstrated to be a more sensitive technique for the diagnosis of cryptococcal meningitis than is examination of CSF for cryptococci by the India ink procedure. Detection of *Histoplasma* antigen in CSF, bronchoalveolar lavage fluid, serum, or urine for diagnosis of *H. capsulatum* infection is available only from the Histoplasmosis Reference Laboratory in Indianapolis, Indiana.

Specimen Processing and Planting

No special processing of specimens is required for isolation of fungi from clinical specimens. Specimens from nonsterile sites are planted onto media containing antibiotics such as chloramphenicol and gentamicin to inhibit bacterial growth; media used for the isolation of dermatophytes may also contain cycloheximide to inhibit yeasts. Media commonly used include inhibitory mold agar and brain-heart infusion agar. A source of fatty acids such as olive oil must be added to media to recover *Malassezia furfur*; clinicians should therefore notify the laboratory when the presence of this organism is suspected.[116] Fungal cultures are generally incubated at 30°C, and until recently, fungal cultures were generally held for 4 weeks and even longer when the presence of a slowly growing mold such as *H.*

capsulatum was suspected.[123] However, it has been shown that shorter periods of incubation suffice for the isolation of most fungal pathogens, depending on the type of specimen and the organisms being sought, and these shorter incubation periods are likely to be used by a growing number of laboratories.[126, 127] Cultures from such sites as the throat, urine, and vagina may routinely be held for just 1 to 2 weeks, with only specimens such as those from the respiratory tract and blood being held for 4 weeks. Thus, if a slowly growing mold such as *H. capsulatum* is suspected, it is useful for the clinician to notify the laboratory.

Significance of Isolation of Fungi from Clinical Specimens

It is often difficult to assess the significance of the isolation of fungi other than dimorphic molds from clinical specimens, particularly if isolated in small quantity from nonsterile sites such as the respiratory tract. It is usually impossible to attach clinical significance to the isolation of *Candida* from pulmonary material other than a lung biopsy because *Candida* can be part of the normal upper respiratory tract flora. Even *C. neoformans* may occasionally be a colonizer and not a pathogen in the respiratory tract.[116] Isolation of opportunistic pathogens such as *Aspergillus* from the respiratory tract of an immunocompromised patient presents a particularly difficult interpretive problem for which no unambiguous guidelines exist. In addition to the clinical and radiographic aspects of each situation, it may be useful to consider (1) whether the organism was seen directly in the specimen, (2) the quantity of organism that grew in culture, and (3) the particular genus or species recovered (*Aspergillus niger,* for example, is less likely to be a pathogen than *Aspergillus fumigatus* or *Aspergillus flavus*[116]) *Penicillium* species other than *P. marneffei* are common laboratory contaminants; their isolation is almost never indicative of disease. However, because many different fungi are capable of causing at least occasional cases of infection, each situation needs to be assessed individually.

Identification of Fungi

Yeasts are identified by performing a simple test initially, such as a germ tube test or a test based on the detection of preformed enzymes to presumptively identify *Candida albicans,* or a rapid urease test and a caffeic acid test for the presumptive identification of *C. neoformans.*[128] Figure 14–6 is a schematic diagram for identification of the various categories of yeast. By using a rapid and inexpensive test such as the germ tube for the presumptive identification of *C. albicans,* the most commonly isolated yeast in the diagnostic laboratory, the laboratory reduces the need for more time-consuming and expensive testing. It has recently been found, however, that another *Candida* species, *Candida dubliniensis,* is also germ tube positive. Although the organism is geographically widespread, and evidently causes disease in individuals infected with human immunodeficiency virus (HIV), the overall frequency of this organism has not yet been established.[129] Both manual kits and automated systems are available for the identification of clinically significant yeasts.[128] A cornmeal agar plate is inoculated along with any of these systems to confirm that the isolate's morphologic features are compatible with the identification. Identification of most molds is based largely on the morphologic features of the organism, but for certain organisms, other features such as the ability to grow at higher temperatures or the need for specific nutritional supplements are also used. For some fungi, assignment to a particular genus may be straightforward, whereas identification to the species level may need a mycologist with expertise in the particular group in question; examples include organisms belonging to the genera *Curvularia* and *Fusarium.* Chemiluminescent probes are available for the identification of isolates of *B. dermatitidis, C. immitis,* and *H. capsulatum.*[128] Like the similar probes for mycobacterial identification, they are intended for use with isolates, not with direct patient specimens; the probe is a DNA probe for organism ribosomal RNA. These probes can be used with either the yeast or mold phases, thus allowing early identification of isolates and obviating the need for conversion of the mold to the

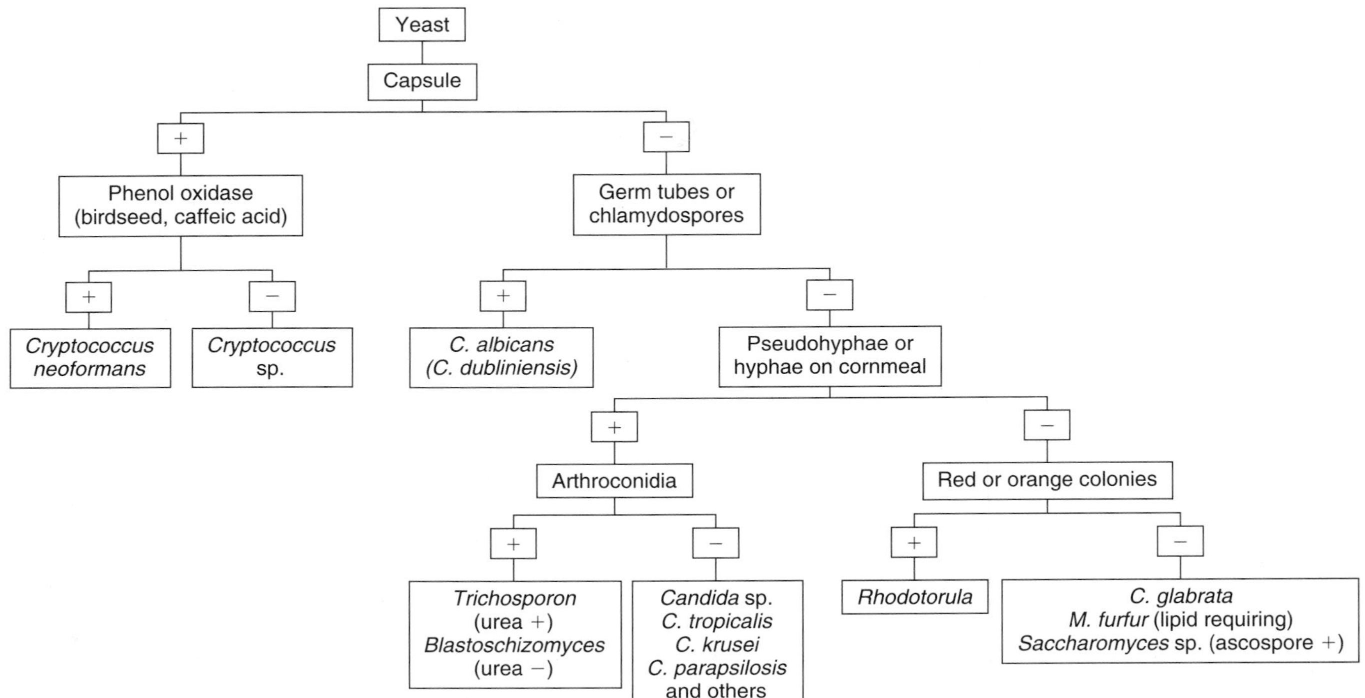

FIGURE 14–6. Schematic diagram for identification of commonly encountered yeasts, excluding dimorphic molds.

yeast phase for *B. dermatitidis* and *H. capsulatum.* Use of these probes also eliminates the need for extensive manipulation of cultures of these hazardous organisms. Exoantigen testing for identification of most of the dimorphic molds can also be done but requires an adequate amount of a mold-phase culture.[128, 130]

Susceptibility Testing

The NCCLS has published a standardized procedure for yeast susceptibility testing.[131] Interpretive guidelines are provided only for flucytosine, fluconazole, and itraconazole; for the azoles, these guidelines are based largely (fluconazole) or entirely (itraconazole) on results with mucosal infections. Correlation of in vitro and in vivo results and determination of the situations in which such susceptibility testing will be of clinical relevance are currently areas of active investigation. Mold susceptibility testing is available from certain reference centers, but no standardized procedure for susceptibility testing of molds has yet been established.

Epidemiology

Molecular techniques such as randomly amplified polymorphic DNA analysis and pulsed-field gel electrophoresis have been applied to yeast isolates for determination of strain relatedness.[132, 133] Such studies, however, are available only from certain specialized centers.

Serology

The utility of serologic determinations for the diagnosis of infection has been investigated for many different fungi. Often, several different methodologies, such as complement fixation and immunodiffusion, have been developed for the same organism. Kits for detection of antibody to certain organisms are commercially available. Testing for the presence of antibody to assist in the diagnosis of invasive disease has been used for blastomycosis, coccidioidomycosis, histoplasmosis, paracoccidioidomycosis, and sporotrichosis.[125] Antibody testing for a variety of other fungal pathogens may be available from research or commercial laboratories but has less well defined utility.[125] Testing for antibody in noninvasive disease has been found useful for the diagnosis of allergic bronchopulmonary aspergillosis and aspergilloma.[125] For details regarding optimal diagnostic methodology for different agents and for problems relating to result interpretation, see the chapters in this text pertaining to the specific organisms, or consult a specialized text such as the *Manual of Clinical Laboratory Immunology.*[125]

VIRUSES

Virology Specimen Collection and Transport

Appropriate specimen collection and transport will vary depending on the specimen site, time of year, and the virus suspected. Many viruses enter through the upper respiratory tract, yet the disease caused by the virus may involve multiple or distant organs. In some cases the optimal site for viral culture or detection may be different from the site at which the virus produces its major clinical impact. Infections with enteroviruses are a good example. Enteroviruses can cause a variety of infections such as aseptic meningitis, myocarditis, exanthems, and conjunctivitis, but the specimens of choice for diagnosis of these enterovirus infections are throat and nasopharyngeal aspirates. Specimen collection based on the suspicion of a specific virus should also be done with caution because a request for a specific viral agent will probably eliminate testing to detect other viruses that may cause the same disease or syndrome. Unlike many other groups of bacterial or fungal pathogens, the time of year is important to keep in mind when making a diagnosis of certain viral diseases. Influenza viruses, which circulate in the winter months, and arboviruses and enteroviruses, which circulate in the summer months, are unlikely to cause infections at other times of the year. Table 14–14 provides a guide for selection of specimens for diagnosis of the more common viral syndromes or specific viral agents. It is important to remember that specimens should not be sent to the virology laboratory with the generalized request for "viral studies." Discussion of the patient's history, signs, and symptoms with the infectious disease physician or the clinical microbiologist should help the caregiver decide on the most likely viral pathogens to suspect, which specimens to collect, and the appropriate laboratory test to order. This information should be included on the requisition accompanying the specimens to the laboratory.

Timing is important when collecting specimens for the detection of viruses; specimens should be collected as early as possible after the onset of symptoms. Enteroviruses are present in the respiratory tract shortly before and after the onset of symptoms, but within a few days the virus can be detected only in stool specimens. Once viral shedding stops, serologic analysis may be the only way of diagnosing the viral pathogen. Acute and convalescent serum specimens collected 2 to 4 weeks apart are recommended. Swab and tissue specimens for viral culture should be placed in a viral transport medium that is buffered and contains protein (serum, albumin, or gelatin) and antibiotics. Because of the presence of antibiotics in viral transport media, separate specimens from the same site are needed if bacterial or fungal cultures are also being requested. Liquid specimens such as CSF, bronchoalveolar lavage fluid, or urine need not be sent in viral transport media. Isolation of virus from sputum, nasopharyngeal washes, or throat swabs can support the clinical diagnosis of a viral respiratory infection.[134] Isolation from bronchoscopic specimens or lung tissue is stronger evidence. Blood for viral diagnostic tests should be sent in a tube containing an anticoagulant. Heparin, ethylenediaminetetraacetic acid, and citrate are all acceptable for the detection of cytomegalovirus (CMV) by culture or antigenemia testing, but citrate should be used if other viruses are to be cultured. Heparin should not be used as an anticoagulant if PCR on blood is to be performed because it is a nonspecific ribonuclease inhibitor.[135] Citrate and ethylenediaminetetraacetic acid are suitable anticoagulants for PCR assays because they are less inhibitory and are easily removed during sample preparation. All specimens for virologic testing should be kept cold after collection and during transport to the laboratory and should be promptly transported to the laboratory. Delays in transport or processing may lead to loss of viral viability or possibly antigen degradation. Specimens should not be frozen unless transport or processing is delayed more than 5 days. Freezing at −70°C is preferable to freezing at −20°C.

Swabs can be used to collect a variety of specimens for viral detection such as from the throat, eye, skin, or rectum. Most fibers, including cotton, Dacron, polyester, and rayon, are acceptable for collection of specimens for viral studies. Calcium alginate has been demonstrated to inactivate HSV and may also act as an inhibitor of PCR and should therefore not be used for viral culture or viral PCR assays.[134, 136] Swabs with metal or plastic shafts are preferable to those with wooden shafts because the latter may cause toxicity in cell cultures.[137]

Laboratory Methods for Diagnosis of Viral Infections

Respiratory Viruses

Although most viral respiratory infections are predominant during the colder months, viruses should be considered in the differential workup of respiratory tract infections throughout the year (see Table 14–14). Cell culture techniques allow detection of a wide range of viral pathogens and can allow detection of dual or mixed viral infections. Diagnostic virology laboratories must use more than one cell line for culture of respiratory viruses because influenza and parainfluenza viruses prefer to replicate in primary cell lines such as RhMK (primary rhesus monkey kidney) cells or heteroploid cell lines

TABLE 14–14 Specimen Collection Guide for Viral Infections

Disease Category and Most Common Viral Agents	Season of Occurrence	Specimen Sources for Viral Detection	Serologic Diagnosis
Upper respiratory tract		Nasopharyngeal swab or wash, nasal wash, throat swab, stool (enterovirus), Stensen's duct (mumps virus)	
Rhinovirus	Y		No
Coronavirus	W, SP		No
Respiratory syncytial virus	W		Yes
Adenovirus	Y		Yes
Influenza virus	W		Yes
Parainfluenza virus	Y		No
Enterovirus	S, F		No
Mumps virus	SP		Yes
Lower respiratory tract		Endotracheal aspirate, bronchial wash, bronchoalveolar lavage fluid, stool (enterovirus)	
Adenovirus	Y		Yes
Influenza virus	W		Yes
Parainfluenza virus	Y		No
Enterovirus	S, F		No
Cytomegalovirus	Y		Yes
Respiratory syncytial virus	W		Yes
Central nervous system			
Meningitis		Throat swab, cerebrospinal fluid, stool (enterovirus), urine (mumps virus), brain biopsy	
Herpes simplex virus type 2	Y		Yes
Mumps virus	SP		Yes
Arboviruses	S, F		Yes
Lymphocytic choriomeningitis virus	Y		Yes
Encephalitis		Throat swab, cerebrospinal fluid, stool (enterovirus), urine (mumps virus), brain biopsy	
Enterovirus	S, F		Yes
Herpes simplex virus type 1	Y		Yes
Cytomegalovirus	Y		Yes
Mumps virus	SP		Yes
Arboviruses	S, F		Yes
Influenza virus	W		Yes
Human polyomavirus (JC virus)	Y		No
Vesicular lesions		Vesicle scraping, vesicle swab, throat swab (varicella-zoster, enterovirus), stool (enterovirus)	
Herpes simplex virus	Y		No
Enterovirus	S, F		No
Varicella-zoster virus	Y (varicella: W, SP)		Yes
Exanthems		Throat swab, urine (measles, rubella), stool (enterovirus), amnionic fluid (parvovirus B19)	
Enterovirus	S, F		No
Parvovirus B19	Y		Yes
Measles virus	Y		Yes
Rubella virus	Y		Yes
Human herpesvirus 6	Y		Yes
Ocular		Conjunctival swab or scraping, throat swab (adenovirus, enterovirus), stool (enterovirus), aqueous or vitreous humor (CMV), blood (CMV)	
Adenovirus	Y		No
Enterovirus	S, F		No
Herpes simplex virus	Y		No
Cytomegalovirus (CMV)	Y		No
Cardiac		Throat swab, stool, pericardial fluid, biopsy	
Enterovirus	S, F		Yes
Gastrointestinal tract		Stool, throat swab (enterovirus)	
Rotavirus	W, SP		No
Adenovirus types 40, 41	Y		No
Norwalk-like viruses	S		No
Enterovirus	S		No
Genital		Vesicle scraping (HSV), endocervical swab, biopsy (HPV)	
Herpes simplex virus (HSV)	Y		No
Human papillomavirus (HPV)	Y		No
Congenital and perinatal disease		Throat swab, urine, skin lesions, cerebrospinal fluid, stool (enterovirus), biopsy, blood	
Cytomegalovirus	Y		Yes
Herpes simplex virus	Y		Yes
Rubella virus	Y		Yes
Varicella-zoster virus	Y		Yes
Enterovirus	S, F		Yes
Post-transplantation syndrome		Biopsy, blood (CMV), urine (CMV, adenovirus, BK virus)	
Adenovirus	Y		Yes
Human polyomavirus (BK virus)	Y		Yes
Cytomegalovirus (CMV)	Y		Yes
Herpes simplex virus	Y		Yes
Human herpesvirus 6	Y		Yes
Epstein-Barr virus	Y		Yes

Abbreviations: F, Fall; S, summer; SP, spring; W, winter; Y, year-round.

such as LLC-Mk2 (rhesus monkey kidney) whereas adenoviruses and respiratory syncytial virus (RSV) prefer to replicate in heteroploid cell lines such as A549 (human lung carcinoma) or Hep-2 (human epidermoid larynx carcinoma). Unfortunately, traditional cell culture techniques often do not provide a diagnosis until the patient is convalescing rather than during the acute stage of illness. Respiratory viruses may take up to 10 days to produce a cytopathic effect in cell culture. Moreover, influenza and parainfluenza viruses may produce little or no visible cytopathic effect and may be detected only after hemadsorption or hemagglutination with guinea pig red blood cells 3 to 7 days after inoculation of the cell culture monolayer. In contrast, some viruses such as RSV produce a distinctive cytopathic effect in continuous cell lines such as HeLa or Hep-2 cells in 1 or 2 days. Most diagnostic virology laboratories also use virus-specific fluorescent antibodies to identify viruses with an uncharacteristic or unrecognizable cytopathic effect in cell culture. Traditional viral cultures are held for 7 to 28 days, depending on the type of viral pathogen being cultured.

Shell vial spin amplification cultures give a more rapid turnaround time than traditional viral cultures do for detection of the more common respiratory viruses. This system uses 1-dram vials that contain cell culture monolayers on 12-mm round coverslips that are immersed in tissue culture media. Specimens are added to the monolayer, centrifuged at low speed, and incubated. Rather than an examination for cytopathic effect, fluorescein-labeled monoclonal antibodies are used to detect viral antigens of replicating viruses. Shell vial cultures are incubated for up to 5 days, but most respiratory viruses can be detected in as little as 24 hours because visual cytopathic effect is not necessary for detection.[138] The shell vial assay for respiratory viruses currently allows detection of influenza A and B, parainfluenza 1, 2, and 3, adenovirus, and RSV. Urine can also be cultured for adenovirus in bone marrow transplant recipients with hemorrhagic cystitis. A pool of monoclonal antibodies to these viruses is first used to detect the presence of a respiratory virus; individual monoclonal antibodies are then used to identify the specific virus.

Rapid identification of RSV can be beneficial because it (1) permits timely cohorting of patients to prevent nosocomial spread of disease and (2) allows prompt initiation of ribavirin therapy if needed. Similarly, rapid identification of influenza A allows early administration of amantadine or rimantadine. In winter months when the incidence of respiratory infections is high and a corresponding increase in hospital admissions for viral respiratory infections is observed, traditional viral cultures and even shell vial spin amplification cultures are not rapid enough for expedient cohorting of patients. Detection of viral antigen provides for more rapid identification of RSV and influenza A; viral antigen tests include DFA assay and EIA. Some laboratories screen specimens directly by DFA performed with a pool of monoclonal antibodies against the common viral respiratory pathogens. Results from these nonculture assays are often available within hours after receipt in the laboratory and may be particularly useful during the peak months of transmission. Because a variety of rapid methods are available for the detection of adenovirus, influenza, parainfluenza, and RSV and because current PCR technology cannot be done on an urgent basis, PCR is not generally recommended for the diagnosis of viral respiratory tract infections.[139] A note of caution when using rapid assays, however, is that most rapid assays target a single viral pathogen and, if used alone, the assay can make a specific diagnosis but will not allow the detection of other viruses. Dual or mixed viral infections have been reported to occur in 5 to 35% of patients.[140] The diagnostic virology laboratory should use rapid methods in conjunction with culture or other assays to allow the detection of a wider range of viruses in each specimen and to detect mixed viral infections.

Childhood Viral Infections

Many of the classic infections of childhood, especially the rash syndromes, are caused by viruses (Table 14–15). Laboratory diagnosis is usually not required for suspected cases of measles, mumps, or rubella unless complications of severe or atypical disease are present. Although virus culture is useful during the acute illness, serologic analysis can provide the diagnosis in retrospect and can also provide information on whether immunity is present. Serologic tests for childhood viral infections are most often performed with commercially available ELISA or immunofluorescence assays. Latex agglutination tests are available for detecting antibodies to VZV and rubella virus. Reference laboratories may offer complement fixation tests for measles, mumps, and VZV. Although VZV can be detected within cells collected from the base of newly formed vesicular lesions, such detection is done more frequently to diagnose zoster than chickenpox. The virus can be cultured by traditional cell culture or shell vial cultures, or VZV-infected cells can be observed directly in specimens by using either the Tzanck test or specific fluorescent antibodies. VZV-specific fluorescent antibody stains are more sensitive than culture and more sensitive and specific than Tzanck smears.[11]

TABLE 14–15 Childhood Rash Syndromes

Disease Name(s)	Disease Number	Etiologic Agent(s)
Rubeola, measles	First disease	Measles virus
Scarlet fever	Second disease	*Streptococcus pyogenes*
Rubella German measles	Third disease	Rubella virus
Duke's disease Filatov-Duke disease Pseudoscarlatina	Fourth disease	Coxsackieviruses Echoviruses
Erythema infectiosum "Slapped cheek disease"	Fifth disease	Parvovirus B19
Roseola Exanthem subitum Roseola infantum	Sixth disease	Human herpesvirus 6, 7
Chickenpox Varicella	None	Varicella-zoster virus
Hand-foot-and-mouth syndrome	None	Coxsackieviruses Echoviruses
Papular-purpuric gloves-and-socks syndrome	None	Parvovirus B19

In addition to the childhood rash syndromes, erythema infectiosum, and papular-purpuric gloves-and-socks syndrome, parvovirus B19 can be a cause of polyarthropathy syndrome, hemolytic disease (primarily in patients with hemolytic anemia or immunocompromise), chronic bone marrow failure, and fetal hydrops.[141] Diagnosis of these manifestations of parvovirus B19 infection in immunocompetent patients can be made by using serologic assays for IgM. Nucleic acid hybridization assays performed on serum have been found to be most helpful for the diagnosis of chronic parvovirus B19 infection.[142] PCR detection on serum or other body fluids is performed by large reference laboratories and is useful for monitoring the response to treatment with immunoglobulin, as well as for the diagnosis of congenital infection.

Enteroviruses are a common cause of mild febrile illness with minimal respiratory or gastrointestinal symptoms and may be accompanied by exanthems, enanthems, myopericarditis, or aseptic meningitis (see Chapter 160). Most infections occur during the summer and early fall in temperate climates, but they are occasionally seen during the rest of the year. Enteroviruses are shed in the stool and oropharynx, often for prolonged periods, so isolation from these sites provides only circumstantial diagnostic evidence. Because of the large number of serotypes,[72] serologic analysis is impractical for the diagnosis of polioviruses, echoviruses, group A coxsackieviruses, and echoviruses. A group-specific serologic test is available for group B coxsackieviruses. Laboratory diagnosis is usually made by the isolation of virus in cell culture. Echoviruses and group B coxsackieviruses usually grow well in primary human or monkey kidney cells and variably in a variety of cell culture strains and continuous cell lines.[143] Group A coxsackieviruses generally grow poorly in cell culture and require inoculation in suckling mouse brain for isolation. Recently, PCR of CSF has been used for the rapid diagnosis of enterovirus-caused aseptic meningitis. Specificity and sensitivity have ranged from 66 to greater than 90%.[144–146]

Gastrointestinal Tract Infections

In addition to the viruses listed in Table 14–14, caliciviruses, astroviruses, and coronaviruses have been associated with diarrhea. Viral agents of diarrhea are not detectable by cell culture. Historically, viral gastrointestinal pathogens have been detected by electron microscopy during investigations of large outbreaks. Rotavirus infections account for approximately 50% of pediatric hospital admissions for diarrhea and dehydration in the cooler months of the year in the United States.[147] Each year, rotavirus epidemics follow a regional sequence from east to west. Outbreaks occur in November and December in the southwestern states and spread to the New England states in April and May.[148] Rapid detection of rotavirus aids not only in the diagnosis of gastroenteritis but also in the identification of infected individuals who may serve as sources of outbreaks in settings such as daycare centers and hospital wards. Commercial kits for the rapid detection of rotavirus antigen in stool specimens are now available and include ELISA, membrane EIA, and latex agglutination formats. Sensitivities range from 90 to 100% for ELISA and 70 to 90% for latex tests.[147] Adenovirus serotypes 40 and 41 are second to rotaviruses as the most common cause of pediatric gastroenteritis. A sensitive commercial EIA is available for the detection of adenovirus serotypes 40 and 41. The application of PCR technology to the detection of gastrointestinal viruses has not yet made its way into diagnostic virology laboratories.

Arboviruses

Arboviruses (*ar*thropod-*bo*rne *viruses*) are not only seasonal but are also regional in distribution as determined by the residence of the specific hematophagous arthropods that transmit the viruses to humans (Table 14–16). More than 500 arboviruses are recognized, and although approximately 150 can cause disease in humans, fewer than 50 are important human or veterinary pathogens worldwide.[149] Arbovirus infections are emerging or resurging throughout the world as a result of changes in public health policy, deemphasis on prevention programs, demographic and societal changes, and genetic changes in pathogens.[150] Diagnosis of infection with an arbovirus can be difficult and delayed because symptoms may range from mild fever to encephalitis. The patient's travel history and exposure are important for laboratory diagnosis of arbovirus infection (see Table 14–16). The availability of direct detection by electron microscopy or immunohistochemical staining is limited by the relatively few experienced laboratory personnel in this specialty and by the scarcity of reagents available for diagnostic testing. The CDC has a battery of monoclonal antibodies for arbovirus antigen detection in peripheral blood mononuclear cells or tissue sections; included in this panel are the viruses listed in Table 14–16, as well as Japanese encephalitis virus, yellow fever virus, Highlands J virus, and Murray Valley encephalitis, among others.[149] Serologic procedures are the primary methods used for laboratory diagnosis of arbovirus infection. Large reference laboratories and state public health laboratories offer immunofluorescence or ELISA testing on serum or CSF for both IgG and IgM antibodies. Detection of IgM antibodies may allow the diagnosis of an arbovirus infection with a single specimen; however, paired acute and convalescent sera collected 2 to 4 weeks apart are recommended. A simple immunoblot assay for IgM and IgG antibody to dengue is useful but is not yet approved for marketing in the United States.

Herpesviruses

The herpesviruses are a diverse group of DNA viruses. CMV, HSV types 1 and 2, and VZV can be easily cultured from most sites by conventional cell culture or in the shell vial assay. In contrast, human herpesvirus 6 (HHV-6), HHV-7, HHV-8, and Epstein-Barr virus (EBV) cannot be cultivated in routine diagnostic virology laboratories. Currently, PCR is the method of choice for the detection of herpesviruses in CSF.[151, 152] In the past, definitive diagnosis of central nervous system infection caused by herpesviruses relied on obtaining a brain biopsy. Because detection in CSF by PCR has been demonstrated to be as sensitive as stain of brain biopsy specimens, CSF PCR is now the recommended test to establish this diagnosis.[151] Traditional laboratory methods for the detection of HSV, CMV, and VZV in CSF, such as cell culture, antigen detection, and CSF or serum antibody detection, are known to be insensitive and are no longer recommended.

In many hospital laboratories, HSV detection may be the only diagnostic virology service offered. Cell culture or the shell vial assay allows detection of HSV in as little as 1 or 2 days. Even more rapid is a detection system that uses a genetically engineered baby hamster kidney cell line in conjunction with an enzyme-linked virus inducible system for the detection of HSV in 16 to 24 hours. The cells in this system contain a plasmid that encodes the *E. coli lacZ* gene (for the enzyme β-galactosidase), which has been engineered to be driven by the promoter of the HSV-1 ribonucleotide reductase gene.[153] The enzyme is synthesized only when cells are infected with HSV types 1 or 2. To detect infected cells an enzyme substrate is added, the enzyme catalyzes the substrate, and a blue color is produced that can be detected by light microscopy. This rapid assay is reported to be as sensitive as traditional cell culture held for 5 to 7 days.[153] Diagnostic laboratories may also detect HSV antigen directly in clinical material with one of several commercially available ELISA, immunofluorescence, or immunoperoxidase kits, the sensitivities of which range from 73 to 94% in comparison to traditional cell culture.[147] The traditional Tzanck smear (scrapings from lesions stained with Giemsa or Wright stain) is still a useful presumptive

TABLE 14–16 Most Common Arboviruses in North America

Virus	Occurrence	Distribution	Vector	Clinical Disease
Eastern equine encephalitis	Sporadic	Atlantic and Gulf Coast, upper New York, Michigan	Mosquito (*Culiseta melanura*)	Encephalitis
Western equine encephalitis	Epidemic	Western United States and Canada	Mosquito (*Culex* spp.)	Encephalitis
St. Louis encephalitis	Epidemic	North America	Mosquito (*Culex* spp.)	Encephalitis
Venezuelan encephalitis	Sporadic	Florida	Mosquito (*Culex* and *Aedes* spp.)	Encephalitis
La Crosse encephalitis	Epidemic	North central and northeast United States	Mosquito (*Aedes triseriatus*)	Encephalitis
Dengue types 1–4	Epidemic	Carribbean	Mosquito (*Aedes* spp.)	Febrile illness and rash, hemorrhagic fever
Colorado tick fever	Frequent	Rocky Mountain States	Tick (*Dermacentor andersoni*)	Febrile illness and rash, encephalitis, hemorrhagic fever

method for rapid diagnosis of HSV skin or mucous membrane lesions, although it does not differentiate between HSV and VZV.

Detection of antibodies to CMV in serum from blood or organ donors and recipients is performed with ELISA or latex agglutination tests. The detection of IgM antibodies to CMV can be used to diagnose acute infection in neonates and pregnant women.[152] CMV antigen detection in tissue sections by immunofluorescence or immunoperoxidase is a valuable complement to and a more sensitive test than histopathologic diagnosis with hematoxylin and eosin staining.[152] Because CMV remains latent after an acute primary infection and can cause recurrent disease in immunosuppressed patients, new methods are being developed to diagnose CMV disease and to monitor anti-CMV therapy in transplant recipients or AIDS patients.[154] Culture methods alone are not useful for the diagnosis of active CMV disease because shedding of CMV in urine or respiratory tract secretions may occur in immunosuppressed patients without development of CMV disease. However, isolation of CMV from the urine or saliva of neonates is still useful for the identification of congenital CMV infection.[154] For transplant patients, detection of CMV in blood by cell culture or by shell vial culture does not provide early enough detection of CMV to allow successful intervention with ganciclovir or other antiviral agents effective against CMV. For this reason, detection of either CMV antigen or CMV DNA in blood is being performed because these assays can detect CMV when the viral load is low, which may be weeks before cultures become positive.[154] For the CMV antigenemia assay, monoclonal antibodies to the pp65 lower matrix protein antigen are used to detect the antigen in CMV-infected leukocytes.

A fluorescent or immunoperoxidase label allows infected cells to be detected and counted (Fig. 14–7). Thus, the CMV antigenemia assay provides quantitative results that can be used either to determine the initiation of antiviral therapy or to monitor viral load during a course of treatment. Unfortunately, the antigenemia assay is not standardized, and different laboratories may examine different numbers of leukocytes and may report either the total number of positive leukocytes or the number of positive leukocytes per differing numbers of total leukocytes examined.[155] The physician must understand how the laboratory performs and reports the assay if interlaboratory comparisons are to be made. Quantitative or semiquantitative PCR assays are thought to be more useful than qualitative PCR assays for the detection of viremia and the diagnosis of disseminated CMV disease.[152] Semiquantitative PCR entails the use of serial dilutions of patient samples followed by PCR, whereas quantitative methods relate the PCR product to an internal control or to an external standard curve.[152] Commercial kits that rely on amplification of the signal rather than CMV DNA itself, such as the branched DNA assay from Chiron Corporation (Emeryville, Calif), are also useful to diagnose CMV disease in immunocompromised hosts. Qualitative PCR assays are adequate for the detection of CMV DNA in aqueous or vitreous humor for the diagnosis of retinitis, in biopsy specimens for demonstrating organ localization, and in other instances in which quantitation is not needed.[154]

Serologic methods are used for the diagnosis of primary EBV infection and for screening and monitoring of nasopharyngeal carcinoma, whereas molecular methods are used to diagnose EBV-associated lymphoma of the brain and EBV involvement in other organ lesions.[156] The most common test for the diagnosis of primary EBV infection, most frequently infectious mononucleosis, is a heterophil antibody test. Heterophil antibodies are IgM antibodies reactive to antigens on heterologous erythrocytes. The antibodies are detected in a variety of assay formats, including detection of lysis of bovine erythrocytes in the presence of complement, agglutination reactions using horse or sheep erythrocytes or antigen-coated latex agglutination particles, and ELISA formats using purified heterophil antigens.[156] A negative heterophil antibody test in the presence of a clinical mononucleosis syndrome should prompt the physician to consider tests for EBV-specific antibodies, CMV, or toxoplasmosis.[157] Specific antibodies used to diagnose EBV infection commonly include IgG and IgM to the viral capsid antigen, antibody to early antigen, and antibody to Epstein-Barr nuclear antigen. Assays to detect EBV-specific antibodies include indirect immunofluorescence, anticomplement immunofluorescence, and ELISA formats. Information concerning the interpretation of serologic tests for EBV can be found in Chapter 128. Reference laboratories offer EBV DNA detection in blood or CSF by PCR and EBV mRNA detection in tissue by in situ hybridization.

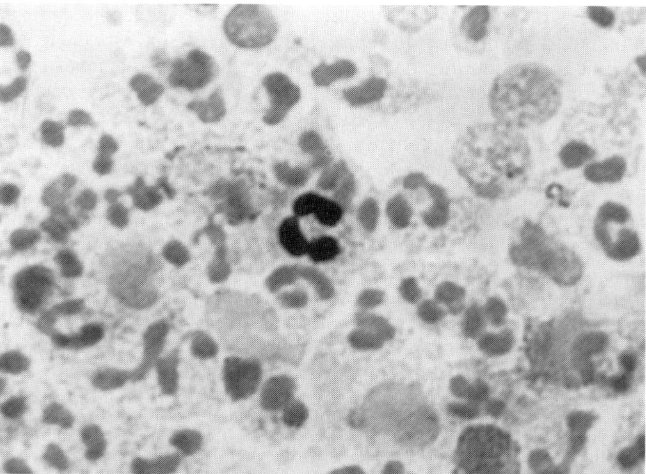

FIGURE 14–7. Positive cytomegalovirus (CMV) antigenemia assay. After staining with mouse monoclonal antibodies to CMV pp65 lower matrix protein and horseradish peroxidase labeled antimouse antibody, a polymorphonuclear leukocyte with CMV antigen localized in the nucleus is clearly seen.

Over the past 10 years three new herpesviruses have been described. HHV-6, which is a cause of exanthem subitum (roseola infantum or sixth disease), has also been associated with an infectious mononucleosis–like syndrome in adults, interstitial pneumonitis, encephalitis, and bone marrow suppression.[158] HHV-6 is postulated to be an opportunistic pathogen in both bone marrow and solid organ transplant recipients.[159] Prompt recognition of HHV-6 disease in transplantation patients may prove to be important because this virus is susceptible to ganciclovir and foscarnet. The virus can be isolated in cell culture, but detection may take 5 to 21 days. A rapid shell vial assay may soon be available that will allow detection within 72 hours.[159] Reference laboratories offer serologic testing for HHV-6 IgG and IgM by both ELISA and immunofluorescence methods. Detection of DNA by PCR is also available and should be performed on serum or plasma rather than leukocytes. Diagnostic methods that cannot distinguish between latent and active infection, such as serum IgG detection or PCR on leukocytes, may be inappropriate or even misleading for the diagnosis of HHV-6 disease.[160] Quantitative PCR, if available, may be more diagnostically useful than qualitative PCR, especially to monitor response to antiviral therapy. HHV-6 has two major variants; the B variant is more frequent, except in patients with AIDS, who are more likely to have variant A.[158] Currently available laboratory tests do not distinguish between variant A or B. HHV-7 may be associated with some cases of exanthem subitum, and HHV-8 has been associated with Kaposi's sarcoma and lymphoma.[158] Serologic assays for HHV-7 are now available from some reference laboratories, but serologic testing for HHV-8 and PCR tests for both viruses are currently restricted to research laboratories.

Hepatitis Viruses

The hepatitis viruses are a group of unrelated DNA and RNA viruses that cause liver disease as their major clinical manifestation.

Laboratory diagnosis of these infections is usually made by serologic testing for a number of different antigenic markers associated with the viruses. Laboratories have tried to make hepatitis diagnosis easier by offering panel or profile testing, depending on patient characteristics: exposure but asymptomatic, symptomatic with acute disease (<6 months), or symptomatic with chronic disease (>6 months) (Table 14–17). The most commonly used methods for serologic diagnosis are ELISA and immunofluorescence assays. The first generation of ELISA tests for hepatitis C lacked sensitivity and specificity, but the second- and third-generation tests have shown greatly improved performance.[161] Similar to HIV testing, immunoblots performed with recombinant antigens (recombinant immunoblot assays) are used to confirm positive sera detected by ELISA. Unfortunately, approximately 10% of recombinant immunoblot assay results are indeterminant and half of the patients with indeterminate results will have detectable viral RNA in their sera.[12] Molecular methods for the detection of hepatitis virus nucleic acids include DNA PCR and the branched DNA assay for hepatitis B virus and reverse transcriptase–PCR for hepatitis C, D, and G viruses. Hepatitis C genotyping by reverse transcriptase–PCR and restriction fragment length polymorphism analysis is also available from large reference laboratories. Details concerning the interpretation of results for hepatitis tests can be found in the chapters discussing acute and chronic hepatitis and the individual chapters for each virus.

Miscellaneous Viruses

The human polyomaviruses BK virus and JC virus infect a high proportion of the general population and remain latent in the kidneys after primary infection.[162] Reactivation can occur when T-cell functions are deficient, for example, in recipients of bone marrow or organ transplants or patients with HIV infection. BK viruria has been implicated as a cause of hemorrhagic cystitis in bone marrow transplant patients, whereas JC virus causes progressive multifocal leukoencephalopathy, which is seen primarily in AIDS patients. Rapid detection of active BK virus may help in the medical management of these patients. Although BK virus can be detected by cytologic examination of exfoliated urinary epithelial cells this method cannot differentiate BK and JC viruses, cytopathic effects caused by other viruses, or changes caused by malignancy.[162] Specific identification of BK virus in urine can be achieved by immunologic staining of exfoliated urinary cells, by ELISA, or by PCR. Serologic testing by hemagglutination inhibition or ELISA for the detection of IgM in serum or CSF may be useful to diagnose active polyomavirus infections. Examination of CSF for JC virus DNA by PCR is the method of choice for the diagnosis of progressive multifocal leukoencephalopathy.[163] A negative PCR result does not rule out the diagnosis of virus progressive multifocal leukoencephalopathy, and for these patients a brain biopsy should be obtained for histopathologic or molecular diagnostic testing.[163]

Although many human papillomavirus (HPV)-induced lesions are benign, certain HPV types have been strongly associated with cervical neoplasia. The assay offered by most laboratories is in situ hybridization performed on paraffin-embedded tissue, with results reported as positive or negative for groups of HPV types: 6/11, 16/18, or 31/33/51. PCR may soon be the method of choice because it has greater sensitivity in that it is capable of detecting as few as 10 to 100 viral genome copies and it is faster and easier to perform than other methods.[164] Over 90% of cervical cancers detected by histologic examination of cervical biopsies are positive for HPV DNA by PCR. HPV can be typed by PCR assays that incorporate specific DNA probes or by sequencing of the PCR product and comparing the sequence with published HPV sequences.

TABLE 14–17 Examples of Test Panels of Serologic Markers Offered by Reference Laboratories for Diagnosis of Asymptomatic and Symptomatic Hepatitis Virus Infections

Hepatitis Exposure Panel (Asymptomatic)	Acute Hepatitis Panel (Symptomatic)	Chronic Hepatitis Panel (Symptomatic)
Anti-HAV (IgG + IgM)	Anti-HAV (IgM)	HBsAg
Anti-HAV (IgM)*	HBsAg	Anti-HBc (IgG + IgM)
HBsAG	Anti-HBc (IgG + IgM)	Anti-HBc (IgM)*
Anti-HBc (IgG + IgM)	Anti-HBc (IgM)*	Anti-HBs
Anti-HBs	Anti-HCV	Anti-HCV
Anti-HCV		

*Assay for IgM is performed if the IgG + IgM assay is positive.
Abbreviations: HAV, Hepatitis A virus; HBc, hepatitis B core antigen; HBsAg, hepatitis B surface antigen; HCV, hepatitis C virus.

Hantavirus infections are zoonoses transmitted to humans through contact with aerosolized rodent excreta containing the virus or through infected rodent bites.[165] Hantaviruses are found worldwide, but hantavirus infections in the United States were not considered a major public health concern until an outbreak of severe pulmonary disease was reported by the New Mexico Department of Public Health in the Four Corners area of New Mexico, Arizona, Colorado, and Utah in 1993. The virus has been cultured by the CDC and the U.S. Army Medical Research Institute of Infectious Disease and is the Sin Nombre virus of the genus Hantavirus in the family Bunyaviridae. Hantaviruses cause two clinical syndromes: hemorrhagic fever with renal syndrome and hantavirus pulmonary syndrome. Detection of IgG and IgM antibodies by ELISA is available at many state health laboratories or by referral by a state laboratory to the CDC; a Western blot assay is available at the University of New Mexico and the University of Alabama at Birmingham.[166] A Hantavirus recombinant immunoblot assay has been jointly developed by the University of New Mexico and the Chiron Corporation. The assay uses membrane-immobilized antigens in a dipstick-like format and requires minimal equipment and 5 hours to perform. The assay has performed well in preliminary studies and will enable field testing by state laboratories for better surveillance and detection of future outbreaks.[166]

Antiviral Susceptibility Testing

Antiviral drugs are now available for the management of infections caused by HIV-1, HSV types 1 and 2, CMV, VZV, influenza A virus, RSV, hepatitis B virus, and hepatitis C virus. The emergence of resistant viruses is inevitable as antiviral agents are used more frequently and widely.[167] Antiviral resistance is defined as a decrease in the susceptibility to an antiviral agent established by in vitro testing and confirmed by genetic analysis of the viral genome and biochemical analysis of the altered enzymes.[168] Clinical failures may not always be due to the presence of a drug-resistant virus. Factors to consider in a patient with a poor clinical response to an antiviral agent include the patient's immunologic status and the pharmacokinetics of the drug in the individual patient (e.g., dose or route of administration).[168] The development of resistance is favored by long-term suppressive therapy, recurrent intermittent therapy, and the use of suboptimal doses of an antiviral agent.[167] Antiviral susceptibility testing is warranted for the following clinical situations: failure of HSV or VZV lesions to resolve or the appearance of new lesions during treatment with acyclovir, progression of CMV disease during ganciclovir therapy, continued shedding or transmission of influenza A virus during treatment or prophylaxis with amantadine or rimantadine, and increased HIV-1 RNA plasma levels or decreased CD4 cell counts in HIV-infected patients during antiretroviral therapy.[167]

Laboratory assays for antiviral susceptibility testing include phenotypic and genotypic assays. Phenotypic assays require growth of the virus in vitro, so viruses for which in vitro culture systems are not available, such as hepatitis B virus, cannot be tested with these assays. Results from phenotypic assays may not be available in a time frame that is clinically relevant because they all require initial propagation of the virus to attain a standard inoculum concentration, followed by growth of the virus in the assay to obtain results. After up to a week of propagation to prepare inoculum, once the assay has been set up, results for HSV may be obtained in 48 hours. For CMV, results may take 8 to 14 days after several weeks of propagation. Results of phenotypic assays are reported as the drug concentration that causes a 50% inhibition in growth of the virus.[167] Phenotypic assays are not standardized, so comparison of results from different laboratories is difficult. The "same" assay may have been performed under different conditions in different laboratories, and interpretive criteria to define whether a virus is sensitive or resistant may vary from laboratory to laboratory.[167] The NCCLS is currently drafting guidelines in an effort to standardize some aspects of virus susceptibility testing beginning with HSV.[169] The most commonly used phenotypic antiviral susceptibility assay is the plaque reduction assay, which measures the ability of varying concentrations of an antiviral agent to inhibit the viral cytopathic effect as the end point. Other end points for phenotypic viral assays that have been developed in an effort to make phenotypic testing more rapid and sensitive include dye uptake by viable (noninfected) cells, DNA hybridization, ELISA, and plaque autoradiography.

Genotypic assays have been developed for rapid detection of mutations that confer antiviral drug resistance.[167] Results from these assays simply report the presence or absence of a mutation known to confer resistance to a specific antiviral agent. Most genotypic assays use PCR to amplify specific viral genes, followed by direct sequencing of the amplified products to detect changes in the sequence known to be associated with resistance to antiviral agents. Genotypic assays are not currently practical for detecting drug resistance in HSV and VZV because of considerable heterogeneity in the thymidine kinase mutations that confer resistance to acyclovir, famciclovir, penciclovir, and valaciclovir.[169] Genotypic assays are useful for detecting resistance in CMV and HIV-1. The major drawback of genotypic assays is that they can detect only resistance caused by known mutations. If resistance to an antiviral agent can be caused by different gene mutations, multiple assays might be needed for optimal detection. Strains with new or different resistance genes would also go undetected, so phenotypic assays will still be required to identify new mutations responsible for antiviral resistance.[169]

REFERENCES

1. Health Care Financing Administration. Medicare, Medicaid and CLIA programs. Regulations implementing the Clinical Laboratory Improvement Amendments of 1988 (CLIA). Fed Register. 1992;57:7002–7186.
2. Elder BL, Hansen SA, Kellogg JA, et al. Verification and Validation of Procedures in the Clinical Microbiology Laboratory. Cumitech 31. Washington, DC: American Society for Microbiology; 1997.
3. Wilson ML. Clinically relevant, cost-effective clinical microbiology. Strategies to decrease unnecessary testing. Am J Clin Pathol. 1997;107:154–167.
4. Pfaller MA, Herwaldt LA. The clinical microbiology laboratory and infection control: Emerging pathogens, antimicrobial resistance, and new technology. Clin Infect Dis. 1997;25:858–870.
5. Mickelsen PA. The use of molecular strain typing has become a standard of practice. Clin Microbiol Newsl. 1997;19:137–142.
6. Busse HJ, Denner EBM, Lubitz W. Classification and identification of bacteria: Current approaches to an old problem. Overview of methods used in bacterial systematics. J Biotechnol. 1996;47:3–38.
7. Miller JM. A Guide to Specimen Management in Clinical Microbiology. Washington, DC: American Society for Microbiology; 1996.
8. Murray PR. ASM Pocket Guide to Clinical Microbiology. Washington, DC: American Society for Microbiology; 1996.
9. Isenberg HD, ed. Essential Procedures for Clinical Microbiology. Washington, DC: American Society for Microbiology; 1998.
10. Murray PR, Baron EJ, Pfaller MA, et al, eds. Manual of Clinical Microbiology, 6th ed. Washington, DC: American Society for Microbiology; 1995.
11. Forbes BA, Sahm DF, Weissfeld AS. Bailey & Scott's Diagnostic Microbiology. St Louis: Mosby; 1998.
12. Koneman EW, Allen SD, Janda WM, et al. Color Atlas and Textbook of Diagnostic Microbiology, 5th ed. Philadelphia: JB Lippincott; 1997.
13. Müller FMC, Hoppe JE, von König CHW. Laboratory diagnosis of pertussis: State of the art in 1997. J Clin Microbiol. 1997;35:2435–2443.
14. Bartlett JG. Invasive diagnostic techniques in pulmonary infections. In: Pennington JE, ed. Respiratory Infections: Diagnosis and Management. New York: Raven; 1989:69–86.
15. Reimer LG, Carroll KC. Role of the microbiology laboratory in the diagnosis of lower respiratory tract infections. Clin Infect Dis. 1998;26:742–748.
16. Gill VJ. Laboratory evaluation of specimens. Ann Intern Med. 1996;124:586–588.
17. Cantral DE, Tape TG, Reed EC, et al. Quantitative culture of bronchoalveolar lavage fluid for the diagnosis of bacterial pneumonia. Am J Med. 1993;95:601–607.
18. Kovacs JA, Ng V, Masur H, et al. Diagnosis of *Pneumocystis carinii* pneumonia: Improved detection in sputum using monoclonal antibodies. N Engl J Med. 1988;318:589–593.
19. Kovacs JA, Gill VJ, Swan JC, et al. Prospective evaluation of a monoclonal antibody in diagnosis of *Pneumocystis carinii* pneumonia. Lancet. 1986;2:1–4.
20. Quinn TC. Diagnosis of atypical pneumonias: *Legionella, Chlamydia,* and *Mycoplasma* infections. Ann Intern Med. 1996;124:591–594.
21. Ieven M, Goossens H. Relevance of nucleic acid amplification techniques for diagnosis of respiratory tract infections in the clinical laboratory. Clin Microbiol Rev. 1997;10:242–256.
22. Reimer LG, Wilson ML, Weinstein MP. Update on detection of bacteremia and fungemia. Clin Microbiol Rev. 1997;10:444–465.
23. Dunne WM, Nolte FS, Wilson ML. Cumitech 1B. In: Hindler JA, ed. Blood Cultures III. Washington, DC: American Society for Microbiology; 1997.
24. Maki DG, Weise CE, Sarafin HW. A semiquantitative culture method for identifying intravenous-catheter related infection. N Engl J Med. 1977;296:1305–1309.
25. Morris AJ, Wilson ML, Mirrett S, Reller LB. Rationale for selective use of anaerobic blood cultures. J Clin Microbiol. 1993;31:2110–2113.
26. Goldstein EJC. Anaerobic bacteremia. Clin Infect Dis. 1996;23:1292–1301.
27. Collignon PJ, Soni N, Pearson IY, et al. Is semiquantitative culture of central vein catheter tips useful in the diagnosis of catheter-associated bacteremia? J Clin Microbiol. 1986;24:532–535.
28. Siegman-Igra Y, Anglim AM, Shapiro DE, et al. Diagnosis of vascular catheter–related bloodstream infection: A meta-analysis. J Clin Microbiol. 1997;35:928–936.
29. Shanholzer CJ, Schaper PJ, Peterson LR. Concentrated Gram stains prepared with a cytospin centrifuge. J Clin Microbiol. 1982;16:1052–1054.
30. Askari S, Cartwright CP. The changing epidemiology of bacterial meningitis: Implications for the clinical laboratory. Clin Microbiol Newsl. 1998;20:33–36.
31. Woods GS, Washington JA II. Comparison of methods for processing dialysate in suspected continuous ambulatory peritoneal–associated peritonitis. Diagn Microbiol Infect Dis. 1987;7:155–157.
32. Pezzlo M. Detection of urinary tract infections by rapid methods. Clin Microbiol Rev. 1988;1:268–280.
33. Dunn BE, Cohen H, Blaser MJ. *Helicobacter pylori.* Clin Microbiol Rev. 1997;10:720–741.
34. Hines J, Nachamkin I. Effective use of the clinical microbiology laboratory for diagnosing diarrheal diseases. Clin Infect Dis. 1996;23(Suppl 1):S97–S101.
35. Aldeen WE, Carroll K, Robison A, et al. Comparison of nine commercially available enzyme-linked immunosorbent assays for detection of *Giardia lamblia* in fecal specimens. J Clin Microbiol. 1998;36:1338–1340.
36. Morris AJ, Wilson ML, Reller LB. Application of rejection criteria for ovum and parasite examinations. J Clin Microbiol. 1992;30:3213–3216.
37. Amsel R, Totten PA, Spiegel CA, et al. Nonspecific vaginitis: Diagnostic criteria and microbial epidemiologic association. Am J Med. 1983;74:14–22.
38. Hale YM, Melton ME, Lewis JS, et al. Evaluation of the PACE 2 *Neisseria gonorrhoeae* assay by three public health laboratories. J Clin Microbiol. 1993;31:458–459.
39. Caliendo AM. Diagnosis of *Chlamydia trachomatis* infection using amplification methods: Can we afford it? Clin Microbiol Newsl. 1998;20:75–78.
40. Baselski VS. The role of molecular diagnostics in the clinical microbiology laboratory. Clin Lab Med. 1996;16:49–60.
41. Longo MC, Bernionger MS, Hartley JL. Use of uracil DNA glycosylase to control carryover contamination in polymerase chain reactions. Gene. 1990;93:125–128.
42. Ballagi-Pordány A, Belák S. The use of mimics as internal standards to avoid false negatives in diagnostic PCR. Mol Cell Probes. 1996;10:159–164.
43. Siebert PD, Larrick JW. PCR mimics: Competitive DNA fragments for use as internal standards in quantitative PCR. Biotechniques. 1993;14:244–249.
44. Cartwright CP, Stock F, Fahle GA, Gill VJ. Comparison of pigment production and motility tests with PCR for reliable identification of intrinsically vancomycin-resistant enterococci. J Clin Microbiol. 1995;33:1931–1933.
45. Doern GV, Ferraro MJ, Brueggemann AB, Ruoff KL. Emergence of high rates of antimicrobial resistance among viridans group streptococci in the United States. Antimicrob Agents Chemother. 1996;40:891–894.
46. Berkowitz FE. The gram-positive bacilli: A review of the microbiology, clinical aspects, and antimicrobial susceptibilities of a heterogeneous group of bacteria. Pediatr Infect Dis J. 1994;13:1126–1138.
47. Franz DR, Jahrling PB, Friedlander AM, et al. Clinical recognition and management of patients exposed to biological warfare agents. JAMA. 1997;278:399–411.
48. Funke G, von Graevenitz A, Clarridge JE, Bernard KA. Clinical microbiology of coryneform bacteria. Clin Microbiol Rev. 1997;10:125–159.
49. Janda WM. *Corynebacterium* species and the coryneform bacteria. Part I: New and emerging species in the genus *Corynebacterium.* Clin Microbiol Newsl. 1998;20:41–52.
50. Janda WM. *Corynebacterium* species and the coryneform bacteria. Part II: Current status of the CDC coryneform groups. Clin Microbiol Newsl. 1998;20:53–66.
51. Weyant RS, Moss CW, Weaver RE, et al. Identification of Unusual Pathogenic Gram-Negative Aerobic and Facultatively Anaerobic Bacteria. 2nd ed. Baltimore: Williams & Wilkins; 1996.
52. NCCLS. Performance Standards for Antimicrobial Disk Susceptibility Tests. 6th

ed. Approved Standard. NCCLS document M2-A6. Wayne, Pa: National Committee for Clinical Laboratory Standards; 1997.
53. NCCLS. Methods for Dilution Antimicrobial Susceptibility Tests for Bacteria That Grow Aerobically. 4th ed. Approved Standard. NCCLS document M7-A4. Wayne, Pa: National Committee for Clinical Laboratory Standards; 1997.
54. Jorgensen JH, Sahm DF. Antimicrobial susceptibility testing: General considerations. In: Murray PR, Baron EJ, Pfaller MA, et al, eds. Manual of Clinical Microbiology. 6th ed. Washington, DC: American Society for Microbiology; 1995:1277–1280.
55. NCCLS. Performance Standards for Antimicrobial Susceptibility Testing. 8th Informational Supplement. NCCLS document M100-S8. Wayne, Pa: National Committee for Clinical Laboratory Standards; 1998.
56. NCCLS. Methods for Antimicrobial Susceptibility Testing of Anaerobic Bacteria. 4th ed. Approved Standard. NCCLS document M11-A4. Wayne, Pa: National Committee for Clinical Laboratory Standards; 1997.
57. NCCLS. Methods for Determining Bactericidal Activity of Antimicrobial Agents. NCCLS document M26-T. Wayne, Pa: National Committee for Clinical Laboratory Standards; 1992.
58. NCCLS. Methodology for the Serum Bactericidal Test. NCCLS document M21-T. Wayne, Pa: National Committee for Clinical Laboratory Standards; 1992.
59. Hindler J. Antimicrobial susceptibility testing. In: Isenberg HD, ed. Essential Procedures for Clinical Microbiology. Washington, DC: American Society for Microbiology; 1998:205–254.
60. Wolfson JS, Swartz MN. Serum bactericidal activity as a monitor of antibiotic therapy. N Engl J Med. 1985;312:968–975.
61. Marshall SA, Wilke WW, Pfaller MA, et al. *Staphylococcus aureus* and coagulase-negative staphylococci from blood stream infections: Frequency of occurrence, antimicrobial susceptibility, and molecular (*mecA*) characterization of oxacillin resistance in the SCOPE program. Diagn Microbiol Infect Dis. 1998;30:205–214.
62. Frebourg NB, Nouet D, Lemée L, et al. Comparison of ATB Staph, Rapid ATB Staph, Vitek, and E-test methods for detection of oxacillin heteroresistance in staphylococci possessing *mecA*. J Clin Microbiol. 1998;36:52–57.
63. Perichon B, Reynolds P, Courvalin P. VanD-type glycopeptide-resistant *Enterococcus faecium* BM4339. Antimicrob Agents Chemother. 1997;41:2016–2018.
64. Eliopoulos GM. Vancomycin-resistant enterococci. Infect Dis Clin North Am. 1997;11:851–865.
65. Jacoby GA. Extended-spectrum β-lactamases and other enzymes providing resistance to oxyimino-β-lactams. Infect Dis Clin North Am. 1997;11:875–887.
66. Coudron PE, Moland ES, Sanders CC. Occurrence and detection of extended-spectrum β-lactamases in members of the family Enterobacteriaceae at a Veterans Medical Center: Seek and you may find. J Clin Microbiol. 1997;35:2593–2597.
67. Cormican MG, Marshall SA, Jones RN. Detection of extended-spectrum β-lactamase (ESBL)-producing strains by Etest ESBL screen. J Clin Microbiol. 1996;34:1880–1884.
68. Swenson JM, Hindler JA, Peterson LR. Special tests for detecting antibacterial resistance. In: Murray PR, Baron EJ, Pfaller MA, et al, eds. Manual of Clinical Microbiology. 6th ed. Washington, DC: American Society for Microbiology; 1995:1356–1367.
69. Richmond JY, McKinney RW, eds. Biosafety in Microbiological and Biomedical Laboratories. 3rd ed. Washington, DC: U.S. Government Printing Office; 1993.
70. Nolte FS, Metchock B. *Mycobacterium*. In: Murray PR, Baron EJ, Pfaller MA, et al, eds. Manual of Clinical Microbiology. 6th ed. Washington, DC: American Society for Microbiology; 1995:400–437.
71. Sandin RL. Polymerase chain reaction and other amplification techniques in mycobacteriology. Clin Lab Med. 1996;16:617–639.
72. Forbes BA. Critical assessment of gene amplification approaches on the diagnosis of tuberculosis. Immunol Invest. 1997;26:105–116.
73. Daniel TM. Antibody and antigen detection for the immunodiagnosis of tuberculosis: Why not? What more is needed? Where do we stand today? J Infect Dis. 1988;158:678–680.
74. Elias J, De Coning JP, Vorster SA, et al. The rapid and sensitive diagnosis of tuberculous meningitis by the detection of tuberculostearic acid in cerebrospinal fluid using gas chromatography–mass spectrometry with selective ion monitoring. Clin Biochem. 1989;22:463–467.
75. Savic B, Sjöbring U, Alugupalli S, et al. Evaluation of polymerase chain reaction, tuberculostearic acid analysis, and direct microscopy for the detection of *Mycobacterium tuberculosis* in sputum. J Infect Dis. 1992;166:1177–1180.
76. Pfyffer GE, Kissling P, Jahn EMI, et al. Diagnostic performance of amplified *Mycobacterium tuberculosis* direct test with cerebrospinal fluid, other nonrespiratory, and respiratory specimens. J Clin Microbiol. 1996;34:834–841.
77. Kent PT, Kubica GP. Public Health Mycobacteriology. A Guide for the Level III Laboratory. Atlanta: US Department of Health and Human Services; 1985.
78. Della-Latta P, Weitzman I. Mycobacteriology. In: Isenberg HD, ed. Essential Procedures for Clinical Microbiology. Washington, DC: American Society for Microbiology; 1998:169–203.
79. Tenover FC, Crawford JT, Huebner RE, et al. The resurgence of tuberculosis: Is your laboratory ready? J Clin Microbiol. 1993;31:767–770.
80. Chiodini RJ. Crohn's disease and the mycobacterioses: A review and comparison of two disease entities. Clin Microbiol Rev. 1989;2:90–117.
81. American Thoracic Society. Diagnosis and treatment of disease caused by nontuberculous mycobacteria. Am J Respir Crit Care Med. 1997;156(Suppl):S1–S25.
82. Weinberger M, Berg SL, Feuerstein IM, et al. Disseminated infection with *Mycobacterium gordonae*: Report of a case and critical review of the literature. Clin Infect Dis. 1992;14:1229–1239.
83. Asnis DS, Bresciani AR, Bhat JG. *Mycobacterium gordonae*: An unusual pathogen causing peritonitis in a patient on chronic ambulatory peritoneal dialysis. Clin Microbiol Newsl. 1996;18:116–119.
84. Harro C, Braden GL, Morris AB, et al. Failure to cure *Mycobacterium gordonae* peritonitis associated with continuous ambulatory peritoneal dialysis. Clin Infect Dis. 1997;24:955–957.
85. Rusconi S, Gori A, Vago L, et al. Cutaneous infection caused by *Mycobacterium gordonae* in a human immunodeficiency virus–infected patient receiving antimycobacterial treatment. Clin Infect Dis. 1997;25:1490–1491.
86. Centers for Disease Control and Infection. Multiple misdiagnoses of tuberculosis resulting from laboratory error—Wisconsin, 1996. MMWR Morb Mortal Wkly Rep. 1997;46:797–801.
87. Witebsky FG, Kruczak-Filipov P. Identification of mycobacteria by conventional methods. Clin Lab Med. 1996;16:569–601.
88. Roberts GD, Böttger EC, Stockman L. Methods for the rapid identification of mycobacterial species. Clin Lab Med. 1996;16:603–615.
89. Esteban J, Fernández-Roblas R, Román A, et al. Catheter-related bacteremia due to *Mycobacterium aurum* in an immunocompromised host. Clin Infect Dis. 1998;26:496–497.
90. Fischer PR, Christenson JC, Pavia AT, et al. Postoperative *Mycobacterium flavescens* infection in a child. Infect Dis Clin Pract. 1997;6:263–265.
91. Tortoli E, Reischl U, Besozzi G, et al. Characterization of an isolate belonging to the newly described species *Mycobacterium hassiacum*. Diagn Microbiol Infect Dis. 1998;30:193–196.
92. Haas WH, Butler WR, Kirschner P, et al. A new agent of mycobacterial lymphadenitis in children: *Mycobacterium heidelbergense* sp. nov. J Clin Microbiol. 1997;35:3203–3209.
93. Domenech P, Jimenez MS, Menendez MC, et al. *Mycobacterium mageritense* sp. nov. Int J Syst Bacteriol. 1997;47:535–540.
94. Shojaei H, Goodfellow M, Magee JG, et al. *Mycobacterium novocastrense* sp. nov., a rapidly-growing photochromogenic mycobacterium. Int J Syst Bacteriol. 1997;47:1205–1207.
95. Floyd MM, Guthertz LS, Silcox VA, et al. Characterization of an SAV organism and proposal of *Mycobacterium triplex* sp. nov. J Clin Microbiol. 1996;34:2963–2967.
96. Hachem R, Raad I, Rolston KVI, et al. Cutaneous and pulmonary infections caused by *Mycobacterium vaccae*. Clin Infect Dis. 1996;23:173–175.
97. NCCLS. Antimycobacterial Susceptibility Testing for *Mycobacterium tuberculosis*; Tentative Standard. NCCLS document M24-T. Wayne, Pa: National Committee for Clinical Laboratory Standards; 1995.
98. Heifets LB. Drug susceptibility testing. Clin Lab Med. 1996;16:641–656.
99. Brown BA, Swenson JM, Wallace RJ Jr. Broth microdilution MIC test for rapidly growing mycobacteria. In: Isenberg HD, ed. Clinical Microbiology Procedures Handbook, v. 1. Washington, DC: American Society for Microbiology; 1994:5.11.1–10.
100. van Embden JDA, Cave MD, Crawford JT, et al. Strain identification of *Mycobacterium tuberculosis* by DNA fingerprinting: Recommendations for a standardized methodology. J Clin Microbiol. 1993;31:406–409.
101. Behr MA, Small PM. Molecular fingerprinting of *Mycobacterium tuberculosis*: How can it help the clinician? Clin Infect Dis. 1997;25:806–810.
102. Wayne LG, Stramek HA. Agents of newly recognized or infrequently encountered mycobacterial diseases. Clin Microbiol Rev. 1992;5:1–25.
103. Zhang Y, Rajagopalan M, Brown BA, et al. Randomly amplified polymorphic DNA PCR for comparison of *Mycobacterium abscessus* strains from nosocomial outbreaks. J Clin Microbiol. 1997;35:3132–3139.
104. Beaman BL, Saubolle MA, Wallace RJ. *Nocardia, Rhodococcus, Streptomyces, Oerskovia,* and other aerobic actinomycetes of medical importance. In: Murray PR, Baron EJ, Pfaller MA, et al, eds. Manual of Clinical Microbiology. 6th ed. Washington, DC: American Society for Microbiology; 1995;379–399.
105. McNeil MM, Brown JM. The medically important aerobic actinomycetes: Epidemiology and microbiology. Clin Microbiol Rev. 1994;7:357–417.
106. Garrett MA, Holmes HT, Nolte FS. Selective buffered charcoal-yeast extract medium for isolation of nocardiae from mixed cultures. J Clin Microbiol. 1992;30:1891–1892.
107. Ruimy R, Riegel P, Carlotti A, et al. *Nocardia pseudobrasiliensis* sp. nov., a new species of nocardia which groups bacterial strains previously identified as *Nocardia brasiliensis* and associated with invasive diseases. Int J Syst Bacteriol. 1996;46:259–264.
108. Wilson RW, Steingrube VA, Brown BA, et al. Recognition of a *Nocardia transvalensis* complex by resistance to aminoglycosides, including amikacin, and PCR–restriction fragment length polymorphism analysis. J Clin Microbiol. 1997;35:2235–2242.
109. Scott MA, Graham BS, Verrall R, et al. *Rhodococcus equi*—an increasingly recognized opportunistic pathogen. Am J Clin Pathol. 1995;103:649–655.
110. Wilson RW, Steingrube VA, Brown BA, et al. Clinical application of PCR–restriction enzyme pattern analysis for rapid identification of aerobic actinomycete isolates. J Clin Microbiol. 1998;36:148–152.
111. Ambaye A, Kohner PC, Wollan PC, et al. Comparison of agar dilution, broth microdilution, disk diffusion, E-test, and BACTEC radiometric methods for antimicrobial susceptibility testing of clinical isolates of the *Nocardia asteroides* complex. J Clin Microbiol. 1997;35:847–852.
112. Lerner PI. Nocardiosis. Clin Infect Dis. 1996;22:891–905.
113. Clark NM, Braun DK, Pasternak A, et al. Primary cutaneous *Nocardia otitidiscaviarum* infection: Case report and review. Clin Infect Dis. 1995;20:1266–1270.
114. Threlkeld SC, Hooper DC. Update on management of patients with *Nocardia*

infection. In: Remington JS, Swartz MA, eds. Current Clinical Topics in Infectious Diseases, v. 17. Cambridge, Mass: Blackwell; 1996:1–23.

115. Louie L, Louie M, Simor AE. Investigation of a pseudo-outbreak of *Nocardia asteroides* infection by pulsed-field gel electrophoresis and randomly amplified polymorphic DNA PCR. J Clin Microbiol. 1997;35:1582–1584.
116. Kwon-Chung KJ, Bennett JE. Medical Mycology. Philadelphia: Lea & Febiger; 1992.
117. Dixon DM, Fromtling RA. Morphology, taxonomy, and classification of the fungi. In: Murray PR, Baron EJ, Pfaller MA, et al, eds. Manual of Clinical Microbiology. 6th ed. Washington, DC: American Society for Microbiology; 1995:699–708.
118. Hadley WK, Ng VL. *Pneumocystis*. In: Murray PR, Baron EJ, Pfaller MA, et al, eds. Manual of Clinical Microbiology. 6th ed. Washington, DC: American Society for Microbiology; 1995:738–748.
119. Thaler M, Pastakia B, Shawker TH, et al. Hepatic candidiasis in cancer patients: The evolving picture of the syndrome. Ann Intern Med. 1988;108:88–100.
120. Koneman EW, Roberts GD. Practical Laboratory Mycology. 3rd ed. Baltimore: Williams & Wilkins; 1985.
121. Larone DH. Medically Important Fungi: A Guide to Identification. 3rd ed. Washington, DC: American Society for Microbiology; 1995.
122. Richmond JY, McKinney RW, eds. Biosafety in Microbiological and Biomedical Laboratories. 3rd ed. Washington, DC: U.S. Government Printing Office; 1993.
123. Merz WG, Roberts GD. Detection and recovery of fungi in clinical specimens. In: Murray PR, Baron EJ, Pfaller MA, et al, eds. Manual of Clinical Microbiology. 6th ed. Washington, DC: American Society for Microbiology; 1995:709–722.
124. Graham DR, Drake C, Barenfanger JE. Recovery of *Histoplasma capsulatum* from BACTEC TB media. J Clin Microbiol. 1996;34:208–209.
125. Kaufman L, Kovacs JA, Reiss E. Clinical immunomycology. In: Rose NR, de Macario EC, Folds JD, et al, eds. Manual of Clinical Laboratory Immunology. 5th ed. Washington, DC: American Society for Microbiology; 1997:585–604.
126. Morris AJ, Byrne TC, Madden JF, et al. Duration of incubation of fungal cultures. J Clin Microbiol. 1996;34:1583–1585.
127. Hove MGM, Woods GL. Duration of fungal culture incubation in an area endemic for *Histoplasma capsulatum*. Diagn Microbiol Infect Dis. 1997;28:41–43.
128. Hazen KC. Mycology and aerobic actinomycetes. In: Isenberg HD, ed. Essential Procedures for Clinical Microbiology. Washington, DC: American Society for Microbiology; 1998:255–360.
129. Sullivan D, Coleman D. *Candida dubliniensis*: Characteristics and identification. J Clin Microbiol. 1998;36:329–334.
130. Walsh TJ, Mitchell TG, Larone DH. *Histoplasma, Blastomyces, Coccidioides,* and other dimorphic fungi causing systemic mycoses. In: Murray PR, Baron EJ, Pfaller MA, et al, eds. Manual of Clinical Microbiology. 6th ed. Washington, DC: American Society for Microbiology; 1995:749–764.
131. NCCLS. Reference Method for Broth Dilution Antifungal Susceptibility Testing of Yeasts; Approved Standard. NCCLS document M27-A. Wayne, Pa: National Committee for Clinical Laboratory Standards; 1997.
132. King D, Rhine-Chalberg J, Pfaller MA, et al. Comparison of four DNA-based methods for strain delineation of *Candida lusitaniae*. J Clin Microbiol. 1995;33:1467–1470.
133. Barchiesi F, Hollis RJ, Del Poeta M, et al. Transmission of fluconazole-resistant *Candida albicans* between patients with AIDS and oropharyngeal candidiasis documented by pulsed-field gel electrophoresis. Clin Infect Dis. 1995;21:561–564.
134. Smith TF. Specimen requirements. In: Specter S, Lancz G, eds. Clinical Virology Manual, 2nd ed. New York: Elsevier; 1992:19–41.
135. Wang J-T, Wang T-H, Sheu J-C, et al. Effects of anticoagulants and storage of blood samples on efficacy of the polymerase chain reaction assay for hepatitis C virus. J Clin Microbiol. 1992;30:750–753.
136. Wadowsky RM, Laus S, Libert T, et al. Inhibition of PCR assay for *Bordetella pertussis* by using calcium alginate fiber and aluminum shaft components of a nasopharyngeal swab. J Clin Microbiol. 1994;32:1054–1057.
137. Lennette DA. Collection and preparation of specimens for virological examination. In: Murray PR, Baron EJ, Pfaller MA, et al, eds. Manual of Clinical Microbiology, 6th ed. Washington, DC: American Society for Microbiology; 1995:868–875.
138. Engler HD, Preuss J. Laboratory diagnosis of respiratory virus infections in 24 hours by utilizing shell vial cultures. J Clin Microbiol. 1997;35:2165–2167.
139. Leven M, Goossens H. Relevance of nucleic acid amplification techniques for diagnosis of respiratory tract infections in the clinical laboratory. Clin Microbiol Rev. 1997;10:242–256.
140. Waner JL. Mixed viral infections: Detection and management. Clin Microbiol Rev. 1994;7:143–151.
141. Mancini AJ. Exanthems in childhood: An update. Pediatr Ann. 1998;27:163–170.
142. Brown KE, Young NS. Parvovirus B19 in human disease. Annu Rev Med. 1997;48:59–67.
143. Dagan R, Menegus MA. A combination of four cell types for rapid detection of enteroviruses in clinical specimens. J Med Virol. 1986;19:219–228.
144. Sawyer M, Holland D, Aintablian N, et al: Diagnosis of enteroviral central nervous system infection by polymerase chain reaction during a large community outbreak. Pediatr Infect Dis J. 1994;13:177–182.
145. Yerly S, Gervaix A, Simonet V, et al. Rapid and sensitive detection of enteroviruses in specimens from patients with aseptic meningitis. J Clin Microbiol. 1996;34:199–201.
146. Pozo F, Casas I, Tenorio A, et al. Evaluation of a commercially available reverse transcription–PCR assay for diagnosis of enteroviral infection in archival and prospectively collected cerebrospinal fluid specimens. J Clin Microbiol. 1998;36:1741–1745.
147. Bruner TA, Fedorko DP. Opportunities for rapid viral diagnosis. Clin Microbiol Newsl. 1993;15:65–69.
148. LeBaron CW, Lew J, Glass RI, et al. Annual rotavirus epidemic patterns in North America. Results of a 5-year retrospective survey of 88 centers in Canada, Mexico, and the United States. JAMA. 1990;264:983–988.
149. Tsai T. Arboviruses. In: Murray PR, Baron EJ, Pfaller MA, et al, eds. Manual of Clinical Microbiology. 6th ed. Washington, DC: American Society for Microbiology; 1995:980–996.
150. Gubler DJ. Resurgent vector-borne diseases as a global health problem. Emerg Infect Dis. 1998;4:442–450.
151. Lakeman FD, Whitley RJ, National Institute of Allergy and Infectious Diseases Collaborative Antiviral Study Group. Diagnosis of herpes simplex encephalitis: Application of polymerase chain reaction to cerebrospinal fluid from brain-biopsied patients and correlation with disease. J Infect Dis. 1995;171:857–863.
152. Ehrnst A. The clinical relevance of different laboratory tests in CMV diagnosis. Scand J Infect Dis Suppl. 1996;100:64–71.
153. Marcon MJ, Salamon D. Traditional and newer approaches to laboratory diagnosis of herpes simplex virus infections. Clin Microbiol Newsl. 1997;19:9–14.
154. Dal Monte P, Lazzarotto T, Ripalti, Landini MP. Human cytomegalovirus infection: A complex diagnostic problem in which molecular biology has induced a rapid evolution. Intervirology. 1997;39:193–203.
155. The TH, Van Den Berg AP, Harmsen MC, et al. The cytomegalovirus antigenemia assay: A plea for standardization. Scand J Infect Dis Suppl. 1995;99:25–29.
156. Linde A. Diagnosis of Epstein-Barr virus–related diseases. Scand J Infect Dis Suppl. 1996;100:83–88.
157. Wolfson WL. Immunology and serology. In: Jacobs DS, Kasten BL, DeMott WR, Wolfson WL, eds. Laboratory Test Handbook, 2nd ed. Baltimore: Williams & Wilkins; 1990:611.
158. Levy JA. Three new human herpesviruses (HHV6, 7, and 8). Lancet. 1997;349:558–562.
159. Singh N, Carrigan DR. Human herpesvirus-6 in transplantation: An emerging pathogen. Ann Intern Med. 1996;124:1065–1071.
160. Lusso P. Human herpesvirus 6 (HHV-6). Antiviral Res. 1996;31:1–21.
161. Wilber JC. Hepatitis C virus. In: Murray PR, Baron EJ, Pfaller MA, et al, eds. Manual of Clinical Microbiology. 6th ed. Washington, DC: American Society for Microbiology; 1995:1050–1055.
162. Arthur RR. Polyomaviruses. In: Lennette EH, ed. Laboratory Diagnosis of Viral Infections. 2nd ed. New York: Marcel Dekker; 1992:613–625.
163. Fong IW, Britton CB, Luinstra KE, et al. Diagnostic value of detecting JC virus DNA in cerebrospinal fluid of patients with progressive multifocal leukoencephalopathy. J Clin Microbiol. 1995;33:484–486.
164. Wieland U, Pfister H. Molecular diagnosis of persistent human papilloma virus infections. Intervirology. 1996;39:145–157.
165. Schmaljohn C, Hjelle B. Hantaviruses: A global disease problem. Emerg Infect Dis. 1997;3:95–104.
166. Mertz GJ, Hjelle BL, Bryan RT. Hantavirus infection. Dis Mon. 1998;44:85–138.
167. Hodinka RL. What clinicians need to know about antiviral drugs and viral resistance. Infect Dis Clin North Am. 1997;11:945–967.
168. Swierkosz EM, Biron KK. Antiviral agents and susceptibility testing. In: Murray PR, Baron EJ, Pfaller MA, et al, eds. Manual of Clinical Microbiology. 6th ed. Washington, DC: American Society for Microbiology; 1995:1415–1423.
169. Lurain NS, Thompson KD. Current methods for antiviral susceptibility testing. Clin Microbiol Newsl. 1997;19:41–45.

SECTION E
ANTI-INFECTIVE THERAPY

Chapter 15

Principles of Anti-infective Therapy

ROBERT C. MOELLERING, JR.

Although the discovery of effective agents to prevent and treat infection caused by bacteria and other pathogenic microorganisms is one of the most important developments of modern medicine, the use of such agents has not been limited to the present era. Substances with anti-infective potential have been applied medically for thousands of years. Indeed, more than 2500 years ago, the Chinese were aware of the therapeutic properties of moldy soybean curd applied to carbuncles, boils, and other infections,[1] and the ancient Greek physicians, including Hippocrates, routinely used substances with antimicrobial activity, including wine, myrrh, and inorganic salts, in their treatment of wounds.[2] Until the discovery of the microbiologic basis of infections in the 19th century, however, the therapy for infections remained strictly empirical. Heavy metals such as arsenic and bismuth were found to be useful against a number of infections, including syphilis, in the early 1900s, but the modern era of chemotherapy did not really begin until the discovery and initial clinical use of the sulfonamides in 1936.[1] This was followed in the 1940s by the discovery of the therapeutic value of penicillin and streptomycin, and by 1950 the "golden age" of antimicrobial chemotherapy was well under way.

It is the result of the relatively recent work in this area since 1936 that forms the basis for this and each of the succeeding chapters on anti-infective therapy. The major emphasis in this chapter is on antibacterial agents, because more data are available on these drugs. However, many of the principles to be discussed can also be applied to the use of antifungal, antiviral, and, to some extent, antiparasitic drugs.

CHOICE OF THE PROPER ANTIMICROBIAL AGENT

In choosing the appropriate antimicrobial agent for therapy for a given infection, a number of important factors must be considered. First, the identity of the infecting organism must be known, or at the very least it must be possible to arrive at a reasonable statistical guess as to its identity on the basis of clinical information. Second, the information about the antimicrobial susceptibility (or potential susceptibility) of the infecting organism must be as accurate as possible. Finally, a series of so-called host factors must be taken into consideration to arrive at the optimal choice of antimicrobial agent. Each of these items is considered in this section.

Identification of the Infecting Organism

Several methods for the rapid identification of pathogenic bacteria in clinical specimens are available. A Gram stain preparation is perhaps the simplest, least expensive, and most useful of all the "rapid methods" of identification of bacterial (and some fungal) pathogens. This technique can be used to identify the presence and morphologic features of microorganisms in body fluids that are normally sterile (cerebrospinal fluid, pleural fluid, synovial fluid, peritoneal fluid, urine). On occasion, Gram staining of a buffy coat preparation of blood reveals phagocytosed organisms in the polymorphonuclear leukocytes of patients with bacteremia or fungemia. Similar preparations of sputum are also helpful in revealing the nature of the infecting organism in patients with bacterial bronchitis or pneumonia.

Gram stain of a stool specimen may produce useful information. The presence of polymorphonuclear leukocytes in the stool also provides a helpful clue to the cause of certain cases of diarrhea. Polymorphonuclear leukocytes are not found in normal stools. When present, they suggest the possibility of a bacterial gastroenteritis such as shigellosis, salmonellosis, or campylobacteriosis or invasive *Escherichia coli* gastroenteritis. Polymorphonuclear leukocytes are not found in the stools of patients with viral gastroenteritis, food poisoning, cholera, and diarrhea due to noninvasive toxigenic *E. coli*.[3] *Campylobacter* may be identified in the stools of patients by its characteristic gull-wing appearance on smears of stool.[4]

Immunologic methods for antigen detection (such as enzyme-linked immunoabsorbent assay [ELISA] or latex agglutination) may also provide clues for the rapid identification of the infecting pathogens. New molecular techniques are also being applied to the detection and identification of antimicrobial agents. The polymerase chain reaction (PCR) has been used to identify RNA or DNA of viruses, bacteria, and other mircroorganisms in the blood of patients,[5,6] and this technique and others, including the use of DNA probes, have proved to be helpful in rapid identification of organisms that have been cultured in the laboratory.[7] At present, however, these techniques are not widely available. Final and definitive identification of pathogenic organisms, therefore, usually requires cultural techniques. It is thus imperative that appropriate specimens be obtained for culture before beginning antimicrobial therapy. Once anti-infective therapy has been started, cultures often are rendered sterile, even though viable organisms remain in the host.

In most cases, it may be impossible to determine the exact nature of the infecting organisms before the institution of antimicrobial therapy. In these cases, the use of bacteriologic statistics may be particularly helpful.[8,9] The term *bacteriologic statistics* refers to the application of knowledge of the organisms most likely to cause infection in a given clinical setting. For example, a person with normal host defense mechanisms who develops cellulitis of the arm after a minor abrasion most likely has an infection due to *Staphylococcus aureus* or group A streptococci, and antimicrobial therapy should be tailored accordingly, even though there is no material available for examination with Gram stain. Similarly, a young child with acute otitis media almost certainly has an infection due either to a virus or to one of four major bacterial pathogens: *Haemophilus influenzae, Streptococcus pneumoniae, Moraxella (Branhamella) catarrhalis*, or a group A streptococcus.

Determination of Antimicrobial Susceptibility of Infecting Organisms

Because different organisms vary in their susceptibility to antimicrobial agents, it is imperative that we have a way to determine the antimicrobial susceptibility of the actual (or presumed) infecting organism or organisms. If the pathogen is isolated from a culture, it can be subjected to direct susceptibility testing, as described in Chapter 14. A number of methods for determining antimicrobial susceptibility are available. The E test, for example, uses diffusion of a continuous concentration gradient of an antimicrobial agent from a plastic strip into an agar medium to yield quantitative measurements of antimicrobial susceptibility.[10]

Quantitative data are also provided by methods that incorporate serial dilutions of antimicrobials in agar-containing or broth culture media. The lowest concentration of the antimicrobial agent that prevents visible growth after an 18- to 24-hour incubation period is the minimal inhibitory concentration (MIC). The minimal bacterial concentration (MBC) or minimal lethal concentration (MLC) may be determined in broth dilution tests by subculturing the containers that show no growth onto antobiotic-free agar-containing media. The lowest concentration of antimicrobial that totally suppresses growth on antibiotic-free media (or results in a 99.9% or greater decline in colony count) after overnight incubation is known as the MBC (or MLC). The aforementioned techniques are based on an 18- to 24-hour incubation period. A variety of "rapid methods" are available as well.[11] These are based on a determination of changes in bacterial growth rates caused by antimicrobial agents and can provide susceptibility in 4 to 8 hours.

Susceptibility testing is particularly important for certain organisms such as *S. aureus* and the various facultative and aerobic gram-negative bacilli. The widespread clinical and agricultural use of antibiotics since the 1930s and 1940s has resulted in the emergence of many strains of bacteria resistant to one or more antimicrobial agents.[12, 13] In most cases in which adequate studies have been done, it appears that the role of antimicrobial agents is to exert selective pressure that results in the emergence of resistant organisms. In some cases the organisms are naturally resistant to the antibiotic used. Examples of this include gram-positive organisms such as staphylococci and streptococci, which are naturally resistant to the polymyxins. Many gram-negative bacilli are naturally resistant to penicillin G, erythromycin, and clindamycin.

In other cases the resistant bacterial strains have acquired genes encoded on transposons or plasmids that enable them to resist antimicrobial inhibition. These genes may provide the organisms with the ability to synthesize enzymes that modify or inactivate the antimicrobial agent; they may result in changes in the bacterial cell's ability to accumulate the antimicrobial agent or may permit the cell to produce metablic enzymes resistant to inhibition by the antimicrobial agent.[12] Examples of each of these mechanisms of resistance are well known. Most strains of *S. aureus* that are resistant to penicillin contain plasmids that enable them to produce an extracellular β-lactamase that hydrolyzes and inactivates penicillin G.[12] Many gram-negative bacilli that are resistant to aminoglycosidic aminocyclitol antibiotics such as streptomycin, kanamycin, tobramycin, gentamicin, and amikacin contain genes on plasmids that code for the production of periplasmic enzymes that catalyze a modification of the aminoglycosidic aminocyclitols by phosphorylation, acetylation, or adenylation.[12] Efflux mechanisms (which may be plasmid or transposon mediated) can cause resistance to tetracyline and other agents in *S. aureus* and gram-negative bacilli.[14] *E. coli* resistant to trimethoprim has been found to contain R factors that enable it to synthesize a new dihydrofolate reductase (the enzyme specifically inhibited by trimethoprim) that is 10,000 times less susceptible to the in vitro effects of trimethoprim than is the host bacteria's own chromosomal enzyme.[12]

The aforementioned developments provide the rationale for performing tests of antimicrobial susceptibility whenever there is reasonable doubt about the susceptibility of a given organism. In certain cases routine susceptibility testing need not be done, but these cases make up an ever-diminishing list. All group A and other β-hemolytic streptococci remain susceptible to the penicillins and cephalosporins; virtually all anaerobes except *Bacteroides* spp. are susceptible to penicillin G. Thus, testing these organisms against the agents listed need not be carried out routinely at the present time. Even a statement such as this is fraught with a certain amount of danger. The discoveries of penicillin-resistant meningococci and pneumococci in South Africa, the emergence of penicillin-resistant gonococci in Asia and Africa, the rapid spread of ampicillin-resistant (and even chloramphenicol-resistant) strains of *H. influenzae* in the United States and Europe, the proliferation of vancomycin-resistant enterococci and staphylococci, and the recent identification of chloramphenicol-resistant meningococci in France and Southeast Asia make us realize that, in time, strains of virtually any organism may be found that are resistant to antimicrobial agents that previously had been effective against them.[15, 16]

It is important to consider geographic differences in patterns of susceptibility of organisms when choosing antimicrobial agents. In many cases, there may be variations in susceptibility patterns between hospitals and the community or among hospitals themselves. The emergence of gram-negative bacilli that are resistant to gentamicin is a good example of this. Most of the aminoglycoside-resistant organisms are found in hospitals, whereas most isolates from nonhospitalized patients remain susceptible to gentamicin.[12, 17]

The possibility of significant geographic variations in antimicrobial susceptibility must be remembered as we examine Table 15–1, which is a compendium of antimicrobial agents of choice for various commonly encountered infectious agents. The data in Table 15–1 are based on material accumulated primarily in the United States and are similar in many aspects to data published periodically in the *Medical Letter on Drugs and Therapeutics.*[18]

Host Factors

It is obviously important to determine the identity and antimicrobial susceptibility of the organism or organisms causing a given infection. However, optimal therapy is impossible unless we also consider a number of host factors that may influence the efficacy and toxicity of antimicrobial agents.[19]

History of Previous Adverse Reactions to Antimicrobial Agents. Simply obtaining an adequate history of previous adverse reactions to drugs may prevent the inadvertent administration of an antimicrobial agent to which the patient is allergic. A failure to do so can have serious (and sometimes fatal) consequences.

Age. The age of the patient is a major factor to consider in the choice of antimicrobial agents. Gastric acidity varies with age. The pH of gastric secretions is higher in young children and does not reach adult levels of acidity until approximately the age of 3 years. At the other end of the age spectrum, there is also a decline in gastric acidity such that gastric achlorhydria is found in 5.3% of people 20 to 29 years of age, in 16% of those 40 to 49, and in 35.4% of those older than 60.[19] The absorption of a number of antimicrobials via the oral route depends on their acid stability and the pH of gastric secretions. Penicillin G is an excellent example of this phenomenon. The oral absorption of penicillin G is markedly reduced by gastric acid. However, in young children and in older achlorhydric patients, the absorption of the drug is markedly enhanced. As a result, various orally administered penicillins will produce high serum levels in young children and in elderly patients who have achlorhydria. It makes no sense to give such a patient the more expensive acid-resistant forms of penicillin such as phenoxymethyl penicillin (penicillin V), since these drugs will not be absorbed any better than the less expensive penicillin G. The absorption of other orally administered β-lactam antibiotics is probably also enhanced in achlorhydric patients; however, evidence is convincing only in the case of the penicillins.[20] Gastric acidity does not always have a negative influence on the absorption of antimicrobials. Drugs that are weak acids such as ketoconazole may be better absorbed at a low pH. Thus, absorption of ketoconazole is impaired by the administration of antacids, cimetidine, or even food.[21]

Renal function, likewise, varies with age. It is relatively diminished in premature and newborn children and reaches "adult levels" between 2 and 12 months of age.[19] Thus, the serum half-lives of drugs that are primarily excreted by the kidneys may be considerably increased in neonates. As a result, doses of antimicrobial agents such

TABLE 15–1 Antimicrobial Agents of Choice

Organism	Antimicrobial of Choice	Alternative Agents
Gram-Positive Cocci		
Staphylococcus aureus		
Non–penicillinase producing	Penicillin	A cephalosporin,* vancomycin, imipenem, erythromycin, neomacrolides,** fluoroquinolone†
Penicillinase producing	A penicillinase-resistant penicillin‡	A cephalosporin,* vancomycin, clindamycin, imipenem, erythromycin, neomacrolides,** fluoroquinolone†
β-Streptococci (groups A, B, C, and G)	Penicillin (some add gentamicin for serious group B streptococcal infections)	A cephalosporin,* erythromycin, vanomycin
α-Streptococci (viridans streptococci)	Penicillin	A cephalosporin,* vancomycin, erythromycin, neomacrolides**
Streptococcus bovis	Penicillin	A cephalosporin,* vancomycin, erythromycin, neomacrolides**
Enterococci (susceptible strains—see Chapter 189 for therapy for infections due to strains with high-level aminoglycoside resistance and/or resistance to penicillin or vancomycin)		
Endocarditis or other serious infection	Penicillin (or ampicillin) plus gentamicin or streptomycin	Vancomycin plus gentamicin or streptomycin
Uncomplicated urinary tract infection	Ampicillin or amoxicillin	Nitrofurantoin, fosfomycin, fluoroquinolone†
Streptococcus pneumoniae	Penicillin	A cephalosporin,* levofloxacin, sparfloxacin, grepafloxacin, trovafloxacin, erythromycin, neomacrolides,** chloramphenicol, vancomycin, cefotaxime or ceftriaxone (penicillin-resistant strains)
Gram-Negative Cocci		
Neisseria meningitidis	Penicillin	Ceftriaxone, cefotaxime, chloramphenicol, cefuroxime, a sulfonamide (some strains)
Neisseria gonorrhoeae		
Non–β-lactamase producing	Penicillin	Spectinomycin, ampicillin, amoxicillin, cefoxitin, ceftriaxone, cefuroxime, cefotaxime, trimethoprim-sulfamethoxazole, cefpodoxime, cefixime, fluoroquinolone†
β-Lactamase producing	Ceftriaxone, cefixime, cefpodoxime	Cefoxitin, cefuroxime, amoxicillin-clavulanate, spectinomycin, cefotaxime, trimethoprim-sulfamethoxazole, fluoroquinolone†
Gram-Negative Bacilli		
Acinetobacter spp. (*mima, herellea*)	Imipenem or meropenem	Ampicillin/sulbactam, fluoroquinolone,† amikacin, trimethoprim-sulfamethoxazole, ceftazidime
Brucella spp.	Doxycycline (± gentamicin or streptomycin)	Doxycycline + rifampin, trimethoprim-sulfamethoxazole + gentamicin, fluoroquinolone + rifampin
Campylobacter jejuni	Erythromycin	Fluoroquinolone,†§ doxycycline, clindamycin, gentamicin, azithromycin, clarithromycin
Enterobacter spp.	Imipenem or meropenem	Cefepime, fluoroquinolone,† ticarillin,/clavulanic acid, piperacillin/tazobactam, gentamicin, tobramycin, piperacillin aztreonam, amikacin, third-generation cephalosporin,‖ cefoperazone
Escherichia coli		
Uncomplicated urinary tract infection	Trimethoprim-sulfamethoxazole or amoxicillin-clavulanate	Fluoroquinolone,† a cephalosporin,* a tetracycline, ampicillin, amoxicillin
Systemic infection	Third-generation cephalosporin,‖ cefoperazone, cefepime	A cephalosporin,* ticarcillin, mezlocillin, piperacillin, gentamicin, tobramycin, kanamycin, amikacin, fluoroquinolone,† imipenem, aztreonam, ampicillin, amoxicillin, ampicillin-sulbactam, ticarcillin-clavulanate, piperacillin-tazobactam
Francisella tularensis	Streptomycin or gentamicin	Doxycycline, chloramphenicol, ciprofloxacin, rifampin
Haemophilus influenzae		
Meningitis	Third-generation cephalosporin‡	Ampicillin (if β-lactamase-negative), chloramphenicol, trimethoprim-sulfamethoxazole, fluoroquinolone†
Other infections	Ampicillin or amoxicillin,¶ amoxicillin-clavulanate, or ampicillin-sulbactam	Trimethoprim-sulfamethoxazole, cefuroxime cefaclor, cefprozil, cefpodoxime, cefixime, cefamandole, sulfisoxazole, fluoroquinolone†
Klebsiella pneumonia	A cephalosporin* (for serious infections, third-generation cephalosporin)‖	Imipenem, meropenem, fluoroquinolone,† aztreonam, trimethoprim-sulfamethoxazole, cefuroxime, cefamandole, amikacin, gentamicin, tobramycin, chloramphenicol, tetracycline
Legionella spp.	Erythromycin ± rifampin or fluoroquinolone†	Azithromycin, clarithromycin, trimethoprim-sulfamethoxazole, doxycycline
Proteus mirabilis	Ampicillin	Trimethoprim-sulfamethoxazole, gentamicin or tobramycin, a cephalosporin,* imipenem, meropenem, aztreonam, ticarcillin, mezlocillin, piperacillin
Other *Proteus* spp. (*P. rettgeri, M. morganii, P. vulgaris*)	Third-generation cephalosporin,‖ cefepime, or fluoroquinolone†	Ampicillin-sulbactam, ticarcilllin clavulanate, piperacillin-tazobactam Ticarcillin, mezlocillin, piperacillin, gentamicin, tobramycin, amikacin, imipenem, meropenem, aztreonam, trimethoprim-sulfamethoxazole

Table continued on following page

TABLE 15-1 Antimicrobial Agents of Choice *Continued*

Organism	Antimicrobial of Choice	Alternative Agents
Providencia spp.	Third-generation cephalosporin,‖ cefepime, or amikacin	Gentamicin, tobramycin, netilmicin, ticarcillin, mezlocillin, piperacillin, ampicillin-sulbactam, ticarcillin clavulanate, piperacillin-tazobactam, imipenem, meropenem, aztreonam, trimethoprim-sulfamethoxazole, fluoroquinolone†
Pseudomonas aeruginosa	Tobramycin or gentamicin plus ticarcillin, azlocillin, mezlocillin, or piperacillin	Fluoroquinolone,† amikacin, imipenem, meropenem, aztreonam, ceftazidime, cefepime
Salmonella spp.	Fluoroquinolone,† ceftriaxone	Chloramphenicol, ampicillin or amoxicillin, trimethoprim-sulfamethoxazole§
Serratia marcescens	Third-generation cephalosporin,‖ imipenem, meropenem, or fluoroquinolone†	Ampicillin-sulbactam, ticarcillin clavulanate, piperacillin-tazobactam, ticarcillin, mezlocillin, piperacillin, imipenem, meropenem, aztreonam, amikacin, gentamicin, tobramycin
Shigella spp.	A fluoroquinolone†	Trimethoprim-sulfamethoxazole, ampicillin, nalidixic acid
Yersinia pestis	Streptomycin or gentamicin	Doxycycline, chloramphenicol, fluoroquinolone†
Anaerobes		
Anaerobic streptococci	Penicillin	Clindamycin, erythromycin, chloramphenicol, a cephalosporin,* tetracycline, vancomycin
Bacteroides spp.		
Oropharyngeal strains	Penicillin	Clindamycin, tetracycline, chloramphenicol, metronidazole, cefoxitin, cefmetazole, cefotetan
Gastrointestinal strains	Metronidazole	Clindamycin, chloramphenicol, cefoxitin, cefotetan, cefmetazole, ticarcillin, piperacillin, mezlocillin, imipenem, meropenem, ticarcillin clavulanate, ampicillin-sulbactam, piperacillin-tazobactam
Clostridium spp.	Penicillin	Doxycycline, erythromycin, chloramphenicol, clindamycin, imipenem, meropenem

*The term *cephalosporin* refers to the first-generation cephalosporins cephalothin, cefazolin, cephapirin, cephradine, cephalexin, cefaclor, and cefadroxil.
†Ciprofloxacin, ofloxacin, levofloxacin, sparfloxacin, grepafloxacin, or trovafloxacin (or, for urinary tract infections, norfloxacin, lomefloxacin, or enoxacin).
‡Methicillin, nafcillin, oxacillin, or dicloxacillin.
§Not approved for this indication by the U.S. Food and Drug Administration.
‖The term *third-generation cephalosporin* refers to ceftriaxone, cefotaxime, ceftizoxime, and ceftazidime.
¶For strains that do not produce β-lactamase.
**The term neomacrolides refers to azithromycin, clarithromycin, and dirythromycin.

as penicillin G and its various semisynthetic derivatives, as well as the aminoglycosides, must be altered in neonates.

Aging results in the decline of a number of physiologic processes, including renal function.[20] It is especially important to realize that creatinine clearance may be significantly reduced in elderly patients even though they have normal blood urea nitrogen or serum creatinine concentrations. In view of this, high doses of the penicillins or cephalosporins must be given with caution to elderly patients to prevent the development of excessively high serum levels that may produce severe neurotoxic reactions such as myoclonus, seizures, and coma.[19, 20] It is likewise possible that other adverse reactions to the penicillins such as reversible neutropenia may be dose related and may occur with increased frequency when high doses of such drugs are given to elderly patients with physiologic renal impairment.[20] This, however, has not been proved. Impaired renal excretion of the aminoglycoside antibiotics may result in elevated serum concentrations, which in turn may be associated with an increasing incidence of ototoxicity in elderly patients.[22]

In addition to the toxicity that may result from impaired renal excretion in neonates and elderly patients, other adverse effects of antimicrobial agents may also be age related.[20, 23] Hepatic function in the neonate is underdeveloped by adult standards. This can result in difficulties if such patients are administered drugs that are normally excreted or inactivated by the liver. Chloramphenicol is inactivated by conjugation to the glucuronide form in the liver. However, in the neonate, hepatic levels of glucuronyl transferase are relatively insufficient. Thus, when neonates are given large doses of chloramphenicol, high serum levels of unconjugated chloramphenicol result. Such high concentrations of unconjugated chloramphenicol are toxic and can result in shock, cardiovascular collapse, and death (the so-called gray syndrome).[19, 24] For this reason, chloramphenicol should be avoided if possible in the neonate. If it is necessary to use the drug, however, it may be administered safely if given in a dosage that has been reduced appropriately for the patient's age.[24, 25]

The sulfonamides compete with bilirubin for binding sites on serum albumin. When given to neonates, they produce increased serum levels of unbound bilirubin that predispose the child to kernicterus.[24, 25] For this reason, these agents should not be administered to neonates. Hyperbilirubinemia per se may be associated with the administration of novobiocin to neonates.[24] This is due to the ability of this drug to inhibit hepatic glucuronyl transferase, which in turn diminishes the ability of the liver to conjugate and excrete bilirubin. Hence, novobiocin should be avoided in newborn infants.

The tetracyclines are avidly bound to developing bone and tooth structures. As they bind to developing teeth, tetracyclines may cause a number of adverse effects, ranging from purplish to brownish discoloration of the teeth to actual enamel hypoplasia.[19, 24] The tetracyclines readily cross the placenta.[26] Thus, when administered during the latter half of pregnancy or from birth to the age of 6 months, they may cause these effects on the deciduous teeth of the infant. From the age of 6 months to 6 to 8 years, similar damage to the permanent teeth may occur. In view of this, tetracycline should be avoided, if possible, in young children.

The quinolone antimicrobials including the newer agents such as ciprofloxacin, norfloxacin, ofloxacin, pefloxacin, and others have been shown to cause cartilage damage and arthropathy in young animals. As a result, they are not currently recommended for use in prepubertal children.[27, 28]

Adverse effects due to a number of antimicrobial agents have been noted to occur with increased incidence in the elderly.[20] In some cases (and perhaps in all if adequately studied), this relationship may be shown to be caused by specific disease states or to impairment of physiologic processes associated with aging, as noted earlier. However, in certain cases no specific factors other than age can be identified. The hepatotoxicity associated with isoniazid administration is a good example of this. A small percentage of patients receiving isoniazid develop toxic hepatitis that may be fatal if not recognized in time.[29] Liver damage from isoniazid almost never occurs in patients younger than 20 years of age. In patients 20 to 34 years of age, the incidence of isoniazid hepatotoxicity is 0.3% and rises steadily with age to reach 2.3% in patients 50 years of age or older.[30] Because of this, it is currently recommended that routine prophylactic use of isoniazid for patients who have positive tuberculin test reactions be limited to people younger than 35, but the risk-benefit ratio of these recommendations is not universally accepted, and recent study suggests that isoniazid prophylaxis has a positive risk-benefit ratio in older patients as long as liver function tests are monitored.[31]

Nephrotoxic reactions to certain antimicrobial agents likewise appear to be more frequent or to occur with lower doses of drugs among the elderly. This has been demonstrated with cephaloridine[32] and colistin[19, 33] and may be true for other nephrotoxic antimicrobials as well.

Finally, hypersensitivity reactions to antimicrobial agents also appear to be more common in elderly than in younger patients.[19] This seems to be due to the fact that older patients are more likely to have been previously exposed and, thus, sensitized to these agents. In addition, prior exposure to drugs such as the aminoglycosidic aminocyclitols, which produce irreversible cochlear damage, can result in cumulative toxicity on repeat exposure.[20]

Genetic or Metabolic Abnormalities. The presence of genetic or metabolic abnormalities may also have a significant effect on the use or toxicity of a given antimicrobial agent. The rate at which isoniazid is conjugated and biologically inactivated by acetylation in the liver is determined genetically.[19] Rapid acetylators are found more commonly among Asian populations, whereas 45 to 65% of U.S. and North European populations are slow acetylators. Several studies have suggested that polyneuritis is seen more frequently as a complication of isoniazid therapy in slow than in rapid acetylators.[19] It was once thought that hepatotoxicity due to isoniazid is related to the conversion of isoniazid to acetylhydrazine and other related hepatotoxic derivatives and is more common among rapid acetylators,[34] but this does not appear to be true.

A number of antimicrobial agents have been shown to be capable of provoking hemolysis in patients with glucose-6-phosphate dehydrogenase (G6PD) deficiency, including the sulfonamides, nitrofurantoin, furazolidone, diaminodiphenylsulfone, and chloramphenicol.[19] Sulfonamides may likewise cause hemolytic reactions in the presence of certain hemoglobinopathies, including hemoglobin Zurich and hemoglobin H.[19]

The presence of metabolic disorders such as diabetes mellitus may also pose problems in antimicrobial therapy. Certain agents such as the sulfonamides (especially the long-acting types) and chloramphenicol can potentiate the hypoglycemic activity of sulfonylurea hypoglycemic agents such as tolbutamide and chlorpropamide.[20] In the case of the sulfonamides, this action may be related to their structural similarity to the sulfonylurea drugs. Chloramphenicol inhibits microsomal enzyme activity in the liver, and this impairs the metabolism of the sulfonylurea hypoglycemic agents. The dextrose load infused with intravenous antibiotics dissolved in dextrose-containing vehicles may be sufficient to produce hyperglycemia and glucosuria in diabetic patients. Another kind of "glucosuria" can occur in patients receiving antimicrobial agents. The cephalosporins, chloramphenicol, isoniazid, nalidixic acid, nitrofurantoin, penicillin, streptomycin, sulfanilimide, and the tetracyclines can all cause false-positive test results when urine sugar levels are determined by a method (e.g., the Benedict test or Clinitest) that measures reducing substances in the urine.[20] Tests that are specific for glucose (i.e., that use glucose oxidase) such as Dextrostix or Labstix are not affected by antimicrobial agents.[35]

The absorption of intramuscularly administered antibiotics may be impaired in diabetic patients. Diabetics with bacterial endocarditis who failed to respond to intramuscular penicillin have been described.[19] Administration of the same dose of penicillin by the intravenous route, however, resulted in bacterial eradication.[19] Because of the potential impaired absorption of intramuscularly administered antimicrobial agents, it is probably prudent to initiate therapy by the intravenous route when using drugs such as the aminoglycosides to treat diabetic patients with gram-negative bacteremia (especially if accompained by hypotension) or other serious infections.

The concomitant administration of chloramphenicol has been noted to delay the reticulocyte response to vitamin B_{12} or iron therapy in patients with pernicious anemia or iron deficiency anemia.[19] As noted previously, patients with pernicious anemia and gastric achlorhydria may exhibit enhanced serum levels of antimicrobials such as penicillin G when chloramphenicol is given by the oral route.

Rifampin may increase the hepatic metabolism and therefore decrease the effect of oral anticoagulants, oral contraceptives, and barbiturates.

Pregnancy. Patients who are pregnant and nursing mothers also pose certain problems in the selection of appropriate antimicrobial agents. All antimicrobial agents cross the placenta in varying degrees.[36, 37] Thus, the use of such agents in pregnant women provides direct exposure of the fetus to the adverse effects of the drug. Although there are few solid data on the teratogenic potential of most antimicrobial agents in humans, experience suggests that certain drugs such as the penicillins (with the possible exception of ticarcillin[38]), the cephalosporins, and erythromycin are unlikely to be teratogenic and are safe for pregnant women to use.[24, 36, 37] Metronidazole and ticarcillin have been shown to be teratogenic in rodents and thus should be avoided in pregnancy.[38, 39] The teratogenic potential of many other drugs in humans, including the fluoroquinolones, rifampin, and trimethoprim, is simply unknown.

A number of antimicrobials have been shown to be deleterious in pregnancy. Tetracycline heads the list. The possible adverse effects of this drug on fetal dentition have already been noted. In addition, pregnant women receiving tetracycline are particularly vulnerable to certain toxic effects, including acute fatty necrosis of the liver, pancreatitis, and probably renal damage.[19] The liver damage may be severe and can result in death. When administered to patients with impaired renal function, these effects may be magnified, particularly if the agent is one of the tetracyclines that is primarily excreted by the kidneys. These adverse effects are dose related and may be more frequent after intravenous administration. Although it has been suggested that tetracyclines may be given to pregnant women by the oral route in doses of 1 g or less per 24 hours, it is probably safer to avoid these agents entirely in pregnancy.[19, 24]

The aminoglycosidic aminocyclitol antibiotics cross the placenta. Thus far fetal toxicity has been reported only for streptomycin when used to treat tuberculosis in pregnant women. Even in that setting, the toxicity has been mild, detectable only by formal vestibular testing or by an audiogram.[40] Psychomotor retardation, myoclonus, and convulsions have been reported in a small uncontrolled series of children whose mothers received isoniazid for tuberculosis during pregnancy.[41] This observation has not been confirmed to date.

Another aspect of drug therapy in pregnancy has been examined. It has been found that serum levels after a given dose of ampicillin are lower in pregnant that in nonpregnant women.[42] This is related to more rapid clearance of the drug and to a greater volume of distribution (probably due to increased plasma volume) in pregnancy, Thus, higher doses of ampicillin are required to achieve therapeutic blood levels in pregnancy. It is likely that these observations will also apply to other antimicrobial agents, but data on this are not available at present.

Virtually all antimicrobial agents appear in measurable concentrations in breast milk when administered in therapeutic doses to nursing women.[43] The amount of drug excreted into breast milk depends on its degree of ionization, its molecular weight, and its solubility in fat and water. Under usual circumstances, the concentrations of antibiotics found in breast milk are quite low. However, even these small amounts may cause significant adverse reactions in the nursing infant. Nalidixic acid and the sulfonamides in breast milk have been shown to cause hemolysis in infants with G6PD deficiency. Sulfonamides in breast milk may be dangerous to premature babies, because even small doses of ingested sulfonamides may produce increased levels of unbound bilirubin by displacing bilirubin from its albumin-binding sites. As noted previously, this predisposes the child to kernicterus.[43] The possibility that antimicrobial agents in breast milk can sensitize newborn children is a theoretical one, but it has not been convincingly demonstrated. Although tetracycline is excreted in breast milk, it is unlikely to produce damage to the nursing child's bones or teeth because the calcium in the milk forms an insoluble chelate with tetracyclines, which is not absorbable by the oral route.[43]

Renal and Hepatic Function. The ability of the patient to metabolize or excrete antimicrobial agents is one of the most important host factors to consider, especially when high serum or tissue concentrations of the administered drugs are potentially toxic. From a practical point of view, this means that one must assess the patient's renal and hepatic function carefully, because these organs serve as the major (and in most cases the *only*) routes of excretion and inactivation of antimicrobials. Renal excretion is the most important route of elimination for most antimicrobial agents.[44–49] Table 15–2 lists the drugs that must be used with particular care in patients with decreased renal function. Doses for these drugs may be found in the chapters dealing with the individual agents and in Chapter 17. In general, agents that require no dosage change in impaired renal function are excreted effectively be extrarenal routes (usually the hepatobiliary system) in patients with renal failure. Their use in normal doses does not result in the appearance of toxic serum levels in this situation, although the urine levels of a number of these agents such as doxycycline, trovafloxacin, and chloramphenicol may be diminished significantly.

Toxic serum levels of the remaining agents may develop if they are used without dosage modification in patients with impaired renal function. Excessive serum levels of penicillin G, carbenicillin, or imipenem may be associated with neuromuscular hyperexcitability, myoclonus, seizures, or coma.[19] Excessive serum levels of semisynthetic penicillins such as carbenicillin and ticarcillin or of cephalothin or moxalactam may cause hemostatic defects in patients with impaired renal failure because of interference with platelet function.[50, 51] Elevated serum levels of aminoglycosidic aminocyclitol antibiotics or vancomycin may result in eighth nerve damage.[22, 49] Neurotoxic reactions including respiratory arrest and death may occur in patients who have excessive serum levels of certain aminoglycosidic aminocyclitols or the polymyxins.[19, 33] Bone marrow suppression may occur in patients with renal failure who receive inappropriately high doses of 5-fluorocytosine.[52] In all the previosuly mentioned situations, the possibility of toxic reactions can be lessened significantly or eliminated if the doses of the antimicrobial agents are appropriately reduced in the presence of renal insufficiency.

TABLE 15–2 Antimicrobial Use in Patients with Varying Degrees of Impaired Renal Function

Function
Antimicrobial agents requiring no dosage change regardless of renal function
Amphotericin B,* azithromycin, cefaclor, cefoperazone, ceftriaxone, chloramphenicol, clindamycin, cloxacillin, dicloxacillin, dirythromycin, doxycycline, erythromycin, grepafloxacin, metronidazole, minocycline, nafcillin, oxacillin, rifampin, trovafloxacin
Antimicrobial agents requiring dosage change only with severe renal failure
Amoxicillin, ampicillin, cefamandole, cefotaxime, cefotetan, cefonicid, cefoxitin, ceftazidime, ceftizoxime, cefuroxime, cephalexin, cephalothin, ciprofloxacin, clarithromycin, ethambutol, isoniazid, levofloxacin, meropenem, methicillin, mezlocillin, nalidixic acid, norfloxacin, ofloxacin, penicillin G, piperacillin, sparfloxacin, trimethoprim-sulfamethoxazole
Antimicrobial agents requiring dosage change with impaired renal function
Amikacin, cefazolin, flucytosine, gentamicin, imipenem, kanamycin, polymyxin B, streptomycin, ticarcillin, tobramycin, vancomycin
Antimicrobial agents contraindicated in renal failure
Cephaloridine, long-acting sulfonamides, methenamine, nitrofurantoin, para-aminosalicyclic acid, tetracyclines (except doxycycline and possibly minocycline)

*Even though amphotericin B is excreted primarily by nonrenal means, this drug must be used with caution in patients with impaired renal function because of its nephrotoxicity.

The tetracyclines (except doxycycline and possibly minocycline) are contraindicated in patients with impaired renal function because the elevated serum levels that result may produce a significant worsening of the uremic state due to their antianabolic effect. Moreover, they may cause enhanced hepatotoxicity in this situation.[19] Cephaloridine and the long-acting sulfonamides should be avoided in this situation because they are potentially nephrotoxic.

Certain antimicrobial agents, including erythromycin, azithromycin, dirythromycin, chloramphenicol, lincomycin, and clindamycin, should be used with caution in patients with impaired hepatic function.[53] These drugs are primarily excreted or detoxified in the liver. Bone marrow suppression due to chloramphenicol is much more likely to occur in patients with impaired hepatic function; because of this, it has been suggested that the dose of chloramphenicol be cut at least in half in patients with cirrhosis and other severe liver disease.[51] The serum half-life of clindamycin is increased in patients with severe liver disease; because of this, the dose should be decreased in this situation. The tetracyclines may produce elevations in serum transaminase levels in patients recovering from viral hepatitis.[19] They should be avoided or used with extreme caution in patients with underlying liver disease. The serum half-lives of both rifampin and isoniazid are prolonged in patients with cirrhosis.[55] Other drugs that should be used with caution or for which serum levels should be monitored in patients with severe liver disease include metronidazole, ketoconazole, miconazole, fluconazole, itraconazole, nitrofurantoin, fusidic acid, and pyrazinamide.[53] It has been suggested that β-lactam antibiotic–induced leukopenia occurs more frequently in patients with impaired hepatic function.[56] Hepatobiliary disease influences antimicrobic therapy in still another way. The biliary concentrations of many antimicrobial agents, including ampicillin and nafcillin, that are normally excreted in high concentration in the bile may be reduced significantly in patients with liver disease or biliary obstruction.[19]

Site of Infection. Of all the host factors to be considered in the choice of an antimicrobial agent, none is more important than the site of infection. The locus of the infectious process determines not only the choice of the agent but also its dose and the route by which it should be administered. For antimicrobial therapy to be effective, an adequate concentration of the drug must be delivered to the site of infection. In most cases, this means that the local concentration of the antimicrobial agent should at least equal the MIC of the infecting organism. Concentrations representing multiples of the MIC are generally believed more likely to be efficacious, but in many cases such local concentrations may be difficult or impossible to achieve. A failure to achieve local concentrations of antibiotics higher than the MIC of the infecting organism may not always be disastrous, however, because there is evidence that subinhibitory concentrations of drugs may produce antimicrobial effects that aid the host defenses against infections. It has been demonstrated clearly that subinhibitory concentrations of antibiotics can alter bacterial morphology,[57] adherence properties,[58] and opsonic requirements[59]; can enhance phagocytosis[60] and can even aid intracellular killing of bacteria by polymorphonuclear leukocytes.[61] This may explain the clinical observation that, on occasion, doses of antimicrobials that produce seemingly inadequate serum levels may still result in clinical cure. In spite of such observations, most infectious disease clinicians feel that optimal therapy requires concentrations of antimicrobials that are above the MIC at the actual site of infection.

Serum concentrations of antimicrobial agents are relatively easy to determine and therefore are often used as a guide in the therapy. However, except in cases of bacteremia, antimicrobial efficacy is more likely determined by the tissue concentration than by the blood level, as noted earlier. Moreover, some agents such as spiromycin and certain macrolides such as azithromycin are effective in vivo despite an inability to achieve serum levels above the MIC of certain organisms.[62] This may be explained by the ability to achieve intracellular and tissue concentrations that far exceed those obtained in serum.[63, 64] Binding to serum proteins may affect both the tissue distribution and the activity of antimicrobial agents in the blood. Although much careful investigation has been done on protein binding, the precise clinical significance of this phenomenon remains to be determined. For example, it has been shown that only the unbound form of a given antimicrobial agent is active in vitro (and presumably also in vivo) against infecting organisms.[65] However, because protein binding is rapidly reversible,[66] the activity of even highly protein-bound agents may not be limited absolutely by protein binding. The penetration of antimicrobial agents into interstitial fluid and lymph is related to protein binding, because only the free form of the agent is able to pass through the capillary wall.[65] Penetration of antibiotics into fibrin clots (which may be analogous to the penetration of the drugs to reach the site of infection in patients with bacterial endocarditis) is likewise related to the amount of unbound antibiotic in the surrounding fluid.[67] Nevertheless, it is often difficult to correlate therapeutic outcome with in vitro susceptibility and protein binding unless several variables are carefully controlled.[68, 69] The reason for this is simply that it is the concentration of antibiotic at the site of infection that is the major determinant in the successful therapy. Such concentrations are often difficult to assess because they are the result of a complex interaction between local factors that may bind, inactivate, or enhance the activity of a given antimicrobial agent. The ability of an antibiotic to pass through membranes by nonionic diffusion is related to its lipid solubility. Thus, lipid-soluble agents such as chloramphenicol, rifampin, trimethoprim, and isoniazid are all more adept at penetrating membranes than are the more highly ionized compounds.[65] These agents rapidly cross the blood-brain barrier and produce better cerebrospinal fluid levels than do more highly ionized compounds such as the aminoglycosidic aminocyclitols. Except in neonates, none of the aminoglycosides produces effective cerebrospinal fluid levels when given parenterally. To be effective for the treatment of meningitis, they must be given via the intrathecal or intraventricular route in adults.[70] This is an excellent example of the importance of the site of infection in determining the most efficacious antimicrobial therapy. For the treatment of bacterial meningitis in adults, we either must choose agents such as chloramphenicol or the third-generation cephalosporins (e,g., cefotaxime, ceftriaxone, or ceftazidime) that cross the blood-brain barrier reasonably well, or we must use high concentrations of parenteral doses of drugs such as penicillin G, ampicillin, or nafcillin that penetrate into the cerebrospinal fluid only with difficulty. Agents such as the aminoglycosidic aminocyclitols and first-generation cephalosporins that produce inadequate cerebrospinal fluid levels even after high-dose parenteral therapy must be administered directly into the cerebrospinal fluid or must be avoided entirely.

The vegetations of bacterial endocarditis, bones, and devitalized tissue represent examples of other areas in which the penetration of antimicrobial agents to the site of infection may be borderline or inadequate. Because of this, high-dose and prolonged parenteral therapy is usually required for the effective treatment of bacterial endocarditis and osteomyelitis. In some cases, we may take advantage of the physiologic handling of antimicrobials to achieve therapeutic success. Agents that are excreted by the liver and are concentrated in the bile such as ampicillin or doxycycline may be more effective in treating cholangitis than are agents such as the first-generation cephalosporins or aminoglycosidic aminocyclitols that are not greatly concentrated in bile. The new fluoroquinolones may owe some of their effectiveness in the treatment of osteomyelitis to their ability to achieve superior concentrations in bone.[71] Likewise, these agents penetrate far more effectively into the prostate than the β-lactams or aminoglycosides, and this undoubtedly accounts for their superior therapeutic efficacy in prostatitis.[72, 73]

Even the achievement of "therapeutic concentrations" of antimicrobial agents at the site of infection may not be sufficient for cure. The reason for this is that a number of local factors may influence the activity of antimicrobial agents. These, too, must be considered in designing an appropriate therapeutic regimen. Aminoglycosidic aminocyclitols and the polymyxins are bound to and inactivated by purulent material.[74] This is one of many reasons why surgical drainage is imperative when treating abscesses with agents such as these. Interestingly, carbenicillin does not lose activity in pus.[74] Although carbenicillin (and other penicillins) may be more active in purulent material, clinical experience strongly suggests that appropriate drainage procedures greatly enhance the efficacy of these agents as well. Although penicillin G, like carbenicillin, is not inactivated by purulent material per se,[65] recent studies suggest that the presence of β-lactamase–producing organisms such as *Bacteroides fragilis* in abscesses may result in local inactivation of penicillin G and other β-lactam antibiotics.[75]

Pencillins and tetracyclines are also bound by hemoglobin and thus may be less effective in the presence of significant hematoma formation.[65] In vitro *Pseudomonas aeruginosa* is protected from the action of the aminoglycosidic aminocyclitols and polymyxins by high concentrations of calcium or magnesium in the culture medium.[76] The clinical significance of this observation, if any, remains to be determined. Local decreases in oxygen tension such as occur in abscesses and intraperitoneal infections may also have an effect on the activity of certain antimicrobial agents. The aminoglycosidic aminocyclitols, for example, are inactive against anaerobes and may also be less effective against facultative organisms under anaerobic conditions because oxygen is required for the transport of these agents into the bacterial cell.[77]

Local alterations in pH such as occur in abscesses and especially in the urine may have an important effect on the activity of a number of antimicrobial agents. Methenamine, nitrofurantoin, novobiocin, and chlortetracycline are more active at an acid pH, whereas alkalinization enhances the activity of erythromycin, azithromycin, dirythromycin, clarithromycin, lincomycin, clindamycin, and the aminoglycosidic aminocyclitol antibiotics. Indeed, the aminoglycosidic aminocyclitols show a marked loss of activity at a low pH. These observations have occasionally been used to advantage in treating patients with urinary tract infections, a situation in which the local pH can be altered by the addition of acidifying or alkalinizing agents.[78, 79]

The presence of foreign bodies also has a profound effect on the activity of antimicrobial agents. Thus, it is often necessary to remove the foreign material to cure an infection in the vicinity of a prosthetic heart valve or joint implant.[80] The mechanism by which foreign bodies potentiate infection is not clear, but they probably cause localized impairment of host defense mechanisms.[81] In addition, the foreign body often serves as a nidus on which organisms can adhere and produce extracellular substances such as glycocalyx or slime that may interfere with phagocytosis and impair the penetration of antibiotics to the underlying organisms.[82] It has also been demonstrated that antimicrobial agents themselves may cause alterations in host defenses. Clinically achievable concentrations of many different agents have been shown to have adverse effects on leukocyte chemotaxis, lymphocyte transformation, monocyte transformation, delayed hypersensitivity, antibody production, phagocytosis, and the microbicidal action of polymorphonuclear leukocytes.[83–89] It is not clear, however, whether any of these effects (largely demonstrated by in vitro studies) are of clinical significance.[89] Nonetheless, the possibility that antimicrobial agents can cause immunosuppression exists, and this fact should discourage the indiscriminate use of antibiotics, especially in patients who are already immunosuppressed because of their underlying disease or because of their concomitant drug therapy.[87] Finally, antimicrobial agents such as the β-lactams that cause rapid lysis of bacteria may also release endotoxins or cell wall components that have potentially deleterious local or systemic effects or both in the host. The local inflammatory consequences of such activity have been clearly defined in experimental models of bacterial meningitis,[90] but their significance in other settings such as gram-negative sepsis remains to be determined.[91]

ANTIMICROBIAL COMBINATIONS

Most infections in humans with normal host defenses can be treated with a single antimicrobial agent, but there are clear-cut (as well as borderline) indications for the use of combinations (usually two) of antimicrobials. Because combinations may provide more broad-spectrum coverage than single agents can, the physician is often tempted to use combinations for the sense of security they provide, even in situations in which they are not indicated. Such inappropriate use of antimicrobial combinations may have significantly deleterious effects. In this section, we examine indications for the use of combinations and the potential disadvantages of this approach to therapy. Although we consider briefly the use of combination therapy in neutropenic patients, this discussion does not attempt to deal with combination therapy in severely immunocompromised patients such as those undergoing organ transplantation or those with severe immunodeficiency states such as occur in patients with human immunodeficiency virus infections. In these settings, under specialized circumstances, clinicians are often forced to use broad-spectrum combinations of antibacterial, antiviral, antifungal, and even, at times, antiparasitic agents.

In Vitro Results of Combination Therapy

When two antimicrobial agents are combined, they may have one of three types of activity against a given organism in vitro: (1) an additive effect (sometimes called an *indifferent effect*), (2) synergism, or (3) antagonism.[92] Two drugs are said to be additive when the activity of the drugs in combination is equal to the sum (or a partial sum) of their independent activities when studied separately. The combined effect of a synergistic pair of antimicrobials is greater than the sum of their independent activities when measured separately. If two drugs are antagonistic, the activity of the combination is less than the sum of their independent effects when measured alone. These concepts are illustrated by "time-kill curves" in Figure 15–1. The various methods useds to determine the in vitro effects of antibiotic combinations are beyond the scope of this chapter but have been reviewed in detail.[93]

Indications for the Clinical Use of Antimicrobial Combinations

Five reasons have been advanced to justify the use of antimicrobial combinations. The first three of these are discussed in detail in other chapters and, therefore, are given only brief mention here.

Prevention of the Emergence of Resistant Organisms. Although the use of antimicrobial agents to prevent the emergence of resistant organisms would seem to be a major indication for the use of such therapy, combination therapy has been clearly documented as effective in preventing resistance only during the treatment of tuberculosis (see Chapters 16 and 240). There is somewhat less epidemiologic evidence in support of this concept as it applies to the use of rifampin for the treatment of nonmycobacterial infections, but it nonetheless appears that one of the major benefits of using rifampin in combination with a second agent for treating staphylococcal infections, for example, is that the combination prevents the rapid emergence of resistance to rifampin, which is evident when this drug is used alone.[94, 95] The effectiveness of combinations of rifampin and a fluoroquinolone for staphylococcal infections of prosthetic implants is likely due in part to the fact that the combination prevents the emergence of resistance to each of the drugs if used alone.[96]

Polymicrobial Infections. In most infections, even those due to more than one organism, a single effective agent can be found. For example, cellulitis due to *S. aureus* and group A streptococci can be treated with a penicillinase-resistant penicillin alone. However, there are certain types of infections due to such a broad variety of organisms that more than one antimicrobial agent may be required to provide adequate coverage. Examples of such infections include intraperitoneal and pelvic infections due to mixed aerobic and anaerobic organisms. However, many of the newer carbapenems and β-lactam–β-lactamase inhibitor combinations have such broad spectra of activity that they can be employed effectively as "monotherapy" for intra-abdominal and pelvic sepsis.[97, 98]

Initial Therapy. In neutropenic patients or other patients with presumed infection in whom the nature of the infection is not clear, it may be reasonable to begin broad-spectrum coverage, usually with two agents such as ticarcillin plus gentamicin or tobramycin while awaiting the results of cultures. In this setting, it is often possible to switch to a single drug after the results of cultures are available (see Chapters 299 and 300). The development of new drugs with broad spectra of activity makes it possible to use a single agent for most cases of initial therapy, but it would be premature to advocate a universal application of this concept at present.[99]

Decreased Toxicity. Many of the drugs used in therapy for infections are potentially toxic (e.g., aminoglycosidic aminocyclitols). Therefore, a major goal of combination therapy has been to reduce the amount of drug required for treatment and, thus, to reduce dose-related toxicity. Unfortunately, at present there are no data from clinical trials that establish beyond doubt that combination therapy with different agents permits a reduction of the drug dose sufficient to reduce dose-related toxicity.

Synergism. The use of synergistic combinations of antimicrobial agents to treat infections due to resistant or relatively resistant organ-

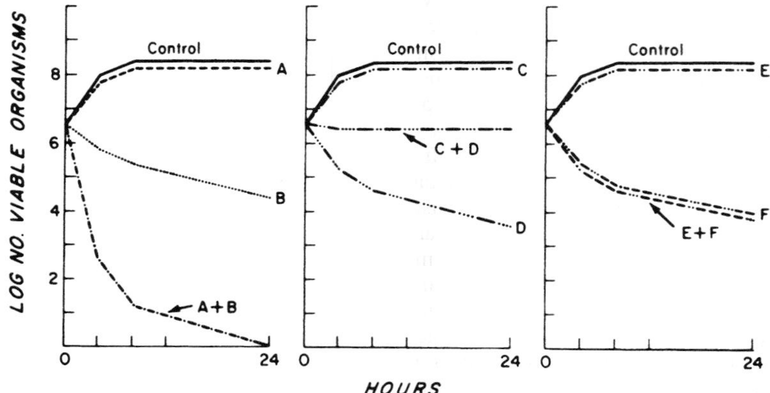

FIGURE 15–1. Antibacterial effects of antibiotic combinations. *Left* (A and B): synergism; *center* (C and D): antagonism; *right* (E and F): indifference (additive). (From Moellering RC Jr. Use and abuse of antibiotic combinations. R I Med J. 1972; 55:341.)

isms represents one of the most appealing ways to use these agents. There are numerous examples of in vitro synergism, but thus far synergistic antimicrobial combinations have proved more effective than are single agents in only a limited number of clinical settings.[100, 101]

Perhaps the best known application of synergistic combinations of antimicrobial agents is for the treatment of enterococcal endocarditis. Treatment of this disease with penicillin alone results in an unacceptable relapse rate because enterococci are relatively resistant to penicillin.[102] Indeed, penicillin alone seems to act as a bacteriostatic and not a bactericidal agent.[103] The addition of an aminoglycoside such as streptomycin or gentamicin results in both in vitro and in vivo synergism and yields clinical cure rates comparable to those achieved for endocarditis caused by less resistant streptococci.[102, 103] Penicillin enhances the uptake of aminoglycosides by enterococci; the result of this interaction is the synergistic killing of the organisms.[104] In recent years some enterococci have been found to be resistant to penicillin-streptomycin, penicillin-kanamycin, and penicillin-amikacin synergism due to high-level resistance (MIC>2000 μg/ml) to streptomycin, to kanamycin, or to both.[105] Strains may resist synergism if they are ribosomally resistant to streptomycin[106] or if they contain plasmid-mediated enzymes that inactivate streptomycin, kanamycin, gentamicin, or amikacin.[107] The prevalence of enterococci with high-level resistance to gentamicin appears to be increasing rapidly.[108–110] Moreover, the use of penicillin-gentamicin therapy in such patients may result in a failure to eradicate the infecting organisms.[111] Therefore, it is important to test for high-level resistance to streptomycin and gentamicin before embarking on a therapeutic regimen for enterococcal endocarditis or meningitis.

Penicillin-streptomycin combinations are also synergistic against viridans streptococci and have been used for the treatment of endocarditis due to these organisms.[101] However, viridans streptococci are usually very susceptible to penicillin, and penicillin alone has been used successfully for treatment of this kind of endocarditis.[112, 113]

A similar type of synergism occurs when semisynthetic penicillinase-resistant penicillins such as nafcillin or oxacillin are combined with gentamicin against *S. aureus*.[114] Thus far there are no data to document that the use of combination therapy for *S. aureus* infections in humans has any advantage over therapy with a penicillin or cephalosporin alone.[115]

Combinations of carbenicillin, ticarcillin, mezlocillin, azlocillin, or piperacillin with gentamicin, tobramycin, or amikacin exhibit synergism against many strains of *P. aeruginosa*.[116, 117] The mechanism of synergism in this setting is similar to that described for enterococci (i.e., enhanced uptake of the aminoglycoside in the presence of the antipseudomonal penicillin). Studies with experimental animals demonstrate convincingly the superiority of such combinations for the treatment of serious *Pseudomonas* infections.[118] Although the information available from limited human trials to date is also consistent with enhanced activity of these combinations for *Pseudomonas* infections, this form of therapy has not been subjected to definitive controlled study.[93] A large prospective (but uncontrolled) study of patients with *Pseudomonas* bacteremia documented an increased survival in patients who received antimicrobial combinations compared with those who received single-drug therapy. Interestingly, the presence or absence of synergism seemed less important than administration of combination therapy in this population.[119]

Synergism occurs by a different mechanism when sulfonamides are combined with trimethoprim. In this case, the two agents are synergistic because they act to inhibit sequential steps in the microbial pathway of folic acid metabolism.[120] As a result, combinations of sulfonamides with trimethoprim are often useful for the treatment of infections due to organisms that may be resistant to sulfonamides alone. A fixed combination of sulfamethoxazole and trimethoprim is available for clinical use and has been shown to be effective for the treatment and prevention of chronic urinary tract infections, even when due to sulfonamide-resistant organisms.[121] The combination has also been shown to be useful for the treatment of typhoid fever and shigellosis caused by organisms resistant to ampicillin, chloramphenicol, or both; for the treatment of infections due to ampicillin-resistant *H. influenzae*; and for therapy for a wide variety of other infections as well.[93, 122–124]

Combinations of amphotericin B with a number of other agents including 5-fluorocytosine, rifampin, and tetracycline have been shown to result in enhanced in vitro antimicrobial activity against fungi.[125] The mechanism of synergism seems to involve damage to the fungal cell envelope by amphotericin B, with resultant enhanced intracellular penetration of 5-fluorocytosine and other agents.[125] Flucytosine and low-dose amphotericin B have been used successfully in treating candidiasis and cryptococcosis when the patient's isolate was susceptible to both drugs.[124, 127]

Synergism and Infections in Impaired Hosts. The clinical applications of antimicrobial combinations discussed thus far have all represented attempts to use a synergistic interaction for enhanced efficacy in the treatment of infections due to relatively resistant organisms. Another use of such therapy is to obtain enhanced antimicrobial activity in the treatment of infections due to susceptible organisms occurring in patients with abnormalities of host defense systems. Several groups have conducted randomized trials of various combinations of two agents chosen from among carbenicillin, ticarcillin, piperacillin, the cephalosporins, gentamicin, tobramycin, and amikacin for the treatment of severe infections in patients with impaired host defense mechanisms. Both Lau and colleagues[128] and Klastersky and associates[129] have demonstrated improved survival rates in patients treated with combinations that were synergistic against the infecting organisms compared with patients who received nonsynergistic combinations. These studies add strong support to the concept that synergistic combinations of antimicrobials may be an important determinant of success in the treatment of serious infections, especially when the infections are caused by gram-negative organisms in patients with impaired host defenses. However, there is no absolute proof that synergistic combinations are more effective in this setting than are single agents that have a sufficiently broad spectrum and that produce sufficiently high serum bactericidal titers against the infecting organisms.[130]

Disadvantages of the Inappropriate Use of Antimicrobial Combinations

Whereas the clinical use of synergistic combinations of antimicrobial agents may have beneficial results as noted earlier, the inappropriate use of antimicrobial combinations may have important adverse effects, three of which are discussed here.

Antagonism. The medical literature contains a large number of reports of in vitro antagonism between antimicrobial agents.[100, 101] In view of this, it is surprising that there are only a few well-documented clinical examples of antagonism. Perhaps the most impressive is the study of Lepper and Dowling,[131] who demonstrated conclusively in 1951 that penicillin is more effective than is the combination of penicillin with chlortetracycline for the treatment of pneumococcal meningitis. The fatality among patients treated with penicillin alone was 21%, whereas that among patients treated with penicillin plus chlortetracycline was 79%. A study of childhood meningitis has also demonstrated the superiority of single-drug therapy. Mathies and associates[132] treated a group of children suffering from bacterial meningitis with either ampicillin alone or a combination of ampicillin, chloramphenicol, and streptomycin. The mortality among 140 children treated with ampicillin alone was 4.3%, whereas the mortality among 124 children receiving the antibiotic combination was 10.5%, a difference that reached statistical significance. There are several other reports of the influence of antagonism on the treatment of urinary tract infections and streptococcal pharyngitis, but none is particularly impressive.[100] Considering the extensive clinical use of antimicrobial combinations and especially in view of the large number of reports of in vitro antagonism, it is surprising that there are so few reports of in vivo antagonism. This may be due in part to the paucity of well-controlled studies in this area or to the reluctance of investigators to report adverse results. Another possible explanation is simply that clinically significant antagonism is not a common event. In most cases, in vitro antagonism results in the loss or partial loss of activity of the most active drug (e.g., the bactericidal activity of such an agent may be reduced to simple bacteriostasis), but the combination still retains some antimicrobial activity. As long as the patient receiving such therapy has normal host defense mechanisms, it is unlikely that adverse effects will be seen. This has been the case in studies using an antagonistic combination of antibiotics (chloramphenicol plus gentamicin) to treat experimental infections due to *Proteus mirabilis* in mice.[133] In healthy mice, in vivo antagonism could not be demonstrated, but after irradiation to render the animals neutropenic, gentamicin alone was more effective than gentamicin plus chloramphenicol. This combination has also been shown to be antagonistic in experimentally produced meningitis due to *P. mirabilis* in rabbits.[134] Thus, it seems that clinically important antagonism is most likely to be manifested in patients with generalized impairment of host defense mechanisms (e.g., in leukemia patients and cancer patients who are neutropenic) or in patients with infections such as meningitis or endocarditis in whom localized host defenses may be inadequate.

The observation of in vivo antagonism in the treatment of bacterial meningitis raised some questions about the recommendations of the use of ampicillin plus chloramphenicol in the initial treatment of childhood meningitis (see Chapter 71), with the initial emergence of ampicillin-resistant strains of *H. influenzae*.[12] Combinations of penicillin plus chloramphenicol were shown to exhibit in vitro antagonism against pneumococci and other organisms.[101] However, this antagonism takes the form of lessened bactericidal activity of penicillin in the presence of chloramphenicol. Because chloramphenicol alone is quite active against the organisms likely to cause childhood meningitis (*H. influenzae, S. pneumoniae, Neisseria meningitidis*) and because there is no evidence that penicillin or ampicillin antagonizes the activity of chloramphenicol, it is not surprising that the use of ampicillin-chloramphenicol therapy for pediatric meningitis did not result in in vivo antagonism when used to treat the organisms listed previously.[101] Moreover, studies documenting the effectiveness of cephalosporins such as cefotaxime and ceftriaxone[135, 136] for childhood meningitis make it unnecessary to continue to use combination therapy in this setting, as does the fact that use of the *H. influenzae* vaccine has virtually eliminated *H. influenzae* as a cause of childhood meningitis in Western countries.

Broad-spectrum β-lactams have been used in combination to obtain broad-spectrum coverage without exposing the patient to the possible toxicity of an agent such as chloramphenicol or an aminoglycosidic aminocyclitol.[137] In some cases, this seems reasonable. However, there is in vitro and in vivo evidence that some β-lactam–β-lactam combinations may be antagonistic against certain organisms such as *Enterobacter*, *Serratia*, or *Pseudomonas*. This antagonism seems to be the result of the induction or derepression of chromosomally mediated β-lactamases by one of the agents, leading to inactivation of the second.[138] The exact clinical significance of this phenomenon is not clear at present, but it must be kept in mind when one considers the clinical use of such combinations. Again, the development of the newest broad-spectrum cephalosporins and β-lactam–β-lactamase inhibitor combinations now renders most earlier combinations obsolete.[99]

Most of the examples of in vitro antagonism are the result of interactions of the antimicrobial agents as they act at a subcellular level on a given microorganism. However, another type of antagonism should also be included in this discussion. This may result from the direct interaction of drugs before they reach the microorganism. If chloramphenicol and erythromycin are inadvertently mixed together in the same parenteral infusion solution, they form insoluble precipitates and hence lose activity. The mixing of penicillins (especially carbenicillin or ticarcillin) with aminoglycosides results in the inactivation of the aminoglycoside.[139] Because the reaction occurs slowly, this is usually not a problem in vivo, provided the drugs are given by separate routes of administration. However, in uremic patients in whom the serum half-life of aminoglycosides is greatly prolonged, in vivo inactivation can occur.[140] The clinical significance of this observation, however, has not yet been elucidated.

Cost. With the possible exception of penicillin G, ampicillin, and certain of the tetracyclines and sulfonamides, antimicrobials are expensive drugs. Thus, the inappropriate use of antimicrobial combinations (when a single agent would be adequate) can add greatly to the cost of the patient's illness.

Adverse Effects. It has been estimated that approximately 5% of the patients receiving an antibiotic in the hospital will experience some sort of adverse reaction that leads to excess length of stay, extra costs, and an almost twofold increased risk of death.[21, 141, 142] Obviously the possibility of such adverse reactions (including hypersensitivity reactions and direct toxic effects) is increased without any enhanced therapeutic benefit when one uses combinations of antimicrobial agents inappropriately. Moreover, when an adverse reaction occurs in a patient receiving more than one drug, it is often difficult to be certain of the agent that caused the reaction. This may mean that treatment with several or all drugs must be stopped. If combination drug therapy is to be used in such a patient, each drug must be tested carefully before use to make certain that it was not the cause of the original adverse reaction. This is time consuming and expensive and may needlessly deprive the patient of the benefits of a useful agent.

CHOICE OF APPROPRIATE ROUTE OF ADMINISTRATION OF ANTIMICROBIAL AGENTS AND EVALUATION OF EFFICACY

Route of Administration

Once the physician has determined the most appropriate drug or drugs with which to treat a given infection, he or she must decide which route of administration to use to obtain maximum benefits from the therapy. In most cases this is a choice between oral and parenteral routes. In general, the oral route of administration is chosen for infections that are mild and can be treated on an outpatient basis. Not all antibiotics can be administered in this way. Drugs such as vancomycin, the polymyxins, the aminoglycosidic aminocyclitols, and amphotericin B are absorbed so poorly form the gastrointestinal tract that they cannot be administered orally to treat systemic infections. When drugs are administered by the oral route, the physician must ascertain that the patient will take them as ordered. The absorption of certain agents such as penicillin G is markedly impaired if taken with meals, whereas the absorption of acid-stable penicillins such as penicillin V is not affected by food or gastric acidity. The concomitant administration of antacids or iron-containing preparations may severely impair the absorption of tetracycline, because this drug forms insoluble chelates in the presence of Mg^{2+}, Ca^{2+}, or Fe^{2+} ions. Antacids and histamine antagonists may also interfere with the absorption of the fluoroquinolones.[143] More detailed information on the oral absorption of antimicrobial agents may be found in the chapters on the individual drugs.

The parenteral route of administration is used for agents that are inefficiently absorbed from the gastrointestinal tract and for the treatment of patients with serious infections in whom higher serum concentrations of antimicrobial agents than can be reliably obtained by the oral route are required. The aminoglycosidic aminocyclitols and polymyxins may be given by intramuscular injection and are well tolerated when given this way. For most infections, adequate serum concentrations are achieved after the intramuscular administration of these drugs.

In life-threatening infections, however, especially in the presence of shock (or in diabetic patients as discussed earlier), intravenous administration is preferred. Intravenous administration allows large doses of drugs to be given with a minimum of discomfort to the patient when high serum concentrations are required for the effective treatment of disease processes such as meningitis, endocarditis, and osteomyelitis.

Whether intravenously administered drugs should be given by continuous infusion or by intermittent bolus infusion remains a matter of controversy. The former method has the advantage of simplicity; because pulses containing very high concentrations of drugs are avoided, it may result in less venous irritation and phlebitis. Studies in animal models suggest that the concentration of drugs such as penicillins and cephalosporins in fibrin clots is related to the peak serum levels achieved. Thus, greater concentrations of drugs are achieved in the clots in the face of intermittent bolus therapy.[144] It has been suggested that these data may be applicable to therapy for infective endocarditis and other infections in which high tissue concentrations of antibiotics are required. More recent evidence, however, strongly suggests that the clinical effectiveness of β-lactam antibiotics is optimal when the concentration of the antimicrobial agent at the site of infection exceeds the MIC of the infecting organism for a prolonged period of time. Because it is easier to maintain such concentrations persistently above the MIC by continuous infusion, these studies lend support to the concept of administering β-lactam antibiotics by continuous infusion for serious systemic infections.[145] On the other hand, antimicrobial agents such as the aminoglycosides exhibit concentration-dependent killing (which is not seen with the β-lactams), and, for this reason, giving these drugs by once-a-day bolus infusion is attractive from a pharmacodynamic point of view.[146] Thus, the high peak levels obtained after bolus dosing cause more rapid killing of the infecting pathogen. Once-a-day dosing of aminoglycosides also leads to lower (or absent) trough levels, which may be advantageous in terms of potential toxicity.[146]

As discussed earlier, the intrathecal or intraventricular route of administration may be necessary for the treatment of meningeal infections with drugs such as the aminoglycosidic aminocyclitols, polymyxins, bacitracin, and possibly vancomycin, all of which cross the blood-brain barrier with considerable difficulty. The parenteral administration of antimicrobial agents results in adequate concentrations in pleural, peritoneal, pericardial, and synovial fluids.[147, 148] Thus, direct instillation of antibiotics into these areas is not necessary.

Monitoring the Response of the Patient to Antimicrobial Therapy

Although several laboratory tests are available to assist in the monitoring of antimicrobial therapy, clinical assessment remains the most important method for determining the efficacy of treatment. It is not uncommon to see patients fail to respond in the face of laboratory studies that suggest adequate therapy is being given and vice versa. The reasons for this may usually be found among the many host factors that affect therapy as described earlier.

Nonetheless, the measurement of serum concentrations of antimicrobial agents and the determination of serum bactericidal titers may be of considerable use in certain circumstances. The major value of the direct determination of serum concentrations of antimicrobial agents is to avoid toxicity from excessive levels of agents such as the aminoglycosidic aminocyclitols, especially in patients with impaired renal or hepatic function. These tests are also useful for determining inadequate serum levels due to insufficient dosing or unusually rapid clearance.

Another method used to monitor the effectiveness of antimicrobial therapy is the serum bactericidal titer (sometimes called the *serum antimicrobial dilution titer*). This test was originally described by Schlichter and MacLean[149] as a guide for effective therapy for subacute bacterial endocarditis. Subsequently this test has been used to monitor therapy in patients with infective endocarditis, osteomyelitis, septic arthritis, empyema, and bacteremia.[129, 150] In this test, serial dilutions of the patient's serum are incubated with an inoculum of the infecting organism; after incubation, the highest dilution that inhibits or kills the organism, or both, is determined. Some investigators feel that a serum bactericidal titer of at least 1:8 can be correlated with a successful therapeutic outcome.[129, 149, 151, 152] A multicenter study has suggested that peak and trough titers of at least 1:64 and 1:32, respectively, are good predictors of a successful therapeutic outcome in patients with infective endocarditis.[153] However, a lack of standardization and a lack of consistency in specifying the point (peak, trough, or midpoint serum levels) at which the test should be done have hindered attempts at more widespread application and evaluation of this test.[154–157]

CONCLUSION

Optimal use of antimicrobial agents demands consideration of a large number of important factors that may influence the choice of an appropriate agent and that determine the most effective dose and route of administration of a drug. A number of these factors have been outlined in this chapter. In the final analysis, sound clinical judgment remains the most important determinant of a successful outcome.

REFERENCES

1. Weinstein L. General considerations. In: Goodman LS, Gilman A, eds. The Pharmacological Basis of Therapeutics. New York: Macmillan; 1970:1154.
2. Majno G. The Healing Hand: Man and Wound in the Ancient World. Cambridge: Harvard University Press; 1975:154, 215.
3. Harris JC, Dupont HL, Hornick RB. Fecal leukocytes in diarrheal illness. Ann Intern Med. 1972;76:697.
4. Ho D, Ault MJ, Ault MA, et al. *Campylobacter* enteritis. Early diagnosis with Gram's stain. Arch Intern Med. 1982;142:1858.
5. Zipeto D, Revello MG, Silini E, et al. Development and clinical significance of a diagnostic assay based on the polymerase chain reaction for detection of human cytomegalovirus DNA in blood samples from immunocompromised patients. J Clin Microbiol. 1992;30:527.
6. Peter J. The polymerase chain reaction: Amplifying our options. Rev Infect Dis. 1991;13:166.
7. Desmond EP. Molecular approaches to the identification of mycobacteria. Clin Microbiol Newslett. 1992;14:145.
8. Weinstein L. Common sense (clinical judgment) in the diagnosis and antibiotic therapy of etiologically undefined infections. Pediatr Clin North Am. 1968;15:141.
9. Moellering RC Jr. A rational approach to the choice of antimicrobial agents in bacterial infections. In: Seminar on Gram-Negative Infections. St Louis: CV Mosby;1974;5.
10. Huang MB, Baker CN, Bannerjee S, Tenover FC. Accuracy of the E test for determining antimicrobial susceptibility of staphylococci, enterococci, *Campylobacter jejuni*, and gram-negative bacteria resistant to antimicrobial agents. J Clin Microbiol. 1992;30:3243.
11. Jorgensen JH. Antibacterial susceptibility tests: Automated or instrument-based methods. In: Balows A, Hausler WJ Jr, Herrmann KL, et al., eds. Manual of Clinical Microbiology. Washington, DC: American Society for Microbiology 1991:1166.
12. Murray BE, Moellering RC, Jr. Patterns and mechanisms of antibiotic resistance. Med Clin North Am. 1978;62:899.
13. Gold HS, Moellering RC Jr. Antimicrobial drug resistance. N Engl J Med. 1996;335:1445.
14. Levy SB. Active efflux mechanisms for antimicrobial resistance. Antimicrob Agents Chemother. 1992;36:695.
15. Ruoff KL. Gram-positive vancomycin-resistant clinical isolates. Clin Microbiol Newslett. 1989;11:1.
16. Moellering RC Jr. Vancomycin-resistant enterococci. Clin Infec Dis. 1998;26:1196.
17. Moellering RC Jr, Kunz LJ, Poitras JW, et al. Microbiologic basis for the rational use of antibiotics, South Med J. 1977;70 (Suppl):8.
18. Abramowicz M, ed. The choice of antibacterial drugs. Med Lett. 1998; 40:33
19. Weinstein L, Dalton AC. Host determinants of response to antimicrobial agents. N Engl J Med. 1968;279:467.
20. Moellering RC Jr. Factors influencing the clinical use of antimicrobial agents in elderly patients. Geriatrics. 1978;33:83.
21. Mannisto PT, Mantyla R, Nykanen S, et al. Impairing effect of food on ketoconazole absorption. Antimicrob Agents Chemother. 1982;21:730.
22. Jackson GG, Arcieri G. Ototoxicity of gentamicin in man: A survey and controlled analysis of clinical experience in the United States. J Infect Dis. 1969;119:432.
23. Calderwood S, Moellering RC Jr. Common adverse effects of antibacterial agents on major organ systems. Surg Clin North Am. 1980;60:65.

24. Moellering RC Jr. Antimicrobial agents in pregnancy and the postpartum period. Clin Obstet Gynecol. 1989;22:277.
25. McCracken GH Jr. Pharmacologic basis for antimicrobial therapy in newborn infants. Am J Dis Child. 1974;128:407.
26. Kline AH, Blattner RJ, Lunin M. Transplacental effect of tetracyclines on teeth. JAMA. 1964;118:178.
27. Hoyer D, Walfson J. Adverse effects of quinolone antibiotics. In: Hooper D, Wolfson J, eds. Quinolone Antimicrobial Agents. Washington, DC: American Society for Microbiology; 1989:249–271.
28. Ball P. The quinolones: History and overview. In: Andriole VT, ed. The Quinolones. San Diego, Calif: Academic Press; 1998:2.
29. Garibaldi RA, Druish RE, Ferebee SH, et al. Isoniazid-associated hepatitis. Am Rev Respir Dis. 1972;106:357.
30. Rose DN, Schechter CB, Silver AL. The age threshold for isoniazid chemoprophylaxis. JAMA. 1986;256:2709.
31. Salpeter SR, Sanders GD, Salpeter EE, et al. Monitored isoniazid prophylaxis for low-risk tuberculin reactors older than 35 years of age: A risk-benefit and cost effectiveness analysis. Ann Intern Med. 1997;127:1051.
32. Foord RD. Cephaloridine, cephalothin and the kidney. J Antimicrob Chemother. 1975;1(Suppl):119.
33. Koch-Weser J, Sidel VW, Federman EB, et al. Adverse effects of sodium colistimethate. Ann Intern Med. 1970;72:857.
34. Van Scoy RE. Antituberculous agents. Mayo Clin Proc. 1977;52:694.
35. Young DS, Thomas DW, Friedman RB, et al. Effects of drugs on clinical laboratory tests. Clin Chem. 1972;18:1041.
36. Hamod KA, Khouzami VA. Antibiotics in pregnancy. In: Nietyl JR, ed. Drug Use in Pregnancy. Philadelphia: Lea & Febiger; 1982:31.
37. Meyer JM, Rodvold KA. Antimicrobials during pregnancy. Infect Med. 1995;12:420.
38. Ticarcillin. Med Lett. 1977;19:17.
39. Is Flagyl dangerous? Med Lett. 1975;17:53.
40. Conway N. Birt BD. Streptomycin in pregnancy: Effect in foetal ear. BMJ. 1965:2:260.
41. Monnet P, Kalb JC, Pujol M. Toxic influence of isoniazid on fetus. Lyon Med. 1967;218:431.
42. Philipson A. Pharmakokinetics of ampicillin during pregnancy. J Infect Dis. 1977;136:370.
43. Vorherr H. Drug excretion in breast milk. Postgrad Med. 1974;56:97.
44. Reeves DS. The effect of renal failure on the pharmacokinetics of antibiotics. J Antimicrob Chemother. 1988;21:5.
45. Jackson EA, McLeod DC. Pharmacokinetics and dosing of antimicrobial agents in renal impairment, part i. Am J Hosp Pharm. 1974;31:36.
46. Jackson EA, McLeod DC. Pharmacokinetics and dosing of antimicrobial agents in renal impairment, part ii. Am J Hosp Pharm. 1974;31:137.
47. Moellering RC Jr, Eliopoulos GM. Principles of anti-infective therapy. In: Stein JH, ed. Internal Medicine. St. Louis: CV Mosby; 1998:1343.
48. Bennett WM, Aronoff GR, Morrison G, et al. Drug prescribing in renal failure: Dosing guidelines for adults. Am J Kidney Dis. 1983;3:155.
49. Cooper K, Bennett WM. Nephrotoxicity of common drugs used in clinical practice. Arch Intern Med. 1987;147:1213.
50. Natelson EA, Brown CH III, Bradshaw MW, et al. Influence of cephalosporin antibiotics on blood coagulation and platelet function. Antimicrob Agents Chemother. 1976;9:91.
51. Neu HC. Adverse effects of new cephalosporins. Ann Intern Med. 1983;98:415.
52. Kaufman CA, Frame PT. Bone marrow toxicity associated with 5-fluorocytosine therapy. Antimicrob Agents Chemother. 1977;11:244.
53. Davey PG. Pharmacokinetics in liver disease. J Antimicrob Chemother. 1988;21:1.
54. Suhrland LG, Weisberger AS. Chloramphenicol toxicity in liver and renal disease. Arch Intern Med. 1963;112:747.
55. Pessayre D, Allemand H, Benhamou J-P. Effets des maladies du foie et des voies biliaires sur le métabolisme des médicaments. Nouv Presse Med. 1977;35:3209.
56. Singh N, Yu VL, Mieles LA, et al. β-Lactam antibiotic–induced leukopenia in severe hepatic dysfunction: Risk factors and implications for dosing in patients with liver disease. Am J Med. 1993;94:251.
57. Lorian V, Atkinson B. Killing of oxacillin-exposed staphylococci in human polymorphonuclear leukocytes. Antimicrob Agents Chemother. 1980;18:807.
58. Ofek IE, Beachey H, Eisenstein BI, et al. Suppression of bacterial adherence by subminimal inhibitory concentration of β-lactam and aminoglycoside antibiotics. Rev Infect Dis. 1979;1:832.
59. Gemmell CG, Peterson PK, Schmeling DJ, et al. Potentiation of opsonization and phagocytosis of *Streptococcus pyogenes* following growth in the presence of clindamycin. J Clin Invest. 1981;67:1249.
60. Friedman HH, Warren GH. Enhanced susceptibility of penicillin-resistant staphylococci to phagocytosis after in vitro incubation with low dose of nafcillin. Proc Soc Exp Biol Med. 1974;146:707.
61. Elliott GR, Peterson PK, Verburg HA, et al. Influence of subinhibitory concentrations of penicillin, cephalothin, and clindamycin on *Staphylococcus aureus* growth in human phagocytic cells. Antimicrob Agents Chemother. 1982;22:781.
62. Moellering RC Jr. Revolutionary changes in the macrolide and azalide antibiotics. Am J Med 1991;91:1s.
63. Smith CR. The spiramycin paradox. J Antimicrob Chemother. 1988;22(Suppl B):141.
64. Foulds G, Johnson RB. Selection of dose regimens of azithromycin. J Antimicrob Chemother. 1993;31(Suppl E):39.
65. Craig WA, Kunin CM. Significance of serum protein and tissue binding of antimicrobial agents. Annu Rev Med. 1976;27:287.
66. Peterson LR, Gerding DN. Interaction of cephalosporins with human and canine serum proteins. J Infect Dis. 1978;137:452.
67. Barza M, Samuelson T, Weinstein L. Penetration of antibiotics into fibrin loci in vivo. II. Comparison of nine antibiotics: Effect of dose and degree of protein binding. J Infect Dis. 1974;129:66.
68. Kunst MW, Mattie H. Cefazolin and cephradine. Relationship between antibacterial activity in vitro and in mice experimentally infected with *Escherichia coli*. J Infect Dis. 1978;137:391.
69. Merrikin DJ, Briant J, Rolinson GN. Effect of protein binding on antibiotic activity in vivo. J Antimicrob Chemother. 1983;11:233.
70. Kaiser AB, McGee ZA. Aminoglycoside therapy of gram-negative bacillary meningitis. N Engl J Med. 1975;293:1215.
71. Lew D, Waldvogel FW. Use of quinolones for treatment of osteomyelitis and septic arthritis. In: Hooper D, Wolfson J, eds. Quinolone Antimicrobial Agents. 2nd ed. Washington, DC: American Society for Microbiology; 1993;371–379.
72. Naber KG. The role of quinolones in the treatment of chronic bacterial prostatitis. In: Hooper D, Wolfson J, eds. Quinolone Antimicrobial Agents. 2nd ed. Washington, DC: American Society for Microbiology; 1993:285.
73. Nicolle L. Use of quinolones in urinary tract infection and prostatitis. In: Andriole VT, ed. The Quinolones. 2nd ed. San Diego, Calif: Academic Press; 1998:183.
74. Bryant RE, Howard D. Interaction of purulent material with antibiotics used to treat *Pseudomonas* infections. Antimicrob Agents Chemother. 1974;6:702.
75. O'Keefe JP, Tally FP, Barza M, et al. Inactivation of penicillin G during experimental infection with *Bacteroides fragilis*. J infect Dis. 1978;137:437.
76. Zimelis VM, Jackson GG. Activity of aminoglycoside antibiotics against *Pseudomonas aeruginosa*. Specificity and site of calcium, and magnesium antagonism. J Infect Dis. 1973;127:663.
77. Bryan LE, Van Den Elzen HM. Streptomycin accumulation in susceptible and resistant strains of *Escherichia coli* and *Pseudomonas aeruginosa*. Antimicrob Agents Chemother. 1976;9:928.
78. Zinner SH, Sabath LD, Casey JI, et al. Erythromycin and alkalinization of the urine in the treatment of urinary tract infection due to gram-negative bacilli. Lancet. 1971;1:1267.
79. Sabath LD, Gerstein DA, Leaf CD, et al. Increasing the usefulness of antibiotics: Treatment of infections caused by gram-negative bacilli. Clin Pharmacol Ther. 1970;11:161.
80. Karchmer AW, Dismukes WE, Buckley MJ, et al. Late prosthetic valve endocarditis. Am J Med. 1978;64:99.
81. Zimmerli W, Waldvogel FA, Vaudaux P, et al. Pathogenesis of foreign body infection: Description and characteristics of an animal model. J Infect Dis. 1982;146:487.
82. Dickinson GM, Bisno AL. Infections associated with indwelling medical devices. Antimicrob Agents Chemother. 1989;33:597.
83. Forsgren A, Schmeling D, Quie PG. Effect of tetracycline on the phagocytic function of human leukocytes. J Infect Dis. 1974;130:412.
84. Seklecki MM, Quintiliani R, Maderazo EG. Aminoglycoside antibiotics moderately impair granulocyte function. Antimicrob Agents Chemother. 1978;13:552.
85. Chaperon EA, Sanders WE Jr. Suppression of lymphoctye responses by cephalosporins. Infect Immun. 1978;19:378.
86. Mandell LA. Effects of antimicrobial and antineoplastic drugs on the phagocytic and microbicidal function of the polymorphonuclear leukocyte. Rev Infect Dis. 1982;4:683.
87. Hauser WE, Remington JS. Effect of antibiotics on the immune response. Am J Med. 1982;72:711.
88. Manzella JP, Clark JK. Effects of moxalactam and cefuroxime on mitogen-stimulated human mononuclear leukocytes. Antimicrob Agents Chemother. 1983;23:360.
89. Daschner FD. Antibiotics and host defense with special reference to phagocytosis by human polymorphonuclear leukocyte function in vivo. Antimicrob Agents Chemother. 1985;27:712.
90. Wispelway B, Lesse AJ, Hansen EJ, et al. *Haemophilus influenzae* lipopolysaccharide-induced blood-brain barrier permeability during experimental meningitis in the rat. J Clin Invest. 1988;82:1339.
91. Evins ME, Pollack M. Effect of antibiotic class and concentration on the release of lipopolysaccharide from *Escherichia coli*. J Infect Dis. 1993;167:1336.
92. Jawetz E. Combined antibiotic action: Some definitions and correlations between laboratory and clinical results. Antimicrob Agents Chemother. 1967;7:203.
93. Eliopoulos GM, Moellering RC Jr. Antimicrobial combinations. In: Lorian V, ed. Antibiotics in Laboratory Medicine. 4th ed. Baltimore: Williams & Wilkins; 1996:330–396.
94. VanderAuwera P, Meunier-Carpentier F, Klastersky J. Clinical study of combination therapy with oxacillin and rifampin for staphylococcal infections. Rev Infect Dis. 1983;5(Suppl 3):515.
95. Karchmer AW, Archer GL, Dimukes WE. Rifampin treatment of prosthetic valve endocarditis due to *Staphylococcus epidermidis*. Rev Infect Dis. 1983;5(Suppl 3):543.
96. Zimmerli W, Widmer AF, Blatter M, et al. Role of rifampin for treatment of orthopedic implant-related staphylococcal infections: A randomized control trial. JAMA. 1998;279:1537.
97. Solomkin JS, Dellinger EP, Christou NV, et al. Results of a multicenter trial comparing imipenem/cilastatin to tobramycin/clindamycin for intra-abdominal infections. Ann Surg. 1990;212:581.
98. Brismar B, Malmborg AS, Tunevall G, et al. Piperacillin-tazobactam versus imi-

penem-cilastatin for treatment of intra-abdominal infections. Antimicrob Agents Chemother. 1992;36:2766.
99. Moellering RC Jr. Antimicrobial combinations. Jpn J Clin Pharmacol Ther. 1993;24:293.
100. Moellering RC Jr. Use and abuse of antibiotic combinations. R I Med J. 1972;55:341.
101. Rahal JJ Jr. Antibiotic combinations: The clinical relevance of synergy and antagonism. Medicine (Baltimore). 1978;57:179.
102. Mandell GL, Kaye D, Levison ME, et al. Enterococcal endocarditis. An analysis of 38 patients observed at the New York Hospital–Cornell Medical Center. Arch Intern Med. 1970;125:258.
103. Moellering RC Jr. Wennersten C, Weinberg AN. Studies on antibiotic synergism against enterococci: I. Bacteriologic studies. J Lab Clin Med. 1971;77:821.
104. Moellering RC Jr. Weinberg AN. Studies on antibiotic synergism against enterococci. II. Effect of various antibiotics on the uptake of ^{14}C-labeled streptomycin by enterococci. J Clin Invest. 1971;50:2580.
105. Moellering RC Jr. Wennersten CBG, Medrek T, et al. Prevalence of high-level resistance to aminoglycosides in clinical isolates of enterococci. Antimicrob Agents Chemother. 1970;10:335.
106. Zimmermann RA, Moellering RC Jr, Weinberg AN. Mechanism of resistance to antibiotic synergism in enterococci. J Bacteriol. 1971;105:873.
107. Krogstad DJ, Korfhagen TR, Moellering RC Jr. et al. Aminoglycoside-inactivating enzymes: An explanation for resistance to penicillin-aminoglycoside synergism in enterococci. J Clin Invest. 1978;62:480.
108. Mederski-Samoraj BD, Murray BE. High-level resistance to gentamicin in clinical isolates of enterococci. J Infect Dis. 1983;147:751.
109. Moellering RC Jr. The entercoccus: High-level resistance to gentamicin and production of beta-lactamase. Clin Microbiol Newslett. 1988;10:129.
110. Moellering RC Jr. The entercoccus—a versatile pathogen. J Infect Chemother. 1997;3:1.
111. Fernandez-Guerrero ML, Barros C, Tudela JLR, et al. Aortic endocarditis caused by gentamicin-resistant *Enterococcus*. Eur J Clin Microbiol. 1988;7:525.
112. Wolfe JC, Johnson WD Jr. Penicillin-sensitive streptococcal endocarditis. Ann Intern Med. 1974;81:178.
113. Karchmer AW, Moellering RC Jr, Maki D, et al. Single antibiotic therapy of streptococcal endocarditis. JAMA. 1979;241:1801.
114. Watanakunakorn C, Glotzbecker C. Enhancement of the effects of antistaphylococcal antibiotics by aminoglycosides. Antimicrob Agents Chemother. 1974;6:802.
115. Korzeniwoski O, Sande MA. The National Collaborative Endocarditis Study Group: Combination antimicrobial therapy for *Staphylococcus aureus* endocarditis in patients addicted to parenteral drugs and in nonaddicts. Ann Intern Med. 1982;97:496.
116. Smith CB, Dans PE, Wilfert JN, et al. Use of gentamicin in combination with other antibiotics. J Infect Dis. 1969;119:370.
117. Eliopoulos GM, Moellering RC Jr. Azlocillin, mezlocillin and piperacillin: New broad-spectrum penicillins. Ann Intern Med. 1982;97:755.
118. Adriole VT. Antibiotic synergy in experimental infection with *Pseudomonas*: II. The effect of carbenicillin, cephalothin or cephanone combined with tobramycin or gentamicin. J Infect Dis. 1974;129:124.
119. Hilf M, Yu VL, Sharp JA, et al. Antibiotic therapy for *Pseudomonas aeruginosa* bacteremia: Outcome correlations in a prospective study of 200 patients. Am J Med. 1989;87:540.
120. Then R. Synergism between trimethoprim and sulfonamides. Science. 1977;197:1301.
121. Harding GKM, Ronald AR. A controlled study of antimicrobial prophylaxis of recurrent urinary tract infections in women. N Engl J Med. 1974;291:597.
122. Gilman RN, Terminel M, Levine MM, et al. Comparison of trimethoprim-sulfamethoxazole and amoxicillin in therapy of chloramphenicol-resistant and chloramphenicol-sensitive typhoid fever. J Infect Dis. 1975;132:630.
123. Chang MJ, Dunkle LM, Van Reken D, et al. Trimethoprim-sulfamethoxazole compared to ampicillin in the treatment of shigellosis. Pediatrics. 1977;59:726.
124. Quintiliani R, Levite RE, Nightingale CH. Potential role of trimethoprim-sulfamethoxazole in the treatment of serious hospital-acquired infections. Rev Infect Dis. 1987;9(Suppl 2):160.
125. Kwan CN, Medoff G, Kobayashi G, et al. Potentiation of the anti-fungal effects of antibiotics by amphotericin B. Antimicrob Agents Chemother. 1972;2:61.
126. Titsworth E, Grunberg E. Chemotherapeutic activity of 5-fluorocytosine and amphotericin B against *Candida albicans* in mice. Antimicrob Agents Chemother. 1973;4:306.
127. Bennett J, Dismukes W, Duma R, et al. A comparison of amphotericin B alone with amphotericin B plus flucytosine in the treatment of cryptoccal meningitis. N Engl J Med. 1979;301:126.
128. Lau WK, Young LS, Block RE, et al. Comparative efficacy and toxicity of amikacin/carbenicillin versus gentamicin/carbenicillin in leukopenic patients. Am J Med. 1977;62:959.
129. Klastersky J, Hensgens C, Meunier-Carpentier F. Comparative effectiveness of combinations of amikacin with penicillin G and amikacin with carbenicillin in gram-negative septicemia: Double-blind clinical trial. J Infect Dis. 1976;134(Suppl):433.
130. Moellering RC Jr. Monotherapy with expanded-spectrum cephalosporins for empiric treatment of serious infections diseases. In: Hoepelman IM, Moellering RC Jr, eds. New Directions in Cephalosporin Therapy: The Expanded Spectrum Cephalosporins. Winchester, UK: Theracom; 1988:49.
131. Lepper MH, Dowling HF. Treatment of pneumococcic meningitis with penicillin compared with penicillin plus aureomycin. Arch Intern Med. 1951;88:489.
132. Mathies AW Jr, Leedom JM, Ivier D, et al. Antibiotic antagonism in bacterial meningitis. Antimicrob Agents Chemother. 1967;7:218.
133. Sande MA, Overton JW. In vivo antagonism between gentamicin and chloramphenicol in neutropenic mice. J Infect Dis. 1973;128:247.
134. Strausbaugh LJ, Sande MA. Factors influencing the therapy of experimental *Proteus mirabilis* meningitis in rabbits. J Infect Dis. 1978;137:251.
135. Schaad UB, Suter S, Gianella-Borradori A, et al. A comparison of ceftriaxone and cefuroxime for the treatment of bacterial meningitis in children. N Engl J Med. 1990;322:141.
136. Del Rio MDL, Chrane D, Shelton S, et al. Ceftriaxone versus ampicillin and chloramphenicol for treatment of bacterial meningitis in children. Lancet. 1983;1:1241.
137. Moellering RC Jr. Rationale for the use of antibiotic combinations. Am J Med. 1983;75(2a):4.
138. Sanders CC. Novel resistance selected by the new expanded spectrum cephalosporins: A concern. J Infect Dis. 1983;147:585.
139. McLaughlin JE, Reeves DS. Clinical and laboratory evidence for inactivation of gentamicin by carbenicillin. Lancet. 1971;1:261.
140. Riff LJ, Jackson GG. Laboratory and clinical conditions for gentamicin inactivation by carbenicillin. Arch Intern Med. 1972;130:887.
141. Seidl LG, Thornton GF, Smith SW, et al. Studies on epidemiology of adverse drug reactions. III. Reactions in patients on general medical service. Bull Johns Hopkins Hosp. 1966;119:299.
142. Classen DC, Pestotnik SL, Evans RC, et al. Adverse drug events in hospitalized patients. JAMA. 1997;277:301.
143. Drusano GL. Pharmacokinetics of quinolone antimicrobial agents. In: Hooper D, Wolfson J, eds. Quinolone Antimicrobial Agents. Washington, DC: American Society for Microbiology; 1989:71–105.
144. Barza M, Brusch J, Bergeron M, et al. Penetration of antibiotics into fibrin loci in vivo. III. Intermittent versus continuous infusion and the effect of probenecid. J Infect Dis. 1974;129:73.
145. Craig WA, Ebert SC. Continuous infusion of β-lactam antibiotics. Antimicrob Agents Chemother. 1992;36:2577.
146. Gilbert DN. Once-daily aminoglycoside therapy. Antimicrob Agents Chemother. 1991;35:399.
147. Nelson JD. Antibiotic concentrations in septic joint effusions. N Engl J Med. 1971;284:349.
148. Gerding DN, Hall WH. The penetration of antibiotics into peritoneal fluid. Bull N Y Acad Med. 1975;51:1016.
149. Schlichter JG, MacLean H. A method of determinig the effective therapeutic level in the treatment of subacute bacterial endocarditis with penicillin. Am Heart J. 1947;34:209.
150. Reller LB, Stratton CW. Serum dilution test for bactericidal activity. II. Standardization and correlation with antimicrobial assays and susceptibility tests. J Infect Dis. 1977;136:196.
151. Carrizosa J, Kaye D. Antibiotic concentrations in serum, serum bactericidal activity, and results of therapy of streptococcal endocarditis in rabbits. Antimicrob Agents Chemother. 1977;12:479.
152. Levy J, Klastersky J. Serum bactericidal test: A review with emphasis on its role in the evaluation of antibiotic combination. In: Klastersky J, Staquet MJ, eds. Combination Antibiotic Therapy in the Compromised Host. New York: Raven; 1982:43.
153. Weinstein MP, Stratton CW, Ackley A, et al. Multicenter collaborative evaluation of a standardized serum bactericidal test as a prognostic indicator in infective endocarditis. Am J Med. 1985;78:262.
154. Pien FD, Vosti KL. Variation in performance of the serum bactericidal test. Antimicrob Agents Chemother. 1974;6:330.
155. Stratton CW, Reller LB. Serum dilution test for bactericidal activity. I. Selection of a physiologic diluent. J Infect Dis. 1977;136:187.
156. Mellors JW, Colmn DL, Andriole VT. Value of the serum bactericidal test in management of patients with bacterial endocarditis. Eur J Clin Microbiol. 1986;5:67.
157. Reller LB. The serum bactericidal test. Rev Infect Dis. 1986;8:803.

Chapter 16

Mechanisms of Bacterial Antibiotic Resistance

STEVEN M. OPAL
KENNETH H. MAYER
ANTONE A. MEDEIROS

MOLECULAR GENETICS OF ANTIBIOTIC RESISTANCE

Genetic variability is essential in order for microbial evolution to occur. Antimicrobial agents exert strong selective pressures on bacterial populations, favoring those organisms that are capable of resisting them.[1, 2] Genetic variability may occur by a variety of mechanisms. Point mutations may occur in a nucleotide base pair, which is referred to as *micro evolutionary change*. These mutations may alter the target site of an antimicrobial agent, interfering with its activity. Point mutations at critical locations on "old" β-lactamase genes (e.g., genes for TEM-1, SHV-1) are primarily responsible for the remarkable array of newly recognized extended-spectrum β-lactamases.[3, 4]

A second level of genomic variability in bacteria is referred to as a *macro evolutionary change* and results in whole-scale rearrangements of large segments of DNA as a single event. Such rearrangements may include inversions, duplications, insertions, deletions, or transposition of large sequences of DNA from one location of a bacterial chromosome or plasmid to another. These whole-scale rearrangements of large segments of the bacterial genome are frequently created by specialized genetic elements known as *transposons* or *insertion sequences*, which have the capacity to move independently as a unit from the rest of the bacterial genome.[2]

A third level of genetic variability in bacteria is created by the acquisition of foreign DNA carried by plasmids, bacteriophages, naked sequences of DNA, or transposable genetic elements. Inheritance of foreign DNA from extrachromosomal elements further contributes to the organism's ability to cope with selection pressures imposed by antimicrobial agents.[5] These mechanisms endow bacteria with the seemingly unlimited capacity to develop resistance to any antimicrobial agent. Recent examples of vancomycin-resistant *Staphylococcus aureus*,[6] multidrug-resistant *Yersinia pestis*,[7] and transferable quinolone resistance in enterobacteria[8] portend an uncertain future for antimicrobial agents in the treatment of infectious diseases. Once an antibiotic resistance gene evolves, this resistance determinant may spread to other bacteria by transformation, transduction, conjugation, or transposition. Favored clones of bacteria may then proliferate in the flora of patients who receive antibiotics. Evidence exists that antibiotic-resistance (R) genes were present in natural environments before the clinical use of antibiotics in medicine.[3, 9] Selection pressures placed on microbial populations by antibiotics favor the expansion of strains that have the capacity to resist the inhibitory effects of antibiotics. These resistant populations then proliferate and spread R genes to other susceptible strains of bacteria. Some R genes may have derived from antibiotic-producing bacteria themselves.[3, 4]

Plasmids

Extrachromosomal elements were present in bacteria before the advent of antibiotics.[10] However, the introduction of antibiotics into clinical medicine over the past 6 decades has created selection pressures that favor the dissemination of R genes via mobile genetic elements (e.g., plasmids, transposons, and other mobile genes). Rapid increases in the spread of antibiotic resistance within and between species often correlate with the dissemination of specific R genes. Plasmids are particularly well adapted to serve as agents of genetic evolution and R-gene dissemination.[11] Plasmids are extrachromosomal genetic elements that are made of circular double-stranded DNA molecules that range from less than 10 to greater than 400 kilobase pairs and are extremely common in bacteria.[12] Although multiple copies of a specific plasmid or multiple different plasmids, or both, may be found in a single bacterial cell, closely related plasmids often cannot coexist in the same cell. This observation has led to a classification scheme of plasmids based upon incompatibility groups.[13]

Plasmids may determine a wide range of functions besides antibiotic resistance, including virulence and metabolic capacities. Plasmids are autonomous, self-reproducing genetic elements that require an origin for replication and genes that facilitate its stable maintenance in host bacteria.[13] Conjugative plasmids require additional genes that can initiate self-transfer.[14]

The transfer of plasmid DNA between bacterial species is a complex process, and thus conjugative plasmids tend to be larger than nonconjugative ones. Some small plasmids may be able to utilize the conjugation apparatus of a coresident conjugative plasmid. Many plasmid-encoded functions enable bacterial strains to persist in the environment by resisting noxious agents, such as heavy metals. For example, mercury released from dental fillings may increase the number of antibiotic-resistant bacteria in the oral flora.[15] Compounds such as hexachlorophene are used as topical bacteriostatic agents, and plasmid-mediated resistance to these agents has increased significantly.[16]

Plasmids may be involved in the dissemination of antibiotic resistance in several ways (Fig. 16–1). A single clone of a specific organism may become resistant by mutation or by the inheritance of a resistance plasmid. The resultant resistant organism may have genes that are particularly well adapted to a specific niche and thus may be able to disseminate widely. The single clone may be responsible for multiple or recurrent, or both, outbreaks of antibiotic resistance. Conjugative plasmids may be transferred from one species to another and result in new outbreaks of antibiotic resistance in previously susceptible species.[17] Transposons create the potential for even wider dissemination of R genes.[18]

Transposable Genetic Elements

Transposons can translocate from one area of the bacterial chromosome to another or between the chromosome and plasmid or bacteriophage DNA. Transposable genetic elements possess a specialized system of recombination that is independent of the generalized recombination system that classically permits recombination of largely homologous sequences of DNA by crossover events (the *rec*A system of bacteria). The *rec*A-independent recombination system of transposable elements usually occurs in a random fashion between nonhomologous sequences of DNA and results in whole-scale modifications of large sequences of DNA as a single event (Fig. 16–2).[1, 5]

There are two types of transposable genetic elements, referred to as *transposons* and *insertion sequences*, that have similar characteristics. Recent evidence from whole-genome sequencing projects indicates that bacterial chromosomes are replete with transposable elements.[19] These mobile sequences probably play an important physiologic role in genetic variation and evolution in procaryotic organisms. Transposons differ from insertion sequences in that they mediate a recognizable phenotypic characteristic such as an antibiotic-resistance marker. Either element can translocate as an independent unit. Both elements are flanked on either end by short identical sequences of DNA in reverse order *(inverted repeats)*. These inverted-repeat DNA termini are essential to the transposition process. Transposons and insertion sequences are incapable of autonomous self-replication and therefore must exist on a replicon such as the chromosome, bacteriophage, or plasmid in order to be replicated and maintained in a bacterial population. A new class of transposable

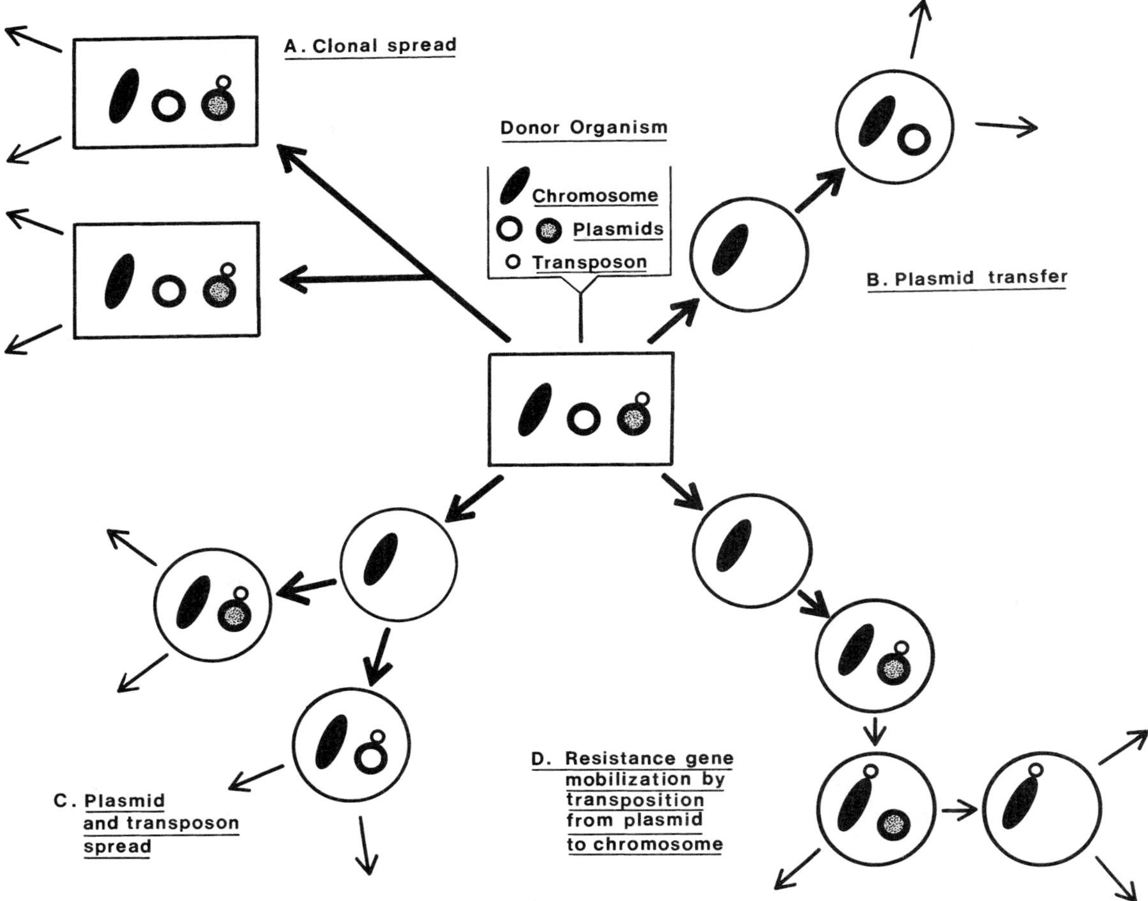

FIGURE 16–1. Examples of the molecular spread of antibiotic resistance. The donor organism has a chromosome, two plasmids, and a transposon. *A*, If it is well adapted to a particular niche, it may remain stable in the environment and continue to replicate itself and thus disseminate through clonal spread. *B*, If the organism comes into close physical contact with another bacterium that may not possess extrachromosomal DNA, attachment between the two cells from different bacterial species may allow for the introduction of one of the plasmids by conjugation. *C*, The donor organism may be able to spread resistance genes through several mechanisms, including the spread of transposons, as well as plasmids. Transposons may be able to hop between plasmids, as shown in *C*, or *D*, they may be able to allow for the mobilization of resistance genes by being transferred on a conjugative plasmid into new bacterial species and then hopping from the plasmid to the chromosome. Some transposons may subsequently become integrated into the host chromosome and be spread as a stable genetic element in the chromosome without any subsequent transfer via plasmid DNA.

elements has been described that has the capability to move from the chromosome of one bacterium to another without becoming incorporated into a plasmid or bacteriophage. These elements are referred to as *conjugative* transposons and have been found primarily in aerobic and anaerobic gram-positive organisms.[20, 21]

Transposition usually results in the localized replication of the transposable element from the original donor sequence of DNA as well as the insertion of a copy of the transposable element into the recipient sequence of DNA (replicative transposition).[1, 2, 5] Transposition is a continuous and ongoing process in bacterial populations. An example of this phenomenon is the spread of a tetracycline-resistance transposon among *Neisseria gonorrhoeae, Mycoplasma hominis*, and *Ureaplasma urealyticum*.[22, 23] Transposons are also essential in the evolution of R plasmids that contain multiple antibiotic-resistance determinants.[18] High-level vancomycin resistance (vanA) in enterococci is mediated by a composite transposon that encodes a series of genes needed to express vancomycin resistance.[24] Single transposons may encode multiple antibiotic-resistance determinants within their inverted-repeat termini as well.[5]

Our recognition of the extent of genetic exchange of antibiotic-resistance determinants between bacteria of different genera and species is expanding.[25, 26] Identical erythromycin-resistance genes occur in streptococci and *Campylobacter*,[27] and enterococci have apparently acquired aminoglycoside[28] and β-lactam[29] resistance from staphylococci. Thus, given the appropriate environmental selection pressures, the ongoing evolution of multiresistant species is inevitable, and prevention will be difficult.[30–32]

DNA Integration Elements

The structural genes that mediate antibiotic resistance are often closely linked and may exist in tandem along the bacterial chromosome or plasmid. Genetic analysis of sequences of DNA adjacent to R genes has revealed that unique integration units often exist near promoter sites.

These integration elements, known as *integrons*,[33] function as recombinational "hot spots" for site-specific recombination events between largely nonhomologous sequences of DNA. The integron provides an integrase function to facilitate this *rec*A-independent recombination and a common integration site consisting of a 59–base pair (bp) sequence of highly conserved DNA. This 59-bp sequence is preserved at the 3′ end of inserted R genes.[34]

Although these integration elements differ structurally and functionally from transposons, they appear to be widespread in bacterial

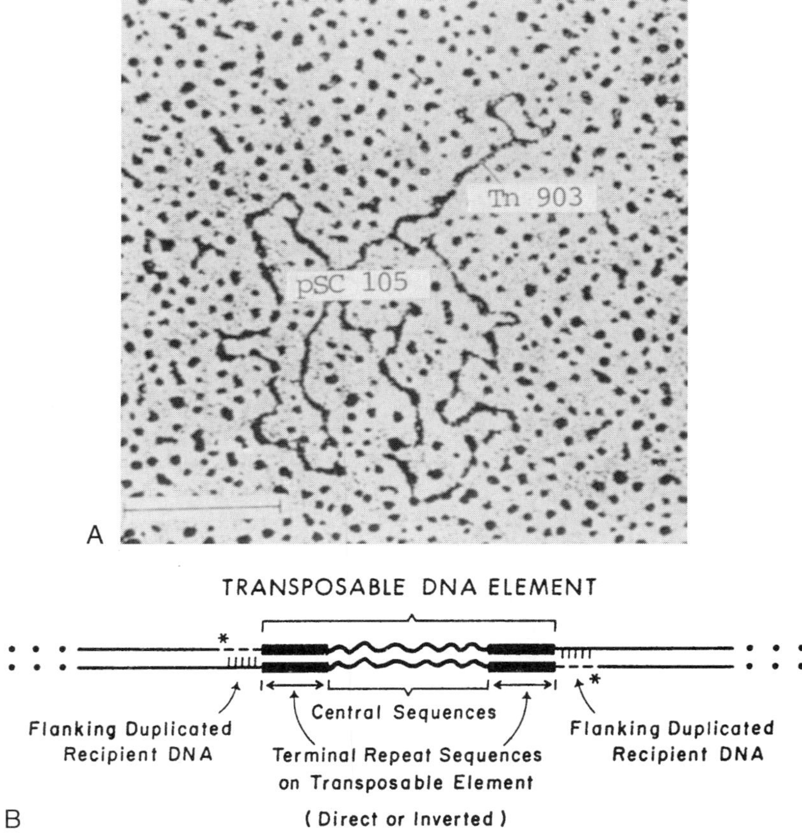

FIGURE 16–2. *A*, Characteristic appearance of a transposon by electron microscopy showing the stem-loop configuration. The kanamycin resistance transposon Tn903 is inserted into a small plasmid (pSC105). Following denaturation, intrastrand annealing of the complementary 1000 base pair, inverted repeat, terminal sequences of the transposon form the stem structure. The kanamycin resistance gene and the genes necessary for transposition are located in the central loop structure. *B*, Structure of a transposable element inserted into a recipient DNA sequence. The transposon (*rectangles* and *wavy lines*) consists of a central sequence containing the phenotypic marker gene(s) (antibiotic resistance gene) and the "transposase" genes. The terminal repeat sequences of the transposon flank the central sequences on both sides. Insertion of the transposon results in single-strand, staggered cuts in the recipient DNA *(asterisks)*. Subsequent gap-filling DNA synthesis and ligation results in duplication of a short sequence of recipient DNA at either end of the transposon.

populations and play an important role in the dissemination of R genes. They provide a convenient site for insertion of R genes from foreign DNA sources. Integrons also serve as expression cassettes for R genes in that an efficient promoter site is provided in close proximity to the 5′ end of the newly inserted DNA sequence. The frequency of transcription of integrated cassettes of R genes depends on the proximity of the gene to the promoter at the 5′ upstream end of the integron. The level of expression of a resistance gene diminishes as the distance between the promoter and the specific R gene cassette increases.[35] Numerous clusters of different R genes have been identified that have evolved through specific insertions into common integrons.[36]

MECHANISMS OF ANTIBIOTIC RESISTANCE

At least eight distinctive mechanisms of antibiotic resistance have been described in bacteria (Table 16–1).[37]

Enzymatic Inhibition

β-Lactamases

Resistance to β-lactam antibiotics is due mainly to the production of β-lactamases, enzymes that inactivate these antibiotics by splitting the amide bond of the β-lactam ring. Numerous β-lactamases exist, encoded either by chromosomal genes or by transferable genes located on plasmids or transposons.[38]

Three evolutionarily distinct classes of β-lactamases have been defined on the basis of amino acid and nucleotide sequence studies.[39] Class A β-lactamases have molecular weights around 29,000, possess a serine residue at their active site, and preferentially hydrolyze penicillins. An example is the TEM-1 β-lactamase, which is widely prevalent in gram-negative bacilli. Class B are metalloenzymes that have a zinc-binding thiol group required for β-lactamase activity. Class C includes the β-lactamase determined by the chromosomal *ampC* gene of *Escherichia coli* K-12, which shares extensive sequence homology with chromosomally mediated β-lactamases of *Shigella* and *Klebsiella* spp. These enzymes are large proteins of molecular weight about 39,000 with mainly cephalosporinase activity. They also have serine at their active site but share little homology with the class A β-lactamases.[40] The tertiary structures of class C β-lactamases show striking similarities to penicillin-binding proteins (PBPs), from which they may have evolved.[41–44] Class D β-lactamases are oxacillin-hydrolyzing enzymes.

Gram-Positive Bacteria. Among the gram-positive bacteria, staphylococci are the major pathogens that produce β-lactamase. Staphylococcal β-lactamases preferentially hydrolyze penicillins. Most are inducible and are excreted extracellularly.[38] The genes that determine staphylococcal β-lactamases are usually carried on small plasmids or transposons. Larger plasmids encoding β-lactamase and other resistances also exist and can transfer by conjugation, not only between strains of *S. aureus* but also between *S. aureus* and *Staphylococcus epidermidis*.[45]

Enterococci produce a plasmid-determined β-lactamase that appears to be of staphylococcal origin.[46, 47] Since the appearance of the first strain in Texas in 1981, β-lactamase–producing enterococci have been found throughout the United States and in South America.[48] The genes often coexist with genes that determine high-level resistance to gentamicin and may occur on transposons as well as on plasmids. Interestingly, these transposons are similar to staphylococcal β-lactamase transposons and may be derived from them.[49]

Gram-Negative Bacteria. Gram-negative bacteria produce a much greater variety of β-lactamases than do gram-positive bacteria. This diversity has led to several classification schemes. A classification by Bush, Jacoby, and Medeiros[50] groups β-lactamases according to

TABLE 16–1 Major Mechanisms of Antibiotic Resistance

Resistance Mechanism	Type of Antibiotic											
	β-Lactams	*Aminoglycosides*	*Chloramphenicol*	*Macrolides*	*Lincosamides*	*Sulfonamides*	*Trimethoprim*	*Tetracyclines*	*Quinolones*	*Vancomycin*	*Rifampin*	*Polymyxin*
Enzymatic inhibition	B	B	P	P	—	—	—	—	—	—	—	—
Membrane impermeability	C	C	P	—	—	C	C	B	—	C	—	C
Active pumping out of antibiotic (efflux)	—	—	—	C	C	—	—	B	C	—	—	—
Alteration of ribosomal target	—	C	C	B	B	—	—	B	—	—	—	—
Alteration of cell wall precursor target	—	—	—	—	—	—	—	—	—	B	—	—
Alteration of target enzymes	C	—	—	—	—	B	B	—	C	—	C	—
Overproduction of target enzyme	—	—	—	—	—	C	C	—	—	—	—	—
Auxotrophs that bypass inhibited steps	—	—	—	—	—	B	B	—	—	—	—	—

Abbreviations: B, Both; C, chromosomally mediated; P, plasmid mediated; —, not yet described.

TABLE 16–2 The Bush-Jacoby-Medeiros Functional Classification Scheme for ß-Lactamases

Group	Enzyme Type	Inhibition by Clavulanate	Molecular Class	No. of Enzymes	Examples†
1	Cephalosporinase	No	C	57	*Enterobacter cloacae* P99 (C), MIR-1 (P)
2a	Penicillinase	Yes	A	20	*Bacillus cereus I, Staphylococcus aureus* (B)
2b	Broad-spectrum	Yes	A	16	SHV-1 (B), TEM-1 (P)
2be	Extended-spectrum	Yes	A	81	*Klebsiella oxytoca* K1 (C), TEM-3 (P), SHV-2 (P)
2br*	Inhibitor-resistant	Diminished	A	13	TEM-30 (IRT-2) (P)
2c	Carbenicillinase	Yes	A	15	AER-1 (C), PSE-1 (P), CARB-3 (P)
2d	Cloxacillinase	Yes	D or A	21	*Streptomyces cacaoi* (C), OXA-1 (P)
2e	Cephalosporinase	Yes	A	19	*Proteus vulgaris* (C), FEC-1 (P)
2f*	Carbapenemase	Yes	A	3	IMI-1 (C), NMC-A (C), Sme-1 (C)
3	Carbapenemase	No	B	15	*Stenotrophomonas maltophilia* L1 (C), IMP-1 (P)
4	Penicillinase	No		7	*Burkholderia cepacia* (C), SAR-2 (P)

*New groups.
†C, Chromosomal; P, plasmid; B, both.
From Bush K, Jacoby GA, Madeiros AA. A functional classification scheme for β-lactamases and its correlation with molecular structure. Antimicrob Agents Chemother. 1995; 39:1211–1233.

substrate profiles and inhibition by clavulanic acid (Table 16–2). The relationships between these functional groups and the β-lactamase classes based on amino acid sequence are shown in Figure 16–3.

β-Lactamases encoded by plasmids are a special concern because the possibility of spread among different strains and different species of pathogens increases. Many types exist.[51] All are produced constitutively and can be grouped into seven broad classes:

1. Broad-spectrum enzymes that hydrolyze benzyl penicillin and cephaloridine at similar rates.
2. Oxacillinases that hydrolyze oxacillin and related penicillins rapidly.
3. Carbenicillinases that break down carbenicillin readily.
4. Extended-spectrum β-lactamases, mutant class A oxyimino-β-lactamases derived from the widely prevalent plasmid-determined TEM, SHV, or OXA β-lactamases.
5. Other class A oxyimino-β-lactamases not related to TEM, SHV, or OXA β-lactamases. Two subgroups in this class consist of six β-lactamases that have high sequence homology with the class A chromosomal β-lactamase of *Klebsiella oxytoca* and two novel β-lactamases, PER-1 and PER-2, that have little sequence similarity to any other known β-lactamases. The former tend to confer resistance to cefuroxime and aztreonam but not to ceftazidime, whereas the latter may confer resistance to ceftibuten, an unusual characteristic for class A β-lactamases.
6. Enzymes that break down cephamycins as well as oxyimino-β-lactams and are resistant to inhibition by clavulanate. The genes that encode these enzymes are similar in nucleotide sequence to chromosomal β-lactamase genes of *Enterobacter cloacae* (two enzymes) or *Citrobacter freundii* (four enzymes). Both types have caused outbreaks in hospitals in Greece and the United States. A group of five enzymes (FOX related) in this class have been isolated only from unique patient isolates so far and have no close nucleotide sequence similarity to any naturally occurring chromosomal β-lactamase outside the group
7. Carbapenemases that confer resistance to imipenem or meropenem. Two plasmid-mediated metalloenzymes have been identified in Japan. One (IMP-1) has spread in several hospitals around Tokyo. Two nonmetallo-β-lactamases, not yet sequenced, that confer resistance to carbapenems have been found in isolates of *Acinetobacter* from Europe and Argentina. Properties of the plasmid-determined β-lactamases are summarized in Table 16–3.

Anaerobic Bacteria. β-Lactamases also contribute to the resistance of anaerobic bacteria to β-lactam antibiotics.[52, 53] The β-lactamases of fusobacteria and clostridia are principally penicillinases.[54, 55] Those produced by *Bacteroides fragilis* are predominantly cephalosporinases, some of which have been found to hydrolyze cefoxitin and imipenem and may be transferable.[56–61] Most of the cephalosporinases are inhibited by clavulanate, sulbactam, or tazobactam. Some isolates

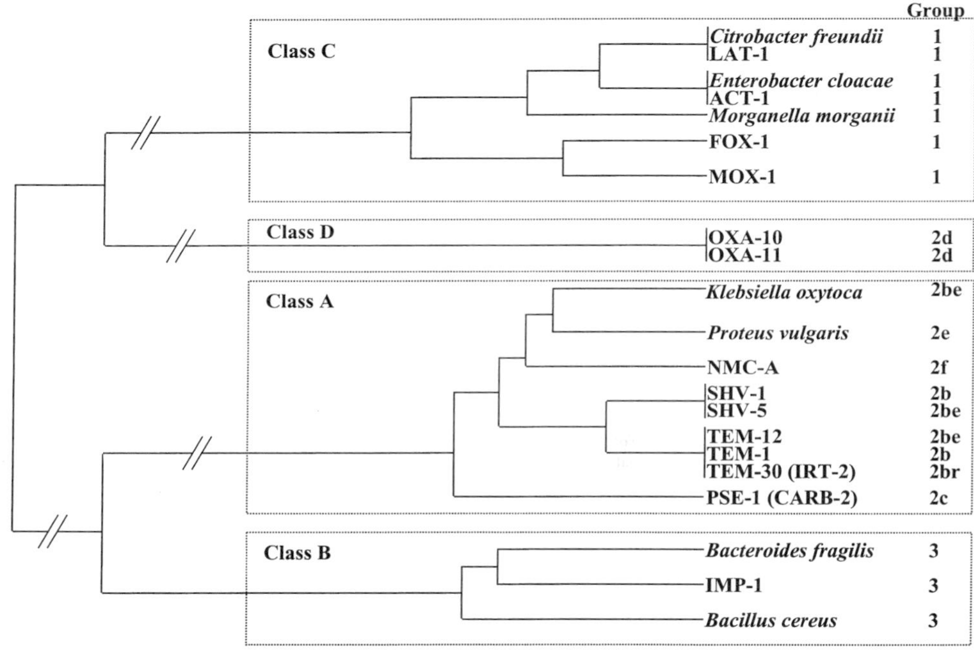

FIGURE 16–3. Correlation between amino acid sequences (Ambler classes) and functional properties of β-lactamases (Bush-Jacoby-Medeiros groups). (Adapted from Philippon A, Dusart J, Doris B, Frère JM. The diversity, structure and regulation of β-lactamases. Cell Mol Life Sci. 1998;54: 341–346.)

TABLE 16–3 Properties of Plasmid-Determined ß-Lactamases

ß-Lactamase	pI	Prevalence	Host Bacteria	Specific Features
1. Broad Spectrum[51]				
HMS-1	5.2	Rare	Enterobacteriaceae	
TEM-1	5.4	Very common	Enterobacteriaceae *Pseudomonas aeruginosa* *Haemophilus influenzae* *Neisseria gonorrhoeae* *Vibrio cholerae*	Most common plasmid-determined ß-lactamase in nearly all bacterial species
TLE-1	5.55	Rare	*Escherichia coli*	Closely related to TEM-1
TEM-2	5.6	Common	Enterobacteriaceae	Differs from TEM-1 by one amino acid, away from binding site
LCR-1	5.85 or 6.5	Rare	*P. aeruginosa*	Not inhibited by clavulanic acid
NPS-1	6.5	Rare	*P. aeruginosa*	Cefsulodin induces conformational change
TLE-2	6.5	Rare	*Klebsiella pneumoniae*	High affinity for cefsulodin and cefotetan
LXA-1	6.7	Uncommon	Enterobacteriaceae	Very low affinity for benzyl penicillin Confers low-level ß-lactam resistance
OHIO-1	7.0	Uncommon	*Enterobacter cloacae* *Serratia marcescens*	Found only in isolates from Ohio Similar to SHV-1
SHV-1 (PIT-2)	7.6	Common	Enterobacteriaceae	Often encoded by chromosomal genes in *K. pneumoniae*
ROB-1	8.1	Uncommon	*H. influenzae* *Haemophilus pleuropneumoniae* *Pasteurella multocida*	Found in both human and animal isolates
2. Oxacillinase[51]				
OXA-9	6.9	Rare	*K. pneumoniae*	Encoded by transposon *Tn 1331*
OXA-3	7.1	Uncommon	Enterobacteriaceae *P. aeruginosa*	
OXA-1	7.4	Common	Enterobacteriaceae *P. aeruginosa*	Second most common type in *E. coli*
OXA-4	7.45	Rare	Enterobacteriaceae	Closely related to OXA-1
OXA-8	7.6?	Rare	?	Encoded by p40Tn2
OXA-5	7.62	Rare	*P. aeruginosa*	
OXA-7	7.65	Rare	*E. coli*	
OXA-6	7.68	Rare	*P. aeruginosa*	
OXA-2	7.7	Common	Enterobacteriaceae *P. aeruginosa*	Second most common type in salmonellae
3. Carbenicillinase[51]				
CARB-4	4.3	Rare	*P. aeruginosa*	Confers resistance to cefsulodin
SAR-1	4.9	Rare	*V. cholerae*	
PSE-4 (CARB-1)	5.3	Uncommon	*P. aeruginosa* Enterobacteriaceae	
BRO-1, BRO-2, BRO-3	Multiple bands (5.3–7.7)	Common	*Brahamella*	Confers resistance to ampicillin and cefaclor Found in *B. catarrhalis* Plasmid location uncertain May be on conjugative transposon
PSE-1 (CARB-2)	5.7	Common	*P. aeruginosa* Enterobacteriaceae	Most common type in *P. aeruginosa*
CARB-3	5.75	Rare	*P. aeruginosa*	
CARB-5	6.3	Rare	*Acinetobacter calcoaceticus*	Susceptible to ticarcillin combined with clavulanate
PSE-3	6.9	Uncommon	*P. aeruginosa* Enterobacteriaceae	
Unnamed (N-29)	6.9 (6.93)	Rare	*Proteus mirabilis*	
4. Extended-Spectrum				
*Class A Oxyimino-β-Lactamases Related to TEM, SHV, or OXA β-Lactamases (Confer Resistance to Cefotaxime, Ceftazidime or Aztreonam)**				
TEM-derived				
TEM-3–TEM-29, TEM-42–TEM-43, TEM-46–TEM-67	5.2–6.5	Nosocomial outbreaks worldwide	*K. pneumoniae* Less common in other Enterobacteriaceae	One to four amino acid substitutions in TEM-1 or TEM-2 active site structure Confer resistance mainly to ceftazidime or aztreonam Susceptible to clavulanate
SHV-derived				
SHV-2–SHV-12	7.0–8.2	Nosocomial outbreaks worldwide	*K. pneumoniae* Less common in other Enterobacteriaceae	One to three amino acid substitutions in SHV-1 active site structure Confer greater resistance to cefotaxime than TEM derivatives
Inhibitor-resistant				
TEM-30–TEM-40, TEM-44–TEM-45	5.2–5.4	Mainly nosocomial isolates from France and Spain	*E. coli*	One to two amino acid substitutions in TEM-1 or TEM-2 active site structure Resistant to inhibition by clavulanate, sulbactam, or tazobactam but often more susceptible to cefazolin than TEM-1
OXA-derived				
OXA-11, OXA-14–OXA-16	6.1–8.0	Nosocomial isolates from Turkey	*P. aeruginosa*	One or two amino acid substitutions in the OXA active site structure
5. Other Class A Oxyimino-β-Lactamases Not Related to TEM, SHV, or OXA β-Lactamases				
Sequence like *Klebsiella oxytoca* chromosomal ß-lactamase (confer resistance to cefuroxime)				
CTX-M-2[230]	5.5	Clinical isolates from Argentina	*Salmonella typhimurium, E. coli, V. cholerae*	Most common oxyimin-β-lactamase in *E. coli* in Argentina
Toho-1[231]	7.8	Clinical isolate from Japan	*E. coli*	
Toho-2[232]	?	Urinary isolate from Japan	lac− *E. coli*	Inhibited better by tazobactam than clavulanate

Table continued on following page

TABLE 16–3 Properties of Plasmid-Determined ß-Lactamases *Continued*

ß-Lactamase	pI	Prevalence	Host Bacteria	Specific Features
MEN-1 (CTX-M-1)[230]	8.4	Clinical isolates from France and Germany	*E. coli*	
CTX-M-3[233]	8.4	Four urinary isolates from hospital in Poland	*E. coli* *Citrobacter freundii*	
CTX-M-4[234]	8.4	Six isolates from Russia	*S. typhimurium*	
PER-related—confer resistance to ceftibuten				
PER-1[235]	5.4	Isolates from university hospitals in several regions of Turkey	*P. aeruginosa* *K. pneumoniae* *Acinetobacter*	Close amino acid sequence similarity only to PER-2 (86% homology)
PER-2[236]	5.4	Isolates from Argentina	*S. typhimurium* Also other Enterobacteriaceae Not in *P. aeruginosa*	Hydrolyzes ceftibuten
6. Class C Cephamycinases (Confer Resistance to Cefoxitin or Cefotetan)				
Sequence like *Enterobacter cloacae* chromosomal ß-lactamase				
MIR-1[101]	8.4	Outbreak in hospital in Providence, R.I.	*K. pneumoniae*	
ACT-1[237]	9.0	Nosocomial isolates from New York City hospital	*E. coli* *K. pneumoniae*	Confers resistance to imipenem in porin-deficient strain
Sequence like *Citrobacter freundii* chromosomal ß-lactamase				
BIL-1[238, 239]	8.8	Burn isolate from child from Pakistan	*E. coli*	
CMY-2[240]	9.0	Urine isolate from patient in Athens, Greece	*K. pneumoniae* *C. freundii*	
SAL-1[241]	9.0	Stool isolate from Nigeria	*Salmonella senftenberg*	
LAT-1[242]	9.4	Nosocomial isolates from Greece	*K. pneumoniae*	
LAT-2[243]	9.4, 9.1, 8.9	Nosocomial isolates from several Greek hospitals	*K. pneumoniae* *E. coli* *Enterobacter aerogenes*	
Sequence like *Morganella morganii* chromosomal ß-lactamase				
MOR-1[244]	?	Clinical isolate	*Salmonella enteritidis*	Encoded by integron-like structure
FOX-related				
FOX-1[245]	6.8 or 7.2	Blood isolate from patient in Buenos Aires hospital	*K. pneumoniae*	No close nucleotide sequence similarity to any naturally occurring chromosomal ß-lactamase
FOX-2[246]	6.7	Urinary isolate from Guatemalan paraplegic	*E. coli*	97% sequence identity with FOX-1
FOX-3[247]	7.25	Vaginal isolate from Italy	*Klebsiella oxytoca*	96% homology with FOX-1
CMY-1[248]	8.0	Wound isolate from Korea	*K. pneumoniae*	89% homology to MOX-1
MOX-1[249, 250]	8.9	Urinary isolate from Nagoya, Japan	*K. pneumoniae*	51% homology with *P. aeruginosa* PAO1, 69% with FOX-1
Unknown source				
CEP-1[251]	8.0	Rare	*P. mirabilis*	Not sequenced
7. Carbapenemases (Confer Resistance to Imipenem or Meropenem)				
Metalloenzymes (class B ß-lactamases)				
IMP-1[104]	9.0	Isolates from several hospitals in Japan	*P. aeruginosa* *S. marcescens* *Alcaligenes xylosoxidans* *Pseudomonas putida* *K. pneumoniae*	Hydrolyzes imipenem Resistant to clavulanate
Unnamed[252, 253]		Wound isolate from Japan	*Bacteroides fragilis*	Encoded on small self-transmissible plasmid Sequence identical to chromosomal CcrA (CfiA) ß-lactamases in *Bacteroides* isolates from United States
Nonmetalloenzymes, not yet sequenced				
ARI-1[106, 107]	6.65	Blood isolate from patient in Scotland	*Acinetobacter baumanii*	Transferred to *Acinetobacter junii* Not inhibited by EDTA
ARI-2[108]	~7.1	Outbreak in Buenos Aires, Argentina Also found in isolates from Europe and Southeast Asia	*Acinetobacter* spp	Inhibited by clavulanate

*For references see Jacoby GA, Bush K. http://www.lahey.org/studies/webt.htm.
Abbreviation: EDTA, Ethylenediaminetetraacetic acid.

of *Bacteroides* produce carbapenemases, metalloenzymes inhibited by EDTA but not clavulanate, that confer resistance to imipenem.

Distribution in Clinical Isolates. The existence of β-lactamase genes on plasmids and transposons ensures that a β-lactamase originally confined to one group of bacteria sooner or later may appear in other groups. The widespread use of antibiotics fosters selection of the resistant organisms that rise in prevalence locally and then spread worldwide. A prime example of this process occurred with the TEM-1 β-lactamase, which has spread from the Enterobacteriaceae to *Haemophilus influenzae*[62] and *N. gonorrhoeae*.[63] Clinical isolates may produce two, and even three, plasmid-determined β-lactamases. In nearly all cases, TEM-1 is one of the β-lactamases produced. A large number of strains from South America and the Far East have had novel or multiple, or both, plasmidic β-lactamases.[51] Curiously, the OXA extended-spectrum β-lactamases and the plasmid-mediated metallocarbapenemase IMP-1 have so far proliferated only in certain regions of Turkey and Japan, respectively.

The success of the pharmaceutical industry in developing new β-lactams resistant to hydrolysis by β-lactamases led to the introduction into clinical use of the third-generation β-lactam antibiotics around 1978 in Europe and 1981 in the United States. These antibiotics were very resistant to hydrolysis by the known plasmid-determined β-lactamases. Then, in 1983 in Germany, isolates of *Klebsiella pneumoniae* and then other Enterobacteriaceae were discovered that produce a plasmid-determined β-lactamase that hydrolyzes cefotaxime, as well as other newer cephalosporins. This new β-lactamase, called SHV-2, derived from a mutation in the well-known SHV-1 β-lactamase commonly found in *Klebsiella*. The mutation resulted in an enhanced affinity of the SHV-1 β-lactamase for cefotaxime.[64] Subsequently, ceftazidime-resistant strains of *K. pneumoniae* producing a novel plasmid-encoded ceftazidime-hydrolyzing β-lactamase, designated CTX-1, were isolated in several French hospitals.[65] Nucleotide sequencing studies showed that this enzyme differed from TEM-2 by only two amino acids. Since then there has been a rapid increase in the number and variety of extended-spectrum β-lactamases.[66] The numbers of derivatives of the TEM and SHV β-lactamases proved to be unique by sequencing have now reached 67 and 12, respectively (see G. Jacoby and K. Bush, http://www.lahey.org/studies/webt.htm).[66, 67] Several (SHV-2, SHV-4, SHV-5, TEM-6) occur in many countries, whereas others seem to occur more commonly in one or two countries. For example, TEM-3 is prevalent in France and TEM-10 and TEM-12 in the United States and England.[66, 68] The varied national patterns of antibiotic use in hospitals probably account for the differences in distribution of these enzymes. Several extended-spectrum β-lactamases derived from OXA enzymes have been found in *Pseudomonas aeruginosa* isolates from Turkey.[69, 70] Most of the clinical isolates that produce extended-spectrum β-lactamases have come from hospitalized patients and have frequently caused nosocomial outbreaks, mostly due to *K. pneumoniae*. Surveys of hospital isolates of *K. pneumoniae* in England,[71] France,[72] and Portugal[73] show that 14 to 16% produce extended-spectrum β-lactamases. In France, the prevalence rose from less than 1% in 1985 to the current level by 1988. Extended-spectrum β-lactamases are also found in nearly all other species of Enterobacteriaceae, but they occur infrequently. In a French survey, 2 to 3% of *Enterobacter* spp. and *K. oxytoca* but only 0.1% of *E. coli* produced extended-spectrum β-lactamases.[72] Surveys of strains isolated since 1988 in England and Portugal also document a low frequency in *E. coli*.[71, 74] Curiously, reports of extended-spectrum β-lactamases in *Proteus mirabilis* have been relatively rare.[75–80] In this species, the spread of extended-spectrum β-lactamases may be limited by a low frequency of plasmid conjugation.[81]

Sporadic nosocomial outbreaks due to strains producing extended-spectrum β-lactamases seem to have led to an endemic problem in some hospitals. Sometimes patients from nursing homes and other long-term care institutions bring such strains into the hospital.[82, 83] Then selection pressure from widespread hospital use of a β-lactam apparently enhances colonization of the digestive or respiratory tracts of other patients, and infection follows.[67, 84] Not surprisingly, outbreaks have often been associated with a prolonged hospital stay, surgery, or the presence of urinary or arterial catheters, especially in patients in intensive care units.[84]

Failure to control outbreaks has resulted in the appearance of new-mutant–type extended-spectrum β-lactamases in the same institution and sometimes in the same patient. For example, in Clermont-Ferrand hospital, eight different extended-spectrum β-lactamases (TEM-3, TEM-5, TEM-8, TEM-12, TEM-24, TEM-16, SHV-4, and SHV-5) have appeared since the first surfaced in 1984.[85] Both plasmid and strain dissemination have occurred. Furthermore, the finding of CAZ-7–producing *K. pneumoniae* and *E. coli* in the same patient led to the discovery that the CAZ-7 and amikacin genes were on a fragment that could translocate to different plasmids. Other extended-spectrum β-lactamase genes (i.e., genes for TEM-3 and TEM-12) are known to reside on transposons.[86–88] TEM-12 arose as the result of a single point mutation in a plasmid bearing the gene for TEM-1 that had been seen 12 years earlier in one hospital.[89] Apparently, single point mutations and recombinations between different β-lactamase genes are yielding new extended-spectrum β-lactamases in the "hot house" environments where these genes are endemic.[89, 90]

Other genetic events may also be contributing to the resistance mediated by extended-spectrum β-lactamases. In many strains producing TEM-6 and other TEM variants, researchers have found IS1-like elements that insert into the promoter of the gene for TEM-6 and increase its strength, causing high-level production of these extended-spectrum β-lactamases.[91] Indeed, even the high-level production of the parent β-lactamase SHV-1 confers resistance to ceftazidime and aztreonam.[92]

Isolates of *E. coli* that produce a new class of TEM-derived plasmid-borne β-lactamase have been found in France, Scotland, and Spain.[93–95] These so-called TRI or IRT β-lactamases confer resistance to β-lactamase inhibitors (clavulanate, sulbactam) but not to the oxyimino-β-lactams such as cefotaxime, aztreonam, and ceftazidime.

β-Lactamases Determined by Chromosomal Genes. Virtually all gram-negative bacteria produce some chromosomally determined β-lactamase. Furthermore, the types of β-lactamases produced are often specific for species and sometimes for subspecies. β-Lactamase activity is frequently very low, particularly in ampicillin-susceptible isolates, but may increase because of either induction or alteration in the number of β-lactamase genes on the chromosome.[96] Also, mutation of genes that regulate induction may lead to constitutive hyperproduction of inducible β-lactamases.[97] Selection of hyperproducer mutants caused the emergence of resistance to third-generation cephalosporins in 19% of patients receiving third-generation cephalosporins for *Enterobacter* bacteremia.[98] Most of the clinically relevant chromosomally determined β-lactamases belonging to Bush group 1 preferentially hydrolyze cephalosporins and are resistant to inhibition by clavulanic acid. They inactivate many of the third-generation β-lactams that are resistant to hydrolysis by most of the plasmid-determined β-lactamases. The metallo-β-lactamases that hydrolyze carbapenems are a growing threat of great concern.[99]

Chromosomally determined β-lactamases nearly always differ in their biochemical properties from the plasmid-determined enzymes. The exception is a chromosomal β-lactamase found in many isolates of *K. pneumoniae* that is indistinguishable from the SHV-1 β-lactamase. It may be that the gene for SHV-1 β-lactamase evolved as a chromosomal gene in *Klebsiella* and was later incorporated into a plasmid.[100] No such ancestral chromosomal gene has been found for the much more common TEM-1 β-lactamase or for any of the other plasmid-determined β-lactamases.

Chromosomal genes have incorporated into plasmids, a long-feared threat. In Providence, Rhode Island, nosocomial isolates of *K. pneumoniae* and *E. coli* were found to produce the MIR-1 β-lactamase, a plasmid-determined *ampC*-type β-lactamase derived from *E. cloacae*.[101] Besides resistance to oxyimino-β-lactams, the strains were also highly resistant to the 7α-methoxy-β-lactams and the clavam and sulfone β-lactamase inhibitors. Recently, nosocomial isolates of *E. coli* and *K. pneumoniae* producing ACT-1, an *E. cloacae*–like plasmid-determined β-lactamase, caused an outbreak in a New York hospital. In addition to resistance to cephamycins and oxyiminocephalosporins, some porin-deficient isolates were resistant to imipenem as well.[94] Plasmid-borne genes determining *ampC*-type β-lactamases from *C. freundii* (CMY-2, BIL-1, SAL-1, LAT-1, and LAT-2), *Morganella morganii* (MOR-1), and *K. oxytoca* (MEN-1, CTX-M-2, CTX-M-3, CTX-M-4, TOHO-1, TOHO-2) have also been found. The plasmids were in strains of *K. pneumoniae* and *E. coli* from France, Greece, and Pakistan, demonstrating that the formidable threat posed by them is already worldwide. The discovery in Japan of a strain of *P. aeruginosa* producing a plasmid-mediated metallo-β-lactamase, IMP-1, that confers resistance to imipenem and all other β-lactams presents an even greater threat.[102] IMP-1 has spread to *Serratia* and other gram-negative bacilli, causing multifocal outbreaks in Japanese hospitals around Tokyo.[103–105] Reports of transferable carbapenemases (apparently nonmetallo-β-lactamases) in *Acinetobacter* isolates from Scotland and Argentina are equally disturbing.[106–108]

Contribution of β-Lactamases to β-Lactam Antibiotic Resistance. The level of antibiotic resistance mediated by a particular β-lactamase in a population of bacteria is determined by several variables. The efficiency of the β-lactamase in hydrolyzing an antibiotic depends on both its rate of hydrolysis (V_{max}) and its affinity for the antibiotic (K_m). Other variables are the amount of β-lactamase produced by the bacterial cell, the susceptibility of the target protein (PBP) to the antibiotic, and the rate of diffusion of the antibiotic into the periplasm of the cell.

Within the bacterial cell, β-lactamases contribute to antibiotic resistance in several ways. The simplest model is that of penicillinase-producing staphylococci in which the bacteria, upon exposure to penicillin, begin to produce β-lactamase, which they excrete extracellularly. Two events then take place concurrently: *(1)* penicillin lyses bacteria, and *(2)* β-lactamase hydrolyzes penicillin. If viable bacterial cells remain after the level of penicillin has fallen below the minimal inhibitory concentration (MIC), regrowth of bacteria occurs.[40]

Another model is exemplified by gram-negative bacilli, which *(1)* produce a β-lactamase that remains trapped in the periplasmic space and *(2)* have no barrier to antibiotic penetration. An example is *H. influenzae* strains that produce the TEM-1 β-lactamase.[109] In both this model and the first one discussed, a marked inoculum effect occurs in that the MIC for a large inoculum (10^6 organisms/ml) may be a thousandfold greater than that for a small inoculum (10^2 organisms/ml). The low level of resistance of single cells has made it possible for ampicillin to cure some infections caused by β-lactamase–producing strains of *H. influenzae* when the inoculum of infecting bacteria was low.

Another model is exemplified by ampicillin resistance of *E. coli* strains that produce the TEM-1 β-lactamase. These bacteria have a barrier to entry of β-lactam molecules (the outer membrane), and they produce a β-lactamase that remains localized to the periplasmic space. In this model, the kinetics are more complicated. The enzyme is strategically situated between the barrier to antibiotic penetration (outer membrane) and the antibiotic targets (penicillin-binding proteins on the cytoplasmic membrane). In this position, the enzyme can sequentially destroy antibiotic molecules as they make their way through the barrier, analogous to a sharpshooter with abundant ammunition who aims at targets passing through a single entry point. As a consequence, high levels of resistance occur with single bacterial cells, unlike the previous example.[40]

Variations on this model occur when the amount of β-lactamase produced increases with exposure to a β-lactam (induction), as occurs in *Enterobacter* and *Pseudomonas* spp. High levels of β-lactamase are produced only after a period of exposure to the inducing antibiotic, and hence resistance may be expressed late. When *Enterobacter* strains are exposed to two β-lactam antibiotics, one of which is a potent inducer (e.g., cefamandole), antagonism between the two antibiotics may result.[110]

Table 16–4 lists mechanisms of resistance to β-lactam antibiotics. Often these mechanisms work in concert and may accumulate in a single patient. An example is a 19-month-old child with aplastic anemia who over 3 months had nine blood isolates of *E. coli*, all derived from a common ancestor, despite multiple courses of antibiotics including ceftazidime.[111] The first isolate produced a TEM-1 β-lactamase but was susceptible to ceftazidime (MIC = 0.25 μg/ml). A subsequent isolate became resistant (MIC of ceftazidime = 32 μg/ml) by acquiring a new plasmid-determined β-lactamase (SHV-1) linked to very efficient promoter and turning off production of an outer membrane porin. An even higher level of resistance (MIC of ceftazidime = >128 μg/ml) occurred when the SHV-1 β-lactamase mutated to form the extended-spectrum β-lactamase, SHV-8, that hydrolyzes ceftazidime much more rapidly. By turning off porin production to slow the rate of entry of ceftazidime into the periplasmic space and producing an extended-spectrum, ceftazidime-inactivating β-lactamase, the infecting *E. coli* utilized two mechanisms synergistically to achieve a high level of resistance to ceftazidime.

Aminoglycoside Resistance–Modifying Enzymes

Among aerobic bacteria, aminoglycoside resistance is most commonly due to modifying enzymes that are coded by genes on plasmids or the chromosome.[112] Several of the aminoglycoside-modifying enzymes have been shown to be carried on transposons.[18]

More than two dozen aminoglycoside-modifying enzymes that have been identified are capable of three general reactions: *N*-acetylation, *O*-nucleotidylation, and *O*-phosphorylation. For each of these general reactions, there are several different enzymes that attack a specific amino or hydroxyl group. The nomenclature for these enzymes lists the molecular site where the modification occurs after the type of enzymatic activity. For example, an aminoglycoside acetyltransferase (AAC) that acts at the 3′ site is designated AAC (3′) (Table 16–5).[45] However, there may be more than one enzyme that will catalyze the same reaction, and thus roman numerals may be necessary (e.g., AAC [3′] - IV).

Enzymatic aminoglycoside resistance is achieved by modification of the antibiotic in the process of transport across the cytoplasmic membrane.[112] Resistance to a particular aminoglycoside is a function of two different rates, that of drug uptake versus that of drug

TABLE 16–4 Mechanisms of Resistance to β-Lactam Antibiotics

- I. Alter target site (PBP, penicillin-binding protein)
  - A. Decrease affinity of PBP for β-lactam antibiotic
    - 1. Modify existing PBP
      - a. Create mosaic PBP
        - (1) Insert nucleotides obtained from neighboring bacteria, e.g., penicillin-resistant *Streptococcus pneumoniae*
      - b. Mutate structural gene of PBP(s), e.g., ampicllin-resistant β-lactamase–negative *Haemophilus influenzae*
    - 2. Import new PBP, e.g., mecA in methicillin-resistant *Staphylococcus aureus*
- II. Destroy β-lactam antibiotic
  - A. Increase production of β-lactamase
    - 1. Acquire more efficient promoter
      - a. Mutate existing promoter
      - b. Import new one
    - 2. Deregulate control of β-lactamase production
      - a. Mutate regulator genes, e.g., *ampD* in "stably derepressed" *Enterobacter cloacae*
  - B. Modify structure of resident β-lactamase
    - 1. Mutate its structural gene, e.g., extended-spectrum β-lactamases in *Klebsiella pneumoniae*
  - C. Import new β-lactamase(s) with different spectrum of activity
- III. Decrease concentration of β-lactam antibiotic inside cell
  - A. Restrict its entry (loss of porins)
  - B. Pump it out (efflux mechanisms)

TABLE 16–5 Aminoglycoside-Modifying Enzymes

Enzymes	Usual Antibiotics Modified	Common Genera
Phosphorylation		
APH(2″)	K, T, G	SA, SR
APH(3′)-I	K	E, PS, SA, SR
APH(3′)-III	K, ±A	E, PS, SA, SR
Acetylation		
AAC(2′)	G	PR
AAC(3)-I	±T, G	E, PS
AAC(3)-III, -IV, or -V	K, T, G	E, PS
AAC(6′)	K, T, ±A	E, PS, SA
Adenylation		
ANT(2″)	K, T, G	E, PS
ANT(4′)	K, T, A	SA

Abbreviations: A, Amikacin; AAC, aminoglycoside acetyltransferase; ANT, aminoglycoside nucleotidyltransferase; APH, aminoglycoside phosphotransferase; E, Enterobacteriaceae; G, gentamicin; K, karamycin; PR, *Providencia-Proteus*; PS, pseudomonids; SA, staphylococci; SR, streptococci; T, tobramycin.

inactivation. An important factor in determining the level of resistance is the affinity of the modifying enzyme for the antibiotic. If an enzyme has a high affinity for the specific aminoglycoside, then drug inactivation can occur at very low concentrations of the enzyme.

The differences in the worldwide distribution of aminoglycoside-modifying enzymes may partially be a function of antibiotic selection pressures and have had profound implications on the choice of antibiotics used at specific medical centers. Aminoglycoside phosphotransferase (APH)(3′) and APH(3″) are widely distributed among gram-positive and gram-negative species worldwide and thus have led to decreased utilization of kanamycin and streptomycin. The gene for aminoglycoside nucleotidyltransferase (ANT)(2″) has been associated with multiple nosocomial outbreaks over the past decade across the United States. The gene for aminoglycoside acetyltransferase—AAC(6′)-I—has been found to be more prevalent in East Asia.[113] The AAC(3) group of enzymes have been responsible for outbreaks of antibiotic resistance in South America, Western Europe, and the United States. Although each outbreak of aminoglycoside-resistant Enterobacteriaceae has its own pattern, the most typical manner of spread has been the appearance of a plasmid-carrying aminoglycoside-resistant strain of *K. pneumoniae* usually carrying the ANT(2″) gene, with subsequent dissemination to other strains of the species and further spread later to other species and genera of Enterobacteriaceae.[114]

Major increases in plasmid-mediated aminoglycoside resistance have been noted among enterococci,[28, 115, 116] initially in the developing world[117] but increasingly in the United States and Europe.[118, 119] The plasmids that carry the aminoglycoside-modifying genes in enterococcal outbreaks are heterogeneous.[120] Their clinical impact is exacerbated by the frequent cotransmission of β-lactamases, resulting in a loss of synergy when combination therapy is employed for serious enterococcal infections. *Staphylococcus aureus* and *S. epidermidis* have become increasingly resistant to aminoglycosides because of the inter- and intraspecies dissemination of plasmid-mediated aminoglycoside-modifying enzymes.[121]

Chloramphenicol Acetyltransferase

Resistance to chloramphenicol in gram-positive and gram-negative organisms is primarily mediated by the inactivating enzyme *chloramphenicol acetyltransferase*. This is an intracellular enzyme that inactivates the drug by 3-*O*-acetylation[122] and is encoded by plasmid-borne or chromosomal genes. Despite homology at the active site of this enzyme, there is considerable diversity between chloramphenicol acetyltransferase enzymes isolated from gram-positive and gram-negative organisms.[123]

Erythromycin Esterase

Although resistance to erythromycin and other macrolides is frequently the result of alteration in the ribosomal target site, several substrate-inactivating enzymes have been characterized.[124] Erythromycin esterases have been isolated from *E. coli* that hydrolyze the lactone ring of the antibiotic and thus result in its inactivation.[125] This is a plasmid-mediated resistance determinant that is constitutively produced and results in high-level resistance to erythromycin (MIC > 2000 μg/ml).[126] Other plasmid-mediated macrolide, lincosamide, streptogramin (MLS)-inactivating enzymes have been described in *Streptococcus hemolyticus* and *S. aureus* that adenylate,[127] acetylate,[128] or hydrolyze[129] substrate. These resistance determinants may limit the utility of oral erythromycin in reducing the aerobic gram-negative flora of the intestinal tract before gastrointestinal surgical procedures.

Alterations of Bacterial Membranes

Outer Membrane Permeability

It was recognized early in the history of antibiotic development that penicillin is effective against gram-positive bacteria but not against gram-negative bacteria.[130] This difference in susceptibility to penicillin is due in large part to the outer membrane, a lipid bilayer that acts as a barrier to the penetration of antibiotics into the cell.[131] Situated outside the peptidoglycan cell wall of gram-negative bacteria, this outer membrane is absent in gram-positive bacteria. The outer portion of this lipid bilayer is composed principally of lipopolysaccharide made up of tightly bound hydrocarbon molecules that impede the entry of hydrophobic antibiotics, such as nafcillin or erythromycin.[132, 133] Agents that disrupt the integrity of the lipopolysaccharide layer, such as polymixin, or mutations that lead to the production of defective lipopolysaccharides result in increased permeability of hydrophobic antibiotics.[134]

The passage of hydrophilic antibiotics through this outer membrane is facilitated by the presence of porins, proteins that are arranged so as to form water-filled diffusion channels through which antibiotics may traverse.[135] Bacteria usually produce a large number of porins; approximately 10^5 porin molecules are present in a single cell of *E. coli*. Bacteria are able to regulate the relative number of different porins in response to the osmolarity of the surrounding media. Thus, in hyperosmolar media, *E. coli* may repress production of the larger porins (OmpF) while continuing to express smaller ones (OmpC).[136]

The rate of diffusion of antibiotics through this outer membrane is a function not only of the numbers and properties of the porin channels but also of the physicochemical characteristics of the antibiotic. Generally, the larger the antibiotic molecule, the more negative charges, and the greater the degree of hydrophobicity, the less likely it is to penetrate through the outer membrane.[131, 137] Small hydrophilic molecules with a zwitterionic charge, such as imipenem, are highly permeable. Conversely, larger highly charged molecules such as carbenicillin are much less permeable.

Mutations resulting in the loss of specific porins can occur in clinical isolates and determine increased resistance to β-lactam antibiotics. For example, a strain of *Salmonella typhimurium* obtained from a perirenal abscess became resistant to multiple cephalosporins during therapy with cephalexin.[138] The parent strain produced both OmpF and OmpC proteins, but the mutant produced only OmpF. The mutant was resistant to β-lactam antibiotics only when tested in media of high osmolarity, comparable to that in the patient's tissues. Under these conditions, the production of the OmpF protein was repressed completely, leaving the microorganism devoid of either species of porin and impermeable to the cephalosporins. Resistance to aminoglycosides and carbapenems emerging during therapy has also been associated with a lack of production of outer membrane proteins.[139, 140] In *P. aeruginosa*, resistance to imipenem appears to be due to an interplay between chromosomal β-lactamase activity and a loss of a specific entry channel, the D2 porin.[141]

Resistance to nalidixic acid and other quinolones has been associated with alterations of outer membrane proteins in *Serratia marcescens*[142] as well as *P. aeruginosa*. However, single-step high-level mutational resistance to nalidixic acid by aerobic gram-negative bacilli occurs with a 10^{-7} frequency, whereas only low-level resistance to the newer quinolones ($<10 \times$ MIC) is usually obtained with a single-step selection of less than 10^{-9}.[143] Plasmid-mediated chloramphenicol resistance due to decreased permeability has been demonstrated in *E. coli*.[144]

Inner Membrane Permeability

The rate of entry of aminoglycoside molecules into bacterial cells is a function of their binding to a usually nonsaturable anionic transporter, whereupon they retain their positive charge and are subsequently "pulled" across the cytoplasmic membrane by the internal negative charge of the cell.[145] This process requires energy and a threshold minimal level of internal negative charge of the cell that has to be present before significant transport occurs *(proton motive force)*.[146] The level of the internal charge that is required may depend on the actual aminoglycoside concentration at a given time. The energy generation or the proton motive force that is required for substrate transport into the cell may be altered in mutants resistant to aminoglycosides.

These aminoglycoside-resistant isolates with altered proton motive force occur rarely but develop in the course of long-term aminoglycoside therapy.[147] These isolates usually have a "small colony" phenotype due to their reduced rate of growth. They may be unstable and revert back to a sensitive phenotype in the absence of selective aminoglycoside pressure. The clinical significance of these isolates is not clear. They may retain some virulence[148] and may rarely cause fatal bacteremia.[149] Because oxidative metabolism is essential for aminoglycoside uptake action, as well as cell growth and development, *Pseudomonas* mutants have been found that have been deficient in specific cytochromes.[145] Resistant mutants with defective electron transport systems have been described in *E. coli, S. aureus*, and *Salmonella* spp. Facultative organisms grown anaerobically are resistant to aminoglycosides because of a marked reduction of the uptake of the antibiotic.[112]

Promotion of Antibiotic Efflux

The major mechanism of resistance to tetracycline found in enteric gram-negative organisms results from the decreased accumulation of tetracycline. This reduced uptake is an energy-dependent process that is related to the generation of an inner membrane protein produced by the tetracycline-resistance determinant. The primary mechanism for the decreased accumulation of tetracycline is mainly active efflux of the antibiotic across the cell membrane.[150, 151] Decreased uptake of tetracycline from the extracellular environment also accounts for decreased accumulation of tetracycline inside resistant cells. These resistance determinants may be found on the chromosome or plasmids and are frequently found on transposable genetic elements. Tetracycline-resistance genes are generally inducible by subinhibitory concentrations of tetracycline.

Active efflux of antimicrobial agents is recognized increasingly as a common mechanism of resistance in many clinically relevant pathogens. Some strains of *E. coli, Shigella*, and other enteric organisms express a membrane transporter system that leads to multidrug resistance by drug efflux.[152] In enteric bacteria, macrolides or quinolones may be inhibited by active efflux.[153, 154]

In some strains of *S. pneumoniae, Staphylococcus pyogenes, S. aureus*, and *S. epidermidis*, an active efflux mechanism causes resistance to macrolides, streptogramins, and azalides.[155] A similar efflux system, encoded by a gene referred to as *mreA* (for *m*acrolide *r*esistance *e*fflux), has been described in group B streptococci.[156] This mechanism of resistance may be more prevalent in community-acquired infections than was generally appreciated. Dissemination of these resistance genes among important bacterial pathogens represents a considerable threat to the usefulness of macrolide antibiotics.

Active efflux mechanisms may also contribute to the full expression of β-lactam resistance in *P. aeruginosa*. Multidrug efflux pumps in the inner and outer membrane of *P. aeruginosa* may act in concert with periplasmic β-lactamases and membrane permeability components to protect the bacterium from β-lactam agents.[157]

Alteration of Ribosomal Target Sites

Resistance to a wide variety of antimicrobial agents, including tetracyclines, macrolides, lincosamides, and the aminoglycosides, may result from alteration of ribosomal binding sites. Failure of the antibiotic to bind to its target site or sites on the ribosome disrupts its ability to inhibit protein synthesis and cell growth. For MLS, this is the principal mechanism of multiple-agent resistance among aerobic and anaerobic gram-positive organisms.[158] Resistance occurs as the result of at least eight classes of methylase enzymes that dimethylate adenine residues on the 23-S ribosomal RNA of the 50-S subunit of the prokaryotic ribosome, disrupting the binding of MLS to the ribosome. Different classes of this resistance determinant may be located on plasmids or on the bacterial chromosome.[159] MLS resistance due to ribosomal methylation has been described in *S. aureus, Streptococcus sanguis, Bacteroides fragilis*, and *Clostridium perfringens*. MLS resistance may be constitutive or inducible by either older macrolides (e.g., erythromycin) or newer azalides. Tetracycline resistance may also occur by a mechanism that interferes with the ability of tetracycline to bind to the ribosome. The ubiquitous *tetM* resistance gene protects the ribosome from tetracycline action. The precise mechanism of action of this resistance gene is unclear at present.[160] The *tetM* determinant is widely dispersed in gram-positive organisms[160] in addition to *Mycoplasma*,[161] *Ureaplasma*,[23] *Campylobacter*,[162] and *Neisseria* spp.[22]

Resistance to aminoglycosides may also be mediated at the ribosomal level. Mutations of the S12 protein of the 30-S subunit have been shown to interfere with binding streptomycin to the ribosome. Ribosomal resistance to streptomycin may be a significant cause of streptomycin resistance among enterococcal isolates.[163] Ribosomal resistance to the 2-deoxystreptamine aminoglycosides (gentamicin, tobramycin, amikacin) appears to be uncommon and may require multiple mutations in that these aminoglycosides appear to bind to several sites on the 30- and 50-S subunits of the prokaryotic ribosome. Ribosomal resistance is often associated with decreased intracellular accumulation of the drug.[164]

Alteration of Cell Wall Precursor Targets

Vancomycin and other glycopeptide antibiotics such as teicoplanin bind to D-alanine-D-alanine, which is present at the termini of peptidoglycan precursors. The large glycopeptide molecules prevent the incorporation of the precursors into the cell wall. Resistance of enterococci to vancomycin has been classified as A, B, or C based on levels of resistance to vancomycin and susceptibility or resistance to teicoplanin.[165]

Strains of *Enterococcus faecium* and *Enterococcus faecalis* with high-level resistance to both vancomycin and teicoplanin have class A resistance. Either vancomycin or teicoplanin can induce resistance in these strains. Class A resistance to glycopeptides transfers by conjugation from *E. faecium* to other gram-positive bacteria,[166] including *E. faecalis*,[167] *S. pyogenes*, and *S. sanguis*, and *Listeria monocytogenes*. The *vanA* gene on the plasmid encodes an inducible protein that is related to the D-alanine-D-alanine ligases involved in cell wall synthesis in *E. coli*.[168] This protein synthesizes peptidoglycan precursors that have a depsipeptide terminus (D-alanine-D-lactate) instead of the usual D-alanine-D-alanine. The modified peptidoglycan binds glycopeptide antibiotics with reduced affinity, thus conferring resistance to vancomycin and teicoplanin.[169, 170]

Strains of *E. faecium* and *E. faecalis* with class B resistance have levels of resistance to vancomycin that range from high (MIC 1024 μg/ml) to low (MIC 4 μg/ml) and are susceptible to teicoplanin. Vancomycin, but not teicoplanin, can induce resistance to both vancomycin and teicoplanin in these strains. The genes determining the vanB phenotype are self-transferrable by conjugation to other *Enterococcus* strains.[171]

All isolates of *Enterococcus gallinarum* and *Enterococcus casseliflavus* possess low-level resistance to vancomycin and are susceptible to teicoplanin (class C phenotype). The resistance is thought to be mediated by a chromosomal gene.[172]

Since 1987, reports from the United States and Japan have documented outbreaks of vancomycin-resistant *S. epidermidis*[173] and *S. aureus*.[6, 174] The resistance patterns have been heterogeneous, and the underlying mechanisms are still being elucidated, but the specter of increasing outbreaks of vancomycin-resistant staphylococci have led the Centers for Disease Control and Prevention to develop interim guidelines to mitigate the spread of this serious nosocomial problem.[175]

Alteration of Target Enzymes

β-Lactams

β-Lactam antibiotics inhibit bacteria by binding covalently to PBPs in the cytoplasmic membrane. These target proteins catalyze the synthesis of the peptidoglycan that forms the cell wall of bacteria.[176] Alterations of PBPs can lead to β-lactam antibiotic resistance.[177]

In gram-positive bacteria, resistance to β-lactam antibiotics may be associated either with a decrease in the affinity of the PBP for the antibiotic[178] or with a change in the amount of PBP produced by the bacterium.[179] Multiple mechanisms appear to be present in some clinical isolates. For example, penicillin-resistant strains of *S. pneumoniae* isolated in South Africa have shown several changes in their PBPs (i.e., decreased affinity of some PBPs, loss of others, and appearance of PBPs not present in the more susceptible cells).[180] The genes that encode these PBPs are mosaics, made up of segments from susceptible pneumococci and segments from resistant commensal streptococci.[181] In *S. aureus*[182–184] and *E. faecium*,[184, 185] additional PBPs may be inducible (i.e., their production is stimulated by exposure of the microorganism to the β-lactam antibiotic). These inducible PBPs have a lower affinity for β-lactam antibiotics, making them less susceptible to inhibition by low concentrations of drug. Changes in the types of PBPs observed in susceptible and resistant strains have also been seen with viridans streptococcal species *Streptococcus mitis*.[186]

Factors that regulate the induction of PBPs are poorly understood. The induction of a low-affinity PBP in methicillin-resistant *S. aureus* occurs to a larger extent when the microorganisms are grown at 32°C rather than at 37°C, conditions known to favor the expression of methicillin resistance.[187] There is evidence that the production of this inducible PBP is under the control of plasmid-borne genes that regulate staphylococcal penicillinase production. The structural gene (*mecA*) that determines the low-affinity PBP of methicillin-resistant *S. aureus* shares extensive sequence homology with a PBP of *E. coli*, and the genes that regulate the production of the low-affinity PBP have considerable sequence homology with the genes that regulate the production of staphylococcal penicillinase.[188] Thus, the production of this low-affinity PBP in methicillin-resistant *S. aureus* may be mediated by a fusion of gene segments from *E. coli* and *S. aureus*. Another gene (*femA*) also influences the expression of methicillin resistance by mechanisms unknown.[189]

The PBPs of β-lactamase–negative penicillin-resistant strains of *N. gonorrhoeae*, *Neisseria meningitidis*, and *H. influenzae* have shown reduced penicillin-binding affinity[190–193] Their PBPs appear to be encoded by hybrid genes containing segments of DNA scavenged from resistant strains of related species, similar to penicillin-resistant pneumococci.[194] Mutations leading to a loss of outer membrane proteins may also be associated with the acquisition of penicillin resistance in non–penicillinase-producing strains of *N. gonorrhoeae*, suggesting that altered permeability may also contribute to the resistance.[195] Permeability changes and decreased affinity of PBPs are mechanisms jointly found in clinical isolates of *P. aeruginosa*[196] and in non–β-lactamase–producing strains of *H. influenzae* as well.[197] Thus, multiple mutations may be necessary in order to effect this type of resistance.

Sulfonamides and Trimethoprim

Sulfonamides compete with para-aminobenzoic acid to bind the enzyme dihydropteroate synthetase, and thereby halt the generation of pteridines and nucleic acids. Sulfonamide resistance may be mediated by the production of a dihydropteroate synthetase that is resistant to binding by sulfonamides.[198] The high prevalence of resistance to sulfonamides among gram-negative bacteria may be attributed to the spread of R plasmids that contain genes that elaborate resistant enzymes. The most common mechanism of transferable trimethoprim resistance occurs in a similar fashion, by making a drug-resistant dihydrofolate reductase.[199] Trimethoprim-resistant dihydrofolate reductases have been found on the chromosome, and multiple forms have been found to be plasmid mediated.[200]

Quinolones

DNA gyrase is necessary for the supercoiling of chromosomal DNA in bacteria in order to have efficient cell division.[201] This enzyme consists of two A subunits encoded by the *gyrA* gene and two B subunits encoded by the *gyrB* gene. Although spontaneous mutations in the *gyrA* locus have resulted in resistance to multiple fluoroquinolones, B-subunit alterations may also affect resistance to these drugs. Mutations in a variety of chromosomal loci have been described that resulted in altered DNA gyrases resistant to nalidixic acid and the newer fluroquinolones in Enterobacteriaceae and *P. aeruginosa*.[202, 203] Many of these mutations involve the substitution of single amino acids at key enzymatic sites that are involved in the generation of the DNA gyrase–bacterial complex.[201, 204] Clinical isolates of *C. freundii* in Japan have been found to be highly resistant to the newer quinolones via alterations in the DNA gyrase.[205] Alterations in the DNA gyrases of clinical isolates of other Enterobacteriaceae, particularly *E. coli*, have been described[206, 207] and are thought to involve a mechanism that is similar to that found in quinolone-resistant *S. aureus* and other gram-positive species. The mechanism responsible for quinolone resistance recently described on a transferable plasmid in *K. pneumoniae* has yet to be defined.[8] It appears that resistance expression in recipients of the R plasmid is facilitated in strains that lack certain outer membrane porins. Transconjugants that have inherited the quinolone-resistance plasmid readily express high-level resistance on progressive exposure to increasing levels of quinolones.

Bypass of Antibiotic Inhibition

Another mechanism for acquiring resistance to specific antibiotics is by the development of auxotrophs, which have growth factor requirements different from those of the wild strain. These mutants require substrates that normally are synthesized by the target enzymes, and thus if the substrates are present in the environment, the organisms are able to grow despite inhibition of the synthetic enzyme. For example, bacteria that lose the enzyme thymidylate synthetase are "thymine dependent" and cannot synthesize thymidylate in the usual way. They therefore require exogenous supplies of thymidine to synthesize thymidylate via salvage pathways and are thus highly resistant to trimethoprim.[208]

CONTROL OF ANTIBIOTIC RESISTANCE

Although the emergence of antibiotic-resistant bacteria has generally been correlated with the rise and fall of specific antibiotic use in clinical practice, the chain of causality is not always clear-cut.[209] Bacterial strains contain complex aggregations of genes that may be linked together. Thus the use of one antibiotic may select for the emergence of resistance to another. Although the development of antibiotic resistance may be inevitable, the rate at which it develops may be diminished by the rational use of antibiotics.[210]

The wider accessibility to computers and the ability to track R genes with molecular techniques have enhanced the ability to track the spread of antibiotic resistance. With the appropriate computerized surveillance, a hospital laboratory may be able to rapidly detect the emergence of a new type of resistance or the presence of a new microbial strain within a specific unit or patient population. Techniques such as restriction endonuclease digestion analyses of microbial genomes and genetic probes of R genes by polymerase chain reaction make it possible to confirm the presence of new genes in the environment. This information may then be correlated with the phenotypic measures determined by the clinical microbiology surveillance system (Fig. 16–4).[211] Utilization of molecular techniques greatly augments surveillance data, since large data sets may obscure subtle changes ("miniepidemics") that may be more amenable to the institution of stringent infection control measures.

The study of the genetics of antibiotic resistance, particularly the awareness of the great mobility of plasmids and transposons, leads one to the conclusion that ultimately each antibiotic used may inexorably alter its microenvironment, creating selective advantages for resistant organisms. Since prokaryotic organisms all contribute to a common "gene pool," favorable genes mediating antibiotic resistance may disseminate among bacterial populations. In less than a decade, newly utilized inexpensive drugs such as trimethoprim have gone from being highly effective in the treatment of dysentery in developing countries to becoming unusable in several of these areas.[212] Other recent examples of the emergence of polyresistant organisms have had clinical significance in the management of outpatient, as well as nosocomial, infections. The increased use of erythromycin for the management of streptococcal pharyngitis in Finland in the 1980s has been paralleled by a dramatic increase in the prevalence of multiresistant streptococci isolated from pharyngeal, as well as blood, cultures.[213] The clinical importance of this finding is that in β-lactam–intolerant or allergic patients, the range of effective antistreptococcal drugs is becoming increasingly limited. Even more worrisome is the specter of multiresistant enterococci as nosocomial pathogens,[214] given their increasing resistance to β-lactams[215] and aminoglycosides,[216] as well as vancomycin[217] and other glycopeptides. Outbreaks of vancomycin-resistant *E. faecalis* and vancomycin-ampicillin–resistant *E. faecium* have occurred in London, New York, Philadelphia, and Providence, Rhode Island.[218–222]

Similar concerns exist regarding the management of staphylococcal infections, given the rapid spread of simultaneous β-lactam, aminoglycoside, and quinolone-resistant isolates.[223–225] Recent reports of vancomycin-resistant *S. aureus* in Japan and the United States suggest that common, invasive, microbial pathogens may become refractory to any chemotherapeutic agent in the future.[6, 226] Rational antibiotic usage policies would suggest the curtailment of the unnecessary use of antibiotics in situations such as animal husbandry, although the causal link between the use of antibiotics for animal growth promotion and their augmentation of the resistance in human pathogens has been disputed.[227] New drug discoveries have allowed us to be one step ahead of the bacterial pathogens. Nonetheless, the rapid evolution of resistance has limited the duration of the effectiveness of specific agents against certain pathogens. The best hope for the future is the development of a greater understanding of how antimicrobial resistance spreads and the implementation of effective infection control strategies.[228] Newer antimicrobial agents have had a substantial impact in decreasing human morbidity and mortality rates over the past half century. It behooves us to expand our surveillance of antibiotic resistance determinants and to exercise caution in dispensing antibiotics in order to maximize their continued efficacy.

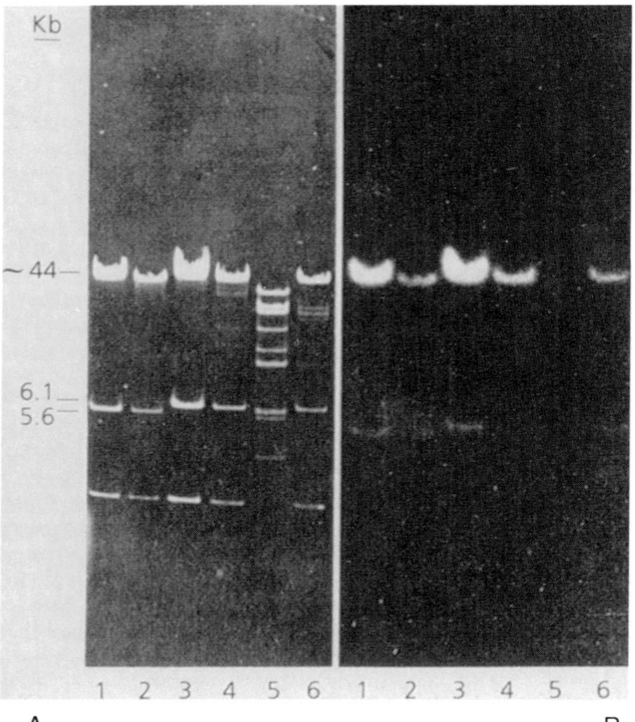

FIGURE 16–4. *A*, Agarose gel of *Eco*RI-digested plasmids derived from four isolates that contain a nosocomial trimethoprim resistance plasmid (known as pBWH10) from a Boston hospital *(lanes 1–4)*. Another nosocomial plasmid from the same hospital that does not contain trimethoprim resistance genes *(lane 5)* and one in which both the trimethoprim resistance and sensitive plasmids are present in the same isolate *(lane 6)* are shown. *B*, To demonstrate that the "fingerprints" from the trimethoprim resistance plasmids in lanes 1–4 and 6 contain the same gene, DNA-DNA hybridization of the same six plasmids was performed using a type II DHFR probe. The probe and the restriction endonuclease analyses helped pinpoint the location and genetic homology of this trimethoprim resistance gene.

REFERENCES

1. Kopecko D. Specialized genetic recombination systems in bacteria: Their involvement in gene expression and evolution. Prog Mol Subcell Biol. 1980;7:135–243.
2. Kopecko DJ. Involvement of specialized recombination in the evolution and expression of bacterial genes. In: Stutgard C, Rozel KR, eds. Plasmids and Transposons. New York: Academic; 1980:165–206.
3. Medeiros AA. Evolution and dissemination of β-lactamases accelerated by generations of β-lactam antibiotics. Clin Infect Dis. 1997;24:S19–S45.
4. Gold HS, Moellering RC, Jr. Antimicrobial-drug resistance. N Engl J Med. 1996;335:1445–1453.
5. Lupski JR. Molecular mechanisms for transposition of drug-resistance genes and other movable genetic elements. Rev Infect Dis. 1987;9:357–368.
6. Hiramatsu K, Aritaka N, Hanaki H, et al. Dissemination in Japanese hospitals of strains of *Staphylococcus aureus* heterogeneously resistant to vancomycin (see Comments). Lancet. 1997;350:1670–1673.
7. Galimand M, Guiyoule A, Gerbaud G, et al. Multidrug resistance in *Yersinia pestis* mediated by a transferable plasmid (see Comments). N Engl J Med. 1997;337:677–680.
8. Martinez-Martinez L, Pascual J, Jacoby GA. Quinolone resistance from a transferable plasmid. Lancet. 1998;351:797–799.
9. Gardner P, Smith DH, Beer H, Moellering R. Recovery of resistance factors from a drug-free community. Lancet. 1969;2:774–776.
10. Datta N. Plasmids as organisms. In: Helinski DR, Cohen SN, Clewell DB, et al. Plasmids in Bacteria. New York: Plenum; 1985:383–395.

11. O'Brien TF, Pla MP, Mayer KH, et al. Intercontinental spread of a new antibiotic resistance gene on an epidemic plasmid. Science. 1985;230:87–88.
12. Timmis KN, Gonzalez-Carrero MI, Sekizaki T, Rojo F. Biological activities specified by antibiotic resistance plasmids. J Antimicrob Chemother. 1986;18(Suppl C):1–12.
13. Nordstrom K. Replication, incompatibility and partition. In: Helinski DR, Cohen SN, Clewell DB, et al. Plasmids in Bacteria. New York: Plenum; 1985:119–123.
14. Thompson R. R plasmid transfer. J Antimicrob Chemother. 1986;18(Suppl C):13–23.
15. Summers AO, Wireman J, Vimy MJ, et al. Mercury released from dental silver fillings provokes an increase in mercury-resistant and antibiotic-resistant bacteria in oral and intestinal floras of primates. Antimicrob Agents Chemother. 1993;37:825–834.
16. Foster TJ. Plasmid-determined resistance to antimicrobial drugs and toxic metal ions in bacteria. Microbiol Rev. 1983;47:361–409.
17. Mayer KH, Hopkins JD, Gilleece ES, et al. Molecular evolution, species distribution, and clinical consequences of an endemic aminoglycoside resistance plasmid. Antimicrob Agents Chemother. 1986;29:628–633.
18. Rubens CE, McNeill WF, Farrar WE, Jr. Evolution of multiple-antibiotic-resistance plasmids mediated by transposable plasmid deoxyribonucleic acid sequences. J Bacteriol. 1979;140:713–719.
19. Blattner FR, Plunkett G, 3rd, Bloch CA, et al. The complete genome sequence of *Escherichia coli* K-12 [Comment]. Science. 1997;277:1453–1474.
20. Franke AE, Clewell DB. Evidence for a chromosome-borne resistance transposon (Tn916) in *Streptococcus faecalis* that is capable of "conjugal" transfer in the absence of a conjugative plasmid. J Bacteriol. 1981;145:494–502.
21. El Solh N, Allignet J, Bismuth R, et al. Conjugative transfer of staphylococcal antibiotic resistance markers in the absence of detectable plasmid DNA. Antimicrob Agents Chemother. 1986;30:161–169.
22. Morse SA, Johnson SR, Biddle JW, Roberts MC. High-level tetracycline resistance in *Neisseria gonorrhoeae* is result of acquisition of streptococcal tetM determinant. Antimicrob Agents Chemother. 1986;30:664–670.
23. Roberts MC, Kenny GE. Dissemination of the tetM tetracycline resistance determinant to *Ureaplasma urealyticum*. Antimicrob Agents Chemother. 1986;29:350–352.
24. Arthur M, Reynolds P, Courvalin P. Glycopeptide resistance in enterococci. Trends Microbiol. 1996;4:401–407.
25. DeFlaun MF, Levy SB. Genes and their various hosts. In. Levy SB, Miller RV. Gene Transfer in the Environment. New York: McGraw-Hill; 1989;1–32.
26. Brisson-Noel A, Arthur M, Courvalin P. Evidence for natural gene transfer from gram-positive cocci to *Escherichia coli*. J Bacteriol. 1988;170:1739–1745.
27. Papadopoulou B, Courvalin P. Dispersal in *Campylobacter* spp. of aphA-3, a kanamycin resistance determinant from gram-positive cocci. Antimicrob Agents Chemother. 1988;32:945–948.
28. Courvalin P, Carlier C, Collatz E. Plasmid-mediated resistance to aminocyclitol antibiotics in group D streptococci. *J Bacteriol*. 1980;143:541–551.
29. Zscheck KK, Hull R, Murray BE. Restriction mapping and hybridization studies of a beta-lactamase-encoding fragment from *Streptococcus (Enterococcus) faecalis*. Antimicrob Agents Chemother. 1988;32:768–769.
30. Courvalin P. Resistance of enterococci to glycopeptides. Antimicrob Agents Chemother. 1990;34:2291–2296.
31. Neu HC. The crisis in antibiotic resistance. Science. 1992;257:1064–1073.
32. Cohen ML. Epidemiology of drug resistance: Implications for a post-antimicrobial era (see Comments). Science. 1992;257:1050–1055.
33. Stokes HW, Hall RM. A novel family of potentially mobile DNA elements encoding site-specific gene-integration functions: Integrons. Mol Microbiol. 1989;3:1669–1683.
34. Cameron FH, Groot Obbink DJ, Ackerman VP, Hall RM. Nucleotide sequence of the AAD(2″) aminoglycoside adenylyltransferase determinant aadB. Evolutionary relationship of this region with those surrounding aadA in R538-1 and dhfrII in R388. Nucleic Acids Res. 1986;14:8625–8635.
35. Collis CM, Hall RM. Expression of antibiotic resistance genes in the integrated cassettes of integrons. Antimicrob Agents Chemother. 1995;39:155–162.
36. Ouellette M, Bissonnette L, Roy PH. Precise insertion of antibiotic resistance determinants into Tn21-like transposons: Nucleotide sequence of the OXA-1 beta-lactamase gene. Proc Natl Acad Sci U S A. 1987;84:7378–7382.
37. Jacoby GA, Archer GL. New mechanisms of bacterial resistance to antimicrobial agents. N Engl J Med. 1991;324:601–612.
38. Medeiros AA. Beta-lactamases. Br Med Bull. 1984;40:18–27.
39. Medeiros AA. Evolution and dissemination of beta-lactamases accelerated by generations of beta-lactam antibiotics. Clin Infect Dis. 1997;24(Suppl 1):S19–S45.
40. Sykes RB, Matthew M. The beta-lactamases of gram-negative bacteria and their role in resistance to beta-lactam antibiotics. J Antimicrob Chemother. 1976;2:115–157.
41. Joris B, Ghuysen J-M, Dive G, et al. The active-site-serine penicillin-recognizing enzymes as members of the *Streptomyces* R61 DD-peptidase family. Biochem J. 1988;250:313–324.
42. Moews PC, Knox JR, Dideberg O, et al. Beta-lactamase of *Bacillus licheniformis* 749/C at 2 Å resolution. Proteins. 1990;7:156–171.
43. Herzberg O. Refined crystal structure of β-lactamase from *Staphylococcus aureus* PC1 at 2.0 Å resolution. J Mol Biol. 1991;217:701–719.
44. Kelly JA, Dideberg O, Charlier P, et al. On the origin of bacterial resistance to penicillin: Comparison of a beta-lactamase and a penicillin target. Science. 1986;231:1429–1431.
45. McDonnell RW, Sweeney HM, Cohen S. Conjugational transfer of gentamicin resistance plasmids intra- and interspecifically in *Staphylococcus aureus* and *Staphylococcus epidermidis*. Antimicrob Agents Chemother. 1983;23:151–160.
46. Murray BE, Mederski-Samoraj B, Foster SK, et al. In vitro studies of plasmid-mediated penicillinase from *Streptococcus faecalis* suggest a staphylococcal origin. J Clin Invest. 1986;77:289–293.
47. Zscheck KK, Murray BE. Genes involved in the regulation of beta-lactamase production in enterococci and staphylococci. Antimicrob Agents Chemother. 1993;37:1966–1970.
48. Murray BE. Beta-lactamase-producing enterococci. Antimicrob Agents Chemother. 1992;36:2355–2359.
49. Rice LB, Marshall SH. Evidence of incorporation of the chromosomal beta-lactamase gene of *Enterococcus-faecalis*-CH19 into a transposon derived from staphylococci. Antimicrob Agents Chemother. 1992;36:1843–1846.
50. Bush K, Jacoby GA, Medeiros AA. A functional classification scheme for β-lactamases and its correlation with molecular structure. Antimicrob Agents Chemother. 1995;39:1211–1233.
51. Medeiros AA. Plasmid-determined beta-lactamases. In: Bryan LE, ed. Handbook of Experimental Pharmacology, v. 91. Berlin: Springer-Verlag; 1989:101–128.
52. Nord CE. Mechanisms of beta-lactam resistance in anaerobic bacteria. Rev Infect Dis. 1986;8(Suppl 5):S543–S548.
53. Appelbaum PC. Patterns of resistance and resistance mechanisms in anaerobes. Clin Microbiol Newslett. 1992;14:49–53.
54. Appelbaum PC, Spangler SK, Pankuch GA, et al. Characterization of a beta-lactamase from *Clostridium clostridioforme*. J Antimicrob Chemother. 1994;33:33–40.
55. Tuner K, Lindqvist L, Nord CE. Purification and properties of a novel beta-lactamase from *Fusobacterium nucleatum*. Antimicrob Agents Chemother. 1985;27:943–947.
56. Cuchural GJ, Jr., Tally FP, Storey JR, Malamy MH. Transfer of beta-lactamase–associated cefoxitin resistance in *Bacteroides fragilis*. Antimicrob Agents Chemother. 1986;29:918–920.
57. Cuchural GJ, Jr., Malamy MH, Tally FP. Beta-lactamase–mediated imipenem resistance in *Bacteroides fragilis*. Antimicrob Agents Chemother. 1986;30:645–648.
58. Hedberg M, Edlund C, Lindqvist L, et al. Purification and characterization of an imipenem hydrolysing metallo-beta-lactamase from *Bacteroides-fragilis*. J Antimicrob Chemother. 1992;29:105–113.
59. Yotsuji A, Minami S, Inoue M, Mitsuhashi S. Properties of novel beta-lactamase produced by *Bacteroides fragilis*. Antimicrob Agents Chemother. 1983;24:925–929.
60. Appelbaum PC, Philippon A, Jacobs MR, et al. Characterization of beta-lactamases from non-*Bacteroides fragilis* group *Bacteroides* spp belonging to seven species and their role in beta-lactam resistance. Antimicrob Agents Chemother. 1990;34:2169–2176.
61. Jacobs MR, Spangler SK, Appelbaum PC. Beta-lactamase production and susceptibility to US and European anaerobic gram-negative bacilli to beta-lactams and other agents. Eur J Clin Microbiol Infect Dis. 1992;11:1081–1093.
62. Medeiros AA, O'Brien TF. Ampicillin-resistant *Haemophilus influenzae* type B possessing a TEM-type beta-lactamase but little permeability barrier to ampicillin. Lancet. 1975;1:716–719.
63. Elwell LP, Roberts M, Mayer LW, Falkow S. Plasmid-mediated beta-lactamase production in *Neisseria gonorrhoeae*. Antimicrob Agents Chemother. 1977;11:528–533.
64. Kliebe C, Nies BA, Meyer JF, et al. Evolution of plasmid-coded resistance to broad-spectrum cephalosporins. Antimicrob Agents Chemother. 1985;28:302–307.
65. Brun-Buisson C, Legrand P, Philippon A, et al. Transferable enzymatic resistance to third-generation cephalosporins during nosocomial outbreak of multiresistant *Klebsiella pneumoniae*. Lancet. 1987;2:302–306.
66. Jacoby GA, Medeiros AA. More extended-spectrum beta-lactamases. Antimicrob Agents Chemother. 1991;35:1697–1704.
67. Naumovski L, Quinn JP, Miyashiro D, et al. Outbreak of ceftazidime resistance due to a novel extended-spectrum beta-lactamase in isolates from cancer patients. Antimicrob Agents Chemother. 1992;36:1991–1996.
68. Sanders CC, Sanders WE. β-Lactam resistance in gram-negative bacteria—global trends and clinical impact. Clin Infect Dis. 1992;15:824–839.
69. Danel F, Hall LMC, Gur D, Livermore DM. OXA-15, an extended-spectrum variant of OXA-2 β-lactamase, isolated from a *Pseudomonas aeruginosa* strain. Antimicrob Agents Chemother. 1997;41:785–790.
70. Danel F, Hall LMC, Gur D, Livermore DM. OXA-14, another extended-spectrum variant of OXA-10 (PSE-2) β-lactamase from *Pseudomonas aeruginosa*. Antimicrob Agents Chemother. 1995;39:1881–1884.
71. Liu PY, Gur D, Hall LMC, Livermore DM. Survey of the prevalence of beta-lactamases amongst 1000 gram-negative bacilli isolated consecutively at the Royal London Hospital. J Antimicrob Chemother. 1992;30:429–447.
72. Sirot DL, Goldstein FW, Soussy CJ, et al. Resistance to cefotaxime and seven other beta-lactams in members of the family Enterobacteriaceae: A 3-year survey in France. Antimicrob Agents Chemother. 1992;36:1677–1681.
73. Ferreira HMN, Sousa JC, Peixe LM. Characterization of the beta-lactamases responsible for the resistance of hospital strains of *Klebsiella pneumoniae* to beta-lactam antibiotics [in Portuguese]. Rev Port Doencas Infecciosas 1992;15:207–209.
74. Sousa JC, Carneiro G, Peixe ML, et al. Characterization of beta-lactamases encoded by pathogenic strains of *Escherichia coli* from Portugal. J Antimicrob Chemother. 1991;27:437–440.
75. Watanabe Y, Yokota T, Higashi Y, et al. In vitro and in vivo transferrable beta-lactam resistance due to a new plasmid-mediated oxyiminocephalosporinase from a clinical isolate of *Proteus mirabilis*. Microbiol Immunol. 1991;35:87–97.

76. Espinasse F, Mariotte S, Labia R, Nicolas MH. Each epidemic cefotaxime (CTX) resistant strain of *Proteus mirabilis* is related to an extended spectrum beta-lactamase. Abstract 1272. In: Program Abstracts of the 32nd Interscience Conference on Antimicrobial Agents and Chemotherapy. Washington, DC: American Society for Microbiology; 1992:323.
77. Rossi MA, Gutkind G, Quinteros M, et al. A *Proteus mirabilis* with a novel extended spectrum beta-lactamase and 6 different aminoglycoside (AG) resistance genes. Abstract 939. In: Program and Abstracts of the 31st Interscience Conference on Antimicrobial Agents and Chemotherapy. Washington, DC: American Society for Microbiology; 1991:255.
78. Mariotte S, Nordmann P, Nicolas MH. Extended-spectrum beta-lactamase in *Proteus mirabilis*. J Antimicrob Chemother. 1994;33:925–935.
79. Bret L, Chanal-Claris C, Sirot D, et al. Chromosomally encoded AmpC-type β-lactamase in a clinical isolate of *Proteus mirabilis*. Antimicrob Agents Chemother. 1998;42:1110–1114.
80. Pitout JDD, Thomson KS, Hanson ND, et al. β-Lactamases responsible for resistance to expanded-spectrum cephalosporins in *Klebsiella pneumoniae, Escherichia coli*, and *Proteus mirabilis* isolates recovered in South Africa. Antimicrob Agents Chemother. 1998;42:1350–1354.
81. Mariotte S, Nordmann P, Nicolas MH. Spread of extended-spectrum beta-lactamases (ES Bla) in *Proteus mirabilis* (P.m.) may be limited by low frequency of plasmid conjugation. Abstract 940. In: Program and Abstracts of the 31st Interscience Conference on Antimicrobial Agents and Chemotherapy. Washington, DC: American Society for Microbiology; 1991:255.
82. Wiener J, Quinn J, Kowalczyk M, et al. Production of TEM-10 beta-lactamase in ceftazidime-resistant (CFZ-R) Enterobacteriaceae from multiple nursing homes (NHs). Abstract 641. In: Program Abstracts of the 32nd Interscience Conference on Antimicrobial Agents and Chemotherapy. Washington, DC: American Society for Microbiology; 1992:217.
83. Schiappa DA, Hayden MK, Matushek MG, et al. Ceftazidime-resistant *Klebsiella pneumoniae* and *Escherichia coli* bloodstream infection: A case-control and molecular epidemiologic investigation. J Infect Dis. 1996;174:529–536.
84. Lucet JC, Chevret S, Decre D, et al. Outbreak of multiply resistant Enterobacteriaceae in an intensive care unit: Epidemiology and risk factors for acquisition. Clin Infect Dis. 1996;22:430–436.
85. Sirot D, deChamps C, Chanal C, et al. Translocation of antibiotic resistance determinants including an extended-spectrum beta-lactamase between conjugative plasmids of *Klebsiella pneumoniae* and *Escherichia coli*. Antimicrob Agents Chemother. 1991;35:1576–1581.
86. Jiang H, Hopkins JD, Zieg J, et al. Origin and transposition of a gene encoding a TEM12 beta-lactamase on pBWH102 and pBWH501 in ceftazidime resistant (CAZ-R) isolates of *Klebsiella pneumoniae* at one U.S. medical center. Abstract 186. In: Program and Abstracts of the 30th Interscience Conference on Antimicrobial Agents and Chemotherapy. Washington, DC: American Society for Microbiology; 1990:117.
87. Heritage J, Hawkey PM, Todd N, Lewis IJ. Transposition of the gene encoding a TEM-12 extended-spectrum beta-lactamase. Antimicrob Agents Chemother. 1992;36:1981–1986.
88. Mabilat C, Lourencaovital J, Goussard S, Courvalin P. A new example of physical linkage between tn1 and tn21—the antibiotic multiple-resistance region of plasmid pCFF04 encoding extended-spectrum beta-lactamase TEM-3. Mol Gen Genet. 1992;235:113–121.
89. Jiang H, Zieg J, O'Brien TF. Observation of the acquisition of an amikacin resistance gene by an endemic nosocomial plasmid encoding a ceftazidime resistance gene. Abstract 442. In: Program Abstracts of the 32nd Interscience Conference on Antimicrobial Agents and Chemotherapy. Washington, DC: American Society for Microbiology; 1992:184.
90. Chanal C, Poupart MC, Sirot D, et al. Nucleotide sequences of CAZ-2, CAZ-6, and CAZ-7 beta-lactamase genes. Antimicrob Agents Chemother. 1992;36:1817–1820.
91. Goussard S, Sougakoff W, Mabilat C, et al. An IS1-like element is responsible for high-level synthesis of extended-spectrum beta-lactamase TEM-6 in Enterobacteriaceae. J Gen Microbiol. 1991;137:2681–2687.
92. Petit A, Ben Yaghlane-bouslama H, Sofer L, Labia R. Does high level production of SHV-type penicillinase confer resistance to ceftazidime in Enterobacteriaceae. FEMS Microbiol Lett. 1992;92:89–94.
93. Thomson CJ, Amyes SGB. TRC-1 — emergence of a clavulanic acid–resistant TEM beta-lactamase in a clinical strain. FEMS Microbiol Lett. 1992;91:113–117.
94. Vedel G, Belaaouaj A, Gilly L, et al. Clinical isolates of *Escherichia coli* producing TRI beta-lactamases: Novel TEM-enzymes conferring resistance to beta-lactamase inhibitors. J Antimicrob Chemother. 1992;30:449–462.
95. Blazquez J, Baquero MR, Canton R, et al. Characterization of a new TEM-type beta-lactamase resistant to clavulanate, sulbactam, and tazobactam in a clinical isolate of *Escherichia coli*. Antimicrob Agents Chemother. 1993;37:2059–2063.
96. Sanders CC. Chromosomal cephalosporinases responsible for multiple resistance to newer beta-lactam antibiotics. Ann Rev Microbiol. 1987;41:573–593.
97. Korfmann G, Sanders CC, Moland ES. Altered phenotypes associated with *ampD* mutations in *Enterobacter cloacae*. Antimicrob Agents Chemother. 1991;35:358–364.
98. Chow JW, Fine MJ, Shlaes DM, et al. Enterobacter bacteremia—clinical features and emergence of antibiotic resistance during therapy. Ann Intern Med. 1991;115:585–590.
99. Livermore DM. Carbapenemases. J Antimicrob Chemother. 1992;29:609–612.
100. Nugent ME, Hedges RW. The nature of the genetic determinant for the SHV-1 beta-lactamase. Molec Gen Genet. 1979;175:239–243.
101. Papanicolaou GA, Medeiros AA, Jacoby GA. Novel plasmid-mediated beta-lactamase (MIR-1) conferring resistance to oxyimino- and alphamethoxy-beta-lactams in clinical isolates of *Klebsiella pneumoniae*. Antimicrob Agents Chemother. 1990;34:2200–2209.
102. Watanabe M, Iyobe S, Inoue M, Mitsuhashi S. Transferable imipenem resistance in *Pseudomonas aeruginosa*. Antimicrob Agents Chemother. 1991;35:147–151.
103. Ito H, Arakawa Y, Ohsuka S, et al. Plasmid-mediated dissemination of the metallo-β-lactamase gene bla_{IMP} among clinically isolated strains of *Serratia marcescens*. Antimicrob Agents Chemother. 1995;39:824–829.
104. Senda K, Arakawa Y, Ichiyama S, et al. PCR detection of metallo-β-lactamase gene (bla_{IMP}) in gram-negative rods resistant to broad-spectrum β-lactams. J Clin Microbiol. 1996;34:2909–2913.
105. Senda K, Arakawa Y, Nakashima K, et al. Multifocal outbreaks of metallo-β-lactamase-producing *Pseudomonas aeruginosa* resistant to broad-spectrum β-lactams, including carbapenems. Antimicrob Agents Chemother. 1996;40:349–353.
106. Scaife W, Young HK, Paton RH, Amyes SGB. Transferable imipenem-resistance in *Acinetobacter* species from a clinical source. J Antimicrob Chemother. 1995;36:585–586.
107. Paton R, Miles RS, Hood J, Amyes SGB. ARI 1: Beta-lactamase-mediated imipenem resistance in *Acinetobacter baumannii*. Int J Antimicrob Agents. 1993;2:81–88.
108. Brown S, Bantar C, Young HK, Amyes SGB. Limitation of *Acinetobacter baumannii* treatment by plasmid-mediated carbapenemase ARI-2. Lancet. 1998;351:186–187.
109. Moxon ER, Medeiros AA, O'Brien TF. Beta-lactamase effect on ampicillin treatment of *Haemophilus influenzae* B bacteremia and meningitis in infant rats. Antimicrob Agents Chemother. 1977;12:461–464.
110. Sanders CC, Sanders WE, Jr, Goering RV. In vitro antagonism of beta-lactam antibiotics by cefoxitin. Antimicrob Agents Chemother. 1982;21:968–975.
111. Rasheed JK, Jay C, Metchock B, et al. Evolution of extended-spectrum beta-lactam resistance (SHV-8) in a strain of *Escherichia coli* during multiple episodes of bacteremia. Antimicrob Agents Chemother. 1997;41:647–653.
112. Bryan LE. Aminoglycoside resistance. In: Bryan LE, ed. Antimicrobial Drug Resistance. Orlando, Academic; 1984:241–277.
113. Shimizu K, Kumada T, Hsieh WC, et al. Comparison of aminoglycoside resistance patterns in Japan, Formosa, and Korea, Chile, and the United States. Antimicrob Agents Chemother. 1985;28:282–288.
114. John JF, Jr, Twitty JA. Plasmids as epidemiologic markers in nosocomial gram-negative bacilli: Experience at a university and review of the literature. Rev Infect Dis. 1986;8:693–704.
115. Horodniceanu T, Bougueleret L, El-Solh N, et al. High-level, plasmid-borne resistance to gentamicin in *Streptococcus faecalis* subsp. *zymogenes*. Antimicrob Agents Chemother. 1979;16:686–689.
116. Mederski-Samoraj BD, Murray BE. High-level resistance to gentamicin in clinical isolates of enterococci. J Infect Dis. 1983;147:751–757.
117. Murray BE, Tsao J, Panida J. Enterococci from Bangkok, Thailand, with high-level resistance to currently available aminoglycosides. Antimicrob Agents Chemother. 1983;23:799–802.
118. Zervos MJ, Kauffman CA, Therasse PM, et al. Nosocomial infection by gentamicin-resistant *Streptococcus faecalis*. An epidemiologic study. Ann Intern Med. 1987;106:687–691.
119. Hoffmann SA, Moellering RC, Jr. The enterococcus: "Putting the bug in our ears." Ann Intern Med. 1987;106:757–761.
120. Patterson JE, Masecar BL, Kauffman CA, et al. Gentamicin resistance plasmids of enterococci from diverse geographic areas are heterogeneous. J Infect Dis. 1988;158:212–216.
121. Lyon BR, Skurray R. Antimicrobial resistance of *Staphylococcus aureus*: Genetic basis. Microbiol Rev. 1987;51:88–134.
122. Gaffney DF, Foster TJ, Shaw WV. Chloramphenicol acetyl transferases determined by R-plasmids from gram (−) bacteria. J Gen Microbiol. 1978;109:351–358.
123. Davies J. General mechanisms of antimicrobial resistance. Rev Infect Dis. 1979;1:23–29.
124. LeClercq R, Courvalin P. Resistance to macrolides, azalides, and streptogramins. In: Neu HC, Young LS, Zinner SH, eds. The New Macrolides, Azalides, and Streptogramins. New York: Dekker; 1993;33–40.
125. Barthelemy P, Autissier D, Gerbaud G, Courvalin P. Enzymatic hydrolysis of erythromycin by a strain of *Escherichia coli*: A new mechanism of resistance. J Antibiot (Tokyo). 1984;37:1692–1696.
126. Andremont A, Gerbaud G, Courvalin P. Plasmid-mediated high-level resistance to erythromycin in *Escherichia coli*. Antimicrob Agents Chemother. 1986;29:515–518.
127. Brisson-Noel A, Delrieu P, Samain D, Courvalin P. Inactivation of lincosaminide antibiotics in *Staphylococcus*. Identification of lincosaminide *O*-nucleotidyltransferases and comparison of the corresponding resistance genes. J Biol Chem. 1988;263:15,880–15,887.
128. Le G'offic F, et al. Plasmid-mediated pristinamycin resistance; PH1A, a pristinamycin 1A hydrolase. Ann Microbiol. 1977;128:417–474.
129. Allignet J, Loncle V, Mazodier P, el Solh N. Nucleotide sequence of a staphylococcal plasmid gene, *vgb*, encoding a hydrolase inactivating the B components of virginiamycin-like antibiotics. Plasmid. 1988;20:271–275.
130. Fleming A. On the antibacterial action of cultures of a penicillium, with special reference to their use in the isolation of *B. influenzae*. Br J Exp Pathol. 1929;10:226–236.
131. Nikaido H. Role of permeability barriers in resistance to beta-lactam antibiotics. Pharmacol Ther. 1985;27:197–231.
132. Labischinski H, Barnickel G, Bradaczek H, et al. High state of order of isolated

bacterial lipopolysaccharide and its possible contribution to the permeation barrier property of the outer membrane. J Bacteriol. 1985;162:9–20.
133. Takeuchi Y, Nikaido H. Physical interaction between lipid A and phospholipids: A study with spin-labeled phospholipids. Rev Infect Dis. 1984;6:488–492.
134. Vaara M. Polymyxin B nonapeptide complexes with lipopolysaccharide (Letter). FEMS Microbiol Lett. 1983;18:117–121.
135. Nikaido H, Vaara M. Molecular basis of bacterial outer membrane permeability. Microbiol Rev. 1985;49:1–32.
136. Hasegawa Y, Yamada H, Mizushima S. Interactions of outer membrane proteins 0-8 and 0-9 with peptidoglycan sacculus of *Escherichia coli* K-12. J Biochem (Tokyo). 1976;80:1401–1409.
137. Yoshimura F, Nikaido H. Diffusion of beta-lactam antibiotics through the porin channels of *Escherichia coli* K-12. Antimicrob Agents Chemother. 1985;27:84–92.
138. Medeiros AA, O'Brien TF, Rosenberg EY, Nikaido H. Loss of OmpC porin in a strain of *Salmonella typhimurium* causes increased resistance to cephalosporins during therapy. J Infect Dis. 1987;156:751–757.
139. Goldstein FW, Gutmann L, Williamson R, et al. In vivo and in vitro emergence of simultaneous resistance to both beta-lactam and aminoglycoside antibiotics in a strain of *Serratia marcescens*. Ann Microbiol. 1983;134A:329–337.
140. Quinn JP, Dudek EJ, DiVincenzo CA, et al. Emergence of resistance to imipenem during therapy for *Pseudomonas aeruginosa* infections. J Infect Dis. 1986; 154:289–293.
141. Livermore DM. Interplay of impermeability and chromosomal beta-lactamase activity in imipenem-resistant *Pseudomonas aeruginosa*. Antimicrob Agents Chemother. 1992;36:2046–2048.
142. Sanders CC, Sanders WE, Jr, Goering RV, Werner V. Selection of multiple antibiotic resistance by quinolones, beta-lactams, and aminoglycosides with special reference to cross-resistance between unrelated drug classes. Antimicrob Agents Chemother. 1984;26:797–801.
143. Hooper DC, Wolfson JS, Ng EY, Swartz MN. Mechanisms of action of and resistance to ciprofloxacin. Am J Med. 1987;82:12–20.
144. Gaffney DF, Cundliffe E, Foster TJ. Chloramphenicol resistance that does not involve chloramphenicol acetyltransferase encoded by plasmids from gram-negative bacteria. J Gen Microbiol. 1981;125:113–121.
145. Bryan LE, Kwan S. Roles of ribosomal binding, membrane potential, and electron transport in bacterial uptake of streptomycin and gentamicin. Antimicrob Agents Chemother. 1983;23:835–845.
146. Mates SM, Eisenberg ES, Mandel LJ, et al. Membrane potential and gentamicin uptake in *Staphylococcus aureus*. Proc Natl Acad Sci U S A. 1982;79:6693–6697.
147. Rusthoven JJ, Davies TA, Lerner SA. Clinical isolation and characterization of aminoglycoside-resistant small colony variants of *Enterobacter aerogenes*. Am J Med. 1979;67:702–706.
148. Musher DM, Baughn RE, Merrell GL. Selection of small-colony variants of Enterobacteriaceae by in vitro exposure to aminoglycosides: Pathogenicity for experimental animals. J Infect Dis. 1979;140:209–214.
149. Funada H, Hattori KI, Kosakai N. Catalase-negative *Escherichia coli* isolated from blood. J Clin Microbiol. 1978;7:474–478.
150. McMurry L, Petrucci RE, Jr, Levy SB. Active efflux of tetracycline encoded by four genetically different tetracycline resistance determinants in *Escherichia coli*. Proc Natl Acad Sci U S A. 1980;77:3974–3977.
151. McMurry LM, Park BH, Burdett V, Levy SB. Energy-dependent efflux mediated by class L (tetL) tetracycline resistance determinant from streptococci. Antimicrob Agents Chemother. 1987;31:1648–1650.
152. Williams JB. Drug efflux as a mechanism of resistance. Br J Biomed Sci. 1996;53:290–293.
153. Ghosh AS, Ahamed J, Chauhan KK, Kundu M. Involvement of an efflux system in high-level fluoroquinolone resistance of *Shigella dysenteriae*. Biochem Biophys Res Commun. 1998;242:54–56.
154. Cohen SP, Hooper DC, Wolfson JS, et al. Endogenous active efflux of norfloxacin in susceptible *Escherichia coli*. Antimicrob Agents Chemother. 1988;32:1187–1191.
155. Sutcliffe J, Tait-Kamradt A, Wandrack L. *Streptococcus pneumoniae* and *Streptococcus pyogenes* resistant to macrolid but sensitive to clindamycin; a common resistance pattern made by an efflux system. Antimicrob Agents Chemother. 1996;40:1817–1824.
156. Clancy J, Dib-Hajj F, Petitpas JW, Yuan W. Cloning and characterization of a novel macrolide efflux gene, *mreA*, from *Streptococcus agalactiae*. Antimicrob Agents Chemother. 1997;41:2719–2723.
157. Srikumar R, Li XZ, Poole K. Inner membrane efflux components are responsible for β-lactam specificity of multidrug efflux pumps in *Pseudomonas aeruginosa*. J Bacteriol. 1997;179:7875–7881.
158. Engel HW, Soedirman N, Rost JA, et al. Transferability of macrolide, lincomycin, and streptogramin resistances between group A, B, and D streptococci, *Streptococcus pneumoniae*, and *Staphylococcus aureus*. J Bacteriol. 1980;142:407–413.
159. Weisblum B. Inducible resistance to macrolides, lincosamides and streptogramin type B antibiotics: The resistance phenotype, its biological diversity, and structural elements that regulate expression—a review. J Antimicrob Chemother. 1985;16(Suppl A):63–90.
160. Burdette V. Streptococcal tetracycline resistance mediated at the level of protein synthesis. J Bacteriol. 1986;165:564–569.
161. Roberts MC, Koutsky LA, Holmes KK, et al. Tetracycline-resistant *Mycoplasma hominis* strains contain streptococcal *tetM* sequences. Antimicrob Agents Chemother. 1985;28:141–143.
162. Taylor DE, Hiratsuka K, Ray H, Manavathu EK. Characterization and expression of a cloned tetracycline resistance determinant from *Campylobacter jejuni* plasmid pUA466. J Bacteriol. 1987;169:2984–2989.
163. Eliopoulos GM, Farber BF, Murray BE, et al. Ribosomal resistance of clinical enterococcal to streptomycin isolates. Antimicrob Agents Chemother. 1984;25:398–399.
164. Ahmad MH, Rechenmacher A, Bock A. Interaction between aminoglycoside uptake and ribosomal resistance mutations. Antimicrob Agents Chemother. 1980;18:798–806.
165. Dutka-Malen S, LeClercq R, Coutant V, et al. Phenotypic and genotypic heterogeneity of glycopeptide resistance determinants in gram-positive bacteria. Antimicrob Agents Chemother. 1990;34:1875–1879.
166. LeClercq R, Derlot E, Weber M, et al. Transferable vancomycin and teicoplanin resistance in *Enterococcus faecium*. Antimicrob Agents Chemother. 1989;33:10–15.
167. Shlaes DM, Bouvet A, Devine C, et al. Inducible, transferable resistance to vancomycin in *Enterococcus faecalis* A256. Antimicrob Agents Chemother. 1989;33:198–203.
168. Nicas TI, Cole CT, Preston DA, et al. Activity of glycopeptides against vancomycin-resistant gram-positive bacteria. Antimicrob Agents Chemother. 1989;33:1477–1481.
169. Bugg TD, Wright GD, Dutka-Malen S, et al. Molecular basis for vancomycin resistance in *Enterococcus faecium* BM4147: Biosynthesis of a depsipeptide peptidoglycan precursor by vancomycin resistance proteins VanH and VanA. Biochemistry. 1991;30:10,408–10,415.
170. LeClercq R, Dutka-Malen S, Brissonnoel A, et al. Resistance of enterococci to aminoglycosides and glycopeptides. Clin Infect Dis. 1992;15:495–501.
171. Quintiliani R, Evers S, Courvalin P. The *van*B gene confers various levels of self-transferable resistance to vancomycin in enterococci. J Infect Dis. 1993;167:1220–1223.
172. LeClercq R, Dutka-Malen S, Duval J, Courvalin P. Vancomycin resistance gene *van*C is specific to *Enterococcus gallinarum*. Antimicrob Agents Chemother. 1992;36:2005–2008.
173. Schwalbe RS, Stapleton JT, Gilligan PH. Emergence of vancomycin resistance in coagulase-negative staphylococci. N Engl J Med. 1987;316:927–931.
174. Centers for Disease Control and Prevention. Reduced susceptibility of *Staphylococcus aureus* to vancomycin—Japan, 1996. MMWR 1997;46:624–635.
175. Hospital Infection Control Practices Advisory Committee (HICPAC). Recommendations for preventing the spread of vancomycin resistance. Infect Control Hosp Epidemiol. 1995;16:105–113.
176. Waxman DJ, Strominger JL. Penicillin-binding proteins and the mechanism of action of beta-lactam antibiotics. Ann Rev Biochem. 1983;52:825–869.
177. Malouin F, Bryan LE. Modification of penicillin-binding proteins as mechanisms of beta-lactam resistance. Antimicrob Agents Chemother. 1986;30:1–5.
178. Williamson R. Resistance of *Clostridium perfringens* to beta-lactam antibiotics mediated by a decreased affinity of a single essential penicillin-binding protein. J Gen Microbiol. 1983;129:2339–2342.
179. Giles AF, Reynolds RE. *Bacillus megaterium* resistance to cloxacillin accompanied by a compensatory change in penicillin binding proteins. Nature. 1979;280:167–168.
180. Hakenbeck R, Tarpay M, Tomasz A. Multiple changes of penicillin-binding proteins in penicillin-resistant clinical isolates of *Streptococcus pneumoniae*. Antimicrob Agents Chemother. 1980;17:364–371.
181. Spratt BG, Dowson CG, Zhang Q-y et al. Mosaic genes, hybrid penicillin-binding proteins, and the origins of penicillin resistance in *Neisseria meningitidis* and *Streptococcus pneumoniae*. In: Pardee A, Campisi J. Perspectives on Cellular Regulation: From Bacteria to Cancer. New York: Wiley-Liss; 1991;73–83.
182. Hartman BJ, Tomasz A. Low-affinity penicillin-binding protein associated with beta-lactam resistance in *Staphylococcus aureus*. J Bacteriol. 1984;158:513–516.
183. Ubukata K, Yamashita N, Konno M. Occurrence of a beta-lactam-inducible penicillin-binding protein in methicillin-resistant staphylococci. Antimicrob Agents Chemother. 1985;27:851–857.
184. Fontana R. Penicillin-binding proteins and the intrinsic resistance to beta-lactams in gram-positive cocci. J Antimicrob Chemother. 1985;16:412–416.
185. Fontana R, Grossato A, Rossi L, et al. Transition from resistance to hypersusceptibility to beta-lactam antibiotics associated with loss of a low-affinity penicillin-binding protein in a *Streptococcus faecium* mutant highly resistant to penicillin. Antimicrob Agents Chemother. 1985;28:678–683.
186. Farber BF, Eliopoulos GM, Ward JI, et al. Multiply resistant viridans streptococci: Susceptibility to beta-lactam antibiotics and comparison of penicillin-binding protein patterns. Antimicrob Agents Chemother. 1977;3(Suppl C):47–51.
187. Sabath LD. Chemical and physical factors influencing methicillin resistance of *Staphylococcus aureus* and *Staphylococcus epidermidis*. J Antimicrob Chemother. 1977;3(Suppl C):47–51.
188. Song MD, Wachi M, Doi M, et al. Evolution of an inducible penicillin-target protein in methicillin-resistant *Staphylococcus aureus* by gene fusion. FEBS Lett. 1987;221:167–171.
189. Berger-Bachi B, Barberis-Maino L, Strassle A, Kayser FH. FemA, a host-mediated factor essential for methicillin resistance in *Staphylococcus aureus*: Molecular cloning and characterization. Mol Gen Genet. 1989;219:263–269.
190. Dougherty TJ, Koller AE, Tomasz A. Penicillin-binding proteins of penicillin-susceptible and intrinsically resistant *Neisseria gonorrhoeae*. Antimicrob Agents Chemother. 1980;18:730–737.
191. Mendelman PM, Chaffin DO, Kalaitzoglou G. Penicillin-binding proteins and ampicillin resistance in *Haemophilus influenzae*. J Antimicrob Chemother. 1990;25:525–534.
192. Dougherty TJ. Genetic analysis and penicillin-binding protein alterations in *Neisse-*

ria gonorrhoeae with chromosomally mediated resistance. Antimicrob Agents Chemother. 1986;30:649–652.
193. Mendelman PM, Campos J, Chaffin DO, et al. Relative penicillin G resistance in *Neisseria meningitidis* and reduced affinity of penicillin-binding protein 3. Antimicrob Agents Chemother. 1988;32:706–709.
194. Spratt BG, Zhang Q-y, Jones DM, et al. Recruitment of a penicillin-binding protein gene from *Neisseria flavescens* during the emergence of penicillin resistance in *Neisseria meningitidis*. Proc Natl Acad Sci USA. 1989;86:8988–8992.
195. Faruki H, Kohmescher RN, McKinney WP, Sparling PF. A community-based outbreak of infection with penicillin-resistant *Neisseria gonorrhoeae* not producing penicillinase (chromosomally mediated resistance). N Engl J Med. 1985;313:607–611.
196. Mirelman D, Nuchamowitz Y, Rubinstein E. Insensitivity of peptidoglycan biosynthetic reactions to beta-lactam antibiotics in a clinical isolate of *Pseudomonas aeruginosa*. Antimicrob Agents Chemother. 1981;19:687–695.
197. Parr TR, Jr, Bryan LE. Mechanism of resistance of an ampicillin-resistant, beta-lactamase-negative clinical isolate of *Haemophilus influenzae* type b to beta-lactam antibiotics. Antimicrob Agents Chemother. 1984;25:747–753.
198. Hamilton-Miller JMT. Resistance to antibacterial agents acting on antifolate metabolism. In: Bryan LE, ed. Antimicrobial Drug Resistance. Orlando: Academic Press; 1984:173–188.
199. Huovinen P. Trimethoprim resistance. Antimicrob Agents Chemother. 1987;31:1451–1456.
200. Steen R, Skold O. Plasmid-borne or chromosomally mediated resistance by Tn7 is the most common response to ubiquitous use of trimethoprim. Antimicrob Agents Chemother. 1985;27:933–937.
201. Wolfson JS, Hooper DC. The fluoroquinolones: Structures, mechanisms of action and resistance, and spectra of activity in vitro. Antimicrob Agents Chemother. 1985;28:581–586.
202. Hane MW, Wood TH. *Escherichia coli* K-12 mutants resistant to nalidixic acid: Genetic mapping and dominance studies. J Bacteriol. 1969;99:238–241.
203. Robillard NJ, Scarpa AL. Genetic and physiological characterization of ciprofloxacin resistance in *Pseudomonas aeruginosa* PAO. Antimicrob Agents Chemother. 1988;32:535–539.
204. Fisher LM, Hopewell R, Oram M, Sreedharan S. The molecular basis of quinolone action and resistance. In: Neu HC, ed. New Antibacterial Strategies. New York: Churchill Livingstone; 1990:177–190.
205. Aoyama H, Fujimaki K, Sato K, et al. Clinical isolate of *Citrobacter freundii* highly resistant to new quinolones. Antimicrob Agents Chemother. 1988;32:922–924.
206. Nakamura S, Nakamura M, Kojima T, Yoshida H. *gyrA* and *gyrB* mutations in quinolone-resistant strains of *Escherichia coli*. Antimicrob Agents Chemother. 1989;33:254–255.
207. Cullen ME, Wyke AW, Kuroda R, Fisher LM. Cloning and characterization of a DNA gyrase A gene from *Escherichia coli* that confers clinical resistance to 4-quinolones. Antimicrob Agents Chemother. 1989;33:886–894.
208. Maskell R, Okubadejo OA, Payne RH, Pead L. Human infections with thymine-requiring bacteria. J Med Microbiol. 1978;11:33–45.
209. McGowan JE, Jr. Antimicrobial resistance in hospital organisms and its relation to antibiotic use. Rev Infect Dis. 1983;5:1033–1048.
210. Levy SB. Resistance to the tetracyclines. In: Bryan LE, ed. Antimicrobial Drug Resistance. Orlando: Academic Press; 1984:192–234.
211. Mayer KH, Hopkins JD, Gilleece ES, et al. Computer-assisted correlations between antibiotypes of clinical isolates and the endonuclease restriction fragment of types of their plasmids. In: Mitsuhasi S, Rosival L, and Krcmery V, eds. Transferrable Antibiotic Resistance; Plasmids and Gene Manipulation. Prague: Czechoslovak Press; 1984:163–169.
212. Murray BE, Alvarado T, Kim KH, et el. Increasing resistance to trimethoprim-sulfamethoxazole among isolates of *Escherichia coli* in developing countries. J Infect Dis. 1985;152:1107–1113.
213. Seppala H, Nissinen A, Jarvinen H, et al. Resistance to erythromycin in group A streptococci (see Comments). N Engl J Med. 1992;326:292–297.
214. Moellering RC, Jr. Emergence of *Enterococcus* as a significant pathogen. Clin Infect Dis. 1992;14:1173–1176.
215. Grayson ML, Eliopoulos GM, Wennersten CB, et al. Increasing resistance to beta-lactam antibiotics among clinical isolates of *Enterococcus faecium*: A 22-year review at one institution. Antimicrob Agents Chemother. 1991;35:2180–2184.
216. Rhinehart E, Smith NE, Wennersten C, et al. Rapid dissemination of beta-lactamase-producing, aminoglycoside-resistant *Enterococcus faecalis* among patients and staff on an infant-toddler surgical ward (see Comments). N Engl J Med. 1990;323:1814–1818.
217. Bugg TD, Dutka-Malen S, Arthur M, et al. Identification of vancomycin resistance protein VanA as a D-alanine:D-alanine ligase of altered substrate specificity. Biochemistry. 1991;30:2017–2021.
218. Rubin LG, Tucci V, Cercenado E, et al. Vancomycin-resistant *Enterococcus faecium* in hospitalized children. Infect Control Hosp Epidemiol. 1992;13:700–705.
219. Karanfil LV, Murphy M, Josephson A, et al. A cluster of vancomycin-resistant *Enterococcus faecium* in an intensive care unit (see Comments). Infect Control Hosp Epidemiol. 1992;13:195–200.
220. Livornese LL, Dias S, Samel C, et al. Hospital-acquired infection with vancomycin-resistant *Enterococcus faecium* transmitted by electronic thermometers. Ann Intern Med. 1992;117:112–116.
221. Uttley AHC, Collins CH. Vancomycin-resistant enterococci. Lancet. 1988;1:57–58.
222. Boyce JM, Opal SM, Chow JW, et al. Outbreak of multidrug-resistant *Enterococcus faecium* with transferable vanB class vancomycin resistance. J Clin Microbiol. 1994;32:1148–1153.
223. Schaefler S. Methicillin-resistant strains of *Staphylococcus aureus* resistant to quinolones. J Clin Microbiol. 1989;27:335–336.
224. Shalit I, Berger SA, Gorea A, Frimerman H. Widespread quinolone resistance among methicillin-resistant *Staphylococcus aureus* isolates in a general hospital. Antimicrob Agents Chemother. 1989;33:593–594.
225. Banerjee SN, Emori TG, Culver DH, et al. Secular trends in nosocomial primary bloodstream infections in the United States, 1980–1989. National Nosocomial Infections Surveillance System. Am J Med. 1991;91:86S–89S.
226. Centers for Disease Control and Prevention. Interim guidelines for prevention and control of staphylococcal infection associated with reduced susceptibility to vancomycin. MMWR Morbid Mortal Wkly Rep. 1997;46:626–635.
227. Holmberg SD, Solomon SL, Blake PA. Health and economic impacts of antimicrobial resistance. Rev Infect Dis. 1987;9:1065–1078.
228. McGowan JE, Jr, Tenover FC. Control of antimicrobial resistance in the health care system. Infect Dis Clin North Am. 1997;11:297–311.
229. Philippon A, Dusart J, Joris B, Frère JM. The diversity, structure and regulation of β-lactamases. Cell Mol Life Sci. 1998;54:341–346.
230. Bauernfeind A, Stemplinger I, Jungwirth R, et al. Sequences of p-lactamase genes encoding CTX-M-1 (MEN-1) and CTX-M-2 and relationship of their amino acid sequences with those of other β-lactamases. Antimicrob Agents Chemother. 1996;40:509–513.
231. Ishii Y, Ohno A, Taguchi H, et al. Cloning and sequence of the gene encoding a cefotaxime-hydrolyzing class a β-lactamase isolated from *Escherichia coli*. Antimicrob Agents Chemother. 1995;39:2269–2275.
232. Ma L, Ishii Y, Ishiguro M, et al. Cloning and sequencing of the gene encoding Toho-2, a class A β-lactamase preferentially inhibited by tazobactam. Antimicrob Agents Chemother. 1998;42:1181–1186.
233. Gniadkowski M, Schneider I, Palucha A, et al. Cefotaxime-resistant Enterobacteriaceae isolates from a hospital in Warsaw, Poland: Identification of a new CTX-M-3 cefotaxime-hydrolyzing β-lactamase that is closely related to the CTX-M-1/MEN-1 enzyme. Antimicrob Agents Chemother. 1998;42:827–832.
234. Gazouli M, Tzelepi E, Sidorenko SV, Tzouvelekis LS. Sequence of the gene encoding a plasmid-mediated cefotaxime-hydrolyzing class A β-lactamase (CTX-M-4): Involvement of serine 237 in cephalosporin hydrolysis. Antimicrob Agents Chemother. 1998;42:1259–1262.
235. Nordmann P, Naas T. Sequence analysis of PER-1 extended-spectrum beta-lactamase from *Pseudomonas aeruginosa* and comparison with class A beta-lactamases. Antimicrob Agents Chemother. 1994;38:104–114.
236. Bauernfeind A, Stemplinger I, Jungwirth R, et al. Characterization of β-lactamase gene bla_{PER-2}, which encodes an extended-spectrum class A β-lactamase. Antimicrob Agents Chemother. 1996;40:616–620.
237. Bradford PA, Urban C, Mariano N, et al. Imipenem resistance in *Klebsiella pneumoniae* is associated with the combination of ACT-1, a plasmid-mediated AmpC β-lactamase, and the loss of an outer membrane protein. Antimicrob Agents Chemother. 1997;41:563–569.
238. Payne DJ, Woodford N, Amyes SGB. Characterization of the plasmid mediated beta-lactamase BIL-1. J Antimicrob Chemother. 1992;30:119–127.
239. Fosberry AP, Payne DJ, Lawlor EJ, Hodgson JE. Cloning and sequence analysis of *bla(BIL-1)*, a plasmid- mediated class C beta-lactamase gene in *Escherichia coli* BS. Antimicrob Agents Chemother. 1994;38:1182–1185.
240. Bauernfeind A, Stemplinger I, Jungwirth R, Giamarellou H. Characterization of the plasmidic β-lactamase CMY-2, which is responsible for cephamycin resistance. Antimicrob Agents Chemother. 1996;40:221–224.
241. Koeck JL, Arlet G, Philippon A, et al. Novel plasmid-mediated ampC-type β-lactamase (SAL-1) in a clinical isolate of *Salmonella senftenberg*. In: Program and Abstracts of the 36th Interscience Conference on Antimicrobial Agents and Chemotherapy. Washington, DC: American Society for Microbiology; 1996:39.
242. Tzouvelekis LS, Tzelepi E, Mentis AF. Nucleotide sequence of a plasmid-mediated cephalosporinase gene (*blaLAT-1*) found in *Klebsiella pneumoniae*. Antimicrob Agents Chemother. 1994;38:2207–2209.
243. Gazouli M, Tzouvelekis LS, Prinarakis E, et al. Transferable cefoxitin resistance in enterobacteria from Greek hospitals and characterization of a plasmid-mediated group 1 β-lactamase (LAT-2). Antimicrob Agents Chemother. 1996;40:1736–1740.
244. Verdet C, Arlet G, Barnaud G, et al. Novel integron carrying *ampC* and *ampR* genes on a plasmid from *Salmonella enteritidis*. Abstract C-125. In: Abstracts of the 37th Interscience Conference on Antimicrobial Agents and Chemotherapy. Washington, DC: American Society for Microbiology; 1997:68.
245. Gonzalez Leiza M, Perez-Diaz JC, Ayala J, et al. Gene sequence and biochemical characterization of FOX-1 from *Klebsiella pneumoniae*, a new AmpC-type plasmid-mediated beta-lactamase with two molecular variants. Antimicrob Agents Chemother. 1994;38:2150–2157.
246. Bauernfeind A, Wagner S, Jungwirth R, et al. A novel class C β-lactamase (FOX-2) in *Escherichia coli* conferring resistance to cephamycins. Antimicrob Agents Chemother. 1997;41:2041–2046.
247. Marchese A, Arlet G, Schito GC, et al. Characterization of FOX-3, an AmpC-type plasmid-mediated β-lactamase from an Italian isolate of *Klebsiella oxytoca*. Antimicrob Agents Chemother. 1998;42:464–467.
248. Bauernfeind A, Stemplinger I, Jungwirth R, et al. Comparative characterization of the cephamycinase bla_{CMY-1} gene and its relationship with other β-lactamase genes. Antimicrob Agents Chemother. 1996;40:1926–1930.
249. Horii T, Arakawa Y, Ohta M, et al. Plasmid-mediated ampC-type beta-lactamase isolated from *Klebsiella pneumoniae* confers resistance to broad-spectrum beta-lactams, including moxalactam. Antimicrob Agents Chemother. 1993;37:984–990.
250. Horii T, Arakawa Y, Ohta M, et al. Characterization of a plasmid-borne and

constitutively expressed *bla(MOX-1)* gene encoding ampC-type beta-lactamase. Gene. 1994;139:93–98.
251. Bobrowski MM, Matthew M, Barth PT, et al. Plasmid-determined beta-lactamase indistinguishable from the chromosomal beta-lactamase of *Escherichia coli*. J Bacteriol. 1976;125:149–157.
252. Bandoh K, Watanabe K, Muto Y, et al. Conjugal transfer of imipenem resistance in *Bacteroides fragilis*. J Antibiot (Tokyo). 1992;45:542–547.
253. Rasmussen BA, Bush K. Carbapenem-hydrolyzing β-lactamases. Antimicrob Agents Chemother. 1997;41:223–232.

Chapter 17

Pharmacokinetics and Pharmacodynamics of Anti-infective Agents

GUY W. AMSDEN
CHARLES H. BALLOW
JOSEPH S. BERTINO, JR.

The purpose of this chapter is to provide the reader with a basic review of pharmacologic terms and concepts. *Pharmacology* is the knowledge base of a compound concerning its history, source, physical and chemical properties, compounding, biochemical and physiologic effects, mechanisms of action and resistance, absorption, distribution, metabolism, excretion, and therapeutic and other uses.[1] *Pharmacokinetics* encompasses all the ways that the body manipulates a drug. This includes absorption, distribution, metabolism, and excretion. In contrast, *pharmacodynamics* describes the biochemical and physiologic effects of the drug and its mechanism of action (Fig. 17–1). The terms defined in this chapter are summarized in Table 17–1.

PHARMACOKINETICS

Pharmacokinetic Modeling

Pharmacokinetic drug data may be analyzed by noncompartmental or compartmental methods. Noncompartmental analysis makes no assumption of the physiologic distribution or elimination of a drug. *Noncompartmental* analysis simply serves as a description of drug behavior in biologic fluids, most commonly serum or plasma. *Compartmental* analysis offers the potential to broaden the appreciation of the drug by providing more insight into physiologic distribution and potential elimination pathways. The latter may be linear, such as renal elimination, or nonlinear, such as may occur during hepatic elimination. Compartmental analysis can best compensate for errors in investigational procedures (i.e., sampling errors, missing values). Furthermore, compartmental analysis is more amenable to population analysis, in which prior information about the pharmacokinetic and pharmacodynamic behaviors of a drug in the target population is incorporated into the analysis.

Compartmental modeling requires exploration of several candidate models (e.g., one-compartment model, two-compartment model), which can be selected initially after visual inspection of the plots of drug concentration versus time. All models are defined by combinations of parameters depending on the route of administration, biologic fluids collected, chemical analyses performed, and other factors. The model that minimizes the statistical error in curve fitting is ultimately selected as the final model. The following sections describe commonly modeled parameters associated with the pharmacokinetic literature.

Absorption

Absorption of a drug occurs anywhere that it is administered, except when it is administered directly into a physiologic fluid compartment (e.g., blood stream, cerebrospinal fluid). This includes intramuscular, subcutaneous, or topical administration as well as absorption from the gastrointestinal tract after oral, rectal, or tube administration. The amount of drug that reaches the systemic circulation is expressed as a percentage of the total amount that could have been absorbed. This percentage is defined as the drug's *bioavailability*, commonly described in the literature by the term "F". It may also be reported as *absolute bioavailability*, a more accurate value that is determined by direct comparison of an intravenous form of the drug with the absorbed form. By definition, most intravenous forms of a drug are 100% bioavailable, because all of the administered dose enters the blood stream. Many other pharmacokinetic values are dependent on F (e.g., clearance, volume of distribution) for drugs that need to be absorbed.

Absorption is a dynamic process. Depending on the form of administration, a drug's absorption, and therefore its bioavailability, can vary. Although a paucity or lack of absorption channels or systems at the site of administration may decrease absorption, this

TABLE 17–1 Pharmacologic Abbreviations and Their Definitions

Category	Abbreviation	Definition
Pharmacokinetics		
Absorption	F	Bioavailability; absolute bioavailability
	Ka	Absorption rate constant
Distribution	V_d	Volume of distribution
	V_d/F	Apparent volume of distribution
	V_{ss}	Volume of distribution at steady state
	V_{ss}/F	Apparent volume of distribution at steady state
	CL_D	Distributional clearance
	CL_D/F	Apparent distributional clearance
Metabolism	Vm	Maximum metabolic capacity (Michaelis-Menten [saturable] metabolism)
	Km	Drug concentration at which the rate that an enzyme system can metabolize the drug is one half of Vm (Michaelis-Menten [saturable] metabolism)
	CYP	Cytochrome P-450 enzyme systems
Elimination	CL_r	Renal clearance
	CL_{nr}	Nonrenal clearance
	CL_{nr}/F	Nonrenal oral clearance
	CL_T	Total clearance
	CL_T/F	Total oral clearance
	$T_{1/2}$	Half-life
Pharmacodynamics		
	MIC_{90}	Minimal inhibitory concentration for 90% of isolates
	EC_{50}	Effective concentration for 50% of all isolates
	IC_{50}	Inhibitory concentration for 50% of isolates
	Cmax/MIC	Ratio of peak antimicrobial serum concentration to MIC (concentration-dependent killers)
	AUC/MIC	Ratio of 24-hour area under the blood antimicrobial concentration versus time curve to (above) MIC ratio
	T>MIC	Time that the blood antimicrobial concentration is higher than the organism's MIC (time-dependent killers)
	SBT	Serum bactericidal titer (concentration)
	PAE	Postantibiotic effect

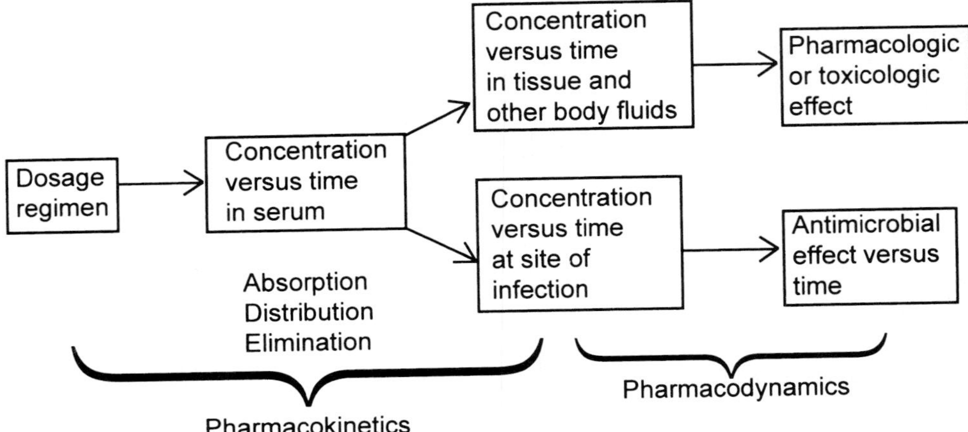

FIGURE 17–1. An overview of the interaction of pharmacokinetics and pharmacodynamics for anti-infective agents. (From Craig WA. Pharmacokinetic/pharmacodynamic parameters: Rationale for antibacterial dosing of mice and men. Clin Infect Dis. 1998;26:1–12.)

may also be caused by the dose administered or the type of absorption channel or system. Many systems can be overwhelmed and go from absorbing everything passed on to them (*nonsaturable absorption*) to absorbing the compound only at a certain rate (*saturable* or *zero-order absorption*). In any case, the rate at which the drug is absorbed is termed the *absorption rate constant (Ka)*.

A factor commonly associated with a decrease in the bioavailability of a drug (i.e., the amount that gets into the systemic circulation) is the first-pass effect. Drugs that are absorbed from the small intestine can be affected by the first-pass effect of the liver, because the circulation leading away from these sites passes through the liver immediately. Drugs administered via other sites (e.g., rectally [variable], intramuscularly, intravenously) usually are not associated with a first-pass effect and can have higher bioavailability because they are not immediately affected by the liver's metabolic capacity.

Other factors that can affect absorption and bioavailability are drug interactions with other compounds or food that may bind the drug and prevent it from being absorbed or a disease state that may adversely affect the site of absorption (i.e., diarrhea, parasites, ileus, ulcerative colitis, corpulence).

Distribution

Distribution of a drug is most commonly described by the *volume of distribution (V_d or V_d/F)*. The volume of distribution is not a real or physiologic volume but rather a value that relates drug concentration in the system to the amount of drug present in that system. Factors that alter the volume of distribution include lipid solubility, partition coefficient of the drug between different types of tissues, blood flow to tissues, pH, and binding to biologic material (e.g., plasma proteins, cellular components).[2]

Drugs with small distribution volumes have limited distribution, whereas drugs with large distribution volumes are extensively distributed throughout the body. For example, a drug with a 5-liter volume of distribution in an adult would be restricted to the circulatory system. If the volume of distribution is between 10 and 20 liters, the drug will distribute into extracellular compartments. If the volume of distribution is on the order of 25 to 30 liters, then intracellular distribution is implied. Distribution volumes of approximately 40 liters suggest distribution within whole body fluid. In rare circumstances, distribution volumes may be measured in hundreds or even thousands of liters. This suggests either "deep" tissue deposition in peripheral compartments (e.g., fat) or extensive binding to biologic structures (e.g., tissue protein, organelles). Once a steady state has been achieved after multiple doses of a medication, the *total volume of distribution* is referred to as the V_{ss}. This value represents the sum of the distribution volumes from each of the identified physiologic compartments.

After intravenous administration of a drug, the concentration rapidly reaches a peak before beginning to decline. Distribution and elimination are two factors that affect the extent of the peak concentration and the rate of decay. Usually distribution is completed sooner than elimination. This results in two phases in the concentration versus time plot (Fig. 17–2). The first phase, or α *phase*, is usually short and represents mixing of the drug throughout the circulatory system and distribution into rapidly equilibrating tissues. The second or β *phase* is usually a reflection of terminal elimination and is the phase from which the terminal half-life ($T_{1/2}$) is calculated. Occasionally, more than two phases may be observed; this usually indicates further distribution into slowly equilibrating tissues.

The rate at which a drug moves from the blood to tissues is described by the *distributional clearance (CL_D or CL_D/F)*. Just as total body clearance describes the volume of blood from which a drug is eliminated per unit time, distributional clearance describes the volume of blood from which a drug is transferred into a tissue or compartment per unit of time. Distributional clearance is a bidirectional process reflecting the equilibrium in movement from blood to tissue and from tissue to blood. Once the drug has moved into a tissue compartment, the local tissue concentration is a function of the amount of drug located in the tissue and the tissue volume of distribution, also known as the *volume of the peripheral compartment (V_p)*. Such volumes can only be estimated by mathematical modeling, because it is unusual to be able to collect biologic specimens from peripheral compartments and then assay the drug concentration.

Metabolism and Biotransformation

Drugs and other compounds are metabolized by a variety of reactions. Although traditionally drug metabolism was thought to occur in the liver, other organs also have the ability to metabolize drugs.

Because drug metabolism requires the presence of enzymes, the principles of Michaelis and Menten can be applied to drug metabolism. Michaelis and Menten demonstrated almost 90 years ago that enzyme systems have a finite capacity to metabolize substrate. Although all routes of drug metabolism are saturable, if the doses and concentrations at the site of metabolism do not exceed the maximum rate of metabolism, the metabolic system will appear to follow linear pharmacokinetics. If the dose exceeds the amount that can be metabolized, drug accumulation can occur, leading to high serum concentrations and high tissue levels. These high levels can result in toxic side effects. If a daily dose is given that is lower than what the body can eliminate, low concentrations may be seen. Such *dose-dependent kinetics* (also called Michaelis-Menten, zero-order, or saturation kinetics) mean that once saturation of the ability to metabolize the drug in a 24-hour period is reached, small dosage increases may produce large, disproportionate increases in serum concentrations.

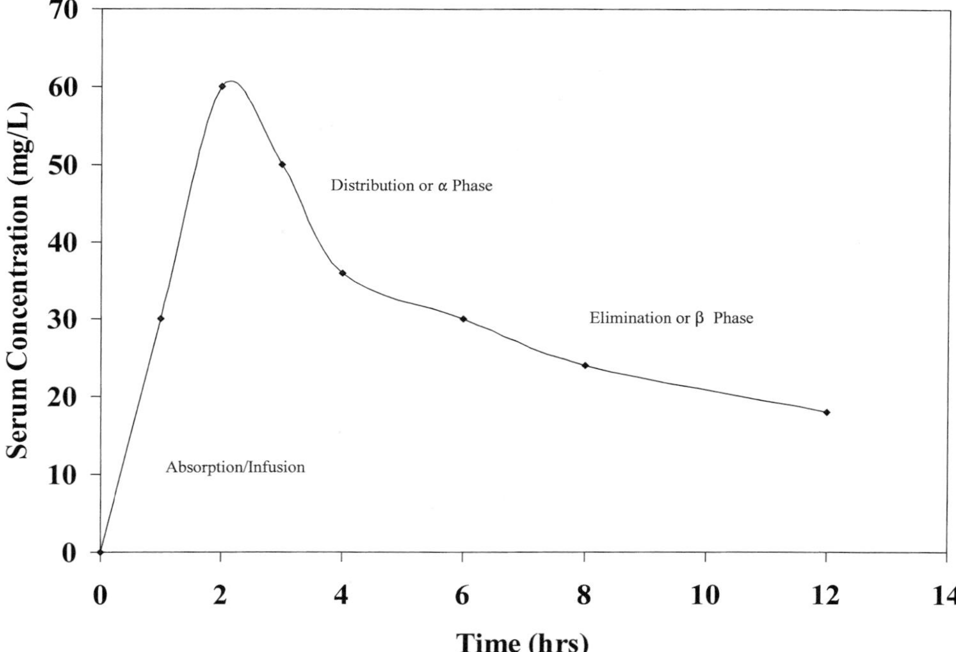

FIGURE 17–2. A graphic example of the serum concentration versus time profile of a typical two-phase or two-compartment drug during the absorptive-infusion, distributive, and elimination phases.

Conversely, if a daily dose is higher than what can be metabolized in a 24-hour period and results in high serum concentrations, small reductions in the dose may cause large reductions in the serum concentration.

Drug metabolism reactions are classified as either phase I or phase II reactions. *Phase I reactions* can inactivate, activate, or convert an active substrate into another active substrate with activity that is higher, lower, or equal to that of the parent compound. Generally, phase I reactions cause inactivation of substrate, with the resulting compound being more polar than the parent. Making the metabolite more polar facilitates its elimination from the body. Phase I reactions include dealkylation, hydroxylation, oxidation, and deamination.

Phase II reactions involve conjugation of the parent compound with larger molecules, which increases the polarity of the parent to ready it for excretion. Phase II reactions need energy to proceed. Although phase II reactions generally lead to inactivation of the parent compound, occasionally conjugation increases the potency of the parent compound. When the conjugated compounds are secreted into the intestine, enzymatic cleavage may occur with release and reabsorption of the active parent compound, a phenomenon known as *enterohepatic recirculation*. Conjugation reactions include glucuronidation, sulfation, and acetylation.

Cytochrome P-450 System. Phase I reactions generally are under the control of the *cytochrome P-450 (CYP) system*. CYP enzymes are heme-containing proteins that are localized in the endoplasmic reticulum of a variety of cell types, most abundantly in the liver. CYP enzymes are controlled by a superfamily of genes that are classified into families according to their amino acid sequences. Each family is further divided into subfamilies. The term "CYP3A4", for example, designates a mammalian enzyme (CYP) family 3, subfamily A, gene 4. Fourteen families of CYPs have been found in mammals, including 26 subfamilies, of which 20 have been mapped in the human genome. Currently, data exist to describe 33 human CYP enzymes in 20 families.[3]

CYP enzymes are affected by a number of factors that stimulate or inhibit their ability to metabolize drugs. Genetic factors have been shown to result in a phenomenon called *polymorphism*. Simply put, this means that individuals vary in their genetically determined ability to metabolize CYP substrate. For some CYP enzymes, such as CYP2D6, distinct "poor" and "extensive" metabolic patterns exist in a population; in a Caucasian population, 4 to 6% are poor metabolizers and the rest are extensive metabolizers. For other CYPs, such as CYP3A, no bimodal distribution or polymorphism has been discovered, but variations in enzyme activity of 10-fold or greater may be seen. These phenomena have important implications for anti-infective agents, for which efficacy against infecting organisms and toxicity to the host are determined by the pharmacokinetics of the agent and its resultant pharmacodynamic effect.

Other factors that have been investigated for their effects on CYP enzymes include sex, disease state, age, and menstrual cycle. In general, differences related to sex and menstrual cycle (i.e., follicular versus luteal phase) have not been observed. Age and disease state effects are not clear, but it may be postulated that cytokines released during acute infection can cause inhibition of CYP activity.

Clinically, effects on the CYP system translate into either inhibition or induction of metabolism. Induction of CYP results in increased production of the protein and a resultant increase in the ability to metabolize specific compounds. An example is the induction by rifampin of CYP3A with a subsequent increase in the metabolism of estrogens. Many inducers of CYP enzymes also induce the phase II conjugation reactions.

Inhibition of CYP occurs through reduction of enzyme production or competition for CYP substrate. Generally, persons with increased enzyme activity exhibit a greater inhibition of the CYP system with an inhibiting agent than do persons with less activity. Enzyme inhibition may result in increased pharmacodynamic effect, with the potential for greater efficacy but also for greater toxicity. This inhibitory process may be used in the clinical setting advantageously. For example, ritonavir can be used to decrease the activity of CYP3A in the gut, allowing greater absorption of saquinavir (through a reduction in the first-pass effect) and thereby reducing the overall cost of therapy.

Quantitation of CYP activity has been performed through the use of genotyping and phenotyping. Genotyping identifies the alleles present in the leukocytes of an individual patient. From this allele identification, a prediction of CYP activity can be made. However, because genetically determined CYP activity is also affected by exogenous influences (e.g., drugs, environmental pollutants, cigarette smoke), phenotyping has shown more promise for determining individual CYP activity. A relatively innocuous agent is administered as a single dose to a subject and either urine, blood, or breath analysis ensues. These techniques, while still investigational, are beginning to be used in the clinical setting in an attempt to optimize drug dosing.

To date, the majority of drugs have been shown to be metabolized by five primary CYP enzymes. In decreasing order of potency for drug metabolism, they are CYP3A, CYP2D6, CYP2C, CYP1A2, and CYP2E1. Although a complete discussion of the CYP system is beyond the scope of this chapter, many of the newer anti-infectives, particularly the antiretroviral agents, can induce or inhibit CYP enzymes, and in many cases they are substrates for CYP enzymes and therefore are affected by changes in CYP activity. A thorough understanding of the CYP system is important to optimize efficacy and minimize toxicity of these agents.

As mentioned, the liver is not the only place in the body where metabolism occurs. Metabolism and detoxification of foreign substances can take place in a number of other systems. As an example, nitrates can be metabolized by substances within vascular tissues, thereby leading to nitrate tolerance.

Elimination

Elimination of a foreign substance from the body occurs via two main mechanisms of excretion. *Renal clearance (CL_r)* describes the rate at which the body eliminates a substance via the kidneys, through various methods including glomerular filtration, tubular secretion, and passive diffusion. Different compounds are eliminated by one or more of these processes, and the degree to which a process is used may depend on the saturation of another process by the compound. Elimination through a dialysis procedure (hemodialysis or peritoneal dialysis) can also be construed as a form of renal elimination, because these processes are acting as an artificial kidney.

Nonrenal clearance (CL_{nr} or CL_{nr}/F) is often thought to denote hepatic clearance of a substance. Although hepatic elimination constitutes the primary route of nonrenal clearance, it may not be the sole method. Rather, nonrenal clearance is a generic term that describes the sum of clearance pathways that do not involve the kidneys. These mechanisms may involve the biliary tree (e.g., ceftriaxone) or the intestine (e.g., azithromycin). Other, uncommon mechanisms can be used, such as elimination of alcohol through the skin and lungs (respiration) and ionization and inactivation of aminoglycosides by the sputum in cystic fibrosis patients with elimination through expectoration.

Renal and nonrenal clearance rates are combined to determine the rate at which a drug is eliminated from the body, known as *total body clearance (CL_T, or CL_T/F for total oral clearance)*. Clearance also affects the *half-life ($T_{1/2}$)*. The half-life of a compound is the amount of time required for the blood concentration of the compound to decrease by half. This time can be as short as minutes or as long as a day or more. Most pharmacologists consider that a *steady-state concentration* of a drug has been achieved once the patient has been taking the drug for a period equal to at least 5 to 7 half-lives (e.g., 5 to 7 days for a drug with a half-life of 24 hours). Similarly, a drug is thought to have been almost completely eliminated once the timespan of 5 to 7 half-lives has passed since the final dose of the drug. It is important for the clinician to realize that half-lives vary from patient to patient and are often reported as ranges. Changes in end-organ function or protein binding can also alter the half-life of a drug.

PHARMACODYNAMICS

Antimicrobial Activity. Pharmacodynamics is the discipline within pharmacology that strives to understand the relationships between drug concentrations and effects, both desirable (e.g., bacterial killing) and undesirable (e.g., side effects).

Desirable effects can be classified as either *static (inhibitory)* or *cidal (lethal)*. Depending on the mechanism of action, an antimicrobial agent may inhibit growth and replication or cause bacterial cell death. Interference in the development of a bacterial cell wall or membrane (e.g., β-lactams, vancomycin) results in cell lysis and death from intolerably high internal osmotic pressure or destruction by autolytic enzymes. Antimicrobials that inhibit nucleic acid (e.g., quinolones) or protein synthesis (e.g., aminoglycosides, macrolides/azalides) also lead ultimately to cell death. In contrast, changes in bacterial physiology, such as inhibition of folic acid synthesis (e.g., sulfonamides), may only cause inhibition of bacterial growth.

Another factor that affects whether a drug is bacteriostatic or bactericidal is the antimicrobial concentration at the site of action. Antimicrobials may be bacteriostatic at low concentrations but bactericidal at high concentrations. Such inhibitory and cidal concentrations have been used to quantitate the activity of an agent against an organism. Most commonly, the *minimum concentration that is inhibitory for 90% of all isolates* of a bacterial species (*MIC_{90}*) and the *inhibitory or effective concentration for 50% of all isolates* of a strain of virus (*IC_{50}* or EC_{50}) have been used. Although these parameters are helpful, they do not provide information on the time course of activity. In addition, they do not provide information on the potential for persistent anti-infective activity after the concentration at the site has dropped below the inhibitory level or on the interaction of the immune system with the drug.

Antimicrobial agents are given in combination for several reasons, including severe or life-threatening infections, empirical therapy when the pathogen is unknown, avoidance of resistance, and the desire for synergistic activity. *Synergism* is defined as activity of two antimicrobials given together that is greater than the sum of activity had the two agents been given separately. For example, β-lactams commonly are given in combination with aminoglycosides to take advantage of synergy against *Pseudomonas* or *Enterococcus* spp. Trimethoprim and sulfamethoxazole are combined to provide synergy through inhibition of sequential steps in folic acid synthesis.

However, combinations of antimicrobial agents may not always be beneficial. *Antagonism* between agents occurs when one agent diminishes the activity of another. β-Lactams require a normally growing bacteria in order to inhibit cell wall synthesis. Concomitant administration with a bacteriostatic agent (e.g., a tetracycline) that inhibits cell growth prevents the β-lactam from exerting its bactericidal activity. In this case, the action of the β-lactam has been antagonized. Concomitant administration of a β-lactam and a β-lactamase inducer may result in induction of β-lactamase synthesis, leading to hyperproduction of enzymes and preventing the antibacterial activity of the β-lactam. Most antimicrobial combinations result in little or no change in activity of the two agents, an interaction termed *indifference*.

Anti-infective pharmacodynamics also take on a much greater meaning, as shown in Figure 17–2.[4] Beyond the effect that the anti-infective has in relation to elimination of the organism, its effects also extend to the development of resistance by the organism to the agent being used for therapy.[5] This has implications not only for the treatment of the patient but for society in general. The use of anti-infective agents therefore has broader implications than use of drugs of other therapeutic classes, in that not just one individual may be affected.

Methodology for the Study of Pharmacodynamic Effects of Anti-infective Agents. Three methodologies have been used to study the pharmacodynamic effects of anti-infective agents: in vitro methodology, animal models, and analysis of human data from retrospective and prospective trials.

In Vitro Models. The traditional model used to study pharmacodynamic effects of anti-infective agents is the "hollow fiber model" system.[6] In this system, broth is used as a growth medium; bacteria are exposed to predetermined concentrations of antibiotics that are "eliminated" from the system in such a manner as to simulate pharmacokinetically determined excretion.[7] Although these models offer ultimate control over bacterial inoculum and drug exposure (in terms of both concentration and time), they do not assess the effects of the immune system on organism killing or growth inhibition.

Animal Models. These models have used a variety of species, often with the animals rendered neutropenic before infection. Animal infectious disease models have been developed to mimic human infections. Animal models allow for frequent sampling of blood and tissue and allow a broad dosage range to be investigated along with a wide range of organism inocula, thereby allowing investigators to study the effects of variation in a single parameter at a time. Problems with animal models include lack of standardization of inocula size (often large inocula are required to produce infection) and the faster rate of drug elimination in animals compared with humans, which leads to the use of unusual dosing regimens in an attempt to mimic human drug exposure.

Human Trials. To date, the majority of human trials reported have been retrospective analyses of prospectively collected data.[8–20] These trials have used three measures of assessment to relate antimicrobial pharmacokinetics to pharmacodynamics: (1) clinical outcome (cure/fail or improved); (2) eradication of bacteria from the site of infection or reduction in virus concentration (load) in blood or other sites, or both; and (3) improvement in surrogate markers of infection such as temperature or leukocyte count. These types of trials suffer from the retrospective nature of their analyses; prospective trials using all three criteria are needed. Most of the retrospective trials that have been published have used one of three antimicrobial pharmacodynamic outcome parameters (discussed later): Cmax/MIC, AUC/MIC, or T>MIC (Fig. 17–3).

Concentration-Dependent Killing Agents. Concentration-dependent killing agents (e.g., fluoroquinolones, aminoglycosides) eliminate bacteria when their concentrations are well above the MIC of the organism. When the ratio of the concentration at the site of infection to the MIC is increased further, greater killing occurs. This is illustrated in Figure 17–4 for tobramycin and ciprofloxacin against *Pseudomonas aeruginosa*.[21] As the ratio of drug concentration to MIC increases from 0.25 to 64, bacterial killing continues to increase. In addition, these agents exhibit postantibiotic effect (discussed later): growth inhibition continues for a varying period after the concentration at the site of the bacteria has dropped below the MIC for the antimicrobial agent. In vivo, the Cmax/MIC ratio—the maximum serum concentration of the drug (Cmax) divided by the MIC—is the clinical correlate used as the pharmacodynamic predictor for outcome for concentration-dependent killing agents. However, in clinical trials, the AUC/MIC ratio—the area under the 24-hour serum concentration curve (AUC) divided by the MIC—has also been correlated with improved outcome.[8–20] This is not surprising, because Cmax and AUC are covariates: when Cmax increases, AUC increases also.

Time-Dependent (Concentration-Independent) Killing Agents. Time-dependent killing agents kill gram-negative bacteria only when the concentration at the site of the bacteria is higher than the MIC of the organism. This is shown for ticarcillin against *P. aeruginosa* in Figure 17–4. Generally, once the concentration at the bacterial site is more than four times higher than the MIC, the additional killing that occurs is modest.

Some authors have attempted to use the time during which the serum drug concentration is greater than the MIC (time above MIC, or *T>MIC*) as the dynamic parameter to predict efficacy for these anti-infectives.[4, 16] One study in the neutropenic mouse model using *Klebsiella pneumoniae* lung infection and treatment with cefotaxime suggested a very strong correlation of 0.94 in terms of reduction of bacterial colony counts versus time above MIC (Fig. 17–5).[22] An additional report of a number of animal studies with *Streptococcus pneumoniae* in which treatment was performed with penicillins or cephalosporins showed that when T>MIC was 20% or less of the dosing interval, mortality was 100%. In contrast a mortality rate of 0 to 10% occurred when serum concentrations were above the MIC for longer than 40 to 50% of the dosing interval.[4, 23]

Time-dependent killing agents include the penicillins, cephalosporins, aztreonam, macrolides/azalides, and clindamycin.

Pharmacodynamic Outcome Parameters

Ratio of Cmax to MIC. The Cmax/MIC ratio has been used in both animal studies and retrospective analyses of clinical trials to predict the outcome of antimicrobial therapy. This pharmacodynamic parameter applies to concentration-dependent killing agents such as aminoglycosides and quinolones. In addition to the prediction of efficacy, the Cmax/MIC ratio has been used in vitro to predict the development of bacterial resistance.[7]

In humans, there have been five studies using Cmax/MIC to predict outcome, four with aminoglycosides and one with levofloxacin. These trials used either clinical response (measured by improvement with therapy or by improvement of surrogate markers) or cure/fail as the outcome measure.

The trial by Keating and colleagues examined neutropenic cancer patients.[8] In this trial, patients were randomly assigned to receive

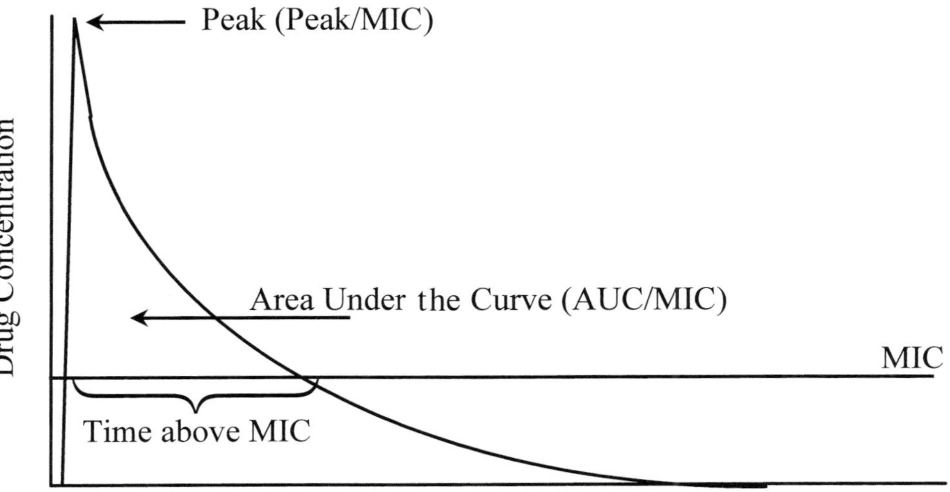

FIGURE 17–3. Common antibiotic pharmacokinetic and minimal inhibitory concentration (MIC) pharmacodynamic relationships.

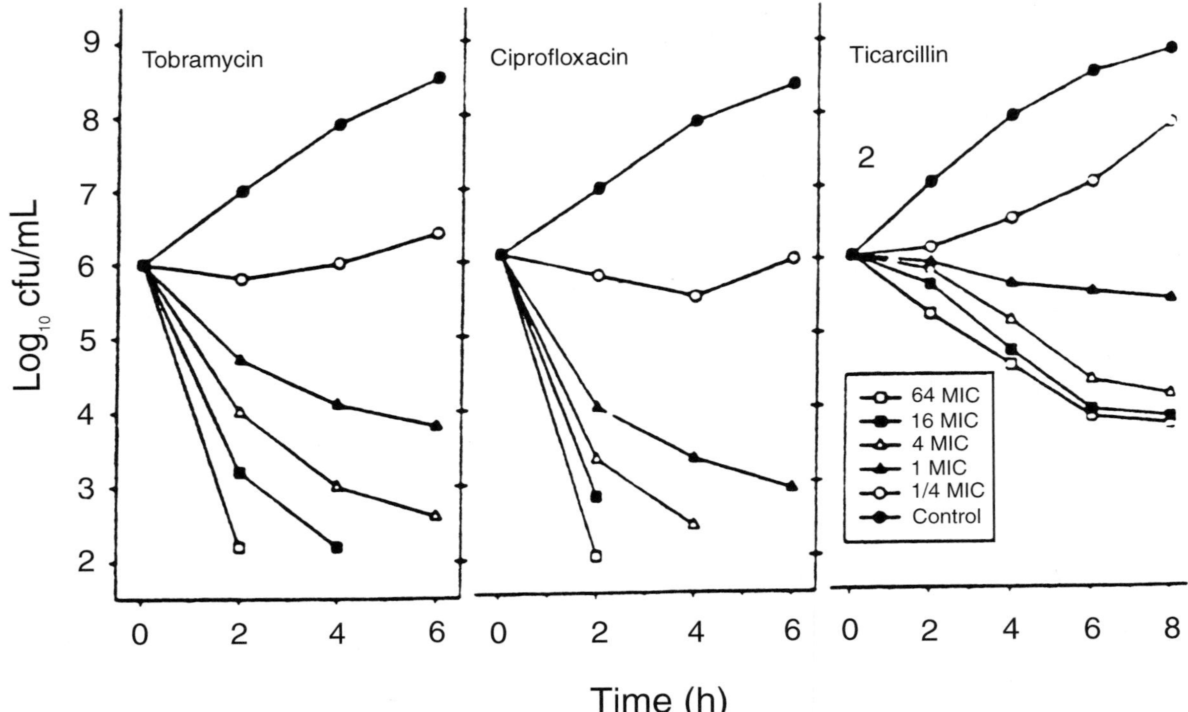

FIGURE 17–4. Time kill curves for *Pseudomonas aeruginosa* ATCC 27853 with exposure to tobramycin, ciprofloxacin, and ticarcillin at concentrations from one fourth to 64 times the minimum inhibitory concentration. (From Craig WA, Ebert SC. Killing and regrowth of bacteria in vitro: A review. Scand J Infect Dis. 1991;74:63–70.)

continuous infusions of one of three aminoglycoside antibiotics plus carbenicillin. When the ratios of aminoglycoside concentration to MIC were examined, a relation was noted for response rate. For mean ratios of 1 to 4, 4 to 10, and higher than 10, response rates were 57%, 67%, and 85%, respectively.

The study by Moore and colleagues is often quoted as the basis

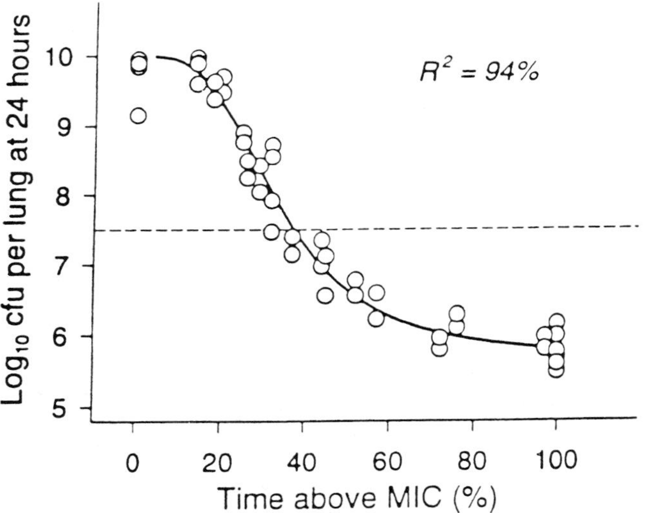

FIGURE 17–5. The relationship of time above the minimal inhibitory concentration and the reduction in bacterial count in a neutropenic mouse model of *Klebsiella pneumoniae* for cefotaxime. (From Craig WA. Interrelationship between pharmacokinetics and pharmacodynamics in determining dosage regimens for broad-spectrum cephalosporins. Diagn Microbiol Infect Dis. 1995;22:89–96.)

for use of a Cmax/MIC target of 10 or higher in the clinical setting.[11] In this retrospective analysis of prospectively collected data, the authors examined 236 patients with a variety of gram-negative infections treated with aminoglycoside antibiotics on an every-8-hour basis. They found that the odds ratio for improved clinical response increased as Cmax/MIC increased, with a mean ratio of 6.6 + 3.9 in patients who responded and 4.6 ± 3.6 in patients who did not respond. However, this trial had a majority of patients with urinary tract infections (approximately 60%). Because aminoglycosides are known to concentrate 5- to 100-fold in the urine, the relation of Cmax to MIC in this study may actually be meaningless. It was impossible to separate patients with other disease states to determine the optimal Cmax/MIC needed to elicit response. In addition, the authors did not consider concurrent antibiotic therapy in their model, so it is difficult to assess the contribution of other antimicrobial agents to the response rate.

An additional study by Deziel-Evans and associates examined a variety of pharmacodynamic predictors in 45 adult patients treated with aminoglycosides.[12] In this trial, a Cmax/MIC ratio greater than 4 was noted to improve clinical response.

A more recent study by Kashuba and coworkers described the relation between Cmax and MIC in 78 patients with documented gram-negative pneumonia.[17] The authors examined cure or failure along with two surrogate markers of infection, temperature and leukocyte count. There was a high cure rate for well-documented gram-negative pneumonia (92%), and no pharmacodynamic variable could be correlated with cure/fail, probably because of the small number of failures. The authors did, however, examine Cmax/MIC in relation to the time required for the patient to become afebrile (≤37.9°C) and the time to normalization of the leukocyte count. As shown by the probability graph in Figure 17–6, a strong relation was noted between Cmax/MIC and time to normalization of fever. A ratio of 10 or higher gave a 90% probability of normalization of temperature by day 7. Similar graphs can be constructed for earlier and later days into therapy. Generally, these probability graphs show

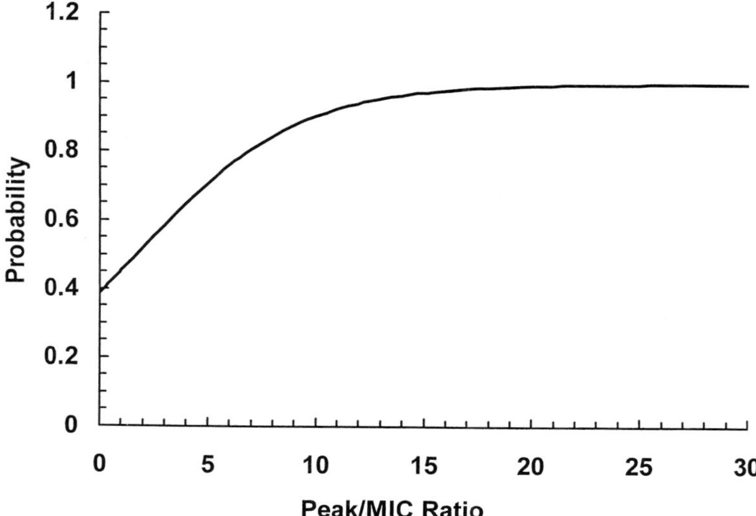

FIGURE 17–6. Probability graph for temperature normalization for Cmax/MIC ratio for aminoglycosides in 78 patients with culture-proven nosocomial gram-negative pneumonia. (From Kashuba et al.,[17] unpublished data.)

that an increased Cmax/MIC ratio yields an earlier and greater chance of surrogate marker normalization. This does not take into account the probability of toxicity with higher Cmax/MIC ratios. A strength of this trial is that the authors statistically analyzed concurrent antibiotic therapy, which was not a significant variable for prediction of surrogate response or cure/fail.

To date, one study has addressed the use of Cmax/MIC with the quinolone levofloxacin. Preston and colleagues examined 134 evaluable patients with bacterial infections of the respiratory or urinary tract or of the skin who were treated with levofloxacin monotherapy.[20] All 134 patients had serum concentrations obtained along with identified microorganisms with an MIC determined. In terms of clinical outcome, Cmax/MIC and AUC/MIC were found to be the most important predictors of outcome; the correlation of these two pharmacodynamic parameters was 0.942. These authors did not find any failures in patients with urinary tract infections, illustrating that Cmax/MIC may not be a valid predictor in patients receiving drugs that concentrate in the urine. In terms of microbiologic response, Cmax/MIC was the most important predictor of bacterial eradication.

These retrospective analyses of prospective data illustrate the potential importance of Cmax/MIC for concentration-dependent killing agents. However, because none of the four trials with aminoglycosides used single daily dosing of these agents, it is not possible to extrapolate these data to support this mode of administration.[24]

In terms of prevention of bacterial resistance, only in vitro data using the hollow fiber model exist relating Cmax/MIC to resistance. The study of Blaser and coworkers examined Cmax/MIC for enoxacin and netilmicin against various gram-negative organisms.[7] Regrowth of organisms occurred in all cultures when enoxacin or netilmicin attained ratios lower than 8. On redosing of these antibiotics after bacterial regrowth, no killing was seen because of the development of resistance. A similar study by Marchbanks and associates, using ciprofloxacin, noted the development of resistant *P. aeruginosa* when the organism was exposed to a Cmax/MIC of 6, compared with no resistance when the Cmax/MIC was 12, even though both regimens showed adequate rates of bacterial killing.[25] These in vitro data suggest that Cmax/MIC ratios may be influential in determining the development of bacterial resistance for aminoglycosides and quinolones. However, these trials suffer from not accounting for the role of the immune system in "cleaning up" small numbers of resistant bacteria before they can become pathogenic.

Although the Cmax/MIC ratios for aminoglycosides and quinolones may be useful, no data to date have examined drug toxicity with higher exposures. A prospective trial to evaluate both efficacy and toxicity with pharmacodynamic dosage adjustments is needed.

Ratio of AUC to MIC. A measure of total exposure of bacteria to an antimicrobial agent is the AUC/MIC. The AUC/MIC ratio encompasses both peak concentration and prolonged exposure, which may be vitally important for drugs with a long $t_{1/2}$. Cmax/MIC and AUC/MIC are difficult to separate in a scientifically designed clinical trial, because when the former ratio is high, the latter usually is high as well. Therefore, both will be found to be statistically predictive of outcome and indistinguishable in terms of which is of primary importance.

Several studies have defined the role of AUC/MIC as a predictor of bacterial or clinical success. An evaluation of various pharmacodynamic predictors of outcome was performed in 74 acutely ill patients, mostly with nosocomial pneumonia, who were treated with ciprofloxacin. AUC/MIC, which represents the inverse serum inhibitory titer over time (SIT^{-1}·T), was identified as the factor most predictive of both clinical and microbiologic success (Fig. 17–7). At an AUC/MIC lower than 125 SIT^{-1}·h ($\log^{10}$ = 2.1 = 125 SIT^{-1}·h), the probabilities of clinical and microbiologic cure were 42% and 26%, respectively, whereas at values greater than 125, the probabilities were 80% and 82%. Moreover, at an AUC/MIC lower than 125, between 125 and 250 ($\log^{10}$ = 2.4 = 250 SIT^{-1}·h), and higher than 250 the median time to eradication was more than 32 days, 6.6 days, and 1.9 days, respectively.[14] A similar analysis was performed for patients experiencing an acute exacerbation of chronic bronchitis treated with grepafloxacin. At an AUC/MIC lower than 75 SIT^{-1}·h, the probability of clinical cure was 71%, whereas with ratios above 175 the probability of cure was 98%.

Time above MIC (T>MIC). This pharmacodynamic parameter measures the time that serum drug concentrations stay higher than the MIC for the organism. This definition usually refers to total drug concentration, although some authors have used free drug concentration in the definition. For intermittent bolus infusions, the parameters T>MIC, AUC/MIC, and Cmax/MIC are interrelated: as T>MIC increases, AUC/MIC and Cmax/MIC do also. Therefore, it may be difficult to separate the importance of these dynamic parameters unless a study compares continuous versus intermittent infusions of antimicrobials.

Animal models have shown that T>MIC is an important pharmacodynamic predictor for penicillins, cephalosporins, carbapenems, monobactams, macrolides, and clindamycin.[4] However, once again, human studies are sparse in defining this parameter as an important

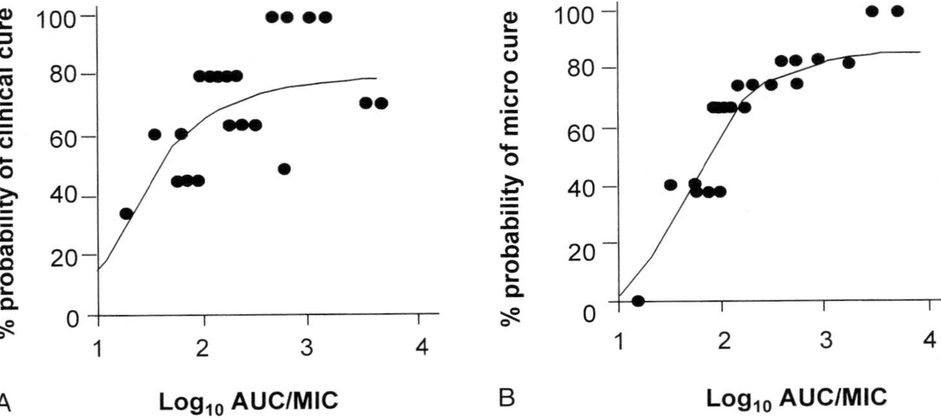

FIGURE 17–7. Relationship between AUC/MIC and clinical (*A*) or microbiologic (*B*) cure in 74 patients with nosocomial pneumonia. (From Forrest A, Nix DE, Ballow CH, et al. Pharmacodynamics of intravenous ciprofloxacin in seriously ill patients. Antimicrob Agents Chemother. 1993;37:1073–1081.)

one. The study of Bodey and colleagues examined the efficacy of intermittent versus continuous infusions of cefamandole plus intermittent infusions of carbenicillin in neutropenic patients.[9] The authors demonstrated a slightly higher response rate in the continuous infusion group, but the difference was not significant. Analysis of a subset of patients with cefamandole-susceptible organisms revealed a significant benefit of continuous versus intermittent infusion, although the patient numbers were small.

Schentag and associates also noted for cefmenoxime that T>MIC correlated better than AUC/MIC for bacterial eradication from the lung.[10]

A retrospective analysis by Craig and Andes attempted to correlate the pharmacodynamics of antibiotics in the treatment of otitis media.[16] Using retrospective data and free drug calculations, the authors examined T>MIC and bacteriologic cure for β-lactams, macrolides, and trimethoprim-sulfamethoxazole. They concluded that an 80 to 85% efficacy rate was achieved when the T>MIC was 40 to 50% of the dosing interval.

Some interesting data are available for staphylococcal infections and vancomycin in pediatric patients. Schaad and colleagues noted that a peak *serum bactericidal titer (SBT)* of 1:8 or greater was associated with cure in 16 of 20 patients.[26] Louria and coworkers noted cure of staphylococcal infections when the SBT was 1:8 or higher (six patients) and failure when it was lower than 1:8 (three patients, although in one, cure was seen after dose escalation).[27]

Therefore, although animal and in vitro data suggest that for certain antibiotics T>MIC is an important pharmacodynamic predictor, few data in human studies exist to support this conclusion.

Postantibiotic Effect. During in vitro testing of antimicrobials, there may be a delay before microorganisms recover and reenter a log-growth period. This phenomenon is termed the *postantibiotic effect*, or *PAE*. The exact duration of the PAE is species and drug dependent. For example, aminoglycosides and fluoroquinolones produce in vitro PAEs against gram-negative bacilli of approximately 2 to 6 hours. β-Lactam antibiotics (with the exception of imipenem) produce little or no PAE against gram-negative organisms under identical experimental conditions but generally induce 2-hour PAEs against gram-positive organisms. Other factors that affect the in vitro PAE include combinations of antimicrobials, antimicrobial concentration, duration of antimicrobial exposure, and pH. Potential factors that may also affect the PAE include size of inoculum, type of growth medium, and bacterial growth phase.

Studies in animal models have verified that PAE is not an artifact of in vitro testing. Investigational animal models that have been studied include a neutropenic mouse thigh model, a rabbit meningitis model, a rat endocarditis model, and a guinea pig pneumonia model. These studies demonstrate that an in vivo PAE exists against gram-negative organisms for aminoglycosides, fluoroquinolones, erythromycin, clindamycin, and tetracycline, but not for β-lactams. As in the in vitro studies, β-lactam agents do produce abbreviated PAEs against gram-positive organisms.

The mechanism of the PAE is unknown. Possible explanations include nonlethal bacterial damage induced by the antimicrobial agent and persistence of the antimicrobial at the site of action. However, when fresh organisms are injected into animals during the PAE period, there is rapid and immediate growth, suggesting that the PAE is not caused by persistence of the drug in tissue.

The presence or absence of a PAE has been used to alter antimicrobial dosing schedules. Theoretically, an agent with a long PAE can be dosed less frequently than an antimicrobial lacking a PAE. Alternatively, an agent with little or no PAE may be most effective if it is given as a continuous infusion, so that the serum concentration always exceeds the MIC. Dosing strategies such as these are theoretical and require clinical investigation in human studies of sufficient size before implementation into clinical practice.

REFERENCES

1. Benet LZ. General Principles: Introduction. In: Hardman JG, Limbird LE, eds. Goodman & Gilman's The Pharmacological Basis of Therapeutics. 9th ed. New York: McGraw-Hill; 1996:1–3.
2. Benet LZ, Kroetz DL, Sheiner LB. Pharmacokinetics: The dynamics of drug absorption, distribution, and elimination. In: Hardman JG, Limbird LE, eds. Goodman & Gilman's The Pharmacological Basis of Therapeutics 9th ed. New York: McGraw-Hill; 1996:3–28.
3. Rendic S, DiCarlo FJ. Human cytochrome-P450 enzymes: A status report summarizing their reactions, substrates, inducers and inhibitors. Drug Metab Rev. 1997;29:413–580.
4. Craig WA. Pharmacokinetic/pharmacodynamic parameters: Rationale for antibacterial dosing of mice and men. Clin Infect Dis. 1998;26:1–12.
5. Thomas JK, Forrest A, Bhavnani SM, et al. Pharmacodynamic evaluation of factors associated with the development of bacterial resistance in acutely ill patients during therapy. Antimicrob Agents Chemother. 1998;42:521–527.
6. Blaser J, Stone BB, Zinner SH. Two compartment kinetic model with multiple artificial capillary units. J Antimicrob Chemother. 15;1985(suppl. A):131–137.
7. Blaser J, Stone BB, Groner MC, et al. Comparative study with enoxacin and netilmicin in a pharmacodynamic model to determine importance of ratio of antibiotic peak concentration to MIC for bacterial activity and emergence of resistance. Antimicrob Agents Chemother. 1987;31:1055–1060.
8. Keating MJ, Bodey GP, Valdivieso M, et al. A randomized comparative trial of three aminoglycosides: Comparison of continuous infusions of gentamicin, amikacin and sisomicin combined with carbenicillin in the treatment of infections in neutropenic patients with malignancies. Medicine (Baltimore). 1979:58:159–170.
9. Bodey GP, Ketchel SJ, Rodriguez V. A randomized study of carbenicillin plus cefamandole or tobramycin in the treatment of febrile episodes in cancer patients. Am J Med. 1979;67:608–611.
10. Schentag JJ, Smith IL, Swanson DJ, et al. Role for dual individualization with cefmenoxime. Am J Med. 1984(suppl 6A):43–50.
11. Moore RD, Lietman PS, Smith CR. Clinical response to aminoglycoside therapy: Importance of the ratio of peak concentration to minimum inhibitory concentration. J Infect Dis. 1987:155:93–99.
12. Deziel-Evans JM, Murphy JE, Job ML. Correlation of pharmacokinetic indices

with therapeutic outcome in patients receiving aminoglycosides. Clin Pharmacol. 1986:5:319–324.
13. Schentag JJ, Nix DE, Adelman MH. Mathematical examination of dual individualization principles (I): Relationships between AUC above MIC and area under the inhibitory curve for cefmenoxime, ciprofloxacin and tobramycin. Ann Pharmacother. 1991:25:1050–1057.
14. Forrest A, Nix DE, Ballow CH, et al. Pharmacodynamics of intravenous ciprofloxacin in seriously ill patients. Antimicrob Agents Chemother. 1993;37:1073–1081.
15. Goss TF, Forrest A, Nix DE, et al. Mathematical examination of dual individualization principles (II): The rate of bacterial eradication at the same area under the inhibitory curve is more rapid for ciprofloxacin than for cefmenoxime. Ann Pharmacother. 1994;28:863–868.
16. Craig WA, Andes D. Pharmacokinetics and pharmacodynamics of antibiotic in otitis media. Pediatr Infect Dis J. 1996;15:255–259.
17. Kashuba ADM, Nafziger AN, Drusano GL, et al. Early optimization of aminoglycoside pharmacokinetic goals reduces time to therapeutic response in gram negative pneumonia. Program and Abstracts 36th Interscience Conference on Antimicrobial Agents and Chemotherapy, September 1996 (Abstract A100).
18. Hyatt JM, Luzier AB, Forrest A, et al. Modeling the response of pneumonia to antimicrobial therapy. Antimicrob Agents Chemother. 1997:41:1269–1274.
19. Forrest A, Chodosh S, Amantea MA, et al. Pharmacokinetics and pharmacodynamics of oral grepafloxacin in patients with acute bacterial exacerbations of chronic bronchitis. J Antimicrob Chemother. 1997;(suppl. A):40:45–57.
20. Preston SL, Drusano GL, Berman AL, et al. Pharmacodynamics of levofloxacin: A new paradigm for early clinical trials. JAMA. 1998;279:125–129.
21. Craig WA, Ebert SC. Killing and regrowth of bacteria in vitro: A review. Scand J Infect Dis. 1991;74:63–70.
22. Craig WA. Interrelationship between pharmacokinetics and pharmacodynamics in determining dosage regimens for broad-spectrum cephalosporins. Diagn Microbiol Infect Dis. 1995:22:89–96.
23. Craig WA. Antimicrobial resistance issues of the future. Diagn Microbiol Infect Dis. 1996;25:213–217.
24. Bertino JS Jr, Rotschafer JC. Single daily dosing of aminoglycosides: A concept whose time has not yet come. Clin Infect Dis. 1997;24:820–823.
25. Marchbanks CR, McKeil JR, Gilbert DH, et al. Dose ranging and fractionation of intravenous ciprofloxacin against *Pseudomonas aeruginosa* and *Staphylococcus aureus* in an in vitro model of infection. Antimicrob Agents Chemother. 1993;37:1756–1763.
26. Schaad UB, McCracken GH Jr, Nelson JD. Clinical pharmacology and efficacy of vancomycin in pediatric patients. J Pediatr. 1980;96:119–126.
27. Louria DB, Kaminski T, Buchman J. Vancomycin in severe staphylococcal infections. Arch Intern Med. 1961;107:225–240.

Chapter 18

Penicillins

HENRY F. CHAMBERS

Penicillin was discovered by Fleming[1] in 1928. Attempts to obtain significant amounts of the agent were initially unsuccessful. The work of Florey, Chain, and associates in 1941 made possible the commercial production of penicillin G. In 1939 Florey at the Sir William Dunn School of Pathology began to work out the isolation, structure, and properties of the compound. In 1940 his group showed that penicillin protected mice experimentally infected with streptococci, and by 1941 these workers had produced enough penicillin to treat a few patients, the first of whom was a British policeman infected with both staphylococci and streptococci. As a result of World War II, production of penicillin was undertaken in the United States. Initial clinical trials at Yale and the Mayo Clinic were so successful that the U.S. Army began to use the material to treat streptococcal, gonococcal, and treponemal infections. As fermentation techniques improved, production of large amounts of pure drug became possible, and by the end of the 1940s, penicillin G was available for general use in the United States.

CHEMISTRY

The basic structure of the majority of commercially available penicillins is a nucleus that consists of a thiazolidine ring—the β-lactam ring—and a side chain (Fig. 18–1). The penicillin nucleus is a condensation of alanine and β-dimethylcysteine. Penicillins currently in use are dextrorotatory and usually exist as sodium or potassium salts. The β-lactam ring is essential for antibacterial activity. The side chain determines in large part the antibacterial spectrum and pharmacologic properties of a particular penicillin. Although biosynthesis of penicillin has been achieved, it has not proved to be a useful technique, and fermentation remains the method of production of penicillin G.

benzylpenicillin

penicillinase (β-lactamase)

benzylpenicilloic acid

1 Thiazolidine ring
2 β-lactam ring

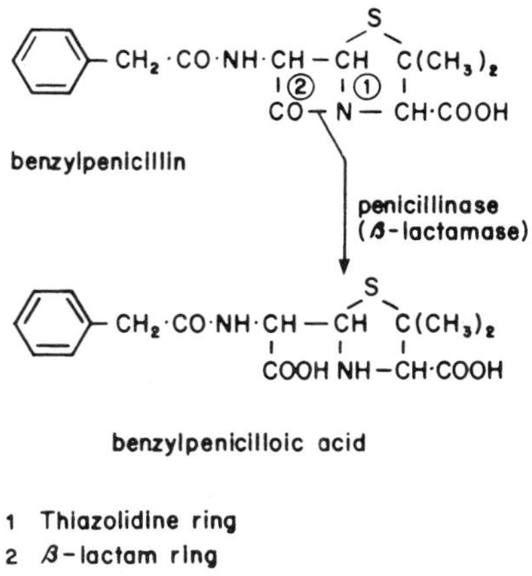

FIGURE 18–1. Structure of penicillin and site of β-lactamase attack.

The appearance of β-lactamase–producing organisms, particularly *Staphylococcus aureus*, prompted studies to develop compounds with resistance to hydrolysis by β-lactamases and also to find agents more active than penicillin G against gram-negative species. In 1959, Batchelor and coworkers[2] isolated the penicillin nucleus, 6-aminopenicillanic acid, from a precursor-depleted fermentation of *Penicillium chrysogenum*. This made possible the production and testing of numerous semisynthetic penicillins, the first of which was methicillin, active against β-lactamase–producing *S. aureus*; followed by ampicillin, active against selected gram-negative bacilli; and carbenicillin which proved to have activity against *Pseudomonas aeruginosa*. Since then, scores of agents with different pharmacologic and antimicrobial properties have been developed.

MECHANISM OF ACTION

Precisely how penicillins kill bacterial cells is not known. Study of the action of penicillins has elucidated many aspects of bacterial physiology, but recent advances suggest that the concept that penicillin kills simply by blocking the last step in cell wall synthesis is a simplistic one. The cell wall of bacteria is assembled in a series of enzymatic steps that involve at least 30 enzymes.

Bacterial Cell Walls

The cell walls of both gram-positive and gram-negative bacteria are held in a rigid manner by peptidoglycan, also called murein sacculus,[3, 4] protecting against osmotic rupture. The cell wall in gram-positive bacteria is a substantial layer 50 to 100 molecules in thickness, whereas the peptidoglycan component of the cell wall in gram-negative bacteria is only one or two molecules thick. An outer lipopolysaccharide layer, which is not found in gram-positive bacteria, is present on top of the peptidoglycan in gram-negative species.

Peptidoglycans are long polysaccharide chains in which *N*-acetylglucosamine (NAG) and *N*-acetylmuramic (NAM) acid alternate in a linear form. Individual chains are cross-linked by short peptides joined in amide linkage to the penultimate D-alanyl group of the *N*-acetylmuramic acid. In gram-negative species the 6-amino group of

This chapter is based in large part on a chapter originally prepared by Dr. Chambers and the late Harold C. Neu.

diaminopimelic acid is linked to the carboxyalanine terminus of another chain.[4] Of interest, the percentage of cross-linking is less in *Escherichia coli* (25%) than in *S. aureus* (90%).[5]

Peptidoglycan synthesis has been divided into three stages. The first is the synthesis of uridine diphosphate (UDP)-NAM-pentapeptide and UDP-NAG. These two compounds are transported across the cytoplasmic membrane by a lipid-soluble carrier that is a C_{55} isoprenyl alcohol phosphate. Transglycosylation of disaccharide monomer into peptidoglycan polymer occurs at this stage. The final reaction is cross-linking the new peptidoglycan into the existing peptidoglycan. In this final reaction a free amino group on the third amino acid (or on the terminal residue of a short peptide chain attached to the third amino acid) of the NAM-pentapeptide of one strand displaces the terminal D-alanine from a pentapeptide of a second strand in a transpeptidation reaction. This transpeptidation reaction is sensitive to inhibition by penicillin. There appear to be distinct transpeptidases, providing for anchoring of new peptidoglycan to old, that cross link special structures and that constitute the cell wall septum. Although there are other penicillin-sensitive reactions, such as the effects on carboxypeptidase, these reactions do not seem to be crucial in gram-negative species. The most telling argument that penicillin inactivates transpeptidases was the stereochemistry modeling performed by Strominger's group,[6] which supports an acyl enzyme intermediate, owing to the structural similarity of penicillin and the acyl–D-alanyl–D-alanine.

Penicillin-Binding Proteins

Bacteria produce four types of penicillin-binding proteins (PBPs), which structurally resemble and probably are derived from serine proteases.[7] High-molecular-weight PBPs (i.e., more than 50 kD) and low-molecular-weight PBPs catalyze transpeptidation and carboxypeptidation reactions of cell wall assembly. Penicillin receptor PBPs transmit a transmembrane signal for induction of β-lactamases. β-Lactamases are PBPs that catalyze hydrolysis of the β-lactam ring, thereby inactivating the drug. PBPs are membrane-bound except for β-lactamases, which may be either secreted or membrane-associated. Transpeptidases form the cross-links in peptidoglycan, and carboxypeptidases possibly are important for modification of peptidoglycan. Both high-molecular-weight and low-molecular-weight PBPs are inhibited by β-lactam antibiotics, which covalently bind by acylation of the active site serine residue. The crucial functions essential for survival of the cell generally reside with high-molecular-weight PBPs. Consequently, it is binding to and inhibition of the high-molecular-weight PBPs that probably are responsible for the antibacterial activity of β-lactam antibiotics.

PBPs of a given organism are numbered according to molecular weight, with the highest-molecular-weight protein being designated PBP 1, the next highest PBP 2, and so on. If what initially seemed to be one PBP (e.g., PBP 2) is subsequently found to be two or more distinct proteins, rather than renumbering all the PBPs, letters are used to differentiate the individual PBPs of similar molecular weight (e.g., PBP 2a, PBP 2b, PBP 2x), or the newly identified PBP may be designated with a prime sign (e.g., PBP 2′). PBPs assigned the same number but produced by different species are not necessarily related or of similar function. The numbering of PBPs for gram-positive bacteria bears no relation to the numbering for gram-negative bacteria.

PBPs account for approximately 1% of membrane proteins. PBPs vary both in amounts present and in the physiologic functions they serve during cell wall assembly. They also differ in their affinities for binding β-lactam antibiotics, which explains at least in part why the β-lactam antibiotics differ in their antibacterial properties and spectrum of activity. Spratt's studies[8, 9] in *E. coli* were the first to elucidate the different functions of PBPs. Inhibition of PBP 1b or a substitute enzyme 1a results in cell lysis. PBP 1 is speculated to be important for cell elongation. Inhibition of PBP 2 results in formation of round cells that eventually lyse, suggesting that PBP 2 has a role in an initial step in cell elongation and in determining the rod shape of *E. coli*. Inhibition of PBP 3 produces long, filamentous cells, indicating that it is important for the ordered process of cross wall formation and cell division. The functions performed by PBPs in other species have not been well defined but presumably also are distinct.

No single PBP species is the target of β-lactam antibiotics, which produce their lethal effect on bacteria by inactivation of multiple PBPs simultaneously.[10] The lethal effect in both gram-positive and gram-negative organisms appears to be cell cycle–dependent, with inhibition of PBPs leading to disruption of a crucial event probably at the time of cell division.[11, 12] Unopposed action of autolysins occurring when PBPs are inhibited by β-lactam antibiotics may also contribute to the antibacterial effect in some organisms.

BACTERIAL RESISTANCE

Three mechanisms account for clinically significant bacterial resistance to β-lactam antibiotics: (1) destruction of antibiotic by β-lactamase, (2) failure of antibiotic to penetrate to PBP targets, and (3) low-affinity binding of antibiotic to PBPs. Of these three mechanisms, β-lactamase destruction of antibiotic is the most important.[13] β-Lactamases, which are a type of PBP, covalently react with the β-lactam bond to form an acyl enzyme intermediate, which undergoes rapid hydrolysis, thereby destroying the activity of the drug. β-Lactamases are classified on the basis of their affinity for β-lactam compounds and amino acid composition (Fig. 18–2). β-Lactamase of staphylococci is plasmid-encoded and inducible by β-lactam antibiotics. Although it may be membrane-bound, staphylococcal β-lactamase, which acts primarily as a penicillinase, is an exoenzyme that is liberated into the surrounding medium, in which it destroys penicillin before it can reach the target PBPs. The activities of methicillin and the isoxazolyl penicillins are due to their stability to staphylococcal β-lactamase.

β-Lactamases of gram-negative bacteria are cell-associated enzymes located in the periplasmic space, which lies between the inner (cytoplasmic) membrane and outer lipopolysaccharide membrane. Thus, gram-negative β-lactamases are concentrated and strategically located to protect the target PBPs from exposure to active β-lactam antibiotics. Gram-negative β-lactamases may be encoded either on the chromosome or on plasmids and may be produced constitutively or as inducible enzymes, with affinity for penicillins or cephalosporins or both types of compounds. All gram-negative species probably contain at least small amounts of β-lactamase. Differences among β-lactam compounds in binding affinity and in susceptibility to hydrolysis by gram-negative β-lactamases and the type of β-lactamase that is produced account for some of the differences in their activities against gram-negative bacteria. For example, carbenicillin is destroyed at a much slower rate than is ampicillin by β-lactamases produced by *Enterobacter cloacae* or *Morganella morganii*; consequently, it is more active.

Gram-positive bacteria lack an outer membrane; consequently, there is no physical barrier that prevents β-lactam antibiotics, which freely diffuse, from reaching the target PBPs. The outer membrane of gram-negative organisms, on the other hand, is an important barrier to drug penetration and an important component of resistance. Small polar molecules (e.g., glucose, essential nutrients, β-lactam antibiotics) cross this barrier through protein channels called porins. Porins constrain entry of molecules into the cell according to size, structure, and charge. β-Lactam antibiotics that satisfy the entry requirements traverse porin channels to the periplasmic space, located between the outer membrane and the cell membrane. The target PBPs, located on the outer surface of cell membrane, are bound once an effective concentration of antibiotic is achieved in the periplasm. Resistance occurs if the concentration of antibiotic in the periplasm is less than that required to bind and inhibit PBPs. The three mechanisms responsible for limiting periplasmic antibiotic concentration, which may work independently but more often operate

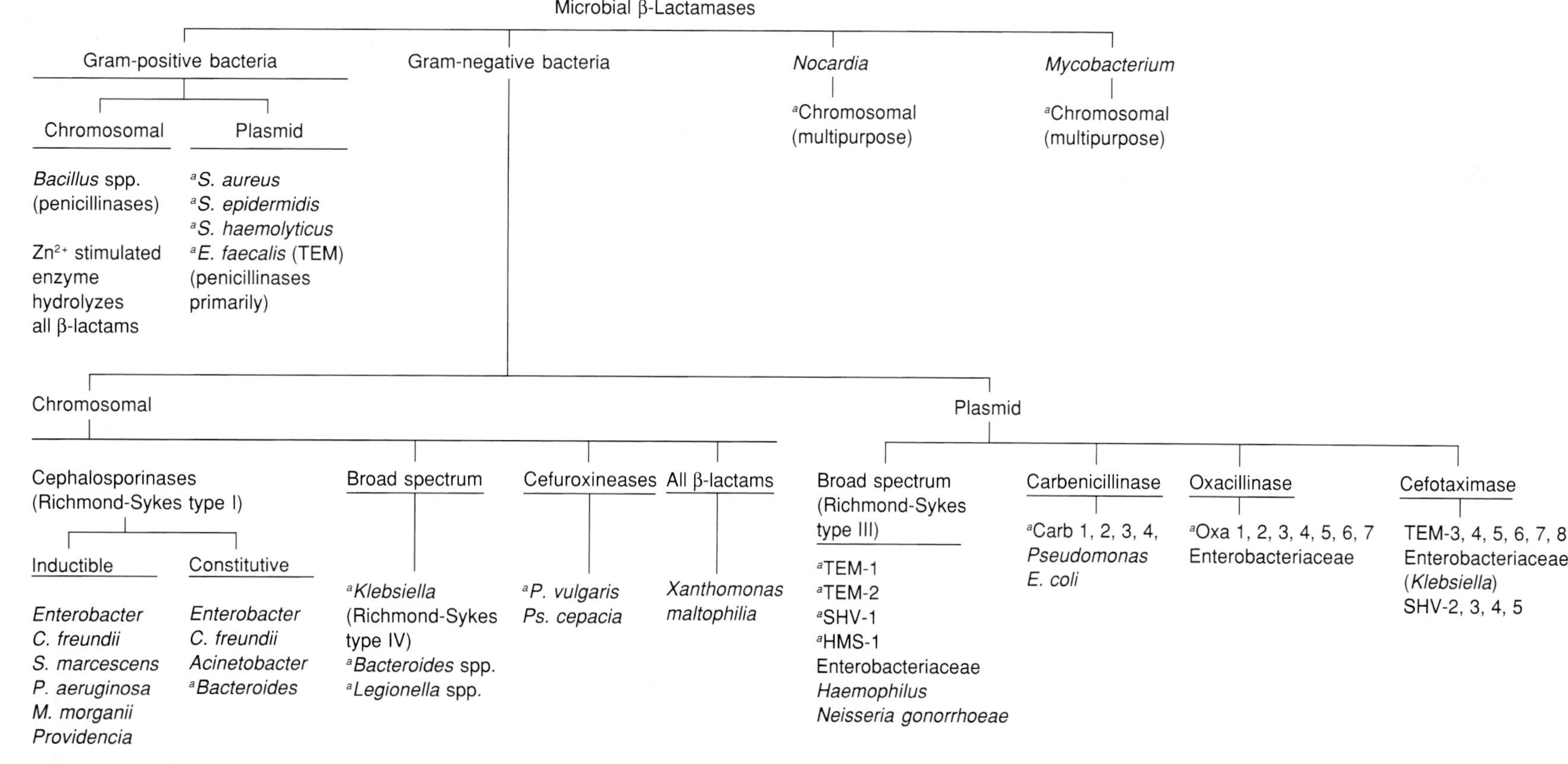

FIGURE 18–2. Diagrammatic representation of β-lactamases. *Abbreviation:* a, Inhibited by clavulanate, sulbactam, and tazobactam.

TABLE 18–1 Classification of Penicillins

	Route(s) of Use	Trade Name(s)
Natural penicillins		
Penicillin G	PO	Pfizerpen
	IM	Wycillin
	IM	Bicillin
Penicillin G potassium or sodium	IV	
Penicillin V	PO	Pen-Vee K, Penicillin VK
Penicillinase-resistant penicillins		
Methicillin	IM, IV	
Nafcillin	IM, IV	Unipen
Isoxazolyl penicillins		
Cloxacillin	PO	
Dicloxacillin	PO	
Flucloxacillin	PO	
Oxacillin	PO, IM, IV	
Aminopenicillins		
Ampicillin	IM, IV	Omipen
Amoxicillin	PO	Amoxil, Wymox
Carboxy- and indanyl penicillins		
Indanyl carbenicillin	PO	Geocillin
Ticarcillin	IM, IV	Ticar
Extended-spectrum ureidopenicillins		
Azlocillin	IM, IV	
Mezlocillin	IM, IV	Mezlin
Piperacillin	IM, IV	Pipracil

Abbreviations: IM, Intramuscular; IV, intravenous; PO, per os (orally).

in tandem, are exclusion of antibiotic by porins, destruction of antibiotic by β-lactamases, which in gram-negative organisms are concentrated in the periplasm, and transport of drug back across the outer membrane.[14] Species differences among the several porins, pumps, β-lactamases, and PBPs that bacteria may produce in conjunction with β-lactam antibiotic structure determine the interaction between bacterial proteins and antibiotic and, ultimately, whether the organism will be susceptible or resistant to that antibiotic. Mutations affecting protein structure or expression may cause a strain that was initially susceptible to a given β-lactam antibiotic to become resistant.

The third general type of resistance mechanism involves production of a PBP that has low affinity for binding of β-lactam antibiotic.[15] Differences in binding of PBPs account for some of the differences in susceptibility of individual bacterial strains to a particular β-lactam antibiotic. Differences in binding of specific β-lactams to target PBPs also account for differences in activity against a single organism or species. For example, staphylococci are susceptible to penicillinase-resistant penicillins because their PBPs have relatively high affinity for these compounds such that significant binding occurs at clinically achievable concentrations. Enterococci, however, are naturally resistant to the penicillinase-resistant penicillins because they produce PBPs with lower affinity, and significant binding occurs only at concentrations above the therapeutic range. Enterococcal PBPs, however, generally have relatively higher affinity for penicillin and ampicillin, and thus they are susceptible to these drugs. Mutations in resident PBP genes that lower binding affinity (as in penicillin-resistant pneumococci or *Neisseria* spp.) or the presence of an extra-low-affinity PBP (e.g., PBP 2a produced by methicillin-resistant staphylococci) can lead to resistance. Multiple mutations affecting more than one PBP gene generally are required to produce resistance, and the probability that several unique mutations would occur simultaneously is remote, suggesting that this mechanism of resistance might not be clinically important. However, the ability of some bacteria to accumulate multiple mutations over time and to transfer mutant genes across species has proved this to be incorrect, as evidenced by the relatively high prevalence of PBP-mediated resistance to penicillins among enterococci, pneumococci, and staphylococci.[16]

CLASSIFICATION

Penicillins can be conveniently divided into classes on the basis of antibacterial activity (Table 18–1), with considerable overlap among the classes. Differences within a class usually are of a pharmacologic nature, although one compound in a class may be more active than another.

The susceptibility patterns of various species of microorganisms are given in Tables 18–2, 18–3, and 18–4. The natural penicillins are most active against non–β-lactamase–producing gram-positive bacteria, anaerobes, and selected gram-negative cocci, such as *Neisseria.* Gram-positive bacteria inhibited by natural penicillins in general are more susceptible to these penicillins than to semisynthetic penicillins.[17–21] Penicillin V (used orally) can be substituted for penicillin G, except against gram-negative species because it is less active than penicillin G against *Neisseria* and *Haemophilus.* Semisynthetic penicillinase-resistant penicillins are the drugs of choice only for penicillin-resistant *S. aureus* and *Staphylococcus epidermidis*, although they also are active against streptococci.[17, 18] Aminopenicillins possess the same spectrum as penicillin G, plus they are more active against gram-negative cocci and members of the family Enterobacteriaceae. Carboxypenicillins such as carbenicillin and ticarcillin are less active than the ureidopenicillins against streptococci and *Hae-*

TABLE 18–2 Usual Minimal Inhibitory Concentrations (MICs) for Penicillins against Cocci

	Mean MIC (μg/ml)							
Organism	*Penicillin G*	*Penicillin V*	*Ampicillin, Amoxicillin*	*Methicillin*	*Oxacillin, Cloxacillin, Dicloxacillin*	*Nafcillin*	*Ticarcillin*	*Azlocillin, Mezlocillin, Piperacillin*
Streptococcus pneumoniae	0.01*	0.02*	0.02*	0.1*	0.04	0.02	0.4	0.02
Streptococcus pyogenes	0.005	0.01	0.02	0.2	0.04	0.02	0.2	0.02
Streptococcus agalactiae	0.005	0.01	0.02	0.2	0.06	0.02	0.2	0.15
Viridans streptococci	0.01	0.01	0.05	0.1	0.1	0.06	0.2	0.12
Enterococcus faecalis	3.0	6.0	1.5†	>25	>25	>25	50	1.5
Peptostreptococcus	0.2	0.5	0.2	2.0	0.6	0.5	0.4	0.8
Staphylococcus aureus								
Penicillinase-negative	0.02	0.02	0.05	1.0	0.3	0.25	1.2	0.8
Penicillinase-positive	>25	>25	>25	2.0	0.4	0.25	25	25
Staphylococcus epidermidis	0.02‡	0.02‡	0.05‡	0.8‡	0.2‡	0.2‡	0.8‡	1.6‡
Neisseria gonorrhoeae§	0.01‡	0.1	0.3‡	12.0	12.0	12.0	0.3‡	0.05‡
Neisseria meningitidis	0.05	0.25	0.05	6.0	6.0	6.0	0.1	0.05

*Rare isolates resistant to penicillin have been found with MIC >5 μg/ml.
†Amoxicillin has a mean MIC of 0.4.
‡Many isolates resistant.
§MIC can range from 0.005 to 100.

TABLE 18–3 Activity of Penicillins against Selected Bacilli and Anaerobic Organisms

Organism	Mean Minimal Inhibitory Concentration (μg/ml)				
	Penicillin G	*Ampicillin, Amoxicillin*	*Oxacillin**	*Ticarcillin†*	*Azlocillin, Mezlocillin, Piperacillin†*
Clostridium perfringens	0.5	0.05	>0.5	0.5	0.05
Corynebacterium diphtheriae	0.1	0.02	>0.1	0.1	1.0
Listeria monocytogenes	0.5	0.5	>4.0	4	0.5
Haemophilus influenzae‡	0.8	0.5	>25	0.5	0.1
Prevotella melaninogenica	0.5	0.5	>25	0.5	0.2
Fusobacterium nucleatum	0.5	0.1	>100	0.5	0.5
Bacteroides fragilis	32	32	>500	64	32

*Oxacillin is used as representative of isoxazolyl penicillins.
†Minor differences do occur.
‡β-Lactamase–producing strains occur and are resistant to the penicillins.

mophilus spp. Carboxypenicillins and ureidopenicillins have activity against gram-negative aerobic rods, such as *P. aeruginosa*, which are resistant to ampicillin. The ureidopenicillins generally are more active against gram-negative bacteria other than *Pseudomonas*, but susceptibility varies from hospital to hospital and from community to community. Many anaerobic gram-positive species are susceptible to the penicillins. Gram-negative anaerobic bacteria are susceptible to most penicillins, with the exception of isolates of *Bacteroides fragilis*, other *Bacteroides* spp., and some *Prevotella* spp., and are inhibited by high levels of penicillin G or the semisynthetic anti-*Pseudomonas* agents—azlocillin, carbenicillin, mezlocillin, piperacillin, and ticarcillin.[20, 22, 23] Strains of *Fusobacterium varium* often are resistant to all penicillins.

PHARMACOLOGIC PROPERTIES

Penicillins differ markedly in their oral absorption (Table 18–5). Penicillin G is acid-labile and has a half-life of less than 20 minutes at pH 2. In contrast, at pH 4 it has a half-life of 1 hour. Methicillin and all the anti-*Pseudomonas* penicillins are acid-labile. However, acid stability is not a guarantee of oral absorption, and there can be major differences in oral absorption of compounds within the same class. Penicillin V is well absorbed even when ingested with food, and the greatest absorption of penicillin V is with the potassium salt. The semisynthetic penicillins except nafcillin are well absorbed. Ampicillin is only partially absorbed, 30 to 60%,[17] whereas amoxicillin is almost totally absorbed.[21] Although carbenicillin is not absorbed, esters of the compound such as indanyl carbenicillin are adequately absorbed to provide urinary concentration to treat urinary tract infections.[23]

The majority of penicillins are absorbed, so they yield peak levels 1 to 2 hours after ingestion. Absorption is delayed to yield peak serum levels 2 to 3 hours after ingestion with food, and peak levels are lower, except for amoxicillin.

Repository forms of penicillin G are available. These are procaine penicillin G and benzathine penicillin G. These are absorbed more slowly from intramuscular sites than are the crystalline salts. Procaine or lidocaine can also be used as a diluent for intramuscular injection of anti-*Pseudomonas* penicillins, but the half-life of these drugs is not prolonged with inclusion of these agents.

Penicillins are bound to protein in varying degrees, ranging from 17% for the aminopenicillins to 97% for dicloxacillin (see Table 18–5). The major protein to which they bind is albumin.[17] Only unbound drug exerts antibacterial activity, because the bound drug is not free to interact with PBPs. However, protein binding is a reversible process, and it is possible for bound penicillin to be released and then to kill bacteria in tissue or in the blood stream. The major mechanism by which these drugs are removed from the body is by excretion as intact molecules via the kidney.[24] Penicillins are metabolized to a minor degree.[25] Even minor differences in metabolism can result in clinically significant differences in half-life in the presence of renal failure. Biliary excretion of penicillins does occur, but it probably is important only for nafcillin and the anti-*Pseudomonas* penicillins.

TABLE 18–4 Activity of Penicillins against Enterobacteriaceae and *Pseudomonas*

Organism	Mean Minimal Inhibitory Concentration (μg/ml)				
	Penicillin G	*Ampicillin, Amoxicillin*	*Oxacillin**	*Ticarcillin*	*Azlocillin,† Mezlocillin, Piperacillin*
Escherichia coli‡	100	3	>1000	6	8
Proteus mirabilis	50	3	>1000	1.5	1
Klebsiella spp.	>400	200	>1000	>400	16
Enterobacter spp.	>500	>500	>1000	50	16
Citrobacter diversus	>500	>100	>1000	12	8
Citrobacter freundii	>500	50	>1000	12	32
Serratia	>500	>500	>1000	100	32
Salmonella‡	10	1.5	>1000	3	4
Shigella‡	20	1.5	>1000	3	8
Proteus vulgaris	>500	>500	>1000	12	16
Providencia	>500	>500	>1000	12	8
Morganella	>500	200	>1000	25	8
Pseudomonas, other	>500	>500	>500	100	>100
Acinetobacter	>500	250	>1000	25	32
Pseudomonas aeruginosa	>500	>500	>1000	50	16*

*Used as representative antistaphylococcal penicillin.
†Some isolates, particularly *Klebsiella*, are resistant to azlocillin but susceptible to mezlocillin and piperacillin.
‡Amoxicillin is twofold more active against *Salmonella* and twofold less active against *Shigella*. Strains containing the TEM plasmid β-lactamase are resistant.

TABLE 18–5 Pharmacokinetic Properties of Penicillins

Antibiotic	Oral Adsorption (%)	Food Decreases Adsorption	Protein Binding (%)	Amount of Dose Metabolized (%)	Serum Level*: Total Drug (μg/ml)	Serum Level*: Free Drug (μg/ml)	Serum $T_{1/2}$ (h)†: Normal (C_{cr} >90 ml/min)	Serum $T_{1/2}$ (h)†: With Renal Failure (C_{cr} <10 ml/min)	Liver Impairment Increases T_i	Na† Content‡ (mEq/g)
Penicillin G	20	Yes	55	20	2	0.9	0.5	10	+	2.7
Penicillin V	60	No	80	55	4	0.8	1	4		
Methicillin	Nil		35	10			0.5	4		3.1
Oxacillin	30	Yes	93	45	6	0.4	0.5	1		
Cloxacillin	50	Yes	94	20	10	0.6	0.5	1	+ +	
Dicloxacillin	50	Yes	97	10	15	0.45	0.5	1.5	+ +	
Nafcillin	Erratic	Yes	87				0.5	1.5	+ + +	
Ampicillin‡	40	Yes	17	10	3.5	2.9	1	8	+ +	3.4
Amoxicillin	75	No	17	10	7.5	6.2	1	8	+	
Indanyl carbenicillin	30	No	50		15	7.5	1.1	15	+ +	
Ticarcillin	Nil		50	15			1.2	15	+ +, 18–20 h	4.7
Mezlocillin	Nil		50				1.1	4	+ +	1.8
Piperacillin	Nil		50				1.3	4	+ +	1.8
Azlocillin	Nil		20				0.8	4	+ +	2.2
Temocillin	Nil		85	10			4	17	+ +	

*After 500-mg dose taken fasting.
†Values have been rounded off to approximate values.
‡Na^+ content based on intravenous preparations.
Abbreviations: C_{cr}, Creatinine clearance; $T_{1/2}$, serum half-life.

The mechanism of excretion of penicillins is via renal tubular cells. Penicillins are rapidly excreted into urine, and hence they have a short half-life, ranging from less than 30 minutes for penicillin to 72 minutes for carbenicillin. The ability of the renal tubular cells to excrete penicillin varies with the agents, but up to 4 g of penicillin G per hour can be excreted. This excretion can be blocked by probenecid, which prolongs the serum half-life of all the penicillins.[26] Probenecid also competes for binding sites on albumin; hence, there is more free drug in the presence of probenecid. Renal excretion of all penicillins in newborns is markedly less than in older children, because tubular function is not fully developed at birth. Hence, the dosage programs for penicillins must be modified when these drugs are given to newborns or low-birth-weight infants.

Reduction in renal function is an important consideration in the administration of certain penicillins (e.g., ticarcillin). If the creatinine clearance is greater than 10 ml/minute, it is necessary to make only minor adjustments in the dosage of other penicillins. In the presence of anuria, reduction in total daily dose of the natural penicillins, of many of the penicillinase-resistant penicillins, and of the aminopenicillins is necessary (Table 18–6).

Peritoneal dialysis removes variable amounts of the penicillins. In general, after peritoneal dialysis only the dosage regimens of ticarcillin need to be adjusted. After hemodialysis it is necessary to replace the dialyzed penicillin G, ampicillin, amoxicillin, ticarcillin, azlocillin, mezlocillin, and piperacillin, but not nafcillin or the isoxazolyl penicillins.

Penicillins are well distributed to most areas of the body such as lung, liver, kidney, muscle, bone, and placenta. The levels of penicillins in abscesses, middle ear, and pleural, peritoneal, and synovial fluids are sufficient in the presence of inflammation to inhibit most susceptible bacteria.[27–30] Most penicillins are relatively insoluble in lipid and penetrate cells relatively poorly. Distribution of all the penicillins to eye, brain, cerebrospinal fluid, or prostate is nil in the absence of inflammation.[31] Inflammation alters normal barriers, permitting entry of penicillins, but more important, it interferes with the anion pump that removes penicillins from areas such as cerebrospinal fluid. Penicillins with low rates of protein binding reach levels in fetal serum equivalent to levels in maternal serum 30 to 60 minutes after injection. In contrast, the highly protein-bound semisynthetic penicillins achieve low concentrations in both amniotic fluid and fetal serum.[32]

Urinary concentrations of all penicillins are high, even in the presence of moderately reduced renal function, but in people with rates of creatinine clearance below 10 ml/minute, the urinary levels may not exceed those in the blood. Cortical and medullary concentrations of penicillins during normal hydration and in hydropenia exceed serum levels.

Most penicillins are actively secreted into the bile, yielding biliary concentrations well in excess of those in serum. The biliary levels of penicillin G, ampicillin, and amoxicillin are at least 10 times those in the serum, and the levels of nafcillin and mezlocillin in bile are as high as 100 times the simultaneous serum level. In the presence of common duct obstruction, the levels of all penicillins in bile are markedly reduced. Because the biliary transport system is a saturable one, with drug doses producing very high serum levels, the biliary levels are not significantly increased over those measured at lower serum levels.

UNTOWARD REACTIONS

The major adverse effects of the penicillins are hypersensitivity reactions, which range in severity from rash to immediate anaphy-

TABLE 18–6 Antibiotic Dosage Change in Renal Disease and after Dialysis

Agent	Dosage Change in Renal Failure*: Creatinine Clearance (30–50 ml/min)	Dosage Change in Renal Failure*: Creatinine Clearance (<10 ml/min)	Dosage Change after Hemodialysis
Penicillin G	NC	1.6 × 10^6 units/6 h	Yes (1.6 × 10^6 units)
Penicillin V	NC	250 mg/6 h	Yes (250 mg)
Methicillin	NC	2 g/8 h	Slight (2 g)
Oxacillin	NC	NC	Slight (as in uremia)
Cloxacillin	NC	NC	Slight (as in uremia)
Dicloxacillin	NC	NC	Slight (as in uremia)
Nafcillin	NC	NC	Slight (as in uremia)
Ampicillin	NC	0.5–1 g/8 h	Yes (500 mg)
Amoxicillin	NC	500 mg/12 h	Yes (250 mg)
Ticarcillin†	2 g/4 h	2 g/12 h	Yes (2 g)
Indanyl carbenicillin†	NC	Avoid	
Azlocillin	NC	3 g/8–12 h	Yes (2 g)
Mezlocillin	NC	3 g/8–12 h	Yes (2 g)
Piperacillin	NC	3 g/8–12 h	Yes (2 g)
Temocillin	1 g/24 h	1 g/48 h	Yes (1 g)

*Refers to maximum dose used.
†Only carbenicillin and ticarcillin need adjustment of dosage after peritoneal dialysis.
Abbreviation: NC, No change.

TABLE 18–7 Adverse Reactions to Penicillins*

Type of Reaction	Frequency (%)	Occurs Most Frequently with*
Allergic		
IgE antibody	0.004–0.4	Penicillin G
Anaphylaxis		
Early urticaria (<72 h)		
Cytotoxic antibody	Rare	Penicillin G
Hemolytic anemia		
Antigen-antibody complex disease	Rare	Penicillin G
Serum sickness		
Delayed hypersensitivity	4–8	Ampicillin
Contact dermatitis		
Idiopathic	4–8	Ampicillin
Skin rash		
Fever		
Late-onset urticaria		
Gastrointestinal	2–5	
Diarrhea	2–5	Ampicillin
Enterocolitis	<1	Ampicillin
Hematologic		
Hemolytic anemia	Rare	Penicillin G
Neutropenia	1–4	Penicillin G Nafcillin Oxacillin Piperacillin
Platelet dysfunction	3	Carbenicillin, ticarcillin
Hepatic		
Elevated serum aspartate transaminase level	1–4	Oxacillin Nafcillin Carbenicillin
Electrolyte disturbance		
Sodium overload	Variable	Ticarcillin
Hypokalemia	Variable	Ticarcillin
Hyperkalemia—acute	Rare	Penicillin G
Neurologic		
Seizures	Rare	Penicillin G
Bizarre sensations		Procaine penicillin
Renal		
Interstitial nephritis	1–2	Methicillin
Hemorrhagic cystitis	Rare	Methicillin

*All the reactions can occur with any of the penicillins.

laxis (Table 18–7) (see Chapter 21).[33, 34] Penicillins are capable of acting as haptens to combine with proteins contaminating the solution or with human protein after the penicillin has been administered to humans. Penicilloyl and penicillanic acid derivatives are the major determinants of penicillin allergy. The penicilloyl determinant, which is produced through opening of the β-lactam ring, thereby allowing amide linkage to body proteins (Fig. 18–3), is the most important antigenic component. Penicillanic acid and derivatives of penicillanic acid are produced when reconstituted penicillins break down in

Penicillin
Penicilloic acid
penicilloylation
Penicillanic acid
protein
Penicilloyl

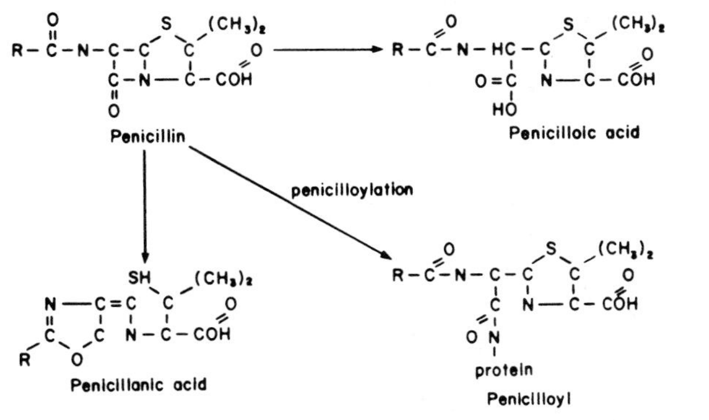

FIGURE 18–3. Mechanisms for formation of antigens from penicillins.

solution owing to acidity or temperature elevation. Minor determinants of allergy are benzyl penicillin itself and sodium benzyl penicilloate, which can either act as sensitizing agents or on their own elicit an allergic reaction.[33, 34] Both major and minor determinants may be involved in anaphylactic reactions, as well as in urticarial reactions. These reactions are mediated by immunoglobulin E (IgE) antibody. Minor determinants are the major cause of anaphylactic reactions. A person who has been sensitized by the hapten-carrier complex can have a reaction to penicillin alone or to penicillin that has formed dimers or polymers in solution. Anaphylactic reactions to penicillins are uncommon, occurring in only 0.2% of 10,000 courses of treatment, with a fatality rate of 0.001% of 100,000 courses.[35] People with atopic dermatitis or allergic rhinitis appear not to be at increased risk of a penicillin reaction.

Serum sickness does occur with penicillins, but it is very uncommon today. It probably is due to IgG antibodies to the benzyl penicilloyl hapten. The illness is characterized by fever, urticaria, joint pains, and angioneurotic edema. Exfoliative dermatitis and Stevens-Johnson syndrome are rare forms of allergic reactions to penicillins. The morbilliform eruptions that develop after penicillin therapy probably are due to IgM antibody to the benzyl penicilloyl hapten and to the minor determinants. In many patients these rashes will disappear, even if the penicillin is continued, owing to the production of IgG-blocking antibody. There is a risk, however, that the rash could progress to generalized desquamation. If an allergic reaction does occur, epinephrine given intramuscularly or intravenously will usually abort the reaction. Antihistamines and corticosteroids have not been shown to be of benefit.

Another allergic reaction to penicillins is that of allergic vasculitis with development of cutaneous and visceral lesions similar to that found with periarteritis nodosa. This reaction is extremely rare.

Hematologic toxicity is rare, although neutropenia has been encountered with the use of all types of penicillins, particularly when large doses are used.[36] The mechanism of the neutropenia is unknown, and white blood cell counts return to normal rapidly if the offending agent is discontinued. Sometimes a lower dose of drug can be used without production of neutropenia. Coombs-positive hemolytic anemia occurs rarely.[37] All penicillins at high concentrations, but particularly carbenicillin and ticarcillin, bind to the adenosine diphosphate receptor site in platelets, preventing normal platelet aggregation. Clinically significant bleeding occurs relatively infrequently.[38]

Renal toxicity from penicillins has varied, ranging from allergic angiitis to interstitial nephritis.[39] Interstitial nephritis occurs most commonly with methicillin but is seen with all penicillins. The clinical syndrome is one of fever, macular rash, eosinophilia, proteinuria, eosinophiluria, and hematuria. Initially the reaction is one of nonoliguric renal failure with a decrease in creatinine clearance and a rise in serum urea nitrogen and serum creatinine concentrations. This reaction can progress to anuria and renal failure. Biopsy specimens of the kidney show an interstitial infiltrate of mononuclear and eosinophilic cells with tubular damage but no glomerular lesions. Discontinuation of the penicillin will result in the return of renal function to normal in most cases.[40]

Administration of massive doses of any penicillin, but most often carbenicillin and ticarcillin, may result in hypokalemia owing to the large dose of nonreabsorbable anion presented to the distal renal tubules, which alters H^+ excretion and secondarily results in K^+ loss.[39]

Central nervous system toxicity in the form of myoclonic seizures can follow administration of massive doses of penicillin G, ampicillin, or methicillin. If there is reduced renal function, the drugs accumulate, and this form of toxicity becomes more likely.[41] Direct instillation of small doses of methicillin, oxacillin, or nafcillin into the ventricles at the time of surgery for placement of atrioventricular shunts has not resulted in seizures. Direct application of penicillin to the cortex will provoke seizure activity.

Gastrointestinal disturbances may follow the use of any of the oral forms but are most pronounced with ampicillin. Enterocolitis due to *Clostridium difficile* has followed the use of each of the penicillins (see Chapter 84). All penicillins used at high doses for prolonged periods will abolish normal bacterial flora, with resulting colonization with resistant gram-negative bacilli or with fungi such as *Candida*. Abnormalities in hepatic function test results such as elevation of the alkaline phosphatase and aminotransferase (transaminase) levels have been reported, most often after the use of oxacillin and carbenicillin.[36, 42] The pathogenesis of the hepatic reaction is unknown. Major hepatic injury is very uncommon, and liver enzymes return to normal values within a few days of stopping therapy.

CLINICAL USE

Table 18–8 lists some uses of penicillins. Penicillin G remains the primary agent for treatment of infections due to *Streptococcus pyogenes*, penicillin-susceptible strains of *Streptococcus pneumoniae*, and enterococci. None of the newer penicillins or agents in other classes has been shown to be more effective. Penicillin-susceptible strains of *S. pneumoniae* are inhibited at concentrations less than 0.1 μg/ml of penicillin G. Other penicillins also are highly active, although minimal inhibitory concentrations (MICs) exceed that of penicillin G.[43] This hierarchy of activity of the penicillins is maintained against penicillin-resistant strains of *S. pneumoniae*, albeit at higher MICs. Penicillin, ampicillin, and amoxicillin are the most active compounds, with MICs rarely exceeding 4 μg/ml, versus MICs of 128 μg/ml or greater for ticarcillin against highly penicillin-resistant strains. Except in pneumococcal meningitis, for which clinical failures with penicillin are well documented, infections caused by penicillin-resistant pneumococci appear to respond to penicillin G.[44] High doses of penicillin G are required to kill off strains of *S. pneumoniae* with intermediate-level (MIC of 0.1 to 1 μg/ml) or

TABLE 18–8 Antimicrobial Spectrum of Penicillin*

Infecting Organism	Penicillin of Choice	Alternative Acceptable Penicillin	Frequency of Resistance to Penicillins (%)
Gram-positive cocci			
Streptococcus pneumoniae	G	V	20–25
Streptococcus pyogenes (A)	G	V	None
Streptococcus agalactiae (B)	G	Ampicillin	None
Viridans streptococci	G		10–20
Streptococcus bovis (D)	G		Rare
Enterococcus faecalis	Ampicillin	Mezlocillin	10–20
Staphylococcus aureus (non–penicillinase-producing)	G	Penicillinase-resistant	Rare†
Staphylococcus aureus (penicillinase-producing)	Penicillinase-resistant		25%‡
Staphylococcus aureus (methicillin-resistant)	None	None	100
Staphylococcus epidermidis	Penicillinase-resistant		80†
Staphylococcus epidermidis (methicillin-resistant)	None	None	100
Gram-negative cocci			
Neisseria meningitidis	G	Ampicillin	Very rare
Neisseria gonorrhoeae	G	Ampicillin	1–40
Gram-positive bacilli			
Bacillus anthracis	G		None
Corynebacterium diphtheriae	G		None
Listeria monocytogenes	Ampicillin	G	None
Anaerobic species			
Peptostreptococcus	G	Ampicillin	None
Actinomyces israelii	G	V	None
Prevotella melaninogenicas	G	C, T	10
Fusobacterium spp.	G	Ampicillin	1–10
Bacteroides fragilis	M, P, A		75
Clostridium spp.	G	Ampicillin	<1
Gram-negative bacilli			
Haemophilus spp.	Ampicillin		5–30
Escherichia coli	Ampicillin		30
Proteus mirabilis	Ampicillin		<5
Salmonella typhi	Ampicillin		20
Salmonella, other spp.	Ampicillin		20
Klebsiella spp.	None		95
Enterobacter spp.	M, P, T		70
Citrobacter freundii	M, P, T		80
Proteus, indole-positive spp.	M, P, T		20
Serratia spp.	M, P, T		90
Pseudomonas aeruginosa	A, P, T		20–30
Pseudomonas, other spp.	None		95
Acinetobacter spp.	T	A, G, P	50
Providencia spp.	M, P, T		20–30
Stenotrophomonas maltophilia	None		95
Other organisms infrequently encountered			
Erysipelothrix spp.	G	Ampicillin	None
Pasteurella multocida	G	Ampicillin*	Rare, <1
Streptobacillus moniliformis	G		None
Spirillum minus	G		None
Treponema pallidum	G		None

*In each case it is assumed that a route of administration would be used that would achieve levels in serum and tissue to eradicate the organism. If there is no entry in the alternate column, it means that an antibiotic in another class would be a more appropriate choice. Amoxicillin can be used in place of ampicillin in all situations except with *Shigellia* infections.
†Most non–penicillinase-producing strains are methicillin-susceptible.
‡Approximate frequency of methicillin-resistant strains among penicillinase-producing strains.
Abbreviations: A, Azlocillin; M, mezlocillin; P, piperacillin; T, ticarcillin.

TABLE 18–9 Dosage of Penicillins

Compound	Dose*		
	Oral	*Intramuscular*	*Intravenous*
Penicillin G			25,000–500,000 units/kg/d, 6 divided doses
Procaine		300,000–600,000 units q12h	
Benzathine		1.2–2.4 million units q15–20d	
Penicillin V	Infant: 50 mg/kg/d, 3 divided doses Adult: 125–500 mg/kg qid		
Ampicillin	25–50 mg/kg/d, 4 divided doses	100–200 mg/kg/d, 4 divided doses	100–300 mg/kg/d, 6 divided doses
Amoxicillin	25–50 mg/kg/d, 2–3 divided doses		
Oxacillin		100 mg/kg/d, 4 divided doses	100–300 mg/kg/d, 6 divided doses
Nafcillin			
Cloxacillin	25–100 mg/kg/d, 4 divided doses		
Dicloxacillin	12–25 mg/kg/d, 4 divided doses		
Ticarcillin		50–100 mg/kg/d, 4 divided doses	50–300 mg/kg/d, 6 divided doses
Indanyl carbenicillin	50–65 mg/kg/d, 4 divided doses		
Azlocillin		50–100 mg/kg/d, 4 divided doses	200–300 mg/kg/d, 4 divided doses
Mezlocillin		50–100 mg/kg/d, 4 divided doses	200–300 mg/kg/d, 4 divided doses
Piperacillin		50–100 mg/kg/d, 4 divided doses	200–300 mg/kg/d, 4 divided doses

*For mg/kg/d (mg/kg/day) the number of doses shown indicates the number of doses into which the total daily dose should be divided.

high-level (MIC of ≥1 mg/ml) resistance to penicillin. For serious pneumococcal infections caused by penicillin-resistant strains, particularly in immunocompromised patients, vancomycin is preferred over a penicillin or other β-lactam antibiotic.[45, 46]

Nearly all *Neisseria meningitidis* strains are susceptible to penicillin G. *Neisseria gonorrhoeae* strains vary in susceptibility to penicillin G; resistance can be due to β-lactamase production, to altered PBPs, or to membrane changes (see Chapter 16). Penicillin G is the drug of choice for treponemal infection in all its forms. Puerperal infections due to anaerobic streptococci or group B streptococci (*Streptococcus agalactiae*), as well as genital clostridial infections, are treated with penicillin G. Infections produced by anaerobic mouth flora including gram-positive and gram-negative cocci and actinomycetes can be treated with penicillin G, although *Prevotella melaninogenica* strains that produce a β-lactamase and are resistant to penicillin are being encountered.

PROPHYLACTIC USE

Penicillins have been used in a number of situations for prevention of infection. Oral administration of 200,000 units of penicillin G or penicillin V every 12 hours has resulted in a significant reduction in recurrences of rheumatic fever. Because of the problems with compliance with oral therapy, intramuscular injections of 1.2 or 2.4 million units of benzathine penicillin given once each month have also been used with excellent results. Outbreaks of streptococcal infection due to *S. pyogenes* have been aborted by the use of oral penicillin G or V given twice a day for 5 days, by single injections of procaine penicillin daily, or by administration of benzathine penicillin.

Ampicillin or amoxicillin has been administered orally to asplenic children or to children with agammaglobulinemia to prevent infections caused by *Haemophilus influenzae* and *S. pneumoniae*. Penicillin prophylaxis has not been of benefit in prevention of meningococcal infection, bacterial infection after viral respiratory infection, or pneumonia after coma, shock, or congestive heart failure.

TABLE 18–10 Dosage of Antibiotics in Newborn Infants

Agent	Infants < 1 wk of Age		Infants 1 wk–1 mo of Age	
	Dose (per kg/d)	*Interval between Doses* (h)	*Dose* (per kg/d)	*Interval between Doses* (h)
Penicillin G	50,000–100,000 units	12	100,000 units	8
Ampicillin	100 mg	12	200 mg	6
Oxacillin	100 mg	12	200 mg	6
Nafcillin	100 mg	12	200 mg	6
Ticarcillin	150 mg	8	300 mg	6
Mezlocillin	75 mg	12	300 mg	6
Azlocillin	75–100 mg	12	300 mg	6

PROPERTIES OF INDIVIDUAL PENICILLINS

Dosages for the penicillins are given in Tables 18–9 and 18–10.

Natural Penicillins

Penicillin G

Penicillin G or benzyl penicillin G (Fig. 18–4) is available as salts for oral and parenteral administration and as repository salts for intramuscular injection. Because of its instability in acid there is no reason to use oral penicillin G, and penicillin V or amoxicillin should be used instead.

Crystalline penicillin G in aqueous solution has been used intramuscularly, subcutaneously, intravenously, and intrathecally. Given intramuscularly as an aqueous solution, penicillin G is very rapidly cleared from the body, and it may be preferable to use a repository form. It is available as sterile dry powder in ampules or vials containing 200,000 to 20 million units per vial. Each million units of penicillin G contain 1.7 mEq of sodium or potassium.

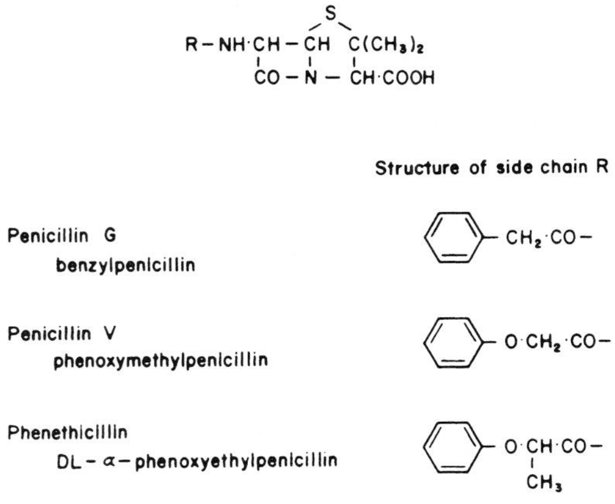

R–NH·CH–CH(S)C(CH₃)₂ / CO–N–CH·COOH

Structure of side chain R

Penicillin G benzylpenicillin: C_6H_5–$CH_2\cdot CO$–

Penicillin V phenoxymethylpenicillin: C_6H_5–$O\cdot CH_2\cdot CO$–

Phenethicillin DL-α-phenoxyethylpenicillin: C_6H_5–$O\cdot CH(CH_3)\cdot CO$–

FIGURE 18–4. Structures of penicillin G and penicillin V.

Repository penicillins provide tissue depots from which the drug is absorbed over hours in the case of procaine penicillin or over days in the case of benzathine penicillin. Repository penicillins are only for intramuscular use and cannot be used intravenously or subcutaneously or to irrigate wounds. Procaine penicillin is a mixture of equal molar parts of procaine and penicillin. Thus, 300,000 units contain 120 mg of procaine. Use of this suspension delays the peak of activity but provides serum and tissue levels for at least 12 hours. Doubling the dose of procaine penicillin given at a single injection site does not double the serum level. To increase the peak level it is necessary to use two body sites, as is done in the treatment of gonorrhea, for example, with 2.4 million units of procaine penicillin given in each buttock.

Benzathine penicillin is a repository form of penicillin, that combines 1 mole of penicillin and 2 moles of an ammonium base. It provides detectable serum levels for 15 to 30 days, depending on the size of the dose. Concentrations of penicillin G in the cerebrospinal fluid after use of benzathine penicillin may be inadequate to treat treponemal infections of the nervous system.

Penicillin V

Phenoxymethyl penicillin (see Fig. 18–4) is available only for oral use as a sodium or a potassium salt in suspension or tablets in doses of 125, 250, and 500 mg. The potassium salt produces higher blood levels than the other salts. Serum levels are from two to five times those obtained with penicillin G. Absorbed penicillin V is handled in the body in similar fashion to that observed for penicillin G. Penicillin V can be substituted for penicillin G in most situations in which it is reasonable to treat an infection by the oral route. However, penicillin V is less active than penicillin G against *Haemophilus, Neisseria*, and enteric organisms. Blood levels after 500 mg given to an adult are equivalent to the levels achieved with 600,000 units of procaine penicillin given intramuscularly. The usual dosage for children is 25 to 50 mg/kg/day and for adults, 1 to 4 g/day. The interval between dosages is 6 to 8 hours.

Penicillinase-Resistant Penicillins (Fig. 18–5)

Methicillin

Methicillin (2,6-dimethoxyphenylpenicillin) was the first of several penicillins developed that are resistant to hydrolysis by staphylococcal β-lactamase.[30] The antibacterial spectrum for each of the several penicillinase-resistant penicillins is identical to that for nafcillin. Nafcillin is active against gram-positive cocci and bacilli, with *Listeria monocytogenes, Enterococcus* spp., and methicillin-resistant strains of staphylococci being important exceptions (the convention is to use the term *methicillin-resistant* to indicate resistance to all penicillinase-resistant penicillins). The basis of methicillin resistance in staphylococci is production of a unique PBP, PBP 2a, which has low affinity for binding methicillin.[47] Although its exact function is not known, PBP 2a probably is a high-molecular-weight transpeptidase that can substitute for the function of antibiotic-bound and inactivated high-affinity PBPs. PBP 2a has low affinity not just for methicillin but for all β-lactam antibiotics; therefore, it confers resistance to this entire class of compounds. Nafcillin inhibits susceptible strains of coagulase-positive and coagulase-negative staphylococci, *S. pyogenes* penicillin-susceptible strains of *S. pneumoniae*, other streptococci, anaerobic gram-positive cocci, and anaerobic gram-positive bacilli. It is inactive against gram-negative organisms. Penicillinase-resistant penicillins are indicated solely for the treatment of infections suspected or proven to be caused by β-lactamase–producing strains of staphylococci that are not methicillin-resistant.

Methicillin is the least active of the penicillinase-resistant penicillins by weight; it is acid-labile and therefore can be administered only parenterally; and it is more likely to cause interstitial nephritis than are the other penicillinase-resistant penicillins. For these reasons, methicillin is no longer used clinically.

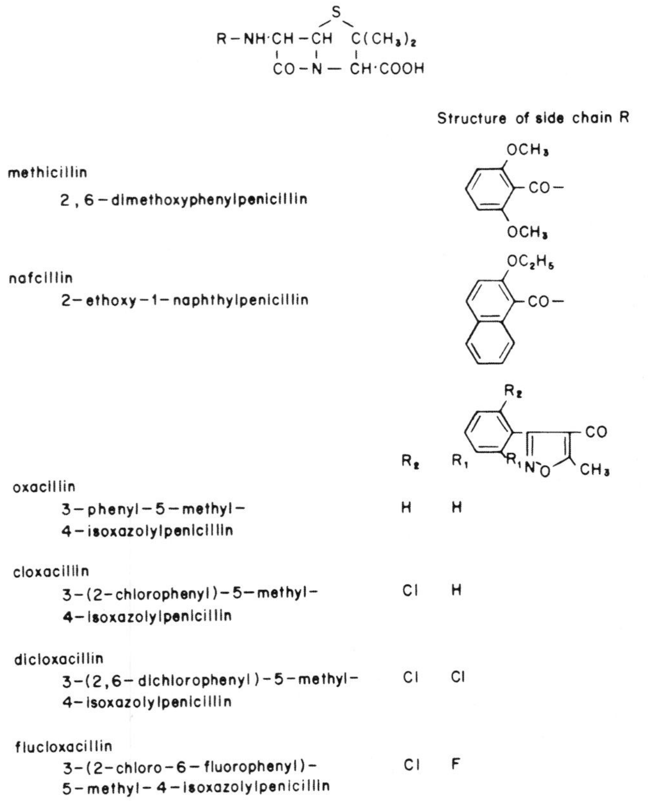

R–NH·CH–CH–S–C(CH$_3$)$_2$ / CO–N–CH·COOH

Structure of side chain R

methicillin
2,6-dimethoxyphenylpenicillin

nafcillin
2-ethoxy-1-naphthylpenicillin

	R_2	R_1
oxacillin 3-phenyl-5-methyl-4-isoxazolylpenicillin	H	H
cloxacillin 3-(2-chlorophenyl)-5-methyl-4-isoxazolylpenicillin	Cl	H
dicloxacillin 3-(2,6-dichlorophenyl)-5-methyl-4-isoxazolylpenicillin	Cl	Cl
flucloxacillin 3-(2-chloro-6-fluorophenyl)-5-methyl-4-isoxazolylpenicillin	Cl	F

FIGURE 18–5. Antistaphylococcal penicillins.

Nafcillin

Nafcillin (2-ethoxy-1-naphthylpenicillin) has more intrinsic activity than methicillin against both staphylococci and streptococci and is also not active against gram-negative bacteria. Nafcillin is highly protein-bound, and its activity in serum is similar to that of methicillin. Although nafcillin is absorbed when taken by mouth, absorption is erratic whether the drug is taken fasting or with food, and hence serum levels are low.[30] Levels after intramuscular injection are low, and the preferred route of administration is intravenous. The antibiotic is primarily excreted by the liver and to a lesser extent by the kidney. Serum levels are elevated and the half-life is prolonged by probenecid. Although nafcillin is available as capsules (250 mg) and as a suspension, cloxacillin or dicloxacillin should be used for oral administration. The usual dosage of nafcillin is 6 to 9 g/day, depending on the severity of the infection, and 100 to 200 mg/kg/day for children.

Isoxazolyl Penicillins

The isoxazolyl penicillins all are stable to staphylococcal β-lactamase and inhibit both penicillin-sensitive and penicillin-resistant staphylococci at mean concentrations of 0.2 to 0.4 μg/ml. Methicillin-resistant staphylococci are resistant to these agents. Isoxazolyl penicillins inhibit streptococci and pneumococci but are virtually inactive against gram-negative bacilli. All are absorbed after oral administration, but absorption is adversely affected by food. There are differences in serum levels among the drugs after oral ingestion, with the serum level of cloxacillin twice that of oxacillin and the levels of dicloxacillin twice that of cloxacillin; all the drugs are highly bound to serum proteins; oxacillin and cloxacillin are equally bound, but dicloxacillin is bound to a greater extent. Thus, actual free serum concentrations of the drugs are greater for cloxacillin and dicloxacillin than oxacillin (see Table 18–5). After intravenous infusion of 1 g over 15 minutes, peak serum levels are 70 to 100 μg/ml, with levels of 25 μg/ml at 1 hour and less than 1 μg/ml at 6 hours. The isoxazolyl penicillins undergo some metabolism but are excreted primarily by the kidney, with slight biliary excretion. Oxacillin undergoes more rapid degradation in the body than does cloxacillin or dicloxacillin.

Oxacillin

Oxacillin is available as a sodium salt for oral use in 250- and 500-mg capsules and as a powder for suspension at 250 mg/5 ml. It should be taken 1 to 2 hours before meals. The daily dosage for adults is 1 to 4 g taken in four parts. The dosage for children is 50 to 100 mg/kg/day taken in four parts. Oxacillin sodium for injection may be given intramuscularly or intravenously. Adult dosage is 2 to 12 g/day and for children, 100 to 300 mg/kg/day given every 4 to 6 hours.

Cloxacillin

Cloxacillin sodium is available in the United States only as an oral solution (125 mg/5 ml) or capsules of 250 and 500 mg. Dosage for children is 50 to 100 mg/kg/day given as four equal doses. Dosage for adults is 1 to 4 g/day given as four equal doses. It yields serum levels similar to those achieved with oxacillin.

Dicloxacillin

Dicloxacillin sodium is available as a suspension (62.5 mg/5 ml) and as capsules of 125 and 250 mg. The dosage for children less than 40 kg is 25 mg/kg/day given as four doses. Some authorities recommend doses as above for cloxacillin. For adults, a dosage of 250 mg to 1 g every 6 hours can be given, depending on the severity of the infection.

Aminopenicillins

The antibacterial activities of all aminopenicillins are similar (Fig. 18–6).[46] They are not stable to β-lactamases of either gram-positive or gram-negative bacteria. The aminopenicillins are only slightly less active than penicillin G against *S. pyogenes*, *S. pneumoniae*, and *S. agalactiae*. They are slightly more active against enterococci. Activity of the compounds against clostridia, *Actinomyces*, corynebacteria, and *N. meningitidis* is equal to that of penicillin G. They are more active than penicillin G against *Listeria monocytogenes*. Sensitivity of *N. gonorrhoeae* (see Chapter 200) varies, ranging from highly sensitive to completely resistant in strains that produce β-lactamase. *H. influenzae* (both typeable and nontypeable strains) and *Haemophilus parainfluenzae* are susceptible, except for the isolates that produce β-lactamases (see Chapters 212 and 213). Strains of *E. coli*, once uniformly susceptible to aminopenicillins, often are resistant due to β-lactamase production. *Shigella sonnei*, many *Salmonella* spp., including many strains of *Salmonella typhi*, are resistant because of β-lactamases. Most *Klebsiella*, *Serratia*, *Acinetobacter*, indole-positive *Proteus*, and *Pseudomonas* spp. and strains of *Bacteroides fragilis* are resistant to the penicillins of this class.

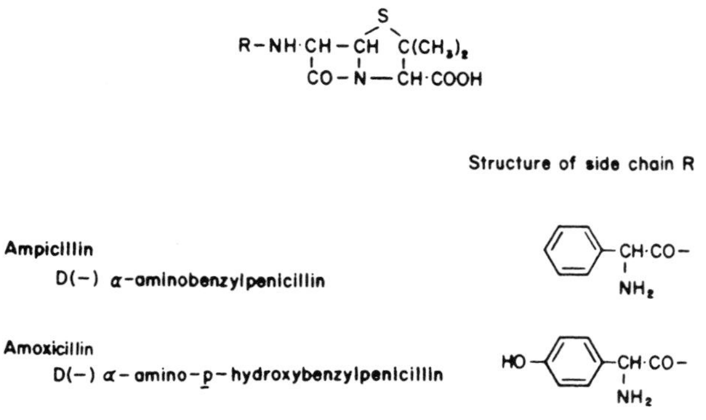

R−NH·CH−CH−S−C(CH$_3$)$_2$ / CO−N—CH·COOH

Structure of side chain R

Ampicillin
D(−) α-aminobenzylpenicillin — C_6H_5−CH(NH$_2$)·CO−

Amoxicillin
D(−) α-amino-p-hydroxybenzylpenicillin — HO−C_6H_4−CH(NH$_2$)·CO−

FIGURE 18–6. Aminopenicillins.

Ampicillin

Ampicillin is moderately well absorbed after oral administration, but peak levels are delayed and lowered if it is ingested with food. Peak blood levels of 3 μg/ml occur 1 to 2 hours after ingestion of 0.5 g. Peak blood levels occur later in diabetic patients with neurologic disease and in patients with renal failure. Drug can be detected in the serum for 4 to 6 hours. After intramuscular injection of 0.5 g, peak levels of 10 μg are achieved in 1 hour and persist for 4 hours. Probenecid increases the magnitude of peak levels and prolongs the period in which the drug can be detected in serum. Ampicillin is well distributed to body compartments and achieves therapeutic concentrations in cerebrospinal fluid and in pleural, joint, and peritoneal fluids in the presence of inflammation after parenteral administration. Urinary levels are high even in the presence of markedly reduced renal function. Peritoneal dialysis is ineffective in removing the drug, but hemodialysis removes approximately 40% in a 6-hour period.

Ampicillin is available for oral use as the sodium salt or as the trihydrate in capsules of 125, 250, and 500 mg; as a suspension of 125 or 250 mg/5 ml; as drops in a formulation of 100 mg/ml; and as 125-mg chewable tablets. It is also prepared as a suspension containing 3.5 g of ampicillin trihydrate and 1 g of probenecid. It is available as ampicillin trihydrate in 2.5-g vials only for intramuscular use. The sodium salt can be used either intramuscularly or intravenously.

Dosage varies with the age of the patient, the status of renal function, and the severity of the disease. For children above 1 month of age the oral dosage is 50 to 100 mg/kg/day in four doses; the intramuscular or intravenous dosage is 100 to 300 mg/kg/day in four or six doses. For adults the oral dosage is 2 to 4 g/day given in divided doses every 6 hours. For severe infection the parenteral dosage is 6 to 12 g/day given in divided doses every 4 hours. See Chapter 20 for a discussion of ampicillin-sulbactam.

Amoxicillin

Amoxicillin differs from ampicillin only in the presence of a hydroxyl group in the para position of the benzene side chain. Its in vitro activity is similar to that of ampicillin. It is significantly better absorbed when given by mouth than is ampicillin.[21] Peak blood levels are from two to two and a half times those achieved with a similar dose of ampicillin, and food does not decrease absorption. Oral amoxicillin produces blood levels similar to those produced by intramuscularly administered sodium ampicillin or ampicillin trihydrate. Urinary excretion of amoxicillin is greater than that of ampicillin. Tissue distribution is similar to that of ampicillin.

Clinical studies with amoxicillin have been extensive, and it has been used in the treatment of otitis media, bronchitis, pneumonia, typhoid, gonorrhea, and urinary tract infections. Among the oral penicillins and cephalosporins, amoxicillin is most likely to achieve serum concentrations that exceed MICs effective against penicillin-resistant strains of *S. pneumoniae*, but clinical data directly supporting efficacy are lacking.[43] In vitro, clavulanate may enhance the activity of amoxicillin against penicillin-resistant strains of pneumococci[48]; however, as with amoxicillin alone, clinical data on efficacy are lacking.

Amoxicillin has been used in a single 3-g dose for therapy of bacterial cystitis in women.[49] It is not useful for treatment of shigellosis. Side effects of amoxicillin are similar to those seen with ampicillin, although diarrhea may be less common than with ampicillin. Usual dosage for children is 20 to 40 mg/kg/day given in three doses every 8 hours, and for adults the dosage is 500 to 750 mg every 12

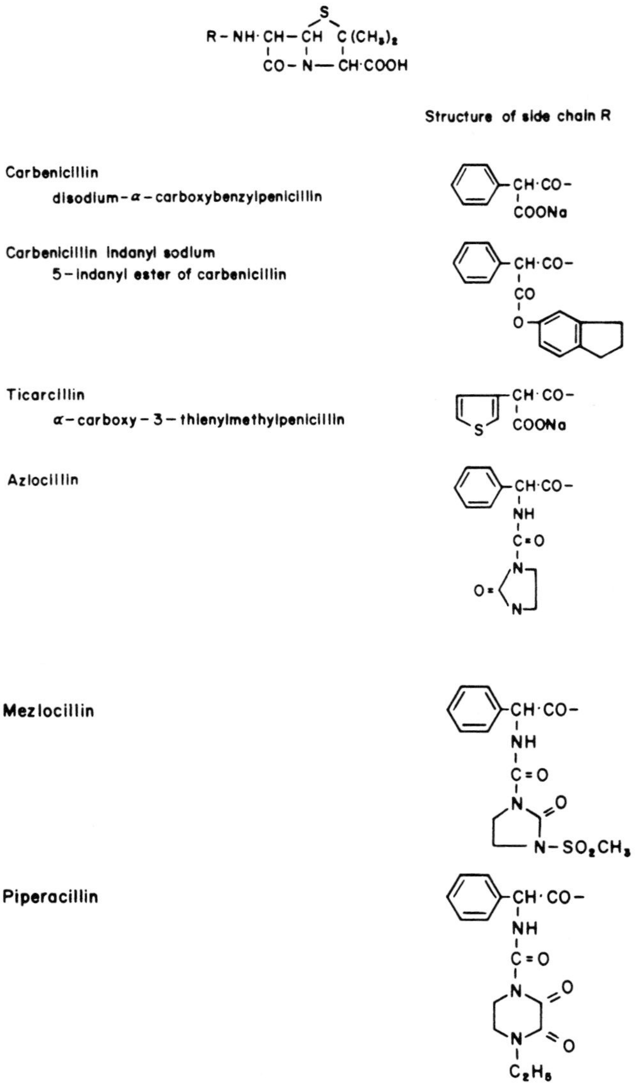

Structure of side chain R

Carbenicillin
disodium-α-carboxybenzylpenicillin

Carbenicillin indanyl sodium
5-indanyl ester of carbenicillin

Ticarcillin
α-carboxy-3-thienylmethylpenicillin

Azlocillin

Mezlocillin

Piperacillin

FIGURE 18–7. Penicillins active against gram-negative bacteria.

hours, although it has been used in doses up to 1 g every 4 hours. It has been useful in pediatric infections, except for shigellosis, and may be preferred to ampicillin. See Chapter 20 for a discussion of amoxicillin-clavulanate.

Carboxypenicillins (Fig. 18–7)

Carbenicillin

Carbenicillin was the first penicillin with activity against *P. aeruginosa* and certain indole-positive *Proteus* spp. that were not susceptible to other penicillins or to the cephalosporins. It is destroyed by β-lactamases of both gram-positive and gram-negative organisms, but it is more stable against hydrolysis by the β-lactamases of species such as *Pseudomonas, Enterobacter, Morganella*, and *Proteus-Providencia* spp., which function primarily as cephalosporinases. Carbenicillin is less active than ampicillin against *S. pyogenes, S. pneumoniae*, and *Enterococcus faecalis*. It is less active than the ureidopenicillins against streptococcal species and *Listeria*. Its activity against *Haemophilus* spp., *N. gonorrhoeae*, and *N. meningitidis* is similar to ampicillin. It has gram-negative activity similar to that of ampicillin against *E. coli, Proteus mirabilis, Salmonella* spp., and *Shigella* spp., but it is inactive against *Klebsiella*. It inhibits some *Enterobacter* and *Serratia* strains and many *B. fragilis* strains, although high concentrations are required. Because of the large doses required, greater potential for toxicity, and the availability of more potent alternatives, it should no longer be used.

Ticarcillin

The antibacterial spectrum for ticarcillin is identical to that for carbenicillin, except that it is from two to four times more active against *P. aeruginosa*. The pharmacokinetics of ticarcillin and carbenicillin are virtually identical, as are the side effects. Ticarcillin is not absorbed by mouth but can be given by intramuscular or intravenous administration. After an intramuscular dose of 1 g, peak serum levels of 20 μg/ml are reached in 1 hour. Serum levels of 150 to 200 μg/ml will be maintained when it is given at dosages of 70 to 100 mg/kg over 1 to 2 hours. Ticarcillin is excreted by renal tubules, but because less is converted to penicilloic acid, its half-life (72 minutes) is longer than that of penicillin G, and it accumulates in the presence of renal failure. Greater accumulation occurs if there is combined hepatic and renal dysfunction. Hemodialysis reduces plasma concentrations. Probenecid delays renal excretion and increases serum concentrations. Tissue distribution is similar to that of ampicillin, but concentrations in the cerebrospinal fluid are not adequate for efficacy against *Pseudomonas*. Side effects are similar to those seen with penicillins. Ticarcillin binds to the adenosine diphosphate (ADP) receptor site on platelets and prevents normal contraction; hence, bleeding occurs on occasion in the presence of high serum levels, such as in the presence of renal failure.

Ticarcillin can be used at dosages of 200 to 300 mg/kg/day. The advantage of ticarcillin over carbenicillin is that it is more active against *Pseudomonas*.[50] Another advantage is that the reduced dose of ticarcillin (with the same therapeutic efficacy) results in less platelet dysfunction and less hypokalemia. See Chapter 20 for a discussion of ticarcillin-clavulanate.

Indanyl Carbenicillin

Indanyl carbenicillin is an α-carboxy ester of carbenicillin. It has no intrinsic activity of its own, but as a sodium ester it is highly acid-stable and relatively well absorbed from the gastrointestinal tract. Ingestion with food may actually enhance absorption. The ester is immediately hydrolyzed to free carbenicillin, and only trace amounts of ester are found in serum or urine. Peak serum levels after 1 g taken orally are 10 μg at 1 to 2 hours. Urine levels are 300 to 1000 μg/ml, with 30% of a dose recovered in the first 6 hours. The compound does not provide adequate serum or tissue levels for efficacy in systemic infections, and it is useful only for the treatment of urinary tract infections. In the presence of decreased renal function, urine levels are lower and may be inadequate to treat *Pseudomonas* infections. Side effects are those of all the penicillins, but gastrointestinal irritation has been a problem in some people. The usual dosage is 1 g every 6 hours for adults. Quinolones have replaced this agent for the treatment of urinary tract infections and prostatitis.

Ureidopenicillins

Azlocillin

Azlocillin is an acyl ureidopenicillin that is 8 to 16 times more active than carbenicillin against *P. aeruginosa* and is less active against indole-positive *Proteus* spp. It has the same activity as ampicillin against streptococcal species.[51] It is destroyed by β-lactamases of both gram-positive and gram-negative bacteria. It is not orally absorbed and must be given by the intravenous route to provide adequate serum levels to treat *Pseudomonas* infection. The half-life is approximately 50 minutes, and administration of 4 g yields peak levels of 285 μg/ml.

Azlocillin shows nonlinear pharmacokinetics. The peak serum concentrations and the area under the drug curve are not proportional; that is, a 4- or 5-g dose produces serum levels that are higher than four or five times the 1-g dose.[52] The drug thus could be administered in larger doses at intervals of 6 hours. Azlocillin also does not accumulate in renal failure to the same degree as do carbenicillin and ticarcillin, because its half-life rises only to 4 hours with creatinine clearances below 7 ml/minute.[53, 54] Azlocillin enters the cerebrospinal fluid in the presence of meningeal inflammation, but levels are only 10% of the serum level. Azlocillin also causes less increase in bleeding time than does carbenicillin, because it apparently has less affinity for the ADP receptor site. Azlocillin is used primarily to treat *Pseudomonas* infections. It has proved to be a useful drug in a variety of clinical situations.[54]

Mezlocillin

Mezlocillin is an acyl ureidopenicillin similar in antibacterial spectrum to carbenicillin and ticarcillin but with some significant differences.[51] It is more active in vitro against *E. faecalis* than either of the aforementioned agents. It inhibits about 75% of *Klebsiella* species at a concentration of 25 μg/ml, whereas less than 5% would be inhibited by 100 μg/ml of carbenicillin.[55] It is also more active than carbenicillin or ticarcillin against *H. influenzae* and is more active than carbenicillin against *B. fragilis*. It is, however, not more resistant to β-lactamase hydrolysis than is carbenicillin; hence, its greater intrinsic activity is due to other factors, such as greater affinity for PBPs and better entry into the bacterial periplasmic space. It acts synergistically against gram-negative bacteria when combined with aminoglycosides. The drug must be given parenterally. Like azlocillin and piperacillin, mezlocillin shows dose-related nonlinear kinetics. Peak serum levels, half-life, and area under the time curve are greater with larger doses. Administration of 4 g produces peak levels of 300 μg/ml.[56] Its half-life increases only to 4 hours in patients in renal failure. Mezlocillin is the least likely of the broad-spectrum penicillins to alter bleeding times. Clinical studies in the United States and Europe have shown that it is an effective agent for treatment of respiratory, urinary, gynecologic, and surgical infections.[54, 57–61] It causes less increase in bleeding time than does carbenicillin. Usual doses have been 12 to 18 g/day for adults.

Piperacillin

Piperacillin is an acyl ureidopenicillin derivative that is similar to ampicillin in activity against gram-positive species.[62] It has excellent activity against streptococcal species and against *Neisseria* and *Haemophilus* and many members of the family Enterobacteriaceae. It also has excellent activity against anaerobic species of both cocci and bacilli. It inhibits 60% of strains of *Pseudomonas* at 3 μg/ml and 90% at 12 μg/ml.[62] It is hydrolyzed by plasmid-mediated β-lactamases of gram-positive and gram-negative bacteria. Its acts synergistically against *Pseudomonas* and against some of the Enterobacteriaceae species when it is combined with aminoglycosides.[62] The human pharmacology of piperacillin is similar to that of azlocillin and mezlocillin.[63–66] Administration of 4 g by the intravenous route produces peak serum drug levels of 300 μg/ml. Piperacillin shows kinetics that are dose-dependent. It accumulates in renal failure to a lesser degree than does carbenicillin, and its half-life is only 4 hours in renal failure.[67] It is removed by hemodialysis.

Piperacillin has shown adverse reactions similar to those for the other penicillins noted earlier. After prolonged administration at high doses, neutropenia has been reported. Alteration of bleeding time and hypokalemia occur but less frequently than with carbenicillin. Clinical studies have shown that it is a useful agent in treatment of a variety of infections.[54, 68–73] It is administered to adults in daily doses of 12 to 18 g. Piperacillin-tazobactam is discussed in Chapter 20.

REFERENCES

1. Fleming A. On the antibacterial action of cultures of a penicillium, with special reference to their use in the isolation of *B. influenzae*. Br J Exp Pathol. 1929;10:226.
2. Batchelor FR, Doyle FP, Naylor JHC, et al. Synthesis of penicillin: 6-Aminopenicillanic acid in penicillin fermentations. Nature. 1959;183:257.
3. Tipper DJ, Wright A. The structure and biosynthesis of bacterial cell walls. In: Sokatch JR, Ornstein LA, eds. The Bacteria, v. 7. New York: Academic Press; 1979:291.
4. Strominger JL. Penicillin-sensitive enzymatic reactions in bacterial cell wall synthesis. Harvey Lect. 1970;64:179.
5. Mirelman D. Biosynthesis and assembly of cell wall peptidoglycan. In: Inouye M, ed. Bacterial Outer Membranes. New York: John Wiley & Sons; 1980:166.
6. Waxman DL, Yocum RR, Stominger JL. Penicillins and cephalosporins are active site–directed acylating agents: Evidence in support of the substrate analogue hypothesis. Philos Trans R Soc Lond [Biol]. 1980;289:257.
7. Ghuysen JM. Serine beta-lactamases and penicillin-binding proteins. Annu Rev Microbiol. 1991;45:37.
8. Spratt BG. Distinct penicillin binding proteins involved in the division, elongation and shape of *Escherichia coli*, K 12. Proc Natl Acad Sci U S A. 1975;72:2999.
9. Spratt BG. Biochemical and genetical approaches to the mechanism of action of penicillin. Philos Trans R Soc Lond [Biol]. 1980;289:273.
10. Georgopapadakou NH, Liu FY. Binding of β-lactam antibiotics to penicillin-binding proteins of *Staphylococcus aureus* and *Streptococcus faecalis* in relation to antibacterial activity. Antimicrob Agents Chemother. 1980;18:834.
11. Spratt BG, Bowler LB, Edelman A, et al. Membrane topology of PBPs 1B and 3 of *E. coli* and the production of water-soluble forms of high molecular weight PBPs. In: Shockman GD, ed. Antibiotic Inhibition of Bacterial Cell Surface Assembly and Function. Washington, DC: American Society for Microbiology; 1988:292.
12. Maidhof H, Johannsen L, Labischinski H, et al. Onset of penicillin-induced bacteriolysis in staphylococci is cell cycle dependent. J Bacteriol. 1989;171:2252.
13. Sykes RB, Matthew M. The β-lactamases of gram-negative bacteria and their role in resistance to β-lactam antibiotics. J. Antimicrob Agents Chemother. 1976;2:115.
14. Li X-Z, Nikaido H, Poole K. Role of MexA-MexB-OprM in antibiotic efflux in *Pseudomonas aeruginosa*. Antimicrob Agents Chemother. 1995;39:1948–1953.
15. Spratt BG. Resistance to antibiotics mediated by target alterations. Science. 1994;264:388–393.
16. Smith JM, Dowson CG, Spratt BG. Localized sex in bacteria. Nature. 1991;349:29.
17. Rolinson GN, Sutherland R. Semisynthetic penicillins. Adv Pharmacol Chemother. 1973;11:152.
18. Marcy SM, Klein JO. The isoxazolyl penicillins: Oxacillin, cloxacillin and dicloxacillin. Med Clin North Am. 1970;54:1127.
19. Finland M, Garner C, Wolcox C, et al. Susceptibility of pneumococci and *Haemophilus influenzae* to antibacterial agents. Antimicrob Agents Chemother. 1976;9:274.
20. Sutter VL, Finegold SM. Susceptibility of anaerobic bacteria to 23 antimicrobial agents. Antimicrob Agents Chemother. 1976;10:736.
21. Neu HC. Antimicrobial activity and human pharmacology of amoxicillin. J Infect Dis. 1974;129(Suppl):S123.
22. Hedberg M, Nord CE. Beta-lactam resistance in anaerobic bacteria: A review. J Chemother. 1996;8:3–16.
23. Tan JS, File TM Jr. Antipseudomonal penicillins. Med Clin North Am. 1995;79:679–693.
24. Eagle H, Newman E. Renal clearance of penicillin F, G, K, and X in rabbits and man. J Clin Invest. 1947;26:903.
25. Cole M, Kening MD, Hewitt VA. Metabolism of penicillins to penicilloic acidosis and 6-aminopenicillanic acid in man and its significance in assessing penicillin absorption. Antimicrob Agents Chemother. 1973;3:463.
26. Gilbaldi M, Swartz MA. Apparent effect of probenecid on the distribution of penicillins in man. Clin Pharmacol Ther. 1968;9:345.
27. Parker RH, Schmid FR. Antibacterial activity of synovial fluid during therapy of septic arthritis. Arthritis Rheum. 1971;14:96.
28. Barza M, Weinstein L. Penetration of antibiotics into fibrin loci in vivo. I. Comparison of penetration of ampicillin into fibrin clots, abscesses and interstitial fluid. J Infect Dis. 1974;129:59.
29. Pancoast SJ, Neu HC. Antibiotic levels in human bone and synovial fluid. Orthop Rev. 1980;9:49.
30. Neu HC. Antistaphylococcal penicillins. Med Clin North Am. 1982;66:51.
31. Fishman RA. Blood-brain and CSF barriers to penicillin and related organic acids. Arch Neurol. 1966;15:13.
32. Depp R, Kind AC, Kirby WMM, et al. Transplacental passage of methicillin and dicloxacillin into the fetus and amniotic fluid. Am J Obstet Gynecol. 1970;197:1054.
33. Levine BB, Redmond AP, Feller MF, et al. Penicillin allergy and the heterogeneous immune response of man to benzylpenicillin. J Clin Invest. 1966;45:1895.
34. Saxon A. Immediate hypersensitivity reactions to β-lactam antibiotics. Rev Infect Dis. 1983;5(Suppl 2):S368.
35. Idsoe O, Gothe T, Wilcox RR, et al. Nature and extent of penicillin side reactions with particular reference to fatalities from anaphylactic shock. Bull WHO. 1968;38:159.

36. Parry MF, Neu HC. The safety and tolerance of mezlocillin. J Antimicrob Chemother. 1982;9(Suppl A):S273.
37. Kerr RO, Cardamone J, Dalmasso AP, et al. Two mechanisms of erythrocyte destruction in penicillin-induced hemolytic anemia. N Engl J Med. 1972;287:1322.
38. Brown CH, Natelson EA, Bradshaw W, et al. The hemostatic defect produced by carbenicillin. N Engl J Med. 1974;291:265.
39. Appel GB, Neu HC. The nephrotoxicity of antimicrobial agents. N Engl J Med. 1977;296:63.
40. Baldwin DS, Levine BB, McCluskey RT, et al. Renal failure and interstitial nephritis due to penicillin and methicillin. N Engl J Med. 1968;279:1245.
41. Bloomer HA, Barton LJ, Maddock RJ Jr. Penicillin-induced encephalopathy in uremic patients. JAMA. 1967;200:121.
42. Wilson FM, Belamavic J, Lauter CB, et al. Anicteric carbenicillin hepatitis. Eight episodes in four patients. JAMA. 1967;232:818.
43. Schreiber JR, Jacobs MR. Antibiotic-resistant pneumococci. Pediatr Clin North Am. 1995;42:519–537.
44. Choi EH, Lee NJ. Clinical outcome of invasive infections caused by penicillin-resistant *Streptococcus pneumoniae* in Korean children. Clin Infect Dis. 1998;26:1346–1354.
45. Friedland IR, McCracken GH. Management of infections caused by antibiotic-resistant *Streptococcus pneumoniae*. N Engl J Med. 1994;331:377–382.
46. Bartlett JG, Breiman RF, Mandell LA, File TM. Community-acquired pneumonia in adults: Guidelines for management. Clin Infect Dis. 1998;26:811–838.
47. Chambers HF. Methicillin resistance in staphylococci: Molecular and biochemical basis and clinical implications. Clin Microbiol Rev. 1997;10:781–791.
48. Martín M, Gómez-Lus ML, Aguilar L, et al. Effect of clavulanic acid and/or polymorphonuclear neutrophils on amoxicillin bactericidal activity against *Streptococcus pneumoniae*. Eur J Clin Microbiol Infect Dis. 1997;16:512–516.
49. Fang LST, Tolokoff-Rubin NE, Rubin RH. Efficacy of single-dose and conventional amoxicillin therapy in urinary tract infection localized by antibody-coated bacteria technique. N Engl J Med. 1978;298:413.
50. Parry MF, Neu HC. Ticarcillin for treatment of serious infections with gram-negative bacteria. J Infect Dis. 1976;134:476.
51. Fu KP, Neu HC. Azlocillin and mezlocillin: New ureido penicillins. Antimicrob Agents Chemother. 1978;13:930.
52. Bergen T. Review of the pharmacokinetics and dose dependency of azlocillin in normal subjects and patients with renal insufficiency. J Antimicrob Agents. 1983;11(Suppl B):101.
53. Whelton A, Stout RL, Delgado FA. Azlocillin kinetics during extracorporeal haemodialysis and peritoneal dialysis. J Antimicrob Chemother. 1983;11(Suppl B):89.
54. Drusano GL, Schimpff SC, Hewitt WL. The acylampicillins: Mezlocillin, piperacillin, and azlocillin. Rev Infect Dis. 1984;6:13.
55. Parry MF, Folta D. The in vitro activity of mezlocillin against community hospital isolates in comparison to other penicillins and cephalosporins. J Antimicrob Chemother. 1983;11(Suppl C):97.
56. Meyers BR, Mendelson MH, Srulevitch-Chin E, et al. Pharmacokinetic properties of mezlocillin in ambulatory elderly subjects. J Clin Pharmacol. 1987;27:678.
57. Pancoast SJ, Jahre JA, Neu HC. Mezlocillin in the therapy of serious infections. Am J Med. 1979;67:747.
58. Issell BF, Bodey GP. Mezlocillin for treatment of infections in cancer patients. Antimicrob Agents Chemother. 1980;17:1008.
59. Melikian V, Wise R, Allum WH, et al. Mezlocillin and gentamicin in the treatment of infections in seriously ill and immunosuppressed patients. J Antimicrob Chemother. 1981;7:657.
60. Faro S, Phillips LE, Baker JL, et al. Comparative efficacy and safety of mezlocillin, cefoxitin, and clindamycin plus gentamicin in post-partum endometritis. Obstet Gynecol. 1987;69:760.
61. Alvarez RD, Kilgore LC, Huddlestone JF. A comparison of mezlocillin versus clindamycin/gentamicin for the treatment of post-caesarean endomyometritis. Am J Obst Gynecol. 1988;158:425.
62. Fu KP, Neu HC. Piperacillin, a new penicillin active against many bacteria resistant to other penicillins. Antimicrob Agents Chemother. 1978;13:358.
63. Bergen T. Overview of acylureidopenicillin pharmacokinetics. Scand J Infect Dis. 1981;29:33.
64. Tjandramaga TB, Mollie A, Verbesselt R, et al. Piperacillin pharmacokinetics after intravenous and intramuscular administration. Antimicrob Agents Chemother. 1978;14:829.
65. Martens MG, Faro S, Feldman S, et al. Pharmacokinetics of the acylureidopenicillins piperacillin and mezlocillin in the post-partum patient. Antimicrob Agents Chemother. 1987;31:2015.
66. Brattstrom C, Malmborg AS, Tyden G. Penetration of clindamycin, cefoxitin, and piperacillin into pancreatic juice in man. Surgery. 1988;103:563.
67. Francke EL, Appel GB, New HC. Pharmacokinetics of intravenous piperacillin in patients undergoing chronic hemodialysis. Antimicrob Agents Chemother. 1979;16:788.
68. Winston DJ, Murphy W, Young LS, et al. Piperacillin therapy for serious bacterial infections. Am J Med. 1980;69:255.
69. Wade JC, Schimpff SC, Newman KA, et al. Piperacillin or ticarcillin plus amikacin: A double blind prospective comparison of empiric antibiotic therapy for febrile granulocytopenic cancer patients. Am J Med. 1981;71:983.
70. Pancoast SJ, Prince AS, Francke EL, et al. Clinical evaluation of piperacillin for therapy of infection. Arch Intern Med. 1981;141:1447.
71. Hemsell DL, Hemsell PG, Heard MC. Piperacillin and a combination of clindamycin and gentamicin for the treatment of hospital and community-acquired acute pelvic infections including pelvic abscess. Surg Gynecol Obstet. 1987;165:223.
72. Menichetti F, Del Favero A, Guerciolini R, et al. Empiric antimicrobial therapy in febrile granulocytopenic patients. Randomized prospective comparison of amikacin plus piperacillin with or without parenteral trimethoprim/sulfamethoxazole. Infection. 1986;14:61.
73. Holmes B, Richard DM, Brodgen RN, et al. Piperacillin: A review of its antibacterial activity, pharmacokinetic properties, and their therapeutic use. Drugs. 1984;28:375.

Chapter 19

Cephalosporins

ADOLF W. KARCHMER

The cephalosporins, among the most widely prescribed antimicrobials, take origin from the work of Giuseppe Brotzu, a professor of the University of Cagliari, Sardinia, in the mid-1940s. Brotzu hypothesized that the apparent periodic clearing of microorganisms from the water in the vicinity of a sewage outlet in the harbor at Cagliari might result from the inhibitory effects of substances produced by another microbe. His search for a microbe producing such a substance in the seawater at the harbor sewage outlet ultimately led to the isolation of a fungus, *Cephalosporium acremonium* (now called *Acremonium chrysogenum*), the first microbial source of a cephalosporin.[1] Brotzu found that the growth of certain gram-positive and gram-negative bacteria was inhibited by this organism. Furthermore, filtrates from cultures of *C. acremonium* seemed to produce antibacterial effects on infections in animals and patients. In fact, Brotzu injected this material into boils and other skin infections with some apparent success and subsequently administered it parenterally to local patients with typhoid fever and brucellosis.[2] In 1948, unable to proceed further with his work on the antimicrobial substance produced by *C. acremonium,* he sent a culture of the organism to Sir Howard Florey at Oxford. There, workers, led by Professor Edward P. Abraham, proceeded to identify several fermentation products of *C. acremonium* that possessed antimicrobial activity.

Three antimicrobial substances were ultimately isolated from cultures of *C. acremonium* by workers at Oxford; one of these gave rise to the cephalosporins. Initially they identified a steroid, called cephalosporin P, with activity against only gram-positive bacteria. Later they found cephalosporin N, a compound with antibacterial activity against gram-negative bacteria. This material was subsequently shown to be a penicillin with an aminocarboxybutyl side chain, and it was renamed penicillin N. Ultimately, a third substance, cephalosporin C, was identified. This material, which was less active against *Salmonella typhi* and staphylococci than penicillin N, was of interest because it was not destroyed by the penicillinase of staphylococci and *Bacillus cereus* and was relatively acid stable.[2] Ultimately cephalosporin C became the foundation upon which our current cephalosporin antimicrobials are constructed.

CHEMISTRY

Cephalosporin C (Fig. 19–1) is a β-lactam compound in which the β-lactam ring is fused to a six-membered dihydrothiazine ring (yielding the cephem nucleus; Fig. 19–2) in contrast to penicillins, in which the comparable unit is a five-membered thiazolidine ring. The knowledge that substitution of different side chains at the 6-acylamino site of the 6-aminopenicillanic acid nucleus resulted in semisynthetic penicillins of increased potency set the stage for attempts to modify cephalosporin C and thus enhance its potency.[3] Acid hydrolysis of cephalosporin C resulted in a 7-aminocephalosporanic acid (7-ACA; see Fig. 19–1) and the basic structure for the future development of the cephalosporins.[4] The basic molecule of the cephalosporins (the fused β-lactam and dihydrothiazine rings) is num-

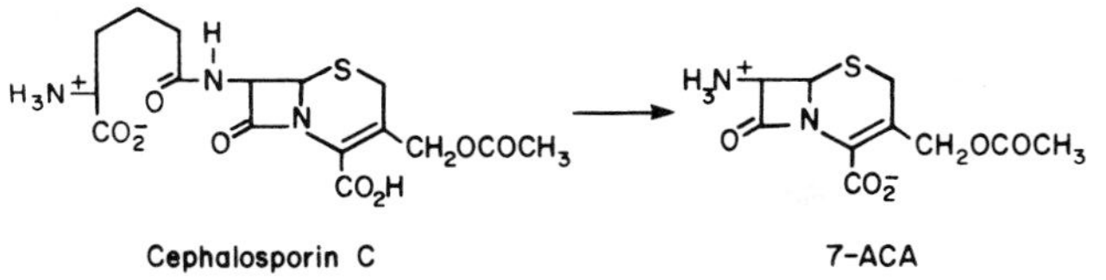

Cephalosporin C → 7-ACA

FIGURE 19–1. Preparation of 7-aminocephalosporanic acid (7-ACA) from cephalosporin C.

bered beginning in the dihydrothiazine ring with the sulfur moiety at position 1 (see Fig. 19–2). There is an unsaturated bond between positions 3 and 4. The modification of this basic structure by substitutions at position 1, by the addition of substituents at position 3 or 7, or by the addition of different acyl side chains from position 7 has given rise to the family of cephalosporin antibiotics. Modifications at position 7 alter antimicrobial activity, whereas substituents added at position 3 predominantly effect changes in metabolic and pharmacokinetic parameters.[5–7]

The factors involved in the net antibacterial activity of β-lactam antibiotics, as well as the resistance of bacteria to these agents, include the ability of the antibiotic to reach its sites of action, the resistance of the antibiotic to destruction by inactivating enzymes (β-lactamases), and the affinity of the agent for its targets. The targets of β-lactam antibiotics are enzymes situated in the bacterial cytoplasmic membrane called *penicillin-binding proteins* (PBPs) that are essential for cell division and survival. Modifications of the cephalosporin nucleus that affect one or more of these factors may alter antimicrobial activity.

The enhanced activity of early cephalosporins against gram-negative bacilli resulted from the presence of a methoxy group at position 7, replacing a hydrogen.[8, 9] Cefoxitin, the initial antibiotic with this structure, was isolated from a culture of *Streptomyces lactamdurans* and is technically a cephamycin.[8] The clinically available cephamycins, which now are synthesized from 7-aminocephalosporanic acid and include cefoxitin, cefotetan, and cefmetazole, are nevertheless considered among the cephalosporins (Fig. 19–3). The addition of the methoxy at position 7, replacing a hydrogen, results in enhanced stability of these compounds to β-lactamases of many gram-negative rods, especially those of *Bacteroides fragilis,* and hence increased antibacterial activity against these organisms.[6–9] However, the substitution for the hydrogen at position 7 results in poor binding of these agents to the PBP of gram-positive cocci.[9] As a consequence of this, the cephamycins have reduced activity against staphylococci and streptococci. Cefuroxime, a true cephalosporin, contains a furyl group on the acyl side and an iminomethoxy at the α-position on this chain. Compared with early cephalosporins, it has increased β-lactamase stability as well as retained activity against streptococci and to a lesser degree against methicillin-susceptible staphylococci.[10, 11]

Further modifications of the acyl side chain at position 7 by the addition of an aminothiazole group resulted in markedly enhanced activity of cephalosporins against many Enterobacteriaceae.[12, 13] The addition of an iminomethoxy group to the α-site of this side chain results in an aminothiazolylmethoxy side chain that confers stability to many of the β-lactamases of gram-negative bacteria while retaining high activity against streptococci and to a lesser degree against methicillin-susceptible *Staphylococcus aureus.*[12–14] The addi-

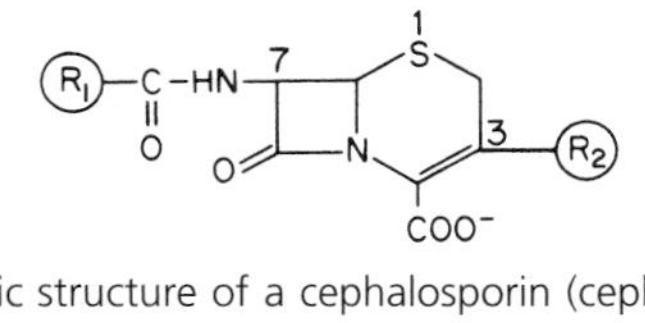

FIGURE 19–2. Basic structure of a cephalosporin (cephem nucleus).

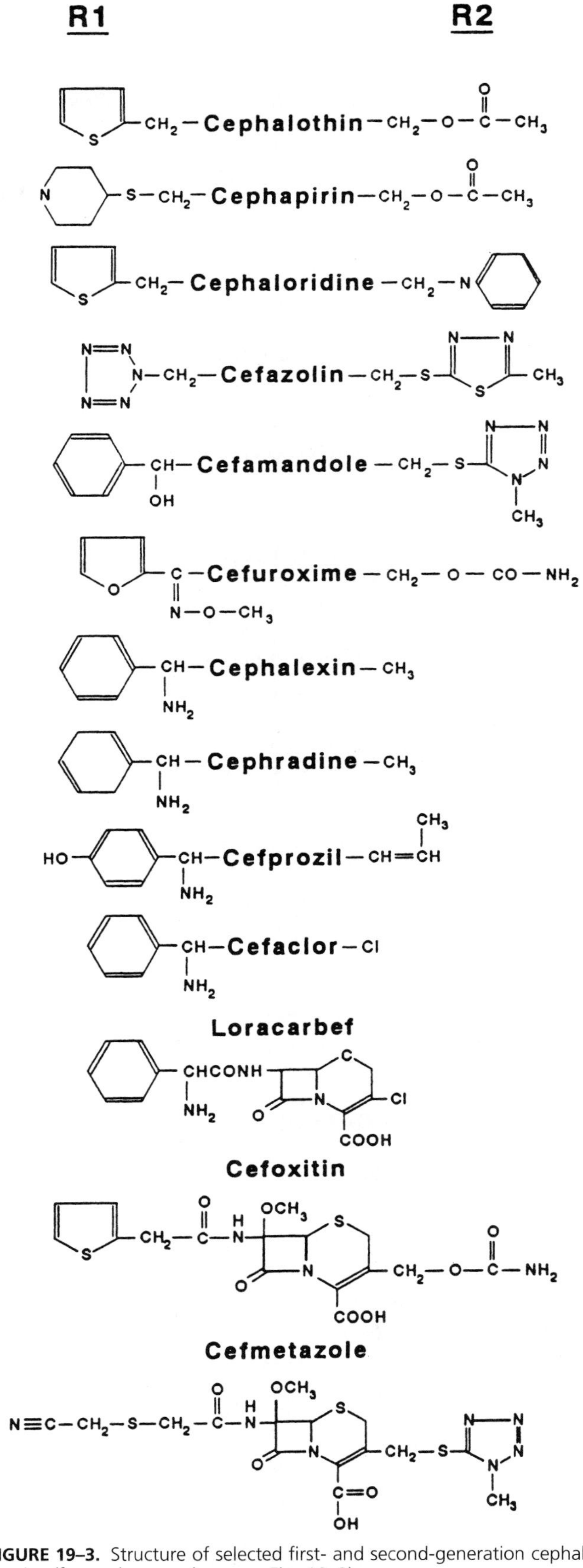

R1 R2

Cephalothin

Cephapirin

Cephaloridine

Cefazolin

Cefamandole

Cefuroxime

Cephalexin

Cephradine

Cefprozil

Cefaclor

Loracarbef

Cefoxitin

Cefmetazole

FIGURE 19–3. Structure of selected first- and second-generation cephalosporins (for cephem nucleus, see Fig. 19–2).

tion of this side chain appears to enhance the penetration of the cephalosporin through the outer cell membrane of gram-negative bacteria and may also increase the affinity of these compounds with PBP.[7] This modification, in conjunction with various substituents at the 3 position of the dihydrothiazine ring, results in cefotaxime, ceftizoxime, and ceftriaxone, used in the United States, and cefmenoxime, which is available in Japan (Fig. 19–4). That these structure-function relationships are sensitive and specific is illustrated by the relative loss of activity against *S. aureus, Escherichia coli,* and *Pseudomonas aeruginosa* that occurs with a shift in the stereoisomer of the methoxy group on the aminothiazolymethoxy side chain of cefotaxime and ceftizoxime. This change in antimicrobial activity is a consequence of a decrease in affinity for PBP rather than a reduction in β-lactamase stability or penetration through the outer cell membrane.[13, 15]

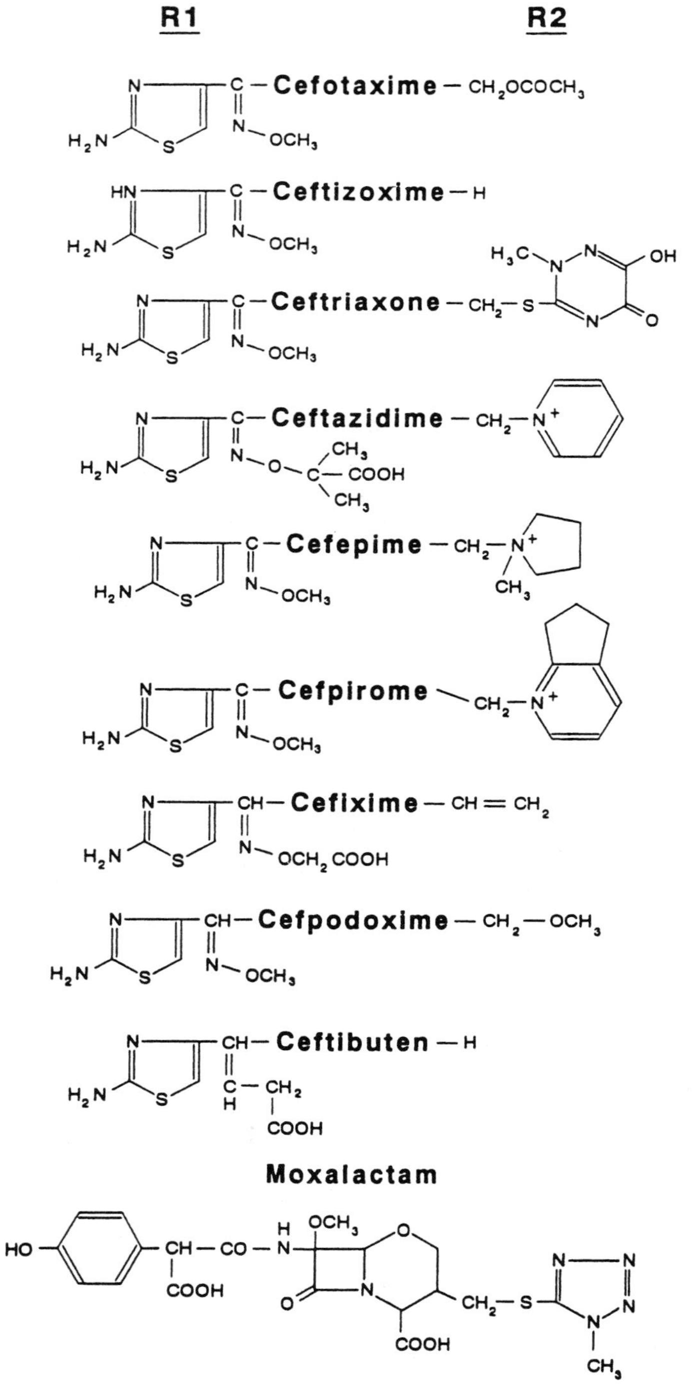

FIGURE 19–4. Structure of selected third-generation cephalosporins (for cephem nucleus, see Fig. 19–2).

The addition of an acidic moiety to the acyl side chain at position 7 enhances activity against *P. aeruginosa.*[7] A propylcarboxy addition to the aminothiazolyl side chain plus a pyridine at position 3 characterizes ceftazidime (see Fig. 19–4), a clinically used cephalosporin active against *P. aeruginosa.*[6, 16–18] Ceftazidime, to a significant degree, retains the antistreptococcal activity of the other aminothiazolyl cephalosporins (cefotaxime, ceftizoxime, ceftriaxone) but has lost its activity against methicillin-susceptible *S. aureus.*[18] This loss of activity is a consequence of reduced binding to staphylococcal PBP.[19] Cefoperazone, with a ureido(-NH-C-H-)2,3 dioxopiperazine on the acyl side chain and a methylthiotetrazole (MTT) moiety at position 3, achieves modest activity against *P. aeruginosa.* Attempts to maintain good activity against streptococci and *S. aureus* while achieving increased activity against β-lactamases–producing gram-negative rods including *P. aeruginosa* and the Enterobacteriaceae with inducible chromosomal β-lactamases (*Enterobacter* spp., *Citrobacter freundii,* and *Serratia* spp.) have involved substitutions at position 3 in aminothiazolylmethoxy cephalosporins. Two such compounds, cefepime and cefpirome, with a pyrolidine and a cyclopentopyridinium moiety at position 3, respectively (see Fig. 19–4), have been evaluated extensively. These dipolar ionic cephalosporins penetrate the gram-negative bacteria outer cell membrane faster than other aminothiazolyl cephalosporins, have good affinity for essential PBP, and have low affinity for many β-lactamases, including the inducible β-lactamases of the Enterobacteriaceae (the latter feature correlates with increased β-lactamase stability).[20]

Major modifications of the cephem nucleus at position 3 have been initiated in the search for useful cephalosporins resulting from alterations of pharmacokinetic features. Cephalexin, the initial cephalosporin absorbed from the gastrointestinal tract, contains an aminobenzyl substituent on the acyl side chain and, importantly for gastrointestinal absorption, a methyl group at position 3 (see Fig. 19–3). Cephradine, which has a cyclohexadine group replacing the phenol group of cephalexin, and cefadroxyl, with a hydroxy aminobenzyl on the acyl side chain, both have a methyl moiety at position 3 (see Fig. 19–3). They are also absorbed from the gastrointestinal tract, suggesting that the simple moiety at position 3, in contrast to the bulky substituents in this position on cephalothin, cephapirin, and cefazolin, has a major impact on bioavailability after ingestion. Cefaclor, which has a chlorine replacing the methyl group at position 3 of cephalexin, and cefprozil, which has a vinyl methyl replacing this methyl group in cefadroxil, are also well absorbed after ingestion. Loracarbef resembles cefaclor; however, it is a carbacephem in which a carbon has replaced the sulfur of the dihydrothiazine ring (see Fig. 19–3). Cefixime, an aminothiazolyl cephalosporin with anticipated activity against a broad group of gram-negative bacteria, has a vinyl group at position 3. The bioavailability after the ingestion of all these compounds is adversely affected by the polarity of the carboxyl group at position 4, a group required for the activity of the β-lactam ring. Esterification of this carboxyl group results in an inactive prodrug that can be cleaved by intestinal mucosal esterases during absorption to liberate an active cephalosporin into the circulation. Cefuroxime axetil and cefpodoxime proxetil are compounds in which esterification of this carboxyl has facilitated gastrointestinal absorption of cephalosporins with an iminomethoxy group as the furyl and aminothiazolyl, respectively.[7, 21, 22] Alteration of the substitution at position 3 may have other pharmacokinetic effects. Markedly enhanced protein binding and a prolonged serum half-life are noted in cefonicid when a sulfamethyl group replaces the methyl group on the MTT moiety at position 3 in cefamandole.[7]

Modifications of the cephalosporin basic unit to achieve a given pharmacokinetic effect may have unanticipated and undesirable con-

TABLE 19–1 Selected Parenteral Cephalosporins by Generation and Dosing Range

Generic Name (Proprietary Name)	Formulation	Dosing Range: Adults: Dose and Interval	Adults: Daily Dose, Severe Infection	Children*: Dose (mg/kg/d) and Interval
First generation				
Cephalothin (Keflin, Seffin)	IV	0.5–2 g q4–6h	6–12 g	75–125 q4–6h
Cefazolin (Ancef, Kefzol)	IV/IM	0.5–1.5 g q6–8h	3–6 g	50–100 q6–8h
Cephapirin (Cefadyl)	IV/IM	0.5–2 g q4–6h	6–12 g	40–80 q4–6h
Cephradine (Velosef)	IV/IM	0.5–2 g q4–6h	4–12 g	50–100 q6h
Second generation				
Cefamandole (Mandol)	IV/IM	0.5–2 g q4–6h	6–12 g	100–150 q4–8h
Cefonicid (Monocid)	IV/IM	0.5–2 g q24h	2 g	40 q24h†
Cefuroxime (Kefurox, Zenacef)	IV/IM	0.75–1.5 g q6–8h	4.5–6 g	100–240 q6–8h
Cephamycins				
Cefoxitin (Mefoxin)	IV/IM	1–2 g q4–6h	6–12 g	80–160 q4–6h
Cefotetan (Cefotan)	IV/IM	1–3 g q12h	4–6 g	40–80 q12h†
Cefmetazole (Zefazone)	IV	2 g q6–12h	8 g	—†
Third generation				
Cefotaxime (Claforan)	IV/IM	1–2 g q4–8h	6–12 g	100–180 q4–6h
Ceftizoxime (Cefizox)	IV/IM	1–4 g q8–12h	6–12 g	150–200 q6–8h
Ceftriaxone (Rocephin)	IV/IM	0.5–2 g q12–24h	2–4 g	50–100 q12–24h
Cefoperazone (Cefobid)	IV/IM	2–4 g q8–12h	6–12 g	100–150 q8–12H†
Ceftazidime (Fortaz, Tazidime, Tazicef)	IV/IM	0.5–2 g q8–12h	6 g	90–150 q8h
Fourth generation				
Cefpirome (not available in United States)	IV/IM	1–2 g q12h	4 g	
Cefepime (Maxipime)	IV/IM	1–2 g q12h	4 g	50 q8h

*Dose for infants in first month of life (neonate) may differ; consult specific reference.
†Pediatric experience limited; not approved for pediatric use.

sequences. The MTT substituent at position 3 of some cephalosporins and cephamycins (cefamandole, cefmenoxime, cefoperazone, moxalactam, cefmetazole, cefotetan) has been associated with prolongation of the prothrombin time and, in association with alcohol consumption, a disulfiramlike reaction.

CLASSIFICATION

Several complex classifications of the cephalosporins using microbiologic, pharmacokinetic, and β-lactamase stability have been proposed. No classification has been entirely suitable; nevertheless, the somewhat arbitrary system that is most widely used combines the parenteral and oral cephalosporins into generations based on their spectrum of microbiologic activity (Tables 19–1 and 19–2). The first-generation compounds have a relatively narrow spectrum of activity focused primarily on the gram-positive cocci. The second-generation cephalosporins have variable activity against gram-positive cocci but have increased activity against gram-negative bacteria. In spite of relatively increased potency against gram-negative aerobic and anaerobic bacilli, the cephamycins are included in the second generation. Those cephalosporins with very marked activity against the gram-negative bacteria are grouped in a third generation; some of these compounds have limited activity against gram-positive cocci, particularly methicillin-susceptible *S. aureus*. Cefsulodin and cefmenoxime,

TABLE 19–2 Selected Oral Cephalosporins by Generation: Formulation and Dosing Range

Generic Name (Proprietary Name)	Formulation	Dosing Range: Adult Dose and Interval	Pediatric Dose (mg/kg/d) and Interval
First generation			
Cephalexin (Keflex, Keftab, Biocef)	0.25, 0.5 g tabs/caps 125, 250 mg/5 ml susp	0.25–1 g q6h	25–100 q6h
Cephradine (Velosef)	0.25–0.5 g caps 125, 250 mg/5 ml susp	0.25–1 g q6h	25–50 q6h
Cefadroxil (Duricef, Ultracef)	0.5, 1.0 g tabs 125, 250, 500 mg/5 ml susp	0.5–1 g q12–24h	30 q12–24h
Second generation			
Cefaclor (Ceclor)	0.25, 0.5 g caps 125, 187, 250, 375 mg/5 ml susp	0.25–0.5 g q8h	40 q8h
(Ceclor CD)	0.375, 0.5 g caps	0.375–0.5 g q12h	
Cefuroxime axetil (Ceftin)	0.125, 0.25, 0.5 g tabs	0.25–0.5 g q12h	30–40 q12h*
Cefprozil (Cefzil)	0.25, 0.5 g caps 125, 250 mg/5 ml susp	0.25–0.5 g q12–24h	30 q12h
Loracarbef (Lorabid)	0.20 g tabs 100, 200 mg/5 ml susp	0.2–0.4 q12h	15–30 q12h*
Third generation			
Cefixime (Suprax)	0.2–0.5 g caps 100 mg/5 ml susp†	0.2 g q12h 0.4 g q24h	8 q12 or 24h
Cefpodoxime proxetil (Vantin)	0.1, 0.2 g tabs 50, 100 mg/5 ml susp	0.2–0.4 q12h‡	10 q12h
Ceftibuten (Cedax)	400 mg caps, 90 or 180 mg/5 ml	0.2–0.4 q12h	9 q24h
Cefdinir (Omnicef)	300 mg caps, 125 mg/5 ml susp	0.3–0.6 q12–24h	7–14 q12–24h

*Higher listed dose recommended for otitis media.
†Higher serum concentrations with suspension.
‡Lower urinary tract infection: cefuroxime axetil, 0.125–0.25 g q12h; loracarbef, 0.2 g qd; cefpodoxime, 0.1 g q12h.

parenterally administered cephalosporins not listed in Table 19–1, are grouped with the third-generation cephalosporins even though the clinically relevant activity of cefsulodin is directed only at *P. aeruginosa*. Several compounds have been considered possibly to merit classification as a fourth generation. These cephalosporins, which include cefepime and cefpirome, have activity against gram-positive cocci and a broad array of gram-negative bacteria, including *P. aeruginosa* and many of the Enterobacteriaceae with inducible chromosomal β-lactamases.

MECHANISM OF ACTION

The antimicrobial activity of the cephalosporins, like that of other β-lactam antibiotics, results at least in part from their ability to interfere with the synthesis of the peptidoglycan component of the bacterial cell wall. The peptidoglycan of the gram-positive bacteria forms an outermost thick permeable structure immediately overlying the cell's cytoplasmic membrane. The analogous component overlying the cytoplasmic membrane of the gram-negative bacteria is relatively thin in comparison. External to the peptidoglycan of gram-negative bacteria and separated from it by the periplasmic space is a complex lipopolysaccharide membrane with interspersed proteins. The peptidoglycans are long polysaccharide chains in which *N*-acetylglucosamine and *N*-acetylmuramic acid residues alternate in a linear form. With the pentapeptide side chain of *N*-acetylmuramic acid residues, these polysaccharide strands are cross-linked into a netlike structure. The *N*-acetylglucosamine and *N*-acetylmuramic acid pentapeptide components of peptidoglycan are synthesized in the cytoplasm and transported across the cytoplasmic membrane. Thereafter, these residues are inserted into the existing cross-linked peptidoglycan as part of cell growth and division by transpeptidases, carboxypeptidases, and endopeptidases. These enzymes, located in the cytoplasmic membrane, are the PBPs and are the site of action for β-lactam antibiotics. Because the amide component of the β-lactam antibiotic is structurally similar to the D-alanyl–D-alanine natural substrate of these enzymes, the antibiotic may bind to the PBP. As a result of its long-lived covalent bond with the β-lactam antibiotic, the PBP is rendered inactive.[23, 24] The PBPs of cells vary structurally, quantitatively, functionally, and in their affinity for β-lactam antibiotics. The effect of a given β-lactam antibiotic on a cell is related to which PBPs are inactivated and to the role of those PBPs in peptidoglycan synthesis and cell survival.[25–29] How cephalosporins and other β-lactam antibiotics exert bactericidal or lytic effects through the inhibition of PBPs is not completely understood.

MECHANISMS OF RESISTANCE

Microbial resistance to cephalosporins, as well as to other β-lactam antibiotics, can be mediated through three mechanisms: alteration of a PBP target that is essential for cell survival, production of β-lactamases that inactivate the cephalosporin, or decreased ability of the antibiotic to reach its PBP target. Often multiple mechanisms may work in concert to render a cell resistant.[30]

Although gram-negative bacteria can utilize the reduced ability of some cephalosporins to penetrate to the PBP target site in order to enhance resistance, this option is not available to gram-positive bacteria. In gram-positive bacteria, the cytoplasmic membrane resides immediately beneath the relatively porous outermost peptidoglycan structure. The peptidoglycan does not exclude molecules the size of cephalosporins; hence, these antibiotics easily reach the PBPs. In contrast, the gram-negative bacteria have a complex outer membrane composed of lipids, polysaccharides, and proteins; this membrane constitutes a significant barrier to cephalosporins and other molecules.[31] Cephalosporins penetrate this outer cell membrane primarily through water-filled channels, called *porins,* that are formed by various outer membrane proteins. The movement of antibiotics through porins is selective based on their size, shape, charge, and hydrophillic properties.[32, 33] Although the relative permeability of this outer membrane for a specific β-lactam antibiotic is an intrinsic feature of the organism, changes in porins as a consequence of exposure to an antimicrobial may reduce penetration further and thus enhance resistance.[34] It is unlikely that porin permeability barriers alone result in the resistance of gram-negative bacteria to cephalosporins.[35] Nevertheless, the rate of a β-lactam antibiotic's penetration through the outer membrane is intrinsically linked to resistance mediated by β-lactamases.[36–38]

Reduced affinity of PBPs for β-lactam antibiotics is a mechanism by which some *Neisseria gonorrhoeae Haemophihes influensae* and *Streptococcus pneumoniae* have become relatively resistant to penicillins or cephalosporins. Methicillin-resistant *S. aureus* produce PBP2′ (also called PBP2a), which has markedly reduced affinity for penicillinase-resistant penicillins and cephalosporins.[33, 39, 40] The ability of this novel PBP to functionally replace essential PBPs that have higher affinity for these antibiotics ultimately mediates the resistance of methicillin-resistant *S. aureus* to all cephalosporins.

Production of β-lactamase is the mechanism by which clinically relevant gram-negative bacteria are most frequently resistant to cephalosporins. These inactivating enzymes are encoded chromosomally or extrachromosomally through plasmids or transposons and may be produced constitutively or induced. β-Lactamases are widely distributed in gram-negative bacteria and are present in some gram-positive bacteria, most notably staphylococci. These enzymes, like the PBPs themselves, belong to a family of serine proteases. The binding of β-lactamase to an antibiotic catalyzes a rapid reaction resulting in hydrolysis at the critical amide bond of the β-lactam ring and antibiotic inactivation. In contrast, on the binding of a β-lactam antibiotic to a PBP, the reaction proceeds slowly or not at all, resulting in effective inactivation of the PBP. The net ability of a β-lactamase to protect a cell from an antibiotic results from a complex interaction of the antibiotic concentration, the stability of the antibiotic to the β-lactamase, the affinity of the antibiotic for the β-lactamase, and the concentration of the β-lactamase in the cell environment.[41] Gram-positive bacteria release β-lactamase directly into their immediate environs. In the presence of a cephalosporin, the survival of otherwise susceptible gram-positive bacteria depends on the collective ability of the cells to inactivate the cephalosporin enzymatically. In fact, most cephalosporins, with the exception of cephaloridine, are poorly hydrolyzed by staphylococcal β-lactamase. The antistaphylococcal effect, therefore, is largely related to the cephalosporin's affinity for essential staphylococcal PBPs. The cephamycins and ceftazidime, which are relatively β-lactamase stable, have reduced antistaphylococcal activity as a consequence of poor affinity for the PBP of *S. aureus.*[6]

β-Lactamase–mediated resistance to cephalosporins among gram-negative bacteria is more complex. In these organisms, β-lactamase is confined to the periplasmic space. The entry of cephalosporins into this space, as noted previously, is regulated by porins. Given suitable affinity for the cephalosporins, both β-lactamase–unstable cephalosporins and ones that are relatively β-lactamase stable can be effectively inactivated by β-lactamases within the confines of the periplasmic space. Reduced penetration of cephalosporins into the periplasmic space enhances the efficiency with which the β-lactamase protects the cell, whereas the converse occurs with increased penetration.[41] Increased production of β-lactamase or production of a new β-lactamase with enhanced affinity may result in resistance to cephalosporins among gram-negative bacilli. High-level production of TEM-1 or SHV-1 β-lactamases, two of the most commonly encountered plasmid-mediated β-lactamases among Enterobacteriaceae, because of increases in the number of gene copies per cell, has been associated with resistance not only to penicillin–β-lactamase inhibitor combinations but also to cephalothin, cefamandole, and cefoperazone.[41, 42] *Enterobacter* spp., *C. freundii, Morganella, Serratia, Providencia,* and *P. aeruginosa* have an inducible chromosomally encoded cephalosporinase (a Bush group 1 AmpC β-lactamase) with sufficient affinity for currently available cephamycins and cephalosporins, including those of the third generation, that it can inactivate these antibiotics in the periplasmic space. The induction or stable derepression of this chromosomal β-lactamase during prior exposure to cephamycins and third-generation cephalosporins results in resistance to all the currently available cephalosporins.[41–44] Emergence of this form of resistance is frequent when infection due to these organisms, particularly *Enterobacter cloacae* and *P. aeruginosa,* are treated with broad-spectrum cephalosporins. Furthermore, this resistance often translates to failure of the β-lactam antibiotic therapy.[43] New plasmid-mediated extended-spectrum β-lactamases (ESBLs) have been discovered. These are derived from a point mutation of TEM-1, TEM-2, or SHV-1 that results in a single amino acid substitution at the enzyme's active site. At least 26 TEM-related and 6 SHV-related distinct EBSLs have been described.[44–47] Although occasionally found in other Enterobacteriaceae, ESBLs have been noted predominantly in *Klebsiella pneumoniae* and *E. coli.* The ESBLs mediate high-level resistance to ceftazidime and aztreonam but also confer reduced susceptibility to other third-generation cephalosporins. Bacteria containing an ESBL do not appear notably resistant to third-generation cephalosporins other than ceftazidime. Consequently, clinical laboratories not testing ceftazidime may overlook strains with ESBLs. Nosocomial outbreaks of infection caused by strains with ESBLs appear to result from both strain and plasmid dissemination. Barring the presence of concurrent mechanisms of resistance, TEM- and SHV-related ESBL strains remain susceptible to imipenem.[45] Plasmids bearing Bush group 1 AmpC β-lactamase genes, which originated from the chromosomal genes of *Enterobacter* spp., *C. freundii,* or *P. aeruginosa,* have now been identified in *K. pneumoniae* and *E. coli* isolated worldwide.[46, 47] Resistance genes for aminoglycosides, chloramphenicol, tetracyclines, and sulfonamides are also present on these plasmids. The epidemiology and spread of these β-lactamase genes is difficult to study. As a consequence, the extent to which this gene has spread is unclear. Nevertheless, among the β-lactams only the carbapenems provide predictable activity against organisms producing these plasmid-mediated β-lactamases.

PHARMACOLOGY

The pharmacologic properties of selected cephalosporins are presented in Table 19–3.[21, 22, 48–51] Absorption of cefuroxime and cefpodoxime from the gastrointestinal tract is facilitated by their formulation as esters; the compounds are cleaved to active drug by intestinal mucosal esterases during absorption. Cefetamef and cefteram, which are investigational aminothiazolyl cephalosporins, have also been esterified to facilitate oral administration. Absorption of esterified cephalosporins is enhanced by administration with food as an apparent consequence of the more prolonged contact with the gastric mucosa that results from a food-associated delay in gastric emptying.[21] The bioavailability of cefpodoxime is decreased by H_2 antagonist and nonabsorbable antacids, presumably due to incomplete dissolution of drug.[21] Cefixime and cefpodoxime are slowly absorbed and reach lower maximal serum concentrations relative to the other orally administered cephalosporins. The oral administration of ceftibuten rapidly generates high peak serum concentrations and is comparable to the absorption of cephalexin.[21, 22] It is recommended that cephalothin and cephapirin, which cause pain when administered intramuscularly, be limited to the intravenous route. The other parenteral

TABLE 19–3 Pharmacologic Properties of the Cephalosporins

Generic Name	Adult Dose for Serious Infection*	Peak Serum Concentration† (μg/ml)	Half-life (h)	Effect of Food on Peak Serum Concentration	Cerebrospinal Fluid Concentration (Range, μg/ml)	Serum Protein Binding (%)	Route of Excretion
First generation							
Cefazolin	1 g q8h	80 (1)	1.8			80	Renal
Cephalothin	1–2 g q4–6h	30 (1)	0.6			71	Renal
Cefadroxil	0.5 g q12h PO	16 (0.5)	1.2	None		20	Renal
Cephalexin	0.5–1 g q6h PO	18 (0.5)	0.9	None		10	Renal
Cephradine	0.5 g q6h PO	18 (0.5)	0.7	None		10	Renal
Second generation							
Cefamandole	1–2 g q4–6h	150 (2)	0.8			75	Renal
Cefonicid	1–2 g q24h	260 (2)	4.5			98	Renal
Cefotetan	2–3 g q12h	230 (2)	3.5			90	Renal
Cefoxitin	2 g q4–6h	150 (2)	0.8			70	Renal
Cefmetazole	2 g q6h	140 (2)	1.1			65	Renal
Cefuroxime	1.5 g q8h	100 (1.5)	1.3		1.1–1.7	35	Renal
Cefaclor	0.25–0.5 g q8h PO	13 (0.5)	0.8	Decreased		25	Renal
Cefuroxime axetil	0.25–0.5 g q12h PO	8–9 (0.5)	1.3	Increased‡		35	Renal
Loracarbef	0.4 g q12h PO	15 (0.4)	1.1	Decreased		35	Renal
Cefprozil	0.5 g q12h PO	10 (0.5)	1.2	None		42	Renal
Third generation							
Cefixime	0.4 g q24h PO	3.9 (0.4)	3.7	None		67	Renal 50%, ? other
Cefpodoxime proxetil	0.4 g q12h PO	4 (0.4)	2.2	Increased‡		40	Renal
Ceftibuten	0.4 g q24h PO	15 (0.4)	2.5	Decreased		63	Renal
Cefdinir	0.6 g q12h PO	2.9 (0.6)	1.7	Slightly decreased		70	Renal
Cefotaxime	2 g q6–8h	130 (2)	1.0		5.6–44	35	Renal
Ceftizoxime	2 g q8–12h	130 (2)	1.7		0.5–29	30	Renal
Ceftriaxone	1–2 g q12h	250 (2)	8.0		1.2–39	83–96	Renal 50%; biliary 40%
Moxalactam	1–2 g q8h	200 (2)	2.2		0.8–33	50	Renal
Cefmenoxime§	2 g q6–8h	100 (2)	1.0			77	Renal
Third-generation cephalosporins with anti-pseudomonad activity							
Cefoperazone	2 g q8–12h	250 (2)	2.0			87–93	Biliary 70%; renal 25%
Ceftazidime	2 g q8h	160 (2)	1.8		0.5–30	17	Renal
Cefpiramide§	1–4 g q12–24h	166 (1)	5.4			94–98	Biliary 80%; renal 20%
Fourth generation							
Cefpirome§	1–2 g q12h	100 (1)	2.0		1.3–7.5	10	Renal
Cefepime	1–2 g q8–12h	130 (2)	2.1		3.3–5.7	20	Renal

*All doses are parenteral unless otherwise stated.
†Level after noted gram amount (in parentheses) of drug given intravenously or, where noted in column 2, orally (PO). Peak serum concentrations reported in the literature vary, depending on the time over which a drug is given and the time of serum sampling. Representative values are noted.
‡H_2 antagonist and nonabsorbable antacids decrease absorption.
§Investigational or not available in United States.

cephalosporins can be administered intravenously or intramuscularly, although the volumes required for administration often limit dosing. The modest discomfort of intramuscular cephalosporin administration has been reduced by adding 1% lidocaine solution to the diluent (see specific package insert). Peak serum concentrations after parenteral administration of cephalosporins are similar; they range between 100 and 150 μg/ml after doses of 2 g.

With a few exceptions, the cephalosporins achieve excellent penetration into tissues and fluid compartments, including lung; female genital tissues; kidney; and synovial, pericardial, peritoneal, and pleural fluids. Cefpiramide, cefoperazone, and ceftriaxone achieve high concentration in bile.[52, 53] Penetration of cephalosporins into the aqueous humor of the eye may be sufficient with high-dose parenteral therapy to allow effective treatment of anterior chamber infection caused by susceptible gram-positive and gram-negative bacteria. Cephalosporins do not achieve significant concentration in the posterior chamber of vitreous humor. For therapeutic purposes, significant penetration into the cerebrospinal fluid occurs only with cefuroxime, cefotaxime, ceftriaxone, ceftizoxime, cefmenoxime, moxalactam, ceftazidime, cefepime and cefpirome. Penetration is less satisfactory with cefoperazone.[53, 54]

Most cephalosporins are excreted through the kidney and hence achieve exceptionally high urine concentrations. The excess urine concentration relative to the minimal inhibitory concentration (MIC) of the usual urinary tract pathogen often allows effective treatment of urinary tract infection with reduced doses. Alternatively, dose adjustments are required with modest to severe renal dysfunction (Table 19–4). Cefoperazone, ceftriaxone, and cefpiramide, with significant biliary excretion, do not require dose adjustment in azotemic patients. The half-life of cefotaxime is not significantly increased with renal failure; however, its desacetyl and other metabolites accumulate significantly. Consequently, reduced cefotaxime dosing is warranted with severe azotemia. Cefoperazone and ceftriaxone are not removed by hemodialysis and do not require additional dosing after dialysis. Severe hepatic disease, even in the absence of ascites and its effect on the volume of distribution, can alter the pharmacokinetics of cefperazone, cefpiramide, and cefotaxime; there is little impact on ceftriaxone.[53, 55, 56] Reduced desacetylation as a result of liver disease may increase the half-life of cefotaxime slightly. In contrast, the half-life of cefoperazone and cefpiramide may increase significantly because of liver disease. In the setting of liver disease, compensatory renal excretion generally occurs. Accumulation of cefoperazone, cefpiramide, ceftriaxone, and cefotaxime is likely to occur in the setting of combined hepatic and renal failure, and dose adjustment is likely to be required.[53, 55]

Cephalosporins with an acetyl group at position 3 on the dihydrothiazine ring (cephalothin, cephapirin, and cefotaxime) undergo in vivo metabolism to a desacetyl form. Although the desacetyl form is a less potent antimicrobial, desacetyl cefotaxime may be synergistic with the parent compound and contribute to cefotaxime's net antibacterial effect.[56]

The interplay of cephalosporin pharmacokinetics in the eradication of bacteria merits consideration in selecting the dose and planning therapy. Cephalosporins do not, in contrast to quinolones and aminoglycosides, exhibit concentration-dependent killing of bacteria. The bactericidal effect of cephalosporins reaches a maximum at four to five times the MIC of the organism. Furthermore, regrowth of bacteria after exposure to cephalosporins occurs promptly; there is a nonexistent or very brief postantibiotic effect for gram-negative bacteria and an abbreviated effect for streptococci and staphylococci. These considerations suggest that the amount of time a cephalosporin is above the MIC of the pathogen at the site of infection is the important pharmacokinetic parameter for enhanced efficacy. A brief time with a high peak concentration followed by a significant period with concentrations below the MIC is not ideal.[57–59] Studies using animal models as well as those correlating pharmacokinetic, microbiologic, and clinical observations in patients support this concept.[60–62]

ADVERSE REACTIONS

The cephalosporins have a highly favorable toxicity profile compared with other antimicrobials. With a few unique exceptions, the adverse events caused by cephalosporins are similar across the group (Table 19–5).

Local Reactions

Thrombophlebitis, a common complication with intravenously administered medications, occurs in 1 to 5% of cephalosporin recipients and is not uniquely associated with a specific agent. Pain at the site of intramuscular injection is not uncommon and can be ameliorated by adding lidocaine to the diluent.

TABLE 19–4 Dosing of Selected Cephalosporins in Patients with Renal Insufficiency*

Agent	Usual Adult Dose in Serious Infection (Parenteral Unless Indicated)	Maintenance Dose (g)/Dosing Interval (h)			Dosing During Dialysis	
		GFR 90–50 ml/min	*GRF 50–10 ml/min*	*GRF <10 ml/min*	*Hemodialysis (g)*†	*CAPD*
Cefazolin	1 g q8h	Usual	0.5–1/8–12	0.5–1/24	0.5–1	0.5 g q12h
Cephalexin	0.5 g q6h PO	Usual	0.5/8–12	0.5/12	0.25	0.25 g q8h
Cephradine	0.5 g q6h PO	Usual	0.5/8	0.25/12	0.5	0.25 g q6h
Cefadroxil	0.5 g q12h PO	Usual	0.5/24	0.5/36	0.5	0.5 g q24h
Cefamandole	2 g q6h	Usual	2/8	1/12	1	1 g q12h
Cefonicid	2 g q24h	Usual	1/24	1/72	None	1 g q72h
Cefotetan	2 g q12h	Usual	2/24	2/48	1	1 g q24h
Cefoxitin	2 g q6h	2/8	2/12	1/12	2	1 g q24h
Cefuroxime	1.5 g q8h	Usual	1.5/12	0.75/24	1.5	0.75 g q24h
Cefuroxime axetil	0.5 g q12h PO	Usual	Usual	0.5/24	0.5	0.5 g q24h
Cefprozil	0.5 g q12h PO	Usual	0.5/24	0.25/24	0.5	0.25 g q12h
Cefaclor	0.5 g q8h PO	Usual	Usual	0.5/12	0.5	0.5 g q8h
Loracarbef	0.4 g q12h PO	Usual	0.4/24	0.4/72	0.4	0.4 g q24h
Cefixime	0.4 g q24h PO	Usual	0.2/24	0.2/24	0.2	0.2 g q24h
Cefdinir	0.3 g q12h PO	Usual	0.3/24	0.3/24	0.3	0.3 g q24h
Cefpodoxime	0.4 g q12h PO	Usual	0.4/24	0.2/24	0.4	0.2 g q24h
Ceftizoxime	2 g q8h	Usual	1/12	0.5/12	1	0.5 g q24h
Cefotaxime	2 g q6–8h	Usual	2/12	2/24	1	1.0 g q24h
Ceftazidime	2 g q8h	Usual	1/12	1/24	1	0.5 g q24h
Cefepime	2 g q12h	Usual	2/16–24	0.5–1/24	1	0.5 g q12h

*Ceftriaxone, cefoperazone: no change in dosing required.
†Supplement given after hemodialysis during maintenance therapy.
Abbreviation: CAPD, Chronic ambulatory peritoneal dialysis; GFR, glomeruler filtration rate.

TABLE 19–5 Adverse Events Associated with Cephalosporins

	Frequency (%)
Hypersensitivity reactions	
Maculopapular rash	1–3
Urticaria	
Pruritis	
Anaphylaxis or angioedema	Rare
Serum sickness (↑ with cefaclor)	
Eosinophilia	1–7
Hematologic reactions	
Reversible neutropenia	<1
Thrombocytosis	2–5
Coombs' test positive (hemolysis is rare)	1–5
Coagulation abnormalities	
Hypoprothrombinemia (related to MTT group)	
Reduced platelet aggregation (moxalactam)	
Gastrointestinal reactions	
Abnormal liver function tests (mild)	1–7
Diarrhea, nonspecific; *Clostridium difficile* related	
Biliary sludge (ceftriaxone-dose related)	20
Nephrotoxicity	
Interstitial nephritis	Rare
Phlebitis	

Abbreviation: MTT, Methylthiotetrazole.

Hypersensitivity Reactions

Hypersensitivity reactions are the most common systemic adverse events encountered with cephalosporin treatment. Nevertheless, immediate (30 to 60 minutes after administration) and accelerated (1 to 72 hours after administration) immunoglobulin E (IgE)-mediated anaphylactic or urticarial reactions are rare (especially with second- and third-generation compounds) relative to the frequency of 0.01% associated with penicillin.[63, 64] Skin rash with or without fever and eosinophilia occurs in 1 to 3% of patients after variable periods of cephalosporin therapy.[64–67] With the exception of an apparent increased incidence of a serum sickness syndrome in children receiving cefaclor, there are no data to indicate that hypersensitivity reactions are more common with any individual cephalosporin.

The cross-reactivity among cephalosporins and between cephalosporins and penicillins has been examined in laboratory and clinical settings; nevertheless, this complex issue remains unresolved.[63, 64] The specific haptens involved in cephalosporin hypersensitivity are not known. The number of potential haptens is quite large, since both side chain and nuclear components of the cephalosporins may participate in the hypersensitivity reaction.[63] Laboratory test systems suggest that cephalosporin derivatives show less cross-reactivity among themselves than do penicillin derivatives but that the cross-reactivity between cephalosporins is greater than between cephalosporins and penicillins.[63] In the absence of information detailing cephalosporin haptenic determinants, these assessments, however, are severely limited. Cephalosporin reactions occur in 1 to 7% of patients with a history of penicillin allergy.[63] Among ceftazidime recipients, for example, 2.7% of patients with a history of penicillin reactions experienced a reaction as contrasted with 1.6% of those with no prior history of penicillin allergy, yielding a relative risk of 1.66 for ceftazidime reactions in persons with a history of penicillin allergy.[64] Additionally, of 99 patients with a history of penicillin allergy and a positive skin test with the major and minor penicillin determinants who received a cephalosporin, only 1 had a reaction.[63] This rate is lower than the 22% reaction rate noted when a similarly defined population was challenged with penicillin.[68] Although the frequency of primary hypersensitivity reactions to cephalosporins is less than for penicillin, they do occur. Furthermore, there is no test system with which to predict who is at risk for these reactions. Skin testing with cephalosporin compounds is unreliable and not recommended. The selection of antibiotic therapy in patients with a history of a reaction to a cephalosporin or penicillin must be guided by the severity of the reaction and the availability of suitable non–β-lactam therapy. Therapy with non–β-lactam antibiotics should be used if severe β-lactam reactions, especially those mediated by IgE, have occurred.[69, 70] If cephalosporin therapy is highly desirable and the allergy history is imprecise, skin test reactivity with penicillolyl polylysine and a minor determinant mixture can be assessed. Reactivity to both reagents may reflect an increased risk of a cephalosporin reaction and may warrant alternative therapy.[70] Although patients with a history of non–IgE-mediated penicillin allergy, even with negative skin tests, are at increased risk of a reaction on receiving a cephalosporin, these reactions are rarely severe, and a cephalosporin can be used, if necessary.[71]

Hematologic Reactions

Eosinophilia occurs in 1 to 7% of cephalosporin recipients and may be noted as an isolated finding. Neutropenia that reverses promptly after the discontinuation of a cephalosporin is seen during prolonged high-dose therapy; the frequency of neutropenia is less than 1%. Approximately 5% of cephalosporin recipients have thrombocytosis. Although a positive reaction to the Coombs test occurs in 3% of patients receiving earlier cephalosporins, hemolytic anemia is very uncommon.[72] Cephalosporins can alter hemostasis mechanisms.[73] Although antibiotic therapy may inhibit the synthesis and absorption of vitamin K by the inhibition of gut flora, hypoprothrombinemia has been associated with the competitive inhibition by the MTT group of the vitamin K–dependent carboxylase that is responsible for converting clotting factors II, VII, IX, and X to their active forms.[74–78] The MTT group, which occupies position 3 in cefamandole, cefoperazone, cefotetan, moxalactam, cefmetazole, and cefmenoxime, may also inhibit, like coumadin, vitamin K 2,3-epoxide reductase, which converts inactive vitamin K to its active form.[76] The frequency of hypoprothrombinemia in recipients of these compounds is variable (range 4 to 68%) and is markedly enhanced by poor nutritional status, debilitation, recent gastrointestinal surgery, and renal failure.[79, 80] Bleeding occurs less frequently and has been associated primarily with moxalactam, cefoperazone, and cefotetan.[79, 81] Vitamin K treatment over 24 to 36 hours restores the prothrombin time to normal. Weekly prophylaxis with vitamin K has been recommended when MTT-bearing cephalosporins are administered to patients at high risk for hypoprothrombinemia. Moxalactam, in addition, reversibly suppresses ADP-induced platelet aggregation with consequent prolongation of the bleeding time.[82] Other cephalosporins do not significantly impair platelet function.

Gastrointestinal Tract Toxicity

Mild elevations in levels of transaminases and alkaline phosphatase have been noted during cephalosporin therapy but rarely necessitate discontinuation of therapy.[67, 71] The frequency of nonspecific antibiotic-associated diarrhea is 2 to 5% in cephalosporin recipients. It is postulated that diarrhea is more frequent with cefoperazone and ceftriaxone as a consequence of biliary excretion and subsequent impact on gastrointestinal flora. Cephalosporin therapy is associated with pseudomembranous or *Clostridium difficile* toxin–related colitis; however, the risk, is not increased for specific cephalosporins or for cephalosporins compared with penicillins or clindamycin. Ceftriaxone has been associated with the formation of sonographically identifiable sludge in the gallbladder and common bile duct. Although commonly asymptomatic, the biliary tract sludge may be associated with symptoms of cholecystitis.[83, 84] Risk factors for ceftriaxone-associated sludge formation, also called *pseudolithiasis,* include childhood, prolonged or high dose (>2 g/day), and biliary stasis (receipt of total parenteral nutrition).[83–85] If the ceftriaxone excreted into the bile and concentrated there exceeds its solubility product it precipitates as crystals of a ceftriaxone-calcium salt.[85] The sludge, which may form in 20 to 45% of patients receiving ceftriaxone 2 g daily, clears between 10 and 60 days after therapy.[83, 86] Occasionally ceftriaxone-calcium crystals may coalesce to form cholelithiasis and precipitate symptomatic disease.[84]

Nephrotoxicity

Nephrotoxicity due to currently available cephalosporins, when they are used in recommended doses, is generally rare. Acute tubular necrosis has occasionally been attributed to extremely high doses of cephalothin or to standard high-dose therapy in elderly patients.[87, 88] Furthermore, cephalothin may enhance the nephrotoxicity of aminoglycosides.[89, 90] Ceftazidime, which shares a pyridine substituent at position 3 with cephaloridine, may cause some decrease in glomerular and tubular function[91]; however, clinically significant nephrotoxicity has not been noted.[66] Interstitial nephritis occurs as an apparent hypersensitivity response to cephalosporins.

Disulfiram-like Reactions

Ingestion of alcohol by patients receiving cephalosporins with the MTT group at position 3 (see "Hematologic Reactions") has been associated with disulfiram-like reactions.[92, 93] These are characterized, depending on severity, by a rapid onset of flushing, tachycardia, headache, sweating, thirst, nausea, vomiting, hypotension, confusion, and blurred vision. The MTT group, the standard configuration of which is similar to that of disulfiram, appears to block alcohol metabolism at the acetaldehyde step. The accumulation of acetaldehyde is associated with these symptoms.

FIRST-GENERATION CEPHALOSPORINS

The first-generation cephalosporins (see Tables 19–1 and 19–2) are very active against gram-positive cocci and have moderate activity against community-acquired *Moraxella catarrhalis, E. coli, Proteus mirabilis* (indole-negative), and *K. pneumoniae* (Tables 19–6 and 19–7).[23, 69–71, 109–113] The antibacterial activity of these agents for other Enterobacteriaceae is unpredictable and should not be assumed. Although active against most of the penicillin-susceptible oral cavity anaerobes, the *B. fragilis* group are resistant. These agents have poor activity against *H. influenzae* and are not active against methicillin-resistant staphylococci, penicillin-resistant pneumococci, and *Enterococcus* spp. Even when in vitro susceptibility tests suggest that cephalosporins are likely to be effective against methicillin-resistant staphylococci, these agents are not effective therapeutically.[114] With the exception of cefazolin, which has slightly enhanced activity for some Enterobacteriaceae, the antibacterial activity of both the oral and the parenteral first-generation cephalosporins is similar.[22, 109–113]

Drugs

Cephalothin (Keflin), now unavailable in the United States, is a parenteral agent that distributes throughout body tissues and fluids with the exception of the cerebrospinal fluid. The acetoxy substituent at position 3 is cleaved from 20 to 30% of the parent compound to form a desacetyl metabolite. Both the desacetyl product and unmetabolized cephalothin are excreted in the urine.

Cefazolin (Ancef, Kefzol) is well tolerated when given intramuscularly or intravenously. Serum concentrations of cefazolin are higher than those achieved with comparable doses of cephalothin, in part because cefazolin has a smaller volume of distribution. Cefazolin is not metabolized; with normal renal function, 80% of the administered dose is excreted through the kidney by glomerular filtration.[115] The antimicrobial spectrum of cefazolin is similar to that of cephalothin, although cefazolin is slightly more potent against *E. coli* and *Klebsiella* spp.[113] Cefazolin is more readily hydrolyzed by staphylococcal β-lactamase than cephalothin.[116, 117] Although this relatively increased β-lactamase vulnerability has not been clearly demonstrated to be clinical significance, some experts prefer cephapirin for the treatment of life-threatening *S. aureus* infections.[118]

Cephapirin (Cefadyl), now unavailable in the United States, a parenterally administered cephalosporin, is very similar to cephalothin in terms of its pharmacokinetics, metabolism, antimicrobial activity, and clinical utility.[111]

Cephalexin (Keflex, Keftab, Biocef) is exceptionally well absorbed from the gastrointestinal tract; maximal serum concentrations of 15 to 18 μg/ml are attained in 1 hour after a 0.5-g oral dose. Ninety percent of the oral dose is excreted in the urine as native drug.

TABLE 19–6 In Vitro Antibacterial Activity of Selected Oral Cephalosporins

	MIC_{90}										
Organism	***Cephalexin***	***Cephradine***	***Cefadroxil***	***Cefaclor***	***Cefprozil***	***Loracarbef***	***Cefuroxime***	***Cefpodoxime***	***Cefixime***	***Ceftibuten***	***Cefdinir‡***
*Strep. pneumoniae**	2	2	2	0.5	0.12	0.5	≤0.06	≤0.06	0.25	4	0.03
Strep. agalactiae	2	2	2	2	0.25	0.5	<0.12	0.12	0.25	16	0.03
B. fragilis	>32	>32	>32	>32	>32	>32	>32	>32	>32	>32	64
P. aeruginosa	>32	>32	>32	>32	>32	>32	>32	>32	>32	>32	>128
Strep. pyogenes	2	2	2	0.5	0.12	0.5	≤0.06	0.06	0.25	2	0.015
Staph. aureus†	4	4	4	4	2	4	4	4	>32	>32	0.5
H. influenzae†	8	16	32	8	8	2	0.5	0.06	0.06	0.06	0.25
N. gonorrhoeae†	2	4	4	1	1	0.12	0.25	0.06	0.06	0.004	0.03
M. catarrhalis†	4	4	4	1	2	1	1.0	0.25	0.06	2	0.12
*E. coli**	>16	>16	>16	>16	2	>16	8	0.5	0.25	0.12	2
C. diversus	4	4	4	0.5	1	0.5	4	0.5	0.06	0.06	0.25
Klebsiella spp.†	>16	>16	>16	>16	>16	>16	2	0.12	0.06	0.03	4
P. mirabilis	16	16	16	1	1	2	2	0.06	0.06	≤0.015	0.12
Salmonella spp.†	>16	>16	>16	16	0	8	4	0.12	0.06	0.06	0.5
Shigella spp.†	>16	>16	>16	16	8	8	2	0.12	≤0.06	≤0.06	0.5
C. freundii	>32	>32	>32	>32	>32	>32	>32	>32	>32	>32	128
E. aerogenes	>32	>32	>32	>32	>32	>32	>32	0.5	2	1	32
E. cloacae	>32	>32	>32	>32	>32	>32	>32	>32	>32	>32	>64
M. morganii	>32	>32	>32	>32	>32	>32	>32	8	8	2	32
P. vulgaris	>32	>32	32	>32	>32	>32	>32	0.12	0.25	0.03	64
P. rettgeri	>32	>32	>32	>32	>32	>32	16	0.03	0.06	0.06	16
P. stuartii	>32	>32	>32	>32	>32	>32	>32	0.5	0.6	0.06	4
Serratia spp.	>32	>32	>32	>32	>32	>32	>32	>32	>32	4	>64

*Penicillin-sensitive isolates.
†ß-Lactamase–producing isolates.
‡Data from ref. 186.
Abbreviation: MIC_{90}, Minimal inhibiting concentration for 90% of strains in μg/ml.
Modified from Neu HC. Oral ß-lactam antibiotics from 1960 to 1993. Infect Dis Clin Pract. 1993; 6:394–404.

TABLE 19–7 In Vitro Antibacterial Activity of Selected Parenteral Cephalosporins*: MIC_{50}/MIC_{90} (μg/ml)*,†

Antibiotic	*S. pyogenes*	*S. pneumoniae*‡	*S. aureus*§	*H. influenzae*¶	*E. coli*	*P. mirabilis*	*K. pneumoniae*	*E. cloacae*	*E. aerogenes*	*C. freundii*	*M. morganii*	*P. aeruginosa*	*B. fragilis*
Cefazolin	0.1/0.1	0.12/0.12	1/1	4/8	<2/16	>2/<2	<2/4	>32/>32	>32/>32	>32/>32	>32/>32	>32/>32	64/>64
Cefamandole	0.06/0.06	0.12/0.12	<0.25/1	16/32	2/16	0.5/1	1/8	32/>64	2>64	2/8	32/64	>32/>32	64/>64
Cefuroxime	<0.03/0.06	0.06/0.12	0.8/4	0.5/2	4/8	<2/<2	2/8	>32/>64	8/>32	4/>32	32/>32	32/>32	64/>64
Cefoxitin	0.5/1	1/2	2/4	1/4	2/8	2/8	2/8	>32/>32	>32/>32	>32/>32	8/8	>32/>32	4/32
Cefotetan	2/4	8/>32	<4/16	4/4	0.12/.48	0.25/0.25	0.12/0.25	8/64	>8/>64	2/64	4/4	>32/>32	8/>64
Cefmetazole	0.5/0.5	1/8	2/4	1/4	1/4	2/4	1/2	>32/>32	4/32	>32/>32	4/8	>32/>32	8/16
Cefotaxime	0.06/0.06	0.01/0.06	2/4	0.06/0.06	0.12/0.12	0.12/0.12	0.12/0.12	0.5/>32	0.12/32	0.25/0.5	0.5/8	16/32	32/>64
Ceftizoxime	0.01/0.01	0.25/0.5	4/16	0.01/0.01	0.25/0.25	0.25/0.25	0.25/0.25	0.25/32	0.25/32	0.25/>32	0.25/2	>32/>32	16/>64
Ceftriaxone	0.01/0.03	0.01/0.06	2/4	0.01/0.01	0.25/0.25	0.25/0.25	0.25/0.25	0.26/>64	0.25/16	0.25/>64	0.25/1	16/>32	32/>64
Ceftazidime	0.12/0.25	0.25/0.5	8/16	0.06/0.12	0.12/0.25	0.12/0.25	0.12/0.5	0.25/>16	0.25/>32	0.05/>16	0.12/4	2/>16	>32/>2
Cefepime	0.02/0.04	0.03/0.06	2/4	0.06/0.12	0.04/0.06	0.04/0.1	0.12/0.25	0.06/2	0.06/0.5	0.05/8	0.03/0.05	<4/16	32/256
Cefpirome	0.02/0.05	0.01/0.06	0.5/1	0.06/0.12	0.12/0.12	0.12/0.12	0.12/0.25	0.12/0.5	0.03/0.12	0.03/0.06	0.12/0.5	4/>16	32/256

*Values are approximations from refs. 18, 20, 94–108, 236.
†Minimal inhibiting concentrations (MICs) for 50 and 90% percent of strains in μg/ml.
‡Penicillin susceptible (MIC <0.1 μg/ml).
§Methicillin susceptible *Staph. aureus*.
¶β-Lactamase producing.

Cephradine (Velosef, oral and parenteral) is similar to cephalexin structurally except that it has a cyclohexidine ring on its acyl side chain where cephalexin has a phenol group. The compound is rapidly absorbed from the intestinal tract, it is not metabolized, and it is rapidly excreted in the urine. Because cephradine is fully bioavailable after oral administration, peak serum concentrations (15 to 18 μg/ml) and the area under the curve after a 0.5-g dose, either oral or intramuscular, are similar.[119]

Cefadroxil (Duricef, Ultracef), the parahydroxy analogue of cephalexin, is almost 100% absorbed after oral administration and has a slightly longer half-life than cephalexin and cephradine (1.1 hour). The more sustained serum and urine concentrations of cefadroxil allow the treatment of less severe infections (skin, pharyngeal, urinary tract) with once- or twice-daily dosing schedules.[22, 109]

Clinical Use

The first-generation cephalosporins are appropriate treatment for *S. aureus* and nonenterococcal streptococcal infections when it is desirable to avoid penicillins. Most commonly, these include skin and soft tissue infection and streptococcal pharyngitis. These antibiotics are not ideal for the treatment of infections that are likely to be caused by *S. pneumoniae, H. influenzae* or *M. catarrhalis* (sinusitis, otitis media, and some lower respiratory tract infections). They may be used for the treatment of community-acquired, uncomplicated urinary tract infection; however, trimethoprim-sulfamethoxazole is more effective and less costly. First-generation cephalosporins are not used to treat infections of the central nervous system and because of their limited activity against gram-negative bacilli are not appropriate choices for empirical therapy of nosocomial infections. Oral first-generation cephalosporins are not effective treatment for infections caused by *Pasturella multocida* (animal bites and scratches).[120] Because of its spectrum of action, favorable toxicity profile, relatively long half-life, modest cost, and proven efficacy, cefazolin is the prophylactic antibiotic of choice for surgical procedures involving foreign body implantation and many clean and clean-contaminated procedures in which there is a relatively high risk of infection.[121, 122] These include cardiac surgery, arterial reconstruction, the insertion of orthopedic devices, head and neck surgery that crosses the oropharyngeal mucosa, high-risk gastroduodenal and biliary tract procedures, vaginal and abdominal hysterectomy, high-risk cesarean sections, and procedures on fresh trauma wounds. Cefazolin alone is not recommended as prophylaxis for colorectal surgery or appendectomy in which *B. fragilis* is a potential pathogen. Also when methicillin-resistant *S. aureus* is a particular threat, cefazolin is not recommended.

SECOND-GENERATION CEPHALOSPORINS

The second-generation cephalosporins should be considered in two groups: the true cephalosporins and the cephamycins (cefoxitin, cefotetan, and cefmetazole; Tables 19–1 and 19–2). In comparison with the first-generation agents, the true cephalosporins in this group include a range of parenteral and oral antibiotics that provide significantly improved activity against *H. influenzae, M. catarrhalis, Neisseria meningitidis,* and *N. gonorrhoeae,* comparable to enhanced activity against staphylococci and nonenterococcal streptococci, and in selected instances increased in vitro activity against some Enterobacteriaceae (see Tables 19–6 and 19–7).[10, 11, 22, 123–129] In comparison with first-generation compounds and the second-generation true cephalosporins, the cephamycins have inferior activity against staphylococci but they, particularly cefotetan, have an enhanced antibacterial effect against selected Enterobacteriaceae. Their activity against *Neisseria* spp. is good. They are noteworthy as the cephems most active against *Bacteroides* spp., particularly *B. fragilis.*[95–98, 130–135] Enterobacteriaceae constituitively producing Bush group1 AmpC β-lactamase, whether the gene remains chromosomal or is on a plasmid, or ESBL are resistant to the second-generation cephalosporins. ESBL-producing strains appear susceptible in vitro to cephamycins, but these agents have not proved reliable when used for the treatment of infection caused by ESBL-producing strains.

Drugs

Cefamandole (Mandol), a parenteral cephalosporin has an MTT group at position 3 and has manifested the associated toxicities. Cefamandole has excellent activity against gram-positive cocci, appearing superior to cefazolin against selected *S. aureus* and coagulase-negative staphylococci. Although cefamandole has improved activity against β-lactamase–negative *H. influenzae,* significant inactivation by β-lactamase renders cefamandole unreliable against TEM-1-plasmid–bearing strains of *H. influenzae.*[123, 125]

Ceforanide (Precef), similar in structure to cefamandole including a modified MTT group at position 3, produces peak serum concentration comparable to those of cefazolin, has a half-life of 2.6 hours, and is excreted unmetabolized in the urine. Except for having reduced activity against *H. influenzae,* its spectrum of antibacterial activity is similar to that of cefamandole. Ceforanide can be administered every 12 hours.

Cefonicid (Monocid), which is structurally and biologically similar to cefamandole, is unique because it is 98% serum protein bound.[129] Although used effectively in once-daily doses, failures have been noted in more serious infection, including *S. aureus* bacteremia.[136] A single preoperative dose of cefonicid reduced the incidence of wound infection in patients undergoing breast surgery or herniorraphy.[137]

Cefuroxime (Kefurox, Zenacef), because of an iminomethoxy group on the acyl side chain, has significantly enhanced stability to the β-lactamases of *H. influenzae* and *N. gonorrhoeae* (TEM-1) and some Enterobacteriaceae, relative to the first-generation cephalosporins and cefamandole. Accordingly, it has notably improved activity against both β-lactamase–positive and –negative *H. influenzae, N. gonorrhoeae,* and *M. catarrhalis* and significantly increased activity against *E. coli, P. mirabilis, Klebsiella* spp., *Citrobacter* spp., and *Morganella*. It does not have good activity against *Proteus vulgaris, Serratia* spp.; and *Providencia* (see Tables 19–6 and 19–7).[10, 11, 22] Although somewhat less potent against *S. aureus,* it is significantly more active against *S. pneumoniae* and *S. pyogenes* than the first-generation cephalosporins.[10, 11, 22] Cefuroxime has provided effective treatment for bacterial meningitis caused by *N. meningitidis, S. pneumoniae,* and *H. influenzae.*[138, 139] However, in a direct randomized comparison to ceftriaxone in the treatment of meningitis in children, cefuroxime was associated with delayed sterilization of the cerebrospinal fluid and a greater frequency of moderate prolonged hearing loss.[86]

Cefprozil (Cefzil) is structurally similar to cefadroxil except that cefprozil contains a vinyl-methyl group at position 3 of the cephem nucleus instead of a methyl group. Because of this difference, cefprozil is more active than the first-generation oral cephalosporins against *S. pneumoniae, S. pyogenes,* other streptococci, *Neisseria* spp., and, to a lesser degree, *S. aureus*. Its activity against *H. influenzae,* both β-lactamase negative and positive strains, is only modestly increased beyond that of cephalexin and cefadroxil; it is comparable to that noted with cefaclor and less than that of cefuroxime. Cefprozil is more active than first-generation cephalosporins against *E. coli, P. mirabilis, Klebsiella* spp., and *Citrobacter* spp.; it is not active against the indole-positive *Proteus, Providencia,* and *Enterobacter* spp. (see Tables 19–6 and 19–7).[22, 119]

Cefuroxime axetil (Ceftin), the acetoxyethyl ester of cefuroxime that is hydrolyzed to the parent compound during absorption, has a bioavailability to 30 to 50% after oral administration. The serum half-life allows twice-daily dosing for mild to moderate infections. Cefuroxime axetil is not available in suspension, and crushed tablets have an unacceptably bitter taste.[140, 141]

Cefaclor (Ceclor), an orally administered cephalosporin, has pharmacokinetic and biologic activities similar to those of cephalexin. Relative to cephalexin, it has moderately increased activity against *H. influenzae, M. catarhhalis, E. coli* and *P. mirabilis*. It is, however, significantly destroyed by the TEM-1 and Bro-1 β-lactamases of some *H. influenzae* and *M. catarrhalis,* respectively.[22, 101] Cefaclor is available in an extended-release formulation, Ceclor CD, which must be taken with food. Peak serum concentrations appear reduced and the area under the concentration curve is similar relative to the same dose of Ceclor.

Loracarbef (Lorabid) is an orally administered carbacephem antibiotic with a carbon at position 1 of the cephem nucleus instead of a sulfur; otherwise, the molecule is structurally similar to cefaclor. Relative to cefaclor, loracarbef has comparable activity against *S. aureus, S. pneumoniae,* and streptococci but has modestly increased activity against *H. influenzae* and *M. catarrhalis* and some Enterobacteriaceae. It is not active in vitro against *Citrobacter, Enterobacter,* indole-positive *Proteus, Providencia,* and *Serratia* spp. Loracarbef is destroyed by the ESBLs.[22, 101, 127] Absorption is more rapid and peak serum concentrations are significantly higher with the suspension formulation than with capsules; food decreases absorption. Azotemia (creatinine clearance <30 ml/minute) increases the half-life to 5 hours, thus warranting dose adjustments. The compound is effectively removed by hemodialysis.[21, 22, 142] Loracarbef is stable in human plasma at body temperature for greater than 100 hours compared with the rapid deterioration of cefaclor.[22, 143]

Cefoxitin (Mefoxin), a cephamycin, is notably resistant to the β-lactamases produced by gram-negative bacilli and is a highly effective inducer of β-lactamase production by some Enterobacteriaceae.[43] Cefoxitin is more active against *E. coli, Klebsiella,* and the indole-negative *Proteus* spp. than first-generation cephalosporins; less active against *H. influenzae* than the second-generation true cephalosporins; and has significantly reduced antibacterial activity against gram-positive cocci compared with first- and second-generation cephalosporins.[130] Cefoxitin is the most potent of the cephalosporins against the *B. fragilis* group. Among *B. fragilis,* resistance to cefoxitin (MIC breakpoint ≥32 μg/ml) ranges from 4 to 31%, whereas resistance among *Bacteroides thetaiotaomicron, Bacteroides distasonis,* and *Bacteroides ovatus* is significantly greater, ranging from 24 to 56%.[96, 98] Cefoxitin has good activity against *N. gonorrhoeae,* including those that produce β-lactamase.

Cefotetan (Cefotan), another cephamycin, has antibacterial activity similar to that of cefoxitin against *B. fragilis* but is less active against the non–*B.fragilis* members of the *B. fragilis* group.[96, 98] Its activity against facultative gram-negative bacilli is greater than that of the second-generation cephalosporins and approaches that of the third-generation agents.[144] It is not active against *Pseudomonas* spp. but is highly effective against *N. gonorrhoeae,* including those that produce β-lactamase. Cefotetan has an MTT group and has been associated with hypoprothrombinemia and bleeding.

Cefmetazole (Zefazone), a cephamycin, is slightly less active against the *B. fragilis* group and moderately more active against some Enterobacteriaceae than is cefoxitin. Cefmetazole is not as potent against gram-negative bacilli as cefotetan, and none of the cephamycins are highly active against the *Enterobacter, Providencia,* indole-positive *Proteus, C. freundi,* or *Serratia* spp.[135] The molecule has an MTT chain at position 3 and has been associated with disulfiram-like reactions when administered after alcohol has been ingested. It does not impair platelet aggregation, as is noted with moxalactam.[145]

Clinical Use

The activity of cefuroxime against *S. pneumoniae, H. influenzae,* and *M. catarrhalis,* including β-lactamase–producing strains of the latter two, has prompted the use of cefuroxime in the treatment of patients hospitalized for community-acquired, presumed bacterial pneumonia.[146, 147] Other serious infections caused by susceptible bacteria, including epiglotitis, complicated sinusitis, bacteremia, soft tissue infection, and uncomplicated urinary tract infection, can also be treated with cefuroxime. Cefuroxime is effective therapy for meningitis due to *H. influenzae, N. meningitidis,* and penicillin-susceptible *S. pneumoniae*. However, as a result of the more advantageous pharmacodynamics of third-generation cephalosporins against these organisms, and particularly for *S. pneumoniae* with decreased penicillin susceptibility, as well as the outcome of a direct clinical comparison, ceftriaxone or cefotaxime are the preferred cephalosporins for use in the therapy of meningitis.[54, 86, 138, 139] Although its spectrum of activity is similar to that of cefuroxime, cefamandole, with less favorable pharmacokinetics, inferior in vitro activity against *H. influenzae,* potential toxicity due to an MTT substituent, and a lack of penetration into the central nervous system, is less widely used. Neither cefamandole nor cefuroxime should be considered for empirical treatment of nosocomial pneumonia or other nosocomial infections that are potentially caused by *Enterobacter, Citrobacter,* indole-positive *Proteus, Providencia, Morganella, Serratia,* or *P. aeruginosa,* which are likely to be resistant intrinsically or through the production of β-lactamases.[41–43]

The oral second-generation cephalosporins, including cefuroxime axetil, cefprozil, cefaclor, and loracarbef, are agents that can be used effectively to treat a spectrum of mild to moderate community-acquired uncomplicated infections.[144–160] Such infections include skin and soft tissue infection and urinary tract infection. In these settings, however, more cost-effective or narrow-spectrum therapy is desirable (e.g., a penicillinase-resistant oral penicillin or cephalexin for skin infection or trimethoprim-sulfamethoxazole for uncomplicated urinary tract infections).

The oral second-generation agents should be used primarily for the treatment of infections of the respiratory tract and its appendages. Trials comparing these agents among themselves, to amoxicillin-clavulanate, and to amoxicillin have not demonstrated a superior agent in a given infection. Based on both clinical and bacteriologic results, shorter courses of second-generation oral cephalosporins are either equivalent or superior to penicillin V for 10 days for the treatment of acute group A, β-hemolytic streptococcal pharyngitis.[161] In the lower respiratory tract, middle ear, and sinuses, the major bacterial pathogens are *S. pneumoniae, H. influenzae,* and *M. catarrhalis.* Pharmacodynamic considerations, that is, selecting and dosing a β-lactam agent so that the antibiotic concentration exceeds the MIC for 90% of the isolates (MIC_{90}) for the pathogen at the site of injection for more than 50% for the dose-to-dose interval, indicate that cefuroxime axetil would be the optimal oral second-generation cephalosporin for empirical therapy of respiratory tract infections.[162, 163] These considerations suggest that cefaclor, loracarbef, and cefprozil are less suitable treatment for infection due to *H. influenzae* and *M. catarrhalis.*[163, 164] All the oral second-generation cephalosporins provide suboptimal treatment for respiratory tract infection caused by penicillin-resistant *S. pneumoniae.*[162] Cefuroxime axetil is an effective alternative to doxycycline and penicillins for the treatment of early (erythema migrans–associated) Lyme disease.[165]

Cefoxitin, cefotetan, and cefmetazole have been demonstrated efficacious in the treatment of intra-abdominal infections, pelvic and gynecologic infections, infected decubitus ulcers, diabetic foot infections, and mixed aerobic-anaerobic soft tissue infections.[131, 166–171] All of these infections represent entities in which facultative gram-negative bacilli and anaerobic organisms, especially *B. fragilis,* are likely to play a prominent role. Although the experience is most extensive with cefoxitin, available comparative trials suggest a similar efficacy for each agent. The clinical significance of the reduced in vitro activity of cefotetan and cefmetazol against the non–*B. fragilis* species in the *B. fragilis* group is not clear. Furthermore, as many as 15% of *B. fragilis* may be resistant to the cephamycin antibiotics. Accordingly, these agents should not be used, in the absence of susceptibility information, to treat life-threatening *B. fragilis* infection. Metronidazole, chloramphenicol, a β-lactam–β-lactamase combination, or imipenem, which are active against virtually all *B. fragilis,* would be preferred in this setting.[95] These cephamycins are not highly active against *S. aureus* and are often inactive in the setting of derepressed Bush 1 chromosomal β-lactamases in Enterobacteriaceae, both of which might be encountered in nosocomial infections.[41–43] Accordingly, these agents should not be considered optimal single-drug therapy when the previously mentioned infections occur in patients who have been hospitalized and received antibiotic therapy. Cefoxitin and cefotetan have been demonstrated to be effective therapy for urogenital gonorrhea but for financial and logistical reasons are not recommended as a therapy of choice.[172, 173] Cefoxitin and cefotetan are effective, in combination with doxycycline, as treatment of pelvic inflammatory disease.[173, 174] Cefoxitin, cefotetan, and cefmetazole have been shown effective and comparable as systemic prophylaxis for surgery performed at various levels of the gastrointestinal tract, for appendectomy, and for selected gynecologic procedures.[121, 171, 175–177] These agents have not been proved superior to cefazolin other than in the setting of colorectal surgery and appendectomy and hence are recommended only in these settings.[121, 122, 177] Although in elective colorectal surgery the benefits of systemic prophylaxis in addition to an oral erythromycinneomycin preoperative bowel preparation have not been fully established, it is common practice to use one of these agents in this setting.[177]

THIRD-GENERATION CEPHALOSPORINS

The third-generation cephalosporins are active against facultative gram-negative bacilli (see Tables 19–6 and 19–7).[70] In addition they have potent antimicrobial activity against *S. pneumoniae* (including those with relative penicillin resistance) *S. pyogenes,* and other streptococci, and, with the exception of ceftazidime, have effective activity against *S. aureus.* They also have excellent activity against *H. influenzae, N. meningitidis, N. gonorrhoeae,* and *M. catarrhalis.* In spite of wide use, these agents have retained an unusually high degree of activity against *E. coli, Klebsiella, P. mirabilis,* indole-positive *Proteus, Providencia,* and *Serratia.*[70, 94, 99, 100, 178] Third-generation cephalosporins may be subdivided based on their activity against *P. aeruginosa*; cefotaxime, ceftizoxime, ceftriaxone, moxalactam (an oxacephem), cefixime, cefpodoxime proxetil, ceftibuten, cefdinir and the investigational agents cefmenoxime, cefodizime, cefetamet, and cefteram lack activity against *P. aeruginosa.* In contrast, antipseudomonal activity is found in cefoperazone, ceftazidime, and the investigational agents cefsulodin and cefpiramide. The third-generation cephalosporins, like all the compounds based on the cephem nucleus, lack activity against *Enterococcus* spp., methicillin-resistant staphylococci, highly penicillin-resistant *S. pneumoniae, Listeria,* and *Stenotrophomonas.* They are variably active against *Acinetobacter.*

The superior broad activity of these agents against the Enterobacteriaceae has recently been challenged by β-lactamase–mediated resistance (see Chapter 16). Chromosomally encoded β-lactamases (Bush group 1 AmpC; see Chapter 16) that are inducible or that can be stably derepressed and that mediate resistance to all cephalosporins have resulted in an increasing number of infections due to *Enterobacter* spp. and *C. freundii.* Although less frequently encountered as causes of infection, *Serratia, Morganella, P. vulgaris* and *Aeromonas* may express resistance to these agents through inducible β-lactamases.[30, 41–44] Additionally, the plasmid-mediated ESBLs, which mediate resistance to third-generation cephalosporins as a consequence of point mutations in the TEM or SHV genes, represent a widening threat to the utility of these agents.[30, 44, 45]

Drugs

Cefotaxime (Claforan) has superior activity against *Strep. pneumoniae, S. pyogenes,* other streptococci, *H. influenzae,* and *Neisseria*; it has modest activity against *S. aureus.* It remains highly potent against *E. coli, P. mirabilis, Klebsiella,* and other Enterobacteriaceae that do not express Bush 1 AmpC β-lactamases or contain ESBLs.[18, 94] Cefotaxime is not active against *P. aeruginosa, Stenotrophomonas,* and non-*aeruginosa* pseudomonads. Cefotaxime's activity against *B. fragilis* is less than that of the cephamycins; nevertheless, 47 to 66% of strains have an MIC below the susceptibility break point.[95, 178] Cefotaxime is metabolized to desacetyl cefotaxime, which although less potent than the parent compound, has a longer half-life and may act synergistically with cefotaxime to allow effective dosing at 8-hour intervals in patients with moderate infections.[179] Cefotaxime reliably enters the cerebrospinal fluid when dosed at 2 g every 4 hours.[54, 139]

Ceftizoxime (Cefizox) shares the pattern of antibacterial activity seen with cefotaxime except that it inhibits a larger percentage of *B. fragilis* (66 to 80%) and is less potent against *Strep. pneumoniae.*[18, 95, 99, 100, 180] Ceftizoxime doses must be adjusted in azotemic patients. Clinically effective cerebrospinal fluid concentrations are achieved with doses of 3 g every 8 hours.[54, 139]

Ceftriaxone (Rocephin) possess antibacterial activity similar to that of cefotaxime.[18, 99, 100, 181] Against several organisms (e.g., *N. gonnorrhoeae N. meningitidis,* and *H. influenzae*) it is the most potent third-generation cephalosporin.[18] Ceftriaxone is 90% protein bound, excreted through both the biliary and urinary tracts, and has a serum half-life of 8 hours. As a consequence, many serious infections can be treated with once-daily dosing; however meningitis should be treated every 12 hours (adults, 2 g every 12 hours; children, 50 mg/kg every 12 hours). Isolated renal or hepatic dysfunction does not require dose adjustment; however, with failure of both organs, dose adjustment is necessary.[53]

Moxalactam (Moxam), an oxacephem with a methoxy group at position 7 similar to the cephamycins, has activity against gram-negative bacteria similar to other third-generation cephalosporins; it, however, is less active against gram-positive cocci than cefotaxime.[53] It inhibits 75 to 85% of *B. fragilis*.[95] Moxalactam has been associated with hypoprothrombinemia related to the MTT group at position 3 and with a platelet-aggregating defect also.[53] The associated coagulopathy has resulted in significant bleeding complications and recommendations that moxalactam not be used.

Cefmenoxime (investigational) is a parenterally administered aminothiazolyl-iminomethoxy cephalosporin with an antibacterial spectrum very similar to those of cefotaxime, ceftizoxime, and ceftriaxone.[6, 18] Cefmenoxime has an MTT group. It is not active against *P. aeruginosa* or *Acinetobacter* and is effective against only 50% of *B. fragilis*.[18]

Cefodizime (investigational), an aminothiazolyl cephalosporin, is administered parenterally, achieving serum concentrations of 100 μg/ml 30 minutes after the intravenous administration of 1 g. It is excreted unchanged in the urine and has a serum half-life of 2.5 to 3.5 hours. The antibacterial activity of cefodizime is similar to that of cefotaxime.[182] Cefodizine enhances the bactericidal activity of neutrophils against both opsonized and nonopsonized bacteria.[183]

Cefixime (Suprax), a third-generation cephalosporin, is administered orally once daily and is highly effective against *S. pyogenes*, penicillin-susceptible *S. pneumoniae, H. influenzae, M. catarrhalis Neisseria*, and many of the Enterobacteriaceae. It has poor activity against *S. aureus*.[21, 22, 184, 185]

Cefpodoxime proxetil (Vantin), an esterified third-generation cephalosporin, is absorbed after oral administration. The microbiologic activity of cefpodoxime is similar to that of cefixime and cefdinir,[186] except cefpodoxime retains moderate antistaphylococcal activity.[22]

Ceftibuten (Cedax), an orally administered third-generation cephalosporin, is rapidly and nearly completely absorbed. Ceftibuten is not active against *S. aureus* and has poor activity against *S. pneumoniae* and *M. catarrhalis*. It is highly active against the Enterobacteriaceae (except those with derepressed Bush 1 AmpC β-lactamase), *H. influenzae* and *Neisseria*. Of note, ceftibuten is not hydrolyzed by some of the ESBLs and remains active against organisms bearing these β-lactamase genes.[22]

Cefdinir (Omnicef) is an orally administered aminothiazolyl hydroximino cephalosporin, with a vinyl group at c-3 like cefixime. It has, as a result of its c-7 substituent, antibacterial activity against the Enterobacteriaceae that is two- to fourfold less than that of cefixime. It is highly active against penicillin-susceptible *S. pneumoniae, H. influenzae S. pyogenes*, and *M. catarrhalis* and this is similar to cefpodoxime.[22, 186, 187] Pharmacodynamic modeling suggests that cefdinir and cefpodoxime would provide effective therapy for bacterial infection of the respiratory tract and its appendages, as has been demonstrated.[161, 163, 188–191] Cefdinir is hydrolyzed by the ESBLs.[22]

Specific Agents with Anti-*Pseudomonas* Activity

Cefoperazone (Cefobid) has modest anti-*Pseudomonas* activity; at least 50% of *P. aeruginosa* are susceptible (MIC ≤ 16 μg/ml). However, cefoperazone is less active than cefotaxime against gram-negative bacteria and gram-positive cocci.[18, 99, 100] Cefoperazone is highly protein bound, has a relatively small volume of distribution, and, although it achieves very high serum concentrations after parenteral administration, does not reliably penetrate into the cerebrospinal fluid.[53, 54] Disulfiram-like reactions and hypoprothrombinemia with bleeding, both consequences of the MTT group at position 3, have been noted in some cefoperazone recipients.[53, 192]

Ceftazidime (Fortaz, Tazidime, Tazicef) is a unique third-generation cephalosporin. It has a low affinity for many inducible β-lactamases and is a weak inducer of β-lactamase itself.[6] It has excellent activity gram-negative bacteria, including *P. aeruginosa*.[18, 70, 99, 100] Ceftazidime has little activity against *B. fragilis* and has poor antistaphylococcal activity.[18, 70, 95, 100] Ceftazidime penetrates into the cerebrospinal fluid and is the treatment of choice for meningitis due to *P. aeruginosa*.[54]

Cefpiramide (investigational) has antipseudomonal activity similar to that of cefoperazone but is less active than other third-generation cephalosporins against Enterobacteriaceae.[197, 198] Like cefoperazone, it is primarily excreted into the biliary tract; renal excretion increases in the presence of liver disease.[52, 55]

Clinical Use

The third-generation cephalosporins are important agents in clinical medicine. Exceptional antimicrobial potency and spectrum of activity, a very acceptable toxicity profile, and, in selected instances, beneficial pharmacokinetics have allowed these compounds to assume a major role in antimicrobial therapy. The unique aspect of the antimicrobial activity of these agents is their superior activity against gram-negative bacilli that are resistant to other β-lactam antibiotics. Because these relatively resistant bacilli are rarely the cause of community-acquired infection, physicians are urged not to use third-generation cephalosporins routinely for community-acquired infections. Third-generation cephalosporins, however, may be beneficial in the treatment of severe community-acquired infections due to less resistant gram-negative bacilli (e.g., *E. coli, P. mirabilis*, and *K. pneumoniae*).

Cefotaxime, ceftizoxime, and ceftriaxone have provided effective treatment for a variety of nosocomial infections caused by susceptible gram-negative bacilli, including pneumonia, wound infection, and complicated urinary tract infection.[199–202] When treatment is instituted empirically in this setting, the potential for infecting pathogens that are resistant to these agents (e.g., stably derepressed *Enterobacter* spp. ESBL-producing Enterobacteriaeae, *P. aeruginosa*, methicillin-resistant *S. aureus*, and enterococci) must be considered and combination antimicrobial therapy or an alternative β-lactam used until microbiologic data allow the design of specific therapy. With the widespread use of potent β-lactam antibiotics capable of inducing or precipitating derepression of chromosomal β-lactamase in *Enterobacter* spp., *C. freundii, Serratia*, and other gram-negative bacilli, it is increasingly likely that nosocomial infections caused by highly β-lactam antibiotic-resistant Enterobacteriaceae will be encountered.[43, 203–205] Third-generation cephalosporins must be used cautiously when empirically treating severely ill patents for nosocomial infection.

The 1990s have witnessed the widespread dissemination of penicillin-ampicillin resistance among the major bacteria causing respiratory tract infections. A very large study of isolates from all geographic regions of the continental United States found 33% of *H. influenzae* and 92% of *M. catarrhalis* resistant to ampicillin and decreased susceptibility or overt resistance to penicillin in 20 and 14% of *S. pneumoniae*, respectively.[206] Ceftriaxone and cefotaxime remain highly active against the susceptible as well as the resistant strains of these bacteria, although occasional highly penicillin-resistant *S. pneumoniae* are relatively resistant to ceftriaxone and cefotaxime also. Antimicrobial activity of the first-, second-, and oral third-generation cephalosporins against penicillin-resistant pneumococci is markedly eroded. As a consequence of these shifts in antimicrobial susceptibility, as well as the occasional other bacteria that cause community-acquired pneumonia, ceftriaxone or cefotaxime, usually in combination with a macrolide or fluoroquinolone, is often used as empirical therapy for the hospitalized patient with severe community-acquired pneumonia.[207]

Cefotaxime, ceftriaxone, and, to a lesser degree, ceftizoxime have been demonstrated to be effective therapy for meningitis caused by *H. influenzae, S. pneumoniae*, and *N. meningitidis* and in children are at least as effective as previously used regimens (ampicillin plus chloramphenicol, ampicillin plus gentamicin).[208–212] Cefotaxime or ceftriaxone is now recommended for treatment of *H. influenzae* meningitis. These two cephalosporins are also effective therapy for meningitis caused by pneumococci that are characterized as either susceptible or relatively resistant to penicillin (MIC 0.1 to 1.0 μg/ml). Because pneumococci causing meningitis can be resistant to penicillin (MIC ≥ 2 μg/ml) and inadequately responsive to cefotaxime or ceftriaxone, vancomycin (with or without ripampin) is added to ceftriaxone or cefotaxime, thus ensuring that empirical therapy for meningitis in children and adults will cover all of the commonly implicated pathogens.[139] These agents have also been proved uniquely effective in the treatment of meningitis due to gram-negative bacilli other than *P. aeruginosa* and *Enterobacter* spp.[213–217] Ceftazidime is the agent of choice for meningitis due to *P. aeruginosa.*[215] Meningitis caused by *Enterobacter* spp. that does not respond to a third-generation cephalosporin may be treated with trimethoprim-sulfamethoxazole or meropenem.[216]

Ceftazidime, because of its unique antipseudomonal activity, should be reserved for the treatment of infections in which the role of *P. aeruginosa* is established or highly likely. Third-generation cephalosporins have been used as part of empirical combination antimicrobial therapy for the febrile neutropenic patient. Because of its antipseudomonal efficacy, ceftazidime is often used in combination with an aminoglycoside for empirical treatment of neutropenic patients.[218] Combination therapy is also advised for the treatment of non-neutropenic patient with severe *P. aeruginosa* infection. Ceftazidime, often as single-drug therapy, has been effective for the treatment of acute exacerbations of chronic pulmonary infection in patients with cystic fibrosis.[218] Cefoperazone, in spite of modest antipseudomonal activity, does not have an important role in the treatment of serious infections caused by *P. aeruginosa.*

Third-generation cephalosporins have become established therapy in specific settings. Ceftriaxone, which remains highly active against both penicillin-resistant and -susceptible strains of *N. gonorrhoeae* is recommended for therapy of all forms of gonococcal infection and pelvic inflammatory disease.[173] Cefixime has been proved effective for uncomplicated anogenital gonorrhea, including that caused by penicillinase-producing strains, and is recommended for single-dose oral therapy.[173, 219] Additionally, single-dose ceftriaxone is recommended therapy for chancroid.[173, 220] Ceftriaxone has been shown to be effective treatment of Lyme disease and is recommended for the treatment of stages of disease with neurologic findings (except isolated Bell's palsy), carditis, arthritis, and refractory late constitutional symptoms.[221, 222] The potent antistreptococcal activity of ceftriaxone and pharmacokinetics allowing once-daily dosing have created a role for ceftriaxone in the outpatient therapy of nonenterococcal penicillin-susceptible streptococcal endocarditis.[223] When treatment with trimethoprim-sulfamethoxazole or a fluoroquinolone is not feasible, acute uncomplicated cystitis or mild uncomplicated pyelonephritis in women can be treated with cefpodoxime proxetil for 7 to 14 days.

Prompted by unusual antibiotic activity against difficult gram-negative pathogens causing complex infections, third-generation cephalosporins have been evaluated and additional therapeutic niches established. Ceftazidime in combination with trimethoprim-sulfamethoxazole has been demonstrated to be more effective than the previous standard therapy for severe infections caused by *Pseudomonas pseudomallei.*[224] Ceftriaxone is an effective therapy for typhoid fever.[225] Third-generation cephalosporins have provided effective therapy for brain abscess caused by gram-negative bacilli, focal salmonella infection, and endocarditis caused by fastidious gram-negative coccobacilli.[226]

FOURTH-GENERATION CEPHALOSPORINS

The fourth-generation cephalosporins are characterized by a C-3′ quaternary ammonium side chain at the 3 position of the cephem nucleus, which because of its positive charge combined with the negative charge on the cephem C-4 carboxylic group, provides zwitterionic properties to the molecule; broad antibacterial activity, including against *P. aeruginosa*; and antibacterial activity against organisms that produce Bush class 1 AmpC β-lactamases. Two compounds from this group, cefepime and cefpirome, have been developed for clinical use. Their zwitterionic nature allows these compounds to rapidly cross the outer membrane of gram-negative bacteria and achieve a significant concentration in the periplasmic space. This feature combined with their relative resistance to hydrolysis by Bush class 1 AmpC β-lactamases and high affinity for PBPs of gram-negative bacilli endows these compounds with uniquely broad activity against the Enterobacteriaceae and *P. aeruginosa,* as well as *H. influenzae* and *Neisseria* spp.[227, 228] Among Enterobacteriaceae that are resistant to ceftazidime, 75 to 80% of isolates remain susceptible to cefpirome or cefepime.[228] These two agents have high affinity for the PBPs of gram-positive bacteria and thus possess excellent antibacterial activity against methicillin-susceptible *S. aureus, Strep. pneumoniae* (including strains relatively resistant to penicillin), and other streptococci. They do not have more significant antibacterial activity against *Listeria monocytogenes,* methicillin-resistant *S. aureus,* and the *B. fragilis* group. Additional fourth-generation compounds are being developed: cefclidin, cefozopran, cefluprenan, and cefoselis.[228] Cefepime and cefpirome are weak inducers of Bush class 1 AmpC β-lactamases and select stably derepressed Enterobacteriaceae less frequently than third-generation cephalosporins, characteristics that may protect against the emergence of resistance among gram-negative bacilli.[105, 227]

Drugs

Cefpirome (not available in the United States) has a cyclopenteno pyridium group at the C-3′ position on the cephen nucleus. It has superior activity against *S. pneumoniae,* other streptococci, methicillin-susceptible *S. aureus, Neisseria, H. influenzae,* and the Enterobacteriaceae.[18, 20, 194, 228] Although 50% of *P. aeruginosa* isolates are inhibited by cefpirome at 6.0 μg/ml, it is less active against these strains than ceftazidime.[194, 208] Cefpirome appears stable to Bush 1 and some extended-spectrum β-lactamases[228] (220). Cefpirome is excreted in the urine and has a half-life of 2 hours. It is cleared by hemodialysis.[195] Limited studies indicated penetration into the cerebrospinal fluid when the meninges are inflamed.[196] Cefpirome has modest activity against *Enterococcus faecalis*; however, the level of activity is likely to be inadequate for therapy.[228]

Cefepime (Maxipime) has superior activity against *Step. pneumoniae, S. pyogenes,* methicillin-susceptible *S. aureus, H. influenzae, Neisseria,* and the Enterobacteriaceae.[106–108] Fifty percent of *P. aeruginosa* are inhibited by cefepime at concentrations less than 8 μg/ml.[20] Pharmacodynamic modeling suggests that dosing at 8-hour intervals, rather than the usual 12-hour intervals, may be desirable when treating severe infection caused by *P. aeruginosa.* Cefepime is resistant to hydrolysis by Bush 1 AmpC β-lactamases and by many ESBLs.[20]

Clinical Use

The clinical use of the fourth-generation cephalosporins, in contrast to those of the third generation, is not fully established. Comparative clinical trials have demonstrated the efficiency of cefpirome and cefepime versus ceftazidime or other appropriate comparators in the treatment of complicated and uncomplicated urinary tract infection, skin and soft tissue infection, gynecologic infection, and other severe bacterial infections.[228, 229] Similarly, the efficacy of each agent has been comparable to that of cefotaxime or ceftriaxone in the treatment of severe community-acquired pneumonia.[228–230] Cefpirome and cefepime each was equivalent to ceftazidime for the treatment of severe nosocomial pneumonia.[228, 231] In the treatment of patients with fever and severe neutropenia, cefpirome and cefepime have been as effective ceftazidime and piperacillin plus gentamicin, respectively.[228, 232] The efficacies of cefepime-amikacin and ceftazidime-amikacin were also comparable in the empirical treatment of fever in neutropenic patients.[233] Cefepime and cefotaxime treatment of acute bacterial meningitis in infants and children were comparable in terms of both mortality rates and neurologic sequelae.[234] Thus, in spite of a broader antibiotic spectrum of activity than third-generation cephalosporins including ceftazidime, treatment with the fourth-generation agents has not yielded superior results. Nevertheless, the microbiologic spectrum of action of cefpirome and cefepime suggests that these agents should be optimally targeted as empirical therapy for nosocomial infections in which an increased frequency of resistant gram-negative bacteria (producing Bush class 1 AmpC β-lactamases) are anticipated. That they might be more effective than other cephalosporins in this setting is suggested by the favorable response to cefepime of infections caused by *Enterobacter* spp. with reduced susceptibility or resistance to ceftazidime.[235]

The major clinical successes of the cephalosporms, particularly third-generation cephalosporins have, led to spectacularly increased utilization of these agents. Frequently, when these agents are administered, the therapeutic of prophylaxis indications are not appropriate and less-broad-spectrum therapy would be equally effective. The relentless pressure of β-lactam antibiotics on the Enterobacteriaceae flora has yielded a prominent array of β-lactamase–producing organisms that are resistant to many of the most potent and previously reliable antimicrobials.[42–44, 46, 47, 193, 203–205] Additionally, these newly resistant gram-negative rods play increasing roles as nosocomial pathogens and agents of secondary infection.[205] Similarly, organisms intrinsically resistant to cephalosporins are emerging as major causes of nosocomial infection. Enhanced infection control efforts and more appropriate utilization of antibiotics are necessary if the clinical efficacy of potent antimicrobials, such as the cephalosporins, is to be maintained.

REFERENCES

1. Abraham EP. Cephalosporins 1945–1986. In: Williams JD, ed. The Cephalosporin Antibiotics. Auckland: Adis Press; 1987:1–14.
2. Abraham EP, Loder PB. Cephalosporin C. In: Flynn EH, ed. Cephalosporins and Penicillins: Chemistry and Biology. New York: Academic Press; 1972:2–26.
3. Rolinson GN. The influence of 6-aminopenicillanic acid on antibiotic development. J Antimicrob Chemother. 1988;22:5–14.
4. Huber FM, Chauvette RR, Jackson BG. Preparative methods for 7-aminocephalosporanic acid and 6-aminopenicillanic acid. In: Flynn EH, ed. Cephalosporins and Penicillins. New York: Academic Press; 1972:27.
5. Neu HC. Structure-activity relations of new beta-lactam compounds and in vitro activity against common bacteria. Rev Infect Dis. 1983;5(Suppl): S319–S337.
6. Neu HC. Relation of structural properties of beta-lactam antibiotics to antibacterial activity. Am J Med. 1985;79(Suppl 2A):2–13.
7. Allan JD, Eliopoulos GM, Moellering RC Jr. Antibiotics: Future directions by understanding structure-function relationships. In: Root RK, Trunkey DD, Sande MA, eds. Contemporary Issues in Infectious Diseases, v. 6. New York: Churchill Livingstone; 1987:263–284.
8. Onishi HR, Daoust DR, Zimmerman SB, et al. Cefoxitin, a semisynthetic cephamycin antibiotic: Resistance to β-lactamase inactivation. Antimicrob Agents Chemother. 1974;5:38–48.
9. Stapley EO, Birnbaum J. Chemistry and microbiological properties of the cephamycins. In: Salton MRJ, Shockman GD, eds. Beta-lactam antibiotics. New York: Academic Press; 1981:327–351.
10. O'Callaghan CH, Sykes RB, Griffith A, et al. Cefuroxime, a new cephalosporin antibiotic: Activity in vitro. Antimicrob Agents Chemother. 1976;9:511–519.
11. Neu HC, Fu KP. Cefuroxime, a β-lactamase–resistant cephalosporin with a broad spectrum of gram-positive and negative activity. Antimicrob Agents Chemother. 1978;13:657–664.
12. Dunn GL. Ceftizoxime and other third generation cephalosporins: Structure-activity relationships. J Antimicrob Chemother. 1982;10(Suppl C):1.
13. Boucourt R, Bormann D, Heymes R, et al. Chemistry of cefotaxime. J Antimicrob Chemother. 1980;6(Suppl A):63–67.
14. Neu HC. β-Lactam antibiotics: Structural relationships affecting in vitro activity and pharmacologic properties. Rev Infect Dis. 1986;8(Suppl 3):S237–S259.
15. Shigi Y, Kojo H, Waksugi M, et al. Differences between ceftizoxime and its stereoisomer in antibacterial activity and affinity for penicillin-binding proteins. Antimicrob Agents Chemother. 1981;19:393–396.
16. Neu HC, Labthavikul P. Antimicrobial activity and beta-lactamase stability of ceftazidime, an aminothiazolyl cephalosporin potentially active against *Pseudomonas aeruginosa*. Antimicrob Agents Chemother. 1982;4:11–18.
17. Phillips I, Warren C, Shannon K, et al. Ceftazidime: In vitro antibacterial activity and susceptibility to beta-lactamases compared with that of cefotaxime, moxalactam, and other beta-lactam antibiotics. J Antimicrob Chemother. 1981;8(Suppl B):13–31.
18. Thornsberry C. Review of in vitro activity of third-generation cephalosporins and other newer beta-lactam antibiotics against clinically important bacteria. Am J Med. 1985;79(Suppl 2A):14–20.
19. Neuman M. Mechanisms of action of beta-lactam antibiotics: Relationship between PBP (penicillin-binding proteins) and autolysis. Drugs Exp Clin Res. 1981;7:363–367.
20. Sanders CC. Cefepime. Clin Infect Dis. 1993;17:369–379.
21. Fassbender M, Lode H, Schaberg T, et al. Pharmacokinetics of new oral cephalosporins, including a new carbacephem. Clin Infect Dis. 1993;16:646–653.
22. Neu HC. Oral β-lactam antibiotics from 1960 to 1993. Infect Dis Clin Pract. 1993;6:394–404.
23. Waxman DJ, Yocum RR, Stominger JL. Penicillins and cephalosporins are active site-directed acylating agents: Evidence in support of the substrate analogue hypothesis. Philos Trans R Soc Lond Biol Sci. 1980;289:257–271.
24. Yocum RR, Rasmussin JR, Strominger SL. Mechanism of action of penicillin: Penicillin activates the active site of *Bacillus stearothermophilus* D-alanine carboxypeptidase. J Biol Chem. 1980;255:3977–3986.
25. Spratt BG. Properties of the penicillin-binding proteins of *Escherichia coli* K12. Eur J Biochem. 1977;72:341–352.
26. Neu HC. Penicillin-binding proteins and role of amdinocillin in causing bacterial cell death. Am J Med. 1983;75(Suppl 2A):9–20.
27. Matsuhashi S, Kamiryo T, Blumberg PM, et al. Mechanism of action and development of resistance to a new amdino penicillin. J Bacteriol. 1974;117:578–587.
28. Waxman DJ, Strominger JL. Penicillin-binding proteins and the mechanism of action of β-lactam antibiotics. Annu Rev Biochem. 1983;52:825–869.
29. Tomasz A. Penicillin-binding proteins and the antibacterial effectiveness of β-lactam antibiotics. Rev Infect Dis. 1986;8(Suppl 3):S260–S278.
30. Pitout JDD, Sanders CC, Sanders WE Jr. Antimicrobial resistance with focus on β-lactam resistance in Gram-negative bacilli. Am J Med. 1997;103:51–59.
31. Nikaido H, Nakae T. The outer membrane of gram-negative bacteria. Adv Microb Physiol. 1979;20:163–250.
32. Yoshimura F, Nikaido H. Diffusion of β-lactam antibiotics through the porin channels of *Escherichia coli* K12. Antimicrob Agents Chemother. 1985;27:84–92.
33. Gutmann L, Williamson R, Collatz E. The possible role of porins in antibiotic resistance. Ann Intern Med. 1984;101:554–557.
34. Hopkins JM, Towner KJ. Enhanced resistance to cefotaxime and imipenem associated with outer membrane protein alterations in *Enterobacter aerogenes*. J Antimicrob Chemother. 1990;25:49–55.
35. Nikaido H. Outer membrane barrier as a mechanism of antimicrobial resistance. Antimicrob Agents Chemother. 1989;33:1831–1836.
36. Richmond MH. Factors influencing the antibacterial action of β-lactam antibiotics. J Antimicrob Chemother. 1978;4(Suppl B):1–14.
37. Bush K, Sykes RB. Interaction of β-lactam antibiotics with β-lactamases as a cause for resistance. In: Bryan LE, ed. Antimicrobial Drug Resistance. Orlando: Academic Press; 1984:1–31.
38. Sawai T, Yamaguchi A, Hiruma R. Effect of interaction between outer membrane permeability and β-lactamase production on resistance to β-lactam agents in gram-negative bacteria. Rev Infect Dis. 1988;10:761–764.
39. Hartman BJ, Tomasz A. Low affinity penicillin binding proteins associated with β-lactam resistance in *Staphylococcus aureus*. J Bacteriol. 1984;158:513–516.
40. Utsui Y, Yokota T. Role of an altered penicillin-binding protein in methicillin and cephem-resistant *Staphylococcus aureus*. Antimicrob Agents Chemother. 1985;28:397–403.
41. Sanders CC. β-Lactamases of gram-negative bacteria: New challenges for new drugs. Clin Infect Dis. 1992;14:1089–1099.
42. Sanders CC, Sanders E Jr. β-Lactam resistance in gram-negative bacteria: Global trends and clinical impact. Clin Infect Dis. 1992;15:824–839.
43. Sanders WE Jr, Sanders CC. Inducible β-lactamases: Clinical and epidemiologic implications for use of newer cephalosporins. Rev Infect Dis. 1988;10:830–838.
44. Medeiros AA. Evolution and dissemination of β-lactamases accelerated by generations of β-lactam antibiotics. Clin Infect Dis. 1997;24(Suppl 1) S19–S45.
45. Jacoby GA, Medeiros AA. More extended-spectrum β-lactamases. Antimicrob Agents Chemother. 1991;35:1697–1704.
46. Thompson KS, Prevain AM, Sanders CC. Novel plasmid mediated β-lactamases in Enterobacteriaceae: Emerging problems for new β lactam antibiotics. Curr Clin Top Infect Dis. 1996;16:151–163.
47. Nordmann P. Trends in β-lactam resistance among Enterobacteriaceae. Clin Infect Dis. 1998;27(Suppl 1) S100–S106.
48. Brogard JM, Conte F. Pharmacokinetics of the new cephalosporins. Antibiot Chemother. 1982;31:145–210.
49. Bergan T. Pharmacokinetic properties of the cephalosporins. In: Williams JD, ed. The Cephalosporin Antibiotics. Auckland: Adis; 1987:89–104.
50. Patel IH, Kaplan SA. Pharmacokinetic profile of ceftriazone in man. Am J Med. 1984;77(Suppl 4G):17–25.
51. Wise R. The pharmacokinetics of the oral cephalosporins—A review. J Antimicrob Chemother. 1990;26(Suppl E):13–20.
52. Brogard JM, Jehl F, Aldoff M, et al. High hepatic excretion in humans of cefpiramide, a new cephalosporin. Antimicrob Agents Chemother. 1988;32:1360–1364.
53. Barriere SL, Flaherty JF. Third generation cephalosporins: A critical evaluation. Clin Pharm. 1984;3:351–373.
54. Cherubin CE, Eng RHK, Norrby R, et al. Penetration of newer cephalosporins into cerebrospinal fluid. Rev Infect Dis. 1989;11:526–548.
55. Demotes-Mainard F, Vincon G, Amouretti M, et al. Pharmacokinetics and protein

binding of cefpiramide in patients with alcoholic cirrhosis. Clin Pharmacol Ther. 1991;49:263–269.

56. Chin NX, Neu HC. Cefotaxime and desacetyl cefotaxime: An example of advantageous antimicrobial metabolism. Diagn Microbiol Infect Dis. 1984;2:215.
57. Craig WA, Ebert SC. Killing and regrowth of bacteria in vitro. A review. Scand J Infect Dis. 1991;74(Suppl):63–70.
58. Bundtzen R, Gerber AU, Cohn D, et al. Post-antibiotic suppression of bacterial growth. Rev Infect Dis. 1981;3:28–37.
59. Vogelman B, Gudmundssun S, Turnidge J, et al. In vivo post-antibiotic effect in thigh infection in neutropenic mice. J Infect Dis. 1988;157:287–289.
60. Vogelman B, Gundmundsson S, Leggett J, et al. Correlation of antimicrobial pharmacokinetic parameters with therapeutic efficacy in an animal model. J Infect Dis. 1988;158:831–847.
61. Leggett J, Fantin B, Ebert S, et al. Comparative antibiotic dose-effect relations at several dosing intervals in murine pneumonitis and thigh infection models. J Infect Dis. 1989;159:281–292.
62. Schentag JJ, Smith IL, Swanson DJ, et al. Role for dual individualization with cefmenoxime. Am J Med. 1984;77(Suppl 6A):43–50.
63. Saxon A, Beall GN, Rohr AS, et al. Immediate hypersensitivity reactions to beta-lactam antibiotics. Ann Intern Med. 1987;107:204–215.
64. Lin R. A perspective on penicillin allergy. Arch Intern Med. 1992;152:930–937.
65. Platt R. Adverse effects of third-generation cephalosporins. J Antimicrob Chemother. 1982;10(Suppl C):135–140.
66. Meyers BR. Comparative toxicities of third-generation cephalosporins. Am J Med. 1985;79(Suppl 2A):96–103.
67. Norrby SR. Side effects of cephalosporins. Drugs. 1987;34(Suppl 2):105–120.
68. Sogn DD, Evans R III, Shepherd GM, et al. Results of the National Institute of Allergy and Infectious Diseases collaborative trial to test the predictive value of skin testing with major and minor penicillin derivatives in hospitalized adults. Arch Intern Med. 1992;152:1025–1032.
69. Moellering RC Jr, Swartz MN. The newer cephalosporins. N Engl J Med. 1976;294:24.
70. Donowitz GR, Mandell GL. Beta-lactam antibiotics. N Engl J Med. 1988;313:490–500.
71. Gustaferro CA, Steckelberg JM. Cephalosporin antimicrobial agents and related compounds. Mayo Clin Proc. 1991;66:1064–1073.
72. Bang N, Kammer RB. Hematologic complications associated with beta-lactam antibiotics. Rev Infect Dis. 1983;5(Suppl 2):S380–S393.
73. Nichols RL, Wikler MA, McDevitt JT, et al. Coagulopathy associated with extended-spectrum cephalosporins in patients with serious infections. Antimicrob Agents Chemother. 1987;31:231–235.
74. Conly JM, Ramotar K, Chubb H, et al. Hypoprothrombinemia in febrile, neutropenic patients with cancer: Association with antimicrobial suppression of intestinal microflora. J Infect Dis. 1984;150:202–212.
75. Lipsky JJ, Lewis JC, Novick WJ Jr. Production of hypoprothrombinemia by moxalactam and 1-methyl-5-thiotetrazole in rats. Antimicrob Agents Chemother. 1984;25:380–381.
76. Bechtold H, Andrassy K, Jahnchen E, et al. Evidence for impaired hepatic vitamin K_1 metabolism in patients treated with *N*-methyl-thiotetrazole cephalosporins. Thromb Haemost. 1984;51:358–361.
77. Barza M, Furie B, Brown AE, et al. Defects in vitamin K–dependent carboxylation associated with moxalactam treatment. J Infect Dis. 1986;153:1166–1169.
78. Agnelli G, Del Favero A, Parise P, et al. Cephalosporin-induced hypoprothrombinemia: Is the *N*-methylthiotetrazole side chain the culprit? Antimicrob Agents Chemother. 1986;29:1108–1109.
79. Sattler FR, Colao DJ, Caputo GM, et al. Cefoperazone for empiric therapy in patients with impaired renal function. Am J Med. 1986;81:229–236.
80. Baxter JG, Marble DA, Whitfield LR, et al. Clinical risk factors for prolonged PT/PTT in abdominal sepsis patients treated with moxalactam or tobramycin plus clindamycin. Ann Surg. 1985;201:96–102.
81. Conjura A, Bell W, Lipsky JJ. Cefotetan and hypoprothrombinemia. Ann Intern Med. 1988;108:643.
82. Weitekamp MR, Caputo GM, Al-Mondhiry HA, et al. The effect of latamoxef, cefotaxime, and cefoperazone on platelet function and coagulation in normal volunteers. J Antimicrob Chemother. 1985;16:95–101.
83. Heim-Duthoy KL, Caperton EM, Pollock R, et al. Apparent biliary pseudolithiasis during ceftriaxone therapy. Antimicrob Agents Chemother. 1990;34:1146–1149.
84. Lopez AJ, O'Keefe P, Morrissey M, et al. Ceftriaxone-induced cholelithiasis. Ann Intern Med. 1991;115:712–714.
85. Park HZ, Lee SP, Schy AL. Ceftiraxone-associated gallbladder sludge: Identification of calcium-ceftiraxone salt as a major component of gallbladder precipitate. Gastroenterology. 1991;100:1665–1670.
86. Schaad UB, Suter S, Gianella-Borradori A, et al. A comparison of ceftiraxone and cefuroxime for the treatment of bacterial meningitis in children. N Engl J Med. 1990;322:141–147.
87. Pasternack DP, Stephen BG. Reversible nephrotoxicity associated with cephalothin therapy. Arch Intern Med. 1975;135:599–602.
88. Barza M. Nephrotoxicity of cephalosporins: An overview. J Infect Dis. 1978;137(Suppl):S60–S73.
89. Wade JC, Petty BG, Conrad G, et al. Cephalothin plus an aminoglycoside is more nephrotoxic than methicillin plus an aminoglycoside. Lancet. 1978;2:604–606.
90. Lutt FC. Cephalosporin and aminoglycoside interactions: Clinical and toxicologic implications. In: Whelton A, Neu HC, eds. The Aminoglycosides: Microbiology, Clinical Use and Toxicology. New York: Marcel Dekker; 1982:387–396.
91. Alestig K, Trollfors B, Anderson R, et al. Ceftazidime and renal function. J Antimicrob Chemother. 1984;13:177–181.
92. Foster RS, Raehl CL, Wilson HD. Disulfiram-like reactions associated with a parenteral cephalosporin. Am J Hosp Pharm. 1980;37:858–859.
93. Buening MK, Wold JS, Israel KS, et al. Disulfiram-like reactions to β-lactams. JAMA. 1981;245:2027.
94. Neu HC. Cephalosporins—Cefotaxime 10 years later, a major drug with continued use. Infection. 1991;19(Suppl 6):S309–S315.
95. Cuchural GH Jr, Tally FP, Jacobus NV, et al. Comparative activities of newer β-lactam agents against members of the *Bacteroides fragilis* group. Antimicrob Agents Chemother. 1990;34:479–480.
96. Appleman MD, Heseltine PNR, Cherubin CE. Epidemiology, antimicrobial susceptibility, pathogenicity, and significance of *Bacteroides fragilis* group organisms isolated at Los Angeles County—University of Southern California Medical Center. Rev Infect Dis. 1991;13:12–18.
97. Jones RN. Microbiologic observations of cefmetazole and other cephamycins. Hosp Ther. 1990;15(Suppl 4):3–15.
98. Lee K, Jang IH, Kim YJ, et al. In vitro susceptibilities of the *Bacteroides fragilis* group to 14 antimicrobial agents in Korea. Antimicrob Agents Chemother. 1992;36:195–197.
99. Jones RN, Pfaller MA, Allen SD, et al. Antimicrobial activity of cefpirome: An update compared to five third-generation cephalosporins against nearly 6000 recent clinical isolates from five medical centers. Diagn Microbiol Infect Dis. 1991;14:361–364.
100. Murray RP, Jones RN, Allen SD, et al. Multilaboratory evaluation of the in vitro activity of 13 β-lactam antibiotics against 1474 clinical isolates of aerobic and anaerobic bacteria. Diagn Microbiol Infect Dis. 1993;16:191–203.
101. Jorgensen JH, Doern GV, Maher LA, et al. Antimicrobial resistance among respiratory isolates of *Haemophilus influenzae, Moraxella catarrhalis*, and *Strepcococcus pneumoniae* in the United States. Antimicrob Agents Chemother. 1990;34:2075–2080.
102. Neu HC, Chin NX, et al. The in vitro activity and beta lactamase stability of cefpirome (HR 810), a pyridine cephalosporin agent active against staphylococci, enterobacteriaceae, and *Pseudomonas aeruginosa*. Infection. 1985;13:146–155.
103. King A, Boothman C, Phillips I. Comparative in vitro activity of cefpirome and cefepime, two new cephalosporins. Eur J Clin Microbiol Infect Dis. 1990;9:677–685.
104. Chin NX, Gu Jin, et al. In vitro activity and β-lactamase stability of GR69153, a new long acting cephalosporin. Antimicrob Agents Chemother. 1991;35:259–266.
105. Neu HC, Chin NX, Jules K, et al. The activity of BMY 28142, a new broad spectrum β-lactamase stable cephalosporin. J Antimicrob Chemother. 1986;17:441–452.
106. Steele HCH, Edwards, Rissing JP. In-vitro activity of BMY 28142, a new aminothiazolyl cephalosporin. J Antimicrob Chemother. 1985;16:463–468.
107. Norden CW, Neiderriter K. In vitro activity of BMY-28142, a new cephalosporin. Chemotherapy. 1987;33:15–17.
108. Masuyoshi S, Hiraoka M, Inoue M, et al. Comparison of the in vitro and in vivo antibacterial activities of cefepime (BMY-28142) with ceftazidime, cefuzonam, cefotaxime and cefmonoxime. Drugs Exp Clin Res. 989;15:1–10.
109. Hartstein AI, Patrick KE, Jones SR, et al. Comparison of pharmacologic antimicrobial properties of cephadroxil and cephalexin. Antimicrob Agents Chemother. 1977;12:93–97.
110. Silver MS, Counts GW, Zeleznik D, et al. Comparison of in vitro antibacterial activity of three oral cephalosporins: Cefaclor, cephalexin and cephadrine. Antimicrob Agents Chemother. 1977;12:591–596.
111. Renzini G, Ravagnan G, Oliva B. In vitro and in vivo microbiological evaluation of cephapirin, a new antibiotic. Chemotherapy. 1975;21:289–296.
112. Klein JO, Eickhoff TC, Tilles JG, et al. Cephalothin: Activity in vitro, absorption and excretion in normal subjects and clinical observations in 40 patients. Am J Med Sci. 1964;248:640–656.
113. Sabath LD, Wilcox C, Garner C, et al. In vitro activity of cefazolin against recent clinical bacterial isolates. J Infect Dis. 1973;128(Suppl):S320–S326.
114. Myers JP, Linneman CC Jr. Bacteremia due to methicillin-resistant *Staphylococcus aureus*. J Infect Dis. 1982;145:532–536.
115. Bergeron MG, Brusch JL, Barza M, et al. Bactericidal activity and pharmacology of cefazolin. Antimicrob Agents Chemother. 1973;4:396–401.
116. Regamey C, Libke RD, Engelking ER, et al. Inactivation of cefazolin, cephaloridine, and cephalothin by methicillin-sensitive and methicillin-resistant strains of *Staphylococcus aureus*. J Infect Dis. 1975;131:291–294.
117. Fong IW, Engelking ER, Kirby WMM. Relative inactivation by *Staphylococcus aureus* of eight cephalosporin antibiotics. Antimicrob Agents Chemother. 1976;9:939–944.
118. Quinn EL, Pohlod D, Madhavan T, et al. Clinical experience with cefazolin and other cephalosporins in bacterial endocarditis. J Infect Dis. 1983;128(Suppl):S386–S391.
119. Neiss E. Cephradine: Summary of preclinical studies and clinical pharmacology. J Irish Med Assoc. 1973;66(Suppl):1–12.
120. Weber DJ, Wolfson JS, Swartz MN, et al. *Pasteurella multocida* infections: Report of 34 cases and review of the literature. Medicine. 1984;63:133–154.
121. Kaiser AB. Antimicrobial prophylaxis in surgery. N Engl J Med. 1986;315:1129–1138.
122. Antimicrobial prophylaxis in surgery. Med Lett. 1993;35:91–94.
123. Sanders CV, Greenberg RN, Marier RL. Cefamandole and cefoxiton. Ann Intern Med. 1985;103:70–78.
124. Fraser DG. Drug therapy reviews: Antimicrobial spectrum, pharmacology and

therapeutic use of cefamandole and cefoxitin. Am J Hosp Pharm. 1979;36:1503–1508.

125. Delgado DG, Crau CJ, Cobbs CG, et al. Clinical and laboratory evaluation of cefamandole in therapy of *Haemophilus* sp. Bronchopulmonary infections. Antimicrob Agents Chemother. 1979;15:807–812.
126. Meyers BR, Hirschman SZ. Antibacterial activity of cefamandole in vitro. J Infect Dis. 1978;137(Suppl):S25–S31.
127. Doern G. In vitro activity of loracarbef and effects of susceptibility test methods. Am J Med. 1992;92(Suppl 6A):75–155.
128. Thornsberry C. Review of the in vitro antibacterial activity of cefprozil, a new oral cephalosporin. Clin Infect Dis. 1992;14(Suppl 2):S189–S194.
129. Actor P. In vitro experience with cefonicid. Rev Infect Dis. 1984;6(Suppl 4):S783–S790.
130. Birnbaum J, Stapley EO, Miller AK, et al. Cefoxitin, a semi-synthetic cephamycin: A microbiologic overview. J Antimicrob Chemother. 1978;4:15–32.
131. Ward A, Richards DM. Cefotetan: A review. Drugs. 1985;30:382–426.
132. Ayres LW, Jones RN, Barry AL, et al. Cefotetan, a new cephamycin. Antimicrob Agents Chemother. 1982;22:859–877.
133. Aldridge KE, Sanders CC, Janney A, et al. Comparison of the activities of penicillin G and new β-lactam antibiotics against clinical isolates of *Bacteroides* species. Antimicrob Agents Chemother. 1984;26:410–413.
134. Goldstein EJC, Citron DM. Annual incidence, epidemiology and comparative in vitro susceptibilities to cefoxitin, cefotetan, cefmetazole and ceftizoxime of recent community-acquired isolates of the *Bacteroides fragilis* group. J Antimicrob Chemother. 1988;26:2361–2366.
135. Jones RN. Review of the in-vitro spectrum and characteristics of cefmetazole (CS = 1170). J Antimicrob Chemother. 1989;12(Suppl D):1–12.
136. Jacob LS, Layne P. Cefonicid: An overview of clinical studies in the United States. Rev Infect Dis. 1984;6(Suppl 4):S791.
137. Platt R, Zaleznik DF, Hopkins CC, et al. Perioperative antibiotic prophylaxis for herniorrhaphy and breast surgery. N Engl J Med. 1990;322:153–160.
138. Marks WA, Stutman HR, Marks MI, et al. Cefuroxime versus ampicillin plus chloramphenicol in childhood bacterial meningitis: A multicenter randomized controlled trial. J Pediatr. 1986;109:123–130.
139. Quagliarello VJ, Scheld WM. Treatment of bacterial meningitis. N Engl J Med. 1997;336:708–716.
140. Harding SM, Williams PEO, Ayrton J. Pharmacology of cefuroxime as the 1-acetoxyethyl ester in volunteers. Antimicrob Agents Chemother. 1984;25:78–82.
141. Sommers D, Wan Wyk M, Williams PEO, et al. Pharmacokinetics and tolerance of cefuroxime axetil in volunteers during repeated dosing. Antimicrob Agents Chemother. 1984;25:344–347.
142. DeSante KA, Zeckel ML: Pharmacokinetic profile of loracarbef. Am J Med. 1992;92(Suppl 6A)16S–25S.
143. Cooper RDG. The carbacephems: A new beta-lactam antibiotic glass. Am J Med. 1992;92(Suppl 6A):2S–6S.
144. Morel C, Vergnaud M, Langeard MM, et al. Cefotetan: Comparative study in vitro against 266 gram-negative clinical isolates. J Antimicrob Chemother. 1983;11(Suppl A):31–36.
145. Peters GR, Metzler CM. The effects of cefmetazole and latamoxef on platelet function in healthy human volunteers. J Antimicrob Chemother. 1989;23(Suppl D):119–123.
146. Pines A, Raafat HH, Khorasani M, et al. Cefuroxime and ampicillin compared in a double-blind study in the treatment of lower respiratory tract infections. Chemotherapy. 1981;27:459–465.
147. Mehtar S, Parr JH, Morgan DJR. A comparison of cefuroxime and cortimoxazole in severe respiratory tract infections. J Antimicrob Chemother. 1982;9:479–484.
148. Schleupner CJ, Anthony WC, Tan J, et al. Blinded comparison of cefuroxime to cefaclor for lower respiratory tract infections. Arch Intern Med. 1988;148:343–348.
149. Dere WH. Acute bronchitis: Results of U.S. and European trials of antibiotic therapy. Am J Med. 1992;92(Suppl 6A):53S–57S.
150. Zeckel ML. Loracarbef (LY163892) in the treatment of actue exacerbations of chronic bronchitis: Results of U.S. and European comparative clinical trials. Am J Med. 1992;92(Suppl 6A):58S–64S.
151. Hyslop DL. Efficacy and safety of loracarbef in the treatment of pneumonia. Am J Med. 1992;92(Suppl 6A):65S–69S.
152. McCarty J. Loracarbef versus penicillin VK in the treatment of streptococcal pharyngitis and tonsillitis in an adult population. Am J Med. 1992;92(Suppl 6A):74S–79S.
153. McCarty J, Ruoff GE, Jacobson KD. Loracarbef (LY163892) versus cefaclor in the treatment of bacterial skin and skin-structure infections in an adult population. Am J Med. 1992;92(Suppl 6A):80S–85S.
154. Hyslop DL, Bischoff W. Loracarbef (LY163892) versus cefaclor and norfloxacin in the treatment of uncomplicated pyelonephritis. Am J Med. 1992;92(Suppl 6A):86S–93S.
155. Stutman HR, Arguedas AG. Comparison of cefprozil with other antibiotic regimens in the treatment of children with acute otitis media. Clin Infect Dis. 1992;14(Suppl 2):S204–S208.
156. McCarty JM, Renteria A. Treatment of pharyngitis and tonsillitis with cefprozil: Review of three multicenter trials. Clin Infect Dis. 1992;14(Suppl 2):S224–S230.
157. Pelletier LL Jr. Review of the experience with cefprozil for the treatment of lower respiratory tract infections. Clin Infect Dis. 1992;14(Suppl 2):S238–S243.
158. Iravani A. Multicenter comparison of safety and efficacy of cefprozil vs. cefaclor in the treatment of acute uncomplicated urinary tract infections. Clin Infect Dis. 1992;14(Suppl 2):S252.
159. Nolen TM. Clinical trials of cefprozil for treatment of skin and skin-structure infections: Rev Clin Infect Dis. 1992;14(Suppl 2):S255–S263.
160. Davies BL, Maesen FDV, Teengs JP. Cefuroxime axetil in acute purulent exacerbations of chronic bronchitis infections. Infection. 1987;15:253–256.
161. Pichichero ME. Evidence for copathogenicity as a mechanism for bacterial resistance. Infect Dis Clin Pract. 1998;7(Suppl 4):S248–S253.
162. Felmingham D. Review of comparative in vitro activity of some oral cephalosporins. Infect Dis Clin. Pract. 1998;7(Suppl 2):S75–S80.
163. Nicolau DP. Pharmacodynamic considerations in oral cephalosporin therapy: Implications for selection and effectiveness. Infect Dis Clin Pract. 1998;7(Suppl 2):S81–S82.
164. Klein JO. Microbiologic efficacy of antibacterial drugs for acute otitis media. Pediatr Infect Dis J. 1993;12:973–975.
165. Nadelman RB, Luger SW, Frank E, et al. Comparison of cefuroxime axetil and doxycycline in the treatment of early Lyme disease. Ann Intern Med. 1992;117:273–280.
166. Poindexter AN III, Sweet R, Ritter M. Cefotetan in the treatment of obstetric and gynecologic infections. Am J Obstet Gynecol. 1986;154:946–950.
167. Lefrock JL, Blais F, Schell RD, et al. Cefoxitin in the treatment of diabetic patients with lower extremity infections. Infect Surg. 1983;2:361–374.
168. Drusano GL, Warren W, Saah AJ, et al. A prospective randomized controlled trial of cefoxitin versus clindamycin-aminoglycoside in mixed anaerobic-aerobic infections. Surg Gynecol Obstet. 1982;154:715–720.
169. Wilson SE, Boswick JA, Duma RJ, et al. Cephalosporin therapy in intraabdominal infections: A multicenter randomized, comparative study of cefotetan, moxalactam and cefoxitin. Am J Surg. 1988;155(Suppl 5A):61–66.
170. Sweet R, Gall SA, Gobbs RS, et al. Multicenter clinical trial comparing cefotetan with moxalactam or cefoxitin as therapy for obstetric gynecologic infections. Am J Surg. 1988;155(Suppl 5A):56–60.
171. Griffith DL, Novak E, Greenwald CA, et al. Clinical experience with cefmetazole sodium in the United States: An overview. J Antimicrob Chemother. 1989;23(Suppl D):21–33.
172. Moran JS, Zenilman JM. Therapy for gonococcal infections: Options in 1989. Rev Infect Dis. 1990;12(Suppl 6):S633–S644.
173. Centers for Disease Control and Prevention. 1998 Guidelines for treatment of sexually transmitted diseases. MMWR Morb Mortal Wkly Rep. 1998;47:RR-1.
174. Peterson HB, Galaid EI, Zenilman JM. Pelvic inflammatory disease: Review of treatment options. Rev Infect Dis. 1990;12(Suppl 6):S656–S664.
175. Orr JW, Varner RE, Kilgore LC, et al. Cefotetan versus cefoxitin as prophylaxis in hysterectomy. Am J Obstet Gynecol. 1986;154:960–963.
176. McGregor JA, French JI, Makowski E. Single dose cefotetan versus multidose cefoxitin for prophylaxis in cesarean section in high risk patients. Am J Obstet Gynecol. 1986;154:955–960.
177. Gorbach SL. The role of cephalosporins in surgical prophylaxis. J Antimicrob Chemother. 1989;23(Suppl D):61–70.
178. Neu HC. Pathophysiologic basis for the use of third-generation cephalosporins. Am J Med. 1990;88(Suppl 4A):3S–11S.
179. Trenholme GM, Schmitt BA, Nelson JA, et al. Comparative study of three different dosing regimens of cefotaxime for gram-negative bacteremia. Diagn Microbiol Infect Dis. 1989;12:107–112.
180. Fu KP, Neu HC. Antibacterial activity of ceftizoxime, a β-lactamase stable cephalosporin. Antimicrob Agents Chemother. 1980;17:583–590.
181. Cleeland R, Squires E. Antimicrobial activity of ceftriaxone, a review. Am J Med. 1984;77:3–11.
182. Jones RN, Barry Al, et al. In vitro activity of evaluation of cefodizime (HR221), a new semisynthetic cephalosporin. Antimicrob Agents Chemother. 1981;20:760–768.
183. Labro MT, Amit N, et al. Cefodizime (HR221) potentiation of human neutrophil oxygen-dependent bactericidal activity. J Antimicrob Chemother. 1987;19:331–341.
184. Neu HC, Chin NX, Labthavikul P. Comparative in vitro activity and β-lactamase stability of FR 17027, a new orally active cephalosporin. Antimicrob Agents Chemother. 1984;26:174–180.
185. Jones RN. Antimicrobial activity spectrum and pharmacokinetics of old and new orally administered cephems. Antimicrob Newslett. 1988;5:1–8.
186. Neu HC, Saha G, Chin NX. Comparative in vitro activity and β-lactamase stability of FK482, a new oral cephalosporin. Antimicrob Agents Chemother. 1989;33:1795–1800.
187. Briggs BN, Jones RN, Erwin ME, et al. In vitro activity evaluations of cefdinir (FK482, CI-983, and PD134393): A novel orally administered cephalosporin. Diagn Microbiol Infect Dis. 1991;14:425–434.
188. Stevens DL. Current concepts in the treatment of strephococcal pharyngitis. Infect Dis Clin Pract. 1998;7(Suppl 2):S86–S89.
189. Adam D. Modern cephalosporins as therapeutics for otitis media. Infect Dis Clin Pract. 1998;7(Suppl 2):S96–S98.
190. Gwaltney JM Jr, Savolainer S, Rivas P, et al. Comparative effectiveness and safety of cefdinir and amoxicillin-clavulanate in the treatment of acute community acquired bacterial sinusitis. Antimicrob Agents Chemother. 1997;41:1517–1520.
191. Drehobl M, Bianchi P, Keyserling CH, et al. Comparison of cefdinir and cefaclor in treatment of community-acquired pneumonia. Antimicrob Agents Chemother. 1997;41:1579–1583.
192. Brogen RN, Carmine A, Heel RC, et al. Cefoperazone, a review of its in vitro antimicrobial activity, pharmacological properties and therapeutic efficacy. Drugs. 1981;22:423–460.
193. Rice LB, Willey SH, Papanicolaou GA, et al. Outbreak of ceftazidime resistance

caused by extended-spectrum β-lactamases at a Massachusetts chronic care facility. Antimicrob Agents Chemother. 1990;34:2193–2199.
194. Schafer V, Shah PM, Doerr HW, et al. In vitro activity of cefpirome against isolates from patients with urinary tract, lower respiratory tract and wound infections. J Antimicrob Chemother. 1992;29(Suppl A):7–12.
195. Meyer BH, Muller FO, Luus HG, et al. Safety, tolerance and pharmacokinetics of cefpirome administered intramuscularly to healthy subjects. J Antimicrob Chemother. 1992;29(Suppl A):63–70.
196. Wolff M, Chavanet P, Kazmierczak A, et al. Diffusion of cefpriome into the cerebrospinal fluid of patients with purulent meningitis. J Antimicrob Chemother. 1992;29(Suppl A):59–62.
197. Pfaller MA, Niles AC, Murray PR. In vitro antibacterial activity of cefpiramide. Antimicrob Agents Chemother. 1984;25:368–372.
198. Fukasawa M, Noguchi H, Okuda T, et al. In vitro antibacterial activity of SM-1652 a new broad-spectrum cephalosporin with anti-pseudomonal activity. Antimicrob Agents Chemother. 1983;3:195–200.
199. Young JPW, Husson JM, Bruch K, et al. The evaluation of efficacy and safety of cefotaxime: A review of 2500 cases. J Antimicrob Chemother. 1980;6(Suppl A):293–300.
200. Daikos GK, Kosmidis J, Giamarellou H, et al. Evaluation of cefotaxime in a hospital with high antibiotic resistance rates. J Antimicrob Chemother. 1980;6(Suppl A):255–261.
201. Scully BE, Neu HC. The use of ceftizoxime in the treatment of critically ill patients infected with multiply antibiotic resistant bacteria. J Antimicrob Chemother. 1982;10(Suppl C):141–150.
202. Eron LJ, Park CH, Goldenberg RI, et al. Ceftriaxone therapy of serious bacterial infections. J Antimicrob Chemother. 1983;12:65–78.
203. Chow JW, Fine MJ, Shlaes DM, et al. *Enterobacter* bacteremia: Clinical features and emergence of antibiotic resistance during therapy. Ann Intern Med. 1991;115:585–590.
204. Jacobson KL, Cohen SH, Inciardi JF et al. The relationship between antecedent antibiotic use and resistance to extended spectrum cephalosporins in group 1 β-lactamase-producing organisms. Clin Infect Dis. 1995;21:1107–1113.
205. D'Agata E, Venkataraman L, DeGirolami P. Multidrug resistant gram-negative bacilli: Epidemiology and risk factors for colonization. Crit Care Med 1998; (In press).
206. Thornsberry C, Ogilvie P, Kahn J, et al. Surveillance of antimicrobial resistance in *Streptococcus pneumoniae, Haemophilus influenzae*, and *Moraxela catarrhalis* in the United States in 1996–97 respiratory season. Diagn Microbial Infect Dis 1997;29:249–257.
207. Bartlett JG, Breiman RF, Mandell LA, et al. Community-acquired pneumonia in adults: Guidelines for management. Clin Infect Dis. 1998;26:811–838.
208. Norrby SR. Role of cephalosporins in the treatment of bacterial meningitis in adults: Overview with special emphasis on ceftazidime. Am J Med. 1985; Suppl 2A:56–61.
209. Jacobs RJ, Wells TG, Steele RW, et al. A prospective randomized comparison of cefotaxime vs ampicillin and chloramphenicol for bacterial meningitis in children. Pediatr Infect Dis. 1986;4:362–368.
210. Barson WJ, Miller MA, Brady MT, et al. Prospective comparative trial of ceftriaxone vs conventional therapy for treatment of bacterial meningitis in children. Pediatr Infect Dis. 1986;4:362–368.
211. Congeni BL. Comparison of ceftriaxone and traditional therapy of bacterial meningitis. Antimicrob Agents Chemother. 1984;25:40–44.
212. Bryan JP, Rocha H, daSilva HR, et al. Comparison of ceftriaxone and ampicillin plus chloramphenicol for therapy of acute bacterial meningitis. Antimicrob Agents Chemother. 1985;28:361–368.
213. Lecour H, Seara A, Miranda AM, et al. Treatment of 160 cases of acute bacterial meningitis with cefotaxime. J Antimicrob Chemother. 1984;14(Suppl B):195–202.
214. Mullaney DT, John JF. Cefotaxime therapy: Evaluation of its effects on bacterial meningitis, CSF drug levels, and bactericidal activity. Arch Intern Med. 1983;143:1705–1708.
215. Fong IW, Tompkins KB. Review of *Pseudomonas aeruginosa* meningitis with special emphasis on treatment with ceftazidime. Rev Infect Dis. 1985;7:604–612.
216. Wolff MA, Young CL, Ramphal R. Antibiotic therapy for enterobacter meningitis: A retrospective review of 13 episodes and review of the literature. Clin Infect Dis. 1983;16:772–777.
217. Viladrich PF, Gudiol F, Linares J, et al. Characteristics and antibiotic therapy of adult meningitis due to penicillin-resistant pneumococci. Am J Med. 1988;84:839–846.
218. Hughes WT, Armstrong D, Bodey GP, et al. Guidelines for the use of antimicrobial agents in neutropenic patients with unexplained fever. J Infect Dis. 1990;161:381–396.
219. Handsfield HH, McCormack WM, Hook EW, et al. A comparison of single-dose cefixime with ceftriaxone as treatment for uncomplicated gonorrhea. N Engl J Med. 1991;325:1337–1341.
220. Schulte JM, Schmid GP. Recommendations for treatment of chancroid, 1993. Clin Infect Dis. 1995;20(Suppl 1):539–546.
221. Dattwyler RJ, Halperin JJ, Pass H, et al. Ceftiraxone as effective therapy in refractory Lyme disease. J Infect Dis. 1987;155:1322–1325.
222. Dattwyler RJ, Halperin JJ, Volkman DJ, et al. Treatment of late Lyme borreliosis—randomized comparison of ceftriaxone and penicillin. Lancet. 1988;1:1191–1194.
223. Francioli P, Etienne J, Hoigne R, et al. Treatment of streptococcal endocarditis with a single daily dose of ceftriaxone sodium for 4 weeks. JAMA. 1992;267:264–267.
224. Sookpranee M, Boonma P, Susaengrat W, et al. Multicenter prospective randomized trial comparing ceftazidime plus co-trimoxazole with chloramphenicol plus doxycycline and co-trimoxazole for treatment of severe melioidosis. Antimicrob Agents Chemother. 1992;158–162.
225. Islam A, Butler T, Nath SK, et al. Randomized treatment of patients with typhoid fever by using ceftriaxone or chloramphenicol. J Infect Dis. 1988;158:742–747.
226. Finch RG. Third-generation cephalosporins in the treatment of rare infections. Am J Med. 1990;88(Suppl 4A):25S–31S.
227. Bryskier A. New concepts in the field of cephalosporins: C-3′ quaternary ammonium cephem (Group IV). Clin Micro Infect. 1997;3(Suppl 1):S1–S6.
228. Garau J, Wilson W, Wood M, Carlet J. Fourth generation cephalosporins: a review of in vitro activity, pharmacokinetics, pharmacodynamics, and clinical utility. Clin Micro Infect. 1997;3(Suppl 1):S87–S101.
229. Hoepelman AI, Kieft H, Aoun M, et al. International comparative study of cefepime and ceftazidime in the treatment of serious bacterial infections. J Antimicrob Chemother. 1993;32(Suppl B):175–186.
230. Zervos M, Nelson M, Cefepime Study Group. Cefepime versus ceftriaxone for empiric treatment of hospitalized patients with community-acquired pneumonia. Antimicrob Agents Chemother. 1998;42:729–733.
231. McCabe R, Chirurgi V, Farkas SA, et al. A new therapeutic option for the treatment of pneumonia. Am J Med. 1996;100(Suppl 6A):60S–67S.
232. Yamamura D, Gucalp R, Carlisle P, et al. Open randomized study of cefepime versus piperacillin-gentamicin for treatment of febrile neutropenic cancer patients. Antimicrob Agents Chemother. 1997;41:1704–1708.
233. Cordonnier C, Herbrecht R, Pico JL, et al. Cefepime/amikacin versus ceftazidime/amikacin as empirical therapy for febrile episodes in neutropenic patients: A comparative study. Clin Infect Dis. 1997;24:41–51.
234. Saez-Llorens X, Castano E, Garcia R, et al. Prospective randomized comparison of cefpemie and cefotaxime for treatment of bacterial meningitis in infants and children. Antimicrob Agents Chemother. 1995;39:937–940.
235. Sanders WE Jr, Tenney JH, Kessler RE. Efficacy of cefepime in the treatment of infections due to multiply resistant *Enterobacter* species. Clin Infect Dis. 1996;23:454–461.
236. Kessler RE, Fung-Tomc J. Susceptibility of bacterial isolates to β-lactam antibiotics from US clinical trials over a 5-year period. Am J Med. 1996;100(Suppl 6A): 13S–19S.

Chapter 20

Other β-Lactam Antibiotics*

HENRY F. CHAMBERS

CARBAPENEMS

Carbapenems are differentiated from penicillins and cephalosporins by a methylene replacement for sulfur in the five-membered α-ring structure, which, as in the cephalosporins, also contains a double bond. They are derivatives of thienamycin, a compound produced by *Streptomyces cattleya.*[1]

Imipenem

Chemistry. In addition to those features shared by other carbapenems, imipenem differs from the conventional β-lactams in the nature and conformation of its side chain. All conventional penicillins and cephalosporins contain an acylamino side chain, whereas imipenem has a hydroxyethyl side chain. Furthermore, the side chain in the conventional β-lactams is in a *cis* configuration, whereas the hydroxyethyl side chain of imipenem is in a *trans* configuration. It is this *trans* conformation that is responsible for the β-lactamase stability of imipenem.

Antibacterial Activity. Imipenem is the *N*-formimidoyl derivative of thienamycin (Fig. 20–1). Imipenem has excellent in vitro activity against aerobic gram-positive species such as the hemolytic streptococci of Lancefield classifications A, B, C, and G, with minimal inhibitory concentration (MIC) values of 0.2 μg/ml or less (Table 20–1).[2, 3] *Streptococcus pneumoniae* organisms are inhibited by less

*This chapter is based, in part, on a chapter originally prepared by Dr. Chambers and the late Harold C. Neu.

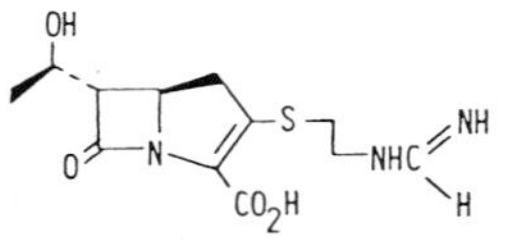

FIGURE 20–1. Imipenem.

than 0.1 μg/ml, and many, but not all, penicillin-resistant strains of *S. pneumoniae* (MIC >4 μg/ml) are inhibited by 1 μg/ml or less. Penicillin-susceptible strains of *Enterococcus faecalis* are inhibited by less than 1.5 μg/ml; however, like penicillin, imipenem is bacteriostatic, not bactericidal, against susceptible enterococci. Non-β-lactamase–producing penicillin-resistant strains of enterococci and *Enterococcus faecium* are resistant to imipenem. *Staphylococcus aureus* and *Staphylococcus epidermidis* are inhibited by less than 0.2 and 1.5 μg/ml, respectively. Methicillin-resistant staphylococci also are resistant to imipenem. *Listeria* and *Bacillus* spp. are inhibited by less than 1 μg/ml.[4]

Most of the Enterobacteriaceae are inhibited by concentrations of imipenem less than or equal to 1 μg/ml. Some *Proteus* strains have MIC values of 2 to 4 μg/ml. *Haemophilus infuenzae* and *Neisseria gonorrhoeae,* including their β-lactamase–producing isolates, are inhibited by less than 0.5 μg/ml.

Pseudomonas aeruginosa, including strains resistant to antipseudomonal penicillins and cephalosporins, are inhibited by 1 to 6 μg/ml.[5] *Stenotrophomonas maltophilia* is resistant, as are many strains of *Burkholderia cepacia*. Most *Acinetobacter* organisms are inhibited by less than 1 μg/ml.

Imipenem inhibits most anaerobic species, including *Bacteroides fragilis*.[6, 7] Most *Clostridium* spp. are inhibited by 1 μg/ml or less, with the exception of *Clostridium difficile,* which is resistant. *Fusobacterium, Actinomyces, Campylobacter,* and *Yersinia* are inhibited by imipenem, and many *Nocardia asteroides* strains are inhibited by 1 μg/ml. It also inhibits *Mycobacterium avium-intracellulare* and some *Legionella* spp.

Mechanism of Action. Imipenem binds with high affinity to high-molecular-weight penicillin-binding proteins (PBPs) of both gram-positive and gram-negative bacteria. It is not hydrolyzed by most β-lactamases, penicillinases, cephalosporinases—plasmid or chromosomally mediated—of *S. aureus, Escherichia coli, Enterobacter cloacae, Citrobacter freundii, Proteus rettgeri, Serratia marcescens, Proteus vulgaris, Klebsiella oxytoca, Pseudomonas aeruginosa, B. cepacia,* and *B. fragilis*. It is hydrolyzed by a *S. maltophilia* β-lactamase, some *Bacillus,* and *Bacteroides* enzymes.

Carbapenems show a postantibiotic effect (PAE) against gram-negative organisms, in contrast to penicillins and cephalosporins and like that of aminoglycosides and fluoroquinolones. The PAE varies by organism and species. It is best seen with *P. aeruginosa* and allows the drug to be administered less frequently than would be expected on the basis of the activity present in serum. This PAE is noted in the presence of nutrient broth, urine, and serum.

Resistance. In *S. maltophilia* there is production of a β-lactamase that hydrolyzes imipenem and other carbapenems. A similar enzyme exists in some *B. cepacia* as well. However, resistance results principally from the absence or loss of an outer membrane protein, referred to as D2, which is in contrast to outer membrane proteins F and C, through which cephalosporins and penicillins traverse the outer membrane of gram-negative organisms. This has been a problem primarily in *P. aeruginosa*. Some hyperproducers of chromosomal β-lactamase in *E. cloacae* have been isolated that are also deficient in outer membrane protein.

Pharmacology. Imipenem is not absorbed after oral ingestion because of its instability in gastric acid. Imipenem is removed from the circulation by glomerular filtration and secretion. It is hydrolyzed by the renal peptidase dehydropeptidase-1, located on the brush border of the proximal renal tubules. To overcome the problem of the destruction of imipenem in urine, cilastatin, a dehydropeptidase inhibitor, is administered in equal amounts to imipenem. Cilastatin has no antibacterial activity nor does it alter the antibacterial activity of imipenem. Cilastatin does not affect zinc metalloenzyme peptidases or angiotensin-converting enzymes. Metabolites of imipenem in the absence of cilastatin are nephrotoxic.

Imipenem is not destroyed in the general circulation and is widely distributed to various body compartments.[8, 9] There is minimal biliary secretion of imipenem, and there is minimal change in bowel flora. In the absence of meningeal inflammation, only minor amounts of imipenem enter the cerebrospinal fluid (CSF). In the presence of meningeal inflamation, CSF levels of 1 to 5 μg/ml have been recorded. Imipenem has a high affinity for brain cells.

After 20 to 30 minutes of infusion of 250 mg imipenem plus 250 mg cilastatin, mean peak serum levels of imipenem are 13 μg/ml. After 500 mg, mean peak serum levels are 33 μg/ml; 1000 mg produces a peak concentration of 52 μg/ml.[10, 11] The half-life of imipenem is 1 hour in healthy people. The serum half-life is 4 hours in patients whose creatinine clearance is less than 10 ml/min. The half-life of cilastatin increases to a much greater extent than does that of imipenem and reaches 16 hours in anuria.[12] Imipenem and cilastatin are removed from the body by hemodialysis, with dialysis half-lives of 2.5 and 3.8 hours, respectively. In the presence of cilastatin, urinary recovery of imipenem is 70% with a 25 to 29% recovery of the metabolites. Fecal elimination of imipenem is less than 1%.[13]

Adverse Reactions. Imipenem has generally been well tolerated.[14] It causes minimal phlebitis when used intravenously. It can cause immediate hypersensitivity,[15] and cross-reactions with penicillins have occurred. No major adverse effects such as diarrhea, pseudomembranous colitis, coagulation abnormalities, nephrotoxicity, or hepatotoxicity have been reported. Rapid infusion of imipenem has produced nausea and emesis in about 1% of patients. About 2 to 4% of imipenem-treated patients have a onefold to twofold elevation of aspartate transaminase (AST), alanine transaminase (ALT), or both. Leukopenia has occurred, but infrequently. No drug interactions have been reported. The most serious toxicity is seizures, an infrequent side effect that occurs most often in patients with underlying central nervous system pathology and in those with decreased renal function in whom dose adjustment has not been made. Seizures have been reported in up to 1.5% of patients, in some studies, although the manufacturer reports an incidence of 0.4%.

Clinical Use. Animal infection studies have demonstrated the utility of imipenem as therapy for staphylococcal endocarditis (but not enterococcal endocarditis, where high relapse rates were noted),[16, 17] for bacteremia caused by *P. aeruginosa* in neutropenic rats,[18] and for pyelonephritis in rats. Similarly, imipenem has been found to be useful in humans in the treatment of bone and soft tissue infections, obstetric and gynecologic infections, complicated urinary tract infections, intra-abdominal sepsis, pneumonia, and endocarditis caused by *S. aureus*.[19–25] Imipenem is effective as a single agent in the treatment of febrile neutropenic patients.[26] Imipenem has activity against *N. asteroides* in vitro and in a murine model of cerebral infection.[27] Clinical experience is limited.[28]

In cystic fibrosis patients receiving imipenem as a single agent for the treatment of pulmonary exacerbations, a significant number of *P. aeruginosa* isolates resistant to imipenem have been encountered.[29] In addition, the treatment of pneumonia caused by *P. aeruginosa* in patients without cystic fibrosis with imipenem as a single agent has had a disappointingly low success rate.[30] These observations suggest that imipenem should not be used alone as therapy for serious pseudomonal infections, particularly those involving the respiratory tract.

The use of imipenem is most appropriate in the treatment of infections caused by cephalosporin-resistant Enterobacteriaceae, particularly *C. freundii* and *Enterobacter* spp.; as empiric therapy in the treatment of serious infections in patients previously treated with multiple antibiotics, because of the high likelihood of encountering organisms resistant to more conventional β-lactams; as a single agent in the treatment of the febrile, neutropenic patient; and in the treatment of polymicrobial infections where otherwise multiple-drug regimens of higher cost and potentially more adverse side effects would be necessary. The recommended dose of imipenem for serious infections is 0.5 g is administered intravenously every 6 to 8 hours for patients with normal renal function. The pediatric dose is 15 to 25 mg/kg every 6 hours. Dosage adjustment is required for patients with creatinine clearance of less than 50 ml/minute.

Meropenem

Chemistry. Meropenem's acyl side chain is in a *cis* position rather than a *trans* position as in penicillin and cephalosporins. However, it has a dimethylcarbanoyl pyrolidiolidyn derivative on position 2 of the ring, in contrast to the *N*-formidyl group present in imipenem. This makes it stable to dihydropeptidase 1.

Mechanism of Action. Excellent penetration into bacteria, high affinity for PBPs, and stability to β-lactamases account for its activity. Studies with *K. pneumoniae, E. coli,* and *Salmonella* spp. using liposomal membranes reconstituted from purified protein porins of outer membranes of *P. aeruginosa* show that meropenem penetrates these gram-negative organisms more readily than does imipenem, accounting for its greater activity against them.[31]

Antibacterial Activity. Meropenem is slightly more active than imipenem against gram-negative organisms. It inhibits *P. aeruginosa* resistant to imipenem by virtue of more rapid entry into these organisms. There is no cross-resistance to ceftazidime or other cephalosporins, nor with the antipseudomonas ureidopenicillins such as piperacillin. Meropenem shows a PAE against *P. aeruginosa* similar to that of imipenem.

Resistance. Like imipenem, meropenem is hydrolyzed, albeit slowly, by β-lactamases such as the zinc-dependent β-lactamase that exists in *S. maltophilia.* It also does not bind to PBPs of *E. faecium,* which uses PBP5 and PBP6 to make cell wall. Because it is more rapidly transported through the D2 porin of gram-negative organisms than is imipenem, resistance caused by permeability is uncommon.

Pharmacology. Meropenem is a dimethylcarbamoyl pyrolidinyl derivative of thienamycin (Fig. 20–2). Its spectrum of antibacterial activity is very similar to that of imipenem (see Table 20–1), with potent activity against a variety of gram-positive species, gram-negative aerobes, and anaerobic species. It is slightly less active than imipenem against gram-positive bacteria but more active against gram-negative organisms, including some imipenem-resistant strains of *P. aeruginosa.*[32]

Meropenem, unlike imipenem, is not significantly degraded by renal tubular dehydropeptidase-1 and therefore does not require coadministration of an inhibitor. Its pharmacology is otherwise very similar to that of imipenem. The mean peak serum concentration with intravenous administration of a single 500-mg dose over 30 minutes is approximately 30 μg/ml in healthy persons and 50 μg/ml in those with end-stage renal disease; half-lives are 1 and 10 hours, respectively. Clearance is linearly proportional to the glomerular filtration rate.[33] Dosage adjustment is required in patients with reduced renal function. The dose need not be adjusted in patients with impaired lever function.[34] Meropenem is removed by hemodialysis and should be administered after each dialysis session. It penetrates inflamed meninges and into bile, bone, synovial fluid, and most tissues. CSF concentrations are approximately 1 to 5 μg/ml.[35]

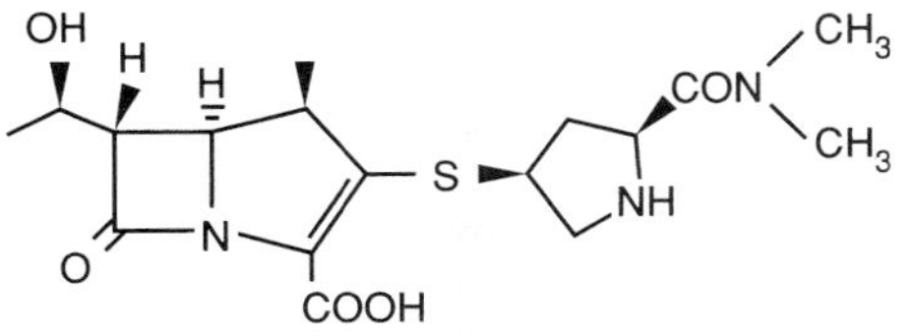

FIGURE 20–2. Meropenem.

TABLE 20–1 Comparative Activity of Imipenem and Meropenem against Aerobic and Anaerobic Bacteria

Organism	MIC$_{90}$ (μg/ml)	
	Imipenem	*Meropenem*
*Staphylococcus aureus**†	0.03	0.3
Coagulase-negative staphylococci*†	0.1	1
Streptococcus pyogenes	0.03	0.1
Streptococcus agalactiae	0.03	0.1
Streptococcus pneumoniae	0.02	0.03
Enterococcus faecalis	2	8
Haemophilus influenzae	2	0.1
Neisseria gonorrhoeae	0.1	0.03
Neisseria meningitidis	0.1	0.01
Listeria monocytogenes	0.3	0.3
*Klebsiella pneumoniae**	0.3	0.1
*Enterobacter cloacae**	1	0.1
*Enterobacter aerogenes**	1	0.1
*Escherichia coli**	0.1	0.03
*Klebsiella oxytoca**	1	0.03
*Aeromonas hydrophila**	8	0.3
Citrobacter freundii	1	0.1
*Citrobacter diversus**	0.5	0.02
*Serratia marcescens**	4	0.1
Proteus marabilis	4	0.1
*Morganella morganii**	4	0.2
*Proteus vulgaris**	4	0.1
Acinetobacter anitratus	0.5	1
*Pseudomonas aeruginosa**	4	2
Stenotrophomonas maltophilia	>50	>50
Burkholderia cepacia	16	32
Bacteroides fragilis	2	1
Prevotella melaninogenicus	0.1	0.1
Clostridium difficile	4	2
Clostridium perfringens	0.1	0.02
Anaerobic gram-positive cocci	0.5	0.3
Campylobacter jejuni	0.03	0.02

*Both β-lactamase- and non-β-lactamase–containing strains.
†Methicillin-susceptible strains; methicillin-resistant strains are also resistant to imipenem and meropenem.

The toxicity profile of meropenem is similar to that of imipenem except that meropenem may be less epileptogenic, permitting the use of higher doses.[36] Meropenem is also less nephrotoxic than imipenem because of its lack of susceptibility to degradation by renal peptidases.

Clinical experience with meropenem indicates that it is therapeutically equivalent to imipenem.[37–39] It has been used successfully to treat pneumonia, meningitis, intra-abdominal infections, bacteremia, urinary tract infections, and febrile episodes in neutropenic patients.[40, 41] It is approved by the U.S. Food and Drug Administration for treatment of serious infections in children 3 months of age and older.[44, 45] As with other antibiotics, single-drug therapy for serious *P. aeruginosa* infections has been accompanied by emergence of resistance to meropenem.[45] Although it is uncertain whether emergence of resistance may be prevented and outcome improved,[46–48] combination therapy should be used whenever possible to treat serious infections caused by *P. aeruginosa.*[49] The recommended adult dose of meropenem for patients with creatinine clearance greater than 50 ml/min is 500 to 1000 mg intravenously every 6 to 8 hours. The pediatric dose is 10 to 20 mg/kg every 6 to 8 hours.

MONOBACTAMS

The development of new methods by Sykes and colleagues[45] to screen large numbers of organisms for the production of β-lactam

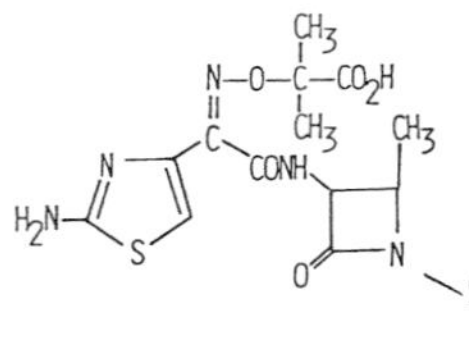

FIGURE 20–3. Aztreonam.

antibiotics showed that a number of bacteria, particularly *Gluconobacter* and *Acinetobacter,* produced monocyclic β-lactam antibiotics with antibacterial activity. From *Chromobacterium violaceum* a monocyclic compound was isolated, and its structure was confirmed. This compound was subsequently modified to yield a highly active therapeutic agent, aztreonam.

Aztreonam

Aztreonam is a monocyclic β-lactam (Fig. 20–3). Aztreonam has no appreciable antibacterial activity against gram-positive or anaerobic bacteria because it does not bind to PBPs in these species. Aztreonam binds primarily to PBP3 in Enterobacteriaceae, *Pseudomonas,* and other gram-negative aerobic organisms. It produces long filamentous structures that are not viable. Aztreonam readily passes through the outer membrane of gram-negative species. It is not hydrolyzed by most plasmid and chromosomal β-lactamases but is hydrolyzed by *K. oxytoca* and *B. cepacia* and by the cefotaxime-hydrolyzing plasmid enzymes.

Antibacterial Activity. Aztreonam inhibits most Enterobacteriaceae at concentrations below 0.5 μg/ml (Table 20–2); some *P. aeruginosa, E. cloacae,* and *C. freundii* strains are resistant. Most *P. aeruginosa* organisms are inhibited by less than 16 μg/ml. Most *B. cepacia* and *S. maltophilia* are resistant, as are many *Acinetobacter* spp.; *Haemophilus* and *Neisseria,* including β-lactamase–producing isolates, are inhibited by less than 0.2 μg/ml. *Yersinia* and *Aeromonas* are inhibited by less than 0.5 μg/ml. In general, the antibacterial activity is minimally affected by inoculum size except for *P. aeruginosa,* and there is no major difference between the MIC and the minimum bactericidal concentration (MBC).[50, 51] Aztreonam acts synergistically with aminoglycosides against *P. aeruginosa* and some Enterobacteriaceae. Enterobacteriaceae and *P. aeruginosa* can be resistant owing to a failure to penetrate the outer membrane, destruction by β-lactamases (i.e., *S. maltophilia*), or a failure to bind to PBPs.

Pharmacokinetics. Aztreonam is not absorbed from the gastrointestinal tract.[52] It is rapidly and completely absorbed after intramuscular administration, with peak serum concentrations attained within 1 hour.[53] A 500-mg intramuscular aztreonam dose produces serum concentrations of 21 to 27 μg/ml at 1 hour, 3.8 to 5.9 μg/ml at 6 hours, and 1.5 to 3.3 μg/ml at 8 hours. After intravenous infusion of a single dose of 0.5, 1, or 2 g of aztreonam in healthy adults over a period of 30 minutes, peak serum concentrations of the drug immediately after completion of the infusion average 55 to 65, 90 to 160, and 200 to 255 μg/ml, respectively. Aztreonam serum concentrations 1 hour after an intramuscular dose are the same as after an intravenous dose.

Aztreonam is widely distributed into body tissues and fluids.[53] Therapeutic levels are present in adipose tissue, bone, gallbladder, liver, lungs, kidney, heart, intestinal tissue, and prostatic tissue. It is also present in saliva, sputum, bronchial secretions, bile, and pericardial, pleural, peritoneal, and synovial fluids.

Aztreonam enters the CSF after intravenous administration, with CSF concentrations at 1 and 4 hours after a 2-g dose of 2 and 3.2 μg/ml, respectively.[54] In neonates and children 3 months to 2 years of age with bacterial meningitis who received a 30 mg/kg dose of aztreonam by intravenous injection over a period of 3 minutes, CSF aztreonam concentrations ranged from 2.1 to 20.8 μg/ml at 0.8 to 4.3 hours after the dose.[55]

Aztreonam is removed from the body primarily by renal mechanisms of glomerular filtration and tubular secretion. No active metabolites have been found in serum or urine. In adults with normal renal and hepatic function, the distribution half-life of aztreonam averages 0.2 to 0.7 hours, and the elimination half-life averages 1.3 to 2.2 hours. The half-life of aztreonam averages 1.7 hours in children 2 months to 12 years of age. In neonates 7 days old and weighing less than 2.5 kg, the half-life of aztreonam averages 5.5 to 9.9 hours.[55]

Serum concentrations of aztreonam are higher and the serum half-life is prolonged in patients with renal impairment.[56] In adults with renal impairment, the half-life of aztreonam averages 3.5, 5.6, 7.8, and 8.5 hours in adults with creatinine clearances of 30 to 80, 10 to 30, 10 or less, and 2 ml/minute, respectively. The half-life of aztreonam is only slightly prolonged in patients with hepatic impairment.

Aztreonam is excreted as unchanged drug by both glomerular filtration and tubular secretion. Approximately 58 to 74% of the dose is excreted unchanged and 1 to 7% as open-ring metabolites.[53] In adults with normal renal function, urinary concentrations of aztreonam after a single intravenous dose of 0.5 or 1 g average 250 to 330 and 710 to 720 μg/ml, respectively, 4 to 6 hours after the dose.[57]

Aztreonam and its renal metabolite are removed by hemodialysis.[56, 58] The serum half-life of aztreonam averages 2.7 hours during hemodialysis and 6 to 8 hours between dialysis sessions. A 4-hour period of hemodialysis removes 25 to 50% of a dose. Aztreonam is removed to a lesser extent by peritoneal dialysis. With a 6-hour dwell time, about 10% of a single 1-g intravenous dose of aztreonam is removed.[58]

TABLE 20–2 In Vitro Activity of Aztreonam

Organism	MIC_{90} (μg/ml)
Escherichia coli	0.25
Klebsiella pneumoniae	1
Klebsiella oxytoca	1
Enterobacter cloacae	16
Enterobacter aerogenes	8
Enterobacter agglomerans	1
Citrobacter freundii	8
Citrobacter diversus	0.25
Serratia marcescens	4
Proteus mirabilis	0.01
Proteus vulgaris	0.12
Proteus rettgeri	0.12
Morganella morganii	0.25
Providencia	0.025
Salmonella enteritidis	0.25
Shigella	0.12
Arizona hinshawii	0.12
Aeromonas hydrophila	0.12
Aeromonas shigelloides	0.12
Yersinia enterocolitica	2
Pasteurella multocida	0.12
Salmonella typhi	0.12
Haemophilus influenzae	0.12
Neisseria gonorrhoeae	0.25
Neisseria meningitidis	0.025
Pseudomonas aeruginosa	16
Stenotrophomonas maltophilia	>128
Pseudomonas, other (*P. diminuta, P. stutzeri, P. fluorescens*)	>128
Burkholderia cepacia	>128
Streptococcus pyogenes	16
Streptococcus pneumoniae	16
Enterococci	>128
Clostridium	>128
Bacteroides spp.	>128

Data from Edwards JR, Turner PJ, Wannop C, et al. In vitro antibacterial activity of SM-7338, a carbapenem antibiotic with stability to dehydropeptidase I. Antimicrob Agents Chemother. 1989;33:215–222; and Sentochnik DE, Eliopoulos GM, Ferraro MJ, et al. Comparative in vitro activity of SM7338, a new carbapenem antimicrobial agent. Antimicrob Agents Chemother. 1989;33:1232–1236.

Adverse Reactions. No major adverse reactions to aztreonam have been reported. Skin rashes have occurred. Neither anaphylaxis nor rashes have occurred after its use in patients with positive skin test reactions to penicillins (see Chapter 21). About 2 to 4% of patients have increases in serum transaminase values two times greater than normal when receiving aztreonam. No hematologic, gastrointestinal, nephrotoxic, or neurotoxic reactions have been noted with this agent.

Clinical Use. Aztreonam has been used for the treatment of a variety of infections such as cystitis, pyelonephritis, lower respiratory tract infections including pneumonia and bronchitis, septicemia, skin and skin structure infections, infections of postoperative wounds or ulcers and burns, intra-abdominal infection including peritonitis, and gynecologic infections including endometritis and pelvic cellulitis caused by gram-negative aerobic bacteria.[59–65] Because of its lack of cross-reactivity with other β-lactam antibiotics, aztreonam can be used safely in patients with serious allergy to penicillins or cephalosporins. The usual dose is 1 to 2 g every 6 to 8 hours intravenously or intramuscularly, with a daily dose for serious infection of 6 g. The drug is not approved for pediatric use but has been given at a dose of 18.75 to 37.5 mg/kg every 6 hours intravenously or intramuscularly.

Because aztreonam has a spectrum of activity limited to aerobic gram-negative bacteria, the drug should not be used alone for empiric therapy in seriously ill patients if there is any possibility that the infection may be caused by gram-positive aerobic bacteria or if a mixed aerobic-anaerobic bacterial infection is suspected. An anti-infective agent effective against the suspected organism or organisms should be used concomitantly. Aztreonam has been used safely and effectively in conjunction with clindamycin, erythromycin, metronidazole, penicillins, and vancomycin.

β-LACTAMASE INHIBITORS

β-Lactamase inhibitors are clavulanic acid and penicillanic acid sulfone derivatives. These compounds, which have weak antibacterial activity, are potent inhibitors of many plasmid-encoded and some chromosomal β-lactamases. These compounds therefore can restore antibacterial activity of amoxicillin, ampicillin, piperacillin, mezlocillin, and cefoperazone, all of which can be destroyed by β-lactamases commonly produced by gram-positive and gram-negative, bacteria (Table 20–3). Although competitive inhibition is seen, β-lactamase inhibitor primarily acts as a suicide substrate that forms a stable intermediate, rendering the enzyme inactive.

Three β-lactamase inhibitors are in clinical use: clavulanic acid, sulbactam, and tazobactam. Each inhibitor is available only as a fixed-combination preparation that includes an active β-lactam antibiotic as the companion agent. There are minor differences in potency, activity, and pharmacology among the β-lactamase inhibitors, but clinically they can be considered therapeutically equivalent except for some *Klebsiella* spp., where clavulanate inhibits isolates resistant to sulbactam and tazobactam. The antibacterial activity of the inhibitor-antibiotic combination is determined by the spectrum of the companion β-lactam antibiotic. The three parenteral combinations—ampicillin-sulbactam, ticarcillin-clavulanate, and piperacillin-tazobactam—although differing in bacterial spectrum and pharmacology, have similar indications, including treatment of pneumonia, complicated skin and skin tissue infections, and intra-abdominal infections.[66, 67]

TABLE 20–3 Activity of Amoxicillin-Clavulanate against Amoxicillin-Resistant Organisms

Organism	Amoxicillin	Augmentin*
Staphylococcus aureus	256	1.0
Staphylococcus epidermidis	256	2.0
Staphylococcus aureus (MRSA)	256	16.0
Haemophilus influenzae	64	0.5
Branhamella catarrhalis	16	0.25
Neisseria gonorrhoeae	128	1.0
Escherichia coli	>256	8.0
Klebsiella pneumoniae	128	4.0
Proteus mirabilis	>256	4.0
Proteus vulgaris	>256	2.0
Bacteroides fragilis	32	0.5
Enterobacter, Citrobacter, Serratia spp. and *Pseudomonas aeruginosa*	>128	>128

*Contains amoxicillin and clavulanate in a 2:1 ratio.

TABLE 20–4 Inhibition of β-Lactamases by β-Lactam Inhibitors

β-Lactamase	Name	Organisms	Inhibited by Clavulanate, Sulbactam, and Tazobactam
Plasmid		*Staphylococcus aureus*	Yes
Plasmid	TEM-1	*Escherichia coli* *Haemophilus* *Neisseria gonorrhoeae* *Salmonella* *Shigella*	Yes
Plasmid	TEM-2	*E. coli*	Yes
Plasmid	TEM-3 to -8	*Klebsiella*	Yes
Plasmid	SHV-1	*Klebsiella*	Yes
Plasmid	SHV-2 to -5	Enterobacteriaceae	Yes
Plasmid	OXA-1, 2, 3	*E. coli*	Variable
Plasmid	PSE-1, 2, 3	*Pseudomonas*	Variable
Chromosomal	Type 1a*	*Enterobacter* *Morganella* *Citrobacter* *Serratia*	No
Chromosomal	Type Id*	*Pseudomonas*	No
Chromosomal	Type IV, K1*	*Klebsiella*	Yes
Chromosomal		*Bacteroides*	Yes
Chromosomal		*Legionella*	Yes
Chromosomal		*Branhamella*	Yes

*Classification based on Richmond MM, Sykes RB. The beta-lactamases of gram-negative bacteria and their possible physiological role. Adv Microb Physiol. 1973;9:31–88.

β-Lactamase inhibitors are most effective against β-lactamases produced by *S. aureus, H. influenzae, Branhamella catarrhalis, Bacteroides* spp., and some Enterobacteriaceae. Chromosomal β-lactamases of *Serratia* spp., *C. freundii, Enterobacter* spp., *P. aeruginosa,* and some Enterobacteriaceae are not inhibited by β-lactamase inhibitors.

β-Lactamase inhibitors are most active against plasmid-encoded β-lactamases, the most common of which is TEM-1, so called for the initials of the original patient from whom the *E coli* β-lactamase containing isolate was derived. There are also TEM-2; oxacillin-hydrolyzing enzymes OXA-1, -2, and -3; sulfhydro-inhibited enzymes SHV-1 and HMS; and PSE-1, -2, -3, and -4, originally thought to be enzymes found only in *Pseudomonas* but now found occasionally in *E. coli.* All of these plasmid enzymes are inhibited, as are the new cefotaxime-ceftazidime–hydrolyzing enzymes TEM-3 through -27 and SHV-2, -3, -4, -5, -7, and -8 (Table 20–4).

Inhibition of chromosomal β-lactamases by β-lactamase inhibitors is variable. The most important chromosomal β-lactamases, which generally are of the Richmond-Sykes class I type (see Fig. 15–2 in Chapter 15) are present in *Acinetobacter, Citrobacter, Enterobacter, Proteus, Pseudomonas,* and *Serratia.*[68] These are inducible enzymes that are not inhibited by β-lactamase inhibitors at clinically useful concentrations. β-Lactamases are produced constitutively by some *Enterobacter, C. freundii,* and *Aeromonas* spp., and these are not inhibited. However, chromosomal β-lactamases of *Legionella* and *Bacteroides* are inhibited by β-lactamase inhibitors, as are some other chromosomally mediated β-lactamases, such as the class IV enzymes produced by *Klebsiella.*[69, 70]

Clavulanate

The β-lactamase inhibitor clavulanate (Fig. 20–4) was found in cultures of *Streptomyces clavuligerus.* It showed only a low level of

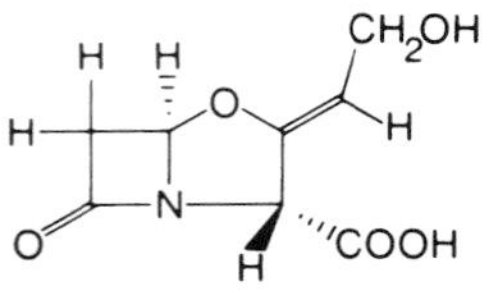

FIGURE 20–4. Clavulanate.

antibacterial action, but, when the compound was combined with penicillin G, inhibition of a *Klebsiella* isolate normally resistant to penicillin was noted. Clavulanate has subsequently been shown to inhibit certain types of β-lactamases from a number of clinically important gram-positive and gram-negative organisms.[71] Clavulanate in combination with amoxicillin is available for oral administration; in a parenteral preparation it is available in many countries, but not in the United States. Clavulanate in combination with ticarcillin is available for intravenous administration in the United States.

Pharmacology. Clavulanate is moderately well absorbed from the gastrointestinal tract, with peak serum levels occurring 40 to 120 minutes after ingestion. Mean peak serum levels for a 62.5-mg dose are 1 μg/ml; for 125 mg, 4 μg/ml; and for 250 mg, 6 μg/ml.[72, 73] Combining clavulanate with amoxicillin does not significantly alter the pharmacologic parameters of either drug. The pharmacokinetics of orally administered clavulanate in children in terms of peak serum levels and plasma half-lives of the drug are similar to those in adults.[74, 75]

The absorption of clavulanate is unaffected by the simultaneous administration of food, milk, or aluminum hydroxide–containing antacids. After intravenous infusion of clavulanate combined with either amoxicillin or ticarcillin, the drug is rapidly distributed. Peak serum concentrations are approximately 11 μg/ml after a 200-mg intravenous dose, with drug detectable to levels of 0.2 μg/ml at 6 hours.[76, 77] Peak serum concentrations of clavulanate in children receiving 5 mg/kg have been 19 μg/ml, with less than 1 μg/ml present at 3 hours.[75]

The serum half-life of clavulanate is slightly less than that of amoxicillin, 0.76 to 1.4 hours. No accumulation of clavulanate occurs until creatinine clearances fall to less than 10 ml/minute.[72] Dose adjustment is made for amoxicillin or ticarcillin. Clavulanate has been shown to be degraded in vivo in animals, with metabolites being excreted via lung, feces, and urine and only 20 to 60% appearing unchanged in urine 6 hours after an oral dose. After a dose of 125 mg of clavulanate, urine levels are 115 to 508 μg/ml for 0 to 2 hours and 45 to 74 μg/ml for 4 to 6 hours.[78]

Clavulanate concentrations of less than 1 μg/ml are achieved in sputum after the oral administration of amoxicillin-clavulanate, but pleural fluid levels are 46 to 91% of peak serum levels. There is rapid penetration of clavulanate into peritoneal fluid, with mean peritoneal fluid levels of clavulanate equaling 66% of serum levels.[76, 79] After 200 mg of clavulanate, peritoneal fluid levels fall to less than 5 μg/ml after about 0.5 hours and to less than 1 μg/ml after about 3 hours. Clavulanate does not penetrate noninflamed meninges, but after large intravenous doses in patients with meningitis CSF levels of clavulanate have been in the range of 1 μg/ml. Clavulanate produces therapeutic levels in bile, middle ear fluid, and tonsil tissue.[79] Clavulanate crosses the placenta and may be found in the cord blood of newborns and in the amniotic fluid, but no clavulanate can be detected in breast milk.

Adverse Reactions. No new or major adverse reactions to the use of clavulanate combined with either amoxicillin or ticarcillin have been reported. The incidence of skin reactions has been similar to that seen when penicillin is used alone. Diarrhea has occurred after the use of 250 mg clavulanate given three times daily, and some nausea has occurred with this dosage program. Parenteral use of amoxicillin-clavulanate and ticarcillin-clavulanate has not caused undue diarrhea.

Amoxicillin-Clavulanate

Amoxicillin-clavulanate (Augmentin) has been used in a number of different clinical settings. The combination has proved useful as therapy for acute otitis media in children that is caused by β-lactamase–producing *H. influenzae* and *B. catarrhalis*.[80] It has also been used to treat sinusitis and, rarely, pharyngitis in persons whose large tonsillar tissue contains β-lactamase–producing *Prevotella melaninogenica*.[80] Amoxicillin-clavulanate has proved useful in lower respiratory tract infections such as exacerbations of bacterial bronchitis or pneumonitis caused by β-lactamase–producing bacteria. It has proved particularly useful to treat bite wounds of human or animal origin. Skin structure infections caused by streptococci and staphylococci have responded to amoxicillin-clavulanate with results comparable to those achieved with oral antistaphylococcal agents and oral cephalosporins.[81] Amoxicillin-clavulanate has been used to treat diabetic foot infections because it has activity against staphylococci, anaerobes, and aerobic gram-negative bacteria. The agent is formulated as 250 to 750 mg of amoxicillin with 125 mg of clavulanate, and dosing is as for the amoxicillin component. The usual dose is 0.25 g (of amoxicillin) every 8 hours to 0.750 g every 12 hours, by mouth. In children the dose is 20 to 45 mg/kg per day in two or three divided doses. The twice-daily formulation (750 mg of amoxicillin and 125 mg of clavulanate by tablet for adults; 400 and 57 mg, respectively, in suspension for children) is as effective as the thrice-daily formulation.[82, 83]

Ticarcillin-Clavulanate

Ticarcillin-clavulanate has been used for treatment of community- and hospital-acquired pneumonia, particularly in cases involving aspiration of oral secretions and aerobic gram-negative bacilli.[84] Intra-abdominal infections and gynecologic infections have been treated successfully, as have skin structure infections and osteomyelitis.[85, 86] When ticarcillin-clavulanate has been used to treat febrile neutropenic patients, it has been necessary to combine it with an aminoglycoside. The usual dose is 3.1 g administered every 4 to 6 hours. The dose should be reduced in patients with creatinine clearance of less than 30 ml/minute (see Chapter 42).

Sulbactam

Sulbactam (Fig. 20–5) is a 6-desaminopenicillin sulfone. Sulbactam is a broader-spectrum β-lactamase inhibitor than clavulanic acid, but it is less potent. Sulbactam does not induce chromosomal β-lactamases, nor does it select for derepressed β-lactamase–producing bacteria. Sulbactam is available in the United States only in combination with ampicillin (Unasyn), in a ratio of 0.5 g of sulbactam per 1 g of ampicillin as a parenteral formulation for intravenous administration.

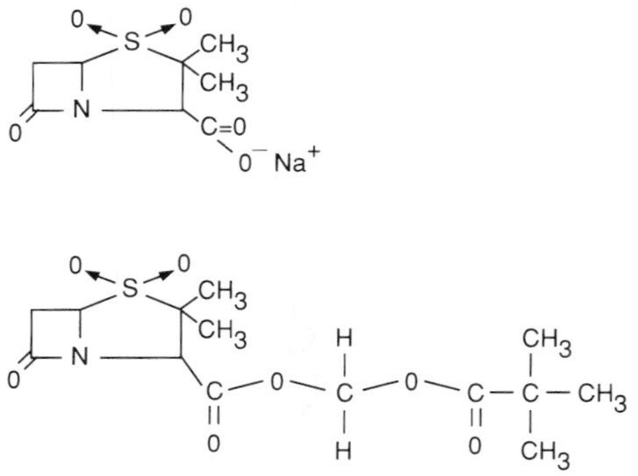

FIGURE 20–5. Sulbactam (*top*) and sulbactam oral ester (*bottom*).

Pharmacology. Sulbactam has pharmacokinetics in humans similar to those of ampicillin.[87, 88] Peak serum levels after intramuscular injections of 0.250 and 0.5 g are 7 and 13 μg/ml, respectively, with a serum half-life of 1.1 to 1.3 hours. After the intravenous infusion of 0.5 g, a peak serum level of 30 μg/ml is achieved, and after 1 g, 68 μg/ml is achieved. The serum half-life is 1 hour. Sulbactam is excreted by the kidney and has a urinary recovery rate of 70 to 80% of a dose. Biliary excretion is minimal, and metabolism is less than 25%. Renal excretion is blocked by probenecid. The half-life is not significantly altered until the creatinine clearance falls to less than 30 ml/min. With clearances between 15 and 30 ml/minute, the half-life is 5.1 hours, with clearances of 5 to 15 it is 9.2 hours, and the half-life in anuric patients is 20 hours. It can be removed by hemodialysis. Concentrations of sulbactam in interstitial fluid and peritoneal secretions are comparable to levels in serum. Penetration of sulbactam into inflamed meninges is low, with levels of 0.1 to 10 μg/ml found in the CSF after an infusion of 1 g.

Adverse Reactions. Clinical studies of the combination of sulbactam plus ampicillin have revealed no major hematologic, renal, hepatic, or central nervous system reactions.[89–91] Diarrhea has not been a major problem after intravenous use. Skin reactions are similar to those found for ampicillin, and there is occasional elevation of transaminase levels.

Clinical Use. Sulbactam-ampicillin and amoxicillin-clavulanate have the same spectrum of antibacterial activity. Sulbactam-ampicillin has been used in the treatment of mixed bacterial infections such as intra-abdominal infections, obstetric and gynecologic infections, and soft tissue and bone infections.[92, 93] It has been used to treat meningitis in infants and children and to treat epiglottitis and selected other pediatric infections.[94, 95] However, the pediatric experience is limited, and third-generation cephalosporins would be preferred in such infections.

Tazobactam

Tazobactam is a penicillanic acid sulfone β-lactamase inhibitor with a structure similar to that of sulbactam (Fig. 20–6). Its spectrum of β-lactamase inhibition is like that of sulbactam, but its potency is more like that of clavulanic acid. It does not induce chromosomal β-lactamases.[96–98] It is available for parenteral administration only in combination with piperacillin (Zosyn) in an 8:1 ratio of piperacillin to tazobactam by weight.

Pharmacology. Mean peak serum concentration after a 30-minute intravenous infusion of 500 mg of tazobactam is 25 μg/ml in healthy subjects.[99] The clearance of tazobactam is primarily renal, and dosage should be adjusted for creatinine clearances of less than 40 ml/minute. Combining tazobactam with piperacillin reduces clearance of tazobactam, but the clearance of piperacillin is not affected. Clearances of piperacillin and tazobactam are similar in subjects with normal renal function. Peak serum concentrations are approximately 50% higher in those with end-stage renal disease.[99] The half-life of tazobactam is 1 hour in subjects with normal renal function, increasing to 3.6 hours (compared with 2 hours for piperacillin) in those with a creatinine clearance of less than 20 ml/minute. The half-life of tazobactam is approximately 7 hours in patients with end-stage renal disease. Hemodialysis removes 31% and 39% of the administered dose of piperacillin and tazobactam, respectively. These differences in pharmacokinetics of piperacillin and tazobactam do not require adjustment of the dose of tazobactam independent of piperacillin; the dose is adjusted based on the pharmacokinetics of piperacillin. Patients undergoing hemodialysis should have the dose of piperacillin-tazobactam administered after dialysis. Negligible amounts of either drug are removed by peritoneal dialysis.

Tissue levels of tazobactam reflect a percent penetration that is similar to that of piperacillin for each tissue type.[100] Tazobactam penetrates inflamed meninges. CSF concentrations of piperacillin and tazobactam were 16% and 32% of simultaneous serum concentrations, respectively, in a rabbit meningitis model.[101]

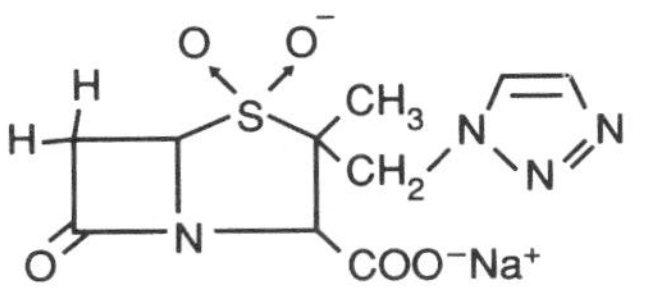

FIGURE 20–6. Tazobactam.

Adverse Reactions. Limited clinical data do not indicate any new or unusual toxicity unique to tazobactam.

Clinical Use. Piperacillin-tazobactam has the broadest spectrum of the three parenteral β-lactamase inhibitor combinations. Published clinical studies have been conducted mainly in adults. Limited experience with this combination for treatment of serious infections in children indicates that it is safe and effective.[102, 103] However, until its role is better defined, other agents are preferred. In general the antibacterial spectrum of piperacillin-tazobactam is similar in vitro to that of ticarcillin-clavulanate. Piperacillin-tazobactam is slightly more active than ticarcillin-clavulanate for some strains (including enterococci), presumably because of the greater intrinsic activity of piperacillin.[96, 98] In clinical trials the efficacy of piperacillin-tazobactam has been equivalent, and occasionally superior, to similarly broad-spectrum comparator drugs (e.g., ticarcillin-clavulanate, imipenem, third-generation cephalosporins) for treatment of pneumonia, skin and soft tissue infections, intra-abdominal infections, polymicrobial infections, and febrile neutropenia in combination with an aminoglycoside.[104–112] Piperacillin-tazobactam should not be used to treat *Pseudomonas* pneumonia because the dose of piperacillin is too low. The adult dose is 12 to 16 g/day of piperacillin (with 1.5 to 2 g/day of tazobactam), administered in divided doses every 6 to 8 hours for creatinine clearance greater than 40 ml/minute.

REFERENCES

1. Kahan JS, Kahan FM, Goegleman R, et al. Thienamycin, a new beta-lactam antibiotic: 1. Discovery, isolation and physical properties. J Antibiot (Tokyo). 1979;32:1–12.
2. Edwards JR, Turner PJ, Wannop C, et al. In vitro antibacterial activity of SM-7338, a carbapenem antibiotic with stability to dehydropeptidase I. Antimicrob Agents Chemother. 1989;33:215–222.
3. Sentochnik DE, Eliopoulos GM, Ferraro MJ, et al. Comparative in vitro activity of SM7338, a new carbapenem antimicrobial agent. Antimicrob Agents Chemother. 1989;33:1232–1236.
4. Jones RN. Review of the in vitro spectrum of activity of imipenem. Am J Med. 1985;78:22–32.
5. Prince AS, Neu HC. Activities of new beta-lactam antibiotics against isolates of *Pseudomonas aeruginosa* from patients with cystic fibrosis. Antimicrob Agents Chemother. 1981;20:545–546.
6. Brown JE, Del Benes VE, Collins CD. In vitro activity of *N*-formimidoyl thienamycin, moxalactam and other new beta-lactam agents against *Bacteroides fragillis:* Contribution of beta-lactamase to resistance. Antimicrob Agents Chemother. 1981;19:248–252.
7. Kesado T, Hashizume T, Ashi Y, et al. Susceptibilities of anaerobic bacteria to *N*-formimidoyl thienamycin (MK0787) and to other antibiotics. Antimicrob Agents Chemother. 1982;21:1016–1022.
8. Norrby SR, Alestig K, Bjauorngard B, et al. Urinary recovery of *N*-formimidoyl thienamycin (MK0787) as affected by coadministration of *N*-formimidoyl thienamycin dehydropeptidase inhibitors. Antimicrob Agents Chemother. 1983;23:300–307.
9. Norrby SR, Alestig K, Ferber F, et al. Pharmacokinetics and tolerance of *N*-formimidoyl thienamycin (MK0787) in humans. Antimicrob Agents Chemother. 1983;23:293–299.
10. Drusano GL, Standiford HC, Ruslamante C, et al. Multiple dose kinetics of imipenem/cilastatin. Antimicrob Agents Chemother. 1984;26:715–721.
11. Drusano GL, Standiford HC. Pharmacokinetic profile of imipenem/cilastatin in normal volunteers. Am J Med. 1985;78:47–53.
12. Berman SJ, Sugihara JG, Nakumara JM, et al. Multiple dose study of imipenem/cilastatin in patients with end-stage renal disease undergoing long-term hemodialysis. Am J Med. 1985;78:105–108.

13. Norrby SR, Rogers JD, Ferber F, et al. Disposition of radio labeled imipenem and cilastatin in normal human volunteers. Antimicrob Agents Chemother. 1985;26:707–714.
14. Calandra GB, Ricci FM, Wang C, et al. Safety and tolerance comparison of imipenem-cilastatin to cephalothin and cefazolin. J Antimicrob Chemother. 1983;12(Suppl D):125–131.
15. Sadon A, Gilden BN, Rohr AS, et al. Immediate hypersensitivity reactions to beta-lactam antibiotics. Ann Intern Med. 1987;127:204–215.
16. Baumgardner JD, Galuser MP. Comparative imipenem treatment of *Staphylococcus aureus* endocarditis in the rat. J Antimicrob Chemother. 1983;12(Suppl D):79–87.
17. Scheld WM, Keely J. Imipenem therapy of experimental *Staphylococcus aureus* and *Streptococcus faecalis* endocarditis. J Antimicrob Chemother. 1983;12(Suppl D):69–78.
18. Johnson De, Calia IM, Snyder MJ, et al. Imipenem therapy of *Pseudomonas aeruginosa* bacteremia in neutropenic rats. J Antimicrob Chemother. 1983;12(Suppl D):89–96.
19. MacGregor RR, Gentry LO. Imipenem/cilastatin in the treatment of osteomyelitis. Am J Med. 1985;78:92–95.
20. Marier RL. Role of imipenem in the treatment of soft tissue infections. Am J Med. 1985;78:140–144.
21. Berkeley AS, Freedman K, Hirsch J, et al. Imipenem/cilastatin in the treatment of obstetric and gynecologic infections. Am J Med. 1985;78:71–76.
22. Cox CE, Corrado ML. Safety and efficacy of imipenem/cilastatin in treatment of complicated urinary tract infections. Am J Med. 1985;78:84–91.
23. Kager L, Nord CE. Imipenem/cilastatin in the treatment of intraabdominal infections: A review of worldwide experience. Rev Infect Dis. 1985;7(Suppl 3):518–521.
24. Salata RA, Gebhart RC, Palmer DL, et al. Pneumonia treated with imipenem/cilastatin. Am J Med. 1985;78:96–101.
25. Dickson G, Rodriguez K, Arcey S, et al. Efficacy of imipenem/cilastatin in endocarditis. Am J Med. 1985;78:109–118.
26. Bodey GP, Alvarez ME, Jones PG, et al. Imipenem/cilastatin as initial therapy for febrile cancer patients. Antimicrob Agents Chemother. 1986;30:211–214.
27. Gombert ME, Aulicino TM, duBouchet L, et al. Therapy of experimental cerebral nocardiosis with imipenem, amikacin, trimethoprim-sulfamethoxazole, and minocycline. Antimicrob Agents Chemother. 1986;30:270–273.
28. Ertl G, Schall K, Kochsiek K. Nocardial endocarditis of an aortic valve prosthesis. Br Heart J. 1987;57:384–386.
29. Krilov LR, Blumer JL, Stern RC, et al. Imipenem/cilastatin in acute pulmonary exacerbations of cystic fibrosis. Rev Infect Dis. 1985;7(Suppl 3):482–489.
30. Acar JF. Therapy for lower respiratory tract infections with imipenem/cilastatin:A review of worldwide experience. Rev Infect Dis. 1985;7:S513–S517.
31. Satake S, Yoshihara E, Nakae T. Diffusion of beta-lactam antibiotics through liposome membranes reconstituted from purified outer membranes of *Pseudomonas aeruginosa*. Antimicrob Agents Chemother. 1990;34:685–690.
32. Iaconis JP, Pitkin DH, Sheikh W, Nadler HL. Comparison of antibacterial activities of meropenem and six other antimicrobials against *Pseudomonas aeruginosa* isolates from North American studies and clinical trials. Clin Infect Dis. 1997;24(Suppl 2):S191–S196.
33. Leroy A, Fillastre JP, Borsa-Lebas F, et al. Pharmacokinetics of meropenem (ICI 194,660) and its metabolite (ICI 213,689) in healthy subjects and in patients with renal impairment. Antimicrob Agents Chemother. 1992;36:2794–2798.
34. Craig WA. The pharmacology of meropenem, a new carbapenem antibiotic. Clin Infect Dis. 1997;24(Suppl 2):S266–S275.
35. Fujii R, Yoshioka H, Fujita K, et al. Pharmacokinetic and clinical studies in the pediatric field. Pediatric study group of meropenem. Jpn J Antibiotics. 1992;45:697–717.
36. Norrby SR. Neurotoxicity of carbapenem antibacterials. Drug Saf. 1996;15:87–90.
37. Garau J, Blanquer J, Cobo L, et al. Prospective, randomised, multicentre study of meropenem versus imipenem/cilastatin as empiric monotherapy in severe nosocomial infections. Eur J Clin Microbiol Infect Dis. 1997;16:789–796.
38. Chang DC, Wilson SE. Meta-analysis of the clinical outcome of carbapenem monotherapy in the adjunctive treatment of intra-abdominal infections. Am J Surg. 1997;174:284–290.
39. Colardyn F, Faulkner KL. Intravenous meropenem versus imipenem/cilastatin in the treatment of serious bacterial infections in hospitalized patients. Meropenem Serious Infection Study Group. J Antimicrob Chemother. 1996;38:523–537.
40. Sugiyama H, Horiuchi A, Hasegawa H, et al. Therapeutic effects of meropenem against severe infections in patients with hematopoietic disorders. Hanshin Study Group of Hematopoietic Disorders and Infection. Jpn J Antibiot. 1992;45:687–696.
41. Kanellakopoulou K, Giamarellou H, Papadothomakos P, et al. Meropenem versus imipenem/cilastatin in the treatment of intraabdominal infections requiring surgery. Eur J Clin Microbiol Infect Dis. 1993;12:449–453.
42. Bradley JS. Meropenem: A new, extremely broad spectrum beta-lactam antibiotic for serious infections in pediatrics. Pediatr Infect Dis J. 1997:16:263–268.
43. Arrieta A. Use of meropenem in the treatment of serious infections in children: Review of the current literature. Clin Infect Dis. 1997;24(Suppl 2):S207–S212.
44. Margaret BS, Drusano GL, Standiford HC. Emergence of resistance to carbapenem antibiotics in *Pseudomonas aeruginosa*. J Antimicrob Chemother. 1989;24(Suppl A):161–167.
45. Sykes RB, Cimarausti CM, Bonner DP, et al. Monocyclic beta-lactam antibiotics produced by bacteria. Nature. 1981;291:489–491.
46. Leibovici L, Paul M, Poznanski O, et al. Monotherapy versus beta-lactam–aminoglycoside combination treatment for gram-negative bacteremia: A prospective, observational study. Antimicrob Agents Chemother. 1997;41:1127–1133.
47. Cometta A, Baumgartner JD, Lew D, et al. Prospective randomized comparison of imipenem monotherapy with imipenem plus netilmicin for treatment of severe infections in nonneutropenic patients. Antimicrob Agents Chemother. 1994;38:1309–1313.
48. Vidal F, Mensa J, Almela M, et al. Epidemiology and outcome of *Pseudomonas aeruginosa* bacteremia, with special emphasis on the influence of antibiotic treatment: Analysis of 189 episodes. Arch Intern Med. 1996;156:2121–2126.
49. Hilf M, Yu VL, Sharp J, et al. Antibiotic therapy for *Pseudomonas aeruginosa* bacteremia: Outcome correlations in a prospective study of 200 patients. Am J Med. 1989;87:540–546.
50. Barry AL, Thornsberry C, Jones RN, et al. Aztreonam: Antibacterial activity, beta-lactamase stability, and interpretive standards and quality control guidelines for disk-diffusion susceptibility tests. Rev Infect Dis. 1985;7(Suppl 4):594–604.
51. Sykes RB, Bonner DP, Bush K, et al. Aztreonam (SQ 26,776), a synthetic monobactam specifically active against aerobic gram-negative bacteria. Antimicrob Agents Chemother. 1982;21:85–92.
52. Swabb EA, Sugerman AA, Stern M. Oral bioavailability of the monobactam aztreonam (SQ 26,776) in healthy subjects. Antimicrob Agents Chemother. 1983;23:548–550.
53. Swabb EA. Review of the clinical pharmacology of the monobactam antibiotic aztreonam. Am J Med. 1985;78(Suppl 2A):11–18.
54. Duma RJ, Berry AJ, Smith SM, et al. Penetration of aztreonam into cerebrospinal fluid of patients with and without inflammed meninges. Antimicrob Agents Chemother. 1984;26:730–733.
55. Stutman HR, Marks MI, Swabb EA. Single-dose pharmacokinetics of aztreonam in pediatric patients. Antimicrob Agents Chemother. 1984;26:196–199.
56. Fillastre JP, Leroy A, Baudoin C, et al. Pharmacokinetics of aztreonam in patients with chronic renal failure. Clin Pharmacokinet. 1985;10:91–100.
57. Scully BE, Swabb EA, Neu HC. Pharmacology of aztreonam after intravenous infusion. Antimicrob Agents Chemother. 1983;24:18–22.
58. Gerig JS, Bolton ND, Swabb EA, et al. Effect of hemodialysis and peritoneal dialysis on aztreonam pharmacokinetics. Kidney Int. 1984;26:308–318.
59. Giamarellou H, Galanakis N, Douzinas E, et al. Evaluation of aztreonam in difficult-to-treat infections with prolonged post-treatment follow-up. Antimicrob Agents Chemother. 1984;26:245–249.
60. Romero-Vivas J, Rodriguez-Creixems M, Bouza E, et al. Evaluation of aztreonam in the treatment of severe bacterial infections. Antimicrob Agents Chemother. 1985;28:222–226.
61. Scully BE, Henry SA. Clinical experience with aztreonam in the treatment of gram-negative bacteremia. Rev Infect Dis. 1985;7(Suppl 4):789–793.
62. Scully BE, Neu HC. Use of aztreonam in the treatment of serious infections due to multiresistant gram-negative organisms, including *Pseudomonas aeruginosa*. Am J Med. 1985;78:251–261.
63. Scully BE, Ores CN, Prince AS, et al. Treatment of lower respiratory tract infections due to *Pseudomonas aeruginosa* in patients with cystic fibrosis. Rev Infect Dis. 1985;7(Suppl):669–674.
64. Simons WJ, Lee TJ. Aztreonam in the treatment of bone and joint infections caused by gram-negative bacilli. Rev Infect Dis. 1985;7(Suppl 4):783–788.
65. Gudiol F, Pallares R, Ariza X, et al. Comparative clinical evaluation of aztreonam versus aminoglycosides in gram-negative septicaemia. J Antimicrob Chemother. 1986;17:661–671.
66. Hart SM, Bailey EM. A practical look at the clinical usefulness of the beta-lactam/beta-lactamase inhibitor combinations. Ann Pharmacother. 1996;30:1130–1140.
67. Wilson, SE, Nord CE. Clinical trials of extended spectrum penicillin/beta-lactamase inhibitors in the treatment of intra-abdominal infections: European and North American experience. Am J Surg. 1995;169(Suppl 5A):21S–26S.
68. Richmond MM, Sykes RB. The beta-lactamases of gram-negative bacteria and their possible physiological role. Adv Microb Physiol. 1973;9:31–88.
69. Neu HC. The contribution of beta-lactamases to bacterial resistance and mechanisms to inhibit beta-lactamases. Am J Med. 1986;79(Suppl 5B):2–12.
70. Neu HC. The role of beta-lactamase inhibitors in chemotherapy. In: Tipper PJ, ed. Antibiotic Inhibitors of Bacterial Cell Wall Biosynthesis. Oxford: Pergamon Press; 1987;241–258.
71. Neu HC, Fu KP. Clavulanic acid:A beta-lactamase-inhibiting beta-lactamase. Antimicrob Agents Chemother. 1978;14:650–655.
72. Munch P, Luthy R, Blaser J, et al. Human pharmacokinetics and CSF penetration of clavulanic acid. J Antimicrob Chemother. 1981;8:29–37.
73. Adam D, Visser I, Koeppe P. Pharmacokinetics of amoxicillin and clavulanic acid administered alone and in combination. Antimicrob Agents Chemother. 1982;22:353–357.
74. Nelson JD, Kusmiesz H, Shelton S. Pharmacokinetics of potassium clavulanate in combination with amoxicillin in pediatric patients. Antimicrob Agents Chemother. 1982;21:681–682.
75. Schaad UB, Casey PA, Copper DL. Single-dose pharmacokinetics of intravenous clavulanic acid with amoxicillin in pediatric patients. Antimicrob Agents Chemother. 1983;23:252–255.
76. Bennett S, Wise R, Weston D, et al. Pharmacokinetics and tissue penetration of ticarcillin combined with clavulanic acid. Antimicrob Agents Chemother. 1983;23:831–834.
77. Scully BE, Chin NX, Neu HC. Pharmacology of ticarcillin combined with clavulanic acid in humans. Am J Med. 1985;79(Suppl 5B):39–43.
78. Jackson D, Cockburn A, Cooper DL, et al. Clinical pharmacology and safety evaluation of Timentin. Am J Med. 1985;79(Suppl 5B):44–55.
79. Walsted RA, Hellum KB, Thurmann-Nielson E, et al. Pharmacokinetics and tissue penetration of Timentin: A simultaneous study of serum, urine, lymph, suction

blister, and subcutaneous treatment fluid. J Antimicrob Chemother. 1986;17(Suppl C):71–80.
80. Kaleida PH, Bluestone DC, Rockette HE, et al. Amoxicillin-clavulanate potassium compared with cefaclor for acute otitis media in infants and children. Pediatr Infect Dis. 1987;6:265–271.
81. Neu HC, ed. Progress and perspectives on beta-lactamase inhibition: A review of Augmentin. Postgrad Med. 1984;3–295.
82. Hoberman A, Paradise JL, Burch DJ, et al. Equivalent efficacy and reduced occurrence of diarrhea from a new formulation of amoxicillin/clavulanate potassium (Augmentin) for treatment of acute otitis media in children. Ped Infect Dis J. 1997;16:463–470.
83. Calver AD, Walsh NS, Quinn PF, et al. Dosing of amoxicillin/clavulanate given every 12 hours is as effective as dosing every 8 hours for treatment of lower respiratory tract infection. Lower Respiratory Tract Infection Collaborative Study Group. Clin Infect Dis. 1997;24:570–574.
84. Neu HC, ed. Beta-lactamase inhibition: Therapeutic advances. Am J Med. 1985;79(Suppl 5B):1–196.
85. Gentry LO, Macko V, Lind R, et al. Ticarcillin plus clavulanic acid (Timentin) therapy for osteomyelitis. Am J Med. 1985;79(Suppl 5B):116–121.
86. Leigh DA, Phillips I, Wise R, eds. Timentin-ticarcillin plus clavulanic acid, a laboratory and clinical perspective. J Antimicrob Chemother. 1986;17(Suppl C):1–244.
87. Foulds G, Stankewich JP, Marshall DC, et al. Pharmacokinetics of sulbactam in humans. Antimicrob Agents Chemother. 1983;23:692–699.
88. Hampel B, Lode H, Bruchnor G, et al. Comparative pharmacokinetics of sulbactam/ampicillin and clavulanic acid/amoxicillin in human volunteers. Drugs. 1988;35(Suppl 7):29–33.
89. Guneren MF. Clinical experience with intramuscular sulbactam/ampicillin in the out-patient treatment of various infections: A multicenter trial. Drugs. 1988;35(Suppl 7):57–68.
90. Dajani AS. Sulbactam/ampicillin in pediatric infections. Drugs. 1988;35(Suppl 7):35–38.
91. Kass EH, Lode H, eds. Enzyme-mediated resistance to beta-lactam antibiotics: A symposium on sulbactam/ampicillin. Rev Infect Dis. 1986;8(Suppl 5):465–650.
92. Reinhardt JF, Johnston L, Ruane P, et al. A randomized, double-blind comparison of sulbactam/ampicillin and clindamycin for the treatment of aerobic and aerobic-anaerobic infections. Rev Infect Dis. 1986;8(Suppl 5):569–575.
93. Hemsell DL, Heard MC, Hemsell PG, et al. Sulbactam/ampicillin versus cefoxitin for uncomplicated and complicated acute pelvic inflammatory disease. Drugs. 1988;35(Suppl 7):39–42.
94. Rodriguez WJ, Kahn WN, Puig N, et al. Sulbactam/ampicillin vs. chloramphenicol/ampicillin for the treatment of meningitis in infants and children. Rev Infect Dis. 1986;8(Suppl 5):620–629.
95. Wald E, Reilly JS, Bluestone CD, et al. Sulbactam/ampicillin in the treatment of acute epiglottitis in children. Rev Infect Dis. 1986;8(Suppl 5):617–619.
96. Fass RJ, Prior RB. Comparative in vitro activity of piperacillin-tazobactam and ticarcillin-clavulanate. Antimicrob Agents Chemother. 1989;33:1268–1274.
97. Aronoff SC, Jacobs MR, Johenning S, Yamabe S. Comparative activities of the β-lactamase inhibitors YTR 830, sodium clavulanate, and sulbactam combined with amoxicillin or ampicillin. Antimicrob Agents Chemother. 1984;26:580–582.
98. Kuck NA, Jacobus NV, Petersen, et al. Comparative in vitro and in vivo activities of piperacillin combined with the β-lactamase inhibitors tazobactam, clavulanic acid, and sulbactam. Antimicrob Agents Chemother. 1989;33:1964–1969.
99. Johnson CA, Halstenson CE, Kelloway JS, et al. Single-dose pharmacokinetics of piperacillin and tazobactam in patients with renal disease. Clin Pharmacol Ther. 1992;51:32–41.
100. Kinzig M, Sörgel F, Brismar B, Nord CE. Pharmacokinetics and tissue penetration of tazobactam and piperacillin in patients undergoing colorectal surgery. Antimicrob Agents Chemother. 1992;36:1997–2004.
101. Kern W, Kennedy S, Sachdeva M, et al. Evaluation of piperacillin-tazobactam in experimental meningitis caused by a beta-lactamase producing strain of K1-positive *Escherichia coli*. Antimicrob Agents Chemother. 1990;34:697–701.
102. Roguin A, Kasis I, Ben-Arush MW, et al. Fever and neutropenia in children with malignant disease. Pediatr Hematol Oncol. 1996;13:503–510.
103. Arguedas A, Sifuentes-Osornio J, Loaiza C, et al. An open, multicenter clinical trial of piperacillin/tazobactam in the treatment of pediatric patients with intra-abdominal infections. J Chemother. 1996;8:130–136.
104. Sanders WE Jr, Sanders CC. Piperacillin/tazobactam: A critical review of the evolving clinical literature. Clin Infect Dis. 1996;22:107–123.
105. Shlaes DM, Baughman R, Boylen CT, et al. Piperacillin/tazobactam compared with ticarcillin/clavulanate in community-acquired bacterial lower respiratory tract infection. J Antimicrob Chemother. 1994;34:565–577.
106. Bryson, HM, Brogden, RN. Piperacillin/tazobactam: A review of its antibacterial activity, pharmacokinetic properties and therapeutic potential. Drugs. 1994;47:506–535.
107. Brismar B, Malmborg AS, Tunevall G, et al. Piperacillin-tazobactam versus imipenem-cilastatin for treatment of intra-abdominal infections. Antimicrob Agents Chemother. 1992;36:2766–2773.
108. Micozzi A, Nucci M, Venditti M, et al. Piperacillin/tazobactam/amikacin versus piperacillin/tazobactam/amikacin/teicoplanin in empirical therapy of neutropenic patients. Eur J Clin Microbiol Infect Dis. 1993;12:1–8.
109. Mouton Y, Leroy D, Beuscart C, et al. Efficacy, safety and tolerance of parenteral piperacillin/tazobactam in the treatment of patients with lower respiratory tract infections. J Antimicrob Chemother. 1993;31(Suppl A):87–95.
110. Tassler H, Cullman W, Elhardt D. Therapy of soft tissue infections with piperacillin/tazobactam. J Antimicrob Chemother. 1993;31(Suppl A):105–112.
111. Eklund RE, Nord CE. A randomized multicenter trial of piperacillin/tazobactam versus imipenem/cilastatin in the treatment of severe intra-abdominal infections. Swedish Study Group. J Antimicrob Chemother. 1993;31(Suppl A):79–85.
112. Niinikoski J, Havia T, Alhava E, et al. Piperacillin/tazobactam versus imipenem/cilastatin in the treatment of intra-abdominal infections. Surg Gynecol Obstet. 1993;176:255–261.

Chapter 21

β-Lactam Allergy

MICHAEL E. WEISS
N. FRANKLIN ADKINSON, JR.

CLASSIFICATION OF β-LACTAM REACTIONS

Since the introduction of penicillin by Fleming in the mid-1940s, the number of β-lactam antibiotics has grown dramatically. Other than allergy, these drugs have remarkably low toxicity when used in moderate doses. In fact, the principal toxicity of β-lactam antibiotics is allergic reactions. The first case of anaphylaxis due to penicillin was reported in 1946,[1] and the first reported death from an allergic reaction was in 1949.[2] Allergic reactions occur in 7 to 40 of every 1000 penicillin treatment courses.[3, 4] Studies have indicated that as many as half of all allergic drug reactions occurring in hospitalized patients are attributable to β-lactam antibiotics.[5] A wide range of allergic reactions have been caused by β-lactam antibiotics. It is possible to classify these reactions by the Gell and Coombs immunopathologic classification system[6]; by Levine's classification system,[7] which is based on time of onset of the reaction; or on the basis of the predominant clinical manifestation.

Gell and Coombs Classification

Gell and Coombs distinguished four types of immunopathologic reactions, all of which have been seen with β-lactam antibiotics (Table 21–1).

Type I—Immediate Hypersensitivity. These reactions result from the interaction of β-lactam antigens with preformed β-lactam–specific immunoglobulin E (IgE) antibodies that are bound to tissue mast cells or circulating basophils via high-affinity IgE receptors. Cross-linking of two or more IgE receptors by β-lactam antigens leads to the release of both preformed mediators (histamine, proteases, and chemotactic factors) and newly formed mediators (prostaglandins, leukotrienes, and platelet-activating factor), which are generated by the metabolism of arachidonic acid.[8] Release of these mediators can lead to urticaria, laryngeal edema, and bronchospasm with or without cardiovascular collapse. Anaphylactic reactions occur in 4 to 15 of every 100,000 penicillin treatment courses.[4–9] Fatality from β-lactam anaphylaxis has been reported to occur once in every 32,000 to 100,000 treatment courses.[4, 9] The use of β-adrenergic antagonists may increase the risk of death if anaphylaxis occurs, because treatment of the anaphylactic reaction is made more difficult.[10] IgE type I acute allergic reactions cause the greatest clinical concern because of the risk of life-threatening anaphylaxis.

Type II—Cytotoxic Antibodies. These reactions result when β-lactam–specific cytotoxic antibodies, usually IgG or IgM, become attached to circulating blood cells or renal interstitial cells that have β-lactam antigens bound to their cell surface. This antigen-antibody interaction activates the complement system, resulting in cell lysis. Type II reactions may also be complement independent. IgG or IgM

TABLE 21–1 Classification of Immunopathologic Reactions According to the Scheme of Gell and Coombs

Type of Reaction	Description	Antibody	Cells	Other	Clinical Reactions
I	Anaphylactic, (reagenic), immediate hypersensitivity	IgE	Basophils, mast cells	—	Anaphylaxis, urticaria
II	Cytotoxic or cytolytic	IgG, IgM	Any cell with isoantigen	C′, RES	Hemolytic anemia, cytopenias, nephritis
III	Immune complex disease	Soluble immune complexes (Ag-Ab)	None directly	C′	Serum sickness, drug fever
IV	"Delayed" or cell-mediated hypersensitivity	None known	Sensitized T lymphocytes	—	Contact dermatitis
Other	Idiopathic		?	?	Maculopapular eruptions
			?	?	Eosinophilia
			?	?	Stevens-Johnson syndrome
			?	?	Exfoliative dermatitis

Abbreviations: Ag-Ab, Antigen-antibody; C′, complement; Ig, immunoglobulin; RES, reticuloendothelial system; ?, immunopathologic mechanism is in doubt.
Modified from Weiss ME, Adkinson NF Jr. Immediate hypersensitivity reactions to penicillin and related antibiotics. Clin Allergy. 1988;18:515–540, with permission.

antibody may bind to β-lactam antigens on cell membranes, resulting in neutrophil or macrophage attachment and activation via IgG or IgM Fc receptors. This opsonization can result in injury to the antigen-laden cell. Examples include hemolytic anemia, leukopenia, thrombocytopenia, and drug-induced nephritis. Long-term, high-dose β-lactam treatment is usually required for this form of allergic reaction to occur.

Type III—Immune Complexes (Arthus Reaction). β-Lactam–specific IgG or IgM antibodies may form circulating complexes with β-lactam antigens. These circulating complexes can fix complement and then lodge in tissue sites, causing serum sickness–like reactions and possibly drug fever. In children, serum sickness is 15 times more likely to occur after administration of cefaclor than after amoxicillin.[11] These reactions typically occur 7 to 14 days after initiation of the β-lactam therapy. The syndrome can occur even after the termination of therapy. Preliminary data, using sera from a small number of patients, suggests that cefaclor serum sickness may be predicted using a microsome metabolite lymphotoxic assay.[12]

Type IV—Cell-Mediated Hypersensitivity. These reactions are not mediated by an antibody but rather by T lymphocytes. A T lymphocyte recognizes the β-lactam antigen through an antigen-specific T-cell receptor. This triggers the T cell to release cytokines that orchestrate an immune response by recruiting and stimulating proliferation of other lymphocytes and mononuclear cells, ultimately causing tissue inflammation and injury. Contact dermatitis is a clinical manifestation of a type IV reaction. The high rate of penicillin-related contact dermatitis (5–10%) in the 1940s led to the discontinuation of its use as a topical antibiotic.

TABLE 21–2 Classification of Allergic Reactions to β-Lactam Antibiotics Based on Their Time of Onset

Reaction Type	Onset (Hours)	Clinical Reactions
Immediate	0–1	Anaphylaxis
		Hypotension
		Laryngeal edema
		Urticaria/angioedema
		Wheezing
Accelerated	1–72	Urticaria/angioedema
		Laryngeal/edema
		Wheezing
Late	>72	Morbilliform rash
		Interstitial nephritis
		Hemolytic anemia
		Neutropenia
		Thrombocytopenia
		Serum sickness
		Drug fever
		Stevens-Johnson syndrome
		Exfoliative dermatitis

Adapted from Levine BB. Immunologic mechanisms of penicillin allergy: A haptenic moel system for the study of allergic diseases of man. N Engl J Med. 1966;275:1115–1125, with permission.

Idiopathic Reactions

Some reactions to β-lactam antibiotics have an obscure pathogenesis and are not included in the Gell and Coombs classification system. These reactions include pruritus, maculopapular (morbilliform) exanthems, erythema multiforme, erythema nodosum, photosensitivity reactions, fixed drug reactions, and exfoliative dermatitis. The very common maculopapular rash appears late in the treatment course in 2 to 3% of penicillin treatments. Rashes induced by ampicillin (and amoxicillin) occur with much greater frequency: 5.2 to 9.5% of treatment courses in uncomplicated cases.[5, 13, 14] When ampicillin or amoxicillin is given during infections with Epstein-Barr virus or cytomegalovirus, or to patients with acute lymphocytic leukemia, a much higher incidence of rash (69 to 100%) occurs.[15]

Other reactions caused by unknown mechanisms include the Stevens-Johnson syndrome, involving rash (usually erythema multiforme) plus involvement of two or more mucous membranes, and Lyell's syndrome, also known as toxic epidermal necrolysis. Patients who have had Stevens-Johnson or Lyell's syndrome associated with

TABLE 21–3 Classification of Reactions to β-Lactam Antibiotics According to Their Predominant Clinical Manifestations

Reaction	Manifestation
Anaphylaxis	Laryngeal edema
	Hypotension
	Bronchospasm
Cutaneous reactions	Urticaria/angioedema
	Vasculitis
	Stevens-Johnson syndrome
	Exfoliative dermatitis
	Contact sensitivity
	Fixed drug eruption
	Toxic epidermal necrolysis
	Pruritus
	Maculopapular (morbilliform) rash
	Erythema multiforme
	Erythema nodosum
	Photosensitivity reactions
Destruction of formed elements of blood	Hemolytic anemia
	Neutropenia
	Thrombocytopenia
Renal reactions	Interstitial nephritis
	Glomerulonephritis
	Nephrotic syndrome
Serum sickness	—
Drug fever	—
Systemic vasculitis	—
Lymphadenopathy	—

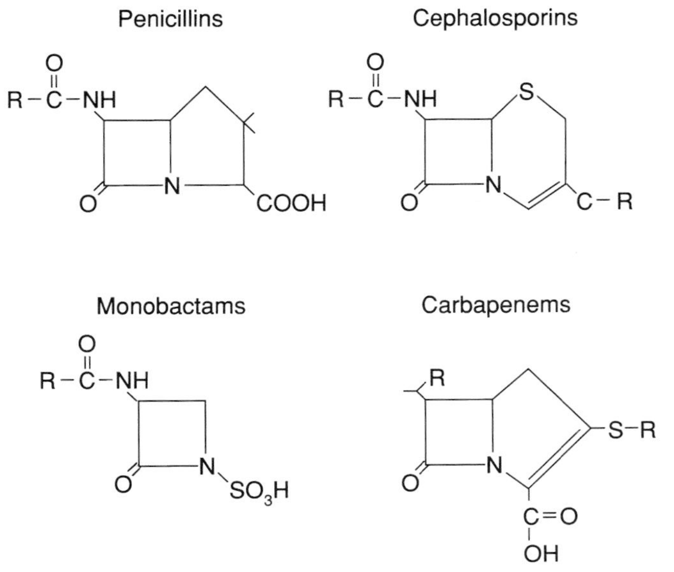

FIGURE 21–1. Structure of four classes of β-lactam antibiotics in use in the United States.

β-lactam antibiotics should not receive β-lactam drugs in the future. Attempts to desensitize patients to the β-lactam antibiotics that caused these syndromes is also not recommended. Pseudoanaphylactic reactions have been observed after intramuscular or inadvertent intravenous injection of procaine penicillin. These reactions are probably caused by a combination of toxic and embolic phenomena from procaine.[16]

Levine's Classification

Levine[7] classified reactions to penicillin according to their time of onset (Table 21–2). Immediate reactions occur within the first hour after β-lactam administration, and they are almost all IgE mediated (anaphylaxis and urticaria). Accelerated reactions occur 1 to 72 hours after initial treatment with β-lactams; they most commonly involve urticaria. Late reactions occur more than 72 hours after onset of therapy. Anaphylaxis does not occur later in the course of continuous β-lactam therapy; maculopapular reactions are most common, but type II, III, and IV reactions also occur during this time frame. Allergic reactions may also be classified according to their predominant clinical manifestations, as listed in Table 21–3.

IMMUNOCHEMISTRY OF β-LACTAM ANTIBIOTICS

Penicillins consist of a β-lactam ring, on which antimicrobial activity depends, and a five-membered thiazolidine ring (Fig. 21–1). Because penicillin is a low-molecular-weight compound (356 Da), it must first covalently combine with tissue macromolecules (presumably proteins) to produce multivalent hapten-protein complexes, which are required for both the induction of an immune response and the later elicitation of an allergic reaction (Fig. 21–2).[17] The most common form of haptenization by penicillin is in the penicilloyl configuration. Because the penicilloyl determinant is the most abundant derivative of penicillin in vivo, it has been labeled the *major determinant*. Although the formation of the penicilloyl group has been shown to occur spontaneously under physiologic conditions, evidence suggests that penicillin haptenization may be facilitated by serum molecules.[18, 19] This reaction occurs with the prototype benzylpenicillin and virtually all semisynthetic penicillins. Penicillin can also be degraded by other metabolic pathways to form additional antigenic determinants.[20] These derivatives are formed in small quantities and stimulate a variable immune response; hence, they have been termed the *minor determinants*. Known precursors of minor determinants of penicillin include benzylpenicillin, its alkaline hydrolysis product (benzylpenicilloate), and an acid hydrolysis product (benzylpenilloate), collectively called the *minor determinant mixture (MDM)*.

Therefore, for penicillin and other β-lactam antibiotics, IgE antibodies can be produced against a number of haptenic determinants (i.e., major and minor determinants). Anaphylactic reactions to peni-

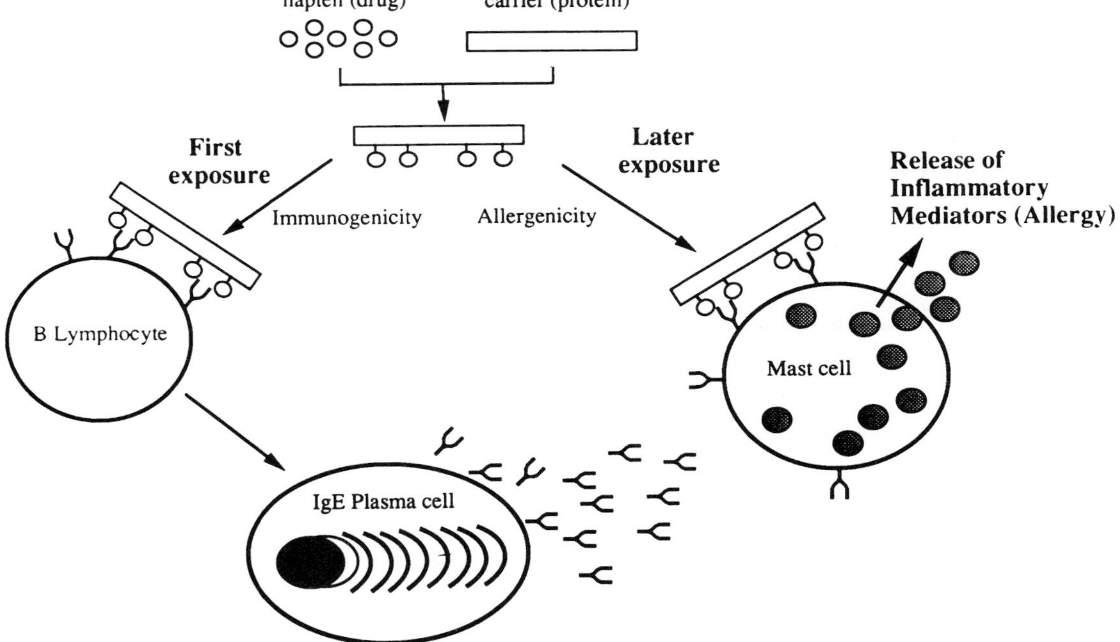

FIGURE 21–2. Illustration of drug hapten combining with carrier molecule to induce IgE antibody production against drug (sensitization). On subsequent exposure, drug combines with IgE antibody on mast cell surface, leading to anaphylactic reaction (immune response).

cillin are usually mediated by IgE antibodies directed against minor determinants, although some anaphylactic reactions have occurred in patients with only penicilloyl-specific IgE antibodies.[7, 20, 21] Accelerated and late urticarial reactions usually are mediated by penicilloyl-specific IgE antibodies (major determinant).[7]

RISK FACTORS FOR β-LACTAM REACTIONS

Immune responses to β-lactam antibiotics occur in only a small percentage of exposed patients, and clinical expression of β-lactam allergy occurs in only a fraction of the patients demonstrating an immune response. The generation of a sustained immune response to a β-lactam antibiotic is probably controlled in part by the genetic makeup of the individual.[22] The half-life of β-lactam IgE antibodies has been shown to range from as short as 10 days to an indeterminately long interval (more than 1000 days).[23] A person whose β-lactam–specific IgE antibody response persists is at greater cumulative risk for allergic reactions to β-lactam antibiotics than one whose IgE antibody quickly disappears.

Parenteral administration of β-lactam antibiotics produces more allergic reactions than oral administration does.[24] However, this may be more related to dose than to route of administration. When higher oral doses are given, as in the treatment of gonorrhea, the incidence of allergic reactions is no different from that seen with intramuscular procaine penicillin at a comparable dose.[25]

A history of atopy (allergic rhinitis, asthma, atopic dermatitis) does not seem to be an independent risk factor for the development of β-lactam allergy,[23, 26] although atopic individuals, especially those with asthma, seem to be predisposed to severe and fatal reactions should anaphylaxis occur.[9]

Persons with a history of penicillin reactions have a fourfold to sixfold increased risk of subsequent reactions to β-lactam antibiotics compared with those without previous reaction histories.[26] The risk is particularly pronounced if the previous reaction was anaphylaxis or urticaria.[23] However, because most serious and fatal allergic reactions to β-lactam antibiotics occur in persons who have never had an allergic reaction, a negative history of β-lactam allergy should not leave lead to a false sense of security. Sensitization in these patients probably occurred from their last therapeutic course of penicillin. A randomized, controlled trial of routine penicillin skin testing in history-negative patients was shown not to be cost-effective, and therefore skin testing at this time is recommended only for patients with a prior history of β-lactam allergy.[27]

In general, the likelihood of sustaining IgE-specific β-lactam antibodies declines with time since the previous reaction. Sullivan and collaborators[28] reported that skin tests done within the first 1 or 2 months after an acute allergic reaction were positive 80 to 90% of the time. Thereafter, there was a time-dependent decline in the rate of positive skin tests, to less than 20% by 10 years.[28] Patients who have had serum sickness–like reactions to β-lactam antibiotics often persist with an intense antibody response and may remain at high risk for allergic reactions for many years.

Despite sparse evidence, it is generally thought that penicillin reactions occur less frequently in children and in elderly persons than in nonelderly adults.[26, 29] Although the frequency of anaphylactic reactions may be less in the elderly, fatal outcomes are more commonly owing to compromised cardiopulmonary reserve.

DIAGNOSING β-LACTAM ALLERGY

An important question facing clinicians is how to assess a patient with a history of β-lactam reaction who has a current clinical need for β-lactam antibiotics. Approximately 5 to 20% of patients give a history of reactions to β-lactam antibiotics. By current medical standards, all of these subjects would be denied therapy with β-lactam antibiotics for the rest of their lives unless further evaluation were undertaken. The most useful single piece of information in assessing an individual's risk for a type I, IgE-mediated reaction (anaphylaxis and urticaria) is the skin test response to major and minor penicillin determinants.

The major (penicilloyl) determinant of penicillin can be assessed by skin testing with pencilloyl-polylysine (PPL). This commercially available skin test reagent (PRE-PEN, Bayer, Spokane, WA) contains multiple penicilloyl molecules synthetically coupled to a weakly immunogenic polylysine carrier. Minor determinants of penicillin are not commercially available in the United States at present, although that this may change in the future. In the meantime, benzylpenicillin alone (10,000 U/ml) can be substituted as a less efficient minor determinant reagent in patients without a history of anaphylactic sensitivity.

Skin testing should first proceed with an epicutaneous (prick-puncture) test for safety. If there is no induration (or systemic symptoms) after 15 minutes, intradermal injections are placed, raising 3- to 4-mm blebs in duplicate on the forearm. Testing should be done with PPL, MDM, a positive control (histamine), and a negative diluent control. The diameter of induration at 15 to 20 minutes is read; if it is greater than 5 mm, the test is considered positive.[30] Antihistamines, tricyclic antidepressants, and adrenergic drugs, all of which may inhibit skin test results, should be discontinued at least 48 hours before skin testing. Antihistamines with long half-lives need to be discontinued for appropriate intervals.

When properly performed with due consideration for preliminary epicutaneous tests and appropriate dilutions, skin testing with penicillin reagents can almost always be accomplished safely. Systemic reactions occur in about 1% of those tested[31, 32]; these are usually mild but can be serious. Therefore, skin tests should be done in the presence of a physician and with immediate access to medications needed to treat anaphylaxis.

In numerous studies in which both PPL and minor determinant skin tests were performed, only 7 to 35% of patients who gave histories of penicillin allergy were skin test positive to either reagent,[33, 34] although one study found a positive skin test rate of 63%.[28] In general, with increasing time since the allergic reaction, the prevalence of positive skin tests to penicillin determinants decreases, although some patients have penicillin antibodies indefinitely.[28, 35] In patients who give a history of penicillin allergy, skin tests confirm that 65 to 93% can safely be given a β-lactam antibiotic. With negative a history of penicillin allergy, the rate of positive skin tests is about 2%.[27, 32]

Extensive worldwide experience involving more than 20,000 patients has shown that persons with a history of penicillin reaction can be retreated safely with penicillin or related antibiotics if intradermal skin tests with PPL and a suitable MDM are negative.[32, 36] When therapeutic doses of penicillin are given to patients with a history of penicillin allergy but negative skin tests to PPL and MDM, IgE-mediated reactions occur in 2 to 15%, depending on the clinical history; such reactions are almost always mild and self-limited. Penicillin anaphylaxis has not been reported in skin test–negative patients in the United States. When penicillin is given after negative skin tests, about 1 to 3% of patients have urticarial or other mild cutaneous reactions.[33] If the major determinant penicillin is used alone as a skin test reagent, approximately 10 to 25% of all potential positive reactions are missed.[28] If benzylpenicillin G, diluted to a concentration of 10,000 U/ml (10^{-2} mol/L) is used as the sole minor determinant, about 5 to 10% of skin test–positive patients are missed.[28] Mendelson and associates[37] studied more than 200 children who had a history of penicillin allergy but were skin test negative to penicillin reagents. After negative skin tests, a 10-day course of oral penicillin was given, and repeat skin testing 1 month later showed that less than 1% of the children became skin test positive to penicillin reagents. In contrast, Parker and colleagues[38] found that 3 (20%) of 15 patients with a history of penicillin allergy who were skin test negative became resensitized (skin tests to penicillin turned positive) after they were treated with high-dose intravenous penicillin in the hospital. Therefore, it may be prudent to retest patients with a history of penicillin allergy who are skin test negative and subsequently treated with penicillin, especially if they are treated with intravenous high-dose penicillin instead of oral agents.

A limited number of skin test–positive patients have been treated with therapeutic doses of penicillin. The risk of an acute immediate or accelerated allergic reaction ranges from about 10% in history-negative subjects to 50 to 70% in history-positive subjects.[33] Therefore, if skin tests are positive, an equally effective, noncross-reacting antibiotic should be substituted if possible. Patients with a history of exfoliative dermatitis, Stevens-Johnson Syndrome, or Lyell's syndrome, reactions that constitute absolute contraindications for penicillin administration, should not be evaluated by skin testing. Skin tests have no predictive value in non–IgE-mediated reactions such as drug fever, serum sickness, cytopenias, interstitial nephritis, contact dermatitis, or maculopapular exanthems. Penicillin skin tests are indeterminate (usually erythema without wheal or discordant duplicates) in about 0.6 to 3% of patients with histories of penicillin allergy.[32, 36] The meaning of such results is unclear.

Type II reactions, such as hemolytic anemias, cytopenias, and interstitial nephritis, usually follow high-dose, long-term β-lactam therapy. Anecdotal experience suggests that short courses of β-lactam therapy in moderate doses can be tolerated by most, if not all, patients with such histories. Penicillin skin testing is important to rule out concomitant type I sensitivity but would not be predictive of type II or type III reactions. If skin tests are negative in these patients and β-lactam antibiotics are strongly indicated, gradual dose escalation under careful medical observation can be prudently attempted. If cytopenia, hemolytic anemia, hematuria, or proteinuria develops, therapy should be promptly stopped and high-dose glucocorticoids administered. However, most subjects can be retreated without recurrence, especially if the history of reaction is remote.

Solid-phase immunoassays such as the radioallergosorbent test (RAST) have been developed to detect serum IgE antibodies directed against the penicilloyl determinant. At present there is no in vitro RAST for minor determinant antibodies.[30] Because it is more time-consuming, more expensive, less sensitive then skin testing for detection of the major determinant IgE antibodies, and presently unavailable for minor determinant antibody detection, the RAST and other in vitro analogues have limited clinical utility at this time.

SEMISYNTHETIC PENICILLINS WITH SPECIAL REFERENCE TO AMPICILLIN/AMOXICILLIN

Semisynthetic penicillins contain the same nuclear structure as benzylpenicillin with differing side chains. Because allergic reactions are thought to be caused by neoantigens formed by interaction of the β-lactam nucleus with native proteins, it has generally been considered unnecessary to skin test with specific derivatives of semisynthetic penicillins. Hapten inhibition theory predicts that antibodies directed against the unmodified side chain will not cause allergic reactions because of overwhelming hapten inhibition from unconjugated univalent drug.[39, 40] Earlier studies showed that skin testing with derivatives of semisynthetic penicillins in addition to benzylpenicillin derivatives were not needed.[41] Blanca and colleagues,[42, 43] in Spain, questioned this dogma and suggested that skin testing with major and minor determinants of benzylpenicillin may not identify all patients with ampicillin/amoxicillin-specific allergy. Silviu-Dan and coworkers[44] subsequently reported that skin testing with derivatives of ampicillin/amoxicillin detected nine patients who otherwise were skin test negative to benzylpenicillin reagents. These nine represented almost half of all skin test–positive persons tested. This study did not provide any information about benzylpenicillin skin test–negative and ampicillin/amoxicillin skin test–positive persons challenged with a β-lactam.

Macy and associates[45] studied 215 patients who had a history of penicillin allergy but negative skin tests to benzylpenicillin reagents. These subjects were given a one-time 250-mg oral challenge dose of amoxicillin. Only 5% had mild reactions, and only 0.9% had possible IgE–mediated reactions. Mendelson and colleagues (personal communication) studied 443 patients with a history of penicillin allergy who were skin test negative to PPL and to an MDM of benzylpenicillin. The 443 patients tolerated a 10-day penicillin challenge, but, when they were given amoxicillin for 10 days, 18.7% had cutaneous reactions. Therefore, amoxicillin/ampicillin seems to have a greater propensity for causing cutaneous allergic reactions. It has been postulated that the diamino acyl side chain contained in ampicillin/amoxicillin more readily allows for the formation of linear polymers of varying lengths, which may explain the higher cutaneous reaction rate seen with ampicillin/amoxicillin.[46] Except for isolated reports from Spain (Blanca and colleagues,[43] Martin and colleagues[47]), there have been no reports of any patient with negative skin tests to PPL and an MDM of benzylpenicillin, subsequently treated with amoxicillin/ampicillin, who had anything more than a cutaneous reaction. Studies in the 1960s showed that patients with late-occurring maculopapular rashes from ampicillin/amoxicillin could safely be retreated with these antibiotics without any increased risk for acute allergic reactions. In such patients, skin testing with PPL and MDM may be useful to rule out concomitant type I, IgE-mediated sensitivity. Studies by Romano and coworkers[48] and by Terrados and associates[49] present preliminary evidence that the maculopapular exanthems seen in some amoxicillin reactions may be related to delayed-type hypersensitivity reactions involving T cells. Diagnostic tests that are presently being evaluated include delayed intradermal skin tests using native amoxicillin, measuring induration at 48 hours, and possibly a patch test using native amoxicillin.

β-LACTAM DESENSITIZATION

Effective, noncross-reacting alternative antibiotics are usually available for patients with positive skin tests to penicillin. If alternative drugs fail, induce unacceptable side effects, or are clearly less effective, then the administration of a β-lactam antibiotic using a desensitization protocol may be justified. Infections in which this may be considered include endocarditis caused by enterococci, brain abscess, bacterial meningitis, and serious infections caused by *Staphylcoccus* or *Pseudomonas* organisms *Listeria* infections, neurosyphilis, or syphilis during pregnancy. Use of a desensitization protocol for penicillin skin test–positive patients markedly reduces the risk of anaphylaxis.

β-Lactam desensitization of patients with prior anaphylactic reactions should be performed only in an intensive care setting. All β-adrenergic antagonists, including ophthalmologic drops, should be discontinued. Asthmatic patients should be under optimal control. An intravenous line should be established, and baseline electrocardiography and spirometry should be performed. Continuous electrocardiogram monitoring should be instituted.

Protocols have been developed for β-lactam desensitization using both the oral and the parenteral route (Tables 21–4 and 21–5).[50] If an oral preparation is available and the patient has a functional gastrointestinal tract, then the oral route may be preferable for desensitization. Results from oral desensitization have shown that approximately one third of patients have a transient allergic reaction during desensitization, and two thirds have a reaction during penicillin treatment after desensitization. These reactions are usually mild and self-limited in nature, but they can be serious.[24]

During desensitization, any dose that causes mild systemic reactions (e.g., pruritus, fleeting urticaria, rhinitis, mild wheezing) should be repeated until the patient tolerates the dose without systemic symptoms or signs. More serious reactions (e.g., hypotension, laryngeal edema, asthma) require appropriate treatment, and if desensitization is continued the dose should be decreased by at least 10-fold and withheld until the patient is stable.[51]

Once desensitized, the patient's treatment with penicillin must not lapse or the risk of an allergic reaction increases. If the patient requires a β-lactam antibiotic in the future and still remains skin test positive to penicillin reagents, desensitization is required again.

TABLE 21–4 Protocol for Oral Desensitization of β-Lactam Antibiotic–Allergic Patients

Step	β-Lactam Drug (mg/ml)	Amount* (ml)	Dose*† (mg)	Cumulative Dose (mg)
1	0.5	0.1	0.05	0.05
2	0.5	0.2	0.10	0.15
3	0.5	0.4	0.20	0.35
4	0.5	0.8	0.40	0.75
5	0.5	1.6	0.80	1.55
6	0.5	3.2	1.60	3.15
7	0.5	6.4	3.20	6.35
8	5.0	1.2	6.00	12.35
9	5.0	2.4	12.00	24.35
10	5.0	4.8	24.00	48.35
11	50.0	1.0	50.00	98.35
12	50.0	2.0	100.00	198.35
13	50.0	4.0	200.00	398.35
14	50.0	8.0	400.00	798.35
15: Observe patient for 30 minutes; then administer 1 g of same agent intravenously.				

*Drug suspension diluted in 30 ml of water for ingestion.
†Interval between doses: 15 minutes.
From Sullivan TJ. Drug allergy. In: Middleton E, Reed C, Ellis E, et al., eds. Allergy: Principles and Practice. 4th ed. St. Louis: CV Mosby; 1993;1523–1534, with permission.

Patients have been maintained on long-term, low-dose oral penicillin therapy (usually two or three times daily) to sustain a chronic state of desensitization.[52]

CROSS-REACTIVITY AMONG β-LACTAM ANTIBIOTICS

Cephalosporins

Like penicillins, cephalosporins possess a β-lactam ring, but the five-membered thiazolidine ring is replaced by a six-membered dihydrothiazine ring (see Fig. 21–1). Shortly after cephalosporins came into clinical use, allergic reactions were reported in penicillin-allergic patients and the question of cross-reactivity between cephalosporins and penicillins was raised.[53] To date, the degree of cross-reactivity between penicillins and cephalosporins remains a matter of considerable uncertainty. Complicating matters, the early cephalosporins were contaminated with trace amounts of penicillin, potentially leading to overestimates of the degree of cross-reactivity. Nevertheless, studies in both animals and humans clearly demonstrated cross-reactivity between penicillins and first-generation cephalosporins when immunoassays and bioassays were used to evaluate IgE, IgM, and IgG antibodies.[55–57] In general, the degree of clinical cross-reactivity is much lower than the in vitro cross-reactivity between penicillins and cephalosporins. Small numbers of penicillin skin test–positive patients have been treated with cephalosporin antibiotics without allergic reactions.[58, 59] Too few cephalosporin skin test–positive individuals have been challenged with cephalosporins to allow estimation of the predictive value of a positive skin test. Major determinant analogues of cephalosporins are not currently available as skin test reagents, so the utility of skin testing for cephalosporin allergy is limited.

The incidence of clinically relevant cross-reactivity between the penicillins and cephalosporins is probably small, but rare cases of life-threatening anaphylactic reactions have occurred. The risk of administering a first-generation cephalosporin to a penicillin skin test–positive patient is lower than that of administering a penicillin antibiotic, but it is not negligible. Antibodies to the second- and third-generation cephalosporins are often directed against the side chains rather than the ring structures, and therefore cross-reactivity with penicillins is less than with first-generation cephalosporins.[50] Patients with positive skin tests to any penicillin reagent probably should not receive cephalosporin antibiotics unless alternative drugs are clearly less desirable. If cephalosporin drugs are to be used, they should be administered with caution and with adequate precautions.

Carbapenems

These are a third class of β-lactam antibiotics of which imipenem is the prototype (see Fig. 21–1). Studies have shown that approximately 50% of penicillin skin test–positive patients have positive skin reactions to analogous imipenem determinants,[60] suggesting appreciable cross-reactivity and indicating that these β-lactam antibiotics are relatively contraindicated in patients with positive penicillin skin tests.

Monobactams

The monobactams are a class of β-lactam antibiotics that contain a monocyclic ring structure rather than the bicyclic structure of the penicillins, cephalosporins, and carbapenems (see Fig. 21–1). The prototype monobactam licensed in the United States is aztreonam. In preclinical studies, negligible cross-reactivity in rabbits and in human subjects between aztreonam and penicillins or cephalosporins was found.[61] When subjects with positive penicillin skin tests were skin tested with analogous aztreonam reagents, appreciable cross-reactivity was not found.[62] In a subsequent trial, 20 patients with a positive penicillin skin test were treated with therapeutic doses of aztreonam, and none had IgE-mediated reactions.[63] Taken together, these data suggest weak cross-reactivity between aztreonam and other β-lactam antibiotics and indicate that aztreonam may be safely administered to most, if not all, penicillin-allergic subjects.

UNANSWERED QUESTIONS

Important clinical questions remain for future research in β-lactam allergy. These include (1) the further elucidation of when side chain–specific allergies may be the cause of β-lactam reactions, (2) the possible identification of genetic factors that predispose to β-lactam allergy, (3) the validation of testing procedures to evaluate clinical cross-reactivity between cephalosporin and penicillin antibiotics, and (4) the potential relation of penicillin allergy to other medication reactions involving structurally unrelated drugs.

TABLE 21–5 Protocol for Parenteral Desensitization of β-Lactam Antibiotic–Allergic Patients

Step	β-Lactam Drug (mg/ml)	Amount* (ml)	Dose*† (mg)	Cumulative Dose (mg)
1	0.1	0.1	0.01	0.01
2	0.1	0.2	0.02	0.03
3	0.1	0.4	0.04	0.07
4	0.1	0.8	0.08	0.15
5	1.0	0.16	0.16	0.31
6	1.0	0.32	0.32	0.63
7	1.0	0.64	0.64	1.27
8	10	0.12	1.20	2.47
9	10	0.24	2.40	4.87
10	10	0.48	4.80	10
11	100	0.10	10	20
12	100	0.20	20	40
13	100	0.40	40	80
14	100	0.80	80	160
15	1000	0.16	160	320
16	1000	0.32	320	640
17	1000	0.64	640	1280
18: Observe patient for 30 minutes; then administer 1 g of same agent intravenously.				

*Doses administered subcutaneously (or intramuscularly or intravenously).
†Interval between doses: 15 minutes.
From Sullivan TJ. Drug allergy. In: Middleton E, Reed C, Ellis E, et al., eds. Allergy: Principles and Practice. 4th ed. St. Louis: CV Mosby; 1993;1523–1534, with permission.

REFERENCES

1. Gorevic PD. Drug-induced autoimmune disease. In: Kaplan A, ed. Allergy. New York: Churchill Livingstone; 1985;480.
2. Schwartz HJ, Sher TH. Anaphylaxis to penicillin in a frozen dinner. Ann Allergy. 1984;52:342–343.
3. Parker CW. Drug therapy (first of three parts). N Engl J Med. 1975;292:511–514.
4. International Rheumatic Fever Study Group. Allergic reactions to long-term benzathine penicillin prophylaxis for rheumatic fever. Lancet. 1993;337:1308–1310.
5. Arndt KA, Jick H. Rates of cutaneous reactions to drugs: A report from the Boston Collaborative Drug Surveillance Program. JAMA. 1976;235:918–922.
6. Gell PGH, Coombs RRA. Classification of allergic reactions responsible for clinical hypersensitivity and disease. In: Gell PGH, Coombs RRA, Hachmann PJ, eds. Clinical Aspects of Immunology. Oxford: Blackwell Scientific Publications; 1975;761–781.
7. Levine BB. Immunologic mechanisms of penicillin allergy: A haptenic model system for the study of allergic diseases of man. N Engl J Med. 1966;275:1115–1125.
8. Ishizaka T. Mechanisms of IgE-mediated hypersensitivity. In: Middleton E Jr, Reed CE, Ellis EF, et al., eds. Allergy: Principles and Practice. St. Louis: CV Mosby; 1988;71–93.
9. Idsoe O, Guthe T, Willcox RR, et al. Nature and extent of penicillin side-reactions, with particular reference to fatalities from anaphylactic shock. Bull World Health Organ 1968;38:159–188.
10. Jacobs RL, Geoffrey WR Jr, Fournier DC, et al. Potentiated anaphylaxis in patients with drug-induced beta-adrenergic blockade. J Allergy Clin Immunol. 1981;68:125–127.
11. Heckbert SR, Stryker WS, Coltin KL, et al. Serum sickness in children after antibiotic exposure: Estimates of occurrence and morbidity in a health maintenance organization population. Am J Epidemiol. 1990;132:336–342.
12. Wheeler JG, Childress SH, Kearns GL. Cefaclor serum sickness: In vitro identification using microsome cytotoxicity and flow cytometry (Abstract). J Allergy Clin Immunol. 1993;91:363.
13. Levine B. Skin rashes with penicillin therapy: Current management. N Engl J Med. 1972;286:42–43.
14. Shapiro S, Siskin V, Slone D, et al. Drug rash with ampicillin and other penicillins. Lancet. 1969;2:7628.
15. Kerns DL, Shira JE, Go S, et al. Ampicillin rash in children: Relationship to penicillin allergy and infectious mononucleosis. Am J Dis Child. 1973;125:187–190.
16. Galpin JE, Chow AW, Yoshikawa TT, et al. "Pseudoanaphylactic" reactions from inadvertent infusion of procaine penicillin G. Ann Intern Med. 1974;81:358.
17. Eisen HN. Hypersensitivity to simple chemicals. In: Lawrence HS, ed. Cellular and Humoral Aspects of the Hypersensitive States. New York: PB Hoeber; 1959;111–116.
18. DiPiro JT, Hamilton RG, Adkinson NF Jr. Facilitation of penicilloation of proteins by serum cofactors (Abstract). J Allergy Clin Immunol. 1990;85:192.
19. Sullivan TJ. Facilitated haptenation of human proteins by penicillin (Abstract). J Allergy Clin Immunol. 1989;83:255.
20. Levine BB, Redmond AP. Minor haptenic determinant-specific reagins of penicillin hypersensitivity in man. Int Arch Allergy. 1969;35:445–455.
21. Levine BB, Redmond AP, Fellner MJ, et al. Penicillin allergy and the heterogeneous immune responses of man to benzylpenicillin. J Clin Invest. 1966;45:1895–1906.
22. Levine BB. Effect of combinations of inbred strain, antigen, and antigen dose on immune responsiveness and reagin production in the mouse: A potential mouse model for immune aspects of human atopic allergy. Int Arch Allergy Appl Immunol. 1970;39:156–171.
23. Adkinson NF Jr. Risk factors for drug allergy. J Allergy Clin Immunol. 1984;74:567–572.
24. Sullivan TJ, Yecies LD, Shatz GS, et al. Desensitization of patients allergic to penicillin using orally administered beta-lactam antibiotics. J Allergy Clin Immunol. 1982;69:275–282.
25. Adkinson NF Jr, Wheeler B. Risk factors for IgE-dependent reactions to penicillin. In: Kerr JW, Ganderton MA, eds. XI International Congress of Allergology and Clinical Immunology. London: MacMillan; 1983;55–59.
26. Sogn DD. Prevention of allergic reactions to penicillin. J Allergy Clin Immunol. 1987;78:1051–1052.
27. Adkinson NF Jr, Spence M, Wheeler B. Randomized clinical trial of routine penicillin skin testing. J Allergy Clin Immunol. 1984;73:163.
28. Sullivan TJ, Wedner HJ, Shatz GS, et al. Skin testing to detect penicillin allergy. J Allergy Clin Immunol. 1981;68:171–180.
29. Sogn DD. Penicillin allergy. J Allergy Clin Immunol. 1984;74:589–593.
30. Adkinson NF Jr. Tests for immunological drug reactions. In: Rose NF, Friedman H, eds. Manual of Clinical Immunology. Washington, DC: American Society for Microbiology; 1986;692–697.
31. Sullivan TJ. Penicillin allergy. In: Lichtenstein LM, Fauci A, eds. Current Therapy in Allergy. St. Louis: CV Mosby; 1985;57–61.
32. Gadde J, Spence M, Wheeler B, et al. Clinical experience with penicillin skin testing in a large inner city STD clinic. JAMA. 1993;270:2456–2463.
33. Weiss ME, Adkinson NF Jr. Immediate hypersensitivity reactions to penicillin and related antibiotics. Clin Allergy. 1988;18:515–540.
34. Pichichero M, Pichichero, D. Diagnosis of penicillin, amoxicillin and cephalosporin allergy: Reliability of examination assessed by skin testing and oral challenge. J Pediatr. 1998;132:137–143.
35. Chandra RK, Joglekar SA, Tomas E. Penicillin allergy: Anti-penicillin IgE antibodies and immediate hypersensitivity skin reactions employing major and minor determinants of penicillin. Arch Dis Child. 1980;55:857–860.
36. Sogn DD, Casale TB, Condemi JJ, et al. Results of the NIAID collaborative clinical trial to test the predictive value of skin testing with major and minor penicillin derivatives in hospitalized adults. Arch Intern Med. 1992;152:1025–1032.
37. Mendelson LML, Ressler C, Rosen JP, et al. Routine elective penicillin allergy skin testing in children and adolescents: Study of sensitization. J Allergy Clin Immunol. 1984;73:76–81.
38. Parker P, Parrinello, JT, Condemi J, et al. Penicillin resensitization among hospitalized patients. J Allergy Clin Immunol. 1991;88:213–217.
39. De Weck AL, Schneider CH. Specific inhibition of allergic reactions to penicillin in man by a monovalent hapten: II. Clinical studies. Int Arch Allergy Immunol. 1972;42:798–815.
40. De Weck AL, Schneider CH. Specific inhibition of allergic reactions to penicillin in man by a monovalent hapten. Int Arch Allergy Immunol. 1972;42:782–797.
41. Warrington RJ, Simons FER, Ho HW, et al. Diagnosis of penicillin allergy by skin testing: The Manitoba experience. CMAJ. 1978;11:787.
42. Blanca M, Vega JM, Garcia J, et al. Allergy to penicillin with good tolerance to other penicillins: Study of the incidence in subjects allergic to betalactams. Clin Exp Allergy. 1990;20:475–481.
43. Blanca M, Perez E, Garcia J, et al. Anaphylaxis to amoxycillin but good tolerance for benzylpenicillin. Allergy. 1988;43:508–510.
44. Silviu-Dan F, McPhillips S, Warrington R. The frequency of skin test reactions to side-chain penicillin determinants. J Allergy Clin Immunol. 1993;91:694–701.
45. Macy E, Richter P, Falkoff R, et al. Clinical aspects of allergic disease: Skin testing with penicilloate and penilloate prepared by an improved method. Amoxicillin oral challenge in patients with negative skin test responses to penicillin reagents. J Allergy Clin Immunol. 1997;100:586–591.
46. Adkinson Jr NF. Side-chain specific beta-lactam allergy. Clin Exp Allergy. 1990;20: 445–447.
47. Martin J, Igea J, Fraj J, et al. Allergy to amoxicillin in patients who tolerated benzylpenicillin, aztreonam, and ceftazidime. Clin Infect Dis. 1992;14:592–593.
48. Romano A, Di Fonso M, Papa G, et al. Evaluation of adverse cutaneous reactions to aminopenicillins with emphasis on those manifested by maculopapular rashes. Allergy. 1995;50:113–118.
49. Terrados S, Blanca M, Garcia J, et al. Nonimmediate reactions to betalactams: Prevalence and role of the different penicillins. Allergy. 1995;50:563–567.
50. Sullivan TJ. Drug allergy. In: Middleton E, Reed C, Ellis E, et al., eds. Allergy: Principles and Practice. 4th ed. St. Louis: CV Mosby; 1993;1523–1534.
51. Adkinson NF Jr. Penicillin allergy. In: Lichtenstein LM, Fauci A, eds. Current Therapy in Allergy, Immunology and Rheumatology. Ontario, Canada: BS Decker; 1983;57–62.
52. Naclerio R, Mizrahi EA, Adkinson NF Jr. Immunologic observations during desensitization and maintenance of clinical tolerance to penicillin. J Allergy Clin Immunol. 1983;71:294–301.
53. Grieco MH. Cross-allergenicity of the penicillins and the cephalosporins. Arch Intern Med. 1967;119:141–146.
54. Pedersen-Bjergaard J. Cephalothin in the treatment of penicillin sensitive patients. Acta Allergol. 1967;12:299–306.
55. Petz L. Immunologic cross-reactivity between penicillins and cephalosporins: A review. J Infect Dis. 1978;137:S74–S79.
56. Shibata K, Atsumi T, Itorivchi Y, et al. Immunological cross-reactivities of cephalothin and its related compounds with benzylpenicillin (penicillin G). Nature. 1966;212:419–420.
57. Abraham GN, Petz LD, Fudenberg HH. Immunohaematological cross-allergenicity between penicillin and cephalothin in humans. Clin Exp Immunol. 1968;3:343–357.
58. Solley GO, Gleich GJ, Van Dellen RG. Penicillin allergy: Clinical experience with a battery of skin-test reagents. J Allergy Clin Immunol. 1982;69:238–244.
59. Saxon A, Beall GN, Rohr AS, et al. Immediate hypersensitivity reactions to beta-lactam antibiotics. Ann Intern Med. 1987;107:204–215.
60. Saxon A. Immediate hypersensitivity reactions to beta-lactam antibiotics. Rev Infect Dis. 1983;5:S368.
61. Adkinson NF Jr, Swabb EA, Sugerman AA. Immunology of the monobactam aztreonam. Antimicrob Agents Chemother. 1984;25:93–97.
62. Saxon A, Hassner A, Swabb EA, et al. Lack of cross-reactivity between aztreonam, a monobactam antibiotic, and penicillin in penicillin-allergic subjects. J Infect Dis. 1984;149:16–22.
63. Adkinson NF Jr, Wheeler B, Swabb EA. Clinical tolerance of the monobactam aztreonam in penicillin allergic subjects (Abstract WS-26-4). Presented at the 14th International Congress of Chemotherapy, June 23–28, 1985. Kyoto, Japan.

Chapter 22

Fusidic Acid

LIONEL A. MANDELL

STRUCTURE

Fusidic acid, a member of the fusidane class, is derived from the fungus *Fusidium coccineum* and is chemically related to the antibiotics helvolic acid and cephalosporin P_1.[1] Despite its steroid-like structure, fusidic acid does not have steroid activity. The sodium salt of fusidic acid, termed *Fucidin,* was developed by Leo Laboratories in Denmark and was first introduced into clinical practice in 1962.

MECHANISM OF ACTION

Fusidic acid is usually bacteriostatic but at higher concentrations may be bactericidal. It exerts its antibacterial effect by inhibiting protein synthesis, but the exact mechanisms by which this inhibition occurs have not been fully elucidated.

Bacterial protein synthesis depends on the translocation of peptidyl–transfer RNA from the ribosomal acceptor site to the peptidyl site. This requires protein elongation factor G and hydrolysis of guanosine triphosphate (GTP). At least part of fusidic acid's action reflects its ability to stabilize ribosome–elongation factor–GTP + inorganic phosphate complexes, thereby inhibiting GTP hydrolysis and blocking elongation of the nascent polypeptide chain.[2]

Resistance to fusidic acid may occur through a variety of mechanisms. Strains of *Staphylococcus aureus* may exhibit chromosome- or plasmid-mediated resistance. Chromosomal mutations, which occur at a frequency of 1 in 10^{-6} to 10^{-7},[3,4] and result in alteration at the target site (i.e., elongation factor G). Plasmid-mediated resistance may be due to reduced permeability to the antibiotic.[5]

ANTIMICROBIAL ACTIVITY

Fusidic acid has an unusual and somewhat unique spectrum of antimicrobial activity. Susceptible organisms include selected aerobes and anaerobes. Although there are no official National Committee for Clinical Laboratory Standards guidelines for in vitro susceptibility testing, a recent study determined the minimal inhibitory concentrations (MICs) and zone diameters for fusidic acid using standard National Committee for Clinical Laboratory Standards methods.[6] The proposed break points for fusidic acid against staphylococci are as follows:

	Minimal Inhibitory Concentration (mg/L)	Zone Diameter (mm)
Susceptible	≤0.25	≥22
Intermediate	0.5–1	>17–<22
Resistant	≥2	≤17

Fusidic acid is most active against *S. aureus* and *Staphylococcus epidermidis,* including strains that are methicillin resistant. Such organisms are generally sensitive to fusidic acid, as there is no cross-resistance between this agent and β-lactam antimicrobials. MICs for methicillin-resistant *S. aureus* range from 0.03 to 0.8 mg/liter, but in one study of bacteremic isolates the MIC_{90} was 0.2 mg/liter.[7] Only a short in vitro postantibiotic effect of 1 to 2 hours has been demonstrated. Fusidic acid is considerably less active against *Staphylococcus saprophyticus* strains and streptococci.

Corynebacteria are generally sensitive, as are *Neisseria gonorrhoeae* and *Meningococcus.* Aerobic gram-negative bacilli appear to be resistant.[3]

With the exception of *Fusobacterium necrophorum,* anaerobic organisms are generally quite sensitive to fusidic acid. Gram-positive anaerobes generally are very susceptible, with MIC_{90} s ranging from 0.25 to 1 mg/liter.[4] MIC_{90} s for *Clostridium difficile* are somewhat higher at 2 mg/liter. Gram-negative anaerobes are a little more variable in their susceptibility. The *Bacteroides* species *B. distasonis, B. ovatus, B. thetaiotaomicron,* and *B. fragilis* exhibit MIC_{90} s ranging from 2 to 16 mg/liter, whereas for the *Prevotella* species *P. buccae, P. oralis,* and *P. melaninogenica* and the *Bacteroides* species *B. ureolyticus* and *B. vulgatus,* MIC_{90} s range from only 0.25 to 1 mg/liter.

MICs are markedly increased in the presence of serum, and antimicrobial activity is also reduced in alkaline media. Reports of the effects of antimicrobial combinations containing fusidic acid have been somewhat inconsistent. In one study of drug combinations involving fusidic acid with either vancomycin or rifampin against isolates of methicillin-resistant *S. aureus,* neither synergy nor antagonism was demonstrated, whereas another study of fusidic acid with rifampin against methicillin-resistant coagulase-positive and coagulase-negative staphylococci suggested some synergistic effect.[8, 9]

Some data suggest that fusidic acid may be active in vitro against mycobacteria.[10] MIC_{90} s of 16 and 30 mg/liter have been reported for *Mycobacterium tuberculosis* and *Mycobacterium bovis*, respectively.

PHARMACOLOGY

Fusidic acid may be used parenterally as an intravenous formulation, or it may be given orally or applied topically. Various formulations, dosages, and frequencies of administration are given in Table 22–1. The sodium salt intravenous formulation may be administered over 2 to 4 hours.

The drug is virtually completely absorbed after oral administration, achieving levels up to 71 mg/liter with repeated thrice-daily dosing. With repeated intravenous infusions, peak plasma concentrations of 123 mg/liter have been recorded. The drug is highly protein bound (95 to 97%), exhibits nonlinear kinetics, and has a half-life of approximately 14 hours. Although the standard frequency of administration has been three times a day, because of the drug's long half-life it has been suggested that dosing could be changed to a twice-daily schedule.[4, 11] This has been our practice for the last 3 years, and it appears to reduce gastrointestinal intolerance without altering efficacy.

TABLE 22–1 Dosage and Administration of Fusidic Acid

Route of Administration	Formulation	Dosage	Frequency of Administration
IV	Sodium fusidate	>50 kg BW, 500 mg*	tid
		<50 kg BW, 7 mg/kg	tid
PO (film-coated tablets)	Sodium fusidate	500 mg	tid
PO (suspension)	Hemihydrate	0–1 yr, 0.3 ml/kg BW	tid
		1–5 yr, 5 ml	tid
		6–12 yr, 10 ml	tid
		Adults, 15 ml	tid
Topical			
Cream (2%)	Fusidic acid		bid
Ointment (2%)	Sodium fusidate		bid
Gel (2%)	Sodium fusidate		bid
Ophthalmic			
Viscous eyedrops (1%)	Fusidic acid		bid

*Five hundred milligrams of sodium fusidate is equivalent to 480 mg of fusidic acid.
Abbreviation: BW, Body weight.

Fusidic acid is widely distributed to such tissues as synovial fluid, bone, subcutaneous fat, kidney, bronchial secretions, cardiac tissue, and aqueous humor.[12] The drug also crosses the placenta.

It is metabolized by the liver and is eliminated primarily by biliary excretion. Approximately 2% of the drug can be recovered unchanged in the stool, but very little is recovered in urine. Dosage modification is not necessary for patients with renal failure or for those on hemodialysis. Little is known about the use of fusidic acid in patients with hepatic impairment, and the drug is probably best avoided in such circumstances.

Fusidic acid also has in vitro and in vivo immunosuppressive functions. The drug has been found to have activity similar to that of cyclosporine and in animal models and in preliminary human trials has been shown to either protect against the development of insulin-dependent diabetes mellitus or have an ameliorating effect on the disease.[13, 15]

ADVERSE REACTIONS

The adverse reactions depend on the route of administration. With the intravenous formulation, thrombophlebitis and reversible jaundice have been noted. Reversible jaundice is also seen with the oral preparation, but to a lesser extent (6% versus 17%).[16]

As the drug is avidly bound to albumin, it competes with bilirubin for binding sites. It should therefore be used with caution, if at all, in newborns, particularly if they are icteric, acidotic, or premature.[17] Oral use is generally well tolerated but has been associated with mild gastrointestinal upset. The ophthalmic preparations may occasionally cause mild to moderate local symptoms such as itching or stinging. A drug-induced reversible immune-mediated thrombocytopenia has been described in which a fusidic acid–dependent platelet-reactive antibody binds platelets but only in the presence of the drug.[18]

CLINICAL USE

Fusidic acid has been used in systemic (intravenous, oral) and topical (ophthalmic, skin preparations) formulations primarily for the treatment of staphylococcal infections. It is not available in the United States, although it may be obtained through compassionate release. The foci of infection, with and without associated bacteremia, have included acute and chronic osteomyelitis, septic arthritis, endocarditis, soft tissue infections including burns, and lower respiratory tract infections in patients with cystic fibrosis.[19–21]

Endocarditis has been treated with some success using fusidic acid in combination with a second drug. Fusidic acid has been given with a penicillinase-resistant semisynthetic penicillin such as flucloxacillin for staphylococcal endocarditis and with erythromycin for endocarditis caused by *Corynebacteria*.[22, 23]

Given the increased incidence of methicillin-resistant *S. aureus* and *S. epidermidis* infections, this drug may offer advantages over currently available agents. Topical use has been limited to external eye infections and superficial skin infections, including erythrasma caused by *Corynebacterium minutissimum.*

Initial concerns about the emergence of resistant strains during therapy led to the practice of combining fusidic acid with a second drug. Resistance may be more likely to occur in the setting of chronic infections if the drug is used alone.[3, 24] However, experience over the past few decades has shown that even when the drug is used alone for the treatment of acute infections, resistance is seen in only zero to 2% of patients, whereas resistance occurs in less than 1% of patients treated with combination therapy.

REFERENCES

1. Godtfredsen W, Roholt K, Tybring L. Fusidin. A new orally active antibiotic. Lancet. 1962;1:928–931.
2. Von Daehne W, Godtfredsen WO, Rasmussen PR. Structure-activity relationships in fusidic acid-type antibiotics. Adv Appl Microbiol. 1979;25:95–146.
3. Verbist L. The antimicrobial activity of fusidic acid. J Antimicrob Chemother. 1990;25(Suppl B):1–5.
4. Steinkraus GE, McCarthy LR. In vitro activity of sodium fusidate against anaerobic bacteria. Antimicrob Agents Chemother. 1979;16:120–122.
5. Shanson DC. Clinical relevance of resistance to fusidic acid in *Staphylococcus aureus*. J Antimicrob Chemother. 1990;25(Suppl B):15–21.
6. Coutant C, Olden D, Bell J, Turnidge J. Disk diffusion interpretive criteria for fusidic acid susceptibility testing of staphylococci by the National Committee for Clinical Laboratory Standards method. Diagn Microbiol Infect Dis. 1996;25:9–13.
7. Van der Auwera P, Godard C, Denis C, et al. In vitro activities of new antimicrobial agents against multiresistant *Staphylococcus aureus* isolated from septicemic patients during a Belgian national survey from 1983 to 1985. Antimicrob Agents Chemother. 1990;34:2260–2262.
8. Foldes M, Munro R, Sorrell TC, et al. In-vitro effects of vancomycin, rifampicin, and fusidic acid, alone and in combination, against methicillin-resistant *Staphylococcus aureus*. J Antimicrob Chemother. 1983;11:21–26.
9. Farber BF, Yee YC, Karchmer AW. Interaction between rifampin and fusidic acid against methicillin-resistant coagulase-positive and -negative staphylococci. Antimicrob Agents Chemother. 1986;30:174–175.
10. Fuursted K, Askgaard D, Faber V. Susceptibility of strains of the mycobacterium tuberculosis complex to fusidic acid. APMIS. 1992;100:663–667.
11. Carr WD, Wall AR, Georgala-Zervogiani S, et al. Fusidic acid tablets in patients with skin and soft tissue infection: A dose-finding study. Eur J Clin Res. 1994;5:87–95.
12. Reeves DS. The pharmacokinetics of fusidic acid. J Antimicrob Chemother. 1987;20:467–476.
13. Nicoletti F, Meroni PL, Bendtzen K. Fusidic acid and insulin-dependent diabetes mellitus. Autoimmunity. 1996;24:187–197.
14. Nicoletti F, Zaconne P, Di Marco R, et al. Effects of sodium fusidate in animal models of insulin-dependent diabetes mellitus and septic shock. Immunology. 1995;85:645–650.
15. Nicoletti F, Di Marco R, Morrone S, et al. Reduction of spontaneous autoimmune diabetes in diabetes-prone BB rats with the novel immunosuppressant fusidic acid. Effect on T-cell proliferation and production of interferon-γ. Immunology. 1994;81:317–321.
16. Eykyn SJ. Staphylococcal bacteremia and endocarditis and fusidic acid. J Antimicrob Chemother. 1990;25(Suppl B):33–38.
17. Brodersen R. Fusidic acid binding to serum albumin and interaction with binding of bilirubin. Acta Paediatr Scand. 1985;74:874–880.
18. El-Kassar N, Kalfon P, Fromont P, et al. Fusidic acid induced acute immunologic thrombocytopenia. Br J Haematol. 1996;93:427–431.
19. O'Brien T, McManus F, MacAuley PH, Ennis JT. Acute haematogenous osteomyelitis. J Bone Joint Surg Br. 1982;64:450–453.
20. Gransden WR, Eykyn SJ, Phillips I. *Staphylococcus aureus* bacteraemia: 400 episodes in St. Thomas's Hospital. BMJ 1984;288:300–303.
21. Wright GLT, Harper J. Fusidic acid and lincomycin therapy in staphylococcal infections in cystic fibrosis. Lancet. 1970;1:9–14.
22. Moy RJD, George RH, de Giovanni JV, Silove ED. Improving survival in bacterial endocarditis. Arch Dis Child. 1986;61:394–399.
23. Jackson G, Saunders K. Prosthetic valve diphtheroid endocarditis treated with sodium fusidate and erythromycin. Br Heart J. 1973;35:931–936.
24. Faber M, Rosdahl VT. Susceptibility to fusidic acid among Danish *Staphylococcus aureus* strains and fusidic acid consumption. J Antimicrob Chemother. 1990;25(Suppl B):7–14.

Chapter 23

Aminoglycosides

DAVID N. GILBERT

Aminoglycoside antibiotics have been an important part of the antibacterial drug arsenal since the 1940s. They demonstrate concentration-dependent bactericidal activity against susceptible organisms. Several members of the aminoglycoside family have predictable in vitro activity against *Pseudomonas aeruginosa* and the vast majority of other aerobic gram-negative bacilli. Some aminoglycosides have useful activity against mycobacteria; one (paromomycin) has been used to treat selected colonic protozoan pathogens, and a related antibiotic, spectinomycin, has been used to treat infection by *Neisseria gonorrhoeae.* The aminoglycoside antimicrobial activity may be additive or synergistic with penicillins or cephalosporins against infection by aerobic gram-negative bacilli or aerobic gram-positive cocci. The prevalence of aminoglycoside resistance has remained low and emergence of bacterial resistance during therapy rare.

The aminoglycoside family shares the potential for nephrotoxicity, ototoxicity, and rarely, neuromuscular blockade. The risk of toxicity may be decreasing as mechanisms are understood, new dosage strategies introduced, concomitant risk factors avoided, and shorter drug courses used. Allergic reactions are rare. With patent expirations, the cost of many aminoglycosides is low. Although new β-lactams and fluoroquinolones share the same antibacterial spectrum, the efficacy of the aminoglycosides and resistance problems with the newer drugs presage a continued need.

NAMES AND SOURCES: INTRODUCTION TO CHEMISTRY

In the 1940s, soil actinomycetes (bacteria) were systematically screened for the elaboration of antimicrobial substances. Streptomycin, the first aminoglycoside found[1] (Table 23–1), was produced by a *Streptomyces* organism, and subsequent drugs were derived from either other *Streptomyces* species or *Micromonospora*.[2, 3] The suffix indicates the source; that is, aminoglycosides with names ending in *mycin* derive directly or indirectly from *Streptomyces,* whereas aminoglycosides with names ending in *micin* derive directly or indirectly from *Micromonospora.*

Neomycin, kanamycin, and gentamicin are fermentation products with two or three chemical constituents. Amikacin, netilmicin, dibekacin, and isepamicin are semisynthetic derivatives of the natural product. Nine aminoglycosides (including spectinomycin) are commercially available at this time in the United States. Sisomicin, dibekacin, and isepamicin are approved for human use in Japan, Europe, and elsewhere.

CHEMISTRY

Structure

All aminoglycosides have an essential six-membered ring with amino-group substituents—hence the name *aminocyclitol* for this structure.[2, 3] The descriptor *aminoglycoside* results from the glycosidic bonds between the aminocyclitol and two or more amino-containing or non–amino-containing sugars. Spectinomycin differs in that it has an aminocyclitol ring but no aminosugars and no glycosidic bonds.

The central aminocyclitol for streptomycin is streptidine, whereas for all other current aminoglycosides it is 2-deoxystreptamine (Fig. 23–1). The standard numbering convention is illustrated in Figure 23–1. Note the counterclockwise numbering of the aminocyclitol ring and the clockwise numbering of linked sugar molecules. Figure 23–1 also illustrates the structural basis of the aminoglycoside subgroups. Neomycin and paromomycin are derived from *Streptomyces* spp. and link to cyclic sugars at positions 4 and 5 of 2-deoxystreptamine. Both drugs contain a distinctive pentose linkage, as well as linkage to two hexose sugars. Note that of the commonly used aminoglycosides, neomycin contains the largest number, six, of free amino groups.

Kanamycin, tobramycin, amikacin, and dibekacin constitute the kanamycin family[3–8] (Table 23–2). All derive from *Streptomyces* spp. and link to cyclic sugars at positions 4 and 6 of 2-deoxystreptamine. Tobramycin is 3′-deoxykanamycin B. Amikacin is kanamycin A with the semisynthetic addition of 2-hydroxy-4-aminobutyric acid to the amino group at position 1 of the aminocyclitol.

Gentamicin is a mixture of three closely related constituents, C_1, C_{1a}, and C_2, elaborated by *Micromonospora* spp. and has glycosidic linkages at positions 4 and 6. Sisomicin is the dihydro analogue of gentamicin C_{1a}; netilmicin is derived from sisomicin by the addition of an ethyl group to the amino group at position 1 of the aminocyclitol.

Aminoglycoside structure-activity relationships are incompletely understood. Removal of amino, hydroxyl, or both groups results in a concomitant loss of both antibacterial activity and toxic potential.[3–5]

Chemical Characteristics

Aminoglycosides are highly soluble in water and insoluble in organic solvents.[9] The latter property correlates with the limited ability of aminoglycosides to cross lipid-containing cellular membranes.

Aminoglycosides have a molecular weight in the range of 445 to 600 daltons.[9] The molecular structure is unchanged by freezing, heating to 100°C for up to 4 hours, or changes in solution pH ranging from 3.0 to 12 over several hours.[10–12] The ionization constants for individual amino groups are difficult to determine. The overall pK_a for gentamicin is about pH 8.4.[9] Hence, at pH 7.4, aminoglycosides have a very high positive charge and are cationic.

The overall positive charge contributes to both antimicrobial activity and toxicity. Antibacterial activity is enhanced in media with an alkaline pH and reduced in media with an acidic pH.[12] The cationic aminoglycosides bind to the lipopolysaccharide of the cell wall of bacteria and to a variety of intracellular and cell membrane anionic molecules (e.g., DNA and phospholipids).[13–17]

Of interest, cationic aminoglycosides interact chemically with β-lactam antibiotics.[18–20] The reaction results in a nucleophilic opening of the β-lactam ring with acylation of an amino group of the aminoglycoside and mutual loss of antibacterial activity. In vitro, gentamicin and tobramycin are inactivated with greater ease than is netilmicin, amikacin, or isepamicin. Perhaps because their dosage is in

TABLE 23–1 The Family of Aminoglycosides in Clinical Use*

Names				
Generic	*Proprietary*	Source	Year Reported	Chemistry
Streptomycin	None	*Streptomyces griseus*	1944	Unique central aminocyclitrol ring
Neomycin	Mycifradin	*Streptomyces fradiae*	1949	Roughly equal proportions of neomycin B and C
Kanamycin	Kantrex	*Streptomyces kanamyceticus*	1957	Mixture of 95% kanamycin A and 5% kanamycin B
Paromomycin	Humatin	*S. fradiae*	1959	Part of the "neomycin" family
Gentamicin	Garamycin	*Micromonospora purpurea* and *Micromonospora echinospora*	1963	Roughly equal proportions of gentamicin C_1, C_{1a}, C_2
Tobramycin	Nebcin	*Streptomyces tenebrarius*	1968	Natural 3′-deoxy derivative of kanamycin B
Amikacin†	Amikin	*S. kanamyceticus*	1972	Semisynthetic derivative of kanamycin A
Netilmicin†	Netromycin	*Micromonospora inyoensis*	1975	*N*-ethyl derivative of sisomicin
Spectinomycin	Trobicin	*Streptomyces spectabilis*	1962	Chemically distinct but closely related to aminoglycosides
Sisomicin‡	Siseptin	*M. inyoensis*	1970	Dehydro analogue of gentamicin C_{1a}
Dibekacin†‡		*S. kanamyceticus*	1971	Dideoxy derivative of kanamycin B
Isepamicin†‡		*M. purpurea*	1978	I-*N*-*S*-α-hydroxy B amino propionyl derivative of gentamicin B

*The drugs are listed by the year in which they were described, with comments on their chemistry.[1–8]
†Semisynthetic aminoglycosides.
‡Approved for human use in countries other than the United States.

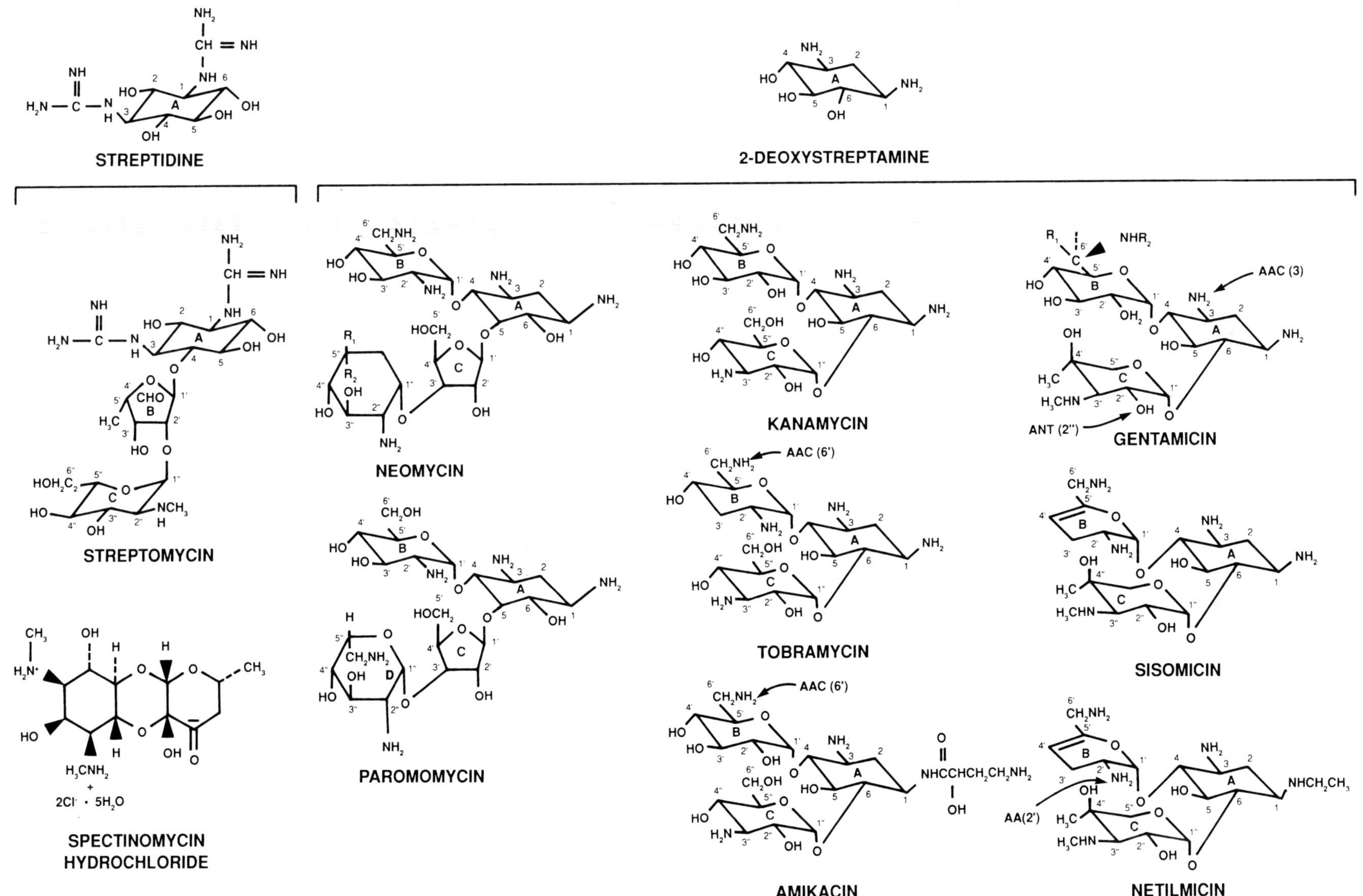

FIGURE 23–1. Chemical structure of the aminoglycosides and spectinomycin. Neomycin contains approximately equal amounts of neomycin B (R_1 = H; R_2 = CH_2NH_2) and neomycin C (R_1 = CH_2NH_2; R_2 = H). Kanamycin is principally kanamycin A, as shown. Gentamicin is gentamicin C complex with roughly equal amounts of C_1 (R_1 = R_2 = CH_3), C_{1a} (R_1 = R_2 = H), and C_2 (R_1 = CH_3; R_2 = H). The sites of action of four inactivating enzymes are shown; three acetyltransferases (AAC [3], AAC [2′], and AAC [6′]) and one adenyltransferase (ANT [2″]).

TABLE 23–2 Chemical Families of Aminoglycoside Antibiotics

Family	Member
Streptomycin	Streptomycin
Kanamycin	Kanamycin A
	Kanamycin B
	Amikacin
	Tobramycin
	Dibekacin
Gentamicin	Gentamicin C_1, C_{1a}, C_2
	Sisomicin
	Netilmicin
	Isepamicin
Neomycin	Neomycin
	Paromomycin
Spectinomycin*	

*An aminocyclitol, no glycosidic bonds.

grams rather than milligrams, the antipseudomonal penicillins (e.g., carbenicillin, ticarcillin, piperacillin, mezlocillin, and azlocillin) are the β-lactams most prone to the reaction. The reaction requires several hours in vitro, so the clinical import is limited. Nonetheless, penicillins and aminoglycosides should not be mixed in the same solution before infusion. Serum specimens for drug level determination from patients receiving both drugs should be assayed immediately or frozen. If patients with renal failure are concomitantly administered an aminoglycoside and an antipseudomonal penicillin, the serum aminoglycoside concentration is reduced 10 to 20% below the levels observed when each drug is administered alone.[21] The interaction is molecule to molecule, and because of the 40-fold difference in dosage, the serum concentration of the penicillin is not noticeably decreased.

Enzymatic Inactivation

Aminoglycosides are subject to modification and loss of antimicrobial activity by enzymes derived from both gram-positive and gram-negative bacterial pathogens.[3, 22, 23] The three classes of enzymes recognized are (1) adenosine triphosphate (ATP)–dependent phosphorylation of a hydroxyl group by a phosphotransferase, (2) ATP-dependent adenylation of a hydroxyl group by a nucleotidyltransferase, or (3) acetyl coenzyme A (CoA)–dependent acetylation of an amino group by an acetyltransferase. Examples of sites of enzyme activity are shown in Figure 23–1. Enzyme modification results in loss of antibacterial activity.

MECHANISM OF ANTIMICROBIAL ACTIVITY

The mechanism of aminoglycoside antibacterial activity is a multifactorial process that includes an initial ionic interaction with the external surface of the cell, two energy-dependent uptake phases, and binding to ribosomes.[24–26] Aminoglycosides bind electrostatically and rapidly to the outer membrane.[27, 28] The binding is passive and non–energy dependent. In gram-negative bacteria, cationic aminoglycosides bind to negatively charged residues in lipopolysaccharide, polar heads of phospholipids, and anionic outer membrane proteins.[15, 25] Aminoglycosides competitively displace the cell wall Mg^{2+} and Ca^{2+} that normally link adjacent lipopolysaccharide molecules.[29, 30] The result is a rearrangement of lipopolysaccharide with subsequent bleeding of the outer membrane, formation of transient holes in the cell wall, and disruption of the cell wall's normal permeability function.[31]

Once across the membrane, the drugs are irreversibly trapped in the cytoplasm of the bacteria. The trapping may be a manifestation of the reactivity of the charged cationic drugs with DNA and other cellular anionic constituents, with subsequent internal coprecipitation.[26, 32, 33] The result is intracellular aminoglycoside concentrations that far exceed external concentrations.

Energy-Dependent Phase

After ionic binding, aminoglycoside uptake can be divided into an energy-dependent initial slow phase (EDP-I) and a subsequent rapid phase (EDP-II).[24–26, 34–36] Both EDP-I and EDP-II are energy dependent. The source of energy is an electrochemical gradient of protons generated by proton extrusion during respiration or by the hydrolysis of ATP.[24] The electrochemical gradient is calculated from the additive effects of the electrical potential difference across the membrane and the proton concentration across the membrane.

The greater the transmembrane electrical potential, the greater the antibacterial effect of the aminoglycoside. The transmembrane electrical potential is decreased in an anaerobic environment, a low external pH, and growth in high-osmolar culture media.[37, 38] Under each of these conditions, aminoglycoside transport is demonstrably reduced, with an associated reduction in antibacterial activity.

The onset of bacterial killing is coincident with the transition from EDP-I to EDP-II.[34, 35] Most bacterial cells have suffered lethal injury before completion of more than 25% of EDP-II uptake.[35] The higher the external concentration of aminoglycoside, the quicker the intracellular drug level reaches concentrations necessary to trigger EDP-II uptake, which in turn forecasts death of the organism.[39]

Aminoglycoside-Ribosome Interaction

Aminoglycosides interfere with the translational accuracy of messenger RNA codons and aminoacyl–transfer RNA anticodons on the small 30S subunit of prokaryotic ribosomes.[40, 41] Aminoglycosides bind to a highly conserved subcomponent of the 30S ribosomal subunit termed the A site of the 16S ribosomal RNA (rRNA). Eukaryotic ribosomes, such as human ribosomes, have a much lower affinity for aminoglycosides. Binding to the decoding region of the bacterial 16S rRNA causes termination and miscoding of protein synthesis with subsequent bacterial death.

The three-dimensional interaction between the aminoglycoside paromomycin and the 27-nucleotide A-site of *Escherichia coli* has been determined by nuclear magnetic resonance spectroscopy.[42] The antibiotic binds in a major deep groove of the rRNA within a pocket created by an adenine-adenine base pair. Of interest, eukaryotes have a guanidine-adenine base pair at the same location. Binding involves the A and B rings of the antibiotic.

The rRNA sequence determinants for aminoglycoside binding are in the process of elucidation. The A-site is formed between nucleotides 1400 and 1500.[43] For paromomycin, an asymmetric internal loop with a bulged nucleotide at position 1492 is necessary.[43, 44] The specifics may differ for tobramycin and other aminoglycosides.[45, 46] Methylation-induced alterations in nucleotide sequencing are expressed by failure of binding and loss of antibacterial activity.

Other naturally occurring RNA species also bind aminoglycosides, and the mechanism may differ from the binding to prokaryote rRNA.[43] Aminoglycosides bind to group I introns, a hammerhead ribozyme, the human immunodeficiency virus Rev response element (core), and the ribozyme derived from the human hepatitis delta virus.[43, 47]

It is accepted that aminoglycosides bind to bacterial ribosomes, and the consequence is a measurable decrease in protein synthesis as a result of misreading of messenger RNA. However, this explanation may be incomplete in that other drugs that inhibit protein synthesis (e.g., chloramphenicol) are only bacteriostatic and not bactericidal.[48] Bacterial death may be multifactorial.[3, 26, 49] Aminoglycoside binding to and alteration of the cell envelope plus ribosomal dysfunction and perhaps other yet unrecognized effects could act in concert to produce a rapid bactericidal result.[49]

AMINOGLYCOSIDE RESISTANCE

Bacteria defend themselves against aminoglycosides by some combination of three mechanisms: alteration in uptake, synthesis of modifying enzymes, or a change in ribosomal binding sites.[22, 23] Enzymatic modification is the most common mechanism.

Enzymatic Modification

Aerobic gram-negative bacteria can alter the aminoglycoside molecule by acetyl CoA–dependent acetylation of an amino group with acetyltransferases (AAC), ATP-dependent adenylation of a hydroxyl group with nucleotidyltransferases (also known as *adenyltransferases*) (ANT), or ATP-dependent phosphorylation of a hydroxyl group with phosphotransferases (APH).[22, 23] More than 50 aminoglycoside-modifying enzymes have been identified.[23] One enzyme, found in staphylococci and enterococci, is a fusion of an acetylating and a phosphorylating enzyme. The combination inactivates all current aminoglycosides except streptomycin and spectinomycin. The terminology for the enzymes and the genes that encode them is confusing in that different systems may be used by different authors.[23, 50, 51]

Enzyme-modified aminoglycoside binds poorly to ribosomes, and the EDP-II of accelerated drug uptake fails to occur; consequently, high-level resistance results.[52] Analysis of the enzymatic resistance mechanisms of thousands of clinical isolates collected worldwide between 1987 and 1993 demonstrates a diverse pattern of enzyme production.[22] Of the AAC group, a family of AAC (6′) enzymes is of particular import because of their ability to modify tobramycin, gentamicin, netilmicin, and amikacin (see Fig. 23–1).

Eight or more genes encode this enzymatic activity. ANT (2″) enzymes result in gentamicin, tobramycin, and dibekacin resistance. At least three encoding genes are involved. APH enzymes produce resistance to neomycin, paromomycin, and kanamycin. Overall, the data suggest that most enzyme-mediated aminoglycoside resistance in gram-negative bacilli is due to more than one gene. Gram-positive cocci, however, may have more homogeneity in genetic resistance. Aminoglycoside resistance surveys on strains collected before 1983 demonstrate a single resistant mechanism (i.e., one aminoglycoside-modifying enzyme).[22] In recent surveys, the majority of resistance strains manifest a combination of several resistance mechanisms. The presence of multiple resistance genes in a single integrin is postulated.

The enzymes encoding aminoglycoside resistance genes are usually found on extrachromosomal bacterial plasmids and transposons. In the laboratory and clinically, resistance genes have been transferred from gram-positive to gram-negative bacteria. For example, a phosphorylating enzyme gene was transferred from enterococci to a *Campylobacter* species.[53] Aminoglycoside genes have been found on both conjugative and nonconjugative plasmids.

Two theories have been presented regarding the origin of aminoglycoside-modifying enzymes.[22] The enzymes may have derived from the organisms that synthesize the aminoglycosides. Such enzymes would provide self-protection against the antibiotic synthesized. Alternatively, the aminoglycoside resistance genes may derive from mutation of genes that encode enzymes involved in normal cellular respiration.

The intracellular location of aminoglycoside-modifying enzymes is debatable. Available data are consistent with localization to the periplasmic space.

No evidence of regulation of the aminoglycoside resistance genes has been reported; gene transcription, with few exceptions, is constitutive. The enzymes are produced in the presence and absence of antibiotic.

Altered Ribosome Binding Sites

The 16S rRNA binding site can be altered as a result of either enzyme activity or mutational modification. Although rRNA methylating enzymes are found in many aminoglycoside-producing organisms, no clinical isolate with this mechanism of resistance has been found.[54] On the other hand, *Mycobacterium tuberculosis* strains resistant as a result of point mutations have been recognized for many years.[23] More recently, a point mutation in the 16S rRNA of *Mycobacterium abscessus* and *Mycobacterium chelonae* was found to encode amikacin resistance.[55]

Altered Aminoglycoside Uptake

Mutant aerobic gram-negative bacilli and staphylococci with reduced uptake of aminoglycosides have been identified.[56] Cross-resistance to all aminoglycosides is seen, but the level of resistance is often less than that resulting from enzymatic modification.[56] In vitro, aminoglycoside concentrations 10 times the minimal inhibitory concentration (MIC) prevent the emergence of mutant populations.[57]

Bacterial chromosomal mutations may result in defect(s) that influence any part of the binding and electrochemical gradient leading to aminoglycoside uptake.[56] Emergence of resistant *Staphylococcus aureus* during aminoglycoside monotherapy is well recognized. The resistant organisms have alterations in their transmembrane electrical potential, electron transport chain, or both. The organisms appear as small colonies on culture plates. Although the small colony variants are often less virulent, they are a mechanism of bacterial persistence during aminoglycoside therapy; after cessation of aminoglycoside treatment, the organism can revert to the original virulent phenotype and cause clinical relapse.[58] Concomitant β-lactam therapy should prevent the problem.[56]

Transient resistance to aminoglycosides is observed after the rapid, early concentration-dependent killing of susceptible bacteria.[28, 59] The refractory state lasts beyond the postantibiotic effective period into the time of regrowth. This phenomenon is termed *adaptive resistance* rather than *emergence of unstable mutants.* It is believed to result from temporary disruption of the energy-dependent phase of aminoglycoside uptake. Adaptive resistance has been documented in vitro, in animal models, and clinically.[60, 61] Of importance, the effect only lasts a few hours. The implications for treatment are discussed later under "Once-Daily Administration."

The non–energy-dependent phases of uptake may lead to resistance based on altered permeability.[39] Alterations in cell wall lipopolysaccharide have been described for *P. aeruginosa.*

Laboratory isolates of *E. coli* resistant to amikacin have been reported that have both impaired aminoglycoside uptake and impaired aminoglycoside phosphorylation.[62] Combined resistance mechanisms have not yet been reported in clinical isolates.

Aminoglycoside-Resistant Enterococci

Enterococci are intrinsically resistant to low concentrations of aminoglycoside (e.g., 4 to 250 μg/ml) because of their anaerobic metabolism.[63] Because aminoglycoside uptake requires aerobic oxidative metabolism, enterococcal low-level resistance is believed to reflect a low level of cell membrane oxidative energization that results in poor active transport of drug.[26, 64] Transport is also influenced by the composition of the cell wall of enterococci.[63]

Acquisition of additional resistance of enterococci to aminoglycosides can result from one or more of three mechanisms: alteration of the target site, interference with drug permeability, or enzymatic inactivation of drug. The first two types result from mutation in the cell chromosome and the third is mediated by plasmids and transposons.

Of concern is rapid dissemination of the bifunctional enzyme 6′-aminoglycoside acetyltransferase (AAC-6′)-2″-aminoglycoside phosphotransferase (APH-2″).[65] The enzyme confers high-level resistance to gentamicin and all other related aminoglycosides with the exception of streptomycin. The gene involved is associated with narrow– and broad–host range conjugative plasmids and transposons. Other enterococcal phosphotransferases result in high-level gentamicin resistance.[66] Some of the same genes and enzymes result in aminoglycoside resistance in methicillin-resistant *S. aureus.*[66]

The difference between low-level and high-level in vitro aminoglycoside resistance has clinical import. The combination of a cell wall–active β-lactam or glycopeptide antibiotic with an aminoglycoside often results in synergistic bactericidal activity.[67] The cell wall–active drug enhances the ability of the aminoglycoside to reach the 16S portion of the ribosome. Resistance enzymes are synthesized constitutively.[67] Hence, clinical resistance is determined by the result of the balance between the rate of drug uptake and binding to the ribosomal target versus the rate of enzymatic modification of the aminoglycoside.

The in vitro method for detecting high-level aminoglycoside resistance was only recently standardized.[68] Agreement has now been reached on test media, inocula, and other pertinent variables. The MIC criteria for streptomycin and gentamicin high-level resistance vary from 500 to 2000 μg/ml, depending on the specifics of the test system used.

Although the in vitro testing is not standardized, reports from around the world indicate that the prevalence of high-level aminoglycoside resistance is 8 to 15% for strains of *Enterococcus faecalis* and 25 to 38% for strains of *Enterococcus faecium*.[69, 70] Because of differences in enzyme substrate specificity, it is desirable to test both gentamicin and streptomycin for high-level resistance.[71]

Clinical Epidemiology of Aminoglycoside Resistance

In vitro resistance of clinical isolates of aerobic gram-negative bacilli to aminoglycosides varies with the specific drug, the target organism, the nature of the patient population and their underlying disease or diseases, and local or regional patterns of physician use of specific aminoglycosides. In 1997, a surveillance system was established at 30 clinical sites in the United States to ascertain the identity and in vitro susceptibility of blood stream bacterial isolates.[72] The four most commonly isolated gram-negative bacilli were quite susceptible to gentamicin, tobramycin, and amikacin[72] (Table 23–3). Note that gentamicin was somewhat less active versus *P. aeruginosa*. Of 1182 clinical isolates of *P. aeruginosa* collected at 16 North American clinical centers, roughly 50% were resistant to gentamicin and 25% were resistant to tobramycin.[73]

The selective use of one aminoglycoside, or of a drug with similar structure, appears to result in an increased prevalence of resistance to the aminoglycoside used.[22] Data suggest that the emergence of resistance is slowest with amikacin and isepamicin.[22, 74–78] For example, 62 aminoglycoside-resistant strains of gram-negative enteric bacteria were isolated over 3 years from two hospitals.[74] One hospital prescribed primarily gentamicin and the other tobramycin. A statistically significant correlation was noted between the aminoglycoside used, the prevalence of drug-modifying enzymes, and the percentage of resistant aerobic gram-negative bacilli. Resistance decreases as drug use falls. In a French hospital, the prevalence of methicillin-resistant *S. aureus* with concomitant gentamicin resistance gradually increased during the 1980s and eventually reached 75% by 1993.[79] After a reduction in gentamicin use and the introduction of infection-control measures, during 1993 to 1995 the percentage of aminoglycoside-resistant, methicillin-resistant *S. aureus* isolates decreased from 75 to 52%. Finally, in Japan the most commonly prescribed aminoglycosides have been members of the kanamycin family (i.e., kanamycin, amikacin, and dibekacin). Of the aminoglycoside-resistant strains from east Asia, 88% were found to have some type of 6′-AAC activity against the kanamycin family of aminoglycosides.[80] Hence, the frequency of aminoglycoside resistance for a specific drug correlates with the frequency of usage of that drug or a closely related aminoglycoside.

In distinction to β-lactams with activity against aerobic gram-negative bacilli, resistance rarely emerges during the course of aminoglycoside therapy. In a study of *Enterobacter* bacteremia in 129 adults, emergence of antimicrobial resistance during 4 to 18 days of therapy occurred in 6 of 31 patients administered a third-generation cephalosporin (19%) and in 1 of 89 patients administered an aminoglycoside (1%) (p = .001).[81] Concomitant administration of an aminoglycoside did not decrease the emergence of resistance to the third-generation cephalosporin. This and other studies document the emergence of cephalosporin-resistant aerobic gram-negative bacilli during therapy; in contrast, the evolution of aminoglycoside resistance appears to require either long periods of exposure or a very large inocula of organisms, as is found in patients with burns or cystic fibrosis.

TABLE 23–3 In Vitro Susceptibility of U.S. Blood Stream Isolates of Aerobic Gram-Negative Bacilli to Aminoglycosides in 1997

Organisms	No. of Isolates	Percent Susceptible to		
		Gentamicin	*Tobramycin*	*Amikacin*
Enterobacter sp.	151	94	94	100
Escherichia coli	769	96	97	96
Klebsiella sp.	311	95	95	99
Pseudomonas aeruginosa	189	90	96	98

Data from Pfaller MA, Jones RN, Doern GV, et al. Bacterial pathogens isolated from patients with bloodstream infection: Frequencies of occurrence and antimicrobial susceptibility patterns from the SENTRY antimicrobial surveillance program (U.S. & Canada, 1997). Antimicrob Agents Chemother. 1998;41:1762–1770.

IN VITRO ANTIMICROBIAL ACTIVITY

Clinical Microbiology

The in vitro spectrum of activity of the aminoglycosides is compared with that of selected β-lactams and fluoroquinolones in Table 23–4.[82] The aminoglycosides demonstrate concentration-dependent bactericidal activity against a broad spectrum of aerobic and facultative gram-negative bacilli. Susceptible organisms in its spectrum of activity range from members of the family Enterobacteriaceae to *Pseudomonas* spp. to *Haemophilus* spp. Methicillin-susceptible but not methicillin-resistant *S. aureus* strains are inhibited. Streptomycin has the greatest activity in vitro against *M. tuberculosis,* whereas amikacin is more active against *Mycobacterium avium-intracellulare* and other atypical mycobacteria. Streptomycin is the drug of choice for *Yersinia pestis* infection, and success with both streptomycin and gentamicin has been reported for *Francisella tularensis* infection. When kanamycin is compared with the other 2-deoxystreptamine aminoglycoside(s), its spectrum is limited by the absence of predictable activity against *P. aeruginosa* and the development of resistant strains of Enterobacteriaceae. Equally important are the other bacteria against which the aminoglycosides have no predictable in vitro activity, such as *Streptococcus pneumoniae, Stenotrophomonas maltophilia, Burkholderia (Pseudomonas) cepacia, Bacteroides* spp., *Clostridium* spp., and other anaerobic organisms. Resistance to aminoglycosides is one characteristic used to identify *S. maltophilia* and *B. cepacia* in clinical specimens. Aminoglycosides have no clinically significant activity against rickettsiae, fungi, *Mycoplasma,* or viruses.

Although the spectrum of activity of streptomycin and kanamycin is limited, the activity spectra of gentamicin, tobramycin, amikacin, and netilmicin are virtually identical. Table 23–4 defines *sensitive* as an in vitro MIC/minimal bactericidal concentration (MBC) that is within the range of blood concentrations achieved clinically with traditional twice- or three-times-daily dosing. Table 23–4 does not indicate relative degrees of in vitro potency. The MIC/MBC of gentamicin against *Serratia* spp. is consistently twofold lower than that of the other aminoglycosides, and the MIC/MBC of tobramycin versus *P. aeruginosa* is also consistently twofold lower than that of the other aminoglycosides. Although tobramycin is more active in animal models of pneumonia, to date no clinical efficacy data have been presented that parallel these in vitro differences.

Aminoglycosides have in vitro activity against *Haemophilus* spp.

TABLE 23–4 Comparison of the "Usual" In Vitro Spectrum of Activity of Aminoglycosides with Other Classes of Antimicrobial Agents against Selected Microorganisms

Organism	Aminoglycosides							ESP						Monobactam	ESC		Carbapenems		FQ		TMP/SMX
	Streptomycin	*Kanamycin*	*Gentamicin*	*Tobramycin*	*Amikacin*	*Netilmicin*	*Spectinomycin*	*Ticarcillin*	*Mezlocillin*	*Piperacillin*	*Amp/Sulb*	*Ticar/Clav*	*Piper/Tazo*	*Aztreonam*	*Ceftriaxone*	*Ceftazidime*	*Imipenem*	*Meropenem*	*Ofloxacin*	*Ciprofloxacin*	
Gram-negative																					
Escherichia coli		+	+	+	+	+	0	+	+	+	+	+	+	+	+	+	+	+	+	+	+
Proteus mirabilis		+	+	+	+	+	0	+	+	+	+	+	+	+	+	+	+	+	+	+	+
Klebsiella sp.		+	+	+	+	+	0	0	+	+	+	+	+	+	+	+	+	+	+	+	+
Enterobacter sp.		0	+	+	+	+	0	±	+	+	+	+	+	+	+	+	+	+	+	+	+
Morganella sp.		+	+	+	+	+	0	+	+	+	+	+	+	+	+	+	+	+	+	+	+
Citrobacter sp.			+	+	+	+	0	+	+	+	+	+	+	+	+	+	+	+	+	+	+
Serratia sp.		+	+	+	+	+	0	+	+	0	+	+	+	+	+	+	+	+	+	+	+
Salmonella sp.								+	+	+	+	+	+	+	+	+	+	+	+	+	
Providencia sp.			+	+	+	+	0	+	+	+	+	+	+	+	+	+	+	+	+	+	
Aetomonas sp.			+	+	+	+	0	+	+	+		+	+	+		+	+	+	+	+	
Acinetobacter sp.			0	±	0			0	0	0	±	+	+	0	+	+	+	+	+	+	0
Pseudomonas aeruginosa		0	+	+	+	+	0	+	+	+	0	+	+	+	0	+	+	+	0	+	0
Burkholderia cepacia		0	0	0	0	0	0	0			0		+	0	+	+	+	+	0	0	+
Stenotrophomonas maltophilia		0	0	0	0	0	0		0	0	0	+	0	0	0	0	0	0	0	0	+
Nesseria gonorrhoeae		0	0	0	0	0	+	+	+	+	+	+	+	+	+	+	+	+	+	+	±
Haemophilus influenzae		+	+	+	+	+	0	0	0	±	+	+	+	+	+	+	+	+	+	+	±
Yersinia pestis	+		+																		
Francisella tularensis	+	+	+																		
Gram-positive																					
Streptococcus pneumoniae		0	0	0	0	0	0	+	+	+	+	+	+	0	+	+	+	+	±	±	+
Staphylococcus aureus (MSSA)		+	+	+	+	+	0	0	0	0	+	+	+	0	+	0	+	+	+	+	+
Staphylococcus aureus (MRSA)		0	0	0	0	0	0	0	0	0	0	0	0	0	0	0	0	0	0	0	0
Miscellaneous																					
Mycobacterium tuberculosis	+	0	0	0	+	0	0	0	0	0	0	0	0	0	0	0	0	0	0	0	0
Mycobacterium avium-intracellulare	0	0	0	0	+	0	0		0	0	0	0	0	0	0	0	+	0	+		0
Bacteroides fragilis	0	0	0	0	0	0	0	0	0	0	+	+	+	0	0	0	+	+	0	0	0

Abbreviations: +, Sensitive (relative degrees of sensitivity are not indicated); ±, variable; 0, resistant; blank, data not available; Amp/Sulb, ampicillin-sulbactam; ESC, representative extended-spectrum cephalosporins; ESP, representative extended-spectrum penicillins; FQ, fluoroquinolones; MRSA, methicillin-resistant *S. aureus*; MSSA, methicillin-sensitive *S. aureus*; Piper/Tazo, piperacillin-tazobactam; Ticar/Clav, ticarcillin-clavulanate; TMP/MSX, trimethoprim-sulfamethoxazole.
Adapted from Gilber DN, Moellering RC, Sande MA. Sanford Guide to Antimicrobial Therapy. 28th ed. Hyde Park, Vt: Antimicrobial Therapy, Inc; 1998.

and *Legionella* spp. but are not used clinically for infections with these organisms. Legionellae are intracellular pathogens, and the intracellular penetration of aminoglycosides is low.[83] Nonetheless, aminoglycosides are used successfully in the treatment of other intracellular infections such as brucellosis, tuberculosis, tularemia, and yersiniosis.[82] In vitro, streptomycin, gentamicin, and to a lesser degree, netilmicin at "therapeutic" concentrations demonstrated bactericidal activity against intracellular *E. coli.*[84]

Only spectinomycin has been used clinically for infections with *N. gonorrhoeae.*[82] Aminoglycosides in combination with other drugs have been successfully used to treat infections with staphylococci, streptococci, enterococci, *Listeria,* and mycobacteria.

Not shown in Table 23–4 is the activity of the aminoglycoside paromomycin against intestinal parasites. Paromomycin is too toxic for parenteral administration. Because the drug is not absorbed from the intestinal tract, it can be used safely as an alternative therapy for infection by *Entamoeba histolytica.*[82] Paromomycin may have some benefit in patients with acquired immunodeficiency syndrome (AIDS) who are infected with the protozoon *Cryptosporidium parvum.*[85]

As Table 23–4 indicates, many extended-spectrum penicillins (with and without a β-lactamase inhibitor), the monobactam aztreonam, the carbapenems, extended-spectrum cephalosporins, and the fluoroquinolones share with aminoglycosides the virtue of in vitro activity against a wide spectrum of fermentative and nonfermentative aerobic gram-negative bacilli. Some differences are apparent when other facets of in vitro antimicrobial sensitivity testing are considered.

Aminoglycosides are little influenced by the size of the test inoculum of bacteria; the MIC for 90% (MIC_{90}) of test strains is unchanged whether the initial inoculum is 10^5 or 10^7 bacteria per milliliter.[12] In contrast, an increase in test inoculum often results in a substantive increase in the MIC_{90} of extended-spectrum penicillins or cephalosporins. Depending on the method used, the percentage of aminoglycoside that is protein bound ranges between 0 and 30 and is considered inconsequential.[86] The higher the cation content of the test medium, the higher the MIC/MBC results versus *P. aeruginosa* and, to a lesser degree, other gram-negative bacilli. Early in the evaluation of gentamicin it was recognized that the Ca^{2+}, Mg^{2+}, and to a lesser extent, sodium concentrations of standard agar culture media varied widely from lot to lot.[87] Broth medium has very low concentrations of Ca^{2+} and Mg^{2+}. Subsequently, test culture media have been standardized as Mueller-Hinton broth supplemented with physiologic concentrations of calcium (50 mg/liter) and magnesium (25 mg/liter).[88] Because netilmicin activity versus *P. aeruginosa* is more influenced by the medium cation concentration than is the activity of other aminoglycosides, some authors recommend separate media with lower cation supplementation for netilmicin MIC testing.[89] No similar standards have been set for the cation content of test agar.[90] Some laboratories incorporate *P*-nitrophenylglycerol into agar susceptibility test media to prevent swarming of *Proteus* organisms *P*-nitrophenylglycerol is reported to increase the MIC of aminoglycosides against strains of *P. aeruginosa.*[91] An alkaline medium will yield an erroneously low MIC, whereas an acid medium will yield an erroneously high MIC.[12]

Urine is known to inhibit the activity of aminoglycosides against urinary tract pathogens. Inhibition is believed to result from the low pH and high osmolality caused by the high salt and glucose concentrations. In addition, present data support the hypothesis that betaines, normally found in urine, permit the expression of increased aminoglycoside resistance.[92] To date, betaine concentrations have not been standardized in test media.

The other drugs listed in Table 23–4 were selected because their spectrum includes activity against aerobic gram-negative bacilli. Note the absence of activity of ampicillin/sulbactam, ceftriaxone, ofloxacin, and trimethoprim-sulfamethoxazole against *P. aeruginosa.*

Time Course of In Vitro Antimicrobial Activity

"Time-kill" curves are not practical for routine susceptibility testing but do illustrate three facets of aminoglycoside antibacterial activity: concentration-dependent killing, the presence of a postantibiotic effect (PAE), and synergism with other drugs.[93]

Aminoglycosides are rapidly bactericidal, and their rate of bacterial killing increases as the antibiotic concentration is increased regardless of the inoculum.[94–96] Standard in vitro test systems have a static drug concentration. In vitro kinetic models allow fluctuations in drug concentration that mimic in vivo pharmacokinetics. For netilmicin and amikacin in the latter model, exposure of test bacteria to the 24-hour aminoglycoside dose as a single bolus with the associated high peak drug concentration resulted in faster killing and a larger magnitude of bactericidal activity than that noted for the same total dose administered in smaller increments at regular intervals.[97, 98] In years past, high concentrations were avoided for fear of toxicity. Now, transient high concentrations are considered a virtue and serve as a part of the rationale for once-daily dosing of aminoglycosides. Of interest, β-lactams do not exhibit concentration-dependent killing; bactericidal activity depends on maintaining drug concentrations at or above the target organism's MIC.[99, 100]

Postantibiotic Effect

The PAE is persistent suppression of bacterial growth after short antimicrobial exposure.[101] PAE can be measured in vitro or in animal models of infection. In vitro, the aminoglycosides consistently demonstrate a PAE that varies from 1 to 3 hours in broth and serum for *P. aeruginosa* and from 0.9 to 2.0 hours for other Enterobacteriaceae.[102] An aminoglycoside PAE can be demonstrated after incubation with *S. aureus* but not after contact with *S. pneumoniae.*[100] The higher the aminoglycoside concentration, the longer the PAE. The smaller the inoculum and the higher the oxygen tension, the longer the PAE.[101–103] The lower the pH of the test medium, the shorter the PAE.[101] For those aerobic or facultative gram-negative rods tested, the combination of a β-lactam and an aminoglycoside resulted in a PAE of the aminoglycoside.[101] An exception is imipenem; imipenem plus tobramycin or gentamicin enhanced the PAE of the aminoglycoside alone.[104, 105] Rifampin was associated with synergistic enhancement of the PAE induced in *P. aeruginosa* by tobramycin.[102]

An aminoglycoside-induced PAE is the second part of the rationale for once-daily dosing of aminoglycosides. The last part is an attenuated risk of toxicity, as discussed later. In contrast, β-lactam antibiotics, other than the carbapenems, have not demonstrated a PAE against aerobic and facultative gram-negative bacilli.[99–103]

In vitro, the tobramycin-induced PAE against *E. coli* correlated with inhibition of protein synthesis but not DNA or RNA synthesis.[106]

Antimicrobial Synergy

The synergy between an aminoglycoside and a cell wall–active antimicrobial (e.g., penicillin, cephalosporin, monobactam, carbapenem, glycopeptide) is a positive interaction.[93–107] The effect of the drugs in combination is greater than the anticipated results based on the effect of each individual drug. In short, the effect is more than additive.

Several laboratory procedures are used to study drug combinations for evidence of synergism. Although cumbersome and labor intensive, only the time-kill curve (or killing curve) method detects and quantifies bactericidal activity. The following comments and the data summarized in Table 23–5 are based on results from time-kill curves.[93] A great many additional studies describe synergism by using "checkerboard" or other techniques that indicate bacteriostatic activity as an end point and are hence excluded from the table.

The mechanism of aminoglycoside synergistic activity may not be the same for all target organisms. Study of the enterococcus indicates that intracellular accumulation of labeled streptomycin is significantly enhanced in the presence of penicillin or other cell wall–active drugs (e.g., bacitracin, vancomycin).[93] Similar enhanced

TABLE 23-5 Selected Examples of In Vitro Synergism of an Aminoglycoside Combined with a Cell Wall–Active Antimicrobial*

Organism	Aminoglycoside(s)	Cell Wall–Active Drug(s)
Enterococci	Streptomycin, kanamycin, gentamicin, tobramycin, netilmicin, sisomicin, amikacin	Penicillin, ampicillin, carbenicillin, nafcillin, vancomycin
Viridans streptococci	Streptomycin	Penicillin
Streptococcus pyogenes	Gentamicin	Penicillin, ampicillin
Staphylococcus aureus, MSSA	Kanamycin, gentamicin, tobramycin, netilmicin, sisomicin	Nafcillin, oxacillin, cephalothin, vancomycin
S. aureus, MRSA		Teicoplanin (+ rifampin)
Staphylococcus epidermidis, MSSE	Gentamicin, tobramycin	Vancomycin (+ rifampin)
S. epidermidis, MRSE		
Enterobacteriaceae	Gentamicin, tobramycin, amikacin	Piperacillin, cephalothin, cefoxitin, cefotaxime
Pseudomonas aeruginosa	Gentamicin, tobramycin, amikacin, netilmicin, sisomicin	Antipseudomonal penicillins,† aztreonam, ceftazidime, imipenem
Listeria monocytogenes	Streptomycin, gentamicin	Penicillin, ampicillin, imipenem
Corynebacteria, group JK	Gentamicin, tobramycin	Vancomycin, teicoplanin

*Inclusion required killing curve data demonstrating bactericidal activity.
†Includes carbenicillin, ticarcillin, mezlocillin, azlocillin, and piperacillin.
Abbreviations: MRSA, Methicillin-resistant *S. aureus*; MSSA, methicillin-sensitive *S. aureus*; MSSE, methicillin-sensitive *S. epidermidis*.
Modified from Eliopoulos GM, Moellering RC. Antimicrobial combinations. In: Lorian V, ed. Antibiotics in Laboratory Medicine. 4th ed. Baltimore: Williams & Wilkins; 1996:330–383.

aminoglycoside uptake in the presence of a cell wall–active drug has been demonstrated with viridans streptococci, *S. aureus,* and *P. aeruginosa.*[93]

The enterococci have been studied extensively since the original description of penicillin-streptomycin synergy in 1947.[108] Subsequently, the concept was extended to viridans streptococci and group B streptococci. Note that no aminoglycoside/cell wall–active drug combination is indicated as effective for methicillin-resistant *S. aureus.* Some laboratories have reported synergy between cephalothin and kanamycin and between high concentrations of either oxacillin or cephalothin and gentamicin.[93] Unfortunately, the latter regimens have not proved useful clinically.

Many time-kill curve studies have documented synergism against *P. aeruginosa* and Enterobacteriaceae.[93, 107] Because of the rapid bactericidal activity of high aminoglycoside concentrations, low to moderate aminoglycoside concentrations are used to detect synergistic activity. The clinical inference might be that lower doses of aminoglycoside could be effectively combined with the cell wall–active drug; from the opposite perspective, higher doses are desirable to maximize the concentration-dependent bactericidal activity of aminoglycosides.

Of equal import, the bactericidal activity of aminoglycosides can be antagonized by bacteriostatic agents such as chloramphenicol and tetracycline.[93] The mechanism is unclear. Postulates include inhibition of the energy-dependent uptake of aminoglycosides and interference with movement of the ribosome along messenger RNA.

ANTIBACTERIAL EFFICACY IN ANIMAL MODELS OF INFECTION

Historical Perspective

An idealistic goal is an animal model that mimics human infection so that the efficacy of aminoglycoside therapy, alone or in combination, can be maximized while simultaneously minimizing the risk of toxicity.[109] In a critical review of the literature published through 1980, the use of aminoglycosides alone was not found very effective in animal models of pyelonephritis, osteomyelitis, endocarditis, peritonitis, and meningitis.[110] Aminoglycosides were more effective in experimental models of pneumonia.[110] In retrospect, the studies reviewed did not consider the influence of dosing regimens, the pretreatment interval, and other variables now recognized to influence therapeutic efficacy. The theoretical value of combined therapy with drugs that have different targets of activity was well known, especially with respect to infections with enterococci; however, cell wall–active drugs with a spectrum of activity that included aerobic gram-negative bacilli have become available only in recent years.

Aminoglycosides Alone

Several infection models have been used to study the influence of aminoglycoside pharmacokinetics on drug efficacy.[99, 101] In the infected mouse thigh model, successful outcome of treatment of aerobic gram-negative rod infection correlated with the presence of granulocytes and with the peak serum aminoglycoside concentration.[99, 101, 102]

The growth of *P. aeruginosa* in thigh muscle increases rapidly in neutropenic mice as opposed to a plateau number of organisms in non-neutropenic animals.[111] Gentamicin therapy results in a rapid and continuing response in normal mice, whereas neutropenic mice display an initial response followed by, despite continued gentamicin therapy, regrowth with organisms resistant to gentamicin. Overgrowth of these small colonies of resistant mutants is prevented by concomitant administration of an active antipseudomonal penicillin (e.g., ticarcillin).

In the neutropenic thigh model, the therapeutic efficacy of aminoglycosides correlated with the peak serum concentration and the area under the concentration curve over time.[112] Because the half-life of aminoglycosides in small animals is short (less than 1 hour), it is possible to separate the influence of the peak serum concentration from the area under the curve.[99] The short drug half-life also predicts a long interval of sub-MIC serum levels, thus implying an in vivo PAE.

The in vivo PAE of aminoglycosides has been studied in at least five animal models.[101, 113, 114] In a study of the neutropenic mouse thigh infected with 15 clinical isolates of Enterobacteriaceae, the in vivo PAE after gentamicin therapy varied from 1.4 to 6.9 hours. In the same model infected with *P. aeruginosa,* increasing the dose of tobramycin fivefold increased the PAE from 2.2 to 7.3 hours.[113] The in vivo PAE is prolonged further in non-neutropenic animals. In experimental thigh infections with *Klebsiella pneumoniae* treated with an aminoglycoside, the PAE ranged from 2.6 hours in granulocytopenic animals to 12.8 hours in non-neutropenic mice.[114] The PAE is more prolonged in renal-impaired neutropenic animals than in neutropenic mice with normal renal function.[114] Guinea pigs with *P. aeruginosa* pneumonia were treated with once-daily tobramycin.[95] Although drug levels were not directly measured, based on assumed serum levels and quantitation of lung bacteria, the PAE is estimated at 12 or more hours.

Animal models are influenced by other factors as well. In a model of *K. pneumoniae* empyema in rabbits, gentamicin alone effected a cure rate of 60%.[115] The cure rate increased to 100% in a shorter time when animals were maintained in a hyperbaric oxygen chamber.[115] The time between experimental infection and treatment had a major influence. In both normal and granulocytopenic mice, a pretreatment interval of 6 or more hours abolished the bactericidal activity of gentamicin against *P. aeruginosa* in the thigh.[116]

In short, current animal data on the efficacy of aminoglycosides alone support the administration of large, appropriately spaced doses rather than frequent small doses. In neutropenic animals, concomitant administration of an active β-lactam antibiotic was necessary to avoid selection of resistant mutants.

Combination Therapy

The organisms in which in vitro synergy can be demonstrated between an aminoglycoside and a cell wall–active antimicrobial are summarized in Table 23–5.[93] Many of the same combinations have been evaluated in animal models of endocarditis, meningitis, pneumonia, peritonitis/bacteremia, pyelonephritis, osteomyelitis, myositis (mouse thigh), subcutaneous infection with and without a foreign body, and more.[93, 110, 117–120] The results can be reviewed by the organ or tissue infected[110] (e.g., endocarditis) or by the etiologic organism.[117] The latter approach is summarized in Table 23–6. In general, when the etiologic organism is susceptible to both the aminoglycoside and the companion drug, antibacterial activity is enhanced. Note the lack of synergy of amikacin plus pefloxacin (a fluorinated quinolone) in a mouse peritonitis model. Although active against different targets, both classes of drugs have an intracellular target; virtually all studies showing effectiveness of combined therapy used a cell wall–active drug (β-lactam or glycopeptide) with the aminoglycoside.

Import of the Dosing Regimen

For drug-organism combinations without a PAE, evidence is increasing in support of β-lactam dosage regimens that maintain serum levels above the MIC for the infecting organism for the entire dosage interval.[99, 100, 121] In contrast, the optimal dosing regimen for aminoglycosides depends on the specific microbial target. For experimental enterococcal endocarditis, antimicrobial activity was best with frequent doses of aminoglycoside.[117, 122] Presumably, both the penicillin and the aminoglycoside must be present at the same time to facilitate aminoglycoside uptake. In contrast, for penicillin-susceptible streptococcal endocarditis, combinations of penicillin and tobramycin are reported to be equally effective regardless of the total daily dose or dosing regimen.[123] The bactericidal activity of penicillin alone is a likely explanation.

For experimental infections with aerobic gram-negative bacilli, a single daily dose of aminoglycoside is reported to be as efficacious as the same total dose divided into multiple administrations.[124] The results are consistent with the known concentration-dependent killing and the long in vivo PAE of aminoglycosides. In neutropenic animals, the PAE of aminoglycosides is much shorter. In contrast, an effective blood level of a β-lactam must be continuously present to ensure efficacy.[100] Of interest, in the neutropenic murine thigh model, the in vivo PAE was prolonged in animals given combination therapy for infections with *S. aureus, E. coli, K. pneumoniae,* and *P. aeruginosa,* provided that both the aminoglycoside and the companion drug demonstrated a PAE when used alone.[125]

Prevention of Emergence of Drug Resistance

The use of an aminoglycoside as part of combination therapy may prevent or delay the emergence of bacteria resistant to either the aminoglycoside or the companion drug. In a series of studies, aminoglycosides were shown to reduce but not fully prevent the emergence of quinolone-resistant strains of Enterobacteriaceae or *P. aeruginosa* in a murine model of peritonitis.[126–128] Of interest, β-lactams were more effective than the aminoglycosides.

As described earlier, the concomitant use of an active β-lactam appears to prevent the emergence of gentamicin-resistant subpopulations in neutropenic animals.[111] Another example is the treatment of *P. aeruginosa* soft tissue infection in the neutropenic mouse with carbenicillin or gentamicin plus carbenicillin.[129] In vivo "synergism" was believed to result from suppression by carbenicillin of the emergence of gentamicin-resistant subpopulations.

TABLE 23–6 Use of Aminoglycosides as Part of Combination Therapy against Selected Bacteria in Animal Models of Infection

Organism	Infection (Animal)	Aminoglycoside	Drug(s) Combined with Aminoglycoside	Results
Enterococcus faecalis	Endocarditis (rat, rabbit)			
Penicillin susceptible		S, G	Penicillin/ampicillin	Combination synergistic
Penicillin resistant		S, G	Vancomycin	Combination synergistic
HLR to streptomycin, kanamycin		G	Penicillin/ampicillin	Combination synergistic
HLR to gentamicin		S	Penicillin/ampicillin	
Enterococcus faecium				
Penicillin susceptible		G	Penicillin	Combination synergistic
Penicillin resistant		G	Penicillin or vancomycin	Penicillin combination failed; vancomycin effective
HLR to vancomycin		G	Teicoplanin	Combination more effective
Viridans streptococci	Endocarditis (rabbit)	S	Penicillin	Combination synergistic
Staphylococcus aureus	Endocarditis (rabbit)			
MSSA		G	Nafcillin	Combination synergistic
MRSA		None	Vancomycin + rifampin	Combination effective
Staphylococcus epidermidis	Endocarditis (rabbit)			
MRSE		G	Vancomycin + rifampin	Triple combination more effective
MGRSE		N, A	Amoxicillin/clavulanic acid	Triple combination effective
Enterobacteriaceae				
Variety of organisms	Peritonitis (mouse)	G, T	Ticarcillin, carbenicillin	Enhanced activity of combination
Escherichia coli	Endocarditis (rabbit)	G	Ceftriaxone + sulbactam	Combination effective
Klebsiella pneumoniae, Pseudomonas aeruginosa, Serratia marcescens	Peritonitis (rats)	A	Imipenem	Enhanced survival with combination
Klebsiella pneumoniae	Pneumonia (neutropenic mice)	G	Ceftazidime	Modest enhanced efficacy
Pseudomonas aeruginosa	Peritonitis (rat, mouse; neutropenic and non-neutropenic)	G, T	Ticarcillin, carbenicillin	Enhanced activity of combination
	Peritonitis (mouse)	A	Pefloxacin	No benefit of combination
	SQ chamber (rabbit)	A	Azlocillin	Combination more effective
	Infected thigh (neutropenic mice)	N	Azlocillin	Combination more effective
	Osteomyelitis (rabbit)	Sis	Carbenicillin	Combination synergistic
	Pneumonia (guinea pig)	T	Ceftazidime	Enhanced activity of combination
Listeria monocytogenes	Meningitis (rabbit)	G	Ampicillin	Enhanced activity of combination

Abbreviations: A, Amikacin; G, gentamicin; HLR, high-level resistance; MGRSE, methicillin/gentamicin-resistant *S. epidermidis;* MRSA, methicillin-resistant *S. aureus;* MRSE, methicillin-resistant *S. epidermidis;* MSSA, methicillin-susceptible *S. aureus;* N, netilmicin; S, streptomycin; Sis, sisomicin; T, tobramycin.
Data from refs. 93, 110, and 117 to 120.

INTRA-ABDOMINAL PERITONITIS OR ABSCESS

Experimental models of intraperitoneal infection differ in that the bacterial inoculum is purposely a polymicrobic mixture of the aerobic and anaerobic flora of the colon. Human or rat pooled colonic content is placed intraperitoneally, and shortly thereafter therapy is initiated.[130] In untreated animals, a two-stage disease develops: in the first few days, 37% of the rats died of acute peritonitis and associated bacteremia; intra-abdominal abscesses developed in all the survivors.[131] The early stage is primarily due to aerobic or facultative gram-negative bacilli; the late stage requires both aerobic and anaerobic gram-negative bacilli. The former includes Enterobacteriaceae and *P. aeruginosa,* whereas the latter is usually due to *Bacteroides fragilis,* especially heavily encapsulated strains.[132]

Treatment of infected animals with gentamicin markedly reduced mortality but had virtually no influence on the incidence of abscess formation.[130–132] Treatment with clindamycin or metronidazole reduced the incidence of abscess formation but had no effect on peritonitis/bacteremia or lethality.[133] Combination therapy reduced both acute mortality and late abscess formation.

The role of enterococci in intra-abdominal infections has been controversial. In the rat model, intraperitoneal implantation of only enterococci and *B. fragilis* resulted in abscess formation.[134] The clinical implications are discussed later.

The efficacy of the aminoglycosides has been surprising. Their activity is significantly reduced at low pH, at low oxygen tension, and in the presence of drug-binding purulent debris.[12–16] The latter conditions characterize the murine intra-abdominal infection model, and yet beneficial aminoglycoside activity is demonstrable.

PHARMACOLOGY

Administration

Aminoglycosides are administered intravenously over a 15- to 30-minute period. If large single daily doses are prescribed, it is reasonable to extend the infusion to 30 to 60 minutes to diminish the theoretical risk of a rapid rise in serum concentration that might precipitate neuromuscular blockade. Aminoglycoside administered intramuscularly is absorbed completely, with maximal serum levels achieved between 30 and 90 minutes.[135] Absorption may be delayed in patients with hypotension and impaired tissue perfusion.

Aminoglycosides are minimally absorbed from the gastrointestinal tract.[136] Nonetheless, instances of deafness have occurred from oral neomycin administered to patients with hepatic encephalopathy and impaired renal function.[137] Also, increased absorption in the presence of concomitant inflammatory bowel disease is of theoretical concern. In contrast, patients with AIDS and severe cryptosporidiosis have ingested large amounts of paromomycin over protracted periods without evidence of toxicity. Other exposures may lead to systemic toxicity. Topical application of aminoglycoside on inflamed skin leads to no or minimal absorption. However, patients with extensive burns or other severe dermal injury may absorb drug and be at risk of toxicity.[138] Aminoglycosides can be instilled into either the pleural space or the peritoneal cavity. Absorption is rapid, with resultant serum concentrations proportionate to the concentration of drug instilled. The use of aminoglycosides in abdominal irrigation solutions is not recommended because rapid absorption with subsequent neuromuscular blockade has been reported.[139] In contrast, aminoglycosides have been administered as a bladder irrigant, as an aerosol, and by direct instillation into the lumbar sac or lateral ventricles without evidence of detectable concentrations in the blood.[140–142]

Distribution

As anticipated for drugs with a low level of protein binding (approximately 10%) and a high level of solubility in water, the aminoglycosides are distributed freely in the vascular space and relatively freely in the interstitial spaces of most tissues.[86] The mean aminoglycoside concentration of interstitial fluids approximates the mean plasma concentration as achieved at steady state after repetitive dosing. Interstitial peak concentrations are lower, oscillations between peak and trough levels are less frequent, and the rate of elimination is slower.[143] In the absence of disease and/or infection, the volume of distribution is 0.2 to 0.3 liter/kg.[144] The volume of distribution increases in edematous states, including ascites, in patients with burns, and in some severe infections. The volume of distribution decreases in obese individuals.[144] Because of their size, polycationic charge, and lipid insolubility, aminoglycosides cross biologic membranes poorly, with the exception of renal tubular cells and perhaps inner ear cells, which have an inherent transport mechanism. The cells of the renal proximal convoluted tubule can concentrate aminoglycosides to levels that exceed those of plasma or interstitial fluid.[145]

Parenteral aminoglycoside administration results in low concentrations of active drug in bronchial secretions.[142] Much higher concentrations can be achieved by administration via aerosol.[146] For success, it is necessary to use an aerosol generator that produces droplets 1 to 3 μm in diameter.

Aminoglycosides traverse the blood–cerebrospinal fluid and blood-brain barriers poorly.[147] Penetration is somewhat better in newborns. Lumbar sac administration yields high local cerebrospinal fluid levels but poor intraventricular levels, whereas intraventricular administration results in high concentrations in both ventricular and spinal fluid.[148, 149] Hence, the intraventricular route is recommended for meningitis caused by aerobic gram-negative bacilli in adults in those rare cases in which this therapy is necessary. In the newborn, intraventricular aminoglycoside is no more effective and perhaps more toxic than the drug given intravenously.[150]

Urine concentrations of aminoglycosides exceed peak plasma levels 25- to 100-fold within 1 hour of drug administration.[151, 152] Because of renal tubular cell absorption and subsequent release, urine concentrations remain above therapeutic levels for several days after a single dose. After termination of a multiple-dose regimen, urine levels remain above therapeutic levels for days, with a terminal half-life of 48 to 200 hours.[152–154]

Aminoglycosides enter synovial fluid easily, with subsequent levels only slightly less than simultaneous serum concentrations.[155] The biliary tract is poorly penetrated by aminoglycosides, with bile drug levels only 30% of concomitant serum concentrations.[156, 157] Aminoglycoside penetration into the tissues of the eye has been studied intensively.[158] Mean vitreous levels are only about 40% of serum levels over a 12-hour period.[159] In humans, subconjunctival injections yield high aqueous humor levels,[160] but neither systemic nor subconjunctival administration in single doses produces reliable levels in the vitreous humor of humans.[161] Direct intravitreal injection is recommended for the treatment of endophthalmitis.[158]

Metabolism

No evidence of in vivo metabolism of the aminoglycosides has been reported.

Excretion

Of a parenteral dose of aminoglycosides, 99% is excreted unchanged by the kidney. Less than 1% is eliminated in the feces and 1% in saliva.[162] Aminoglycosides undergo glomerular filtration. In animals, approximately 5% binds to the brush border of renal proximal tubular cells and is reabsorbed.[145, 163–165] Tubular cell handling of the drug is discussed later under "Toxicity." Reabsorbed drug is returned to the tubular lumen and excreted. With normal renal function in adults, more than 90% of an administered dose is recovered in urine unchanged during the first 24 hours.[162, 166] The remainder is slowly recycled to the tubular lumen, with a tissue half-life of 30 to 700

TABLE 23–7 Estimated Frequency of Serious Clinical Adverse Reactions after Administration of Aminoglycoside Antibiotics*

Adverse Reaction	Estimated Frequency (%)
Nephrotoxicity	0–50[177–184]
Ototoxicity	
Cochlear	0–62[176, 185–188]
Vestibular	0–19[176, 187–190]
Neuromuscular blockade	Exceedingly rare[191]

*See the text for an explanation of the large range.

hours.[166, 167] Drug can be detected in urine for 20 days or longer after discontinuation of therapy.

Pharmacokinetics

All the aminoglycosides have similar pharmacokinetics. The pharmacokinetics occurs in three interrelated phases.[168] The first (α or distributive) phase is the result of drug distribution from the vascular to the extravascular space. This phase occurs with a half-life of 15 to 30 minutes.[168] It is suggested that "peak" aminoglycoside serum levels be checked 30 minutes after the end of an intravenous infusion. Because the drug is often infused over a 15- to 30-minute period, it is convenient to request that the serum sample be collected 1 hour after the start of the drug administration.

The second (or β) phase of elimination results from excretion of drug from plasma and the extravascular space. The second phase is determined by the glomerular filtration rate and is hence of greatest import in clinical dosage regimens. In adults and infants older than 6 months with normal renal function, the half-lives of all the aminoglycosides are similar and range from 1.5 to 3.5 hours.[169–172] The half-life in infants younger than 1 week or in low-birth-weight premature infants can be 8 to 11 hours. The half-life in neonates who weigh over 2 kg is roughly 5 hours.[173] The half-life is shortened in febrile illnesses and progressively prolonged with any process that decreases renal function. Prolongation of the half-life in the elderly is the result of age-related decrements in renal function.[174]

The third (or γ) phase is the prolonged and slow elimination of drug that has accumulated in the kidney. The third phase is not considered in dosage calculations. Clinical dosing procedures are presented in later sections.

TOXICITY

With the exception of the aminocyclitol spectinomycin, aminoglycoside antibiotics share the potential for causing injury to the renal proximal convoluted tubules, damage to the cochlea and/or vestibular apparatus, and neuromuscular blockade[139, 175, 176] (Table 23–7). The inherent toxicity and relative toxic potential of the aminoglycosides correlate with their positive electrical charge at physiologic pH.[9] At intracellular sites, the pH is lower and the drugs are more cationic.

Also important are untoward effects that are encountered rarely. Hypersensitivity reactions are uncommon, and the aminoglycosides do not provoke inflammation. Hence, phlebitis at intravenous infusion sites is rare; intramuscular injection sites do not become painful; instillation into the pleural space, abdominal cavity, and cerebrospinal fluid causes no irritation; and incorporation of an aminoglycoside into methyl methacrylate prosthetic joint cement is well tolerated over protracted periods. The aminoglycosides are not hepatotoxic, do not induce photosensitivity, and have no identified adverse influence on hematopoiesis or the coagulation cascade.

Nephrotoxicity

Experimental Nephrotoxicity

Pathogenesis. Attempts to elucidate the mechanism or mechanisms of aminoglycoside-induced injury to renal proximal tubular cells have used isolated enzyme systems, cell membrane vesicles, tissue culture of tubular cells, isolated perfused kidneys, and animal models with and without active infection. A role for a genetic predisposition is suggested by differences in susceptibility among rats, rabbits, and other animals and among inbred strains of a specific animal.[192]

Based on current accumulated knowledge, a postulate of the pathophysiology of renal tubular damage can be constructed (Fig. 23–2), thereby summarizing a large body of research. It has been suggested that the aminoglycosides bind to specific receptors and then undergo endocytosis via the same mechanism used to "scavenge" amino acids, small peptides, and perhaps polyamines from the glomerular filtrate.[193, 194] Alternatively, binding may reflect an electrostatic interaction between the cationic aminoglycoside and the anionic membrane phosphatidylinositol.[195] Interaction of drug with the cells lining the S_1 and S_2 portions of the proximal convoluted tubules is manifested by an increase in the excretion of brush border enzymes; this enzymuria occurs after a single dose of drug and hence is too sensitive to use as a practical clinical marker of toxicity.[196, 197] Also, a rapid increase is seen in calcium and, to a lesser extent, magnesium excretion.[198]

Aminoglycosides bind to megalin in clathrin-coated pits.[195] Megalin is an anionic protein that binds multiple cationic ligands.[199, 200] Existing data support rapid intracellular movement of the aminoglycoside-megalin complex to the Golgi apparatus within 15 minutes and subsequently to the ribosomes of the endoplasmic reticulum.[201, 202] This localization correlates with the rapid decrease observed in protein synthesis.[203]

Aminoglycoside-megalin complexes also fuse with lysosome membranes.[195] Lysosome localization is observed after an hour or more. Dissociation occurs and megalin returns to the cell membrane. Lysosome interaction results in deposition of osmiophilic membrane–appearing material in a layered whorl-like pattern that vaguely resembles myelin by electron microscopy—hence the term *myeloid body* (also called *cytosegresomes*).[15] These alterations in plasma membrane and lysosomal membrane phospholipids have been referred to as aminoglycoside-induced phospholipidosis.[15] In intact animals, myeloid bodies can be found in voided urine, presumably as a result of lysosomal excretion. Myeloid bodies may result from inhibition of lysosomal enzymes by aminoglycosides.[15] Myeloid bodies are not unique to aminoglycosides; they occur after the administration of a wide variety of other cationic amphophilic drugs.[204]

Aminoglycosides cause dysfunction of a variety of other cellular organelles and enzymes. It is unclear whether these "toxicities" represent primary sites of injury or secondary dysfunction in a damaged or injured cell. Ribosome, mitochondria, and membrane Na^+,K^+-ATPase functional abnormalities are reported.[203, 205–207] Irre-

TABLE 23–8 Variables Reported to Increase or Decrease the Severity of Experimental Aminoglycoside Nephrotoxicity

Factors That Increase Severity of Injury	Factors That Reduce Severity of Injury
More toxic aminoglycoside	Less toxic aminoglycoside[211, 212]
Frequent dosing[213]	Once-daily dosing[213, 214]
Old male Fischer rats[215]	Young female Sprague-Dawley rats[216]
Infected, volume- and sodium-depleted, acidotic rats[217, 218]	Uninfected euvolemic, role of alkalosis unclear[217–220]
Hypokalemia[221, 222]	Thyroid hormone[223]
Experimental liver disease[223–225]	Calcium loading[226–229]
Drugs	Induced diabetes mellitus[230, 231]
Vancomycin, teicoplanin[232–234]	Drugs
Methoxyflurane[237]	Extended-spectrum penicillins*[235, 236]
Cyclosporine[248, 249]	Polyaspartic acid[238–247]
Cisplatin[251]	? Cephalothin[250]
Magnesium depletion	

*For example, carbenicillin, ticarcillin, mezlocillin, piperacillin.

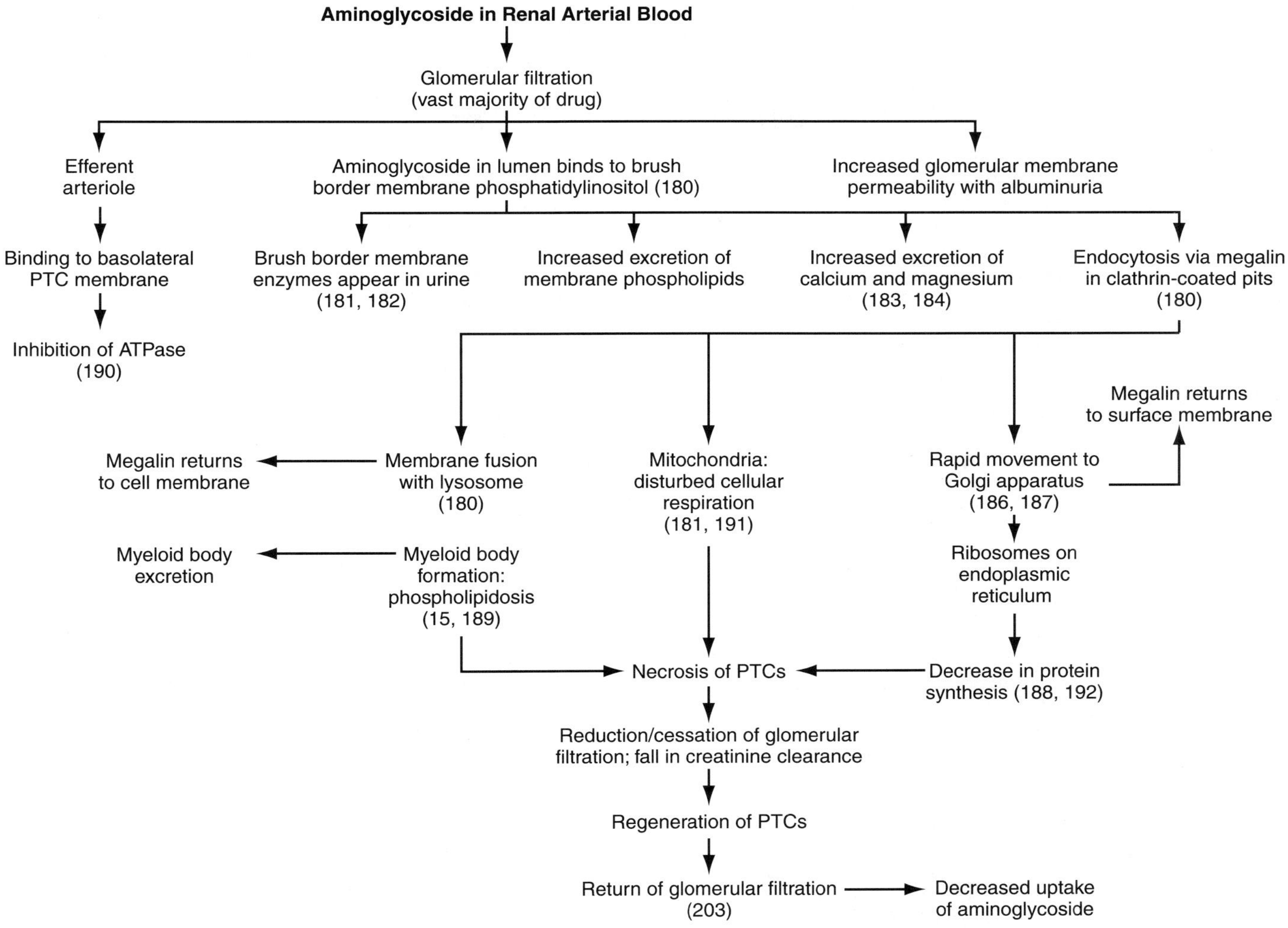

FIGURE 23–2. A proposed pathway of the handling of aminoglycosides by the renal proximal tubular cells (PTCs). Numbers in parentheses are references.

versible cell death is associated with changes in the intracellular compartmentalization of calcium.[204]

No consensus has been reached regarding how injury or death of proximal tubular cells results in a fall in the glomerular filtration rate. Theories include (1) a release of vasoconstrictive hormones affecting the afferent arterioles, (2) backleak of waste products across damaged epithelium, (3) cellular debris obstructing individual nephrons, and (4) a change in glomerular fenestrae with a decrease in the glomerular ultrafiltration coefficient.[208] One or a combination of these mechanisms may be operative.

Whatever the mechanism(s), the cell is relatively resistant. In intact animals purposely given toxic doses, several days of drug administration is necessary before functional or anatomic evidence of toxicity occurs. Furthermore, aminoglycoside-induced renal tubular necrosis is reversible. Remarkably, the tubular cells can regenerate despite continued administration of the aminoglycoside.[209] In addition, the regenerated cells selectively decrease the endocytosis of aminoglycosides.[210]

Variables. Animal models, particularly rat models, have been studied to delineate variables that may have clinical import or to elucidate the pathophysiology. Selected examples are summarized in Table 23–8. A hierarchy of nephrotoxic potential exists among the aminoglycosides.[211, 212] Neomycin is the most toxic aminoglycoside, and parenteral administration is precluded. Streptomycin is the least nephrotoxic, perhaps because the drug does not accumulate in the renal cortex. The influence of dosage regimens has been tested in multiple types of animals administered a variety of aminoglycosides. For a given total daily dose of a specific drug, the magnitude of toxicity is greatest when the dose is divided into multiple small increments and least when given as a single daily dose.[213, 214] Older animals either are more susceptible to injury or have a reduced capacity for cellular regeneration.[215] The enhanced susceptibility of male rats is of interest inasmuch as retrospective analysis of clinical studies suggests an increased susceptibility of human females.[216, 252, 253] Depletion of vascular volume, sodium, or both and systemic acidosis worsen renal injury, but volume or salt loading does not prevent or lessen renal injury.[217, 218] The influence of an induced alkalosis is unclear; some studies suggest blunting of renal injury, whereas another demonstrated marked kidney calcification.[217, 219, 220] Potassium depletion worsens and potassium loading attenuates renal injury.[224] The mechanism may relate to changes in Na^+,K^+-ATPase activity.[222] A similar mechanism is suggested for the reduced renal injury observed after thyroid administration.[254] Loop diuretics may amplify toxicity via volume depletion, hypokalemia, or acceleration of drug uptake by renal cells.[255]

Dietary calcium loading ameliorates gentamicin-induced acute renal failure and the associated decline in mitochondrial function.[226–228] The mechanism of protection remains unclear.[229]

The influence of experimental liver disease on aminoglycoside nephrotoxicity is unclear. One report describes amplification of drug-induced renal injury by experimental extrahepatic cholestasis.[223] A second study found no influence of experimental cirrhosis on the severity of aminoglycoside nephrotoxicity.[224] The accumulated clinical data indicate that concomitant liver disease is a risk factor for nephrotoxicity.[225]

Animals with streptozotocin-induced experimental diabetes are reported to have attenuated aminoglycoside nephrotoxicity.[230, 231] The mechanism and clinical relevance of this observation are unclear.

Various drugs influence the severity of experimental aminoglycoside nephrotoxicity. Vancomycin and the related drug teicoplanin amplify experimental aminoglycoside nephrotoxicity.[232, 233] Neither drug alone exhibits a toxic potential. Of interest, vancomycin interacts with the kidney at sites other than the proximal tubular cell.[234] Extended-spectrum penicillins lower the risk of kidney injury.[235] Some data suggest that the protection is the result of the high sodium content of the penicillin salts.[236]

Polymers of aspartic acid dramatically reduce renal tubular injury despite the accumulation of very high renal concentrations of aminoglycoside.[238–247] It is postulated that the anionic polyaspartic acid complexes the cationic aminoglycoside in cytoplasmic vacuoles and thereby precludes movement of aminoglycoside to an intracellular site or sites of toxicity.[246] Despite the dramatic results in animal models, at present little interest has been shown in clinical evaluation of these drugs.

Although differences were noted between species, animal experiments with an aminoglycoside plus cephalothin, cefazolin, or cefamandole indicate either no effect or an attenuation of nephrotoxicity when compared with those using an aminoglycoside plus placebo.[250] These results contrast with clinical studies suggesting amplification of toxicity with some cephalosporins.

TABLE 23–9 Risk Factors for Clinical Aminoglycoside Nephrotoxicity

Factors That Increase Risk of Toxicity	Factors That Decrease Risk of Toxicity
Patient factors	Patient factors
Older patients	Younger patients
Preexisting renal disease	Normal renal function
Female gender[252]; male gender[182]	Normotensive
Volume depletion, hypotension	No hepatic dysfunction
Hepatic dysfunction[225, 260]	Aminoglycoside factors
Aminoglycoside factors	No recent aminoglycoside therapy
Recent aminoglycoside therapy	With smaller doses
With larger doses	Treatment less than 3 days
Treatment lasting 3 or more days	Drug choice, e.g., tobramycin[180]
Drug choice, e.g., gentamicin[180]	Once-daily dosing[124, 259]
Frequent dosing interval[124, 259]	Concomitant drugs
Concomitant drugs	Extended-spectrum penicillins[264, 265]
Vancomycin[261–263]	
Amphotericin B	
Furosemide	
Clindamycin	
Piperacillin	
Cephalosporins[197, 264–266]	
Methoxyflurane[267]	
Foscarnet	
Intravenous radiocontrast agents	

Data from refs. 178, 182, 252, and 253, in addition to the references in the table.

Clinical Nephrotoxicity

The reported incidence of nephrotoxicity varies from 0 to 50%, with most reports in the 5 to 25% range[177–184] (see Table 23–8). The variability results from differences in the definition of nephrotoxicity, the frequency of and the particular tests used to measure renal function, and the clinical setting in which the drugs are administered. The incidence in a small group of healthy young volunteers who received a single daily infusion of tobramycin for 11 days was zero; the incidence in infected older patients with multisystem disease and exposure to other potential nephrotoxins ranged as high as 35 to 50%.[177, 178, 256] In prospective randomized studies with definitions of nephrotoxicity that reflect a substantive decrement in the glomerular filtration rate in seriously ill patients, the reported incidence of nephrotoxicity varied between 5 and 10% of patient courses.[179–184]

In studies of the etiology of acute renal failure, medication-induced renal injury is reported as a major cause. In an analysis of more than 2000 hospitalized patients, almost 100 experienced renal insufficiency, and seven episodes were attributed to aminoglycoside therapy.[257]

In general, the aminoglycoside-induced decrement in the glomerular filtration rate is small. Most patients have a nonoliguric fall in creatinine clearance; progression to dialysis-dependent oliguric-anuric renal failure is rare. As in animal models, the tubular injury is reversible, and in a few patients, recovery of renal function has been documented despite continued administration of the aminoglycoside.[258]

Reported risk factors for aminoglycoside nephrotoxicity are summarized in Table 23–9.[177, 178, 252, 253, 259] The factors listed can be grouped as relating to the patient, to the aminoglycoside, and to the influence of the selected concomitant drug. Many of the factors identified in clinical trials concur with data from animal models of nephrotoxicity. Female gender was identified as a risk factor in one study but not confirmed in others.[177, 183, 184, 252] In a retrospective analysis, male gender was a risk factor.[182] Reported clinical studies with cephalosporins do not include an aminoglycoside-only group of patients, and hence it is not possible to ascertain whether the cephalosporins had no influence on or increased or decreased the risk of nephrotoxicity. Based on the urinary excretion of tubular cell brush border enzymes, ceftazidime increased the enzymuria seen with gentamicin alone in human volunteers.[197]

The correlation of increased risk of toxicity with age, preexisting renal disease, or both may be misleading. It is unclear whether a risk exists when the dosing regimen is adjusted for a preexisting decrease in the glomerular filtration rate.

Hypotensive patients, especially those with septic shock or sepsis syndrome, have an increased incidence of renal insufficiency. The role of aminoglycosides is unclear in that infection-related low perfusion, consumptive coagulopathy, cytokine-mediated endothelial damage, and other factors may be etiologic in the fall in the glomerular filtration rate.

Liver disease was identified as a risk factor in the retrospective analysis of two large clinical trials and was then validated in two additional prospective trials.[225] Further support derives from a retrospective review of aminoglycoside treatment in patients with biliary obstruction, cholangitis, or both.[260]

The significance of recent aminoglycoside therapy is hard to define. In animals, the pattern of injury is cyclic. Administration of more aminoglycoside during the renal saturation phase may increase risk, whereas risk may be decreased if more drug is given when the tubular cells are in a regenerative phase.

Clinical trial data support the notion of a need for several days of therapy to cause nephrotoxicity of clinical consequence. In contrast, accidental massive overdosage of 1 day or less has not resulted in acute tubular necrosis.[268, 269]

In the rat model of nephrotoxicity, tobramycin was found to be less nephrotoxic than gentamicin.[212] This hypothesis was tested in a randomized prospective clinical trial. The results indicated a lower incidence of nephrotoxicity in tobramycin recipients, but controversy surrounds the study methods and data interpretation.[180] The results of subsequent trials were mixed. Amikacin and gentamicin were found to be equivalent with respect to the risk of nephrotoxicity.[179] One study reported a lower incidence of renal injury in netilmicin recipients than in patients administered tobramycin.[183]

Based on 26 published clinical trials and 8 meta-analyses of those trials, a single daily dose of aminoglycoside appears to be a safe and efficacious treatment method.[259] Single daily dosing does not prevent drug toxicity but may reduce the risk. This subject is amplified later.

The influence of concomitant drugs is difficult to interpret in patients with serious or complex disease states who are receiving multiple pharmaceuticals. Nonetheless, the majority of studies suggest an increased risk of a fall in the glomerular filtration rate when the drugs listed in Table 23–9 are administered concomitantly with aminoglycosides.[177, 178, 182, 252, 253] The data are not always conclusive in that many studies suffer from the absence of a matched patient population given only an aminoglycoside. Three prospective studies, one of which was double blind, found the combination of cephalothin plus aminoglycoside more nephrotoxic than a penicillin derivative plus an aminoglycoside.[264–266] Subsequent multiple logistic regression risk factor analysis identified a variety of cephalosporins as risk factors. These results are consistent with ceftazidime enhancement of gentamicin enzymuria in normal volunteers.[197] Two studies evaluated concomitant vancomycin administration; one analysis included a control group that received only an aminoglycoside.[261, 262] Both studies indicated that vancomycin was a risk factor. In children, vancomycin was not found to be a risk factor.[263]

In febrile neutropenic patients administered gentamicin or tobramycin plus carbenicillin or ticarcillin, the reported incidence of nephrotoxicity is 2 to 6% as compared with 10 to 15% or higher when the aminoglycoside is combined with other β-lactam antibiotics.[264, 265] Of interest, a recent risk factor analysis found an increased risk with concomitant piperacillin but not carbenicillin or ticarcillin.[236] The authors speculated that the lower sodium content of piperacillin may explain the difference.[236]

The identification of some concomitant drugs as risk factors intuitively made sense because a drug may have its own inherent potential kidney toxicity (e.g., amphotericin B), some drugs may act indirectly by altering intravascular volume or electrolyte concentrations (e.g., furosemide), some are of theoretical concern because of their own inherent toxicity potential (e.g., foscarnet, intravenous radiocontrast agents), and some statistically identified risk factors defy explanation at present (e.g., clindamycin). Finally, it should be noted that two drugs that amplify aminoglycoside experimental nephrotoxicity, cyclosporine and cisplatin, do not appear to increase the risk of clinical nephrotoxicity in their clinical application.[248–251, 270, 271]

If deterioration in renal function occurs, it is advisable to discontinue aminoglycoside therapy. Spontaneous recovery occurs within a few days in the absence of other nephrotoxins, hypotension, renal cortical necrosis of another etiology, or other clinical factors. Progression to anuric renal failure is uncommon. In patients in whom it is inadvisable to discontinue therapy (e.g., those with *P. aeruginosa* endocarditis), the aminoglycoside dosage is adjusted and therapy continued. Recovery of renal function concomitant with continued aminoglycoside therapy has been reported.[258]

Serum Levels and Nephrotoxicity

Note that serum levels are not included as a risk factor, although they are frequently identified as such.[182, 252, 253] In experimental animals and presumably in patients, the higher the dose of aminoglycoside, the higher the serum levels, the greater the area under the time-concentration curve, and the greater the risk of toxicity. Measurement of peak serum concentrations is indicated to ensure that enough drug was given for antibacterial efficacy and to avoid a large overdosage. Trough levels are measured to ensure adequacy of renal clearance of drug. A high trough concentration is a reflection of impaired renal clearance of drug and indicates a need to adjust the dosage regimen as discussed later.

Ototoxicity

Aminoglycoside antibiotics may cause cochlear and vestibular damage in both experimental animals and humans. Streptomycin-induced hearing loss and dizziness were included in the first clinical report of the drug's efficacy.[272] Ototoxicity is of particular concern because it is usually irreversible and can appear after the end of treatment and repeated exposure engenders cumulative risk.[176] Because the target sites of injury are small and buried in bone, studies dealing with pathophysiology are fewer in number than those addressing nephrotoxicity. A given patient may suffer just cochlear damage or just vestibular damage, or rarely, both organs are injured. Of interest, it is unusual to have both ototoxicity and nephrotoxicity in the same patient; in addition, it is unusual to have both cochlear and vestibular toxicity in the same patient.

Cochlear Toxicity

Incidence. Few recipients of aminoglycoside therapy complain of hearing loss, and yet the reported incidence is as high as 62% when asymptomatic high-frequency audiograms are performed repeatedly.[185] An overall incidence is quoted as 3 to 14%.[186]

Normal sound perception extends to frequencies of 20 kHz. The outer hair cells in the basal turn of the cochlea are most susceptible to aminoglycoside damage; the basal turn is the site of detection of high-frequency sound.[176] Perception of human speech requires sound detection in the 0.3- to 3-kHz range. Even in the speech frequency range, a loss of hearing threshold of 25 to 30 dB is necessary before the patient is aware of the deficit. Hence, considerable cochlear damage can occur without patient recognition. Furthermore, detection is difficult in ill patients with impaired cognition. Finally, many audiometers do not test frequencies above 8 kHz.

Another problem in ascertaining incidence is the absence of a universally accepted definition for drug-induced ototoxicity. A commonly used definition is an increase in auditory threshold of 15 dB or greater at any of two or more frequencies.[176]

Controlled data on cochlear toxicity are sparse. In healthy adult male volunteers administered kanamycin sulfate, cochlear toxicity developed in 17%.[273] In contrast, ototoxicity was reported in 7.4% of infected patients treated with cefotaxime.[178] Also as a comparison, hearing deficits developed in 15 of 27 patients admitted to the hospital without exposure to antimicrobials or other known ototoxins.[274] In a series of prospective clinical studies that examined the efficacy and toxicity of gentamicin, tobramycin, and amikacin in combination with β-lactam antibiotics, 22% of the aminoglycoside recipients had documented audiometric toxicity; all but one patient had hearing loss at 4 or 8 kHz.[275] Frequencies over 8 kHz were not tested. In a different study of 53 subjects administered gentamicin, tobramycin, or amikacin for at least 4 days who were tested at frequencies up to 20 kHz, 33 of the 53 patients suffered either a 20-dB or greater loss at one frequency, a 10-dB or greater loss at two consecutive frequencies, or loss of response at three consecutive frequencies.[185] Of the ears with damage, 62% demonstrated hearing loss initially at or above 9 kHz.[185] Loss was unilateral in 55% and bilateral in 45% of patients. Treatment ranged from 4 to 32 days, and hearing loss was initially detected after a mean of 9 days of therapy.

Pathophysiology. The site of aminoglycoside toxicity is the outer hair cells of the organ of Corti.[176, 276] The specifics of the interaction are unclear. In experimental animals, aminoglycosides can be detected in inner ear fluid, but the concentration never exceeds serum levels.[276] Inner ear tissues are saturated with gentamicin roughly 3 hours after administration, but cochlear damage, as measured by brain stem evoked potentials, requires 3 weeks of daily injections.[276, 277]

As in renal proximal tubular cells, lysosomal changes (myeloid bodies) are visible within the hair cells of treated animals. Attempts to study intracellular trafficking are consistent with endocytotic uptake and lysosomal accumulation.[278, 279] To date, the role of megalin in ototoxicity has not been described.

The intracellular target of toxicity is unknown. One postulate is that gentamicin complexes with iron and that this complex produces toxic free radicals.[280] A second hypothesis proposes aminoglycoside overactivation of glutamate receptors on cochlear synapses.[281]

Hair cell loss has been considered irreversible. However, recent animal studies in nonmammals and mammals document the potential for regeneration.[282–284]

Inherited Risk. The greatest risk may be a genetic predisposition. Numerous families are reported wherein deafness developed in multiple members after receiving an aminoglycoside.[285, 286] Likewise, macaque and patas monkeys differ markedly in their susceptibility to cochlear toxicity.[285]

Multiple family pedigrees have been studied.[285, 286] In three Chinese families, a specific mutation was identified in the 12S mitochondrial rRNA. The mitochondrial locus is consistent with a matrilineal pattern of inheritance. The abnormality is an A-to-G substitution at nucleotide position 1555. The same A-to-G substitution has been reported in Japanese families, Mongolian families, and an Israeli-Arab kindred. Forty-one ethnically diverse U.S. patients were studied after aminoglycoside-induced deafness developed; 7 (17%) of the patients had the nucleotide 1555 A-to-G mutation.[285] Of clinical import, four of the seven had a family history of aminoglycoside-induced ototoxicity. In three of the patients, hearing loss was delayed for several years. To date, no reports of genetic predisposition to aminoglycoside vestibular or renal toxicity have appeared.

In vitro constructs of normal and mutant 12S rRNA have been reported.[287] The mutant rRNA bound aminoglycosides, whereas the normal construct did not. Of interest, the binding was tighter for the clinically more toxic drugs (paromomycin, neomycin) than for the others tested (gentamicin, tobramycin).[287]

Other Risk Factors. Risk factors have been assessed in animal models of cochlear injury. Many of the results parallel those observed in the rat model of nephrotoxicity. To wit, toxicity is related to the dose and duration of aminoglycoside therapy.[288] A hierarchy of toxic potential has been established, with neomycin being the most toxic, followed in descending order by gentamicin, tobramycin, amikacin, and netilmicin.[288] Drug structure makes a difference. Streptomycin's potential to cause neurosensory hearing loss is well known. Changing an aldehyde group of streptomycin to an alcohol yields dihydrostreptomycin. Dihydrostreptomycin has little cochlear toxicity but causes damage to the vestibular apparatus.

Concomitant "loop" diuretics, vancomycin, and loud ambient noise increase the risk of toxicity.[289–291] Once-daily dosing decreases the risk when compared with the same total daily dose administered at frequent intervals or by continuous infusion.[292]

Risk factor analysis of human trials is difficult to assess in that patients were not studied for high-frequency hearing loss and baseline data cannot be obtained with confidence in ill, febrile patients. Nonetheless, retrospective stepwise discriminant analysis of 135 patients enrolled in prospective double-blind clinical trials of aminoglycoside therapy identified treatment duration, associated bacteremia, hypovolemia, degree of temperature elevation, and liver dysfunction as risk factors.[189] One group used multivariate analysis and identified only age as a risk factor.[190] With the currently available data, it is difficult to ascertain measurable differences in the risk of cochlear toxicity between gentamicin, tobramycin, amikacin, and netilmicin.[186, 293] In one study, netilmicin was found to be less cochleotoxic than tobramycin.[183] The development of renal impairment for whatever reason and failure to lower the aminoglycoside daily dose or to discontinue aminoglycoside therapy result in higher serum levels, greater perilymph drug concentrations, and an increased risk of toxicity.[294]

Clinical Features. Cochlear toxicity may be unilateral or bilateral.[187, 188, 294] Injury may occur days to weeks after termination of drug administration. Cochlear injury may be independent of nephrotoxicity. The cumulative dose and duration of therapy are more important than serum concentrations.

The risk of either cochlear or vestibular toxicity is greater in patients with renal impairment.[294] The use of neomycin, regardless of the route of administration (e.g., oral, intraperitoneal, topical on open wounds, or bladder irrigation), is particularly hazardous.[294]

High-frequency hearing loss can occur with no symptoms. Conversational hearing loss can occur without warning. Some patients complain of tinnitus or a sensation of "fullness in the ears," which may represent early injury.

Vestibular Toxicity

The target of drug toxicity is the type I hair cell of the summit of the ampullar cristae.[295] The true incidence of vestibular toxicity in ill patients is virtually impossible to determine.[187, 188] Because vestibular injury can be compensated by visual and proprioceptive cues, patients can suffer considerable injury before the appearance of symptoms or clinical findings. Suspicion is raised at the bedside by complaints of nausea, vomiting, and vertigo.[296] Symptoms are exacerbated in the dark, when the eyes are closed, or in other situations that block compensatory pathways. Nystagmus may be evident. Systematic surveillance of patients with electronystagmography is seldom performed; in one clinical study using electronystagmographic surveillance, abnormalities were found in 4 to 6% of patients receiving gentamicin or amikacin.[183, 184] Over time, symptoms abate, presumably because of compensatory mechanisms. In addition, hair cell regeneration is possible and has been demonstrated in a chinchilla animal model.[297]

Prevention

When aminoglycoside therapy is indicated, the risk of ototoxicity can be minimized by as short a duration of therapy as is clinically appropriate and by periodic assessments of renal function to avoid rising serum concentrations. If high-frequency audiometric testing is available, the patient's mental state allows valid responses to auditory stimuli, and a treatment duration of more than 4 days is likely, it seems reasonable to serially monitor the ability of the patient to hear high-frequency sound.

Neuromuscular Blockade

Neuromuscular blockade after aminoglycoside administration is a rare but serious and potentially lethal adverse effect. Neuromuscular blockade has been described in patients administered neomycin, streptomycin, kanamycin, tobramycin, gentamicin, amikacin, on netilmicin.[191] In general, blockade has occurred in clinical situations in which a disease state or a concomitant drug interferes with neuromuscular transmission.[191] A rapid rise in serum drug concentrations is also a risk factor.

Clinical manifestations of blockade may include weakness of respiratory musculature, flaccid paralysis, and dilated pupils.[191] Deep tendon reflexes may be absent, hypoactive, or present. Drug exposure may have been a result of intraperitoneal, intravenous, intramuscular, intrapleural, oral, topical, or retroperitoneal administration.[191] Both in vitro and in vivo, the greater the positive charge, the greater the propensity to cause blockade; hence, neomycin is the most potent of the aminoglycosides.[298]

The risk of blockade is amplified in patients also administered D-tubocurarine, succinylcholine, on similar agents.[191] Hypomagnesemia, hypocalcemia, and perhaps calcium channel blockers amplify the risk.[299] Patients with infant botulism are at risk.[300] Reports are conflicting regarding the risk in patients with myasthenia gravis.[301, 302]

Blockade results from inhibition of the presynaptic release of acetylcholine and blockage of postsynaptic receptor sites of acetylcholine. Aminoglycosides can prevent internalization of calcium into the presynaptic region of the axon.[303] Calcium internalization must occur before acetylcholine release. The drugs also blunt the response of postsynaptic receptors to acetylcholine. Neomycin is more apt to inhibit presynaptic release, whereas streptomycin and netilmicin are the most active drugs at the postsynaptic site.[304, 305] The neuromuscular blockade is rapidly reversed by the intravenous administration of calcium gluconate.[306] The response to neostigmine has been variable.

Blockade is preventable by intravenously infusing aminoglycoside over a period of 20 to 30 minutes or more, especially in patients administered large doses once per day. No clear indication is recognized for instillation of high concentrations of aminoglycoside into the peritoneal cavity or pleural space.

CLINICAL INDICATIONS

The clinical indications for aminoglycosides are divided into empirical, specific, and prophylactic categories. Empirical and specific uses are respectively summarized in Tables 23–10 and 23–11.

Empirical Therapy

The aminoglycosides (gentamicin, tobramycin, amikacin) are effective in the empirical treatment of infections suspected of being due to aerobic gram-negative bacilli, including *P. aeruginosa*. Aminoglycosides have in vitro activity against *S. aureus*, but resistant small colony variants appear within 24 hours unless a concomitant antistaphylococcal β-lactam or vancomycin is administered. Activity against *Enterococcus* spp. requires a concomitant active penicillin or vancomycin. It is emphasized that aminoglycosides have no practical activity against pneumococci or anaerobic organisms. For reasons of anticipated spectrum of activity or to achieve an additive or synergistic effect, aminoglycosides are often combined with a β-lactam antibiotic, vancomycin, or a drug active against anaerobic bacteria. Except for selected mycobacterial infections, there is no reason to combine an aminoglycoside with a fluoroquinolone.

Other classes of antimicrobials, alone or in combination, may be equally efficacious in the empirical treatment of the infections listed in Table 23–10. Examples include the antipseudomonal penicillins (e.g., piperacillin), a penicillin combined with a β-lactamase inhibitor (e.g., ampicillin-sulbactam, ticarcillin–clavulanic acid, piperacillin-tazobactam), the extended-spectrum cephalosporins (e.g., ceftriaxone, ceftazidime), a carbapenem (e.g., imipenem-cilastatin, meropenem), or the fluorinated quinolones (e.g., ciprofloxacin, trovafloxacin).

The efficacy of empirical aminoglycoside therapy is documented

TABLE 23–10 Examples of Empirical Indications for Aminoglycosides

Type of Infection	Example(s)	Initial Use in Combination with Other Antimicrobials
Bacteremia, possible[178–184]	Fever without obvious source	Yes
Burn wound[307]	Burn wound infection	Yes
Endocarditis, infective[308]	Streptococcal, enterococcal, staphylococcal	Yes
Intra-abdominal[133, 309, 310]	Appendicitis, diverticulitis, cholecystitis, peritonitis	Yes
Meningitis[147, 148, 150]	Post-trauma, postoperative	Yes
Neutropenia and fever[311, 312]	Postchemotherapy	Yes
Ocular[158, 161]	Endophthalmitis	Yes
Osteomyelitis/septic arthritis[83, 313–315]	Postoperative or post-trauma	Yes
Otitis[82, 313, 316, 317]	Malignant external otitis in a diabetic	Yes
Pneumonia[82, 313, 318]	Respirator-associated pneumonia	Yes
Pyelonephritis[82, 313]	Patients with chronic Foley catheter infection	Yes
Sexually transmitted disease[319]	Pelvic inflammatory disease	Yes
Skin–subcutaneous tissue[82]	Infected diabetic foot	Yes

Data from refs. 82, 93, 178, 293, 313, and 320, in addition to the references in the table.

TABLE 23–11 Specific Indications for Aminoglycosides

Pathogen	Aminoglycoside	Drugs Used in Combination
Aerobic gram-negative bacilli		
Klebsiella spp.[321]	A, G, N, T	App, ESC
Enterobacter aerogenes[81, 322, 323]	A, G, N, T	APP, ESC
Serratia marcescens[324]	G	APP, ESC
Pseudomonas aeruginosa[325–327]	T	APP, APC
Francisella tularensis	St, G	No
Brucella abortus[328, 329]	G or St	Doxycycline
Yersinia pestis[330]	St, G	No
Vibrio vulnificus[331]	A, G, N, T	ESC
Aerobic gram-positive cocci		
Viridans streptococci	G	Penicillin G
Enterococcus faecalis	G	Penicillin G
Staphylococcus aureus	G	Nafcillin
Staphylococcus epidermidis	G	Vancomycin (rifampin)
Neisseria gonorrhoeae[319]	Sp	No
Mycobacterium avium-intracellulare[332]	A	Multiple
Mycobacterium tuberculosis	St	Multiple
Entamoeba histolytica[333]	P	No
Cryptosporidium parvum[333]	P	No

Abbreviations: A, Amikacin; APC, antipseudomonal cephalosporin; APP, antipseudomonal penicillin; ESG, extended-spectrum cephalosporin; G, gentamicin; N, netilmicin; P, paromomycin; Sp, spectinomycin; St, streptomycin; T, tobramycin.
Data from refs. 82 and 308, in addition to the references in the table.

in published symposia describing the results of clinical trials that served as the basis for licensure, as well as in subsequent trials that compared one aminoglycoside with another or with a β-lactam.[178–184, 293, 320, 334–339] In febrile neutropenic patients, a high failure rate was experienced after monotherapy with an aminoglycoside, and hence, the aminoglycosides are administered in combination with a β-lactam antibiotic active against aerobic gram-negative bacilli.[311, 312]

The need for inclusion of an aminoglycoside in the empirical treatment of intra-abdominal infections may be decreasing.[309, 310] Clinical trials indicate that extended-spectrum penicillins and cephalosporins, β-lactams in combination with a β-lactamase inhibitor, and fluoroquinolones can substitute for the activity of aminoglycosides against aerobic gram-negative bacilli.[309, 310] In some studies, the failure rate of the aminoglycoside combination regimen was statistically higher than that of monotherapy or a combination that did not include an aminoglycoside.[340–342] Aminoglycoside failures were theorized as being due to the relative resistance of gram-negative organisms functioning as facultative anaerobes, to failure to achieve "therapeutic" peak serum levels rapidly, or to both. Some investigators have expressed concern that the aminoglycosides may be more efficacious in the 5 to 18% of patients whose initial cultures yield *P. aeruginosa* or *Enterobacter* spp.[309] The weight of evidence suggests that the virulence of *Enterococcus* is insufficient to warrant inclusion of an aminoglycoside in empirical therapy.[310] An exception may be patients with underlying valvular heart disease.

Specific Therapy

After 1 or 2 days, when the patient is stabilized, the disease process is better understood, and the results of culture(s) performed on admission are available, it may be possible to increase the specificity of the patient's antimicrobial therapy (see Table 23–11). If *P. aeruginosa* is isolated, an aminoglycoside is often continued with an antipseudomonal penicillin (e.g., ticarcillin) or an antipseudomonal cephalosporin (e.g., ceftazidime).[82, 313] Occasionally, rifampin may be added to combination therapy.[325] In a non-neutropenic patient with a urinary tract infection of mild severity, monotherapy with an aminoglycoside may suffice. Because of greater activity in vitro and in animal models, tobramycin is the preferred aminoglycoside for *P. aeruginosa* infection. Because gentamicin displays greater in vitro activity against *Serratia* spp., gentamicin is preferred when *Serratia* is the pathogen. For other aerobic gram-negative bacilli, amikacin, gentamicin, netilmicin, and tobramycin appear to be of equivalent efficacy.

Streptomycin and gentamicin have proved efficacious in the treatment of plague and tularemia, as has gentamicin plus doxycycline in the treatment of brucellosis.[82, 313, 328–330] Other aminoglycosides may be effective, but no experience with their use has been reported.

The aminoglycosides are most often used in combination therapy as indicated in Table 23–11. With an increasing armamentarium of drugs of different classes that have predictable activity against aerobic gram-negative bacilli, it is now possible and often advisable to discontinue aminoglycoside therapy after 2 or 3 days. Such a strategy takes advantage of the efficacy of aminoglycosides and, because of the short duration of therapy, minimizes the risk of aminoglycoside toxicity. Initiating empirical therapy with one of the nonaminoglycoside drugs is another treatment strategy. The emergence of resistant Enterobacteriaceae during the first few days of therapy with extended-spectrum cephalosporins is a concern.[81] It is theorized that this problem is inoculum dependent and hence less likely to occur after a few days of aminoglycoside or combined therapy including an aminoglycoside.

Prophylaxis

Genitourinary and gastrointestinal surgical procedures place the patient at risk of enterococcal bacteremia. If the patient has underlying valvular heart disease, antimicrobial prophylaxis with the combination of ampicillin and gentamicin is recommended.[343] Vancomycin is substituted for ampicillin in penicillin-allergic patients.

The risk of infection after elective colectomy is reduced by mechanical cleansing of the bowel plus the oral administration of neomycin and erythromycin.[344] One gram of each is given three times during the 18 to 24 hours before surgery.

DOSING OF AMINOGLYCOSIDES

The aminoglycosides are licensed for multiple administrations per day to patients with normal renal function, that is, twice a day for streptomycin and amikacin and three times a day for gentamicin, tobramycin, netilmicin, and amikacin. As an alternative, aminoglycosides can be administered once a day. Both methods will be described as they apply to adults. Dosing in the pediatric population and in other selected circumstances is reviewed separately.

Multiple Daily Dosing

Loading Dose

The treatment regimen is divided into an initial (loading) dose and maintenance doses (Table 23–12). The purpose of the initial dose is to rapidly achieve a "therapeutic" peak plasma concentration. The targeted range of peak levels represents a compromise between the efficacy that correlates with higher concentrations and the desirability of excreting potentially toxic drug before the next dose. The indicated trough levels reflect the intent to maintain trough concentrations at or above the MIC for the majority of susceptible aerobic gram-negative bacilli for the entire dosage interval.

Calculation of the loading dose is based on ideal body weight in kilograms as derived from the following formulas:

Females: 45 kg + 2.3 kg/inch of height over 5 ft

Males: 50 kg + 2.3 kg/inch of height over 5 ft

The loading dose is independent of renal function. The peak serum level obtained is dependent on the volume of distribution. Because the volume of distribution is less in adipose tissue than in lean body mass, the initial dose is adjusted in patients with an actual body weight that is more than 30% above ideal weight. The ideal body weight is added to 40% of the excess weight and the total used as a basis for calculating the loading dose: ideal body weight + 0.4 (total body weight − ideal body weight).[144] Adjustment for excess adiposity is of particular import in the "morbidly" obese.[348]

Volume of distribution is increased in patients with severe burns, ascites, other edematous states, and at least in theory, any disease process that results in a capillary "leak" syndrome. The volume of distribution of aminoglycosides is reported as 0.2 to 0.3 liter/kg.[345] Conversely, dehydration or muscle wasting decreases the apparent volume of distribution. The latter conditions vary widely from patient to patient and hour to hour in critically ill patients.[345] Hence, it is recommended that after either the initial dose or the first maintenance dose a "peak" serum drug level be obtained.

A rough estimate of the predicted serum level (micrograms per milliliter) can be calculated from the following formula:

$$\frac{\text{Dose (mg/kg)} \times \text{kg body weight}}{\text{Volume distribution (liter/kg)} \times \text{kg body weight}}$$

The definition of the time of a target peak drug level varies from author to author.[347, 349] For the clinician, a precise definition is not necessary. For patients treated intravenously, the loading dose is infused over a 15- to 30-minute period. Ideally, peak serum levels are obtained 30 minutes after the end of the infusion. Such careful timing is often not feasible or practical, and it is acceptable and easier to time the serum collection for 1 hour from the start of the 15- to 30-minute infusion. After intramuscular administration, serum is collected 1 hour later. The ranges of desired peak and trough concentrations are summarized in Table 23–12.

Maintenance Dose

Calculation of the maintenance dosage regimen requires an estimation of renal function inasmuch as aminoglycoside excretion correlates directly with glomerular filtration. Glomerular filtration falls

TABLE 23–12 Suggested Loading Doses, Maintenance Doses, and Desirable Serum Concentrations of Aminoglycosides Administered Multiple Times per Day to Adult Patients with an Estimated Creatinine Clearance above 90 ml/min

Drug*	Loading Dose	Daily Maintenance Dose		Desired Serum Concentrations (μg/ml)	
		Total mg/kg	*Divided as mg/kg*	*Peak*	*Trough*
Gentamicin	2	5.1	1.7 q8h	4–10	1–2
Tobramycin	2	5.1	1.7 q8h	4–10	1–2
Netilmicin	2	6	2 q8h	4–10	1–2
Amikacin	7.5	15	7.5 q12h	15–30	5–10
Streptomycin†	7.5	15	7.5 q12h	15–30	5–10

*All drugs, including streptomycin, can be given intramuscularly or intravenously.
†Maximum daily dose, 2.0 g; 1.0 g intramuscularly (or intravenously) can be administered daily for tuberculosis.
Data from refs. 245 to 347.

normally with aging and as a result of some disease states. The glomerular filtration rate is reflected by the endogenous creatinine clearance. The endogenous creatinine clearance (C_{cr}) is estimated by the equation of Cockcroft and Gault[350]:

$$C_{cr} = \frac{(140 \times \text{age})(\text{weight in kg})}{\text{Serum creatinine} \times 72}$$

To adjust for females, the calculated creatinine clearance is multiplied by 0.85.

Disease states that result in significant loss of muscle mass are associated with low serum creatinine values. In such patients, the estimated creatinine clearance formula may seriously overestimate the glomerular clearance of aminoglycosides. As such, it is suggested that the minimum serum creatinine concentration used in the formula just presented be 0.8 μg/ml.[351]

Normal Renal Function. Suggested loading doses, maintenance doses, and desirable serum concentrations in patients with an estimated creatinine clearance above 90 ml/minute are summarized in Table 23–12.[82, 345, 347, 349] It is desirable to measure peak and trough serum aminoglycoside levels after the first or second maintenance dose and adjust the maintenance dosage accordingly. Subsequently, serum creatinine should be measured every 3 to 5 days. If the creatinine level is stable, it is not necessary to repeat serum aminoglycoside measurements. If renal function changes, the dosage is recalculated, and serum levels are repeated after initiation of the new regimen.

Peak serum aminoglycoside levels are obtained to ensure that enough drug was administered for therapeutic efficacy. Data from infected animals and analysis of clinical trial data support the correlation between high peak levels and antibacterial efficacy.[95, 124, 318, 352, 353]

Among other risk factors, the larger the total daily dose and the longer the duration of therapy, the greater the risk of renal toxicity and ototoxicity.[202, 242, 246, 288, 289] Trough levels are a measure of renal function, as is the serum creatinine concentration, and do not predict nephrotoxicity per se. If the dosage calculation is in error and the dosage administered exceeds renal excretory capacity, the overdosage is reflected by a high trough concentration. Individualized pharmacokinetic dosing has been used in some medical centers. It has not been convincing proved that customized dosing reduces the incidence of nephrotoxicity.[246, 354–356]

Impaired Renal Function. The two general methods of dosage adjustment are either continuation of the same dose and extending the dosage interval or reduction of the dose and continuing the every-8-hour dosage interval for gentamicin-tobramycin and every-12-hour dosage interval for amikacin. Extension of the dosage interval is favored in that higher peak levels are achieved with enhanced bactericidal activity. Suggested intervals are summarized by the degree of renal impairment in Table 23–13.

Alternatively, after a loading dose, the maintenance dose can be decreased while maintaining the standard dosage interval at every 8 to 12 hours.[357, 358] The maintenance dose is calculated as follows:

$$(\text{Estimated } C_{Cr}) \times \frac{(\text{mg/kg maintenance dose used for } C_{Cr} \text{ over 80 ml/minute})}{(100)}$$

Recall that serum creatinine concentrations below 0.8 mg/dl may overestimate renal clearance of gentamicin.[351]

Dosing of Dialysis Patients. Patients with end-stage renal disease are usually assisted via either hemodialysis or continuous ambulatory peritoneal dialysis. Critically ill patients may require continuous arteriovenous hemofiltration. All three procedures enhance the clearance of aminoglycosides. The suggested amount of supplementation is summarized in Table 23–13. The data in Table 23–13 do not refer to the use of aminoglycosides in the treatment of peritonitis complicating continuous ambulatory peritoneal dialysis; the latter is discussed later.

The supplements suggested for patients undergoing hemodialysis are based on the assumption that roughly two thirds of circulating aminoglycoside will be removed per hemodialysis. However, aminoglycoside clearance can vary widely depending on the characteristics of the dialysis membrane, duration of dialysis, patient blood pressure during dialysis, and other variables. Hence, it is suggested, especially in critically ill patients, that a peak serum aminoglycoside concentration be determined after the postdialysis dose of aminoglycoside.

Continuous arteriovenous hemofiltration is used with increasing frequency in the management of critically ill patients with acute renal failure.[359–361] Depending on variables that relate to both the patient and the filter, continuous hemofiltration results in the equivalent of a creatinine clearance of between 10 and 50 ml/minute. The filtered fluid is continuously replaced by administration of parenteral fluid. For example, it is suggested that gentamicin be given as a separate infusion, once daily in a dosage of 2.5 mg/kg body weight. With this dosage, the peak serum concentration should be in the range of 8 to 12 μg/ml and the trough level (at the end of 24 hours) between 1 and 2 μg/ml. Because of individual variability, serum levels should be measured. Suggested doses for tobramycin, netilmicin, and amikacin are summarized in Table 23–13.

Once-Daily Administration

Premise

The concept of once-daily aminoglycoside therapy evolved from three separate but related observations.[124] First, experimental nephrotoxicity and ototoxicity were less severe in animals administered a daily dose of drug as a single injection as opposed to the same daily dosage administered in two or three divided doses. Animals given a single daily dose accumulated less drug in the renal cortex. The same result was observed in patients who agreed to receive an

TABLE 23–13 Multiple Daily Dosing Method: Adjustment of Dosage of Aminoglycoside Antibiotics in Patients with Variable Degrees of Impaired Renal Function via the Method of Prolongation of the Dosage Interval*

Drug	Maintenance Dose for Normal Renal Function (mg/kg)	Dosage Interval Based on Estimated Creatinine Clearance (ml/min)				Supplement after Hemodialysis† (mg/kg)	Supplement during CAVH† (mg/kg/day)	Supplement during CAPD (mg lost/liter of dialysate/day)
		80–90	*50–80*	*10–50*	*<10*			
Gentamicin	1.7 q8h	q12h	q12–24h	q24–48h	q48–72h	1–2	2.5	3–4‡
Tobramycin	1.7 q8h	q12h	q12–24h	q24–48h	q48–72h	1–2	2.5	3–4‡
Netilmicin	2 q8h	q12h	q12–24h	q24–48h	q48–72h	2	2.5	3–4‡
Amikacin	7.5 q12h	q12h	q12–24h	q24–48h	q48–72h	5–7	4.0	15–20§

*Also shown are suggested doses of aminoglycoside for patients requiring hemodialysis and continuous arteriovenous hemofiltration (CAVH) and dosages to treat peritonitis in patients maintained by continuous ambulatory peritoneal dialysis (CAPD).
†The rate and absolute amount of drug removed are influenced by a variety of host disease and dialysis-related factors. In critically ill patients, serum aminoglycoside levels should be monitored.
‡Replace (intravenously) the 3 to 4 mg lost per liter of dialysate per day: e.g., 8 liter/day × 4 mg/liter = 32 mg/day.
§Replace (intravenously) the 15 to 20 mg lost per liter of dialysate per day: e.g., 8 liter/day × 20 mg/liter = 160 mg/day.

aminoglycoside before elective nephrectomy. Patients given standard doses every 8 hours had lower renal tissue concentrations of tobramycin, netilmicin, and amikacin than those in recipients given an equivalent amount of drug by continuous intravenous infusion.[362, 363] Second, the aminoglycosides demonstrate a PAE against aerobic gram-negative bacilli both in vitro and in vivo.[101, 113, 114] The duration of the PAE is greater the higher the peak aminoglycoside concentration. In animals, the duration of the PAE is much longer in intact animals than in animals rendered neutropenic. Finally, once-daily dosing obviates concern over the adaptive resistance phenomenon. During the period of undetectable aminoglycoside at the end of the once-daily dosage interval, the adaptive resistance phenomenon disappeared in vitro, in an animal model of endocarditis, and in the sputum of patients with cystic fibrosis.[364–366] Hence, the serum level of aminoglycoside can fall below the MIC for the pathogenic bacteria without loss of efficacy. Third, antibacterial efficacy of the aminoglycosides is enhanced with high peak drug concentrations.[94, 101] Thus, once-a-day dosing offers the potential of both reducing the risk of ototoxicity and nephrotoxicity and not sacrificing antibacterial efficacy.

Once-daily therapy proved safe and efficacious in infected animal models. Nephrotoxicity was delayed in onset and less severe in rats with subcutaneous abscesses given once-daily doses than in rats given multiple daily doses.[367] In guinea pigs with pneumonia secondary to *P. aeruginosa,* once-daily dosing was as efficacious as multiple daily doses.[95] In neutropenic animals, once-daily aminoglycoside therapy was less efficacious unless the drug was combined with a β-lactam active against *P. aeruginosa.*[95]

Two small groups of healthy volunteers received a single dose of aminoglycoside. No evidence of nephrotoxicity or ototoxicity was detected.[256, 368, 369]

Clinical Trials

Clinical trials of once-daily aminoglycoside therapy were initially understandably cautious, that is, small numbers of patients, low doses, and infections of modest severity. In early trials in the 1970s and 1980s, adults with urinary tract infections, cystic fibrosis, and pelvic inflammatory disease were treated.[124, 214, 370] Now, the results of more than 50 clinical trials have been reported, including 31 prospective randomized trials deemed suitable for 8 published meta-analyses.[371–409] The controlled trials plus experience with large numbers of patients not part of controlled trials include treatment of all the commonly encountered infections and in virtually all patient populations: neonates,[410–412] children,[382, 384, 400, 413] elderly,[387, 399, 401] febrile neutropenic patients,[373, 393, 395, 401] critically ill patients,[374, 382, 401] and patients with variable levels of renal insufficiency.[380, 401, 414, 415] The overview of the large, published, extensively analyzed patient experience is that once-daily aminoglycoside administration[416]

1. Is as efficacious as the traditional multiple-dose method (see later for exceptions).
2. May lower but not eliminate the risk of drug-induced nephrotoxicity and ototoxicity.
3. Is simpler, less time consuming, and more cost-effective than multiple-dose regimens.[417, 418]
4. Should not be used in patients with enterococcal endocarditis.[415, 419]
5. Needs further study in selected patient populations, for example, pregnancy, cystic fibrosis (see later), meningitis from aerobic gram-negative bacilli, osteomyelitis.[415, 420]
6. Does not worsen neuromuscular function even in critically ill ventilated patients. Nonetheless, rapid intravenous infusion should be avoided.[421]

Single-Daily-Dose Regimens

At present, no consensus has been reached regarding the details of a once-daily dosing regimen. The two methods used most often are summarized in Tables 23–14, 23–15, and 23–16 and are discussed in the following sections.

Total Daily Dose—Normal Renal Function. Normal renal function is defined as an estimated creatinine clearance of 80 ml/minute. This calculation may be invalid in patients with reduced muscle mass reflected by a serum creatinine level of 0.5 mg/dl.

One approach uses the sum of the Food and Drug Administration–approved multiple-dose regimens; for example, gentamicin or tobramycin is approved for up to 1.7 mg/kg per dose for three doses per day for a total daily dose of 5.1 mg/kg/day (see Table 23–14).[401, 422] For netilmicin the total would be 6.0 mg/kg/day and for amikacin,

TABLE 23–14 Suggested Once-Daily Dosage Regimens of Gentamicin and Tobramycin in Patients with Estimated Creatinine Clearance between 20 and 100 mg/min and Every-Other-Day Regimens for Creatinine Clearance below 20 ml/min*

Est CrCl† (ml/min)	Dosage Interval (h)	Dose (mg/kg)	$T_{1/2}$ (h)	Estimated Serum Level (μ/ml) at			
				1 h	*12 h*	*18 h*	*24 h*
100	24	5 (7)‡	2.5	20 (28)	1.0 (1.4)	<1	<1
90	24	5 (7)	3.1	20 (28)	2.0 (2.3)	<1	<1
80	24	5 (7)	3.4	20 (28)	2.5 (2.9)	<1	<1
70	24	4 (5.5)	3.9	16	2.0	<1	<1
60	24	4 (5.5)	4.5	16	3.0	1.5	<1
50	24	3.5 (5.0)	5.3	14	3.5	1.0	<1
40	24	2.5 (3.5)	6.5	10	3.0	1.5	<1
30	24	2.5 (3.5)	8.4	10	4.0	2.5	1.5
				1 h	*24 h*	*36 h*	*48 h*
20	48	4.0 (5.5)	11.9	16	4.0	2.0	1.0
10	48	3.0 (4.0)	20.4	12	5.0	3.0	2.0
0§ (hemodialysis)	48	2.0 (4.0)	69.3	8	7.0	6.0	5.0

*Predicted peak and trough serum levels are shown. Peak levels are calculated as follows:

$$\frac{\text{mg/kg administered} \times \text{kg body wt.}}{V_D\ (\text{L/kg}) \times \text{kg body weight}}$$

Trough levels are calculated from peak concentration and published half-life ($T_{1/2}$) in hours at varying levels of renal function (V_D, volume of distribution).
†The estimated creatinine clearance assumes a minimum serum creatinine of 0.8 mg/dl.
‡Initial 7-mg/kg dose recommended for patients with anticipated increased volume of drug distribution—see the text.
§Example values are for patient receiving hemodialysis every other day. The actual peak depends on the efficiency of dialysis. The dose is given postdialysis.
Data from Gilbert DN, Lee BL, Dworkin RJ, et al. A randomized comparison of the safety and efficacy of one-daily gentamicin or thrice-daily gentamicin in combination with ticarcillin-clavulanate. Am J Med. 1998;105:182–191; and Gilbert DN, Bennett WM. Use of antimicrobial agents in renal failure. Infect Dis Clin North Am. 1989;3:517–531.

TABLE 23–15 Suggested Once-Daily Dosage Regimens of Netilmicin, Amikacin, Kanamycin, and Streptomycin in Patients with Estimated Creatinine Clearance between 20 and 90 ml/min and Every-Other-Day Regimen for Creatinine Clearance below 20 mg/min*

Est CrCl† (ml/min)	Dosage Interval (h)	Dose (mg/kg)	$T_{1/2}$ (h)	Estimated Serum Level (μg/ml) at 1 h	12 h	18 h	24 h
Netilmicin							
90	24	6.5	3.1	26	2	<1	<1
70	24	5.0	3.9	20	2.5	1.0	<1
50	24	4.0	5.3	16	4	1	<1
30	24	2.0	8.4	8	3	2	1
				1 h	*24 h*	*36 h*	*48 h*
20	48	3.0	11.9	13	3.0	1.5	0.75
10	48	2.5	20.4	10	4.0	3	2
0‡ (hemodialysis)	48	2.0	69.3	8	7.0	6	5
Amikacin, kanamycin, streptomycin				*1 h*	*12 h*	*18 h*	*24 h*
90	24	15	3.1	60	6.0	<1	<1
70	24	12	3.9	48	9.0	2.5	<1
50	24	7.5	5.3	30	7.0	3.5	1.0
30	24	4.0	8.4	20	7.5	5.0	3.0
				1 h	*24 h*	*36 h*	*48 h*
20	48	7.5	11.9	30	7.5	3.3	1.6
10	48	4.0	20.4	16	12	5.0	3.0
0‡ (hemodialysis)	48	3.0	69.3	20	16	15	12

*Predicted peak and trough serum levels are shown. Peak levels are calculated as follows:

$$\frac{\text{mg/kg administered} \times \text{kg body wt.}}{V_D\ (\text{l/kg}) \times \text{kg body weight}}$$

Trough levels are calculated from peak concentration and published half-life ($T_{1/2}$) in hours at varying levels of renal function (V_D, volume of distribution).
†The estimated creatinine clearance assumes a minimum serum creatinine of 0.8 mg/dl.
‡Example values are for patient receiving hemodialysis every other day. The actual peak depends on the efficiency of dialysis. The dose is given postdialysis.
Data from Gilbert DN, Bennett WM. Use of antimicrobial agents in renal failure. Infect Dis Clin North Am. 1989;3:517–531.

15 mg/kg/day (see Table 23–15).[422] The advantage of this method is confidence that the serum level will fall below 1 μg/ml between 12 and 18 hours after the dose and hence lower the risk of nephrotoxicity. The disadvantage is the potential failure of achieving the targeted peak serum concentration (for gentamicin-tobramycin) of 16 to 24 μg/ml because of an increased volume of drug distribution as encountered in patients with edematous states (e.g., congestive heart failure, ascites) or "leaky" capillaries as a result of bacteremia. In one clinical study that included a high percentage of critically ill patients, the peak serum gentamicin concentration after the first dose of 5.1 mg/kg was below 16 μg/ml in 48% of the patients.[401]

A second method increases the daily dose of gentamicin or tobramycin to 7 mg/kg/day to increase the average peak serum concentration and hence further facilitate concentration-dependent bactericidal activity (see Table 23–16).[414, 415] The higher dose has a clear advantage in patients with an increased volume of drug distribution, and neuromuscular blockade has not been reported. No controlled studies have compared 5 versus 7 mg/kg/day of gentamicin or tobramycin, but clinical experience with the 7-mg/kg/day dosage is substantial.[414, 415] With the exception of patients with cystic fibrosis, the clinical use of single doses of amikacin or netilmicin exceeding the licensed total daily dose has not been reported. Neonates and patients with cystic fibrosis have altered aminoglycoside kinetics and are discussed separately. As for multiple daily dosing, the dose calculation is based on ideal body weight with an adjustment for obesity if needed (see earlier).

For critically ill patients, it is recommended that the initial dose of gentamicin or tobramycin be 7 mg/kg, with confirmation of a peak serum level between 16 and 24 μg/ml. Assuming clinical improvement and continued normal renal function, the dose could be decreased to 5.1 mg/kg/day during the first few days of therapy.

TABLE 23–16 Alternative Once-Daily Aminoglycoside Dosage Regimen Based on Constant Dose and Interval Prolongation

Estimated Creatinine Clearance (ml/min)	Administer 7 mg/kg at Time Interval (h) as Indicated
≥60	Every 24 h
40–60	Every 36 h
20–40	Every 48 h
<20	After initial dose, monitor blood levels. Readminister when level <1 μg/ml

Adapted from Nicolau DP, Freeman CD, Belliveau PP, et al. Experience with a once-daily aminoglycoside program administered to 2184 adult patients. Antimicrob Agents Chemother 1995;39:650–655; Freeman CD, Nicolau DP, Belliveau PP, et al. Once-daily dosing of aminoglycosides: Review and recommendations for clinical practice. J Antimicrob Chemother 1997;39:677–686.

Total Daily Dose—Abnormal Renal Function. Dosing in patients with reduced renal function and, hence, decreased drug clearance is unsettled. One method gradually lowers the daily dose proportionate to the fall in creatinine clearance (see Tables 23–14 and 23–15). The dosage interval is maintained at 24 hours for patients, with an estimated creatinine clearance between 30 and 80 ml/minute with prolongation to every 48 hours when the creatinine clearance falls below 30 ml/minute. Note that for creatinine clearances of 40 ml/minute or less, the theoretical advantage of once-daily dosing is gone; that is, the peak serum level is 10 μg/ml and drug is detectable in serum throughout the 24-hour dosing interval. This dose reduction method has the advantage of convenient timing of doses and maintaining some time period of no detectable drug in serum for patients with mild to moderate renal impairment.

The second method prolongs the dosage interval without altering the total daily dosage[414, 415] (see Table 23–16). The published tables are based on a gentamicin-tobramycin daily dosage of 7 mg/kg. The advantage is achievement of high peak serum levels regardless of the degree of impairment in renal function. One disadvantage is implementation of an every-36-hour dosage interval in patients with an estimated creatinine clearance between 40 and 60 ml/minute. Perhaps more substantive is the longer duration of high aminoglycoside levels and the theoretical concern that the risk of nephrotoxicity and ototoxicity may be increased.

Summary of Once-Daily Dosing Regimens

Subject to data from controlled trials, I prefer a total daily dosage that achieves targeted peak serum concentrations for a given level of renal function. For patients with an expanded volume of distribution, the first few daily doses should be larger as indicated in Table 23–14. For prolonged treatment in patients with normal renal function, for example, osteomyelitis, 5 mg/kg/day for gentamicin-tobramycin, 6 mg/kg/day for netilmicin, and 15 mg/kg/day for amikacin should be efficacious.

When renal function is impaired, the total daily dose may be reduced or the dosage interval prolonged. On practical and theoretical grounds, the former method is preferred pending new data.

Serum Level Monitoring with Once-Daily Regimens

It is necessary to obtain serum levels early in a course of therapy. Peak serum levels are obtained to ensure efficacy; trough serum levels are obtained to reduce the risk of toxicity. In critically ill patients, a peak level should be obtained after the first dose. The serum is collected 60 minutes after the start of a 30- to 45-minute infusion. Alternatively, serum can be obtained later postinfusion and a formula used to back-calculate an idealized peak serum concentration.

The timing of determining trough serum levels has not been standardized. I have found 18 hours after dosing to be convenient; the goal in patients with creatinine clearance values of 70 ml/minute is a trough level of less than 1 μg/ml (undetectable) (see Table 23–14). If the estimated creatinine clearance is between 40 and 60 ml/minute, a reasonable target is a serum level of less than 1 μg/ml 23 to 24 hours after the dose.

Another approach, based on a 7-mg/kg fixed daily dosage, uses serum drawn between 6 and 14 hours after a dose. The serum level is applied to a nomogram to determine the recommended fixed-dose dosage interval.[414, 415]

In patients with stable renal function who require more than 3 days of therapy, additional serum levels are not needed. It is recommended that serum creatinine levels be measured once or twice per week. A change in creatinine concentration leads to a change in dosage and the need to revalidate serum levels.

Special Circumstances

Children

The pharmacokinetics of aminoglycosides in newborns and infants differs from that in adults in at least two ways.[173, 423] The renal clearance of aminoglycosides is reduced in newborns with a resultant prolongation of the half-life and need for a reduction in the aminoglycoside dosage.[423] The half-life is even further prolonged in low-birth-weight infants. By 7 days in newborns with normal birth weight, the serum half-life is approaching adult values.

Furthermore, the volume of distribution of aminoglycosides is larger, as a percentage of body weight, in newborns than in adults. This larger volume of distribution compensates, but only in a modest way, for the reduction in renal clearance. Because of the unpredictable pharmacokinetics, particularly in low-birth-weight newborns, it is necessary to obtain peak and trough serum levels.

Multiple-daily-dose regimens for the three most commonly used aminoglycosides are presented in Table 23–17. Note that neither kanamycin nor streptomycin is listed in Table 23–17, the former because of the frequency of resistance among Enterobacteriaceae and the latter because of the risk of ototoxicity. Nonetheless, streptomycin therapy may prove necessary in patients with multidrug-resistant tuberculosis.

TABLE 23–17 Multiple-Daily-Dose Regimens of Aminoglycosides Based on Postconceptual Age

Aminoglycoside (IV, IM)	Dosage (mg/kg) and Time Interval of Administration Based on Gestational Age Plus Weeks of Life			
	≤26	*27–34*	*35–42*	*≥43*
Amikacin	7.5 q24h	7.5 q18h	10 q12h	10 q8h
Gentamicin	2.5 q24h	2.5 q18h	2.5 q12h	2.5 q8h
Tobramycin	2.5 q24h	2.5 q18h	2.5 q12h	2.5 q8h

Data from Hickey SM, McCracken GH Jr. Antibacterial therapeutic agents. In: Feigin RD, Cherry JD, eds. Textbook of Pediatric Infectious Diseases. 4th ed. Philadelphia: WB Saunders; 1998: 2614–2649.

Experience is limited with once-daily dosing. Gentamicin administered at 5 mg/kg once daily was as effective as 2.5 mg/kg twice daily in 11 neonates.[410] Netilmicin given as 6 mg/kg once daily was reported effective in 21 neonates.[417] In an open randomized study of children aged 3 months to 16 years, 4.5 mg/kg/day of gentamicin was equally effective given once a day or in three divided doses.[400] Similarly, no toxicity was encountered with once-daily amikacin in neonates.[412]

Cystic Fibrosis

Patients with advanced cystic fibrosis suffer airway colonization with *P. aeruginosa*. As the disease progresses, such patients have an increased frequency of episodes of tracheobronchitis and pneumonia necessitating treatment with a combination of antipseudomonal β-lactam antibiotics and aminoglycosides.[424]

Aminoglycoside therapy in patients with cystic fibrosis is complicated by altered pharmacokinetics, reduced antibacterial effect, and the risk of ototoxicity (especially cochlear toxicity) because of the need for chronic therapy. Patients with cystic fibrosis demonstrate altered aminoglycoside kinetics by some combination of an increase in glomerular clearance, a shortened serum half-life, and an increased volume of distribution.[425] The antibacterial activity of aminoglycosides is hampered by the need for higher drug doses, by the difficulty ensuring drug delivery to organisms embedded in tenacious mucus, and perhaps by the reduced rate of replication of the bacteria.[424] A high percentage of patients with end-stage cystic fibrosis and the need of nearly continuous aminoglycoside therapy over months suffer severe cochlear damage and deafness.[426] For unclear reasons, nephrotoxicity and vestibular toxicity are uncommon.

Parenteral Therapy. Because of altered drug kinetics, the dosage of drug must be increased to achieve targeted serum concentrations. For multiple-daily-dose regimens of tobramycin or gentamicin, the recommended initial dose is 3.3 mg/kg every 8 hours. The peak serum levels achieved are variable and often necessitate dosage adjustment. The suggested dose for amikacin is 35 mg/kg every 12 hours. Tobramycin is usually selected because of somewhat lower MICs versus *P. aeruginosa*.

Once-daily intravenous therapy is an alternative approach. The dosages used in four published studies are summarized in Table 23–18.[214, 428–430] No reduction in efficacy or toxicity was reported, but

TABLE 23–18 Once-Daily Aminoglycoside Therapy for Cystic Fibrosis Patients. Summary of Reported Effective Dosage Regimens

Study	Aminoglycoside	Dosage, mg/kg/d	Mean Peak Serum Level, μg/ml (range)
Powell[199]	Tobramycin	11	62
Bates[429]	Tobramycin	11.9 ± 1.9	43 (40–65)
Smith[428] and Wagner[422]	Netilmicin	8	47 (29–60)
Canis[430]	Amikacin	35	121 ± 37

all studies were of short duration. The suggested dosage regimens result in the desired high ratios of peak serum level to *P. aeruginosa* MIC, and serum levels of aminoglycoside were less than 1 μg/ml for 12 or more hours of the 24-hour dosage interval.

Aerosol Therapy. Aerosol therapy has many advantages: the prospect of higher concentrations of drug in sputum, less systemic exposure to drug, patient self-administration at home, and improvement in lung function coincident with a reduced burden of *P. aeruginosa*. When compared with placebo, 600 mg of tobramycin in saline delivered via nebulizer three times per day improved pulmonary function and reduced the sputum density of *P. aeruginosa* over a 28-day study period.[431] The dosage recommended by the Food and Drug Administration for both adults and children 6 years and older is 300 mg via one of two approved nebulizers twice a day for 28 days.[432] After 28 days, inhaled tobramycin therapy ceases for 28 days and then the cycle repeats. Efficacy data have not been established for patients colonized with *Burkholderia (Pseudomonas) cepacia*.

Ten minutes after inhalation, sputum tobramycin concentrations are variable but range up to several thousand micrograms per milliliter. Within 2 hours after the dose, sputum concentrations are approximately 14% of the levels found 10 minutes after inhalation.[432]

Absorption into serum is low. The average serum drug concentration 1 hour after inhalation was 1.0 μg/ml with a range of 0.2 to 3.0 μg/ml.[433] Ototoxicity has not been reported, but transient tinnitus occurred in a few individuals during clinical trials. Nephrotoxicity has not been observed. Inhaled therapy is expensive: roughly $2000 for the drug per 28-day cycle plus the expense of the nebulizer.

Infective Endocarditis

No reported clinical trials have compared aminoglycoside dosage frequency in patients with infective endocarditis. Based on in vitro studies and animal models of endocarditis, some tentative generalizations are possible.[415, 419] The antibacterial effect of aminoglycosides against *Enterococcus* spp. requires the continuous presence of both a cell wall–active β-lactam antibiotic (e.g., ampicillin) and an aminoglycoside. Hence, once-daily dosing does not seem justified. Assuming in vitro susceptibility and evidence of clinical response, the current consensus recommendation of an American Heart Association–sponsored expert committee is penicillin G plus gentamicin, 3 mg/kg/day (assuming normal renal function) divided into an every-8-hour dosage schedule, for viridans streptococcal and enterococcal endocarditis.[308]

Endocarditis from aerobic gram-negative bacilli is exceedingly rare. Some success is reported with the combination of an aminoglycoside and a cell wall–active β-lactam antibiotic.[434]

Peritonitis during Continuous Ambulatory Peritoneal Dialysis

Aminoglycosides are often used in peritoneal dialysis fluid to treat peritoneal dialysis–associated peritonitis resulting from aminoglycoside-susceptible organisms.[435] This method of drug administration is not recommended for patients with systemic infection. The aminoglycoside is added to the peritoneal dialysis fluid. It may be added in a "therapeutic" concentration to each bag of dialysis fluid, or the aminoglycoside may be added in a higher concentration to only one of the usual four daily exchanges of peritoneal dialysis fluid (Table 23–19). The once-a-day regimen is analogous to once-daily parenteral aminoglycoside therapy.

Spectinomycin and Gonorrhea

Spectinomycin is used exclusively to treat gonococcal infections.[319] It is not effective in the treatment of infections with *Treponema pallidum* or *Chlamydia trachomatis*. The drug does not achieve therapeutic concentrations in saliva and hence does not eliminate pharyngeal gonococci. The drug is neither nephrotoxic nor ototoxic. Spectinomycin is effective in the treatment of uncomplicated urethral, cervical, or disseminated gonorrhea. It is an alternative therapy in patients allergic to penicillin or in patients infected with penicillinase-producing strains of gonococci. For infection of the cervix or urethra, the dose is 2 g given as a single intramuscular injection. For gonococcemia, the suggested dose is 2 g intramuscularly every 12 hours for 3 days. No intravenous form of the drug is available.

TABLE 23–19 Dosage of Aminoglycosides Added to Dialysis Bags to Treat Continuous Ambulatory Peritoneal Dialysis–Associated Peritonitis

	Dose	
Drug	***Intermittent Method: Dose Added to One Bag/day (mg/kg)***	***Continuous Method: mg Drug/L Added to All Bags (mg/L)***
Amikacin	2	Loading dose: 25 Maintenance dose: 12
Gentamicin, netilmicin, tobramycin	0.6	Loading dose: 8 Maintenance dose: 4

Data from Keane WF, Everett ED, Golper TA, et al. Peritoneal dialysis related peritonitis treatment recommendations. 1993 update. Perit Dial Int 1993;13:14–28.

REFERENCES

1. Waksman SA, Schatz AI. Present status of streptomycin therapy. Lancet. 1946;66:77–78.
2. Piepersberg W. Molecular biology, biochemistry, and fermentation of aminoglycoside antibiotics. In: Strohl WR, ed. Biotechnology of Antibiotics. 2nd ed. New York: Marcel Dekker; 1997:81–163.
3. Davies JE. Aminoglycoside-aminocyclitol antibiotics and their modifying enzymes. In: Lorian V, ed. Antibiotics in Laboratory Medicine. 3rd ed. Baltimore: Williams & Wilkins; 1991:691–713.
4. Umezawa S, Tsuchiya T. Total synthesis and chemical modification of the aminoglycoside antibiotics. In: Umezawa H, Hooper IR, eds. Aminoglycoside Antibiotics. New York: Springer-Verlag; 1982:37.
5. Price KE, Godfrey JC. Effect of structural modifications on the biological properties of aminoglycoside antibiotics containing 2-deoxystreptamine. Adv Appl Microbiol. 1974;18:191–307.
6. Price KE. Aminoglycoside research 1975–1985: Prospects for development of improved agents. Antimicrob Agents Chemother. 1986;29:543–548.
7. Nagabhushan TL, Miller GH, Weinstein MJ. Structure-activity relationships in aminoglycoside-aminocyclitol antibiotics. In: Whelton A, Neu HC, eds. The Aminoglycosides. New York: Marcel Dekker; 1982:3–27.
8. Leitner F, Price KE. Aminoglycosides under development. In: Whelton A, Neu HC, eds. The Aminoglycosides. New York: Marcel Dekker; 1982:29–64.
9. Berdy J, Aszalos A, Bostian M, et al. CRC Handbook of Antibiotic Compounds. v 1. Carbohydrate Antibiotics. Boca Raton, Fla: CRC Press; 1980.
10. Weinstein MJ, Wagman GH, Oden EM, et al. Biological activity of the antibiotic components of the gentamicin complex. J Bacteriol. 1967;94:789–790.
11. Gilbert DN, Kohlhepp SJ. New sodium hydroxide digestion method for measurement of renal tobramycin concentrations. Antimicrob Agents Chemother. 1986;30:361–365.
12. Moellering RC Jr. In vitro antibacterial activity of the aminoglycoside antibiotics. Rev Infect Dis. 1983;5(Suppl):S212–S232.
13. Rocque WJ, Fesik SW, Haug A, et al. Polycation binding to isolated lipopolysaccharide from antibiotic-hypersusceptible mutant strains of *Escherichia coli*. Antimicrob Agents Chemother. 1988;32:308–313.
14. Vandaux P, Waldvogel FA. Gentamicin inactivation in purulent exudates: Role of cell lysis. J Infect Dis. 1980;142:586–593.
15. Laurent G, Kishore BK, Tulkens PM. Aminoglycoside-induced renal phospholipidosis and nephrotoxicity. Biochem Pharmacol. 1990;40:2383–2392.
16. Ramphal R, Lhermitte M, Filliat M, et al. The binding of antipseudomonas antibiotics to macromolecules from cystic fibrosis sputum. J Antimicrob Chemother. 1988;22:483–490.
17. Bataillon V, Lhermitte M, Lafitte J-JH, et al. The binding of amikacin to macromolecules from the sputum of patients suffering from respiratory diseases. J Antimicrob Chemother. 1992;29:499–508.
18. McLaughlin JE, Reeves DS. Clinical and laboratory evidence for inactivation of gentamicin by carbenicillin. Lancet. 1971;1:261–264.
19. Pickering LK, Rutherford I. Effect of concentration and time upon inactivation of tobramycin, gentamicin, netilmicin, mezlocillin, and piperacillin. J Pharmacol Exp Ther. 1981;217:345–349.
20. Walterspiel JN, Feldman S, Van R, et al. Comparative inactivation of isepamicin, amikacin, and gentamicin by nine beta-lactams and two beta-lactamase inhibitors, cilastatin and heparin. Antimicrob Agents Chemother. 1991;35:1875–1878.

21. Halstenson CE, Wong MU, Herman CS, et al. Effect of concomitant administration of piperacillin on the dispositions of isepamicin and gentamicin in patients with end-stage renal disease. Antimicrob Agents Chemother. 1992;36:1832–1836.
22. Muller GH, Sabetelli FJ, Hare RS, et al. The most frequent aminoglycoside resistance mechanisms—changes with time and geographic area: A reflection of aminoglycoside usage patterns? Clin Infect Dis. 1997;24(Suppl 1):S46–S62.
23. Davies J, Wright GD. Bacterial resistance to aminoglycoside antibiotics. Trends Microbiol. 1997;5:234–238.
24. Bryan LE, Kawan S. Roles of ribosomal binding, membrane potential, and electron transport in bacterial uptake of streptomycin and gentamicin. Antimicrob Agents Chemother. 1983;23:835–845.
25. Taber HW, Muller JP, Arrow AS. Bacterial uptake of aminoglycoside antibiotics. Microbiol Rev. 1987;51:439–457.
26. Hancock RE, Bellido F. Antibiotic uptake: Unusual results for unusual molecules. J Antimicrob Chemother. 1992;29:235–239.
27. Hurwitz C, Rosano CL, Landau JV. Kinetics of loss of viability of *Escherichia coli* exposed to streptomycin. J Bacteriol. 1962;83:1210–1216.
28. Jackson GE, Lolans VT, Daikos GL. The inductive role of ionic binding in the bactericidal and postexposure effects of aminoglycoside antibiotics with implications for dosing. J Infect Dis. 1990;162:408–413.
29. Hancock REW. Alterations in outer membrane permeability. Annu Rev Microbiol. 1984;38:237–264.
30. Peterson AA, Hancock REW, McGroarty EJ. Binding of polycationic antibiotics and polyamines to lipopolysaccharides of *Pseudomonas aeruginosa.* J Bacteriol. 1985;164:1256–1261.
31. Martin NL, Beveridge TJ. Gentamicin interaction with *Pseudomonas aeruginosa.* Antimicrob Agents Chemother. 1986;29:1079–1087.
32. Moskowitz M. Differences in precipitability of nucleic acids with streptomycin and dihydrostreptomycin. Nature. 1963;200:335–337.
33. Nichols WW, Young SN. Respiration-dependent uptake of dihydrostreptomycin by *Escherichia coli.* Its reversible nature and lack of evidence for a uniport process. Biochem J. 1985;228:505–512.
34. Hancock REW. Aminoglycoside uptake and mode of action with special reference to streptomycin and gentamicin. I. Antagonists and mutants. J Antimicrob Chemother. 1981;8:249–276.
35. Hancock REW. Aminoglycoside uptake and mode of action with special reference to streptomycin and gentamicin. II. Effects of aminoglycosides on cells. J Antimicrob Chemother. 1981;8:429–445.
36. Bryan LE. Mechanisms of action of aminoglycoside antibiotics. In: Root RK, Sande MA, eds. Contemporary Issues in Infectious Diseases, v. 1, New Dimensions in Antimicrobial Therapy. New York: Churchill Livingstone; 1984:17–36.
37. Damper PD, Epstein W. Role of the membrane potential in bacterial resistance to aminoglycoside antibiotics. Antimicrob Agents Chemother. 1981;20:803–808.
38. Mates SM, Patel L, Kaback HR, et al. Membrane potential in anaerobically growing *Staphylococcus aureus* and its relationship to gentamicin uptake. Antimicrob Agents Chemother. 1983;23:526–530.
39. Nicas TI, Hancock REW. Outer membrane protein H1 of *Pseudomonas aeruginosa:* Involvement in adaptive and mutational resistance to ethylenediamine tetraacetate, polymyxin B, and gentamicin. J Bacteriol. 1980;143:872–878.
40. Noller HF. Ribosomal RNA and translation. Annu Rev Biochem. 1991;60:191–227.
41. Purohit P, Stern S. Interactions of a small RNA with antibiotic and RNA ligands of the 30S subunit. Nature. 1994;370:659–662.
42. Fourmy D, Recht MI, Blanchard SC, et al. Structure of the A site of *Escherichia coli* 16S ribosomal RTNA complexed with an aminoglycoside antibiotic. Science. 1996;274:1367–1371.
43. Wallis MG, Schroeder R. The binding of antibiotics to RNA. Prog Biophys Mol Biol. 1997;67:141–154.
44. Fourmy D, Recht MI, Puglisi JD. Binding of neomycin-class aminoglycoside antibiotics to the A-site of 16S rRNA. J Mol Biol. 1998;277:347–362.
45. Cho J, Hamasaki K, Rando RR. The binding site of a specific aminoglycoside binding RNA molecule. Biochemistry. 1998;37:4985–4992.
46. Jiang J, Suri AK, Fiala R, et al. Saccharide-RNA recognition in an aminoglycoside antibiotic-RNA aptamer complex. Chem Biol. 1997;4:35–50.
47. Hermann T, Westhoff E. Aminoglycoside binding to the hammerhead ribozyme: A general model for the interaction of cationic antibiotics with RNA. J Mol Biol. 1998;276:903–912.
48. Davis BB. The lethal action of aminoglycosides. J Antimicrob Chemother. 1988;22:1–3.
49. Kodurugamuwa JL, Lam JS, Beveridge TJ. Interaction of gentamicin with the A band and B band lipopolysaccharides of *Pseudomonas aeruginosa* and its possible lethal effect. Antimicrob Agents Chemother. 1993;37:715–721.
50. Novick RP, Clowes RC, Cohen SN, et al. Uniform nomenclature for bacterial plasmids: A proposal. Bacteriol Rev. 1976;40:168–189.
51. Vanhoof R, Hannecart-Polcorni E, Content J. Nomenclature of genes encoding aminoglycoside-modifying enzymes. Antimicrob Agents Chemother. 1998;42:483.
52. Dickie P, Bryan LE, Pickard MA. Effect of enzymatic adenylation on dihydrostreptomycin accumulation in *Escherichia coli* carrying an R-factor: Model explaining aminoglycoside resistance by inactivating mechanisms. Antimicrob Agents Chemother. 1978;14:569–580.
53. Brisson-Noel A, Athur M, Courvalin P. Evidence for natural gene transfer from gram-positive cocci to *Escherichia coli.* J Bacteriol. 1988;170:1739–1745.
54. Cundliffe E. How antibiotic producing organisms avoid suicide. Annu Rev Microbiol. 1989;43:207–233.
55. Prammananan T, Sander P, Brown BA, et al. A single 16S ribosomal RNA substitution is responsible for resistance to amikacin and other 2-deoxystreptamine aminoglycosides in *Mycobacterium abscessus* and *Mycobacterium chelonae.* J Infect Dis. 1998;177:1573–1581.
56. Bryan LE. Aminoglycoside resistance. In: Bryan LE, ed. Antimicrobial Drug Resistance. Orlando, Fla: Academic Press; 1984:241–277.
57. Blaser J. Efficacy of once- and thrice-daily dosing of aminoglycosides in in vitro models of infection. J Antimicrob Chemother. 1991;27(Suppl C):21–28.
58. Rusthoven JJ, Davies TA, Lerner SA. Clinical isolation and characterization of aminoglycoside-resistance small colony variants of *Enterobacter aerogenes.* Am J Med. 1979;67:702–706.
59. Daikos GL, Jackson GG, Lolans VT, et al. Adaptive resistance to aminoglycoside antibiotics from first-exposure down-regulation. J Infect Dis. 1990;162:414–420.
60. Xiong Y-Q, Caillon J, Kergueris MF, et al. Adaptive resistance of *Pseudomonas aeruginosa* induced by aminoglycosides and killing kinetics in a rabbit endocarditis model. Antimicrob Agents Chemother. 1997;41:823–826.
61. Barclay ML, Begg EJ, Chambers ST, et al. Adaptive resistance to tobramycin in *Pseudomonas aeruginosa* lung infection in cystic fibrosis. J Antimicrob Chemother. 1996;37:1155–1164.
62. Perlin MH, Lerner SA. High-level amikacin resistance in *Escherichia coli* due to phosphorylation and impaired aminoglycoside uptake. Antimicrob Agents Chemother. 1986;29:216–224.
63. Moellering RC. The enterococcus: A classic example of the impact of antimicrobial resistance on therapeutic options. J Antimicrob Chemother. 1991;28:1–12.
64. Bryan LE, Kowand SK, Van Den Elzen HM. Mechanism of aminoglycoside antibiotic resistance in anaerobic bacteria. *Clostridium perfringens* and *Bacteroides fragilis.* Antimicrob Agents Chemother. 1979;15:7–13.
65. Simjee S, Gill MJ. Gene transfer, gentamicin resistance, and enterococci. J Hosp Infect. 1997;36:249–259.
66. Thompson PR, Hughes DW, Wright GD. Regiospecificity of aminoglycoside phosphotransferase from enterococci and staphylococci. Biochemistry. 1996;35:8686–8695.
67. Leclercq R. Enterococci acquire new kinds of resistance. Clin Infect Dis. 1997;24(Suppl 1):S80–S84.
68. Swenson JM, Ferraro MJ, Salim DF, et al. Multilaboratory evaluation of screening methods for detection of high-level aminoglycoside resistance in enterococci. National Committee for Clinical Laboratory Standards Study Group on Enterocci. J Clin Microbiol. 1995;33:3008–3018.
69. Tripodi MF, Rambaldi A, Utili R, et al. Resistance to aminoglycosides and other antibiotics among clinical isolates of enterococcus species. New Microbiol. 1995;18:319–323.
70. Vandamme P, Vercauteren E, Lammens C, et al. Survey of enterococcal susceptibility patterns in Belgium. J Clin Microbiol. 1996;34:2572–2576.
71. Bhattacharya M, Warren JR. Treatment of infections due to enterococci with high-level gentamicin resistance and streptomycin susceptibility. Clin Infect Dis. 1993;16:330–331.
72. Pfaller MA, Jones RN, Doern GV, et al. Bacerial pathogens isolated from patients with bloodstream infection: Frequencies of occurrence and antimicrobial susceptibility patterns from the SENTRY antimicrobial surveillance program (U.S. & Canada, 1997). Antimicrob Agents Chemother. 1998;42:1762–1770.
73. Iaconis JP, Pitkin DH, Sheikh W, et al. Comparison of antibacterial activities of meropenem and six other antimicrobials against *Pseudomonas aeruginosa* isolates from North American studies and clinical trials. Clin Infect Dis. 1997;24(Suppl 2):S191–S196.
74. Busch-Sorensen C, Sonmezoglu M, Frimodt-Moller N, et al. Aminoglycoside resistance mechanism in Enterobacteriaceae and *Pseudomonas* spp from two Danish hospitals: Correlation with type of aminoglycoside used. APMIS. 1996;104:763–768.
75. Gerding DN, Larson TA, Hughes RA, et al. Aminoglycoside resistance and aminoglycoside usage: Ten years experience in one hospital. Antimicrob Agents Chemother. 1991;35:1284–1290.
76. King JW, White MC, Todd JR, et al. Alterations in the microbial flora and in the incidence of bacteremia at a university hospital after adoption of amikacin as the sole formulary aminoglycoside. Clin Infect Dis. 1992;14:908–915.
77. Hesseling PB, Mouton WL, Henning PA, et al. A prospective study of long-term use of amikacin in a pediatrics department. S Afr Med J. 1990;768:192–195.
78. Friedland IR, Funk E, Khoosal M, et al. Increased resistance to amikacin in a neonatal unit following intensive amikacin usage. Antimicrob Agents Chemother. 1992;36:1596–1600.
79. Aubry-Damon H, Legrand P, Brun-Buisson C et al. Re-emergence of gentamicin-susceptible strains of methicillin-resistance *Staphylococcus aureus*: Roles of an infection control program and changes in aminoglycoside use. Clin Infect Dis. 1997;25:647–653.
80. Shimizu K, Jumada T, Hseih W-C, et al. Comparison of aminoglycoside resistance patterns in Japna, Formosa, Korea, Chile, and the U.S. Antimicrob Agents Chemother. 1985;28:282–288.
81. Chow JW, Fine MJ, Shlaes DM, et al. *Enterobacter* bacteremia: Clinical features and emergence of antibiotic resistance during therapy. Ann Intern Med. 1991;115:585–590.
82. Gilbert DN, Moellering RC, Sande MA. Sanford Guide to Antimicrobial Therapy. 28th ed. Hyde Park, Vt: Antimicrobial Therapy; 1998.
83. Hand WL, King-Thompson NL. Contrasts between phagocyte antibiotic uptake and subsequent intracellular bactericidal activity. Antimicrob Agents Chemother. 1986;29:135–140.
84. Utili R, Adinolfi LE, Dillilo M, et al. Activity of aminoglycosides against phagocytosed bacteria. J Antimicrob Chemother. 1991;28:897–904.

85. Goodgame RW. Understanding intestinal spore-forming protozoa: Cryptosporidia, *Isospora,* and *Cyclospora.* Ann Intern Med. 1996;124:429–441.
86. Craig WA, Suh B. Protein binding and the antimicrobial effects: Methods for the determination of protein binding. In: Lorian V, ed. Antibiotics in Medicine. 3rd ed. Baltimore: Williams & Wilkins; 1991:367–402.
87. Gilbert DN, Kutscher E, Ireland P, et al. Effect of the concentrations of magnesium and calcium on the in vitro susceptibility of *Pseudomonas aeruginosa* to gentamicin. J Infect Dis. 1971;124:537–544.
88. Reller LB, Schoenknecht FD, Kenny MA, et al. Antibiotic susceptibility testing of *Pseudomonas aeruginosa*: Selection of a control strain and criteria for magnesium and calcium content in media. J Infect Dis. 1974;130:454–463.
89. Barry AL, Miller GH, Thornsberry C, et al. Influence of cation supplements on activity of netilmicin against *Pseudomonas aeruginosa* in vitro and in vivo. Antimicrob Agents Chemother. 1987;31:1514–1518.
90. Barry AL. Procedures and theoretical considerations for testing antimicrobial agents in agar media. In: Lorian V, ed. Antibiotics in Laboratory Medicine. 3rd ed. Baltimore: Williams & Wilkins; 1991:3–8.
91. Ward PB, Palladino S, Looker JC, et al. P-nitrophenylglycerol in susceptibility testing media alters the MICs of antimicrobials for *Pseudomonas aeruginosa.* J Antimicrob Chemother. 1993;31:489–496.
92. Peddie BA, Chambers ST. Effects of betaines and urine on the antibacterial activity of aminoglycosides. J Antimicrob Chemother. 1993;31:481–488.
93. Eliopoulos GM, Moellering RC. Antimicrobial combinations. In: Lorian V, ed. Antibiotics in Laboratory Medicine. 4th ed. Baltimore: Williams & Wilkins; 1996:330–383.
94. Vogelman B, Craig WA. Kinetics of antimicrobial activity. J Pediatr. 1986;108: 835–840.
95. Kapusnik JE, Hackbarth CJ, Chambers HF, et al. Single, large daily dosing vs intermittent dosing of tobramycin for treating experimental *Pseudomonas aeruginosa* pneumonia. J Infect Dis. 1988;158:7–12.
96. Gerber AU, Fellder-Segessenmann C. In vivo assessment of in vitro killing patterns of *Pseudomonas aeruginosa.* J Antimicrob Chemother. 1985;15(Suppl A):201–206.
97. Blaser JB, Stone B, Zinner SH. Efficacy of intermittent versus continuous administration of netilmicin in a two-compartment in vitro model. Antimicrob Agents Chemother. 1985;27:343–349.
98. Dudley MN, Zinner SH. Single daily dosing of amikacin in an in vitro model. J Antimicrob Chemother. 1991;27(Suppl C):15–19.
99. Drusano GL. Role of pharmacokinetics in the outcome of infections. Antimicrob Agents Chemother. 1988;32:289–297.
100. Craig WA, Ebert SC. Continuous infusion of beta-lactams. Antimicrob Agents Chemother. 1992;36:2577–2583.
101. Craig WA, Gudmundsson S. Postantibiotic effect. In: Lorain V, ed. Antibiotics in the Laboratory. 4th ed. Baltimore: Williams & Wilkins; 1996:296–329.
102. Fantin B, Ebert S, Leggett J, et al. Factors influencing the duration of in vivo postantibiotic effect for aminoglycosides against gram-negative bacilli. J Antimicrob Chemother. 1990;27:829–386.
103. Craig WA, Ebert SC. Killing and regrowth of bacteria in vitro: A review. Scand J Infect Dis Suppl. 1991;74:63–70.
104. Gudmundsson S, Erlendsdottir H. The impact of drug combinations on the postantibiotic effect (PAE). In: Programs and Abstracts of the 28th Interscience Conference on Antimicrobial Agents and Chemotherapy. Abstract 773. Washington, DC: American Society for Microbiology; 1988:246.
105. Hessen MT, Pitsakis PG, Levison ME. Absence of a postantibiotic effect in experimental *Pseudomonas endocarditis* treated with imipenem, with or without gentamicin. J Infect Dis. 1988;158:542–548.
106. Barmada S, Kohlhepp S, Leggett J, et al. Correlation of tobramycin-induced inhibition of protein synthesis with postantibiotic effect in *Escherichia coli.* Antimicrob Agents Chemother. 1993;27:2678–2683.
107. Holm SE. Interaction between β-lactam and other antibiotics. Rev Infect Dis. 1986;8(Suppl 3):S305–S314.
108. Hunter TH. Use of streptomycin in the treatment of bacterial endocarditis. Am J Med. 1947;2:436–442.
109. Zak O, O'Reilly T. Animal models in the evaluation of antimicrobial agents. Antimicrob Agents Chemother. 1991;35:1527–1531.
110. Andriole VT. Aminoglycoside antibiotics: Antibacterial efficacy in animal models of infection. J Infect Dis. 1983;5(Suppl 2):S233–S249.
111. Vastola AP, Brandel J, Craig WA. Selection of aminoglycoside-resistant variants of *Pseudomonas aeruginosa* in an in vivo model. J Infect Dis. 1982;146:691–697.
112. Gerber AU, Feller-Segessenmann C. In vivo assessment of in vitro killing patterns of *Pseudomonas aeruginosa.* J Antimicrob Chemother. 1985;15:201–206.
113. Vogelman B, Gudmundsson S, Turnidge J, et al. In vivo postantibiotic effect in a thigh infection in neutropenic mice. J Infect Dis. 1988;157:287–298.
114. Craig WA. Post-antibiotic effects in experimental infection models: Relationship to in vitro phenomena and to treatment of infections in man. J Antimicrob Chemother. 1993;31(Suppl D):S149–S158.
115. Sohet I, Yellin A, Meyerovitch J, et al. Pharmacokinetics and therapeutic efficacy of gentamicin in an experimental pleural empyema rabbit model. Antimicrob Agents Chemother. 1987;31:982–985.
116. Gerber AU, Grestes U, Segesseman C, et al. The impact of the pre-treatment interval on antimicrobial efficacy in a biological model. J Antimicrob Chemother. 1993;31(Suppl D):S29–S39.
117. Fantin B, Carbon C. In vivo antibiotic synergism. Contribution of animal models. Antimicrob Agents Chemother. 1992;36:907–912.
118. Chavanet P, Colin F, Muggeo E, et al. The in vivo activity of co-amoxiclav with netilmicin against experimental methicillin and gentamicin resistant *Staphylococcus epidermidis* infection in rabbits. J Antimicrob Chemother. 1993;31:129–138.
119. Trautman M, Bruckner O, Marre R, et al. Comparative efficacy of ciprofloxacin, ceftazidime and gentamicin, given alone or in combination, in a model of experimental septicemia due to *Klebsiella pneumoniae* in neutropenic mice. Infection. 1988;16:49–53.
120. Chadwick EK, Shulman ST, Yogev R. Correlation of antibiotic synergy in vitro and in vivo: Use of an animal model of neutropenic gram-negative sepsis. J Infect Dis. 1986;154:670–675.
121. Craig WA. Pharmacokinetic/pharmacodynamic parameters: Rationale for antibacterial dosing of mice and men. Clin Infect Dis. 1998;26:1–10.
122. Marangos MN, Nicolau DP, Quintiliani R, et al. Influence of gentamicin dosing interval on the efficacy of penicillin-containing regimens in experimental *Enterococcus faecalis* endocarditis. J Antimicrob Chemother. 1997;39:519–522.
123. Fantin B, Pangon B, Potel G, et al. Ceftriaxone-netilmicin combination in single-daily-dose treatment of experimental *Escherichia coli* endocarditis. Antimicrob Agents Chemother. 1989;33:767–770.
124. Gilbert DN. Once daily aminoglycoside therapy. Antimicrob Agents Chemother. 1991;35:339–405.
125. Gudmundsson S, Einarsson S, Erlendstotter H, et al. The postantibiotic effect of antimicrobial combinations in a neutropenic murine thigh infection model. J Antimicrob Chemother. 1993;31(Suppl D):S177–S191.
126. Michea Hamzehpour M, Auckenthaler R, Regamey P, et al. Resistance occurring after fluoroquinolone therapy of experimental *Pseudomonas aeruginosa* peritonitis. Antimicrob Agents Chemother. 1987;31:1803–1808.
127. Michea-Hamzehpour M, Pechere JC, Marchou B, et al. Combination therapy: A way to limit emergence of resistance? Am J Med. 1986;80(Suppl 6B):S138–S142.
128. Pechere JC, Marchou B, Michea-Hamzehpour M, et al. Emergence of resistance after therapy with antibiotics used alone or combined in a murine model. J Antimicrob Chemother. 1986;17(Suppl A):S11–S18.
129. Gerber AU, VaStola AP, Brandel J, et al. Selection of aminoglycoside-resistant variants of *Pseudomonas aeruginosa* in an in vivo model. J Infect Dis. 1982;146:691–697.
130. Weinstein WM, Onderdonk AB, Bartlett JG, et al. Antimicrobial therapy of experimental intra-abdominal sepsis. J Infect Dis. 1975;132:282–286.
131. Weinstein WM, Onderdonk AB, Bartlett JG, et al. Experimental intra-abdominal abscesses in rats: Development of an experimental model. Infect Immun. 1974;10:1250–1255.
132. Onderdonk AB, Kasper DL, Cisneros RL, et al. The capsular polysaccharide of *Bacteroides fragilis* as a virulence factor: Comparison of the pathogenic potential of encapsulated and unencapsulated strains. J Infect Dis. 1977;136:82–89.
133. Nichols RL, Smith JW. Wound and intra-abdominal infections: Microbiological considerations and approaches to treatment. Clin Infect Dis. 1993;16(Suppl 4):S266–S277.
134. Onderdonk AB, Bartlett JG, Louie T, et al. Microbial synergy in experimental intra-abdominal abscess. Infect Immun. 1976;13:22–26.
135. Barza M, Lauermann M. Why monitor serum levels of gentamicin? Clin Pharmacokinet. 1978;3:202–215.
136. Kunin CM, Chalmers TC, Leevy CM, et al. Absorption of orally administered neomycin and kanamycin. N Engl J Med. 1960;262:380–385.
137. Breen KJ, Bryant RE, Levinson JD, et al. Neomycin absorption in man. Ann Intern Med. 1972;76:211–218.
138. Bamford MFM, Jones LF. Deafness and biochemical imbalance after burns treatment with topical antibiotics in young children. Arch Dis Child. 1978;53:326–329.
139. Pittinger CB, Adamson R. Antibiotic blockade of neuromuscular function. Annu Rev Pharmacol. 1972;12:169–184.
140. Chamberlain G, Needham P. The absorption of antibiotics from the bladder. J Urol. 1976;116:172–173.
141. Lifschitz MI, Denning CR. Safety of kanamycin aerosol. Clin Pharmacol Ther. 1971;12:91–95.
142. Odio W, VanLeier E, Klastersky J. Concentrations of gentamicin in bronchial secretions after intramuscular and endotracheal administration. J Clin Pharmacol. 1975;15:518–524.
143. Van Etta LL, Kravitz GR, Russ TE, et al. Effect of method of administration on extravascular penetration of four antibiotics. Antimicrob Agents Chemother. 1982;21:873–880.
144. Schwartz SN, Pazin GJ, Lyon JA, et al. A controlled investigation of the pharmacokinetics of gentamicin and tobramycin in obese subjects. J Infect Dis. 1978;138:499–505.
145. Kunar MJ, Mak LL, Lietman PS. Localization of ^{3}H-gentamicin in the proximal renal tubule of the mouse. Antimicrob Agents Chemother. 1979;15:131–133.
146. Ramsey BW, Dorkin HL, Eisenberg JD, et al. Efficacy of aerosolized tobramycin in patients with cystic fibrosis. N Engl J Med. 1993;328:1740–1746.
147. Rahal JJ Jr, Hyams PJ, Simberkoff MS, et al. Combined intrathecal and intramuscular gentamicin for gram-negative meningitis. N Engl J Med. 1974;290:1394–1398.
148. Kaiser AB, McGee ZA. Aminoglycoside therapy of gram-negative bacillary meningitis. N Engl J Med. 1975;293:1215–1220.
149. Wirt TC, McGee ZA, Oldfield EH, et al. Intraventricular administration of amikacin for complicated gram-negative meningitis and ventriculitis. J Neurosurg. 1979;50:95–99.
150. Cracken GH Jr, Mize S, Threlkeld N. Intraventricular gentamicin therapy in gram-negative bacillary meningitis of infancy. Lancet. 1980;1:787–791.
151. Wood MJ, Farrell W. Comparison of urinary excretion of tobramycin and gentamicin in adults. J Infect Dis. 1976;134(Suppl):S133–S136.

152. Kahlmeter G, Kamme G. Prolonged excretion of gentamicin in a patient with unimpaired renal function. Lancet. 1975;1:286.
153. Kahlmeter G. Netilmicin: Clinical pharmacokinetics and aspects of dosage schedules. An overview. Scand J Infect Dis. 1980;23:74–81.
154. Laskin OL, Longstreth JA, Smith CR, et al. Netilmicin and gentamicin multidose kinetics in normal subjects. Clin Pharmacol Ther. 1983;34:644–650.
155. Dee TH, Kozin F. Gentamicin and tobramycin penetration into synovial fluid. Antimicrob Agents Chemother. 1977;12:548–549.
156. Pitt HA, Roberts RB, Johnson WD Jr. Gentamicin levels in the human biliary tract. J Infect Dis. 1973;127:299–302.
157. Mendelson J, Portnoy J, Sigman H. Pharmacology of gentamicin in the biliary tract of humans. Antimicrob Agents Chemother. 1973;4:538–541.
158. Baum J. Infections of the eye. Clin Infect Dis. 1995;21:479–488.
159. Barza M, Kane A, Baum J. Comparison of the effects of continuous and intermittent systemic administration on the penetration of gentamicin into infected rabbit eyes. J Infect Dis. 1983;147:144–148.
160. Gorden TB, Cunningham RD. Tobramycin levels in aqueous humor after subconjunctival injection in humans. Am J Ophthalmol. 1982;93:107–110.
161. Rubenstein E, Goldfarb J, Keren G, et al. The penetration of gentamicin into the vitreous humor in man. Invest Ophthalmol Vis Sci. 1983;24:637–639.
162. Wilson TW, Mahon WA, Inaba T, et al. Elimination of tritiated gentamicin in normal human subjects and in patients with severely impaired renal function. Clin Pharmacol Ther. 1973;14:815–822.
163. Collier VU, Lietman PS, Mitch WE. Evidence for luminal uptake of gentamicin in perfused rat kidney. J Pharmacol Exp Ther. 1979;210:247–251.
164. Silberblatt FJ, Kuehn C. Autoradiography of gentamicin uptake by the rat proximal tubular cell. Kidney Int. 1979;15:335–345.
165. Beauchamp D, Gourde P, Bergeron MG. Subcellular distribution of gentamicin in proximal tubular cells, determined by immunogold labeling. Antimicrob Agents Chemother. 1991;35:2173–2179.
166. Fabre J, Rudhardt M, Blanchard P, et al. Persistence of sisomicin and gentamicin in renal cortex and medulla compared with other organs and serum of rats. Kidney Int. 1976;10:444–449.
167. Schentag JJ, Jusko WJ: Renal clearance and tissue accumulation of gentamicin. Clin Pharmacol Ther. 1977;22:364–370.
168. Laskin OL, Longstreth JA, Smith CR, et al. Netilmicin and gentamicin multidose kinetics in normal subjects. Clin Pharmacol Ther. 1983;34:644–650.
169. Gyselynck A-M, Forrey A, Cutler R. Pharmacokinetics of gentamicin: Distribution and plasma and renal clearance. J Infect Dis. 1971;124(Suppl):S70–S76.
170. Plantier J, Forrey AW, O'Neill MA, et al. Pharmacokinetics of amikacin in patients with normal or impaired renal function: Radioenzymatic acetylation assay. J Infect Dis. 1976;134(Suppl):S323–S330.
171. Barza M, Brown RB, Shen D, et al. Predictability of blood levels of gentamicin in man. J Infect Dis. 1975;132:165–174.
172. Clarke JT, Libke RD, Regamey C, et al. Comparative pharmacokinetics of amikacin and kanamycin. Clin Pharmacol Ther. 1974;15:610–616.
173. McCracken GH, Freij BJ. Clinical pharmacology of antimicrobial agents. In: Remington JS, Klein JO, eds. Infectious Diseases of the Fetus and Newborn Infant. 3rd ed. Philadelphia: WB Saunders; 1990:1020–1076.
174. Welling PG, Baumueller A, Lau CC, et al. Netilmicin pharmacokinetics after single intravenous doses to elderly male patients. Antimicrob Agents Chemother. 1977;12:328–334.
175. Swan SK. Aminoglycoside nephrotoxicity. Semin Nephrol. 1997;17:27–33.
176. Brummett RE, Fox KE. Aminoglycoside-induced hearing loss in humans. Antimicrob Agents Chemother. 1989;33:797–800.
177. Kahlmeter G, Dahlager JI: Aminoglycoside toxicity—a review of clinical studies published between 1975 and 1982. J Antimicrob Chemother. 1984;13(Suppl A): S9–S22.
178. Lietman PS, Smith CR. Aminoglycoside nephrotoxicity in humans. Rev Infect Dis. 1983;5(Suppl 2):S284–S292.
179. Smith CR, Baughman KL, Edwards CQ, et al. Controlled comparison of amikacin and gentamicin. N Engl J Med. 1977;296:349–353.
180. Smith CR, Lipsky JJ, Laskin OL, et al. Double-blind comparison of the nephrotoxicity and auditory toxicity of gentamicin and tobramycin. N Engl J Med. 1980;302:1106–1109.
181. Smith CR, Ambinder R, Lipsky JJ, et al. Cefotaxime compared with nafcillin plus tobramycin for serious bacterial infections. Ann Intern Med. 1984;101:469–477.
182. Bertino JS, Booker LA, Franck PA, et al. Incidence of and significant risk factors for aminoglycoside-associated nephrotoxicity in patients dosed by using individualized pharmacokinetic monitoring. J Infect Dis. 1993;167:173–179.
183. Lerner AM, Cone LA, Jansen W, et al. Randomized, controlled trial of the comparative efficacy, auditory toxicity and nephrotoxicity of tobramycin and netilmicin. Lancet. 1983;1:1123–1126.
184. Lerner SA, Schmitt BA, Seligsohn R, et al. Comparative study of ototoxicity and nephrotoxicity in patients randomly assigned treatment with amikacin and gentamicin. Am J Med. 1986;80(Suppl 5B):S98–S104.
185. Fausti SA, Henry JA, Schaffer HI, et al. High-frequency audiometric monitoring for early detection of aminoglycoside ototoxicity. J Infect Dis. 1992;165:1026–1032.
186. Govaerts PJ, Claes PH, DeHeyring PHV, et al. Aminoglycoside-induced ototoxicity. Toxicol Lett. 1990;52:227–251.
187. Bendush CL. Ototoxicity: Clinical considerations and comparative information. In: Whelton A, Neu HC, eds. The Aminoglycosides. New York: Marcel Dekker; 1982:452–486.
188. DeOliveira JAA. Audiovestibular Toxicity of Drugs. v. 1, 2. Boca Raton, Fla: CRC Press; 1989.
189. Moore RD, Smith CR, Lietman PS. Risk factors for the development of auditory toxicity in patients receiving aminoglycosides. J Infect Dis. 1984;149:23–30.
190. Gatell JM, Ferran F, Araujo V, et al. Univariate and multivariate analyses of risk factors predisposing to auditory toxicity in patients receiving aminoglycosides. Antimicrob Agents Chemother. 1987;31:1383–1387.
191. Snavely SR, Hodges GR. The neurotoxicity of antibacterial agents. Ann Intern Med. 1984;101:92–104.
192. Reinhard MK, Hottendorf GH, Powell FD. Differences in the sensitivity of Fischer and Sprague-Dawley rats to aminoglycoside nephrotoxicity. Toxicol Pathol. 1991;19:66–71.
193. Kirschbaum BB. Interactions between renal brush border membranes and "polyamines." J Pharmacol Exp Ther. 1984;229:409–416.
194. Kaloyanides GJ, Ramsammy LS. Possible role of altered polyamine metabolism in gentamicin toxicity in OK cells. Contrib Nephrol. 1993;101:199–205.
195. Molitaris BA. Cell biology of aminoglycoside nephrotoxicity: Newer aspects. Curr Opin Nephrol Hypertens. 1997;63:384–388.
196. Scherberich JE, Mondorf WA. Nephrotoxic potential of antiinfective drugs as assessed by tissue-specific proteinuria of renal antigens. Int J Clin Pharmacol Ther. 1998;36:153–158.
197. Nix DE, Thomas JK, Symonds WT, et al. Assessment of the enzymuria resulting from gentamicin alone and combination of gentamicin with various β-lactam antibiotics. Ann Pharmacother. 1997;31:696–703.
198. Foster JE, Harpur ES, Garland HO. An investigation of the acute effect of gentamicin on the renal handling of electrolytes in the rat. J Pharmacol Exp Ther. 1992;281:38–43.
199. Christensen EI, Birn J, Verroust P, et al. Megalin-mediated endocytosis in renal proximal tubule. Ren Fail. 1998;20:191–199.
200. Moestrup SK, Shiying C, Vorum H, et al. Evidence that epithelial glycoprotein 330/
megalin mediates uptake of polybasic drugs. J Clin Invest. 1995;96:1404–1413.
201. Sandoval R, Molitoris BA. Intracellular trafficking of gentamicin: Endoplasmic reticulum (ER) and Golgi associations (Abst). J Am Soc Nephrol. 1995;6:1003.
202. Kohlhepp S, Bennett J, Leggett J, et al. Computerized fluorescent videomicroscopy demonstration of the renal cell handling of tobramycin in vitro. In: Programs and Abstracts of the 29th Interscience Conference on Antimicrobial Agents and Chemotherapy. Abstract 293. Washington, DC: American Society for Microbiology; 1989:385.
203. Bennett WM, Mela-Riker L, Houghton DC, et al. Microsomal protein synthesis inhibition: An early manifestation of gentamicin nephrotoxicity. Am J Physiol. 1988;2255:F265–F269.
204. Gilbert DN, Bennett WM. Progress in the elucidation of aminoglycoside nephrotoxicity. Contemp Issues Infect Dis. 1984;1:121–152.
205. Lipsky JJ, Lietman PS. Neomycin inhibition of adenosine triphosphate: Evidence for a neomycin-phospholipid interaction. Antimicrob Agents Chemother. 1980;18:532–535.
206. Sastrasink M, Weinberg JM, Humes HD. The effect of gentamicin on calcium uptake by renal mitochondria. Life Sci. 1982;30:2309–2315.
207. Loveless MO, Kohlhepp SJ, Gilbert DN. The influence of aminoglycoside antibiotics on the in vitro function of rat liver ribosomes. J Lab Clin Med. 1984;103: 94–303.
208. Appel GB. Aminoglycoside nephrotoxicity. Am J Med. 1990;88(Suppl C): S16–S20.
209. Gilbert DN, Houghton DC, Bennett WM, et al. Reversibility of gentamicin nephrotoxicity in rats: Recovery during continuous drug administration. Proc Soc Exp Biol Med. 1979;160:99–103.
210. Sundin DP, Meyer C, Dahl R, et al. Cellular mechanism of aminoglycoside tolerance in long-term gentamicin treatment. Am J Physiol. 1997;272:C1309–C1318.
211. Luft FC, Bennett WM, Gilbert DN. Experimental aminoglycoside nephrotoxicity: Accomplishments and future potential. Rev Infect Dis. 1983;5(Suppl 2):S268–S293.
212. Gilbert DN, Plamp C, Starr P, et al. Comparative nephrotoxicity of gentamicin and tobramycin in rats. Antimicrob Agents Chemother. 1979;13:34–40.
213. Bennett WM, Plamp CE, Gilbert DN, et al. The influence of dosage regimen on experimental gentamicin nephrotoxicity: Dissociation of peak serum levels from renal failure. J Infect Dis. 1979;140:576–580.
214. Powell SH, Thompson WL, Luthe MA, et al. Once daily vs continuous aminoglycoside dosing: Efficacy and toxicity in animal and clinical studies of gentamicin, netilmicin, and tobramycin. J Infect Dis. 1983;147:918–923.
215. Beauchamp D, Gourde P, Thereault G, et al. Age-dependent gentamicin experimental nephrotoxicity. J Pharmacol Exp Ther. 1992;260:444–449.
216. Bennett WM, Parker RA, Elliott WB, et al. Sex: A determinant of susceptibility to gentamicin nephrotoxicity in the rat. J Infect Dis. 1982;145:370–373.
217. Elliott WB, Parker RA, Houghton DC, et al. Effect of sodium bicarbonate and ammonium chloride ingestion in experimental gentamicin nephrotoxicity in rats. Res Commun Pathol Pharmacol. 1980;28:483–496.
218. Bennett WM, Hartnett MN, Gilbert D, et al. Effect of sodium intake on gentamicin nephrotoxicity in the rat. Proc Soc Exp Biol Med. 1976;151:736–738.
219. Peterson LN, Borzecki JS. Inhibition of tobramycin reabsorption in nephron segments by metabolic alkalosis. Kidney Int. 1990;37:1492–1499.
220. Chiu PJS, Miller GH, Long JF, et al. Renal uptake and nephrotoxicity of gentamicin during urinary alkalinization in rats. Clin Exp Pharmacol Physiol. 1979;6:317–326.
221. Thompson JR, Simonsen R, Spindler MA, et al. Protective effect of KCl loading in gentamicin nephrotoxicity. Am J Kidney Dis. 1990;15:583–591.

222. Rodriquez HJ, Hogan WC, Hellman RN, et al. Mechanism of activation of renal Na^+-K^+-ATPase in the rat: Effects of potassium loading. Am J Physiol. 1980;238:F315–F323.
223. Vakil N, Abu-Alfa A, Mujais SK. Gentamicin nephrotoxicity in extrahepatic cholestasis: Modulation by dietary calcium. Hepatology. 1989;9:519–524.
224. Camps J, Sola X, Rimola A, et al. Comparative study of aminoglycoside nephrotoxicity in normal rats and rats with experimental cirrhosis. Hepatology. 1988;8: 837–844.
225. Lietman PS. Liver disease, aminoglycoside antibiotics, and renal dysfunction. Hepatology. 1988;4:966–968.
226. Bennett WM, Elliott WC, Houghton DC, et al. Reduction of experimental gentamicin nephrotoxicity in rats by dietary calcium loading. Antimicrob Agents Chemother. 1982;22:508–512.
227. Quarum ML, Houghton DC, Gilbert DN, et al. Increasing dietary calcium moderates experimental gentamicin nephrotoxicity. J Lab Clin Med. 1984;103:104–114.
228. Humes HD, Sastrasinh M, Weinberg JM. Calcium is a competitive inhibitor of gentamicin—renal membrane binding interactions and dietary calcium supplementation protects against gentamicin nephrotoxicity. J Clin Invest. 1984;73:134–147.
229. Ernst S. Model of gentamicin-induced nephrotoxicity and its amelioration by calcium and thyroxine. Med Hypotheses. 1989;30:195–202.
230. Teixeira RB, Kelley J, Alpert H, et al. Complete protection from gentamicin-induced acute renal failure in the diabetes mellitus rat. Kidney Int. 1982;21: 600–612.
231. Elliott WB, Houghton DC, Gilbert DN, et al. Experimental gentamicin nephrotoxicity: Effect of streptozotocin-induced diabetes. J Pharmacol Exp Ther. 1985;233:264–270.
232. Wood CA, Kohlhepp SJ, Kohnen PW, et al. Vancomycin enhancement of experimental tobramycin nephrotoxicity. Antimicrob Agents Chemother. 1985;30:20–24.
233. Kohlhepp SJ, Gilbert DN, Kohnen PW, et al. Teicoplanin enhancement of experimental tobramycin nephrotoxicity (Abstract). In: Proceedings of the 31st Interscience Conference on Antimicrobial Agents Chemotherapy. Washington, DC: American Society for Microbiology; 1991.
234. Golper TA, Noonan HM, Elzinga L, et al. Vancomycin pharmacokinetics, renal handling and non-renal clearance in normal human subjects. Clin Pharmacol Ther. 1988;43:565–570.
235. English J, Gilbert DN, Kohlhepp SJ, et al. Attenuation of experimental tobramycin nephrotoxicity by ticarcillin. Antimicrob Agents Chemother. 1985;276:897–902.
236. Sabra R, Branch RA. Role of sodium in protection by extended spectrum penicillins against tobramycin-induced nephrotoxicity. Antimicrob Agents Chemother. 1990;340:1020–1025.
237. Barr GA, Mazze RI, Cousins MJ, et al. An animal model for combined methoxyflurane and gentamicin nephrotoxicity. Br J Anaesth. 1973;45:306–331.
238. Williams PD, Hottdenford GH. Inhibition of renal membrane binding and nephrotoxicity of gentamicin by polyasparagine and polyaspartic acid in the rat. Res Commun Chem Pathol Pharmacol. 1985;47:317–320.
239. Gilbert DN, Wood CA, Kohlhepp SJ, et al. Polyaspartic acid prevents experimental aminoglycoside nephrotoxicity. J Infect Dis. 1989;159:945–953.
240. Swan SK, Kohlhepp SJ, Kohnen PW, et al. Long-term protection of polyaspartic acid in experimental gentamicin nephrotoxicity. Antimicrob Agents Chemother. 1991;35:2591–2595.
241. Gilbert DN, Kohlhepp SJ, Swan SK, et al. Pharmacologic limits of polyaspartic acid's protective effect on experimental gentamicin nephrotoxicity. Antimicrob Agents Chemother. 1993;37:347–348.
242. Swan SK, Gilbert DN, Kohlhepp SJ, et al. Duration of the protective effect of polyaspartic acid on experimental gentamicin nephrotoxicity. Antimicrob Agents Chemother. 1992;36:2556–2558.
243. Ramsammy LS, Josepovitz C, Lane BP, et al. Polyaspartic acid protects against gentamicin nephrotoxicity in the rat. J Pharmacol Exp Ther. 1989;250:149–153.
244. Beauchamp D, Laurent G, Maldague P, et al. Protection against gentamicin-induced early renal alterations (phospholipidosis and increased DNA synthesis) by coadministration of poly-L-aspartic acid. J Pharmacol Exp Ther. 1990;255:858–866.
245. Kishore BK, Ibrahim S, Lambrict P, et al. Comparative assessment of poly-L-aspartic and poly-L-glutamic acids as protectants against gentamicin-induced renal lysosomal phospholipidosis, phospholipiduria and cell proliferation in rats. J Pharmacol Exp Ther. 1992;262:424–432.
246. Kohlhepp SJ, McGregor D, Gilbert DN. Determinants of the in vitro interaction of polyaspartic acid and aminoglycoside antibiotics. J Pharmacol Exp Ther. 1992;263:1464–1470.
247. Ramsammy L, Josepovitz C, Lane B, et al. Polyaspartic acid inhibits gentamicin-induced perturbations of phospholipid metabolism. Am J Physiol. 1990; 58:C1141–C1149.
248. Whiting PH, Simpson JG. The enhancement of cyclosporin-A induced nephrotoxicity by gentamicin. Biochem Pharmacol. 1983;32:2025–2028.
249. Ryffel B, Muller AM, Mihatsch MJ. Experimental cyclosporine nephrotoxicity: Risk of concomitant chemotherapy. Clin Nephrol. 1988;25(Suppl 1):S121–S125.
250. Luft FC. Cephalosporin and aminoglycoside interactions: Clinical and toxicologic implications. In: Whelton A, Neu HC, eds. The Aminoglycosides. New York: Marcel Dekker; 1982:387–399.
251. Jongejan HTM, Provoost AP, Molenaar JC. Potentiated nephrotoxicity of cisplatin when combined with amikacin comparing young and adult rats. Pediatr Nephrol. 198;31:290–295.
252. Moore RD, Smith CR, Lipsky JJ, et al. Risk factors for nephrotoxicity in patients treated with aminoglycosides. Ann Intern Med. 1984;100:352–357.
253. Sawyers CL, Moore RD, Lerner SA, et al. A model for predicting nephrotoxicity in patients treated with aminoglycosides. J Infect Dis. 1985;153:1062–1068.
254. Cronin RE, Newman JA. Protective effect of thyroxine but not parathyroidectomy on gentamicin nephrotoxicity. Am J Physiol. 1985;248:F332–F339.
255. Adelman RD, Spangler WL, Beasom F, et al. Furosemide enhancement of experimental gentamicin nephrotoxicity: Comparison of functional and morphological changes with activities of urinary enzymes. J Infect Dis. 1979;140:342–352.
256. Petty BG, Baumgardner JY, Leitman PS. Comparison of the renal effects of single vs. thrice daily dosing in healthy volunteers (Abstract). In: Proceedings of the 26th Interscience Conference on Antimicrobial Agents and Chemotherapy. Washington DC: American Society of Microbiology; 1986.
257. Hou SH, Bushinsky DA, Wish JB, et al. Hospital-acquired renal insufficiency: A prospective study. Am J Med. 1983;74:243–248.
258. Trollfors B. Gentamicin-associated changes in renal function reversible during continued treatment. J Antimicrob Chemother. 1983;12:285–287.
259. Gilbert DN. Meta-analyses are no longer required for determining the efficacy of single daily dosing of aminoglycosides. Clin Infect Dis. 1997;24:816–819.
260. Desai TK, Tsang T-K. Aminoglycoside nephrotoxicity in obstructive jaundice. Am J Med. 1988;85:47–50.
261. Farber BF, Moellering RC. Retrospective study of the toxicity of preparations of vancomycin from 1974–1981. Antimicrob Agents Chemother. 1983;23:138–141.
262. Rybak MJ, Albrecht LM, Boike SC, et al. Nephrotoxicity of vancomycin alone and with an aminoglycoside. J Antimicrob Chemother. 1990;25:679–687.
263. Nahata MC. Lack of nephrotoxicity in pediatric patients receiving vancomycin and aminoglycoside therapy. Chemotherapy. 1987;33:302–304.
264. The EORTC International Antimicrobial Therapy Project Group. Three antibiotic regimens in the treatment of infection in febrile granulocytopenic patients with cancer. J Infect Dis. 1978;137:14–29.
265. Klastersky J, Hensgens C, Debusscher I. Empiric therapy for cancer patients: Comparative study of ticarcillin-tobramycin, ticarcillin-cephalothin, and cephalothin-tobramycin. Antimicrob Agents Chemother. 1975;7:640–645.
266. Wade JC, Smith CR, Petty BG, et al. Cephalothin plus an aminoglycoside is more nephrotoxic than methicillin plus an aminoglycoside. Lancet. 1978;3:604–606.
267. Mazze RI, Cousins MJ. Combined nephrotoxicity of gentamicin and methoxyflurane in man. Br J Anaesth. 1973;45:394–398.
268. Green FJ, Lavelle KJ, Aronoff GR, et al. Management of amikacin overdose. Am J Kidney Dis. 1981;1:110–112.
269. Ho PW, Pien FD, Kominami N. Massive amikacin "overdose." Ann Intern Med. 1979;91:227–228.
270. Cooper B, Creger RJ, Soegiarso W, et al. Renal dysfunction during high-dose cisplatin therapy and autologous hematopoietic stem cell transplantation: Effect of aminoglycoside therapy Am J Med. 1993;94:497–504.
271. Leach CT, Kuhls TL, Brill JE, et al. Use of aminoglycosides during cyclosporine A immunosuppression after liver transplantation in children. Pediatr Infect Dis J. 1989;8:354–357.
272. Hinshaw HC, Feldman WH. Streptomycin in treatment of clinical tuberculosis: A preliminary report. Proc Staff Meet Mayo Clin. 1945;20:313–318.
273. Sataloff J, Wagner S, Menduke H. Kanamycin ototoxicity in healthy men. Arch Otolaryngol. 1964;80:413–417.
274. Davey PG, Jabeen F, Harpur ES, et al. The use of pure-tone audiometry in the assessment of gentamicin auditory toxicity. Br J Audiol. 1982;16:151–154.
275. Moore RD, Smith CR, Lietman PS. Risk factors for the development of auditory toxicity in patients receiving aminoglycosides. J Infect Dis. 1984;149:23–30.
276. Hutchin T, Cortopassi G. Proposed molecular and cellular mechanism of aminoglycoside ototoxicity. Antimicrob Agents Chemother. 1994;38:2517–2520.
277. Tran Ba Huy P, Bernard P, Schacht J. Kinetics of gentamicin uptake and release in the rat. Comparison of inner ear tissues and fluids with other organs. J Clin Invest. 1986;77:1492–1500.
278. de Groot JCMJ, Meeuwsen F, Ruizendaal WE, et al. Ultrastructural localization of gentamicin in the cochlear. Hear Res. 1990;50:35–42.
279. Hashino E, Shero M, Salvi RJ. Lysosomal targeting and accumulation of aminoglycoside antibiotics in sensory hair cells. Brain Res. 1997;777:75–85.
280. Song B-B, Schacht J. Variable efficacy of radical scavengers and iron chelators to attenuate gentamicin ototoxicity in guinea pig in vivo. Hear Res. 1996;94:987–993.
281. Basile AS, Huang J-M, Zie C, et al. *N*-methyl-D-aspartate antagonists limit aminoglycoside antibiotic–induced hearing loss. Nat Med. 1996;2:1338–1343.
282. Hashino E, Tanaka Y, Salvi RJ, et al. Hair cell regeneration in the adult budgerigar after kanamycin ototoxicity. Hear Res. 1992;59:46–58.
283. Lombarte A, Yan HY, Popper AN, et al. Damage and regeneration of hair cell ciliary bundles in a fish ear following treatment with gentamicin. Hear Res. 1993;64:166–174.
284. Forge A, Li L, Corwin JT, et al. Ultrastructural evidence for hair cell regeneration in the mammalian inner ear. Science. 1993;259:1616–1621.
285. Fischel-Ghodsian N, Prezant TR, Chaltraw WE, et al. Mitochondrial gene mutation is a significant predisposing factor in aminoglycoside ototoxicity. Am J Otolaryngol. 1997;18:173–178.
286. Pandya A, Xia X, Raduaabazar J, et al. Mutation in the mitochondrial 12S rRNA gene in two families from Mongolia with matrilineal aminoglycoside ototoxicity. J Med Genet. 1997;34:169–172.
287. Hamasaki K, Rando RR. Specific binding of aminoglycoside to a human rRNA construct based on a DNA polymorphism which causes aminoglycoside-induced deafness. Biochemistry. 1997;36:12323–12328.
288. Brummett RE, Fox KE. Studies of aminoglycoside ototoxicity in animal models. In: Whetton A, Neu HC, eds. The Aminoglycosides: Microbiology, Clinical Use and Toxicology. New York: Marcel Dekker; 1982:419–451.
289. Brummett RE, Bendrick T, Himes D. Comparative ototoxicity of bumetani'

and furosemide when used in combination with kanamycin. J Clin Pharmacol. 1981;21:628–636.
290. Brummett RE, Fox KE. Vancomycin- and erythromycin-induced hearing loss in humans. Antimicrob Agents Chemother. 1989;33:791–796.
291. Brummett RE, Fox KE, Kempton JB. Quantitative relationships of the interaction between sound and kanamycin. Arch Otolaryngol Head Neck Surg. 1992;118: 498–500.
292. Tran Ba Huy PT, Deffrennes D. Aminoglycoside ototoxicity: Influence of dosage regimen on drug uptake and correlation between membrane binding and some clinical features. Acta Otolaryngol. 1988;105:511–515.
293. Buring JE, Evans DA, Mayrent SL, et al. Randomized trials of aminoglycoside antibiotics: Quantitative overview. Rev Infect Dis. 1988;10:951–957.
294. Manian FA, Stone WJ, Alford R: Adverse antibiotic effects associated with renal insufficiency. Rev Infect Dis. 1990;12:236–249.
295. Amiko M, Bagger-Sjoback D, Wersall J, et al. Gentamicin binding to the isolated crista ampullaris of the guinea pig. Res Commun Chem Pathol Pharmacol. 1982;37:333–342.
296. Minor LB. Gentamicin-induced bilateral vestibular hypofunction. JAMA. 1998;279:541–544.
297. Tanyeri H, Lopez I, Vicente H. Histologic evidence for hair cell regeneration after ototoxic cell destruction with local application of gentamicin in the chinchilla crista ampullaris. Hear Res. 1995;89:194–202.
298. Talbot PA. Potentiation of aminoglycoside-induced neuromuscular blockade by protons in vitro and in vivo. J Pharmacol Exp Ther. 1987;241:686–694.
299. Del-Pozo E, Baezem JM. Effects of calcium channel blockers on neuromuscular blockade induced by aminoglycoside antibiotics. Eur J Pharmacol. 1986;128:49–54.
300. Gay CT, Marks WA, Riley HD Jr, et al. Infantile botulism. South Med J. 1988;81:457–460.
301. Sanders DB, Kim YI, Howard JR Jr, et al. Intercostal muscle biopsy studies in myasthenia gravis: Clinical correlations and the direct effects of drugs and myasthenic serum. Ann N Y Acad Sci. 1981;377:544–566.
302. Hokkanen E. The aggravating effect of some antibiotics on the neuromuscular blockade in myasthenia gravis. Acta Neurol Scand. 1964;40:346–352.
303. Wright JM, Collier B. The effects of neomycin upon transmitter release and action. J Pharmacol Exp Ther. 1977;200:576–587.
304. Lee C, DeSilva AJ. Acute and subchronic neuromuscular blocking characteristics of streptomycin: A comparison with neomycin. Br J Anaesth. 1979;51:431–434.
305. Caputy AJ, Kim YI, Sanders DB. The neuromuscular blocking effects of therapeutic concentrations of various antibiotics on normal rat skeletal muscle: A quantitative comparison. J Pharmacol Exp Ther. 1981;217:369–378.
306. Antibiotic-induced paralysis of the mouse phrenic nerve–hemidiaphragm preparation, and reversibility by calcium and by neostigmine. Anesthesiology. 1978;48:418–424.
307. Warren S, Burke JF. Infection and burn wounds: Evaluation and management. Curr Clin Top Infect Dis. 1991;11:206–217.
308. Wilson WR, Karchmer AW, Dajani AS, et al. Antibiotic treatment of adults with infective endocarditis due to streptococci, enterococci, staphylococci and HACEK microorganisms. JAMA. 1995;274:1706–1173.
309. Ho JL, Barza M. Role of aminoglycoside antibiotics in the treatment of intra-abdominal infection. Antimicrob Agents Chemother. 1987;31:485–491.
310. Gorbach SL. Treatment of intra-abdominal infections. J Antimicrob Chemother. 1993;31(Suppl A):S67–S78.
311. Hughes WT, Armstrong D, Bodey GP, et al. 1997 Guidelines for the use of antimicrobial agents in neutropenic patients with unexplained fever. Clin Infect Dis. 1997;25:551–573.
312. Pizzo PA. Management of fever in patients with cancer and treatment-induced neutropenia. N Engl J Med. 1993;328:1323–1332.
313. Choice of antibacterials. Med Lett. 1998;40:33–42.
314. Ho G Jr. Bacterial arthritis. Curr Opin Rheumatol. 1992;4:509–515.
315. Lew DP, Waldvogel FA. Osteomyelitis. N Engl J Med. 1997;336:999–1007.
316. Giamarellou H. Malignant otitis externa: The therapeutic evolution of a lethal infection. J Antimicrob Chemother. 1992;30:745–751.
317. Hospital-acquired pneumonia in adults: Diagnosis, assessment of severity, initial antimicrobial therapy and preventative strategies. Am J Respir Crit Care Med. 1995;153:1711–1725.
318. Craig WA, Andes D. Aminoglycosides are useful for severe respiratory tract infections. Semin Respir Infect. 1997;12:271–277.
319. 1998 Guidelines for treatment of sexually transmitted diseases. MMWR Morb Mortal Wkly Rep. 1998;47(Suppl RR-1):1–116.
320. Neu HC. Clinical use of aminoglycosides. In: Whelton A, Neu HC, eds. The Aminoglycosides. New York: Marcel Dekker; 1982:611–628.
321. Korvick JA, Bryan CS, Farber B, et al. Prospective observational study of *Klebsiella* bacteremia in 230 patients: Outcome for antibiotic combinations versus monotherapy. Antimicrob Agents Chemother. 1992;36:2639–2644.
322. Tunkel AR, Fisch MJ, Schlein A, et al. Enterobacter endocarditis. Scand J Infect Dis. 1992;24:233–240.
323. Bodey GP, Elting LS, Rodriquez S. Bacteremia caused by *Enterobacter*: 15 years of experience in a cancer hospital. Rev Infect Dis. 1991;13:550–558.
324. Saito H, Elting L, Bodey GP, et al. *Serratia* bacteremia: Review of 118 cases. Rev Infect Dis. 1989;11:912–920.
325. Korvick JA, Peacock JE, Muder RR, et al. Addition of rifampin to combination antibiotic therapy for *Pseudomonas aeruginosa* bacteremia: Prospective trial using the Zelen protocol. Antimicrob Agents Chemother. 1992;36:620–625.
326. Rolston KV, Bodey GP. *Pseudomonas aeruginosa* infection in cancer patients. Cancer Invest. 1992;10:43–59.
327. Saha V, Stansfield R, Masterton R, et al. The treatment of *Pseudomonas aeruginosa* meningitis—old regime or newer drugs? Scand J Infect Dis. 1993;25:81–83.
328. Montejo JM, Alberok I, Glez-Zarate P, et al. Open randomized trial of six antimicrobial regimens in the treatment of human brucellosis. Clin Infect Dis. 1993;16:671–676.
329. Young EJ. An overview of brucellosis. Clin Infect Dis. 1995;21:283–290.
330. Cleri DJ, Verualeo JR, Lombardi LJ, et al. Plague pneumonia caused by *Yersinia pestis*. Semin Respir Infect. 1997;12:12–23.
331. Chuang YC, Yuan CY, Liu CY, et al. *Vibrio vulnificus* infection in Taiwan: Report of 28 cases and review of clinical manifestations and treatment. Clin Infect Dis. 1992;15:271–276.
332. Jorup-Ronstrom C, Julander I, Petrini B. Efficacy of triple drug regimen of amikacin, ethambutol and rifabutin in AIDS patients with symptomatic *Mycobacterium avium* complex infection. J Infect. 1993;26:67–70.
333. Drugs for parasitic infections. Med Lett Drugs Ther. 1998;40:1–12.
334. Jackson GG, Finland M, eds. International Symposium on Gentamicin. J Infect Dis. 1969;119:341–540.
335. Finland M, Hewitt WL, eds. Second International Symposium on Gentamicin. J Infect Dis. 1971;124(Suppl):S1–S300.
336. Finland M, Neu HC, eds. Tobramycin. J Infect Dis. 1976;134(Suppl):S1–S234.
337. Hewitt WL, Young LS. Symposium perspective. Am J Med. 1977;62:863–867.
338. Netilmicin. Based on a symposium, Vienna, Austria, 28 August 1983. J Antimicrob Chemother. 1984;13(Suppl A):S1–S83.
339. Gruenwaldt G, Marget W, Weuta H. New aspects of aminoglycoside therapy: Sisomicin extended summarizes of papers presented at a symposium May 6–7, 1977, Geneva, Switzerland. Infection. 1979;7(Suppl 3):S241–S304.
340. Solomkin JS, Dellinger EP, Christou NV, et al. Results of a prospective and double-blind trial of new beta-lactams in the treatment of appendicitis. Antimicrob Agents Chemother. 1990;28:639–642.
341. Williams RR, Hotchkin D. Aztreonam plus clindamycin versus tobramycin plus clindamycin in the treatment of intra-abdominal infections. Rev Infect Dis. 1991;13(Suppl 7):S629–S633.
342. Bubrick MP, Heim-Duthoy KL, Yellin AE, et al. Ceftazidime/clindamycin versus tobramycin/clindamycin in the treatment of intra-abdominal infections. Am Surg. 1990;56:613–617.
343. Dajani AS, Taubert KA, Wilson W, et al. Prevention of bacterial endocarditis. Recommendations by the American Heart Association. JAMA. 1997;277:1794–1801.
344. Gorbach SL. Antimicrobial prophylaxis for appendectomy and colorectal surgery. Rev Infect Dis. 1991;13(Suppl 10):S815–S820.
345. Aronoff GR, ed. Drug Prescribing in Renal Failure. 4th ed. Philadelphia: American College of Physicians; 1998.
346. Hickling KG, Begg EJ, Perry RE, et al. Serum aminoglycoside clearance is predicted as poorly by renal aminoglycoside clearance as by creatinine clearance in critically ill patients. Crit Care Med. 1991;19:1041–1047.
347. McCormack JP, Jewesson PJ. A critical reevaluation of the "therapeutic range" of aminoglycoside. Clin Infect Dis. 1992;14:320–329.
348. Voytovich RM, Massaro MJ, Titus DL, et al. An aminoglycoside dosing regimen in a morbidly obese patient (Letter). DICP. 1990;24:100–102.
349. Edwards C, Bent AJ, Venables CW, et al. Sampling time for serum gentamicin levels. J Antimicrob Chemother. 1992;29:575–578.
350. Cockcroft DW, Gault MH. Prediction of creatinine clearance from serum creatinine. Nephron. 1976;16:31–41.
351. Reichley RM, Ritchie DJ, Bailey TC. Analysis of various creatinine clearance formulas in predicting gentamicin elimination in patients with low serum creatinine. Pharmacotherapy. 1995;15:625–630.
352. Moore RD, Lietman PS, Smith CR. Clinical response to aminoglycoside therapy: Importance of the ratio of peak concentration to minimal inhibitory concentrations. J Infect Dis. 1987;155:93–99.
353. Noone P, Rogers BT. Pneumonia caused by coliforms and *Pseudomonas aeruginosa*. J Clin Pathol. 1976;29:652–656.
354. Spector R, Park GD, Johnson GF, et al. Therapeutic drug monitoring. Clin Pharmacol Ther. 1988;43:345–53.
355. McInnes GT. The value of therapeutic drug monitoring to the practising physician—an hypothesis in need of testing. Br J Clin Pharmacol. 1989;278:281–284.
356. Matzke GR, Lucarotti RL, Shapiro HS. Controlled comparison of gentamicin and tobramycin nephrotoxicity. Am J Nephrol. 1983;3:11–17.
357. Sarubbi FA, Hull H. Amikacin serum concentrations: Prediction of levels and dosage guidelines. Ann Intern Med. 1978;89:612–618.
358. Maderazo EG, Sun H, Jay GT. Simplification of antibiotic dose adjustments in renal insufficiency: The DREM system. Lancet. 1992;340:767–770.
359. Golper TA, Wedel SK, Kaplan AA, et al. Drug removal during continuous arteriovenous hemofiltration: Theory and clinical observations. Int J Artif Organs. 1985;2:307–312.
360. Bickley SK. Drug dosing during continuous hemofiltration. Clin Pharmacol. 1988;7:198–206.
361. Reetze-Bonorden P, Bohler J, Keller E. Drug dosage in patients during continuous renal replacement therapy. Clin Pharmacokinet. 1993;24:362–379.
362. Verpooten GA, Giuliano RA, Verbist L, et al. Once-daily dosing decreases renal accumulation of gentamicin and netilmicin. Clin Pharmacol Ther. 1989;45:22–27.
363. De Broe ME, Verbist L, Verpooten GA. Influence of dosage schedule on renal cortical accumulation of amikacin and tobramycin in man. J Antimicrob Chemother. 1991;27(Suppl C):S41-S47.
364. Karlowsky J, Zhanel GG, Davidson RJ et al. Postantibiotic effect in *Pseudomonas*

aeruginosa following single and multiple aminoglycoside exposures in vitro. J Antimicrob Chemother. 1994;33:937–947.
365. Xiong Y, Caillon J, Kergueris MF et al. Adaptive resistance of *Pseudomonas aeruginosa* induced by aminoglycosides and killing kinetics in a rabbit endocarditis model. Antimicrob Agents Chemother. 1997;41:823–826.
366. Barclay ML, Begg EJ, Chambers ST, et al. Adaptive resistance to tobramycin in *Pseudomonas aeruginosa* lung infection in cystic fibrosis. J Antimicrob Chemother. 1996;37:1155–1164.
367. Wood CA, Norton DR, Kohlhepp SJ, et al. The influence of tobramycin dosage regimen on nephrotoxicity, ototoxicity and antibacterial efficacy in a rat model of subcutaneous abscess. J Infect Dis. 1988;158:13–22.
368. Pierre C, Blanchet F, Seta N, et al. Tolerance of once daily dosing of netilmicin and teicoplanin alone or in combination in healthy volunteers. Clin Pharmacol Ther. 1988;44:458–466.
369. Proctor L, Petty B, Lietman P, et al. Study of potential vestibulotoxic effects of one daily versus thrice daily administrations of tobramycin. Laryngoscope. 1987;97:1443–1449.
370. Labovitz E, Levison ME, Kaye D. Single-dose daily gentamicin therapy in urinary tract infection. Antimicrob Agents Chemother. 1974;6:465–470.
371. Klastersky J, Prevost JM, Meunier-Carpentier F, et al. Comparative trials of single dose vs twice daily sisomicin in bacteriuric patients. J Clin Pharmacol. 1997;17:520–528.
372. Nordstrom L, Ringberg H, Cronberg S, et al. Does administration of an aminoglycoside in single daily dose affect its efficacy and toxicity? J Antimicrob Chemother. 1990;25:159–173.
373. Hansen M, Achen F, Carstensen C, et al. Once- versus thrice-daily dosing of netilmicin in febrile immunocompromised patients: A randomized, controlled study of efficacy and safety. J Drug Dev. 1988;1(Suppl 3):S119–S124.
374. Muijsken MA, Vreeede RW, Van Dijk WC, et al. A randomized clinical study of efficacy and safety of once daily versus conventional dosing of netilmicin in patients with severe infections. J Drug Dev. 1988;1(Suppl 3):S145–S146.
375. Tulkens PM, Clerckx-Braun F, Donnez J, et al. Safety and efficacy of aminoglycosides once-a-day: Experimental data and randomized, controlled evaluation in patients suffering from pelvic inflammatory disease. J Drug Dev. 1988;1(Suppl 3):S71–S83.
376. Hollender LF, Bahnini J, DeManzini N, et al. A multicentric study of netilmicin once daily versus thrice daily in patients with appendicitis and other intra-abdominal infections. J Antimicrob Chemother. 1989;23:773–783.
377. Mauracher EH, Lau WY, Kartowisastro H, et al. Comparison of once-daily and thrice-daily netilmicin regimens in serious system infections: A multicenter study in six Asian countries. Clin Ther. 1989;11:604–613.
378. Strum AW. Netilmicin in the treatment of gram-negative bacteremia: Single daily versus multiple daily dosage. J Infect Dis. 1989;159:931–937.
379. DeVries PJ, Verkooyen RP, Leguit P, et al. Prospective randomized study of once-daily versus thrice-daily netilmicin regimens in patients with intra-abdominal infections. Eur J Clin Microbiol Infect Dis. 1990;9:161–168.
380. Ter Braak EW, deVried PJ, Bouter KP, et al. Once-daily dosing regimen for aminoglycoside plus B-lactam combination therapy of serious bacterial infections: Comparative trial with netilmicin plus ceftriaxone. Am J Med. 1990;89:58–66.
381. Giamarellou H, Yiallouros K, Petrikkos G, et al. Comparative kinetics and efficacy of amikacin administered once or twice daily in the treatment of systemic gram-negative infections. J Antimicrob Chemother. 1991;27(Suppl C):S73–S79.
382. Marik PE, Lipman J, Kobilski S, et al. A prospective randomized study comparing once- versus twice-daily amikacin dosing in critically ill adult and pediatric patients. J Antimicrob Chemother. 1991;28:753–764.
383. Van de Auwera P, Meunier J, Ibrahim S, et al. Pharmacodynamic and toxicity of netilmicin (5 mg/kg/day) given once daily or in three divided doses to cancer patients with urinary tract infections. Antimicrob Agents Chemother. 1991;35: 640–647.
384. Vigano A, Prinicipi N, Brivio L, et al. Comparison of 5 mg of netilmicin per kilogram of body weight once daily versus 2 mg per kilogram thrice daily for treatment of gram-negative pyelonephritis in children. Antimicrob Agents Chemother. 1992;36:1499–1503.
385. Gonzalez P, Aguado JM, Martin MA, et al. Once-daily aminoglycoside dosing (Letter). Lancet. 1993;341:895.
386. Maller R, Ahrne H, Holmen, et al. Once- versus twice-daily amikacin regimen. Efficacy and safety in systemic gram-negative infections. J Antimicrob Chemother. 1993;31:939–948.
387. Vanhaeverbeek M, Siska G, Douchamps J, et al. Comparison of the efficacy and safety of amikacin once or twice-a-day in the treatment of severe gram-negative infections in the elderly. Int J Clin Pharmacol Ther Toxicol. 1993;31:153–156.
388. Gibson J, Johnson L, Snowson L, et al. Single daily ceftriaxone and tobramycin in the empirical management of febrile neutropenic patients: A randomized trial. Int J Hematol. 1993;58:63–72.
389. Mendes da Costa P, Kaufman L. Amikacin once daily plus metronidazole versus amikacin twice daily plus metronidazole in colorectal surgery. Hepatogastroenterology. 1992;39:350–354.
390. Fan ST, Lau WY, Teoh-Chan CH, et al. Once daily administration of netilmicin compared with thrice daily, both in combination with metronidazole, in gangrenous and perforated appendicitis. J Antimicrob Chemother. 1988;22:69–74.
391. Prins JM, Buller HP, Kuijper EJ, et al. Once versus thrice daily gentamicin in patients with serious infection. Lancet. 1993;341:335–339.
392. Raz R, Adawi M, Romano S. Intravenous administration of gentamicin once daily versus thrice daily in adults. Eur J Clin Microb Infect Dis. 1995;14:88–91.
393. Rozdzinsk E, Kern WV, Reichle A, et al. Once-daily versus thrice-daily dosing of netilmicin in combination with beta-lactam antibiotics as empirical therapy for febrile neutropenic patients. J Antimicrob Chemother. 1993;31:585–598.
394. Ibrahim S, Derde MP, Kaufman et al. Safety pharmacokinetics and efficacy of once-a-day netilmicin and amikacin versus their conventional schedules in patients suffering from pelvic inflammatory disease. Ren Fail. 1990;12:199–203.
395. International Antimicrobial Therapy Cooperative Group of the European Organization for Research and Treatment of Cancer. Efficacy and toxicity of single daily doses of amikacin and ceftriaxone versus multiple daily doses of amikacin and ceftazidime for infection in patients with cancer and granulocytopenia. Ann Intern Med. 1993;199:584–593.
396. Maller R, Isaksson B, Nilsson L, et al. A study of amikacin given once versus twice daily in serious infections. J Antimicrob Chemother. 1998;22:75–79.
397. Vreede D. Infections by gram-negative bacilli. In: Humoral Defense of the Host and Antimicrobial Therapy. Utrecht: Drukkerij Elinkwijg BV; 1988:143–165.
398. Blaser J, Simmen HP, Thrunheer U, et al. Nephrotoxicity, high frequency ototoxicity, efficacy and serum kinetics of once versus thrice daily dosing of netilmicin in patients with serious infections. J Antimicrob Chemother. 1995;36:803–814.
399. Koo J, Tight R, Rajkumar V, et al. Comparison of once-daily versus pharmacokinetic dosing of aminoglycosides in elderly patients. Am J Med. 1996;101:177–183.
400. Elhanan K, Siplovich L, Ra R. Gentamicin once-daily versus thrice-daily in children. J Antimicrob Chemother. 1995;35:327–332.
401. Gilbert DN, Lee BL, Dworkin RJ, et al. A randomized comparison of the safety and efficacy of once-daily gentamicin or thrice-daily gentamicin in combination with ticarcillin-clavulanate. Am J Med. 1998;105:182–191.
402. Bailey TC, Little JR, Littenberg B, et al. A meta-analysis of extended interval dosing versus multiple daily dosing of aminoglycosides. Clin Infect Dis. 1997;24:786-795.
403. Ali MZ, Goetz B. Meta-analysis of the relative efficacy and toxicity of once-daily versus multiple daily dosing of aminoglycosides. Clin Infect Dis. 1997;24:796–809.
404. Hatala R, Dinh TT, Cook DJ. Once-daily aminoglycoside dosing for immunocompromised adults: A systematic review. Clin Infect Dis. 1997;24:810–815.
405. Barza M, Ioannidis JPA, Cappelleri JC, et al. Single or multiple daily doses of aminoglycosides: A meta-analysis. BMJ. 1996;312:338–345.
406. Munckhof WJ, Grayson JL, Turnide JD. A meta-analysis of studies on the safety and efficacy of aminoglycosides given either once daily or as divided doses. J Antimicrob Chemother. 1996;37:645–663.
407. Hatala R, Dinh T, Cook DJ. Once-daily aminoglycoside dosing in immunocompetent adults: A meta-analysis. Ann Intern Med. 1996;124:717–725.
408. Galloe AM, Gaudal N, Christensen HR, et al. Aminoglycosides: Single or multiple daily dosing: A meta-analysis on efficacy and safety. Eur J Clin Pharmacol. 1995;48:39–43.
409. Ferriols-Lisart R, Alos-Alminana M. Effectiveness and safety of once-daily aminoglycosides: A meta-analysis. Am J Health Syst Pharm. 1996;53:1141–1150.
410. Hayani KC, Hatzopoulos FK, Frank AL, et al. Pharmacokinetics of once-daily dosing of gentamicin in neonates. J Pediatr. 1997;131:76–80.
411. Wagner BP, Pfenninger J. Once daily dosing of netilmicin in neonatal and pediatric intensive care. Intensive Care Med. 1994;20:365–367.
412. Langhendries JP, Battisti O, Bertrand O, et al. Once-a-day administration of amikacin in neonates: Assessment of nephrotoxicity and ototoxicity. Dev Pharmacol Ther. 1993;20:220–230.
413. Vigano A, Principi N, Brivio L, et al. Comparison of 5 mg of netilmicin per kilogram of body weight once daily versus 2 mg per kilogram thrice for treatment of gram negative pyelonephritis in children. Antimicrob Agents Chemother. 1992;36:1499–503.
414. Nicolau DP, Freeman CD, Bellineau PP, et al. Experience with a once-daily aminoglycoside program administered to 2184 adult patients. Antimicrob Agents Chemother. 1995;39:650–655.
415. Freeman CD, Nicolau DP, Belliveau PP, et al. Once-daily dosing of aminoglycosides: Review and recommendations for clinical practice. J Antimicrob Chemother. 1997;39:677–686.
416. Gilbert DN. Editorial response: Meta-analyses are no longer required for determining the efficacy of single daily dosing of aminoglycosides. Clin Infect Dis. 1997;24:816–819.
417. Ettlinger JJ, Bedford KA, Lovering AM, et al. Pharmacokinetics of once-a-day netilmicin (6 mg/kg) in neonates. J Antimicrob Chemother. 1996;38:499–505.
418. Mithani H, Brown G, Economic impact of once-daily versus conventional administration of gentamicin and tobramycin. Pharmacoeconomics. 1996;10:494–503.
419. Marangos MN, Nicolau DP, Quintiliani R, et al. Influence of gentamicin dosing interval on the efficacy of penicillin-containing regimens in experimental *Enterococcus faecalis* endocarditis. J. Antimicrob Chemother. 1997;39:519–522.
420. Akmed H, Paris MM, Trujililo M, et al. Once-daily gentamicin therapy for experimental *Escherichia coli* meningitis. Antimicrob Agents Chemother. 1997;41: 49–53.
421. Wong J, Brown G. Does once-daily dosing of aminoglycosides affect neuromuscular function? J Clin Pharm Ther. 1996;21:407–411.
422. Gilbert DN, Bennett WM. Use of antimicrobial agents in renal failure. Infect Dis Clin North Am. 1989;3:517–531.
423. Hickey SM, McCracken GH Jr. Antibacterial therapeutic agents. In: Feigin RD, Cherry JD, eds. Textbook of Pediatric Infectious Diseases. 4th ed. Philadelphia: WB Saunders; 1998:2614–1649.
424. Denton M, Wilcox MH. Antimicrobial treatment of pulmonary colonization and infection by *Pseudomonas aeruginosa* in cystic fibrosis patients. J Antimicrob Chemother. 1997;40:468–474.
425. Zebner R, Quinn JP. Antimicrobials in cystic fibrosis: Emergence of resistance and implications for treatment. Semin Respir Infect. 1992;7:210–217.

426. Mulherin D, Fahy J, Grant W, et al. Aminoglycoside-induced ototoxicity in patients with cystic fibrosis. Ir J Med Sci. 1991;160:173–175.
427. Touw DJ, Vinks AATMM, Heyerman HGM, et al. Prospective evaluation of a dose prediction algorithm for intravenous tobramycin in adolescent and adult patients with cystic fibrosis. Ther Drug Monit. 1996;18:118–123.
428. Smith DL, Stableforth DE, Geddes AM. Evaluation of a once-daily netilmicin regimen in the treatment of cystic fibrosis. J Antimicrob Chemother. 1994;33: 191–193.
429. Bates RD, Nahata MC, Jones JW. Pharmacokinetics and safety of tobramycin after once-daily administration in patients with cystic fibrosis. Chest. 1997;112:1208–1213.
430. Canis F, Husson MO, Turck D, et al. Pharmacokinetics and bronchial diffusion of single daily dose amikacin in cystic fibrosis patients. J Antimicrob Chemother. 1997;39:431–433.
431. Ramsey BW, Dorkin HL, Eisenberg JD, et al. Efficacy of aerosolized tobramycin in patients with cystic fibrosis. N Engl J Med. 1993;328:1740–1746.
432. Package insert prescribing information for Tobramycin Solution for Inhalation. Pathogenesis Corporation, Seattle, Wash; January 1998.
433. Touw DJ, Jacobs FAH, Brimicombe RW, et al. Pharmacokinetics of aerosolized tobramycin in adult patients with cystic fibrosis. Antimicrob Agents Chemother. 1997;41:184–187.
434. Levine DP, Crane LR, Zervos MJ. Bacteremia in narcotic addicts at the Detroit Medical Center: II. Infectious endocarditis: A prospective comparative study. Rev Infect Dis. 1986;8:374.
435. Keane WF, Everett ED, Golper TA, et al. Peritoneal dialysis related peritonitis treatment recommendations. 1993 update. Perit Dial Int. 1993;13:14–28.

Chapter 24

Tetracyclines and Chloramphenicol

HAROLD C. STANDIFORD

TETRACYCLINES

All the tetracyclines are primarily bacteriostatic at therapeutic concentrations and have a broad spectrum that includes gram-positive, gram-negative, aerobic, and anaerobic bacteria, spirochetes, mycoplasmas, rickettsiae, chlamydiae, and some protozoans. The analogues can be divided into three groups based on differences in their pharmacology: (1) the short-acting compounds chlortetracycline, oxytetracycline, and tetracycline; (2) an intermediate group consisting of demeclocycline and methacycline; and (3) the more recently discovered, longer-acting compounds doxycycline and minocycline. Although several other derivatives have been developed called *glycylcyclines,* which have activity against tetracycline-resistant bacteria, none are available at this time.[1]

Structure, Derivation, Nomenclature, and Brand Names

Unlike the fortuitous discovery of penicillin by Fleming, the first tetracycline, chlortetracycline, was discovered by screening organisms obtained from the soil for their antimicrobial properties. Benjamin M. Duggar, a meticulous mycologist in his seventies, noted unusual antimicrobial activity from organisms that formed a golden yellow colony.[2] He designated the organism *Streptomyces aureofaciens* (L. *aurum,* "golden") and named the product *Aureomycin.* Oxytetracycline was derived from *Streptomyces rimosus* in 1950, and tetracycline was produced by the catalytic dehalogenation of chlortetracycline in 1953. The two long-acting compounds were derived semisynthetically: doxycycline in 1966 and minocycline in 1967. The generic names of the analogues are determined by the substitutions on the basic structure of tetracycline, which consists of a hydronaphthacene nucleus containing four fused rings (Fig. 24–1). The compounds currently available in the United States and their major brand names, doses, and costs are listed in Table 24–1. Of these, tetracycline HCl and doxycycline have emerged as the most useful clinically. Chlortetracycline (Aureomycin), the first member of the family, is no longer available except for topical use, and methacycline (Rondomycin) has been withdrawn from the market.

Mechanism of Action

The tetracyclines enter bacteria by passive diffusion through porins in gram-negative bacteria and are probably accumulated by a ΔpH-dependent process.[3–4] Once within the cell, they reversibly bind primarily to the 30S ribosomal subunit at a position that blocks the binding of the aminoacyl–transfer RNA to the acceptor site on the messenger RNA–ribosome complex.[5] This prevents the addition of new amino acids into the growing peptide chain. The tetracyclines also inhibit protein synthesis in mammalian cells, particularly in mitochondrial ribosomes, but apparently are not in sufficient concentration in these structures to produce severe toxicity.[6]

In Vitro Activity

The antimicrobial spectra of all the tetracyclines are almost identical. Some differences, however, in the degree of activity against these organisms do exist among the analogues. In general, the lipophilic congeners are more active than those that are more hydrophilic. It follows, therefore, that minocycline is the most active of the analogues, closely followed by doxycycline. The minimal inhibitory concentration of the more hydrophilic congeners oxytetracycline and tetracycline are two- to fourfold higher against many bacteria and are the least-active analogues. Despite these differences, for cost reasons it is recommended that tetracycline be used in the clinical microbiology laboratory to evaluate susceptibility for all the analogues.[7] Minimal inhibitory concentrations of tetracycline and doxycycline for many aerobic bacteria are given in Table 24–2. For the

TABLE 24–1 The Names, Preparations, and Usual Adult Oral Dosages for the Tetracyclines Currently Available in the United States

Generic Name (Major Brand Name, Company)*	Oral Preparations	Usual Adult Oral Dosage
Short-acting†		
Oxytetracycline (Terramycin, Pfizer)	Capsules: 125, 250 mg	500 mg q6h
Tetracycline HCl‡	Capsules: 100, 250, 500 mg Syrup: 125 mg/5 ml	500 mg q6h
Intermediate		
Demeclocycline HCl (Declomycin, Lederle)	Capsules: 150 mg Tablets: 150, 300 mg	300 mg q12h
Long-acting§		
Doxycycline (Vibramycin, Pfizer)	Capsules (hyclate): 50, 100 mg Tablets: 50, 100 mg Syrup (calcium): 50 mg/5 ml Syrup (monohydrate): 25 mg/5 ml	200 mg (or 100 mg q12h for first day), then 100 mg q24h‖
Minocycline (Minocin, Lederle)	Capsules and tablets: 50, 100 mg Suspension: 50 mg/5 ml	200 mg, then 100 mg q12h

*Many other brands are available for some of the analogues.
†The short-acting tetracyclines are also available for intravenous administration at usual doses of 500 mg every 6 to 12 hours not to exceed 2 g daily. However, most prefer doxycycline for this route of administration. Preparation combined with a local anesthetic agent can be given intramuscularly, but these are not recommended.
‡Tetracycline is also available as a tetracycline phosphate complex (Tetrex, Bristol) intended to enhance absorption, but its superiority has not been established.
§The longer-acting agents can be given intravenously in the same doses that are recommended for oral therapy. Doxycycline is available at 100 or 200 mg per vial and minocycline at 100 mg per vial.
‖The treatment schedules for sexually transmitted diseases and for Lyme disease use 100 mg twice daily.

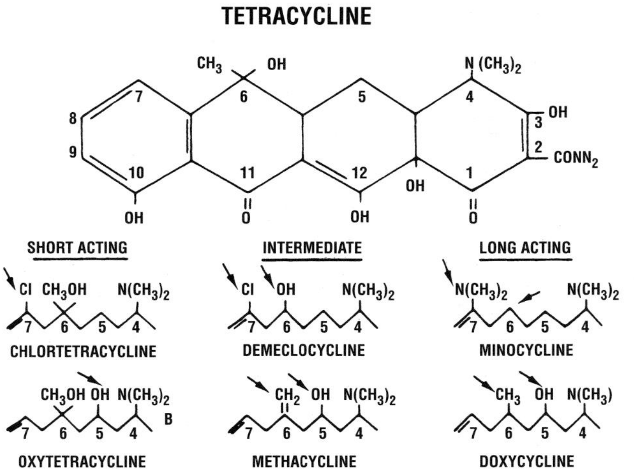

FIGURE 24–1. Chemical structure of the tetracyclines. The analogues differ from tetracycline at the fifth, sixth, or seventh position, as indicated by the arrows.

activities of the other analogues, the reader is referred to the extensive work from the laboratory of Finland and colleagues.[8–10]

Although many of the aerobic and facultative anaerobic organisms are within the spectrum of the tetracyclines, more effective agents are available for the treatment of infections caused by most of these bacteria. Pneumococci and *Haemophilus influenzae* can be inhibited by concentrations of tetracyclines achieved in the serum, and this provides a rationale for their use in sinusitis and acute exacerbations of chronic bronchitis.[11] However, pneumococci resistant to penicillin are generally more resistant to tetracyclines, although doxycycline is the more active congener.[12, 13] Gonococci and meningococci are extremely susceptible; unfortunately, gonococci resistant to penicillin G also tend to be resistant to tetracycline.[14, 15] In most cases, *Escherichia coli* acquired outside the hospital setting can be inhibited by concentrations achieved in the urine, if not the serum. Tetracyclines, therefore, are useful agents for the treatment of acute, uncomplicated, urinary tract infections and the acute urethral syndrome. *Pseudomonas pseudomallei* organisms are generally sensitive, and this has therapeutic importance, as does the high degree of susceptibility of *Brucella* spp.[16, 17] *Vibrio cholerae, Vibrio vulnificus,* and other vibrios are generally susceptible, and the tetracyclines are important for therapy for diseases caused by this group of organisms.[18] Although *Campylobacter* spp. are generally susceptible, a high percentage of resistant isolates has been noted in some countries.[19–21] Therefore, it is not the drug of choice for infections caused by these bacteria. *Shigella* organisms have become increasingly resistant.[22] *Mycobacterium marinum* is susceptible and appears to respond clinically.[23]

The tetracyclines have activity against many anaerobic organisms (Table 24–3).[24] Their activity against *Actinomyces* is particularly relevant clinically. Doxycycline is more active against *Bacteroides fragilis* than tetracycline is, but other agents are preferred for infections caused by this organism. The activity of the tetracyclines against anaerobic bacteria, however, may be partially responsible for the effectiveness of the neomycin-tetracycline combination and doxycycline alone as alternative oral presurgical bowel preparations.[25, 26] Many pathogenic spirochetes are susceptible, including *Borrelia burgdorferi,* the agent of Lyme disease.[27] Other organisms generally inhibited by this group of antibiotics include rickettsiae, chlamydiae, mycoplasmas, and, to a limited degree, protozoans (*Plasmodium* spp. and *Entamoeba histolytica*).[28]

Bacteria develop resistance to the tetracyclines predominantly by

TABLE 24–2 Minimal Inhibitory Concentration of Tetracycline and Doxycycline for Common Aerobic and Facultative Anaerobic Bacteria

Organism	No. of Strains	Antibiotic	Cumulative Percentage Inhibited by Indicated Concentrations (μg/ml)				
			0.4	*0.8*	*1.6*	*3.2*	*6.4*
Gram-positive							
Staphylococcus aureus	56	Tetracycline	0	2	20	65	67
		Doxycycline	2	25	63	65	68
*Streptococcus pyogenes**	63	Tetracycline	10	50	80	87	90
		Doxycycline	56	90	90	95	95
Streptococcus pneumoniae†	35	Tetracycline	70	96	96	100	—
		Doxycycline	100	—	—	—	—
Group B streptococci	12	Tetracycline	0	0	50	50	50
		Doxycycline	0	50	50	50	50
Enterococcus	36	Tetracycline	0	0	0	0	10
		Doxycycline	0	0	0	0	10
Gram-negative‡							
Neisseria gonorrhoeae§	25	Tetracycline	5	60	85	88	100
		Doxycycline	60	75	80	92	100
Neisseria meningitidis‖	10	Tetracycline	0	50	—	100	—
		Doxycycline	0	—	50	—	100
Haemophilus influenzae	15	Tetracycline	0	0	0	33	87
		Doxycycline	0	0	60	93	100
Escherichia coli	48	Tetracycline	0	0	0	5	35
		Doxycycline	0	0	0	5	35
Klebsiella pneumoniae	17	Tetracycline	0	0	0	0	5
		Doxycycline	0	0	0	0	12
Enterobacter spp.	10	Tetracycline	0	10	30	50	70
		Doxycycline	0	0	0	0	10
Pseudomonas pseudomallei	10	Tetracycline	0	0	60	100	—
Campylobacter jejuni	172	Tetracycline	44	62	74	81	84
	107	Doxycycline	68	74	79	80	86
Shigella spp.	213	Tetracycline	0	10	12	50	50

*More recent series indicate that 20 to 40% of *Strep. pyogenes* have become resistant to the tetracyclines.
†Tetracycline-resistant *Strep. pneumoniae* strains are more common in some areas. Those strains resistant to penicillin tend to be resistant to the tetracyclines.
‡*Proteus mirabilis*, indole-positive *Proteus* spp., and *P. aeruginosa* are generally resistant to 25 μg/ml.
§Gonococci resistant to penicillin G also tend to be resistant to tetracycline.[14, 15]
‖The minimal inhibitory concentration of minocycline for meningococci is 1.6 μg/ml (range, 0.8 to 1.6 μg/ml).
Data from refs. 8–10, 16, 19, 22. Organisms should be considered susceptible if the minimal inhibitory concentrations are 4 μg/ml or less. A moderate susceptibility range of up to 8 μg/ml may be useful for the treatment of urinary tract infections.[7]

TABLE 24–3 Minimal Inhibitory Concentrations of Tetracycline and Doxycycline for Common Anaerobic Bacteria*

Organism	No. of Strains	Antibiotic	Cumulative Percentage Susceptible to Indicated Concentration (μg/ml)				
			0.5	*1.0*	*2.0*	*4.0*	*8.0*
Gram-positive							
Peptococcus	59	Tetracycline	25	29	36	36	37
Peptostreptococcus	29	Tetracycline	38	41	48	52	72
		Doxycycline	45	45	66	79	97
Streptococci, anaerobic and microaerophilic	10	Tetracycline	50	60	70	90	90
		Doxycycline	70	90	90	90	100
Eubacterium	17	Tetracycline	24	59	65	65	77
		Doxycycline	59	65	77	82	88
Propionibacterium	12	Tetracycline	58	75	83	83	83
		Doxycycline	75	83	83	92	92
Clostridium perfringens	9	Tetracycline	22	22	56	67	67
		Doxycycline	67	67	67	78	89
Other clostridia	33	Tetracycline	36	46	49	52	61
		Doxycycline	49	52	61	68	82
Actinomyces	16	Tetracycline	56	69	94	94	94
		Doxycycline	63	69	94	100	—
Gram-negative							
Gram-negative cocci	26	Tetracycline	54	69	73	73	73
		Doxycycline	58	69	73	81	96
Fusobacterium	34	Tetracycline	94	97	97	97	97
		Doxycycline	94	94	94	94	100
Bacteroides fragilis	76	Tetracycline	25	40	40	42	46
		Doxycycline	41	42	50	75	88
Prevotella melaninogenica	67	Tetracycline	75	76	79	87	94
		Doxycycline	75	78	90	96	97
Other *Bacteroides* spp.	72	Tetracycline	33	35	43	50	60
Selenomonas		Doxycycline	40	43	53	68	79

*An organism with a minimal inhibitory concentration of 4 μg/ml or less should be considered susceptible.
Modified from Sutter VL, Finegold SM. Susceptibility of anaerobic bacteria to 23 antimicrobial agents. Antimicrob Agents Chemother. 1976;10:736.

preventing the accumulation of tetracycline within the cell. This is accomplished by decreasing the influx or increasing the ability of the cell to export the antibiotic.[4, 29] Rarely, the tetracyclines are inactivated biologically or altered chemically by resistant bacteria; oxidative destruction has been found in a few species.[29–35] Resistance to one tetracycline usually implies resistance to all, although there are marked differences in the degree of resistance among species. The resistance among bacteria can be mediated by transferable resistance plasmids. The tetracyclines have been widely used in feeds to promote growth in animals. This may be a major factor in providing selective antibiotic pressure for the spread of plasmid-mediated resistance to these and other antibiotics.[36–38]

Pharmacology

Serum levels achieved by usual oral doses in adults are given in Figure 24–2. Absorption occurs primarily in the proximal small bowel and produces peak serum concentrations 1 to 3 hours after administration. The commonly used 500-mg therapeutic dose of tetracycline gives a serum level of 4 μg/ml, the highest of all the short-acting analogues.[39] Doxycycline and minocycline (200 mg) achieve serum levels of about 2.5 μg/ml, slightly higher than levels attained by the larger therapeutic doses of the intermediate agents.[40–44]

After the intravenous administration of 500 mg, serum levels of the short-acting agents (not shown) are approximately 8 μg/ml at 30 minutes and decrease to 2 to 3 μg/ml by 5 hours.[45] Intravenous injection of the usual 200-mg loading dose of the long-acting agents doxycycline and minocycline produces serum levels of approximately 4 μg/ml at 30 minutes. Once tissue distribution occurs for the long-acting analogues, the levels are almost identical to the concentrations achieved orally.[40, 46] Thrombophlebitis is a frequent complication of the intravenous preparations. Intramuscular preparations are available for the short-acting compounds but are not recommended because of the severe pain produced on injection, even when they are mixed with local anesthetics.

Some of the pharmacokinetic properties of the tetracyclines are compared in Table 24–4. The high levels obtained orally with tetracycline compared with other short-acting agents are due primarily to better absorption from the gastrointestinal tract. The long-acting analogues doxycycline and minocycline are absorbed almost completely; thus, high serum levels are achieved with relatively small doses.[40–41] The tetracyclines can be differentiated into three groups on the basis of their different half-lives. Doxycycline has the longest of all and allows therapeutic levels to be maintained with a single

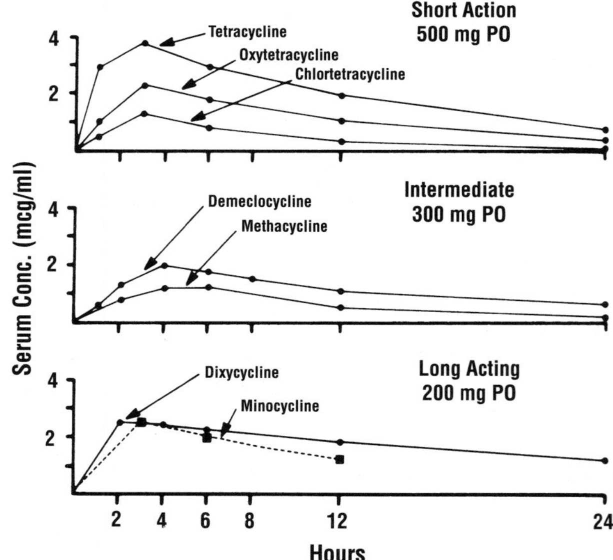

FIGURE 24–2. Serum levels achieved with the usually recommended oral doses of the tetracyclines. Chlortetracycline and methacycline are no longer available for oral or parenteral administration. (Data from refs. 39–43.)

TABLE 24-4 Pharmacokinetic Features of the Tetracyclines*

Antibiotic	Gastrointestinal Absorption (%)	Half-Life (h)	Renal Clearance† (ml/min/1.73 m²)	Urinary Recovery (%)	Apparent Volume of Distribution† (Liters)	Protein Binding‡ (%)
Short-acting						
Oxytetracycline	58	9	99	70	128	35
Tetracycline	77	8	74	60	108	65
Intermediate						
Demeclocycline	66	12	35	39	121	91
Methacycline	58	14	31	60	79	90
Long-acting						
Doxycycline	93	18	20	42	50	93
Minocycline	95	16	9	6	60	76

*The pharmacokinetic values vary considerably from laboratory to laboratory. These values were selected in most instances because comparative data were available from reliable investigators.
†After single-dose intravenous administration.
‡Ultrafiltration technique.
Data from refs. 40–45 and 45–48.

daily dose, although twice-daily regimens are frequently recommended.[40] The 8-hour half-life of tetracycline suggests that the dosage interval could be 8 hours for this antibiotic when it is used to treat minor infections.[45] The half-lives of the compounds are determined mainly by the rate of excretion by the kidneys. Chlortetracycline is an exception: it has a short half-life despite a slow rate of clearance as a result of the marked instability of the compound in vitro as well as in vivo.[45] Adequate therapeutic concentrations of all the tetracyclines, with the possible exception of chlortetracycline and minocycline, are achieved in the urine for the treatment of urinary tract infections caused by sensitive organisms. The degree of protein binding of the analogues is variable, depending on the methods used for the determination, but it tends to be greater for the intermediate- and long-acting compounds.[46–48] This may be one of the factors that determines their slow rate of renal excretion. The apparent volume of distribution for most of the tetracyclines is greater than that of extracellular body water, thus indicating sequestration in tissues, presumably the liver.[45] Minocycline and doxycycline have the smallest volume of distribution, another factor that tends to enhance their serum levels.[46]

Tissue Distribution

The tetracyclines can be found in small amounts in many tissues and fluids, including the lung, liver, kidney, brain, sputum, and mucosal fluid. For tetracycline, the levels in the cerebral spinal fluid are approximately 10 to 26% of the serum levels,[49, 50] whereas concentrations in synovial fluid and the maxillary sinus mucosa approach serum levels.[51, 52] All the tetracyclines are concentrated in unobstructed bile and produce levels in this fluid 5 to 20 times those obtained in the serum. It has been suggested that lipid solubility is a primary determinant for the diffusion in many tissues. Minocycline, followed by doxycycline, is more lipophilic at a physiologic pH than are the other drugs. This may explain why minocycline reaches sufficient concentrations in saliva and tears to eradicate the meningococcal carrier state, whereas the other tetracyclines do not.[53, 54] The tetracyclines cross the placenta and accumulate in fetal bone and teeth and therefore should not be given during pregnancy.[55, 56] They are excreted in breast milk; however, concentrations in the infant's serum are below detectability.[57]

Renal and Hepatic Insufficiency

The tetracyclines should not be used in patients with renal failure. Doxycycline, the only exception, is excreted in the gastrointestinal tract under these circumstances. Neither the half-life nor the therapeutic dose of this antibiotic varies with alterations in renal function.[58] The tetracyclines are slowly removed by hemodialysis but not effectively by peritoneal dialysis. Hepatic disease is not known to cause elevated serum levels of the tetracyclines. However, they should be used very cautiously in such situations, because they have been noted to cause hepatic toxicity.

Assay

The tetracyclines can be measured by a number of different techniques. These include bioassay using *Bacillus cereus* as the test organism, by high-performance liquid chromatographic procedures, or by direct fluorescent chemical analysis,[59–61] but monitoring of serum levels during therapy is rarely indicated.

Toxicity

Skin and Allergy

Hypersensitivity reactions including anaphylaxis, urticuria, periorbital edema, fixed drug eruptions, and morbilliform rashes occur with tetracyclines but are not common.[62–64] A patient who is allergic to one analogue should be considered to be allergic to all. There are a number of recent reports of a systemic lupus erythematosus–like syndrome reported in association with minocycline. These patients have antinuclear antibody. Symptoms disappear in most patients when the antibiotic is discontinued and recur when rechallenged.[65–67] Photosensitivity reactions consisting of a red rash on areas exposed to sunlight that is frequently associated with onycholysis are most common in patients receiving demeclocycline but occur with all analogues.[68, 69] They appear to be a toxic rather than an allergic reaction. Prolonged administration of minocycline has been noted rarely to cause nail, skin, and scleral pigmentation, which is usually reversible, as well as an asymptomatic black pigmentation of the thyroid.[70, 71] A blue or blue-black discoloration of the gums also has been reported; this appears to be secondary to bone pigmentation, which is visible through the oral mucosal tissues. The pigmentation is permanent.[72, 73]

Teeth and Bones

A gray-brown to yellow discoloration of the teeth has been noted in some communities in 80% of the children taking tetracyclines.[74] This side effect is permanent and may be associated with hypoplasia of the enamel[68, 75] and depression of skeletal growth in premature infants.[76] The darkening effect of tetracyclines on permanent teeth appears to be related to the total dose of the antibiotic administered. In a retrospective study, cosmetically noticeable but mild darkening of the permanent teeth occurred in 3 of 14 children receiving five courses of tetracycline, whereas 4 of 6 children receiving eight courses had moderate darkening of the enamel.[77] Primary teeth generally show more darkening than do the larger, thicker, and more opaque permanent teeth. Since there is some variability in staining with similar tetracycline exposure, it is prudent not to administer these agents to pregnant women and to children up to the age of 8 years, the period when tooth enamel is being formed. For this reason, the Food and Drug Administration has withdrawn from the market the concentrated liquid dosage forms (drops) specifically intended for pediatric use.[78] It is not unreasonable, however, to administer a single course of tetracycline therapy to young children for specifically defined indications when the alternative regime may produce more severe toxicity. Thus, the tetracyclines may be indicated for children suspected of having Rocky Mountain spotted fever who can tolerate oral medications. Doxycycline binds less with calcium than do other tetracyclines and may cause dental changes less frequently in children.[79]

Gastrointestinal Symptoms

The tetracyclines are irritative substances and frequently produce gastrointestinal symptoms after oral administration. Esophageal ulcerations that are manifested as retrosternal pain exacerbated by swallowing have been clearly documented after tetracycline and doxycycline administration. In most cases, the patients were taking the capsules with little or no fluid just before going to bed. A word of caution to the patient is indicated in order to prevent this toxicity. The complication may also occur in patients with esophageal obstruction or motility disorders.[80, 81] Nausea, vomiting, and epigastric distress are dose related and limit the dose of most of the analogues. The administration of food with doxycycline, minocycline, or oxytetracycline may ameliorate some of these symptoms, but food seriously decreases the absorption of the other tetracyclines. Diarrhea is most often associated with analogues that are poorly absorbed and appears to be related to alterations in the enteric flora. Doxycycline produces less of an effect on bowel flora than does tetracycline.[82] The diarrhea usually subsides when treatment with the antibiotic is stopped, but prolonged symptoms due to pseudomembranous colitis have been reported.[83] Tetracycline also has been noted, rarely, to cause pancreatitis with or without overt liver disease.[84]

Liver

The hepatoxicity of the tetracyclines, first described in patients receiving intravenous chlortetracycline but now described with other analogues, appears pathologically as a fine droplet fatty metamorphosis and results in a high mortality.[85, 86] The administration of less than 2 g/day intravenously is not associated with liver dysfunction or injury except in pregnant women, who are particularly at risk,[87] and in patients with an excessive serum level due to renal failure.[88] This toxicity is rarely reported with doxycycline.[89, 90]

Renal Function

The tetracyclines aggravate preexisting renal failure by inhibiting protein synthesis, which increases the azotemia from amino acid metabolism.[91] Nephrogenic diabetes insipidus is produced by demeclocycline, a side effect that has been used therapeutically to reverse chronic inappropriate antidiuretic hormone secretion;[92] renal failure has complicated its use for this purpose in patients with cirrhosis.[93] Outdated tetracycline has produced a reversible Fanconi-like syndrome with renal tubular acidosis, but tetracycline formulations producing this syndrome have been modified. It is unlikely that this complication will recur.[58]

Nervous and Sensory Systems

Vertigo is a side effect unique to minocycline. Symptoms of lightheadedness, loss of balance, dizziness, and tinnitus usually begin on the second and third days of therapy and have been noted more frequently in women (70%) than in men (28%). The symptoms are reversible within several days after the discontinuation of therapy with the antibiotic, but this side effect has seriously limited the use of minocycline.[94] Benign intracranial hypertension (pseudotumor cerebri) has been described in infants and adults with many of the analogues.[95, 96]

Superinfection

Colonization by tetracycline-resistant organisms is a frequent occurrence during tetracycline therapy and is generally of little clinical significance. Rarely, a fulminating diarrhea resulting from *Clostridium difficile* pseudomembranous colitis or staphylococcal enteritis may occur after oral or parenteral therapy.[97, 98] More often and less serious, oral or vaginal monaliasis complicates treatment, a complication that may require specific therapy.

Significant Food and Drug Interactions

Food adversely affects the absorption of tetracycline, chlortetracycline, methacycline, and demeclocycline. Doxycycline and minocycline absorption decreases by less than 20%, which does not appear to be important clinically.[99, 100] All the tetracyclines form complexes with divalent or trivalent cations. Therefore, absorption is markedly decreased when these drugs are administered simultaneously with calcium, magnesium, and aluminum in antacids; milk; iron and iron-containing tonics; multivitamins; didanosine; or sucralfate. Administration of the drugs should be spaced by 2 hours.[101, 102] Sodium bicarbonate also has an adverse effect on absorption and should not be administered simultaneously.[103] Cimetidine has been shown to decrease the absorption of tetracycline, but this is unlikely to be significant in the clinical situation.[104] Carbamazepine (Tegretol), diphenylhydantoin, and barbiturates decrease the normal half-life of doxycycline to almost one half by increasing the hepatic metabolism of the antibiotic.[105, 106] Chronic ethanol ingestion has also resulted in a shorter half-life of doxycycline but not tetracycline, presumably also through the induction of hepatic microsomal enzymes.[107] Methoxyflurane anesthesia may cause nephrotoxicity when administered with tetracyclines.[108] It has been suggested that this adverse interaction occurs with the newer, less nephrotoxic fluorinated anesthetic agents as well.[109] The use of these antibiotics concurrently with diuretics produces an elevated blood urea nitrogen level, although the exact mechanism has not been determined.[110] It has been reported that women receiving oral contraceptives have become pregnant while receiving tetracycline. This may be caused by the reduction in bacterial hydrolysis of conjugated estrogen in the intestine.[111, 112] Women should be advised to use an additional form of birth control. The tetracyclines may potentiate the effects of oral anticoagulants, making careful monitoring of prothrombin times essential.

There is in vitro antagonism when anti-infective agents that are primarily inhibitory are combined with cidal agents. This appears to account for the poor outcome in the treatment of pneumococcal meningitis with penicillin and tetracycline. Whether it can be generalized to other indications is not known.[113]

Indications

The tetracyclines are the drugs of choice or effective alternative therapy for a wide variety of bacterial, chlamydial, mycoplasmal, and rickettsial infections (Table 24–5).[114–116] The use of minocycline for early (within the first year of disease) rheumatoid arthritis is of note as is the use of intrapleural tetracycline for the control of malignant pleural effusions.[117–119] The tetracyclines have no role in the treatment of viral or fungal diseases. Tetracycline or doxycycline can be used interchangeably for most of these indications. However, compliance may be better with doxycycline since it can be taken twice daily without regard to meals, and cost is no longer an important factor. Doxycycline is preferred by most when intravenous administration is required.

TABLE 24–5 Major Therapeutic Indications for the Tetracyclines*

Major Indications	Effective Alternative Therapy
Borrelia burgdorferi (Lyme disease, early)	Acne, severe
Borrelia recurrentis (relapsing fever)	*Actinomyces israelii* (actinomycosis)
Brucellosis (with gentamicin in seriously ill patients)	Anthrax
Calymmatobacterium granulomatis (granuloma inguinale)	*Bartonella henselae* and *quintana*
Chlamydial infections	*Campylobacter fetus, jejuni*
Chlamydia pneumoniae (TWAR strain)	Chronic bronchitis (acute exacerbation)
Epididymitis, acute (sexually transmitted form)	*Clostridium tetani*
Inclusion conjunctivitis (adult)	*Eikenella corrodens*
Lymphogranuloma venereum	*Francisella tularensis* (tularemia)
Ornithosis, psittacosis	*Legionella* spp. (doxycycline ± rifampin)
Trachoma	*Leptospira* (leptospirosis)
Urethral, endocervical, or rectal infections in adults	*Leptotrichia buccalis*
Ehrlichia	*Mycobacterium leprae* (minocycline)
Helicobacter pylori (plus metronidazole plus bismuth subsalicylate)	*Mycobacterium marinum* (minocycline)
Pelvic inflammatory disease (acute, in combination with other antibiotics) (doxycycline)	*Mycoplasma pneumoniae*
Pseudomonas mallei (glanders) (streptomycin with a tetracycline)	*Nocardia* (minocycline)
Rickettsial infections (some prefer chloramphenicol for severe infections)	*Pasteurella multocida*
Q fever	*Pseudomonas pseudomallei* (melioidosis) (doxycycline with TMP/SMX and chloramphenicol)
Rickettsial pox	Rat-bite fever (*Spirillum minus, Streptococcus moniliformis*)
Rocky Mountain spotted fever	*Stenotrophomanas maltophilia* (minocycline)
Typhus fever	*Treponema pallidum* (syphillis)
Urethritis, nonspecific	*Treponema pertenue* (yaws, nasopalatal)
Urethral syndrome, acute	*Ureaplasma urealyticum*
Vibrio cholerae (cholera)	*Yersinina pestis* (plague)
Vibrio parahaemolyticus	**Alternative Prophylaxis**
Vibrio vulnificus	Oral bowel preparation for intestinal surgery (tetracycline in combination with neomycin or doxycycline alone)
	Meningococcal disease prophylaxis (minocycline)

*Unless specified, tetracycline and doxycycline can be considered interchangeable.
Abbreviation: TMP/SMX, Trimethoprim-sulfamethoxazole.

CHLORAMPHENICOL

Soon after chloramphenicol was released in the United States in 1949, reports linked this highly effective agent with aplastic anemia, and it quickly fell into disfavor. The increased awareness of the pathogenicity of anaerobic organisms and the development of ampicillin-resistant *H. influenzae* accounted for a brief resurgency. However, the availability of other agents has dramatically reduced the need for this antibiotic. Because it is effective, readily available (often over the counter), and inexpensive, it is still used as first-line therapy for enteric fever and other infections in many parts of the world. In the United States and other developed nations, chloramphenicol remains a useful antibiotic, but only as alternative therapy in seriously ill patients or for patients infected with very antibiotic-resistant organisms.

Structure, Derivation, Brand Names, and Preparations

Like the early tetracyclines, chloramphenicol was discovered by screening organisms for their antimicrobial activity. Isolated independently by Burkholder from a mulched field near Caracas, Venezuela[120] and by workers at the University of Illinois from compost,[121] the organism producing the active compound was named *Streptomyces venezuelae.*[122] The structure of chloramphenicol is shown in Figure 24–3. It was the first antibiotic whose chemical synthesis was economically and technically practical for large-scale production.[123] In many countries, chloramphenicol is available in 250-mg capsules (Chloromycetin, Parke-Davis), suspension 150 mg/5 ml (Chloromycetin Palmitate), and as a parenteral formulation (Chloromycetin Sodium Succinate, 1-g powder). Generic formulations are also available. It also is available as Chloromycetin ophthalmic ointment 1%; Chloromycetin ophthalmic 25 mg (powder to prepare ophthalmic solution) and Chloromycetin Otic (drops). In the United States, Parke-Davis discontinued manufacturing the oral Chloromycetin Kapseals (250 mg) in 1995 and the Chloromycetin Palmitate in 1991. No oral products are currently available in the United States. In March 1998, Parke-Davis sold their remaining line to Monarch Pharmaceuticals (David Rhodes, Medical Affairs, Parke-Davis, personal communication).

Thiamphenical, not available in the United States, is an analogue in which the *p*-nitro group on the benzene ring is replaced by a methylsulfonyl group. Its spectrum of activity is similar to that of chloramphenicol, but it has not been reported to cause aplastic anemia.

Mechanism of Action

Chloramphenicol appears to enter the cell by an energy-dependent process.[124] Once within the cell, it inhibits protein synthesis. This is accomplished by reversibly binding to the larger 50-S subunit of the 70-S ribosome at a locus that prevents the attachment of the amino acid–containing end of the aminoacyl–transfer RNA to its binding region. Without this attachment, the association of the amino acid substrate with peptidyltransferase does not occur and peptide bond formation is prevented.[3] This block in protein synthesis produces a static effect against most sensitive microorganisms. However, chloramphenicol is bactericidal against some meningeal pathogens such as *H. influenzae, Streptococcus pneumoniae,* and *Neisseria meningitidis* but not group B streptococci or enteric gram-negative bacilli at concentrations that can be achieved therapeutically.[125–127] Although mammalian cells contain primarily 80-S ribosomes that are unaffected by chloramphenicol, the mitochondria do contain 70-S particles. The effect of chloramphenicol on these has been suggested as a cause for the dose-related bone marrow suppression of the compound but not the idiosyncratic aplastic anemia.[128]

In Vitro Activity

Chloramphenicol is extremely active against a variety of organisms, including bacteria, spirochetes, rickettsiae, chlamydiae, and mycoplasmas. The percent of strains of bacteria inhibited at various concentrations of antibiotic is listed in Table 24–6. Most of the gram-positive and gram-negative aerobic bacteria are inhibited by concentrations easily achieved in the serum of patients, but more active or less toxic therapeutic agents are available for most of these pathogens.[9, 10, 16, 24, 123, 129–133] Salmonellae including *Salmonella typhi* are generally susceptible.[131] In the United States, resistant strains occasionally occur,[134] but imported strains may be highly resistant. The three most common organisms causing meningitis in childhood *(H. influenzae, Strep. pneumoniae,* and *N. meningitidis)* are highly susceptible,[10, 135, 136] although rare resistant strains of each species have been reported. The overall rate of *H. influenzae* resistance among clinical strains in the United States is approximately 0.6%.[137] Indeed, strains of *H. influenzae* that cause clinical infections and are resistant to both chloramphenicol and ampicillin have been isolated in several parts of the world.[138–140] These resistant isolates are rare in the United States and Canada but rather frequent in Spain.[141–143] Chloramphenicol is one of the most active antibiotics against anaerobic bacteria including the *B. fragilis* group, but other agents have

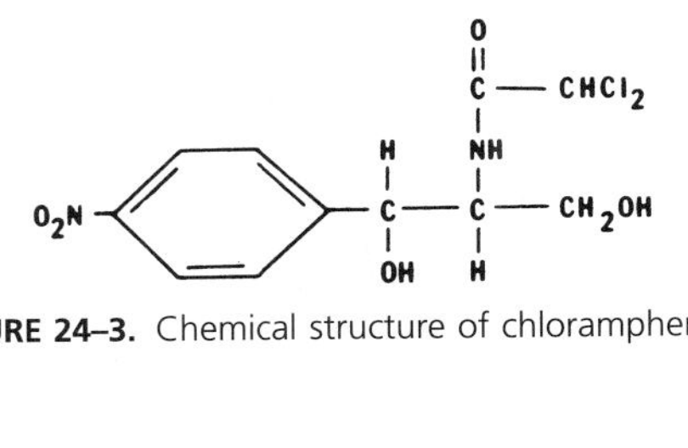

FIGURE 24–3. Chemical structure of chloramphenicol.

TABLE 24–6 Activity of Chloramphenicol against Selected Bacteria*

Bacteria	No. of Strains	Cumulative Percentage Inhibited at Indicated Concentration (μg/ml)				
		0.4	*0.8*	*1.6*	*3.2*	*6.4*
Aerobic bacteria						
Gram-positive						
Stapholococcus aureus	291	0	0	0	5	55
Staph. aureus (methicillin-resistant)	22	0	0	0	0	20
Streptococcus pyogenes	303	0	0	20	92	99
Streptococci, group B	146	0	0	0	85	99
Viridans streptococci	193	0	0	0	60	90
Enterococci	382	0	0	0	0	0
Streptococcus pneumoniae	78	—	—	—	50	100
Gram-negative						
Haemophilus influenzae	17	—	—	50	100	—
Neissera meningitidis	7	—	50	—	100	—
Neissera gonorrhoeae	106	5	52	97	100	—
Escherichia coli	71	0	0	5	30	75
Klebsiella pneumoniae	35	0	0	6	70	75
Enterobacter	10	0	0	0	10	20
Serratia marcescens	111	0	0	0	5	—
Proteus mirabilis	209	0	0	0	20	60
Proteus (indole-positive)	32	0	0	0	10	40
Salmonella typhi	81	0	0	0	50	95
S. paratyphi A	31	—	—	—	28	97
Shigella spp.	44	—	20	30	75	90
Vibrio cholerae	64	—	—	—	—	84
Brucella spp.	25	0	0	28	92	100
Pseudomonas aeruginosa	11	0	0	0	0	0
P. pseudomallei	10	0	0	0	0	50
Bordetella pertussia	31	20	45	85	97	99
Anaerobic bacteria						
Gram-positive						
Peptococcus spp.	145	8	25	67	97	98
Peptostreptococcus spp.	72	11	37	63	96	100
Propionibacterium acnes	16	12	31	94	100	—
Eubacterium lentum	14	14	14	28	71	100
Clostridium perfringens	34	0	0	15	100	—
Clostridium spp.	17	12	12	53	88	100
Gram-negative						
Veillonella spp.	13	23	46	85	100	—
Bacteroides fragilis	195	0	1	2	23	98
Prevotella melaninogenica	29	14	31	93	96	100
Fusobacterium spp.	18	39	44	56	89	100

*The National Committee for Laboratory Standards recommends that 8 μg/ml or less be considered susceptible, 16 μg/ml intermediate and 32 μg/ml or greater be considered resistant. For *Haemophilus*, ≥2 μg/ml are sensitive, 4 μg/ml intermediate and ≥8 μg/ml resistant. For testing *S. pneumoniae* the breakpoints are ≤4, 8, and ≥ 16 μg/ml.[7]
Data from refs. 8–10, 12, 20, 123, and 129–147.

become more important clinically to treat infections caused by these bacteria.[24, 144–147]

Bacteria develop resistance to chloramphenicol by becoming impermeable to the drug or by producing an enzyme, acetyltransferase, that acetylates the antibiotic to an inactive diacetyl derivative.[148, 149] This latter mechanism has been R factor mediated and has been responsible for widespread epidemics of chloramphenicol-resistant typhoid fever and *Shigella* dysentery in Central and South America, Vietnam, India, and other countries.[150–153] It has been suggested that the unrestricted over-the-counter sales of chloramphenicol in the countries involved may be an important factor that provides antibiotic pressure for the development of these resistant strains.[152, 153] In the United States, chloramphenicol resistance in *Salmonella* has been traced to the use of chloramphenicol on dairy farms.[38]

Pharmacology

Chloramphenicol serum levels achieved by different routes of administration and with different product forms are listed in Figure 24–4. Chloramphenicol in the encapsulated form is well absorbed from the gastrointestinal tract and results in peak serum levels of 12 μg/ml of active antibiotic after a 1-g dose.[154, 155] Since it is a very bitter substance, aqueous solutions may not be accepted by children. A tasteless suspension in the form of chloramphenicol palmitate is available in some countries. This preparation must be hydrolyzed in the intestine to produce active chloramphenicol. Although earlier formulations sometimes produced erratic serum levels, the bioavailability of chloramphenicol palmitate in the current formulation is the same as in the capsules and is effective for children with *H. influenzae* meningitis (A. J. Glazko, Warner-Lambert/Parke-Davis Pharmaceutical Research Division, Ann Arbor, Michigan, personal communication).[156, 157] In the United States, the oral preparations are no longer available. Practitioners must resort to using the intravenous preparation orally; pharmacokinetic data is meager. In one patient receiving an oral dose equivalent to 1 g of chloramphenicol monosuccinate diluted in a glass of milk, peak serum levels at 2 hours were 4.3 μg/ml by microbiologic assay compared with 5.0 μg/ml in three volunteers receiving the compound intravenously and assayed by the same methodology. If oral therapy is required using this intravenous formulation, assays are essential.[158]

The intravenous preparation of the drug is the soluble but inactive chloramphenicol succinate ester that is rapidly hydrolized within the body to biologically active chloramphenicol.[159] This preparation produces active chloramphenicol levels in the serum that are 70% of those obtained after oral administration due to incomplete hydrolysis.[154] Bhutta and colleagues found consistently lower serum levels when treating typhoid fever compared with other diseases with intravenous chloramphenicol in children and suggested a dose of 75 mg/kg/day instead of 50 mg/kg/day to compensate.[160] Intramuscular injection is well tolerated and in most studies produces peak serum levels and areas under the serum-level curve similar to those of intravenous administration.[161–164] In adults with enteric fever, how-

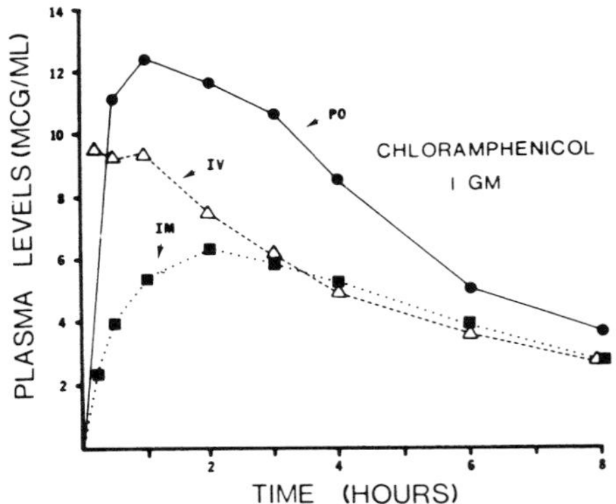

FIGURE 24–4. Plasma levels of active chloramphenicol achieved with 1 g of chloramphenicol administrated orally (Chloromycetin Kapseals) and with chloramphenicol sodium succinate intravenously (IV) and intramuscularly (IM). (Modified from Glazko AJ, Dill WA, Kinkel AW, et al. Absorption and excretion of parenteral doses of chloramphenicol sodium succinate in comparison with peroral doses of chloramphenicol [Abstract]. Clin Pharmacol Ther. 1977;21:104.)

ever, peak concentrations of only one half to two thirds of those obtained by the intravenous route were obtained, and this was associated with a delayed therapeutic response and increased relapse rate of typhoid fever.[165, 166] Since 30% of the unhydrolyzed inactive succinate ester is found in the urine regardless of which parenteral route is used, the lower serum levels produced by intramuscular injection appear to be due to delayed absorption of the ester from the site of injection rather than to decreased hydrolysis.[154, 166] The intramuscular route should be used cautiously.

Chloramphenicol is metabolized primarily by the liver, where it is conjugated with glucuronic acid, and it is excreted in this inactive form by the kidney. The findings of other metabolites in the serum suggests that some biotransformation takes place by oxidation and reduction as well.[167] Only about 5 to 10% of the administered dose is recovered in the urine as biologically active chloramphenicol. Nevertheless, in the absence of renal disease, concentrations of 150 to 200 μg/ml of active drug are achieved, which is sufficient to treat urinary tract infections if necessary. Urinary concentrations are markedly diminished, however, in patients with renal failure.[168]

The use of chloramphenicol in children has led to a better understanding of its pharmacokinetics. It is clear that there is a wide variation in the metabolism and excretion in that age group. Dosage requirements may vary threefold in children of the same age, with even greater variation noted in newborn and young infants. Because newborns metabolize the antibiotic at a slow rate, the initial dose for those younger than 1 week should be 25 mg/kg every 24 hours and for infants from 1 to 4 weeks old, 25 mg/kg every 12 hours instead of the usual 50 mg/kg/day divided into 6-hour dosing intervals for older children and adults. However, the wide variation makes monitoring serum levels imperative.[164, 169, 170]

Chloramphenicol has a half-life in adults of 4.1 hours after single intravenous injections, is not highly bound to protein (25 to 50%), and has an apparent volume of distribution of 100 liters.[123, 154, 171] The antibiotic diffuses well into many tissues and body fluids. Kramer and associates have shown levels in the brain to be 36 μg/ml, whereas corresponding serum levels were 4 μg/ml.[172] These high levels may reflect the antibiotic's high degree of lipid solubility in conjunction with low protein binding and small molecular size.[173] Levels in the cerebrospinal fluid even without inflamed meninges are generally 30 to 50% of serum concentrations, much higher than those of most other antibiotics.[123] Therapeutic levels are obtained in pleural, ascitic, and synovial fluids.[123, 174] In the aqueous humor, levels are approximately 50% of those in the serum,[175] but studies in rabbits and humans suggest that topical administration may be more efficient in providing high aqueous concentrations.[176, 177] Subconjunctival injections are not satisfactory.[178] The antibiotic crosses the placenta to the fetal circulation but produces negligible amounts in the amniotic fluid. Only small amounts of active chloramphenicol are recovered in the bile (0.14% of a 1-g dose).[123]

Renal and Hepatic Insufficiency

The half-life of biologically active chloramphenicol in patients with renal disease differs only slightly from that of healthy subjects, whereas its metabolites increase markedly. However, the dose should not be modified if therapeutic levels of the active drug are to be maintained. Fortunately, the metabolites do not appear to be as toxic as the active compound. Neither peritoneal nor hemodialysis alters serum levels sufficiently to require dose alterations.[171, 179]

Patients with hepatic failure, as evidenced by jaundice or ascites, conjugate chloramphenicol at a slower rate. Serum levels of active chloramphenicol increase to levels capable of bone marrow suppression.[180] The regimen suggested for adults with hepatic insufficiency is an initial 1-g loading dose followed by 500 mg every 6 hours. The course of therapy should be limited when possible to 10 to 14 days and levels should be monitored.

Assay

Because of the narrow therapeutic/toxic ratio, it is important to monitor serum levels of this antibiotic, particularly in newborn and premature infants, in patients with hepatic disease, and in patients taking interacting drugs. There are a number of very effective assays that can be used, including bioassays, radioenzymatic assays, competitive enzyme-linked immunoassays, and high-performance chromotography.[61, 181–189] Serum levels in most cases should be maintained between 10 and 25 μg/ml.

Toxicity

Hematologic

The most important toxic effects of chloramphenicol occur in the bone marrow. The effects can be divided into two types. The first is a reversible bone marrow depression due to a direct pharmacologic effect of the antibiotic as a result of inhibition of mitochondrial protein synthesis. It is manifested by reticulocytopenia, anemia, leukopenia, thrombocytopenia, or any combination thereof. There is an increase in serum iron levels in association with a reduced uptake of radioactive iron by the red blood cells, thus indicating diminished hemoglobin synthesis. The bone marrow reveals vacuolization of the erythyroid and myeloid precursors, but these changes are not specific for chloramphenicol. This type of toxicity is extremely common, occurs during the course of therapy, and is dose related.[190] It is more likely to occur in patients receiving 4 g/day or more or in patients in whom serum levels are above 25 μg/ml, a level that may occur in patients with severe liver disease who are receiving usual doses. It is reversible when treatment with the antibiotic is discontinued.[191]

The second type of toxicity is a rare but generally fatal "idiosyncratic" response that is most frequently manifested as aplastic anemia.[192] Indeed, at one time chloramphenicol toxicity was the most common cause of this syndrome. According to the best epidemiologic studies in the United States, aplastic anemia occurs once in 24,500 to 40,800 patients who receive the antibiotic, a risk about 13 times greater than that for aplastic anemia in the general population.[193] The aplastic anemia most commonly occurs weeks to months after the completion of therapy and is not necessarily dose related. It appears that this toxic effect is caused by a mechanism different from the direct bone marrow suppression previously described. Although the pathogenesis of this idiosyncratic response is not known, there have been several observations and theories that suggest the toxicity is very complex, involving interactions of the host and toxic intermediates of the antibiotic. This type of toxicity has occurred in identical twins, which suggests a genetic predisposition.[194] Morley and coworkers have observed that mice given chloramphenicol after treatment with busulfan had a progressive decrease in the number of pluripotential stem cells, whereas control mice did not,[195] suggesting that the aplastic anemia might result in patients with unrecognized preexisting residual marrow damage either genetic or acquired. In 1967, Holt observed that the aplastic anemia occurred only after oral administration of the antibiotic.[196] He postulated that the fatal reaction may be caused by the absorption of toxic products produced by enzymatic degradation of chloramphenicol, perhaps as a result of specific types of bacteria colonizing the gut of affected people. Supporting this hypothesis, Jimenez and colleagues have shown that one of chloramphenicol's metabolites, dehydrochloramphenicol, is 10- to 20-fold more cytotoxic than chloramphenicol yet is only one third as effective in inhibiting protein synthesis,[197] thus suggesting that this metabolite and perhaps others may play a significant role in this toxicity. These toxic metabolites may undergo further metabolic transformation in the bone marrow with on-site production of toxic intermediates.[198, 199] Although the number of cases reported is greater after oral therapy, a number of cases of aplastic anemia from parenteral chloramphenicol even after the administration of eyedrops have also been reported.[200, 201] These latter cases have received considerable debate but are very rare; estimates of serious hematologic toxicity appear to be no more than 3 in 442,543 patients and most likely much less.[202, 203] In a review of 426 cases of aplastic anemia, none of the patients used chloramphenicol eye drops.[204]

Although most cases of aplastic anemia from chloramphenicol become apparent after the completion of therapy, it should be emphasized that 22% of the cases occur concurrently with antibiotic administration.[192, 201] Whether some of these episodes can be prevented by checking the blood counts of patients is not known. Until the pathogenesis of the toxicity is clearly understood, it is recommended that a complete blood count be obtained on a twice-a-week basis from all patients receiving chloramphenicol. If the white blood cell count decreases below 2500/mm^3, it is desirable to discontinue treatment with the antibiotic if the clinical condition allows. It should be recognized, however, that low numbers of white blood cells may occur in illnesses for which chloramphenicol is used, such as typhoid fever.

Also of concern are the reports of childhood leukemia after the use of chloramphenicol. Although these cases generally follow the aplastic anemia, a population-based case-control interview study of 309 childhood leukemia cases and 618 age- and sex-matched controls showed a significant dose-response relation between chloramphenicol and the risk of both acute lymphocytic and nonlymphocytic leukemia, particularly after treatment for greater than 10 days in children without prior aplastic anemia. Until this is more clearly defined, it seems prudent to change therapy as quickly as possible to alternate agents when organisms prove susceptible to other equally effective and less toxic antibiotics.[205]

Chloramphenicol may also produce a hemolytic anemia in patients with the Mediterranean form of glucose-6-phosphate dehydrogenase deficiency. This apparently does not occur with the milder A type glucose-6-phosphate dehydrogenase deficiency, which is the most common form in blacks.[206]

Gray Baby Syndrome

The gray baby syndrome of neonates is characterized by abdominal distention, vomiting, flaccidity, cynosis, circulatory collapse, and death. The side effect results from a diminished ability of neonates to conjugate chloramphenicol and to excrete the active form in the urine.[207] If chloramphenicol is necessary in premature infants and neonates, the dose should be reduced to 25 mg/kg/day and the antibiotic levels should be monitored. This syndrome has also been recognized in toddlers and after accidental overdoses in adults.[208, 209] It is generally associated with serum concentrations of chloramphenicol of greater than 50 μg/ml and may present with unexplained metabolic acidosis.[210] Large-volume exchange transfusions or charcoal hemoperfusion have been used to accelerate drug removal. This syndrome is due in part to impaired myocardial contractility related to direct interference of myocardial tissue respiration and oxidative phosphorylatation.[211–214]

Optic Neuritis

Optic neuritis resulting in decreased visual acuity has been described in patients receiving prolonged chloramphenicol therapy.[215] The symptoms are generally reversible, but loss of vision has occurred. Other neurologic sequelae such as peripheral neuritis, headache, depression, ophthalmoplegia, and mental confusion have also been described.

Other Types

Hypersensitivity reactions (including rashes and drug fevers) and anaphylaxis are rare. Herxheimer-like responses during therapy for syphilis, brucellosis, and typhoid fever have been observed. Symptoms involving the gastrointestinal tract, including nausea, vomiting and diarrhea, glossitis, and stomatitis, occur but have not been a major problem. Bleeding due to decreased vitamin K synthesis has resulted from prolonged administration.

Significant Drug Interactions

Chloramphenicol prolongs the half-life of tolbutamide, chlorpropamide, phenytoin, cyclophosphamide, and warfarin (Coumadin), apparently by inhibiting hepatic microsomal enzymes.[216–219] Severe toxicity and death have occurred. Phenytoin, rifampin, and phenobarbital have been observed to decrease the serum concentration and increase the total body clearance of chloramphenicol, perhaps by inducing hepatic microsomal enzymes. Serum concentrations should be monitored when these drugs are administered concurrently.[220, 221] The physician should be on the alert for toxicity from other agents that

TABLE 24–7 Indications for Chloramphenicol*

Indications	Comments
Therapy of Choice	
None†	
Effective Alternative Therapy	
Bacterial meningitis	For penicillin-allergic patients.
Haemophilus influenzae	
Streptococcus pneumoniae	
Neisseria meningitidis	
Brain abscess	
Chlamydia psittaci (psittacosis)	
Clostridium perfringens	
Ehrlichiosis	
Rickettsial infections	Preferred by some when patients require parenteral therapy, during pregnancy, and for young children
Rocky Mountain spotted fever	
Typhus (murine)	
Scrub typhus	
Tick-bite fever	
Q fever	
Pseudomonas mallei	Used with streptomycin
Pseudomonas pseudomallei (melioidosis, acute)	Used with doxycycline
Typhoid fever and invasive salmonellosis	Strains in some areas may be chloramphenicol-resistant; not used for gastroenteritis or carrier state.
Vibrio vulnificus cellulitis and/or sepsis	
Yersinia pestis	

*The usual recommended adult dose is 50 mg/kg/day. Some prefer 75 mg/kg/day for the treatment of typhoid fever. For infections of the central nervous system, 100 mg/kg/day is suggested. See text for pediatric doses.

†In some countries, chloramphenicol remains the standard for the therapy of typhoid fever.

are metabolized by the liver when administering this agent and should monitor serum levels when these drugs are administered concurrently. Chloramphenicol may delay the response of anemias to iron, folic acid, and vitamin B_{12}.[222]

Chloramphenicol is primarily a bacteriostatic agent and will antagonize in vitro the bactericidal activity of the penicillins, cephalosporins, and aminoglycoside antibiotics. This has doubtful clinical significance in most instances. However, care should be exercised in the use of such combinations for infections that require bactericidal activity for efficacy such as for infections in the granulocytopenic host or in the treatment of endocarditis.[223] In the treatment of meningitis, the bacteriostatic activity of chloramphenicol against group B streptococci and its in vitro antagonism with ampicillin against this organism are of concern and should be considered in selecting therapy when this organism is likely to be a pathogen.[127]

Indications

The clinical indications for the use of chloramphenicol are listed in Table 24–7. With the possible exception of typhoid fever in areas where cost and availability make it the primary therapy, it is no longer the drug of choice for any specific infection. The third-generation cephalosporins have superseded chloramphenicol for the treatment of bacterial meningitis in infants and children, though chloramphenicol is still used for the treatment of meningitis in the penicillin-allergic patients.[224] Occasionally, the antibiotic is useful when the differential diagnosis includes both meningococcemia and Rocky Mountain spotted fever, diseases that may be difficult to distinguish on clinical characteristics. Of note is the occasional use of chloramphenicol for the treatment of infections caused by multiply resistant organisms, although its use for meningitis caused by penicillin-resistant pneumococcus has been discouraging.[224–228]

REFERENCES

1. Tally FT, Ellestad GA, Testa RT. Glycylcyclines: A new generation of tetracyclines. J Antimicrob Chemother. 1995;35:449–452.
2. Finland M. Twenty-fifth anniversary of the discovery of Aureomycin: The place of the tetracyclines in antimicrobial therapy. Clin Pharmacol Ther. 1974;15:3.
3. Yamaguchi A, Onmori H, Kaneko-Ohdera M, et al. ΔpH-dependent accumulation of tetracycline in *Escherichia coli.* Antimicrob Agents Chemother. 1991;35:53.
4. Chopra I, Hawkey PM, Hinton M. Tetracyclines, molecular and clinical aspects. J Antimicrob Chemother. 1992;29:245–277.
5. Craven GR, Gavin R, Fanning T. The transfer RNA binding site of the 30 S ribosome and the site of tetracycline inhibition. Symp Quant Biol. 1969;34:129.
6. Bread NS, Armentrout SA, Weisberger AS. Inhibition of mammalian protein synthesis by antibiotics. Pharmacol Rev. 1969;21:213.
7. National Committee for Clinical Laboratory Standards. Sixth Informational Supplement: Performance Standards for Antimicrobial Susceptibility Testing: Approved Standard. NCCLS publication M2-AS, M2-A3, and MH-A3. Villanova, Pa: NCCLS; 1995.
8. Steigbigel NH, Reed CR, Finland M. Susceptibility of common pathogenic bacteria to seven tetracycline antibiotics in vitro. Am J Med Sci. 1968;255:179.
9. Finland M. Changing patterns of susceptibility of common bacterial pathogens to antimicrobial agents. Ann Intern Med. 1972;76:1009.
10. Sabath LD, Stumpf LL, Wallace SJ, et al. Susceptibility of *Diplococcus pneumoniae, Haemophilus influenzae,* and *Neisseria meningitidis* to 23 antibiotics. Antimicrob Agents Chemother. 1970;10:53–56.
11. Neu HC. A symposium on the tetracyclines: A major appraisal. Introduction. Bull N Y Acad Med. 1978;54:141.
12. Poulsen RK, Knudsen JC, Petersen MB. In vitro activity of 6 macrolides, clindamycin, and tetracycline on *Streptococcus pneumoniae* with different penicillin susceptibilities. APMIS. 1996;104:227–233.
13. Shea KW, Cunha BA. Doxycycline activity against penicillin-resistant *Streptococcus pneumoniae.* Chest. 1995;108:1775–1776.
14. Centers for Disease Control. Antibiotic-resistant strains of *Neisseria gonorrhoeae.* MMWR Morb Mortal Wkly Rep. 1987;36(Suppl 55)1–18.
15. Sparling PF. Antibiotic resistance in *Neisseria gonorrhoeae.* Med Clin North Am. 1972;56:1133.
16. Eickhoff TC, Bennett JV, Hayes PS, et al. *Pseudomonas pseudomallei* susceptibility to chemotherapeutic agents. J Infect Dis. 1970;121:95.
17. Farrell ID, Hinchliffe PM, Robertson L. Susceptibility of *Brucella* spp. to tetracycline and its analogues. J Clin Pathol. 1976;29:1097.
18. Morris JG Jr., Black RE. Cholera and other vibrioses in the United States. N Engl J Med. 1985;312:343–350.
19. Karmali MA, DeGrandis S, Fleming PC. Antimicrobial susceptibility of *Campylobacter jejuni* with special reference to resistance patterns of Canadian isolates. Antimicrob Agents Chemother. 1981;19:593.
20. Chow AW, Patten V, Dominick B. Susceptibility of *Campylobacter fetus* to twenty-two antimicrobial agents. Antimicrob Agents Chemother. 1978;13:416.
21. Michel J, Rogol M, Dickman D. Susceptibility of clinical isolates of *Campylobacter jejuni* to sixteen antimicrobial agents. Antimicrob Agents Chemother. 1983;23:796.
22. Gordon RC, Thompson TR, Carlson W, et al. Antimicrobial resistance of shigellae isolated in Michigan. JAMA. 1975;231:1159.
23. Wallace RJ, Wiss K. Susceptibility of *Mycobacterium marinum* to tetracyclines and aminoglycosides. Antimicrob Agents Chemother. 1981;20:610.
24. Sutter VL, Finegold SM. Susceptibility of anaerobic bacteria to 23 antimicrobial agents. Antimicrob Agents Chemother. 1976;10:736.
25. Washington JA, Dearing WH, Judd ES, et al. Effect of preoperative antibiotic regimen on development of infection after intestinal surgery: Prospective, randomized, double-blind study. Ann Surg. 1974;180:567.
26. Hojer H, Wetterfors J. Systemic prophylaxis with doxycycline in surgery of the colon and rectum. Ann Surg. 1978;187:362.
27. Johnson SE, Klein GP, Schmid GP, et al. Susceptibility of the Lyme disease spirochete to seven antimicrobial agents. Yale J Biol Med. 1984;57:549–553.
28. Pang LW, Limsomwong N, Boudreau EF, et al. Doxycycline prophylaxis for falciparum malaria: Lancet. 1987;1:1161–1164.
29. Schnappinger D, Hillen W. Tetracyclines: Antibiotic action, uptake, and resistance mechanisms. Arch Microbiol. 1996;165:359–369.
30. Benveniste R, Davies J. Mechanisms of antibiotic resistance in bacteria. Annu Rev Biochem. 1973;42:471.
31. Sompolinsky D, Zemira S. Plasmid-determined resistance to tetracycline. Microbios. 1981;30:109.
32. Park BH, Hendricks M, Malamy MH, et al. Cryptic tetracycline resistance determinant (class F) isolated from *Bacteroides fragilis* mediates resistance in *Escherichia coli* by actively reducing tetracycline accumulation. Antimicrob Agents Chemother. 1987;31:1739–1743.
33. Roberts MC, Kenny GE, Tet M. Tetracycline resistance determinants in *Ureaplasma urealyticum.* Antimicrob Agents Chemother. 1986;29:350–2.
34. Burdett V. Purification and characterization of Tet(M), a protein that renders ribosomes resistant to tetracycline. J Biol Chem. 1991;266:2872–2877.
35. Manavathu EK, Fernandez CL, Cooperman BS, Taylor DE. Molecular studies on the mechanism of tetracycline resistance mediated by Tet(O). Antimicrob Agents Chemother. 1990;34:71–77.
36. Rapoport MI, Calia FM. The use of antibiotics in animal feeds. JAMA. 1974;229:1212.
37. VanLeeuwen WJ, VanEmbden J, Guinee PAM, et al. Decrease in drug resistance in *Salmonella* in the Netherlands. Antimicrob Agents Chemother. 1979;16:237.
38. Spika JS, Waterman SH, Soo Hoo GW, et al. Chloramphenicol-resistant *Salmonella newport* traced through hamburger to dairy farms. N Engl J Med. 1987;316: 565–570.
39. Finland M, Garrod LP. Demethylchlortetracycline. BMJ. 1960;2:959.
40. Fabre J, Milek E, Kalfopoulos P, et al. The kinetics of tetracyclines in man: Digestive absorption and serum concentrations. In: Doxycycline (Vibramycin): A Compendium of Clinical Evaluation. New York: Pfizer Laboratories; 1973:13–18.
41. Lederle Laboratories. Minocin: Minocycline. Pearl River, NY: Lederle Laboratories; 1975.
42. Rosenblatt JE, Barrett JE, Brodie JL, et al. Comparison of in vitro activity and clinical pharmacology of doxycycline with other tetracyclines. Antimicrob Agents Chemother. 1966;6:134–141.
43. Kirby WMM, Roberts CE, Burdick RE. Comparison of two new tetracyclines with tetracycline and demethylchlortetracycline. Antimicrob Agents Chemother. 1961;286–292.
44. Fabre J, Pitton JS, Junz JP, et al. Distribution and excretion of doxycycline in man. Chemotherapia. 1966;11:73.
45. Kunin CM, Dornbush AC, Finland M. Distribution and excretion of four tetracycline analogues in normal young men. J Clin Invest. 1959;38:1950.
46. MacDonald H, Kelley RG, Allen ES, et al. Pharmacokinetic studies on minocycline in man. Clin Pharmacol Ther. 1973;14:852.
47. Kunin CM. Comparative serum binding distribution and excretion of tetracycline and a new analogue methacycline. Proc Soc Exp Biol Med. 1962;110:311.
48. Bennett JV, Mickewait JS, Barrett JE, et al. Comparative serum binding of four tetracyclines under simulated in vivo conditions. Antimicrob Agents Chemother. 1965;5:180–182.
49. Wood WS, Kipnis GP. The concentrations of tetracycline, chlortetracycline and oxytetracycline in the cerebrospinal fluid after intravenous administration. In: Welch H, Marti-Ibanez F, eds. Antibiotics Annual, 1953–1954. New York: Medical Encyclopedia; 1953:98–101.
50. Yim CW, Flynn NM, Fitzgerald FT. Penetration of oral doxycycline into the cerebrospinal fluid of patients with latent or neurosyphilis. Antimicrob Agents Chemother. 1985;28:347.
51. Parker RH, Schmid F. Antimicrobial activity of synovial fluid during therapy of septic arthritis. Arthritis Rheum. 1971;14:96.
52. Lundberg C, Malmburg A, Ivemark BI. Antibiotic concentrations in relation to structural changes in maxillary sinus mucosa following intramuscular or peroral treatment. Scand J Infect Dis. 1974;6:187.
53. Fabre J, Milek E, Kalopoulos P, et al. The kinetics of tetracyclines in man. II. Excretion, penetration in normal and inflammatory tissues, behavior in renal insufficiency and hemodialysis. In: Doxycycline (Vibramycin): A Compendium of Clinical Evaluations. New York: Pfizer Laboratories; 1973:19–28.

54. Hoeprich PD, Warshauer DM. Entry of four tetracyclines into saliva and tears. Antimicrob Agents Chemother. 1974;5:330.
55. LeBlanc AL, Perry JE. Transfer of tetracycline across the human placenta. Tex Rep Biol Med. 1967;25:541.
56. Czeizel AE, Rockenbauer M. Teratogenic study of doxycycline. Obstet Gynecol. 1997;89:524–528.
57. Briggs GG, Freeman RK, Yaffe SJ. Drugs in pregnancy and lactation. 4th ed. Baltimore: Williams & Wilkins; 1994:808–811.
58. Whelton A. Tetracyclines in renal insufficiency: Resolution of a therapeutic dilemma. Bull N Y Acad Med. 1978;54:223.
59. Bennett JV, Brodie JL, Benner EJ, et al. Simplified accurate method for antibiotic assay of clinical specimens. Appl Microbiol. 1966;14:170.
60. Ray A, Newton V. Use of high-performance liquid chromatography to monitor for stability of tetracycline and chlortetracycline in susceptibility determination. Antimicrob Agents Chemother. 1991;35:1264–1266.
61. Klassen MK, Edberg SC. Measurement of antibiotics in human body fluids: Techniques and significance. In: Lorian V (ed). Antibiotics in Laboratory Medicine. 4th ed. Baltimore: Williams & Wilkins; 1996:230–295.
62. Csonka GW, Rosedale N, Walkden L. Balanitis due to fixed drug eruption associated with tetracycline therapy. Br J Vener Dis. 1970;47:42.
63. Fellner MJ, Baer RL. Anaphylactic reaction to tetracycline in a penicillin-allergic patient: Immunologic studies. JAMA. 1965;192:997.
64. Furey WW, Tan C. Anaphylactic shock due to oral demethylchlortetracycline. Ann Intern Med. 1969;70:357.
65. Byrne PAC, Williams BD, Pritchard MH. Minocycline-related lupus. Br J Rheumatol. 1994;33:674–676.
66. Gough A, Chapman S, Wagstaff K, et al. Minocycline induced autoimmune hepatitis and systemic lupus erythematosus-like syndrome. BMJ. 1996;312: 169–172.
67. Singer SJ, Piazza-Hepp TD, Girardi LS, Moledina NR. Lupus-like reaction associated with minocycline. JAMA. 1997;277:295–296.
68. Carey BW. Photodynamic response of a new tetracycline. JAMA. 1960;172:1196.
69. Frost P, Weinstein GD, Gomez EC. Phototoxic potential of minocycline and doxycycline. Arch Dermatol. 1972;105:681.
70. Angeloni VL, Salasche SJ, Ortiz R. Nail, skin and scleral pigmentation induced by minocycline. Cutis. 1987;40:229–233.
71. Atwood HD, Dennet X. A black thyroid and minocycline treatment. BMJ. 1976;2:1109.
72. Siller GM, Tod MA, Savage NW. Minocycline-induced oral pigmentation. J Am Acad Dermatol. 1994;30:350–354.
73. Odell EW, Hodgson RP, Haskell R. Oral presentation of minocycline-induced black bone disease. Oral Surg Oral Med Oral Pathol Oral Radiol Endod. 1995;79:459–461.
74. Brearley LJ, Storey E. Tetracycline-induced tooth changes: Part 2. Prevalence, localization and nature of staining in extracted deciduous teeth. Med J Aust. 1968;2:714.
75. Witkop CJ, Wolf RO. Hypoplasia and intrinsic staining of enamel following tetracycline therapy. JAMA. 1963;185:1008.
76. Cohan S, Bevelander G, Tiamsic T. Growth inhibition of prematures receiving tetracycline. Am J Dis Child. 1963;105:453.
77. Grossman ER, Walcheck A, Freedman H. Tetracycline and permanent teeth: The relationship between doses and tooth color. Pediatrics. 1971;47:567.
78. Department of Health Education and Welfare. Tetracycline pediatric drops to be withdrawn from the market. FDA Drug Bull. 1978;8:23.
79. Forti G, Benincori C. Doxycycline and the teeth. Lancet. 1969;1:782.
80. Schneider R. Doxycycline esophageal ulcers. Am J Dig Dis. 1977;22:805.
81. Winckler K. Tetracycline ulcers of the oesophagus: Endoscopy, histology, and reoentgenology in two cases, and review of the literature. Endoscopy. 1981;13:225.
82. Hinton NA. The effect of oral tetracycline HCl and doxycycline on the intestinal flora. Curr Ther Res. 1970;12:341.
83. Gorbach SL, Bartlett JG. Anaerobic infections. N Engl J Med. 1974;290:1289.
84. Elmore MF, Rogge JD. Tetracycline induced pancreatitis. Gastroenterology. 1981;81:1134.
85. Lepper MH, Wolfe CK, Zimmerman HJ, et al. Effect of large doses of Aureomycin on human liver. Arch Intern Med. 1951;88:271.
86. Schultz JC, Adamson JS Jr, Workman WW, et al. Fatal liver disease after intravenous administration of tetracycline in high doses. N Engl J Med. 1963;269:999.
87. Whalley PJ, Adams RH, Combes B. Tetracycline toxicity in pregnancy: Liver and pancreatic dysfunction. JAMA. 1964;189:357.
88. Damjanov I, Arnold R, Faour M. Tetracycline toxicity in a non-pregnant woman. JAMA. 1968;204:934.
89. Vial T, Biour M, Descotes J, Trepo C. Antibiotic-associated hepatitis: Update from 1990. Ann Pharmacother. 1997;31:304–320.
90. Hunt CM, Washington K. Tetracycline-induced bile duct paucity and prolonged cholestasis. Gastroenterology. 1994;107:1844–1847.
91. Shils ME. Renal disease and the metabolic effects of tetracycline. Ann Intern Med. 1963;58:389.
92. Forrest JN, Cox M, Hong C, et al. Superiority of demeclocycline over lithium in the treatment of chronic syndrome of inappropriate secretion of antidiuretic hormone. N Engl J Med. 1978;298:173.
93. Carrilho F, Bosch J, Arroyo V, et al. Renal failure associated with demeclocycline in cirrhosis. Ann Intern Med. 1977;87:195.
94. Fanning WL, Gump DW, Sofferman RA. Side effects of minocycline: A double blind study. Antimicrob Agents Chemother. 1977;11:712.
95. Koch-Weser J, Gilmore EB. Benign intracranial hypertension in an adult after tetracycline therapy. JAMA. 1967;200:345.
96. Walters BNJ, Gubbay SS. Tetracycline and benign intracranial hypertension: Report of five cases. BMJ. 1981;282:19.
97. Jackson GG, Haight TH, Kass EH, et al. Tetramycin therapy of pneumonia: Clinical and bacteriologic studies in 91 cases. Ann Intern Med. 1951;35:1175.
98. Lundsgaard-Hansen P, Senn A, Roos B, et al. Staphylococcal enteritis: Report of six cases with two fatalities after intravenous administration of *N.*-(pyrrolidinomethyl) tetracycline. JAMA. 1960;173:1008.
99. Leyden JJ. Absorption of minocycline hydrochloride and tetracycline hydrochloride: Effect of food, milk, and iron. J Am Acad Dermatol. 1985;12:308–312.
100. MacArthur CG, Johnson AJ, Allen ES, et al. The absorption and sputum penetration of doxycycline. J Antimicrob Chemother. 1978;4:509–514.
101. Neuvonen PJ, Gothoni G, Hackman R, et al. Interference of iron with the absorption of tetracycline in man. BMJ 1970;4:532.
102. Gugler R, Allgayer H. Effects of antacids on the clinical pharmacokinetics of drugs: An update. Clin Pharmacokinet. 1990;18:210–219.
103. Bar WH, Adir J, Garrettson L. Decrease of tetracycline in man by sodium bicarbonate. Clin Pharmacol Ther. 1971;12:779.
104. Fisher P, House F, Inns P, et al. Effect of cimetidine on the absorption of orally administered tetracycline. Br J Clin Pharmacol. 1980;9:153.
105. Neuvonen PJ, Pentitila O. Interaction between doxycycline and barbiturates. BMJ. 1974;1:535.
106. Pentitla O, Neuvonen PJ, Lehtovaara R. Interaction between doxycycline and some antiepileptic drugs. BMJ. 1974;2:470.
107. Neuvonen PJ, Penttila O, Roos M. Effect of long-term alcohol consumption on the half-life of tetracycline and doxycycline in man. Int J Clin Pharmacol. 1976;14:303.
108. Kuzucu EY. Methoxyflurane, tetracycline and renal failure. JAMA. 1970;211:1162.
109. Semel JD. Renal failure and multiple organ toxicity associated with tetracycline operative prophylaxis. Infect Surg. 1988;June:405–408.
110. Boston Collaborative Drug Surveillance Program. Tetracycline and drug-attributed rises in blood urea nitrogen. JAMA. 1972;220:377.
111. Bacon JF, Chenfield GM. Pregnancy attributable to interaction between tetracycline and oral contraceptives. BMJ. 1980;280:293.
112. Hansen PD. Drug Interactions. 5th ed. Philadelphia: Lea & Febiger; 1985:239.
113. Lepper MH, Dowling HF. Treatment of pneumococcol meningitis with penicillin compared with penicillin plus aureomycin. Arch Intern Med. 1951;88:489.
114. Raoult D, Drancourt M. Antimicrobial therapy of rickettsial diseases. Antimicrob Agents Chemother. 1991;35:2457–2462.
115. Centers for Disease Control and Prevention. 1998 Guidelines for treatment of sexually transmitted diseases. MMWR. 1998;47:1–116.
116. Montecalvo, MA, Horowitz H, Wormser GP, et al. Effect of novobiocin-containing antimicrobial regimens on infection and colonization with vancomycin-resistant *Enterococcus faecium.* Antimicrob Agents Chemother. 1995;39:794.
117. O'Dell JR, Haure CE, Palmer W, et al. Treatment of early rheumatoid arthritis with minocycline or placebo: Results of a randomized, double-blind, placebo-controlled trial. Arthritis Rheum. 1997;40:794–796.
118. Pillemer SR, Fowler SE, Tilley BC, et al. Meaningful improvement criteria sets in a rheumatoid arthritis clinical trial. MIRA trial group. Minocycline in rheumatoid arthritis. Arthritis Rheum. 1997;40:419–425.
119. Walker-Renard PB, Vaughan LM, Sahn SA. Chemical pleurodesis for malignant pleural effusions. Ann Intern Med. 1994;120:56–64.
120. Ehrlich J, Bartz QR, Smith RM, et al. Chloromycetin, a new antibiotic from a soil actinomycete. Science. 1947;106:417.
121. Carter HE, Gottliebb D, Anderson HW. Comments and communications. Science. 107;113:947.
122. Ehrlich J, Gottlieb D, Burkholder PR, et al. *Streptomyces venezuelae,* N sp, the source of chloromycetin. J Bacteriol. 1948;56:467.
123. Woodward TE, Wisseman CL. Chloromycetin (Chloramphenicol). New York: Medical Encyclopedia; 1958.
124. Abdel-Sayed S. Transport of chloramphenicol into sensitive strains of *Escherichia coli* and *Pseudomonas aeruginosa.* J Antimicrob Chemother. 1987;19:7–20.
125. Turk DC. A comparison of chloramphenicol and ampicillin as bactericidal agents for *Haemophilus influenzae* type B. J Med Microbiol. 1977;10:127.
126. Rahal JJ, Simberkoff MS. Bactericidal and bacteriostatic action of chloramphenicol against meningeal pathogens. Antimicrob Agents Chemother. 1979;16:13.
127. Weeks JL, Mason EO Jr, Baker CJ. Antagonism of ampicillin and chloramphenicol for meningeal isolates of group B streptococci. Antimicrob Agents Chemother. 1981;20:281.
128. Roodyn DB, Wilkie D. The Biogenesis of Mitochondria. London: Methuen; 1968.
129. McGowan JE, Garner C, Wilcox C, et al. Antibiotic susceptibility of gram negative bacilli isolated from blood cultures: Results of tests with 35 agents and strains from 169 patients at Boston City Hospital during 1972. Am J Med. 1974;57:225.
130. Yow EM, Spink WW. Experimental studies on the action of streptomycin, Aureomycin and Chloromycetin on *Brucella.* J Clin Invest. 1949;28:871.
131. Robertson RP, Wahab MFA, Raasch FO. Evaluation of chloramphenicol and ampicillin in *Salmonella* enteric fever. N Engl J Med. 1968;278:171.
132. Rubinstein E, Shainberg B. In vitro activity of cinoxacin, ampicillin, and chloramphenicol against *Shigella* and non-typhoid *Salmonella.* Antimicrob Agents Chemother. 1977;11:577.
133. Wells EB, Chang SM, Jackson GG, et al. Antibiotic spectrum of *Hemophilus pertussis.* J Pediatr. 1950;36:752.
134. Cherubin CE, Neu HC, Rahal JJ, et al. Emergence of resistance to chloramphenicol in *Salmonella.* J Infect Dis. 1977;135:807.

135. Long SS, Phillips SE. Chloramphenicol-resistant *Haemophilus influenzae*. J Pediatr. 1976;90:1030.
136. Mathies AW Jr. Penicillins in the treatment of bacterial meningitis. *J R Coll Physicians Lond.* 1972;6:139.
137. Doern GV, Jorgensen JH, Thornsberry C, et al. Prevalance of antimicrobial resistance among clinical isolates of *Haemophilus influenzae*: A collaborative study. Diagn Microbiol Infect Dis. 1986;4:95–107.
138. MacMahon P, Sills J, Hall E, et al. *Haemophilus influenzae* type B resistant to both chloramphenicol and ampicillin in Britain. BMJ. 1982;24:1229.
139. Bergeron MC, Claveau S, Simard P. Limited in vitro activity of cefamandole against 100 beta-lactamase and non–beta-lactamase-producing *Haemophilus influenzae* strains: Comparison of moxalactam, chloramphenicol and ampicillin. Antimicrob Agents Chemother. 1981;19:101.
140. Kenny JF, Isburg CD, Michaels RH. Meningitis due to *Haemophilus influenzae* type b resistant to both ampicillin and chloramphenicol. Pediatrics. 1980;66:14.
141. Campos J, Garcia-Tornel S, San Feliu I. Susceptibility studies of multiply resistant *Haemophilus influenzae* isolated from pediatric patients and contacts. Antimicrob Agents Chemother. 1984;25:706.
142. Williams JD, Mossdeen F. Antibiotic resistance in *Haemophilus influenzae*. Epidemiology, mechanisms, and therapeutic possibilities. Rev Infect Dis. 1986;8(Suppl 5):555–561.
143. Kabani A, Joffe A, Jadavji T. *Haemophilus influenzae* type B resistant to ampicillin and chloramphenicol. Pediatr Infect Dis J. 1991;9:681.
144. Martin WJ, Gardner M, Washington JA II. In vitro antimicrobial susceptibility of anaerobic bacteria isolated from clinical specimens. Antimicrob Agents Chemother. 1972;1:148.
145. Cuchural GJ Jr, Talley FP, Jacobus NV, et al. Susceptibility of the *Bacteroides fragilis* group in the United States: Analysis by site of isolation. Antimicrob Agents Chemother. 1988;32:717–722.
146. Finegold SM, Wexler HM. Therapeutic implications of bacteriologic findings in mixed aerobic-anaerobic infections. Antimicrob Agents Chemother. 1988;32: 611–616.
147. Snydman DR, McDermott L, Cuchural G Jr, et al. Analysis of trends in antimicrobial resistance patterns among clinical isolates of *Bacteroides fragilis* group species from 1990 to 1994. Clin Infect Dis. 1996;23(Suppl 1):S54–S65.
148. Okamoto S, Mizuno D. Mechanism of chloramphenicol and tetracycline resistance in *Escherichia coli*. J Gen Microbiol. 1964;35:125.
149. Okamoto S, Suzuki Y. Chloramphenicol-, dihydrostreptomycin-, and kanamycin-inactivating enzymes from multiple drug-resistant *Escherichia coli* carrying episome "R." Nature. 1965;208:1301.
150. Gangarosa EJ, Bennett JV, Wyatt C, et al. An epidemic-associated episome? J Infect Dis. 1972;126:215.
151. Butler T, Linh NN, Arnold K, et al. Chloramphenicol-resistant typhoid fever in Vietnam associated with R-factor. Lancet. 1973;2:983.
152. Editorial: Drug resistance in salmonellas. Lancet. 1982;1:1391.
153. Halder KK, Dalal BS, Ghose E, Samyal S. Chloramphenicol resistant *Salmonella typhi*: The cause of recent outbreak of enteric fever in Calcutta. Indian J Pathol Microbiol. 1992;35:11–17.
154. Glazko AJ, Dill WA, Kinkel AW, et al. Absorption and excretion of parenteral doses of chloramphenicol sodium succinate in comparison with peroral doses of chloramphenicol (Abstract). Clin Pharmacol Ther. 1977;21:104.
155. Bartelloni PJ, Calia FM, Minchew BH, et al. Absorption and excretion of two chloramphenicol products in humans after oral administration. Am J Med Sci. 1969;258:203.
156. Pickering LK, Hoecker JL, Kramer WG, et al. Clinical pharmacology of two chloramphenicol preparations in children: Sodium succinate (IV) and palmitate (oral) esters. J Pediatr. 1980;96:757.
157. Tuomen EI, Powell KR, Marks MI, et al. Oral chloramphenicol in the treatment of *Haemophilus influenzae* meningitis. J Pediatr. 1981;99:968.
158. Glazko AJ, Carnes HE, Kazenko A, et al. Chloramphenicol. Antibiotics Annual, 1957–1958. New York: Medical Encyclopedia; 1958:792–802.
159. McCrumb FR, Snyder MJ, Hicken WJ. The use of chloramphenicol acid succinate in the treatment of acute infections. In: Welch H, Marti-Ibanez F, eds. Antibiotics Annual, 1957–1958. New York: Medical Encyclopedia; 1958:837–841.
160. Bhutta ZA, Niazi SK, Suria A. Chloramphenicol clearance in typhoid fever. Implications for therapy. Indian J Pediatr. 1992;59:213–219.
161. Ross S, Puig JR, Zarembra EA. Chloramphenicol acid succinate (sodium salt); some preliminary clinical and laboratory observations in infants and children. In: Welch H, Marti-Ibanez F, eds.: Antibiotics Annual, 1957–1958. New York: Medical Encyclopedia; 1958:803–820.
162. McCrumb FR Jr, Snyder MJ, Hicken WJ. The use of chloramphenicol acid succinate in the treatment of acute infections. In: Welch H, Marti-Ibanez F, eds. Antibiotics Annual, 1957–1958. New York: Medical Encyclopedia; 1958:837.
163. Shann F, Linnenmann V, MacKenzie A, et al. Absorption of chloramphenicol sodium succinate after intramuscular administration in children. N Engl J Med. 1985;313:410–414.
164. Smith AL, Weber A. Pharmacology of chloramphenicol. Pediatr Clin North Am. 1983;30:209–336.
165. DuPont HL, Hornick RB, Weiss CF, et al. Evaluation of chloramphenicol acid succinate therapy of induced typhoid fever and Rocky Mountain spotted fever. N Engl J Med. 1970;282:53.
166. Acharya GP, Davis TME, Ho M, et al. Factors affecting the pharmacokinetics of parenteral chloramphenicol in enteric fever. J Antimicrob Chemother. 1997;40: 91–98.
167. Holt DE, Hurley R, Harvey D. A reappraisal of chloramphenicol metabolism: Detection and quantification of metabolites in the sera of children. J Antimicrob Chemother. 1995;35:115–127.
168. Lindberg AA, Nilsson LH, Bucht H, et al. Concentration of chloramphenicol in the urine and blood in relation to renal function. BMJ. 1966;2:724.
169. Kauffman RE, Miceti JN, Strebel L, et al. Pharmacokinetics of chloramphenicol and chloramphenicol succinate in infants and children. J Pediatr. 1981;98:315.
170. Kauffman RE, Thirumoorthi MC, Buckley JA, et al. Relative bioavailability of intravenous chloramphenicol succinate and oral chloramphenicol palmitate in infants and children. J Pediatr. 1981;99:363.
171. Kunin CM. A guide to use of antibiotics in patients with renal disease. Ann Intern Med. 1967;67:151.
172. Kramer PW, Griffith RS, Campbell RL, et al. Antibiotic penetration of the brain: A comparative study. J Neurosurg. 1969;31:295.
173. Braude AI: Antimicrobial Drug Therapy. Philadelphia: WB Saunders; 1976:82.
174. Rapp GF, Griffith RS, Hebble WM. The permeability of traumatically inflamed synovial membrane to commonly used antibiotics. J Bone Joint Surg Am. 1966;48:1534.
175. Abraham RK, Burnett HH. Tetracycline and chloramphenicol studies on rabbit and human eyes. Arch Ophthalmol. 1955;54:641.
176. Beasley H, Boltralik JJ, Baldwin HA. Chloramphenicol in aqueous humor after topical application. Arch Ophthalmol. 1975;93:184.
177. George FJ, Hanna C. Ocular penetration of chloramphenicol. Arch Ophthalmol. 1977;95:879.
178. McPherson SD Jr, Presley GD, Crawford JR. Aqueous humor assays of subconjunctival antibiotics. Am J Ophthalmol. 1968;66:430.
179. Kunin CM, Glazko AJ, Finland M. Persistence of antibiotics in blood of patients with acute renal failure. II. Chloramphenicol and its metabolic products in the blood of patients with severe renal disease or hepatic cirrhosis. J Clin Invest. 1959;38:1498.
180. Suhrland LG, Weisberger AS. Chloramphenicol toxicity in liver and renal disease. Arch Intern Med. 1963;112:161.
181. Louie TJ, Tally FP, Bartlett JG, et al. Rapid microbiological assay for chloramphenicol and tetracyclines. Antimicrob Agents Chemother. 1976;9:874.
182. Jorgensen JH, Alexander GA. Rapid bioassay for chloramphenicol in the presence of other antibiotics. Am J Clin Pathol. 1981;76:474.
183. Lietman PS, White TJ, Shaw WV. Chloramphenicol: An enzymological microassay. Antimicrob Agents Chemother. 1976;10:347.
184. Smith AL, Smith DH. Improved enzymatic analysis of chloramphenicol. Clin Chem. 1978;24:1452.
185. Aravind MK, Miceli JN, Kauffman RE, et al. Simultaneous measurements of chloramphenicol and chloramphenicol succinate in body fluids utilizing HPLC. J Chromatogr. 1980;221:176.
186. Nahata MC, Powell DA. Simultaneous determination of chloramphenicol and its succinate ester by high-performance liquid chromatography. J Chromatogr. 1981;223:247.
187. Cambell GS, Mageau RP, Schwab B, et al. Detection and quantitation of chloramphenicol by competitive enzyme-linked immunoassay. Antimicrob Agents Chemother. 1984;25:205–211.
188. Abou-Khalil S, Abou-Khalil WH, Masoud AM, et al. High-performance liquid chromatographic determination of chloramphenicol and four analogues using reductive and oxidative electrochemical and ultraviolet detection. J Chromatogr. 1987;417:111–119.
189. Schwartz JC, Castro DT, Ayo S, et al. A commercial enzyme immunoassay method (EMIT) compared with liquid chromatography and bioassay methods for measurement of chloramphenicol. Clin Chem. 1988;34:1872–1875.
190. Yunis AA. Chloramphenicol-induced bone marrow suppression. Semin Hematol. 1973;10:225.
191. Scott JL, Finegold SM, Belkin GA, et al. A controlled double-blind study of the hematologic toxicity of chloramphenicol. N Engl J Med. 1965;272:1137.
192. Best WR. Chloramphenicol-associated blood dyscrasias. A review of cases submitted to the American Medical Association Registry. JAMA. 1967;201:181.
193. Wallerstein RO, Condit PK, Kasper CK, et al. Statewide study of chloramphenicol therapy and fatal aplastic anemia. JAMA. 1969;208:2045.
194. Nagao T, Mauer AM. Concordance for drug-induced aplastic anemia in identical twins. N Engl J Med. 1969;281:7.
195. Morley A, Trainor K, Remes J. Residual marrow damage: Possible explanation for idiosyncrasy to chloramphenicol. Br J Haematol. 1976;32:525.
196. Holt R. The bacterial degradation of chloramphenicol. Lancet. 1967;1:1259.
197. Jimenez JJ, Arimura GK, Abou-Khalil WH, et al. Chloramphenicol-induced bone marrow injury: Possible role of bacterial metabolites of chloramphenicol. Blood. 1987;70:1180–1185.
198. Jimenez JJ, Jimenez JG, Daghistani D, Yunis AA. Interaction of chloramphenicol and metabolites with colony stimulating factors: Possible role in chloramphenicol-induced bone marrow injury. Am J Med Sci. 1990;300:350–3.
199. Yunis AA. Chloramphenicol toxicity: 25 years of research. Am J Med. 1989;87(3N):44N–48N.
200. Plaut ME, Best WR. Aplastic anemia after parenteral chloramphenicol: Warning renewal (Letter). N Engl J Med. 1982;306:1486.
201. Daum RS, Cohen DL, Smith AL. Fatal aplastic anemia following apparent "dose-related" chloramphenicol toxicity. J Pediatr. 1979;94:403.
202. Lancaster T, Stewart AM, Jick H. Risk of serious hematological toxicity with use of chloramphenicol eye drops in a British general practice database. BMJ. 1998;316:667.
203. Doona M, Walsh JB. Use of chloramphenicol as topical eye medication: Time to cry halt (Editorial) (see comments)? BMJ. 1995;310:1217–1218.

204. Wiholm BE, Kelly JP, Kaufman D, et al. Relation of aplastic anaemia to use of chloramphenicol eye drops in two international case-control studies. BMJ. 1998;316:666.
205. Shu XO, Linet MS, Gao RN, et al. Chloramphenicol use and childhood leukaemia in Shanghai. Lancet. 1987;2:934–937.
206. Beutler E. Glucose 6-phosphate dehydrogenase deficiency. In: Williams WJ, Beutler E, Erslev AJ, et al, eds. Hematology. New York: McGraw-Hill; 1977:466.
207. Burns LE, Hodgman JE, Cass AB. Fatal circulatory collapse in premature infants receiving chloramphenicol. N Engl J Med. 1959;261:1318.
208. Craft AW, Brocklebank JT, Hey EN, et al. The "grey toddler:" Chloramphenicol toxicity. Arch Dis Child. 1974;49:235.
209. Thompson WL, Anderson SE, Lipsky JJ, et al. Overdoses of chloramphenicol. JAMA. 1975;234:149.
210. Evans LS, Kleiman MB. Acidosis as a presenting feature of chloramphenicol toxicity. J Pediatr. 1986;108:475–477.
211. Fripp RR, Carter MC, Werner JC, et al. Cardiac function and acute chloramphenicol toxicity. J Pediatr. 1983;103:487–490.
212. Suarez CR, Ow EP. Chloramphenicol toxicity associated with severe cardiac dysfunction. Pediatr Cardiol. 1992;13:48–51.
213. Stevens DC, Kleinman MB, Lietman PS, et al. Exchange transfusion in acute chloramphenicol toxicity. J Pediatr. 1981;99:651.
214. Freundlick M, Cynamon H, Tamer A, et al. Management of chloramphenicol intoxication in infancy by charcoal hemoperfusion. J Pediatr. 1983;103:485.
215. Chloramphenicol blindness (Editorial). BMJ. 1965;1:1511.
216. Christensen LK, Skovsted L. Inhibition of drug metabolism by chloramphenicol. Lancet. 1969;2:1397.
217. Petitpierre B, Fabre J. Chlorpropamide and chloramphenicol. Lancet. 1970;1:789.
218. Rose JQ, Choi HK, Schentag JJ. Intoxication caused by interaction of chloramphenicol and phenytoin. JAMA. 1977;237:2630.
219. Faber OK, Mouridsen HT, Skovsted L, et al. The effect of chloramphenicol and sulphaphenazole on the biotransformation of cyclophosphamide in man. Br J Clin Pharmacol. 1975;2:281.
220. Powell DA, Nahata MC, Durrell DC, et al. Interactions among chloramphenicol, phenytoin and phenobarbital in a pediatric patient. J Pediatr. 1981;98:1001.
221. Prober CG. Effect of rifampin on chloramphenicol levels. N Engl J Med. 1985;312:788–789.
222. JiJi RM, Gangarosa EJ, de la Macorra F. Chloramphenicol and its sulfamoyl analogue. Report of reversible erythropoietic toxicity in healthy volunteers. Arch Intern Med. 1963;11:70.
223. Sande MA, Overton JW. In vivo antagonism between gentamicin and chloramphenicol in neutropenic mice. J Infect Dis. 1973;128:247.
224. Klass PE, Klein JO. Therapy of bacterial sepsis, meningitis and otitis media in infants and children: 1992 poll of directors of programs in pediatric infectious diseases. Pediatr Infect Dis J. 1992;11:702–705.
225. Norris AH, Reilly JP, Edelstein PH, et al. Chloramphenicol for the treatment of vancomycin-resistant enterococcal infections. Clin Infect Dis. 1995;20:1137–1144.
226. Messick CR, Pendland SL. In vitro activity of chloramphenicol alone and in combination with vancomycin, ampicillin, or RP 59500 (quinupristin/dalfopristin) against vancomycin-resistant enterococci. Diagn Microbiol Infect Dis. 1997;29:203–205.
227. Mundlein E, von Baum H, Geiss HK, et al. Life-threatening infection with multiresistant *Staphylococcus epidermidis* in a patient with end-stage renal disease: Cure with chloramphenicol and quinupristin/dalfopristin (RP 59500). Infection. 1997;25:252–254.
228. Bradley JS, Scheld WM. The challenge of penicillin-resistant *Streptococcus pneumoniae* meningitis: Current antibiotic therapy in the 1990s. Clin Infect Dis. 1997;24(Suppl 2):S213–S221.

Chapter 25

Rifamycins

BARRY M. FARR

Rifampin is a semisynthetic derivative of rifamycin B, a macrocyclic antibiotic compound produced by the mold *Streptomyces mediterranei*. First isolated from fermentation culture of a soil isolate in 1957, rifamycins were named for a then-current French movie, *Rififi*.[1] Rifampin, which is the 3,4-methylpiperazinyliminomethyl derivative of rifamycin SV, is more soluble and active in vitro than is its parent compound (Fig. 25–1).[2] Rifampin is a zwitterion (inner salt) that is soluble in acidic aqueous solution, is even more soluble in organic solvents, and displays remarkable diffusion through lipids.[3]

MECHANISM OF ACTION

The rifamycins exert a bactericidal effect by inhibition of DNA-dependent RNA polymerase at the β-subunit, which prevents chain initiation but not elongation.[4] Mammalian mitochondrial RNA synthesis is not impaired at clinically achievable concentrations.

PHARMACOLOGY

Rifampin is available in the United States as a capsule of orange-red powder and as a solution for intravenous infusion. The oral preparation is almost completely absorbed from the gastrointestinal tract to yield peak plasma concentrations of approximately 7 to 10 μg/ml (range, 4 to 32) within 1 to 4 hours after the ingestion of 600 mg in adults or 10 mg/kg of body weight in children. Higher doses such as 1200 mg in adults result in a similar, more-than-proportional increase in the peak (≥30 μg/ml) serum concentration, because such doses exceed the biliary transport maximum (Tm) for the excretion of rifampin.[5] The area under the curve shows a similar, more-than-proportional increase after saturation of the biliary Tm, which usually occurs with doses between 300 and 450 mg. For this reason, a single daily dose 450 mg or greater results in higher area-under-the-curve values for rifampin than do divided doses totaling the same amount.

The recommended dosage is usually 10 to 20 mg/kg (600 mg maximum) in a single daily administration. A 1% weight/volume oral suspension containing 10 mg/ml may be prepared by mixing the contents of four 300-mg capsules with 120 ml of any of several commercially available syrups according to the directions in the package insert or the *Physicians' Desk Reference*.[6] It should not be cosuspended with other antituberculosis agents such as isoniazid or pyrazinamide, or with ascorbic acid, because such cosuspensions are associated with a significant decline in detectable concentrations of the drugs.[7] Fixed-dose combinations with isoniazid or pyrazinamide, or both, in a capsule or tablet have not resulted in impaired absorption, however, and can be used to prevent ill-advised monotherapy of tuberculosis.[8] An oral desensitization protocol for rifampin was adapted from one devised for penicillin and used successfully in treating patients with previous cutaneous hypersensitivity reactions to rifampin.[9]

Dosage adjustment is unnecessary in renal failure, but rifampin should be avoided or used with caution (perhaps at a lower dosage) in patients with hepatic dysfunction. Food with a high fat concentration interferes with absorption, lowering and delaying peak blood levels.[10] Para-aminosalicylic acid also interferes with absorption. In one study, absorption was found to be diminished in patients with acquired immunodeficiency syndrome (AIDS) and D-xylose malabsorption.[11]

The drug is 80% protein bound in serum and distributes into a volume calculated to be 160% of body weight. Plasma clearance is through hepatic uptake, deacetylation to an active metabolite, and biliary excretion. Deacetylation diminishes reabsorption and increases fecal excretion, but there is significant enterohepatic circula-

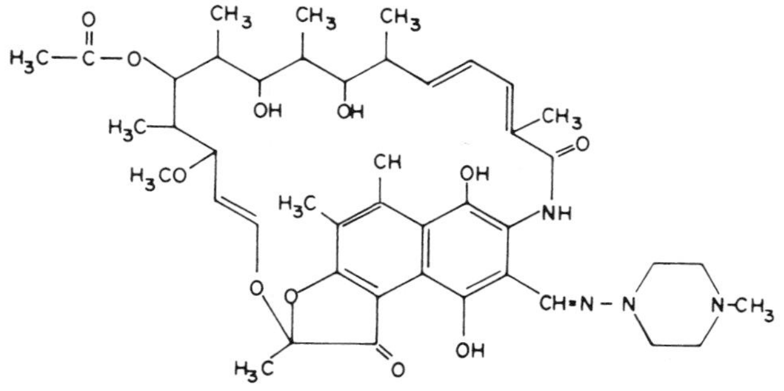

FIGURE 25–1. Structure of rifampin.

tion. The half-life is initially 2 to 5 hours, but it decreases by 40% during the first 2 weeks of therapy because of enhanced biliary excretion. Slow acetylators of isoniazid have an accelerated clearance of rifampin. From 6 to 30% of a dose is excreted in the urine. Probenecid does not consistently affect rifampin serum levels. Renal excretion is reduced in elderly patients, but serum levels remain similar to those in young adults because of hepatic clearance.[12] Pharmacokinetics in pediatric patients are similar to those in adults.[13] The intravenous preparation yields higher peak concentrations of about 27 μg/ml but otherwise similar pharmocokinetics.[14]

Rifampin penetrates well into almost all body tissues. In lung, liver, bile, cholecystic wall, and urine, it achieves concentrations that exceed peak blood levels.[15] Peak concentrations average 300 to 350 μg/ml in urine.[5] The concentration in tears is similar to that in serum, and salivary concentrations are about 20% of those in serum. It achieves therapeutic levels in pleural exudate, sputum,[5] ascites, cavity fluid, milk, urinary bladder wall, skin blister fluid,[16] and soft tissues. It penetrates bone, with higher levels being reached in the presence of osteomyelitis.[15] Aqueous humor concentrations ranged from 0.2 to 1.3 μg/ml after a single oral dose of 600 mg in patients undergoing cataract removal.[17] In a rabbit model, mean concentrations in the vitreous were approximately half those measured in the aqueous humor.[18] Cerebrospinal fluid levels of zero to 0.5 μg/ml have been achieved in healthy people, and higher levels (up to 1.3 μg/ml) have been observed during meningitis after a standard oral dosage of 600 mg/day. Rifampin has also been shown to penetrate and sterilize abscess fluid more readily than do most other antibiotics with similar antibacterial activity.[19, 20] This may relate both to the drug's high lipid solubility and to its relatively unusual ability to enter living phagocytes and kill intracellular bacteria.[3, 16, 20]

ANTIMICROBIAL ACTIVITY

Rifampin exhibits bactericidal activity against a wide range of organisms (Table 25–1).[21, 22] It is extremely active against staphylococci (both coagulase-positive and coagulase-negative strains) and is also effective against other gram-positive cocci. It is active against the pulmonary pathogen *Rhodococcus equi*, which is usually resistant to penicillin.[23] *Neisseria meningitidis, Neisseria gonorrhoeae*, and *Haemophilus influenzae* are the most sensitive gram-negative species. Rifampin has less activity than do tetracycline, chloramphenicol, or aminoglycosides against most gram-negative aerobic bacilli.

Rifampin is the most active agent known against the various species and strains of *Legionella*, being clearly more active than erythromycin, the drug of choice for legionellosis.[22] It is as active as vancomycin in vitro against *Clostridium difficile*, the organism associated with pseudomembranous colitis.

Mycobacterium tuberculosis has remained quite sensitive to rifampin, with most epidemiologic surveys finding less than 4% initial resistance to the drug.[24–26] *Mycobacterium ulcerans* is equally sensitive. A spiropiperidyl rifamycin called *rifabutin* (ansamycin) has potent in vitro activity against many mycobacteria, including the *Mycobacterium avium-intracellulare* complex and *Mycobacterium fortuitum*,[27] as do the new derivatives, the benzoxazinorifamycins.[28]

The rifamycins possess antiviral and possible antitumor activity but have not proved clinically useful at usual therapeutic levels. Rifampin is among the most active agents against *Chlamydia*, including *Chlamydia trachomatis* (lymphogranuloma venereum and non–lymphogranuloma venereum strains) and *Chlamydia psittaci*.[29] *Ureaplasma urealyticum* and *Treponema pallidum* are usually resistant. Rifampin has shown synergy with amphotericin B in vitro and in animal models of infection with fungal species such as *Histoplasma capsulatum, Aspergillus* spp.,[30] and *Fusarium proliferatum*[31] and also with itraconazole against *Cryptococcus neoformans*.[32] The clinical significance of this, if any, is unclear.

Bacteria rapidly develop resistance to rifampin in vitro or in vivo due to mutations altering the β-subunit of the DNA-dependent RNA polymerase. These mutations may occur at many different sites in

TABLE 25–1 Susceptibility of Various Bacteria to Rifampin

Species (n)	MICs (μg/ml) Range (Mode)	MIC_{50}	MIC_{90}
Gram-positive bacteria			
Staphylococcus aureus (26)	0.008–0.015 (0.015)	0.015	0.015
Staphylococcus epidermidis (25)	0.004–0.015 (0.015)	0.015	0.015
Group A streptococci (25)	0.03–0.12 (0.12)	0.12	0.12
Group B streptococci (25)	0.25–1 (1)	1.0	1.0
Streptococcus pneumoniae (28)	0.06–32 (0.06)	0.12	4.0
Viridans group			
Streptococci (34)	0.03–8 (0.06)	0.06	0.12
Enterococcus faecalis (16)	1.0–8 (2)	2.0	8.0
Haemophilus influenzae (26)	0.5–64 (1)	1.0	1.0
Neisseria gonorrhoeae (29)	0.06–2 (0.25)	0.25	0.5
Neisseria meningitidis (26)	0.015–1 (0.015)	0.03	0.5
Listeria monocytogenes (40)	≤0.12–0.25 (≤0.12)	≤0.12	0.25
Mycobacterium fortuitum (18)	16.0–>64 (>64)	>64	>64
Mycobacterium chelonae (15)	>64 (>64)	>64	>64
Gram-negative bacteria			
Escherichia coli (15)	8–16 (8)	8	16
Klebsiella pneumoniae (14)	16–32 (32)	32	32
Enterobacter agglomerans (14)	8–64 (32)	32	64
Enterobacter cloacae (13)	16–64 (32)	64	64
Enterobacter aerogenes (15)	16–64 (32)	32	64
Citrobacter freundii (4)	32 (32)	32	32
Citrobacter diversus (4)	32 (32)	32	32
Proteus mirabilis (15)	4–8 (4)	4	8
Proteus vulgaris (17)	8–32 (32)	16	32
Morganella morganii (15)	8–32 (32)	16	32
Providencia rettgeri (15)	8–64 (8, 16)	16	32
Providencia stuartii (15)	4–16 (8)	8	16
Serratia marcescens (15)	32–64 (64)	64	64
Acinetobacter spp. (15)	4–16 (8)	8	8
Pseudomonas aeruginosa (17)	32–>64 (32)	32	64
Pseudomonas spp. (12)	4–>64 (8)	8	32

Abbreviation: MIC, Minimal inhibitory concentration.
From Thornsberry C, Hill BC, Swenson JM, et al. Rifampin. Spectrum of antibacterial activity. Rev. Infect. Dis. 1983; 5(Suppl): 412.

the RNA polymerase and lead to various degrees of resistance to rifampin.[33] Approximately 1 out of every 10^{11} tubercle bacilli is a resistant mutant. A national survey of 3313 isolates in the first quarter of 1991 found the incidence of rifampin resistance among previously untreated tuberculous patients to be 3.5% compared with 9% of patients previously treated for tuberculosis. The rates of isoniazid resistance in this same survey were much higher, 8.2 and 21.5% for untreated and previously treated patients, respectively.[26]

The mutation rate to rifampin resistance among other bacteria is higher than that for *M. tuberculosis* (e.g., *Staphylococcus aureus*, 10^{-7}; *Streptococcus* spp., 10^{-7}; *H. influenzae* type B, 10^{-7}; meningococci, 10^{-7}; and *Escherichia coli*, 10^{-8}).[21, 34] Except for short-term meningitis prophylaxis, rifampin should not be used alone because of this rapid development of resistance during monotherapy.

ADVERSE EFFECTS

Short-term meningitis prophylaxis with rifampin has been associated with mild, reversible symptoms in 20 to 25% of recipients compared with about 10% of placebo recipients.[35, 36] The symptoms reported most frequently have been dizziness, drowsiness, abdominal pain, diarrhea, nausea, vomiting, headache, visual change, pruritus, and rash. Each of these symptoms usually occurs in less than 5 to 10% of recipients.[36] An orange-red discoloration of urine and permanent staining of soft contact lenses may also occur with such brief regimens.

Chronic daily therapy is associated with a mild, usually self-limited maculopapular rash in up to 5% of patients. More severe rashes such as exfoliative dermatitis and toxic epidermal necrolysis have been rarely reported as being associated with rifampin.[37, 38] Fixed drug eruptions have also been rarely reported.[39] Gastrointestinal complaints are noted by 1 to 2% of patients. Rantitidine, 150 mg twice daily, was shown in a randomized trial to reduce the frequency of gastrointestinal complaints with rifampin therapy without altering rifampin serum concentrations.[40] An asymptomatic elevation of serum enzyme levels is observed in up to 14% of adult patients,[21] and overt hepatitis in 1% of patients receiving rifampin with combination antituberculous therapy excluding isoniazid and in 2.6% of patients receiving both rifampin and isoniazid.[41] The addition of isoniazid to rifampin therapy increases the risk of hepatitis, but the combination is usually considered acceptably safe in the absence of prior liver disease.[42] Hepatotoxicity is more common with advanced age, alcoholism, and malnutrition.[43] Hepatic enzyme abnormalities tend to normalize in asymptomatic patients without treatment adjustment.[44] In a recent national survey, 14 of 430 children treated with rifampin and isoniazid for tuberculosis (3.3%) were reported to have hepatotoxic reactions.[45] In a study of rifampin (15 mg/kg/day) and higher-dose isoniazid (15 to 20 mg/kg/day) therapy for children with severe tuberculosis, 36 of 44 developed an elevation of hepatic enzyme levels during therapy, and one child died of hepatitis.[46] A meta-analysis of seven pediatric studies showed that the combination of isoniazid with rifampin resulted in a significantly higher rate of clinical hepatitis (6.9%) than did isoniazid alone (0.2%).[41] Some patients develop cholestatic jaundice with rifampin therapy.[47] Rifampin causes an increase in serum bile acid levels and can cause slight elevations of serum bilirubin concentrations that return to normal during the first week of therapy in the absence of hepatitis. This increase in bilirubin levels appears to be due to a competitive inhibition of hepatic bilirubin metabolism.[41]

Acute renal failure has been reported during daily therapy and has occasionally required dialysis.[48] The renal failure has been related to a variety of different mechanisms, including interstitial nephritis, glomerulonephritis, and massive hemolysis.[49, 50] Light-chain proteinuria has been reported to occur in a majority of patients receiving rifampin without apparent ill effect, but in the setting of dehydration these proteins may contribute to the development of a cast nephropathy and acute renal failure on this basis.[51, 52]

Intermittent administration (less than twice per week) and high individual dosages (greater than or equal to 1200 mg) have been associated with an increased incidence of side effects. A flulike syndrome with fever, chills, and myalgias may develop in up to 20% of patients after several months of intermittent therapy and correlates with the presence of antirifampin antibodies.[53] These patients may develop eosinophilia, interstitial nephritis, acute tubular necrosis, thrombocytopenia, hemolytic anemia, and even shock.[54–56] Acute massive hemolysis is rarely associated with such flulike reactions after intermittent therapy, in which case nausea, vomiting, flank pain, and brown turbid urine may be observed; most patients with massive hemolysis develop acute renal failure.[57–60] Anaphylaxis has been rarely reported with systemic therapy[61] but was recently reported in four patients at a French hospital where surgeons washed surgical wounds with a rifampin-containing solution (three orthopedic cases and one urethrotomy).[62]

Various effects of rifampin on the central nervous system have been reported, including rare cases of organic brain syndrome. Pseudomembranous colitis has been observed in animal models after rifampin administration to animals colonized with a rifampin-resistant strain of *C. difficile*. Pseudomembranous colitis has rarely occurred with rifampin-resistant *C. difficile* during rifampin therapy. This appears to be a very rare side effect with only a few reports of such an association despite widespread chronic use of rifampin in antituberculous chemotherapy.[63–65] Pancreatitis has been reported in rare cases. One case of hemorrhagic gastritis has been reported that responded to cessation of rifampin therapy and recurred with readministration.[66] Patients have survived overdoses of up to 12 g, turning "lobster red" for several days; facial or periorbital edema, pruritus of the head, and vomiting each occur in a majority of cases of the "red man syndrome" after an overdose.[67, 68]

Rifampin causes a reduction in 25-hydroxycholecalciferol levels without changing the levels of 1,25-dihydroxycholecalciferol or parathyroid hormone, and osteomalacia has been mentioned as a possible side effect with long-term treatment. It causes increased deiodination and biliary clearance of thyroxine and lowers the serum concentration of thyroxine. The serum concentration of triiodothyronine remains normal.

Immunosuppression has been an alleged side effect of rifampin therapy. Contradictory studies have found diminished or normal antibody responses to various antigens such as sheep red blood cells, pneumococcal vaccine, and tetanus toxoid. Some workers have suggested blunted cell-mediated immunity with a diminished response to phytohemagglutinin in vitro, whereas others have shown no change in response to phytohemagglutinin, concanavalin A, pokeweed mitogen, or purified protein derivative. Skin tests with purified protein derivative have not been consistently altered by rifampin therapy, and no ill effect from this possible immunosuppression in the form of opportunistic infection or an inability to heal tuberculosis has been reported.[69] Rifampin readily crosses the placenta and has caused teratogenic effects in rodents treated with high doses; such effects have not been observed in humans, except in patients with severe tuberculosis, but during pregnancy rifampin should only be used for severe tuberculous infections.[70]

DRUG INTERACTIONS

Rifampin competitively inhibits the hepatic uptake of several compounds such as cholecystografin and sulfobromophthalein. Rifampin is one of the most potent inducing agents for intestinal and hepatic microsomal enzymes,[71, 72] leading to reduced oral bioavailability and to a decreased serum half-life for a number of compounds including prednisone, norethisterone, digitoxin, quinidine, ketoconazole, and the sulfonylureas (Table 25–2).[73–77] These effects have been reported to cause decreased efficacy of oral contraceptive agents, relapse of arrhythmias during quinidine therapy, decompensation of heart failure during digoxin or digitoxin therapy, and exacerbation of diabetes during oral hypoglycemic therapy. Rifampin also reduces the efficacy of warfarin, causing a reduction in the prothrombin time in patients anticoagulated with this drug. Patients receiving glucocorticoid therapy for Addison's disease or asthma have relapsed, and transplant patients receiving cyclosporine therapy have developed acute rejection when given rifampin. Hypothyroid patients receiving replacement L-thyroxine may require an increased dosage.[76]

Aluminum hydroxide–containing antacids were associated with significantly lower rifampin peak concentrations in one randomized trial.[78] Rifampin significantly decreases the serum concentrations of ketoconazole, which in turn may decrease rifampin concentrations[79]; the U.S. Food and Drug Administration has advised against using this

TABLE 25–2 Medications for Which Serum Concentrations Are Decreased through Enhancement of Hepatic or Intestinal Metabolism by Rifampin*

Amprenavir	Estrogens	Phenytoin
Barbiturates	Fluconazole	Propafenone
Chloramphenicol	Haloperidol	Propranolol
Cimetidine	Indinavir	Quinidine
Clarithromycin	Itraconazole	Ritonavir
Clofibrate	Ketoconazole	Saquinavir
Contraceptive, oral	Levothyroxine	Sulfonylureas
Corticosteroids	Lorcainide	Tertatolol
Cyclosporine	Losartan	Tocainide
Dapsone	Metoprolol	Theophylline
Delavirdine	Methadone	Thyroxine
Digitoxin	Midazolam	Triazolam
Digoxin	Mexiletine	Verapamil
Diltiazem	Nelfinavir	Warfarin
Diazepam	Nifedipine	Zidovudine
Disopyramide	Nitrazepam	Zolpidem
Doxycycline	Nortryptyline	Zopiclone
Efavirenz	Novobiocin	

*See Strayhorn and colleagues[310] and Rizak[311] for a complete list.

drug combination.[80] Trimethoprim-sulfamethoxazole administration results in increased rifampin levels.[81, 82]

THERAPEUTIC USES

Mycobacterial Infections

The unique pharmacology and bactericidal activity of rifampin have revolutionized chemotherapy for pulmonary tuberculosis, with rifampin-containing treatment courses of 6 to 9 months yielding cure rates equal to those achieved with 18 months of regimens without rifampin.[83] The regimen of choice for uncomplicated pulmonary or extrapulmonary tuberculosis (e.g., involving lymph nodes, pleura, or meninges) is now 6 months of daily rifampin (15 mg/kg/day; maximum, 600 mg) and isoniazid (10 mg/kg/day; maximum, 300 mg), with daily pyrazinamide being added for the first 2 months.[84–91] In most areas, a fourth drug, ethambutol or streptomycin, is recommended until susceptibility to isoniazid and rifampin is documented.[92] Therapy of tuberculosis with 2 months of isoniazid, rifampin, pyrazinamide, and sometimes ethambutol followed by 7 months of isoniazid and rifampin therapy was evaluated in 89 patients with human immunodeficiency virus infection; 52 of 54 had sputum cultures revert to negative within 3 months, and no relapses occurred during 916 patient-months of follow-up.[93] Combinations excluding rifampin have resulted in relapse rates exceeding 20% with such short courses.[94, 95] Almost half of patients with pulmonary tuberculosis resistant to rifampin and isoniazid remain sputum culture–positive despite multidrug therapy for years.[96] Tuberculous meningitis was successfully treated in a patient with hepatic failure using combination therapy including intraventricular administration of rifampin to avoid hepatic side effects.[97] Twice-weekly supervised administration after daily therapy for 2 to 8 weeks has been successful in noncompliant patients.[98, 99] It should be emphasized that rifampin monotherapy is contraindicated in mycobacterial disease, as illustrated by one study in which 5 of 11 tuberculous patients developed rifampin-resistant isolates within 3 months when receiving rifampin alone.[100] The American Thoracic Society has recommended the use of rifampin (with or without ethambutol) as prophylactic therapy for infected contacts of persons with known isoniazid-resistant tuberculosis.[84] In one study, isoniazid prophylaxis showed no benefit in this situation with 3 (7.9%) of 38 patients receiving isoniazid developing active disease compared with 6 (8.6%) of 71 refusing therapy. By contrast, rifampin prophylaxis was associated with no failures (zero of 49 receiving rifampin and zero of 37 receiving rifampin plus isoniazid).[101] In another study, none of 157 adolescents exposed to an isoniazid-resistant strain developed tuberculosis after rifampin prophylaxis compared with seven expected cases in the absence of prophylaxis.[102] For rifampin-resistant organisms pyrazinamide plus either ciprofloxacin or ofloxacin has been suggested.

Rifampin-containing regimens have proved useful in therapy for *M. avium-intracellulare*,[103–106] *Mycobacterium kansasii*,[107, 108] *Mycobacterium xenopi*,[109] *Mycobacterium marinum*,[110] and Calmette-Guérin bacillus infections.[111, 112]

Rifampin kills *Mycobacterium leprae* faster than do the sulfones. If used in patients with lepromatous leprosy, however, it should be combined with dapsone to prevent the development of resistance. The multidrug regimens recommended by the World Health Organization for adults are as follows: (1) for multibacillary leprosy, rifampin, 600 mg monthly (supervised); dapsone, 100 mg daily; and clofazimine, 300 mg monthly (supervised) and 50 mg daily for at least 2 years and until skin smear negativity if possible; and (2) for paucibacillary leprosy, rifampin, 600 mg monthly (supervised); and dapsone, 100 mg daily.[113] Monthly rifampin doses may be given without producing the flulike side effects seen more frequently with weekly rifampin administration.[114, 115]

Meningitis Prophylaxis

Rifampin has been approved by the Food and Drug Administration for prophylaxis in close contacts of patients with meningococcal meningitis at a daily dose of 10 mg/kg (600 mg maximum) for 4 days. As an alternative dose, the Centers for Disease Control and Prevention recommends 600 mg every 12 hours for 2 days for adults and 10 mg/kg every 12 hours for 2 days for children. Rifampin has been shown to eradicate meningococci from the nasopharynx in approximately 90% of carriers.[116–119] Sulfadiazine was formerly recommended for meningococcal prophylaxis, but up to 70% of recent meningococcal isolates are resistant to sulfa. Minocycline is also an effective prophylactic agent, but it is associated with a higher incidence of side effects, especially vestibular symptoms.[120] Studies have suggested the efficacy of oral ciprofloxacin (1 to 10 doses) and also of a single intramuscular injection of ceftriaxone (250 mg for adults, 125 mg for children younger than 15 years).[121, 122] A large outbreak of group C meningococcal meningitis was effectively controlled by mass rifampin prophylaxis after vaccination failed to stop the outbreak.[123] A randomized trial compared the use of oral rifampin and ciprofloxacin for eradication of nasopharyngeal carriage of *N. meningitidis* in contacts of patients with meningococcal meningitis but provided ceftraxone therapy to all children younger than 2 years and to pregnant women. Eradication at 2 weeks was confirmed in 97.7% receiving rifampin, 91.1% receiving a single dose of ciprofloxacin, and 97.6% receiving ceftraxone, suggesting that the drugs had comparable efficacy.[124]

Epidemiologic studies of *H. influenzae* type B meningitis have shown a high incidence of secondary disease among preschool contacts.[125] Secondary disease attack rates for this group have been approximately 1%, which yields a relative risk approximately 600 times that of the general population.[126] Rifampin at a single daily dose of 20 mg/kg (up to a maximal dose of 600 mg) for 4 days has been shown to eradicate *H. influenzae* from the nasopharynx in over 90% of carriers and to reduce significantly the risk of secondary infection.[35] It has been recommended that families with unvaccinated children younger than 4 years exposed to another member of the household with invasive *H. influenzae* type B disease (e.g., meningitis, epiglottitis, or pneumonia) take rifampin prophylaxis.[126, 127] The age below which child household contacts and their families should receive prophylaxis has been debated. All agree that prophylaxis should be given when there are children younger than 2 years, and some recommend prophylaxis when there are children younger than 4 years (see Chapter 212).[126–129] Pregnant family members should not take rifampin prophylaxis. Day care center staff (excluding pregnant women) and day care classmates of a child with such disease have also been advised to take rifampin prophylaxis if any of the exposed classmates are younger than 2 years. Some authorities recommend prophylaxis after a single case in a day care center, whereas others have advocated instituting prophylaxis only if a second case occurs within 60 days.[127, 130] Failure to provide simultaneous rifampin prophylaxis to all day care center contacts including those who have received *Haemophilus* B polysaccharide vaccine has been associated with persistent colonization of children in the center and subsequent cases of disease.[131] The prophylaxis should be given as rapidly as possible after identification of the index case, since a majority of secondary cases appear to occur in the week after the onset of the index case. Index cases with invasive *H. influenzae* disease should also be given the same rifampin regimen before hospital discharge because of the 1 per-rate of recurrent systemic disease in index cases after therapy and also the risk of exposing other children to the organism.[132] Attempts to eradicate nasopharyngeal carriage with other drugs active against *H. influenzae*, including ampicillin and trimethoprim-sulfamethoxazole, have been less successful; data regarding the efficacy of quinolones and third-generation cephalosporins for this indication are not yet available.

Endocarditis

The use of rifampin in the treatment of staphylococcal endocarditis remains an unsettled and controversial issue.[133] Rifampin was shown to be superior to therapy with vancomycin, gentamicin, or β-lactams in an experimental model of *Staphylococcus epidermidis* endocarditis in rabbits.[134] In another rabbit model of *Staph. epidermidis* endocarditis, rifampin plus teicoplanin proved more effective therapy than either agent alone.[135] A retrospective series of 75 cases of prosthetic valve endocarditis due to *Staph. epidermidis*, the most common cause of prosthetic valve endocarditis, suggested a trend toward higher survival ($p = 0.10$) in patients receiving rifampin (900 to 1200 mg/day) or an aminoglycoside plus vancomycin as opposed to vancomycin alone.[136] The only randomized trial of rifampin therapy in endocarditis compared patients with prosthetic valve endocarditis due to methicillin-resistant *Staph. epidermidis* who were treated with vancomycin (30 mg/kg/day) and rifampin (300 mg every 8 hours) or with vancomycin and rifampin (same doses) plus gentamicin (3 mg/kg/day). The cure rate was 77% with the two-drug regimen and 85% with the three-drug regimen. Rifampin resistance developed in six patients receiving the two-drug regimen compared with none receiving the three-drug regimen.[137] A separate study identified three patients in whom rifampin resistance developed during therapy for prosthetic valve *Staph. epidermidis* endocarditis with rifampin plus vancomycin.[138]

Several patients with endocarditis due to *Staph. aureus* have been reported to respond only after the addition of rifampin to nafcillin or vancomycin.[21, 139, 140] Some in vitro studies with *Staph. aureus*, however, have suggested that rifampin frequently results in antagonism when added to oxacillin or ciprofloxacin therapy.[141, 142] Rifampin therapy for experimental endocarditis due to *Staph. aureus* in rabbits has been examined by Sande and Johnson[19] and Zak and associates.[143] In one study, the combination of rifampin with penicillin was antagonistic in vitro against a strain of *Staph. aureus*, and there was a trend toward slower sterilization of vegetations with the rifampin combination than with penicillin alone. Sterilization of renal abscesses, however, occurred faster in the group receiving the rifampin combination than in the group receiving penicillin alone despite in vitro antagonism. It was suggested that this was due to rifampin's unique ability to penetrate and sterilize abscess fluid and living polymorphonuclear neutrophil leukocytes.

In a subsequent study using the same animal model and a methicillin-sensitive strain of *Staph. aureus*, it was found that rifampin plus cloxacillin was additive or synergistic in four of five different regimens studied; the only regimen showing antagonism combined a high dose of cloxacillin (100 mg/kg) with a low dose of rifampin (2 mg/kg).[143]

A combination of oral rifampin with ciprofloxacin (intravenous for 1 week and oral thereafter) was studied for 4-week therapy of right-sided endocarditis with a cure of all 10 patients who completed therapy.[144] A study of this combination in a rabbit model of *Staph. aureus* endocarditis found it to be as effective as vancomycin and to result in a lower rate of resistance to ciprofloxacin developing during combination therapy than with monotherapy, but also noted that the combination was less effective than ciprofloxacin alone in reducing vegetation counts with one of the two strains tested.[145] An in vitro study also raised concern about antagonism between ciprofloxacin and rifampin when combined for *Staph. aureus*.[141] Early development of resistance has been reported during therapy of right-sided *Staph. aureus* endocarditis with this combination from one hospital.[146] A randomized trial of 1 month of oral therapy with rifampin and ciprofloxacin versus 1 month of intravenous therapy with oxacillin or vancomycin coupled with gentamicin for the first 5 days was conducted in injection drug users with possible right-sided endocarditis. The therapy failed in 1 (5.2%) of 19 receiving oral therapy versus 3 (12%) of 25 receiving parenteral therapy ($p = 0.62$). Drug toxicity was more common with parenteral therapy (62%) than with oral therapy (3%), mostly due to elevated liver enzymes in patients receiving oxacillin.[147]

Kapusnik and colleagues have concluded that rational treatment of staphylococcal endocarditis might involve initial therapy with a β-lactam or vancomycin alone or in combination with an aminoglycoside,[148] which should result in rapid elimination of organisms from vegetations. They suggest the addition of rifampin for cases in which myocardial or metastatic abscesses are detected, while emphasizing the necessity of surgical drainage of abscesses.[148] Adding rifampin after several days of effective therapy with nafcillin or vancomycin plus gentamicin might be less likely to result in the development of rifampin resistance because the titer of organisms exposed to rifampin should then be lower.

The problem of methicillin-resistant *Staph. aureus* (MRSA) endocarditis has been studied in a rabbit model by Bayer and Lam,[149] who found that a combination of rifampin (20 mg/kg/day) plus vancomycin (30 mg/kg/day) was significantly more effective than was either drug alone in eliminating organisms from the valve and curing the animal. Rifampin resistance developed in 2 of 4 animals that were sacrificed after treatment with rifampin alone but was not found in any of the 21 animals given the combination.[149] Another study of MRSA endocarditis in a rabbit model found that ampicillin-sulbactam combined with rifampin was as effective as vancomycin even though neither ampicillin-sulbactam nor rifampin alone was effective.[150] One retrospective study of treatment of MRSA endocarditis in drug-addicted patients did not demonstrate a higher cure rate for rifampin-containing regimens than for vancomycin alone, but such studies are likely to be biased, with only the more severely ill patients receiving rifampin. Randomized trials are needed to assess accurately the efficacy of rifampin for endocarditis due to MRSA.

The problem of rifampin resistance developing during therapy for endocarditis that has been noted with methicillin-resistant *Staph. epidermidis* has also been observed with MRSA during treatment with rifampin and vancomycin.[151, 152] Acar and colleagues reported that two of three patients with *Staph. aureus* endocarditis in whom therapy with another regimen had failed developed rifampin resistance when rifampin was added to either vancomycin or pristinamycin.[140] It has been suggested by the results of one study that although rifampin resistance may develop in the presence of a β-lactam such as nafcillin in vitro, the rate of developing such resistance is lower with this combination than with rifampin alone; in contrast, this study found that vancomycin did not suppress the emergence of rifampin resistance when incubated with rifampin in vitro.[153] The results of other studies, however, have suggested that incubation of vancomycin with rifampin in vitro can suppress the emergence of rifampin resistance.[154, 155]

The efficacy of rifampin in *Staph. aureus* endocarditis will have to be demonstrated by randomized controlled trials. One small randomized trial of vancomycin compared with vancomycin plus rifampin for endocarditis due to MRSA showed slow clearance of bacteremia in both groups and no trend toward benefit for the combination.[156] It would appear reasonable to consider using rifampin in cases with renal, myocardial, splenic, or cerebral abscess formation or because of failure of conventional therapy. If rifampin were to be added, an optimal regimen would probably include at least two other drugs such as gentamicin and either nafcillin or vancomycin to minimize the probability of developing rifampin resistance during therapy.

The value of serum bactericidal titers and of in vitro synergy studies of antibiotic combinations including rifampin are of unclear value. Serum bactericidal titers have not been clearly demonstrated to predict the clinical outcome in patients with endocarditis,[157] and in vitro studies of rifampin and vancomycin or nafcillin with large batteries of staphylococcal isolates have produced inconsistent results in different laboratories, with most studies finding indifference for a majority of isolates.[158–165] Synergy studies performed with the same strain of *Staph. aureus* and the same concentrations of antibiotics have yielded directly contradictory results using checkerboard and time-kill methods.[158, 161, 166] Faster sterilization of renal abscesses has been shown in one animal model when a combination of rifampin and penicillin was administered despite in vitro evidence of antagonism.

One theme that has emerged from several synergy studies is that lower ratios of the concentration of rifampin to the concentration of oxacillin appear to be less bactericidal in vitro. Since the highest peak concentrations and area-under-the-curve values are achieved by administering a single large daily dose of rifampin (e.g., ≥600 mg for an adult),[5] this approach may be more effective than smaller divided doses would be.

Rifampin (300 mg orally twice daily) has also been recommended in combination with vancomycin and gentamicin for the treatment of endocarditis due to *Corynebacterium* spp.[167] One case of endocarditis due to psittacosis was refractory to several other antibiotics but subsequently responsive to rifampin.[168] Rifampin has activity against *Coxiella burnetii*, the cause of Q fever endocarditis, and has been used in combination with doxycycline or with fluroroquinolones. Although randomized trials have not been done, the currently favored regimen is doxycycline plus a fluoroquinolone for at least 3 years.[169, 170]

Tolerant Staphylococci

Staphylococci with an antibiotic minimal bactericidal concentration much greater than the minimal inhibitory concentration (MIC) (minimal bactericidal concentration ≥ 32 × MIC) are said to be tolerant to the antibiotic in question. Tolerance to nafcillin or vancomycin, or both, has been described in several cases of persistent staphylococcal infection. The addition of rifampin has led to improved serum bactericidal levels and the successful treatment of such infections in several cases.[171, 172] No randomized trials of such therapy for this indication are available.

Staphylococcal Carriage and Furunculosis

Rifampin has been shown to reduce the rate of staphylococcal nasal colonization markedly,[173–175] whereas systemic penicillinase-resistant penicillins or intranasal gentamicin cream has not eradicated nasal carriage.[176] Mandell and Sande (unpublished data) have used cloxacillin plus rifampin to eradicate nasal carriage and interrupt the course of recurrent furunculosis. Its role in preventing staphylococcal infections in dialysis patients continues to be studied.[177] Methicillin-resistant staphylococcal nasal carriage in nosocomial epidemics has been successfully eradicated by using a combination of rifampin plus vancomycin, trimethoprim-sulfamethoxazole, minocycline, novobiocin, or nasal mupirocin ointment.[176, 178–182]

Methicillin-Resistant Staphylococcal Infection

Methicillin-resistant infections should be treated with vancomycin, to which they are uniformly sensitive. There are no data to support the routine addition of rifampin to vancomycin therapy, but if there is inadequate response to vancomycin alone, then the addition of gentamicin or rifampin, or both, should be considered. The development of rifampin resistance has been reported during therapy for MRSA infections with vancomycin plus rifampin,[140, 152] and the addition of gentamicin to the regimen may help to prevent the development of rifampin resistance.[137]

Streptococcal Carriage

Chronic pharyngeal carriage of *Streptococcus pyogenes* in children has sometimes resulted in multiple courses of antibiotic therapy for apparent streptococcal pharyngitis with each new cold because of continuing positive cultures after completion of each course of therapy, and even has resulted in tonsillectomy. Eradication of carriage is not usually medically indicated for chronic carriers, but when carriage eradication is desired, rifampin, 10 mg/kg orally twice daily for 4 days, plus benzathine penicillin has been shown to eradicate *Strep. pyogenes* in 93% of cases.[183] Such therapy for the eradication of *Strep. pyogenes* was tried in patients with psoriasis, with apparent benefit to their skin disease,[184] but a randomized trial including 20 patients showed no benefit.[185]

Group B streptococci are the leading cause of sepsis and meningitis in neonates, and efforts to eradicate colonization are now being studied. A recent study of the treatment of experimentally exposed infant rats showed that rifampin plus penicillin eradicated group B streptococci in 80% of the animals, a significantly higher rate than for either drug alone.[186] Clinical data are not available.

Osteomyelitis and Septic Arthritis

Experimental animal data suggest that rifampin combined with another antistaphylococcal drug such as nafcillin or vancomycin provides better results than does single-drug therapy for chronic staphylococcal osteomyelitis, even when the drug combination is antagonistic in vitro.[187, 188] In a rat model, azithromycin plus rifampin showed synergy against *Staph. aureus* osteomyelitis, being slightly more active than a clindamycin-rifampin combination even though azithromycin alone was ineffective.[189] Controlled trials are necessary to confirm these data in human infection, however. The only randomized trial evaluating a rifampin-containing regimen in chronic staphylococcal osteomyelitis was halted after the enrollment of 18 patients: there was a trend toward a higher rate of favorable response in the group receiving rifampin and nafcillin (8 of 10) compared with the group receiving nafcillin alone (4 of 8). The difference was not statistically significant (p = 0.2), but because of the small sample size, the statistical power was only 40% for detecting significance in the 30% higher rate of response that was observed.[190]

An uncontrolled trial of rifampin combined with ciprofloxacin or a β-lactam antibiotic for therapy of streptococcal or staphylococcal orthopedic implant infection reported a success rate of 82%.[191] In a rabbit model of orthopedic device–related infection using a slime-producing strain of *Staph. epidermidis* inoculated into a hole drilled through the intercondylar notch before placement of a stainless steel screw, the highest cure rate after 2 weeks was with vancomycin and rifampin (90%), followed by minocycline and rifampin (70%), minocycline alone (20%) and vancomycin alone (0%).[192]

Rifampin is not part of the usual regimen for staphylococcal arthritis, but it has been added with success in occasional patients initially refractory to nafcillin alone;[193] however, rifampin resistance developed in one patient due to MRSA treated with vancomycin and rifampin.[153]

Legionella Infection

Both *Legionella pneumophila* and *Legionella micdadei* are sensitive to rifampin. It has been suggested that rifampin be added to erythromycin for patients with legionnaires' disease when the illness does not respond to erythromycin alone, but data from randomized trials are lacking. In vitro studies show that the combination of erythromycin with rifampin or pefloxacin is more active than erythromycin alone.[194]

Brucellosis

Rifampin has been shown to be superior to tetracycline in therapy for experimental brucellosis in rodents, and there have been several case reports of successful therapy for human infections.[195] In one uncontrolled study, relapses occurred after rifampin monotherapy, thus suggesting the need for combination therapy if rifampin is used.[196] Another case series identified 2 relapses in 10 cases treated with rifampin alone, 1 relapse after tetracycline and streptomycin therapy in 56 cases, and no relapses after tetracycline and rifampin therapy in 40 cases.[197] Four randomized trials comparing tetracycline (or doxycycline) regimens containing either rifampin or streptomycin consistently found that a significantly higher proportion of the rifampin recipients failed therapy or relapsed compared with streptomycin recipients.[198–201] A more recent randomized trial with 61 patients compared doxycycline and rifampin with ofloxacin plus rifampin; only one failure (in the ofloxacin group) and one relapse in each group were found.[202] Rifampin resistance has also developed during such therapy and has been documented during clinical relapse. Several studies of rifampin and doxycycline therapy for patients with neurobrucellosis have suggested a high rate of efficacy, with relapse rates between zero and 10%.[203]

Rickettsia: Mediterranean Spotted Fever

Rifampin has activity against *Rickettsia conorii*, the agent of Mediterranean spotted fever, and was shown to be effective clinically although with slower resolution of symptoms than with doxycycline, the drug of choice.[204] *Coxiella burnetii* infection (Q fever) has been treated successfully with rifampin, but doxycycline and fluoroquinolones are the preferred treatment at this time.[170]

Infection Occurring in Patients with Chronic Granulomatous Disease of Childhood

Rifampin has been shown to kill living intracellular staphylococci in neutrophils from healthy people and from patients with chronic granulomatous disease.[205] One patient with an axillary staphylococcal abscess responded dramatically to the addition of rifampin after months of unsuccessful therapy with vancomycin, nafcillin, and gentamicin.[206]

Infected Cerebrospinal Fluid Shunts, Vascular Grafts, and Implants

Cerebrospinal fluid shunt infections have responded to the addition of rifampin in several cases after an initial failure with multiple-drug therapy excluding rifampin.[207–210] Data from controlled trials of prophylactic therapy are lacking, but a randomized trial of rifampin-trimethoprim prophylaxis at the time of shunt placement showed a trend favoring this approach (12% infection rate versus 19% among placebo recipients).[211] A meta-analysis has shown significantly lower infection rates with antimicrobial prophylaxis.[212] Another study suggested that cerebrospinal fluid shunts impregnated with rifampin and clindamycin were less likely to become infected.[213]

Three patients with *Staph. epidermidis* infections of a penile prosthesis were successfully treated by removal of the prosthesis and 72 hours of continuous irrigation of the corpora cavernosa with rifampin before the insertion of a new prosthesis.[214] Therapy with rifampin plus clindamycin for aortic Dacron grafts experimentally infected with *Staph. aureus* was found to cure the infection in seven of seven dogs compared with five of seven dogs in which infection was cured with cefazolin therapy.[215] Data from clinical trials are not available.

A rat model of chronic *Staph. aureus* foreign body infection using subcutaneous tissue cages showed that a combination of vancomycin with fleroxacin and rifampin was superior to regimens with fewer drugs.[216] An in vitro model of *Staph. epidermidis* biofilm on a foreign body showed that rifampin was the only drug of 35 tested with significant activity against organisms in a biofilm and that adding an agent with cell wall activity (e.g., vancomycin or a β-lactam) resulted in synergistic activity against the biofilm.[217]

Prevention of vascular graft infections using rifampin-impregnated grafts has been investigated.[218–223] In a sheep model, 2 of 10 rifampin-impregnated Dacron grafts became infected compared with 6 of 8 regular grafts.[224] Some high-risk patients have had rifampin-impregnated grafts implanted without complications.[225] When an infant suffered sternal infection and ventricular septal patch dehiscence after a truncus arteriosus repair, the recurrent defect was successfully repaired with a rifampin-impregnated gelatin-sealed Dacron patch.[226]

Catheter Infections

Prevention of vascular catheter-related blood stream infection is an important goal because of significant morbidity and mortality.[227] Patients receiving interleukin-2 were significantly less likely to develop catheter-related bacteremia while taking oral rifampin and novobiocin prophylaxis (6%) then when taking no prophylaxis (41%) ($p = 0.04$).[228] Catheters coated with rifampin and minocycline have been shown to prevent blood stream infection in an experimental rabbit model[229] and in a randomized trial in patients.[230]

Cutaneous Leishmaniasis

When a patient with *Leishmania mexicana amazonensis* refractory to previous antileishmanial therapy was treated with rifampin and isoniazid for intercurrent mycobacterial infection, the cutaneous leishmaniasis improved.[231] Several uncontrolled case series have suggested that rifampin may be effective in 80% of patients with this disease,[232, 233] but controlled trials are lacking.[234]

Urinary Tract Infection

A number of studies have been conducted that show the efficacy of rifampin in the treatment of urinary tract infections. Rifampin resistance has arisen with monotherapy, but combination therapy with trimethoprim has resulted in cure rates that are comparable to those of trimethoprim-sulfamethoxazole.[235] Rifampin combined with trimethoprim has been used with success in eradicating persistent, relapsing infections of the kidney or prostate.[235] Rifampin combinations are not the drug of choice for infections of the urinary tract but may be considered when conventional therapy fails.

Urethritis

Although not a first-line drug for gonococcal urethritis, rifampin (900 mg) plus erythromycin (1 g) as a single oral dose has been shown to cure 95% of patients with gonorrhea, with equivalent efficacy against penicillinase-producing *N. gonorrhoeae* strains.[236, 237] Despite excellent activity against chlamydia in vitro, a single dose of rifampin in combination with erythromycin showed poor efficacy in the treatment of chlamydial urethritis.[237]

Rhodococcus Infection

Rhodococcus equi is a common equine pathogen that has recently been described as a rare cause of human pneumonia with cavity formation in 69%. Almost all cases have occurred in immunocompromised patients, including AIDS patients.[238] Optimal therapy in foals has been with rifampin combined with erythromycin. This regimen has been used successfully in patients as has vancomycin and vancomycin combined with rifampin. Therapy is recommended for 2 to 6 months.[239]

Chancroid

Rifampin has good activity against *Haemophilus ducreyi*, the causative agent of chancroid, and has been shown effective in treatment.[240] However, intramuscular ceftriaxone and oral erythromycin are the treatments of choice.[241]

Infections Due to *Pseudomonas aeruginosa* and Other Aerobic Gram-Negative Bacilli

Most isolates of *Pseudomonas aeruginosa* are relatively resistant to rifampin, with MICs ranging from 32 to 64 μg/ml. Occasional isolates of *P. aeruginosa*, however, are also resistant to available β-lactams, aminoglycosides, or both. In vitro data have suggested synergy of rifampin with ticarcillin and tobramycin, with impenem and ciprofloxacin, and with ceftazidime or cefpirome and an aminoglycoside against such resistant strains even when some strains were resistant to all three individual drugs.[242, 243] There are case reports of patients refractory to conventional therapy who have responded dramatically after the addition of rifampin to their regimen, suggesting that rifampin may be of value in combination therapy for such infections.[244] Rifampin combined with imipenem has also shown in vitro synergy against *P. aeruginosa* and *Enterobacter* spp. and an additive effect against *Serratia marcescens*; in vitro synergy was also shown for the combination of rifampin, imipenem, and ciprofloxacin against each of these three species.[245] Data from clinical trials are needed regarding the use of rifampin in such combination therapy. One randomized trial of rifampin added to β-lactam and aminoglycoside therapy for *Pseudomonas* bacteremia showed a lower rate of breakthrough bacteremia and of relapse in the rifampin group, but there was no significant difference in the survival rate.[246] An uncontrolled series of rifampin combined with ciprofloxacin for 6 to 12 weeks of therapy for malignant external otitis found that 10 of 11 were cured.[247]

Rhinoscleroma, a granulomatous disease of the nose due to *Klebsiella rhinoscleromatis*, can be effectively treated with rifampin administered orally or as a topical ointment.[248] Brazilian purpuric fever, a life-threatening infection preceded by conjunctivitis, is caused by *H. influenzae* biogroup *aegyptius*, which was eradicated from the conjunctiva by oral rifampin (20 mg/kg/d for 4 days) in 100% of patients in one study.[249]

Anaerobic Infections

Data from experimental animal models suggest that rifampin is as effective as metronidazole in the prevention of abscess formation and eradication of *Bacteroides fragilis* after intraperitoneal injection of the organism. Clinical data are not available.[250, 251]

Rifampin is highly active against *C. difficile* and has been used in combination with vancomycin to interrupt relapsing pseudomembranous colitis successfully in one series.[252] Rifampin plus bacitracin showed synergy against 85% of 55 strains in one study.[253]

Meningitis

Rifampin has been used successfully in the therapy of several cases of meningitis refractory to other available antibiotics. *Chryseobacterium meningosepticum* is a rare cause of meningitis and occurs primarily in neonates but sometimes in adults after surgery. Most strains are susceptible to trimethoprim-sulfamethoxazole, imipenem, minocycline, and rifampin.[254] Rifampin has been used successfully as part of combination therapy with one or more of these other agents in curing such patients.[232, 255] Randomized trials of such therapy are not available.

Rifampin was also added to the regimen of a patient with *H. influenzae* meningitis who had not responded clinically to therapy with chloramphenicol or subsequently with ampicillin and trimethoprim-sulfamethoxazole. The patient responded dramatically after the addition of rifampin.[256] A similar success was reported with rifampin and vancomycin therapy of previously unresponsive enterococcal meningitis.[257]

Prophylaxis of Infection during Neutropenia

The addition of rifampin to ciprofloxacin or ofloxacin therapy for prevention of infection in neutropenic patients has been evaluated and shown to result in significantly lower rates of gram-positive infection than when a quinolone alone was used. The rate of neutropenic fever, however, was reduced in only one of three studies.[258–260]

Rabies

A study of experimental rabies infection in mice suggested that rifampin might have some activity, but these findings require confirmation.[261]

OTHER RIFAMYCINS

Rifapentine

Rifapentine is a cyclopentyl rifamycin with antibacterial[262, 263] and antimycobacterial[264, 265] activity similar to those of rifampin but has a longer half-life of approximately 14 to 18 hours in animals (rat, mouse, and rabbit).[266] Sixty-five percent of an oral dose of 10 mg/kg is absorbed by such animals; its hepatic metabolism, biliary excretion, and wide distribution throughout body tissues are each similar to that of rifampin, as is its marked induction of hepatic microsomal oxidase activity,[267, 268] which has also been documented in humans.[269] This drug appears to be several times more active against *M. tuberculosis* and *M. leprae* than rifampin is, and its longer half-life may facilitate therapy by allowing less frequent administration. Twice-weekly rifapentine was as effective as daily rifampin in a randomized trial of combination therapy of pulmonary tuberculosis.[270] It was more active against *M. avium* in vitro and in a murine model than was rifampin.[271, 272]

Rifabutin

Rifabutin is a semisynthetic spiropiperidyl derivative of rifamycin S that shows good activity against most species of mycobacteria, including all rifampin-sensitive *M. tuberculosis* strains and about one third of rifampin-resistant strains; strains highly resistant to rifampin are usually resistant to rifabutin. Rifabutin shows better activity against the *M. avium-intracellulare* complex of organisms than rifampin; it inhibits 81% of these strains at a concentration of 1.0 μg/ml compared with only 6% being inhibited by rifampin at this concentration.[273]

Rifabutin is absorbed from the gastrointestinal tract, with a peak level of 0.49 μg/ml about 4 hours after ingestion of 300 mg in an adult. The serum half-life is 16 hours, and protein binding is 20%. The drug is taken up by all tissues and especially concentrated in the lungs, where levels may be 10-fold higher than in serum. Both hepatic and renal clearances occur as with other rifamycins. Rifabutin has less of an effect on hepatic microsomal enzyme activity than rifampin has, but significant interactions still occur. Rifabutin serum concentrations are significantly increased by ritonavir, clarithromycin, ketoconazole, and fluconazole.[274, 275] The rates and types of side effects from rifabutin appeared to be comparable to those of rifampin in early studies,[273] but subsequent studies have shown a significantly higher rate of uveitis. When receiving long-term rifabutin, 5.7% of patients developed uveitis at 300 mg/day, compared with 38% at 600 mg/day.[276] This uveitis is associated with a noninfectious hypopyon and responds to topical corticosteroid therapy even while rifabutin therapy is continued.[277] Nine of 10 patients with AIDS-related complex developed arthralgia or arthritis when treated with more than 1050 mg/day. Two of these developed uveitis and mouth ulcers at a dose of 1800 mg/day.[278]

Rifabutin was ineffective as monotherapy in open trials for the treatment of *M. avium-intracellulare* disease in patients with AIDS,[279, 280] but daily rifabutin has proved effective in preventing *M. avium* complex disease in AIDS patients although not as effective as weekly azithromycin or the combination of the two drugs, which was most effective but also associated with significantly more adverse effects.[281] Rifabutin, ethambutol, and clarithromycin were significantly more effective than rifampin, ethambutol, clofazimine, and ciprofloxacin in the treatment of *M. avium* complex bacteremia.[282]

Rifabutin therapy for patients with newly diagnosed cavitary pulmonary tuberculosis had significantly less effect on bacilli in cavities than did rifampin in one randomized trial.[283] In another randomized trial, rifampin (600 mg/day) was compared with rifabutin (300 mg/day) as part of combination therapy of pulmonary tuberculosis; rates of success, adverse effects, and relapse were equivalent in the two groups.[284] Rifabutin has been somewhat effective in combination therapy of various mycobacteria resistant to rifampin.[285, 286] One study suggests that rifabutin may be an effective preventive agent against *Cryptosporidium parvum* infection in AIDS patients.[287]

Bezoxazinorifamycins

The benzoxazinorifamycins, a group of newly synthesized rifamycin derivatives, exhibited MICs more than 64-fold lower than those of rifampin against *M. tuberculosis, M. kansasii, M. scrofulaceum, M. avium*, and *M. intracellulare*.[288] Rifampin-resistant *M. tuberculosis* showed MICs eightfold lower than those for rifampin, and *M. fortuitum* and *Mycobacterium chelonae* had MICs equal to those for rifampin.[288] One benzoxazinorifamycin, KRM-1648, had MICs for *M. avium-intracellulare* ranging from 0.004 to 0.0625, lower than those of rifampin, rifabutin, and eight other antituberculous agents tested.[28] KRM-1648 administered in a nude mouse leprosy model was significantly more active than rifampin at equivalent oral doses of 1 mg/kg or 3 mg/kg twice weekly.[289] Against *M. avium*, KRM-1648 MIC values were 32 to 128 times lower than for rifampin.[290]

Rifaximin

Rifaximin is a new rifamycin derivative that has only negligible oral absorption. After the administration of 1600 mg to 13 subjects, biliary concentrations could be detected in only 6, and concentrations were more than fivefold lower than those expected for a similar dose of rifampin.[291] The drug has been used primarily in Italy, with studies suggesting efficacy in uncomplicated diverticulitis, small bowel overgrowth syndrome, and hepatic encephalopathy.[292–295] In randomized trials, rifaximin has been as effective as neomycin or lactulose in lowering blood ammonia levels in patients with hepatic encephalopathy.[296–298] It has also been used to treat pyogenic skin infections successfully in a cream formulation.[299]

NONINFECTIOUS DISEASES

Rifampin has been used successfully to decrease pruritus in patients with primary biliary cirrhosis.[300–302] The drug also has immunomodulatory effects and has been studied for use in a number of conditions. Oral rifampin was given to eight rheumatoid arthritis patients without clear response.[303] Rifampin has been injected into the peripheral joints of patients with ankylosing spondylitis with reported decreases in erythrocyte sedimentation rate and Schober's test measurements, but no randomized trial has been done.[304] An open trial of rifampin injection into joints affected by hemophilic synovitis resulted in responses described as excellent in 40 and good in 8.[305]

Rifabutin and ethambutol were given to 10 patients with recurrent Crohn's disease without clinical or pathologic improvement.[306] A randomized trial of 2 years of antituberculous therapy also showed no significant benefit.[307]

Antitumor activity has also been reported. One study showed additive effects of rifampin and tamoxifen against biliary tract carcinoma cell lines in vitro.[308] Another study reported prolonged remission in patients with acute myelogenous leukemia receiving rifampin.[309]

REFERENCES

1. Sensi P. History of the development of rifampin. Rev Infect Dis. 1983;5(Suppl):402.
2. Sensi P, Maggi N, Furesz S, et al. Chemical modifications and biological properties of rifamycins. Antimicrob Agents Chemother. 1966;6:699.
3. Mandell GL. Interaction of intraleukocytic bacteria and antibiotics. J Clin Invest. 1973;52:1673.
4. Wehrli W, Knusel F, Schmid K, et al. Interaction of rifamycin with bacterial RNA polymerase. Proc Natl Acad Sci U S A. 1968;61:667.
5. Acocella G. Pharmacokinetics and metabolism of rifampin in humans. Rev Infect Dis. 1983;5(Suppl):428.
6. Krukenberg CC, Mischler PG, Massad N, et al. Stability of 196 rifampin suspensions prepared in five syrups. Am J Hosp Pharm. 1986;43:2225–2228.
7. Stewart HI, Perkin DP, Donald PR. Stability of isoniazid, rifampin and pyrazinamide in suspensions used for the treatment of tuberculosis in children. Pediatr Infect Dis J. 1991;10:827–831.
8. Moulding T, Dutt AK, Reichman LB. Fixed-dose combinations of antituberculous medications to prevent drug resistance. Ann Intern Med. 1995:122:951–954.
9. Matz J, Borish LC, Routes JM, Rosenwasser LJ. Oral desensitization to rifampin and ethambutol in mycobacterial disease. Am J Respir Crit Care Med. 1994;149:815–817.
10. Purohit SD, Gupta ML, Gupta PR. Dietary constituents and rifampicin absorption. Tubercle. 1987;68:151.
11. Sahai J, Gallicano K, Swick L, et al. Reduced plasma concentrations of antituberculosis drugs in patients with HIV infection. Ann Intern Med. 1997;127:289–293.
12. Advenier C, Gobert C, Houin G, et al. Pharmacokinetic studies of rifampicin in the elderly. Ther Drug Monit. 1983;5:61–65.
13. Koup JR, Williams-Warren J, Viswanathan CT, et al. Pharmacokinetics of rifampin in children. II. Oral bioavailability. Ther Drug Monit. 1986;8:17–22.
14. Roup JR, Williams-Warren J, Weber A, et al. Pharmacokinetics of rifampin in children. I. Multiple dose intravenous infusion. Ther Drug Monit. 1986;8:11–16.
15. Furesz S. Chemical and biological properties of rifampicin. Antibiot Chemother. 1970;16:316.
16. Solberg CO, Halstensen A, Digranes A, et al. Penetration of antibiotics into human leukocytes and dermal suction blisters. Rev Infect Dis. 1983;5:S468.
17. Outman WR, Levitz RE, Hill DA, et al. Intraocular penetration of rifampin in humans. Antimicrob Agents Chemother. 1992;36:1575–1576.
18. Wong KW, D'Amico DJ, Oum BS, et al. Intraocular penetration of rifampin after oral administration. Graefes Arch Clin Exp Ophthalmol. 1990;228:40–43.
19. Sande MA, Johnson ML. Antimicrobial therapy of experimental endocarditis caused by *Staphylococcus aureus*. J Infect Dis. 1975;131:367.
20. Mandell GL, Vest TK. Killing of intraleukocytic *Staphylococcus aureus* by rifampin: In vitro and in vivo studies. J Infect Dis. 1972;125:486.
21. Farr BM, Mandell GL. Rifampin. Med Clin North Am. 1982;66:157.
22. Thornsberry C, Hill BC, Swenson JM, et al. Rifampin: Spectrum of antibacterial activity. Rev Infect Dis. 1983;5(Suppl):412.
23. Prescott JF. *Rhodococcus equi*: An animal and human pathogen. Clin Microb Rev. 1991;4:20–34.
24. Collins CH, Yates MD. Low incidence of rifampin resistant tubercle bacilli. Thorax. 1982;37:526.
25. Cauthen GM, Kilburn JO, Kelly GD, et al. Resistance to anti-tuberculosis drugs in patients with and without prior treatment: Survey of 31 state and large city laboratories, 1982–1986. Am Rev Respir Dis. 1988;137:260.
26. Bloch AB, Cauthen GM, Onorato IM, et al. Nationwide survey of drug-resistant tuberculosis in the United States (see comments). JAMA. 1994;271:665–671.
27. Woodley CL, Kilburn JO. In vitro susceptibility of *Mycobacterium avium* complex and *Mycobacterium tuberculosis* strains to a spiro-piperidyl rifamycin. Am Rev Respir Dis. 1982;126:586.
28. Tomioka H, Saito H, Fujii K, et al. In vitro antimicrobial activity of benzoxazinorifamycin, KRM-1648, against *Mycobacterium avium* complex, determined by the radiometric method. Antimicrob Agents Chemother. 1993;37:67–70.
29. Schachter J. Rifampin in chlamydial infections. Rev Infect Dis. 1983;5(Suppl):562.
30. Medoff G. Antifungal action of rifampin. Rev Infect Dis. 1983;5(Suppl):614.
31. Barrios NJ, Kirkpatrick DV, Murciano A, et al. Successful treatment of disseminated *Fusarium* infection in an immunocompromised child. Am J Pediatr Hematol Oncol. 1990;12:319–324.
32. Tucker RM, Denning DW, Hanson LH, et al. Interaction of azoles with rifampin, phenytoin, and carbamazepine: In vitro and clinical observations. Clin Infect Dis. 1992;14:165–174.
33. Wehrli W. Rifampin: Mechanisms of action and resistance. Rev Infect Dis. 1983;5(Suppl):407.
34. Yogev R, Melick C, Glogowski W. In vitro development of rifampin resistance in clinical isolates of *Haemophilus influenzae* type B. Antimicrob Agents Chemother. 1982;21:387.
35. Band JD, Fraser DW, Ajello G, et al. Prevention of *Hemophilus influenzae* type b disease. JAMA. 1984;251:2381–2386.
36. Band JD, Fraser DW. Adverse effects of two rifampicin dosage regimens for the prevention of meningococcal infection. Lancet. 1984;1:101.
37. Goldin HM, Schweitzer WJ, Bronson DM. Rifampin and exfoliative dermatitis. Ann Intern Med. 1987;107:789.
38. Okano M, Kitano Y, Igarashi T. Toxic epidermal necrolysis due to rifampicin. J Am Acad Dermatol. 1987;17:303.
39. Mimouni A, Hodak E, Mimouni M. Fixed drug eruption following rifampin treatment. DICP 1990;24:947–948.
40. Purohit SD, Johri SC, Gupta PR, et al. Ranitidine-rifampicin interaction. J Assoc Physicians India 1992;40:308–310.
41. Steele MA, Burk RF, DesPrez RM. Toxic hepatitis with isoniazid and rifampin. A meta-analysis. Chest. 1991;99:465–471.
42. Mandell GL, Sande MA. Drugs used in the chemotherapy of tuberculosis and

leprosy. In: Goodman AG, Goodman LS, Gilman A, eds. The Pharmacological Basis of Therapeutics. 6th ed. New York: Macmillan; 1980:1203–1206.
43. Gendrel D, Nardou M, Mouba JF, et al. Hepatotoxicity of the combination of isoniazid rifampicin in African children. Role of malnutrition and HB virus. Arch Fr Pediatrie. 1989;46:645–648.
44. Van den Brande P, van Steenbergen W, Vervoort G, Demedts M. Aging and hepatotoxicity of isoniazid and rifampin in pulmonary tuberculosis. Am J Respir Crit Care Med. 1995;152:1705–1708.
45. O'Brien RJ, Long MW, Cross FS, et al. Hepatotoxicity from isoniazid and rifampin among children treated for tuberculosis. Pediatrics. 1983;72:491–499.
46. Tsagaropoulou-Stinga H, Mataki-Emmanouilidou T, Karida-Kavalioti S, et al. Hepatotoxic reactions in children with severe tuberculosis treated with isomazid-rifampin. Pediatr Infect Dis. 1985;4:270–273.
47. Taillan B, Chichmanian RM, Fuzibet JG, et al. Jaundice caused by rifampicin: 3 cases. Rev Med Int. 1989;10:409–411.
48. Qunibi WY, Godwin J, Eknoyan G. Toxic nephropathy during continuous rifampin therapy. South Med J. 1980;73:791.
49. Grosset J, Leventis S. Adverse effects of rifampin. Rev Infect Dis. 1983;5(Suppl):440.
50. Murray AN, Cassidy MJD, Templecamp C. Rapidly progressive glomerulonephritis associated with rifampicin therapy for pulmonary tuberculosis. Nephron. 1987;46:373.
51. Soffer O, Nassar VH, Campbell WG, Jr. Light chain cast nephropathy and acute renal failure associated with rifampin therapy. Am J Med. 1987;82:1052.
52. Winter RJD, Banks RA, Collins CMP, et al. Rifampicin induced light chain proteinuria and renal failure. Thorax. 1984;39:952.
53. Poole G, Stradling P, Worlledge S. Potentially serious side-effects of high dose twice weekly rifampicin. Postgrad Med J. 1971;47:742–747.
54. Girling DJ, Hitze HL. Adverse reactions to rifampicin. Bull WHO. 1979;57:45.
55. Fahal IH, Williams PS, Clark RE, et al. Thrombotic thrombocytopenic purpura due to rifampicin. BMJ 1992;304:882.
56. Lee CH, Lee CJ. Thrombocytopenia—a rare but potentially serious side effect of initial daily and interrupted use of rifampicin. Chest. 1989;96:202–203.
57. Tahan SR, Diamond JR, Blank JM, et al. Acute hemolysis and renal failure with rifampicin-dependent antibodies after discontinuous administration. Transfusion. 1985;25:124–127.
58. Pereira A, Sanz C, Cervantes F, et al. Immune hemolytic anemia and renal failure associated with rifampicin-dependent antibodies with anti-I specificity. Ann Hematol. 1991;63:56–58.
59. Levine M, Collin K, Kassen BO. Acute hemolysis and renal failure following discontinuous use of rifampin. DICP 1991;25:743–744.
60. Gupta A, Sakhuja V, Gupta KL, et al. Intravascular hemolysis and acute renal failure following intermittent rifampin therapy. Int J Lepr Other Mycobact Dis. 1992;60:185–188.
61. Harland RW, Lindblom SS, Munnell MO. Anaphylaxis from rifampin. Am J Med. 1992;92:581–582.
62. Cardot E, Tillie-Leblond I, Jeannin P, et al. Anaphylactic reaction to local administration of rifamycin SV. J Allergy Clin Immunol. 1995;95:1–7.
63. Fekety R, O'Connor R, Silva J. Rifampin and pseudomembranous colitis. Rev Infect Dis. 1983;5(Suppl):524–527.
64. Miller DL, Sedlack JD, Holt RW. Perforation complicating rifampin-associated pseudomembranous enteritis. Arch Surg. 1989;124:1082.
65. Byrd RP, Jr, Roy TM, Ossorio MA, Fields CL. Delayed onset of pseudomembranous colitis after rifampin therapy. South Med J. 1997;90:644–646.
66. Zargar SA, Thapa BR, Sahni A, et al. Rifampicin-induced upper gastrointestinal bleeding. Postgrad Med J. 1990;66:310–311.
67. Bolan G, Laurie RE, Broome CV. Red man syndrome: Inadvertent administration of an excessive dose of rifampin to children in a day-care center. Pediatrics. 1986;77:633.
68. Holdiness RM. A review of the redman syndrome and rifampicin overdosage. Med Toxicol Adverse Drug Exp. 1989;4:444–451.
69. Humber DP, Nsanzumuhire H, Aluoch HA, et al. Controlled double-blind study of the effect of rifampin on humoral and cellular immune responses in patients with pulmonary tuberculosis and in tuberculosis contacts. Am Rev Respir Dis. 1980;122:425.
70. Snider DE, Jr, Layde PM, Johnson MW, et al. Treatment of tuberculosis during pregnancy. Am Rev Respir Dis. 1980;122:65.
71. Ohnhaus EE, Kirchhof B, Peheim E. Effect of enzyme induction on plasma lipids using antipyrine, phenobarbital, and rifampicin. Clin Pharmacol Ther. 1979;25:591.
72. Kolars JC, Schmiedlin-Ren P, Schuetz JD, et al. Identification of rifampin-inducible P450IIIA4 (CYP3A4) in human small bowel enterocytes. J Clin Invest. 1992;90:1871–1878.
73. Twum-Barima Y, Carruthers SG. Quinidine-rifampin interaction. N Engl J Med. 1981;304:1466.
74. Brass C, Galgiani JN, Blaschke TF, et al. Disposition of ketoconazole, an oral antifungal, in humans. Antimicrob Agents Chemother. 1982;21:151.
75. Baciewicz AM, Self TH, Bekemeyer WB. Update on rifampin drug interactions. Arch Intern Med. 1987;147:565.
76. Baciewicz AM, Self TH. Rifampin drug interactions. Arch Intern Med. 1984;144:1667–1671.
77. Isley WL. Effect of rifampin therapy on thyroid function tests in a hypothyroid patient on replacement L-thyroxine. Ann Intern Med. 1987;107:517.
78. Gupta PR, Mehta YR, Gupta ML, et al. Rifampin-aluminum antacid interaction. J Assoc Physicians India 1988;36:363–364.
79. Pilheu JA, Galati MR, Yunis AS, et al. Pharmacokinetic interaction of ketoconazole, isoniazid and rifampicin. Med Buenos Aires 1989;49:43–47.
80. Borcherding SM, Baciewicz AM, Self TH. Update of rifampin drug interactions. II. Arch Intern Med 1992;152:711–716.
81. Malhi R, Uppal R, Sharma PL. Drug interaction between rifampicin, isoniazid and cotrimoxazole in rabbits. Hum Exp Toxicol. 1992;11:105–107.
82. Bhatia RS, Uppal R, Malhi R, et al. Drug interaction between rifampicin and cotrimoxazole in patients with tuberculosis. Hum Exp Toxicol. 1991;10:419–421.
83. British Thoracic Association: A controlled trial of six months chemotherapy in pulmonary tuberculosis. Second report: Results during the 24 months after the end of chemotherapy. Am Rev Respir Dis. 1982;126:460.
84. American Thoracic Society/CDC. Treatment of tuberculosis and tuberculous infection in adults and children. Am Rev Respir Dis. 1986;134:355–363.
85. McCarthy OR, Rudd RM. Six months' chemotherapy for lymph node tuberculosis. Respir Med. 1989;83:425–427.
86. Reis FJ, Bedran MB, Moura JA, et al. Six-month isoniazid-rifampin treatment for pulmonary tuberculosis in children. Am Rev Respir Dis. 1990;142:996–999.
87. Ormerod LP, McCarthy OR, Rudd RM, et al. Short course chemotherapy for pulmonary tuberculosis. Respir Med. 1991;85:291–294.
88. Agounitestane D, Chiheb M, Khaled S, et al. A therapeutic trial of a combination of 3 essential drugs in a short course of chemotherapy in tuberculosis. Results 6 months after the end of treatment. Rev Mal Respir. 1990;7:209–213.
89. Chatterjee G, Kaur S, Sharma VK, et al. Bacillemia in leprosy and effect of multidrug therapy. Leprosy Rev. 1989;60:197–201.
90. Alarcon F, Escalante L, Perez Y, et al. Tuberculous meningitis. Short course of chemotherapy. Arch Neurol. 1990;47:1313–1317.
91. Dutt AK, Moers D, Stead WW. Tuberculous pleural effusion: 6-month therapy with isoniazid and rifampin. Am Rev Respir Dis. 1992;145:1429–1432.
92. Initial therapy for tuberculosis in the era of multidrug resistance. MMWR. 1993;42:1–8.
93. Jones BE, Otaya M, Antoniskis D, et al: A prospective evaluation of antituberculosis therapy in patients with immunodeficiency virus infection. Am J Resp Crit Care Med. 1994;150:1499–1502.
94. Felten MK. Importance of rifampicin in combined daily/intermittent chemotherapy for tuberculosis. S Afr Med J. 1989;75:524–526.
95. Balasubramanian R, Sivasubramanian S, Vijayan VK, et al. Five year results of a 3-month and two 5-month regimens for the treatment of sputum-positive pulmonary tuberculosis in south India. Tubercle. 1990;71:253–258.
96. Goble M, Iseman MD, Madsen LD, et al. Treatment of 171 patients with pulmonary tuberculosis resistant to isoniazid and rifampin. N Engl J Med. 1993;328:527–532.
97. Vincken W, Meysman M, Verbeelen D, et al. Intraventricular rifampicin in severe tuberculous meningo-encephalitis. Eur Respir J. 1992;5:891–893.
98. Castelo A, Jardim JR, Goihman S, et al. Comparison of daily and twice-weekly regimens to treat pulmonary tuberculosis. Lancet. 1989;2:1173–1176.
99. Cohn DL, Catlin BJ, Peterson KL, et al. A 62-dose, 6 month therapy for pulmonary and extrapulmonary tuberculosis: A twice-weekly, directly observed, and cost-effective regimen. Ann Intern Med. 1990;112:407–414.
100. Baronti A, Lukinovich N. A pilot trial of rifampicin in tuberculosis. Tubercle. 1968;49:180.
101. Polesky A, Farber HW, Gottlieb DJ, et al. Rifampin preventive therapy for tuberculosis in Boston's homeless. Am J Respir Crit Care Med. 1996;154:1473–1477.
102. Villarino ME, Ridzon R, Weismuller PC, et al. Rifampin preventive therapy for tuberculosis infection: Experience with 157 adolescents. Am J Respir Crit Care Med. 1997;155:1735–1738.
103. Hunter AM, Campbell IA, Jenkins PA, et al. Treatment of pulmonary infections caused by mycobacteria of the *Mycobacterium avium-intracellulare* complex. Thorax. 1981;36:326.
104. Baron EJ, Young LS. Amikacin, ethambutol, and rifampin for treatment of disseminated *Mycobacterium avium-intracellulare* infections in patients with acquired immune deficiency syndrome. Diagn Microbiol Infect Dis. 1986;5:215–220.
105. Chiu J, Nussbaum J, Bozzette S, et al. Treatment of disseminated *Mycobacterium avium* complex infection in AIDS with amikacin, ethambutol, rifampin, and ciprofloxacin. California Collaborative Treatment Group. Ann Intern Med. 1990;113:358–361.
106. Dautzenberg B, Tuffot C, Mignon A, et al. Rifabutin in combination with clofazimine, isoniazid and ethambutol in treatment of AIDS patients with infections due to opportunistic mycobacteria. Tubercle. 1991;72:168–175.
107. Ahn CH, Lowell JR, Ahn SS, et al. Chemotherapy for pulmonary disease due to *Mycobacterium kansasii*: Efficacies of some individual drugs. Rev Infect Dis. 1981;3:1028.
108. Helm U, Kaustova J, Kubin M, et al. Susceptibility of *Mycobacterium kansasii* to ethambutol and its combination with rifamycins, ciprofloxacin and isoniazid. Eur J Clin Microbiol Infect Dis. 1992;11:51–54.
109. Bogaerts Y, Elinck W, van Renterghem D, et al. Pulmonary disease due to *Mycobacterium xenopi*: Report of two cases. Eur J Respir Dis. 1982;63:298.
110. Donta ST, Smith PW, Levitz RE, et al. Therapy of *Mycobacterium marinum* infections. Arch Intern Med. 1986;146:902–904.
111. Kallenius G, Moller E, Ringden O, et al. The first infant to survive a generalized BCG infection. Acta Paediatr Scand. 1982;71:161.
112. Izumi AK, Matsunaga J. BCG vaccine-induced lupus vulgaris. Arch Dermatol. 1982;118:171.
113. Gilbody JS. Impact of multidrug therapy on the treatment and control of leprosy. Int J Leprosy 1991;59:458–478.
114. Yawalkar SJ, McDougall AC, Longuillon J, et al. Once monthly rifampicin plus daily dapsone in initial treatment of lepromatous leprosy. Lancet. 1982;1:1119.

115. Bullock WE. Rifampin in the treatment of leprosy. Rev Infect Dis. 1983;5(Suppl):606–613.
116. Deal WB, Sanders E. Efficacy of rifampin in treatment of meningococcal carriers. N Engl J Med. 1969;281:641–645.
117. Devine LF, Rhode SL, Pierce WE. Rifampin: Effect of two-day treatment on the meningococcal carrier state and the relationship to the levels of drug in sera and saliva. Am J Med Sci. 1971;261:79–83.
118. Weidmer CE, Dunkel TB, Pettyjohn FS, et al. Effectiveness of rifampin in eradicating the meningococcal carrier state in a relatively closed population: Emergence of resistant strains. J Infect Dis. 1971;124:172–178.
119. Beaty HN. Rifampin and minocycline in meningococcal disease. Rev Infect Dis. 1983;5(Suppl):451–458.
120. Jacobson JA, Daniel B. Vestibular reactions associated with minocycline. Antimicrob Agents Chemother. 1975;8:453–456.
121. Schwartz B, Al-Ruwais A, A'Ashi J, et al. Comparative efficacy of ceftriax-one and rifampicin in eradicating pharyngeal carriage of group A *Neisseria meningitidis*. Lancet. 1988;1:1239–1242.
122. Pugsley MP, Dworzack DL, Horowitz EA, et al. Efficacy of ciprofloxacin in the treatment of nasopharyngeal carriers of *Neisseria meningitidis*. J Infect Dis. 1987;156:211–213.
123. Pearce MC, Sheridan JW, Jones DM, et al. Control of group C meningococcal disease in Australian aboriginal children by mass rifampicin chemoprophylaxis and vaccination. Lancet. 1995;346:20–23.
124. Cuevas LE, Kazembe P, Mughogho GK, et al. Eradication of nasopharyngeal carriage of *Neisseria meningitidis* in children and adults in rural Africa: A comparison of ciprofloxacin and rifampicin. J Infect Dis. 1995;171:728–731.
125. Broome CV, Mortimer EA, Katz SL, et al. Use of chemoprophylaxis to prevent the spread of *Hemophilus influenzae* B in day-care facilities. N Engl J Med. 1987;316:1226–1228.
126. Update: Prevention of *Haemophilus influenzae* type b disease. MMWR. 1986;35:170–180.
127. Brunnel PA, Bass JW, Daum RS, et al. Revision of recommendation for use of rifampin prophylaxis of contact of patients with *Haemophilus influenzae* infection. Pediatrics. 1984;74:301–302.
128. Respiratory and Special Pathogens Epidemiology Branch (CDC): Prevention of secondary cases of *Haemophilus influenzae* type B disease. MMWR. 1982;31:672.
129. American Academy of Pediatrics. Report of the Committee on Infectious Diseases. 22nd ed. Elk Grove Village, Ill: American Academy of Pediatrics; 1991:220–229.
130. Dashefsky B, Wald E, Li K. Management of contacts of children in day care with invasive *Haemophilus influenzae* type b disease. Pediatrics. 1986;78:939–940.
131. Wilde J, Adler SP. Molecular epidemiology of *Haemophilus influenzae* type B: Failure of rifampin prophylaxis in a day care center. Pediatr Infect Dis. 1986;5:505–508.
132. Cates KL, Krause PJ, Murphy TV, et al. Second episodes of *Haemophilus influenzae* type b disease following rifampin prophylaxis of the index patients. Pediatr Infect Dis J. 1987;6:512–515.
133. Sande MA. The use of rifampin in treatment of nontuberculous infections. Rev Infect Dis. 1983;5(Suppl):399.
134. Vazquez GJ, Archer GL. Antibiotic therapy of experimental *Staphylococcus epidermidis* endocarditis. Antimicrob Agents Chemother. 1980;17:280–285.
135. Tuazon CU, Washburn D. Teicoplanin and rifampicin singly and in combination in the treatment of experimental *Staphylococcus epidermidis* endocarditis in the rabbit model. J Antimicrob Chemother. 1987;20:233–237.
136. Karchmer AW, Archer GL, Dismukes WE. *Staphylococcus epidermidis* causing prosthetic valve endocarditis: Microbiological and clinical observations as guides to therapy. Ann Intern Med. 1983;48:447.
137. Karchmer AW, Archer GA. Methicillin-resistant *Staphylococcus epidermidis* (SE) prosthetic valve (PV) endocarditis (E): A therapeutic trial. Abstract 476. In: Program and Abstracts of the Twenty-fourth Interscience Conference on Antimicrobial Agents and Chemotherapy, October 8–10, 1984.
138. Chamovitz B, Bryant RE, Gilbert D, et al. Prosthetic valve endocarditis caused by *Staphylococcus epidermidis*. JAMA. 1985;253:2867–2868.
139. Swanberg L, Tuazon CU. Rifampin in the treatment of serious staphylococcal infections. Am J Med Sci. 1984;287:49–54.
140. Acar JF, Goldstein EW, Duval J. Use of rifampin for the treatment of serious staphylococcal and gram-negative bacillary infections. Rev Infect Dis. 1983;5(Suppl)502–506.
141. Roder BL, Gutschik E. In-vitro activity of ciprofloxacin combined with either fusidic acid or rifampicin against *Staphylococcus aureus*. J Antimicrob Chemother. 1989;23:347–352.
142. Moretti MV, Fiorio M, Pasticci MB, et al. Killing rate and serum bactericidal activity of oxacillin, rifampin and ciprofloxacin against *Staphylococcus aureus*. Microbiologica. 1989;12:297–306.
143. Zak O, Scheld M, Sande M. Rifampin in experimental endocarditis due to *Staphylococcus aureus* in rabbits. Rev Infect Dis. 1983;5(Suppl):481–490.
144. Dworkin RJ, Lee BL, Sande MA, et al. Treatment of right-sided *Staphylococcus aureus* endocarditis in intravenous drug users with ciprofloxacin and rifampicin. Lancet. 1989;2:1071–1073.
145. Kaatz GW, Seo SM, Barriere SL, et al. Ciprofloxacin and rifampin, alone and in combination, for therapy of experimental *Staphylococcus aureus* endocarditis. Antimicrob Agents Chemother. 1989;33:1184–1187.
146. Tebas P, Martinez Ruiz R, Roman F, et al. Early resistance to rifampin and ciprofloxacin in the treatment of right-sided *Staphylococcus aureus* endocarditis. J Infect Dis. 1991;163:204–205.
147. Heldman AW, Hartert TV, Ray SC, et al. Oral antibiotic treatment of right-sided staphylococcal endocarditis in injection drug users: Prospective randomized comparison with parenteral therapy. Am J Med. 1996;101:68–76.
148. Kapusnik JE, Parenti F, Sande M. The use of rifampicin in staphylococcal infections—a review. J Antimicrob Chemother. 1984;13:61–66.
149. Bayer AS, Lam K. Efficacy of vancomycin plus rifampin in experimental aortic-valve endocarditis due to methicillin-resistant *Staphylococcus aureus*: In vitro–in vivo correlations. J Infect Dis. 1985;151:157–165.
150. Chambers HF, Kartalija M, Sande M. Ampicillin, sulbactam, and rifampin combination treatment of experimental methicillin-resistant *Staphylococcus aureus* endocarditis in rabbits. J Infect Dis. 1995;171:897–902.
151. Eng RHK, Smith SM, Tillem M, et al. Rifampin resistance. Development during the therapy of methicillin-resistant *Staphylococcus aureus* infection. Arch Intern Med. 1985;145:146–148.
152. Simon GL, Smith RH, Sande MA. Emergence of rifampin-resistant strains of *Staphylococcus aureus* during combination therapy with vancomycin and rifampin: A report of two cases. Rev Infect Dis. 1983;5(Suppl):507–508.
153. Eng RHK, Smith SM, Buccini FJ, et al. Differences in ability of cell-wall antibiotics to suppress emergence of rifampicin resistance in *Staphylococcus aureus*. J Antimicrob Chemother. 1985;15:201–207.
154. Hackbarth CJ, Chambers HF, Sande MA. Serum bactericidal activity of rifampin in combination with other antimicrobial agents against *Staphylococcus aureus*. Antimicrob Agents Chemother. 1986;29:611–613.
155. Foldes M, Munro R, Sorrell TC, et al. In-vitro effects of vancomycin, rifampicin, and fusidic acid, alone and in combination, against methicillin-resistant *Staphylococcus aureus*. J Antimicrob Chemother. 1983;11:21–26.
156. Levine DP, Fromm BS, Reddy BR. Slow response to vancomycin or vancomycin plus rifampin in methicillin-resistant *Staphylococcus aureus* endocarditis. Ann Intern Med. 1991;115:674–680.
157. Coleman DL, Horwitz RI, Andriole VT. Association between serum inhibitory and bactericidal concentrations and therapeutic outcome in bacterial endocarditis. Am J Med. 1982;73:260–267.
158. Traczewski MM, Goldmann DA, Murphy P. In vitro activity of rifampin in combination with oxacillin against *Staphylococcus aureus*. Antimicrob Agents Chemother. 1983;23:571.
159. Watanakunakorn C, Guerriero JC. Interaction between vancomycin and rifampin against *Staphylococcus aureus*. Antimicrob Agents Chemother. 1981;19:1089.
160. Walsh TJ, Auger P, Tatem BA, et al. Novobiocin and rifampicin in combination against methicillin-resistant *Staphylococcus aureus*: An in-vitro comparison with vancomycin plus rifampicin. J Antimicrob Chemother. 1986;17:75–82.
161. Varaldo PE, Debbia E, Schito GC. In vitro activity of teichomycin and vancomycin alone and in combination with rifampin. Antimicrob Agents Chemother. 1983;23:402–406.
162. Zinner SH, Lagast H, Klastersky J. Antistaphylococcal activity of rifampin with other antibiotics. J Infect Dis. 1981;144:365–371.
163. Van der Auwera P, Klastersky J. In vitro study of the combination of rifampin with oxacillin against *Staphylococcus aureus*. Rev Infect Dis. 1983;5(Suppl):509–514.
164. Van der Auwera P, Klastersky J. Bactericidal activity and killing rate of serum in volunteers receiving teicoplanin alone or in combination with oral or intravenous rifampin. Antimicrob Agents Chemother. 1987;31:1002–1005.
165. Ho JL, Klempner MS. In vitro evaluation of clindamycin in combination with oxacillin rifampin or vancomycin against *Staphylococcus aureus*. Diun Microbiol Infect Dis. 1986;4:133.
166. Bayer AS, Morrison JO. Disparity between timed-kill and checkerboard methods for determination of in vitro bactericidal interactions of vancomycin plus rifampin versus methicillin-susceptible and resistant *Staphylococcus aureus*. Antimicrob Agents Chemother. 1984;26:220–223.
167. Sande MA, Scheld WM. Combination antibiotic therapy of bacterial endocarditis. Ann Intern Med. 1980;92:390.
168. Jariwalla AG, Davies BH, White J. Infective endocarditis complicating psittacosis: Response to rifampicin. BMJ. 1980;280:155.
169. Raoult D. Treatment of Q fever. Antimicrob Agents Chemother. 1993;37:1733–1736.
170. Levy PY, Drancourt M, Etienne J, et al. Comparison of different antibiotic regimens for therapy of 32 cases of Q fever endocarditis. Antimicrob Agents Chemother. 1991;35:533–537.
171. Faville RJ, Zaske DE, Kaplan EL, et al. *Staphylococcus aureus* endocarditis: Combined therapy with vancomycin and rifampin. JAMA. 1978;240:1963.
172. Simmons NA. Synergy and rifampicin. J Antimicrob Chemother. 1977;3:109.
173. Wheat LJ, Kohler RB, White AL, et al. Effect of rifampin on nasal carriers of coagulase-positive staphylococci. J Infect Dis. 1981;144:177.
174. Wheat LJ, Kohler RB, Luft PC, et al. Long term studies of the effect of rifampin on nasal carriage of coagulase-positive staphylococci. Rev Infect Dis. 1983;5(Suppl):459–462.
175. McNally TP, Lewis MR, Brown DR. Effect of rifampin and bacitracin on nasal carriers of *Staphylococcus aureus*. Antimicrob Agents Chemother. 1984;25:422–426.
176. Locksley RM, Cohen ML, Quinn TC, et al. Multiply antibiotic-resistant *Staphylococcus aureus*: Introduction, transmission, and evolution of nosocomial infection. Ann Intern Med. 1982;97:317.
177. Zimmerman SW, Johnson CA. Rifampin use in peritoneal dialysis. Peritoneal Dialysis Int. 1989;9:241–243.
178. Ward TT, Winn RE, Hartstein AL, et al. Observations relating to an interhospital outbreak of methicillin resistant *Staphylococcus aureus*: Role of antimicrobial therapy in infection control. Infect Control. 1981;2:453.
179. Ellison H, Judson PN, Peterson LC, et al. Oral rifampin trimethoprim-sulfa-

methoxazole therapy in symptomatic carriers of methicillin-resistant *Staphylococcus aureus* infections. West J Med. 1984;140:735–740.
180. Pearson JW, Christiansen KJ, Annear DI, et al. Control of methicillin-resistant *Staphylococcus aureus* (MRSA) in an Australian metropolitan teaching hospital complex. Med J Aust. 1985;142:103–108.
181. Darouiche R, Wright C, Hamill R, et al. Eradication of colonization by methicillin-resistant *Staphylococcus aureus* by using oral minocycline-rifampin and topical mupirocin. Antimicrob Agents Chemother. 1991;35:1612–1615.
182. Arathoon EG, Hamilton JR, Hench CE, et al. Efficacy of short courses of oral novobiocin-rifampin in eradicating carrier state of methicillin-resistant *Staphylococcus aureus* and in vitro killing studies of clinical isolates. Antimicrob Agents Chemother. 1990;34:1655–1659.
183. Tanz RR, Shulman ST, Barthel MJ, et al. Penicillin plus rifampin eradicates pharyngeal carriage of group A streptococci. J Pediatr. 1985;106:876–880.
184. Rosenberg EW, Noah PW, Zanolli MD, et al. Use of rifampin with penicillin and erythromycin in the treatment of psoriasis. J Am Acad Dermatol. 1986;14:761–764.
185. Vincent F, Ross JB, Dalton M, et al. A therapeutic trial of the use of penicillin V or erythromycin with or without rifampin in the treatment of soriasis. J Am Acad Dermatol. 1992;26:458–461.
186. Millard DD, Shulman ST, Yogev R. Rifampin and penicillin for the elimination of group B streptococci in nasally colonized infant rats. Pediatr Res. 1985;19:1183–1186.
187. Norden CW, Shaffer M. Treatment of experimental chronic osteomyelitis, due to *Staphylococcus aureus* with vancomycin and rifampin. J Infect Dis. 1983;147:352.
188. Dworkin R, Modin G, Kunz S, et al. Comparative efficacies of ciprofloxacin, pefloxacin, and vancomycin in combination with rifampin in a rat model of methicillin-resistant *Staphylococcus aureus* chronic osteomyelitis. Antimicrob Agents Chemother. 1990;34:1014–1016.
189. O'Reilly T, Kunz S, Sande E, et al. Relationship between antibiotic concentration in bone and efficacy of treatment of staphylococcal osteomyelitis in rats: Azithromycin compared with clindamycin and rifampin. Antimicrob Agents Chemother. 1992;36:2693–2697.
190. Norden CW, Bryant R, Palmer D, et al. Chronic osteomyelitis caused by *Staphylococcus aureus*: Controlled clinical trial of nafcillin therapy and nafcillin-rifampin therapy. South Med J. 1986;79:947–951.
191. Widmer AF, Gaechter A, Ochsner PE, et al. Antimicrobial treatment of orthopedic implant-related infections with rifampin combinations. Clin Infect Dis. 1992;14:1251–1253.
192. Isiklar ZU, Darouiche RO, Landon GC, Beck T. Efficacy of antibiotics alone for orthopaedic device related infections. Clin Orthop. 1996;332:184–189.
193. Beam TR. Sequestration of *Staphylococcus aureus* at an inaccessible focus. Lancet. 1979;2:227.
194. Dournon E, Mayaud C, Wolff M, et al. Comparison of the activity of three antibiotic regimens in severe legionnaires' disease. J Antimicrob Chemother. 1990;26(Suppl B):129–139.
195. Jacobs F, Abramowicz D, Vereerstraeten P, et al. *Brucella* endocarditis: The role of combined medical and surgical treatment. Rev Infect Dis. 1990;12:740–744.
196. LLoren-Terol J, Busquets RM. Brucellosis treated with rifampicin. Arch Dis Child. 1980;55:486.
197. Shehabi A, Shakir K, el-Khateeb M, et al. Diagnosis and treatment of 106 cases of human brucellosis. J Infect. 1990;20:5–10.
198. Ariza J, Gudiol P, Pallares R, et al. Comparative trial of rifampin-doxycycline versus tetracycline-streptomycin in the therapy of human brucellosis. Antimicrob Agent Chemother. 1985;28:548–551.
199. Colmenero Castillo JD, Hernandez Marquez S, Reguera Iglesias JM, et al. Comparative trial of doxycycline plus streptomycin versus doxycycline plus rifampin for the therapy of human brucellosis. Chemotherapy. 1989;35:146–152.
200. Solera J, Medrano F, Rodriguez M, et al. A comparative therapeutic and multicenter trial of rifampicin and doxycycline versus streptomycin and doxycycline in human brucellosis. Med Clin. 1991;96:649–653.
201. Ariza J, Guidol F, Pallares R, et al. Treatment of human brucellosis with doxycycline plus rifampin or doxycycline plus streptomycin. A randomized, double-blind study. Ann Intern Med. 1992;117:25–30.
202. Akova M, Uzun O, Akalin HE, et al. Quinolones in treatment of human brucellosis: Comparative trial of ofloxacin-rifampin versus doxycycline-rifampin. Antimicrob Agents Chemother. 1993;37:1831–1834.
203. Perez MAH, Rodriguez BA, Garcia AP, et al. Treatment of nervous system brucellosis with rifampin and doxycycline (Letter). Neurology. 1986;36:1408–1409.
204. Bella F, Espejo E, Uriz S, et al. Randomized trial of 5-day rifampin versus 1-day doxycycline therapy for Mediterranean spotted fever. J Infect Dis. 1991;164: 433–434.
205. Ezer G, Soothill JF. Intracellular bactericidal effect of rifampicin in both normal and chronic granulomatous disease polymorphs. Arch Dis Child. 1974;49:463.
206. Lorber B. Rifampin in chronic granulomatous disease. N Engl J Med. 1980;303:111.
207. Archer G, Tenenbaum JM, Haywood HB. Rifampin therapy of *S. epidermidis*: Use in infections from indwelling artificial devices. JAMA. 1978;240:751.
208. Bolton WK, Sande MA, Normansell DE, et al. Ventriculojugular shunt nephritis with *Corynebacterium bovis.* Am J Med. 1975;59:417.
209. Ring JC, Cates KL, Belani KK, et al. Rifampin for CSF shunt infection caused by coagulase-negative staphylocci. J Pediatr. 1979;95:317.
210. O'Keefe PT, Bayston R. Pneumococcal meningitis in child with ventriculoperitoneal shunt. J Infect. 1991;22:77–79.
211. Walters BC, Goumnerova L, Hoffman HJ, et al. A randomized controlled trial of perioperative rifampin/trimethoprim in cerebrospinal fluid shunt surgery. Childs Nerv Sys. 1992;8:253–257.
212. Langley JM, LeBlanc JC, Drake J, Milner R. Efficacy of antimicrobial prophylaxis in placement of cerebrospinal fluid shunts: meta-analysis. Clin Infect Dis. 1993;17:98–103.
213. Bayston R, Lambert E. Duration of protective activity of cerebrospinal fluid shunt catheters impregnated with antimicrobial agents to prevent bacterial catheter-related infection. J Neurosurg. 1997;87:247–251.
214. Teloken C, Souto JC, Da Ros C, et al. Prosthetic penile infection: "Rescue procedure" with rifamycin. J Urol. 1992;148:1905–1906.
215. Wakefield TW, Schaberg DR, Pierson CL, et al. Treatment of established prosthetic vascular graft infection with antibiotics preferentially concentrated in leukocytes. Surgery. 1987;102:8–14.
216. Chuard C, Herrmann M, Vaudaux P, et al. Successful therapy of experimental chronic foreign-body infection due to methicillin-resistant *Staphylococcus aureus* by antimicrobial combinations. Antimicrob Agents Chemother. 1991;35:2611–2616.
217. Gagnon RF, Richards GK, Wisenfeld L. *Staphylococcus epidermidis* biofilms: Unexpected outcome of double and triple antibiotic combinations with rifampin. ASAIO Trans. 1991;37:M158–M160.
218. Colburn MD, Moore WS, Chvapil M, et al. Use of an antibiotic-bonded graft for in situ reconstruction after prosthetic graft infections. J Vasc Surg. 1992;16:651–660.
219. Freyrie A, Curti T, Rodio M, et al. Interaction between vascular prostheses and rifampicin in the prevention of the grafts infection. An experimental study. Int Angiol. 1992;11:113–116.
220. Lundell A, Bergqvist D, Lindblad B, et al. The acute thrombogenicity of an infection-resistant rifampicin-soaked Dacron graft: An experimental study in sheep. 1992;6:403–407.
221. Goeau-Brissonniere O, Leport C, Bacourt F, et al. Prevention of vascular graft infection by rifampin bonding to a gelatin-sealed Dacron graft. Ann Vasc Surg. 1991;5:408–412.
222. Chervu A, Moore WS, Gelabert HA, et al. Prevention of graft infection by use of prostheses bonded with a rifampin/collagen release system. J Vasc Surg. 1991;14:521–525.
223. Avramovic Jr, Fletcher JP. Rifampicin impregnation of a protein-sealed Dacron graft: An infection-resistant prosthetic vascular graft. Aust N Z J Surg. 1991;61:436–440.
224. Avramovic J, Fletcher JP. Prevention of prosthetic vascular graft infection by rifampicin impregnation of a protein-sealed Dacron graft in combination with parenteral cephalosporin. J Cardiovasc Surg. 1992;33:70–74.
225. Strachan CJ, Newsom SW, Ashton TR. The clinical use of an antibiotic-bonded graft. Eur J Vasc Surg 1991;5:627–632.
226. French BG, Chard RB, Sholler GF, Cartmill TB. Salvage of infected truncus repair using rifampicin-impregnated gelatin-sealed graft. Ann Thorac Surg. 1994;57: 754–755.
227. Farr BM. Catheter related *Staphylococcus aureus.* In: Catheter Related Infections. Seifert H, Jansen B, Farr BM, eds., New York: Marcel Dekker; 1997:59–78.
228. Raad II, Hachem RY, Abi-Said D, et al. A prospective crossover randomized trial of novobiocin and rifampin prophylaxis for the prevention of intravascular catheter infections in cancer patients treated with interleukin-2. Cancer. 1998;82:403–411.
229. Raad I, Darouiche R, Hachem R, et al. The broad-spectrum activity and efficacy of catheters coated with minocycline and rifampin. J Infect Dis. 1996;173:418–424.
230. Raad I, Darouiche R, Dupuis J, et al. Central venous catheters coated with minocycline and rifampin for the prevention of catheter-related colonization and bloodstream infections. A randomized, double-blind trial. The Texas Medical Center Catheter Study Group. Ann Intern Med. 1997;127:267–274.
231. Peters W, Shaw JJ, Lainson R, et al. Potentiating action of rifampicin and isomazid against *Leishmania mexicana amazonensis.* Lancet. 1981;1:1122.
232. Even-Paz Z, Weinrauch L, Livshin R, et al. Rifampicin treatment of cutaneous leishmaniasis. Int J Dermatol. 1982;21:110.
233. Joshi RK, Nambiar PM. Dermal leishmaniasis and rifampicin. Int J Dermatol. 1989;28:612–614.
234. Conti R, Parenti P. Rifampin therapy for brucellosis, *Flavobacterium meningitis,* and cutaneous leishmaniasis. Rev Infect Dis. 1983;5(Suppl):600–605.
235. Brumfitt W, Dixson S, Hamilton-Miller JMT. Use of rifampin for the treatment of urinary tract infections. Rev Infect Dis. 1983;5(Suppl):573–582.
236. Desudchit P, Nunthapisud P, Rukjutitum S, et al. Rifampicin-erythromycin combination for the treatment of gonococcal urethritis in men. Southeast Asian J Trop Med Public Health. 1984;15:360–363.
237. Oriel JD, Ridway GL, Goldmeir D, et al. Treatment of gonococcal urethritis in men with a rifampicin-erythromycin combination. Sex Transm Dis. 1982;9:208–211.
238. Lasky J, Pulkingham N, Powers M, et al. *Rhodococcus equi* causing human pulmonary infection: Review of 29 cases. South Med J. 1991;84:1217–1220.
239. Gray B. Case report: *Rhodococcus equi* pneumonia in a patient infected by the human immunodeficiency virus. Am J Med Sci. 1992;303:180–183.
240. Plummer PA, Nsanze H, D'Costa LJ, et al. Short-course and single-dose antimicrobial therapy for chancroid in Kenya: Studies with rifampin alone and in combination with trimethoprim. Rev Infect Dis. 1983;5(Suppl):565–572.
241. Treatment of sexually transmitted diseases. Med Lett. 1988;30:5–10.
242. Kumar A, Wofford-McQueen R, Gordon RC. Ciprofloxacin, imipenem and rifampicin: In-vitro synergy of two and three drug combinations against *Pseudomonas cepacia.* J Antimicrob Chemother. 1989;23:831–835.
243. Zuravleff JJ, Yu VL, Yee RB. Ticarcillin-tobramycin-rifampin: In vitro synergy of the triplet combination against *Pseudomonas aeruginosa.* J Lab Clin Med. 1983;101:896–902.

244. Yu VL, Zuravleff JJ, Peacock JE, et al. Addition of rifampin to carboxypenicillin-aminoglycoside combination for the treatment of *Pseudomonas aeruginosa* infection: Clinical experience with four patients. Antimicrob Agents Chemother. 1984;26:575–577.
245. Chin NX, Heu HC. Synergy of imipenen, a novel carbapenem, and rifampin and ciprofloxacin against *Pseudomonas aeruginosa, Serratia marcescens* and *Enterobacter* species. Chemotherapy. 1987;33:183–188.
246. Korvick JA, Peacock JE, Jr, Muder RR, et al. Addition of rifampin to combination antibiotic therapy for *Pseudomonas aeruginosa* bacteremia: Prospective trial using the Zelen protocol. Antimicrob Agents Chemother. 1992;36:620–625.
247. Rubin J, Stoehr G, Yu VL, et al. Efficacy of oral ciprofloxacin plus rifampin for treatment of malignant external otitis. Arch Otolaryngol Head Neck Surg. 1989;115:1063–1069.
248. Gamea AM, el-Tatawi FA. The effect of rifampicin on rhinoscleroma: An electron microscopic study. J Laryngol Otol. 1990;104:722–777.
249. Perking BA, Tondella ML, Bortolotto IM, et al. Comparative efficacy of oral rifampin and topical chloramphenicol in eradicating conjunctival carriage of *Haemophilus influenzae* biogroup *aegyptius*. Pediatr Infect Dis J. 1992;11:717–721.
250. Fu KP, Lasinski ER, Zoganas HC, et al. Therapeutic efficacy and pharmacokinetic properties of rifampicin in a *Bacteroides fragilis* intra-abdominal abscess. J Antimicrob Chemother. 1984;14:633–640.
251. Fu KP, Lasinski ER, Zoganas HC, et al. Efficacy of rifampicin in experimental *Bacteroides fragilis* and *Pseudomonas aeruginosa* mixed infections. J Antimicrob Chemother. 1985;15:579–585.
252. Buggy BP, Fekety R, Silva J, Jr. Therapy of relapsing *Clostridium difficile* associated diarrhea and colitis with the combination of vancomycin and rifampin. J Clin Gastroenterol. 1987;9:155–159.
253. Bacon AE, McGrath S, Fekety R, et al. In vitro synergy studies with *Clostridium difficile*. Antimicrob Agents Chemother. 1991;35:582–583.
254. Bloch KC, Nadarajah R, Jacobs R. Chryseobacterium meningosepticum: An emerging pathogen among immunocompromised adults. Report of 6 cases and literature review. Medicine. 1997;76:30–41.
255. Hirsh BE, Wong B, Kiehn TE, et al. A case of *Flavobacterium meningosepticum* bacteremia in an adult with acute leukemia. Use of rifampin to clear persistent infection. Diagn Microbiol Infect Dis. 1986;4:65–69.
256. Lewis MA, Priestley BL. Addition of rifampicin in persistent *Haemophilus influenzae* type B meningitis. 1986;292:448–449.
257. Ryan JL, Pachner A, Andriole VT, et al. Enterococcal meningitis: Combined vancomycin and rifampin therapy. Am J Med. 1980;68:449–451.
258. Bow EJ, Mandell LA, Louie TJ, et al. Quinolone-based antibacterial chemoprophylaxis in neutropenic patients: Effect of augmented gram-positive activity on infectious morbidity. National Cancer Institute of Canada Clinical Trials Group. Ann Intern Med. 1996;125:183–190.
259. Hidalgo M, Hornedo J, Lumbreras C, et al. Lack of ability of ciprofloxacin-rifampin prophylaxis to decrease infection-related morbidity in neutropenic patients given cytotoxic therapy and peripheral blood stem cell transplants. Antimicrob Agents Chemother. 1997;41:1175–1177.
260. Gilbert C, Meisenberg B, Vredenburgh J, et al. Sequential prophylactic oral and empiric once-daily parenteral antibiotics for neutropenia and fever after high-dose chemotherapy and autologous bone marrow support. J Clin Oncol. 1994;12:1005–1011.
261. Zubovich IK, Votyakov VI, Mishaeva NP. Rifampicin protective action in experimental rabies infection of albino mice. Antibiot Khimioter. 1989;34:123–125.
262. Varaldo PE, Debbia E, Schito GC. In vitro activities of rifapentine and rifampin, alone and in combination with six other antibiotics, against methicillin-susceptible and methicillin-resistant staphylococci of different species. Antimicrob Agents Chemother. 1985;27:615–618.
263. Korvic J, Yu VL, Sharp JA. Interaction of rifampicin or rifapentine with other agents against *Pseudomonas aerugionosa*. J Antimicrob Chemother. 1987;19: 847–848.
264. Dickinson JM, Mitchison DA. In vitro properties of rifapentine (MDL473) relevant to its use in intermittent chemotherapy of tuberculosis. Tubercle. 1987;68:113–118.
265. Bermudez LEM, Wu M, Young LS. Intracellular killing of *Mycobacterium avium* complex by rifapentine and liposome-encapsulated amikacin. J Infect Dis. 1987;156:510–513.
266. Assandri A, Ratti B, Cristina T. Pharmacokinetics of rifapentine, a new long lasting rifamycin, in the rat, the mouse and the rabbit. J Antibiot (Tokyo). 1984;37:1066–1073.
267. Durand DV, Hampden C, Boobis AR, et al. Induction of mixed function oxidase activity in man by rifapentine (MDL473), a long-acting rifamycin derivative. Br J Clin Pharmacol. 1986;21:1–7.
268. Liw DY, Wang YS. Inductive effects of rifapentine on mice hepatic mixed function oxidase system. Methods Find Exp Clin Pharmacol. 1990;12:109–113.
269. Vital Durand D, Hampden C, Boobis AR, et al. Induction of mixed function oxidase activity in man by rifapentine (MDL473), a long-acting rifamycin derivative. Br J Clin Pharmacol. 1986;21:1–7.
270. He GJ. A comparative study of rifapentine treatment and three years follow-up on initial pulmonary tuberculous (in Chinese). Chung-Hua Chieh Ho Ho Hu Hsi Tsa Chih (Chin J Tuberc Respir Dis). 1993;16:73–76, 122.
271. Klemens SP, Cynamon MH. Activity of rifapentine against *Mycobacterium avium* infection in beige mice. J Antimicrob Chemother. 1992;29:555–561.
272. Heifets LB, Lindholm-Levy PJ, Flory MA. Bactericidal activity in vitro of various rifamycins against *Mycobacterium avium* and *Mycobacterium tuberculosis*. Am Rev Respir Dis. 1990;141:626–630.
273. O'Brien RJ, Lyle MA, Snider DE. Rifabutin (ansamycin LM 427): A new rifamycin-S derivative for the treatment of mycobacterial diseases. Rev Infect Dis. 1987;9:519–530.
274. Cato A, 3rd, Cavanaugh J, Shi H, et al. The effect of multiple doses of ritonavir on the pharmacokinetics of rifabutin. Clin Pharmacolo Thera. 1998;63:414–421.
275. Iatsimirskaia E, Tulebaev S, Storozhuk E, et al. Metabolism of rifabutin in human enterocyte and liver microsomes: Kinetic parameters, identification of enzyme systems, and drug interactions with macrolides and antifungal agents. Clin Pharmacol Ther. 1997;61:554–562.
276. Shafran SD, Singer J, Zarowny DP, et al. A comparison of two regimens for the treatment of *Mycobacterium avium* complex bacteremia in AIDS: Rifabutin, ethambutol, and clarithromycin versus rifampin, ethambutol, clofazimine, and ciprofloxacin. Canadian HIV Trials Network Protocol 010 Study Group. N Engl J Med. 1996;335:377–383.
277. Saran BR, Maguire AM, Nichols C, et al. Hypopyon uveitis in patients with acquired immunodeficiency syndrome treated for systemic *Mycobacterium avium* complex infection with rifabutin. Arch Ophthalmol. 1994;112:1159–1165.
278. Siefal FP, Eilbott D, Burger H, et al. Dose-limiting toxicity of rifabutin in AIDS-related complex: Syndrome of arthralgia/arthritis. AIDS. 1990;4:433–441.
279. Hawkins CC, Gold JWM, Whimbey E, et al. *Mycobacterium avium* complex infections in patients with the acquired immunodeficiency syndrome. Ann Intern Med. 1986;105:184–188.
280. Masur H, Tuazon C, Gill V, et al. Effect of combined clofazimine and ansamycin therapy on *Mycobacterium avium-Mycobacterium intracellulare* bacteremia in patients with AIDS. J Infect Dis. 1987;155:126–129.
281. Havlir DV, Dube MP, Sattler FR, et al. Prophylaxis against disseminated *Mycobacterium avium* complex with weekly azithromycin, daily rifabutin, or both. California Collaborative Treatment Group. N Engl J Med. 1996;335:392–398.
282. Shafran SD, Singer J, Zarowny DP, et al. A comparison of two regimens for the treatment of *Mycobacterium avium* complex bacteremia in AIDS: rifabutin, ethambutol, and clarithromycin versus rifampin, ethambutol, clofazimine, and ciprofloxacin. Canadian HIV Trials Network Protocol 010 Study Group. N Engl J Med. 1996;335:377–383.
283. Chan SL, Yew WW, Ma WK, et al. The early bactericidal activity of rifabutin measured by sputum viable counts in Hong Kong patients with pulmonary tuberculosis. Tubercle Lung Dis. 1992;73:33–38.
284. McGregor MM, Olliaro P, Wolmarans L, et al. Efficacy and safety of rifabutin in the treatment of patients with newly diagnosed pulmonary tuberculosis. Am J Respir Crit Care Med. 1996;154:1462–1467.
285. Pretet S, Lebeaut A, Parrot R, et al. Combined chemotherapy including rifabutin for rifampicin and isoniazid resistant pulmonary tuberculosis. Eur Respir J. 1992;5:680–684.
286. Anonymous. Rifabutine in the treatment of mycobacterial infections resistant to rifampicin. Preliminary results. Rev Mal Respir. 1989;6:335–342.
287. Holmberg SD, Moorman AC, Von Bargen JC, et al. Possible effectiveness of clarithromycin and rifabutin for cryptosporidiosis chemoprophylaxis in HIV disease. HIV Outpatient Study (HOPS) Investigators. JAMA. 1998;279:384–386.
288. Saito H, Tomioka H, Sato K, et al. In vitro antimycobacterial activities of newly synthesized benzoxazinorifamycins. Antimicrob Agents Chemother. 1991;35: 542–547.
289. Gidoh M, Tsutsumi S, Yamane T, et al. Bactericidalaction at low doses of a new rifamycin derivative, 3′-hydroxy-5′-(4-isobutyl-1-piperazinyl) benzoxazinorifamycin (KRM01648) on *Mycobacterium leprae* inoculated into footpads of nude mice. Leprosy Rev. 1992;63:319–328.
290. Yamamoto Y, Saito H, Tomioka KH, et al. In vitro and in vivo activities of KRM-1648, a newly synthesized benzoxazinorifamycin, against *Mycobacterium marinum*. Int J Med Microbiol Virol Parasitol Infect Dis. 1992;277:204–209.
291. Verardi S, Verardi V. Bile rifaximin concentration after oral administration in patients undergoing cholecystectomy. Farmaco. 1990;45:131–135.
292. Iosca N, Ferrieri A. The rifaximin therapy and prophylaxis of episodes of acute diverticulitis. Recent Prog Med. 1993;84:49–53.
293. Corazza GR, Sorge M, Strocchi A, et al. Non-absorbable antibiotics and small bowel bacterial overgrowth. Italian J Gastrol. 1992;24:4–9.
294. Papi C, Camarri E. Non-absorbable antibiotics in the treatment of diverticular disease of the colon. Italian J Gastrol. 1992;24:19–22.
295. Di Febo G, Claabrese C, Matassoni F. New trends in non-absorbable antibiotics in gastrointestinal disease. Italian J Gastrol. 1992;24:10–13.
296. Pedretti G, Calzetti C, Missale, et al. Rifaximin versus neomycin on hyperammoniemia in chronic portal system encephalopathy of cirrhotics. A double-blind, randomized trial. Italian J Gastrol. 1991;23:175–178.
297. Bucci L, Palmieri GC. Double-blind, double-dummy comparison between treatment with rifaximin and lactulose in patients with medium to severe degree hepatic encephalopathy. Curr Med Res Opin. 1993;13:109–118.
298. Miglio F, Valpiani D, Rossellini SR, Ferrieri A. Rifaximin, a non-absorbable rifamycin, for the treatment of hepatic encephalopathy. A double-blind, randomised trial. Curr Med Res Opin. 1997;13:593–601.
299. Palazzini E, Palmerio B. Treatment of pyogenic skin infections with rifaximin cream. Riv Eur Sci Med Farmacol. 1993;15:87–92.
300. Bachs L, Pares A, Elena M, et al. Effects of long-term rifampicin administration in primary biliary cirrhosis. Gastrology 1992;102:2077–2080.
301. Podesta A, Lopez P, Terg R, et al. Treatment of pruritus of primary biliary cirrhosis with rifampin. Dig Dis Sci. 1991;36:216–220.
302. Cynamon HA, Andres JM, Iafrate RP. Rifampin relieves pruritus in children with cholestatic liver disease. Gastroenterology. 1990;98:1013–1016.
303. Gabriel SE, Conn DL, Luthra H. Rifampin therapy in rheumatoid arthritis. J Rheumatol. 1990;17:163–166.

304. Caruso I, Cazzola M, Santandrea S. Clinical improvement in ankylosing spondylitis with rifamycin SV infiltrations of peripheral joints. J Int Med Res. 1992;20:171–181.
305. Caviglia HA, Fernandez-Palazzi F, Maffei E, et al. Chemical synoviorthesis for hemophilic synovitis. Clin Orthop. 1997;343:30–36.
306. Rutgeerts P, Geboes K, Vantrappen G, et al. Rifabutin and ethambutol do not help recurrent Crohn's disease in the neoterminal ileum. J Clin Gastroenterol. 1992;15:24–28.
307. Swift GL, Srivastava ED, Stone R, et al. Controlled trial of anti-tuberculous chemotherapy for two years in Crohn's disease. Gut. 1994;35:363–368.
308. West CM, Reeves SJ, Brough W. Additive interaction between tamoxifen and rifampicin in human biliary tract carcinoma cells. Cancer Lett. 1990;55:159–163.
309. Burghouts J, Haanen C. A possible role of rifampicin in prolonging remission duration in acute myelogenous leukemia. Scand J Haematol. 1986;36:376–378.
310. Strayhorn VA, Baclewicz AM, Self TH. Update on rifampin drug interactions. III. (Review). Arch Intern Med. 1997;157:2453–2458.
311. Rizak MA. Handbook of Adverse Drug Interactions. New Rochelle, NY: Medical Letter; 1998.

Chapter 26

Metronidazole

SYDNEY M. FINEGOLD

DESCRIPTION

Metronidazole was introduced in 1959 for the treatment of *Trichomonas vaginalis* infections. It is now known to be effective against most infections involving anaerobic bacteria and against certain other parasitic infections. Metronidazole diffuses well into all tissues, including the central nervous system. It is well tolerated and has the best bactericidal activity of all drugs active against anaerobic bacteria.

Metronidazole is a nitroimidazole drug with the chemical formula 1-(2-hydroxyethyl)-2-methyl-5-nitroimidazole. It has a low molecular weight, 171.

SPECTRUM OF ACTIVITY, RESISTANCE

Table 26–1 summarizes the activity of metronidazole against 793 strains of anaerobic and microaerophilic bacteria. Note that virtually all the organisms tested were inhibited by 16 μg/ml or less except for one third of gram-positive non–spore-forming bacilli and 7% of *Capnocytophaga* spp. Metabolites are found in serum and urine, and Sutter[1] found that the hydroxy metabolite of metronidazole was slightly less active than the parent compound against many anaerobes but had equivalent or better activity against some. The acid metabolite has poor activity against anaerobes. In general, studies by other workers have given comparable results in terms of the in vitro activity of metronidazole. Wüst[2] found that seven strains of *Propionibacterium acnes* required 100 μg/ml for inhibition. Werner and associates[3] also noted that the hydroxy metabolite of metronidazole is roughly comparable in activity to the parent compound. Only about 25% of strains of *Actinomyces* and *Propionibacterium propionicum* are susceptible to metronidazole at achievable levels. Rosenblatt and Edson[4] noted somewhat less activity against anaerobic gram-positive cocci (a minimal inhibitory concentration for 70% of strains [MIC_{70}] of 6.25 and an MIC_{90} of 25 μg/ml or more). *P. acnes* was highly resistant. *Actinobacillus actinomycetemcomitans* and *Eikenella corrodens* are typically resistant, and one fourth of *Sutterella wadsworthensis* strains are resistant. The study by Chow and associates[5] found significantly more resistance to metronidazole among anaerobes than was indicated by the studies previously cited.

Also sensitive to metronidazole are *Treponema pallidum*, oral spirochetes, *Campylobacter fetus*, *Gardnerella vaginalis*, and *Helicobacter pylori*. In certain animal models, *Escherichia coli* may be inhibited by metronidazole when it is present together in a mixture with *Bacteroides fragilis*. However, in another animal model[6] there was no activity against *E. coli*. We have noted decreased counts of *E. coli* initially present together with anaerobes in the bypassed loop of patients with ileal bypass for obesity who were treated with metronidazole for "bypass enteropathy."

Trichomonas vaginalis, *Giardia lamblia*, and *Entamoeba histolytica* are usually susceptible to metronidazole.

Resistance to metronidazole develops rarely, and a combination of several mechanisms may be required for emergence of high-level resistance.[7] Failure to test metronidazole susceptibility under strict anaerobic conditions has led to reports of false resistance. Although both plasmid-mediated and chromosomally mediated resistance have been described, their transfer to metronidazole-sensitive *Bacteroides* spp. does not yet appear to be a problem.[8] Resistant strains identified include one strain each of *B. fragilis*, *Bacteroides distasonis*, what was originally described as *Bacteroides melaninogenicus* subsp. *melaninogenicus* and *Bacteroides bivius*. Phillips and coworkers[9] noted that they had seen occasional marginally resistant isolates of *B. bivius* (now called *Prevotella bivia*), *Bacteroides ureolyticus*, and perhaps *B. melaninogenicus* (now called *Prevotella melaninogenica*). Tally and colleagues[10] studied a metronidazole-resistant strain of *B. fragilis*. They found that the uptake of metronidazole by cells was slower than in a sensitive strain. Also, the rate of reduction of metronidazole was four times less than with a sensitive control strain, possibly due to decreased nitroreductase activity. Although rare, case reports suggest that resistant organisms may develop in patients receiving therapy, and this could lead to a clinical relapse of infection.[11, 12] *T. vaginalis* may become resistant to metronidazole, and several case reports have described recalcitrant vaginal trichomoniasis caused by resistant strains.[13–15]

MODE OF ACTION

Mechanism of Action

It is convenient to think of the action of the drug as occurring in four successive steps:[16] (1) the entry of the drug into the bacterial cell, (2) reductive activation, (3) the toxic effect of the reduced

TABLE 26–1 Activity of Metronidazole against Anaerobic and Microaerophilic Bacteria

Bacteria	No. Strains	Cumulative Percentage Susceptible to Indicated Concentration (μg/ml)			
		4	*8*	*16*	*32*
*Bacteroides fragilis**	161	90	99	100	—
B. melaninogenicus†	60	98	100	—	—
Other *Bacteroides, Prevotella,* and *Selenomonas* spp.	154	95	98	100	—
Fusobacterium spp.	65	100	—	—	—
Anaerobic gram-negative cocci	24	92	96	100	—
Anaerobic gram-positive cocci	124	98	—	—	—
Clostridium perfringens	18	94	100	—	—
Other *Clostridium* spp.	73	97	99	—	100
Gram-positive nonsporulating bacilli	87	57	60	62	66
Capnocytophaga spp.	27	52	70	93	—

*Includes all species of the *B. fragilis* group.
†Includes *Prevotella melaninogenica* (formerly *Bacteroides melaninogenicus*) and *Porphyromonas* (formerly *Bacteroides asaccharolyticus* subsp.).
From Sutter VL. In vitro susceptibility of anaerobic and microaerophilic bacteria to metronidazole and its hydroxy metabolite. In: Finegold SM, George WL, Rolfe RD, eds. Proceedings of the First United States Metronidazole Conference, Tarpon Springs, Fla, February 1982. New York: Biomedical Information Corp; 1982:61.

intermediate product or products, and (4) the release of inactive end products. A key feature is reduction of the nitro group of the drug; the drug acts as a preferential electron acceptor, being reduced by low–redox potential electron transport proteins (ferredoxin-like and flavodoxin-like). Reduction of the drug decreases the intracellular concentration of unchanged drug, thus maintaining a gradient that drives the uptake and generates compounds that are toxic to the cell. The toxicity is due to short-lived intermediate compounds or free radicals that produce damage by interaction with DNA and possibly other macromolecules. The cytotoxic intermediates decompose into nontoxic and inactive end products, including acetamide and 2-hydroxethyl oxamic acid.

Metabolic Products

As noted before, the hydroxy derivative of metronidazole has significant antianaerobic activity; it is more active than metronidazole is on *G. vaginalis.* The acid derivative of metronidazole has relatively little activity, less than one tenth as much as metronidazole against *B. fragilis* and *Trichomonas.*[16] The drug is also conjugated; the glucuronide has no activity on *Trichomonas* and is not taken up.[16]

Bactericidal Activity

Metronidazole is a potent bactericidal agent. It typically kills organisms at the same concentration or within one twofold dilution of that required for inhibition.[17] Under reduced conditions, metronidazole has a rapid onset of bactericidal activity. Killing rates are not affected by the inoculum size, nutritional requirements, or growth rate.[18, 19]

Bartlett and coworkers[20] found metronidazole to be the most effective drug in a *B. fragilis* subcutaneous abscess model in mice even when treatment was delayed for 8 to 120 hours after challenge.

PHARMACOLOGY

When given orally, metronidazole is absorbed rapidly and almost completely. Serum levels are similar during the elimination phase after equivalent doses by the intravenous and oral routes. Blood levels are proportional to the administered dose. The standard intravenous dosage regimen that has been used in the United States consists of a loading dose of 15 mg/kg of body weight followed by 7.5 mg/kg every 6 hours. This results in peak and trough steady-state plasma levels averaging 25 and 18 μg/ml, respectively. There is very little protein binding of metronidazole. The half-life is 8 hours. Absorption of metronidazole is not affected by the ingestion of food, but peak levels may be markedly delayed. Metronidazole is absorbed after vaginal administration, but peak serum levels (mean, 1.2 μg/ml) and bioavailability (20%) are lower than by oral or intravenous administration.[21] Absorption after rectal administration is quite good, although peak serum levels occur approximately 3 hours after insertion. Serum levels have generally been low after the use of vaginal suppositories and vaginal gel and after the application of gel to skin lesions such as acne rosacea. Metronidazole is rapidly transferred across the placenta; peak serum levels in the fetus are equivalent to maternal levels after intravenous administration to pregnant women.[22]

There is a large apparent volume of distribution of metronidazole that is equivalent to about 80% of body weight; it reaches all tissues and fluids. Therapeutic levels are achieved in amniotic fluid, polymorphonuclear leukocytes, the unobstructed biliary tract, pancreas, alveolar bone, cerebrospinal fluid and brain abscess contents, cord blood, pleural empyema fluid, peritoneal fluid, hepatic abscesses, middle ear discharge, middle ear mucosa, breast milk, pelvic tissues (concentrations attained in the myometrium and fallopian tubes are nearly the same as concomitant serum levels), colonic mucosa, saliva, seminal fluid, and vaginal secretions. Levels achieved in the aqueous humor were between one third and one half those attained in the serum.[23]

During metabolization of metronidazole, five major products are formed. The most important one is the hydroxy derivative. In addition, there is an acid metabolite, acetylmetronidazole, metronidazole glucuronide, and the glucuronide conjugate of hydroxy metronidazole. A sulfate conjugate may also be found on occasion. Metronidazole and particularly its metabolites are eliminated primarily in the urine (60 to 80% of the dose). From 6 to 15% is excreted in the feces.

The elimination half-life of metronidazole in patients with no renal function is the same as in healthy people. However, the hydroxy metabolite may accumulate in patients with absent renal function, and, although dosage adjustment is usually not considered necessary in the absence of hepatic disease, consideration might be given to dosage adjustment in patients initially receiving large doses. Metronidazole and its metabolites are rapidly removed by hemodialysis; the elimination half-life of metronidazole is reduced to 2.6 hours. Dose reduction is generally not necessary in patients undergoing chronic ambulatory peritoneal dialysis.[24] In patients with impaired hepatic function, even without concomitant renal function impairment, the plasma clearance of metronidazole is delayed. Although data are limited, pharmacokinetic studies in patients with significant liver disease suggest that doses should be reduced by at least 50% in this patient population.[25]

ADMINISTRATION AND DOSAGE

Table 26–2 gives dosage recommendations and routes of administration for the major indications for metronidazole therapy. The intravenous route is recommended initially for seriously ill patients. Since oral therapy gives blood levels comparable to those achieved by the intravenous route, one may switch when conditions warrant.

As noted, the standard regimen in the United States for intravenous administration has been a loading dose of 15 mg/kg of body weight followed by a maintenance schedule of 7.5 mg/kg every 6 hours. Clearly, the half-life of the drug would warrant administration at longer intervals such as every 8 or even every 12 hours. The manufacturer recommends that intravenous infusions be administered over a period of 1 hour. However, a number of foreign investigators have administered the drug in as little as 20 minutes without any apparent adverse effects. The maximal daily dose recommended is 4 g.

After reconstitution, metronidazole hydrochloride should be diluted with intravenous fluid to a concentration not exceeding 8 mg/ml and should be neutralized to pH 6 to 7 with sodium bicarbonate before administration. There is also a metronidazole intravenous solution (Flagyl IV RTU), a ready-to-use isotonic solution that does not require dilution or buffering before infusion.

The duration of therapy varies according to the entity being treated. Certain recommendations are made in Table 26–2. For serious infections, however, one may often need to treat the patient for 2 to 4 weeks or longer.

TABLE 26–2 Major Indications for Metronidazole: Administration and Dosage

Indication	Route of Administration	Dosage
Susceptible anaerobic infections	IV	Loading dose of 15 mg/kg, then 7.5 mg/kg q6h
	PO	1–2 g/d in 2–4 doses q6–12h
Bacterial vaginosis	PO	500 mg bid for 7 d
	Intravaginal	5 g of 0.75% intravaginal gel bid × 5 d
Trichomonas vaginitis	PO	250–500 mg tid for 7 d *or* 1.5 to 2 g in single dose
Amebiasis (intestinal or extraintestinal)	IV or PO	750 mg tid for 10 d
Giardiasis	PO	250 mg bid or tid for 5–7 d *or* 2 g/d for 3 d

Comments regarding dosage in patients with impaired renal or hepatic function, or both, are presented in the earlier section on pharmacology.

ADVERSE REACTIONS, PRECAUTIONS

In general, metronidazole is well tolerated. There is an interesting report of an accidental 10-fold overdose on three occasions in a preterm neonate that resulted in a peak serum level of 140 mg/liter and a level of 40 mg/liter 33.75 hours later but with no clinical signs of toxicity.[26] The more commonly encountered major and minor adverse reactions are listed in Table 26–3. There may also be furring of the tongue; glossitis; stomatitis; dry mouth; headache; fever; dizziness; syncope; vertigo; impaired sleep; states of confusion, excitation, or depression; and occasionally overgrowth of *Candida* in the oral cavity or vagina. Thrombophlebitis has been reported with intravenous infusion but is seldom seen now with proper buffering of the preparation. There is one report of an immediate rhinoconjunctivitis. No significant irritant or sensitization reactions have been reported with topical formulations. Gastrointestinal side effects include nausea, epigastric distress, anorexia, and, less commonly, vomiting, diarrhea, or pancreatitis. Although pseudomembranous colitis has been reported rarely with metronidazole therapy, the drug has proved effective therapeutically for this condition and is comparable to vancomycin in effectiveness. The most serious adverse effects are those involving the central nervous system. These are rare unless prolonged therapy or large doses, or both, are used, but peripheral neuropathy has been described in an individual who received repeated short courses of the drug. There is one report of metronidazole-induced psychosis of 2 weeks' duration. If abnormal neurologic symptoms are observed, treatment with the drug must be discontinued immediately. Metronidazole should be used with caution in people with a history of seizures or other central nervous system disorders. The peripheral neuropathy is generally reversible but may take a considerable period of time to resolve.

There has been concern about mutagenicity in the Ames *Salmonella* mutant system and carcinogenicity of metronidazole. Reduction of the nitro group of the compound is necessary for both antibacterial and mutagenic activity. Mutagenic activity has been detected in the urine of patients receiving 750 mg/day of metronidazole. When a mutant *Salmonella* strain that did not possess nitroreductase was used in the mutagenic testing system, metronidazole could not be demonstrated to be a mutagen. Thus, not the drug itself but rather one or more reduction products of it is mutagenic. Some protozoa, bacteria (including facultative anaerobes), and fungi possess nitroreductase activity. Eukaryotic tissues have very little nitroreductase activity. It has been suggested that during metronidazole therapy some reduction products of the drug might escape from the bacterial cells and serve as mutagens to the host's mammalian tissue. However, these active derivatives are very short lived and either promptly bind to macromolecules within the bacterial cell or are promptly reduced to compounds that are not mutagenic or carcinogenic. The drug has been studied specifically for mutagenic potential in eukaryotic test systems (human lymphocytes in vitro and lymphocytes of patients receiving metronidazole therapy) with conflicting results. No chromosomal aberrations or sister chromatid exchanges could be detected in vitro with metronidazole or its metabolites in concentrations of 1000 to 10,000 μg/ml. No lymphocyte abnormalities were noted in patients receiving a short course of metronidazole therapy.[27] On the other hand, Elizondo and coworkers[28] reported a significant increase in lymphocyte chromatid and isochromatid breaks. Metronidazole has shown tumorigenic activity in several studies in mice involving lifetime (or almost lifetime) oral administration. Female rats given metronidazole over long periods (sometimes for life) had a significant increase in neoplasms, especially mammary tumors, compared with controls. Interestingly, in one study drug-fed rats lived longer than controls did. Two lifetime studies in hamsters were negative (see Finegold[29]). Acetamide has been found in the urine of patients receiving metronidazole, and prolonged feeding of high doses of this compound to rats has produced hepatocarcinomas.[30] A study in rats with the dimethylhydrazine model for colon neoplasia showed that the addition of metronidazole on a long-term basis had an apparent cocarcinogenic effect.[31] As Condon notes in the discussion of this paper, the dimethylhydrazine tumor model is relatively specific and may not be readily extrapolated to humans.[31] Indeed, in another study looking at bile salt–induced colorectal cancer in rats, metronidazole administration appeared to reduce the carcinogenic effect of sodium deoxycholate.[32]

Long-term follow-up of a cohort of 771 women who received metronidazole therapy for the treatment of vaginal trichomoniasis during the 1960s has not shown an increased incidence of malignancy.[33] It should be recognized that these patients received relatively low doses of the drug for brief periods of time (7 to 10 days). A larger study with 5222 metronidazole user-nonuser pairs, with a median follow-up of 12.6 years, also failed to show an association between metronidazole use and cancer.[34] A report raises the possibility of carcinogenicity in three patients with Crohn's disease who had received prolonged therapy with metronidazole;[35] these observations remain anecdotal, and further studies are clearly needed. Although metronidazole appears to be safe, the long-term effects of high-dose prolonged therapy are not completely known, and such usage should be avoided if other alternatives are available.

Metronidazole crosses the placental barrier, and concerns have been raised about possible teratogenic effects in light of the evidence for mutagenicity in bacterial systems. To date, there has been little evidence for this in animal models. Studies in pregnant women who had received metronidazole during pregnancy for the treatment of vaginal trichomoniasis have not shown an increased incidence of stillbirths, small-for-age infants, premature infants, or teratogenicity.[36] A meta-analysis failed to find any relationship between metronidazole exposure during the first trimester of pregnancy and birth defects.[37] Nevertheless, the use of metronidazole during pregnancy should be reserved for situations in which it is clearly needed. Metronidazole during the first trimester should be avoided. Because metronidazole is excreted into breast milk, nursing should be discontinued during and for 2 days after therapy with metronidazole.

There is some evidence that the use of metronidazole contributes to the risk of vancomycin-resistant enterococcal infection or colonization. This is true to a greater extent for vancomycin use and is true for other drugs active against anaerobic bacteria (e.g., imipenem, clindamycin, ampicillin-sulbactam).

TABLE 26–3 Adverse Effects Related to Metronidazole Therapy

Major adverse reactions (rare)
Seizures, encephalopathy
Cerebellar dysfunction, ataxia
Peripheral neuropathy
Disulfiram reaction with alcohol
Potentiation of effects of warfarin
Pseudomembranous colitis
Pancreatitis, mild
Minor adverse reactions
Minor gastrointestinal disturbances
Reversible neutropenia
Metallic taste
Dark or red-brown urine
Maculopapular rash, urticaria; rarely, pustular eruption
Urethral, vaginal burning
Gynecomastia

Drug Interactions, Interference with Laboratory Tests

In patients ingesting alcohol, metronidazole may cause reactions similar to those produced by disulfiram. Patients should be advised not to drink alcohol when taking this drug. Metronidazole inhibits the metabolism of warfarin and other oral coumarin-type anticoagulants.

Therefore, if concomitant use is needed, the dosage of the anticoagulant should be reduced to maintain the desired prothrombin time.

Metronidazole interferes with certain chemical analyses for the serum enzyme glutamic oxaloacetic transaminase, which results in falsely low or negative values.

EFFECT ON NORMAL FECAL FLORA

In persons who have a healthy gastrointestinal tract and are not receiving other drugs, metronidazole has very little effect on the fecal flora.[38] This is thought to be due to the drug's being rapidly reduced by the bowel flora under the usual anaerobic conditions in the colon. Why this reduction would not have an impact on the organisms carrying out the reduction, as it does in the course of treating infections, is not at all clear. In patients on high-dosage regimens, in patients with diarrhea, and in patients receiving certain other antimicrobial agents concurrently, there may be a significant impact of metronidazole on the fecal flora. For example, when oral neomycin or kanamycin (active primarily against nonanaerobes) is given with metronidazole, there is a significant negative impact on both the anaerobic and aerobic flora. Thus, it has been feasible to use metronidazole for therapy in certain conditions such as ileal bypass enteropathy and for preoperative "bowel preparation" along with an oral aminoglycoside.

CLINICAL USES

Parasitic Infections

Metronidazole has been used successfully for therapy for *Trichomonas* vaginitis for many years. A topical preparation is available (see Chapters 95 and 270). It is also an effective agent for therapy of amebic liver abscess and has been used with generally good results in intestinal amebiasis. The drug is also effective against giardiasis, being at least as active as quinacrine for this purpose. Metronidazole has been used effectively in treating *Dientamoeba fragilis* infections in children.

Some workers have felt that metronidazole has been effective in *Balantidium coli* infection and in infection due to *Dracunculus medinensis,* but these indications are certainly not well established. Metronidazole has been used in the treatment of cutaneous leishmaniasis, although it appears to be less effective than other available agents.[39]

Anaerobic Infections

As suggested by the spectrum of activity of metronidazole, this drug is useful for the vast majority of anaerobic infections. Certainly, actinomycosis is one notable exception, and infections with *P. acnes,* which are uncommon, would be another. There is one other setting in which metronidazole may represent less than optimal therapy—anaerobic infections of the lower respiratory tract. Data from Sanders and colleagues[40] show a relatively high rate of suboptimal response. Most treatment failures had mixed infections with aerobic bacteria as well as anaerobes. The addition of penicillin G or ampicillin for mixed infections involving streptococci, pneumococci, or *Haemophilus influenzae* or the addition of erythromycin in the case of a penicillin-allergic patient would likely provide an excellent regimen. In the case of aspiration pneumonia involving aerobic or facultative gram-negative bacilli or *Staphylococcus aureus,* or all of these, other appropriate therapy to cover these agents would be needed along with metronidazole. Many anaerobic infections are mixed with aerobic or facultative bacteria, of course, and particularly in sicker patients, therapy aimed at both categories of organisms is desirable.

The excellent distribution of metronidazole throughout the body, including the central nervous system, and the impressive bactericidal activity of this compound, even against organisms that are not actively multiplying, make it an excellent choice for a number of serious infections, including brain abscess and other central nervous system infections involving anaerobes, endocarditis due to anaerobic bacteria, and, perhaps, any anaerobic infection of serious nature in patients who are immunocompromised.

The *B. fragilis* group of organisms is the one most commonly encountered in anaerobic infections overall. A number of medical centers have been encountering varied degrees of resistance of the *B. fragilis* group to clindamycin. Thus, metronidazole may become an even more important part of the armamentarium for the management of anaerobic infections. It should be noted, however, that in intra-abdominal infections, in which *B. fragilis* is almost always involved, comparative studies failed to show any significant difference among metronidazole, clindamycin, chloramphenicol, ticarcillin, or cefoxitin;[18] most of these were used together with an aminoglycoside.

The resistance of a number of clostridia other than *Clostridium perfringens* to cefoxitin and clindamycin again suggests that metronidazole might have an advantage in selected intra-abdominal and obstetric and gynecologic infections. However, there are no specific data to back up this point.

Metronidazole has been useful against other types of anaerobic infections, including bacteremia, infections of bones and joints, soft tissue infections, oral and dental infections, and head and neck infections. Metronidazole has also provided good results in the therapy for bacterial vaginosis, a condition in which various anaerobes or *G. vaginalis,* or both, may be important.[41, 42] As noted elsewhere, it has been effective in the management of pseudomembranous colitis due to *Clostridium difficile.* Limited studies have shown that fecal levels of metronidazole (up to 1212 μg/g dry weight and 24.2 μg/g wet weight of feces) may be attained by using either an oral or a parenteral route in patients with active colitis.[43, 44] The parenteral route may be especially useful in patients who have *C. difficile*–induced toxic megacolon and are unable to take oral medications. *H. pylori* is clearly linked to peptic ulcer disease; metronidazole, in combination with various other agents such as tetracycline or other antibiotics, bismuth subsalicylate, other bismuth compounds, histamine H_2 receptor antagonists or proton pump inhibitors appears to be effective therapy and markedly decreases the incidence of relapse.[45] Moreover, such therapy has led to regression of gastric lymphoma of mucosa-associated lymphoid tissue (see Chapter 205). Another important entity for which metronidazole has been very useful is periodontal disease, including severe and refractory cases. The drug has been effective both systemically and topically, in conjunction with scaling or surgery. A clinical study suggests that metronidazole may be more effective than penicillin for antimicrobial therapy for tetanus.[46] Metronidazole is not a suitable alternative to penicillin for syphilis.

Other Therapeutic Uses

Metronidazole has been used experimentally in very high doses as a hypoxic cell sensitizer in radiotherapy for malignancy. It has been useful in a number of types of bowel bacterial overgrowth syndromes such as for complications of jejunoileal bypass for obesity[47] and dysfunction of the continent ileostomy,[48] for pouchitis after pouch construction for ulcerative colitis, and for the prevention of intrahepatic cholestasis associated with total parenteral nutrition.[49] Although not everyone agrees, it appears that metronidazole has had a beneficial effect in Crohn's disease by producing a lessening of diarrhea (in patients with colonic involvement) and promoting the healing of perianal lesions and erythema nodosum.[50, 51] Prolonged use of the drug, however, may result in a significant incidence of metronidazole-induced peripheral neuropathy,[52] and concerns have been raised about possible carcinogenic effects of the drug.[34]

Metronidazole is beneficial in the treatment of acne rosacea whether used orally or topically.[53] It has also been useful in perioral dermatitis, childhood granulomatous periorificial dermatitis, demodicidosis (apparently due to a *Demodex* mite), decubitus ulcers, and malodorous infected malignant processes. An intriguing report[54] noted striking decreases in serum cholesterol and triglyceride levels in patients receiving metronidazole for other indications. Only short courses of therapy were used. There is no information as to the mechanism of this effect.

Prophylactic Use

Several groups have carried out prospective controlled studies of metronidazole, alone or in combination with other agents, for prophylaxis in patients undergoing elective colonic surgery, gynecologic surgery, or emergency appendectomy. In the case of appendectomy, a perforated appendix is an indication for therapy rather than prophylaxis, and in uncomplicated appendicitis the frequency of postoperative infection is quite low. In general, however, in these studies metronidazole has appeared to be as effective as other effective prophylactic agents. It should be kept in mind, however, that the prophylactic use of metronidazole is not an approved indication for the drug in the United States.

Finally, it should be appreciated that not all of the prophylactic trials have found metronidazole effective. Metronidazole was not effective prophylactically in one study of hysterectomy[55] and in one study of appendectomy for nonperforated appendicitis.[56]

REFERENCES

1. Sutter VL. In vitro susceptibility of anaerobic and microaerophilic bacteria to metronidazole and its hydroxy metabolite. In: Finegold SM, George WL, Rolfe RD, eds. Proceedings of the First United States Metronidazole Conference, Tarpon Springs, Fla, February 1982. New York: Biomedical Information Corp; 1982;61.
2. Wüst J. Susceptibility of anaerobic bacteria to metronidazole, ornidazole, and tinidazole and routine susceptibility testing by standardized methods. Antimicrob Agents Chemother. 1977;11:631.
3. Werner H, Schädler G, Krasemann C. In vitro activity of azlocillin, metronidazole and its hydroxy metabolite against anaerobes. Arzneimittelforsch Drug Res. 1983;33:574.
4. Rosenblatt JE, Edson RS. Metronidazole. Mayo Clin Proc. 1983;58:154.
5. Chow AW, Bednorz D, Guze LB. Susceptibility of obligate anaerobes to metronidazole: An extended study of 1,054 clinical isolates. In: Finegold SM, McFadzean JA, Roe FJC, eds. Metronidazole. Proceedings of the International Metronidazole Conference, Montreal, May 1976. Princeton, NJ: Excerpta Medica; 1977:286.
6. Reznikov M, McDonald PJ. Effect of metronidazole on *Escherichia coli* in the presence of *Bacteroides fragilis*: An investigation in mice. Chemotherapy. 1983;29:225.
7. Rasmussen BA, Bush K, Tally FP. Antimicrobial resistance in *Bacteroides*. Clin Infect Dis. 1993;16:S390–S400.
8. Reysset G, Haggoud A, Sebald M. Genetics of resistance of *Bacteroides* species to 5-nitroimidazole. Clin Infect Dis. 1993;16:S401–S403.
9. Phillips I, Warren C, Taylor E, et al. The antimicrobial susceptibility of anaerobic bacteria in a London teaching hospital. J Antimicrob Chemother. 1981;8:17.
10. Tally FP, Snydman DR, Shimell MJ, et al. Mechanisms of antimicrobial resistance of *Bacteroides fragilis*. In: Phillips I, Collier J, eds. Metronidazole. Proceedings of the Second International Symposium on Anaerobic Infections, Geneva, April 1979. London: The Royal Society of Medicine and Academic Press. New York: Grune & Stratton; 1979:19.
11. Ingham HR, Eaton S, Venables CW, et al. *Bacteroides fragilis* resistant to metronidazole after long-term therapy. Lancet. 1978;1:214.
12. Sprott MS, Ingham HR, Hickman JE, et al. Metronidazole-resistant anaerobes. Lancet. 1983;1:1220.
13. Krajden S, Lossick JG, Wilk E, et al. Persistent *Trichomonas vaginalis* infection due to a metronidazole-resistant strain. Can Med Assoc J. 1986;134:1373–1374.
14. Müller M, Meingassner JG, Miller WA, et al. Three metronidazole-resistant strains of *Trichomonas vaginalis* from the United States. Am J Obstet Gynecol. 1980;138:808–812.
15. Dombrowski MP, Sokol RJ, Bronsteen RA. Intravenous therapy of metronidazole-resistant *Trichomonas vaginalis*. Obstet Gynecol. 1987;69:524–525.
16. Müller M. Mode of action of metronidazole on anaerobic bacteria and protozoa. In: Proceedings of the North American Metronidazole Symposium on Anaerobic Infections, Scottsdale, Ariz, October 1981. Surgery. 1983;93:165.
17. Nastro LJ, Finegold SM. Bactericidal activity of five antimicrobial agents against *Bacteroides fragilis*. J Infect Dis. 1972;126:104.
18. Tally FP, Sullivan CE. Metronidazole: In vitro activity, pharmacology and efficacy in anaerobic bacterial infections. Pharmacotherapy. 1981;1:28.
19. Corrodi P, Busch DF, Sutter VL, et al. Factors affecting the in vitro antibacterial activity of metronidazole. In: Finegold SM, McFadzean JA, Roe FJC, eds. Metronidazole. Proceedings of the International Metronidazole Conference, Montreal, May 1976. Princeton, NJ: Excerpta Medica; 1977:299.
20. Bartlett JG, Dezfulian M, Joiner K. Relative efficacy and critical interval of antimicrobial agents in experimental infections involving *Bacteroides fragilis*. Arch Surg. 1983;118:181.
21. Fredricsson B, Hagström B, Nord C-E, et al. Systemic concentrations of metronidazole and its main metabolites after intravenous, oral and vaginal administration. Gynecol Obstet Invest. 1987;24:200–207.
22. Visser AA, Hundt HKL. The pharmacokinetics of a single intravenous dose of metronidazole in pregnant patients. J Antimicrob Chemother. 1984;13:279–283.
23. Mattila J, Nerdrum K, Rouhiainen H, et al. Penetration of metronidazole and tinidazole into the aqueous humor in man. Chemotherapy. 1983;29:188.
24. Guay DR, Meatherall RC, Baxter H, et al. Pharmacokinetics of metronidazole in patients undergoing continuous ambulatory peritoneal dialysis. Antimicrob Agents Chemother. 1984;25:306–310.
25. Lau AH, Evans R, Chang C-W, et al. Pharmacokinetics of metronidazole in patients with alcoholic liver disease. Antimicrob Agents Chemother. 1987;31:1662–1664.
26. Lentelink MB, de Vries TW, van Dijk KN. Accidental metronidazole overdose in a preterm newborn. Clin Pharmacokinet. 1997;32:496–497.
27. Lambert B, Lindblad A, Lindsten J, et al. Genotoxic effects of metronidazole in human lymphocytes in vitro and in vivo. In: Phillips I, Collier J, eds. Metronidazole. Proceedings of the Second International Symposium on Anaerobic Infections, Geneva, April 1979. London: The Royal Society of Medicine and Academic Press. New York: Grune & Stratton; 1979:229.
28. Elizondo G, Gonsebatt ME, Salazar AM, et al. Genotoxic effects of metronidazole. Mutat Res. 1996;370:75–80.
29. Finegold SM. Metronidazole. Ann Intern Med. 1980;93:585.
30. Koch RL, Chrystal EJT, Beaulieu BB, et al. Acetamide—A metabolite of metronidazole formed by the intestinal flora. Biochem Pharmacol. 1979;28:3611.
31. Sloan DA, Fleiszer DM, Richards GK, et al. Increased incidence of experimental colon cancer associated with long-term metronidazole therapy. Am J Surg. 1983;145:66.
32. Rainey JB, Maeda M, Williams C, et al. The cocarcinogenic effect of intrarectal deoxycholate in rats is reduced by oral metronidazole. Br J Cancer. 1984;49:631–636.
33. Beard CM, Noller KL, O'Fallon WM, et al. Cancer after exposure to metronidazole. Mayo Clin Proc. 1988;63:147–153.
34. Falagas ME, Walker AM, Jick H, et al. Late incidence of cancer after metronidazole use: A matched metronidazole user/nonuser study. Clin Infect Dis 1998;26:384–388.
35. Krause JR, Ayuyang HQ, Ellis LD. Occurrence of three cases of carcinoma in individuals with Crohn's disease treated with metronidazole. Am J Gastroenterol. 1985;80:978–982.
36. Robbie MO, Sweet RL. Metronidazole use in obstetrics and gynecology: A review. Am J Obstet Gynecol. 1983;145:865–881.
37. Caro-Patón T, Carvajal A, Martin de Diego I, et al. Is metronidazole teratogenic? A meta-analysis. Br J Clin Pharmacol. 1997;44:179–182.
38. Lewis RP, Wideman P, Sutter VL, et al. The effect of metronidazole on human fecal flora. In: Finegold SM, McFadzean JA, Roe FJC, eds. Metronidazole. Proceedings of the International Metronidazole Conference, Montreal, May 1976. Princeton, NJ: Excerpta Medica; 1977:307.
39. Chong H. Oriental sore. A look at trends in and approaches to the treatment of leishmaniasis. Int J Dermatol. 1986;25:615–623.
40. Sanders CV, Hanna BJ, Lewis AC, et al. The use of metronidazole in the treatment of anaerobic pleuropulmonary infections. In: Phillips I, Collier J, eds. Metronidazole. Proceedings of the Second International Symposium on Anaerobic Infections, Geneva, April 1979. London: The Royal Society of Medicine and Academic Press. New York: Grune & Stratton, 1979:83.
41. Swedberg J, Steiner JF, Deiss F, et al. Comparison of single-dose vs one-week course of metronidazole for symptomatic bacterial vaginosis. JAMA. 1985;254:1046–1049.
42. Biswas NJ. Bacterial vaginosis. Clin Obstet Gynecol. 1993;36:166–176.
43. Kleinfeld DI, Sharpe RJ, Donta ST. Parenteral therapy for antibiotic-associated pseudomembranous colitis. J Infect Dis. 1988;157:389.
44. Bolton RP, Culshaw MA. Faecal metronidazole concentrations during oral and intravenous therapy for antibiotic associated colitis due to *Clostridium difficile*. Gut. 1986;27:1169–1172.
45. Freeman CD, Klutman NE, Lamp KC. Metronidazole. A therapeutic review and update. Drugs. 1997;54:679–708.
46. Ahmadsyah I, Salim A. Treatment of tetanus: An open study to compare the efficacy of procaine penicillin and metronidazole. BMJ. 1985;291:648–650.
47. Drenick EJ. Extraintestinal complications of jejunoileal bypass for obesity. In: Finegold SM, George WL, Rolfe RD, eds. Proceedings of the First United States Metronidazole Conference, Tarpon Springs, Fla, February 1982. New York: Biomedical Information Corp; 1982:371.
48. Kelly DG, Phillips SF, Kelly KA, et al. Dysfunction of the continent ileostomy: Clinical features and bacteriology. Gut. 1983;24:193.
49. Capron J-P, Herve M-A, Gineston J-L, et al. Metronidazole in prevention of cholestasis associated with total parenteral nutrition. Lancet. 1983;1:446.
50. Gilat T. Metronidazole in Crohn's disease (Editorial). Gastroenterology. 1982;83:702.
51. Bernstein CN, Shanahan F. Metronidazole in Crohn's disease: What's the score? Gastroenterology. 1992;102:1435–1436.
52. Duffy LF, Daum F, Fisher SE, et al. Peripheral neuropathy in Crohn's disease patients treated with metronidazole. Gastroenterology. 1985;88:681–684.
53. Nielsen PG. Metronidazole treatment in rosacea. Int J Dermatol. 1988;27:1–5.

54. Davis JL, Schultz TA, Mosley CA. Metronidazole lowers serum lipids. Ann Intern Med. 1983;99:43.
55. Vincelette J, Finkelstein F, Aoki FY, et al. Double-blind trial of perioperative intravenous metronidazole prophylaxis for abdominal and vaginal hysterectomy. In: Proceedings of the North American Metronidazole Symposium on Anaerobic Infections, Scottsdale, Ariz, October 1981. Surgery. 1983;93:185.
56. Keiser TA, MacKenzie RL, Feld R, et al. Prophylactic metronidazole in appendectomy: A double-blind controlled trial. In: Proceedings of the North American Metronidazole Symposium on Anaerobic Infections, Scottsdale, Ariz, October 1981. Surgery. 1983;93:201.

Chapter 27

Macrolides and Clindamycin

NEAL H. STEIGBIGEL

The macrolide antibiotics (erythromycin, azithromycin, clarithromycin, and others) and the lincosamide antibiotics (lincomycin and clindamycin) are chemically unrelated but possess many similar biologic properties in terms of mechanisms of action and resistance, antimicrobial activity, and clinical pharmacology. Erythromycin, the macrolide in longest use, has several primary indications in therapy and is sometimes useful as an alternative to penicillin G. It is one of the safest antibiotics in clinical use, although it may be associated with some important drug interactions. Azithromycin and clarithromycin have some advantages over erythromycin in their antimicrobial activity, pharmacokinetics, and fewer gastrointestinal side effects and in the treatment of certain opportunistic infections related to the acquired immunodeficiency syndrome (AIDS). Some of the macrolides possess interesting anti-inflammatory activities. Preliminary clinical studies of macrolides in patients with coronary artery disease have shown tantalizing results, which must be confirmed. One hypothesis is that the effect is related to activity against *Chlamydia pneumoniae* which is associated with coronary artery disease. Clindamycin has been restricted in use by its potential gastrointestinal toxicity but remains particularly important in the treatment of certain anaerobic infections. Lincomycin is now mainly of historic interest.

ERYTHROMYCIN

Derivation, Chemistry, and Preparations

Erythromycin was derived in 1952 from a strain of *Streptomyces erythreus* obtained from soil from the Philippines. The structure (Fig. 27–1) consists of a 14-member macrocyclic lactone ring—therefore the class name *macrolide*—attached to two sugar moieties, desosamine and cladinose. Erythromycin base is poorly soluble in water, has a pK of 8.8, is rapidly inactivated by gastric acid, and is often inconsistently absorbed after oral administration. Pharmaceutical preparations for oral use have been made with an aim to diminish destruction by gastric acid and to promote better absorption. Six preparations for oral use are available: enteric-coated tablets (Ilotycin, E-Mycin, Ery-Tab, Robimycin, and generics), enteric-coated pellets in capsules (ERYC), and "film"-coated tablets of the base (Filmtab, Abbott); stearate salt (formed in association with the amino group on desosamine), available as film-coated tablets (Erythrocin, other brand names, and generics); ethylsuccinate ester (formed with the hydroxyl group on desosamine), available in tablet, chewable, and liquid forms (Erythrocin, EryPed, EES); lauryl sulfate salt of the propionyl ester (the estolate), available in tablet, capsule, or liquid forms (Ilosone). There are two water-soluble salts of erythromycin prepared for intravenous use, erythromycin gluceptate and erythromycin lactobionate. The drug is not given intramuscularly because of pain on injection. Erythromycin base is also available in 1.5% and 2% topical solutions, gels, and creams for treatment of acne vulgaris and in an ophthalmic ointment for treatment of bacterial conjunctivitis and prevention of neonatal gonococcal and chlamydial conjunctivitis.

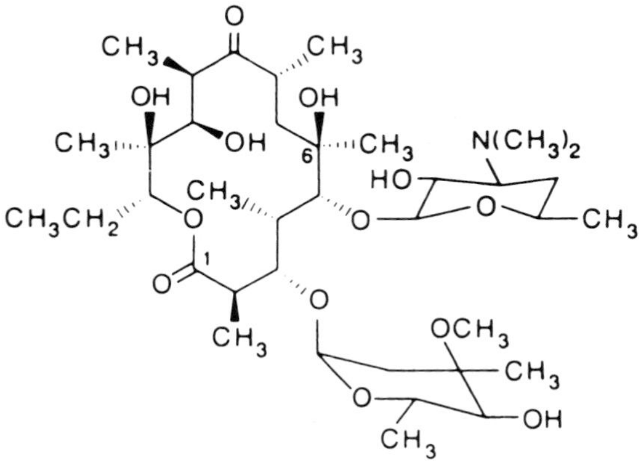

FIGURE 27–1. Erythromycin base.

Mechanisms of Action

Erythromycin inhibits RNA-dependent protein synthesis at the step of chain elongation in susceptible prokaryotic organisms. A single molecule of the antibiotic reversibly binds to the 50S ribosomal subunit, resulting in blockage of the transpeptidation and/or translocation reactions.[1–3] It is suggested that the macrolide binds to the peptidyl donor (P) site and by competition interferes with the translocation of the peptide chain from the acceptor to the donor site. Erythromycin may also promote dissociation of peptidyl-tRNA from the ribosomes.[4] Studies in *Escherichia coli* have demonstrated that erythromycin also inhibits the formation of the 50S ribosomal subunit.[5] In some bacteria erythromycin interferes with the ribosomal binding of other macrolides, lincomycin, and chloramphenicol, suggesting common or overlapping binding sites for these antibiotics.

Antimicrobial Activity and Mechanisms of Resistance

The antimicrobial activity of erythromycin is broad in spectrum, being exhibited against gram-positive and gram-negative bacteria, including actinomycetes and mycobacteria, as well as against treponemes, mycoplasmas, *Chlamydia,* and rickettsiae. Depending on drug concentration, bacterial species, phase of growth, and density of the inoculum, erythromycin may be primarily bacteriostatic or bactericidal. Bacterial killing is favored by higher antibiotic concentrations, lower bacterial density, and rapid growth.[6] The activity of erythromycin, which is a weak base, increases markedly with increasing pH over the range 5.5 to 8.5 for both gram-positive and gram-negative bacteria,[7, 8] possibly reflecting increased entry into the bacterial cell of the un-ionized drug that is more plentiful at the higher pH.

The in vitro susceptibilities of potential pathogens to erythromycin are listed in Table 27–1.[9–24] Erythromycin shows high activity against the majority of pneumococci and group A streptococci isolated in the United States; however, resistant clinical isolates have been increasingly encountered worldwide, especially in *Streptococcus pneumoniae* and particularly, in the latter species, if the strain shows resistance to penicillin.[21, 22, 25–41] The incidence of erythromycin resistance among clinical isolates of *S. pneumoniae* in Spain doubled from 7.6% in 1988 to 15.2% in 1992.[27] Reports from the United States (1995–1998) indicated that 10 to 15% of pneumococci were resistant to erythromycin, clarithromycin, and azithromycin. Approximately 40% of strains showing intermediate resistance to penicillin (minimal inhibitory concentration [MIC], 0.12 to 1.0 μg/ml) and

TABLE 27–1 In Vitro Susceptibilities to Erythromycin, Azithromycin, and Clarithromycin

	Erythromycin		Azithromycin		Clarithromycin	
Organism	*MIC$_{50}$*	*MIC$_{90}$*	*MIC$_{50}$*	*MIC$_{90}$*	*MIC$_{50}$*	*MIC$_{90}$*
Streptococcus pneumoniae						
Penicillin-susceptible (MIC ≤ 0.06 μg/ml	0.06	0.06	0.06	0.125	0.03	0.06
Penicillin-intermediate (MIC 0.12–1.0 μg/ml)	0.03	0.06	0.06	0.125	0.03	0.03
Penicillin-resistant (MIC ≥2.0 μg/ml)	0.06	>128	0.125	>128	0.03	>128
Streptococcus pyogenes	0.03–0.12	0.03–4	0.12–1	0.12–4	0.012–0.03	0.012–2
Streptococcus agalactiae	0.03–0.12	0.03–0.25	0.12–0.5	0.12–0.5	0.03–0.12	0.03–0.25
Viridans streptococci	0.06	>3.1	8	16	—	>1.6
Enterococcus spp.	1.5	>100	8	>32	0.5–1	>32
Staphylococcus aureus						
Methicillin-sensitive	0.12–0.5	>128	0.12–1	>128	0.06–0.25	>128
Methicillin-resistant	>128	>128	>128	>128	>128	>128
Staphylococcus epidermidis	8–32	>128	16	>128	4	>128
Corynebacterium diphtheriae	0.02	3.1	—	—	—	—
Listeria monocytogenes	0.25–0.5	0.5–4	1–2	2–4	0.12–0.25	0.12–2
Moraxella catarrhalis	0.12–0.5	0.25–2	<0.015–0.12	0.03–0.5	0.06–0.25	0.12–1
Haemophilus influenzae	1–8	2–32	0.25–4	0.25–4	1–8	2–16
Bordetella pertussis	—	0.03	0.015	0.06–0.12	—	0.03
Neisseria gonorrhoeae	0.12–0.5	0.25–2	<0.025–0.12	0.03–0.25	0.125–0.25	0.25–2
Neisseria meningitidis	0.4	1.6	0.06	0.12	—	—
Campylobacter jejuni	0.5–2	1–4	0.25	0.12–0.5	0.5–2	1–8
Helicobacter pylori	0.12	0.25	0.25	0.25	0.03	0.03
Mycoplasma pneumoniae	0.004–0.01	0.004–0.02	0.01–0.03	0.01–0.12	0.004–0.5	0.03–0.5
Chlamydia trachomatis	0.06–1	0.06–2	0.03–0.06	0.12–0.25	0.004–0.06	0.008–0.125
Chlamydia pneumoniae	0.25	0.50	0.25	0.50	0.06	0.50
Legionella pneumophila	0.1–1	0.5–2	0.12–0.5	0.25–2	0.12–0.25	0.25
Bacterioides fragilis	2–8	4–32	2–3.2	2–8	1–2	2–8
Peptococcus, Peptostreptococcus	<0.12–2	2–>32	0.25–1	2–4	0.25–2	4–>32
Clostridium perfringens	1	1	0.25–0.78	0.25–0.78	0.25–0.5	0.5–2
Proprionibacterium acnes	<0.03	<0.03–0.03	<0.004–0.015	0.03–0.15	<0.03–0.03	0.03–0.25

MIC$_{50}$ (MIC$_{90}$), minimal inhibitory concentration for 50% (90%) of isolates (μg/ml); values are the ranges reported in referenced publications.

about 60 to 65% of penicillin-resistant strains (MIC, ≥ 2.0 μg/ml) were resistant to those macrolides.[22, 28, 29, 29a] *S. pneumoniae* strains demonstrate complete cross-resistance among the macrolides,[21, 30–32] but cross-resistance extending from the macrolides to clindamycin is variable, depending on whether the resistance mechanism is of the MLS$_B$ or M phenotype (see later discussion).[30–34] The M phenotype is the predominant one in the United States for *S. pneumoniae;* it is associated with low levels of erythromycin resistance (MIC, 1–32 μg/ml) and usually does not extend to clindamycin.[29a, 34] The MLS$_B$ phenotype for *S. pneumoniae* is associated with a high level of erythromycin resistance (MIC, ≥ 256 μg/ml)[29a] and generally is associated with clindamycin resistance.

In a study in Japan, 60% of strains of group A streptococci isolated from infected children were highly resistant to erythromycin and lincomycin.[35] Almost all of these resistant strains were of type 12, and erythromycin had been widely used to treat respiratory infections in Japan in the several years before the study. A survey of 474 group A streptococcal strains isolated from patients in Oklahoma in 1980 indicated that 5% had MIC to erythromycin by microtiter broth dilution of 1 μg/ml or more.[36] In Finland, where there had been a great increase in the use of erythromycin in the 1980s through 1991, resistance to that antibiotic was found in up to 44% of clinical isolates of group A streptococci from some communities in 1990.[37] However, nationwide policies in Finland reduced the use of macrolides for respiratory and skin infections in outpatients after 1991 and erythromycin resistance among clinical isolates steadily dropped, from 16.5% in 1992 to 8.6% in 1996.[38] In contrast, erythromycin resistance in *Streptococcus pyogenes* rose in Italy from 5.1% in 1993 to 25.9% in 1995.[39] Despite the emergence of macrolide resistance by *S. pyogenes* in some areas, resistance to those antibiotics remains at less than 5% in most countries.[40] As with *S. pneumoniae,* there is cross-resistance among the macrolides by *S. pyogenes*; however, resistance does not usually extend to clindamycin.[31, 32, 41]

The emergence of resistance to erythromycin encountered in clinical isolates of these organisms from patient populations treated with this antibiotic is consistent with in vitro studies of pneumococci and streptococci subcultured sequentially in the presence of erythromycin, which demonstrate the selection of erythromycin resistance and often cross-resistance to other macrolides. Similar in vitro results are obtained with staphylococci[42] Although resistance to erythromycin by *Staphylococcus aureus* may be selected by its use in hospitals,[43] most methicillin-sensitive clinical isolates remain sensitive to this agent.[29, 44] However, there is always a potential for the emergence, during treatment in an individual patient, of erythromycin resistance by *S. aureus.*[43, 45, 46] These strains may demonstrate the emergence of one-step high-level resistance to erythromycin alone, or they may show cross-resistance to other macrolides and to lincomycin and clindamycin. In addition, staphylococci isolated from patients treated with erythromycin may exhibit a phenomenon called *dissociated resistance* by Garrod.[47] Only a small proportion of the population of such staphylococcal isolates exhibit resistance when grown in large concentrations of erythromycin; however, in the presence of lower concentrations of erythromycin almost the entire population demonstrates resistance to erythromycin, to other macrolides, and often to the lincosamide antibiotics. In the absence of erythromycin these organisms appear sensitive to these antibiotics. Methicillin-resistant strains of *S. aureus* are almost always resistant to erythromycin.[48]

The majority of strains of the "viridans" group of streptococci, *Listeria monocytogenes,* and *Corynebacterium diphtheriae* show appreciable susceptibility to erythromycin. However, 39.4% of viridans streptococci isolated from blood cultures from neutropenic cancer patients in Spain during the period 1988–1994 demonstrated resistance to erythromycin, clarithromycin, and azithromycin, with resistance most likely in penicillin-resistant strains.[23] Many strains of *Clostridium perfringens* may be only moderately sensitive.[49] Appreciable in vitro activity has been demonstrated against *Actinomyces israelii, Mycobacterium scrofulaceum,* and *Mycobacterium kansaii*[50] and against *Nocardia asteroides* when combined with ampicillin.[51]

With gram-negative bacteria, erythromycin displays relatively consistent and useful activity against *Neisseria meningitidis, Neisseria gonorrhoeae,* and *Bordetella pertussis*[9] and somewhat lower activity against *Haemophilus influenzae.*[52] Strains of *N. gonorrhoeae* that are resistant to erythromycin, with MICs up to 32 μg/ml, are occasionally encountered.[53] High bacteriostatic and bactericidal activity is demonstrated against more than 90% of strains of *Campylobacter jejuni.*[11] Erythromycin has activity against some species of gram-negative anaerobes, but *Bacteroides fragilis* strains are usually resistant.[54] The Enterobacteriaceae are usually resistant, except as the pH rises to 8.5.[8]

The extensive spectrum of activity of erythromycin is also demonstrated by its clinically useful activity against such diverse organisms as *Treponema pallidum, Legionella pneumophila,*[10] *Mycoplasma pneumoniae, Ureaplasma urealyticum,* some strains of *Rickettsia, Chlamydia trachomatis,* and *Chlamydia pneumoniae.* Erythromycin is about 50 times more potent against *M. pneumoniae* than is tetracycline.[55] Erythromycin-resistant variants of *M. pneumoniae* have been isolated in the laboratory and from a patient.[56] Extracellular and intracellular *L. pneumophila* strains show substantial susceptibility to erythromycin, but clarithromycin and azithromycin and more potent.[57–59]

Resistance to erythromycin may result from a number of causes. First, decreased permeability of the cell envelope to the drug is exhibited by the Enterobacteriaceae; cell-free systems and protoplasts of these organisms are susceptible to the drug.[44, 60, 61] This intrinsic resistance is also exhibited by *Pseudomonas* spp. and *Acinetobacter* spp. Second, plasmid-mediated erythromycin resistance in *Staphylococcus epidermidis* and *S. aureus* caused by active efflux of the drug has also been described.[44] That resistance mechanism is encoded by the *msra* gene and is carried out by an adenosine triphosphatase–binding protein working together with additional transmembrane domains to complete the transporter functions.[62] A different efflux system for erythromycin and other 14- and 15-membered macrolides, but not 16-membered macrolides, lincosamides or analogues of streptogramin B (called the M phenotype), has been elucidated in erythromycin-resistant strains of *S. pyogenes* (encoded by the *mefa* gene), *S. pneumoniae* (encoded by the *mefe* gene) and group C streptococci (encoded by the *mefa* or *mefe* genes).[31, 32, 34, 41, 63]

In a third resistance mechanism, alteration in a single 50S ribosomal protein of the receptor site confers resistance to erythromycin and sometimes to other macrolides, lincomycin, and clindamycin; in some but not all strains this is associated with a decreased binding affinity for erythromycin.[3] This one-step high-level resistance is the result of chromosomal mutation; has been demonstrated in some strains of *Bacillus subtilis, S. pyogenes, Campylobacter* spp., and *E. coli;* and probably occurs in *S. aureus.*

Fourth, alteration in the 23S ribosomal RNA of the 50S ribosomal subunit by methylation of adenine, at a defined position[64, 65] is associated with resistance to erythromycin and most other macrolides (M), lincocasamides (L, lincomycin, and clindamycin), and streptogramin type B (S_B). This pattern of resistance, referred to as *MLS_B phenotype,* is mediated by the *erm* gene (*erma, ermb, ermc, ERMTR*) on plasmids or transposons on chromosomes. The resistance results from decreased binding of the antibiotics to their overlapping targets on the ribosome, which is probably altered in conformation by methylation. It can be exhibited by strains of *S. aureus*, streptococci (including *S. pneumoniae*), *Enterococcus* spp., *C. diphtheriae, Campylobacter* spp., *B. fragilis, C. perfringens, Listeria* spp., *M. pneumoniae*, and *Legionella* spp. This phenomenon may be constitutive or inducible by subinhibitory concentrations of erythromycin that bring about induction of the methylating enzyme. The inducible mechanism seems to explain the phenomenon of dissociated resistance already described.

Finally, enzymatic inactivation of erythromycin and some other 14- and 15- membered ring macrolides by esterases or a phosphotransferase in strains of Enterobacteriaceae with high-level resistance has been demonstrated.[44] The esterase genes (*erea* and *ereb*) are probably encoded by a plasmid-mediated determinant.[44] An erythromycin esterase has also been found in a clinical strain of *S. aureus.*[66]

Polymerase chain reaction methods have been developed that allow for relatively rapid detection of the different mechanisms of macrolide resistance among clinical isolates.[67]

Other Activities of Erythromycin

Erythromycin and other 14-member ring macrolides have a gastrointestinal motility-stimulating effect.[68, 69] In this regard, erythromycin acts as a motilin receptor agonist in the gut and gallbladder.[70] These prokinetic effects are being studied for their potential in the treatment of gastroparesis.[71, 72]

There has been appreciable interest in the anti-inflammatory activities of erythromycin and other macrolides. These include interference with oxidant production by neutrophils, acceleration of neutrophil apoptosis, suppression of the release of proinflammatory cytokines, and promotion of the release of nitric oxide from endothelial cells.[73–76] The L-cladinose moiety at position 3 in the lactone ring was found to be the key structure making for the reduction of oxidant production by neutrophils.[73]

Clinical Pharmacology

The peak serum levels obtained after single doses of various erythromycin preparations are given in Table 27–2.[9, 54, 77, 78] Erythromycin base is subject to destruction by gastric acid, and preparations of the base have been made with an acid-resistant coating to delay dissolution of the drug until it reaches the small bowel. The esters and ester salts of erythromycin are more acid stable, form a stable suspension in water, and are tasteless. These characteristics are used in the liquid suspension for children. Erythromycin base (absorbed intact), stearate (absorbed as the base), and ethylsuccinate (absorbed both as the intact ester and as the free base after hydrolysis in the intestine) are usually absorbed more completely in the fasting state, although one study demonstrated increased absorption of a stearate preparation when it was taken with a meal.[78] After absorption, about 45% of the ethylsuccinate preparation is present in the serum as the inactive ester and about 55% as the active base.

Average serum levels achieved under fasting conditions with these preparations are similar; however, results with the base may be erratic. Erythromycin base has become available in a capsule containing enteric-coated granules; this preparation is promoted as giving more uniform absorption,[79, 81] but some enteric-coated tablets may provide similar blood levels.[80] The absorption of the estolate is not affected by food, and the resulting peak serum level consists of both free base (20 to 30%, active form) and estolate (70 to 80%, much less active); the level of base achieved is similar to that achieved by the other oral preparations taken in comparable doses in the fasting state. The clinical significance of the much less active esterified form of the drug that is present in serum in appreciable concentration is controversial. It would seem that in treatment of infections of only moderate severity by organisms highly sensitive to erythromycin (e.g., *S. penumoniae, S. pyogenes, M. pneumoniae*), differences in therapeutic results using the various oral preparations would be insignificant. Limited clinical comparisons confirm that suspicion.[82] However, in the treatment of group A streptococcal pharyngitis in children, substantially higher rates of bacteriologic eradication and lower rates of gastrointestinal side effects have been reported with the estolate preparation in comparison with the ethylsuccinate formulation.[83] Intravenous preparations of erythromycin achieve appreciably higher serum levels and should be used to treat serious infections requiring erythromycin.

Erythromycin is distributed through total body water.[84] Values given for protein binding vary from 40 to 90%; however, the significance of such binding is speculative.[85] The drug persists in tissues longer than in the blood. The ratios of tissue or body fluid concentrations to simultaneous serum concentrations (usually at peak) are as follows: aqueous humor, 0.3; ascites, 0.4; bile, 28; middle ear exudate in otitis media, 0.3 to 0.7; pleural fluid, 0.7; prostatic fluid, 0.4; cerebrospinal fluid without meningitis, 0 to 0.02, with meningitis, 0.05 to 0.1; infected maxillary paranasal sinus, 0.4 to 0.8; tonsil, 0.3. Concentrations achieved in the middle ear in otitis media are adequate to treat pneumococcal and group A streptococcal infections

TABLE 27-2 Serum Levels of Erythromycin in Adults

Preparation	Dose (mg)	Route	Peak Serum Level	
			Hours After Dose	*Concentration* (μg/ml)
Base	250	Oral	4	0.3–1.0*
	500			0.3–1.9
Stearate	250 (fasting)	Oral	3	0.2–1.3
	500 (fasting)		3	0.4–1.8
	500 (after food)		3	0.1–0.4†
Ethylsuccinate	500	Oral	0.5–2.5	1.5‡ (0.6§)
Estolate	250	Oral	2–4	1.4–1.7
	500		3.5–4	4.2‡ (1.1§)
Lactobionate	200	Intravenous	Immediately	3–4
	500		1	9.9
Gluceptate	250	Intravenous	Immediately	3.5–10.7
	1000		1	9.9

*Somewhat higher levels reported with some enteric-coated preparation after repeated doses.[79, 80]
†One study demonstrated higher levels (to 2.8 μg/ml) with dose taken during a meal.[78]
‡Total drug (inactive ester and free base).
§Free base.

involving sensitive strains of these species but are not adequate to consistently eradicate *H. influenzae.*[86, 87] High concentrations of erythromycin are achieved in alveolar macrophages[88] and polymorphonuclear leukocytes[89] compared with those in extracellular fluid.

There are very limited data on concentrations of erythromycin achieved in the cerebrospinal fluid of patients with meningitis which suggest that large parenteral doses may be effective against meningeal infection by highly susceptible organisms such as *S. pneumoniae.*[90] Limited data from patients with septic arthritis suggest poor penetration of synovial fluid. Erythromycin is transferred across the placenta; fetal serum concentrations are about 2% of those in maternal serum, but higher concentrations accumulate in fetal tissue and amniotic fluid.[91] The drug is excreted in breast milk.

Up to 4.5% of an oral dose and 15% of a parenteral dose of erythromycin are recoverable in the urine.[9] Urine concentrations after oral doses are often high but quite variable. Erythromycin is concentrated by the liver and excreted into the bile in high concentrations; however, only about 1.5% of the dose of the base and 0.2% of the ester can be recovered from bile in the first 8 hours, and some of this is reabsorbed from the intestine.[92] The higher serum levels achieved by the estolate have been attributed to both better absorption and lower biliary excretion. After an oral dose, large concentrations of the antibiotic are found in feces, probably representing ingested drug that was never absorbed as well as some that was excreted in bile. A large proportion of absorbed drug cannot be accounted for by urinary or biliary excretion or by tissue binding and may be inactivated in the liver by demethylation.[93]

The normal serum half-life of erythromycin is 1.4 hours, and appreciable serum levels are maintained for 6 hours. In anuric patients, the half-life is only prolonged to about 5 hours, and for that reason dosage reduction in patients with renal failure is generally not necessary.[94] Erythromycin is not removed by peritoneal dialysis or hemodialysis.

Adverse Reactions

Erythromycin is one of the safest antibiotics in clinical use. Untoward reactions caused by the drug itself, except for pseudomembranous colitis and ventricular arrhythmias (with intravenous use), are not life-threatening and, with the exception of the irritative reactions, they are rare.

1. Irritative reactions include dose-related abdominal cramps, nausea, vomiting, diarrhea, and gas; these reactions occur more commonly in children and young adults than in older persons and may be associated with either intravenous or oral administration. They result from the motility-stimulating effects of erythromycin discussed previously. Enteric coating of erythromycin base in the form of pellets in a capsule (e.g., ERYC) does not reduce the common dose-related gastrointestinal side effects of oral erythromycin.[95] Thrombophlebitis with intravenous use can be decreased by appropriate dilution of the dose in at least 250 ml of solution and by avoidance of rapid infusions (infusion over about 45 to 60 minutes).

2. Allergic reactions include skin rash, fever, and eosinophilia.

3. Cholestatic hepatitis occurs rarely,[96] almost always with the estolate preparation and chiefly in adults.[97] The syndrome typically begins after 20 days of therapy, but more rapidly in those previously treated, and consists of nausea, vomiting, and abdominal pain followed by jaundice, fever, and abnormal liver function tests consistent with cholestatic hepatitis. These findings are sometimes accompanied by rash, leukocytosis, and eosinophilia. The abnormalities usually clear within days to a few weeks after the drug is stopped but may return rapidly on rechallenge. The syndrome appears to represent a hypersensitivity reaction to the specific structure of the estolate compound.[98] However, hepatocyte toxicity induced by the drug or its metabolites and allergy to altered hepatocyte components, may be contributory.[99] Milder forms of the syndrome occur with the estolate and may be more common in pregnant women.[100] It must be distinguished from false-positive serum glutamic-oxaloacetic transaminase (AST) elevations that occur in patients taking the estolate.[101] The latter may be found when AST is determined by colorimetric procedures rather than by an enzymatic method and seems to result from an interfering substance present in the blood in association with estolate administration. Reversible hepatotoxicity, including jaundice, has occurred with the stearate salt and with the ethylsuccinate ester of erythromycin.[102–104]

4. Transient hearing loss has been reported rarely in association with the use of large intravenous doses of erythromycin lactobionate or large doses of oral erythromycin.[105, 106] This may occur more commonly in elderly patients with renal insufficiency.[107–109] The ototoxicity depends on the serum concentration of the drug.[110]

5. Polymorphic ventricular tachycardia with QT prolongation (torsade de pointes) has been rarely reported in association with treatment with intravenous erythromycin.[111, 112] The drug has been shown to effect repolarization in the isolated heart and to block electrical current in guinea pig ventricular myocytes in a way consistent with the observed arrhythmia.[113] The possibility for interaction with potential-lengthening drugs (class Ia and III antiarrythmics) and for increased risk in the presence of electrolyte abnormality or prolonged QT interval should be kept in mind.

6. Superinfection, especially of the gastrointestinal tract or vagina, with *Candida* species or gram-negative bacilli may occur, as with other antibiotics.

7. Pseudomembranous colitis caused by overgrowth of toxinproducing *Clostridium difficile* occurs rarely with the use of erythromycin.[114, 115]

TABLE 27–3 Potentially Clinically Significant Drug Interactions Produced by Macrolides*

Drug	Interactions
Erythromycin	Alfentanil, astemizole, buspirone, bromocriptine, carbamazepine, cisapride, clomipramine plus respiradone, clozapine, colchicine, cyclosporine, digoxin, disopyramide, ergot alkaloids, felodipine, loratadine, lovastatin, methylprednisolone, midazolam, phenytoin, quinidine, tacrolimus (FK506), terfenadine,[120] theophylline, triazolam, valproate, warfarin
Clarithromycin	Carbamazepine, cisapride, cyclosporine,[121] digoxin, pimozide, rifampin, rifabutin, ritonavir, terfenadine,[120] zidovudine
Azithromycin	Cyclosporine (one case)

*Interactions generally lead to increased levels of the listed drugs caused by interaction of the macrolide with CYP-450 hepatic metabolism. Exceptions are digoxin, in which the raised levels are caused by interference with digoxin inactivation by gut flora, and zidovudine, in which serum concentrations may be decreased by unknown mechanisms. Rifampin and vifabutin may lower the levels of clarithromycin, and clarithromycin may raise the levels of rifampin and rifabutin.
Modified from Rizack MA. The Medical Letter Handbook of Adverse Drug Interactions. New Rochelle, NY: The Medical Letter on Drugs and Therapeutics; 1999.

Drug Interactions

Incompatibility during administration between intravenous preparations of erythromycin and other drugs has been reported; the latter include vitamin B complex and vitamin C, cephalothin, tetracycline, chloramphenicol, colistin, heparin, metraminol, and diphenylhydantoin.

Erythromycin may produce interactions with other drugs by interfering with their hepatic metabolism through the cytochrome P-450 enzyme (CYP3A subclass) system.[116, 117] This may occur because erythromycin metabolites are capable of forming inactive complexes with cytochrome P-450 enzymes.[117, 118] The resulting raised level of drug may result in serious toxicity (Table 27–3).[119] For example, elevations of terfenadine or astemizole serum concentrations have led to serious ventricular arrhythmias, and the same phenomenon with midazolam has led to unconsciousness.

Erythromycin can increase the bioavailability of digoxin by interfering with its inactivation by gut flora.[116] Erythromycin may inhibit the assay organism used in some determinations of serum folic acid. Sequential use of erythromycin and clindamycin should be avoided when possible because of the potential for the development of cross-resistance or dissociated resistance.

Uses of Erythromycin

Erythromycin has a few indications for use as the drug of choice and some important applications as an alternative drug to penicillin G (Table 27–4).[122] When given to adults by the oral route, preparations other than the estolate are generally preferable because they have less risk of cholestatic hepatitis. Absorption, particularly with the enteric-coated base, stearate, or ethylsuccinate preparations taken in the fasting state or before meals, is usually adequate. The estolate preparation should be particularly avoided during pregnancy, when hepatotoxicity may be more common.[100] When higher serum levels are needed in more severe infections requiring erythromycin therapy, the drug should be given intravenously.

Treatment of *M. pneumoniae* infection with erythromycin, as with tetracycline, shortens the clinical course of the infection; radiologic clearing of pulmonary lesions occurs earlier with erythromycin.[123] Clinical experience and studies in vitro and in guinea pigs suggest that erythromycin is very effective in treating pneumonia caused by *L. pneumophila* or *Legionella micdadei.*[10, 57, 59, 124, 125] The use of erythromycin in combination with rifampin is now favored, especially in severe cases.[57, 59] Azithromycin, clarithromycin and the fluoroquinolones are somewhat more active than erythromycin in vitro and appear to be at least as effective clinically.[58, 59] Early treatment of pertussis with erythromycin is associated with both

TABLE 27–4 Major Indications for Use of Erythromycin

Infections in Which Erythromycin Is the Drug of First Choice	Erythromycin Dosage for Adults	Alternative Drug
Mycoplasma pneumoniae infections	0.5 g tid–qid po*,† for 14–21 d	A fluoroquinolone
Legionella pneumonia	0.5–1.0 g qid po* (± rifampin)‡ for 10–21 d	Doxycycline ± rifampin, or trimethoprim-sulfamethoxazole
Diphtheria§	Carrier state: 500 mg qid po for 10 d	Pencillin G
	Disease*: followed by oral for 10 d	Penicillin G
Pertussis	0.5 g qid po	Trimethoprim-sulfamethoxazole
Chlamydia trachomatis pneumonia or conjunctivitis	10 mg/kg qid po	Sulfisoxazole‖
Prevention of infection after colorectal surgery	1 g po each of neomycin and erythromycin base at 1, 2, and 11 PM on the day before 8 AM surgery (combined with vigorous purgation over the 2 d before surgery)	Parenteral cephalosporin
Campylobacter jejuni gastroenteritis	250 mg qid po¶	A tetracycline
Bacillary angiomatosis	250–500 mg qid po for at least 8 wk; with visceral involvement, several months of therapy is used	Doxycycline
Infections in Which Erythromycin Is an Important Alternative Drug	**Erythromycin Dosage for Adults**	**Drug of First Choice**
Groups A, C, G streptococcal infection	250–500 mg qid po*, **	Penicillin G
Streptococcus pneumoniae infection	250–500 mg qid po*, ††	Penicillin G, ceftriaxone, or cefotaxime
C. pneumoniae (TWAR) infection	0.5 g tid–qid po*	A tetracycline
Rheumatic fever prophylaxis	250 mg bid po	Penicillin G
Anthrax	500 mg qid* for 10 d‡‡	Penicillin G
Lymphogranuloma venereum	500 mg qid po for 21 d	Tetracycline
Chancroid	500 mg qid po for 7 d	Azithromycin or ceftriaxone
Chlamydia trachomatis urethritis, cervicitis	500 mg qid po for 7 d	Azithromycin or tetracycline
Acne vulgaris	250 mg qid po or topical preparation	Tetracycline po and a number of topical drugs

*Intravenous therapy (2–4 g/d) should be used in serious illness or when oral therapy is not possible or reliable.
†Clarithromycin, azithromycin, and tetracyclines are also considered drugs of first choice.
‡Clarithromycin, azithromycin, and fluoroquinolones are also considered drugs of first choice.
§Antitoxin is essential primary therapy for disease.
‖Only for infants >4 wk old.
¶A fluoroquinolone is also a drug of choice.
**Treatment should be continued for 10 d for group A.
††Resistance to macrolides is increasing and is frequent in penicillin-resistant strains.
‡‡Therapy may need to continue for prolonged periods until vaccination is completed in those infected by the pulmonary route.

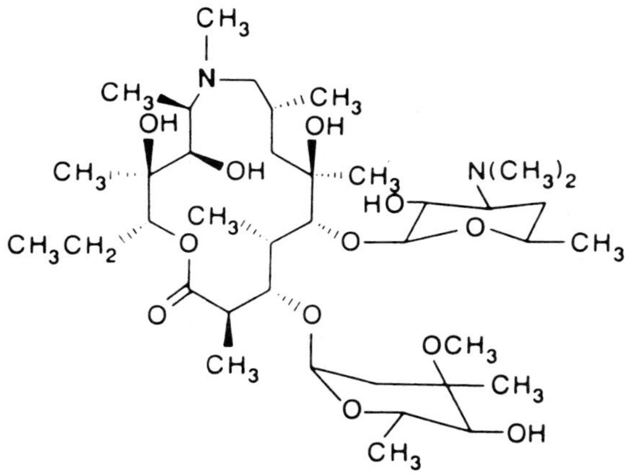

FIGURE 27–2. Azithromycin base.

clinical improvement and a reduction in secondary transmission in households.[126] Erythromycin treatment of patients with gastroenteritis caused by *C. jejuni* hastens the eradication of the organism from the feces but does not appear to alter the clinical course of uncomplicated infection when therapy begins 4 days or more after the onset of symptoms.[127] However, earlier treatment of young children with acute dysentery associated with *C. jejuni* has been shown to shorten the course of diarrhea and fecal excretion of the organism.[128] Nevertheless, in an institutional setting in Thailand, where *C. jejuni* strains were frequently resistant to erythromycin in vitro, early treatment of infants with diarrhea caused by this organism was not beneficial.[129] Treatment of infants with erythromycin for pneumonia caused by *C. trachomatis* appears to speed recovery and eradication of the shedding of organisms.[130] Erythromycin base given orally together with neomycin on the day before colorectal surgery and combined with vigorous purgation is about as effective as parenteral cephalosporin administration just before surgery in decreasing the incidence of septic complications.[131] No advantage has been demonstrated for the use of a combination of oral and intravenous antibiotics.[132] In the presence of bowel obstruction or when there is need for emergency surgery, the parenteral antibiotic regimen should be used.[122] Erythromycin has become the drug of choice in treating bacillary angiomatosis in patients with AIDS.[133]

Although erythromycin continues to be useful in the treatment of community-acquired respiratory infections, its usefulness has become more limited in areas in which the incidence of penicillin-resistant pneumococci has become substantial. Such strains are often resistant to erythromycin, as discussed.[22, 28, 29] The results of treating syphilis with erythromycin during pregnancy must be considered uncertain at best; fetal syphilis may not be eradicated,[134] and this treatment is no longer recommended when pregnant women with syphilis have a history of penicillin allergy.[135] Erythromycin may occasionally be useful in treating urinary tract infections caused by gram-negative bacilli that might otherwise require the use of more toxic agents.[136] Urine pH must generally be raised to 8.0 or above to achieve effective activity at urinary concentrations against the gram-negative bacilli. A comparative study involving a small number of children with cholera, who were all treated with rehydration solutions, showed that erythromycin or trimethoprim-sulfamethoxazole was effective and superior to treatment without an antimicrobial agent.[137] Erythromycin may be used as an alternative antibiotic in the treatment of anthrax and in infections by *M. catarrhalis* and *Eikenella corrodens*. Erythromycin is not consistently effective in treatment of infections caused by *H. influenzae*,[86, 87] and in vitro studies suggest resistance by some strains of *C. perfringens*.[49] In view of the availability of more effective alternative drugs, erythromycin should not be used alone in the treatment of deep-seated staphylococcal infections because of the potential for the emergence of resistant strains during therapy.[42, 45, 46]

Diffuse panbronchiolitis, a chronic inflammatory disease of the airways, particularly encountered in Japan, is associated with an increase in survival in patients treated with erythromycin.[137a] The beneficial effect is generally attributed to the anti-inflammatory activity of the macrolide.

AZITHROMYCIN AND CLARITHROMYCIN

There has been a search for newer macrolides that have better oral absorption, longer half-life, fewer gastrointestinal side effects, and a greater antimicrobial spectrum of activity than erythromycin. Azithromycin (CP-62,993), clarithromycin (A-56268), and some newer investigational agents have some of these properties.

Derivation, Chemistry, and Preparations

Azithromycin is derived from erythromycin, differing in having a methyl-substituted nitrogen in its 15-member lactone ring (Fig. 27–2). It is therefore an azalide antibiotic. Clarithromycin, having a 14-member ring structure, is produced by modifying position C6 of the lactone ring of erythromycin to possess a methoxy group (Fig. 27–3). These changes increase the stability of these compounds in gastric acid, improving absorption by the oral route.[16]

Azithromycin is available in capsules for oral use as azithromycin dihydrate equivalent to 250 mg of azithromycin, in tablets of 600 mg, as a powder for oral suspension, and in vials of 500 mg for intravenous infusion. Clarithromycin is provided in 250- or 500-mg film-coated tablets and as granules for oral suspension.

Mechanisms of Action and Resistance

Limited studies suggest that azithromycin, clarithromycin, and erythromycin bind to the same receptor on the bacterial 50S ribosomal subunit and inhibit RNA-dependent protein synthesis by the same mechanism.[15, 138] Azithromycin has greater activity than the 14-member macrolides erythromycin and clarithromycin against gram-negative bacteria (especially for *Moraxella catarrhalis* and *H. influenzae*) and therefore appears to better penetrate the outer envelope of those organisms.[18] Like other macrolides, azithromycin and clarithromycin are generally considered to be bacteriostatic agents; however, bactericidal activity is easily demonstrated in vitro against such species as *S. pyogenes, S. pneumoniae*, and *H. influenzae*.[15, 18, 138, 139] In vitro activity of the new macrolides increases with rising pH, as with erythromycin.

Mechanisms of resistance to azithromycin or clarithromycin are the same as or similar to those for erythromycin. There is complete cross-resistance between erythromycin, azithromycin, and clarithromycin for gram-positive organisms showing resistance to erythromycin by the MLS_B phenotype, because the methylation mechanism already described operates for all of the 14- and 15-member macro-

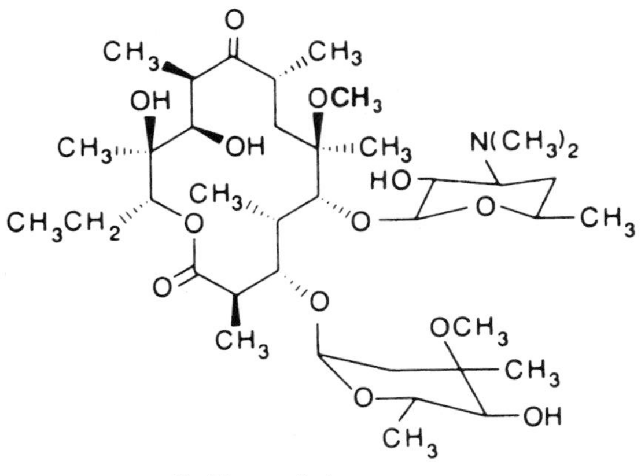

FIGURE 27–3. Clarithromycin base.

lides.[64, 138] Cross-resistance among the 14- and 15-membered macrolides is also characteristic of the M phenotype that is the result of an efflux system for the drugs and is found in some strains of *S. pyogenes* and *S. pneumoniae*. Clarithromycin-resistant strains of *Helicobacter pylori* with point mutations in the 23S rRNA genes that presumably result in diminished binding of the drug to the ribosomal target have been isolated from patients with peptic ulcer disease treated with that antibiotic.[140] Further studies with such strains suggest that horizontal transfer of the mutated gene can occur.[141] Similar point mutations in the 23S rRNA gene associated with macrolide resistance in *Mycobacterium avium* complex have been selected in patients undergoing clarithromycin or azithromycin monotherapy for disseminated infections.[142]

Antimicrobial Activity

Clarithromycin is highly active against gram-positive bacteria, being twofold to fourfold more active than erythromycin against most streptococci, including *S. pneumoniae* and *S. pyogenes*, and methicillin-sensitive *S. aureus*.[15, 16] However, azithromycin is about twofold to fourfold less active than erythromycin against those organisms.[15, 16] Streptococci and staphylococci that are resistant to erythromycin are resistant to clarithromycin and azithromycin.[15, 18, 143] The emergence of macrolide resistance in clinical isolates of *S. pneumoniae* and *S. pyogenes* was discussed in the section on erythromycin. Almost all methicillin-resistant staphylococci are resistant to the new macrolides.[15, 17] The activity of clarithromycin against many gram-negative bacteria is similar to that of erythromycin,[15, 143] although it is slightly more active against *M. catarrhalis*. An active metabolite of clarithromycin, 14-hydroxyclarithromycin, has slightly greater activity than the parent compound against *H. influenzae* and *M. catarrhalis* and is additive in vitro the activity of clarithromycin.[143] Azithromycin is more active than erythromycin or clarithromycin against gram-negative bacteria, especially against *H. influenzae* and *M. catarrhalis*.[15, 16] The greater activity of azithromycin against the Enterobacteriaceae is of questionable clinical significance. However, it is of interest that prolonged incubation of *Pseudomonas aeruginosa* strains with macrolides at clinically achieveable concentrations is associated with decreased viability and diminished protein synthesis.[144] Azithromycin is the most potent in that regard.

Azithromycin and clarithromycin have equal or slightly better in vitro activities than erythromycin against *L. pneumophila*.[15, 58] In guinea pigs infected with *L. pneumophila*, azithromycin was found to be more effective in treatment than clarithromycin or erythromycin.[145, 146] All three of those macrolides have good activity against *M. pneumoniae* and *C. pneumoniae*.[15, 17, 18, 20, 24, 143] Both of the new macrolides have significantly greater activity than erythromycin against *C. trachomatis*, *U. urealyticum*,[15] and somewhat greater activity for *B. burgdorferi*.[15, 18, 143]

The macrolides show little activity against *Mycobacterium tuberculosis*. In contrast, clarithromycin shows substantial activity against *Mycobacterium leprae* and is superior in this respect to erythromycin and azithromycin.[15, 143]

Clarithromycin and azithromycin have appreciable activities against *M. avium* complex. Clarithromycin is about fourfold more active than azithromycin against this organism in vitro[147] and is somewhat more active in slowing its replication in infected human macrophages.[148] However, macrolide-resistant populations of *M. avium* emerge frequently after treatment of experimentally infected beige mice with clarithromycin or azithromycin.[149] Both of these macrolides also have significant and approximately equal activity against *Toxoplasma gondii* in tissue culture systems.[150, 151]

Aside from their antimicrobial activity, the interesting and potentially useful anti-inflammatory actions of the macrolides were discussed in the section on erythromycin.

Clinical Pharmacology

Clarithromycin is well absorbed after oral administration, with or without food, and is approximately 50% bioavailable.[15] Mean peak serum concentrations in the steady state with oral doses of 250 and 500 mg every 12 hours are 1 and 2 to 3 μg/ml, respectively. The elimination half-lives for those two regimens are 3 to 4 and 5 to 7 hours, respectively. Clarithromycin is appreciably metabolized in the liver by oxidation and hydrolysis to a number of compounds, accounting for a recovery of 78%. The major metabolite, 14-hydroxyclarithromycin, has antibacterial activity and accounts for 20% of the metabolites.[15] With the 250-mg oral dose given every 12 hours, about 20% of the drug is excreted into the urine unchanged and 10 to 15% as the hydroxy metabolite. With the 500-mg dose given at the same interval, about 30% is excreted into the urine unchanged and 10 to 15% as the major metabolite. At higher doses there is some nonlinearity of half-life, apparently because of saturation of metabolic mechanisms with a higher proportion of unchanged drug eliminated in the urine.[15] About 65 to 70% of the drug is bound to protein in the serum. With renal insufficiency involving creatinine clearances of less than 30 ml/min, there is a marked increase in half-life of clarithromycin.[143] Dose adjustment is suggested in patients with severe renal failure, including recommendations for a 500-mg loading dose followed by 250 mg once or twice daily depending on the type of infection being treated.[143] In the face of severe hepatic disease, there is an increase in the renal clearance of clarithromycin associated with a decrease in metabolic clearance, to the extent that no dosage adjustment is recommended at present.[143]

Clarithromycin is widely distributed and penetrates well into various tissues, generally exceeding peak maximum serum levels by severalfold.[143] Concentrations of clarithromycin and its 14-hydroxy metabolite in middle ear fluids of children with acute otitis media exceeded the plasma concentrations by approximately ninefold and fourfold, respectively, 12 hours after the sixth dose when the drug was given every 12 hours.[152] Concentrations generally exceed the MIC of most strains of middle ear pathogens, except for highly penicillin-resistant *S. pneumoniae*. Limited data indicate minimal penetration of clarithromycin and its 14-hydroxy metabolite into cerebrospinal fluid in patients without meningitis.[153] The levels achieved were below the MIC for the usual pathogens associated with bacterial meningitis and were 1 to 2% of the corresponding plasma levels. Clarithromycin, like the other macrolides, penetrates well into phagocytic cells.[154]

The oral bioavailability of azithromycin after a single 500-mg dose is 37%.[155] Food decreases the absorption by 50%; therefore, the dose should be taken at least 1 hour before or 2 hours after a meal.[156] The drug should not be taken simultaneously with magnesium- or aluminum-containing antacids, which decrease the rate of absorption and therefore the peak serum concentration but do not change the extent of absorption (area under the curve).[157] The maximum serum concentration achieved after a single 500-mg oral dose was 0.41 μg/ml; after a 500-mg loading dose on day 1 followed by 250 mg daily for four additional days, it was 0.24 μg/ml; after 500 mg twice on day 1 followed by 500 mg daily for five additional days, it was 0.62 μg/ml.[15] Protein binding of azithromycin in serum varies between 7 and 50% depending on the drug concentration.[15] Azithromycin is widely distributed in tissues, and for most the drug concentration exceeds that in serum by 10- to 100-fold,[155] particularly in sputum and lung. Very high concentrations were found in alveolar macrophages and neutrophils.[158] The extensive tissue uptake of azithromycin has been attributed to cell uptake of this basic compound into relatively acidic lysosomes because of ionic trapping.[158] Very low concentrations were noted in cerebrospinal fluid in patients without meningitis and in the aqueous humor of the uninflamed eye.[159] However, appreciable concentrations of azithromycin have been detected in the brains of patients undergoing resections of brain tumors after they received 500 mg orally.[159] The average half-life in many tissues is between 2 and 4 days,[155] so that it is estimated that significant antibacterial activity against many pathogens persists in tissue for at least 5 days after a 5-day course of treatment.[155] The average terminal half-life is 68 hours, consistent with a slow release of drug from tissues followed by elimination from the vascular compartment. About 6% of an oral dose appears as unchanged drug in the urine within 1 week of administration, and another small proportion is metabolized to inactive compounds, particularly by demethylation.[155] Most of the drug that is absorbed remains unmetabolized and is probably eliminated in feces by way of biliary excretion and possibly transintestinal elimination.[155] Biliary concentrations of azithromycin are higher than in the serum, and most of the drug in the bile is unchanged.[155] There are no data available on dose adjustments required with severe renal or hepatic failure.

Adverse Reactions

Adverse reactions to clarithromycin and azithromycin at the usual doses have been rare.[15, 16, 156] The most common complaints are gastrointestinal (diarrhea, nausea, abdominal pain), and discontinuance of therapy is rarely required. This is in contrast to the relatively common abdominal complaints encountered with erythromycin, which not infrequently lead to cessation of therapy.[15, 16] Abnormalities in liver function and complaints of headache and dizziness are occasionally encountered in patients treated with clarithromycin or azithromycin. With the high doses of these drugs used in the treatment of *M. avium*-complex, tinnitus, dizziness and reversible hearing loss have been reported.[133, 160] Rarely, severe allergic reactions have occurred with the use of azithromycin. One case of ventricular tachycardia that was probably caused by clarithromycin has been reported.[161] Acute psychosis or "mania" has been noted in a few patients receiving clarithromycin.[162, 163] High doses of clarithromycin in animals have been associated with teratogenic effects.

Drug Interactions

Clarithromycin has been reported to be associated with increased concentrations of several drugs that undergo hepatic metabolism by the CYP3A system (see Table 27–3).[119] As with erythromycin, these interactions can lead to serious toxicity. It is not yet clear whether the clarithromycin interactions can occur with all the drugs that interact with erythromycin, but a conservative clinical approach would be to consider that potential. These interactions with the hepatic metabolism of other drugs have not been documented with azithromycin, which does not appear to induce or bind and inactivate the CYP-450 enzymes, probably because of its differing azalide structure.[117, 118, 120]

Clarithromycin may decrease the serum concentration of zidovudine by unknown mechanisms when the two drugs are taken at the same time.[164] However, in another study, with a somewhat different design, there was no significant alteration of zidovudine bioavailability in volunteers with AIDS who took the two drugs 2 hours apart.[165]

Clarithromycin, like erythromycin, may occasionally lead to digoxin toxicity, probably by diminishing the bacterial metabolism of digoxin in the gut.[166]

Uses of Clarithromycin and Azithromycin

Clarithromycin and azithromycin were as effective as other commonly used antimicrobial agents when employed in randomized multicenter trials for the treatment of pharyngitis, sinusitis, community-acquired pneumonia, (including *M. pneumoniae* and *C. pneumoniae* pneumonia), and skin infections.[15, 16, 29, 167, 168] In those studies, direct comparisons of the effectiveness of azithromycin with clarithromycin were not made. Azithromycin administered for 5 days or clarithromycin for 7 to 10 days for the treatment of acute otitis media in children has been effective.[169–171] Side effects, mostly gastrointestinal, were more common with clarithromycin in those studies, but the two macrolides were not directly compared. As with other antimicrobial agents, bacterial meningitis may develop during oral therapy with macrolides for otitis media in children, particularly when the susceptibility of the pathogen is not optimal and spinal fluid penetration of the drug is limited.[172] The dosage of clarithromycin recommended for adults for those conditions is 250 mg orally twice daily for 7 to 14 days, except with sinusitis or bronchitis caused by *H. influenzae*, in which case 500 mg twice daily is suggested. The recommended azithromycin dosage for the same conditions in adults is 500 mg orally on day 1 and 250 mg on days 2 through 5 for a 5-day course of therapy. The 5-day course is used because of the prolonged persistence of good concentrations of azithromycin in tissues.[15] At present, the consideration to use these newer agents for those aforementioned conditions must balance the potential advantages of a low incidence of side effects and infrequent dosing with the disadvantages of no increased effectiveness and a higher cost. Azithromycin can be given effectively for a shorter duration than clarithromycin and seems to be associated with fewer gastrointestinal disturbances, especially in children. However, the increasing incidence of macrolide resistance by *S. pneumoniae*, especially in strains showing penicillin resistance,[22, 28, 29] now raises a caution regarding the use of any macrolide alone for the empirical treatment of pneumonia, especially in seriously ill patients in whom *S. pneumoniae* is a potential etiologic agent.

In a study involving a small number of children with pertussis in Japan, a 5-day course of azithromycin and a 7-day course of clarithromycin were as effective in eradicating *B. pertussis* from cultures 1 week after treatment as in historical control subjects who had been treated with erythromycin, for 2 weeks.[173]

Although the macrolides, including the newer agents, are becoming less reliable in the treatment of pneumococcal pneumonia, clarithromycin and azithromycin show increasing promise in the treatment of *Legionella* pneumonia.[57, 59] Azithromycin showed superior results in an animal model of that infection,[145, 146] and its lower likelihood of drug interactions compared with the other macrolides gives it a potential advantage, especially in the treatment of immunodeficient patients, who often are receiving multiple medications, including those undergoing hepatic metabolism by the CYP-450 system. The suggested dosage of azithromycin for this condition for adults is 500 mg orally or intravenously for 5 to 10 days.[59]

Clarithromycin (500 mg orally twice daily) or azithromycin (500 mg orally once daily) in addition to ethambutol with or without rifabutin are now considered the drugs of choice in the treatment of disseminated *M. avium* complex infections in patients with AIDS.[122, 133] The use of the macrolides alone is often associated with clinical relapse and the emergence of macrolide-resistant organisms.[141] In AIDS patients with $CD4^+$ T-lymphocyte counts lower than 100 cells/mm^3, prophylaxis of disseminated *M. avium* complex infection with clarithromycin (500 mg orally once or twice daily) or azithromycin (1200 mg orally once weekly) is effective.[174, 175] Clarithromycin prophylaxis of this condition has been demonstrated to increase survival.[174] In patients who develop disseminated infection despite prophylaxis, macrolide-resistant isolates are frequent.

A single oral dose of azithromycin (20 mg/kg) is highly effective in treating trachoma and has become the treatment of choice.[122, 176] A singe oral 1-g dose of azithromycin has been as effective as a 1-week course of doxycycline in the treatment of *C. trachomatis* urethritis and cervicitis[177] and acute nongonococcal urethritis (caused by *C. trachomatis* or *U. urealyticum*) in men.[178] Azithromycin (1-g single oral dose) is as effective as ceftriaxone (250 mg intramuscular dose) in treating chancroid.[179]

The majority of patients with peptic ulcer disease can now be cured with short courses of antimicrobial agents combined with an acid-reducing agent, often together with a bismuth salt.[122, 180, 181] Clarithromycin (500 mg orally daily) with either metronidazole, amoxicillin, or tetracycline given for 7 days, together with the aforementioned drugs, is very effective. Failure is often associated with primary resistance by *H. pylori* strains to one of these antimicrobials (relatively common to metronidazole and rare to clarithromycin in several studies) or with the emergence of secondary resistance, which occurs more frequently if only one antimicrobial agent is used or if two are used in the presence of primary resistance to one of them.[182, 183] One study suggests the effectiveness of azithromycin (500 mg daily) and metronidazole given for 3 days, together with lansoprazole, a proton pump inhibitor, for 7 days.[184]

Azithromycin is an effective alternative to ciprofloxacin in the treatment of *Campylobacter* enteritis, but in some areas azithromycin-resistant strains are common.[185, 186] Azithromycin treatment for 5 days was found to be as effective as ciprofloxacin in the treatment of shigellosis in a randomized controlled trial and can be considered a good alternative therapy for that condition.[122, 187]

Clarithromycin has been used effectively in a variety of mycobacterial infections other than tuberculosis and infections caused by *M. avium* complex. It can serve as an alternative in treating infections caused by *Mycobacterium chelonei*, *Mycobacterium fortuitum*, *Mycobacterium genavense*, and *M. kansasii.*[122, 188] In deep-seated infections and in immunocompromised patients with these infections, it is suggested that therapy be carried out with more than one active agent to decrease the chance for the emergence of resistant strains.[189] Clarithromycin has had a limited trial suggesting its effectiveness in treating leprosy and can serve as an alternative drug for that disease.[122, 188]

A few studies suggest that clarithromycin (500 mg twice daily for 21 days) or azithromycin (for 7 to 10 days) is effective in treating most cases of early Lyme disease.[190–192] One of those studies demonstrated that azithromycin (500 mg daily for 7 days) was less effective than amoxicillin (500 mg three times daily for 20 days).[192]

A human volunteer study suggested that azithromycin has potential in the prevention of chloroquine-resistant *Plasmodium falciparum* infection.[193]

In an uncontrolled study, nine patients with AIDS and chronic cryptosporidiosis were treated with azithromycin at a variety of doses for 30 to 360 days (mean, 129 days) and in seven there was a "complete" clinical response, with a major decrease (five patients) or eradication (2 patients) of parasites in the stool.[194] However, in another limited study of azithromycin, given for shorter periods for the same condition, results were poor.[195] With the availability in some communities of highly active antiretroviral therapy for AIDS, the relative role of a drug with activity against cryptosporidia in improving diarrheal disease in these patients needs to be interpreted with data from appropriate control groups.

There has been great interest in the potential role of chronic infections (especially those caused by *C. pneumoniae*) in potentiating atherosclerosis and vascular thromboses, including coronary artery disease.[196, 197] One study in a small number of men who had survived myocardial infarction demonstrated a significant decrease in subsequent adverse cardiovascular events in those who had substantial titers of antibody to *C. pneumoniae* and were given azithromycin (500 mg daily for 3 or 6 days), compared with a similar group of men who were not treated with azithromycin.[198] Studies involving larger numbers of individuals are needed to confirm those results. Assuming a real effect of the macrolide on such cardiac events, it is uncertain whether the result is related to its antimicrobial activity, its anti-inflammatory activity on atheromata or thrombogenesis (discussed in the section on the antimicrobial activity of erythromycin), both of these activities, or other unknown effects.

Dirithromycin

Dirithromycin, a semisynthetic 14-membered macrolide antibiotic, is a prodrug that is rapidly converted by nonenzymatic hydrolysis after intestinal absorption to erythromycylamine. The latter differs from erythromycin by having an amino group instead of a carbonyl group at the C9 position of the lactone ring. Dirithromycin became available for pharmaceutical use in the United States in 1995 and is provided in 250-mg enteric-coated tablets. Its mechanism of action is the same as that of the other macrolides. The antimicrobial activity of dirithromycin against gram-positive bacteria is about the same or half that of erythromycylamine, which is usually fourfold to eightfold less active than erythromycin against *S. pneumoniae, H. influenzae*, and *M. catarrhalis.*[199–201] Strains of *H. influenzae* are often resistant to achievable serum concentrations of dirithromycin.[201] Dirithromycin is less active than erythromycin against *L. pneumophila, M. pneumoniae*, and *C. pneumoniae.*[199, 202, 203] There is complete cross-resistance between erythromycin and dirithromycin.

Erythromycylamine, the active product of hydrolysis of the prodrug after absorption, reaches peak serum concentrations in 4 to 5 hours, achieving levels lower than those of other macrolides (< 1 μg/ml).[199] About 10% of an oral dose is bioavailable. The drug is widely distributed and achieves much higher levels in tissue than in serum. There are no data on cerebrospinal fluid penetration. Erythromycylamine and a smaller amount of dirithromycin, are eliminated in the bile and feces, with a half-life of 30 to 44 hours. About 2% of the orally administered dose is recovered in the urine. There is little or no hepatic metabolism, and slow elimination allows once-daily dosing, with 500 mg suggested in adults.

In a limited number of studies, dirithromycin was similar to erythromycin in clinical and bacteriologic effectiveness in the treatment of community-acquired pneumonia caused by *S. pneumoniae, H. influenzae, L. pneumophila, M. pneumoniae*, or *C. pneumoniae.*[200, 204] The drug was also effective in treating acute bacterial exacerbations of bronchitis, streptococcal pharyngitis, and skin and soft tissue infections.

The adverse effects of dirithromycin have mainly been limited to gastrointestinal symptoms, especially abdominal pain and nausea, probably similar in incidence to those associated with erythromycin. Dirithromycin does not inhibit the CYP-450 hepatic enzyme system and has not been implicated in the drug interactions typical of erythromycin in relation to that system.[201, 205] Its limited in vitro antimicrobial activity and the clinical studies of effectiveness preclude a recommendation for its widespread use.

Other Macrolides

Trioleandomycin, an ester of the 14-member ring macrolide oleandomycin, is still marketed although it has no advantages over erythromycin and may occasionally cause cholestatic hepatitis. It is a potent inhibitor of the cytochrome P-450 enzyme system.[118] Roxithromycin is a 14-member ring macrolide that like dirithromycin, has a modification at the C9 position. It is an investigational drug in the united states, with some-what less or similar in vitro antibacterial activity compared with erythromycin but with a longer half-life.[16, 199] In a double-blind, randomized, placebo-controlled trial in patients with unstable angina or non–Q-wave myocardial infarction, those who received roxithromycin, 150 mg orally twice daily for 3 to 30 days, had significantly decreased rates of severe recurrent ischemia, acute myocardial infarction, or death from cardiac ischemia when assessed at day 31.[206] The results were attributed by the authors of the report to an antichlamydial or an anti-inflammatory effect of the macrolide on atheromata.

LINCOMYCIN AND CLINDAMYCIN

Derivation, Chemistry, and Preparations

Lincomycin was isolated in 1962 from an organism, *Streptomyces lincolnensis*, obtained from soil near Lincoln, Nebraska. Many of its biologic properties are similar to those of erythromycin, but it is chemically unrelated, consisting of an amino acid linked to an amino sugar (Fig. 27–4). Chemical modification provided clindamycin (7-chloro-7-deoxy-lincomycin) (see Fig. 27–4) with increased antibactetrans-L-4-n-propyl hygrinic acid

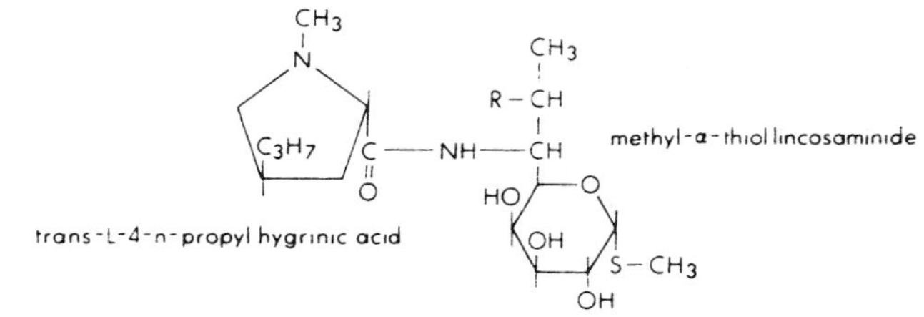

methyl-α-thiol lincosaminide

FIGURE 27–4. The lincosamide antibiotics. Lincomycin, R = OH; clindamycin, R = Cl.

rial potency and absorption after oral administration.[207] Because there are no therapeutic advantages for lincomycin over clindamycin, the discussion here concentrates on the latter, although both are still marketed as pharmaceuticals. Both are weak bases that are readily water soluble when provided as salts.

Lincomycin (Lincocin) is available as the hydrochloride salt in 250- and 500-mg capsules and syrup for oral administration and in solution (300 mg/ml) for parenteral use. Clindamycin (Cleocin) is prepared as the hydrochloride salt of the base in 75-, 150-, and 300-mg capsules and of the palmitate ester for pediatric suspension. It is supplied as the phosphate ester for intramuscular or intravenous use (150 mg/ml). It is also available in a topical solution, gel, and lotion for the treatment of acne vulgaris, and in a concentration of 2% in a vaginal cream for the treatment of bacterial vaginosis.

Mechanism of Action

The lincosamide antibiotics have, in susceptible organisms, the same or overlapping 50S ribosomal binding sites as those for the macrolides and chloramphenicol, and they may compete with these drugs for binding.[3] Protein synthesis is inhibited primarily in early chain elongation by interference with the transpeptidation reaction,[1, 3] possibly by blocking of the P (peptidyl donor) site. Like the macrolides, the lincosamide antibiotics may also stimulate the dissociation of peptidyl-tRNA from ribosomes.

Antimicrobial Activity and Mechanisms of Resistance

In vitro susceptibilities to clindamycin are given in Table 27–5.[13, 207, 208] Clindamycin is more potent than lincomycin but similar in degree of activity to erythromycin against staphylococci, pneumococci, *S. pyogenes*, and streptococci of the "viridans" group. However, although erythromycin demonstrates at least moderate activity against *Enterococcus, H. influenzae*, and *N. meningitidis*, clindamycin is generally inactive against these organisms at clinically achievable concentrations. In contrast, clindamycin shows significantly greater activity than erythromycin against most clinically significant anaerobic bacteria, particularly *B. fragilis*,[209, 210] and some erythromycin-resistant strains of *S. aureus*.[211] Clindamycin has been one of the most active antibiotics available against *B. fragilis*. In a survey of nine hospitals in the United States that provided 750 strains of the *B. fragilis* group in 1981, 6% of isolates were resistant to clindamycin (MIC >4 μg/ml by an agar dilution method); this represented 0 to 13% of strains in individual institutions.[13] In a similar survey by the same group involving eight centers and 678 isolates of the *B. fragilis* group collected in 1984 and 1985, 5% were resistant to clindamycin, representing 0 to 10% of the strains in individual institutions.[208] Of the species belonging to the *B. fragilis* group, clindamycin resistance was found in 5% of *B. fragilis*, 10% of *Bacteroides thetaiotaomicron*, 15% of *Bacteroides vulgatus*, 6% of *Bacteroides distasonis*, and 7% of *Bacteroides ovatus*.[208] There has been a reduction in the degree of susceptibility of the *B. fragilis* group to clindamycin in recent years.[212] A 1994 report on 2800 clinical strains of the *B. fragilis* group collected over a 5-year period from a variety of sites in the United States showed 14% to be resistant to clindamycin.[213] During approximately the same period, 579 clinical isolates of the *B. fragilis* group collected from three Canadian hospitals showed 7.3% of *B. fragilis* strains and 9.4% of non-*fragilis* strains to be resistant to clindamycin.[214] However, in Denmark, clindamycin resistance was documented in only 3% of *B. fragilis* group strains collected in 1990–1991 at several laboratories.[215] Resistance to clindamycin by that group of organisms is significantly more likely when the infection is acquired in hospital or when the patient has received prior antimicrobial therapy.[216] Clindamycin resistance to anaerobes can show substantial variations among hospitals as well as across geographic regions.[217] Resistance to clindamycin by anaerobes also includes 10 to 20% of clostridial species other than *C. perfringens*, about 10 to 20% of peptostreptococci and peptococci, and most *Fusobacterium varium* strains.[209, 210] All the Enterobacteriaceae are resistant to clindamycin.

TABLE 27–5 In Vitro Susceptibilities to Clindamycin

Organism	Minimal Inhibitory Concentration (μg/ml) Range	Median
Streptococcus pneumoniae	0.002–0.04*	0.01
Streptococcus pyrogenes	0.02–0.1*	0.04
Viridans streptococci	0.005–0.04*	0.02
Enterococcus	12.5–>100	100
Staphylococcus aureus	0.04–>100	0.1
Staphylococcus epidermidis	0.1–>100	0.1
Clostridium perfringens	<0.1–8	0.8
Neisseria gonorrhoeae	0.01–6.3	3.1
Neisseria meningitidis	6.3–25	12.5
Haemophilus influenzae	0.4–50	12.5
Bacteriodes fragilis group	<0.125–>256	0.25
Bacteroides melaninogenicus	≤0.1–1	<0.1
Fusobacterium spp.	≤0.5*	≤0.5
Peptococcus spp.	≤0.1–>100	≤0.5
Peptostreptococcus spp.	≤0.1–0.8	≤0.5
Mycoplasma pneumoniae	1.6–3.1	3.1

*Occasional clinical isolates are more resistant.

Clindamycin provides high activity against pneumococci and group A streptococci; however, clinical isolates showing resistance to clindamycin and erythromycin have been increasingly reported from different areas, as already discussed in the section on erythromycin. However, in the United States most macrolide-resistant *S. pneumoniae* and *S. pyogenes* strains are of the M phenotype, which does not show cross-resistance to clindamycin.[31, 32, 34, 41] One study of isolates of *S. pneumoniae* from middle ears and nasal sinuses of infected children in Houston showed that more than 90% of strains that had in vitro susceptibilities to penicillin classified as intermediate or highly resistant were sensitive to clindamycin.[218] Of 63 clinical isolates of *S. pyogenes* in Germany, none was resistant to clindamycin.[219]

The antibacterial activity of clindamycin against *S. pyogenes* displays several characteristics that have the potential to be clinically advantageous and are less prominently demonstrated or absent with the penicillin family. Subinhibitory concentrations of clindamycin diminish encapsulation of group A streptococci,[220] production of M protein,[221] pyrogenic exotoxin A and promitogenic activity[222] in broths of *S. pyogenes*. In a mouse model of *S. pyogenes* myositis, clindamycin administration was more effective than penicillin in limiting bacterial growth and bringing about survival.[223, 224]

In most hospitals at present, the majority of isolates of *S. aureus* are sensitive to lincomycin or clindamycin.[225–227] However, resistance occurs in 12 to 34% of strains especially in those that are methicillin resistant or are isolated from inpatients.[225, 227, 228] Lincomycin or clindamycin resistance has been reported in 20 to 84% of methicillin-resistant strains[225, 228] and in 50% of erythromycin-resistant strains[229] of *S. aureus*. Cross-resistance of *S. aureus* between lincomycin and clindamycin is complete. The MICs of clindamycin and erythromycin in vitro are generally similar for *S. aureus* strains that are sensitive to both agents; however, resistance can be selected in vitro by serial subculture in the presence of subinhibitory concentrations of either drug, and it occurs slowly for clindamycin and more rapidly for erythromycin.[211, 230] In contrast, strains that are sensitive to clindamycin and resistant to erythromycin can be rapidly selected for clindamycin resistance by serial subculture on clindamycin. Consistent with these in vitro observations, the emergence of clindamycin-resistant *S. aureus* has been noted in clindamycin-treated patients, in particular when the organisms had demonstrated erythromycin resistance at the onset of treatment i.e., dissociated resistance of Garrod, described previously.[211, 230] Clindamycin resistance, often crossing to erythromycin, has also emerged from treated patients infected with *S. aureus* that were initially sensitive to erythromycin.[231]

The antibacterial activity of lincomycin and clindamycin has been shown, in limited in vitro studies, to be bactericidal for *S. pneumoniae, S. pyogenes*, and *S. aureus*. Its killing activity is similar to that of erythromycin and therefore probably varies with the concentration, bacterial species, and inoculum. It is more slowly bactericidal for *S. aureus* than are the penicillins,[232] and it is inconsistently bactericidal for *B. fragilis.*[233]

Clindamycin has substantial in vitro activity against *T. gondii* in infected human fibroblasts.[234]

There are several mechanisms of resistance to the lincosamide antibiotics. First, alteration in a single 50S ribosomal protein of the receptor site confers resistance to erythromycin and often to the lincosamides[3]; this mechanism was previously discussed for erythromycin. Second, alteration in the 23S ribosomal RNA of the 50S ribosomal subunit by methylation of adenine[64] has also been discussed. It is usually plasmid mediated and provides the MLS_B type of resistance, which includes that exhibited by some strains of *S. aureus* and *B. fragilis* to clindamycin. Third, resistance is conferred through inactivation of lincomycin and clindamycin by a few isolates of staphylococci (including *S. aureus*) that possess a plasmid-mediated 3-lincomycin 4-clindamycin 0-nucleotidyltransferase that catalyzes the nucleotidylation of the hydroxyl group in position 4 of clindamycin.[44, 235] This adenylation of the lincosamides is associated with high-level resistance to lincomycin, but clindamycin resistance may not be detected by routine methods. The adenylation of clindamycin is associated with impaired bactericidal activity and decreased activity at high inoculum levels. The nucleotide sequences of the plasmid-mediated genes, *lin A* and *lin A'*, which encode for the inactivating enzymes, have been determined. Finally, Enterobacteriaceae, *Pseudomonas* spp., and *Acinetobacter* spp. are intrinsically resistant to clindamycin, apparently because of poor permeability of the cellular outer envelope to the drug.[44]

Clinical Pharmacology

Peak serum levels achieved after oral administration of clindamycin occur earlier and are at least twice as high as those of lincomycin. Absorption of clindamycin is about 90% and is slightly delayed, but not decreased, by ingestion of food, whereas that of lincomycin is markedly decreased.[207] Mean peak serum concentrations of clindamycin in adults after single oral doses of 150 and 300 mg occur at 1 hour and are 2.5 and 3.6 μg/ml, respectively; at 6 hours they are 0.7 and 1.1 μg/ml, respectively. The esters clindamycin palmitate in suspension for oral use and clindamycin phosphate for parenteral use are absorbed as the inactive ester and are rapidly hydrolyzed in the blood to the active base. After intramuscular administration, which causes little pain, mean peak serum levels are reached in 3 hours and are about 6 μg/ml after a 300-mg dose and 9 μg/ml after a 600-mg dose; at 12 hours they are 0.7 and 0.9 μg/ml, respectively.[236] In adult healthy volunteers, immediately after 20- to 45-minute intravenous infusions of 600, 900, or 1200 mg of clindamycin phosphate, serum levels of base are 10, 11, and 14 μg/ml, respectively. Higher levels after intravenous infusion have been reported in infected patients under treatment.[237] Dose regimens of intravenous clindamycin using 900 mg every 8 hours or 600 mg every 6 hours are considered acceptable.[238]

Limited studies have demonstrated good penetration of most tissues by the lincosamides, except for clinically insignificant entry of clindamycin into the cerebrospinal fluid, even with meningitis.[239] The concentration in bone compared with serum is particularly high.[240] Clindamycin administered to pregnant women readily passes the placental barrier and enters fetal blood and tissues.[91] Clindamycin is actively transported into polymorphonuclear leukocytes and macrophages[241] and is present in relatively high concentrations, compared with peak serum levels, in experimental abscesses.[242]

The normal half-life of clindamycin is 2.4 hours. Most of the absorbed drug is metabolized, probably by the liver, to products with variable antibacterial activity, including *N*-demethyl-clindamycin (more active than the parent compound) and clindamycin sulfoxide (less active), which have been detected in bile and urine but not in serum.[236] High bioactivity is found in bile, mostly as the *N*-demethyl metabolite; this represents a minor route of excretion and accounts for the activity assayed in feces after parenteral administration.[236, 243] Clindamycin activity in feces persists for at least 5 days after 48 hours of parenteral administration and is associated with a major reduction in the population of sensitive bacteria in the colon that lasts for up to 14 days.[244] Clindamycin concentration in bile is markedly diminished or absent when the common bile duct is obstructed.[245] High clindamycin bioactivity, also mostly in the *N*-demethyl form, is found in the urine and persists for up to 4 days after a single dose, suggesting slow release from tissues.[237] Accurate data on the proportion of absorbed clindamycin that is excreted in the urine are not available because of the variable activity of the metabolites and their unknown proportions in urine.

The half-life of clindamycin is increased from 2.4 to about 6 hours in patients with severe renal failure, and peak blood levels after parenteral administration are about twice those in healthy people.[246] If modified at all, parenteral doses should be halved in such patients. Some prolongation of clindamycin activity in serum is noted in patients with severe liver disease.[247] Appreciable dose modification should be made when there is concomitant severe renal and hepatic disease in the same patient. Neither hemodialysis nor peritoneal dialysis removes significant amounts of clindamycin.

Adverse Reactions

1. Allergic reactions include a variety of rashes, fever, and rare cases of erythema multiforme and anaphylaxis.

2. Diarrhea occurs in up to 20% of patients and is more common with oral administration. However, the major toxicity of lincomycin and clindamycin that now appreciably limits their use is the occurrence of pseudomembranous colitis caused by a toxin secreted by *C. difficile* that overgrows in the presence of these antibiotics.[248–250] This has been reported to occur in 0.01 to 10% of clindamycin-treated patients.[210, 251] The syndrome may occur in association with administration of other antibiotics but does so less frequently; it is not related to the dose and may occur after oral or parenteral therapy. It has been reported after the use of clindamycin vaginal cream in a patient being treated for bacterial vaginosis.[252] The variable incidence of colitis in different reports has been ascribed to different diagnostic methods and the variable epidemiology of *C. difficile.*[210, 251, 253] Studies suggest that variabilities in the presence of humoral immunity (antitoxin) among individual patients account for some of the differences in susceptibility or recurrence of this infection.[254] It may begin during or as long as several weeks after a course of lincomycin or clindamycin therapy and is characterized by diarrhea, sometimes bloody, with fever and cramps and the appearance of yellow-white

plaques on the colonic mucosa, seen by proctoscopy. The toxin of *C. difficile* can be detected in the stool of almost all patients with antibiotic-associated pseudomembranous colitis and in about 20% of patients with antibiotic-associated diarrhea by a cytotoxicity assay using tissue culture cells.[115, 253, 255] The cytotoxic effect can be prevented by neutralization of the toxin in the stool extract with *Clostridium sordelli* antitoxin. The syndrome can be protracted and may end fatally. Prompt cessation of the antibiotic is essential. Use of antiperistaltic drugs should be avoided because they may worsen the condition. Vancomycin given by mouth and oral metronidazole are effective in treatment.[256] Metronidazole is preferred to limit the selective pressure that potentiates the emergence of vancomycin-resistant enterococci in the environment. Passive and active immunization against the *C. difficile* toxins hold promise for the future.[254] Relapse after treatment may occur when the immune reaction has been inadequate.

3. Hepatotoxicity: Minor reversible elevation of transaminase levels, unassociated with other evidence of liver abnormality, has been commonly observed in patients receiving clindamycin, especially by the parenteral route. Some of these may have been false-positive reactions associated with colorimetric rather than specific enzymatic measurements.[207] However, rare cases of frank hepatotoxicity, including jaundice associated with hepatocellular damage, have been observed.[257]

4. Isolated cases of reversible neutropenia, thrombocytopenia, and agranulocytosis associated with lincomycin or clindamycin therapy have been reported; their relation to the administration of the antibiotic was uncertain.

5. Hypotension, electrocardiographic changes, and, rarely, cardiopulmonary arrest have occasionally been reported when large intravenous doses of lincomycin were given rapidly. These effects have not been reported with clindamycin.

6. Local irritative reactions are rare with these drugs. Intramuscular or intravenous administration is generally well tolerated.

Drug Interactions

Clindamycin may block neuromuscular transmission and may enhance the action of other blocking agents.[258] Clindamycin phosphate in solution is physically incompatible with ampicillin, diphenylhydantoin, barbiturates, aminophylline, calcium gluconate, and magnesium sulfate.

Uses of Clindamycin

The higher activity and absorption properties of clindamycin compared with lincomycin, along with no greater potential for toxicity, favors the former in all indications for use of these antibiotics. The lincosamides have been used in a variety of infections, often with good effect; however, the appreciation of the potential for serious or even fatal toxicity with pseudomembranous colitis and the availability of safer alternative antibiotics should now generally limit the use of clindamycin to a few indications,[122] as follows.

The most important use of clindamycin is in the treatment of infections that are outside of the central nervous system and are likely to involve *B. fragilis* or other penicillin-resistant anaerobic bacteria. These particularly involve polymicrobial intra-abdominal or gynecologic pelvic infections.[210] Clindamycin is likely to be beneficial where there is spillage of fecal flora associated with tissue damage, as in cases involving bowel damage or perforation. In these situations, studies of experimental animal models and patients with infection suggest that clindamycin decreases the likelihood of abscess formation involving fecal organisms, especially *B. fragilis*.[259, 260] In these conditions, clindamycin is administered together with an aminoglycoside, third-generation cephalosporin, or aztreonam because additional activity is required against Enterobacteriaceae. The beneficial effect of clindamycin in preventing or ameliorating morbidity from fecal abscess formation or other infections appears to be superior to that of penicillin, cephalothin, or aminoglycosides.[259, 261] However, in comparative trials of therapy for intra-abdominal or pelvic sepsis, clindamycin, cefoxitin, metronidazole, imipenem, meropenem, ticarcillin-clavulanic acid, and chloramphenicol have shown similar effectiveness.[210, 262–264] Although increasing resistance by the *B. fragilis* group to clindamycin has been reported,[212–214] there has not been good documentation correlating that with clinical failure of treatment,[265] probably because of the complex nature of those infections, which are usually polymicrobial and often are treated with broad-spectrum regimens combined with mechanical drainage.

Clindamycin may offer some advantage over penicillin G in the treatment of anaerobic bronchopulmonary infections,[264] and, in addition, it may serve as an alternative in patients who are allergic to penicillin. In a prospective, randomized study of 39 patients with community-acquired putrid lung abscess, clindamycin was more effective than penicillin in the time until eradication of fever and fetid sputum and in the "overall response" to treatment.[267] The study involved small numbers of patients and had some flaws in the analysis,[268] however, the superiority of clindamycin for some patients was demonstrated and may relate to observations that 15 to 25% of anaerobic pulmonary infections involve β-lactamase–producing strains of *B. fragilis, B. melaninogenicus, Prevotella ruminicola*, and *Bacteroides ureolyticus*, which are resistant to penicillin.[210, 268] Another similar study also demonstrated a higher failure rate with penicillin than with clindamycin and attributed it to penicillin-resistant anaerobes.[269] That study was problematic in that penicillin oral therapy was used to complete the course of treatment of some patients in the penicillin group. Nevertheless, clindamycin may be preferable for treatment of this condition, particularly in seriously ill patients and in those who have responded poorly to penicillin.

Clindamycin is useful as an alternative to penicillin in treatment of *C. perfringens* infections. Clindamycin was more effective than penicillin in reducing mortality in a mouse model of *C. perfringens* gas gangrene and in vitro in suppressing the alpha toxin activity produced by that organism.[270, 271]

Clindamycin may sometimes be useful as an alternative to a penicillin in the treatment of staphylococcal infections. However, its more limited bactericidal rate for staphylococci than that of the penicillins, and particularly the real potential for the emergence of clindamycin-resistant strains in treated patients, are disadvantages. The latter problem, noted especially but not only with erythromycin-resistant strains, appreciably limits its effectiveness as therapy for deep-seated staphylococcal infections, particularly endocarditis.[231] Vancomycin or a cephalosporin is usually a better alternative to the penicillins for the latter. Although high concentrations of clindamycin are achieved in bone, an advantage of clindamycin for the treatment of osteomyelitis has not been established.[240]

The topical solution of clindamycin may be used to treat acne vulgaris.[272] However, pseudomembranous colitis associated with the use of topical clindamycin has been reported.[273] In the treatment of bacterial vaginosis, clindamycin vaginal cream (2%) appears to be similar in efficacy and in the incidence of side affects to oral metronidazole (both used for 7 days).[274, 275] The case report of *C. difficile* colitis associated with clindamycin vaginal cream has already been noted.[252]

Clindamycin is effective in treating experimental animals and when combined with pyrimethamine in treating patients with toxoplasmosis of the central nervous system.[276, 277] A randomized, controlled study found pyrimethamine-clindamycin therapy for that condition in AIDS patients to be less effective in preventing relapses, compared with a pyrimethamine-sulfadiazine regimen.[278]

Clindamycin in combination with primaquine is an effective and well-tolerated regimen for the treatment of mild and moderately severe *Pneumocystis carinii* pneumonia in patients with AIDS.[279, 280] A comparative trial showed the regimen to be equally effective as trimethoprim with sulfamethoxazole or trimethoprim with dapsone.[281]

Clindamycin in combination with quinine is effective in the treatment of falciparum malaria.[122, 282] That regimen used for 4 days was found to be superior to quinine used alone for 7 days in a randomized trial in Gabonese children with severe disease.[283] The same combination has also been reported to be useful in the treatment of babesiosis.[122, 284]

Several studies have suggested that the coexistence of β-lactamase–producing *S. aureus* or *Bacteroides* spp, and group A streptococci may be associated with the failure of penicillin to eradicate the latter, resulting in recurrent tonsillitis. These studies suggest that recurrence rates may be lowered when clindamycin is used.[285, 286] In a more recent study, patients with group A streptococcal pharyngitis in whom the organisms with the same T protein type persisted (in some with symptoms and signs as well) after 10 days of treatment with phenoxymethyl penicillin were randomly allocated to retreatment for 10 days with phenoxymethyl penicillin or clindamycin.[287] Group A streptococci were not recovered from any of the patients receiving clindamycin, but the same T type was cultured from 64% of those retreated with the penicillin. However, widespread use of clindamycin for this common problem is likely to lead to a substantial number of cases of pseudomembranous colitis, as well as selection for clindamycin-resistant strains of group A streptococci.

Although penicillin has been the traditional drug of choice for the treatment of group A streptococcal infections, clindamycin must be considered as potentially more effective in serious soft tissue infections, based on data, already discussed, from the treatment of experimental infections in mice and the effectiveness of that agent compared with penicillin in decreasing the in vitro production of several of the virulence factors of the pathogen. However, there are, as yet, no data from clinical trials to substantiate such an advantage for clindamycin, and, because some strains of *S. pyogenes* may be resistant to clindamycin, that drug should be use in combination with penicillin for the empiric treatment of life-threatening group A streptococcal infections, until sensitivity data are available.[122] Limited in vitro data suggest that the addition of penicillin to clindamycin does not antagonize the bactericidal effects of the latter.[288]

The dosage of clindamycin for adults depends on the site and severity of infection and the condition of the patient. Oral doses are usually 150 to 300 mg every 6 hours, and parenteral doses, given every 6 to 12 hours, usually total 600 to 2700 mg/day, occasionally higher.

REFERENCES

1. Pestka S. Inhibitors of protein synthesis. In: Weissbach H, Pestka S, eds. Molecular Mechanisms of Protein Biosynthesis. New York: Academic Press; 1977:467.
2. Goldman RC, Fesik SW, Doran CC. Role of protonated and neutral forms of macrolides in binding to ribosomes from gram-positive and gram-negative bacteria. Antimicrob Agents Chemother. 1990;34:426–431.
3. Tai PC, Daris BD. The actions of antibiotics on the ribosome. In: Greenwood D, O'Grady F, eds. The Scientific Basis of Antimicrobial Chemotherapy. Cambridge: Cambridge University Press; 1985:41–68.
4. Mazzei T, Mini E, Novelli A, et al. Chemistry and mode of action of macrolides. J Antimicrob Chemother. 1993;31 (SupplC):1–9.
5. Chittum HS, Champney WS. Erythromycin inhibits the assembly of the large ribosomal submit in growing *Escherichia coli* cells. Curr Microbiol. 1995;30: 273–279.
6. Haight TH, Finland M. Observations on mode of action of erythromycin. Proc Soc Exp Biol Med. 1952;81:188–193.
7. Haight TH, Finland M. The antibacterial action of erythromycin. Proc Soc Exp Biol Med. 1952;81:175–183.
8. Sabath LD, Gerstein DA, Loder PB, et al. Excretion of erythromycin and its enhanced activity in urine against gram-negative bacilli with alkalinization. J Lab Clin Med. 1968;72:916–923.
9. Washington JA II, Wilson WR. Erythromycin: A microbial and clinical perspective after 30 years of clinical use:I. Mayo Clin Proc. 1984;60:189–203; II. 1985;60: 271–278.
10. Edelstein PM, Meyer RD. Susceptibility of *Legionella pneumophila* to twenty antimicrobial agents. Antimicrob Agents Chemother. 1980;18:403–408.
11. Vanhoff R, Gordts B, Dierickx R, et al. Bacteriostatic and bactericidal activities of 24 antimicrobial agents against *Campylobacter fetus* subsp. *jejuni*. Antimicrob Agents Chemother. 1980;18:118–121.
12. Kuo C, Wang S, Grayston T. Antimicrobial activity of several antibiotics and a sulfonamide against *Chlamydia trachomitis* organisms in cell culture. Antimicrob Agents Chemother. 1977;12:80–83.
13. Tally FP, Cuchural GJ, Jacobus NV, et al. Susceptibility of the *Bacteroides fragilis* group in the United States in 1981. Antimicrob Agents Chemother. 1983;23: 536–540.
14. Ahmad F, McLeod DT, Croughan MJ, et al. Antimicrobial susceptibility of *Branhamella catarrhalis* isolates from bronchopulmonary infections. Antimicrob Agents Chemother. 1984;26:424–425.
15. Piscitelli SC, Danziger LH, Rodvold KA. Clarithromycin and azithromycin: New macrolide antibiotics. Clin Pharm. 1992;11:137–152.
16. Bahal N, Nahata MC. The new macrolide antibiotics: Azithromycin, clarithromycin, dirithromycin, and roxithromycin. Ann Pharmacother. 1992;26:46–55.
17. Neu HC. The development of macrolides: Clarithromycin in perspective. J Antimicrob Chemother. 1991;27(Suppl 4):1–9.
18. Neu HC. Clinical microbiology of azithromycin. Am J Med. 1991;91(Suppl 3A):12S–18S.
19. Waites KB, Cassell GH, Canupp KC, et al. In vitro susceptibilities of mycoplasmas and ureaplasmas to new macrolides and aryl-fluoroquinolones. Antimicrob Agents Chemother. 1988;32:1500–1502.
20. Renaudin H, Bebear C. Comparative in vitro activity of azithromycin, clarithromycin, erythromycin and lomefloxacin against *Mycoplasma pneumoniae*, *Mycoplasma hominis* and *Ureaplasma urealyticum*. Eur J Clin Microb Infect Dis. 1990;9:838–841.
21. Ednie LM, Visalli MA, Jacobs MR, et al. Comparative activities of clarithromycin, erythromycin and azithromycin against penicillin-susceptible and penicillin-resistant pneumococci. Antimicrob Agents Chemother. 1996;40:1950–1952.
22. Thornsberry C, Ogilvie P, Kahn J, et al. Surveillance of antimicrobial resistance in *Streptococcus pneumoniae*, *Hemophilus influenzae*, and *Moraxella catarrhalis* in the United States in 1996–1997 respiratory season. Diagn Microb Infect Dis. 1997;29:249–257.
23. Alcaide F, Carratala J, Linares J, et al. In vitro activities of eight macrolide antibodies and RP-59500 (quinupristin-dalfopristin) against viridans group streptococci isolated from blood of neutropenic cancer patients. Antimicrob Agents Chemother. 1996;40:2117–2120.
24. Welsh L, Gaydos C, Quinn TC. In vitro activities of azithromycin, clarithromycin, erythromycin, and tetracycline against 13 strains of *Chlamydia pneumoniae*. Antimicrob Agents Chemother. 1996;40:212–214.
25. Sanders E, Foster MT, Scott D. Group A beta-haemolytic streptococci resistant to erythromycin and lincomycin. N Engl J Med. 1968;278:538–540.
26. Dixon JM. *Pneumococcus* resistant to erythromycin and lincomycin. Lancet. 1967;1:573.
27. Moreno S, Garcia-Leoni E, Cercenado E, et al. Infections caused by erythromycin-resistant *Streptococcus pneumoniae*: Incidence, risk factors, and response to therapy in a prospective study. Clin Infect Dis. 1995;20:1195–1200.
28. Hoffman J, Cetron MS, Farley MM, et al. The prevalence of drug-resistant *Streptococcus pneumoniae* in Atlanta. N Engl J Med. 1995;333:481–486.
29. Bartlett JG, Brieman RF, Mandell LA, et al. Community-acquired pneumonia in adults: Guidelines for management. Clin Infect Dis. 1998;26:811–838.

29a. Corso A, Severina EP, Petruk VF, et al. Molecular characterization of penicillin-resistant *Streptococcus pneumoniae* isolates causing respiratory disease in the United States. Microb Drug Resist. 1998;4:328–337.

30. Poulsen PL, Knudsen JD, Petersen MB, et al. In vitro activity of six macrolides, clindamycin and tetracycline on *Streptococcus pneumoniae* with different penicillin susceptibilities. APMIS 1996;104:227–233.
31. Sutcliffe J, Tait-Kamradt A, Wondrack L. *Streptococcus pneumoniae* and *Streptococcus pyogenes* resistant to macrolides but sensitive to clindamycin: A common resistance pattern mediated by an efflux system. Antimicrob Agents Chemother. 1996;40:1817–1824.
32. Tait-Kamradt A, Clancy J, Cronan M, et al. mefE is necessary for the erythromycin-resistant M phenotype in *Streptococcus pneumoniae*. Antimicrob Agents Chemother. 1997;41:2251–2255.
33. Jones RN, Cormican MG, Wanger A. Clindamycin resistance among erythromycin-resistant *Streptococcus pneumoniae*. Diagn Microbiol Infect Dis. 1996;25:201–204.
34. Widdowson CA, Klugman KP. Emergence of the M phenotype of erythromycin-resistant pneumococci in South Africa. Emerg Infect Dis. 1998;4:277–281.
35. Maruyama S, Yoshioka H, Fujita K, et al. Sensitivity of group A streptococci to antibiotics. Am J Dis Child. 1979;133:1143–1145.
36. Istre GR, Welch DF, Marks MI, et al. Susceptibility of group A beta-hemolytic *Streptococcus* isolates to penicillin and erythromycin. Antimicrob Agents Chemother. 1981;20:244–246.
37. Seppala H, Nissinen A, Jarvinen H, et al. Resistance to erythromycin in group A streptococci. N Engl J Med. 1992;326:292–297.
38. Seppala H, Klaukka T, Vuopio-Varkila J, et al. The effect of changes in the consumption of macrolide antibiotics on erythromycin resistance in Group A streptococci in Finland. Finnish Study Group for Antimicrobial Resistance. N Engl J Med. 1997;337:441–446.
39. Cornaglia G, Ligozzi M, Mazzariol A, et al. Rapid increase of resistance to erythromycin and clindamycin in *Streptococcus pyogenes* in Italy, 1993–1995. The Italian Surveillance Group for Antimicrobial Resistance. Emerg Infect Dis. 1996;2:339–342.
40. Kaplan EL. Recent evaluation of antimicrobial resistance in beta-hemolytic streptococci. Clin Infect Dis. 1997;24(Suppl 1):S89–S92.
41. Clancy J, Pettipas J, Dib-Hajj F, et al. Molecular cloning and functional analysis of a novel macrolide-resistance determinant, mefA, from *Streptococcus pyogenes*. Mol Microbiol. 1996;22:867–879.
42. Haight TH, Finland M. Resistance of bacteria to erythromycin. Proc Soc Exp Biol Med. 1952;81:183–188.

43. Lepper MH, Dowling HF, Jackson GG, et al. Effect of antibiotic usage in the hospital on the incidence of antibiotic-resistant strains among personnel carrying staphylococci. J Lab Clin Med. 1953;42:832.
44. Leclercq R, Courvalin P. Intrinsic and unusual resistance to macrolides, lincosamide, and streptogramin antibiotics in bacteria. Antimicrob Agents Chemother. 1991;35:1273–1276.
45. Griffith RS, Black HR. Erythromycin. Med Clin North Am. 1970;54:1199–1215.
46. Haight TH, Finland M. Laboratory and clinical studies on erythromycin. N Engl J Med. 1952;247:227–232.
47. Garrod LP. The erythromycin group of antibiotics. Br Med J. 1957;2:57–63.
48. Mapple PAC, Hamilton-Miller JMT, Brumfitt W. World-wide antibiotic resistance in methicillin-resistant *Staphylococcus aureus*. Lancet. 1989;1:537–539.
49. Sapico FL, Kwok Y, Sutter V, et al. Standardized antimicrobial disc susceptibility testing of anaerobic bacteria: In vitro susceptibility of *Clostridium perfringens* to nine antibiotics. Antimicrob Agents Chemother. 1972;2:320–325.
50. Molavi A, Weinstein L. In vitro activity of erythromycin against atypical mycobacteria. J Infect Dis. 1971;123:216–219.
51. Finland M, Bach MC, Garner C, et al. Synergistic action of ampicillin against *Nocardia asteroides:* Effect of time of incubation. Antimicrob Agents Chemother. 1974;5:344–353.
52. Fernandes PB, Hardy D, Bailer R, et al. Susceptibility testing of macrolide antibiotics against *Hemophilus influenzae* and correlation of in vitro results with in vivo efficacy in a mouse septicemia model. Antimicrob Agents Chemother. 1987;31:1243–1250.
53. Ehret JM, Nims LJ, Judson FN. A clinical isolate of *Neisseria gonorrhoeae* with in vitro resistance to erythromycin and decreased susceptibility to azithromycin. Sex Transm Dis. 1996;23:270–272.
54. Kucers A. Chloramphenicol, erythromycin, vancomycin, tetracyclines. Lancet. 1982;2:425–429.
55. Jao RL, Finland M. Susceptibility of *Mycoplasma pneumoniae* to 21 antibiotics in vitro. Am J Med Sci. 1967;253:639–650.
56. Niitu Y, Hasegawa S, Kubota H. In vitro development of resistance to erythromycin, other macrolide antibiotics, and lincomycin in *Mycoplasma pneumoniae*. Antimicrob Agents Chemother. 1974;5:513–519.
57. Edelstein PH. Antimicrobial chemotherapy for Legionnaires' disease: A review. Clin Infect Dis. 1995;21(Suppl 3):S265–S276.
58. Segreti J, Meyer P, Kepell K. In vitro activity of macrolides against intracellular *Legionella pneumophila*. Diagn Microbiol Infect Dis. 1996;25:123–126.
59. Stout JE, Yu VL. Legionellosis. N Engl J Med. 1997;337:682–687.
60. Mao JC-H, Putterman M. Accumulation in gram-positive and gram-negative bacteria as a mechanism of resistance to erythromycin. J Bacteriol. 1968;95:1111–1117.
61. Taubeneck U. Susceptibility of *Proteus mirabilis* and its stable L-forms to erythromycin and other macrolides. Nature. 1962;196:195–196.
62. Ross JI, Eady EA, Cove JH, et al. Minimal functional system required for expression of erythromycin resistance by msrA in *Staphylococcus aureus* RN4220. Gene. 1996;183:143–148.
63. Kataja J, Seppala H, Skurnik M, et al. Different erythromycin resistance mechanisms in Group C and Group G streptococci. Antimicrob Agents Chemother. 1998;42:1493–1494.
64. Leclercq R, Courvalin P. Bacterial resistance to macrolide, lincosamide, and streptogramin antibiotics by target modification. Antimicrob Agents Chemother. 1991;35:1267–1272.
65. Weisblum B. Erythromycin resistance by ribosome modification. Antimicrob Agents Chemother. 1995;39:577–585.
66. Wondrack L, Massa M, Yang BV, et al. Clinical strain of *Staphylococcus aureus* inactivates and causes efflux of macrolides. Antimicrob Agents Chemother. 1996;40:992–998.
67. Sutcliffe J, Grebe T, Tait-Kamradt A, et al. Detection of erythromycin-resistant determinants by PCR. Antimicrob Agents Chemother. 1996;40:2562–2566.
68. Itoh Z, Suzuki T, Nakaya M, et al. Gastrointestinal motor-stimulating activity of macrolide antibiotics and analysis of their side effects on the canine gut. Antimicrob Agents Chemother. 1984;26:863–869.
69. Itoh Z, Suzuki T, Nakaya M, et al. Structure–activity relation among macrolide antibiotics in initiation of interdigestive migrating contractions in the canine gastrointestinal tract. Am J Physiol. 1985;11:G320–G325.
70. Catnach SM, Fairclough PD. Erythromycin and the gut. Gut. 1992;33:397–401.
71. Annese V, Lombardi G, Frusciante V, et al. Cisapride and erythromycin prokinetic effects in gastroparesis due to type 1 (insulin-dependent) diabetes mellitus. Aliment Pharmacol Ther. 1997;11:599–603.
72. Brand RM, Quigley EM. Transdermal delivery of erythromycin lactobionate: Implications for the therapy of gastroparesis. Aliment Pharmacol Ther. 1997;11:589–592.
73. Abdelghaffar H, Vazifeh D, Labro MT. Erythromycin A-derived macrolides modify the functional activities of human neutrophils by altering the phospholipase D-phosphatidate phosphorylase transduction pathway: L-Cladinose is involved both in alterations of neutrophil functions and modulation of this transductional pathway. J Immunology. 1997;159:3995–4005.
74. Aoshiba K, Nagai A, Konno K. Erythromycin shortens neutrophil survival by accelerating apotosis. Antimicrob Agents Chemother. 1995;39:872–877.
75. Takizawa H, Desaki M, Ohtoshi T, et al. Erythromycin suppresses interleukin 6 expression by human bronchial epithelial cells: A potential mechanism of its anti-inflammatory action. Biochem Biophys Res Commun. 1995;210:781–786.
76. Mitsuyama T, Hidaka K, Furuno T, et al. Release of nitric-oxide and expression of constitutive nitric oxide synthase of human endothelial cells: Enhancement by a 14-membered ring macrolide. Mol Cell Biochem. 1998;181:157–161.
77. Bechtol LD, Stephens VC, Pugh CT, et al. Erythromycin esters: Comparative in vivo hydrolysis and bioavailability. Curr Ther Res. 1976;20:610–622.
78. Malmborg A. Effect of food on absorption of erythromycin. A study of two derivatives, the stearate and the base. J Antimicrob Chemother. 1979;5:591–599.
79. McDonald PJ, Mather LE, Story MJ. Studies on absorption of a newly developed enteric-coated erythromycin base. J Clin Pharmacol. 1977;17:601–606.
80. DiSanto AR, Chodos DJ. Influence of study design in assessing food effects on absorption of erythromycin base and erythromycin stearate. Antimicrob Agents Chemother. 1981;20:190–196.
81. Yakatan GJ, Rasmussen CE, Feis PJ, et al. Bioinequivalence of erythromycin ethylsuccinate and enteric-coated erythromycin pellets following multiple oral doses. J Clin Pharmacol. 1985;25:36–42.
82. Janicki RS, Garnham JC, Worland MC, et al. Comparison of erythromycin ethylsuccinate, stearate and estolate treatments of group A streptococcus infections of the upper respiratory tract. Clin Pediatr (Phila). 1975;14:1098–1107.
83. Ginsburg CM, McCracken GH Jr, Crow SD, et al. Erythromycin therapy for group A streptococcal pharyngitis: Results of a comparative study of the estolate and ethylsuccinate formulation. Am J Dis Child. 1984;138:536–539.
84. Osono T, Umezawa H. Pharmacokinetics of macrolides, lincosamides and streptogramins. J Antimicrob Chemother. 1985;16(Suppl A):151–66.
85. Welling PG. The esters of erythromycin. J Antimicrob Chemother. 1979;5:633–634.
86. Bass JW, Steele RW, Wiebe RA, et al. Erythromycin concentrations in middle ear exudates. Pediatrics. 1971;48:417–422.
87. Howard JE, Nelson JD, Clahsen J, et al. Otitis media of infancy and early childhood. Am J Dis Child. 1976;130:965–970.
88. Hand WL, Corwin RW, Steinberg TH, et al. Uptake of antibiotics by human alveolar macrophages. Am Rev Respir Dis. 1984;129:933–937.
89. Miller MF, Martin JR, Johnson P, et al. Erythromycin uptake and accumulation by human polymorphonuclear leukocytes and efficacy of erythromycin in killing ingested *Legionella pneumophila*. J Infect Dis. 1984;149:714–718.
90. Romansky MJ, Nasou JP, Davis DS, et al. The treatment of 171 patients with erythromycin, including 132 with bacterial pneumonia. Antibiotics Annual. New York: Medical Encyclopedia; 1956;1955–1956:48.
91. Phillipson A, Sabath LD, Charles D. Transplacental passage of erythromycin and clindamycin. N Engl J Med. 1973;288:1219–1221.
92. Hammond JB, Griffith RS. Factors affecting the absorption and biliary excretion of erythromycin and two of its derivatives in humans. Clin Pharmacol Ther. 1961;2:308–312.
93. Mao JC-H, Tardrew PL. Demethylation of erythromycin by rabbit tissues in vitro. Biochem Pharmacol. 1965;14:1049–1058.
94. Kunin CM. A guide to use of antibiotics in patients with renal disease. Ann Intern Med. 1967;67:151–158.
95. Ellsworth AJ, Christensen DB, Volpone-McMahon MT. Prospective comparison of patient tolerance to enteric-coated vs nonenteric-coated erythromycin. J Fam Pract. 1990;31:265–270.
96. Inman WHW, Rawson NSB. Erythromycin isolate and jaundice. BMJ. 1983;286:1954–1955.
97. Braun P. Hepatotoxicity of erythromycin. J Infect Dis. 1969;119:300–306.
98. Tolman KG, Sannella JJ, Freston JW. Chemical structure of erythromycin and hepatotoxicity. Ann Intern Med. 1974;81:58–60.
99. Pessayre D, Larrey D, Funck-Brentano C, et al. Drug interactions and hepatitis produced by some macrolide antibiotics. J Antimicrob Chemother. 1985;16(Suppl A):181–194.
100. McCormack WM, George H, Donner A, et al. Hepatotoxicity of erythromycin estolate during pregnancy. Antimicrob Agents Chemother. 1977;12:630–635.
101. Sabath LD, Gerstein DA, Finland M. Serum glutamic oxalacetic transaminase: False elevation during administration of erythromycin. N Engl J Med. 1968;279:1137–1139.
102. Sullivan D, Csuka ME, Blanchard B. Erythromycin ethylsuccinate hepatotoxicity. JAMA. 1980;243:1074.
103. Auckenthaler RW, Zwahlen A, Waldvogel FA. Macrolides. In: Peterson, PK, Verhoef J, eds. The Antimicrobial Agents Annual, v. 2. Amsterdam: Elsevier; 1987:120.
104. Carson JL, Strom BL, Duff A. Acute liver disease associated with erythromycins, sulfanomides, and tetracyclines. Ann Intern Med. 1993;119:576–583.
105. Karmody CS, Weinstein L. Reversible sensorineural hearing loss with intravenous erythromycin lactobionate. Ann Otol Rhinol Laryngol. 1977;86:9–11.
106. Eckman MR, Johnson T, Riess R. Partial deafness after erythromycin (Letter). N Engl J Med. 1975;292:649.
107. Mery JP, Kanfer A. Ototoxicity of erythromycin in patients with renal insufficiency (Letter). N Engl J Med. 1979;301:944.
108. Taylor R, Schofield IS, Ramos JM, et al. Ototoxicity of erythromycin in peritoneal dialysis patients (Letter). Lancet. 1981;2:935–936.
109. Haydon RC, Thaelin JW, Davis WE. Erythromycin ototoxicity: Analysis and conclusions based on 22 case reports. Otolaryngol Head Neck Surg. 1984;92: 678–684.
110. Swanson DJ, Sung RJ, Fine MJ, et al. Erythromycin ototoxicity: Prospective assessment with serum concentrations and audiograms in a study of patients with pneumonia. Am J Med. 1992;92:61–68.
111. Schoenenberger RA, Haefel WE, Weiss P, et al. Association of intravenous erythromycin and potentially fatal ventricular tachycardia with Q-T prolongation (torsades de pointes). BMJ. 1990;300:1375–1376.
112. Katapadik K, Kostandy G, Katapadi M, et al. A review of the erythromycin-induced malignant tachyarrhythmia torsade de pointes: A case report. Angiology. 1997;48:821–826.
113. Daleau P, Lessard E, Grouleau MF, et al. Erythromycin blocks the rapid component of the delayed rectifier potassium current and lengthens repolarization of guinea pig ventricular myocytes. Circulation. 1995;91:3010–3016.

114. Gantz NM, Zawacki JK, Dickerson J, et al. Pseudomembranous colitis associated with erythromycin. Ann Intern Med. 1979;91:866–867.
115. Bartlett JG. Antimicrobial agents implicated in *Clostridium difficile* toxin-associated diarrhea or colitis. Johns Hopkins Med J. 1981;149:6–9.
116. Ludden TM. Pharmacokinetic interactions of the macrolide antibiotics. Clin Pharmacokinet. 1985;10:63–79.
117. Amsden GW. Macrolides versus azalides: A drug interaction update. Ann Pharmacother. 1995;29:906–917.
118. Periti P, Mazzei T, Mini E, et al. Pharmacokinetic drug interactions of macrolides. Clin Pharmacokinet. 1992;23:106–131.
119. Rizack MA. The Medical Letter Handbook of Adverse Drug Interactions. New Rochelle, N.Y.: The Medical Letter on Drugs and Therapeutics; 1999.
120. Honig PK, Wortham DC, Zamani K, et al. Comparison of the effect of the macrolide antibiotics erythromycin, clarithromycin and azithromycin on steady-state pharmacokinetics and electrocardiographic parameters. Drug Invest. 1994;7:148–156.
121. Spicer ST, Liddle C, Chapman JR, et al. The mechanism of cyclosporine toxicity induced by clarithromycin. Br J Clin Pharm. 1997;43:194–196.
122. Handbook of Antimicrobial Therapy. The Medical Letter on Drugs and Therapeutics. New Rochelle, NY: Medical Letter; 1998.
123. Rasch JR, Mogabgab WJ. Therapeutic effect of erythromycin on *Mycoplasma pneumoniae* pneumonia. Antimicrob Agents Chemother. 1965;5:693–699.
124. Kirby BD, Snyder KM, Myer RD, et al. Legionnaires' disease: Report of sixty-five nosocomially acquired cases and review of the literature. Medicine (Baltimore). 1980;59:188–205.
125. Muder RF, Yu VL, Zuravleff MS. Pneumonia due to the Pittsburgh pneumonia agent: New clinical perspective with a review of the literature. Medicine (Baltimore). 1983;62:120–128.
126. Sprauer MA, Cochi SL, Zell ER, et al. Prevention of secondary transmission of pertussis in households with early use of erythromycin. Am J Dis Child. 1992;146:177–181.
127. Anders BJ, Lauer BA, Paisley JW, et al. Double-blind placebo controlled trial of erythromycin for treatment of *Campylobacter* enteritis. Lancet. 1982;1:131–132.
128. Salazar-Lindo E, Sack B, Chea-Woo E, et al. Early treatment with erythromycin of *Campylobacter jejuni*-associated dysentery in children. J Pediatr. 1986;109: 355–360.
129. Taylor DN, Blaser MJ, Escheverria P. Erythromycin-resistant *Campylobacter* infections in Thailand. Antimicrob Agents Chemother. 1987;31:438–442.
130. Beem MD, Saxon E, Tipple MA. Treatment of chlamydial pneumonia of infancy. Pediatrics. 1979;63:198–203.
131. Clarke JS, Condon RE, Fenton LJ, et al. Preoperative oral antibiotics reduce septic complications of colon operations: Results of prospective randomized, double-blind clinical study. Ann Surg. 1977;186:251–259.
132. Stellato TA, Danziger LH, Gordon N, et al. Antibiotics in elective colon surgery: A randomized trial of oral, systemic, and oral/systemic antibiotics for prophylaxis. Ann Surg. 1990;56:251–254.
133. Bartlett JG. Medical Management of HIV infection. Baltimore: Port City Press; 1998.
134. Fenton LJ, Light IJ. Congenital syphilis after maternal treatment with erythromycin. Obstet Gynecol. 1976;47:492–949.
135. Centers for Disease Control and Prevention. 1998 guidelines for treatment of sexually transmitted diseases. MMWR Morb Mortal Wkly Rep. 1998;47(RR-1): 41,46.
136. Zinner SK, Sabath LD, Casey JI, et al. Erythromycin and alkalinization of the urine in treatment of urinary tract infections due to gram-negative bacilli. Lancet. 1971;1:1267–1268.
137. Kabir I, Khan WA, Haider R, et al. Erythromycin and trimethoprim-sulphamethoxazole in the treatment of cholera in children. J Diarrhoeal Dis Res. 1996;14:243–247.
137a. Kudoh S, Azuma A, Yamamoto M, et al. Improvement of survival in patients with diffuse panbronchiolitis treated with lower-dose erythromycin. Am J Respir Crit Care Med. 1998;157:1829–1832.
138. Retsema J, Giraud A, Schelkly W, et al. Spectrum and mode of action of azithromycin (CP-62,993), a new 15-membered-ring macrolide with improved potency against gram-negative organisms. Antimicrob Agents Chemother. 1987;31:1939–1947.
139. Fernardes PB, Bailer R, Swanson R, et al. In vitro and in vivo evaluation of A-56268 (TE-031), a new macrolide. Antimicrob Agents Chemother. 1986;30: 865–873.
140. Versalovic J, Shortridge D, Kibler K, et al. Mutations in 23S rRNA are associated with clarithromycin resistance in *Helicobacter pylori*. Antimicrob Agents Chemother. 1996;40:477–480.
141. Taylor DE, Ge Z, Purych D, et al. Cloning and sequence analysis of two copies of a 23S rRNA gene from *Helicobacter pylori* and association of clarithromycin resistance with 23S rRNA mutations. Antimicrob Agents Chemother. 1997;41:2621–2628.
142. Nash KA, Inderleid CB. Genetic basis of macrolide resistance in *Mycobacterium avium* isolated from patients with disseminated disease. Antimicrob Agents Chemother. 1995;39:2625–2630.
143. Hardy DJ, Guay DRP, Jones RN. Clarithromycin, a unique macrolide: A pharmacokinetic, microbiological, and clinical overview. Diagn Microbiol Infect Dis. 1992;15:39–53.
144. Tateda K, Ishii Y, Matsumoto T, et al. Direct evidence for antipseudomonal activity of macrolides: Exposure-dependent bactericidal activity and inhibition of protein synthesis by erythromycin, clarithromycin and azithromycin. Antimicrob Agents Chemother. 1996;40:2271–2275.
145. Fitzgeorge RB, Featherstone ASR, Baskerville A. Efficacy of azithromycin in the treatment of guinea pigs infected with *Legionella pneumophila* by aerosol. J Antimicrob Chemother. 1990;25(Suppl A):101–108.
146. Fitzgeorge RB, Lever S, Baskerville A. A comparison of efficacy of azithromycin and clarithromycin in oral therapy of experimental airborne Legionnaire's disease. J Antimicrob Chemother. 1993(Suppl E):171–176.
147. Naik S, Ruck R. In vitro activities of several new macrolide antibiotics against *Mycobacterium avium* complex. Antimicrob Agents Chemother. 1989;33:1614–1616.
148. Perronne C, Gikas A, Truffot-Pernot C, et al. Activities of sparfloxacin, azithromycin, temafloxacin and rifapentine compared with that of clarithromycin against multiplication of *Mycobacterium avium* complex within human macrophages. Antimicrob Agents Chemother. 1991;35:1356–1359.
149. Bermudez LE, Petrofsky M, Kolonoski P, et al. Emergence of *Mycobacterium avium* populations resistant to macrolides during experimental chemotherapy. Antimicrob Agents Chemother. 1998;42:180–183.
150. Derouin F, Chastang C. Activity in vitro against *Toxoplasma gondii* of azithromycin and clarithromycin alone and with pyrimethamine (Letter). J Antimicrob Chemother. 1990;25:708–711.
151. Chang HR, Pechere JCF. In vitro effects of four macrolides (roxithromycin, spiramycin, azithromycin [CP-62,693], and A-56268) on *Toxoplasma gondii*. Antimicrob Agents Chemother. 1988;32:524–529.
152. Gan VN, McCarty JM, Chu SY, et al. Penetration of clarithromycin into middle ear fluid of children with acute otitis media. Pediatr Infect Dis J. 1997;16:39–43.
153. Sanche S, Williams K, Stein K. Cerebrospinal fluid penetration of clarithromycin and 14-hydroxyclarithromycin. (Abstract 728). Presented at the Thirty-third Interscience Conference on Antimicrobial Agents and Chemotherapy, New Orleans, La., October, 1993.
154. Anderson R, Joone G, van Rensburg CEJ. An in vitro evaluation of the cellular uptake and intraphagocytic bioactivity of clarithromycin (A56268, TE-031), a new macrolide antimicrobial agent. J Antimicrob Chemother. 1988;22:923–933.
155. Schentag JJ, Ballow CH. Tissue directed pharmacokinetics. Am J Med. 1991;91(Suppl 3A):5S–11S.
156. Hopkins S. Clinical toleration and safety of azithromycin. Am J Med. 1991;91(Suppl 3A):40S–45S.
157. Foulds G, Hilligoss DM, Henry EB, et al. The effects of antacid or cimetidine on the serum concentrations of azithromycin. J Clin Pharmacol. 1991;31:164–167.
158. Ballow CH, Amsden GW. Azithromycin: The first azalide antibiotic. Ann Pharmacother. 1992;26:1253–1261.
159. Jaruratanasirikul S, Hortiwakul R, Tantisarasart T, et al. Distribution of azithromycin into brain tissue, cerebrospinal fluid, and aqueous humor of the eye. Antimicrob Agents Chemother. 1996;40:825–826.
160. Wallace RJ Jr, Brown BA, Griffith DE. Drug intolerance to high dose clarithromycin among elderly patients. Diagn Microbial Infect Dis. 1993;16:215–221.
161. Kundu S, Williams SR, Nordt SP. Clarithromycin-induced ventricular tachycardia. Ann Emerg Med. 1997;30:542–544.
162. Nightingale SD, Koster FT, Mertz GJ, et al. Clarithromycin-induced mania in two patients with AIDS. Clin Infect Dis. 1995;20:1563–1564.
163. Cone LA, Sneider RA, Nazemi R, et al. Mania due to clarithromycin therapy in a patient who was not infected with human immunodeficiency virus. Clin Infect Dis. 1996;22:595–596.
164. Polis MA, Piscitelli SC, Vogel S, et al. Clarithromycin lowers plasma zidovudine levels in persons with human immunodeficiency virus infection. Antimicrob Agents Chemother. 1997;41:1709–1714.
165. Vance E, Watson-Bitar M, Gustavson L, et al. Pharmacokinetics of clarithromycin and zidovudine in patients with AIDS. Antimicrob Agents Chemother. 1995;39:1355–1360.
166. Nawarskas JJ, McCarthy DM, Spinler SA. Digoxin toxicity secondary to clarithromycin therapy. Ann Pharmacother. 1997;31:864–866.
167. Clarithromycin and azithromycin. Med Lett Drugs and Ther. 1992;34:45–47.
168. Hammerschlag MR. Antimicrobial susceptibility and therapy of infections caused by *Chlamydia pneumoniae*. Antimicrob Agents Chemother. 1994;38:1873–1878.
169. McCarty J. A multicenter, open label trial of azithromycin for the treatment of children with acute otitis media. Pediatr Infect Dis J. 1996;15(Suppl 9):S10–S14.
170. Aronovitz G. A multicenter, open label trial of azithromycin vs. amoxicillin/clavulanate for the management of acute otitis media in children. Pediatr Infect Dis J. 1996;15(Suppl 9):S15–S19.
171. Pukander JS, Jero JP, Kaprio EA, et al. Clarithromycin vs. amoxicillin suspensions in the treatment of pediatric patients with acute otitis media. Pediatr Infect Dis J. 1993;12(Suppl 3):S118–S121.
172. Reid R Jr, Bradley JS, Hindler J. Pneumococcal meningitis during therapy of otitis media with clarithromycin. Pediatr Infect Dis J. 1995;14:1104–1105.
173. Aoyama T, Sunakawa K, Iwata S, et al. Efficacy of short-term treatment of pertussis with clarithromycin and azithromycin. J Pediatr. 1996;129:761–764.
174. Pierce M, Crampton S, Henry D, et al. A randomized trial of clarithromycin as prophylaxis against disseminated *Mycobacterium avium* complex infection in patients with advanced acquired immunodeficiency syndrome. N Engl J Med. 1996;335:384–391.
175. Havlir DV, Dube MP, Sattler FR, et al. Prophylaxis against disseminated *Mycobacterium avium* complex with weekly azithromycin, daily rifabutin, or both. N Engl J Med. 1996;335:392–398.
176. Tabbara KF, Abu-el-Asrar A, al-Omar O, et al. Single-dose azithromycin in the treatment of trachoma: A randomized controlled study. Ophthalmology. 1996;103:852–856.
177. Martin DH, Mroczkowski TF, Dalu ZA, et al. A controlled trial of a single dose of azithromycin for the treatment of chlamydial urethritis and cervicitis. N Engl J Med. 1992;327:921–5.

178. Stamm WE, Hicks CB, Martin DH, et al. Azithromycin for empirical treatment of the nongonococcal urethritis syndrome in men. JAMA. 1995;274:545–549.
179. Martin DH, Sargent SJ, Wendel GD Jr, et al. Comparison of azithromycin and ceftriaxole for the treatment of chancroid. Clin Infect Dis. 1995;21:409–414.
180. Blaser MJ. *Helicobacter pylori* and gastric diseases. BMJ. 1998;316:1507–1510.
181. Lind T, Veldhuyzen van Zanten S, Unge P, et al. Eradication of *Helicobacter pylori* using one-week triple therapies combining omeprazole with two antimicrobials: The MACH I Study. Helicobacter. 1996;1:138–144.
182. Tompkins DS, Perkins J, Smith C. Failed treatment of *Helicobacter pylori* infection associated with resistance to clarithromycin. Helicobacter. 1997;2:185–187.
183. Buckley MJ, Xia HX, Hyde DM, et al. Metronidazole resistance reduces efficacy of triple therapy and leads to secondary clarithromycin resistance. Dig Dis Sci. 1997;42:2111–2115.
184. Caselli M, Trevisani L, Tursi A, et al. Short-term low dose triple therapy with azithromycin, metronidazole and lansoprazole appears highly effective for the eradication of *Helicobacter pylori*. Eur J Gastroenterol Hepatol. 1997;9:45–48.
185. Kuschner RA, Trofa AF, Thomas RJ, et al. Use of azithromycin for the treatment of *Campylobacter enteritis* in travelers to Thailand, an area where ciprofloxacin resistance is prevalent. Clin Infect Dis. 1995;21:536–541.
186. Murphy GS, Echeverria P, Jackson LR, et al. Ciprofloxacin and azithromycin-resistant *Campylobacter* causing travelers' diarrhea in U.S. troops deployed in Thailand in 1994. Clin Infect Dis. 1996;22:868–869.
187. Khan WA, Seas C, Dhar U, et al. Treatment of shigellosis: V. Comparison of azithromycin and ciprofloxacin. A double-blind, randomized controlled trial. Ann Intern Med. 1997;126:697–703.
188. Kurers A, Crowe SM, Grayson ML, et al. The Use of Antibiotics: A Clinical Review of Antibacterial, Antifungal and Antiviral Drugs. 5th ed. Oxford: Butterworth-Heinemann; 1997:648.
189. Tehas P, Sultan F, Wallace RJ Jr, et al. Rapid development of resistance to clarithromycin following monotherapy for disseminated *Mycobacterium chelonae* infection in a heart transplant patient. Clin Infect Dis. 1995;20:443–444.
190. Dattwyler RJ, Grunwaldt E, Luft BJ. Clarithromycin in treatment of early Lyme disease: A pilot study. Antimicrob Agents Chemother. 1996;40:468–469.
191. Strle F, Ruzic E, Cimperman J. Erythema migrans: Comparison of treatment with azithromycin, doxycycline and phenoxymethyl penicillin. J Antimicrob Chemother. 1992;30:543–550.
192. Luft BJ, Dattwyler RJ, Johnson RC, et al. Azithromycin compared with amoxicillin in the treatment of erythema migrans: A double-blind, randomized, controlled trial. Ann Intern Med. 1996;124:785–791.
193. Anderson SL, Berman J, Kuschner R, et al. Prophylaxis of *Plasmodium falciparum* malaria with azithromycin administered to volunteers. Ann Intern Med. 1995;123:771–773.
194. Dionisio D, Orsi A, Serrantino G, et al. Chronic cryptosporidiosis in patients with AIDS: Stable remission and possible eradication after long-term low dose azithromycin. J Clin Pathol. 1998;51:138–142.
195. Blanshard C, Shanson DC, Gazzard BG. Pilot studies of azithromycin, letrazuril and paromomycin in the treatment of cryptosporidiosis. Int J STD AIDS. 1997;8:124–129.
196. Lip GYH, Beevers G. Commentary. Can we treat coronary artery disease with antibiotics? Lancet. 1997;350:378–379.
197. Danesh J, Collins R, Peto R. Chronic infection and coronary heart disease: Is there a link? Lancet. 1997;350:430–436.
198. Gupta S, Leatham EW, Carrington D, et al. Elevated *Chlamydia pneumoniae* antibodies, cardiovascular events, and azithromycin in male survivors of myocardial infarction. Circulation. 1997;96:404–407.
199. Bryskier A, Butzler J-P. Macrolides. In: O'Grady F, Lambert HP, Finch RG, et al., eds. Antibiotic and Chemotherapy: Antinfective Agents and Their Use in Therapy. 7th ed. New York: Churchill Livingstone; 1997:377–393.
200. Visalli MA, Jacobs MR, Applebaum PC. Susceptibility of penicillin-susceptible and -resistant pneumococci to dirithromycin compared with susceptibilities to erythromycin, azithromycin, clarithromycin, roxithromycin, and clindamycin. Antimicrob Agents Chemother. 1997;41:1867–1870.
201. Dirithromycin. Med Lett Drugs Ther. 1995;37:109–110.
202. Stout JE, Arnold B, Yu VL. Activity of azithromycin, clarithromycin, roxithromycin, dirithromycin, quinupristin/dalfopristin and erythromycin against *Legionella* species by intracellular susceptibility testing in HL-60 cells. J Antimicrob Chemother. 1998;41:289–291.
203. Roblin PM, Kutlin A, Sokolovskaya N, et al. In vitro activity of dirithromycin against *Chlamydia pneumoniae*. J Antimicrob Chemother. 1997;39:647–649.
204. Jacobson K. Clinical efficacy of dirithromycin in pneumonia. J Antimicrob Chemother. 1993;32(Suppl C):121–129.
205. Watkins VS, Polk RE, Stotka JL. Drug interactions of macrolides: Emphasis on dirithromycin. Ann Pharmacother. 1997;31:349–356.
206. Gurfinkel E, Bozovich G, Daroca A, et al for the ROXIS Study Group. Ramdomized trial of roxithromycin in non-Q-wave coronary syndromes: ROXIS pilot study. Lancet. 1997;350:404–407.
207. McGehee RF Jr, Smith CB, Wilcox C, et al. Comparative studies of antibacterial activity in vitro and absorption and excretion of lincomycin and clindamycin. Am J Med Sci. 1968;256:279–292.
208. Cuchural GJ Jr, Tally FP, Jacobus NV, et al. Susceptibility of the *Bacteroides fragilis* group in the United States: Analysis by site of isolation. Antimicrob Agents Chemother. 1988;32:717–722.
209. Sutter VL: In vitro susceptibility of anaerobes: Comparison of clindamycin and other antimicrobial agents. J Infect Dis. 1977;135(Suppl):S7–S12.
210. Bartlett JG. Anti-anaerobic antibacterial agents. Lancet. 1982;2:478–481.
211. McGehee RF, Barrett FF, Finland M. Resistance of *Staphylococcus aureus* to lincomycin, clindamycin and erythromycin. Antimicrob Agents Chemother. 1969;1968:392–397.
212. Snydman DR, McDermott L, Cuchural GJ Jr, et al. Analysis of trends in antimicrobial resistance patterns among clinical isolates of *Bacteroides fragilis* group species from 1990 to 1994. Clin Infect Dis. 1996;23(Suppl 1):S54–S65.
213. Aldridge KE, Gelfand M, Reller LB, et al. A five-year multicenter study of the susceptibility of the *Bacteroides fragilis* group isolates to cephalosporins, cephamins, penicillins, clindamycin, and metronidazole in the United States. Diagn Microb Infect Dis. 1994;18:235–241.
214. Turgeon P, Turgeon V, Gourdeau M, et al. Longitudinal study of susceptibilities of species of the *Bacteroides fragilis* group to five antimicrobial agents in three medical centers. Antimicrob Agents Chemother. 1994;38:2276–2279.
215. Bremmelgaard A, Jansen JE, Justesen T, et al. Antibiotic sensitivity of the *Bacteroides fragilis* group in Denmark. Danish study group. APMIS. 1993;101:727–731.
216. Dalmau D, Cayouette M, Lamothe F, et al. Clindamycin resistance in the *Bacteroides fragilis* group: Association with hospital-acquired infections. Clin Infect Dis. 1997;24:874–877.
217. Rasmussen BA, Bush K, Tally FP. Antimicrobial resistance in anaerobes. Clin Infect Dis. 1997;24(Suppl 1):S110–S120.
218. Nelson CT, Mason EO Jr, Kaplan SL. Activity of oral antibiotics in middle ear and sinus infections caused by penicillin-resistant *Streptococcus pneumoniae*: Implications for treatment. Pediatr Infect Dis J. 1994;13:585–589.
219. Troub WH, Leonhard B. Comparative susceptibility of clinical group A,B,C,F and G beta-hemolytic streptococci isolates to 24 antimicrobial drugs. Chemotherapy. 1997;43:10–20.
220. Brook I, Gober AE, Leyva F. In vitro and in vivo effects of penicillin and clindamycin on expression of group A beta-hemolytic streptococcal capsule. Antimicrob Agents Chemother. 1995;39:1565–1568.
221. Gemmell CG, Peterson PK, Schmeling D, et al. Potentiation of opsonization and phagocytosis of *Streptococcus pyogenes* following growth in the presence of clindamycin. J Clin Invest. 1981;67:1249–1256.
222. Sriskandan S, McKee A, Hall L, et al. Comparative effects of clindamycin and ampicillin on superantegenic activity of *Streptococcus pyogenes*. J Antimicrob Chemother. 1997;40:275–277.
223. Stevens DL, Gibbons AE, Bergstrom R, et al. The Eagle effect revisited: Efficacy of clindamycin, erythromycin and penicillin in the treatment of streptococcal myositis. J Infect Dis. 1988;158:23–28.
224. Stevens DL, Yan S, Bryant AE. Penicillin-binding protein expression at different growth stages determines penicillin efficacy in vitro and in vivo: An explanation for the inoculum effect. J Infect Dis. 1993;167:1401–1405.
225. Reeves DS, Holt HA, Phillips I, et al. Activity of clindamycin against *Staphylococcus aureus* and *Staphylococcus epidermidis* from four UK centres. J Antimicrob Chemother. 1991;27:469–474.
226. McKitrick JC. Antibiotic susceptibility data from the microbiology laboratory for bacterial isolates from 1997 (by the Kirby-Bauer method). Bronx, NY: Montefiore Medical Center; 1998.
227. Speller DC, Johnson AP, James D, et al. Resistance to methicillin and other antibiotics in isolates of *Staphylococcus aureus* from blood and cerebrospinal fluid, England and Wales, 1989–1995. Lancet. 1997;350:323–325.
228. Barrett FF, McGehee RF Jr, Finland M. Methicillin resistance *Staphylococcus aureus* at Boston City Hospital. N Engl J Med. 1968;279:441–448.
229. Desmyter J, Reybrouck G. Lincomycin sensitivity of erythromycin-resistant staphylococci. Chemotherapia. 1964;9:183–189.
230. Duncan IBR. Development of lincomycin resistance by staphylococci. Antimicrob Agents Chemother. 1967;1968:723–729.
231. Watanakunakorn C. Clindamycin therapy of *Staphylococcus aureus* endocarditis: Clinical relapse and development of resistance to clindamycin, lincomycin and erythromycin. Am J Med. 1976;60:419–425.
232. Sande MA, Johnson ML. Antimicrobial therapy of experimental endocarditis caused by *Staphylococcus aureus*. J Infect Dis. 1975;131:367–375.
233. Nastro LJ, Finegold SM. Bactericidal activity of five antimicrobial agents against *Bacteroides fragilis*. J Infect Dis. 1972;126:104–107.
234. Pfefferkorn ER, Nothnagel RF, Borotz SE. Parasiticidal effect of clindamycin on *Toxoplasma gondii* grown in cultured cells and selection of a drug resistant mutant. Antimicrob Agents Chemother. 1992;36:1091–1096.
235. Leclercq R, Brisson-Noel A, Duval J, et al. Phenotypic expression and genetic heterogeneity of lincosamide inactivation in *Staphylococcus* spp. Antimicrob Agents Chemother. 1987;31:1887–1891.
236. DeHaan RM, Metzler CM, Schellenberg D, et al. Pharmacokinetic studies of clindamycin phosphate. J Clin Pharmacol. 1973;13:190–209.
237. Fass RJ, Salow S. Clindamycin: Clinical and laboratory evaluations of parenteral therapy. Am J Med Sci. 1972;263:369–382.
238. Townsend RJ, Baker RP. Pharmacokinetic comparison of three clindamycin phosphate dosing schedules. Drug Intell Clin Pharmacol. 1987;21:279–281.
239. Panzer JD, Brown DC, Epstein WL, et al. Clindamycin levels in various body tissues and fluids. J Clin Pharmacol. 1972;12:259–262.
240. Nicholas P, Meyers BR, Levy RN. Concentrations of clindamycin in human bone. Antimicrob Agents Chemother. 1975;8:220–221.
241. Prokesch RC, Hand WL. Antibiotic entry into human polymorphonuclear leukocytes. Antimicrob Agents Chemother. 1982;23:373–380.
242. Joiner KA, Lowe BR, Dzink JL, et al. Antibiotic levels in infected and sterile subcutaneous abscesses in mice. J Infect Dis. 1981;143:487–494.
243. McCall CE, Steigbigel NH, Finland M. Lincomycin: Activity in vitro and absorption and excretion in normal young men. Am J Med Sci. 1967;254:144–155.

244. Kager L, Liljeqvist L, Malmborg AS, et al. Effect of clindamycin prophylaxis on the colonic microflora in patients undergoing colorectal surgery. Antimicrob Agents Chemother. 1981;20:736–740.
245. Brown RB, Martyak SN, Barza M, et al. Penetration of clindamycin phosphate into the abnormal human biliary tract. Ann Intern Med. 1976;84:168–170.
246. Joshi A, Stein R. Altered serum clearance of intravenously administered clindamycin phosphate in patients with uremia. J Clin Pharmacol. 1974;14:140–144.
247. Williams DN, Crossley K, Hoffman C, et al. Parenteral clindamycin phosphate: Pharmacology with normal and abnormal liver function and effect on nasal staphylococci. Antimicrob Agents Chemother. 1975;7:153–158.
248. Rifkin GD, Fekety FR, Silva J Jr, et al. Antibiotic-induced colitis: Implication of a toxin neutralized by *Clostridium sordellii* antitoxin. Lancet. 1977;11:1103–1106.
249. Bartlett JG, Chang TW, Gurwith M, et al. Antibiotic-associated pseudomembranous colitis due to toxin-producing clostridia. N Engl J Med. 1978;298:531–534.
250. Kelly CP, LaMont JT. *Clostridium difficile* infection. Annu Rev Med. 1998;49: 375–390.
251. Tedesco FJ. Clindamycin and colitis: A review. J Infect Dis. 1977;135(Suppl): S95–S98.
252. Meadowcroft AM, Diaz PR, Latham GS. *Clostridium difficile* toxin—induced colitis after use of clindamycin phosphate vaginal cream. Ann Pharmacother. 1998;32:309–311.
253. Knoop FC, Owens M, Crocker IC. *Clostridium difficile*: Clinical disease and diagnosis. Clin Microbiol Rev. 1993;6:251–265.
254. Salcedo J, Keater S, Pothoulakis C, et al. Intravenous immunoglobulin therapy for severe *Clostridium difficile* colitis. Gut. 1997;41:366–370.
255. Vargas SO, Horensky D, Onderdonk AB. Evaluation of a new enzyme immunoassay for *Clostridium difficile* toxin A. J Clin Pathol. 1997;50:996–1000.
256. Bartlett JG. Management of *Clostridium difficile* infection and other antibiotic-associated diarrhoeas. Eur J Gastroenterol Hepatol. 1996;8:1054–1061.
257. Elmore M, Rissing JP, Rink L, et al. Clindamycin-associated hepatotoxicity. Am J Med. 1974;57:627–630.
258. Fogdall RP, Miller RD. Prolongation of a pancuronium-induced neuromuscular blockade by clindamycin. Anesthesiology. 1974;41:407–408.
259. Thadepalli H, Gorbach SL, Broido PW, et al. Abdominal trauma, anaerobes, and antibiotics. Surg Gynecol Obstet. 1973;137:270–276.
260. Weinstein WM, Onderdonk AB, Bartlett JG, et al. Antimicrobial therapy of experimental intra-abdominal sepsis. J Infect Dis. 1975;132:282–286.
261. diZerega G, Yonekura L, Roy S, et al. A comparison of clindamycin-gentamicin and penicillin-gentamicin in the treatment of post-cesarean section endometritis. Am J Obstet Gynecol. 1979;134:238–242.
262. Solomkin JS, Dellinger EP, Christou NV, et al. Results of a multicenter trial comparing imipenem/cilastatin to tobramycin/clindamycin for intrabdominal infections. Ann Surg. 1990;212:581–591.
263. Sirinek KR, Levine BR. A randomized trial of ticarcillin and clavulanate versus gentamicin and clindamycin in patients with complicated appendicitis. Surg Gynecol Obstet. 1992;172(Suppl):30–35.
264. Condon RE, Walker AP, Sirinek KR, et al. Meropenem versus tobramycin plus clindamycin for treatment of intraabdominal infections: Results of a prospective, randomized, double-blind clinical trial. Clin Infect Dis. 1995;21:544–550.
265. Bartlett JG. Intra-abdominal sepsis. Med Clin North Am. 1995;79:599–617.
266. Bartlett JG, Gorbach SL. Treatment of aspiration pneumonia and primary lung abscess: Penicillin F vs. clindamycin. JAMA. 1975;234:936–937.
267. Levison ME, Mangura CT, Lorber B, et al. Clindamycin compared with penicillin for the treatment of anaerobic lung abscess. Ann Intern Med. 1983;98:466–471.
268. Bartlett JG, Gorbach SL. Penicillin or clindamycin for primary lung abscess? (Editorial). Ann Intern Med. 1983;98:546–548.
269. Gudiol F, Manresa F, Pallares R, et al. Clindamycin vs penicillin for anaerobic lung infections: High rate of penicillin failures associated with penicillin-resistant *Bacteroides melaninogenicus*. Arch Intern Med. 1990;150:2525–2529.
270. Stevens DL, Maier KA, Laine BM, et al. Comparison of clindamycin, rifampin, tetracycline, metronidazole, and penicillin for efficacy in prevention of experimental gas gangrene due to *Clostridium perfringens*. J Infect Dis. 1987;155:220–228.
271. Stevens DL, Maier KA, Miller JE. Effect of antibiotics on toxin production and viability of *Clostridium perfringens*. Antimicrob Agents Chemother. 1987;31: 213–218.
272. Leyden JJ, Shalita AR, Saatjian GD, et al. Erythromycin 2% gel in comparison with clindamycin phosphate 1% solution in acne vulgaris. J Am Acad Dermatol. 1987;16:822–827.
273. Parry MF, Rha CK. Pseudomembranous colitis caused by topical clindamycin phosphate. Arch Dermatol. 1986;122:583–584.
274. Andres FJ, Parker R, Hosein I. Clindamycin vaginal cream versus oral metronidazole in the treatment of bacterial vaginosis: A prospective double-blind clinical trial. South Med J. 1992;85:1077–1080.
275. Schmitt C, Sobel JD, Meriwether C. Bacterial vaginosis: Treatment with clindamycin cream versus oral metronidazole. Obstet Gynecol. 1992;79:1020–1023.
276. Hofflin JM, Remington JS. Clindamycin in a murine model of toxoplasmic encephalitis. Antimicrob Agents Chemother. 1987;31:492–496.
277. Dannemann B, McCutchan JA, Israelski D, et al. Treatment of toxoplasmic encephalitis in patients with AIDS: A randomized trial comparing pyrimethamine plus clindamycin to pyrimethamine plus sulfadiazine. The California Collaborative Treatment Group. Ann Intern Med. 1992;116:33–43.
278. Katlama C, DeWit S, O'Doherty E, et al. Pyrimethamine-clindamycin vs. pyrimethamine-sulfadiazine as acute and long term therapy for toxoplasimic encephalitis in patients with AIDS. Clin Infect Dis. 1996;22:268–275.
279. Black JR, Feinberg J, Murphy RL, et al. Clindamycin and primaquine as primary treatment for mild and moderately severe *Pneumocystis carinii* pneumonia in patients with AIDS. Eur J Clin Microbiol Infect Dis. 1991;10:204–207.
280. Norskin GA, Murphy RL, Black JR, et al. Salvage therapy with clindamycin/primaquine for *Pneumocystis carinii* pneumonia. Clin Infect Dis. 1992;14:183–188.
281. Safrin S, Finkelstein DM, Feinberg, J et al. Comparison of three regimens for treatment of mild to moderate *Pneumocystis carinii* pneumonia in patients with AIDS: A double-blind, randomized trial of oral trimethoprim-sulfamethoxazole, dapsone-trimethoprim, and clindamycin-primaquine. ACTG 108 Study Group. Ann Intern Med. 1996;124:792–802.
282. el Wakeel ES, Homeida MM, Ali HM, et al. Clindamycin in the treatment of falciparum malaria in Sudan. Am J Trop Med Hyg. 1985;34:1065–1068.
283. Kremsner PG, Radloff P, Metzger W, et al. Quinine plus clindamycin improves chemotherapy of severe malaria in children. Antimicrob Agents Chemother. 1995;39:1603–1605.
284. Wittner M, Rowin KS, Tanowitz HB, et al. Successful chemotherapy of transfusion babesiosis. Ann Intern Med. 1982;96:601–604.
285. Brook I, Hirokawa R. Treatment of patients with a history of recurrent tonsillitis due to group A beta-hemolytic streptococci: A prospective randomized study comparing penicillin, erythromycin and clindamycin. Clin Pediatr. 1985;24: 331–336.
286. Jensen JH, Larsen SB. Treatment of recurrent acute tonsillitis with clindamycin. An alternative to tonsillectomy? Clin Otolaryngol. 1991;16:498–500.
287. Orrling A, Stjernquist-Desatnik A, Schalen C, et al. Clindamycin in persisting streptococcal pharyngotonsillitis after penicillin treatment. Scand J Infect Dis. 1994;26:535–541.
288. Stevens DL, Madaras-Kelly KJ, Richards DM. In vitro antimicrobial effects of various combinations of penicillin and clindamycin against four strains of *Streptococcus pyogenes*. Antimicrob Agents Chemother. 1998;42:1266–1268.

Chapter 28

Vancomycin, Teicoplanin, and the Streptogramins: Quinupristin and Dalfopristin

ROBERT FEKETY

VANCOMYCIN

Structure

Vancomycin is a complex soluble glycopeptide that has a molecular weight of approximately 1450 Da. It is similar to teicoplanin and several other glycopeptides that are still investigational but is unrelated to other antibiotics. When vancomycin was first introduced, commercial preparations contained as much as 30% of another substance of unknown nature that probably contributed to its side effects.[1, 2] Current preparations are highly purified (although not completely pure) and appear to be less toxic than the early preparations.

Derivation and Nomenclature

Vancomycin (Vancocin, Lilly; Vancomycin HCl, Lederle) is a narrow-spectrum bactericidal antibiotic obtained from *Streptomyces orientalis*. Introduced in 1956 because of its effectiveness against penicillin-resistant staphylococci, it was relegated because of its toxicity to the role of alternate therapy when methicillin became available. With the spread of methicillin-resistant *Staphylococcus aureus* (MRSA) in the United States, vancomycin underwent a marked increase in frequency of use and became the drug of choice for the treatment of these infections in seriously ill, hospitalized patients. Vancomycin given by the oral route is also highly effective in the treatment of severe antibiotic-associated colitis caused by *Clostridium difficile*. In 1989, vancomycin-resistant enterococci (VRE) emerged as important nosocomial pathogens in the United States. Strains of *S. aureus* that were intermediately resistant to vancomycin (VIRSA) were detected in many Japanese hospitals in 1996[3, 4] and in the United States in 1997.[5] VRE and VIRSA have raised serious concerns about the continued effectiveness of vancomycin in the treatment of these infections.

Mechanism of Action

Vancomycin inhibits synthesis and assembly of the second stage of cell wall peptidoglycan polymers by complexing with their D-alanyl-D-alanine precursor, which fits into a "pocket" in the vancomycin molecule, thereby preventing its binding to the peptidoglycan terminus that is the target of transglycolase and transpeptidase enzymes. In addition, vancomycin may impair RNA synthesis and injure protoplasts by altering the permeability of their cytoplasmic membrane. The unique multiple mechanisms of the action of vancomyin may have contributed to the observed low frequency of development of resistance until recently. Rapidly and tightly bound to target organisms, vancomycin exerts a bactericidal effect without a lag period but acts only on multiplying organisms. Vancomycin continues to exert its antibacterial activity after concentrations fall below inhibitory levels, with a postantibiotic effect of about 2 hours.[6]

Antimicrobial Activity

Until recently, *S. aureus* and *Staphylococcus epidermidis* were both highly susceptible to vancomycin. Concentrations of 1 to 5 mg/liter or less were almost invariably inhibitory, even with isolates resistant to methicillin, and most of these organisms were killed at about the same concentrations. Rare strains required 10 to 20 mg/liter for inhibition; up to 20% of strains were deficient in autolysins and relatively tolerant to the bactericidal action of vancomycin.[7, 8] Biofilms of slime, produced particularly on plastic foreign bodies by *S. epidermidis*, can impair penetration of vancomycin to the sites of lodgment of organisms and also may be responsible for tolerance to its bactericidal effect and for treatment failure.[9]

In 1987, it was reported that certain coagulase-negative staphylococci were showing resistance to vancomycin.[10] Some strains of at least two species, *Staphylococcus haemolyticus* and *S. epidermidis*, have been reported to have minimal inhibitory concentrations (MICs) and minimum bactericidal concentrations (MBCs) that are increased fourfold, to 8 and 12 mg/liter, respectively, and the MBC with heavy inocula may be as high as 32 mg/liter. These organisms were also resistant to teicoplanin. These strains of coagulase-negative staphylococci have been associated with failure of treatment with glycopeptide antimicrobials until infected foreign bodies or cardiac valves were removed.

As mentioned, VIRSA strains with heterogeneous, intermediate resistance to vancomycin were first detected in Japan in 1996 and were soon found to have spread widely to many hospitals there.[3, 4] MICs of vancomycin for these organisms ranged from 8 to 16 mg/liter; MBCs were similar. This report was soon followed by the detection of VIRSA in the United States and Europe.[5, 11] VIRSA isolates were usually cross-resistant to teicoplanin, with MICs of 8 to 16 mg/liter, and susceptible only to pristinamycin, trimethoprim-sulfamethoxazole, and arbekacin.[4, 11] Thus far, it does not seem that VIRSA have acquired genes for Van A, Van B, or Van C from vancomycin-resistant enterococci. Instead, it appears that VIRSA are resistant because of excessive production of cell wall material, possibly penicillin-binding protein 2 (PBP2), with formation of multicellular aggregates that clump and prevent access of vancomycin to its target sites. Patients infected with VIRSA frequently have been treated unsuccessfully with repeated courses of vancomycin; in addition, intravascular or peritoneal dialysis catheters are often present at the site of the infection and need to be removed. Standard clinical laboratory disk-diffusion susceptibility tests are not highly reliable for the detection of VIRSA strains, which may also appear initially to be coagulase-negative.[11]

Streptococcus pyogenes, group B streptococci, *Corynebacterium jeikeium*, *C. difficile*, and both penicillin-resistant and susceptible strains of *Streptococcus pneumoniae* are highly susceptible to vancomycin. *Listeria monocytogenes*, anaerobic or microaerophilic streptococci, *Clostridium perfringens* and most other clostridia, *Bacillus anthracis*, actinomycetes, lactobacilli, diphtheroids, *Corynebacterium diphtheriae*, other corynebacteria including CDC-D2, *Neisseria gonorrhoeae*, and *Neisseria meningitidis* are usually susceptible.[12, 13] Viridans streptococci, *Streptococcus agalactiae*, *Streptococcus bovis*, and, until the late 1980s, *Enterococcus faecalis* (formerly *Streptococcus faecalis*) and *Enterococcus faecium* (formerly *Streptococcus faecium*) isolates were usually inhibited at concentrations of vancomycin attainable in serum, but few if any enterococcus isolates were killed at concentrations below 100 mg/liter.[12, 13] Nutritionally deficient variants of streptococci may be killed by vancomycin alone.[14] In the past, 40 to 70% of *Enterococcus* isolates showed a synergistic bactericidal effect when vancomycin was combined with streptomycin or gentamicin, and the combination of vancomycin plus gentamicin was almost always bactericidal at attainable concentrations[15, 16] unless so-called high-level gentamicin-resistant isolates (MIC >500 mg/liter) were implicated.[17] Vancomycin and gentamicin are also synergistic against most susceptible strains of viridans streptococci, *S. bovis*, methicillin-sensitive and methicillin-resistant *S. aureus*, and up to 50% of *S. epidermidis* strains. The combination of vancomycin and rifampin is usually synergistic against *S. epidermidis* but is much less often synergistic against *S. aureus*, and in fact is often antagonistic toward this organism. Vancomycin-resistant isolates of *S. bovis*,[18] *E. faecalis*,[19] *E. faecium*,[19] *Enterococcus gallinarum*,[20] *Enterococcus casseliflavus*, *Pediococcus*, and *Leukonostoc* spp. (which may be misidentified as streptococci) have been detected.[21] Plasmids transferable to other gram-positive organisms and containing DNA coding for vancomycin resistance have been identified in strains of *E. faecium* and *E. faecalis* that are highly resistant to vancomycin and teicoplanin.

At least three gene complexes and three types of resistance (Van A, Van B, and Van C) of enterococci to vancomycin have been identified. Van A is the most common type; Van A resistance is induced by either vancomycin or teicoplanin and may be plasmid encoded.[22, 23] Van A strains are resistant to both vancomycin and teicoplanin. The genes for Van A resistance have been cloned and have been found to be part of a cluster of at least seven genes responsible for synthesis of peptidoglycan cell wall precursors containing a pentapeptide ending with D-alanine-D-lactate instead of the usual D-alanyl-D-alanine terminus. Reduced affinity of glycopeptides for this depsipeptide confers resistance to the antibiotic.[24] Vancomycin resistance genes can also be encoded on a transposon.[25] Van B strains demonstrate inducible synthesis of a 39.5-kD cytoplasmic membrane protein termed Van B. This protein is inducible by vancomycin[26] but not by teicoplanin.[27] Van B strains are vancomycin resistant and teicoplanin susceptible. Van C strains demonstrate low-level vancomycin resistance but are susceptible to teicoplanin. Van C is constitutive and chromosomally encoded.[28–30]

Genes encoding vancomycin resistance have been conjugatively transferred from enterococci to *S. aureus* in the laboratory,[31] and there is concern, largely because of widespread indiscriminate use of vancomycin, that this will soon occur in nature, although so far this fear has not been confirmed. Prolonged or indiscriminate nosocomial use of vancomycin and teicoplanin, when given by either the oral or the intravenous route, seems to have been important in encouraging the emergence of glycopeptide-resistant enterococci in the United States, and in Europe avoparcin, a glycopeptide-like substance used as an animal feed supplement, has played a similar role. The clinical, epidemiologic, and microbiologic aspects of the complex and increasingly important area of vancomycin resistance have been reviewed by Murray.[32]

There is no cross-resistance between vancomycin and unrelated antibiotics, and significant resistance to vancomycin rarely if ever develops during therapy. Cross-resistance with teicoplanin occurs but is variable. Antibacterial activity of vancomycin varies little between pH 6.5 and pH 8. Some *N. gonorrhoeae* isolates are susceptible and may be missed on culture when vancomycin-containing selective media such as Thayer-Martin are used. *Flavobacterium meningosepticum* (gram-negative) and some *N. meningitidis* isolates are also susceptible at attainable concentrations (between 16 and 25 mg/liter), but other gram-negative bacilli, mycobacteria, fungi, and *Bacteroides* spp. are not susceptible. One report indicated that *Borrelia burgdorferi* isolates are inhibited at low concentrations of vancomycin (0.5 to 2 mg/liter) and killed at only slightly higher concentrations and that vancomycin is synergistic with penicillin G at low concentrations against this organism.[33]

Pharmacology

Administration. After being dissolved in sterile water, vancomycin should be given intravenously in 100 to 250 ml of 5% dextrose or 0.9% saline solution over at least 60 minutes.[1] It can also be given by continuous intravenous drip, but intermittent infusion is preferred. Rapid or bolus administration is dangerous, especially if 1-g doses are used, probably because it causes histamine release by basophils and mast cells,[34] resulting in flushing (the "red-man" or "red-neck" syndrome), anaphylactoid reactions, hypotension, and even cardiac arrest; this is rarely seen except shortly after the rapid administration of vancomycin.[12, 34] Antihistamines may help to prevent this. Hydrocortisone (20 mg) can be added to infusions to reduce side effects, but the mixture may precipitate at high concentrations. Heparin and vancomycin also can precipitate at high concentrations, and they should not be infused simultaneously through the same intravenous line.[35] Because of pain on injection, no satisfactory intramuscular preparation of vancomycin is available. Vancomycin is absorbed poorly from the gastrointestinal tract, even when the colon is inflamed, and it is nontoxic when used orally for treatment of severe clostridial enterocolitis[1, 34–38] or for prevention of infection in leukopenic cancer patients.[39]

Distribution, Excretion, and Protein Binding. Vancomycin is eliminated from the body almost exclusively by glomerular filtration, although a small amount may be metabolized by the liver and appear in active form in the bile. From 80 to 90% of an administered dose appears in the urine within 24 hours. The half-life of vancomycin in serum is 6 to 8 hours in persons with normal renal function. In anuric patients, it may be prolonged to about 9 days, and the drug may be detected in serum for as long as 21 days after a single 1-g dose.[40, 41] From 10 to 55% is protein bound in serum; this is believed to have a negligible effect on clinical results.

Concentrations in Body Fluids and Tissues. Trough serum levels after intravenous administration of 500 mg of vancomycin to adults range from 6 to 10 mg/liter, with an average of 8 mg/liter after repeated dosing. Peak levels of up to 50 mg/liter may be seen, depending on how soon the blood is drawn after the infusion. When 1 g is given slowly intravenously, peak (1 hour after infusion) and trough levels of 20 to 50 mg/liter and 5 to 12 mg/liter, respectively, are achieved; these are considered desirable and appropriate concentrations. Some clinicians monitor only trough concentrations and attempt to keep these in the range of about 10 to 12 mg/liter,[42] but some patients with severe obesity, infections necessitating a bactericidal effect, or less susceptible organisms may not achieve adequate peak levels (25 to 35 mg/liter or more) when dosing is based only on trough levels. Urinary concentrations usually range from 100 to 300 mg/liter. When vancomycin is given orally in a dose of 500 mg four times daily, concentrations of 1000 to 9000 mg/liter may be found in stools, but only trace amounts are ordinarily found in serum.[12, 13, 37] Concentrations as high as therapeutic ones have occasionally been found in the serum of anuric patients given the drug orally for treatment of colitis.[43] When 125 mg is given orally, stool concentrations range from 100 to 800 mg/liter. When vancomycin is given intravenously, concentrations of up to 100 mg/liter may be found in stools of some patients, but the drug is undetectable in stools of most patients[13]; for this reason, the intravenous route alone is not recommended for treatment of colitis.

Vancomycin is not found in cerebrospinal fluid (CSF) of persons without meningitis, but bactericidal levels (from less than 1 to 7 mg/liter) have been found in the CSF of most (but not all) patients with meningitis. Small supplemental amounts (3 to 5 mg) may be given intrathecally for the treatment of meningitis, particularly if there is no response after 48 hours of intravenous therapy.[44] A larger intrathecal dose may be needed for less susceptible organisms, such as flavobacteria. Vancomycin is irritating when injected into serous or synovial cavities, and peritonitis has been reported after direct instillation.[45] Adequate concentrations are reached in pleural, pericardial, synovial, ascitic, and abscess fluids after intravenous administration, but only low levels are found in bile.[12]

An intravenous loading dose of 1.0 g (15 mg/kg) vancomycin in 100 to 250 ml of normal saline or dextrose solution may be given to adults over a 1-hour period, regardless of renal function. If renal function is normal, this dose can be repeated every 12 hours (the mean elimination half-life of vancomycin from plasma is 4 to 6 hours). Alternatively, 7.5 mg/kg can be infused every 6 hours. Dosing is based on actual body weight, and many morbidly obese patients with serious infections may not respond until their dose is adjusted upward so as to obtain conventional peak therapeutic levels (25 to 35 mg/liter).

The mean elimination half-life of vancomycin in anephric patients is 7.5 days. Because the kidney is the only significant organ of elimination of vancomycin, high and potentially toxic serum levels can be attained in patients with renal insufficiency unless subsequent dosage is reduced appropriately.[39, 41–46] To achieve a mean therapeutic concentration of 20 mg/liter in serum of adults with renal impairment, an easily remembered formula can be used to estimate maintenance dosage: the daily parenteral dose of vancomycin in milligrams should be approximately 150 plus 15 times the creatinine clearance in milliliters per minute.[41, 42] Another strategy is to give 1 g every 36 hours when the serum creatinine concentration is 1.5 to 5 mg/100 ml and 1 g every 10 to 14 days when it is greater than 5 mg/100 ml. As little as 1 g may yield effective serum concentrations for 7 to 14 days in anuric patients.[41] There are nomograms that may be more accurate and effective than these simple rules for dosing patients with renal failure.[45–48] Most nomograms (such as the one shown in Fig. 28–1) are designed to provide steady-state trough concentrations of 8 to 12 mg/liter[47] and are probably the most accurate dosing methods.[49] In difficult situations, serum concentrations should be monitored, although the data supporting this practice are meager.[39, 41, 45, 50]

Because hemodialysis does not remove significant amounts of vancomycin (although peritoneal dialysis can),[32, 34, 38] it is a common practice to dose patients with renal failure with 1 g vancomycin weekly, since about 150 mg is removed each day in the average adult by nonrenal mechanisms. Use of newer, more permeable (high-flux) hemodialysis membranes can result in a significant but transient decrease in serum concentrations because of binding to the polyacronitrile membrane,[51] but transfer of the drug from tissues back to blood with a rebound in vancomycin levels occurs, and therapeutic concentrations may still be present for 1 week.[52] Hemofiltration is also efficient at removing vancomycin and is useful in managing overdosage in patients with renal failure.[53] Serum levels should be monitored at frequent, regular intervals in dialyzed, uremic, or seriously ill patients to ascertain that safe yet adequate concentrations are present. Cardiopulmonary bypass is associated with a fall in serum concentrations because of dilution.[54] When it is used prophylactically, a preoperative vancomycin dose of 15 mg/kg is needed before bypass surgery, and 10 mg/kg should be given after bypass surgery if renal function is normal. Pediatric dosing is discussed later.

Toxicity and Adverse Reactions

With the purified preparations now available, adverse reactions seem to be much less frequent than when vancomycin was first introduced.

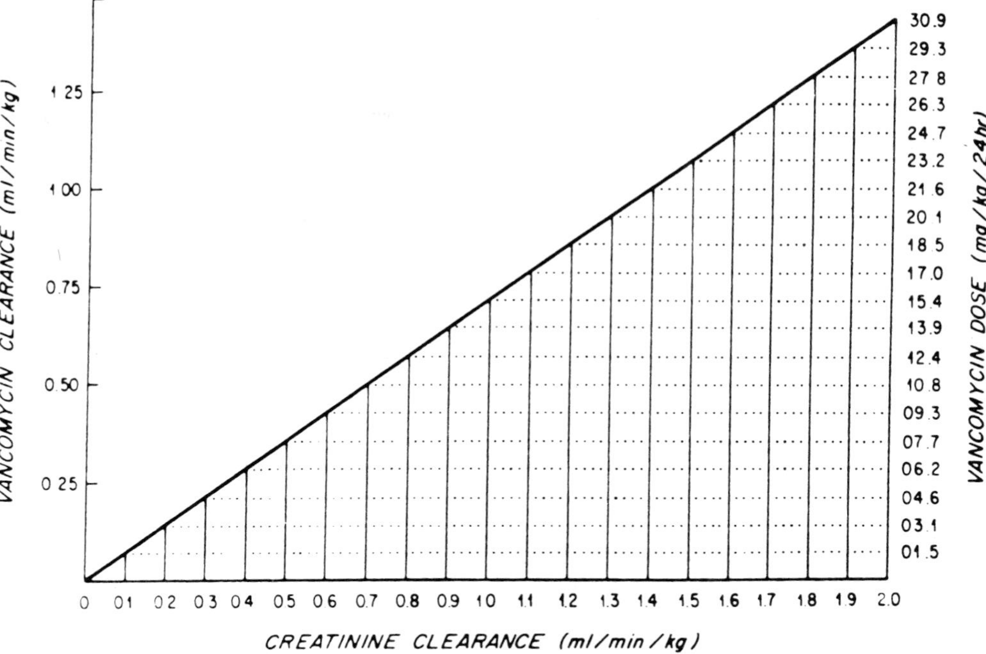

FIGURE 28–1. Dosage nomogram for vancomycin in patients with impaired renal function. The nomogram is not valid for functionally anephric patients receiving dialysis. For such patients, the dose is 1.9 mg/kg per day. (From Moellering RC, Krogstad DJ, Greenblatt DJ. Vancomycin therapy in patients with impaired renal function: A nomogram for dosage. Ann Intern Med. 1981;94:343–346.)

The most common side effects are fever, chills, and phlebitis at the site of the infusion. These occur less often if the drug is infused slowly in a large volume of fluid. Tingling and flushing of the face, neck, and thorax are often experienced (i.e., the red-neck or red-man syndrome), especially if 1-g doses are given[34, 55] and the drug is infused very rapidly[56]; this is thought to be related to histamine release secondary to local hyperosmolarity and not to allergic hypersensitivity. Maculopapular or diffuse erythematous rashes, presumably caused by hypersensitivity, occur in 4 to 5% of patients, and although they may persist for weeks despite discontinuation of vancomycin in patients with marked renal failure, they may respond to steroid or antihistamine therapy. Shock has occurred after rapid intravenous infusion of the drug, especially during surgery. Reversible leukopenia, thrombocytopenia, or eosinophilia sometimes develops,[57] and lacrimation has also been reported.[34] One case of antibiotic-induced *C. difficile* colitis has been reported after intravenous use of vancomycin,[58] and there are other cases that have not been reported.

An important adverse reaction to vancomycin is neurotoxicity, which is manifested primarily by auditory nerve damage and hearing loss. Tinnitus and high-tone hearing loss are often an antecedent to deafness, which is infrequent when serum concentrations are maintained below 30 mg/liter and more common when they are in the range of 80 mg/liter or higher. Hearing occasionally improves after the drug is discontinued, but it usually continues to deteriorate and the loss becomes permanent.[59, 60] Nephrotoxicity was relatively common with early, impure preparations of vancomycin, especially when they were given in high doses; it was usually transient or reversible. With appropriate doses selected through monitoring of renal function and serum concentrations, nephrotoxicity is now uncommon,[60–62] and it is usually transient or reversible unless multiple courses are given, high and toxic levels are achieved, or aminoglycosides are also given. Although the preparations of vancomycin now available are purified and are no longer appreciably nephrotoxic, high doses given by the parenteral route should be avoided, and serum levels should be carefully monitored when other nephrotoxic drugs are being given. The risk of nephrotoxicity appears to be enhanced even with normally safe levels when drugs such as aminoglycosides or ethacrynic acid are given concomitantly.

Drug Interactions

Vancomycin is incompatible with many other drugs in intravenous solutions, especially chloramphenicol, adrenal corticosteroids, and methicillin. Heparin (at very high concentrations) may inactivate vancomycin in intravenous solutions and can be responsible for persistence of bacteremia.[35] Vancomycin is not stable enough for use with Infusaid and certain other implantable pumps.[63]

Major Uses and Doses

The usual intravenous dose of vancomycin for adults with normal renal function is 1 g (15 mg/kg) every 12 hours or 500 mg (6.5 to 8 mg/kg) every 6 hours. In severely ill patients with normal renal function, especially patients with obesity or meningitis, 1 g may be given every 8 hours for 2 to 3 days until the infection is under control. Dosing should be based on actual body weight. Morbidly obese patients with severe infections may require high doses, based on total body weight, creatinine clearance, and the monitoring of serum levels.[64] Various dosage regimens have been proposed for pediatric use. For newborn infants, 15 mg/kg may be given slowly every 12 hours intravenously during the first week of life or every 8 hours in those 8 to 30 days of age; 10 mg/kg every 6 hours is recommended for older infants and children and 15 mg/kg every 6 hours for infants and children with staphylococcal central nervous system infections. Monitoring of serum levels is desirable, especially in preterm infants.[65] A continuous intravenous drip may be used.[66, 67]

Oral doses of 125 to 500 mg four times per day have been used for treatment of adults with *C. difficile* colitis (but without ileus), with equivalent results.[68] For infants and children with *C. difficile* colitis, an oral dose of 500 mg/1.73 m^2 every 6 hours has been recommended.[69] Oral therapy is much more reliable than intravenous therapy for treatment of *C. difficile* colitis. Serum concentrations of vancomycin are usually negligible after oral administration, even when the colon is inflamed.

The intravenous dosage must be reduced in the presence of renal impairment and may be monitored to achieve peak serum concentrations no higher than 30 to 40 mg/liter and troughs ranging from 5 to 10 mg/liter.[50] If a continuous infusion is used, a steady-state concentration of 15 mg/liter seems desirable.[44, 45, 58, 70] Evidence indicates that impaired liver function may also delay elimination of vancomycin and require dosage modification.[71]

Vancomycin for parenteral use should be reserved primarily for serious MRSA infections. Intravenous vancomycin is the therapy of choice for serious staphylococcal infections in patients with methicillin-oxacillin-nafcillin-cephalosporin–resistant organisms and patients who cannot be given these primary drugs.[12, 61, 72–76] It has also become the most reliable and popular therapy for serious intravenous catheter or device-related coagulase-negative staphylococcal infections.[77]

All strains of coagulase-positive MRSA have been susceptible to low concentrations of vancomycin, but clinical responses in MRSA endocarditis may be slow and may require 1 week or longer. Rare isolates show clinically significant tolerance (MBC >16 times MIC) to its bactericidal action.[8, 72, 75, 78] When treatment of serious MRSA infections with vancomycin alone has failed, addition of gentamicin, rifampin, or both may be successful. Rifampin appears especially attractive because it penetrates into leukocytes, serous cavities, and other closed spaces; gentamicin may be synergistic with vancomycin. Because antagonism occurs occasionally with some of these combinations of antimicrobials,[72] they should not be used routinely, and some experts believe that serum bacteriostatic and bactericidal levels should be monitored as a guide to therapy when they are used. When vancomycin is used to treat adults in conjunction with an aminoglycoside, some experts believe the dosage of vancomycin should rarely exceed 0.5 g every 8 hours.[61] Methicillin-resistant *S. epidermidis* endocarditis involving a prosthetic valve is best treated with the usual doses of vancomycin for at least 4 weeks in combination with rifampin, plus an aminoglycoside (the latter for the first 2 weeks),[76] assuming the isolate is susceptible to them. This regimen is also useful for managing other serious staphylococcal infections involving a foreign body that cannot be removed and for treatment of diphtheroid endocarditis.

Survival rates of 60 to 75% have been achieved with vancomycin in patients with staphylococcal endocarditis or bacteremia.[1, 12] Survival in patients aged 70 years or older is about 50%. The usual duration of therapy is 4 to 6 weeks. Success rates of 75% or greater have been reported with vancomycin in patients with pneumonia, parotitis, or meningitis. Although vancomycin penetrates into the central nervous system in most ill patients in amounts adequate to treat meningitis and shunt infections, this is not always the case,[44] and removal of foreign bodies or supplemental intraventricular or intrathecal instillation of vancomycin may be required in patients with a poor response.[78–80] CSF concentrations need not be greater than about 25 mg/liter, so intrathecal doses of 5 to 20 mg every 24 hours are usually adequate. Penicillin-resistant *S. pneumoniae* isolates are usually susceptible to the inhibitory effects of vancomycin, although the concentrations needed for a bactericidal effect may be fourfold to eightfold higher than inhibitory ones and they may not be achievable in the CSF or ventricles of the brain. Penetration into the spinal fluid may be further impaired if adrenal corticosteroids are used and when inflammation subsides. About 40% of adults treated with vancomycin for pneumococcal meningitis were reported to experience therapeutic failure,[81] but they did respond to therapy with cefotaxime or ceftriaxone. Vancomycin should probably be reserved in meningitis for patients with allergies to other drugs or with organisms resistant to them.

Vancomycin is the treatment of choice for patients with *E. faecalis* endocarditis who are allergic to penicillin. In this setting it should be given along with an aminoglycoside, because vancomycin is rarely bactericidal by itself against these organisms.[15, 16, 82, 83] Bactericidal synergism between gentamicin and vancomycin was uniformly demonstrated until recently with most susceptible enterococci,[17, 84] so gentamicin is preferable to streptomycin, which is not synergistic with as many as 40% of these organisms; conversely, streptomycin is only occasionally more active than gentamicin. Laboratory studies of synergism with the patient's organism or by Schlichter's tests of the bactericidal activity of the patient's serum may be helpful in determining the best treatment regimen. A vancomycin dose of 0.5 g every 8 hours intravenously plus either streptomycin, 0.5 g every 12 hours intramuscularly, or gentamicin, 60 to 80 mg (1 mg/kg) every 8 hours intravenously, for 4 to 6 weeks is recommended for adults with normal renal function. More vigorous or prolonged therapy may be needed for complicated cases, such as when a prosthetic valve is infected. Such patients should be monitored closely for signs of ototoxicity or nephrotoxicity, and drug dosages should be carefully adjusted for patients with renal failure. Viridans streptococcal or *S. bovis* endocarditis may be treated with vancomycin alone if the MBC for the isolate is no more than 10 mg/liter; otherwise vancomycin should be combined with streptomycin, gentamicin, or another aminoglycoside.[12, 61] Again, monitoring of serum bactericidal activity may be helpful when bactericidal sensitivity tests in combination are not available.

Other serious infections with resistant organisms that have been responsive to vancomycin include *Corynebacterium* endocarditis in patients with prosthetic valves and *F. meningosepticum* meningitis.[12, 44, 79] Vancomycin has been considered the drug of choice for treatment of acute staphylococcal pseudomembranous enterocolitis, which is now an uncommon disease. In two series of cases, 67 of 72 patients were cured of the disease (93%).[36, 85] Vancomycin was usually given orally, 500 mg diluted in water every 6 hours for adults.

Orally administered vancomycin is considered the drug of choice by most investigators for treating seriously ill patients with antibiotic-associated *C. difficile* (pseudomembranous) colitis, although metronidazole is less expensive and is usually effective in mild or moderately ill patients.[86] In addition, metronidazole may be less likely than vancomycin to promote the spread of VRE, VIRSA, and other resistant organisms. *C. difficile* is occasionally resistant to metronidazole, but it is always susceptible to vancomycin. Treatment failures are very rare with vancomycin unless treatment is delayed.[36, 43, 86, 87] Vancomycin dosages of either 125 or 500 mg four times daily have been effective, and the lower and less expensive dose seemed to be as good as the larger one[68] in most patients. Vancomycin is also highly effective in treating relapses of colitis caused by *C. difficile*,[79] but neither it nor metronidazole reliably kills the spores of the organism and eradicates the *C. difficile* carrier state.[88]

Vancomycin is best given orally for treatment of colitis, because it is needed to inhibit toxin production within the lumen of the bowel and not for inhibition of the organism in tissues.[79] Intravenous vancomycin by itself is not reliable for treatment of colitis, because adequate concentrations are seldom achieved within the lumen of the colon when it is given by the intravenous route. In patients with ileus, vancomycin should be given orally or by nasogastric tube in doses of 500 mg every 6 hours, or by a catheter inserted via a colonoscope to the proximal cecum.[89, 90] A solution containing 200 to 500 mg vancomycin per liter can be used in the latter situation. Vancomycin (in full parenteral doses) plus metronidazole may also be given intravenously in this difficult situation. Even though little vancomycin will be absorbed from the intestinal tract,[89] serum levels should be monitored to prevent toxicity when it is administered by both routes. For patients with ileus, the drug has also been given by enema, via an ileostomy or colostomy, by a long intestinal tube inserted nasogastrically and passed to the distal ileum or cecum, or via a catheter inserted per rectum with a colonoscope to the proximal cecum. Many patients with severe ileus or toxic megacolon ultimately require an emergency colectomy.

Staphylococcal peritonitis occurring during peritoneal dialysis can be treated with intravenous vancomycin alone. One gram given intravenously yields peritoneal fluid concentrations greater than 5 mg/liter for 1 week or longer in this setting.[45, 56] Others have noted that peritoneal dialysis removes vancomycin from the blood and have recommended instilling vancomycin into the peritoneal cavity to a concentration of 25 mg/liter in addition to parenteral vancomycin to ensure good levels in peritoneal fluid.[91] In fact, it may be possible to treat staphylococcal peritonitis in patients undergoing chronic peritoneal dialysis solely by the intraperitoneal administration of vancomycin at a concentration of 50 mg/liter in the dialysate.[91, 92] However, vancomycin given intraperitoneally may be irritating,[93] and organisms protected by a biofilm on the catheter may be clinically tolerant to the bactericidal effect of vancomycin and therefore responsible for relapse.[9] The addition of rifampin to vancomycin for treatment of refractory staphylococcal peritonitis in chronic dialysis may be synergistic and curative.[94]

According to an American Heart Association's Advisory Committee,[95, 96] vancomycin is useful for the prevention of bacterial endocarditis in patients who are allergic to penicillin and undergoing dental or respiratory tract procedures. The mechanism of prevention is thought to be either the bactericidal action of vancomycin or its ability to interfere with the adherence of the organism to the endocardium. One gram may be given slowly intravenously within 60 minutes before the start of the procedure; no repeat dose is necessary. For genitourinary or gastrointestinal surgery or instrumentation (after which enterococcal endocarditis may develop), vancomycin can be given for prophylaxis in a similar manner, along with gentamicin, 1.5 mg/kg; these doses may be repeated once 8 to 12 hours later.[95] Vancomycin can be used prophylactically for insertion of prosthetic valves, with an initial intravenous dose of 15 mg/ml given over 1 hour just before surgery, followed by 10 mg/kg immediately after bypass surgery (if renal function is normal),[54] along with 1.7 mg/kg gentamicin before surgery and 8 hours later. The efficacy of this regimen has not been proved, but it is designed to prevent *S. aureus*, *S. epidermidis*, and enterococcal and coliform infections of the prosthesis or sternum. Vancomycin is often included in empirical therapy for febrile neutropenic patients, but unless there is good evidence to suggest the presence of a staphylococcal infection, its use probably should not be routine[97] but should be reserved instead for documented infections.

Vancomycin has been used in prophylactic oral nonabsorbable antibiotic regimens designed to prevent endogenous infections in patients with cancer or leukemia.[39] Such patients also seem to experience a lower rate of *C. difficile* colitis complicating their chemotherapy. Otherwise, these regimens are probably of no value unless protective environments and leukocyte transfusions are available and used, and they may encourage the development of resistance.

Vancomycin has been used prophylactically in patients receiving chronic dialysis to prevent staphylococcal infections, but this has resulted in the emergence of vancomycin-resistant enterococci and serious enterococcal infections.[20]

There has been a marked resurgence in the use of vancomycin in the last two decades. Many new indications for its use have been established, and much new information has been accumulated. However, because of the emergence of resistance, there is little reason for optimism, and vancomycin must be used more judiciously than ever before. Excellent, detailed reviews of vancomycin and its use have been published.[61, 98]

TEICOPLANIN

Teicoplanin (formerly teichomycin A) is a glycopeptide antibiotic derived from the fermentation products of *Actinoplanes teichomyceticus*.[99] Although widely used in Europe for treatment of gram-positive infections, teicoplanin is still investigational in the United States. Teicoplanin is a complex of six analogues having the same linear heptapeptide base, an aglycone containing aromatic amino acids, D-mannose, and *N*-acetyl-D-glycosamine as sugars; it has a molecular weight ranging from 1562 to 1891 Da.

Teicoplanin is chemically similar to vancomycin, but it has important differences that are responsible for the unique physical and chemical properties of the complex.[100] It has greater lipophilicity than vancomycin, which results in rapid and excellent tissue and intracellular phagocyte penetration. Other characteristics are a long elimination half-life, slow release from tissues, and water solubility at physiologic pH. It has few if any inactive metabolites.[101]

Mechanism of Action and Pharmacokinetics

Teicoplanin has an antibacterial spectrum and a mechanism of action similar to those of vancomycin. It is usually bactericidal (except for certain enterococci), although tolerance has been observed to its bactericidal action. Staphylococci and enterococci that are resistant to vancomycin are usually resistant to teicoplanin. The development of resistance during treatment has not been reported. Teicoplanin impairs cell wall synthesis by inhibiting polymerization of peptidoglycan in a way similar to that of vancomycin, but at different sites from those inhibited by β-lactams.[102–104] It does this by forming a complex with the terminal D-alanyl-D-alanine precursor, which fits into a "pocket" in the teicoplanin molecule. It has an elimination half-life of 40 to 70 hours after intravenous administration, a disappearance curve that fits both a two- and a three-compartment model, and a volume of distribution of 0.5 to 0.8 liter/kg.[105, 106] In contrast to the low degree of protein binding of vancomycin, that of teicoplanin is as high as 90%,[104] which may account for its slow renal clearance.

Because of its long half-life, it can be given intramuscularly or intravenously once per day.[107] Provided in 200-mg vials, it has usually been given in a daily intravenous dose of 2 to 3 mg/kg after a loading dose of 6 mg/kg (400 mg).[108] Higher doses may be needed and can be given with better results but with greater toxicity.[101] When single intravenous injections of 3 or 6 mg/kg were given rapidly (over 5 minutes) to healthy volunteers, peak plasma concentrations of 53 and 112 mg/liter were observed, and concentrations of 2.1 and 4.2 μg/ml were observed at 24 hours. Similar concentrations were seen after intramuscular dosing with 3 mg/kg. With these doses, serum levels greater than the MIC_{90} for susceptible organisms were sustained for at least 24 hours after a single injection. When 3 mg/kg was given to volunteers at a constant rate over 30 minutes, peak concentrations were about 22 mg/liter. After six intramuscular doses of 200 mg (3 mg/kg) over a 5-day period, absorption was still rapid and the peak level was 2.8 mg/liter at 1 hour, 5.8 mg/liter at 2 hours, and 7.1 mg/liter at 4 hours. After the last injection, mean peak levels of 12.1 mg/liter were reached. Trough levels at 24 hours on days 2 through 6 were approximately 5.4 to 7.3 mg/liter,[106] and the calculated elimination half-life was about 99 hours. Urinary concentrations ranged from 16 to 156 mg/liter from days 1 through 7. About 80% of the drug was eliminated in urine.[107] Teicoplanin administered orally was not significantly absorbed from the intestinal tracts of rats, dogs, or human volunteers. In humans, 40% of the administered dose was present in feces in a microbiologically active form.[102]

In patients with renal impairment, serum concentrations are related to creatinine clearance, which can be used for adjusting the dosage.[108, 109] Teicoplanin is exchanged bidirectionally across the peritoneum, but it is not removed by hemodialysis.[108, 109] In one study, only 2.7% of a parenterally administered dose was found in feces over the next 8 days.[107] Although the evidence suggests that teicoplanin penetrates tissues well, the penetration of teicoplanin into bone, peritoneal fluid, and CSF needs more study. Teicoplanin is well tolerated by children. A dose of 10 mg/kg per day has been recommended for children and 6 mg/kg per day for neonates.[110]

Antibacterial Activity

Teicoplanin has excellent bactericidal activity against gram-positive organisms, including *S. pneumoniae*, *S. pyogenes*, and many other streptococci, *E. faecalis*, *S. aureus* (both penicillinase-producing and methicillin-resistant organisms), *S. epidermidis*, *Clostridium* species, *C. jeikeium*, *Propionibacterium acnes*, and *L. monocytogenes*.[111–113] Inhibitory concentrations range from 0.025 to 3.1 mg/liter. Some strains of *S. epidermidis* and *S. haemolyticus* are relatively resistant to teicoplanin but susceptible to vancomycin.[113, 114] Against many susceptible organisms, teicoplanin is two to four times more active than vancomycin. Teicoplanin is the more active antimicrobial against *E. faecalis*, but, like vancomycin, it is rarely bactericidal for this species. Teicoplanin cross-resistance occurs in isolates of *E. faecalis* and *E. faecium* with Van A resistance and can arise rapidly in patients infected with Van B–resistant *E. faecalis* who are treated with vancomycin. Teicoplanin resistance is not inducible by teicoplanin exposure of Van B–resistant isolates. Teicoplanin is more active than vancomycin against *C. difficile*, but it is even more highly bound by cholestyramine.[115] It is not active against gram-negative organisms, including *Neisseria*, *Mycobacterium* spp., and fungi. Teicoplanin does not give rise to stably resistant mutants in vitro, and it shows no cross-resistance with nonglycopeptide antibiotics, except for aminoglycosides. Like vancomycin, teicoplanin can be synergistic with rifampin or aminoglycosides against staphylococci, enterococci, other streptococci, or *Listeria*.[104, 116–119]

Toxicity

Teicoplanin has been well tolerated when given to humans either intramuscularly or intravenously. Unlike vancomycin, it produces only mild pain at the site of injection. After slow intravenous infusion, it has not caused thrombophlebitis[120] or adverse effects on platelet function or coagulation.[121] Studies with 100 human volunteers showed no untoward effects at doses of up to 7.5 mg/kg. When given by rapid intravenous infusion to 310 hospitalized patients with infections, significant adverse effects were uncommon (2%), and no patient developed flushing or the red-man or red-neck syndrome,[115] although the latter has been seen. However, ototoxicity has been reported.[122–124]

Clinical Uses

Teicoplanin is potentially an effective alternate to vancomycin, with the advantage of less frequent dosing (once per day) and, because of its greater potency and therapeutic ratio, less nephrotoxicity and ototoxicity. It may be useful for patients who have had neutropenic or allergic reactions to vancomycin.[11] Possible uses for teicoplanin include the treatment of serious gram-positive infections, including endocarditis caused by MRSA, pneumonia, septicemia, soft tissue infections, urinary tract infections, and osteomyelitis.[125–127] It was more effective than vancomycin in a rabbit model of MRSA endocarditis.[128] Clinical cures were seen in 96% of 88 patients treated with 200 to 400 mg teicoplanin once daily for coagulase-negative staphylococcal infections and in 79 to 91% of 1781 patients with various other gram-positive infections.[129, 130] These included MRSA infections, pneumonia, endocarditis,[125] septicemia, and joint infections. Some of these patients developed ototoxicity or nephrotoxicity, but many of them had also received an aminoglycoside.[123, 124]

Given once daily (400 mg) for treatment of mild MRSA infections, teicoplanin was comparable to vancomycin in efficacy. When serious MRSA infections were treated with teicoplanin, 200 to 800 mg/day, in some cases supplemented with another antibiotic, the cure rate was 75%. When patients with deep-seated staphylococcal infections were treated with maintenance doses of 200 mg/day, only 44% were cured.[131] Treatment failure was related to the presence of foreign bodies and poor tissue concentrations. The high degree of protein binding of teicoplanin may have been an important factor in these low-dose treatment failures. Doses of 400 mg/day or more are probably needed for successful treatment of severe infections. In combination with an aminoglycoside, teicoplanin could be a suitable alternative to ampicillin, penicillin G, or vancomycin for treatment of serious or refractory enterococcal infections.[132] It could be useful for prophylaxis of endocarditis in penicillin-allergic patients or when vancomycin or other antibiotics are not tolerated.[125] However, when used once daily for prophylaxis in cardiac surgery, teicoplanin was associated with a higher than expected number of sternal wound and urinary tract infections.[133] Other potential indications include shunt infections and treatment of gram-positive peritonitis in patients undergoing chronic dialysis.[134, 135] Finally, oral administration of teicoplanin may be an alternative for treatment of *C. difficile* colitis or necrotizing staphylococcal enterocolitis. Twenty-two patients with *C. difficile*–associated diarrhea or colitis were treated via the oral route with teicoplanin (400 to 600 mg/day for 10 days). All patients treated with teicoplanin remained asymptomatic after discontinuation of treatment, but 3 of 23 evaluable patients given vancomycin developed recurrences.[136]

Its potential for safe and effective once-daily dosing by either the intramuscular or the intravenous route will make teicoplanin a useful addition to the antibiotic armamentarium if further clinical studies substantiate its safety and efficacy. Preliminary data suggest caution in its use alone at doses of 400 mg/day or less in patients with endocarditis or other serious deep-seated staphylococcal infections. A review of 200 publications indicated that teicoplanin needs to be given in significantly larger doses (10 to 12 mg/kg) than initially thought necessary to maximize clinical efficacy and that its lower incidence of side effects at these dosages, compared with vancomycin, is clinically negligible.[137]

QUINUPRISTIN AND DALFOPRISTIN: SYNERGISTIC DERIVATIVES OF THE STREPTOGRAMIN PRISTINAMYCIN

Structure, Derivation, and Nomenclature

Quinupristin and dalfopristin are derived from the streptogramins pristinamycin IA and IIB; they are macrolactones that belong to the antibiotic family of macrolides-lincosamides-streptogramins. Like other natural streptogramins, pristinamycins are highly water insoluble and can be administered only orally. Pristinamycin has been marketed outside of the United States for 25 years, primarily for the oral treatment of staphylococcal infections including MRSA, enterococcal infections, and other gram-positive coccal infections. Its in vitro activity includes almost all aerobic and anaerobic gram-positive cocci, including many of those that are resistant to macrolides, β-lactams, and glycopeptides. It does not exhibit cross-resistance with other anti-infective agents. Pristinamycin is relatively nontoxic, and no serious adverse drug reactions to it have been reported.

The quinupristin and dalfopristin components of natural pristinamycin were isolated, and methanesulfonate derivatives were made that have the antibacterial activity of pristinamycin and are water soluble and injectable. Quinupristin is derived from pristinamycin IA and is a peptide macrolactone classed as a streptogramin A; dalfopristin is derived from pristinamycin IIB and is a polyunsaturated macrolactone streptogramin B. Each derivative by itself exerts limited antibacterial activity, but together they have markedly increased activity as a result of synergy. They are present in a fixed 30:70 ratio in a preparation known as quinupristin-dalfopristin (formerly RP 59500), which is named Synercid. Like their natural counterparts, they are synergistic and together have in vitro activity equivalent to that of pristinamycin.[138]

Quinupristin-dalfopristin has been investigated in clinical trials primarily to determine its efficacy and safety in the treatment of adults with vancomycin- and teicoplanin-resistant *E. faecium* and other gram-positive coccal infections, including complicated skin and skin structure infections, septicemia, and hospital-acquired pneumonia. It is available for parenteral use only.

Mechanism of Action

Quinupristin and dalfopristin inhibit bacterial protein synthesis by irreversibly binding to different sites on the 50S bacterial ribosomal subunit to form a stable quinupristin-ribosome-dalfopristin tertiary complex. Quinupristin inhibits peptide chain elongation, whereas dalfopristin directly interferes with peptidyl transferase.[138, 139]

Resistance to streptogramins can occur by at least three mechanisms.[136] The most important one is a plasmid-mediated target modification that confers resistance to macrolides, lincosamides, and quinupristin by methylation of their common binding site; this does not affect susceptibility to dalfopristin. Infrequently, resistance is mediated by drug-modifying enzymes or efflux. It is also possible that when resistance to only one of the components of quinupristin-dalfopristin occurs, the organism may continue to be inhibited but not killed. Rare forms of macrolide-lincosamide-streptogramin B resistance can affect the activity of quinupristin-dalfopristin, but at present these strains are uncommon.[140–142] During clinical trials of treatment of vancomycin-resistant *E. faecium*, resistance has developed in vitro and in three patients; resistance also occurred during treatment of a patient with *S. aureus* bacteremia.[138, 140]

Antimicrobial Activity In Vitro. Quinupristin-dalfopristin is often bactericidal as well as bacteriostatic, and it has demonstrated synergistic activity with other antimicrobials against a wide variety of gram-positive bacteria.[138, 140–150] An MIC of 2 mg/liter or less usually indicates susceptibility. Both vancomycin-susceptible *E. faecium* (MIC_{90}, 4 mg/liter; range, 0.25 to 4 mg/liter) and Van A– and Van B–resistant *E. faecium* (MIC_{90}, 1 to 4 mg/liter; range, 0.06 to 32 mg/liter) are susceptible.[144–147] Quinupristin-dalfopristin is primarily bacteriostatic or only slowly bactericidal for *E. faecium*, an organism that is often resistant to those aminoglycosides that otherwise could produce bactericidal synergy with it.[144–150] The addition of 0.5 mg/liter of ciprofloxacin significantly reduced the modal MIC of quinupristin-dalfopristin for vancomycin-resistant *E. faecium* to 0.015 mg/liter in one study, but not in another.[144, 148]

Quinupristin-dalfopristin has only limited bacteriostatic activity against *E. faecalis* (MIC_{90}, 4 to 32 mg/liter) and poor bactericidal activity. Intrinsic resistance of *E. faecalis*, primarily to the dalfopristin component, appears to be responsible for the lower in vitro activity of quinupristin-dalfopristin toward it, compared with its efficacy against *E. faecium*.[138, 142, 147] *S. aureus* strains had an MIC_{90} of 1 to 2 mg/liter, including strains resistant to erythromycin and methicillin, and the majority of strains were killed at similar concentrations. MRSA strains are highly susceptible (MIC_{90}, 1 to 2 mg/liter), and bactericidal concentrations are only slightly higher.[148] Other susceptible organisms include coagulase-negative staphylococci (MIC_{90}, 2 mg/liter); *S. pneumoniae*, including penicillin-resistant strains (MIC_{90}, 2 mg/liter); viridans streptococci (MIC_{90}, 0.5 to 2.0 mg/liter depending on the species); and *S. pyogenes*.

Quinupristin-dalfopristin is also active in vitro against *Leukonostoc* spp., *Lactobacillus* spp., *Pediococcus*, *Bacteroides* spp., *Prevotella/Porphyromonas* spp., *L. monocytogenes* (MIC_{90}, 1.6 mg/liter), *C. jeikeium* (MIC_{90}, 0.2 mg/liter), and the respiratory pathogens *Legionella* spp., *Mycoplasma pneumoniae*, and *Moraxella (Branhamella) catarrhalis*. It also has some in vitro activity against *N. gonorrhoeae*, *N. meningitidis*, *Chlamydia trachomatis*, *Mycoplasma hominis*, and *Ureaplasma urealyticum*.[136, 151, 152] *Haemophilus influenzae* is only moderately susceptible (MIC_{90}, 4 to 8 mg/liter).[153]

Pharmacology

Administration. The usual recommended dose of quinupristin-dalfopristin for treatment of serious nosocomial infections is 7.5 mg/kg of actual body weight administered intravenously in a 5% glucose-dextrose solution over a period of 60 minutes every 8 to 12 hours for 7 to 10 days.[136, 154, 155] This has usually required a peripheral or, more often, a central venous catheter. There is a straight-line correlation between dose and mean area under the concentration-time curve.[154] Mean half-life ranged from 1.27 to 1.53 hours. The postantibiotic effect after 30 minutes of exposure to 5 mg/liter of quinupristin-dalfopristin was 5 to 7.5 hours for most staphylococci, 7.9 hours for *S. pneumoniae*, and longer than 18 hours for *S. pyogenes*.[136] Preliminary data indicate that doses of 4.5 to 6 mg/kg given every 12 hours are effective in the treatment of *S. pneumoniae* pneumonia and lower-limb erysipelas. Some patients with serious infections caused by resistant pathogens (VRE, MRSA) were treated for longer periods (mean, 18 ± 11 and 23.5 ± 14 days in two studies). No dose adjustment was needed in elderly patients, obese patients, patients with renal impairment, or patients undergoing peritoneal dialysis. Experience with a limited number of pediatric patients suggests no dosage adjustment is required for them.[155]

Distribution, Excretion, and Protein Binding. In rats and monkeys, quinupristin-dalfopristin undergoes rapid elimination from the blood and wide tissue distribution.[136, 153] It does not penetrate the central nervous system or cross the placenta to any significant degree. Both compounds are eliminated primarily in bile into feces; quinupristin-dalfopristin is rapidly converted in the liver to several active metabolites. Biliary excretion into feces is the primary route of elimination for both parent compounds and their metabolites. Urinary excretion accounts for approximately 15 to 19% of quinupristin-dalfopristin.[136] By ultracentrifugation, the serum binding of 32 mg/liter quinupristin-dalfopristin was 90%.[154] Quinupristin-dalfopristin is taken up by macrophages, where concentrations may be 30 to 50 times the extracellular concentration, and is active intracellularly.[152] After intravenous administration, both compounds are rapidly cleared from the blood of humans, with elimination half-lives of approximately 1 hour for quinupristin, and 0.75 hour for dalfopristin. The pharmacokinetic profile of quinupristin is dose independent, and so is that of dalfopristin when they are considered together.[154]

Concentrations in Body Fluids and Tissues. The mean peak blood concentration in 18 human volunteers at the end of a 1-hour infusion of quinupristin-dalfopristin at a dose of 5 mg/kg was 4 mg/liter dalfopristin and 1.0 mg/liter quinupristin; at a dose of 10 mg/kg it was 5.5 and 2.0 mg/liter, respectively, and at 15 mg/kg it was 7.5 and 3.5 mg/liter, respectively. There was a linear relation between dose and mean area under the serum concentration curve.[154]

Toxicity and Adverse Reactions

In clinical trials, the most common adverse event was inflammation, pain, and/or phlebitis at the injection site; nausea, vomiting, diarrhea, arthralgia, myalgia, muscle weakness, and rash have also been seen. Increases in serum creatinine, thrombocytopenia, and anemia occur but are less common in patients treated with quinupristin-dalfopristin than in those treated with comparable drugs; eosinophilia, increases in direct and conjugated bilirubin, and increases in γ-glutamyl transferase were more common with quinupristin-dalfopristin. In uncontrolled trials, increases in serum potassium and phosphorus and decreases in bicarbonate, chloride, and sodium occurred.[136]

Drug Interactions

One patient was reported whose cyclosporine blood concentration tripled (from 80 to 105 ng/ml to 261 to 291 ng/ml) 2 to 3 days after initiation of quinupristin-dalfopristin therapy. After discontinuation of quinupristin-dalfopristin, the cyclosporine concentrations decreased and its dosage was returned to the initial levels.[156] This experience suggests that cyclosporine concentrations should be monitored, and dosing adjustment is recommended when these medications are given at the same time.

Major Uses

Quinupristin-dalfopristin has been evaluated in five trials involving 2000 patients and also in compassionate or emergency use programs for patients for whom there was no alternative therapy. It has been used in this way primarily in adults with vancomycin- or teicoplanin-resistant *S. faecium* infections, complicated skin and skin structure infections, intra-abdominal infections, hospital-acquired pneumonia, urinary tract infections, bone and joint infections, endocarditis, catheter-related bacteremia, and bacteremia of unknown origin. Considering the fact that most patients treated with quinupristin-dalfopristin were critically ill and had serious infections, the antimicrobial was relatively well tolerated and the clinical results seemed good. Because of its unique spectrum of activity against multiple-drug–resistant gram-positive pathogens, including *S. aureus* and *E. faecium*, it is indicated primarily for treatment of serious, refractory infections caused by such pathogens.

Bryson and Spencer[141] found that 67% of 95 evaluable patients with vancomycin-resistant gram-positive infections or intolerance of vancomycin showed improvement with eradication of infection. Linden and colleagues[157] compared the clinical and bacteriologic responses of 20 patients with vancomycin-resistant *E. faecium* (VREF) bacteremia treated with quinupristin-dalfopristin with a historical cohort of 42 patients treated for VREF infections with other agents. In-hospital mortality was high in both groups, but VREF-associated mortality was significantly lower in the quinupristin-dalfopristin group (5 versus 17 patients, $p = 0.05$).

Rubenstein and Bompart[158] reviewed available clinical reports concerning more than 250 patients treated on a compassionate basis with quinupristin-dalfopristin for serious MRSA or VREF systemic or bloodstream infections. Quinupristin-dalfopristin was discontinued because of adverse events in only 7.3% of patients, and it produced clearance of bacteremia (71%) or clinical cure or improvement in the majority of the critically ill patients.[158]

Furlong and Rakowski[159] reported on their experience with a remarkable patient with prosthetic valve endocarditis caused by two strains of enterococci having both Van A and Van B resistance patterns. She was cured clinically and microbiologically by treatment for 10 weeks with quinupristin-dalfopristin after having failed valve replacement plus teicoplanin therapy. These reports suggest that quinupristin-dalfopristin will be a useful addition to the therapeutic armamentarium.

Finally, in order to delay the emergence of resistance to quinupristin-dalfopristin, this needed new antimicrobial should be judiciously reserved for treatment of serious, life-threatening, systemic infections for which there is no alternative therapy. As the old adage relates, "The more you use it, the quicker you lose it."

REFERENCES

1. Alexander MR. Review of vancomycin after 15 years of use. Drug Intell Clin Pharm. 1974;8:520.
2. Perkins HR, Nieto M. The chemical basis for the action of the vancomycin group of antibiotics. Ann N Y Acad Sci. 1974;235:348.
3. Hiramatsu K, Hanaki H, Ino T. Methicillin-resistant *Staphylococcus aureus* clinical strain with reduced vancomycin susceptibility. J Antimicrob Chemother. 1997;40:135–136.
4. Hiramatsu K, Aritaka N, Hanaki H, et al. Dissemination in Japanese hospitals of strains of *Staphylococcus aureus* heterogeneously resistant to vancomycin. Lancet. 1997;350:1670–1673.
5. Centers for Disease Control and Prevention. *Staphylococcus aureus* with reduced susceptibility to vancomycin—United States, 1997. MMWR Morb Mortal Wkly Rep 1997;46:765–766.
6. Craig WA, Vogelman B. The post-antibiotic effect. Ann Intern Med. 1987;106: 900–902.
7. Gopal V, Bisno AL, Silverblatt FJ. Failure of vancomycin treatment in *Staphylococcus aureus* endocarditis: In vivo and in vitro observations. JAMA. 1976;236:1604.
8. Sabath L, Wheeler N, Laverdiere M, et al. A new type of penicillin resistance in *Staphylococcus aureus*. Lancet. 1977;1:443.
9. Evans RC, Holmes CJ. Effect of vancomycin hydrochloride on *Staphylococcus epidermidis* biofilm associated with silicone elastomer. Antimicrob Agents Chemother. 1987;31:889–894.
10. Schwalke RS, Stapleton JT, Gilligan PH. Emergence of vancomycin resistance in coagulase-negative staphylococci. N Engl J Med. 1987;316:927–931.
11. Ploy M, Grelaud C, Martin C. First clinical isolate of vancomycin intermediate *Staphylococcus aureus* resistance in a French hospital. Lancet. 1998;351:1212–1213.
12. Geraci JE. Vancomycin. Mayo Clin Proc. 1977;52:631.
13. Geraci JE, Heilman FR, Nichols DR, et al. Some laboratory and clinical experiences with a new antibiotic, vancomycin. Proc Staff Meet Mayo Clin. 1956;31:564.
14. Reimer LG. Measurement of serum bactericidal activity and use of vancomycin for treatment of nutritionally variant streptococcal bacteremia. Diagn Microbiol Infect Dis. 1987;6:319–322.
15. Watanakunakorn C, Bakie C. Synergism of vancomycin-gentamicin and vancomycin-streptomycin against enterococci. Antimicrob Agents Chemother. 1973;4:120.
16. Harwick HJ, Kalmanson GM, Guze LB. In vitro activity of ampicillin or vancomycin combined with gentamicin or streptomycin against enterococci. Antimicrob Agents Chemother. 1973;4:383.
17. Mederski-Samoraj BD, Murray BE. High level resistance to enterococci in clinical isolates of staphylococci. J Infect Dis. 1983;147:751–757.
18. Poyart C, Pierre C, Quesne G, et al. Emergence of vancomycin resistance in the genus *Streptococcus*: Characterization of a van B transferable determinant in *Streptococcus bovis*. Antimicrob Agents Chemother. 1997;41:24–29.
19. Utley AC, Collins CH, Naidoo J, et al. Vancomycin-resistant enterococci. Lancet. 1988;1:57–58.
20. Kaplan AH, Gilligan PH, Facklam RR. Recovery of resistant enterococci during vancomycin prophylaxis. J Clin Microb. 1988;26:126–128.
21. Rubin LG, Velozzi E, Shapiro J, et al. Infection with vancomycin-resistant "streptococci," due to *Leuconostoc* species. J Infect Dis. 1988;157:216.
22. Leclercq R, Deriot E, Weber M, et al. Transferable vancomycin and teicoplanin resistance in *Enterococcus faecium*. Antimicrob Agents Chemother. 1989;33:10–15.
23. Leclercq R, Deriot E, Duval J, et al. Plasmid-mediated resistance to vancomycin and teicoplanin in *Enterococcus faecium*. N Engl J Med. 1988;319:157–161.
24. Leclercq R, Dutka-Malen S, Brisson-Noel A, et al. Resistance of enterococci to aminoglycosides and glycopeptides. Clin Infect Dis. 1992;15:495–501.
25. Arthur M, Molinas C, Depardieu F, et al. Characterization of Tn 1546, a Tn-3 related transposon conferring glycopeptide resistance to synthesis of depsipeptide peptidoglycan precursors in *Enterococcus faecium* BM4147. J Bacteriol. 1993;175:117–127.
26. Williamson R, Al-Obeid S, Shlaes JH, et al. Inducible resistance to vancomycin in *Enterococcus faecium* D366. J Infect Dis. 1989;159:1095–1104.
27. Al-Obeid S, Collatz E, Gutmann L. Mechanism of resistance to vancomycin in *Enterococcus faecium* D366 and *Enterococcus faecalis* A256. Antimicrob Agents Chemother. 1990;34:252–256.
28. Vincent S, Minkler P, Bincziewski B, et al. Vancomycin resistance in *Enterococcus gallinarum*. Antimicrob Agents Chemother. 1992;36:1392–1399.
29. Shlaes DM, Etter L, Gutmann L. Synergistic killing of vancomycin-resistant enterococci of classes A, B, and C by combinations of vancomycin, penicillin, and gentamicin. Antimicrob Agents Chemother. 1991;35:776–779.
30. Vincent S, Knight RG, Green M, et al. Vancomycin susceptibility and identification of motile enterococci. J Clin Microbiol. 1991;29:2335–2337.
31. Noble W, Virani Z, Cree R. Co-transfer of vancomycin and other resistance genes from *Enterococcus faecalis* NCTC 12201 to *Staphylococcus aureus*. FEMS Microbiol Lett. 1992;72:195–198.
32. Murray B. Vancomycin-resistant enterococci. Am J Med. 1997;101:284–293.
33. Dever L, Jorgensen JH, Barbour A. In vitro activity of vancomycin against the spirochete *Borrelia burgdorferi*. Antimicrob Agents Chemother. 1993;37:1115–1121.
34. Polk RE, Healy DP, Schwartz LB, et al. Vancomycin and the red-man syndrome: Pharmacodynamics of histamine release. J Infect Dis. 1988;157:502–507.
35. Barg NL, Fekety R, Supena R. Persistent staphylococcal bacteremia in an intravenous drug abuser. Antimicrob Agents Chemother. 1986;29:209–211.
36. Khan MY, Hall WH. Staphylococcal enterocolitis: Treatment with oral vancomycin. Ann Intern Med. 1966;65:1.
37. Tedesco F, Markham R, Gurwith M, et al. Oral vancomycin for antibiotic-associated pseudomembranous colitis. Lancet. 1978;2:226–228.
38. Silva J, Batts DH, Fekety R, et al. Treatment of *Clostridium difficile* colitis and diarrhea with vancomycin. Am J Med. 1981;71:815–822.
39. Bodey G. Oral antibiotic prophylaxis in protected environment units: Effect of nonabsorbable and absorbable antibiotics on the fecal flora. Antimicrob Agents Chemother. 1972;1:343.
40. Lindholm DD, Murray JS. Persistence of vancomycin in the blood during renal failure and its treatment by hemodialysis. N Engl J Med. 1966;274:1047.
41. Eykyn S, Phillip I, Evans J. Vancomycin for staphylococcal shunt infections in patients on regular hemodialysis. BMJ. 1970;3:80.
42. Rice TL. Simplified dosing and monitoring of vancomycin for the burn care clinician. Burns. 1992;18:355–361.
43. Spitzer PC, Eliopoulos GM. Systemic absorption of enteral vancomycin in a patient with pseudomembranous colitis. Ann Intern Med. 1984;100:533–534.
44. Hawley HB, Gump DW. Vancomycin therapy of bacterial meningitis. Am J Dis Child. 1973;126:261.
45. Ayus JC, Enkas JF, Tong TG, et al. Peritoneal clearance and total body elimination of vancomycin during chronic intermittent peritoneal dialysis. Clin Nephrol. 1979;11:129–132.
46. Nielsen HE, Hansen JE, Korsager B, et al. Renal excretion of vancomycin in kidney disease. Acta Med Scand. 1975;197:261.
47. Moellering RC, Krogstad DJ, Greenblatt DJ. Vancomycin therapy in patients with impaired renal function: A nomogram for dosage. Ann Intern Med. 1981;94: 343–346.
48. Matzke G, Kovarik JM, Rybak MJ, et al. Evaluation of the vancomycin clearance: Creatinine-clearance relationship for predicting vancomycin dosage. Clin Pharmacol. 1985;4:311–315.
49. Cantú TG, Yamanaka-Yuen NA, Lietman PS. Serum vancomycin concentrations: Reappraisal of their clinical value. Clin Infect Dis. 1994;18:533–543.
50. Moellering RC. Monitoring serum vancomycin levels: Climbing the mountain because it is there? (Editorial). Clin Infect Dis. 1994;78:544–546.
51. Quale JM, O'Halloran JJ, De Vincenzo N, et al. Removal of vancomycin by high-flux hemodialysis membranes. Antimicrob Agents Chemother. 1992;36:1424–1426.
52. Bohler J, Reeza-Bonorden P, Keller E, et al. Rebound of plasma vancomycin levels after haemodialysis with highly permeable membranes. Eur J Clin Pharmacol. 1992;42:635–640.

53. Matzke GR, O'Connell MB, Collins AJ, et al. Disposition of vancomycin during hemofiltration. Clin Pharmacol Ther. 1986;40:425–430.
54. Austin TW, Leake J, Coles JC, et al. Vancomycin blood levels during cardiac surgery. Cardiol J Surg. 1981;24:423–425.
55. Healy DP, Polk RE, Garson ML, et al. Comparison of steady-state pharmacokinetics of two dosage regimens of vancomycin in normal volunteers. Antimicrob Agents Chemother. 1987;31:393–397.
56. Newfield P, Roizen MF. Hazards of rapid administration of vancomycin. Ann Intern Med. 1979;91:581.
57. Mordenti J, Ries C, Brooks GF, et al. Vancomycin-induced neutropenia complicating bone marrow recovery in a patient with leukemia. Case report and a review of the literature. Am J Med. 1986;30:333–335.
58. Miller SN, Ringler RP. Vancomycin-induced pseudomembranous colitis. J Clin Gastroenterol. 1987;9:114–115.
59. Traber PG, Levine DP. Vancomycin ototoxicity in a patient with normal renal function. Ann Intern Med. 1981;95:458–460.
60. McHenry MC, Gavan TL. Vancomycin. Pediatr Clin North Am. 1983;30:31–47.
61. Geraci JE, Hermans PE. Vancomycin. Mayo Clin Proc. 1983;58:88–91.
62. Appel GB, Neu HC. The nephrotoxicity of antimicrobial agents. N Engl J Med. 1977;296:722.
63. Greenberg RN, Saud AMK, Kennedy DJ, et al. Instability of vancomycin in Infusaid drug pump model 100. Antimicrob Agents Chemother. 1987;31:610–611.
64. Blovin RA, Bauer LA, Miller DD, et al. Vancomycin pharmacokinetics in normal and morbidly obese subjects. Antimicrob Agents Chemother. 1982;21:575–580.
65. Nagvi SH, Kennan WJ, Reichley RM, et al. Vancomycin pharmacokinetics in small, seriously ill infants. Am J Dis Child. 1986;140:107–110.
66. Riley HD. Vancomycin and novobiocin. Med Clin North Am. 1970;54:1277.
67. Schaad VB, McCracken GH, Nelson JD. Clinical pharmacology and efficacy of vancomycin in pediatric patients. J Pediatr. 1980;96:119–126.
68. Fekety R, Silva J, Kauffman C, et al. Treatment of *C. difficile* antibiotic-associated colitis with oral vancomycin: Comparison of two dosage regimens. Am J Med. 1989;86:15–19.
69. Batts DH, Martin D, Holmes R, et al. Treatment of antibiotic-associated *Clostridium difficile* diarrhea with oral vancomycin. J Pediatr. 1980;97:151–153.
70. Rotschafer JC, Crossley K, Zaski DE, et al. Pharmacokinetics of vancomycin: Observations in 28 patients and dosage recommendations. Antimicrob Agents Chemother. 1982;22:391–394.
71. Brown N, Ho DHW, Fong KL, et al. Effects of hepatic function on vancomycin clinical pharmacology. Antimicrob Agents Chemother. 1983;23:603–609.
72. Watanakunakorn C. Treatment of infections due to methicillin-resistant *Staphylococcus aureus*. Ann Intern Med. 1982;97:376–378.
73. Myers JP, Linnemann CC. Bacteremia due to methicillin-resistant *Staphylococcus aureus*. J Infect Dis. 1982;4:532–536.
74. Sorrell TC, Packham DR, Shanker S, et al. Vancomycin therapy for methicillin-resistant *Staphylococcus aureus*. Ann Intern Med. 1982;97:344–350.
75. Levine DP, Cushing R, Jim J, et al. Community-acquired methicillin-resistant *Staphylococcus aureus* endocarditis in the Detroit Medical Center. Ann Intern Med. 1982;97:330–338.
76. Karchmer AW, Archer GL, Dismukes WE. *Staphylococcus epidermidis* causing prosthetic-valve endocarditis: Microbiologic and clinical observations as guides to therapy. Ann Intern Med. 1983;98:447–455.
77. Ena J, Dick RW, Jones RN, et al. The epidemiology of intravenous vancomycin usage in a university hospital: A 10-year study. JAMA. 1993;269:598–602.
78. Sutherlan GE, Palitang EG, Marr JJ, et al. Sterilization of Ommaya reservoir by instillation of vancomycin. Am J Med. 1981;71:1068–1070.
79. Gump DW. Vancomycin for treatment of bacterial meningitis. Rev Infect Dis. 1981;3:S289–S292.
80. Swayne RS, Rampling A, Newsom SWB. Intraventricular vancomycin for treatment of shunt-associated ventriculitis. J Antimicrob Chemother. 1987;19:249–253.
81. Viladrich PF, Gudiol F, Linares J, et al. Evaluation of vancomycin for therapy of adult pneumococcal meningitis. Antimicrob Agents Chemother. 1991;35:2467–2472.
82. Westenfelder GO, Paterson PY, Reisberg BE, et al. Vancomycin-streptomycin synergism in enterococcal endocarditis. JAMA. 1973;223:37.
83. Harwick HJ, Kalmanson GM, Guze LB. Pyelonephritis: XVII. Comparison of combinations of vancomycin, ampicillin, streptomycin, and gentamicin in the treatment of enterococcal infection in the rat. J Infect Dis. 1974;129:358.
84. Zervos MJ, Kauffman CA, Therasse PM, et al. Nosocomial infection by gentamicin-resistant *Streptococcus faecalis*. Ann Intern Med. 1987;106:687–691.
85. Esposito AL, Gleckman RA: Vancomycin, a second look. JAMA. 1977;238:1756.
86. Teasley DG, Gerding DN, Olson MM, et al. Prospective randomised trial of metronidazole versus vancomycin for *Clostridium difficile*–associated diarrhea and colitis. Lancet. 1983;2:1043–1046.
87. Fekety R, Silva J, Armstrong J, et al. Treatment of antibiotic-associated enterocolitis with vancomycin. Rev Infect Dis. 1981;3:S273–S281.
88. Tedesco FJ. Treatment of recurrent antibiotic-associated pseudomembranous colitis. Am J Gastroenterol. 1982;77:220–221.
89. Johnson S, Homann SR, Bettin KM, et al. Treatment of asymptomatic *Clostridium difficile* carriers (fecal excretors) with vancomycin: A randomized, placebo controlled trial. Ann Intern Med. 1992;117:297–302.
90. Pasic M, Carrel T, Opravil M, et al. Systemic absorption after local intracolonic vancomycin in pseudomembranous colitis (Letter). Lancet. 1993;342:443.
91. Pasic M, Jost R, Carrel T, et al. Intracolonic vancomycin for pseudomembranous colitis (Letter). N Engl J Med. 1993;329:583.
92. Nielsen HE, Sorensen I, Hansen HE. Peritoneal transport of vancomycin during peritoneal dialysis. Nephron. 1979;24:274–277.
93. Morse GD, Farolino DF, Apicella MA, et al. Comparative study of intraperitoneal and intravenous vancomycin pharmacokinetics during continuous ambulatory peritoneal dialysis. Antimicrob Agents Chemother. 1987;31:173–177.
94. Piraino B, Bernardini J, Johnston J, et al. Chemical peritonitis due to intraperitoneal vancomycin. Perit Dial Bull. 1987;7(Suppl):S59.
95. Buggy BP, Schaberg DR, Swartz RD. Intraleukocytic sequestration as a cause of persistent *Staphylococcus aureus* peritonitis in continuous ambulatory peritoneal dialysis. Am J Med. 1984;76:1035–1040.
96. Kaye D. Prophylaxis for infective endocarditis: An update. Ann Intern Med. 1986;104:419–423.
97. Kaplan EL, Anthony BF, Bisno A, et al. Prevention of bacterial endocarditis. Circulation. 1977;56:139A–143A.
98. Rubin M, Hathorn JW, Marshall D, et al. Gram-positive infections and the use of vancomycin in 550 episodes of fever and neutropenia. Ann Intern Med. 1988;108:30–35.
99. Wise RI, Kory M, eds: Reassessments of vancomycin—a potentially useful antibiotic. Rev Infect Dis. 1981;3:S199–S300.
100. Williams AH, Gruneberg RN. Teicoplanin. J Antimicrob Chemother. 1984;14: 441–448.
101. Parenti F. Structure and mechanism of action of teicoplanin. J Hosp Infect. 1986;7(Suppl A):79–83.
102. Neville LD, Baillod R, Grady D, et al. Teicoplanin in patients with chronic renal failure on dialysis: Microbiological and pharmacokinetic aspects. Int J Clin Pharmacol Res. 1987;7:485–490.
103. Somma S, Gastaldo L, Corti A: Teicoplanin, a new antibiotic from *Actinoplanes teichomyceticus* nov sp. Antimicrob Agents Chemother. 1984;26:917–923.
104. Greenwood D. Microbiological properties of teicoplanin. J Antimicrob Agents Chemother. 1988;21(Suppl A):1–13.
105. Parenti F. Glycopeptide antibiotics. J Clin Pharmacol. 1988;28:136–140.
106. McNulty CAM, Garden GMF, Wise R, et al. The pharmacokinetics and tissue penetration of teicoplanin. J Antimicrob Chemother. 1985;16:743–749.
107. Verbist L, Tjandramaga B, Hendrickx B, et al. In vitro activity and human pharmacokinetics of teicoplanin. Antimicrob Agents Chemother. 1984;12:119–128.
108. Buniva G, DelFavero A, Bernareggi A, et al. Pharmacokinetics of ^{14}C-teicoplanin in healthy volunteers. J Antimicrob Chemother. 1988;21(Suppl A):23–28.
109. Bonati M, Traina GL, Rosiva R, et al. Pharmacokinetics of a single intravenous dose of teicoplanin in subjects with various degrees of renal impairment. Antimicrob Chemother. 1988;21(Suppl A):29–37.
110. Presterl E, Graninger W, Georgapoulos A. The efficacy of teicoplanin in the treatment of endocarditis caused by gram-positive bacteria. J Antimicrob Chemother. 1993;31:755–766.
111. Tarral E, Jehl F, Tarral A, et al. Pharmacokinetics of teicoplanin in children. J Antimicrob Chemother. 1988;21(Suppl A):47–51.
112. Domart Y, Pierre C, Clair B, et al. Pharmacokinetics of teicoplanin in critically ill patients with various degrees of renal impairment. Antimicrob Agents Chemother. 1987;31:1600–1604.
113. Bauernfeind A. Teichomycin and AM-715 activity on staphylococci and enterococci in comparison to other antibiotic agents (Abstract). Program and Abstracts of the Twenty-first Interscience Conference on Antimicrobial Agents and Chemotherapy. Chicago: American Society for Microbiology, November 1981.
114. Jadeja L, Fainstein V, LeBlanc B, et al. Comparative in vitro activities of teichomycin and other antibiotics against JK diphtheroids. Antimicrob Agents Chemother. 1983;24:145–146.
115. Greenwood D. Microbiological properties of teicoplanin. J Antimicrob Chemother. 1988;21(Suppl A):1–3.
116. Felmingham D, Solomonides K, O'Hare MD, et al. The effect of medium and inoculum on the activity of vancomycin and teicoplanin against coagulase-negative staphylococci. J Antimicrob Chemother. 1987;10:609–619.
117. Pantosti A, Luzzi I, Cardine R, et al. Comparison of the in vitro activities of teicoplanin and vancomycin against *Clostridium difficile* and their interactions with cholestyramine. Antimicrob Agents Chemother. 1985;28:847–848.
118. Van der Auwera P, Klastersky J. Bactericidal activity and killing rate of serum in volunteers receiving vancomycin or teicoplanin with and without amikacin given intravenously. J Antimicrob Chemother. 1987;19:623–635.
119. Van der Auwera P, Joly P. Comparative in-vitro activities of teicoplanin, vancomycin, coumermycin and ciprofloxacin, alone and in combination with rifampicin or LM427, against *Staphylococcus aureus*. J Antimicrob Chemother. 1987;19: 313–320.
120. Watanakunakorn C. In-vitro activity of teicoplanin alone and in combination with rifampicin, gentamicin or tobramycin against coagulase-negative staphylococci. J Antimicrob Chemother. 1987;19:439–443.
121. Tuazon CU, Washburn D. Teicoplanin and rifampicin singly and in combination in the treatment of experimental *Staphylococcus epidermidis* endocarditis in the rabbit model. J Antimicrob Chemother. 1987;20:233–237.
122. Shanson DC, Todayon M. Activity of teicoplanin compared with vancomycin alone, and combined with gentamicin, against penicillin tolerant viridans streptococci and enterococci causing endocarditis. J Hosp Infect. 1986;7(Suppl A):65–72.
123. Agnelli G, Longetti M, Guerciolini R, et al. Effects of the new glycopeptide antibiotic teicoplanin on platelet function and blood coagulation. Antimicrob Agents Chemother. 1987;31:1609–1612.
124. Williams AH, Gruneberg RN, Webster A, et al. Teicoplanin in the treatment of infection caused by gram-positive organisms. J Hosp Infect. 1986;7(Suppl A): 101–103.

125. Stille W, Sietzen W, Dieterich HA, et al. Clinical efficacy and safety of teicoplanin. J Antimicrob Chemother. 1988;21(Suppl A):69–79.
126. Maher ER, Hollman A, Gruneberg RN. Teicoplanin induced ototoxicity in Down's syndrome. Lancet. 1986;1:613.
127. Drabu YJ, Walsh B, Blakemore PH, et al. Teicoplanin in infections caused by methicillin-resistant staphylococci. J Antimicrob Chemother. 1988;21(Suppl A):89–92.
128. Schlemmer B, Falkman H, Boudjadja A, et al. Teicoplanin for patients allergic to vancomycin. N Engl J Med. 1988;318:1127–1128.
129. Chambers HF, Rusnak NG, Hackbarth CJ, et al. Treatment of *Staphylococcus aureus* endocarditis in rabbits with teichomycin (Abstract). Program and Abstracts of the 23rd Interscience Conference on Antimicrobial Agents and Chemotherapy. Las Vegas: American Society for Microbiology, October 1983.
130. Lewis P, Garaud JJ, Parenti F. A multicentre open clinical trial of teicoplanin in infections caused by gram-positive bacteria. J Antimicrob Chemother. 1988;21(Suppl A):61–67.
131. Harding I, Garaud JJ. Teicoplanin in the treatment of infections caused by coagulase-negative staphylococci. J Antimicrob Chemother. 1988;21(Suppl A):93–103.
132. Galanakis N, Giamarellou H, Vlachogiannis N, et al. Poor efficacy of teicoplanin in treatment of deep-seated staphylococcal infections. Eur J Clin Microbiol Infect Dis. 1988;7:130–134.
133. Schmib JL. Efficacy of teicoplanin for enterococcal infections: 63 cases and review. Clin Infect Dis. 1992;15:302–306.
134. Wilson APR, Treasure T, Gruneberg RN, et al. Antibiotic prophylaxis in cardiac surgery: A prospective comparison of two dosage regimens of teicoplanin with combination of flucloxacillin and tobramycin. J Antimicrob Chemother. 1988;21:213–233.
135. Neville LO, Baillod RA, Brumfitt W, et al. Efficacy and safety of teicoplanin in gram-positive peritonitis in patients on peritoneal dialysis. J Antimicrob Chemother. 1988;21(Suppl A):123–131.
136. Bowley JA, Pickering SJ, Scantlebury AJ, et al. Intraperitoneal teicoplanin in the treatment of peritonitis associated with continuous ambulatory peritoneal dialysis. J Antimicrob Chemother. 1988;21(Suppl A):133–139.
137. deLalla F, Privitera G, Rinaldi E, et al. Treatment of *Clostridium difficile*–associated disease with teicoplanin. Antimicrob Agents Chemother. 1989;33:1125–1127.
138. Phillips G, Golledge CL. Vancomycin and teicoplanin: Something old, something new. Med J Aust. 1992;156:537.
139. Synercid® Investigator's Brochure. Collegeville, Pa: Rhone Poulenc Rorer, October 27, 1993.
140. Aumercier M, Bouhallab S, Capmau M, et al. RP 59500: A proposed mechanism for its bactericidal activity. J Antimicrob Chemother. 1992;30(Suppl A):9–14.
141. Bryson H, Spencer C. Quinupristin/dalfopristin. Drugs. 1996;52:406–415.
142. Soussy CJ, Acar J, Cluzel R, et al. A collaborative study of the in vitro sensitivity to RP59500 of bacteria isolated in seven hospitals in France. J Antimicrob Chemother. 1992;30(Suppl A):53–58.
143. Fantin B, Leclercq R, Garry L, et al. Influence of inducible cross-resistance to macrolides, lincosamides and streptogramin B-type antibiotics in *Enterococcus faecium* on activity of quinupristin/dalfopristin in vitro and in rabbits with experimental endocarditis. Antimicrob Agents Chemother. 1997;41:931–935.
144. Chow J, Davidson A, Sanford E, et al. Superinfection with *Enterococcus faecalis* during quinupristin/dalfopristin therapy. Clin Infect Dis. 1997;24:91–92.
145. Bonilla H, Perri M, Kauffman C, et al. Comparative in vitro activity of quinupristin/dalfopristin against multidrug resistant *Enterococcus faecium*. Diagn Microbiol Infect Dis. 1996;25:127–131.
146. Bouanchaud D. In-vitro and in-vivo antibacterial activity of quinupristin/dalfopristin. J Antimicrob Chemother. 1997;39(Suppl A):15–21.
147. Finch R. Antibacterial activity of quinupristin/dalfopristin: Rationale for clinical use. Drugs. 1996;51(Suppl 1):31–37.
148. Hill R, Smith C, Sayed-Akhavani M, et al. Bactericidal and inhibitory activity of quinupristin/dalfopristin against vancomycin and gentamicin resistant *Enterococcus faecium*. J Antimicrob Chemother. 1997;39(Suppl A):23–28.
149. Nicas T, Zeckel M, Braun D. Beyond vancomycin: New therapies to the challenge of glycopeptide resistance. Trends Microbiol. 1997;5:240–249.
150. Mouton J, Enctz H, den Hollander J, et al. In vitro activity of quinupristin/dalfopristin compared with other widely used antibiotics against strains isolated from patients with endocarditis. J Antimicrob Chemother. 1997;39(Suppl A):75–80.
151. Bebear C, Bouanchaud DH. A review of the in-vitro activity of quinupristin/dalfopristin against intracellular pathogens and mycoplasmas. J Antimicrob Chemother. 1997;39(Suppl A):59–62.
152. Moore L, Schneider B, Holloway W. Minimal inhibitory concentrations and minimal bactericidal concentrations of quinupristin/dalfopristin against clinical isolates of *Corynebacterium jeikeium* and *Listeria monocytogenes*. J Antimicrob Chemother. 1997;39(Suppl A):67–68.
153. Jorgensen J, McElmeel M. Activity of quinupristin/dalfopristin and its components against *Haemophilus influenzae*. J Antimicrob Chemother. 1997;39(Suppl A):69–73.
154. Griswold M, Lomaestro B, Briceland L. Quinupristin/dalfopristin (RP59500): An injectable streptogramin combination. Am J Health Syst Pharm. 1996;53:2045–2053.
155. Bergeron M, Montay G. The pharmacokinetics of quinupristin/dalfopristin in laboratory animals and in humans. J Antimicrob Chemother. 1997;39(Suppl A):129–138.
156. Stamatakis M, Richards J. Interaction between quinupristin/dalfopristin and cyclosporine. Ann Pharmacother. 1997;31:576–578.
157. Linden P, Pasculle A, McDevitt D, et al. Effect of quinupristin/dalfopristin on the outcome of vancomycin-resistant *Enterococcus faecium* bacteraemia: Comparison with a control cohort. J Antimicrob Chemother. 1997;39(Suppl A):145–151.
158. Rubinstein E, Bompart F. Activity of quinupristin/dalfopristin against gram-positive bacteria: Clinical application and therapeutic potential. J Antimicrob Chemother. 1997;39(Suppl A):139–143.
159. Furlong W, Rakowski T. Therapy with RP 59500 (quinupristin/dalfopristin) for prosthetic valve endocarditis due to enterococci with VanA/VanB resistance patterns. Clin Infect Dis. 1997;25:163–164.

Chapter 29

Oxazolidinones

GERALD R. DONOWITZ

The oxazolidinones are a class of antibiotics prepared by organic synthesis. In 1978, a patent was issued to the E.I. DuPont de Nemours and Company, Inc., for a series of 5-(halomethyl)-3-aryl-2-oxazolidinones that had antimicrobial activity against plant pathogens. Further manipulation of the molecule led to the development of two agents that displayed activity against human pathogens.[1] These two agents, DuP 105 and DuP 721, were orally absorbed and displayed activity against a variety of streptococcal and staphylococcal species comparable to that of vancomycin and β-lactam agents. Further manipulation of these compounds has led to the development of two agents presently under investigation for clinical use, eperezolid (PNU-100592) and linezolid (PNU-100766).

CHEMICAL STRUCTURE

The basic molecular structure of the oxazolidinones is shown in Figure 29–1. Initial chemical manipulation included the incorporation of a piperazine moiety into the basic structure at site A. Antibacterial activity has been increased by the addition of a hydroxyacetyl group to the heterocyclic nitrogen at site B.[2] Further antibacterial activity was derived by fluorine substitution at the phenyl 3-position. Only the enantiomers with a 5S acetamidomethyl configuration have antibacterial activity. The molecular structures of eperezolid and linezolid are shown in Figure 29–1. The unique chemical structure of the compound makes cross-resistance with more commonly used compounds unlikely.

MECHANISM OF ACTION

The oxazolidinones are inhibitors of protein synthesis and are bacteriostatic against a variety of bacteria. The mechanism of activity is thought to be unique and involves the inhibition of an early step in protein synthesis.[3, 4] These agents bind to the 50S ribosome. Binding is competitively inhibited by chloramphenicol and lincomycin, which suggests either shared or overlapping binding sites. However, unlike chloramphenicol or lincomycin, the oxazolidinones do not interfere with peptide elongation or termination of translation. It has been shown that they do not inhibit the formation of initiator tRNA (*N*-formyl-methionyl-tRNA).[5] It has been hypothesized that these agents bind to the 50S ribosome at a site near the 30S ribosome interface and that such binding results in changes that prevent the 30S initiation complex from forming the 70S initiation complex. The initiation of protein synthesis is thereby blocked.

ANTIMICROBIAL ACTIVITY

Linezolid and eperezolid possess activity against gram-positive organisms, including methicillin-resistant strains of *Staphylococcus*

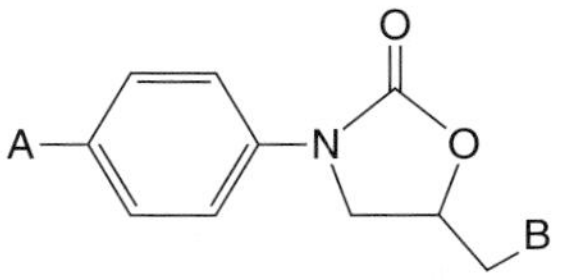

Basic oxazolidinone structure

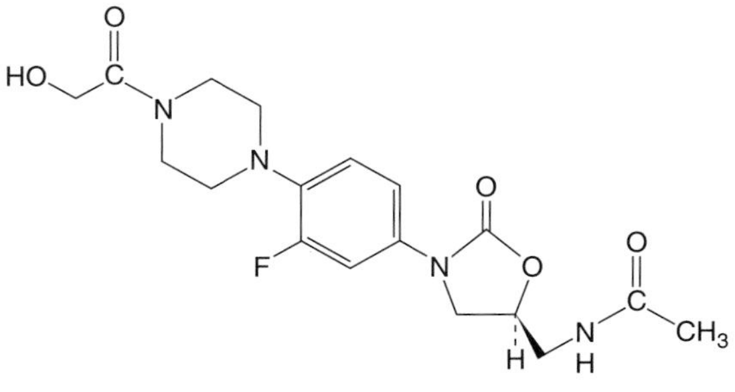

Eperezolid

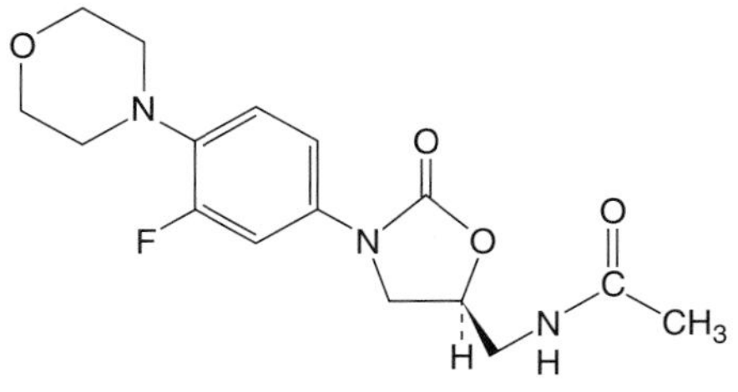

Linezolid

FIGURE 29–1. Structure of oxazolidinones.

aureus, coagulase-negative staphylococci, vancomycin-resistant strains of *Enterococcus* species, and penicillin-resistant strains of *Streptococcus pneumoniae*[3, 6–16] (Table 29–1). In general, eperezolid was slightly more active against staphylococci than linezolid was and approximately twofold more active against enterococci. At a breakpoint of 4 μg/ml, both drugs displayed activity similar to that of vancomycin and in addition were active against vancomycin-resistant strains of enterococci.

Both agents are effective in vitro against *Clostridium, Prevotella, Peptostreptococcus,* and *Mycobacterium tuberculosis,* including strains resistant to the usual antituberculosis agents.[3]

TABLE 29–1 In Vitro Activity of Eperezolid and Linezolid

Organism	Eperezolid	Linezolid
Staphylococcus aureus		
Methicillin sensitive	3.2*	3.6
Methicillin resistant	3.4	3.3
Staphylococcus epidermidis		
Methicillin sensitive	1.3	1.9
Methicillin resistant	1.1	2.0
Streptococcus pneumoniae		
Penicillin sensitive	0.5	1
Penicillin intermediate	0.5	1
Penicillin resistant	0.5	1
Enterococcus faecium		
Vancomycin sensitive	1.4	2.6
Vancomycin resistant	2	3
Enterococcus faecalis		
Vancomycin sensitive	2.3	2.5
Vancomycin resistant	2	3
Streptococcus pyogenes	0.5	0.5
Streptococcus agalactiae	2	4
Bacillus species	1	1
Corynebacterium	0.5	0.5

*Values given are the minimal inhibitory concentrations of drug in micrograms per liter at which 90% of strains are inhibited, or MIC_{90}, and are averages of cumulative data from refs. 3 and 9–18.

PHARMACOLOGY

The published human data involve linezolid. Absorption after ingestion is rapid, with peak serum levels occurring at 1 to 2 hours. With oral doses of 400 and 625 mg three times daily, mean plasma levels of 12.38 and 26.44 μg/ml, respectively, have been observed.[17, 18] The elimination half-life is approximately 5.5 hours. Trough values are approximately 4 μg/ml with the doses studied. About 30% of the drug is eliminated unchanged in urine.[19]

Intravenous dosing at 500 and 625 mg twice daily maintains serum levels above 4 μg/ml throughout the dosing interval.[20] Protein binding of the oxazalidinones is 6% for eperezolid and 31% for linezolid.[6]

UNTOWARD REACTIONS

Volunteer studies and preliminary evaluation of phase II studies have shown that linezolid is relatively safe.[21] Approximately 60% of volunteers noted some "digestive event" while taking the drug, most of which involved a discoloration of the tongue. Folliculitis was reported by about 21% of volunteers. In addition, linezolid has been shown to be a relatively weak reversible inhibitor of human monoamine oxidase.[7] Analysis of phase II trials suggests that headache and diarrhea were the most commonly reported events.

CLINICAL USE

Phase II trials are presently under way to examine the usefulness of linezolid in skin and soft tissue infections, as well as pneumonia. Initial review of data suggests that the drug may be effective in both conditions.[21] The activity of these agents and favorable pharmacokinetic and toxicity profiles suggest that agents of this class may be useful in the treatment of infections caused by resistant strains of enterococci, pneumococci, and staphylococci. They may also be useful as a part of combination therapy for resistant strains of *M. tuberculosis.*

REFERENCES

1. Slee AM, Wuonola MA, McRipley RJ, et al. Oxazolidinones, a new class of synthetic antibacterial agents: In vitro and in vivo activities of DuP1O5 and DuP721. Antimicrob Agents Chemother. 1987;31:1791–1797.
2. Brickner SJ, Hutchinson DK, Barbachyn MR, et al. Synthesis and antibacterial activity of U-100592 and U-100766, two oxazolidinone antibacterial agents for the potential treatment of multidrug-resistant gram-positive bacterial infections. J Med Chem. 1996;39:673–679.
3. Dresser LD, Rybek MJ. The pharmacologic and bacteriologic properties of oxazolidinones, a new class of synthetic antimicrobials. Pharmacotherapy. 1998;18:456–462.
4. Lin AH, Murray RW, Vidmar TJ, Marotti KR. The oxazolidinone eperezolid binds to the 50s ribosomal subunit and competes with binding of chloramphenicol and lincomycin. Antimicrob Agents Chemother. 1997;41:2127–2131.
5. Shinabarger DL, Marotti KR, Murray RW, et al. Mechanism of action of oxazolidinones: Effects of linezolid and eperezolid on translation reactions. Antimicrob Agents Chemother. 1997;41:2132–2136.
6. Zurenko GE, Yagi BH, Schaadt RD, et al. In vitro activities of U-100592 and U-100766, novel oxazolidinone antibacterial agents. Antimicrob Agents Chemother. 1996;40:839–845.
7. Martin JP, Herberg JT, Slatter JG, Dupuls MJ. Although a novel microtiter-plate assay demonstrates that linezolid (PNU-100766) is a weak, competitive (reversible) inhibitor of human monoamine oxidase (MAO A) no clinical evidence of MAO A inhibition in clinical trials has been observed. Abstract A-85. Presented at the Thirty-eighth Annual Interscience Conference on Antimicrobial Agents and Chemotherapy, San Diego, September 1998.

8. Jorgensen JH, McElmeel ML, Trippy CW. In vitro activities of the oxazolidinone antibiotics U-100592 and U-100766 against *Staphylococcus aureus* and coagulase-negative *Staphylococcus* species. Antimicrob Agents Chemother. 1997;41:465–467.
9. Rybak MJ, Cappelletty DM, Moldovan T, et al. Comparative in vitro activities and post-antibiotic effects of the oxazolidinone compounds eperezolid (PNU-100592) and linezolid (PNU-100766) versus vancomycin against *Staphylococcus aureus* and *Enterococcus faecium.* Antimicrob Agents Chemother. 1998;42:721–724.
10. Jones RN, Johnson DM, Erwin ME. In vitro antimicrobial activities and spectra of U-100592 and U-0100766, two novel fluorinatal oxazolidinones. Antimicrob Agents Chemother. 1996;40:720–726.
11. Kaatz GW, Seo SM. In vitro activities of oxazolidinone compounds U-100592 and U-100766 against *Staphylococcus aureus* and *Staphylococcus epidermidis.* Antimicrob Agents Chemother. 1996;40:799–801.
12. Mulazimoglu L, Drenning SD, Yu VL. In vitro activities of two novel oxazolidinones (U-100592 and U100766), a new fluoroquinolone (trovafloxacin), and dalfopristin-quinupristin against *Staphylococcus aureus* and *Staphylococcus epidermidis.* Antimicrob Agents Chemother. 1996;40:2428–2430.
13. Mason EO Jr, Lamberth LB, Kaplan SL. In vitro activities of oxazolidinones U1005992 and U100766 against penicillin-resistant and cephalosporin-resistant strains of *Streptococcus pneumoniae.* Antimicrob Agents Chemother. 1996;40:1039–1040.
14. Eliopoulos GM, Wennersten CB, Gold HS, Moellering RC Jr. In vitro activities of new oxazolidinone antimicrobial agents against enterococci. Antimicrob Agents Chemother. 1996;40:1745–1747.
15. Spangler SK, Jacobs MR, Appelbaum PC. Activities of RPR 10692 (a new oral streptogramin), cefditoren (a new oral cephalosporin), two new oxazolidinones (U1005592 and 100766), and other oral and parenteral agents against 203 penicillin-susceptible and -resistant pneumococci. Antimicrob Agents Chemother. 1996;40:481–484.
16. Piper KE, Rouse MS, Patel R, et al. In vitro activity of linezolid against vancomycin resistant enterococci, methicillin-resistant *Staphylococcus aureus* and penicillin-resistant pneumococci. Abstract E-124. Presented at the Thirty-eighth Annual Interscience Conference on Antimicrobial Agents and Chemotherapy, San Diego, September 1998.
17. Stalker DJ, Wajszczuk CP, Batts DH. Linezolid safety, tolerance, pharmacokinetics following oral dosing twice daily for 14.5 days. Abstract A-115. Presented at the Thirty-seventh Interscience Conference on Antimicrobial Agents and Chemotherapy, Toronto, Ontario, Canada, Sept–Oct 1997.
18. Schaadt RD, Batts DH, Daley-Yates PT, et al. Serum inhibitory titers and serum bactericidal titers for human subjects receiving multiple doses of the antibacterial oxazolidinones eperezolid and linezolid. Diagn Microbiol Infect Dis. 1997;28:201–204.
19. Feenstra KL, Slatter JG, Stalher DJ, et al. Metabolism and excretion of the oxazolidinone antibiotic linezolid (PNU 100766) following oral administration of [^{14}C] PNU 100766 to healthy human volunteers. Abstract A-53. Presented at the Thirty-eighth Annual Interscience Conference on Antimicrobial Agents and Chemotherapy, San Diego, September 1998.
20. Stalker DJ, Wajszczuk CP, Batts DH. Linezolid safety, tolerance, and pharmacokinetics after intravenous dosing twice daily for 7.5 days. Abstract A-116. Presented at the Thirty-seventh Interscience Conference on Antimicrobial Agents and Chemotherapy, Toronto, Ontario, Canada, Sept–Oct 1997.
21. Batts D. Safety and efficacy of linezolid in phase II studies. Oxazolidinones: A new class of antibiotic. Presented at the Eighth International Congress on Infectious Diseases, Industry-sponsored symposium, Boston, May 1998, 27–29.

Chapter 30

Sulfonamides and Trimethoprim

STEPHEN H. ZINNER
KENNETH H. MAYER

The modern era of antimicrobial chemotherapy began in 1932 with the first reports by Gerhard Domagk of the protective activity of prontosil against murine streptococcal infections. This drug was an outgrowth of the German dye industry and had been commercially available since the early 20th century. Prontosil (sulfachrysoidine) exerted its antibacterial activity through the release in vivo of para-aminobenzenesulfonamide (sulfanilamide). This was the first antibacterial agent used in the United States, in an unsuccessful attempt, in July 1935, to treat a 10-year-old girl late in the course of meningitis and sepsis caused by *Haemophilus influenzae.*[1] During the late 1930s, the basic sulfanilamide compound was modified to remove unpleasant side effects and expand its spectrum of activity. More recent modifications resulted in compounds of specific usefulness, for example, in urinary infections (those compounds that are highly soluble) or within the gastrointestinal tract (nonabsorbable sulfonamides).

Trimethoprim is a 2,4-diamino-pyrimidine and, as such, inhibits the enzyme dihydrofolate reductase, resulting in interference in folic acid and subsequent pyrimidine synthesis in the bacterial cell. Trimethoprim is one of several such compounds synthesized and studied by Hitchings and coworkers in the 1950s and 1960s. The use of trimethoprim as a potentiator of sulfonamide activity was introduced by Bushby and Hitchings[2] in 1968. In the subsequent decade the combination of trimethoprim-sulfamethoxazole (TMP-SMX) was introduced clinically and gained a place in the chemotherapy for many infectious diseases. These agents, available in a fixed drug combination, show true antibacterial synergism against a wide variety of organisms.

SULFONAMIDES

Structure

The clinically useful sulfonamides are derived from sulfanilamide, which is similar in structure to para-aminobenzoic acid (PABA), a factor required by bacteria for folic acid synthesis (Fig. 30–1).

A free amino group at the 4-carbon position is associated with enhanced activity. Increased activity due to increased PABA inhibition is associated with substitutions at the sulfonyl radical (SO_2), which is attached to the 1 carbon, as seen with sulfadiazine, sulfisoxazole, and sulfamethoxazole, all of which are more active than the parent compound, sulfanilamide. The nature of these substitutions determines other pharmacologic properties of the drug such as absorption, solubility, and gastrointestinal tolerance. Substitutions at the 4-amino group result in decreased absorption from the gastrointestinal tract (e.g., phthalylsulfathiazole).

Derivation and Nomenclature

Since the introduction of sulfonamides into clinical medicine, dozens of compounds have been used. However, relatively few survive today. They can be classified as (1) short- or medium-acting sulfonamides, (2) long-acting sulfonamides, (3) sulfonamides limited to the gastrointestinal tract, and (4) topical sulfonamides.

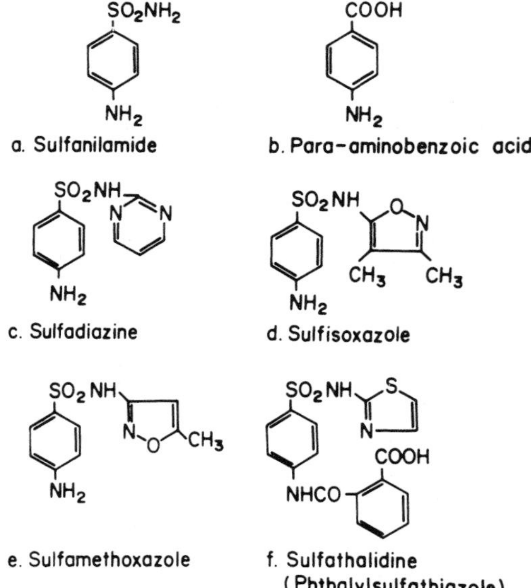

FIGURE 30–1. *A–F,* Structural formulas of selected sulfonamides.

Short- or Medium-Acting Sulfonamides. Sulfisoxazole (*United States Pharmacopeia* [USP]; sulphafurazole, *British Pharmacopeia* [BP]; 3,4-dimethyl-5-sulfanilamidoisoxazole; Gantrisin) is a highly soluble drug especially useful in urinary tract infections. Sulfamethoxazole USP (5-methyl-3-sulfanilamidoisoxazole; Gantanol) is somewhat less soluble than sulfisoxazole and yields higher blood levels. It is the sulfonamide most frequently combined with trimethoprim. Sulfadiazine USP (2-sulfanilamidopyridine; Microsulfon) is highly active, attains high blood and cerebrospinal fluid levels, and is associated with low protein binding and lower solubility than the drugs previously described. Sulfamethizole USP (2-sulfanilamide-5-methyl-1:3:4-thiazole; Thiosulfil) is used for urinary tract infections. Sulfadimidine and sulfacarbamide are available in the United Kingdom.

Short-acting sulfonamides are also available in several combinations. Sulfisoxazole and sulfamethoxazole have been combined with phenazopyridine, a urinary analgesic, as Azo Gantrisin and Azo Gantanol or Azo-Urizole and Microsul-A. Phenazopyridine is also present with sulfamethizole and sulfadiazine in Suladyne.

Long-Acting Sulfonamides. Sulfamethoxypyridazine (3-sulfanilamido-5-methoxy-pyridazine) and sulfameter [4-amino-*N*-(5-methoxy-2-pyrimidinyl)] benzene-sulfonamide are no longer available for single-daily-dose therapy, since they were associated with hypersensitivity reactions such as Stevens-Johnson syndrome. Neither sulfadimethoxine (Madribon) nor any other long-acting sulfonamides other than sulfadoxine are currently available in the United States.

Sulfadoxine, originally known as sulformethoxine (*N*′-[5,6-dimethoxy-4-pyrimidyl]sulfanilamide) is a very long-acting sulfonamide that, combined with pyrimethamine, is available as Fansidar. Sulfadoxine has a half-life of 100 to 230 hours and reaches a peak serum level of 51 to 76 μg/ml 2.5 to 6 hours after an oral dose of 500 mg. Fansidar is active in the treatment and prophylaxis of malaria caused by chloroquine-resistant *Plasmodium falciparum.*[3] Because of the unknown teratogenic potential of pyrimethamine, Fansidar should not be recommended for prophylaxis of pregnant women, and its use has been associated with Stevens-Johnson syndrome. Also, some strains of *P. falciparum* from Southeast Asia and South America may be resistant.

Sulfonamides Limited to the Gastrointestinal Tract. Sulfaguanidine (*N*′-amidinosulfanilamide), sulfasuxidine (2-[para-succinylsulfanilamido]-thiazole, succinylsulfathiazole), and sulfathalidine (2[para-phthalyl-sulfanilamido]-thiazole) are relatively poorly absorbed from the gastrointestinal tract. They have been used in the past to suppress the susceptible bowel flora before surgery.

Salicylazosulfapyridine (sulfasalazine, Azulfidine) is a sulfonamide derivative used in the treatment of ulcerative colitis. This drug is absorbed in its parent form as sulfapyridine, and significant blood levels of this compound are measurable.

Topical Sulfonamides. Mafenide acetate (para-aminomethylbenzene sulfonamide, Sulfamylon cream) is available for use in the topical treatment of burns. However, its use has been limited by metabolic acidosis caused by carbonic anhydrase inhibition. Silver sulfadiazine (Silvadene cream) has fewer side effects and is used extensively for burns.[4] Here the sulfonamide acts primarily as a vehicle for release of silver ions that exert an antibacterial effect. Outbreaks of silver-resistant infections in burn units may ultimately limit its usefulness.[5, 6] Various combinations of other sulfonamides are available as vaginal creams or suppositories (e.g., Sultrin vaginal cream and tablets, Trysul vaginal cream, AVC cream and suppositories).

There are a variety of ophthalmic ointments and solutions of sulfacetamide sodium USP (a highly soluble sulfonamide) available for use in the treatment of conjunctivitis caused by susceptible bacteria and as adjunctive therapy for trachoma (e.g., Bleph-10, Cetamide, Blephamide, Sulamyd).

Mechanisms of Action

Although a wide variety of chemical modifications of the sulfonamides have been synthesized, all basically share the same mechanism of action. The sulfonamides are bacteriostatic in that they inhibit bacterial growth by interfering with microbial folic acid synthesis. More specifically, sulfonamides inhibit competitively the incorporation of PABA into tetrahydropteroic acid,[7–9] and they in turn may be incorporated into dihydropteroate.[10] Sulfonamides may have a higher affinity for the microbial enzyme tetrahydropteroic acid synthetase than the natural substrate PABA. Richmond[11] suggested that sulfonamides may act on bacterial repressor genes or by feedback inhibition to decrease formation of new enzyme. The ultimate result of decreased folic acid synthesis is a decrease in bacterial nucleotides, with subsequent inhibition of bacterial growth.

Antimicrobial Activity In Vitro

Sulfonamides exhibit in vitro inhibitory activity against a broad spectrum of gram-positive and gram-negative bacteria as well as *Actinomyces, Chlamydia, Plasmodium* and *Toxoplasma* (Table 30–1). The in vitro antimicrobial sensitivity of sulfonamides is strongly influenced by the size of the inoculum and the composition of the test medium, High concentrations of PABA and thymidine inhibit sulfonamide activity.

Antimicrobial Resistance

Resistance to sulfonamides is widespread and increasingly common in both community and nosocomial strains of bacteria, including streptococci, staphylococci, Enterobacteriaceae, *Neisseria* spp., and *Pseudomonas* spp.[12, 13] Cross-resistance among different sulfonamides is common.

Organisms may develop resistance or partial resistance by mutation, resulting in either microbial overproduction of PABA[14] or structural change in dihydropteroate synthetase that produces an enzyme with lowered affinity for sulfonamide.[15] PABA overproduction has been implicated in resistant strains of *Neisseria gonorrhoeae* and *Staphylococcus aureus*[14, 16]; altered dihydropteroate synthetase has been found in strains of *Escherichia coli.*[17] Resistance also may be

TABLE 30–1 In Vitro Activity of Sulfonamides against Representative Organisms

Organism	Range of MIC* (μg/ml)
Gram-positive organisms	
Staphylococcus aureus	8–64
Streptococcus pneumoniae	4–128
Streptococcus pyogenes	0.5–16
Enterococcus faecalis	25–250
Corynebacterium diphtheriae	25–75
Listeria monocytogenes	3–75
Bacillus anthracis	12–100
Gram-negative organisms	
Escherichia coli	4–64
Klebsiella spp.	8–128
Proteus mirabilis	8–128
Serratia marcescens	25–>1000
Salmonella spp.	16–128
Shigella spp.	2–32
Haemophilus influenzae	1–16
Neisseria gonorrhoeae	4–32
Neisseria meningitidis	0.25–>10
Pseudomonas aeruginosa	>100–200
Other organisms	
Chlamydia trachomatis	0.1
Nocardia asteroides	2–16

*Minimal inhibitory concentration (MIC). Range is expressed for a variety of sulfonamide compounds. The acquisition of plasmids may increase MICs.
Data from Garrod et al.,[29] Bushby,[30] and Bach et al.[31]

mediated by plasmids that code for the production of drug-resistant enzymes, such as dihydropteroate synthetase,[18] or decrease bacterial cell permeability to sulfonamides.[19] Plasmid transfer can occur in the gastrointestinal tract and in vitro and has been seen especially with multiple species of Enterobacteriaceae.[20]

Transformational exchanges of dihydropteroate synthetase among *Neisseria* spp. raise the specter of wider dissemination of sulfonamide resistance by chromosomal and plasmid genes.[21] Sulfonamide resistance genes also have been found in a common *Pseudomonas aeruginosa* integron, which may be facilitating the spread of resistance among aerobic gram-negative bacilli.[22] More than one resistance mechanism may be operating simultaneously.[23]

Plasmid-mediated sulfonamide resistance has greatly increased in recent years, often in conjunction with trimethoprim resistance. More than one fourth of the uropathogens and one half of the clinical *Shigella* isolates studied in Sweden,[24] England,[12, 25] and the United States[26] were sulfonamide resistant. *Salmonella* resistance to sulfonamides has also increased in the United States,[27] often in conjunction with resistance to other antibiotic classes. The increase in sulfonamide-resistant *Haemophilus ducreyi* in Asia and Africa has been associated with a plasmid related to those found in Enterobacteriaceae.[28]

Pharmacology

Routes of Administration. Sulfonamides are usually administered orally, although sulfadiazine and sulfisoxazole are available for use as intravenous or subcutaneous preparations. These latter forms are used rarely, if at all. Sulfacetamide is available as ophthalmic preparations; silver sulfadiazine and mafenide acetate are applied topically in burn patients and are associated with significant absorption of sulfonamide percutaneously. Vaginal preparations are available for topical application.

Absorption. Most of the short- and medium-acting sulfonamides are absorbed rapidly and almost completely in the un-ionized state from the small intestine and stomach. Compounds with *N*-1 substitutions are absorbed poorly, as are more acidic compounds (e.g., phthalylsulfathiazole; see Fig. 30–1*F*). Long-acting sulfonamides also are absorbed rapidly but have a much slower excretion rate. Topical sulfonamides are absorbed and may be detectable in blood.

Distribution. The sulfonamides generally are well distributed throughout the body, entering the cerebrospinal fluid and synovial, pleural, and peritoneal fluids with concentrations approaching 80% of serum levels. Blood and tissue levels are related to the degree of protein binding (Table 30–2) and lipid solubility. Sulfonamides administered in pregnancy readily cross the placenta and are present in the fetal blood and amniotic fluid.[33]

Excretion. Acetylation and glucuronidation occur in the liver, and free and metabolized drug appears in the urine. Glomerular filtration is probably a route of excretion, although partial reabsorption and active tubular secretion also are involved, especially at low creatinine clearance rates. Urinary excretion is more rapid for those sulfonamides with low pKa values (e.g., sulfamethizole, sulfisoxazole), and alkalinization of the urine increases excretion by this route. Plasma half-lives vary widely; they are related inversely to lipid solubility and directly to pKa values but are not clearly related to the degree of protein binding.[32] Small amounts of sulfonamides are found in bile, human milk, prostatic secretions, saliva, and tear.

Protein Binding and Blood or Tissue Levels. Sulfonamides are bound variably and not irreversibly to plasma albumin, and the bound drug is inactive (see Table 30–2). Levels obtainable in cerebrospinal and other body fluids are inversely related to the degree of protein binding. The amount of free drug in plasma is directly related to pKa.[32]

Use in Renal Insufficiency. Sulfonamides can be used in renal failure, but therapeutic serum levels will persist longer because of reduced excretion, and the dosage must be reduced and the interval between doses extended in proportion to the degree of renal impairment. Protein binding of sulfonamides is decreased in severe renal insufficiency.[34] The *N*-4 acetylated metabolite of sulfonamides can accumulate in patients with renal failure, especially during prolonged therapy. This derivative loses its antibacterial effect but still may have toxic properties. Plasma levels of sulfonamide should be measured every 3 days, and peak concentrations of sulfamethoxazole should be less than 120 μg/ml.

Toxicity and Adverse Reactions

Sulfonamides can cause nausea, vomiting, diarrhea, rash, fever, headache, depression, jaundice, hepatic necrosis, drug-induced lupus,[35] and a serum sickness–like syndrome. Earlier, less soluble compounds (sulfadiazine, sulfathiazole) used in excessively high doses were associated with crystalluria and tubular deposits of sulfonamide crystals. These complications could be minimized by maintenance of high urine flow and alkalinization of the urine. This complication usually is not seen with modern, soluble sulfonamides. Tubular necrosis, interstitial nephritis, or necrotizing angiitis may be associated rarely with sulfonamide sensitivity. Acute pancreatitis has been attributed to sulfonamide.[36]

More serious adverse reactions caused by sulfonamides may include acute hemolytic anemia sometimes related to a deficiency in erythrocyte glucose-6-phosphate dehydrogenase [G6PD], aplastic anemia, agranulocytosis, thrombocytopenia, and leukopenia. In one study, G6PD-deficient patients who received trimethoprim-sulfamethoxazole did not have hemolytic reactions during therapy.[37]

Sulfonamides should not be administered during the last month of pregnancy because they compete for bilirubin-binding sites on plasma albumin and may increase fetal blood levels of unconjugated bilirubin, increasing the risk of kernicterus. Also, because of the immature fetal acetyltransferase system, blood levels of free sulfonamide may be increased, further adversely affecting the risk of kernicterus.[32]

Finally, significant hypersensitivity reactions can occur with sulfonamides administered via any route. The most important of these are erythema nodosum, erythema multiforme (including Stevens-Johnson syndrome), drug eruption, vasculitis similar to periarteritis nodosa, and anaphylaxis. One report suggests that cutaneous reactions including toxic epidermal necrolysis may be related to an

TABLE 30–2 Levels in Blood, Cerebrospinal Fluid (CSF), Plasma Half-Life, and Protein Binding of Some Sulfonamides

Drug	Peak Blood Level* (μg/ml)	Level in CSF (%)	Plasma Half-Life (hs)	Protein Binding (%)
Sulfadiazine	30–60	40–80	17	45
Sulfisoxazole	40–50	30–50	5–6	92
Sulfamethoxazole	80–100	25–30	11	70
Sulfadoxine	50–75	20–30	100–230	80–98

*Approximate free sulfonamide level after a 2-g oral dose.
Data from Anand[32] and Garrod et al.[29]

inherited constitutional defect in detoxification of metabolites.[38] Long-acting sulfonamides have been associated with fatal hypersensitivity reactions, especially in children, and this severely limits their use. Locally applied sulfonamides (e.g., to skin) may be associated with any of these adverse reactions. The acute onset of hypotension and fever rarely has been associated with trimethoprim-sulfamethoxazole therapy in human immunodeficiency virus (HIV) infection.[39] Although the reaction resembles immunoglobulin E–mediated anaphylaxis, the specific cause and allergen are not clearly known.[40]

Drug Interactions

Sulfonamides may displace from albumin-binding sites drugs such as warfarin, thus increasing the effective activity of the displaced drug. Anticoagulant dosage therefore should be reduced during sulfonamide therapy. Sulfonamides also displace methotrexate from its bound protein, thereby increasing methotrexate toxicity. An increased hypoglycemic effect of chlorpropamide and tolbutamide may occur during sulfonamide therapy, possibly because of the same mechanism or structural similarities. Sulfonamides may potentiate the action of some thiazide diuretics, phenytoin, and uricosuric agents. Conversely, sulfonamides themselves can be displaced from binding sites by indomethacin, phenylbutazone, salicylates, probenecid, and sulfinpyrazone, resulting in increased sulfonamide activity.

The activity of sulfonamides may be decreased by procaine and other local anesthetics derived from PABA. Methenamine compounds should not be used with sulfonamides because of the formation of insoluble urinary precipitates. Intravenous solutions of sulfonamides are physically incompatible with chloramphenicol, aminoglycosides, lincomycin, methicillin, tetracyclines, vancomycin, norepinephrine, insulin, procaine, Ringer's lactate solution, and others. Sulfonamides may decrease protein-bound iodine and ^{131}I uptake and may produce false-positive Benedict tests for urine glucose and false-positive sulfosalicylic acid tests for urine proteins.[41, 42]

Major Clinical Use

Sulfonamides are used primarily in the treatment of acute urinary tract infections, but increasing resistance has diminished their effectiveness. Most first episodes of infection in the unobstructed urinary tract are caused by *E. coli* that are often sensitive to sulfonamides. Sulfisoxazole is administered orally in a usual dosage of 1 g four times daily. Because the infecting organism of any urinary tract infection may or may not be sensitive to sulfonamides, the choice of therapy should be based on appropriate sensitivity tests (see Chapter 62).

Sulfonamides are also quite effective in the treatment of infections caused by *Nocardia asteroides*. Therapy must include 4 to 6 g or more daily after a loading dose of 4 g and should be continued for 4 to 6 months or longer if necessary (see Chapter 244). Sulfonamides may be useful in combination with other antimycobacterial drugs for the management of infections caused by rifampin-resistant *Mycobacterium kansasii*.[43]

Sulfonamides are effective for prophylaxis against recurrent attacks of rheumatic fever associated with group A β-hemolytic streptococcal infections, but they are not effective as therapy for established streptococcal pharyngitis or in the eradication of these organisms from the upper respiratory tract.[44] Sulfonamide prophylaxis of close contacts of patients with meningitis caused by *Neisseria meningitidis* is effective if the infecting organism is known to be sulfonamide sensitive; the adult dose for sulfadiazine is 1 g every 12 hours for 2 days. However, rifampin or ciprofloxacin is preferred.

Long-term sulfisoxazole therapy has been efficacious in the management of chronic otitis media.[45] Sulfonamides have been used to treat toxoplasmosis in patients with or without acquired immunodeficiency syndrome (AIDS) and chloroquine-sensitive or chloroquine-resistant *P. falciparum* malaria (with pyrimethamine). Melioidosis, dermatitis herpetiformis, lymphogranuloma venereum, and chancroid have responded to sulfonamides. Nongonococcal urethritis due to *Chlamydia*, but not that due to *Ureaplasma urealyticum*, responds well to sulfonamide therapy (see Chapter 94). Sulfasalazine is used in the treatment of inflammatory bowel diseases.[46] Currently, sulfonamides are used most frequently in combination with trimethoprim (see later discussion).

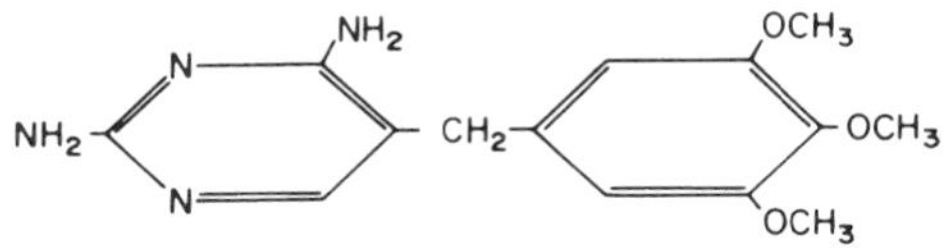

TRIMETHOPRIM

(2,4-diamino-5-(3′,4′,5′-trimethoxybenzyl)pyrimidine)

FIGURE 30–2. Chemical structure of trimethoprim.

TRIMETHOPRIM

Structure and Derivation

Trimethoprim is a 2,4-diamino-5-(3′,4′,5′-trimethoxybenzyl) pyrimidine (Fig. 30–2). This drug was synthesized by Bushby and Hitchings[2] as a dihydrofolate reductase inhibitor thought to potentiate the activity of sulfonamides by sequential inhibition of folic acid synthesis. In the United States, trimethoprim is now available as a single agent and in combination with sulfamethoxazole (cotrimoxazole) (see later discussion). Trimethoprim does have antibacterial activity of its own.

Mechanism of Action

Trimethoprim owes its activity to powerful inhibition of bacterial dihydrofolate reductase, which is the enzyme step after the step in folic acid synthesis blocked by sulfonamides. Trimethoprim is 50,000 to 100,000 times more active against bacterial dihydrofolate reductase than against the human enzyme. Trimethoprim interferes with the conversion of dihydrofolate to tetrahydrofolate, the precursor of folinic acid and ultimately of purine and DNA synthesis (Fig. 30–3). The sequential blockage of the same biosynthetic pathway by sulfonamides and trimethoprim results in a high degree of synergistic activity against a wide spectrum of microorganisms. Humans do not synthesize folic acid but require it in their diet, and therefore human purine synthesis is not affected significantly by the enzyme inhibition of trimethoprim.[47, 48]

Antimicrobial Activity

Trimethoprim is quite active in vitro against many gram-positive cocci and most gram-negative rods except for *P. aeruginosa* and *Bacteroides* spp. (Table 30–3). *Treponema pallidum, Mycobacterium tuberculosis, Mycoplasma* spp., and most anaerobes are resistant. Thymidine inhibits the in vitro activity of trimethoprim, but the

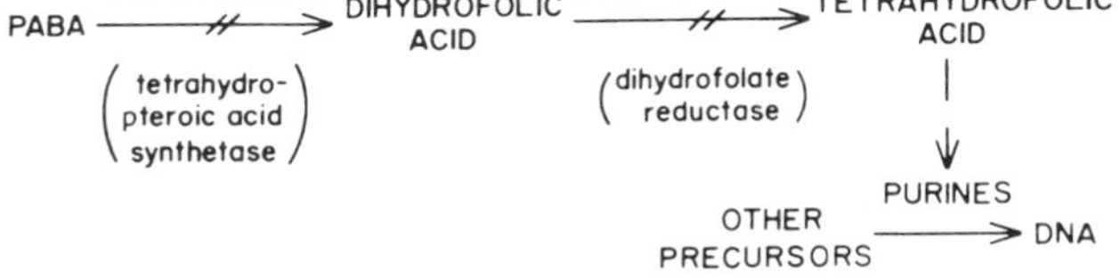

PABA —SULFONAMIDES (tetrahydropteroic acid synthetase)→ DIHYDROFOLIC ACID —TRIMETHOPRIM (dihydrofolate reductase)→ TETRAHYDROFOLIC ACID → PURINES; OTHER PRECURSORS → DNA

FIGURE 30–3. Action of sulfonamides and trimethoprim on the metabolic pathway of bacterial folic acid synthesis.

TABLE 30–3 In Vitro Activity of Trimethoprim against Representative Organisms

Organism	MIC Alone* (μg/ml)	MIC with Sulfamethoxazole (μg/ml, 1:20)†
Gram-positive organisms		
Staphylococcus aureus	0.15–2	0.04–1.6
Staphylococcus epidermidis	0.02	—
Streptococcus pneumoniae	0.004–5	0.05–1.5
Streptococcus pyogenes	0.02–1	0.015–0.4
Enterococcus faecalis	0.15–0.5	0.015–0.4†
Corynebacterium diphtheriae	0.15–0.5	0.05–0.15
Listeria monocytogenes	0.05–1.5	0.015–0.15
Clostridium perfringens	2–50	—
Propionibacterium acnes	0.07	—
Gram-negative organisms		
Escherichia coli	0.01–>5	0.005–>5
Klebsiella spp.	0.15–5	0.05–3.1
Proteus mirabilis	0.15–1.5	0.05–0.15
Serratia marcescens	0.8–50	0.4–50
Salmonella spp.	0.01–0.4	0.05–0.15
Shigella spp.	0.4–0.8	0.02–0.5
Citrobacter freundii	0.2	—
Vibrio cholerae	0.2	—
Haemophilus influenzae	0.1–12.5	0.004–50
Neisseria gonorrhoeae	0.2–128	0.15–3.1
Neisseria meningitidis	3.1–50	0.01–1.6
Pseudomonas aeruginosa	50–1000	3.1–100
Burkholderia cepacia	1–2	—
Stenotrophomonas maltophilia	1–>32	1–>32
Bacteroides fragilis	≥4.0	—
Other organisms		
Nocardia asteroides	3–100	1.5
Chlamydia trachomatis	20	—

*MIC varies with the method, inoculum size, and media used. Acquisition of residence plasmids may increase MICs.

†Minimal bactericidal concentration may be much higher.[52]

Abbreviation: MIC, Minimal inhibitory concentration.

Data from refs. 29–31 and 49–51.

addition of thymidine phosphorylase or 5% lysed horse blood to Mueller-Hinton or other sensitivity media removes this inhibition. The minimal inhibitory concentration (MIC) varies considerably with the medium used.[53] Trimethoprim alone has excellent in vitro activity against *H. influenzae* (most strains have MIC ≤0.25 μg/ml), *S. aureus,* and *Streptococcus pyogenes* (MICs ≤2 μg/ml).[54]

Potentiation of the action of trimethoprim is seen in combination with sulfamethoxazole (see Table 30–3). Antibacterial synergism has been demonstrated in vitro for trimethoprim and polymyxins[55] and for trimethoprim and aminoglycosides against some gram-negative bacilli.[56] The combination TMP-SMX is active in vitro against many isolates of *S. aureus,*[57] *S. pyogenes, Streptococcus pneumoniae, E. coli, Proteus mirabilis, Shigella* spp., *Salmonella* spp., *Burkholderia cepacia, Malleomyces pseudomallei, Yersinia enterocolitica, N. gonorrhoeae,*[58] and *Stenotrophomonas maltophilia.* Studies of children in areas of high incidence of penicillin-resistant pneumococci showed TMP-SMX resistance in 40% of isolates.[59] Similar resistance rates for TMP-SMX were found in an area of Mexico with low rates of penicillin resistance.[60]

Variable bactericidal effects have been noted when enterococci are tested against TMP-SMX.[52] The susceptibility of Enterobacteriaceae may vary greatly between locations and within the same location from year to year, owing to the spread of trimethoprim-resistant plasmids and transposons.[58] Almost all strains of *P. aeruginosa* are resistant in vitro to TMP-SMX.[57]

Trimethoprim combined with sulfamethoxazole or dapsone has been effective in the treatment of *Pneumocystis carinii* pneumonia in immunocompromised patients (see later discussion). *Listeria monocytogenes,*[61] *Moraxella catarrhalis,*[62] and atypical mycobacteria[63] have been shown to be susceptible to the combination TMP-SMX.

The optimal ratio for in vitro synergism of trimethoprim and sulfamethoxazole in combination is 1:20, but this ratio does not always obtain in vivo. The synergism seen depends somewhat on the sensitivity of the organism to each drug.

Resistance to Trimethoprim. Bacteria may develop trimethoprim resistance by several mechanisms, which can be chromosomal or plasmid mediated. Clinical resistance has increased. In one hospital in France,[58] trimethoprim-resistant Enterobacteriaceae (MIC ≥4 μg/ml) increased from 18 to 25% of isolates. A decrease in the ratio of strains resistant to both sulfamethoxazole and trimethoprim compared with strains resistant only to trimethoprim may reflect an increase in independent trimethoprim resistance, and this might be a useful monitoring parameter in hospitals.[64] Concomitant resistance to sulfonamides has increased greatly in East Asia.

Trimethoprim resistance may be caused by changes in cell permeability, loss of bacterial drug-binding capacity, and overproduction of or alterations in dihydrofolate reductase. Clinically the most important mechanism is plasmid-mediated dihydrofolate reductases that are resistant to trimethoprim.[65, 66]

Distinctive dihydrofolate reductases have been described in Enterobacteriaceae, *P. aeruginosa,* and *S. aureus.*[67, 68] They are frequently plasmid mediated[57, 58, 66–68] and may be disseminated by highly mobile transposons (such as Tn7) with wide host-species ranges.[69] Outbreaks caused by trimethoprim-resistant conjugative plasmids have been noted in Western and Eastern Europe,[66, 67, 69, 70] East Asia,[71] South America,[72] and the United States.[72, 73] Many of the outbreaks occurred in immunocompromised hosts, associated with resistance to multiple other antibiotic groups. Two groups of mutations in dihydrofolate reductase genes of *S. pneumoniae* were reported from South Africa. These changes were highly conserved and might have resulted from recombination by transformation.[74]

Local increases in trimethoprim resistance, particularly among Enterobacteriaceae, have been especially marked in developing countries,[75] with up to 20% of nosocomial clinical isolates resistant to trimethoprim. Also, fecal isolates from outpatient settings and day-care centers are increasingly resistant to trimethoprim.[76] With more than one third of the *E. coli* and *Salmonella* isolates resistant to trimethoprim in several South American and Asian nations, the use of this low-cost agent for the treatment of urinary tract infections and serious enteric infections is imperiled. Whether the clinical use of trimethoprim alone in some countries has resulted in increasing resistance to the combination is unclear. Monitoring of data from the Netherlands revealed that almost one half of Dutch *Shigella sonnei* isolates were resistant to TMP-SMX.[77] Concomitant trimethoprim and sulfonamide resistance may limit the utility of the combination against methicillin-resistant *S. aureus* and *Staphylococcus epidermidis.*[78]

Permeability changes may occur in the bacterial cell and result in resistance to both trimethoprim and sulfonamides. Thymine-requiring auxotrophs may also account for clinically significant resistance to both drugs. These mutants lack thymidylate synthetase and are probably less virulent than are sensitive strains.[79]

Pharmacology

Routes of Administration. Trimethoprim is available as 100-mg tablets for oral use. Trimethoprim is absorbed readily and almost completely from the gastrointestinal tract. Peak serum levels appear 1 to 4 hours after ingestion of 100 mg and approach 1 μg/ml. The coadministration of sulfamethoxazole does not affect the rate of absorption of serum levels of trimethoprim.

Trimethoprim is also available in fixed combination with sulfamethoxazole in a ratio of 1:5 for oral use (trimethoprim, 80 mg; sulfamethoxazole, 400 mg; Bactrim, Septra). Double-strength and quarter-strength pediatric tablets are available, as is an oral suspension containing 40 mg trimethoprim and 200 mg sulfamethoxazole per 5 ml. Intravenous trimethoprim (16 mg/ml) plus sulfamethoxazole (80 mg/ml) is available. When administered intravenously, 10 ml or 160 mg trimethoprim (with 800 mg sulfamethoxazole) produces a peak serum trimethoprim concentration of 3.4 μg/ml in 1 hour. After repeated doses, the peak trimethoprim concentration may approach 9 μg/ml.[80] Similar peak levels may be reached with oral therapy, but at 2 to 4 hours after administration.[81, 82]

Distribution. Trimethoprim is widely distributed in tissues and may appear in kidney, lung, and sputum in higher concentrations than in plasma, as well as in bile, saliva, human breast milk, and seminal fluid.[83] Trimethoprim is also found in prostatic fluid at two to three times the serum concentration, but lower levels may be present in patients with chronic prostatitis.[84] Cerebrospinal fluid concentrations are about 40% of serum levels.

Metabolism and Excretion. Approximately 60 to 80% of an administered dose of trimethoprim is excreted in the urine via tubular secretion within 24 hours. The remainder of the drug is excreted by the kidney in one of four oxide or hydroxyl derivatives. The urinary metabolites are bacteriologically inactive.[80] Trimethoprim is also excreted in the bile. The serum half-life ranges from 9 to 11 hours in healthy subjects and is prolonged in patients with renal insufficiency. Unlike sulfamethoxazole, the excretion rate of trimethoprim is increased with acidification of the urine, and serum protein binding (65 to 70%) does not decrease significantly with increasing degrees of uremia.[34] Urine concentrations in healthy subjects (60 to 1000 μg/ml) are usually in excess of the MIC of most urinary pathogens.[34] TMP-SMX can be given in the usual doses to patients with creatinine clearances of 30 ml/min or greater. One half of the usual daily dose can be given to patients with creatinine clearances of 15 to 30 ml/min, but TMP-SMX is not recommended for use in patients with clearances lower than 15 ml/min.[34, 85, 86] Both trimethoprim and non-acetylated sulfamethoxazole are removed by hemodialysis.[34] Patients needing chronic peritoneal dialysis can receive the equivalent of one double-strength TMP-SMX tablet every 48 hours.

Toxicity and Side Effects

The toxic and undesired effects of TMP-SMX include all those discussed previously for sulfonamides. Nausea, vomiting, diarrhea, anorexia, and hypersensitivity reactions are the most common.[87] Hospitalization rates are 5.6 and 2.8 per 100,000 discharges for drug-related skin disorders and hematologic reactions, respectively.[88] Rash and other adverse reactions including hypouricemia (after high-dose therapy)[89] and Sweet's syndrome (acute febrile neutrophilic dermatosis)[90] have been noted frequently in patients with AIDS.[91, 92] In one report, 40% of HIV-infected children had adverse reactions including erythema multiforme, neutropenia, and Stevens-Johnson syndrome.[93] Patients have been desensitized successfully with the use of oral regimens.[94, 95] Also, in patients with AIDS, transient diffuse pulmonary infiltrates and hypotension have been described after reexposure to TMP-SMX.[96, 97] In addition, impaired folate utilization may be seen in humans with prolonged administration. This usually manifests as a megaloblastic marrow, with hypersegmented polymorphonuclear leukocytes. Also leukopenia, thrombocytopenia, and granulocytopenia may be seen. One study suggested that this occurs in 1 case per 18,000 prescriptions and that elderly patients are at greater risk.[98] The administration of folinic acid usually prevents or treats effectively the antifolate effects of trimethoprim, and the latter drug's antibacterial efficacy is not impaired except possibly against enterococci. Pseudomembranous colitis has been described with TMP-SMX but is uncommon.[99] Renal dysfunction may occur in patients with preexisting renal disease, but this is reversible with dose reduction. Hyperkalemia also has been noted, especially after high doses and in patients with renal insufficiency,[100–102] and TMP-SMX may cause an increase in measured serum creatinine.[103] Drug-induced hepatitis has been reported,[104] and prolonged cholestasis with pruritis may occur rarely.[105] Fulminant hepatic failure and pancreatitis have been reported.[106] TMP-SMX–induced meningitis has been described,[107, 108, 113] and meningoencephalitis confirmed by magnetic resonance imaging has been reported.[109] Renal tubular acidosis has been reported in children undergoing treatment for acute lymphocytic leukemia.[110] Drug-induced hypoglycemia occurs infrequently,[111, 112] and rhabdomyolysis has been described in an HIV-infected patient.[113] Anterior uveitis and retinal hemorrhage have been described with trimethoprim alone and in combination with sulfamethoxazole,[114] as have reversible myopia and angle-closure glaucoma.[115]

Drug Interactions. Active levels of phenytoin may be increased markedly by TMP-SMX.[116] Also, concomitant administration of TMP-SMX and methotrexate results in decreased renal clearance of free methotrexate.[117] Severe pancytopenia may result.[117] Reversible inhibition of tubular creatinine excretion may be caused by trimethoprim in the presence of cyclosporine.[118] Serum rifampin levels may rise during concomitant therapy with TMP-SMX.[119] Through its inhibition of cytochrome P-450, fluconazole may decrease hypersensitivity reactions to TMP-SMX caused by hydroxylamine or other metabolites.[120] Although TMP-SMX may inhibit metabolism of some antiretroviral drugs, including lamivudine, saquinavir, and delavirdine,[121] the effect is minimal and does not require adjustment of antiretroviral drug dosage.

Trimethoprim Plus Other Antimicrobial Agents

Other sulfonamides, such as sulfamoxole, sulfadiazine, sulfadimidine, and sulfametrol, have been combined with trimethoprim, but more clinical studies are needed to recommend their use over the currently administered combination.[122–124] Trimethroprim-sulfadiazine was reported to be less likely to accumulate in the kidneys of elderly patients with impaired renal function than is TMP-SMX.[123] Combinations of trimethoprim with other agents such as rifampin,[125] polymyxin,[55] amikacin,[126, 127] and metronidazole[128] have been suggested or used. Extensive clinical experience with these combinations is lacking. Reports suggest that trimethoprim-dapsone is more efficacious for the treatment of *P. carinii* pneumonia than is dapsone alone.[91, 129]

Clinical Use

Urinary Tract Infections. TMP-SMX is useful in the treatment of recurrent or chronic urinary tract infections caused by sensitive organisms. Many Enterobacteriaceae are sensitive to the combined action of these drugs. The combination is also effective in acute pyelonephritis and cystitis (see Chapter 62), although either antibiotic alone could be appropriate for susceptible isolates.

Because trimethoprim accumulates in prostatic secretions, TMP-SMX is often effective in bacterial prostatitis,[84] as well as in orchitis and epididymitis caused by susceptible bacteria.

The usual dosage in an adult for the treatment of acute prostate or urinary infection is two tablets every 12 hours or one double-strength tablet every 12 hours. The pediatric dose for urinary tract infection is 150 to 185 mg/m^2 for trimethoprim and 750 to 925 mg/m^2 for sulfamethoxazole daily in two divided doses. Single-dose therapy with one or two double-strength tablets may be effective in some women with uncomplicated lower urinary tract infection,[130] but a trial suggested that 7 days of TMP-SMX was better than single-dose ofloxacin and was equivalent to 3-day treatment with the quinolone.[131] However, in patients with chronic tissue-invasive urinary tract infections, longer-term therapy of up to 6 weeks may be required.[132]

TMP-SMX has been shown to be useful in the long-term suppressive therapy of adults and children with chronic or recurrent urinary infections, and extremely low doses (one-half to one tablet at bedtime or every other night) are effective.[133] This approach has been effective in preventing recurrent urinary tract infections in children with vesicoureteral reflux.[134] Postcoital prophylactic TMP-SMX effectively reduces recurrent urinary tract infections related to intercourse.[135] Trimethoprim is thought to achieve effective concentrations in the vaginal secretions, and it is believed by some that it exerts its protective effect on reducing the number of recurrent infections in this manner despite the fact that TMP-SMX–resistant organisms may be present in the vaginal and stool flora.[136] Trimethoprim alone is effective therapy for uncomplicated and recurrent urinary infections in women. Usual doses are 100 to 200 mg twice daily,[136, 137] and nightly doses of 100 mg may be effective suppressive therapy.[137, 138] Trimethoprim alone has been thought by some to be preferable to the combination TMP-SMX for acute urinary tract infections and possibly for other infections as well.[139] However, trimethoprim-resistant organisms may increase with extended use.

Respiratory Tract Infections. TMP-SMX is effective in the treatment of acute bronchitis and pneumonitis caused by sensitive organisms, although it is not the treatment of choice for any single organism. TMP-SMX may be as effective as tetracyclines in the reduction of acute exacerbations in patients with chronic bronchitis,[139, 140] but full doses should be used. Although not usually considered for use in seriously ill patients with pneumonia, intravenously administered TMP-SMX may be effective in patients with infections caused by susceptible gram-negative bacteria.[141]

TMP-SMX may be as effective as ampicillin for the treatment of otitis media,[142] and it is effective in otitis externa[143] and sinusitis even with a 3-day course.[144] Also, 10-day treatment with TMP-SMX was equivalent to a single intramuscular dose of ceftriaxone in a large study of acute otitis media with effusion in children.[145] Ampicillin-resistant strains of *H. influenzae* and *M. catarrhalis* may be susceptible. TMP-SMX plus prednisone produced short- but not long-term resolution of this condition.[146, 147]

Gastrointestinal Infections. Although antibiotics per se prolong the carrier state in acute gastroenteritis caused by *Salmonella* spp., TMP-SMX may be effective in eliminating chronic *Salmonella* carriage, including carriage of *Salmonella typhi,* especially in patients older than 2 years of age. Typhoid fever also may be treated successfully with this combination, although the development of resistant strains has been increasingly reported.[58, 75] TMP-SMX is effective in shigellosis,[148] especially that caused by ampicillin-resistant strains; however, susceptibility testing is necessary given reports of plasmid-mediated outbreaks of resistant organisms.[149] Intravenous administration may be necessary for patients with some of these infections. TMP-SMX also may be effective in the treatment of diarrhea caused by enteropathogenic *E. coli* and in the treatment and prophylaxis of traveler's diarrhea with or without loperamide[150, 151] if the prevalence of resistant strains in the area to be visited is low. The combination may be a useful adjunct to fluids in the treatment of cholera[152]; however, plasmid-mediated trimethoprim resistance has been reported in East Asia.[153]

Sexually Transmitted Diseases. TMP-SMX may be effective in the treatment of uncomplicated gonorrhea when used in several dosage regimens (e.g., 2 tablets orally twice daily for 5 days, 4 tablets for 2 days, and a single dose of 8 tabs).[154, 155] For pharyngeal gonorrhea, especially that caused by penicillinase-producing *N. gonorrhoeae,* 9 tablets per day for 5 days had been recommended, but these regimens are no longer included in the Centers for Disease Control and Prevention guidelines for treatment of sexually transmitted diseases. Almost one half of the *N. gonorrhoeae* that were chromosomally resistant to penicillin in one study were resistant to TMP-SMX as well.[156] Nongonococcal urethritis caused by *Chlamydia trachomatis* may be treatable with the combination, but its activity is a result of the sulfonamide.[157] The combination is also effective therapy for chancroid and lymphogranuloma venereum. It is ineffective for syphilis. Trimethoprim plus sulfametrole has been successful as a single-dose regimen for chancroid,[124] but in recent years *H. ducreyi* resistance has increased significantly in East Africa, an endemic area.[158]

Other Infections. TMP-SMX is useful against brucellosis (long-term therapy for 6 weeks),[159] biliary tract infections, acute and chronic osteomyelitis,[160] periodontal infection,[161] paracoccidioidomycosis,[162] and nocardiosis.[163, 164] Successful responses to combination therapy have been described for melioidosis[165] and *B. cepacia* bacteremia.[166] Trimethoprim and sulfonamides have been used successfully in Whipple's disease,[167, 168] *S. maltophilia* infection,[169, 170] and Wegener's granulomatosis alone or as adjunctive therapy, but clinical responses vary with disease stage.[171, 172] TMP-SMX can be used to treat infections caused by *Mycobacterium chelonei, Mycobacterium fortuitum,* and *Cyclospora cayetanensis.*

Intravenous TMP-SMX has been useful in treating gram-negative rod bacteremia and staphylococcal bacteremia and endocarditis, although other agents may be preferred.[128, 173, 174] Reports have described nosocomial *S. aureus* infections with TMP-SMX–resistant strains.[175] TMP-SMX plus extended spectrum β-lactams, aminoglycosides, or both provides effective broad-spectrum antimicrobial coverage in the management of febrile neutropenic patients.[176, 177] Meningitis due to susceptible organisms may be successfully treated,[178, 179] but other agents are usually preferred. The combination may be effective in meningitis caused by *L. monocytogenes.*[61] Lyme disease has been treated successfully by the combination of TMP-SMX and roxithromycin.[180] One daily dose of TMP-SMX given for 5 days/week may prevent spontaneous bacterial peritonitis in patients with cirrhosis.[181]

The *Mycobacterium* species *kansasii, marinum,* and *scrofulaceum* are inhibited in vitro by TMP-SMX, and several clinical successes have been reported, often in combination with other agents.[43, 63, 182] TMP-SMX is being studied in combination with isoniazid and rifampin in the treatment of leprosy.[183]

Trimethoprim plus sulfalene and TMP-SMX have been used in the treatment of susceptible *P. falciparum* infections, although these combinations are not very active against multiply-resistant strains. HIV-infected patients with *Isospora belli* enteritis have had clinical responses after receiving TMP-SMX[184]; however, relapse after treatment is common, necessitating chronic suppressive therapy. The drug combination has been shown to decrease the duration of oocyst excretion in children with *C. cayetanensis* infection,[185] but TMP-SMX has no activity against other related coccidial parasites, such as *Cryptosporidium parvum.*

TMP-SMX is active against *Toxoplasma gondii* in vitro[186] and has been used clinically[187] but is not superior to first-line therapy with pyrimethamine-sulfadiazine. In preliminary studies, low doses (trimethoprim, 160 mg; sulfamethoxazole, 800 mg) appear promising for the prophylaxis of *T. gondii* infection in HIV-infected toxoplasma antibody-positive patients.[188]

Pneumocystis carinii *Infections.* TMP-SMX has been highly efficacious in the treatment of *P. carinii* pneumonia in immunocompromised patients with and without AIDS[91, 189–191] (see Chapter 260). Patients with AIDS frequently respond to therapy but have a higher incidence of adverse reactions, particularly neutropenia and rash. Although the toxicities are different, the efficacy and rate of drug reactions associated with systemic pentamidine are comparable.[192] Patients were more likely to manifest a hypersensitivity reaction while receiving TMP-SMX if they were less immunocompromised (i.e., had higher CD4-positive T-lymphocyte counts) and were treated for longer than 2 weeks, suggesting a role for intact cell-mediated immunity in the pathogenesis of these reactions.[193] The toxicities of a 3-week course of parenteral TMP-SMX for *P. carinii* pneumonia may be decreased if serum trimethoprim levels are monitored and maintained between 5 and 8 μg/ml.[194] Trimethoprim also has been used successfully with dapsone for treatment of mild to moderate *P. carinii* pneumonia.[129]

TMP-SMX has been used successfully for primary and secondary chemoprophylaxis of *P. carinii* pneumonia[91, 195, 196] and is generally selected as the first-line agent, but chronic use may be limited by toxicities such as rash or leukopenia.[39, 40] AIDS patients receiving *P. carinii* prophylaxis with TMP-SMX had fewer serious bacterial infections than those who received aerosolized pentamidine.[197, 198]

In randomized studies, trimethoprim, 160 mg, plus sulfamethoxazole, 800 mg, given daily was more effective than monthly aerosolized pentamidine for prophylaxis after an initial episode of *P. carinii* pneumonia,[199] and half of this daily dose was more efficacious in patients with less than 200 CD4+ cells/mm^3 and no prior *P. carinii* pneumonia.[200] *P. carinii* pneumonia prophylaxis in conjunction with antiretroviral therapy has been associated with enhanced survival in patients with AIDS.[201]

Prophylactic Therapy in Immunocompromised Patients. Several studies have presented evidence of a striking reduction in gram-negative rod bacteremia in neutropenic patients treated prophylactically with TMP-SMX (2 tablets twice daily or more until stools are free of Enterobacteriaceae), compared with untreated control neutropenic patients.[202, 203] Other studies have not universally shown benefit in preventing bacteremia in neutropenic patients with acute myelocytic leukemia.[204] Oral prophylaxis with TMP-SMX decreased the incidence of serious bacterial infections in patients with multiple myeloma.[205] TMP-SMX plus colistin compared favorably to ciprofloxacin except for gram-negative rod bacteremia in a prophylactic trial,[206] but in another study it was less effective than penicillin G in preventing viridans group streptococcal bacteremia.[207] TMP-SMX may prolong recovery from induction chemotherapy-induced neutropenia, as has been reported in some but not all studies,[208] and it may be associated with *C. difficile*–related diarrhea[209] or with the emergence of resistant organisms.[210] Its effective prophylactic use in chronic granulomatous disease has been reported.[211]

Trimethoprim Use in Pregnancy. The teratogenicity of trimethoprim in humans is not clearly defined, but this drug is not recommended for use in pregnancy. It is, however, well tolerated in pediatric populations.[212]

REFERENCES

1. Carithers HA. The first use of an antibiotic in America. Am J Dis Child. 1974;128:207–211.
2. Bushby SRM, Hitchings GH. Trimethoprim, a sulphonamide potentiator. Br J Pharmacol Chemother. 1968;33:72–90.
3. Pearson RD, Hewlett EL. Use of pyrimethamine-sulfadoxine (Fansidar) in prophylaxis against chloroquine-resistant *Plasmodium falciparum* and *Pneumocystis carinii*. Ann Intern Med. 1987;106:714–718.
4. Ballin JC. Evaluation of a new topical agent for burn therapy. Silver sulfadiazine (Silvadene). JAMA. 1974;230:1184–1185.
5. Mayer KH, Hopkins JD, Gilleece ES, et al. Molecular evolution, species distribution, and clinical consequences of an endemic aminoglycoside resistance plasmid. Antimicrob Agents Chemother. 1986;29:628–633.
6. McHugh G, Moellering RC Jr, Hopkins CC, et al. *Salmonella typhimurium* resistant to silver nitrate, chloramphenicol and ampicillin: A new threat in burn units? Lancet. 1975;1:235–240.
7. Woods DD. Relation of p-aminobenzoic acid to mechanism of action of sulphanilamide. Br J Exp Pathol. 1940;21:74–90.
8. Fildes P. Rational approach to research in chemotherapy. Lancet. 1940;1:955–957.
9. Miller AK, Bruno P, Berglund RM. The effect of sulfathiazole on the in vitro synthesis of certain vitamins by *Escherichia coli*. J Bacteriol. 1947;54:9.
10. Brown GH. The biosynthesis of pteridines. Adv Enzymol. 1971;35:35–77.
11. Richmond MH. Structural analogy and chemical reactivity in the action of antibacterial compounds. In: Biochemical Studies of Antimicrobial Drugs. Proceedings of the Sixteenth Symposium of the Society of General Microbiology. London: Cambridge University Press; 1966:301.
12. Hamilton-Miller JMT. Mechanisms and distribution of bacterial resistance to diaminopyrimidines and sulphonamides. J Antimicrob Chemother. 1979;5(Suppl B):61–73.
13. Mennish ML, Salam MA, Hossain MA, et al. Antimicrobial resistance of *Shigella* isolates in Bangladesh, 1983–1990: Increasing frequency of strains multiply resistant to amipicillin, trimethoprim-sulfamethoxazole, and nalidixic acid. Clin Infect Dis. 1992;14:1055–1060.
14. Landy M, Larkun NW, Oswald EJ, et al. Increased synthesis of p-aminobenzoic acid associated with the development of resistance in *Staphylococcus aureus*. Science. 1943;97:265–267.
15. Wolf B, Hotchkiss RD. Genetically modified folic acid synthesising enzymes in *Pneumococcus*. Biochemistry. 1940;2:145–150.
16. Landy M, Gerstung RB. p-Aminobenzoic acid synthesis by *Neisseria gonorrhoeae* in relation to clinical and cultural sulfonamide resistance. J Bacteriol. 1944;47:448.
17. Swedberg G, Castenssos S, Sköld O. Characterization of mutationally altered dihydropteroate synthase and its ability to form a sulfonamide-containing dihydrofolate analog. J Bacteriol. 1979;137:129–136.
18. Sköld O: R-factor mediated resistance to sulfonamides by a plasmid-borne, drug resistant dihydropteroate synthase. Antimicrob Agents Chemother. 1976;9:49–54.
19. Kabins SA, Panse MV, Cohen S. Role of R-factor and bacterial host in sulfonamide resistance mediated by R-factor in *Escherichia coli*. J Infect Dis. 1971;123:158–168.
20. Watanabe T. Infective heredity of multiple drug resistance in bacteria. Bacteriol Rev. 1963;27:87–115.
21. Radstrom P, Fermer C, Kristiansen BE, et al. Transformational exchanges in the dihydropteroate synthase gene of *Neisseria meningitidis:* A novel mechanism for acquisition of sulfonamide resistance. J Bacteriol. 1992;174:6386–6393.
22. Bissonnette L, Roy PH. Characterization of InO of *Pseudomonas aeruginosa* plasmid pVS1, an ancestor of integrons of multiresistance plasmids and transposons of gram-negative bacteria. J Bacteriol. 1992;174:1248–1257.
23. Then RL. Mechanisms of resistance to trimethoprim, the sulfonamides and trimethoprim-sulfamethoxazole. Rev Infect Dis. 1982;4:261–269.
24. Hansson HB, Walder M, Juhlin I. Susceptibility of shigellae to mecillinam, nalidixic acid, trimethoprim, and five other antimicrobial agents. Antimicrob Agents Chemother. 1981;19:271–274.
25. Davies JR, Farrant WN, Uttley AHC. Antibiotic resistance of *Shigella sonnei*. Lancet. 1970;2:1157–1160.
26. Gordon RC, Thompson TR, Carlson W, et al. Antimicrobial resistance of shigellae isolated in Michigan. JAMA. 1975;231:1159–1164.
27. Ryder RW, Blake PA, Murlin AC, et al. Increase in antibiotic resistance among isolate of salmonella in the United States, 1967–1975. J Infect Dis. 1980;142:485–491.
28. Albritton WL, Brunton JL, Slaney L, Maclean I. Plasmid-mediated sulfonamide resistance in *Haemophilus ducreyi*. Antimicrob Agents Chemother. 1982;21:159–166.
29. Garrod LP, Lambert HP, O'Grady F. Antibiotic and Chemotherapy. 4th ed. Edinburgh and London: Churchill Livingstone; 1973.
30. Bushby SRM. Trimethoprim-sulfamethoxazole: In vitro microbiologic aspects. J Infect Dis. 1973;128:S442–S62.
31. Bach MC, Finland M, Gold W, et al. Susceptibility of recently isolated pathogenic bacteria to trimethoprim and sulfamethoxazole separately and combined. J Infect Dis. 1973;128:S508–S533.
32. Anand N. Sulfonamides and sulfones. In: Corcoran JW, Hahn FE, eds. Antibiotics III: Mechanism of Action of Antimicrobial and Antitumor Agents. Berlin: Springer-Verlag; 1975:668.
33. Sparr RA, Pritchard JA. Maternal and newborn distribution and excretion of sulfamethoxypyridazine (Kynex). Obstet Gynecol. 1958;12:131–134.
34. Craig WA, Kunin CM. Trimethoprim-sulfamethoxazole: Pharmacodynamic effects of urinary pH and impaired renal function. Ann Intern Med. 1973;78:491–497.
35. Price EJ, Venables PJ. Drug-induced lupus. Drug Safety. 1995;12:283.
36. Bartels RH, van der Spek JA, Oosten HR. Acute pancreatitis due to sulfamethoxazole-trimethoprim. South Med J. 1992;85:1006–1007.
37. Markowitz N, Saravolatz LD. Use of trimethoprim-sulfamethoxazole in a glucose-6-phosphate dehydrogenase-deficient population. Rev Infect Dis. 1987;9:S218–S225.
38. Wolkenstein P, Charue D, Laurent P, et al. Metabolic predisposition to cutaneous adverse drug reactions: Role in toxic epidermal necrolysis caused by sulfonamides and anticonvulsants. Arch Dermatol. 1995;131:544.
39. Kelly JW, Dooley DP, Lattuada CP, et al. A severe, unusual reaction to trimethoprim-sulfamethoxazole in patients infected with human immunodeficiency virus. Clin Infect Dis. 1992;14:1034–1039.
40. Johnson MP, Goodwin SD, Shands JW Jr. Trimethoprim-sulfamethoxazole anaphylactoid reactions in patients with AIDS: Case reports and literature review. Pharmacotherapy. 1990;10:413–416.
41. Dunea G, Freedman P. Proteinuria. JAMA. 1968;203:973–984.
42. Stockley IH. Drug Interactions. 2nd ed. Oxford: Blackwell Scientific Publications; 1991.
43. Ahn CH, Wallace RJ Jr, Steel LC, et al. Sulfonamide-containing regimens for disease caused by rifampin-resistant *Mycobacterium kansasii*. Am Rev Respir Dis. 1987;135:10–16.
44. Gerber MA. Antibiotic resistance: relationship to persistence of group A streptococci in the upper respiratory tract. Pediatrics. 1996;97:971.
45. Bernard PA, Stenstrom RJ, Feldman W, et al. Randomized controlled trial comparing long-term sulfonamide therapy to ventilation tubes for otitis media with effusion. Pediatrics. 1991;88:215–222.
46. Peppercorn MA. Sulfasalazine: Pharmacology, clinical use, toxicity, and related new drug development. Ann Intern Med. 1984;3:377–384.
47. Burchall JJ. Trimethoprim and pyrimethamine. In: Corcoran JW, Hahn FE, eds. Antibiotics III: Mechanism of Antimicrobial and Antitumor Agents. Berlin: Springer-Verlag; 1975:304.
48. Hitchings GT. The biochemical basis for the antimicrobial activity of septrin. In: Bernstein LS, Salter AJ, eds. Trimethoprim/sulphamethoxazole in Bacterial Infections. Edinburgh and London: Churchill Livingstone; 1973:7–16.
49. Phillips I, Warren C. Activity of sulfamethoxazole and trimethoprim against *Bacteroides fragilis*. Antimicrob Agents Chemother. 1976;9:736–740.
50. Trehane JD, Day J, Yeo CK, et al. Susceptibility of chlamydiae to chemotherapeutic agents. In: Hobsen D, Holmes KK, eds. Nongonococcal Urethritis and Related Infections. Washington, DC: American Society for Microbiology; 1977:214–222.
51. Moody MR, Young VM. In vitro susceptibility of *Pseudomonas cepacia* and

Pseudomonas maltophilia to trimethoprim and trimethoprim-sulfamethoxazole. Antimicrob Agents Chemother. 1975;7:836–839.

52. Najjar A, Murray BE. Failure to demonstrate a consistent in vitro bactericidal effect of trimethoprim-sulfamethoxazole against enterococci. Antimicrob Agents Chemother. 1987;31:808–810.
53. Dornbusch K, Moore WB. The effects of different media on the response of bacteria to sulphonamides and trimethoprim using the disc-diffusion method and regression line analysis. In: Bernstein LS, Salter AJ, eds. Trimethoprim/Sulphamethoxazole in Bacterial Infections. Edinburgh and London: Churchill Livingstone; 1973:39–51.
54. Eliopoulos GM, Wennersten CB: In vitro activity of trimethoprim alone compared with trimethoprim-sulfamethoxazole and other antimicrobials against bacterial species associated with upper respiratory tract infections. Diag Microbiol Infect Dis. 1997;29:33.
55. Simmons NA. Colistin, sulphamethoxazole and trimethoprim in synergy against gram-negative bacilli. J Clin Pathol. 1970;23:757–764.
56. Parsley TL, Provonchee RB, Glicksman C, et al. Synergistic activity of trimethoprim and amikacin against gram-negative bacilli. Antimicrob Agents Chemother. 1977;12:349–354.
57. Bushby SRM. Sensitivity patterns and use of a combined disc of trimethoprim-sulphamethoxazole. In: Bernstein LS, Salter AJ, eds. Trimethoprim/Sulphamethoxazole in Bacterial Infections. Edinburgh and London: Churchill Livingstone; 1973:31–38.
58. Goldstein FW, Papadopoulou B, Acar JF. The changing of trimethoprim resistance in Paris, with a review of worldwide experience. Rev Infect Dis. 1986;8:725–737.
59. Mainous AG 3rd, Evans ME, Hueson WJ, et al. Patterns of antibiotic-resistant *Streptococcus pneumoniae* in children in a day-care setting. J Fam Pract. 1998;46:142.
60. Miranda Novales MG, Solorzano Santos, F, Guiscaafre Gallardo H, et al. *Streptococcus pneumoniae*: Low frequency of penicillin resistance and high resistance to trimethoprim-sulfamethoxazole in nasopharyngeal isolates from children in a rural area in Mexico. Arch Med Res. 1997;28:559.
61. Armstrong RW, Slater B. *Listeria monocytogenes* meningitis treated with trimethoprim-sulfamethoxazole. Pediatr Infect Dis J. 1986;5:712–713.
62. Doern GV, Brueggemann AB, Pierce AG, et al. Prevalence of antimicrobial resistance among 723 outpatient clinical isolates of *Moraxella catarrhalis* in the United States in 1994 and 1995: Results of a 30-center national surveillance study. Antimicrob Agents Chemother. 1996;40:2884.
63. Wallace RJ Jr, Swanson JM, Silcox VA, et al. Treatment of nonpulmonary infections due to *Mycobacterium fortuitum* and *Mycobacterium chelonei* based on in vitro susceptibility. J Infect Dis. 1985;152:500–514.
64. O'Brien TF, Acar JF, Altmann G, et al. Laboratory surveillance of synergy between and resistance to trimethoprim and sulfonamides. Rev Infect Dis. 1982;4:351–357.
65. Burchall JJ, Pelwell L, Fling ME. Molecular mechanisms of resistance to trimethoprim. Rev Infect Dis. 1982;4:246–254.
66. Houvinen P. Trimethoprim resistance. Antimicrob Agents Chemother. 1987;31:1451–1456.
67. Goldstein FW, Labigne-Roussel A, Gerbaud G, et al. Transferable plasmid-mediated antibiotic resistance in *Acinetobacter.* Plasmid. 1983;10:138–147.
68. Jorgensen JH. Update on mechanisms and prevalence of antimicrobial resistance in *Haemophilus influenzae*. Clin Infect Dis. 1992;14:1119–1123.
69. Steen R, Sköld O. Plasmid-borne or chromosomally mediated resistance by Tn7 is the most common response to ubiquitous use of trimethoprim. Antimicrob Agents Chemother. 1985;27:933–937.
70. Bratoeva MP, Jorh JF, Barg NL. Molecular epidemiology of trimethoprim-resistant *Shigella boydii* serotype 2 strains from Bulgaria. J Clin Microbiol. 1992;30:1428–1431.
71. Goldstein FW, Chumpitaz JC, Guevara JM, et al. Plasmid-mediated resistance to multiple antibiotics in *Salmonella typhi*. J Infect Dis. 1986;153:261–266.
72. O'Brien TF, Hopkins JD, Gilleece ES, et al. Molecular epidemiology of antibiotic resistance in *Salmonella* from animals and human beings in the United States. N Engl J Med. 1982;307:1–6.
73. Mayer KH, Fling ME, Hopkins JD, et al. Trimethoprim resistance in multiple genera of Enterobacteriaceae at a U.S. hospital: Spread of the type II dihydrofolate reductase gene by a single plasmid. J Infect Dis. 1985;5:783–789.
74. Adrian PV, Klugman KP. Mutations in the dihydrofolate reductase gene of trimethoprim-resistant isolates of *Streptococcus pneumoniae*. Antimicrob Agents Chemother. 1997;41:2406.
75. Murray BE, Alvardo T, Kim K-H, et al. Increasing resistance to trimethoprim-sulfamethoxazole among isolates of *Escherichia coli* in developing countries. J Infect Dis. 1985;152:1107–1113.
76. Reves RR, Fong M, Pickering LK, et al. Risk factors for fecal colonization with trimethoprim-resistant and multiresistant *Escherichia coli* among children in day-care centers in Houston, Texas. Antimicrob Agents Chemother. 1990;34:1429–1434.
77. Voogd CE, Schot CS, van Leeuwen WJ, et al. Monitoring of antibiotic resistance in shigellae isolated in The Netherlands 1984–1989. Eur J Clin Microbiol Infect Dis. 1992;11:164–167.
78. Then RL, Kohl I, Burdeska A. Frequency and transferability of trimethoprim sulfonamide resistance in methicillin-resistant *Staphylococcus aureus* and *Staphylococcus epidermidis*. J Chemother. 1992;4:67–71.
79. Smith HW, Tucker JF. The virulence of trimethoprim resistant thymine-requiring strains of Salmonella. J Hyg (Lond). 1976;76:97–108.
80. Grose WE, Bodey GP, Loo TL. Clinical pharmacology of intravenously administered trimethoprim-sulfamethoxazole. Antimicrob Agents Chemother. 1979;15:447–451.
81. Bach MC, Gold O, Finland M. Absorption and urinary excretion of trimethoprim, sulfamethoxazole, and trimethoprim-sulfamethoxazole: Results with single doses in normal young adults and preliminary observations during therapy with trimethoprim-sulfamethoxazole. J Infect Dis. 1973;128:S584–S598.
82. Kaplan SA, Weinfeld RE, Abruzzo CW, et al. Pharmacokinetic profile of trimethoprim-sulfamethoxazole in man. J Infect Dis. 1973;128:S547–S555.
83. Pater RB, Welling PG. Clinical pharmacokinetics of co-trimoxazole (trimethoprim/sulfamethoxazole). Clin Pharmacokinet. 1980;5:405–423.
84. Meares EM Jr. Prostatitis: Review of pharmacokinetics and therapy. Rev Infect Dis. 1982;4:475–483.
85. Welling PG, Craig WA, Amidon GL, et al. Pharmacokinetics of trimethoprim and sulfamethoxazole in normal subjects and in patients with renal failure. J Infect Dis. 1974;128(Suppl):556–566.
86. Salter AJ. Trimethoprim-sulfamethoxazole: An assessment of more than 12 years of use. Rev Infect Dis. 1982;4:196–236.
87. Jick H. Adverse reactions to trimethoprim-sulfamethoxazole in hospitalized patients. Rev Infect Dis. 1982;4:426–428.
88. Myers MW, Jick H. Hospitalization for serious blood and skin disorders following cotrimoxazole. Br J Clin Pharmacol. 1997;43:649.
89. Chertow GM, Seifter JL, Christiansen CL, O'Donnell WJ. Trimethoprim-sulfamethoxazole and hypouricemia. Clin Nephrol. 1996;46:193.
90. Walker DC, Cohen PR. Trimethoprim-sulfamethoxazole-associated acute febrile neutrophilic dermatosis: Case report and review of drug-induced Sweet's syndrome. J Am Acad Dermatol. 1996;34:918.
91. Masur H, Kovacs JA. Treatment and prophylaxis of *Pneumocystis carinii* pneumonia. In: Moellering RC Jr, ed. Infectious Disease Clinics of North America (Medical Management of AIDS). Philadelphia: WB Saunders; 1988:419–428.
92. van der Ven AJ, Koopmans PP, Vree TB, et al. Adverse reaction to cotrimoxazole in HIV infection. Lancet. 1991;338:431–433.
93. Reider MJ, King SM, Read S. Adverse reactions to trimethoprim-sulfamethoxazole among children with human immunodeficiency virus infection. Pediatr Infect Dis J. 1997;16:1028.
94. Kalanadhabhatta V, Muppidi D, Sahni H, et al. Successful oral desensitization to trimethoprim-sulfamethoxazole in acquired immune deficiency syndrome. Ann Allergy Asthma Immunol. 1996;77:394.
95. Gluckstein D, Ruskin J. Rapid oral desensitization to trimethoprim-sulfamethoxazole (TMP-SMZ): Use in prophylaxis for *Pneumocystis carinii* pneumonia in patients with AIDS who were previously intolerant to TMP-SMZ. Clin Infect Dis. 1995;20:849.
96. Silvestri RC, Jensen WA, Zibrak JD, et al. Pulmonary infiltrates and hypoxemia in patients with the acquired immunodeficiency syndrome re-exposed to trimethoprim-sulfamethoxazole. Am Rev Respir Dis. 1987;136:1003–1004.
97. Kelly JW, Dooley DP, Lattuada CP, et al. A severe, unusual reaction to trimethoprim-sulfamethoxazole in patients infected with human immunodeficiency virus. Clin Infect Dis. 1992;14:1034–1039.
98. Keisu M, Wiholm BE, Palmblad J. Trimethoprim-sulphamethoxazole–associated blood dyscrasias: Ten years experience of the Swedish spontaneous reporting system. J Intern Med. 1990;228:353–356.
99. Cameron A, Thomas M. Pseudomembranous colitis and co-trimoxazole. BMJ. 1977;1:1321.
100. Alappan R, Perazella MA, Buller GK. Hyperkalemia in hospitalized patients treated with trimethoprim-sulfamethoxazole. Ann Intern Med. 1996;124:316.
101. Hsu I, Wordell CJ. Hyperkalemia and high-dose trimethoprim/sulfamethoxazole. Ann Pharmacother. 1995;29:427.
102. Perazella MA, Mahnensmith RL. Trimethoprim-sulfamethoxazole: Hyperkalemia is an important complication regardless of dose. Clin Nephrol. 1996;46:187.
103. Trollfors B, Wahl M, Alestig K. Co-trimoxazole, creatinine and renal function. J Infect. 1980;2:221.
104. Vial T, Biour M, Descotes J, Trepo C. Antibiotic-associated hepatitis: Update from 1990. Ann Pharmacother. 1997;31:204.
105. Kowdley KV, Keefe EB, Fawaz KA. Prolonged cholestasis due to trimethoprim-sulfamethoxazole. Gastroenterology. 1992;102:2148–2150.
106. Alberti-Flor JJ, Hernandez ME, Ferrer JP, et al. Fulminant liver failure and pancreatitis associated with the use of sulfamethoxazole-trimethoprim. Am J Gastroenterol. 1989;84:1577–1579.
107. Escalante A, Stimmler MM. Trimethoprim-sulfamethoxazole induced meningitis in systemic lupus erythematosus. J Rheumatol. 1992;19:800–802.
108. Derhes SJ. Trimethoprim-induced aseptic meningitis, JAMA. 1984;252:2865–2867.
109. Blumenfeld H, Cha JH, Cudkowicz ME. Trimethoprim and sulfonamide-associated meningoencephalitis with MRI correlates. Neurology. 1996;36:556.
110. Murphy JL. Renal tubular acidosis in children treated with trimethoprim-sulfamethoxazole during therapy for acute lymphoid leukemia. Pediatrics. 1992;89:1072–1074.
111. Northrop CV, Shepherd SM, Abbuhl S. Sulfonamide-induced iritis. Am J Emerg Med. 1996;14:577.
112. Lee AJ, Maddix DS. Trimethoprim/sulfamethoxazole-induced hypoglycemia in a patient with acute renal failure. Ann Pharmacother. 1997;31:727.
113. Anders HJ, Bogner JR, Goebel FD. Mild rhabdomyolysis after high-dose trimethoprim-sulfamethoxazole in a patient with HIV infection. Eur J Med Res. 1997;2:198.
114. Kristinsson JK, Hannesson OB, Sveinsson O. Bilateral anterior uveitis and retinal haemorrhages after administration of trimethoprim. Acta Ophthalmol Scand. 1997;75:314.
115. Postel EA, Assalian A, Epstein DL. Drug-induced transient myopia and angle-

closure glaucoma associated with supraciliary choroidal effusion. Am J Ophthalmol. 1996;122:110.
116. Hansen JM, Kampmann JP, Siersback-Nielsen K, et al. The effect of different sulfonamides on phenytoin metabolism in man. Acta Med Scand. 1979;624(Suppl):106–110.
117. Ferrazzini G, Klein J, Sulh H, et al. Interaction between trimethoprim-sulfamethoxazole and methotrexate in children with leukemia. J Pediatr. 1990;117:823–826.
118. Maki DG, Fox BC, Kuntz J, et al. A prospective, randomized, double-blind study of trimethoprim-sulfamethoxazole for prophylaxis of infection in renal transplantation: Side effects of trimethoprim-sulfamethoxazole, interaction with cyclosporine. J Lab Clin Med. 1991;119:11–24.
119. Bhatia RS, Uppal R, Malhi R, et al. Drug interaction between rifampicin and cotrimoxazole in patients with tuberculosis. Hum Exp Toxicol. 1991;10:419–421.
120. Gill HJ, Maggs JL, Madden S, et al. The effect of fluconazole and ketoconazole on the metabolism of sulphamethoxazole. Br J Clin Pharmacol. 1996;42:347.
121. Taburet AM, Singlas E: Drug interactions with antiviral drugs. Clin Pharmacokinet. 1996;30:385.
122. Bernstein LS. Combination of trimethoprim with sulfonamides other than sulfamethoxazole. Rev Infect Dis. 1982;4:411–418.
123. Bergan T, Allgulander S, Fellner H. Pharmacokinetics of co-trimazine (sulphadiazine plus trimethoprim) in geriatric patients. Chemotherapy. 1986;32:478–485.
124. Dylewski J, D'Costa LJ, Nsanze H, et al. Single dose therapy with trimethoprim-sulfametrol for chancroid in females. Sex Transm Dis. 1986;13:166–168.
125. Alvarez S, DeMaria A Jr, Kulkarni R, et al. Interactions of rifampin and trimethoprim in vitro. Rev Infect Dis. 1982;4:390–401.
126. Zinner SH, Lagast H, Kasry A, et al. Synergism of trimethoprim combined with aminoglycosides in vitro and in serum of volunteers. Eur J Clin Microbiol. 1982;1:144–148.
127. Engervall P, Gunther G, Ljungman P, et al. Trimethoprim-sulfamethoxazole plus amikacin versus ceftazidime monotherapy as empirical treatment in patients with neutropenia and fever. Scand J Infect Dis. 1996;28:297.
128. Salter AJ. Trimethoprim-sulfamethoxazole in treatment of severe infections. Rev Infect Dis. 1982;4:338–350.
129. Glatt A, Chirgwin K. *Pneumocystis carinii* pneumonia in human immunodeficiency virus-infected patients. Arch Intern Med. 1990;150:271–279.
130. Tolkoff-Rubin NE, Weber D, Fang LST, et al. Single dose therapy with trimethoprim-sulfamethoxazole for urinary infection in women. Rev Infect Dis. 1982;4:444–448.
131. Hooton TM, Johnson C, Winter C, et al. Single-dose and three-day regimens of ofloxacin versus trimethoprim-sulfamethoxazole for acute cystitis in women. Antimicrob Agents Chemother. 1991;35:1479–1483.
132. Gleckman R, Crowley M, Natsios GA. Treatment of recurrent invasive urinary tract infections of men. N Engl J Med. 1979;301:878–880.
133. Harding GKM, Ronald AR, Nicolle LE, et al. Long-term antimicrobial prophylaxis for recurrent urinary tract infection in women. Rev Infect Dis. 1982;4:438–443.
134. Hori C, Hiraoka M, Tsukahara H, et al. Intermittent trimethoprim-sulfamethoxazole in children with vesicoureteral reflux. Pediatr Nephrol. 1997;11:328.
135. Stapleton A, Latham RH, Johnson C, et al. Postcoital antimicrobial prophylaxis for recurrent urinary tract infection: A randomized, double-blind, placebo-controlled trial. JAMA. 1990;264:703–706.
136. Brumfitt W, Pursell R. Double-blind trial to compare ampicillin, cephalexin, co-trimoxazole and trimethoprim in treatment of urinary infection. BMJ. 1972;2:673–674.
137. Iravani A, Richard GA, Baer H. Treatment of uncomplicated urinary tract infection with trimethoprim versus sulfisoxazole with special reference to antibody-coated bacteria and faecal flora. Antimicrob Agents Chemother. 1981;19:842–850.
138. Stamm WE, Counts GW, Wagner KR, et al. Antimicrobial prophylaxis of recurrent urinary tract infections. Ann Intern Med. 1980;92:770–775.
139. Amyes SGB, Doherty CJ, Wonnacott S. Trimethoprim and co-trimoxazole: A comparison of the use in respiratory tract infections. Scand J Infect Dis. 1986;18:561–566.
140. Pandy GJ. Trimethoprim/sulphamethoxazole and doxycycline in acute exacerbations of chronic bronchitis in general practice: A comparative study. Med J Aust. 1979;1:264–266.
141. Schmidt U, Sen P, Kapila R, et al. Clinical evaluation of intravenous trimethoprim sulfamethoxazole for serious infections. Rev Infect Dis. 1982;4:332–337.
142. Shurin PA, Pelton SI, Donner A, et al. Trimethoprim-sulfamethoxazole compared with ampicillin in the treatment of acute otitis media. J Pediatr. 1980;96:1081–1087.
143. Yelland MJ. The efficacy of oral cotrimoxazole in the treatment of otitis externa in general practice. Med J Aust. 1993;158:697.
144. Williams JW Jr, Holleman DR Jr, Samsa GP, et al. Randomized controlled trial of 3 vs 10 days of trimethoprim/sulfamethoxazole for acute maxillary sinusitis. JAMA. 1995;273:1015.
145. Barnett ED, Teele DW, Klein JO, et al. Comparison of ceftriaxone and trimethoprim-sulfamethoxazole for acute otitis media. Pediatrics. 1997;99:23.
146. Daly K, Giebink GS, Batalden PB, et al. Resolution of otitis media with effusion with the use of a stepped treatment regimen of trimethoprim-sulfamethoxazole and prednisone. Pediatr Infect Dis J. 1991;10:500–506.
147. Giebink GS, Batalden PB, Le CT, et al. A controlled trial comparing three treatments for chronic otitis media with effusion. Pediatr Infect Dis J. 1990;9:33–40.
148. Nelson JD, Kusmiesz H, Shelton S. Oral or intravenous trimethoprim-sulfamethoxazole therapy for shigellosis. Rev Infect Dis. 1982;4:546–550.
149. Bannatyne RM, Toma S, Cheung R, et al. Resistance to trimethoprim and other antibiotics in Ontario shigellae (Letter). Lancet. 1980;1:425–426.
150. DuPont HL, Reves RR, Galindo E, et al. Treatment of travelers' diarrhea with trimethoprim/sulfamethoxazole and with trimethoprim alone. N Engl J Med. 1982;307:841–844.
151. Ericsson CD, Nicholls-Vasquez I, DuPont HL, et al. Optimal dosing of trimethoprim-sulfamethoxazole when used with loperamide to treat traveler's diarrhea. Antimicrob Agents Chemother. 1992;36:2821–2824.
152. Kabir I, Khan WA, Haider R, et al. Erythromycin and trimethoprim-sulphamethoxazole in the treatment of cholera in children. J Diarrhoeal Dis Res. 1996;14:243.
153. Threlfall EJ, Rowe B, Huq I. Plasmid-encoded multiple antibiotic resistance in *Vibrio cholerae* El Tor from Bangladesh (Letter). Lancet. 1980;1:1247–1248.
154. Svindland HB. Treatment of gonorrhoea with sulphamethoxazole-trimethoprim. Lack of effect on concomitant syphilis. Br J Vener Dis. 1973;49:50–53.
155. Rahim G. Single dose treatment of gonorrhoea with cotrimoxazole: A report on 1,223 cases. Br J Vener Dis. 1975;51:179–182.
156. Centers for Disease Control and Prevention. Chromosomally mediated resistant *Neisseria gonorrhoeae*—United States. MMWR Morb Mortal Wkly Rep. 1984;33:408–410.
157. Hammerschlag MR. Activity of trimethoprim-sulfamethoxazole against *Chlamydia trachomatis* in vitro. Rev Infect Dis. 1982;4:500–505.
158. Bogaerts J, Kestens L, Martinez Tello W, et al. Failure of treatment for chancroid in Rwanda is not related to human immunodeficiency virus infection: In vitro resistance of *Haemophilus ducreyi* to trimethoprim-sulfamethoxazole. Clin Infect Dis. 1995;20:924.
159. Shehabi A, Shakir K, el-Khateeb M, et al. Diagnosis and treatment of 106 cases of human brucellosis. J Infect 1990;20:5–10.
160. Bajpai J, Chaturvedi SN, Khanuja SPS. Chemotherapy of acute bone and joint infections. Int Surg. 1977;62:172–174.
161. Lakshamanan CDS. Comparative evaluation of cotrimoxazole and demeclocycline in periodontal bacterial infection (Abstract 128). J Dent Res. 1976;55(Spec Iss):D137.
162. Mahgoub ES. Medical management of mycetoma. Bull WHO. 1976;54:303.
163. Wallace RJ, Septimus EJ, Williams JH, et al. Use of trimethoprim-sulfamethoxazole for the treatment of infections due to *Nocardia*. Rev Infect Dis. 1982;4:315–325.
164. Javaly K, Horowitz HW, Wormser GP. Nocardiosis in patients with human immunodeficiency virus infection. Report of 2 cases and review of the literature. Medicine. 1992;71:128–138.
165. Morrison IM. Chronic melioidosis. Proc R Soc Med. 1970;63:239–249.
166. Neu HC, Garvey GJ, Bleach MP. Successful treatment of *Pseudomonas cepacia* endocarditis in a heroin addict with trimethoprim-sulfamethoxazole. J Infect Dis. 1973;128(Suppl):768–770.
167. Viteri AL, Greene JF Jr, Chandler JB Jr. Whipple's disease, successful response to sulfamethoxazole-trimethoprim. Am J Gastroenterol. 1981;75:309–314.
168. Durand DV, Lecomte C, Cathebras P, et al. Whipple disease: Clinical review of 52 cases. Medicine (Baltimore). 1997;76:170.
169. Munoz JL, Garcia MI, Munoz S, et al. Activity of trimethoprim/sulfamethoxazole plus polymyxin B against multiresistant *Stenotrophomonas maltophilia*. Eur J Clin Microbiol. Infect Dis. 1996;15:879.
170. Gutierrez Rodero F, Masia MM, Cortes J, et al. Endocarditis caused by *Stenotrophomonas maltophilia*: Case report and review. Clin Infect Dis. 1966;23:1261.
171. Stegeman CA, Cohen Tervaert JW, de John PE, et al. Trimethoprim-sulfamethoxazole (co-trimoxazole) for the prevention of relapses of Wegener's granulomatosis: Dutch co-trimoxazole Wegener study group. N Engl J Med. 1996;335:16.
172. Reinhold-Keller E, De Groot K, Rudert H, et al. Response to trimethoprim/sulfamethoxazole in Wegener's granulomatosis depends on the phase of disease. QJM. 1996;89:15.
173. Geddes AM, Ball AP, Farrell ID. Co-trimoxazole for the treatment of serious infections. J Antimicrob Chemother. 1979;5(Suppl B):221–230.
174. Quintiliani R, Levitz RE, Nightingale CH. Potential role of trimethoprim-sulfamethoxazole in the treatment of serious hospital-acquired infections. Rev Infect Dis. 1987;9:S160–S165.
175. Alonso R, Padilla B, Sanchez-Carrillo C, et al. Outbreak among HIV-infected patients of *Staphylococcus aureus* resistant to cotrimoxazole and methicillin. Infect Control Epidemiol. 1997;18:617.
176. Young LS, Hindler J. Use of trimethoprim-sulfamethoxazole singly and in combination with other antibiotics in immunocompromised patients. Rev Infect Dis. 1987;9:S177–S181.
177. Engervall PA, Stiernstedt GT, Gunther GC, et al. Trimethoprim-sulfamethoxazole plus amikacin as first-line therapy and imipenem/cilastatin as second empirical therapy in febrile neutropenic patients with hematological disorders. J Chemother. 1992;4:99–106.
178. Levitz RE, Quintiliani R. Trimethoprim-sulfamethoxazole for bacterial meningitis. Ann Intern Med. 1984;100:881–890.
179. Markowitz N, Quinn EL, Saravolatz LD. Trimethoprim-sulfamethoxazole compared with vancomycin for the treatment of *Staphylococcus aureus* infection. Ann Intern Med. 1992;117:390–398.
180. Gasser R, Reisinger E, Sedij B, et al. Oral treatment of late Lyme borreliosis with a combination of roxithromycin and co-trimoxazole: A pilot study on 18 patients. Acta Medica Austriaca. 1996;23:99.
181. Singh N, Gayowski AT, Yu VL, et al. Trimethoprim-sulfamethoxazole for the prevention of spontaneous bacterial peritonitis in cirrhosis: A randomized trial. Ann Intern Med. 1995;122:595.
182. Wallace RJ, Wissk, Bushby MB, et al. In vitro activity of trimethoprim and

sulfamethoxazole against nontuberculosis mycobacteria. Rev Infect Dis. 1982;4:326–331.
183. Freerksen E, Alvarenga AE, Legguizamo O, et al. A new short-term combination therapy of leprosy. Chemotherapy. 1991;37:353–363.
184. Gellin BG, Soave R. Coccidian infections in AIDS. Toxoplasmosis, cryptosporidiosis, and isosporiasis. Med Clin North Am. 1992;76:205–234.
185. Madico G, McDonald J, Gilman RH, et al. Epidemiology and treatment of *Cyclospora cayetanensis* infection in Peruvian children. Clin Infect Dis 1997;24:977–981.
186. Israelski DM, Remington JS. Toxoplasmic encephalitis in patients with AIDS. In: Moellering RC Jr, ed. Infectious Disease Clinics of North America (Medical Management of AIDS). Philadelphia: WB Saunders; 1988:429–450.
187. Canessa A, DelBono V, De Leo P, et al. Cotrimoxazole therapy of *Toxoplasma gondii* encephalitis in AIDS patients. Eur J Clin Microbiol Infect Dis. 1992;11:125–130.
188. Carr A, Tindall B, Brew BJ, et al. Low dose trimethoprim-sulfamethoxazole prophylaxis for toxoplasmic encephalitis in patients with AIDS. Ann Intern Med. 1992;117:106–111.
189. Kovacs JA, Masur H. Prophylaxis for *Pneumocystis carinii* pneumonia in patients infected with human immunodeficiency virus. Clin Infect Dis. 1992;14:1005–1009.
190. Davey RT, Masur H. Recent advances in the diagnosis, treatment, and prevention of *Pneumocystis carinii* pneumonia. Antimicrob Agents Chemother. 1990;34:499–504.
191. Sattler FR, Feinberg J. New developments in the treatment of *Pneumocystis carinii* pneumonia. Chest. 1992;101:451–457.
192. Klein NC, Duncanson FP, Lenox TH, et al. Trimethoprim-sulfamethoxazole versus pentamidine for *Pneumocystis carinii* pneumonia in AIDS patients: Results of a large prospective randomized treatment trial. AIDS. 1992;6:301–305.
193. Carr A, Swanson C, Penny R, et al. Clinical and laboratory markers of hypersensitivity to trimethoprim-sulfamethoxazole in patients with *Pneumocystis carinii* pneumonia and AIDS. J Infect Dis. 1993;167:180–185.
194. Sattler FR, Cowan R, Nielsen DM. Trimethoprim/sulfamethoxazole compared with pentamidine for treatment of *Pneumocystis carinii* pneumonia in acquired immunodeficiency syndrome: Prospective, noncrossover study. Ann Intern Med. 1988;109:280–287.
195. Hughes WT, Smith BL. Intermittent chemoprophylaxis for *Pneumocystis carinii* pneumonia. Antimicrob Agents Chemother. 1983;24:300–305.
196. Anonymous. Recommendations for prophylaxis against *Pneumocystis carinii* pneumonia for adults and adolescents infected with human immunodeficiency virus. MMWR Morb Mortal Wkly Rep. 1992;41:1–11.
197. Tabet SR, Krone MR, Hooton TM, et al. Bacterial infections in adult patients hospitalized with AIDS: Case-control study of prophylactic efficacy of trimethoprim-sulfamethoxazole versus aerosolized pentamidine. Int J STD AIDS. 1997;8:563.
198. Edge MD, Rimland D. Community-acquired bacteremia in HIV-positive patients: Protective benefit of co-trimoxazole. AIDS. 1996;10:1635.
199. Hardy WD, Feinberg J, Finkelstein DM, et al. A controlled trial of trimethoprim-sulfamethoxazole or aerosolized pentamidine for secondary prophylaxis of *Pneumocystis carinii* pneumonia in patients with the acquired immunodeficiency syndrome. AIDS Clinical Trials Group Protocol 021. N Engl J Med. 1992;327:1842–1848.
200. Schneider MM, Hoepelman IM, Eeftininck Schattenkerk JK, et al. A controlled trial of aerosolized pentamidine or trimethoprim-sulfamethoxazole as primary prophylaxis against *Pneumocystis carinii* pneumonia in patients with human immunodeficiency virus infection. The Dutch AIDS Treatment Group. N Engl J Med. 1992;327:1836–1841.
201. Chaisson RE, Keruly J, Richman DD, et al. *Pneumocystis* prophylaxis and survival in patients with advanced human immunodeficiency virus infection treated with zidovudine. The Zidovudine Epidemiology Group. Arch Intern Med. 1992;152:2009–2013.
202. Gurwith M, Brunton J, Lank B, et al. A prospective controlled investigation of prophylactic trimethoprim/sulfamethoxazole in hospitalized granulocytopenic patients. Am J Med. 1979;66:248–256.
203. Gualtieri RJ, Donowitz GR, Kaiser DC, et al. Double-blind randomized study of prophylactic trimethoprim/sulfamethoxazole in granulocytopenic patients with hematologic malignancies. Am J Med. 1983;74:934–940.
204. EORTC International Antimicrobial Therapy Project Group. Trimethoprim-sulfamethoxazole in the prevention of infection in neutropenic patients. J Infect Dis. 1984;150:372–379.
205. Oken MM, Pomeroy C, Weisdorf D, et al. Prophylactic antibiotics for the prevention of early infection in multiple myeloma. Am J Med. 1996;100:624.
206. Donnelly JP, Masschmeyer G, Daenen S. Selective oral antimicrobial prophylaxis for the prevention of infection in acute leukaemia—Ciprofloxacin versus co-trimoxazole plus colistin. The EORTC-Gnotobiotic Project Group. Eur J Cancer. 1992;28A:873–878.
207. Guiot HF, van der Meer JW, van den Broek PJ, et al. Prevention of viridans-group streptococcal septicemia in oncohematologic patients: A controlled comparative study on the effect of penicillin G and cotrimoxazole. Ann Hematol. 1992;64:260–265.
208. Wade JC, de Jongh CA, Newman KA, et al. Selective antimicrobial modulations as prophylaxis against infection during granulocytopenia: Trimethoprim-sulfamethoxazole vs. nalidixic acid. J Infect Dis. 1983;147:624–634.
209. Lew MA, Kehoe K, Ritz J, et al. Ciprofloxacin versus trimethoprim/sulfamethoxazole for prophylaxis of bacterial infections in bone marrow transplant recipients: A randomized, controlled trial. J Clin Oncol. 1995;13:239.
210. Ward TT, Thomas RG, Fye CL, et al. Trimethoprim-sulfamethoxazole prophylaxis in granulocytopenic patients with acute leukemia: Evaluation of serum antibiotic levels in a randomized, double-blind, placebo-controlled Department of Veterans Affairs Cooperative Study. Clin Infect Dis. 1993;17:323.
211. Margolis DM, Melnick DA, Alling DW, Gallin JI. Trimethoprim-sulfamethoxazole prophylaxis in the management of chronic granulomatous disease. J Infect Dis. 1990;162:723–726.
212. Overturf GD. Use of trimethoprim-sulfamethoxazole in pediatric infections: Relative merits of intravenous administration. Rev Infect Dis. 1987;9:S168–S173.

Chapter 31

Quinolones

DAVID C. HOOPER

The first member of the quinolone class of antimicrobial agents, nalidixic acid, is a 1,8-naphthyridine structure that was identified by Lesher and associates in 1962 among the by-products of chloroquine synthesis. Oxolinic acid and cinoxacin were also developed in the 1970s, but it was the identification in the 1980s of the fluorine- and piperazinyl-substituted derivatives with substantially greater potency and expanded spectrum that began a resurgence in the development and a rapid and steady expansion of this class of compounds. A broad spectrum of activity, good oral absorption, and overall good tolerability have resulted in extensive clinical use of the newer fluoroquinolones.

CHEMICAL STRUCTURES

All current quinolone derivatives in clinical use have a dual ring structure with a nitrogen at position 1, a carbonyl group at position 4, and a carboxyl group attached to the carbon at the 3 position of the first ring (Fig. 31–1). Several different dual ring structures have been developed (Fig. 31–2). Quinolones themselves have a carbon at position 8 in the second ring, and naphthyridines contain a nitrogen at position 8. Compounds based on other ring structures such as the cinnoline (nitrogens at positions 1 and 2) and pyridopyrimidine (nitrogens at positions 1, 6, and 8) rings have had fewer derivatives in clinical use in the United States. Derivatives with any of these ring structures, however, are commonly referred to as *quinolones,* and, for simplicity, the numbering of the positions in the ring follow the convention used for the quinolone ring. The 2-pyridones, which have a related dual ring structure in which the nitrogen is located at the junction of the two rings, have been developed, but no members of this group are in clinical use.

Nalidixic acid is a 1,8-naphthyridine with 1-ethyl and 7-methyl substituents (see Fig. 31–1). Oxolinic acid (quinolone ring) (Fig. 31–1) and cinoxacin (cinnoline ring) (not shown in Fig. 31–1) also have 1-ethyl substituents, as well as a dioxolo ring bridging positions 6 and 7. Potency is greatly improved by the addition of a fluorine at position 6, and potency against gram-negative bacteria is further enhanced by the addition of a piperazinyl (norfloxacin, enoxacin, ciprofloxacin), methyl-piperazinyl (pefloxacin, ofloxacin, lomefloxacin, fleroxacin, temafloxacin, grepafloxacin, gatifloxacin), or dimethyl-piperazinyl (sparfloxacin) substituent at position 7. Methyl substituents on the piperazine ring may result in improved oral bioavailability. These structural features are common to most of the newer quinolone derivatives now in clinical use. Pyrrolidinyl substituents at position 7 (clinafloxacin) enhance activity against gram-positive bacteria, as do dual-ring structures derived from the pyrrolidinyl ring (trovafloxacin, moxifloxacin, sitafloxacin). Some newer compounds retain the 1-ethyl substituent found in nalidixic acid or contain a similar structure (fleroxacin, 1-fluoroethyl). The

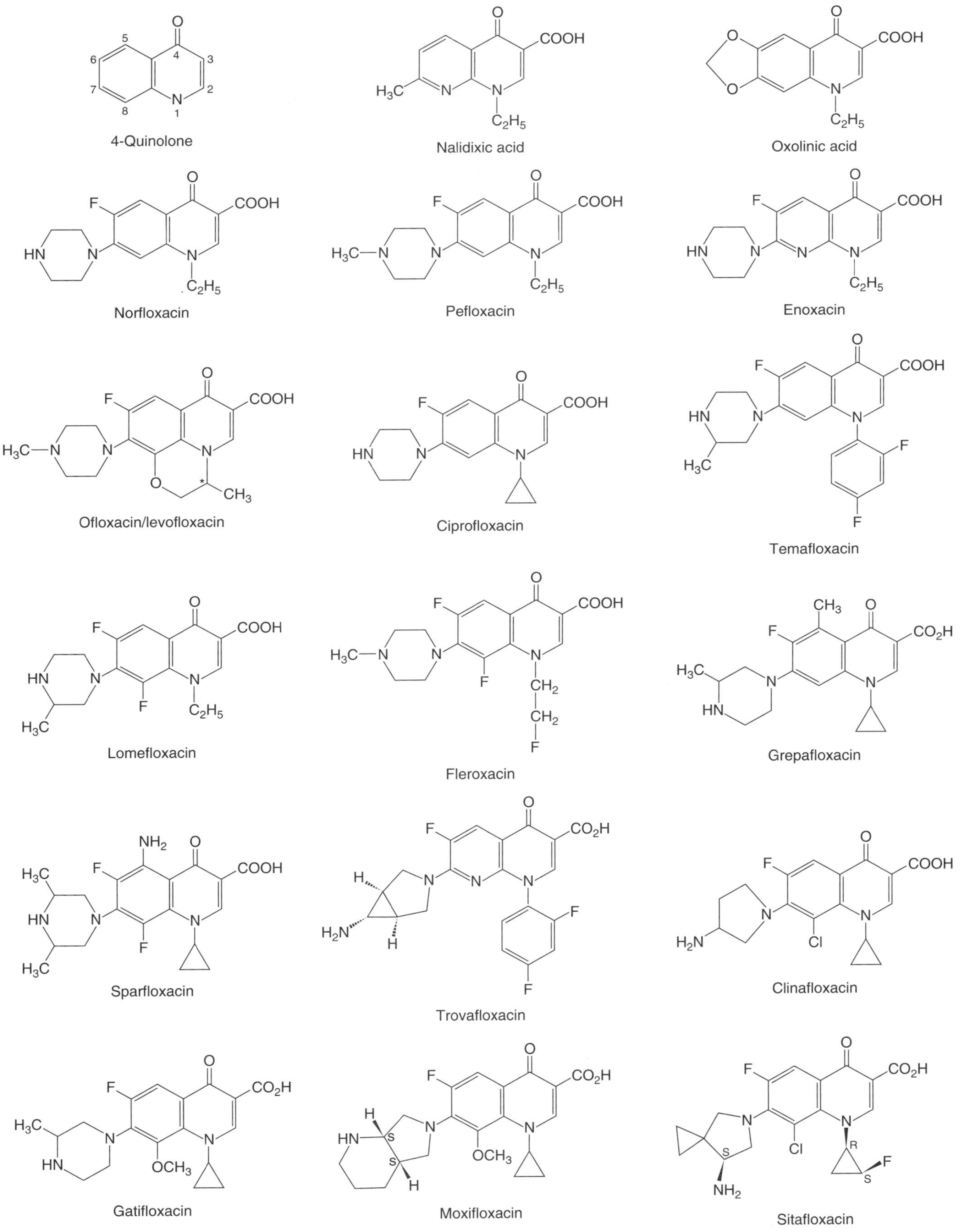

4-Quinolone

Nalidixic acid

Oxolinic acid

Norfloxacin

Pefloxacin

Enoxacin

Ofloxacin/levofloxacin

Ciprofloxacin

Temafloxacin

Lomefloxacin

Fleroxacin

Grepafloxacin

Sparfloxacin

Trovafloxacin

Clinafloxacin

Gatifloxacin

Moxifloxacin

Sitafloxacin

FIGURE 31–1. Quinolone ring structure and numbering and structures of selected quinolones in clinical use or under development.

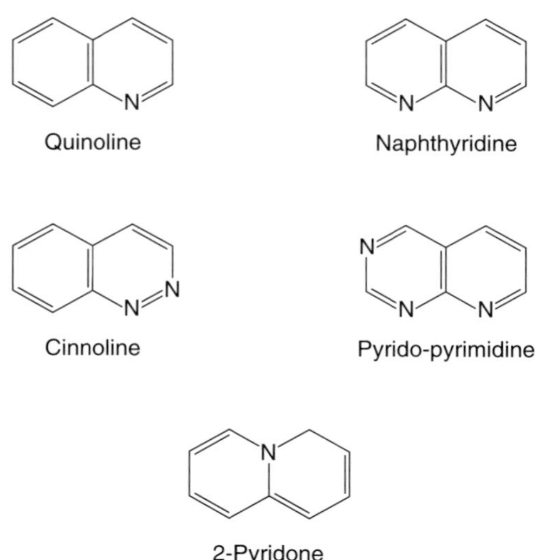

FIGURE 31–2. Dual ring structures that constitute different members of the quinolone and related classes of antimicrobials.

1-cyclopropyl group has been used in a number of compounds (ciprofloxacin, sparfloxacin, gatifloxacin, moxifloxacin) because of its major effect on potency. Additional structures placed at the 1 position include the 1-difluorophenyl group of temafloxacin and trovafloxacin and the additional ring structure bridging positions 1 and 8 of ofloxacin and levofloxacin. The asymmetric carbon present in this latter ring results in stereoisomers; ofloxacin is a racemic mixture of both stereoisomers, and levofloxacin is the more active of the two isomers. At position 5, replacement of the hydrogen by an amino group (sparfloxacin) or a methyl group (grepafloxacin) results in some enhancement of activity against gram-positive bacteria. At position 8, the addition of halide (chlorine in clinafloxacin, fluorine in sparfloxacin and sitafloxacin) or a methoxy group (gatifloxacin, moxifloxacin) enhances activity against anaerobic bacteria.

Quinolones have been chemically linked to cephalosporins. Desacetylcefotaxime has been attached to the 3-carboxyl group of fleroxacin (Ro 23-9424)[1] and ciprofloxacin (Ro 24-6392)[2] by an ester linkage and to the piperazine group of ciprofloxacin by tertiary-amino (Ro 24-8138) and carbamate (Ro 24-4383)[2] linkages. The intact ester-linked molecules appear to function as cephalosporins, but spontaneous or β-lactamase–enhanced cleavage of the ester results in the release of active quinolone. The more stable intact amino- and carbamate-linked derivatives, however, appear to have activities characteristic of both component classes of compounds, and activity was further enhanced in a β-lactamase–producing strain, which may enhance release of the quinolone moiety.[2] Structure-activity relationships of the quinolone class have been reviewed.[3, 4]

MECHANISM OF ACTION

The quinolones rapidly inhibit bacterial DNA synthesis, an event that is followed by rapid bacterial cell death. The molecular events that underly these actions are understood in part, but key details remain to be defined.[5]

Quinolones inhibit the enzymatic activities of two members of the topoisomerase class of enzymes, DNA gyrase and topoisomerase IV, and promote the cleavage of DNA in these enzyme-DNA complexes. DNA gyrase, which was first recognized as a target of quinolones, is an essential bacterial enzyme composed of two A and two B subunits, products of *gyrA* and *gyrB* genes, respectively.[6] DNA gyrase catalyzes the introduction of negative superhelical twists into closed covalently circular chromosomal and plasmid DNA within the bacterial cell. The superhelical state of intracellular DNA is regulated by the actions of DNA gyrase and topoisomerase I, which removes DNA superhelical twists but is not inhibited by quinolones. DNA superhelicity affects the initiation of DNA replication and transcription of many genes. DNA gyrase is also responsible for removing positive superhelical twists that accumulate ahead of the DNA replication fork. These activities result from the enzyme's coordinated breaking of both strands of duplex DNA, passage of another segment of DNA through the break, and resealing of the break, a mechanism that defines type 2 topoisomerases.[7]

Quinolones also inhibit the activities of topoisomerase IV, another type 2 topoisomerase that is composed of two subunits encoded by the *parC* and *parE* genes. Topoisomerase IV and DNA gyrase are structurally related; *parC* is homologous to *gyrA,* and *parE* is homologous to *gyrB.*[8] Topoisomerase IV resolves interlinked (catenated) daughter DNA molecules that are the products of completion of a round of DNA replication to allow their segregation into daughter cells. Thus, DNA gyrase and topoisomerase IV have distinct essential roles in bacterial DNA replication.[9]

Quinolones appear to function by trapping or stabilizing the enzyme-DNA complexes after strand breakage and before resealing of DNA. This trapped complex appears to function as a cellular poison, possibly by generating a DNA break that the cell is able to repair only poorly.[10] Quinolones have been shown to bind specifically to the complex of DNA gyrase and DNA rather than to DNA gyrase alone.[11] The importance of the interaction of quinolones with the gyrase-DNA complex for the antibacterial activities of the quinolones in *Escherichia coli* is indicated by the identification of bacterial single *gyrA* or *gyrB* mutants that are resistant to quinolones and produce gyrase-DNA complexes with reduced quinolone binding (see the section on mechanisms of resistance).[12] In contrast to the information for *E. coli,* for *Staphylococcus aureus* and *Streptococcus pneumoniae,* interactions of quinolones with topoisomerase IV have been shown to determine antibacterial activity by the identification of *parC* (*grlA* in *Staph. aureus*) and *parE* (*grlB* in *S. aureus*) single mutants that have reduced quinolone activity.[13] Based on studies of mutants of this type, a general pattern has emerged. For many gram-negative bacteria, DNA gyrase is the primary quinolone target, and for many gram-positive bacteria, topoisomerase IV is the primary target, with the other enzyme being the secondary target in both cases. There are exceptions, however, that depend on the quinolone studied.[14] These patterns appear to result from the relative sensitivities of these two topoisomerases to a given quinolone, with the most sensitive enzyme defining the primary target of a particular quinolone.[15] Some quinolones under development appear to have similar potencies against both DNA gyrase and topoisomerase IV in some bacterial species.

Quinolone inhibition of bacterial DNA replication and bacterial killing may be dissociated under some conditions, suggesting that events in addition to the initial interaction of quinolones with the topoisomerase-DNA complex may be required for cell killing. In particular, inhibitors of RNA and protein synthesis reduce the bactericidal activity of some quinolones but do not affect their ability to inhibit bacterial DNA synthesis.[16] Thus, inhibition of bacterial DNA synthesis per se is not sufficient to account for bacterial killing, and possibly newly synthesized gene products may also be necessary. This effect may account for the observations that at high concentrations of quinolones, which also secondarily inhibit protein synthesis, cell killing is reduced.

The nature of the gene products (in addition to DNA gyrase and topoisomerase IV) that contribute to killing, however, has yet to be defined. The gene products in the RecA-SOS DNA repair and recombination system, the expression of which is known to be induced by the damage to bacterial DNA caused by quinolones, appear to function at least in part to repair quinolone-induced DNA damage, because *rec* mutants with defective function are hypersusceptible to killing by quinolones.[17] Certain *hip* mutants exhibit a *h*igher fraction of *p*ersisters, or surviving cells, after treatment with bactericidal antimicrobial agents without exhibiting major differences in the concentrations of drug that inhibit bacterial growth. The *hipA* mutants selected for reduced killing by ampicillin have alterations in the cell wall and are also killed less well by quinolones, and the *hipQ* mutants selected for reduced killing by quinolones also exhibit selective reduced killing by β-lactams.[18] The nature of the *hipA* and *hipQ* gene products is not known, but the overlap in reduced killing by both β-lactams and quinolones suggests that after the interaction of these classes of drugs with their different targets, there may be common overlapping pathways that are necessary for bacterial lethality. One possibility, as yet unproved, is that induction of cell autolysins is necessary for killing by both classes of drugs.

Differences among quinolones in the magnitude of bacterial killing in the presence of rifampin (an inhibitor of RNA synthesis), phosphate-buffered saline, and anaerobiasis have led to the suggestions that some quinolones may have more than one mechanism of killing,[19] but the molecular events underlying these phenomena are not yet understood, except that killing is dependent on drug interaction with DNA gyrase and topoisomerase IV.

Eukaryotic cells also contain topoisomerases, and eukaryotic topoisomerase II, which is a homodimeric enzyme, has limited primary amino acid sequence homology with DNA gyrase and topoisomerase IV.[20] Current antibacterial quinolones have only minimal activity against mammalian topoisomerase II,[21] but other quinolone structures (containing a 7-hydroxyphenyl substituent or an isothiazolo ring bridging positions 2 and 3) have been shown to have substantially enhanced potency against the mammalian enzyme.[22, 23]

MECHANISMS OF ACQUIRED BACTERIAL RESISTANCE

Bacteria acquire resistance to quinolones by spontaneously occurring mutations in chromosomal genes that either alter the target enzymes—DNA gyrase and topoisomerase IV—or alter the drug's permeation across the bacterial cell membranes.[24] No specific quinolone-degrading or quinolone-inactivating enzymes have been identified, but certain fungi (*Gloeophyllum striatum*) have been shown to degrade quinolones by metabolic pathways.[25] Plasmid-mediated quinolone resistance has been identified in clinical isolates of *Klebsiella pneumoniae,* but the mechanism and prevalence of this resistance have not been defined.[26]

Resistant chromosomal mutants may be selected in the laboratory by plating bacteria on drug-containing agar. The frequency of occurrence of spontaneous mutants differs with the selecting drug concentration and the drug. For gram-negative bacteria selected with the newer fluoroquinolones, frequencies range, in general, from 10^{-6} or higher at twofold above the minimal inhibitory concentration (MIC) to undetectable ($<10^{-10}$) at 16- to 32-fold above the MIC. With a similar selection with nalidixic acid, mutants are detected more frequently. This difference results in part from the ability of certain mutations to confer higher levels of resistance to nalidixic acid than to other quinolones. Serial passage of bacteria on increasing concentrations of quinolones selects mutants with high levels of resistance resulting from the additive effects of several mutations.[27]

Alterations in the A subunit of DNA gyrase that cause quinolone resistance have been defined in a substantial number of clinical and laboratory isolates of *E. coli.* These alterations are clustered between amino acids 67 and 106 in the amino terminus of the A protein near the active site of the enzyme (tyrosine-122).[7] In particular, changes in serine-83 (to leucine or tryptophan) are most common and cause the largest increment in resistance as well as reduced binding of the drug to the gyrase-DNA complex in vitro.[12] Leucine-83 causes a 128-fold increase in resistance to nalidixic acid but lesser increases in resistance to the newer fluoroquinolones (16- to 32-fold), thus likely accounting for the greater ease of selection of resistant mutants with nalidixic acid. Similar changes in the A subunit have been associated with resistance in many species of gram-negative bacteria. Single amino acid changes in the midportion of the gyrase B protein have also been found to cause lower levels of resistance to nalidixic acid and fluoroquinolones.[28]

Resistance mutations in the *parC* gene of topoisomerase IV in *Staph. aureus* and *Strep. pneumoniae* have been most commonly found at position 80 in which a wild-type serine (homologous to serine-83 of DNA gyrase) is replaced by phenylalanine or tyrosine. These mutations cause eightfold increases in resistance to several fluoroquinolones. Resistance mutations have also been found less commonly in the *parE* gene.

Stepwise increasing resistance occurs by sequential mutations in the *gyrA* (or *gyrB*) and *parC* (or *parE*) genes, with the first target mutation occurring in a gene for the more sensitive target enzyme. The level of susceptibility of the first-step mutant is then usually determined by the intrinsic level of sensitivity of the secondary target enzyme. A second mutation in a gene for the secondary target then further increases resistance to the level that is determined by the already-mutant primary enzyme target. This finding implies that the drug concentration above which two mutations will be required to select resistance will decrease to the extent that the similarity of sensitivities of DNA gyrase and topoisomerase IV to a given quinolone approach the same value. In the most highly resistant clinical strains of both gram-positive and gram-negative bacteria, one or more mutations in each of the *gyrA* and *parC* genes have commonly been found.

The routes of quinolone permeation across the bacterial cell membranes are not fully defined, but the hydrophilic congeners appear to diffuse across the gram-negative bacterial outer membrane through porin channels. In *E. coli* and *Pseudomonas aeruginosa,* resistance mutations in genes that affect the expression of outer membrane proteins have been described.[29–31] In both cases resistance cannot be explained by reduced diffusion alone, and reduced drug accumulation in some mutants is energy-dependent, being abolished by agents that collapse the proton-motive force. In *E. coli* resistance of Mar mutants, which exhibit reduced porin channels, is dependent on the AcrAB efflux pump, which is linked to the TolC outer membrane protein.[32] In *P. aeruginosa,* resistance has been shown to be caused by increased expression of one of several sets of three genes that appear to encode an efflux pump in the inner membrane, a periplasm-spanning protein, and a linked outer membrane protein (e.g., MexAB-OprM).[33] Resistance in many mutants of this type is pleiotropic with additional low levels of resistance to tetracycline, chloramphenicol, and some β-lactams.[27]

In gram-positive bacteria, which lack an outer membrane, overexpression of endogenous efflux pumps has also been shown to cause low-level quinolone resistance. The *Staph. aureus norA* gene encodes a hydrophobic membrane protein with 12 membrane-spanning segments and with similarities to other drug transport proteins such as TetA, the tetracycline efflux transporter.[34] Cloned *norA* causes resistance to hydrophilic quinolones in *E. coli* and *Staph. aureus,* and a resistance mutation in the promoter region upstream of *norA* on the *Staph. aureus* chromosome is associated with increased levels of *norA* mRNA. Energized everted inner membrane vesicles from *E. coli* containing cloned *norA* also exhibit saturable norfloxacin uptake that is dependent on the pH gradient across the membrane,[35] suggesting that NorA protein functions as a quinolone efflux transporter energetically coupled in antiport with the proton gradient across the cell membrane. Recent data also suggest that *Strep. pneumoniae* also exhibits efflux-mediated quinolone resistance.[36] Quinolones vary in the extent to which their activity is affected by expression of various efflux pumps in both gram-negative and gram-positive bacteria, with more hydrophobic drugs being less affected, although other features of drug structure may also be important.[37]

ANTIMICROBIAL ACTIVITY

Current quinolones are most active against aerobic gram-negative bacilli, particularly members of the family Enterobacteriaceae and *Haemophilus* spp., and against gram-negative cocci such as *Neisseria* spp. and *Moraxella* (*Branhamella*) *catarrhalis* (Table 31–1).[38, 39] Relative to nalidixic acid, the fluoroquinolones also have additional

TABLE 31-1 Activity of Selected Quinolones against Selected Gram-Negative, Mycoplasmal, and Chlamydial Pathogens In Vitro

Organism	Representative MIC_{90} (Range) (μg/ml)											
	Nalidixic Acid	*Ciprofloxacin*	*Norfloxacin*	*Enoxacin*	*Ofloxacin*	*Pefloxacin*	*Lomefloxacin*	*Fleroxacin*	*Sparfloxacin*	*Levofloxacin*	*Grepafloxacin*	*Trovafloxacin*
Acinetobacter spp.	32–256	0.25–2 (0.25–>128)	(8–64)	1–2	0.25–1 (0.25–>128)	(1–8)	4	0.5–4 (0.5–32)	0.06–1 (0.06–16)	0.4–16 (0.12–16)	0.4–>4	0.03–16
Aeromonas spp.	0.5	≤0.06 (≤0.06–0.25)	0.03	0.06	0.03–0.5 (0.03–1)	0.03	0.12	0.12–0.25 (0.12–1)	≤0.12 (≤0.12–1)	(0.12–1)	0.5	0.03–0.06
Burkholderia cepacia	16	2 (0.5–16)	8 (8–50)	25 (16–25)	3.1 (3–32)	—	16 (16)	4 (4–16)	1 (1)	2–8	—	0.25–32
Campylobacter jejuni	8	(0.12–0.78)	(0.25–2)	(1–32)	(0.12–2)	0.5	(0.125–1)	0.5	0.12–0.25	0.4	—	—
Chlamydia pneumoniae	—	1–2	—	—	1	—	4	2	0.5	—	0.12–0.5	1
Chlamydia trachomatis	—	1–3.1	≥16	6.3	0.5–1.6	—	2–3.1	(1.5–6.3)	0.06	—	0.12	0.016–0.063
Citrobacter spp.	8	0.12 (≤0.03–6.25)	0.5 (≤0.25–50)	0.5 (0.25–1.56)	0.5 (0.1–25)	0.4–1	0.5 (0.12–25)	0.12 (≤0.06–25)	0.5 (0.6–2)	0.12–6.25	0.12–1.56	0.06–16
Enterobacter aerogenes	8	0.06 (≤0.03–0.25)	0.5 (0.2–2)	0.25	0.25 (0.12–1)	0.25	0.5 (≤0.25–1)	0.12–0.25	0.12 (0.12–0.5)	0.06–0.25	0.06–1	0.06–0.12
Enterobacter cloacae	8	0.12 (≤0.3–0.5)	0.5 (<0.25–2)	0.5 (0.1–1)	0.25 (0.1–1)	0.5	0.5 (≤0.25–1)	0.25	0.25 (0.12–0.5)	0.12–0.78	0.12–0.5	0.06–1
Escherichia coli	4	≤0.06 (≤0.01–0.25)	0.12 (0.01–0.5)	0.25 (0.03–2)	0.12 (0.02–1)	0.12–0.25	0.2 (0.06–1)	0.1 (0.03–2)	≤0.06 (≤0.03–0.1)	0.05–0.12	0.03–0.12	0.03–4
Haemophilus influenzae	1	(≤0.008–≤0.06)	0.06	0.12	(≤0.06–0.5)	0.06	≤0.06–0.12)	(≤0.06–1)	≤0.06	0.025–0.06	0.008–0.0125	0.015–0.03
Klebsiella spp.	8–16	0.12 (0.02–1)	0.5 (0.2–2)	1 (0.5–2)	0.25 (0.12–1)	2 (0.5–2)	1 (0.2–6.25)	0.5 (0.12–6.25)	0.12 (≤0.03–1)	0.1–3.1	0.1–4	0.06–1
Legionella spp.	1	≤0.12	(0.2–2)	0.2	≤0.06	—	≤0.06	≤0.06	≤0.06	(0.03–0.25)	0.008–0.25	0.008–0.06
Moraxella catarrhalis	2	(≤0.03–0.25)	0.4	0.06	(0.06–0.5)	0.25	(≤0.1–1)	(0.25–2)	(0.01–0.12)	0.06–0.12	0.015–0.06	≤0.015–0.06
Morganella morganii	8	0.06 (0.01–6.25)	0.12 (≤0.06–25)	0.5 (≤0.12–1.56)	0.25 (0.1–12.5)	(0.25–4)	0.25 (0.25–12.5)	0.12 (<0.06–12.5)	0.5 (0.25–1)	0.12–6.25	0.125–0.4	0.25–2
Mycoplasma hominis	>256	0.5–2	8–16	8	1–2	4	2	2	≤0.06	—	0.06–0.125	0.03
Mycoplasma pneumoniae	—	(1–8)	12	8	(0.78–2)	4	4–8	4	(0.1–0.25)	—	0.25–0.5	0.12
Neisseria gonorrhoeae	1	0.01	0.06	0.25	0.06	0.06	0.12	0.2	≤0.06	0.015–0.1	0.006–0.025	0.015–0.25
Neisseria meningitidis	0.5	(0.008–0.12)	0.03	0.03	(≤0.06–0.4)	0.03	(≤0.06–0.42)	(≤0.03–0.25)	≤0.06	—	0.008	0.008
Proteus mirabilis	8	0.06 (≤0.03–0.39)	0.1 (0.12–0.5)	0.5 (0.25–1.56)	0.5 (0.12–1)	0.25	0.5–1	0.5 (≤0.12–0.5)	≤0.06	0.06–0.25	0.25–0.5	0.25–4
Proteus vulgaris	8	0.06 (0.01–0.25)	0.1 (0.12–0.5)	0.5 (0.25–2)	0.25 (0.06–0.5)	0.25	0.5 (0.25–1)	0.12 (≤0.12–0.25)	0.5–1	0.2–0.5	0.25–0.78	0.25–0.5
Providencia rettger	16	1 (0.03–2)	2 (0.25–3.1)	1 (0.5–6.25)	1 (0.5–8)	0.5	4 (1.6–6.2)	0.5 (0.12–1)	0.5 (0.25–2)	0.5–3.1	0.5–>4	0.5
Providencia stuartii	32	0.5 (0.125–2)	2 (≤0.25–2)	1–2	1 (1–8)	(4)	1 (1–4)	1 (0.5–2)	0.5 (0.2–2)	0.25–1	0.5–>4	0.5–2
Pseudomonas aeruginosa	16	0.5 (0.25–8)	2 (2–16)	4 (3–32)	2 (2–>50)	2	4 (4–>50)	2 (2–>50)	(1.6–8)	2–50	0.5–>4	1–8
Salmonella spp.	2–4	≤0.06	≤0.06 (≤0.06–0.25)	0.12–0.25	0.12–0.25	0.12	0.25	≤0.12–0.25	≤0.06	0.12	0.06–0.12	0.03–0.12
Serratia marcescens	≥100	0.25 (0.06–12.5)	1 (≤0.25–50)	2 (1–25)	1 (0.5–25)	1 (1–8)	2 (0.25–25)	0.5 (0.25–25)	1 (0.12–12.5)	0.12–12.5	0.25–8	0.25–4
Shigella spp.	8	≤0.03	≤0.06–0.12	(0.06–0.25)	(0.06–0.78)	0.25	(0.06–0.25)	≤0.125	≤0.06	0.1	0.03	≤0.015–0.06
Stenotrophomonas maltophilia	16	2 (2–25)	4 (4–>64)	8 (3–16)	3.1 (3–>25)	4	8 (8–>25)	3 (3–25)	(0.5–>2)	2–25	0.78–2	0.5–4
Yersinia enterocolitica	2	≤0.06	≤0.12	0.12–0.25	(0.06–0.25)	0.25	(≤0.06–0.25)	(≤0.06–2)	≤0.06	—	0.03–0.25	0.03–0.06

Abbreviation: MIC_{90}, Minimal inhibitory concentration for 90% of strains.
Data from refs. 38 and 39.

activity against gram-negative bacilli such as *P. aeruginosa* (Table 31–1) and against staphylococci (Table 31–2). Ciprofloxacin remains the most potent marketed fluoroquinolone against gram-negative bacteria. For norfloxacin, ciprofloxacin, ofloxacin, lomefloxacin, and enoxacin, activity against streptococci and many anaerobes is limited (Tables 31–2 and 31–3). Newer agents released in the United States, levofloxacin, sparfloxacin, grepafloxacin, and trovafloxacin, and agents under development (clinafloxacin, gatifloxacin, moxifloxacin, sitafloxacin, and others), however, have greater potency against these organisms. For the fluoroquinolones that are used for treatment of infections outside the urinary tract, the MICs listed in Table 31–1 should be interpreted in relation to peak drug concentrations in serum that range from 1.1 to 6.4 μg/ml (with usual dosing) and in relation to drug concentrations in urine that are manyfold higher for most quinolones except those that are largely excreted by nonrenal mechanisms (see the section on pharmacology). For highly susceptible organisms, MICs may be 10- to 30-fold below achievable serum concentrations.

Fluoroquinolones also have activity against mycobacteria (see Table 31–3).[40] Ciprofloxacin, ofloxacin, fleroxacin, levofloxacin, and sparfloxacin are active against *Mycobacterium tuberculosis, Mycobacterium fortuitum, Mycobacterium kansasii,* and some strains of *Mycobacterium chelonae* but have only fair or poor activity against *Mycobacterium avium-intracellulare.* Ofloxacin and pefloxacin have activity against *Mycobacterium leprae* in animal models.

Other bacteria are also inhibited by quinolones in vitro (see Table 31–1). Ciprofloxacin, ofloxacin, levofloxacin, sparfloxacin, grepafloxacin, and trovafloxacin all have activity against the agents of atypical pneumonias, including *Legionella pneumophila, Mycoplasma pneumoniae,* and *Chlamydia pneumoniae,* and against genital pathogens such as *Chlamydia trachomatis, Ureaplasma urealyticum,* and *Mycoplasma hominis. Treponema pallidum* is resistant to ofloxacin in animal models, and no other quinolone has been shown to have activity against this spirochete.

Trovafloxacin among available quinolones and gatifloxacin, moxifloxacin, clinafloxacin, and sitifloxacin among quinolones under development all have increased potency against anaerobes. This activity along with enhanced gram-positive activity and substantial retention of the gram-negative activity of ciprofloxacin results in compounds of exceptionally broad spectrum, similar to that of the carbapenems.

Activity in vitro is reduced in the presence of urine but generally not in the presence of serum. Activity is also reduced at pH values below 7 and in the presence of magnesium concentrations at 8 to 16 mM. Both these factors often contribute to the reduced quinolone activity observed in the presence of urine. Low pH and elevated concentrations of magnesium are associated with reduced drug accumulation in *E. coli.*[29]

Minimal bactericidal concentrations of quinolones are usually within two- to fourfold of the MIC, and the magnitude of bacterial killing increases with further increases in drug concentration, reaching a maximum at about 30-fold above the MIC. Above this maximal killing concentration, paradoxical reductions in killing are observed and are associated with additional inhibition of protein synthesis by high concentrations of quinolones.[19]

The postantibiotic effect is the period of time required for bacteria surviving a brief exposure to an antimicrobial agent to resume growth. Although the postantibiotic effect may be relevant in estimating the proper interval for drug dosing, its clinical importance, which may be greatest in patients with compromised host defenses, has not been proved. For quinolones, the duration of the postantibiotic effect has been in the range of 1 to 2 hours and tends to increase with increasing drug concentrations and length of drug exposure.

Combinations of quinolones with other antimicrobial agents have been extensively studied, and interactions with β-lactams and aminoglycosides as measured by fractional inhibitory or bactericidal concentrations or time-kill curve studies have generally been found to be indifferent or additive.[39, 41] Synergistic interactions were found in a minority of strains, although for *P. aeruginosa* in some studies synergy with ciprofloxacin in combination with imipenem or azlocillin were seen in a substantial minority, 30 to 50%, of strains. Antagonistic interactions of quinolones with other antimicrobial agents have been rare. Rifampin reduced the bactericidal activity of ciprofloxacin and pefloxacin against *Staph. aureus* in some studies.[42]

PHARMACOLOGY

Absorption

The quinolones are well absorbed from the upper gastrointestinal tract, with bioavailability exceeding 50% for all compounds and approaching 100% for several (Table 31–4).[43–46] Peak concentrations in serum are usually attained within 1 to 3 hours of administering a dose. Food does not substantially reduce quinolone absorption but may delay the time to reach peak drug concentrations in serum.[47, 48] Enteral feedings given orally, however, may reduce absorption.[49] Absorption is good when ciprofloxacin is given by nasogastric or jejunostomy tube[50] but may be decreased by concurrent enteral feedings given through these tubes.[49]

Peak fluoroquinolone concentrations in serum after a 200- to 500-mg dose range from 1.1 μg/ml for sparfloxacin to 6.4 μg/ml for levofloxacin (see Table 31–4). A 1-g dose of nalidixic acid produces concentrations of 20 to 50 μg/ml of serum. Drug binding to serum proteins is generally low, around 15 to 30%, with the exception of trovafloxacin, which is approximately 75% bound to serum proteins. The intravenous formulation of trovafloxacin (alatrofloxacin) is an alanine ester of trovafloxacin that is promptly converted to the parent compound by serum esterases.

Distribution in Tissues

The volumes of distribution of quinolones are high and in most cases exceed the volume of total body water (see Table 31–4), indicating accumulation in some tissues. Concentrations in prostate tissue, stool, bile, lung, and neutrophils and macrophages usually exceed serum concentrations (Table 31–5). Concentrations in urine and kidney tissue are high for quinolones with a major renal route of elimination (all except sparfloxacin, grepafloxacin, and trovafloxacin). Concentrations of quinolones in saliva, prostatic fluid, bone, and cerebrospinal fluid are usually lower than drug concentrations in serum.

Penetration into ascitic fluid in patients with liver failure has been found for pefloxacin (72% of serum concentration) and ofloxacin (120%).[51] Penetration into human breast milk has also been documented for ciprofloxacin, ofloxacin, and pefloxacin.[52]

Elimination

The terminal half-lives of elimination from serum range from 3 hours for norfloxacin and ciprofloxacin to 20 hours for sparfloxacin, allowing twice- or once-daily dosing (Table 31–6; see also Table 31–4). The principal routes of elimination differ among quinolones. Cinoxacin, ofloxacin, and lomefloxacin are eliminated predominantly by the kidneys; and nalidixic acid, pefloxacin, sparfloxacin, grepafloxacin, and trovafloxacin are eliminated predominantly by nonrenal pathways. Most other quinolones have mixed excretion by both renal and nonrenal routes.

Renal clearance of norfloxacin, ciprofloxacin, ofloxacin, enoxacin, and lomefloxacin exceeds glomerular filtration rates, indicating net tubular secretion. In support of tubular secretion, renal clearances of norfloxacin and ciprofloxacin are reduced by probenecid, but drug accumulation does not occur. In contrast, the renal clearance of pefloxacin and fleroxacin is below or equal to the glomerular filtration rate, suggesting net tubular reabsorption.[53]

Hepatic metabolism accounts for the majority of the elimination of pefloxacin and nalidixic acid. In these cases, however, active metabolites contribute to antibacterial effects. The desmethylpiperazinyl derivative of pefloxacin is norfloxacin, and hydroxynalidixic

TABLE 31-2 Activity of Selected Quinolones against Selected Gram-Positive Bacteria In Vitro

Organism	Representative MIC^{90} (Range) (μg/ml)											
	Nalidixic Acid	***Ciprofloxacin***	***Norfloxacin***	***Enoxacin***	***Ofloxacin***	***Pefloxacin***	***Lomefloxacin***	***Fleroxacin***	***Sparfloxacin***	***Levofloxacin***	***Grepafloxacin***	***Trovafloxacin***
Staphylococcus aureus	100	0.5 (0.25–2)	2 (1–4)	2 (2–4)	0.5 (0.1–2)	0.5 (0.1–2)	2 (0.5–4)	1 (0.125–4)	0.12 (0.006–0.25)	0.5–0.8 (0.25–32)	0.12–>4	0.03–4
Coagulase-negative staphylococci	100	0.5 (≤0.1–>2)	2 (0.5–>4)	2 (0.5–4)	1 (0.25–2)	1 (0.5–4)	2 (0.5–4)	1 (0.5–8)	0.12 (0.03–>4)	0.2–8	0.12–>4	0.06–>4
Streptococcus pneumoniae	>128	2 (0.78–6.2)	16 (4–>16)	16 (8–16)	2 (1–8)	12 (8–16)	8 (4–16)	8 (8–25)	0.5 (0.25–1)	1–3.13	0.12–0.4	0.125–0.25
Streptococcus pyogenes	>100	1 (0.5–4)	4 (2–16)	>8	2 (1–4)	8 (8–16)	8 (4–12.5)	8 (4–12.5)	1 (0.5–2)	0.5–2	0.25–0.5	0.06–0.5
Streptococcus agalactiae	>128	2 (0.5–4)	16 (4–16)	>8	2 (2–4)	32	16 (8–32)	8 (≥8)	0.5 (0.5–2)	1–2	0.5	0.25–0.5
Streptococcus bovis	—	4 (1–4)	>8	>8	4 (2–4)	—	—	>8	—	—	—	(0.12–0.25)
Streptococcus spp.	>64	2 (0.5–4)	16 (4–32)	32 (8–32)	4 (1–6.2)	>12.5	8 (4–16)	4–8	1 (0.25–1)	1–2	0.25–0.5	0.06–0.5
Enterococcus faecalis	>64	2 (0.5–4)	8 (4–32)	8 (8–16)	4 (2–6.2)	4–8	8 (4–16)	8 (8–>16)	1 (0.25–1)	1–3.1	0.4–4	0.25–8
Enterococcus faecium	>64	4 (2–8)	≥12.5	32	6.2 (2–16)	—	8	8	1 (0.5–4)	3.1	—	1–>16
Listeria monocytogenes	>64	2 (0.5–2)	8 (4–16)	8–16	2–4	6–8	6.2–8	8 (4–>16)	2 (1–4)	1	—	0.25–0.5
Corynebacterium spp.	—	1 (0.05–128)	4 (4–>128)	8 (4–>128)	1 (0.5–64)	8 (8–>128)	>12.5	2 (1–32)	0.25 (0.25–64)	(0.12–4)	—	0.06–8
Bacillus spp.	—	0.25 (0.12–1)	1 (1)	1 (0.5–1)	0.5 (0.5)	—	—	0.5–1	0.25	—	—	≤0.015–0.12
Nocardia spp.	>128	(1.4–>25)	64	32	(2.6–>25)	64	—	64	—	—	—	—

Abbreviation: MIC_{90}, Minimal inhibitory concentration for 90% of strains.
Data from refs. 38 and 39.

TABLE 31–3 Activity of Selected Quinolones against Selected Anaerobic Bacteria and Mycobacteria In Vitro

Organism	Representative MIC_{90} (Range) (μg/ml)											
	Nalidixic Acid	*Ciprofloxacin*	*Norfloxacin*	*Enoxacin*	*Ofloxacin*	*Pefloxacin*	*Lomefloxacin*	*Fleroxacin*	*Sparfloxacin*	*Levofloxacin*	*Grepafloxacin*	*Trovafloxacin*
Bacteroides fragilis	512	4–128	>128	32	2–12.5	16	8–64	≥16	1–2	4–6.25	0.5–12.5	0.25–>8
Bacteroides spp.	512	1–32	128	16	2–32	—	8–32	2–64	4	(0.5–64)	—	0.5–4
Fusobacterium spp.	256	2–8	16	32	2–16	32	16	16	—	1	1–4	0.25–4
Clostridium spp.	256	1–16	2	32	1–8	1	16	2–32	4	(0.12–4)	—	0.5–2
Clostridium perfringens	64	0.5–8	8	16	0.5–8	8	2–8	1–4	0.5–2	0.25	0.5–2	0.12–0.5
Clostridium difficile	>128	8–25	128	128	12.5–16	64	≥32	16–32	6.25	—	1–50	1–4
Anaerobic gram-positive cocci	256–512	2–6.25	16–64	2–8	2–8	16	4–25	8–12.5	1–4	1–8	1–4	0.25–1
Mycobacterium tuberculosis	—	1	8	>5	0.8–1.3	8	4	≤0.5	0.2	0.5–1	3.1	32
Mycobacterium avium complex	—	16	≥16	>256	10–100	>64	—	16	12.5	(1–8)	12.5	64
Mycobacterium chelonae	—	8	>16	—	>20	>64	—	>32	6.25–>100	(1–4)	≥100	—
Mycobacterium fortuitum	—	0.3	2	—	1–3.1	2	—	≤0.5	1.56	0.25	25	—
Mycobacterium kansasii	—	1	8	≥5	1–3.1	4	—	≤0.5	—	0.25	25	—

Abbreviation: MIC_{90}, Minimal inhibitory concentrations for 90% of strains.
Data from refs. 38–40.

TABLE 31–4 Pharmacokinetics of Selected Quinolones

Quinolone	Dose (mg)	C_{max} (μg/ml)	Half-life (h)	Bioavailability (%)	V_D (liters)	Cl_r (ml/min)	Renal Excretion* (%)
Norfloxacin	400 PO	1.5	3.3	50	—	234	27
Ciprofloxacin	500 PO	2.4	4	70	358	358	40
	400 IV	4.6	5–6	—	147	300	—
Ofloxacin	400 PO	4.6	4–5	95	102	195	73
	400 IV	5.5	6	—	102	190	—
Levofloxacin	500 PO	5.7	6–8	99	102	116	77
	500 IV	6.4	6–8	—	91	99	—
Pefloxacin	400 PO	3.2	10.5	95	112	13	11†
	400 IV	5.8	11	—	134	20	—
Enoxacin	400 PO	2.3	4.9	88	175	193	44
Lomefloxacin	400 PO	3.5	7.8	95	133	189	66
Fleroxacin	400 PO	4.3	11.2	92	97	53	50‡
Sparfloxacin	200 PO	1.1	20	92	273	25	10
Grepafloxacin	600 PO	2.2	15.7	70	355	47	<10
Trovafloxacin	200 PO	3.1	12.2	88	—	9	6
Alatrofloxacin	200 IV	3.1	11.7	—	91	10	6

*Cumulative percentage of dose in urine after 24 hours.
†After 84 hours.
‡After 72 hours.
Abbreviations: C_{max}: Maximal serum concentration; Cl_r: renal clearance; IV, intravenous; PO, by mouth; V_D: volume of distribution.
Data from manufacturers and refs. 39, 43–45, 221–228.

acid is more active than its parent compound. These metabolites and inactive glucuronide conjugates linked to the 3-carboxyl group are excreted in the urine. Conversion of norfloxacin, ciprofloxacin, enoxacin, and fleroxacin to less active metabolites accounts for 10 to 20% of elimination. There is minimal hepatic biotransformation (<10%) of ofloxacin and lomefloxacin. Hepatic metabolism and biliary excretion are the principal routes of elimination of sparfloxacin (90% of dose, largely by glucuronidation), grepafloxacin (65% of dose; metabolism by cytochrome P-450 isozyme 1A2), and trovafloxacin (largely biliary excretion of unchanged drug; 25% glucuronidation; minimal metabolism). In addition to glucuronide conjugates and desmethylpiperazinyl derivatives, other metabolites of quinolones that have been identified have had predominantly alterations of the piperazine ring, including *N*-oxide, *N*-sulfo, *N*-formyl, and desethylene derivatives.[44, 53, 54]

Transintestinal secretion has been identified after the intravenous administration of ciprofloxacin and accounts for about 10 to 15% of drug excretion.[44]

Dosage Adjustments in Renal and Hepatic Insufficiency

As expected from differences in the routes of excretion, increases in drug half-lives in the presence of severe renal insufficiency are greatest for ofloxacin (four- to fivefold) and least for pefloxacin, grepafloxacin, and trovafloxacin (no change), with other quinolones exhibiting intermediate effects (about twofold) (see Table 31–6). To prevent excessive drug accumulation, dosage reduction (an increase in the dose interval from 12 to 24 hours or halving the daily dose for those quinolones normally given once daily) is indicated at creatinine clearances below 50 ml/min for ofloxacin and levofloxacin and below 30 ml/min for norfloxacin, ciprofloxacin, enoxacin, and lomefloxacin. No dosage reduction is indicated for nalidixic acid, pefloxacin, grepafloxacin, and trovafloxacin. Because its glucuronide conjugates may accumulate in the presence of renal failure, the dose of sparfloxacin is reduced below a creatinine clearance of 50 ml/min. Clearance by hemodialysis is low (≤14% of plasma clearance) for norfloxacin, ciprofloxacin, ofloxacin, and enoxacin and is slightly greater (28%) for pefloxacin. Similarly, peritoneal dialysis contributes little to the clearance of ciprofloxacin and ofloxacin.[55]

Despite its hepatic metabolism by glucuronidation, reduction in the dose of sparfloxacin is not recommended for patients with hepatic insufficiency. For pefloxacin but not norfloxacin, ciprofloxacin, and ofloxacin, threefold increases in the half-lives were seen in some patients with cirrhosis, but there was substantial variation.[51] Changes in renal function that accompany severe liver disease may, however, affect ciprofloxacin and ofloxacin elimination to a lesser extent. In patients with severe liver disease, reduction of the pefloxacin dose (possibly a twofold increase in the dose interval) with monitoring of drug levels in serum may be indicated. Reductions in the dose of trovafloxacin (from 300 mg to 200 mg every 24 hours or from 200 mg to 100 mg every 24 hours) are recommended for patients with Child-Pugh class A and B cirrhosis. Grepafloxacin is contraindicated in the presence of hepatic failure.

TABLE 31–5 Body Tissues, Fluids, and Cells in Which Quinolone Concentrations Exceed Quinolone Concentrations in Serum

Site	Fold Increment
Prostate tissue	0.9–2.3
Feces	100–1000
Bile	2–20
Lung tissue	1.6–6
Macrophages and neutrophils	2–>100

Interactions with Other Drugs

When coadministered by mouth with aluminum-, magnesium-, or, to a lesser extent, calcium-containing antacids, quinolones have markedly reduced oral bioavailability, presumably because of the formation of cation-quinolone complexes that are poorly absorbed.[56] Sucralfate, which contains large numbers of aluminum ions, also reduces the absorption of quinolones. Although staggering doses of antacids and quinolones may reduce this interaction, there is sufficient variability to suggest that this maneuver may not be fully reliable in an individual patient. Generally H_2-receptor antagonists and proton-pump inhibitors do not have important effects on the absorption of quinolones, with the exceptions that ranitidine reduces enoxacin absorption by 60% and omeprazole reduces trovafloxacin absorption by 17%.[57] Concurrent administration of quinolones with $FeSO_4$, multivitamin-mineral regimens containing zinc, and the buffered formulation of dideoxyinosine have also been reported to reduce quinolone absorption.[58] Nutritional supplements given by nasogastric tube may reduce the absorption of quinolones given concurrently by the same route, likely because these supplements also contain multivalent cations such as iron and zinc.

TABLE 31–6 Dosage of Quinolones in Patients with Normal and Reduced Renal Function

Quinolone	Normal Renal Function		Renal Failure with GFR (ml/min)		Removal by Dialysis
	Oral	*Intravenous*	*10–50*	*<10*	
Nalidixic acid	500–1000 mg q6h	—	No change	No change	
Cinoxacin	250 mg q6h	—	1× dose q12h	1× dose q24h	
Norfloxacin	400 mg q12h	—	1× dose q24h	1× dose q24h	No (H, P)
Ciprofloxacin	250–750 mg q12h	200–400 mg q12h	1× dose q18h	1× dose q24h	No (H, P)
Ofloxacin	200–400 mg q12h	200–400 mg q12h	1× dose q24h	1/2× dose q24h	No (H, P)
Pefloxacin	400 mg q12h	400 mg q12h	No change	No change	No (H)
Enoxacin	200–400 mg q12h	—	1/2× dose q12h	1/2× dose q24h	No (H)
Lomefloxacin	400 mg q24h	—	1/2× dose q24h	1/2× dose q24h	No (H)
Sparfloxacin	400 mg loading dose, then 200 mg q24h	—	400 mg loading dose, then 1× dose q48h	—	No data
Levofloxacin	500 mg q24h	500 mg q24h	1/2× dose q24h	1/2× dose q48h	No (H, P)
Grepafloxacin	400–600 mg q24h	—	No change	No change	No data
Trovafloxacin	200–300 mg q24h	200–300 mg q24h	No change	No change	No (H)

Abbreviations: GFR: Glomerular filtration rate; H: hemodialysis; P: peritoneal dialysis; 1×: 100%; 1/2×: 50%.

For intravenous formulations of ciprofloxacin and pefloxacin, precipitates have been reported when these quinolones were infused through the same intravenous tubing with aminophylline, amoxicillin with and without clavulanate, or flucloxacillin. Separate infusions are indicated.

Quinolones vary in the extent to which they impair the elimination of the methylxanthines theophylline and caffeine. The effects appear to result from inhibition by some quinolones of hepatic cytochrome P-450 isozyme 1A2, which is involved in theophylline and caffeine metabolism. Enoxacin exhibits the greatest effect and may produce two- to threefold increases in theophylline concentrations in serum associated with a 40 to 65% reduction in total theophylline clearance without alterations in renal clearance of theophylline.[56] Similar effects of a lesser magnitude are seen with grepafloxacin (30% increase in maximal serum concentrations of theophylline), ciprofloxacin (30% reduction in clearance and 20 to 90% increases in serum concentrations of theophylline), and pefloxacin (30% reduction in clearance), but norfloxacin, ofloxacin, levofloxacin, fleroxacin, lomefloxacin, sparfloxacin, and trovafloxacin had little or no effect (2 to 11% increases in serum concentrations of theophylline).[59, 60] In patients receiving enoxacin, grepafloxacin, or ciprofloxacin in combination with theophylline, serum levels of theophylline should be monitored and reductions in the dose of theophylline considered. No such adjustments should be needed in patients receiving theophylline concurrently with other fluoroquinolones.

Nonsteroidal anti-inflammatory drugs (NSAIDs) may affect the central nervous system stimulant effects of quinolones. Seizures were reported in a group of Japanese patients receiving enoxacin and the NSAID fenbufen. Potentiation of seizures by combinations of quinolones and NSAIDs has also been reported in animals. Assays of the displacement of the inhibitory neurotransmitter γ-aminobutyric acid (GABA) or a related molecule from GABA receptors in rat brain tissue have demonstrated displacement of GABA by quinolones and enhancement of this displacement by fenbufen and by theophylline. Patients receiving quinolones with NSAIDs should be cautioned about and monitored for these potential adverse effects.

Interactions with other drugs have been studied less extensively. Rifampin appears not to affect the pharmacokinetics of ciprofloxacin. Ciprofloxacin and pefloxacin appear to have little effect on the pharmacokinetics of cyclosporine in some but not all studies. Although probenecid reduces the renal clearance of norfloxacin and fleroxacin, no quinolone accumulation occurs. The effect of probenecid might be predicted to be greater with quinolones such as ofloxacin and lomefloxacin for which renal clearance includes tubular secretion and is the predominant mode of clearance, but data are lacking. Enoxacin and ciprofloxacin have been shown to reduce the clearance of the less active *R*-enantiomer of warfarin, but had no clinically important effect on the more active *S*-enantiomer.[61] Concomitant administration of morphine decreases maximal serum concentrations of oral trovafloxacin by 46%.

CLINICAL USES

Earlier quinolones such as nalidixic acid, oxolinic acid, and cinoxacin were used almost exclusively for the treatment of urinary tract infections, although nalidixic acid was also used for the treatment of shigellosis. With the development of the more potent fluoroquinolones, a broader array of infections can now be treated with members of the fluoroquinolone class.

Urinary Tract Infections

Although the low pH and magnesium concentrations present in urine may reduce quinolone activity, the concentrations of many quinolones in urine are usually sufficient to provide substantial therapeutic ratios of urinary drug concentration to the MIC of most urinary pathogens. Lower urinary concentrations are expected with sparfloxacin, grepafloxacin, and trovafloxacin because of their predominantly nonrenal clearance.

For uncomplicated urinary tract infections, usually in symptomatic young women with cystitis caused by highly susceptible organisms such as *E. coli,* most quinolones are likely to be highly effective when given for brief courses of 3 to 10 days,[62] and norfloxacin, ciprofloxacin, and ofloxacin have been found to be comparable to trimethoprim-sulfamethoxazole.[63] Usually the lowest dose in the dosage range (see Table 31–6) is sufficient for the treatment of these infections. Three-day regimens of norfloxacin and lomefloxacin result in cure rates of 81 to 96%.[64] Limited data on single-dose therapies with ciprofloxacin, ofloxacin, and norfloxacin indicate eradication in 75 to 96% of patients.[65, 66] Single-dose norfloxacin (800 mg) was equivalent to a 3-day regimen for *E. coli* infections,[67] but for *Staphylococcus saprophyticus* infections, a 7-day regimen is preferred because of failures with shorter courses.[68, 69] Women with uncomplicated pyelonephritis given norfloxacin or ofloxacin for 7 to 10 days have bacteriologic cure rates comparable to those with trimethoprim-sulfamethoxazole. For prophylaxis of recurrent infections in women, norfloxacin (200 mg at bedtime) was highly effective and superior to nitrofurantoin,[70] and low doses of ofloxacin (100 mg), norfloxacin (200 mg), and ciprofloxacin (125 mg) taken after coitus have also been effective as prophylaxis.[71]

Complicated urinary tract infections occurring in men and in patients from catheters or structural or functional abnormalities of the urinary tract are often caused by more resistant pathogens and have a higher frequency of relapse and reinfection. Bacteriologic cure rates for ciprofloxacin were superior to those for trimethoprim-sulfamethoxazole and aminoglycosides shortly after completion of a

7- to 10-day course, but the low fractions of patients who continued to have sterile urine were similar by 4 to 6 weeks after therapy.[63, 72] The superiority of lomefloxacin (400 mg daily) over trimethoprim-sulfamethoxazole both given for 14 days in eradication of bacteriuria was shown at initial post-therapy evaluation, and differences at late follow-up were sustained in the subset of male patients.[73] Sparfloxacin (200 mg loading dose followed by 100 mg daily) and ciprofloxacin (500 mg twice daily) given for 10 to 14 days were equivalent in clinical response, but eradication of bacteriuria was lower for sparfloxacin, possibly reflecting its lower concentrations in urine.[74] In collected noncomparative trials, infections caused by *P. aeruginosa* were eradicated in 70% of patients given ciprofloxacin and 83% given norfloxacin. Development of bacterial resistance has been associated with therapeutic failure in about 2% of patients overall, but resistance rates (10 to 20%) may be higher for *P. aeruginosa* infections. In patients with bladder dysfunction due to spinal cord injury who used intermittent suprapubic taps or self-catheterization for bladder emptying, ciprofloxacin (100 mg at bedtime) reduced episodes of infection about 10-fold relative to placebo.[75] Whereas infections in the placebo group represented a mixture of enteric and nonenteric bacteria and enterococci, breakthrough infections in the ciprofloxacin group were largely nonenteric bacteria, particularly *P. aeruginosa,* which were often resistant.

Prostatitis

Fluoroquinolones concentrate in prostatic tissue with lower levels in prostatic fluid. In one small comparative study of men with predominantly *E. coli* infections, norfloxacin given for 4 to 6 weeks was superior (92% eradication) to trimethoprim-sulfamethoxazole (67% eradication) at 1 month follow-up.[76] In open studies, similar courses of norfloxacin, ciprofloxacin, and ofloxacin have produced eradication rates of 67 to 91% at follow-up ranging from 1 to 13 months. With 2-week courses of therapy and infections caused by less susceptible organisms such as *P. aeruginosa* and enterococci, failures appear to be more frequent.[63, 77] No published data are available on use of trovafloxacin for the treatment of prostatitis.

Sexually Transmitted Diseases

Quinolones have activity in vitro against the major sexually transmitted pathogens, *Neisseria gonorrhoeae, C. trachomatis,* and *Haemophilus ducreyi,* but appear to lack activity against *T. pallidum.*

Uncomplicated gonococcal urethritis and cervicitis are effectively eradicated by single doses of quinolones (norfloxacin, 800 mg; ciprofloxacin, 250 mg; ofloxacin, 400 mg; fleroxacin, 400 mg; sparfloxacin, 200 mg; grepafloxacin, 400 mg; trovafloxacin, 100 mg.[78–82] Rectal and pharyngeal infections have also been cured in 99 and 88% of patients, respectively. Single doses of ciprofloxacin (500 mg) or ofloxacin (400 mg) are considered as alternative regimens for the treatment of gonorrhea at genital and nongenital sites in the guidelines from the Centers for Disease Control and Prevention.[83] Small numbers of patients with gonococcal salpingitis have been cured with 10- to 14-day courses of sequential intravenous and oral ciprofloxacin or oral ofloxacin,[84, 85] and intravenous regimens of ciprofloxacin (400 mg every 12 hours) or ofloxacin (400 mg every 12 hours) may be used for disseminated infection with a switch to oral therapy after improvement to complete a 1-week course.[83]

Single doses of quinolones are ineffective for genital chlamydial infections.[78] Seven-day courses of therapy with norfloxacin and ciprofloxacin and a 3-day course of sparfloxacin have also had unacceptably low response rates, but 7-day courses of ofloxacin and sparfloxacin were comparable to a similar course of doxycycline for the treatment of chlamydial infections and nongonococcal urethritis,[86–89] and ofloxacin (300 mg twice daily for 7 days) is a recommended alternative regimen.[83] There are only limited data on the use of ofloxacin for the treatment of patients with chlamydial salpingitis.[85]

In patients with chancroid, *H. ducreyi* was eradicated from genital ulcers by ciprofloxacin (500 mg twice daily for 3 days) and enoxacin (400 mg twice daily for 3 doses) in 93% of patients, a result comparable to that with trimethoprim-sulfamethoxazole.[90] The ciprofloxacin regimen is an option for the treatment of chancroid in the Centers for Disease Control and Prevention guidelines.[83]

For treatment of pelvic inflammatory disease, a syndrome with mixed microbiology including gonococci, chlamydiae, enteric bacteria, and anaerobes, clinical response rates for ofloxacin (400 mg twice daily for 10 days) and cefoxitin (2 g intravenously once) plus doxycycline (100 mg twice daily for 10 days) were similar, and ofloxacin was highly effective in eradicating gonococci and chlamydia.[91] Ciprofloxacin (250 mg twice daily) plus clindamycin (300 mg three times daily) given for 14 days was also comparable to ceftriaxone plus doxycycline with high clinical cure rates.[92] The Centers for Disease Control and Prevention now recommends a combination of ofloxacin (400 mg twice daily) and metronidazole (500 mg twice daily) given for 14 days as a preferred oral regimen for the treatment of pelvic inflammatory disease.[83] Two cases of gonococcal septic arthritis have responded to ciprofloxacin. For bacterial vaginosis, ofloxacin was less effective than metronidazole.[93] Data on the treatment of syphilis with quinolones in humans are inadequate, but in animal models, ofloxacin has failed.

Gastrointestinal and Abdominal Infections

All bacterial pathogens known to cause gastroenteritis are generally susceptible to quinolones in vitro. Although fecal material may decrease the activity of quinolones, drug concentrations in feces are exceedingly high. The penetration of quinolones into macrophages (see Table 31–5) may also be important for their effectiveness in systemic *Salmonella* infections.

In traveler's diarrhea, which is often caused by enterotoxigenic *E. coli* and *Shigella* spp., norfloxacin (400 mg twice daily for 3 days) or ciprofloxacin (500 mg twice daily for 5 days), with therapy begun shortly after the onset of diarrhea, have shortened the duration of loose stools by 1 to 3 days relative to placebo and have been comparable to trimethoprim-sulfamethoxazole.[94, 95] When given as prophylaxis to travelers, quinolones have produced protection rates that ranged from 68 to 92% compared with placebo controls, although the routine use of quinolones or other antimicrobials is not recommended for the prevention of diarrhea in travelers.[96] Contingency treatment at the onset of diarrhea is preferred for travelers, and with this approach, norfloxacin (400 mg twice daily for 3 days)[97] and ciprofloxacin (500 mg single dose)[98] were shown to shorten diarrhea by 1 to 3 days relative to placebo, with the largest benefit seen with patients with *Campylobacter jejuni* infection given norfloxacin.

In patients with shigellosis, 5-day courses of norfloxacin, ciprofloxacin, and ofloxacin have been highly effective. The addition of loperamide to ciprofloxacin may further shorten the duration of diarrhea.[99] Even a single dose of ciprofloxacin (750 mg) may be effective in shigellosis, except those cases caused by *Shigella dysenteriae* type 1.[100] In patients with *Salmonella* and *C. jejuni* infections, symptoms may be shortened with ciprofloxacin or norfloxacin, but the eradication of stool carriage of *Salmonella* is often transient[101, 102] although not necessarily prolonged.[103] Clinical and microbiologic failures have been associated with the development of resistant *C. jejuni* in some[104, 105] but not all studies.[103] Norfloxacin (400 mg twice daily for 3 days) has been shown to be superior to trimethoprim-sulfamethoxazole, a single dose of doxycycline, and placebo in shortening diarrhea in patients with cholera,[106, 107] and 3 days of ciprofloxacin (250 mg every day) and a standard tetracycline (500 mg four times daily) regimen were comparable.[108] In patients with diarrhea caused by *Yersinia enterocolitica, Plesiomonas shigelloides,* and *Aeromonas* spp., quinolones have eradicated the organisms from stool but have not yet been clearly shown to shorten clinical illness.[63]

In noncomparative studies of patients with enteric fever caused predominantly by *Salmonella typhi,* ciprofloxacin cured 92% of patients and ofloxacin cured 96% percent, with resolution of fever within 5 days.[109, 110] Three- to 5-day courses of ofloxacin (200 mg twice daily; 10 mg/kg daily in pediatric patients) have been highly effective and in adults shown to be superior to ceftriaxone given for 3 days for patients with enteric fever.[111, 112] Relapses have been reported in some patients with acquired immunodeficiency syndrome and bacteremic nontyphoidal *Salmonella* infections. Because of their effectiveness in short-course regimens and the common occurrence of resistance to other antimicrobials in *S. typhi* isolates in some areas of the developing world, ciprofloxacin or ofloxacin are now considered the agents of choice for treatment of patients with enteric fever. Chronic fecal carriage of *S. typhi* has been eradicated in 83 to 93% of small numbers of patients, including a few with gallstones, given norfloxacin, ciprofloxacin, or ofloxacin for 4 weeks.[113, 114]

Although active against *Helicobacter pylori* in vitro, quinolones have failed to eradicate this organism from gastric mucosa, and failures have been associated with the acquisition of quinolone resistance.[63] Data are quite limited on the use of quinolones for the treatment of biliary tract infections. In a single small study, 83% of patients with cholecystitis and cholangitis, most associated with *E. coli* bacteremia, responded to intravenous and then oral ciprofloxacin therapy.[115] For patients with complicated intra-abdominal infections due to disruption of the integrity of the gastrointestinal tract, a mixture of anaerobes and facultative gram-negative aerobes with or without enterococci are usually involved. In a randomized, double-blind trial, ciprofloxacin (400 mg intravenously every 12 hours or 500 mg orally every 12 hours) plus metronidazole (500 mg intravenously or orally every 6 hours) was compared with imipenem (500 mg every 6 hours) for patients with complicated infections largely due to disease of the colon, small bowel, and appendix. Ciprofloxacin and metronidazole were given either entirely intravenously or with a switch to orally after an initial response. Clinical outcomes were highly similar in all three arms of the study. There was, however, regardless of treatment, a significantly higher rate of treatment failure if enterococci were isolated from the site of infection (28%) than if they were not (14%),[116] suggesting that additional agents active against enterococci should be considered if culture results dictate. Trovafloxacin, which has activity against gram-negative bacilli similar to that of ciprofloxacin and additional activity against anaerobic bacteria, has been approved in the United States as a single treatment of intra-abdominal infections, and preliminary unpublished data suggest clinical response rates similar to those of imipenem followed by amoxicillin-clavulanate.

The use of quinolones in peritonitis has been evaluated most in patients undergoing chronic ambulatory peritoneal dialysis and in patients with cirrhosis. Oral ofloxacin (300 mg daily) and ciprofloxacin (500 mg daily) have cured episodes of peritonitis in chronic ambulatory peritoneal dialysis patients, but failures in infections caused by the common coagulase-negative staphylococci have occurred. Higher concentrations of ciprofloxacin have been achieved by adding drug to the dialysate (20 to 50 μg/ml) with outcomes similar to those with standard regimens of intraperitoneal vancomycin plus gentamicin.[117] In patients with cirrhosis at high risk for recurrent spontaneous bacterial peritonitis, norfloxacin (400 mg daily) given as prophylaxis reduced recurrences by threefold.[118] Ciprofloxacin (750 mg given once weekly) has also been effective.[119] Prolonged use of norfloxacin was, however, later associated with increasing occurrence of quinolone-resistant bacteria.[120] Thus, the risks of selecting resistant enteric bacteria must also be considered before embarking on prolonged use in prophylaxis.

Respiratory Tract Infections

A range of respiratory tract pathogens is susceptible to a number of quinolones in vitro. *Haemophilus influenzae, M. catarrhalis,* and enteric gram-negative bacilli are highly susceptible. Ciprofloxacin and ofloxacin also have activity against the agents of atypical pneumonias, *M. pneumoniae, C. pneumoniae,* and *L. pneumophila,* and against *Staph. aureus* and *M. tuberculosis.* Least susceptible among common pathogens is *Strep. pneumoniae,* but levofloxacin, sparfloxacin, grepafloxacin, and trovafloxacin have improved activity.

Patients with acute bacterial exacerbations of chronic bronchitis have been treated with many different quinolones, which have generally been effective in eradicating *H. influenzae* from sputum.[39, 121, 122] In studies with ciprofloxacin, eradication rates for *Strep. pneumoniae* and *P. aeruginosa* were lower, and some failures have been associated with the development of bacterial resistance. In comparative trials, clinical responses have usually been similar to or better than those with ampicillin, amoxicillin, or cefaclor. In a randomized community-based study, ciprofloxacin (500 mg orally twice a day) resulted in similar clinical outcomes compared with usual treatments (agents chosen at the discretion of the investigator and dominated by macrolides, cefuroxime, and amoxicillin with or without clavulanate) but was somewhat more expensive, except in those patients with the greatest frequency of recurrent episodes, for whom ciprofloxacin was more cost-effective.[123] Microbiologic eradication rates were not determined. For more recently released quinolones with enhanced pneumococcal activity, in randomized comparative trials, clinical and microbiologic outcomes were similar for sparfloxacin (200 mg loading dose, then 100 mg daily) versus amoxicillin-clavulanate,[124] levofloxacin (500 mg daily) versus cefuroxime axetil,[125] and grepafloxacin (400 to 600 mg daily) versus amoxicillin.[126] In these studies, eradication of pneumococci from sputum was reported in 24 of 27 (89%) patients given sparfloxacin, 14 of 16 (88%) given levofloxacin, and 79 of 82 (96%) given grepafloxacin. Grepafloxacin and ciprofloxacin were also comparable in clinical outcomes, but ciprofloxacin appeared less effective in eradicating pneumococci from sputum in a small subset of patients.[127] Comparison of 5-day courses of trovafloxacin (200 mg every day), trovafloxacin (100 mg every day), and amoxicillin (500 mg three times daily) found similar rates of clinical success and bacteriologic eradication.[127a] There was a trend for better eradication of *H. influenzae* with trovafloxacin at both doses, but eradication of pneumococci was somewhat lower with the 100 mg dose of trovafloxacin (75 to 86%) than in either of the other two arms (95 to 100%).

In patients with community-acquired pneumonias, ciprofloxacin and ofloxacin have consistently eradicated *H. influenzae* and *M. catarrhalis.*[39] Cures of pneumococcal pneumonias, including a few cases with bacteremia, have been reported with intravenous and then oral ciprofloxacin[128] or ofloxacin[129, 130] and with oral ofloxacin alone,[131] but some failures with both drugs have occurred, and pneumococcal bacteremia has developed during ciprofloxacin therapy of pneumonia.[63] For newer quinolones, similar or better clinical and microbiologic efficacies relative to a range of comparison agents have been reported. Sparfloxacin (400 mg loading dose, then 200 mg daily) has been compared with high-dose amoxicillin (1 gm three times daily),[131a] high-dose amoxicillin plus ofloxacin,[132] and roxithromycin[133] with similar response rates overall. Clinical responses to sparfloxacin in the subgroups with pneumococci isolated from sputum were also generally comparable to those with comparison agents: sparfloxacin 71 of 80 (89%) versus amoxicillin 59 of 65 (91%),[131a] sparfloxacin 11 of 14 (79%) versus amoxicillin plus ofloxacin 9 of 11 (82%),[132] and sparfloxacin 25 of 26 (96%) versus roxithromycin 14 of 15 (93%).[133] Levofloxacin intravenous and/or oral (500 mg daily) produced somewhat higher clinical success (95% versus 90%) and microbiologic eradication rates (98% versus 88%) compared with ceftriaxone intravenous and/or oral cefuroxime axetil (with optional erythromycin or doxycycline).[134] Clinical responses in the group with pneumococcal infection were also similar (levofloxacin 30 of 30 [100%] versus ceftriaxone/cefuroxime 31 of 33 [94%]). Grepafloxacin (600 mg daily) produced similar clinical responses to amoxicillin (500 mg three times daily) overall and in the subgroup with pneumococci isolated from sputum (grepafloxacin 15 of 17 [88%] amoxicilllin versus 8 of 12 [67%]).[135] Trovafloxacin (200 mg daily) produced somewhat higher rates of clinical success (91% versus 81%, $p = 0.01$) than high-dose amoxicillin, and there was a trend toward higher eradication of pneumococci by trovafloxacin (20 of 20 [100%] versus 17 of 21 [81%]).[135a] Only three studies have included patients with pneumococcal pneumonia and bacteremia with generally good responses in the small numbers of patients treated with sparfloxacin (20 of 24 [83%]),[131a] levofloxacin (9 of 9 [100%]),[134] or trovafloxacin (4 of 4 [100%]).[135a]

Among atypical pneumonias, small numbers of patients with pneumonias caused by *Legionella,*[136, 137] *Mycoplasma,*[39] and *C. pneumoniae*[138] have also responded to ciprofloxacin and ofloxacin, but some apparent failures were seen in patients with *M. pneumoniae* and *C. pneumoniae* infection treated with ofloxacin.[130] Clinical responses to sparfloxacin and roxithromycin in patients with *M. pneumoniae* or *C. pneumoniae* infections were similar (26 of 27 [96%] for sparfloxacin versus 27 of 30 [90%]) for roxithromycin,[133] and clinical responses to levofloxacin in patients with *C. pneumoniae* (46 of 47), *M. pneumoniae* (19 of 19), and *L. pneumophila* (5 of 5) infection diagnosed serologically were high.[134] Similarly clinical responses to trovafloxacin were generally high in patients with infection with *M. pneumoniae* (16 of 17), *C. pneumoniae* (22 of 29), or *L. pneumophila* (6 of 6).[135a] Interpretation of clinical responses in patients with *M. pneumoniae* and *C. pneumoniae* pneumonia is difficult, however, because of improvement that may occur without antimicrobials.

Hospital-acquired pneumonias, which are commonly caused by gram-negative bacilli, have responded to intravenous ciprofloxacin[63, 139] and ofloxacin,[129] and responses to ciprofloxacin correlated with the level of susceptibility of the infecting organism, with better bacteriologic responses in infections caused by *Haemophilus* spp. and members of the Enterobacteriaceae than in infections caused by the less susceptible *P. aeruginosa.* For hospitalized patients with severe pneumonia, ciprofloxacin in a high dose (400 mg intravenously every 8 hours) was compared with imipenem (1000 mg intravenously every 8 hours) in a multicenter, randomized, double-blind trial.[140] Most of the patients (78%) had nosocomial pneumonia and were mechanically ventilated (79%). Clinical and microbiologic response rates were somewhat higher in the ciprofloxacin (69 and 69%) than in the imipenem (56 and 59%) group, and bacterial eradication rates were highest for members of the Enterobacteriaceae. Substantially poorer responses in both treatment groups were seen in patients with *P. aeruginosa* infection, and for both *P. aeruginosa* and *Staph. aureus,* persistence in sputum was substantial (60 to 67% and 35% of patients, respectively) and was associated with the development of resistance. For these reasons, combination therapy and the use of maximal approved doses of ciprofloxacin (750 mg orally every 12 hours or 400 mg intravenously every 12 hours to every 8 hours) may be preferred when quinolones are used in patients with *P. aeruginosa* infection.

Mild to moderate respiratory exacerbations in patients with cystic fibrosis and *P. aeruginosa* in sputum respond clinically to oral ciprofloxacin (750 mg twice daily) and ofloxacin (400 mg twice daily) similarly to conventional parenteral therapies that use an antipseudomonal β-lactam and tobramycin.[63] In patients with more severe exacerbations, however, conventional parenteral combination therapy may be superior. Rarely is *P. aeruginosa* eliminated from sputum by any regimen in patients with cystic fibrosis. Rotating the use of different regimens may reduce the selective pressure for the persistence of resistant bacteria that may emerge with either type of regimen.

Invasive otitis externa in diabetic patients is usually caused by *P. aeruginosa* and may respond to oral ciprofloxacin (750 mg twice daily) given for 6 weeks.[63] No studies comparing quinolones with conventional parenteral therapies have been reported.

Bone and Joint Infections

The prolonged antimicrobial therapy usually employed for bone and joint infections is facilitated by effective oral agents, and quinolones may fill this role in some cases.[141] For the treatment of chronic osteomyelitis, there have been noncomparative trials using ciprofloxacin, ofloxacin, or pefloxacin in which the treatment was usually for 6 or more weeks and the follow-up was for at least 6 months after the completion of therapy.[39, 63] Clinical cures after oral ciprofloxacin (750 mg twice daily) therapy were 75% overall in infections in which gram-negative bacilli predominated, and similar rates of cure were reported in the smaller subgroups of patients with *P. aeruginosa* and methicillin-susceptible *Staph. aureus* (MSSA) infections. Failures were associated with incomplete débridement, the presence of foreign bodies, and the development of resistance in *P. aeruginosa, Staph. aureus,* and *Serratia marcescens.* Three months of treatment with ciprofloxacin produced a cure rate of 60% in one study of osteomyelitis in the feet of diabetic patients.[142] Calcaneal osteochondritis due to nail puncture wounds of the foot is often due to *P. aeruginosa.* Local débridement in combination with ciprofloxacin (400 mg intravenously every 12 hours, then 750 mg orally twice daily) given for 14 days appears to be highly effective for this condition with cures in all 18 patients with *P. aeruginosa* infection and two with *Staph. aureus* infection.[143]

In four small comparative trials, ciprofloxacin (750 mg twice daily) and ofloxacin (400 mg twice daily) have generally produced apparent rates of cure similar to those of conventional parenteral therapies using β-lactams with or without an aminoglycoside,[63, 144] but the power of these studies to detect differences between the regimens has been small. For ofloxacin, cures of MSSA infections were 80% (10 of 12), but cures of *P. aeruginosa* infections were only 25% (1 of 4).[144]

For septic arthritis of prosthetic joints, standard therapy involves staged prosthesis removal, prolonged antibiotic treatment, and prosthesis reimplantation. Infections of prosthetic joints due to *Staph. aureus* and coagulase-negative staphylococci have been treated with ofloxacin (200 mg orally three times daily) plus rifampin (900 mg daily) for 6 to 9 months using the standard approach as well as retention of the prosthesis in patients for whom removal was not possible.[145] With prolonged follow-up after the completion of therapy, response rates were high in patients following the standard approach (81 to 93%) and unexpectedly high in the patients with retained prostheses (54 to 70%). Similar results have been reported for ciprofloxacin plus rifampin that also document the importance of rifampin in the antimicrobial regimen, since failure rates were high when ciprofloxacin was used alone.[146] Ceftazidime (1.5 g every 12 hours) given for 6 weeks plus ciprofloxacin (500 mg orally every 8 hours) given for 6 months also appeared to cure *P. aeruginosa*–infected orthopedic implants without prosthesis removal.[147]

There are few other data on the treatment of septic arthritis with quinolones, most often with ciprofloxacin, ofloxacin,[39] or fleroxacin.[148] Infections caused by *N. gonorrhoeae* and *E. coli* have responded to oral therapy. Failures have been seen in infections of prosthetic joints and infections caused by *Staph. aureus* and *P. aeruginosa.*

Skin and Soft Tissue Infections

Quinolones have been evaluated as treatment for skin and soft tissue infections.[149]

Comparisons of oral ciprofloxacin (750 mg twice daily)[150] and ofloxacin (400 mg twice daily)[151] with intravenous cefotaxime given for 9 days to patients with mixed infections in which gram-negative bacilli predominated showed similar rates of clinical and bacteriologic efficacy (80 to 90%) in both cases. For treatment of uncomplicated skin and soft tissue infections in which *Staph. aureus* and *Strep. pyogenes* predominated, levofloxacin (500 mg daily) and ciprofloxacin (500 mg twice daily) had similar clinical efficacy (98 versus 94%, respectively), but levofloxacin was significantly more effective in eradicating *Staph. aureus.*[152] In these and noncomparative studies[39] failures have been seen with infections caused by *P. aeruginosa* (11%), streptococci (6%), and *Staph. aureus* (5%) and have been associated with the development of resistant organisms, which for *P. aeruginosa* may be more frequent in diabetic patients.[149] In diabetic foot infections without osteomyelitis, the overall rate for complete healing using ciprofloxacin alone was 50%.[142] The use of additional antimicrobial agents with activity against anaerobes should be considered in these patients. Other studies have shown similar rates of clinical and bacteriologic response to oral fleroxacin (400 mg daily) and amoxicillin-clavulanate in patients in whom staphylococcal infections with skin abscesses and ulcers and impetigo predominated.[153] Published data on the use of trovafloxacin for treatment of diabetic foot infections are not yet available.

For patients with uncomplicated cellulitis or pyodermas in whom staphylococci and streptococci are the most likely pathogens, conventional therapies with penicillin, semisynthetic penicillins, and cephalosporins, either oral or parenteral, remain the therapies of choice. For infections with methicillin-resistant *Staph. aureus* (MRSA) for which the quinolones were initially hoped to be valuable oral therapies, the rapid emergence of quinolone resistance has become a particular problem, and resistance is now highly prevalent in many medical centers.[154] Thus, vancomycin remains the therapy of choice for MRSA infections.

Other Uses

There are limited data on the use of quinolones for the treatment of mycobacterial infections. In patients with multidrug-resistant pulmonary tuberculosis, ofloxacin (300 or 800 mg daily) has been used in combination with other second-line agents with sputum conversions and apparent clinical cures,[155] but in cases in which ofloxacin was the only active drug, there was failure of sputum conversion and the development of ofloxacin resistance.[155, 156] Ciprofloxacin (750 mg orally daily) has been compared with rifampin when used together with three other agents, isoniazid, pyrazinamide, and streptomycin, for short-course (6 month) therapy. Somewhat poorer responses were seen in the ciprofloxacin-containing regimen than in the rifampin-containing regimen (3 of 18 [17%] versus 1 of 17 [6%] bacteriologic relapses).[157] Ciprofloxacin (750 mg daily) combined with rifampin and isoniazid was also associated with a slower rate of conversion of sputums to negative and a higher rate of relapse than a regimen of isoniazid, rifampin, pyrazinamide, and ethambutol, a difference that was particularly apparent in the group of patients with human immunodeficiency virus infection.[158] Thus, ciprofloxacin appears to be less effective than first-line antituberculous agents, but its activity and that of ofloxacin may be valuable when second-line agents are needed because of resistance to first-line agents.

For nontuberculous mycobacteria, ciprofloxacin (750 mg twice daily or 500 mg three times daily) has been used in three-drug (with clarithromycin plus amikacin)[159] and four-drug (with rifampin, ethambutol, and clofazimine)[160] regimens in patients with AIDS and *M. avium-intracellulare* complex bacteremia. Improvement in symptoms occurred with both regimens, but clearance of bacteremia appeared better with the clarithromycin-containing three-drug regimen.[161] In cutaneous *M. fortuitum* infections, ciprofloxacin used alone was followed by relapse and the development of drug resistance,[63] but ofloxacin has been used successfully in some sternotomy infections caused by *M. fortuitum.*[162] Preliminary studies have also documented bactericidal activity in vivo and clinical improvement in patients with lepromatous leprosy given ofloxacin (400 mg daily) and pefloxacin (800 mg daily).[163]

For patients with bacteremias, intravenous ciprofloxacin and ofloxacin have been effective in cases caused by enteric gram-negative bacilli, although responses have been poor for *P. aeruginosa* bacteremias when these drugs were used in relatively low doses of 200 mg twice daily.[164, 165] In neutropenic patients with fever, ciprofloxacin in combination with aminoglycosides produced defervescence and cure of documented infections comparably to standard β-lactam–aminoglycoside combinations,[166] but ciprofloxacin monotherapy was less effective than such combinations,[166] and should not be used. Although lower doses were used in some studies, in patients with normal renal function doses no less than 400 mg of ciprofloxacin twice daily would be preferred.[168] The use of quinolones in this setting should be cautious and should be considered principally as an alternative regimen when there are reasons for not choosing standard regimens with combinations of β-lactams and aminoglycosides.

Oral ciprofloxacin (500 mg twice daily), ofloxacin (300 mg twice daily), and norfloxacin (400 mg twice daily) given as prophylaxis in neutropenic patients have consistently reduced the occurrence of gram-negative bacteremia and in some cases prolonged the time to first fever, but breakthrough gram-positive bacteremias have occurred, particularly streptococcal bacteremias in bone marrow transplant recipients.[169, 170] Ciprofloxacin and ofloxacin appear superior to norfloxacin,[171, 172] with lower rates of gram-negative and, in the case of ofloxacin, streptococcal bacteremias. The addition of penicillin to norfloxacin therapy reduced breakthrough streptococcal bacteremias,[173] and the addition of rifampin to ofloxacin therapy reduced staphylococcal bacteremias.[172] In a feasibility study, highly selected low-risk patients with neutropenia and fever (expected duration of neutropenia of 7 days or less, clinical stability, reliable for compliance, and close follow-up) were randomized to inpatient and outpatient management, both groups receiving ofloxacin (400 mg orally twice daily).[174] Two thirds or more of patients had negative cultures of blood, urine, stool, and throat. Resolution of fever without a change of therapy occurred equivalently in the two groups (77 to 78% of episodes), but 21% of outpatients subsequently required admission to the hospital. One early death occurred in an outpatient, but overall death rates (4% of outpatients versus 2% of inpatients) were similar. Further studies are needed to define risk criteria and optimal regimens.

There is limited experience in using quinolones for the treatment of endocarditis. One study has reported good responses in intravenous drug abusers with right-sided MSSA endocarditis who complied with the full course of ciprofloxacin (300 mg intravenously twice daily for 1 week, then 750 mg orally twice daily for 3 weeks) plus rifampin (300 mg orally twice daily for 4 weeks).[175] An additional study compared 28 days of inpatient therapy with ciprofloxacin (750 mg orally twice daily) plus rifampin (300 mg orally twice daily) versus intravenous oxacillin plus gentamicin or vancomycin plus gentamicin (given for the first 5 days) for similar patients, with similar response rates for the two regimens when patients were evaluated at 6 to 7 days after the completion of therapy.[176] Drug resistance, however, has occurred in this setting, and there have been failures in patients with left-sided MSSA endocarditis. There have been a number of single case reports of patients with gram-negative bacillary endocarditis whose infections have been suppressed with oral quinolones, but there have been failures. The use of quinolones for endocarditis should currently be limited to circumstances in which established therapies are not possible.

Quinolones vary in their penetration across the blood-brain barrier into cerebrospinal fluid. In the presence of meningeal inflammation, concentrations in cerebrospinal fluid have reached as high as 39, 90, and 60% of serum concentrations for ciprofloxacin, ofloxacin, and pefloxacin, respectively. Trovafloxacin achieves cerebrospinal fluid concentrations that are 25% of those in serum in the absence of meningeal inflammation. In two small studies of patients with predominantly gram-negative bacillary meningitis, pefloxacin (800 mg intravenously every 12 hours) cured 12 of 16 neurosurgical patients, many of whom had failed to respond to β-lactam therapies,[177] and ciprofloxacin (200 mg intravenously every 12 hours) cured 18 of 20 similar patients.[178] Treatment of *P. aeruginosa* meningitis with ciprofloxacin may require very high doses in some patients (800 mg every 8 hours).[179] The use of these quinolones for the treatment of meningitis should only be considered in those circumstances in which standard therapies are not possible or have failed. For the eradication of nasopharyngeal carriage of *N. meningitidis,* which is indicated in the setting of close contact with patients with meningococcal meningitis, ciprofloxacin (750 mg) or ofloxacin (400 mg) given as a single dose has been highly effective,[180, 181] and ciprofloxacin had efficacy similar to those of rifampin (600 mg twice daily for 2 days) and ceftriaxone (2 g intramuscularly).[182]

Quinolones have been used for the treatment of a variety of other infections in small numbers of patients. A few patients with tularemia have responded to ciprofloxacin,[183] and several patients with cat-scratch disease improved more rapidly after ciprofloxacin treatment than might be expected without treatment.[184] Patients with Mediterranean spotted fever caused by *Rickettsia conorii* and Q fever caused by *Coxiella burnetii* may respond to ciprofloxacin or ofloxacin, but doxycycline remains the preferred therapy.[185] Attempts to treat patients with brucellosis with quinolones have been complicated by a high frequency of relapses,[186] but a combination of ofloxacin (400 mg daily) and rifampin (600 mg daily) for 6 weeks resulted in a low relapse rate and was comparable to doxycycline plus rifampin.[187] Patients with falciparum malaria have had inconsistent responses to quinolones.[188, 189]

PROBLEMS WITH QUINOLONE RESISTANCE DURING CLINICAL USE

The development of bacterial resistance among pathogens during the clinical use of quinolones is predicted to occur more often in settings in which there are large numbers of bacteria at the site of infection and the therapeutic index at this site is below 8,[190] because spontaneous chromosomal resistance mutations causing resistance increments of four- to eightfold for fluoroquinolones may occur at frequencies of 10^{-8} to 10^{-10}. Therapeutic indices below 8 are more likely in infections caused by less susceptible pathogens such as *P. aeruginosa* and *Staph. aureus* and at sites of infection at which drug delivery or host eradication mechanisms may be compromised and in patients who receive inadequate drug doses.

General surveys of resistance patterns occurring over time have found resistance to increase after the introduction of fluoroquinolones and to occur most often with *Pseudomonas* spp. and staphylococci and in soft tissue infections and infections associated with foreign bodies.[191, 192] In some medical centers, ciprofloxacin resistance has increased markedly (to over 90%) among MRSA but not MSSA strains. Resistance appears to have been selected in patients colonized with MRSA and given ciprofloxacin for other infections.[193] Clonal dissemination may also contribute to the spread of resistance during outbreaks. A similar difference between methicillin-resistant and methicillin-susceptible strains has been seen for ciprofloxacin resistance in coagulase-negative staphylococci, and in this setting cross-selection by exposure to other antibiotics in addition to direct quinolone selection appears to augment ciprofloxacin resistance in methicillin-resistant strains, which are usually also multidrug-resistant.[194]

Increasing fluoroquinolone resistance has also been noted among strains of *C. jejuni* in the Netherlands, Finland, and Spain (from 0 to 30%),[195] and clinical and microbiologic failures associated with the acquisition of resistance have been reported in some small studies.[104] Fluoroquinolone use in animals has also been associated with rising resistance in animal isolates, raising the risk that fluoroquinolones will be ineffective for human infections acquired from zoonotic sources.[196] Surprisingly, resistance has also occurred in *E. coli,* a usually highly susceptible pathogen, in two settings. Among strains causing urinary tract infections in Spain and France, resistance rose to 8 to 14% and was associated with quinolone use, complicated infections, and the use of urinary catheters.[197, 198] Resistance in *E. coli* was also seen in blood stream isolates from patients in cancer centers who had received fluoroquinolones as prophylaxis during periods of neutropenia. Resistance was associated with fluoroquinolone use and was shown to occur in different strains, likely representing selection from the endogenous reservoir of *E. coli* in the gastrointestinal tract.[199, 200] Fluoroquinolone resistance in *N. gonorrhoeae* has also become substantial in some countries in the Far East, and outbreaks of strains with reduced susceptibility also have been reported in some areas of the United States. In one outbreak, reduced susceptibility was associated with reduced rates of positive Gram stains of urethral discharge, thereby likely resulting in decreased detection and enhanced spread.[201] Resistance should be monitored, and strategies for minimizing its occurrence, including focused quinolone use, should be considered to avoid compromising the future utility of the fluoroquinolones. The inverse relationship between quinolone concentration and the frequency of selection of resistant mutants in vitro and in vivo[202, 203] also argues that underdosing of quinolones should be avoided to minimize opportunities for the selection of resistant bacteria.

ADVERSE EFFECTS

In an analysis of 56 double-blind randomized trials in which fluoroquinolones were compared with placebo or other antimicrobial agents, most studies found similar adverse effect profiles.[204] In six studies, there were significantly fewer adverse events with fluoroquinolones relative to the comparison agent (ciprofloxacin versus trimethoprim-sulfamethoxazole and ampicillin; norfloxacin versus trimethoprim-sulfamethoxazole and cefadroxil; ofloxacin versus erythromycin). Conversely, adverse events were more frequent with the fluoroquinolone in seven studies (ciprofloxacin versus doxycycline; norfloxacin versus placebo; temafloxacin versus cefadroxil; fleroxacin versus amoxicillin and placebo). In a number of instances, increasing doses and durations of therapy were associated with higher rates of adverse effects.

The most frequent category of adverse effect involves the gastrointestinal tract, occurring in 3 to 17% of patients reported in clinical trials. In most patients anorexia, nausea, vomiting, and abdominal discomfort when they occur are mild. An unpleasant taste, a side effect that is dose-related, has been reported by 9 to 17% of patients receiving grepafloxacin.[60] Diarrhea is less frequent, and antibiotic-associated colitis has been rare, possibly because most current quinolones have little or no effect on the anaerobic bowel flora. Trovafloxacin, which has activity against anaerobes, however, was reported by the manufacturer to be associated with diarrhea in only 2% of patients.

The next most frequent category of adverse effects involves the central nervous system, occurring in 0.9 to 11% of patients. Symptoms of mild headache and dizziness have predominated followed by insomnia and alterations in mood. Dizziness has been reported by the manufacturer in up to 11% of patients receiving trovafloxacin at 200 mg orally daily. Hallucinations, delirium, and seizures are rare with fluoroquinolones. Seizures may have resulted in some but not all cases from theophylline accumulation or from the ability of theophylline and NSAIDs to augment the ability of quinolones to displace GABA from its receptors.[205]

Allergic and skin reactions have occurred in 0.4 to 2.2% of patients in clinical trials. Unspecified rashes have been most frequent. Phototoxicity reactions also occur in some patients after exposure to ultraviolet A (320 to 400 nm) light and appear to be more frequent with lomefloxacin, pefloxacin, fleroxacin, and sparfloxacin.[206–210] All these agents except pefloxacin have a halide substituent at the 8 position, which is known to increase phototoxicity. Drug fever, urticaria, angioedema, vasculitis, serum sickness–like syndromes, and anaphylactoid reactions have been uncommon. Acute interstitial nephritis likely allergic in origin also occurs infrequently and has been associated with eosinophiluria but generally not crystalluria. Infiltrates of lymphocytes and eosinophils have been found in the renal interstitium on renal biopsies.

Arthropathy with cartilage erosions and noninflammatory effusions occurs in the weight-bearing joints of juvenile animals given quinolones. Experience with the use of quinolones in children has increased, particularly in children with cystic fibrosis given ciprofloxacin. These children and others receiving nalidixic acid, norfloxacin, and ciprofloxacin have only uncommonly had joint symptoms, which have been reversible.[211, 212] Studies to identify subclinical cartilage damage by nuclear magnetic resonance imaging of joints of treated children have also been negative.[213] In cystic fibrosis patients given pefloxacin, however, arthralgia and joint swelling developed in 14%.[214] Tendinitis with tendon rupture has been reported uncommonly in adults given norfloxacin, ofloxacin, and pefloxacin.[215] Because of concerns about cartilage toxicity in children, quinolones have not been recommended for routine pediatric use, but there is an evolving view based on the absence of human arthropathy seen over the past decade of fluoroquinolone use that in some children, particularly those with cystic fibrosis, the benefit of quinolones outweighs what appears to be a small short-term risk of joint toxicity, and expanded pediatric use of quinolones is under consideration.[212, 216]

QT-interval prolongation of a similar magnitude to that seen with erythromycin has been reported on the electrocardiograms of patients receiving sparfloxacin, and there have been rare (3 of 750,000) cases of ventricular arrhythmias associated with its use.[217] Grepafloxacin also prolongs the QT interval but substantially less than sparfloxacin. This effect has not been reported with other marketed quinolones.

Leukopenia and eosinophilia generally occur in less than 1% of patients, and mild elevations in serum transaminase levels occur in less than 1 to 3% of patients receiving quinolones; these abnormalities are rarely of sufficient severity to require the cessation of therapy. Asymptomatic transaminase elevations (≥ threefold normal) were reported in one study late in the course of therapy of 13 of 140 patients (9%) receiving trovafloxacin for 28 days for treatment of chronic prostatitis (manufacturer's data). These abnormalities resolved within 1 to 2 months after cessation of trovafloxacin. After marketing of trovafloxacin, however, there have been reports of rare (n >100, reporting incidence of 1 in 18,000 prescriptions) but serious hepatic reactions in patients receiving 2 to 14 days or more of trovafloxacin. Among these reactions were 14 cases of acute liver failure strongly associated with exposure to trovafloxacin, with 5 deaths and 4 patients requiring liver transplantation. These reports led the U.S. Food and Drug Administration to make recommendations that initial therapy with trovafloxacin be limited to inpatient use for serious and life- or limb-threatening infections including nosocomial pneumonia, community-acquired pneumonia, complicated intra-abdominal infections, and complicated skin infections when the benefits of therapy are felt to outweigh the risks.[217a]

Several months after the release of temafloxacin for clinical use in the United States, the U.S. Food and Drug Administration through its postmarketing surveillance mechanism received reports of hemolytic anemia in patients given temafloxacin. Subsequent investigations identified patients receiving temafloxacin who developed hemolysis, renal failure, and thrombocytopenia with or without disseminated intravascular coagulation, with an estimated reporting incidence of 1 in 5000 prescriptions. These occurrences led the manufacturer to remove temafloxacin from the market.[218] In patients given other quinolones, hemolytic anemia, occasionally associated with renal failure, coagulation abnormalities, or both have been reported to the Food and Drug Administration, but the reporting incidence was far lower than that with temafloxacin. The mechanisms of these rare but severe toxic effects are not known.

Safety in pregnancy has not been established for any of the quinolones, but studies of babies born to women exposed to norfloxacin or ciprofloxacin during the first trimester have not identified any increased teratogenic risk.[219, 220] In one prospective case-control study comparing 200 women exposed to fluoroquinolones and 200 women exposed to known nonembryotoxic antibiotics, there were no differences in birth defects, spontaneous abortions, prematurity, or fetal distress, but a higher rate of therapeutic abortions, suggesting that concerns about teratogenic risks may exceed the actual risks.[220] Because quinolones are excreted in breast milk, they should be avoided in nursing mothers.

REFERENCES

1. Jones RN, Barry AL, Thornsberry C. Antimicrobial activity of Ro 23-9424, a novel ester-linked codrug of fleroxacin and desacetylcefotaxime. Antimicrob Agents Chemother. 1989;33:944–950.
2. Georgopapadakou NH, Bertasso A. Mechanisms of action of cephalosporin 3′-quinolone esters, carbamates, and tertiary amines in *Escherichia coli.* Antimicrob Agents Chemother. 1993;37:559–565.
3. Mitscher LA, Devasthale P, Zavod R. Structure-activity relationships. In: Hooper DC, Wolfson JS, eds. Quinolone antimicrobial agents. 2nd ed. Washington, DC: American Society for Microbiology; 1993:3–51.
4. Asahina Y, Ishizaki T, Suzue S. Recent advances in structure activity relationships in new quinolones. Prog Drug Res. 1992;38:57–106.
5. Hooper DC, Wolfson JS. Mechanisms of quinolone action and bacterial killing. In: Hooper DC, Wolfson JS, eds. Quinolone antimicrobial agents. 2nd ed. Washington, DC: American Society for Microbiology; 1993:53–75.
6. Wang JC. DNA topoisomerases. Annu Rev Biochem. 1996;65:635–692.
7. Reece RJ, Maxwell A. DNA gyrase: Structure and function. Crit Rev Biochem Mol Biol. 1991;26:335–375.
8. Kato J, Nishimura Y, Imamura R, et al. New topoisomerase essential for chromosome segregation in *E. coli.* Cell. 1990;63:393–404.
9. Ullsperger C, Cozzarelli NR. Contrasting enzymatic activities of topoisomerase IV and DNA gyrase from *Escherichia coli.* J Biol Chem. 1996;271:31,549–31,555.
10. Drlica K, Zhao XL. DNA gyrase, topoisomerase IV, and the 4-quinolones. Microbiol Rev. 1997;61:377–392.
11. Shen LL, Kohlbrenner WE, Weigl D, Baranowski J. Mechanism of quinolone inhibition of DNA gyrase. Appearance of unique norfloxacin binding sites in enzyme-DNA complexes. J Biol Chem. 1989;264:2973–2978.
12. Willmott CJ, Maxwell A. A single point mutation in the DNA gyrase A protein greatly reduces binding of fluoroquinolones to the gyrase-DNA complex. Antimicrob Agents Chemother. 1993;37:126–127.
13. Ng EY, Trucksis M, Hooper DC. Quinolone resistance mutations in topoisomerase IV: Relationship of the *flqA* locus and genetic evidence that topoisomerase IV is the primary target and DNA gyrase the secondary target of fluoroquinolones in *Staphylococcus aureus.* Antimicrob Agents Chemother. 1996;40:1881–1888.
14. Pan XS, Fisher LM. Targeting of DNA gyrase in *Streptococcus pneumoniae* by sparfloxacin: Selective targeting of gyrase or topoisomerase IV by quinolones. Antimicrob Agents Chemother. 1997;41:471–474.
15. Blanche F, Cameron B, Bernard FX, et al. Differential behaviors of *Staphylococcus aureus* and *Escherichia coli* type II DNA topoisomerases. Antimicrob Agents Chemother. 1996;40:2714–2720.
16. Dietz WH, Cook TM, Goss WA. Mechanism of action of nalidixic acid on *Escherichia coli.* III. Conditions required for lethality. J Bacteriol. 1966;91:768–773.
17. McDaniel LS, Rogers LH, Hill WE. Survival of recombination-deficient mutants of *Escherichia coli* during incubation with nalidixic acid. J Bacteriol. 1978;134:1195–1198.
18. Wolfson JS, Hooper DC, McHugh GL, et al. Mutants of *Escherichia coli* K-12 exhibiting reduced killing by both quinolone and beta-lactam antimicrobial agents. Antimicrob Agents Chemother. 1990;34:1938–1943.
19. Lewin CS, Morrissey I, Smith JT. The mode of action of quinolones: The paradox in activity of low and high concentrations and activity in the anaerobic environment. Eur J Clin Microbiol Infect Dis. 1991;10:240–248.
20. Lynn R, Giaever G, Swanberg SL, Wang JC. Tandem regions of yeast DNA topoisomerase II share homology with different subunits of bacterial gyrase. Science. 1986;233:647–649.
21. Hussy P, Maass G, Tummler B, et al. Effect of 4-quinolones and novobiocin on calf thymus DNA polymerase alpha primase complex, topoisomerases I and II, and growth of mammalian lymphoblasts. Antimicrob Agents Chemother. 1986;29:1073–1078.
22. Hooper DC. Quinolone mode of action—new aspects. Drugs. 1993;45(Suppl 3):8–14.
23. Gootz TD, Osheroff N. Quinolones and eukaryotic topoisomerases. In: Hooper DC, Wolfson JS, eds. Quinolone antimicrobial agents. 2nd ed. Washington, DC: American Society for Microbiology; 1993:139–160.
24. Hooper DC, Wolfson JS. Mechanisms of bacterial resistance to quinolones. In: Hooper DC, Wolfson JS, eds. Quinolone antimicrobial agents. 2nd ed. Washington, DC: American Society for Microbiology; 1993:97–118.
25. Wetzstein HG, Schmeer N, Karl W. Degradation of the fluoroquinolone enrofloxacin by the brown rot fungus *Gloeophyllum striatum:* Identification of metabolites. Appl Environ Microbiol. 1997;63:4272–4281.
26. Martínez-Martínez L, Pascual A, Jacoby GA. Quinolone resistance from a transferable plasmid. Lancet. 1998;351:797–799.
27. Hooper DC, Wolfson JS, Souza KS, et al. Genetic and biochemical characterization of norfloxacin resistance in *Escherichia coli.* Antimicrob Agents Chemother. 1986;29:639–644.
28. Yoshida H, Bogaki M, Nakamura M, et al. Quinolone resistance–determining region in the DNA gyrase *gyrB* gene of *Escherichia coli.* Antimicrob Agents Chemother. 1991;35:1647–1650.
29. Hooper DC, Wolfson JS, Souza KS, et al. Mechanisms of quinolone resistance in *Escherichia coli*: Characterization of *nfxB* and *cfxB,* two mutant resistance loci decreasing norfloxacin accumulation. Antimicrob Agents Chemother. 1989;33:283–290.
30. Cohen SP, McMurry LM, Levy SB. *marA* locus causes decreased expression of OmpF porin in multiple-antibiotic-resistant (Mar) mutants of *Escherichia coli.* J Bacteriol. 1988;170:5416–5422.
31. Okazaki T, Hirai K. Cloning and nucleotide sequence of the *Pseudomonas aeruginosa nfxB* gene, conferring resistance to new quinolones. FEMS Microbiol Lett. 1992;76:197–202.
32. Okusu H, Ma D, Nikaido H. AcrAB efflux pump plays a major role in the antibiotic resistance phenotype of *Escherichia coli* multiple-antibiotic-resistance (Mar) mutants. J Bacteriol. 1996;178:306–308.
33. Poole K, Tetro K, Zhao QX, et al. Expression of the multidrug resistance operon *mexA-mexB-oprM* in *Pseudomonas aeruginosa: mexR* encodes a regulator of operon expression. Antimicrob Agents Chemother. 1996;40:2021–2028.
34. Yoshida H, Bogaki M, Nakamura S, et al. Nucleotide sequence and characterization of the *Staphylococcus aureus norA* gene, which confers resistance to quinolones. J Bacteriol. 1990;172:6942–6949.

35. Ng EY, Trucksis M, Hooper DC. Quinolone resistance mediated by *norA*: Physiologic characterization and relationship to *flqB*, a quinolone resistance locus on the *Staphylococcus aureus* chromosome. Antimicrob Agents Chemother. 1994;38:1345–1355.
36. Zeller V, Janoir C, Kitzis MD, et al. Active efflux as a mechanism of resistance to ciprofloxacin in *Streptococcus pneumoniae*. Antimicrob Agents Chemother. 1997;41:1973–1978.
37. Takenouchi T, Tabata F, Iwata Y, et al. Hydrophilicity of quinolones is not an exclusive factor for decreased activity in efflux-mediated resistant mutants of *Staphylococcus aureus*. Antimicrob Agents Chemother. 1996;40:1835–1842.
38. Eliopoulos GM, Eliopoulos CT. Activity in vitro of the quinolones. In: Hooper DC, Wolfson JS, eds. Quinolone antimicrobial agents. 2nd ed. Washington, DC: American Society for Microbiology; 1993:161–193.
39. Wolfson JS, Hooper DC. Fluoroquinolone antimicrobial agents. Clin Microbiol Rev. 1989;2:378–424.
40. Leysen DC, Haemers A, Pattyn SR. Mycobacteria and the new quinolones. Antimicrob Agents Chemother. 1989;33:1–5.
41. Eliopoulos GM, Eliopoulos CT. Ciprofloxacin in combination with other antimicrobials. Am J Med. 1989;87:17S–22S.
42. Hackbarth CJ, Chambers HF, Sande MA. Serum bactericidal activity of rifampin in combination with other antimicrobial agents against *Staphylococcus aureus*. Antimicrob Agents Chemother. 1986;29:611–613.
43. Mant TG. Multiple-dose pharmacokinetics of lomefloxacin: Rationale for once-a-day dosing. Am J Med. 1992;92:26S–32S.
44. Lode H, Hoffken G, Boeckk M, et al. Quinolone pharmacokinetics and metabolism. J Antimicrob Chemother. 1990;26(Suppl B):41–49.
45. Nightingale CH. Overview of the pharmacokinetics of fleroxacin. Am J Med. 1993;94:38S–43S.
46. Flor S. Pharmacokinetics of ofloxacin. An overview. Am J Med. 1989;94:24S–30S.
47. Sorgel F, Kinzig M. Pharmacokinetics of gyrase inhibitors. Part 1. Basic chemistry and gastrointestinal disposition. Am J Med. 1993;94:44S–55S.
48. Staib AH, Beermann D, Harder S, et al. Absorption differences of ciprofloxacin along the human gastrointestinal tract determined using a remote-control drug delivery device (HF-capsule). Am J Med. 1989;87:66S–69S.
49. Healy DP, Brodbeck MC, Clendening CE. Ciprofloxacin absorption is impaired in patients given enteral feedings orally and via gastrostomy and jejunostomy tubes. Antimicrob Agents Chemother. 1996;40:6–10.
50. Yuk JH, Nightingale CH, Sweeney KR, et al. Relative bioavailability in healthy volunteers of ciprofloxacin administered through a nasogastric tube with and without enteral feeding. Antimicrob Agents Chemother. 1989;33:1118–1120.
51. Montay G, Gaillot J. Pharmacokinetics of fluoroquinolones in hepatic failure. J Antimicrob Chemother. 1990;26(Suppl B):61–67.
52. Giamarellou H, Kolokythas E, Petrikkos G, et al. Pharmacokinetics of three newer quinolones in pregnant and lactating women. Am J Med. 1989;87:49S–51S.
53. Sorgel F, Kinzig M. Pharmacokinetics of gyrase inhibitors. Part 2. Renal and hepatic elimination pathways and drug interactions. Am J Med. 1993;94:56S–69S.
54. Outman WR, Nightingale CH. Metabolism and the fluoroquinolones. Am J Med. 1989;87:37S–42S.
55. Fillastre JP, Leroy A, Moulin B, et al. Pharmacokinetics of quinolones in renal insufficiency. J Antimicrob Chemother. 1990;26(Suppl B):51–60.
56. Radandt JM, Marchbanks CR, Dudley MN. Interactions of fluoroquinolones with other drugs: Mechanisms, variability, clinical significance, and management. Clin Infect Dis. 1992;14:272–284.
57. Teng RL, Dogolo LC, Willavize SA, et al. Effect of Maalox and omeprazole on the bioavailability of trovafloxacin. J Antimicrob Chemother. 1997;39:93–97.
58. Polk RE, Healy DP, Sahai J, et al. Effect of ferrous sulfate and multivitamins with zinc on absorption of ciprofloxacin in normal volunteers. Antimicrob Agents Chemother. 1989;33:1841–1844.
59. Robson RA. The effects of quinolones on xanthine pharmacokinetics. Am J Med. 1992;92:22S–25S.
60. Stahlmann R, Schwabe R. Safety profile of grepafloxacin compared with other fluoroquinolones. J Antimicrob Chemother. 1997;40:83–92.
61. Israel DS, Stotka J, Rock W, et al. Effect of ciprofloxacin on the pharmacokinetics and pharmacodynamics of warfarin. Clin Infect Dis. 1996;22:251–256.
62. Wolfson JS, Hooper DC. Treatment of genitourinary tract infections with fluoroquinolones: Activity in vitro, pharmacokinetics, and clinical efficacy in urinary tract infections and prostatitis. Antimicrob Agents Chemother. 1989;33:1655–1661.
63. Hooper DC, Wolfson JS. Fluoroquinolone antimicrobial agents. N Engl J Med. 1991;324:384–394.
64. Nicolle LE, Dubois J, Martel AY, et al. Treatment of acute uncomplicated urinary tract infections with 3 days of lomefloxacin compared with treatment with 3 days of norfloxacin. Antimicrob Agents Chemother. 1993;37:574–579.
65. Raz R, Rottensterich E, Hefter H, et al. Single-dose ciprofloxacin in the treatment of uncomplicated urinary tract infection in women. Eur J Clin Microbiol Infect Dis. 1989;8:1040–1042.
66. Pfau A, Sacks TG. Single dose quinolone treatment in acute uncomplicated urinary tract infection in women. J Urol. 1993;149:532–534.
67. Saginur R, Nicolle LE. Single-dose compared with 3-day norfloxacin treatment of uncomplicated urinary tract infection in women. Canadian Infectious Diseases Society Clinical Trials Study Group. Arch Intern Med. 1992;152:1233–1237.
68. The Urinary Tract Infection Study Group. Coordinated multicenter study of norfloxacin versus trimethoprim-sulfamethoxazole of symptomatic urinary tract infections. J Infect Dis. 1987;155:170–177.
69. Raz R, Rottensterich E, Leshem Y, Tabenkin H. Double-blind study comparing 3-day regimens of cefixime and ofloxacin in treatment of uncomplicated urinary tract infections in women. Antimicrob Agents Chemother. 1994;38:1176–1177.
70. Raz R, Boger S. Long-term prophylaxis with norfloxacin versus nitrofurantoin in women with recurrent urinary tract infection. Antimicrob Agents Chemother. 1991;35:1241–1242.
71. Pfau A, Sacks TG. Effective postcoital quinolone prophylaxis of recurrent urinary tract infections in women. J Urol. 1994;152:136–138.
72. Fang GD, Brennen C, Wagener M, et al. Use of ciprofloxacin versus use of aminoglycosides for therapy of complicated urinary tract infection: Prospective, randomized clinical and pharmacokinetic study. Antimicrob Agents Chemother. 1991;35:1849–1855.
73. Nicolle LE, Louie TJ, Dubois J, et al. Treatment of complicated urinary tract infections with lomefloxacin compared with that with trimethoprim-sulfamethoxazole. Antimicrob Agents Chemother. 1994;38:1368–1373.
74. Naber KG, Di Silverio F, Geddes A, Guibert J. Comparative efficacy of sparfloxacin versus ciprofloxacin in the treatment of complicated urinary tract infection. J Antimicrob Chemother. 1996;37:135–144.
75. Biering-Sørensen F, Høiby N, Nordenbo A, et al. Ciprofloxacin as prophylaxis for urinary tract infection: Prospective, randomized, cross-over, placebo controlled study in patients with spinal cord lesion. J Urol. 1994;151:105–108.
76. Sabbaj J, Hoagland VL, Cook T. Norfloxacin versus co-trimoxazole in the treatment of recurring urinary tract infections in men. Scand J Infect Dis Suppl. 1986;48:48–53.
77. Schaeffer AJ, Darras FS. The efficacy of norfloxacin in the treatment of chronic bacterial prostatitis refractory to trimethoprim-sulfamethoxazole and/or carbenicillin. J Urol. 1990;144:690–693.
78. Hooper DC, Wolfson JS. Treatment of genitourinary tract infections with fluoroquinolones: Clinical efficacy in genital infections and adverse effects. Antimicrob Agents Chemother. 1989;33:1662–1667.
79. Thorpe EM Jr, Schwebke JR, Hook EW III, et al. Comparison of single-dose cefuroxime axetil with ciprofloxacin in treatment of uncomplicated gonorrhea caused by penicillinase-producing and non–penicillinase-producing *Neisseria gonorrhoeae* strains. Antimicrob Agents Chemother. 1996;40:2775–2780.
80. Moi H, Morel P, Gianotti B, et al. Comparative efficacy and safety of single oral doses of sparfloxacin versus ciprofloxacin in the treatment of acute gonococcal urethritis in men. J Antimicrob Chemother. 1996;37(Suppl A):115–122.
81. Hook EW III, McCormack WM, Martin D, et al. Comparison of single-dose oral grepafloxacin with cefixime for treatment of uncomplicated gonorrhea in men. Antimicrob Agents Chemother. 1997;41:1843–1845.
82. Jones RB, Schwebke J, Thorpe EM Jr, et al. Randomized trial of trovafloxacin and ofloxacin for single-dose therapy of gonorrhea. Am J Med. 1998;104:28–32.
83. Anonymous. 1998 Guidelines for treatment of sexually transmitted diseases. MMWR 1998;47:1–118.
84. Crombleholme WR, Schachter J, Ohm-Smith M, et al. Efficacy of single-agent therapy for the treatment of acute pelvic inflammatory disease with ciprofloxacin. Am J Med. 1989;87:142S–147S.
85. Wendel GDJ, Cox SM, Bawdon RE, et al. A randomized trial of ofloxacin versus cefoxitin and doxycycline in the outpatient treatment of acute salpingitis. Am J Obstet Gynecol. 1991;164:1390–1396.
86. Boslego JW, Hicks CB, Greenup R, et al. A prospective randomized trial of ofloxacin vs. doxycycline in the treatment of uncomplicated male urethritis. Sex Transm Dis. 1988;15:186–191.
87. Hooton TM, Batteiger BE, Judson FN, et al. Ofloxacin versus doxycycline for treatment of cervical infection with *Chlamydia trachomatis*. Antimicrob Agents Chemother. 1992;36:1144–1146.
88. Kitchen VS, Donegan C, Ward H, et al. Comparison of ofloxacin with doxycycline in the treatment of non-gonococcal urethritis and cervical chlamydial infection. J Antimicrob Chemother. 1990;26(Suppl D):99–105.
89. Phillips I, Dimian C, Barlow D, et al. A comparative study of two different regimens of sparfloxacin versus doxycycline in the treatment of non-gonococcal urethritis in men. J Antimicrob Chemother. 1996;37(Suppl A):123–134.
90. Naamara W, Plummer FA, Greenblatt RM, et al. Treatment of chancroid with ciprofloxacin. A prospective, randomized clinical trial. Am J Med. 1987;82:317–320.
91. Martens MG, Gordon S, Yarborough DR, et al. Multicenter randomized trial of ofloxacin versus cefoxitin and doxycycline in outpatient treatment of pelvic inflammatory disease. South Med J. 1993;86:604–610.
92. Arredondo JL, Diaz V, Gaitan H, et al. Oral clindamycin and ciprofloxacin versus intramuscular ceftriaxone and oral doxycycline in the treatment of mild-to-moderate pelvic inflammatory disease in outpatients. Clin Infect Dis. 1997;24:170–178.
93. Covino JM, Black JR, Cummings M, et al. Comparative evaluation of ofloxacin and metronidazole in the treatment of bacterial vaginosis. Sex Transm Dis. 1993;20:262–264.
94. Wiström J, Jertborn M, Hedstrom SA, et al. Short-term self-treatment of travellers' diarrhoea with norfloxacin: A placebo-controlled study. J Antimicrob Chemother. 1989;23:905–913.
95. Ericsson CD, Johnson PC, DuPont HL, et al. Ciprofloxacin or trimethoprim-sulfamethoxazole as initial therapy for travelers' diarrhea. A placebo-controlled, randomized trial. Ann Intern Med. 1987;106:216–220.
96. DuPont HL, Ericsson CD. Prevention and treatment of traveler's diarrhea. N Engl J Med. 1993;328:1821–1827.
97. Mattila L, Peltola H, Siitonen A, et al. Short-term treatment of traveler's diarrhea with norfloxacin: A double-blind, placebo-controlled study during two seasons. Clin Infect Dis. 1993;17:779–782.
98. Salam I, Katelaris P, Leigh-Smith S, Farthing MJG. Randomised trial of single-dose ciprofloxacin for travellers' diarrhoea. Lancet. 1994;344:1537–1539.
99. Murphy GS, Bodhidatta L, Echeverria P, et al. Ciprofloxacin and loperamide in the treatment of bacillary dysentery. Ann Intern Med. 1993;118:582–586.

100. Bennish ML, Salam MA, Khan WA, Khan AM. Treatment of shigellosis. III. Comparison of one- or two-dose ciprofloxacin with standard 5-day therapy. A randomized, blinded trial. Ann Intern Med. 1992;117:727–734.
101. Neill MA, Opal SM, Heelan J, et al. Failure of ciprofloxacin to eradicate convalescent fecal excretion after acute salmonellosis: Experience during an outbreak in health care workers. Ann Intern Med. 1991;114:195–199.
102. Wiström J, Jertborn M, Ekwall E, et al. Empiric treatment of acute diarrheal disease with norfloxacin. A randomized, placebo-controlled study. Swedish Study Group. Ann Intern Med. 1992;117:202–208.
103. Dryden MS, Gabb RJE, Wright SK. Empirical treatment of severe acute community-acquired gastroenteritis with ciprofloxacin. Clin Infect Dis. 1996;22:1019–1025.
104. Goodman LJ, Trenholme GM, Kaplan RL, et al. Empiric antimicrobial therapy of domestically acquired acute diarrhea in urban adults. Arch Intern Med. 1990;150:541–546.
105. Petruccelli BP, Murphy GS, Sanchez JL, et al. Treatment of travelers' diarrhea with ciprofloxacin and loperamide. J Infect Dis. 1992;165:557–560.
106. Bhattacharya SK, Bhattacharya MK, Dutta P, et al. Double-blind, randomized, controlled clinical trial of norfloxacin for cholera. Antimicrob Agents Chemother. 1990;34:939–940.
107. Dutta D, Bhattacharya SK, Bhattacharya MK, et al. Efficacy of norfloxacin and doxycycline for treatment of *Vibrio cholerae* 0139 infection. J Antimicrob Chemother. 1996;37:575–581.
108. Gotuzzo E, Seas C, Echeverria P, et al. Ciprofloxacin for the treatment of cholera: A randomized, double-blind, controlled clinical trial of a single daily dose in Peruvian adults. Clin Infect Dis. 1995;20:1485–1490.
109. Wang F, Gu XJ, Zhang MF, Tai TY. Treatment of typhoid fever with ofloxacin. J Antimicrob Chemother. 1989;23:785–788.
110. Uwaydah AK, al Soub H, Matar I. Randomized prospective study comparing two dosage regimens of ciprofloxacin for the treatment of typhoid fever. J Antimicrob Chemother. 1992;30:707–711.
111. Smith MD, Duong NM, Hoa NT, et al. Comparison of ofloxacin and ceftriaxone for short-course treatment of enteric fever. Antimicrob Agents Chemother. 1994;38:1716–1720.
112. Hien TT, Bethell DB, Hoa NTT, et al. Short course of ofloxacin for treatment of multidrug-resistant typhoid. Clin Infect Dis. 1995;20:917–923.
113. Gotuzzo E, Guerra JG, Benavente L, et al. Use of norfloxacin to treat chronic typhoid carriers. J Infect Dis. 1988;157:1221–1225.
114. Ferreccio C, Morris JGJ, Valdivieso C, et al. Efficacy of ciprofloxacin in the treatment of chronic typhoid carriers. J Infect Dis. 1988;157:1235–1239.
115. Chrysanthopoulos CJ, Skoutelis AT, Starakis JC, et al. Use of ciprofloxacin in biliary sepsis. Infection. 1988;16:249–250.
116. Solomkin JS, Reinhart HH, Dellinger EP, et al. Results of a randomized trial comparing sequential intravenous oral treatment with ciprofloxacin plus metronidazole to imipenem cilastatin for intra-abdominal infections. Ann Surg. 1996;223:303–315.
117. Friedland JS, Iveson TJ, Fraise AP, et al. A comparison between intraperitoneal ciprofloxacin and intraperitoneal vancomycin and gentamicin in the treatment of peritonitis associated with continuous ambulatory peritoneal dialysis (CAPD). J Antimicrob Chemother. 1990;26:77–81.
118. Gines P, Rimola A, Planas R, et al. Norfloxacin prevents spontaneous bacterial peritonitis recurrence in cirrhosis: Results of a double-blind, placebo-controlled trial. Hepatology. 1990;12:716–724.
119. Rolachon A, Cordier L, Bacq Y, et al. Ciprofloxacin and long-term prevention of spontaneous bacterial peritonitis: Results of a prospective controlled trial. Hepatology. 1995;22:1171–1174.
120. Dupeyron C, Mangeney N, Sedrati L, et al. Rapid emergence of quinolone resistance in cirrhotic patients treated with norfloxacin to prevent spontaneous bacterial peritonitis. Antimicrob Agents Chemother. 1994;38:340–344.
121. Gotfried MH, Ellison WT. Safety and efficacy of lomefloxacin versus cefaclor in the treatment of acute exacerbations of chronic bronchitis. Am J Med. 1992;92:108S–113S.
122. Ulmer W. Fleroxacin versus amoxicillin in the treatment of acute exacerbation of chronic bronchitis. Am J Med. 1993;94:136S–141S.
123. Grossman R, Mukherjee J, Vaughan D, et al. A 1-year community-based health economic study of ciprofloxacin vs usual antibiotic treatment in acute exacerbations of chronic bronchitis—The Canadian Ciprofloxacin Health Economic Study Group. Chest. 1998;113:131–141.
124. Allegra L, Konietzko N, Leophonte P, et al. Safety and efficacy of sparfloxacin in the treatment of acute exacerbations of chronic obstructive pulmonary disease: A double-blind, randomised, parallel, multicentre study. J Antimicrob Chemother. 1996;37:93–104.
125. DeAbate CA, Russell M, McElvaine P, et al. Safety and efficacy of oral levofloxacin versus cefuroxime axetil in acute bacterial exacerbation of chronic bronchitis. Respir Care. 1997;42:206–213.
126. Langan CE, Cranfield R, Breisch S, Pettit R. Randomized, double-blind study of grepafloxacin versus amoxycillin in patients with acute bacterial exacerbations of chronic bronchitis. J Antimicrob Chemother. 1997;40:63–72.
127. Chodosh S, Lakshminarayan S, Swarz H, Breisch S. Efficacy and safety of a 10-day course of 400 or 600 milligrams of grepafloxacin once daily for treatment of acute bacterial exacerbations of chronic bronchitis: Comparison with a 10-day course of 500 milligrams of ciprofloxacin twice daily. Antimicrob Agents Chemother. 1998;42:114–120.
127a. O'Doherty B, Daniel R, the Trovafloxacin Bronchitis Study Group. Treatment of acute exacerbations of chronic bronchitis: Comparison of trovafloxacin and amoxicillin in a multicentre, double-blind, double-dummy study. Eur J Clin Microbiol Infect Dis. 1998;17:441–446.
128. Chrysanthopoulos CJ, Starakis JC, Skoutelis AT, et al. Sequential intravenous/oral therapy with ciprofloxacin in severe infection. Am J Med. 1989;87:225S–227S.
129. Gentry LO, Rodriguez-Gomez G, Kohler RB, et al. Parenteral followed by oral ofloxacin for nosocomial pneumonia and community-acquired pneumonia requiring hospitalization. Am Rev Respir Dis. 1992;145:31–35.
130. Plouffe JF, Herbert MT, File TM Jr, et al. Ofloxacin versus standard therapy in treatment of community-acquired pneumonia requiring hospitalization. Antimicrob Agents Chemother. 1996;40:1175–1179.
131. Sanders WE Jr, Morris JF, Alessi P, et al. Oral ofloxacin for the treatment of acute bacterial pneumonia: Use of a nontraditional protocol to compare experimental therapy with "usual care" in a multicenter clinical trial. Am J Med. 1991;91:261–266.
131a. Aubier M, Verster R, Reganney C, et al. Once-daily sparfloxacin versus high-dosage amoxicillin in the treatment of community-acquired, suspected pneumococcal pneumonia in adults. Clin Infect Dis. 1998;26:1312–1320.
132. Portier H, May T, Proust A, et al. Comparative efficacy of sparfloxacin in comparison with amoxycillin plus ofloxacin in the treatment of community-acquired pneumonia. J Antimicrob Chemother. 1996;37:83–91.
133. Örtqvist Å, Valtonen M, Cars O, et al. Oral empiric treatment of community-acquired pneumonia—a multicenter, double-blind, randomized study comparing sparfloxacin with roxithromycin. Chest. 1996;110:1499–1506.
134. File TM Jr, Segreti J, Dunbar L, et al. A multicenter, randomized study comparing the efficacy and safety of intravenous and/or oral levofloxacin versus ceftriaxone and/or cefuroxime axetil in treatment of adults with community-acquired pneumonia. Antimicrob Agents Chemother. 1997;41:1965–1972.
135. O'Doherty B, Dutchman DA, Pettit R, Maroli A. Randomized, double-blind, comparative study of grepafloxacin and amoxycillin in the treatment of patients with community-acquired pneumonia. J Antimicrob Chemother. 1997;40:73–81.
135a. Trémolières F, de Kock F, Pluck N, et al. Trovafloxacin versus high-dose amoxicillin (1 g three times daily) in the treatment of community-acquired bacterial pneumonia. Eur J Clin Microbiol Infect Dis. 1998;17:447–453.
136. Mouton Y, Leroy O, Beuscart C, et al. Efficacy of intravenous ofloxacin: A French multicentre trial in 185 patients. J Antimicrob Chemother. 1990;26(Suppl D):115–121.
137. Unertl KE, Lenhart FP, Forst H, et al. Ciprofloxacin in the treatment of legionellosis in critically ill patients including those cases unresponsive to erythromycin. Am J Med. 1989;87:128S–131S.
138. Lipsky BA, Tack KJ, Kuo CC, et al. Ofloxacin treatment of *Chlamydia pneumoniae* (strain TWAR) lower respiratory tract infections. Am J Med. 1990;89:722–724.
139. Peloquin CA, Cumbo TJ, Nix DE, et al. Evaluation of intravenous ciprofloxacin in patients with nosocomial lower respiratory tract infections. Impact of plasma concentrations, organism, minimum inhibitory concentration, and clinical condition on bacterial eradication. Arch Intern Med. 1989;149:2269–2273.
140. Fink MP, Snydman DR, Niederman MS, et al. Treatment of severe pneumonia in hospitalized patients: Results of a multicenter, randomized, double-blind trial comparing intravenous ciprofloxacin with imipenem-cilastatin. Antimicrob Agents Chemother. 1994;38:547–557.
141. Gentry LO. Oral antimicrobial therapy for osteomyelitis. Ann Intern Med. 1991;114:986–987.
142. Peterson LR, Lissack LM, Canter K, et al. Therapy of lower extremity infections with ciprofloxacin in patients with diabetes mellitus, peripheral vascular disease, or both. Am J Med. 1989;86:801–808.
143. Raz R, Miron D. Oral ciprofloxacin for treatment of infection following nail puncture wounds of the foot. Clin Infect Dis. 1995;21:194–195.
144. Gentry LO, Rodriguez-Gomez G. Ofloxacin versus parenteral therapy for chronic osteomyelitis. Antimicrob Agents Chemother. 1991;35:538–541.
145. Drancourt M, Stein A, Argenson JN, et al. Oral rifampin plus ofloxacin for treatment of *Staphylococcus*-infected orthopedic implants. Antimicrob Agents Chemother. 1993;37:1214–1218.
146. Zimmerli W, Widmer AF, Blatter M, et al. Role of rifampin for treatment of orthopedic implant–related staphylococcal infections: A randomized controlled trial. Foreign-Body Infection (FBI) Study Group. JAMA. 1998;279:1537–1541.
147. Brouqui P, Rousseau MC, Stein A, et al. Treatment of *Pseudomonas aeruginosa*–infected orthopedic prostheses with ceftazidime-ciprofloxacin antibiotic combination. Antimicrob Agents Chemother. 1995;39:2423–2425.
148. Putz PA. A pilot study of oral fleroxacin given once daily in patients with bone and joint infections. Am J Med. 1993;94:177S–181S.
149. Gentry LO. Review of quinolones in the treatment of infections of the skin and skin structure. J Antimicrob Chemother. 1991;28(Suppl C):97–110.
150. Gentry LO, Ramirez-Ronda CH, Rodriguez-Noriega E, et al. Oral ciprofloxacin vs parenteral cefotaxime in the treatment of difficult skin and skin structure infections. A multicenter trial. Arch Intern Med. 1989;149:2579–2583.
151. Gentry LO, Rodriguez-Gomez G, Zeluff BJ, et al. A comparative evaluation of oral ofloxacin versus intravenous cefotaxime therapy for serious skin and skin structure infections. Am J Med. 1989;87:57S–60S.
152. Nichols RL, Smith JW, Gentry LO, et al. Multicenter, randomized study comparing levofloxacin and ciprofloxacin for uncomplicated skin and skin structure infections. South Med J. 1997;90:1193–1200.
153. Tassler H. Comparative efficacy and safety of oral fleroxacin and amoxicillin/clavulanate potassium in skin and soft tissue infections. Am J Med. 1993;94:159S–165S.
154. Trucksis M, Hooper DC, Wolfson JS. Emerging resistance to fluoroquinolones in staphylococci: An alert. Ann Intern Med. 1991;114:424–426.
155. Yew WW, Kwan SY, Ma WK, et al. In-vitro activity of ofloxacin against *Mycobacterium tuberculosis* and its clinical efficacy in multiply resistant pulmonary tuberculosis. J Antimicrob Chemother. 1990;26:227–236.

156. Tsukamura M, Nakamura E, Yoshii S, Amano H. Therapeutic effect of a new antibacterial substance ofloxacin (DL8280) on pulmonary tuberculosis. Am Rev Respir Dis. 1985;131:352–356.
157. Mohanty KC, Dhamgaye TM. Controlled trial of ciprofloxacin in short-term chemotherapy for pulmonary tuberculosis. Chest. 1993;104:1194–1198.
158. Kennedy N, Berger L, Curram J, et al. Randomized controlled trial of a drug regimen that includes ciprofloxacin for the treatment of pulmonary tuberculosis. Clin Infect Dis. 1996;22:827–833.
159. De Lalla F, Maserati R, Scarpellini P, et al. Clarithromycin-ciprofloxacin-amikacin for therapy of *Mycobacterium avium–Mycobacterium intracellulare* bacteremia in patients with AIDS. Antimicrob Agents Chemother. 1992;36:1567–1569.
160. Kemper CA, Meng TC, Nussbaum J, et al. Treatment of *Mycobacterium avium* complex bacteremia in AIDS with a four-drug oral regimen. Rifampin, ethambutol, clofazimine, and ciprofloxacin. The California Collaborative Treatment Group. Ann Intern Med. 1992;116:466–472.
161. Shafran SD, Singer J, Zarowny DP, et al. A comparison of two regimens for the treatment of *Mycobacterium avium* complex bacteremia in AIDS: Rifabutin, ethambutol, and clarithromycin versus rifampin, ethambutol, clofazimine, and ciprofloxacin. N Engl J Med. 1996;335:377–383.
162. Yew WW, Kwan SY, Ma WK, et al. Ofloxacin therapy of *Mycobacterium fortuitum* infection: Further experience. J Antimicrob Chemother. 1990;25:880–881.
163. Grosset JH, Ji BH, Guelpa-Lauras CC, et al. Clinical trial of pefloxacin and ofloxacin in the treatment of lepromatous leprosy. Int J Lepr Other Mycobact Dis. 1990;58:281–295.
164. Bouza E, Diaz-Lopez MD, Bernaldo de Quiros JC, Rodriguez-Creixems M. Ciprofloxacin in patients with bacteremic infections. The Spanish Group for the Study of Ciprofloxacin. Am J Med. 1989;87:228S–231S.
165. Regamey C, Steinbach-Lebbin C. Severe infections treated with intravenous ofloxacin: A prospective clinical multicentre Swiss study. J Antimicrob Chemother. 1990;26(Suppl D):107–114.
166. Chan CC, Oppenheim BA, Anderson H, et al. Randomized trial comparing ciprofloxacin plus netilmicin versus piperacillin plus netilmicin for empiric treatment of fever in neutropenic patients. Antimicrob Agents Chemother. 1989;33:87–91.
167. Meunier F, Zinner SH, Gaya H, et al. Prospective randomized evaluation of ciprofloxacin versus piperacillin plus amikacin for empiric antibiotic therapy of febrile granulocytopenic cancer patients with lymphomas and solid tumors. The European Organization for Research on Treatment of Cancer International Antimicrobial Therapy Cooperative Group. Antimicrob Agents Chemother. 1991;35:873–878.
168. Echols RM. The selection of appropriate dosages for intravenous ciprofloxacin. J Antimicrob Chemother. 1993;31:783–787.
169. Winston DJ. Use of quinolone antimicrobial agents in immunocompromised patients. In: Hooper DC, Wolfson JS, eds. Quinolone antimicrobial agents. 2nd ed. Washington, DC: American Society for Microbiology; 1993;435–471.
170. Jansen J, Cromer M, Akard L, et al. Infection prevention in severely myelosuppressed patients: A comparison between ciprofloxacin and a regimen of selective antibiotic modulation of the intestinal flora. Am J Med. 1994;96:335–341.
171. Anonymous. Prevention of bacterial infection in neutropenic patients with hematologic malignancies. A randomized, multicenter trial comparing norfloxacin with ciprofloxacin. The GIMEMA Infection Program. Gruppo Italiano Malattie Ematologiche Maligne dell'Adulto. Ann Intern Med. 1991;115:7–12.
172. Bow EJ, Mandell LA, Louie TJ, et al. Quinolone-based antibacterial chemoprophylaxis in neutropenic patients: Effect of augmented gram-positive activity on infectious morbidity. Ann Intern Med. 1996;125:183–190.
173. Broun ER, Wheat JL, Kneebone PH, et al. Randomized trial of the addition of gram-positive prophylaxis to standard antimicrobial prophylaxis for patients undergoing autologous bone marrow transplantation. Antimicrob Agents Chemother. 1994;38:576–579.
174. Malik IA, Khan WA, Karim M, et al. Feasibility of outpatient management of fever in cancer patients with low-risk neutropenia: Results of a prospective randomized trial. Am J Med. 1995;98:224–231.
175. Dworkin RJ, Lee BL, Sande MA, Chambers HF. Treatment of right-sided *Staphylococcus aureus* endocarditis in intravenous drug abusers with ciprofloxacin and rifampin. Lancet. 1989;2:1071–1072.
176. Heldman AW, Hartert TV, Ray SC, et al. Oral antibiotic treatment of right-sided staphylococcal endocarditis in injection drug users: Prospective randomized comparison with parenteral therapy. Am J Med. 1996;101:68–76.
177. Segev S, Rosen N, Joseph G, et al. Pefloxacin efficacy in gram-negative bacillary meningitis. J Antimicrob Chemother. 1990;26(Suppl B):187–192.
178. Schonwald S, Beus I, Lisic M, et al. Ciprofloxacin in the treatment of gram-negative bacillary meningitis. Am J Med. 1989;87:248S–249S.
179. Wong-Beringer A, Beringer P, Lovett MA. Successful treatment of multidrug-resistant *Pseudomonas aeruginosa* meningitis with high-dose ciprofloxacin. Clin Infect Dis. 1997;25:936–937.
180. Dworzack DL, Sanders CC, Horowitz EA, et al. Evaluation of single-dose ciprofloxacin in the eradication of *Neisseria meningitidis* from nasopharyngeal carriers. Antimicrob Agents Chemother. 1988;32:1740–1741.
181. Gilja OH, Halstensen A, Digranes A, et al. Use of single-dose ofloxacin to eradicate tonsillopharyngeal carriage of *Neisseria meningitidis.* Antimicrob Agents Chemother. 1993;37:2024–2026.
182. Cuevas LE, Kazembe P, Mughogho GK, et al. Eradication of nasopharyngeal carriage of *Neisseria meningitidis* in children and adults in rural Africa: A comparison of ciprofloxacin and rifampicin. J Infect Dis. 1995;171:728–731.
183. Syrjala H, Schildt R, Raisainen S. In vitro susceptibility of *Francisella tularensis* to fluoroquinolones and treatment of tularemia with norfloxacin and ciprofloxacin. Eur J Clin Microbiol Infect Dis. 1991;10:68–70.
184. Holley HP Jr. Successful treatment of cat-scratch disease with ciprofloxacin. JAMA. 1991;265:1563–1565.
185. Raoult D, Drancourt M. Antimicrobial therapy of rickettsial diseases. Antimicrob Agents Chemother. 1991;35:2457–2462.
186. Lang R, Rubinstein E. Quinolones for the treatment of brucellosis. J Antimicrob Chemother. 1992;29:357–360.
187. Akova M, Uzun O, Akalin HE, et al. Quinolones in treatment of human brucellosis: Comparative trial of ofloxacin-rifampin versus doxycycline-rifampin. Antimicrob Agents Chemother. 1993;37:1831–1834.
188. McClean KL, Hitchman D, Shafran SD. Norfloxacin is inferior to chloroquine for falciparum malaria in northwestern Zambia: A comparative clinical trial. J Infect Dis. 1992;165:904–907.
189. Watt G, Shanks GD, Edstein MD, et al. Ciprofloxacin treatment of drug-resistant falciparum malaria. J Infect Dis. 1991;164:602–604.
190. Blaser J, Stone BB, Groner MC, Zinner SH. Comparative study with enoxacin and netilmicin in a pharmacodynamic model to determine importance of ratio of antibiotic peak concentration to MIC for bactericidal activity and emergence of resistance. Antimicrob Agents Chemother. 1987;31:1054–1060.
191. Parry MF, Panzer KB, Yukna ME. Quinolone resistance. Susceptibility data from a 300-bed community hospital. Am J Med. 1989;87:12S–16S.
192. Kresken M, Wiedemann B. Development of resistance to nalidixic acid and the fluoroquinolones after the introduction of norfloxacin and ofloxacin. Antimicrob Agents Chemother. 1988;32:1285–1288.
193. Blumberg HM, Rimland D, Carroll DJ, et al. Rapid development of ciprofloxacin resistance in methicillin-susceptible and -resistant *Staphylococcus aureus.* J Infect Dis. 1991;163:1279–1285.
194. Pegues DA, Colby C, Hibberd PL, et al. The epidemiology of resistance to ofloxacin and oxacillin among clinical coagulase-negative staphylococcal isolates: Analysis of risk factors and strain types. Clin Infect Dis. 1998;26:72–79.
195. Reina J, Borrell N, Serra A. Emergence of resistance to erythromycin and fluoroquinolones in thermotolerant *Campylobacter* strains isolated from feces 1987–1991. Eur J Clin Microbiol Infect Dis. 1992;11:1163–1166.
196. Endtz HP, Ruijs GJ, van Klingeren B, et al. Quinolone resistance in campylobacter isolated from man and poultry following the introduction of fluoroquinolones in veterinary medicine. J Antimicrob Chemother. 1991;27:199–208.
197. Aguiar JM, Chacon J, Canton R, Baquero F. The emergence of highly fluoroquinolone-resistant *Escherichia coli* in community-acquired urinary tract infections. J Antimicrob Chemother. 1992;29:349–350.
198. Ena J, López-Perezagua MD, Martínez-Peinado C, et al. Emergence of ciprofloxacin resistance in *Escherichia coli* isolates after widespread use of fluoroquinolones. Diagn Microbiol Infect Dis. 1998;30:103–107.
199. Carratala J, Fernandez-Sevilla A, Tubau F, et al. Emergence of fluoroquinolone-resistant *Escherichia coli* in fecal flora of cancer patients receiving norfloxacin prophylaxis. Antimicrob Agents Chemother. 1996;40:503–505.
200. Kern WV, Andriof E, Oethinger M, et al. Emergence of fluoroquinolone-resistant *Escherichia coli* at a cancer center. Antimicrob Agents Chemother. 1994;38:681–687.
201. Gordon SM, Carlyn CJ, Doyle LJ, et al. The emergence of *Neisseria gonorrhoeae* with decreased susceptibility to ciprofloxacin in Cleveland, Ohio: Epidemiology and risk factors. Ann Intern Med. 1996;125:465–470.
202. Thomas JK, Forrest A, Bhavnani SM, et al. Pharmacodynamic evaluation of factors associated with the development of bacterial resistance in acutely ill patients during therapy. Antimicrob Agents Chemother. 1998;42:521–527.
203. Drusano GL, Johnson DE, Rosen M, Standiford HC. Pharmacodynamics of a fluoroquinolone antimicrobial agent in a neutropenic rat model of *Pseudomonas* sepsis. Antimicrob Agents Chemother. 1993;37:483–490.
204. Hooper DC, Wolfson JS. Adverse effects. In: Hooper DC, Wolfson JS, eds. Quinolone antimicrobial agents. 2nd ed. Washington, DC: American Society for Microbiology; 1993:489–512.
205. Halliwell RF, Davey PG, Lambert JJ. Antagonism of $GABA_A$ receptors by 4-quinolones. J Antimicrob Chemother. 1993;31:457–462.
206. Norrby SR. Side-effects of quinolones: Comparisons between quinolones and other antibiotics. Eur J Clin Microbiol Infect Dis. 1991;10:378–383.
207. Stahlmann R. Safety profile of the quinolones. J Antimicrob Chemother. 1990;26(Suppl D):31–44.
208. Rizk E. The U.S. clinical experience with lomefloxacin, a new once-daily fluoroquinolone. Am J Med. 1992;92:130S–135S.
209. Rubinstein E. Safety profile of sparfloxacin in the treatment of respiratory tract infections. J Antimicrob Chemother. 1996;37:145–160.
210. Ferguson J. Fluoroquinolone photosensitization: A review of clinical and laboratory studies. Photochem Photobiol. 1995;62:954–958.
211. Adam D. Use of quinolones in pediatric patients. Rev Infect Dis. 1989;11(Suppl 5):S1113–S1116.
212. Burkhardt JE, Walterspiel JN, Schaad UB. Quinolone arthropathy in animals versus children. Clin Infect Dis. 1997;25:1196–1204.
213. Schaad UB, Wedgwood J. Lack of quinolone-induced arthropathy in children. J Antimicrob Chemother. 1992;30:414–416.
214. Pertuiset E, Lenoir G, Jehanne M, et al. Joint tolerance of pefloxacin and ofloxacin in children and adolescents with cystic fibrosis (in French). Rev Rhum Maladies Osteo-Articulaires. 1989;56:735–740.
215. Zabraniecki L, Negrier I, Vergne P, et al. Fluoroquinolone induced tendinopathy: Report of 6 cases. J Rheumatol. 1996;23:516–520.
216. Schaad UB, Abdus Salam M, Aujard Y, et al. Use of fluoroquinolones in pediatrics: Consensus report of an International Society of Chemotherapy commission. Pediatr Infect Dis J. 1995;14:1–9.
217. Jaillon P, Morganroth J, Brumpt I, Talbot G. Overview of electrocardiographic and

cardiovascular safety data for sparfloxacin. J Antimicrob Chemother. 1996;37:161–167.
217a. Lumpkin MM. Public health advisory. U.S. Food and Drug Administration, 9 June 1999.
218. Blum MD, Graham DJ, McCloskey CA. Temafloxacin syndrome: Review of 95 cases. Clin Infect Dis. 1994;18:946–950.
219. Berkovitch M, Pastuszak A, Gazarian M, et al. Safety of the new quinolones in pregnancy. Obstet Gynecol. 1994;84:535–538.
220. Loebstein R, Addis A, Ho E, et al. Pregnancy outcome following gestational exposure to fluoroquinolones: A multicenter prospective controlled study. Antimicrob Agents Chemother. 1998;42:1336–1339.
221. Vance-Bryan K, Guay DR, Rotschafer JC. Clinical pharmacokinetics of ciprofloxacin. Clin Pharmacokinet. 1990;19:434–461.
222. Frydman AM, Le Roux Y, Lefebvre MA, et al. Pharmacokinetics of pefloxacin after repeated intravenous and oral administration (400 mg bid) in young healthy volunteers. J Antimicrob Chemother. 1986;17(Suppl B):65–79.
223. Fish DN, Chow AT. The clinical pharmacokinetics of levofloxacin. Clin Pharmacokinet. 1997;32:101–119.
224. Montay G. Pharmacokinetics of sparfloxacin in healthy volunteers and patients: A review. J Antimicrob Chemother. 1996;37:27–39.
225. Child J, Andrews JM, Wise R. Pharmacokinetics and tissue penetration of the new fluoroquinolone grepafloxacin. Antimicrob Agents Chemother. 1995;39:513–515.
226. Vincent J, Venitz J, Teng R, et al. Pharmacokinetics and safety of trovafloxacin in healthy male volunteers following administration of single intravenous doses of the prodrug, alatrofloxacin. J Antimicrob Chemother. 1997;39:75–80.
227. Teng RL, Liston TE, Harris SC. Multiple-dose pharmacokinetics and safety of trovafloxacin in healthy volunteers. J Antimicrob Chemother. 1996;37:955–963.
228. Guay DR, Opsahl JA, McMahon FG, et al. Safety and pharmacokinetics of multiple doses of intravenous ofloxacin in healthy volunteers. Antimicrob Agents Chemother. 1992;36:308–312.

Chapter 32

Urinary Tract Agents: Nitrofurantoin and Methenamine

DAVID C. HOOPER

Two antimicrobial agents in clinical use are employed exclusively for treatment or prophylaxis of urinary tract infections because of their pharmacologic and chemical properties. At tolerated doses, nitrofurantoin achieves adequate concentrations only in kidney tissues and urine. Methenamine, which lacks antimicrobial activity itself, becomes active only after chemical degradation in acidic bladder urine to generate its active breakdown product, formaldehyde.

NITROFURANTOIN

Chemical Structure

Nitrofurantoin (*N*-[5-nitro-2-furfurylidene]-1-aminohydantoin) is a weak acid (pK_a 7.2) (Fig. 32–1) and a member of a group of synthetic nitrofuran compounds that also includes furazolidone, which is available in Europe but not the United States. Three oral formulations of nitrofurantoin were developed. A microcrystalline form was introduced in 1953, and a macrocrystalline form (Macrodantin, Procter & Gamble) has been available since 1967. Capsules (Mylan) and an oral suspension (Furadantin, Dura) are now available.

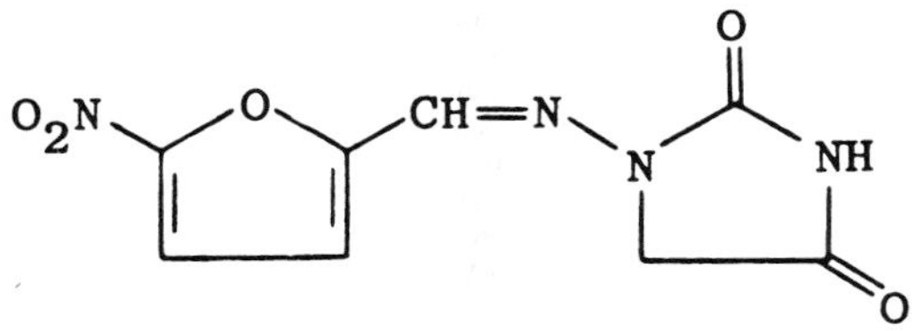

O_2N … CH=N … N … NH … O … O

FIGURE 32–1. Chemical structure of nitrofurantoin.

Mechanisms of Drug Action and Bacterial Resistance

The mechanism of action of nitrofurantoin is poorly understood, but activity in many cases appears to require enzymatic reduction within the bacterial cell.[1] The reduced derivatives appear to be capable of binding to ribosomal proteins. Nitrofurans have been shown to inhibit the synthesis of inducible enzymes by blocking translation[2] and also to inhibit bacterial respiration and pyruvate metabolism. Recently, antibacterial activity has been shown under conditions in which nitroreductase activity was inhibited, suggesting that nitrofurantoin may act in part without reduction to active metabolites.[3] The nitrofurans, like the quinolones, appear to damage bacterial DNA,[4] and they induce bacterial DNA repair systems.[5] Mutants with defective DNA repair functions are hypersusceptible.[6] Nitrofurantoin may antagonize the bactericidal activity of quinolones against *Proteus* and *Enterobacter*.[7] The principal drug action that determines the bactericidal activity of nitrofurantoin, however, remains to be defined.

Resistant strains of *Escherichia coli* with chromosomal or plasmid-mediated resistance have been associated with inhibition of nitrofuran reductase enzyme activity, thereby decreasing the production of the active derivative(s).[8–10] In clinical use, however, the emergence of nitrofurantoin-resistant variants from initially susceptible pathogens has been rare despite many years of clinical use of this agent.[11]

Spectrum of Activity

Susceptibility breakpoints are based on urinary concentrations of nitrofurantoin and have been correlated with eradication of bacteriuria in patients with urinary tract infections.[12, 13] Bacterial strains with a minimum inhibitory concentration (MIC) of 32 μg/ml or less are considered clinically susceptible. For strains having an MIC of 64 μg/ml, clinical responses may be more variable.[14] MIC values of greater than 500 μg/ml are uniformly correlated with clinical failure.[12] On the basis of these criteria, more than 90% of clinical strains of *E. coli, Citrobacter* spp., *Staphylococcus saprophyticus,* and *Enterococcus faecalis* are susceptible. Group B streptococci are also usually susceptible. In contrast, only a minority of strains of *Enterobacter* spp. (20 to 50%), *Klebsiella* spp. (45%), and *Enterococcus faecium* (50%) are susceptible, and members of the genera *Proteus, Providencia, Morganella, Serratia, Acinetobacter,* and *Pseudomonas* are almost always resistant.[13, 14] These patterns of susceptibility have generally remained stable in our hospital and others.[15]

Other organisms that are uncommonly associated with urinary tract infections but may be susceptible to nitrofurantoin in vitro include *Salmonella* spp., *Shigella* spp., *Staphylococcus aureus,* coagulase-negative staphylococci, *Streptococcus pneumoniae, Streptococcus pyogenes, Corynebacterium* spp., and *Bacteroides* spp.[16–18]

Pharmacology

Absorption. The completeness of absorption of orally administered nitrofurantoin as determined from drug recovery in the urine is about 40 to 50% and absorption is enhanced when the drug is taken with food.[19] Absorption occurs principally and rapidly in the small intestine. Two formulations of nitrofurantoin differ in the rate of drug absorption. The slower rate of dissolution and absorption of the macrocrystalline form relative to the microcrystalline form was associated with a lower occurrence of gastrointestinal adverse effects, a minimal reduction in overall absorption (36% versus 43%), and no change in efficacy (see later on). Although parenteral preparations of nitrofurantoin have been evaluated, they are not generally available for clinical use.

Distribution. Serum concentrations of nitrofurantoin are low or undetectable (≤1 μg/ml) with standard oral doses of 100 mg four times daily. After administration of intravenous nitrofurantoin, serum half-life has been estimated to be 30 minutes or less. In animals given intravenous nitrofurantoin, a high volume of distribution (0.7 liter/kg) suggested drug distribution into extracellular and intracellular compartments, but enzymatic degradation of nitrofurantoin in situ is thought to contribute to low drug levels in most tissues.[19, 20] Therapeutic concentrations are not detected in prostatic secretions,[21] and only low concentrations have been detected in human breast milk.[22] Nitrofurantoin concentrations in bile may be equal to or greater than those in serum.[19] Drug concentrations in urine are substantial (50 to 250 μg/ml) and exceed the MIC for susceptible organisms.[23]

Excretion. Nitrofurantoin is eliminated predominantly in the urine. Renal elimination involves glomerular filtration, tubular secretion, and tubular reabsorption.[19] Tubular handling is by the weak acid transport system. Reabsorption is decreased in the presence of alkaline urine, because at alkaline pH the equilibrium of nonionized and ionized drug is shifted toward the ionized form, which diffuses back across the renal tubular epithelium less well than the nonionized form. Urine alkalinization does not enhance antibacterial activity in the urine, however, because nitrofurantoin may be less active at alkaline pH.[11] In patients with renal failure, nitrofurantoin excretion is decreased in proportion to decreases in creatinine clearance, and urinary drug concentrations become subtherapeutic.[24] In severe renal failure, there may also be modest increases in serum concentrations of nitrofurantoin (≤6 μg/ml).[24] Thus, nitrofurantoin should not be used in patients with renal insufficiency (creatinine clearance of <40 ml/min).

With normal renal function, metabolism and biliary excretion are minor pathways of nitrofurantoin elimination that are less well understood.[19] No dosage adjustment is required in patients with liver disease without alterations in renal function.

Dosing. For therapy of established urinary tract infections, nitrofurantoin is given orally at 50 to 100 mg four times daily. For use as prophylaxis for recurrent urinary tract infections, it is usually given as 50 to 100 mg once daily.

Clinical Uses

Nitrofurantoin is indicated only for the treatment and prophylaxis of urinary tract infections.

Acute Uncomplicated Cystitis

In earlier noncomparative studies, bacteriologic and clinical responses in patients with acute uncomplicated cystitis ranged from 61 to 100%,[11] although in a number of these studies, follow-up periods were brief. Infections caused by *E. coli* generally responded well, and infections caused by *Proteus* spp. and *P. aeruginosa* responded poorly if at all. When given for 7 days to young women, nitrofurantoin and trimethoprim (200 mg PO once daily) produced similar rates of eradication of infections caused by *E. coli* (66/78 [84%] versus 72/77 [93%]) and *S. saprophyticus* (7/8 [87%] versus 10/12 [83%]), but the smaller numbers of infections caused by *Klebsiella* spp. and *Proteus* spp. responded better to trimethoprim.[25] With 3-day courses of therapy for acute cystitis in young women, nitrofurantoin (100 mg qid) produced cure rates at 6-weeks follow-up evaluation similar to those of cefadroxil and amoxicillin (61%) but lower than that of trimethoprim-sulfamethoxazole (82%).[26] Persistence of bacteriuria was also lower for trimethoprim-sulfamethoxazole (noted in 3% of patients) than for nitrofurantoin (in 16%). In both studies, suppression of potential pathogens in the periurethral, vaginal, and rectal flora occurred significantly more often with trimethoprim than with nitrofurantoin, a finding that may have contributed to the higher success rate noted in the trimethoprim-sulfamethoxazole group. A modified-release formulation of nitrofurantoin that can be given twice daily was comparable to trimethoprim-sulfamethoxazole for treatment of women with uncomplicated cystitis in a general practice population.[27] Nitrofurantoin has also been used for treatment of lower urinary tract infections in pregnant women[28] and children.[17] In young girls with cystitis, responses to nitrofurantoin given for 3 days were similar to responses to a 7-day course.[29] At present, 15 to 20% of urinary isolates causing acute uncomplicated cystitis may be resistant to nitrofurantoin, and responses to this agent in infections caused by susceptible pathogens may be less satisfactory than responses to trimethoprim-sulfamethoxazole or fluoroquinolones.[28] Thus, nitrofurantoin should be considered an alternative rather than a first-line therapeutic agent for this clinical syndrome.

Acute Uncomplicated Pyelonephritis and Complicated Urinary Tract Infections

Patients with acute pyelonephritis respond inconsistently to nitrofurantoin, and bacteremias have occurred during nitrofurantoin treatment, presumably because serum concentrations are inadequate.[11] Thus, nitrofurantoin should not be used for treatment of patients with pyelonephritis. In addition, complicated urinary tract infections, which are defined as those associated with structural or functional abnormalities of the urinary tract, are often associated with pyelonephritis and are often caused by pathogens resistant to nitrofurantoin. In general, nitrofurantoin is not indicated for treatment of these infections, and it is specifically contraindicated in cases that are complicated by resistant pathogens, pyelonephritis, renal failure, or prostatic infection. An earlier study of older men with recurring bacteriuria showed that nitrofurantoin given for long-term suppressive therapy reduced recurrences of bacteriuria by about 40% relative to placebo,[30] but drugs that penetrate the prostate (trimethoprim or fluoroquinolones) are more likely to eradicate bacteriuria in these patients.

Prophylaxis of Recurrent Urinary Tract Infections

In young women with two or more episodes of symptomatic bacteriuria within 12 months, once-daily nitrofurantoin (100 mg) was highly effective and comparable to trimethoprim-sulfamethoxazole (40 to 200 mg) in preventing recurrent urinary tract infections without emergence of resistant organisms.[31] Infections recurred at the same rate when prophylaxis was stopped after 6 months. In two trials in a more heterogeneous population of women with a history of four or more symptomatic urinary tract infections in the preceding 12 months, nitrofurantoin (50 to 100 mg at bedtime) was comparable to cefaclor (250 mg at bedtime)[32] or norfloxacin (200 mg at bedtime)[33] in increasing the interval between symptomatic episodes (five- to seven-fold). In both trials, nitrofurantoin was somewhat less well tolerated than the comparison agent.

For women in whom recurrence of infection is associated with sexual intercourse, a single dose of nitrofurantoin (100 mg) taken shortly after intercourse has also been highly effective in preventing symptomatic infection.[34] Postcoital prophylaxis was also effective in pregnant women with a history of recurrent urinary tract infections before pregnancy.[35] Nitrofurantoin has reduced the rates of bacteriuria in patients undergoing intermittent catheterization in some[36] but not all[37] studies. Antimicrobial prophylaxis is not of value in patients with long-term indwelling catheters.[28]

Adverse Effects

Gastrointestinal and Skin Reactions

The overall tolerability of nitrofurantoin is determined by gastrointestinal adverse effects, the rates of which are dose-related and differ for the two formulations.[23] In a randomized, double-blind comparison, the microcrystalline formulation (100 mg four times daily) was associated with adverse effects (predominantly nausea or vomiting) in 39% of patients, compared with 17% of patients receiving the macrocrystalline formulation in the same dose.[38] Slower dissolution of the macrocrystalline formulation is thought to be responsible for its lower frequency of gastrointestinal side effects.

Rashes, presumably of an allergic nature, have been reported in about 1% of hospitalized patients receiving nitrofurantoin.[17] Other less common but more serious toxic effects of nitrofurantoin have received considerable attention.[17, 23]

Pulmonary Reactions

Pulmonary reactions have been classified into acute, subacute, and chronic forms[17] and in the United States appear to occur at a frequency of 1 or fewer cases per 100,000 courses of treatment.[23] The chronic form of pulmonary reactions appears to be less common than the acute form, at least in part because fewer patients receive the extended courses of therapy that precede the chronic form.

The acute reaction appears to be a reversible hypersensitivity phenomenon and may occur within hours to weeks of drug exposure, with a shorter time to onset of symptoms after drug reexposure.[39, 40] The clinical presentation is characterized by the rapid onset of fever, cough, dyspnea, and myalgia. These symptoms are usually accompanied by peripheral blood eosinophilia (in 83% of cases) and lower lobe infiltrates (in 94%) with (in 20%) or without pleural effusions on chest radiographs. Alveolar exudates, interstitial inflammation, and vasculitis have been found on lung biopsy. In addition, rash, pruritus, chest discomfort, and sputum production may also be present. Improvement is generally rapid after discontinuation of the drug, and acute reactions do not generally progress to the chronic form.

It is not clear whether the subacute and chronic forms of nitrofurantoin pulmonary reactions are distinct from each other except for onset after 1 and 6 or more months of drug therapy, respectively.[40] These reactions are thought to result from toxic effects on the lung, possibly related to oxidant injury of the type that has been demonstrated in rat lung explants treated with nitrofurantoin.[41] In both the subacute and chronic forms, clinical features include the gradual onset of progressive nonproductive cough and dyspnea and interstitial infiltrates on chest radiographs. Fever is variably present. Eosinophilia is uncommon, but abnormalities on liver function testing may be seen in up to 40% of patients, and positive results on assays for antinuclear antibodies have been reported.[39] Regression often occurs with discontinuation of nitrofurantoin, but in the more chronic cases, irreversible pulmonary fibrosis and fatal reactions have occurred. A beneficial effect of corticosteroid therapy has not been convincingly demonstrated in patients with the chronic form of nitrofurantoin pulmonary reactions.

Hepatic Reactions

Hepatic reactions appear to occur with a frequency similar to that of the chronic form of pulmonary reactions.[42] In some cases, findings have included both hepatitis and pulmonary infiltrates.[43] Acute hepatitis with or without cholestasis associated with short-term use of nitrofurantoin is generally self-limited and reversible.[44] Prolonged use of nitrofurantoin, however, has been associated with chronic active hepatitis, cirrhosis, and death.[43] In such cases, hyperglobulinemia and antinuclear antibodies were commonly present, but eosinophilia was an inconsistent finding.

Hematologic Reactions

Hemolytic anemia has occurred rarely in patients receiving nitrofurantoin and most often, but not always, in those with deficiency of glucose-6-phosphate dehydrogenase (G6PD).[23, 45] Decreases in cellular NADPH in such patients result in diminished cellular levels of reduced glutathione. Nitrofurantoin may inhibit glutathione reductase, further compromising the ability of the cell to generate reduced glutathione,[46] and it may also generate the release of superoxide from oxyhemoglobin in the presence of oxygen,[47] thereby further contributing to oxidant stresses.[17] Patients with deficiencies in enolase and glutathione peroxidases have developed nitrofurantoin-induced hemolysis as well. Folic acid–responsive megaloblastic anemia has also been reported.[48] Eosinophilia is seen as a feature of the acute pulmonary reactions and some hepatic reactions, but leukopenia and aplastic anemia have been only rarely reported.

Peripheral Neuropathy

A peripheral sensorimotor neuropathy of unclear mechanism has been reported uncommonly and less often than have been pulmonary reactions. Neuropathy has been seen in patients receiving nitrofurantoin for prolonged periods as well as in patients with renal failure.[23, 42] The onset of neuropathy is often insidious, with the occurrence of paresthesias and dysesthesias in a stocking-and-glove distribution. Distal weakness with centripetal spread may also occur.[49] Histopathologic findings have included demyelination and axonal degeneration.[50] The reversibility of the deficits after cessation of drug therapy may be slow and variable.

Uses in Pediatrics and in Pregnancy

Toxic effects of nitrofurantoin appear to be similar in children and adults,[51] but the drug is not recommended for use in neonates. It may be used for treatment of urinary tract infections in pregnancy when clearly indicated but should not be used at term.[7, 28] Nitrofurantoin crosses the placenta, but very low concentrations are reached in amniotic fluid.[52] Although it is mutagenic in some bacterial tests in vitro,[53] results of tests for teratogenicity and carcinogenicity in animals have been negative.[7, 23] Reviews of adverse events in a total of 165 pregnant patients who received nitrofurantoin therapy in each of the three trimesters of pregnancy found no increased incidence of fetal loss or fetal abnormality over that in the population in general.[54, 55] Healthy infants with G6PD deficiency have been born to mothers treated with nitrofurantoin during pregnancy.[23]

METHENAMINE

Chemical Structure

Methenamine (hexamethylenetetramine) (Fig. 32–2) is available as a salt of mandelic acid (α-hydroxybenzene acetic acid) (Mandelamine, Warner Chilcott; Uroquid-Acid, Beach) or hippuric acid (benzoylamino-acetic acid) (Urex, 3M) or without these acids (Urised, Polymedica; Prosed, Star).

Mechanism of Action and Antimicrobial Activity

Methenamine itself has little antibacterial activity, but at acid pH, each molecule of methenamine that is hydrolyzed generates four molecules of ammonia and six molecules of formaldehyde[56, 57]:

$$(N_4[CH_2])_6 + 6H_2O + 4H^+ \leftrightarrow 4NH_4^- + 6HCHO$$

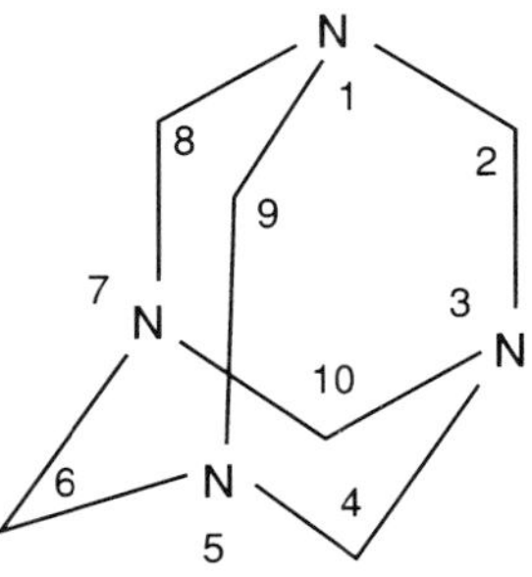

FIGURE 32–2. Chemical structure of methenamine. Numbers are conventional designations of atom positions.

Increasing concentrations of H^+ and diffusional loss of NH_3 drive the reaction to the right. Formaldehyde, the active product, is a nonspecific denaturant of proteins and nucleic acids and has broad-spectrum antimicrobial activity. Free formaldehyde concentrations above 25 μg/ml may be bactericidal. Microbial resistance to formaldehyde has not been described.[56] Antimicrobial activity in urine is correlated with urinary concentrations of formaldehyde.[58] Although formaldehyde has activity against *Proteus* spp., an alkaline urine may be generated by the urease activity of these organisms, preventing conversion of methenamine to formaldehyde. Inhibitors of urease may prevent this effect in laboratory simulations of *Proteus* growing in urine.[59] Hippuric and mandelic acids themselves have only limited antibacterial activity at concentrations achieved with usual doses of their respective methenamine salts.[60]

Pharmacology

Absorption and Distribution. Methenamine itself is rapidly absorbed after oral administration, and 82 to 88% is recovered in the urine of normal volunteers in the 24 hours after a 1-g dose,[61] indicating excellent bioavailability. Methenamine may be partially degraded in the presence of gastric acid before absorption.[62] This degradation is avoided with enteric-coated formulations, but absorption is slower. The volume of distribution (0.56 liter/kg) is relatively high, suggesting broad distribution in tissues. Methenamine crosses the placenta, and concentrations in breast milk are similar to those in plasma.[63]

Excretion. The half-life of elimination of methenamine from serum is 3 to 4 hours with normal renal function. Renal clearance is 95% of total clearance from serum, indicating a predominant renal route of excretion.[61] Hippuric and mandelic acids are also excreted renally by both glomerular filtration and tubular secretion.[57, 64] The extent to which methenamine and hippuric and mandelic acids accumulate in patients with renal failure is not known.

Factors Affecting Formaldehyde Concentrations in Urine. The concentration of formaldehyde in bladder urine determines antimicrobial activity and is a function of (1) methenamine concentrations in urine, (2) the rate of hydrolysis of methenamine to formaldehyde, and (3) the rate of urine loss from the bladder by voiding or drainage. At constant rates of renal clearance, methenamine concentrations in urine decrease with increasing urine volumes, but with repetitive dosing, concentrations above 150 μg/ml are usually maintained.[61] Conversion of methenamine to formaldehyde occurs as a first-order reaction, with higher rates of conversion in the presence of higher concentrations of methenamine.[65] The relative rate constant for conversion increases with decreasing urine pH and is 13-fold higher at pH 5.2 than at pH 6.5[65]; no hydrolysis occurs above pH 6.8. At methenamine concentrations of 1000 μg/ml, the time needed to generate formaldehyde concentrations in excess of 25 μg/ml is more than 6 hours at pH 6.5, 3 hours at pH 5.85, and 1.5 to 2 hours at pH 5.6.[66] At such concentrations of formaldehyde, bacterial exposure for at least 2 hours appears to be necessary for antibacterial activity. Thus, increases in the frequency of voiding or bladder drainage will reduce antibacterial effects by removing formaldehyde and by reducing the time of exposure of bladder bacteria to formaldehyde.[67] For these reasons, methenamine is ineffective in the presence of indwelling bladder catheters and may be ineffective when intermittent catheterization is performed frequently. Similarly, the brief time in which methenamine resides in the renal tissues and the upper urinary tract obviates efficacy in pyelonephritis.

Acidification of the Urine during Methenamine Treatment. Maintaining urinary pH below 6 is necessary for generating antibacterial activity from methenamine, and in many patients, urine pH is sufficiently low without additional measures. The amounts of hippuric and mandelic acids given with usual doses of methenamine hippurate and methenamine mandelate, however, do not contribute importantly to urine acidification.[62] Ascorbic acid has been given to aid urine acidification, but doses as high as 12 g per day may be required.[57] The value of acetohydroxamic acid, an inhibitor of urease, as an adjunctive agent in patients with an alkaline urine associated with *Proteus* infection is suggested by in vitro data[59] but is unclear in vivo.

Dosing. With equimolar mixtures of methenamine and their respective acids, 1 g of methenamine mandelate contains 480 mg methenamine, and 1 g of methenamine hippurate contains 440 mg of methenamine. For adults and children over 12 years, methenamine mandelate and methenamine hippurate are usually given in a dose of 1 g PO twice daily, but up to 4 g per day (1 g four times daily) may be given. For children between 6 and 12 years, the dose is 500 mg to 1 g twice daily. An oral suspension (methenamine mandelate, 500 mg/5 ml and 250 mg/5 ml) is available for younger children; for children less than 6 years old, the usual dose is 250 mg per 30 lb body weight PO four times daily.

Clinical Uses

The efficacy of methenamine for treatment of established cystitis has not been adequately documented in comparative clinical trials, and methenamine is not effective for treatment of pyelonephritis. Methenamine thus should not be used for treatment of established urinary tract infections.

Methenamine has been shown, however, to be effective for suppression or prophylaxis of recurrent lower urinary tract infections. In a double-blind, placebo-controlled, crossover trial in young, otherwise healthy women with recurrent cystitis, 1 g of methenamine hippurate twice daily reduced recurrent symptomatic infections by 73%.[68] A similar significant reduction (56%) was seen in another comparative study of a similar population of young women and girls given methenamine mandelate (500 mg four times daily) and ascorbic acid (2 g daily).[69] Trimethoprim-sulfamethoxazole (40 to 200 mg at bedtime), however, was significantly better than methenamine in reducing the frequency of recurrent infections in this study,[69] as was trimethoprim alone in another study.[70] Trimethoprim-sulfamethoxazole was more effective than methenamine in reducing periurethral colonization with gram-negative bacilli, a potential reservoir of recurring pathogens.[69] Although less well tolerated, nitrofurantoin was also more effective than methenamine hippurate in preventing symptomatic infections in another trial.[71]

Methenamine has also prevented episodes of recurring bacteriuria in children[72, 73] and has suppressed chronic bacteriuria in men.[30] It has not been shown, however, that methenamine is superior to other agents such as trimethoprim-sulfamethoxazole for these uses.

Attempts to prevent recurring infections in patients with indwelling bladder catheters by use of methenamine have not been successful,[74] as might be expected because sufficient concentrations of formaldehyde cannot be generated under these conditions. The results of prophylaxis in patients undergoing intermittent catheterization have been variable.[74, 75] In a double-blind, randomized, placebo-controlled trial in patients with neurogenic bladders undergoing bladder retraining, urinary acidification was augmented with ammonium chloride in the methenamine group (both agents given as 1 g every 6 hours), and catheterization (usually every 6 hours), voiding, and drinking schedules were specifically controlled. Over the 21 days of the study, bacteriuria occurred at a significantly lower rate in the methenamine group—53% (9 of 17 patients)—than in the placebo group—86% (19 of 22 patients).[75] For patients undergoing intermittent catheterization for longer periods, however, antimicrobial regimens may only delay episodes of bacteriuria. The effectiveness of methenamine-containing regimens is probably inversely related to the frequency of catheterization and voiding.

Adverse Effects

Methenamine is generally well tolerated,[57, 69] and in double-blind studies,[75] side effects have been few, mild, and reversible, and the incidence of such effects is comparable to that reported with placebo.

In nonblinded studies, most commonly encountered have been gastrointestinal side effects (nausea, vomiting) and rashes or pruritus.[57] Symptoms of bladder irritation have been reported in patients with sterile urine receiving methenamine suppression.[30] With high doses of methenamine, increased gastrointestinal intolerance and hemorrhagic cystitis[76] may occur, possibly related to increased local concentrations of formaldehyde.

Methenamine salts may predispose to the development of urate crystals in the urine of patients with gout and may cause precipitation of sulfonamides in the urine of patients concurrently receiving these drugs.

Because conversion of methenamine to formaldehyde also releases ammonia, methenamine should be avoided in patients with hepatic insufficiency. The safety of methenamine itself in patients with renal failure is unclear; because of the potential risk of increasing systemic acidosis, acidifying agents should be avoided in such patients.[77] Limited data suggest that methenamine may be given safely in the second and third trimesters of pregnancy.[78]

REFERENCES

1. McCalla DR, Reuvers A, Kaiser C. Mode of action of nitrofurazone. J Bacteriol. 1970;104:1126–1134.
2. Herrlich P, Schweiger M. Nitrofurans, a group of synthetic antibiotics, with new mode of action: Discrimination of specific messenger RNA classes. Proc Natl Acad Sci U S A. 1976;73:3386–3390.
3. McOsker CC, Fitzpatrick PM. Nitrofurantoin: mechanism of action and implications for resistance development in common uropathogens. J Antimicrob Chemother. 1994;33(suppl. A):23–30.
4. Tu Y, McCalla DR. Effect of activated nitrofurans on DNA. Biochim Biophys Acta. 1975;402:142–149.
5. Rahman MdS, Pal AK, Chatterjee SN. Induction of SOS like responses by nitrofurantoin in *Vibrio cholerae* El Tor cells. Arch Microbiol. 1993;159:98–100.
6. Jenkins ST, Bennett PM. Effect of mutations in deoxyribonucleic acid repair pathways on the sensitivity of *Escherichia coli* K-12 strains to nitrofurantoin. J Bacteriol. 1976;125:1214–1216.
7. Shah S, Greenwood D. Interactions between antibacterial agents of the quinolone group and nitrofurantoin. J Antimicrob Chemother. 1988;21:41–48.
8. McCalla DR, Kaiser C, Green MHL. Genetics of nitrofurazone resistance in *Escherichia coli*. J Bacteriol. 1978;133:10–16.
9. Breeze AS, Obaseiki-Ebor EE. Nitrofuran reductase activity in nitrofurantoin-resistant strains of *Escherichia coli* K-12: some with chromosomally determined resistance and others carrying R-plasmids. J Antimicrob Chemother. 1983;12:543–547.
10. Breeze AS, Obaseiki-Ebor EE. Transferable nitrofuran resistance conferred by R-plasmids in clinical isolates of *Escherichia coli*. J Antimicrob Chemother. 1983;12:459–467.
11. Richards WA, Riss E, Kass EH, et al. Nitrofurantoin. Clinical and laboratory studies in urinary tract infections. Arch Intern Med. 1955;96:437–450.
12. Winn WR, Silton J, Finegold SM. In vitro sensitivity to nitrofurantoin compared with clinical bacteriological response. Antimicrob Agents Chemother. 1965;582–590.
13. Turck M, Ronald AR, Petersdorf RG. Susceptibility of Enterobacteriaceae to nitrofurantoin correlated with eradication of bacteriuria. Antimicrob Agents Chemother. 1967;446–452.
14. Barry AL. Nitrofurantoin susceptibility test criteria. J Antimicrob Chemother. 1990;25:711–713.
15. Bulger RJ, Larson E, Sherris JC. Decreased incidences of resistance to antimicrobial agents among *Escherichia coli* and *Klebsiella-Enterobacter:* Observations in a university hospital over a 10 year period. Ann Intern Med. 1970;72:65–71.
16. Schroeder SA, Terry PM, Bennett JV. Antibiotic resistance and transfer factor in *Salmonella,* United States 1967. JAMA. 1968;205:903–906.
17. Gleckman R, Alvarez S, Joubert DW. Drug therapy reviews: Nitrofurantoin. Am J Hosp Pharm. 1979;36:342–351.
18. Brumfitt W, Reynolds AV, Hamilton-Miller JMT. Activity of nitrofurantoin and nifuratel against anaerobic gram-negative bacilli (Letter). Lancet. 1975;1:460.
19. Conklin JD. The pharmacokinetics of nitrofurantoin and its related bioavailability. Antibiot Chemother. 1978;25:233–252.
20. Schmidt FH. Inactivation of nitrofuran derivatives by mammalian tissue. Klin Wochenschr. 1966;44:653–654.
21. Dunn BL, Stamey TA. Antibacterial concentrations in prostatic fluid, 1-nitrofurantoin. J Urol. 1967;97:505–507.
22. Varsano I, Fischl J, Shochet SB. The excretion of orally ingested nitrofurantoin in human milk. J Pediatr. 1973;82:886–887.
23. D'Arcy PF. Nitrofurantoin. Drug Intell Clin Pharm. 1985;19:540–547.
24. Sachs J, Geer J, Noell P, et al. Effect of renal function on urinary recovery of orally administered nitrofurantoin. N Engl J Med. 1968;278:1032–1035.
25. Iravani A, Richard GA, Baer H. Trimethoprim once daily vs. nitrofurantoin in treatment of acute urinary tract infections in young women, with special reference to periurethral, vaginal, and fecal flora. Rev Infect Dis. 1982;4:378–387.
26. Hooton TM, Winter C, Tiu F, Stamm WE. Randomized comparative trial and cost analysis of 3-day antimicrobial regimens for treatment of acute cystitis in women. JAMA. 1995;273:41–45.
27. Spencer RC, Moseley DJ, Greensmith MJ. Nitrofurantoin modified release versus trimethoprim or co-trimoxazole in the treatment of uncomplicated urinary tract infection in general practice. J Antimicrob Chemother. 1994;33(suppl A):121–129.
28. Stamm WE, Hooton TM. Management of urinary tract infections in adults. N Engl J Med. 1993;329:1328–1334.
29. Lohr JA, Hayden GF, Kesler RW, et al. Three-day therapy of lower urinary tract infections with nitrofurantoin macrocrystals: A randomized clinical trial. J Pediatr. 1981;99:980–983.
30. Freeman RB, Smith WM, Richardson JA, et al. Long-term therpay for chronic bacteriuria in men. U.S. Public Health Service Cooperative Study. Ann Intern Med. 1975;83:133–147.
31. Stamm WE, Counts GW, Wagner KF, et al. Antimicrobial prophylaxis of recurrent urinary tract infections. A double-blind, placebo-controlled trial. Ann Intern Med. 1980;92:770–775.
32. Brumfitt W, Hamilton-Miller JMT. A comparative trial of low dose cefaclor and macrocrystalline nitrofurantoin in the prevention of recurrent urinary tract infection. Infection. 1995;23:98–102.
33. Brumfitt W, Hamilton-Miller JMT, Smith GW, Al-Wali W. Comparative trial of norfloxacin and macrocrystalline nitrofurantoin (Macrodantin) in the prophylaxis of recurrent urinary tract infection in women. Q J Med. 1991;81:811–820.
34. Vosti KL. Recurrent urinary tract infections. Prevention by prophylactic antibiotics after sexual intercourse. JAMA. 1975;231:934–940.
35. Pfau A, Sacks TG. Effective prophylaxis for recurrent urinary tract infections during pregnancy. Clin Infect Dis. 1992;14:810–814.
36. Anderson RU. Prophylaxis of bacteriuria during intermittent catheterization of acute neurogenic bladder. J Urol. 1980;123:364–366.
37. Kuhlemeier KV, Stover SL, Lloyd LK. Prophylactic antibacterial therapy for preventing urinary tract infections in spinal cord injury patients. J Urol. 1985;134:514–517.
38. Kalowski S, Radford N, Kincaid-Smith P. Crystalline and macrocrystalline nitrofurantoin in the treatment of urinary-tract infection. N Engl J Med. 1974;290:385–387.
39. Holmberg L, Boman G. Pulmonary reactions to nitrofurantoin. 447 cases reported to the Swedish Adverse Drug Reaction Committee 1966–1976. Eur J Respir Dis. 1981;62:180–189.
40. Sovijärvi ARA, Lemola M, Stenius B, et al. Nitrofurantoin-induced acute, subacute and chronic pulmonary reactions. A report of 66 cases. Scand J Respir Dis. 1977;58:41–50.
41. Martin WJ III. Nitrofurantoin: Evidence for the oxidant injury of lung parenchymal cells. Am Rev Respir Dis. 1983;127:482–486.
42. Holmberg L, Boman G, Böttiger LE, et al. Adverse reactions to nitrofurantoin. Analysis of 921 reports. Am J Med. 1980;69:733–738.
43. Sharp JR, Ishak KG, Zimmerman HJ. Chronic active hepatitis and severe hepatic necrosis associated with nitrofurantoin. Ann Intern Med. 1980;92:14–19.
44. Goldstein LI, Ishak KG, Burns W. Hepatic injury associated with nitrofurantoin therapy. Am J Digest Dis. 1974;19:987–998.
45. Gait JE. Hemolytic reactions to nitrofurantoin in patients with glucose-6-phosphate dehydrogenase deficiency: Theory and practice. DICP Ann Pharmacother. 1990;24:1210–1213.
46. Buzard JA, Kopko F, Paul MF. Inhibition of glutathione reductase by nitrofurantoin. J Lab Clin Med. 1960;56:885–890.
47. Dershwitz M, Novak RF. Studies of the mechanism of nitrofurantoin-mediated red cell toxicity. J Pharmacol Exp Therapeut. 1982;222:430–434.
48. Shah RR, Wade G. Reappraisal of the risk/benefit of nitrofurantoin: Review of toxicity and efficacy. Adverse Drug React Acute Poisoning Rev. 1989;8:183–201.
49. Toole J, Parrish M. Nitrofurantoin polyneuropathy. Neurology. 1973;23:554–559.
50. Yiannikas C, Pollard JD, McLeod JG. Nitrofurantoin neuropathy. Aust N Z J Med. 1981;11:400–405.
51. Corragio MJ, Gross TP, Roscelli JD. Nitrofurantoin toxicity in children. Pediatr Infect Dis J. 1989;8:163–166.
52. Perry JE, LeBlanc AL. Transfer of nitrofurantoin across the human placenta. Tex Rep Biol Med. 1967;25:265–269.
53. Wang CY, Benson RC Jr, Bryan GT. Mutagenicity for *Salmonella typhimurium* of urine obtained from humans receiving nitrofurantoin. J Natl Cancer Inst. 1977;58:871–873.
54. Hailey FJ, Fort H, Williams JC, et al. Foetal safety of nitrofurantoin macrocrystals therapy during pregnancy: A retrospective analysis. J Int Med Res. 1983;11:364–369.
55. Kass EH. Pyelonephritis and bacteriuria: A major problem in preventive medicine. Ann Intern Med. 1962;56:46–53.
56. Duca CJ, Scudi JV. Some antibacterial properties of mandelamine (methenamine mandelate). Proc Soc Exp Biol Med. 1947;66:123–126.
57. Gleckman R, Alvarez S, Joubert DW, et al. Drug therapy reviews: Methenamine mandelate and methenamine hippurate. Am J Hosp Pharm. 1979;36:1509–12.
58. Gandelman AL. Methenamine mandelate: Antimicrobial activity in urine and correlation with formaldehyde levels. J Urol. 1967;97:533–536.
59. Musher DM, Griffith DP, Templeton BG. Further observations on the potentiation of the antibacterial effect of methenamine by acetohydroxamic acid. J Infect Dis. 1976;133:564–567.
60. Hamilton-Miller JMT, Brumfitt W. Methenamine and its salts as urinary tract antiseptics. Variables affecting the antibacterial activity of formaldehyde, mandelic acid, and hippuric acid in vitro. Invest Urol. 1977;14:287–291.
61. Klinge E, Männistö P, Mäntylä R, et al. Pharmacokinetics of methenamine in healthy volunteers. J Antimicrob Chemother. 1982;9:209–216.
62. Mayrer AR, Andriole VT. Urinary tract antiseptics. Med Clin North Am. 1982;66:199–208.

63. Allgén L-G, Holmberg G, Persson B, et al. Biological fate of methenamine in man. Absorption, renal excretion and passage into umbilical cord blood, amniotic fluid and breast milk. Acta Obstet Gynecol Scand. 1979;58:287–293.
64. Knoefel PK, Huang KC. Biochemorphology of renal tubular transport: Hippuric acid and related substances. J Pharmacol Exp Ther. 1959;126:296–303.
65. Strom JG, Jun HW. Effect of urine pH and ascorbic acid on the rate of conversion of methenamine to formaldehyde. Biopharmaceut Drug Dispos. 1993;14:61–69.
66. Musher DM, Griffith DP. Generation of formaldehyde from methenamine: Effect of pH and concentration, and antibacterial effect. Antimicrob Agents Chemother. 1974;6:708–711.
67. Musher DM, Griffith DP, Richie Y. The generation of formaldehyde from methenamine. Effect of urinary flow and residual volume. Invest Urol. 1976;13:380–382.
68. Cronberg S, Welin C-O, Henriksson L, et al. Prevention of recurrent acute cystitis by methenamine hippurate: Double blind controlled crossover long term study. BMJ. 1987;294:1507–1508.
69. Harding GKM, Ronald AR. A controlled study of antimicrobial prophylaxis of recurrent urinary tract infection in women. N Engl J Med. 1974;291:597–601.
70. Kasanen A, Junnila SYT, Kaarsalo E, et al. Secondary prevention of recurrent urinary tract infections. Comparison of the effect of placebo, methenamine hippurate, nitrofurantoin and trimethoprim alone. Scand J Infect Dis. 1982;14:293–296.
71. Brumfitt W, Cooper J, Hamilton-Miller JMT. Prevention of recurrent urinary tract infections in women: A comparative trial between nitrofurantoin and methenamine hippurate. J Urol. 1981;126:71–74.
72. Holland NH, West CD. Prevention of recurrent urinary tract infections in girls. Am J Dis Child. 1963;105:560–567.
73. Elo J, Sarna S, Ahava K, et al. Methenamine hippurate in urinary tract infections in children: Prophylaxis, treatment and side effects. J Antimicrob Chemother. 1978;4:355–365.
74. Vainrub B, Musher DM. Lack of effect of methenamine in suppression of, or prophylaxis against, chronic urinary tract infection. Antimicrob Agents Chemother. 1977;12:625–629.
75. Kevorkian CG, Merritt JL, Ilstrup DM. Methenamine mandelate with acidification: An effective urinary antiseptic in patients with neurogenic bladder. Mayo Clin Proc. 1984;59:523–529.
76. Ross RR, Conway GF. Hemorrhagic cystitis following accidental overdose of methenamine mandelate. Am J Dis Child. 1970;119:86–87.
77. Kasanen A, Mustakallio EK, Koskinen EH. Methenamine hippurate in the treatment of urinary tract infections. Ann Clin Res. 1974;6:279–284.
78. Furness MB, McDonald PJ, Beasley NV. Urinary antiseptics in asymptomatic bacteriuria of pregnancy. N Z Med J. 1974;81:417–419.

Chapter 33

Topical Antibacterials

ALLAN R. TUNKEL

Topical antibacterial therapy has several advantages over oral or parenteral administration of antibacterial agents (Table 33–1).[1] After the application of small amounts of compounds directly to an infection or wound, very high local drug concentrations are achieved. This broadens the in vitro spectrum of the antibacterial agent, permitting the use of compounds that might be too toxic if large amounts or systemic administration were required. After topical administration, the drug first enters the skin as the target organ, a variable quantity is distributed throughout the body, and then it is eliminated. Concentrations of a topical antibacterial decline from the skin surface to the subcutis, the opposite of which occurs after systemic administration.[2] Therefore, topical administration is favored if the pathologic process is in the epidermis or papillary dermis. For infection in the lower dermis or subcutis, one needs to determine whether topical antibacterial administration yields the necessary drug concentrations to eradicate the infection effectively. Mixtures of antibacterial agents can also be used, and this leads to synergistic effects and may delay the selection of resistant microorganisms. The following section reviews the general uses of topical antibacterial agents in the therapy and prevention of infections. Although topical agents are also effective in the therapy of eye and ear infections, these indications are reviewed in Chapters 98 and 50.

TABLE 33–1 Advantages of Topical Antibacterial Therapy

Ease of administration
Lower potential for adverse reactions
Lower risk of noncompliance
Delivery of high drug concentrations to site of infection
Decreased risk of bacterial resistance or cross-resistance
Cost savings*

*Depends on agent used.

GENERAL USES OF TOPICAL ANTIBACTERIALS

Disinfecting the Skin

Some topical antibacterial agents are very effective at decreasing the number of bacteria on the skin. The ideal agent should have the following properties: a broad antimicrobial spectrum; rapid bactericidal activity; persistent activity on the skin; an absence of irritating, allergic, or toxic reactions; an absence of systemic absorption; activity in the presence of body fluids (e.g., blood); and cosmetic acceptance.[1] Unfortunately, no single compound fulfills all these criteria. Depending on the specific clinical situation, however, only certain properties may be required. For example, for repeated hand washings (e.g., by medical personnel), a lack of irritation and persistence of activity are essential properties. In contrast, for preparation of operative sites, rapid bactericidal activity is needed.

Several topical antibacterial agents have been used as skin disinfectants. Alcohols are rapidly bactericidal but have a transient action and are irritating, especially with repeated use or when applied to damaged skin. This contrasts with chlorhexidine, a cationic biguanide that derives its activity by causing disruption of microbial cell membranes and precipitation of cell contents; it is the most ideal agent for skin cleaning and surgical scrubs. Its valuable properties include persistent activity on the skin when used regularly, rapid bactericidal activity, a broad antibacterial spectrum, little evidence of irritancy or allergy, activity in the presence of body fluids, and minimal absorption. Hexachlorophene, despite its remarkable persistence on the skin when used regularly, has lost favor as a skin disinfecting agent. It does not have a very effective gram-negative spectrum, and absorption, with resultant toxicity (especially in newborns), has been a concern. Iodophors (e.g., povidone-iodine) are organic complexes consisting of iodine and a carrier (e.g., polyvinylpyrrolidone) that slowly liberate iodine on reduction. These agents have a broad antimicrobial spectrum, although antibacterial activity does not persist on the skin and iodophors may be inactivated by body fluids. Their microbicidal effects are the result of cell wall penetration, oxidation, and substitution of microbial contents with free iodine. The iodophors are widely used for preoperative skin preparation, hand scrubbing, and the treatment and prevention of skin infections.[1]

Prophylaxis of Infection in Clean Wounds

When a wound leads to disruption in epidermal integrity (i.e., secondary to abrasions, cuts, or bites), one can consider the application of a topical antibacterial agent to prevent infection from developing. However, no antibacterial formulation has ever been proved to be efficacious in the prophylaxis of clean wounds because so few clean wounds become infected. Studies of topical preparations (e.g., neomycin, alone or in combination with bacitracin or polymyxin, or both) have shown efficacy in the prevention of infection in some circumstances, although these studies have been criticized because of the absence of control groups.[3] Controlled studies are unlikely to be performed, however, because the number of patients required to be studied would be extremely large. To avoid the difficulties in performing a large, randomized controlled trial, a human skin infection model was developed to test the efficacy of topical antibiotic formulations in the prophylaxis of minor skin infections.[3] After the induction of abrasion-type wounds in human volunteers, the wounds were inoculated with either 10^5 *Staphylococcus aureus* or 10^7 *Streptococcus pyogenes* and covered with an impermeable dressing for 6 hours. Both neomycin and bacitracin were highly effective in preventing infection with both *S. aureus* and *S. pyogenes* compared with the bland ointment vehicle. The treated wounds did not develop pus and reepithelialized within 3 to 5 days. Other investigators have also found that use of either topical neomycin-bacitracin-polymyxin ointment or bacitracin alone enhanced epidermal healing of wounds[4, 5] and significantly reduced streptococcal skin colonization and subsequent infection of small skin traumas in children.[6] In one placebo-controlled trial, the efficacy of a novel topical antimicrobial gel containing cetrimide, bacitracin, and polymyxin B was studied in the prevention of infections in minor wounds.[7] The preparation showed therapeutic action and reduced the incidence of clinical infection from 12.5 to 1.6%.

Despite these studies, the efficacy of topical antibacterials in the prevention of infections in clean wounds and wound healing remains questionable. The use of topical antibacterials for a few days in superficial wounds until the integrity of the epidermis is reestablished has been recommended, since the longer the epidermal barrier remains defective, the more likely infection is to occur. An important principle is that the agent do no harm and not be irritating, toxic, sensitizing, or lead to the development of organisms resistant to therapeutically important antimicrobial agents.

Prophylaxis of Infection in Operative Wounds

There is good evidence from both controlled and uncontrolled trials that topical antibacterials are efficacious in the prevention of postoperative wound infections; a significant decrease in wound infections has been reported in treated patients. In one study involving more than 6000 cases over a 4-year period,[8] a declining rate of infection was documented with the increased use of a neomycin-bacitracin-polymyxin spray during operations. When the neomycin-bacitracin-polymyxin spray was compared with no prophylaxis in 851 surgical wounds,[9] a significant decrease in wound infection was noted in the treatment group. Other investigators have noted similar results in prospective, randomized clinical trials,[2] indicating the importance of preoperative topical antibacterials in the prophylaxis of operative wounds. The iodophors (e.g., povidone-iodine) are currently the most commonly used topical agents for preoperative skin preparation, producing a rapid, significant reduction in skin microbial counts.[10]

Prophylaxis of Catheter-Related Infections

Many authorities have recommended the use of topical antibacterial agents for prophylaxis against bacterial colonization of central and peripheral intravascular catheter sites,[11] although the efficacy of this practice in the prevention of catheter-associated bacteremia remains unclear. In one prospective evaluation of 827 random catheter insertions employing three regimens of catheter care (neomycin-bacitracin-polymyxin at insertion and every 48 hours versus iodophor ointment at insertion and every 48 hours versus no ointment), no differences in catheter-acquired sepsis (two patients in each group) or local inflammation (38.9 versus 41.9 versus 41.7%, respectively) were noted.[12] The only differences were in semiquantitative cultures of catheter tips, with 6 positive cultures in the neomycin-bacitracin-polymyxin group, 10 in the iodophor group, and 18 in the no-treatment group. In contrast, a randomized controlled trial of the use of povidone-iodine in the prevention of infection in subclavian vein hemodialysis catheters found that povidone-iodine was associated with a significant decrease in the incidence of septicemia (5 versus 18%; $p < .02$).[13] Another study comparing skin preparation with either 2% chlorhexidine, 70% alcohol, or 10% povidone-iodine found that chlorhexidine was superior to the other two disinfectants in the reduction of both local infection and catheter-related bacteremias.[14] Finally, a newly available antiseptic solution (composed of 0.25% chlorhexidine gluconate, 0.025% benzalkonium chloride, and 4% benzyl alcohol) was more effective than 10% povidone-iodine for insertion site care of short-term central venous and arterial catheters[15]; this effect appeared related to a more efficacious prevention of gram-positive bacterial infections. Further studies are needed, however, to determine the optimal regimen for the prophylaxis of catheter-related infections.

Therapy of Pyodermas

The major pyoderma in which topical antibacterials have been utilized is impetigo. Impetigo is a superficial infection of the skin caused by group A streptococci (see Chapter 186) or *S. aureus,* or both. Bullous impetigo is usually caused by *S. aureus.* One of the goals of antimicrobial therapy in impetigo is to prevent the spread of infection to uninvolved skin.[1] Early uncontrolled and controlled trials of topical antibacterial therapy in patients with impetigo suggested the efficacy of topical antibacterials, although other studies found that systemic antimicrobial therapy was more efficacious.[16] Despite this controversy, it appears that systemic antimicrobial therapy is somewhat superior to topical therapy in the management of streptococcal pyoderma, with swifter healing and fewer failures. However, topical therapy may be used early in infection when the number of lesions is small and there is a reasonable chance that these agents will be scrupulously and skillfully applied.[16] Exclusions to the use of topical antibacterials in pyodermas include the following: bullous impetigo (because the pathogenesis of this exfoliative infection may lead to continuing infection, rapid spread, or recurrence, or all of these, unless *S. aureus* is promptly eradicated); extensive pyoderma, regardless of the clinical form or bacterial cause; and children with poststreptococcal pyodermal nephritis and their infected contacts.[17] However, systemic antimicrobial therapy for streptococcal pyoderma does not guarantee the prevention of poststreptococcal glomerulonephritis,[16] although prompt eradication of nephritogenic streptococci may lessen the risk of spread to others, with the subsequent prevention of secondary cases. A newer topical antibacterial, mupirocin, has been shown to be as efficacious as systemic antibiotics in the therapy of limited impetigo (see later).

Topical antibacterial agents may have some efficacy in the therapy of secondary pyodermas, although the available studies generally did not include control groups.[16] Despite organism eradication, the underlying process persisted. Therefore, cure, in the sense of complete healing, was not achieved. Since topical antibacterials can lower the bacterial colony counts in acute dermatitis, the use of these agents in combination with topical glucocorticoids is a logical treatment regimen.[1] There is no role for topical antibacterials in the treatment of erysipelas, cellulitis, or furuncles; erythrasma may respond.

Prophylaxis of Infection in Burn Wounds

Prevention of infection in the burned patient is extremely difficult since burn wound sites are favorable for bacterial overgrowth, the epidermal barrier is often defective for extended periods of time, and the patients are in the hospital where multiple antibiotic-resistant organisms are found.[1] Frequent débridement and the establishment of an epidermis, or a surrogate such as skin graft or skin substitute, are essential for the prevention of infection. As a result of the pathogenesis and pathophysiology of the burn wound, the delivery of systemic antimicrobial therapy to the deepest, most severely ischemic areas of the wound cannot be relied on because gradient diffusion from the wound periphery is the sole means of access.[18] The use of topical antibacterial agents for burned patients is well established. Before the development of effective topical burn wound chemotherapy, burn wound sepsis was diagnosed as the principal cause of death in 60% of burn patients who died[19]; the use of mafenide acetate has reduced to 28% the incidence of burn wound sepsis as a cause of death. After administration, high antimicrobial concentrations are found on the wound surface where the risk of bacterial contamination is the greatest. In patients with deep, extensive wounds, dense bacterial colonization, particularly by gram-positive cocci, often occurs within 24 hours; aerobic gram-negative bacilli typically appear within 3 to 7 days. If this initial bacterial colonization is not treated, deeper spread and ultimate systemic invasion of pathogenic bacteria can occur. Therefore, topical antibacterial therapy should be initiated as soon as possible to delay or prevent these processes.

There is evidence that effective topical antibacterial therapy delays colonization of the burn wound for a variable period (measured in days, not weeks); maintains the wound bacterial density at lower levels than can otherwise be achieved and for appreciable intervals (measured in weeks); and tends to result in a relatively homogeneous and less diverse wound flora than would otherwise be expected.[18] The specific antimicrobial agent chosen for topical therapy should have a broad in vitro spectrum of activity against gram-positive cocci (staphylococci, streptococci, and enterococci) and the aerobic gram-negative flora (including *Pseudomonas aeruginosa*). Ideally the agent should penetrate the eschar but may be absorbed so it must have low toxicity[20]; the agent must also remain active in the presence of serum and necrotic debris. Furthermore, with increasing use of cultured skin grafts in the therapeutic approach to the burned patient, topical antibacterials may be required to prevent microbial colonization and destruction of grafts containing cultured skin cells.[21] Successful use of topical agents prevents the bacterial conversion of superficial burns to deeper injury, results in spontaneous healing of wounds that initially appeared clinically to be full thickness, and decreases the frequency of episodes of systemic sepsis.[18] Specific topical agents for use in burned patients are discussed in Chapter 310.

Treatment of Acne Vulgaris

Topical antibacterials are helpful for inflammatory acne.[22, 23] The proliferation of *Propionibacterium acnes* is considered critical for the development of inflammatory lesions. The blocked follicles become an ideal anaerobic culture medium filled with nutrients in the form of lipid substrates; *P. acnes* metabolize the lipid, producing free fatty acids, and this may be the triggering mechanism that leads to retention hyperkeratosis and microcomedo formation. Benzoyl peroxide exerts its effects by bacteriostatic activity on the proliferation of *P. acnes*.[24] Oxygen is liberated when the drug is decomposed by cysteine in the skin, and bacterial proteins are thus oxidized. After 2 weeks of daily application, a 10% benzoyl peroxide preparation reduces concentrations of free fatty acids by about 50% and *P. acnes* by about 98%, comparable to the results obtained with the use of many antibiotics after 4 weeks of use.

Topical antibiotics are also used almost universally by dermatologists for the treatment of acne vulgaris.[22, 23, 25] These agents also exert their beneficial effects by decreasing the population of *P. acnes* in the follicle, although not as effectively or rapidly as benzoyl peroxide,[26] and also inhibit the production of proinflammatory mediators by organisms that are not killed.[22] Preparations containing clindamycin and erythromycin are most commonly used[22, 23]; topical tetracyclines have also been utilized but are less effective than either clindamycin or erythromycin. Topical azelaic acid, a dicarboxylic acid derivative that is bacteriostatic against *P. acnes*, has been shown to reduce colony counts of *P. acnes* to about the same degree as clindamycin. However, the most effective topical antibacterial regimen against *P. acnes* is probably the combination of benzoyl peroxide and erythromycin. A recent randomized 10-week trial comparing the efficacy of benzoyl peroxide 5%–erythromycin 3% gel with erythromycin 4%–zinc 1.2% solution in 72 acne vulgaris patients revealed that both inflammatory lesions and comedones showed a significantly greater percentage reduction from baseline in those patients receiving the benzoyl peroxide 5%–erythromycin 3% combination[27]; both physician and patient efficacy evaluations were also more favorable for this regimen.

Strains of *P. acnes* have emerged that are less sensitive to the antimicrobial agents used to treat acne. Several studies have been performed to assess the clinical significance of this antimicrobial resistance and to monitor the acquisition of resistant strains during therapy[28]; in these trials, topical antibacterials were used alone or in combination with either zinc or benzoyl peroxide. Generally these studies have demonstrated a marked reduction in the colony counts of *P. acnes,* although there was emergence of antimicrobial-resistant strains. Combinations of benzoyl peroxide and erythromycin have a greater in vivo activity against *P. acnes* than erythromycin alone and bring about clinical improvement in acne patients who have high numbers of erythromycin-resistant strains.[29] The significance of this phenomenon, however, requires further study.

Elimination of *Staphylococcus aureus* Nasal Carriage

Approximately 20 to 40% of healthy persons carry *S. aureus* in their anterior nares.[30] In hospitalized patients, serious infection caused by *S. aureus* may occur from autoinoculation onto susceptible sites or transfer of organisms from another patient or staff member who is a carrier.[31–33] Attempts to control these outbreaks have included methods to eradicate nasal carriage of offending staphylococci by means of systemic or topical antimicrobial agents; recolonization is frequent, however, and the development of resistance has been reported. Numerous topical antibacterial agents have been utilized in the nasal eradication of *S. aureus,* with varied degrees of success (see later).

SPECIFIC TOPICAL ANTIBACTERIALS

Numerous topical antibacterial agents are available for clinical use in various concentrations, vehicles, and mixtures (Table 33–2). The following sections review in detail the more common topical antibacterials in general use. Antimicrobial agents such as clindamycin, erythromycin, tetracycline, and gentamicin, although used as topical agents, are covered in other chapters of this book and not discussed here.

Bacitracin

Mechanism of Action. Bacitracin is a polypeptide antibiotic produced by *Bacillus subtilis.* There are three bacitracins subgrouped as A, B, and C; subgroup A is the major constituent of commercial preparations.[34] Bacitracin contains a thiazolidine ring and peptide side chains. After administration, it forms a complex with C55-phenol pyrophosphate, a component of the bacterial cell wall. This molecule acts as a carrier involved in the transfer of polysaccharides, peptidoglycans, and lipopolysaccharides to the growing cell wall. Thus, formation of the bacterial cell wall is stunted.

In Vitro Spectrum of Activity. The spectrum of activity of bacitracin is primarily against gram-positive organisms: staphylococci, streptococci, corynebacteria, and clostridia.[34] Development of resistance to bacitracin is rare, although it has been reported in *S. aureus.*

Clinical Uses. Topical bacitracin has been used for many years, although its efficacy in controlled clinical trials has never been shown. In impetigo, bacitracin ointment was shown to be 80% effective in clearing pathogenic organisms,[17] although slow or delayed healing was noted in one third of those patients cured. Bacitracin was least effective for bullous impetigo, in which four of six patients continued to develop new lesions, requiring systemic erythromycin therapy. Furthermore, in a recent trial comparing topical bacitracin to topical mupirocin or oral cephalexin for the treatment of impetigo, the treatment failed in most patients (six of nine) treated with bacitracin.[35] Bacitracin has also been evaluated in the eradication of nasal carriage of *S. aureus,* although its efficacy has never been shown.[36, 37] One study demonstrated a lack of efficacy of bacitracin in the nasal eradication of staphylococci when compared with oral rifampin.[38] For topical use, bacitracin is often formulated with neomycin or polymyxin B, or both (see Table 33–2).

Adverse Effects. Toxicity with bacitracin is minimal. Minor skin irritation may occur. Cases of anaphylaxis have been reported after the topical administration of bacitracin to open lesions[34, 39–41]; these patients had multiple previous exposures to the drug. Ready access

TABLE 33–2 Selected Topical Antibacterial Agents in Clinical Use

Topical Antibacterial (Trade Name)	Concentrations	Frequency	Indications
Azeleic acid (Azelex)	20% cream	2 times daily	Acne vulgaris
Benzoyl peroxide	2.5–10%	1–2 times daily	Acne vulgaris
Clindamycin (Cleocin)*	1%, 2%	2 times daily	Acne vulgaris; bacterial vaginosis
Erythromycin (A/T/S; Emgel; Erycette; T-Stat; Theramycin; Erygel; Erymax)	2%	2 times daily	Acne vulgaris
Erythromycin–benzoyl peroxide (Benzamycin)	3%–5%	2 times daily	Acne vulgaris
Fusidic acid (Fucidin)†	2%	3 times daily	Skin infections; eradication of nasopharyngeal carriage of *Staphylococcus aureus*
Gentamicin (Garamycin)	0.1%	3–4 times daily	Skin infections
Mafenide (Sulfamylon)	—	2 times daily	Burns
Metronidazole (MetroGel, MetroCream)	0.75%	2 times daily	Inflammatory pustules, papules, and rosacea; bacterial vaginosis
Mupirocin (Bactroban)	2% ointment	3 times daily	Skin infections; elimination of nasopharyngeal carriage of *Staph. aureus*
Neomycin-dexamethasone (NeoDecadron)	3.5 mg/g–0.1%	3–4 times daily	Corticosteroid-responsive dermatoses with secondary infection
Nitrofurazone (Furacin)	0.2%	1 time daily	Burns; skin grafting
Polymyxin B–bacitracin–neomycin (Neosporin)‡	5000 units/g–400 units/g–3.5 mg/g	1–3 times daily	Prevention of infection in minor cuts, scrapes, burns
Polymyxin B–neomycin–hydrocortisone (Cortisporin)	10,000 units/g–3.5 mg/g–0.5%	2–4 times daily	Corticosteroid-responsive dermatoses with secondary infection
Silver sulfadiazine (SSD; Silvadene)	1%	1–2 times daily	Burns
Tetracycline (Topicycline)	3%	2 times daily	Acne vulgaris

*The 2% formulation is recommended for bacterial vaginosis.
†Not licensed in the United States.
‡Maximal strength formulation contains 10,000 units/g polymyxin B, 500 units/g bacitracin, and 3.5 mg/g neomycin.

to the systemic circulation appears to be a prerequisite for the development of anaphylaxis from this externally applied agent. Rarely, an allergic contact dermatitis has been reported.[42] Since bacitracin and polymyxin B are both derived from *Bacillus* spp., cross-reactivity between the two agents may occur.[43]

Neomycin

Mechanism of Action. Neomycin is an aminoglycoside antibiotic isolated from cultures of *Streptomyces fradiae.*[34] The mechanism of action involves inhibition of protein synthesis by binding to the 30-S subunit of the bacterial ribosome, leading to misreading of the genetic code; neomycin may also inhibit the bacterial DNA polymerase.

In Vitro Spectrum of Activity. Neomycin has in vitro activity against many gram-positive and gram-negative bacteria, including *Escherichia coli, Haemophilus influenzae, Proteus* spp., *S. aureus,* and *Serratia* spp. *Pseudomonas aeruginosa* is generally resistant.[44] There is minimal in vitro activity against streptococci, although at the high concentrations achieved on the skin, *S. pyogenes* organisms are probably killed by topical neomycin preparations.[1] Resistance to neomycin has been reported in both gram-positive and gram-negative bacteria[16, 34] and can be plasmid mediated; resistance to other aminoglycosides such as kanamycin and gentamicin may be on the same plasmid.

Clinical Uses. Neomycin is widely used in combination with other antibiotics, antifungals, and corticosteroids because of its availability, relatively low cost, and perceived efficacy.[3, 16] There are few well-controlled clinical trials documenting the efficacy and safety of topical neomycin.[17] Neomycin has been shown to enhance reepithelialization in wound healing.[5] However, in view of its well-documented contact sensitivity, possible systemic toxicity, and cross-reactivity with other antibiotics, and because of the emergence of resistance, it is difficult to recommend the use of topical neomycin in the treatment of superficial skin infections.[34]

Adverse Reactions. Neomycin is not absorbed through intact skin, although application to denuded or damaged epithelium can lead to sensitization and systemic toxicity.[44] After systemic absorption, neomycin is excreted by the kidney. Patients with decreased renal function may develop ototoxicity that is irreversible and may progress after discontinuation of the drug. Allergic contact sensitivity is widely reported with a prevalence of 1 to 6% and an incidence of 3 to 6%.[15, 44, 45] The incidence of hypersensitivity, as assessed by patch testing, in 390 patients with suspected contact dermatitis to topical medications, was approximately 36%.[46] Sensitivity is most likely to occur with chronic use on inflamed skin. Sensitivity to neomycin was reported in 49% of patients with a history of allergy to any topical agent.[34] Neomycin may also cause mast cell degranulation and histamine release.

Polymyxin B

Mechanism of Action. Polymyxin B is isolated from the aerobic gram-positive rod *Bacillus polymyxa,* a soil organism.[47] The polymyxins are cationic branched cyclic decapeptides that destroy bacterial membranes with a surface detergent-like mechanism by interacting with membrane phospholipids and increasing cellular permeability.

In Vitro Spectrum of Activity. The spectrum of activity of polymyxin B is almost exclusively limited to gram-negative organisms.[47] The agent is bactericidal against gram-negative organisms such as *P. aeruginosa, Proteus mirabilis,* and *Serratia marcescens*; some *Proteus* and *Serratia* may be resistant. There is no in vitro activity against gram-positive organisms. Although *Pseudomonas* is usually sensitive, the in vitro activity of polymyxin B against *Pseudomonas* is promptly neutralized by divalent cations at concentrations in body fluids. Organisms resistant to polymyxin B have cell walls that prevent access of the drug to the bacterial cell membrane. There is no cross-resistance with other antimicrobial agents, and resistance rarely develops during therapy.

Clinical Uses. Polymyxin B is used primarily in the prevention and treatment of minor skin infections.[47] It is most often added to neomycin and bacitracin (see earlier) to broaden coverage against gram-negative organisms.

Adverse Effects. Because polymyxin B binds to cell membranes with very high affinity, there is little systemic absorption and few reactions even when applied to open wounds. Contact sensitization has been reported.[43]

Mupirocin

Structure and Mechanism of Action. Mupirocin has a unique chemical structure unlike that of any other antimicrobial agent (Fig. 33–1).[48–51] It contains a short fatty acid side chain (9-hydroxy-nonanoic acid) linked to monic acid by an ester linkage. Mupirocin is formulated in a bland water-miscible ointment base consisting of polyethylene glycol 400 and polyethylene glycol 3350. Mupirocin used to be called *pseudomonic acid* because its major metabolite is derived from submerged fermentation by *Pseudomonas fluorescens.*[52] Pseudomonic acid A represents 90 to 95% of the pseudomonic acid family and is responsible for most of the antibacterial activity; three other minor metabolites of similar chemical structure and antimicrobial spectrum have been denoted as pseudomonic acids B, C, and D.[48] Mupirocin inhibits bacterial RNA and protein synthesis by binding to bacterial isoleucyl–transfer RNA (tRNA) synthetase, which catalyzes the formation of isoleucyl-tRNA from isoleucine and tRNA.[48–52] This prevents the incorporation of isoleucine into protein chains of the bacterial cell wall, leading to the arrest of protein synthesis. Because of this unique mechanism of action, mupirocin does not crossreact with other antimicrobial agents.

In Vitro Spectrum of Activity. The antibacterial spectrum of mupirocin is shown in Table 33–3.[48, 52, 53] Mupirocin is bacteriostatic at low concentrations near the minimal inhibitory concentration (MIC) for *S. aureus,* but bactericidal at concentrations achieved by topical administration (20,000 μg/ml with the 2% formulation) after 24 to 36 hours of exposure.[48, 53, 54] It is highly active in vitro against methicillin-resistant strains of *S. aureus* (MRSA), staphylococcal strains resistant to other antibacterials (e.g., penicillin, streptomycin, neomycin, erythromycin, fusidic acid, lincomycin, chloramphenicol, and tetracycline), and streptococci that are associated with primary and secondary skin infections.[48] The exception to the antistreptococcal activity of mupirocin is the enterococcus.[53] Mupirocin is inactive in vitro against *P. aeruginosa,* anaerobes, fungi, and the Enterobacteriaceae. An important feature of mupirocin's antibacterial spectrum is its weaker in vitro activity against the normal skin flora (e.g., *Micrococcus, Corynebacterium,* and *Propionibacterium* spp.), which are part of the skin's natural defense against infection. The in vitro antibacterial activity of mupirocin is greatest at an acidic pH, which is advantageous because of the low pH of the skin; in one study, mupirocin was four- to eightfold more active in vitro at pH 6 than at pH 7.[53]

Long-term therapy with mupirocin can lead to the development of resistant staphylococci,[48, 52, 55, 56] an effect that is irreversible. Staphylococcal isolates with low- or intermediate-level resistance have MICs in the range of 8 to 32 μg/ml, whereas isolates with MICs above 256 μg/ml demonstrate high-level resistance. This resistance can be induced in *S. aureus* by subculturing the organisms onto media containing increasing concentrations of the drug.[52] Naturally occurring clones of staphylococci with low-level resistance to mupirocin have been described,[51, 55] although their clinical significance is unclear since the concentration of mupirocin in ointment exceeds 20,000 μg/ml. High-level mupirocin resistance has emerged in both MRSA and *Staphylococcus epidermidis,* associated with clinical

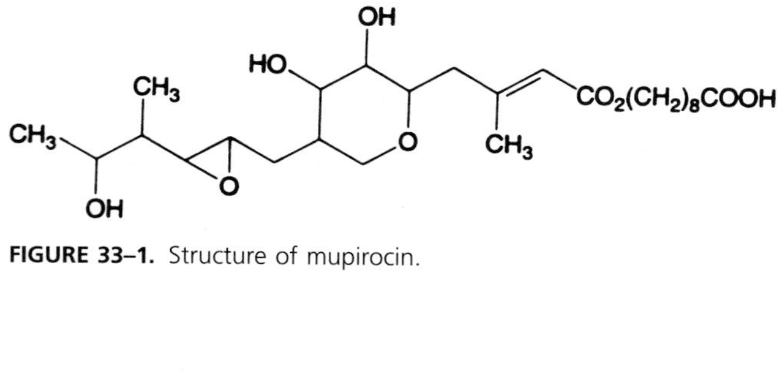

FIGURE 33–1. Structure of mupirocin.

TABLE 33–3 Antibacterial Activity of Mupirocin against Selected Bacteria

Organism and Strain	MIC (μg/ml)
Gram-positive cocci	
Streptococcus pyogenes 421	0.12
Streptococcus pneumoniae 1959	0.12
Staphylococcus aureus ATCC 25923	0.25
Staphylococcus epidermidis 54815	0.5
Streptococcus agalactiae 9579	0.5
Streptococcus sanguis	1
Peptostreptococcus anaerobius 3395	32
Enterococcus faecium 98-D	32
Enterococcus faecalis I	64
Peptococcus prevotii 372.5	>128
Micrococcus luteus ATCC 9341	>128
Gram-positive bacilli	
Bacillus subtilis ATCC 6633	0.12
Erysipelothrix rhusiopathiae	8
Listeria monocytogenes NCTC 5348	8
Clostridium difficile 12328	32
Clostridium sporogenes 532	32
Bacillus anthracis NCTC 8234	64
Corynebacterium hofmannii M8	64
Corynebacterium xerosis 9755	>128
Corynebacterium jekeium	>128
Propionibacterium acnes 10162	>128
Gram-negative cocci	
Neisseria gonorrhoeae WHO V	0.05
Neisseria meningitidis 1990	0.05
Moraxella catarrhalis 1502	0.2
Gram-negative bacilli	
Bordetella pertussis 2420	0.02
Haemophilus influenzae Q1	0.12
Pasteurella multocida 1633	0.25
Proteus vulgaris X	64
Enterobacter cloacae 10005	64
Enterobacter aerogenes T660	128
Citrobacter freundii W18	128
Escherichia coli NCTC 10418	128
Klebsiella pneumoniae A	128
Proteus mirabilis 889	128
Serratia marcescens US9	1600
Morganella morganii F	6400
Pseudomonas aeruginosa R3	6400
Bacteroides fragilis BC4	>6400

Abbreviation: MIC, Minimal inhibitory concentration.

Data from Pappa KA. The clinical development of mupirocin. J Am Acad Dermatol. 1990; 22:873–879; Leyden JJ. Mupirocin: A new topical antibiotic. Semin Dermatol. 1987;6:48–54; and Sutherland R, Boon RJ, Griffin KE, et al. Antibacterial activity of mupirocin (pseudomonic acid), a new antibiotic for topical use. Antimicrob Agents Chemother. 1985;27:495–498.

treatment failure.[56, 57] In one study,[56] resistance emerged in three patients treated with mupirocin for months and, in addition, from patients never treated with mupirocin, suggesting the possibility of cross-infection. In another study of 144 patients with epidermolysis bullosa, many of whom received continuous application of mupirocin for as long as 4 consecutive years, five isolates of *S. aureus* were resistant to mupirocin[48]; four of the five patients with resistant isolates had a less favorable response to mupirocin and required systemic antistaphylococcal therapy. Most mupirocin-resistant staphylococcal isolates have been found in patients with chronic skin infections, many of whom had been treated with prolonged courses of mupirocin.[51]

Several mechanisms have been advanced to explain mupirocin resistance in staphylococci. Low-level resistance is likely mediated by altered access to binding sites on isoleucyl-tRNA synthetase, whereas high-level resistance appears to be mediated by a transferable plasmid on the *mupA* gene that codes for a modified isoleucyl-tRNA synthetase.[51, 58] It has been suggested that high-level resistance may have evolved by the conjugate transfer of plasmids from enterococci,[59–61] which are inherently resistant to mupirocin; conjugate transfer of high-level mupirocin resistance has also been observed among coagulase-negative staphylococci.[62] A recent study has demonstrated that two different isoleucyl-tRNA synthetase enzymes are present in highly mupirocin-resistant *S. aureus* isolates (MIC ≥ 512 μg/ml), whereas only a chromosomally encoded isoleucyl-tRNA synthetase was detected in strains expressing intermediate levels of resistance (MIC between 8 and 256 μg/ml).[63]

Pharmacokinetics. After systemic administration, mupirocin is immediately metabolized to monic acid, which is bacteriologically inactive and rapidly eliminated (plasma half-life of <30 minutes).[50] Mupirocin is not appreciably absorbed after topical administration to intact skin. In one study, a mean of 0.24% of applied radiolabeled ointment was absorbed through intact skin after 24 hours of occlusion.[64] Greater penetration of mupirocin is expected in damaged or diseased skin. Any drug that is absorbed, however, is converted to monic acid, formed by deesterification of mupirocin at the ester linkage between the side chain and the nucleus, and rapidly eliminated in the urine.[34] Skin can also metabolize mupirocin to its inactive metabolite, but at a rate below 3%. Therefore, because only small amounts of mupirocin penetrate skin and equally small amounts are degraded, most of the drug is available to act at skin level. Because mupirocin is highly protein bound (approximately 95%), its activity decreases in the presence of serum.[48]

Clinical Uses. Mupirocin is used primarily in skin infections such as impetigo and folliculitis, which are usually caused by *S. aureus* and *S. pyogenes.* In trials of mupirocin alone in the therapy of impetigo (772 evaluable patients),[65–71] clinical cure rates ranged from 81 to 100% and bacterial elimination rates from 67 to 100%. Several trials have shown mupirocin to be more effective in the treatment of impetigo than its polyethylene glycol vehicle, which also has antibacterial activity. Clinical cure and bacterial elimination rates have ranged from 85 to 100% and 80 to 95%, respectively, for mupirocin versus 12 to 84% and 12 to 63%, respectively, for the vehicle.[52, 65, 72–74] Since impetigo is a self-limiting condition, bacteriologic results are a more appropriate assessment of efficacy since elimination of pathogens can be used to ascertain infection resolution. In eight comparative trials of mupirocin versus several other topical antibacterials (neomycin, fusidic acid, chlortetracycline, polymyxin B–bacitracin–neomycin),[65, 75–78] six found mupirocin to be the more effective agent. Multiple studies have also compared topical mupirocin to systemic antibiotics (erythromycin, cloxacillin, dicloxacillin, flucloxacillin, ampicillin, cephalexin) in the therapy of impetigo, in which topical mupirocin was as, or more, effective than the oral agent.[35, 65, 79–86] In many of these studies, however, the entry criteria excluded patients who, in the judgment of the investigator, had too many lesions to allow reliable compliance with topical therapy.[87] No studies have shown that topical therapy is as effective as systemic antimicrobial therapy for the treatment of widespread, extensive lesions.

Mupirocin is effective for the treatment of secondarily infected eczema, burns, lacerations, and leg ulcers. In one study in which 33 centers contributed a total of 1030 cases,[52] mupirocin ointment produced significantly better bacteriologic and clinical responses than its vehicle in the treatment of secondary skin infections. Of 851 evaluable patients with 1131 pathogens, mupirocin eliminated 87% (505/583) of pathogens versus only 53% (288/548) with the vehicle. In a double-blind, vehicle-controlled study, mupirocin successfully eradicated 85% of *S. aureus* in 33 patients compared with a 6% eradication rate in the vehicle-treated group[88]; for all pathogens, the success rate of mupirocin versus the vehicle was 69% versus 14%, respectively. Comparative trials have also demonstrated the efficacy of mupirocin compared with other topical antibacterials and systemic antimicrobial agents in the treatment of secondary skin infections.[77, 79, 80, 86]

Mupirocin can also eliminate nasal carriage of *S. aureus.* In four blinded, placebo-controlled trials conducted in health care workers with *S. aureus* nasal carriage,[89–92] virtually all persons treated with mupirocin were initially cleared of the carrier state compared with a zero to 18% rate of clearance after treatment with placebo; in one of the studies, a corresponding effect on the eradication of hand carriage at 72 hours of therapy was also found.[90] However, relapse after therapy occurred in 19 to 59% of persons after 4 to 12 weeks of evaluation. Relapses could have resulted from reinoculation of the nares with staphylococci from an untreated site (e.g., skin, perineum, rectum) or by reinfection with new staphylococcal strains after the completion of therapy. Mupirocin has been evaluated in acute carrier outbreaks of epidemic MRSA colonization.[93–98] Mupirocin was effective in clearing MRSA from nearly all patients and staff, although these studies were uncontrolled and it is difficult to know whether the development of negative cultures in these patients can be attributed to therapy with mupirocin or to a transient carrier state. Recently, mupirocin has been evaluated in the control of MRSA in facilities for rehabilitation and long-term care.[99, 100] Mupirocin was effective in the elimination of chronic nasal MRSA colonization, although in one study transient recolonization occurred in about 44% of patients.[100] In another study of 65 patients colonized with MRSA at a Veterans Affairs long-term care facility, mupirocin (applied to the nares for the first 7 months and to the nares and wounds for the second 5 months) rapidly eliminated MRSA at treated sites in most patients by the end of the first week.[101] Despite weekly maintenance mupirocin therapy, 40% of patients had recurrence of MRSA colonization. In contrast, a 5-day treatment course of mupirocin of all infants, colonized and noncolonized, and parents of and personnel working with colonized infants in a neonatal intensive care unit, failed to eradicate the organism.[102] Nasal mupirocin was also studied in immunocompetent staphylococcal carriers who experienced recurrent skin infections.[103] Monthly application reduced the incidence of nasal colonization, which, in turn, lowered the risk of skin infection, although the small size of the study precluded the authors from making definitive recommendations for the management of recurrent furunculosis and folliculitis in staphylococcal carriers. Well-controlled clinical trials are needed to clarify these issues.

The development of mupirocin resistance in MRSA has become a problem after widespread use of nasal mupirocin. In one study at a Veterans Affairs long-term care facility where patients were treated with nasal mupirocin for 1 year, mupirocin-resistant MRSA organisms were identified in 11% of patients.[101] In another study, resistance among MRSA after the use of nasal mupirocin increased from 2.7 to 65% from 1990 to 1993[104]; a resistance rate of 63% was also observed in a study of MRSA strains in Rio de Janeiro where there was extensive use of topical mupirocin.[105] In contrast, in another study of blanket use of intranasal mupirocin for outbreak control and long-term prophylaxis of endemic MRSA colonization in an open ward, no mupirocin resistance was observed.[106] However, despite conflicting results from clinical trials, prolonged use of nasal mupirocin in controlled outbreaks of MRSA colonization should be discouraged; it should be used primarily in outbreak situations and not in facilities with endemic MRSA colonization.[51, 107, 108]

Adverse Effects. Mupirocin is not associated with substantial toxicity in humans because of its very low affinity for mammalian isoleucyl-tRNA synthetase. The propylene glycol base may irritate mucous membranes and eroded skin. There is minimal potential for inducing allergic contact dermatitis; only two cases have been reported.[109] The drug is not phototoxic. Local effects such as itching, stinging, or rash have been reported when mupirocin is used on broken skin or mucous membranes. No photosensitivity reactions have occurred. In experimental rat and rabbit models, mupirocin has been shown to be without teratogenic effects, embryotoxicity, or effects on fertility and reproduction in doses up to 160 mg/kg/day.[52] Prolonged use may lead to overgrowth of nonsusceptible organisms such as fungi.

Fusidic Acid

Mechanism of Action. Fusidic acid is isolated from culture media of the fungus *Fusidium coccineum.*[34] Chemically it is a carboxylic acid belonging to the group of tetracycline triterpenes. Fusidic acid is lipophilic. It penetrates intact epidermis at approximately the same rate as glucocorticoids and penetrates both intact and damaged skin. Fusidic acid inhibits bacterial protein synthesis primarily by interfering with elongation factor G (translocase) (see Chapter 22).[110]

In Vitro Spectrum of Activity. Fusidic acid has a narrow antibacterial spectrum, mainly against gram-positive bacteria; there is an exceptionally high in vitro activity against *S. aureus* (MIC range of 0.04 to 0.16 μg/ml). There is also in vitro activity against corynebacteria and clostridia. Streptococci are 100 times less sensitive (MIC range of 4.2 to 16 μg/ml) to fusidic acid when compared with staphylococci, but at concentrations given topically it is efficacious against both organisms. Reports from Europe have documented staphylococcal resistance to fusidic acid,[111, 112] although general levels of resistance have remained low (about 1 to 2%).[113] In one report of 8176 *S. aureus* strains isolated from cases of bacteremia during the years 1963 to 1987 in Denmark, 1% or less of strains were resistant to fusidic acid (MIC ≥2 μg/ml).[114] After topical use of fusidic acid, a rate of staphylococcal resistance of 43% has been reported, although other authors have not observed the emergence of resistance.[113] In vitro evidence suggests that resistance to *S. aureus* is less likely to occur after exposure to high concentrations of fusidic acid, reflecting the situation with topical use.

Clinical Uses. Fusidic acid has the remarkable ability to penetrate both intact and damaged skin, making it useful for treating deep infections such as paronychia or boils.[34] It also penetrates crust and cellular debris seen in impetigo and pyoderma. In comparative trials of fusidic acid for the therapy of primary and secondary skin infections, fusidic acid has been found to be equivalent or inferior to mupirocin.[65] In one study, the combination of topical fusidic acid plus oral co-trimoxazole was found to be as efficacious as topical mupirocin in the eradication of nasal carriage of MRSA.[115] The drug is unavailable in the United States but has been used in Europe and Canada.

Adverse Effects. Because the structure of fusidic acid differs markedly from that of other antibiotics, it is unlikely to produce cross-sensitivity. There are a few reports of contact sensitivity. Although the ring structure of fusidic acid is remarkably similar to that of the glucocorticoids, there is no evidence of suppressive activity on the pituitary axis.

REFERENCES

1. Feingold DS. Antibacterial agents. In: Fitzpatrick TB, Eisen AZ, Wolff K, et al., eds. Dermatology in General Medicine. 3rd ed. New York: McGraw-Hill; 1987;2550–2552.
2. Kaye ET, Kaye KM. Topical antibacterial agents. Infect Dis Clin North Am. 1995;9:547–559.
3. Leyden JJ, Sulzberger MB. Topical antibiotics and minor skin trauma. Am Fam Physician. 1981;23:121–125.
4. Geronemus RG, Mertz PM, Eaglstein WH. Wound healing—The effects of topical antimicrobial agents. Arch Dermatol. 1979;115:1311–1314.
5. Eaglstein WH, Mertz P, Alvarez OM. Effect of topically applied agents on healing wounds. Clin Dermatol. 1984;2:112–115.
6. Maddox JS, Ware JC, Dillon HC Jr. The natural history of streptococcal skin infection. Prevention with topical antibiotics. J Am Acad Dermatol. 1985;13:207–212.
7. Langford JH, Artemi P, Benrimoj SI. Topical antimicrobial prophylaxis in minor wounds. Ann Pharmacother. 1997;31:559–563.
8. Forbes GB. Staphylococcal infection of operation wounds with special reference to topical antibiotic prophylaxis. Lancet. 1961;2:505–507.
9. Fielding G, Rao A, Davis NC, et al. Prophylactic topical use of antibiotics in surgical wounds: A controlled clinical trial using "polybactrin." Med J Aust. 1965;2:159–161.
10. Larson E. Guideline for use of topical antimicrobial agents. Am J Hosp Infect. 1988;16:253–266.
11. Pearson ML, the Hospital Infection Control Practices Advisory Committee. Guideline for prevention of intravascular-device-related infections. Infect Control Hosp Epidemiol. 1996;17:438–473.
12. Maki DG, Band JD. A comparative study of polyantibiotic and iodophor ointments in prevention of vascular catheter-related infection. Am J Med. 1981;70:739–744.
13. Levin A, Mason AJ, Jindal KK, et al. Prevention of hemodialysis subclavian vein catheter infections by topical povidone-iodine. Kidney Int. 1991;40:934–938.
14. Maki DG, Ringer M, Alvarado CJ. Prospective randomised trial of povidone-iodine, alcohol, and chlorhexidine for prevention of infection associated with central venous and arterial catheters. Lancet. 1991;338:339–343.
15. Mimoz O, Pieroni L, Lawrence C, et al. Prospective, randomized trial of two antiseptic solutions for prevention of central venous or arterial catheter colonization and infection in intensive care unit patients. Crit Care Med. 1996;24:1818–1823.
16. Leyden JJ, Kligman AM. Rationale for topical antibiotics. Cutis. 1978;22:515–528.
17. Dillon HC Jr. Topical and systemic therapy for pyodermas. Int J Dermatol. 1980;19:443–451.
18. Monafo WW, Freedman B. Topical therapy for burns. Surg Clin North Am. 1987;67:133–145.
19. Pruitt BA Jr, McManus AT, Kim SH, Goodwin CW. Burn wound infections: Current status. World J Surg. 1998;22:135–145.
20. Andreassi L, Flori L. Pharmacologic treatment of burns. Clin Dermatol. 1992;9:453–458.
21. Boyce ST, Warden GD, Holder IA. Noncytotoxic combinations of topical antimicrobial agents for use with cultured skin substitutes. Antimicrob Agents Chemother. 1995;39:1324–1328.
22. Leyden JJ. Therapy for acne vulgaris. N Engl J Med. 1997;336:1156–1162.
23. Weiss JS. Current options for the topical treatment of acne vulgaris. Pediatr Dermatol. 1997;14:480–488.
24. Shalita AR, Leyden JE Jr, Pochi PE, et al. Acne vulgaris. J Am Acad Dermatol. 1987;16:410–412.
25. Schachner L, Pestana A, Kittles C. A clinical trial comparing the safety and efficacy of a topical erythromycin-zinc formulation with a topical clindamycin formulation. J Am Acad Dermatol. 1990;22:489–495.
26. Swinyer LJ, Baker MD, Swinyer TA, et al. A comparative study of benzoyl peroxide and clindamycin phosphate for treating acne vulgaris. Br J Dermatol. 1988;119:615–622.
27. Chu A, Huber FJ, Plott RT. The comparative efficacy of benzoyl peroxide 5%/erythromycin 3% gel and erythromycin 4%/zinc 1.2% solution in the treatment of acne vulgaris. Br J Dermatol. 1997;136:235–238.
28. Thiboutot DM. Acne. An overview of clinical research findings. Dermatol Clin. 1997;15:97–109.
29. Eady EA, Bojar RA, Jones CE, et al. The effects of acne treatment with a combination of benzoyl peroxide and erythromycin on skin carriage of erythromycin-resistant propionibacteria. Br J Dermatol. 1996;134:107–113.
30. Williams RE. Healthy carriage of *Staphylococcus aureus*: Its prevalence and importance. Bacteriol Rev. 1963;27:56–71.
31. Boyce JC. Methicillin-resistant *Staphylococcus aureus*. Infect Dis Clin North Am. 1989;3:901–913.
32. Duckworth GJ, Lothian JL, Williams JD. Methicillin-resistant *Staphylococcus aureus*: Report of an outbreak in a London teaching hospital. J Hosp Infect. 1988;11:1–15.
33. Thompson RL, Cabezudo I, Wenzel RP. Epidemiology of nosocomial infection caused by methicillin-resistant *Staphylococcus aureus*. Ann Intern Med. 1982;97:309–317.
34. Winkelman W, Gratton D. Topical antibacterials. Clin Dermatol. 1989;7:156–162.
35. Bass JW, Chan DS, Creamer KM, et al. Comparison of oral cephalexin, topical mupirocin and topical bacitracin for treatment of impetigo. Pediatr Infect Dis J. 1997;16:708–710.
36. Yu VL, Goetz A, Wagener M, et al. *Staphylococcus aureus* nasal carriage and infection in patients on hemodialysis. Efficacy of antibiotic prophylaxis. N Engl J Med. 1986;315:91–96.
37. Bryan CS, Wilson RS, Meade P, et al. Topical antibiotic ointments for staphylococcal nasal carriers: Survey of current practices and comparison of bacitracin and vancomycin ointments. Infect Cont. 1980;1:153–156.
38. McAnally TP, Lewis MR, Brown DR. Effect of rifampin and bacitracin on nasal carriers of *Staphylococcus aureus*. Antimicrob Agents Chemother. 1984;25:422–426.
39. Schecter JF, Wilkinson RD, Del Carpio J. Anaphylaxis following the use of bacitracin ointment. Arch Dermatol. 1984;120:909–911.
40. Dyck ED, Vadas P. Anaphylaxis to topical bacitracin. Allergy. 1997;52:870–871.
41. Lin FL, Woodmansee D, Patterson R. Near-fatal anaphylaxis to topical bacitracin ointment. J Allergy Clin Immunol. 1998;101:136–137.
42. Binnick AN, Clendenning WE. Bacitracin contact dermatitis. Contact Dermatol. 1978;4:180–181.
43. Fisher AA. Adverse reactions to bacitracin, polymyxin, and gentamicin sulfate. Cutis. 1983;32:510–512.
44. MacDonald RH, Beck M. Neomycin: A review with particular reference to dermatological usage. Clin Exp Dermatol. 1983;8:249–258.
45. Gette MT, Marks JG Jr, Maloney ME. Frequency of postoperative allergic contact dermatitis to topical antibiotics. Arch Dermatol. 1992;128:365–367.
46. Bajaj AK, Gupta SC. Contact hypersensitivity to topical antibacterial agents. Int J Dermatol. 1986;25:103–105.
47. Hoeprich PD. The polymyxins. Med Clin North Am. 1970;54:1251–1265.
48. Pappa KA. The clinical development of mupirocin. J Am Acad Dermatol. 1990;22:873–879.
49. Parenti MA, Hatfield SM, Leyden JJ. Mupirocin: A topical antibiotic with a unique structure and mechanism of action. Clin Pharmacol. 1987;6:761–770.
50. Casewell MW, Hill RLR. Mupirocin ("pseudomonic acid")—A promising new topical antimicrobial agent. J Antimicrob Chemother. 1987;19:1–5.
51. Bradley SF. Effectiveness of mupirocin in the control of methicillin-resistant *Staphylococcus aureus*. Infect Med. 1993;10:23–31.
52. Leyden JJ. Mupirocin: A new topical antibiotic. Semin Dermatol. 1987;6:48–54.
53. Sutherland R, Boon RJ, Griffin KE, et al. Antibacterial activity of mupirocin (pseudomonic acid), a new antibiotic for topical use. Antimicrob Agents Chemother. 1985;27:495–498.
54. Casewell MW, Hill RLR. In vitro activity of mupirocin against clinical isolates of *Staphylococcus aureus*. J Antimicrob Chemother. 1985;15:523–531.
55. Eltringham I. Mupirocin resistance and methicillin-resistant *Staphylococcus aureus* (MRSA). J Hosp Infect. 1997;35:1–8.

56. Rahman M, Noble WC, Cookson B. Mupirocin-resistant *Staphylococcus aureus*. Lancet. 1987;2:387.
57. Smith GE, Kennedy CTC. *Staphylococcus aureus* resistant to mupirocin. J Antimicrob Chemother. 1988;21:141–142.
58. Capobianco JO, Doran CC, Goldman RC. Mechanism of mupirocin transport into sensitive and resistant bacteria. Antimicrob Agents Chemother. 1989;33:156–163.
59. Noble WC, Rahman M, Cookson B, et al. Transferable mupirocin-resistance. J Antimicrob Chemother. 1988;22:771–772.
60. Rahman M, Noble WC, Cookson B. Transmissible mupirocin resistance in *Staphylococcus aureus*. Epidemiol Infect. 1989;102:261–270.
61. Cookson BD. Mupirocin resistance in staphylococci. J Antimicrob Chemother. 1990;25:497–503.
62. Udo EE, Jacob LE, Mokadas EM. Conjugate transfer of high-level mupirocin resistance from *Staphylococcus haemolyticus* to other staphylococci. Antimicrob Agents Chemother. 1997;41:693–695.
63. Gilbart J, Perry CR, Slocombe B. High-level resistance in *Staphylococcus aureus*: Evidence for two distinct isoleucyl-tRNA synthetases. Antimicrob Agents Chemother. 1993;37:32–38.
64. Ward A, Campoli-Richards DM. Mupirocin: A review of its antibacterial activity, pharmacokinetic properties and therapeutic use. Drugs. 1986;32:425–444.
65. Booth JH, Benrimoj SI. Mupirocin in the treatment of impetigo. Int J Dermatol. 1992;31:1–9.
66. Wuite J, Davies BI, Go M, et al. Pseudomonic acid: A new topical antimicrobial agent. Lancet. 1983;2:394.
67. Wuite J, Davies BI, Go MJ, et al. Pseudomonic acid, a new antibiotic for topical therapy. J Am Acad Dermatol. 1985;12:1026–1031.
68. Buchvald J. An evaluation of topical mupirocin in moderately severe primary and secondary skin infections. J Int Med Res. 1988;16:66–70.
69. Phillips LM, Yogev R, Esterly NB. The efficacy of mupirocin (pseudomonic acid) in the treatment of pyoderma in children. Pediatr Emerg Care. 1985;1:180–183.
70. Bork K, Brauers J, Kresken M. Efficacy and safety of 2% mupirocin ointment in the treatment of primary and secondary skin infections—An open multicentre trial. Br J Clin Pract. 1989;43:284–288.
71. De la Brassinne M, De Bersaques J, Vossaert K, et al. Efficacy of mupirocin 2% ointment in skin infection: Belgian prospective open multicentre study. Dermatologica. 1988;177:397–400.
72. Eells LD, Mertz PM, Piovanetti Y, et al. Topical antibiotic treatment of impetigo with mupirocin. Arch Dermatol. 1986;122:1273–1276.
73. Colin M, Avon P. Comparative double-blind evaluation of a new topical antibacterial agent, mupirocin, compared with placebo in the treatment of skin and soft tissue infections. Pharmatherapeutica. 1988;5:198–203.
74. Orecchio RM, Mischler TW. A double-blind multiclinic comparative trial of mupirocin topical and its vehicle in the treatment of bacterial skin infections. Curr Ther Res. 1986;39:82–86.
75. Wilkinson RD, Carey WD. Topical mupirocin versus topical neosporin in the treatment of cutaneous infections. Int J Dermatol. 1988;27:514–515.
76. White DG, Collins PO, Rowsell RB. Topical antibiotics in the treatment of superficial skin infections in general practice: A comparison of mupirocin with sodium fusidate. J Infect. 1989;18:221–229.
77. Gilbert M. Topical 2% mupirocin versus 2% fusidic acid ointment in the treatment of primary and secondary skin infections. J Am Acad Dermatol. 1989;20:1083–1087.
78. Morley PA, Munot LD. A comparison of sodium fusidate ointment and mupirocin ointment in superficial skin sepsis. Curr Med Res Opin. 1988;11:142–148.
79. Dux PH, Fields L, Pollock D. 2% topical mupirocin versus systemic erythromycin and cloxacillin in primary and secondary skin infections. Curr Ther Res. 1986;40:933–940.
80. Gratton D. Topical mupirocin versus oral erythromycin in the treatment of primary and secondary skin infections. Int J Dermatol. 1987;26:472–473.
81. Goldfarb J, Crenshaw D, O'Horo J, et al. Randomized clinical trial of topical mupirocin versus oral erythromycin for impetigo. Antimicrob Agents Chemother. 1988;32:1780–1783.
82. Barton LL, Friedman AD, Sharkey AM, et al. Impetigo contagiosa. III. Comparative efficacy of oral erythromycin and topical mupirocin. Pediatr Dermatol. 1989;6:134–138.
83. McLinn S. Topical mupirocin vs. systemic erythromycin treatment for pyoderma. Pediatr Infect Dis J. 1988;7:785–790.
84. Mertz PM, Marshall DA, Eaglstein WH, et al. Topical mupirocin treatment of impetigo is equal to oral erythromycin therapy. Arch Dermatol. 1989;125:1069–1073.
85. Arrendondo JL. Efficacy and tolerance of topical mupirocin compared with oral dicloxacillin in the treatment of primary skin infections. Curr Ther Res. 1987;41:121–127.
86. Welsh O, Saenz C. Topical mupirocin compared with oral ampicillin in the treatment of primary and secondary skin infections. Curr Ther Res. 1987;41:114–120.
87. Leyden JJ. Review of mupirocin ointment in the treatment of impetigo. Clin Pediatr. 1992;31:549–553.
88. Breneman DL. Use of mupirocin ointment in the treatment of secondarily infected dermatoses. J Am Acad Dermatol. 1990;22:886–892.
89. Casewell MW, Hill RLR. Elimination of nasal carriage of *Staphylococcus aureus* with mupirocin ("pseudomonic acid")—A controlled study. J Antimicrob Chemother. 1986;17:365–372.
90. Reagan DR, Doebbeling BN, Pfaller MA, et al. Elimination of coincident *Staphylococcus aureus* nasal and hand carriage with intranasal application of mupirocin calcium ointment. Ann Intern Med. 1991;114:101–106.
91. Scully BE, Briones F, Gu JW, et al. Mupirocin treatment of nasal staphylococcal colonization. Arch Intern Med. 1992;152:353–356.
92. Fernandez C, Gaspar C, Torrellas A, et al. A double-blind, placebo-controlled clinical trial to evaluate the safety and efficacy of mupirocin calcium ointment for eliminating nasal carriage of *Staphylococcus aureus* among hospital personnel. J Antimicrob Chemother. 1995;35:399–408.
93. Dacre JE, Emmerson AM, Jenner EA. Nasal carriage of gentamicin and methicillin-resistant *Staphylococcus aureus* treated with topical pseudomonic acid. Lancet. 1983;2:1036.
94. Davies EA, Emmerson AM, Hogg GM, et al. An outbreak of infection with methicillin-resistant *Staphylococcus aureus* in a special care baby unit: Value of topical mupirocin and of traditional methods of infection control. J Hosp Infect. 1987;1:120–128.
95. Dacre J, Emmerson AM, Jenner EA. Gentamicin-methicillin–resistant *Staphylococcus aureus*: Epidemiology and containment of an outbreak. J Hosp Infect. 1986;7:130–136.
96. Hill RLR, Duckworth GJ, Casewell MW. Elimination of nasal carriage of methicillin-resistant *Staphylococcus aureus* with mupirocin during a hospital outbreak. J Antimicrob Chemother. 1988;22:377–384.
97. Vandenbroucke-Grauls CM, Frenay HME, van Klingeren B, et al. Control of epidemic methicillin-resistant *Staphylococcus aureus* in a Dutch university hospital. Eur J Clin Microbiol Infect Dis. 1991;10:6–11.
98. Barrett SP. The value of nasal mupirocin in containing an outbreak of methicillin-resistant *Staphylococcus aureus* in an orthopedic ward. J Hosp Infect. 1990;15:137–142.
99. Dariouche R, Wright C, Hamill R, et al. Eradication of colonization by methicillin-resistant *Staphylococcus aureus* by using oral minocycline-rifampin and topical mupirocin. Antimicrob Agents Chemother. 1991;35:1612–1615.
100. Cederna JE, Terpenning MS, Ensberg M, et al. *Staphylococcus aureus* nasal colonization in a nursing home: Eradication with mupirocin. Infect Control Hosp Epidemiol. 1990;11:13–16.
101. Kauffman CA, Terpenning MS, He X, et al. Attempts to eradicate methicillin-resistant *Staphylococcus aureus* from a long-term-care facility with use of mupirocin ointment. Am J Med. 1993;94:371–378.
102. Back NA, Linnemann CC Jr, Staneck JL, et al. Control of methicillin-resistant *Staphylococcus aureus* in a neonatal intensive-care unit: Use of intensive microbiologic surveillance and mupirocin. Infect Control Hosp Epidemiol. 1996;17:227–231.
103. Raz R, Miron D, Colodner R, et al. A 1-year trial of nasal mupirocin in the prevention of recurrent staphylococcal nasal colonization and skin infection. Arch Intern Med. 1996;156:1109–1112.
104. Miller MA, Dascal A, Portnoy J, et al. Development of mupirocin resistance among methicillin-resistant *Staphylococcus aureus* after widespread use of nasal mupirocin ointment. Infect Control Hosp Epidemiol. 1996;17:811–813.
105. Dos Santos KRN, de Souza L, Filho PPG. Emergence of high-level mupirocin resistance in methicillin-resistant *Staphylococcus aureus* isolated from Brazilian university hospitals. Infect Control Hosp Epidemiol. 1996;17:813–816.
106. Mayall B, Martin R, Keenan AM, et al. Blanket use of intranasal mupirocin for outbreak control and long-term prophylaxis of endemic methicillin-resistant *Staphylococcus aureus* in an open ward. J Hosp Infect. 1996;32:257–266.
107. Neu HC. The use of mupirocin in controlling methicillin-resistant *Staphylococcus aureus*. Infect Control Hosp Epidemiol. 1990;11:11–12.
108. Muder RR. Mupirocin and MRSA: Current status. Infect Med. 1993;10:21–22.
109. Zappi E, Brancaccio RR. Allergic contact dermatitis from mupirocin ointment. J Am Acad Dermatol. 1997;36:266.
110. Verbist L. The antimicrobial activity of fusidic acid. J Antimicrob Chemother. 1990;25:1–5.
111. Anderson JD. Fusidic acid: New opportunities with an old antibiotic. Can Med Assoc J. 1980;122:765–769.
112. Ayliffe AJ, Green W, Livingston R, et al. Antibiotic-resistant *Staphylococcus aureus* in dermatology and burn wards. J Clin Pathol. 1977;30:40–44.
113. Shanson DC. Clinical relevance of resistance to fusidic acid in *Staphylococcus aureus*. J Antimicrob Chemother. 1990;25:15–21.
114. Faber M, Rosdahl VT. Susceptibility to fusidic acid among Danish *Staphylococcus aureus* strains and fusidic acid consumption. J Antimicrob Chemother. 1990;25:7–14.
115. Parras F, del Carmen Guerrero M, Bouza E, et al. Comparative study of mupirocin and oral co-trimoxazole plus topical fusidic acid in eradication of nasal carriage of methicillin-resistant *Staphylococcus aureus*. Antimicrob Agents Chemother. 1995;39:175–179.

Chapter 34

Antimycobacterial Agents

RICHARD J. WALLACE, JR.

Drugs for mycobacterial infections are discussed in three groups: those primarily for the treatment of infections caused by *Mycobacterium tuberculosis,* drugs for nontuberculous *(atypical)* mycobacterial infections, and agents principally for the treatment of leprosy.

Approaches to antituberculous chemotherapy have been affected by the recent spread of multidrug-resistant *M. tuberculosis* (MDR-TB), defined as resistance to at least isoniazid (INH) and rifampin,[1–4] and by the special impact on *M. tuberculosis* of those infected with the human immunodeficiency virus (HIV).[5, 6]

MDR-TB strains having various combinations of resistance to INH, rifampin, streptomycin, or ethambutol have necessitated the use of drugs that were considered second-line agents, as well as drugs that must be administered by injection.[2] The list of agents active against MDR-TB is quite limited, emphasizing both the need for universal supervised therapy[7] and the need for new antituberculous agents.[8]

MDR-TB infections are of increased concern in persons immunologically disabled by HIV with or without acquired immunodeficiency syndrome (AIDS) because the host contribution to controlling the infection is severely diminished. HIV-infected individuals have a number of other special problems. They are especially prone to adverse drug reactions.[9] The susceptibility of protease inhibitors to hepatic metabolism induced by rifampin has introduced the need for finding new treatment alternatives that exclude rifampin.[10] In addition, malabsorption of antituberculous drugs can occur in AIDS patients.[11]

The advent of AIDS has also greatly increased the prevalence and severity of *Mycobacterium avium-intracellulare* and other nontuberculous mycobacterial infections, especially in their disseminated forms. Fortunately, the new macrolide-azalide group, rifabutin, and the fluorinated quinolones appear to be active against many of these mycobacteria, even in patients with markedly impaired cell-mediated immune defenses. The effects of HIV and AIDS on leprosy and its chemotherapy do not appear to be as great as expected.

Traditionally, antimicrobials for tuberculosis have been classified as *first-line* drugs, having superior efficacy with acceptable toxicity, and *second-line* drugs, having either less efficacy, greater toxicity, or both. Several excellent reviews of antimycobacterial agents and therapy are available,[12–17] including guidelines for therapy of MDR-TB.[17]

Antituberculous drugs differ in their mechanism of bactericidal action and in their delivery to tuberculous lesions.[12] Four first-line agents—INH, rifampin, streptomycin, and ethambutol—are active against the large populations of tubercle bacilli in cavities. Streptomycin, other aminoglycosides, and capreomycin penetrate cells poorly and are inactive at acidic pH. Pyrazinamide (PZA), inactive at the neutral or slightly alkaline pH that may occur extracellularly, is active only in acidic environments. Slowly replicating organisms in necrotic foci are killed by rifampin and somewhat less readily by INH.

First-line antituberculous agents, except ethambutol, are bactericidal. The bactericidal activities of both INH and rifampin against tubercle bacilli in cavitary, intracellular, or necrotic foci provide the basis for the efficacy of short-course INH-rifampin regimens. A combination of three bactericidal agents active against intracellular organisms—INH, rifampin, and PZA—is fundamental for the standard 6-month regimen currently recommended for drug-susceptible disease in the United States. A residual population consisting of virtually nonreplicating dormant tubercle bacilli within necrotic foci is especially difficult to eradicate, perhaps explaining the minimum of approximately 4 months of therapy needed even in persons with competent immune defenses.

FIRST-LINE ANTITUBERCULOUS DRUGS

Isoniazid

Derivation and Structure. Isoniazid, isonicotinic acid hydrazide (INH), a synthetic agent, was introduced in 1952.

Mechanism of Action. Isoniazid is bactericidal against actively growing *M. tuberculosis* and bacteriostatic against nonreplicating organisms. It acts by inhibition of synthetic pathways of mycolic acid, an important constituent of mycobacterial cell walls. It also likely inhibits the catalase-peroxidase enzyme.

Antimicrobial Activity and Resistance. Against *M. tuberculosis,* 0.025 to 0.05 μg/ml of INH is inhibitory, and higher concentrations are bactericidal against replicating organisms. When INH is administered alone, resistance tends to emerge. Initially susceptible isolates become resistant in over 70% of cases treated with INH monotherapy for 3 months. Resistance results from selection under antimicrobic pressure of resistant mutants of *M. tuberculosis* that number 1 in 10^6 among untreated bacillary populations. Large populations like the 10^9 to 10^{10} bacilli in pulmonary cavities are especially likely to contain significant numbers of inherently resistant tubercle bacilli. Low-level INH resistance is most commonly associated with point mutations or short deletions within the catalase-peroxidase gene *(katG),* which still produces some enzymatic activity, whereas high-level resistance is associated with major deletions within the gene with loss of all enzymatic activity.[18–19] Resistance in the regulatory region of a second gene involved in mycolic acid synthesis *(inhA)* also confers INH resistance.[18, 19] INH resistance (primary resistance) was 7.8% in 1995 among more than 13,000 isolates in the United States,[4] with higher rates encountered in selected populations including immigrants from areas such as Southeast Asia and Central America, where resistance is more common.[1–4, 20]

Pharmacology. INH is well absorbed orally or intramuscularly and is distributed throughout the body. Cerebrospinal fluid (CSF) levels are generally about 20% of plasma concentrations but may approach plasma levels in the presence of meningeal inflammation. Coadministration with vitamin C appears to inactivate INH suspensions markedly.[21]

Metabolism of INH occurs initially by liver *N*-acetyltransferase. Diminished acetylation capacity is inherited as an autosomal recessive trait that varies from a 5% prevalence rate in Canadian Eskimos to 83% in Egyptians. Ten to 15% of Asians are "slow" acetylators, as are 58% of American whites. Six hours after a 4 mg/kg oral dose, slow acetylators exhibit plasma INH levels of more than 0.8 μg/ml and rapid acetylators of less than 0.2 μg/ml.[13] The striking bimodal distribution of plasma half-lives of INH depending on acetylator status generally does not affect the outcome with daily therapy, because plasma levels are maintained well above inhibitory concentrations. Metabolically altered INH is principally excreted in urine along with lesser amounts of unaltered drug. Dosage modification in renal insufficiency is not usually necessary, but in significant hepatic failure a dosage reduction to 150 to 200 mg/day is recommended for slow acetylators. Table 34–1 summarizes dosage modifications for INH and other antituberculous drugs in hepatic or renal failure.

Adverse Reactions

Hepatitis. INH has infrequent major toxicities, most notably hepatitis. Approximately 15% of INH recipients have minor asymptomatic elevations in serum aspartate aminotransferase levels that usually resolve with continued therapy. An appreciation of the incidence of major INH hepatotoxicity was gained after the results of a large prophylactic trial were reported in 1978 in which 19 of 2321 recipients developed serious hepatitis and 2 died.[22] Hepatotoxicity can

TABLE 34-1 Need for Dosage Modification for Commonly Used Antituberculous Drugs in Hepatic or Renal Failure

Antimicrobial Drug	Modify in Hepatic Failure	Modify in Renal Failure
Isoniazid	Yes	Minor
Pyrazinamide	Yes	Yes
Ethambutol	No	Yes
Rifampin	Yes	No
Rifabutin	Yes	No
Amikacin	No	Yes
Capreomycin	No	Yes
Kanamycin	No	Yes
Streptomycin	No	Yes
Quinolones	No	Yes
Para-aminosalicylic acid	No	Yes
Ethionamide	Yes	No
Cycloserine	No	Yes

occur at any time but is most likely 4 to 8 weeks after treatment is begun. INH hepatotoxicity is clearly correlated with age, presumably due to a diminished capacity for repair of INH-induced hepatocellular damage in the elderly. Undernutrition may also play a role in the expression of INH hepatotoxicity.[23] Hepatotoxicity is increased in alcoholic patients with preexisting liver damage,[22] in pregnant women,[24] and in combination with acetaminophen.[25] Histologically, hepatocellular damage can progress to submassive necrosis. Although endemic viral hepatitis has been considered a possible factor contributing to INH hepatotoxicity,[26, 27] INH has been safely administered to some with acute hepatitis[28] and prophylactically to persons chronically infected with hepatitis B.[29, 30] Educating patients about the recognition of symptoms of INH-induced liver disease is key in preventing its progression. The value of routine monitoring of serum hepatic enzyme concentrations remains controversial except in high-risk patients such as elderly ones.[31] Patients should be advised to discontinue INH therapy at the onset of symptoms consistent with incipient hepatitis, such as nausea, loss of appetite, and dull midabdominal pain. Generally, hepatotoxicity subsides after INH discontinuation. Cautious readministration of INH after a resolution of hepatitis has been reported to be well tolerated and safe.[32] Recognition of the frequency and severity[33] of INH hepatotoxicity has not curtailed therapeutic usage but has led to a revision of "prophylactic" indications with special caution indicated in those, especially black women, older than 35 years.[34]

Neurotoxicity. Peripheral neuropathy has been described in 17% of recipients of 6 mg/kg/day of INH but is less frequent when adults receive the standard dose of 300 mg/day. Poor nutrition or underlying alcoholism, diabetes mellitus, or uremia predisposes to neuropathy, which is more frequent in slow acetylators who have higher plasma levels of unaltered drug. Increased pyridoxine excretion is promoted by INH. Pyridoxine, 10 to 50 mg daily, can ameliorate the neuropathy without interfering with the antimycobacterial effect.

INH-induced central nervous system toxicity can produce aberrations ranging from memory loss to psychosis or seizures. Particular caution is indicated when administering INH to those with convulsive disorders. Optic neuropathy has been reported. Toxic central nervous system reactions are not necessarily related to pyridoxine deficiency but have responded to its administration.[13]

Hypersensitivity Reactions. Fever, which may be sustained or "spiking," skin eruptions, or hematologic abnormalities can occur. INH recipients can develop positive antinuclear antibody reactions, and rarely manifest a lupus-like syndrome that is reversible on discontinuation of the INH.

Miscellaneous Adverse Reactions. INH-associated arthritic disorders have included Dupuytren's contracture and shoulder-hand syndrome. Pellagra can occur in malnourished INH recipients.[13, 35] Pyridoxine deficiency–related anemia can occur in children or adults.[36]

Overdose. Accidental ingestion of INH by children or ingestion during a suicide attempt may result in metabolic acidosis, hyperglycemia, seizures, and coma. High-dose pyridoxine usually reverses these toxicities.

Significant Drug Interactions. Phenytoin (Dilantin) toxicity is potentiated by INH. Mental changes, nystagmus, and ataxia can result, especially in slow acetylators whose high INH levels inhibit phenytoin metabolism. Theophylline toxicity has been reported with coadministration of INH. Combined INH and rifampin therapy predisposes to elevation of plasma hepatic enzymes. Plasma INH concentrations are increased by para-aminosalicylic acid (PAS) through interference with acetylation.

Usage. INH is indicated for all clinical forms of tuberculosis. It is used alone for preventive therapy or "chemoprophylaxis" for selected purified protein derivative skin test reactors at high risk for developing disease. INH has not been categorized for pregnancy but should be given with caution.

Availability and Dosage. INH is available generically (tablets, syrup, injectable solutions) and under brand names—INH tablets or Nydrazid injectable solution. Dosage forms include 100 and 300 mg tablets; syrup containing 10 mg/ml; 100 mg/ml solution for parenteral injection; and combination capsules combining 150 mg of INH with 300 mg of rifampin (Rifamate) or tablets of 50 mg with 120 mg of rifampin and 300 mg of PZA (Rifater). The usual adult dosage is 5 mg/kg/day (preferably 300 mg once daily). A higher dosage (10 mg/kg/day) has been recommended for special situations such as meningitis and for infants and children.

With the move toward the use of directly observed therapy for all patients, twice-weekly high-dose INH (15 mg/kg orally) is combined with rifampin (600 mg orally) and PZA (50 mg/kg, not to exceed 3 g) after an initial period of daily drug therapy for drug-susceptible isolates. For areas with a greater than 5% risk of drug-resistant tuberculosis, these drugs are combined with streptomycin (25 to 30 mg/kg intramuscularly) or ethambutol (50 mg/kg orally) twice weekly until susceptibilities are available. A reliable urine test is available to confirm INH ingestion.[37]

Although the preferred parenteral route is intramuscular injection, INH for injection can be administered safely intravenously.[38]

Rifampin

Derivation and Structure. Rifampin (termed *rifampicin* in the United Kingdom) is a semisynthetic derivative of a complex macrocyclic antibiotic, rifamycin B, produced by *Streptomyces mediterranei.* It was introduced for clinical trials in tuberculosis in 1967.

Mechanism of Action. Rifampin inhibits DNA-dependent RNA polymerase; human RNA polymerase is insensitive.

Antimicrobial Activity and Resistance. Rifampin is bactericidal against actively replicating *M. tuberculosis* to a degree comparable to INH with minimal inhibitory concentrations of 0.005 to 0.2 μg/ml. It is also active against intracellular, slowly replicating bacilli and somewhat against nearly dormant organisms in necrotic foci. Unlike other two-drug combinations, rifampin plus INH sterilizes tissues in experimental murine tuberculosis. Rifampin's efficacy is indicated in susceptible pulmonary tuberculosis by sputum conversion 2 weeks earlier with rifampin-containing regimens than with regimens without the drug. Resistance emerges rapidly if the drug is given as monotherapy. Primary resistance among isolates of *M. tuberculosis* is currently 3% in the United States, but more than 10% in Southeast Asia and some Central American countries. Approximately 95% of resistance to rifampin results from a point mutation or deletion within an 81-bp region of the gene encoding the β-subunit of RNA polymerase *(rpoB).*[19, 39] Rifampin resistance coupled with resistance to INH and other antituberculous agents now characterizes many MDR-TB isolates.[2]

Pharmacology. Rifampin is well absorbed orally, yielding peak plasma concentrations of 7 to 8 μg/ml after a dose of 600 mg. It is widely distributed throughout the body. CSF concentrations range from undetectable to 0.5 μg/ml in healthy persons and reach 50% of plasma concentrations with meningeal inflammation. Rifampin's high lipid solubility enhances phagosomal penetration. Rifampin is deacetylated to an active form that undergoes biliary excretion and enterohepatic recirculation. Due to autoinduction of rifampin metabolism (cytochrome P-450–coupled),[40] biliary excretion increases with continued therapy. Induction of rifampin's metabolism with consequent reduction in its half-life and plasma concentrations becomes maximal after approximately 6 doses.[41] Excretion is primarily into the gastrointestinal tract, with lesser amounts in the urine. The plasma concentration and urinary excretion increase in hepatic failure. Probenecid blocks hepatic uptake, causing decreased biliary excretion. Liver failure requires a moderate dosage reduction, but the full dosage can be given in renal insufficiency. Rifampin is removed by hemodialysis or peritoneal dialysis.[42]

Adverse Reactions. Minor adverse reactions are rather frequent with rifampin, but in only 6 of 372 patients taking the drug for 20 weeks was cessation of therapy necessary because of adverse effects.[43]

Hepatitis. Rifampin's major adverse effect is hepatotoxicity, which reportedly caused 16 deaths in 500,000 recipients.[13] Minimal abnormalities in liver function tests are common in those taking rifampin and usually resolve, possibly because of autoinduction of its metabolism even with continuation of the drug. Characteristically, elevations of bilirubin and alkaline phosphatase levels result, whereas elevation of hepatocellular enzyme concentrations can be caused by rifampin, INH, or both. Alcoholic patients with preexisting liver damage appear to be especially prone to rifampin-induced liver reactions.

Effects on Immune Parameters. Rifampin has widespread effects on humoral and cell-mediated immunity, but they appear to be of no clinical significance.

Hypersensitivity Reactions. Flushing, fever, pruritus without rash, urticaria, cutaneous vasculitis, eosinophilia, thrombocytopenia, hemolysis, or renal failure due to interstitial nephritis can occur because of rifampin. A systemic flulike syndrome, at times associated with thrombocytopenia, has been described almost exclusively with intermittent, high-dose therapy. Regimens of 600 mg of rifampin twice weekly have infrequently produced the flulike syndrome.

Miscellaneous Adverse Reactions. Widespread distribution of rifampin is reflected in an orange color appearing in urine, feces, saliva, sputum, pleural effusions, tears, soft contact lenses, sweat, semen, and CSF. With overdosage, a "red man syndrome" of skin discoloration has been described. Gastrointestinal upset is frequent but is usually ameliorated by a temporary reduction in dosage.

Significant Drug Interactions. By induction of microsomal cytochrome P-450–mediated enzymatic activities, rifampin causes increased hepatic metabolism of many substances. Rifampin interaction with more than 100 drugs has been described.[44–46] A partial compilation of this expanding list of compounds is given in Table 34–2. The recent introduction of the protease inhibitors for the treatment of HIV infection has complicated the treatment of tuberculosis in this setting. Because rifampin induces metabolism of the protease inhibitors, rifampin should not be coadministered with these agents.[10, 47]

Competition for excretion with contrast agents used for biliary tract imaging may cause failure to visualize the gallbladder. Probenecid interferes with renal excretion, whereas PAS may interfere with gastrointestinal absorption.

Usage. Rifampin is indicated for treatment of all forms of pulmonary and extrapulmonary tuberculosis. It is generally recommended for chemoprophylaxis when INH cannot be used and in combination with PZA is effective in HIV-positive patients for prophylaxis when given for only 2 months.[48] Rifampin is a category C drug, and should be used with caution in pregnancy.

TABLE 34–2 Commonly Used Compounds Having Rifampin-Induced Reduction in Plasma Concentrations

Antimicrobials	Hormonal Agents
Chloramphenicol	Estrogens
Clarithromycin	Oral contraceptives
Fluconazole	Prednisone-glucocorticoids
Itraconazole	Miscellaneous
Ketoconazole	Barbiturates
Indinavir	Cyclosporine
Nelfinavir	Diazepam
Retonavir	Haloperidol
Saquinavir	Methadone
Cardiovascular Agents	Nortriptyline
Coumadin	Phenytoin
Digitoxin	Sulfonylurea
Digoxin	Theophylline
Diltiazem	
Metoprolol	
Propanolol	
Quinidine	
Tocainide	
Verapamil	

Availability and Dosage. Rifampin is supplied in the United States as Rifadin, available in 150- or 300-mg capsules and in combination 300-mg capsules with 150-mg INH (Rifamate) or in 120-mg tablets with 50-mg INH and 300 mg of PZA (Rifater). Rifampin for intravenous infusion (600 mg/vial, Rifadin) should not be used intramuscularly. The usual oral dosage is 600 mg once daily for adults and 10 to 20 mg/kg/day for children (not to exceed 600 mg/day). Twice weekly 900- or 1200-mg dosage regimens have largely been abandoned due to toxic reactions. A 600-mg twice-weekly schedule generally has been well tolerated. Rifampin from opened capsules can be suspended (usually 10 mg/ml) in simple or flavored sugar syrups that should not include ascorbic acid, which can inactivate rifampin.[21] Suspensions can be refrigerated up to 2 weeks.

Pyrazinamide

Derivation and Structure. PZA is a synthetic pyrazine analogue of nicotinamide.

Mechanism of Action. The mechanism of action of PZA remains unknown.

Antimicrobial Activity and Resistance. PZA is bactericidal for tubercle bacilli at 12.5 μg/ml. Its optimal activity appears to be against semidormant organisms in an acid pH environment, like that existing intracellularly in phagolysosomes. Despite good activity at acid pH in vitro and inhibitory concentrations within monocytes,[49] PZA exhibits low activity alone in pretreated macrophages.[50] Resistance rapidly evolves if PZA is used alone. Primary resistance is seen in less than 1% of isolates, but nearly 50% of INH-rifampin–resistant MDR-TB isolates are PZA-resistant.[2] Most isolates resistant to PZA have mutations in the gene encoding pyrazinamidase *(pncA)* (Table 34–3).[51, 52] This results in the loss of pyrazinamidase activity, an enzyme that converts PZA to the active form of pyrazinoic acid.

Pharmacology. Well-absorbed orally, PZA is widely distributed throughout the body, attaining concentrations above that needed to inhibit tubercle bacilli. Peak plasma concentrations are approximately 50 μg/ml, with a half-life of 12 hours, making once-daily or less frequent dosing practical. PZA crosses inflamed meninges and has been recommended in combination regimens for tuberculous meningitis.[53] It is metabolized by the liver, and metabolic products, including principally pyrazinoic acid, are excreted mainly by the kidneys, requiring dosage modification in renal failure. PZA is dialyzable so that supplemental dosage may be advisable after dialysis sessions.[42]

TABLE 34-3 Mechanism of Action and Recognized Mutational Resistance in Commonly Used Antituberculous Agents

Drug	Mechanism of Action	Site of Mutational Resistance (gene)
Isoniazid	Inhibits mycolic acid synthesis	*inhA* (regulatory region) (mycolic acid gene)
	Catalase-peroxidase enzyme	*katG* (catalase-peroxidase gene)
Rifampin	Inhibits RNA polymerization	β-subunit *rpoB* (RNA polymerase gene)
Pyrazinamide	Unknown	*pncA* (pyrazinamidase gene)
Ethambutol	Inhibits cell wall synthesis (blocks arabinosyl transferase)	*embB* (gene for arabinosyl transferase enzyme)
Streptomycin	Inhibits protein synthesis	*rpsL* (gene for ribosomal S12 protein); 16-S ribosomal RNA gene
Amikacin	Inhibits protein synthesis	16-S ribosomal RNA gene (? amikacin-binding site)
Capreomycin	Inhibits cell wall synthesis	Unknown
Quinolones	Inhibits DNA structure	*gyrA* (gyrase A gene)

Adverse Reactions. The most common side effects are nausea and vomiting. Hepatotoxicity occurred in nearly 15% of PZA recipients in early trials that employed dosages of 40 to 50 mg/kg/day for prolonged periods. Current regimens of 20 to 35 mg/kg/day are much safer.[54] Patients with preexisting liver disease should have symptoms and hepatic function tests monitored closely. Other adverse reactions (1% of patients or less) include interstitial nephritis,[55] rhabdomyolysis with myoglobinuric renal failure,[56] nonincapacitating polymyalgia, photosensitivity, and rash. Asymptomatic urate retention occurs in 50% of PZA recipients.[54]

Significant Drug Interactions. There are no significant drug interactions with PZA.

Usage. PZA is included as an essential component of multidrug 6-month short-course chemotherapy.[12, 17, 54] Without PZA for the first 2 months, relapse rates are unacceptable.[55] Efficacy with its administration as infrequently as once weekly makes PZA suitable for directly observed therapy regimens. PZA is a class C drug and should be used with caution in pregnancy.

Availability and Dosage. PZA is available in 500-mg tablets, or as 300-mg tablets in combination with INH (50 mg) and rifampin (120 mg) (Rifater). Dosage is 20 to 35 mg/kg/day (often 1.5 to 2.0 g) orally once or in two divided doses. PZA has been well tolerated in a twice-weekly dosage of 50 mg/kg (not to exceed 3 g/day) for short-course regimens. It has even been administered safely once weekly in a dose of 90 mg/kg.

Ethambutol

Derivation and Structure. Ethambutol (ethylenediiminobutanol) was discovered in 1961 among synthetic compounds screened for antituberculous activity.

Mechanism of Action. Ethambutol inhibits arabinosyl transferase enzymes that are involved in arabinogalactan and lipoarabinomannan biosynthesis within the cell wall.[57]

Antimicrobial Activity and Resistance. Ethambutol is bacteriostatic in vitro or within macrophages[49] at concentrations of 1 μg/ml against susceptible strains of *M. tuberculosis.* Primary ethambutol resistance in the United States is only 2%.[4] Ethambutol's principal role has been as a "companion" drug to curtail resistance. However, resistance rates as high as 80% for ethambutol in INH-rifampin–resistant isolates from New York City apparently indicate limited utility against MDR-TB.[2] Ethambutol resistance relates to point mutations in the arabinosyl transferase enzyme EmbB, which is coded for by the *embB* gene.[58]

Pharmacology. Ethambutol administered orally is 75 to 80% absorbed, yielding peak plasma concentrations of 5 μg/ml after a dose of 25 mg/kg. It is distributed throughout the body, including the CSF. Although little ethambutol crosses normal meninges, levels 10 to 50% of those in plasma occur in CSF with meningeal inflammation. After conversion of approximately 25% of absorbed ethambutol to inactive metabolites, 80% of the parent together with metabolites is excreted in urine. Consequently, it becomes necessary to modify the dosage in significant renal failure.

Adverse Reactions

Neuropathy. The major toxicity of ethambutol is neuropathy. Peripheral neuropathy is infrequent; retrobulbar neuritis is more common. Characteristically, patients complain of bilateral blurry vision and are found to have impairment of visual acuity and red-green color vision. Common in association with high-dose (50 mg/kg/day) therapy with prolonged administration, and more common with 25 mg/kg/day than with 15 mg/kg/day dosing, retrobulbar neuritis is usually slowly reversible. Visual loss has rarely occurred in elderly persons receiving as little as 15 mg/kg/day.[59] Recipients of ethambutol should be instructed to report symptoms of blurry vision promptly and to discontinue the drug until confirmatory visual testing can be done. Visual acuity and red-green color perception testing is recommended at baseline, whenever a change in visual symptoms occurs, and every 4 to 6 weeks in those taking 25 mg/kg/day. Monthly testing in patients on 15 mg/kg can be useful in establishing the range of visual abnormalities in those already visually impaired.

Miscellaneous Adverse Reactions. Gastrointestinal intolerance is infrequent. Hyperuricemia occurs because of decreased renal uric acid excretion. Hypersensitivity reactions are rare and include dermatitis, arthralgias, and fever.

Significant Drug Interactions. There are no significant drug interactions with ethambutol.

Usage. Ethambutol is commonly included as the fourth drug along with INH, rifampin, and PZA in patients with tuberculosis at high risk of drug resistance. It is also routinely used in treatment regimens for patients with isolates resistant to INH or rifampin, or both. Ethambutol has no detectable effects on the fetus but has no pregnancy classification.

Availability and Dosage. Ethambutol is available as ethambutol hydrochloride (Myambutol) supplied in 100- or 400-mg tablets. The usual dosage is 15 to 25 mg/kg/day initially, followed after 60 days by 15 mg/kg/day as a single daily dose.

Streptomycin

Derivation, Structure, and Pharmacology. Streptomycin, an aminoglycoside antibiotic introduced in the 1940s, was the first drug to reduce tuberculosis mortality. Its structure, mechanism of action, and pharmacology are covered in other chapters. Briefly, intramuscular injection of 1 g yields peak plasma concentrations of 25 to 45 μg/ml. It is virtually excluded from the CNS.

Antimicrobial Activity and Resistance. Streptomycin is bactericidal against *M. tuberculosis* in vitro but is inactive against intracellular tubercle bacilli. Concentrations of 4 to 10 μg/ml of plasma are inhibitory. The rapid emergence of resistance to streptomycin was quickly recognized as a consequence of single-drug therapy. Approximately 1 in 10^6 tubercle bacilli is spontaneously resistant to streptomycin. Primary resistance to streptomycin is seen most often in patient populations having a high incidence of INH resistance. In MDR-TB outbreaks, approximately 80% of INH-rifampin–resistant isolates are also streptomycin-resistant.[2] Streptomycin resistance relates to mutational changes involving ribosomal binding protein or the ribosomal binding site.[19, 60, 61] Isolates resistant to streptomycin are not cross-resistant to amikacin, kanamycin, or capreomycin.

Adverse Reactions. Streptomycin toxicity is like that of other aminoglycoside antibiotics but with less renal and auditory toxicity and greater vestibular toxicity than more commonly used aminoglycosides. Patients receiving streptomycin should be instructed to be aware of tinnitus, decreased hearing, and problems with balance, and they should be instructed to notify their caregiver immediately if such reactions occur.

Significant Drug Interactions. There are no significant drug interactions with streptomycin.

Usage. Streptomycin is indicated as the fourth drug along with INH, rifampin, and PZA in patients at significant risk for drug resistance. It is also used for multidrug therapy of susceptible resistant tuberculosis. Dosages of greater than 1 g per day should be avoided. Dosage reduction is indicated in patients older than 50 years, those with low body weight, and those in whom renal function is impaired. Special care must be taken when streptomycin is used in combination with other nephrotoxic or ototoxic drugs. It is a category D drug in pregnancy because of fetal ototoxicity.

Availability and Dosage. Streptomycin sulfate for intramuscular injection is provided in 1-g single-injection vials. The recommended dosage in adults with normal renal function is 0.5 to 1 g daily to 1 g twice weekly. Children receive 20 to 40 mg/kg/day in divided doses every 12 hours. Streptomycin is available in the United States, but its supply has been interrupted in the past.

SECOND-LINE ANTITUBERCULOUS DRUGS

Rifabutin

Derivation, Pharmacology. Several spiropiperidyl rifamycins have activity against mycobacteria, including *M. tuberculosis, M. avium-intracellulare* complex, and *Mycobacterium fortuitum.*[62–66] Rifabutin (Mycobutin), a derivative of rifamycin-S, is more active in vitro and more effective on a weight basis in experimental murine tuberculosis than is rifampin.[65] The mechanism of action is inhibition of RNA polymerase, as it is with rifampin. It has a long plasma half-life (45 hours) in humans and marked tissue tropism, producing tissue concentrations fivefold to 10-fold greater than in serum. Peak serum concentrations of rifampin (5 to 10 μg/ml) are fivefold to 10-fold higher than those of rifabutin (0.5 μg/ml).[67]

Adverse Reactions. A polymyalgia syndrome, a yellowish-tan discoloration of the skin *(pseudojaundice),* and anterior uveitis have occurred in patients taking rifabutin, usually at doses exceeding 300 mg daily.[68, 69] Almost all persons with these side effects have also been receiving clarithromycin, fluconazole, or ritonavir. Symptoms of uveitis include ocular pain and blurred vision. Neutropenia occurs infrequently when rifabutin is used to treat tuberculosis but has been reported in one third of patients receiving therapy for pulmonary *M. avium* complex disease.[70] The incidence of rash, hepatitis, and gastrointestinal distress appears comparable to that with rifampin. It also can produce an orange-red discoloration of urine, saliva, tears, and contact lenses similar to that of rifampin.

Significant Drug Interactions. Rifabutin induces the hepatic cytochrome P-450 system, but only about 50% of that seen with rifampin. This induction produces lowered serum levels of numerous drugs normally metabolized in the liver, including the protease inhibitors. Concurrent administration of retonavir and saquinavir with rifabutin is not recommended for this reason.[71] Rifabutin is also metabolized by this same system, so enzyme inhibitors such as the protease inhibitors, fluconazole, and clarithromycin increase plasma rifabutin concentrations.[67, 71]

Usage. Rifabutin appears as effective as rifampin in the treatment of drug-susceptible tuberculosis,[72, 73] but experience with it is limited. In patients on protease inhibitors for HIV infection, rifabutin at 150 mg is recommended in place of rifampin 600 mg because it has less effect on the metabolism of the protease inhibitors.[10] Rifabutin's potential for treatment of MDR-TB is under investigation.[74, 75] Approximately 25% of rifampin-resistant tuberculosis strains are inhibited by low concentrations of rifabutin.

Other Rifamycins

With the microbiologic success of rifabutin but problems with low serum levels and complex adverse reactions, investigators are studying other rifamycin compounds. The two most promising agents are rifapentine[76,77, 77a] and KRM-1648.[78] In the study leading to licensure in 1998, rifapentine, 600 mg twice weekly, was compared with rifampin, 450 to 600 mg, when both were given with daily isoniazid, pyrazinamide, and ethambutol for 2 months, followed by rifapentine, 600 mg, plus isoniazid weekly or rifampin, 450 to 600 mg, plus isoniazid twice weekly. Results at 6 months follow-up were comparable, although the rifapentine relapse rate was slightly higher (10% vs. 5%).[77a] Twice weekly followed by once weekly rifapentine, 600 mg, is the recommended regimen. When given with a fatty meal, peak blood levels following the administration of 600 mg rifapentine are 15 μg/ml of native drug and 6 μg/ml of 25-desacetyl rifapentine, the active metabolite. The half-life of both compounds is 13 hours. It appears to be a more potent inducer of the cytochrome P-50 system than rifabutin but less than rifampin. The drug probably should be avoided in HIV-positive patients because of interaction with protease inhibitors and the unexplained development of rifamycin monoresistance in some patients.[79] The drug is available as Priftin in 150-mg tablets. KRM-1648 is not yet approved by the U.S. Food and Drug Administration (FDA).

Quinolones

Mechanism of Action. Emerging outbreaks of MDR-TB[1–3] have stimulated the investigation of new fluorinated quinolones for their activity against mycobacteria.[80–86] Some are bactericidal against *M. tuberculosis,* presumably by inhibition of its DNA gyrase at concentrations within achievable serum levels.[81]

Antimicrobial Activity and Resistance. Ciprofloxacin and ofloxacin inhibit 90% of strains of susceptible tubercle bacilli at concentrations of 0.5 and 1.0 μg/ml, respectively.[82–84] Fluoroquinolones, particularly sparfloxacin,[85] have produced additive effects with other antituberculous drugs in vitro and in animals. Clinical trials of ofloxacin in combination with INH and rifampin indicate activity comparable to that of ethambutol.[86] Ofloxacin used alone in a dose of 300 mg/day in patients having MDR-TB has produced decreases in sputum colony counts, with sputum conversion in 26%.[87] In nonconverters, ofloxacin resistance emerged. Usage as a single agent in animal models or in human trials with inactive drugs has led to the rapid emergence of resistance. Resistance appears to result from mutations in the genes responsible for DNA configuration (DNA gyrase).[19, 88]

Usage. Quinolones are now routinely incorporated into treatment regimens for MDR-TB along with other agents. The usual dosage is ciprofloxacin 750 mg or ofloxacin 400 mg, both given twice daily.

Capreomycin, Amikacin, Kanamycin, Viomycin

Capreomycin, amikacin, kanamycin, and viomycin are considered as a group because all are administered by intramuscular or intravenous injection, have similar pharmacokinetics and toxicities, and are excreted by the renal route. These drugs have been used principally as alternative agents for MDR-TB. All have additive ototoxicity and nephrotoxicity and in that regard should be given cautiously, just like streptomycin or other aminoglycosides.

Capreomycin

Antimicrobial Activity and Resistance. Capreomycin, a polypeptide antibiotic obtained from *Streptomyces capreolus,* is active against *M.*

tuberculosis, including most MDR-TB strains,[2] at concentrations of 1 to 50 μg/ml (usually 10 μg/ml). Average peak plasma concentrations of 30 μg/ml are achievable. There is no cross-resistance between streptomycin and capreomycin,[89] but some isolates resistant to kanamycin or amikacin are cross-resistant to capreomycin. The site of mutational change resulting in capreomycin resistance is unknown.

Adverse Reactions. Capreomycin can cause hearing loss, tinnitus, and decreased renal function but is considered less toxic than amikacin, viomycin, and especially kanamycin.

Significant Drug Interactions. There are no significant drug interactions with capreomycin.

Usage. Capreomycin has emerged as the first-line injectable agent in multidrug regimens for the treatment of drug-resistant tuberculosis, especially when there is streptomycin resistance.

Availability and Dosage. Capreomycin sulfate is supplied as Capastat. The dosage is the same as with streptomycin, with a range of 500 mg to 1 g deep intramuscularly five times weekly for 2 to 4 months in those younger than 50 years and having normal renal function. The dose is thereafter reduced to 1 g two to three times weekly. It is a category C pregnancy drug.

Amikacin

Antimicrobial Activity and Resistance. In vitro and in animals, amikacin is among the most active aminoglycosides against *M. tuberculosis.* There is limited experience with amikacin in human tuberculosis. Because of its expense and greater toxicity, it is generally considered the third-line agent after streptomycin and capreomycin for the treatment of MDR-TB. It has generally replaced kanamycin in the United States. Resistance to amikacin and kanamycin results from an A-to-G change at base pair 1408 of the 16-S ribosomal RNA gene.[90]

Adverse Reactions. Common side effects include tinnitus, hearing loss, and nonoliguric renal failure. Hypersensitivity events are rare.

Usage. Amikacin is an alternative injectable agent for the treatment of resistant *M. tuberculosis* infections. The customary dose is 7 to 10 mg/kg (not to exceed 1 g) five times weekly. Because most pathology laboratories can determine blood levels of amikacin but not kanamycin, streptomycin, or capreomycin, amikacin is especially suited when parenteral therapy is required in patients with renal failure or in elderly patients with preexisting hearing loss. It is a category D drug in pregnancy.

Kanamycin

Kanamycin is an aminoglycoside that has activity against most strains of streptomycin-resistant tubercle bacilli. Except for its lower cost, kanamycin offers no advantage over amikacin in combination therapy and has substantial ototoxicity. In addition, serum levels are not readily available.

Availability and Dosage. Kanamycin sulfate is available as Kantrex, 0.5 g/2 ml, 1 g/3 ml, or 75 mg/2 ml (pediatric formulation) for intramuscular injection. The usual dose is 10 mg/kg generally limited to 500 mg/day in adults because of ototoxicity.

Viomycin

Viomycin is a complex basic polypeptide antibiotic for injection.[14] Many strains of MDR-TB appear to be susceptible.[2] Cross-resistance to viomycin and capreomycin occurs frequently; cross-resistance to viomycin and kanamycin occurs less frequently.[89] Viomycin is not available in the United States but is included because of its activity against most MDR-TB strains.[2]

Para-aminosalicylic Acid

Derivation, Structure, and Pharmacology. As a calcium or sodium salt, this synthetic compound inhibits the growth of tubercle bacilli by the impairment of folate synthesis. PAS is incompletely absorbed orally. A 4-g dose yields plasma concentrations of 70 to 80 μg/ml. Eighty-five percent of absorbed PAS is excreted in urine as various metabolic products.

Adverse Reactions. Chief among PAS side effects is gastrointestinal intolerance, which is often severe and results in poor compliance. PAS can cause reversible drug-induced lupus-like reactivity and, when given as the sodium salt, sodium overload. It can produce lymphoid hyperplasia, and recipients can develop mononucleosis-like syndromes with fever, rash, hepatosplenomegaly, occasionally toxic hepatitis, and adenopathy. Hypersensitivity to PAS is frequent.

Usage. PAS has retained a limited role in multidrug therapy in developing countries because of its low cost. However, it is becoming less favored because of poor compliance and primary resistance. Its use in the United States is limited to the treatment of MDR-TB.

Availability and Dosage. PAS in the United States is available from the Centers for Disease Control and Prevention. Dosage forms include 500-mg tablets or 4-g resin packets. The usual dosage is 10 to 12 g/day in three or four divided doses for adults (6 to 8 g/day of the sodium-potassium–free ascorbate) and, in children, 200 to 300 mg/kg/day in divided doses.

Cycloserine

Derivation, Mechanism of Action. Initially a fermentation product, cycloserine is now synthesized. By virtue of inhibiting cell wall synthesis, cycloserine possesses antimicrobial activity against a broad range of prokaryotic organisms including mycobacteria. From 5 to 20 μg/ml inhibits susceptible *M. tuberculosis* in vitro.

Pharmacology. Cycloserine is readily absorbed orally, producing peak plasma concentrations of 20 to 50 μg/ml. Widely distributed among tissues, no blood-brain barrier exists to cycloserine.[13] Little of the drug is metabolized, and approximately two thirds is excreted unchanged by the kidneys.

Adverse Reactions. Cycloserine can cause peripheral neuropathy or CNS dysfunction, including confusion, irritability, somnolence, headache, nervousness, vertigo, dysarthria, and seizures. Behavioral alterations include severe depression with suicidal ideation. Cycloserine is contraindicated in patients with a history of seizures or those with severe underlying depression.

Usage. Cycloserine is one of several alternatives for re-treatment regimens or for treatment of primary drug-resistant *M. tuberculosis.* It does not appear to have great activity against MDR-TB strains.[2] It is classified as a category C drug in pregnancy.

Availability and Dosage. Cycloserine is provided in the United States as Seromycin in 250-mg pulvules. The usual dosage is 500 to 1000 mg/day in two divided doses, with 500 mg/day commonly used.

Ethionamide

Derivation, Mechanism of Action, and Resistance. Ethionamide, a derivative of isonicotinic acid, was first synthesized in 1956. It is tuberculostatic at 0.6 to 2.5 μg/ml against susceptible strains, presumably by inhibition of oxygen-dependent mycolic acid synthesis.[91] The mechanism of ethionamide resistance is unknown, but some isolates are resistant to both INH and ethionamide and harbor mutations in the region of the *inhA* gene, which is involved in mycolic acid biosynthesis.[19]

Pharmacology. Ethionamide is absorbed well orally, yielding peak plasma concentrations of 20 μg/ml. It is widely distributed and penetrates both normal and inflamed meninges to yield CSF concentrations equivalent to those in plasma. It is metabolized by the liver, with metabolites renally excreted. Ethionamide interferes with INH acetylation.

Adverse Reactions. Gastrointestinal distress with nausea and vomiting frequently leads to poor compliance and drug discontinuance. Various neurologic disorders have been caused by ethionamide, including peripheral neuropathy and psychiatric disturbances. Neurologic side effects have been reported to be alleviated by pyridoxine or nicotinamide. Reversible hepatotoxicity occurs in approximately 5% of ethionamide recipients. A hypersensitivity-type rash and poor diabetic control are infrequent complications.

Usage. Ethionamide is among the agents that can be chosen for the treatment of resistant tuberculosis. It appears to be active against most MDR-TB isolates.[2] Its usage is limited by a high frequency of severe gastrointestinal intolerance.

Availability and Dosage. Ethionamide is available in the United States as Trecator-SC in 250-mg coated tablets. The initial dosage is 250 mg twice daily (or as a single dose at bedtime), which is increased by 250 mg daily until 1 g/day in divided doses is reached. Usually, 500 to 750 mg is the maximal tolerated dose.

β-Lactams

All mycobacteria produce β-lactamase. Several β-lactamase–resistant β-lactam antibiotics or combinations of a β-lactam with β-lactamase inhibitors such as clavulanic acid are active in vitro against *M. tuberculosis*[92, 93] and various nontuberculous mycobacteria.[94] Unfortunately, activity of β-lactam agents against intracellular mycobacteria is generally poor.[49, 95] In concentrations as high as 50 μg/ml in a macrophage model, ceforanide, active in vitro, was unable to inhibit tubercle bacilli.[49] Similarly, cefotaxime, ceftizoxime, and cefoperazone lack intracellular activity against *M. avium-intracellulare* strains that have in vitro activity.[95] However, cefoxitin and imipenem-cilastatin have proved efficacious in *M. fortuitum* and *Mycobacterium abscessus* infections,[96] giving hope that β-lactamase–stable β-lactam antibiotics with activity against resistant *M. tuberculosis* strains could be developed.[97]

Amithiozone

Amithiozone (thiacetazone), a thiosemicarbazole, is active against many strains of *M. tuberculosis.*[13, 14] Because of its low cost, amithiozone has been employed as a first-line drug, particularly in East Africa.[14] However, because of severe toxicity in HIV-infected recipients there, clinical usage no longer appears appropriate.[6, 9]

MAJOR DRUGS FOR THE TREATMENT OF NONTUBERCULOUS MYCOBACTERIAL INFECTIONS

Nontuberculous (atypical or environmental) mycobacteria vary greatly in susceptibility to antimicrobics. Some, such as *Mycobacterium kansasii,* are susceptible to agents used principally for the treatment of tuberculosis; others, such as *M. fortuitum* and *Mycobacterium chelonae,* respond to antibiotics used more commonly for pyogenic bacterial infections; and still others, especially *M. avium-intracellulare,* are broadly resistant. Choosing appropriate therapy for nontuberculous infections is further confounded because methodologies for susceptibility testing have yet to be standardized.[98] However, chemotherapy for nontuberculous mycobacterial infections based on susceptibility results is now feasible for many species. An important exception is that susceptibility testing has no clinically predictive value in infections due to *M. avium-intracellulare* except for the newer macrolide clarithromycin.[47]

Macrolides

Antimicrobial Activity and Resistance. Pretreatment strains of *M. kansasii, Mycobacterium scrofulaceum, Mycobacterium marinum, Mycobacterium haemophilum, Mycobacterium malmoense, M. avium-intracellulare, M. chelonae,* and *M. abscessus* (formerly *M. chelonae* subsp. *abscessus*) are susceptible to achievable therapeutic concentrations of the newer macrolides, clarithromycin and azithromycin. This has resulted in a dramatic change in therapy of nontuberculous mycobacteria with a macrolide now part of the treatment regimen for most species. Clarithromycin inhibits almost all species with the exception of 20% of *M. fortuitum* and most *Mycobacterium simiae* at 4 μg/ml or less.[99, 100] Initial therapeutic results have indicated that these agents are clinically efficacious as well, including against both pulmonary and disseminated *M. avium-intracellulare* infections.[101–105] Both macrolides have proved efficacious for the prevention of disseminated *M. avium* infection in patients with AIDS.[106, 107] These agents should not be used as monotherapy because of the rapid emergence of resistance, which results from a point mutation at adenine 2058 or 2059 on the 23-S ribosomal RNA, the presumed macrolide-binding site, and produces cross-resistance to all macrolides.[108, 109]

Pharmacology. Clarithromycin is metabolized in the liver, and significant concentrations of the 14-OH metabolite are detectable in the serum.[110] Clarithromycin is also excreted in part by the kidneys, and a reduction in dosage is required in elderly patients and with renal failure.

Adverse Reactions. The most common side effects are nausea, vomiting, and diarrhea, which are dose related.[111] A toxic hepatitis occurs with daily doses above 1.0 g and is associated with elevated levels of alkaline phosphatase and γ-glutamyl transferase.[111] Temporary hearing loss may also occur with high doses, more commonly with azithromycin.[112]

Significant Drug Interactions. Clarithromycin is metabolized by the cytochrome P-450 enzyme system, and serum levels are dramatically reduced by enzyme inducers such as rifampin.[110] Clarithromycin is an inhibitor of the P-450 enzyme system, and its use results in increased serum levels and potential increased toxicities of multiple drugs metabolized by these enzymes, including rifabutin,[68, 69] carbamazepine, cisapride, astemizole, terfenadine, and theophylline. Clarithromycin inhibits the metabolism of protease inhibitors as well.[71] In contrast, azithromycin is not metabolized by the cytochrome P-450 system and has no significant drug interactions.

Dosage. The usual therapeutic doses are 500 mg twice daily for clarithromycin and 250 mg once daily for azithromycin. For disseminated *M. avium* prophylaxis, the dosage of azithromycin is 1200 mg once a week.[107]

Rifampin

Antimicrobial Activity. Rifampin is employed for the treatment of many nontuberculous mycobacterial infections. In vitro, 93 to 100% of strains of *M. kansasii, M. marinum,* and *M. haemophilum* are inhibited by 0.25 to 1.0 μg/ml.[47, 113, 114] Other species are much less susceptible. Only one half of *M. scrofulaceum* or *M. avium-intracellulare* strains are inhibited in vitro by 4 to 16 μg/ml of rifampin. Synergy between rifampin and other agents has been demonstrable for a number of species in vitro. Its role as a single agent is discouraged because resistance will occur.[114]

Pharmacology, Adverse Events, Significant Drug Interactions. See the earlier discussion in the section on tuberculosis.

Usage. The excellent response of *M. kansasii* infections to rifampin-containing regimens has made rifampin a recommended component of most treatment regimens.[47] For patients with HIV infection on protease inhibitors, rifabutin (150 mg/day) or clarithromycin (500 mg twice daily) is recommended over rifampin,[47] because of its lesser effect on the cytochrome P-450 system.

Rifabutin

Antimicrobial Activity. Rifabutin is inhibitory against 90% of strains of *M. avium-intracellulare* at a concentration of 2 μg/ml.[65, 66] It is concentrated severalfold in tissue and, like rifampin, has gastrointestinal toxicity as its most common adverse effect. Rifabutin at a dose of 300 mg/day has been shown to reduce by 50% the incidence and rate of dissemination of *M. avium-intracellulare* infections in AIDS patients having CD4 counts of less than 200,[115] although it is probably not as effective as the newer macrolides.

Pharmacology, Adverse Events, Significant Drug Interactions. See the earlier discussion in the section on tuberculosis.

Usage. Rifabutin is used in place of rifampin in patients on protease inhibitors, although it is not recommended with saquinavir or retonavir.[71] Rifabutin is routinely recommended in the multidrug regimen for treatment of *M. avium-intracellulare* lung disease.[47] However, for disseminated disease in patients with AIDS, a recent placebo-controlled study showed that through 16 weeks of follow-up, a dose of 300 mg daily added nothing over clarithromycin and ethambutol alone.[116]

Aminoglycosides

Aminoglycoside antibiotics have been used extensively for the treatment of nontuberculous mycobacterial infections. Among *M. kansasii* strains, 86% demonstrated streptomycin susceptibility, as did 93% of *M. scrofulaceum* strains. Forty-four percent of strains of *M. avium-intracellulare* have been streptomycin susceptible. *M. fortuitum* complex isolates are resistant.

Amikacin is the most active aminoglycoside against the nontuberculous mycobacteria.[47, 117–119] However, marked variability exists between mycobacterial species in susceptibility to amikacin. Virtually all strains of *M. marinum, M. kansasii,* and *M. fortuitum* are susceptible to 4 μg/ml or less,[113, 118, 119] whereas isolates of *M. chelonae, M. abscessus,* and *M. avium-intracellulare* are more resistant but are usually inhibited by 8 to 32 μg/ml of amikacin.[118, 119] Tobramycin is the most active aminoglycoside against isolates of *M. chelonae.*[118, 119] Other aminoglycosides are less active and are generally not clinically useful.

Mutational resistance to amikacin is rare, probably because of relatively high toxicity, which limits therapy. Resistance has been described with *M. abscessus* and results from the same 16-S ribosomal RNA mutation described with *M. tuberculosis.*[90, 120]

Ethambutol

Ethambutol has good in vivo activity against *M. avium* complex and is included as part of most treatment regimens for these organisms.[47] It also has activity against most other slowly growing nontuberculous mycobacteria, including *M. kansasii, M. marinum,* and *Mycobacterium xenopi.* Species of rapidly growing mycobacteria are all highly resistant with the exception of the *Mycobacterium smegmatis* group.

LESS FREQUENTLY USED MISCELLANEOUS ANTIMICROBIALS FOR TREATMENT OF NONTUBERCULOUS MYCOBACTERIA

Isoniazid

Drugs such as INH used principally for treatment of *M. tuberculosis* were evaluated relatively early for their activity against nontuberculous mycobacteria. INH inhibits nearly 90% of strains of *M. kansasii* at concentrations of 1 to 5 μg/ml, as contrasted to only 10 to 30% of *M. avium-intracellulare* strains. At present, INH is included routinely in the therapy of *M. kansasii* in the United States,[47] *M. xenopi,* and *Mycobacterium szulgai.* It has generally been replaced by more active agents for therapy of other species, including *M. avium-intracellulare.*

Tetracyclines

Approximately 50% of isolates of the rapidly growing species *M. fortuitum* and 20% of *M. chelonae* are tetracycline susceptible.[119] Minocycline and doxycycline are two- to fourfold more active than tetracycline[118] and have been effective in therapy when the isolates were susceptible in vitro.[96] Minocycline and doxycycline are also active against *M. marinum*[113, 121, 122] and have been used successfully in *M. marinum* infections.[47, 121]

Sulfonamides

Sulfamethoxazole is active against *M. fortuitum* but not against *M. chelonae* or *M. abscessus.*[118, 119] Localized infections have been cured with sulfamethoxazole alone or in combination with trimethoprim.[96] *Mycobacterium marinum* infections have responded to therapy with trimethoprim-sulfamethoxazole,[47] but strains are susceptible in vitro only against a low inoculum.[122]

Both *M. marinum* and *M. kansasii* exhibit very similar drug susceptibilities. Sulfamethoxazole is also active against isolates of *M. kansasii.* It has been curative in combination regimens used for the treatment of rifampin-resistant *M. kansasii* infections.[114]

Limited experience indicates some in vitro activity and clinical efficacy of sulfonamides against *Mycobacterium terrae* complex, *M. haemophilum, M. simiae,* and *M. avium-intracellulare.*[47]

Clofazimine

Discussed more fully later in the section "Drugs for Treatment of Leprosy (Hansen's Disease)," clofazimine (Lamprene) possesses in vitro activity against *M. chelonae, M. abscessus,* and *M. avium-intracellulare.* Most strains are inhibited by 1.6 to 2.0 μg/ml.[64, 123] Clinical experience with clofazimine in therapy against *M. avium* in AIDS has been disappointing.[64]

Quinolones

The newer fluorinated quinolones (ciprofloxacin, ofloxacin, sparfloxacin) have in vitro activity against a number of nontuberculous mycobacteria at achievable serum levels.[81, 82, 84, 119, 124] *Mycobacterium fortuitum* strains are the most susceptible, with ciprofloxacin MICs of 0.25 μg/ml or less and good responses clinically.[124] A number of species are inhibited by intermediate concentrations of ciprofloxacin (1 to 4 μg/ml). These include *M. chelonae* (25%), *M. malmoense, M. marinum, M. xenopi, M. kansasii, M. haemophilum,* and some strains of *M. avium-intracellulare.* The clinical efficacy of the quinolones for these species has yet to be established. Resistance to ciprofloxacin after monotherapy has been described[124] and presumably involves the same DNA gyrase mutations observed with quinolone resistance with *M. tuberculosis.*[88]

β-Lactams

All mycobacteria produce β-lactamase, although it can be difficult to detect in *M. avium* complex. β-Lactams or combinations of β-lactam–β-lactamase inhibitor have been shown to be active or useful clinically, however, only for the *M. fortuitum* complex. Cefoxitin, cefmetazole, and imipenem-cilastatin are active in vitro against approximately 80% of *M. fortuitum* strains and most isolates of *M. abscessus* at clinically achievable plasma concentrations.[94, 125]

Susceptibility Tests

In vitro susceptibility of nontuberculous mycobacterial drugs is no guarantee of therapeutic efficacy. Previously cited failures of clofazimine in *M. avium-intracellulare* infections indicate limitations in extrapolating in vitro data to clinical experience. As a rule, favorable therapeutic results are likely when drugs are used to which nontuberculous mycobacteria are susceptible in vitro, and poor outcomes can be anticipated when there is in vitro resistance. Least predictable are outcomes of *M. avium-intracellulare* infections, for which routine susceptibility testing is *not* recommended.[47]

DRUGS FOR TREATMENT OF LEPROSY (HANSEN'S DISEASE)

Background

The special parasite-host relationship of *Mycobacterium leprae* (Hansen's bacillus), characterized by persistence of the organism in tissue for years, has mandated prolonged chemotherapy to prevent relapse. For years, chemotherapy for leprosy mainly consisted of dapsone alone, which produced gratifying clinical results and was affordable. However, because of monotherapy, resistance of leprosy bacilli, both secondary and now primary, has become a problem worldwide.[126] Currently, multidrug therapy is the rule for both multibacillary and paucibacillary disease. The principal agents used in therapeutic multidrug regimens are dapsone, rifampin, and clofazimine.

Dapsone

Derivation and Structure. Dapsone (diaminophenyl sulfone) a synthetic compound, was demonstrated to be effective in rat leprosy in 1941 and soon thereafter was used successfully in human trials.

Mechanism of Action. Sulfones inhibit bacterial dihydropteroate synthase, as do sulfonamides, and presumably inhibit *M. leprae* by the same mechanism.

Antimicrobial Activity. By mouse footpad inoculation, as little as 0.003 μg/ml of dapsone is estimated to inhibit multiplication of *M. leprae*. Dapsone has been described as "weakly bactericidal" for susceptible leprosy bacilli. In humans, it has been estimated that 99.9% of bacillary populations are killed after 3 to 4 months of dapsone therapy.[127] In lepromatous (multibacillary) patients on monotherapy, secondary dapsone resistance often emerges 5 to 24 *years* after commencing therapy.[128] Before the usage of current standard multidrug regimens, secondary resistance occurred in approximately 20% of cases.

Pharmacology. Dapsone is well absorbed orally. Distributed throughout body fluids, tissue concentrations are approximately 2 μg/ml. The plasma half-life of dapsone is 21 to 44 hours, with some drug retention for up to 3 weeks. Dapsone becomes acetylated, with 70 to 80% excreted as metabolites in urine. The dosage should be reduced accordingly in renal failure.

Adverse Reactions. An oxidant drug, dapsone produces dose-dependent hemolysis, which is not of clinical consequence in patients without a hematologic disorder taking dapsone 50 to 100 mg daily. Hemolysis is greatly enhanced in patients with glucose-6-phosphate dehydrogenase deficiency, especially in its severe forms. Gastrointestinal intolerance occurs with resulting anorexia, nausea, or vomiting. Hematuria, fever, pruritus, skin rashes, and granulocytopenia can occur.

Dapsone is now being used in AIDS patients as prophylaxis and treatment of *Pneumocystis pneumoniae* pneumonia. These patients usually have preexisting anemia, making dapsone-induced hemolysis less well tolerated. Conversion of up to 20% of erythrocyte hemoglobin to methemoglobin can occur with dapsone doses of 100 mg daily. Although methemoglobinemia is usually asymptomatic, it may become of clinical consequence if the patient develops hypoxemia from lung disease. Rash is common in this patient population. In one study using dapsone, 100 mg daily, for prophylaxis, 33 of 47 patients discontinued the drug.[129]

In leprosy patients, reactions with dapsone may be difficult to extricate from the reactions attendant with the disease itself.[130] A sulfone syndrome occurring 5 to 6 weeks after the initiation of therapy can be characterized by fever, jaundice, dermatitis, and lymphadenopathy—a presentation not unlike that of infectious mononucleosis.[131] During initial dapsone therapy, erythema nodosum leprosum reactions commonly become manifest in those with multibacillary disease.

Usage. Dapsone and rifampin are the principal therapeutic agents for the treatment of both multibacillary and paucibacillary *M. leprae* infections. Usage in pneumocystosis is discussed in Chapter 260. Dapsone is also useful in dermatatitis herpetiformis, a subject beyond the scope of this chapter.

Availability and Dosage. Dapsone is available generically in tablets of 25 or 100 mg. The adult daily dosage is 100 mg, and for children it is 1 to 1.5 mg/kg/day. It is administered daily for 6 months in paucibacillary disease and for a minimum of 2 years in multibacillary disease.

Rifampin

Mechanism of Action and Resistance. The mechanism of action of rifampin is presumed to be inhibition of *M. leprae* DNA-dependent RNA polymerase that produces a relatively rapid bactericidal effect. Its inhibitory concentration of human strains of *M. leprae* tested in mice is 0.3 μg/ml. Acquired rifampin resistance is caused by mutational changes in RNA polymerase.[132]

Usage. Clinical usage of rifampin has confirmed that it is more bactericidal by several orders of magnitude than all other antileprosy drugs either alone or in combination. It is considered the only rapidly bactericidal drug against *M. leprae*. Using a skin biopsy assay, a single 1500-mg dose of rifampin was determined to reduce the viability of leprosy bacilli to undetectable levels by 3 to 5 days.[133] Despite such a dramatic impact on numbers of tissue *M. leprae,* rifampin must be employed with one or more companion drugs to prevent the development of resistance.[127] The high cost of rifampin has discouraged daily usage in economically disadvantaged regions. However, once-monthly therapy with 600 to 1200 mg of rifampin in combination drug regimens has produced satisfactory clinical responses with a minimum of adverse reactions.[134] Current recommendations are that rifampin be administered in a single monthly supervised dose of 600 mg. This dosage is continued for 6 months in paucibacillary disease and for a minimum of 2 years in multibacillary disease. In the United States, rifampin is given as a 600-mg daily dose in both of the settings described. Reversal and erythema nodosum leprosum reactions with rifampin have been comparable or less severe than with sulfones alone.

Clofazimine (Lamprene)

Derivation and Structure. Clofazimine is a phenazine dye.

Mechanism of Action and Antimicrobial Activity. Clofazimine's precise mechanism of action is unknown. Highly lipophilic and bound to mycobacterial DNA, clofazimine is weakly bactericidal against *M. leprae*. Its action may relate to iron chelation with resulting production of nascent oxygen radicals intracellularly.[135] The inhibitory concentration of clofazimine in mouse tissue is between 0.1 and 1 mg/kg. A delay of some 50 days ensues before tissue antimicrobic activity can be demonstrated in humans.

Pharmacology. Clofazimine pharmacokinetics are complex. Absorption is quite variable, with 9 to 74% of an administered dose appearing in feces. Oral administration results in plasma concentrations of 0.4 to 3 μg/ml with a half-life of approximately 70 days. Clofazimine is widely distributed throughout reticuloendothelial tissues, especially liver, spleen, lung, adrenals, adipose tissue, and skin lesions. Red-orange phagocytized crystals of clofazimine are observed microscopically in macrophages. It is largely unmetabolized and subsequently slowly excreted with less than 1% in urine. Biliary excretion appears to be the major route of excretion. Excretion also occurs in breast milk. Dosage of 100 mg/day has been calculated to result eventually in a total accumulation of at least 10 g in human tissue.

Adverse Reactions. Gastrointestinal intolerance (anorexia, diarrhea, abdominal pain) is the most common therapy-limiting side effect and is generally dose related. Dry mouth and skin may occur. Skin pigmentation is quite common, resulting from drug accumulation and producing red-brown to nearly black discoloration, especially in dark-skinned persons.

Usage. Clofazimine's current role is principally in combination with rifampin and dapsone for multibacillary disease. It is also used in combination for sulfone-resistant infections and for individuals who are sulfone-intolerant, usually because of severe sulfone-associated erythema nodosum leprosum or reversal reactions. Such reactions occur much less often with clofazimine than with dapsone,[136] possibly because of anti-inflammatory properties of clofazimine.

Availability and Dosage. Clofazimine is supplied in 50- and 100-mg capsules. For multibacillary disease, it is administered in a dosage of 50 mg/day for a minimum of 2 years in combination with rifampin and dapsone. A dapsone alternative dosage has usually been 100 to 300 mg/day.

Additional or Second-Line Drugs

Thiacetazone (Amithiozone)

Thiacetazone's efficacy is greater in tuberculoid (paucibacillary) than in lepromatous (multibacillary) disease. It can be administered when sulfones are not tolerated. Considerable cross-resistance occurs with sulfones. Thiacetazone is unavailable in the United States.

Ethionamide and Prothionamide

Ethionamide (Trecator-SC) is described in the section "Second-Line Antituberculous Drugs." It and its congener prothionamide (not available in the United States) possess similar pharmacokinetics and dosing and provide alternatives to clofazimine in multidrug regimens for multibacillary disease in those who are unable to tolerate clofazimine or refuse it because of skin pigmentation. Ethionamide and prothionamide are apparently weakly bactericidal against *M. leprae.* Ethionamide is provided in 250-mg tablets. The usual dosage is 250 mg daily. Both agents are expensive and cause considerable gastrointestinal intolerance and occasional hepatitis.

Other Substituted Rifamycins

Rifabutin (Mycobutin) and rifapentine (Priftin) are substituted rifamycins active against *M. leprae.* Both were recently approved by the Food and Drug Administration in the United States. In mice, these compounds are even more active than rifampin,[137] which raises interest in their use, especially in intermittent regimens.

Other Sulfones

Acedapsone. Acedapsone (4,4′-diacetyldiaminodiphenyl sulfone) is a long-acting intramuscular repository derivative of dapsone. The parent compound possesses little activity against *M. leprae* but is metabolized into active dapsone. Its half-life is 46 days, and that of the derived dapsone is 43 days.[138] A 300-mg intramuscular dose maintains dapsone levels in volunteers above the inhibitory concentration for *M. leprae* for approximately 100 days. Microbiologic and clinical responses are somewhat slower than those for daily dapsone. Long-term studies with acedapsone by injection five times yearly have yielded encouraging results. Acedapsone shows promise especially in regions where, or in patients in whom, long-term oral therapy is not practical.

Sulfoxone. Less well absorbed and more expensive than dapsone, sulfoxone, a disubstituted sulfone, may be better tolerated gastrointestinally. It is formulated in 165-mg enteric-coated tablets, with a usual daily dosage of 300 mg.[13]

Newer Agents. Several other agents have shown promising activity against *M. leprae* in mouse foot pad models and early clinical trials. Among these are included minocycline (Minocin),[139] clarithromycin (Biaxin),[139] and fluorinated quinolones—perfloxacin, ofloxacin (Floxin),[140, 141] and especially sparfloxacin.[141] Their roles in replacing drugs in existing multidrug regimens remain to be determined, although none of these agents appear to be as bactericidal against *M. leprae* as rifampin. Current efforts with these newer agents are also focusing on short-course therapy[142] rather than the current standard 2-year regimens.

Chemotherapy-Associated Reactions in Leprosy

Febrile reactions in leprosy can be ameliorated with acetylsalicylic acid (aspirin) in conventional dosage. Immunologic reactions are common during chemotherapy. "Reversal" reactions associated with swelling and edema in preexisting skin lesions or peripheral neuropathy in more severe reactions usually occur in the first year of therapy. Corticosteroids such as prednisone 40 to 80 mg/day initially with subsequent tapering of dosage have been reasonably efficacious for reversal reactions.

For patients with erythema nodosum leprosum reactions, thalidomide in an initial dosage of 400 mg daily may be the treatment of choice. Its beneficial effect for these reactions appears to be mediated by the inhibition of tumor necrosis factor-α.[143] It should be tapered over the first week, with a maintenance dose of 50 to 100 mg/day. Thalidomide is commercially available for the treatment of leprosy, but its usage is tightly regulated. Because of its marked teratogenicity, thalidomide should never be administered to women of childbearing age. In patients with erythema nodosum leprosum for whom thalidomide is unacceptable, high-dose prednisone offers an alternative. Patients who manifest puzzling or severe reactions are best managed by specialists such as those at the Hansen's Disease Clinic in Carville, La.[130]

REFERENCES

1. Frieden TR, Sterling T, Pablos-Méndez A, et al. The emergence of drug-resistant tuberculosis in New York City. N Engl J Med. 1993;328:521–526.
2. Goble M, Iseman MD, Madsen LA, et al. Treatment of 171 patients with pulmonary tuberculosis resistant to isoniazid and rifampin. N Engl J Med. 1993;328:527–532.
3. Centers for Disease Control and Prevention. Outbreak of multidrug-resistant tuberculosis at a hospital—New York City, 1991. MMWR Morb Mortal Wkly Rept. 1993;42:427–434.
4. Pablos-Méndez A, Raviglione MC, Laszlo A, et al. Global surveillance for antituberculosis-drug resistance, 1994–1997. N Engl J Med. 1998;338:1641–1649.
5. Laraque F, Riley LW. Tuberculosis in HIV-infected patients. AIDS Reader. 1992;(Sept-Oct):171–180.
6. Eriki PP, Okera A, Aisu T, et al. The influence of human immunodeficiency virus infection on tuberculosis in Kampala, Uganda. Am Rev Respir Dis. 1991;143:185–187.
7. Iseman MD, Cohn DL, Sbarbaro JA. Directly observed treatment of tuberculosis. N Engl J Med. 1993;328:576–578.
8. Sensi P. Approaches to the development of new antituberculosis drugs. Rev Infect Dis. 1989;11(Suppl 2):S467–S470.
9. Pozniak AL, MacLeod GA, Mahari M, et al. The influence of HIV status on

single and multiple drug reactions to antituberculous therapy in Africa. AIDS. 1992;6:809–814.
10. Centers for Disease Control and Prevention. Impact of HIV protease inhibitors on the treatment of HIV-infected tuberculosis patients with rifampin. MMWR Morb Mortal Wkly Rep. 1996;45:921–925.
11. Gordon SM, Horsburgh CR, Peloquin CA, et al. Low serum levels of oral antimycobacterial agents in patients with disseminated *Mycobacterium avium* complex disease. J Infect Dis. 1993;168:1559–1562.
12. Bass JB, Jr, Farer LS, Hopewell PC, et al. Treatment of tuberculosis and tuberculosis infection in adults and children. American Thoracic Society Statement. Am J Respir Crit Care Med. 1994;149:1359–1374.
13. Mandell GL, Sande MA. Drugs used in the chemotherapy of tuberculosis and leprosy. In: Gilman AS, Rall TW, Nies AS, et al, eds. The Pharmacological Basis of Therapeutics. 8th ed. New York: Pergamon; 1990:1146–1164.
14. Kucers A, Bennett NM. Drugs mainly for tuberculosis. Part III. In: The Use of Antibiotics. 4th ed. Philadelphia: JB Lippincott; 1987:1351–1437.
15. Davidson PT, Hahn QL. Drug treatment of tuberculosis—1992. Drugs. 1992;43:651–673.
16. Starke JR. Current chemotherapy for tuberculosis in children. Infect Dis Clin North Am. 1992;6:215–238.
17. Centers for Disease Control and Prevention. Initial therapy for tuberculosis in the era of multidrug resistance. Recommendations of the Advisory Council for the Elimination of Tuberculosis. MMWR Morb Mortal Wkly Rep. 1993;42:1–8.
18. Musser JM, Kapur V, Williams DL, et al. Characterization of the catalase-peroxidase gene *(katG)* and *inhA* locus in isoniazid-resistant and -susceptible strains of *Mycobacterium tuberculosis* by automated DNA sequencing: Restricted array of mutations associated with drug resistance. J Infect Dis. 1996;173:196–202.
19. Musser JM. Antimicrobial agent resistance in mycobacteria: Molecular genetic insights. Clin Microbiol Rev. 1995;8:496.
20. Ormerod LP, Harrison JM, Wright PA. Drug resistance trends in *Mycobacterium tuberculosis*: Blackburn 1985–89. Tubercle. 1990;71:283–285.
21. Seifart HI, Parkin DP, Donald PR. Stability of isoniazid, rifampin and pyrazinamide in suspensions used for the treatment of tuberculosis in children. Pediatr Infect Dis J. 1991;10:827–831.
22. Kopanoff DE, Snider DE, Caras GJ. Isoniazid-related hepatitis. Am Rev Respir Dis. 1978;117:991–1001.
23. Krishnaswamy K, Prasad CE, Murthy KJ. Hepatic dysfunction in undernourished patients receiving isoniazid and rifampicin. Trop Geogr Med. 1991;43:156–160.
24. Franks AL, Binkin NJ, Snider DE, Jr, et al. Isoniazid hepatitis among pregnant and postpartum Hispanic patients. Public Health Rep. 1989;104:151–155.
25. Murphy R, Swartz R, Watkins PB. Severe acetaminophen toxicity in a patient receiving isoniazid. Ann Intern Med. 1990;113:799–800.
26. Wu JC, Lee SD, Yeh PF, et al. Isoniazid-rifampin-induced hepatitis in hepatitis B carriers. Gastroenterology. 1990;98:502–504.
27. Kumar A, Misra PK, Mehotra R, et al. Hepatotoxicity of rifampin and isoniazid. Is it all drug-induced hepatitis? Am Rev Respir Dis. 1991;143:1350–1352.
28. Deshpande DV, Nachne D, Koyande D, et al. Anti-tubercular treatment in patients with hepatitis. J Assoc Physicians India. 1991;143:1350–1352.
29. McGlynn KA, Lustbader ED, Sharrar RE, et al. Isoniazid prophylaxis in hepatitis B carriers. Am Rev Respir Dis. 1986;134:666–668.
30. Gangadharam PRJ. Isoniazid, rifampin, and hepatotoxicity. Am Rev Respir Dis. 1986;133:963–965.
31. Woo J, Chan HS. Therapeutic problems in the management of elderly patients with tuberculosis. Adverse Drug React Toxicol Rev. 1992;11:13–18.
32. Ansari MM, Beg MH, Haleem S. Hepatitis in patients with surgical complications of pulmonary tuberculosis. Indian J Chest Dis Allied Sci. 1991;33:133–138.
33. Centers for Disease Control and Prevention. Severe isoniazid-associated hepatitis—New York, 1991–1993. MMWR Morb Mortal Wkly Rep. 1993;42:545–547.
34. Jordan TJ, Lewit EM, Reichman LB. Isoniazid preventive therapy for tuberculosis. Decision analysis considering ethnicity and gender. Am Rev Respir Dis. 1991;144:1357–1360.
35. Ishii N, Nishibara Y. Pellagra encephalopathy among tuberculous patients: Its relation to isoniazid therapy. J Neurol Neurosurg Psychiatry. 1985;48:628–634.
36. Pellock JM, Howell J, Kendig EL, Jr, et al. Pyridoxine deficiency in children treated with isoniazid. Chest. 1985;87:658–661.
37. Schraufnagel DE, Stoner R, Whiting E, et al. Testing for isoniazid. An evaluation of the Arkansas method. Chest. 1990;98:314–316.
38. Koestner JA, Jones LK, Polk WH, et al. Prolonged use of intravenous isoniazid and rifampin. Drug Intell Clin Pharm. 1989;23:48–50.
39. Telenti A, Imboden P, Marchesi F, et al. Detection of rifampicin-resistance mutations in *Mycobacterium tuberculosis*. Lancet 1993;341:647–650.
40. Venkatesan K. Pharmacokinetic drug interactions with rifampin. Clin Pharmacokinet. 1992;22:47–65.
41. Immanuel C, Jayasankar K, Narayana AS, et al. Induction of rifampicin metabolism during treatment of tuberculous patients with daily and fully intermittent regimens containing the drug. Indian J Chest Dis Allied Sci. 1989;31:251–257.
42. Woo J, Leung A, Chan K, et al. Pyrazinamide and rifampicin regimens for patients on maintenance dialysis. Int J Artif Organs. 1988;11:181–185.
43. Newman R, Doster BE, Murray FJ, et al. Rifampin in initial treatment of pulmonary tuberculosis. A US Public Health Service tuberculosis therapy trial. Am Rev Respir Dis. 1974;109:216–232.
44. Mehta M, ed. Physicians' Desk Reference Guide to Drug Interactions, Side Effects, Indications. Montvale, NJ: Medical Economics Data; 1992:797–799.
45. Strayhorn VA, Baciewicz AM, Self TH. Update on rifampin drug interactions. III. Arch Intern Med. 1997;157:2453–2458.
46. Borcherding SM, Baciewicz AM, Self TH. Update on rifampin drug interactions. II. Arch Intern Med. 1992;152:711–716.
47. Wallace RJ, Jr, Glassroth J, Griffith DE, et al. American Thoracic Society Statement: Diagnosis and treatment of disease caused by nontuberculous mycobacteria. Am Rev Respir Crit Care Med. 1997;156:S1–S25.
48. Gordin F, et al. Abstract LB5. Prevention and treatment of opportunistic infections. Presented at the 5th Retrovirus Conference, Washington, DC, 1998.
49. Crowle AJ. Studies of antituberculosis chemotherapy with an in vitro model of human tuberculosis. Semin Respir Infect. 1986;1:262–264.
50. Rastogi N, Potar M, David HL. Pyrazinamide is not effective against intracellularly growing *Mycobacterium tuberculosis*. Antimicrob Agents Chemother. 1987;31:287.
51. Scorpio A, Lindholm-Levy P, Heifets L, et al. Characterization of *pncA* mutations in pyrazinamide-resistant *Mycobacterium tuberculosis*. Antimicrob Agents Chemother. 1997;41:540–543.
52. Sreevatsan S, Pan X, Zhang Y, et al. Mutations associated with pyrazinamide resistance in *pncA* of *Mycobacterium tuberculosis* complex organisms. Antimicrob Agents Chemother. 1997;41:636–640.
53. Donald PR, Seifart H. Cerebrospinal fluid pyrazinamide concentrations in children with tuberculous meningitis. Pediatr Infect Dis J. 1988;7:469–471.
54. Zierski M, Bek E. Side effects of drug regimens used in short-course chemotherapy for pulmonary tuberculosis. A controlled clinical study. Tubercle. 1980;61:41–49.
55. Ssanwijarja S, Kauffmann RH, te Velde J, et al. Tubulointerstitial nephritis associated with pyrazinamide. Neth J Med. 1989;34:40–46.
56. Namba S, Igari T, Nishiyama K, et al. A case of pyrazinamide-associated myoglobinuric renal failure. Jpn J Med. 1991;30:468–472.
57. Belanger AE, Besra GS, Ford ME, et al. The *embAB* genes of *Mycobacterium avium* encode an arabinosyl transferase involved in cell wall arabinan biosynthesis that is the target for the antimycobacterial drug ethambutol. Proc Natl Acad Sci U S A. 1996;93:11,919–11,924.
58. Alcaide F, Pfyffer GE, Telenti A. Role of *embB* in natural and acquired resistance to ethambutol in mycobacteria. Antimicrob Agents Chemother. 1997;41:2270–2273.
59. Chatterjee VK, Buchanan OR, Friedman AI, et al. Ocular toxicity following ethambutol in standard dosage. Br J Dis Chest. 1986;80:288–291.
60. Meier A, Sander P, Schaper K-J, et al. Correlation of molecular resistance mechanisms and phenotypic resistance levels in streptomycin-resistant *Mycobacterium tuberculosis*. Antimicrob Agents Chemother. 1996;40:2452–2454.
61. Honoré N, Cole ST. Streptomycin resistance in mycobacteria. Antimicrob Agents Chemother. 1994;38:238–242.
62. Dautzenberg B, Castellani P, Pellegrin J-L, et al. Early bactericidal activity of rifabutin versus that of placebo in treatment of disseminated *Mycobacterium avium* complex bacteremia in AIDS patients. Antimicrob Agents Chemother. 1996;40:1722–1725.
63. Heifets LB, Iseman MD, Lindholm-Levy PJ, et al. Determination of ansamycin MICs for *Mycobacterium avium* complex in liquid medium by radiometric and conventional methods. Antimicrob Agents Chemother. 1985;28:570–575.
64. Masur H, Tuazon C, Gill V, et al. Effect of combined clofazimine and ansamycin therapy on *Mycobacterium avium–Mycobacterium intracellulare* bacteremia in patients with AIDS. J Infect Dis. 1987;155:127–129.
65. O'Brien RJ, Lyle MA, Snider DE, Jr. Rifabutin (ansamycin LM 427): A new rifamycin-S derivative for the treatment of mycobacterial diseases. Rev Infect Dis. 1987;9:519–530.
66. Woodley CL, Kilburn JO. In vitro susceptibility of *Mycobacterium avium* complex and *Mycobacterium tuberculosis* strains to a spiro-piperidyl rifamycin. Am Rev Respir Dis. 1992;126:586–587.
67. Blaschke TF, Skinner MH. The clinical pharmacokinetics of rifabutin. Clin Infect Dis. 1996;22(Suppl 1):S15–S22.
68. Shafran SD, Deschenes J, Phillips P, et al. Uveitis and pseudojaundice during a regimen of clarithromycin, rifabutin, and ethambutol. N Engl J Med. 1994;330:438–439.
69. Frank MO, Graham MB, Wispelway B. Rifabutin and uveitis. N Engl J Med. 1994;330:868.
70. Griffith DE, Brown BA, Girard WM, et al. Adverse events associated with high-dose rifabutin in macrolide-containing regimens for the treatment of *Mycobacterium avium* complex lung disease. Clin Infect Dis. 1995;21:594–598.
71. Flexner C. HIV-protease inhibitors. N Engl J Med. 1998;338:1281–1291.
72. Grassi C, Peona V. Use of rifabutin in the treatment of pulmonary tuberculosis. Clin Infect Dis. 1996;22(Suppl 1):S50–S54.
73. Chan SL, Yew WW, Ma WK, et al. The early bactericidal activity of rifabutin measured by sputum viable counts in Hong Kong patients with pulmonary tuberculosis. Tubercle Lung Dis. 1992;73:33–38.
74. Hong Kong Chest Service/British Medical Research Council. A controlled study of rifabutin and an uncontrolled study of ofloxacin in the re-treatment of patients with pulmonary tuberculosis resistant to isoniazid, streptomycin and rifampicin. Tubercle Lung Dis. 1992;73:59–67.
75. Pretet S, Lebaeaut A, Parrot R, et al and the Group for the Study and Treatment of Resistant Mycobacterial Infections. Combined chemotherapy including rifabutin for rifampicin and isoniazid resistant pulmonary tuberculosis. Eur Respir J. 1992;5:680–684.
76. Grosset J, Lounis N, Truffot-Pernot C, et al. Once-weekly rifapentine-containing regimens for treatment of tuberculosis in mice. Am J Respir Crit Care Med. 1998;157:1436–1440.
77. Tam CM, Chan SL, Lam CW, et al. Rifapentine and isoniazid in the continuation

phase of treating pulmonary tuberculosis. Am J Respir Crit Care Med. 1998;157:1726–1733.

77a. Rifapentine—a long acting rifamycin for tuberculosis. Med Lett. 1999;41:21–22.

78. Klemens SP, Cynamon MH. Activity of KRM-1648 in combination with isoniazid against *Mycobacterium tuberculosis* in murine model. Antimicrob Agents Chemother. 1996;40:298–301.

79. Vernon A, Khan A, Bozeman L, et al. Update on US Public Health Service (USPHS) Study 22: A trial of once weekly isoniazid (NIH) and rifapentine (RPT) in the continuation phase of TB treatment. The USPHS Rifapentine Trial Group. Am J Respir Crit Care. 1998;157(S):A467.

80. Yew WW, Kwan SY, Ma WK, et al. In-vitro activity of ofloxacin against *Mycobacterium tuberculosis* and its clinical efficacy in multiply resistant pulmonary tuberculosis. J Antimicrob Chemother. 1990;26:227–236.

81. Leysen DC, Haemers A, Pattyn SR. Mycobacteria and the new quinolones. Antimicrob Agents Chemother. 1989;33:1–5.

82. Gay JD, DeYoung DR, Roberts GD. In vitro activities of norfloxacin and ciprofloxacin against *Mycobacterium tuberculosis, M. avium* complex, *M. chelonei, M. fortuitum,* and *M. kansasii.* Antimicrob Agents Chemother. 1984;26:94–96.

83. Chen CH, Shih JF, Lindholm-Levy PJ, et al. Minimal inhibitory concentrations of rifabutin, ciprofloxacin, and ofloxacin against *Mycobacterium tuberculosis* isolated before treatment of patients in Taiwan. Am Rev Respir Dis. 1989;140:987–989.

84. Caekenberghe DV. Comparative in vitro activities of ten fluoroquinolones and fusidic acid against *Mycobacterium* spp. J Antimicrob Chemother. 1990;26:381–386.

85. LaLande V, Truffot-Pernot C, Paccaly-Moulin A, et al. Powerful bactericidal activity of sparfloxacin (AT-4140) against *Mycobacterium tuberculosis* in mice. Antimicrob Agents Chemother. 1993;37:407–413.

86. Kohno S, Koga H, Kaku M, et al. Prospective comparative study of ofloxacin or ethambutol for the treatment of pulmonary tuberculosis. Chest. 1992;102:1815–1818.

87. Tsukamura M, Nakamura E, Yoshii S, et al. Therapeutic effect of new antibacterial substance ofloxacin (DL 8280) on pulmonary tuberculosis. Am Rev Respir Dis. 1985;131:352–356.

88. Takiff HE, Salazar L, Guerrero C, et al. Cloning and nucleotide sequence of *Mycobacterium tuberculosis gyrA* and *gyrB* genes and detection of quinolone resistance mutations. Antimicrob Agents Chemother. 1994;38:773–780.

89. McClatchy JK, Kanes W, Davidson PT, et al. Cross-resistance in *M. tuberculosis* to kanamycin, capreomycin, and viomycin. Tubercle. 1977;58:29–34.

90. Alangaden GJ, Kreiswirth BN, Aouad A, et al. Mechanism of resistance to amikacin and kanamycin in *Mycobacterium tuberculosis.* Antimicrob Agents Chemother. 1998;42:1295–1297.

91. Quemard A, Laneelle G, Lacave C. Mycolic acid synthesis: A target for ethionamide in mycobacteria? Antimicrob Agents Chemother. 1992;36:1316–1321.

92. Cynamon MH, Palmer GS. In vitro activity of amoxicillin in combination with clavulanic acid against *Mycobacterium tuberculosis.* Antimicrob Agents Chemother. 1983;24:429–431.

93. Chambers HF, Kocagöz T, Sipit T, et al. Activity of amoxicillin/clavulanate in patients with tuberculosis. Clin Infect Dis. 1998;26:874–877.

94. Wallace RJ, Jr, Brown BA, Onyi GO. Susceptibilities of *Mycobacterium fortuitum* biovar *fortuitum* and the two subgroups of *Mycobacterium chelonae* to imipenem, cefmetazole, cefoxitin, and amoxicillin-clavulanic acid. Antimicrob Agents Chemother. 1991;35:773–775.

95. Nozawa RT, Kato H, Yokota T, et al. Susceptibility of intra- and extracellular *Mycobacterium avium-intracellulare* to cephem antibiotics. Antimicrob Agents Chemother. 1985;27:132–134.

96. Wallace RJ, Jr, Swenson JM, Silcox VA, et al. Treatment of nonpulmonary infections due to *Mycobacterium fortuitum* and *Mycobacterium chelonei* on the basis of in vitro susceptibilities. J Infect Dis. 1985;152:500–514.

97. Kernodle DS. Editorial Response: β-Lactam drugs and tuberculosis. Clin Infect Dis. 1998;26:878–879.

98. Hawkins JE, Wallace RJ, Jr, Brown BA. Antibacterial susceptibility tests: mycobacteria. In: Balows A, ed. Manual of Clinical Microbiology. 5th ed. Washington, DC: American Society for Microbiology; 1991:1138–1152.

99. Brown BA, Wallace RJ, Jr, Onyi GO. Activities of clarithromycin against eight slowly growing species of nontuberculous mycobacteria, determined by using a broth microdilution MIC system. Antimicrob Agents Chemother. 1992;36:1987–1990.

100. Brown BA, Wallace RJ, Jr, Onyi GO, et al. Activities of four macrolides, including clarithromycin, against *Mycobacterium fortuitum, Mycobacterium chelonae,* and *Mycobacterium chelonae*-like organisms. Antimicrob Agents Chemother. 1992;36:1987–1990.

101. Laing RBS, Wynn RF, Leen CLS. New antimicrobials against *Mycobacterium marinum* infection. Br J Dermatol 1994;131(6):914.

102. Wallace RJ, Jr, Tanner D, Brennan PJ, et al. Clinical trial of clarithromycin for cutaneous (disseminated) infection due to *Mycobacterium chelonae.* Ann Intern Med. 1993;119:482–486.

103. Saubolle MA, Kiehn TE, White MH, et al. *M. haemophilum*: Microbiology and expanding clinical and geographic spectra of disease in humans. Clin Microbiol Rev. 1996;9:435–447.

104. Dautzenberg B, Truffot C, Legris S, et al. Activity of clarithromycin against *Mycobacterium avium* infection in patients with the acquired immune deficiency syndrome. A controlled clinical trial. Am Rev Respir Dis. 1991;144:564–569.

105. Young LS, Wiviott L, Wu M, et al. Azithromycin for treatment of *Mycobacterium avium-intracellulare* complex infection in patients with AIDS. Lancet. 1991;338:1107–1109.

106. Pierce M, Crampton S, Henry D, et al. A randomized trial of clarithromycin as prophylaxis against disseminated *Mycobacterium avium* complex infection in patients with advanced acquired immunodeficiency syndrome. N Engl J Med. 1996;335:384–391.

107. Oldfield EC, III, Fessel J, Dunne MW, et al. Once weekly azithromycin therapy for prevention of *Mycobacterium avium* complex infection in patients with AIDS: A randomized, double-blind, placebo-controlled multicenter trial. Clin Infect Dis. 1998;26:611–619.

108. Meier A, Kirschner P, Springer B, et al. Identification of mutations in 23S rRNA gene of clarithromycin-resistant *Mycobacterium intracellulare.* Antimicrob Agents Chemother. 1994;38:381–384.

109. Wallace RJ, Jr, Meier A, Brown BA, et al. Genetic basis for clarithromycin resistance among isolates of *Mycobacterium chelonae* and *Mycobacterium abscessus.* Antimicrob Agents Chemother. 1996;40:1676–1681.

110. Wallace RJ, Jr, Brown BA, Griffith DE, et al. Reduced serum levels of clarithromycin in patients treated with multidrug regimens including rifampin or rifabutin for *Mycobacterium avium–M. intracellulare* infection. J Infect Dis. 1995;171:747–750.

111. Brown BA, Wallace RJ, Jr, Griffith DE, et al. Clarithromycin-induced hepatotoxicity. Clin Infect Dis. 1995;20:1073–1074.

112. Brown BA, Griffith DE, Girard W, et al. Relationship of adverse events to serum drug levels in patients receiving high-dose azithromycin for mycobacterial lung disease. Clin Infect Dis. 1997;24:958–964.

113. Sanders WJ, Wolinsky E. In vitro susceptibility of *Mycobacterium marinum* to eight antimicrobial agents. Antimicrob Agents Chemother. 1980;18:529–531.

114. Wallace RJ, Jr, Dunbar D, Brown BA, et al. Rifampin-resistant *Mycobacterium kansasii.* Clin Infect Dis. 1994;18:736–743.

115. Nightingale SD, Cameron DW, Gordin FM, et al. Two controlled trials of rifabutin prophylaxis against *Mycobacterium avium* complex infection in AIDS. N Engl J Med. 1993;329:828–833.

116. Gordin F, et al. A placebo-controlled trial of rifabutin added to a regimen of clarithromycin and ethambutol in the treatment of *M. avium* complex (MAC) bacteremia. Abstract B/9. Presented at the 12th World AIDS Conference, Geneva, Switzerland, 1998.

117. Nozawa RT, Kato H, Yokota T. Intra- and extracellular susceptibility of *Mycobacterium avium-intracellulare* complex to aminoglycoside antibiotics. Antimicrob Agents Chemother. 1984;26:841–844.

118. Swenson JM, Thornsberry C, Silcox VA. Rapidly growing mycobacteria: Testing of susceptibility to 34 antimicrobial agents by broth microdilution. Antimicrob Agents Chemother. 1982;22:186–192.

119. Swenson JM, Wallace RJ, Jr, Silcox VA, et al. Antimicrobial susceptibility of five subgroups of *Mycobacterium fortuitum* and *Mycobacterium chelonae.* Antimicrob Agents Chemother. 1985;28:807–811.

120. Prammananan T, Sander P, Brown BA, et al. A single 16S ribosomal RNA substitution is responsible for resistance to amikacin and other 2-deoxystreptamine aminoglycosides in *Mycobacterium abscessus* and *Mycobacterium chelonae.* J Infect Dis. 1998;177:1573–1581.

121. Donta ST, Smith PW, Levitz RE, et al. Therapy of *Mycobacterium marinum* infections. Use of tetracyclines vs rifampin. Arch Intern Med. 1986;146:902–904.

122. Stone MS, Wallace RJ, Jr, Swenson JM, et al. Agar disk elution method for susceptibility testing of *Mycobacterium marinum* and *Mycobacterium fortuitum* complex to sulfonamides and antibiotics. Antimicrob Agents Chemother. 1983;24:486–493.

123. Gangadharam PRJ, Candler ER. Activity of some antileprosy compounds against *Mycobacterium intracellulare* in vitro. Am Rev Respir Dis. 1977;115:705–708.

124. Wallace RJ, Jr, Bledsole G, Sumter G, et al. Activities of ciprofloxacin and ofloxacin against rapidly growing mycobacteria with demonstration of acquired resistance following single-drug therapy. Antimicrob Agents Chemother. 1990;34:65–70.

125. Cynamon MH, Palmer GS. In vitro susceptibility of *Mycobacterium fortuitum* to *N*-formidoyl thienamycin and several cephamycins. Antimicrob Agents Chemother. 1982;22:1079–1081.

126. Public Health Service Centers for Disease Control and Prevention. Increase in prevalence of leprosy caused by dapsone-resistant *Mycobacterium leprae.* MMWR Morb Mortal Wkly Rep. 1982;30:637–638.

127. Hastings RC, Franzblau SG. Chemotherapy of leprosy. Annu Rev Pharmacol Toxicol. 1988;28:231–245.

128. Pearson JMH, Rees RJW, Waters MFR. Sulphone resistance in leprosy. A review of one hundred proven clinical cases. Lancet. 1975;2:69–72.

129. Blum RA, Miller LA, Gaggini LC, Cohn DL. Comparative trial of dapsone versus trimethoprim/sulfamethoxazole for primary prophylaxis of *Pneumocystis carinii* pneumonia. J Acquir Immune Defic Syndr. 1992;5:341–347.

130. Case records of the Massachusetts General Hospital. Weekly clinicopathological exercises. Case 49–1985. Erythema nodosum leprosum reaction in patient with lepromatous leprosy. N Engl J Med. 1985;313:1464–1472.

131. Adverse reactions to dapsone (Editorial). Lancet. 1981;2:184–185.

132. Honore N, Cole ST. Molecular basis of rifampin resistance in *Mycobacterium leprae.* Antimicrob Agents Chemother. 1993;37:414–418.

133. Shepard CC, Levy L, Fasal P. Further experience with the rapid bactericidal effect of rifampin on *Mycobacterium leprae.* Am J Trop Med Hyg. 1974;23:1120–1124.

134. Yawalkar SJ, Languillon J, Hajra SK, et al. Once-monthly rifampicin plus dapsone in initial treatment of lepromatous leprosy. Lancet. 1982;1:1199–1202.

135. Niwa Y, Sakance T, Miyachi Y, et al. Oxygen metabolism in phagocytes of leprotic patients: Enhanced endogenous superoxide dismutase activity and hydroxyl radical generation by clofazimine. J Clin Microbiol 1984;20:837–842.

136. US Leprosy Panel. Spaced clofazimine therapy of lepromatous leprosy. Am J Trop Med Hyg. 1976;25:437–444.
137. Pattyn SR. Rifabutin and rifapentine compared with rifampin against *Mycobacterium leprae* in mice. Antimicrob Agents Chemother. 1987;31:134.
138. Peters JH, Murray JF, Gordon GR, et al. Acedapsone treatment of leprosy patients: Response versus drug disposition. Am J Trop Med Hyg. 1977;26:127–136.
139. Ji B, Jamet P, Perani EG, et al. Powerful bactericidal activities of clarithromycin and minocycline against *Mycobacterium leprae* in lepromatous leprosy. J Infect Dis. 1993;168:188–190.
140. Ji B, Perani EG, Petinom C, et al. Clinical trial of ofloxacin alone and in combination with dapsone plus clofazimine for treatment of lepromatous leprosy. Antimicrob Agents Chemother. 1994;38:662–667.
141. Gelber RH, Iranmanesh A, Murray L, et al. Activities of various quinolone antibiotics against *Mycobacterium leprae* in infected mice. Antimicrob Agents Chemother. 1992;36:2522–2527.
142. Ji B, Jamet P, Sow S, et al. High relapse rate among lepromatous leprosy patients treated with rifampin plus ofloxacin daily for 4 weeks. Antimicrob Agents Chemother. 1997;41:1953–1956.
143. Sampaio EP, Kaplan G, Miranda A. The influence of thalidomide on the clinical and immunologic manifestation of erythema nodosum leprosum. J Infect Dis. 1993;168:404–414.

Chapter 35

Antifungal Agents

DAVID A. STEVENS
JOHN E. BENNETT

Both topical and systemic antifungal agents are discussed in this chapter, with an emphasis on pharmacology. Agents used to treat pneumocystosis are discussed in Chapter 39 because so many of the drugs used for this organism, now classified among the fungi, are also used to treat parasitic infections. Indications for treatment, dose and duration of therapy, and other details of treating pneumocystosis and other mycoses are discussed in Part III of this text and are not covered in depth here.

TOPICAL AGENTS

Topical Agents for Cutaneous Use

Use of topical agents is confined to infections of the epidermis, hair, nails, and cornea (Table 35–1). This form of application is not effective in deeper cutaneous infections such as sporotrichosis, blastomycosis, or chromomycosis. The choice between treating superficial infections with a topical or systemic agent depends on the fungus and on the site and extent of the lesion. For example, topical therapy is rarely used for ringworm of the scalp, nails, or extensive *Trichophyton rubrum* lesions of the trunk. The efficacy of topical agents in ringworm of the beard or in chronic noninflammatory sole and palm lesions also tends to be poor. Among the topical agents, the choice of formulation is important. Creams or solutions are preferred for fissured or inflamed intertriginous areas such as on the toe webs, groin, or scrotum. Use of powder, whether administered by a shake container or aerosol, is confined to mild lesions in those same areas or for preventive therapy in patients with repeated relapses of tinea pedis. Sprays are not recommended for the face. None of the preparations for cutaneous use should be applied to the vagina or eye. Secondary bacterial infection requires ancillary measures. Despite some antibacterial effect of the imidazoles in vitro, none of the antifungals included here have useful antibacterial activity.

The plethora of agents used for topical application necessitates that older agents with limited indications, such as iodine, sulfur, and gentian violet, not be discussed. Undecylenic acid and its salts, even though widely used in nonprescription formulations, have too little efficacy to warrant further comment. Although a list of over-the-counter (nonprescription) drugs would also include tolnaftate, clotrimazole, and miconazole, other agents can be expected to be added. Changes regarding which formulations of antifungal agents are marketed in combination with corticosteroids or antibacterial agents are also frequent. Details of the treatment of cutaneous mycoses are given in Chapter 257.

Salicylic and Benzoic Acids (Whitfield's Ointment). Salicylic acid is widely used in topical preparations as a keratolytic agent, often combined with other agents. The ointment marketed for nonprescription use in ringworm usually contains 3% salicylic acid and 6% benzoic acid. Although Whitfield's ointment can be used for mild tinea pedis, the occlusive effects of the ointment and mild irritation of the salicylic acid make the undiluted preparation inappropriate for inflamed or macerated toe webs or scrotal infections. Except for its low cost, there is little to recommend the use of Whitfield's ointment in ringworm.

Allylamines and Benzylamines. Allylamines, including naftifine and terbinafine, are synthetic compounds that inhibit squalene epoxidase, an enzyme essential for the synthesis of ergosterol (Fig. 35–1). Naftifine and terbinafine are available as 1% creams and are effective for the treatment of tinea pedis, tinea cruris, and tinea corporis. Butenafine, available as a 1% cream, is a benzylamine structurally related to the allylamines and has the same spectrum and clinical use.

Azoles. Azoles are synthetic compounds and include two classes, imidazoles and triazoles. The latter are named for the presence of three nitrogens in the azole ring, imidazoles having only two (see Fig. 35–1). The primary mechanism of action of azoles is inhibition of C-14α demethylase, an enzyme required for the synthesis of ergosterol. At the high concentrations that might be achieved topically, these agents directly damage the cytoplasmic membrane. The antifungal spectrum is extremely broad in vitro but often only fungistatic. Clinical efficacy has been demonstrated in ringworm of the body, foot, hand, and perineum, as well as in cutaneous candidiasis and tinea versicolor.

Morpholine Derivatives. Not listed in Table 35–1, amorolfine is available in some European countries as a 5% nail lacquer and a 0.25% cream. Based on limited data, use may be similar to that for topical azoles.

Polyenes. A large number of macrolide polyene antibiotics are known and have broad-spectrum antifungal activity in vitro. Topically, they are useful only against *Candida,* not ringworm. The hypertrophic skin lesions of chronic mucocutaneous candidiasis do not respond to these antibiotics, although macerated or intertriginous lesions typically respond well. These polyenes are derived by biosynthesis from aerobic actinomycetes, are poorly soluble in water, and share a common mechanism of action. Their antifungal activity depends on binding to membrane sterols such as ergosterol and thereby increasing membrane permeability. Other pharmacologic properties are discussed later. Nystatin and amphotericin B are available for topical use in the United States.

Topical Agents for Vaginal Use

Vulvovaginal candidiasis is a common disease that can cause substantial chronic discomfort. Both tablets and creams are marketed for once-a-day use, preferably at bedtime to facilitate retention. If candidiasis has extended onto the vulva or perineum, creams that can be applied topically as well as vaginally may have an advantage over tablets. Cream dispensers are designed to administer 5 g per use. The differences between creams and vaginal troches are less important than correct insertion deep in the vagina. During pregnancy, manual insertion of tablets is preferred to the use of a vaginal applicator. Persistence of drug in vaginal secretions long after application appears to enhance activity, particularly with azoles. Some

TABLE 35–1 Topical Treatment of Superficial Mycoses*

Drug (Trade Name)	Prescription Required	Formulation					Indications	
		Solution or Spray	*Lotion*	*Cream*	*Ointment*	*Powder*	*Ringworm*	*Candidiasis*
Azoles								
Clotrimazole (Fungoid, Lotromin, Mycelex)	No	+	+	+	0	0	+	+
Econazole (Spectazole)	Yes	0	0	+	0	0	+	+
Ketoconazole (Nizoral)	Yes	+	0	+	0	0	+	+
Miconazole (Micatin, Monistat-Derm)	No	+	+	+	0	+	+	+
Oxiconazole (Oxistat)	Yes	0	+	+	0	0	+	+
Sulconazole (Exelderm)	Yes	+	0	+	0	0	+	?
Polyenes								
Amphotericin B (Fungizone)	Yes	0	+	+	+	0	0	+
Nystatin (Mycostatin, Nilstat, Mykinac, Pedi-Dri)	Yes	0	0	+	+	+	0	+
Other								
Butenafine HCl (Mentax)	Yes	0	0	+	0	0	+	0
Ciclopirox (Loprox)	Yes	0	+	+	0	0	+	+
Haloprogin (Halotex)	Yes	0	0	+	0	0	+	+
Naftifine (Naftin)	Yes	0	0	+	+	+	+	0
Terbinafine (Lamisil)	Yes	0	0	+	0	0	+	0
Tolnaftate (Aftate, NP-27, Tinactin, Ting)	No	+	0	+	0	+	+	0
Undecylenate (Cruex, Desenex Antifungal)	No	+	0	+	+	+	+	0

*Formulations and over-the-counter sales reflect only the U.S. practice and are subject to change. Compounds that have formulations available without prescription often have other preparations that require prescription.

FIGURE 35–1. Structures of the major antifungal agents.

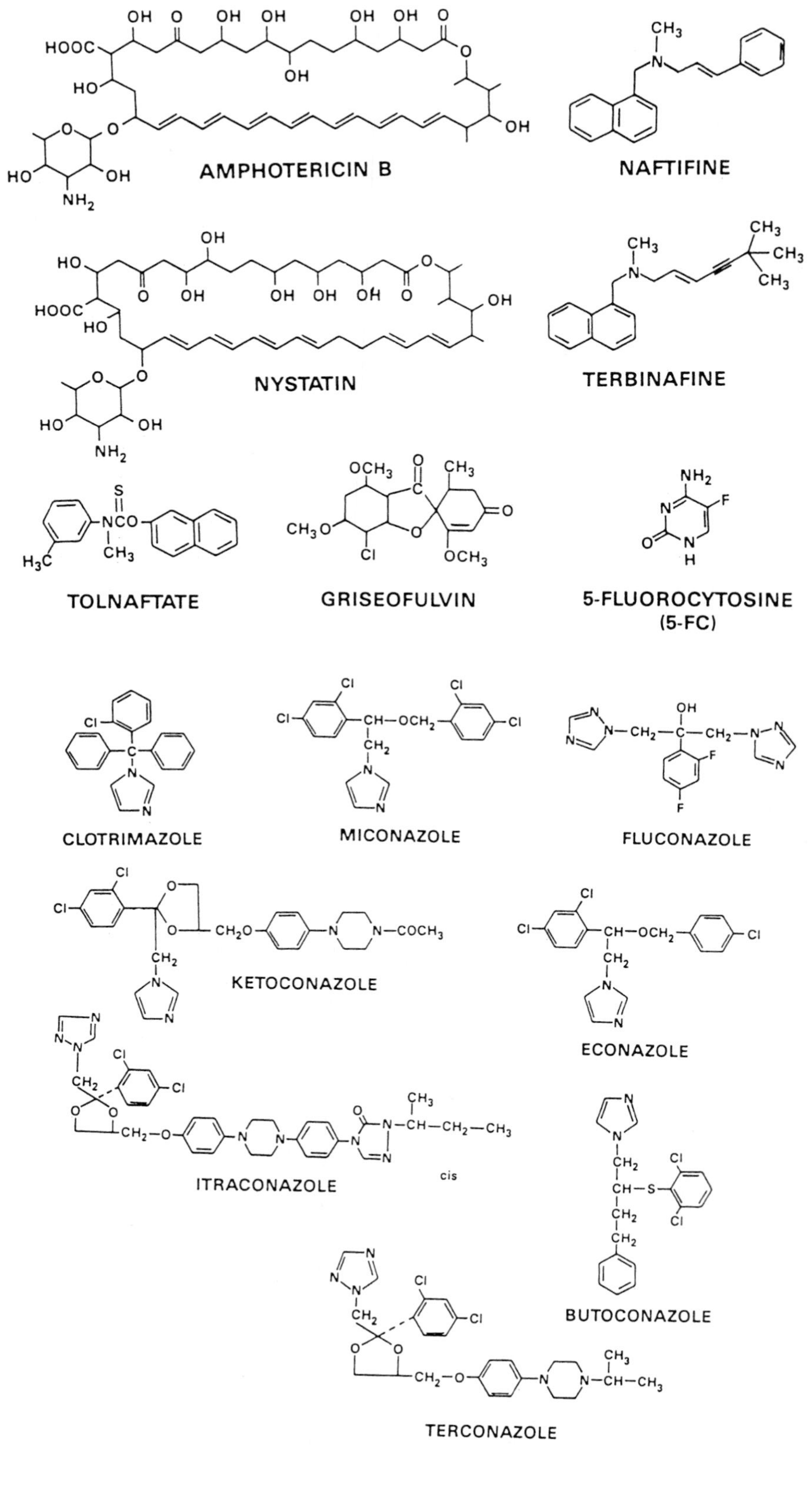

AMPHOTERICIN B

NAFTIFINE

NYSTATIN

TERBINAFINE

TOLNAFTATE

GRISEOFULVIN

5-FLUOROCYTOSINE (5-FC)

CLOTRIMAZOLE

MICONAZOLE

FLUCONAZOLE

KETOCONAZOLE

ECONAZOLE

ITRACONAZOLE

BUTOCONAZOLE

TERCONAZOLE

preparations have a patient package insert with a clear set of instructions. The duration of therapy is longer for polyene troches than for the imidazoles, which has led to increasing use of the latter class. Most of the studies of imidazoles have shown short-term efficacy of roughly 80 to 90% if high-risk patients are excluded, such as patients relapsing from recent treatment.[1] Although a fecal reservoir may be one source of relapse, the evidence of efficacy of oral nystatin to enhance therapy or prevent relapse is unconvincing.

Adverse effects of vaginal therapy are few. Allergy to any one imidazole probably precludes the use of other imidazoles. Local irritation or burning, rarely a serious problem, does vary among preparations. Some systemic absorption, generally less than 10% of the dose, has been documented for many of the vaginal imidazoles and may be a general phenomenon. Systemic absorption is of theoretical interest in that it might cause birth defects during the first trimester of pregnancy or alter the metabolism of other medications taken by the patient. However, none of these consequences have been observed. Systemic absorption of vaginal polyenes probably does not occur. The base used in some formulations may weaken some latex products such as condoms or diaphragms. A list of agents currently available for vaginal use in the United States is given in Table 35–2. The list of topical vaginal preparations available without a prescription is constantly expanding. Over-the-counter azoles account for approximately 80% of vaginal azole sales, which suggests that many women try these agents before seeking medical attention.

ORAL THERAPY FOR SUPERFICIAL MYCOSES

Agents for the Treatment of Oral and Esophageal Candidiasis (Thrush)

Nystatin (Mycostatin, Nilstat, and generic), named for New York State, is produced by *Streptomyces noursei.* The drug is available as an oral suspension of 100,000 units/ml. Adults should swish 5 to 10 ml around in the mouth three times per day. Swallowing the suspension rather than expectorating it may help treat subclinical esophageal candidiasis in immunosuppressed patients. Nystatin suspension is not absorbed from the gastrointestinal tract and, except for its bitter taste, is remarkably free of adverse effects. Nystatin pastilles (troches) can be held in the mouth until they dissolve. Oral amphotericin B is available as a suspension in the United States and as tablets overseas. This suspension is well tolerated and is less bitter than nystatin.[1a] The recommended dose is 1 ml (100 mg) four times daily. As with nystatin suspension, it is most effective when used after meals and at bedtime. Swishing in the mouth for 3 to 4 minutes before swallowing is preferred to enhance mucosal contact. An alternative topical agent is clotrimazole troches. These pleasant-tasting 10-mg tablets are effective in oral thrush when used five times per day. Each tablet should not be chewed, but kept in the mouth until it dissolves. Although some absorption occurs after the drug is swallowed, no adverse effects or systemic efficacy occurs. Oral ketoconazole, 200 to 400 mg/day, is also effective in oral candidiasis. The 400-mg dose is recommended for patients in the late stages of acquired immunodeficiency syndrome (AIDS). These patients absorb ketoconazole less well because they have reduced gastric acidity. Fluconazole, 100 to 400 mg once daily, is more effective than ketoconazole in AIDS patients with oropharyngeal or esophageal candidiasis, possibly because fluconazole is reliably absorbed even in the absence of gastric acid.[2] Chronic administration of fluconazole has led to azole-resistant oropharyngeal candidiasis in patients in the late stages of AIDS.[3] Intravenous amphotericin B remains a useful drug in patients with esophageal candidiasis who fail fluconazole therapy.

TABLE 35–2 Topical Treatment of *Candida* Vulvovaginitis

Drug	Representative Trade Names	Dose*	Duration (Days)
Azoles			
Creams and ointments			
Butoconazole 2%	Femstat	5 g	3 or 6†
Clotrimazole 1%	Gyne-Lotrimin,‡ Mycelex-7‡	5 g	7–14
Miconazole 2%	Monistat 7‡	5 g	7
Terconazole 0.4%	Terazole 7	5 g	7
Tioconazole 6.5%	Vagistat-1	4.6 g	1
Tablets or suppositories			
Clotrimazole	Gyne-Lotrimin,‡ Mycelex-7‡	100 mg	7§
Clotrimazole	Gyne-Lotrimin, Mycelex-G	500 mg	1
Miconazole	Monistat 7‡	100 mg	7
Miconazole	Monistat 3‡	200 mg	3
Terconazole	Terazole 3	80 mg	3
Polyenes			
Suppository			
Nystatin	Mycostatin, Nilstat	100,000 units	14

*All medications given at bedtime. Dose of cream refers to total weight, including excipient.
†Duration for pregnant patients.
‡Preparations available in the United States without prescription.
§Alternatively, two tablets may be used each night for 3 nights.
Adapted from Kwon-Chung KJ, Bennett JE. Medical Mycology. Philadelphia: Lea & Febiger; 1992:98–99.

Oral Therapy for Superficial Cutaneous Infections

Systemic therapy for ringworm of the scalp, beard, and nails is preferred to topical therapy. Chronic noninflammatory ringworm of the soles and palms, as well as extensive ringworm of the trunk or groin, may also require systemic therapy. Griseofulvin is usually effective and has a low incidence of side effects. Candidiasis of the nail or skin, particularly of the groin, can closely resemble ringworm and does not respond to griseofulvin. Itraconazole and terbinafine have supplanted griseofulvin for the treatment of tinea corporis, onychomycosis, and tinea capitis. These drugs are incorporated into the proximal, growing edge of the nail, and healthy, drug-containing nail gradually replaces infected nail in a distal direction. Replacement of the diseased with healthy nail can be very slow, often 10 months for a toenail. Because terbinafine and itraconazole accumulate in the growing nail, shorter courses, such as 4 months for a toenail, can produce reasonable cure rates and relapse rates of 50% or less.[4–7] Daily therapy with itraconazole, 200 mg, or terbinafine, 250 mg, is the most effective regimen, but double-dose itraconazole (400 mg) for 1 week of each month is a cost-effective alternative[6] (see Chapter 257).

Griseofulvin. Griseofulvin, derived from a species of *Penicillium,* is active against ringworm but not against *Candida* or tinea versicolor. It is poorly active topically but reaches the skin and hair after ingestion. Absorption is favored by reducing the particle size and perhaps by ingestion with a fatty meal. A microcrystalline form (generic, Fulvicin-U/F, Grifulvin V, and Grisactin) is available as 125-, 250-, and 500-mg tablets, plus a pediatric suspension of 125 mg/5 ml. The ultramicrocrystalline form (Fulvicin P/G, Gris-PEG, and Grisactin Ultra) comes in 125-, 165-, 250-, and 330-mg tablets. The two forms have comparable efficacy. Griseofulvin is metabolized in the liver with a serum half-life of 24 to 36 hours. Blood levels can be depressed by phenobarbital therapy and may require increasing the griseofulvin dose. Conversely, metabolism of warfarin anticoagulants is increased by griseofulvin. Central nervous system effects of ethanol ingestion are magnified by griseofulvin. Adverse reactions to griseofulvin are uncommon. Headache may be observed early in therapy but usually disappears with continued use. Allergic reactions can occur, apparently unrelated to penicillin allergy. Hepatotoxic reactions have been observed in patients with acute intermittent porphyria. Gastrointestinal intolerance and photosensitivity have been observed. Safety during pregnancy has not been established.

The usual daily dose is 500, 750, or 1000 mg daily for the microcrystalline drug, with children receiving 10 mg/kg. The 500-mg/day dose is reserved for mild infections and small adults. A dose of 330 mg daily is recommended for the ultramicrocrystalline form. Either preparation can be given once daily at the end of a meal, but dividing the dose into twice-daily administration may help maintain therapeutic levels in the epidermis and is recommended for refractory infections.

Ketoconazole and Itraconazole. The pharmacologic properties of the oral agents ketoconazole and itraconazole are discussed later. Both drugs are effective for ringworm, chronic mucocutaneous candidiasis, and tinea versicolor. Itraconazole, despite its cost, has become favored over ketoconazole for superficial mycoses because of the latter drug's endocrine side effects and rare, but potentially lethal hepatotoxicity. Itraconazole has a number of drug interactions but is a safe drug, a major consideration during the long duration required to treat onychomycosis.

Terbinafine. The oral agent terbinafine, an allylamine structurally related to naftifine, is effective in treatment of ringworm, including onychomycosis, and is comparable to azoles and superior to griseofulvin.[7] It is 99% protein-bound. Terbinafine is metabolized in the liver and has an initial half-life of 12 hours. The drug accumulates in skin, nails, and fat. Probably because of its accumulation in fat and subsequent release, terbinafine persists in plasma for 4 to 8 weeks after dosing and has a terminal half-life of 200 to 400 hours. Clearance is slower in the presence of liver or renal impairment. Rifampin markedly increases and cimetidine modestly decreases terbinafine clearance, and cyclosporine clearance is slightly enhanced. Side effects, principally gastrointestinal and taste complaints, rarely limit therapy. Hepatitis is an uncommon side effect.

Systemic Therapy for *Candida* Vulvovaginitis

Ketoconazole, Itraconazole, and Fluconazole. Ketoconazole at 400 mg daily for 5 days is effective for the treatment of *Candida* vulvovaginitis but is not approved for this use by the Food and Drug Administration (FDA) and is no longer recommended. The potential hepatotoxicity even with a 5-day course and the concern about fetal malformation have prevented widespread acceptance of this regimen. Fluconazole is approved by the FDA for this use, is given as a single dose, and has a better safety record than ketoconazole does, which makes it the preferred oral regimen. Both drugs can be used during menstruation and are convenient. A single 150-mg dose provides a cure rate as good as that of topical azole therapy.[8] Rare reports of infants with severe craniofacial bone and cardiac abnormalities who were born to mothers taking long term 400- to 800-mg daily doses of fluconazole serve as a cautionary note that fluconazole, even as a single dose, is not an appropriate drug for vulvovaginal candidiasis during pregnancy. In one study, itraconazole, 400 mg on 1 day, gave results equivalent to those after fluconazole, 50 mg daily for 3 days.[9] Itraconazole is not approved by the FDA for use in *Candida* vulvovaginitis. Itraconazole and fluconazole are both pregnancy class C.

TREATMENT OF DEEP MYCOSIS

Amphotericin B

Mechanism of Action. Amphotericin B is produced by *Streptomyces nodosus*. The drug is a lipophilic, rodlike molecule (Fig. 35–1) that exerts its antifungal effect by insertion into the fungal cytoplasmic membrane, probably orienting as head-to-tail oligomers perpendicular to the plane of the membrane.[10] The drug exists as aggregates in the cytoplasmic membrane and is closely bound to sterols such as ergosterol. Amphotericin B causes membrane permeability to increase. At lower drug concentrations, K^+ channel activity is increased.[11] At higher concentrations, pores 40 to 105 nm in size are formed in the membrane. Loss of intracellular potassium and other molecules impairs fungal viability. The onset of action is rapid and unrelated to the growth rate, consistent with the concept that the drug acts at preformed sites and no metabolic processing is required before a target is exposed. Amphotericin B also has effects on oxidation that may enhance antifungal activity. Although modest degrees of amphotericin B resistance can be selected under drug pressure in vitro, such strains have altered membrane sterols, reduced growth rates, and decreased virulence. Most clinical isolates of *Candida* spp., particularly *Candida lusitaniae,* that have been less susceptible to amphotericin B have been isolated from mucocutaneous surfaces or urine and may not be capable of causing deep infection.[12] Correlation of antifungal activity in *Candida*-infected mice with in vitro susceptibility depends on assay conditions.

Amphotericin B Deoxycholate. Amphotericin B deoxycholate (ABD) is insoluble in water at physiologic pH. The drug is marketed for intravenous use as a powder containing amphotericin B, 50 mg, sodium deoxycholate, 41 mg, and sodium phosphate buffer, 25.2 mg. Although a clear yellow solution forms when the powder is hydrated, the colloidal nature of ABD is easy to demonstrate. If a filter with a 0.22-μ pore diameter is placed in the infusion line, considerable drug is removed by the filter. The addition of electrolyte will aggregate the colloids, so the solution becomes cloudy when saline or sodium bicarbonate is added to an ABD solution. All currently available lipid-complexed amphotericin B formulations also must be infused in 5% dextrose with no electrolytes added. Infusion bottles need not be protected from light as older product brochures advocated.

Lipid-Complexed Amphotericin B. Three amphotericin B formulations are available in the United States: amphotericin B colloidal dispersion (ABCD, Amphotec), amphotericin B lipid complex (ABLC, Ablecet), and liposomal amphotericin B (AmBisome).[13] All three result in lower kidney concentrations in animals and are less nephrotoxic than ABD. All generally require higher doses in experimental animals to achieve the same therapeutic effect as ABD. Acute febrile infusion-related reactions can occur with all three preparations early in the course of therapy but are generally less than seen with ABD, with the notable exception of ABCD. Randomized clinical trials comparing ABD with any of the lipid-complexed formulations are needed. Randomized comparisons have been in febrile neutropenic patients. The other comparative studies have been heavily flawed and almost uninterpretable historical analyses. These anecdotal studies suggest that in infections outside the central nervous system, the lipid-complexed amphotericins can provide an effect equal but not superior to that of ABD, albeit at a higher dose. The place of lipid-complexed amphotericin B is to replace ABD in patients in whom unacceptable nephrotoxicity has developed or whose renal function is so borderline that they are unlikely to tolerate a therapeutic ABD regimen. Cost remains a critical issue in prescribing a lipid-complexed amphotericin B, with a therapeutic dose of ABCD and ABLC currently costing about 30-fold and AmBisome 60-fold more than ABD.

ABCD, which contains cholesterol sulfate in equimolar amounts to amphotericin B, forms disklike colloidal particles about 122 ± 48 nm in diameter. Like ABD, it forms a clear yellow solution when hydrated. However, the pharmacokinetics of ABCD differ substantially, with much lower serum concentrations and, in animals, higher liver amphotericin B concentrations. A randomized prospective, double-blind comparison of ABD, 0.8 mg/kg/day and ABCD, 4 mg/kg/day was done in neutropenic patients whose fever had not abated after 72 hours of antibacterial therapy.[14] Efficacy was the same in the 98 patients receiving ABCD as in the 95 receiving ABD, with 53 and 58%, respectively, becoming afebrile after 48 hours and 14 versus 15% having a suspected or documented mycosis emerge during amphotericin B therapy. Acute febrile reactions were significantly more common with ABCD than ABD, with hypoxia developing in 15 versus 3%. The percentage of patients having amphotericin B therapy discontinued because of some toxicity was the same in the two arms (14 versus 15%), with the ABD discontinuations much more often being due to azotemia. Herbrecht has reviewed the manufacturer's data on toxicity and noted that use of the drug was discontinued because of adverse events in 12.2%, about half of which were infusion-related events.[15] Nephrotoxicity has been minimal, even up to the maximal tolerable dose of 7.5 mg/kg. At 8 mg/kg, three of five patients had rigors, chills, and hypotension.[16] Analysis of the company's data from treating 82 patients with suspected or proven aspergillosis demonstrated nephrotoxicity in only 8%.[17] Problems in study design and data collection prevent assessment of efficacy in aspergillosis from that study. Because the company's data were largely confined to patients who had received prior ABD, the FDA approved ABCD only for one indication, invasive aspergillosis in patients in whom renal impairment precludes the use of ABD or in whom ABD therapy has failed. The recommended dose for adults and children is 3 to 4 mg/kg once daily infused as 0.6 mg/ml at a rate of 1 mg/kg/hour. The infusion can be speeded to a duration of 2 hours for patients who tolerate the drug well. Premedication with acetaminophen has not been studied prospectively but should be considered.

ABLC is a complex of almost equimolar concentrations of amphotericin B and lipid, the latter being a 7:3 mixture of dimyristoylphosphatidylcholine and dimyristoylphosphatidylglycerol. The drug is shipped as a cloudy suspension with particles 1.6 to 11 μm in diameter (an erythrocyte is 7 μm in diameter). Particle shape is not globular but ribbon-like. The manufacturer provides a device for the pharmacy to filter out aggregates larger than 5 μm before dispensing in 5% dextrose solution. Serum concentrations are about one fifth those of ABD at the same dose, but the recommended dose is fivefold higher than that of ABD, that is, 5 mg/kg once daily infused as 1.0 mg/ml over a 2-hour period. If longer infusion times are used, the bottle should be shaken to resuspend the particles. Data on efficacy come from the manufacturer's open-label, noncomparative study of 556 patients who had received prior ABD.[18] Only 291 were considered to have a documented mycosis and had sufficient data to evaluate the drug's therapeutic effect. If all the mycoses are considered together, a complete response to ABLC was judged to have occurred in 25% and a partial response in 32%. The study design did not permit an estimate of efficacy for any mycosis, but failure in three of six patients with cryptococcal meningitis raised the question of whether ABLC is suitable for central nervous system infections. ABLC provided fewer conversions of cerebrospinal fluid cultures to negative in a randomized comparison with ABD in cryptococcal meningitis, although the ABLC-treated patients appeared to be sicker at the start and a variety of regimens were used, including low and intermittent dosing.[19] The drug is approved by the FDA for the treatment of patients with "invasive fungal infections" who have failed to respond to or have become intolerant of ABD. Toxicity has been similar to that of ABD, but much less frequent.

AmBisome is a unilamellar liposome about 55 to 75 nm in diameter that contains roughly one molecule of amphotericin B per nine molecules of lipid. The latter is a mixture of hydrogenated soy lecithin-cholesterol-distearoylphosphatidylglycerol in a 10:5:4 ratio. Unlike the other lipid-complexed amphotericins, serum concentrations are not lower than those obtained with the same dose of ABD. Data on efficacy in mycoses come from retrospective case reviews of patients not responding to or intolerant of ABD.[20] The European Organization for Research and Treatment of Cancer conducted a prospective randomized comparison of 1 and 3 mg/kg AmBisome in 120 patients with proven and probable aspergillosis.[21] Of the 87 evaluable patients, responses were the same in the 41 receiving 1 mg/kg as the 46 receiving 4 mg/kg. No subset of patients could be found in whom the higher, more expensive dose was more effective. Unlike the other lipid-complexed amphotericins, several case series describe favorable responses in cryptococcal meningitis.[22] Three prospective randomized studies, in both adults and children, have compared AmBisome with ABD in neutropenic patients with fever not responsive to 96 hours of antibacterial antibiotics. The U.S. study compared 343 patients receiving 1.5 to 6.0 mg/kg AmBisome daily and 344 adults receiving 0.3 to 1.2 mg/kg ABD daily.[22a] Even though some patients received subtherapeutic doses of ABD, the two regimens had identical efficacy. A subset analysis of possible and proven mycoses emerging during therapy has proved difficult to interpret because the numbers were small and the infections occurred over a range of doses. A report of two combined studies in Europe that compared ABD, 1 mg/kg with AmBisome, 3 mg/kg, also found equal efficacy in neutropenic patients failing 96 hours of antibacterial therapy.[23] No difference was noted in mycoses emerging during empirical therapy. Both studies showed that AmBisome caused less nephrotoxicity and less severe hypokalemia than ABD did. AmBisome is approved in the United States for empirical treatment of neutropenic patients at a recommended dose of 3 mg/kg daily. The drug is also approved at a recommended dose of 3 to 5 mg/kg for patients with cryptococcosis, candidiasis, or aspergillosis who are intolerant to or fail to respond to ABD. Infusion as 1 to 2 mg/ml over a 2-hour period is recommended. Infusion intervals can be shortened to 60 minutes for patients in whom the treatment is well tolerated, but short infusions can be accompanied by dyspnea with chest tightness or hypoxia.[24] AmBisome is the only lipid-complexed amphotericin B formulation that does not contraindicate the use of an in-line filter, although pore size should be at least 1.0 μm.

Some hospitals have been mixing ABD with Intralipid (Pharmacia), a parenteral fat emulsion, at an ABD concentration of 1 to 2 mg/ml of lipid for intravenous infusion. Less nephrotoxicity in adults has been observed with this preparation at a dose of 1 mg/kg daily than with infusions of ABD in 5% dextrose.[25] No advantage was found in children.[25a] Serum amphotericin B concentrations were also lower with the fat emulsion, which raises the possibility that amphotericin B was simply aggregating in the fat emulsion but the cloudiness could not be perceived in the milky-looking lipid.

Pharmacology. Concentrations of amphotericin B in biologic fluids have usually been measured by bioassay,[26] but high-pressure liquid chromatography,[27] immunoassay,[28] and radiometric respirometry[29] have been described. Despite the proliferation of methods, routine determination of amphotericin B serum, urine, or cerebrospinal fluid concentrations has no definite clinical value. Nonetheless, amphotericin B assays have revealed some remarkable pharmacologic properties of this drug. When colloidal amphotericin B is admixed in serum, desoxycholate separates from amphotericin B, and more than 95% of the latter binds to serum proteins, principally to β-lipoprotein. Presumably the drug is bound to the cholesterol carried on this protein. Most of the drug leaves the circulation promptly, perhaps bound to cholesterol-containing cytoplasmic membranes. Amphotericin B is stored in the liver and other organs; the drug appears to reenter the circulation slowly. Most of the drug is degraded in situ, with only a small percentage being excreted in urine or bile. Blood levels are uninfluenced by hepatic or renal failure. Hemodialysis does not alter blood levels, except in an occasional patient with lipemic plasma who may be losing drug by adherence to the dialysis membrane. Concentrations of amphotericin B in fluid from inflamed areas, such as pleura, peritoneum, joint, vitreous humor, and aqueous humor, are roughly two thirds of the trough serum level. Cord blood from one infant contained an amphotericin B concentration of 0.37 μg/ml, half the simultaneous maternal trough blood level. Amphotericin B penetrates poorly into either normal or inflamed meninges, saliva, bronchial secretions, brain, pancreas, muscle, bone, vitreous humor, or normal amniotic fluid. Urine concentrations are similar to serum concentrations. Peak serum concentrations with conventional intravenous doses are roughly 0.5 to 2.0 μg/ml but rapidly fall initially to slowly approach a plateau of roughly 0.2 to 0.5 μg/ml.[26] The initial half-life is about 24 hours; the β-phase half-life is roughly 15 days. Serum concentrations can be detected for at least 7 weeks after the end of therapy, presumably reflecting release from cell membranes. The drug also has complex immunomodulatory properties, potentially of clinical significance but presently undefined.

Toxicity of Amphotericin B Deoxycholate

Nephrotoxicity. ABD causes a dose-dependent decrease in the glomerular filtration rate. The direct vasoconstrictive effect of amphotericin B on afferent renal arterioles results in reduced glomerular and renal tubular blood flow.[30] Other primary or secondary effects on the kidney include potassium, magnesium, and bicarbonate wasting and decreased erythropoietin production. Permanent loss of renal function is related to the total dose, not the level of temporary azotemia, and is due to destruction of renal tubular cells, disruption of tubular basement membrane, and loss of functioning nephron units. Saline loading, such as infusion of 1 liter of saline before ABD, has been associated with reduced nephrotoxicity in some studies but not others.[31] Potassium wasting often requires supplemental oral or intravenous potassium. Renal tubular acidosis from bicarbonate wasting rarely requires base replacement, but other drugs and diseases that promote acidosis may act synergistically.

Azotemia caused by amphotericin B is often worse in patients taking other nephrotoxic drugs such as cyclosporine or aminoglycosides. Hypotension, intravascular volume depletion, renal transplantation, and other preexisting renal disease all magnify the management problems associated with amphotericin B–induced azotemia.

Early in a course of amphotericin B, azotemia may increase rapidly, often falls a little, and then stabilizes after several days. Adults with no other renal disease will have an average serum creatinine level of 2 to 3 mg/dl at therapeutic doses, and therapy should not be withheld unless azotemia exceeds this level. Attempting to give amphotericin B to an adult without causing azotemia will usually lead to inadequate therapy.

Other Chronic Toxicity. Nausea, anorexia, and vomiting are common. Phlebitis occurs if peripheral vein catheters are used. Normocytic normochromic anemia occurs gradually and is associated with decreased plasma erythropoietin levels. The hematocrit rarely falls below 20 to 25% unless other causes of anemia are present. Rarely, thrombocytopenia, modest leukopenia, arrhythmias, coagulopathy, hemorrhagic enteritis, tinnitus, vertigo, encephalopathy, seizures, hemolysis, or dysesthesia of the soles of the feet may be observed.

Acute Reactions. About 30 to 45 minutes after beginning the first few amphotericin B infusions, chills, fever, and tachypnea may occur, peak in 15 to 30 minutes, and slowly abate over a period of 2 to 4 hours. A patient with underlying cardiac or pulmonary disease may have hypoxemia. These reactions are less common in young children or patients receiving adrenal corticosteroids. Subsequent infusions of the same dose cause progressively milder reactions. Premedication with acetaminophen or the addition of hydrocortisone, 25 to 50 mg, to the infusion solution can diminish the reactions. Meperidine given early in a chill can shorten the rigor. Concern about this kind of reaction in an unstable patient had led some physicians to use a test dose of 1 mg given over a 15-minute period to assess the subsequent reaction over 1 hour before deciding whether the next dose should be a full therapeutic dose of at least 0.5 mg/kg or an intermediate dose. Whether or not a test dose is given, patients with rapidly progressive mycoses should receive a full therapeutic dose within 24 hours, without any delay entailed by test or intermediate doses. Equally important, this reaction should not be mistaken for anaphylaxis or otherwise considered a contraindication to further amphotericin B. Allergic reactions to amphotericin B are extremely rare.

Administration. ABD is infused in 5% dextrose over a 2- to 4-hour infusion interval. Infusion 1 hour in duration appears to generally be safe for persons who have tolerated slower infusions and may be advantageous for outpatient therapy.[32, 33] Early in the course of therapy, fever is more pronounced with infusion intervals of only 45 minutes than infusion lasting 4 hours.[34] Rapid infusion in patients with severely compromised renal function may lead to acute, marked hyperkalemia and ventricular fibrillation.

Once therapy is well under way, patients receiving a stable daily dose may be changed to a double dose on alternate days to reduce the frequency of infusion-associated toxicity, particularly anorexia, and as a convenience for outpatient therapy. Doses above 1.5 mg/kg are not generally given on this schedule because the toxicity of such infusions is not well described. This strategy does not have a substantial effect on toxicity. A common misconception is that amphotericin B may be switched to alternate-day administration at the same dose as daily therapy. This dosage results in reduced trough serum concentrations and may lead to serious underdosing.

Dosage. Daily ABD doses of 0.3 mg/kg often suffice for esophageal candidiasis. A dose of 0.5 mg/kg is appropriate for blastomycosis, disseminated histoplasmosis, and extracutaneous sporotrichosis. Patients with cryptococcal meningitis are generally given doses of 0.6 to 0.8 mg/kg; those with coccidioidomycosis may require doses of 1 mg/kg. Patients with mucormycosis or invasive aspergillosis are given daily doses of 1 to 1.5 mg/kg until improvement is clearly present. Doses of 0.5 to 1.0 mg/kg are often used in neutropenic patients receiving empirical amphotericin B (see Chapter 300).[35] Local instillation of amphotericin B into cerebrospinal fluid, joints, or pleura is rarely indicated. One exception is coccidioidal meningitis, which is treated with intrathecal amphotericin B because it may produce superior results, particularly in the long term, although with far greater toxicity than seen with systemic azole therapy. Intraocular administration for fungal endophthalmitis is occasionally used; doses of 10 μg appear to avoid retinal toxicity. Corneal baths with 1 mg/ml in sterile water are useful for fungal keratitis but are irritating. Bladder irrigation with 50 μg/ml in sterile water is useful for patients with *Candida* cystitis and a Foley catheter, particularly as preparation for transurethral resection of the prostate or bladder surgery. Equivalent results may be obtained with oral fluconazole.

Flucytosine

Flucytosine (5-fluorocytosine, Ancobon) is the fluorine analogue of a normal body constituent, cytosine (see Fig. 35–1). Flucytosine is moderately soluble in water, very stable in dry storage, and marketed as 250- and 500-mg capsules. Absorption from the gastrointestinal tract is rapid and complete, and approximately 90% is excreted unchanged in the urine. Protein binding is barely measurable.[36] Cerebrospinal fluid concentrations approximate 74% of simultaneous serum concentrations. Limited data suggest that it also penetrates well into aqueous humor, joints, bronchial secretions, peritoneal fluid, brain, bile, and bone. The drug is readily cleared by hemodialysis[36] and peritoneal dialysis.

The half-life of the drug in the serum of patients with normal renal function is 3 to 5 hours and higher in newborns. Abnormal hepatic function has no influence, but decreased renal function prolongs the half-life.

The mechanism of flucytosine's antifungal action appears to be by deamination to 5-fluorouracil and then conversion through several steps to 5-fluorodeoxyuridylic acid monophosphate, a noncompetitive inhibitor of thymidylate synthetase,[37] which interferes with DNA synthesis. Additional mechanisms of action may also be operative.

Flucytosine is usually administered at 150 mg/kg/day in four divided doses. Patients with a serum creatinine level of 1.7 mg/dl or greater usually require dose reduction. As an approximation, the total daily dose should be reduced to 75 mg/kg with a creatinine clearance of 26 to 50 ml/minute and to 37 mg/kg when the creatinine clearance is 13 to 25 ml/minute.[38] Ideally, the blood level should be measured in azotemic patients 2 hours after the last dose and immediately before the next dose. These values should range between 20 and 100 μg/ml. Patients requiring hemodialysis may be given a single postdialysis dose of 37.5 mg/kg. Further doses are adjusted by blood level. Reliable biologic,[39] enzymatic,[40] and physical[41] methods are available to assay flucytosine, even in the presence of amphotericin B.

Flucytosine given alone to patients with normal renal, hematologic, and gastrointestinal function is associated with very infrequent adverse effects, including rash, diarrhea, and in about 5%, hepatic dysfunction. In the presence of azotemia such as that caused by concomitant amphotericin B, leukopenia, thrombocytopenia, and enterocolitis may appear and can be fatal. These complications seem to be far more frequent among patients whose flucytosine blood levels attain and especially if they exceed 100 to 125 μg/ml.[38] Patients receiving flucytosine whose renal function is changing should have their serum flucytosine concentrations determined as often as twice per week and the leukocyte count, platelet count, alkaline phosphatase, and aminotransferase levels at a similar frequency. Patients in whom loose stools or dull abdominal pain suddenly develops or who have laboratory evidence consistent with flucytosine toxicity should have their flucytosine blood levels determined and consideration given to withholding therapy with the drug until the situation is clarified. Patients with bone marrow and gastrointestinal toxicity from flucytosine often tolerate the drug at reduced dosage. Patients with rash or hepatotoxicity have not been rechallenged. Uncommonly, vomiting, bowel perforation, confusion, hallucinations, headache, sedation, and euphoria have been reported. Flucytosine is teratogenic for rats and is contraindicated in pregnancy.

Conversion of flucytosine to 5-fluorouracil within the human body occurs in sufficient degree to be a possible explanation for toxicity to bone marrow and the gastrointestinal tract.[42] It is possible that the drug may be secreted into the colon, where flucytosine becomes deaminated by intestinal bacteria and is reabsorbed as 5-fluorouracil.[43]

Flucytosine has a beneficial effect in patients with cryptococcosis,[44] candidiasis, and chromomycosis. It is not the drug of choice for any infection because its clinical efficacy in the first two mycoses is inferior to that of amphotericin B and because primary drug resistance is not common in *Candida* infection and secondary drug resistance is common in all three infections. Drug resistance arising during therapy is usually profound and accompanied by clinical deterioration. Mechanisms for the drug resistance may include altered phosphorylation steps, loss of deaminase, and decreased permeability to the drug. This problem has been significant enough to cause flucytosine to be used largely in combination with amphotericin B.

Flucytosine and amphotericin B are at least additive in their effects in vitro and in mice experimentally infected with doubly sensitive isolates of *Candida* and *Cryptococcus*. Results with *Aspergillus* are contradictory.[45, 46] In animals, the combination has never been better than an optimum dose of amphotericin B alone. Flucytosine permitted a lower dose of amphotericin B to be used to gain the same therapeutic effect, and amphotericin B prevented the emergence of secondary drug resistance. The same advantages have been confirmed in two large multicenter studies of cryptococcal meningitis.[47] Experience with candidiasis remains limited.[48]

Flucytosine is more difficult to manage in patients with diminished bone marrow reserve. Leukopenia and diarrhea are difficult to manage in patients with AIDS, as is leukopenia and thrombocytopenia in patients after bone marrow transplantation or patients with leukemia or other hematologic malignancies. Oral flucytosine may not be reliably ingested by patients who are confused or vomiting. Intravenous flucytosine is no longer available in the United States but is used at the same dose as the capsule formulation. The incidence of diarrhea or leukopenia is not lower with intravenous administration.

Flucytosine resistance has occurred, albeit uncommonly, during combination therapy. Use of the combination in such patients incurs the risk of toxicity without evidence that flucytosine adds to the therapeutic effect. Whenever flucytosine is used to treat a patient who has received that drug before, the isolate should be tested for susceptibility. In most laboratories, a minimal inhibitory concentration of 20 μg/ml or less is considered susceptible.

Imidazoles

The imidazole ring (see Fig. 35–1) confers antifungal activity on a variety of synthetic organic compounds. Unlike the 5-nitroimidazoles such as metronidazole, activity against bacteria and protozoa, although measurable, has not been clinically significant. Most of the imidazoles reaching clinical trials have had similar in vitro activity against a broad range of superficial and deep pathogens.[49] Methods for in vitro susceptibility testing are becoming standardized; such standardization will facilitate the establishment of breakpoints between susceptibility and resistance in vitro, which should correlate with clinical response.[50]

N-substitution of imidazoles has created a family of drugs called triazoles that have the same mechanism of action as imidazoles, a similar or broader spectrum of activity, and less effect on human sterol synthesis. Both imidazoles and triazoles inhibit C-14α demethylation of lanosterol in fungi by binding to one of the cytochrome P-450 enzymes, which leads to the accumulation of C-14α methylsterols and reduced concentrations of ergosterol, a sterol essential for a normal fungal cytoplasmic membrane. Inhibition of cytochrome P-450 also decreases the synthesis of testosterone and cortisol in mammals. By studying cytochrome P-450 inhibition in vitro, new drugs can be selected that have better antifungal specificity. Some azoles, in addition to blocking ergosterol synthesis, have an immediate effect of damaging the fungal cytoplasmic membrane.

Newer triazoles have properties that make them preferable to ketoconazole—not only less hormonal inhibition but also fewer drug interactions, a parenteral formulation, a broader spectrum, better distribution into body fluids, less gastrointestinal distress, and less hepatotoxicity. The ideal triazole has not arrived because none has all these properties yet and resistance to azoles in previously susceptible species is emerging. Resistance mechanisms include altered or increased C-14α demethylase and increased drug efflux. Development of fluconazole resistance has been documented in *C. albicans,* and increased resistance has been seen in *Candida glabrata. Candida krusei, C. glabrata, Candida norvegensis,* and *Candida inconspicua* are intrinsically more resistant to azoles.[50a] Increased isolation of *C. glabrata* and *C. krusei* has been observed in patients receiving long-term azoles. Isolates resistant to fluconazole are variably cross-resistant to itraconazole and ketoconazole.[51]

Ketoconazole

The synthetic agent ketoconazole differs from its closely related congener miconazole in its solubility at pH less than 3. Solubility in acidic aqueous solutions is conferred in large part by the basic piperazine ring.

Ketoconazole is metabolized in the liver and excreted as inactive drug in bile and, to a small extent, in urine.[49] Very little biologically active drug appears in urine. Serum protein binding exceeds 90%. The drug is not removed significantly by hemodialysis or peritoneal dialysis. Decreased renal or hepatic function does not alter plasma drug levels. Based on studies of oral ingestion by volunteers, the initial half-life is approximately 2 hours, with a β-phase half-life of about 9 hours commencing 8 to 12 hours after ingestion.

Oral absorption of ketoconazole varies among different individuals. Serious gastrointestinal disease such as the graft-versus-host reaction[52] may lead to low blood levels. H_2 receptor blocking agents or other inhibitors of gastric acid secretion such as omeprazole should not be given to patients taking ketoconazole because blood levels of the latter drug are drastically reduced. Citrus fruit juices or cola beverages administered with ketoconazole improve absorption in hypochlorhydric patients. Antacids can be given to patients taking ketoconazole but should follow ketoconazole by 1 to 2 hours. Rifampin causes a substantial lowering of ketoconazole blood levels, probably by accelerating metabolism. Isoniazid possibly has the same effect. Occasional patients have had elevated phenytoin or oral anticoagulant levels while taking ketoconazole. Cyclosporine blood levels should be monitored during ketoconazole therapy because these levels usually increase and cause nephrotoxicity. Penetration into cerebrospinal fluid is very poor, even in the presence of inflammation. Low concentrations are found in vaginal secretions, saliva, and breast milk, but penetration into inflamed joints is better.

Ketoconazole is available as scored 200-mg tablets. When used as two tablets daily (400 mg), the drug is effective in chronic mucocutaneous candidiasis, coccidiodomycosis, histoplasmosis, paracoccidioidomycosis, and blastomycosis in nonimmunosuppressed hosts.[53] Therapy is continued for 6 to 12 months or longer, when the response is slow, to prevent relapse. Improvement may require weeks to months to be evident. Although the dose can be advanced to 600 or 800 mg daily in patients not responding to therapy, more evidence of increased toxicity than increased efficacy has been observed.[54, 55] If the mycosis involves the meninges, ketoconazole requires doses exceeding 400 mg/day and produces limited efficacy.

Ketoconazole has limited value in nonmeningeal cryptococcosis and is of no value in meningeal cryptococcosis. Some patients with chromoblastomycosis and cutaneous sporotrichosis will respond, but itraconazole would be preferred. Ketoconazole has been used in Old World leishmaniasis and was useful in *Leishmania major* but not in *Leishmania tropica* or *Leishmania aethiopica* infections (see Chapter 265). Studies on New World leishmaniasis are not encouraging.

Aspergillosis does not respond to ketoconazole. Additionally, there is concern, based on experience with mice, that subsequent use of amphotericin B may be antagonized.[56] The agents of mucormycosis have all been resistant to imidazoles and triazoles in vitro, thus discouraging clinical use for that indication.

The most frequent toxic effects of ketoconazole are anorexia, nausea, and vomiting. These reactions occurred in 17% of 71 patients taking 400 mg/day and in 29% of those receiving 800 mg/day.[53] Gastrointestinal distress is most common when the drug is first begun and can be partially controlled by taking the tablets with food. Dividing doses above 400 mg/day has not been recommended because hormonal suppression is prolonged. Ketoconazole causes a dose-dependent depression in serum testosterone- and adrenocorticotropic hormone–stimulated cortisol response.[57, 58] Although this effect is reversible after a 24-hour period at 400 mg once daily, doses of 800 to 1200 mg/day cause a profound enough effect to have prompted trials in the treatment of Cushing's syndrome and prostatic cancer. Hypertension has been seen in a few of these high-dose patients in association with increased mineralocorticoid precursors. Gynecomastia and oligospermia in men and menstrual irregularities in women may also be seen during prolonged therapy. Allergic rash has been seen in 10% of patients. Pruritus occurs with equal frequency, sometimes associated with a complaint of dry skin. Perhaps the most grave complication of ketoconazole therapy is hepatitis.[59] Fortunately, this complication is quite rare and is estimated to appear in 1 in 15,000 exposed individuals. Asymptomatic slight elevation of transaminase levels occurs in 5 to 15% and is generally transient. This event is distinguished from the potentially lethal hepatitis by the presence of symptoms and the progressive course. Ketoconazole-associated hepatitis begins as anorexia, malaise, nausea, and vomiting. Abnormalities of either or both serum transaminase and alkaline phosphatase become increasingly profound and are soon accompanied by jaundice. Eighty percent of cases occur within the first 3 months, but onset can occur at any time. Progression can be surprisingly swift. Patients should be instructed to discontinue ketoconazole therapy if they experience the aforementioned symptoms and to call their physician. If hepatotoxicity is suspected, serum transaminase and alkaline phosphatase levels should be measured within 1 to 2 days of discontinuing therapy. Rechallenge should be done with great caution. Some authorities have recommended that liver function be measured periodically.[59] This procedure does not protect a patient who has a rapid onset of hepatitis in the interval between tests but does require that all patients with abnormalities be contacted to inquire about symptoms and to arrange for repeat testing.

Itraconazole (Sporanox)

Pharmacology. Itraconazole is marketed as a 100-mg capsule and an oral suspension of 100 mg per 10 ml in cyclodextrin, an oligosaccharide ring. The ring entraps the hydrophobic, water-insoluble drug and releases it at the lipid-rich gut lining for absorption. The solution makes possible delivery of the drug through a nasogastric tube in intubated patients and makes dosing of infants and small children more convenient. A parenteral formulation is under clinical trial. Oral absorption of the capsule is significantly enhanced by food, although absorption of the solution is best on an empty stomach.[60] Bioavailability of the capsule is 55% when ingested after breakfast, and the area under the time-concentration curve is increased 30% with the solution and food and a further 25 to 30% with the solution in a fasting state.[61–64] In fasting AIDS patients, coadministration of a cola beverage with itraconazole capsules increases the area under the plasma concentration-time curve by 38%.[65] Peak levels with either preparation are achieved 4 to 6 hours after a dose. Steady state is achieved only after 13 to 15 days, at which time the β-elimination half-life is about 19 to 22 hours. Absorption of the capsules in patients with AIDS is about half that in normal volunteers.[66] Absorption of the capsule is markedly depressed in bone marrow transplant recipients, probably because of hypochlorhydria, mucositis, and graft-versus-host intestinal changes, but the depressed absorption can be alleviated by using the solution.[60] For deep mycoses, an initial itraconazole dose of 200 mg three times per day is recommended for the first 3 days to give high serum and tissue levels initially. Hydroxyitraconazole, a metabolite of itraconazole, appears in blood in amounts roughly twice that of the parent drug and has antifungal activity and pharmokinetics similar to those of the parent compound.[67] Bioassays of itraconazole give much higher concentrations than high-pressure liquid chromatography does, the difference depending on the susceptibility of the bioassay organism to hydroxyitraconazole. Tissue, pus, and bronchial secretion concentrations of itraconazole are generally higher than plasma concentrations, but cerebrospinal fluid concentrations are usually unmeasurable, even in patients with meningitis. Ocular levels are low. Saliva concentrations persist for 8 hours after the solution and provide a possible benefit in treating oral disease or eradicating oral colonization. The drug is metabolized in the liver and excreted in feces as metabolites. Fifty to 64% of the cyclodextrin administered is secreted intact in feces, with most of the remainder broken down by gut bacteria amylases; less than 0.5% is absorbed. No significant amount of bioactive itraconazole appears in urine. Plasma concentrations do not increase in patients with renal insufficiency or decrease with hemodialysis. The half-life is prolonged in those with cirrhosis. About 99% of serum itraconazole is bound to plasma proteins.

Adverse Effects. The most common adverse effect is dose-related nausea and abdominal discomfort, but symptoms rarely necessitate stopping therapy.[67a] Dividing the dose into twice-daily administration improves tolerance and absorption. Hypokalemia and edema may occur at 400 mg/day or higher doses. Allergic rash is seen occasionally. Therapy is contraindicated during pregnancy and in nursing mothers. Unlike ketoconazole, itraconazole does not appear to be hepatotoxic and does not suppress adrenal or testicular function at the dosages recommended. Flavoring in the solution ameliorates the unpleasant taste of cyclodextrin. Diarrhea, nausea, and other gastrointestinal complaints are more frequent with the solution. This increased toxicity is probably due to the osmotic effect or bile salt complexing by unmetabolized cyclodextrin.

Interactions. Blood levels are reduced by about half in patients taking drugs that decrease gastric acidity, such as H_2 blockers and drugs blocking the gastric proton pump.[68] Simultaneous ingestion of itraconazole with antacids and, most likely, with buffered didanosine decreases absorption. Rifampin, rifabutin, isoniazid, phenytoin, carbamazepine, phenobarbital, and cisapride decrease itraconazole blood levels. Itraconazole decreases rifampin blood levels and increases blood levels of the antihistamines terfenadine[69] and astemizole, potentially causing polymorphic ventricular tachycardia (torsades de pointes), as well as increasing levels of cisapride, warfarin, benzodiazepines, hepatic hydroxymethylglutaryl coenzyme A reductase cholesterol-lowering agents,[70] dihydropyridine calcium channel blockers,[71] digoxin, quinidine, cyclosporine, tacrolimus, methylprednisolone, human immunodeficiency virus (HIV) protease inhibitors (ritonavir, indinavir), and vinca alkaloids (vincristine, vinblastine).[72]

Indications. This oral triazole is useful for treatment of blastomycosis,[73] histoplasmosis,[73] coccidioidomycosis (including meningeal disease), paracoccidioidomycosis, sporotrichosis,[74, 75] ringworm, including onychomycosis,[76] tinea versicolor, and aspergillosis.[77] Itraconazole is also useful for the prevention of relapse in AIDS patients with disseminated histoplasmosis.[78] The solution shows promise for the treatment of oral and esophageal candidiasis when used at 100 to 200 mg daily.[79, 80] *L. major* infections respond poorly.[81]

Fluconazole (Diflucan)

Pharmacology. Fluconazole is well absorbed from the gastrointestinal tract.[82] After ingestion of fluconazole, more than 80% of the drug can be found in the circulation. Of the oral dose, 60 to 75% appears unchanged in the urine and 8 to 10% appears unchanged in the feces. Oral absorption is not decreased in patients with AIDS or patients taking H_2 blocking agents.[83] Only 11% of serum fluconazole is protein-bound. Concentrations of fluconazole in cerebrospinal fluid are approximately 70% of simultaneous blood levels, whether or not the meninges are inflamed and the drug penetrates into the brain. Penetration into saliva, sputum, urine, and other body fluids has also been excellent.[81] The half-life in patients with normal renal function is 27 to 34 hours and increases to 59 and 98 hours in groups with creatinine clearances of 35 and 14 ml/minute, respectively. According to the manufacturer, the normal dose should be reduced to 50% when the creatinine clearance is reduced to 50 ml/minute and to 25% when creatinine clearance is below 20 ml/minute. A loading dose of twice the daily dose is recommended. Patients receiving hemodialysis should have one daily dose after each session. A dose of 6 mg/kg every 3 days has been advocated for premature infants in the first week of life, with dosing every 2 days during the second week of life.[84]

Drug Interactions. Fluconazole can cause significant increases in the blood level of phenytoin, glipizide, glyburide, tolbutamide, warfarin, rifabutin,[85] or cyclosporine. This interaction is most obvious in adults given 400 mg daily or in azotemic patients given lower doses. Rifampin lowers fluconazole blood levels by about one fourth.[86]

Side Effects. Adverse effects are uncommon.[87] Even with chronic therapy, including doses exceeding 400 mg/day, headache, hair loss, and anorexia were the most common symptoms, each occurring in 3% of patients, whereas 10% had rises in aspartate aminotransferase levels. Alopecia is reversible, even in some instances when the drug is continued at lower doses.[88] Neurotoxicity has been described after heroic doses of 2000 mg daily. Rarely, anaphylaxis after the first dose or Stevens-Johnson syndrome has been observed.

Administration. Fluconazole is currently available in 50-, 100-, 150-, and 200-mg tablets, a powder for oral suspension, and an intravenous formulation of either 200 or 400 mg, both as 2 mg/ml. The much higher price of the intravenous drug makes the tablets preferred. Local instillation into the cerebrospinal fluid, bladder, or another site is unnecessary because of excellent penetration of the drug into body compartments.

Indications

Candidiasis. Fluconazole, 50 to 100 mg once daily, is one of the most effective agents for the treatment of oropharyngeal candidiasis. Daily doses of 100 to 400 mg are recommended for esophageal candidiasis.[2] A single dose of 150 mg is approximately as effective as topical treatment of vulvovaginal candidiasis. Patients with candidemia who are not neutropenic or otherwise seriously immunosuppressed respond as well to intravenous fluconazole therapy as to amphotericin B, provided that they do not have fluconazole-resistant *Candida* species.[89] Changing potentially infected central intravenous catheters in such patients is an important part of therapy. In a small number of patients with *Candida* endocarditis, long-term fluconazole therapy has been used to prevent relapse after amphotericin B therapy.[90] For immunosuppressed patients and rapidly progressing or severely ill patients with deep candidiasis, amphotericin B remains the drug of choice.

Cryptococcal Meningitis. Fluconazole has been used for the initial treatment of AIDS patients with cryptococcal meningitis who are neurologically intact and judged to have a good prognosis.[91] Many authorities recommend amphotericin B or amphotericin B plus flucytosine for at least the first 2 weeks. Therapy can be changed to fluconazole, 400 mg daily for 2 months, if the patient has remained clinically stable. The propensity of AIDS patients to relapse has led to life-long maintenance therapy with fluconazole, 200 mg daily.[92] Itraconazole capsules, 200 mg daily, are inferior to fluconazole, 200 mg daily, for maintenance therapy.[93] Thus far, relapse because of fluconazole resistance has been rare. Fluconazole is effective for the eradication of genitourinary foci. For initial treatment, fluconazole at doses of 800 mg[94] or given with flucytosine[95] has been advocated, but insufficient data exist to recommend these regimens (see Chapter 253). For patients without AIDS, fluconazole is useful for those who have completed a course of amphotericin B and seem to have a high risk of relapse. At present, virtually no studies have defined the dose and duration of fluconazole for non-AIDS patients with cryptococcosis.

Other Mycoses. Fluconazole is useful for coccidioidal meningitis and is approximately as effective as other azoles for disseminated nonmeningeal coccidioidomycosis, although doses exceeding 400 mg daily may be required and relapse rates may be higher.[96] Cutaneous sporotrichosis,[97] ringworm, histoplasmosis,[98] and blastomycosis may respond, but the results are inferior to those with itraconazole. Fluconazole is not indicated for aspergillosis, mucormycosis, or pseudallescheriasis.

Prophylaxis in Neutropenic Patients. In a multicenter trial, administration of fluconazole, 400 mg daily, decreased the incidence of death from deep mycoses in bone marrow transplant recipients, most of whom had received allogeneic transplants, from 10 per 177 placebo recipients to 1 per 179 fluconazole recipients.[99] All the protection afforded seemed to be in deep candidiasis, not aspergillosis. This result was confirmed in a similar study of bone marrow transplant recipients.[100] Fluconazole resulted in decreased use of empirical amphotericin B in one study[100] but not the other.[99] Reduction in deep mycoses has not been convincingly demonstrated in other groups such as patients with acute leukemia.[101, 102] Nor has an effect of overall survival been demonstrated, perhaps because death from deep candidiasis is now uncommon in patients with leukemia. In most studies, fluconazole prophylaxis has decreased the incidence of mucocutaneous candidiasis, but this complication can also be diagnosed readily and treated when present.

Prophylaxis in Patients with Acquired Immunodeficiency Syndrome. Fluconazole, 200 or 400 mg once per week, has reduced the incidence of oral and vulvovaginal candidiasis in patients with advanced HIV infection, but this regimen has not been demonstrated to prevent histoplasmosis, cryptococcosis, or esophageal candidiasis in this population.[103, 104] Prophylaxis with 200 mg daily does reduce the incidence of oropharyngeal and esophageal candidiasis, as well as cryptococcosis in patients with a CD4 count below $200/mm^3$ Cost, lack of effect on survival, and the possibility of azole resistance has led the U.S. Public Health Service Infectious Disease Society of America advisory committee to recommend against fluconazole prophylaxis in AIDS patients. Fluconazole is an alternative to itraconazole for maintenance therapy in AIDS patients with prior disseminated histoplasmosis.[105]

Investigational Agents

Triazoles

Voriconazole (UK-109,496) expands the antifungal spectrum of fluconazole to include *Aspergillus.* Voriconazole has an oral bioavailability of at least 80%. Both tablets and an intravenous formulation in sulfobutylcyclodextrin are being used in clinical trials. Voriconazole has a half-life of 6 hours in most subjects but a longer half-life in a small percentage of white persons. Blood levels are about 1 to

10 μg/ml. The drug is metabolized in the liver, with no significant amounts of bioactive drug found in the urine. Significant drug interactions include rifampin, rifabutin, phenytoin, cyclosporine, and prednisolone. Toxicity has been largely confined to transient ocular symptoms at the time of peak blood levels. Doses of 200 to 400 mg every 12 hours intravenously or orally are being used in clinical trials. Two randomized studies to compare amphotericin B with voriconazole are in progress. One is a study of invasive aspergillosis in severely immunocompromised patients, and the other is a study of empirical treatment of fever in neutropenic patients not responding to antibacterial therapy.

Other new triazoles include SCH 56592 and BMS 207147.

Lipopeptides

MK-0991 is a semisynthetic derivative of pneumocandin B0, a fermentation product of *Zalerion arboricola*. The mechanism of action of this class of antifungal is inhibition of β1,3 glucans in the fungal cell wall. The spectrum includes *Candida* and *Aspergillus* species, as well as the cyst form of *Pneumocystis carinii.* MK-0991 is metabolized in the liver with a plasma half-life of 9 to 10 hours. The drug is given intravenously once every 24 hours, currently at a dose of 50 mg. Hepatotoxicity has been seen at higher doses. Cyclosporine but not tacrolimus has increased MK-0991 levels by 50%. A randomized comparison of amphotericin B and MK-0991 in candidemia and an open study of aspergillosis are under way.

LY 303366 and FK 463 are other investigational lipopeptide antifungals.

Other Agents

Drugs still being evaluated in vitro include sordarins, which inhibit protein synthesis by their effect on fungal elongation factor 2, nikkomycins, which inhibit chitin synthesis, and various peptides with unknown mechanisms of action. Immunomodulators hold promise, but insufficient data exist to determine where and how these drugs might be used.[106, 107]

REFERENCES

1. Doering PL, Santiago TM. Drugs for treatment of vulvovaginal candidiasis: Comparative efficacy of agents and regimens. Ann Pharmacother. 1990;24:1078–1083.
1a. Stevens DA, ed. Role of oral amphotericin B in the management of oral candidiasis. J Mycol Med. 1996;7(Suppl II):1–48.
2. Laine L, Dretler RH, Conteas CN, et al. Fluconazole compared with ketoconazole for the treatment of *Candida* esophagitis in AIDS. Ann Intern Med. 1992;117:655–660.
3. Quereda C, Polanco AM, Giner C, et al. Correlation between in vitro resistance to fluconazole and clinical outcome of oropharyngeal candidiasis in HIV-infected patients. Eur J Clin Microbiol Infect Dis. 1996;15:30–37.
4. Bonifaz A, Carrasco-Gerard E, Saul A. Itraconazole in onychomycosis: Intermittent dose schedule. Int J Dermatol. 1997;36:70–72.
5. Havu V, Brandt H, Heikkila H, et al. A double-blind, randomized study comparing itraconazole pulse therapy with continuous dosing for the treatment of toe-nail onychomycosis. Br J Dermatol. 1997;136:230–234.
6. Brautigam M, Nolting S, Schope RE, Weidinger G. German randomized double-blind multicentre comparison of terbinafine and itraconazole for the treatment of toenail tinea infection. Br J Dermatol. 1996;134 (Suppl 46):S18–S21.
7. Elewski BE. Onchomycosis: Pathogenesis, diagnosis, and management. Clin Microbiol Rev. 1998;11:415–429.
8. Multicentre study group. Treatment of vaginal candidiasis with a single dose of fluconazole. Eur J Clin Microbiol Infect Dis. 1988;7:364–367.
9. Rees T, Phillips R. Multicenter comparison of one-day oral therapy with fluconazole or itraconazole in vaginal candidiasis. Int J Gynaecol Obstet. 1992;37:33–38.
10. Balakrishnan AR, Easwaran KRK. CD and NMR studies on the aggregation of amphotericin-B in solution. Biochim Biophys Acta. 1993;1148:269–277.
11. Hsu S, Burnette RR. The effect of amphotericin B on the K channel activity of MDCK cells. Biochim Biophys Acta. 1993;1152:189–191.
12. Merz WG. *Candida lusitaniae*: Frequency of recovery, colonization, infection, and amphotericin B resistance. J Clin Microbiol. 1984;20:1994–1995.
13. Wong-Beringer A, Jacobs RA, Gugliemo JB. Lipid formulations of amphotericin B: Clinical efficacy and toxicities. Clin Infect Dis. 1998;27:603–618.
14. White MH, Bowden RE, Sandler ES, et al. Randomized, double-blind clinical trial of amphotericin B colloidal dispersion vs amphotericin B in the empirical treatment of fever and neutropenia. Clin Infect Dis. 1998;27:296–302.
15. Herbrecht R. Safety of amphotericin B colloidal dispersion. Eur J Clin Microbiol Infect Dis. 1997;16:74–80.
16. Bowden RA, Cays M, Gooley T, et al. Phase I study of amphotericin B colloidal dispersion for the treatment of invasive fungal infections after marrow transplant. J Infect Dis. 1996;173:1208–1215.
17. White MH, Anaissie EJ, Kusne S, et al. Amphotericin B colloidal dispersion vs. amphotericin B as therapy for invasive aspergillosis. Clin Infect Dis. 1997;24:635–642.
18. Walsh TJ, Hiemenz JW, Seibel NL, et al. Amphotericin B lipid complex for invasive fungal infections: Analysis of safety and efficacy in 556 cases. Clin Infect Dis. 1998;26:1383–1396.
19. Sharkey PK, Graybill JR, Johnson ES, et al. Amphotericin B lipid complex compared with amphotericin B in the treatment of cryptococcal meningitis in patients with AIDS. Clin Infect Dis. 1996;22:315–321.
20. Ng TT, Denning DW. Liposomal amphotericin B (AmBisome) therapy in invasive fungal infections. Evaluation of United Kingdom compassionate use data. Arch Intern Med. 1995;155:1093–1098.
21. Ellis M, Spence D, De Pauw B, et al. An EORTC international multicenter randomized trial (EORTC Number 19923) comparing two dosages of liposomal amphotericin for treatment of invasive aspergillosis. Clin Infect Dis. 1998;27:1406–1412.
22. Viviani MA, Rizzardini G, Tortorano AM, et al. Lipid-based amphotericin B in the treatment of cryptococcosis. Infection. 1994;22:136–142.
22a. Walsh TJ, Finberg RW, Arndt C, et al. Liposomal amphotericin B for empirical therapy in patients with persistent fever and neutropenia. N Engl J Med. 1999;340:764–771.
23. Prentice HG, Hann IM, Herbrecht R, et al. A randomized comparison of liposomal versus conventional amphotericin B for the treatment of pyrexia of unknown origin in neutropenic patients. Br J Haematol. 1997;98:711–718.
24. Johnson MD, Drew H, Perfect JR. Chest discomfort associated with liposomal amphotericin B: Report of three cases and review of the literature. Pharmacotherapy. 1998;18:1053–1061.
25. Chavanet PY, Garry I, Charlier N, et al. Trial of glucose versus fat emulsion in preparation of amphotericin for use in HIV infected patients with candidiasis. BMJ. 1992;305:921–925.
25a. Nath CE, Shaw PJ, Gunning R, et al. Amphotericin B in children wtih malignant disease: A comparison of the toxicities and pharmacokinetics of amphotericin B administered in dextrose versus lipid emulsion. Antimicrob Agents Chemother. 1999;43:1417–1423.
26. Bindschadler DD, Bennett JE. A pharmacologic guide to the clinical use of amphotericin B. J Infect Dis. 1969;120:427.
27. Mayhew JW, Fiore C, Murray T, et al. An internally standardized assay for amphotericin B in tissues and plasma. J Chromatogr. 1983;274:271.
28. Cleary JD, Chapman SW, Hardin TC, et al. Amphotericin B enzyme-linked immunoassay for clinical use: Comparison with bioassay and HPLC. Ann Pharmacother. 1997;31:39–44.
29. Merz WG, Fay D, Thumar B, et al. Susceptibility testing of filamentous fungi to amphotericin B by a rapid radiometric method. J Clin Microbiol. 1984;19:54.
30. Sawaya BP, Weihprecht H, Campbell WE, et al. Direct vasoconstriction as a possible cause of amphotericin B–induced nephrotoxicity in rats. J Clin Invest. 1991;87:2097–2107.
31. Anderson CM. Sodium chloride treatment of amphotericin B nephrotoxicity. Standard of care? West J Med. 1995;162:313–317.
32. Cruz JM, Peacock JE Jr, Loomer L, et al. Rapid intravenous infusion of amphotericin B: A pilot study. Am J Med. 1992;93:123–130.
33. Drutz DJ. Rapid infusion of amphotericin B: Is it safe, effective and wise? Am J Med. 1992;93:119–121.
34. Ellis ME, Al-Hokail AA, Clink HM, et al. Double blind randomized study of the effect of infusion rates on toxicity of amphotericin B. Antimicrob Agents Chemother. 1992;36:172–179.
35. Pizzo PA. Management of fever in patients with cancer and treatment-induced neutropenia. N Engl J Med. 1993;328:1323–1332.
36. Block ER, Bennett JE, Livoti LG, et al. Flucytosine and amphotericin B: Hemodialysis effects on the plasma concentration and clearance. Ann Intern Med. 1974;80:613.
37. Diasio RB, Bennett JE, Myers CE. Mode of action of 5-fluorocytosine. Biochem Pharmacol. 1978;27:703.
38. Stamm AM, Diasio RB, Dismukes WE, et al. Toxicity of amphotericin B plus flucytosine in 194 patients with cryptococcal meningitis. Am J Med. 1987;83:236–242.
39. Kaspar RL, Drutz DJ. Rapid, simple bioassay for 5-fluorocytosine in the presence of amphotericin B. Antimicrob Agents Chemother. 1975;7:462.
40. Huang CM, Kroll MH, Ruddel M, et al. An enzymatic method for 5-fluorocytosine. Clin Chem. 1988;34:59–62.
41. Harding SA, Johnson GF, Solomon HM. Gas chromatographic determination of 5-fluorocytosine in human serum. Clin Chem. 1976;22:772.
42. Diasio RB, Lakings DE, Bennett JE. Evidence for conversion of 5-fluorocytosine to 5-fluorouracil in humans. Possible factor in 5-fluorocytosine clinical toxicity. Antimicrob Agents Chemother. 1978;14:903.
43. Harris BE, Manning BW, Federle TW, et al. Conversion of 5-fluorocytosine to 5-fluorouracil by human intestinal microflora. Antimicrob Agents Chemother. 1986;29:44–48.
44. Hospenthal D, Bennett J. Flucytosine monotherapy for cryptococcosis. Clin Infect Dis. 1998;27:260–264.
45. Kitahara M, Seth UK, Medoff G, et al. Activity of amphotericin B, 5-fluorocytosine and rifampin against six clinical isolates of *Aspergillus.* Antimicrob Agents Chemother. 1976;9:915.

46. Polak A, Scholer HJ, Wall M. Combination therapy of experimental candidiasis and aspergillosis in mice. Chemotherapy. 1982;28:461.
47. Dismukes WE, Cloud GC, Gallis HA, et al. Treatment of cryptococcal meningitis with combination amphotericin B and flucytosine for four as compared with six Cweeks. N Engl J Med. 1987;317:334–341.
48. Smego RA, Perfect JR, Durack DT. Combined therapy with amphotericin B and 5-fluorocytosine for *Candida* meningitis. Rev Infect Dis. 1984;6:791–801.
49. Heel RC, Brogden RN, Carmine A, et al. Ketoconazole: A review of its therapeutic efficacy in superficial and systemic fungal infections. Drugs. 1982;23:1.
50. Rex JH, Pfaller MA, Galgiani JN, et al. Development of interpretive breakpoints for antifungal susceptibility testing: Conceptual framework and analysis of in vitro–in vivo correlation data for fluconazole, itraconazole, and candida infections. Subcommittee on Antifungal Susceptibility Testing of the National Committee for Clinical Laboratory Standards. Clin Infect Dis. 1997;24:235–247.
50a. Rex JH, Rinaldi MG, Pfaller MA. Resistance of Candida species, to fluconazole. Antimicrob Agents Chemother. 1995;39:1–8.
51. Stevens DA, Stevens JA. Cross-resistance phenotypes of fluconazole-resistant *Candida* species: Comparison of methods, results with 655 clinical isolates. Diagn Micro Infect Dis. 1996;26:145–148.
52. Van HV, Piens MA, Archimbaud E, et al. Serum levels of ketoconazole in bone marrow transplanted patients. Nouv Rev Fr Hematol. 1983;25:241–244.
53. NIAID Mycoses Study Group. Treatment of blastomycosis and histoplasmosis with ketoconazole. Results of a prospective randomized clinical trial. Ann Intern Med. 1985;103:861–872.
54. Galgiani JN, Stevens DA, Graybill JR, et al. Ketoconazole therapy of progressive coccidioidomycosis. Comparison of 400 and 800 mg doses and observations at higher doses. Am J Med. 1988;84:603–610.
55. Sugar AM, Alsip SG, Galgiani JN, et al. Pharmacology and toxicity of high-dose ketoconazole. Antimicrob Agents Chemother. 1987;31:1874–1878.
56. Schaffner A, Frick PG. The effect of ketoconazole on amphotericin B in a model of disseminated aspergillosis. J Infect Dis. 1985;151:902–910.
57. Pont A, Graybill JR, Craven PC, et al. High-dose ketoconazole therapy and adrenal and testicular function in humans. Arch Intern Med. 1984;144:2150–2153.
58. Stevens DA. Ketoconazole metamorphosis: An antimicrobial becomes an endocrine drug. Arch Intern Med. 1985;145:813–815.
59. Lewis JH, Zimmerman HJ, Benson GD, et al. Hepatic injury associated with ketoconazole therapy. Gastroenterology. 1984;86:503–513.
60. Stevens DA. Itraconazole in cyclodextrin solution. Pharmacotherapy. 1999;19:603–611.
61. Barone JA, Moskovitz BL, Guarnieri J, et al. Enhanced bioavailability of itraconazole in hydroxypropyl B-cyclodextrin solution versus capsules in healthy volunteers. Antimicrob Agents Chemother. 1998;42:1862–1865.
62. De Repentigny L, Ratelle J, Leclerc JM, et al. Repeated-dose pharmacokinetics of an oral solution of itraconazole in infants and children. Antimicrob Agents Chemother. 1998;42:404–408.
63. Saag M. Itraconazole oral solution: Pharmacokinetics and absorption. AIDS Patient Care STD. 1997;11(Suppl 1):S16–S21.
64. Reynes J, Bazin C, Ajana F, et al. Pharmacokinetics of itraconazole (oral solution) in two groups of human immunodeficiency virus–infected adults with oral candidiasis. Antimicrob Agents Chemother. 1997;41:2554–2558.
65. Lange D, Pavao JH, Jacqmin P, et al. The effect of coadministration of a cola beverage on the bioavailability of itraconazole in patients with acquired immunodeficiency syndrome. Curr Ther. 1997;58:202–212.
66. Smith D, Van De Velde V, Woestenborghs R, et al. The pharmacokinetics of oral itraconazole in AIDS patients. J Pharm Pharmacol. 1992;44:618–619.
67. Hostetler JS, Heykants J, Clemons KV, et al. Discrepancies in bioassay and chromatography determinations explained by metabolism of itraconazole to hydroxyitraconazole: Studies of interpatient variations in concentrations. Antimicrob Agents Chemother. 1993;37:2224–2227.
67a. Tucker RM, Haq Y, Denning DW, et al. The toxicity of itraconazole in 189 patients on chronic therapy. J Antimicrob Chemother. 1990;26:561–566.
68. Lim SG, Sawyer AM, Sercombe J, et al. Short report: The absorption of fluconazole and itraconazole under conditions of low intragastric acidity. Aliment Pharmacol Ther. 1993;7:317–321.
69. Crane JK, Shih H. Syncope and cardiac arrhythmia due to an interaction between itraconazole and terfenadine. Am J Med. 1993;95:445–446.
70. Neuvonen PJ, Jalava KM. Itraconazole drastically increases plasma concentrations of lovastatin and lovastatin acid. Clin Pharmacol Ther. 1996;60:54–61.
71. Jalava KM, Olkkola KT, Neuvonen PJ. Itraconazole greatly increases plasma concentrations and effects of felodipine. Clin Pharmacol Ther. 1997;61:410–415.
72. Buggia I, Zecca M, Alessandrino EP, et al. Itraconazole can increase systemic exposure to busulfan in patients given bone marrow transplantation. Anticancer Res. 1996;16:2083–2088.
73. Mangino JE, Pappas PG. Itraconazole for the treatment of histoplasmosis and blastomycosis. Int J Antimicrob Agents. 1995;5:219–225.
74. Badley AD, Van Scoy RE. Long term follow-up of multifocal osteoarticular sporotrichosis treated with itraconazole. Clin Infect Dis. 1996;23:394–395.
75. Sharkey-Mathis PK, Kauffman CA, Graybill JR, et al. Treatment of sporotrichosis with itraconazole. Am J Med. 1993;95:279–285.
76. Van Hecke E, Van Cutsem J. Double-blind comparison of itraconazole with griseofulvin in the treatment of tinea pedis and tinea manuum. Mycoses. 1998;31:641–649.
77. Stevens DA, Lee JY. Analysis of compassionate use itraconazole therapy for invasive aspergillosis by the NIAID Mycoses Study Group criteria. Arch Intern Med. 1997;157:1857–1862.
78. Hecht FM, Wheat J, Korzun AH, et al. Itraconazole maintenance treatment for histoplasmosis in AIDS: A prospective, multicenter trial. J Acquired Immune Defic Syndr Hum Retrovirol. 1997;16:100–107.
79. Wilcox CM, Darouiche RO, Laine L, et al. A randomized, double-blind comparison of itraconazole oral solution and fluconazole tablets in the treatment of esophageal candidiasis. J Infect Dis. 1997;176:227–232.
80. Graybill JR, Vazquez J, Darouiche RO, et al. Randomized trial of itraconazole oral solution for oropharyngeal candidiasis in HIV/AIDS patients. Am J Med. 1998;104:33–39.
81. Momeni AZ, Jalayer T, Emamjomeh M, et al. Treatment of cutaneous leishmaniasis with itraconazole. Arch Dermatol. 1996;132:784–786.
82. Zervos M, Meunier F. Fluconazole (Diflucan): A review. Int J Antimicrob Agents. 1993;3:147–170.
83. DeMuria D, Forrest A, Rich J, et al. Pharmacokinetics and bioavailability of fluconazole in patients with AIDS. Antimicrob Agents Chemother. 1993;37:2187–2192.
84. Saxen H, Hoppu K, Pohjavuori M: Pharmacokinetics of fluconazole in very low birth weight infants during the first two weeks of life. Clin Pharmacol Ther. 1993;54:269–277.
85. Trapnell CB, Narang PK, Li R, Lavelle JP. Increased plasma rifabutin levels with concomitant fluconazole therapy in HIV-infected patients. Ann Intern Med. 1996;124:573–576.
86. Baciewicz AM, Baciewicz FA: Ketoconazole and fluconazole drug interactions. Arch Intern Med. 1993;153:1970–1976.
87. Stevens DA, Diaz M, Negroni R, et al. Safety evaluation of chronic fluconazole therapy. Chemotherapy. 1997;43:371–377.
88. Diaz M, Negroni R, Montero-Crei F, et al. A Pan-American 5-year study of fluconazole therapy for deep mycoses in the immunocompetent host. Clin Infect Dis. 1992;14(Suppl. 1):S68–S76.
89. Rex J, Bennett JE, Sugar AM, et al. A randomized trial comparing fluconazole with amphotericin B for the treatment of candidemia in patients without neutropenia. N Engl J Med. 1994;331:1325–1330.
90. Czwerwiec FS, Bilsker MS, Kamerman ML, et al. Long-term survival after fluconazole therapy of candidal prosthetic valve endocarditis. Am J Med. 1993;94:545–546.
91. Saag MS, Powderly WG, Cloud GA, et al. Comparison of amphotericin B with fluconazole in the treatment of acute AIDS-associated cryptococcal meningitis. N Engl J Med. 1992;326:83–89.
92. Van der Horst CM, Saag MS, Cloud GA, et al. Treatment of cryptococcal meningitis associated with the acquired immunodeficiency syndrome. N Engl J Med. 1997;337:15–21.
93. Powderly WG, Saag MS, Cloud GA, et al. A controlled trial of fluconazole or amphotericin B to prevent relapse of cryptococcal meningitis in patients with the acquired immunodeficiency syndrome. N Engl J Med. 1992;326:793–798.
94. Haubrich RH, Haghighat D, Bozzette SA, et al. High-dose fluconazole for treatment of cryptococcal disease in patients with human immunodeficiency virus infection. J Infect Dis. 1994;170:238–242.
95. Larsen RA, Bozzette SA, Jones BE, et al. Fluconazole combined with flucytosine for treatment of cryptococcal meningitis in patients with AIDS. Clin Infect Dis. 1994;19:741–745.
96. Catanzaro A, Galgiani JN, Levine BE, et al. Fluconazole in the treatment of pulmonary and non-meningeal coccidioidomycosis. Amer J Med. 1995;98:249–256.
97. Castro LGM, Belda W Jr, Cuce LC, et al. Successful treatment of sporotrichosis with oral fluconazole: A report of three cases. Br J Dermatol. 1993;128:352–356.
98. McKinsey DS, Kauffman CA, Pappas PG, et al. Fluconazole therapy for histoplasmosis. Clin Infect Dis. 1996;23:996–1001.
99. Goodman JL, Winston DJ, Greenfield RA, et al. A controlled trial of fluconazole to prevent fungal infections in patients undergoing bone marrow transplantation. N Engl J Med. 1992;326:845–851.
100. Slavin MA, Osborne B, Adams R, et al. Efficacy and safety of fluconazole prophylaxis for fungal infections after marrow transplantation—a prospective, randomized, double-blind study. J Infect Dis. 1995;171:1545–1552.
101. Menichetti F, Del Favero A, Martino P, et al. Preventing fungal infection in neutropenic patients with acute leukemia: Fluconazole compared with oral amphotericin B. Ann Intern Med. 1994;120:913–918.
102. Winston DJ, Chandrasekar PH, Lazarus HM, et al. Fluconazole prophylaxis of fungal infections in patients with acute leukemia. Ann Intern Med. 1993;118:495–503.
103. Havlir DV, Dube MP, et al. Prophylaxis with weekly versus daily fluconazole for fungal infections in patients with AIDS. Clin Infect Dis. 1998;27:1369–1375.
104. Schuman P, Capps L, Peng G, et al. Weekly fluconazole for the prevention of mucosal candidiasis in women with HIV infection. Ann Intern Med. 1997;126:689–696.
105. Norris S, Wheat J, McKinsey D, et al. Prevention of relapse of histoplasmosis with fluconazole in patients with the acquired immunodeficiency syndrome. Am J Med. 1994;96:504–508.
106. Stevens DA. Combination immunotherapy and antifungal chemotherapy. Clin Infect Dis. 1998;26:1266–1269.
107. Rowe JM. Treatment of acute myeloid leukemia with cytokines. Effect on duration of neutropenia and response to infections. Clin Infect Dis. 1998;26:1290–1294.

Chapter 36

Antiviral Drugs (Other Than Antiretrovirals)

FREDERICK G. HAYDEN

GENERAL PRINCIPLES

Antiviral drugs with proven therapeutic (Table 36–1) and prophylactic effectiveness are available for a number of common and some life-threatening viral infections. In part as a response to human immunodeficiency virus (HIV) infection and its sequelae, the search for new antiviral agents and therapeutic approaches for managing viral diseases continues to intensify. More than two dozen antiviral agents are approved for use in the United States, and a number of others are in advanced clinical development. This chapter reviews antiviral agents used for infections caused by viruses other than HIV. Anti-retroviral drugs are reviewed in Chapter 115.

Mechanisms of Action

Chemotherapeutic agents for viral infections can be categorized into three broad groups: agents that directly inactivate intact viruses (virucides); those that inhibit viral replication at the cellular level (antivirals); and those that augment or modify the host response to infection (immunomodulators). Virucidal agents may cause direct inactivation in a single step, examples including detergents, organic solvents such as ether or chloroform, and ultraviolet light, or in multiple steps, as with photodynamic inactivation. However, such interventions have not proved clinically useful in the treatment of mucocutaneous herpes simplex virus (HSV) infections. Treatments that destroy both host tissues and virus simultaneously, such as cryotherapy, laser, or podophyllin treatment of warts, are useful only in discrete mucocutaneous infections. One potential use of virucidal agents may be in preventing transmission of certain viral infections.

Antivirals. Because viral replication depends primarily on host cell metabolic functions, useful antiviral agents must inhibit virus-specific events, such as attachment to the cell, uncoating of the viral genome, or assembly of progeny virions, or preferentially inhibit virus-directed (as contrasted to host cell–directed) macromolecular synthesis. Consequently, antiviral agents typically have a restricted spectrum of activity. Although many compounds exist that exhibit antiviral activity in vitro, most affect some host cell function and are associated with low therapeutic ratios or unacceptable toxicity in humans. Most current antivirals target viral nucleic acid synthesis. In addition, because these agents inhibit ongoing replication at the host cell level, replication may resume when the drug is removed. Similarly, current antiviral agents are not effective in the elimination of nonreplicating or latent viruses.

Susceptibility assays for viruses are not standardized, and results depend on various factors including the assay system, cell line, viral inoculum, and laboratory.[1] Several commercial laboratories offer sensitivity testing of selected herpesviruses and of HIV.

Host Immune Responses. Intact host immunologic responses remain essential for recovery from virus infections. Immunosuppression resulting from organ transplantation, cancer chemotherapy, or HIV infection has been associated with high rates of recrudescent or chronic viral infections. Antiviral prophylaxis and preemptive therapy have become standard practice in immunocompromised patients such as bone marrow and solid organ transplant recipients.[2] Responses to antiviral treatment may be delayed, and the risk of selecting drug-resistant viruses may be higher in such patients. In addition, some antiviral agents may blunt host immune responses by direct immunosuppressive effects[3] or by altering humoral and cellular immune responses indirectly through reductions in viral antigen exposure. Factors other than inhibition of viral replication alone are important in treating certain viral diseases, such as orofacial HSV infections or rhinovirus colds in normal hosts and cytomegalovirus (CMV) pneumonia in bone marrow transplant recipients, in which it has been possible to demonstrate antiviral effects without clinical benefit.

Immunomodulating agents used to treat viral infections include those that replace deficient host immune responses (e.g., exogenous antibody in chronic echovirus infection, cytotoxic T lymphocytes in CMV infection of marrow transplant recipients) and those that enhance endogenous ones. Chemical agents that appear to augment cell-mediated immune responses have been used with variable success and remain largely investigational. One topical immune response modifier, imiquimod, has shown clinically useful effects in genital papillomavirus infections.[4]

Drug Resistance

Drug-resistant viruses have been recognized increasingly during clinical use of various antiviral agents.[5] Indeed, the laboratory selection of a drug-resistant strain of virus implies that the drug has a specific antiviral mechanism. The development of resistance results from mutations within the viral genome, and the presence of selective drug pressure leads to the emergence of a resistant virus population. Resistant subpopulations often exist naturally in clinical isolates, but spontaneous mutations may also arise during drug exposure. Single-nucleotide mutations leading to critical amino acid substitutions in a target protein are often sufficient to cause antiviral resistance.

The possibility of drug resistance is usually recognized because of a lack of clinical and virologic response to treatment. However, clinical failures of antiviral therapy may involve drug-sensitive viruses in immunocompromised hosts who are unable to resolve infection. Factors favoring the emergence of resistant variants include high viral replicative load, as in infections with chronic or high-titer replication; high intrinsic viral mutation rate, which is generally greater in RNA than in DNA viruses; and degree of selective drug pressure, which is higher with prolonged or repeated courses of drug therapy. Consequently, most drug-resistant viruses, (including HSV, varicella-zoster virus [VZV], CMV, and HIV-1), are recovered from immunocompromised patients; influenza A virus is an exception.[6]

The consequences of the emergence of resistance may include a reduction or alteration (e.g., different clinical syndromes) in viral pathogenicity, although such viruses appear to be able to cause severe disease in immunocompromised hosts. Whether resistant variants are at some biologic disadvantage with respect to transmissibility, ability to establish chronic or latent infection, or persistence in the absence of selective drug pressure depends on the particular virus and drug.

Drug Administration

Clinical efficacy depends on achieving effective antiviral concentrations at the site of infection, usually adequate intracellular concentrations of an agent or its active metabolites. Many antivirals, particularly nucleoside analogues, are inactive until they are metabolized within the cell to phosphorylated derivatives, which compete with natural nucleoside for viral and sometimes host cell enzymes. The state of activation or stage of differentiation of the cell can affect the intracellular pools of the phosphorylated antiviral and its competing natural substrate and thereby affect inhibitory activity and toxicity.[7]

Human pharmacokinetic studies that define absorption, stability in body fluids, tissue and cellular distribution, and metabolic fate of antiviral drugs are important in selecting proper dose. Because predictive relationships between the drug concentrations that are active

TABLE 36–1 Antiviral Agents of Established Therapeutic Effectiveness

Viral Infection	Drug	Route	Usual Dosage
Cytomegalovirus			
Retinitis	Ganciclovir	IV	5 mg/kg/12 h in 1-h infusion for 14–21 d*
	Cidofovir	IV	5 mg/kg once weekly × 2 then every other wk
	Formivirsen	Intravitreal	330 μg every 2 wk
	Foscarnet	IV	60 mg/kg/8 h in 1–2 h infusion for 14–21 d†
Pneumonia	Ganciclovir	IV	5 mg/kg/12 h in 1-h infusion *plus* IV immunoglobulin for 14–21 d‡
Hepatitis viruses			
Chronic hepatitis C	Interferon-α-2b	SC/IM	3 MU 3 times weekly for 24 weeks
	plus Ribavirin§	PO	1000–1200 mg/d depending on weight
Chronic hepatitis B	Interferon-α-2b	SC/IM	5 MU/d or 10 MU 3 times weekly for 16 wk
	Lamivudine‖	PO	100 mg/d
Herpes simplex virus			
Genital herpes			
First episode	Acyclovir	PO¶	200 mg 5 times daily or 400 mg tid for 10 d
	Famciclovir	PO	250 mg tid for 7–10 d
	Valacyclovir	PO	1 g bid for 10 d
Recurrence	Acyclovir	PO	200 mg 5 times daily or 400 mg tid for 5 d
	Famciclovir	PO	125 mg bid for 5 d
	Valacyclovir	PO	500 mg bid for 5 d
Suppression**	Acyclovir	PO	400 mg bid or 200 mg tid for up to 5 y
	Valacyclovir	PO	500 or 1000 mg PO qd for up to 1 y
	Famciclovir	PO	250 mg PO bid for up to 1 y
Encephalitis	Acyclovir††	IV	10 mg/kg/8h in 1-h infusion for 14–21 d
Mucocutaneous disease in immunocompromised hosts	Acyclovir‡‡	IV	5 mg/kg/8h for 7–14 d§§
		PO	400 mg 5 times daily for 7–14 d
	Penciclovir	IV	5 mg/kg/8–12h for 7 d
	Famciclovir	PO	500 mg bid for 7 d
Orolabial herpes	Penciclovir 1%	Topical	q2h while awake for 4 d
Neonatal	Acyclovir‖‖	IV	10–20 mg/kg/8 h for 10–21 d
Keratoconjunctivitis	Trifluridine¶¶		1 drop of 1% solution topically, q2h up to 9 drops/d
	Vidarabine		1/2 inch ribbon of 3% ointment 5 times daily
Influenza virus	Oseltamivir	PO	75 mg bid for 5 d
	Zanamivir	Aerosol	10 mg bid by inhaler for 5 d
Influenza A virus	Amantadine	PO	100 mg bid for 5 d for treatment***
	Rimantadine	PO	200 mg/d for 5 d for treatment†††
Papillomavirus			
Condyloma acuminatum	Interferon-α-2b‡‡‡	Intralesional	1 mu/0.1 ml injected in up to 5 warts
Respiratory syncytial virus	Ribavirin	Aerosol	Aerosol treatment 12 to 18 h/d for 3 to 7 d§§§
Varicella-zoster virus			
Varicella in normal children	Acyclovir	PO	20 mg/kg up to 800 mg qid for 5 d
Varicella in immunocompromized hosts	Acyclovir	IV	500 mg/8h for 7–10 d
Herpes zoster in immunocompromised hosts	Acyclovir**	IV	10 mg/kg/8h in 1-h infusion for 7 d‖‖‖
Herpes zoster in normal hosts	Acyclovir	PO	800 mg 5 times daily for 7–10 d
	Valacyclovir	PO	1 g tid for 7 d
	Famciclovir	PO	500 mg tid for 7 d

*In AIDS and in other highly immunocompromised patients, chronic suppression with a daily infusion of 5 mg/kg given 7 d/wk or 6 mg/kg given 5 d/wk is recommended after acute treatment. These doses are also approved for prevention of CMV disease in transplant recipients. Dose reduction is required for creatinine clearance <80 ml/min. An intraocular insert is also available.
†Chronic suppression with daily infusion of 90 to 120 mg/kg over 2 h is recommended after initial treatment in AIDS patients. Use of metered infusion pump to maintain dosing at maximum of 1 mg/kg/min and close monitoring of renal function with dose reduction for creatinine clearance <1.6 ml/min/kg are required.
‡Not approved by FDA for this indication. In bone marrow transplantation patients, combined use of ganciclovir and intravenous immunoglobulin is necessary for therapeutic benefit.
§Combination therapy is approved for patients with compensated liver disease who have relapsed after interferon therapy and also for initial treatment.
‖Safety and effectiveness have not been established beyond 1 y of therapy.
¶For severe initial genital herpes and in patients unable to tolerate oral medicines, IV acyclovir 5 mg/kg/8 h for 5–7 d is recommended.
**Famciclovir 500 mg bid and valacyclovir 500 mg bid have been effective in reducing recurrences in HIV-infected persons.
††Vidarabine 15 mg/kg/d as an IV infusion over 12 to 24 h is a less effective alternative.
‡‡In acyclovir-resistant in HSV or VZV infections, IV foscarnet 40 mg/kg/8 h appears beneficial. Duration of therapy depends on the clinical response. For limited cutaneous infections in immunocompromised patients, 5% acyclovir ointment can be applied to lesions every 3 h up to 6 times daily for 7 d (about 1/2-inch ribbon per 4 square inches), using a finger cot or glove.
§§Dose reductions are indicated for creatinine clearance <50 ml/min. Pediatric dosage is 250 mg/m²/8 h IV for 7–14 d.
‖‖Not approved by the FDA for this indication. For premature infants, 20 mg/kg/d in two divided doses is advised. Vidarabine 15–30 mg/kg/d as an IV infusion over 12 to 24 hours is an FDA-approved alternative.
¶¶An ophthalmic ointment of 3% acyclovir is available in some countries. Idoxuridine 0.1% solution, q1h while awake and q2h at night, or 0.5% ointment 5 times/day is a less effective alternative. Treatment of HSV ocular infections should be supervised by an ophthalmologist.
***The maximum recommended dose for older adults is 100 mg/d. Dose reductions are indicated for creatinine clearance <80 ml/min. The recommended pediatric dose is 4.4 mg/kg/d up to a maximum of 150 mg/d. For prophylaxis, daily dose must be given for period at risk (2–6 wk).
†††Pediatric dose is 5 mg/kg up to maximum of 150 mg/d. For prophylaxis, daily dose must be given for period at risk.
‡‡‡Other interferons are also approved for this indication.
§§§Reservoir concentration of 20 mg/ml. Requires special aerosol-generating device available from manufacturer and expert respiratory therapy monitoring for administration.
‖‖‖Dose reductions are indicated for creatinine clearance <50 ml/min. Pediatric dosage is 500 mg/m²/8 h for 7–10 d. Vidarabine 10 mg/kg/d as IV infusion over 12 to 24 hours is a less effective alternative.
Abbreviations: IM, Intramuscular; IV, intravenous; PO, oral; SC, subcutaneous.

in vitro, those that are achieved in blood or other body fluids, and the clinical response have not been established for most antiviral agents, pharmacodynamic studies that examine correlations of in vivo antiviral activity, dose, and kinetics are particularly useful. Although animal models are useful in the testing of antiviral agents, they may differ from the corresponding human infection in regard to pathogenesis, drug susceptibility of the virus, drug pharmacology, or toxicity.

Topical application of an antiviral agent to the cornea, skin, mucus membranes, or respiratory tract is intended to provide high concentrations at the site of infection and to avoid the possible toxicity of systemic administration. However, topically applied drugs must be able to penetrate such barriers as stratified epithelium or local secretions to reach the site of active viral replication.

The combined use of antiviral agents with different mechanisms of action has been studied as a means of increasing antiviral activity,

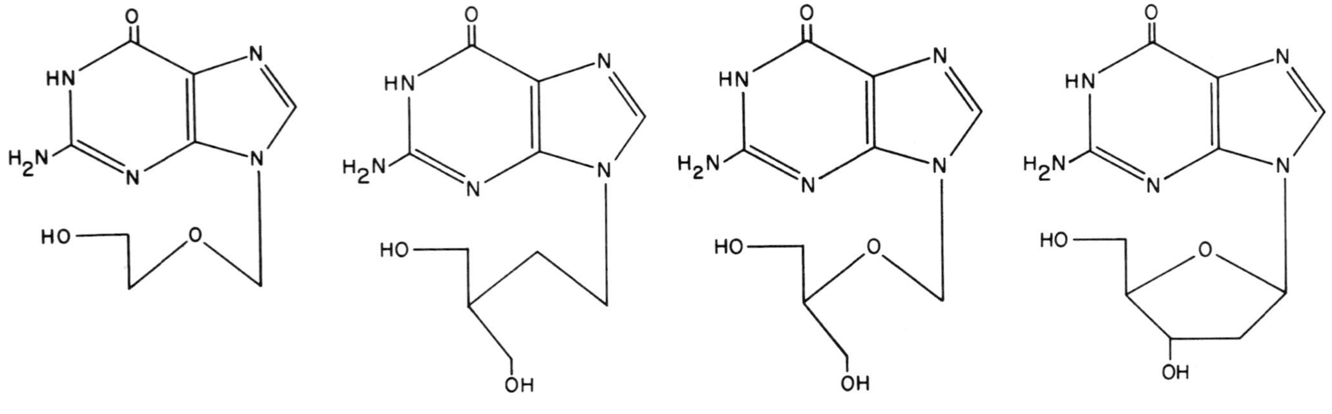

ACYCLOVIR PENCICLOVIR GANCICLOVIR DEOXYGUANOSINE

FIGURE 36–1. Chemical structures of acyclovir, penciclovir, ganciclovir, and the nucleoside deoxyguanosine.

reducing drug dosage and the associated risk of toxicity, and preventing or modifying the development of drug resistance. Viral isolates from treated patients may be genetically heterogeneous with respect to mixtures of sensitive and resistant viruses or viruses with different resistance mutations, so that combinations may be able to provide broader activity than single agents. In addition, individual drugs may act preferentially on different cell types or in different tissues. Combination therapy is the standard of care in HIV infection and is likely to become increasingly used in other viral infections.

ACYCLOVIR AND VALACYCLOVIR

Spectrum

Acyclovir (9-[(2-hydroxyethoxy)methyl]-9H-guanine) (acycloguanosine, Zovirax) is a deoxyguanosine analogue that has an acyclic side chain lacking the 3′-hydroxyl group instead of the cyclic base of natural nucleosides (Fig. 36–1). Valacyclovir (Valtrex) is the L-valyl ester prodrug of acyclovir. Acyclovir's clinically useful antiviral spectrum is limited to herpesviruses. It is approximately 10 times more potent against HSV-1 and -2 than against VZV, and it is even less active against CMV (Table 36–2).[8–11] Acyclovir inhibits the replication of Epstein-Barr virus (EBV) in productively infected cells but does not affect latent or persistent infection.[12] Acyclovir has shown antiviral activity in experimental HSV infection when administered topically, parenterally, or orally and in simian varicella when given systemically.[8] Enhanced anti-herpesvirus activity occurs when acyclovir is given in combination with interferons and other antiviral agents in vitro and in animal models.[8]

Growth of uninfected mammalian cells is generally unaffected by high acyclovir concentrations. Acyclovir (20 μg/ml) does not reproducibly alter cell-mediated immune responses of human peripheral blood leukocytes or affect human granulocyte progenitor cell growth in vitro.[3, 13]

TABLE 36–2 Representative In Vitro Inhibitory Concentrations of Acyclic Nucleosides and Nucleotides for Clinical Isolates of Herpesviruses in Human Cells

Virus	Inhibitory Concentration (μg/ml)			
	Acyclovir	*Penciclovir*	*Ganciclovir*	*Cidofovir*
Herpes simplex virus 1	0.02–0.9	0.2–0.6	0.05–0.6	0.4–3
Herpes simplex virus 2	0.3–2.2	0.3–2.4	0.05–0.6	0.4–3
Varicella-zoster virus	0.8–4.0	0.9–4.0	0.4–10	0.25
Cytomegalovirus	2–57	52	0.2–2.8	0.2–0.9
Epstein-Barr virus	1.6	—	1.5	<0.03

Data from refs. 17–20, 203, 291–293, 335–339, 559, 560

Mechanism of Action

Acyclovir is the prototype of a group of antiviral agents that are activated by viral thymidine kinase (TK) to become inhibitors of viral DNA polymerase and block viral DNA synthesis.[9, 14] Acyclovir uptake and intracellular phosphorylation to the monophosphate derivative are facilitated by HSV TK.[14] Cellular enzymes convert the monophosphate to acyclovir triphosphate, which is present in 40- to 100-fold higher concentrations in HSV-infected than in uninfected cells. Acyclovir triphosphate competitively inhibits viral DNA polymerase, and to a much smaller extent cellular DNA polymerases, with respect to deoxyguanosine triphosphate.[15] Acyclovir triphosphate is also incorporated into viral DNA, where it acts as a chain terminator because of the lack of the 3′-hydroxyl group. Formation of a complex between the terminated DNA template containing acyclovir and the enzyme may lead to irreversible inactivation of the DNA polymerase.[16] The DNA polymerases of various herpesviruses differ in their degree of inhibition by acyclovir triphosphate; the polymerases of EBV and CMV appear to be especially sensitive.[17]

Resistance

Acyclovir-resistant HSV, often defined by an in vitro inhibitory concentration greater than 1 to 3 μg/ml, can be readily selected by passage in the presence of acyclovir and also is present in native virus populations with an estimated frequency of 1 in 10^{-3} to 10^{-4} virions.[18] One study found that 40% of HSV isolates from untreated patients contain acyclovir-resistant variants, accounting for at least 1% of the total virus population.[19] Three basic resistance mechanisms have been identified: absent or low production of viral TK, altered TK substrate specificity (e.g., phosphorylation of thymidine but not of acyclovir), and altered viral DNA polymerase. Changes in these viral enzymes relate to point mutations or base insertions or deletions in the corresponding genes.[20] The most common mechanism found in clinical HSV isolates is deficient TK activity.[21, 22] Such variants are cross-resistant to other agents activated by viral TK (e.g., penciclovir, ganciclovir). Less commonly, resistant isolates have altered TK activity, and DNA polymerase mutants are rare in clinical strains. Heterogeneous mixtures are not uncommonly found.

The prevalence of acyclovir-resistant HSV isolates in immunocompetent hosts is generally less than 1%, but it is approximately 6 to 8% in immunocompromised patients.[23–25] Resistant HSV can be recovered from 11 to 17% of patients with the acquired immunodeficiency syndrome (AIDS) and transplantation patients receiving acyclovir treatment for 2 weeks or longer.[26] Most isolates recovered during oral suppressive therapy have sensitive phenotypes.[27, 28] After chronic acyclovir suppression of genital HSV, the frequency of resistant HSV (3.5%) is comparable to that before treatment or in unexposed patients.[29] In contrast, progressive HSV disease associated with recovery of acyclovir-resistant virus and poor response to acyclovir therapy is well recognized in immunocompromisd patients.[24, 25] Painful ulcerating perirectal lesions, often indolent and necrotizing, caused by HSV-2 represent the most common pattern in AIDS patients, and orofacial disease due to HSV-1 is most common in transplantation patients. The risk factors include degree of immunosuppression, size of lesions, and repeated or prolonged use of acyclovir for treatment rather than prophylaxis.

Most TK-deficient mutants of HSV are less neurovirulent than wild-type strains and less able to be reactivated from latency in animal models, although they may cause extensive mucocutaneous disease in immunocompromised hosts.[18] TK-altered or polymerase mutants have variable or minimal decrease in pathogenicity. Recurrent genital HSV caused by a TK-altered variant has occurred in an immunocompromised host.[30] No proven person-to-person spread of resistant HSV has been documented, and recurrences after cessation of acyclovir are usually caused by sensitive virus. However, in AIDS patients, persistent shedding of resistant HSV at the site of initial infection and recurrences with acyclovir-resistant variants have been found in the absence of selective drug pressure.[31] Visceral disease is uncommon, but keratouveitis, meningoencephalitis, and pneumonitis have occurred with resistant variants.[26, 32, 33]

Depending on the degree of immunosuppression, resistant HSV infections may undergo spontaneous healing during or after cessation of acyclovir therapy. In patients with progressive disease, intravenous foscarnet therapy is effective, but vidarabine is not.[31] High-dose, continuous infusion of acyclovir,[34] topically applied trifluridine, topical interferon (IFN)-α2 alone or in combination with topical trifluridine,[35] and topical cidofovir[36] have been used in small numbers of patients. Ganciclovir is not active against TK-deficient mutants.

Acyclovir resistance in VZV isolates, associated with 20- to 40-fold increases in inhibitory concentrations, is usually related to mutations in VZV TK with inability to phosphorylate acyclovir, or, less often, to mutations in viral DNA polymerase. Such isolates are very uncommon[37] but have been recovered from HIV-infected children and adults with chronic (months), disseminated, hyperkeratotic or verrucous papular lesions that failed to heal with intravenous acyclovir.[38] Invasive disease with resistant variants occurs.[39] Chronic suppressive therapy with subtherapeutic doses of acyclovir appears to be a risk factor. Intravenous foscarnet also appears to be effective for acyclovir-resistant VZV infections.[40]

Pharmacokinetics

The bioavailability of oral acyclovir is low (15 to 21%) and decreases with increasing doses.[41, 42] Peak plasma concentrations average 0.4 to 0.8 μg/ml after 200-mg oral doses[43] and increase to about 1.6 μg/ml with 800-mg doses.[44] Bioavailability is lower in transplantation patients, in whom doses of 400 mg provide peak levels of 0.7 to 0.9 μg/ml.[45] A liquid suspension has somewhat lower oral bioavailability; peak plasma concentrations average 1.0 μg/ml in children receiving doses of 600 mg/m^2.[46] Peak and trough plasma concentrations at the end of a 1-hour infusion average 9.8 and 0.7 μg/ml after administration of 5 mg/kg in 8 hours and 20.7 and 2.3 μg/ml after 10 mg/kg in 8 hours, respectively.

After oral administration, valacyclovir is rapidly and almost completely (>99%) converted to acyclovir.[47, 48] This is the result of first-pass enzymatic hydrolysis in the liver and intestine by an enzyme designated valacyclovir hydrolase. The relative bioavailability of acyclovir is three to five times greater after ingestion of the prodrug valacyclovir. The absolute bioavailability averages 54%.[49] Peak plasma levels of valacyclovir are 0.4 μg/ml or less after 1000-mg doses. Peak plasma acyclovir levels average 5.0 and 8.5 μg/ml after doses of 1000 and 2000 mg, respectively. Total acyclovir exposure is similar to that seen with intravenous acyclovir, although peak plasma concentrations are twofold to fourfold lower.[50] In elderly adults, peak plasma concentrations increase 15 to 20% and overall acyclovir exposure increases 30 to 50%,[47] probably because of reduced renal clearance in this population.

Acyclovir is distributed widely in body fluids. Plasma protein binding is less than 20%. Cerebrospinal fluid concentrations are approximately one half of plasma values.[42] After oral administration, salivary concentrations average 13% of plasma levels, but concentrations in vaginal secretions range from 15 to 170% of those in plasma.[43] Zoster vesicular fluid levels are similar to those in plasma. Aqueous humor levels average 37% of concurrent plasma values.[51] Concentrations in breast milk average more than three times higher than those in serum.[52] Plasma levels in newborns are similar to maternal ones, and amniotic fluid and placental concentrations are several-fold higher.[53] Percutaneous absorption of acyclovir after topical administration appears to be low.

The mean plasma elimination half-life ($T_{1/2}$) of acyclovir is about 2.5 to 3 hours (range, 1.5 to 6.3 hours) in adults with normal renal function; it is slightly longer (3.8 hours) in neonates and increases to 19.5 hours in anuric patients.[41, 42, 53, 54] Renal excretion of unmetabolized acyclovir by glomerular filtration and tubular secretion accounts for 60 to 91% of an administered dose, whereas less than 15% is excreted as 9-carboxymethoxymethylguanine and/or minor metabolites.[55] Dosage reduction is indicated in patients with a creatinine clearance of less than 50 ml/min (Table 36–3). Acyclovir is readily hemodialyzable, and plasma concentrations are reduced by about 60% during 6 hours of hemodialysis.[56, 57] Peritoneal dialysis is much less efficient in removing acyclovir,[58] so dosing supplementation is not needed during continuous ambulatory peritoneal dialysis. Bioavailability is about 61% after intraperitoneal dosing.[59]

Interactions

Severe somnolence and lethargy may occur with combinations of zidovudine and acyclovir.[60] Concomitant use of cyclosporine and probably of other nephrotoxic agents enhances the risk of nephrotoxicity. Probenecid decreases the renal clearance and prolongs the plasma $T_{1/2}$. By competing for the organic acid secretory pathway, acyclovir may decrease the renal clearance of other drugs eliminated by active renal secretion, such as methotrexate.[42] Thiazide diuretics do not alter acyclovir pharmacokinetics.[47]

Toxicity

Topical acyclovir may cause transient burning when it is applied to genital lesions. The polyethylene glycol base of topical acyclovir

TABLE 36–3 Acyclovir Dose Adjustments Suggested for Patients with Impaired Renal Function

Creatinine Clearance (ml/min/1.73 m^2)	Intravenous		Oral*	
	Standard Dose (%)	*Dosing Interval (hs)*	*Dose*	*Dosing Interval (hs)*
>50	100	8	800	4
25–50	100	12	800	4
10–25	100	24	800	4
0–10†	50	24	800	12‡

*Oral acyclovir dose adjustments are needed for severe renal insufficiency. Recommendations are based on high-dose oral regimen (4000 mg/d). For low-dose (1000 mg/d) oral regimen, the suggested dose is 200 mg q12h for creatinine clearance <10 ml/min/1.73m^2.

†An alternative in patients with end-stage renal disease is administration of 14% of standard dose q8h after loading with 37% of the standard dose. For posthemodialysis administration, 60–100% of standard dose should be used.[56] An intravenous dosage of 2.5 mg/kg/d has been suggested in continuous ambulatory peritoneal dialysis patients.

‡In dialysis-dependent patients, a further dose reduction to 200 mg/12 h and 400 mg after dialysis is recommended to avoid toxic levels. A dose of 800 mg PO q24h has been suggested for those on continuous ambulatory peritoneal dialysis.[561]

Adapted from Blum MR, Liao SH, de MP. Overview of acyclovir pharmacokinetic disposition in adults and children. Am J Med. 1982;73:186–192; Laskin OL, Longstreth JA, Whelton A, et al. Effect of renal failure on the pharmacokinetics of acyclovir. Am J Med. 1982;73:197–201, with permission from Excerpta Medica, Inc..

may cause mucosal irritation and is not approved for intravaginal use. Acyclovir cream uncommonly causes allergic contact dermatitis.[8]

Intravenous acyclovir is generally well tolerated,[8, 61] although inflammation, phlebitis, and, rarely, vesicular eruption[62] can occur at the injection site after extravasation of the alkaline solution (pH 9 to 11). Uncommon side effects include rash, diaphoresis, hematuria, hypotension, headache, and nausea. Approximately 1 to 4% of patients receiving intravenous acyclovir have manifested neurotoxicity, characterized by lethargy, confusion, obtundation, tremor, myoclonus, hallucinations, delirium, seizures, extrapyramidal signs, autonomic instability, and/or coma.[63–66] Diffuse electroencephalographic abnormalities and increased cerebrospinal fluid concentrations of myelin basic protein may occur. Symptoms of neurotoxicity usually develop within 1 to 3 days after starting treatment. Most of these patients have acute renal dysfunction or preexisting renal disease, and neurotoxicity occurs in association with high serum acyclovir concentrations (>25 μg/ml). Neurotoxicity occurs uncommonly after oral administration and after prolonged therapy without changes in renal function. Neurologic side effects usually resolve within several days after drug concentrations decrease.[60] Hemodialysis may be useful in severe cases.[58]

Reversible renal dysfunction has been observed in approximately 5% of patients, and a higher proportion of children, treated with intravenous acyclovir.[8, 64] Acyclovir can cause a crystalline nephropathy and, rarely, interstitial nephritis.[67] Acyclovir solubility decreases to 2.5 mg/ml at 37°C, and crystalluria has been described in adult and pediatric patients.[68] Obstructive nephropathy may be manifested by nausea, emesis, flank pain, and increasing azotemia. Bolus infusion, dehydration, preexisting renal insufficiency, high doses, and high acyclovir plasma levels are risk factors. Nephrotoxicity usually resolves with drug cessation and volume expansion.

Oral acyclovir has been associated infrequently with nausea, diarrhea, rash, and headache and uncommonly with renal insufficiency or neurotoxicity. Immediate hypersensitivity reactions to acyclovir are rare but may be managed with oral desensitization.[69] Long-term acyclovir suppression for frequently recurring genital or mucocutaneous infections is safe during over 5 years of continuous use,[70] and no adverse effects on sperm production or peripheral blood lymphocyte cytogenetics have been detected.[71, 72] However, chronic oral acyclovir can cause neutropenia in infants.[73] No excess frequency of abnormalities has been recognized in infants born to women exposed to acyclovir during pregnancy, but the number of instances monitored is insufficient to reach definitive conclusions about safety during pregnancy.[74] High-dose valacyclovir (8 g/day) is associated with gastrointestinal intolerance, azotemia, and possibly thrombotic microangiopathy in AIDS patients[75] and with confusion and hallucinations in transplant patients.[75a] Tolerance at lower doses is comparable to that of acyclovir.

Acyclovir has shown mutagenic activity in some in vitro assays at high concentrations, but no significant immunosuppressive activity, carcinogenicity, or teratogenicity has been noted in animal studies. High doses decrease spermatogenesis and cause testicular atrophy in animals.

Clinical Studies

Acyclovir is currently the agent of choice for management of many types of HSV and VZV infections because of its efficacy, safety, and ease of administration (see Table 36–1).[9] Valacyclovir is comparably effective in most of the conditions in which acyclovir is used and offers more convenient dosing regimens at higher cost.

Herpes Simplex Virus. Acyclovir by various routes is effective in initial genital HSV infections.[76–79] Topical acyclovir is less effective than oral or intravenous administration, and its use is discouraged. Intravenous acyclovir markedly reduces viral shedding, time to healing, and duration of symptoms in patients hospitalized with severe primary genital HSV infections.[76] In outpatients, oral acyclovir (200 mg five times daily for 10 days) is associated with significant reductions in virus shedding, symptoms, and time to healing.[77, 78] Higher doses of oral acyclovir do not increase efficacy,[79] and valacyclovir (1 g twice daily for 10 days) is comparable to acyclovir in efficacy and tolerability for treating a first episode genital herpes.[80] None of these regimens has been associated with consistent reductions in the risk of recurrent genital lesions. Acyclovir therapy decreases the humoral and cellular immune response to HSV after first-episode genital herpes.[81, 82] Higher oral doses (400 mg five times daily for 10 days) provide similar benefit in first-episode HSV proctitis.[83]

In recurrent genital HSV infections, patient-initiated oral acyclovir (200 mg five times daily for 5 days) during the prodrome or at the first sign of lesions is associated with reductions of 1.5 to 2 days in the duration of shedding and time to healing.[78, 84] Valacyclovir (500 mg twice daily for 5 days) is comparable to acyclovir and superior to placebo in the treatment of recurrent genital herpes.[85, 86] Topical acyclovir offers no significant clinical benefit in this condition. In patients with frequently recurring genital herpes, long-term oral acyclovir (400 to 1000 mg/day in divided doses) reduces the frequency of clinical recurrences by about 90%, protects 65 to 85% of patients from recurrence, and reduces the frequency of subclinical viral shedding and viral DNA detectability.[70, 87–89] Doses of 400 mg twice daily are effective for longer than 5 years. Once-daily or weekend-only use of acyclovir is inadequate, whereas once-daily valacyclovir appears to be effective and well tolerated.[90] Asymptomatic shedding may occur during suppression, and rare cases of transmission to sexual partners have occurred.[91] After cessation of acyclovir, patients generally return to their previous pattern of recurrent infection. Oral acyclovir suppression reduces recurrences during late pregnancy and may reduce cesarean delivery rates after first-episode genital herpes during pregnancy.[92, 93]

Long-term suppression may be useful in other patients with disabling recurrences of herpes whitlow or HSV-related erythema multiforme. In patients with recurrent herpes labialis or ocular HSV disease, oral acyclovir (400 mg twice daily) reduces the number of recurrences by about one half.[94, 95] In patients with a history of sun-induced recurrences, short-term prophylaxis (400 to 800 mg twice daily) inconsistently reduces the risk of recurrence.[96, 97] Short-term prophylaxis during outbreaks in daycare centers may be effective in preventing primary infections in children,[98] but the efficacy of post-exposure prophylaxis remains to be established.

In recurrent orolabial HSV infections, topical acyclovir ointment is not associated with clinical benefit. Topical acyclovir cream, not available in the United States, may be more effective. Oral acyclovir (200 to 400 mg five times daily for 5 days) provides only modest clinical benefit in recurrent orolabial herpes but appears to be therapeutically efficacious in recurrent whitlow.[99, 100] Acyclovir (15 mg/kg five times daily to a maximum of 200 mg/dose for 7 days) is beneficial for treating HSV gingivostomatitis in children,[101] and chronic suppression reduces cutaneous recurrences after neonatal infection. Acyclovir combined with prednisone is superior to prednisone alone for the treatment of Bell's palsy.[102]

Systemic acyclovir in various regimens has been used successfully for both prevention and treatment of mucocutaneous HSV infections in immunosuppressed patients.[29, 103–107] Intravenous acyclovir (250 mg/m² given over 8 to 12 hours), begun before transplantation and continuing for several weeks, is highly effective in reducing the incidence of HSV disease in seropositive bone marrow transplant recipients.[103] For patients who can tolerate oral medications, oral acyclovir (400 mg five times daily for 5 weeks) is effective in marrow transplantation patients,[105] and long-term oral acyclovir (400 mg three times daily for 6 months) also reduces the risk of VZV infection.[104] Low doses of oral acyclovir (200 mg every 6 to 8 hours) appear to be effective in renal transplantation patients[106] and other immunosuppressed hosts and during periods of intense chemotherapy.

In immunocompromised patients with established mucocutaneous HSV infection, intravenous acyclovir (250 mg/m² every 8 hours for 7 days) shortens healing time, duration of pain, and virus shedding,[2, 108] although recurrences are common after cessation of therapy. Oral acyclovir (800 mg five times daily) is also effective.[109] Intravenous acyclovir may be beneficial in cases of viscerally disseminating HSV in pregnant women and transplantation patients.[110, 111]

In HSV encephalitis, acyclovir reduces mortality to 19 to 28%, compared with 50 to 54% with vidarabine.[9] In neonates, in immunosuppressed patients, and, rarely, in apparently healthy persons, early relapse of encephalitis may follow initial acyclovir therapy,[112] so that longer courses of treatment may be warranted. Acyclovir also appears to be effective in the acute retinal necrosis syndrome.[113]

Varicella-Zoster Virus Infections. Intravenous acyclovir is effective for varicella and herpes zoster in immunocompromised patients. It also appears to be effective in varicella pneumonia or encephalitis in previously healthy adults.[114] In immunocompromised patients with herpes zoster, intravenous acyclovir (500 mg/m^2 every 8 hours for 7 days) reduces the risk of cutaneous dissemination and visceral complications, compared with placebo.[115] In immunosuppressed children with varicella, intravenous acyclovir reduces the risk of visceral complications and time to full crusting.[116, 117] Early relapse of infection may occur after cessation of therapy, and treatment may be ineffective in visceral disease. Early treatment with oral acyclovir (800 mg five times daily for 7 days) may be effective in children.[118]

High-dose oral acyclovir is effective treatment for herpes zoster in older adults, for zoster ophthalmicus, and, if begun within 24 hours after rash onset, for varicella in children,[119] adolescents,[120] and adults.[121] In children, acyclovir's effects include reductions of about 1 day in fever and 15 to 30% in the severity of other illness measures, so routine use in uncomplicated varicella is not recommended.[122] In adults with varicella, oral acyclovir (800 mg five times daily for 7 days), initiated within 24 hours after the onset of rash, reduces fever and the time to total crusting of lesion by approximately 2 days; it does not affect the course of illness if begun later.[121] Postcontact prophylaxis with oral acyclovir (40 mg/kg daily in divided doses), beginning 9 to 11 days after exposure, may reduce the risk of varicella in household contacts.[123]

In immunocompetent older adults with herpes zoster, intravenous acyclovir reduces virus shedding, time to healing of skin lesions, and duration of acute pain.[124] Oral acyclovir (800 mg five times daily for 7 to 10 days) also reduces acute pain and healing time in older adults, if treatment can be initiated within 72 hours after rash onset, and particularly within 1 or 2 days.[2, 44] Lower doses and later initiation of therapy are ineffective. A reduction in ocular complications, particularly keratitis and anterior uveitis, occurs with oral acyclovir treatment of zoster ophthalmicus.[125] However, no consistent effect on the incidence or severity of postherpetic neuralgia has been found.[126] Compared with acyclovir, oral valacyclovir (1 g three times daily for 7 days) speeds resolution of zoster-associated pain and decreases the frequency of persistent pain.[127]

Other Viruses. Acyclovir is therapeutically ineffective in established CMV infections. High-dose intravenous acyclovir (500 mg/m^2 every 8 hours), beginning 5 days before allogenic bone marrow transplantation and continuing for 30 days afterward, is associated with an approximate 50% lower risk of CMV disease and improved survival in CMV-seropositive patients.[128] This approach is not effective for recipients of autologous marrow.[129] High-dose oral acyclovir for 3 months also reduces the risk of CMV disease in renal and liver transplant recipients but appears to be less effective than ganciclovir.[2, 130–132] It has not proved effective in liver transplant recipients receiving OKT3 therapy or in lung transplantation patients. High-dose acyclovir has been reported to provide a modest survival benefit in advanced HIV infection, although this remains controversial.[133] High-dose valacyclovir (2 g four times daily), but not acyclovir, reduces CMV disease risk in advanced HIV infection but is less well tolerated and is associated with higher mortality.[75] Valacyclovir prophylaxis (2 g qid for 90 days) reduces the risk of CMV disease and of graft rejection in renal transplant recipients, including CMV seronegative recipients of seropositive grafts.[75a]

In infectious mononucleosis acyclovir is associated with transient suppression of salivary EBV excretion but no important effects on illness parameters.[134] High-dose acyclovir is not effective in patients with the chronic fatigue syndrome.[135] Some cases of severe EBV infection or EBV-related lymphoproliferation may respond to acyclovir.[136, 137] EBV-related oral hairy leukoplakia regresses with oral acyclovir treatment.[138]

Acyclovir is useful in managing herpes virus B (cercopithecine herpesvirus 1) exposures and infections.[107] High intravenous doses are recommended for treating established herpes virus B infections. Neither intravenous nor oral acyclovir enhances the response to IFN in patients with chronic hepatitis B.[139] Long-term acyclovir does not reduce neurologic deterioration in multiple sclerosis.[140]

AMANTADINE AND RIMANTADINE

Spectrum

Amantadine (1-adamantanamine hydrochloride) (Symmetrel) and rimantadine (alpha-methyl-1-adamantane methylamine hydrochloride) (Flumadine) are symmetric tricyclic amines (Fig. 36–2) that specifically inhibit the replication of influenza A viruses at low concentrations (<1.0 μg/ml). By plaque assay, inhibitory concentrations of the drugs range from 0.1 to 0.4 μ/ml for human influenza A viruses, including H1N1, H2N2, and H3N2 subtypes.[141, 142] Rimantadine is 4 to 10 times more active than amantadine in vitro. Higher concentrations (10 to 50 μ/ml) have in vitro inhibitory activity against other enveloped viruses, including parainfluenza, influenza B, rubella, and dengue, but these concentrations are not achievable clinically and can be cytotoxic and immunosuppressive in vitro. Inhibition of hepatitis C virus HCV replication in humans has been reported.[143]

These agents have both prophylactic and therapeutic activity in experimental influenza A virus infection of animals after oral or parenteral dosing.[144] Amantadine and ribavirin combinations show enhanced antiviral and therapeutic effects in vitro and in experimental influenza. Rimantadine exhibits enhanced antiviral activity in combination with ribavirin, interferon, zanamivir, or protease inhibitors.[145–147]

Mechanism of Action

Amantadine and rimantadine share two concentration-dependent mechanisms of antiviral action.[148] Low concentrations inhibit the ion channel function of the M2 protein of influenza A viruses, which affects two different stages in virus replication.[148, 149] The primary effect involves inhibition of viral uncoating or disassembly of the virion during endocytosis. For H7-subtype viruses, a late effect on viral assembly is presumably mediated through altered pH regulation of the trans-Golgi network. Amantadine and rimantadine block ion permeation and prevent M2-mediated changes in pH. This action probably accounts for both inhibition of the acid-mediated dissociation of the matrix protein from the ribonucleoprotein complex within

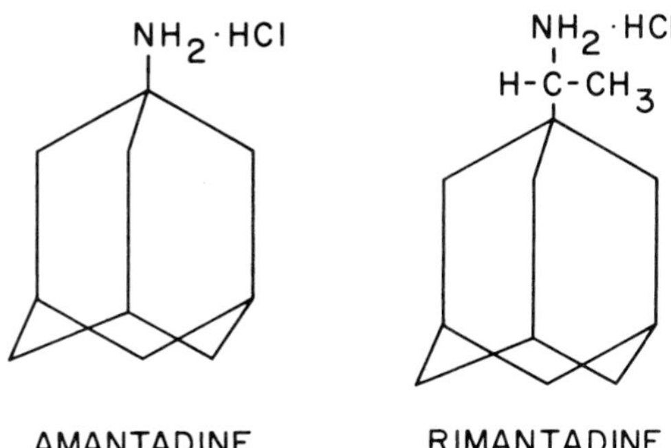

FIGURE 36–2. Chemical structures of amantadine hydrochloride and rimantadine hydrochloride.

endosomes early in replication and potentiation of pH-induced alterations in the hemagglutinin during its transport late in infection.

Amantadine and rimantadine are also concentrated in the lysosomal fraction of mammalian cells. Drug-mediated increases in lysosomal pH may inhibit virus-induced membrane fusion events and account for the broader antiviral spectrum at higher concentrations. In contrast, the selective anti–influenza A virus effects are quickly lost after removal of the drug from the surrounding medium, which suggests that drug must be present in extracellular fluid early in the replicative cycle.[150]

Resistance

Contemporary epidemic strains have been drug sensitive,[141, 151] but resistant virus is readily selected by virus passage in the presence of drug.[152] Resistance with more than 100-fold increases in inhibitory concentrations has been associated with single amino acid substitutions at critical sites in the transmembrane region of the M2 protein.[148] Amantadine and rimantadine share cross-susceptibility or cross-resistance. In avian models resistant viruses are virulent, genetically stable, and able to compete with wild-type virus, so that transmission of drug-resistant virus may occur after cessation of drug use.[153, 154]

Up to 30% of drug-treated children and adults shed resistant virus by the fifth day of therapy.[155] Immunocompetent persons shedding resistant virus resolve their illness promptly,[156] whereas prolonged shedding may occur in immunocompromised hosts.[157] Transmission of resistant virus, associated with failure of drug prophylaxis, has been documented in household contacts of rimantadine-treated index cases[158] and in nursing home residents receiving amantadine.[159] Resistant variants can cause typical influenza illness. It is prudent to avoid contact between treated patients and susceptible high-risk contacts and to avoid use of both treatment (specifically of young children) and postexposure prophylaxis in the same household.

Ribavirin and the neuraminidase inhibitors zanamivir and GS4071 are active in vitro against amantadine- and rimantadine-resistant strains.

Pharmacokinetics

Amantadine. Amantadine is well absorbed after oral administration of capsule, tablet, or syrup forms.[160–162] Steady-state peak plasma concentrations average 0.5 to 0.8 μg/ml with a 100-mg twice daily regimen in healthy young adults. Elderly persons require only one half of the weight-adjusted dose needed for young adults to achieve equivalent trough plasma levels of 0.3 μ/ml.[161] Plasma protein binding of amantadine is about 67% and amantadine's volume of distribution is large. Nasal secretion and salivary levels of amantadine approximate those found in the serum. Cerebrospinal fluid levels are about one half of those in plasma, and amantadine is excreted in breast milk.

Amantadine is excreted unmetabolized in the urine through glomerular filtration and probably through tubular secretion.[163] The plasma $T_{1/2}$ is about 12 to 18 hours but ranges widely. Because of age-related declines in renal function, $T_{1/2}$ increases up to twofold in the elderly,[160] and even more in patients with impaired renal function.[163] In patients with creatinine clearance less than 10 ml/min, the $T_{1/2}$ may be as long as 30 days. Dose reductions are required in renal insufficiency (Table 36–4). Amantadine is inefficiently cleared in hemodialysis patients, and additional doses are not required.[163, 164] Monitoring of plasma concentrations in such patients is desirable but impractical.

Rimantadine. Rimantadine is well but slowly absorbed, with the time to peak plasma concentration averaging 2 to 6 hours.[165, 166] Absorption does not appear to be decreased by food. With multiple doses of 100 mg twice daily, the steady-state peak and trough plasma concentrations in healthy adults are approximately 0.4 to 0.5 and 0.2 to 0.4 μg/ml, respectively.[167] In infants receiving doses of 3 mg/kg each day, steady-state peak serum levels range from 0.1 to 0.6 μg/ml.[168] No important age-related changes in pharmacokinetics have been found in healthy elderly adults or in children.[169, 170] However, steady-state plasma concentrations in elderly nursing home residents receiving 100 mg twice daily average more than twofold higher (mean, 1.2 μg/ml) than those observed in healthy adults, which indicates the need for lower doses in such patients.[171] Plasma protein binding is about 40%. Rimantadine has a very large volume of distribution, and concentrations in nasal mucus average 50% higher than those in plasma.[170]

TABLE 36–4 Amantadine Dosage Regimens for Prophylaxis and Alterations in Renal Failure

Condition	Suggested Dose
No renal insufficiency	
Children, 1–9 y	4.4 mg/kg/d in 2 divided doses, up to 150 mg/d
Ages 10–64 y	100 mg twice daily
Ages ≥ 65 y	100 mg (1.4 mg/kg) once daily*
Creatinine clearance (ml/min/1.73 m²)†	
≥80	100 mg (1.4 mg/kg) twice daily
79–35	Once daily
34–25	q2d
24–15	q3d
<15	q7d

*Use weight-adjusted dosing for smaller patients (< 50 kg). Doses of 1.4 mg/kg/d have been suggested.[161]

†Based on adult dose of 200 mg/d. Proportionate reductions should be made for older adults receiving lower doses.

From Wu MJ, Ing TS, Soung LS, et al. Amantadine hydrochloride pharmacokinetics in patients with impaired renal function. Clin Nephrol. 1982; 17:19–23.

In contrast to amantadine, rimantadine undergoes extensive metabolism by hydroxylation, conjugation, and glucuronidation before renal excretion.[160, 170, 172, 173] The plasma $T_{1/2}$ of rimantadine averages 24 to 36 hours, approximately twofold longer than that of amantadine. No clinically important differences in pharmacokinetics are found in patients with chronic liver disease without significant hepatocellular dysfunction.[174] In hemodialysis patients with severe renal failure, the clearance of rimantadine is decreased by 40% and the $T_{1/2}$ is about 55% longer.[172] Dose reductions by one half (e.g., 100 mg/day) are recommended for marked hepatic or renal insufficiency (creatinine clearance <10 ml/min). Hemodialysis removes only a small amount of rimantadine, so supplemental doses are not required.

Interactions

The central nervous system (CNS) effects of amantadine appear to be increased by concomitant ingestion of antihistamines or anticholinergic drugs. Concurrent use of trimethoprim-sulfamethoxazole or of triamterene-hydrochlorothiazide has been associated with CNS toxicity due to decreased renal clearance in several cases.[175] Cimetidine is asociated with 15 to 20% increases and aspirin or acetaminophen with 10% decreases in plasma rimantadine concentrations, but such changes are unlikely to be of significance.[173] Patients receiving either amantadine or rimantadine along with drugs affecting CNS function (e.g., antihistamines, antidepressants, minor tranquilizers) should be monitored closely.

Toxicity

Oral amantadine and rimantadine do not appear to cause clinically important renal, hepatic, or hematopoietic toxicity.[176] In the setting of renal insufficiency or high doses, serious neurotoxic reactions, including tremor, seizures, or coma; cardiac arrhythmias; and death can occur in association with high amantadine plasma concentrations (1.0 to 5.0 μg/ml).[177, 178] Neurotoxic reactions may be transiently reversed by physostigmine administration, and lidocaine has been used to treat ventricular arrhythmias. Long-term amantadine ingestion has been associated with livedo reticularis, peripheral edema, orthostatic hypotension, and, rarely, congestive heart failure, vision loss, or urinary retention. Patients with preexisting seizure disorders may develop an increased frequency of major motor seizures during amantadine use, and dose reductions are advised.[179] Rimantadine may also cause exacerbations of seizures. Psychiatric side effects in patients with Parkinson's disease and psychotic exacerbations in patients with schizophrenia may occur with addition of amantadine.[180] Rash and leukopenia have been described rarely.

The most common side effects related to amantadine ingestion are minor, dose-related gastrointestinal and CNS complaints. These include nervousness, lightheadedness, difficulty concentrating, insomnia, and loss of appetite or nausea.[181] CNS side effects occur in approximately 5 to 33% of amantadine recipients at doses of 200 mg/day but are significantly less frequent with rimantadine. When used for influenza prophylaxis, doses of 200 mg/day are associated with excess withdrawals in 6 to 11% of recipients because of drug side effects.[187, 188] Doses of 100 mg/day are better tolerated and may be protective against influenzal illness.[182] Amantadine dose reductions are required in older adults (100 mg/day) because of decreased renal function, but 20 to 40% experience side effects even at this lower dose.[183, 184] Trough steady-state plasma concentrations greater than 0.45 μg/ml and peak concentrations greater than 1.0 μg/ml are associated with an increased risk of CNS side effects.[185, 186] Complaints typically develop within the first week of administration, often resolve despite continued ingestion, and are promptly reversible on discontinuation of the drug.

Rimantadine administration is associated with dose-related side effects similar to those observed with amantadine, although the risk of CNS side effects is lower with rimantadine at doses of 200 or 300 mg/day.[187–189] During prophylaxis, excess withdrawal rates are usually less than 5%.[176, 190] However, conventional 200 mg/day doses are associated with higher plasma levels and side effect rates in elderly nursing home residents.[171]

The clinical observations of dry mouth, pupillary dilation, toxic psychosis, and urinary retention in acute amantadine overdose suggest that anticholinergic activity is present in humans. Amantadine demonstrates activity on the adrenergic nervous system by affecting accumulation, release, and reuptake of catecholamines in the CNS and in the peripheral nervous system. Ventricular irritability occurs in animals given high doses of amantadine, and malignant ventricular arrhythmia after amantadine overdose has been described in humans.[177]

Amantadine is teratogenic and embryotoxic in rodents. Rimantadine is not mutagenic in vitro and does not appear to cause teratogenic effects in rabbits or rats. Birth defects have been reported after amantadine exposure during pregnancy,[191] and the safety of either drug has not been established in pregnancy.

Clinical Studies

The clinical usefulness of amantadine and rimantadine is limited to the prevention and treatment of influenza A virus infections.[181, 187, 189, 192] Both drugs, at a dose of 200 mg/day in adults, are about 70 to 90% protective against clinical illness caused by various influenza A subtypes, including pandemic strains.[193] Prophylaxis is effective in preventing nosocomial influenza and possibly in curtailing nosocomial outbreaks.[179] Protection appears to be additive to that provided by vaccine.[194] Rimantadine administration to school-aged children (5 mg/kg/day) decreases the risk of influenza A illness in recipients and possibly in their family contacts.[195] However, postexposure prophylaxis with these drugs provides inconsistent protection to family contacts, in part depending on whether ill index children are treated.[158] Doses of 100 mg/day appear to be protective against influenza A illness and are well-tolerated in adults.[182, 196]

Amantadine and rimantadine are also effective therapies in uncomplicated influenza A illness,[156, 189, 197, 198] but it remains uncertain whether treatment reduces the risk of complications in high-risk patients or is useful in patients with established pulmonary complications. When begun within 1 to 2 days after onset of symptoms, doses of 200 mg/day reduce the duration of fever and systemic complaints by 1 to 2 days and in some studies decrease the duration of virus shedding, compared with placebo. Treated persons are also able to resume usual activities more rapidly.[156, 189] In illness caused by H3N2-subtype influenza viruses, certain abnormalities of peripheral airways function, but not of airway hyperreactivity, resolve more quickly in amantadine-treated patients. Therapeutic benefits occur in elderly influenza patients treated with rimantadine.[198] In children with influenza A H3N2 subtype infection, rimantadine treatment is associated with lower symptom burden, fever, and viral titers during the first 2 days of treatment, compared with acetaminophen administration, but rimantadine-treated children have more prolonged shedding of virus.[199] Treatment generally does not appear to affect immune responses to infection but may blunt secretory antibody levels.[200] The optimal dose and duration of therapy have not been established in children for either agent.

Intermittent aerosol administration of amantadine or rimantadine appears to be therapeutically useful in uncomplicated influenza.[201] An injectable formulation of either drug is not available. Amantadine (100 mg twice daily for 6 months) may reduce HCV RNA levels and aminotransferase levels in some patients with chronic hepatitis C not responsive to IFN therapy.[143] Further studies are in progress.

CIDOFOVIR

Spectrum

Cidofovir (HPMPC) (Vistide) is an acyclic phosphonate nucleotide analogue of deoxycytidine monophosphate (Fig. 36–3) with inhibitory activity against human herpesviruses, including EBV, human herpesvirus-6 (HHV-6), and HHV-8, and other DNA viruses, including papilloma-, polyoma-, pox-, and adenoviruses.[202–204] In vitro inhibitory concentrations range from less than 0.2 to 0.7 μg/ml for CMV,[205] 0.4 to 33 μg/ml for HSV,[206] and 0.02 to 17 μg/ml for adenoviruses.[207] Because activation does not depend on virus-specified enzymes, cidofovir is inhibitory for acyclovir-resistant, TK-deficient or TK-altered HSV strains and ganciclovir-resistant CMV strains with UL97 mutations. TK mutants of HSV show up to 20-fold enhanced susceptibility to cidofovir compared with wild-type HSV, because mutant viruses induce smaller elevations in competing deoxycytidine triphosphate (dCTP) pools in infected cells.[208] In vitro, cidofovir shows synergistic inhibition of CMV in combination with ganciclovir or foscarnet.[209] The prolonged intracellular half-life of the diphosphate is associated with persistent antiviral activity and enables infrequent dosing regimens. Single doses are effective in animal models of HSV, simian varicella, and poxvirus infec-

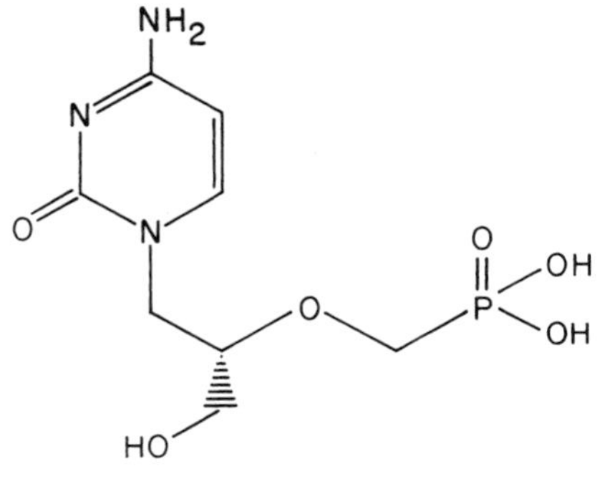

CIDOFOVIR

FIGURE 36–3. Chemical structure of cidofovir.

tions.[210–212] Topical cidofovir is active against ocular adenovirus infection in rabbits but is associated with local irritation.[213]

Mechanism of Action

Cidofovir inhibits viral DNA synthesis. Cidofovir is metabolized intracellularly to its active diphosphate form by cellular enzymes, and the levels of phosphorylated metabolites are similar in infected and uninfected cells. The diphosphate acts as both a competitive inhibitor with respect to dCTP and an alternative substrate for viral DNA polymerase. Incorporation of cidofovir slows chain elongation and abrogates it if two consecutive cidofovir molecules are introduced. The diphosphate has a prolonged intracellular half-life, averaging 17 to 65 hours depending on the cell type, and competitively inhibits CMV and HSV DNA polymerase at concentrations 8- to 600-fold lower than those inhibitory for human DNA polymerases.[214, 215] An adduct with prolonged intracellular half-life (>2 days) may serve as a reservoir of drug.

Resistance

CMV isolates with reduced susceptibility to cidofovir and cross-resistance to ganciclovir have been selected by in vitro passage. Highly ganciclovir-resistant clinical isolates of CMV that possess DNA polymerase mutations plus UL97 mutations show cross-resistance to cidofovir in vitro. Some foscarnet-resistant CMV isolates show cross-resistance to cidofovir, and triple-drug–resistant variants with DNA polymerase point mutations have been described.[216] The development of resistance to cidofovir as a result of cidofovir therapy appears to be uncommon and low level (Leightfold change in susceptibility).[205, 217] Reduced susceptibility to cidofovir in vitro, resulting from prior ganciclovir therapy, may not predict clinical progression.[217]

Pharmacokinetics

Oral bioavailability is low (<5%). After intravenous infusion, plasma levels are proportional to dose and decline in a biphasic pattern, with a terminal $T_{1/2}$ that averages about 2.6 hours.[218] The volume of distribution approximates total body water. Cidofovir is cleared by the kidney via glomerular filtration and active tubular secretion. More than 90% of the dose is recovered unchanged in the urine, and no significant metabolism has been recognized in humans. Less than 6% is protein bound. High-dose probenicid (2 g 3 hours before and 1 g 2 and 8 hours after each infusion) reduces renal clearance by blocking tubular secretion of cidofovir and increases blood levels. At cidofovir doses of 5 mg/kg, peak plasma concentrations increase from 11.6 to 26.1 μg/ml after addition of probenicid. Penetration into the cerebrospinal fluid or eye has not been well characterized. After application of cidofovir gel, systemic absorption is minimal (peak plasma concentrations, <0.5 μg/ml) and is related to lesion size.[206] The effects of renal insufficiency or dialysis on pharmacokinetics are unknown.

Interactions

Probenicid but not cidofovir alters zidovudine pharmacokinetics, and zidovudine doses should be reduced on administration days. Concomitant therapy with other nephrotoxic agents is contraindicated during cidofovir therapy, and an interval of at least 7 days is recommended after aminoglycoside, intravenous pentamidine, amphotericin B, foscarnet, nonsteroidal anti-inflammatory drug, or contrast dye exposure.

Toxicity

Dose-related nephrotoxicity is the principal side effect of intravenous cidofovir.[203] It is characterized by proximal tubular dysfunction including proteinuria, azotemia, glycosuria, metabolic acidosis, and, uncommonly, Fanconi's syndrome. Concomitant oral probenicid and vigorous saline prehydration reduce, whereas prior foscarnet therapy and concurrent use of other nephrotoxic agents increase, the risk of renal toxicity. On maintenance doses of 5 mg/kg every other week, approximately 50% of patients develop proteinuria and 15% have elevated serum creatinine. Neutropenia occurs in approximately 20%, and regular monitoring of neutrophil counts is necessary. Fever, nausea, emesis, diarrhea, headache, rash, asthenia, anterior uveitis, and ocular hypotony may occur with combined therapy with cidofovir and probenicid.[218a] Maintenance is withdrawn in approximately 25 to 35% of patients because of intolerance. Dose reductions are indicated for minor rises in serum creatinine (0.3 to 0.4 mg/dl) and cessation of administration for greater creatinine rises or development of proteinuria of 3+ or higher.

Topical application is associated with dose-related application site reactions (burning, pain, pruritus) in up to one third of patients and occasionally with ulceration, but no evidence of systemic toxicity has been reported.[206] Intravitreal cidofovir may cause iritis, vitreitis, reduced intraocular pressure, and visual loss.[219]

Preclinical studies indicate that cidofovir has mutagenic, gonadotoxic, embryotoxic, and teratogenic effects. Because cidofovir is associated with tumors in rats, this agent is considered a potential human carcinogen. It may cause infertility in humans and is contraindicated during pregnancy.

Clinical Studies

Intravenous cidofovir is approved for the treatment of CMV retinitis in AIDS patients. Its efficacy and tolerability have not been proved in other CMV syndromes or in non-HIV infected patients. Intravenous cidofovir (5 mg/kg once a week for 2 weeks followed by every-other-week dosing) significantly increases the time to progression of CMV retinitis in previously untreated patients and in those failing or intolerant of ganciclovir and foscarnet therapy.[209, 220, 221] Maintenance doses of 5 mg/kg every other week are more effective but less well tolerated than 3 mg/kg doses.[222] Clearance of viruria but not viremia has been demonstrated.[223] Intravenous cidofovir has been used anecdotally to treat acyclovir-resistant mucocutaneous HSV infection.[224] Studies of intravenous cidofovir in progressive multifocal leukoencephalopathy and in Kaposi's sarcoma are in progress. Topical cidofovir gel formulated in polyethylene glycol (once daily for 5 days) reduces pain, virus shedding, and lesion healing time in HIV-infected patients with acyclovir-resistant mucocutaneous HSV infections.[206] Intralesional cidofovir induces remissions in adults with respiratory papillomatosis,[209] and topical cidofovir is under study for the treatment of anogenital warts. Intravitreal cidofovir injection may be effective for treatment of CMV retinitis[219] but is contraindicated because of toxicity. An ophthalmic formulation is being studied in adenoviral keratoconjunctivitis.

PENCICLOVIR AND FAMCICLOVIR

Spectrum

Penciclovir (9-[4-hydroxy-3-hydroxymethylbut-1-yl] guanine) is an acyclic guanosine analogue (see Fig. 36–1) similar to acyclovir in its spectrum of activity and potency against herpesviruses (see Table 36–2).[225, 226] Famciclovir (Famvir) is the diacetyl ester of 6-deoxy penciclovir and lacks antiviral activity. Because of its dependence on viral TK for initial phosphorylation, penciclovir is inactive against TK-deficient strains of HSV or VZV but may be active against some TK-altered or polymerase mutants that are resistant to acyclovir and some foscarnet-resistant HSV isolates.[227, 228] Penciclovir is also inhibitory for hepatitis B virus (HBV) and shows synergistic inhibition in combination with lamivudine in vitro.[229, 230] Topical, parenteral, and oral penciclovir and oral famciclovir are active in experimental HSV infections.[231]

Mechanism of Action

Penciclovir is an inhibitor of viral DNA synthesis. In infected cells penciclovir is preferentially phosphorylated to its active form, penciclovir triphosphate, which serves as a competitive inhibitor of viral DNA polymerase.[232] Unlike acyclovir, it is not an obligate chain terminator. Although penciclovir triphosphate is approximately 100-fold less potent in inhibiting viral DNA polymerase than acyclovir triphosphate, it is present in much higher concentrations and for more prolonged periods in infected cells. The prolonged intracellular $T_{1/2}$ of penciclovir-triphosphate, which ranges from 7 to 20 hours, is associated with a sustained antiviral effect in cell culture and in animal models.[233] This effect may allow for infrequent dosing during clinical use. Although not preferentially phosphorylated in HBV-infected cells, penciclovir triphosphate is also a potent inhibitor of HBV DNA polymerase-reverse transcriptase.[234]

Resistance

Penciclovir-resistant variants of HSV selected by in vitro passage have mutations in viral TK or DNA ploymerase. Acyclovir-resistant, TK-deficient mutants are resistant to penciclovir, but TK mutants with altered substrate specifically may retain susceptibility.[235] DNA polymerase mutations confer only twofold to fourfold reductions in susceptibility.[236] Emergence of resistance during clinical use has been very low to date.[237, 238] Resistance of HBV to penciclovir is associated with point mutations in viral DNA polymerase and has occurred in liver transplant recipients receiving famciclovir suppression.[239]

Pharmacokinetics

Famciclovir is a prodrug that is well absorbed orally and rapidly converted to penciclovir by deacetylation and oxidation of the purine. This occurs during and after absorption through the intestinal wall and in the liver.[225] Although poorly absorbed itself, the bioavailability of penciclovir averages 77% after oral administration of famciclovir.[240] Little or no famciclovir is detectable in blood or urine. Penciclovir is less than 20% bound to plasma proteins. The volume of distribution is approximately double that of body water. After single 250- and 500-mg doses of oral famciclovir, the peak plasma concentration of penciclovir averages 1.6 to 1.9 and 2.7 to 4.0 μg/ml, respectively.[240] Food reduces peak plasma concentrations but does not significantly alter overall bioavailability. After intravenous infusion of penciclovir (10 mg/kg), peak plasma levels average 12 μg/ml.[241]

The plasma $T_{1/2}$ of penciclovir averages 2 to 3 hours, and approximately 70% is recovered unchanged in the urine.[241] About 5% is excreted as the 6-deoxy precursor. Its rapid renal clearance suggests elimination by both filtration and active tubular secretion. Nonrenal clearance accounts for about 30% of dose, primarily by fecal excretion of penciclovir and its 6-deoxy precursor. The plasma elimination rate is reduced approximately fourfold and penciclovir exposure is increased 10-fold in those with severe renal failure (creatinine clearance, <30 ml/minute).[242] Dose reductions are indicated in moderate or advanced renal failure (Table 36–5). In patients with compensated liver disease, peak plasma levels are reduced by approximately 40%, but overall penciclovir exposure is unchanged and dose adjustments are not necessary.[242] Elderly adults have approximately 40% higher penciclovir exposure because of lower renal clearance.

Interactions

No clinically important drug interactions have been identified to date. Famciclovir does not interact pharmacokinetically with cimetidine, theophylline, allopurinol, digoxin, or zidovudine.[243, 244]

Toxicity

Oral famciclovir is well tolerated but may be associated with headache, nausea, and diarrhea.[245] The frequencies of such complaints are generally comparable to those seen with placebo or acyclovir. Urticaria, rash, and, predominantly in the elderly, hallucinations or confusional states have been reported. Neutropenia and elevated transaminase values occur in less than 5% of patients. Famciclovir reduces spermatogenesis and fertility in rodents and dogs, but long-term administration (1 year) does not affect spermatogenesis in men.[246] No teratogenic effects have been observed in animals, but safety during pregnancy has not been established. Very high penciclovir concentrations are mutagenic, and long-term administration of high-dose famciclovir is associated with mammary tumors in rats but not in mice. The clinical significance of these observations is uncertain.

Topical penciclovir, which is formulated in 40% propylene glycol and a cetomacrogol base, is associated with application site reactions at low rates (approximately 1%), comparable to the vehicle.

TABLE 36–5 Dose Adjustment of Famciclovir for Renal Insufficiency

Standard Dose and Interval*	Creatinine Clearance (ml/min)†	Adjusted Dose and Interval
500 mg q8h or q 12h	40–59	500 mg q12h
	20–39	500 mg q24h
	<20	250 mg q24h
250 mg q12h	≥40	250 mg q12h
	20–39	125 mg q12h
	<20	125 mg q24h
125 mg q12h	≥40	125 mg q12h
	20–39	125 mg q24h
	<20	125 mg q24h

*Dosing is based on manufacturers' recommendations.
†For hemodialysis patients, give the adjusted dose for creatinine clearance <20 ml/min after dialysis.

Clinical Studies

Topical penciclovir and oral famciclovir are approved for clinical use in the United States, and intravenous penciclovir has been approved in some countries. In immunocompetent persons with recurrent orolabial HSV, topical 1% penciclovir cream (applied every 2 hours while awake for 4 days) shortens healing time and symptoms by 0.5 to 1.0 days compared with placebo.[247] Oral famciclovir (250 mg three times daily for 5 to 10 days) is as effective as acyclovir in treating first-episode genital herpes.[248] In patients with recurrent genital HSV, patient-initiated famciclovir treatment (125 mg twice daily for 5 days) reduces healing time and symptoms by approximately 1 day compared with placebo.[249] Suppressive therapy (250 mg twice daily) for up to 1 year is effective and well tolerated in persons with frequent recurrences, but single daily doses are not as effective.[237, 250] Famciclovir suppression (500 mg twice daily) reduces clinical HSV recurrences and asymptomatic viral shedding in HIV-infected persons.[238] Famciclovir (500 mg twice daily for 7 days) is comparable to acyclovir (400 mg five times daily) in the treatment of mucocutaneous HSV infections in HIV-infected patients.[251] Intravenous penciclovir (5 mg/kg every 8 or 12 hours for 7 days) is comparable to intravenous acyclovir in efficacy and tolerance for treatment of HSV infections in non–HIV-infected, immunocompromised hosts.[252]

In immunocompetent adults with herpes zoster of 3 days' duration or less, famciclovir (500 mg three times daily for 10 days) is at least as effective as acyclovir (800 mg five times daily) and superior to placebo in reducing both acute manifestations and the duration of postherpetic neuralgia, particularly in patients older than 50 years of age.[253, 254] Famciclovir is comparable to acyclovir in the treatment of ophthalmic herpes zoster.[254a] Famciclovir is also comparable to high-dose oral acyclovir in the treatment of zoster in immunocompromised patients.[255]

Famciclovir is associated with dose-related reductions in HBV DNA and transaminase levels in patients with chronic hepatitis B and appears to be additive in anti-HBV effects when combined with interferon.[256, 257] Famciclovir has been used to treat recurrent HBV infection after liver transplantation, with reductions in HBV DNA levels for longer than 1 year in some patients.[258, 259]

FOMIVIRSEN

Fomivirsen (ISIS 2922, Vitravene) is a 21-nucleotide phosphorothioate oligonucleotide that inhibits human CMV replication through an antisense mechanism. It is the first antisense therapy to be approved by the US Food and Drug Administration. Fomivirsen is complementary to a sequence in the messenger RNA transcripts of the major immediate early region 2 of CMV, which encodes proteins responsible for regulation of viral gene expression. Other mechanisms of antiviral action may include non-antisense, sequence-dependent inhibition of virus replication and sequence-independent inhibition of virus absorption to virus cell.[259a] With persistent in vitro passage it has been possible to isolate CMV clones with 10-fold less susceptibility to inhibition of replication.[295b]Fomivirsen, because of its novel mechanism of antiviral action, retains activity against CMV strains that are resistant to ganciclovir, foscarnet, or cidofovir.

Fomivirsen is administered by intravitreal injection. In animals it is cleared from the vitreous over a course of 7 to 10 days by a combination of tissue distribution and metabolism. Retinal levels are detectable within hours after injection and increase over 3 to 5 days. The major route of elimination from the eye is metabolism by exonucleases. Approximately 40% of fomivirsen is bound to proteins. Human clinical ocular pharmacokinetic studies have not been completed. Data on oncogenicity and carcinogenicity are not available.

Fomivirsen is indicated for the intravitreal treatment of CMV retinitis in HIV-infected patients who are intolerant of, have not responded to, or have contraindications to other treatments. Injection of 330 μg every 2 weeks is associated with significant delays in time to progression.[259c] Ocular inflammations, including iritis and vitritis, occur in approximately one quarter of patients but respond to topical corticosteroids. Increased intraocular pressure has been commonly reported and needs to be monitored. Fomivirsen is not recommended for use in patients who have recently been treated with cidofovir because of the increased risk of ocular inflammation.

FOSCARNET

Spectrum

Foscarnet (trisodium phosphonoformate) (Foscavir) is an inorganic pyrophosphate analogue (Fig 36–4) that is inhibitory for herpesviruses and HIV.[260, 261] In vitro inhibitory concentrations vary widely among clinical isolates but are generally 100 to 300 μmol/liter for CMV and 80 to 200 μmol/liter for HSV, VZV, EBV, and HHV-8.[262] Foscarnet is inhibitory for most ganciclovir-resistant CMV and acyclovir-resistant HSV and VZV strains. Combinations of foscarnet and ganciclovir or acyclovir synergistically inhibit CMV infection in vitro.[263] Foscarnet also acts synergistically with zidovudine in inhibiting HIV replication.[264]

Concentrations of 500 to 1000 μmol/liter reversibly inhibit the proliferation and/or cellular DNA synthesis of uninfected cells. Foscarnet is active in animal models of herpesvirus and hepadnavirus infection.[260, 261]

Mechanism of Action

Unlike nucleosides, foscarnet does not undergo significant intracellular metabolism and directly inhibits herpesvirus DNA polymerase or

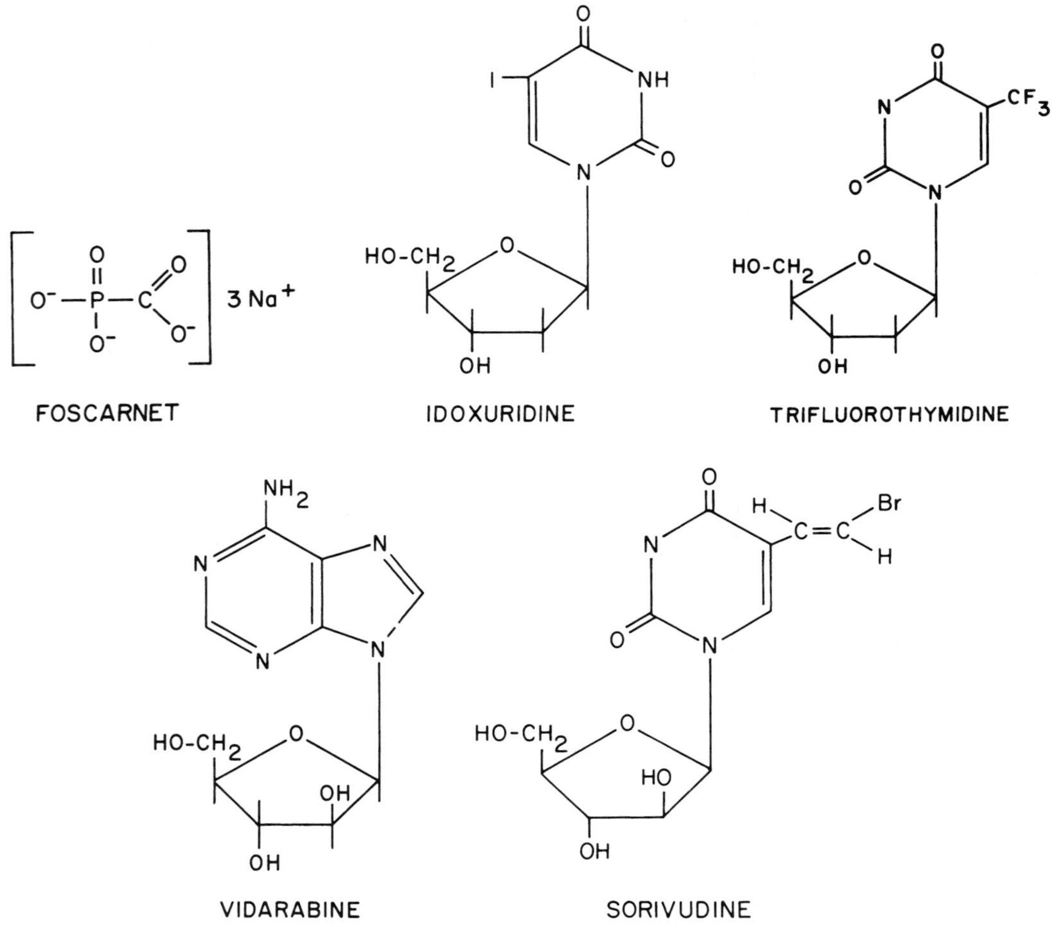

FOSCARNET IDOXURIDINE TRIFLUOROTHYMIDINE

VIDARABINE SORIVUDINE

FIGURE 36–4. Chemical structures of antiherpesvirus antiviral agents: foscarnet, idoxuridine, trifluorothymidine, vidarabine, and sorivudine.

HIV reverse transcriptase. Foscarnet reversibly blocks the pyrophosphate binding site of the viral polymerase in a noncompetitive manner with respect to deoxynucleotide triphosphates (dNTPs) and inhibits cleavage of pyrophosphate from dNTP.[260, 261, 265] Concentrations that inhibit cell-free viral polymerases are many times lower than those required for inhibition of viral replication in cell culture, and cellular uptake is slow. Foscarnet's selectivity relates to its 100-fold greater inhibitory effects against herpesvirus DNA polymerases or HIV reverse transcriptase, compared with cellular DNA polymerase-α.[265]

Resistance

Resistance to foscarnet is caused by point mutations in DNA polymerase of HSV and CMV or in reverse transcriptase of HIV.[260, 266, 267] CMV resistance, defined by in vitro inhibitory concentrations greater than 400 μmol/liter, occurs in less than 5% of patients.[268] Resistant clinical isolates of HSV, VZV, and CMV show threefold to eightfold increases in inhibitory concentrations and may be associated with poor response to foscarnet treatment. Progressive retinitis and CNS disease have occurred with foscarnet-resistant CMV strains.[266, 269] Some foscarnet-resistant CMV infections respond to ganciclovir or cidofovir. Foscarnet resistance in HIV, associated with a reduction of about 10-fold in susceptibility, can phenotypically reverse zidovudine resistance.[270]

Pharmacokinetics

Oral bioavailability is low, averaging 7 to 9%.[271] After an infusion of 60 mg/kg every 8 hours, peak and trough plasma concentrations range broadly but average approximately 450 to 575 and 80 to 150 μmol/liter, respectively. Peak concentrations range from 490 to 2600 μmol/liter after doses of 90 mg/kg/day. Plasma protein binding is about 15%. Cerebrospinal fluid concentrations vary widely but average 66% of plasma values at steady state.[272] Vitreous concentrations average 1.4 times higher than concurrent plasma ones.[273]

Foscarnet is eliminated by renal mechanisms, and more than 80% of the dose is excreted as unmetabolized drug by glomerular filtration and probably by tubular secretion. Plasma clearance decreases proportionately with creatinine clearance, and dose adjustments are indicated for small decreases in renal function (Table 36–6). Probenecid does not affect renal excretion. Plasma elimination is complex, with two initial $T_{1/2}$ values totaling approximately 4 to 8 hours and a prolonged terminal $T_{1/2}$ averaging 18 to 88 hours. This appears to relate to bone deposition, which accounts for an estimated 15 to 20% of a dose. Foscarnet is removed by hemodialysis, and plasma levels decrease by about 50% with a 3-hour run.[274] Dosing after dialysis is recommended. Peritoneal dialysis clears foscarnet to a limited extent.[275]

TABLE 36–6 Foscarnet Dose Reduction in Renal Insufficiency

Creatinine Clearance (ml/min/kg)	Induction Dose* (mg/kg/8h)	Maintenance Dose* (mg/kg/d)	
≥ 1.6	60	90	120
1.5	57	90	120
1.4	53	78	104
1.3	49	78	104
1.2	46	75	100
1.1	42	75	100
1.0	39	71	94
0.9	35	71	94
0.8	32	63	84
0.7	28	63	84
0.6	25	57	76
0.5	21	57	76
0.4	18	57	76

*Dosing based on manufacturer's recommendations.

Interactions

Administration of foscarnet with amphotericin B[276] or other nephrotoxic agents (e.g., aminoglycosides, intravenous pentamidine, intravenous acyclovir, cyclosporine) may cause enhanced renal toxicity. The risk of symptomatic hypocalcemia is increased by concomitant intravenous pentamidine. Foscarnet and zidovudine do not affect each other's clearance,[277] but the risk of anemia is higher with the combination.

Toxicity

Nephrotoxicity with azotemia, mild proteinuria, and sometimes acute tubular necrosis are the major dose-limiting side effect.[261, 278] Approximately one third of patients develop significant renal impairment (serum creatinine 2.0 mg/dl or greater). Increases in serum creatinine usually occur during the second week of therapy and are reversible within 2 to 4 weeks after cessation in most patients. High doses, rapid or continuous infusion, dehydration, and concurrent use of nephrotoxic drugs are risk factors. Saline loading appears to reduce the risk of nephrotoxicity.[278] Crystalluria, renal tubular acidosis, nephrogenic diabetes insipidus, and interstitial nephritis have also been described.[279]

Metabolic abnormalities are common and include both hypocalcemia (15 to 35%) and hypercalcemia, hypophosphatemia and hyperphosphatemia, hypomagnesemia (15 to 44%), and hypokalemia (10 to 16%).[280] Hypocalcemia due to chelation and decreased serum ionized calcium may cause paresthesias, arrhythmias, tetany, seizures, and other CNS disturbances.[281] Intravenous foscarnet should be administered at a fixed rate (maximum, 1 mg/kg/minute) by infusion pump, to minimize the possibility of acute metabolic abnormalities. Renal function and electrolytes need to be monitored closely, and multiple dose adjustments are often required during induction therapy (see Table 36–6).

CNS side effects include headache in about one fourth of patients, tremor, irritability, seizures in up to 10%, and hallucinosis. Other reported side effects are fever in 65% of patients, rash, diarrhea in 30%, nausea or emesis in up to one half, abnormal liver function tests, anxiety, fatigue, and painful genital ulcerations.[280] These ulcerations may be caused by high urinary foscarnet concentrations and usually resolve within weeks after therapy is stopped. Although anemia may develop in 20 to 50% of AIDS patients and granulocytopenia in a smaller fraction, foscarnet is less myelosuppressive than ganciclovir. Heart block and electrocardiographic changes occur in 5% or less of patients. Oral foscarnet causes dose-related gastrointestinal disturbances, particularly diarrhea.[271]

Preclinical studies indicate that high concentrations are mutagenic and that foscarnet may cause tooth and skeletal developmental anomalies in animals. Safety in pregnancy or in childhood is uncertain.

Clinical Studies

Intravenous foscarnet is approved for treatment of CMV retinitis in AIDS patients and of acyclovir-resistant mucocutaneous HSV infections. With the usual foscarnet regimen (60 mg/kg every 8 hours for 14 to 21 days followed by chronic maintenance at 90 to 120 mg/kg/day), about 90% of retinitis patients experience clinical stabilization and a smaller portion cease CMV excretion.[261, 282, 283] An induction regimen of 100 mg/kg twice daily also is effective but is associated with a higher risk of penile ulceration.[284] Maintenance doses of 120 mg/kg/day appear to be more effective in prolonging survival and controlling retinitis.[285] Compared with ganciclovir, one study found that foscarnet provides comparable control of CMV retinitis in AIDS patients but improved survival, although patients had to be switched from foscarnet more than three times as often because of side effects.[286] In patients with persistently active or relapsed retinitis, combined foscarnet (90 mg/kg/day) and ganciclovir (5 mg/kg/day) delay progression significantly longer than higher doses of either single agent.[287] In non-neutropenic patients, most practitioners still initiate therapy with ganciclovir because of its more predictable toxicities and lower cost. Intravitreal foscarnet has been used.[288]

Foscarnet appears to be effective in treating ganciclovir-resistant CMV retinitis and other syndromes.[282, 289] Foscarnet is effective in treating CMV gastrointestinal and pulmonary infections in AIDS patients,[290] but not in treating CMV pneumonia in bone marrow transplantation patients.[260] Foscarnet prophylaxis may be effective in preventing CMV disease in marrow transplantation patients but should not be used in combination with amphotericin B or cyclosporine because of the risk of severe nephrotoxicity.[276]

In acyclovir-resistant mucocutaneous HSV infections, lower doses (40 mg/kg every 8 hours) are associated with complete healing in about 75% of patients.[31] Other dose regimens (e.g., 90 mg/kg every 12 hours) appear to be effective. Foscarnet also appears to be effective in acyclovir-resistant VZV infections in AIDS patients.[40] In recurrent orolabial or genital herpes infections of immunocompetent hosts, topically applied foscarnet is not associated with reproducible clinical benefits.[260, 291]

In AIDS patients, foscarnet administration significantly reduces p24 antigen and HIV RNA levels without clear increases in CD4 T-cell counts.[292, 293] Foscarnet use may reduce the risk of Kaposi's sarcoma in HIV-infected persons with CMV disease.[294, 295]

GANCICLOVIR

Spectrum

Ganciclovir (9-[1,3-dihydroxy-2-propoxymethyl] guanine) (DHPG, Cytovene) is a deoxyguanosine analogue that differs from acyclovir in that it has an additional hydroxymethyl group on the acyclic side chain (see Fig. 36–1). This agent has inhibitory activity against herpesviruses (see Table 36–2), but its unique characteristic is potent inhibition of CMV replication.[296–299] Inhibitory concentrations are 10- to more than 50-fold lower than acyclovir for human CMV strains. Combinations of ganciclovir and foscarnet synergistically inhibit CMV replication in vitro.[263] Ganciclovir antagonizes the anti-HIV activity of didanosine and zidovudine in vitro,[300] and zidovudine antagonizes the anti-CMV effects of ganciclovir,[301, 302] but the clinical significance of these observations is unknown. Concentrations of less than 10 μg/ml also inhibit adenovirus replication in vitro,[303] and inhibition of HBV occurs in vivo.[304] Systemic ganciclovir is effective at relatively low dosages in animal models of CMV and HSV infections.[305, 306]

Although high concentrations are needed to inhibit the growth of uninfected cells, inhibitory concentrations for human bone marrow progenitor cells are similar to those that are inhibitory for CMV replication.[307] Inhibition of human lymphocyte proliferative responses to mitogen and antigen occurs at concentrations of 1 to 10 μg/ml, so immune responses requiring active DNA synthesis may be depressed at therapeutic ganciclovir concentrations.[3] Cells transformed by viral TK are readily killed on ganciclovir exposure, and this antitumor strategy is being explored.

Mechanism of Action

Ganciclovir inhibits viral DNA synthesis.[296, 298] Intracellular ganciclovir is phosphorylated to the monophosphate derivative by a virus-induced enzyme, the viral TK during HSV infection, and by a viral protein kinase encoded by the UL97 gene during CMV infection.[308–310] Ganciclovir diphosphate and triphosphate are formed through the action of cellular enzymes. At least 10-fold higher concentrations of ganciclovir triphosphate are present in CMV-infected than in uninfected cells.[311] Intracellular ganciclovir triphosphate concentrations are also more than 10-fold higher than those of acyclovir triphosphate in CMV-infected cells, and the intracellular $T_{1/2}$ of ganciclovir triphosphate is prolonged (16.5 to more than 24 hours).[308, 312] These differences may account in part for ganciclovir's greater anti-CMV activity and explain how single daily doses are effective in suppressing human CMV infections.

Ganciclovir triphosphate is a competitive inhibitor of deoxyguanosine triphosphate (dGTP) incorporation into DNA and preferentially inhibits viral more than host cellular DNA polymerases. Incorporation of ganciclovir triphosphate into viral DNA causes a slowing and subsequent cessation of viral DNA chain elongation.[313] Unlike acyclovir, ganciclovir is not an obligate chain terminator, and continued viral DNA synthesis results in intranuclear accumulation of short, noninfectious viral DNA fragments.[314] Ganciclovir is incorporated into both host cell and viral DNA.

Resistance

Resistance in CMV isolates, often defined by inhibitory concentrations greater than 2 to 3 μg/ml in vitro, has been related to two mechanisms: reduced intracellular ganciclovir phosphorylation caused by point mutations or deletions in the phosphotransferase encoded by the UL97 gene[315] and point mutations in viral DNA polymerase.[316] Most resistant clinical isolates with fourfold to 20-fold increases in inhibitory concentrations have impaired phosphorylation[317] and usually remain susceptible to forcarnet and cidofovir. Some have DNA polymerase mutations that may confer reduced susceptibility to forcarnet and cidofovir. Highly resistant CMV strains (inhibitory concentrations greater than 10 μg/ml) are associated with both UL97 and polymerase alterations[318] and appear after prolonged therapy.[216, 310]

Ganciclovir resistance has been recognized clinically by progressive disease and persistent CMV viremia despite therapy.[282, 319, 320] One survey found that 8% of 72 AIDS patients had progressive disease and shed resistant CMV after 3 months or more of continuous ganciclovir therapy; 38% of those shedding virus after 3 months had resistant isolates.[320] Emergence of resistance, sometimes within several weeks, also occurs with ganciclovir use in transplantation patients.[321, 322] The transmissibility of ganciclovir-resistant CMV strains is undefined, but patients with such strains may have invasive disease, including retinitis, polyradiculopathy, or pneumonia.[319, 323] Foscarnet therapy may benefit patients with ganciclovir-resistant CMV infections.[282, 289]

Ganciclovir is more than 40 times less active against acyclovir-resistant, TK-deficient HSV strains than against wild-type strains.[297, 298]

Pharmacokinetics

The oral bioavailability of ganciclovir is about 5% under fasting conditions. Food increases the bioavailability to 6 to 9% so dosing with meals is recommended.[324, 325] Peak and trough plasma levels average about 0.9 to 1.2 and 0.2–0.5 μg/ml, respectively, on an oral regimen of 1000 mg every 8 hours. After intravenous administration of 5 mg/kg doses, peak and trough plasma concentrations average 8 to 11 and 0.6 to 1.2 μg/ml, respectively.[296, 326, 327] After oral dosing, drug exposure is approximately 70% of that occurring after a single 5 mg/kg intravenous dose. Subcutaneous and intramuscular administration are too irritating for clinical use. A valine ester prodrug that provides high oral bioavailability of ganciclovir is under development.

Plasma protein binding is only 1 to 2%. After intravenous dosing, aqueous, vitreous, and subretinal fluid levels are similar to those in serum.[273, 328] Cerebrospinal fluid levels are 24 to 70%, and brain tissue levels are 38% of those in plasma.[327] The plasma $T_{1/2}$ averages 2 to 4 hours in patients with normal renal function but increases almost linearly as creatinine clearance declines.[329] Plasma $T_{1/2}$ may increase to 28 to 40 hours in those with severe renal insufficiency (serum creatinine >4.5 mg/dl). Most ganciclovir is eliminated unmetabolized by renal excretion (>90% of dose) by both glomerular filtration and tubular secretion. Dose reductions are necessary in patients with creatinine clearance of less than 80 ml/min (Table 36–7). A single hemodialysis session reduces the plasma levels of

TABLE 36-7 Ganciclovir Dose Adjustments in Renal Insufficiency

Creatinine Clearance (ml/min/1.73 m²)	IV Dose (mg/kg)*	Dosing Interval (h)	Oral dose (mg)	Interval
≥70	5	12	1,000‡	tid
50–69	2.5	12	1,500	qd
25–49	2.5	24	1,000	qd
10–24	1.25	24	500	qd
<10†	1.25	tiw	500	tiw

*The optimal maintenance dose in renal impairment is not known but once daily dosing with proportionate reductions (50%) in total dose are recommended. Based on manufacturing recommendations.
†A maximum dose of 1.25 mg/kg/tiw is suggested for persons on hemodialysis. Dosing should be done after completion of dialysis.
‡For children with renal insufficiency, a daily dose in milligrams per kilogram equaling the estimated glomerular filtration rate has been suggested.[362]

ganciclovir by approximately 50 to 60%, and dosing after dialysis is recommended.[329, 330]

The intravitreal ganciclovir implant is designed to release drug at a rate of approximately 1 μg/hour over a period of 5 to 8 months.[331]

Interactions

Concurrent oral ganciclovir doubles the overall exposure to didanosine, increases zidovudine exposure by a much smaller extent, and may increase the risk of didanosine concentration-related toxicities.[332] Ganciclovir exposure is reduced about 20% when it is ingested 2 hours after but not simultaneously with didanosine. Zidovudine[333, 334] and probably other cytotoxic agents increase the risk of ganciclovir-induced myelosuppression, as do nephrotoxic agents that impair ganciclovir excretion. Probenecid and possibly acyclovir reduce renal clearance of ganciclovir. In animals, zidovudine but not amphotericin B, ketoconazole, dapsone, or trimethoprim-sulfoxazole antagonizes the anti-CMV effects of ganciclovir.[301, 335] Renal dysfunction may occur in patients given concurrent ganciclovir and either amphotericin B or cyclosporine, and ganciclovir may increase cyclosporine levels.

Toxicity

Myelosuppression is the principal dose-limiting toxicity of ganciclovir. The most common adverse events are neutropenia in about 40% and thrombocytopenia in 15 to 20% AIDS patients receiving intravenous ganciclovir.[296, 326] The risk of these toxicities is substantially lower in transplantation patients. Neutropenia occurs in approximately one fourth of those receiving oral ganciclovir. Neutropenia is most commonly observed during the second week of treatment and is reversible in most patients within 1 week after drug cessation. Treatment should be temporarily discontinued if the absolute neutrophil count falls below 500 cells/mm³. Recombinant granulocyte-macrophage colony-stimulating factor may be useful in treating ganciclovir-induced neutropenia.[336]

CNS side effects, ranging in severity from headache, to behavioral changes with confusion or psychosis, to convulsions and coma, have been described in 5 to 15% of patients. About one third of patients receiving intravenous ganciclovir interrupt or prematurely stop therapy because of bone marrow or CNS toxicity. In addition, twofold to fourfold higher rates of azotemia occur in transplant recipients receiving intravenous ganciclovir prophylaxis.[337] Oral ganciclovir prophylaxis is also associated with mild nephrotoxicity.[338]

Anemia, rash, fever, liver function test abnormalities, nausea or vomiting, and eosinophilia have also been reported. Phlebitis at the infusion site may be caused by the alkaline pH of the solution. In the event of massive overdosage, hemodialysis and hydration may be effective in reducing plasma ganciclovir levels. Placement of the intravitreal insert may be associated with visual changes, hemorrhage, infection, and retinal detachment.

Ganciclovir is mutagenic, carcinogenic, immunosuppressive, and causes irreversible reproductive toxicity in animals and possibly humans.[296] Teratogenicity, embryotoxicity, testicular atrophy, and bone marrow hypocellularity have been observed in animals at ganciclovir dosages comparable to those used in humans.

Clinical Studies

Ganciclovir is currently approved for treatment and chronic suppression of CMV retinitis in immunocompromised patients and prevention of CMV disease in transplantation patients. Because of its toxicity, ganciclovir use has been limited to patients with life-threatening or sight-threatening CMV infections. With initial or induction intravenous doses of 2.5 mg/kg every 8 hours or 5 mg/kg every 12 hours for 10 to 21 days, about 85% of CMV retinitis patients improve or stabilize their disease.[296, 339–341] Ganciclovir is comparable to foscarnet in initial control of retinitis.[286] Fundoscopic improvement is usually evident by 10 to 14 days. Approximately 90% of treated patients have a conversion of blood cultures to negative in 7 to 15 days. Almost all AIDS patients who respond to initial ganciclovir treatment relapse within weeks without suppressive therapy.[326, 341] High doses of intravenous ganciclovir (30 to 35 mg/kg/week), but not low doses (10 to 20 mg/kg/week), are effective for chronic suppression. Oral ganciclovir suppression (1 g three times daily) appears to be comparably effective to intravenous dosing.[342] Retinal detachments are common during long-term follow-up.[343] Combined ganciclovir and foscarnet is superior to monotherapy and may be effective when single agent therapy fails.[287] Intraocular sustained-release ganciclovir implants[344, 345] and repeated intravitreal injections are effective in controlling retinitis but do not prevent CMV disease in the other eye or in other sites.

Clinical improvement and virologic responses are also seen in CMV pneumonia and gastrointestinal infections in AIDS patients and in solid organ transplant recipients.[326, 341, 346] CNS syndromes respond less predictably and may progress despite therapy.[347] In biopsy-proven CMV colitis in AIDS patients, ganciclovir (5 mg/kg every 12 hours for 14 days) is associated with significant antiviral effects, stabilization of weight loss, and lower incidence of extracolonic CMV disease but no differences in symptoms compared with placebo.[348] In bone marrow transplant recipients, virologic responses but no reduction in mortality occur in patients with CMV pneumonia treated with ganciclovir alone or in combination with corticosteroids. In contrast, ganciclovir combined with intravenous immunoglobulin or CMV immunoglobulin reduces the mortality rate among bone marrow transplantation patients with CMV pneumonia, from 80 to 90% to 30 to 50%.[349, 350] No significant clinical benefit is found in gastrointestinal infection in marrow transplant recipients with ganciclovir monotherapy.[351] Usefulness in treating congenital CMV disease is under study.

Intravenous ganciclovir prophylaxis appears to be effective and reasonably well tolerated in preventing CMV disease in bone marrow[352, 353] and solid organ transplant recipients.[36, 337] Preemptive ganciclovir treatment (5 mg/kg every 12 hours for 7 to 14 days followed by 5 mg/kg/day until day 100 to 120 after transplantation) when CMV is isolated from bronchoalveolar lavage fluid[352] or from other body sites[353] is highly effective in preventing CMV pneumonia and appears to reduce mortality in bone marrow transplant recipients. In seropositive bone marrow transplantation patients, initiation of ganciclovir at the time of engraftment also markedly reduces CMV shedding and disease rates but does not improve survival, in part because of neutropenia-related infections.[354, 355]

Short-term ganciclovir administration after transplantation reduces the risk of CMV disease in seropositive allograft recipients undergoing heart, lung, or liver transplantation.[2, 337, 356] More prolonged administration (to day 100) provides protection against late-onset CMV disease.[365a] When ganciclovir is administered preemptively during anti-lymphocyte antibody treatment for periods up to 2 weeks, the incidence of CMV disease is reduced more than three fold in seropositive allograft recipients.[357] Ganciclovir prophylaxis is also effective in preventing HSV infection[355] and results in clearance of EBV from oropharyngeal secretions, although a rapid rebound in excretion occurs after cessation of therapy.[358]

Oral ganciclovir (1 g three times daily to day 98) markedly reduces the risk of invasive CMV disease in liver transplant recipients, including the high-risk group comprising seronegative recipients of seropositive donors.[338] Ganciclovir (1 g three times daily for 12 weeks) is also effective in renal transplant recipients.[359] Oral ganciclovir (1 g every 8 hours) also appears to decrease incidence of disease in HIV-infected patients with CD4 T-cell counts lower than 100 cells/mm^3,[360] although not when administered with didanosine.[361]

Intravenous ganciclovir reduces biochemical abnormalities and HBV DNA levels by 90% in post-transplantation HBV infection.[304] Topical 0.15% ganciclovir ophthalmic gel is comparable to acyclovir ointment in treating HSV keratitis.[362]

IDOXURIDINE

Idoxuridine (5-iodo-2′-deoxyuridine) (IDU, Herplex), is an iodinated thymidine analogue (see Fig. 36–4) that inhibits replication of various DNA viruses in vitro, particularly herpesviruses and poxviruses.[363] Plaque production by most clinical isolates of HSV type 1 is inhibited by concentrations of 2 to 10 μg/ml. Idoxuridine's antiviral mechanism of action is not completely defined, but the phosphorylated derivatives interfere with various enzyme systems. The triphosphate inhibits viral DNA synthesis and is incorporated into both viral and cellular DNA. Resistance to idoxuridine readily develops under laboratory conditions[364] and occurs in viral isolates recovered from idoxuridine-treated patients with HSV keratitis.

In humans, extremely low plasma concentrations of idoxuridine (0.1 to 0.4 ppm) are detected in about one half of patients treated topically with 40% idoxuridine in the penetration-enhancing agent dimethylsulfoxide (DMSO). Idoxuridine is also teratogenic, mutagenic, tumor-promoting, and immunosuppressive in preclinical testing. DMSO is teratogenic and can cause adverse ocular effects in laboratory animals.

In the United States, idoxuridine is approved only for topical treatment of HSV keratitis, whereas idoxuridine in DMSO is available in Europe for treatment of herpes labialis, genitalis, and zoster. In ocular HSV infections, topical idoxuridine is more effective in epithelial infections, especially initial episodes, than in stromal infections.[365, 366] Adverse reactions include pain, pruritus, inflammation, or edema involving the eye or lids and, rarely, allergic reactions.

Topical idoxuridine alone is ineffective in mucocutaneous herpesvirus infections. Frequent topical application of 5 to 40% idoxuridine dissolved in DMSO appears to hasten healing and shorten pain duration in localized herpes zoster. Topical 30% idoxuridine in DMSO may shorten the duration of viral shedding in recurrent or primary genital HSV infections, but it does not reduce the duration of symptoms or healing time.[367] Topical 15% idoxuridine in DMSO reduces the duration of pain and healing time in recurrent herpes labialis.[368] Mild local burning and aftertaste are common after topical application of DMSO, and headache, dizziness, sedation, nausea, and localized and generalized dermatitis have also been reported.

INTERFERONS

Classification

Since their discovery in 1957 as mediators of the phenomenon of viral interference (i.e., inhibition of growth of one virus by another) IFNs have become recognized as potent cytokines that are associated with complex antiviral, immunomodulating, and antiproliferative actions.[369] IFNs are proteins that are synthesized by eukaryotic cells in response to various inducers and that in turn cause biochemical changes leading to a nonselective antiviral state in exposed cells of the same species. Formally designated on the basis of the cell types from which they were derived, three major classes of human IFNs are currently recognized (Table 36–8). Each type is immunologically distinct and has different producer cells, inducers, and biologic effects, as well as unique physicochemical characteristics.[369–370a]

IFN-α and IFN-β are produced by almost all cells in response to viral infection and a variety of other stimuli, including double-stranded RNA, bacteria, protozoa, mycoplasmas, polyanions, several low-molecular-weight organic compounds, and certain cytokines and growth factors such as interleukin-1 (IL-1), IL-2, and tumor necrosis factor. IFN-γ production is restricted to T lymphocytes and natural killer cells responding to antigenic stimuli, mitogens, and certain cytokines such as IL-2. The principal antiviral interferons, IFN-α and IFN-β, are approximately 30% homologous at the amino acid level. Human IFN-α is actually a family of multiple species that share a high degree of amino acid sequence homology (>70%) but have differing in vitro antiviral and biologic effects on human cells.[371] Compared with IFN-α/β, IFN-γ has less antiviral activity but more potent immunoregulatory effects, particularly with respect to macrophage activation, expression of class II major histocompatibility complex antigens, and mediation of local inflammatory responses. IFNs in clinical use include those produced by recombinant DNA techniques and native ones purified from stimulated leukocytes or other cells (see Table 36–8).

TABLE 36–8 Nomenclature and Classification of Human Interferons

Characteristic	Class α	Class β	Class γ
Former designations	Type 1, leukocyte	Type 1, fibroblast	Type II, immune
No. species	>24	1*	1
No. amino acids	165–172	166	143
Apparent molecular weight (kD)†	16–27.6	20–23	15.5–25
Disulphide bonds	2	1	0
Glycosylation	Variable‡	Yes	Yes
Acid stability (pH 2)	Stable§	Stable	Labile
Chromosome coding for receptor	21	21	6
Commercial formulations	rIFN-α-2b (Intron A) rIFN-α-2a (Roferon A) Le-IFN-αn3 (Alferon N) Ly-IFN-αn1 (Wellferon) rIFNalfacon-1(Infergen)	rIFN-β-1b (Betaseron) rIFN-β-1a (Avonex)	rIFN-γ-1b (Actimmune) rIFN-γ (Immuneron)

*Interleukin-6 (also designated IFN-β-2) has negligible antiviral effects and functions primarily as a β-cell differentiation factor (BSF-2). It has minimal sequence homology with classical IFN-β and is encoded by a different chromosome (12).

†Range of molecular weight relates to posttranslation modifications including formation of dimers, glycosylation, protein-binding. Molecular weight of nonglycosylated recombinant IFN-α is approximately 19.5 kD.

‡Generally not, but several minor species are glycosylated.

§Acid-labile IFN-α species occur in certain pathologic states, including human immunodeficiency virus infection, systemic lupus erythematosus, rheumatoid arthritis, and pemphigus.

Abbreviations: IFN, Interferon; Le, leukocyte-derived; Ly, lymphoblastoid cell–derived; r, recombinant.

Adapted from Zoon KC. Human interferons: Structure and function. In: Anonymous. Interferon 9. London: Academic Press; 1987:1–12; Greenberg SB. Human interferon in viral diseases (Review). Infect Dis Clin North Am. 1987;1:383–423.

Mechanisms of Action

A wide range of animal viruses are sensitive to the antiviral actions of IFNs, although many DNA viruses are relatively insensitive and considerable differences in potency exist among viruses and assay systems.[372] IFN activity is usually measured in terms of antiviral effects in cell culture. Typically, one unit of IFN activity is the amount present in a sample dilution that causes a 50% reduction in virus replication or expression in certain cell lines; this is generally expressed as international units (IU) relative to National Institutes of Health or World Health Organization reference standards.

IFNs are not directly antiviral but cause elaboration of effector proteins in exposed cells, which contribute to a state of viral resistance.[373–375] The initial step involves IFN binding to specific cell surface receptors, which are shared between IFN-α and IFN-β but are different for IFN-γ. The IFN receptor is part of a JAK-STAT signaling complex, which activates transcription factors that bind selectively to approximately 100 IFN-regulated genes.[376, 377] The onset of IFN antiviral action is rapid, and IFN exposure leads to production of more than two dozen cellular proteins. Depending on the virus and cell type, IFN's antiviral effects are mediated through inhibition of viral penetration or uncoating, synthesis or methylation of messenger RNA (mRNA), translation of viral proteins, and/or viral assembly and release.

Among IFN-induced proteins are unique 2′-5′oligoadenylate [2-5(A)] synthetases and the protein kinase PKR, either of which can inhibit protein synthesis in the presence of double-stranded RNA. The 2-5(A) synthetase produces adenylate oligomers, which activate a latent cellular endoribonuclease (Rnase L) to cleave both cellular and viral single-stranded RNAs. PKR selectively phosphorylates and inactivates a protein involved in protein synthesis, eukaryotic initiation factor 2 (eIF-2). PKR is also a transducer for activation of the transcription factor NF-κB.[378] IFN may also block mRNA capping by inhibiting *trans*-methylation reactions. IFN induction of a phosphodiesterase, which cleaves a portion of transfer RNA and thereby prevents peptide elongation, also contributes to the inhibition of protein synthesis. IFN also induces the soluble form of the low-density lipoprotein receptor inhibitory for rhabdovirus assembly,[379] and the MxA protein, a guanosine triphosphatase with activity against orthoviruses and certain RNA viruses.[380] Induction of nitric oxide synthase appears to mediate a substantial antiviral effect of IFN-γ.[381] Increased levels of 2-5(A) activity and MxA protein or mRNA in peripheral leukocytes are also used as a marker for IFN exposure or endogenous release.[380]

Except possibly for the Mx proteins and influenza viruses and for 2-5(A) synthetase/RNase L and picornaviruses, no consistent correlations exist between induction of a particular enzyme and resistance to specific viruses across a range of cell types.[373–375] A particular virus may be inhibited at several steps, and the principal inhibitory effect differs among virus families. In addition, certain viruses are able to counter IFN effects by blocking production or activity of selected IFN-inducible proteins.[374, 375] For example, the NS5A protein of HCV represses the function of the IFN-induced PKR.[382] IFN exposure may also reduce the expression of certain cellular genes, including selected oncogenes and those involved in collagen synthesis.

Complex interactions exist between IFNs and other parts of the immune system.[370a, 383] For example, IFN-γ enhances the expression of IL-2 receptors on T lymphocytes, and IL-2 modulates IFN-γ production. The induction of cytotoxic T-lymphocyte responses appears to require both IL-2 and IFN-γ. IFN-α is produced by macrophages and also can modify macrophage functions, increasing phagocytosis and cytolytic activity. The effects of IFN include inhibiting delayed-type hypersensitivity responses, inhibiting lymphocyte blastogenesis, and prolonging survival of allogeneic grafts; increasing production of proinflammatory cytokines; enhancing (low concentration) or suppressing (high concentration) antibody formation; increasing natural killer cell activity and antibody-dependent cellular cytotoxicity; enhancing phagocytic and cytolytic activity of macrophages; inhibiting macrophage migration; increasing the expression of major histocompatibility antigens on cell surfaces; inhibiting the growth of intracellular parasites; augmenting immunoglobulin E (IgE)–mediated histamine release; increasing the expression of Fc receptors on lymphocytes and accessory cells; interfering with attachment of hormones and certain toxins to ganglioside receptors on the cell membrane; inhibiting growth of rapidly dividing cells; and enhancing differentiation (low concentration) or inhibiting differentiation (high concentration) of cells.

IFNs may ameliorate viral infections by exerting direct antiviral effects and by modifying the immune response to infection. For example, IFN-induced expression of major histocompatibility complex antigens may contribute to the antiviral actions of IFN by enhancing the lytic effects of cytotoxic T lymphocytes. IFN titers generally appear at the sites of viral replication just after peak titers of virus and before humoral antibody responses. In contrast to resolution of viral infection, IFNs may mediate some of the systemic symptoms associated with viral infections and contribute to immunologically mediated tissue damage in certain viral diseases.[384] High IFN titers are usually followed by a reduction of virus titers, although persistently elevated IFN titers have been recognized in certain chronic and acute viral infections (e.g., hemorrhagic fevers). Unusual acid-labile IFN-α has been observed in patients with certain autoimmune disorders and AIDS, in which its presence appears to predict disease progression.[385, 386]

Pharmacokinetics

The prolonged biologic effects of IFN are not easily related to serum concentrations or other conventional pharmacokinetic parameters. After intramuscular or subcutaneous injection of IFN-α absorption exceeds 80%.[387, 388] Plasma levels are dose-related, peaking at 4 to 8 hours and returning to baseline by 18 to 36 hours. Levels of 2-5(A) synthetase in peripheral blood mononuclear cells, which have been used as an index of biologic responsiveness to IFN, show increases beginning at 6 hours and lasting through 4 days after a single dose.[389] An antiviral state in these cells is detectable at 1 hour, peaks at 24 hours, and slowly decreases to baseline by 6 days after injection. Absorption of IFN-α is more variable, and intramuscular or subcutaneous injections of IFN-β result in negligible plasma levels, although increases in 2-5(A) synthetase may occur. Oral administration does not result in detectable serum IFN levels or increases in 2-5(A) synthetase activity in peripheral blood mononuclear cells.[390]

After systemic administration, low levels of IFN are detected in respiratory secretions, cerebrospinal fluid, eye, and brain. After intravenous dosing cerebrospinal fluid levels average less than 1% of serum concentrations.[391] IFN-α is relatively stable in most body fluids, whereas IFN-β and IFN-α appear to lose activity readily. However, it is unknown whether measurable IFN levels at a particular site accurately reflect its antiviral or other biologic activities.

After intravenous dosing, both IFN-α and IFN-β are cleared rapidly in a complex fashion. Leukocyte and recombinant IFN-α species have a plasma $T_{1/2}$ of approximately 2 to 4 hours. The clearance of IFN includes inactivation by various body fluids, cellular uptake, and metabolism by body organs, primarily the kidney and to some extent the liver, heart and skeletal muscle, and lung. Negligible biologically active IFN is excreted in the urine.

Interactions

IFN and its inducers reduce the metabolism of various drugs by the hepatic cytochrome P-450–dependent mixed-function oxidase system and significantly increase plasma $T_{1/2}$ and levels of drugs such as theophylline. IFNs may increase the neurotoxic, hematotoxic, or cardiotoxic effects of other drugs.

Toxicity

Both purified natural and recombinant IFNs are associated with dose-related immediate and late-onset toxicities.[392, 393] Adverse effects are generally mild and reversible at doses of less than 5 million IU(MU)/day.[388] Intramuscular and subcutaneous injection of IFN doses of 1 to 2 MU or more usually are associated with an acute influenza-like syndrome including fever, chills, headache, myalgia, arthralgia, nausea, vomiting, and diarrhea, especially during the first week of therapy. Symptoms begin several hours after administration; fever may range higher than 40°C but usually resolves within 12 hours. Tolerance develops in most patients within several weeks. Febrile responses can be moderated by pretreatment with various antipyretics. Up to one half of patients receiving intralesional therapy for genital warts experience the influenza-like illness. Intralesional IFN also causes discomfort at the injection site and leukopenia. Local reactions consisting of tenderness and erythema also occur after subcutaneous injection, and intranasal IFN causes local irritation.

Major toxicities that limit dose and duration of therapy are bone marrow suppression with granulocytopenia and thrombocytopenia; neurotoxicity manifested by somnolence, confusion, behavioral disturbance, electroencephalographic changes, and, rarely, seizures[394]; reversible neurasthenia with profound fatigue and anorexia, weight loss, and myalgia; thyroid dysfunction and autoimmune thyroiditis; and cardiotoxicity with hypotension, arrhythmias, and reversible cardiomyopathy.[395] Psychiatric disturbance and depression are more common in patients with preexisting disorders but can also occur in those without previous mental illness. Elevations in hepatic enzymes and triglycerides and retinopathy are common.[396] Alopecia, psoriasis, vitiligo, lichen planus, proteinuria, renal insufficiency, interstitial nephritis, autoantibody formation, bacterial infections, and hepatotoxicity occur.[397]

The development of serum neutralizing antibodies to exogenous IFNs varies with the IFN type, dose, and route of administration, but may be more common with IFN-α-2a.[398] Neutralizing antibodies may be associated infrequently with loss of clinical responsiveness.[388] Those directed against recombinant IFN-α may or may not cross-react with natural IFN-α or other recombinant species, and patients with antibodies against one recombinant IFN-alfa subtype may respond to natural IFN-α.

IFN may impair fertility and alter hormone levels in females. IFN is an abortifacient in monkeys at high doses, and safety during pregnancy is not established.

Clinical Studies

Clinical use of IFNs has been limited by relative lack of potency, side effects, and the availability of competing antiviral agents. Depending on the IFN type, recombinant and natural IFN-α (see Table 36–9) are approved in the United States for treatment of condyloma acuminatum, chronic hepatitis C, chronic hepatitis B, Kaposi's sarcoma in HIV-infected patients, and other malignancies. IFN-β is approved for management of multiple sclerosis, and recombinant IFN-γ for treatment of chronic granulomatous disease.

Hepatitis B Virus. Chronic HBV infections are associated with deficient IFN production and often with decreased responsiveness to IFN. HBV polymerase is able to inhibit cellular responses to IFN-α and IFN-γ in vitro.[399] In patients with chronic hepatitis B, parenteral administration of various IFNs is associated with loss of HBV DNA, loss of hepatitis B early antigen (HBeAg) and development of anti-HBeAg antibody, and biochemical and histologic improvement in about 25 to 40% of patients.[388, 400] Lasting responses require moderately high IFN doses and prolonged administration (about 5 MU/day or 10 MU three times/week for 4 to 6 months). Responses with seroconversion to anti-HBeAg are usually associated with transaminase elevations and often a hepatitis-like illness during the second or third month of therapy, presumably related to immune clearance of infected hepatocytes. An increased risk of clinical deterioration exists in patients with poor or decreasing hepatic synthetic function, and lower doses have been suggested for such patients. Factors associated with reduced response rates include high plasma HBV DNA levels (>200 pg/ml), long-standing infection, male gender, low transaminase levels (less than two times the upper limit of normal), inactive histology, immunosuppressive therapy, and HIV infection.

Remissions in chronic hepatitis B induced by IFN are sustained in more than 80% of patients and are frequently followed by later loss of hepatitis B surface antigen (HBsAg) and improved long-term clinical outcomes.[401–404] Patients with anti-HBeAg and precore mutants of HBV may have higher relapse rates.[405] IFN-γ is less effective than IFN-α/β, and combinations do not appear to enhance antiviral effects.[406, 407] Some nonresponders to IFN-α may respond to a course of IFN-β.[408] Despite possible short-term enhancement of antiviral effects by combinations of systemic IFN-α with acyclovir or corticosteroid pretreatment, no dual therapies have yet emerged as providing long-term benefit or reductions in toxicity.[139, 409]

IFN may improve HBV-associated nephrotic syndrome and glomerulonephritis in some patients.[410, 411] Antiviral effects and improvements occur in about one half of patients with chronic hepatitis D,[412] but relapse is common unless HbsAg disappears. Long-term treatment (12 months or longer) at doses used for chronic HBV may result in sustained improvement.[413] IFN does not appear beneficial in acute HBV or hepatitis D virus infections.

Hepatitis C Virus. In chronic HCV infection, subcutaneous IFN-α (3 MU three times/weekly for 6 months) is associated with an approximate 50% rate of serum aminotransferase normalization.[414–416] Biochemical response is associated with loss of detectable serum HCV RNA in 75% or more of patients,[417] but more than 50% of responding patients have virologic and usually biochemical relapse 1 to 2 months after treatment is stopped. Those with normal aminotransferase levels and negative HCV RNA at 6 months after therapy have long-term biochemical and histologic improvement,[418] whereas persistent HCV RNA is predictive of hepatitis relapse.[419, 420] Prolonged treatment (up to 18 months) or possibly higher doses (5 or 10 MU three times weekly) may increase sustained response rates.[421] The recommended duration of treatment is 12 months.[422] Combined IFN and oral ribavirin therapy significantly increases sustained virologic responses compared with monotherapy, especially in those with high HCV RNA levels.[414, 423, 424] The combination is superior to monotherapy for both initial treatment and retreatment after failure of IFN monotherapy. IFN treatment may benefit HCV-associated cryoglobulinemia and glomerulonephritis.[425, 426]

Younger age (<45 years), shorter disease duration (<5 years), absence of cirrhosis, and low serum levels of HCV RNA ($<10^5$ copies/ml) are predictors of response to IFN.[414] Differences in genotype (1a, 1b, and 4) or in mutations within an IFN sensitivity-determining region of the NS5A gene influence response in some patient populations.[427–429] Concurrent hepatitis G virus infection does not influence response and itself may resolve with IFN in a minority of patients.[430] Patients who do not respond to IFN within 3 months do not benefit from continued therapy. Patients with autoimmune chronic hepatitis, who may have false-positive enzyme immunoassay tests for anti-HCV antibodies, can worsen if treated with IFN.[431] Safety and efficacy remain to be established in uncompensated liver disease. In patients with compensated HCV-related cirrhosis, IFN therapy (6 MU three times weekly for 12 to 24 weeks) appears to reduce the risk of hepatocellular carcinoma.[432, 433] IFN administration during acute HCV infection may reduce the risk of chronicity.[434] Combined IFN and ribavirin but not IFN alone appear to reduce the risk of recurrent HCV infection after liver transplantation.[435]

Herpesviruses. Although IFN is associated with antiviral effects, no consistent reductions in symptoms or lesion duration have been observed with topical or systemic IFN treatment of genital herpes.[372, 436, 437] Topical application of IFN-α in several formulations modestly reduces viral shedding and symptom duration in recurrent genital herpes. Topical IFN appears to have some activity in combination with trifluridine in drug-resistant mucocutaneous HSV infections. In superficial HSV keratitis, combined administration of topical IFN-α with trifluridine or acyclovir appears to be more effective than single-agent therapy.[372]

In localized herpes zoster in cancer patients, early treatment with high-dose IFN-α (about 36 MU/day for 5 to 7 days) reduces the risk of cutaneous or visceral dissemination and possibly the severity of postherpetic neuralgia.[438] Lower doses and shorter duration of therapy are less effective, and systemic reactions are frequent. In older adults with acute herpes zoster, treatment with intramuscular IFN-α (10 MU/day) is similar to intravenous acyclovir in lesion and symptom resolution but is associated with more side effects.[439] IFN is not effective in preventing CMV infection in bone marrow recipients or in treating CMV pneumonia.

Human Immunodeficiency Virus. HIV-infected patients frequently have detectable IFN levels, and plasma inhibitors of IFN activity are often present during AIDS.[385, 386] IFN-α and IFN-γ inhibit HIV replication in vitro,[372] and synergistic inhibition occurs in combination with zidovudine and other antiretroviral agents. High doses of IFN-α induce 10 to 40% response rates in patients with Kaposi's sarcoma without benefitting concurrent herpesvirus infections or immune functions.[440] IFN treatment is associated with dose-related antiretroviral effects, particularly in early-stage infection, but also with adverse effects.[441] IFN-α (3 MU three times weekly) combined with zidovudine is more effective than zidovudine alone in symptomatic infection.[442] IFN appears to benefit HIV-related thrombocytopenia[443] and eosinophilc cellulitis. In vitro resistance to IFN has been described in HIV isolates.[444]

Papillomavirus. Both intralesional and systemic administration of IFN produce some regression of anogenital warts,[372, 445–448] but more cost-effective and better tolerated modalities are adequate in most patients. In refractory condylomata acuminata, intralesional injection of various natural and recombinant IFNs is associated with complete clearance of injected warts in 36 to 62% of patients.[4] Response rates are twofold to threefold higher than those observed in placebo recipients, but uninjected warts do not respond. Responding patients generally show lesion involution within 4 weeks and maximal responses at 4 to 12 weeks after initiating therapy. Complete responders have relatively low relapse rates (21 to 25%) during short-term follow-up. Responsiveness is poor in HIV-infected patients and those with chronic lesions. Intralesional IFN may enhance the response to topical podophyllin[445] and other local therapies.[4] Mild to moderate systemic side effects (8 to 10% dropout rate), discomfort at injection site, and leukopenia (up to 30%) are common with intralesional IFN.

Plantar warts are poorly responsive to intramuscular IFN, but verruca vulgaris may respond to intralesional IFN-α.[449] Responses to intralesional and systemic IFN have also been observed in the rare human papillomavirus–related condition of epidermodysplasia verruciformis. Systemic IFN may provide adjunctive benefit in recurrent juvenile laryngeal papillomatosis. The majority of children have some initial decrease in lesions, but recurrence rates are high after cessation of therapy, and the long-term response to parenteral IFN-α is variable.[450–452] Laryngeal disease in older patients appears to be more responsive.

Respiratory Viruses. Except for adenovirus, IFN has broad-spectrum antiviral activity against respiratory viruses in vitro.[453] In experimentally induced infections in humans, intranasal administration of leukocyte or recombinant IFN-α is protective against rhinovirus, coronavirus, respiratory syncytial virus (RSV), and, to a lesser extent, influenza virus infections.[454, 455] However, under natural conditions, prophylactic intranasal IFN-α is protective only against rhinovirus colds,[456, 457] and chronic use is limited by the occurrence of nasal side effects. Intranasal IFN-α is therapeutically ineffective in established rhinovirus colds.[458]

LAMIVUDINE

Lamivudine (3TC, Epivir) is a nucleoside reverse trancriptase inhibitor that is discussed in more detail in Chapter 115 on Antiretroviral Therapy. The triphosphate moiety is also a potent inhibitor of the RNA-dependent DNA polymerase of HBV, and oral lamivudine is active in animal models of hepadnavirus infection.

Resistance

Resistance to lamivudine in HBV is associated with a more than 40-10^4-fold reduced in vitro susceptibility.[458a, b] Several patterns of mutations (codons 552 and 528) result in reduced lamivudine sensitivity and associated changes in the YMDD motiff of HBV DNA polymerase. Viruses bearing YMDD mutations are less replication competent in vitro than wild-type HBV.[458c] Mutant virus begins to appear after 6 months of therapy, and the frequency increases progressively with continued drug administration. The cumulative frequency of emergence of resistance is 16 to 32% after 1 year in chronic hepatitis B but is higher in post-transplant infections.[458d] Resistance may be associated with diminished treatment response manifested by the return of HBV DNA and sometimes biochemical deterioration.[458a, d]

Clinical Studies

In patients with chronic HBV infection, lamivudine is associated with dose-related, reversible decreases in serum HBV DNA levels.[458e, f] Doses of 100 mg/day for 1 year suppress HBV DNA levels by 98%, normalize aminotransferase levels in most patients, reduce hepatic inflammation and fibrosis in more than 50%, but lead to HbeAg seroconversion in only 15 to 17% of patients.[458d] The effects of more prolonged therapy and combinations are under study. Significant post-treatment aminotransferase elevations (>500 IU/ml) occur in about 15% of patients after stopping lamivudine. Higher doses cause sustained reductions of HBV replication in HIV-infected persons.[458g] Some dually infected patients with chronic hepatitis B develop recurrent hepatitis when lamivudine is stopped. Administration before and after liver transplantation appears useful in preventing or suppressing recurrent HBV infection.[458h] The use of lamivudine in chronic HBV infection is discussed in more detail in Chapter 103, Chronic Hepatitis.

RIBAVIRIN

Spectrum

Ribavirin (1-β-D-ribofuranosyl-1,2,4-thiazole-3-carboxamide) (Virazole, Rebetol) is a guanosine analogue (Figure 36–5) in which both the base and the D-ribose sugar are necessary for antiviral activity.[459] Ribavirin inhibits the in vitro replication of a wide range of RNA and DNA viruses, including myxo-, paramyxo-, arena-, bunya-, RNA tumor, herpes, adeno-, pox- and retroviruses.[459–462] By plaque assay, inhibitory concentrations range from 3 to 10 μg/ml for influenza, parainfluenza, and RSV.[460, 461] Ribavirin antagonizes the anti–HIV-1 effects of zidovudine but enhances the activity of purine dideoxynucleosides.[463]

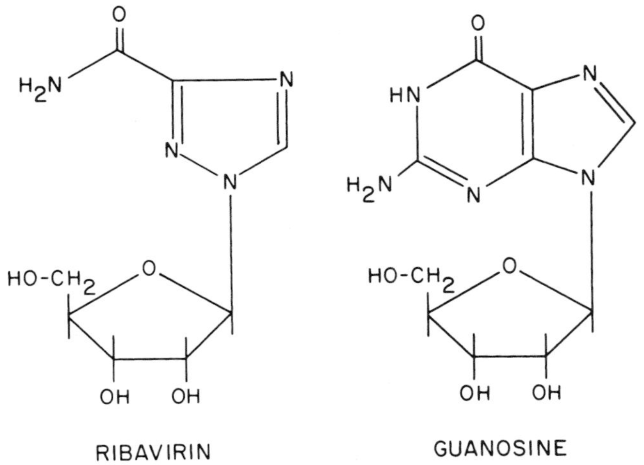

RIBAVIRIN GUANOSINE

FIGURE 36–5. Chemical structures of ribavirin and the nucleoside guanosine.

Low concentrations of ribavirin (1 to 10 μg/ml) reversibly inhibit macromolecular synthesis and the proliferation of certain rapidly dividing, uninfected cells.[3] Ribavirin suppresses nucleic acid synthesis in quiescent and mitogen-stimulated human lymphocytes in vitro[3, 464] but does not adversely affect polymorphonuclear leukocyte functions.[465] Inhibition of mast cell secretory responses occurs after in vitro ribavirin exposure.[466]

Aerosol administration is more effective than parenteral dosing in animal models of influenza and RSV infection.[467, 468] Parenteral ribavirin has antiviral and therapeutic activity in animal models of Lassa virus, other arenaviruses, and bunyavirus infections.[462, 469] Combinations of ribavirin with immunoglobulin in RSV infection[470] and with amantadine or rimantadine in influenza A infection[471] show enhanced antiviral activity.

Mechanism of Action

The antiviral mechanism of action of ribavirin is not fully defined but relates to alteration of cellular nucleotide pools and of viral messenger RNA formation.[459] Intracellular phosphorylation to the mono-, di-, and triphosphate derivatives is mediated by host cell enzymes. In both uninfected and RSV-infected cells, the predominant derivative (>80%) is the triphosphate, which is rapidly lost with an intracellular $T_{1/2}$ of less than 2 hours.[472]

Ribavirin monophosphate competitively inhibits inosine-5′-phosphate dehydrogenase and interferes with the synthesis of guanosine triphosphate and therefore with nucleic acid synthesis. Decreased concentrations of competing guanosine could potentiate other antiviral effects. Ribavirin triphosphate may inhibit influenza virus RNA polymerase activity and competitively inhibit the guanosine triphosphate–dependent 5′-capping of viral messenger RNA. Ribavirin triphosphate appears to inhibit the initiation and particularly the elongation of capped mRNA primer fragments by the influenza virus polymerase complex.[473] Ribavirin diphosphates and triphosphates also inhibit HIV reverse transcriptase activity.[474]

Ribavirin has immunosuppressive effects in experimental animals and shows therapeutic activity against transplantable virus-induced tumors and autoimmune diseases.[475, 476]

Resistance

In contrast to other nucleoside analogues, resistance to ribavirin has not been recognized, except for Sindbis virus.[477] No ribavirin-resistant RSV have been detected during aerosol therapy of children.[478]

Pharmacokinetics

After oral administration, bioavailability averages 33 to 45% in adults and children.[479–481] After single oral doses of 600, 1200, or 2400 mg, peak plasma concentrations occur at 1 to 2 hours and average 1.3, 2.5, and 3.2 μg/ml, respectively. Tenfold higher peak plasma levels occur 0.5 hours after intravenous administration of equivalent doses.[479] Plasma concentrations average approximately 24 μg/ml and 17 μg/ml after intravenous doses of 1000 and 500 mg, respectively, in patients with Lassa fever.[482] At steady state, cerebrospinal fluid levels are about 70% of those in plasma.[480]

The disposition of ribavirin is complex. The β-phase $T_{1/2}$ is about 2 hours, but a prolonged terminal-phase $T_{1/2}$ of 18 to 36 hours is also present.[479] Ribavirin triphosphate concentrates in erythrocytes with an erythrocyte:plasma ratio of 40:1 or greater, and erythrocyte levels gradually decrease with an apparent $T_{1/2}$ of 40 days. Renal excretion accounts for approximately 40% of ribavirin's clearance, and hepatic metabolism appears to be an important route of elimination. After oral administration, about 4% is recovered unchanged in the urine and 39% is excreted as the 1,2,4-triazole-3-carboxamide metabolite.[481] Hemodialysis and hemofiltration remove small amounts of drug.[483]

With aerosol administration, plasma levels increase with the duration of exposure. Peak plasma levels range from 0.5 to 2.2 μg/ml after 8 hours exposure and from 0.8 to 3.3 μg/ml after 20 hours in pediatric patients.[482] Respiratory secretion levels often exceed 1000 μg/ml and persist with a half-life of 1.4 to 2.5 hours. A special aerosol generator (SPAG-2, ICN Pharmaceuticals) is needed to produce particles of proper aerodynamic size to reach the lower respiratory tract. Revised estimates indicate that the delivered dose is twice as high in infants (1.8 mg/kg/hour) than in adults and that various other factors influence dosage.[484]

Toxicity

Systemic ribavirin causes dose-related anemia because of extravascular hemolysis and, at higher doses, suppression of bone marrow release of erythroid elements.[462, 485] Reversible increases of serum bilirubin (in up to one quarter of recipients), serum iron, and uric acid concentrations occur during short-term oral administration. Chronic oral ribavirin courses reverse hemoglobin falls of 2 to 3 g/dl in most recipients and increases in reticulocytes by 4 weeks of therapy. Severe anemia may require dose reduction or cessation. Other reported side effects include pruritus, rash, nausea, depression, and cough or respiratory symptoms.[486] Bolus intravenous infusion may cause rigors.[487] Aerosolized ribavirin may cause mild conjunctival irritation, rash, bronchospasm, reversible deterioration in pulmonary function, and, rarely, acute water intoxication.[488] No adverse hematologic effects have been associated with aerosolized ribavirin.

Ribavirin exposure may occur in health care workers working in the environment of aerosol-treated infants.[489–492] Health care worker exposure is higher during delivery by oxygen hood than by ventilator or vacuum-exhausted hood systems.[491] Use of aerosol containment systems except during mechanical ventilation, turning off the aerosol generator before providing routine care, and use of protective equipment have been recommended.[492]

When ribavirin is used in conjunction with mechanical ventilation, in-line filters, modified circuitry, and frequent monitoring are required to prevent plugging of ventilator valves and tubing with precipitates of ribavirin.[493, 494] The possible effects of such modifications on drug delivery to the lower respiratory tract are undefined.

In preclinical studies, ribavirin is teratogenic, embryotoxic, mutagenic, tumor-promoting, and possibly gonadotoxic.[485] Its use is relatively contraindicated during pregnancy, and pregnant women should not directly care for patients receiving ribavirin aerosol.

Clinical Studies

Ribavirin aerosol is approved in the United States for treatment of RSV bronchiolitis and pneumonia in hospitalized children, and oral ribavirin is approved for treatment of chronic hepatitis C in combination with IFN. Aerosolized ribavirin (12 to 22-hour exposure daily for 3 to 6 days) variably shortens the duration of virus shedding and improves certain clinical measures in infants hospitalized with RSV pneumonia, including high-risk infants with bronchopulmonary dysplasia or congenital heart disease.[478, 495] In infants receiving mechanical ventilation for RSV-related respiratory failure, no consistent benefits on duration of ventilatory support or mortality have been documented.[495–497] Intermittent, high-dose therapy (2-hour exposures three times daily for 5 days) is well tolerated and may be as effective as prolonged exposure.[498]

Use of aerosol ribavirin is limited by concerns regarding its efficacy, ease of administration, risk of occupational exposure, and cost. The American Academy of Pediatrics suggests that treatment may be considered in infants at high risk for serious RSV disease (e.g., complicated congenital heart disease, chronic lung disease, immunodeficiency states), those hospitalized with severe illness, and those at increased risk of deterioration (e.g., age <6 weeks).[499] Decreased RSV-specific serum neutralizing antibody titers, as well as diminished nasopharyngeal secretion RSV-specific IgE and IgA responses, may occur in ribavirin-treated children.[500] No long-term adverse or beneficial effects of ribavirin therapy have been documented in children.[501] Combinations of aerosol ribavirin and intravenous immunoglobulin appear to be beneficial in treating RSV pneumonia in immunocompromised patients,[502] whereas intravenous ribavirin is ineffective in bone marrow transplantation patients.[503]

Intravenous and aerosolized ribavirin have been used to treat severe influenza virus infections.[504, 505] Aerosolized ribavirin is associated with inconsistent reductions in viral titers and illness measures in adults with uncomplicated influenza A or B virus infection.[504, 506] Oral doses of 1.0 g/day have no activity in uncomplicated influenza,[472] whereas a high-dose oral regimen may provide clinical benefit.[507] Intravenous or aerosolized ribavirin, or both, have also been used in immunosuppressed patients with severe parainfluenza, measles, vaccinia, or adenovirus infections with uncertain clinical benefits, if any.[508–512]

In patients with Lassa fever who are at high risk of death because of elevated serum aspartate aminotransferase levels or high-titer viremia, intravenous (4 g/day) or oral ribavirin significantly reduces mortality, especially when therapy is initiated during the first 6 days of illness.[513] High-dose intravenous ribavirin reduces mortality and the risk of oliguria or hemorrhage in hemorrhagic fever with renal syndrome[514] and has also been associated with benefit in Argentine, Sabia, and Bolivian hemorrhagic fevers.[515, 516] Oral ribavirin appears to be beneficial in treating Crimean-Congo hemorrhagic fever[517] and has been used for prophylaxis in contacts of those patients and in Lassa fever.[518] Intravenous ribavirin is being tested in treatment of hantavirus pulmonary syndrome (see Chapter 154). In HIV-infected patients, chronic oral ribavirin at tolerable doses has no consistent benefits on CD4T-lymphocyte counts or HIV RNA levels.[519]

In adults with chronic hepatitis C, long-term oral ribavirin therapy (600 mg twice daily) reversibly reduces serum transaminase elevations, hepatic inflammation on biopsy, and fatigue without significantly affecting serum HCV RNA concentrations.[486, 520] The mechanism of this benefit is uncertain. The addition of oral ribavirin (500 to 600 mg twice daily) to a 24-week course of IFN-α-2b (3 MU three times weekly) therapy significantly increases the frequency of sustained biochemical and virologic response after cessation of therapy, specifically in those with higher baseline blood HCV RNA levels, compared with IFN monotherapy.[423] Increases in sustained responses also occur in those nonresponsive to or relapsing after previous interferon therapy.[424] Combined ribavirin and IFN treatment followed by maintenance oral ribavirin has been used to control disease in recurrent HCV infection after liver transplantation,[435] and other studies are in progress.

TRIFLURIDINE

Trifluridine (triflurothymidine, 5-trifluoromethyl-2′-deoxyuridine) (Viroptic) is a fluorinated pyrimidine nucleoside (see Fig. 36–4) that has in vitro inhibitory activity against HSV types 1 and 2, CMV, vaccinia, and, to lesser extent, certain adenoviruses.[521, 522] Concentrations of 0.2 to 10 μg/ml inhibit replication of herpesviruses, including acyclovir-resistant strains.[35]

Its antiviral mechanism of action involves inhibition of viral DNA synthesis. Trifluridine monophosphate irreversibly inhibits thymidylate synthetase, and the triphosphate competitively inhibits DNA polymerases with respect to thymidine triphosphate.[521] Trifluridine is incorporated into viral and, to a lesser extent, cellular DNA and also inhibits cellular DNA synthesis at relatively low concentrations. It also exhibits mutagenic, teratogenic, and antineoplastic activities in experimental systems. Trifluridine-resistant HSV with altered TK substrate specificity can be selected on laboratory passage.[364] The clinical significance of this observation is uncertain.

Trifluridine's clinical use is limited to topical therapy for HSV infections, and it is approved in the United States for treatment of primary keratoconjunctivitis and recurrent epithelial keratitis due to HSV types 1 and 2[365, 366, 521] (see Table 36–1). Topical trifluridine is more active than idoxuridine in HSV ocular infections, but trials comparing its efficacy with that of topical vidarabine have generally found no important differences.[523] Topical trifluridine is effective in some patients who have not responded clinically to idoxuridine or vidarabine. Adverse reactions include discomfort on instillation, palpebral edema, and, uncommonly, hypersensitivity reactions, irritation, and superficial punctate or epithelial keratopathy.

Topical trifluridine also appears to benefit some patients with acyclovir-resistant HSV cutaneous infections.[524] Combinations of trifluridine and IFN-α synergistically inhibit HSV replication in vitro and have been used to treat both ocular and drug-resistant mucocutaneous HSV infections.[35, 525]

VIDARABINE

Vidarabine (9-β-D-ribofuranosyladenine) (ara-A, adenine arabinoside, Vira-A) is an analogue of adenosine (see Fig. 36–4), which has in vitro antiviral activity against herpes-, pox-, rhabdo-, and some RNA tumor viruses.[526] Vidarabine inhibits in vitro replication idoxuridine- or acyclovir-resistant HSV and VZV strains. Plaque formation by most HSV and VZV strains is completely inhibited by 3.0 μg/ml or less of vidarabine.

Vidarabine inhibits viral DNA synthesis. Vidarabine is phosphorylated by cellular enzymes to the triphosphate derivative, which competitively inhibits the activity of viral, and to a lesser extent cellular, DNA polymerases. Vidarabine triphosphate is incorporated into both cellular and viral DNA, where it may act as a chain terminator. Vidarabine triphosphate inhibits other enzyme systems, including ribonucleoside reductase, RNA polyadenylation, and *S*-adenosylhomocysteine hydrolase. Resistant variants resulting from mutations in viral DNA polymerase can be selected under laboratory conditions, but drug resistance is not a recognized clinical problem.

Little systemic absorption occurs after ophthalmic application. Absorbed vidarabine is rapidly converted to its hypoxanthine metabolite (araHx) which has 30 to 50-fold less antiviral activity. Excretion of vidarabine and araHx occurs by the kidneys.

Vidarabine has been shown to be mutagenic, teratogenic, and oncogenic in preclinical testing. Hypersensitivity reactions, including pruritus, erythema, ocular pain, and foreign body sensation may occur after ocular application. Other reported effects include photophobia, keratitis after exposure to ultraviolet light, and increased lacrimation.

The intravenous formulation of vidarabine, which was useful in certain life-threatening herpes virus infections, was discontinued by the manufacturer in 1992. Vidarabine's use is restricted to an ophthalmic ointment. In HSV keratoconjunctivitis, topical vidarabine is superior to idoxuridine[365, 366] (see Table 36–1) and is effective in patients who cannot receive idoxuridine because of allergy, toxicity, or drug resistance.

AGENTS OF INVESTIGATIVE INTEREST

A large number of viral infections exist for which no effective antiviral treatment is available, either because of lack of an agent with sufficient potency and selectivity or because active viral replication is not be central to the pathogenesis of disease manifestations. Many agents have problems with drug-related toxicities, poor oral bioavailability, or high cost. Although several antivirals can suppress reactivations of infection, none can eradicate viral latency. Gene inhibition therapy (e.g., antisense oligonucleotides, ribozymes) may be able to accomplish this goal. One such agent (Fomivirsen) has been approved for intravitreal injection treatment of CMV retinitis and was discussed in a previous section.

Current investigation is focused heavily on antiretroviral agents, and a substantial number of candidate agents are in clinical trials (Table 36–9). In addition to agents with improved pharmacokinetic properties, greater potency, or improved toxicity profiles, the use of

TABLE 36–9 Representative New Antiviral Agents of Clinical Investigative Interest

Drug	Class	Principal Spectrum	Target of Antiviral Action	Preclinical	Clinical
Sorivudine (BV-ara U)	Cytidine nucleoside analogue	VZV, HSV-1	DNA polymerase	High protein binding (>95%); principal metabolite (bromovinyl uracil) inhibits dihydropyrimidine dehydrogenase; oncogenic in animals	High oral bioavailability; more effective than acyclovir in zoster of HIV-infected persons; deaths due to potentiation of 5-fluorouracil toxicity
Zanamivir	Sialic acid analogue	Influenza A, B	Neuraminidase—inhibits release of virus and spread in respiratory tract	Active topically in animal models of influenza	When inhaled is effective for treatment and prophylaxis of acute influenza; excellent tolerance
Oseltamivir (GS4104, GS4071)	Carbocyclic sialic acid analogue	Influenza A, B	Neuraminidase—inhibits release of virus and spread in respiratory tract	Ethylester prodrug (GS4104) is active orally in animal models of influenza	Oral GS4104 is effective for prophylaxis and treatment of acute influenza; mild gastrointestinal intolerance
Pleconaril	Oxadiozole derivative	Enteroviruses Rhinoviruses	VP1 of capsid—inhibits attachment, uncoating	Active orally in animal models of systemic/CNS enterovirus disease	Oral pleconaril is effective in enteroviral meningitis and experimental human coxsackievirus A21 infection
Intercellular adhesion molecule-1	Soluble cell receptor	Rhinoviruses	Receptor decoy—blocks attachment	Active intranasally in chimpanzees	Protective effect in experimental human infection
Lobucavir	Guanine nucleoside analogue	Herpes virus, HBV	DNA polymerase	Oncogenic in animals	Active orally in treating recurrent orolabial and genital HSV in immunocompetent patients; studies in CMV and chronic HBV in progress
Entecavir (BMS-200475)	Guanine nucleoside analogue	HBV	DNA polymerase	Potent oral activity in animal models of hepadnavirus infection; prolonged intracellular half-life	High oral bioavailability and prolonged program $T_{1/2}$ (60 h) in humans
Moribavir (1263W94)	Benzimidazole derivative	CMV, EBV	DNA synthesis inhibition via UL97 protein kinase inhibition	Novel mode of action; high protein binding	Good oral bioavailability (>50%) and anti-CMV effects; limited CNS penetration

Abbreviations: CMV, Cytomegalovirus; CNS, central nervous system; EBV, Epstein-Barr virus; HBV, hepatitis B virus; HIV, human immunodeficiency virus; HSV, herpes simplex virus; $T_{1/2}$, elimination half-life; VZV, varicella-zoster virus.

drug combinations is receiving greater emphasis. The areas in which advances are likely to provide more effective treatments include the identification of new viral targets (e.g., virus-specific enzymes, regulatory proteins); new drug delivery techniques to improve pharmacokinetic properties or target particular tissues; use of agents to modulate the effects of immunopathologic responses or host inflammatory mediators; and the use of immunomodulators or specific immunotherapies (e.g. monoclonal antibodies, therapeutic vaccines). Investigational agents likely to be considered for approval by the U.S. Food and Drug Administration in the near future are reviewed in what follows.

LOBUCAVIR

Lobucavir (carbocyclic oxetanocin-G, cyclobut-G) is a synthetic cyclobutane nucleoside analogue with in vitro inhibitory activity against a broad range of herpesviruses, HBV, and HIV (Fig. 36–6).

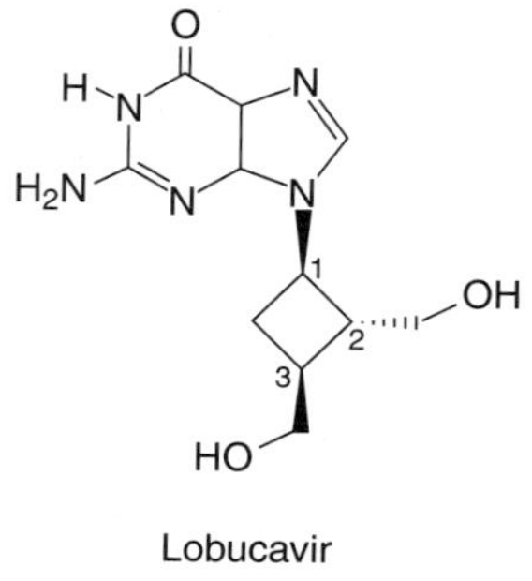

Lobucavir

FIGURE 36–6. Chemical structure of lobucavir.

Concentrations of approximately 0.5 μg/ml inhibit CMV and HBV replication,[527] whereas lower concentrations of 0.01 to 0.02 μg/ml are inhibitory for HSV and VZV in cell cultures. Depending on the cell type, cytotoxicity is observed at concentrations of about 8 μg/ml or higher. Lobucavir is less active against ganciclovir-resistant CMV and about 25-fold less inhibitory for TK-deficient, acyclovir-resistant HSV strains. Oral lobucavir is active in animal models of HSV, CMV, and hepadnavirus infection.[528]

Lobucavir inhibits viral DNA synthesis. It is preferentially phosphorylated in HSV-infected cells to the active triphosphate; much lower concentrations of lobucavir triphosphate accumulate in CMV-infected and in uninfected human cells. The intracellular $T_{1/2}$ of the triphosphate is prolonged (10 hours or longer). Like acyclovir, lobucavir triphosphate is a potent inhibitor of HSV DNA polymerase and serves as an alternative substrate with respect to dGTP.[529] In addition, the triphosphate is a potent inhibitor of CMV and HBV polymerases.[530] CMV DNA polymerase has a greater affinity for lobucavir triphosphate than the natural substrate dGTP. Higher concentrations inhibit cellular DNA polymerases. Incorporation of lobucavir appears to cause DNA chain termination, although very low amounts are incorporated internally into cellular DNA.

Lobucavir is formulated as oral capsules and for intravenous administration. Following intravenous dosing, the plasma $T_{1/2\,elim}$ averages about 2 hours, and approximately 80% of the drug is recovered unchanged in the urine. Tubular secretion plays an important role in excretion. The oral bioavailability of lobucavir is dose-dependent, averaging about 25 to 40% at doses of 200 mg or less, but decreasing at higher doses. Doses of 200 mg provide maximum plasma concentrations of 0.3 to 0.6 μg/ml. A high fat meal does not affect bioavailability, so that lobucavir can be administered with food or fasting. It has low serum protein binding (<10%).

The preclinical toxicity profile of lobucavir is similar to that of ganciclovir. Lobucavir is mutagenic in several genotoxicity assays and causes both bone marrow suppression and testicular degeneration in animals. Gastrointestinal tract and pulmonary inflammation have also been observed in dogs. Although not teratogenic in animals, lobucavir should be regarded as a male reproductive toxin. Its carcinogenic potential is under study. In humans, oral lobucavir has been associated with headache, insomnia, and gastrointestinal upset but no serious end-organ toxicities to date. Intravenous and less often oral administration may cause transaminase elevations. Neutropenia has been observed uncommonly.

Since entering clinical trials in 1992, oral lobucavir has shown antiviral activity in CMV- and HBV-infected patients and clinical benefits in HSV infections of immunocompetent hosts. Doses of 200 and 400 mg four times a day are associated with suppression of CMV viruria in HIV-infected persons,[531] but clinical efficacy data are not available. One month dosing of 200 mg twice or four times daily causes a more than 100-fold reduction in serum HBV DNA levels in chronically infected patients that returned to baseline after cessation of dosing.[532] Studies of long-term administration are in progress. Oral doses of 200 mg twice a day shorten healing times and pain in patients with recurrent genital herpes.[533] Lobucavir is being studied in other herpesvirus diseases but is an experimental agent at present.

PLECONARIL

Pleconaril (3-[3,5 dimethyl-4[[3-(3-methyl-5-isoxazoyl)propyl]-oxy]phenyl]-5-(trifluo romethyl)-1,2,4-oxadiazole) is an orally active antipicornavirus agent in advanced clinical development. Pleconaril inhibits picornavirus replication by binding to a specific hydrophobic pocket within the viral capsid and preventing viral attachment and/or uncoating of the genome. In cell culture, pleconaril inhibits replication of more than 90% of the most commonly isolated enterovirus serotypes at concentrations less than 0.07 μg/ml and approximately 80% of rhinovirus serotypes at concentrations of 0.34 μg/ml or lower (Investigator's Brochure, Pleconaril, ViroPharma, Inc, 1997). Pleconaril is active in murine models of severe coxsackievirus infection and can prevent the development of signs in coxsackievirus A9–exposed mice. In rats, radiolabeled pleconaril and/or its metabolites achieve concentrations in the nasal epithelium and CNS that are several–fold higher than those in blood. Preclinical studies have found no evidence of genotoxicity, fetal toxicity, or teratogenicity.

After oral administration in adults, the time required to reach maximal plasma concentrations is 1.5 to 5 hours, and the terminal $T_{1/2\,elim}$ averages 25 hours. Peak plasma concentrations average 1.1 and 2.4 μg/ml after doses of 200 and 400 mg, respectively, and then drop relatively rapidly to levels of approximately one tenth of the maximum plasma concentration within 12 hours. Modest accumulation occurs in the plasma with repetitive dosing. Ingestion in the fed state significantly increases plasma concentrations. Single oral doses of 5 mg/kg in children provide maximum plasma concentrations of 1.3 μg/ml and approximately 40% lower overall drug exposure owing to a larger volume of distribution and more rapid clearance. The plasma $T_{1/2\,elim}$ averages about 6 hours in children.

Pleconaril is poorly water soluble (<0.2 μg/ml) and is supplied in an oral suspension containing 40 mg/ml of pleconaril, medium-chain triglyceride, and surfactants. Pleconaril has been generally well tolerated; the most common adverse events after ingestion have been headache, nausea, diarrhea, stomach upset, and discomfort. These have occurred at frequencies comparable to those observed in placebo recipients. No serious end-organ toxicity has been recognized to date. Administration of oral pleconaril before and after experimental coxsackievirus A21 infection reduced peak viral titers by more than 100-fold and protected against illness.[534] In adults with enteroviral meningitis, pleconaril treatment resulted in significant shortening of illness duration, time to headache resolution, and reduction in use of analgesics, compared with placebo.[535] Clinical studies of hand-foot-and-mouth disease, picornaviral respiratory tract disease, and severe or life-threatening enteroviral syndromes such as chronic enteroviral meningoencephalitis in agammaglobulinemic patients and neonatal sepsis are in progress.

ZANAMIVIR AND OSELTAMIVIR

Zanamivir (4-gluanidino-neu5Ac2en or GG167 [Relenza]) is a sialic acid analogue (Fig. 36–7) that is a potent and specific inhibitor of the neuraminidases of influenza A and B viruses.[536] GS4071 is a transition state analogue of sialic acid cleavage that has a similar antiviral spectrum and potency.[537, 538] Oseltamivir (GS4104) is the ethyl ester prodrug of GS4071 (see Fig. 36–7). Both zanamivir and GS4071 competitively and reversibly interact with the active enzyme site to inhibit neuraminidase activity at low concentrations. For example, zanamivir inhibits purified influenza neuraminidases at 0.6 to 8 nM in vitro, whereas a much broader range of concentrations (0.002–>10 μM) inhibits influenza A and B virus replication in cell culture.[539] Zanamivir and GS4071 are not cytotoxic and inhibit neuraminidases from mammalian sources or other pathogens only at 10^6-fold higher concentrations. Because they target a different protein of the virus, zanamivir and GS4071 inhibit replication of amantadine and rimantadine resistant strains. Topical zanamivir and oral oseltamivir are active in murine and ferret models of influenza.[538, 540, 541]

Influenza neuraminidase cleaves terminal sialic acid residues and destroys the receptors recognized by viral hemagglutinin. This action is essential for release of virus from infected cells, prevention of viral aggregates, and spread within the respiratory tract.[542] Viruses resistant to inhibition by zanamivir or GS4071 following in vitro passage have mutations in the viral hemagglutinin and/or neuraminidase.[543] Hemagglutinin variants generally have mutations in or near the receptor binding site that make them less dependent on neuraminidase action for release from cells in vitro. One of these variants retained full susceptibility to zanamivir in vivo.[539] Hemagglutinin variants are cross-resistant to other neuraminidase inhibitors. Neuraminidase variants contain mutations in the active enzyme site that diminish binding of zanamivir (Glu119Gly, Ala, or Asp) or alter part of the catalytic triad (Arg292Lys). GS4071 is inhibitory for zanamivir-resistant variants with Glu119 mutations but is much less active than zanamivir against Arg292 variants. The altered neuraminidases have reduced activity or stability, and the mutated viruses have decreased infectivity in animals.[544] Resistance emergence has not been documented with zanamivir in immunocompetent hosts to date. One combined hemagglutinin and neuraminidase mutant has been recovered from an immunocompromised child with prolonged virus excretion despite receiving nebulized zanamivir.[545] Oral oseltamivir

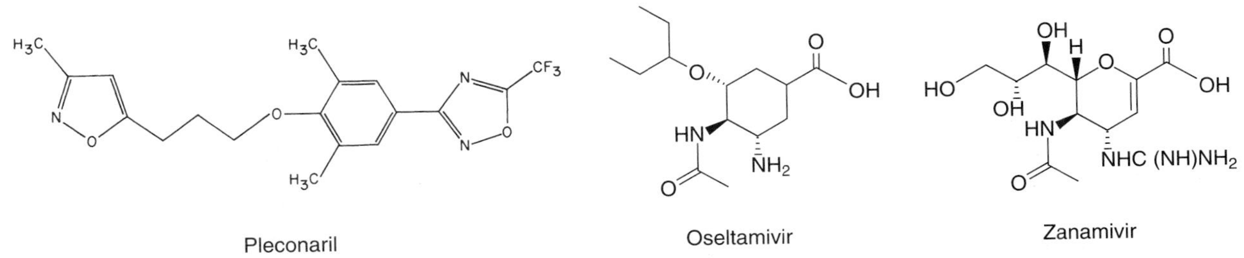

Pleconaril

Oseltamivir

Zanamivir

FIGURE 36–7. Chemical structures of pleconaril and the neuraminidase inhibitors oseltamivir and zanamivir.

therapy has been associated with recovery of viruses with diminished neuraminidase susceptibility in about 1 to 2% of recipients.

The oral bioavailability of zanamivir is low (<5%), and most clinical trials have used intranasal or dry powder inhalation delivery. Following intravenous dosing, the plasma $T_{1/2\,elim}$ of zanamivir averages 1.6 hours, and about 90% is eliminated unchanged in the urine.[546] Following inhalation of the dry powder, approximately 15% is deposited in the lower respiratory tract and the remainder in the oropharynx.[547] Bioavailability averages about 20%, and plasma levels are detectable but low. The proprietary inhaler device for delivering zanamivir is breath-actuated and requires a cooperative patient.

Oral oseltamivir is cleaved by esterases in the gastrointestinal tract or blood and provides good bioavailability of the active parent GS4071 (estimated ~80%).[548] The time to maximum plasma concentrations is about 3 to 4 hours. Very low blood levels of GS4104 are detectable. Administration with food may delay absorption slightly but does not decrease bioavailability. Doses of 100 mg provide plasma concentrations of 0.3 to 0.5 μg/ml. Following oral administration of oseltamivir, the plasma $T_{1/2\,elim}$ of GS4071 averages 7 to 9 hours. Both the prodrug and parent are eliminated primarily unchanged through the kidney. Distribution is not well characterized in humans, but peak bronchoalveolar lavage levels are similar to plasma levels in animals.[549] No clinically significant drug interactions have been recognized for either drug.

Topically applied zanamivir and oral oseltamivir are generally well tolerated, and no serious end-organ toxicity has been found for either agent. For zanamivir, no bronchospasm or local irritation has been recognized, and the frequencies of complaints are not significantly different from those in placebo recipients.[550, 551] Tolerance in uninfected asthmatic patients assessed by pulmonary function testing and in influenza-infected cardiopulmonary patients has been good. Oral oseltamivir is associated with nausea, discomfort, and, less often, emesis in a minority of influenza-infected patients. Gastrointestinal complaints are usually mild in intensity, transient despite continued dosing, and ameliorated by administration with food. Preclinical studies of zanamivir found no evidence of mutagenic, teratogenic, or oncogenic effects. High-dose oseltamivir causes renal tubular mineralization in mice and impaired parturition in female mice.

Intranasal or intravenous zanamivir and oral oseltamivir are highly protective against experimental human influenza, and early treatment is associated with reductions in viral titers, symptoms, and middle ear pressure abnormalities.[552–555] Inhaled zanamivir and oral oseltamivir are both therapeutically beneficial in acute influenza in previously healthy adults, and they shorten the time to illness resolution by 1 to 3 days compared with placebo.[550, 551, 556] Inhaled zanamivir is associated with more rapid recovery and reduced complications in influenza patients with underlying cardiopulmonary disorders. Oral oseltamivir may also reduce complications in previously healthy adults with influenza. Prophylactic administration of once-daily inhaled zanamivir and oral oseltamivir are both effective in reducing the likelihood of developing febrile illness during influenza season.[557, 558] Treatment studies in children, hospitalized patients, and the elderly and prevention studies in families and nursing home residents are in progress with these agents.

REFERENCES

1. Newton AA. Tissue culture methods for assessing antivirals and their harmful effects. In: Field HJ, ed. Antiviral Agents: The Development and Assessment of Antiviral Chemotherapy. Boca Raton, Fla: CRC Press; 1988:23–67.
2. Rubin RH, Tolkoff-Rubin NE. Antimicrobial strategies in the care of organ transplant recipients. Antimicrob Agents Chemother. 1993;37:619–624.
3. Heagy W, Crumpacker C, Lopez PA, Finberg RW. Inhibition of immune functions by antiviral drugs. J Clin Invest. 1991;87:1916–1924.
4. Beutner KR, Ferenczy A. Therapeutic approaches to genital warts. Am J Med. 1997;102:28–37.
5. Richman DD, ed. Antiviral Drug Resistance. Chichester: John Wiley & Sons Ltd; 1996.
6. Houde M, Arora DJ. Human influenza virus neuraminidase, but not hemagglutinin, induces murine macrophage interleukin 1 in vivo and in vitro [published erratum appears in Immunol Lett 1989;23:79]. Immunol Lett. 1989;22:41–46.
7. Sommadossi JP. Nucleoside analogs: similarities and differences. Clin Infect Dis. 1993;16(Suppl 1):S7–S15.
8. Wagstaff AJ, Faulds D, Goa KL. Aciclovir: A reappraisal of its antiviral activity, pharmacokinetic properties and therapeutic efficacy (Review). Drugs. 1994;47:153–205.
9. Whitley RJ, Gnann JJ. Acyclovir: A decade later [published erratum appears in N Engl J Med. 1993;328:671]. N Engl J Med. 1992;327:782–789.
10. Biron KK, Elion GB. In vitro susceptibility of varicella-zoster virus to acyclovir. Antimicrob Agents Chemother 1980;18:443–447.
11. Lang DJ, Cheung KS. Effectiveness of acycloguanosine and trifluorothymidine as inhibitors of cytomegalovirus infection in vitro. Am J Med. 1982;73:49–53.
12. Lin JC, Smith MC, Cheng YC, et al. Epstein-Barr virus: Inhibition of replication by three new drugs. Science. 1983;221:578–579.
13. Wingard JR, Hess AD, Stuart RK, et al. Effect of several antiviral agents on human lymphocyte functions and marrow progenitor cell proliferation. Antimicrob Agents Chemother. 1983;23:593–597.
14. Elion GB. History, mechanism of action, spectrum and selectivity of nucleoside analogs. In: Mills J, Corey L, eds. Antiviral Chemotherapy: New Directions for Clinical Application and Research. New York: Elsevier; 1986:118–137.
15. Derse D, Cheng YC, Furman PA, et al. Inhibition of purified human and herpes simplex virus-induced DNA polymerases by 9-(2-hydroxyethoxymethyl)guanine triphosphate: Effects on primer-template function. J Biol Chem. 1981;256:11447–11451.
16. Furman PA, St. Clair MA, Spector T. Acyclovir triphosphate is a suicide inactivator of the herpes simplex virus DNA polymerase. J Bio Chem. 1984;259:9575–9579.
17. Pagano JS, Datta AK. Perspectives on interactions of acyclovir with Epstein-Barr and other herpes viruses. Am J Med. 1982;73:18–26.
18. Chatis PA, Crumpacker CS. Resistance of herpesviruses to antiviral drugs (Review). Antimicrob Agents Chemother. 1992;36:1589–1595.
19. Parris DS, Harrington JE. Herpes simplex virus variants restraint to high concentrations of acyclovir exist in clinical isolates. Antimicrob Agents Chemother. 1982;22:71–77.
20. Gaudreau A, Hill E, Balfour HH, et al. Phenotypic and genotypic characterization of acyclovir-resistant herpes simplex viruses from immunocompromised patients. J Infect Dis. 1998;178:297–303.
21. Nugier F, Colin JN, Aymard M, et al. Occurrence and characterization of acyclovir-resistant herpes simplex virus isolates: Report on a two-year sensitivity screening survey. J Med Virol. 1992;36:1–12.
22. Hill EL, Hunter GA, Ellis MN. In vitro and in vivo characterization of herpes simplex virus clinical isolates recovered from patients infected with human immunodeficiency virus. Antimicrob Agents Chemother. 1991;35:2322–2328.
23. Christophers J, Clayton J, Craske J, et al. Survey of resistance of herpes simplex virus to acyclovir in northwest England. Antimicrob Agents Chemother. 1998;42:868–872.
24. Erlich KS, Mills J, Chatis P, et al. Acyclovir-resistant herpes simplex virus infections in patients with the acquired immunodeficiency syndrome. N Engl J Med. 1989;320:293–296.
25. Wade JC, McLaren C, Meyers JD. Frequency and significance of acyclovir-resistant herpes simplex virus isolated from marrow transplant patients receiving multiple courses of treatment with acyclovir. J Infect Dis. 1983;148:1077–1082.
26. Englund JA, Zimmerman ME, Swierkosz EM, et al. Herpes simplex virus resistant to acyclovir: A study in a tertiary care center. Ann Intern Med. 1990;112:416–422.
27. Straus SE, Takiff HE, Seidlin M, et al. Suppression of frequently recurring genital herpes: A placebo-controlled double-blind trial of oral acyclovir. N Engl J Med. 1984;310:1545–1550.
28. Lehrman SN, Douglas JM, Corey L, et al. Recurrent genital herpes and suppressive oral acyclovir therapy: Relation between clinical outcome and in-vitro drug sensitivity. Ann Intern Med. 1986;104:786–790.
29. Fife KH, Crumpacker CS, Mertz GJ, et al. Recurrence and resistance patterns of herpes simplex virus following cessation of ≥6 years of chronic suppression with acyclovir: Acyclovir Study Group. J Infect Dis. 1994;169:1338–1341.
30. Kost RG, Hill EL, Tigges M, et al. Brief report: Recurrent acyclovir-resistant genital herpes in an immunocompetent patient. N Engl J Med. 1993;329:1777–1782.
31. Safrin S, Crumpacker C, Chatis P, et al. A controlled trial comparing foscarnet with vidarabine for acyclovir-resistant mucocutaneous herpes simplex in the acquired immunodeficiency syndrome: The AIDS Clinical Trials Group. N Engl J Med. 1991;325:551–555.
32. Sonkin PL, Baratz KH, Frothingham R, et al. Acyclovir-resistant herpes simplex virus keratouveitis after penetrating keratoplasty. Ophthalmology. 1992;99:1805–1808.
33. Ljungman P, Ellis MN, Hackman RC, et al. Acyclovir-resistant herpes simplex virus causing pneumonia after marrow transplantation. J Infect Dis. 1990;162:244–248.
34. Engel JP, Englund JA, Fletcher CV, et al. Treatment of resistant herpes simplex virus with continuous-infusion acyclovir. JAMA. 1990;263:1662–1664.
35. Birch CJ, Tyssen DP, Tachedjian G, et al. Clinical effects and in vitro studies of trifluorothymidine combined with interferon-alpha for treatment of drug-resistant and -sensitive herpes simplex virus infections. J Infect Dis. 1992;166:108–112.
36. Winston DJ, Wirin D, Shaked A, et al. Randomised comparison of ganciclovir and high-dose acyclovir for long-term cytomegalovirus prophylaxis in liver-transplant recipients. Lancet. 1995;346:69–74.
37. Cole NL, Balfour HJ. Varicella-zoster virus does not become more resistant to acyclovir during therapy. J Infect Dis. 1986;153:605–608.
38. Jacobson MA, Berger TG, Fikrig S, et al. Acyclovir-resistant varicella-zoster virus infection after chronic oral acyclovir therapy in patients with the acquired immunodeficiency syndrome (AIDS). Ann Intern Med. 1990;112:187–191.

39. Snoeck R, Gerard M, Sadzot-Delvaux C, et al. Meningoradiculoneuritis due to acyclovir-resistant varicella-zoster virus in a patient with AIDS (Letter). J Infect Dis. 1993;168:1330–1331.
40. Safrin S, Berger TG, Gilson I, et al. Foscarnet therapy in five patients with AIDS and acyclovir-resistant varicella-zoster virus infection. Ann Intern Med. 1991;115:19–21.
41. Blum MR, Liao SH, de MP. Overview of acyclovir pharmacokinetic disposition in adults and children. Am J Med. 1982;73:186–192.
42. Laskin OL. Clinical pharmacokinetics of acyclovir. Clin Pharmacokinet. 1983;8:187–201.
43. Van DB, Connor JD, Wyborny C, et al. Pharmacokinetics of orally administered acyclovir in patients with herpes progenitalis. Am J Med. 1982;73:172–175.
44. McKendrick MW, McGill JI, White JE, et al. Oral acyclovir in acute herpes zoster. BMJ Clin Res Ed. 1986;293:1529–1532.
45. Wade JC, Newton B, Flournoy N, et al. Oral acyclovir for prevention of herpes simplex virus reactivation after marrow transplantation. Ann Intern Med. 1984;100:823–828.
46. Sullender WM, Arvin AM, Diaz PS, et al. Pharmacokinetics of acyclovir suspension in infants and children. Antimicrob Agents Chemother. 1987;31:1722–1726.
47. Wang LH, Schultz M, Weller S, et al. Pharmacokinetics and safety of multiple-dose valaciclovir in geriatric volunteers with and without concomitant diuretic therapy. Antimicrob Agents Chemother. 1996;40:80–85.
48. Weller S, Blum MR, Doucette M, et al. Pharmacokinetics of the acyclovir pro-drug valaciclovir after escalating single- and multiple-dose administration to normal volunteers. Clin Pharmacol Ther. 1993;54:595–605.
49. Soul-Lawton J, Seaber E, On N, et al. Absolute bioavailability and metabolic disposition of valaciclovir, the L-valyl ester of acyclovir, following oral administration to humans. Antimicrob Agents Chemother. 1995;39:2759–2764.
50. Beutner KR, Friedman DJ, Forszpaniak C, et al. Valacyclovir compared with acyclovir for improved therapy for herpes zoster in immunocompetent adults. Antimicrob Agents Chemother. 1995;39:1546–1553.
51. Hung SO, Patterson A, Rees PJ. Pharmacokinetics of oral acyclovir (Zovirax) in the eye. Br J Ophthalmol. 1984;68:192–195.
52. Meyer LJ, de MP, Sheth N, et al. Acyclovir in human breast milk. Am J Obstet Gynecol. 1988;158:586–588.
53. Frenkel LM, Brown ZA, Bryson YJ, et al. Pharmacokinetics of acyclovir in the term human pregnancy and neonate. Am J Obstet Gynecol. 1991;164:569–576.
54. Hintz M, Connor JD, Spector SA, et al. Neonatal acyclovir pharmacokinetics in patients with herpes virus infections. Am J Med. 1982;73:210–214.
55. de MP, Good SS, Krasny HC, et al. Metabolic fate of radioactive acyclovir in humans. Am J Med. 1982;73:215–220.
56. Laskin OL, Longstreth JA, Whelton A, et al. Effect of renal failure on the pharmacokinetics of acyclovir. Am J Med. 1982;73:197–201.
57. Krasny HC, Liao SH, de Miranda P, et al. Influence of hemodialysis on acyclovir pharmacokinetics in patients with chronic renal failure. Am J Med. 1982;73:202–204.
58. Davenport A, Goel S, Mackenzie JC. Neurotoxicity of acyclovir in patients with end-stage renal failure treated with continuous ambulatory peritoneal dialysis. Am J Kid Dis. 1992;20:647–649.
59. Burgess ED, Gill MJ. Intraperitoneal administration of acyclovir in patients receiving continuous ambulatory peritoneal dialysis. J Clin Pharmacol. 1990;30:997–1000.
60. Cooper DA, Pehrson PO, Pedersen C, et al. The efficacy and safety of zidovudine alone or as cotherapy with acyclovir for the treatment of patients with AIDS and AIDS-related complex: A double-blind randomized trial. European-Australian Collaborative Group. AIDS. 1993;7:197–207.
61. Keeney RE, Kirk LE, Bridgen D. Acyclovir tolerance in humans. Am J Med. 1982;73:176–181.
62. Sylvester RK, Ogden WB, Draxler CA, et al. Vesicular eruption: A local complication of concentrated acyclovir infusions. JAMA. 1986;255:385–386.
63. Wade JC, Meyers JD. Neurologic symptoms associated with parenteral acyclovir treatment after marrow transplantation. Ann Intern Med. 1983;98:921–925.
64. Bean B, Aeppli D. Adverse effects of high-dose intravenous acyclovir in ambulatory patients with acute herpes zoster. J Infect Dis. 1985;151:362–365.
65. Feldman S, Rodman J, Gregory B. Excessive serum concentrations of acyclovir and neurotoxicity. J Infect Dis. 1988;157:385–388.
66. Haefeli WE, Schoenenberger RA, Weiss P, et al. Acyclovir-induced neurotoxicity: Concentration-side effect relationship in acyclovir overdose (Review). Am J Med. 1993;94:212–215.
67. Rashed A, Azadeh B, Abu RH. Acyclovir-induced acute tubulo-interstitial nephritis. Nephron. 1990;56:436–438.
68. Sawyer MH, Webb DE, Balow JE, et al. Acyclovir-induced renal failure: Clinical course and histology. Am J Med. 1988;84:1067–1071.
69. Henry RE, Wegmann JA, Hartle JE, et al. Successful oral acyclovir desensitization. Ann Allergy. 1993;70:386–388.
70. Goldberg LH, Kaufman R, Kurtz TO, et al. Long-term suppression of recurrent genital herpes with acyclovir: A 5-year benchmark. Acyclovir Study Group. Arch Dermatol. 1993;129:582–587.
71. Clive D, Corey L, Reichman RC, et al. A double-blind, placebo-controlled cytogenetic study of oral acyclovir in patients with recurrent genital herpes. J Infect Dis. 1991;164:753–757.
72. Douglas JJ, Davis LG, Remington ML, et al. A double-blind, placebo-controlled trial of the effect of chronically administered oral acyclovir on sperm production in men with frequently recurrent genital herpes. J Infect Dis. 1988;157:588–593.
73. Kimberlin D, Powell D, Gruber W, et al. Administration of oral acyclovir suppressive therapy after neonatal herpes simplex virus disease limited to the skin, eyes and mouth: Results of a phase I/II trial. Pediatr Infect Dis J. 1996;15:247–254.
74. Anonymous. Pregnancy outcomes following systemic prenatal acyclovir exposure–June 1, 1984–June 30, 1993. MMWR Morb Mortal Wkly Rep. 1993;42:806–809.
75. Feinberg JE, Hurwitz S, Cooper D, et al. A randomized, double-blind trial of valaciclovir prophylaxis for cytomegalovirus disease in patients with advanced human immunodeficiency virus infection. AIDS Clinical Trials Group Protocol 204/Glaxo Wellcome 123-014 International CMV Prophylaxis Study Group. J Infect Dis. 1998;177:48–56.
75a. Lowance D, Neumayer H, Legendre CM, et al: Valacyclovir for the prevention of cytomegalovirus disease after renal transplantation. N Engl J Med. 1999;340:1462–1470.
76. Corey L, Fife KH, Benedetti JK, et al. Intravenous acyclovir for the treatment of primary genital herpes. Ann Intern Med. 1983;98:914–921.
77. Bryson YJ, Dillon M, Lovett M, et al. Treatment of first episodes of genital herpes simplex virus infection with oral acyclovir: A randomized double-blind controlled trial in normal subjects. N Engl J Med. 1983;308:916–921.
78. Nilsen AE, Aasen T, Halsos AM, et al. Efficacy of oral acyclovir in the treatment of initial and recurrent genital herpes. Lancet. 1982;2:571–573.
79. Wald A, Benedetti J, Davis G, et al. A randomized, double-blind, comparative trial comparing high- and standard-dose oral acyclovir for first-episode genital herpes infections. Antimicrob Agents Chemother. 1994;38:174–176.
80. Fife KH, Barbarash RA, Rudolph T, et al. Valaciclovir versus acyclovir in the treatment of first-episode genital herpes infections: Results of an international, multicenter, double-blind, randomized clinical trial. The Valaciclovir International Herpes Simplex Virus Study Group. Sex Transm Dis. 1997;24:481–486.
81. Lafferty WE, Brewer LA, Corey L. Alteration of lymphocyte transformation response to herpes simplex virus infection by acyclovir therapy. Antimicrob Agents Chemother. 1984;26:887–891.
82. Bernstein DI, Lovett MA, Bryson YJ. The effects of acyclovir on antibody response to herpes simplex virus in primary genital herpetic infections. J Infect Dis. 1984;150:7–13.
83. Rompalo AM, Mertz GJ, Davis LG, et al. Oral acyclovir for treatment of first-episode herpes simplex virus proctitis. JAMA. 1988;259:2879–2881.
84. Reichman RC, Badger GJ, Mertz GJ, et al. Treatment of recurrent genital herpes simplex infections with oral acyclovir: A controlled trial. JAMA. 1984;251:2103–2107.
85. Bodsworth NJ, Crooks RJ, Borelli S, et al. Valaciclovir versus aciclovir in patient initiated treatment of recurrent genital herpes: A randomised, double blind clinical trial. International Valaciclovir HSV Study Group. Genitourinary Medicine. 1997;73:110–116.
86. Spruance SL, Tyring SK, Degregorio B, et al. A large-scale, placebo-controlled, dose-ranging trial of peroral valaciclovir for episodic treatment of recurrent herpes genitalis. Valaciclovir HSV Study Group. Arch Intern Med. 1996;156:1729–1735.
87. Douglas JM, Critchlow C, Benedetti J, et al. A double-blind study of oral acyclovir for suppression of recurrences of genital herpes simplex virus infection. N Engl J Med. 1984;310:1551–1556.
88. Mindel A, Faherty A, Carney O, et al. Dosage and safety of long-term suppressive acyclovir therapy for recurrent genital herpes. Lancet. 1988;1:926–928.
89. Wald A, Corey L, Cone R, Hobson A, et al. Frequent genital herpes simplex virus 2 shedding in immunocompetent women: Effect of acyclovir treatment. J Clin Invest. 1997;99:1092–1097.
90. Reitano M, Tyring S, Lang W, et al. Valacyclovir for the suppression of recurrent genital herpes simplex virus infection: A large-scale dose range—finding study. J Infect Dis. 1998;178:603–610.
91. Rooney JF, Felser JM, Ostrove JM, et al. Acquisition of genital herpes from an asymptomatic sexual partner. N Engl J Med. 1986;314:1561–1564.
92. Scott LL, Sanchez PJ, Jackson GL, et al. Acyclovir suppression to prevent cesarean delivery after first-episode genital herpes. Obstet Gynecol. 1996;87:69–73.
93. Brocklehurst P, Kinghorn G, Carney O, et al. A randomized placebo controlled trial of suppressive acyclovir in late pregnancy in women with recurrent genital herpes infection. Br J Obstet Gynaecol. 1998;105:275–280.
94. Rooney JF, Straus SE, Mannix ML, et al. Oral acyclovir to suppress frequently recurrent herpes labialis: A double-blind, placebo-controlled trial. Ann Intern Med. 1993;118:268–272.
95. The Herpetic Eye Disease Study Group. Acyclovir for the prevention of recurrent herpes simplex virus eye disease. N Engl J Med 1998;339:300–306.
96. Spruance SL, Hamill ML, Hoge WS, et al. Acyclovir prevents reactivation of herpes simplex labialis in skiers. JAMA. 1988;260:1597–1599.
97. Raborn GW, Martel AY, Grace MG, et al. Oral acyclovir in prevention of herpes labialis: A randomized, double-blind, multi-centered clinical trial. Oral Surg Oral Med Oral Pathol Oral Radiol Endod. 1998;85:55–59.
98. Kuzushima K, Kudo T, Kimura H, et al. Prophylactic oral acyclovir in outbreaks of primary herpes simplex virus type 1 infection in a closed community. Pediatrics. 1992;89:379–383.
99. Gill MJ, Bryant HE. Oral acyclovir therapy of recurrent herpes simplex virus type 2 infection of the hand. Antimicrob Agents Chemother. 1991;35:382–383.
100. Spruance SL, Stewart JC, Rowe NH, et al. Treatment of recurrent herpes simplex labialis with oral acyclovir. J Infect Dis. 1990;161:185–190.
101. Amir J, Harel L, Smetana Z, et al. Treatment of herpes simplex gingivostomatitis with aciclovir in children: A randomised double blind placebo controlled study. BMJ. 1997;314:1800–1803.
102. Adour KK, Ruboyianes JM, Von DG, et al. Bell's palsy treatment with acyclovir and prednisone compared with prednisone alone: A double-blind, randomized, controlled trial. Ann Otol Rhinol Laryngol. 1996;105:371–378.
103. Saral R, Burns WH, Laskin OL, et al. Acyclovir prophylaxis of herpes-simplex-virus infections. N Engl J Med. 1981;305:63–67.
104. Lundgren G, Wilczek H, Lonnqvist B, et al. Acyclovir prophylaxis in bone marrow transplant recipients. Scand J Infect Dis Suppl. 1985;47:137–144.

105. Gluckman E, Lotsberg J, Devergie A, et al. Prophylaxis of herpes infections after bone-marrow transplantation by oral acyclovir. Lancet. 1983;2:706–708.
106. Seale L, Jones CJ, Kathpalia S, et al. Prevention of herpesvirus infections in renal allograft recipients by low-dose oral acyclovir. JAMA. 1985;254:3435–3438.
107. Holmes GP, Chapman LE, Stewart JA, et al. Guidelines for the prevention and treatment of B-virus infections in exposed persons: The B Virus Working Group. Clin Infect Dis. 1995;20:421–439.
108. Wade JC, Newton B, McLaren C, et al. Intravenous acyclovir to treat mucocutaneous herpes simplex virus infection after marrow transplantation: A double-blind trial. Ann Intern Med. 1982;96:265–269.
109. Shepp DH, Newton BA, Dandliker PS, et al. Oral acyclovir therapy for mucocutaneous herpes simplex virus infections in immunocompromised marrow transplant recipients. Ann Intern Med. 1985;102:783–785.
110. Klein NA, Mabie WC, Shaver DC, et al. Herpes simplex virus hepatitis in pregnancy: Two patients successfully treated with acyclovir (Review). Gastroenterology. 1991;100:239–244.
111. Kusne S, Schwartz M, Breinig MK, et al. Herpes simplex virus hepatitis after solid organ transplantation in adults. J Infect Dis. 1991;163:1001–1007.
112. Kimura H, Aso K, Kuzushima K, et al. Relapse of herpes simplex encephalitis in children. Pediatrics. 1992;89:891–894.
113. Palay DA, Sternberg PJ, Davis J, et al. Decrease in the risk of bilateral acute retinal necrosis by acyclovir therapy. Am J Ophthalmol. 1991;112:250–255.
114. Haake DA, Zakowski PC, Haake DL, et al. Early treatment with acyclovir for varicella pneumonia in otherwise healthy adults: Retrospective controlled study and review. Rev Infect Dis. 1990;12:788–798.
115. Balfour HJ, Bean B, Laskin OL, et al. Acyclovir halts progression of herpes zoster in immunocompromised patients. N Engl J Med. 1983;308:1448–1453.
116. Prober CG, Kirk LE, Keeney RE. Acyclovir therapy of chickenpox in immunosuppressed children: A collaborative study. J Pediatr. 1982;101:622–625.
117. Nyerges G, Meszner Z, Gyarmati E, et al. Acyclovir prevents dissemination of varicella in immunocompromised children. J Infect Dis. 1988;157:309–313.
118. Meszner Z, Nyerges G, Bell AR. Oral acyclovir to prevent dissemination of varicella in immunocompromised children. J Infect. 1993;26:9–15.
119. Dunkle LM, Arvin AM, Whitley RJ, et al. A controlled trial of acyclovir for chickenpox in normal children [see comments]. N Engl J Med. 1991;325:1539–1544.
120. Balfour HJ, Rotbart HA, Feldman S, et al. Acyclovir treatment of varicella in otherwise healthy adolescents: The Collaborative Acyclovir Varicella Study Group [see comments]. J Pediatr. 1992;120:627–633.
121. Wallace MR, Bowler WA, Murray NB, et al. Treatment of adult varicella with oral acyclovir: A randomized, placebo-controlled trial [see comments]. Ann Intern Med. 1992;117:358–363.
122. Anonymous. American Academy of Pediatrics Committee on Infectious Diseases: The use of oral acyclovir in otherwise healthy children with varicella [published erratum appears in Pediatrics 1993;91:858]. Pediatrics. 1993;91:674–676.
123. Lin TY, Huang YC, Ning HC, et al. Oral acyclovir prophylaxis of varicella after intimate contact. Pediatr Infect Dis J. 1997;16:1162–1165.
124. Bean B, Braun C, Balfour HJ. Acyclovir therapy for acute herpes zoster. Lancet. 1982;2:118–121.
125. Cobo LM, Foulks GN, Liesegang T, et al. Oral acyclovir in the treatment of acute herpes zoster ophthalmicus. Ophthalmology. 1986;93:763–770.
126. McKendrick MW, McGill JI, et al. Lack of effect of acyclovir on postherpetic neuralgia. BMJ. 1989;298:431.
127. Beutner KR, Friedman DJ, Forszpaniak C, et al. Valaciclovir compared with acyclovir for improved therapy for herpes zoster in immunocompetent adults. Antimicrob Agents Chemother 1995;39:1546–1553.
128. Meyers JD, Reed EC, Shepp DH, et al. Acyclovir for prevention of cytomegalovirus infection and disease after allogeneic marrow transplantation. N Engl J Med. 1988;318:70–75.
129. Boeckh M, Gooley TA, Reusser P, et al. Failure of high-dose acyclovir to prevent cytomegalovirus disease after autologous marrow transplantation. J Infect Dis. 1995;172:939–943.
130. Vasquez EM, Sanchez J, Pollak R, et al. High-dose oral acyclovir prophylaxis for primary cytomegalovirus infection in seronegative renal allograft recipients. Transplantation. 1993;55:448–450.
131. Bailey TC, Ettinger NA, Storch GA, et al. Failure of high-dose oral acyclovir with or without immune globulin to prevent primary cytomegalovirus disease in recipients of solid organ transplants. Am J Med. 1993;95:273–278.
132. Badley AD, Seaberg EC, Porayko MK, et al. Prophylaxis of cytomegalovirus infection in liver transplantation: A randomized trial comparing a combination of ganciclovir and acyclovir to acyclovir. NIDDK Liver Transplantation Database. Transplantation. 1997;64:66–73.
133. Ioannidis JP, Collier AC, Cooper D, et al. Clinical efficacy of high-dose acyclovir in patients with human immunodeficiency virus infection: A meta-analysis of randomized individual patient data. J Infect Dis. 1998;178:349–359.
134. Tynell E, Aurelius E, Brandell A, et al. Acyclovir and prednisolone treatment of acute infectious mononucleosis: A multicenter, double-blind, placebo-controlled study. J Infect Dis. 1996;174:324–331.
135. Straus SE, Dale JK, Tobi M, et al. Acyclovir treatment of the chronic fatigue syndrome: Lack of efficacy in a placebo-controlled trial. N Engl J Med. 1988;319:1692–1698.
136. Schooley RT, Carey RW, Miller G, et al. Chronic Epstein-Barr virus infection associated with fever and interstitial pneumonitis: Clinical and serologic features and response to antiviral chemotherapy. Ann Intern Med. 1986;104:636–643.
137. Sullivan JL, Byron KS, Brewster FE, et al. Treatment of life-threatening Epstein-Barr virus infection with acyclovir. Am J Med. 1982;73:262–266.
138. Resnick L, Herbst JS, Ablashi DV, et al. Regression of oral hairy leukoplakia after orally administered acyclovir therapy. JAMA. 1988;259:384–388.
139. Berk L, Schalm SW, de MA, et al. Failure of acyclovir to enhance the antiviral effect of alpha lymphoblastoid interferon on HBe-seroconversion in chronic hepatitis B: A multi-centre randomized controlled trial. J Hepatol. 1992;14:305–309.
140. Lycke J, Svennerholm B, Hjelmquist E, et al. Acyclovir treatment of relapsing-remitting multiple sclerosis: A randomized, placebo-controlled, double-blind study. J Neurol. 1996;243:214–224.
141. Hayden FG, Cote KM, Douglas RGJ. Plaque inhibition assay for drug susceptibility testing of influenza viruses. Antimicrob Agents Chemother. 1980;17:865–870.
142. Browne MJ, Moss MY, Boyd MR. Comparative activity of amantadine and ribavirin against influenza virus in vitro: Possible clinical relevance. Antimicrob Agents Chemother. 1983;23:503–505.
143. Smith JP. Treatment of chronic hepatitis C with amantadine. Dig Dis Sci. 1997;42:1681–1687.
144. Hayden FG. Animal models of influenza virus infection for evaluation of antiviral agents. In: Zak O, Sande MA, eds. Experimental Models in Antimicrobial Chemotherapy. London: Academic Press; 1986:353–371.
145. Hayden FG. Combinations of antiviral agents for treatment of influenza virus infections. J Antimicrob Chemother 1986;18(Suppl B):177–183.
146. Zhirnov OP. High protection of animals lethally infected with influenza virus by aprotinin-rimantadine combination. J Med Virol. 1987;21:161–167.
147. Madren LK, Shipman C Jr, Hayden FG. In vitro inhibitory effects of combinations of anti-influenza agents. Antiviral Chemistry and Chemotherapy. 1995;6:109–113.
148. Hay AJ. Amantadine and rimantadine: Mechanisms. In: Richman DD, ed. Antiviral Drug Resistance. New York: John Wiley & Sons; 1996:43.
149. Pinto LH, Holsinger LJ, Lamb RA. Influenza virus M2 protein has ion channel activity. Cell. 1992;69:517–528.
150. Richman DD, Hostetler KY, Yazaki PJ, et al. Fate of influenza A virion proteins after entry into subcellular fractions of LLC cells and the effect of amantadine. Virology. 1986;151:200–210.
151. Belshe RB, Burk B, Newman F, et al. Resistance of influenza A virus to amantadine and rimantadine: Results of one decade of surveillance. J Infect Dis. 1989;159: 430–435.
152. Oxford JS, Galbraith A. Antiviral activity of amantadine: A review of laboratory and clinical data (Review) Pharmacol Ther. 1980;11:181–262.
153. Bean WJ, Threlkeld SC, Webster RG. Biologic potential of amantadine-resistant influenza A virus in an avian model. J Infect Dis. 1989;159:1050–1056.
154. Webster RG, Kawaoka Y, Bean WJ, et al. Chemotherapy and vaccination: A possible strategy for the control of highly virulent influenza virus. J Virol. 1985;55:173–176.
155. Hayden FG. Amantadine and rimantadine—clinical aspects. In: Richman DD, ed. Antiviral Drug Resistance. Chichester: John Wiley & Sons Ltd; 1996:59–77.
156. Hayden FG, Sperber SJ, Belshe RB, et al. Recovery of drug-resistant influenza A virus during therapeutic use of rimantadine. Antimicrob Agents Chemother. 1991;35:1741–1747.
157. Englund JA, Champlin RE, Wyde PR, et al. Common emergence of amantadine and rimantadine resistant influenza A viruses in symptomatic immunocompromised adults. Clin Infect Dis. 1998;26:1418–1424.
158. Hayden FG, Belshe RB, Clover RD, et al. Emergence and apparent transmission of rimantadine-resistant influenza A virus in families. N Engl J Med. 1989;321:1696–1702.
159. Mast EE, Harmon MW, Gravenstein S, et al. Emergence and possible transmission of amantadine-resistant viruses during nursing home outbreaks of influenza A (H3N2). Am J Epidemiol. 1991;134:988–997.
160. Hayden FG, Minocha A, Spyker DA, et al. Comparative single-dose pharmacokinetics of amantadine hydrochloride and rimantadine hydrochloride in young and elderly adults [published erratum appears in Antimicrob Agents Chemother 1986;30:579]. Antimicrob Agents Chemother. 1985;28:216–221.
161. Aoki FY, Sitar DS. Amantadine kinetics in healthy elderly men: Implications for influenza prevention. Clin Pharmacol Ther. 1985;37:137–144.
162. Aoki FY, Sitar DS. Clinical pharmacokinetics of amantadine hydrochloride (Review). Clin Pharmacokinet. 1988;14:35–51.
163. Horadam VW, Sharp JG, Smilack JD, et al. Pharmacokinetics of amantadine hydrochloride in subjects with normal and impaired renal function. Ann Intern Med. 1981;94:454–458.
164. Soung LS, Ing TS, Daugirdas JT, et al. Amantadine hydrochloride pharmacokinetics in hemodialysis patients. Ann Intern Med. 1980;93:46–49.
165. Wills RJ, Choma N, Buonpane G, et al. Relative bioavailability of rimantadine HCl tablet and syrup formulations in healthy subjects. J Pharm Sci. 1987;76:886–888.
166. Wills RJ, Rodriguez LC, Choma N, et al. Influence of a meal on the bioavailability of rimantadine HCl. J Clin Pharmacol. 1987;27:821–823.
167. Wills RJ, Farolino DA, Choma N, et al. Rimantadine pharmacokinetics after single and multiple doses. Antimicrob Agents Chemother. 1987;31:826–828.
168. Nahata MC, Brady MT. Serum concentrations and safety of rimantadine in paediatric patients. Eur J Clin Pharmacol. 1986;30:719–722.
169. Anderson EL, Van VLP, Bartram J, et al. Pharmacokinetics of a single dose of rimantadine in young adults and children. Antimicrob Agents Chemother. 1987;31:1140–1142.
170. Tominack RL, Wills RJ, Gustavson LE, et al. Multiple-dose pharmacokinetics of rimantadine in elderly adults. Antimicrob Agents Chemother. 1988;32:1813–1819.
171. Patriarca PA, Kater NA, Kendal AP, et al. Safety of prolonged administration of rimantadine hydrochloride in the prophylaxis of influenza A virus infections in nursing homes. Antimicrob Agents Chemother. 1984;26:101–103.
172. Capparelli EV, Stevens RC, Chow MS, et al. Rimantadine pharmacokinetics in healthy subjects and patients with end-stage renal failure. Clin Pharmacol Ther. 1988;43:536–541.

173. Wills RJ. Update on rimantadine's clinical pharmacokinetics. J Respir Dis. 1989;10(Suppl):S20–S25.
174. Wills RJ, Belshe R, Tomlinsin D, et al. Pharmacokinetics of rimantadine hydrochloride in patients with chronic liver disease. Clin Pharmacol Ther. 1987;42:449–454.
175. Speeg KV, Leighton JA, Maldonado AL. Toxic delirium in a patient taking amantadine and trimethoprim-sulfamethoxazole. Am J Med Sci. 1989;298: 410–412.
176. Soo W. Adverse effects of rimantadine: Summary from clinical trials. J Respir Dis. 1989;10(Suppl):S26–S31.
177. Sartori M, Pratt CM, Young JB. Torsade de Pointe: Malignant cardiac arrhythmia induced by amantadine poisoning. Am J Med. 1984;77:388–391.
178. Pimentel L, Hughes B. Amantadine toxicity presenting with complex ventricular ectopy and hallucinations. Pediatr Emerg Care. 1991;7:89–92.
179. Atkinson WL, Arden NH, Patriarca PA, et al. Amantadine prophylaxis during an institutional outbreak of type A (H1N1) influenza. Arch Intern Med. 1986;146:1751–1756.
180. Nestelbaum Z, Siris SG, Rifkin A, et al. Exacerbation of schizophrenia associated with amantadine. Am J Psychiatry. 1986;143:1170–1171.
181. Douglas RGJ. Prophylaxis and treatment of influenza. N Engl J Med. 1990;322:443–450.
182. Reuman PD, Bernstein DI, Keefer MC, et al. Efficacy and safety of low dosage amantadine hydrochloride as prophylaxis for influenza A. Antiviral Res. 1989;11:27–40.
183. Degelau J, Somani SK, Cooper SL, et al. Occurrence of adverse effects and high amantadine concentrations with influenza prophylaxis in the nursing home. J Am Geriatr Soc. 1990;38:428.
184. Stange KC, Little DW, Blatnik B. Adverse reactions to amantadine prophylaxis of influenza in a retirement home. J Am Geriatr Soc. 1991;39:700–705.
185. Hayden FG, Hoffman HE, Spyker DA. Differences in side effects of amantadine hydrochloride and rimantadine hydrochloride relate to differences in pharmacokinetics. Antimicrob Agents Chemother. 1983;23:458–464.
186. Arden NH, Patriarca PA, Fasano MB, et al. The roles of vaccination and amantadine prophylaxis in controlling an outbreak of influenza A (H3N2) in a nursing home. Arch Intern Med. 1988;148:865–868.
187. Dolin R, Reichman RC, Madore HP, et al. A controlled trial of amantadine and rimantadine in the prophylaxis of influenza A infection. N Engl J Med. 1982;307:580–584.
188. Pettersson RF, Hellstrom PE, Penttinen K, et al. Evaluation of amantadine in the prophylaxis of influenza A (H1N1) virus infection: A controlled field trial among young adults and high-risk patients. J Infect Dis. 1980; 142:377–383.
189. Van Voris LP, Betts RF, Hayden FG, et al. Successful treatment of naturally occurring influenza A/USSR/77 H1N1. JAMA. 1981;245:1128–1131.
190. Levin M. Experience with amantadine and rimantadine in children. J Respir Dis. 1998;8:S60–S66.
191. Pandit PB, Chitayat D, Jefferies AL, et al. Tibial hemimelia and tetralogy of Fallot associated with first trimester exposure to amantadine. Reprod Toxicol. 1994;8:89–92.
192. Wintermeyer SM, Nahata MC. Rimantadine: A clinical perspective. Ann Pharmacother. 1995;29:299–310.
193. Hayden FG. Antivirals for pandemic influenza. J Infect Dis. 1997;176(Suppl 1):S56–S61.
194. Libow LS, Neufeld RR, Olson E, et al. Sequential outbreak of influenza A and B in a nursing home: efficacy of vaccine and amantadine. J Am Ger Soc. 1996;44:1153–1157.
195. Crawford SA, Clover RD, Abell TD, et al. Rimantadine prophylaxis in children: A follow-up study. Pediatr Infect Dis J. 1988;7:379–383.
196. Brady MT, Sears SD, Pacini DL, et al. Safety and prophylactic efficacy of low-dose rimantadine in adults during an influenza A epidemic. Antimicrob Agents Chemother. 1990;34:1633–1636.
197. Younkin SW, Betts RF, Roth FK, et al. Reduction in fever and symptoms in young adults with influenza A/Brazil/78 H1N1 infection after treatment with aspirin or amantadine. Antimicrob Agents Chemother. 1983;23:577–582.
198. Betts RF, Treanor JJ, Graman PS, et al. Antiviral agents to prevent or treat influenza in the elderly. J Respir Dis. 1987;8(Suppl):S56–S59.
199. Hall CB, Dolin R, Gala CL, et al. Children with influenza A infection: Treatment with rimantadine. Pediatrics. 1987;80:275–282.
200. Clover RD, Waner JL, Becker L, et al. Effect of rimantadine on the immune response to influenza A infections. J Med Virol. 1991;34:68–73.
201. Hayden FG, Zlydnikov DM, Iljenko VI, et al. Comparative therapeutic effect of aerosolized and oral rimantadine HCl in experimental human influenza A virus infection. Antiviral Res. 1982;2:147–153.
202. Hitchcock MJ, Jaffe HS, Martin JC, et al. Cidofovir, a new agent with potent anti-herpesvirus activity. Antiviral Chemistry and Chemotherapy. 1996;7:115–127.
203. Safrin S, Cherrington JM, Jaffe HS. Clinical uses of cidofovir. Rev Med Virol. 1997;7:145–156.
204. Andrei G, Snoeck R, Vandeputte M, de CE: Activities of various compounds against murine and primate polyomaviruses. Antimicrob Agents Chemother. 1997;41:587–593.
205. Cherrington JM, Miner R, Hitchcock MJ, et al. Susceptibility of human cytomegalovirus to cidofovir is unchanged after limited in vivo exposure to various regimens of drug. J Infect Dis. 1996;173:987–992.
206. Lalezari J, Schacker T, Feinberg J, et al. A randomized, double-blind, placebo-controlled trial of cidofovir gel for the treatment of acyclovir-unresponsive mucocutaneous herpes simplex virus infection in patients with AIDS. J Infect Dis. 1997;176:892–898.
207. Gordon YJ, Romanowski E, Araullo-Cruz T, et al. Inhibitory effect of (S)-HPMPC, (S)-HPMPA, and 2′-nor-cyclic GMP on clinical ocular adenoviral isolates is serotype-dependent in vitro. Antiviral Res. 1991;16:11–16.
208. Mendel DB, Barkhimer DB, Chen MS. Biochemical basis for increased susceptibility to cidofovir of herpes simplex viruses with altered or deficient thymidine kinase activity. Antimicrob Agents Chemother. 1995;39:2120–2122.
209. Safrin S, Cherrington JM, Jaffe HS. Clinical uses of cidofovir. Rev Med Virol. 1997;7:145–156.
210. Soike KF, Huang JL, Zhang JY, et al. Evaluation of infrequent dosing regimens with (S)-1-[3-hydroxy-2-(phosphonylmethoxy)propyl]-cytosine (S-HPMPC) on simian varicella infection in monkeys. Antiviral Res. 1991;16:17–28.
211. Yang H, Datema R. Prolonged and potent therapeutic and prophylactic effects of (S)-1-[(3-hydroxy-2-phosphonylmethoxy)propyl]cytosine against herpes simplex virus type 2 infections in mice. Antimicrob Agents Chemother. 1991;35:1596–1600.
212. Huggins JW, Smee DF, Martinez MJ, et al. Cifofovir (HPMPC) treatment of monkeypox (Abstract 118). Antiviral Res. 1998;37:A73.
213. de OB, Stevenson D, LaBree L, et al. Evaluation of cidofovir (HPMPC, GS-504) against adenovirus type 5 infection in vitro and in a New Zealand rabbit ocular model. Antiviral Res. 1996;31:165–172.
214. Ho HT, Woods KL, Bronson JJ, et al. Intracellular metabolism of the antiherpes agent (S)-1-[3-hydroxy-2-(phosphonylmethoxy)propyl]cytosine. Mol Pharmacol. 1992;41:197–202.
215. Hitchcock MJ, Jaffe HS, Martin JC, et al. Cidofovir, a new agent with potent anti-herpesvirus activity. Antiviral Chemistry and Chemotherapy. 1996;7:115–127.
216. Tatarowicz WA, Lurain NS, Thompson KD. A ganciclovir-resistant clinical isolate of human cytomegalovirus exhibiting cross-resistance to other DNA polymerase inhibitors. J Infect Dis. 1992;166:904–907.
217. Cherrington JM, Fuller MD, Larry PD, et al. In vitro antiviral susceptibilities of isolates from CMV retinitis patients receiving first or second line cidofovir therapy: Relationship to clinical outcome. J Infect Dis. 1998;178:1821–1825.
218. Cundy KC, Petty BG, Flaherty J, et al. Clinical pharmacokinetics of cidofovir in human immunodeficiency virus-infected patients. Antimicrob Agents Chemother. 1995;39:1247–1252.
218a. Neau D, Renaud-Rougier MB, Viallard JF, et al. Intravenous cidofovir-induced iritis. Clin Infect Dis. 1999;28:157–158.
219. Kirsch LS, Arevalo JF, Chavez DE, et al. Intravitreal cidofovir (HPMPC) treatment of cytomegalovirus retinitis in patients with acquired immune deficiency syndrome [published erratum appears in Ophthalmology 1995;102:702]. Ophthalmology. 1995;102:533–542.
220. Lalezari JP, Stagg RJ, Kuppermann BD, et al. Intravenous cidofovir for peripheral cytomegalovirus retinitis in patients with AIDS: A randomized, controlled trial. Ann Intern Med. 1997;126:257–263.
221. Lalezari J, Holland GN, Kramer F, et al. Randomized, controlled study of the safety and efficacy of intravenous cidofovir for the treatment of relapsing cytomegalovirus retinitis in patients with AIDS. J Acquir Immune Def Syndr Hum Retrovirol. 1998;17:339–344.
222. Anonymous. Parenteral cidofovir for cytomegalovirus retinitis in patients with AIDS: The HPMPC peripheral cytomegalovirus retinitis trial. A randomized, controlled trial. Studies of Ocular Complications of AIDS Research Group in Collaboration with the AIDS Clinical Trials Group. Ann Intern Med. 1997;126:264–274.
223. Polis MA, Spooner KM, Baird BF, et al. Anticytomegaloviral activity and safety of cidofovir in patients with human immunodeficiency virus infection and cytomegalovirus viruria. Antimicrob Agents Chemother. 1995;39:882–886.
224. Lalezari JP, Drew WL, Glutzer E, et al. Treatment with intravenous (S)-1-[3-hydroxy-2-(phosphonylmethoxy)propyl]-cytosine of acyclovir-resistant mucocutaneous infection with herpes simplex virus in a patient with AIDS. J Infect Dis. 1994;170:570–572.
225. Vere Hodge RA. Review: Antiviral portraits series, number 3. Famciclovir and penciclovir: The mode of action of famciclovir including its conversion to penciclovir. Antiviral Chemistry and Chemotherapy. 1993;4:67–84.
226. Weinberg A, Bate BJ, Masters HB, et al. In vitro activities of penciclovir and acyclovir against herpes simplex virus types 1 and 2. Antimicrob Agents Chemother. 1992;36:2037–2038.
227. Talarico CL, Phelps WC, Biron KK. Analysis of the thymidine kinase genes from acyclovir-resistant mutants of varicella-zoster virus isolated from patients with AIDS. J Virol. 1993;67:1024–1033.
228. Boyd MR, Kern ER, Safrin S. Penciclovir: A review of its spectrum of activity, selectivity and cross-resistance pattern. Antiviral Chemistry and Chemotherapy 1993;4:3–11.
229. Colledge D, Locarnini S, Shaw T. Synergistic inhibition of hepadnaviral replication by lamivudine in combination with penciclovir in vitro [see comments]. Hepatology. 1997;26:216–225.
230. Korba BE, Boyd MR. Penciclovir is a selective inhibitor of hepatitis B virus replication in cultured human hepatoblastoma cells. Antimicrob Agents Chemother. 1996;40:1282–1284.
231. Thackray AM, Field HJ. Famciclovir and valaciclovir differ in the prevention of herpes simplex virus type 1 latency in mice: A quantitative study. Antimicrob Agents Chemother 1998;42:1555–1562.
232. Earnshaw DL, Bacon TH, Darlison SJ, et al. Mode of antiviral action of penciclovir in MRC-5 cells infected with herpes simplex virus type 1 (HSV-1), HSV-2, and varicella-zoster virus. Antimicrob Agents Chemother. 1992;36:2747–2757.
233. Goldthorpe SE, Boyd MR, Field HJ. Effects of penciclovir and famciclovir in a murine model of encephalitis induced by intranasal inoculation of herpes simplex virus type 1. Antiviral Chemistry and Chemotherapy. 1992;3:37–47.
234. Shaw T, Mok SS, Locarnini SA. Inhibition of hepatitis B virus DNA polymerase by enantiomers of penciclovir triphosphate and metabolic basis for selective inhibition of HBV replication by penciclovir. Hepatology. 1996;24:996–1002.

235. Pelosi E, Mulamba GB, Coen DM. Penciclovir and pathogenesis phenotypes of drug-resistant herpes simplex virus mutants. Antiviral Res. 1998;37:17–28.
236. Chiou HC, Kumura K, Hu A, et al. Penciclovir-resistance mutations in the herpes simplex virus DNA polymerase gene. Antiviral Chemistry and Chemotherapy. 1995;6:281–288.
237. Mertz GJ, Loveless MO, Levin MJ, et al. Oral famciclovir for suppression of recurrent genital herpes simplex virus infection in women: A multicenter, double-blind, placebo-controlled trial. Collaborative Famciclovir Genital Herpes Research Group. Arch Intern Med. 1997;157:343–349.
238. Schacker T, Hui-lin H, Koelle DM, et al. Famciclovir for the suppression of symptomatic and asymptomatic herpes simplex virus reactivation in HIV-infected persons. Ann Intern Med. 1998;128:21–28.
239. Aye TT, Bartholomeusz A, Shaw T, et al. Hepatitis B virus polymerase mutations during antiviral therapy in a patient following liver transplantation. J Hepatol. 1997;26:1148–1153.
240. Perry CM, Wagstaff AJ. Famciclovir: A review of its pharmacological properties and therapeutic efficacy in herpesvirus infections (Review) Drugs. 1995;50:396–415.
241. Fowles SE, Pierce DM, Prince WT, et al. The tolerance to and pharmacokinetics of penciclovir (BRL 39,123A), a novel antiherpes agent, administered by intravenous infusion to healthy subjects. Eur J Clin Pharmacol. 1992;43:513–516.
242. Boike SC, Pue M, Audet PR, et al. Pharmacokinetics of famciclovir in subjects with chronic hepatic disease. J Clin Pharmacol. 1994;34:1199–1207.
243. Daniels S, Schentag JJ. Drug interaction studies and safety of famciclovir in healthy volunteers: A review. Antiviral Chemistry and Chemotherapy 1993;4:57–64.
244. Siederer S, Scott S, Fowles S, et al. Lack of interaction between steady-state digoxin and famciclovir (Abstract A33). Abstracts of the 36th Interscience Conference on Antimicrobial Agents and Chemotherapy. New Orleans, 1996.
245. Saltzman R, Jurewicz R, Boon R. Safety of famciclovir in patients with herpes zoster and genital herpes. Antimicrob Agents Chemother. 1994;38:2454–2457.
246. Sacks SL, Sasadeusz JJ, Shafran SD. Effect of long-term famciclovir treatment on sperm parameters in patients with recurrent genital herpes (Abstract 22.022). Eighth International Congress on Infectious Diseases, Boston, Mass. 1998.
247. Spruance SL, Rea TL, Thoming C, et al. Penciclovir cream for the treatment of herpes simplex labialis: A randomized, multicenter, double-blind, placebo-controlled trial. Topical Penciclovir Collaborative Study Group. JAMA. 1997;277:1374–1379.
248. Loveless M, Sacks SL, Harris RJ. Famciclovir in the management of first-episode genital herpes. Infect Dis Clin Pract. 1997;6:512–516.
249. Sacks SL, Aoki FY, Diaz-Mitoma F, et al. Patient-initiated, twice-daily oral famciclovir for early recurrent genital herpes: A randomized, double-blind multicenter trial. Canadian Famciclovir Study Group [see comments]. JAMA. 1996;276:44–49.
250. Diaz-Mitoma F, Sibbald RG, Shafran SD. Oral famciclovir for the suppression of recurrent genital herpes: A randomized controlled trial. JAMA. 1998;280:887–892.
251. Frechette G, Romanowski B. Efficacy and safety of famciclovir for the treatment of HSV infections in HIV+ patients (Abstract F083). Canadian Conference on HIV/AIDS Research, May 22, 1997.
252. Lazarus HM, Belanger R, Candoni A, et al. Efficacy and safety of penciclovir (PCV) for the treatment of HSV infections in immunocompromised (IC) patients (Abstract H72). Abstracts of the 37th Interscience Conference on Antimicrobial Agents and Chemotherap 1997.
253. Tyring S, Barbarash RA, Nahlik JE, et al. Famciclovir for the treatment of acute herpes zoster: Effects on acute disease and postherpetic neuralgia. A randomized, double-blind, placebo-controlled trial. Collaborative Famciclovir Herpes Zoster Study Group [see comments]. Ann Intern Med. 1995;123:89–96.
254. Degreef H, Famciclovir Herpes Zoster Clinical Study Group. Famciclovir, a new oral antiherpes drug: Results of the first controlled clinical study demonstrating its efficacy and safety in the treatment of uncomplicated herpes zoster in immunocompetent patients. Int J Antimicrob Agents 1994;4:241–246.
254a. Tyring S, Engst R, Lassonde MTS, et al. Famciclovir for the treatment of ophthalmic herpes zoster (HZO). Abstracts of the 38th Interscience Conference on Antimicrobial Agents and Chemotherapy. San Diego, 1998;21 (Abstract LB-3).
255. Tyring S, Belanger R, Bezwoda W, et al. The efficacy and safety of famciclovir (FCV) for the treatment of herpes zoster (HZ) in immunocompromised (IC) patients (Abstract). Abstracts of the 20th International Congress of Chemotherapy, June 29–July 3, 1997.
256. Marques AR, Lau DT, McKenzie R, et al. Combination therapy with famciclovir and interferon-alpha for the treatment of chronic hepatitis B. J Infect Dis. 1998;178:1483–1487.
257. Singh N, Gayowski T, Wannstedt CF, et al. Pretransplant famciclovir as prophylaxis for hepatitis B virus recurrence after liver transplantation. Transplantation. 1997;63:1415–1419.
258. Haller GW, Bechstein WO, Neuhaus R, et al. Famciclovir therapy for recurrent hepatitis B virus infection after liver transplantation. Transpl Int. 1996;9(Suppl 1):S210–S212.
259. Cirelli R, Herne K, McCrary M, et al. Famciclovir: Review of clinical efficacy and safety. Antiviral Res. 1996;29:141–151.
259a. Anderson KP, Fox MC, Brown-Driver V, et al. Inhibition of human cytomegalovirus immediate-early gene expression by an antisense oligonucleotide complementary to immediate-early RNA. Antimicrob Agents Chemother. 1996;40:2004–2011.
259b. Mulamba GB, Hu A, Azad RF, et al. Human cytomegalovirus mutant with sequence-dependent resistance to the phosphorothioate oligonucleotide fomivirsen (ISIS 2922). Antimicrob Agents Chemother. 1998;42:971–973.
259c. Muccioli C, Goldstein D, Johnson DW. Fomivirsen safety and efficacy in the treatment of CMV retinitis: A phase 3, controlled multicenter study comparing immediate versus delayed treatment. Abstracts of the 5th Conference on Retroviruses and Opportunistic Infections. Chicago, 1998.
260. Oberg B: Antiviral effects of phosphonoformate (PFA, foscarnet sodium) (Review) Pharmacol Ther. 1989;40:213–285.
261. Chrisp P, Clissold SP. Foscarnet. A review of its antiviral activity, pharmacokinetic properties and therapeutic use in immunocompromised patients with cytomegalovirus retinitis. Drugs. 1991;41:104–129.
262. Kedes DH, Ganem D. Sensitivity of Kaposi's sarcoma-associated herpesvirus replication to antiviral drugs: Implications for potential therapy. J Clin Invest. 1997;99:2082–2086.
263. Manischewitz JF, Quinnan GJ, Lane HC, et al. Synergistic effect of ganciclovir and foscarnet on cytomegalovirus replication in vitro. Antimicrob Agents Chemother. 1990;34:373–375.
264. Eriksson BF, Schinazi RF. Combinations of 3′-azido-3′-deoxythymidine (zidovudine) and phosphonoformate (foscarnet) against human immunodeficiency virus type 1 and cytomegalovirus replication in vitro. Antimicrob Agents Chemother. 1989;33:663–669.
265. Crumpacker CS. Mechanism of action of foscarnet against viral polymerases (Review) Am J Med. 1992;92:3S–7S.
266. Safrin S, Kemmerly S, Plotkin B, et al. Foscarnet-resistant herpes simplex virus infection in patients with AIDS. J Infect Dis. 1994;169:193–196.
267. Baldanti F, Underwood MR, Stanat SC, et al. Single amino acid changes in the DNA polymerase confer foscarnet resistance and slow-growth phenotype, while mutations in the UL97-encoded phosphotransferase confer ganciclovir resistance in three double-resistant human cytomegalovirus strains recovered from patients with AIDS. J Virol. 1996;70:1390–1395.
268. Jabs DA, Dunn JP, Enger C, et al. Cytomegalovirus retinitis and viral resistance: Prevalence of resistance at diagnosis, 1994. Cytomegalovirus Retinitis and Viral Resistance Study Group. Arch Ophthalmol. 1996;114:809–814.
269. Read RC, Vilar FJ, Smith TL. AIDS-related herpes simplex virus encephalitis during maintenance foscarnet therapy. Clin Infect Dis. 1998;26:513–514.
270. Tachedjian G, Mellors J, Bazmi H, et al. Zidovudine resistance is suppressed by mutations conferring resistance of human immunodeficiency virus type 1 to foscarnet. J Virol. 1996;70:7171–7181.
271. Noormohamed FH, Youle MS, Higgs CJ, et al. Pharmacokinetics and absolute bioavailability of oral foscarnet in human immunodeficiency virus-seropositive patients. Antimicrob Agents Chemother. 1998;42:293–297.
272. Hengge UR, Brockmeyer NH, Malessa R, et al. Foscarnet penetrates the blood-brain barrier: Rationale for therapy of cytomegalovirus encephalitis. Antimicrob Agents Chemother. 1993;37:1010–1014.
273. Arevalo JF, Gonzalez C, Capparelli EV, et al. Intravitreous and plasma concentrations of ganciclovir and foscarnet after intravenous therapy in patients with AIDS and cytomegalovirus retinitis. J Infect Dis. 1995;172:951–956.
274. MacGregor RR, Graziani AL, Weiss R, et al. Successful foscarnet therapy for cytomegalovirus retinitis in an AIDS patient undergoing hemodialysis: Rationale for empiric dosing and plasma level monitoring. J Infect Dis. 1991;164:785–787.
275. Alexander AC, Akers A, Matzke GR, et al. Disposition of foscarnet during peritoneal dialysis. Ann Pharmacother. 1996;30:1106–1109.
276. Reusser P, Gambertoglio JG, Lilleby K, et al. Phase I-II trial of foscarnet for prevention of cytomegalovirus infection in autologous and allogeneic marrow transplant recipients [see comments]. J Infect Dis. 1992;166:473–479.
277. Aweeka FT, Gambertoglio JG, van der Horst C, et al. Pharmacokinetics of concomitantly administered foscarnet and zidovudine for treatment of human immunodeficiency virus infection (AIDS Clinical Trials Group protocol 053). Antimicrob Agents Chemother. 1992;36:1773–1778.
278. Deray G, Martinez F, Katlama C, et al. Foscarnet nephrotoxicity: Mechanism, incidence and prevention. Am J Nephrol. 1989;9:316–321.
279. Navarro JF, Quereda C, Gallego N, et al. Nephrogenic diabetes insipidus and renal tubular acidosis secondary to foscarnet therapy. Am J Kidney Dis. 1996;27:431–434.
280. Jayaweera DT. Minimising the dosage-limiting toxicities of foscarnet induction therapy (Review). Drug Saf. 1997;16:258–266.
281. Jacobson MA, Gambertoglio JG, Aweeka FT, et al. Foscarnet-induced hypocalcemia and effects of foscarnet on calcium metabolism. J Clin Endocrinol Metab. 1991;72:1130–1135.
282. Jacobson MA, Drew WL, Feinberg J, et al. Foscarnet therapy for ganciclovir-resistant cytomegalovirus retinitis in patients with AIDS. J Infect Dis. 1991;163:1348–1351.
283. Palestine AG, Polis MA, De Smet MD, et al. A randomized, controlled trial of foscarnet in the treatment of cytomegalovirus retinitis in patients with AIDS [see comments]. Ann Intern Med. 1991;115:665–673.
284. Katlama C, Dohin E, Caumes E, et al. Foscarnet induction therapy for cytomegalovirus retinitis in AIDS: Comparison of twice-daily and three-times-daily regimens. J Acquir Immune Def Syndr. 1992;5(Suppl 1):S18–S24.
285. Jacobson MA, Causey D, Polsky B, et al. A dose-ranging study of daily maintenance intravenous foscarnet therapy for cytomegalovirus retinitis in AIDS. J Infect Dis. 1993;168:444–448.
286. Anonymous. Mortality in patients with the acquired immunodeficiency syndrome treated with either foscarnet or ganciclovir for cytomegalovirus retinitis: Studies of Ocular Complications of AIDS Research Group, in collaboration with the AIDS Clinical Trials Group [published erratum appears in N Engl J Med 1992;23:326:1172]. N Engl J Med. 1992;326:213–220.
287. Anonymous. Combination foscarnet and ganciclovir therapy vs monotherapy for the treatment of relapsed cytomegalovirus retinitis in patients with AIDS: The Cytomegalovirus Retreatment Trial. The Studies of Ocular Complications of AIDS Research Group in Collaboration with the AIDS Clinical Trials Group. Arch Ophthalmol. 1996;114:23–33.

288. Lieberman RM, Orellana J, Melton RC. Efficacy of intravitreal foscarnet in a patient with AIDS. N Engl J Med. 1994;330:868–869.
289. Drobyski WR, Knox KK, Carrigan DR, et al. Foscarnet therapy of ganciclovir-resistant cytomegalovirus in marrow transplantation. Transplantation. 1991;52:155–157.
290. Youle M, Chanas A, Gazzard B. Treatment of acquired immune deficiency syndrome (AIDS)-related pneumonitis with foscarnet: A double-blind placebo controlled study. J Infect 1990;20:41–50.
291. Lawee D, Rosenthal D, Aoki FY, et al. Efficacy and safety of foscarnet for recurrent orolabial herpes: A multicentre randomized double-blind study. CMAJ 1988;138:329–333.
292. Jacobsen MA, van der Horst C, Causey DM, et al. In vivo additive antiretroviral effect of combined zidovudine and foscarnet therapy for human immunodeficiency virus infection (ACTG Protocol 053). J Infect Dis. 1991;163:1219–1222.
293. Bergdahl S, Jacobsson B, Moberg L, et al. Pronounced anti-HIV-1 activity of foscarnet in patients without cytomegalovirus infection. J Acquir Immune Def Synd Hum Retrovirol. 1998;18:51–53.
294. Glesby MJ, Hoover DR, Weng S, et al. Use of antiherpes drugs and the risk of Kaposi's sarcoma: Data from the Multicenter AIDS Cohort Study. J Infect Dis. 1996;173:1477–1480.
295. Jones JL, Hanson DL, Chu SY, et al. AIDS-associated Kaposi's sarcoma. Science. 1995;267:1078–1079.
296. Faulds D, Heel RC. Ganciclovir: A review of its antiviral activity, pharmacokinetic properties and therapeutic efficacy in cytomegalovirus infections (Review). Drugs. 1990;39:597–638.
297. Field AK, Davies ME, DeWitt C, et al. 9-([2-Hydroxy-1-(hydroxymethyl)ethoxy]-methyl)guanine: A selective inhibitor of herpes group virus replication. Proc Nat Acad Sci U S A. 1983;80:4139–4143.
298. Smee DF, Martin JC, Verheyden JP, et al. Anti-herpesvirus activity of the acyclic nucleoside 9-(1,3-dihydroxy-2-propoxymethyl)guanine. Antimicrob Agents Chemother. 1983;23:676–682.
299. Plotkin SA, Drew WL, Felsenstein D, et al. Sensitivity of clinical isolates of human cytomegalovirus to 9-(1,3-dihydroxy-2-propoxymethyl)guanine. J Infect Dis. 1985;152:833–834.
300. Medina DJ, Hsiung GD, Mellors JW. Ganciclovir antagonizes the anti-human immunodeficiency virus type 1 activity of zidovudine and didanosine in vitro. Antimicrob Agents Chemother. 1992;36:1127–1130.
301. Feng JS, Crouch JY, Tian PY, et al. Zidovudine antagonizes the antiviral effects of ganciclovir against cytomegalovirus infection in cultured cells and in guinea pigs. Antiviral Chemistry and Chemotherapy. 1993;4:19–25.
302. Freitas VR, Fraser-Smith EB, Chiu S, et al. Efficacy of ganciclovir in combination with zidovudine against cytomegalovirus in vitro and in vivo. Antiviral Res. 1993;21:301–315.
303. Taylor DL, Jeffries DJ, Taylor-Robinson D. The susceptibility of adenovirus infection to the anti-cytomegalovirus drug, ganciclovir (DHPG). FEMS Microbiol Lett. 1988;49:337–341.
304. Gish RG, Lau JY, Brooks L, et al. Ganciclovir treatment of hepatitis B virus infection in liver transplant recipients. Hepatology. 1996;23:1–7.
305. Shanley JD, Morningstar J, Jordan MC. Inhibition of murine cytomegalovirus lung infection and interstitial pneumonitis by acyclovir and 9-(1,3-dihydroxy-2-propoxymethyl)guanine. Antimicrob Agents Chemother. 1985;28:172–175.
306. Fong CK, Cohen SD, McCormick S, et al. Antiviral effect of 9-(1,3-dihydroxy-2-propoxymethyl)guanine against cytomegalovirus infection in a guinea pig model. Antiviral Res. 1987;7:11–23.
307. Sommadossi JP, Carlisle R. Toxicity of 3′-azido-3′-deoxythymidine and 9-(1,3-dihydroxy-2-propoxymethyl)guanine for normal human hematopoietic progenitor cells in vitro. Antimicrob Agents Chemother. 1987;31:452–454.
308. Smee DF, Boehme R, Chernow M, et al. Intracellular metabolism and enzymatic phosphorylation of 9-(1,3-dihydroxy-2-propoxymethyl)guanine and acyclovir in herpes simplex virus-infected and uninfected cells. Biochem Pharmacol. 1985;34:1049–1056.
309. Sullivan V, Talarico CL, Stanat SC, et al. A protein kinase homologue controls phosphorylation of ganciclovir in human cytomegalovirus-infected cells [published errata appear in Nature 1992;3;359:85 and 1993;23–30;366:756]. Nature. 1992;358:162–164.
310. Littler E, Stuart AD, Chee MS. Human cytomegalovirus UL97 open reading frame encodes a protein that phosphorylates the antiviral nucleoside analogue ganciclovir. Nature. 1992;358:160–162.
311. Freitas VR, Smee DF, Chernow M, et al. Activity of 9-(1,3-dihydroxy-2-propoxymethyl)guanine compared with that of acyclovir against human, monkey, and rodent cytomegaloviruses. Antimicrob Agents Chemother. 1985;28:240–245.
312. Biron KK, Stanat SC, Sorrell JB, et al. Metabolic activation of the nucleoside analog 9-[(2-hydroxy-1-(hydroxymethyl)ethoxy]methyl)guanine in human diploid fibroblasts infected with human cytomegalovirus. Proc Nat Acad Sci U S A. 1985;82:2473–2477.
313. Reid R, Mar EC, Huang ES, et al. Insertion and extension of acyclic, dideoxy, and ara nucleotides by herpesviridae, human alpha and human beta polymerases: A unique inhibition mechanism for 9-(1,3-dihydroxy-2-propoxymethyl)guanine triphosphate. J Biol Chem. 1988;263:3898–3904.
314. Hamzeh FM, Lietman PS. Intranuclear accumulation of subgenomic noninfectious human cytomegalovirus DNA in infected cells in the presence of ganciclovir. Antimicrob Agents Chemother. 1991;35:1818–1823.
315. Chou S, Guentzel S, Michels KR, et al. Frequency of UL97 phosphotransferase mutations related to ganciclovir resistance in clinical cytomegalovirus isolates. J Infect Dis. 1995;172:239–242.
316. Lurain NS, Thompson KD, Holmes EW, et al. Point mutations in the DNA polymerase gene of human cytomegalovirus that result in resistance to antiviral agents. J Virol. 1992;66:7146–7152.
317. Stanat SC, Reardon JE, Erice A, et al. Ganciclovir-resistant cytomegalovirus clinical isolates: Mode of resistance to ganciclovir. Antimicrob Agents Chemother. 1991;35:2191–2197.
318. Smith IL, Cherrington JM, Jiles RE, et al. High-level resistance of cytomegalovirus to ganciclovir is associated with alterations in both the UL97 and DNA polymerase genes. J Infect Dis. 1997;176:69–77.
319. Erice A, Chou S, Biron KK, et al. Progressive disease due to ganciclovir-resistant cytomegalovirus in immunocompromised patients. N Engl J Med. 1989;320:289–293.
320. Drew WL, Miner RC, Busch DF, et al. Prevalence of resistance in patients receiving ganciclovir for serious cytomegalovirus infection. J Infect Dis. 1991;163:716–719.
321. Wolf DG, Yaniv I, Honigman A, et al. Early emergence of ganciclovir-resistant human cytomegalovirus strains in children with primary combined immunodeficiency. J Infect Dis. 1998;178:535–538.
322. Rosen HR, Benner KG, Flora KD, et al. Development of ganciclovir resistance during treatment of primary cytomegalovirus infection after liver transplantation. Transplantation. 1997;63:476–478.
323. Tokumoto JI, Hollander H. Cytomegalovirus polyradiculopathy caused by a ganciclovir-resistant strain. Clin Infect Dis. 1993;17:854–856.
324. Lavelle J, Follansbee S, Trapnell CB, et al. Effect of food on the relative bioavailability of oral ganciclovir. J Clin Pharmacol. 1996;36:238–241.
325. Anderson RD, Griffy KG, Jung D, et al. Ganciclovir absolute bioavailability and steady-state pharmacokinetics after oral administration of two 3000-mg/d dosing regimens in human immunodeficiency virus- and cytomegalovirus-seropositive patients. Clin Ther. 1995;17:425–432.
326. Laskin OL, Cederberg DM, Mills J, et al. Ganciclovir for the treatment and suppression of serious infections caused by cytomegalovirus. Am J Med. 1987;83:201–207.
327. Fletcher C, Sawchuk R, Chinnock B, et al. Human pharmacokinetics of the antiviral drug DHPG. Clin Pharmacol Ther. 1986;40:281–286.
328. Kuppermann BD, Quiceno JI, Flores-Aguilar M, et al. Intravitreal ganciclovir concentration after intravenous administration in AIDS patients with cytomegalovirus retinitis: Implications for therapy. J Infect Dis. 1993;168:1506–1509.
329. Sommadossi JP, Bevan R, Ling T, et al. Clinical pharmacokinetics of ganciclovir in patients with normal and impaired renal function. Rev Infect Dis. 1988;10(Suppl 3):S507–S514.
330. Swan SK, Munar MY, Wigger MA, et al. Pharmacokinetics of ganciclovir in a patient undergoing hemodialysis. Am J Kidney Dis. 1991;17:69–72.
331. Marx JL, Kapusta MA, Patel SS, et al. Use of the ganciclovir implant in the treatment of recurrent cytomegalovirus retinitis. Arch Ophthalmol. 1996;114:815–820.
332. Cimoch PJ, Lavelle J, Pollard R, et al. Pharmacokinetics of oral ganciclovir alone and in combination with zidovudine, didanosine, and probenecid in HIV-infected subjects. J Acquir Immune Def Syndr Hum Retrovirol. 1998;17:227–234.
333. Jacobson MA, de Miranda P, Gordon SM, et al. Prolonged pancytopenia due to combined ganciclovir and zidovudine therapy (Letter). J Infect Dis. 1988;158:489–490.
334. Hochster H, Dieterich D, Bozzette S, et al. Toxicity of combined ganciclovir and zidovudine for cytomegalovirus disease associated with AIDS: An AIDS Clinical Trials Group Study. Ann Intern Med. 1990;113:111–117.
335. Freitas VR, Fraser-Smith EB, Matthews TR. Efficacy of ganciclovir in combination with other antimicrobial agents against cytomegalovirus in vitro and in vivo. Antiviral Res. 1993;20:1–12.
336. Hardy WD. Combined ganciclovir and recombinant human granulocyte-macrophage colony-stimulating factor in the treatment of cytomegalovirus retinitis in AIDS patients. J Acquir Immune Def Syndr. 1991;4(Suppl 1):S22–S28.
337. Merigan TC, Renlund DG, Keay S, et al. A controlled trial of ganciclovir to prevent cytomegalovirus disease after heart transplantation. N Engl J Med. 1992;326:1182–1186.
338. Gane E, Saliba F, Valdecasas GJC, et al. Randomized trial of efficacy and safety of oral ganciclovir in the prevention of cytomegalovirus disease in liver-transplant recipients. Lancet. 1997;350:1729–1733.
339. Anonymous. Treatment of serious cytomegalovirus infections with 9-(1,3-dihydroxy-2-propoxymethyl)guanine in patients with AIDS and other immunodeficiencies: Collaborative DHPG Treatment Study Group. N Engl J Med. 1986;314:801–805.
340. Holland GN, Sidikaro Y, Kreiger AE, et al. Treatment of cytomegalovirus retinopathy with ganciclovir. Ophthalmology. 1987;94:815–823.
341. Drew WL. Cytomegalovirus infection in patients with AIDS (Review). Clin Infect Dis. 1992;14:608–615.
342. Drew WL, Ives D, Lalezari JP, et al. Oral ganciclovir as maintenance treatment for cytomegalovirus retinitis in patients with AIDS: Syntex Cooperative Oral Ganciclovir Study Group. N Engl J Med. 1995;333:615–620.
343. Freeman WR, Henderly DE, Wan WL, et al. Prevalence, pathophysiology, and treatment of rhegmatogenous retinal detachment in treated cytomegalovirus retinitis. Am J Ophthal. 1987;103:527–536.
344. Marx JL, Kapusta MA, Patel SS, et al. Use of the ganciclovir implant in the treatment of recurrent cytomegalovirus retinitis. Arch Ophthalmol. 1996;114:815–820.
345. Musch DC, Martin DF, Gordon JF, et al. Treatment of cytomegalovirus retinitis with a sustained-release ganciclovir implant. The Ganciclovir Implant Study Group. N Engl J Med. 1997;337:83–90.
346. Crumpacker CS. Ganciclovir. N Engl J Med. 1996;335:721–729.

347. Berman SM, Kim RC. The development of cytomegalovirus encephalitis in AIDS patients receiving ganciclovir. Am J Med. 1994;96:415–419.
348. Dieterich DT, Kotler DP, Busch DF, et al. Ganciclovir treatment of cytomegalovirus colitis in AIDS: A randomized, double-blind, placebo-controlled multicenter study. J Infect Dis. 1993;167:278–282.
349. Reed EC, Bowden RA, Dandliker PS, et al. Treatment of cytomegalovirus pneumonia with ganciclovir and intravenous cytomegalovirus immunoglobulin in patients with bone marrow transplants. Ann Intern Med. 1988;109:783–788.
350. Emanuel D, Cunningham I, Jules-Elysee K, et al. Cytomegalovirus pneumonia after bone marrow transplantation successfully treated with the combination of ganciclovir and high-dose intravenous immune globulin. Ann Intern Med. 1988;109:777–782.
351. Reed EC, Wolford JL, Kopecky KJ, et al. Ganciclovir for the treatment of cytomegalovirus gastroenteritis in bone marrow transplant patients. A randomized, placebo-controlled trial. Ann Intern Med. 1990;112:505–510.
352. Schmidt GM, Horak DA, Niland JC, et al. A randomized, controlled trial of prophylactic ganciclovir for cytomegalovirus pulmonary infection in recipients of allogeneic bone marrow transplants: The City of Hope-Stanford-Syntex CMV Study Group [see comments]. N Engl J Med. 1991;324:1005–1011.
353. Goodrich JM, Mori M, Gleaves CA, et al. Early treatment with ganciclovir to prevent cytomegalovirus disease after allogeneic bone marrow transplantation. N Engl J Med. 1991;325:1601–1607.
354. Winston DJ, Ho WG, Bartoni K, et al. Ganciclovir prophylaxis of cytomegalovirus infection and disease in allogeneic bone marrow transplant recipients: Results of a placebo-controlled, double-blind trial. Ann Intern Med. 1993;118:179–184.
355. Goodrich JM, Bowden RA, Fisher L, et al. Ganciclovir prophylaxis to prevent cytomegalovirus disease after allogeneic marrow transplant. Ann Intern Med. 1993;118:173–178.
356. Duncan SR, Paradis IL, Dauber JH, et al. Ganciclovir prophylaxis for cytomegalovirus infections in pulmonary allograft recipients. Am Rev Respir Dis. 1992;146:1213–1215.
357. Hibberd PL, Tolkoff-Rubin NE, Conti D, et al. Preemptive ganciclovir therapy to prevent cytomegalovirus disease in cytomegalovirus antibody-positive renal transplant recipients: A randomized controlled trial. Ann Intern Med. 1995;123:18–26.
358. Preiksaitis JK, Diaz-Mitoma F, Mirzayans F, et al. Quantitative oropharyngeal Epstein-Barr virus shedding in renal and cardiac transplant recipients: Relationship to immunosuppressive therapy, serologic responses, and the risk of posttransplant lymphoproliferative disorder. J Infect Dis. 1992;166:986–994.
359. Brennan DC, Garlock KA, Singer GG, et al. Prophylactic oral ganciclovir compared with deferred therapy for control of cytomegalovirus in renal transplant recipients. Transplantation. 1997;64:1843–1846.
360. Spector SA, McKinley GF, Lalezari JP, et al. Oral ganciclovir for the prevention of cytomegalovirus disease in persons with AIDS. Roche Cooperative Oral Ganciclovir Study Group [see comments]. N Engl J Med. 1996;334:1491–1497.
361. Brosgart CL, Louis TA, Hillman DW, et al. A randomized, placebo-controlled trial of the safety and efficacy of oral ganciclovir for prophylaxis of cytomegalovirus disease in HIV-infected individuals: Terry Beirn Community Programs for Clinical Research on AIDS. AIDS. 1998;12:269–277.
362. Hoh HB, Hurley C, Claoue C, et al. Randomised trial of ganciclovir and acyclovir in the treatment of herpes simplex dendritic keratitis: A multicentre study. Br J Ophthal. 1996;80:140–143.
363. Prusoff WH. Idoxuridine or how it all began. In: DeClercq E, ed. Clinical Use of Antiviral Drugs. Boston: Martinus Nijhoff; 1988:15–24.
364. Fardeau C, Langlois M, Mathys B, et al. Emergence of cross-resistant herpes simplex virus following topical drug therapy in rabbit keratitis. Curr Eye Res. 1991;10(Suppl):151–158.
365. Kaufman HE. The treatment of herpetic eye infections with trifluridine and other antivirals. In: DeClercq E, ed. Clinical Use of Antiviral Drugs. Boston: Martinus Nijhoff; 1988:25–38.
366. Pavan-Langston D. Major ocular viral infections. In: Galasso GJ, Whitley RJ, Merigan TC, eds. Antiviral Agents and Viral Diseases of Man. New York: Raven Press; 1990:183–233.
367. Silvestri DL, Corey L, Holmes KK. Ineffectiveness of topical idoxuridine in dimethyl sulfoxide for therapy for genital herpes. JAMA. 1982;248:953–959.
368. Spruance SL, Stewart JC, Freeman DJ, et al. Early application of topical 15% idoxuridine in dimethyl sulfoxide shortens the course of herpes simplex labialis: A multicenter placebo-controlled trial. J Infect Dis. 1990;161:191–197.
369. Baron S, Coppenhaver DH, Doanzani F. Introduction to the interferon system. In: Baron S, ed. Interferon: Principles and Medical Applications. Galveston, TX: UTMN; 1992:1–15.
370. Zoon KC. Human interferons: Structure and function. In: Anonymous. Interferon 9. London: Academic Press; 1987:1–12.
370a. Dianzani F, Antonelli G. Mechanisms of action of the interferons: Biological basis. In: Stuart-Harris R, Penny R, eds. Clinical Applications of the Interferons. London: Chapman & Hall; 1997:20–31.
371. Finter NB. Why are there so many subtypes of alpha-interferons? In: Marcus PI, ed. Journal of Interferon Research. New York: Mary Ann Liebert Publishers; 1991:185–194.
372. Greenberg SB. Human interferon in viral diseases (Review). Infect Dis Clin North Am. 1987;1:383–423.
373. Staeheli P. Interferon-induced proteins and the antiviral state. Adv Virus Res. 1990;38:147–200.
374. Sen GC, Ransohoff RM. Interferon-induced antiviral actions and their regulation. Adv Virus Res. 1993;42:57–102.
375. Sen GC, Lengyel P. The interferon system: A bird's eye view of its biochemistry. J Biol Chem. 1992;267:5017–5020.
376. Pfeffer LM, Mullersman JE, Pfeffer SR, et al. STAT3 as an adapter to couple phosphatidylinositol 3-kinase to the IFNAR1 chain of the type I interferon receptor. Science. 1997;276:1418–1420.
377. Ransohoff RM. Cellular responses to interferons and other cytokines: The JAK-STAT paradigm. N Engl J Med. 1998;338:616–618.
378. Maran A, Maitra RK, Kumar A, et al. Blockage of NF-kappa B signaling by selective ablation of an mRNA target by 2-5A antisense chimeras. Science. 1994;265:789–792.
379. Fischer DG, Tal N, Novick D, et al. An antiviral soluble form of the LDL receptor induced by interferon. Science. 1993;262:250–253.
380. Roers A, Hochkeppel HK, Horisberger MA, et al. MxA gene expression after live virus vaccination: A sensitive marker for endogenous type I interferon. J Infect Dis. 1994;169:807–813.
381. Karupiah G, Xie QW, Buller RM, et al. Inhibition of viral replication by interferon-gamma-induced nitric oxide synthase. Science. 1993;261:1445–1448.
382. Gale MJ, Korth MJ, Tang NM, et al. Evidence that hepatitis C virus resistance to interferon is mediated through repression of the PKR protein kinase by the nonstructural 5A protein. Virology. 1997;230:217–227.
383. Heremans H, Billiau A. Interferons and the cytokine network: Role in thymic and pituitary physiology, in endotoxin-induced shock, and in cachexia. In: Baron S, ed. Interferon: Principles and Medical Applications. Galveston, Tex: UTMB; 1992:361–371.
384. Hooks JJ, Detrick B: The interferon system and disease. In: Pfeffer LM, ed. Mechanisms of Interferon Actions. Boca Raton: CRC Press; 1987:113–328.
385. Ikossi-O'Connor MG, Chadha KC, et al. Interferon inactivator(s) in patients with AIDS and AIDS-unrelated Kaposi's sarcoma. Am J Med. 1986;81:783–785.
386. Ambrus JL, Poiesz BJ, Lillie MA, et al. Interferon and interferon inhibitor levels in patients infected with varicella-zoster virus, acquired immunodeficiency syndrome, acquired immunodeficiency syndrome-related complex, or Kaposi's sarcoma, and in normal individuals. Am J Med. 1989;87:405–407.
387. Wills RJ. Clinical pharmacokinetics of interferons. Clin Pharmacokinet. 1990;19:390–399.
388. Haria M, Benfield P. Interferon-alpha-2a: A review of its pharmacological properties and therapeutic use in the management of viral hepatitis (Review) Drugs. 1995;50:873–896.
389. Barouki FM, Witter FR, Griffin DE, et al. Time course of interferon levels, antiviral state, 2′,5′-oligoadenylate synthetase and side effects in healthy men. J Interferon Res. 1987;7:29–39.
390. Witt PL, Goldstein D, Storer BE, et al. Absence of biological effects of orally administered interferon-beta ser. J Interferon Res. 1992;12:411–413.
391. Smith RA, Norris F, Palmer D, et al. Distribution of alpha interferon in serum and cerebrospinal fluid after systemic administration. Clin Pharmacol Ther. 1985;37:85–88.
392. Quesada JR. Toxicity and side effects of interferons. In: Baron S, ed. Interferon: Principles and Medical Applications. Galveston, TX: UTMB; 1992;426–432.
393. Renault PF, Hoofnagle JH. Side effects of alpha interferon. Semin Liver Dis. 1989;9:273–277.
394. McDonald EM, Mann AH, Thomas HC. Interferons as mediators of psychiatric morbidity: An investigation in a trial of recombinant alpha-interferon in hepatitis-B carriers. Lancet. 1987;2:1175–1178.
395. Deyton LR, Walker RE, Kovacs JA, et al. Reversible cardiac dysfunction associated with interferon alfa therapy in AIDS patients with Kaposi's sarcoma [see comments]. N Engl J Med. 1989;321:1246–1249.
396. Kawano T, Shigehira M, Uto H, et al. Retinal complications during interferon therapy for chronic hepatitis C. Am J Gastroenterol. 1996;91:309–313.
397. Bayraktar Y, Bayraktar M, Gurakar A, et al. A comparison of the prevalence of autoantibodies in individuals with chronic hepatitis C and those with autoimmune hepatitis: The role of interferon in the development of autoimmune diseases. Hepato-Gastroenterol. 1997;44:417–425.
398. Antonelli G, Currenti M, Turriziani O, et al. Neutralizing antibodies to interferon-alpha: Relative frequency in patients treated with different interferon preparations. J Infect Dis. 1991;163:882–885.
399. Foster GR, Ackrill AM, Goldin RD, et al. Expression of the terminal protein region of hepatitis B virus inhibits cellular responses to interferons alpha and gamma and double-stranded RNA [published erratum appears in Proc Natl Acad Sci U S A 1995;11;92:3632]. Proc Nat Acad Sci U S A. 1991;88:2888–2892.
400. Hoofnagle JH, Di Bisceglie AM. Drug therapy: The treatment of chronic viral hepatitis. N Engl J Med. 1997;336:347–356.
401. Korenman J, Baker B, Waggoner J, et al. Long-term remission of chronic hepatitis B after alpha-interferon therapy. Ann Intern Med. 1991;114:629–634.
402. Perrillo RP, Schiff ER, Davis GL, et al. A randomized, controlled trial of interferon alfa-2b alone and after prednisone withdrawal for the treatment of chronic hepatitis B: The Hepatitis Interventional Therapy Group [see comments]. N Engl J Med. 1990;323:295–301.
403. Niederau C, Heintges T, Lange S, et al. Long-term follow-up of HBeAg-positive patients treated with interferon alfa for chronic hepatitis B. N Engl J Med. 1996;334:1422–1427.
404. Lau DT, Everhart J, Kleiner DE, et al. Long-term follow-up of patients with chronic hepatitis B treated with interferon alfa. Gastroenterology. 1997;113:1660–1667.
405. Fattovich G, McIntyre G, Thursz M, et al. Hepatitis B virus precore/core variation and interferon therapy. Hepatology. 1995;22:1355–1362.
406. Di BM, Rustgi VK, Kassianides C, et al. Therapy of chronic hepatitis B with recombinant human alpha and gamma interferon. Hepatology. 1990;11:266–270.
407. Kakumu S, Ishikawa T, Mizokami M, et al. Treatment with human gamma interferon of chronic hepatitis B: Comparative study with alpha interferon. J Med Virol. 1991;35:32–37.

408. Ruiz-Moreno M, Fernandez P, Leal A, et al. Pilot Interferon-beta trial in children with chronic hepatitis B who had previously not responded to interferon-alpha therapy. Pediatrics. 1997;99:222–225.
409. Perrillo RP, Brunt EM. Hepatic histologic and immunohistochemical changes in chronic hepatitis B after prolonged clearance of hepatitis B e antigen and hepatitis B surface antigen. Ann Intern Med. 1991;115:113–115.
410. Lisker-Melman M, Webb D, Di BM, et al. Glomerulonephritis caused by chronic hepatitis B virus infection: Treatment with recombinant human alpha-interferon. Ann Intern Med. 1989;111:479–483.
411. Lai KN, Li PK, Lui SF, et al. Membranous nephropathy related to hepatitis B virus in adults. N Engl J Med. 1991;324:1457–1463.
412. Farci P, Mandas A, Coiana A, et al. Treatment of chronic hepatitis D with interferon alfa-2a. N Engl J Med. 1994;330:88–94.
413. Haria M, Benfield P. Interferon-alpha-2a: A review of its pharmacological properties and therapeutic use in the management of viral hepatitis (Review) Drugs. 1995;50:873–896.
414. Hoofnagle JH, Di Bisceglie AM. Drug therapy: The treatment of chronic viral hepatitis. N Engl J Med. 1997;336:347–356.
415. Di Bisceglie AM, Martin P, Kassianides C, et al. Recombinant interferon alfa therapy for chronic hepatitis C: A randomized, double-blind, placebo-controlled trial. N Engl J Med. 1989;321:1506–1510.
416. Davis GL, Balart LA, Schiff ER, et al. Treatment of chronic hepatitis C with recombinant interferon alfa: A multicenter randomized, controlled trial. Hepatitis Interventional Therapy Group. N Engl J Med. 1989;321:1501–1506.
417. Shindo M, Di BM, Cheung L, et al. Decrease in serum hepatitis C viral RNA during alpha-interferon therapy for chronic hepatitis C. Ann Intern Med. 1991;115:700–704.
418. Marcellin P, Boyer N, Gervais A, et al. Long-term histologic improvement and loss of detectable intrahepatic HCV RNA in patients with chronic hepatitis C and sustained response to interferon-alpha therapy. Ann Intern Med. 1997;127:875–881.
419. Chemello LMP, Cavalletto LM, Casarin CM, et al. Persistent hepatitis C viremia predicts late relapse after sustained response to interferon-alpha in chronic hepatitis C. Ann Intern Med. 1996;124:1058–1060.
420. Shindo M, Arai K, Sokawa Y, Okuno T. Hepatic hepatitis C virus RNA as a predictor of a long-term response to interferon-alpha therapy [see comments]. Ann Intern Med. 1995;122:586–591.
421. Poynard T, Bedossa P, Chevallier M, et al. A comparison of three interferon alfa-2b regimens for the long-term treatment of chronic non-A, non-B hepatitis: Multicenter Study Group [see comments] [published erratum appears in N Engl J Med; 1996:25;334:1143]. N Engl J Med. 1995;332:1457–1462.
422. Management of Hepatitis C. NIH Consensus Statement 15(3), 1-41. 3-24-1997.
423. McHutchison JG, Gordon SC, Schiff ER, et al. Interferon alfa-2b alone or in combination with ribavirin as initial treatment for chronic hepatitis C. Hepatitis Interventional Therapy Group. N Engl J Med 1998;339:1485–1492.
424. Davis GL, Esteban-Mur R, Rustgi V, et al. Interferon alfa-2b alone or in combination with ribavirin for the treatment of relapse of chronic hepatitis C. International Hepatitis Interventional Therapy Group. N Engl J Med. 1998;339:1493–1499.
425. Johnson RJ, Gretch DR, Yamabe H, et al. Membranoproliferative glomerulonephritis associated with hepatitis C virus infection. N Engl J Med. 1993;328:465–470.
426. Misiani R, Bellavita P, Fenili D, et al. Interferon alfa-2a therapy in cryoglobulinemia associated with hepatitis C virus. N Engl J Med. 1994;330:751–756.
427. Polyak SJ, McArdle S, Liu SL, et al. Evolution of hepatitis C virus quasispecies in hypervariable region 1 and the putative interferon sensitivity-determining region during interferon therapy and natural infection. J Virol. 1998;72:4288–4296.
428. Enomoto N, Sakuma I, Asahina Y, et al. Mutations in the nonstructural protein 5A gene and response to interferon in patients with chronic hepatitis C virus 1b infection. N Engl J Med. 1996;334:77–81.
429. Herion D, Hoofnagle JH. The interferon sensitivity determining region: All hepatitis C virus isolates are not the same. Hepatology. 1997;25:769–771.
430. Martinot M, Marcellin P, Boyer N, et al. Influence of hepatitis G virus infection on the severity of liver disease and response to interferon-alpha in patients with chronic hepatitis C. Ann Intern Med. 1997;126:874–881.
431. Papo T, Marcellin P, Bernuau J, et al. Autoimmune chronic hepatitis exacerbated by alpha-interferon. Ann Intern Med. 1992;116:51–53.
432. Nishiguchi S, Kuroki T, Nakatani S, et al. Randomised trial of effects of interferon-alpha on incidence of hepatocellular carcinoma in chronic active hepatitis C with cirrhosis. Lancet. 1995;346:1051–1055.
433. International Interferon-α Hepatocellular Carcinoma Study Group: Effect of interferon-alpha on progression of cirrhosis to hepatocellular carcinoma: A retrospective cohort study. Lancet. 1998;351:1535–1539.
434. Omata M, Yokosuka O, Takano S, et al. Resolution of acute hepatitis C after therapy with natural beta interferon. Lancet. 1991;338:914–915.
435. Bizollon T, Palazzo U, Ducerf C, et al. Pilot study of the combination of interferon alfa and ribavirin as therapy of recurrent hepatitis C after liver transplantation. Hepatology. 1997;26:500–504.
436. Eron LJ, Toy C, Salsitz B, Scheer RR, et al. Therapy of genital herpes with topically applied interferon. Antimicrob Agents Chemother. 1987;31:1137–1139.
437. Lebwohl M, Sacks S, Conant M, et al. Recombinant alpha-2 interferon gel treatment of recurrent herpes genitalis. Antiviral Res. 1992;17:235–243.
438. Winston DJ, Eron LJ, Ho M, et al. Recombinant interferon alpha-2a for treatment of herpes zoster in immunosuppressed patients with cancer. Am J Med. 1988;85:147–151.
439. Duschet P, Schwarz T, Soyer P, et al. Treatment of herpes zoster: Recombinant alpha interferon versus acyclovir. Int J Dermatol. 1988;27:193–197.
440. Krown SE. The role of interferon in the therapy of epidemic Kaposi's sarcoma (Review) Semin Oncol. 1987;14:27–33.
441. Berglund O, Engman K, Ehrnst A, et al. Combined treatment of symptomatic human immunodeficiency virus type 1 infection with native interferon-alpha and zidovudine. J Infect Dis. 1991;163:710–715.
442. Husak R, Goerdt S, Orfanos CE. Interferon alfa treatment of a patient with eosinophilic cellulitis and HIV infection. N Engl J Med. 1997;337:641–642.
443. Marroni M, Gresele P, Landonio G, et al. Interferon-alpha is effective in the treatment of HIV-1-related, severe, zidovudine-resistant thrombocytopenia: A prospective, placebo-controlled, double-blind trial. Ann Intern Med. 1994;121:423–429.
444. Edlin BR, St. Clair MH, Pitha PM, et al. In-vitro resistance to zidovudine and alpha-interferon in HIV-1 isolates from patients: Correlations with treatment duration and response [published erratum appears in Ann Intern Med 1992;15;117:879]. Ann Intern Med. 1992;117:457–460.
445. Douglas JJ, Eron LJ, Judson FN, et al. A randomized trial of combination therapy with intralesional interferon alpha 2b and podophyllin versus podophyllin alone for the therapy of anogenital warts. J Infect Dis. 1990;162:52–59.
446. Reichman RC, Oakes D, Bonnez W, et al. Treatment of condyloma acuminatum with three different interferon-alpha preparations administered parenterally: A double-blind, placebo-controlled trial. J Infect Dis. 1990;162:1270–1276.
447. Anonymous. Randomized placebo-controlled double-blind combined therapy with laser surgery and systemic interferon-alpha 2a in the treatment of anogenital condylomata acuminatum. The Condylomata International Collaborative Study Group. J Infect Dis. 1993;167:824–829.
448. Frazer IH, McMillan AJ. Papillomatosis and condylomata acuminata. In: Stuart-Harris R, Penny R, eds. Clinical Applications of the Interferons. London: Chapman & Hall; 1997:79–90.
449. Berman B, Davis-Reed L, Silverstein L, et al. Treatment of verrucae vulgaris with alpha 2 interferon. J Infect Dis. 1986;154:328–330.
450. Healy GB, Gelber RD, Trowbridge AL, et al. Treatment of recurrent respiratory papillomatosis with human leukocyte interferon: Results of a multicenter randomized clinical trial. N Engl J Med. 1988;319:401–407.
451. Lusk RP, McCabe BF, Mixon JH. Three-year experience of treating recurrent respiratory papilloma with interferon. Ann Otol Rhinol Laryngol. 1987;96:158–162.
452. Leventhal BG, Kashima HK, Mounts P, et al. Long-term response of recurrent respiratory papillomatosis to treatment with lymphoblastoid interferon alfa-n1: Papilloma Study Group. N Engl J Med. 1991;325:613–617.
453. Sperber SJ, Hayden FG. Comparative susceptibility of respiratory viruses to recombinant interferons-alpha 2b and -beta. J Interferon Res. 1989;9:285–293.
454. Hayden FG. Intranasal interferons for control of respiratory viral infections. In: Revel M, ed. Clinical Aspects of Interferons. Boston: Kluwer Academic Publishers; 1988:3–16.
455. Higgins PG, Barrow GI, Tyrrell DA, et al. The efficacy of intranasal interferon alpha-2a in respiratory syncytial virus infection in volunteers. Antiviral Res. 1990;14:3–10.
456. Hayden FG, Albrecht JK, Kaiser DL, et al. Prevention of natural colds by contact prophylaxis with intranasal alpha 2-interferon. N Engl J Med. 1986;314:71–75.
457. Douglas RM, Moore BW, Miles HB, et al. Prophylactic efficacy of intranasal alpha 2-interferon against rhinovirus infections in the family setting. N Engl J Med. 1986;314:65–70.
458. Hayden FG, Kaiser DL, Albrecht JK. Intranasal recombinant alfa-2b interferon treatment of naturally occurring common colds. Antimicrob Agents Chemother. 1988;32:224–230.
458a. Bartholomew MM, Jansen RW, Jeffers LJ, et al. Hepatitis B virus resistance to lamivudine given for recurrent infection after orthotopic liver transplantation. Lancet. 1997;349:20–22.
458b. Allen MI, Deslauriers M, Andrews CW, et al. Indentification and characterization of mutations in hepatitis B virus resistant to lamivudine. Lamivudine Clinical Investigation Group. Hepatology. 1998;27:1670–1677.
458c. Melegari M, Scaglioni PP, Wands JR. Hepatitis B virus mutants associated with 3TC and famciclovir administration are replication defective. Hepatology. 1998;27:628–633.
458d. Lai CL, Chien RN, Leung N, et al. A one-year trial of lamivudine for chronic hepatitis B. N Engl J Med. 1998;339:61–68.
458e. Dienstag JL, Perrillo RP, Schiff ER, et al. A preliminary trial of lamivudine for chronic hepatitis B infection. N Engl J Med. 1995;333:1657–1661.
458f. Lai CL, Ching CK, Tung AK, et al. Lamivudine is effective in suppressing hepatitis B virus DNA in Chinese hepatitis B surface antigen carriers: A placebo-controlled trial. Hepatology. 1997;25:241–244.
458g. Benhamou Y, Katlama C, Lunel F, et al. Effects of lamivudine on replication of hepatitis B virus in HIV-infected men. Ann Intern Med. 1996;125:705–712.
458h. Grellier L, Mutimer D, Ahmed M, et al. Lamivudine prophylaxis against reinfection in liver transplantation for hepatitis B cirrhosis [published erratum appears in Lancet 1997 Feb 1;349(9048):364]. Lancet. 1996;348:1212–1215.
459. Gilbert BE, Knight V. Biochemistry and clinical applications of ribavirin (Review) Antimicrob Agents Chemother. 1986;30:201–205.
460. Hruska JF, Bernstein JM, Douglas RJ, et al. Effects of ribavirin on respiratory syncytial virus in vitro. Antimicrob Agents Chemother. 1980;17:770–775.
461. Browne MJ. Comparative inhibition of influenza and parainfluenza virus replication by ribavirin in MDCK cells. Antimicrob Agents Chemother. 1981;19:712–715.
462. Huggins JW. Prospects for treatment of viral hemorrhagic fevers with ribavirin, a broad-spectrum antiviral drug. Rev Infect Dis. 1989;11(Suppl 4):S750–S761.
463. Baba M, Pauwels R, Balzarini J, et al. Ribavirin antagonizes inhibitory effects of pyrimidine 2′,3′-dideoxynucleosides but enhances inhibitory effects of purine 2′,3′-dideoxynucleosides on replication of human immunodeficiency virus in vitro. Antimicrob Agents Chemother. 1987;31:1613–1617.
464. Peavy DL, Koff WC, Hyman DS, et al. Inhibition of lymphocyte proliferative responses by ribavirin. Infect Immun. 1980;29:583–589.

465. Steele RW, Crosby DL, Pilkington NJ, et al. Effects of ribavirin on neutrophil function. Am J Med Sci. 1988;295:503–506.
466. Marquardt DL, Gruber HE, Walker LL. Ribavirin inhibits mast cell mediator release. J Pharmacol Exp Ther. 1987;240:145–149.
467. Hruska JF, Morrow PE, Suffin SC, et al. In vivo inhibition of respiratory syncytial virus by ribavirin. Antimicrob Agents Chemother. 1982;21:125–130.
468. Wyde PR, Wilson SZ, Petrella R, et al. Efficacy of high dose-short duration ribavirin aerosol in the treatment of respiratory syncytial virus infected cotton rats and influenza B virus infected mice. Antiviral Res. 1987;7:211–220.
469. Jahrling PB, Hesse RA, Eddy GA, et al. Lassa virus infection of rhesus monkeys: Pathogenesis and treatment with ribavirin. J Infect Dis. 1980;141:580–589.
470. Gruber WC, Wilson SZ, Throop BJ, et al. Immunoglobulin administration and ribavirin therapy: Efficacy in respiratory syncytial virus infection of the cotton rat. Pediatr Res. 1987;21:270–274.
471. Hayden FG. Combination antiviral therapy for respiratory virus infections. Antiviral Res. 1996;29:45–48.
472. Smee DF, Matthews TR. Metabolism of ribavirin in respiratory syncytial virus-infected and uninfected cells. Antimicrob Agents Chemother. 1986;30:117–121.
473. Wray SK, Gilbert BE, Knight V. Effect of ribavirin triphosphate on primer generation and elongation during influenza virus transcription in vitro. Antiviral Res. 1985;5:39–48.
474. Fernandez-Larsson R, Patterson JL. Ribavirin is an inhibitor of human immunodeficiency virus reverse transcriptase. Mol Pharmacol. 1990;38:766–770.
475. Peavy DL, Powers CN, Knight V. Inhibition of murine plaque-forming cell responses in vivo by ribavirin. J Immunol. 1981;126:861–864.
476. Potter CW, Phair JP, Vodinelich L, et al. Antiviral, immunosuppressive and antitumour effects of ribavirin. Nature. 1976;259:496–497.
477. Scheidel LM, Durbin RK, Stollar V. Sindbis virus mutants resistant to mycophenolic acid and ribavirin. Virology. 1987;158:1–7.
478. Hall CB, McBride JT, Walsh EE, et al. Aerosolized ribavirin treatment of infants with respiratory syncytial viral infection. A randomized double-blind study. N Engl J Med. 1983;308:1443–1447.
479. Laskin OL, Longstreth JA, Hart CC, et al. Ribavirin disposition in high-risk patients for acquired immunodeficiency syndrome. Clin Pharmacol Ther. 1987;41:546–555.
480. Connor E, Morrison S, Lane J, et al. Safety, tolerance, and pharmacokinetics of systemic ribavirin in children with human immunodeficiency virus infection. Antimicrob Agents Chemother. 1993;37:532–539.
481. Paroni R, Del PM, Borghi C, Sirtori CR, et al. Pharmacokinetics of ribavirin and urinary excretion of the major metabolite 1,2,4-triazole-3-carboxamide in normal volunteers. Int J Clin Pharmacol Ther Toxicol. 1989;27:302–307.
482. Connor JD, Hintz M, Van Dyke R. Ribavirin pharmacokinetics in children and adults during therapeutic trials. In: Smith RA, Knight V, Smith J, eds. Clinical Applications of Ribavirin. Orlando, FL: Academic Press; 1984:107–123.
483. Kramer TH, Gaar GG, Ray CG, et al. Hemodialysis clearance of intravenously administered ribavirin. Antimicrob Agents Chemother. 1990;34:489–490.
484. Knight V, Yu CP, Gilbert BE, et al. Estimating the dosage of ribavirin aerosol according to age and other variables. J Infect Dis. 1988;158:443–448.
485. Hillyared IW. The preclinical toxicology and safety of ribavirin. In: Smith RA, Kirkpatrick W, eds. Ribavirin: A Broad Spectrum Antiviral Agent. Smith New York: Academic Press; 1980:59.
486. Di Bisceglie AM, Conjeevaram HS, Fried MW, et al. Ribavirin as therapy for chronic hepatitis C: A randomized, double-blind, placebo-controlled trial. Ann Intern Med. 1995;123:897–903.
487. Fisher-Hoch SP, Gborie S, Parker L. Unexpected adverse reactions during a clinical trial in rural West Africa. Antiviral Rev. 1992;19:139–147.
488. Titus BJ, Perez AF, Arcala BI. Water intoxication after nebulised tribavirin. Lancet. 1995;345:1116.
489. Rodriguez WJ, Bui RH, Connor JD, et al. Environmental exposure of primary care personnel to ribavirin aerosol when supervising treatment of infants with respiratory syncytial virus infections. Antimicrob Agents Chemother. 1987;31:1143–1146.
490. Gladu JM, Ecobichon DJ. Evaluation of exposure of health care personnel to ribavirin. J Toxicol Environ Health. 1989;28:1–12.
491. Bradley JS, Connor JD, Compogiannis LS, et al. Exposure of health care workers to ribavirin during therapy for respiratory syncytial virus infections. Antimicrob Agents Chemother. 1990;34:668–670.
492. Shults RA, Baron S, Decker J, et al. Health care worker exposure to aerosolized ribavirin: Biological and air monitoring. J Occup Environ Med. 1996;38:257–263.
493. Frankel LR, Wilson CW, Demers RR, et al. A technique for the administration of ribavirin to mechanically ventilated infants with severe respiratory syncytial virus infection. Crit Care Med. 1987;15:1051–1054.
494. Outwater KM, Meissner HC, Peterson MB. Ribavirin administration to infants receiving mechanical ventilation. Am J Dis Child. 1988;142:512–515.
495. Randolph AG, Wang EE. Ribavirin for respiratory syncytial virus lower respiratory tract infection: A systematic overview. Arch Pediatr Adolesc Med. 1996;150:942–947.
496. Moler FW, Steinhart CM, Ohmit SE, Stidham GL. Effectiveness of ribavirin in otherwise well infants with respiratory syncytial virus–associated respiratory failure. Pediatric Critical Study Group. J Pediatr. 1996;128:422–428.
497. Smith DW, Frankel LR, Mathers LH, et al. A controlled trial of aerosolized ribavirin in infants receiving mechanical ventilation for severe respiratory syncytial virus infection. N Engl J Med. 1991;325:24–29.
498. Englund JA, Piedra PA, Jefferson LS, et al. High-dose, short-duration ribavirin aerosol therapy in children with suspected respiratory syncytial virus infection. J Pediatr. 1990;117:313–320.
499. Committee on Infectious Diseases. Reassessment of the indications for ribavirin therapy in respiratory syncytial virus infections: American Academy of Pediatrics Committee on Infectious Diseases. Pediatrics. 1996;97:137–140.
500. Rosner IK, Welliver RC, Edelson PJ, et al. Effect of ribavirin therapy on respiratory syncytial virus-specific IgE and IgA responses after infection. J Infect Dis. 1987;155:1043–1047.
501. Long CE, Voter KZ, Barker WH, et al. Long term follow-up of children hospitalized with respiratory syncytial virus lower respiratory tract infection and randomly treated with ribavirin or placebo. Pediatr Infect Dis J. 1997;16:1023–1028.
502. Whimbey E, Champlin RE, Englund JA, et al. Combination therapy with aerosolized ribavirin and intravenous immunoglobulin for respiratory syncytial virus disease in adult bone marrow transplant recipients. Bone Marrow Transplant. 1995;16:393–399.
503. Lewinsohn DM, Bowden RA, Mattson D, et al. Phase I study of intravenous ribavirin treatment of respiratory syncytial virus pneumonia after marrow transplantation. Antimicrob Agents Chemother. 1996;40:2555–2557.
504. Knight V, Gilbert BE. Ribavirin aerosol treatment of influenza (Review) Infect Dis Clin North Am. 1987;1:441–457.
505. Ray CG, Icenogle TB, Minnich LL, et al. The use of intravenous ribavirin to treat influenza virus-associated acute myocarditis [published erratum appears in J Infect Dis 1989;160:564]. J Infect Dis. 1989;159:829–836.
506. Bernstein DI, Reuman PD, Sherwood JR, et al. Ribavirin small-particle-aerosol treatment of influenza B virus infection. Antimicrob Agents Chemother. 1988;32:761–764.
507. Stein DS, Creticos CM, Jackson GG, et al. Oral ribavirin treatment of influenza A and B. Antimicrob Agents Chemother. 1987;31:1285–1287.
508. Wendt CH, Weisdorf DJ, Jordan MC, et al. Parainfluenza virus respiratory infection after bone marrow transplantation. N Engl J Med. 1992;326:921–926.
509. Kaplan LJ, Daum RS, Smaron M, et al. Severe measles in immunocompromised patients (Review) JAMA. 1992;267:1237–1241.
510. Gururangan S, Stevens RF, Morris DJ. Ribavirin response in measles pneumonia. J Infect. 1990;20:219–221.
511. Maslo C, Girard PM, Urban T, et al. Ribavirin therapy for adenovirus pneumonia in an AIDS patient. Am J Respir Crit Care Med. 1997;156:1263–1264.
512. Kesson AM, Ferguson JK, Rawlinson WD, et al. Progressive vaccinia treated with ribavirin and vaccinia immune globulin. Clin Infect Dis. 1997;25:911–914.
513. McCormick JB, King IJ, Webb PA, et al. Lassa fever: Effective therapy with ribavirin. N Engl J Med. 1986;314:20–26.
514. Huggins JW, Hsiang CM, Cosgriff TM, et al. Prospective, double-blind, concurrent, placebo-controlled clinical trial of intravenous ribavirin therapy of hemorrhagic fever with renal syndrome. J Infect Dis. 1991;164:1119–1127.
515. Kilgore PE, Ksiazek TG, Rollin PE, et al. Treatment of Bolivian hemorrhagic fever with intravenous ribavirin. Clin Infect Dis. 1997;24:718–722.
516. Enria DA, Maiztegui JI. Antiviral treatment of Argentine hemorrhagic fever. Antiviral Res. 1994;23:23–31.
517. Fisher-Hoch SP, Khan JA, Rehman S, et al. Crimean-Congo haemorrhagic fever treated with oral ribavirin. Lancet. 1995;346:472–475.
518. Holmes GP, McCormick JB, Trock SC, et al. Lassa fever in the United States: Investigation of a case and new guidelines for management [see comments]. N Engl J Med. 1990;323:1120–1123.
519. Japour AJ, Lertora JJ, Meehan PM, et al. A phase-I study of the safety, pharmacokinetics, and antiviral activity of combination didanosine and ribavirin in patients with HIV-1 disease. AIDS Clinical Trials Group 231 Protocol Team. J Acquir Immune Def Syndr Hum Retrovirol. 1996;13:235–246.
520. Bodenheimer HJ, Lindsay KL, Davis GL, et al. Tolerance and efficacy of oral ribavirin treatment of chronic hepatitis C: A multicenter trial. Hepatology. 1997;26:473–477.
521. Carmine AA, Brogden RN, Heel RC, et al. Trifluridine: a review of its antiviral activity and therapeutic use in the topical treatment of viral eye infections. Drugs. 1982;23:329–353.
522. Spector SA, Tyndall M, Kelley E. Inhibition of human cytomegalovirus by trifluorothymidine. Antimicrob Agents Chemother. 1983;23:113–118.
523. van Bijsterveld OP, Post H. Trifluorothymidine versus adenine arabinoside in the treatment of herpes simplex keratitis. Br J Ophthalmol. 1980;64:33–36.
524. Kessler HA, Hurwitz S, Farthing C, et al. Pilot study of topical trifluridine for the treatment of acyclovir-resistant mucocutaneous herpes simplex disease in patients with AIDS (ACTG 172): AIDS Clinical Trials Group. J Acquir Immune Def Syndr Hum Retrovirol. 1996;12:147–152.
525. de Koning EW, van Bijsterveld OP, Cantell K. Combination therapy for dendritic keratitis with human leucocyte interferon and trifluorothymidine. Br J Ophthalmol. 1982;66:509–512.
526. Whitley R, Alford C, Hess F, et al. Vidarabine: A preliminary review of its pharmacological properties and therapeutic use. Drugs. 1980;20:267–282.
527. Nagahata T, Kitagawa M, Matsubara K. Effect of oxetanocin G, a novel nucleoside analog, on DNA synthesis by hepatitis B virus virons. Antimicrob Agents Chemother. 1994;38:707–712.
528. Mariod PL, Colonno RJ. Evaluation of BMS-200475 and lobucavir in the duck model of hepatitis B virus infection. Abstract H-49. Abstracts of the 38th Interscience Conference on Antimicrobial Agents and Chemotherapy, 1998;329.
529. Terry BJ, Cianci CW, Hagen ME. Inhibition of herpes simplex virus type 1 DNA polymerase by [1R(1 alpha,2 beta,3 alpha)]-9-[2,3-bis(hydroxymethyl]cyclobutyl] guanine. Mol Pharmacol. 1991;40:591–596.
530. Izuta S, Shimada N, Kitagawa M, et al. Inhibitory effects of triphosphate derivatives of oxetanocin G and related compounds on eukaryotic and viral DNA polymerases and human immunodeficiency virus reverse transcriptase. J Biochem. 1992;112:81–87.
531. Lalezari J, Drew WL, Jordan C. In vivo anti-CMV activity and safety of oral lobucavir in HIV-infected patients (protocol AI459-007). Abstract 301. Abstracts of the 4th Conference on Retroviruses and Opportunistic Infections, 1997.

532. Sherman M, Chan R, Kwan S, et al. Lobucavir treatment for chronic hepatitis B infection: A placebo-controlled phase 1/2 study. Abstract H-32. Abstracts of the 37th Interscience Conference on Antimicrobial Agents and Chemotherapy, 1997;219.
533. Wilber R, Buffington D, Tyring S, et al. Efficacy and safety of oral lobucavir (LBV) in patients with recurrent genital herpes. Abstract H-86. Abstracts of the 38th Interscience Conference on Antimicrobial Agents and Chemotherapy, 1998;339.
534. Schiff GM, Sherwood JR: Oral Efficacy of VP 63843. Abstracts of the 36th Interscience Conference on Antimicrobial Agents and Chemotherapy 1996; 171 (Abstract H43).
535. Weiner LB, Rotbart HA, Mynhardt JH, et al. Treatment of enterovirus meningitis with pleconaril (VP 63843), an antipicornaviral agent. 37th ICAAC Program Addendum 1997; 14 (Abstract LB-27).
536. von Itzstein M, Wu WY, Kok GB, et al. Rational design of potent sialidase-based inhibitors of influenza virus replication. Nature. 1993;363:418–423.
537. Kim CU, Lew W, Williams MA, et al. Influenza neuraminidase inhibitors possessing a novel hydrophobic interaction in the enzyme active site: Design, synthesis, and structural analysis of carbocyclic sialic acid analogues with potent anti-influenza activity. J Am Chem Soc. 1997;119:681–690.
538. Mendel DB, Tai CY, Escarpe PA, et al. Oral administration of a prodrug of the influenza virus neuraminidase inhibitor GS4071 protects mice and ferrets against influenza infection. Antimicrob Agents Chemother. 1998;42:640–646.
539. Woods JM, Bethell RC, Coates JA, et al. 4-Guanidino-2,4-dideoxy-2,3-dehydro-*N*-acetylneuraminic acid is a highly effective inhibitor both of the sialidase (neuraminidase) and of growth of a wide range of influenza A and B viruses in vitro. Antimicrob Agents Chemother. 1993;37:1473–1479.
540. Sidwell RW, Huffman JH, Barnard DL, et al. Inhibition of influenza virus infections in mice by GS4104, an orally effective influenza virus neuraminidase inhibitor. Antiviral Res. 1998;37:107–120.
541. Calfee DP, Hayden FG. New approaches to influenza chemotherapy. Neuraminidase inhibitors. Drugs. 1998;56:537–553.
542. Colman PM. Influenza virus neuraminidase: Structure, antibodies, and inhibitors. Protein Science. 1994;3:1687–1696.
543. Mendel DB, Sidwell RW. Influenza virus resistance to neuraminidase inhibitors. Drug Resistance Updates. 1998;1:184–189.
544. Gubareva LV, Robinson MJ, Bethell RC, Webster RG. Catalytic and framework mutations in the neuraminidase active site of influenza viruses that are resistant to 4-guanidino-Neu5Ac2en. J Virol. 1997;71:3385–3390.
545. Gubareva LV, Matrosovich MN, Brenner MK, et al. Evidence for zanamivir resistance in an immunocompromised child infected with influenza B virus. J Infect Dis. 1998;178:1257–1262.
546. Waghorn SL, Goa KL. Zanamivir. Drugs. 1998;55:722–725.
547. Newman SP, Brown J, Pickford M, et al. Deposition pattern in the respiratory tract of the neuraminidase inhibitor zanamivir: A gamma scintigraphic study. Abstract H-134. Abstracts of the 37th Interscience Conference on Antimicrobial Agents and Chemotherapy, 1997;237.
548. Wood ND, Aitken M, Sharp S, Evison H. Tolerability and pharmacokinetics of the influenza neuraminidase inhibitor Ro-64-0802 (GS4071) following oral administration of the prodrug Ro-64-0796 (GS4104) to healthy male volunteers. Abstract A-123. Abstracts of the 37th Interscience Conference on Antimicrobial Agents and Chemotherapy, 1997;25.
549. Eisenberg G, Bidgood A, Lynch G, et al. Penetration of GS4071, a novel influenza neuraminidase inhibitor, into rat bronchoalveolar lining fluid following oral administration of the prodrug GS4104. Antimicrob Agents Chemother. 1997;41:1949–1952.
550. Hayden FG, Osterhaus ADME, Treanor JJ, et al. Efficacy and safety of the neuraminidase inhibitor zanamivir in the treatment of influenza virus infections. N Engl J Med. 1997;337:874–879.
551. MIST Study Group. Randomized trial of efficacy and safety of inhaled zanamivir in treatment of influenza A and B virus infections. Lancet. 1998;352:1877–1881.
552. Hayden FG, Treanor JJ, Betts RF, et al. Safety and efficacy of the neuraminidase inhibitor GG167 in experimental human influenza. JAMA. 1996;275:295–299.
553. Walker JB, Hussey EK, Treanor JJ, et al. Effects of the neuraminidase inhibitor zanamivir on otologic manifestations of experimental human influenza. J Infect Dis. 1997;176:1417–1422.
554. Hayden FG, Lobo M, Treanor JJ, et al. Efficacy and tolerability of oral GS4104 for early treatment of experimental influenza in humans. Abstract LB-26. Abstracts of the 37th Interscience Conference on Antimicrobial Agents and Chemotherapy, 1997;14.
555. Calfee DP, Peng AW, Cass L, et al. Protective efficacy of intravenous zanamivir in experimental human influenza. Abstract H-58. Abstracts of the 38th Interscience Conference on Antimicrobial Agents and Chemotherapy, 1998;332.
556. Treanor JJ, Vrooman PS, Hayden FG, et al. Efficacy of oral GS4104 in treating acute influenza. Abstract LB-4. Final Program, Abstracts and Exhibits Addendum: 38th Annual Intercontinental Conference on Antimicrobial Agents and Chemotherapy. San Diego, 1998;1998;21.
557. Hayden FG, Atmar RL, Schilling M, et al. Safety and efficacy of oral GS4104 in long-term prophylaxis of natural influenza. Abstract LB-6. Final Program, Abstracts and Exhibits Addendum: 38th Annual Intercontinental Conference on Antimicrobial Agents and Chemotherapy, San Diego, 1998;1998;22 (Abstract LB-7).
558. Monto AS, Robinson DP, Herlocher L, et al. Efficacy and safety of zanamivir in prevention of influenza among healthy adults. Final Program, Abstracts and Exhibits Addendum: 38th Annual Intercontinental Conference on Antimicrobial Agents and Chemotherapy, San Diego, 1998.
559. Cherrington JM, Miner R, Hitchcock MJ, et al. Susceptibility of human cytomegalovirus to cidofovir is unchanged after limited in vivo exposure to various regimens of drug. J Infect Dis. 1996;173:987–992.
560. Mendel DB, Barkhimer DB, Chen MS. Biochemical basis for increases in susceptibility to cidofovir of herpes simplex viruses with altered or deficient thymidine kinase activity. Antimicrob Agents Chemother. 1995;39:2120–2122.
561. Stathoulopoulou F, Almond MK, Dhillon S, et al. Clinical pharmacokinetics of oral acyclovir in patients on continuous ambulatory peritoneal dialysis. Nephron. 1996;74:337–341.
562. Filler G, Lampe D, von BA, et al. Prophylactic oral ganciclovir after renal transplantation-dosing and pharmacokinetics. Pediatr Nephrol. 1998;12:6–9.

Chapter 37

Immunomodulators

MICHAEL O. FRANK
GERALD L. MANDELL

Traditional strategies for the treatment and prevention of infectious diseases have centered on antimicrobial agents and vaccines, and both have produced considerable success. Yet many infections remain a difficult problem. Treatment may be complicated by a compromised immune system resulting from either an underlying disease or the treatment thereof. In these circumstances it may be helpful to enhance the activity of the immune system. In contrast, there are situations such as sepsis in which the body's defense systems have gone awry with an overzealous release of inflammatory cytokines, and here a dampening of activation may be beneficial.

Immunomodulators are also known as *biologic response modifiers* or *biologic therapeutics*. Fauci defined an immunomodulator as "a biological or nonbiological substance that directly influences a specific immune function or modifies one or more components of the immunoregulatory network to achieve an indirect effect on a specific immune function."[1] The immunoregulatory network is a complex and intricate system involving a wide variety of cell types and cytokines. As knowledge of this system grows, rational approaches to modulating its activity are becoming possible. In the near future combinations of cytokines, antibodies, and synthetic compounds may be used to "fine tune" the immune response, adjusting it as needed for a given infection. Many of these products are expensive, and cost-effectiveness is an important determinant of use.

Immunomodulators can be divided into five main groups: (1) naturally occurring cytokines, including the colony-stimulating factors (CSFs), interferons (IFNs), and thymic hormones; (2) monoclonal antibodies and receptor antagonists that block inflammatory cytokines; (3) immunoglobulins, used either as replacements in immunoglobulin-deficient patients or as true immunomodulators to upregulate or downregulate the immune response; (4) corticosteroids at higher than physiologic replacement doses; and (5) synthetic compounds with immunomodulatory effects, such as pentoxifylline, thalidomide, and imiquimod. Agents used to treat sepsis, such as antibodies to endotoxin and to inflammatory cytokines and interleukin-1 (IL-1) receptor antagonists, are discussed in Chapter 63.

This chapter focuses on agents that have been used to manipulate the immune system for the treatment or prevention of infection. There are many potentially useful immunomodulators that have undergone only in vitro or animal model experiments. Because of the complex interactions of the various components of the immune response, in vitro data often do not correlate with in vivo results. Furthermore, animal models, although useful for preliminary testing, have a number of limitations affecting their applicability to human disease states.[2] Therefore, this discussion is limited to agents that have undergone (or are currently undergoing) clinical trials in humans. Table 37–1 lists those immunomodulators that have been approved by the U.S. Food and Drug Administration (FDA) for the prevention or treatment of infections.

TABLE 37–1 U.S. Food and Drug Administration–Approved Uses of Immunomodulators to Treat Infection

Generic Names	Brand Names	Indications
Granulocyte colony-stimulating factor (filgrastim)	Neupogen	Prevention of infection in neutropenia caused by chemotherapy or bone marrow transplantation or in congenital, cyclic, or idiopathic neutropenia
Granulocyte-macrophage colony-stimulating factor (sargramostim)	Leukine	Prevention of infection after bone marrow or peripheral stem cell transplantation or after chemotherapy for acute myelogenous leukemia in patients older than 55 years of age
Interferon alfa		Treatment of Kaposi's sarcoma in the acquired immunodeficiency syndrome (AIDS), of chronic hepatitis B and C, and of genital or perianal warts
Interferon alfa-2a	Roferon-A	
Interferon alfa-2b	Intron A	
Interferon alfacon-1	Infergen	
Interferon alfa-n3	Alferon-N	
Intravenous immunoglobulin	Gamimune	Prevention of infection in patients with primary antibody-deficiency syndromes, after bone marrow transplantation, and in children with AIDS
	Gammagard	
	Gammar	
	Iveegam	
	Polygam	
	Sandoglobulin	
	Venoglobulin	
Imiquimod	Aldara	Treatment of genital or perianal warts

COLONY-STIMULATING FACTORS

CSFs are a group of naturally occurring glycoproteins that are involved in the production, differentiation, survival, and activation of the myeloid line of blood cells. At present there are seven known CSFs with differing degrees of relative activity on the various cell types: granulocyte colony-stimulating factor (G-CSF), granulocyte-macrophage colony-stimulating factor (GM-CSF), macrophage colony-stimulating factor (M-CSF), IL-3, IL-5, thrombopoietin, and erythropoietin. Erythropoietin stimulates growth of red blood cells and thrombopoietin that of megakaryocytes. IL-5 stimulates growth of eosinophils and basophils, and IL-3, which was formerly known as multicolony-stimulating factor, appears to be a stimulator of multiple cell lineages.

Granulocyte Colony-Stimulating Factor

G-CSF is a 174-amino-acid glycoprotein that predominantly affects the neutrophil cell line. It is available in recombinant form with the generic name filgrastim and the brand name Neupogen (Amgen) in the United States and outside the United States as lenograstim. Lenograstim differs from filgrastim in that it is produced in Chinese hamster ovary cells and is glycosylated, whereas filgrastim is produced in *Escherichia coli* and is nonglycosylated. Clinical trials have shown similar benefits and adverse effects for lenograstim and filgrastim.[3] The most immediate effect of G-CSF is actually a transient decrease in neutrophil count 5 to 60 minutes after administration; this is followed by a sustained dose-dependent rise in neutrophil levels over a 5- to 6-day course. Neutrophil counts stabilize or decrease slightly if G-CSF is continued for a 2-week course and return to baseline in 4 to 7 days after its discontinuation. The increase in neutrophil count is primarily caused by an increase in the rate of production with a shortened maturation time; no change in the half-life of neutrophils in circulation has been noted. At doses higher than 10 μg/kg/day, slight increases in monocyte and lymphocyte counts are also seen, and doses greater than 30 μg/kg/day for 2 weeks have been associated with small decreases in number of platelets.[4]

The first FDA-approved use of G-CSF was in neutropenia after cancer chemotherapy, where the risk of infection is related to both the degree and the duration of neutropenia. In a randomized, double-blind, placebo-controlled trial in patients receiving cytotoxic chemotherapy for small cell lung cancer, G-CSF was given for 8 to 13 days, beginning the day after the last dose of chemotherapy. G-CSF reduced the severity and duration of neutropenia and also decreased the incidence of fever, infections, hospitalization and antibiotic use, the duration of antibiotic use, and the duration of hospitalization. There was no effect on mortality. The benefit was sustained over several cycles of chemotherapy.[5] There are now many other studies showing similar benefits of G-CSF in neutropenia (for reviews see Nemunaitis[6] and Lifton and Bennett[7]), although only one study has shown a benefit in overall survival.[8]

Because of its high cost and the lack of a survival benefit, the routine use of G-CSF after chemotherapy has been controversial.[9] In 1994, the American Society of Clinical Oncology published recommendations regarding the use of CSFs after chemotherapy.[10] These recommendations included reserving G-CSF for use in patients receiving chemotherapy regimens associated with a 40% or higher rate of febrile neutropenia, or in patients with additional risk factors including previous episodes of febrile neutropenia. There is no clinical evidence to support the theoretical concern that use of G-CSF may increase relapse rates when used in patients with leukemia. In a study of elderly leukemia patients, G-CSF did not reduce infections.[11]

G-CSF has also been used after both allogeneic and autologous bone marrow transplantation, where it was found to increase the rate of recovery of neutrophils and to shorten the duration of parenteral antibiotics and the time in isolation, without affecting rates of graft-versus-host (GVH) disease, relapse, or graft failure.[6, 12, 13] An economic analysis of the use of G-CSF after autologous bone marrow transplantation suggested a reduction of 3% in overall costs compared with usual care.[14]

Neutropenia is relatively common in human immunodeficiency virus (HIV) infection, especially in patients receiving zidovudine or ganciclovir. When an alternative therapy cannot be used, G-CSF may raise the neutrophil count sufficiently to allow continuation of these medications. In 14 patients with acquired immunodeficiency syndrome (AIDS), G-CSF produced a dose-dependent rise in neutrophil levels, with continuation of zidovudine, without affecting CD4 or p24 antigen levels.[15] G-CSF may also be useful in neutropenia associated with HIV in general. In a prospective, randomized, but open-label trial of more than 200 patients, G-CSF decreased rates of neutropenia and bacterial infections and days of hospitalization and antibiotics.[16] However, most of the patients were not receiving prophylaxis for *Mycobacterium avium* complex (MAC), which was the most common infection seen. HIV viral loads were measured in a subset of patients and were not different between the two groups. There is also a report of an HIV-infected patient with refractory oral aphthous ulcers that responded to treatment with G-CSF.[17]

Other neutropenic states in which G-CSF has been found to raise neutrophil counts and decrease infections, hospitalizations, and days of antibiotics include cyclic neutropenia, idiopathic neutropenia, and congenital chronic neutropenia.[6, 18, 19] G-CSF is often used with antibiotics for treatment (as opposed to prevention) of febrile neutropenia, although there are no controlled data for its use in this setting. There are case reports of the use of G-CSF together with antifungal therapy for treatment of fungal infections complicating neutropenia.[20, 21] Whether G-CSF would be of benefit in non-neutropenic patients with serious infections (e.g., in diabetic patients, burn patients, fungal infections, postoperative infections) is not known, and investigation of these potential uses is underway. G-CSF has been studied in 37 patients after liver transplantation.[22] Compared with historical controls, the G-CSF–treated patients had decreased episodes of sepsis, sepsis-related mortality, and acute rejection. G-CSF plus antibiotics and débridement resulted in more rapid healing than placebo plus antibiotics and débridement for severe foot infections in patients with diabetes mellitus.[23]

G-CSF has been studied in treatment of pneumonia in a phase III double-blind, placebo-controlled, multicenter study. A total of 756 patients with acute community-acquired pneumonia were enrolled and were given either placebo or 300 μg G-CSF daily for an average of 4 days in addition to antibiotics. There was no effect on mortality (6.1% with G-CSF versus 6.4% with placebo). However, there were 14 episodes of the acute respiratory distress syndrome in the placebo group and only 4 in the G-CSF group ($p = .017$). There was an indication of benefit in the subset of 261 patients with multilobar pneumonia, with 17.1% of the placebo group developing organ dysfunction or empyema and only 5.8% of the G-CSF group developing these complications. Studies of the efficacy of G-CSF for multilobar pneumonia and pneumonia with sepsis syndrome are underway.[24]

Dosage. The recommended dosage of G-CSF for high-risk patients after cytotoxic cancer chemotherapy is 5 μg/kg/day subcutaneously or intravenously, starting the day after the last chemotherapy dose, with subsequent individualized adjustment of dosage depending on response. After bone marrow transplantation, the manufacturer recommends administering a dose of 10 μg/kg/day subcutaneously or intravenously until the absolute neutrophil count is greater than 1000/mm^3 for 3 consecutive days, then reducing the dose to 5 μg/kg/day, and discontinuing if the neutrophil count remains greater than 1000/mm^3. For treatment of cyclic or idiopathic neutropenia, the initial dosage is 5 μg/kg/day subcutaneously. For congenital neutropenia, which often requires higher doses, treatment should begin at 6 μg/kg twice daily. Maintenance treatment is generally required for these conditions, and the dosage should be individualized based on the response. In patients with neutropenia and HIV infection, lower doses are often sufficient; an initial dose can be 1 μg/kg/day subcutaneously, with increases up to 10 μg/kg/day as needed. Maintenance doses should be adjusted based on neutrophil counts; often less than 1 μg/kg/day or administration only two to three times per week is necessary to maintain an absolute neutrophil count greater than 1000/mm^3. For example, in the HIV study with more than 200 patients, the median dose of G-CSF necessary to maintain a neutrophil count higher than 2000/mm^3 was 300 μg twice weekly.[16]

Adverse Effects. G-CSF is usually well tolerated. Bone pain is the most common adverse effect, occurring in about 20% of patients.[5] It is usually mild and transient and can be treated with simple analgesics. Other adverse effects have included mild local erythema and swelling at sites of injection; asymptomatic elevations of lactate dehydrogenase, alkaline phosphatase, and leukocyte alkaline phosphatase; splenomegaly (in up to one third of children receiving chronic therapy for chronic neutropenia—only 10% of these were symptomatic); and isolated reports of Sweet's syndrome and leukocytoclastic vasculitis.[25]

Granulocyte-Macrophage Colony-Stimulating Factor

GM-CSF is a 127-amino-acid glycoprotein available as a recombinant product with the generic name sargramostim. The FDA-approved form of recombinant human GM-CSF is a yeast product manufactured by Immunex and marketed as Leukine. Other forms of recombinant GM-CSF include molgramostim from *E. coli* and regramostim from mammalian cells. GM-CSF raises counts of monocytes and eosinophils, in addition to neutrophils, in peripheral blood. As with G-CSF, a transient decrease in leukocytes is seen immediately after administration. Unlike G-CSF, GM-CSF does not appear to shorten the maturation time of neutrophils but prolongs their half-life in the circulation and increases their rate of production. A transient decrease in platelets has also been seen, especially at higher doses.[4]

GM-CSF was first shown to be beneficial in patients undergoing autologous bone marrow transplantation. When given for 3 weeks after bone marrow transplantation for lymphoid malignancies, GM-CSF accelerated neutrophil recovery and shortened the duration of antibiotic administration and hospitalization.[26] There was no change in the frequency of infection or fever and no effect on survival. GM-CSF may also be useful after bone marrow transplantation for other (nonlymphoid) malignancies or in peripheral stem cell transplantation.[27] A placebo-controlled trial in patients undergoing peripheral stem cell transplantation for lymphoma found that GM-CSF decreased the duration of neutropenia and the incidence of bacterial infections and enhanced engraftment, without affecting relapse or survival rates.[28] Several additional studies have now confirmed the benefit of GM-CSF in autologous bone marrow or peripheral stem cell transplantation.[6]

Whether GM-CSF is beneficial in allogeneic bone marrow transplantation is less clear, especially when donor and recipient are unrelated. There has been a theoretical concern that GM-CSF therapy may result in an increased incidence of GVH disease, but this has not been documented. Several small studies of GM-CSF in allogeneic bone marrow transplantation have not consistently shown a benefit.[29] In studies of transplantations between human leukocyte antigen (HLA)–identical siblings, one trial found a difference in outcome depending on the regimen used for prevention of GVH disease. In patients who received cyclosporine and prednisone, GM-CSF shortened the time to engraftment and decreased the incidence of early infection (compared with historical controls) without affecting the incidence of GVH disease. However, in patients who received cyclosporine and methotrexate, a minimal effect on neutrophil recovery was noted.[30] Prospective randomized, placebo-controlled trials have now been performed using GM-CSF in cases of matched sibling allogeneic bone marrow transplantation[6]; the largest of these found reductions in incidence of bacteremia and infections overall, with no change in rates of GVH disease, relapse, or survival.[31]

Like G-CSF, GM-CSF has been used for neutropenia after chemotherapy for solid tumors, with decreases in duration of neutropenia, number of infections, and length of hospitalizations.[32, 33] In patients receiving chemotherapy for leukemia, a decreased incidence of infection was seen in one study with the use of G-CSF,[34] but not in another study involving only elderly patients.[35]

The use of GM-CSF in patients with AIDS has been controversial because of early data showing increased HIV replication in monocytes stimulated with GM-CSF in vitro and increased p24 antigen levels in some patients treated with GM-CSF. However, it appears that this may be offset by the concomitant use of antiretroviral therapy. GM-CSF increases intracellular concentrations of zidovudine, the combination appears to be synergistic in inhibiting HIV replication in vitro, and in vivo no effect on HIV levels as measured by the polymerase chain reaction was noted.[3, 36, 37] GM-CSF does raise numbers of neutrophils, monocytes, and eosinophils in patients with AIDS, and in some patients functional neutrophil defects have also been corrected with administration of GM-CSF.[38] Use of GM-CSF has been reported as adjunctive therapy in eight patients with AIDS and disseminated MAC infection[39] and in two patients with AIDS and cryptococcal meningitis.[40]

The potential use of GM-CSF in the treatment of other infections is also being investigated. The addition of GM-CSF to antibiotics for treatment of febrile neutropenia was evaluated in a prospective randomized trial of 107 cancer patients. Although there was a significant improvement in response rate with GM-CSF among the evaluable patients, the difference was not significant in an intention-to-treat analysis.[41] The combination of GM-CSF, granulocyte transfusions, and amphotericin B was used successfully to treat invasive *Candida* infection in one patient after bone marrow transplantation[42] and disseminated *Fusarium* infection in another patient after chemotherapy for relapse of leukemia.[43] GM-CSF was also used to treat frequent infections in two children with glycogen storage disease type 1b, although continued administration resulted in severe reactions in one patient.[44] Both GM-CSF and G-CSF have undergone preliminary investigation as combination therapy with IFN to treat chronic infections with hepatitis B virus (HBV) and hepatitis C virus (HCV).[45, 46]

Dosage. A variety of dosing regimens (generally 0.3 to 10 μg/kg/day) have been used in studies. The current manufacturer's (Immunex) recommendation for use in bone marrow transplantation is a dose of 250 μg/m²/day, given as a 2- to 4-hour intravenous infusion starting 2 to 4 hours after bone marrow infusion and continuing until the absolute neutrophil count is greater than 1500/mm³ for three consecutive days. The same daily dose and duration is recommended after peripheral stem cell transplantation, given intravenously over 24 hours or subcutaneously beginning immediately after stem cell infusion, and after induction chemotherapy for leukemia, beginning 4 days after completion of chemotherapy.

Adverse Effects. Toxicity is more common and more severe than for G-CSF, is dose related, and is greater with intravenous than with subcutaneous administration. A first-dose reaction can occur, with flushing, tachycardia, hypotension, dyspnea, hypoxemia, myalgias, and nausea and vomiting. Other adverse effects include fever and chills (especially with doses higher than 3 μg/kg), lethargy, bone pain, anorexia, and rash; although these occur in one half or more of patients who received GM-CSF, they are also common after bone marrow transplantation, and the true incidence attributable to GM-CSF is difficult to determine. In some placebo-controlled studies of GM-CSF, adverse effect rates have been similar to those seen with placebo. At doses greater than 20 μg/kg/day, fluid retention, pleural and pericardial effusions, and venous thrombosis may occur. Reactivation of idiopathic thrombocytopenic purpura, rheumatoid arthritis, autoimmune thyroiditis, and hemolysis have also been reported.[4]

Macrophage Colony-Stimulating Factor

M-CSF is a glycoprotein that stimulates production of the monocyte-macrophage line and enhances monocyte and macrophage activity in vitro. It has received interest primarily as a possible adjunctive treatment for fungal infections.[47] A phase 1 trial of recombinant human M-CSF in patients with invasive fungal infections after bone marrow transplantation has been reported.[48] Doses ranged from 100 to 2000 μg/m²/day intravenously. The only significant toxicity reported was transient dose-related thrombocytopenia. There was no apparent effect on incidence of GVH disease or change in numbers of neutrophils, monocytes, or lymphocytes. Of the 12 evaluable patients, 6 had resolution of fungal infections, which was thought to be a better response rate than that of historical controls. After the completion of this trial, the authors treated an additional 22 patients and pooled the two sets of results for comparison with historical controls.[49] Significant improvement in survival was noted, but only in the subgroup of patients with Karnofsky scores higher than 20 and *Candida* infections. M-CSF is available in Japan in highly purified but not recombinant form. There it has indications for use in allogeneic bone marrow transplantation, acute myelogenous leukemia, and ovarian cancer chemotherapy, and is administered at a rate of 8 million IU/day intravenously for 14 days.

INTERFERONS

IFNs are protein cytokines produced by cells in response to a variety of stimuli, including viral infections and certain intracellular organisms and bacterial toxins. IFNs play a complex role in the immune response, often augmenting the effects of interleukins. There are three main classes of IFNs: IFN-α and IFN-β are produced by many cell types but primarily by leukocytes and fibroblasts, respectively; IFN-γ is produced by T lymphocytes. Although there is overlap and even synergism in activities, IFN-α and IFN-β are primarily antiviral interferons, whereas IFN-γ is more effective as an activator of macrophages. Interferon beta-1b is approved for therapy of relapsing-remitting multiple sclerosis.

Interferon-α

The antiviral activity of IFN-α is discussed in Chapter 36. IFN-α is not a single molecular entity; there are at least 25 different subtypes of IFN-α, and their various activities and roles are still being elucidated. At present there are four forms available for clinical use. Recombinant interferon alfa-2a (Roferon-A; Roche) and interferon alfa-2b (Intron A; Schering), which differ by only one amino acid, and natural interferon alfa-n3 (Alferon-N; Purdue Frederick), which is purified from human leukocytes and consists of a mixture of subtypes of IFN-α, have been approved and available for several years. A new form of IFN-α, interferon alfacon-1 (Infergen; Amgen) was approved in 1997; not occurring naturally, it was bioengineered based on a "consensus" amino acid sequence representing the most common sequences found in the natural IFN-α types studied to date. IFN-α is approved for use in chronic HBV and HCV infections, condyloma acuminatum, and Kaposi's sarcoma in AIDS and is being investigated for many other infections including HIV and viral upper respiratory tract infections.

IFN-α has become a standard part of management of chronic HBV and HCV infections.[50, 51] In chronic hepatitis B, several studies have shown a benefit from parenteral IFN-α, if given in sufficient doses for a long enough period (see Chapters 102, 103, and 131). The largest early study included 169 patients and found that 5 million U/day (but not 1 million U/day) of IFN-α for 16 weeks resulted in loss of hepatitis B early antigen (HBeAg) and HBV DNA from serum and histologic and biochemical improvement in about 40% of patients.[52] Furthermore, the remissions are often of long duration, as shown by a follow-up study at the National Institutes of Health. Of 23 patients who had responded to the treatment described, 3 relapsed, all within 1 year. After a mean follow-up period of 4.3 years, the other 20 patients remained asymptomatic with no HBV DNA detectable by blot hybridization, and 13 of the 20 had become negative for the HBV surface antigen (HBsAg).[53] The likelihood of response is said to be lower in men and in patients with more prolonged infection, coincident HIV infection, or little inflammatory response as assessed by liver enzymes and histology.[54] Longer follow-up is needed to prove that treatment of chronic hepatitis B reduces the incidence of cirrhosis and hepatocellular carcinoma and improves survival, although one published decision analysis suggested that it should.[55] Responses to IFN therapy in patients with concurrent hepatitis D are much less likely to be sustained.[56, 57]

Interferon alfa-2b has also produced beneficial responses in chronic HCV infection (see Chapters 102, 103, and 143). When it was given at a dose of 2 to 3 million U three times a week subcutaneously or intravenously for 6 months, improvement in liver enzymes and histology was seen in about half of the patients in two studies. In contrast to the situation with HBV infection, however, relapse is common, occurring in 51% of the patients in one study[58] and 90% in the other[59] by 6 months after completion of therapy. Several additional studies of IFN-α in hepatitis C have been performed, some with higher dosages or longer duration of treatment; in general, sustained responses have been reported in less than 30% of patients.[50, 51, 60] The combination of IFN-α and ribavirin has been shown to be more effective for treatment of chronic HCV infection.[60a, 60b] The combination of interferon alfa-2b with ribavirin in a single injection has been marketed for patients at least 18 years old with compensated liver disease who have relapsed after previous IFN therapy.

IFN-α is effective for condyloma acuminatum (genital warts) caused by human papillomavirus (see Chapter 133). Intralesional interferon alfa-2b, 1 to 5 million U (1 million U in each wart, up to five warts at a time) three times a week for 3 weeks, was effective for 60 to 70% of patients with recurrences after use of other therapeutic modalities.[61] In addition, systemically administered IFN-α may be an effective adjunctive therapy for recurrent respiratory papillomatosis.[62] IFN-α has been studied as therapy for the common cold (see Chapter 46). As a nasal spray for prophylaxis, IFN-α was able to decrease upper respiratory tract infections caused by rhinovirus but not those caused by coronaviruses, influenza viruses, or parainfluenza viruses.[63, 64] Used alone, however, IFN nasal spray itself causes rhinitis. Combinations of antiviral drugs with IFN-α may prove useful in a variety of viral infections. A combination of topical trifluorothymidine and IFN-α was reported to be effective in three AIDS patients with severe cutaneous herpes simplex virus infection refractory to acyclovir and foscarnet.[65] A case report describes successful use of IFN-α with foscarnet to treat severe acyclovir-resistant perianal herpes simplex in a patient with AIDS.[66]

A phase 1 study of a combination of interferon alfa-2b and IL-2 in 17 HIV-infected patients with counts of CD4-positive T lymphocytes lower than 200/mm^3 has been reported.[67] In the study, the maximal tolerated dose of IFN-α ranged from 5 to 15 million U/day. Twelve patients then had IL-2 added at doses of 3 to 12 million U/day. Transient increases in CD4 counts were seen, but only nine patients were able to complete the 21-day course of therapy. Toxicities included pancreatitis, cytopenias, mental status changes, elevated liver enzymes, and flu-like symptoms.

The major adverse effects of systemically administered IFN-α are dose related. An influenza-like syndrome of fever, headache, myalgia and arthralgia, nausea, and anorexia is seen in almost all patients; pretreatment with acetaminophen or a nonsteroidal anti-inflammatory agent can lessen its severity, and tolerance to these effects often develops after a few weeks, especially at doses of less than 10 million U daily.[25] At higher doses, bone marrow suppression (seen in 3 to 69% of patients, depending on dose), neuropsychiatric problems (most commonly depression, paresthesias, or change in mental status and seen in about one fifth of patients), and elevated liver enzymes (frequency of 10 to 80%) can also result. Intralesional IFN has caused local discomfort and inflammation and mild systemic effects, especially with a higher number of injections given concurrently.

Interferon-γ

The early finding that administration of recombinant human IFN-γ to three patients with chronic granulomatous disease resulted in increased bactericidal activity of the patients' monocytes against *Staphylococcus aureus*[68] led to a multicenter, double-blind, placebo-controlled trial.[69] This study enrolled 128 patients, half of whom received 50 μg/m^2 IFN-γ subcutaneously three times a week. The treatment group developed significantly fewer serious infections (14 of 63 patients, compared with 30 of 65 patients given placebo; the total number of infections was 20 in the interferon group and 56 in the placebo group). This benefit was seen regardless of age, use of prophylactic antibiotics, or mode of inheritance. No change in superoxide production by phagocytes from treated patients could be demonstrated, making the mechanism of the benefit unclear. Toxicity was not thought to be serious, requiring withdrawal of only four patients from the treatment group. The major adverse effects noted were fever (in 52% of patients), headache (33%), chills (14%), and erythema at the injection site (14%). The results of long-term follow-up of 30 patients have been reported and show continued favorable effects.[70]

IFN-γ has been investigated as adjunctive therapy in several chronic infections caused by intracellular organisms. Badaro and coworkers[71] reported that IFN-γ at a dose of 100 to 400 μg/m^2/day intramuscularly for 10 to 40 days given with pentavalent antimony was successful in six of eight patients with visceral leishmaniasis previously unresponsive to pentavalent antimony alone and in eight of nine patients previously untreated. An update of their experience added another 22 patients (14 refractory, 8 untreated) with severe pancytopenia and splenomegaly.[72] Although 7 patients required retreatment after relapse (6 of these were in the refractory group), the overall response rate was 17 of 22, with follow-up now at longer than 1 year. The authors stated that these response rates were significantly better than those of historical controls, but no prospective, randomized, controlled study has yet been done. IFN-γ plus meglumine antimonate was effective for cutaneous leishmaniasis.[73]

Lepromatous leprosy is a chronic indolent infection associated with decreased production of IFN-γ and macrophage activation. Administration of IFN-γ can increase the response of macrophages to *Mycobacterium leprae* and increase clearance of bacteria from skin samples.[74] MAC is another intracellular organism that causes chronic disseminated infection, especially in AIDS patients. Because T cells from AIDS patients are deficient in production of IFN-γ (although their mononuclear phagocytes respond normally to it), IFN-γ is being studied for treatment of opportunistic infections. Squires and colleagues[75] reported on six AIDS patients with MAC bacteremia treated with IFN-γ. Although the patients treated with IFN-γ alone experienced only a minimal transient benefit, the three patients being treated concurrently with antimicrobials displayed decreases in the level of bacteremia. Holland and associates[76] studied seven HIV-negative patients with disseminated MAC or *Mycobacterium kansasii* infection refractory to a multidrug antibiotic regimen, who had low levels of IFN-γ. When IFN-γ, 50 μg/m^2 subcutaneously three times weekly, was added to the antimycobacterial agents, all seven patients had dramatic clinical improvement.[76]

INTERLEUKINS

Interleukins are a family of immune system cytokines with a variety of effects on various cell types. They serve primarily as a communication network between inducer and effector cells of the immune response. The number of identified interleukins is currently 17; the activities of many of these are only beginning to be elucidated. A description of all of these cytokines is beyond the scope of this discussion but can be found elsewhere.[77–79]

Interleukin-1

Clinical interest in IL-1 has centered on mechanisms to dampen its augmentation of the inflammatory response in sepsis (see Chapter 63) and on IL-1 as a nonspecific adjunctive therapy for bacterial infections.[80]

Interleukin-2

Recombinant human IL-2 is approved for the treatment of metastatic renal cell carcinoma under the generic name aldesleukin and the brand name Proleukin (Chiron). IL-2 shares many of the same effects as IFN-γ and has been used to treat some of the same infections. In three patients with disseminated cutaneous leishmaniasis given intralesional injections of 10 μg recombinant IL-2 at 48-hour intervals for 14 days, significant reductions in numbers of amastigotes were seen, and in two of the patients, sites became sterile by culture.[81] In leprosy, 10 μg IL-2 intradermally (in the skin of the back) enhanced cell-mediated immunity and decreased the number of organisms in lesions; adverse effects included nontender axillary lymphadenopathy and local site inflammation.[82]

In a randomized, prospective trial of 60 patients with HIV infection and CD4 counts greater than 200/mm^3, IL-2 was administered at a dose of 18 million U/day by continuous infusion for 5 days every 2 months for a 1-year period to half of the patients.[83] Both treatment and control groups received antiretroviral therapy. Whereas there was no difference between the groups in levels of plasma HIV RNA, the IL-2 group responded with significantly greater CD4 counts (mean increase of 36.7 versus a decrease of 4.8 cells/mm^3/month for the control group). Adverse effects resulted in study withdrawal for 17% of the IL-2 patients and included constitutional symptoms (in 90% of patients), elevated bilirubin and liver enzymes, cytopenias, and hypothyroidism. The AIDS Clinical Trials Group is conducting a study of subcutaneous administration of lower doses of IL-2 with antiretroviral therapy in patients with HIV infection.

IL-2 is being used (often with lymphokine-activated killer cells) as immunotherapy for malignancies.[84] This therapy in cancer patients has been associated with an increased incidence of staphylococcal infections,[85] although one paper suggests that the increased risk can be adequately dealt with through patient screening, rigorous monitoring, and liberal use of antibiotics for suspected infections.[86] It has been postulated that the increased infections are caused by IL-2–induced elevations of tumor necrosis factor (TNF) with a consequent defect in neutrophil chemotaxis; dexamethasone lowered TNF levels and prevented this defect.[87]

Interleukin-12

IL-12 is produced predominantly by macrophages and B lymphocytes and regulates activation and cytotoxicity of T cells and natural killer cells.[88] It appears to play a critical role in defense against infection by many different intracellular organisms and is being investigated as adjunctive therapy for mycobacterial and leishmanial infections.[79] IL-12 is also being studied with antiretroviral therapy in several clinical trials for HIV infection being conducted by the AIDS Clinical Trials Group.

IMMUNOGLOBULINS

Commercially available preparations of immunoglobulin are derived from human blood; formulations are available for intravenous use in addition to the traditional intramuscular route. There are currently eight preparations of intravenous immunoglobulin marketed in the United States: Gamimune N, from Bayer; Gammagard S/D, from Hyland; Gammar-P, from Centeon; Iveegam, from Immuno-US; Polygam S/D, marketed by the American Red Cross and manufactured by Hyland with plasma from Red Cross donors; Sandoglobulin, marketed by Novartis and manufactured by the Swiss Red Cross; and Venoglobulin-I and Venoglobulin-S, from Alpha Therapeutics. They are prepared by somewhat different methods and have different additives for stabilization, but for most situations they are thought to be therapeutically equivalent.[25, 89–92] All are prepared from plasma from at least 1000 donors per lot and contain more than 90% intact IgG with normal ratios of IgG subclasses. All donated plasma is tested for HIV antibody, HBsAg, and elevated alanine aminotransferase before it is used. In the early 1990s, there were several reports of HCV transmission by intravenous immunoglobulin products.[93–95] Gammagard S/D, Polygam S/D, and Venoglobulin-S undergo a solvent-detergent procedure step in their preparation to reduce the risk of viral contamination. The FDA is requiring manufacturers who do not use a solvent-detergent procedure to test their donated plasma for HCV RNA before use.[25]

One of the oldest uses for immunoglobulin is to provide specific antibodies that the recipient is lacking. This is the rationale for its intramuscular use in travelers to prevent hepatitis A and for the use of products such as varicella-zoster virus immunoglobulin, HBV immunoglobulin, tetanus immunoglobulin, and rabies immunoglobulin in selected patients. The same reasoning has been applied in the well-accepted use of intravenous immunoglobulin in the primary immunoglobulin deficiencies, including X-linked agammaglobulinemia, common variable immunodeficiency, severe combined immunodeficiency, X-linked immunodeficiency with hyperimmunoglobulinemia M, Wiskott-Aldrich syndrome, and ataxia-telangiectasia.[89]

Despite normal or even high serum immunoglobulin levels, infants and young children with AIDS often have decreased antibody responses and a corresponding increased incidence of bacterial and viral infections. An early double-blind, placebo-controlled study demonstrated fewer serious infections and hospitalizations in the treatment group among children whose CD4 count was still higher than 200/mm^3.[96] Because the majority of the study was conducted before zidovudine therapy and *Pneumocystis carinii* pneumonia prophylaxis became widespread, the applicability of these results to present practice is questionable. Another prospective, randomized, controlled trial in HIV-infected children receiving zidovudine showed a benefit from the use of intravenous immunoglobulin, but only in children not receiving trimethoprim-sulfamethoxazole prophylaxis.[97] A randomized but open-label trial of intravenous immunoglobulin in 127 adults with HIV infection demonstrated a delay in time to serious infection but no difference in number of infections overall or in mortality.[98] Again the relevance to today's practice can be questioned, because only 25% of study patients were taking trimethoprim-sulfamethoxazole and zidovudine was the only antiretroviral agent used.

In the period after bone marrow transplantation, immunoglobulin appears to play an immunomodulatory role in addition to providing antibodies.[99] In a randomized, controlled trial of bone marrow transplantation patients, administration of 500 mg/kg intravenous immunoglobulin weekly to day 90 and then monthly to day 360 decreased the incidences of acute GVH disease, interstitial pneumonia in cytomegalovirus (CMV)–seropositive patients, gram-negative septicemia, and local infection.[100] There were no overall differences in mortality or relapse rates. However, there were significantly fewer deaths from transplant-related causes in the immunoglobulin-treated group among HLA-identical transplantation patients. The benefit of standard immunoglobulin in prevention of CMV disease after bone marrow transplantation appears to be equivalent to that seen with the use of CMV hyperimmune globulin.[101, 102] Immunoglobulin also reduced the incidence of clinical CMV infection after kidney transplantation.[101]

Two studies have found immunoglobulin to be helpful when given with ganciclovir for the treatment of CMV pneumonia after bone marrow transplantation. One study used 400 mg/kg of CMV immunoglobulin given intravenously on days 1, 2, and 7 and 200 mg/kg on days 14 and 21 in addition to ganciclovir in 25 patients and achieved a 52% survival rate, compared with 15% for historical controls.[103] The other study used 500 mg/kg standard immunoglobulin given intravenously every other day for 20 days, then twice a week for 4 weeks, plus ganciclovir, and documented recurrence-free survival in 7 of 10 patients at a median follow-up of 10 months, compared with no survival in historical controls given ganciclovir alone (2 patients), CMV hyperimmune globulin alone (5 patients), or standard immunoglobulin alone (4 patients).[104]

Intravenous immunoglobulin has been shown to be beneficial in preventing infection in patients with chronic lymphocytic leukemia, although the cost-effectiveness of this treatment was challenged by Weeks and colleagues,[105] who calculated that each patient would gain only 0.8 quality-adjusted days per year with no change in life expectancy and that it would cost $6 million for each quality-adjusted life-year gained.

Premature infants are another group that may benefit from administration of immunoglobulin, since there is little transplacental transfer of IgG before 32 weeks' gestation. This question has been addressed in two double-blind trials, the first involving 588 premature neonates who were randomly assigned (with stratification for birth weight) to receive either placebo or periodic infusions of immunoglobulin. The treatment group had fewer infections and fewer days of hospitalization for infection, but there was no difference in morbidity, mortality, or mean duration of hospitalization.[106] A much larger multicenter trial, however, failed to find any benefit from the use of intravenous immunoglobulin in premature infants.[107]

Another double-blind study evaluated the use of immunoglobulin for prevention of infection in high-risk postsurgical patients.[108] The study had three arms—placebo, standard immunoglobulin, and hyperimmune globulin with high titers of antibody to *Salmonella minnesota* R595 lipopolysaccharide—each given intravenously weekly for up to 4 weeks while the patient was in the surgical intensive care unit. A decrease in infections in the standard immunoglobulin group, compared with the placebo group, was noted, with the decrease caused primarily by fewer episodes of pneumonia (particularly pneumonia caused by gram-negative organisms). Shorter stays in the intensive care unit and in the hospital were also found in the standard immunoglobulin group compared with the placebo group. However, the rate of infection in the hyperimmune group was not different from that in the placebo group, which is difficult to explain since hyperimmune globulin would be expected to be at least as effective as standard immunoglobulin. Furthermore, there was no difference between the groups in rates of systemic infection, shock, or death. In burn patients, a nonrandomized trial of prophylactic use of plasma containing high titers of antilipopolysaccharide IgG reported a decrease in burn wound colonization by gram-negative bacteria, but no difference in incidence of bacteremia, antibiotic use, time to healing of wounds, or mortality.[109]

Pyrogenic exotoxins such as streptococcal pyrogenic exotoxin A and toxic shock syndrome toxin-1 play a central role in the pathogenesis of the streptococcal and staphylococcal toxic shock syndromes. In vitro studies showing the ability of immunoglobulin to neutralize these toxins have raised the hope that it may be useful in management of these life-threatening conditions.[110, 111] An increasing number of case reports have suggested clinical benefit from the use of intravenous immunoglobulin as adjunctive therapy for streptococcal toxic shock syndrome (see Chapter 186).[112–115] Intravenous immunoglobulin and aspirin is considered the standard of care for the treatment of Kawasaki syndrome (see Chapter 288).[116] The mechanism of action is unclear, but in vitro work contributes further evidence to the hypothesis of neutralization of a bacterial toxin.[110, 116]

At present, intravenous immunoglobulin is approved by the FDA only for treatment of immune thrombocytopenic purpura, primary antibody immunodeficiency, and AIDS in children, and after bone marrow transplantation. Expert panel recommendations for use in other conditions have been published.[92] The recommended dosage of intravenous immunoglobulin for primary immunodeficiency is 100 to 400 mg/kg, depending on the preparation used, given monthly. If the resulting clinical response or serum level of IgG is inadequate, the dosage can be increased or the interval between doses can be decreased. One study, however, suggested that higher doses did not confer additional protection.[117] For bone marrow transplantation, the recommended dosage is 500 mg/kg given on days 7 and 2 before transplantation and then weekly to day 90 after transplantation. Adverse effects of intravenous immunoglobulin are seen in less than 10% of patients and are usually related to the rate of administration. Headache is the most common adverse effect; others include myalgias, arthralgias, fatigue, and malaise. Immunoglobulin is contraindicated in patients with selective IgA deficiency, because these patients may have anti-IgA antibodies and immunoglobulin preparations contain small amounts of IgA. Rarely, intravenous immunoglobulin causes hypotension with fever, diaphoresis, chest tightness, and other manifestations of anaphylaxis. This reaction is more common when the recommended rate of infusion is exceeded and in patients with hypogammaglobulinemia or agammaglobulinemia who have not received prior immunoglobulin infusion or who have received an infusion within the preceding 8 weeks. Aseptic meningitis has been reported primarily in patients receiving high doses for autoimmune disease.

GLUCOCORTICOSTEROIDS

Glucocorticosteroids have marked anti-inflammatory activity on a variety of immune cell types and are potent suppressors of the immune response. When used for infectious diseases, the situation is usually such that an overactive immune response is contributing to the pathology of the infection rather than containing it. A dramatic example occurs in AIDS patients with pneumonia due to *P. carinii,* who often experience worsening oxygenation initially after appropriate antimicrobial therapy. This effect is thought to be secondary to the increased inflammatory response to the dying organisms. Several studies have shown that, in patients with moderate to severe hypoxia, glucocorticosteroid therapy initiated within 72 hours of initiation of antibiotics increases oxygenation and decreases the incidence of respiratory failure and mortality (see Chapters 109 and 260).[118]

In general, steroids are not helpful (and may even be harmful) in septic shock or gram-negative sepsis (see Chapter 63).[119] Severe typhoid fever with shock may be an exception, based on a randomized, double-blind, placebo-controlled trial carried out in Indonesia.[120] Patients with typhoid fever with shock or mental status changes received either placebo or very high doses of dexamethasone (3 mg/kg followed by 1 mg/kg every 6 hours for eight doses). Mortality in the dexamethasone group was 10%, versus 56% in the placebo group, a statistically significant difference. Of note, all patients were treated with chloramphenicol, and there were no intensive care unit facilities available. Bacterial meningitis is another area with some controversy regarding use of steroids. Although use of steroids in children with meningitis caused by *Haemophilus influenzae* is now well accepted, their use in adults or with other bacteria is less straightforward (see Chapter 71).

Complications of tuberculosis are often included as indications for steroid therapy. Tuberculous meningitis is typically a basilar meningitis with considerable inflammation and consequent risk of hydrocephalus. An open-label prospective study in Egypt, in which intramuscular isoniazid, ethambutol, and streptomycin were used to treat tuberculous meningitis, found that dexamethasone as adjunctive therapy decreased morbidity and mortality.[121] One recommended dosing schedule for patients with increased intracranial pressure, focal neurologic deficits, or change in mental status due to tuberculous meningitis is 60 mg prednisone daily for 1 to 2 weeks, then tapered over 4 to 6 weeks.[122] In tuberculous pericarditis, drainage may be necessary to prevent tamponade, and inflammation with scarring can lead to later constriction. A randomized trial in Transkei, South Africa, found that prednisolone as adjunctive therapy for tuberculous pericarditis resulted in faster clinical improvement and decreased mortality.[123] The dosage used in the trial was 60 mg prednisolone daily for 4 weeks, then tapered over the next 7 weeks (see Chapter 240).

INFLAMMATORY CYTOKINE BLOCKERS IN SEPSIS

A variety of compounds with blocking activity against various inflammatory cytokines are being investigated for use in sepsis. These include monoclonal antibodies against endotoxin and TNF, soluble receptors for IL-1 and TNF, IL-1 receptor antagonist, and others. The lack of efficacy of tested agents in clinical trials prompts the question of whether an adequate understanding of the complex processes involved and of the appropriate biologic targets and patient population for successful immunomodulator therapy in sepsis has yet been achieved.[124–126] The treatment of sepsis is discussed in Chapter 63.

OTHER AGENTS

Imiquimod is a heterocyclic amine that stimulates production of IFN-α and other cytokines. It is available as a 5% cream with the brand name Aldara (3M Pharmaceuticals) for topical treatment of genital and perianal condyloma acuminatum. Multicenter double-blind, vehicle-controlled trials have shown the 5% cream to give wart clearance rates that are significantly higher than those achieved with the cream vehicle control (50 to 71% versus 4 to 14%).[127–129] As with other treatments for warts, recurrences are common. The most common adverse effect is a local reaction including erythema, erosion, and flaking, which occurs in up to 61% of patients; however, only 1% of patients discontinued use of the drug because of adverse effects. Patients should apply the cream to their warts three times per week at bedtime, leaving it for 6 to 10 hours before washing it off, for a maximum of 16 weeks.

Pentoxifylline is a methylxanthine derivative that in vitro decreases the production of TNF by monocytes stimulated with endotoxin and also counteracts some of the effects of TNF and other inflammatory cytokines on neutrophils.[130] On the basis of efficacy in a murine model of malaria, pentoxifylline was studied as therapy for severe falciparum malaria and found to be ineffective.[131] Pentoxifylline has been evaluated for prevention of renal insufficiency in bone marrow transplantation patients receiving amphotericin B and cyclosporine A,[132] for prevention of transplant-related toxicities after bone marrow transplantation,[133, 134] and in the treatment of diffuse idiopathic pneumonia complicating bone marrow transplantation.[135] In a prospective, controlled trial, 51 patients with severe sepsis were studied. Intravenous pentoxifylline improved cardiopulmonary dysfunction but did not change mortality.[136] Pentoxifylline is also being investigated as a potential immunomodulator in patients with HIV infection.[137]

Thalidomide is a drug that is making a comeback as a result of its recently appreciated value as an immunomodulator. Thalidomide selectively inhibits the production of TNF-α in human peripheral blood mononuclear cells.[138] Its efficacy is well established in patients who have developed erythema nodosum leprosum while being treated for lepromatous leprosy.[139] Thalidomide has also been shown to be effective in the treatment of two of the complications of HIV infection, namely wasting and aphthous ulcers. Reyes-Teran and associates conducted a randomized, double-blind, placebo-controlled trial of thalidomide in 28 patients with HIV infection who had experienced a weight loss of more than 10% over the previous 6 months.[140] Patients were all receiving antiretroviral therapy and had no known active opportunistic infections. Over the 12-week period of the study, the group treated with thalidomide (100 mg four times daily) was significantly more likely to gain weight (eight subjects, versus one in the placebo arm). The median weight change between baseline and 12 weeks was a gain of 4.05 kg in the thalidomide-treated group and a loss of 1.30 kg in the placebo-treated group ($p = .0001$). In another study to examine the nature of the weight gain produced by thalidomide, HIV-infected subjects who completed a 14-day course of thalidomide while consuming a constant level of calories demonstrated reduced urinary nitrogen excretion, unchanged resting energy expenditure, and expansion of lean tissue mass.[141]

The AIDS Clinical Trials Group performed a randomized, double-blind, placebo-controlled study of thalidomide (200 mg daily) for treatment of oral aphthous ulcers in patients with HIV infection.[142] This study was terminated early after an interim analysis found a significantly better response rate in the thalidomide group. By 4 weeks of treatment, 90% of the subjects in the thalidomide group had at least a partial response, and 55% had a complete response, compared with 25% and 7%, respectively, in the placebo group. Enthusiasm for these results is tempered, however, by the finding that patients in the thalidomide group also had a significantly greater increase in their HIV viral load, although the study was done before the use of highly active antiretroviral therapy became standard (median HIV RNA at baseline was 83,300 copies/ml in the placebo group and 120,600 copies/ml in the thalidomide group). An open-label trial of the same dose of thalidomide showed a similar success rate in HIV-infected patients with idiopathic esophageal ulcers.[143]

In the above studies, the most common adverse effects of thalidomide were sedation (24 to 79%) and rash (also 24 to 79%). Other adverse effects included constipation and dry mouth. Peripheral neuropathy is a common adverse effect of long-term thalidomide use, and the severe teratogenicity of thalidomide is well known. Thalidomide is currently marketed only for the treatment of leprosy but is also available in the United States through compassionate use programs by two manufacturers, Andrulis Pharmaceuticals (301-827-2335) and Celgene Corporation (800-801-8328).

Thymosin-α₁, a 28-amino-acid protein that has been sequenced and synthesized, is one of a group of peptides produced by the thymus with effects on the neuroendocrine and immune systems; among these effects are induction of the cytokines IL-1, IL-2, IFN-α, and IFN-γ. Thymosin-α_1 has been compared with placebo and with interferon-alfa for the treatment of chronic hepatitis B. In a pilot study, patients receiving thymosin-α_1, 900 μg/m^2 subcutaneously administered twice weekly for 6 months, had significantly increased clearance of HBV DNA, decreased transaminase levels, and improved histology compared with those given placebo.[144] In a larger trial, thymosin-α_1, 900 μg/m^2 subcutaneously twice weekly, was compared with interferon-alfa, 5 million U subcutaneously three times weekly, for the treatment of chronic hepatitis B in 33 patients with positive tests for both anti-HBe antibody and HBV DNA.[145] At the end of the 6-month treatment period, 29% of the thymosin group and 44% of the IFN group had achieved a complete response with normalization of the alanine transaminase value and clearing of HBV DNA. After 6 months of follow-up, a complete response was seen in 41% of the thymosin group and 25% of the interferon group. The differences were not statistically significant at either timepoint. Thymosin-α_1 was much better tolerated than interferon, with only two patients (12%) reporting local reactions and no reported systemic adverse effects. An open-label study assessed the combination of lymphoblastoid interferon-alfa and thymosin-α_1 in 15 patients with chronic hepatitis B, 11 of whom had failed standard therapy with interferon alfa-2b. Patients were treated for 6 months and then monitored for an additional 12 months. Three of the 4 interferon-naïve patients and 6 of the 11 interferon-experienced patients had documented normalization of alanine transaminase levels and clearance of HBV DNA at the end of the study.[146]

Thymosin-α_1 has had less success in treatment of chronic hepatitis C, with one small, randomized, blinded, placebo-controlled trial showing no benefit with the same dosing used in the hepatitis B trials.[147] The combination of lymphoblastoid interferon-alfa and thymosin-α_1 was also studied in an open-label trial in 15 patients with hepatitis C. After 1 year of treatment, 73% of patients had cleared serum HCV RNA; 40% remained negative for HCV RNA 6 months after completion of treatment.[148] The combination of thymosin-α_1 and polyethylene glycol–modified IL-2 (PEG-IL-2) was studied in 12 patients with HIV infection and CD4 counts of 50 to 250/mm^3. Patients tolerated both therapies well, but no additional increase in CD4 count was seen with the combination therapy beyond that produced by the PEG-IL-2 infusions alone.[149]

REFERENCES

1. Fauci AS. Immunomodulators in clinical medicine. Ann Intern Med. 1987;106:421–433.
2. Roilides E, Pizzo PA. Modulation of host defenses by cytokines: Evolving adjuncts in prevention and treatment of serious infections in immunocompromised hosts. Clin Infect Dis. 1992;15:508–524.
3. Frampton JE, Yarker YE, Goa KL. Lenograstim: A review of its pharmacological properties and therapeutic efficacy in neutropenia and related clinical settings. Drugs. 1995;49:767–793.
4. Lieschke GJ, Burgess AW. Granulocyte colony-stimulating factor and granulocyte-macrophage colony-stimulating factor. N Engl J Med. 1992;327:28–35, 99–106.
5. Crawford J, Ozer H, Stoller R, et al. Reduction by granulocyte colony-stimulating factor of fever and neutropenia induced by chemotherapy in patients with small-cell lung cancer. N Engl J Med. 1991;325:164–170.
6. Nemunaitis J. A comparative review of colony-stimulating factors. Drugs. 1997;54:709–729.
7. Lifton R, Bennett JM. Clinical use of granulocyte-macrophage colony-stimulating factor and granulocyte colony-stimulating factor in neutropenia associated with malignancy. Hematol Oncol Clin North Am. 1996;10:825–839.
8. Fischer JR, Manegold C, Bulzebruck H, et al. Induction chemotherapy with and without recombinant human granulocyte colony-stimulating factor support in lo-

cally advanced stage IIIA/B non-small cell lung cancer. Semin Oncol. 1994;21(suppl 3):20–27.
9. Croockewit AJ, Koopmans PP, de Pauw BE. Should hematopoietic growth factors routinely be given concurrently with cytotoxic chemotherapy? Clin Pharmacol Ther. 1996;59:1–6.
10. Miller LL, Ozer H, et al. American Society of Clinical Oncology recommendations for the use of hematopoietic colony-stimulating factors: Evidence-based, clinical practice guidelines. J Clin Oncol. 1994;12:2471–2508.
11. Dombret H, Chastang C, Fenaux P, et al. A controlled study of recombinant human granulocyte colony-stimulating factor in elderly patients after treatment for acute myelogenous leukemia. N Engl J Med. 1995;332:1678–1683.
12. Masaoka T, Takaku F, Kato S, et al. Recombinant human granulocyte colony-stimulating factor in allogeneic bone marrow transplantation. Exp Hematol. 1989;17:1047–1050.
13. Sheridan WP, Morstyn G, Wolf M, et al. Granulocyte colony-stimulating factor and neutrophil recovery after high-dose chemotherapy and autologous bone marrow transplantation. Lancet. 1989;2:891–895.
14. Souetre E, Qing W, Penelaud PF. Economic analysis of the use of recombinant human granulocyte colony stimulating factor in autologous bone marrow transplantation. Eur J Cancer. 1996;32A:1162–1165.
15. Kimura S, Matsuda J, Ikamatsu S, et al. Efficacy of recombinant human granulocyte colony-stimulating factor on neutropenia in patients with acquired immune deficiency syndrome. AIDS. 1990;4:1251–1255.
16. Kuritzkes DR, Parenti D, Ward DJ, et al. Filgrastim prevents severe neutropenia and reduces infective morbidity in patients with advanced HIV infection: Results of a randomized, multicenter, controlled trial. AIDS. 1998;12:65–74.
17. Manders SM, Kostman JR, Mendez L, et al. Thalidomide-resistant HIV-associated aphthae successfully treated with granulocyte colony-stimulating factor. J Am Acad Dermatol. 1995;33:380–382.
18. Donadieu J, Boutard P, Bernatowska E, et al. A European phase II study of recombinant human granulocyte colony-stimulating factor (lenograstim) in the treatment of severe chronic neutropenia in children. Eur J Pediatr. 1997;156:693–700.
19. Dale DC, Bonilla MA, Davis MW, et al. A randomized controlled phase III trial of recombinant human granulocyte colony-stimulating factor (filgrastim) for treatment of severe chronic neutropenia. Blood. 1993;81:2496–2502.
20. Gonzalez CE, Couriel DR, Walsh TJ. Disseminated zygomycosis in a neutropenic patient: Successful treatment with amphotericin B lipid complex and granulocyte colony-stimulating factor. Clin Infect Dis. 1997;24:192–196.
21. Bouza E, Munoz P, Vega L, et al. Clinical resolution of *Scedosporium prolificans* fungemia associated with reversal of neutropenia following administration of granulocyte colony-stimulating factor. Clin Infect Dis. 1996;23:192–193.
22. Foster PF, Mital D, Sankary HN, et al. The use of granulocyte colony-stimulating factor after liver transplantation. Transplantation. 1995;59:1557–1563.
23. Gough A, Clapperton M, Rolando N, et al. Randomised placebo-controlled trial of granulocyte-colony stimulating factor in diabetic foot infection. Lancet. 1997;350:855–859.
24. Andresen J, Movahed H, Nelson S. Filgrastim (r-metHuG-CSF) in pneumonia. In: Morstyn G, Dexter T, Foot MA, ed. Filgrastim in Clinical Practice. 2nd ed. New York: Marcel Dekker; 1998;429–446.
25. American Hospital Formulary Service. AHFS Drug Information. Bethesda, Maryland: American Society of Hospital Pharmacists; 1998.
26. Nemunaitis J, Rabinowe SN, Singer JW, et al. Recombinant granulocyte-macrophage colony-stimulating factor after autologous bone marrow transplant for lymphoid cancer. N Engl J Med. 1991;324:1173–1178.
27. Peters WP. Use of cytokines during prolonged neutropenia associated with autologous bone marrow transplantation. Rev Infect Dis. 1991;13:993–996.
28. Advani R, Chao NJ, Horning SJ, et al. Granulocyte-macrophage colony-stimulating factor (GM-CSF) as an adjunct to autologous hemopoietic stem cell transplantation for lymphoma. Ann Intern Med. 1992;116:183–189.
29. Fleischman RA. Southwestern internal medicine conference: Clinical use of hematopoietic growth factors. Am J Med Sci. 1993;305:1248–1273.
30. Nemunaitis J, Buckner CD, Appelbaum FR, et al. Phase I/II trial of recombinant human granulocyte-macrophage colony-stimulating factor following allogeneic bone marrow transplantation. Blood. 1991;77:2065–2071.
31. Nemunaitis J, Rosenfeld C, Ash R, et al. Phase III randomized, double-blind placebo-controlled trial of rhGM-CSF following allogeneic bone marrow transplantation. Bone Marrow Transplant. 1995;15:949–954.
32. Antman KS, Griffin JD, Elias A, et al. Effect of recombinant human granulocyte-macrophage colony-stimulating factor on chemotherapy-induced myelosuppression. N Engl J Med. 1988;319:593–598.
33. Riikonen P, Saarinen UM, Makipernaa A, et al. Recombinant human granulocyte-macrophage colony-stimulating factor in the treatment of febrile neutropenia: A double blind placebo-controlled study in children. Pediatr Infect Dis J. 1994;13:197–202.
34. Rowe JM, Aandersen JW, Mazza JJ, et al. A randomized placebo controlled phase III study of granulocyte-macrophage colony-stimulating factor in adult patients (>55 to 70 years of age) with acute myelogenous leukemia: A study of the Eastern Cooperative Oncology Group (E1490). Blood. 1995;86:457–462.
35. Stone RM, Berg DT, George SL, et al. Granulocyte-macrophage colony-stimulating factor after initial chemotherapy for elderly patients with primary acute myelogenous leukemia. N Engl J Med. 1995;332:1671–1677.
36. Davison FD, Kaczmarski RS, Pozniak A, et al. Quantification of HIV by PCR in monocytes and lymphocytes in patients receiving antiviral treatment and low dose recombinant human granulocyte macrophage colony stimulating factor. J Clin Pathol. 1994;47:855–857.
37. Scadden DT, Pickus O, Hammer SM, et al. Lack of in vivo effect of granulocyte-macrophage colony-stimulating factor on human immunodeficiency virus type 1. AIDS Res Hum Retroviruses. 1996;12:1151–1159.
38. Baldwin GC, Gasson JC, Quon SG, et al. Granulocyte-macrophage colony stimulating factor enhances neutrophil function in acquired immunodeficiency syndrome patients. Proc Natl Acad Sci U S A. 1988;85:2763–2766.
39. Kemper CA, Bermudez LE, Deresinski SC. Immunomodulatory treatment of *Mycobacterium avium* complex bacteremia in patients with AIDS by use of recombinant granulocyte-macrophage colony-stimulating factor. J Infect Dis. 1998;177:914–920.
40. Price DA, Klein JL, Fisher M, et al. Potential role for granulocyte-macrophage colony-stimulating factor in the treatment of HIV-associated cryptococcal meningitis (Letter). AIDS. 1997;11:693–694.
41. Anaissie EJ, Vartivarian S, Bodey GP, et al. Randomized comparison between antibiotics alone and antibiotics plus granulocyte-macrophage colony-stimulating factor (*Escherichia coli*-derived) in cancer patients with fever and neutropenia. Am J Med. 1996;100:17–23.
42. Montgomery B, Bianco JA, Jacobsen A, et al. Localization of transfused neutrophils to site of infection during treatment with recombinant human granulocyte-macrophage colony-stimulating factor and pentoxifylline. Blood. 1991;78:533–534.
43. Spielberger RT, Falleroni MJ, Coene AJ, et al. Concomitant amphotericin B therapy, granulocyte transfusions, and GM-CSF administration for disseminated infection with *Fusarium* in a granulocytopenic patient. Clin Infect Dis. 1993;16:528–530.
44. Hurst D, Kilpatrick L, Becker J, et al. Recombinant human GM-CSF treatment of neutropenia in glycogen storage disease-1b. Am J Pediatr Hematol Oncol. 1993;15:71–76.
45. Van Thiel DH, Friedlander L, Kania RJ, et al. A preliminary experience with GM-CSF plus interferon in patients with HBV and HCV resistant to interferon therapy. J Viral Hepat. 1997;4(Suppl 1):101–106.
46. Pardo M, Castillo I, Navas S, et al. Treatment of chronic hepatitis C with cirrhosis with recombinant human granulocyte colony-stimulating factor plus recombinant interferon-alpha. J Med Virol. 1995;45:439–444.
47. Nemunaitis J. Use of macrophage colony-stimulating factor in the treatment of fungal infections. Clin Infect Dis. 1998;26:1279–1281.
48. Nemunaitis J, Meyers JD, Buckner CD, et al. Phase I trial of recombinant human macrophage colony-stimulating factor in patients with invasive fungal infections. Blood. 1991;78:907–913.
49. Nemunaitis J, Dorcy KS, Appelbaum FR, et al. Long-term follow-up of patients with invasive fungal disease who received adjunctive therapy with recombinant human macrophage colony-stimulating factor. Blood. 1993;82:1422–1427.
50. Saracco G, Rizzetto M. A practical guide to the use of interferons in the management of hepatitis virus infections. Drugs. 1997;53:74–85.
51. Rothstein KD, Munoz SJ. Interferon and other therapies for hepatitis B and hepatitis C infections. Clin Lab Med. 1996;16:465–491.
52. Perillo RP, Schiff ER, Davis GL, et al. A randomized controlled trial of interferon α-2b alone and after prednisone withdrawal for the treatment of chronic hepatitis B. N Engl J Med. 1990;323:295–301.
53. Korenman J, Baker B, Waggoner J, et al. Long-term remission of chronic hepatitis B after alpha-interferon therapy. Ann Intern Med. 1991;114:629–634.
54. Martin P, Friedman LS. Therapies for hepatitis B: Current status and future possibilities. In: Block T, ed. Innovations in Antiviral Development and the Detection of Virus Infection. New York: Plenum Press; 1992;111–120.
55. Wong JB, Koff RS, Tine F, et al. Does interferon therapy for chronic hepatitis B reduce the risks of developing cirrhosis and hepatocellular carcinoma? Ann Intern Med. 1995;122:664–675.
56. Farci P, Mandas A, Coiana A, et al. Treatment of chronic hepatis D with interferon alfa-2a. N Engl J Med. 1994;330:88–94.
57. Gaudin JL, Faure P, Codinot H, et al. The French experience of treatment of chronic type D hepatitis with a 12 month course of IFN alpha-2b: Results of a randomized, controlled trial. Liver. 1995;15:45–52.
58. Davis BL, Balart LA, Schiff ER, et al. Treatment of chronic hepatitis C with recombinant interferon alpha: A multicenter, randomized, controlled trial. N Engl J Med. 1989;321:1501–1506.
59. Di Bisceglie AM, Martin P, Kassianides C, et al. Recombinant interferon alpha therapy for chronic hepatitis C: A randomized double-blind placebo-controlled trial. N Engl J Med. 1989;321:1506–1510.
60. Tong MJ, Reddy RK, Lee WM, et al. Treatment of chronic hepatitis C with consensus interferon: A multicenter randomized controlled trial. Hepatology. 1997;26:747–754.
60a. McHutchison JG, Gordon SC, Schiff ER, et al. Interferon alfa-2b alone or in combination with ribavirin as initial treatment for chronic hepatitis C. N Engl J Med. 1998;339:1485–1492.
60b. Davis GL, Esteban-Mur R, Rustgi V, et al. Interferon alfa-2b alone or in combination with ribavirin for the treatment of relapse of chronic hepatitis C. N Engl J Med. 1998;339:1493–1499.
61. Reichman RC, Oakes D, Bonnez W, et al. Treatment of condyloma acuminatum with three different alpha interferon preparations administered parenterally: A double-blind, placebo-controlled trial. J Infect Dis. 1990;162:1270–1276.
62. Leventhal BG, Kashima HK, Mounts P, et al. Long-term response of recurrent respiratory papillomatosis to treatment with lymphoblastoid interferon α-n1. N Engl J Med. 1991;325:613–617.
63. Hayden FG, Albrecht JK, Kaiser DL, et al. Prevention of natural colds by contact prophylaxis with intranasal alpha 2-interferon. N Engl J Med. 1986;314:71–75.

64. Douglas RM, Moore BW, Miles HB, et al. Prophylactic efficacy of intranasal alpha 2 interferon against rhinovirus infections in the family setting. N Engl J Med. 1986;314:65–70.
65. Birch CJ, Tyssen DP, Tachedjian G, et al. Clinical effects and in vitro studies of trifluorothymidine combined with interferon-alpha for treatment of drug-resistant and sensitive herpes simplex virus infections. J Infect Dis. 1992;166:108–112.
66. Borrego L, Castro I, Adela F, et al. Treatment of acyclovir-resistant perianal herpetic ulceration with intramuscular interferon alfa. Arch Dermatol. 1996;132:1157–1158.
67. Schnittman SM, Vogel S, Baseler M, et al. A phase I study of interferon-α2b in combination with interleukin-2 in patients with human immunodeficiency virus infection. J Infect Dis. 1994;169:981–989.
68. Sechler JMG, Malech HL, White CJ, et al. Recombinant human interferon gamma reconstitutes defective phagocyte function in patients with chronic granulomatous disease of childhood. Proc Natl Acad Sci U S A. 1988;85:4874–4878.
69. The International CGD Cooperative Study Group. A controlled trial of interferon-gamma to prevent infection in chronic granulomatous disease. N Engl J Med. 1991;324:509–516.
70. Bemiller LS, Roberts DH, Starko KM, et al. Safety and effectiveness of long-term interferon gamma therapy in patients with chronic granulomatous disease. Blood Cells Mol Dis. 1995;21:239–247.
71. Badaro R, Falcoff E, Badaro FS, et al. Treatment of visceral leishmaniasis with pentavalent antimony and interferon gamma. N Engl J Med. 1990;322:16–21.
72. Badaro R, Johnson WD. The role of interferon-gamma in the treatment of visceral and diffuse cutaneous leishmaniasis. J Infect Dis. 1993;167(Suppl 1):S13–S17.
73. Arana BA, Navim TR, Arana FE, et al. Efficacy of a short course (10 days) of high-dose meglumine antimonate with or without interferon-γ in treating cutaneous leishmaniasis in Guatemala. Clin Infect Dis. 1994;18:381–384.
74. Kaplan G. Recent advances in cytokine therapy in leprosy. J Infect Dis. 1993;17(Suppl 1):S18–S22.
75. Squires KE, Brown ST, Armstrong D, et al. Interferon-gamma treatment for *Mycobacterium avium-intracellulare* complex bacillemia in patients with AIDS. J Infect Dis. 1992;166:686–687.
76. Holland SM, Eisenstein EM, Kuhns DB, et al. Treatment of refractory disseminated nontuberculous mycobacterial infection with interferon gamma. N Engl J Med. 1994;330:1348–1355.
77. Curfs JHAJ, Meis JFGM, Hoogkamp-Korstanje JAA. A primer on cytokines: Sources, receptors, effectors, and inducers. Clin Microbiol Rev. 1997;10:742–780.
78. Liles WC, Van Voorhis WC. Review: Nomenclature and biologic significance of cytokines involved in inflammation and the host immune response. J Infect Dis. 1995;172:1573–1580.
79. DiPiro JT. Cytokine networks with infection: Mycobacterial infections, leishmaniasis, human immunodeficiency virus infection, and sepsis. Pharmacotherapy. 1997;17:205–223.
80. Vogels MTE, Van der Meer JWM. Use of immune modulators in nonspecific therapy of bacterial infections. Antimicrob Agents Chemother. 1992;36:1–5.
81. Akuffo H, Kaplan G, Kiessling R, et al. Administration of recombinant interleukin-2 reduces the local parasite load of patients with disseminated cutaneous leishmaniasis. J Infect Dis. 1990;161:775–780.
82. Kaplan G, Britton WJ, Hancock GE, et al. The systemic influence of recombinant interleukin-2 in the manifestations of lepromatous leprosy. J Exp Med. 1991;173:993–1006.
83. Kovacs JA, Vogel S, Albert JM, et al. Controlled trial of interleukin-2 infusions in patients infected with the human immunodeficiency virus. N Engl J Med. 1996;335:1350–1356.
84. Rosenberg SA, Lotze MT, Muul LM, et al. A progress report on the treatment of 157 patients with advanced cancer using lymphokine-activated killer cells and interleukin-2 or high dose interleukin-2 alone. N Engl J Med. 1987;316:889–897.
85. Syndman DR, Sullivan B, Gill M, et al. Nosocomial sepsis associated with interleukin-2. Ann Intern Med. 1990;112:102–107.
86. Pockaj BA, Topalian SL, Steinberg SM, et al. Infectious complications associated with interleukin-2 administration: A retrospective review of 935 treatment courses. J Clin Oncol. 1993;11:136–147.
87. Mier JW, Vachino G, Klemper MS, et al. Inhibition of interleukin-2–induced tumor necrosis factor release by dexamethasone: Prevention of an acquired neutrophil chemotaxis defect and differential suppression of interleukin-2–associated side effects. Blood. 1990;76:1933–1940.
88. Brunda MJ. Interleukin-12. J Leukoc Biol. 1994;55:280–288.
89. Buckley RH, Schiff RI. The use of intravenous immune globulin in immunodeficiency diseases. N Engl J Med. 1991;325:110–117.
90. Stiehm ER. New uses for intravenous immune globulin. N Engl J Med. 1991;325:123–125.
91. Dickler HB, Gelfand EW. Current perspectives on the use of intravenous immunoglobulin. Adv Intern Med. 1996;41:641–680.
92. Ratko TA, Burnett DA, Foulke GE, et al. Recommendations for off-label use of intravenously administered immunoglobulin preparations. JAMA. 1995;273:1865–1870.
93. Bjoro K, Froland SS, Yuru Z, et al. Hepatitis C infection in patients with primary hypogammaglobulinemia after treatment with contaminated immune globulin. N Engl J Med. 1994;331:1607–1611.
94. Schiff R. Transmission of viral infections through intravenous immune globulin. N Engl J Med. 1994;331:1649–1650.
95. Centers for Disease Control and Prevention. Outbreak of hepatitis C associated with intravenous immunoglobulin administration—United States, October 1993–June 1994. MMWR Morb Mortal Wkly Rep 1994;43:505–509.
96. National Institutes of Child Health and Human Development Intravenous Immunoglobulin Study Group. Intravenous immune globulin for the prevention of bacterial infections in children with symptomatic human immunodeficiency virus infection. N Engl J Med. 1991;325:73–80.
97. Spector A, Gelber RD, McGrath N, et al. Controlled trial of intravenous immune globulin for the prevention of serious bacterial infections in children receiving zidovudine for advanced human immunodeficiency virus infection. N Engl J Med. 1994;331:1181–1187.
98. Kiehl MG, Stoll R, Broder M, et al. A controlled trial of intravenous immune globulin for the prevention of serious infections in adults with advanced human immunodeficiency virus infection. Arch Intern Med. 1996;156:2545–2550.
99. Barnes RA. Immunotherapy and immunoprophylaxis in bone marrow transplantation. J Hosp Infect. 1995;30(Suppl):223–231.
100. Sullivan KM, Kopecky KJ, Jocom J, et al. Immunomodulatory and antimicrobial efficacy of intravenous immunoglobulin in bone marrow transplantation. N Engl J Med. 1990;323:705–712.
101. Berkman SA, Lee ML, Gale RP. Clinical uses of intravenous immunoglobulins. Ann Intern Med. 1990;112:278–292.
102. Bass EB, Power NR, Goodman SN, et al. Efficacy of immune globulin in preventing complications of bone marrow transplantation: A meta-analysis. Bone Marrow Transplant. 1993;12:273–282.
103. Reed EC, Bowden RA, Dandliker PS, et al. Treatment of cytomegalovirus pneumonia with ganciclovir and intravenous cytomegalovirus immunoglobulin in patients with bone marrow transplants. Ann Intern Med. 1988;109:783–788.
104. Emanuel D, Cunningham I, Jules-Elysee K, et al. Cytomegalovirus pneumonia after bone marrow transplantation successfully treated with the combination of ganciclovir and high-dose intravenous immune globulin. Ann Intern Med. 1988;198:777–782.
105. Weeks JC, Tierney MR, Weinstein MC. Cost effectiveness of prophylactic intravenous immune globulin in chronic lymphocytic leukemia. N Engl J Med. 1991;325:81–86.
106. Baker CJ, Melish ME, Hall RT, et al. Intravenous immune globulin for the prevention of nosocomial infection in low-birth-weight neonates. N Engl J Med. 1992;327:213–219.
107. Fanaroff AA, Korones SB, Wright LL, et al. A controlled trial of intravenous immune globulin to reduce nosocomial infections in very-low-birth-weight infants. N Engl J Med. 1994;331:1107–1113.
108. The Intravenous Immunoglobulin Collaborative Study Group. Prophylactic intravenous administration of standard immune globulin as compared with core-lipopolysaccharide immune globulin in patients at high risk of postsurgical infection. N Engl J Med. 1992;327:234–240.
109. Jones EB. Prophylactic anti-lipopolysaccharide freeze-dried plasma in major burns: A double blind controlled trial. Burns. 1995;21:267–272.
110. Takei S, Arora YK, Walker SM. Intravenous immunoglobulin contains specific antibodies inhibitory to activation of T cells by staphylococcal toxin superantigens. J Clin Invest. 1993;91:602–607.
111. Bohach GA, Hovde CJ, Handley JP, Schlievert PM. Cross-neutralization of staphylococcal and streptococcal pyrogenic toxins by monoclonal and polyclonal antibodies. Infect Immun. 1988;56:400–404.
112. Perez CM, Kubak BM, Cryer HG, et al. Adjunctive treatment of streptococcal toxic shock syndrome using intravenous immunoglobulin: Case report and review. Am J Med. 1997;102:111–113.
113. Barry W, Hudgins L, Donta ST, Pesanti EL. Intravenous immunoglobulin therapy for toxic shock syndrome. JAMA. 1992;267:3315–3316.
114. Yong JM. Necrotising fasciitis (Letter). Lancet. 1994;343:1427.
115. Lamothe F, D'Amico P, Ghosn P, et al. Clinical usefulness of intravenous human immunoglobulins in invasive group A streptococcal infections: Case report and review. Clin Infect Dis. 1995;21:1469–1470.
116. Dwyer JM. Manipulating the immune system with immune globulin. N Engl J Med. 1992;326:107–116.
117. Pruzanski W, Sussman G, Dorian W, et al. Relationship of the dose of intravenous gammaglobulin to the prevention of infections in adults with common variable immunodeficiency. Inflammation. 1996;20:353–359.
118. The National Institutes of Health–University of California Expert Panel for Corticosteroids as Adjunctive Therapy for Pneumocystis Pneumonia. Consensus statement on the use of corticosteroids as adjunctive therapy for *Pneumocystis* pneumonia in the acquired immunodeficiency syndrome. N Engl J Med. 1990;323:1500–1504.
119. McGowan JE, Chesney PJ, Crossley KB, et al. Guidelines for the use of systemic glucocorticosteroids in the management of selected infections. J Infect Dis. 1992;165:1–13.
120. Hoffman SL, Punjabi NH, Kumala S, et al. Reduction of mortality in chloramphenicol-treated severe typhoid fever by high-dose dexamethasone. N Engl J Med. 1984;310:82–88.
121. Girgis NI, Farid Z, Kilpatrick ME, et al. Dexamethasone adjunctive treatment for tuberculous meningitis. Pediatr Infect Dis J. 1991;10:179–183.
122. Molavi A, Lefrock JL. Tuberculous meningitis. Med Clin North Am. 1985;69:315–331.
123. Strang JIG, Gibson DG, Nunn AJ, et al. Controlled trial of prednisolone as adjuvant in treatment of tuberculous constrictive pericarditis in Transkei. Lancet. 1987;2:1418–1422.
124. Cross AS. Antiendotoxin antibodies: A dead end? Ann Intern Med. 1994;121:58–59.
125. Cohen J, Heumann D, Glauser MP. Do monoclonal antibodies and anticytokines still have a future in infectious diseases? Am J Med. 1995;99(Suppl 6A):45S–53S.

126. Warren HS. Strategies for the treatment of sepsis. N Engl J Med. 1997;336:952–953.
127. Beutner KR, Tyring SK, Trofatter KF, et al. Imiquimod, a patient-applied immune-response modifier for treatment of external genital warts. Antimicrob Agents Chemother. 1998;42:789–794.
128. Edwards L, Beutner K, Tyring S, et al. Comparison of results from two vehicle controlled clinical trials evaluating topical imiquimod for the treatment of genital/perianal warts. Clinical Dermatology 2000 International Congress, Vancouver, British Columbia, May 28–31, 1996.
129. 3M Pharmaceuticals. Prescribing information for Aldara (imiquimod) 5% Cream, 1997.
130. Sullivan GW, Carper HT, Novick WJ, et al. Inhibition of the inflammatory action of interleukin-1 and tumor necrosis factor (alpha) on neutrophil function by pentoxifylline. Infect Immun. 1988;56:1722–1729.
131. Looareesuwan S, Wilairatana P, Vannaphan S, et al. Pentoxifylline as an ancillary treatment for severe falciparum malaria in Thailand. Am J Trop Med Hyg. 1998;58:348–353.
132. Bianco JA, Almgren J, Kern DL, et al. Evidence that oral pentoxifylline reverses acute renal dysfunction in bone marrow transplant recipients receiving amphotericin B and cyclosporine. Transplantation. 1991;51:925–927.
133. Bianco JA, Appelbaum FR, Nemunaitis J, et al. Phase I–II trial of pentoxifylline for the prevention of transplant-related toxicities following bone marrow transplantation. Blood. 1991;78:1205–1211.
134. Kalhs P, Lechner K, Stockschlader M, et al. Pentoxifylline did not prevent transplant-related toxicity in 31 consecutive allogeneic bone marrow transplant recipients. Blood. 1992;80:2683.
135. Bianco JA, Appelbaum FR, Bakke L, et al. A phase II study of intravenous pentoxifylline for the treatment of diffuse idiopathic pneumonia in marrow transplant recipients. In: Mandell GL, Novick WJ Jr, eds. Proceedings of a Workshop: Pentoxifylline, Leukocytes, and Cytokines. Somerville, New Jersey: Hoechst-Roussel Pharmaceuticals; 1992;57–67.
136. Staubach K, Schröder J, Stüber F, et al. Effect of Pentoxifylline in severe sepsis. Arch Surg 1998;133:94–100.
137. Clerici M, Piconi S, Balotta C, et al. Pentoxifylline improves cell-mediated immunity and reduces human immunodeficiency virus (HIV) plasma viremia in asymptomatic HIV-seropositive persons. J Infect Dis. 1997;175:1210–1215.
138. Sampaio EP, Sarno EN, Gallily R, et al. Thalidomide selectively inhibits tumor necrosis factor alpha production by stimulated human monocytes. J Exp Med. 1991;173:699–703.
139. Sampaio EP, Kaplan G, Miranda A, et al. The influence of thalidomide on the clinical and immunological manifestation of erythema nodosum leprosum. J Infect Dis. 1993:168:408–414.
140. Reyes-Teran G, Sierra-Madero JG, Martinez del Cerro V, et al. Effects of thalidomide on HIV-associated wasting syndrome: A randomized, double-blind, placebo-controlled clinical trial. AIDS. 1996;10:1501–1501.
141. Haslett P, Hempstead M, Seidman C, et al. The metabolic and immunologic effects of short-term thalidomide treatment of patients infected with the human immunodeficiency virus. AIDS Res Hum Retroviruses. 1997;13:1047–1054.
142. Jacobson JM, Greenspan JS, Spritzler J, et al. Thalidomide for the treatment of oral aphthous ulcers in patients with human immunodeficiency virus infection. N Engl J Med. 1997;336:1487–1493.
143. Alexander LN, Wilcox CM. A prospective trial of thalidomide for the treatment of HIV-associated idiopathic esophageal ulcers. AIDS Res Hum Retroviruses. 1997;13:301–304.
144. Mutchnick MG, Appelman HD, Chung HT, et al. Thymosin treatment of chronic hepatitis B: A placebo-controlled pilot trial. Hepatology. 1991;14:409–415.
145. Andreone P, Cursaro C, Gramenzi A, et al. A randomized controlled trial of thymosin-alpha1 versus interferon alfa treatment in patients with hepatitis B e antigen antibody– and hepatitis B virus DNA–positive chronic hepatitis B. Hepatology. 1996;24:774–777.
146. Rasi G, Mutchnick MG, Di Virgilio D, et al. Combination low-dose lymphoblastoid interferon and thymosin α_1 therapy in the treatment of chronic hepatitis B. J Viral Hepatitis. 1996;3:191–196.
147. Andreone P, Cursaro C, Gramenzi A, et al. A double-blind, placebo-controlled, pilot trial of thymosin alpha 1 for the treatment of chronic hepatitis C. Liver. 1996;16:207–210.
148. Rasi G, Di Virgilio D, Mutchnick MG, et al. Combination thymosin α_1 and lymphoblastoid interferon treatment in chronic hepatitis C. Gut. 1996;39:679–683.
149. Ramachandran R, Katzenstein DA, Winters MA, et al. Polyethylene glycol-modified interleukin-2 and thymosin alpha 1 in human immunodeficiency virus type 1 infection. J Infect Dis. 1996;173:1005–1008.

Chapter 38

Hyperbaric Oxygen

JEAN MARIE MULINDE
ELLIS S. CAPLAN

As defined by the Undersea and Hyperbaric Medicine Society, hyperbaric medicine is "a therapeutic technique using air or other gas mixtures at greater-than-atmospheric pressure for short intervals, over days or months, to treat various disease states." Albert Behnke, in 1939, reported the first clinical use of hyperbaric oxygen (HBO) therapy using intermittent inhalation of 100% oxygen under pressure to treat decompression sickness.[1] It was not until 1967, however, that HBO treatment of "the bends" was officially accepted, and it has since become the standard worldwide.[1] The first non–diving-related use of HBO was by Boerema in 1956,[1] when he used a large pressurized operating room to perform procedures requiring the interruption of circulation to the brain and other vital organs, operations that would otherwise have been impossible in the pre–heart-lung bypass era. A number of similar operating chambers were built in the United States and United Kingdom, but with the development of effective cardiopulmonary bypass equipment, by the mid-1970s they became obsolete for this indication.[1] In the interim, however, hyperbaric practitioners (frequently nonphysicians) began treating a wide variety of conditions with HBO, often making claims without sound scientific foundation. In 1977, in response to concerns about the misuse of HBO therapy, the Undersea and Hyperbaric Medicine Society produced a report defining those conditions for which animal experiments and clinical series showed that HBO treatment was beneficial, and these disorders became eligible for reimbursement by third-party payers. This report has been updated every 2 to 3 years and currently recognizes 12 disorders that are reimbursable for HBO treatment (Table 38–1).[2]

EQUIPMENT

HBO can be delivered through monoplace or multiplace chambers. Monoplace chambers are essentially Plexiglas tubes that are continuously flooded with 100% oxygen at pressures up to 3 ATA. Ports for hemodynamic monitoring, electrocardiographs, intravenous infusions, oxygen monitoring, and respirator management are available, and the controls for chamber operation are on the unit. The advantages of monoplace units are decreased expenses and a limited need for space; the disadvantages include a decreased access to the patient and an increased risk of fire in the chamber because the entire internal environment is flooded with 100% oxygen. Multiplace chambers accommodate from 2 to 14 patients and their attendants (Fig.

TABLE 38–1 Disorders Approved for Treatment with Hyperbaric Oxygen

Infectious disease related
Gas gangrene
Necrotizing fasciitis
Osteomyelitis
Noninfectious disease related
Decompression sickness
Air or gas embolism
Carbon monoxide and cyanide poisoning
Radiation osteonecrosis
Exceptional blood loss anemia
Crush injury
Selected problem wounds
Smoke inhalation
Skin grafts and flaps

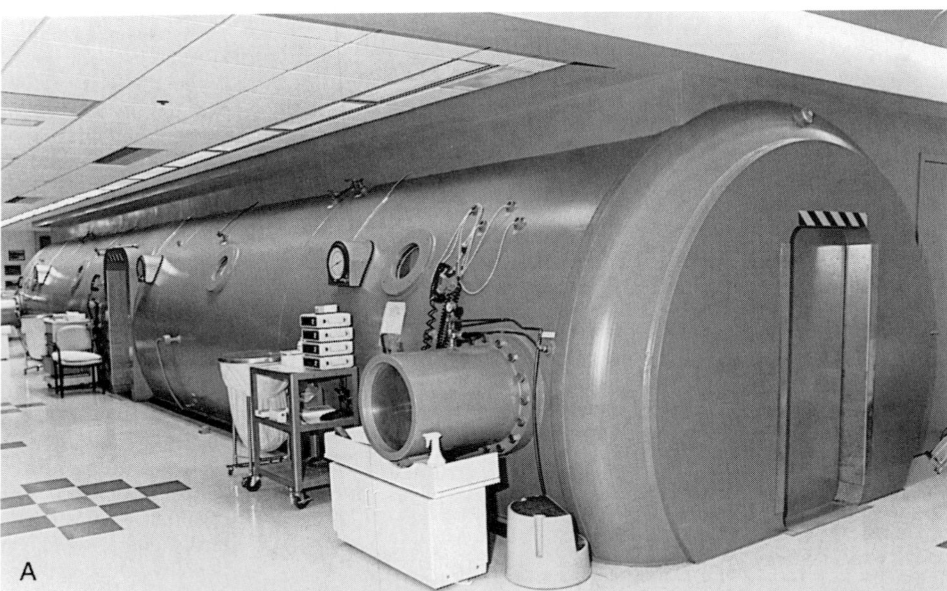

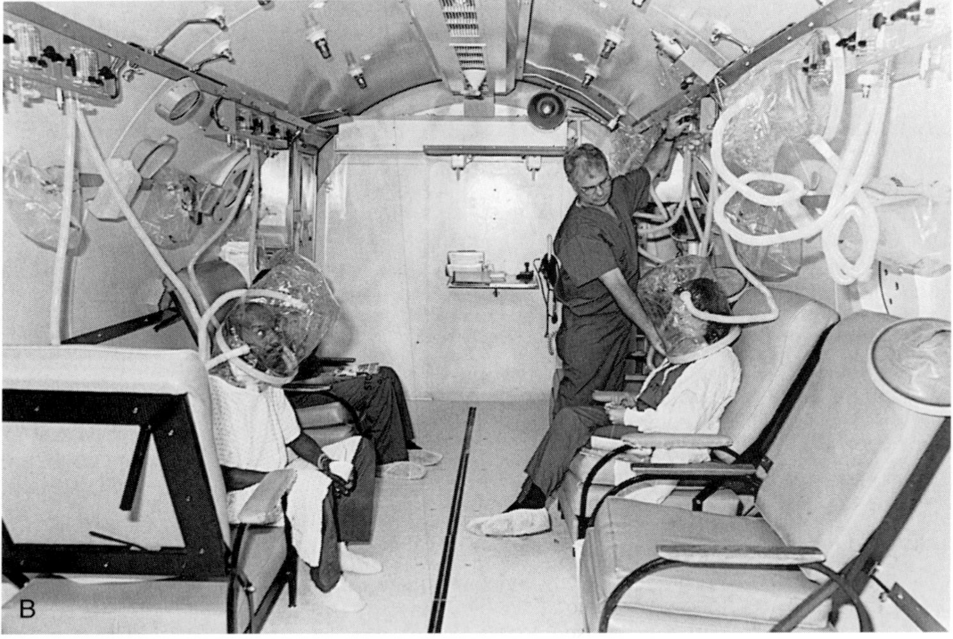

FIGURE 38–1. *A,* Hyperbaric chamber at the RA Cowley Shock Trauma Center. *B,* Patients fitted with hoods in the hyperbaric chamber, RA Cowley Shock Trauma Center.

38–1*A*). A chamber pressure of up to 6 ATA is provided by air, and the patient breathes 100% oxygen via a closely fitting hood or mask or, if mechanically ventilated, through the ventilator circuit (see Fig. 38–1*B*). Advantages of the multiplace chamber include ready access to patients by the inside attendant and the ability to provide pressures of up to 6 ATA. Disadvantages include the large expense of such a unit and the potential for attendants to experience nitrogen-saturation illness.

PHYSIOLOGY

HBO has two basic physiologic effects. The first is the reduction of bubble size; this phenomenon is governed by Boyle's law, which states that the volume of gas in an enclosed space is inversely proportional to the pressure exerted on it. It is this reduction of bubble size that is important in the treatment of iatrogenic air embolism and in nitrogen saturation illness ("the bends"). The second physiologic effect of HBO is increased partial pressure of oxygen in body tissues. When air is inspired under normal pressure, 98.4% of the available oxygen is bound to hemoglobin and the remaining portion is dissolved in plasma.[3] For each increased atmosphere of pressure, an additional 2.3 vol% of oxygen is dissolved in plasma. At 3 ATA, the most common pressure used, more than 6 vol% of oxygen is carried by plasma. Because approximately 5 vol% is required for adequate tissue oxygenation, inspired 100% oxygen at 3 ATA provides enough oxygen in plasma alone to support life and can raise peripheral tissue oxygen tensions measured through the skin from 40 to over 2200 mmHg.[3]

The dramatic increase in tissue oxygenation by HBO results in a number of local tissue effects. These effects include an increased ability of leukocytes to kill some bacteria[4] and exert a bacteriostatic effect on others[5–7]; the direct killing of some anaerobic bacteria[8] and the inhibition of formation of clostridial α-toxin[9, 10]; the stimulation of fibroblast growth, which results in increased collagen formation and resultant neovascularization[11–13]; and the inhibition of neutrophil adherence to ischemic vessel walls, a reduction in postischemic vasoconstriction, and reduced lipid peroxidation (vasoconstriction and lipid peroxidation are key components of ischemic tissue injury).[14–16]

ADVERSE EFFECTS

The most common adverse effects associated with HBO are barotrauma of the middle ear, cranial sinuses, or teeth. Auditory barotrauma occurs in less than 1% of patients and rarely permanently curtails treatment.[17] The occurrence of auditory barotrauma may be minimized by careful screening of individuals for their ability to clear their ears and may be minimized with the use of decongestants. For those who display an inability to clear their ears or for those who are obtunded, needle myringotomy or tympanotomy tube placement provides a simple solution. Lung barotrauma is a potentially more severe adverse effect of HBO. Pulmonary barotrauma is of particular concern in asthmatic patients, those with chronic obstructive lung disease, and those with lung cysts or bullae, because they are at increased risk of developing a pneumothorax during decompression.[3] Although rare, oxygen toxicity is also a potential risk, occurring in 1 in 10,000 patient therapies.[2] When present, oxygen toxicity usually manifests as symptoms involving the central nervous system, which range from agitation to generalized seizures. The risk is minimized by adhering to well-defined guidelines for time and pressure limits. Additional adverse effects of HBO include a reversible myopia, resulting from a direct toxic effect of oxygen on the lens, and cataract formation.[18] A summary of adverse effects is presented in Table 38–2.

TABLE 38–2 Complications and Side Effects of Hyperbaric Oxygen Treatment

Barotrauma of ear	Seizures
Sinus squeeze	Numb fingers
Visual refractive changes	Pulmonary oxygen toxicity
Dental problems	Chamber fire
Pneumothorax	

HYPERBARIC OXYGEN THERAPY IN INFECTIOUS DISEASES

Clostridial Myonecrosis

HBO serves a number of important functions in the treatment of clostridial myonecrosis. At 3-ATA oxygen, Van Unnik demonstrated that the production of α-toxin ceases.[9] Since α-toxin, a lecithinase C, is believed to be responsible for tissue destruction and shock, a clear theoretical benefit is evident. Van Unnik also demonstrated the arrest of clostridial growth with 3-ATA oxygen. Bacterial growth and toxin production resumed, however, on return to a normal environment. Other in vitro studies support the finding of a bacteriostatic effect by HBO but have found that the addition of blood or muscle to culture media inhibits this effect of HBO because a catalase present in blood and muscle protects the bacteria from the effects of oxygen,[8, 10, 19–21] suggesting that for HBO therapy to provide optimal results, blood and necrotic tissue should be débrided from the wound.

Brummelkamp first reported the use of HBO for the treatment of clostridial myonecrosis in 1961.[22] He described four patients with clostridial myonecrosis whose disease was progressing despite surgery and antibiotic therapy; HBO therapy produced a rapid and dramatic improvement in their clinical condition, and all patients survived. Since 1961, there have been many reports of the treatment of clostridial myonecrosis with HBO in both experimental animal models[8, 10, 23–26] and human disease.[27–32] A review of 20 clinical series, including a total of more than 1200 patients in whom HBO was used, reported a cumulative mortality of 23%.[29] Although there has never been a controlled, randomized study of the use of HBO for clostridial myonecrosis in humans, historical data suggest a mortality of 45% without HBO.[33] In perhaps the most well designed in vivo study to date, Demello and colleagues reported on the use of HBO in the treatment of gas gangrene in a dog model.[24] They showed that survival increased from 70% in animals treated with surgery and antibiotics alone to 95% with the addition of HBO to surgery and antimicrobial therapy.

The timing of HBO in the treatment of clostridial myonecrosis is somewhat controversial. If readily available, an initial treatment before surgery may help to delineate the surviving tissue and decrease the production of α-toxin, resulting in a patient who is more hemodynamically stable. If HBO therapy cannot be administered within 24 hours of the onset of disease, initial surgical débridement should be performed with subsequent transfer of the patient to a facility providing HBO. The recommended HBO treatment protocol for clostridial myonecrosis is 100% oxygen at 3 ATA for 90 minutes (with appropriate air breaks), two to three times daily, for 5 to 7 days.[34] In addition to HBO and surgical débridement, appropriate antibiotic therapy is essential. Antimicrobials recommended for the treatment of clostridial myonecrosis include penicillin G, clindamycin, and metronidazole. It has been our clinical experience, at R Adams Cowley Shock Trauma Center, that these infections frequently also involve aerobic gram-negative rods and that additional gram-negative coverage is appropriate pending culture data.

Necrotizing Fasciitis

Necrotizing fasciitis is a rapidly progressing infection of the skin, underlying subcutaneous soft tissues, and fascia without muscle involvement. Bacteriologically, these infections may be divided into two groups: those caused by a single aerobic species such as *Streptococcus pyogenes* and more commonly those that are polymicrobial, involving both anaerobes and aerobes. Although resuscitation, surgical débridement, and antibiotic therapy are considered the mainstays of therapy for necrotizing fasciitis, HBO therapy is often used as adjunctive therapy. The rationale for the use of HBO includes the reversal of tissue hypoxia, enhanced neutrophil function, a direct toxic effect on selected bacteria, and enhanced activity of certain antimicrobial agents.[35] Although carefully controlled trials of HBO for the treatment of necrotizing fasciitis in humans have not been performed and some authors refute the role of HBO for the treatment of necrotizing fasciitis,[36] studies in animals[24, 37–41] and other retrospective clinical studies have reported efficacy.[42] Riseman and associates retrospectively described 29 adults with necrotizing fasciitis.[42] Those patients receiving HBO, despite being more seriously ill at the time of presentation, had a lower mortality rate (23 versus 66% in those not receiving HBO) and required fewer surgical débridements (1.16 versus 3.25 in those not receiving HBO).[42] If utilized, it is recommended that HBO begin after the first surgical débridement and that three sessions be given within the first 24 hours, consisting of 3-ATA 100% oxygen for 90 minutes (with appropriate air breaks) followed by twice-daily sessions until granulation is obtained.[43]

Refractory Osteomyelitis

Mader and coworkers, in a rabbit model of *Staphylococcus aureus* osteomyelitis, showed the oxygen tension in osteomyelitic bone to be 23 mmHg.[4] At 23 mmHg, there was a reduced ability of phagocytes to kill bacteria compared with killing in normal bone at an oxygen tension of 45 mmHg. When the rabbits were subjected to 100% oxygen at 2 ATA, the oxygen tension in osteomyelitic bone increased to 109 mmHg and phagocytic killing of *S. aureus* was restored. Thus Mader concluded that for osteomyelitic bone, HBO therapy allows the return of intramedullary oxygen tensions to normal or supranormal levels, resulting in normalization of phagocytic killing. Work by other authors suggests that similarly enhanced phagocytic killing may also be the mechanism by which HBO is beneficial in *Staphylococcus epidermidis, Pseudomonas aeruginosa,* and *Escherichia coli* osteomyelitis.[44]

HBO therapy should be viewed as adjunctive therapy to surgical débridement and antibiotic therapy in patients with refractory osteomyelitis (defined as failure after standard surgical débridement and at least 6 weeks of appropriate antibiotic therapy). Although there has not been a placebo-controlled, double-blind study of the use of HBO in osteomyelitis, animal data[45] and clinical experience[46–48] suggest benefit. Davis studied 38 patients with refractory osteomyelitis treated with débridement, antimicrobial therapy, and adjunctive HBO; this combination therapy was successful in 34 patients.[48] In another study, no benefit of HBO was found when patients treated with surgical débridement and antibiotics were compared with those with surgical débridement, antibiotics, and HBO.[49] However, because more than 90% of patients in the control group were cured, there is some question as to whether these patients truly had refractory osteomyelitis.[18] The recommended protocol for adjunctive HBO therapy for refractory osteomyelitis is 2.4 ATA for 95 minutes with appropriate air breaks. Sessions are usually once daily for at least 15 days.[44]

Mucormycosis

Traditional therapy for mucormycosis includes control of underlying predisposing conditions, aggressive surgical débridement, and administration of high-dose amphotericin B. Adjunctive HBO therapy may offer additional benefit. Oxygen-based free radicals are believed to be responsible for the fungistatic and fungicidal effects of HBO.[35] Additionally, HBO may potentiate the antifungal effect of amphotericin B by reversing tissue hypoxia.[35] In a review of 145 cases of rhino-orbital-cerebral mucormycosis, 24 patients with bilateral disease (a situation associated with increased mortality) were identified.[50] In 18 patients who received standard treatment with amphotericin B, surgery, or both, the mortality was 78%, whereas the mortality in six patients treated with standard therapy in addition to HBO was 17%. The role of HBO in the treatment of mucormycosis remains uncertain.

Human Immunodeficiency Virus

In 1993, Reillo published a study that looked at the effect of HBO on debilitating fatigue and decreased immunologic function related to human immunodeficiency virus–acquired immunodeficiency disease.[51] Twenty-five patients positive for human immunodeficiency virus and with CD4 counts of 500 mm^3 or less and Karnofsky performance scales of 75% or less were studied. Patients were assessed and serum samples were obtained monthly for 12 months. Although specific values were not supplied, Reillo states that "all patients had significant improvements in energy levels, as measured by the Karnofsky Performance Scale." Sixty percent of the patients had a decrease in the total CD8 count and stabilization or improvement in CD4/CD8 ratios (only 20% of patients were reported to be receiving antiretroviral therapy). In addition, platelet and hematocrit levels were noted to have increased, weight rose or stabilized in all patients, and the level of tumor necrosis factor reportedly decreased in 13 patients. Although HBO therapy cannot be recommended for human immunodeficiency virus–acquired immunodeficiency disease based on the limited data presented by Reillo, further investigation may be warranted.

REFERENCES

1. Kindwall EP. Uses of hyperbaric oxygen therapy in the 1990s. Clev Clin J Med. 1992;59:517–528.
2. Thom SR. Hyperbaric Oxygen Therapy: A Committee Report. Bethesda, Md: Undersea and Hyperbaric Medicine Society; 1994.
3. Tabrah FI, Tanner R, Vega R, Batkin S. Baromedicine today—rational uses of hyperbaric oxygen therapy. Hawaii Med J. 1994;53:112–119.
4. Mader TJ, Brown GL, Guckian JC, et al. A mechanism for the amelioration by hyperbaric oxygen of experimental staphylococcal osteomyelitis in rabbits. J Infect Dis. 1980;142:915–922.
5. Boehme DE. Oxygen and toxicity inhibition of amino acid biosynthesis. Nature. 1976;262:418–420.
6. Brown OR. Reversible inhibition of *Escherichia coli* by hyperoxia. Microbiology. 1972;5:7–16.
7. Park MK, Muhvich KH, Myers RAM, Marzella L. Hyperoxia prolongs the aminoglycoside-induced postantibiotic effect in *Pseudomonas aeruginosa*. Antimicrob Agents Chemother. 1991;35:691–695.
8. Hill GB, Osterhout S. Experimental effects of hyperbaric oxygen on selected clostridial species. I. In vitro studies. J Infect Dis. 1972;125;17–25.
9. Van Unnik AJM. Inhibition of toxin production in *Clostridium perfrigens* in vitro by hyperbaric oxygen. Antonie Van Leeuwenhoek. 1965;31:181–186.
10. Kaye D. Effect of hyperbaric oxygen on clostridia in vitro and in vivo. Proc Soc Exp Biol Med 1967;124:360–366.
11. Prockop DJ, Kivirikko KI, Tuderman L, Guzman NA. The biosynthesis of collagen and its disorders. N Engl J Med. 1979;301:13–23.
12. Hunt TK. The physiology of wound healing. Ann Emerg Med. 1988;17:1265–1273.
13. Hunt TK, Pai MP. The effect of varying ambient oxygen tensions on wound metabolism and collagen synthesis. Surg Gynecol Obstet. 1972;135:561–567.
14. Zamboni WA, Roth AC, Russell RC, et al. The effect of acute hyperbaric oxygen therapy on axial pattern skin flap survival when administered during and after total ischemia. J Reconstr Microsurg. 1989;5:343–347.
15. Thom SR. Leukocytes in carbon monoxide-mediated brain oxidative injury. Toxicol Appl Pharmacol 1993;123:234–247.
16. Zamboni WA, Roth AC, Russell RC, et al. Morphologic analysis of the microcirculation during perfusion of ischemic skeletal muscle and the effect of hyperbaric oxygen. Plast Reconstr Surg. 1993;91:1110–1123.
17. Thom SR. Hyperbaric oxygen therapy. J Intensive Care Med. 1989;4:58–74.
18. Tibbles PM, Edelsberg JS. Hyperbaric-oxygen therapy. N Engl J Med. 1996;334:1642–1648.
19. Brown IW, Cox BG, eds. In Vitro and In Vivo Experimental Effects of Hyperbaric Oxygen on *Clostridium perfringens*. Washington DC: National Academy of Science, National Research Council Publication 1404. 1966:538–543.
20. Wada J, Iwa T, eds. The Effect of Hyperbaric Oxygen on the Germination and Toxin

Production of *Clostridium perfringens* Spores, Baltimore: Williams & Wilkins; 1969:276–281.
21. Nuckolls JG, Osterhout SS. The effect of hyperbaric oxygen on anaerobic bacteria. Clin Res. 1964;12:244.
22. Brummelkamp WH, Hogendijk J, Boerema I. Treatment of anaerobic infections (clostridial myositis) by drenching the tissues with oxygen under high atmospheric pressure. Surgery. 1961;49:299–302.
23. Glover JL, Mendelson J, Heitkamp DH. Effects of hyperbaric oxygenation on rabbits with *Clostridium perfringens* infection. J Trauma. 1964;4:642–651.
24. Demello FJ, Haglin JJ, Hitchcock CR. Comparative study of experimental *Clostridium perfringens* infection in dogs treated with antibiotics, surgery, and hyperbaric oxygen. Surgery. 1973;73:936–941.
25. Muhvich KH, Anderson LH, Mehm WJ. Evaluation of antimicrobials combined with hyperbaric oxygen in a mouse model of clostridial myonecrosis. J Trauma. 1994;36:7–10.
26. Stevens DL, Bryant AE, Adams K, et al. Evaluation of therapy with hyperbaric oxygen for experimental infection with *Clostridium perfringens*. Clin Infect Dis. 1993;17:231–237.
27. Unsworth IP, Shap PA. Gas gangrene. An 11-year review of 73 cases managed with hyperbaric oxygen. Med J Aust. 1984;1430:256–259.
28. Darke SG, King AM, Slack WK. Gas gangrene and related infection: Classification, clinical features and etiology, managements and mortality. A report of 88 cases. Br J Surg. 1977;64:104–112.
29. Rudge FW. The role of hyperbaric oxygenation in the treatment of clostridial myonecrosis. Mil Med. 1993;158:80–83.
30. Keogh G, Unsworth I, Vowels M, et al. Spontaneous *Clostridium septicum* myonecrosis in congenital neutropenia. Aust N Z J Surg. 1994;64:574–575.
31. Bush GW, Clements RH, Phillips M, et al. *Clostridium perfringens* sepsis with intravascular hemolysis following laparoscopic cholecystectomy: A newly reported complication. Am Surg. 1996;62:326–327.
32. Rich RS, Salluzzo RF. Spontaneous clostridial myonecrosis with abdominal involvement in a nonimmunocompromised patient. Ann Emerg Med. 1993;22:1477–1480.
33. Hitchock CR, Demello FJ, Haglin JJ. Gangrene infection. New approaches to an old disease. Surg Clin North Am. 1975;55:1403–1410.
34. Brown RB, Sands M. Infectious disease indications for hyperbaric oxygen therapy. Compr Ther. 1995;21:663–667.
35. Park MK, Muhvich KH, Myers RAM, et al. Effects of hyperbaric oxygen in infectious diseases: Basic mechanisms. In: Kindwall EP, ed. Hyperbaric Medicine Practice. Flagstaff, Ariz: Best; 1994:141–172.
36. Shupack A, Shoshani O, Goldenberg I, et al. Necrotizing fasciitis: An indication for hyperbaric oxygenation therapy? Surgery. 1995;118:873–878.
37. Zamboni WA, Mazolewski PJ, Erdmann D, et al. Evaluation of penicillin and hyperbaric oxygen in the treatment of streptococcal myositis. Ann Plast Surg. 1997;39:131–136.
38. Thom SR, Lauerman MW, Hart GW. Intermittent hyperbaric oxygen therapy for reduction of mortality in experimental polymicrobial sepsis. J Infect Dis. 1986;154:504–510.
39. Park MK, Myers RAM, Marzella L. Oxygen tensions and infection: Modulation of microbial growth, activity of antimicrobial agents, and immunologic responses. Clin Infect Dis. 1992;14:720–740.
40. Hirn M, Niinikoski J, Lehtonen OP. Effect of hyperbaric oxygen and surgery on experimental gas gangrene. Eur Surg Res 1992;24:356–362.
41. Stevens DL, Bryant AE, Adams K, et al. Evaluation of therapy with hyperbaric oxygen for experimental infection with *Clostridium perfringens*. Clin Infect Dis. 1993;17:231–237.
42. Riseman JA, Zamboni WA, Curtis A, et al. Hyperbaric oxygen therapy for necrotizing fasciitis reduced mortality and the need for debridements. Surgery. 1990;108:847–850.
43. Baker DJ. Selected aerobic and anaerobic soft tissue infections—diagnosis and the use of hyperbaric oxygen as an adjunct. In: Kindwall EP, ed. Hyperbaric Medicine Practice. Flagstaff, Ariz: Best; 1994:395–418.
44. Britt M, Calhoun J, Mader TJ, et al. The use of hyperbaric oxygen in the treatment of osteomyelitis. In: Kindwall EP, ed. Hyperbaric Medicine Practice. Flagstaff, Ariz: Best; 1994:419–427.
45. Mader TJ, Guckian JC, Glass DL, et al. Therapy with hyperbaric oxygen for experimental osteomyelitis due to *Staphylococcus aureus* in rabbits. J Infect Dis. 1978;138:312–318.
46. Depenbusch FL, Thompson RE, Hart GB. The use of hyperbaric oxygen in the treatment of refractory osteomyelitis: A preliminary report. J Trauma. 1972;12:807–812.
47. Morrey BF, Dunn JM, Heimbach RD, et al. Hyperbaric oxygen and chronic osteomyelitis. Clin Orthop. 1979;144:121–127.
48. Davis JC, Heckman JD, DeLee JC, et al. Chronic non-hematogenous osteomyelitis treated with adjuvant hyperbaric oxygen. J Bone Joint Surg Am. 1986;68:1210–1217.
49. Esterhai JL, Pisarello J, Brighton CT, et al. Adjunctive hyperbaric oxygen therapy in the treatment of chronic refractory osteomyelitis. J Trauma. 1987;27:763–768.
50. Yohai RA, Bullock JD, Aziz AA, et al. Survival factors in rhino-orbital-cerebral mucormycosis. Surv Ophthalmol. 1994;39:3–22.
51. Reillo MR. Hyperbaric oxygen therapy for the treatment of debilitating fatigue associated with HIV/AIDS. Journal Assoc Nurses AIDS Care. 1993;4:33–38.

Chapter 39

Agents Active against Parasites and *Pneumocystis carinii*

RICHARD D. PEARSON

A comprehensive discussion of antiparasitic chemotherapy must take into account the large number of parasites that can infect humans, the complexity of their life cycles, differences in their metabolism, and the wide array of drugs that have been developed to treat them. Taxonomically, parasites are divided into protozoa and helminths.[1–4] The protozoa are unicellular. Helminths are multicellular and have highly developed neuromuscular systems, digestive tracts, reproductive organs, and integuments. It is not surprising that many drugs that are effective against helminths are not active against protozoa, and vice versa. Although taxonomists have placed *Pneumocystis carinii* closer to fungi than protozoa, so many antiparasitic drugs are useful against *P. carinii* that treatment of pneumocystosis is included in this chapter instead of the chapter on antifungal agents.

The susceptibility of the parasites to chemotherapeutic agents correlates to some degree with their taxonomy and metabolism (Table 39–1). The parasites can be grouped along those parameters. Protozoa that inhabit the gastrointestinal lumen and vagina form one group. Although they arise from several taxonomic classes,[1] they share a common microenvironment and in many instances have similar metabolic adaptations. Included in this group are amebae of the superclass Rhizopodia, the luminal flagellates of the class Zoomastigophorea, and ciliates of the class Kinetofragminophorea. The second major group includes members of the phylum Apicomplexa. These protozoa are important causes of morbidity and mortality worldwide. They include *Plasmodium* spp., which cause malaria; *Babesia* spp. and the coccidians *Toxoplasma gondii, Cyclospora* spp., *Isospora belli, Cryptosporidium parvum*; and the microsporidia, *Encephalitozoon intestinalis, Enterocytozoon bieneusi*, and others. The coccidians have emerged as important pathogens in persons with the acquired immunodeficiency syndrome (AIDS). The third group of protozoan pathogens include flagellates of the class Zoomastigophorea, family Trypanosomidiae. They are arthropod-borne and cause leishmaniasis, Chagas' disease, and African sleeping sickness.

The susceptibility of helminths also correlates with their taxonomy. The helminths can be divided into nematodes (roundworms),[2] which can be subdivided into those that live in the lumen of the intestine and those that reside in tissue; trematodes (flukes); and cestodes (tapeworms).[3, 4] Chemotherapeutic agents are often active against multiple genera within these groups.

The discussion of antiparasitic drugs that follows is arranged according to these taxonomic groups. Some drugs are active against pathogens in more than one group. This is particularly true for praziquantel, which is active against a broad spectrum of trematodes and cestodes; albendazole, with activity against nematodes and larval cestodes; and ivermectin, with activity against many nematodes as well as blood-sucking arthropods. Drugs that have a broad spectrum of activity are discussed in the context of their primary indications.

The dosage and duration of therapy for specific parasitic diseases as recommended by the *Medical Letter on Drugs and Therapeutics*[5] and adverse effects of some antiparasitic drugs are provided in Tables 39–2 and 39–3, respectively. Not all of these drugs are licensed or available through pharmacies in the United States. Some (marked with an asterisk) can be obtained only from the manufacturer or from the Drug Service at the Centers for Disease Control and Prevention (CDC), Atlanta, Georgia. Others (marked with two asterisks) are not available in the United States but are discussed because they are used elsewhere in the world or hold promise for the future.

Text continued on page 516

TABLE 39–1 Spectrum of Activity of the Major Antiparasitic and Antipneumocystis Drugs Licensed for Use in the United States, Available in the United States from the Manufacturer or from the CDC Drug Service, Centers for Disease Control and Prevention (*), or Not Currently Available in the United States (**)

Drug	Indications
***Amoebae, Intestinal and Vaginal Flagellates, and* Balantidium coli**	
Metronidazole	*Entamoeba histolytica* (invasive disease) *Entamoeba polecki* *Trichomonas vaginalis* *Blastocystis hominis* *Giardia lamblia* *Balantidium coli* (alternative)
Iodoquinol	*E. histolytica* (luminal infection) *Dientamoeba fragilis* *B. hominis* *B. coli* (alternative)
Diloxanide furoate**	*E. histolytica* (asymptomatic and luminal infection) *E. polecki* (luminal infection)
Paromomycin	*E. histolytica* (asymptomatic and luminal infection) *D. fragilis* *Cryptosporidium* (may be effective)
Furazolidone	*G. lamblia* (alternative)
Tetracycline	*B. coli* *D. fragilis*
Amphotericin B	*Naegleria* spp. (used with miconazole and rifampin) *Leishmania* spp. (liposome-encapsulated amphotericin B is approved for the treatment of visceral leishmaniasis)
Plasmodium *spp. (Malaria)*	
Chloroquine	Suppressive prophylaxis and treatment of the asexual erythrocytic phase of susceptible *Plasmodium vivax, Plasmodium ovale, Plasmodium malariae,* and susceptible *Plasmodium falciparum*
Primaquine	Radical cure of the exoerythrocytic hypnozoites of *P. vivax* and *P. ovale*
Quinine	Treatment of chloroquine-resistant *P. falciparum;* effective against asexual erythrocytic phase of other *Plasmodium* spp.
Quinidine	Treatment of chloroquine-resistant *P. falciparum* when parenteral therapy is required; effective against asexual erythrocytic phase
Mefloquine	Prophylaxis and occasionally treatment of chloroquine-resistant *P. falciparum;* effective against asexual erythrocytic phase of other *Plasmodium* spp.
Tetracycline	Used with quinine to treat asexual erythrocytic state of chloroquine-resistant *P. falciparum* in Southeast Asia
Doxycycline	Used alone for suppressive prophylaxis or with quinine for treatment of chloroquine-resistant *P. falciparum*
Artemisinin derivatives (Qinghaosu)**	Treatment of *Plasmodium* spp. in the asexual erythrocytic phase, including chloroquine-resistant *P. falciparum*
Halofantrine**	Treatment of *Plasmodium* spp. in the asexual erythrocytic phase, including chloroquine-resistant *P. falciparum* (alternative)
Pyrimethamine/short-acting sulfonamides	Used with quinine to treat asexual erythrocytic phase of chloroquine-resistant *P. falciparum* acquired in areas where resistance is not common
Pyrimethamine-sulfadoxine (Fansidar)	Presumptive treatment of chloroquine-resistant *P. falciparum* in areas where isolates remain sensitive
Proguanil**	Used with chloroquine or atovoquone for suppressive prophylaxis of chloroquine-resistant *P. falciparum* (failures occur with chloroquine/proguanil)
Other Apicomplexa (Toxoplasmosis, Isosporiasis, Cyclosporiasis)	
Pyrimethamine plus sulfadiazine	*T. gondii*
Trimethoprim-sulfamethoxazole (cotrimoxazole)	*Pneumocystis carinii* *Isospora belli* *Cyclospora cayatanensis*
Clindamycin	Used with steroids for treatment of ocular *T. gondii* in immunocompetent hosts; used with pyrimethamine for *T. gondii* encephalitis in persons with AIDS who cannot tolerate sulfonamides Used with quinine for treatment of *Babesia* spp. Used with quinine for *P. falciparum* (alternative)
Spiramycin*	*T. gondii* during pregnancy and in the neonate
Pneumocystis carinii	
Atovaquone	*P. carinii*—treatment of mild to moderate disease (alternative)
Dapsone	*P. carinii*—with trimethoprim for treatment of mild to moderate disease (alternative); with or without trimethoprim for prophylaxis Also used for *T. gondii* (with pyrimethamine) and *Mycobacterium leprae*
Trimethoprim-sulfamethoxazole	*P. carinii*—treatment or prophylaxis
Pentamadine isethionate	*P. carinii*—treatment, IV (alternative); prophylaxis, aerosolized (alternative)
Primaquine and clindamycin	*P. carinii*—treatment of mild to moderate disease (alternative)
Trimetrexate with folinic acid	*P. carinii*—treatment (alternative)
Members of the Family Trypanosomatidae (Leishmaniasis, Chagas' Disease, African Trypanosomiasis)	
Eflornithine*	*Trypanosoma brucei gambiense* (hemolymphatic and late disease with nervous system involvement)
Suramin*	*T. b. gambiense* and *Trypanosoma brucei rhodesiense* (hemolymphatic stage)
Melarsoprol B*	*T. b. gambiense* and *T. b. rhodesiense* (late disease with central nervous system involvement)
Nifurtimox*	*Trypanosoma cruzi*
Benznidazole**	*T. cruzi*
Stibogluconate sodium*	*Leishmania* spp.
Meglumine antimonate**	*Leishmania* spp.
Amphotericin B deoxycholate	*Leishmania* spp. (alternative)
Liposome-encapsulated amphotericin B	Visceral leishmaniasis
Pentamidine isethionate	*T. b. gambiense* and *T. b. gambiense* (alternative for use in the hemolymphatic stage) *Leishmania* spp. (alternative)

TABLE 39–1 Spectrum of Activity of the Major Antiparasitic and Antipneumocystis Drugs Licensed for Use in the United States, Available in the United States from the Manufacturer or from the CDC Drug Service, Centers for Disease Control and Prevention (*), or Not Currently Available in the United States (**) *Continued*

Drug	Indications
Helminthic Diseases: Nematodes (Roundworms)	
Mebendazole	*Ascaris lumbricoides*
	Ancylostoma duodenale
	Necator americanus
	Trichuris trichiura
	Enterobius vermicularis
	Capillaria philippinensis
	Moniliformis moniliformis (alternative)
	Mansonella perstans
	Angiostrongylus cantonensis
	Trichostrongylus spp. (alternative)
	Trichinella spiralis (recommended by some; used with steroids)
	Visceral larva migrans (alternative)
Albendazole	*A. lumbricoides*
	A. duodenale
	N. americanus
	E. vermicularis
	T. trichiura (alternative)
	Cutaneous larva migrans
	Visceral larva migrans (alternative)
	Gnathostoma spinigerum
	Trichostrongylus spp. (alternative)
	C. philippinensis (alternative)
Thiabendazole	*S. stercoralis*
	Cutaneous larva migrans (effective topically)
	Angiostrongylus costaricensis (alternative)
Pyrantel pamoate	*E. vermicularis*
	A. lumbricoides
	A. duodenale
	N. americanus
	Trichostrongylus spp.
Piperazine citrate	*A. lumbricoides* (alternative)
Diethylcarbamazine	*Wuchereria bancrofti*
	Brugia malayi
	Mansonella streptocerca
	Loa loa
	Tropical eosinophilia
	Visceral larva migrans
Ivermectin	*Onchocerca volvulus*
	S. stercoralis
	Cutaneous larva migrans
	M. streptocerca
	Mansonella ozzardi
	Also scabies
Metronidazole	*Dracunculus medinensis*
Helminthic Diseases: Trematodes (Flukes) and Cestodes (Tapeworms)	
Praziquantel	*Schistosoma* spp.
	Clonorchis sinensis
	Opisthorchis viverrini
	Paragonimus westermani
	Fasciolopsis buski
	Heterophyes heterophyes
	Metagonimus yokogawai
	Metorchis conjunctus
	Nanophyetus salmincola
	Taenia solium (adult worm and cysticercosis)
	Taenia saginata
	Diphyllobothrium latum
	Hymenolepis nana
	Dipylidium caninum
Metrifonate	*Schistosoma haematobium* (alternative)
Oxamniquine	*Schistosoma mansoni* (alternative)
Bithionol	*Fasciola hepatica*
	P. westermani (alternative)
Niclosamide	*D. latum*
	T. saginata
	T. solium (adult stage, alternative)
	Hymenolepis nana (alternative)
	D. caninum
Albendazole	Cysticercosis
	Echinococcus granulosus
	Echinococcus multilocularis
	C. sinensis

TABLE 39–2 Drugs for Treatment of Parasitic Infections and Pneumocystosis

Infection	Drug	Adult Dosage	Pediatric Dosage
Acanthamoeba **keratitis**			
Drug of choice:	See footnote 1		
AMEBIASIS (*Entamoeba histolytica*)			
asymptomatic			
Drug of choice:	Iodoquinol	650 mg tid × 20 d	30–40 mg/kg/d (max. 2 g) in 3 doses × 20d
	or Paromomycin	25–35 mg/kg/d in 3 doses × 7d	25–35 mg/kg/d in 3 doses × 7d
Alternative:	Diloxanide furoate	500 mg tid × 10d	20 mg/kg/d in 3 doses × 10d
mild to moderate intestinal disease			
Drug of choice[2]:	Metronidazole	500–750 mg tid × 10d	35–50 mg/kg/d in 3 doses × 10d
	or Tinidazole[3]	2 g/d × 3d	50 mg/kg (max. 2 g) qd × 3d
severe intestinal disease, hepatic abscess			
Drug of choice[2]:	Metronidazole	750 mg tid × 10d	35–50 mg/kg/d in 3 doses × 10d
	or Tinidazole[3]	600 mg bid or 800 mg tid × 5d	50 mg/kg or 60 mg/kg (max. 2 g) qd × 5d
AMEBIC MENINGOENCEPHALITIS, PRIMARY			
Naegleria			
Drug of choice:	Amphotericin B[4, 5]	1 mg/kg/d IV, uncertain duration	1 mg/kg/d IV, uncertain duration
Acanthamoeba			
Drug of choice:	See footnote 6		
ANCYLOSTOMA caninum (Eosinophilic enterocolitis)			
Drug of choice:	Mebendazole	100 mg bid × 3d	100 mg bid × 3d
	or Pyrantel pamoate[5]	11 mg/kg (max. 1 g) × 3d	11 mg/kg (max. 1 g) × 3d
	or Albendazole[5]	400 mg once	400 mg once
Ancylostoma duodenale, see HOOKWORM			
ANGIOSTRONGYLIASIS			
Angiostrongylus cantonensis			
Drug of choice[7]:	Mebendazole[5]	100 mg bid × 5d	100 mg bid × 5d
Angiostrongylus costaricensis			
Drug of choice:	Mebendazole	200–400 mg tid × 10d	200–400 mg tid × 10d
Alternative:	Thiabendazole[5]	75 mg/kg/d in 3 doses × 3d (max. 3 g/d)[8]	75 mg/kg/d in 3 doses × 3d (max. 3 g/d)[8]
ANISAKIASIS (*Anisakis*)			
Treatment of choice:	Surgical or endoscopic removal		
ASCARIASIS (*Ascaris lumbricoides,* roundworm)			
Drug of choice:	Mebendazole	100 mg bid × 3d or 500 mg once	100 mg bid × 3d or 500 mg once
	or Pyrantel pamoate[5]	11 mg/kg once (max. 1 g)	11 mg/kg once (max. 1 g)
	or Albendazole[5]	400 mg once	400 mg once
BABESIOSIS (*Babesia spp.*)			
Drugs of choice[9]:	Clindamycin[5]	1.2 g bid IV or 600 mg tid PO × 7d	20–40 mg/kg/d PO in 3 doses × 7d
	plus quinine	650 mg tid PO × 7d	25 mg/kg/d in 3 doses × 7d
BALANTIDIASIS (*Balantidium coli*)			
Drug of choice:	Tetracycline[5, 10]	500 mg qid × 10d	40 mg/kg/d (max. 2 g) in 4 doses × 10d
Alternatives:	Iodoquinol[5]	650 mg tid × 20d	40 mg/kg/d in 3 doses × 20d
	Metronidazole[5]	750 mg tid × 5d	35–50 mg/kg/d in 3 doses × 5d
BAYLISASCARIASIS (*Baylisascaris procyonis*)			
Drug of choice:	See footnote 11		
BLASTOCYSTIS *hominis* infection			
Drug of choice:	See footnote 12		
CAPILLARIASIS (*Capillaria philippinensis*)			
Drug of choice:	Mebendazole[5]	200 mg bid × 20d	200 mg bid × 20d
Alternative	Albendazole[5]	400 mg daily × 10d	400 mg daily × 10d
Chagas' disease, see TRYPANOSOMIASIS			
Clonorchis sinensis, see FLUKE infection			
CRYPTOSPORIDIOSIS (*Cryptosporidium*)			
Drug of choice[13]:	Paromomycin[5]	25–35 mg/kg/d in 3 or 4 doses	
CUTANEOUS LARVA MIGRANS (creeping eruption, dog and cat hookworm)			
Drug of choice:	Thiabendazole	Topically[14]	Topically[14]
	or Ivermectin[5]	150–200 μg/kg once	150–200 μg/kg once
	or Albendazole[5]	400 mg daily × 3d	400 mg daily × 3d
CYCLOSPORA infection			
Drug of choice:	Trimethoprim-sulfamethoxazole[5, 15]	TMP 160 mg, SMX 800 mg bid × 7d	TMP 5 mg/kg, SMX 25 mg/kg bid × 7d
CYSTICERCOSIS, see TAPEWORM infection			

TABLE 39-2 Drugs for Treatment of Parasitic Infections and Pneumocystosis *Continued*

Infection	Drug	Adult Dosage	Pediatric Dosage
***DIENTAMOEBA** fragilis* infection			
Drug of choice:	Iodoquinol	650 mg tid × 20 d	40 mg/kg/d (max. 2 g) in 3 doses × 20d
	or Paromomycin[5]	25–30 mg/kg/d in 3 doses × 7d	25–30 mg/kg/d in 3 doses × 7d
	or Tetracycline[5, 10]	500 mg qid × 10d	40 mg/kg/d (max. 2 g) in 4 doses × 10d
Diphyllobothrium latum, see TAPEWORM infection			
***DRACUNCULUS** medinensis* (guinea worm) infection			
Drug of choice:	Metronidazole[5,16]	250 mg tid × 10d	25 mg/kg/d (max. 750 mg) in 3 doses × 10d
Echinococcus, see TAPEWORM infection			
Entamoeba histolytica, see AMEBIASIS			
***ENTAMOEBA** polecki* infection			
Drug of choice:	Metronidazole[5]	750 mg tid × 10d	35–50 mg/kg/d in 3 doses × 10d
***ENTEROBIUS** vermicularis* (pinworm) infection			
Drug of choice:	Pyrantel pamoate	11 mg/kg once (max. 1 g); repeat in 2 wk	11 mg/kg once (max. 1 g); repeat in 2 weeks
	or Mebendazole	100 mg once; repeat in 2 wk	100 mg once; repeat in 2 weeks
	or Albendazole[5]	400 mg once; repeat in 2 wk	400 mg once; repeat in 2 weeks
Fasciola hepatica, see FLUKE infection			
FILARIASIS			
Wuchereria bancrofti, Brugia malayi			
Drug of choice[17, 18]:	Diethylcarbamazine[19]	Day 1: 50 mg, p.c. Day 2: 50 mg tid Day 3: 100 mg tid Days 4 through 14: 6 mg/kg/d in 3 doses	Day 1: 1 mg/kg, p.c. Day 2: 1 mg/kg tid Day 3: 1–2 mg/kg tid Days 4 through 14: 6 mg/kg/d in 3 doses
Loa loa			
Drug of choice[18, 20]:	Diethylcarbamazine[19]	Day 1: 50 mg, oral, p.c. Day 2: 50 mg tid Day 3: 100 mg tid Days 4 through 21: 9 mg/kg/d in 3 doses	Day 1: 1 mg/kg, oral, p.c. Day 2: 1 mg/kg tid Day 3: 1–2 mg/kg tid Days 4 through 21: 9 mg/kg/d in 3 doses
Mansonella ozzardi			
Drug of choice:	See footnote 21		
Mansonella perstans			
Drug of choice:	Mebendazole[5]	100 mg bid × 30d	
Mansonella streptocerca			
Drug of choice:	Ivermectin	150 μg/kg once	
	or Diethylcarbamazine	6 mg/kg/d × 14d	
Tropical Pulmonary Eosinophilia (TPE)			
Drug of choice:	Diethylcarbamazine	6 mg/kg/d in 3 doses × 14d	6 mg/kg/d in 3 doses × 14d
Onchocerca volvulus (River blindness)			
Drug of choice:	Ivermectin[22]	150 μg/kg once, repeated every 6 to 12 mo	150 μg/kg once, repeated every 6 to 12 mo
FLUKE, hermaphroditic, infection			
***Clonorchis sinensis* (Chinese liver fluke)**			
Drug of choice:	Praziquantel	75 mg/kg/d in 3 doses × 1d	75 mg/kg/d in 3 doses × 1d
	or Albendazole	10 mg/kg × 7d	
***Fasciola hepatica* (sheep liver fluke)**			
Drug of choice[23]:	Bithionol	30–50 mg/kg on alternate days × 10–15 doses	30–50 mg/kg on alternate days × 10–15 doses
	or Triclabendazole	10 mg/kg once	
***Fasciolopsis buski, Heterophyes heterophyes, Metagonimus yokogawai* (intestinal flukes)**			
Drug of choice:	Praziquantel[5]	75 mg/kg/d in 3 doses × 1d	75 mg/kg/d in 3 doses × 1d
***Metorchis conjunctus* (North American liver fluke)[24]**			
Drug of choice:	Praziquantel[5]	75 mg/kg/d in 3 doses × 1 d	75 mg/kg/d in 3 doses × 1 d
Nanophyetus salmincola			
Drug of choice:	Praziquantel[5]	60 mg/kg/d in 3 doses × 1d	60 mg/kg/d in 3 doses × 1d
***Opisthorchis viverrini* (Southeast Asian liver fluke)**			
Drug of choice:	Praziquantel	75 mg/kg/d in 3 doses × 1d	75 mg/kg/d in 3 doses × 1d
***Paragonimus westermani* (lung fluke)**			
Drug of choice:	Praziquantel[5]	75 mg/kg/d in 3 doses × 2d	75 mg/kg/d in 3 doses × 2d
Alternative[25]:	Bithionol	30–50 mg/kg on alternate days × 10–15 doses	30–50 mg/kg on alternate days × 10–15 doses
GIARDIASIS (*Giardia lamblia*)			
Drug of choice:	Metronidazole[5]	250 mg tid × 5d	15 mg/kg/d in 3 doses × 5d
Alternatives:[26]	Tinidazole[2]	2 g once	50 mg/kg once (max. 2 g)
	Furazolidone	100 mg qid × 7–10d	6 mg/kg/d in 4 doses × 7–10d
	Paromomycin[5,27]	25–35 mg/kg/d in 3 doses × 7d	

TABLE 39–2 Drugs for Treatment of Parasitic Infections and Pneumocystosis *Continued*

Infection	Drug	Adult Dosage	Pediatric Dosage
GNATHOSTOMIASIS (*Gnathostoma spinigerum*)			
Treatment of choice[28]:	Surgical removal		
	or Albendazole[5]	400 mg bid × 21d	
HOOKWORM infection (*Ancylostoma duodenale, Necator americanus*)			
Drug of choice:	Mebendazole	100 mg bid × 3d or 500 mg once	100 mg bid × 3d or 500 mg once
	or Pyrantel pamoate[5]	11 mg/kg (max. 1 g) × 3d	11 mg/kg (max. 1 g) × 3d
	or Albendazole[5]	400 mg once	400 mg once
Hydatid cyst, see TAPEWORM infection			
Hymenolepis nana, see TAPEWORM infection			
ISOSPORIASIS (*Isospora belli*)			
Drug of choice:	Trimethoprim-sulfamethoxazole[5, 29]	160 mg TMP, 800 mg SMX qid × 10d, then bid × 3 wk	
LEISHMANIASIS (*L. mexicana, L. tropica, L. major, L. braziliensis, L. donovani, L. infantum*)			
Drug of choice:	Sodium stibogluconate	20 mg Sb/kg/d IV or IM × 20–28d[30]	20 mg Sb/kg/d IV or IM × 20–28d[30]
	or Meglumine antimonate	20 mg Sb/kg/d × 20–28d[30]	20 mg Sb/kg/d × 20–28d[30]
Alternatives[31]:	Amphotericin B[5]	0.5 to 1 mg/kg by slow infusion daily or every 2d for up to 8 wk	0.5 to 1 mg/kg by slow infusion daily or every 2d for up to 8 wk
	or Lipid-encapsulated Amphotericin B	15–20 mg/kg total dose over 5 or more days	15–20 mg/kg total dose over 5 or more days
	Pentamidine isethionate[5]	2–4 mg/kg daily or every 2d for up to 15 doses[32]	2–4 mg/kg daily or every 2d for up to 15 doses[32]
	Paromomycin	Topically twice daily × 15d[33]	
LICE infestation (*Pediculus humanus, capitis, Phthirus pubis*)[34]			
Drug of choice:	1% Permethrin	Topically	Topically
	or 0.5% Malathion	Topically	Topically
Alternatives:	Pyrethrins with piperonyl butoxide	Topically[35]	Topically[35]
	Ivermectin[5, 36]	200 µg/kg oral once	200 µg/kg oral once
Loa loa, see FILARIASIS			
MALARIA, Treatment of (*Plasmodium falciparum, P. ovale, P. vivax,* and *P. malariae*)			
Chloroquine-resistant *P. falciparum*[37]			
ORAL			
Drugs of choice:	Quinine sulfate	650 mg q8h × 3–7 d[38]	25 mg/kg/d in 3 doses × 3–7 d[38]
	plus		
	doxycycline[5, 10]	100 mg bid × 7d	2 mg/kg/d × 7d
	or plus		
	pyrimethamine-sulfadoxine[39]	3 tablets at once on last day of quinine	<1 yr: 1/4 tablet 1–3 yr: 1/2 tablet 4–8 yr: 1 tablet 9–14 yr: 2 tablets
	or plus		
	clindamycin[5]	900 mg tid × 5d	20–40 mg/kg/d in 3 doses × 5d
Alternatives[40]:	Mefloquine[41,42]	1250 mg once[43]	25 mg/kg once[44] (<45 kg)
	Halofantrine[45]	500 mg q6h × 3 doses; repeat in 1 wk[46]	8 mg/kg q6h × 3 doses (<40 kg); repeat in 1 week[46]
	Atovaquone[5]	1000 mg qd × 3d	11–20 kg: 250 mg, 21–30 kg: 500 mg, 31–40 kg: 750 mg
	plus		
	proguanil[47]	400 mg qd × 3d	11–20 kg: 100 mg, 21–30 kg: 200 mg, 31–40 kg: 300 mg
	or **plus** doxycycline[5,10]	100 mg bid × 3d	2 mg/kg/d × 3d
	Artesunate	4 mg/kg/d × 3d	
	plus		
	mefloquine	1250 mg once[43]	
Chloroquine-resistant *P. vivax*[48]			
Drug of choice:	Quinine sulfate	650 mg q8h × 3–7d[38]	25 mg/kg/d in 3 doses × 3–7d[38]
	plus		
	doxycycline[5,10]	100 mg bid × 7d	2 mg/kg/d × 7d
	or **plus**		
	pyrimethamine-sulfadoxine[39]	3 tablets at once on last day of quinine	<1 yr: 1/4 tablet 1–3 yr: 1/2 tablet 4–8 yr: 1 tablet 9–14 yr: 2 tablets
	or Mefloquine	1250 mg once[43]	25 mg/kg once (<45 kg)[44]
All *Plasmodium* except Chloroquine-resistant *P. falciparum*[37] **and Chloroquine-resistant *P. vivax***[48]			
ORAL			
Drug of choice:	Chloroquine phosphate[49]	1 g (600 mg base), then 500 mg (300 mg base) 6 hr later, then 500 mg (300 mg base) at 24 and 48 hr	10 mg base/kg (max. 600 mg base), then 5 mg base/kg 6 hr later, then 5 mg base/kg at 24 and 48 hr

TABLE 39–2 Drugs for Treatment of Parasitic Infections and Pneumocystosis *Continued*

Infection	Drug	Adult Dosage	Pediatric Dosage
All *Plasmodium*			
PARENTERAL			
Drug of choice[50]:	Quinidine gluconate[51, 52]	10 mg/kg loading dose (max. 600 mg) in normal saline slowly over 1 to 2 hr, followed by continuous infusion of 0.02 mg/kg/min until oral therapy can be started	Same as adult dose
	or		
	Quinine dihydrochloride[51,52]	20 mg/kg loading dose IV in 5% dextrose over 4 hr, followed by 10 mg/kg over 2–4 hr q8h (max. 1800 mg/d) until oral therapy can be started	Same as adult dose
Alternative:	Artemether[53]	3.2 mg/kg IM, then 1.6 mg/kg qd	Same as adult dose
Prevention of relapses: *P. vivax* and *P. ovale* only			
Drug of choice:	Primaquine phosphate[54, 55]	26.3 mg (15 mg base)/d × 14d or 79 mg (45 mg base)/wk × 8 wk	0.3 mg base/kg/d × 14d
MALARIA, Prevention of[56, 57]			
Chloroquine-sensitive areas			
Drug of choice:	Chloroquine phosphate[58]	500 mg (300 mg base), once/wk[59]	5 mg/kg base once/wk, up to adult dose of 300 mg base
Chloroquine-resistant areas			
Drug of choice:	Mefloquine[42, 58, 60]	250 mg once/wk[59]	<5 kg: no data 5–9 kg: 1/8 tablet 10–19 kg: 1/4 tablet 20–30 kg: 1/2 tablet 31–45 kg: 3/4 tablet >45 kg: 1 tablet
	or Doxycycline[10, 58]	100 mg daily[61]	2 mg/kg/d, up to 100 mg/d[10]
	or Primaquine[5, 55, 62]	0.5 mg/kg base daily	Same as adult
Alternatives:	Chloroquine phosphate[58]	Same as above	Same as above
	plus pyrimethamine-sulfadoxine[39] for presumptive treatment[63]	Carry a single dose (3 tablets) for self-treatment of febrile illness when medical care is not immediately available	<1 yr: 1/4 tablet 1–3 yr: 1/2 tablet 4–8 yr: 1 tablet 9–14 yr: 2 tablets
	or **plus** proguanil[64]	200 mg daily	<2 yr: 50 mg daily 2–6 yr: 100 mg 7–10 yr: 150 mg >10 yr: 200 mg
MICROSPORIDIOSIS			
Ocular (*Encephalitozoon hellem, Encephalitozoon cuniculi, Vittaforma corneae* [*Nosema corneum*])			
Drug of choice[65]:	Albendazole[5]	400 mg bid	
Intestinal (*Enterocytozoon bieneusi, Encephalitozoon [Septata] intestinalis*)			
Drug of choice[66]:	Albendazole[5]	400 mg bid	
Disseminated (*E. hellem, E. cuniculi, E. intestinalis, Pleistophora sp.*)			
Drug of choice[67]:	Albendazole[5]	400 mg bid	
Mites, see SCABIES			
MONILIFORMIS *moniliformis* infection			
Drug of choice:	Pyrantel pamoate[5]	11 mg/kg once, repeat twice, 2 wk apart	11 mg/kg once, repeat twice, 2 wk apart
***Naegleria* species,** see AMEBIC MENINGOENCEPHALITIS, PRIMARY			
Necator americanus, see HOOKWORM infection			
OESOPHAGOSTOMUM *bifurcum*			
Drug of choice:	See footnote 68		
Onchocerca volvulus, see FILARIASIS			
Opisthorchis viverrini, see FLUKE infection			
Paragonimus westermani, see FLUKE infection			
Pediculus capitis, P. humanus, Phthirus pubis, see LICE			
Pinworm, see ENTEROBIUS			

TABLE 39-2 Drugs for Treatment of Parasitic Infections and Pneumocystosis *Continued*

Infection	Drug	Adult Dosage	Pediatric Dosage
***PNEUMOCYSTIS** carinii* pneumonia[69]			
Drug of choice:	Trimethoprim-sulfamethoxazole	TMP 15 mg/kg/d, SMX 75 mg/kg/d, oral or IV in 3 or 4 doses × 14–21d	Same as adult dose
Alternatives:	Pentamidine	3–4 mg/kg IV qd × 14–21 d	Same as adult dose
	Trimetrexate	45 mg/m² IV qd × 21 d	
	plus folinic acid	20 mg/m² PO or IV q6h × 21 d	
	Trimethoprim[5]	5 mg/kg PO tid × 21 d	
	plus dapsone[5]	100 mg PO qd × 21 d	
	Atovaquone	750 mg bid PO × 21 d	
	Primaquine[5, 55]	30 mg base PO qd × 21 d	
	plus clindamycin[5]	600 mg IV q6h × 21 d, or 300–450 mg PO q6h × 21 d	
Primary and secondary prophylaxis			
Drug of choice:	Trimethoprim-sulfamethoxazole	1 tab (single or double strength) PO qd or 1 DS tab 3×/wk	TMP 150 mg/m², SMX 750 mg/m² in 2 doses PO on 3 consecutive d/wk
Alternatives:	Dapsone[5]	50 mg PO bid, or 100 mg PO qd	2 mg/kg (max. 100 mg) PO qd
	Dapsone[5]	50 mg PO qd or 200 mg each wk	
	plus pyrimethamine[70]	50 mg or 75 mg PO each wk	
	Pendamidine aerosol	300 mg inhaled monthly via Respirgard II nebulizer	>5 yr: same as adult dose
	Atovaquone[5]	750 mg bid	
Roundworm, see ASCARIASIS			
SCABIES (*Sarcoptes scabiei*)			
Drug of choice:	5% Permethrin	Topically	Topically
Alternatives:	Ivermectin[5]	200 μg/kg PO once	200 μg/kg PO once
	10% Crotamiton	Topically	Topically
SCHISTOSOMIASIS (*Bilharziasis*)			
S. haematobium			
Drug of choice:	Praziquantel	40 mg/kg/d in 2 doses × 1d	40 mg/kg/d in 2 doses × 1d
S. japonicum			
Drug of choice:	Praziquantel	60 mg/kg/d in 3 doses × 1d	60 mg/kg/d in 3 doses × 1d
S. mansoni			
Drug of choice:	Praziquantel	40 mg/kg/d in 2 doses × 1d	40 mg/kg/d in 2 doses × 1d
Alternative:	Oxamniquine[71]	15 mg/kg once[72]	20 mg/kg/d in 2 doses × 1d[72]
S. mekongi			
Drug of choice:	Praziquantel	60 mg/kg/d in 3 doses × 1d	60 mg/kg/d in 3 doses × 1d
Sleeping sickness, see TRYPANOSOMIASIS			
STRONGYLOIDIASIS (*Strongyloides stercoralis*)			
Drug of choice[73, 74]:	Ivermectin	200 μg/kg/d × 1–2d	200 μg/kg/d × 1–2d
Alternative:	Thiabendazole	50 mg/kg/d in 2 doses (max. 3 g/d) × 2d[8]	50 mg/kg/d in 2 doses (max. 3 g/d) × 2d[8]
TAPEWORM infection—**Adult (intestinal stage)**			
***Diphyllobothrium latum* (fish), *Taenia saginata* (beef), *Taenia solium* (pork), *Dipylidium caninum* (dog)**			
Drug of choice:	Praziquantel[5]	5–10 mg/kg once	5–10 mg/kg once
***Hymenolepis nana* (dwarf tapeworm)**			
Drug of choice:	Praziquantel[5]	25 mg/kg once	25 mg/kg once
—Larval (tissue stage)			
***Echinococcus granulosus* (hydatid cyst)**			
Drug of choice[75, 76]:	Albendazole	400 mg bid × 28 d, repeated as necessary	15 mg/kg/d × 28 d, repeated as necessary
Echinococcus multilocularis			
Treatment of choice:	See footnote 77		
***Cysticercus cellulosae* (cysticercosis)**			
Drug of choice[78]:	Albendazole	400 mg bid × 8–30d, repeated as necessary	15 mg/kg/d (max. 800 mg) in 2 doses × 8–30d, repeated as necessary
	or Praziquantel[5]	50 mg/kg/d in 3 doses × 15d	
Alternative:	Surgery		
Toxocariasis, see VISCERAL LARVA MIGRANS			
TOXOPLASMOSIS (*Toxoplasma gondii*)[79]			
Drugs of choice[80]:	Pyrimethamine[81]	25–100 mg/d × 3–4 wk	2 mg/kg/d × 3d, then 1 mg/kg/d (max. 25 mg/d) × 4 wk[82]
	plus sulfadiazine	1–1.5 g qid × 3–4 wk	100–200 mg/kg/d × 3–4 wk
Alternative[83]:	Spiramycin	3–4 g/d	50–100 mg/kg/d × 3–4 wk
TRICHINOSIS (*Trichinella spiralis*)			
Drugs of choice:	Steroids for severe symptoms		
	plus mebendazole[5, 84]	200–400 mg tid × 3d, then 400–500 mg tid × 10d	
TRICHOMONIASIS (*Trichomonas vaginalis*)			
Drug of choice[85]:	Metronidazole	2 g once; or 250 mg tid or 375 mg bid PO × 7d	15 mg/kg/d orally in 3 doses × 7d
	or Tinidazole[3]	2 g once	50 mg/kg once (max. 2 g)

TABLE 39–2 Drugs for Treatment of Parasitic Infections and Pneumocystosis *Continued*

Infection	Drug	Adult Dosage	Pediatric Dosage
TRICHOSTRONGYLUS infection			
Drug of choice:	Pyrantel pamoate[5]	11 mg/kg once (max. 1 g)	11 mg/kg once (max. 1 g)
Alternative:	Mebendazole[5]	100 mg bid × 3d	100 mg bid × 3d
	or Albendazole[5]	400 mg once	400 mg once
TRICHURIASIS (*Trichuris trichiura,* whipworm)			
Drug of choice:	Mebendazole	100 mg bid × 3d or 500 mg once	100 mg bid × 3d or 500 mg once
Alternative:	Albendazole[5]	400 mg once[86]	400 mg once[86]
TRYPANOSOMIASIS			
T. cruzi **(American trypanosomiasis, Chagas' disease)**			
Drug of choice:	Nifurtimox[87]	8–10 mg/kg/d in 3–4 doses × 90–120d	1–10 yr: 15–20 mg/kg/d in 4 doses × 90d; 11–16 yr: 12.5–15 mg/kg/d in 4 doses × 90d
Alternative:	Benznidazole	5–7 mg/kg/d × 30–90d	Up to 12 yr: 10 mg/kg/d in 2 doses × 30–90d
T. brucei gambiense, T. b. rhodesiense **(African trypanosomiasis, sleeping sickness) hemolymphatic stage**			
Drug of choice:	Suramin	100–200 mg (test dose) IV, then 1 g IV on days 1, 3, 7, 14, and 21	20 mg/kg on days 1, 3, 7, 14, and 21
	or Eflornithine	See footnote 88	
Alternative:	Pentamidine isethionate[5]	4 mg/kg/d IM × 10d	4 mg/kg/d IM × 10d
Late disease with CNS involvement			
Drug of choice:	Melarsoprol[89]	2–3.6 mg/kg/d IV × 3 d; after 1 wk 3.6 mg/kg/d IV × 3d; repeat again after 10–21 d	18–25 mg/kg total over 1 mo; initial dose of 0.36 mg/kg IV, increasing gradually to max. 3.6 mg/kg at intervals of 1–5 d for total of 9–10 doses
	or Eflornithine	See footnote 88	
Alternatives (*T.b. gambiense* only):	Tryparsamide	One injection of 30 mg/kg (max. 2 g) IV every 5d to total of 12 injections; may be repeated after 1 mo	
	plus suramin	One injection of 10 mg/kg IV every 5d to total of 12 injections; may be repeated after 1 mo	
VISCERAL LARVA MIGRANS[90] **(Toxocariasis)**			
Drug of choice:	Diethylcarbamazine[5]	6 mg/kg/d in 3 doses × 7–10d	6 mg/kg/d in 3 doses × 7–10d
Alternatives:	Albendazole	400 mg bid × 3–5d	400 mg bid × 3–5d
	Mebendazole[5]	100–200 mg bid × 5d	100–200 mg bid × 5d
Whipworm, see TRICHURIASIS			
Wuchereria bancrofti, see FILARIASIS			

1. Trophozoites and cysts of *Acanthamoeba* from infected corneas, contact lenses, and their cases are susceptible *in vitro* to chlorhexidine, polyhexamethylene biguanide, propamidine, pentamidine, diminazine and neomycin and, especially, to combinations of these drugs (J Hay et al, Eye, 8:555, 1994). For treatment of keratitis, oral itraconazole plus topical miconazole (Y Ishabashi et al, Am J Ophthalmol, 109:121, 1990) or topical 0.02% polyhexamethylene biguanide (PHMB) plus 0.1% propamidine isethionate (*Brolene*) have been successful (IGM Duguid et al, Ophthalmology, 104:1587, 1997). PHMB is available as *Baquacil* (Zeneca), a swimming pool disinfectant (E Yee and TK Winarko, Am J Hosp Pharm. 50:2523, 1993).
2. Treatment should be followed by a course of iodoquinol or paromomycin in the dosage used to treat asymptomatic amebiasis.
3. A nitro-imidazole similar to metronidazole, but not marketed in the USA, tinidazole appears to be at least as effective as metronidazole and better tolerated. Ornidazole, a similar drug, is also used outside the USA. Higher dosage is for hepatic abscess.
4. Naegleria infections have been treated successfully with amphotericin B, rifampin and chloramphenicol (A Wang et al, Clin Neurol Neurosurg, 95:249, 1993), amphotericin B, oral rifampin and oral ketoconazole (N Poungvarin et al, J Med Assoc Thailand, 74:112, 1991), or amphotericin B alone (RL Brown, Arch Intern Med, 152:1330, 1992).
5. An approved drug, but considered investigational for this condition by the U.S. Food and Drug Administration.
6. Strains of *Acanthamoeba* isolated from fatal granulomatous amebic encephalitis are usually susceptible *in vitro* to pentamidine, ketoconazole (*Nizoral*), flucytosine (*Ancobon*) and (less so) to amphotericin B. One patient with disseminated infection was treated successfully with intravenous pentamidine isethionate, topical chlorhexidine and 2% ketoconazole cream followed by oral itraconazole (CA Slater et al, N Engl J Med, 331:85, 1994).
7. Antiparasitic drugs can provoke neurologic symptoms, and most patients recover spontaneously without them. Analgesics, corticosteroids, and careful removal of CSF at frequent intervals can relieve symptoms (J Koo et al, Rev Infect Dis, 10:1155, 1988). Albendazole, levamisole (*Ergamisol*), or ivermectin have been used successfully in animals.
8. This dose is likely to be toxic and may have to be decreased.
9. Atovaquone suspension, 750 mg bid., plus azithromycin, 500 to 1000 mg daily, may be effective when quinine and clindamycin fail (M Wittner et al, Am J Trop Med Hyg, 55:219, 1996). Exchange transfusion has been used in severely ill patients with high (>10%) parasitemia (V Iacopino and T Earnhart, Arch Intern Med, 150:1527, 1990). One report indicates that azithromycin, 500–1000 mg daily, plus quinine may also be effective (LM Weiss et al, J Infect Dis, 168:1289, 1993). Concurrent use of pentamidine and trimethoprim-sulfamethoxazole has been reported to cure an infection with *B. divergens* (D Raoult et al, Ann Intern Med, 107:944, 1987).
10. Use of tetracyclines is contraindicated in pregnancy and in children less than 8 years old.
11. Drugs that could be tried include albendazole, mebendazole, thiabendazole, levamisole (*Ergamisol*) and ivermectin. Steroid therapy may be helpful, especially in eye and CNS infections. Ocular baylisascariasis has been treated successfully using laser photocoagulation therapy to destroy the intraretinal larvae.
12. Clinical significance of these organisms is controversial, but metronidazole 750 mg tid × 10d or iodoquinol 650 mg tid × 20d anecdotally has been reported to be effective (PFL Boreham and D Stenzel, Adv Parasitol, 32:2, 1993; JS Keystone; EK Markell, Clin Infect Dis, 21:102 and 104, 1995).
13. Infection is self-limited in immunocompetent patients. Duration of treatment is uncertain.
14. HD Davies et al, Arch Dermatol, 129:588, 1993.
15. HIV-infected patients may need higher dosage and long-term maintenance (JW Pape et al, Ann Intern Med, 121:654, 1994).
16. Not curative, but decreases inflammation and facilitates removing the worm. Mebendazole 400–800 mg/d for 6d has been reported to kill the worm directly.
17. A single dose of ivermectin, 20–200 μg/kg, is effective for treatment of microfilaremia but does not kill the adult worm. Use of single doses of ivermectin 200–400 μg/kg and albendazole 400 mg has been more effective than ivermectin alone (DG Addiss et al, Lancet, 350:480, 1997).
18. Antihistamines or corticosteroids may be required to decrease allergic reactions due to disintegration of microfilariae in treatment of filarial infections, especially those caused by *Loa loa*.
19. For patients with no microfilariae in the blood, full doses can be given from day one.
20. In heavy infections with *Loa loa,* rapid killing of microfilariae can provoke an encephalopathy. Ivermectin or albendazole has been used to reduce microfilaremia (Y Martin-Prevel et al, Am J Trop Med Hyg, 48:186, 1993; AD Klion et al, J Infect Dis, 168:202, 1993; J Gardon et al, Trans R Soc Trop Med Hyg, 91:593, 1997). Apheresis has been reported to be effective in lowering microfilarial counts in patients heavily infected with *Loa loa* (EA Ottesen, Infect Dis Clin North Am, 7:619, 1993). Diethylcarbamazine, 300 mg once weekly, has been recommended for prevention of loiasis (TB Nutman et al, N Engl J Med, 319:752, 1988).
21. Diethylcarbamazine has no effect. Ivermectin, 6 mg once, has been effective (DD Chadee et al, Ann Trop Med Parasitol, 90:645, 1996).
22. Annual treatment with ivermectin 150 μg/kg can prevent blindness due to ocular onchocerciasis (D Mabey et al, Ophthalmology, 103:1001, 1996).
23. Unlike infections with other flukes, *Fasciola hepatica* infections may not respond to praziquantel. Triclabendazole (*Fasinex* – Novartis), a veterinary fasciolide, has been safe and effective (W Apt et al, Am J Trop Med Hyg, 52:532, 1995).
24. JD MacLean et al, Lancet, 347:154, 1996.

TABLE 39–2 Drugs for Treatment of Parasitic Infections and Pneumocystosis *Continued*

25. Unpublished data indicate triclabendazole (*Fasinex*), a veterinary fasciolide, may be effective in a dosage of 5 mg/kg once daily for 3 days or 10 mg/kg twice in one day.
26. Albendazole 400 mg daily × 5d may be effective (A Hall and Q Nahar, Trans R Soc Trop Med Hyg, 87:84, 1993). Bacitracin zinc or bacitracin 120,000 U bid for 10 days may also be effective (BJ Andrews et al, Am J Trop Med Hyg, 52:318, 1995).
27. Not absorbed; may be useful for treatment of giardiasis in pregnancy.
28. Ivermectin has been reported to be effective in animals (MT Anantaphruti et al, Trop Med Parasitol, 43:65, 1992).
29. In sulfonamide-sensitive patients, pyrimethamine 50–75 mg daily has been effective (JP Ackers, Semin Gastrointest Dis, 8:33, 1997).
30. May be repeated or continued. A longer duration may be needed for some forms of visceral leishmaniasis.
31. Some studies indicate that *L. donovani* resistant to sodium stibogluconate or meglumine antimonate may respond to lipid-encapsulated amphotericin B (JD Berman, Clin Infect Dis, 24:684, 1997; S Sundar et al, Ann Intern Med, 127:133, 1997; L diMartino et al, J Pediatr, 131:271, 1997). the combination of aminosidine (chemically identical to paromomycin) and sodium stibogluconate has been used to cure kala-azar (CP Thakur et al, Trans R Soc Trop Med Hyg, 89:219, 1995) and diffuse cutaneous leishmaniasis caused by *L. aethiopica* (S Teklemariam et al, Trans R Soc Trop Med Hyg, 88:334, 1994).
32. 4 mg/kg qod × 15 doses for *L. donovani;* 2 mg/kg qod × 7 or 3 mg/kg qod × 4 doses for cutaneous disease.
33. A formulation of 15% paromomycin sulfate and 12% methylbenzethonium chloride in soft white paraffin topically has been reported to be effective in some patients against cutaneous leishmaniasis due to *L. major* (O Ozgoztasi and I Baydar, Int J Dermatol, 36:61, 1997).
34. For infestation of eyelashes with crab lice, use petrolatum.
35. A second application is recommended one week later to kill hatching progeny.
36. Medical Letter, 39:6, 1997.
37. Chloroquine-resistant *P. falciparum* occur in all malarious areas except Central America west of the Panama Canal Zone, Mexico, Haiti, the Dominican Republic, and most of the Middle East (chloroquine resistance has been reported in Yemen, Oman and Iran).
38. In Southeast Asia, relative resistance to quinine has increased and the treatment should be continued for seven days.
39. *Fansidar* tablets contain 25 mg of pyrimethamine and 500 mg of sulfadoxine. Resistance to pyrimethamine-sulfadoxine has been reported from Southeast Asia, the Amazon basin, sub-Saharan Africa, Bangladesh and Oceania.
40. For treatment of multiple-drug-resistant *P. falciparum* in Southeast Asia, especially Thailand, where resistance to mefloquine and halofantrine is frequent, a 7-day course of quinine and tetracycline is recommended (G Watt et al, Am J Trop Med Hyg, 47:108, 1992). Artesunate plus mefloquine (C Luxemburger et al, Trans R Soc Trop Med Hyg, 88:213, 1994), artemether plus mefloquine (J Karbwang et al, Trans R Soc Trop Med Hyg, 89:296, 1995) or mefloquine plus doxycycline are also used to treat multiple-drug-resistant *P. falciparum.*
41. At this dosage, adverse effects including nausea, vomiting, diarrhea, dizziness, disturbed sense of balance, toxic psychosis and seizures can occur. Mefloquine is teratogenic in animals and has not been approved for use in pregnancy, but mefloquine prophylaxis appears to be safe when used during the second half of pregnancy and possibly during early pregnancy as well (BL Smoak et al, J Infect Dis, 175:831, 1997). It should not be given together with quinine or quinidine, and caution is required in using quinine or quinidine to treat patients with malaria who have taken mefloquine for prophylaxis. The pediatric dosage has not been approved by the FDA. Resistance to mefloquine has been reported in some areas, such as the Thailand-Myanmar border, where 25 mg/kg should be used.
42. In the USA, a 250-mg tablet of mefloquine contains 228 mg mefloquine base. Outside the USA, each 275-mg tablet contains 250 mg base.
43. 750 mg followed 12 hours later by 500 mg.
44. 15 mg/kg followed 8–12 hours later by 10 mg/kg.
45. May be effective in multiple-drug-resistant *P. falciparum* malaria, but treatment failures and resistance have been reported, and the drug has caused lengthening of the PR and QTc intervals and fatal cardiac arrhythmias. It should not be used for patients with cardiac conduction defects. Cardiac monitoring is recommended. Variability in absorption is a problem; halofantrine should not be taken one hour before to two hours after meals because food increases its absorption.
46. A single 250-mg dose can be used for repeat treatment in mild to moderate infections (JE Touze et al, Lancet, 349:255, 1997).
47. PD Radloff et al, Lancet 347:1511, 1996; S Looareesuwan et al, Am J Trop Med Hyg, 54:62, 1997; FEC de Alencar et al, J Infect Dis, 175:1544, 1997. Atovaquone plus proguanil is available outside the USA in a combination tablet (250 mg atovaquone, 100 mg proguanil) as *Malarone.*
48. *P. vivax* with decreased susceptibility to chloroquine has been reported in Papua-New Guinea, Indonesia, Myanmar, India, Irian Jaya and the Solomon Islands.
49. If chloroquine phosphate is not available, hydroxychloroquine sulfate is as effective; 400 mg of hydroxychloroquine sulfate is equivalent to 500 mg of chloroquine phosphate.
50. Exchange transfusion has been helpful for some patients with high-density (>10%) parasitemia, altered mental status, pulmonary edema or renal complications (KD Miller et al, N Engl J Med, 321:65, 1989).
51. Continuous EKG, blood pressure and glucose monitoring are recommended, especially in pregnant women and young children.
52. Quinidine may have greater antimalarial activity than quinine. The loading dose should be decreased or omitted in those patients who have received quinine or mefloquine. If more than 48 hours of parenteral treatment is required, the quinine or quinidine dose should be reduced by 1/3 to 1/2.
53. NJ White, N Engl J Med, 335:800, 1996.
54. Some relapses have been reported with this regimen, especially in strains from Southeast Asia; relapses should be treated with a second 14-day course of 30 mg base/day.
55. Primaquine phosphate can cause hemolytic anemia, especially in patients whose red cells are deficient in glucose-6-phosphate dehydrogenase. This deficiency is most common in African, Asian, and Mediterranean peoples. Patients should be screened for G-6-PD deficiency before treatment. Primaquine should not be used during pregnancy.
56. No drug regimen guarantees protection against malaria. If fever develops within a year (particularly within the first two months) after travel to malarious areas, travelers should be advised to seek medical attention. Insect repellents, insecticide-impregnated bed nets and proper clothing are important adjuncts for malaria prophylaxis.
57. In pregnancy, chloroquine prophylaxis has been used extensively and safely; the safety of other prophylactic antimalarial agents in pregnancy is less clear. Therefore, travel during pregnancy to chloroquine-resistant areas should be discouraged. See footnote 37.
58. For prevention of attack after departure from areas where *P. vivax* and *P. ovale* are endemic, which includes almost all areas where malaria is found (except Haiti), some experts prescribe in addition primaquine phosphate 15 mg base (26.3 mg)/d or, for children, 0.3 mg base/kg/d during the last two weeks of prophylaxis. Others prefer to avoid the toxicity of primaquine and rely on surveillance to detect cases when they occur, particularly when exposure was limited or doubtful. See also footnotes 54 and 55.
59. Beginning one week before travel and continuing weekly for the duration of stay and for four weeks after leaving.
60. The pediatric dosage has not been approved by the FDA, and the drug has not been approved for use during pregnancy. However, it has been reported to be safe for prophylactic use during the second half of pregnancy and possibly during early pregnancy as well (BL Smoak et al, J Infect Dis, 176:831, 1997). Women should take contraceptive precautions while taking mefloquine and for two months after the last dose. Mefloquine is not recommended for patients with cardiac conduction abnormalities. Patients with a history of seizures or psychiatric disorders should probably avoid mefloquine (Medical Letter, 32:13, 1990). Resistance to mefloquine has been reported in some areas, such as Thailand; in these areas, doxycycline should be used for prophylaxis. In children less than eight years old, proguanil plus sulfisoxazole has been used (KN Suh and JS Keystone, Infect Dis Clin Pract, 5:541, 1996).
61. Beginning one day before travel and continuing for the duration of stay and for four weeks after leaving. Use of tetracyclines is contraindicated in pregnancy and in children less than eight years old. Doxycycline can cause gastrointestinal disturbances, vaginal moniliasis and photosensitivity reactions.
62. Several studies have shown that daily primaquine provides effective prophylaxis against chloroquine-resistant *P. falciparum* (WR Weiss et al, J Infect Dis, 171:1569, 1995; DJ Fryauff et al, Lancet, 346:1190, 1995).
63. In areas with strains resistant to pyrimethamine-sulfadoxine, atovaquone plus proguanil or doxycycline can also be used for presumptive treatment.
64. Proguanil (*Paludrine*—Wyeth Ayerst, Canada; Zeneca, England), which is not available in the USA but is widely available in Canada and overseas, is recommended mainly for use in Africa south of the Sahara. Prophylaxis is recommended during exposure and for four weeks afterwards. Proguanil has been used in pregnancy without evidence of toxicity (PA Phillips-Howard and D Wood, Drug Saf, 14:131, 1996).
65. Ocular lesions due to *E. hellem* in HIV-infected patients have responded to fumagillin eyedrops prepared from *Fumidil-B,* a commercial product (Mid-Continent Agrimarketing, Inc., Olathe, Kansas, 1-800-547-1392) used to control a microsporidial disease of honey bees (MC Diesenhouse, Am J Ophthalmol, 115:293, 1993). For lesions due to *V. corneae,* topical therapy is generally not effective and keratoplasty may be required (RM Davis et al, Ophthalmology, 97:953, 1990).
66. Octreotide (*Sandostatin*) has provided symptomatic relief in some patients with large volume diarrhea. Oral fumagillin (see footnote 65) has been effective in treating *E. bieneusi* (J-M Molina et al, AIDS, 11:1603, 1997), but has been associated with thrombocytopenia.
67. J-M Molina et al, J Infect Dis, 171:245, 1995. There is no established treatment for *Pleistophora.*
68. Albendazole or pyrantel pamoate may be effective (HP Krepel et al, Trans R Soc Trop Med Hyg, 87:87, 1993).
69. In severe disease with room air $PO_2 \leq 70$ mmHg or Aa gradient ≥35 mmHg, prednisone should also be used (S Gagnon et al, N Engl J Med, 323:1444, 1990; E Caumes et al, Clin Infect Dis, 18:319, 1994).
70. Plus leucovorin 25 mg with each dose of pyrimethamine.
71. Oxamniquine has been effective in some areas in which praziquantel is less effective (FF Steima et al, J Infect Dis, 176:304, 1997). Oxamniquine is contraindicated in pregnancy.
72. In East Africa, the dose should be increased to 30 mg/kg, and in Egypt and South Africa, 30 mg/kg/d × 2d. Some experts recommend 40–60 mg/kg over 2–3 days in all of Africa (KC Shekhar, Drugs, 42:379, 1991).
73. In immunocompromised patients or disseminated disease, it may be necessary to prolong or repeat therapy or use other agents.
74. Ivermectin is not FDA-approved for disseminated strongyloidiasis, and thiabendazole may be preferred.
75. Some patients may benefit from or require surgical resection of cysts (RK Tomplins, Mayo Clin Proc, 66:1281, 1991). Praziquantel may be useful preoperatively or in case of spill during surgery.
76. Percutaneous drainage with ultrasound guidance plus albendazole therapy has been effective for management of hepatic hydatid cyst disease (MS Khuroo et al, N Engl J Med, 337:881, 1997).
77. Surgical excision is the only reliable means of treatment. Some reports have suggested use of albendazole or mebendazole (W Hao et al, Trans R Soc Trop Med Hyg, 88L340, 1994; WHO Group, Bull WHO, 74:231, 1996).
78. Corticosteroids should be given for two to three days before and during drug therapy for neurocysticercosis. Any cysticercocidal drug may cause irreparable damage when used to treat ocular or spinal cysts, even when corticosteroids are used (AC White, Jr, Clin Infect Dis, 24:101, 1997). An ophthalmic examination should be done before treatment.
79. In ocular toxoplasmosis, corticosteroids should also be used for an anti-inflammatory effect on the eyes.

TABLE 39–2 Drugs for Treatment of Parasitic Infections and Pneumocystosis *Continued*

80. To treat CNS toxoplasmosis in HIV-infected patients, some clinicians have used pyrimethamine 50 to 100 mg daily after a loading dose of 200 mg with a sulfonamide and, when sulfonamide sensitivity developed, have given clindamycin 1.8 to 2.4 g/d in divided doses instead of the sulfonamide (JS Remington et al, Lancet, 338:1142, 1991; BJ Luft et al, N Engl J Med, 329:995, 1993). Atovaquone plus pyrimethamine appears to be an effective alternative in sulfa-intolerant patients (JA Kovacs et al, Lancet, 340:637, 1992). For primary prophylaxis in HIV patients with <100 CD4 cells, either trimethoprim-sulfamethoxazole, pyrimethamine plus dapsone or pyrimethamine plus sulfisoxazole can be used (USPHS/IDSA, Clin Infect Dis, 25 suppl 3:S313, 1997). Pyrimethamine plus folinic acid should be considered in HIV patients with <100 CD4 counts who are intolerant to trimethoprim-sulfamethoxazole (C Leport et al, J Infect Dis, 173:91, 1996).
81. Plus leucovorin 10 mg with each dose of pyrimethamine.
82. Congenitally infected newborns should be treated with pyrimethamine every two or three days and a sulfonamide daily for about one year (JS Remington and G. Desmonts in JS Remington and JO Klein, eds, *Infectious Disease of the Fetus and Newborn Infant*, 4th ed, Philadelphia:Saunders, 1995, page 140).
83. For prophylactic use during pregnancy. If it is determined that transmission has occurred *in utero*, therapy with pyrimethamine and sulfadiazine should be started.
84. Albendazole or flubendazole (not available in the USA) may also be effective.
85. Sexual partners should be treated simultaneously. Metronidazole-resistant strains have been reported; higher doses of metronidazole for longer periods or use of tinidazole are sometimes effective against these strains (J Lossick, Rev Infect Dis, 12:S665, 1990). Desensitization has been recommended for patients allergic to metronidazole (MD Pearlman et al, Am J Obstet Gynecol, 174:934, 1996).
86. In heavy infection, it may be necessary to extend therapy to 3 days.
87. The addition of gamma interferon to nifurtimox for 20 days in a limited number of patients and in experimental animals appears to have shortened the acute phase of Chagas' disease (RE McCabe et al, J Infect Dis, 163:912, 1991).
88. Eflornithine is highly effective in *T.b. gambiense* and variably effective in *T.b. rhodesiense* infections, but remaining supply (only available from WHO) is very limited. Some clinicians have given 400 mg/kg/d IV in 4 divided doses for 14 days, followed by oral treatment with 300 mg/kg/d for 3–4 wks (F Milford et al, Lancet, 340:652, 1992).
89. In frail patients, begin with as little as 18 mg and increase the dose progressively. Pretreatment with suramin has been advocated for debilitated patients. Corticosteroids have been used to prevent arsenical encephalopathy (J Pepin et al, Trans R Soc Trop Med Hyg, 89:92, 1995).
90. For severe symptoms or eye involvement, corticosteroids can be used in addition.

From Drugs for treatment of parasitic infections. Med Lett Drugs Ther. 1998; 40:1–12.

TABLE 39–3 Manufacturers and Adverse Effects of Some Antiparasitic Drugs*

ALBENDAZOLE—*Albenza* (SmithKline Beecham)
Occasional: abdominal pain; reversible alopecia; increased serum transaminase activity; migration of *Ascaris* through mouth and nose
Rare: leukopenia; rash; renal toxicity

‡**AMINOSIDINE**—See Paromomycin

‡**ARTEMETHER**—*Artenam* (Arenco, Belgium)
Occasional: neurological toxicity; possible increase in length of coma; increased convulsions; prolongation of QTc interval

‡**ARTESUNATE**—(Guilin No. 1 Factory, People's Republic of China)
Occasional: ataxia; slurred speech; neurological toxicity; possible increase in length of coma; increased convulsions; prolongation of QTc interval

ATOVAQUONE—*Mepron* (Glaxo-Wellcome); ‡*Malarone* (with proguanil)
Frequent: rash; nausea
Occasional: diarrhea

BACITRACIN—many manufacturers
Frequent: nephrotoxicity
Occasional: rash
Rare: anaphylaxis

‡**BACITRACIN-ZINC**—(Apothekernes Laboratorium A.S., Oslo, Norway)

‡**BENZNIDAZOLE**—*Rochagan* (Roche, Brazil)
Frequent: allergic rash; dose-dependent polyneuropathy; gastrointestinal disturbances; psychic disturbances

§**BITHIONOL**—*Bitin* (Tanabe, Japan)
Frequent: photosensitivity reactions; vomiting; diarrhea; abdominal pain; urticaria
Rare: leukopenia; toxic hepatitis

CHLOROQUINE HCl and CHLOROQUINE PHOSPHATE—*Aralen* (Sanofi Wintrop), others
Occasional: pruritus; vomiting; headache; confusion; depigmentation of hair; skin eruptions; corneal opacity; weight loss; partial alopecia; extraocular muscle palsies; exacerbation of psoriasis, eczema, and other exfoliative dermatoses; myalgias, photophobia
Rare: irreversible retinal injury (especially when total dosage exceeds 100 grams); discoloration of nails and mucous membranes; nerve-type deafness; peripheral neuropathy and myopathy; heart block; blood dyscrasias; hematemesis

CROTAMITON—*Eurax* (Westwood-Squibb)
Occasional: rash; conjunctivitis

DAPSONE—(Jacobus)
Frequent: rash; transient headache; GI irritation; anorexia; infectious mononucleosis-like syndrome
Occasional: cyanosis due to methemoglobinemia and sulfhemoglobinemia; other blood dyscrasias, including hemolytic anemia; nephrotic syndrome; liver damage; peripheral neuropathy; hypersensitivity reactions; increased risk of lepra reactions; insomnia; irritability; uncoordinated speech; agitation; acute psychosis
Rare: renal papillary necrosis; severe hypoalbuminemia; epidermal necrolysis; optic atrophy; agranulocytosis; neonatal hyperbilirubinemia after use in pregnancy

†**DIETHYLCARBAMAZINE CITRATE USP**—*Hetrazan* (Wyeth-Ayerst)
Frequent: severe allergic or febrile reactions in patients with microfilariae in the blood or the skin; GI disturbances
Rare: encephalopathy

‡**DILOXANIDE FUROATE**—*Furamide* (Boots, England)
Frequent: flatulence
Occasional: nausea; vomiting; diarrhea
Rare: diplopia, dizziness; urticaria; pruritus

†**EFLORNITHINE** (Difluoromethylornithine, DFMO)—*Ornidyl* (Hoechst Marion Roussel)
Frequent: anemia; leukopenia
Occasional: diarrhea; thrombocytopenia; seizures
Rare: hearing loss

‡**FLUBENDAZOLE**—similar to mebendazole

FURAZOLIDONE—*Furoxone* (Roberts)
Frequent: nausea; vomiting
Occasional: allergic reactions, including pulmonary infiltration, hypotension, urticaria, fever, vesicular rash; hypoglycemia; headache
Rare: hemolytic anemia in G-6-PD deficiency and neonates; disulfiram-like reaction with alcohol; MAO-inhibitor interactions; polyneuritis

‡**HALOFANTRINE**—*Halfan* (SmithKline Beecham)
Occasional: diarrhea; abdominal pain, pruritus; serious prolongation of QTc and PR interval

IODOQUINOL—*Yodoxin* (Glenwood), others
Occasional: rash; acne; slight enlargement of the thyroid gland; nausea; diarrhea; cramps; anal pruritus
Rare: optic neuritis; optic atrophy, loss of vision, peripheral neuropathy after prolonged use in high dosage (for months); iodine sensitivity

IVERMECTIN—*Stromectol* (Merck)
Occasional: Mazzotti-type reaction seen in onchocerciasis, including fever, pruritus, tender lymph nodes, headache, and joint and bone pain
Rare: hypotension

‡**MALATHION**—*Prioderm*
Occasional: local irritation

MEBENDAZOLE—*Vermox* (Janssen)
Occasional: diarrhea; abdominal pain; migration of *Ascaris* through mouth and nose
Rare: leukopenia; agranulocytosis; hypospermia

MEFLOQUINE—*Lariam* (Roche)
Frequent: vertigo; lightheadedness; nausea; other gastrointestinal disturbances; nightmares; visual disturbances; headache; insomnia
Occasional: confusion
Rare: psychosis; hypotension; convulsions; coma; paresthesias

‡**MEGLUMINE ANTIMONATE**—*Glucantime* (Rhône-Poulenc Rorer, France)
Similar to sodium stibogluconate

§**MELARSOPROL**—*Arsobal* (Rhône-Poulenc Rorer)
Frequent: myocardial damage; albuminuria; hypertension; colic; Herxheimer-type reaction; encephalopathy; vomiting; peripheral neuropathy
Rare: shock

Table continued on following page

TABLE 39–3 Manufacturers and Adverse Effects of Some Antiparasitic Drugs* *Continued*

METRONIDAZOLE—*Flagyl* (Searle), others
Frequent: nausea; headache; anorexia; metallic taste
Occasional: vomiting; diarrhea; insomnia; weakness; dry mouth; stomatitis; vertigo; tinnitus; paresthesias; rash; dark urine; urethral burning; disulfiram-like reaction with alcohol; candidiasis
Rare: seizures; pseudomembranous colitis; ataxia; leukopenia; peripheral neuropathy; pancreatitis; encephalopathy

§**NIFURTIMOX**—*Lampit* (Bayer, Germany)
Frequent: anorexia; vomiting; weight loss; loss of memory; sleep disorders; tremor; paresthesias; weakness; polyneuritis
Rare: convulsions; fever; pulmonary infiltrates and pleural effusion

‡**ORNIDAZOLE**—*Tiberal* (Hoffman-LaRoche, Switzerland)
Occasional: dizziness; headache; gastrointestinal disturbances
Rare: reversible peripheral neuropathy

OXAMNIQUINE—*Vansil* (Pfizer)
Occasional: headache; fever; dizziness; somnolence; nausea; diarrhea; rash; insomnia; hepatic enzyme changes; ECG changes; EEG changes; orange-red discoloration of urine
Rare: seizures; neuropsychiatric disturbances

PAROMOMYCIN—*Humatin* (Parke-Davis); aminosidine (topical and parenteral formulations not available in USA)
Frequent: GI disturbances with oral use
Occasional: eighth-nerve damage (mainly auditory) and renal damage when aminosidine is given IV; vertigo; pancreatitis

PENTAMIDINE ISETHIONATE—*Pentam 300, NebuPent* (Fujisawa)
Frequent: hypotension; hypoglycemia often followed by diabetes mellitus; vomiting; blood dyscrasias; renal damage; pain at injection site; GI disturbances
Occasional: may aggravate diabetes; shock; hypocalcemia; liver damage; cardiotoxicity; delirium; rash
Rare: Herxheimer-type reaction; anaphylaxis; acute pancreatitis; hyperkalemia; ventricular arrhythmias

PERMETHRIN—*Nix* (Glaxo-Wellcome), *Elimite* (Allergan), *Lyclear* (Canada)
Occasional: burning; stinging; numbness; increased pruritus; pain; edema; erythema; rash

PRAZIQUANTEL—*Biltricide* (Bayer)
Frequent: abdominal pain; diarrhea; malaise; headache; dizziness
Occasional: sedation; fever; sweating; nausea; eosinophilia
Rare: pruritus; rash; edema; hiccup

PRIMAQUINE PHOSPHATE USP
Frequent: hemolytic anemia in G-6-PD deficiency
Occasional: neutropenia; GI disturbances; methemoglobinemia
Rare: CNS symptoms; hypertension; arrhythmias

‡**PROGUANIL**—*Paludrine* (Wyeth Ayerst, Canada, Zeneca, England); *Malarone* (with atovaquone)
Occasional: oral ulceration; hair loss; scaling of palms and soles; urticaria
Rare: hematuria (with large doses); vomiting; abdominal pain; diarrhea (with large doses); thrombocytopenia

PRANTEL PAMOATE—*Antiminth* (Pfizer)
Occasional: GI disturbances; headache; dizziness; rash; fever

PYRETHRINS and PIPERONYL BUTOXIDE—*RID* (Pfizer), others
Occasional: allergic reactions

PYRIMETHAMINE USP—*Daraprim* (Glaxo-Wellcome)
Occasional: blood dyscrasias; folic acid deficiency
Rare: rash; vomiting; convulsions; shock; possibly pulmonary eosinophilia; fatal cutaneous reactions with **pyrimethamine-sulfadoxine** (*Fansidar*)

QUININE SULFATE—many manufacturers
‡**QUININE DIHYDROCHLORIDE**
Frequent: cinchonism (tinnitus, headache, nausea, abdominal pain, visual disturbance)
Occasional: deafness; hemolytic anemia; other blood dyscrasias; photosensitivity reactions; hypoglycemia; arrhythmias; hypotension; drug fever
Rare: blindness; sudden death if injected too rapidly

§**SODIUM STIBOGLUCONATE**—*Pentostam* (Glaxo-Wellcome, England)
Frequent: muscle and joint pain; fatigue; nausea; transaminase elevations; T-wave flattening or inversion; pancreatitis
Occasional: weakness; abdominal pain; liver damage; bradycardia; leukopenia; thrombocytopenia; rash; vomiting
Rare: diarrhea; pruritus; myocardial damage; hemolytic anemia; renal damage; shock; sudden death

†**SPIRAMYCIN**—*Rovamycine (Rhône-Poulenc Rorer)*
Occasional: GI disturbances
Rare: allergic reactions

§**SURAMIN SODIUM**—(Bayer, Germany)
Frequent: vomiting; pruritus; urticaria; paresthesias; hyperesthesia of hands and feet; photophobia; peripheral neuropathy
Occasional: kidney damage; blood dyscrasias; shock; optic atrophy

THIABENDAZOLE—*Mintezol* (Merck)
Frequent: nausea; vomiting; vertigo; headache; drowsiness; pruritus
Occasional: leukopenia; crystalluria; rash; hallucination and other psychiatric reactions; visual and olfactory disturbance; erythema multiforme
Rare: shock; tinnitus; intrahepatic cholestasis; convulsions; angioneurotic edema; Stevens-Johnson syndrome

‡**TINIDAZOLE**—*Fasigyn* (Pfizer)
Occasional: metallic taste; nausea; vomiting; rash

‡**TRICLABENDAZOLE**—*Fasinex* (Novartis Agribusiness)

TRIMETREXATE (with "leucovorin rescue") *Neutrexin* (US Bioscience)
Occasional: rash; peripheral neuropathy; bone marrow depression; increased serum aminotransferase activity

‡**TRYPARSAMIDE**
Frequent: nausea; vomiting
Occasional: impaired vision; optic atrophy; fever; exfoliative dermatitis; allergic reactions; tinnitus

*Drug interactions are generally not included here; see the current edition of *The Medical Letter Handbook of Adverse Drug Interactions.*
†Available in the USA only from the manufacturer.
‡Not available in the USA.
§Available from the CDC Drug Service, Centers for Disease Control and Prevention, Atlanta, Georgia 30333; 404-639-3670 (evenings, weekends, or holidays: 404-639-2888).
From Drugs for treatment of parasitic infections. Med Lett Drugs Ther. 1998; 40:1–12.

DRUGS ACTIVE AGAINST LUMINAL PROTOZOA: AMEBAE, INTESTINAL AND VAGINAL FLAGELLATES, AND CILIATES

Metronidazole and Other Nitroimidazoles

Metronidazole (Fig. 39–1), tinidazole,** and ornidazole** have selective activity against numerous anaerobic protozoa and bacteria. Only metronidazole, 2-methyl-5-nitroimidazole-1-ethanol, has been licensed in the United States. It is recommended for the treatment of invasive enterocolitis and liver abscess due to *Entamoeba histolytica*[6, 7–10] and *Entamoeba polecki* infections,[11] enteritis due to *Giardia lamblia*,[12, 13] and vaginitis due to *Trichomonas vaginalis*.[14, 15] It is considered an alternative drug for the treatment of *Blastocystis hominis*[16] and *Balantidium coli*.[17]

FIGURE 39–1. Metronidazole.

Metronidazole kills the trophozoites of *E. histolytica* in the intestine and in tissue, but it does not invariably eradicate the cysts.[7–10] A luminally active agent is required for that purpose and to treat asymptomatic cyst passers, as discussed later. Metronidazole resistance has been documented in some strains of *T. vaginalis*.[18] Metronidazole has been used as empiric therapy for presumptive protozoal enterocolitis in areas of the world where laboratory facilities are insufficient to provide a specific diagnosis.[19] Although metronidazole has the approval of the US Food and Drug Administration (FDA) only for the treatment of amebiasis and trichomoniasis, this does not prevent physicians from using it for other diseases, such as giardiasis, for which data support its efficacy.[20] Finally, metronidazole is recommended for the treatment of the guinea worm, *Dracunculus medinensis*,[21] but its clinical effects are attributed to a reduction in inflammation rather than to a direct effect on the worm. The use of metronidazole for the treatment of anaerobic bacterial infections is summarized in Chapter 26.

Metronidazole is available as 250-, 375-, and 500-mg tablets and 750-mg extended release tablets for oral use and in vials with 500 mg of lyophilized powder for parenteral administration. When it is administered orally, 90 to 95% is absorbed[22, 23]; peak serum levels are reached within 1 hour. Metronidazole has limited plasma protein binding. It is widely distributed throughout the body and penetrates well into tissues, abscesses, fluid compartments, vaginal secretions, bone, central nervous system, and breast milk.[24, 25] The elimination half-life is 6.2 to 11.5 hours. Metronidazole is extensively metabolized in the liver. The principal metabolites result from oxidation of side chains and glucuronide formation and are excreted via the kidney. Although renal failure prolongs the half-life of these metabolites, the hepatic metabolism is such that the drug dosage need not be modified during renal failure; however, it should be adjusted in liver failure and in persons with severe malnutrition.[26]

Metronidazole is activated in anaerobic organisms by reduction of the 5-nitro group through a sequence of intermediate steps involving microbial electron transport proteins of low redox potential.[27] This results in a concentration gradient across the membrane of the parasite and permits accumulation of high concentrations of the reduced compound within the cell. Metronidazole acts as an electron sink, depriving the anaerobe of reducing equivalents. Furthermore, the reduced form of metronidazole causes loss of the helical structure of DNA, strand breakage, and impaired template function.[28, 29]

Gastrointestinal side effects include nausea, vomiting, diarrhea, and a metallic aftertaste. They are less common with the low doses (250 mg three times daily) recommended for giardiasis than with the high doses (750 mg three times daily) used for amebiasis. Other, less frequent side effects include headache, dizziness, dry mouth, stomatitis, rash, urethral burning, vaginal or oral candidiasis, and reversible neutropenia.[30] Side effects are seldom severe enough to cause discontinuation of the drug. The urine of some persons may become red or brown owing to the presence of metabolites. Metronidazole can potentiate the anticoagulant effects of coumarin.[31] Rarely, patients treated with metronidazole experience peripheral neuropathy, paresthesia, tinnitus, vertigo, seizures, ataxia, psychotic disorders, or encephalopathy.[32] Acute pancreatitis has been reported.[33] Alcohol in beverages or medications must be avoided because of the disulfiram (Antabuse)-like effects of metronidazole and the potential of a life-threatening reaction.[34]

The potential role of metronidazole in human carcinogenesis and birth defects has been debated. Although metronidazole is mutagenic for certain strains of *Salmonella typhimurium*,[35] and human urine contains metabolites that are carcinogenic in rodents,[36] long-term follow-up of persons who have been treated with metronidazole have failed to demonstrate an increased prevalence of cancer.[37–39] Although it has not been approved or recommended for use during pregnancy, treatment with oral metronidazole during pregnancy has not been associated with birth defects.[40, 41]

Tinidazole and ornidazole, two other 5-nitroimidazole derivatives, have amebicidal, giardiacidal, and trichomonicidal activity similar to that of metronidazole.[7, 8, 42, 43] Tinidazole has activity against some but not all strains of metronidazole-resistant *T. vaginalis*.[18, 44] A single 2-g dose of tinidazole is effective for the treatment of giardiasis.[45] Both tinidazole and ornidazole are well absorbed orally, have good tissue penetration, and are widely distributed in the body. Tinidazole and ornidazole have half-lives of 14 and 12 to 13 hours, respectively.[46, 47] They are excreted primarily in urine, 50% of tinidazole and 96% of ornidazole in the form of metabolites. These drugs have a favorable side effect profile when compared with metronidazole. Reported side effects include anorexia, headache, and dizziness.

Paromomycin (Aminosidine)

Paromomycin, like other aminoglycoside antibiotics, is poorly absorbed after oral administration and reaches high concentrations in the lumen of the colon. It is used for the treatment of asymptomatic intestinal amebiasis, for the eradication of *E. histolytica* cysts in persons with intestinal or extraintestinal amebiasis who are treated with metronidazole,[48, 49] and for treatment of *Dientamoeba fragilis* infection. Paromomycin temporarily eliminates diarrhea in approximately 60% of persons with human immunodeficiency virus (HIV) infection and cryptosporidiosis.[50, 51] Paromomycin in a cream has been used to treat refractory trichomoniasis[52]; it has been applied topically with methylbenzethonium chloride in the treatment of cutaneous leishmaniasis caused by *Leishmania major*,[53, 54] and it has been administered systemically in a limited number of persons to treat visceral leishmaniasis.[54, 55]

Paromomycin is available in 250-mg capsules. Like other aminoglycoside antibiotics, it binds to 30S ribosomal RNA in the aminoacyl-tRNA site, resulting in inhibition of protein synthesis. Side effects are primarily gastrointestinal and include nausea, vomiting, abdominal cramps, and diarrhea in some patients. Paromomycin is potentially ototoxic and nephrotoxic when administered parenterally. Although little is absorbed from the gastrointestinal tract, oral paromomycin is contraindicated in persons with renal failure. Pancreatitis was reported in a patient with AIDS and cryptosporidiosis who received paromomycin.[56]

Iodoquinol

Iodoquinol (diiodohydroxyquin), a halogenated oxyquinoline (5,7-diiodo-8-quinolinol), is a luminally active agent used to eradicate cysts in persons with asymptomatic *E. histolytica* infection or after metronidazole administration in persons with invasive intestinal or extraintestinal disease. Iodoquinol is also recommended for the treatment of *D. fragilis* and *B. hominis*, and it is used as an alternative drug for the treatment of *B. coli*.

Iodoquinol is available in 210- and 650-mg tablets. It is poorly absorbed and best tolerated if given with meals. The mechanism of action is not known. Side effects include headache, diarrhea, nausea, vomiting and abdominal pain, fever, itching, seizures, and encephalopathy.[57, 58] Occasionally, the drug is associated with iodine dermatitis (iodine toxicoderma). The high iodine content (63%) can interfere with the results of thyroid function tests for months after completion of therapy. Iodoquinol is contraindicated in persons with iodine intolerance. A related compound, iodochlorhydroxyquin, gained notoriety as a cause of subacute myelooptic neuropathy and was discontinued. Optic nerve damage or inflammation and peripheral neuropathy may occur with prolonged high doses of iodoquinol as well. The dosage regimen recommended for amebic disease (see Table 39–2) avoids these complications, but the recommended doses and duration of therapy should never be exceeded.[5, 24]

Diloxanide Furoate**

Diloxanide furoate, a substituted acetanilide, 4-(*N*-methyl-2,2-dichloroacetamido)phenyl-2-furoate, is a luminally active agent used for the treatment of asymptomatic *E. histolytica* infection[59–62] and to eradicate cysts after treatment of invasive disease with metronidazole. It is ineffective in the treatment of extraintestinal amebiasis. Diloxanide furoate is hydrolyzed by intestinal esterases, releasing diloxanide, which is absorbed. Delayed or reduced absorption of the ester results in higher concentrations in the large intestine and the desired luminal effect.

Diloxanide furoate is formulated in 500-mg tablets. In experimental animals, 60 to 90% of the drug is excreted in the urine within 48 hours.[49] Excretion in the feces accounts for 4 to 9%. Diloxanide is amebicidal at low concentrations, but the mechanism of action is unknown. There are rarely serious side effects at the recommended dosage. The most common untoward effect is flatulence.[63] Mild gastrointestinal complaints may also occur. The low cost of the drug makes it an excellent alternative for the treatment of asymptomatic intestinal amebic infections in developing countries.

Furazolidone

Furazolidone, 3-[(5-nitro-2-furanyl)methylene-amino]-2-oxazolidinone, is a nitrofuran derivative. Like other nitrofurans, it acts by damaging DNA. It is the only anti-*Giardia* drug available as a liquid, and it is commonly used for the treatment of giardiasis in children.[64, 65] It is as effective as metronidazole. Furazolidone also has some activity against *I. belli* and a variety of enteropathogenic bacteria. Although not curative, it has been shown to provide symptomatic relief in AIDS patients with diarrhea who are infected with *E. bieneusi*.[66]

Furazolidone is available as a suspension containing 50 mg/15 ml and as 100-mg tablets. Despite earlier reports to the contrary, furazolidone is well absorbed; more than 65% is recovered in the urine in the form of metabolites.[67] Common side effects include nausea, vomiting, diarrhea, and fever.[68] Some of the metabolites are brown and may discolor the urine. Other rare side effects are hypotension, urticaria, serum sickness, hypersensitivity reactions, and mood disorders.[69] A mild to moderate hemolysis may occur in patients with glucose-6-phosphate dehydrogenase (G6PD) deficiency. As with metronidazole, alcohol should not be ingested because furazolidone has disulfiram-like activity. It is also a monoamine oxidase inhibitor. Furazolidone should not be administered to mothers who are breast-feeding or to neonates, because hemolytic anemia due to glutathione instability may occur.

DRUGS USED AGAINST MALARIA, TOXOPLASMOSIS, CRYPTOSPORIDIOSIS, CYCLOSPORIASIS AND PNEUMOCYSTOSIS

The four *Plasmodium* spp. that infect humans are responsible for an estimated 300 to 500 million new cases of malaria worldwide annually, and between 1.5 and 2.7 million deaths[70] (see Chapter 264). An estimated 47% of the world's population living in 100 countries are a risk.[70] Countries in tropical Africa account for more than 90% of the total cases and mortality. The resistance of *Plasmodium falciparum* and, more recently, *Plasmodium vivax* to antimalarials has complicated prophylaxis and treatment.[71]

As travel has increased, so has the exposure of nonimmune hosts to malaria. Every year more than 1 million Americans visit tropical or subtropical areas where they may be exposed. More than 1000 cases of malaria are diagnosed in the United States or one of its territories each year.[72] Prophylaxis is effective, but the evolution of drug resistance continues to pose problems.[71, 73] The erythrocytic stage of malaria is the most susceptible to chemotherapy. Most drugs are not active against exoerythrocytic plasmodia. Sporozoites are resistant to all currently available drugs.

T. gondii is ubiquitous throughout the world. Although acquired infection is usually asymptomatic or mild, *T. gondii* is a major cause of birth defects. It is also an important cause of encephalitis in persons with AIDS.[74, 75] *C. parvum, I. belli*, and the microsporidia have emerged as important enteric pathogens among persons with AIDS.[76] *Cryptosporidium* also has increasingly been recognized as a cause of sporadic and epidemic diarrhea in immunocompetent hosts.[77] *Cyclospora cayetanensis* has been associated with diarrhea in residents of developing areas, travelers, and Americans who have eaten imported raspberries from Central America.[78] Drugs used in the treatment of these infections are described in the following sections.

Aminoquinolines Used for the Prophylaxis and Treatment of Malaria

Chloroquine. Chloroquine (Fig. 39–2), 7-chloro-4-(4-diethylamino-1-methylbutylamino)-quinoline, the best known of the 4-aminoquinolines, is active against the erythrocytic stages of susceptible *Plasmodium* spp. It was once the mainstay of antimalarial chemotherapy and prophylaxis, but the widespread emergence of chloroquine-resistant *P. falciparum* in Africa, Southeast Asia, India, and South America has limited its use.[79] Although still geographically restricted, chloroquine-resistant *P. vivax* have been identified in Papua New Guinea, India, Irian Jaya, the Solomon Islands, Indonesia, Myanmar, and Guyana.[80–83] Chloroquine has also been used for the treatment of rheumatoid arthritis and systemic lupus erythematosus. Hydroxychloroquine has a spectrum of antimalarial activity similar to that of chloroquine and has been used for prophylaxis.

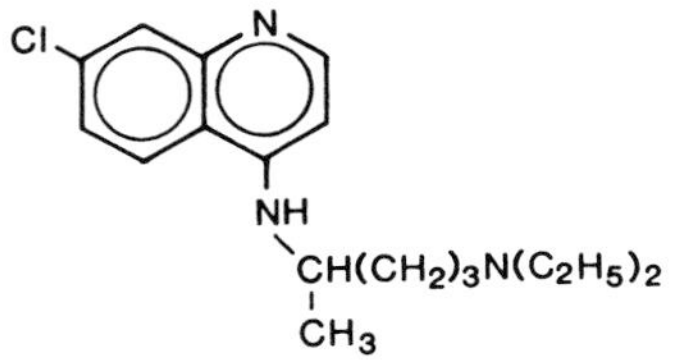

FIGURE 39–2. Chloroquine.

Chloroquine phosphate is available as a bitter white medication, which is dispensed in tablets containing 250 or 500 mg of the salt (150- and 300-mg base, respectively). Chloroquine is rapidly absorbed after oral ingestion and is slowly excreted.[84] The therapeutic blood concentration is reached within 2 or 3 hours. Chloroquine is widely distributed throughout the body and is relatively concentrated in the liver, spleen, kidneys, and erythrocytes. It is metabolized by alkylation in the liver, but approximately 50% of the parent drug is excreted in the urine. The half-life is 4 days, which allows for once-weekly administration for prophylaxis.[85, 86] Approximately 50% of chloroquine is protein bound. The renal status of the patient does not affect the amount used for acute malaria, but prophylactic doses should be reduced for those with reduced renal function.[86]

Chloroquine is a dibasic compound. It is concentrated in the acidic vacuoles of intraerythrocytic parasites.[87–92] The concentration in parasitized erythrocytes is 100-fold higher than in nonparasitized ones.[87] In erythrocytes with schizonts, the concentration of chloroquine is 600-fold higher than in plasma. Chloroquine has a marked and rapid effect on the hemoglobin-containing digestive vesicles of asexual erythrocytic parasites. With therapy there is fusion of adjacent vesicles, followed by sequestration of the fused vesicles and their malaria pigment into a large autophagic vacuole.[88, 89]

Ferriprotoporphyrin IX, a product of hemoglobin degradation by the parasite, damages membranes and inhibits a variety of parasitic enzymes in its soluble form. *Plasmodium* spp. protect themselves from the toxic effects of this molecule by the activity of a heme polymerase that incorporates ferriprotoporphyrin IX into an insoluble, nontoxic crystalline material.[90] Chloroquine and hydroxychloroquine inhibit this enzyme.

Chloroquine-resistant plasmodia transport chloroquine out of intraparasitic compartments more rapidly than susceptible strains and maintain lower chloroquine concentrations in their acid vesicles.[92] There is experimental evidence that this situation can be reversed by drugs that block calcium channels,[93, 94] but the high concentrations required in vivo have prevented such a treatment from being used clinically.

Chloroquine is relatively well tolerated when it is used for chemoprophylaxis or treatment of susceptible *Plasmodium* spp. Oral administration is preferred. Temporary side effects include headache, nausea, vomiting, blurred vision, dizziness, fatigue, and confusion.[84, 86] Some Africans experience pruritus, which responds to an antihistamine. Rare side effects include depigmentation of hair, corneal opacities, weight loss, insomnia, leukopenia, myalgias, exacerbation of psoriasis, and exfoliative dermatoses. Extremely rare reactions include blood dyscrasias, peripheral neuropathy, nerve deafness, myopathy, arrhythmia, heart block, toxic psychosis, and photophobia. Permanent retinal damage has occurred with long-term, high-dose therapy administered to persons with collagen vascular diseases.[95] Chloroquine is relatively contraindicated in persons with retinal disease, psoriasis, or porphyria.

Chloroquine can also be given by intravenous infusion, but it must be administered slowly and with great caution.[84, 96] The intravenous formulation is available in the United States. Respiratory depression, hypotension, cardiovascular collapse, and seizures can follow excessively rapid parenteral administration. Heart block and cardiac arrest are thought to be caused by a direct toxic effect on the myocardium of high plasma chloroquine concentrations. It is recommended that oral administration be substituted for parenteral administration as soon as possible.[84]

Deaths from chloroquine toxicity have followed accidental ingestion by children, in adults who habitually self-medicate, and in persons attempting suicide. The ingestion of as little as 5 g of chloroquine can be fatal. Therapy includes mechanical ventilation and other supportive measures. Although diazepam has been recommended, its efficacy in this setting has not been documented.[97]

Chloroquine was implicated in severe cochleovestibular abnormalities in the fetus of a mother taking high doses for the treatment of systemic lupus erythematosus.[98] There has been no association between chloroquine administered in antimalarial doses and fetal abnormalities.[86]

Primaquine. Primaquine (Fig. 39–3), an 8-aminoquinoline, 8-(4-amino-1-methylbutylamino)-6-methoxyquinoline, is the only drug available that has activity against the exoerythrocytic, hypnozoite forms of *P. vivax* and *Plasmodium ovale* that reside in the liver.[99] It is administered after chloroquine treatment of acute *P. vivax* or *P. ovale* infection and after prophylaxis with chloroquine or other drugs in persons who have had substantial exposure to *P. vivax* or *P. ovale*.[100] Relapses occur in a variable percentage of persons after primaquine therapy because of tolerant *P. vivax*. Such strains were initially reported from the Western Pacific; more recent reports have suggested decreasing sensitivity to primaquine in areas of Southeast Asia, Africa, and Latin America. Relapses after conventional primaquine therapy can be treated with higher doses or for longer periods of time.[101–105] Daily primaquine has been used experimentally in a limited number of persons as prophylaxis against *P. falciparum*. Primaquine has gametocytocidal activity against all four *Plasmodium* spp. that infect humans, but that is not of clinical significance. Primaquine in combination with clindamycin has been used for the treatment of mild to moderately severe *P. carinii* pneumonia.[106] The combination has also been used for prophylaxis against *P. carinii*, but it is less effective than trimethoprim-sulfamethoxazole or dapsone.[107]

Primaquine phosphate is supplied in tablets containing 26.3 mg of the salt, which is equivalent to 15 mg of the base. It has a bitter taste. Tablets may be crushed and added to sweet liquid or fruit to make it more palatable. The dosage is usually expressed in terms of the base. Primaquine is readily absorbed when taken orally. Plasma concentrations reach a peak at 6 hours and decline to undetectable levels by 24 hours.

The mechanism of action is uncertain, but primaquine is fully active only after metabolism by the host. The nature of the active metabolites is not clear. Based on studies with pamoquine,** the first of this series of drugs, they are thought to affect both the mitochondrial electron transport chain and pyrimidine synthesis.[88] Primaquine also selectively inhibits the formation of functional cellular transport vesicles in vitro.[108]

The major toxicity with primaquine is hemolysis in persons with G6PD deficiency.[109, 110] There are more than 100 million people worldwide with this deficiency (approximately 1% of males in the Middle East, 5% of Chinese males, and 10% of black males). G6PD deficiency is rare in whites. It is recommended that persons be tested for G6PD deficiency before primaquine is prescribed. Administration of primaquine should be discontinued if darkening of the urine or a fall in hematocrit is noted. For persons with the more mild African form of G6PD deficiency, a dose of 45 mg (base) weekly for 8

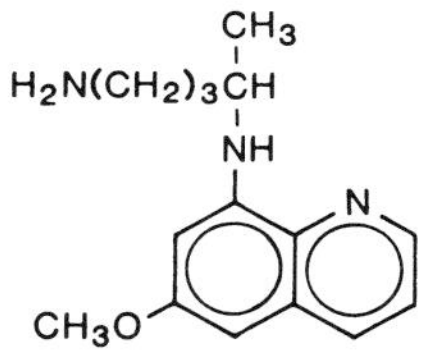

CH_3
$H_2N(CH_2)_3CH$
NH
N
CH_3O

FIGURE 39–3. Primaquine.

weeks has been used.[111] For patients with the more severe Mediterranean variety, 30 mg weekly for 30 weeks has been used.[110]

Apart from the potential for hemolysis, primaquine is usually well tolerated.[86] Abdominal cramps, epigastric distress, and nausea occur in some patients. Mild anemia, cyanosis (methemoglobinemia, with primaquine alone or in combination with dapsone[112]), and leukocytosis are observed in some persons given higher doses. Rare complications include granulocytopenia or agranulocytosis, hypertension, and arrhythmias.

Cinchona Alkaloids: Quinine and Quinidine

Quinine. Quinine (Fig. 39–4), a cinchona alkaloid, was the first successful agent for the treatment of malaria.[84] It acts rapidly against asexual erythrocytic stages of all four *Plasmodium* spp. that infect humans. After the introduction of chloroquine the use of quinine fell, but with the widespread emergence of chloroquine-resistant *P. falciparum* its use increased dramatically.[84] Decreasing sensitivity to quinine has emerged in isolates of *P. falciparum* in Southeast Asia, and there have been reports of decreased sensitivity in West Africa as well.[113, 114]

Quinine sulfate is supplied as 260- and 325-mg tablets and in capsules of 200, 300, and 325 mg. It has a very bitter taste. Quinine is rapidly absorbed after oral administration and reaches peak levels in 1 to 3 hours. Peak serum concentrations after a dose of 10 mg/kg are 7 to 17 μg/ml; side effects can be seen at concentrations greater than 10 μg/ml.[86] Quinine is formulated for parenteral use as quinine dihydrochloride** in 2-ml ampules containing 300 mg/ml. The parenteral preparation is no longer available in the United States, but it is used in other countries. Intravenous quinidine, its dextrostereoisomer, is effective and available in the United States and elsewhere. It is considered the drug of choice for the parenteral treatment of complicated *P. falciparum* infections.[5, 115]

Quinine is metabolized in the liver and excreted in the urine, mainly as metabolites.[116] Only 20% of the drug is excreted unchanged.[117] It is not as avidly bound to tissues as chloroquine and has a shorter half-life of 5 to 15 hours. Malaria is associated with a reduction in the systemic clearance of quinine that is proportional to the severity of disease. The elimination half-life is prolonged by approximately 50% in persons with malaria.[118] Monitoring of blood levels is recommended for persons with impaired renal or hepatic function, and dose reduction is necessary in those with severe renal impairment.[119]

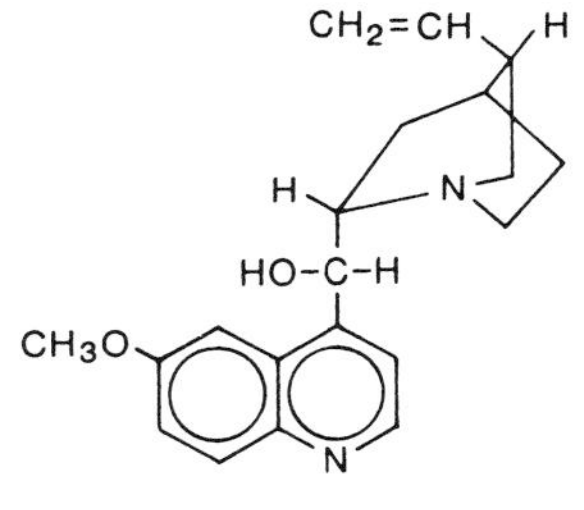

$CH_2=CH$ H
H N
HO-C-H
CH_3O
N

FIGURE 39–4. Quinine.

The exact mechanism of action of quinine as an antimalarial is unknown, but, like chloroquine, it may act at the level of the hemoglobin-containing digestive vesicles of intraerythrocytic parasites. Quinine and other quinolinemethanols bind to high-density lipoproteins in the serum and may be transported into plasmodium-infected erythrocytes via a pathway for the uptake of exogenous phospholipids.[92] There is speculation that they may act on specific parasite proteins. Quinine can intercalate into DNA, but this does not appear to be its primary mode of action.

Quinine has the poorest therapeutic-to-toxic ratio of all of the antimalarial drugs.[115] The side effects are collectively referred to as *cinchonism* and include tinnitus, temporary hearing loss, headache, dysphoria, nausea, vomiting, and mild visual disturbances.[84] These alterations are dose related and reversible. Other, less common side effects include rash, urticaria, angioedema of the face, pruritus, agranulocytosis, hepatitis, and, rarely, massive hemolysis in persons with falciparum malaria (blackwater fever).[119–121] Quinine has a curare-like effect on skeletal muscle and is used for the treatment of nocturnal leg cramps. It can result in respiratory depression in patients with myasthenia gravis.

An important adverse effect in patients with severe *P. falciparum* malaria is hypoglycemia, which is caused in part to the parasites' consumption of glucose and by the release of insulin from the pancreas by quinine.[122] It can be treated and prevented by the administration of intravenous glucose.

Quinine can cause hemolysis in patients with G6PD deficiency. It can stimulate uterine contractions and may produce abortion if given in high doses. However, quinine has been used successfully to treat seriously ill women with malaria during the third trimester of pregnancy.[123] Quinine must be used cautiously by the intravenous route, because rapid intravenous infusion may cause shock as a result of myocardial depression and peripheral vasodilatation. Overdoses are associated with convulsions, coma, delirium, depressed respiration, circulatory collapse, and death.

Quinidine. Quinidine is the dextrostereoisomer of quinine. Quinidine gluconate is now considered the drug of choice in the United States and elsewhere for persons requiring parenteral treatment of chloroquine-resistant falciparum malaria.[115] A major advantage of parenteral quinidine over parenteral quinine is that it is available because of its role in the treatment of cardiac arrhythmias. The efficacy of parenteral quinidine in the treatment of severe falciparum malaria is well established.[124–132]

Quinidine gluconate is available for intravenous administration. The half-life is 12.8 hours. Electrocardiographic changes including prolonged Q-Tc intervals are common, but life-threatening arrhythmias are rare if proper doses are used. Hypotension may occur if the infusion is too rapid. The rate of infusion, blood pressure, and electrocardiograms of persons receiving intravenous quinidine should be monitored closely,[127] preferably in an intensive care setting.

4-Quinoline-Carbinolamines (Quinoline-Methanols): Mefloquine

Mefloquine (Fig. 39–5) is a quinoline-methanol derived chemically from quinine. Like quinine and chloroquine, mefloquine is a blood schizonticidal drug and has no effect on exoerythrocytic schizonts or gametocytes.[86] Used in a single weekly dose, it is effective in prophylaxis against all four *Plasmodium* spp. that infect humans, including chloroquine-resistant and pyrimethamine-sulfadoxine–resistant isolates of *P. falciparum*.[128–131] Mefloquine can also be used for the treatment of acute chloroquine-resistant falciparum malaria. Resistance to mefloquine has been increasingly reported, initially in Thailand and other Southeast Asian areas, and later in West Africa and South America.[131–137]

Mefloquine is available only for oral administration. It is slowly and incompletely absorbed.[138] It is widely distributed in the body; 99% of the drug is protein bound. It has a long half-life in humans, ranging from 6 to 23 days, with a mean of 14 days. Mefloquine is given weekly at an adult dose of 250 mg for malaria prophylaxis. When used for the treatment of acute malaria, it can be administered as a single dose of 1250 mg or in divided doses of 750 mg followed in 12 hours by 500 mg. It is extensively metabolized and excreted through bile and feces. Mefloquine concentrates on red blood cell membranes and seems to interfere with the food vacuoles of *Plasmodium* spp. in a manner similar to that of quinine.[139] Mefloquine has been administered as a suspension via a nasogastric tube to unconscious patients with cerebral malaria. Absorption was rapid, with an absorption half-life of 1.5 hours. Plasma mefloquine levels were higher than 200 ng/ml within 3 hours.[140]

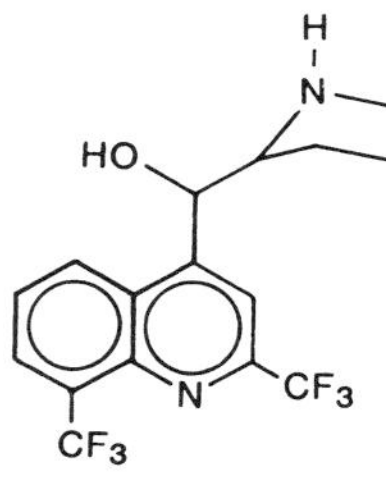

H N HO CF3 N CF3

FIGURE 39–5. Mefloquine.

Mefloquine is generally well tolerated by travelers using it for prophylaxis; mild side effects such as nausea, dizziness, and vivid dreams are relatively common. More severe neuropsychiatric reactions such as seizures, acute psychosis, anxiety neurosis, and disturbances of the sleep-wake cycle have been estimated to occur in 0.5% of users after treatment doses.[141] They are less common with prophylactic doses, but do occur and have sparked debate over the risk-benefit ratio of mefloquine for prophylaxis.[142, 143] Mefloquine is contraindicated in persons with a history of epilepsy or psychiatric disorders.

Mefloquine can cause alterations in cardiac conduction. Sinus bradycardia and sinus arrhythmia are common during therapy, but in the absence of other cardiac medications these changes are transient and benign. Sudden death was reported after a single dose of mefloquine in a patient with cardiac disease taking propranolol. Patients with cardiac conduction abnormalities, particularly those who are taking drugs that alter cardiac conduction (e.g., β-blockers), should not receive mefloquine.

Other isolated adverse effects include exfoliative dermatitis and the Stevens-Johnson syndrome, agranulocytosis, cutaneous vasculitis, and parasthesias.[144–148] Mefloquine has antibiotic activity and kills the live *Salmonella typhi* (Ty21a) oral vaccine at concentrations achieved enterally. Consequently, administration of that vaccine should be separated in time from administration of mefloquine.[149] Mefloquine has not been observed to cause birth defects in humans,[150] but it is teratogenic in animals at high doses. It is advisable for women to avoid taking the drug while pregnant unless the benefit is deemed to outweigh the risk. Because of its long half-life, women should be advised to use contraceptive measures for 2 months after the last dose of mefloquine. Despite initial concerns, mefloquine does not appear to adversely affect fine motor coordination or spatial discrimination and can be prescribed for persons whose activities involve those skills.[151]

Artemisinin Derivatives (Qinghaosu)**

Artemisinin and its derivatives, artemether, artesunate, and arteether, are sesquiterpene lactones derived from the wormwood plant *Artemisia annua*. Qinghaosu, an extract of the plant, has been used for centuries as a traditional Chinese medication for febrile illnesses and is known to have activity against *Plasmodium* species, the free-living ameba *Naegleria fowleri*, and the trematodes *Schistosoma japonicum*, *Schistosoma mansoni*, and *Clonorchis sinensis*. Artemisinin and its derivatives represent an exciting breakthrough in the treatment of multiple-drug–resistant falciparum malaria.[131, 152–154] They result in more rapid parasitologic clearance then the aminoquinoline antimalarials and have comparable efficacy against susceptible strains. They are relatively cheap to produce and are well tolerated. Their short half-lives limit their potential for prophylaxis. To date, the lack of detailed data on their pharmacology and toxicity have precluded approval by Western regulatory agencies.[131, 152]

Artemisinin and its derivatives are endoperoxide-containing compounds. Although their mode of action is not fully understood, it is thought that in the presence of intraparasitic iron they are converted to free radicals and other intermediates, which alkylate malaria proteins or damage membranes.[155] They act rapidly, arresting parasite development and preventing cytoadherence and rosetting, both thought to be important pathophysiologic mechanisms in severe falciparum malaria.

Depending on the derivative, the compounds are available for enteral, intravenous, or intramuscular administration. They are cleared rapidly from the circulation.[156] Delivery of artemisinin by suppository represents a potentially major advantage in treating severe malaria in patients who cannot take oral medications and are treated in settings where injections cannot be given.[154] Artemisinin derivatives are frequently administered with mefloquine.

Experience to date suggests that they are better tolerated than quinine or treatment doses of mefloquine in patients with acute falciparum malaria. Adverse effects have been infrequent and mild.[152] They have included decreases in reticulocyte and neutrophil counts, elevated liver transaminases, abdominal pain, diarrhea, and drug fever. No severe adverse effects occurred among more than 4000 patients enrolled in early clinical studies. Contact dermatitis is well documented with sesquiterpene lactones,[157] and there are case reports of cerebellar dysfunction in persons treated with artesunate for acute malaria.[158] Experience in animals suggests that neurotoxicity may occur if these compounds are administrated chronically at high doses.[159] Clinical isolates resistant to artemisinin, mefloquine, and halofantrine have been reported from Africa.[160]

Tetracycline and Doxycycline

Tetracycline has been used with quinine to treat acute falciparum malaria acquired in areas where *P. falciparum* is resistant to chloroquine, pyrimethamine, and sulfonamides.[5, 161] Daily doses of doxycycline, a long-acting tetracycline, have been used prophylactically as an alternative to weekly chloroquine and mefloquine and in areas where there is chloroquine- and mefloquine-resistant *P. falciparum*.[162, 163] Daily doxycycline is administered while persons are exposed and for 4 weeks after they leave the endemic area.

Tetracyclines are well absorbed orally. Their pharmacology is discussed in Chapter 24. They inhibit protein synthesis in prokaryotic ribosomes. It is likely that they inhibit protein synthesis in *Plasmodium* spp. in a similar manner.[88] The most common untoward effects are gastrointestinal. Photosensitivity occurs in approximately 3% of recipients and can be an important problem for travelers exposed to the sun in the tropics. *Candida* vaginitis can complicate tetracycline use in women, and pseudomembranous colitis due to *Clostridium difficile* can develop, particularly in the elderly. Finally, the tetracyclines are contraindicated during pregnancy and for children younger than 8 years of age. They are concentrated in bone and teeth and may cause dental staining, hypoplasia of dental enamel, and impaired bone growth in a fetus or young child.

Halofantrine**

Halofantrine is a 9-phenanthrenemethanol with activity against chloroquine-sensitive and chloroquine-resistant *P. falciparum* and *P. vivax*. It is a blood schizontocide with activity against the intraerythrocytic stages of *Plasmodium* spp. It has no activity against gametocytes or the extraerythrocytic stage. Halofantrine has been used primarily for the treatment of falciparum malaria in areas where chloroquine and sulfonamide-pyrimethamine resistance is found. Cross-resistance between halofantrine and mefloquine has been documented.[164] The use of halofantrine has been limited since the publication of reports that it can induce rare but life-threatening cardiac effects, including prolongation of the Q-Tc interval, torsade de pointes, and fatal arrhythmias.[165, 166]

Halofantrine is available only in oral form. The recommended dose for the treatment of acute falciparum malaria in adults and children weighing more than 40 kg is three 500-mg doses given at 6-hour intervals. A second course after 7 days is recommended in patients who have had minimal or no previous exposure to malaria. In patients weighing less than 40 kg, three doses of 8 mg/kg are given at 6-hour intervals. Halofantrine has poor and variable absorption, but peak serum levels are increased up to 10-fold when the drug is taken with a fatty meal. It is excreted mainly in the feces, with an elimination half-life of 1 to 2 days, and 3 to 5 days for its active metabolite.[164] The mechanism of action is poorly understood. Possibilities include inhibition of ferriprotoporphyrin IX sequestration, inhibition of a proton pump present at the host-parasite interface, and mitochondrial damage.[164]

Halofantrine occasionally causes abdominal pain, vomiting, diarrhea, headache, pruritus, or rash. Prolongation of the Q-T interval and fatal ventricular arrhythmia can occur.[165, 166] Use is contraindicated in pregnant and lactating women.

Dihydrofolate Reductase Inhibitors and Sulfonamides

The diaminopyrimidine dihydrofolate reductase inhibitors, pyrimethamine and trimethoprim, have been used alone or, more commonly, in conjunction with sulfonamides for the prevention and treatment of malaria,[86, 88, 128, 162] *I. belli* infection,[167] toxoplasmosis,[168–170] and *P. carinii* pneumonia.[171, 172] They act at sequential steps in the folic acid cycle. *Plasmodium* spp., and presumably other sensitive parasites, carry out pyrimidine synthesis de novo, and folic acid derivatives are essential cofactors. Unlike mammalian cells, these parasites cannot use preformed pyrimidines obtained through salvage pathways.

Pyrimethamine is more active than trimethoprim in inhibiting the dihydrofolate reductases of *Plasmodium* spp. and *T. gondii*. Conversely, trimethoprim has greater activity against bacteria. Both of these drugs have some inhibitory effect on mammalian dihydrofolate reductase. This is more of a problem with pyrimethamine than with trimethoprim. Trimetrexate, a low-molecular-weight, lipid-soluble dihydrofolate reductase inhibitor, can be used for treatment of pneumocystosis and is also active against *T. gondii*.[173] For treatment of *P. carinii*, trimetrexate is given in a dose of 45 mg/m^2 once daily over 60 to 90 minutes. The usual course of treatment is 21 days. To prevent potentially fatal bone marrow toxicity, leucovorin must be administered concurrently as 20 mg/m^2 intravenously over 5 to 10 minutes every 6 hours, or orally four times a day, and continued for 72 hours after the last dose of trimetrexate. Patients must be monitored closely for hematologic toxicity.

Pyrimethamine and Short-Acting Sulfonamides. Pyrimethamine (Fig. 39–6), a 2,4-diaminopyrimidine, was once widely used on a weekly basis for malaria prophylaxis and with sulfadiazine and quinine for the treatment of acute chloroquine-resistant *P. falciparum* malaria, but its usefulness has been limited by the widespread emergence of resistant *P. falciparum* and *P. vivax*.[162, 174]

Pyrimethamine and sulfadiazine are the treatment of choice for

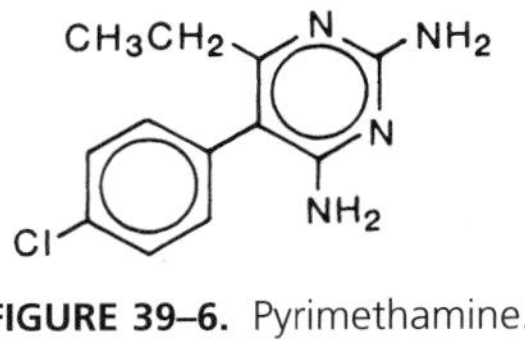

FIGURE 39–6. Pyrimethamine.

toxoplasmosis.[168–172] The majority of immunocompetent persons who acquire *T. gondii* have mild or asymptomatic, self-limited infections and do not require treatment. In immunocompromised persons, including those with AIDS, *Toxoplasma* encephalitis is life-threatening and therapy with pyrimethamine and sulfonamides for prolonged periods is recommended.[168, 170] In persons who cannot tolerate sulfonamides, clindamycin or atovaquone may be used as alternatives with pyrimethamine.[175, 176] Pyrimethamine is also used with sulfisoxazole or dapsone for primary prophylaxis against *T. gondii* in HIV-infected patients with CD4 T-lymphocyte counts lower than 100 cells/mm^3.[177] Congenital toxoplasmosis is treated with pyrimethamine and sulfonamides.[171, 172] The optimal treatment of acute toxoplasmosis during pregnancy is uncertain; pyrimethamine is contraindicated, at least for the first trimester, and sulfonamides cannot be used close to the time of delivery because they displace bilirubin from binding sites on albumin. Spiramycin,* a macrolide, is an alternative, but it is not licensed for use in the United States.[178]

Pyrimethamine is well absorbed orally; the half-life is 4 to 6 days.[179] It is extensively metabolized; less than 3% of the drug is excreted unchanged in the urine in 24 hours. Pyrimethamine acts preferentially to inhibit the parasite's dihydrofolate reductase. It is approximately 1000-fold more active against the parasite's dihydrofolate reductase than the human enzyme.[180]

Pyrimethamine is tolerated at a dose of 25 mg/week, which has been used for malaria prophylaxis. Blood dyscrasias, rash, vomiting, seizures, and shock are all rare side effects. Bone marrow suppression with neutropenia, anemia, and thrombocytopenia are seen with the higher doses used for the treatment of toxoplasmosis (50 to 100 mg/day). Careful follow-up with complete blood counts is necessary, but concurrent administration of folinic acid usually prevents these complications. Pyrimethamine is teratogenic in animals and is contraindicated during the first 16 weeks of pregnancy.[181, 182] It has been used to treat pregnant women with primary toxoplasmosis after this period, but concern remains about its safety. Some experts have argued that there has been no unequivocal documentation of pyrimethamine-associated birth defects at the dose levels used for malaria prophylaxis.[183, 184]

Sulfonamides decrease the activity of dihydropteroate synthetase and reduce the binding of *p*-aminobenzoic acid to this enzyme in several members of the Apicomplexa. The sulfonamides are described in detail in Chapter 30. They are well absorbed orally. The most common untoward effects are allergic reactions and gastrointestinal complaints. Allergic reactions include fever and rash. Less common are toxic epidermal necrolysis, erythema multiforme, Stevens-Johnson syndrome, hepatitis, pneumonitis, bone marrow depression, and serum sickness.[185] Untoward effects are encountered in approximately 60% of persons with AIDS and *Toxoplasma* encephalitis who receive sulfonamides and pyrimethamine.[169] They include fever, skin rash, bone marrow suppression, and hepatotoxicity. When they are severe enough to result in discontinuation of sulfonamides, clindamycin or atovaquone can be administered with pyrimethamine.[175–177]

Fansidar (Pyrimethamine and Sulfadoxine). Fansidar (each tablet contains pyrimethamine 25 mg and sulfadoxine 500 mg) is used for the treatment of chloroquine-resistant falciparum malaria. It was previously recommended as prophylaxis for travelers to areas with chloroquine-resistant *P. falciparum*,[162] but it is seldom used for prophylaxis today because it can elicit life-threatening allergic reactions. In addition, pyrimethamine and sulfonamide resistance have emerged in many areas. Fansidar was also administered as prophylaxis against *P. carinii* pneumonia in patients with AIDS, but serious untoward allergic reactions were encountered.[185, 186]

Sulfadoxine, like pyrimethamine, is well absorbed from the gastrointestinal tract. Its half-life is 5 to 9 days.[179] The severe reactions observed with Fansidar have been attributed to sulfadoxine. Fatalities with prophylactic Fansidar have occurred in 1 in 11,000 to 1 in 26,000 users.[185] Most of the severe cutaneous reactions, including toxic epidermal necrolysis, erythema multiforme, and the Stevens-Johnson syndrome, have occurred soon after the start of prophylaxis, usually within the first 5 weeks.[185] Other serious but unusual side effects with sulfadoxine include serum sickness, bone marrow suppression, hepatitis, hepatic granuloma, and pneumonitis.

Trimethoprim-Sulfamethoxazole (Cotrimoxazole). The combination of trimethoprim-sulfamethoxazole has been used widely used for the treatment of bacterial infections and *P. carinii* pneumonia[171] (see Chapter 30). It is also effective for several parasitic diseases. Prophylactic administration of trimethoprim-sulfamethoxazole in persons with AIDS and low CD4$^+$ T-cell counts has been shown to protect against the development of *T. gondii* encephalitis as well as *P. carinii* pneumonia.[172, 177] Trimethoprim-sulfamethoxazole is also the treatment of choice for gastroenteritis caused by *I. belli.* Although usually a self-limited illness in immunocompetent hosts, *I. belli* can cause severe, chronic gastroenteritis in patients with AIDS. Relapses are common after therapy in patients with AIDS (up to 50%). They can be prevented by suppressive therapy with trimethoprim-sulfamethoxazole.[167]

Both trimethoprim and sulfamethoxazole are well absorbed when administered orally. Peak blood levels are reached in 1 to 4 hours. The half-lives are similar: 10 to 12 hours for trimethoprim and 9 to 11 hours for sulfamethoxazole.[186] Excretion is through the kidney; renal failure prolongs the half-lives of both drugs. Trimethoprim has greater lipid solubility than sulfamethoxazole, and its apparent volume of distribution is five to six times greater. As a result, the drugs are formulated at a trimethoprim:sulfamethoxazole ratio of 1:5. Single-strength tablets contain 80 mg trimethoprim and 400 mg sulfamethoxazole; double-strength tablets have 160 mg trimethoprim and 800 mg sulfamethoxazole. The combination is also available in suspension for oral use, containing 40 mg trimethoprim and 200 mg sulfamethoxazole per 5 ml for children. For intravenous use, trimethoprim-sulfamethoxazole is available as a solution containing 16 mg trimethoprim and 80 mg sulfamethoxazole per milliliter.

In patients without AIDS, common side effects include gastrointestinal upset (4%) and skin reactions (3%).[187] Rare adverse reactions include agranulocytosis, aplastic anemia, acute interstitial nephritis, Stevens-Johnson syndrome, jaundice, headaches, depression, and hallucinations.[188] Malnourished persons receiving prolonged therapy may require concomitant therapy with folinic acid to prevent megaloblastic anemia. The drug combination is not recommended during pregnancy.

For unknown reasons, patients with AIDS have an unusually high incidence of severe adverse reactions when given sulfonamides. Approximately 65% experience significant drug-related symptoms with trimethoprim-sulfamethoxazole, some of which are severe enough to result in discontinuation of therapy.[189, 190] These adverse reactions include neutropenia, fever, and rashes in up to one half of these patients and thrombocytopenia, intolerable gastrointestinal effects, and hepatitis in one tenth.

Dapsone. Dapsone, a sulfone that has been widely used in the treatment of leprosy, has been administered in combination with pyrimethamine for prophylaxis against malaria. It is marketed as maloprim,** a combination of pyrimethamine 25 mg and dapsone 100 mg, for malaria prophylaxis. Dapsone with trimethoprim is used as an alternative to trimethoprim-sulfamethoxazole for the treatment of mild to moderate *P. carinii* pneumonia,[171] and dapsone alone can be used for prophylaxis.[172] Dapsone and pyrimethamine have also been used in HIV patients with low CD4 T-cell counts to prevent *T. gondii* encephalitis.[177]

Like the sulfonamides, dapsone interferes with folic acid metabolism by competitively inhibiting dihydropteroate synthetase. Dapsone is available in 25-mg and 100-mg tablets. It is well absorbed after oral administration and is widely distributed in tissues. About 70 to 80% of the drug is bound to plasma proteins. After acetylation and deacetylation, the drug is excreted in the urine as glucuronide or sulfate conjugates. The half-life is variable but averages 25 to 27 hours.

Serious side effects of dapsone include hemolytic anemia, methemoglobinemia, and bone marrow suppression. Very rarely, when maloprim has been used in high doses, fatal agranulocytosis has occurred.[191] Uncommon side effects include peripheral neuropathy, anorexia, vomiting, vertigo, blurred vision, tinnitus, fever, headache, pruritus, psychosis, hematuria, and skin rash. Pulmonary eosinophilia was attributed to maloprim in one report.[192] Dapsone is contraindicated in patients with G6PD deficiency. Complete blood counts should be performed periodically for patients receiving dapsone and pyrimethamine.

Proguanil.** Proguanil, also known as chloroguanide, was the first agent found to inhibit plasmodial dihydrofolate reductase. The elucidation of its mechanism of action led to the synthesis of the diaminopyrimidines pyrimethamine and trimethoprim.[193] Daily proguanil has been used with weekly chloroquine as prophylaxis against chloroquine-resistant *P. falciparum* in travelers to East Africa, but failures occur because of parasite resistance.[194] Proguanil acts too slowly to be used alone for the treatment of acute malaria. More recently, proguanil has been used successfully in combination with atovaquone (Malarone) for prophylaxis against *P. falciparum* malaria.[195–197]

Proguanil is formulated in 100-mg tablets. It is slowly absorbed after oral administration. It reaches peak serum concentrations in 2 to 4 hours, and the serum levels decline to practically zero by 24 hours. It must be taken daily to provide effective prophylaxis. The concentration of proguanil in erythrocytes is six times that in plasma. Approximately 40 to 60% is excreted in the urine and 10% in the feces. It is the metabolite 2,4-diamino-1-*p*-chlorophenyl-1,6-dihydro-6,6-dimethyl-1,3,5-triazine that inhibits plasmodial dihydrofolate reductase.

Proguanil is usually well tolerated at the daily doses used for malaria prophylaxis, but hematologic effects have been reported on rare occasion.[198] At higher levels, proguanil can produce nausea, vomiting, abdominal pain, and diarrhea. Excessive amounts have been associated with hematuria, proteinuria, and renal casts.

Atovaquone. Hydroxynaphthoquinones have been known to have antimalarial activity since World War II, but problems with poor absorption and rapid metabolism limited their use.[199] Atovaquone, a newer member of the class, is an exception (Fig. 39–7). Atovaquone has activity against *Plasmodium* spp. Early experience suggested that there was a high relapse rate when it was used alone for treatment. More recent studies of the combination of atovaquone plus proguanil (Malarone) suggest that it is effective for both prophylaxis and treatment of *P. falciparum* malaria.[195–197, 200] Atovaquone can be used as an alternative to trimethoprim-sulfamethoxazole for the treatment of mild to moderately severe *P. carinii* pneumonia.[201] The combination of atovaquone and pyrimethamine has also been used to treat toxoplasmosis and for long-term suppression in persons with AIDS who cannot tolerate sulfonamides.[176, 202–203]

Atovaquone is available in tablet or oral suspension. The bioavailability is low after oral administration. It is enhanced by administration of the drug with a fatty meal. Atovaquone is highly lipophilic and protein bound. The half-life is 2.2 to 3.2 days. More than 90% of the drug is eliminated in the feces. The measurable concentration in cerebrospinal fluid is low. Rifampin reduces atovaquone serum concentrations by 50%, whereas fluconazole and prednisolone each raise steady-state atovaquone concentrations by 20%. Atovaquone is generally well tolerated. Side effects include fever, skin rash, cough, nausea, vomiting, diarrhea, headache, and insomnia.

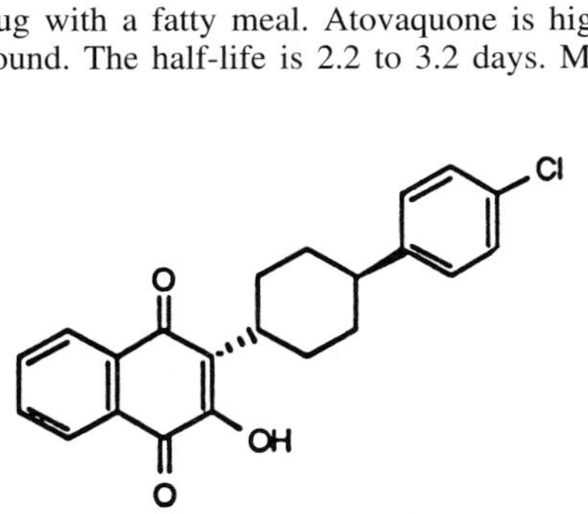

FIGURE 39–7. Atovaquone.

Antibacterial Antibiotics Active against Apicomplexa

Clindamycin. Clindamycin has activity against several protozoa and *P. carinii*. The combination of clindamycin plus pyrimethamine can be used for treatment or suppression of toxoplasmosis in persons who cannot tolerate the standard regimen of pyrimethamine plus sulfadiazine.[204, 205] Clindamycin has also been used along with prednisone for the treatment of ocular toxoplasmosis in immunocompetent patients.[206, 207] It has relatively good penetration into the eye and inhibits replication of *T. gondii*. Although the outcome of therapy has been good, there are no prospective, double-blind studies comparing the efficacy of clindamycin with the combination of pyrimethamine and a sulfonamide. Clindamycin has been used with quinine for the treatment of chloroquine-resistant falciparum malaria. The combination is the treatment of choice for symptomatic human babesiosis.[208] Finally, clindamycin with primaquine is used as an alternative to trimethoprim-sulfamethoxazole for the treatment of *P. carinii* pneumonia.[106]

The pharmacokinetics and untoward effects of clindamycin are discussed in Chapter 27. The major concern is the development of pseudomembranous colitis, a side effect that increases in incidence with patient age.

Spiramycin.* Spiramycin, another macrolide antibiotic, has been widely used as an additive in animal feeds. It is active against *T. gondii*, but it has not yet been licensed in the United States. Spiramycin has been used to treat primary toxoplasmosis acquired during pregnancy.[178, 209] In one study, only 3.7% of fetuses became infected in mothers who received spiramycin after acquiring toxoplasmosis during the first 16 weeks of pregnancy.[178] It has also been used for the treatment of congenital toxoplasmosis in newborns.[210] One important, although rare, potential complication in neonates, is Q-Tc prolongation with associated life-threatening ventricular arrhythmias.[211]

Azithromycin. Azithromycin (see Chapter 27) has activity against *T. gondii* and has been used with pyrimethamine for treatment and suppression of *Toxoplasma* encephalitis in a limited number of persons with AIDS.[212, 213] Preliminary data suggest that daily azithromycin may be effective in malaria prophylaxis.[214, 215]

DRUGS FOR TREATMENT OF LEISHMANIASIS, AFRICAN TRYPANOSOMIASIS, AND CHAGAS' DISEASE

Members of the genera *Trypanosoma* and *Leishmania* are important pathogens. *Trypanosoma brucei gambiense* and *Trypanosoma brucei rhodesiense* cause African sleeping sickness. In the case of African trypanosomiasis, the early hemolymphatic stage of disease has traditionally been treated with suramin or pentamidine isethionate. Neither of these compounds reaches therapeutic levels in the central nervous system. Once central nervous system involvement is documented, melarsoprol B, a toxic trivalent arsenical, is the treatment of choice. Eflornithine, an inhibitor of ornithine decarboxylase, is effective in patients with hemolymphatic and central nervous system *T. b. gambiense* infection, but it is not active against *T. b. rhodesiense*. Eflornithine is less toxic but more costly than conventional therapy. The supplies of the drug are now very limited.

The therapeutic situation is worse with *Trypanosoma cruzi*, the cause of Chagas' disease in Central and South America. The drugs currently used for therapy, nifurtimox and benznidazole, are variably effective and are frequently associated with sufficient toxicity to necessitate their discontinuation. Efforts continue to identify more effective, less toxic alternatives.

Various *Leishmania* spp. produce cutaneous, mucosal, or visceral leishmaniasis. Visceral leishmaniasis has emerged as an important opportunistic infection among persons with HIV in southern Europe. The pentavalent antimonials, stibogluconate sodium and meglumine antimonate, have been widely used for the treatment of leishmaniasis, but resistance is increasingly recognized and persons with mucosal or diffuse cutaneous leishmaniasis often respond poorly.

Liposome-encapsulated amphotericin B (AmBisome) is effective for the treatment of visceral leishmaniasis and has been approved by the U.S. Food and Drug Administration for that indication. Conventional amphotericin B deoxycholate and pentamidine isethionate are effective, but more toxic, alternatives. A number of other forms of therapy have been studied. Topical paromomycin with methylbenzethonium chloride has been used successfully to treat cutaneous leishmaniasis caused by *L. major.*

Suramin*

Suramin is a nonmetallic compound that is effective for the treatment of the hemolymphatic stage of African trypanosomiasis.[216] It has been used on occasion as prophylaxis against *T. b. gambiense* in persons working in highly endemic areas. Suramin also has some activity against adult *Onchocerca volvulus*, but ivermectin is the drug of choice for onchocerciasis.

Suramin sodium is a white microcrystalline powder that is readily soluble in water.[63] It is dispensed in 1.0-g vials for parenteral administration. It cannot be given orally. Suramin binds to plasma proteins and persists at low levels in the serum for up to 3 months after infusion. There seems to be negligible metabolism of the drug. Suramin does not penetrate the central nervous system, which limits its usefulness to the hemolymphatic stage of African trypanosomiasis.

Its mechanism of action is uncertain, but suramin is known to inhibit many enzymes, even at low concentrations. It is polyanionic and forms firm complexes with proteins. The antitrypanosomal activity of suramin correlates with its inhibition of glycerol-3-phosphate oxidase and glycerol-3-phosphate dehydrogenase, two parasite enzymes that are involved in energy metabolism.[217]

Suramin causes a variety of untoward effects.[218] Immediate reactions include nausea, vomiting, shock, loss of consciousness, and occasionally death. Fever and urticaria may also occur. Later reactions, which appear up to 24 hours after administration, include fever, papular rash, exfoliative dermatitis, stomatitis, paresthesias of the palms and soles, photophobia, lacrimation, palpebral edema, and hyperesthesia. These may be followed by renal dysfunction with albuminuria, hematuria, and renal casts. Other reactions include diarrhea and severe prostration. Jaundice, hemolytic anemia, and agranulocytosis are rare. The frequency and severity of side effects are more severe in malnourished hosts.[63] Suramin is relatively contraindicated in persons with preexisting kidney or liver disease.

Melarsoprol*

Melarsoprol, or Mel B, is a trivalent arsenical used for the treatment of central nervous system trypanosomiasis. It is also effective in treatment of the hemolymphatic phase, but it is too toxic to be recommended in that setting.

Melarsoprol is only slightly soluble in water, but it is readily soluble in propylene glycol, in which it is dispensed as a 3.6% weight/volume solution.[63] Melarsoprol is administered intravenously. A small but sufficient amount of the drug penetrates the central nervous system, where it can have a lethal effect on trypanosomes. Data indicate that the drug enters the parasite via an adenosine transporter; resistant strains lack this transport system.[219] Arsenicals react avidly with sulfhydryl groups and thereby interact with and inactivate enzymes. This is the most likely mechanism of action against trypanosomes and the cause of its toxicity in humans. Melarsoprol may act differentially on parasite pyruvate kinase, which is a terminal glycolytic enzyme.[220] Melarsoprol is oxidized to a nontoxic or less toxic pentavalent metabolite that is excreted.

Melarsoprol is a highly toxic drug.[221] Febrile reactions are common and may be accompanied by hypertension, abdominal pain, vomiting, and arthralgia. Reactive encephalopathy is the most serious side effect; it has been reported to cause death in approximately 6% of recipients.[222, 223] It usually appears in the first 3 or 4 days of therapy. The clinical manifestations include headache, dizziness, mental dullness, confusion, and ataxia with progression to obtundation and seizures. The pathophysiology is thought to be an immune response to trypanosomal antigens that are released during therapy.[224] Data suggest that the administration of corticosteroids can reduce the incidence of encephalopathy and mortality during treatment.[223] Less common untoward effects include hemorrhagic encephalopathy and agranulocytosis. A Guillain-Barré–like syndrome has also been described.[225] Allergic reactions including rash may complicate subsequent courses of therapy. On occasion, the appearance of numerous casts in the urine or evidence of hepatotoxicity necessitates a modification of therapy. Severe hemolysis can occur in patients with G6PD deficiency. The gastrointestinal side effects can be reduced by administering the drug slowly to fasting patients. Melarsoprol therapy can precipitate erythema nodosum in patients who have leprosy.

Eflornithine*

Eflornithine (DL-α-difluoromethylornithine) is effective in the treatment of African sleeping sickness caused by *T. b. gambiense*, even in patients with advanced central nervous system dlsease.[226–228] Although it is less toxic than melarsoprol, it is more expensive and supplies are very limited.[229, 230] Eflornithine is not effective in east African sleeping sickness caused by *T. b. rhodesiense*.[231]

Eflornithine hydrochloride can be administered intravenously or orally; 80% of the drug is excreted unchanged in the urine.[63, 231] Serum levels during administration of 20 g/day by intravenous infusion approach 1200 nmol/ml; oral administration of 5 g every 4 hours produces levels of approximately 500 nmol/ml. The ratio of cerebrospinal fluid to serum concentration ranges from 0.09 to 0.45. The highest cerebrospinal fluid levels are found in persons with the most severe central nervous system involvement. Eflornithine is an enzyme-activated, irreversible inhibitor of the enzyme ornithine decarboxylase, which is involved in the first step in the polyamine pathway. Polyamines play an essential role in the growth, differentiation, and replication of the trypanosomatids.

In comparison with the other drugs used to treat African trypanosomiasis, eflornithine is relatively well tolerated. Adverse effects are usually mild and reversible. They include anemia, thrombocytopenia, leukopenia, nausea, vomiting, diarrhea, and transient hearing loss.

Nifurtimox*

Nifurtimox, 4-[(5-nitrofurfurylidene)amino]-3-methylthiomorpholine-1,1-dioxide, a nitrofuran, is used for the treatment of acute Chagas' disease.[232, 233] It can reduce the duration of symptoms of acute disease, and it decreases mortality resulting from myocarditis and meningoencephalitis. The level and duration of parasitemia are also reduced. However, in clinical trials there have been significant numbers of treatment failures. There also seems to be geographic variation in responsiveness. Treatment has been found to be most effective in Argentina and Chile, but therapy in Brazil and in some other countries has been less successful. Prolonged therapy for 120 days is recommended, but it is not unusual for a treatment course to be terminated prematurely because of drug toxicity. The effectiveness of nifurtimox in the treatment of patients with the indeterminate phase or chronic Chagas' disease has not been documented. Nifurtimox has been used in a limited number of cases to treat arseno-resistant *T. b. gambiense* sleeping sickness with some success, but toxicity and relapses were common.[234, 235]

Nifurtimox is well absorbed orally, but marked first-pass metabolism results in low serum and tissue concentrations. The elimination half-life is 2 to 4 hours.[236] Nifurtimox is active against both trypomastigote and amastigote forms of *T. cruzi*. The trypanocidal action is thought to relate to the ability of nifurtimox to form reactive oxygen radicals that are toxic to the parasite.[233]

Toxicity occurs in 40 to 70% of persons who receive nifurtimox. This is probably caused at least in part, by free radical formation and oxidative damage to host tissues.[237] Most of the symptoms are related to the gastrointestinal tract and the central and peripheral nervous systems. Nifurtimox seems to be better tolerated by children than by adults. Nausea, vomiting, abdominal pain, anorexia, and weight loss are common and may require premature termination of therapy. Neurologic sequelae include restlessness, disorientation, insomnia, twitching, paresthesias, polyneuritis, weakness, and stiffness. Convulsions may occur. Rashes, neutropenia, and decreased sperm counts have also been reported. The side effects are usually reversible with discontinuation of the drug, but they frequently pose a therapeutic dilemma given the prolonged course of therapy that is necessary.

Benznidazole**

Benznidazole, a nitroimidazole derivative, is another relatively toxic drug used for the treatment of Chagas' disease.[232, 238] It seems to be similar to nifurtimox in efficacy,[238] although recent reports suggest that benznidazole may be effective in eradicating *T. cruzi* in some patients with indeterminate or chronic infection.[239, 240] Benznidazole is administered orally for 30 to 90 days for Chagas' disease. Therapy is often limited by polyneuropathy, rash, gastrointestinal disturbances, or neuropsychiatric effects.

Pentavalent Antimony: Stibogluconate Sodium* and Meglumine Antimonate**

The term *leishmaniasis* refers to the spectrum of clinical syndromes produced by *Leishmania* spp. Two pentavalent antimonials, stibogluconate sodium and meglumine antimonate, have been widely used for the treatment of leishmaniasis.[241] The compounds are of comparable efficacy and toxicity when administered on the basis of their pentavalent antimony content. Stibogluconate is the only pentavalent antimonial available in the United States. It has been extensively studied and widely used in Africa and India.[242–244] Meglumine antimonate is used in francophone countries and in Central and South America.

The efficacy of the pentavalent antimonials varies with the leishmanial syndrome and the causative *Leishmania* species (see Chapter 265). Treatment failures have become increasingly common in some areas. Some of the resistance appears to be acquired, arising from subcurative therapy resulting in selection of resistant parasite strains.[245] Relapses are common in persons with AIDS, suggesting that human immune responses also play a role in the clinical response. Experience with recombinant interferon-γ indicates that it is a useful adjunct when administered with pentavalent antimony in patients with visceral leishmaniasis who fail to respond to pentavalent antimony alone and in patients with diffuse cutaneous leishmaniasis.[246–248]

Sodium stibogluconate is available in sterile aqueous solution for parenteral administration. The standard recommended dose is 20 mg of pentavalent antibody per kilogram of body weight per day. Pentostam is supplied in 10-ml bottles; each milliliter contains 330 mg of drug, which is equivalent to 100 mg of pentavalent antimony. Meglumine antimoniate is available in 5-ml bottles, with 85 mg of antimony per milliliter. These drugs are prescribed on the basis of their antimony content. They can be administered intramuscularly but are usually given intravenously, either undiluted over a 5-minute period or diluted in 50 ml of 5% dextrose in water or saline and administered over 20 minutes.

The antimony concentration in blood is best described by a three-compartment model, with a short initial distribution phase followed by biexponential elimination, primarily through the kidneys.[249–251] The mean half-lives for the elimination phases have been reported to be 1.7 and 33 hours after intravenous administration and 2 and 766 hours after the drug is given intramuscularly. The slow terminal elimination phase may be caused by conversion of pentavalent to trivalent antimony. The latter may be responsible for the toxicity seen with long-term, high-dose therapy. The mechanism of action is uncertain. Pentavalent antimony is concentrated in cells of reticuloendothelial origin. It appears to affect parasite metabolism.

The pentavalent antimonials are relatively well tolerated.[241–243, 250, 251] Common adverse effects include abdominal pain, nausea, vomiting, malaise, headache, increased transaminase levels, nephrotoxicity, weakness, myalgias, arthralgias, fever, skin rash, cough, and pneumonitis, but these seldom prevent completion of the treatment course. Pancreatic enzymes are frequently elevated, and clinically significant pancreatitis occurs in some recipients.[252, 253] Dose-related changes are observed in the electrocardiogram. The most common are non-specific ST-T wave changes and a prolonged Q-Tc interval. Rarer but more serious effects include atrial and ventricular arrhythmias. Sudden death has been associated with doses higher than recommended. The use of pentavalent antimony is relatively contraindicated in patients with myocarditis, hepatitis, pancreatitis, or renal failure.

Pyrazolopyrimidines (Allopurinol and Allopurinol Ribonucleoside**)

Allopurinol, allopurinol riboside, and other purine analogues have activity against *Leishmania* spp.[254–256] and *T. cruzi*. Reports of their clinical efficacy have varied. The metabolism of purines in trypanosomatids differs significantly from that in humans. The trypanosomatids rely on salvage pathways to obtain purine analogues, whereas humans synthesize purines de novo. Pyrazolopyrimidines, like allopurinol, inhibit *Leishmania* spp. and *T. cruzi* in vitro and in animal models in vivo. Allopurinol was shown in a small number of cases to be effective when administered with stibogluconate sodium to persons with visceral leishmaniasis who failed to respond to stibogluconate sodium alone.[257] In one randomized, controlled trial, oral allopurinol was as effective in treating cutaneous leishmaniasis due to *Leishmania panamensis* as Pentostam,[258] but other investigators have observed failures with allopurinol.[259]

Amphotericin B and Ketaconazole

Amphotericin B deoxycholate has been used as an alternative drug for the treatment of visceral, cutaneous, and mucosal leishmaniasis for years.[260, 261] AmBisome is as effective as amphotericin B deoxycholate or pentavalent antimony in the treatment of visceral leishmaniasis, and it is less toxic.[262–267] AmBisome is the first drug to receive FDA approval for the treatment of visceral leishmaniasis. Amphotericin B cholesterol dispersion also appears to be effective, but it has not been as extensively studied.[268] Amphotericin binds to sterols and probably damages the surface membrane of *Leishmania* organisms, as it does to a number of fungi. Amphotericin B has also been used with miconazole and rifampin to treat amebic encephalitis caused by *Naegleria* spp. The pharmacokinetics and toxicity of amphotericin are summarized in Chapter 34.

Ketoconazole, an imidazole antifungal drug, has activity against some *Leishmania* spp., such as *Leishmania mexicana*, but not others, such as *Leishmania (Viannia) braziliensis*. The use of ketoconazole in patients with cutaneous and visceral disease has produced variable results.[269–273] Itraconazole has also been variably effective.[274–279]

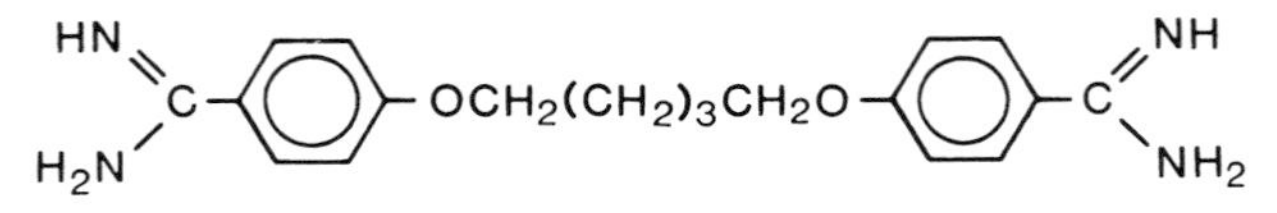

FIGURE 39–8. Pentamidine.

Pentamidine

Pentamidine isethionate (Fig. 39–8) is a diamidine that is used for the treatment of the hemolymphatic stage of *T. b. gambiense* or *T. b. rhodesiense* infection,[280, 281] as an alternative for the treatment of leishmaniasis in persons who fail pentavalent antimony,[282, 283] for secondary prophylaxis in those with HIV and visceral leishmaniasis,[284, 285] and for prophylaxis and treatment of *P. carinii* in persons with AIDS who cannot tolerate sulfonamides.[286, 287] Aerosolized pentamidine has been used for the prevention of *P. carinii* pneumonia, but it is less effective than trimethoprim-sulfamethoxazole, and its administration can result in environmental contamination.[288, 289]

Pentamidine isethionate is a white powder that is water soluble; each 1.74 mg contains 1 mg of pentamidine base.[290] It is available for intramuscular, intravenous, or aerosol administration. Intramuscular injections are frequently complicated by pain, swelling, and sterile abscesses at the administration site. Pentamidine is now most commonly given intravenously after being diluted in 100 to 250 ml of 5% dextrose in water. It must be administered slowly over 1 to 2 hours.[291] Pentamidine is highly tissue bound and is excreted slowly over an extended period. It does not penetrate well into the central nervous system.

The mechanism of action has not been defined. Pentamidine is known to bind to DNA in a nonintercalative manner.[292] It interacts selectively with trypanosomal kinetoplast DNA, resulting in swelling and loss of structure of the kinetoplast.[293] Pentamidine also inhibits RNA polymerase,[294] ribosomal function,[295] and synthesis of nucleic acids, proteins, and phospholipids.[296] It decreases the amount of membrane phospholipids, thereby altering cytoplasmic and mitochondrial membranes.[297] It affects polyamine synthesis by decreasing the activity of ornithine decarboxylase.[298] It can inhibit folic acid synthesis,[299] but this does not appear to be its mode of action. It can also inhibit trypsin and related proteases.[300] At high concentrations, pentamidine impairs oxygen consumption.[301]

The administration of pentamidine isethionate by the intravenous or the intramuscular route is associated with toxicity in 50% of patients.[301] Adverse effects include tachycardia, nausea, vomiting, dizziness, rash, facial flushing, breathlessness, and a metallic taste. Severe hypotension may result after rapid intravenous infusion.[291] Hypoglycemia has been reported during therapy in 6 to 9% of persons treated in the United States.[302–304] Hypoglycemia can be severe and life-threatening, and it may even occur after the completion of therapy. It is probably caused by a direct toxic effect of pentamidine on pancreatic beta cells.[305, 306] Hypoglycemia can be followed by the development of insulin-dependent diabetes mellitus. Severe hypoglycemia may be controlled with diazoxide, but it is not known whether this treatment prevents the subsequent development of diabetes mellitus.

Reversible renal failure occurs in approximately 25% of persons who receive pentamidine.[303] Although severe renal failure has been reported in a few patients, it was impossible to attribute the renal toxicity solely to pentamidine because of the concurrent administration of other nephrotoxic agents. Other adverse effects of pentamidine include leukopenia and thrombocytopenia, increased transaminase levels, fever, hypocalcemia, hyperkalemia, confusion, hallucinations, and, rarely, Q-Tc prolongation and cardiac arrhythmias, particularly torsades de pointes. Rare cases of fatal pancreatitis have been reported in patients with AIDS who received pentamidine.[307, 308]

Aerosolized pentamidine is better tolerated than parenterally administered pentamidine and has been used for prevention of *P. carinii* pneumonia in persons with AIDS. Only a small amount of drug reaches the systemic circulation. Untoward effects include a metallic taste, pharyngeal irritation, and bronchospasm, the last occurring particularly in patients with a history of asthma or chronic obstructive pulmonary disease. Pretreatment with inhaled bronchodilators helps reduce bronchospasm. Aerosolized pentamidine is less effective for those with underlying bullous or obstructive lung disease. In addition, patients receiving prophylaxis with inhaled pentamidine are at increased risk for development of extrapulmonary pneumocystosis. Finally, aerosol pentamidine raises environmental safety concerns for health care workers, because of both exhaled drug and the potential of exposure to pathogens such as *Mycobacterium tuberculosis*. All patients for whom aerosolized pentamidine is prescribed should be screened for tuberculosis before therapy begins.

DRUGS FOR TREATMENT OF INTESTINAL NEMATODES (ROUNDWORMS)

The intestinal nematodes remain prevalent in areas of the world where sanitation is poor. As many as 80% of rural inhabitants in some developing areas may be infected with one or more species. *Enterobius vermicularis* is common in the United States. In North America and Europe, intestinal helminths are most likely to be encountered among immigrants from endemic areas or occasionally in returning travelers who have had intense local exposure.

Mebendazole

Mebendazole (Fig. 39–9), a synthetic benzimidazole, methyl 5-benzoylbenzimidazole-2-carbamate, has been widely used for the treatment of intestinal nematodes. *E. vermicularis* responds to a single dose of 100 mg with a repeat dose given after 2 weeks.[309] Mebendazole is also effective against *Ascaris lumbricoides, Necator americanus, Ancylostoma duodenale*, and *Trichuris trichiura*. Treatment with a single dose is effective against *A. lumbricoides*, but twice-daily administration for 3 days is recommended for the hookworms and *T. trichiura*.[309–311] Albendazole, which is more effective as a single dose, has replaced mebendazole in community treatment programs. The effect of mebendazole on *Strongyloides stercoralis* is variable[312–314]; ivermectin is the treatment of choice. Mebendazole has been used at high doses, 200 mg twice a day for 20 days, for the treatment of *Capillaria philippinensis*, an uncommon but important cause of chronic malabsorption in Southeast Asia.[309]

Mebendazole is active against adult *Trichinella spiralis* and has some activity against invading larvae.[315, 316] Although no data are available for humans, mebendazole has been used effectively to treat experimental trichinosis and is now recommended for the treatment of human trichinosis. Steroids are administered concomitantly. Mebendazole has activity against two filaria species, *Loa loa* and *Mansonella perstans*.[317, 318] At 100 mg twice a day for 30 days, it is considered the drug of choice for *M. perstans*,[317] against which diethylcarbamazine is not active. Diethylcarbamazine remains the treatment of choice for *L. loa*. Mebendazole has some activity against *Taenia* spp.,[319] but praziquantel and niclosamide are more effective.

Mebendazole has been used at very high doses for prolonged periods to treat *Echinococcus granulosus* and *Echinococcus multilocularis*, but albendazole is superior.[320–332] The major anthelmintic metabolite of albendazole, albendazole sulfoxide, attains higher serum and cyst concentrations than mebendazole.[326–328]

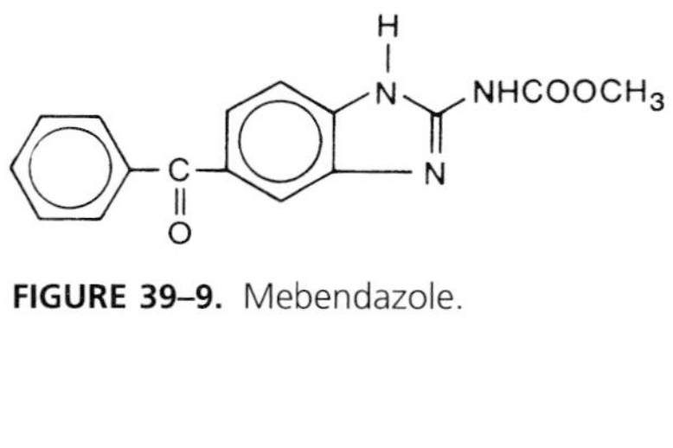

FIGURE 39–9. Mebendazole.

Mebendazole is dispensed in 100-mg tablets. It is only slightly soluble in water and is poorly absorbed from the gastrointestinal tract.[309] This contributes to its low frequency of side effects but limits its usefulness in treating tissue larvae. Up to 10% of an orally administered dose of mebendazole is recovered within 48 hours in the urine. Most of the drug excreted by the kidney is the decarboxylated metabolite. Mebendazole selectively binds to helminthic β-tubulin,[329] prevents microtubule assembly in susceptible helminths, and inhibits glucose uptake.[330] Parasite immobilization and death follow, but it can take several days for susceptible nematodes to be cleared from the gastrointestinal tract. Mebendazole also inhibits the development of the ova of hookworms and *T. trichiura*.

Side effects are uncommon when mebendazole is used at low doses (100 mg twice a day for 3 days) for the treatment of the common intestinal helminths.[309, 330] Transient abdominal pain and diarrhea occur in a small number of persons, usually those with large parasite burdens. Migration of adult *A. lumbricoides* to the nose or mouth occurs occasionally. Mebendazole produces embryotoxicity and teratogenicity in animals; it is therefore contraindicated during pregnancy.

At the high doses used for the treatment of echinococcal cysts, systemic side effects such as alopecia, liver enzyme abnormalities, and transient bone marrow suppression with severe but reversible neutropenia have been observed.[309, 331, 332] The leukocyte count should be monitored closely after initiation of high-dose therapy; neutropenia is usually observed within the first 30 days. Accidental poisoning in one infant was associated with respiratory arrest, tachyarrhythmia, and seizures.[333]

Albendazole

Albendazole (Fig. 39–10), methyl-5-*N*-propoxythio-2-benzimidazole carbamate) has an exceptionally broad spectrum of antiparasitic activity. Albendazole has been widely used throughout the world in individuals and in community-based treatment programs for intestinal nematode infections. It has the advantage of being effective when given as a single dose for the treatment of *A. lumbricoides*, the hookworms *A. duodenale* and *N. americanus*, and, to a lesser extent, *T. trichiura*.[334–347] Periodic treatment at 4- to 6-month intervals with albendazole has been shown to improve the nutritional status, growth, and function of malnourished children infected with multiple species of intestinal helminths.[338–340] Albendazole is also effective against *E. vermicularis*. It has been used successfully for the treatment of cutaneous[341–343] and visceral larva migrans,[344] gnathostomiasis,[345] *C. philippinensis*,[346] mixed hookworm and *Oesophagostomum* infections,[347] *T. spiralis*,[348] *M. perstans*,[349] and *C. sinensis*.[350] Multiple doses have been used to treat *S. stercoralis*, but failures occur.[351, 352]

Albendazole has activity against *G. lamblia*,[353, 354] but it is not currently recommended for the treatment of giardiasis. It has been used successfully for the treatment of intestinal and disseminated microsporidiosis caused by *Encephalitozoon* species in persons with AIDS.[355–358] Given empirically to African patients with HIV infection and persistent diarrhea of more than 3 weeks' duration, albendazole resulted in a significant reduction in days of diarrhea and led to remission in approximately a quarter of those treated.[359]

High-dose, prolonged therapy with albendazole (cycles of 400 mg twice a day for 28 days, followed by 14 days of rest, for a minimum of three cycles) has emerged as the best approach for the medical treatment of *Echinococcus granulosus, Echinococcus multilocularis*, and *Echinococcus vogeli*.[322, 327, 328, 360, 361] It is estimated that approximately one third of persons with echinococcosis can be cured with albendazole, and an additional 50% show improvement.[360, 361] Preoperative administration of albendazole decreases the viability of liver hydatid cysts and reduces the likelihood of peritoneal implantation if cyst contents are spilled during surgery.[362]

Albendazole has also been used successfully for the treatment of neurocysticercosis. Although it has not been compared with praziquantel in a double-blind, controlled manner, albendazole seems

H_3C … S … N, NH, OCH$_3$, O

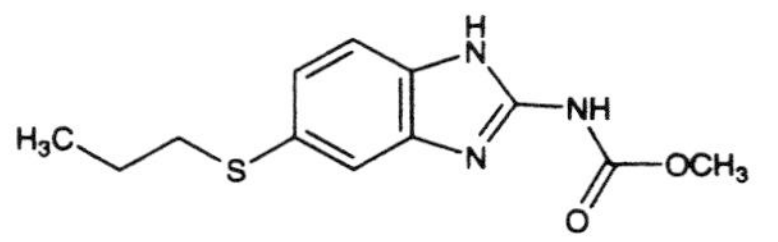

FIGURE 39–10. Albendazole.

to produce higher response rates.[363–374] Corticosteroids are usually administered concurrently to control the inflammatory response elicited by the release of parasite antigens. Albendazole has been used successfully to treat some patients with subarachnoid and ventricular cysticercosis,[371–374] but not all respond. Albendazole has variable activity against adult *Taenia* species in the human gastrointestinal tract.[375, 376]

Albendazole is a white, odorless powder that is dispensed as 400-mg tablets.[361] It is practically insoluble in water; absorption is enhanced when the drug is taken with a fatty meal.[361] Albendazole undergoes extensive first-pass metabolism in the liver, and only albendazole sulfoxide, which is primarily responsible for the systemic anthelmintic effects, is detectable in serum. Sulfoxidation of albendazole also occurs in the gut.[377] Albendazole sulfoxide reaches peak levels in 2.0 to 2.4 hours and has a half-life of 10 to 15 hours.[361, 378] Plasma levels of albendazole sulfoxide at steady state show great individual variability. Drug concentrations in the central nervous system are approximately 40% that of serum.[379] Concurrent administration of dexamethasone increases the levels of albendazole by approximately 50%.[380] The concentration of albendazole sulfoxide in echinococcal cysts is approximately 25% of the serum concentration. The bile appears to be the major route of elimination, and enterohepatic recirculation occurs. Albendazole, like other benzimidazoles, binds to β-tubulin, inhibits its assembly into microtubules,[381] and impairs the uptake of glucose leading to the depletion of glycogen stores in helminths. It also inhibits helminthic-specific fumarate reductase.[382]

Albendazole is usually well tolerated when given as a single 400-mg dose for the treatment of intestinal nematodes. Diarrhea, abdominal discomfort, rash, or migration of *Ascaris* through the nose or mouth can occur. On rare occasions it has been associated with fever, rash, the Stevens-Johnson syndrome, or pseudomembranous colitis.[383, 384] High-dose, prolonged therapy for echinococcal disease or neurocysticercosis is occasionally complicated by serum transaminase elevation, bone marrow suppression with anemia, neutropenia or thrombocytopenia, or, less commonly, alopecia.[361, 385, 386] Liver enzymes and complete blood counts should be measured at least every 2 weeks. Liver and bone marrow toxicity are reversible with discontinuation of the drug. Occasionally gastrointestinal disturbances, headache, or dizziness occur. In view of the potential teratogenicity of benzimidazole compounds, albendazole is contraindicated during pregnancy.

Thiabendazole

Thiabendazole, 2-(4′-thiazolyl)-1H-benzimidazole, is a potent anthelminthic drug,[387] but its use has been limited by its high frequency of untoward effects. Thiabendazole is active against a number of adult nematodes that infect the gastrointestinal tract and against larvae in tissues. It is much better absorbed than mebendazole. The most common indication for thiabendazole has been the treatment of *S. stercoralis*[388] or *Strongyloides fuelleborni*[389] infection, but ivermectin, which is equally effective but less toxic, is now recommended. Thiabendazole has also been used to treat *Trichostrongylus* spp. infections,[390] visceral larva migrans,[387] and trichinosis, but there are now less toxic alternatives.[5, 394, 395] Although thiabendazole is active against the hookworms *A. lumbricoides, E. vermicularis*, and, to a lesser extent, *T. trichiura*,[387] mebendazole and albendazole have higher response rates and are far better tolerated. Thiabendazole is effective when applied topically or taken orally for cutaneous larva migrans.[394, 395] It is widely used as a fungicide and food preservative and in veterinary practice.[396, 397]

Thiabendazole is available in 500-mg tablets and as an oral suspension of 500 mg/5 ml. It is rapidly absorbed after oral administration; peak concentrations occur in plasma about 1 hour after treatment.[330] It is recommended that the drug be given with meals. No parenteral preparation is available, which poses a problem for critically ill patients with disseminated *S. stercoralis* infection who cannot take oral medications. Most of the drug is excreted in urine within 24 hours as 5-hydroxythiabendazole conjugated as the glucuronide or as the sulfate. The precise mechanism of action is not known. Like other benzimidazoles, thiabendazole binds to β-tubulin and prevents microtubule formation and glucose uptake.[398] It also inhibits fumarate reductase in susceptible helminths.[393]

Approximately half of the persons who receive thiabendazole experience one or more side effects, most commonly nausea, anorexia, vomiting, and dizziness.[330] Less frequent are diarrhea, epigastric pain, pruritus, drowsiness, giddiness, and headache. Rare side effects include tinnitus, abnormal sensation in the eyes, numbness, decreased pulse and blood pressure, elevated liver enzymes, and progressive bile duct injury.[330, 399] Seizures were reported in a child with Down syndrome.[400] Transient neutropenia has been observed in some patients. Allergic manifestations such as fever, facial flush, angioneurotic edema, lymphadenopathy, perianal rash, and skin rashes also occur; some or all of these may be caused by the release of parasite antigens. Thiabendazole can give urine an asparagus-like odor. Crystalluria has been observed.

Because of the central nervous system effects, activities requiring alertness should be avoided during therapy. The drug should be used with caution in persons with hepatic disease or decreased hepatic function. Thiabendazole has been found to be genotoxic in both in vitro and in vivo assays,[401] and it is contraindicated in pregnant women. Thiabendazole increases the half-life of theophylline and was associated with theophylline toxicity and severe nausea and vomiting when the two were administered concurrently.[402]

Pyrantel Pamoate

Pyrantel pamoate is effective against *E. vermicularis*. It can also be used to treat *A. lumbricoides, N. americanus, A. duodenale*, and *Moniliformis moniliformis*.[403–407] Treatment with pyrantel pamoate resulted in increased appetite and growth in children infected with *A. lumbricoides*.[408] Pyrantel pamoate is an alternative to mebendazole for the treatment of *Trichostrongylus* spp. It is not active against *T. trichiura*, but oxantel**, an m-oxyphenol derivative that has not been licensed in the United States, is.

Pyrantel is available as a suspension (250 mg of pyrantel base/5 ml). It is poorly absorbed; less than 15% is excreted in the urine as the parent drug or metabolite.[405, 406, 409] Pyrantel acts as an agonist at nicotinic acetylcholine receptors of sensitive nematodes. It functions as a depolarizing neuromuscular blocking agent that results in a short period of calcium-dependent stimulation followed by irreversible paralysis of the worm.[410, 411] Pyrantel also inhibits acetylcholinesterases.

Pyrantel pamoate has minimal toxicity at the oral doses used to treat intestinal helminths. Mild, transient gastrointestinal symptoms, headache, drowsiness, insomnia, or dizziness are occasionally encountered. The metabolites of pyrantel pamoate are mutagenic in bacteria. Pyrantel pamoate has not been studied in pregnancy, and it is not recommended for pregnant women or children younger than 1 year of age. Pyrantel and piperazine, which produces hyperpolarization with a reduction in spike wave activity in helminthic muscle cells, appear to be mutually antagonistic and should not be used together.[406, 407]

Piperazine**

Piperazine citrate was once widely used for the treatment of *A. lumbricoides*. It has been replaced in the United States and most other areas by mebendazole, albendazole, or pyrantel pamoate, which are less toxic. Piperazine also has activity against *E. vermicularis*. The piperazine moiety has been incorporated into a number of compounds that have a broad range of pharmacologic activity. Some substituted piperazines are central serotonin agonists; others depress monosynaptic spinal cord excitation, block chloride channels, have antioxidant effects, display antiarrhythmic activity, or act as vasodilators. One of the derivatives, diethylcarbamazine, is effective against filaria, as discussed later.

Piperazine is well absorbed orally.[330] Some of the drug is metabolized; the remainder is excreted in the urine. Piperazine causes flaccid paralysis of susceptible intestinal helminths. It acts as a low-potency agonist at extrasynaptic γ-aminobutyric acid–gated chloride channels in nematode muscle.[412] Activation of these receptors gives rise to an increase in chloride conductance. There is hyperpolarization and suppression of spontaneous action potentials.[413] Worms are paralyzed and excreted alive, usually without migrating.

Piperazine is generally well tolerated. On occasion, there are gastrointestinal symptoms, transient neurologic side effects, or urticarial reactions. Lethal overdoses have been associated with convulsions and respiratory depression. Epileptic activity may be exaggerated, so piperazine is contraindicated in persons with a history of seizures.[414] Neurotoxicity has also been observed in persons with impaired renal function. Visual disturbances, ataxia, and hypotonia occur rarely.[415] Piperazine has been used during pregnancy without apparent adverse effects, but it has not been thoroughly evaluated in this setting. Although adverse dermatologic reactions are rare, rashes have been reported with piperazine and compounds containing the piperazine moiety.[416]

DRUGS FOR TREATMENT OF SYSTEMIC NEMATODES

Diethylcarbamazine*

Diethylcarbamazine (Fig. 39–11) is a piperazine derivative, *N,N*-diethyl-4-methyl-1-piperazinecarboxamide dihydrogen citrate. It results in the rapid death of microfilaria of *Wuchereria bancrofti, Brugia malayi*, and *Brugia timori*, the three lymphatic-dwelling filaria that infect humans.[417–422] The annual administration of a single dose of diethylcarbamazine to persons with lymphatic filariasis reduces microfilaremia by 90%, and in combination with a single dose of ivermectin by 99%.[419, 420] A major reduction in microfilaremia has also been observed with the administration of diethylcarbamazine-medicated salt.[419, 420] Field studies have confirmed that reductions in microfilarial load and prevalence can interrupt transmission.[417] Diethlycarbamazine is variably effective against adult *W. bancrofti*[423] and, although not well documented, probably has some macrofilaricidal action against *B. malayi* and *B. timori* as well. It is currently the drug of choice for all three species. Males with hydroceles before treatment have demonstrated improvement 1 year after starting therapy,[419] but the chronic lymphatic damage that results in elephantiasis is not reversed. Mass treatment campaigns have been associated with a decrease in the frequency of advanced hydroceles.[418]

Diethylcarbamazine has been used successfully to treat persons with pulmonary infiltrates with eosinophilia in the tropics, because this syndrome is in many instances caused by microfilaria in the lungs.[424] Diethylcarbamazine kills the microfilaria of *L. loa*, but severe adverse reactions, including encephalopathy caused by the

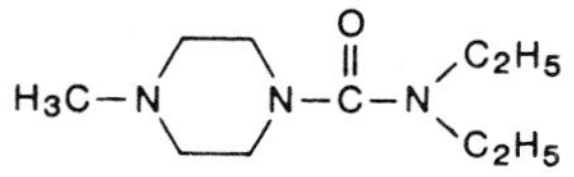

$H_3C{-}N(\text{piperazine ring})N{-}C(=O){-}N(C_2H_5)_2$

FIGURE 39–11. Diethylcarbamazine.

release of parasite antigens, can occur in persons with heavy microfilarial burdens.[5, 425] Diethylcarbamazine has no effect against *Mansonella ozzardi* or *Mansonella perstans*[5, 426, 427]; it has been used to treat visceral larva migrans, but with variable success.[428, 429]

Ivermectin replaced diethylcarbamazine for the treatment of onchocerciasis. Diethylcarbamazine rapidly kills microfilaria of *O. volvulus* in the skin and eye, but the resulting inflammatory reaction can cause severe damage.[430–432] Ocular complications may be permanent and include visual field constriction, optic nerve damage, chorioretinitis, anterior uveitis, and punctate keratitis.[430–435] Diethylcarbamazine does not kill adult *O. volvulus*, and microfilaria reaccumulate after therapy.[433] Ivermectin is associated with a slower reduction of microfilaria in the eye and much less toxicity. It has replaced diethylcarbamazine for the treatment of onchocerciasis. Diethylcarbamazine is also widely used in veterinary practice to kill *Dirofilaria immitis*, the dog heartworm.

Diethylcarbamazine is available in 50-mg tablets.[330] It is readily absorbed from the gastrointestinal tract. Peak blood levels are reached in 1 to 2 hours; the serum half-life is approximately 8 hours.[436] The parent compound and its metabolites are cleared through the kidney.[437, 438] Diethylcarbamazine is distributed equally throughout all body compartments except adipose tissue, and there is little accumulation even after repeated doses are given.

The drug seems to affect microfilariae in multiple ways. First, it is associated with a decrease in helminthic muscle activity, which leads eventually to immobilization of the worm.[439] The piperazine moiety may result in hyperpolarization, causing the observed paralysis.[330] Second, the drug appears to alter the surface membranes of microfilariae, resulting in enhanced killing by the host's immune system.[440, 441] Diethylcarbamazine has also been shown to enhance the adherence properties of eosinophils and polymorphonuclear leukocytes,[442] and there is evidence to suggest that human platelets may contribute to the antimicrofilarial effects.[443] Diethylcarbamazine has effects on arachidonic acid metabolism and inhibits parasite eicosanoid production.[411, 444] It also disrupts microtubules and inhibits their formation in vitro.[445]

Untoward effects include those produced directly by the drug and inflammatory reactions that follow the release of filarial antigens. Common reactions include headache, malaise, weakness, arthralgia, anorexia, nausea, and vomiting. The gastrointestinal effects are usually dose related. Acute psychotic reactions have been reported but are rare.

Systemic and ocular reactions occur when diethylcarbamazine is used to treat onchocerciasis. They include severe pruritus, edema of the skin, fever, hypotension, heightened eosinophilia, lymphadenopathy, splenomegaly, and proteinuria.[434, 435] The elicitation of such reactions by even low doses of diethylcarbamazine is the basis for the Mazzotti test,[446] which has been used to diagnose onchocerciasis but is potentially dangerous. In *W. bancrofti* and *B. malayi* infections, localized swellings or nodules may develop along lymphatics, and there may be accompanying lymphadenitis.[435] Transient hydrocele formation or lymphedema may be observed. Serious reactions including encephalopathy, presumably caused by release of parasite antigens, have been observed in persons treated with diethylcarbamazine who had heavy *L. loa* burdens.[447]

Ivermectin

Ivermectin is the 22,23-dihydro derivative of ivermectin B1, a macrocyclic lactone produced by the actinomycete *Streptomyces avermitilis*.[448] It is active at low doses against a large number of nematodes and blood-sucking arthropods that parasitize humans and animals.

Ivermectin is the treatment of choice for human onchocerciasis.[430–433, 449–457] It kills microfilariae in the skin and produces a gradual reduction in the eye. The systemic and ocular inflammatory responses that occur after treatment are much less severe than with diethylcarbamazine. In mass community-based treatment programs ivermectin has proved safe, acceptable to indigenous populations, and effective in reducing microfilarial loads and the prevalence of onchocerciasis.[449–457] Although ivermectin does not kill adult *O. volvulus*, it inhibits oviposition. Successive annual treatments are associated with a progressive decline in the microfilarial burden.[458, 459]

Ivermectin kills microfilariae of *W. bancrofti* and *B. malayi*.[460–463] In persons with lymphatic filariasis, annual therapy with a single dose of ivermectin reduces blood microfilaria by 90%, and coadministration with diethylcarbamazine or albendazole, by 99%.[417, 418] Despite a profound effect on blood microfilaremia, ivermectin has no observable activity on the viability of adult *W. bancrofti* or *B. malayi*.[464] Ivermectin kills microfilariae of *L. loa*.[465, 466] In persons with high concentrations of *L. loa*, treatment may be associated with encephalopathy, presumably because of the release of antigens in the central nervous system. Ivermectin is also active against microfilariae of *Mansonella streptocerca* and *M. ozzardi*, but not *M. perstans*.[5, 467]

Ivermectin has activity against a number of nematodes.[352, 448] It has emerged as the treatment of choice for strongyloidiasis.[468–470] It is as effective as thiabendazole against *S. stercoralis* but has fewer untoward effects. Ivermectin is also effective in the treatment of cutaneous larva migrans.[471, 472] It is active against the human intestinal pathogens *A. lumbricoides* and *E. vermicularis*, variably effective against *T. trichiura*, and not effective for the hookworms.[448, 471]

Ivermectin administered orally is useful in the treatment of scabies.[471, 473, 474] A single dose is usually effective in immunocompetent persons, but multiple doses are often necessary in persons with HIV and crusted scabies. Ivermectin is widely used in veterinary practice for the treatment of helminthic and arthropod infestations.

Ivermectin is odorless and colorless and has been effective when administered as a single oral dose. Peak serum concentrations are reached 4 to 5 hours after an oral dose, and the elimination half-life is 50 to 60 hours.[475] It is highly protein bound.[476] It is concentrated in the liver and adipose tissues. Only a small percentage of the drug is excreted in the urine; the rest is excreted in the stool. Ivermectin potentiates the opening of glutamate-gated chloride channels that are found only in nematodes and arthropods. The result is an influx of chloride ions. In nematodes this is associated with paralysis of the pharyngeal pumping motion.[477]

Ivermectin is well tolerated. The initiation of therapy in persons with onchocerciasis can be complicated by fever, pruritus, tender lymphadenopathy, headache, arthralgias, myalgia, and cutaneous edema caused by the release of microfilarial antigens, but the side effects are less frequent and less severe than those of diethylcarbamazine.[430–433, 449–457, 478, 479] Similar symptoms can occur with the treatment of other filarial diseases. The administration of ivermectin to some patients with high burdens of *L. loa* microfilaremia has been associated with the development of encephalopathy. Cases have been reported during mass treatment programs for onchocerciasis in areas of Africa where *L. loa* is coendemic.[480, 481] In cattle, 30 times the recommended dose of ivermectin was tolerated without signs of toxicity, but death occurred at 40 times the recommended dose. No teratogenicity has been reported in animals. In a study of 203 children born to women inadvertently treated during pregnancy, no increase in the rate of birth defects was observed, but ivermectin is not approved for use during pregnancy.[482]

DRUGS FOR TREATMENT OF PLATYHELMINTHS: TREMATODES (FLUKES) AND CESTODES (TAPEWORMS)

Praziquantel

Praziquantel (Fig. 39–12), 2-[cyclohexylcarbonyl-(1,2,3,6,7,11β)-hexyahydro-4H-pyrazino [2,1-α]isoquinolin-4-one], is a heterocyclic prazino-isoquinoline derivative with a broad spectrum of activity against trematodes and cestodes.[483–490] Praziquantel is highly effective against all *Schistosoma* spp. that infect humans.[483–490] It has even been effective in the treatment of schistosomiasis of the central nervous system.[491, 492] The possibility of praziquantel-tolerant *S. mansoni* has been suggested by decreased cure rates in a focus in

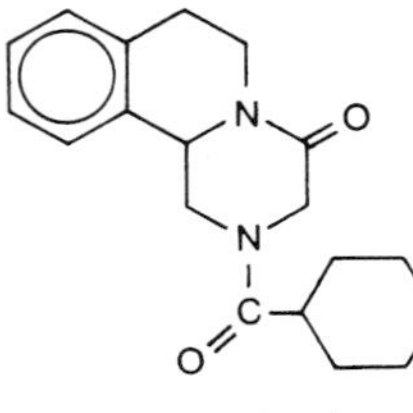

FIGURE 39–12. Praziquantel.

northern Senegal,[493] but frank praziquantel resistance has not been confirmed.

Praziquantel is also the drug of choice for the liver flukes *C. sinensis*, *Opisthorchis viverrini*, and *Metorchis conjunctus*; the lung flukes *Paragonimus westermani*, *Paragonimus kellicoti*, and other *Paragonimus* spp.; and the intestinal flukes *Heterophyes heterophyes*, *Fasciolopsis buski*, *Metagonimus yokogawai*, and *Nanophyetus salmincola*.[5, 483–485, 494] Only against the liver fluke *Fasciola hepatica* have praziquantel failures been frequent.[495, 496]

Praziquantel is also active against adult and larval forms of the cestodes.[483–485] It has been used successfully for the treatment of parenchymal neurocysticercosis due to *Taenia solium*.[363, 366, 368, 369, 394, 497–500] Although not compared in a blinded, controlled manner, albendazole appears to be more effective and is administered in a shorter course. Praziquantel is often ineffective when there is subarachnoid involvement, cysticercal meningitis, or cysts in the ventricular system,[501, 502] although it has been effective in some cases in which albendazole has failed. Praziquantel is contraindicated in persons with intraocular cysticerci.[503, 504] Praziquantel is highly effective in the treatment of intestinal *T. solium, Taenia saginata, Diphyllobothrium latum, Diphyllobothrium pacificum, Hymenolepis nana*, and *Dipylidium caninum* infections.[5, 483–485, 505] Praziquantel is not effective in the treatment of human hydatid disease, but it is active against adult *Echinococcus* spp. in the canine gastrointestinal tract. Although it damages protoscolices in hydatids, the germinal layer is not destroyed.[506, 507]

Praziquantel is dispensed as 600-mg tablets that contain a mixture of its two enantiomers.[508, 509] The drug is crystalline, colorless, and almost insoluble in water. Variability has been reported in the bioavailability of different praziquantel preparations.[510] A peak serum concentration of 1 μm/ml is reached 1 to 2 hours after an oral dose of 50 mg/kg body weight of the standard preparation is administered.[483–485] Praziquantel is approximately 80% protein bound. There is pronounced first-pass metabolism.[511, 512] Approximately 80% of praziquantel is excreted in the urine in 4 days; 90% of that amount is excreted within the first 24 hours. The remainder is excreted in the feces. The pharmacokinetics of the drug are not significantly altered in patients undergoing hemodialysis. The concentration of praziquantel in the cerebrospinal fluid is approximately 14 to 24% of the concentration of free plus protein-bound drug in the plasma.[513] Plasma levels are decreased by approximately 50% in patients with neurocysticercosis receiving dexamethasone, which is problematic because corticosteroids are often administered concurrently with praziquantel to reduce cerebral edema.[514] In contrast, the concurrent administration of praziquantel with cimetidine increases the plasma level of praziquantel by approximately 100%.[515]

Praziquantel is rapidly taken up by flukes and tapeworms. It is uniformly distributed in these organisms and is not metabolized. It damages the integument and increases the permeability to calcium ions.[516–519] In adult schistosomes, an influx of calcium is followed by tetanic contraction and paralysis of the musculature. The initial effects are rapid and associated with intense vacuolation of the tegument.[517] Adult worms are then swept to the liver, where they are attacked by phagocytes. Praziquantel results in exposure of parasite antigens, including actin, on the surface of adult schistosomes; this facilitates the host immune response.[520, 521] In the tapeworm *Hymenolepis diminuta*, praziquantel causes calcium release from endogenous stores, leading to massive contraction of the worm.[522] Expulsion from the gastrointestinal tract follows. The tegument of the neck of the tapeworm develops blebs, but the scolex and proglottids appear to be unaffected.

Praziquantel is generally well tolerated.[483–485] Reactions are common but are usually mild and transient. They are often caused by responses that follow the release of worm antigens. The most common are nausea, vomiting, abdominal pain, dizziness, headache, and lassitude. Only rarely is vomiting severe. Exudative polyserositis with respiratory failure was reported in one patient.[523] Urticarial reactions have been observed during the treatment of paragonimiasis.[524] Intense abdominal pain and bloody diarrhea have occurred in patients with heavy *S. mansoni* infections.[525–527] Increased intracranial pressure, cerebral edema, and inflammation have been observed during the treatment of neurocysticercosis. Corticosteroids are usually administered concomitantly in that setting.[528, 529]

There has been no evidence of mutagenicity or teratogenicity with praziquantel in humans, but there is some evidence to suggest that it could have comutagenic effects. Fetal death was observed when high-dose praziquantel was administered to pregnant rats early in gestation.[530] Praziquantel is contraindicated during pregnancy. It is excreted in breast milk. It is recommended that women not nurse on the day that praziquantel is given or for 72 hours thereafter. Cimetidine, ketaconazole, and miconazole inhibit the metabolism of praziquantel and increase serum levels.[531]

Metrifonate**

Metrifonate, an organophosphate that is transformed nonenzymatically in humans to dichlorvos, is a potent inhibitor of acetylcholinesterase. It is used as an alternative to praziquantel for the treatment of *Schistosoma haematobium*.[514, 532] Metrifonate has comparable efficacy, and has been used successfully in mass treatment programs.[533–536]

Metrifonate is well absorbed after oral ingestion.[537] When given to humans, it produces a 95% decrease in plasma cholinesterase activity within 6 hours. Plasma activity usually returns to normal relatively quickly. Erythrocyte cholinesterase is inhibited to approximately 50% of pretreatment values, but it takes 2 to 2.5 months for it to return to normal.[537] Although its mechanism of action against *S. haematobium* is uncertain, it may act by inhibiting tegumental acetylcholine receptors that mediate glucose transport.[538]

Metrifonate is usually well tolerated, but mild vertigo, lassitude, nausea, vomiting, and occasionally bronchospasm have been reported. A limitation for large-scale treatment programs is that metrifonate is usually administered in three doses at 2-week intervals, which can result in poor compliance and reduced efficacy.[539] In contrast, praziquantel is administered in 1 day. Persons treated with metrifonate should not receive neuromuscular blocking agents or be exposed to insecticides with anticholinesterase effects for at least 48 hours after treatment.

Oxamniquine**

Oxamniquine, a tetrahydroquinoline, is an alternative to praziquantel for the treatment of *S. mansoni* infections.[540–545] It has been used successfully in mass treatment programs and in a focus of *S. mansoni* infection where the response to praziquantel was unusually poor.[493] The sensitivity of *S. mansoni* to oxamniquine varies in different geographic regions. Higher doses are recommended in many areas of Africa.

Oxamniquine is dispensed in 250-mg capsules. It is well absorbed orally, and the parent drug and its metabolites are excreted in the urine. Peak plasma concentrations are achieved 1 to 4 hours after dosing, and the elimination half-life is 2.2 hours.[546] It is given as a single dose. Oxamniquine produces marked tegumental alterations in treated adult schistosomes that appear 4 to 8 days after treatment.[547] The tegumental changes seen after praziquantel treatment are much

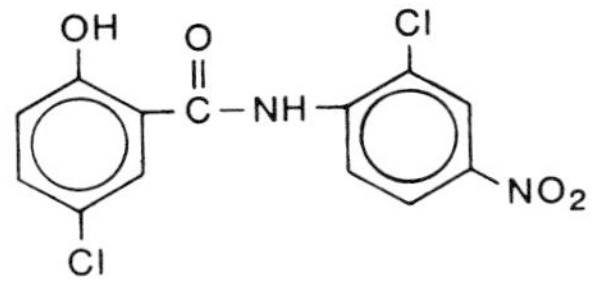

FIGURE 39–13. Niclosamide.

more rapid. An enzyme in *S. mansoni* may be responsible for activation of the drug.[548] Side effects include dizziness, which occurs in 40% of the treated population, drowsiness, headache, fever, diarrhea, rash, hepatic enzyme elevations, electrocardiographic changes, electroencephalographic changes and orange to red discoloration of the urine. Convulsions and neuropsychiatric disturbances occur rarely. Oxamniquine should not be used in persons with epilepsy. It is contraindicated during pregnancy.

Bithionol*

Bithionol is the drug of choice for treatment of *F. hepatica* and is an alternative to praziquantel for the treatment of paragonimiasis.[549, 550] It is administered orally, usually on alternate days, for 10 to 15 doses. It is frequently associated with urticaria, photosensitivity reactions, and gastrointestinal complaints, including vomiting, diarrhea, and abdominal pain. These reactions may be caused, in part or solely, by the release of worm antigens. Leukopenia and toxic hepatitis are rare complications.

Niclosamide**

Niclosamide, *N*-(2′-chloro-4′-nitrophenyl)-5-chloro-salicylamide (Fig. 39–13), given as a single dose, is active against a number of adult tapeworms that reside in the human gastrointestinal tract.[551, 552] It kills *T. saginata*, the beef tapeworm; *T. solium*, the pork tapeworm; *D. latum*, the fish tapeworm; *H. nana*, the dwarf tapeworm; and *D. caninum*, the dog tapeworm. Finally, niclosamide is a molluscicide and is used in large scale snail control programs.

Although niclosamide kills *T. solium*, treatment results in the disintegration of the adult tapeworm and release of viable ova, raising the theoretical possibility of autoinfection. Praziquantel is preferred for *T. solium* because it is active against larvae as well as adults and could prevent cysticercosis if ova hatched. If niclosamide is used, it is often followed by a purge to reduce the theoretical risk of autoinfection. In the case of *H. nana*, praziquantel is effective when administered as a single dose, whereas niclosamide must be administered daily for 6 days.

Niclosamide is very poorly absorbed.[551] It is supplied in 500-mg vanilla-flavored tablets, which should be chewed thoroughly and then washed down with water. The anthelmintic mechanisms of niclosamide are not completely understood. The drug appears to uncouple oxidative phosphorylation in the scolex and proximal segments of the adult tapeworm and to stimulate adenosine triphosphatase activity of mitochondria, resulting in death of the worm and rapid disintegration of the scolex.[553] Niclosamide is free of side effects except for occasional mild gastrointestinal complaints, lightheadedness, and, rarely, rash. Niclosamide has been observed to be genotoxic in vitro,[554] but because little is absorbed the risk to humans is probably small.

REFERENCES

1. Smith DF, Parsons M. Molecular Biology of Parasitic Protozoa. Oxford: IRL Press at Oxford University Press; 1996.
2. Freeman DO. Immunopathogenetic Aspects of Disease Induced by Helminth Parasites. Basel: Karger; 1997.
3. Neva FA, Brown HW. Basic Clinical Parasitology. Norwalk, Conn: Appleton & Lange; 1994.
4. Guerrant RL, Weller PF, Walker DH. Tropical Infectious Diseases: Principles, Pathogens and Practice. Philadelphia: WB Saunders; 1999.
5. Drugs for treatment of parasitic infections. Med Lett Drugs Ther. 1998;40:1–12.
6. Powell SJ, Wilmot AJ, Elsdon-Dew R. Further trials of metronidazole in amoebic dysentery and amoebic liver abscess. Ann Trop Med Parasitol. 1967;61:511–514.
7. Welsh JS, Rowsell BJ, Freeman C. Treatment of intestinal amoebiasis and giardiasis: Efficacy of metronidazole and tinidazole compared. Med J Aust. 1978;1:469–471.
8. Spillman R, Ayala SC, DeSanchez CE. Double blind test of metronidazole and tinidazole in the treatment of asymptomatic *Entamoeba histolytica* and *Entamoeba hartmanni* carriers. Am J Trop Med Hyg. 1976;25:549–551.
9. Thoren K, Hakansson C, Bergstrom T, et al. Treatment of asymptomatic amebiasis in homosexual men: Clinical trials with metronidazole, tinidazole, and diloxanide furoate. Sex Transm Dis. 1990;17:72–74.
10. Irusen EM, Jackson TF, Simjee AE. Asymptomatic intestinal colonization by pathogenic *Entamoeba histolytica* in amebic liver abscess: Prevalence, response to therapy and pathogenic potential. Clin Infect Dis. 1992;14:889–893.
11. Salaki JS, Shirey JL, Strickland GT. Successful treatment of symptomatic *Entamoeba polecki* infection. Am J Trop Med Hyg. 1979;28:190–193.
12. Wolfe MS. Giardiasis. N Engl J Med. 1978;298:319–321.
13. Lerman SJ, Walker RA. Treatment of giardiasis: Literature review and recommendations. Clin Pediatr. 1982;21:409–414.
14. Lossick JG. Treatment of sexually transmitted vaginosis/vaginitis. Rev Infect Dis. 1990;12(Suppl)6:S665–S681.
15. Lossick JG, Kent HL. Trichomoniasis: Trends in diagnosis and management. Am J Obstet Gynecol. 1991;165:1217–1222.
16. Wolfe MS. *Blastocystis hominis* infection. In: Strickland GT, ed. Hunter's Tropical Medicine. 6th ed. Philadelphia: WB Saunders; 1984:513.
17. Walzer PD, Judson FN, Murphy KB, et al. Balantidiasis outbreak in Truk. Am J Trop Med Hyg. 1973;22:33–41.
18. Hamed KA, Studemeister AE. Successful response of metronidazole-resistant trichomonal vaginitis to tinidazole: A case report. Sex Transm Dis. 1992;19:339–340.
19. Dupont HL, Sullivan PS. Giardiasis: The clinical spectrum, diagnosis and therapy. Pediatr Infect Dis. 1986;5:S131–S138.
20. Weniger BG, Schantz PM. Praziquantel and refugee health. JAMA. 1984;251:2391–2392.
21. Sharma VP, Rathore HS, Sharma MM. Efficacy of metronidazole in dracunculiasis: A clinical trial. Am J Trop Med Hyg. 1979;28:658–660.
22. Houghton GW, Smith J, Thorpe PS, et al. The pharmacokinetics of oral and intravenous metronidazole in man. J Antimicrob Chemother. 1979;5:621–623.
23. McGilveray IJ, Midha KK, Loo JCK, et al. The bioavailability of commercial metronidazole formulations. Int J Clin Pharmacol. 1978;16:110–115.
24. Norris SM, Ravdin JI. The pharmacology of antiamebic drugs. In: Ravdin JI, ed. Amebiasis: Human Infection by *Entamoeba histolytica*. New York: Wiley; 1988:734–740.
25. Lau AH, Lam NP, Piscitelli SC, et al. Clinical pharmacokinetics of metronidazole and other nitroimidazole anti-infectives. Clin Pharmacokinet. 1992;23:328–364.
26. Lares-Asseff I, Cravioto J, Santiago P, et al. Pharmacokinetics of metronidazole in severely malnourished and nutritionally rehabilitated children. Clin Pharmacol Ther. 1992;51:42–45.
27. Lindmark DG, Müller M. Antitrichomonad action, mutagenicity, and reduction of metronidazole and other nitroimidazoles. Antimicrob Agents Chemother. 1976;10:476–482.
28. Knight RC, Skolimowski IM, Edwards DI. The interaction of reduced metronidazole with DNA. Biochem Pharmacol. 1978;27:2089–2093.
29. LaRusso NF, Tomasz M, Müller M, et al. Interaction of metronidazole with nucleic acids in vitro. Mol Pharmacol. 1977;13:872–882.
30. Lefebvre Y, Hesseltine HC. The peripheral white blood cells and metronidazole. JAMA. 1965;194:15–18.
31. Kazmier FJ. A significant interaction between metronidazole and warfarin. Mayo Clin Proc. 1976;51:782–784.
32. Kusumi RK, Plouffe JF, Wyatt RH, et al. Central nervous system toxicity associated with metronidazole therapy. Ann Intern Med. 1980;93:59–60.
33. Friedman GD, Selby JV. How often does metronidazole induce pancreatitis? Gastroenterology. 1990;98:1702–1703.
34. Cina SJ, Russell RA, Conradi SE. Sudden death due to metronidazole/ethanol interaction. Am J Forensic Med Pathol. 1996;17:343–346.
35. Rosenkranz HS, Speck WT. Studies on the significance of the mutagenicity of metronidazole for *Salmonella typhimurium*. In: Finegold SM, ed. Metronidazole: Proceedings of the International Metronidazole Conference, Montreal, Quebec, Canada, May 26–28, 1976. Princeton, NJ: Excerpta Medica; 1977:119–125.
36. Koch RL, Beaulieu BB Jr, Chrystal EJT, et al. A metronidazole metabolite in human urine and its risk. Science. 1981;211:398–400.
37. Beard CM, Noller KL, O'Fallon WM, et al. Lack of evidence for cancer due to use of metronidazole. N Engl J Med. 1979;301:519–522.
38. Friedman GD. Cancer after metronidazole (Letter). N Engl J Med. 1980;302:519.
39. Falagas ME, Walker AM, Ruthazer R, et al. Late incidence of cancer after metronidazole use: A matched metronidazole user/nonuser study. Clin Infect Dis. 1998;26:384–388.
40. Czeizel AE, Rockenbauer M. A population based case-control teratologic study of oral metronidazole treatment during pregnancy. Br J Obstet Gynecol. 1998;105:322–327.

41. Caro-Paton T, Carvajal A, Martin de Diego I, et al. Is metronidazole teratogenic? A meta-analysis. Br J Clin Pharmacol. 1997;44:179–182.
42. Bassily S, Farid Z, El-Masry NA, et al. Treatment of intestinal *E. histolytica* and *G. lamblia* with metronidazole, tinidazole and ornidazole: A comparative study. J Trop Med Hyg. 1987;90:9–12.
43. Nigam P, Kapoor KK, Kumar A, et al. Clinical profile of giardiasis and comparison of its therapeutic response to metronidazole and tinidazole. J Assoc Physicians India. 1991;39:613–615.
44. Narisi EM, Secor WE. In vitro effect of tinidazole and furazolidone on metronidazole-resistant *Trichomonas vaginalis*. Antimicrob Agents Chemother. 1996;40:1121–1125.
45. Gupta JP, Jain AK, Nanivadekar AS. Efficacy of tinidazole (Fasigyn) in giardiasis by parasitologic, biochemical, and gut transit studies. Indian J Gastroenterol. 1989;8:103–104.
46. Goldman P. The development of 5-nitroimidazoles for the treatment and prophylaxis of anaerobic bacterial infections. J Antimicrob Chemother. 1982;10(Suppl A):23–33.
47. Rossignol JF, Maisonneuve H, Cho YW. Nitroimidazoles in the treatment of trichomoniasis, giardiasis, and amebiasis. Int J Clin Pharmacol Ther Toxicol. 1984;22:63–72.
48. Simon M, Shookhoff HB, Terner H, et al. Paromomycin in the treatment of intestinal amebiasis: A short course of therapy. Am J Gastroenterol. 1967;48:504–511.
49. Soderman WA Jr. Amebiasis (Clinical Seminar). Am J Dig Dis. 1971;16:51–60.
50. Fichtenbaum CJ, Ritchie DJ, Powderly WG. Use of paromomycin for the treatment of crytosporidiosis in patients with AIDS. Clin Infect Dis. 1993;16:298–300.
51. Blanshard C, Shanson DC, Gazzard BG. Pilot studies of azithromycin, letrazuril and paromomycin in the treatment of cryptosporidiosis. Intern J STD AIDS. 1997;8:124–129.
52. Nyirjesy P, Sobel JD, Weitz MV, et al. Difficult-to-treat trichomoniasis: Results with paromomycin cream. Clin Infect Dis. 1998;26:986–988.
53. el-On J, Halevy S, Grunwald MH, et al. Topical treatment of old world cutaneous leishmaniasis caused by *Leishmania major*: A double-blind control study. J Am Acad Dermatol. 1992;27:227–231.
54. Berman JD. Human leishmaniasis: Clinical, diagnostic, and chemotherapeutic developments in the last 10 years. Clin Infect Dis. 1997;24:684–703.
55. Jha TK, Olliaro P, Thakur CP, et al. Randomised controlled trial of aminosidine (paromomycin) vs sodium stibogluconate for treating visceral leishmaniasis in North Bihar, India. BMJ. 1998;316:1200–1205.
56. Tan WW, Chapnick EK, Abter EI, et al. Paromomycin-asociated pancreatitis in HIV-related cryptosporidiosis. Ann Pharmacother. 1995;29:22–24.
57. Fisher AK, Walter FG, Szabo S. Iodoquinol associated seizures and radiopacity. J Toxicol Clin Toxicol. 1993;31:113–120.
58. Oakley GP Jr. The neurotoxicity of the halogenated hydroxyquinolines. JAMA. 1973;225:395–397.
59. Wolfe MS. The treatment of intestinal protozoal infections. Med Clin North Am. 1982;66:707–720.
60. Krogstad DJ, Spencer HC Jr, Healy GR. Amebiasis. N Engl J Med. 1978;298:262–265.
61. Pehrson P, Bengtsson E. Treatment of non-invasive amoebiasis: A comparison between tinidazole alone and in combination with diloxanide furoate. Trans R Soc Trop Med Hyg. 1983;77:845–846.
62. Wolfe MS. Nondysenteric intestinal amebiasis: Treatment with diloxanide furoate. JAMA. 1973;224:1601–1604.
63. Tracey JW, Webster LT Jr. Drugs used in the chemotherapy of protozoal infections: Trypanosomiasis, leishmaniasis, amebiasis, giardiasis, trichomoniasis, and other protozoal infections. In: Hardman JG, Limbird LE, eds. Goodman & Gilman's Pharmacological Basis of Therapeutics. 9th ed. New York: McGraw-Hill; 1996:987–1008.
64. Smith JW, Wolfe MS. Giardiasis. Annu Rev Med. 1980;31:373–383.
65. Craft JC, Murphy T, Nelson JD. Furizolidone and quinacrine: Comparative study of therapy for giardiasis in children. Am J Dis Child. 1981;135:164–166.
66. Dionision D, Manneschi LI, Di Lollo S, et al. *Enterocytozoon bieneusi* in AIDS: Symptomatic relief and parasite changes after furazolidone. J Clin Pathol. 1997;50:472–476.
67. White AH. Absorption, distribution, metabolism, and excretion of furazolidone: A review of the literature. Scand J Gastroenterol. 1989;169(Suppl):4–10.
68. Altamirano A, Bondani A. Adverse reactions to furazolidone and other drugs: A comparative review. Scand J Gastroenterol. 1989;169(Suppl): 70–80.
69. Elliott AM, Klaus BD, Morth DS, Martin HP. Furazolidone-induced mood disorder during treatment of refractory giardiasis in a patient with AIDS. Clin Infect Dis. 1998;26:1015.
70. Anonymous. World malaria situation in 1994. Part I–III. Wkly Epidemiol Rec. 1997;72:269–274, 277–283, 285–290.
71. White NJ. The treatment of malaria. N Engl J Med. 1996;335:800–806.
72. Kachur SP, Reller ME, Barber AM, et al. Malaria surveillance—United States, 1994. MMWR Morb Mortal Wkly Rep. 1997;46:1–18.
73. Lobel HO, Kozarsky PE. Update on prevention of malaria for travelers. JAMA. 1997;278:1767–1771.
74. Garly ML, Peterson E, Pedersen C, et al. Toxoplasmosis in Danish AIDS patients. Scand J Infect Dis. 1997;29:597–600.
75. Wong B, Gold JWM, Brown AE, et al. Central-nervous-system toxoplasmosis in homosexual men and parenteral drug abusers. Ann Intern Med. 1984;100:36–42.
76. Pozio E, Rezza G, Boschinin A, et al. Clinical cryptosporidiosis and human immunodeficiency virus (HIV)-induced immunosuppression: Findings from a longitudinal study of HIV-positive and HIV-negative former injection drug users. J Infect Dis 1997;176:969–975.
77. Morris RD, Naumova EN, Griffiths JK. Did Milwaukee experience waterborne cryptosporidiosis before the large documented outbreak in 1993? Epidemiology. 1998;9:264–270.
78. Herwaldt BL, Ackers ML. An outbreak in 1996 of cyclosporiasis associated with raspberries: The Cyclospora Working Group. N Engl J Med. 1997;336:1548–1556.
79. Centers for Disease Control and Prevention. Health Information for International Travel 1996. HHS publication no. (CDC) 97–8280. Washington DC, US Department of Health and Human Services, 1996.
80. Collignon P. Chloroquine resistance in *Plasmodium vivax*. J Infect Dis. 1991;164:222–223.
81. Schwartz IK, Lackritz EM, Patchen LC. Chloroquine-resistant *Plasmodium vivax* from Indonesia. N Engl J Med. 1991;324:927.
82. Marlar-Than, Myat-Phone-Kyam, Aly-Yu-Soe, et al. Development of resistance to chloroquin by *Plasmodium vivax* in Myanmar. Trans R Soc Trop Med Hyg. 1995;89:307–308.
83. Phillips EJ, Keystone JS, Kain KC. Failure of combined chloroquine and high-dose primaquine therapy for *Plasmodium vivax* malaria acquired in Guyana, South America. Clin Infect Dis. 1996;23:1171–1173.
84. Krogstad DJ, Herwaldt BL, Schlesinger PH. Antimalarial agents: Specific treatment regimens. Antimicrob Agents Chemother. 1988;32:957–961.
85. Brohult J, Rombo L, Sirleaf V, et al. The concentration of chloroquine in serum during short and long term malaria prophylaxis with standard and "double" dosage in non-immunes: Clinical implications. Ann Trop Med Parasitol 1979;73:401–405.
86. Tracey JW, Webster LT Jr. Drugs used in the chemotherapy of protozoal infections: Malaria. In: Hardman JG, Limbird LE, eds. Goodman and Gilman's Pharmacological Basis of Therapeutics. 9th ed. New York: McGraw-Hill; 1996:965–985.
87. Andrews P, Haberkorn A, Thomas H. Antiparasitic drugs: Mechanisms of action, pharmacokinetics, and in vitro and in vivo assays of drug activity. In: Lorian V, ed. Antibiotics in Laboratory Medicine. 2nd ed. Baltimore: Williams & Wilkins; 1986:282–345.
88. Warhurst DC. Antimalarial drugs: Mode of action and resistance. J Antimicrob Chemother. 1986;18(Suppl B):51–59.
89. Warhurst DC, Homewood CA, Baffaley VC. The chemotherapy of rodent malaria: XX. Autophagic vacuole formation in *Plasmodium berghei* in vitro. Ann Trop Med Parasitol. 1974;68:265–281.
90. Slater AFG, Cerami A. Inhibition by chloroquine of a novel heme polymerace enzyme activity in malaria trophozoites. Nature. 1992;355:167–169.
91. Krogstad DJ, Schlesinger PH. Acid-vesicle function, intracellular pathogens and the action of chloroquine against *Plasmodium falciparum*. N Engl J Med. 1987;317:542–549.
92. Foley M, Tilley L. Quinoline antimalarials: Mechanism of action and resistance. Int J Parasitol. 1997;27:231–240.
93. Kyle DE, Milhous WK, Rossan RN. Reversal of *Plasmodium falciparum* resistance to chloroquine in Panamanian *Aotus* monkeys. Am J Trop Med Hyg. 1993;48:126–133.
94. Martin SK, Oduola AMJ, Milhous WK. Reversal of chloroquine resistance in *Plasmodium falciparum* by verapamil. Science. 1987;235:899–901.
95. Marks JS. Chloroquine retinopathy: Is there a safe daily dose? Ann Rheum Dis. 1982;41:52–58.
96. White NJ, Watt G, Bergvist Y, et al. Parenteral chloroquine for treating falciparum malaria. J Infect Dis. 1987;155:192–201.
97. Clemessy JL, Taboulet P, Hoffman JR, et al. Treatment of acute chloroquine poisoning: A 5-year experience. Crit Care Med. 1996;24:1189–1195.
98. Hart CW, Naunton RF. The ototoxicity of chloroquine phosphate. Arch Otolaryngol. 1964;80:407–412.
99. Saxena AK, Saxena M. Advances in chemotherapy of malaria. Prog Drug Res. 1986;30:221–280.
100. Looareesuwan S, White NJ, Chittamas S, et al. High rate of *Plasmodium vivax* relapse following treatment of falciparum malaria in Thailand. Lancet 1987;2:1052–1055.
101. Arias AE, Corredor A. Low response rate of Columbian strains of *Plasmodium vivax* to classical antimalarial therapy. Trop Med Parasitol. 1989;40:21–23.
102. Luzzi GA, Warrell DA, Barnes AJ, et al. Treatment of primaquine resistant *Plasmodium vivax* malaria. Lancet. 1992;340:310.
103. Looareesuwan S, Buchachart K, Wilairatanan P, et al. Primaquine-tolerant vivax malaria in Thailand. Ann Trop Med Parasitol. 1997;91:939–943.
104. Smoak BL, DeFraites RF, Magill AJ, et al. *Plasmodium vivax* infections in U.S. Army troops: Failure of primaquine to prevent relapse in studies from Somalia. Am J Trop Med Hyg. 1997;56:231–234.
105. Collins WE, Jeffery GM. Primaquine resistance in *Plasmodium vivax*. Am J Trop Med Hyg. 1996;55:243–249.
106. Safrin S, Finkelstein DM, Feinberg J, et al. Comparison of three regimens for treatment of mild to moderate *Pneumocystis carinii* pneumonia in patients with AIDS: A double-blind, randomized trial of oral trimethoprim-sulfamethoxazole, dapsone-trimethoprim, and clindamycin-primaquine. ACTG 108 Study Group. Ann Intern Med. 1996;124:792–802.
107. Barber BA, Pegram PS, High KP. Clindamycin/primaquine as prophylaxis for *Pneumonocystis carinii* pneumonia. Clin Infect Dis. 1996;23:718–722.
108. Hiebsch RR, Raub TJ, Wattenberg BW. Primaquine blocks transport by inhibiting the formation of functional transport vesicles. J Biol Chem. 1991;266:20323–20328.
109. Kellermeyer RW, Tarlov AR, Brewer GJ, et al. Hemolytic effect of therapeutic

drugs: Clinical considerations of the primaquine-type hemolysis. JAMA. 1962;180:388–394.

110. Clyde DF. Clinical problems associated with the use of primaquine as a tissue schizontocidal and gametocytocidal drug. Bull World Health Organ. 1981;59:391–395.

111. Alving AS, Johnson CF, Tarlov AR, et al. Mitigation of the haemolytic effect of primaquine and enhancement of its action against exoerythrocytic forms of the Chesson strain of *Plasmodium vivax* by intermittent regimens of drug administration: A preliminary report. Bull World Health Organ. 1960;22:621–631.

112. Sin DD, Shafran SD. Dapsone- and primaquine-induced methemoglobinemia in HIV-infected individuals. J Acquir Immune Defic Syndr Hum Retrovirol. 1996;12:477–481.

113. Brasseur P, Kouamouo J, Moyou-Somo R, et al. Multi-drug resistant falciparum malaria in Cameroon in 1987–1988: I. Stable figures of prevalence of chloroquine- and quinine-resistant isolates in the original foci. Am J Trop Med Hyg. 1992;46:1–7.

114. Lege-Oguntoye L, Abua JU, Werblinska B, et al. Chloroquine-resistant *Plasmodium falciparum* with reduced sensitivity in vitro to mefloquine and quinine in Zaria, Northern Nigeria. J Trop Med Hyg. 1991;94:73–75.

115. Anonymous. Treatment of severe *Plasmodium falciparum* malaria with quinidine gluconate: Discontinuation of quinine from the CDC drug service. MMWR Morb Mortal Wkly Rep. 1991;40:240–241.

116. Brodie BB, Baer JE, Craig LC. Metabolic products of the cinchona alkaloids in human urine. J Biol Chem. 1951;188:567–581.

117. White NJ, Looareesuwan S, Warrell DA, et al. Quinine pharmacokinetics and toxicity in cerebral and uncomplicated falciparum malaria. Am J Med. 1982;73:564–572.

118. Krishna S, White NJ. Pharmacokinetics of quinine, chloroquine and amodiaquine: Clinical implications. Clin Pharmacokinet. 1996;30:263–299.

119. Canfield CJ, Miller LH, Bartelloni PJ, et al. Acute renal failure in *Plasmodium falciparum* malaria. Arch Intern Med. 1968;122:199–203.

120. Punukollu RC, Kumar S, Mullen KD. Quinine hepatotoxicity: An underrecognized or rare phenomenon? Arch Intern Med. 1990;150:1112–1113.

121. Mathur S, Dooley J, Scheuer PJ. Quinine induced granulomatous hepatitis and vasculitis. BMJ. 1990;300:613.

122. White JN, Warrell DA, Chanthavanich P, et al. Severe hypoglycemia and hyperinsulinemia in falciparum malaria. N Engl J Med. 1983;309:61–66.

123. Phillips RE, Looareesuwan S, White NJ, et al. Quinine pharmacokinetics and toxicity in pregnant and lactating women with falciparum malaria. Br J Clin Pharmacol. 1986;21:677–683.

124. Phillips RE, Warrell DA, White NJ, et al. Intravenous quinidine for the treatment of severe falciparum malaria. N Engl J Med. 1985;312:1273–1278.

125. Rudnitsky G, Miller KD, Padua T, et al. Continuous-infusion quinidine gluconate for treating children with severe *Plasmodium falciparum* malaria. J Infect Dis. 1987;155:1040–1043.

126. Miller KD, Greenberg AE, Campbell CC. Treatment of severe malaria in the United States with a continuous infusion of quinidine gluconate and exchange transfusion. N Engl J Med. 1989;321:65–70.

127. Swerdlow CD, Yu JO, Jacobsen E, et al. Safety and efficacy of intravenous quinidine. Am J Med. 1983;75:36–42.

128. Botero D, Restrepo M, Montoya A. Prospective double-blind trial of two different doses of mefloquine plus pyrimethamine-sulfadoxine compared with pyrimethamine-sulfadoxine alone in the treatment of falciparum malaria. Bull World Health Organ. 1985;63:731–737.

129. De Sousa JM, Sheth UK, Oliveira RMG, et al. An open, randomized, phase III clinical trial of mefloquine and of quinine plus sulfadoxime-pyrimethamine in the treatment of symptomatic falciparum malaria in Brazil. Bull World Health Organ. 1985;63:603–609.

130. Tin F, Hlaing N, Tun T, et al. Falciparum malaria treated with a fixed combination of mefloquine, sulfadoxine and pyrimethamine: A field study in adults in Burma. Bull World Health Organ. 1985;63:727–730.

131. Nosten F, Price RN. New antimalarials: A risk-benefit analysis. Drug Saf. 1995;12:264–273.

132. Oduola AM, Sowunmi A, Milhous WK, et al. Innate resistance to new antimalarial drugs in *Plasmodium falciparum* from Nigeria. Trans R Soc Trop Med Hyg. 1992;86:123–126.

133. Wongsrichanalai C, Webster HK, Wimonwattrawatee T, et al. Emergence of multidrug-resistant *Plasmodium falciparum* in Thailand: In vitro tracking. Am J Trop Med Hyg. 1992;47:112–116.

134. Hopperus Buma AP, van Thiel PP, Hobel HO, et al. Long-term malaria chemoprophylaxis with mefloquine in Dutch marines in Cambodia. J Infect Dis. 1996;173:1506–1509.

135. Nosten F, ter Kuile F, Chongsuphajaisiddhi T, et al. Mefloquine-resistant falciparum malaria on the Thai-Burmese border. Lancet. 1991;337:1140–1143.

136. Brasseur P, Kouamouo J, Moyou-Somo R, et al. Multi-drug resistant falciparum malaria in Cameroon in 1987–1988: II. Mefloquine resistance confirmed in vitro and in vivo and its correlation with quinine resistance. Am J Trop Med Hyg. 1992;46:8–14.

137. Oduola AMJ, Milhous WK, Salako LA, et al. Reduced in-vitro susceptibility to mefloquine in West African isolates of *Plasmodium falciparum*. Lancet. 1987;2:1304–1305.

138. Desjardins RW, Pamplin CL III, von Bredow J, et al. Kinetics of a new antimalarial, mefloquine. Clin Pharmacol Ther. 1979;26:372–379.

139. Jacobs GH, Aikawa M, Milhous WK, et al. An ultrastructural study of the effects of mefloquine on malaria parasite. Am J Trop Med Hyg. 1987;36:9–14.

140. Chanthavanich P, Looareesuwan S, White NJ, et al. Intragastric mefloquine is absorbed rapidly in patients with cerebral malaria. Am J Trop Med Hyg. 1985;34:1028–1036.

141. Weinke T, Trautmann M, Held T, et al. Neuropsychiatric side effects after the use of mefloquine. Am J Trop Med Hyg. 1991;45:86–91.

142. Barrett PJ, Emmins PD, Clarke PD, et al. Comparison of adverse events associated with use of mefloquine and combination of chloroquine and proguanil as antmalarial prophylaxis: Postal and telephone survey of travellers. BMJ. 1996;313:525–528.

143. Croft AM, Clayton TC, World MJ. Side effects of mefloquine prophylaxis for malaria: An independent randomized controlled trial. Trans R Soc Trop Med. 1997;91:199–203.

144. Olson PE, Kennedy CA, Morte PD. Parasthesias and mefloquine prophylaxis. Ann Intern Med. 1992;117:1058–1059.

145. Van den Enden E, Gompel AV, Colebunders R, et al. Mefloquine induced Stevens-Johnson syndrome. Lancet. 1991;337:683.

146. Hennequin C, Bouree P, Halfon P. Agranulocytosis during treatment with mefloquine. Lancet. 1991;337:984.

147. Martin GJ, Malone JL, Ross EV. Exfoliative dermatitis during malarial prophylaxis with mefloquine. Clin Infect Dis. 1993;16:341.

148. White AC Jr, Gard DA, Sessoms SL. Cutaneous vasculitis associated with mefloquine. Ann Intern Med. 1995;123:894.

149. Horowitz H, Carbonaro CA. Inhibition of *Salmonella typhi* oral vaccine strain, Ty21a, by mefloquine and chloroquine. J Infect Dis. 1992;166:1462–1464.

150. Vanhauwere B, Maradit H, Kerr L. Post-marketing surveillance of prophylactic mefloquine (Lariam) use in pregnancy. Am J Trop Med Hyg. 1998;58:17–21.

151. Schlagenhauf P, Lobel H, Steffen R, et al. Tolerance of mefloquine by Swiss Air trainee pilots. Am J Trop Med Hyg. 1997;56:235–240.

152. Hien TT, White NJ. Qinghaosu. Lancet. 1993;341:603–607.

153. Tran TH, Day NP, Nguyen HP, et al. A controlled trial of artemether or quinine in Vietnamese adults with severe falciparum malaria. N Engl J Med. 1996;335:76–83.

153a. Seaton RA, Trevett AJ, Wembri JP, et al. Randomized comparison of intramuscular artemether and intravenous quinine in adult, Melanesian patients with severe or complicated *Plasmodium falciparum* malaria in Papua New Guinea. Ann Trop Med Parasitol. 1998;92:133–139.

154. Wilairatana P, Viriyavejakul P, Looareesuwan S, et al. Artesunate suppositories: An effective treatment for severe falciparum malaria in rural areas. Ann Trop Med Parasitol. 1997;91:891–896.

155. Meshnick SR, Taylor TE, Kamchonwongpaisan S. Artemisinin and the antimalarial endoperoxides: From herbal remedy to targeted chemotherapy. Microbiol Rev. 1996;60:301–315.

156. Batty KT, Thu LT, Davis TM, et al. A pharmacokinetic and pharmacodynamic study of intravenous vs oral artesunate in uncomplicated malaria. Br J Clin Pharmacol. 1998;45:123–129.

157. Warshaw EM, Zug KA. Sesquiterpene lactone allergy. Am J Contact Dermat. 1996;7:1–23.

158. Miller LG, Panosian CB. Ataxia and slurred speech after artesunate treatment for falciparum malaria. N Engl J Med. 1997;336:1328.

159. Brewer TG, Grate SJ, Peggins JO, et al. Fatal neurotoxicity of arteether and artemether. Am J Trop Med Hyg. 1994;51:251–259.

160. Basco LA, Le Bras J. In vitro activity of artemisinin derivatives against African isolates and clones of *Plasmodium falciparum*. Am J Trop Med Hyg. 1993;49:301–307.

161. Meek SR, Doberstyn EB, Gaüzère BA, et al. Treatment of falciparum malaria with quinine and tetracycline or combined mefloquine/sulfadoxine/pyrimethamine on the Thai-Kampuchean border. Am J Trop Med Hyg. 1986;35:246–250.

162. Lobel HO, Kozarsky PE. Update on prevention of malaria for travelers. JAMA. 1997;278:1767–1771.

163. Ohrt C, Richie TL, Widjaja H, et al. Mefloquine compared with doxycycline for the prophylaxis of malaria in Indonesian soldiers: A randomized, double-blind, placebo-controlled trial. Ann Intern Med. 1997;126:963–972.

164. Bryson HM, Goa KL. Halofantrine: A review of its antimalarial activity, pharmacokinetic properties and therapeutic potential. Drugs. 1992;43:236–258.

165. Touze JE, Fourcade L, Peyron F, et al. Is halofantrine still advisable in malaria attacks? Am Trop Med Parasitol. 1997;91:867–873.

166. Matson PA, Luby SP, Redd SC, et al. Cardiac effects of standard-dose halofantrine therapy. Am J Trop Med Hyg. 1996;54:229–231.

167. Pape JW, Verdier RI, Johnson WD. Treatment and prophylaxis of *Isospora belli* infection in patients with the acquired immunodeficiency syndrome. N Engl J Med. 1989;320:1044–1047.

168. Luft BJ, Conley F, Remington JS. Outbreak of central-nervous-system toxoplasmosis in Western Europe and North America. Lancet. 1983;1:781–784.

169. Haverkos HW. Assessment of therapy for toxoplasma encephalitis: The TE study group. Am J Med. 1987;82:907–914.

170. Luft BJ, Remington JS. Toxoplasmic encephalitis. J Infect Dis. 1988;157:1–6.

171. Deresinski SC. Treatment of *Pneumocystis carinii* pneumonia in adults with AIDS. Semin Respir Infect. 1997;12:79–97.

172. Ioannidis JP, Cappelleri JC, Skolnik PR, et al. A meta-analysis of the relative efficacy and toxicity of *Pneumocystis carinii* prophylactic regimens. Arch Intern Med. 1996;156:177–188.

173. Kovacs JA, Allegra CJ, Chabner BA, et al. Potent effect of trimetrexate, a lipid-soluble antifolate, on *Toxoplasma gondii*. J Infect Dis. 1987;155:1027–1032.

174. Wang P, Read M, Sims PF, et al. Sulfadoxine resistance in the human malaria parasite *Plasmodium falciparum* is determined by mutations in dihydropteroate synthetase and an additional factor associated with folate utilization. Mol Microbiol. 1997;23:979–986.

175. Luft BJ, Hafner R, Korzun AH, et al. Toxoplasmic encephalitis in patients with the acquired immunodeficiency syndrome: Members of the ACTG077p/ANRS009 Study Team. N Engl J Med. 1993;329:995–1000.
176. Kovacs JA. Efficacy of atovaquone in treatment of toxoplasmosis in patients with AIDS: The NIAID-Clinical Center Intramural AIDS Program. Lancet. 1992;340:637–638.
177. Anonymous. 1997 USPHS/IDSA guidelines for the prevention of opportunistic infections in persons infected with human immunodeficiency virus: Disease-specific recommendations. USPHS/IDSA Prevention of Opportunistic Infections Working Group. Clin Infect Dis. 1997;25(Suppl 3):S313–S315.
178. Daffos F, Forestier F, Capella-Pavlovsky M, et al. Prenatal management of 746 pregnancies at risk for congenital toxoplasmosis. N Engl J Med. 1988;318:271–275.
179. Weidekamm E, Plozza-Nottebrock H, Forgo I, et al. Plasma concentrations of pyrimethamine and sulfadoxine and evaluation of pharmacokinetic data by computerized curve fitting. Bull World Health Organ. 1982;60:115–122.
180. Jaffe JJ. Dihydrofolate reductase in parasitic protozoa and helminths. In: Van den Bossche H, ed. Biochemistry of Parasites. London: Academic Press; 1972:219–233.
181. Hayama T, Kokue E. Use of the Goettingen miniature pig for studying pyrimethamine teratogenesis. Crit Rev Toxicol. 1985;14:403–421.
182. Petter C, Bourbon J. Foetal red cell macrocytosis induced by pyrimethamine: Its teratogenic role. Experientia. 1975;31:369–370.
183. Pyrimethamine combinations in pregnancy. Lancet. 1983;2:1005–1007.
184. Harpey JP, Darbois Y, LeFèbvre G. Teratogenicity of pyrimethamine (Letter). Lancet. 1983;2:399.
185. Miller KD, Lobel HO, Satriale RF, et al. Severe cutaneous reactions among American travelers using pyrimethamine-sulfadoxine (Fansidar) for malaria prophylaxis. Am J Trop Med Hyg. 1986;35:451–458.
186. Navin TR, Miller KD, Satriale RF, et al. Adverse reactions associated with pyrimethamine-sulfadoxine prophylaxis for *Pneumocystis carinii* infections in AIDS (Letter). Lancet. 1985;1:1332.
187. Jick H. Adverse reactions to trimethoprim-sulfamethoxazole in hospitalized patients. Rev Infect Dis. 1982;4:426–428.
188. Pratt WB, Fekety R. The antimetabolites. In: The Antimicrobical Drugs. New York: Oxford University Press; 1986:229–251.
189. Gordin FM, Simon GL, Wofsy CB, et al. Adverse reactions to trimethoprim-sulfamethoxazole in patients with the acquired immunodeficiency syndrome. Ann Intern Med. 1984;100:495–499.
190. Small CB, Harris CA, Friedland GH, et al. The treatment of *Pneumocystis carinii* pneumonia in the acquired immunodeficiency syndrome. Arch Intern Med. 1985;145:837–840.
191. Cook GC. Prevention and treatment of malaria. Lancet. 1988;1:32–37.
192. Begbie S, Burgess KR. Maloprim-induced pulmonary eosinophilia. Chest. 1993;103:305–306.
193. Rollo IM. The mode of action of sulphonamides, proguanil and pyrimethamine on *Plasmodium gallinaceum*. Br J Pharmacol Chemother. 1955;10:208–214.
194. Barnes AJ, Ong ELC, Dunbar EM, et al. Failure of chloroquine and proguanil prophylaxis in travellers to Kenya. Lancet. 1991;338:1338–1339.
195. Lell B, Lucner D, Ndjave M, et al. Randomised placebo-controlled study of atovaquone plus proguanil for malaria prophylaxis in children. Lancet. 1998;351:709–713.
196. Gay F, Bustos D, Traore B, et al. In vitro response of *Plasmodium falciparum* to atovaquone and correlation with other antimalarials: Comparison between African and Asian strains. Am J Trop Med Hyg. 1997;56:315–317.
197. de Alencar FE, Cerutti C Jr, Durlacher RR, et al. Atovaquone and proguanil for the treatment of malaria in Brazil. J Infect Dis. 1997;175:1544–1547.
198. Ericksson B, Bjorkman A, Keisu M. How safe is proguanil? A post-marketing investigation of side effects. Scand J Infect Dis. 1991;23:489–493.
199. Hudson AT. Atovaquone: A novel broad-spectrum anti-infective drug. Parasitol Today. 1993;9:66.
200. Chiodini PL, Conlon CP, Hutchinson DB, et al. Evaluation of atovaquone in the treatment of patients with uncomplicated *Plasmodium falciparum* malaria. J Antimicrob Chemother. 1995;36:1073–1078.
201. Anonymous. Atovaquone for *Pneumocystis* pneumonia. Med Lett Drugs Ther. 1993;35:28–29.
202. Araujo FG, Lin T, Remington JS. The activity of atovaquone (566C80) in murine toxoplasmosis is markedly augmented when used in combination with pyrimethamine or sulfadiazine. J Infect Dis. 1993;167:494–497.
203. Katlama C, Mouthon B, Gourdon D, et al. Atovaquone as long-term suppressive therapy for toxoplasmic encephalitis in patients with AIDS and multiple drug intolerance: Atovaquone Expanded Access Group. AIDS. 1996;10:1107–1112.
204. Behbahani R, Moshfeghi M, Baxter JD. Therapeutic approaches for AIDS-related toxoplasmosis. Ann Pharmacol. 1995;29:760–768.
205. Danneman B, McCutchan A, Isrealski D, et al. Treatment of toxoplasmic encephalitis in patients with AIDS: A randomized trial comparing pyrimethamine plus clindamycin to pyrimethamine plus sulfadiazine. Ann Intern Med. 1992;116:33.
206. Lakhanpal V, Schocket SS, Nirankari VS. Clindamycin in the treatment of toxoplasmic retinochoroiditis. Am J Ophthalmol. 1983;95:605–613.
207. Ferguson JG Jr. Clindamycin therapy for toxoplasmosis. Ann Ophthalmol. 1981;13:95–100.
208. Anonymous. Clindamycin and quinine treatment for *Babesia microti* infections. MMWR Morb Mortal Wkly Rep. 1983;32:65–66.
209. Vergani P, Ghidini A, Ceruti P, et al. Congenital toxoplasmosis: Efficacy of maternal treatment with spiramycin alone. Am J Reprod Immunol. 1998;39:335–340.
210. Mombro M, Perathoner C, Leone A, et al. Congenital toxoplasmosis: 10-Year follow-up. Eur J Pediatr. 1995;154:645–649.
211. Stramba-Badiale M, Nador F, Porta N, et al. QT interval prolongation and risk of life-threatening arrhythmias during toxoplasmosis prophylaxis with spiramycin in neonates. Am Heart J. 1997;133:108–111.
212. Nasta P, Chiodera S. Azithromycin for relapsing cerebral toxoplasmosis in AIDS. AIDS. 1997;11:1188.
213. Chang HR. The potential role of azithromycin in the treatment or prophylaxis of toxoplasmosis. Int J STD AIDS. 1996;4(Suppl 1):18–22.
214. Anderson SL, Berman J, Kuschner R, et al. Prophylaxis of *Plasmodium falciparum* malaria with azithromycin administered to volunteers. Ann Intern Med. 1995;123:771–773.
215. Andersen SL, Oloo AJ, Goron DM, et al. Successful double-blinded, randomized, placebo-controlled field trial of azithromycin and doxycycline as prophylaxis for malaria in western Kenya. Clin Infect Dis. 1998;26:146–150.
216. Pepin J, Milord F. The treatment of human African trypanosomiasis. Adv Parasitol. 1994;33:1–47.
217. Fairlamb AH, Bowman IB. *Trypanosoma brucei*: Suramin and other trypanocidal compounds. Effects on *sn*-glycerol-3 phosphate oxidase. Exp Parasitol. 1977;43:353–361.
218. Anderson J, Fuglsang H, de C Marshall TF. Effects of suramin on ocular onchocerciasis. Tropenmed Parasitol. 1976;27:279–296.
219. Carter NS, Fairlamb AH. Arsenical-resistant trypanosomes lack an unusual adenosine transporter. Nature. 1993;361:173–175.
220. Flynn IW, Bowman IBR. Further studies on the mode of arsenicals on trypanosome pyruvate kinase (Abstract). Trans R Soc Trop Med Hyg. 1969;63:121.
221. Robertson DHH. Chemotherapy of African trypanosomes. Practitioner. 1962;188:80–83.
222. Arrox JOL. Melarsoprol and reactive encephalopathy in *Trypanosoma brucei rhodesiense*. Trans R Soc Trop Med Hyg. 1987;81:192.
223. Pepin J, Milord F, Khonde AN, et al. Risk factors for encephalopathy and mortality during melarsoprol treatment of *Trypanosoma brucei gambiense* sleeping sickness. Trans R Soc Trop Med Hyg. 1995;89:92–97.
224. Pepin J, Milord F. African trypanosomiasis and drug induced encephalopathy: Risk factors and pathogenesis. Trans R Soc Trop Med Hyg. 1991;85:222–224.
225. Gherardi RK, Chariot P, Vanderstigel M, et al. Organic arsenic induced Guillain-Barré–like syndrome due to melarsoprol: A clinical, electrophysiological and pathological study. Muscle Nerve. 1990;13:637–645.
226. Taelman H, Schechter PJ, Marcelis L, et al. Difluoromethylornithine: An effective new treatment of Gambian trypanosomiasis. Am J Med. 1987;82:607–614.
227. Di Bari C, Pastore G, Roscigno G, et al. Late-stage African trypanosomiasis and eflornithine (Letter). Ann Intern Med. 1986;105:803–804.
228. Van Nieuwenhove S, Schechter PJ, Declercg J, et al. Treatment of gambiense sleeping sickness in the Sudan with oral DFMO (DL-α-difluoromethylornithine), an inhibitor of ornithine decarboxylase: First field trial. Trans R Soc Trop Med Hyg. 1985;79:692–698.
229. Milord F, Pepin J, Loko L, et al. Efficacy and toxicity of eflornithine for treatment of *Trypanosoma brucei gambiense* sleeping sickness. Lancet. 1992;340:652–655.
230. Politi C, Carrin G, Evans D, et al. Cost-effectiveness analysis of alternative treatments of African gambiense trypanosomiasis in Uganda. Health Econ. 1995;4:273–287.
231. Bacchi CJ, Nathan HC, Livingston T, et al. Differential susceptibility to DL-α-difluoromethylornithine in clinical isolates of *Trypanosoma brucei rhodesiense*. Antimicrob Agents Chemother. 1990;34:1183–1188.
232. Marr JJ, Docampo R. Chemotherapy for Chagas' disease: A perspective of current therapy and considerations for future research. Rev Infect Dis. 1986;8:884–903.
233. Docampo R, Morena SNJ. Free radical metabolites in the mode of action of chemotherapeutic agents and phagocytic cells on *Trypanosoma cruzi*. Rev Infect Dis. 1984;6:223–238.
234. Pepin J, Milord F, Mpia B, et al. An open clinical trial of nifurtimox for arseno-resistant *Trypanosoma brucei gambiense* sleeping sickness in Zaire. Trans R Soc Trop Med Hyg. 1989;83:514–517.
235. Pepin J, Milord F, Meurice F, et al. High-dose nifurtimox for arseno-resistant *Trypanosoma brucei gambiense* sleeping sickness: An open trial in central Zaire. Trans R Soc Trop Med Hyg. 1992;86:254–256.
236. Paulos C, Paredes J, Vasquez I, et al. Pharmacokinetics of a nitrofuran compound, nifurtimox, in healthy volunteers. Int J Clin Pharmacol Ther Toxicol. 1989;27:454–457.
237. Moreno SNJ, Palmero DJ, de Palmero KE, et al. Stimulation of lipid peroxidation and ultrastructural alterations by nifurtimox in mammalian tissues. Medicina (B Aires). 1980;40:553–559.
238. Apt W, Arribada A, Arab F, et al. Clinical trial of benznidazole and an immunopotentiator against Chagas' disease in Chile (Letter). Trans R Soc Trop Med Hyg. 1986;80:1010.
239. de Andrade AL, Zicker E, de Oliveira RM, et al. Randomised trial of efficacy of benznidazole in treatment of early *Trypanosoma cruzi* infection. Lancet. 1996;1407–1413.
240. Coura JR, de Abreu LL, Willcox HP, et al. [Comparative controlled study on the use of benznidazole, nifurtimox and placebo, in the chronic form of Chagas' disease, in a field area with interrupted transmission: I. Preliminary evaluation.] Rev Soc Bras Med Trop. 1997;30:139–144.
241. Pearson RD, Navin TR, Sousa AQ, et al. Leishmaniasis. In: Kass EH, Platt R, eds. Current Therapy in Infectious Diseases. Toronto: BC Decker; 1990: 384–389.
242. Anabwani GM, Ngira JA, Dimiti G, et al. Comparison of two dosage schedules of

sodium stibogluconate in the treatment of visceral leishmaniasis in Kenya. Lancet. 1983;1:210–212.

243. Report of a WHO Expert Committee. The leishmaniases: WHO Technical Report Series 701. Geneva: World Health Organization; 1984.
244. Ballou WR, McClain JB, Gordon DM, et al. Safety and efficacy of high-dose sodium stibogluconate therapy of American cutaneous leishmaniasis. Lancet. 1987;2:13–16.
245. Grogl M, Thomason TN, Franke ED. Drug resistance in leishmaniasis: Its implications in systemic chemotherapy of cutaneous and mucocutaneous disease. Am J Trop Med Hyg. 1992;47:117–126.
246. Badaro R, Johnson WJ. The role of interferon gamma in the treatment of visceral and diffuse cutaneous leishmaniasis. J Infect Dis. 1993;167(Suppl 1): S13–S17.
247. Harms G, Zwingenberger K, Sandkamp B, et al. Immunotherapy of visceral leishmaniasis: A pilot trial of sequential treatment with recombinant interferon-gamma and pentavalent antimony. J Interferon Res. 1993;13:39–41.
248. Bottasso O, Cabrini J, Falcoff R. Successful treatment of an antimony-resistant American mucocutaneous leishmaniasis: A case report. Arch Dermatol. 1992;128:996–997.
249. Chulay JD, Fleckenstein L, Smith DH. Pharmacokinetics of antimony during treatment of visceral leishmaniasis with sodium stibogluconate or meglumine antimonate. Trans R Soc Trop Med Hyg. 1988;82:69–72.
250. Berman JD. Human leishmaniasis: Clinical, diagnostic, and chemotherapeutic developments in the last 10 years. Clin Infect Dis. 1997;24:684–703.
251. Herwaldt BL, Berman JD. Recommendations for treating leishmaniasis with sodium stibogluconate (Pentostam) and review of pertinent clinical studies. Am J Trop Med Hyg. 1992;46:296–306.
252. Donovan KL, White AD, Cooke DA, et al. Pancreatitis and palindromic arthropathy with effusions associated with sodium stibogluconate treatment in a renal transplant recipient. J Infect. 1990;21:107–110.
253. Halim MA, Alfurayh O, Kalin ME, et al. Successful treatment of visceral leishmaniasis with allopurinol plus ketoconazole in a renal transplant recipient after the occurrence of pancreatitis due to stibogluconate. Clin Infect Dis. 1993;16:397–399.
254. Marr JJ, Berens RL. Pyrazolopyrimidine metabolism in the pathogenic trypanosomatides. Mol Biochem Parasitol. 1983;7:339–356.
255. Neal RA, Croft SL, Nelson DJ. Anti-leishmanial effect of allopurinol ribonucleoside and the related compounds, allopurinol, thiopurinol, thiopurinol ribonucleoside, and of formycin B, sinefungin and the lepidine WR 6026. Trans R Soc Trop Med Hyg. 1985;79:122–128.
256. Kager PA, Rees PH, Wellde BT, et al. Allopurinol in the treatment of visceral leishmaniasis. Trans R Soc Trop Med Hyg. 1981;75:556–559.
257. Croft SL, Neal RA. The effect of allopurinol ribonucleoside and formycin B on *Trypanosoma cruzi* infections in mice. Trans R Soc Trop Med Hyg. 1985;79: 517–518.
258. Martinez S, Marr JJ. Allpurinol in the treatment of American cutaneous leishmaniasis. N Engl J Med. 1992;326:741–744.
259. Herwaldt BL, Neva FA, Berman JD. Allopurinol in the treatment of American cutaneous leishmaniasis. N Engl J Med. 1992;327:498–499.
260. Mishra M, Biswas UK, Jha DN, et al. Amphotericin versus pentamidine in antimony-unresponsive kala-azar. Lancet. 1992;340:1256–1257.
261. Thakur CP, Sinha GP, Pandey AK, et al. Daily versus alternate-day regimen of amphotericin B in the treatment of kala-azar: A randomized comparison. Bull World Health Organ. 1994;72:931–936.
262. Torre-Cisneros J, Villanueva JL, Kindelan JM, et al. Successful treatment of antimony-resistant visceral leishmaniasis with liposomal amphotericin B in patients infected with human immunodeficiency virus. Clin Infect Dis. 1993;17:625–627.
263. Gokhale PC, Kshiragar NA, Khan MU, et al. Successful treatment of resistant visceral leishmaniasis with liposomal amphotericin B. Trans R Soc Trop Med Hyg. 1994;88:228.
264. Davidson RN, di Martino L, Gradoni L, et al. Liposomal amphotericin B (AmBisome) in Mediterranean visceral leishmaniasis: A multi-centre trial. Q J Med. 1994;87:75–81.
265. di Martiono L, Ramondi F, Scotti S, et al. Efficacy and tolerability of liposomal amphotericin B in Italian infants with visceral leishmaniasis. Trans R Soc Trop Med Hyg. 1993;87:477.
266. Seaman J, Boer C, Wilkerson R, et al. Liposomal amphotericin B (AmBisome) in the treatment of complicated kala-azar under field conditions. Clin Infect Dis. 1995;21:188–193.
267. Sundar S, Agrawal, NK, Sinha PR, et al. Short-course, low-dose amphotericin B lipid complex therapy for visceral leishmaniasis unresponsive to antimony. Ann Intern Med. 1997;127:133–137.
268. Berman JD, Ksionski G, Chapman WL, et al. Activity of amphotericin B cholesterol dispersion (Amphocil) in experimental visceral leishmaniasis. Antimicrob Agents Chemother. 1992;36:1978–1980.
269. Saenz RE, Paz H, Berman JD. Efficacy of ketoconazole against *Leishmania braziliensis panamensis* cutaneous leishmaniasis. Am J Med. 1990;89:147–155.
270. Navin TR, Arana BA, Arana FA, et al. Placebo-controlled clinical trial of sodium stibogluconate (Pentostam) versus ketoconazole for treating cutaneous leishmaniasis in Guatemala. J Infect Dis. 1992;165:528–534.
271. Wali JP, Aggarwal P, Gupta U, et al. Ketoconazole in the treatment of antimony- and pentamidine-resistant kala-azar. J Infect Dis. 1992;166:215–216.
272. Wali JP, Aggarwal P, Gupta U, et al. Ketoconazole in treatment of visceral leishmaniasis. Lancet. 1990;336:810–811.
273. Sundar S, Kumar K, Singh VP. Ketoconazole in visceral leishmaniasis. Lancet. 1990;336:1582.
274. Piałoux G, Hennequin C, Dupont B, et al. Cutaneous leishmaniasis in an AIDS patient: Cure with itraconazole. J Infect Dis. 1990;162:1221–1222.
275. Dogra J, Aneja N, Behari Lal B, et al. Cutaneous leishmaniasis in India: Clinical experience with itraconazole (R51 211 Janssen). Int J Dermatol. 1990;29:661–662.
276. Albanese G, Giorgetti P, Santagostino L, et al. Cutaneous leishmaniasis: Treatment with itraconazole. Arch Dermatol. 1989;125:1540–1542.
277. Akuffo H, Dietz M, Teklemariam S, et al. The use of itraconazole in the treatment of leishmaniasis caused by *Leishmania aethiopica*. Trans R Soc Trop Med Hyg. 1990;84:532–534.
278. Al-Fouzan AS, Al Saleh QA, Najeem NM, et al. Cutaneous leishmaniasis in Kuwait: Clinical experience with itraconazole. Int J Dermatol. 1991;30:519–521.
279. Guderian RH, Chico ME, Rogers MD, et al. Placebo controlled treatment of Ecuadorian cutaneous leishmaniasis. Am J Trop Med Hyg. 1991;45:92–97.
280. Doua F, Miezan TW, Sanon Singaro JR, et al. The efficacy of pentamidine in the treatment of early-late stage *Trypanosoma brucei gambiense* trypanosomiasis. Am J Trop Med Hyg. 1996;55:586–588.
281. Pepin J, Khonde N. Relapses following treatment of early-stage *Trypanosoma brucei gambiense* sleeping sickness with a combination of pentamidine and suramin. Trans R Soc Trop Med Hyg. 1996;90:183–186.
282. Jha TK. Evaluation of diamidine compound (pentamidine isethionate) in the treatment of resistant cases of kala-azar occurring in North Bihar, India. Trans R Soc Trop Med Hyg. 1983;77:167–170.
283. Kager PA, Rees PH, Manguyu FM, et al. Clinical and haematological and parasitological response to treatment of visceral leishmaniasis. Trop Geogr Med. 1984;36:21–35.
284. Lustig V, Karger PA, Meenhorst PL. Treatment of visceral leishmaniasis in a patient with AIDS with antimony and gamma-interferon: Remission and prevention of relapse by maintenance therapy with weekly pentamidine. Neth. J Med. 1995;47:66–69.
285. Perez-Molina JA, Lopez-Velez R, Montilla P, et al. Pentamidine isethionate as secondary prophylaxis against visceral leishmaniasis in HIV-positive patients. AIDS. 1996;10:237–238.
286. Deresinski SC. Treatment of *Pneumocystis carinii* pneuomonia in adults with AIDS. Semin Respir Dis. 1997;12:79–97.
287. Bozzette SA, Finkelstein DM, Spector SA, et al. A randomized trial of three antipneumocystis agents in patients with advanced human immunodeficiency virus infection: NIAID AIDS Clinical Trials Group. N Engl J Med. 1995;332:693–699.
288. Ross JJ, Langen MC, Stallen PC, et al. Pentamidine aerosols and environmental contamination: Health-care worker risk. Pharm World Sci. 1996;18:148–152.
289. Balmes JR, Estacio PL, Quinlan P, et al. Respiratory effects of occupational exposure to aerosolized pentamidine. J Occup Environ Med. 1995;37:145–150.
290. Pearson RD, Hewlett EL. Pentamidine for the treatment of *Pneumocytis carinii* pneumonia and other parasitic diseases. Ann Intern Med. 1985;103:782–786.
291. Navin TR, Fontaine RE. Intravenous versus intramuscular administration of pentamidine (Letter). N Engl J Med. 1984;311:1701–1702.
292. Williamson J. Effects of trypanosides on the fine structure of target organisms. Pharmacol Ther. 1979;7:445–512.
293. Croft SL, Brazil RP. Effect of pentamidine isethionate on the ultrastructure and morphology of *Leishmania mexicana amazonensi* in vitro. Ann Trop Med Parasitol. 1982;76:37–43.
294. Waring MJ. The effects of antimicrobial agents on ribonucleic acid polymerase. Mol Pharmacol. 1965;1:1–13.
295. Wallis OC. The effect of pentamidine on ribosomes of the parasitic flagellate *Crithidia (Strigomonas) oncopelti*. J Protozool. 1966;13:234–239.
296. Gutteridge WE. Some effects of pentamidine di-isethionate on *Crithidia fasciculata*. J Protozool. 1969;16:306–311.
297. Basselin M, Robert-Gero M. Alterations in membrane fluidity, lipid metabolism, mitochondrial activity and lipophosphoglycan expression in pentamidine-resistant *Leishmania*. Parasitol Res. 1998;84:78–83.
298. Basselin M, Badet-Denisot MA, Lawrence F, et al. Effects of pentamidine on polyamine level and biosynthesis in wild-type, pentamidine-treated, and pentamidine-resistant *Leishmania*. Exp Parasitol. 1997;85:274–282.
299. Waalkes TP, Makulu DR. Pharmacologic aspects of pentamidine. Natl Cancer Inst Monogr. 1976;43:171–177.
300. Geratz JD. Inhibitory effect of aromatic diamidines on trypsin and enterokinase. Experientia. 1969;25:1254–1255.
301. Hill GC, Hutner SH. Effect of trypanocidal drugs on terminal respiration of *Crithidia fasciculata*. Exp Parasitol. 1968;22:207–212.
302. Walzer PD, Perl DP, Krogstad DJ, et al. *Pneumocystis carinii* pneumonia in the United States: Epidemiologic, diagnostic, and clinical features. Ann Intern Med. 1974;80:83–93.
303. Western KA, Perera DR, Schultz MG. Pentamidine isethionate in the treatment of *Pneumocystis carinii* pneumonia. Ann Intern Med. 1970;73:695–702.
304. Assan R, Perrone C, Assan D, et al. Pentamidine-induced derangements of glucose homeostasis: Determinant roles of renal failure and drug accumulation. A study of 128 patients. Diabetes Care. 1995;18:47–55.
305. Bouchard P, Sai P, Reach G, et al. Diabetes mellitus following pentamidine-induced hypoglycemia in humans. Diabetes. 1982;31:40–45.
306. Osei K, Falko JM, Nelson KP, et al. Diabetogenic effect of pentamidine: In vitro and in vivo studies in a patient with malignant insulinoma. Am J Med. 1984;77:41–46.
307. Girgis I, Gualberti J, Langan L, et al. A prospective study of the effect of I.V. pentamidine therapy on ventricular arrhythmias and QTc prolongation in HIV-infected patients. Chest. 1997;112:646–653.
308. O'Brien JG, Dong BJ, Coleman RL, et al. A 5-year retrospective review of adverse

drug interactions and their risk factors in human immunodeficiency virus-infected patients who were receiving intravenous pentamidine therapy for *Pneumocystis carinii* pneumonia. Clin Infect Dis. 1997;24:854–859.

309. Keystone JS, Murdoch JK. Mebendazole. Ann Intern Med. 1979;91:582–586.
310. Tankhiwale SR, Kudade AL, Sarmah HC, et al. Single dose therapy of ascariasis: A randomized comparison of mebendazole and pyrantel. J Commun Dis. 1989;21:71–74.
311. Nontasut P, Singhasivanon V, Prarinyanuparp V, et al. Effect of single-dose albendazole and single-dose mebendazole on *Necator americanus*. Southeast Asian J Trop Med Public Health. 1989;20:237–242.
312. Abadi K. Single dose mebendazole therapy for soil-transmitted nematodes. Am J Trop Med Hyg. 1985;34:129–133.
313. Pelletier LL Jr, Baker CB. Treatment failures following mebendazole therapy for chronic strongyloidiasis. J Infect Dis. 1987;156:532–533.
314. Wilson KH, Kauffman CA. Persistent *Strongyloides stercoralis* in a blind loop of the bowel: Successful treatment with mebendazole. Arch Intern Med 1983;143:357–358.
315. Levin ML. Treatment of trichinosis with mebendazole. Am J Trop Med Hyg. 1983;32:980–983.
316. Hess JA, Chandrasekar PH, Mortiere M, et al. Comparative efficacy of ketoconazole and mebendazole in experimental trichinosis. Antimicrob Agents Chemother. 1986;30:953–954.
317. Van Hoegaerden M, Ivanoff B, Flocard F, et al. The use of mebendazole in the treatment of filariasis due to *Loa loa* and *Mansonella perstans*. Ann Trop Med Parasitol. 1987;81:275–282.
318. Van Hoegaerden M, Flocard F. Mebendazole treatment of loiasis (Letter). Lancet. 1985;1:1278.
319. Cruz AC. Treatment of human taeniasis in the Philippines: A review. Southeast Asian J Trop Med Public Health. 1991;22(Suppl):271–274.
320. Bartoloni C, Tricerri A, Guidi L, et al. The efficacy of chemotherapy with mebendazole in human cystic echinococcosis: Long-term follow-up of 52 patients. Ann Trop Med Parasitol. 1992;86:249–256.
321. Messaritakis J, Psychou P, Nicolaidou P, et al. High mebendazole doses in pulmonary and hepatic hydatid disease. Arch Dis Child. 1991;66:532–533.
322. Wilson JF, Rausch RL, McMahon BJ, et al. Parasiticidal effect of chemotherapy in alveolar hydatid disease: Review of experience with mebendazole and albendazole in Alaskan Eskimos. Clin Infect Dis. 1992;15:234–249.
323. Luder J, Witassek F, Weigand K, et al. Treatment of cystic echinococcosis *(Echinococcus granulosus)* with mebendazole: Assessment of bound and free drug levels in cyst fluid and of parasite vitality in operative specimens. Eur J Clin Pharmacol. 1985;28:279–285.
324. Smego DR, Smego RA Jr. Hydatid cyst: Preoperative sterilization with mebendazole. South Med J. 1986;79:900–901.
325. Sayek I, Cakmakci M. The effect of prophylactic mebendazole in experimental peritoneal hydatidosis. Surg Gynecol Obstet. 1986;163:351–353.
326. Todorov T, Mechkov G, Vutova K, et al. Factors influencing the response to chemotherapy in human cystic echinococcosis. Bull World Health Organ. 1992;70:347–358.
327. Todorov T, Vutova K, Mechkov G, et al. Chemotherapy of human cystic echinococcosis: Comparative efficacy of mebendazole and albendazole. Ann Trop Med Parasitol. 1992;86:59–66.
328. Morris DL. Pre-operative albendazole therapy for hydatid cyst. Br J Surg. 1987;74:805–806.
329. Gill JH, Lacey E. The kinetics of mebendazole binding to *Haemonchus contortus* tubulin. Int J Parasitol. 1992;22:939–946.
330. Tracy JW, Webster LT Jr. Drugs used in the chemotherapy of helminthiasis. In: Hardman JG, Limbird LE, eds. Goodman and Gilman's Pharmacologic Basis of Therapeutics. 9th ed. New York: McGraw-Hill; 1996:1009–1026.
331. Levin MH, Weinstein RA, Axelrod JL, et al. Severe, reversible neutropenia during high-dose mebendazole therapy for echinococcosis. JAMA. 1983;249:2929–2931.
332. Fernández-Bañares F, González-Huix F, Xiol X, et al. Marrow aplasia during high dose mebendazole treatment. Am J Trop Med Hyg. 1986;35:350–351.
333. el Kalla S, Menon NS. Mebendazole poisoning in infancy. Ann Trop Paediatr. 1990;10:313–314.
334. Bassily S, El-Masry NA, Trabolsi B, et al. Treatment of ancylostomiasis and ascariasis with albendazole. Ann Trop Med Parasitol. 1984;78:81–82.
335. Jagota SC. Albendazole, a broad-spectrum anthelmintic, in the treatment of intestinal nematode and cestode infections: A multicenter study in 480 patients. Clin Ther. 1986;8:226–231.
336. Raccurt CP, Lambert MT, Bouloumie J, et al. Evaluation of the treatment of intestinal helminthiases with albendazole in Djohong (North Cameroon). Trop Med Parasitol. 1990;41:46–48.
337. Norhayati M, Oothuman P, Azizi O, et al. Efficacy of single dose albendazole on the prevalence and intensity of infection of soil-transmitted helminths in Orang Asli children in Malaysia. Southeast Asian J Trop Med Public Health. 1997;28:563–569.
338. Stephenson LS, Latham MC, Adams EJ, et al. Weight gain of Kenyan school children infected with hookworm, *Trichuris trichiura*, and *Ascaris lumbricoides* is improved following once- or twice-yearly treatment with albendazole. J Nutr. 1993;123:656–665.
339. Stephenson LS, Latham MC, Kinoti SN, et al. Improvements in physical fitness of Kenyan schoolboys infected with hookworm, *Trichuris trichiura* and *Ascaris lumbricoides* following a single dose of albendazole. Trans R Soc Trop Med Hyg. 1990;84:277–282.
340. Albonico M, Smith PG, Ercole E, et al. Rate of reinfection with intestinal nematodes after treatment of children with mebendazole or albendazole in a highly endemic area. Trans R Soc Trop Med Hyg. 1995;89:538–541.
341. Davies HD, Sakuls P, Keystone JS. Creeping eruption: A review of clinical presentation and management of 60 cases presenting to a tropical disease unit. Arch Dermatol. 1993;129:588–591.
342. Jones SK, Reynolds NJ, Oliwiecki S, et al. Oral albendazole for the treatment of cutaneous larva migrans. Br J Dermatol. 1990;122:99–101.
343. Rizzitelli G, Scarabelli G, Veraldi S. Albendazole: A new therapeutic regimen in cutaneous larva migrans. Int J Dermatol. 1997;36:700–703.
344. Sturchler D, Schubarth P, Gualzata M, et al. Thiabendazole vs. albendazole in treatment of toxocariasis: A clinical trial. Ann Trop Med Parasitol. 1989;83: 473–478.
345. Kraivichian P, Kulkumthorn M, Yingyourd P, et al. Albendazole for the treatment of human gnathostomiasis. Trans R Soc Trop Med Hyg. 1992;86:418–421.
346. Chichino G, Bernuzzi AM, Bruno A, et al. Intestinal capillariasis *(Capillaria philippinensis)* acquired in Indonesia: a case report. Am J Trop Med Hyg. 1992;47:10–12.
347. Krepel HP, Haring T, Baeta S, et al. Treatment of mixed *Oesophagostomum* and hook worm infection: Effect of albendazole, pyrantel pamoate, levamisole and thiabendazole. Trans R Soc Trop Med Hyg. 1993;87:87–89.
348. Cabie A, Bouchaud O, Houze S, et al. Albendazole versus thiabendazole as therapy for trichinosis: A retrospective study. Clin Infect Dis. 1996;22:1033–1035.
349. Lipani F, Caramello P, Biglino A, Sacchi C. Albendazole for the treatment of *Mansonella perstans* filariasis. Trans R Soc Trop Med Hyg. 1997;91:221.
350. Liu YH, Wang XG, Gao P, et al. Experimental and clinical trial of albendazole in the treatment of *Clonorchiasis senensis*. Chin Med J (Engl). 1991;104:27–31.
351. Chanthavanich P, Nontasut P, Prarinyanuparp V, et al. Repeated doses of albendazole against strongyloidiasis in Thai children. Southeast Asian J Trop Med Public Health. 1989;20:221–226.
352. Marti H, Haji HJ, Savioli L, et al. A comparative trial of a single-dose ivermectin versus three days of albendazole for treatment of *Strongyloides stercoralis* and other soil-transmitted helminth infections in children. Am J Trop Med Hyg. 1996;55:477–481.
353. Hall A, Nahar Q. Albendazole as a treatment for infections with *Giardia duodenalis* in children in Bangladesh. Trans R Soc Trop Med Hyg. 1993;87:84–86.
354. Misra PK, Kumar A, Agarwal V, et al. A comparative clinical trial of albendazole versus metronidazole in children with giardiasis. Indian Pediatr. 1995;32:779–782.
355. Blanshard C, Ellis DS, Tovey DG, et al. Treatment of intestinal microsporidiosis with albendazole in patients with AIDS. AIDS. 1992;6:311–313.
356. Molina JM, Chastang C, Goguel J, et al. Albendazole for treatment and prophylaxis of microsporidiosis due to *Encephalitozoon intestinalis* in patients with AIDS: A randomized double blind controlled trial. J Infect Dis. 1998;177:1373–1377.
357. Molina JM, Oksenhendler E, Beauvais B, et al. Disseminated microsporidiosis due to *Septata intestinalis* in patients with AIDS: Clinical features and response to albendazole therapy. J Infect Dis. 1995;171:245–249.
358. Dore GJ, Marriott DJ, Hing MC, et al. Disseminated microsporidiosis due to *Septata intestinalis* in nine patients infected with the human immunodeficiency virus: Response to therapy with albendazole. Clin Infect Dis. 1995;21:70–76.
359. Kelly P, Lungu F, Keane E et al. Albendazole chemotherapy for treatment of diarrhoea in patients with AIDS in Zambia: A randomized double blind controlled trial. BMJ. 1996;312:1187–1191.
360. Horton RJ. Albendazole in treatment of human cystic echinococcosis: 12 Years of experience. Acta Trop. 1997;64:79–93.
361. Eskazole: Clinical and Technical Review. SmithKline Beecham Pharmaceuticals. 1990:A1–B28.
362. Aktan AO, Yalin R. Preoperative albendazole treatment for liver hydatid disease decreases the viability of the cyst. Eur J Gastroenterol Hepatol. 1996;8:877–879.
363. Sotelo J, del Brutto OH, Penagos P, et al. Comparison of therapeutic regimen of anticysticercal drugs for parenchymal brain cysticercosis. J Neurol. 1990;237: 69–72.
364. Escobedo F, Penagos P, Rodriguez J, et al. Albendazole therapy for neurocysticercosis. Arch Intern Med. 1987;147:738–741.
365. Meneghelli UG, Martinelli AL, Bellucci AD, et al. Polycystic hydatid disease *(Echinococcus vogeli)*: Treatment with albendazole. Ann Trop Med Parasitol. 1992;86:151–156.
366. Takayanagui OM, Jardim E. Therapy for neurocysticercosis: Comparison between albendazole and praziquantel. Arch Neurol. 1992;49:290–294.
367. Sanchez M, Suastegui R, Gonzalez-Esquivel D, et al. Pharmacokinetic comparison of two albendazole dosage regimens in patients with neurocysticercosis. Clin Neuropharmacol. 1993;16:77–82.
368. Cruz M, Cruz I, Horton J. Clinical evaluation of albendazole and praziquantel in the treatment of cerebral cysticercosis. Southeast Asian J Trop Med Public Health. 1991;22(Suppl):279–283.
369. Cruz M, Cruz I, Horton J. Albendazole versus praziquantel in the treatment of cerebral cysticercosis: Clinical evaluation. Trans R Soc Trop Med Hyg. 1991;85:244–247.
370. Cruzi I, Cruz ME, Carrasco F, et al. Neurocysticercosis: Optimal dose treatment with albendazole. J Neurol Sci. 1995;133:152–154.
371. del Brutto OH, Sotelo J, Aguirre R, et al. Albendazole therapy for giant subarachnoid cysticerci. Arch Neurol. 1992;49:535–538.
372. del Brutto OH, Sotelo J. Albendazole therapy for subarachnoid and ventricular cysticercosis: Case report. J Neurosurg. 1990;72:816–817.
373. del Brutto OH. Albendazole therapy for subarachnoid cysticerci: Clinical and neuroimaging analysis of 17 patients. J Neurol Neurosurg Psychiatry. 1997;62: 659–661.

374. Proano JV, Madrazo I, Garcia L, et al. Albendazole and praziquantel treatment in neurocysticercosis of the fourth ventricle. J Neurosurg. 1997;87:29–33.
375. Chung WC, Fan PC, Lin CY, et al. Poor efficacy of albendazole for the treatment of human taeniasis. Int J Parasitol. 1991;21:269–270.
376. de Kaminsky RG. Albendazole treatment for human taeniasis. Trans R Soc Trop Med Hyg. 1991;85:648–650.
377. Lawrenz A, Eglit S, Kroker R. The metabolism of albendazole in the isolated perfused intestine of rats. DTW Dtsch Tierarztl Wochenschr. 1992;99:416–418.
378. Jung H, Hurtado M, Sanchez M, et al. Clinical pharmacokinetics of albendazole in patients with brain cysticercosis. J Clin Pharmacol. 1992;32:28–31.
379. Jung H, Hurtado M, Sanchez M, et al. Plasma and CSF levels of albendazole and praziquantel in patients with neurocysticercosis. Clin Neuropharmacol. 1990;13:559–564.
380. Jung H, Hurtado M, Medina MT, et al. Dexamethasone increases plasma levels of albendazole. J Neurol. 1990;237:279–280.
381. Ireland CM, Gull K, Gutteridge WE, et al. The interaction of benzimidazole carbamates with mammalian microtubule protein. Biochem Pharmacol. 1979;28:2680–2682.
382. Barrowman MH. The fumarate reductase system as a site of anthelmintic attack in *Ascaris suum*. Biosci Rep. 1984;4:879–883.
383. Dewerdt S, Machet L, Jan-Lamy V et al. Stevens-Johnson syndrome after albendazole. Acta Derma Venereol. 1997;77:411.
384. Shah V, Marino C, Altice FL. Albendazole-induced pseudomembranous colitis. Am J Gastroenterol. 1996;91:1453–1454.
385. Morris DL, Smith PG. Albendazole in hydatid disease: Hepatocellular toxicity. Trans R Soc Trop Med Hyg. 1987;81:343–344.
386. Pilar Garcia-Muret M, Sitjas D, Tuneu L, et al. Telogen effluvium associated with albendazole (Letter). Int J Dermatol. 1990;29:669–670.
387. Campbell WC, Cuckler AC. Thiabendazole in the treatment and control of parasitic infections in man. Tex Rep Biol Med. 1969;27(Suppl 2):665–692.
388. Berk SL, Verghese A, Alvarez S, et al. Clinical and epidemiological features of strongyloidiasis: A prospective study in rural Tennessee. Arch Intern Med. 1987;147:1257–1261.
389. Barnish G, Barker J. An intervention study using thiabendazole suspension against *Strongyloides fuelleborni*-like infections in Papua New Guinea. Trans R Soc Trop Med Hyg. 1987;81:60–63.
390. Gordon HM. Thiabendazole: A highly effective anthelminthic for sheep. Nature. 1961;191:1409–1410.
391. Campbell WC, Denham DA. Chemotherapy. In: Campbell WC, ed. *Trichinella* and trichinosis. New York: Plenum Press; 1983:335–366.
392. Hennekeuser HH, Pabst K, Poeplau W, et al. Thiabendazole for the treatment of trichinosis in humans. Tex Rep Biol Med. 1969;27(Suppl 2):581–596.
393. Criado Fornelio A, Rodriguez Caabeiro F, Jimenez Gonzalez A. The mode of action of some benzimidazole drugs on *Trichinella spiralis*. Parasitology. 1987;95:61–70.
394. Jelinek T, Maiwald H, Nothdurft HD, et al. Cutaneous larva migrans in travelers: Synopsis of histories, symptoms, and treatment of 98 patients. Clin Infect Dis. 1994;19:1062–1066.
395. Davies HD, Sakuls P, Keystone JS. Creeping eruption: A review of clinical presentation and management of 60 cases presenting to a tropical medicine unit. Arch Dermatol. 1993;129:588–591.
396. Lewis DJ, Thorpe SA, Reynolds SL. The carry-through of residues of thiabendazole, tecnazene and chlorpropham from potatoes following manufacture into potato crisps and jacket potato crisps. Food Addit Contam. 1996;13:21–29.
397. Bushway RJ. Complementation of direct-infection high-performance liquid chromatography and enzyme-linked immunosorbent assay for the analysis of thiabendazole in fruit juices and concentrates. J Chromatogr. 1996;754:431–435.
398. Jasra N, Sanyal SN, Khera S. Effect of thiabendazole and fenbendazole on glucose and carbohydrate metabolism in *Trichuris globulosa*. Vet Parasitol. 1990;35: 201–209.
399. Manivel JC, Bloomer JR, Snover DC. Progressive bile duct injury after thiabendazole administration. Gastroenterology. 1987;93:245–249.
400. Tchao P, Templeton T. Thiabendazole-associated grand mal seizures in a patient with Down syndrome. J Pediatr. 1983;102:317–318.
401. De Pargament MDM, de Vinuesa ML, Larripa I. Mutagenic bioassay of certain pharmacological drugs: I. Thiabendazole (TBZ). Mutat Res. 1987;188:1–6.
402. Schneider D, Gannon R, Sweeney K, et al. Theophylline and antiparasitic drug interactions: A case report and study of the influence of thiabendazole and mebendazole on theophylline pharmacokinetics in adults. Chest. 1990;97:84–87.
403. Austin WC, Courtney W, Danilewicz JC, et al. Pyrantel tartrate, a new anthelmintic effective against infections of domestic animals. Nature. 1966;212:1273–1274.
404. Bumbalo TS, Fugazzoto DJ, Wyczalek JV. Treatment of enterobiasis with pyrantel pamoate. Am J Trop Med Hyg. 1969;18:50–52.
405. Tankhiwale SR, Kukade AL, Sarmah HC, et al. Single dose therapy of ascariasis: A randomized comparison of mebendazole and pyrantel. J Commun Dis. 1989;21:71–74.
406. Aubry ML, Cowell P, Davey MJ, et al. Aspects of the pharmacology of a new anthelminthic: Pyrantel. Br J Pharmacol. 1970;38:332–344.
407. Eyre P. Some pharmacodynamic effects of the nematocides: Methyridine, tetramisole and pyrantel. J Pharm Pharmacol. 1970;22:26–36.
408. Hadju V, Stephenson LS, Abadi K, et al. Improvements in appetite and growth in helminth-infected schoolboys three and seven weeks after a single dose of pyrantel pamoate. Parasitology. 1996;113:497–504.
409. Rollo IM. Drugs used in the chemotherapy of helminthiasis. In: Gilman AG, Goodman LS, Gilman A, eds. The Pharmacological Basis of Therapeutics. 6th ed. New York: Macmillan; 1980:1013–1037.
410. Ganguly B, Awasthi PK, Singhal KC. Regulation of cholinomimetic action of pyrantel pamoate by calcium channels in *Setaria cervi*. Indian J Physiol Pharmacol. 1996;40:245–248.
411. Martin RJ, Robertson AP, Bjorn H. Target sites of anthelmintics. Parasitology. 1997;114(Suppl):S111–S114.
412. Martin RJ. (γ-Aminobutyric acid- and piperazine-activated single-channel currents from *Ascaris suum* body muscle. Br J Pharmacol. 1985;84:445–461.
413. Saz HJ, Bueding E. Relationships between anthelminthic effects and biochemical and physiological mechanisms. Pharmacol Rev. 1966;18:871–894.
414. Nickey LN. Possible precipitation of petit mal seizures with piperazine citrate. JAMA. 1966;195:1069–1070.
415. Parsons AC. Piperazine neurotoxicity: "Worm wobble." BMJ. 1971;4:792.
416. Wright S, Harman RRM. Ethylenediamine and piperazine sensitivity. BMJ. 1983;287:463–464.
417. Ottesen EA, Duke BO, Karam M, et al. Strategies and tools for the control/ elimination of lymphatic filariasis. Bull World Health Organ. 1997;75:491–503.
418. Bockarie JJ, Alexander ND, Hyun P, et al. Randomized community-based trial of annual single-dose diethylcarbamazine with or without ivermectin against *Wuchereria bancrofti* infection in human beings and mosquitoes. Lancet. 1998;351: 162–168.
419. Meyrowitsch DW, Simonsen PE, Makunde WH. Mass diethylcarbamazine chemotherapy for control of bancroftian filariasis through community participation: Comparative efficacy of a low monthly dose and medicated salt. Trans R Soc Trop Med Hyg. 1996;90:74–79.
420. Reddy GS, Venkateswaralu N. Mass administration of DEC-medicated salt for filariasis control in the endemic population of Karaikal, south India: Implementation and impact assessment. Bull World Health Organ. 1996;74:85–90.
421. Hakim SL, Vythilingam I, Marzukhi MI, et al. Single-dose diethylcarbamazine in the control of periodic brugian filariasis in peninsular Malaysia. Trans R Soc Trop Med Hyg. 1995;89:686–689.
422. Partono F. Treatment of elephantiasis in a community with timorian filariasis. Trans R Soc Trop Med Hyg. 1985;79:44–46.
423. Noroes J, Dreyer G, Santos A, et al. Assessment of the efficacy of diethylcarbamazine on adult *Wuchereria bancrofti* in vivo. Trans R Soc Trop Med Hyg. 1997;91:78–81.
424. Ong RK, Doyle RL. Tropical pulmonary eosinophilia. Chest. 1998;113:1673–1679.
425. Hawking F. Chemotherapy of filariasis. Antimicrob Agents Chemother. 1980;30:135–162.
426. Chadee DD, Tilluckdharry CC, Rawlins SC, et al. Mass chemotherapy with diethylcarbamazine for the control of Bancroftian filariasis: A twelve-year follow-up in northern Trinidad, including observations on *Mansonella ozzardi*. Am J Trop Med Hyg. 1995;52:174–176.
427. Bartholomew CF, Nathan MD, Tikasingh ES. The failure of diethylcarbamazine in the treatment of *Mansonella ozzardi* infections. Trans R Soc Trop Med Hyg. 1978;72:423–424.
428. Wiseman RA, Woodruff AW, Pettitt LE. The treatment of toxocaral infection: Some experimental and clinical observations. Trans R Soc Trop Med Hyg. 1971;65:591–598.
429. Megnaval JF. Comparative efficacy of diethylcarbamazine and mebendazole for the treatment of human toxocariasis. Parasitology. 1995;110:529–533.
430. Taylor HR. Recent developments in the treatment of onchocerciasis. Bull World Health Organ. 1984;62:509–515.
431. Lariviere M, Vingtain P, Aziz M, et al. Double-blind study of ivermectin and diethylcarbamazine in African onchocerciasis patients with ocular involvement. Lancet. 1985;2:174–177.
432. Diallo S, Aziz MA, Lariviere M, et al. A double-blind comparison of the efficacy and safety of ivermectin and diethylcarbamazine in a placebo controlled study of Senegalese patients with onchocerciasis. Trans R Soc Trop Med Hyg. 1986;80: 927–934.
433. Dadzie KY, Bird AC, Awadzi K, et al. Ocular findings in a double-blind study of ivermectin versus diethylcarbamazine versus placebo in the treatment of onchocerciasis. Br J Ophthalmol. 1987;71:78–85.
434. Greene BM, Taylor HR, Brown EJ, et al. Ocular and systemic complications of diethylcarbamazine therapy for onchocerciasis: Association with circulating immune complexes. J Infect Dis. 1983;147:890–897.
435. Ottesen EA. Description, mechanisms and control of reactions to treatment in the human filariases. Ciba Found Symp. 1987;127:265–283.
436. Hawking F. Chemotherapy of filariasis. In: Schnitzer RJ, Hawking F, eds. Experimental Chemotherapy, v. 1. New York: Academic Press; 1963:893–912.
437. Rée GH, Hall AP, Hutchinson DBA, et al. Plasma levels of diethylcarbamazine in man. Trans R Soc Trop Med Hyg. 1978;71:542–543.
438. Faulkner JK, Smith KJ. Dealkylation and *N*-oxidation in the metabolism of 1-diethyl-carbamyl-4-methylpiperazine in the rat. Xenobiotica. 1972;2:59–68.
439. Langham ME, Kramer TR. The in vitro effect of diethylcarbamazine on the motility and survival of *Onchocerca volvulus* microfilariae. Tropemed Parasitol. 1980;31:59–66.
440. Hawking F. Diethylcarbamazine and new compounds for the treatment of filariasis. Adv Pharmacol Chemother. 1979;16:129–194.
441. Van den Bossche H. A look at the mode of action of some old and new antifilarial compounds. Ann Soc Belg Med Trop. 1981;16:287–296 (cited in Ref. 387).
442. King CH, Greene BM, Spagnuolo PJ. Diethylcarbamazine citrate, an antifilarial drug, stimulates human granulocyte adherence. Antimicrob Agents Chemother. 1983;24:453–456.
443. Cesbron J-V, Capron A, Vargaftig BB, et al. Platelets mediate the action of diethylcarbamazine on microfilariae. Nature. 1987;325:533–536.

444. Kanesa-thasan N, Douglas JG, Kazura JW. Diethylcarbamazine inhibits endothelial and microfilarial prostanoid metabolism in vitro. Mol Biochem Parasitol. 1991;49:11–20.
445. Fujimaki Y, Ehara M, Kimura E, et al. Diethylcarbamazine, antifilarial drug, inhibits microtubule polymerization and disrupts preformed microtubules. Biochem Pharmacol. 1990;39:851–856.
446. Francis H, Awadzi K, Ottesen EA. The Mazzotti reaction following treatment of onchocerciasis with diethylcarbamazine: Clinical severity as a function of infection intensity. Am J Trop Med Hyg. 1985;34:529–536.
447. Carme B, Boulesteix J, Boutes H, et al. Five cases of encephalitis during treatment of loiasis with diethylcarbamazine. Am J Trop Med Hyg. 1991;44:684–690.
448. Campbell WC, Fisher MH, Stapley EO, et al. Ivermectin: A potent new antiparasitic agent. Science. 1983;221:823–828.
449. Taylor H, Pacque M, Munoz B, et al. Impact of mass treatment of onchocerciasis with ivermectin on the transmission of infection. Science. 1990;250:116.
450. Dadzie KY, Remme J, De Sole G. Changes in ocular onchocerciasis after two rounds of community-based ivermectin treatment in a holo-endemic onchocerciasis focus. Trans R Soc Trop Med Hyg. 1991;85:267–271.
451. Taylor HR, Semba RD, Newland HS, et al. Ivermectin treatment of patients with severe onchocerciasis. Am J Trop Med Hyg. 1989;40:494–500.
452. Abiose A, Jones BR, Cousens SN, et al. Reduction in the incidence of optic nerve disease with annual ivermectin to control onchocerciasis. Lancet. 1993;341:130–135.
453. Pacque M, Munoz B, Greene BM, et al. Safety of and compliance with community-based ivermectin therapy. Lancet. 1990;335:1377–1380.
454. Pacque M, Munoz B, Greene BM, et al. Community-based treatment of onchocerciasis with ivermectin: Safety, efficacy, and acceptibility of yearly treatment. J Infect Dis. 1991;163:381–385.
455. Somo R, Ngosso A, Dinga JS, et al. A community-based trial of ivermectin for onchocerciasis control in the forest of southwest Cameroon: Clinical and pathologic findings after three treatments. Am J Trop Med Hyg. 1993;48:9–13.
456. Collins RC, Gonzalez-Peralta C, Castro J, et al. Ivermectin: Reduction in prevalence and infection intensity of *Onchocerca volvulus* following biannual treatments in five Guatemalan communities. Am J Trop Med Hyg. 1992;47:156–169.
457. Pacque M, Greene BM, Munoz B, et al. Ivermectin therapy: A 5-year follow-up. J Infect Dis. 1991;164:1035–1036.
458. Duke BOL, Pacque MC, Munoz B, et al. Viability of adult *Onchocerca volvulus* after six 2-weekly doses of ivermectin. Bull World Health Organ. 1991;69:163–168.
459. Plaisier AP, Alley ES, Boatin BA, et al. Irreversible effects of ivermectin on adult parasites in onchocerciasis patients in the Onchocerciasis Control Programme in West Africa. J Infect Dis. 1995;172:204–210.
460. Kumaraswami V, Ottesen EA, Vijayasekaran V, et al. Ivermectin for the treatment of *Wuchereria bancrofti* filariasis: Efficacy and adverse reactions. JAMA. 1988;259:3150–3153.
461. Ottesen EA, Vijayasekaran V, Kumaraswami V, et al. A controlled trial of ivermectin and diethylcarbamazine in lymphatic filariasis. N Engl J Med. 1990;322:1113–1117.
462. Mak JW, Navaratnam V, Grewel JS, et al. Treatment of subperiodic *Brugia malayi* infection with a single dose of ivermectin. Am J Trop Med Hyg. 1993;48:591–596.
463. Addiss DG, Eberhard ML, Lammie PJ, et al. Comparative efficacy of clearing-dose and single-dose ivermectin and diethylcarbamazine against *Wuchereria bancrofti* microfilaremia. Am J Trop Med Hyg. 1993;48:178–185.
464. Dreyer G, Addiss D, Noroes J, et al. Ultrasonographic assessment of the adulticidal efficacy of repeat high-dose ivermectin in bancroftian filariasis. Trop Med Int Health. 1996;1:427–432.
465. Kombila M, Duong TH, Ferrer A, et al. Short- and long-term action of multiple doses of ivermectin on loiasis microfilaremia. Am J Trop Med Hyg. 1998;58: 258–260.
466. Gardon J, Kamgno J, Folefack G, et al. Marked decrease in *Loa loa* microfilaremia six and twelve months after a single dose of ivermectin. Trans R Soc Trop Med Hyg. 1997;91:593–594.
467. Fischer P, Bamuhiiga J, Buttner DW. Treatment of human *Mansonella streptocerca* infection with ivermectin. Trop Med Int Health. 1997;2:191–199.
468. Naquira C, Jimenez G, Guerra JG, et al. Ivermectin for human strongyloidiasis and other intestinal helminths. Am J Trop Med Hyg. 1989;40:304–309.
469. Lyagoubi M, Datry A, Mayorga R, et al. Chronic persistent strongyloidiasis cured by ivermectin. Trans R Soc Trop Med Hyg. 1992;86:541.
470. Ashraf M, Gue CL, Baddour LM. Case report: Strongyloidiasis refractory to treatment with ivermectin. Am J Med Sci. 1996;311:178–179.
471. Ottesen EA, Campbell WC. Ivermectin in human medicine. J Antimicrob Chemother. 1994;34:195–203.
472. Caumes E, Carriere J, Datry A, et al. A randomized trial of ivermectin versus albendazole for the treatment of cutaneous larva migrans. Am J Trop Med Hyg. 1993;49:641–644.
473. Meinking TL, Taplin D, Hermida JL, et al. The treatment of scabies with ivermectin. N Engl J Med. 1995;333:26–30.
474. Taplin D, Meinking TL. Treatment of HIV-infected scabies with emphasis on the efficacy of ivermectin. Semin Cutan Med Surg. 1997;16:235–240.
475. Okonkwo PO, Ogbuokiri JE, Ofoegbu E, et al. Protein binding and ivermectin estimations in patients with onchocerciasis. Clin Pharmacol Ther. 1993;53: 426–429.
476. Klotz U, Ogbuokiri JE, Okonkwo PO. Ivermectin binds avidly to plasma proteins. Eur J Clin Pharmacol. 1990;39:607–608.
477. Brownlee DJ, Holden-Dye L, Walker RJ. Actions of the anthelmintic ivermectin on the pharyngeal muscle of the parasite nematode, *Ascaris suum*. Parasitology. 1997;115:553–561.
478. Chijioke CP, Okonkwo PO. Adverse events following ivermectin therapy for onchocerciasis. Trans R Soc Trop Med Hyg. 1992;86:284–286.
479. Baraka OZ, Khier MM, Ahmed KM, et al. Community based distribution of ivermectin in eastern Sudan: Acceptability and early post-treatment reactions. Trans R Soc Trop Med Hyg. 1995;89:316–318.
480. Boussinesq M, Gardon J, Gardon-Wendel N, et al. Three probable cases of *Loa loa* encephalopathy following ivermectin treatment for onchocerciasis. Am J Trop Med Hyg. 1998;58:461–469.
481. Gardon J, Gardon-Wendel N, Demanga-Ngangue, et al. Serious reactions after mass treatment of onchocerciasis with ivermectin in an area endemic for *Loa loa* infection. Lancet. 1997;350:18–22.
482. Pacque M, Munoz B, Poetschke G, et al. Pregnancy outcome after inadvertent ivermectin treatment during community-based distribution. Lancet. 1990;336:1486–1489.
483. King CH, Mahmoud AA. Drugs five years later: Praziquantel. Ann Intern Med. 1989;110:290–296.
484. Pearson RD, Wilson ME. Role of praziquantel in the treatment of helminthic diseases. Int Med Specialist. 1986;7:183–204.
485. Wegner DHG. The profile of the trematodicidal compound praziquantel. Arzneimittelforschung. 1984;34:1132–1136.
486. Latham MC, Stephenson LS, Kurz KM, et al. Metrifonate or praziquantel treatment improves physical fitness and appetite of Kenyan schoolboys with *Schistosoma haematobium* and hookworm infections. Am J Trop Med Hyg. 1990;43:170–179.
487. Kimura E, Moji K, Uga S, et al. Effects of *Schistosoma haematobium* infection on mental test scores of Kenyan school children. Trop Med Parasitol. 1992;43: 155–158.
488. King CH, Muchiri E, Ouma JH, et al. Chemotherapy-based control of schistosomiasis hematobia: IV. Impact of repeated annual chemotherapy on prevalence and intensity of *Schistosoma haematobium* infection in an endemic area of Kenya. Am J Trop Med Hyg. 1991;45:498–508.
489. Simarro PP, Sima FO, Mir M, et al. Effect of repeated targeted mass treatment with praziquantel on the prevalence, intensity of infection and morbidity due to *Schistosoma intercalatum* in an urban community in equatorial Guinea. Trop Med Parasitol. 1991;42:167–171.
490. Homeida MA, el Tom I, Nash T, et al. Association of the therapeutic activity of praziquantel with the reversal of Symmers' fibrosis induced by *Schistosoma mansoni*. Am J Trop Med Hyg. 1991;45:360–365.
491. Watt G, Adapon B, Long GW, et al. Praziquantel in treatment of cerebral schistosomiasis. Lancet. 1986;2:529–532.
492. Richards F Jr, Sullivan J, Ruiz-Tiben E, et al. Effect of praziquantel on the eggs of *Schistosoma mansoni*, with a note on the implications for managing central nervous system schistosomiasis. Ann Trop Med Parasitol. 1989;83:465–472.
493. Stelma FF, Sall S, Daff B, et al. Oxamniquine cures *Schistosoma mansoni* infection in a focus in which cure rates with praziquantel are unusually low. J Infect Dis. 1997;176:304–307.
494. Fritsche TR, Eastburn RL, Wiggins LH, et al. Praziquantel for treatment of human *Nanophyetus salmincola (Troglotrema salmincola)* infection. J Infect Dis. 1989;160:896–899.
495. Farid Z, Trabolsi B, Boctor F, et al. Unsuccessful use of praziquantel to treat acute fascioliasis in children. J Infect Dis. 1986;154:920–921.
496. Farag HF, Ragab M, Salem A, et al. A short note on praziquantel in human fascioliasis. J Trop Med Hyg. 1986;89:79–80.
497. Botero D, Castano S. Treatment of cysticercosis with praziquantel in Columbia. Am J Trop Med Hyg. 1982;31:811–821.
498. De Ghetaldi LD, Norman RM, Douville AW Jr. Cerebral cysticercosis treated biphasically with dexamethasone and praziquantel. Ann Intern Med. 1983;99: 179–181.
499. Sotelo J, Torres B, Rubio-Donnadieu F, et al. Praziquantel in the treatment of neurocysticercosis: Long-term follow-up. Neurology. 1985;35:752–755.
500. Norman RM, Kapadia C. Cerebral cysticercosis: Treatment with praziquantel. Pediatrics. 1986;78:291–294.
501. Vasconcelos D, Cruz-Segura H, Mateos-Gomez H, et al. Selective indications for the use of praziquantel in the treatment of brain cysticercosis. J Neurol Neurosurg Psychiatry. 1987;50:383–388.
502. Joubert J. Cysticercal meningitis: A pernicious form of neurocysticercosis which responds poorly to praziquantel. S Afr Med J. 1990;77:528–530.
503. Santos R, Chavarria M, Aguirre AE. Failure of medical treatment in two cases of intraocular cysticercosis. Am J Ophthalmol. 1984;97:249–250.
504. Kestelyn P, Taelman H. Effect of praziquantel on intraocular cysticercosis: A case report. Br J Ophthalmol. 1985;69:788–790.
505. Groll E. Praziquantel for cestode infections in man. Acta Trop (Basel). 1980;37:293–296.
506. Heath DD, Lawrence SB. The effect of mebendazole and praziquantel on the cysts of *Echinococcus granulosus, Taenia hydatigena*, and *T. ovis* in sheep. N Z Vet J. 1978;26:11–15.
507. Marshall I, Edwards GT. The effects of sustained release praziquantel on the survival of protoscolices of *Echinococcus granulosus equinus* in laboratory mice. Ann Trop Med Parasitol. 1982;76:649–651.
508. Irie Y, Utsunomiya H, Tanaka M, et al. *Schistosoma japonicum* and *S. mansoni*: Ultrastructural damage in the tegument and reproductive organs after treatment with levo- and dextropraziquantel. Am J Trop Med Hyg. 1989;41:204–211.
509. Staudt U, Schmahl G, Blaschke G, et al. Light and scanning electron microscopy studies on the effects of the enantiomers of praziquantel and its main metabolite on *Schistosoma mansoni* in vitro. Parasitol Res. 1992;78:392–397.
510. Kaojarern S, Nathakarnkikool A, Suvanakoot U. Comparative bioavailability of praziquantel tablets. DICP. 1989;23:29–32.

511. Mandour ME, el Turabli H, Homeida MM, et al. Pharmacokinetics of praziquantel in healthy volunteers and patients with schistosomiasis. Trans R Soc Trop Med Hyg. 1990;84:389–393.
512. Leopold G, Ungethum W, Groll E, et al. Clinical pharmacology in normal volunteers of praziquantel, a new drug against schistosomes and cestodes: An example of a complex study covering both tolerance and pharmacokinetics. Eur J Clin Pharmacol. 1978;14:281–291.
513. Thomas H, Andrews P, Mehlhorn H. New results on the effect of praziquantel in experimental cysticercosis. Am J Trop Med Hyg. 1982;31:803–810.
514. Vazquez ML, Jung H, Sotelo J. Plasma levels of praziquantel decrease when dexamethasone is given simultaneously. Neurology. 1987;37:1561–1562.
515. Jung H, Medina R, Castro N, et al. Pharmacokinetic study of praziquantel administered alone and in combination with cimetidine in a single-day therapeutic regimen. Antimicrob Agents Chemother. 1997;41:1256–1259.
516. Andrews P. Praziquantel: Mechanisms of anti-schistosomal activity. Pharmacol Ther. 1985;29:129–156.
517. Xiao S-H, Friedman PA, Catto BA, et al. Praziquantel-induced vesicle formation in the tegument of male *Schistosoma mansoni* is calcium dependent. J Parasitol. 1984;70:177–179.
518. Gardner DR, Brezden BL. The sites of action of praziquantel in smooth muscle of *Lymnaea stagnalis*. Can J Physiol Pharmacol. 1984;62:282–287.
519. Ruenwongsa P, Hutadilok N, Yuthavong Y. Stimulation of Ca^{2+} uptake in the liver fluke *Opisthorchis viverrini* by praziquantel. Life Sci. 1983;32:2529–2534.
520. Harnett W, Kusel JR. Increased exposure of parasite antigens at the surface of adult *Schistosoma mansoni* exposed to praziquantel in vitro. Parasitology. 1986;93:401–405.
521. Linder E, Thors C. *Schistosoma mansoni*: Praziquantel-induced tegumental lesion exposes actin on surface spines and allows binding of actin depolymerizing factor, gelsolin. Parasitology. 1992;105:71–79.
522. Prichard RK, Bachmann R, Hutchinson GW, et al. The effect of praziquantel on calcium in *Hymenolepis diminuta*. Mol Biochem Parasitol. 1982;5:297–308.
523. Azher M, el-Kassimi FA, Wright SG, et al. Exudative polyserositis and acute respiratory failure following praziquantel therapy. Chest. 1990;98:241–243.
524. Johnson RJ, Jong EC, Dunning SB, et al. Paragonimiasis: Diagnosis and the use of praziquantel in treatment. Rev Infect Dis. 1985;7:200–206.
525. Polderman AM, Gryseels B, Gerold JL, et al. Side effects of praziquantel in the treatment of *Schistosoma mansoni* in Maniema, Zaire. Trans R Soc Trop Med Hyg. 1984;78:752–754.
526. Farid Z, Wallace CK. Schistosomiasis and praziquantel (Letter). Ann Intern Med. 1983;99:883.
527. Watt G, Baldovino PC, Castro JT, et al. Bloody diarrhoea after praziquantel therapy. Trans R Soc Trop Med Hyg. 1986;80:345–346.
528. Markwalder K, Hess K, Valavanis A, et al. Cerebral cysticercosis: Treatment with praziquantel. Am J Trop Med Hyg. 1984;33:273–280.
529. Sotelo J, Escobedo F, Rodriguez-Carbajal J, et al. Therapy of parenchymal brain cysticercosis with praziquantel. N Engl J Med. 1984;310:1001–1007.
530. Montero R, Ostrosky P. Genotoxic activity of praziquantel. Mutat Res. 1997;387:123–139.
531. Diekmann HW, Schneidereit M, Overbosch D. Inhibitory effects of cimetidine, ketoconazole and miconazole on the metabolism of praziquantel. Acta Leidensia. 1989;57:217–228.
532. Cioli D, Pica-Mattoccia L, Archer S. Antischistosomal drugs: Past, present ...and future? Pharmacol Ther. 1995;68:35–38.
533. Davis A, Bailey DR. Metrifonate in urinary schistosomiasis. Bull World Health Organ. 1969;41:209–224.
534. Omer AHS, Teesdale CH. Metrifonate trial in the treatment of various presentations of *Schistosoma haematobium* and *S. mansoni* infections in the Sudan. Ann Trop Med Parasitol. 1978;72:145–150.
535. Feldmeier H, Doehring E, Daffala AA, et al. Efficacy of metrifonate in urinary schistosomiasis: Comparison of reduction of *Schistosoma haematobium* and *S. mansoni* eggs. Am J Trop Med Hyg. 1982;31:1188–1194.
536. Aden Abdi Y, Gustafsson LL. Field trial of the efficacy of a simplified and standard metrifonate treatment of *Schistosoma haematobium*. Eur J Clin Pharmacol. 1989;37:371–374.
537. Nordgren I, Bengtsson E, Holmstedt B, et al. Levels of metrifonate and dichlorvos in plasma and erythrocytes during treatment of schistosomiasis with Bilarcil. Acta Pharmacol Toxicol. 1981;49(Suppl V):79–86.
538. Camacho M, Agnew A. Schistosoma: Rate of glucose import is altered by acetylcholine interaction with tegumental acetylcholine receptors and acetylcholinesterase. Exp Parasitol. 1995;81:584–591.
539. Aden Abdi Y, Gustafsson LL. Poor patient compliance reduces the efficacy of metrifonate treatment of *Schistosoma haematobium* in Somalia. Eur J Clin Pharmacol. 1989;36:161–164.
540. Katz N, Zicker F, Pereira JP. Field trials with oxamniquine in a schistosomiasis mansoni-endemic area. Am J Trop Med Hyg. 1977;26:234–237.
541. Omer AHS. Oxamniquine for treating *Schistosoma mansoni* infection in Sudan. BMJ. 1978;2:163–165.
542. Kilpatrick ME, Farid Z, Bassily S, et al. Treatment of schistosomiasis mansoni with oxamniquine: Five years' experience. Am J Trop Med Hyg. 1981;30:1219–1222.
543. Butterworth AE, Sturrock RF, Ouma JH, et al. Comparison of different chemotherapy strategies against *Schistosoma mansoni* in Machakos District, Kenya: Effects on human infection and morbidity. Parasitology. 1991;103:339–355.
544. Gryseels B, Nkulikyinka L. Two-year follow-up of *Schistosoma mansoni* infection and morbidity after treatment with different regimens of oxamniquine and praziquantel. Trans R Soc Trop Med Hyg. 1989;83:219–228.
545. Katz N, Rocha RS, de Sousa CP, et al. Efficacy of alternating therapy with oxamniquine and praziquantel to treat *Schistosoma mansoni* in children following failure of first treatment. Am J Trop Med Hyg. 1991;44:509–512.
546. Kokwaro GO, Taylor G. Oxamniquine pharmacokinetics in healthy Kenyan African volunteers. East Afr Med J. 1991;68:359–364.
547. Fallon PG, Fookes RE, Wharton GA. Temporal differences in praziquantel and oxamniquine-induced tegumental damage in adult *Schistosoma mansoni*: Implications for drug-antibody synergy. Parasitology. 1996;112:47–58.
548. Pica-Mattoccia L, Novi A, Cioli D. Enzymatic basis for the lack of oxamniquine activity in *Schistosoma haematobium* infections. Parasitol Res. 1997;83:687–689.
549. Bassiouny HK, Soliman NK, el-Daly SM, et al. Human fascioliasis in Egypt: Effect of infection and efficacy of bithionol treatment. J Trop Med Hyg. 1991;94:333–337.
550. Kim JS. Treatment of *Paragonimus westermani* infections with bithionol. Am J Trop Med Hyg. 1970;19:940–942.
551. Pearson RD, Hewlett EL. Niclosamide therapy for tapeworm infections. Ann Intern Med. 1985;102:550–551.
552. Perera DR, Western KA, Schultz MG. Niclosamide treatment of cestodiasis: Clinical trials in the United States. Am J Trop Med Hyg. 1970;19:610–612.
553. Hecht VG, Gloxhuber C. Experimentelle Untersuchungen mit *N*-(2′-Chlor-4′-Nitrophenyl)-5-Chlorsalicylamid, einem neuen Bandwurmmittel: 2. Mitteilung: Toxikologische Untersuchungen. Arzneimittelforschung. 1960;10:884–885.
554. de la Torre RA, de la Rua Barcelo R, Hernandez G, et al. Genotoxic effects of niclosamide in *Aspergillus nidulans*. Mutat Res. 1989;222:337–341.

Chapter 40

Antimicrobial Management and Cost Containment

NEIL O. FISHMAN

The potential for the misuse and abuse of antibiotics was recognized shortly after their introduction into the medical armamentarium in the early 1940s. The introduction of new antibiotics during the next decade increased the inappropriate use of these agents. In his review of the subject in 1956, Jawetz was the first to recognize the problems caused by the attractiveness of new antibiotics to physicians, the exaggerated claims by the pharmaceutical industry, and the enormous impact that promotion by the drug companies had on medical practice.[1] Antimicrobial drugs are the second most commonly used class of drugs in the United States, second only to neurologic agents. Studies have demonstrated that at least one third of all hospitalized patients receive a course of antimicrobial therapy and that approximately 50% of this use is unnecessary or otherwise inappropriate.[2–7] Antibiotic expenditures can account for as much as 30 to 50% of a hospital's total drug budget.[8–10] The rise in the use of antimicrobial agents has resulted in expenditures of greater than $7 billion in the United States. An additional $4 billion is used for treatment of nosocomial infections due to antibiotic-resistant bacteria.[11]

Among the unwanted consequences of antimicrobial therapy are adverse reactions, the emergence of drug-resistant microorganisms, predisposition to secondary infections, and the increased cost of medical care. Broad-spectrum antimicrobial therapy is held responsible, at least in part, for the rising incidence of serious nosocomial infections due to methicillin-resistant *Staphylococcus aureus*, glycopeptide-resistant *S. aureus*, vancomycin-resistant enterococci, extended-spectrum β-lactamase–producing Enterobacteriaceae, and fungi,[12–14] as well as the proliferation of penicillin-resistant pneumococci as a cause of community-acquired upper and lower respiratory tract infections. Therefore, it is not surprising that a number of methods for facilitating more appropriate use of antimicrobials have been developed, including (1) educational programs, sometimes incorporating feedback of information obtained from antimicrobial audits; (2) administrative measures, such as limiting the antimicrobials in a hospital's formulary, using standardized order forms, and requiring justification for the use of particular agents; (3) concurrent monitoring of antimicrobial usage with intervention when misuse is identified; and (4) computer-assisted selection of antibiotics.[15, 16] The potential benefits of such programs are somewhat intuitive and include more discriminate use of new agents, decreased development of antimicrobial resistance, improved education of physicians, improved outcomes in patients (such as decreased drug toxicity and a decreased length of stay), increased nursing availability for direct patient care, and cost containment resulting from a decrease in both direct drug expenditures and associated costs. In this chapter, we review the various antimicrobial management strategies that have been reported in the literature, summarize the clinical and institutional outcomes of these efforts, and end with recommendations for the development, implementation, and funding of a successful antimicrobial management and cost-containment program.

PHILOSOPHY OF ANTIMICROBIAL USE

To address the problem of inappropriate antimicrobial usage, we first must understand the constraints under which physicians work and the pressures that are exerted on them to prescribe drugs. The prescription of antibiotics has become more of a psychological or philosophic endeavor than a scientific exercise. Several factors have been identified that lead to inappropriate use of antimicrobial agents.[17, 18] These include

1. Good intentions. The physician is motivated to give the best treatment, often without regard to cost or the spectrum of activity of the chosen agent.
2. Inappropriate dosing. Some physicians believe that if a small amount of drug is effective, greater and more prolonged administration may be better.
3. Inappropriate prophylaxis. Approximately 30% of patients who receive antibiotics during a hospitalization are given the drugs for a variety of prophylactic purposes, despite limited data supporting the efficacy of such practices. In addition, antimicrobial prophylaxis is continued for greater than 48 hours in 80% of cases.[19]
4. Use of multiple antimicrobial agents or broad-spectrum combinations to cover uncommon organisms. This approach, generalized from management of the neutropenic febrile patient, is often used as a substitute for appropriate diagnostic evaluation.
5. Pressure from the patient to be treated with an antimicrobial agent (most active in adult and pediatric outpatient settings).
6. Time constraints. It is much more time consuming for physicians to explain why they are not prescribing an antibiotic than it is simply to write the prescription.
7. Cost and availability of radiographic studies and diagnostic tests in relation to the ready solution offered by drugs. This varies with practice setting and may be more operative in community hospitals.
8. Inadequacy of the physician's knowledge of diagnostic procedures and management of patients with infectious diseases. This is becoming more important in an era of increasingly complex infectious disease issues, such as acquired immunodeficiency syndrome and infections in oncology patients, transplant recipients, and other immunocompromised hosts.[20]
9. Malpractice considerations and fear of litigation.
10. Easy solutions provided by pharmaceutical manufacturers. The industry exploits the physicians fear of failure and takes advantage of the previously described concerns and problems by offering expensive and often inappropriate panaceas supported by heavy promotion.

In this environment, many physicians feel that antimicrobial control programs impose unnecessary or even deleterious constraints on the practice of medicine.[15] Furthermore, prescribers fail to appreciate that antimicrobial use has significant microbiologic and ecologic consequences that extend beyond the individual patient under their care and can affect their entire practice population.[21] This skepticism most likely arises from the perception that there is a lack of documented efficacy of management programs across varied health care settings, a paucity of direct evidence demonstrating an improvement in clinical outcomes, limited physician time or incentive to pursue such efforts, and a weak causal link between the emergence of resistance and antibiotic use patterns.[22] Although there are no large multicenter randomized controlled trials to address these questions, the preponderance of evidence supports the implementation of such efforts.

ANTIMICROBIAL MANAGEMENT STRATEGIES

As noted, a number of methodologies have been employed to address these issues in an attempt to curb soaring antimicrobial expenditures and to limit the adverse consequences of inappropriate antimicrobial therapy. The various strategies are listed in Table 40–1. In a 1983 survey of 112 hospitals associated with medical schools, Klapp and Ramphal found that 62 of 108 respondents had some form of direct control of antimicrobial usage, either through requirements for authorization by a specialist or through restriction of acceptable indications for the use of particular agents.[23] Implementation has remained relatively stable during the subsequent 15 years. In a 1998 study performed by the Society of Infectious Diseases Pharmacists, 60 respondents from among 225 members indicated some form of antimicrobial management, with a mean of approximately 4.5 different strategies constituting each program.[24] However, a survey of the 47 hospitals participating in phase 3 of Project ICARE (Intensive Care Antimicrobial Resistance Epidemiology) revealed that 62% of participants did not have any restriction mechanisms implemented, supporting the widespread skepticism toward such efforts.[25] John and Fishman recently published a critical review of antimicrobial management strategies that summarized the results of 37 programs and evaluated the strengths and weaknesses of each approach.[26] The emphasis of the programs that were reviewed is illustrated in Figure 40–1. We now consider the data supporting major strategies.

Educational Programs

Although education has long been considered one of the hallmarks of the activities of the infectious diseases physician, it is the least rigorously studied intervention. A variety of approaches have been used over the years, including staff conferences, lectures by visiting professors (grand rounds), clinical pharmacy consultations, drug-utilization evaluations, newsletters, and the development of clinical pathways or guidelines.[27] Inasmuch as there are significant ongoing deficiencies in physicians' knowledge concerning antibiotics and

TABLE 40–1 Antimicrobial Management Strategies
Educational programs
Direct interaction
Performance evaluation
Formal seminars
Newsletters
Antimicrobial formulary restriction
Prior-approval programs
Telephone approval
Antibiotic order forms
Automatic stop orders
Direct interaction
Simple chart entry
Therapeutic substitution and streamlining programs
Costing of items in clinical microbiology laboratory
Purchase plans
Computer-assisted management programs
Antibiotic rotation
Multidisciplinary approaches

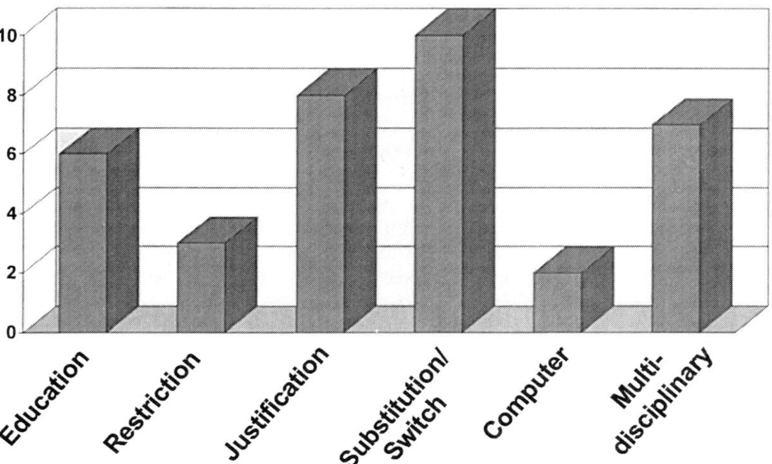

FIGURE 40–1. Emphasis of 37 antimicrobial management programs. (Adapted from John JF, Fishman NO. Programmatic role of the infectious diseases physician in controlling antimicrobial costs in the hospital. Clin Infect Dis. 1997; 24:471.)

inappropriate use remains a problem,[28, 29] it is reasonable to assume that education alone is not an effective method to achieve a long-term impact on prescribing practices. Educational programs are difficult to assess because of the complex nature of educational variables, the diverse nature of various efforts, the lack of standardized feedback, and the intricacy of the infectious diseases decision-making process. Nonetheless, several generalizations can be culled from the existing literature. Individual instruction by an antibiotic-utilization expert appears to be the most successful educational strategy, whereas utilization review is less useful.[26] Contemporaneous interventions have a greater impact than those removed from the original antibiotic order by space and time. However, in the absence of continuous reinforcement, all results extinguish rapidly.[30, 31] Therefore, although education should be the cornerstone of any antimicrobial management program, this approach should not be used as the sole intervention strategy.

Antimicrobial Formulary Restriction

Limiting the availability of agents on formulary is the most direct method to influence antimicrobial utilization; it is a simple way to prohibit the use of newer more expensive antibiotics in favor of older equally effective drugs.[32] The Infectious Diseases Society of America established guidelines for formulary development in 1987 with recommendations to (1) restrict the formulary to the minimal number of agents necessary for effective therapy; (2) eliminate duplicate agents within each class; (3) consider susceptibility patterns of nosocomial pathogens; (4) restrict certain agents on the basis of special indications, toxicity, or excess costs; and (5) conduct periodic reviews. The antimicrobial formulary should be a dynamic, and not a static, document.[33]

One of the landmark studies in this area was published by Woodward and colleagues.[34] Use of a restricted formulary resulted in cost savings of $34,597 per month for restricted agents and $24,620 per month for all antibiotics ($p < 0.03$), with no adverse impact on the clinical outcomes of patients with bacteremia or a variety of other infections. Before implementation, unnecessarily expensive agents were prescribed 37% of the time, compared with just 2% of the time during the study period. Therefore, they were able to demonstrate that the restriction of certain agents could result in significant cost savings without decreasing the quality of patient care. Conversely, a study by Himmelberg and associates evaluated the impact of removing long-standing formulary restrictions at a university hospital.[35] Antimicrobial expenditures escalated by 103% during the study. Imipenem-cilastatin accounted for the greatest proportion of the increase, with costs rising from $44,423 to $126,332 annually, whereas expenditures for unrestricted drugs did not change appreciably. Although the study was not designed to test this hypothesis, the results imply that the increase was due to unnecessary use of formerly restricted agents and not substitution of drugs. Antimicrobial formulary restriction is a simple and effective means of controlling drug costs without resulting in adverse patient outcomes and should be included in most antimicrobial management schemes.

Prior-Approval Programs

Multiple innovative prior-approval or justification approaches have been designed to improve the utilization of antibiotics. These include telephone-approval mechanisms, antibiotic order forms, automatic stop orders, direct interaction with an antimicrobial management team, implementation of control categories, and simple chart entry.

McGowan and Finland were the first to use telephone calls for justification by prescribers and approval by infectious diseases physicians to limit the use of systemic antimicrobial agents.[36] Most approvals were given by telephone, and formal consultation was generally not required. Chloramphenicol prescription rates demonstrated the most dramatic results of this program, with annual usage decreasing from 20,000 to 3000 g. Recco and colleagues were the first to demonstrate the economic impact of a prior-approval program.[37] These researchers also utilized a telephone-approval mechanism, but disagreements necessitated consultation with an infectious diseases physician. A concomitant educational program was implemented as well. Antimicrobial expenditures decreased by $131,826 during the first year, and savings were sustained during the initial 3 years reported in the study. Additionally, inappropriate use of antibiotics was curtailed significantly. Antibiotic order forms also have effected similar improvements in the use of anti-infectives for empirical and prophylactic purposes.[38] However, order forms should be used in conjunction with a restricted formulary, and the forms should be reviewed regularly to document reporting accuracy.

The final landmark study in this category was conducted by Coleman and colleagues and was the first effort to critically analyze reductions in antibiotic expenditures in a long-term fashion among many different clinical syndromes.[39] They collected baseline data for 18 months before instituting four categories of restricted usage (cephalosporins, penicillins, aminoglycosides, and miscellaneous agents) and maximal dosage guidelines for seven drugs. Additionally, a review of treatment plans was required before the pharmacy could distribute drugs. The program yielded savings of $7600 per month ($91,200 annually). The doses and cost of antibiotics decreased for pneumonia, urinary tract infection, and septicemia, but increased for cellulitis. The cost per treatment day, the cost per admission, the total number of doses, and the percentage of the reimbursement rate as set by the United States Health Care and Financing Administration all differed significantly from those in the prestudy period. The length of therapy did not differ between the pre- and postrestriction intervals. The most significant decreases in use were seen with cefoxitin and clindamycin, whereas the largest increases were demonstrated with ticarcillin-clavulanate and cefotetan.

Obviously, enforcement of a prior-approval program can be difficult, and the process may be viewed as a punitive exercise. Therefore, it is important to stress that the major goal of such efforts is to improve the care of patients. Although these strategies are the most onerous to prescribing physicians, they undoubtedly are the most effective single interventions to improve usage patterns and to control the antimicrobial budget.[26]

Therapeutic Substitution and Streamlining Programs

In private practices, infectious diseases physicians are not enthusiastic about policies restricting antibiotics because of concerns that the policies will place them in a policing role and thereby damage their traditional referral patterns.[40] Therapeutic-substitution and streamlining programs may offer a less dictatorial option; however, they are less likely to be as strictly enforced as formulary restriction and prior-approval programs. The two most common approaches involve the substitution of a member of a class of drugs with a less expensive therapeutic equivalent, and the change to a different class of agents, frequently with the aim of switching from parenteral to oral therapy. The benefits of switch therapy have been well documented in the management of pulmonary infections. Studies demonstrate significant savings in drug costs, as well as decreased lengths of stay.[41] One report also identified an unexpected cost avoidance associated with a decreased incidence of catheter-related infections.[42]

Quintiliani and colleagues at Hartford Hospital have been leaders in the area of streamlining programs, incorporating a variety of these strategies.[43] Additionally, they have introduced innovative altered-dosing schemes based on pharmacodynamic principles. For example, 4 g of piperacillin administered every 8 hours has preferable pharmacodynamics compared with 5 g of mezlocillin given every 8 hours. This switch would yield cost savings of approximately $17,000 annually.[44] However, it is difficult to generalize the findings in this area because reports frequently focus on different specific agents and the interventions vary significantly from study to study.

Nonetheless, a streamlining program at Maine Medical Center has been evaluated in a randomized controlled trial, with promising results.[45] Patients receiving 1 or more of 10 designated parenteral antibiotics for 3 days or more were randomized to either an intervention or a control group. The intervention group received antibiotic-related suggestions from a team consisting of an infectious diseases fellow and a clinical pharmacist. Sixty-two (49%) of the intervention group patients received a total of 74 recommendations, and 84% of these were implemented. The majority involved changes in the choice of antibiotic, dosing regimen, or route of administration. Antibiotic charges were $400 less per patient in the intervention group, extrapolating to annual savings of $390,000. Furthermore, there was no difference in clinical outcomes between the two groups. Despite these intriguing findings, it is important to remember that overall therapeutic substitution and streamlining programs generally are less efficient as a sole antimicrobial management strategy. However, they are effective adjuncts to restriction and prior-approval programs.

Computer-Assisted Management Programs

The computer has the potential to be the ultimate method for antibiotic stewardship and education. Computer order entry affords a unique opportunity for instantaneous feedback, education, and alteration in prescription patterns. A group of researchers headed by Burke and Classen at the LDS Hospital in Salt Lake City have been the leaders in developing this field.[46] They developed a computerized decision-support program that is linked to computer-based patient records. The program presents epidemiologic information, detailed information, and warnings and assists in the selection of anti-infective regimens and courses of therapy for patients.

The system has been prospectively studied for 1 year in a 12-bed intensive care unit.[16] When compared with the management of patients admitted to the same unit during the 2 years before the intervention period, computer-assisted antimicrobial selection led to significant reductions in orders for drugs to which the patient had reported allergies (35 versus 146; $p < 0.01$), excess drug dosages (87 versus 405; $p < 0.01$), and mismatches of antibiotic susceptibility (12 versus 206, $p < 0.01$). There were also marked reductions in the mean number of days of excessive drug dosage and in adverse events caused by antimicrobial agents. Additionally, those patients treated with regimens that were recommended by the computer program demonstrated significant reductions in anti-infective costs, total hospital costs, and the length of stay compared with the control groups. This computer-assisted management program can improve the quality of patient care and reduce costs. Unfortunately, the results cannot be generalized inasmuch as the program is not readily available to other institutions. However, the approaches taken and lessons learned during the development of this system should be used as a paradigm for the design of similar programs.

Multidisciplinary Approaches

The review by John and Fishman readily demonstrates that multidisciplinary programs offer the best potential for sustained improvements in both clinical and economic outcomes.[26] Annualized cost savings with or without the inclusion of estimates of cost avoidance began at $7440 for programs with a single target but increased to $483,032 for comprehensive multidisciplinary efforts. These savings can be sustained for greater than 3 years.[47] Furthermore, approaches that utilized four or more strategies appeared to be the most effective. For example, the Antimicrobial Management Program at Hartford Hospital emphasizes formulary streamlining reinforced by formulary restriction and review, antibiotic order forms, and educational efforts.[32] Additionally, such programs tend to be more readily accepted because they involve input from a variety of hospital services, including the departments of infectious diseases, clinical pharmacy, infection control, clinical microbiology, nursing, and hospital administration. The team approach supports the implementation of multiple strategies and offers the best option for sustained success.[48] The survey by the Society of Infectious Diseases Pharmacists indicates that most centers are taking this approach when designing management efforts (Fig. 40–2).[24]

OUTCOMES OF ANTIMICROBIAL MANAGEMENT PROGRAMS

In assessing whether comprehensive antimicrobial management programs are effective, one must consider both clinical and institutional (economic) outcomes. Although the preponderance of evidence supports the positive impact of such efforts, it is important to recognize that the literature likely presents a skewed view of this topic since negative studies are underrepresented.

Clinical Outcomes

The best evidence for improved clinical outcomes resulting from an antimicrobial management strategy comes from the computerized antibiotic assistant at LDS Hospital in Salt Lake City that was discussed earlier.[16] Additional data come from a retrospective review before and after the initiation of a prior-approval program at Indiana University Medical Center.[49] In this review, Frank and coworkers found statistically significant decreases in the rates of enterococcal bacteremia (0.34 versus 0.16 events per 1000 patient-days), selected

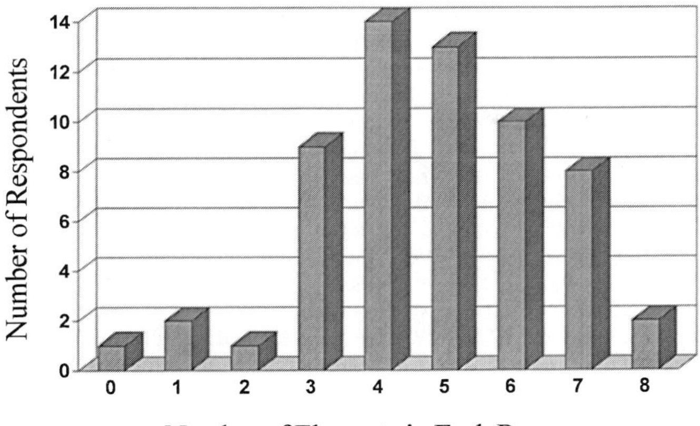

FIGURE 40–2. Distribution of the number of different strategies employed by antimicrobial management programs responding to the Society of Infectious Diseases Pharmacists antibiotic management survey. (From Society of Infectious Diseases Pharmacists homepage. http://165.6.9.23.)

gram-negative bacteremias (0.26 versus 0.11), methicillin-resistant *S. aureus* colonization or infection (0.66 versus 0.20), and *Stenotrophomonas* colonization or infection (0.35 versus 0.17). The program also resulted in a decrease in antimicrobial expenditures from $2,486,902 to $1,701,522. The effort resulted in improved clinical outcomes in the form of significant decreases in rates of selected nosocomial infections due to resistant organisms coupled with substantial cost savings.

Further support can be found in the results of a randomized controlled trial designed to assess the clinical and economic outcomes of a comprehensive antimicrobial management program compared with usual practice at the Hospital of the University of Pennsylvania.[50] A summary of the results of the univariate analysis is shown in Table 40–2. The program resulted in an improved cure rate, a decreased failure rate, and more appropriate use of antimicrobial agents as judged by adherence to institutional guidelines. There also was a trend toward decreased emergence of resistant nosocomial pathogens. Although a large multicenter trial of various interventions is lacking, the majority of published evidence demonstrates a beneficial impact of antimicrobial management programs on patient outcomes.

Economic Outcomes

It is clear from the discussion of antimicrobial management strategies that most published reports demonstrate successful cost containment. However, if savings are calculated as a function of pharmacy expenditures, they tend to plateau over time; this likely is a function of improved antimicrobial-utilization practices and sustained benefits of the program. In order to address this issue, Kinky and colleagues developed a probability-pathway model to calculate both the direct and the indirect cost savings of a management program.[50] In this model, total cost was defined as the sum of drug expenditures, microbiology costs, bed costs, and the costs of infectious diseases consultations; additional costs accrued if the initial antibiotic regimen failed. The median drug costs per recommendation were $50 lower for the antimicrobial management program compared with usual practice, and total costs were $379 lower per recommendation. Using the probability-pathway model, this annualizes to savings of $363,000 in antibiotic expenditures and $2.7 million in total costs.

TABLE 40–2 Clinical Outcomes of a Comprehensive Antimicrobial Management Program

Outcome	AMP (n = 96)	UP (n = 96)	RR (95% CI)
Cure	52 (54%)	34 (35%)	1.50 (1.10–2.10)
Failure	5 (5%)	18 (19%)	0.17 (0.07–0.43)
Appropriate	86 (90%)	30 (31%)	2.90 (2.10–3.90)
Resistance	1 (1%)	9 (9%)	0.13 (0.02–1.0)

Abbreviations: AMP, Antimicrobial management program; CI, confidence intervals; RR, risk ratio; UP, usual practice.
Adapted from Kinky DE, Gross R, Morgan AS, et al. Clinical and economic outcomes of a comprehensive antimicrobial management program (Abstract). Clin Infect Dis. 1998;27:926.

DO ANTIMICROBIAL MANAGEMENT PROGRAMS PREVENT THE EMERGENCE OF RESISTANCE?

The effectiveness of antimicrobial control as a means to prevent the emergence of resistance has been reviewed in detail. Available studies are suggestive but not conclusive about the efficacy of this approach.[51, 52] The shortcomings of published studies include the presence of selection biases, a small sample size, a limitation to single institutions, and a failure to control for confounding variables.[21] However, recent limited data suggest benefits from attention to inappropriate antimicrobial utilization.

White and colleagues instituted a prior-authorization program in response to an epidemic of multidrug-resistant *Acinetobacter,* in the surgical intensive care unit of their institution, that did not respond to routine infection-control interventions. Susceptibilities to all β-lactam and fluoroquinolone antibiotics increased, with dramatically increased susceptibilities in isolates recovered in intensive care units, increased susceptibilities in isolates recovered in other inpatient sites, and little change in susceptibilities in isolates recovered in outpatient sites.[53] These changes occurred despite a lack of variation in infection-control practices. Additionally, antimicrobial expenditures decreased by 32%, and neither patient outcomes nor the length of hospital stay were compromised.

Additional support of a positive correlation between limiting antibiotic use and preventing the emergence of resistance can be found in the Finnish experience with group A streptococci.[54] In the early 1990s, there was an increase in erythromycin resistance among this organism in Finland. In response, nationwide recommendations were issued that called for reductions in the use of macrolides for respiratory and skin infections in outpatients. Consumption of macrolide antibiotics decreased from 2.40 defined daily doses per 1000 inhabitants per day in 1991 to 1.38 in 1992 (p = 0.007). The change in consumption was followed by a steady decrease in the frequency of erythromycin resistance among group A streptococcal isolates from throat swabs and pus samples.

These reports are preliminary, but promising. They suggest that attention to antimicrobial use may produce a favorable impact on the emergence of resistance. Further work is needed to evaluate the role that infection control and community factors play in other institutions, including acute care settings and long-term care facilities.[21]

ADDITIONAL QUESTIONS

It is not clear whether homogeneity in antibiotic prescribing is good or bad. Several authors have suggested that reducing the heterogeneity in antimicrobial use may be more harmful than beneficial.[20, 55] If this is the case, clinical guidelines, formulary systems, and antimicrobial restriction may promote the emergence of resistant organisms. These concerns have led to the suggestion that antibiotics be rotated or cycled in the various hospital units. Guidelines have been developed,[56] but there are few data available to help assess the potential impact of such schemes.

Kollef and colleagues switched empirical therapy of suspected gram-negative infections in cardiac surgery from ceftazidime to ciprofloxacin at 6-month intervals. Subsequently, they demonstrated a decrease in the incidence of ventilator-associated pneumonia from 11.6 to 6.7%; pneumonia caused by antibiotic-resistant gram-negative bacilli decreased from 4 to 0.9%. Although there was a trend toward a lower incidence of bacteremia with resistant gram-negative organisms, the total incidence of bacteremia did not decline.[57] Additionally, the use of postoperative antibiotics did not decrease despite fewer suspected and proven infections during the study period; this may indicate an increase in inappropriate use. Many more questions are engendered than answered in this study. At least one additional report failed to exhibit any benefit of a rotation scheme.[58] The identification of the correct antibiotics to be cycled, the duration of cycles, and the preferred order of rotation all remain unknown. There is little evidence to support the routine rotation or cycling of antimicrobial agents.

DESIGN AND IMPLEMENTATION

A summary of guidelines for the design and implementation of a successful antimicrobial management program is listed in Table 40–3 and described in this section.[26]

1. Define the philosophy of the program. This may seem to be a trivial step, but the initial approach defined at this early time is likely to form the foundation for the success or failure of the program. Although most physicians generally understand that resistance is important, increasing in scope, and costly, they do not necessarily agree that the care of individual patients affects this issue. However, antibiotic misuse more often results from inadequate information than from inappropriate behavior.[20] Therefore, physicians are more likely to respond to a program designed to "improve" antibiotic use or patient care, rather than to an effort to "restrict" or "control" antimicrobials or solely to decrease costs. Most physicians will alter their behavior to improve the quality of patient care. (J. E. McGowan, Jr, personal communication.)
2. Gather baseline data concerning antimicrobial expenditures, antimicrobial-utilization patterns, and susceptibilities of nosocomial and community pathogens. Benchmark the antimicrobial budget to equivalent institutions.
3. Define the structure of participation in the antimicrobial management program. An example of a comprehensive program is diagrammed in Figure 40–3. The minimal-requirements for an effective team include an infectious diseases physician, an infectious diseases clinical pharmacist, the director of clinical microbiology, and the hospital epidemiologist.
4. Develop a budget for all official positions and operating costs.
5. Involve hospital administrators early in the design and implementation process, and clarify budgetary issues. Agree upon a formula to calculate cost savings. It may be prudent to involve managed care organizations in these discussions if they are at risk for pharmacy costs. The support of key officials is critical to the success of the program. Physicians are more likely to comply with a health system effort rather than with an infectious diseases or pharmacy program that may be perceived to have predominantly financial motives. Maintain an open dialogue with chief administrative personnel and update them frequently concerning the progress of the program.

TABLE 40–3 Guidelines for the Design and Implementation of an Antimicrobial Management Program

Define philosophy of program
Gather baseline data
Define structure of program
Develop budget
Meet with hospital administrators
Evaluate antimicrobial formulary for redundancy
Develop and publish guidelines for antimicrobial use
Define intervention strategies
Develop mechanisms to arbitrate disagreements
Develop innovative educational methods
Develop and maintain database
Continuously reevaluate program

6. Evaluate the antimicrobial formulary for redundancy and seek competitive bidding between therapeutic equivalents.
7. Develop and publish guidelines for antibiotic use and empirical antimicrobial therapy. Recommendations should be based on local susceptibility profiles. Additionally, establish appropriate dosing and dosage intervals based on disease-state and pharmacokinetic principles. This step is critical to the success of the program. Involve key personnel from all departments when designing the guidelines in order to build consensus for the program. Be willing to compromise on certain issues, but demand that all recommendations be evidence based. It is also worthwhile to consider multimedia formats. For example, we have posted our guidelines on the Internet and have included links to relevant articles, as well as other educational materials.[59] It is also useful to publish reports of antimicrobial susceptibility and price lists along with the clinical guidelines.
8. Define the strategies that the program will use. As previously discussed, multidisciplinary efforts offer the greatest potential for sustained improvements. However, interventions must be tailored to the character of the institution. For example, telephone-approval mechanisms are less likely to be successful at a community hospital staffed by busy private practitioners. Begin with a focus on the most frequently used and most costly agents.
9. Develop mechanisms to arbitrate disagreements. A discussion between the prescriber and the director of the program is usually sufficient, if the director has administrative time to handle these issues. A mandatory infectious diseases consultation is another viable option.
10. Develop innovative educational methods. We have found the Internet to be a useful tool in this regard.[59] Information systems personnel may be helpful in incorporating guidelines, recommendations, or reminders into the hospital computer network.
11. Develop and maintain a database to follow clinical and institutional outcomes.
12. Continuously reevaluate the program, paying particular attention to changes in susceptibility profiles and patterns of use. Drug-utilization evaluations should be a part of this process. Reformulate the program as indicated to address problems as they arise. This should be a dynamic process that is responsive to the needs of prescribers and their patients.

FUNDING

It is clear from the data presented previously that the cost savings from comprehensive antimicrobial management efforts can easily offset the budget of the program. Minimal requirements include support by a part-time physician and a full-time clinical pharmacist. New salary lines for antimicrobial management are beginning to emerge nationally.[26] There are three options for support: (1) defined compensation; (2) payment on a time basis for consultative services; and (3) negotiation for a percentage of the cost savings. Toward this end, it is critical to gather baseline data and to define a formula to calculate cost savings before implementing a program. The method and amount of compensation will vary with the size and setting of the program. Managed care organizations may offer additional options for funding, particularly if the program expands to the ambulatory setting or oversees devices used to treat infections.

THE FUTURE

Health care is changing. Providers are challenged to deliver high-quality care in an increasingly cost-constrained environment. This requires limiting cost-increasing technology while improving patient and population health outcomes. Although the data are limited, comprehensive antimicrobial management programs have the potential to decrease costs while improving both patient and institutional outcomes. However, further work is needed to clearly identify the relationship between antimicrobial use and the emergence of resis-

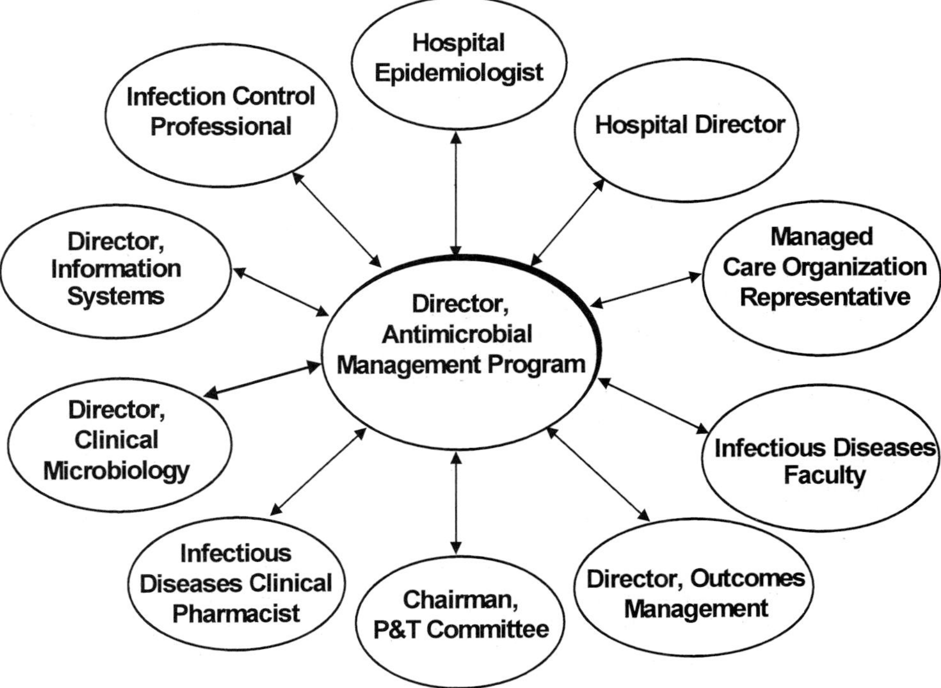

FIGURE 40–3. Organizational structure of a comprehensive antimicrobial management program. (Adapted from John JF Jr, Fishman NO. Programmatic role of the infectious diseases physician in controlling antimicrobial costs in the hospitals. Clin Infect Dis. 1997;24:471.)

tance in a way that colleagues will appreciate and accept.[60] Relevant studies will require sufficient statistical power to describe baseline resistance, to deal with limits of random variation, and to control for a multitude of confounding variables (personal communication, J. E. McGowan, Jr.). It is likely that a multicenter trial will be necessary to accomplish these tasks.

In addition, we also must begin to focus on issues of antimicrobial use and the emergence of resistance throughout the entire health care system. As these systems expand and become a prominent feature of medical practice in the United States, it is no longer sufficient to consider infection solely in the context of the acute care hospital. Rather, health care must be viewed in the larger context of acute care, extended care, and ambulatory components of the integrated delivery system.[21] Therefore, future efforts to improve the use of antimicrobial agents and studies to document efficacy must be expanded to include these arenas.

REFERENCES

1. Jawetz E. Antimicrobial chemotherapy. Annu Rev Microbiol. 1956;10:85.
2. Achong MR, Hauser BA, Krusky JL. Rational and irrational use of antibiotics in a Canadian teaching hospital. Can Med Assoc J. 1977;116:256.
3. Kunin CM, Tupasi T, Craig WA. Use of antibiotics: A brief exposition of the problem and some tentative solutions. Ann Intern Med. 1973;79:555.
4. Kunin CM. The responsibility of the infectious disease community for the optimal use of antimicrobial agents. J Infect Dis. 1985;151:388.
5. Maki DG, Schuna AA. A study of antimicrobial misuse in a university hospital. Am J Med Sci. 1978;275:271.
6. Roberts AW, Visconti JA. The rational and irrational use of systemic antimicrobial drugs. Am J Hosp Pharm. 1972;29:828.
7. Scheckler WE, Bennett JV. Antibiotic use in seven community hospitals. JAMA. 1970;213:264.
8. Col NF, O'Connor RW. Estimating world-wide current antibiotic usage; report of task force. 1. Rev Infect Dis. (Suppl) 1987;9:S232.
9. Craig WA, Sarver KP. Antimicrobial usage in the USA. In: Williams JD, Geddes AM, eds. Chemotherapy, v. 4. New York: Plenum; 1976:293.
10. Craig WA, Uman SJH, Shaw WR, et al. Hospital use of antimicrobial drugs: Survey of 19 hospitals and results of antimicrobial control programs. Ann Intern Med. 1978;89:793.
11. Office of Technology Assessment USC. Impacts of Antibiotic-Resistant Bacteria. Washington, DC: Government Printing Office; 1995.
12. McGowan JE Jr. Antimicrobial resistance in hospital organisms and its relation to antibiotic use. Rev Infect Dis. 1983;5:1033.
13. McGowan JE Jr. Changing etiology of nosocomial bacteremia and fungemia and other hospital-acquired infections. Rev Infect Dis. 1985;7(Suppl):S357.
14. Archibald L, Phillips L, Monnet D, et al. Antimicrobial resistance in isolates from inpatients and outpatients in the United States: Increasing importance of the intensive care unit. Clin Infect Dis. 1997;24:211.
15. Dunagan WC, Medoff G. Formulary control of antimicrobial usage: What price freedom? Diagn Microbiol Infect Dis. 1993;16:265.
16. Evans RS, Pestotnik SL, Classen DC, et al. A computer-assisted management program for antibiotics and other antiinfective agents. N Engl J Med. 1998;338:232.
17. Kunin CM. Problems in antibiotic usage. In: Mandell GL, Douglas RG Jr, Bennett JE, eds. Principles and Practice of Infectious Diseases. 3rd ed. New York: Churchill Livingstone; 1990;427.
18. Centers for Disease Control and Prevention. Defining the public health impact of drug-resistant *Streptococcus pneumoniae:* Report of a working group. MMWR Morb Mortal Wkly Rep. 1996;45(RR-1):1–14.
19. Shapiro M, Townsend TR, Rosner B, Kass EH. Use of antimicrobial drugs in general hospitals: Patterns of prophylaxis. N Engl J Med. 1979;301:351.
20. Burke JP. Antibiotic resistance—squeezing the balloon? JAMA. 1998;280:1270.
21. McGowan JE Jr, Tenover FC. Control of antimicrobial resistance in the health care system. Infect Dis Clin North Am. 1997;11:297.
22. Phillips I. Lessons from the past: A personal view. Clin Infect Dis. 1998;27(Suppl):S2.
23. Klapp DL, Ramphal R. Antibiotic restriction in hospitals associated with medical schools. Am J Hosp Pharm. 1983;40:1957.
24. Society of Infectious Diseases Pharmacists homepage. http://165.6.9.23.
25. Fridkin SK, Lawton RM, Gaynes RP, et al. Antimicrobial control practices at 47 US hospitals: Are we doing enough (Abstract)? Clin Infect Dis. 1998;27:1049.
26. John JF, Fishman NO. Programmatic role of the infectious diseases physician in controlling antimicrobial costs in the hospital. Clin Infect Dis. 1997;24:471.
27. Kunin CM, Johansen KS, Worning AM, Daschner FD. Report of a symposium on use and abuse of antibiotics worldwide. Rev Infect Dis. 1990;12:12.
28. Neu HC, Howrey SP. Testing the physician's knowledge of antibiotic use: Self-assessment and learning via videotape. N Engl J Med. 1975;293:1291.
29. Barclay LP, Hation RH, Doering PL, Shands JW. Physicians' perceptions and knowledge of drag costs: Results of a survey. Formulary. 1995;30:268.
30. Gilbert DN, Eubanks NM, Jackson JM. The effects of monitoring the use of gentamicin in a community hospital. J Med Educ. 1978;53:129.
31. Jones SR, Pannell J, Barks J, et al. The effect of an educational program upon hospital antibiotic use. Am J Med Sci. 1977;273:79.
32. Crowe HM, Quintiliani R. Antibiotic formulary selection. Med Clin North Am. 1995;79:463.
33. Marr JJ, Moffet HL, Kunin CM. Guidelines for improving the use of antimicrobial agents in hospitals: A statement by the Infectious Diseases Society of America. J Infect Dis. 1987;157:869.
34. Woodward RS, Medoff G, Smith MD, Gray JL III. Antibiotic cost savings from

formulary restrictions and physician monitoring in a medical school–affiliated hospital. Am J Med. 1987;83:817.
35. Himmelberg CJ, Pleasants RA, Weber DJ, et al. Use of antimicrobial drugs before and after removal of a restriction policy. Am J Hosp Pharm. 1991;48:1220.
36. McGowan JE Jr, Finland M. Usage of antibiotics in a general hospital: Effect of requiring justification. J Infect Dis. 1974;130:165.
37. Recco RA, Gladstone JL, Friedman SA, Gerken EH. Antibiotic control in a municipal hospital. JAMA. 1979;241:2283.
38. Durbin WA Jr, Lapidas B, Goldmann DA. Improved antibiotic usage following introduction of a novel prescription system. JAMA. 1981;246:1796.
39. Coleman RW, Rodondi LC, Kaubisch S, et al. Cost-effectiveness of prospective and continuous parenteral antibiotic control: Experience at the Palo Alto Veterans Affairs Medical Center from 1987 to 1989. Am J Med. 1991;90:439.
40. Pelletier LL Jr. Hospital usage of parenteral antimicrobial agents: A gradated utilization review and cost containment program. Infect Control. 1985;6:226.
41. Ehrenkranz NJ, Nerenberg DE, Shultz JM, Slater KC. Intervention to discontinue parenteral antimicrobial therapy in patients hospitalized with pulmonary infections: Effect on shortening patient stay. Infect Control Hosp Epidemiol. 1992;13:21.
42. Ramirez JA. Switch therapy in community-acquired pneumonia. Diagn Microbiol Infect Dis. 1995;22:219.
43. Nightingale CH, Quintiliani R, Nicolau DP. Intelligent dosing of antimicrobials. In: Remington JS, Swartz MN, eds. Current Clinical Topics in Infectious Diseases, v. 14. Boston: Blackwell Scientific; 1994:252.
44. Quintiliani R, Nightingale CH, Sullivan MC. Use of pharmacodynamic concepts in developing a cost-effective dosing method for piperacillin. Clin Ther. 1993;15(Suppl):S44.
45. Fraser GL, Stogsdill P, Dickens JD Jr, et al. Antibiotic optimization: An evaluation of patient safety and economic outcomes. Arch Intern Med. 1997;157:1689.
46. Evans RS, Classen DC, Pestotnik SL, et al. Improving empiric antibiotic selection using computer decision support. Arch Intern Med. 1994;154:878.
47. Fletcher CV, Metzler D, Borchardt-Phelps P, Rodman JH. Patterns of antibiotic use and expenditures during 7 years at a university hospital. Pharmacotherapy. 1990;10:199.
48. Schentag JJ, Ballow CH, Fritz AL, et al. Changes in antimicrobial agent usage resulting from interactions among clinical pharmacy, the infectious diseases division, and the microbiology laboratory. Diagn Microbiol Infect Dis. 1993;16:255.
49. Frank MO, Batteiger BE, Sorensen SJ, et al. Decrease in expenditures and selected nosocomial infections following implementation of an antimicrobial-prescribing improvement program. Perform Quality Health Care. 1997;5:180.
50. Kinky DE, Gross R, Morgan AS, et al. Clinical and economic outcomes of a comprehensive antimicrobial management program (Abstract). Clin Infect Dis. 1998;27:926.
51. McGowan JE Jr. Do intensive hospital antibiotic control programs prevent the spread of antibiotic resistance? Infect Control Hosp Epidemiol. 1994;15:478.
52. McGowan JE Jr, Gerding DN. Does antibiotic restriction prevent resistance? New Horiz. 1996;4:370.
53. White AC Jr, Atmar RL, Wilson J, et al. Effects of requiring prior authorization for selected antimicrobials: Expenditures, susceptibilities, and clinical outcomes. Clin Infect Dis. 1997;25:230.
54. Seppala H, Klaukka T, Vuopio-Varkila J, et al. The effect of changes in the consumption of macrolide antibiotics on erythromycin resistance in group A streptococci in Finland. N Engl J Med. 1997;337:441.
55. Schentag JJ, Hyatt JM, Carr JR, et al. Genesis of methicillin-resistant *Staphylococcus aureus* (MRSA), how treatment of MRSA infections has selected for vancomycin-resistant *Enterococcus faecium*, and the importance of antibiotic management and infection control. Clin Infect Dis. 1998;26:1204.
56. Sanders WEJ, Sanders CC. Circumventing antibiotic resistance in specialized hospital units. Clin Microbiol Infect. 1997;3:272.
57. Kollef MH, Vlasnik J, Sharpless L, et al. Scheduled change of antibiotic classes: A strategy to decrease the incidence of ventilator-associated pneumonia. Am J Crit Care Med. 1997;156:1040.
58. Moss W, Beers C, McFarlane G, et al. Impact of antibiotic cycling on infection and colonization with antibiotic-resistant bacteria in a pediatric ICU (abstract). Clin Infect Dis. 1998;27:963.
59. Fishman N, Morgan A, Green S, Edelstein PH. Guidelines for antimicrobial therapy at the hospital of the University of Pennsylvania, 1998 ed. 18 February 1998. Available at http://www.med.upenn.edu/bugdrug/.
60. Moellering RC Jr. Antibiotic resistance: Lessons for the future. Clin Infect Dis. 1998;27(Suppl):S135.

Chapter **41**

Outpatient Intravenous Antibiotic Therapy

ALAN D. TICE

BACKGROUND

Intravenous therapy was developed in hospitals and was considered an exclusively hospital procedure until 1974, when Rucker reported the outpatient treatment of respiratory infections in cystic fibrosis patients with intravenous antibiotics.[1] Since then, outpatient care has evolved to include provision of intravenous antibiotics, parenteral nutrition, and chemotherapy in patients' homes, in infusion clinics, and in physicians' offices.

The growth of outpatient parenteral antimicrobial therapy (OPAT) has been largely attributable to rising costs of hospitalization, which currently average a thousand dollars per day.[2] This economic stimulus aside, however, home care offers a number of quality-of-life advantages over hospitalization, including the presence of family and friends, privacy, and home-cooked food. For children and some elderly people, the hospital can be a particularly stressful and frightening environment. Outpatient care requires greater involvement of the patient and family in the treatment process, resulting in improved understanding of the disease. This participatory approach to medical care fosters greater appreciation of the health care process, reduces the likelihood of future infections, and contributes to a positive clinical outcome.

The managed care industry is very much interested in OPAT and outpatient care in general because it provides an unusual opportunity to reduce costs while improving the quality of care and patient satisfaction.[3] However, the outpatient setting represents a challenge to today's physicians, who are no longer familiar with medical care beyond the confines of the hospital and their offices.[4] Now, as patient care moves more and more into the community, OPAT offers models for clinicians to consider in the treatment of their patients with serious infections who need intravenous antibiotics yet are otherwise able to be treated at home. Many of these patients are able to return to work or school during OPAT and hence can earn as well as save money.[5, 6] OPAT may also reduce the morbidity, mortality, and cost of nosocomial infections.

MODELS OF DELIVERY

There are three basic models of delivery of OPAT: the visiting nurse, the infusion center, and self-administration (Table 41–1).[7] The visiting nurse model is effective when there is an established home care agency that can provide medication at home under the supervision of a nurse. A home visit may be very revealing in regard to the underlying diseases and social problems of the patient but has become expensive compared with the other models. An infusion center can be established in almost any setting, including a physician's office, a clinic, or a hospital emergency department, or it may be freestanding. Such centers offer the ready availability of physicians and nurses as well as a supply of medications and equipment should there be a problem with vascular access or the need to change the antibiotic. The self-administration model has been made possible through the use of reliable vascular access catheters and infusion devices that can be programmed to administer medications as reliably as in the hospital and for days at a time.

INFECTIONS TREATED

The list of diseases amenable to OPAT is long (Table 41–2), but the study of this form of therapy is limited.[8] As OPAT has evolved, the

TABLE 41–1 Models of Outpatient Parenteral Antibiotic Therapy

Model	Advantages	Disadvantages
Visiting nurse	Home evaluation	Cost of nurse's time and travel
	Supervised drug administration	Concerns with privacy
Infusion center	Medical staff on hand	Cost of facility
	Access to medications and devices	Patient's travel to clinic
	Supervised administration	
Self-administration	Reduced facility cost	Patient and/or caregiver training
	Patient autonomy	Compliance
		Unsupervised administration

question of which infections can be treated has become more a matter of which cannot. In fact, it seems that virtually every infection that requires intravenous antibiotic therapy can be treated outside the hospital for at least part of the therapeutic course. However, some infections require initial hospitalization.[8, 9] For example, patients with meningitis, endocarditis, or possible sepsis should be hospitalized immediately on presentation. If they have a good response to initial treatment, however, even they can often be discharged to complete the course of therapy as outpatients.

Central nervous system infections are of particular concern because of the potential for neurologic injury and the need for prompt, high-dose antibiotic therapy. Seizures are an added concern for patients with a brain abscess, who should receive prophylactic anticonvulsant therapy. Children with meningitis who have had a good clinical response can safely complete their therapy at home if they meet specific criteria.[10]

Bacterial endocarditis was one of the first infections to be treated on an outpatient basis given the requirement for 4 to 6 weeks of intravenous therapy. Although a number of studies have reported the safety and effectiveness of OPAT for endocarditis, some precautions and questions remain.[11] A number of potentially complicating factors may discourage, if not contraindicate, the use of OPAT for endocarditis. These may include *Staphylococcus aureus* infection, particularly on the left side of the heart; conduction abnormalities; the development of a thrombus with a potential for embolus; and heart failure requiring early surgical intervention.[12–15]

Osteomyelitis is another infection for which OPAT has been useful.[16] It also often requires a prolonged course of intravenous therapy in patients who are otherwise well. Osteomyelitis was first treated in the hospital with early discharge after surgical intervention. In many communities, however, patients may be started directly on OPAT with elective admissions only if surgery is indicated or the patient fails to respond to outpatient care. Although some of the new oral quinolones have replaced intravenous therapy for gram-negative osteomyelitis, bacteria resistant to oral antimicrobials and gram-positive organisms remain a challenge. Studies that equate oral and intravenous therapy for osteomyelitis are not yet convincing, particularly where *S. aureus* is involved.[17] Surgical intervention is always an important consideration if there is a sequestrum, necrotic tissue, or inadequate blood supply, but it may be prudent to begin OPAT a few days before surgery in the face of an acute infection.

TABLE 41–2 Infections Amenable to Outpatient Parenteral Antibiotic Therapy

Hospitalize first	Chronic infections
Meningitis	Osteomyelitis
Endocarditis	Diabetic foot infections
Suspected sepsis	Sinusitis
Acute infections	HIV-related infections
Cellulitis	Cytomegalovirus
Wound infections	*Pneumocystis carinii*
Pneumonia	Chronic fungal infections
Pyelonephritis	

Abbreviation: HIV, Human immunodeficiency virus.

Although classic chronic and recurrent osteomyelitis has largely been eliminated with appropriate medical and surgical management, infections related to implanted devices and materials are increasing.[18] These often involve coagulase-negative staphylococci, which are usually resistant to oral antimicrobials and require prolonged courses of intravenous vancomycin therapy. Prosthetic joint infections often require removal of the hardware followed by several weeks of intravenous therapy before and after a new joint is placed.[19, 20] OPAT is also possible in this situation, as a person may be able to get along without a functioning joint for a few weeks.

The epidemic of human immunodeficiency virus (HIV) infection with associated opportunistic infections has provided another impetus for home therapy. Many acquired immunodeficiency syndrome (AIDS) patients have staunchly refused hospitalization and challenged the medical community to provide therapies at home that would previously have been administered only in hospitals. These patients are often willing to take any risk to be treated at home. Thus, diseases such as cryptococcal meningitis and systemic or retinal cytomegalovirus infections, which require intravenous therapy, have been treated for much of their course on an outpatient basis. Cytomegalovirus infection has responded well to intravenous ganciclovir, foscarnet, and, more recently, cidofovir, which has the advantage that it can be given intravenously every other week. Prolonged courses of amphotericin B can also be given on an outpatient basis if oral antifungals are not sufficient or active; this treatment is commonly given in an infusion center three times a week rather than every day, which makes OPAT much more tolerable. Pentamidine has been administered in patients' homes but should be provided only according to careful and reliable protocols.[21]

Lower respiratory infections and sinusitis may also benefit from intravenous antibiotic therapy. For community-acquired pneumonia, it has been common practice to admit patients for intravenous antibiotic therapy. According to recent studies, however, many of those patients do not require hospitalization, and for those who do, inhospital days can be reduced if OPAT programs are available in the community.[22, 23] Furthermore, patients with community-acquired pneumonia would prefer to be treated at home if it is safe to do so.[24, 25] The new risk-stratification system proposed by Fine and others[26] may prove useful in distinguishing patients who are sick enough to require hospitalization from those who are not. The Infectious Diseases Society of America has published guidelines for the management of community-acquired pneumonia that may also be useful in deciding on admission.[27]

Serious skin and soft tissue infections have traditionally been treated in the hospital for a few days with intravenous therapy, particularly if surgical débridement is necessary. However, many can be treated entirely in the outpatient setting with a dose of intravenous antibiotics administered at the initial evaluation and a follow-up examination the next day.[28, 29] There are some limitations, however, in treating one of the most challenging soft tissue infections, the diabetic foot infection. Poor outcomes are seldom due to a failure of the antibiotic but rather to other factors such as inadequate perfusion, neuropathy, hypoglycemia, and poor compliance. These patients should be offered hospitalization early and then considered for OPAT when they are stable and the infection is responding to therapy.[30]

ANTIMICROBIAL USE

The first decision to be made regarding antimicrobial use in OPAT is whether or not a patient needs intravenous therapy. Although some oral antibiotics have been found equivalent to intravenous agents, good comparative studies are lacking. Moreover, there is a continued need for some parenteral antibiotics, such as vancomycin, for which there is no oral equivalent. The antibiotics selected for use in the outpatient setting may be different from those administered to closely supervised hospital patients.[31] Outpatient drugs should be safe and

TABLE 41–3 Antibiotics Suitable for Outpatient Parenteral Antibiotic Therapy

Once-Daily Antibiotics	Less Than Once Daily
Ceftriaxone	Amphotericin B
Aminoglycosides	Teicoplanin
Vancomycin (in elderly patients)	Cidofovir
Azithromycin*	
New quinolones*	

*These may be given orally.

well tolerated, with long half-lives. They should be tailored specifically to the infection, which calls for early identification and antibiotic-susceptibility testing of the pathogen. Finally, the agents must be stable after mixing, a particularly important consideration for patients self-administering premixed medications over 3 to 4 days.[9]

The less often a drug needs to be administered, the more convenient it is for OPAT. Ceftriaxone has been a very useful drug for OPAT because its 8-hour half-life makes it effective in once-daily dosing for most types of infection.[32–35] Despite a relatively short half-life of 2 hours, the aminoglycosides' pharmacodynamics also permit once-a-day administration.[31, 36] A single daily dose is sufficient for some of the new quinolones,[36, 37] as well as for azithromycin, which has a tissue half-life of 30 hours.[38]

Some newer antimicrobials can be dosed even less frequently than daily. Teicoplanin's prolonged half-life permits a dosing schedule of every other day, or three times a week.[39, 40] Intravenous cidofovir appears to be useful in the treatment and suppression of cytomegalovirus infections when given only each week or two.[41] Table 41–3 lists medications that can be given once a day or less frequently.

It is also important to assess organ function before initiating antimicrobial therapy. With renal failure, vancomycin may need to be dosed only once per week.[42] Moreover, given the gradual decline in renal function with age, elderly patients may also do well with once-daily dosing of vancomycin.[43, 44]

Once-daily administration is an obvious advantage for any of the delivery models. However, some antibiotics that have a shorter half-life but are relatively stable may be administered by a battery-powered, computer-operated portable infusion device programmed to deliver doses at selected intervals. These pumps can also be used for continuous infusion of antibiotics, which may be the most effective way to deliver cell wall–active antibiotics such as the penicillins and some of the cephalosporins.[45–47]

A word of caution is needed in regard to the first dose of an intravenous antibiotic. Given an anaphylaxis incidence of approximately 1 in 700 to 800 patients,[48] there is a risk if the first dose is given in the home or outside a medical setting without ready access to medical personnel and emergency equipment. Although some nurses take epinephrine and antihistamine kits to the home, it is generally recommended that the first dose of antibiotic be given in a hospital, emergency department, or physician's office equipped for emergencies.[8] Thereafter, the chances of a life-threatening reaction developing are much smaller, although anaphylactoid reactions have been reported to occur during the course of therapy.[49]

How long to continue parenteral therapy remains a question to be decided by the clinician. Some diseases, such as otitis media in children, gonorrhea, and streptococcal pharyngitis, require only a single dose of ceftriaxone for good clinical and culture responses.[50–52] Once there is a good clinical response to parenteral therapy some patients may be "switched" to an oral antimicrobial to complete the course of therapy.[53–55] Optimal management of antimicrobials requires close physician follow-up for clinical response as well as toxicity.

TECHNOLOGY

A variety of new devices have facilitated outpatient therapy. Because vascular access is essential for OPAT, and nurses are not readily available to examine or restart intravenous infusions in patients' homes, a reliable intravenous line is essential. Plastic peripheral catheters are an improvement over steel needles in patient comfort and results. Central lines have made prolonged courses of intravenous therapy easier and more reliable. A variety of these lines have been developed to facilitate OPAT.[56, 57] One of the most interesting and practical is the peripherally inserted central catheter (PICC), which is inserted into an antecubital vein and passed into the superior vena cava. A peripherally inserted central catheter line should be considered for patients whose course of intravenous medication is planned for more than a week, particularly if the medication is likely to cause phlebitis or the patient already has poor venous access. Central lines can lead to a variety of complications, but the risk of infection seems to be particularly low with peripherally inserted central catheter lines and comparable to that of peripheral catheters in some series.[58–61]

Infusion devices can also simplify an outpatient antibiotic program. Gravity drip systems are increasingly being replaced by syringe pumps, which provide a consistent flow and require less patient training, with little added expense. The use of these pumps also reduces plastic waste, as the syringe is used to both mix and infuse the medication. Battery-driven, computer-operated pumps are advantageous for use in patients who require a prolonged course of therapy or frequent dosing, such as every-4-hour infusions, and for those who have difficulty manipulating the intravenous equipment. The device can administer antimicrobials automatically without interfering with patients' daily routines or sleep.[62] It can also be programmed to give antimicrobials by continuous infusion, which may be as effective as or more effective than intermittent dosing for the penicillins and cephalosporins.[45] Pump-driven continuous infusion may also be less costly in terms of nursing staff time and the amount of antibiotic needed to maintain a level above the minimal inhibitory concentration of the bacteria.[63]

PATIENT SELECTION

Not every patient is a candidate for OPAT despite increasing economic incentives for early hospital discharge or avoidance of hospitalization altogether. As these pressures mount, it is important that physicians understand the risks and limits of outpatient therapy. The responsibility to admit or discharge a patient from the hospital rests with the physician who signs the order, as does the decision to use an OPAT program. However, the physician may know little of what it really means to send a patient home with a serious infection. Because doctors are far less involved in home visits and outpatient management than they were in previous generations,[4, 64] they must trust home-infusion-provider organizations whose quality may vary significantly. Payers and insurance companies may select home health agencies based on charges alone.[65] The physician needs to know the quality of the home care program to be used and to compare its program with guidelines from the Infectious Disease Society of America.[8] If the quality of OPAT care will not be as good as that in the hospital, the patient should stay in the hospital.

The criteria for the selection of patients should be carefully assessed (Table 41–4).[8, 9, 66, 67] The patients must be stable in regard to their diseases. Although it may be possible to treat the presenting infections with OPAT, the patient may have other conditions, such as diabetes, heart failure, or renal failure, that preclude home care. Nursing needs are also an important consideration, particularly if there is limited home support and expertise. Patients must also be evaluated for their physical, emotional, and mental abilities to perform the procedures required for OPAT. Both patients and their families or caretakers should be informed about OPAT and assessed as to their willingness to participate. Patients should have the option of remaining hospitalized despite pressure from insurance companies for early discharge. The home situation and environment should also be considered. Patients with good family support who live in safe environments are the best candidates. In general, a patient who does

TABLE 41–4 Criteria for Selection of Patients

Infection	Risk of complications
	Oral therapy not reasonable
Other diseases	Clinical status
	Nursing needs
Patient assessment	Clinically stable
	Willing to participate
	Physically and mentally able
	Substance abuse
Home situation	Family or caregiver support
	Transportation
	Emergency service
	Telephone
	Running water
	Refrigeration
Reimbursement	Restrictions
	Patient's responsibility

not have a social support system, a safe home environment with a telephone, and ready access to transportation should not be sent home. A skilled nursing facility might be a better alternative.

Once the physician and the intravenous therapy nurse have selected a patient for OPAT, the insurance company should be approached for authorization and to see what restrictions it may have in terms of exclusive contracts and coverage of particular items, such as infusion devices. The payer may control the choice of the provider, drug, delivery model, and technology that can be used.

If a physician is to provide outpatient intravenous therapy through his or her office, a number of factors must be considered. Although it is a time-honored tradition to administer limited courses of intramuscular antibiotics in the office, prolonged courses of intravenous antibiotics are more difficult, challenging, and expensive. There should be policies and procedures in place to ensure the quality of medications and care provided.[8] Table 41–5 lists recommendations to assess the quality of an infusion center.

Physicians who work with infusion providers outside their practices should consider a number of additional factors, outlined in the Infectious Diseases Society of America guidelines (see Table 41–6). The physician remains responsible for the patient's care, even though it may be outside the hospital and, in some respects, outside the physician's control. It is therefore important that the physician develop a good working relationship with the infusion provider, and good lines of communication with the team members.[68] Continued quality assurance and quality improvement measures should be an essential part of the OPAT program and will be increasingly required for accreditation and compensation.[49, 69]

MONITORING PATIENTS

The physician's role does not end with the development of the treatment plan and discharge of the patient from the hospital. It is particularly important that the physician remain involved with the patient's care, periodically assess the patient for a response to the antibiotic, and look for adverse drug reactions. Ongoing management of the patient's other medical problems, which are often present, may also be necessary.

TABLE 41–5 Outpatient Parenteral Antibiotic Therapy Requirements for Infusion Center Model

Health care team	Physician
	Nurse
	Pharmacist
Communications	Physician, nurse, and pharmacist always available
	System for rapid communication with patient, and among team members
Written policies and procedures	Outline of responsibilities of team members
	Information on admission of patient
	Criteria for selection of patient
	Materials for patient education

Adapted from Williams DN, Rehm SJ, Tice AD, et al. Practice guidelines for community-based parenteral anti-infective therapy. Clin Infect Dis. 1997; 25:787–801.

TABLE 41–6 Criteria for Evaluating Outpatient Parenteral Antibiotic Therapy Programs

Medical director or adviser knowledgeable about infectious diseases and OPAT
Defined roles for prescribing physician in relation to case management, medical director, nurse, and pharmacist
Standards for nurse, pharmacist, physician, and other patient care personnel in regard to training, experience, and licensure
Accreditation status in regard to providing OPAT
Policies regarding
- Frequency of physician's and nurse's clinical assessment of patient
- Staffing and on-call policies
- Frequency of clinical status reports to physicians
- Report of laboratory results to physicians within 24 h
- Rapid reporting of patient's problems and critical laboratory values

Willingness to share quality and outcome information
Willingness to share charge information regarding individual patients
Information about
- Anti-infective preparation and dispensing
- Vascular access systems and care
- Infusion device care
- Monitoring guidelines for laboratory studies
- Waste disposal

Patient education and resource materials
- Instructions for emergency situations
- Information about anti-infective use and possible adverse effects
- Understanding of potential risks and problems and patient's responsibilities in regard to OPAT

System for ongoing quality assurance and outcome monitoring

Abbreviation: OPAT, Outpatient parenteral antibiotic therapy.

The schedule of visits to the physician and periodic laboratory studies should be established with the initial treatment plan.[8, 49] The standard for monitoring by the physician is once or twice weekly, but daily for patients who are unstable, and less frequently for those who are stable but undergoing a prolonged course of intravenous antimicrobials such as with ganciclovir for a cytomegalovirus infection. The risk of phlebitis and central line infections is also significant, requiring close monitoring of vascular access devices.[58–60] Although the clinical course of patients on OPAT is usually one of improvement, the potential for drug toxicity increases. This seems to be true for the renal and vestibular toxicities associated with the aminoglycosides, which are most likely to develop several weeks into the course of therapy.[70, 71] Leukopenia may also occur several weeks after the initiation of therapy with penicillins, cephalosporins, or vancomycin.[69, 72] Thus, even though the infection may be responding well, the potential for antibiotic toxicities requires increasing vigilance.

A reliable system for follow-up of patients started on OPAT may have additional benefits. Many patients are admitted to hospitals for 1 or 2 day courses of intravenous antimicrobial therapy. Many of these patients can be started on OPAT in the emergency room, then sent home if they can be assured of seeing a physician the next morning.

FUTURE OF OUTPATIENT PARENTERAL ANTIBIOTIC TREATMENT

The need for intravenous antibiotic therapy will continue despite the availability of new oral antibiotics that are increasingly active and now are required to be effective at once-daily dosing to remain competitive. Further investigations are needed of intramuscular versus intravenous medication and of an early "switch" to oral antibiotics. As patients are increasingly treated in the community instead of in the hospital, it behooves physicians to develop knowledge of and expertise in home and outpatient therapy.

REFERENCES

1. Rucker RW, Harrison GM. Outpatient intravenous medications in the management of cystic fibrosis. Pediatrics. 1974;54:358–360.
2. American Hospital Association. Hospital Statistics. Chicago: Healthcare InfoSource; 1998.
3. Tice AD, Slama TG, Berman S, et al. Managed care and the infectious diseases specialist. Clin Infect Dis. 1996;23:341–368.
4. Meyer GS, Gibbons RV. House calls to the elderly—a vanishing practice among physicians. N Engl J Med. 1997;337:1815–1820.
5. Poretz DM, Eron LJ, Goldenberg RI, et al. Intravenous antibiotic therapy in an outpatient setting. JAMA. 1982;248:336–339.
6. Williams DN. Home intravenous anti-infective therapy (HIVAT)—do the benefits outweigh the risks? Drug Saf. 1996;14:1–7.
7. Tice AD, Nolet BR. Delivery models for outpatient parenteral antimicrobial therapy. A Special Report from Scientific American Medicine. Outpatient Parenteral Antimicrobial Therapy: Current Status. Proceedings of an OPAT Advisory Board Meeting, May 16–18, 1996, Chicago, Ill. Published July 1997.
8. Williams DN, Rehm SJ, Tice AD, et al. Practice guidelines for community-based parenteral anti-infective therapy. Clin Infect Dis. 1997;25:787–801.
9. Tice AD. Handbook of Outpatient Parenteral Therapy for Infectious Diseases. New York: Scientific American; 1997.
10. Bradley JS. Meningitis. Hosp Pract. 1993;28(Suppl 2):15–19.
11. Francioli P, Etienne J, Hoigne R, et al. Treatment of streptococcal endocarditis with a single daily dose of ceftriaxone sodium for 4 weeks. Efficacy and outpatient treatment feasibility (Comment). JAMA. 1992;267:264–267.
12. Stamboulian D. Outpatient treatment of endocarditis in a clinic-based program in Argentina. Eur J Clin Microbiol Infect Dis. 1995;14:16–22.
13. Sexton DJ, Tenenbaum MJ, Wilson WR, et al. Ceftriaxone once daily for four weeks compared with ceftriaxone plus gentamicin once daily for two weeks for treatment of endocarditis due to pencillin-susceptible streptococci. Endocarditis Treatment Consortium Group. Clin Infect Dis. 1998;27:1470–1474.
14. Rehm SJ. Outpatient intravenous antibiotic therapy for endocarditis. Infect Dis Clin North Am. 1998;12:879–901.
15. Kunkel MJ. Outpatient treatment of endocarditis. A Special Report from Scientific American Medicine. Outpatient Parenteral Antimicrobial Therapy: Current Status. Proceedings of an OPAT Advisory Board Meeting, May 16–18, 1996, Chicago, Ill. Published July 1997.
16. Tice AD. Outpatient parenteral antimicrobial therapy for osteomyelitis. Infect Dis Clin North Am. 1998;12:903–919.
17. Lew DP, Waldvogel FA. Quinolones and osteomyelitis: State-of-the-art. Drugs. 1995;49(Suppl 2):100–111.
18. Lew DP, Waldvogel FA. Osteomyelitis. N Engl J Med. 1997;336:999–1007.
19. Thornhill TS. Delayed exchange reimplantation for infected total knee arthroplasty. In: Lotke PA, ed. Knee Arthroplasty (Master Techniques in Orthopaedic Surgery). New York: Raven; 1995:253–272.
20. Karchmer AW. Editorial response: Salvage of infected orthopedic devices. Clin Infect Dis. 1998;27:714–716.
21. Gross R, Graziani AL, Laufer D. Adverse effects of the use of intravenous pentamidine in the home. Infect Dis Clin Pract. 1996;5:456–458.
22. Fine MJ, Hough LJ, Medsger AR, et al. The hospital admission decision for patients with community-acquired pneumonia. Arch Intern Med. 1997;157:36–44.
23. Fine MJ, Medsger AR, Stone RA, et al. The hospital discharge decision for patients with community-acquired pneumonia. Arch Intern Med. 1997;157:47–56.
24. Coley CM, Li Y-H, Medsger AR, et al. Preferences for home vs hospital care among low-risk patients with community-acquired pneumonia. Arch Intern Med. 1996;156:1565–1571.
25. Strandvik B, Hjelte L, Malmborg AS, Widen B. Home intravenous antibiotic treatment of patients with cystic fibrosis. Acta Paediatr. 1992;81:340–344.
26. Fine MJ, Auble TE, Yealy DM, et al. A prediction rule to identify low-risk patients with community-acquired pneumonia. N Engl J Med. 1997;336:243–250.
27. Bartlett JG, Breiman RF, Mandell LA, File TM. Community-acquired pneumonia in adults: Guidelines for management. Clin Infect Dis. 1998;26:811–838.
28. Deery II HG. Outpatient parenteral anti-infective therapy for skin and soft-tissue infections. Infect Dis Clin North Am. 1998;12:935–949.
29. Powers RD. Infections of skin and soft tissue. Outpat Parent Antimicrob Ther Curr Status. 1997;65–68.
30. Fox HR, Karchmer AW. Management of diabetic foot infections, including the use of home intravenous antibiotic therapy. Clin Podiatr Med Surg. 1996;13:671–682.
31. Craig WA. Kinetics of antibiotics in relation to effective and convenient outpatient parenteral therapy. Int J Antimicrob Agents. 1995;5:19–22.
32. Bradley JS. Once-daily ceftriaxone in the outpatient treatment of paediatric infections. Chemotherapy. 1991;37(Suppl 3):3–6.
33. Poretz DM, Woolard D, Eron LJ, et al. Outpatient use of ceftriaxone: A cost-benefit analysis. Am J Med. 1984;77:77–83.
34. Tice AD. Once-daily ceftriaxone outpatient therapy in adults with infections. Chemotherapy. 1991;37(Suppl 3):7–10.
35. Blumer J. Pharmacokinetics of ceftriaxone. Hosp Pract. 1991;26:7–13.
36. MacGowan AP, Bowker KE. Pharmacodynamics of antimicrobial agents and rationale for their dosing. J Chemother. 1997;9:64–73.
37. Teng R, Harris SC, Nix DE, et al. Pharmacokinetics and safety of trovafloxacin (CP-99,219), a new quinolone antibiotic, following administration of single oral doses to healthy male volunteers. J Antimicrob Chemother. 1995;36:385–394.
38. Luke DR, Foulds G, Cohen SF, Levy B. Safety, toleration, and pharmacokinetics of intravenous azithromycin. Antimicrob Agents Chemother. 1996;40:2577–2581.
39. Graninger W, Wenisch C, Wiesenger E, et al. Experience with outpatient intravenous teicoplanin therapy for chronic osteomyelitis. Eur J Clin Microbiol Infect Dis. 1995;14:11–15.
40. Graninger W, Presterl E, Wenisch C, et al. Management of serious staphylococcal infections in the outpatient setting. Drugs. 1997;54:21–28.
41. Lea AP, Bryson HM. Cidofovir. Drugs. 1997;52:225–230.
42. Livornese LL, Benz RL, Ingerman MJ, Santoro J. Antibacterial agents in renal failure. Infect Dis Clin North Am. 1995;9:591–614.
43. Gleckman RA. Antibiotic concerns in the elderly: A clinician's perspective. Infect Dis Clin North Am. 1995;9:575–590.
44. Guay DRP, Vance-Bryan K, Gilliland SS, et al. Comparison of vancomycin pharmacokinetics in hospitalized elderly and young patients using a Bayesian forecaster. J Clin Pharmacol. 1993;33:918–922.
45. Craig WA. Continuous infusion of beta-lactam antibiotics. Antimicrob Agents Chemother. 1992;36:2577–2583.
46. Visser LG, Arnouts P, van Furth R, et al. Clinical pharmacokinetics of continuous intravenous administration of penicillins. Clin Infect Dis. 1993;17:491–495.
47. Benko AS, Cappelletty DM, Kruse JA, Rybak MJ. Continuous infusion (ci) versus intermittent administration (ib) of ceftazidime (caz) in critically ill patients with suspected gram-negative infection (Abstract). ICAAC-35th Annual. 1995.
48. Boston Collaborative Drug Surveillance Program. Drug-induced anaphylaxis. JAMA. 1973;224:613–615.
49. Kunkel MJ. Outcomes measurement in OPAT: A Special Report from Scientific American Medicine. Outpatient Parenteral Antimicrobial Therapy: Current Status. Proceedings of an OPAT Advisory Board Meeting, May 16–18, 1996, Chicago, Ill. Published July 1997.
50. Pichichero ME, Cohen R. Shortened course of antibiotic therapy for acute otitis media, sinusitis and tonsillopharyngitis. Pediatr Infect Dis J. 1997;16:680–695.
51. Hoang KD, Pollack CV. Antibiotic use in the emergency department. IV. Single-dose therapy and parenteral-loading dose therapy. J Emerg Med. 1996;14:619–628.
52. Powers RD. The role of the emergency department in OPAT. A Special Report from Scientific American Medicine. Outpatient Parenteral Antimicrobial Therapy: Current Status. Proceedings of an OPAT Advisory Board Meeting, May 16–18, 1996, Chicago, Ill. Published July 1997.
53. Hamilton-Miller JMT. Switch therapy: The theory and practice of early change from parenteral to non-parenteral antibiotic administration. Clin Microbiol Infect. 1996;2:12–19.
54. Ramirez JA, Srinath L, Ahkee S, et al. Early switch from intravenous to oral cephalosporins in the treatment of hospitalized patients with community-acquired pneumonia. Arch Intern Med. 1995;155:1273–1276.
55. Ahkee S, Smith S, Newman D, et al. Early switch from intravenous to oral antibiotics in hospitalized patients with infections: A 6-month prospective study. Pharmacotherapy. 1997;17:569–575.
56. Gilbert DN, Dworkin R, Raber SR, Leggett JE. Outpatient parenteral antimicrobial-drug therapy. N Engl J Med. 1997;337:829–838.
57. Mortlock NJ, Schleis TG. Outpatient parenteral antimicrobial therapy technology. Infect Dis Clin North Am. 1998;12:861–878.
58. Tice AD, Kunkel MJ, Sullivan DR, et al. Complications of PICC line use in outpatient care (Abstract). Presented at Infectious Diseases Society of America Annual Meeting. San Francisco, Sept. 16–18, 1995.
59. Gilbert D, Jackson JM, Leggett JE, Dworkin R. Complications of 252 peripherally-inserted central catheters (picc) in 216 consecutive patients (Abstract). Presented at The Infectious Diseases Society of America Annual Meeting. New Orleans, Oct. 16–18, 1993.
60. Maki DG. Infections caused by intravascular devices used for infusion therapy: Pathogensis, prevention, and management. In: Bisno AL, Waldvogel FA, eds. Infections Associated with Indwelling Medical Devices. 2nd ed. Washington, DC: American Society for Microbiology; 1994:155–212.
61. Herbst SL, Kaplan LK, McKinnon BT. Vascular access devices: Managing occlusions and related complications in home infusion. Infusion. 1998;4:1–32.
62. Schleis TG, Tice AD. Selecting infusion devices for use in ambulatory care. Am J Health Syst Pharm. 1996;53:868–877.
63. Hitt CM, Nightingale CH, Quintiliani R, Nicolau DP. Cost comparisons of single daily IV dose of ceftriaxone versus continuous infusion of cefotaxime (Abstract). Am J Health Syst Pharm. 1997;54.
64. Campion EW. Can house calls survive? N Engl J Med. 1997;337:1840–1841.
65. Birnbaum HG, Tang M. The home infusion therapy/relative benefit index: Summary of an analysis using insurance claims data. Med Care. 1998;36:757–765.
66. Nolet BR. Patient selection in outpatient parenteral antimicrobial therapy. Infect Dis Clin North Am. 1998;12:835–847.
67. Montalto M. An audit of patients admitted for home intravenous therapy directly from the emergency department. Int J Clin Pract. 1997;51:433–437.
68. Tice AD. The importance of teamwork for outpatient parenteral antibiotic therapy. Int J Antimicrob Agents. 1995;5:13–17.
69. Kunkel MJ. Quality assurance. Hosp Pract. 1993;28(Suppl 1):33–38.
70. Ferriols-Lisart R, Alos-Alminana M. Effectiveness and safety of once-daily aminoglycosides: A meta-analysis. Am J Health Syst Pharm. 1996;53:1141–1150.
71. Koo J, Tight R, Rajkumar V, Hawa Z. Comparison of once-daily versus pharmacokinetic dosing of aminoglycosides in elderly patients. Am J Med. 1996;101:177–183.
72. Hoffman-Terry ML, Fraimow HS, Fox TR, et al. Adverse effects of outpatient parenteral antibiotic therapy. Am J Med. 1999;106:44–49.

Chapter 42

Tables of Antimicrobial Agent Pharmacology

GUY W. AMSDEN

In addition to the tables of pharmacology, this chapter also provides tables of generic and trade names for antimicrobial agents; the antimicrobial "family" classification is also specified to help the reader locate information in subsequent tables. Tables of commonly available dosage forms for the majority of marketed anti-infectives are included as well.

DOSING GUIDELINES

The selection of an appropriate dose of an antimicrobial agent is based on information such as the site of infection, the identity of the infecting organism and its known or presumed antibiotic susceptibility, dose-related drug toxicity, and the patient's ability to eliminate the drug.

Generally, *dosage* selections from the upper end of the range are recommended for severe, life-threatening infections (sepsis, meningitis). Infections due to organisms with intermediate susceptibility—that is, those with high minimal inhibitory concentrations (MICs)—should also prompt the use of the higher dosages.

The lowest dosages are used for urinary tract infections, or when the isolated pathogen is extremely susceptible to the antimicrobial. A sizable range in dosing *intervals* exists for some antimicrobial agents, with the longer duration between doses appropriate for less severe infections in which a critical threshold level in serum or other site of infection (e.g., central nervous system) is not mandatory, or when the drug concentrates significantly at the site of infection (urine, bile). Lower dosages are also appropriate when the patient has impairment in the function of excreting organs.

Dosing recommendations may change. To prevent dosing errors, the recommendations in this chapter should be compared with those presented on the most recent package labeling.

DOSAGE ADJUSTMENT FOR RENAL IMPAIRMENT

Drug half-life in *adults* with impaired renal function and changes related to dialysis procedures (hemodialysis or peritoneal dialysis) are summarized for the user. An alternative to the elongation of the interval between doses is reduction of the daily dose given at the "usual" dosing interval (as described by Bennett and colleagues; see Bibliography). Antimicrobial serum levels should be selected and patient-specific dosage adjustments made on the basis of these determinations when appropriate.

Unless otherwise stated, the doses indicated for hemodialysis should supplement "anuric doses." The route of administration for the usual adult dose is parenteral unless the oral route is specified.

With the increasing use of chronic ambulatory peritoneal dialysis (CAPD), drug addition to the dialysate solution with direct instillation into the peritoneal cavity is becoming a widely used method of drug delivery. Generally, the amount of drug added to the dialysate solution approximates the target serum concentration. For example, 5 mg of gentamicin is added to each liter of dialysate solution to achieve the desired serum level of 5 μg/ml. A loading dose given intravenously may be appropriate for severely ill patients, as the addition method is based on steady-state concentrations, and it may not achieve these values for several doses.

BODY FLUID CONCENTRATIONS

In determining the appropriateness of a particular antibiotic for a given site of infection, the ultimate concentration of a drug at the site of infection as compared with the MIC for the infecting organism is crucial. To be able to interpret this information, the clinician must know the basic pharmacokinetic and pharmacodynamic properties of each agent or type of agent. For example, whereas β-lactams and aminoglycosides have extracellular concentrations that are in relative equilibrium with serum concentrations, macrolides and quinolones concentrate in extracellular sites as well as in phagocytic cells.

TABLE 42–1 Generic-Trade Names of Antibacterial Agents

Generic Name	Trade Name	Class
Abacavir	Ziagen	Antiretroviral
Acyclovir	Zovirax	Antiviral
Acyclovir sodium	Zovirax	Antiviral
Alatrofloxacin	Trovan IV	Fluoroquinolone
Albendazole	Zentel	Antiparasitic
Amantadine hydrochloride	Symadine Symmetrel	Antiviral
Amdinocillin	Coactin	Penicillin
Amikacin sulfate	Amikin	Aminoglycoside
Aminosalicylate sodium	P.A.S. Tubasal	Antimycobacterial
Amithiozone	Panthrone Tibione	Antimycobacterial
Amoxicillin	Amoxil Polymox Trimox Wymox	Penicillin
Amoxicillin + clavulanate potassium	*Augmentin	Penicillin + β-lactamase inhibitor
Amphotericin B	Fungizone	Antifungal
Amphotericin B cholesteryl sulfate complex	Amphotec	Antifungal
Amphotericin B lipid complex	Abelcet AmBisome	Antifungal
Ampicillin	Omnipen	Penicillin
Ampicillin sodium	Omnipen-N Polycillin-N Totacillin-N	Penicillin

Table continued on following page

TABLE 42–1 Generic-Trade Names of Antibacterial Agents *Continued*

Generic Name	Trade Name	Class
Ampicillin trihydrate	Polycillin Principen Totacillin *Polycillin-PRB *Probampacin	Penicillin
Ampicillin + probenecid	*Polycillin-PRB *Probampacin	Penicillin + tubular secretion inhibitor
Ampicillin + sulbactam	*Unasyn	Penicillin + β-lactamase inhibitor
Apalcillin	——	Penicillin
Atovaquone	Mepron	Antiparasitic
Azithromycin	Zithromax, Z-Pak Sumamed	Azalide
Azlocillin	Azlin	Penicillin
Aztreonam	Azactam	Monobactam
Bacampicillin hydrochloride	Spectrobid	Penicillin
Bacitracin	Baci-IM	Polypeptide
Bithionol	Bitin, Lorothidol	Antiparasitic
Butoconazole nitrate	Femstat 3	Antifungal
Capreomycin sulfate	Capastat	Polypeptide
Carbenicillin indanyl sodium	Geocillin	Penicillin
Carbol-fuchsin	——	Antifungal
Cefaclor	Ceclor	Cephalosporin
Cefadroxil	Duricef Ultracef	Cephalosporin
Cefamandole nafate	Mandol	Cephalosporin
Cefazolin sodium	Kefzol Ancef Zolicef	Cephalosporin
Cefdinir	Omnicef	Cephalosporin
Cefepime	Maxipime	Cephalosporin
Cefixime	Suprax	Cephalosporin
Cefmetazole sodium	Zefazone	Cephalosporin
Cefonicid sodium	Monocid	Cephalosporin
Cefoperazone sodium	Cefobid	Cephalosporin
Ceforanide	Precef	Cephalosporin
Cefotaxime sodium	Claforan	Cephalosporin
Cefotetan disodium	Cefotan	Cephalosporin
Cefoxitin sodium	Mefoxin	Cephalosporin
Cefpodoxime proxetil	Vantin	Cephalosporin
Cefprozil	Cefzil	Cephalosporin
Cefsulodin	Cefomonil	Cephalosporin
Ceftazidime	Fortaz Tazidime Ceptaz Pentacef Tazicef	Cephalosporin
Ceftibuten	Cedax	Cephalosporin
Ceftizoxime sodium	Cefizox	Cephalosporin
Ceftriaxone sodium	Rocephin	Cephalosporin
Cefuroxime axetil	Ceftin Zinnat	Cephalosporin
Cefuroxime sodium	Kefurox Zinacef	Cephalosporin
Cefuzonam	Cosmosin	Cephalosporin
Cephalexin	Cefanex Keflex Keflet	Cephalosporin
Cephalexin hydrochloride	Keftab	Cephalosporin
Cephaloglycin	Kafocin	Cephalosporin
Cephalothin sodium	Keflin	Cephalosporin
Cephapirin sodium	Cefadyl	Cephalosporin
Cephradine	Velosef	Cephalosporin
Chloramphenicol	Chloromycetin	Chloramphenicol
Chloramphenicol palmitate	Chloromycetin Palmitate	Chloramphenicol
Chloramphenicol sodium succinate	Chloromycetin Sodium Succinate	Chloramphenicol
Chloroquine hydrochloride	Aralen HCl	Antimalarial
Chloroquine phosphate	Aralen Phosphate	Antimalarial
Ciclopirox	Loprox	Antifungal
Cidofovir	Vistide	Antiviral
Cinoxacin	Cinobac	Quinolone
Ciprofloxacin hydrochloride	Cipro	Fluoroquinolone
Ciprofloxacin lactate	Cipro IV	Fluoroquinolone
Clarithromycin	Biaxin Biclar Klacid LA Klaricid XL Zeclar	Macrolide
Clinafloxacin		Fluoroquinolone
Clindamycin hydrochloride	Cleocin	Lincosamide
Clindamycin palmitate hydrochloride	Cleocin Pediatric	Lincosamide
Clindamycin phosphate	Cleocin Phosphate	Lincosamide

TABLE 42–1 Generic-Trade Names of Antibacterial Agents *Continued*

Generic Name	Trade Name	Class
Clioquinol	*Ala-Quin	Antifungal
	*Corque	
Clofazimine	Lamprene	Antimycobacterial
Clotrimazole	Mycelex	Antifungal
	Lotrimin	
	Lotrisone	
	Gyne-Lotrimin	
	FemCare	
	Cruex	
	Desenex	
	Fungoid	
Cloxacillin sodium	Cloxapen	Penicillin
	Tegopen	
Co-trimoxazole	*Bactrim	Folate antagonists
	*Cotrim	
	*Septra	
	*Sulfatrim	
	*Sulfoxaprim	
	*Uroplus	
Colistimethate sodium	Coly-Mycin M	Polymixin
Colistin sulfate	Coly-Mycin S	Polymixin
Cyclacillin	Cyclapen	Penicillin
Cycloserine	Seromycin	Antimycobacterial
Dapsone	—	Sulfone
Delavirdine	Rescriptor	Antiretroviral
Demeclocycline hydrochloride	Declomycin	Tetracycline
Dicloxacillin sodium	Dynapen	Penicillin
	Dycill	
	Pathocil	
Didanosine	Videx	Antiretroviral
Dideoxycytidine (ddC) (also *zalcitabine*)	Hivid	Antiretroviral
Diethylcarbamazine	Hetrazan	Antiparasitic
Diloxanide furoate	Furamide	Antiparasitic
Dirithromycin	Dynabac	Macrolide
Doxycycline calcium	Vibramycin	Tetracycline
Doxycycline hyclate	Doxy Caps	Tetracycline
	Vibra-Tabs	
	Doryx	
	Doxy	
Doxycycline monohydrate	Vibramycin	Tetracycline
	Monodox	
Econazole nitrate	Spectazole	Antifungal
Efavirenz	Sustiva	Antiretroviral
Enoxacin	Penetrex	Fluoroquinolone
Erythromycin	ERYC	Macrolide
	PCE	
	E-Mycin	
	Ery-Tab	
	Robimycin	
	E-Base	
Erythromycin estolate	Ilosone	Macrolide
Erythromycin ethylsuccinate	EryPed, E.E.S.	Macrolide
Erythromycin ethylsuccinate + sulfisoxazole acetyl	*Eryzole	Macrolide + sulfonamide
	*E.S.P.	
	*Pediazole	
	*Sulfimycin	
Erythromycin gluceptate	Ilotycin	Macrolide
Erythromycin lactobionate	Erythrocin	Macrolide
Erythromycin stearate	Erythrocin	Macrolide
	Wyamycin	
Ethambutol hydrochloride	Myambutol	Antimycobacterial
Ethionamide	Trecator	Antimycobacterial
Flomoxef	Flumarin	Cephalosporin
Flucloxacillin	Floxapen	Penicillin
Fluconazole	Diflucan	Antifungal
Flucytosine	Ancobon	Antifungal
Foscarnet sodium	Foscavir	Antiviral
Fosfomycin tromethamine	Monurol	Urinary anti-infective
Furazolidone	Furoxone	Antiprotozoal
Ganciclovir sodium	Cytovene	Antiviral
Gatifloxacin	—	Fluoroquinolone
Gentamicin sulfate	Garamycin	Aminoglycoside
	Storz-G	
	Jenamicin	
Gentian violet	—	Antifungal
Grepafloxacin	Raxar	Fluoroquinolone
	Vaxar	

Table continued on following page

TABLE 42–1 Generic-Trade Names of Antibacterial Agents *Continued*

Generic Name	Trade Name	Class
Griseofulvin	Grisactin Grifulvin V Fulvicin U/F Fulvicin P/G Grisactin Ultra Gris-PEG	Antifungal
Halofantrine	Halfan	Antiparasitic
Hetacillin	Versapen, Versapen K	Penicillin
Hydroxychloroquine sulfate	Plaquenil Sulfate	Antimalarial
Imipenem + cilastatin	*Primaxin	Carbapenem + enzyme inhibitor
Indinavir	Crixivan	Protease inhibitor
Interferon alfa-2a recombinant	Roferon-A	Antiviral
Interferon alfa-2b recombinant	Intron A	Antiviral
Interferon alfa-N3	Alferon N	Antiviral
Iodoquinol	Yodoxin M/Diquinol Yodoquinol Yodoxin	Amebicide
Isepamicin	Vizax	Aminoglycoside
Isoniazid	Laniazid Tubizid Nydrazid	Antimycobacterial
Isoniazid + rifampin	*Rifamate *Rimactane/INH	Antimycobacterial
Itraconazole	Sporanox	Antifungal
Ivermectin	Mectizan	Antiparasitic
Josamycin	Josalid	Macrolide
Kanamycin sulfate	Kantrex	Aminoglycoside
Ketoconazole	Nizoral	Antifungal
Lamivudine (3TC)	Epivir	Antiretroviral
Levofloxacin	Levaquin	Fluoroquinolone
Lincomycin hydrochloride	Lincocin	Lincosamide
Linezolid		Oxazolidone
Lomefloxacin hydrochloride	Maxaquin	Fluoroquinolune
Loracarbef	Lorabid	Carbacepham
Mafenide	Sulfamylon	Sulfonamide
Mebendazole	Vermox	Anthelmintic
Mefloquine	Lariam	Antiparasitic
Meglumine antimonate	Glucantime	Antiparasitic
Melarsoprol B	Mel B, Arsobal	Antiparasitic
Meropenem	Merrem	Carbapenem
Methenamine hippurate	Hiprex Urex	Urinary anti-infective
Methenamine mandelate	Mandelamine	Urinary anti-infective
Methicillin sodium	Staphcillin	Penicillin
Metronidazole	Flagyl Metric Protostat Metro	Nitroimidazole
Mezlocillin sodium	Mezlin	Penicillin
Miconazole	Monistat Micatin	Antifungal
Minocycline hydrochloride	Minocin	Tetracycline
Moxalactam	Moxam	Cephalosporin
Moxifloxacin	——	Fluoroquinolone
Mupirocin	Bactroban	Pseudomonic acid
Nafcillin sodium	Unipen Nafcil Nallpen	Penicillin
Naftifine	Naftin	Antifungal
Nalidixic acid	NegGram	Quinolone
Nelfinavir	Viracept	Protease inhibitor
Neomycin sulfate	Neo-Tabs Neo-fradin Neo-Rx Powder Mycifradin	Aminoglycoside
Netilmicin sulfate	Netromycin	Aminoglycoside
Nevirapine	Viramune	Antiretroviral
Niclosamide	Niclocide	Anthelmintic
Nifurtimox	Bayer 2502, Lampit	Antiparasitic
Niridazole	Ambilhar	Antiparasitic
Nitrofurantoin	Macrodantin Macrobid Furadantin	Urinary anti-infective
Norfloxacin	Noroxin	Fluoroquinolone
Novobiocin sodium	Albamycin	——
Nystatin	Nystat-Rx Nilstat Mycostatin	Antifungal
Ofloxacin	Floxin	Fluoroquinolone
Oxacillin sodium	Bactocill Prostaphlin	Penicillin

TABLE 42–1 Generic-Trade Names of Antibacterial Agents *Continued*

Generic Name	Trade Name	Class
Oxamniquine	Vansil	Anthelmintic
Oxiconazole nitrate	Oxistat	Antifungal
Oxolinic acid	Utibid	Quinolone
Oxytetracycline	*Terramycin	Tetracycline
Oxytetracycline hydrochloride	Terramycin	Tetracycline
	Urobiotic	
Para-aminosalicylic acid	PAS, Para, Parasal, Rezipas	Antimycobacterial
Paromomycin sulfate	Humatin	Amebicide
Pefloxacin	Peflacine	Fluoroquinolone
Penicillin G benzathine	Bicillin L-A	Penicillin
	Permapen	
Penicillin G + phenoxymethyl penicillin	Kesso-pen	Penicillin
Penicillin G potassium	Pfizerpen	Penicillin
Penicillin G procaine	Crysticillin	Penicillin
	Pfizerpen-AS	
	Wycillin	
+ penicillin G benzathine	*Bicillin C-R	
Penicillin G sodium		Penicillin
Penicillin V potassium	Beepen-VK	Penicillin
	Betapen-VK	
	Pen-Vee K	
	V-Cillin K	
	Veetids	
	Ledercillin VK	
	Robicillin VK	
Pentamidine isethionate	NebuPent	Antiprotozoal
	Pentam	
Phenazopyridine + sulfisoxazole	*Azo Gantrisin	Urinary analgesic + sulfonamide
Phenethicillin potassium	Darcil, Paxipen, Synicillin	Penicillin
Piperacillin sodium	Pipracil	Penicillin
Piperacillin sodium + tazobactam	*Zosyn	Penicillin + β-lactamase inhibitor
Piperazine citrate	——	Anthelmintic
Polymyxin B sulfate	Aerosporin	Polymyxin
Polymyxin B sulfate + neomycin sulfate	*Neosporin	Polymyxin + aminoglycoside
Praziquantel	Biltricide	Anthelmintic
Primaquine phosphate	——	Antimalarial
Proguanil	Paludrine	Antiparasitic
Pyrantel pamoate	Antiminth	Anthelmintic
	Reese's Pinworm	
Pyrazinamide	—	Antimycobacterial
Pyrimethamine	Daraprim	Antimalarial
	*Fansidar	
Pyrimethamine + sulfadoxine	*Fansidar	Antimalarial + sulfonamide
Quinacrine hydrochloride	Atabrine Hydrochloride	Anthelmintic
Quinine sulfate	Legatrin	Antimalarial
	Quin-Amino	
	Quinaminoph	
	Quinamm	
	Quindan	
	Quiphile	
	*M-KYA	
	*Q-Vel	
Quinupristin + dalfopristin	*Synercid	Streptogramin
Ribavirin	Virazole	Antiviral
Rifabutin	Mycobutin	Antimycobacterial
Rifampin	Rifadin	Antituberculosis
	Rimactane	
Rifampin + isoniazid	*Rifamate	Antimycobacterial
	*Rimactane/INH	
Rifapentine	Priftin	Antituberculosis
Rimantadine	Flumadine	Antiviral
Ritonavir	Norvir	Protease inhibitor
Roxithromycin	Rulid	Macrolide
Saquinavir	Invirase	Protease inhibitor
	Fortovase	
Silver sulfadiazine	Silvadene	Sulfonamide
Sparfloxacin	Zagam	Fluoroquinolone
Spectinomycin hydrochloride	Trobicin	Aminocyclitol
Spiramycin	Rovamycin	Macrolide
	Rovamycine	
	Dicorvin	
Stavudine (d4T)	Zerit	Antiretroviral
Stibogluconate	Pentostam	Antiparasitic
Streptomycin sulfate	——	Aminoglycoside
Sulfadiazine + sulfamerazine + sulfamethazine	*Triple Sulfa	Sulfonamide

Table continued on following page

TABLE 42–1 Generic-Trade Names of Antibacterial Agents *Continued*

Generic Name	Trade Name	Class
Sulfabenzamide + sulfacetamide + sulfathiazole	*Dayto Sulf *Gyne-Sulf *Sulfa-Gyn *Sultrin *Triple Sulfa *Trysul *V.V.S.	Sulfonamide
Sulfadiazine	Microsulfon	Sulfonamide
Sulfadoxine + pyrimethamine	*Fansidar	Antiparasitic
Sulfamethizole	Thiosulfil Forte *Urobiotic	Sulfonamide
Sulfamethoxazole	Gantanol Urobak	Sulfonamide
Sulfamethoxazole + phenazopyridine	*Azo Gantanol	Sulfonamide + urinary analgesic
Sulfanilamide	AVC	Sulfonamide
Sulfasalazine	Azulfidine	Sulfonamide
Sulfisoxazole	Gantrisin	Sulfonamide
Sulfisoxazole + phenazopyridine	*Azo Gantrisin *Azo-Sulfisoxazole	Sulfonamide
Sulfisoxazole acetyl	Gantrisin	Sulfonamide
Sulfisoxazole acetyl + erythromycin ethylsuccinate	*Eryzole *E.S.P. *Pediazole *Sulfimycin	Sulfonamide + macrolide
Suramin	Germanin	Antiparasitic
Teicoplanin	Targocid	Glycopeptide
Terbinafine	Lamisil	Antifungal
Terconazole	Terazol	Antifungal
Tetracycline	Sumycin	Tetracycline
Tetracycline hydrochloride	Achromycin V Panmycin Robitet Sumycin Tetralan	Tetracycline
Thiabendazole	Mintezol	Anthelmintic
Ticarcillin disodium	Ticar	Penicillin
Ticarcillin disodium + clavulanate potassium	*Timentin	Penicillin + β-lactamase inhibitor
Tobramycin inhalation solution	Tobi	Aminoglycoside
Tobramycin sulfate	Nebcin	Aminoglycoside
Tolnaftate	Tinactin	Antifungal
Trifluridine	Viroptic	Antiviral
Trimethoprim	Proloprim Trimpex	Folate antagonist
Trimethoprim + sulfamethoxazole	*Bactrim *Septra	Folate antagonist
Trisulfapyrimidines	Terfonyl	Sulfonamide
Troleandomycin	Tao	Macrolide
Trovafloxacin	Trovan	Fluoroquinolone
Valacyclovir	Valtrex Zelitrex	Antiviral
Vancomycin hydrochloride	Vancocin Lyphocin Vancoled Vancor	Glycopeptide
Vidarabine	Vira-A	Antiviral
Voriconazole		Antifungal
Viomycin	Vinactane, Viocin	Antimycobacterial
Zalcitabine	Hivid	Antiretroviral
Zidovudine	Retrovir	Antiretroviral
Zidovudine + lamivudine	*Combivir	Antiretroviral

*Combination product.

TABLE 42–2 Trade-Generic Names of Antibacterial Agents

Trade Name	Generic Name	Class
Abelcet	Amphotericin B lipid complex	Antifungal
Achromycin V	Tetracycline hydrochloride	Tetracycline
Aerosporin	Polymyxin B sulfate	Polymixin
*Ala-Quin	Clioquinol	Antifungal
Albamycin	Novobiocin sodium	—
Ambilhar	Niridazole	Antiparasitic
AmBisome	Amphotericin B lipid complex	Antifungal
Amikin	Amikacin sulfate	Aminoglycoside
Amoxil	Amoxicillin	Penicillin
Amphotec	Amphotericin B cholesteryl sulfate complex	Antifungal

TABLE 42–2 Trade-Generic Names of Antibacterial Agents *Continued)*

Trade Name	Generic Name	Class
Ancef	Cefazolin sodium	Cephalosporin
Ancobon	Flucytosine	Antifungal
Antiminth	Pyrantel pamoate	Anthelmintic
Aralen Hydrochloride	Chloroquine hydrochloride	Antimalarial
Aralen Phosphate	Chloroquine phosphate	Antimalarial
Arsobal	Melarsoprol B	Antiparasitic
Atabrine Hydrochloride	Quinacrine hydrochloride	Anthelmintic
*Augmentin	Amoxicillin + clavulanate potassium	Penicillin + β-lactamase inhibitor
AVC	Sulfanilamide	Sulfonamide
Azactam	Aztreonam	Monobactam
Azlin	Azlocillin	Penicillin
*Azo Gantrisin	Sulfisoxazole + phenazopyridine	Sulfonamide + urinary analgesic
*Azo-Sulfisoxazole	Sulfisoxazole + phenazopyridine	Sulfonamide + urinary analgesic
Azulfidine	Sulfasalazine	Sulfonamide
Baci-IM	Bacitracin	Polypeptide
Bactocill	Oxacillin sodium	Penicillin
*Bactrim	Co-trimoxazole	Folate antagonist
Bactroban	Mupirocin	Pseudomonic acid
Beepen-VK	Penicillin V potassium	Penicillin
Betapen-VK	Penicillin V potassium	Penicillin
Biaxin	Clarithromycin	Macrolide
Bicillin L-A	Penicillin G benzathine	Penicillin
*Bicillin C-R	Penicillin G benzathine + penicillin G procaine	Penicillin
Biclar	Clarithromycin	Macrolide
Biltricide	Praziquantel	Anthelmintic
Bitin	Bithionol	Antiparasitic
Capastat Sulfate	Capreomycin sulfate	Polypeptide
Ceclor	Cefaclor	Cephalosporin
Cedax	Ceftibuten	Cephalosporin
Cefanex	Cephalexin	Cephalosporin
Cefizox	Ceftizoxime sodium	Cephalosporin
Cefobid	Cefoperazone sodium	Cephalosporin
Cefomonil	Ceftazidime	Cephalosporin
Cefotan	Cefotetan disodium	Cephalosporin
Ceftin	Cefuroxime axetil	Cephalosporin
Cefzil	Cefprozil	Cephalosporin
Ceptaz	Ceftazidime	Cephalosporin
Chloromycetin	Chloramphenicol	Chloramphenicol
Chloromycetin Palmitate	Chloramphenicol palmitate	Chloramphenicol
Chloromycetin Sodium Succinate	Chloramphenicol sodium succinate	Chloramphenicol
Cinobac	Cinoxacin	Quinolone
Cipro	Ciprofloxacin hydrochloride	Fluoroquinolone
Cipro IV	Ciprofloxacin lactate	Fluoroquinolone
Claforan	Cefotaxime Sodium	Cephalosporin
Cleocin	Clindamycin hydrochloride	Lincosamide
Cleocin Pediatric	Clindamycin palmitate hydrochloride	Lincosamide
Cleocin Phosphate	Clindamycin phosphate	Lincosamide
Cloxapen	Cloxacillin sodium	Penicillin
Coactin	Amdinocillin	Penicillin
Coly-Mycin M	Colistimethate sodium	Polymyxin
Coly-Mycin S	Colistin sulfate	Polymyxin
*Combivir	Zidovudine + lamivudine	Antiretroviral
*Corque	Clioquinol	Antifungal
Cosmosin	Cefuzonam	Cephalosporin
*Cotrim	Co-trimoxazole	Folate antagonist
Crixivan	Indinavir	Protease inhibitor
Cruex	Clotrimazole	Antifungal
Crysticillin	Penicillin G procaine	Penicillin
Cyclapen	Cyclacillin	Penicillin
Cytovene	Ganciclovir sodium	Antiviral
Daraprim	Pyrimethamine	Antimalarial
Darcil	Phenethicillin potassium	Penicillin
*Dayto Sulf	Sulfabenzamide + sulfacetamide + sulfathiazole	Sulfonamide
Declomycin	Demeclocycline hydrochloride	Tetracycline
Desenex	Clotrimazole	Antifungal
Dicorvin	Spiramycin	Macrolide
Diflucan	Fluconazole	Antifungal
Diquinol	Iodoquinol	Amebicide
Doryx	Doxycycline hyclate	Tetracycline
Doxy	Doxycycline hyclate	Tetracycline
Doxy Caps	Doxycycline hyclate	Tetracycline
Duricef	Cefadroxil	Cephalosporin
Dycill	Dicloxacillin sodium	Penicillin
Dynabac	Dirithromycin	Macrolide
Dynapen	Dicloxacillin sodium	Penicillin
E.E.S.	Erythromycin ethylsuccinate	Macrolide
E-Base	Erythromycin	Macrolide
E-Mycin	Erythromycin	Macrolide
Epivir	Lamivudine	Antiretroviral

Table continued on following page

TABLE 42–2 Trade-Generic Names of Antibacterial Agents *Continued*

Trade Name	Generic Name	Class
ERYC	Erythromycin	Macrolide
EryPed	Erythromycin ethylsuccinate	Macrolide
Ery-Tab	Erythromycin	Macrolide
Erythrocin	Erythromycin lactobionate Erythromycin stearate	Macrolide
*Eryzole	Erythromycin ethylsuccinate + sulfisoxazole acetyl	Macrolide + sulfonamide
*E.S.P.	Erythromycin ethylsuccinate + sulfisoxazole acetyl	Macrolide + sulfonamide
*Fansidar	Sulfadoxine + pyrimethamine	Antiparasitic
FemCare	Clotrimazole	Antifungal
Flagyl	Metronidazole	Nitroimidazole
Floxapen	Flucloxacillin	Penicillin
Floxin	Ofloxacin	Fluoroquinolone
Flumadine	Rimantadine	Antiviral
Flumarin	Flomoxef	Cephalosporin
Fortaz	Ceftazidime	Cephalosporin
Fortovase	Saquinavir	Protease inhibitor
Foscavir	Foscarnet sodium	Antiviral
Fulvicin P/G	Griseofulvin	Antifungal
Fulvicin U/F	Griseofulvin	Antifungal
Fungizone	Amphotericin B	Antifungal
Fungoid	Clotrimazole	Antifungal
Furadantin	Nitrofurantoin	Urinary anti-infective
Furamide	Diloxanide furoate	Antiparasitic
Furoxone	Furazolidone	Antiprotozoal
Gantanol	Sulfamethoxazole	Sulfonamide
Gantrisin	Sulfisoxazole Sulfisoxazole acetyl	Sulfonamide
Garamycin	Gentamicin sulfate	Aminoglycoside
Geocillin	Carbenicillin indanyl sodium	Penicillin
Germanin	Suramin	Antiparasitic
Glucantime	Meglumine antimonate	Antiparasitic
Grifulvin V	Griseofulvin	Antifungal
Grisactin	Griseofulvin	Antifungal
Grisactin Ultra	Griseofulvin	Antifungal
Gris-PEG	Griseofulvin	Antifungal
Gyne-Lotrimin	Clotrimazole	Antifungal
*Gyne-Sulf	Sulfabenzamide + sulfacetamide + sulfathiazole	Sulfonamide
Halfan	Halofantrine	Antiparasitic
Hetrazan	Diethylcarbamazine	Antiparasitic
Hiprex	Methenamine hippurate	Urinary anti-infective
Hivid	Zalcitabine	Antiretroviral
Humatin	Paromomycin sulfate	Amebicide
Ilosone	Erythromycin estolate	Macrolide
Ilotycin	Erythromycin gluceptate	Macrolide
Intron A	Interferon alfa-2b recombinant	Antiviral
Invirase	Saquinavir	Protease inhibitor
Jenamicin	Gentamicin sulfate	Aminoglycoside
Josalid	Josamycin	Macrolide
Kafocin	Cephaloglycin	Cephalosporin
Kantrex	Kanamycin sulfate	Aminoglycoside
Keflet	Cephalexin	Cephalosporin
Keflex	Cephalexin	Cephalosporin
Keftab	Cephalexin hydrochloride	Cephalosporin
Kefurox	Cefuroxime sodium	Cephalosporin
Kefzol	Cefazoline sodium	Cephalosporin
Klacid LA	Clarithromycin	Macrolide
Klaricid XL	Clarithromycin	Macrolide
Lamisil	Terbinafine	Antifungal
Lampit	Nifurtimox	Antiparasitic
Lamprene	Clofazimine	Antimycobacterial
Laniazid	Isoniazid	Antimycobacterial
Ledercillin VK	Penicillin V potassium	Penicillin
Legatrin	Quinine sulfate	Antimalarial
Levaquin	Levofloxacin	Fluoroquinolone
Lincocin	Lincomycin hydrochloride	Lincosamide
Loprox	Ciclopirox	Antifungal
Lorabid	Loracarbef	Carbacepham
Lorothidol	Bithionol	Antiparasitic
Lotrimin	Clotrimazole	Antifungal
Lotrisone	Clotrimazole	Antifungal
Lyphocin	Vancomycin hydrochloride	Glycopeptide
Macrobid	Nitrofurantoin	Urinary anti-infective
Macrodantin	Nitrofurantoin	Urinary anti-infective
Mandelamine	Methenamine mandelate	Urinary anti-infective
Mandol	Cefamandole nafate	Cephalosporin
Maxaquin	Lomefloxacin hydrochloride	Fluoroquinolone
Maxipime	Cefepime hydrochloride	Cephalosporin
Mectizan	Ivermectin	Antiparasitic
Mefoxin	Cefoxitin sodium	Cephalosporin
Mel B	Melarsoprol B	Antiparasitic

TABLE 42–2 Trade-Generic Names of Antibacterial Agents *Continued*

Trade Name	Generic Name	Class
Mepron	Atovaquone	Antiparasitic
Merrem	Meropenem	Carbapenem
Metric	Metronidazole	Nitroimidazole
Metro	Metronidazole	Nitroimidazole
Mezlin	Mezlocillin sodium	Penicillin
Micatin	Miconazole	Antifungal
Microsulfon	Sulfadiazine	Sulfonamide
Minocin	Minocycline hydrochloride	Tetracycline
Mintezol	Thiabendazole	Anthelmintic
Monistat	Miconazole	Antifungal
Monocid	Cefonicid sodium	Cephalosporin
Monodox	Doxycycline monohydrate	Tetracycline
Monurol	Fosfomycin tromethamine	Urinary anti-infective
Moxam	Moxalactam	Cephalosporin
Myambutol	Ethambutol hydrochloride	Antimycobacterial
Mycelex	Clotrimazole	Antifungal
Mycifradin Sulfate	Neomycin sulfate	Aminoglycoside
Mycobutin	Rifabutin	Antimycobacterial
Mycostatin	Nystatin	Antifungal
*M-KYA	Quinine sulfate	Antimalarial
Nafcil	Nafcillin sodium	Penicillin
Naftin	Naftifine	Antifungal
Nallpen	Nafcillin sodium	Penicillin
Nebcin	Tobramycin sulfate	Aminoglycoside
NebuPent	Pentamidine isethionate	Antiprotozoal
NegGram	Nalidixic acid	Quinolone
Neo-fradin	Neomycin sulfate	Aminoglycoside
Neo-Rx Powder	Neomycin sulfate	Aminoglycoside
Neo-Tabs	Neomycin sulfate	Aminoglycoside
*Neosporin	Polymyxin B sulfate + neomycin sulfate	Polymyxin + aminoglycoside
Netromycin	Netilmicin sulfate	Aminoglycoside
Niclocide	Niclosamide	Anthelmintic
Nilstat	Nystatin	Antifungal
Nizoral	Ketoconazole	Antifungal
Noroxin	Norfloxacin	Fluoroquinolone
Nydrazid	Isoniazid	Antimycobacterial
Nystat-Rx	Nystatin	Antifungal
Omnicef	Cefdinir	Cephalosporin
Omnipen	Ampicillin	Penicillin
Omnipen-N	Ampicillin sodium	Penicillin
Oxistat	Oxiconazole nitrate	Antifungal
Paludrine	Proguanil	Antiparasitic
Panmycin	Tetracycline hydrochloride	Tetracycline
Panthrone	Amithiozone	Antimycobacterial
Para	Para-aminosalicylic acid	Antimycobacterial
Parasal	Para-aminosalicylic acid	Antimycobacterial
P.A.S.	Aminosalicylate sodium	Antimycobacterial
Pathocil	Dicloxacillin sodium	Penicillin
Paxipen	Phenethicillin potassium	Penicillin
PCE	Erythromycin	Macrolide
*Pediazole	Erythromycin ethylsuccinate + sulfisoxazole acetyl	Macrolide + sulfonamide
Peflacine	Pefloxacin	Fluoroquinolone
Penetrex	Enoxacin	Fluoroquinolone
Pentacef	Ceftazidime	Cephalosporin
Pentam	Pentamidine isethionate	Antiprotozoal
Pentostam	Stibogluconate	Antiparasitic
Pen-Vee K	Penicillin V potassium	Penicillin
Permapen	Penicillin G benzathine	Penicillin
Pfizerpen	Penicillin G potassium	Penicillin
Pfizerpen-AS	Penicillin G procaine	Penicillin
Pipracil	Piperacillin sodium	Penicillin
Plaquenil Sulfate	Hydroxychloroquine sulfate	Antimalarial
Polycillin	Ampicillin trihydrate	Penicillin
Polycillin-N	Ampicillin sodium	Penicillin
*Polycillin-PRB	Ampicillin trihydrate + probenecid	Penicillin + tubular secretion inhibitor
Polymox	Amoxicillin	Penicillin
Precef	Ceforanide	Cephalosporin
Priftin	Rifapentine	Antituberculosis
*Primaxin	Imipenem/cilastatin	Carbapenem + enzyme inhibitor
Principen	Ampicillin trihydrate	Penicillin
*Probampacin	Ampicillin trihydrate + probenecid	Penicillin + tubular secretion inhibitor
Proloprim	Trimethoprim	Folate antagonist
Prostaphlin	Oxacillin sodium	Penicillin
Protostat	Metronidazole	Nitroimidazole
*Q-Vel	Quinine sulfate	Antimalarial
Quin-Amino	Quinine sulfate	Antimalarial
Quinaminoph	Quinine sulfate	Antimalarial

Table continued on following page

TABLE 42–2 Trade-Generic Names of Antibacterial Agents *Continued*

Trade Name	Generic Name	Class
Quinamm	Quinine sulfate	Antimalarial
Quindan	Quinine sulfate	Antimalarial
Quiphile	Quinine sulfate	Antimalarial
Raxar	Grepafloxacin	Fluoroquinolone
Reese's Pinworm	Pyrantel pamoate	Anthelmintic
Rescriptor	Delavirdine	Antiretroviral
Retrovir	Zidovudine	Antiretroviral
Rezipas	Para-aminosalicylic acid	Antimycobacterial
Rifadin	Rifampin	Antimycobacterial
*Rifamate	Rifampin + isoniazid	Antimycobacterial
Rimactane	Rifampin	Antimycobacterial
*Rimactane/INH	Rifampin + isoniazid	Antimycobacterial
Robicillin VK	Penicillin V potassium	Penicillin
Robimycin	Erythromycin	Macrolide
Robitet	Tetracycline hydrochloride	Tetracycline
Rocephin	Ceftriaxone sodium	Cephalosporin
Rovamycin	Spiramycin	Macrolide
Rovamycine	Spiramycin	Macrolide
Rulid	Roxithromycin	Macrolide
*Septra	Co-trimoxazole	Folate antagonist
Seromycin	Cycloserine	Antimycobacterial
Silvadene	Silver sulfadiazine	Sulfonamide
Spectazole	Econazole nitrate	Antifungal
Spectrobid	Bacampicillin hydrochloride	Penicillin
Sporanox	Itraconazole	Antifungal
Staphcillin	Methicillin sodium	Penicillin
Storz-G	Gentamicin sulfate	Aminoglycoside
Streptomycin sulfate	Streptomycin sulfate	Aminoglycoside
*Sulfa-Gyn	Sulfabenzamide + sulfacetamide + sulfathiazole	Sulfonamide
Sulfamylon	Mafenide	Sulfonamide
*Sulfatrim	Co-trimoxazole	Folate antagonist
*Sulfimycin	Erythromycin ethylsuccinate + sulfisoxazole acetyl	Sulfonamide + macrolide
*Sulfoxaprim	Co-trimoxazole	Folate antagonist
*Sultrin Triple Sulfa	Sulfabenzamide + sulfacetamide + sulfathiazole	Sulfonamide
Sunamed	Azithromycin	Azalide
Sumycin	Tetracycline hydrochloride Tetracycline	Tetracycline
Suprax	Cefixime	Cephalosporin
Sustiva	Efaverenz	Antiretroviral
Symadine	Amantadine hydrochloride	Antiviral
Symmetrel	Amantadine hydrochloride	Antiviral
*Synercid	Quinupristin + dalfopristin	Streptogramin
Synicillin	Phenethicillin potassium	Penicillin
Tao	Troleandomycin	Macrolide
Targocid	Teicoplanin	Glycopeptide
Tazicef	Ceftazidime	Cephalosporin
Tazidime	Ceftazidime	Cephalosporin
Tegopen	Cloxacillin sodium	Penicillin
Terazol	Terconazole	Antifungal
Terfonyl	Trisulfapyrimidines	Sulfonamide
Terramycin	Oxytetracycline hydrochloride Oxytetracycline	Tetracycline
Tetralan	Tetracycline hydrochloride	Tetracycline
Thiosulfil Forte	Sulfamethizole	Sulfonamide
Tibione	Amithiozone	Antimycobacterial
Ticar	Ticarcillin disodium	Penicillin
*Timentin	Ticarcillin disodium + clavulanate potassium	Penicillin + β-lactamase inhibitor
Tinactin	Tolnaftate	Antifungal
Tobi	Tobramycin inhalation solution	Aminoglycoside
Totacillin	Ampicillin trihydrate	Penicillin
Totacillin-N	Ampicillin sodium	Penicillin
Trecator	Ethionamide	Antimycobacterial
Trimox	Amoxicillin	Penicillin
Trimpex	Trimethoprim	Folate antagonist
*Triple Sulfa	Sulfadiazine + sulfamerazine + sulfamethazine Sulfabenzamide + sulfacetamide + sulfathiazole	Sulfonamide
Trobicin	Spectinomycin hydrochloride	Aminocyclitol
Trovan	Trovafloxacin	Fluoroquinolone
Trovan IV	Alatrofloxacin	Fluoroquinolone
*Trysul	Sulfabenzamide + sulfacetamide + sulfathiazole	Sulfonamide
Tubasal	Aminosalicylate sodium	Antimycobacterial
Tubizid	Isoniazid	Antimycobacterial
Ultracef	Cefadroxil	Cephalosporin
*Unasyn	Ampicillin + sulbactam	Penicillin + β-lactamase inhibitor
Unipen	Nafcillin sodium	Penicillin
Urex	Methenamine hippurate	Urinary anti-infective
Urobak	Sulfamethoxazole	Sulfonamide
*Uroplus	Co-trimoxazole	Folate antagonist
Vancocin	Vancomycin hydrochloride	Glycopeptide
Vancoled	Vancomycin hydrochloride	Glycopeptide
Vancor	Vancomycin hydrochloride	Glycopeptide

TABLE 42–2 Trade-Generic Names of Antibacterial Agents *Continued*

Trade Name	Generic Name	Class
Vansil	Oxamniquine	Anthelmintic
Vantin	Cefpodoxime proxetil	Cephalosporin
Vaxar	Grepafloxacin	Fluoroquinolone
V-Cillin K	Penicillin V potassium	Penicillin
Veetids	Penicillin V potassium	Penicillin
Velosef	Cephradine	Cephalosporin
Vermox	Mebendazole	Anthelmintic
Versapen	Hetacillin	Penicillin
Versapen K	Hetacillin	Penicillin
Vibramycin	Doxycycline calcium	Tetracycline
Vibramycin	Doxycycline monohydrate	Tetracycline
Vibra-Tabs	Doxycycline hyclate	Tetracycline
Videx	Didanosine	Antiretroviral
Vinactane	Viomycin	Antimycobacterial
Viocin	Viomycin	Antimycobacterial
Vira-A	Vidarabine	Antiviral
Viracept	Nelfinavir	Protease inhibitor
Viramune	Nevirapine	Antiretroviral
Virazole	Ribavirin	Antiviral
Viroptic	Trifluridine	Antiviral
Vistide	Cidofovir	Antiviral
Vizax	Isepamicin	Aminoglycoside
*V.V.S.	Sulfabenzamide + sulfacetamide + sulfathiazole	Sulfonamide
Wyamycin S	Erythromycin stearate	Macrolide
Wycillin	Penicillin G procaine	Penicillin
Wymox	Amoxicillin	Penicillin
Yodoquinol	Iodoquinol	Amebicide
Yodoxin	Iodoquinol	Amebicide
Zagam	Sparfloxacin	Fluoroquinolone
Zeclar	Clarithromycin	Macrolide
Zefazone	Cefmetazole sodium	Cephalosporin
Zelitrex	Valacyclovir	Antiviral
Zentel	Albendazole	Antiparasitic
Zerit	Stavudine	Antiretroviral
Ziagen	Abacavir	Antiretroviral
Zinacef	Cefuroxime sodium	Cephalosporin
Zinnat	Cefuroxime axetil	Cephalosporin
Zithromax	Azithromycin	Azalide
Zolicef	Cefazolin sodium	Cephalosporin
*Zosyn	Piperacillin sodium + tazobactam	Penicillin + β-lactamase inhibitor
Zovirax	Acyclovir sodium Acyclovir	Antiviral
Z-Pak	Azithromycin	Azalide

*Combination product.

TABLE 42–3 Dosage Forms: Penicillins

Drug	Formulations		
	Oral		
	Tablets/Capsules (mg)	*Liquid (mg/ml)*	***Parenteral (g)***
Amoxicillin	125*, 250*, 250, 500	50/1, 125/5, 250/5	
Amoxicillin/clavulanate	125*, 250*, 250, 500, 875	125/5, 250/5	1.2
Ampicillin	125*, 250, 500	100/1, 125/5, 250/5, 500/5	0.125, 0.25, 0.5, 1, 2, 10
Ampicillin/sulbactam	375		1.5, 3
Azlocillin			2, 3, 4
Bacampicillin	400, 800	125/5	
Carbenicillin			1, 2, 5, 10, 20, 30
Carbenicillin indanyl sodium	382		
Cloxacillin	250, 500	125/5	0.25, 0.5, 1, 2
Cyclacillin	250, 500	125/5, 250/5	
Dicloxacillin	125, 250, 500	62.5/5	
Methicillin			1, 2, 4, 6, 10
Mezlocillin			1, 2, 3, 4
Nafcillin	250, 500	250/5	0.5, 1, 2, 10
Oxacillin	250, 500	250/5	0.25, 0.5, 1, 2, 4, 10
Penicillin G[a]	0.2 MU, 0.25 MU, 0.4 MU, 0.5 MU, 0.8 MU, 4 MU	0.2 MU/5, 0.25 MU/5, 0.5 MU/5	0.3 MU, 0.5 MU, 1 MU, 5 MU, 10 MU, 20 MU
Penicillin G benzathine			0.3 MU, 0.6 MU, 1.2 MU, 2.4 MU
Penicillin G procaine			0.3 MU, 0.6 MU, 1.2 MU, 2.4 MU
Penicillin V potassium	250, 300, 500	125/5, 250/5, 300/5	
Piperacillin			2, 3, 4, 40
Piperacillin/tazobactam			2.25, 3.375, 4.5
Ticarcillin			1, 3, 6, 20, 30
Ticarcillin/clavulanate			3.1, 31

*Chewable tablets.
[a]400,000 IU = 0.4 MU = 250 mg.

TABLE 42–4 Dosage Forms: Cephalosporins

Drug	Formulations		
	Oral		
	Tablets/Capsules (mg)	*Liquid (mg/ml)*	***Parenteral (g)***
First-Generation Agents			
Cefadroxil	250, 500, 1000	125/5, 250/5, 500/5, 500/10	
Cefazolin			0.25, 0.5, 1, 2, 5, 10
Cephalexin	250, 500, 1000	125/5, 250/5, 375/5, 500/5	
Cephalothin			1, 2, 4, 10, 20
Cephapirin			0.5, 1, 2, 4, 20
Cephradine	250, 500, 1000	125/5, 250/5	0.25, 0.5, 1
Second-Generation Agents			
Cefaclor	250, 375*, 500, 500*	125/5, 187/5, 250/5, 375/5	
Cefamandole			0.5, 1, 2, 10
Cefmetazole			0.25, 0.5, 1, 2
Cefonicid			0.5, 1
Cefotetan			0.5, 1, 2, 10
Cefoxitin			0.5, 1, 2, 10
Cefprozil	250, 500	125/5, 250/5	
Cefuroxime	125, 250, 500	125/5, 250/5	0.25, 0.75, 1.5, 7.5
Third-Generation Agents			
Cefdinir	300	125/5	
Cefixime	50, 100, 200, 400	100/5	
Cefoperazone			0.25, 0.5, 1, 2, 10
Cefotaxime			0.5, 1, 2
Cefpodoxime	100, 200	50/5, 100/5	
Ceftazidime			0.25, 0.5, 1, 2, 6, 10
Ceftibuten	218, 400, 435	90/5, 98/5, 180/5, 196/5	
Ceftizoxime			0.5, 1, 2
Ceftriaxone			0.25, 0.5, 1, 2, 10
Moxalactam			1, 2, 10
Fourth-Generation Agent			
Cefepime			0.5, 1, 2

*Sustained-release formulation.

TABLE 42–5 Dosage Forms: Miscellaneous β-Lactams

Drug	Formulations		
	Oral		
	Tablets/Capsules (mg)	*Liquid (mg/ml)*	***Parenteral (g)***
Aztreonam			0.5, 1, 2
Imipenem			0.25, 0.5, 1
Meropenem			0.25, 0.5, 1
Loracarbef	200, 400	100/5, 200/5	

TABLE 42–6 Dosage Forms: Aminoglycosides

Drug	Formulations		
	Oral		
	Tablets/ Capsules (mg)	*Liquids (mg/ml)*	***Parenteral (g)***
Amikacin			0.1, 0.25, 0.5, 1
Gentamicin			0.01, 0.04, 0.08, 0.8
Kanamycin	500		0.075, 0.5, 1
Neomycin	350, 500	125/5	0.5
Netilmicin			0.05, 0.15, 0.2, 2
Spectinomycin		400/5, 2000/1, 4000/1	
Streptomycin			1
Tobramycin			0.02, 0.06, 0.08, 1.2, 2

TABLE 42–7 Dosage Forms: Tetracyclines

Drug	Formulations: Oral — Tablets/Capsules (mg)	Formulations: Oral — Liquid (mg/ml)	Formulations: Parenteral (g)
Demeclocycline	75, 150, 300		
Doxycycline	50, 100, 100*	25/5, 50/5	0.1, 0.2
Methacycline	150, 300		
Minocycline	50, 100	50/5	0.1
Oxytetracycline	250		0.05
Tetracycline	250, 500	125/5	0.1, 0.25, 0.5

*Sustained-release formulation.

TABLE 42–8 Dosage Forms: Azalides, Macrolides, Lincosamides, Chloramphenicol, and Metronidazole

Drug	Formulations: Oral — Tablets/Capsules (mg)	Formulations: Oral — Liquid (mg/ml)	Formulations: Parenteral (g)
Macrolides			
Azithromycin	250, 600, 1000	100/5, 200/5	0.5
Clarithromycin	250, 500	125/5, 250/5	
Dirithromycin	250		
Erythromycin base	125, 250, 250*, 333, 333*, 500, 500*		
Erythromycin stearate	250, 500	125/5, 250/5	
Erythromycin ethylsuccinate	200†, 400	100/2.5, 200/5, 400/5	
Erythromycin lactobionate			0.5, 1
Erythromycin gluceptate			0.25, 0.5, 1
Erythromycin estolate	125†, 250†, 250, 500	100/1, 125/1, 125/5, 150/5, 250/1, 250/5	
Roxithromycin	150, 300		
Lincosamides			
Clindamycin	75, 150, 300	75/5	0.15, 0.3, 0.6, 0.9
Lincomycin	250, 500		0.3, 0.6
Miscellaneous			
Chloramphenicol	250		1
Metronidazole	250, 375, 500, 750*		0.5

*Sustained-release formulation.
†Chewable tablets.

TABLE 42–9 Dosage Forms: Miscellaneous Agents

Drug	Formulations: Oral — Tablets/Capsules (mg)	Formulations: Oral — Liquid (mg/ml)	Formulations: Parenteral (g)
Colistimethate			0.15
Vancomycin	125, 250	1 g, 10 g	0.5, 1, 5, 10
Fusidic acid	250	246/5	

TABLE 42–10 Dosage Forms: Sulfonamides and Trimethoprim

	Formulations		
	Oral		
Drug	*Tablets/Capsules (mg)*	*Liquid (mg/ml)*	***Parenteral** (g)*
Trimethoprim-sulfamethoxazole	80/400, 160/800	40/200/5	0.080/0.400, 0.160/0.800, 0.480/2.400
Trimethoprim	100, 200		
Sulfisoxazole	500	500/5	
Sulfamethoxazole	500, 1000	500/5	
Sulfamethizole	500		
Sulfacytine	250		
Sulfadiazine	500		
Sulfadoxine (with pyrimethamine)	500		
Sulfasalazine	500, 500*	250/5	
Dapsone	25, 100		

*Sustained-release formulation.

TABLE 42–11 Dosage Forms: Quinolones

	Formulations		
	Oral		
Drug	*Tablets/Capsules (mg)*	*Liquids (mg/ml)*	***Parenteral** (g)*
Cinoxacin	250, 500		
Ciprofloxacin	100, 250, 500, 750	50/1, 100/1	0.2, 0.4
Enoxacin	200, 400		
Grepafloxacin	200		
Levofloxacin	250, 500		0.25, 0.5
Lomefloxacin	400		
Nalidixic acid	250, 500, 1000	250/5	
Norfloxacin	400		
Ofloxacin	100, 200, 300, 400		0.2, 0.4
Sparfloxacin	200		
Trovafloxacin	100, 200		0.2, 0.3

TABLE 42–12 Dosage Forms: Urinary Anti-infectives

	Oral Formulations	
Drug	*Tablets/Capsules (mg)*	*Liquids (mg/ml)*
Methenamine mandelate	500, 1000	500/5
Nitrofurantoin	25, 50, 100	5/1

TABLE 42-13 Dosage Forms: Antimycobacterial Agents

Drug	Formulations		
	Oral		
	Tablets/Capsules (mg)	Liquid (mg/ml)	Parenteral (g)
Capreomycin			1
Clofazimine	50, 100		
Cycloserine	250		
Ethambutol	100, 400		
Ethionamide	250		
Isoniazid	50, 100, 300	50/5	0.1
Para-aminosalicylic acid	400, 500, 500*		
Pyrazinamide	500		
Rifabutin	150		
Rifampin	150, 300, 450, 600	100/5	0.6
Streptomycin			1

*Sustained-release formulation.

TABLE 42-14 Dosage Forms: Antifungal Agents

Drug	Formulations		
	Oral		
	Tablets/Capsules (mg)	Liquid (mg/ml)	Parenteral (g)
Amphotericin B	100	100/1	0.05
Amphotericin B cholesteryl sulfate complex			0.05, 0.1
Amphotericin B lipid complex			5 mg/ml
Amphotericin B liposomal			0.05
Fluconazole	50, 100, 150, 200	50/5, 200/5	0.2, 0.4
Flucytosine	200, 250, 500		0.25
Griseofulvin	125, 165, 250, 330, 500	125/5	
Itraconazole	100	10/1	
Ketoconazole	200	20/1	
Nystatin	200,000 U, 500,000 U	100,000 U/1	
Pentamidine			0.2, 0.3
Terbinafine	250		

TABLE 42-15 Dosage Forms: Antiviral Agents

Drug	Formulations		
	Oral		
	Tablets/Capsules (mg)	Liquid (mg/ml)	Parenteral (g)
Acyclovir	200, 400, 800	200/5	0.5, 1
Amantadine	100	50/5	
Cidofovir			0.375
Delavirdine	100		
Famciclovir	125, 250, 500		
Foscarnet			6, 12
Ganciclovir	250		0.5
Indinavir	200, 400		
Lamivudine	150		
Nelfinavir	250		
Nevirapine	200		
Ribavirin			6[a]
Ritonavir	100	80/1	
Saquinavir	200		
Stavudine	15, 20, 30, 40		
Valacyclovir	500, 556, 1000		
Vidarabine			1
Zalcitabine	0.375, 0.75		
Zidovudine	100, 300	50/5	0.2

[a]For inhalation.

TABLE 42–16 Pharmacology: Penicillins

Drug (% oral absorption)	Drug Concentrations Achieved with Specific Doses			Dosage Recommendations						
		Measured Levels (μg/ml)		Adults			Children		Newborns (Parenteral)	
	Dose (g)	Serum (peak)	Urine (peak or range)	Oral	Parenteral	Serious Infection (daily dose)	Oral	Parenteral	Up to 1 wk	1–4 wk
Amdinocillin	10 mg/kg	50	1260		10 mg/kg q4–6h			10 mg/kg q4–6h (not approved)		
Amoxicillin* (74–92)	0.25 PO† 0.5 PO†	3.5–5.0 5.5–11.0		0.25–0.5 g q8h		1.5 g	6.7–13.3 mg/kg q8h[c]			
Amoxicillin clavulanate	0.25 PO 0.5 PO	3.7–4.8 6.0–9.7	381	0.25–0.5 g q8h		1.5 g	6.6–13.3 mg/kg q8h[d]			
Ampicillin* (30–55)	0.25 PO† 0.5 PO† 2.0 IV	1.8–2.9 3–6 47.6		0.25–0.5 g q6h	0.5–2 g q4–6h	4 g PO; 12 g IV	6.25–25[e] mg/kg q6h	6.25–25 mg/kg q6h[f]	25 mg/kg q12h	25 mg/kg q8h
Ampicillin/sulbactam	1.5 IV 3.0 IV	40–71 109–150			1.5–3.0 g q6h	12 g		25–50 mg/kg q6h		
Apalcillin	2 IV[g]	208	835							
Azlocillin (minimal)	2 IV[g] 3 IV[g]	165 214	 2200–8100		2–4 g q4–6h	24 g		75 mg/kg q6h (not approved)[f]	Not recommended	
Bacampicillin[i] (80–98)	0.4 PO 0.8 PO 1.6 PO	5.8–8.3 12.0–15.9 18.6–20.1		0.4–1.6 g q12h		3.2 g	12.5–25 mg/kg q12h			
Carbenicillin	1 IV 3 IV[j]	45–71 278	1000 4165		5–6 g q4h	30 g		25–100 mg/kg q4–6h	66.7–100 mg/kg q8h	400 mg/kg/day q6–8h
Carbenicillin indanyl sodium (30–40)	0.382 PO	6.5	0.576–1.13[k]	0.382–0.764 g q6h		3 g				
Cloxacillin* (37–60)	0.5 PO	6.9–15		0.25–1.0 g q6h		4 g	12.5–25 mg/kg q6h			
Cyclacillin	0.25 PO 0.5 PO	6–7 11–12		0.25–0.5 g q6h		2 g	12.5–25 mg/kg q6h			
Dicloxacillin* (35–76)	0.5 PO	10–18		0.125–0.5 g q6h		2 g	3.125–6.25[e] mg/kg q6h			
Hetacillin[l]	0.225 PO 0.45 PO	1.7–2.1 2.5–2.7		0.225–0.45 g q6h		1.8 g	5.6–11.25 mg/kg q6h			
Methicillin	1 IV[j] 1 IM 2 IM	59.8 9–18 13.8			1–2 g q4–6h	12 g		25–100 mg/kg q4–6h[m]	25–50 mg/kg q12h	25–50 mg/kg q8h
Mezlocillin	1 IV[j] 2 IV[j] 5 IV[j]	64–143 161–364 199–597	 4000		3–4 g q4–6h	24 g		50–75 mg/kg q4h	75 mg/kg q12h	75 mg/kg q6–8h[n]
Nafcillin* (36)	1 PO 1 IM 0.5 IV[j]	7.7 7.6 40		0.5–1 g q6h	0.5–2 g q4–6h	4 g PO; 12 g IV	12.5–25 mg/kg q6h[e]	12.5–25 mg/kg q6h[e]	25 mg/kg q8–12h[o]	25 mg/kg q6–8h[n]
Oxacillin* (30–35)	0.25 PO 0.5 PO 0.5 IV	1.65 2.6–3.9 52–63		0.5–1 g q4–6h	0.5–2 g q4–6h	4 g PO; 12 g IV	12.5–25 mg/kg q6h[e]	12.5–50 mg/kg q6h[e]	25–50 mg/kg q8–12h[o]	25–50 mg/kg q6–8h[n]
Penicillin G* (15–30)	400,000 U PO 2 mU q2h IV	0.5 U/ml[p] 20		0.5–1 g q6h	1–4 mU q4–6h	4 g PO/24mU IV	25,000–90,000 U/kg/d in 3–6 doses	25,000–400,000 U/kg/d q4–6h[q]	50,000–150,000 U/kg/d q8–12h[o]	75,000–200,000 U/kg/d q6–8h[n]
Penicillin G benzathine	1.2 mU IM	0.15 U/ml			0.6–1.2 mU IM q12h	2.4 mU		0.6 mU IM × 1[c]		50,000 U/kg IM × 1
Penicillin G procaine	0.6 mU IM 1.2 mU IM	1.6 1.95			0.6–1.2 mU IM q12h	4.8 mU		25,000–50,000 U/kg/d IM[q]		50,000 U/kg/day IM
Penicillin V* potassium (60–73)	0.25 PO 0.5 PO	2.3–2.7 4.9–6.3		0.25–0.5 g q6h		2 g	25,000–100,000 U/kg/d in 3–6 doses			
Piperacillin	2 IV[j] 4 IV[j] 6 IV[j]	159–615 389–484 695–849	 8500 14,100		3–4 g q4–6h	24 g		50 mg/kg q4h[q]		
Piperacillin/tazobactam	3.375 IV[g] 4.5 IV[g]	209 224			3.375–4.5 g q6–8h	13.5 g				
Temocillin	0.5 IV[j] 1 IV[j] 2 IV[j]	78 160 236	100–500		0.5–1 g q12h					
Ticarcillin	1 IV[j] 2 IV[j] 3 IV[j]	70–100 200–218 257	 650–2500[k]		3 g q4–6h	18 g		200–300 mg/kg/d q4–6h[e]	75 mg/kg q8–12h[o]	75 mg/kg q8h if <2 kg; 100 mg/kg q8h if >2 kg
Ticarcillin/clavulanate	3.1 IV	324	1500		3.1 g q4–8h	18.6 g		50 mg/kg q4–6h		

*Decreased rate and/or extent of absorption when given with food.
†Fasting.
[a]Specified dose is supplemental to that after hemodialysis.
[b]Inflamed meninges.
[c]Children <20–27 kg.
[d]Children <40 kg should not receive the 250-mg film-coated tablet.
[e]Children <40–50 kg.
[f]16.7–33.3 mg/kg q4h for meningitis.
[g]Infusion over 15–30 min.
[h]Mean concentration.
[i]100% of bacampicillin is metabolized to ampicillin.
[j]IV push (over 2–10 min).
[k]Over 3 hours.
[l]Hetacillin is rapidly converted to ampicillin.
[m]Depending on severity of infection.
[n]q6h if >2 kg; q8h if <2 kg.
[o]q8h if >2 kg; q12h if <2 kg.
[p]Higher when given with probenecid.
[q]Dosage should not exceed adult dosage.
Abbreviations: Cl_{Cr}, Creatinine clearance; CSF, cerebrospinal fluid; HD, hemodialysis; PD, peritoneal dialysis.

Serum Half-life (h)				Standard Dose with Dosing Intervals in Renal Impairment					Dosage with Dialysis		Body Fluid Concentrations				
With Normal and Anuric Cl_{Cr} Values (ml/min)		*With Dialysis*		*Usual Adult Dose*	*For Cl_{Cr} Ranges (ml/min)*				*After HD*[a]	*During PD (daily dose)*	*CSF/ Serum (%)*[b]	*Newborn Serum/ Maternal Serum (%)*	*Breast Milk/ Maternal Serum (%)*	*Bile/ Serum (%)*	*Aqueous Humor/ Serum (%)*
>80	*<10*	*HD*	*PD*		*>80*	*80–50*	*50–10*	*<10 (anuric)*							
0.8–1	3.4–5.6	1.8		10 mg/kg	4h	4h	6–8h	8h	10 mg/kg					400	
0.7–1.4	7.4–21			0.25–0.5 g	8h	8h	8–12h	12–16h	0.25–0.5 g		5–10	25–33	5	100–3000	Negligible
1.1–1.3	7.5			0.25–0.5 g	8h	8h	12h	12–24h	0.25 g				Low		
0.7–1.4	7.4–21			0.5–2 g	4–6h	4–6h	8h	12h	0.5–2 g	1–4 g		100	11	100–3000	2–8
1	9			1.5–3.0 g	6–8h	6–8h	8–12h	24h							
1.5–2															
1	5	1.5–2.6		2–4 g	4–6h	4–6h	8h	12h	3 g		13.3[h]				
0.7–1.4	7.4–21			0.4–1.6 g	12h	12h	12h					65–75	1.7–3.6	17	
0.78–1	9.4–23.4	6	4.2–7.4	5–6 g	4h	4h	2–3 g q6h	Avoid	0.75–2 g	2 g q6–12h	9.4[i]	50–100	0.4	50–75	Up to 3
0.78–1	9.4–23.4														
0.4–0.8	0.8–2.3			0.5–1 g	6h	6h	6h	6h	Usual regimen	Usual regimen					
				0.25–0.5 g	6h	6h	12–24h	24h							
0.6–0.8	1–2.2	1–2.2	1–2.2	0.125–0.5 g	6h	6h	6h	6h	Usual regimen	Usual regimen	Minimal	0–10		5–8	
0.3				0.225–0.45 g	6h										
0.4–0.5	4–6	4–6	4–6	1–2 g	4–6h	6h	8h	12h			10	50–100		≥100	Negligible
0.71–1.3	1.6–14		1.6–14	3–4 g	4–6h	4–6h	8h	2 g q8h	2–3 g	3 g q12h	1.2–11.7	70–500	Low	1000	
0.5–1.5	1.8–2.8	1.8–2.8	1.8–2.8	0.5–2 g	4–6h	4–6h	4–6h	4–6h	Usual regimen	Usual regimen	9–20	10–15		≥100	Negligible
0.3–0.8	0.5–2	0.5–2	0.5–2	0.5–2 g	4–6h	4–6h	4–6h	4–6h	Usual regimen	Usual regimen		10–15	≤3.5	20–30	0
0.4–0.9	6–20		6–20	1–4 mU	4–6h	4–6h	4–6h	0.5–2 mU q4–6h	500,000 U		0–10	100	6	200–800	
days											Minimal				
24				0.6–1.2 mU	12h	12h	12h	12h							
0.5	7–10			0.25–0.5 g	6h	6h	6h	6h	0.25 g						
0.6–1.3	2.1–6		2.1–6	3–4 g	4–6h	4–6h	8h	12h	1 g, then 2 g q8h				1	3000–6000	
0.7–1.1	1.9–3.5			2.5–4.5 g	6–8h	6–8h								>100	
4.5–5	18–27	4.5		0.5–1 g	12h	12h	12–24h	36–48h	0.5 g						
0.93–1.3	13.5–16.2			3 g	4–6h	4–6h	6–8h	2 g q12h	3 g, then 2 g q12h	3 g q12h	39				
1.1–1.5	8.5			3.1 g	4–6h	4–6h	2–3.1 g q6–8h	2 g q12h	3.1 g	3.1 g q12h			Low		

TABLE 42–17 Pharmacology: Cephalosporins

Drug (% oral absorption)	Drug Concentrations Achieved with Specific Doses			Dosage Recommendations						
		Measured Levels (μg/ml)		*Adults*			*Children*		*Newborns (Parenteral)*	
	Dose (g)	*Serum (peak)*	*Urine (peak or range)*	*Oral*	*Parenteral*	*Serious Infection (daily dose)*	*Oral*	*Parenteral*	*Up to 1 wk*	*1–4 wk*
First-Generation Agents										
Cefadroxil (100)	0.5 PO 1 PO	10–18 24–35	1800	0.5–1 g q12–24h		2 g	30 mg/kg/d q12h			
Cefazolin	1 IV 1 IM	188 64–76	 4000		0.5–2 g q8h	6 g		25–100 mg/kg/d q6–8h		
Cephalexin (100)	0.25 PO 0.5 PO	9 15–18	 2000	0.25–1 g q6h		2 g	25–100 mg/kg/d in 4 doses			
Cephalothin	1 IM 1 IV	15–21 30	2500		0.5–2 g q4–6h	12 g		80–160 mg/kg/d q6h		
Cephapirin	1 IV	67	2560		0.5–2 g q4–6h	12 g		40–80 mg/kg/d q6h		
Cephradine* (>90)	0.25 PO 0.5 PO 1 IV	9 15–18 86	1600 3200	0.25–1.0 g q6h	0.5–2 g q4–6h	2 g PO; 8 g IV	25–100 mg/kg/d q6 *or* 12h	50–100 mg/kg/d q6h		
Second-Generation Agents										
Cefaclor* (≥52)	0.25 PO 0.5 PO	5–7 13–15	600 900	0.25–0.5 g q8h		1.5 g	20–40 mg/kg/d q8h[c]			
Cefamandole	1 IV[d] 2 IV[d] 3 IV[d]	139 214 534	750 1400		0.5–2 g q4–8h	8 g		50–150 mg/kg/d q4–8h[e]		
Cefmetazole					2 g q6–12h	8 g				
Cefonicid	7.5 mg/kg IV[d] 0.5 IV 1 IV	95–156 91 221	1020		0.5–2 g q24h	2 g				
Cefotetan	1 IV[d] 2 IV[d]	142–179.6 237	1400–2000 3500–4000		1–2 g q12h	4 g		40–60 mg/kg/d q12h		
Cefoxitin	1 IM 1 IV[d] 2 IV[d]	22–24 110–125 221	3000		1–2 g q6–8h	8 g		80–160 mg/kg/d q4–8h[f]		
Cefprozil (95)	0.25 PO 0.5 PO 1 PO	5.6–6.8 8.2–10.4 15.5–19.9	250 1000 2900	0.25–0.5 g q12–24h		1 g	15 mg/kg q12h			
Cefuroxime (37–52)[g]	0.5 PO 0.75 IV[h]	7 51.1	1150	0.125–0.5 g q12h	0.75–1.5 g q8h	1 g PO; 4.5 g IV	0.125–0.25 g q12h[i]	50–100 mg/kg/d q6–8h[j]		10 mg/kg q12h (not approved)
Third-Generation Agents										
Cefdinir* (36)	0.2 PO 0.6 PO	0.7–1.7 2.4		0.3–0.6 g q12–24h		0.6 g	14 mg/kg/d			
Cefixime* (30–50)	0.4 PO tabs 0.4 PO susp	3.7 4.6	15.7–305 15.7–305	0.4 g q24h		0.4 g	8 mg/kg/d q24h			
Cefoperazone	1 IV[h] 2 IV[h]	153 253	 2200		1–2 g q6–12h	12 g		25–100 mg/kg q12h (not approved)		25–100 mg/kg q12h (not approved)
Cefotaxime	0.5 IM 1 IV[d] 2 IV[d]	11.7–11.9 102.4 214.1	90–3261		0.5–2 g q8–12h	12 g		50–200 mg/kg/d q4–8h	50 mg/kg q12h	50 mg/kg q6–8h
Cefpodoxime[l] (50)	0.1 PO 0.2 PO 0.4 PO	1.4 2.3 3.9	60	0.1–0.4 g q12h		0.8 g	5 mg/kg q12h[m]			
Ceftazidime[o]	0.5 IV[h] 1 IV[h] 2 IV[h]	42 69 159–185.5			1–2 g q8–12h	6 g		25–50 mg/kg q8h	30–50 mg/kg q8h[p]	30 mg/kg q8h
Ceftibuten (80)	0.4 PO	15		0.2–0.4 q12–24h		0.6 g	9 mg/kg/d			
Ceftizoxime	1 IV[h] 2 IV 3 IV	84.4 131.8 221.1	>6000		1–3 g q6–8h	12 g		33–50 mg/kg q6–8h[f]		
Ceftriaxone	1 IV[h] 2 IV[h] 2 IV[q]	123.2–150.7 223–276 216–281	504–995		0.5–2 g q12–24h	4 g		50–100 mg/kg/d q12–24h	50 mg/kg q24h	50–75 mg/kg q24h[r]
Moxalactam	1 IV[h] 2 IV[d]	60–100 150–200	2100 4200		0.5–4 g q8–12h[s]	12 g[s]		50 mg/kg q6–8h[s,t]	50 mg/kg q12h[s,t]	50 mg/kg q8h[s,t]
Fourth-Generation Agent										
Cefepime	1 IV 2 IV	81.7 163.9			0.5–2 g q8–12h	6 g		50 mg/kg q8–12h		

*Decreased rate and/or extent of absorption when given with food.
[a]Specified dose is supplemental to that after hemodialysis.
[b]Inflamed meninges.
[c]Should not exceed 1 g.
[d]IV push (over 2–10 min).
[e]Dosage should not exceed adult dosage.
[f]Should not exceed 12 g.
[g]52% after food.
[h]Infusion over 15–30 min.
[i]0.125 g q12h for children <2 yr.
[j]200–240 mg/kg/d q6–8h for meningitis.
[k]Microbiologic activity in hepatic bile/microbiologic activity in serum.

Serum Half-life (h)				Standard Dose with Dosing Intervals in Renal Impairment					Dosage with Dialysis		Body Fluid Concentrations				
With Normal and Anuric Cl_{Cr} Values (ml/min)		*With Dialysis*		*Usual Adult Dose*	*For Cl_{Cr} Ranges (ml/min)*										
>80	*<10*	*HD*	*PD*		*>80*	*80–50*	*50–10*	*<10 (anuric)*	*After HD*[a]	*During PD (daily dose)*	*CSF/ Serum (%)*[b]	*Newborn Serum/ Maternal Serum (%)*	*Breast Milk/ Maternal Serum (%)*	*Bile/ Serum (%)*	*Aqueous Humor/ Serum (%)*
1.1–2	20–25			0.5–1 g	12–24h	12–24h	0.5 g q12–24h	0.5 q36h	0.5–1 g			50	0.9–1.9	22	
1.2–2.2	18–36			0.5–2 g	8h	8h	0.5–1 g q8–12h	0.5–1 g q18–24h	0.25–0.5 g		1–4	35–69	3	29–300	<1.7
0.5–1.2	5–30			0.25–1 g	6h	6h	8–12h	24–48h	0.25–1 g		Minimal	60	2	216	11
0.5–0.9	3–8			0.5–2 g	4–6h	4–6h	1–1.5 g q6h	0.5 g q8h	0.5–2 g	≤6 mg/L of dialysate	1.2–5.6	16–41		22–172	4
0.6–0.9	2.4			0.5–2 g	4–6h	6h	8h	12h	7.5–15 mg/kg before, then 12h after			60	7		
0.7–2	8–15			0.25–1.0 g	6h	6h	0.5 g q6h	0.25 g q12h	0.25 before, then 12 and 36–48h after	0.5 g q6h	≤1	9–22	14–20	10–400	5–9
0.5–1	2.8			0.25–0.5 g	8h	8h	8h	8h	0.25–0.5 g				2	≥60	1–3
0.5–2.1	12.3–18			0.5–2 g	4–8h	6h	8h	0.5–1 g q12h	0.5–1 g		2		2.4	300–400	1.5
1.2				1–2 g	6–12h	12h	16–24h	48h							
3.5–5.8	50–60			0.5–2 g	24h	8–25 mg/kg q24h	4–15 mg/kg q24–48h	3–15 mg/kg q3–5d	None				<1	<10	0.2
2.8–4.6	12–30			1–2 g	12h	12h	24h	48h	25% on non-dialysis days, 50% on dialysis days				2.3	2–21	
0.7–1.1	13–22			1–2 g	6–8h	8–12h	12–24h	0.5–1 g q12–48h	1–2 g		2.8	100	≤3	280	4–7
0.9–1.5	5.9			0.25–0.5 g	12–24h	12–24h	50% q12–24h	50% q12–24h							
1–2	20			0.125–0.5 g PO 0.75–1.5 g IV	12h 8h	12h 8h	12h 8–12h	0.25 g q24h 0.75 g q24h	0.75 g	15 mg/kg after dialysis	17–88	20–33	≤3	35–80	10–14
1.1–4.4				0.3–0.6 g	12–24h										
2.4–4	11.5	7		0.4 g	24h	24h	0.3 g q24h	48h	None			15–50			
1.6–2.6	2–2.5			1–2 g	6–12h	6–12h	6–12h	6–12h	Dose after dialysis		1.8–3.1	20–50	≤1.5	800–1200	1–6
0.9–1.7				0.5–2 g	8–12h	8–12	12–24h	24h	0.5–2 g		27		Up to 3–8	15–75[k]	0.5–4
1.9–3.2	9.8			0.1–0.4 g	12h	12h	24h[n]	24h	Usual dose 3×wk					102–127	
1.4–2	11.9–35			1–2 g	8–12h	8–12h	12–24h	0.5 g q24–48h	1 g load then 1 g after dialysis	0.5 g q24h or 250 mg/2L of dialysate	20–40		7	13–54	3–12
1.5–2.9	18–29		16	0.2–0.4 g	12–24h	12–24h	24h	0.1 g q24h	0.4 g	0.2 g q24h			Neg.		
1.4–1.8	25–35			1–3 g	6–8h	0.5–1.5 g q8h	0.25–1 g q12h	0.5 g q24h	Dose after dialysis	3 g q48h	22.5	28–33	1–6	34–82	3.6–6
5.4–10.9	12.2–18.2	12.2–18.2	12.2–18.2	0.5–2 g	12–24h	12–24h	12–24h	12–24h	None		16–32	18–25	3–4	200–500	
2	20	4	16.7	0.5–4 g	8–12h	3 g q8h	2–3 g q12h	1 g q12–24h	1–2 g	0.5 g q18–24h	4–55	30–40	2.7	152–224	1–16
2	13.5	13.5	19	0.5–2 g	8–12h	12–24h	24h	0.25–0.5 g q24h	0.25 g	1–2 g q48h			0.5 mg/1 L of milk		

[l]Should be given with food to increase absorption.
[m]No more than 400 mg/d for otitis or 100 mg/d for pharyngitis/tonsillitis.
[n]Cl_{Cr} <30 ml/min.
[o]Arginine component not approved for children <12 yr.
[p]30–50 mg/kg q12h for <2 kg; 30 mg/kg q8h for >2 kg.
[q]2 g q24h at steady state.
[r]50 mg/kg/d for <2 kg; 50–75 mg/kg/d for >2 kg.
[s]Bleeding time should be monitored in patients receiving more than 4 g/d for more than 3 d. Prophylactic vitamin K, 10 mg/wk, should be given to patients receiving moxalactam.
[t]For meningitis due to gram-negative organisms in children, the manufacturer recommends an initial loading dose of 100 mg/kg.
Abbreviations: Cl_{Cr}, Creatinine clearance; CSF, cerebrospinal fluid; HD, hemodialysis; PD, peritoneal dialysis.

TABLE 42–18 Pharmacology: β-Lactams Other Than Those in Tables 42–16 and 42–17

	Drug Concentrations Achieved with Specific Doses			**Dosage Recommendations**						
		Measured Levels (μg/ml)		***Adults***			***Children***		***Newborns (Parenteral)***	
Drug (% oral absorption)	***Dose (g)***	*Serum (peak)*	*Urine (peak or range)*	*Oral*	*Parenteral*	*Serious Infection (daily dose)*	*Oral*	*Parenteral*	*Up to 1 wk*	*1–4 wk*
Aztreonam	1 IV[c] 2 IV[c]	90–164 204–255	3000–3500		1–2 g q6h	6 g		30–50 mg/kg q6–12h (not approved)		30–50 mg/kg q6–12h (not approved)
Carumonam	1 2	190 300			0.5–2 g q8h					
Imipenem	0.25 IV[c] 0.5 IV[c] 1 IV[c]	14–24 21–58 41–83	50 100 ≥100		0.5–1 g q6h	2 g		15–25 mg/kg q6h (not approved)		
Meropenem	0.5 IV[c] 1.0 IV[c]	26 55–62			0.5–2 g q8–12h	6 g		20–40 mg/kg q8h		
Loracarbef* (90)	0.2 PO cap 0.4 PO cap 0.4 PO	8 14 17		0.2–4 g q12–24h		0.8 g	15–30 mg/kg/d q12h			

*Decreased rate and/or extent of absorption when given with food.
[a]Specified dose is supplemental to that in hemodialysis.
[b]Inflamed meninges.
[c]IV infusion over 15–30 min.
[d]2.7 h during dialysis/7–9 h between dialysis sessions.
Abbreviations: Cl_{Cr}, Creatinine clearance; CSF, cerebrospinal fluid; HD, hemodialysis; PD, peritoneal dialysis.

Serum Half-life (h)				Standard Dose with Dosing Intervals in Renal Impairment					Dosage with Dialysis		Body Fluid Concentrations				
With Normal and Anuric Cl_{Cr} Values (ml/min)		*With Dialysis*		*Usual Adult Dose*	*For Cl_{Cr} Ranges (ml/min)*										
>80	*<10*	*HD*	*PD*		*>80*	*80–50*	*50–10*	*<10 (anuric)*	*After HD*[a]	*During PD (daily dose)*	*CSF/ Serum (%)*[b]	*Newborn Serum/ Maternal Serum (%)*	*Breast Milk/ Maternal Serum (%)*	*Bile/ Serum (%)*	*Aqueous Humor/ Serum (%)*
1.3–2.2	6–9	2.7 7.9[d]		1–2 g	6h	8–12h	12–18h	24h	1/8 initial dose	Usual initial dose, then 1/4 usual dose at usual intervals	3–52		0.1–0.6	115–405	5–14
1.3–1.7	11.3			0.5–2 g	8h	8–12h	12–24h	0.25–1 g q24h			3				
0.8–1	3.5			0.5–1 g	6h	0.5 g q6–8h	0.5 g q8–12h	0.25–0.5 g q12h	0.25–0.5 g after, then q12h		1–10			Minimal	3
0.8–1	6–20			0.5–2 g	8–12h	8–12h	0.5–1 g q12h	0.5 g q24h	0.5 g		12			40	
1	32	4		0.2–0.4 g	12–24h	12–24h	24–48h	3–5 d	0.2–0.4 g						

TABLE 42–19 Pharmacology: Aminoglycosides

	Drug Concentrations Achieved with Specific Doses			Dosage Recommendations						
		Measured Levels (µg/ml)		*Adults*			*Children*		*Newborns (Parenteral)*	
Drug (% oral absorption)	***Dose (g)***	*Serum (peak)*	*Urine (peak or range)*	*Oral*	*Parenteral*	*Serious Infection (daily dose)*	*Oral*	*Parenteral*	*Up to 1 wk*	*1–4 wk*
Amikacin[c]	0.5 IM 7.5 mg/kg IV[d]	38 17–25	832		15 mg/kg/d q8–12h[e]	15 mg/kg		15 mg/kg/d q8–12h[e]	Not approved	Not approved
Gentamicin[g]	1 mg/kg IM 1 mg/kg IV[h]	4–7.6 4–7.6	113–423		3–5 mg/kg/d q8h[e]	3–5 mg/kg		3–7.5 mg/kg/d q8h[e]	2.5 mg/kg q12h[e]	7.5 mg/kg/d q8h[e]
Isepamicin	15 mg/kg IV[d] 1.0 IM	51 38			8–15 mg/kg q24h	15 mg/kg			7.5 mg/kg q24h[i]	7.5 mg/kg q12h[i]
Kanamycin[c] (1)	7.5 mg/kg IM 7.5 mg/kg IV[d]	22 22			15 mg/kg/d q8–12h[e]	1.5 g		15 mg/kg/d q8–12h[e]	15–20 mg/kg/d q12h[e, j]	15 mg/kg/d q8–12h[e]
Neomycin[k] (3)	4 g PO	2.5–6.1		50 mg/kg/ d q6h		3 g PO				
Netilmicin[l]	2 mg/kg IV[d] 2 mg/kg IM	16.6 7			4–6.5 mg/kg/d q8–12h[e]	3.9 mg/kg		3–7.5 mg/kg/d q8–12h[e]	4–6.5 mg/kg/d q12h[e, j]	4–6.5 mg/kg/d q12h[e, m]
Spectinomycin	2 g IM	100			2 g IM/d	2 g		Not approved	Not approved	Not approved
Streptomycin[n]	0.5 g IM 1 g IM	5–12 25–50	400 ≥1000		0.5–1 g q12h	1 g		20–40 mg/kg/d q6–12h		
Tobramycin[g]	1 mg/kg IM 1 mg/kg IV[d]	4–6 4–6	75–100		3–5 mg/kg/d q8h[e]	3–5 mg/kg		3–6 mg/kg/d q8h[e]	≤4 mg/kg/d q12h[e]	3–5 mg/kg/d q8h[e]

[a]Specified dose is supplemental to that in hemodialysis.
[b]Inflamed meninges.
[c]Desired concentrations: peak 15–30 µg/ml; trough <5–10 µg/ml.
[d]Infused over 30–60 min.
[e]The dosing strategy for aminoglycosides involves the use of ideal (lean) body weight (IBW) for dosage calculation. In obese patients, this approach would result in serum aminoglycoside concentrations less than expected. Alternative dosing recommendations have been proposed that account for the change in drug distribution volume with obesity:

1. Lean body weight + 40% of excess weight, defined as total body weight (TBW) minus IBW (J Infect Dis. 1978;138:499–505).
2. IBW + 58% of excess weight (TBW − IBW) (Clin Pharmacol Ther. 1979;26:508).
3. IBW + 38% of excess weight (TBW − IBW) (Am J Hosp Pharm. 1980;37:519–522).

[f]Dosing at Cl_{Cr} ≤10 ml/minute should be assisted with serum concentrations.
[g]Desired concentrations: peak 4–10 µg/ml; trough <2 µg/ml.
[h]Infused over 2 h.
[i]q24h for infants <16 days old; q12h for those ≥16 days old.
[j]15 mg/kg/d q12h for ≤ 2 kg; 20 mg/kg/d q12h for >2 kg.
[k]Parenteral administration of neomycin is no longer recommended.
[l]Desired concentrations: peak 6–12 µg/ml; trough <2 µg/ml.
[m]For premature or full-term infants <6 weeks of age.
[n]Desired concentrations: peak 5–25 µg/ml; trough <5 µg/ml.
Abbreviations: Cl_{Cr}, Creatinine clearance; CSF, cerebrospinal fluid; HD, hemodialysis; PD, peritoneal dialysis.

Serum Half-life (h)				Standard Dose with Dosing Intervals in Renal Impairment					Dosage with Dialysis		Body Fluid Concentrations				
With Normal and Anuric Cl_{Cr} Values (ml/min)		*With Dialysis*		*Usual Adult Dose*	*For Cl_{Cr} Ranges (ml/min)*							*Newborn Serum/ Maternal Serum (%)*	*Breast Milk/ Maternal Serum (%)*		
>80	*<10*	*HD*	*PD*		*>80*	*80–50*	*50–10*	*<10 (anuric)*	*After HD*[a]	*During PD (daily dose)*	*CSF/ Serum (%)*[b]			*Bile/Serum (%)*	*Aqueous Humor/ Serum (%)*
2–3	30–86			5–7.5 mg/kg	8h	8–12h	12–48h	≥48h[f]	2.5–3.75 mg/kg	2.5 mg/kg/d	15–24	20		30	Minimal
2–3	24–60			1–1.7 mg/kg	8h	8–12h	12–48h	≥48h[f]	1.0–1.7 mg/kg	1 mg/2 L of dialysate removed	10–30	30–40		30–60	Minimal
2–2.5				8 mg/kg	24h	24h	48–72h	96h							
2–4	27–80			7.5 mg/kg	8–12h	8–12h	12–48h	≥48h[f]	4–5 mg/kg	3.75 mg/kg/d	43	50	35		Minimal
2–3	12–24														Minimal
2–2.5	30			2–2.2 mg/kg	8h	8–12h	12–48h	≥48h[f]	2 mg/kg		21–26				Minimal
1.2–2.8				2 g	24h	24h	24h	24h							Minimal
2–3	Up to 110			0.5–1 g	12h	7.5 mg/kg q24h	7.5 mg/kg q24–72h	7.5 mg/kg q72–96h	0.5 g		20	10–40	<25	40–300	Minimal
2–3	5–70			1–1.7 mg/kg	8h	8–12h	12–48h	≥48h	1 mg/kg	1 mg/2 L of dialysate removed	14–23	50		10–20	18

TABLE 42–20 Pharmacology: Tetracyclines[a]

Drug (% oral absorption)	Drug Concentrations Achieved with Specific Doses			Dosage Recommendations						
		Measured Levels (μg/ml)		*Adults*			*Children*		*Newborns (Parenteral)*	
	Dose (g)	*Serum (peak)*	*Urine (peak or range)*	*Oral*	*Parenteral*	*Serious Infection (daily dose)*	*Oral*	*Parenteral*	*Up to 1 wk*	*1–4 wk*
Chlortetracycline[d] (30)	0.25 PO 0.5 PO	1.5–2.5 7	320	As for tetracycline		2 g	As for tetracycline		Not recommended	
Demeclocycline (60–80)	0.15 PO 0.3 PO	0.9–1.2 1.5–1.7		0.6 g/d q6–12h		0.6 g	6.6–13.2 mg/kg/d q6–12h		Not recommended	
Doxycycline (90–100)	0.1 PO 0.1 IV[f]	1.5–2.1 2.5		0.1 g q12h	0.1 g q12h	0.2 g	2.2 mg/kg q12–24h	2.2 mg/kg q12–24h	Not recommended	
Methacycline[d] (58)	0.15 PO 0.3 PO	1.3 2.4		0.15 g q6h *or* 0.3 g q12h		1.2 g	6.6–13.2 mg/kg/d q6–12h		Not recommended	
Minocycline (90–100)	0.2 PO	2–3.5		0.1 g q12h	0.1 g q12h	0.2 g	2 mg/kg q12h	2 mg/kg q12h	Not recommended	
Oxytetracycline[d] (60)	0.25 PO 0.5 PO	1.3–1.4 4–4.2		1–2 g/d q6h	0.25 g IM q24h	2 g	25–50 mg/kg/d q6h	15–25 mg/kg/d q8–12h[g]	Not recommended	
Tetracycline[d] (75–80)	0.25 PO 0.5 PO 0.5 PO[h]	1.5–2.2 3–4.3 2–5		0.25–0.5 g q6h		2 g	25–50 mg/kg/d q6–12h		Not recommended	

[a]The tetracyclines cause a brown discoloration of the teeth and may retard the growth of bone in the human fetus and children. The American Academy of Pediatrics recommends that tetracyclines be used in children who are 9 years of age or older.
[b]Specified dose is supplemental in hemodialysis.
[c]Inflamed meninges.
[d]All tetracyclines should be given 1 hour before or 2 hours after meals.
[e]Patients in the convalescent stage of poliomyelitis.
[f]Infused over 60 minutes.
[g]No more than 250 mg/d.
[h]At steady-state.

Serum Half-life (h)				**Standard Dose with Dosing Intervals in Renal Impairment**					**Dosage with Dialysis**		**Body Fluid Concentrations**				
With Normal and Anuric Cl_{Cr} Values (ml/min)		***With Dialysis***			***For Cl_{Cr} Ranges (ml/min)***										
>80	*<10*	*HD*	*PD*	***Usual Adult Dose***	*>80*	*80–50*	*50–10*	*<10 (anuric)*	***After HD***[b]	***During PD (daily dose)***	***CSF/ Serum (%)***[c]	***Newborn Serum/ Maternal Serum (%)***	***Breast Milk/ Maternal Serum (%)***	***Bile/ Serum (%)***	***Aqueous Humor/ Serum (%)***
5.6	6.8–11			0.25–0.5 g	6h	Not recommended					2–6[e]		40	333	
10–17	42–68			0.15–0.3 g	6–12h	Not recommended					Minimal		70	200–3200	10–30
14–24	18–30	18–30		0.1 g	12h	12h	12h	12h	0.1 g q12h	0.1 g q12h	26		30–40	200–3200	10–13
7–15	Up to 44			0.15–0.3 g	6–12h	Not recommended									
11–26	12–30			0.1 g	12h	12h	12h	12h	0.1 g q12h	0.1 g q12h		77	8–26	200–3200	17
6–10	47–66			0.25–0.5 g PO 0.25 g IM	6h 24h	6h 24h	Use doxycycline				Minimal		20–140	200–3200	
6–12	57–120			0.25–0.5 g	6h	6h	Use doxycycline				7	60–70	25–150	200–3200	9–11

TABLE 42-21 Pharmacology: Azalides, Macrolides, Lincosamides, Chloramphenicol, and Metronidazole

	Drug Concentrations Achieved With Specific Doses			Dosage Recommendations						
		Measured Levels (μg/ml)		Adults			Children		Newborns (Parenteral)	
Drug (% oral absorption)	***Dose (g)***	*Serum (peak)*	*Urine (peak or range)*	*Oral*	*Parenteral*	*Serious Infection (daily dose)*	*Oral*	*Parenteral*	*Up to 1 wk*	*1–4 wk*
Azithromycin[c] (35–40)	0.5 PO 0.5 IV	0.09–0.44 3.63	8.64–26.8	0.5 g q24h × 3 d	0.5 g q24h	0.5 g	5–12 mg/kg/d	10–12 mg/kg/d[d]		
Clarithromycin (50–55)	0.25 PO[e] 0.5 PO[e] 0.5 PO[e]	1 2–3 1[f]		0.25–0.5 g q12h		1 g	7.5 mg/kg q12h (not approved)			
Dirithromycin[g] (6–14)	0.5 PO	0.3–0.4	Minimal	0.5 g q24h		0.5 g	0.5 g q24h[h]			
Erythromycin base[i, j]	0.25 PO	0.1–2		0.25–0.5 g q6h		2 g	30–50 mg/kg/d q6h			
Erythromycin stearate[j]	0.25 PO	0.1–2		0.25–0.5 g q6h		2 g	30–50 mg/kg/d q6h			
Erythromycin ethyl succinate[j]	0.4 PO	0.1–2		0.4 g q6h		2 g	30–50 mg/kg/d q6h			
Erythromycin lactobionate[k, l]	0.2 IV	3–4			0.5–1 g q6h	4 g		15–20 mg/kg/d q6h		
Erythromycin gluceptate[k]	0.2 IV	3–4			15–20 mg/kg/d q6h	4 g		15–20 mg/kg/d q6h		
Erythromycin estolate[j]	0.25 PO	0.1–2[m]		0.25–0.5 g q6h		2 g	30–50 mg/kg/d q6h			
Josamycin (>90)	0.5 PO 0.5 PO[e]	0.65 1.64	200–400	0.5–1 g q8–12h		3 g	30–75 mg/kg/d q6–12h			
Roxithromycin	0.15 PO 0.3 PO	6 10		0.15–0.3 g q12–24h		0.3 g	5–7.5 mg/kg/d q12h			
Spiramycin (33–40)	1 PO 2 PO 0.5 IV	0.96 1.65 2.28		1 g q6–12h	0.5–1 g q8h	4–5 g				
Clindamycin[i] (90)	0.15 PO 0.6 IV[n]	1.9–3.9 10		0.15–0.3 g q6h	0.3–0.9 g q6–8h	1.2 g PO; 2.7 g IV	8–25 mg/kg/d q6–8h	15–40 mg/kg/d q6–8h	15 mg/kg/d q6–8h[o]	15–20 mg/kg/d q6–8h[o]
Lincomycin[i] (20–30)	0.5 PO 0.6 IM 0.6 IV[p]	1.8–5.3 9.3–18.5 15.9–20.9		0.5 g q6–8h	0.6–1 g q8–12h	8 g	30–60 mg/kg/d q6–8h	10–20 mg/kg/d q8–12h	Not indicated	
Chloramphenicol[q] (75–90)	1 PO 1 PO[e] 1 IV	11 18 4.9–12		0.25–0.75 g q6h	0.25–1 g q6h	4 g	50–100 mg/kg/d q6h	50–100 mg/kg/d q6h	25 mg/kg/d q24h[r]	50 mg/kg/d q12–24h[s]
Metronidazole[i] (80)	0.25 PO 7.5 mg/kg[e]	4.6–6.5 26		0.25–7.5 g q8h	0.5 g q6h	30 mg/kg				

[a] Specified dose is supplemental to that in hemodialysis.
[b] Inflamed meninges.
[c] Decreased extent of absorption of capsule formulation only when given with food.
[d] No studies to support; extrapolated from adult conversion.
[e] At steady state.
[f] Of 14-hydroxyclarithromycin (active metabolite).
[g] Must be given with food.
[h] Not approved for children <12 years of age.
[i] Denotes decreased rate and/or extent of absorption when given with food.
[j] Erythromycin and its derivatives have varying degrees of bioavailability (18 to 45%).
[k] Oral erythromycin therapy should replace IV therapy as soon as possible.
[l] Owing to the local irritative effects, the drug must not be administered rapidly by direct IV injection (IV push).
[m] Higher serum concentrations have been reported in patients taking erythromycin estolate versus other derivatives.
[n] Over 20 min.
[o] When IV clindamycin is given to neonates and infants, organ system functions should be monitored.
[p] When given over 2 h.
[q] Chloramphenicol dosage should be administered to maintain serum concentrations of 10–25 mg/L for peak and 5–10 mg/L for trough.
[r] <2 wk.
[s] >2 wk.
Abbreviations: Cl_{Cr}, Creatinine clearance; CSF, cerebrospinal fluid; HD, hemodialysis; PD, peritoneal dialysis.

Serum Half-life (h)				**Standard Dose with Dosing Intervals in Renal Impairment**					**Dosage with Dialysis**		**Body Fluid Concentrations**				
With Normal and Anuric Cl_{Cr} Values (ml/min)		*With Dialysis*		*Usual Adult Dose*	*For Cl_{Cr} Ranges (ml/min)*				*After HD*[a]	*During PD (daily dose)*	*CSF/ Serum (%)*[b]	*Newborn Serum/ Maternal Serum (%)*	*Breast Milk/ Maternal Serum (%)*	*Bile/Serum (%)*	*Aqueous Humor/ Serum (%)*
>80	*<10*	*HD*	*PD*		*>80*	*80–50*	*50–10*	*<10 (anuric)*							
68	68	68	68	0.5 g	24h	24h	24h	24h	24h	24h					
5–7				0.25–0.5 g	12h	12h	12–24h	24h			Minimal		30	7000	
20–50	20–50	20–50		0.5 g	24h	24h	24h	24h	Usual regimen	Usual regimen					
1.5–2	6			0.25–0.5 g	6h	6h	6h	6h	Usual regimen	Usual regimen	2–13	5–20	50		
1.5–2	6			0.25–0.5 g	6h	6h	6h	6h	Usual regimen	Usual regimen	2–13	5–20	50		
1.5–2	6			0.4 g	6h	6h	6h	6h	Usual regimen	Usual regimen	2–13	5–20	50		
1.5–2	6			0.5–1 g	6h	6h	6h	6h	Usual regimen	Usual regimen	2–13	5–20	50		
1.5–2	6			15–20 mg/ kg/d	6h	6h	6h	6h	Usual regimen	Usual regimen	2–13	5–20	50		
1.5–2	6			0.25–0.5 g	6h	6h	6h	6h	Usual regimen	Usual regimen	2–13	5–20	50		
0.9–2				0.5–1 g	6–12h	6–12h									
12	≈12			0.15–0.3 g	12–24h	12–24h	12–24h	24–48h				30–40	0.05		50–200
5–6				0.5–1 g	6–12h									>100	
2–3	2–3.5			0.15–3 g PO 0.3–0.9 g IV	6h 6–8h	6h 6–8h	6h 6–8h	6h 6–8h	Usual regimen	Usual regimen	Minimal	46	38–50	250–300	
4–6.4	10			0.5 g PO 0.6–1 g IV	6–8h 8–12h	6–8h 8–12h	6–8h 8–12h	24h 24–36h			18	25	13	250–400	8.75
1.5–4.1	3–7		3–7	0.25–0.75 g PO 0.25 g IV	6h 6h	6h 6h	6h 6h	6h 6h	Schedule dose post HD	Usual regimen	45–89	30–80	100		
6–14	8–15		8–15	0.25–0.75 g PO 0.5 g IV	8h 6h	8h 6h	8h 6h	8h 6h	Usual regimen	Usual regimen	≥100	97	100	100	33–50

TABLE 42–22 Pharmacology: Miscellaneous Gram-Positive Agents and Polymixins/Fusidic Acid

	Drug Concentrations Achieved with Specific Doses			**Dosage Recommendations**						
		Measured Levels ($\mu g/ml$)		***Adults***			***Children***		***Newborns (Parenteral)***	
Drug (% oral absorption)	***Dose (g)***	*Serum (peak)*	*Urine (peak or range)*	*Oral*	*Parenteral*	*Serious Infection (daily dose)*	*Oral*	*Parenteral*	*Up to 1 wk*	*1–4 wk*
Colistimethate[c]	0.15 g IM	5–7.5	200–270	5–15 mg/kg/d q8h[d]	2.5–5 mg/kg/d q6–12h	5 mg/kg	5–15 mg/kg/d q8h[d]	2.5–5 mg/kg/d q6–12h	Not recommended	
Polymyxin B[e]	20,000–40,000 U/kg IM	1–8			15,000–25,000 U/kg/d q12h			15,000–25,000 U/kg/d q12h	Not recommended	
Vancomycin (minimal)	1 g IV	25		0.5–2 g/d q6–8h	1 g q12h	1 g PO; 2 g IV	40 mg/kg/d q6–8h[g]	40 mg/kg/d q6–12h	15 mg/kg load, then 10 mg/kg q12h	10 mg/kg q8h
Teicoplanin	3 mg/kg IV[h] 6 mg/kg IV[h]	53 112			0.2–0.4 g q24h			10 mg/kg q24h	6 mg/kg q24h (preliminary)	6 mg/kg q24h (preliminary)
Fusidic acid	0.5 g PO	14–38[i]	<1	0.5–1 g q8h	0.58 g q8h[j]		6.6–16.6 mg/kg q8h	6.6 mg/kg q8h		
Quinupristin-dalfopristin SCH 27899 (Ziracin)	7 mg/kg IV 6 mg/kg IV	5 49–55			7.5 mg/kg q8–12h 1–12 mg/kg/d[k]	22.5 mg/kg/d		7.5 mg/kg q8h		
Linezolid				0.375–0.625 g q12h[k]						

[a]Specified dose is supplemental to that in hemodialysis.
[b]Inflamed meninges.
[c]Colistimethate is the sulfamethyl derivative of colistin; colistin is absorbed to some extent in infants.
[d]Of colistin.
[e]Bioavailability can be up to 10% in infants.
[f]For Cl_{Cr} of 5–20 ml/min, dose should be 7500–12,500 U/kg/d q12h.
[g]Not to exceed 2 g/d.
[h]5-min infusion.
[i]Accumulation occurs with multiple doses of 0.5 g given q8h; a mean serum concentration of 71 $\mu g/ml$ has been reported after 96 h of therapy.
[j]Diethanolamine fusidate, 580 mg, is equivalent to 500 mg sodium fusidate.
[k]Based on early phase I studies.
Abbreviations: Cl_{cr}, Creatinine clearance; CSF, cerebrospinal fluid; HD, hemodialysis; PD, peritoneal dialysis.

Serum Half-life (h)				**Standard Dose with Dosing Intervals in Renal Impairment**					**Dosage with Dialysis**		**Body Fluid Concentrations**				
With Normal and Anuric Cl_{Cr} Values (ml/min)		***With Dialysis***		***Usual Adult Dose***	***For Cl_{Cr} Ranges (ml/min)***				***After HD***[a]	***During PD (daily dose)***	***CSF/ Serum (%)***[b]	***Newborn Serum/ Maternal Serum (%)***	***Breast Milk/ Maternal Serum (%)***	***Bile/Serum (%)***	***Aqueous Humor/ Serum (%)***
>80	*<10*	*HD*	*PD*		*>80*	*80–50*	*50–10*	*<10 (anuric)*							
1.5–8	48–72			2.5–5 mg/kg/d IV	6–12h	2.5–3.8 mg/kg/d q12h	2.5 mg/kg/d q12–24h	1.5 mg/kg q36h			Minimal	50	18		25–30
4.3–6	48–72			15,000–25,000 U/kg/d	12h	12h	12h[f]	2250–3750 U/kg/d q12h			Minimal				
4–6	44.1–406.4			15 mg/kg	12h	See nomogram in Chapter 28			1 g/wk	0.5–1 g/wk	7.21			50	Minimal
40–70	125	163		0.4 g 0.5–1 g PO	24h 8h	48h 8h	48h 8h	72h 8h							
1.3–1.5										10–20 mg/kg/d q12h					
8.6				1–12 mg/kg[k]	24h	24h									
5.5				0.375–0.625 g[k]	12h	12h									

TABLE 42-23 Pharmacology: Sulfonamides and Trimethoprim

	Drug Concentrations Achieved with Specific Doses			**Dosage Recommendations**						
		Measured Levels (μg/ml)		***Adults***			***Children***		***Newborns (Parenteral)***	
Drug (% oral absorption)	***Dose (g)***	*Serum (peak)*	*Urine (peak or range)*	*Oral*	*Parenteral*	*Serious Infection (daily dose)*	*Oral*	*Parenteral*	*Up to 1 wk*	*1–4 wk*
Trimethoprim-sulfamethoxazole* (85)	0.16/0.8 PO 0.16/0.8 IV	1–2/40–60[c] 9/105[e]		0.16/0.8 g q12–24h	3–5 mg/kg q6–8h[d]	1.2 g IV[d]	6–12 mg/kg/d q6–12h[d]	6–12 mg/kg/d q6–12h[d]	Not recommended	
Trimethoprim (80)	0.1 PO 0.2 PO	1 2	30–160	0.1 g q12h		0.2 g	4 mg/kg/d q12h[g]			
Sulfisoxazole* (70–90)	2–4 PO 2–4 IM	11.2–25 11.2–25		0.5–1 g q6h	25 mg/kg q6h	4 g	120–150 mg/kg/d q4–6h		Not recommended	
Sulfamethoxazole* (70–90)	2 PO	50–120		1 g q8–12h		2 g	50–60 mg/kg/d q12h		Not recommended	
Sulfamethizole* (70–90)	2 PO	60		0.5–1 g q6–8 h		6 g	30–45 mg/kg/d q6h		Not recommended	
Sulfacytine* (70–90)	0.25 PO	17	420	0.5 g load, then 0.25 g q6h		1 g	Not recommended		Not recommended	
Sulfadiazine* (70–90)	3 PO	50		2–4 g/d q4–8h		4 g	120–150 mg/kg/d q4–6h	100 mg/kg/d q6–8h	Not recommended	
Sulfadoxine[h]* (70–90)	0.5 PO[i]	51–76		1 tablet qwk or 2 tablets qwk		1.5 g	By age[j]		Not recommended	
Sulfasalazine (10–15)	2 PO	14/21[k]		0.5–1 g q4–6h		4 g[l]	30–60 mg/kg/d q4–8h		Not recommended	
Sulfaphenazole* (70–90)	2 PO	100–150		1 g q12h		2 g	66 mg/kg, then 33 mg/kg q12h		Not recommended	
Dapsone	0.2 PO	0.1–7[c]		0.05–0.1 g q24h		0.1 g	1–2 mg/kg/d q24h			

*Decreased rate and/or extent of absorption when given with food.
[a]Specified dose is supplemental to that in hemodialysis.
[b]Inflamed meninges.
[c]At steady state.
[d]Based on the trimethoprim component.
[e]Uninflamed meninges.
[f]Amniotic fluid concentrations (μg/ml).
[g]Not approved for children <12 years of age.
[h]For malaria prophylaxis. The first dose should be given 1–2 d before departure to an endemic area and the course continued throughout the stay and 4–6 wk thereafter.
[i]One tablet = 500 mg sulfadoxine and 25 mg pyrimethamine.
[j]Under 4 years: ¼ tablet weekly or ½ tablet every other week; 4–8 years: ½ tablet weekly or 1 tablet every other week; 9–14 years: ¾ tablet weekly or 1½ tablets every other week.
[k]Sulfasalazine/sulfapyridine.
[l]Although doses up to 12 g have been administered, a daily dosage exceeding 4 g is associated with an increased incidence of adverse effects.
[m]Sulfapyridine.
Abbreviations: Cl_{Cr}, Creatinine clearance; CSF, cerebrospinal fluid; HD, hemodialysis; PD, peritoneal dialysis.

Serum Half-life (h)				**Standard Dose with Dosing Intervals in Renal Impairment**					**Dosage with Dialysis**		**Body Fluid Concentrations**				
With Normal and Anuric Cl_{Cr} Values (ml/min)		***With Dialysis***		***Usual Adult Dose***	***For Cl_{Cr} Ranges (ml/min)***										
>80	*<10*	*HD*	*PD*		*>80*	*80–50*	*50–10*	*<10 (anuric)*	***After HD[a]***	***During PD (daily dose)***	***CSF/ Serum (%)[b]***	***Newborn Serum/ Maternal Serum (%)***	***Breast Milk/ Maternal Serum (%)***	***Bile/Serum (%)***	***Aqueous Humor/ Serum (%)***
8–15/ 7–12	24/22–50			3–5 mg/kg IV[d]	6–12h	18h	24h	Avoid	4–5 mg/kg[d]	0.16/0.8 g q48h	50/40[e]	80/50[f]	125/10	100–200/ 40–70	10–45/ 20–30
8–15	24			0.1 g	12h	12h	18–24h	Avoid			30–50	70–100	100	100	10
3–7	6–12			1–2 g	6h	6h	1 g q8–12h	1 g q12–24h			8–57[e]	≥50	10	40–70	20–30
7–12	22–50			1 g	8–12h						25–30	≥50			
4–8	58			0.5–1 g	6–8h							≥50			
4–8				0.25 g	6h							≥50			
17	34			0.5–1 g	4–6h						50–80	≥50			
100–231				0.5 g PO 1 g PO	qwk q2wk							≥50			
7.6/10.4[k]				0.5–1 g	4–6h							≥50	30–60[m]		
				1 g	12h							≥50			
20–30				0.05–0.1 g	24h	24h	24h						69		

TABLE 42–24 Pharmacology: Quinolones and Urinary Anti-infectives

Drug (% oral absorption)	Drug Concentrations Achieved with Specific Doses			Dosage Recommendations						
	Dose (g)	Measured Levels (μg/ml)		Adults			Children		Newborns (Parenteral)	
		Serum (peak)	*Urine (peak or range)*	*Oral*	*Parenteral*	*Serious Infection (daily dose)*	*Oral*	*Parenteral*	*Up to 1 wk*	*1–4 wk*
Quinolones										
Cinoxacin (97)	0.25 PO 0.5 PO	8 16	400	0.25 g q6h *or* 0.5 g q12h[c]		1				
Ciprofloxacin* (50–85)	0.5 PO 0.75 PO 0.4 IV[f]	1.6–2.9 2.5–4.3 4.6	350	0.25–0.75 g q12h	0.2–0.4 g q8–12h	1.5 g PO/1.2 IV	25 mg/kg/d q12h	3.2–12.5 mg/kg/d q12h		
Clinafloxacin	0.2 PO 0.2 IV	1.8 1.7–1.9		0.1–0.2 g q12h	0.2–0.4 g q12h	1.2 g	0.1 g q12h[h]			
Enoxacin* (80–90)	0.4 PO 0.6 PO 0.2 IV	2.8–3.6 4 1.8	250–300 337	0.4 g q12h	0.4 g q12h	0.8 g				
Gatifloxacin	0.4 PO 0.6 PO	4.2 5.7		0.4–0.6 g q24h		0.6 g				
Grepafloxacin (70)	0.4 PO	1.2–1.5	15[j]	0.4–0.6 g q24h		0.6 g				
Levofloxacin (99)	0.5 PO 0.5 IV[f]	5.7 6.2		0.25–0.5 g q24h	0.25–0.5 g q24h	0.5 g				
Lomefloxacin (>95)	0.2 PO 0.4 PO	2.1 3–4.7	170	0.4 g q24h		0.4 g				
Nalidixic acid* (100)	1 PO	20–40		1 g q6h		4 g				
Norfloxacin* (30–50)	0.4 PO	1.3–1.9	≥200	0.4 g q12h		0.8 g				
Ofloxacin* (85–100)	0.4 PO 0.2 PO 0.4 IV[f]	2.9–5.6 1.5–2.7 4	200	0.2–0.4 g q12h	0.2–0.4 g q12h	0.8 g				
Oxolinic acid (poor)	0.75 PO	0.9–3.6	45–100	0.75 q12h[c]		2 g				
Pefloxacin (98)	0.4 PO 0.4 IV[f]	3.8–5.6 5.8	100–115	0.4 q12–24h						
Sparfloxacin (92)	0.4 PO	1–2		0.4 g on day 1, 0.2 g q24h		0.4 g				
Trovafloxacin (88–90)	0.2 PO 0.3 PO 0.3 IV[f]	2.3 2.9 3.6		0.1–0.2 g q24h	0.2–0.3 g q24h	0.3 g	3 mg/kg q24h	3 mg/kg q24h		
Urinary Anti-infectives										
Methenamine mandelate[m]	1 PO		40 (formaldehyde)	1 g q6h[c]		4 g	12.5–18.75 mg/kg q6h[c]		Not recommended	
Methenamine hippurate[m]	1 PO	70–100 μmol/L	≈50 (formaldehyde)	1 g q12h[c]		2 g	12.5–25 mg/kg q12h[c]		Not recommended	
Nitrofurantoin (good but variable)	0.1 PO	<2	50–150	0.05–0.1 g q6–8h		0.4 g	5–7 mg/kg/d q6h		Not recommended	

*Decreased rate and/or extent of absorption when given with food.
[a]Specified dose is supplemental to that in hemodialysis.
[b]Inflamed meninges.
[c]Use primarily for the treatment of urinary tract infections.
[d]Use during pregnancy not recommended.
[e]Animal pharmacology studies indicate the presence of drug in the milk of lactating rats receiving oral doses of cinoxacin. Human data are not currently available.
[f]Infused over 60 min.
[g]3.2 h during dialysis/5.8 h in between sessions.
[h]Case report.
[i]For Cl_{Cr} of <30 ml/min; for >30 ml/min, use normal dose.
[j]12–24 h after dose.
[k]Ineffective urinary concentrations expected with compromised renal function.
[l]8–12 h during dialysis/13–48 h in between sessions.
[m]Usually coadministered with an acidifying agent to convert the methenamine salts in urine to ammonia and bactericidal formaldehyde (pH ≤5.5). Mandelic acid and hippuric acid are mildly antiseptic and contribute to urine acidification.
[n]Methenamine penetrates a number of body fluids, including bile and CSF. This penetration proves clinically inconsequential because negligible amounts of formaldehyde are generated at physiologic pH.
[o]Nitrofurantoin accumulates in the serum of patients with a Cl_{Cr} of <60 ml/min, which leads to systemic toxicity.
[p]Although only small amounts of nitrofurantoin have been detected in breast milk, the drug could cause hemolytic anemia in a G-6-PD–deficient infant exposed in this manner.
Abbreviations: Cl_{Cr}, Creatinine clearance; CSF, cerebrospinal fluid; HD, hemodialysis; PD, peritoneal dialysis.

Serum Half-life (h)				**Standard Dose with Dosing Intervals in Renal Impairment**					**Dosage with Dialysis**		**Body Fluid Concentrations**				
With Normal and Anuric Cl_{Cr} Values (ml/min)		*With Dialysis*		*Usual Adult Dose*	*For Cl_{Cr} Ranges (ml/min)*						*CSF/ Serum (%)*[b]	*Newborn Serum/ Maternal Serum (%)*	*Breast Milk/ Maternal Serum (%)*	*Bile/Serum (%)*	*Aqueous Humor/ Serum (%)*
>80	*<10*	*HD*	*PD*		*>80*	*80–50*	*50–10*	*<10 (anuric)*	*After HD*[a]	*During PD (daily dose)*					
1.5	8.4	3–4.4		0.25–0.5 g	6–12h	0.25 g q8h	0.25 g q12–24h	Not recommended				Avoid[d]	<100 (18–78)[e]		
3–5	5–10	3.2/5.8[g]		0.25–0.75 g PO 0.2–0.4 g IV	12h 8–12h	12h 8–12h	0.25–0.5 q12h 12–24	0.25–0.5 q18h 0.2–0.4 q18–24h	0.25–0.5 g q24h	0.25–0.5 g q24h	11–46			2800–4500	3–22
5				0.2–0.4 g IV; 0.1–0.2 g PO	12h	12h	12h	50% q12h			76				
5–7	40	9.8		0.2–0.4 g	12h	12h	0.1–0.2 g q12h[i]	0.1–0.2 g q12h			67			900	
7															
15.7				0.1–0.6 g	24h								Unsafe	5666	
6–8				0.25–0.5 g	24h	24h	24–48h	48h	0.25 g q48h	0.25 g q48h	15		100		
7–8.5	21			0.4 g	24h	24h	0.2 g q24h	0.2 g q24h	0.4 g load, then 0.2 g q24h					700	
1.1–2.5	21			1 g	6h	6h	6h	Avoid[k]			Minimal				
2.3–4	7.6			0.4 g	12h	12h	24h	24h						1000	
4–8	16.9–28.4	8–12/ 13–48[l]		0.2–0.4 g PO/IV	12h	12h	24h	0.1–0.2 g q24h	0.2 g load, then 0.1 g q24h		28–87		96–112	210–1886	
6–7				0.75 g	12h		Not recommended	Not recommended[k]						200–300	
8–12	11–15										52–58			200–600	
16–30				0.4 g load, then 0.2 g	24h	24h	48h	48h							
9–13	9–13	9–13		0.1–0.3 g	24h	24h	24h	24h			25			1540	
3–6				1 g	6h	6h	Avoid[k]				No effect[n]			No effect[n]	No effect[n]
3–6				1 g	12h	12h	Avoid[k]				No effect[n]	50	70–100	No effect[n]	No effect[n]
0.3	1			0.05–0.1 g	6h	6h	Avoid[k,o]					100	<25[p]	200–400	

TABLE 42–25 Pharmacology: Antimycobacterial Agents

	Drug Concentrations Achieved with Specific Doses			**Dosage Recommendations**						
		Measured Levels (μg/ml)		***Adults***			***Children***		***Newborns (Parenteral)***	
Drug (% oral absorption)	***Dose (g)***	*Serum (peak)*	*Urine (peak or range)*	*Oral*	*Parenteral*	*Serious Infection (daily dose)*	*Oral*	*Parenteral*	*Up to 1 wk*	*1–4 wk*
Capreomycin[c]	1 IM	20–47			1 g IM q24h[d]	1 g		10–20 mg/kg/d q24h (not approved)		10–20 mg/kg/d q24h (not approved)
Clofazimine* (45–70)	0.1 PO[e]	0.7[f]		0.1 g q24h		0.1 g				
Cycloserine[h] (70–90)	0.25 PO	10		0.25–0.5 g q12h		1 g	10–20 mg/kg/d q12h			
Ethambutol (75–80)	25 mg/kg PO	2–5		15 mg/kg q24h		15 mg/kg	10–15 mg/kg q24h (not recommended)			
Ethionamide (80)	1 PO	20		0.25–0.5 g q12h		1 g	15–20 mg/kg/d q24h[i] (not approved)			
Isoniazid†[j]	7 mg/kg PO	4.5/1[k]		0.3 g q24h	0.3 g IM q24h	0.3 g	10–20 mg/kg/d q12–24h	10–20 mg/kg/d q12–24h		
Para-aminosalicylic acid	4 PO	76–104		150 mg/kg/d q6–12h		12 g	150–360 mg/kg/d q6–8h[l]			
Pyrazinamide	0.5 PO	9–12		15–30 mg/kg q24h		2 g	30 mg/kg/d q12–24h (not approved)			
Rifabutin (≥20)	0.3 PO	0.375		0.3 g q24h		0.3 g	(not approved)	Not approved	Not approved	Not approved
Rifampin (100)	0.6 PO 0.6 IV[m]	7 17.5		0.6 g q24h	0.6 g q24h	0.6 g	10–20 mg/kg/d q12–24h			
Streptomycin	1 IM	25–50	≥1000		1 g IM q24h	1 g		20–40 mg/kg/d q24h		
Viomycin					1 g q12h 2×/wk	2 g				

*Should be taken with food.
†Decreased rate and/or extent of absorption when given with food.
[a]Specified dose is supplemental to that in hemodialysis.
[b]Inflamed meninges.
[c]Pharmacokinetics similar to those of streptomycin.
[d]Administer for 60–120 d followed by 1 g q 2–3×/wk.
[e]In leprosy patients.
[f]At steady state.
[g]8-d serum half-life/70-d tissue half/life.
[h]Dosage should be adjusted to maintain plasma concentrations <30 μg/ml.
[i]Limited evidence suggests that 20 mg/kg daily given as a single dose in children is more likely to produce CSF concentrations exceeding the MIC of 2.5 μg/ml for *Mycobacterium tuberculosis.*
[j]To minimize the risk of polyneuritis from isoniazid-induced pyridoxine deficiency, pyridoxine (15–50 mg) is often given concurrently.
[k]4.5 μg/ml in slow inactivators/1.0 μg/ml in rapid inactivators.
[l]Should not exceed the adult dose.
[m]Infused over 30 min.
[n]Desirable serum concentrations: peak 5–25 μg/ml; trough <5 μg/ml.
Abbreviations: Cl_{Cr}, Creatinine clearance; CSF, cerebrospinal fluid; HD, hemodialysis; MIC, minimal inhibitory concentration; PD, peritoneal dialysis.

Serum Half-life (h)				Standard Dose with Dosing Intervals in Renal Impairment					Dosage with Dialysis		Body Fluid Concentrations				
With Normal and Anuric Cl_{Cr} Values (ml/min)		*With Dialysis*		*Usual Adult Dose*	*For Cl_{Cr} Ranges (ml/min)*				*After HD*[a]	*During PD (daily dose)*	*CSF/ Serum (%)*[b]	*Newborn Serum/ Maternal Serum (%)*	*Breast Milk/ Maternal Serum (%)*	*Bile/ Serum (%)*	*Aqueous Humor/ Serum (%)*
>80	*<10*	*HD*	*PD*		*>80*	*80–50*	*50–10*	*<10 (anuric)*							
4–6	29.4–55.5			1 g	24h	24h	7.5 mg/kg q24–48h	7.5 mg/kg 2×/wk						Minimal	
8D/70D[g]				0.1 g	8h	8h	8h	8h							
10				0.25–0.5 g	12h	12h	24h	0.25 g q24h			80–100	100	72		
3.3	≥7			15–25 mg/kg	24h	15 mg/kg q24h	15 mg/kg q24–36h	15 mg/kg q48h	15 mg/kg/d	15 mg/kg/d	25–50	≈100			
3	9			0.25–0.5 g	12h	12h	12h	5 mg/kg q24h			100				
0.5–4	2–10			0.3 g PO/IM	24h	24h	24h	½ dose in slow acetylators	5 mg/kg	Daily dose after dialysis	100	High	100		
1	23			3 g	6–8h						10–50				
10–16				15–30 mg/kg	24h	24h	24h	12–20 mg/kg q24h			100				
16–69				0.3 g	24h	24h									
2–5	2–5	Minimal change		0.6 g	24h	24h	24h	24h			10–20	33	20–60	10,000	
2–3	Up to 110			1 g[n]	24h	7.5 mg/kg/d q24h	7.5 mg/kg/d q24–72h	7.5 mg/kg/d q72–96h	0.5 g		20	10–40	<25	40–300	
				1g	12 2 ×/wk						Poor				

TABLE 42–26 Pharmacology: Antifungal Agents

	Drug Concentrations Achieved with Specific Doses			Dosage Recommendations						
		Measured Levels (μg/ml)		*Adults*			*Children*		*Newborns (Parenteral)*	
Drug (% oral absorption)	***Dose (g)***	*Serum (peak)*	*Urine (peak or range)*	*Oral*	*Parenteral*	*Serious Infection (daily dose)*	*Oral*	*Parenteral*	*Up to 1 wk*	*1–4 wk*
Amphotericin B (poor)	0.03 IV[c] 0.05 IV[c]	1 2			0.25–1 mg/kg q24h[d, e]	1 mg/kg[f]		0.25–1 mg/kg q24–48h[d]	0.1–1 mg/kg/d[d]	0.1–1 mg/kg/d[d]
Fluconazole (≥90)	0.4 PO 0.1 IV[g]	6.72 3.86–4.96		0.05–0.4 g q24h	0.05–0.4 g q24h	0.4 g				
Flucytosine*[h] (75–90)	2 PO	30–45		50–150 mg/kg/d q6h		150 mg/kg	50–150 mg/kg/d q6h			
Griseofulvin (50/>50)[i]	0.5/0.25 PO[i]	0.4–2/0.4–2		0.5–1 g q24h/ 0.33–0.66 g q24h		1 g	15 mg/kg/d q24h			
Itraconazole (99.8)[j, k]	0.2 PO[l]	2.3/3.5[m]		0.2–0.4 g q24h		0.4 g				
Ketoconazole[k]	0.2 PO	4.2		0.2–0.4 g q12–24h		0.8 g	5–10 mg/kg/d q12–24h			
Miconazole (50)	0.522 IV[o]	6			0.4–1.2 q8h	3.6 g		20–40 mg/kg/d q8h		
Nystatin (minimal)	All doses	Not detectable		0.4–1 mU q8h		2 mU	0.4–0.6 mU q6h		0.1 mU q6h	0.1 mU q6h
Pentamidine	4 mg/kg IV	0.5			4 mg/kg/d	4 mg/kg		4 mg/kg/d		
Terbinafine (80)				0.125–0.5 g q12–24h		0.5 g				

*Decreased rate and/or extent of absorption when given with food.
[c]Infused over several hours
[d]A test dose of 1 mg infused over 15 minutes is often given to assess febrile reactions prior to proceeding to higher doses
[e]Should be administered by slow infusion; rapid IV infusion should be avoided since potentially serious adverse effects (e.g., hypotension, hypokalemia, arrhythmias, shock) may occur
[f]Or 1.5 mg/kg every other day
[g]Infused over 30 minutes; ascertained on day 6–7
[h]Peak concentrations should be above 25 μg/ml to avoid development of resistance but should not exceed 100–120 μg/ml to avoid side effects
[i]Microsize/ultramicrosize
[j]When given with meals
[k]Gastric acid suppressing agents decrease bioavailability to <5%
[l]Taken 2× day for 15 days
[m]Parent drug/active metabolite (hydroxyitraconazole)
[n]Half-life extends as dosing continues
[o]Infused over 15 minutes
[p]Triphasic elimination: alpha = 0.4h; beta = 2.1h; gamma = 24.1h

Serum Half-life (h)				Standard Dose with Dosing Intervals in Renal Impairment					Dosage with Dialysis		Body Fluid Concentrations				
With Normal and Anuric Cl_{Cr} Values (ml/min)		*With Dialysis*		*Usual Adult Dose*	*For Cl_{Cr} Ranges (ml/min)*										
>80	*<10*	*HD*	*PD*		*>80*	*80–50*	*50–10*	*<10 (anuric)*	*After HD*[a]	*During PD (daily dose)*	*CSF/ Serum (%)*[b]	*Newborn Serum/ Maternal Serum (%)*	*Breast Milk/ Maternal Serum (%)*	*Bile/ Serum (%)*	*Aqueous Humor/ Serum (%)*
24 or more	24 or more			0.25–1 mg/kg	24h	24h	24h	24h	Usual regimen	Usual regimen	3	50			25
20–50	48			0.05–0.4 g	24h	24h	50% of dose	25% of dose			50–94				
3–6	30–250			37 mg/kg	6h	6h	12–24h	15–25 mg/kg q24h	20–37.5 mg/kg		60–100				
24	24			0.5–1 g/0.33–0.66 g	24h/24h	24h/24h	24h/24h	24h/24h				80			
21–60[n]				0.2–0.4 g	24h	24h					<10				
8	8			0.2–0.4 g	12–24h	12–24h	12–24h	12–24h	Usual regimen	Usual regimen	Minimal			Minimal	≈10
0.4–24.1[p]	0.4–24.1[p]			0.4–1.2 g	8h	8h	8h	8h		<3–48					
				0.4–1 mU	8h	8h	8h	8h							
9	9	9	9	4 mg/kg	24h	24h	24h	24h	4 mg/kg q24h						
22–30				0.125–0.25 g	12–24h	12–24h							Unsafe		

TABLE 42-27 Pharmacology: Antiviral Agents

	Drug Concentrations Achieved with Specific Doses			Dosage Recommendations						
		Measured Levels (μg/ml)		*Adults*			*Children*		*Newborns (Parenteral)*	
Drug (% oral absorption)	***Dose (g)***	*Serum (peak)*	*Urine (peak or range)*	*Oral*	*Parenteral*	*Serious Infection (daily dose)*	*Oral*	*Parenteral*	*Up to 1 wk*	*1–4 wk*
Abacavir (76–100)	0.4 PO	3.3		0.6–1.2 g q8–12h		1.2 g				
Acyclovir (15–30)[a]	0.2 PO[b] 0.8 PO[b] 5 mg/kg IV[c]	0.83 1.61 7.7		0.2–0.8 g 2–5/d	5–12 mg/kg q8h	4 g PO; 30 mg/kg IV	0.2 g for 5/d	25–50 mg/kg/d q8h		
Adefovir (12)	1 mg/kg IV	4		0.125 g q24h	1–3 mg/kg/d					
Amantadine (85–90)	0.1 PO[d]	0.302		0.1 g q12h		0.2 g	5–8 mg/kg/d q12h			
Cidofovir	10 mg/kg IV	24			5 mg/kg qwk[d]	5 mg/kg				
Delavirdine (60–100)	0.4 PO[b]	30[e]		0.4 g q8h		1.2 g	0.4 g q8h[f]			
Didanosine* (21–43)	33 mg/kg	29.8[e]		0.125–0.25 g q12h		12 mg/kg/d	Dose based on BSA[h]			
Efavirenz	0.2 PO[b] 0.6 PO[b]	2.0 4.5		0.2–0.6 g q24h		0.6 g				
Famciclovir (75–77)	0.5 PO 0.75 PO	3.3–3.4 5.1–5.3		0.125–0.75 g q8–12h		2.25 g				
Foscarnet	0.09 IV[b]	218[e]			60 mg/kg q8h[i]	120–180 mg/kg				
Ganciclovir	5 mg/kg IV[c]	6.6–8.3			5 mg/kg q12h[j]	5 mg/kg maintenance		5 mg/kg q12h[j]		
Indinavir	0.8 PO[b, g]	251–12,617[k]		0.8 g q8h		2.4 g				
Lamivudine (82–87)	2–8 mg/kg PO	1.725–5.815		0.15–0.3 g q12h		0.6 g	4 mg/kg q12h[l]			
Nelfinavir[m]				0.75 g q8h[m]		2.25 g	20–30 mg/kg q8h[m]			
Nevirapine	0.2 PO 0.4 PO	1.5–2.5 2.9–3.4		0.2 g q12h		0.4 g	0.2 mg/m² q12h[n]			
Ribavirin	0.82 mg/kg/h[o] 0.82 mg/kg/h[p]	0.275 1.1		Aerosol[q]			Aerosol[r]			
Ritonavir (80)[s]	0.6 PO 1.2 PO	5 11.2		0.6 g q12h		1.2 g				
Saquinavir[m]	0.6 PO	0.066		0.6–1.2 g q8h[u]		7.2 g				
Stavudine (80)	4 mg/kg PO	4.2		0.04 g q12h		2 mg/kg/d	2 mg/kg/d[w]			
Valacyclovir (55)	2 PO[b]	8.49		1 g q8–12h						
Vidarabine	10 mg/kg IV	0.2–0.4/3–6[y]			10–15 mg/kg/d over 12 h	15 mg/kg		10–15 mg/kg/d over 12 h	15–30 mg/kg/d over 12 h	15–30 mg/kg/d over 12 h
Zalcitabine* (70–88)[g]	0.0005 PO 0.005 PO	0.0076 0.079		0.75 mg q8h[aa]		2.25 mg	0.75 mg q8h[bb]			
Zanamivir (10, intranasal)				6.4 mg q4–12h nasally						
Zidovudine (50–76)[cc]	0.25 PO[b] 5 mg/kg IV[i]	0.62 1.6–2.7		0.2 g q4h[dd]	1–2 mg/kg q4h[ee]	0.6 g	180 mg/m² q6h			

*Decreased rate and/or extent of absorption when given with food.
[a]Bioavailability decreases as dosage is increased.
[b]At steady state.
[c]Infused over 1 h.
[d]qwk × 2 wk, then q2wk.
[e]micromol/L.
[f]For children 13 years of age or older.
[g]In HIV-infected patients.
[h]Solution doses for children: for BSA 1–1.4 m²: 125 mg q12h; for BSA 0.8–1 m²: 94 mg q12h; for BSA 0.5–0.7 m²: 62 mg q12h; for BSA 0.4 m²: 31 mg q12h (manufacturer recommendations; optimum dosage has not been elucidated).
[i]For 14–21 d as initial induction therapy, then 90 mg/kg q24h as maintenance.
[j]For 14–21 d as induction therapy, then 5 mg/kg q24h.
[k]nMol.
[l]Over 12 years of age: 150 mg q12h.
[m]Give with food.
[n]Over 9 years of age: 120 mg/m².
[o]Inhaled over 5 h each day for 3 d.
[p]Inhaled over 8 h each day for 3 d.
[q]Mist of 190 μg/L via SPAG-2 aerosol generator; rate of 12.5 L mist/min × 16–18 h/day 1 of influenza A or B infection; then × 12h/d on days 2 and 3; then × 4h on day 4 (not approved in United States).
[r]Mist of 190 μg/L via SPAG-2 aerosol genertor; rate of 12.5 L mist/min × 12–18 h/d for 3–7 d.
[s]In animals.
[t]Following administration for 4–7 wk in AIDS or ARC patients.
[u]Lower dose for saquinavir mesylate.
[v]600 mg q8h for saquinavir mesylate and 1200 mg q8h for plain saquinavir (Fortovase).
[w]Children >30 kg should receive adult dosage.
[x]Half-life of valacyclovir is less than 30 min but its metabolite acyclovir has a half-life of 2.5–3.6 h.
[y]Vidarabine/ara-hypoxanthine (less active metabolite).
[z]With normal meninges.
[aa]Should be coadministered with zidovudine 200 mg q8h.
[bb]In children 13 years of age or at least 30 kg.
[cc]Reaches systemic circulation as unchanged drug.
[dd]For 1 month; then can be decreased to 100 mg q4h in symptomatic HIV-infected patients.
[ee]An IV dose of 1 mg/kg q4h is equivalent to an oral dose of 100 mg q4h.
[ff]In asymptomatic patients.
Abbreviations: AIDS, Acquired immunodeficiency syndrome; ARC, AIDS-related complex; BSA, body surface area; Cl_{Cr}, creatinine clearance; CSF, cerebrospinal fluid; HD, hemodialysis; HIV, human immunodeficiency virus; PD, peritoneal dialysis.

Serum Half-life (h)				Standard Dose with Dosing Intervals in Renal Impairment					Dosage with Dialysis		Body Fluid Concentrations				
With Normal and Anuric Cl_{Cr} Values (ml/min)		*With Dialysis*		*Usual Adult Dose*	*For Cl_{Cr} Ranges (ml/min)*				*After HD*[a]	*During PD (daily dose)*	*CSF/ Serum (%)*[b]	*Newborn Serum/ Maternal Serum (%)*	*Breast Milk/ Maternal Serum (%)*	*Bile/ Serum (%)*	*Aqueous Humor/ Serum (%)*
>80	*<10*	*HD*	*PD*		*>80*	*80–50*	*50–10*	*<10 (anuric)*							
0.8–1.5				0.6–1.2 g	8–12h										
2.1–3.5	19.5		Minimal change	0.2–0.8 g PO 5–12 mg/kg IV	2–5 ×/d 8h	2–5 ×/d 8h	2–5 ×/d 12–24h	0.2–0.8 g q24h 2.5–6 mg/kg q24h	0.5 g	2.5 mg/kg/d	50		≥100		37
1.6				0.125 g PO; 1–3 mg/kg IV	24h	24h									
15–20	170	7–10.3 d		0.1 g	12h	24h	0.1–0.2 g 2–3 ×/wk	0.1–0.2 g qwk			50				
2.5				5 mg/kg	qwk	qwk	Do not use	Do not use	Do not use	Do not use					
2–11				0.4 g	8h						0.4				
1.3–1.6	4.5			0.167–0.375 g	12h	12h			No suppl but give normal dose after HD		12–85				
60											1.19				
2–2.3				0.125–0.75 g	8–12h	8–12h	12–24h	24–48h							
36–196				60 mg/kg	8h	8h					7–39				
2.53–3.6	10			5 mg/kg	12h	2.5 mg/kg q12h	2.5 mg/kg q24h	1.25 mg/kg q24h	1.25 mg/kg q24h		41				40
1.5–2				0.8 g	8h			0.05 g q24h					Unsafe		
3–7				0.15–0.3 g	12h	12h	24h								
3.5–5	3.5–5	3.5–5	3.5–5	0.75–1 g	8h	8h	8h	8h	None	Normal					
40	40			0.2 g	12h	12h	12h	12h							
24–36									None		70[t]				
3–3.5				0.6 g	12h				None						
13				0.6 or 1.2 g[v]	8h						Negative				
0.9–1.6	≥8			0.04 g	12h	12h	0.02 g q12–24h	0.02 g q24h			16–97				
2.5–3.6[x]				0.5–1 g	8–12h	8–12h	12–24h	24h	0.5–1 g	Normal			Unsafe		
1.5/3.3				15 mg/kg/d	Over 12 h	Over 12 h	Over 12 h	10 mg/kg/d Over 12 h	Schedule after HD		33–35[z]				
0.5–3	8.5			0.75 g	8h	8h	12h	24h			9–37	9–37			
3.4				6.4 mg	4–12h										
0.8–1.9	1.4			0.1 g[ff]	4h	4h	6h	6h			15–98	100			

TABLE 42–28 Adverse Drug Interactions Involving Antimicrobial Agents

Interacting Drugs	Adverse Effect	Probable Mechanism
Acyclovir with		
Aminoglycosides	Increased nephrotoxicity and/or neurotoxicity	Mechanism not established
Narcotics	Increased meperidine effect	Decreased renal excretion
Probenecid	Possible increased acyclovir toxicity	Decreased renal excretion
Zidovudine	Increased neurotoxicity (profound drowsiness and lethargy)	Additive
Amantadine with		
Anticholinergics	Hallucinations, confusion, nightmares	Mechanism not established
Antihistamines	Increased CNS adverse reactions	Additive anticholinergic effects
CNS stimulants	Additive CNS-stimulant effects	Mechanism not established
Triamterene	CNS toxicity	Decreased renal clearance
Trimethoprim	CNS toxicity	Decreased renal clearance
Aminoglycoside antibiotics with		
Acyclovir	Increased nephrotoxicity and/or neurotoxicity	Additive
Amphotericin B	Nephrotoxicity	Synergism
Anticoagulants, oral	Potentiation of anticoagulation effects	Decreased GI absorption or synthesis of vitamin K
Bacitracin	Increased nephrotoxicity	Additive
Bumetanide	Increased ototoxicity	Additive
Capreomycin	Increased nephrotoxicity and/or neurotoxicity	Additive
Carboplatin	Increased ototoxicity	Additive
Cephalosporins	Increased nephrotoxicity	Mechanism not established
Cidofovir	Increased nephrotoxicity	Additive
Cisplatin	Increased nephrotoxicity	Mechanism not established
Colistimethate	Increased nephrotoxicity and/or neurotoxicity	Additive
Cyclosporine	Increased renal toxicity	Possibly additive or synergistic
Digoxin	Probable decreased digoxin effect with oral gentamicin or neomycin	Decreased absorption
Ethacrynic acid	Increased ototoxicity	Additive
Furosemide	Increased ototoxicity and nephrotoxicity	Additive
Magnesium sulfate	Increased neuromuscular blockade	Additive
Methotrexate	Possible increased methotrexate toxicity with kanamycin	Mechanism not established
	Possible decreased methotrexate effect with oral aminoglycosides	Decreased absorption
Methoxyflurane	Increased nephrotoxicity	Additive
Miconazole	Possible decreased tobramycin concentration	Mechanism not established
Neuromuscular blocking agents	Neuromuscular blockade	Additive
NSAIDs	Possible aminoglycoside toxicity in preterm infants with indomethacin given for patent ductus closure	Decreased renal clearance
Penicillins	Decreased aminoglycoside effect with high concentrations of carbenicillin or ticarcillin	Inactivation
	Falsely low aminoglycoside levels	In vitro inactivation
Polymyxins	Increased nephrotoxicity; neuromuscular blockade	Additive
Tacrolimus	Increased nephrotoxicity	Additive
Vancomycin	Possible increased nephrotoxicity and ototoxicity	Additive
Aminosalicylic acid (PAS) with		
Anticoagulants, oral	Enhanced hypoprothrombinemic effects	Mechanism not established
Ammonium chloride	Increased probability of crystalluria	Acidification of urine
BCG vaccine	Negates BCG effect	Negates immune response
Digoxin	Decreased digoxin effect	Decreased absorption with time
Diphenhydramine	Decreased effect of PAS	Decreases GI absorption
Ethionamide	GI distress/hepatotoxicity	Additive
Isoniazid	Increased isoniazid serum concentrations	Decreased metabolism
Probenecid	Increased PAS toxicity	Decreased renal excretion
Rifampin	Rifampin effectiveness may be decreased; separate doses by 8–12 hr	Decreased GI absorption due to excipient bentonite
Amphotericin B with		
Aminoglycoside antibiotics	Nephrotoxicity	Synergism
Antineoplastics	Possible increased renal toxicity, bronchospasm, and hypotension	Mechanism not established
Capreomycin	Increased nephrotoxicity	Additive
Cidofovir	Increased nephrotoxicity	Additive
Cisplatin	Increased nephrotoxicity	Additive
Colistin	Increased nephrotoxicity	Additive
Corticosteroids	Increased hypokalemia	Additive
Cyclosporine	Increased renal toxicity	Possible synergism
Digitalis glycosides	Increased digitalis toxicity	Hypokalemia
Imidazole antifungals	Possible antagonism in animal models	Mechanism not established
Methoxyflurane	Increased nephrotoxicity	Additive
Neuromuscular blocking agents	Increased neuromuscular blocking effect	Hypokalemia
Pentamidine	Increased nephrotoxicity	Additive
Polymyxins	Increased nephrotoxicity	Additive
Tacrolimus	Increased nephrotoxicity	Additive
Vancomycin	Increased nephrotoxicity	Additive
Zidovudine	Potential for increased myelotoxicity and nephrotoxicity	Mechanism not established

TABLE 42–28 Adverse Drug Interactions Involving Antimicrobial Agents *Continued*

Interacting Drugs	Adverse Effect	Probable Mechanism
Azithromycin with		
Aluminum/magnesium antacids	Decreased peak concentrations; does not affect overall absorption	Mechanism not established
Digoxin	Increased digoxin concentrations	Destruction of intestinal *Eubacterium lentum* in 10% of digoxin patients
Aztreonam with		
Chloramphenicol	Possible in vitro antagonism; administer a few hours apart	Mechanism not established
Bacitracin with		
Aminoglycosides	Increased nephrotoxicity	Additive
Anesthetics	Potentiation of neuromuscular blocking effects	Additive
Neuromuscular blocking drugs	Potentiation of neuromuscular blocking effects	Additive
Polymyxins	Increased nephrotoxicity	Additive
Capreomycin with		
Aminoglycosides	Increased nephrotoxicity and/or ototoxicity	Additive
BCG vaccine	Negates BCG effect	Negates immune response
Colistin	Increased nephrotoxicity	Additive
Polymyxin B	Increased nephrotoxicity	Additive
Vancomycin	Increased nephrotoxicity and/or ototoxicity	Additive
Cephalosporins with		
Alcohol	Disulfiram-like effect with cefamandole, cefmetazole, cefotetan, cefoperazone, and moxalactam; also with cefonicid in animals, but not shown in humans	Inhibition of intermediary metabolism of alcohol
Aminoglycoside antibiotics	Increased nephrotoxicity	Mechanism not established
Ampicillin	In vitro antagonism with ceftazidime versus group B streptococci and *Listeria*	Mechanism not established
Anticoagulants, oral	Possible increased anticoagulant effect with moxalactam, cefamandole, cefmetazole, or cefoperazone	Mechanism not established
Aspirin	Possible increased bleeding risk with moxalactam	Additive
Chloramphenicol	In vitro antagonism	Mechanism not established
Colistin	Increased nephrotoxicity	Additive
Diuretics	Increased nephrotoxicity with some cephalosporins	Mechanism not established
Ethacrynic acid	Increased nephrotoxicity	Mechanism not established
Furosemide	Increased nephrotoxicity	Mechanism not established
Heparin	Possible increased bleeding risk with moxalactam	Additive
Penicillins	Possible increased cefotaxime toxicity with azlocillin in patients with renal impairment	Decreased excretion
Polymyxins	Increased nephrotoxicity	Additive
Probenecid	Higher and prolonged cephalosporin concentrations	Competitive inhibition of tubular secretion
Salicylates	Decreased cefixime concentrations and AUCs	Displacement from protein-binding sites
Vancomycin	Increased nephrotoxicity	Additive
Chloramphenicol with		
Acetaminophen	Possible decreased chloramphenicol effect	Increased metabolism
Anticoagulants (oral)	Increased dicumarol effect	Decreased metabolism
Aminoglycosides	In vitro antagonism; not seen in vivo	Mechanism not established
Aztreonam	Antagonism; administer chloramphenicol separately a few hours later	Mechanism not established
Barbiturates	Increased barbiturate effect; decreased chloramphenicol effect	Decreased metabolism Increased metabolism
Cephalosporins	Antagonism	Mechanism not established
Cimetidine	Aplastic anemia	Possibly additive or synergistic
Cyclophosphamide	Decreased cyclophosphamide effect	Decreased clearance
Etomidate	Prolonged anesthesia	Decreased metabolism
Folic acid	Delayed response to folic acid	Mechanism not established
Hypoglycemics, sulfonylurea	Increased hypoglycemic effect	Mechanism not established
Iron	Delayed response to iron	Mechanism not established
Lincomycin	Decreased lincomycin effect	Target site antagonism
Penicillins	In vitro antagonism; not seen in vivo	Mechanism not established
Phenytoin/fosphenytoin	Increased phenytoin toxicity Possible increased chloramphenicol toxicity	Decreased metabolism Mechanism not established
Rifampin/rifabutin	Decreased chloramphenicol effect	Increased metabolism
Vitamin B_{12}	Delayed response to vitamin B_{12}	Mechanism not established
Chloroquine with		
Ampicillin	Decreased ampicillin effect	Decreased bioavailability
Aurothioglucose	Blood dyscrasias	Additive
Cholestyramine	Decreased effect	Decreased bioavailability
Cimetidine	Increased toxicity	Decreased clearance
Cyclosporine	Increased cyclosporine toxicity	Decreased clearance
Magnesium antacids	Decreased efficacy	Decreased bioavailability
Methotrexate	Decreased methotrexate efficacy	Increased clearance

Table continued on following page

TABLE 42–28 Adverse Drug Interactions Involving Antimicrobial Agents *Continued*

Interacting Drugs	Adverse Effect	Probable Mechanism
Chloroquine with *Continued*		
Rabies vaccine	Decreased vaccine effect	Interference with the antibody response
Ritonavir	Increased chloroquine toxicity	Decreased metabolism
Succinylcholine	Increased neuromuscular blockade	Decreased clearance
Clarithromycin with		
Anticoagulant, oral	Hypoprothrombinemia potentiated	Possible decreased metabolism
Astemizole	Increased Q-T interval and possible arrhythmias	Decreased antihistamine metabolism
Benzodiazepines	Increased CNS toxicity	Decreased metabolism
Carbamazepine	Increased carbamazepine toxicity	Possible decreased metabolism
Cimetidine	Decreased clarithromycin concentrations	Prolonged absorption
Cisapride	Increased cardiotoxicity	Decreased metabolism
Clindamycin	In vitro antagonism; not documented clinically	Mechanism not established
Corticosteroids	Increased effect and possible toxicity of methylprednisolone	Decreased excretion
Cyclosporine	Increased cyclosporine toxicity	Probably decreased metabolism
Delavirdine	Increased clarithromycin toxicity	Decreased metabolism
Digoxin	Increased digoxin effect	Decreased gut metabolism and increased absorption
Disopyramide	Increased disopyramide concentrations, Q-T interval prolongation and polymorphic ventricular tachycardia	Mechanism not established
Ergot alkaloids	Increased ergot toxicity	Mechanism not established
Phenytoin	Possible increased or decreased effect	Altered metabolism
Rifampin/rifabutin	Decreased clarithromycin concentrations/ increased rifamycin toxicity	Increased/decreased metabolism
Ritonavir	Increased clarithromycin toxicity	Decreased metabolism
Saquinavir	Increased saquinavir concentrations	Decreased metabolism
Tacrolimus	Increased tacrolimus toxicity	Decreased metabolism
Terfenadine	Prolonged Q-T interval and possible arrhythmias	Decreased antihistamine metabolism
Theophylline	Increased theophylline effect and possible toxicity	Decreased metabolism
Zidovudine	Decreased zidovudine concentrations and AUCs with clarithromycin	Mechanism not established
Clindamycin with		
Neuromuscular blocking agents	Increased neuromuscular blockade	Additive
Saquinavir	Increased clindamycin toxicity	Decreased metabolism
Clofazimine with		
Dapsone	Possible decrease or nullification of clofazimine's anti-inflammatory activity	Opposing effects on neutrophil motility and lymphocyte transformation
Isoniazid	Increased clofazimine serum and urine concentrations and decreased skin concentrations	Mechanism not established
Phenytoin	Decreased efficacy	Increased phenytoin clearance
Rifampin	Decreased rate of absorption, time to reach peak, and AUC of rifampin	Mechanism not established
Colistimethate: same as for *Polymyxin B*		
Cycloserine with		
Alcohol	Increased alcohol effect or convulsions	Mechanism not established
Anticoagulants, oral	Increased effect	Mechanism not established
Ethionamide	Increased neurotoxicity	Additive
Isoniazid	CNS effects, dizziness, drowsiness	Mechanism not established
	Increased neurotoxicity	Additive
Phenytoin	Increased phenytoin concentrations	Inhibition of hepatic metabolism
Dapsone with		
Aniline	Increased risk of hemolysis in G-6-PD–deficient patients	Additive
Clofazimine	Decrease in or nullification of clofazimine's antiinflammatory effects	Opposing effects on neutrophil motility and lymphocyte transformation in vitro
Delavirdine	Increased dapsone toxicity	Decreased metabolism
Didanosine	Increased incidence of PCP recurrence	Mechanism not established
Folic acid antagonists	Increased risk of hematologic toxicity	Additive
Naphthalene	Increased risk of hemolysis in G-6-PD–deficient patients	Additive
Niridazole	Increased risk of hemolysis in G-6-PD–deficient patients	Additive
Nitrite	Increased risk of hemolysis in G-6-PD–-deficient patients	Additive
Nitrofurantoin	Increased risk of hemolysis in G-6-PD–deficient patients	Additive
Phenylhydrazine	Increased risk of hemolysis in G-6-PD–deficient patients	Additive
Primaquine	Increased risk of hemolysis in G-6-PD–deficient patients	Additive
Pyrimethamine	Increased risk of hematologic toxicity	Additive
Rifampin/rifabutin	Decreased dapsone serum concentrations	Hepatic enzyme induction

TABLE 42–28 Adverse Drug Interactions Involving Antimicrobial Agents *Continued*

Interacting Drugs	Adverse Effect	Probable Mechanism
Dapsone with *Continued*		
Saquinavir	Increased dapsone toxicity	Decreased metabolism
Trimethoprim	Increased dapsone serum concentrations; increased risk of adverse effects	Mechanism not established
Zidovudine	Increased risk of hematologic toxicity	Additive
Didanosine with		
Benzodiazepines	Increased confusion	Mechanism not established
Co-trimoxazole	Increased risk of pancreatitis	Additive
Dapsone	Increased incidence of PCP recurrence	Antacids necessary for antiviral absorption may have impeded absorption
Delavirdine	Decreased delavirdine/didanosine effect	Mechanism not established
Ganciclovir	In vitro antiretroviral antagonism	Mechanism not established
Indinavir	Decreased indinavir effect	Decreased bioavailability
Itraconazole	Decreased itraconazole effect	Decreased bioavailability
Ketoconazole	Decreased absorption; administer ≥2 hr before didanosine	Antacids necessary for didanosine administration raise gastric pH too high for ketoconazole absorption
Pentamidine	Increased risk of pancreatitis	Additive
Quinolones	Decreased absorption; decreased serum concentration of the quinolones	Concomitant antacids bind quinolones and prevent absorption
Tetracyclines	Decreased absorption; decreased serum concentration of the tetracyclines	Concomitant antacids bind tetracyclines and prevent absorption
Zalcitabine	Increased neurotoxicity	Additive
Erythromycins with		
Alfentanil	Increased alfentanil toxicity	Decreased metabolism
Anticoagulants, oral	Hypoprothrombinemia potentiated	Possible decreased metabolism
Astemizole	Cardiotoxicity	Decreased metabolism
Benzodiazepines	Increased benzodiazepine toxicity	Decreased metabolism
Bromocriptine	Increased toxicity	Increased bioavailability
Carbamazepine	Increased carbamazepine toxicity	Possible decreased metabolism
Cisapride	Cardiotoxicity	Decreased metabolism
Clindamycin	Antagonism	Target site competition
Clozapine	Increased clozapine toxicity	Decreased metabolism
Corticosteroids	Increased effect and possible toxicity of methylprednisolone	Decreased excretion
Cyclosporine	Increased cyclosporine toxicity	Probably decreased metabolism
Digoxin	Increased digoxin effect	Decreased gut metabolism and increased absorption
Disopyramide	Cardiac arrhythmias	Decreased metabolism
Ergot alkaloids	Increased ergot toxicity	Mechanism not established
Felodipine	Increased toxicity	Decreased metabolism
HMG-CoA reductase inhibitors	Increased risk of rhabdomyolysis	Decreased clearance
Loratadine	Increased loratadine toxicity	Decreased metabolism
Phenytoin	Possible increased or decreased effect	Altered metabolism
Ritonavir	Increased erythromycin toxicity	Decreased metabolism
Tacrolimus	Increased tacrolimus toxicity	Decreased metabolism
Terfenadine	Cardiotoxicity	Decreased metabolism
Theophylline	Increased theophylline effect and possible toxicity	Decreased metabolism
Trimetrexate	Increased trimetrexate toxicity	Decreased metabolism
Valproic acid	Increased valproic acid toxicity	Decreased metabolism
Vinblastine	Increased vinblastine toxicity	Decreased metabolism
Zafirlukast	Decreased zafirlukast effect	Mechanism not established
Ethionamide with		
Aminosalicylic acid	Increased GI distress/hepatotoxicity	Mechanism not established
BCG vaccine	Negates BCG effect	Negates immune response
Cycloserine	Increased neurotoxicity	Additive
Ethambutol	Increased ethambutol toxicity	Mechanism not established
Isoniazid	Increased neurotoxicity	Additive
Pyrazinamide	Increased hepatotoxicity	Additive
Rifampin/rifabutin	Increased hepatotoxicity	Additive
Fluconazole with		
Amitriptyline	Increased amitriptyline toxicity	Decreased metabolism
Amphotericin B	Possible antagonism in animal models	Mechanism not established
Astemizole	Prolonged Q-T interval and possible arrhythmias	Inhibition of antihistamine metabolism
Benzodiazepines	Increased CNS toxicity	Decreased metabolism
Cimetidine	Decreased fluconazole effect	Decreased bioavailability
Cisapride	Increased risk of cardiotoxicity	Decreased metabolism
Coumarin anticoagulants	Increased prothrombin times	Mechanism not established
Cyclosporine	Increased cyclosporine concentrations	Mechanism not established
Dihydropyridines	Increased dihydropyridine toxicity	Decreased metabolism
HMG-CoA reductase inhibitors	Increased risk of rhabdomyolysis	Mechanism not established
Phenytoin	Increased phenytoin concentrations	Decreased metabolism
Quetiapine fumarate	Possible increased quetiapine concentrations	Decreased metabolism

Table continued on following page

TABLE 42–28 Adverse Drug Interactions Involving Antimicrobial Agents *Continued*

Interacting Drugs	Adverse Effect	Probable Mechanism
Fluconazole with *Continued*		
Rifampin/rifabutin	Decreased fluconazole concentrations	Mechanism not established
Sulfonylureas	Increased plasma concentrations and decreased metabolism of tolbutamide, glyburide, and glipizide	Decreased metabolism
Tacrolimus	Increased tacrolimus toxicity	Decreased metabolism
Terfenadine	Prolonged Q-T interval and possible arrhythmias	Inhibition of antihistamine metabolism
Thiazides	Increased fluconazole concentrations and AUC	Decreased renal clearance
Zidovudine	Increased zidovudine concentrations	Decreased metabolism
Fluoroquinolones with		
Antacids	Decreased fluoroquinolone effect with aluminum or magnesium antacids	Decreased absorption
Anticoagulants, oral	Prolonged prothrombin times	Mechanism not established
BCG vaccine	Negates BCG effect	Negates immune response
Chloramphenicol	Inhibition in vitro of norfloxacin bactericidal activity	Mechanism not established
Cyclosporine	Increased risk of nephrotoxicity; increased serum cyclosporine concentrations	Mechanism not established
Didanosine	Decreased fluoroquinolone effect	Decreased GI absorption
Iron	Decreased serum fluoroquinolone concentrations	Decreased GI absorption
Nitrofurantoin	Decreased norfloxacin activity	In vitro antagonism
NSAIDs	Possible increased risk of CNS stimulation	Mechanism not established
Pirenzepine	Decreased rate of fluoroquinolone absorption	Mechanism not established
Probenecid	Increased serum concentrations of quinolones; prolonged AUCs	Decreased tubular secretion
Rifampin/rifabutin	Inhibition in vitro of norfloxacin bactericidal activity	Mechanism not established
Riluzole	Increased risk of riluzole toxicity	Decreased elimination
Scopolamine	Decreased rate of fluoroquinolone absorption	Mechanism not established
Sucralfate	Decreased serum fluoroquinolone concentrations	Decreased GI absorption
Tetracycline	Inhibition in vitro of norfloxacin bactericidal activity	Mechanism not established
Theophylline	Possible theophylline toxicity	Decreased metabolism
Zinc	Decreased serum fluoroquinolone concentrations	Decreased GI absorption
Foscarnet with		
Acyclovir	Increased nephrotoxicity	Additive
Cidofovir	Increased nephrotoxicity	Additive
Co-trimoxazole	Increased nephrotoxicity	Additive
Pentamidine	Increased nephrotoxicity; increased hypocalcemia	Additive
Probenecid	Increased foscarnet serum concentrations; increased possibility of adverse effects	Decreased tubular secretion
Suramin	Increased nephrotoxicity	Additive
Furazolidone with		
Alcohol	Disulfiram-like effect	Either inhibition of aldehyde dehydrogenase or inhibition of monoamine oxidase
Antidepressants	Increased adverse effects	Additive
Sympathomimetics	Hypertensive crisis	Increased norepinephrine availability
Ganciclovir with		
Aminoglycosides	Increased nephrotoxicity	Additive
Amphotericin B	Increased nephrotoxicity; replication inhibition of rapidly dividing host cells	Additive; additive
Co-trimoxazole	Replication inhibition of rapidly dividing host cells	
Cyclosporine	Increased nephrotoxicity	
Cytotoxic antineoplastics	Replication inhibition of rapidly dividing host cells	Additive
Dapsone	Replication inhibition of rapidly dividing host cells	Additive
Didanosine	In vitro antiretroviral antagonism	
Flucytosine	Replication inhibition of rapidly dividing host cells	Additive
Imipenem	Generalized seizures	
Immunosuppressives	Increased suppression of bone marrow and immune system	Mechanism not established
Nucleoside analogues	Replication inhibition of rapidly dividing host cells	Additive
Pentamidine	Replication inhibition of rapidly dividing host cells	Mechanism not established
Probenecid	Increased ganciclovir concentrations; prolonged AUC	Additive
Pyrimethamine	Replication inhibition of rapidly dividing host cells	Additive
Taerolimus	Increased risk of nephrotoxicity	

TABLE 42–28 Adverse Drug Interactions Involving Antimicrobial Agents *Continued*

Interacting Drugs	Adverse Effect	Probable Mechanism
Ganciclovir with *Continued*		
Zidovudine	In vitro antiretroviral antagonism; increased risk of hematologic toxicity	Additive
		Decrease in tubular secretion
		Additive
		Additive
		Mechanism not established; additive
Griseofulvin with		
Alcohol	Increased alcohol effects, tachycardia and flushing	Mechanism not established
Anticoagulants, oral	Decreased anticoagulant effect	Mechanism not established
Contraceptives, oral	Decreased contraceptive effect	Increased metabolism
Phenobarbital	Decreased griseofulvin concentrations	Decreased absorption or hepatic enzyme induction
Hydroxychloroquine with		
Digoxin	Increased digoxin effect	Mechanism not established
Imipenem with		
Aztreonam	Antagonism	β-Lactamase induction
Cephalosporins	Antagonism	β-Lactamase induction
Chloramphenicol	Antagonism; administer a few hours after imipenem	Mechanism not established
Extended-spectrum penicillins	Antagonism	β-Lactamase induction
Ganciclovir	Generalized seizures	Mechanism not established
Isoniazid with		
Alcohol	Increased incidence of hepatitis	Mechanism not established
	Decreased isoniazid effect in some alcoholic patients	Increased metabolism
Aluminum antacids	Decreased isoniazid effect	Decreased absorption
Aminosalicylic acid	Increased isoniazid concentrations	Reduced acetylation
Anticoagulants, oral	Possible increased anticoagulant effect	Decreased metabolism
Benzodiazepines	Pharmacologic effects of benzodiazepines may be increased; documented for diazepam and triazolam	Decreased metabolism
BCG vaccine	Vaccine may be ineffective	Isoniazid inhibits multiplication of BCG
Carbamazepine	Increased toxicity of both drugs	Altered metabolism
Cycloserine	CNS effects, dizziness, drowsiness	Mechanism not established
Disulfiram	Psychotic episodes, ataxia	Altered dopamine metabolism
Enflurane	Possible nephrotoxicity	Increased metabolism of enflurane causes increased fluoride concentration
Ethionamide	Increased CNS adverse effects	Additive
Itraconazole	Decreased itraconazole activity	Increased metabolism
Ketoconazole	Decreased ketoconazole effect	Decreased concentration
Phenytoin/fosphenytoin	Increased phenytoin toxicity	Decreased metabolism
Rifampin/rifabutin	Possible increased isoniazid hepatotoxicity	Possible increased toxic metabolites
Itraconazole with		
Amphotericin B	In vitro antagonism	Mechanism not established
Antacids	Possible decreased itraconazole bioavailability	Mechanism not established
Anticoagulants, oral	Increased anticoagulant effect	Decreased metabolism
Astemizole	Possible prolongation of Q-T interval and arrhythmias	Decreased antihistamine metabolism
Barbiturates	Decreased itraconazole effect	Increased metabolism
Benzodiazepines	Increased CNS effects	Decreased metabolism
Carbamazepine	Decreased itraconazole effect	Increased metabolism
Cisapride	Increased risk of cardiotoxicity	Decreased metabolism
Cyclosporine	Possible increase in cyclosporine concentrations	Mechanism not established
Didanosine	Decreased itraconazole effect	Decreased bioavailability
Digoxin	Increased digoxin toxicity	Decreased metabolism
Dihydropyridines	Increased dihydropyridine effect	Decreased metabolism
Histamine H_2 antagonists	Decreased itraconazole bioavailability	Decreased gastric acidity
HMG-CoA reductase inhibitors	Increased risk of rhabdomyolysis	Decreased metabolism
Omeprazole/lansoprazole	Decreased itraconazole bioavailability	Decreased gastric acidity
Phenytoin	Decreased itraconazole effect	Increased metabolism
Rifampin/rifabutin	Decreased systemic bioavailability of itraconazole	Hepatic enzyme induction
Tacrolimus	Increased tacrolimus toxicity	Decreased metabolism
Terfenadine	Possible prolongation of Q-T interval and arrhythmias	Decreased antihistamine metabolism
Ketoconazole with		
Alcohol	Possible disulfiram-like reaction	Mechanism not established
Antacids	Decreased ketoconazole effect	Decreased absorption
Anticoagulants, oral	Increased anticoagulant effect	Mechanism not established
Astemizole	Prolonged Q-T interval and possible arrhythmias	Inhibition of antihistamine metabolism
Benzodiazepines	Increased CNS toxicity	Decreased metabolism
Carbamazepine	Increased carbamazepine toxicity	Decreased metabolism
Cisapride	Increased risk of cardiotoxicity	Decreased metabolism
Corticosteroids	Increased methylprednisolone effect	Decreased metabolism

Table continued on following page

TABLE 42–28 Adverse Drug Interactions Involving Antimicrobial Agents *Continued*

Interacting Drugs	Adverse Effect	Probable Mechanism
Ketoconazole with *Continued*		
Cyclosporine	Increased concentration of cyclosporine in blood	Mechanism not established
Delavirdine	Increased delavirdine concentrations	Mechanism not established
Didanosine	Decreased ketoconazole effect	Decreased absorption
Dihydropyridines	Increased dihydropyridine effect	Decreased metabolism
Donepezil	Increased cholinomimetic effects	Decreased metabolism
Histamine H_2 antagonists	Possible decreased antifungal effect	Decreased absorption
Hepatotoxic agents	Increased hepatotoxicity	Additive
HMG-CoA reductase inhibitors	Increased risk of rhabdomyolysis	Decreased metabolism
Indinavir	Increased indinavir toxicity	Decreased metabolism
Isoniazid	Decreased ketoconazole effect	Decreased blood concentrations
Loratadine	Increased loratadine concentrations	Decreased metabolism
Omeprazole/lansoprazole	Decreased ketoconazole bioavailability	Decreased gastric acidity
Phenytoin	Altered effects of one or both drugs	Altered metabolism
Quetiapine fumarate	Increased risk of quetiapine toxicity	Decreased metabolism
Rifampin/rifabutin	Decreased rifampin and ketoconazole effects	Decreased blood concentrations
Ritonavir	Increased ketoconazole concentrations	Decreased metabolism
Saquinavir	Increased saquinavir concentrations	Decreased metabolism
Tacrolimus	Increased tacrolimus toxicity	Decreased metabolism
Terfenadine	Prolonged Q-T interval and possible arrhythmias	Inhibition of antihistamine metabolism
Theophylline	Decreased theophylline concentrations	Mechanism not established
Lamivudine with		
Nelfinavir	Increased lamivudine concentrations	Decreased clearance
Sulfonamides	Increased lamivudine concentrations	Decreased clearance
Trimethoprim	Increased lamivudine concentrations	Decreased clearance
Zidovudine	Increased zidovudine concentrations	Mechanism not established
Mebendazole with		
Carbamazepine	Decreased mebendazole concentrations	Hepatic microsomal enzyme induction
Phenytoin	Decreased mebendazole concentrations	Hepatic microsomal enzyme induction
Methenamine with		
Sulfonamides	Increased risk of crystalluria; formation of formaldehyde-sulfamethazole precipitate	Acidification of the urine
Metronidazole with		
Alcohol	Mild disulfiram-like symptoms	Possible inhibition of intermediary metabolism of alcohol
Anticoagulants, oral	Increased anticoagulant effect	Decreased metabolism
Astemizole	Possible prolongation of the Q-T interval and arrhythmias	Decreased antihistamine metabolism
Azathioprine	Transient neutropenia	Mechanism not established
Barbiturates	Decreased metronidazole effect with phenobarbital	Probably increased metabolism
Carbamazepine	Increased carbamazepine toxicity	Decreased metabolism
Cimetidine	Possible increased metronidazole toxicity	Decreased metabolism
Disulfiram	Organic brain syndrome	Mechanism not established
Fluorouracil	Transient neutropenia	Mechanism not established
Lithium	Lithium toxicity	Mechanism not established
Terfenadine	Possible prolongation of the Q-T interval and arrhythmias	Decreased antihistamine metabolism
Miconazole with		
Aminoglycosides	Possible decreased tobramycin concentration	Mechanism not established
Amphotericin B	Possible antagonism in vitro	Mechanism not established
Anticoagulants, oral	Increased anticoagulant effect	Mechanism not established
Astemizole	Prolonged Q-T interval and possible arrhythmias	Inhibition of antihistamine metabolism
Cisapride	Increased cardiotoxicity	Decreased metabolism
Cyclosporine	Increased nephrotoxicity	Decreased metabolism
Hypoglycemics, sulfonylurea	Severe hypoglycemia	Mechanism not established
Phenytoin	Increased phenytoin toxicity	Decreased metabolism
Terfenadine	Prolonged Q-T interval and possible arrhythmias	Inhibition of antihistamine metabolism
Nalidixic acid with		
Antacids	Decreased nalidixic acid serum concentrations	Impaired absorption
Anticoagulants, oral	Increased anticoagulant effect	Displacement from binding sites
Nevirapine with		
Cimetidine	Increased nevirapine concentrations	Decreased metabolism
Clarithromycin	Increased nevirapine concentrations	Decreased metabolism
Erythromycin	Increased nevirapine concentrations	Decreased metabolism
Indinavir	Decreased indinavir concentrations	Increased metabolism
Ketoconazole	Increased nevirapine concentrations	Decreased metabolism
Rifamycins	Decreased nevirapine concentrations	Increased metabolism
Ritonavir	Decreased ritonavir concentrations	Increased metabolism
Zidovudine	Decreased zidovudine concentrations	Increased metabolism
Nitrofurantoin with		
Antacids	Possible decreased nitrofurantoin effect	Decreased absorption
Fluoroquinolones	In vitro antagonism of quinolone activity	Mechanism not established

TABLE 42–28 Adverse Drug Interactions Involving Antimicrobial Agents *Continued*

Interacting Drugs	Adverse Effect	Probable Mechanism
Nitrofurantoin with *Continued*		
Probenecid	Increased nitrofurantoin serum concentrations	Inhibition of renal excretion
Sulfinpyrazone	Increased nitrofurantoin serum concentrations	Inhibition of renal excretion
Para-aminosalicylic acid: see *Aminosalicylic acid*		
Pentamidine with		
Aminoglycosides	Increased nephrotoxicity	Additive
Amphotericin B	Increased nephrotoxocity	Additive
Capreomycin	Increased nephrotoxicity	Additive
Cidofovir	Increased nephrotoxicity	Additive
Colistin	Increased nephrotoxicity	Additive
Cisplatin	Increased nephrotoxicity	Additive
Foscarnet	Hypocalcemia	Mechanism not established
Grepafloxacin	Increased cardiotoxicity	Additive
Methoxyflurane	Increased nephrotoxicity	Additive
Polymyxins	Increased nephrotoxicity	Additive
Sparfloxacin	Increased cardiotoxicity	Additive
Vancomycin	Increased nephrotoxicity	Additive
Piperazine with		
Chlorpromazine	Seizures	Mechanism not established
Pyrantel pamoate	Decreased piperazine and pyrantel pamoate activity	Antagonism
Polymyxin B with		
Aminoglycoside antibiotics	Increased nephrotoxicity; increased neuromuscular blockade	Additive
Neuromuscular blocking agents	Increased neuromuscular blockade	Additive
Parenteral quinidine	Increased neurotoxicity	Additive
Parenteral quinine	Increased neurotoxicity	Additive
Vancomycin	Increased nephrotoxicity	Additive
Primaquine with		
Aurothioglucose	Increased blood dyscrasias	Additive
Quinacrine	Increased toxicity to the antimalarial primaquine	Additive
Ritonavir	Increased primaquine concentrations	Decreased metabolism
Protease inhibitors (except ritonavir) with		
Astemizole	Increased cardiotoxicity	Decreased metabolism
Barbiturates	Decreased protease inhibitor effect	Increased metabolism
Benzodiazepines	Increased CNS toxicity	Decreased metabolism
Carbamazepine	Decreased protease inhibitor effect	Increased metabolism
Cisapride	Increased cardiotoxicity	Decreased metabolism
Clarithromycin	Increased protease inhibitor toxicity	Decreased metabolism
Delavirdine	Increased protease inhibitor toxicity, increased hepatotoxicity, decreased delavirdine effect	Mechanism not established
Dihydropyridines	Increased dihydropyridine toxicity	Decreased clearance
Ergot derivatives	Increased ergot toxicity	Decreased metabolism
Ketoconazole	Increased protease inhibitor toxicity	Decreased metabolism
Phenytoin	Decreased protease inhibitor effect	Increased metabolism
Rifampin/rifabutin	Decreased protease inhibitor effect/increased rifamycin toxicity	Increased/decreased metabolism
Ritonavir	Increased protease inhibitor toxicity	Decreased metabolism
Terfenadine	Increased cardiotoxicity	Decreased metabolism
Pyrantel pamoate with		
Piperazine	Decreased pyrantel pamoate and piperazine activity	Antagonism
Theophylline	Increased theophylline toxicity	Decreased metabolism
Quinacrine with		
Alcohol	Possible disulfiram-like reaction	Accumulation of acetaldehyde
Aurothioglucose	Increased blood dyscrasias	Additive
Hepatotoxic agents	Possible increased hepatotoxicity	Additive
Primaquine	Increased primaquine toxicity	Release from tissue binding sites causing marked increase in primaquine concentrations
Quinine with		
Acetazolamide	Increased quinine serum concentrations; increased toxicity	Decreased clearance from increased urinary pH
Aluminum antacids	Decreased quinine serum concentrations	Decreased absorption
Anticoagulants, oral	Potentiation of hypoprothrombinemic effects	Hepatic suppression of synthesis of vitamin K–dependent clotting factors
Astemizole	Increased cardiotoxicity	Decreased metabolism
Aurothioglucose	Increased blood dyscrasias	Additive
Cimetidine	Decreased quinine clearance; prolonged AUCs	Hepatic enzyme inhibition
Digoxin/digitoxin	Increased digoxin/digitoxin concentrations	Mechanism not established
Flecainide	Increased flecainide toxicity	Decreased metabolism
Heparin	Decreased anticoagulant effect	Mechanism not established
Mefloquine	Increased cardiac events	Additive

Table continued on following page

TABLE 42–28 Adverse Drug Interactions Involving Antimicrobial Agents *Continued*

Interacting Drugs	Adverse Effect	Probable Mechanism
Quinine with *Continued*		
Neuromuscular blocking agents	Potentiation of neuromuscular blocking effects	Additive
Ritonavir	Increased quinine toxicity	Decreased metabolism
Sodium bicarbonate	Increased quinine serum concentrations; increased toxicity	Decreased clearance from increased urinary pH
Ribavirin with		
Zalcitabine	In vitro retroviral antagonism	Mechanism not established
Zidovudine	In vitro retroviral antagonism	Mechanism not established
Rifamycins with		
Analgesics	Possible decreased concentrations and activity	Increased metabolism
Anticoagulants, oral	Possible decreased concentrations and activity	Increased metabolism
Anticonvulsants	Possible decreased concentrations and activity	Increased metabolism
Atovaquone	Decreased atovaquone effect	Increased metabolism
Barbiturates	Possible decreased concentrations and activity	Increased metabolism
BCG vaccine	Negates BCG effect	Negates immune response
Beta blockers	Possible decreased concentrations and activity	Increased metabolism
Cardiac glycosides	Possible decreased concentrations and activity	Increased metabolism
Chloramphenicol	Possible decreased concentrations and activity	Increased metabolism
Clarithromycin	Decreased clarithromycin concentrations/ increased rifamycin toxicity	Increased/decreased metabolism
Clofibrate	Possible decreased concentrations and activity	Increased metabolism
Contraceptives, oral	Possible decreased concentrations and activity	Increased metabolism
Corticosteroids	Possible decreased concentrations and activity	Increased metabolism
Cyclosporine	Possible decreased concentrations and activity	Increased metabolism
Dapsone	Possible decreased concentrations and activity	Increased metabolism
Delavirdine	Decreased delavirdine concentrations/increased rifamycin toxicity	Increased/decreased metabolism
Diazepam	Possible decreased concentrations and activity	Increased metabolism
Digitalis	Decreased digitoxin and digoxin effect	Increased metabolism
Dihydropyridines	Decreased dihydropyridine effect	Increased metabolism
Disopyramide	Possible decreased concentrations and activity	Increased metabolism
Doxycycline	Decreased doxycycline effect	Increased metabolism
Estrogens	Decreased estrogen concentrations	Hepatic enzyme induction
Ethionamide	Increased hepatotoxicity	Additive
Fluconazole	Decreased fluconazole effect	Increased metabolism
HMG-CoA reductase inhibitors	Decreased HMG effect	Increased metabolism
Hypoglycemics, oral	Possible decreased concentrations and activity	Increased metabolism
Indinavir	Decreased indinavir effect	Increased metabolism
Isoniazid	Possible increased hepatotoxicity	Possible increased toxic metabolites
Itraconazole	Decreased itraconazole effect	Increased metabolism
Ketoconazole	Possible decreased concentrations and activity	Increased metabolism
Mexiletine	Possible decreased concentrations and activity	Increased metabolism
Narcotics	Possible decreased concentrations and activity	Increased metabolism
Nelfinavir	Decreased nelfinavir effect	Increased metabolism
Nevirapine	Decreased nevirapine effect	Increased metabolism
Progestins	Possible decreased concentrations and activity	Increased metabolism
Quinidine	Possible decreased concentrations and activity	Increased metabolism
Ritonavir	Decreased ritonavir effect/increased rifamycin toxicity	Increased/decreased metabolism
Saquinavir	Decreased saquinavir effect/increased rifamycin toxicity	Increased/decreased metabolism
Tacrolimus	Decreased tacrolimus effect	Increased metabolism
Terbinafine	Decreased terbinafine effect	Increased metabolism
Theophylline	Possible decreased concentrations and activity	Increased metabolism
Verapamil	Possible decreased concentrations and activity	Increased metabolism
Zidovudine	Decreased zidovudine concentrations/AUCs	Mechanism not established
Ritonavir with		
Amiodarone	Increased amiodarone toxicity risk	Decreased metabolism
Antihypoglycemics, oral	Increased hypoglycemia risk	Decreased metabolism
Anticoagulants, oral	Increased anticoagulant response risk	Decreased metabolism
Astemizole	Increased cardiotoxicity	Decreased metabolism
Atovaquone	Decreased efficacy of atovaquone	Increased metabolism
Benzodiazepines	Increased CNS toxicity risk	Decreased metabolism
Beta blockers	Increased beta blocker toxicity risk	Decreased metabolism
Bupropion	Increased seizure risk	Decreased metabolism
Carbamazepine	Decreased ritonavir efficacy/increased carbamazepine toxicity	Increased/decreased metabolism
Cisapride	Increased cardiotoxicity	Decreased metabolism
Clarithromycin	Increased macrolide toxicity risk	Decreased metabolism
Clozapine	Increased risk of clozapine toxicity	Decreased metabolism
Cyclosporine	Increased cyclosporine toxicity risk	Decreased metabolism
Dihydropyridines	Increased dihydropyridine toxicity risk	Decreased metabolism
Diltiazem	Increased diltiazem toxicity risk	Decreased metabolism
Disopyramide	Increased risk of disopyramide toxicity	Decreased metabolism
Doxorubicin	Increased risk of doxorubicin toxicity	Decreased metabolism
Encainide	Increased risk of encainide toxicity	Decreased metabolism
Erythromycin	Increased risk of macrolide toxicity	Decreased metabolism
Flecainide	Increased risk of flecainide toxicity	Decreased metabolism
HMG-CoA reductase inhibitors	Increased risk of rhabdomyolysis	Decreased metabolism
Nefazodone	Increased risk of nefazodone toxicity	Decreased metabolism
Nelfinavir	Increased risk of nelfinavir toxicity	Decreased metabolism

TABLE 42–28 Adverse Drug Interactions Involving Antimicrobial Agents *Continued*

Interacting Drugs	Adverse Effect	Probable Mechanism
Ritonavir with *Continued*		
Phenytoin	Decreased ritonavir effect/increased phenytoin toxicity	Increased/decreased metabolism
Rifampin/rifabutin	Decreased ritonavir efficacy	Increased metabolism
Risperidone	Increased risk of risperidone toxicity	Decreased metabolism
Saquinavir	Increased risk of saquinavir toxicity	Decreased metabolism
SSRI antidepressants	Increased risk of SSRI toxicity	Decreased metabolism
Tacrolimus	Increased risk of tacrolimus toxicity	Decreased metabolism
Tamoxifen	Increased risk of tamoxifen toxicity	Decreased metabolism
Terfenadine	Increased risk of cardiotoxicity	Decreased metabolism
Theophylline	Decreased efficacy	Increased clearance
Tramadol	Increased risk of tramadol toxicity	Decreased metabolism
Tricyclic antidepressants	Increased risk of tricyclic toxicity	Decreased metabolism
Valproic acid	Decreased efficacy of valproic acid	Increased clearance
Verapamil	Increased risk of verapamil toxicity	Decreased metabolism
Zolpidem	Increased risk of zolpidem toxicity	Decreased metabolism
Spectinomycin with		
Lithium	Increased lithium toxicity	Decreased renal excretion
Sulfadoxine/pyrimethamine with		
Aurothioglucose	Increased hematologic toxicity	Additive
Lorazepam	Mild hepatotoxicity	Mechanism not established
PABA	Decreased pyrimethamine effect	Interference with pyrimethamine action
Sulfonamides	Increased toxicity	Additive
Trimethoprim	Increased toxicity	Additive
Sulfonamides with		
Antibiotics	Altered action of sulfasalazine	Alteration of intestinal flora
Anticoagulants, oral	Increased anticoagulant effect	Decreased metabolism and displacement from binding sites
Barbiturates	Increased thiopental effect	Decreased albumin binding
Chloroprocaine	Possible antagonism of sulfonamide action	Competition for PABA site
Cyclosporine	Decreased cyclosporine effect with sulfamethazine	Possible increased metabolism
Digoxin	Possible decreased digoxin effect with sulfasalazine	Decreased digoxin absorption
Folic acid	Decreased absorption, metabolism, and concentrations with sulfasalazine	Inhibition of hepatic folate metabolism, intestinal transport of folic acid, and jejunal brush-border folate conjugase
Hypoglycemics, sulfonylurea	Increased hypoglycemic effect	Mechanism not established
Iron	Decreased sulfasalazine serum concentrations	Chelation
Lamivudine	Increased lamivudine toxicity	Competition for renal clearance
Methenamine	Crystallization of sulfonamides in the urine; precipitate of formaldehyde-sulfamethizole	Acidification of the urine
Methotrexate	Possible increased methotrexate toxicity	Decreased renal clearance and displacement from binding
Monoamine oxidase inhibitors	Possible increased phenelzine toxicity with sulfisoxazole	Decreased metabolism
PABA	Possible antagonism of sulfonamide action	Competition for PABA site
Paraldehyde	Crystallization of sulfonamides in the urine	Acidification of the urine
Phenytoin	Increased phenytoin effect, except possibly with sulfisoxazole	Decreased metabolism
Piperocaine	Possible antagonism of sulfonamide action	Competition for PABA site
Procaine	Possible antagonism of sulfonamide action	Competition for PABA site
Propoxycaine	Possible antagonism of sulfonamide action	Competition for PABA site
Sulfinpyrazone	Increased serum sulfonamide concentrations	Displacement from protein-binding sites and inhibition of tubular secretion
Tetracaine	Possible antagonism of sulfonamide action	Competition for PABA site
Thiopental	Increased thiopental effect; decreased dose necessary when given with sulfisoxazole	Plasma protein-binding competition
Tetracyclines with		
Alcohol	Decreased doxycycline effect in alcoholic patients	Increased metabolism
Aminoglycosides	In vitro antagonism; no in vivo support	Mechanism not established
Antacids, oral	Decreased oral tetracycline effects	Decreased tetracycline absorption
Anticoagulants, oral	Increased anticoagulant effect	Mechanism not established
Antidepressants, tricyclic	Localized hemosiderosis with amitriptyline and minocycline	Possible synergism
Barbiturates	Decreased doxycycline effect	Increased metabolism
Bismuth subsalicylate	Decreased tetracycline effect	Decreased absorption
Carbamazepine	Decreased doxycycline effect	Increased metabolism
Contraceptives, oral	Decreased contraceptive effect	Possible decreased enterohepatic circulation of estrogen
Digoxin	Increased digoxin effect	Decreased gut metabolism and increased absorption
Iron, oral	Decreased tetracycline effect, but not with doxycycline; decreased iron effect	Decreased absorption
Kaolin/pectin	Decreased concentrations of tetracyclines	Decreased absorption
Lithium	Increased lithium toxicity	Decreased renal excretion

Table continued on following page

TABLE 42–28 Adverse Drug Interactions Involving Antimicrobial Agents *Continued*

Interacting Drugs	Adverse Effect	Probable Mechanism
Tetracyclines with *Continued*		
Methotrexate	Possible increased risk of methotrexate toxicity	Mechanism not established
Methoxyflurane	Increased nephrotoxicity	Displacement from binding
Molindone	Decreased tetracycline effect	Calcium as an excipient inhibits absorption
Penicillins	In vitro antagonism; rare in vivo support for this	Mechanism not established
Phenformin	Increased lactic acidosis	Possible decreased phenformin excretion
Phenytoin	Decreased doxycycline effect	Increased metabolism
Rifampin/rifabutin	Possible decreased doxycycline effect	Increased metabolism
Theophylline	Possible theophylline toxicity	Mechanism not established
Zinc sulfate	Decreased tetracycline effect	Decreased absorption
Thiabendazole with		
Theophylline	Increased theophylline toxicity	Decreased metabolism
Trimethoprim with		
ACE inhibitors	Hyperkalemia	Reduced potassium clearance
Amiloride	Trimethoprim may potentiate hyponatremia caused by concomitant use of amiloride with thiazide diuretics	Additive
Azathioprine	Leukopenia	Mechanism not established
Cyclosporine	Increased nephrotoxicity	Synergism
Dapsone	Increased dapsone toxicity	Altered clearance
Digoxin	Possible increased digoxin effect	Decreased renal excretion and possibly decreased metabolism
Methotrexate	Increased methotrexate toxicity	Decreased clearance
Phenytoin	Increased phenytoin serum concentrations with increased risk of phenytoin toxicity; increased risk of folate deficiency	Inhibition of hepatic metabolism; additive
Thiazide diuretics	Trimethoprim may potentiate hyponatremia caused by concomitant use of amiloride with thiazide diuretics	Additive
Vancomycin with		
Aminoglycosides	Possible increased nephrotoxicity and ototoxicity	Possibly additive
Amphotericin B	Increased nephrotoxicity	Additive
Bacitracin	Increased nephrotoxicity	Additive
Cephalosporins	Increased nephrotoxicity	Additive
Cisplatin	Increased nephrotoxicity	Additive
Colistin	Increased nephrotoxicity	Additive
Digoxin	Possible decreased digoxin effect	Possibly decreased absorption
Paromomycin	Increased nephrotoxicity	Additive
Polymyxins	Increased nephrotoxicity	Additive
Warfarin	Increased risk of bleeding	Mechanism not established
Vidarabine with		
Allopurinol	Increased neurotoxicity	Decreased metabolism
Theophylline	Increased theophylline effect	Decreased metabolism
Zalcitabine with		
Aminoglycosides	Increased risk of peripheral neuropathy	Decreased clearance of zalcitabine
Amphotericin B	Increased risk of peripheral neuropathy	Decreased clearance of zalcitabine
Chloramphenicol	Increased risk of peripheral neuropathy	Additive
Cimetidine	Increased zalcitabine toxicity	Decreased clearance
Cisplatin	Increased risk of peripheral neuropathy	Additive
Co-trimoxazole	Increased risk of pancreatitis	Additive
Dapsone	Increased risk of peripheral neuropathy	Additive
Didanosine	Increased risk of peripheral neuropathy	Additive
Disulfiram	Increased risk of peripheral neuropathy	Additive
Ethionamide	Increased risk of peripheral neuropathy	Additive
Foscarnet	Increased risk of peripheral neuropathy	Decreased clearance of zalcitabine
Glutethimide	Increased risk of peripheral neuropathy	Additive
Gold	Increased risk of peripheral neuropathy	Additive
Hydralazine	Increased risk of peripheral neuropathy	Additive
Iodoquinol	Increased risk of peripheral neuropathy	Additive
Metronidazole	Increased risk of peripheral neuropathy	Additive
Nitrofurantoin	Increased risk of peripheral neuropathy	Additive
Pentamidine	Increased risk of pancreatitis	Additive
Phenytoin	Increased risk of peripheral neuropathy	Additive
Ribavirin	Increased risk of peripheral neuropathy; in vitro antiretroviral antagonism	Additive; mechanism not established
Vincristine	Increased risk of peripheral neuropathy	Additive
Zidovudine with		
Acetaminophen	Granulocytopenia	Mechanism not established
Acyclovir	Neurotoxicity	Mechanism not established
Amphotericin B	Increased risk of nephrotoxicity and hematologic toxicity	Mechanism not established
Antimycobacterials	Possible increased risk of hematologic toxicity	Possible inhibition of zidovudine glucuronidation
Aspirin	Possible increased risk of hematologic toxicity	Possible inhibition of zidovudine glucuronidation

TABLE 42–28 Adverse Drug Interactions Involving Antimicrobial Agents *Continued*

Interacting Drugs	Adverse Effect	Probable Mechanism
Zidovudine with *Continued*		
Cimetidine	Possible increased risk of hematologic toxicity	Possible inhibition of zidovudine glucuronidation
Clarithromycin	Decreased zidovudine concentrations and AUCs	Mechanism not established
Cytotoxic/myelosuppressive agents	Increased risk of hematologic toxicity	Additive
Dapsone	Increased neutropenia	Additive
Flucytosine	Increased neutropenia	Additive
Ganciclovir	In vitro antiretroviral antagonism; increased risk of hematologic toxicity	Mechanism not established; additive
Indomethacin	Possible increased risk of hematologic toxicity	Possible inhibition of zidovudine glucuronidation
Interferon alpha	Increased neutropenia	Additive
Interferon beta	Increased hematologic toxicity	Decreased glucuronidation
Lorazepam	Possible increased risk of hematologic toxicity	Possible inhibition of zidovudine glucuronidation
Nephrotoxic agents	Increased risk of toxicity	Increased serum concentrations; decreased clearance
Nucleoside analogues	Increased risk of hematologic toxicity	Additive
Probenecid	Increased and prolonged zidovudine serum concentration	Inhibition of glucuronidation and/or reduces renal excretion
Ribavirin	In vitro antiretroviral antagonism	Mechanism not established
Rifamycins	Decreased zidovudine efficacy	Mechanism not established
Valproic acid	Increased zidovudine concentrations	Decreased metabolism

Abbreviations: ACE, Angiotensin-converting enzyme; AUC, area under the serum or plasma concentration–time curve; BCG, Calmette-Guérin bacillus; CNS, central nervous system; GI, gastrointestinal; G-6-PD, glucose-6-phosphate dehydrogenase; HMG-CoA, 3-hydroxy-3-methyl-glutaryl–coenzyme A; NSAID, nonsteroidal anti-inflammatory drug; PABA, para-aminobenzoic acid; PAS, para-aminosalicylic acid; PCP, *Pneumocystis carinii* pneumonia; SSRI, selective serotonin reuptake inhibitor.

BIBLIOGRAPHY

Amsden GW, Ballow CH, Schentag JJ. Population pharmacokinetic methods to optimize antibiotic effects. Drug Invest. 1993;5:256–268.

Bennett WM, Arnoff GR, Morrison G, et al. Drug prescribing in renal failure; dosing guidelines for adults. Am J Kidney Dis. 1983;3:155–193.

Nix DE, Goodwin SD, Peloquin CA, et al. Antibiotic tissue penetration and its relevance: Models of tissue penetration and their meaning. Antimicrob Agents Chemother. 1991;35:1947–1952.

Nix DE, Goodwin, SD, Peloquin CA, et al. Antibiotic tissue penetration and its relevance: Impact of tissue penetration on infection response. Antimicrob Agents Chemother. 1991;35:1953–1959.

Schentag JJ. Correlation of pharmacokinetic parameters to efficacy of antibiotics: Relationships between serum concentrations, MIC values, and bacterial eradication in patients with gram-negative pneumonia. Scand J Inf Dis. 1991;74(Suppl):218–234.

P A R T II

Major Clinical Syndromes

SECTION A
FEVER

Chapter 43

Temperature Regulation and the Pathogenesis of Fever

PHILIP A. MACKOWIAK

The oldest known written reference to fever exists in Akkadian cuneiform inscriptions from the sixth century BC, which appear to have been derived from an ancient Sumerian pictogram of a flaming brazier used to symbolize both fever and the local warmth of inflammation.[1] Theoretical constructs concerned with the pathogenesis of fever did not emerge until several centuries later, when hippocratic physicians proposed that body temperature, and physiologic harmony in general, involved a delicate balance between four corporal humors—blood, phlegm, black bile, and yellow bile.[2] Fever was believed to result from an excess of yellow bile, a concept in concert with the fact that many infections of that era caused both fever and jaundice. During the Middle Ages, demonic possession was added to the list of mechanisms thought to be responsible for fever. By the 18th century, Harvey's discovery of the circulation of blood and the birth of clinical chemistry led iatrophysicists and iatrochemists to hypothesize alternatively that body heat and fever result from friction associated with the flow of blood through the vascular system and from fermentation and putrefaction occurring in the blood and intestines.[3] Ultimately, as a result of the work of Claude Bernard, the metabolic processes occurring within the body came to be recognized as the source of body heat. Subsequent work established that body temperature is tightly controlled within a narrow range by mechanisms regulating the rate at which such heat is allowed to dissipate from the body.

The origin of the practice of monitoring body temperature as an aid to diagnosis is uncertain. The oldest known references to devices used to measure temperature date to the first or second century BC, when Philo of Byzantium and Hero of Alexandria are believed to have invented several such devices.[4] It is reasonably certain that Galileo manufactured a primitive (air) thermometer at about the time he assumed the chair in mathematics at Padua in 1592.[5] However, thermometry was not fully assimilated into medical practice until 1868, when Carl Reinhold August Wunderlich published an opus magnus entitled *Das Verhalten der Eigenwärme in Krankenheiten* (*The Course of Temperature in Diseases*).[6]

Through *Das Verhalten der Eigenwärme in Krankenheiten,* Wunderlich gave 37°C (98.6°F) special significance with respect to normal body temperature.[7] He described the diurnal variation of body temperature and, in the process, alerted clinicians to the fact that "normal body temperature" is actually a temperature range, rather than a specific temperature. In an analysis of a series of clinical thermometric measurements, the size of which has never been equaled (estimated to have included some 1 million observations in as many as 25,000 subjects), Wunderlich posited 38°C (100.4°F) as the upper limit of the normal range and in so doing, proffered one of the first quantitative definitions of fever.

In spite of the fact that Wunderlich's work was published over a century ago and was based primarily on axillary measurements generally taken no more often than twice daily, it has survived almost verbatim in modern concepts of clinical thermometry. Interestingly, recent tests conducted with one of Wunderlich's thermometers suggest that his instruments may have been calibrated by as much as 1.4 to 2.2°C (2.6 to 4.0°F) higher than today's instruments.[7] As a result, at least some of Wunderlich's cherished dictums regarding body temperature (e.g., the special significance of 37°C [98.6°F]) have had to be revised.[8]

TERMINOLOGY

Of the many definitions of fever promulgated over the centuries, the one proposed by the International Union of Physiological Sciences Thermal Commission in 1987[9] is the one most consistent with current concepts. It defines *fever* as "a state of elevated core temperature, which is often, but not necessarily, part of the defensive responses of multicellular organisms (host) to the invasion of live (microorganisms) or inanimate matter recognized as pathogenic or alien by the host." The *febrile response* (of which fever is a component) is a complex physiologic reaction to disease, involving a cytokine-mediated rise in the core temperature, the generation of acute-phase reactants, and the activation of numerous physiologic, endocrinologic, and immunologic systems. The rise in temperature during fever is to be distinguished from that occurring during episodes of hyperthermia. Unlike fever, *hyperthermia* involves an unregulated rise in body temperature, in which pyrogenic cytokines are not directly involved and against which standard antipyretics are ineffective. It represents a failure of thermoregulatory homeostasis, in which there is either uncontrolled heat production, inadequate heat dissipation, or defective thermoregulation.

In the clinical setting, fever is typically defined as a pyrogen-mediated rise in body temperature above the normal range. Although useful as a descriptor for the febrile patient, the definition ignores the fact that a rise in body temperature is but one component of this multifaceted response. This standard clinical definition is further flawed, because it implies that "body temperature" is a single entity when, in fact, it is a pastiche of many different temperatures, each representative of a particular body part, and each varying throughout the day in response to both activities of daily living and the influence of endogenous diurnal rhythms.

CLINICAL THERMOMETRY

For over a century, the thermometer has been preeminent among clinical instruments used to distinguish health from disease and to monitor the course of illness. Unfortunately, thermometric measurements are influenced by a host of variables, all too frequently ignored when interpreting the significance of clinical temperature readings.

Observer Variability

Although generally simple to perform, thermometric measurements involve a number of basic technical details, which if not attended to, can invalidate any effort to obtain a reliable estimate of body temperature. Few physicians, for example, ever take the time to ensure the reliability or proper calibration of thermometers used in clinical examinations. And yet, Abbey and colleagues[10] found that a quarter of mercury-in-glass thermometers obtained from four different manufacturers were inaccurate after 8 months of use or storage.

Likewise, proper positioning of the temperature probe in the appropriate anatomic site is all too often given less than careful attention. Erickson has reported that oral thermometric readings vary by as much as 0.95°C (1.7°F) from the rear sublingual pocket to the area beneath the frenum in the anterior floor of the mouth.[11] Interestingly, regional differences in readings obtained within the oral cavity were more pronounced with electronic than with mercury thermometers, perhaps because of differences in the dwell times required when taking measurements with the two types of thermometers. It is also pertinent, in this regard, that studies performed earlier in the 20th century indicated that from the anus inward, the temperature gradually rises, reaching its apogee at a depth of approximately 2.5 inches (6.4 cm), and then gradually falls as the probe is advanced beyond 6 inches (15.2 cm).[12] More recent studies, however, found no significant differences between temperature readings obtained with rectal probes inserted to depths of 5, 9, and 13 cm.[13]

With today's electronic thermometers, equilibration times are relatively brief and, hence, are thought not to influence the results of clinical thermometric measurements. As noted earlier, this conclusion is not necessarily justified. With mercury thermometers, opinions regarding proper placement times have varied from 2 to 12 minutes for axillary recordings and 1 to 9 minutes for rectal readings.[14, 15] In a series of studies, Nichols and Kucha determined that 1 to 12 minutes are required for equilibration of mercury-in-glass thermometers during measurements of oral temperature.[16] In these studies, only 13% of the temperature readings reached their maximum after 3 minutes, whereas 90% did so after 8 minutes.

Anatomic Variability

Although clinicians frequently regard temperature readings from various anatomic sites as equivalent approximations of "body temperature,"[1] no one temperature characterizes the thermal status of the human body. This is because the body has many different temperatures, each representative of a particular body part. Nevertheless, within the body, there are two basic thermal compartments worthy of special consideration—the core and the shell.

The shell, which consists of skin and subcutaneous fat, insulates the core from the external environment. *The core,* of which the viscera are a major component, although insulated by the shell, has temperature gradients of its own, resulting from differences in the metabolic rates and blood flow patterns of the various organs contained therein. Even during baseline conditions, organs with higher metabolic rates have slightly higher temperatures than those with lower metabolic rates; in general, tissues close to the skin have lower temperatures than those at deeper locations.[18] Although such differences are normally small, during vigorous exercise, muscle temperatures rise markedly in comparison with less metabolically active organs. During shock and under extreme environmental conditions, regional anatomic variations in temperature may also be exaggerated.

Rectal measurements have long been regarded as the most practical and accurate means of obtaining routine estimates of core temperature. Benzinger and Benzinger, however, have pointed out that no known thermoregulatory system exists at this particular anatomic site.[18] Rectal temperature readings are consistently higher than those obtained at other sites (even pulmonary artery blood), which some authorities have suggested might be due to heat generated as a result of the metabolic activity of fecal bacteria.[19] However, an early study showed no significant decrease in the rectal temperature after a reduction in the colonic bacterial content.[19] There is also concern that stool in the rectum acts as a heat sink to delay or mitigate changes in the rectal temperature, particularly so if the thermometer is inserted directly into stool.[20] During shock, perfusion of the rectum may be markedly impaired, causing the rectal temperature to lag significantly behind a rapidly rising or falling core temperature.[21] For this reason, Houdas and Ring have concluded that the rectal temperature provides a reliable approximation of the core temperature only if the patient is in thermal balance.[22] In neonates, even in the absence of shock, the rectal temperature (measured by standard technique) has been reported to correlate poorly with the core temperature (as measured by a deep rectal probe).[23] Although generally safe, such measurements are associated with a small risk of rectal perforation—especially in neonates and very young infants[24, 25] and if proper infection control measures are not followed, may be a source of nosocomial infection.[26]

Of the three sites most commonly used for clinical thermometric measurement (rectum, mouth, and tympanic membrane), *the mouth* is usually preferred, because it is accessible, responds promptly to changes in the core temperature, and has a long tradition of use in monitoring body temperature in clinical practice. The temperature of the sublingual pocket may be especially relevant clinically, because its main artery is a branch of the external carotid artery and, like its parent artery, responds quickly to changes in the core temperature.[19] However, because oral temperature measurements require the cooperation of the subject being examined, not all patients (e.g., young children, uncooperative adults, and intubated individuals) are amenable to such measurements. A pacifier containing temperature-sensitive crystals has been marketed as a novel and convenient way of measuring the oral temperature in infants. Unfortunately, in clinical tests, the device identified only 10% of febrile infants correctly, labeling seven of eight infants with rectal temperatures of 102°F (38.9°C) or greater incorrectly as afebrile.[27]

It has long been suspected that the ingestion of hot or cold food or beverages and smoking influence oral temperature readings. In a study of 22 healthy young adults, Rabinowitz and associates showed that mastication and smoking both cause significant and persistent increases in the oral temperature, whereas drinking ice water causes a significant but much more transient decrease in the oral temperature (Fig. 43–1).[28]

There is controversy regarding the effect of tachypnea on the accuracy of oral thermometric readings. In studies employing electronic thermometers, Tandberg and Sklar obtained average rectal temperature readings that were 0.96°F (0.6°C) higher than simultaneous oral temperatures in patients with respiratory rates of 20/minute or less compared with 1.67°F (1.0°C) higher in patients with respiratory rates of greater than 20/minute.[29] A more recent study of 78 subjects by Neff and coworkers that controlled for open- and closed-mouth breathing and used tympanic rather than rectal temperature as a reference concluded that sublingual temperature changes do not correlate with the respiratory rate or depth but do depend on whether the mouth is opened or closed.[30] As noted earlier, the probe location and equilibration time are two additional variables that can alter the results of oral temperature measurements.

In theory, the *tympanic membrane* (TM) is an ideal site for measuring core temperature, because it is perfused by a tributary of the artery supplying the body's thermoregulatory center.[31] This fact, and the ease with which TM measurements can be obtained using modern infrared TM thermometers, have made these instruments the thermometers of choice in many clinics and intensive care units. There are two basic types of infrared TM thermometers. One type detects radiant energy emitted from the TM and portions of the ear canal, processes the information, and then displays a value representing tissue temperature in the ear canal (unadjusted mode).[32] The other displays an (adjusted) estimate of the core temperature (e.g., pulmonary arterial blood temperature) based on comparison data obtained from selected study samples. Readings obtained using the former type of TM thermometer tend to be lower than simultaneously obtained oral readings, whereas those obtained with the latter type are generally higher.[31] Unfortunately, numerous studies of many different TM thermometers have shown that although convenient, such instruments tend to give highly variable readings that correlate poorly with simultaneously obtained oral or rectal readings.[28, 32–35]

Although Wunderlich's monumental treatise on clinical thermometry was based primarily on *axillary measurements,* recent experience indicates that the axillary temperature provides a reasonable approximation of body temperature in the neonate, but not in the older child

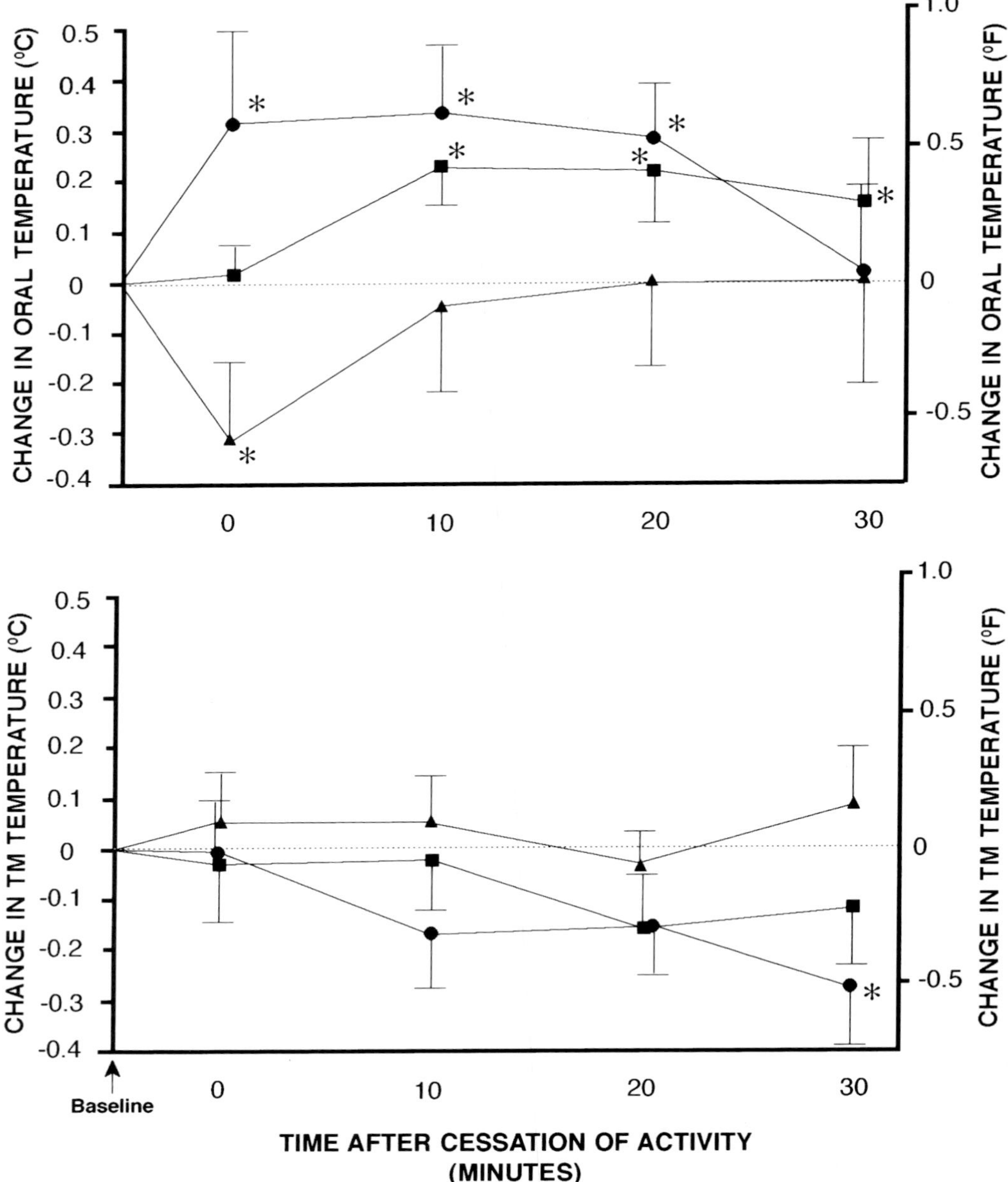

FIGURE 43–1. Effect of mastication (●), cigarette smoking (■), and drinking ice water (▲) on oral *(top)* and tympanic membrane *(bottom)* temperature readings. Each curve depicts the results (mean ± standard error) of 16 to 19 data sets. An *asterisk* indicates a value significantly different from that of the baseline (Bonferroni-adjusted $P < .05$). Measurements related to the three activities were obtained after 5 minutes of chewing gum in a seated position, immediately after smoking an entire cigarette over 5 minutes, and immediately after ingestion of 250 ml of an ice/water slurry, respectively. (From Rabinowitz RP, Cookson ST, Wasserman SS, Mackowiak PA. Effects of anatomic site, oral stimulation and body position on estimates of body temperature. Arch Intern Med. 1996;156:777–780.)

or adult. In studies of core (deep rectal), anus, axillary, and skin temperature measurements in the newborn, Mayfield and associates observed that axillary measurements obtained with a mercury thermometer are as reliable as rectal temperature measurements.[23] Buntain and colleagues have also reported that in the neonate, axillary temperature measurements are sufficiently accurate to replace rectal measurements if a mercury-in-glass thermometer is used with an axillary dwell time of 5 minutes or more.[36] Schiffman has shown a similarly good correlation between axillary and rectal temperature measurements taken with mercury thermometers.[37]

Loudon, on the other hand, has shown that in older children, axillary temperature measurements with mercury thermometers vary from 1.6°C (2.6°F) lower to 0.6°C (1°F) higher than simultaneous oral measurements.[38] Nichols and colleagues have reported that in adults, even with 12-minute dwell times, axillary temperatures exhibit differences of 0 to 2.5°C (0 to 4.2°F) compared with oral temperature readings.[39] Furthermore, they noted that whereas 90% of rectal temperature readings reached their zenith at 4 minutes and 28% of oral readings reached their zenith at 5 minutes, only 18% of axillary readings reached a maximum at 5 minutes. Following a similar experience in children, Ogren has concluded that axillary temperature readings may be misleading and should be abandoned in the outpatient setting.[40]

Several studies have shown that monitoring the *skin temperature* using temperature-sensitive crystals incorporated into plastic strips placed on the forehead is an insensitive technique for detecting elevations in the core temperature.[41, 42] The detection of fever by palpation is similarly insensitive. Bergeson and Steinfield found that 42% of 138 febrile children (as defined by a "body temperature" of 38°C or greater) were judged to be afebrile by nurse assistants using palpation to detect fever.[43] Only 1.8% of over 1000 afebrile children were judged to be febrile using this same technique. In an evaluation of a mother's ability to assess the temperature of her child by palpation, Banco and Veltri found mothers to have a sensitivity of 73.9% and a specificity of 85.6% for detecting fever of greater than 38°C (100.4°F).[44] Thus, palpation by mothers was more sensitive than that by nurse assistants but was less specific for detecting the febrile state. Finally, Bonadio and coworkers have reported that among infants younger than 2 months of age presenting to the emergency room with a history of fever, those in whom fever had been documented at home by rectal thermometer were twice as likely to be febrile on presentation or during hospitalization than those whose fever had been documented by palpation alone (92 versus 46%; $p < 0.001$).[45]

Because the temperature of the rectum, mouth, and tympanic membrane are related but not identical, it would be useful to have a reliable formula *for converting data from one site to that of another.* In a recent study of healthy, young adults, Rabinowitz and associates determined that on average, rectal readings exceed concurrent oral readings by 0.4°C (0.8°F) and exceed TM readings (obtained with the IVAC CORE) by 0.8°C (1.6°F).[28] However, these relationships were extremely variable. Their findings concerning the relationship between rectal and oral readings were in agreement with those of several earlier investigations.[46, 47] Their findings with respect to the relationship between oral and TM readings, however, differed from earlier reports,[20] which had generally shown TM readings to be higher than simultaneously obtained oral measurements. This discrepancy most likely reflected the fact that unadjusted-mode TM thermometers, like the IVAC CORE, generally give lower readings than adjusted-mode TM thermometers, such as those used in earlier studies.[32]

Togawa has reported that on average, in a resting healthy adult, the core temperature (pulmonary artery) is 0.4°C (0.7°F) higher than the oral temperature and 0.2°C (0.4°F) lower than the rectal temperature, however, again with considerable individual variability.[48] Anagnostakis and coworkers have concluded in studies comparing rectal and axillary temperatures in infants that because of a similarly high degree of variability, no standard factor can be developed for converting axillary to rectal temperatures.[49] Thus, using a temperature reading from one anatomic site to predict the temperature at another must be done with caution.

Physiologic Variables

Wunderlich and Seguin[50] believed that "old" people have lower body temperatures than younger persons, and their views in this regard were corroborated by Howel[51] in a report published in the *Lancet* in 1948. There is also a substantial body of data suggesting that thermoregulation is impaired in elderly persons because of various effects of aging on the autonomic nervous system.[52] Nevertheless, more recent work has not shown lower average core temperatures among healthy elderly subjects (mean age 80.3 years; range 62 to 99 years) than among healthy younger people.[53] Comparisons of simultaneous oral, axillary, and rectal temperature readings from such subjects have shown lower average oral and axillary readings in elderly persons but comparable average rectal temperatures in elderly and young subjects.

It has long been known that women exhibit increases in body temperature of about 0.5°C (0.9°F) at the time of ovulation.[22] Wunderlich and Seguin also maintained that women have slightly higher normal temperatures than men overall and often show greater and more sudden changes in temperature.[50] Two more recent studies have corroborated Wunderlich and Seguin's former but not latter observation.[8, 54]

Body temperature, like most physiologic functions, exhibits circadian rhythmicity that is linked to the sleep-wake cycle.[55] During normal sleep-wake cycles (i.e., asleep during the night and awake during the day), the core temperature reaches its zenith in the late afternoon or early evening and its nadir in the early morning.[8] Adaptation to night shift work causes a reversal of this pattern. Therefore, when interpreting clinical thermometric measurements, it is important to consider not only the time of the measurement and the site at which the temperature was taken, but also the sleep-wake cycle of the subject being studied.

In addition to these physiologic variables, exercise, digestion, underlying disorders such as chronic renal failure, shock, and local inflammation at the site of the thermometric measurement (e.g., proctitis, external otitis, or stomatitis) may alter thermoregulatory responses or local temperatures, or both. It has, for example, been shown that the core temperature varies by as much as 3°C (36°C to 39°C) in states ranging from sleep to moderately high levels of sustained exercise, and this continuum of body temperature is related to a continuum of activity.[56] Although never systematically studied, it is also possible that body temperature varies according to the time of year or local climate. It is pertinent in this regard that Cheng and Partridge have shown that bundling and warm environments can elevate rectal temperatures of newborns to the febrile range.[57]

Normal "Body" Temperature

A survey of physicians' perceptions of body temperature published in 1995 indicated widespread confusion regarding key features of the human body temperature.[17] Seventy-five percent of 268 physicians and medical students surveyed gave 37°C (98.6°F) as their definition of *normal body temperature.* An additional 13% defined the normal temperature as a narrow range of temperatures about a mean of 37°C (98.6°F). Only 10 (4%) subjects in the group as a whole specified a particular body site (e.g., oral or rectal) for temperature measurements in their definition. Ninety-eight percent believed that the normal temperature varies during the day, with quantitative estimates of such diurnal variability ranging from 0.2°C (0.4°F) to 2.8°C (5°F) (mean ± SD = 0.8 ± 0.4°C [1.6 ± 0.8°F]). Estimates of the lower and upper ends of the normal temperature range varied between 32.8°C (91°F) and 37.2°C (99°F) and 36.7°C (98.0°F) and 39°C (102.2°F), respectively. Temperatures used to define fever (i.e., the lower end of the febrile range) varied between 36.9°C (98.5°F) and 40°C (104°F). Seventy-nine percent of the subjects believed that body temperature normally reaches its zenith in the evening and its nadir in the morning. However, fewer medical students (72%) than graduate physicians (85%) believed this to be the case ($p = 0.01$).

The origin of these perceptions of body temperature is uncertain, but in all likelihood lies among the writings of Carl Wunderlich, who, in 1868, published a book on clinical thermometry that many regard to this day as the definitive work on the subject.[6] Unfortunately, several of Wunderlich's dictums concerning body temperature, like the perceptions of modern-day physicians, appear to be in error.

A 1992 descriptive analysis of 700 baseline oral temperature observations from 148 healthy men and women found a range of 35.6°C (96.0°F) to 38.2°C (100.8°F), an overall mean of 36.8 ± 0.4°C (98.2 ± 0.7°F), a median of 36.8°C (98.2°F), and a mode of 36.7°C (98.0°F); 37°C (98.6°F) accounted for only 56 of the 700 (8%) oral temperature observations recorded (Fig. 43–2).[8] The mean temperature varied diurnally with a 6 AM nadir and a 4 to 6 PM apogee (Fig. 43–3). The maximal temperature (as reflected by the 99th percentile) varied from a low of 37.2°C (98.9°F) at 6 AM to a high of 37.7°C (99.9°F) at 4 PM. Comparison of initial temperature recordings obtained on admission to the research ward in which these observations were recorded with ones obtained the same hour the day after admission revealed no significant difference in variability (F tests for individual studies, $p \geq 0.12$). Age did not significantly influence temperature within the age range studied (18 to 40 years) (linear regression, $p = 0.99$).

Women had a slightly higher average oral temperature than men (36.9°C [98.4°F] versus 36.7°C [98.1°F]; t test, $p < 0.001$, $df = 698$) but did not exhibit greater average diurnal temperature oscillations than male counterparts (0.56°C [1.0°F] versus 0.54°C [0.97°F]). Black subjects exhibited a slightly higher mean temperature and slightly lower average diurnal temperature oscillations than white subjects (36.8°C [98.2°F] versus 36.7°C [98.1°F] and 0.51°C [0.93°F] versus 0.61°C [1.09°F], respectively); these differences approached, but did not quite reach, statistical significance (t test, $p = 0.06$,

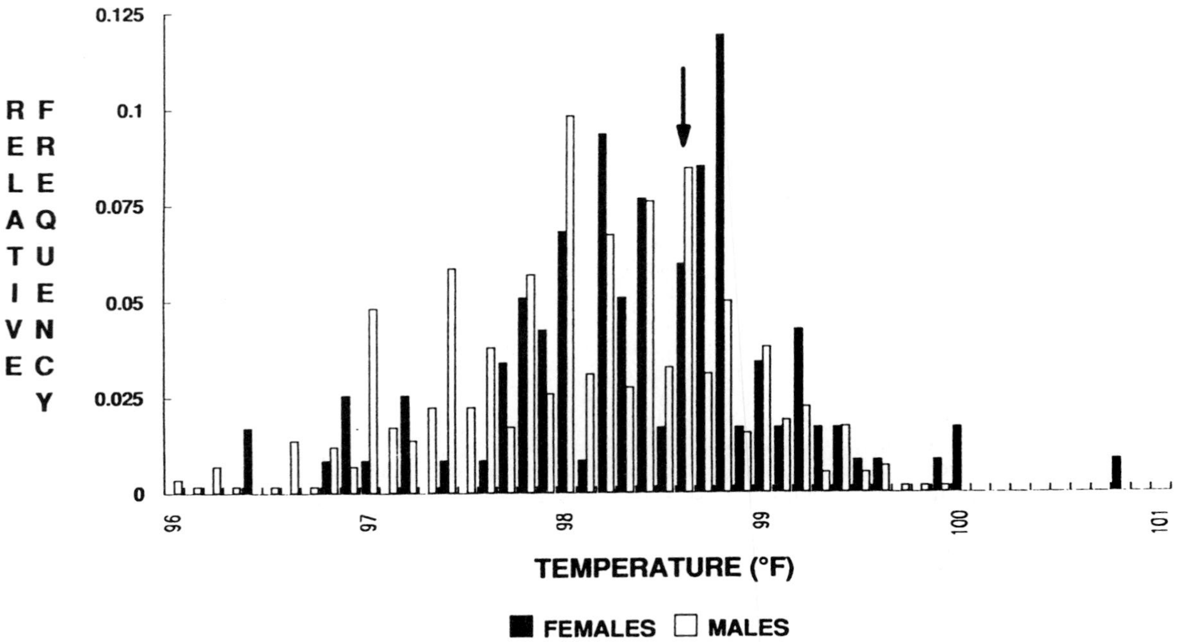

FIGURE 43–2. Frequency distribution of 700 baseline oral temperatures obtained during 2 consecutive days of observation in 148 healthy young volunteers. *Arrow* indicates location of 98.6°F (37°C). (From Mackowiak PA, Wasserman SS, Levine MM. A critical appraisal of 98.6°F, the upper limit of the normal body temperature, and other legacies of Carl Reinhold August Wunderlich. JAMA 1992;268:1578–1580.)

df = 698). Oral temperature recordings of smokers did not differ significantly from those of nonsmokers. There was a statistically significant linear relationship between temperature and pulse rate (regression analysis, $p < 0.001$) with an average increase in heart rate of 4.4 beats/minute for each 1°C (2.44 beats/minute for each 1°F) rise in temperature over the range of temperatures examined (96.0°F to 100.8°F).

According to Wunderlich and Seguin, "When the organism (man) is in a normal condition, the general temperature of the body maintains itself at the physiologic point: 37°C = 98.6°F."[50] Although several investigations since Wunderlich and Seguin's have recorded mean temperatures of normal adult populations closer to 36.6°C (98.0°F),[58] Wunderlich and Woodman's intimation that 37°C (98.6°F) is the most normal of temperatures[59] persists to this day, not only in lay thinking, but in medical writing as well.[60–63] The special significance accorded 37°C (98.6°F) is perhaps best illustrated by the 1990 edition of *Stedman's Medical Dictionary,* which defines fever as "a body temperature above the normal of 37°C (98.6°F)."[64]

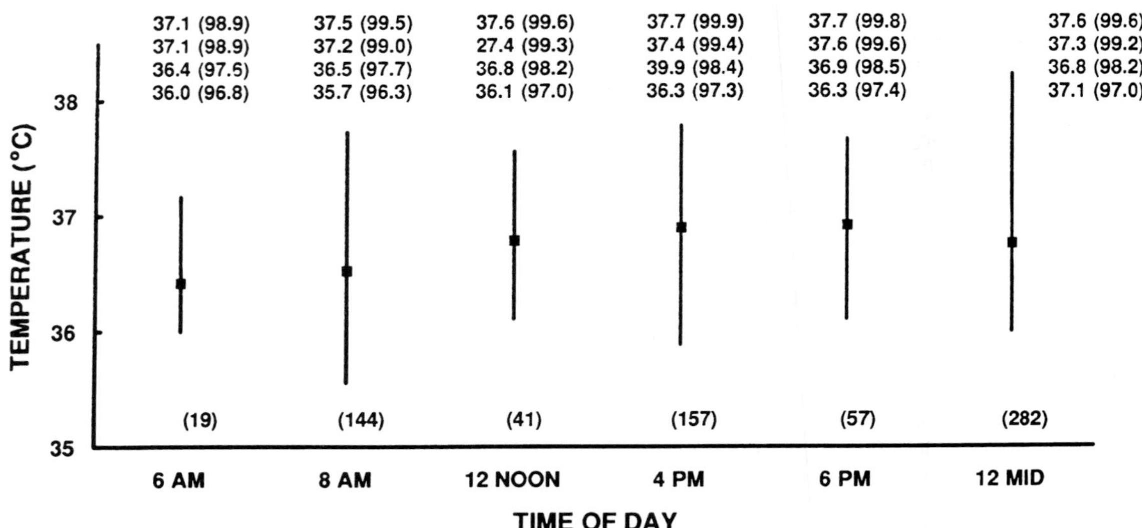

FIGURE 43–3. Mean oral temperatures and temperature ranges in 148 healthy young volunteers according to time of day. The four temperatures shown at each sample time are the 99th percentile (*top*), the 95th percentile (*second*), the mean (*third*), and the fifth percentile (*bottom*) for each sample set. The numbers in parentheses on the x axis indicate the number of observations analyzed at each sample time. (From Mackowiak PA, Wasserman SS, Levine MM. A critical appraisal of 98.6°F, the upper limit of the normal body temperature, and other legacies of Carl Reinhold August Wunderlich. JAMA 1992;268:1578–1580.)

The data reviewed earlier suggest that 37°C (98.6°F) has no special significance vis-à-vis body temperature in healthy young adults when such temperature is measured orally using modern thermometers. In the population examined, 37°C (98.6°F) was not the overall mean temperature, the mean temperature of any of the time periods studied, the median temperature, or the single most frequent temperature recorded. Furthermore, it did not fall within the 99.9% confidence limits for the sample mean (36.7°C to 36.8°C; 98.1°F to 98.2°F).

Wunderlich and Seguin regarded 38.0°C (100.4°F) as the upper limit of normal body temperature and by extrapolation, any temperature greater than 38.0°C (100.4°F) as fever.[50] Modern medical textbooks differ in their definition of the upper limit of normal oral temperature. Published values include 37.1°C (98.8°F) and 38°C (100.4°F) in textbooks of physiology,[65, 66] 37.2°C (99.0°F) in *Harrison's Principles of Internal Medicine,*[67] and 37.4°C (99.4°F) in a 1991 monograph on fever.[68] As noted earlier, a widely used medical dictionary defines this same upper limit as 37°C (98.6°F).[64]

The source of the confusion over what constitutes the upper limit of normal body temperature in all likelihood derives from individual variability, which limits the application of mean values derived from population studies to individual subjects, and the fact that the maximal oral temperature, like the mean temperature, exhibited by a population varies according to the time of day and the site at which temperature measurements are taken. Because of such variability, no single temperature can be designated as the upper limit of normal. In the study population considered earlier, 37.2°C (98.9°F) was the maximal oral temperature (i.e., the 99th percentile) recorded at 6 AM, whereas at 4 PM, the maximal oral temperature observed reached 37.7°C (99.9°F). Thus, these data suggest that when modern thermometers are used to monitor oral temperature in young or middle-aged adults, fever is most appropriately defined as an early-morning temperature of 37.2°C (99.0°F) or greater or a temperature of 37.8°C (100°F) or greater at any time during the day.

Wunderlich wrote in 1868 that "[temperature] oscillates even in healthy persons according to time of day by 0.5°C = 0.9°F." The next year Wunderlich and Reeve wrote, "The lowest point is reached in the morning hours between two and eight, and the highest in the afternoon between four and nine."[69] Modern authorities have generally concurred with the observations of Wunderlich and associates on such matters.[61, 67] However, Tauber has suggested that the amplitude of diurnal variation might be as high as 1°C (1.8°F).[62] The data described earlier are more consistent with the views of Wunderlich and colleagues. Nevertheless, the subjects examined in that study exhibited considerable individual variability, with some having daily temperature oscillations as wide as 1.3°C (2.4°F) and others having oscillations as narrow as 0.1°C (0.2°F).

According to Wunderlich and Seguin, women have slightly higher normal temperatures than men and often show greater and more sudden changes of temperature.[50] In a study of nine healthy young adults (six male and three female), Dinarello and Wolff corroborated both observations.[70] The investigation described earlier, which did not control for the effects of ovulation on thermal observations, was only able to corroborate the former observation of Wunderlich and Seguin.[8]

It has been maintained for over a century that elderly persons have lower body temperatures than younger persons.[50] A study reported in the *Lancet* in 1948 by Howel seemed to substantiate this belief.[71] Although there are considerable data suggesting that thermoregulation is impaired in elderly persons because of various effects of aging on the autonomic system,[72] as noted previously, more recent investigation has not shown lower average core temperatures among healthy elderly persons than among healthy young people.[53]

Some authors believe that the first temperature reading obtained on admission to a hospital can be falsely elevated, because stress, in the broadest sense, has the capacity to elevate body temperature.[50, 68] The University of Maryland study described previously did not find evidence that the first temperature reading obtained after admission to a research study unit was any less reliable than measurements obtained at later times.[8] Maryland investigators, however, could not be certain that stress levels at the time of admission to their unit were comparable to levels of stress experienced by patients at the time of admission to a hospital.

As a result of work conducted earlier this century,[73, 74] it is widely believed that the heart rate increases 10 beats/minute for each 1°F rise in body temperature. More recent data presented earlier indicate that the heart rate increases only 2.44 beats/minute for each 1°F rise in temperature.[8] The difference between the earlier and more recent investigations most likely reflects the fact that in the latter instance, subjects were afebrile and were examined seated, whereas those examined in earlier investigations were mostly febrile and rested reclining on a couch for 20 minutes before examination.

The normal range of body temperature in children is not well delineated. Lorin has written that the range is higher in children than in adults and that a decrease toward adult levels begins at about 1 year of age, continues through puberty, and stabilizes at 13 to 14 years of age in girls and 17 to 18 years of age in boys.[75] He offers as documentation of his views on the matter a 1937 publication by Bayley and Stolz.[76] Unfortunately, these early investigators did not control for variables such as the time of day, bundling, and the thermometer dwell time, each of which might have significantly affected the results of their survey. It has also been maintained that the circadian rhythm that characterizes body temperature in the adult is less evident in the first few months of life, is well established by the second birthday, and tends to be more pronounced during childhood than during adulthood.[75] This concept, like many concerned with the normal temperature of children, is difficult to substantiate with published data.

THERMOREGULATION

Heat is derived from biochemical reactions occurring in all living cells.[77] At the mitochondrial level, energy derived from the catabolism of metabolites such as glucose is used in oxidative phosphorylation to convert adenosine diphosphate to adenosine triphosphate (ATP). At rest, more than half of the body's heat is generated as a result of the inefficiency of the biochemical processes that convert food energy into the free energy pool (e.g., ATP). Even if no external work is being performed, heat is, nevertheless, generated as a result of both internal work (e.g., peristalsis, myocardial contractions, and the circulation of blood) and biochemical reactions involved in maintaining the structural and functional integrity of the various organ systems (i.e., the utilization and resynthesis of ATP). When external work is performed, additional heat is generated as a by-product of skeletal muscle contractions.

In adult humans and most other large mammals, shivering is the primary means by which heat production is enhanced. Nonshivering thermogenesis is more important in smaller mammals, newborns (including humans), and cold-acclimated mammals.[77, 78] Although several tissues (e.g., the heart, respiratory muscles, and adipose tissue) contribute to the process, brown adipose tissue has been most closely associated with nonshivering thermogenesis. This highly specialized form of adipose tissue located near the shoulder blades, neck, adrenals, and deep blood vessels is characterized by its brownish color, a profuse vascular system, and an abundance of mitochondria.[77, 79]

Heat generated primarily in vital organs lying deep within the body core, is distributed throughout the body via the circulatory system. In response to input from the nervous system, the circulatory system determines both the temperature of the various body parts and the rate at which heat is lost from body surfaces to the environment (by conduction, convection, radiation, and evaporation).[80] In a warm environment, or in response to an elevation in the core temperature due to exercise, cutaneous blood flow increases so that heat is transported from the core to be dissipated at the skin surface. Simultaneous activation of sweat glands enhances such heat loss via evaporation. In anesthetized animals, increases in cutaneous blood flow in response to hypothalamic warming are offset by concomitant reductions in gastrointestinal blood flow.[81] In a cold environment or in response to a decrease in the core temperature, cutaneous blood flow normally decreases as a means of conserving heat within the body core.

No single center within the nervous system controls body temperature. Rather, thermoregulation is a process that involves a continuum of neural structures and connections extending from the hypothalamus and limbic system through the lower brain stem and reticular formation to the spinal cord and sympathetic ganglia (Fig. 43–4).[77] Nevertheless, an area of the brain located in and near the rostral hypothalamus appears to play a pivotal role in the process of thermoregulation. Although generally referred to as the "preoptic region," it actually includes the medial and lateral aspects of the preoptic area, anterior hypothalamus, and septum. Numerous studies extending over 60 years have established that neurons located in this region are thermosensitive and exert at least partial control over physiologic and behavioral thermoregulatory responses.[80, 82]

Many, although not all, thermophysiologists believe that the temperature-sensitive, preoptic region "regulates" body temperature by integrating thermal input signals from thermosensors in the skin and core areas (including the central nervous system).[83] One of the more widely held theories is that such integration involves a designated thermal setpoint for the preoptic region that is maintained by a system of negative feedback. According to this theory, if the preoptic temperature rises above its setpoint, for whatever reason (e.g., during exercise), heat-loss responses are activated to lower the body temperature and return the temperature of the preoptic region to the thermal setpoint (e.g., 37°C).[84] The thermal setpoint of a particular heat-loss response is thus the maximal temperature tolerated by the preoptic region before the heat-loss response is evoked. If, on the other hand, the preoptic temperature falls below its thermal setpoint (e.g., as a result of cold exposure), various heat-retention and heat-production responses are activated to raise body temperature and with it, the

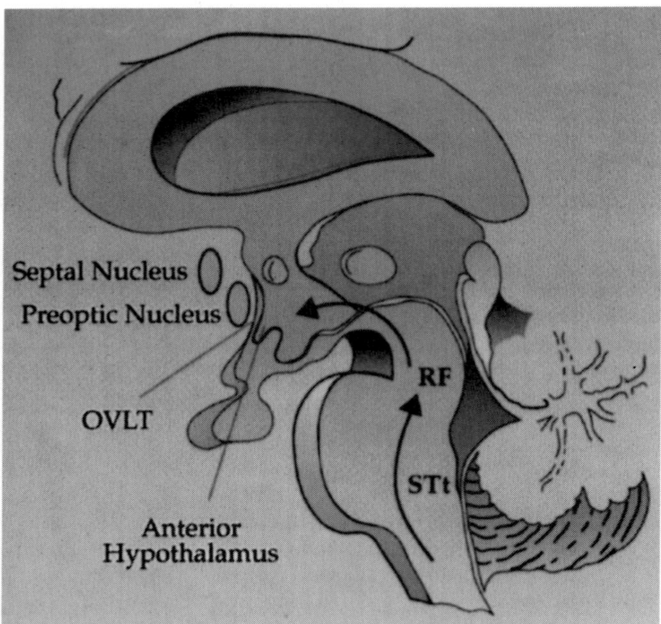

FIGURE 43–4. Saggital view of the brain and upper spinal cord showing the multisynaptic pathway of skin and spinal thermoreceptors through the spinothalamic tract (STt) and reticular formation (RF) to the anterior hypothalamus, preoptic region, and the septum. (From Mackowiak PA. Concepts of fever. Arch Intern Med. 1998;158:1870–1881.)

temperature of the preoptic region to its thermal setpoint. The thermal setpoint of a particular heat-production response is thus the minimal temperature tolerated by the preoptic region before the response is evoked.

Although a convenient explanation of the means by which temperature elevations are coordinated during fever, the concept of a single, central setpoint temperature is regarded by many thermal physiologists as oversimplified. At least some physiologists prefer to think of body temperature as regulated within a narrow range of temperatures by a composite setpoint of several thermosensitive areas and several different thermoregulatory responses.[85–87]

A variety of endogenous substances and drugs appear to affect temperature regulation by altering the activity of hypothalamic neurons. Perhaps the best examples of such substances are the pyrogenic cytokines discussed later. These are released by phagocytic leukocytes in response to a wide array of stimuli and have the capacity to raise the thermoregulatory center's thermal setpoint. Whether they cross the blood-brain barrier to do so[88, 89] or act by evoking the release of other mediators (e.g., prostaglandin E_2) in circumventricular organs, such as the organum vasculosum laminae terminalis,[88] is uncertain. Whatever the precise endogenous mediators of fever, their primary effect appears to be to decrease the firing rate of preoptic warm-sensitive neurons, leading to the activation of responses designed to decrease heat loss and increase heat production.

ENDOGENOUS PYROGENS

Pyrogens have traditionally been divided into two general categories: those that originate outside the body (exogenous pyrogens) and those that are derived from host cells (endogenous pyrogens). Exogenous pyrogens are, for the most part, microorganisms, and toxins or other products of microbial origin, whereas endogenous pyrogens are host cell–derived (pyrogenic) cytokines that are the principal central mediators of the febrile response.[90] According to current concepts, exogenous pyrogens, regardless of their physicochemical structure, initiate fever by inducing host cells (primarily macrophages) to produce endogenous pyrogens. Such concepts not withstanding, certain endogenous molecules also have the capacity to induce endogenous pyrogens. These include, among others, antigen-antibody complexes in the presence of complement,[91, 92] certain androgenic steroid metabolites,[93–95] inflammatory bile acids,[96] complement,[97] and various lymphocyte-derived molecules.[98, 99]

Complete understanding of the function of individual pyrogenic cytokines has been hampered by the fact that one cytokine often influences the expression of other cytokines or their receptors, or both, and may also induce more distal comediators of cytokine-related bioactivities (e.g., prostaglandins and platelet-activating factor).[100] In short, cytokines function within a complex regulatory network, in which information is conveyed to cells by combinations, and perhaps sequences, of a host of cytokines and other hormones.[101] Like the words of human communication, individual cytokines are basic units of information. On occasion, a single cytokine, like a single word, may communicate a complete message. More often, however, complete messages received by cells probably resemble sentences, in which combinations and sequences of cytokines convey information. Because of such interactions, it has been difficult to ascertain the direct in vivo bioactivities of particular cytokines. Nevertheless, several cytokines have in common the capacity to induce fever. Based on this characteristic, they have been codified together as so-called pyrogenic cytokines.

The list of currently recognized pyrogenic cytokines includes, among others, interleukin-1 (IL-1 [IL-1α and IL-β]), tumor necrosis factor-α (TNF-α), IL-6, and interferon-γ (IFN-γ) (Table 43–1).[102–110] Even among these few cytokines, complex relationships exist, with certain members upregulating the expression of other members or their receptors in certain situations and downregulating them in others.[100] The four major pyrogenic cytokines have monomeric molecular masses that range from 17 to 30 kDa. Undetectable under

TABLE 43-1 Biological Characteristics of the Principal Pyrogenic Cytokines

Pyrogenic Cytokine	Aliases	Cell Source	Expression: Upregulated by	Expression: Downregulated by	Effect on Other Pyrogenic Cytokines	Biologic Activities
Interleukin-1 (IL-1)	Endogenous pyrogen Leukocyte endogenous pyrogen Lymphocyte-activating factor Mononuclear factor Catabolin Osteoclast-activating factor Hematopoietin-1 Melanoma growth inhibition factor Tumor inhibitory factor-2	Astrocytes Endothelial cells Keratinocytes Monocytes Macrophages Dendrites Fibroblasts	TNF-α IFN-γ GM-CSF Zymosan LPS IL-1 C5a Leukotrienes PMA	IL-4 IL-6 IL-10 TGF-β Corticosteroids PGE_2 Retinoic acid	↑ IL-6 ↑ TNF-α ↑ IL-1	IL-2 and IL-2R induction Thymocyte costimulation Fibroblast activation Induction of acute-phase response T-cell activation Costimulation of B-cell proliferation and differentiation CTL augmentation, LAK induction Induction of endothelial adhesion molecules Enhancement of phagocyte microbial killing Acceleration of wound healing
Tumor necrosis factor-α (TNF-α)	Cachectin	Monocytes Macrophages Eosinophils Neutrophils Lymphocytes Astrocytes Endothelial cells Mast cells Kupffer cells NK cells Certain tumors	Bacteria Viruses Fungi Protozoa LPS Staph. TSSTI IL-1 IL-2 TNF-α IFNs GM-CSF PAF Substance P Anti-TCR Tumor cells PMA	Corticosteroids Cyclosporin A PGE_2 IL-4 IL-6 IL-10 TGF-β Vitamin D_3	↑ TNF-α ↑ IL-1 ↑ IL-6	Septic shock Enhancement of phagocyte microbial killing Tumor necrosis Cachexia Anorexia Endothelial and epithelial MHC, adhesion molecule induction Osteoclast activation B-cell differentiation CTL induction
Interleukin-6 (IL-6)	Interferon-β2 B-cell stimulatory factor-2 Hybridoma/plasmacytoma growth factor Hepatocyte-stimulating factor Cytotoxic T-cell differentiation factor Macrophage granulocyte–inducing factor 2A	Monocytes Macrophages Lymphocytes Fibroblasts Endothelial cells Epithelial cells Keratinocytes Bone marrow stroma Certain tumors	LPS IL-1 TNF IFN-β Calcium ionophore Mitogenic lectin + PMA Viruses	Corticosteroids Estrogens	↓ TNF-α ↓ IL-1	B-cell growth, differentiation, and IgG synthesis Myeloma proliferation CTL induction Acute-phase response Thymocyte costimulation Weak antiviral activity Megakaryocyte maturation Neuronal differentiation Enhancement of IL-3–dependent stem cell proliferation
Interferon-γ (IFN-γ)	Type II interferon Immune interferon	T cells NK cells	Mitogenic lectins IL-1 IL-2	Corticosteroids Cyclosporin A Vitamin D_3	↑ TNF-α ↑ IL-1	Macrophage priming Antiviral activity TNF activity enhancement MHC induction NK activity enhancement Enhancement of endothelial ICAM-1 expression Inhibition of IL-4 induced B-cell responses B cell differentiation and IgG2a secretion

Abbreviations: anti-TCR, Anti–T-cell receptor; C5a, complement component C5a; CTL, cytotoxic T lymphocyte; GM-CSF, granulocyte-monocyte colony-stimulating factor; ICAM, intracellular adhesion molecule; LAK, lymphokine-activated killer; LPS, (bacterial) lipopolysaccharide; MHC, major histocompatibility complex; NK, natural killer; PAF, platelet-activating factor; PGE, prostaglandin E; PMA, phorbol myristate acetate; Staph. TSST1, staphylococcal toxic shock syndrome toxin-1; TGF-β, transforming growth factor-beta; ↑, enhanced expression; ↓, reduced expression.

Adapted from Hasday and Goldblum in Mackowiak PA, Barlett JG, Borden EC, et al. Recent advances and lingering dogma (Symposium Summary). Clin Infect Dis. 1997;25:119–138.

basal conditions in healthy subjects, they are produced by many different tissues in response to appropriate stimuli. Once released, pyrogenic cytokines have short intravascular half-lives. They are pleiotropic, in that they interact with receptors present on many different host cells. They are active in picomolar quantities, induce maximal cellular responses even at low receptor occupancy, and exert local (autocrine-paracrine) as well as systemic (endocrine) effects.[100]

It has been theorized, although not yet proved, that interactions between pyrogenic cytokines and their receptors in the preoptic region of the anterior hypothalamus activates phospholipase A_2, liberating plasma membrane arachidonic acid as a substrate for the cyclooxygenase pathway. Some cytokines might do so by increasing cyclooxygenase expression directly, causing liberation of the arachidonate metabolite prostaglandin E_2. Because this small lipid molecule easily diffuses across the blood-brain barrier, it is thought by some to be the local mediator that actually activates thermosensitive neurons. Although not yet widely accepted, some studies indicate that thermal information involved in the febrile response might also be transmitted from the periphery to the thermoregulatory center via peripheral nerves.[111]

Extensive work with pyrogenic cytokines over the last 2 decades has provided a hypothetic model for the febrile response (Fig. 43–5).[112] Nevertheless, our understanding of this process remains incomplete and largely speculative. As indicated previously, it is not yet clear whether circulating cytokines cross the blood-brain barrier or have to be produced within the central nervous system in order to activate thermosensitive neurons; or if each of the pyrogenic cytokines is capable of raising the thermoregulatory setpoint independently or must exert this effect through some common pathway (e.g., IL-6, as suggested by Dinarello[90]; see Fig. 43–3); or if prostaglandin E_2 or other local mediators are a sine qua non of the febrile response; or what determines the magnitude of expression of individual cytokines in response to various stimuli; or how the upper limit of the febrile range is set.[100]

TNF-α and IL-1 have pivotal roles during the induction phase of the febrile response[113] but are also expressed throughout the response.[114] A small but growing body of data suggests that temperatures near the upper end of the febrile range influence the production of such cytokines.[115–126] However, such effects are highly dependent on experimental conditions.

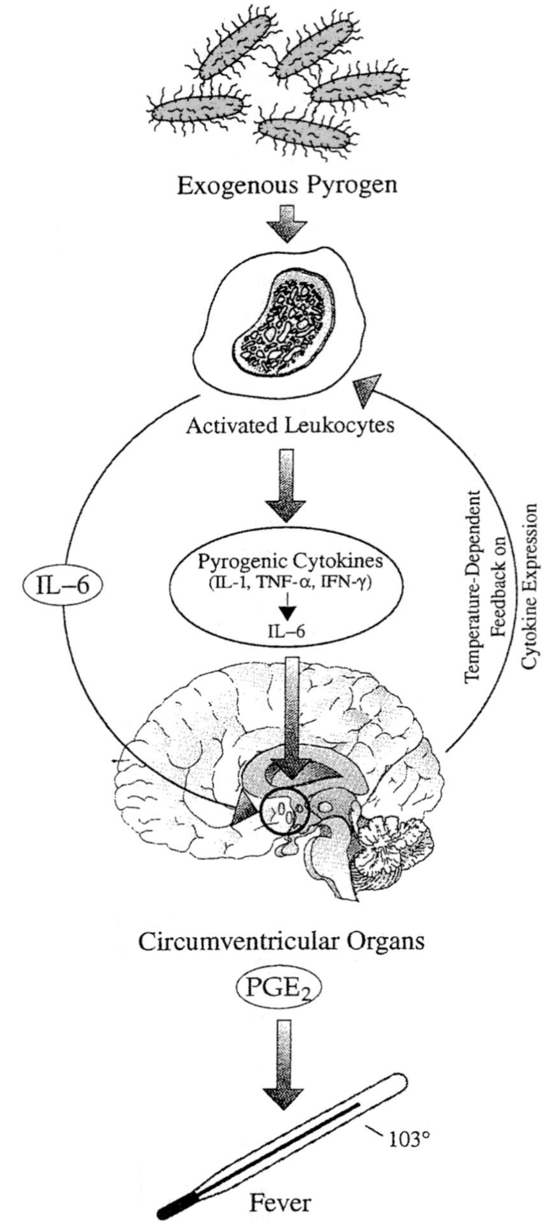

FIGURE 43–5. Hypothetical model for the febrile response. (From Boulant JA. Thermoregulation. In: Mackowiak PA, ed. Fever. Basic Mechanisms and Management. 2nd ed. Philadelphia: Lippincott-Raven; 1997:35–58.)

ACUTE-PHASE RESPONSE

As noted previously, a cytokine-mediated rise in the core temperature is but one of many features of the febrile response. Numerous other physiologic reactions, collectively referred to as the *acute-phase response,* are mediated by members of the same group of pyrogenic cytokines that activate the thermal response of fever.[101] Such reactions include somnolence, anorexia, changes in plasma protein synthesis, and altered synthesis of hormones such as corticotropin-releasing hormone, glucagon, insulin, corticotropin, cortisol, adrenal catecholamines, growth hormone, thyroid-stimulating hormone, thyroxin, aldosterone, and arginine vasopressin. Inhibition of bone formation, negative nitrogen balance, gluconeogenesis, and altered lipid metabolism are also seen during the acute-phase response, as are decreases in serum concentrations of zinc and iron and increases in the concentration of copper. Hematologic alterations[127] involved in the acute-phase response include leukocytosis, thrombocytosis, and decreased erythropoiesis (resulting in an *anemia of chronic inflammation*).[128] Stimuli capable of inducing an acute-phase response include bacterial and (to a lesser extent) viral infections, trauma, malignant neoplasms, burns, tissue infarction, immunologically mediated and crystal-induced inflammatory states, strenuous exercise, and childbirth.[101, 129] Data also suggest that major depression,[130] schizophrenia,[131] and psychological stress[132] are capable of inducing an acute-phase response.

Traditionally, the phrase *acute-phase response* has been used to denote changes in plasma concentrations of a number of secretory proteins derived from hepatocytes. *Acute-phase proteins,* of which there are many (Table 43–2),[101] exhibit either increased synthesis (*positive* acute-phase proteins) or decreased synthesis (*negative* acute-phase proteins) during the acute-phase response.

Many of the acute-phase proteins are believed to modulate inflammation and tissue repair.[133] A major function of C-reactive protein (CRP), for example, is presumed to involve binding of phosphocholine on pathogenic microorganisms, as well as phospholipid constituents on damaged or necrotic host cells. Through such binding, CRP might both activate the complement system and promote phagocyte adherence, thereby initiating the process by which pathogenic microbes or necrotic cells are cleared from the host. Such activities are most likely potentiated by CRP-induced production of

TABLE 43–2 The Acute-Phase Proteins

Positive Acute-Phase Proteins*	
C-reactive protein	Ferritin
Serum amyloid A	Phospholipase A_2
Haptoglobin	Plasminogen activator inhibitor-1
α_1-Acid glycoprotein	Fibronectin
α_1-Protease inhibitor	Hemopexin
Fibrinogen	Pancreatic secretory trypsin inhibitor
Ceruloplasmin	Inter-alpha protease inhibitor
Complement (C3 and C4)	Mannose-binding protein
C-1 esterase inhibitor	Lipopolysaccharide-binding protein
C4b-binding protein	
α_2-macroglobulin	
Negative Acute-Phase Proteins†	
Albumin	Transferrin
Transthyretin	α_2-HS glycoprotein

*Proteins exhibiting increased plasma concentrations during the acute-phase response.
†Proteins exhibiting decreased plasma concentrations during the acute-phase response.
Adapted from Kushner I, Rzewnicki DL. The acute phase response. In: Mackowiak PA, ed. Fever, Basic Mechanisms and Management. 2nd ed. Philadelphia: Lippincott-Raven; 1997:165–176.

inflammatory cytokines[134] and tissue factor[135] by monocytes. Nevertheless, the ultimate function of CRP is uncertain, in that several in vivo studies have shown it to have anti-inflammatory properties.[136–138]

Another of the major human acute-phase protein, serum amyloid A, has been reported to potentiate adhesiveness and chemotaxis of phagocytic cells and lymphocytes.[139] There is also evidence that macrophages bear specific binding sites for serum amyloid A, that serum amyloid A–rich, high-density lipoproteins mediate the transfer of cholesterol to macrophages at sites of inflammation,[140] and that serum amyloid A enhances low-density lipoprotein oxidation in arterial walls.[141]

Complement components, many of which are acute-phase reactants, modulate chemotaxis, opsonization, vascular permeability, and vascular dilation and have cytotoxic effects as well.[101] Haptoglobin, hemopexin, and ceruloplasmin are all antioxidants. It is, therefore, reasonable to assume that, like the antiproteases, α_1-antichymotrypsin, and C-1 esterase inhibitor, they play important roles in modulating inflammation. However, the functional capacity of such proteins is broad. There is also a growing literature concerned with the acute-phase protein lipopolysaccharide-binding protein, which appears both to enhance and to neutralize the biologic activity of lipopolysaccharide.[142]

Although closely associated with fever, the acute-phase response is not an invariable component of the febrile response.[101] Some febrile patients (e.g., those with certain viral infections) have normal blood levels of CRP. Moreover, patients with elevated blood levels of CRP are not always febrile. The acute-phase response, like the febrile response, is a complex response consisting of numerous integrated, though separately regulated, components. The particular components expressed in response to a given disease process more than likely reflects the specific cytokines induced by the disease.

ENDOGENOUS CRYOGENS

Hippocrates maintained that "heat is the immortal substance of life endowed with intelligence. . . . However, heat must also be refrigerated by respiration and kept within bounds if the source or principle of life is to persist; for if refrigeration is not provided, the heat will consume itself."[143] Modern-day clinicians also generally subscribe to the notion that the febrile range has an upper limit but do not agree on a precise temperature defining this limit.[17] The lack of a consensus in this regard is understandable, owing to the fact that "body" temperature profiles exhibit considerable individual, anatomic, and diurnal variability. For this reason, the upper limit of the febrile range cannot be defined as a single temperature applicable to all body sites of all people at all times during the day. Nevertheless, the febrile response is a regulated physiologic response, in which the temperature is maintained within a specific range, the upper limit of which almost never exceeds 41°C, regardless of the cause of the fever or the site at which the temperature measurements are taken.[144] The physiologic necessity of this upper limit is supported by considerable experimental data demonstrating adverse physiologic consequences of core temperatures of greater than 41 to 42°C (107.6°F).[145]

The mechanisms regulating fever's upper limit have yet to be fully characterized. They could lie with the intrinsic properties of the neurons themselves or involve the release of endogenous antipyretic substances that antagonize the effects of pyrogens on thermosensitive neurons. With regard to the former possibility, plots of the firing rates of neurons coordinating thermoregulatory responses and heat production tend to converge at 42°C (107.6°F) (Fig. 43–6).[145] At this temperature, the sustained firing rates of warm-sensitive neurons reach their zenith and cannot be increased further in response to higher temperatures. Similarly, the firing rates of cold-sensitive neurons reach their nadir at 42°C (107.6°F) and cannot decrease further, even if the temperature continues to increase. Thus, regardless of the pyrogen concentration, thermosensitive neurons appear to be incapable of providing additional thermoregulatory signals once the temperature reaches 42°C (107.6°F).

These same thermosensitive neurons are influenced by a variety of endogenous substances, at least some of which appear to function as endogenous cryogens.[145] One such substance is arginine vasopressin. Studies from several laboratories employing a variety of animal models have established that arginine vasopressin is present in the fibers and terminals of the ventral septal area of the hypothalamus, is released into the ventral septal area during fever, reduces fever by its action at type 1 vasopressin receptors when introduced into the ventral septal area, and, when inhibited, prolongs fever.[146–148]

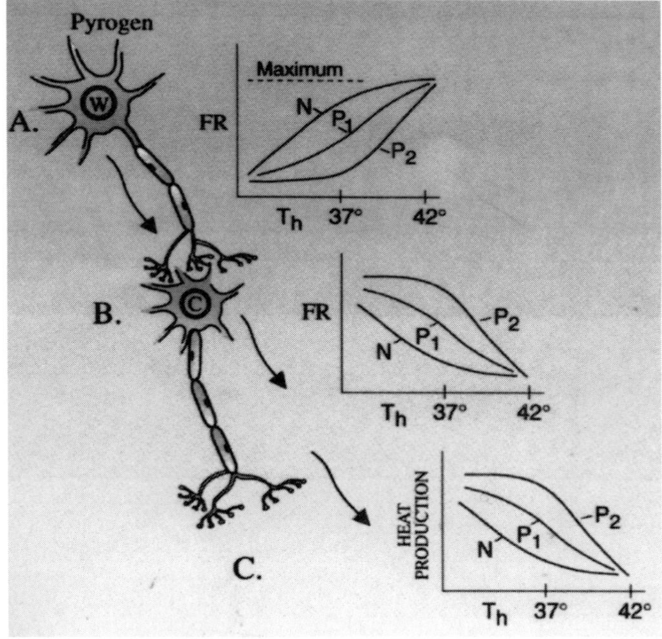

FIGURE 43–6. Model showing responses (*A* and *B*) of neuronal firing rates (FR) in the preoptic region and anterior hypothalamus and whole-body metabolic heat production (*C*) during changes in hypothalamic temperature (T_h). Thermosensitivity is reflected by the slope of each plot. The letters inside the cells indicate a warm-sensitive (w) neuron and a cold-sensitive (c) neuron. With increases in T_h, warm-sensitive neurons raise their FRs, and heat production decreases. Pyrogens inhibit (−) the FRs of warm-sensitive neurons, thereby resulting in accelerated FRs of cold-sensitive neurons and increased heat production. The plots show FR and heat production responses during normal conditions in the absence of pyrogens (N) and in the presence of low concentrations (P_1) and high concentrations (P_2) of pyrogens. (From Mackowiak PA, Boulant JA. Fever's glass ceiling. Clin Infect Dis. 1996;22:525–536.)

α-Melanocyte–stimulating hormone (α-MSH) is another neuropeptide exhibiting endogenous antipyretic activity.[149] Unlike some of the other antipyretic peptides, α-MSH has not been identified in fibers projecting into the ventral septal area.[150] It does, nevertheless, reduce pyrogen-induced fever when administered to experimental animals in doses below those having an effect on the basal body temperature.[151–155] When given centrally, α-MSH is more than 25,000 times more potent as an antipyretic than acetaminophen.[149] Repeated central administration of α-MSH does not induce tolerance to its antipyretic effect.[156] In addition, injection of anti–α-MSH antiserum into the cerebral ventricles augments the febrile response of experimental animals to IL-1.[157]

Numerous neurochemicals appear to have the capacity to influence the hypothalamic control of body temperature. Because some of these lower the body temperature even in the absence of fever, they are more appropriately termed *hypothermic* agents than *antipyretic* agents. In some of the earliest work in this area, Feldberg and Myers observed that in cats, intracerebroventricular injections of adrenalin and noradrenalin cause a fall in body temperature, whereas injections of serotonin cause the temperature to rise.[158] Based on these observations, they proposed that the regulation of body temperature involves a balance between the release of catecholamines (inducing heat loss) and serotonin (activating heat production) in the anterior hypothalamus. More recent data suggest that the basis of setpoint determination by the thermoregulatory network is considerably more complex.[159]

Glucocorticoids and their inducers (corticotropin-releasing hormone and corticotropin) inhibit the synthesis of pyrogenic cytokines such as IL-6 and TNF-α.[160–162] Through such effects, they are believed to exert inhibitory feedback on lipopolysaccharide (LPS)-induced fever.[163] Lipocortin 1, a putative mediator of glucocorticoid function, has also been shown to inhibit the pyrogenic actions of IL-1 and IFN.[164] Injection of CRH into the third ventricle of experimental animals produces similar antipyretic effects.[165]

Thyrotropin-releasing hormone,[166] gastric-inhibitory peptide,[167] neuropeptide Y,[168] and bombesin,[169] likewise, exhibit cryogenic properties under certain conditions. Of these, bombesin has exhibited the highest potency, in that it consistently produces hypothermia associated with changes in heat dissipation and heat production when injected into the preoptic area/anterior hypothalamus of conscious goats and rabbits.[169–171] Bombesin is believed to exert its hypothermic effect by decreasing the sensitivity of warm-sensitive neurons.[171]

Pyrogenic cytokines, the mediators of the febrile response, might themselves have a role in determining fever's upper limit. There is, for instance, experimental evidence indicating that under certain conditions (e.g., intracerebral injection of recombinant human TNF-α in Zucker rats, TNF-α acts to lower, rather than to raise, body temperature.[172, 173] Thus, it is possible that at certain concentrations or in the appropriate physiologic milieu, pyrogenic cytokines function paradoxically as endogenous cryogens.

A growing body of literature indicates that the release of pyrogenic cytokines such as IL-1 is followed by increased shedding of soluble receptors for such cytokines, which function as endogenous inhibitors of these pyrogens.[174] In the case of IL-1, a 22- to 25-kDa molecule identified in supernatants of human monocytes blocks binding of IL-1 to its receptors.[175] The IL-1 receptor antagonist is structurally related to IL-1α and IL-1β[176] and binds to both type I and type II receptors on various target cells without inducing a specific biologic response.[177, 178] Shedding of soluble receptors of TNF-α that bind to circulating TNF-α and thereby inhibit binding to cell-associated receptors has also been described.[179–183] The precise biologic function of such circulating receptor antagonists and soluble receptors is not known. However, it is possible that one function is to serve as a natural braking system for the febrile response.

RISK-BENEFIT CONSIDERATIONS

Questions concerning fever's risk-benefit quotient have generated considerable controversy.[184] The controversy arises because of data indicating both potentiating and inhibitory effects of the response on resistance to infection. As a result, there is as yet no consensus as to the appropriate clinical situations (if any) in which fever or its mediators should be suppressed.

Data illustrating fever's beneficial effects originate from several sources. Studies of the phylogeny of fever have shown the response to be widespread within the animal kingdom.[185] With few exceptions, mammals, reptiles, amphibians, and fish, as well as several invertebrate species, have been shown to elevate the core temperature in response to a challenge with microorganisms or other known pyrogens (Fig. 43–7). It has been assumed, although not established conclusively, that such elevations in temperature are the poikilothermic corollary of fever. The prevalence of such "febrile responses" has been offered as some of the strongest evidence that fever is an adaptive response, based on the argument that the metabolically expensive increase in body temperature that accompanies the febrile response would not have evolved and been so faithfully preserved within the animal kingdom unless fever had some net benefit to the host.

Further evidence of fever's beneficial effects can be found in numerous investigations demonstrating enhanced resistance of animals to infection with increases in body temperature within the physiologic range.[185] In classic studies involving experimental infection of the reptile *Dipsosaurus dorsalis* with *Aeromonas hydrophila,* Kluger and associates demonstrated a direct correlation between body temperature and survival.[186, 187] They also showed in their model that suppression of the febrile response with sodium salicylate is

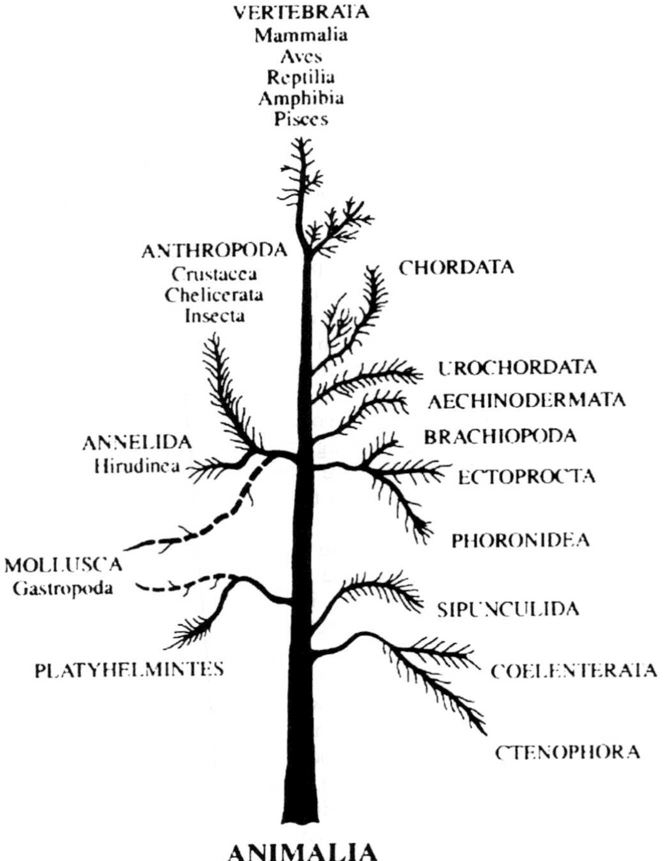

FIGURE 43–7. Evolutionary tree of animals. A febrile response has been documented in the vertebrata, arthropoda, and annelida. These observations suggest that the febrile response evolved more than 400,000,000 years ago at about the time evolutionary lines leading to arthropods and annelids diverged.

associated with a substantial increase in mortality.[187] Covert and Reynolds corroborated these findings in an experimental model involving goldfish.[188]

In mammalian experimental models, increasing the body temperature by artificial means has been reported to enhance the resistance of mice to herpes simplex virus,[189] poliovirus,[190] coxsackie B virus,[191] rabies virus,[192] and *Cryptococcus neoformans*[193] but to decrease resistance to *Streptococcus pneumoniae.*[194] Increased resistance of rabbits to *S. pneumoniae*[195] and *C. neoformans,*[196] dogs to herpesvirus,[197] piglets to gastroenteritis virus,[198] and ferrets to influenza virus[199] has also been observed after the induction of artificial fever. Unfortunately, because raising the body temperature by artificial means does not duplicate the physiologic alterations that occur during fever in homeotherms (and, indeed, entails a number of opposite physiologic responses[200]), data obtained using mammalian experimental models must be interpreted with caution when used to understand the febrile response.

Clinical data supporting an adaptive role for fever have accumulated slowly. Like animal data, clinical data include evidence of both beneficial effects of fever and adverse effects of antipyretics on the outcome of infections. In a retrospective analysis of 218 patients with gram-negative bacteremia, Bryant and associates reported a positive correlation between maximal temperature on the day bacteremia was diagnosed and survival.[201] A similar relationship has been observed in patients with polymicrobial sepsis and mild (but not severe) underlying diseases.[202] In an examination of factors influencing the prognosis of spontaneous bacterial peritonitis, Weinstein and coworkers identified a positive correlation between a temperature reading of greater than 38°C (100.4°F) and survival.[203]

It has been reported that children with chickenpox who are treated with acetaminophen have a longer time to total crusting of lesions than placebo-treated controls.[204] Stanley and colleagues have reported that adults infected with rhinovirus exhibit more nasal viral shedding when they receive aspirin than when given placebo.[205] Furthermore, Graham and colleagues have reported a trend toward a longer duration of rhinovirus shedding in association with antipyretic therapy and have shown that the use of aspirin or acetaminophen is associated with suppression of the serum neutralizing antibody response and with increased nasal symptoms and signs.[206] These data, like those reviewed in the preceding paragraph, are subject to several interpretations and do not prove a causal relationship between fever and improved prognosis during infection. Nevertheless, they are consistent with such a relationship and when considered in concert with the phylogeny of the febrile response and the animal data summarized earlier, constitute strong circumstantial evidence that fever is an adaptive response in most situations.

Whereas the foregoing investigations examined the relationship between the elevation of the core temperature and the outcome of infection, others have considered the endogenous mediators of the febrile response. In such studies, all four of the major pyrogenic cytokines have been shown to have immune-potentiating capabilities, which might theoretically enhance resistance to infection (see Table 43–1).[100, 207] In vitro and in vivo investigations of these cytokines have provided evidence of a protective effect of IFN, TNF-α, or IL-1, or all of these, against *Plasmodium,*[208–210] *Toxoplasma gondii,*[211] *Leishmania major,*[212] *Trypanosoma cruzi,*[213] and *Cryptosporidium.*[214]

Several reports have also shown enhancement of resistance to viral[215–217] and bacterial infections[218, 219] by pyrogenic cytokines. Treatment of normal and granulocytopenic animals with IL-1 has been shown to prevent death in some gram-positive and gram-negative bacterial infections.[219] However, IL-1 is effective only if administered an appreciable time (e.g., 24 hours) before the initiation of infections having rapidly fatal courses. In less acute infections, IL-1 administration can be delayed until shortly after the infectious challenge. Such observations suggest that those physiologic effects of the febrile response that enhance resistance to infection might be limited to localized infections or systemic infections of only mild to moderate severity.

The febrile response's potential for harm is reflected in a recent flurry of reports suggesting that IL-1, TNF-α, IL-6, and IFN mediate the physiologic abnormalities of certain infections. Although proof of an adverse effect of fever on the clinical outcome of these infections has yet to be established, the implication is that if pyrogenic cytokines contribute to the pathophysiologic burden of infections, both the mediators themselves and the febrile response are potentially deleterious.

The most persuasive evidence in this regard derives from studies of gram-negative bacterial sepsis.[220] It has long been suspected that bacterial LPS is involved in the pathophysiology of the syndrome. Purified LPS induces a spectrum of physiologic abnormalities that are similar to those occurring in patients with gram-negative bacterial sepsis. In experimental animals, challenge with LPS causes TNF-α and IL-1 to be released into the blood stream coincident with the appearance of signs of sepsis.[221] Furthermore, patients with the septic syndrome have detectable levels of circulatory TNF-α, IL-1, and IL-6 independent of culture-documented infection, and such levels correlate inversely with survival.[222] IL-1, alone or in combination with other cytokines, induces many of the same physiologic abnormalities (e.g., fever, hypoglycemia, shock, and death) seen after the administration of purified LPS.[223] In a murine experimental model for septic shock, IFN administered before or as long as 4 hours after LPS challenge increases mortality, whereas pretreatment with anti-IFN antibody significantly reduces mortality.[224] In several investigations, the adverse effects of gram-negative bacterial sepsis or LPS injections, or both, have been attenuated by pretreating experimental animals with IL-1 antagonists[225, 226] and monoclonal antibodies directed against TNF-α.[227, 228] Furthermore, animals rendered tolerant to TNF-α by repeated injections of the recombinant cytokine are protected against the hypotension, hypothermia, and lethality of gram-negative bacterial sepsis.[229]

Together, these observations have led to a growing conviction that pyrogenic cytokines are central mediators of the clinical and humoral manifestations of gram-negative bacterial sepsis and have generated intense interest, although little progress,[230] in the clinical application of antagonists of such cytokines. Similar data suggest that pyrogenic cytokines might mediate at least some of the systemic or local, or both, manifestations of gram-positive bacterial infections,[221, 231, 232] acquired immunodeficiency syndrome,[233] spirochetal infections,[234, 235] meningitis,[236] the adult respiratory distress syndrome,[233, 237] suppurative arthritis,[238] and mycobacteriosis.[239]

ANTIPYRETIC THERAPY

Although clinicians have long had at their disposal effective means of lowering the core temperature in febrile patients, the actual benefit of such reductions in temperature is still uncertain. Moreover, it has yet to be shown in humans that increases in the core temperature encountered during fever are harmful per se. Certainly, during the course of heat stroke and other forms of hyperthermia, the core temperature can, and frequently does, rise to levels that are inherently harmful.[240] However, as discussed previously, such levels are almost never reached during fever's regulated rise in temperature, which rarely exceeds 41°C (105.8°F) in humans.[146] Nevertheless, whereas healthy volunteers have been reported to withstand core temperatures of 42°C (107.6°F) for periods of as long as 4 hours without apparent ill effect,[241] the possibility remains that in certain patients, even the relatively modest increases in core temperature encountered during fever are deleterious and should, therefore, be suppressed.

One such category of patients includes children—primarily between the ages of 3 months and 5 years. In such children, seizures have been reported to occur during episodes of fever at a frequency of as high as 14% in selected populations.[242] Although most children with febrile seizures have temperatures of 39°C (102.2°F) or more at the time of their seizure,[243] many tolerate even higher fevers at later dates without convulsing.[244] Unfortunately, antipyretic therapy has not been shown to protect against recurrences of febrile seizures in the few controlled trials conducted thus far (see later).[245]

It has also been suggested that patients with underlying cardiovascular or pulmonary disorders might be especially susceptible to the adverse effects of fever, because of metabolic demands imposed by the elevated temperature.[246] Such demands are particularly high during the chill phase if shivering is present, as evidenced by increases in the sympathetic tone,[200] oxygen consumption, respiratory minute volume, and respiratory quotient.[247] As a result of the associated increase in metabolic demand, the chill phase of fever might be expected to add to the burden of cardiac or pulmonary disorders. Although this possibility has been offered as justification for antipyretic therapy in patients with these disorders, the risk-benefit ratio of such therapy has yet to be determined.

Antipyretic therapy might also be justified, at least in theory, if fever's metabolic cost exceeded its physiologic benefit, if the treatment provided symptomatic relief without adversely affecting the course of the febrile illness, or if the toxicologic costs (side effects) of the antipyretic regimen were appreciably lower than its beneficial effects. Unfortunately, although clinicians have long argued the validity of each of these propositions as justification for antipyretic therapy, few scientific data exist to support any of these arguments.

Antipyretic drugs can be grouped into three general categories based on their mechanisms of action. These include corticosteroids, aspirin and the other nonsteroidal anti-inflammatory agents (NSAIAs), and acetaminophen. Each exerts its effects at different points in the febrile response pathway.

Although not generally used for antipyresis, corticosteroids suppress fever through both direct and indirect mechanisms. They block the transcription of pyrogenic cytokines and inducible cyclooxygenase via interactions involving the glucocorticoid receptor.[90, 248] They downregulate the synthesis of cytokine receptors,[248] and by inducing lipocortin-1, they secondarily inhibit the activity of phospholipase A_2, a critical enzyme in the prostaglandin synthetic pathway.[248]

Acetaminophen, aspirin, and the other NSAIAs all block the conversion of arachidonic acid to prostaglandins such as prostaglandin E_2 by inhibiting cyclooxygenase (also known as prostaglandin synthetase).[248] This effect is thought to be critical to their antipyretic activity, in that production of prostaglandin E_2 at key sites within the hypothalamus is widely regarded as a crucial step in the process by which the physiologic cascade responsible for raising the core temperature during the febrile response is activated (see Fig. 43–5).[249]

Physical Methods of Antipyresis

A variety of physical techniques are used to cool febrile patients. These include sponging with various solutions (e.g., tepid water or alcohol), the application of ice packs or cooling blankets, and exposure to circulating fans (most often in conjunction with sponging). In contrast to antipyretic drugs, external cooling lowers the temperature of febrile patients by overwhelming effector mechanisms that have been evoked by an elevated thermoregulatory setpoint, rather than by lowering that setpoint. Therefore, unless concomitant antipyretic agents are used, or shivering is inhibited by other pharmacologic means, external cooling is vigorously opposed in the febrile patient by thermoregulatory mechanisms endeavoring to maintain the elevated body temperature.

Physical methods of antipyresis promote heat loss by conduction, convection, and evaporation. Evaporative methods have traditionally been touted as the most effective physical means of promoting heat loss in febrile patients, because such methods are deemed to be least likely to induce shivering.[250] However, carefully designed comparative trials have not yet established any one physical method of antipyresis as superior.

Direct comparisons of pharmacologic and physical methods of antipyresis are, likewise, all but nonexistent. In the only extant controlled study, Wenzel and Werner reported that salicylates reduced the second phase of endotoxin-induced fever in rabbits, whereas abdominal cooling increased heat production and did not lower the core temperature unless the animals were simultaneously exposed to environmental hyperthermia.[251] Neither antipyretic modality abolished the initial febrile response.

The few available clinical studies of the efficacy of physical methods of antipyresis have differed in their conclusions. Interpretation of the results of these studies has been difficult, because pharmacologic agents have almost invariably been administered concomitantly with external cooling. Steele and coworkers found acetaminophen (in age-adjusted dosages ranging from 80 to 320 mg) and sponging to be equally effective in lowering fever in children admitted to a pediatric hospital because of fever.[252] However, when combined, the two modalities produced more rapid cooling than either alone. By contrast, Newman found that tepid-water sponging in combination with acetaminophen (5 to 10 mg/kg) was no more effective than acetaminophen alone in lowering the temperature of febrile children.[253] O'Donnell and colleagues have concluded that in adults, although hypothermia blanket therapy adds little to the action of pharmacologic agents in lowering temperature, it induces wider temperature fluctuations and more episodes of rebound hyperthermia.[250]

Diagnostic Considerations

Numerous investigators have observed a direct correlation between the height of fevers and the rate of serious bacterial infections in children, with the maximal incidence of such infections at temperatures in excess of 40°C (104°F).[254–257] It has also been suggested that the response of a fever to antipyretic therapy might have diagnostic implications, in that a drop in temperature or improvement in the appearance of a febrile child, or both, generally indicates that the fever is not due to a serious illness.[258] This conclusion, however, is not supported by numerous investigations comparing the temperature response of bacteremic and nonbacteremic infections to antipyretic therapy in children.[259–264]

Several studies have suggested that an antipyretic response to NSAIAs can distinguish fevers of infectious origin from those due to cancer by virtue of the fact that the latter fevers are more readily suppressed by such agents. Naproxen was the first such agent to be studied in this regard.[265] Subsequent randomized comparisons have shown naproxen, indomethacin, and diclofenac to be equally effective in inhibiting cancer-induced fever,[266] although the sensitivity and specificity of the "naproxen test" for differentiating neoplastic from infectious fevers are not yet known. Nor is it known why NSAIAs might be more effective in reducing fever due to cancer than that due to infection.

Benefits versus Risks

Two critical assumptions are made when prescribing antipyretic therapy. One is that fever is, at least in part, noxious, and the other is that suppressing fever will reduce if not eliminate fever's noxious effects. Neither assumption has been validated experimentally. In fact, there is considerable evidence that fever is an important defense mechanism that contributes to the host's ability to resist infection.[267] However, even if fever (or its mediators) does adversely affect the course of certain disorders, as for example bacterial sepsis,[184] it does not necessarily follow that inhibiting fever using current modes of antipyretic therapy will obviate this effect, especially if such therapy has intrinsic toxicity of its own.

One of the reasons commonly given to justify suppressing fever is that the metabolic cost of fever exceeds its clinical benefit. In fact, the metabolic cost of fever is substantial, especially during the chill phase of the response with its shivering-induced increase in metabolic rate, nonepinephrine-mediated peripheral vasoconstriction, and increased arterial blood pressure.[200] Because of the potential adverse consequences of these metabolic effects on cardiovascular and pulmonary function, fever has been attacked with particular vigor in patients with underlying cardiovascular and pulmonary diseases.[268] Although antipyretic therapy has theoretical merit in this regard (if it does not induce shivering[269]), the detrimental effects of fever and the salutary effects of antipyretic therapy have yet to be critically evaluated.

External cooling, which is widely used in critically ill patients to suppress fevers unresponsive to antipyretic drugs, has been shown to decrease oxygen consumption by as much as 20% if shivering is prevented by therapeutic paralysis (Fig. 43–8).[269] If shivering is not inhibited, external cooling causes a rise, rather than a fall, in oxygen consumption.[269] Perhaps more important to febrile patients with underlying cardiovascular disease, external cooling has the capacity to cause vasospasm of diseased coronary arteries by inducing a cold pressor response.[270, 271] For all these reasons, it has been suggested that a more rational strategy for treating fevers unresponsive to antipyretic drugs is to *warm* rather than to *cool* selected skin surfaces, thereby reducing the vasoconstriction and shivering thresholds dictated by the elevated hypothalamic thermal setpoint, and, in turn, effecting a decrease in the core temperature.[272]

Unfortunately, certain antipyretic drugs also appear to cause coronary vasoconstriction in patients with coronary artery disease. Friedman and associates observed significant increases in the mean arterial pressure, coronary vascular resistance, and myocardial arteriovenous oxygen difference after intravenous indomethacin (0.5 mg/kg) in such patients.[273] Coronary blood flow decreased simultaneously from 181 ± 29 to 111 ± 14 ml/min ($p < 0.05$). Thus, in this investigation, myocardial oxygen demand increased in the face of a fall in coronary blood flow after indomethacin administration. The authors believe that indomethacin's vasoconstrictor effect most likely relates to its capacity to block the synthesis of vasodilatory prostaglandins.

Antipyretic therapy is also commonly administered to enhance the comfort of the patient.[268] General experience with antipyretic drugs, which are for the most part also analgesic agents, seems to support this contention. However, carefully controlled efficacy studies have not yet established the validity of this contention. Moreover, the relative cost of such symptomatic relief, in terms of drug toxicity and adverse effects of antipyretic agents on the course of the illness responsible for the fever have never been determined. The importance of such information is underscored by reports that acetaminophen prolongs the time to crusting of lesions in children with chickenpox[204] and that both acetaminophen and aspirin increase viral shedding and nasal signs and symptoms while suppressing the serum neutralizing antibody response in adults with rhinovirus infections.[205, 206]

Antipyretic therapy is also occasionally given to prevent febrile seizures in children, and to prevent or to reverse fever-induced mental dysfunction in frail elderly patients. As illustrated in Figure 43–9, Beisel and coworkers have shown that aspirin (in combination with propoxyphene) ameliorates fever-induced decrements in mental work performance in young volunteers infected with sand fly fever virus, even in the face of only partial relief of either the fever or other symptoms of the illness.[274] In view of these observations, antipyretic therapy might be expected to have a beneficial effect on fever-induced mental dysfunction in frail elderly patients. However, studies designed to test this hypothesis have not yet been reported.

Unfortunately, antipyretic therapy does not appear to be effective in preventing febrile seizures.[245] Camfield and colleagues conducted a randomized double-blind study comparing single-daily-dose phenobarbital plus antipyretic instruction to placebo plus antipyretic instruction to prevent recurrent seizure after an initial simple febrile seizure.[275] In children treated with both phenobarbital and antipyretics, the febrile seizure recurrence rate was 5%, whereas in those given placebo with antipyretics, the rate was 25%, suggesting that a single daily 5 mg/kg dose of phenobarbital is more effective than counseling parents about antipyretic therapy in preventing recurrent febrile seizures. More recently, acetaminophen has been given to children with fever as prophylaxis against febrile seizure recurrences. Whether given in moderate dosage (10 mg/kg/dose four times a day)[276] or in relatively high doses (15 to 20 mg/kg/dose every 4 hours),[277] acetaminophen failed to reduce the rate of febrile seizure recurrence.

Finally, there has been mounting interest in the use of certain

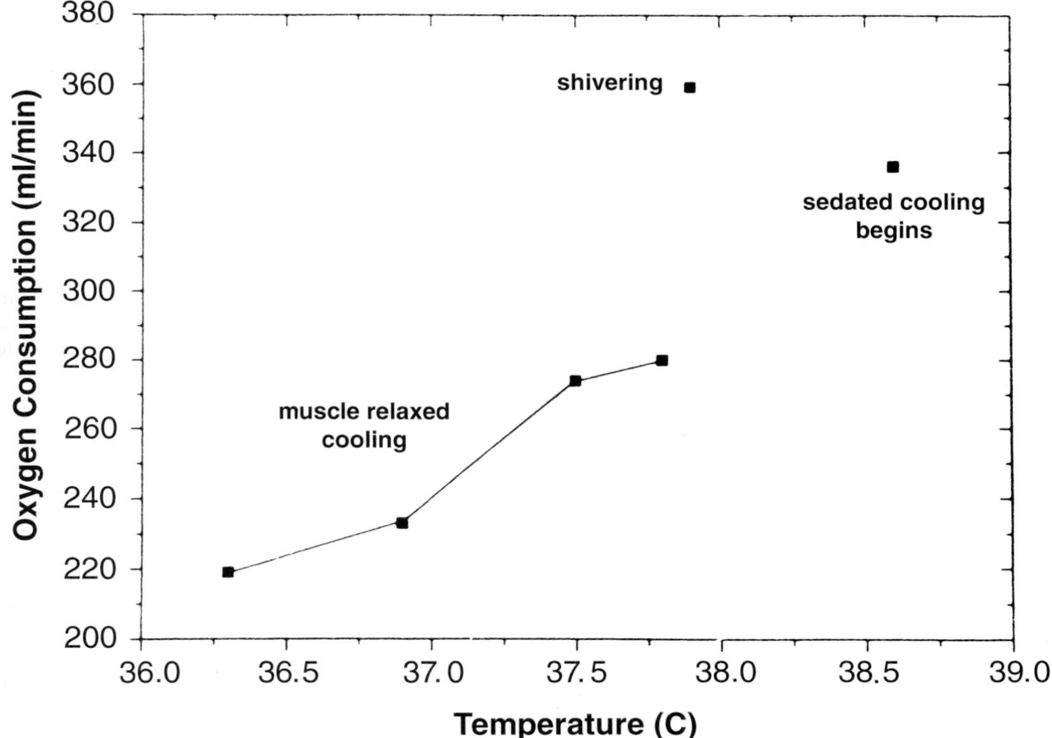

FIGURE 43–8. Effect of external cooling on oxygen consumption (Vo_2) in a febrile critically ill patient. With cooling from 38.6 to 37.9°C, the patient began to shiver and exhibited an increase in Vo_2 from 336 to 359 ml/minute. Once shivering had been inhibited by therapeutic paralysis, subsequent cooling was associated with a progressive fall in Vo_2. (From Manthous CA, Hall JB, Olson D, et al. Effect of cooling on oxygen consumption in febrile critically ill patients. Am J Respir Crit Care Med. 1995;151:10–14.)

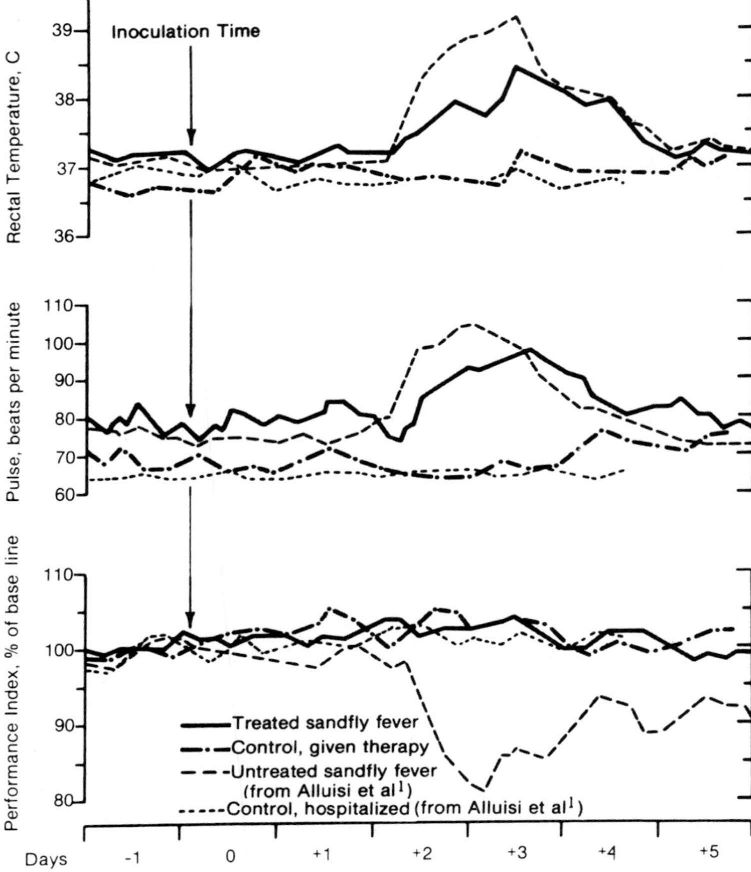

FIGURE 43–9. Effect of therapy with aspirin and propoxyphene on temperature, pulse rate, and mental work performance in experimentally-induced sandfly fever. (From Beisel WR, Morgan BB Jr, Bartelloni PJ, et al. Symptomatic therapy in viral illness. A controlled study of effects on work performance. JAMA. 1974;228:581–584.)

antipyretic drugs to modulate the activity of pyrogenic cytokines during bacterial sepsis.[278] In some animal models of sepsis, antipyretic drugs that inhibit cyclooxygenase confer protection when given soon after bacterial challenge, presumably by blunting the adverse effects of TNF-α and IL-1. In a large clinical trial, Bernard and associates reported that 48 hours of intravenous therapy with the cyclooxygenase inhibitor ibuprofen lowered the core temperature, heart rate, oxygen consumption, and lactic acid blood levels but did not decrease the incidence of organ failure or mortality at 30 days.[279] Thus, in spite of promising results obtained in some experimental models, antipyretic agents have not yet been shown to be of value clinically in the treatment of bacterial sepsis.

Indications

Although clinicians have resorted to various forms of antipyretic therapy since time immemorial, there is a dearth of scientific data concerning the actual benefits and relative risks of such treatments.[280] Nevertheless, several tentative conclusions regarding antipyretic therapy seem warranted in light of the limited data available. It is clear, for instance, that short courses of approved doses of standard antipyretic drugs carry a low risk of toxicity. Most of these drugs have analgesic as well as antipyretic properties. Therefore, if not otherwise contraindicated (e.g., aspirin in young children because of the risk of Reye's syndrome), such drugs can be prescribed to provide symptomatic relief in febrile patients, to reduce the metabolic demands of fever in patients with underlying cardiovascular and pulmonary disorders, and, possibly, to prevent or alleviate fever-induced mental dysfunction in elderly patients. To minimize antipyretic-induced fluctuations in temperature (as well as the risk of recurrent shivering with its associated increased metabolic demands), antipyretic agents should be administered to febrile patients at regular intervals that preclude abrupt recurrences of fever, rather than as needed for temperatures above some arbitrary level. Whenever such medications are prescribed, it should also be recognized that each carries its own risk of toxicity and might prolong the course of the illness responsible for the fever while reducing the intensity of its symptoms.

In view of the capacity of external cooling measures to induce a cold pressor response, it is questionable whether this form of antipyretic therapy should ever be administered to febrile patients (much less to intensive care unit patients for whom it is so frequently prescribed). If external cooling is used to treat fever, care must be taken to prevent shivering, because of its associated increased oxygen consumption. Unfortunately, even if shivering is prevented, there is no guarantee that a cold pressor response will be averted. In view of indomethacin's capacity to cause coronary vasoconstriction in patients with coronary artery disease, NSAIAs should be used cautiously to suppress fever in such patients.

REFERENCES

1. Majno G. The Healing Hand. Man and Wound in the Ancient World. Cambridge: Harvard University Press; 1975;57.
2. Galen. Opera omnia. In: Siegel RE ed. Galen's System of Physiology and Medicine, v. 11. New York:Krager, 1968.
3. Atkins E. Fever: Its history, cause and function. Yale J Biol Med. 1982;55:283–287.
4. Berger RL, Clem TR, Harden VA, Mangum BW. Historical development and newer means of temperature measurements in biochemistry. Methods Biochem Anal. 1984;269–331.
5. Bolton HC. Evolution of the Thermometer 1592–1743. Easton, Pa: Chemical. 1900:18, 98.
6. Wunderlich C. Das Verhalten der Eigenwärme in Krankenheiten. Leipzig: Otto Wigard, 1868.

7. Mackowiak PA, Worden G. Carl Reinhold August Wunderlich and the evolution of clinical thermometry. Clin Infect Dis. 1994;18:458–467.
8. Mackowiak PA, Wasserman SS, Levine MM. A critical appraisal of 98.6°F, the upper limit of the normal body temperature, and other legacies of Carl Reinhold August Wunderlich. JAMA. 1992;268:1578–1580.
9. IUPS Thermal Commission. Glossary of terms for thermal physiology. 2nd ed. Pflugers Arch. 1987;410:567–587.
10. Abbey JC, Anderson AS, Close EL, et al. How long is that thermometer accurate? Am J Nurs. 1978;78:1375–1376.
11. Erickson RS. Thermometer placement for oral temperature measurement in febrile adults. Int J Nurs Stud. 1976;13:199–208.
12. Mead J, Bonmarito L. Reliability of rectal temperatures as an index of internal body temperature. J Appl Physiol. 1949;2:97–109.
13. Abrams RM, Royston JP. Some properties of rectum and vagina as sites for basal body temperature measurement. Fertil Steril. 1981;35:313–316.
14. Middleton D. Nursing 1. Oxford: Blackwell Scientific; 1983:43–45.
15. Nichols GA, Ruskin MM, Glor BAK, Kelly WH. Oral, axillary and rectal temperature determinations and relationships. Nurs Res. 1966;15:307–310.
16. Nichols GA, Kucha DH. Oral measurements. Am J Nurs. 1972;72:1091–1093.
17. Mackowiak PA, Wasserman SS. A study of physicians' perceptions of body temperature in health and disease. South Med J. 1995;88:934–938.
18. Benzinger M, Benzinger TH. National Bureau of Standards Fifth Symposium on Temperature. Pittsburgh: Instrument Society of America; 1971:2080–2102.
19. Blainey CG. Site selection in taking body temperature. Am J Nurs. 1974;74:1859–1861.
20. Lorin MI. Measurement of body temperature. Semin Pediatr Infect Dis. 1993;4:4–8.
21. Buck SH, Zaritsky AL. Occult core hyperthermia complicating cardiogenic shock. Pediatrics. 1989;83:782–783.
22. Houdas Y, Ring EFJ. Human body temperature. New York: Plenum; 1982:57–141.
23. Mayfield SR, Bhatia J, Nakamura KT, et al. Temperature measurement in term and preterm neonates. J Pediatr. 1984;104:271–275.
24. Fonkalsrud E, Clathworthy HW. Accidental perforation of the colon and rectum in newborn infants. N Engl J Med. 1965;272:1097–1100.
25. Horwitz MA, Bennett JV. Nursery outbreak of peritonitis with pneumoperitonium probably caused by thermometer induced perforation. Am J Epidemiol. 1976;104:632–644.
26. McAllister TA, Roud JA, Marshall A, et al. Outbreak of *Salmonella eimsbuettel* in newborn infants spread by rectal thermometers. Lancet. 1986;1:1262–1264.
27. Banco L, Jayashekaramurthy S, Graffam J. The inability of a temperature sensitive pacifier to identify fevers in ill infants. Am J Dis Child. 1988;142:171–172.
28. Rabinowitz RP, Cookson ST, Wasserman SS, Mackowiak PA. Effects of anatomic site, oral stimulation and body position on estimates of body temperature. Arch Intern Med. 1996;156:777–780.
29. Tandberg D, Sklar D. Effect of tachypnea on the estimation of body temperature by an oral thermometer. N Engl J Med. 1983;308:945–946.
30. Neff J, Ayoub J, Longman A, Noyes A. Effect of respiratory rate, respiratory depth, and open versus closed mouth breathing on sublingual temperature. Res Nurs Health. 1989;12:195–202.
31. Klein DG, Mitchell C, Petrinec A, et al. A comparison of pulmonary artery, rectal, and tympanic membrane temperature measurements in the ICU. Heart Lung. 1993;22:435–441.
32. Erickson RA, Kirklin SK. Comparison of ear-based, bladder, oral and axillary methods for core temperature measurement. Crit Care Med. 1993;21:1528–1534.
33. Freed GL, Fraley JK. Lack of agreement of tympanic membrane temperature assessments with conventional methods in a private setting. Pediatrics. 1992;89:384–386.
34. Stewart JV, Webster D. Re-evaluation of the tympanic thermometer in the emergency department. Ann Emerg Med. 1992;21:158–161.
35. Peterson-Smith A, Barber N, Coody DK, et al. Comparison of aural infrared with traditional rectal temperatures in children from birth to age three years. J Pediatr. 1994;125:83–85.
36. Buntain WI, Pregler M, O'Brien PC, et al. Axillary versus rectal temperature: A comparative study. J Louisiana State Med Soc. 1977;129:5–8.
37. Schiffman RF. Temperature monitoring in the neonate: A comparison of axillary and rectal temperatures. Nurs Res. 1982;31:274–277.
38. Loudon ISL. On taking the temperature in the mouth and axilla. Lancet. 1957;268:233–235.
39. Nichols GA, Kulvi RL, Life HR, et al. Measuring oral and rectal temperatures of febrile children. Nurs Res. 1972;21:261–264.
40. Ogren JM. The inaccuracy of axillary temperatures measured with an electronic thermometer. Am J Dis Child. 1990;144:109–111.
41. Reisinger KS, Kao J, Grant DM. Inaccuracy of the clinitemp skin thermometer. Pediatrics. 1979;64:4–6.
42. Scholefield JH, Gerber MA, Dwyer P. Liquid crystal forehead temperature strips. Am J Dis Child. 1982;136:198–201.
43. Bergeson PS, Steinfeld HJ. How dependable is palpation as a screening method for fever? Clin Pediatr. 1974;13:350–351.
44. Banco L, Veltri D. Ability of mothers to subjectively assess the presence of fever in their children. Am J Dis Child. 1984;138:976–978.
45. Bonadio WA, Hegenbarth M, Zachariason M. Correlating reported fever in young infants with subsequent temperature patterns and rate of serious bacterial infections. Pediatr Infect Dis J. 1990;9:158–160.
46. Linder FE, Carmichael HY. A biometric study of the relation between oral and rectal temperatures in normal and schizophrenic subjects. Hum Biol. 1935;7:24–46.
47. Tanner JM. The relationship between the frequency of the heart, oral temperature and rectal temperature in man at rest. J Physiol. 1951;115:391–409.
48. Togawa T. Body temperature measurement. Clin Phys Physiol Meas. 1985;6(2):83–108.
49. Anagnostakis D, Matsaniotis N, Grafakos S, Sarafidou E. Rectal-axillary temperature difference in febrile and afebrile infants and children. Clin Pediatr. 1993;32:268–272.
50. Wunderlich KRA, Seguin E. Medical thermometry and human temperature. New York: William Wood; 1871.
51. Howell TH. Normal temperatures in old age. Lancet. 1948;1:517–519.
52. Weitzman ED, Moline ML, Czeisler CA, Zimmerman JC. Chronobiology of aging: Temperature, sleep-wake rhythms, and entrainment. Neurobiol Aging. 1982;3:299–309.
53. Jones SR. Fever in the elderly. In: Mackowiak PA, ed. Fever: Basic mechanisms and management. New York: Raven; 1991:233–242.
54. Dinarello CA, Wolff SM. Pathogenesis of fever in man. N Engl J Med. 1978;298:607–612.
55. Stephenson LA. Circadian timekeeping. In: Mackowiak PA, ed. Fever, Basic Mechanisms and Management. 2nd ed. Philadelphia: Lippincott-Raven; 1997:59–77.
56. Webb P. Daily activity and body temperature. Eur J Appl Physiol. 1993;66:174–177.
57. Cheng TL, Partridge JC. Effect of bundling and high environmental temperature on neonatal body temperature. Pediatrics. 1993;92:238–240.
58. Horvath SM, Menduke H, Piersol GM. Oral and rectal temperatures of man. JAMA 1950;144:1562–1565.
59. Wunderlich CA, Woodman WB. On the temperature in diseases: A manual of medical thermometry. London, England: New Sydenham Society; 1871:71.
60. Beutler B, Beutler SM. Pathogenesis of fever. In: Wyngaarden JB, Smith LH Jr, eds. Cecil Textbook of Medicine. 19th ed. Philadelphia: WB Saunders; 1992:1568–1571.
61. Dinarello CA, Wolff SM. Pathogenesis of fever. In: Mandell GL, Douglas RG Jr, Bennett JE. Principles and Practice of Infectious Diseases. 3rd ed. New York: Churchill Livingstone; 1990:462–469.
62. Tauber MG. Fever of unknown origin. In: Stein JH, ed. Internal Medicine. 3rd ed. Boston: Little Brown; 1990:1240–1246.
63. Thomas CL, ed. Taber's Cyclopedic Medical Dictionary. 16th ed. Philadelphia: FA Davis; 1989:665.
64. Hensyl WR, ed. Stedman's Medical Dictionary. 25th ed. Baltimore: Williams & Wilkins; 1990:574.
65. Guyton AC. Textbook of Medical Physiology. 8th ed. Philadelphia: WB Saunders; 1991:6.
66. Brengelmann GL. Body temperature regulation. In: Patton HD, Fuchs AF, Hille B, et al, eds. Textbook of Physiology. Philadelphia: WB Saunders; 1989:1584–1585.
67. Petersdorf RG. Control of body temperature. In: Wilson JW, Braunwald E, Isselbacher KJ, et al, eds. Harrison's Principles of Internal Medicine. 12th ed. New York: McGraw-Hill; 1991:2194–2200.
68. Dominguez EA, Musher DM. Clinical thermometry. In: Mackowiak PA, ed. Fever: Basic Mechanisms and Managements. New York: Raven; 1991:71–81.
69. Wunderlich CA, Reeve JC. The course of the temperature in diseases: A guide to clinical thermometry. Am J Med Sci. 1869;57:425–447.
70. Dinarello C, Wolff S. Pathogenesis of fever in man. N Engl J Med. 1978;298:607–612.
71. Howel TH. Normal temperature in old age. Lancet. 1948;1:517–518.
72. Weizman ED, Moline ML, Czeiler CA, Zimmerman JC. Chronobiology of aging: temperature, sleep-wake rhythms, and intrainment. Neurobiol Aging. 1982;3:299–309.
73. Lyon DM. The relation of pulse-rate to temperature in febrile conditions. Q J Med. 1927;20:205–218.
74. Tanner JM. The relationship between the frequency of the heart, oral temperature and rectal temperature in man at rest. J Physiol. 1951;115:391–409.
75. Lorin MI. Fever: Pathogenesis and treatment. In: Feigin RD and Cherry JD, eds. Textbook of Pediatric Infectious Diseases. 4th ed. Philadelphia: WB Saunders; 1998:89.
76. Bayley N, Stolz HR. Maturational changes in rectal temperatures of 61 infants from 1 to 36 months. Child Dev. 1937;8:195–206.
77. Boulant JA. Thermoregulation. In: Mackowiak PA, ed. Fever. Basic Mechanisms and Management. 2nd ed. Philadelphia: Lippincott-Raven; 1997:35–58.
78. Bruck K. Heat balance and the regulation of body temperature. In: Schmidt RF, Thews G, eds. Human Physiology. Berlin: Springer-Verlag, 1983:531–547.
79. Stanier MW, Mount LE, Bligh J. Energy Balance and Temperature Regulation. Cambridge: Cambridge University Press, 1984.
80. Boulant JA. Hypothalamic control of thermoregulation: Neurophysiological basis. In: Morgane PJ, Pankepp J, eds. Handbook of the Hypothalamus, v. 3, pt A. New York: Marcel Dekker; 1980:1–82.
81. Schonung W, Wagner H, Jessen C, Simon E. Differentiation of cutaneous and intestinal blood flow during hypothalamic heating and cooling in anesthetized dogs. Pflugers Arch. 1971;328:145–154.
82. Boulant JA. Hypothalamic neurons regulating body temperature. In: Fregly MJ, Blatteis CM, eds. APS Handbook of Physiology, Section 4: Environmental Physiology. New York: Oxford University Press; 1996:105–126.
83. Hammel HT, Jackson DC, Stolwijk JAJ, et al. Temperature regulation by hypothalamic proportional control with an adjustable set point. J Appl Physiol. 1963;18:1146–1154.
84. Hammel HT. Neurons and temperature regulation. In: Yamamoto WS, Brobeck JR,

eds. Physiological Controls and Regulations. Philadelphia: WB Saunders; 1965:71–97.

85. Sawka MN, Wenger CB. Physiological responses to acute exercise-heat stress. In: Pandolf KB, Sawka MN, Gonzalez RR, eds. Human Performance Physiology and Environmental Medicine at Terrestrial Extremes. Indianapolis: Benchmark; 1988:97–151.
86. Bligh J. Temperature Regulation in Mammals and Other Vertebrates. Amsterdam: North Holland; 1973.
87. Benzinger TH, Kitzinger C, Pratt AW. The human thermostat. In: Hardy JD, ed. Temperature—Its Measurement and Control in Science and Industry, v. 3, pt 5: Biology and Medicine, New York: Reinhold; 1963:637–665.
88. Stitt JT. Prostaglandin E as the mediator of the febrile response. Yale J Biol Med. 1986;59:137–149.
89. Mitchell D, Laburn HP, Cooper KE, et al. Is prostaglandin E the neural mediator of the febrile response? The case against a proven obligatory role. Yale J Biol Med. 1986;59:159–168.
90. Dinarello CA. Cytokines as endogenous pyrogens. In: Mackowiak PA, ed. Fever. Basic Mechanisms and Management. 2nd ed. Philadelphia: Lippincott-Raven; 1997:87–116.
91. Mickenberg ID, Snyderman R, Root RK, et al. The relationship of complement consumption to immune fever. J Immunol. 1971;107:1466–1476.
92. Arend WP, Joslin FG, Massoni RJ. Effects of immune complexes on production by human monocytes of interleukin 1 or an interleukin 1 inhibitor. J Immunol. 1985;134:3868–3875.
93. Dillard GM, Bodel P. Studies on steroid fever. II. Pyrogenic and anti-pyrogenic activity in vitro of some endogenous steroids of man. J Clin Invest. 1970;49:2418–2426.
94. Kappas A, Hellman L, Fukushima DK, Gallagher TF. The pyrogenic effect of etiocholanolone (Letter). J Clin Endocrinol Metab. 1957;17:451–453.
95. Wolff SM, Kimball HR, Perry S, et al. The biological properties of etiocholanolone. Ann Intern Med. 1967;67:1268–1295.
96. Bondy PK, Bodel P. Mechanism of action of pyrogenic and antipyretic steroids in vitro. In: Wolstenholme GEW, Birch J, eds. Pyrogens and Fever. Edinburgh: Churchill Livingstone; 1971:101–13.
97. Goodman MG, Chenoweth DE, Weigle WO. Induction of interleukin 1 secretion and enhancement of humoral immunity by binding of human C5a to macrophage surface C5a receptors. J Exp Med. 1982;156:912–917.
98. Bernheim HA, Block LH, Francis L, Atkins E. Release of endogenous pyrogen-activating factor from concanavalin A–stimulated human lymphocytes. J Exp Med. 1980;152:1811–1816.
99. Dinarello CA. Demonstration of a human pyrogen-inducing factor during mixed leukocyte reactions. J Exp Med. 1981;153:1215–1224.
100. Mackowiak PA, Barlett JG, Borden EC, et al. Fever: Recent advances and lingering dogma (Symposium Summary). Clin Infect Dis. 1997;25:119–138.
101. Kushner I, Rzewnicki DL. The acute phase response. In: Mackowiak PA, ed. Fever, Basic Mechanisms and Management. 2nd ed. Philadelphia: Lippincott-Raven; 1997:165–176.
102. Dinarello CA, Wolff SM. The role of interleukin-1 in disease. N Engl J Med. 1993;328:106–113.
103. Dinarello C. The interleukin-1 family: 10 years of discovery. FASEB J. 1994;8:1314–1325.
104. Dinarello C. Interleukin-1. Adv Pharmacol. 1994;25:21–51.
105. Fiers W. Tumor necrosis factor: Characterization at the molecular, cellular and in vivo level. FEBS Lett. 1991;285:199–212.
106. Vassalli P. The pathophysiology of tumor necrosis factors. Annu Rev Immunol. 1992;10:411–452.
107. Tracey K, Cerami A. Tumor necrosis factor: A pleiotropic cytokine and therapeutic target. Annu Rev Med. 1994;45:491–503.
108. Brach M, Herrman F. Interleukin 6: Presence and future. Int J Clin Lab Res. 1992;22:143–151.
109. Lotz M. Interleukin-6. Cancer Invest. 1993;11:731–742.
110. Jones T. Interleukin-6, an endocrine cytokine. Clin Endocrinol. 1994;40:703–713.
111. Blatteis CM, Sehic E. Prostaglandin E_2: A putative fever mediator. In: Mackowiak PA, ed. Fever. Basic Mechanisms and Management. 2nd ed. Philadelphia: Lippincott-Raven; 1997:117–145.
112. Mackowiak PA. Concepts of fever. Arch Intern Med. 1998;158:1870–1881.
113. Kluger M. Fever: Role of pyrogens and cryogens. Physiol Rev. 1991;71:93–127.
114. Michie HR, Manague KR, Spriggs DR, et al. Detection of circulating tumor necrosis factor after endotoxin administration. N Engl J Med. 1988;318:1481–1486.
115. Klostergaard J, Barta M, Tomasovic SP. Hyperthermic modulation of tumor necrosis factor–dependent monocyte/macrophage tumor cytotoxicity in vitro. J Biol Res Mod. 1989;8:262–277.
116. Tomasovic SP, Klostergaard J. Hyperthermic modulation of macrophage-tumor cell interactions. Ca Met Rev. 1989;8:215–229.
117. Fouqueray B, Philippe C, Amrani A, et al. Heat shock prevents lipopolysaccharide-induced tumor necrosis factor-α synthesis by rat mononuclear phagocytes. Eur J Immunol. 1992;22:2983–2987.
118. Snyder Y, Guthrie ML, Evans GF, Zuckerman SH. Transcriptional inhibition of endotoxin-induced monokine synthesis following heat shock in murine peritoneal macrophages. J Leuko Biol. 1992;51:181–187.
119. Valasco S, Tarlow M, Olsen K, et al. Temperature-dependent modulation of lipopolysaccharide-induced interleukin-1β and tumor necrosis factor-α expression in cultured human astroglia by dexamethasone and indomethacin. J Clin Invest. 1991;87:1674–1680.
120. Kappel M, Diamant M, Hansen MB, et al. Effects of in vitro hyperthermia on the proliferative response of blood mononuclear cell subsets, and detection of interleukins 1 and 6, tumor necrosis factor-alpha and interferon-gamma. Immunology. 1991;73:304–308.
121. Ensor JE, Wiener SM, McCrea KA, et al. Differential effects of hyperthermia on macrophage interleukin-6 and tumor necrosis factor-α expression. Am J Physiol. 1994;266:C967–C974.
122. Ensor JE, Crawford EK, Hasday JD. Warming macrophages to febrile range destabilizes tumor necrosis factor-α mRNA without inducing heat shock. Am J Physiol. 1995;269:C1140–C1146.
123. Weiner S, Hasday JD. Temperature dependence of monocyte cytokine release. FASEB J. 1991;5:A626.
124. Costa J, DeTolla L, Piper J, et al. Effects of febrile range temperature on cytokine expression in lipopolysaccharide-challenged mice. FASEB J. 1995;9:A960.
125. Aderka D, Le J, Vilcek J. IL-6 inhibits lipopolysaccharide-induced tumor necrosis factor production in cultured human monocytes, U937 cells, and in mice. J Immunol. 1989;143:3517–3523.
126. Cross AS, Sadoff JC, Kelly N, et al. Pretreatment with recombinant murine tumor necrosis factor α/cachectin and murine interleukin 1α protects mice from lethal bacterial infection. J Exp Med. 1989;169:2021–2027.
127. Trey J, Kushner I. The acute phase response and the hematopoietic system: The role of cytokines. Crit Rev Oncol Hematol. 1995;21:1–18.
128. Schilling RF. Anemia of chronic disease: A misnomer. Ann Intern Med. 1991;115:572–573.
129. Ernst E, Saradeth T, Achhammer G. n-3 fatty acids and acute-phase proteins. Eur J Clin Invest. 1991;21:77–82.
130. Joyce PR, Hawes CR, Mulder RT, et al. Elevated levels of acute phase plasma proteins in major depression. Biol Psychiatry. 1992;32:1035–1041.
131. Ganguli R, Yang Z, Shurin G, et al. Serum interleukin-6 concentration in schizophrenia: Elevation associated with duration of illness. Psychiatry Res. 1994;51:1–10.
132. LeMay LG, Vander AJ, Kluger MJ. The effects of psychological stress on plasma interleukin-6 activity in rats. Phys Behav. 1990;47:957–961.
133. Volanakis JE. Acute phase proteins. In: McCarty DJ, Koopman WJ, eds. Arthritis and Allied Conditions. A Textbook of Rheumatology. Malvern, Pa: Lea & Febiger; 1993:469–477.
134. Ballou SP, Lozanski G. Induction of inflammatory cytokines release from cultured human monocytes by C-reactive protein. Cytokine. 1992;4:361–368.
135. Cermak J, Key NS, Bach RR, et al. C-reactive protein induces human peripheral blood monocytes to synthesize tissue factor. Blood. 1993;82:513–520.
136. Tilg H, Vannier E, Vachine G, et al. Antiinflammatory properties of hepatic acute phase proteins: Preferential induction of interleukin 1 (IL-1) receptor antagonist over IL-1β synthesis by human peripheral blood mononuclear cells. J Exp Med. 1993;178:1629–1636.
137. Dobrinich R, Spagnuolo PJ. Binding of C-reactive protein to human neutrophils: Inhibition of respiratory burst activity. Arthritis Rheum. 1991;34:1031–1038.
138. Ahmed N, Thorley R, Xia D, et al. Transgenic mice expressing rabbit C-reactive protein exhibit diminished chemotactic factor-induced alveolitis. Am J Respir Crit Care Med. 1996;153:1141–1147.
139. Xu L, Badolato R, Murphy WJ, et al. A novel biologic function of serum amyloid A–induction of T lymphocyte migration and adhesion. J Immunol. 1995;155:1184–1190.
140. Kisilevsky R, Subrahmanyan L. Serum amyloid A changes high density lipoprotein's cellular affinity. Lab Invest. 1992;66:778.
141. Berliner JA, Navab M, Fogelman AM, et al. Atherosclerosis: Basic mechanisms—oxidation, inflammation, and genetics. Circulation. 1995;91:2488–2496.
142. Wurfel MM, Monks BG, Ingalls RR, et al. Targeted deletion of the lipopolysaccharide (LPS)-binding protein gene leads to profound suppression of LPS responses ex vivo, whereas in vivo responses remain intact. J Exp Med. 1997;186:2051–2056.
143. May MT. Galen on the Usefulness of the Parts of the Body. Ithaca, NY: Cornell University Press; 1968:50–53.
144. DuBois EF. Why are fever temperatures over 106°F rare? Am J Med Sci. 1949;217:361–368.
145. Mackowiak PA, Boulant JA. Fever's glass ceiling. Clin Infect Dis. 1996;22:525–536.
146. Pittman QJ, Wilkinson MF. Central arginine vasopressin and endogenous antipyresis. Can J Physiol Pharmacol. 1992;70:786–790.
147. Pittman QJ, Poulin P, Wilkinson, MF. Role of neurohypophysial hormones in temperature regulation. Ann N Y Acad Sci. 1993;689:375–381.
148. Kasting N. Criteria for establishing a physiological role for brain peptides. A case in point: The role of vasopressin in thermoregulation during fever and antipyresis. Brain Res Rev. 1989;14:143–153.
149. Lipton JM. Disorders of temperature control. In: Rieder P, Kopp N, Pearson J. An Introduction to Neurotransmission in Health and Disease. Oxford, England: Oxford University Press; 1990:119–123.
150. Zeisberger E. The role of septal peptides in thermoregulation and fever. In: Bligh J, Voigt K, eds. Thermoreception and Temperature Regulation. Berlin: Springer-Verlag; 1990:273–283.
151. Glyn JR, Lipton JM. Hypothermic and antipyretic effects of centrally administered ACTH (− 24) and α-melanotropin. Peptides. 1981;2:177–187.
152. Glyn-Ballinger JR, Bernardini GL, Lipton JM. α-MSH injected into the septal region reduces fever in rabbits. Peptides. 1983;4:199–203.
153. Lipton JM, Whisenant JD, Gean JT. Hypothermia produced by peripheral and central injections of chlopromazine in aged rabbits. Brain Res Bull. 1979;4:297–300.

154. Murphy MT, Lipton JM. Peripheral administration of α-MSH reduces fever in older and younger rabbits. Peptides. 1982;13:775–779.
155. Murphy MT, Richard DB, Lipton JM. Antipyretic potency of centrally administered α-melanocyte stimulating hormone. Science. 1983;221:192–193.
156. Deeter LB, Martin LW, Lipton JM. Antipyretic effect of central alpha-MSH summates with that of acetaminophen or ibuprofen. Brain Res Bull. 1989;23:573–575.
157. Shih ST, Lipton JM, McCann SM. Central administration of α-MSH antiserum augments fever in the rabbit. Am J Physiol. 1986;250:R803–R808.
158. Feldberg W, Meyers RD. A new concept of temperature regulation by amines in the hypothalamus. Nature 1963;200:1325.
159. Bligh J. Cells, cell-talk and mammalian homeothermy. In: Bligh J, Voigt K, eds. Thermoreception and Temperature Regulation. Berlin, Germany: Springer-Verlag; 1990:163–173.
160. Morrow LE, McClellan JL, Conn CA, Kluger MJ. Glucocorticoids alter fever and IL-6 responses to psychological stress and to lipopolysaccharide. Am J Physiol. 1993;225:R151–R156.
161. Luedke CE, Cerami A. Interferon-gamma overcomes glucocorticoid suppression of cachectin/tumor necrosis factor biosynthesis by murine macrophages. J Clin Invest. 1990;86:1234–1240.
162. Nakano T, Ohara O, Teraoka H, Arita H. Glucocorticoids suppress group II phospholipase A_2 production by blocking mRNA synthesis and post-transcriptional expression. J Biol Chem. 1990;265:12,745–12,748.
163. Alexander DP, Bashore RA, Britton HG, Forsling MA. Maternal and fetal arginine vasopressin in the chronically catheterised sheep. Biol Neonate. 1974;25:242–248.
164. Carey F, Forder M, Edge D, et al. Lipocortin 1 fragment modifies pyrogenic actions of cytokines in rats. Am J Physiol. 1990;259:R266–R269.
165. Bernadini GL, Lipton JM, Clark WG. Intracerebroventricular and septal injections of arginine vasopressin are not antipyretic in the rabbitt. Peptides. 1983;4:195–198.
166. Riedel W. Role of thyroid-stimulating hormone (TSH) in endogenous antipyresis and evidence of extrahypothalamic thyroid-stimulating neurons (TSN) in rabbits. Pflugers Arch 1987;408(Suppl):R49.
167. Bahendeka SK, Moor RE, Tomkin GH, Buchanan KD. Gastric inhibitory polypeptide, dietary-induced thermogenesis and obesity. Can J Physiol Pharmacol. 1987;65:1242–1247.
168. Stanley BG, Leibowitz SF. Neuropeptide Y. Stimulation of feeding and drinking by injection into the paraventricular nucleus. Life Sci. 1984;35:2635–2642.
169. Jansky L, Vybiral S, Moravec J, et al. Neuropeptides and temperature regulation. J Therm Biol. 1986;11:79–83.
170. Schmid H, Pierau Fr-K. Long-term modulation of hypothalamic neurons by neuropeptides. In: Bligh J, Voigt K, eds. Thermoregulation and Temperature Regulation. Berlin, Germany: Springer-Verlag; 1990:53–63.
171. Gale CC, McCreery BR. Mechanism of bombesin hypothermia. Fed Proc. 1979;38:997.
172. Holt SJ, Grimble RF, York DA. Tumor necrosis factor-α and lymphotoxin have opposite effects on sympathetic efferent nerves to brown adipose tissue by direct action in the central nervous system. Brain Res. 1989;497:183–186.
173. Shih ST, Khorram O, Lipton JM, McCann SM. Central administration of α-MSH antiserum augments fever in the rabbit. Am J Physiol. 1986;250:R803–R806.
174. Sivo J, Salkowski CA, Politis AD, Vogel SN. Differential regulation of LPS-induced IL-1β and IL-1 receptor antagonist mRNA by IFNα and IFNγ in murine peritoneal macrophages. J Endotox Res. 1994;1:30–36.
175. Seckinger P, Lowenthal JW, Williamson K, et al. A urine inhibitor of interleukin-1 activity that blocks ligand binding. J Immunol. 1987;139:1546–1549.
176. Eisenberg SP, Brewer MT, Verderber E, et al. Interleukin-1 receptor antagonist is a member of the interleukin-1 gene family: Evolution of a cytokine control mechanism. Proc Natl Acad Sci U S A. 1991;88:5232–5236.
177. Dripps DJ, Brandhuber BJ, Thompson RC, Eisenberg SP. Interleukin-1 (IL-1) receptor antagonist binds to the 80-k Da IL-receptor but does not initiate IL-1 signal transduction. J Biol Chem. 1991;266:10,331–10,336.
178. Dripps DJ, Verderber E, Ng Rk, et al. Interleukin-1 receptor antagonist binds to the type II interleukin-1 receptor on B cells and neutrophils. J Biol Chem. 1991;266:20,311–20,315.
179. Engelmann H, Aderka D, Rubinstein M, et al. A tumor necrosis factor binding protein purified to homogeneity from human urine protects cells from tumor necrosis factor toxicity. J Biol Chem. 1989;264:11,974–11,980.
180. Olsson I, Lantx M, Nilsson E, et al. Isolation and characterization of a tumor necrosis factor binding protein from urine. Eur J Haematol. 1989;42:270–275.
181. Engleman H, Novick D, Wallach D. Two tumor necrosis factor–binding proteins from human urine. J Biol Chem. 1990;265:1531–1536.
182. Brockhaus M, Schoenfeld HJ, Schlaeger EJ, et al. Identification of two types of tumor necrosis factor receptors on human cell lines by monoclonal antibodies. Proc Natl Acad Sci U S A. 1990;87:3127–3131.
183. Porteu F, Nathan C. Shedding of tumor necrosis factor receptors by activated human neutrophils. J Exp Med. 1990;172:599–607.
184. Mackowiak PA. Fever: Blessing or curse? A unifying hypothesis. Ann Intern Med. 1994;120:1037–1040.
185. Kluger MJ, Kozat W, Conn CA, et al. The adaptive value of fever. In: Mackowiak PA, ed. Fever: Basic Mechanisms and Management. Philadelphia: Lippincott-Raven; 1997:255–266.
186. Kluger MJ, Ringler DH, Anver MR. Fever and survival. Science. 1975;188:166–168.
187. Bernheim HA, Kluger MJ. Fever: Effect of drug-induced antipyresis on survival. Science. 1976;193:237–239.
188. Covert JR, Reynolds WW. Survival value of fever in fish. Nature. 1977;267:43–45.
189. Schmidt JR, Rasmussen AF Jr. The influence of environmental temperature on the course of experimental herpes simplex infection. J Infect Dis. 1960;107:356–360.
190. Lwoff A. Factors influencing the evolution of viral diseases at the cellular level and in the organism. Bacteriol Rev. 1959;23:109–124.
191. Walker DL, Boring WD. Factors influencing host-virus interactions. III. Further studies on the alteration of coxsackie virus infection in adult mice by environmental temperature. J Immunol. 1958;80:39–44.
192. Bell JF, Moore GJ. Effects of high ambient temperature on various stages of rabies virus infection in mice. Infect Immun. 1974;10:510–515.
193. Kuhn LR. Effect of elevated body temperature on cryptococcus in mice. Proc Soc Exp Biol Med. 1949;71:341–343.
194. Eiseman B, Mallette WG, Wotkyns RS, et al. Prolonged hypothermia in experimental pneumococcal peritonitis. J Clin Invest. 1956;35:940–946.
195. Rich AR, McKee CM. The mechanism of a hitherto unexplained form of native immunity to the type III pneumococcus. Bull Johns Hopkins Hosp. 1936;59:171–207.
196. Kuhn LR. Growth and viability of *Cryptococcus hominis* at mouse and rabbit body temperatures. Proc Soc Exp Biol Med. 1939;41:573–574.
197. Carmichael LE, Barnes FD. Effect of temperature on growth of canine herpes virus in canine kidney cell and macrophage cultures. J Infect Dis. 1969;120:664–668.
198. Furuchi S, Shimizu Y. Effect of ambient temperatures on multiplication of attenuated transmissable gastroenteritis virus in the bodies of newborn piglets. Infect Immun. 1976;13:990–992.
199. Toms GL, Davies JA, Woodward CG, et al. The relation of pyrexia and nasal inflammatory response to virus levels in nasal washings of ferrets infected with influenza viruses of differing virulence. Br J Exp Pathol. 1977;588:444–458.
200. Greisman SE. Cardiovascular alterations during fever. In: Mackowiak PA, ed. Fever: Basic Mechanisms and Management. New York: Raven; 1991:143–165.
201. Bryant RE, Hood AF, Hood CE, Koenig MG. Factors affecting mortality of gram-negative rod bacteremia. Arch Intern Med. 1971;127:120–128.
202. Mackowiak PA, Browne RH, Southern PM Jr, Smith JW. Polymicrobial sepsis; analysis of 184 cases using log linear models. Am J Med Sci. 1980;280:73–80.
203. Weinstein MR, Iannini PB, Staton CW, Eichoff TC. Spontaneous bacterial peritonitis. A review of 28 cases with emphasis on improved survival and factors influencing prognosis. Am J Med. 1978;64:592–598.
204. Dorn TF, DeAngelis C, Baumgardner RA, et al. Acetaminophen: More harm than good for chicken pox? J Pediatr. 1989;114:1045–1048.
205. Stanley ED, Jackson GG, Panusarn C, et al. Increased viral shedding with aspirin treatment of rhinovirus infection. JAMA. 1975;231:1248–1251.
206. Graham MH, Burrell CJ, Douglas RM, et al. Adverse effects of aspirin, acetaminophen, and ibuprofen on immune function, viral shedding, and clinical status in rhinovirus-infected volunteers. J Infect Dis. 1990;162:1277–1282.
207. Dinarello CA. Endogenous pyrogens. The role of cytokines in the pathogenesis of fever. In: Mackowiak PA, ed. Fever: Basic Mechanisms and Management. New York: Raven; 1991:23–47.
208. Mellouk S, Green SJ, Nacy CA, Hoffman SL. IFN-γ inhibits development of *Plasmodium berghei* exoerythrocytic stages in hepatocytes by an L-arginine–dependent effector mechanism. J Imunol. 1991;146:3971–3976.
209. Naotunne TDS, Karunaweera ND, Del Giudice G, et al. Cytokines kill malaria parasites during infection crisis: Extracellular complementary factors are essential. J Exp Med. 1991;173:523–529.
210. Curfs JHAJ, Van Der Meer JWM, Sauerwein RW, Eling WMC. Low dosages of interleukin 1 protect mice against lethal cerebral malaria. J Exp Med. 1990;172:1287–1291.
211. Woodman JP, Dimier IH, Bout DT. Human endothelial cells are activated by IFN-γ to inhibit *Toxoplasmosis gondii* replication. Inhibition is due to a different mechanism from that existing in mouse macrophages and human fibroblasts. J Immunol. 1991;147:2019–2023.
212. Liew FY, Li Y, Millott S. Tumor necrosis factor α synergizes with IFN-γ in mediating killing of *Leishmania major* through the induction of nitric oxide. J Immunol. 1990;145:4306–4310.
213. Torrico F, Heremans H, Rivera MT, et al. Endogenous IFN-γ is required for resistance to acute *Trypanosoma cruzi* infection in mice. J Immunol. 1991;146:3626–3632.
214. Ungar BVP, Kao T-C, Burris JA, Finkelman FD. *Cryptosporidium* infection in an adult mouse model. Independent roles for IFN-γ and $CD4^+$ T lymphocytes in protective immunity. J Immunol. 1991;147:1014–1022.
215. Sambhi SK, Kohonen-Corish MRJ, Ramshaw IA. Local production of tumor necrosis factor encoded by recombinant vaccinia virus is effective in controlling viral replication in vivo. Proc Natl Acad Sci U S A. 1991;88:4025–4029.
216. Feduchi E, Carrasco L. Mechanism of inhibition of HSV-1 replication by tumor necrosis factor and interferon. Virology. 1991;180:822–825.
217. Strijp HAG, Van Der Tol ME, Miltenburgh LAM, et al. Tumor necrosis factor triggers granulocytes to internalize complement-coated virus particles. Immunology. 1991;73:77–82.
218. Hedges S, Anderson P, Lidin-Janson G, et al. Interleukin-6 response to deliberate colonization of the human urinary tract with gram-negative bacteria. Infect Immun. 1991;59:421–427.
219. Vogels MTE, Vander Meer JWM. Use of immune modulators in nonspecific therapy of bacterial infections. Antimicrob Agents Chemother. 1992;36:1–5.
220. Bernheim HA, Bodel T, Askenase PW, Atkins E. Effects of fever on host defense mechanisms after injection of the lizard *Diposaurus dorsalis*. Br J Exp Pathol. 1978;59:76–84.
221. Dinarello CA. The proinflammatory cytokines interleukin-1 and tumor necrosis

factor and treatment of the septic shock syndrome. J Infect Dis. 1991;163:1177–1184.
222. Casey LC, Balk RA, Bone RC. Plasma cytokine and endotoxin levels correlate with survival in patients with the sepsis syndrome. Ann Intern Med. 1993;119:771–778.
223. Johnson J, Brigman KL, Jesmok G, Meyrick B. Morphologic changes in lungs of anesthesized sheep following intravenous infusion of recombinant tumor necrosis factor α^{1-3}. Am Rev Respir Dis. 1991;144:179–186.
224. Heinzel FP. The role of IFN-γ in the pathology of experimental endotoxemia. J Immunol. 1990;145:2920–2924.
225. Henricson BE, Neta R, Vogel SN. An interleukin-1 receptor antagonist blocks lipopolysaccharide-induced colony-stimulating factor production and early endotoxin tolerance. Infect Immun. 1991;59:1188–1191.
226. Ohlsson K, Björk P, Bergenfeldt M, et al. Interleukin-1 receptor antagonist reduces mortality from endotoxin shock. Nature. 1990;348:550–552.
227. Opal SM, Cross AS, Sadoff JC, et al. Efficacy of antilipopolysaccharide and anti–tumor necrosis factor monoclonal antibodies in a neutropenic rat model of pseudomonas sepsis. J Clin Invest. 1991;88:885–890.
228. Overbeek BP, Veringa EM. Role of antibodies and antibiotics in aerobic gram-negative septicemia: Possible synergism between antimicrobial treatment and immunotherapy. Rev Infect Dis. 1991;13:751–760.
229. Alexander HR, Sheppard BC, Jensen JC, et al. Treatment with recombinant tumor necrosis factor-alpha protects rats against lethality, hypotension, and hypothermia of gram-negative sepsis. J Clin Invest. 1991;88:34–39.
230. Fisher CJ Jr, Agosti JM, Opal SM, et al. Treatment of septic shock with tumor necrosis factor receptor: Fc fusion protein. N Engl J Med. 1996;334:1697–1702.
231. Freudenberg MA, Galanos C. Tumor necrosis factor alpha mediates lethal activity of killed gram-negative and gram-positive bacteria in D-galactosamine–treated mice. Infect Immun. 1991;59:2110–2115.
232. Gibson RL, Redding GJ, Henderson WR, Truog WE. Group B streptococcus induces tumor necrosis factor in neonatal piglets. Effect of the tumor necrosis factor inhibitor pentoxifylline on hemodynamics and gas exchange. Am Rev Respir Dis. 1991;143:598–604.
233. Birx DL, Redfield RR, Tencer K, et al. Induction of interleukin-6 during human immunodeficiency virus infection. Blood. 1990;76:2303–2310.
234. Radolf JD, Norgard MV, Brandt ME, et al. Lipoproteins of *Borrelia burgdorferi* and *Treponema pallidum* activate cachectin/tumor necrosis factor synthesis. Analysis using a CAT reporter construct. J Immunol. 1991;147:1968–1974.
235. Habicht GS, Katona LI, Benach JL. Cytokines and the pathogenesis of neuroborreliosis: *Borrelia burgdorferi* induces glioma cells to secrete interleukin-6. J Infect Dis. 1991;164:568–574.
236. Jacobs RF, Jabor DR. The immunology of sepsis and meningitis-cytokine biology. Scand J Infect Dis Suppl. 1990;73:7–15.
237. Jenkins JK, Carey PD, Byrne K, et al. Sepsis-induced lung injury and the effects of ibuprofen pretreatment. Analysis of early alveolar events via repetitive bronchoalveolar lavage. Am Rev Respir Dis. 1991;143:155–161.
238. Saez-Llorens X, Jafara HS, Olsen KD, et al. Induction of suppurative arthritis in rabbits by *Haemophilus* endotoxin, tumor necrosis factor-α, and interleukin-1β. J Infect Dis. 1991;163:1267–1272.
239. Rook GAW, Al Attiyah R. Cytokines and the Koch phenomenon. Tubercle. 1991;72:13–20.
240. Mackowiak PA. Editorial response: Assaulting a physiological response. Clin Infect Dis. 1997;24:1214–1216.
241. Neymann CA, Osborne SL. Artificial fever. Am J Syphilis Neurol. 1934;18–34.
242. Lessell S, Torres JM, Kurland LT. Seizure disorders in a Guamanian village. Arch Neurol. 1962;7:37–44.
243. Aicardi J. Febrile convulsions. In: Aicardi J, ed. Epilepsy in children. 2nd ed. New York: Raven; 1994;253–275.
244. Lennox-Buchthal MA. Febrile convulsions—a reappraisal. Amsterdam: Elsevier; 1973:1–138.
245. Rosman NP. Febrile convulsions. In: Mackowiak PA, ed. Fever. Basic Mechanisms and Management. 2nd ed. Philadelphia: Lippincott-Raven; 1997:267–277.
246. Styrt B, Sugarman B. Antipyresis and fever. Arch Intern Med. 1990;150:1589–1597.
247. Horwath SM, Spurr GB, Hutt BK, Hamilton LH. Metabolic cost of shivering. J Appl Physiol. 1956;8:595–602.
248. Vane JR, Botting RM. New insights into the mode of action of anti-inflammatory drugs. Inflamm Res. 1995;44:1–10.
249. Blatteis CM, Sehic E. Prostaglandin E2: A putative fever mediator. In: Mackowiak PA, ed. Fever: Basic mechanisms and management. 2nd ed. Philadelphia: Lippincott-Raven; 1997:17–145.
250. O'Donnell J, Axelrod P, Fisher C, Lorber B. Use and effectiveness of hypothermia blankets for febrile patients in the intensive care unit. Clin Infect Dis. 1997;24:1208–1213.
251. Wenzel C, Werner J. Physical versus pharmacological counter-measures. Eur J Appl Physiol. 1988;57:81–88.
252. Steele RW, Tanaka PT, Lara RP, Bass JW. Evaluation of sponging and of oral antipyretic therapy to reduce fever. J Pediatr. 1970;77:824–829.
253. Newman J. Evaluation of sponging to reduce body temperature in febrile children. Can Med Assoc J. 1985;132:641–642.
254. McCarthy PL, Grundy GW, Spiesel SZ, Dolan TF. Bacteremia in children: An outpatient clinical review. Pediatrics. 1976;57:861–868.
255. McGowan JE, Bratton L, Klein JO, Finland M. Bacteremia in febrile children seen in a "walk-in" pediatric clinic. N Engl J Med. 1973;288:1309–1312.
256. Teele DW, Pelton SI, Grant MJ, et al. Bacteremia in febrile children under 2 years of age: Results of cultures of blood of 600 consecutive febrile children seen in a "walk-in" clinic. J Pediatr. 1975;87:227–230.
257. Bonadio WA, Romine K, Gyuro J. Relationship of fever magnitude to rate of serious bacterial infections in neonates. J Pediatr. 1990;116:733–735.
258. McCarthy PL. Fever in infants and children. In: Mackowiak PA, ed. Fever. Basic Mechanisms and Management, 2nd ed. Philadelphia: Lippincott-Raven; 1997:351–362.
259. Toney SB, Henretig F, Fleisher G, et al. Temperature response to antipyretic therapy in children. Relationship to occult bacteremia. Am J Emerg Med. 1985;3:190–192.
260. Baker MD, Fosarelli PD, Carpenter RO. Childhood fever: Correlation of diagnosis with temperature response to acetaminophen. Pediatrics. 1987;80:315–318.
261. Yamamoto LT, Wigder HN, Fligner DJ, et al. Relationship of bacteremia to antipyretic therapy in febrile children. Pediatr Emerg Care. 1987;3:223–227.
262. Weisse ME, Miller G, Brien JH. Fever response to acetaminophen in viral vs. bacterial infections. Pediatr Infect Dis J. 1987;6:1091–1094.
263. Baker RC, Tiller T, Bausher JC, et al. Severity of disease correlated with fever reduction in febrile infants. Pediatrics. 1989;83:1016–1019.
264. Mazur LJ, Jones TM, Kozinetz CA. Temperature response to acetaminophen and risk of occult bacteremia: A case-control study. J Pediatr. 1989;115:888–891.
265. Chang JC, Gross HM. Utility of naproxen in the differential diagnosis of fever of undetermined origin in patients with cancer. Am J Med. 1984;76:597–603.
266. Tsavaris N, Zinelis A, Karabelis A, et al. A randomized trial of the effect of three nonsteroidal antiinflammatory agents in ameliorating cancer-induced fever. J Intern Med. 1990;228:451–455.
267. Kluger MJ, Kozak W, Conn CA, et al. The adaptive value of fever. In: Mackowiak PA, ed. Fever. Basic Mechanisms and Management. 2nd ed. Philadelphia: Lippincott-Raven; 1997:255–266.
268. Isaacs SN, Axelrod PI, Lorber B. Antipyretic orders in a university hospital. Am J Med. 1990;88:31–35.
269. Manthous CA, Hall JB, Olson D, et al. Effect of cooling on oxygen consumption in febrile critically ill patients. Am J Respir Crit Care Med. 1995;151:10–14.
270. Raizner AE, Chahine RA, Ishimori T, et al. Provocation of coronary artery spasm by the cold pressor test. Hemodynamic, arteriographic and quantitative arteriographic observations. Circulation. 1980;62:925–932.
271. Nobel EG, Gang P, Gordon JB, et al. Dilation of normal and construction of atherosclerotic coronary arteries caused by the cold pressor test. Circulation. 1987;77:43–52.
272. Lenhardt R, Kurz A, Sessler DI. Thermoregulation and hyperthermia. Acta Anaesthesiol Scand Suppl. 1996;109:34–38.
273. Friedman PL, Brown EJ Jr, Gunther S, et al. Coronary vasoconstrictor effect of indomethacin in patients with coronary artery disease. N Engl J Med. 1981;305:1171–1175.
274. Beisel WR, Morgan BB Jr, Bartelloni PJ, et al. Symptomatic therapy in viral illness. A controlled study of effects on work performance. JAMA. 1974;228:581–584.
275. Camfield PR, Camfield CS, Shapiro SH, et al. The first febrile seizure—antipyretic instruction plus either phenobarbital or placebo to prevent recurrence. J Pediatr. 1980;5:719–737.
276. Uhari M, Rantala H, Vainionpää L, et al. Effect of acetaminophen and of low intermittent doses of diazepam on prevention of recurrences of febrile seizures. J Pediatr. 1995;126:991–995.
277. Schnaiderman D, Lahat E, Sheefer T, et al. Antipyretic effectiveness of acetaminophen in febrile seizures: Ongoing prophylaxis versus sporadic usage. Eur J Pediatr. 1993;152:747–749.
278. Warren HS. Strategies for the treatment of sepsis. N Engl J Med. 1997;336:952–953.
279. Bernard GR, Wheeler AP, Russell JA, et al. The effects of ibuprofen on the physiology and survival of patients with sepsis. N Engl J Med. 1997;336:912–918.
280. Mackowiak PA, Plaisance KI. The benefits and risks of antipyretic therapy. Ann N Y Acad Sci. 1998;856:214–223.

Chapter 44

Fever of Unknown Origin

PHILIP A. MACKOWIAK
DAVID T. DURACK

Most fevers are both brief and self-limited and do not require extensive diagnostic investigation or specific therapy. Some fevers are manifestations of more serious illnesses, most of which can be readily diagnosed and effectively treated. A small but important subgroup of fevers are both persistent and difficult to diagnose. Such fevers have fascinated and frustrated clinicians since the earliest days of clinical thermometry.[1] They have generated a welter of publications over the years—the two most important of which, from a historical perspective, have been the classic treatises *Prolonged and Perplexing Fevers* by Keefer and Leard in 1955[2] and *Fever of Unknown Origin: Report on 100 Cases* by Petersdorf and Beeson in 1961.[3]

TERMINOLOGY

In the United States, the term *fever of unknown origin* (FUO) has generally been used to describe this special group of fevers.[4] In other countries, *pyrexia of unknown origin* is more commonly used.[5]

The first formal definition of FUO to attain broad acceptance was one proposed by Petersdorf and Beeson 4 decades ago: "fever higher than 38.3°C (101°F) on several occasions, persisting without diagnosis for at least 3 weeks in spite of at least 1 week's investigation in hospital."[3] Later investigators have modified and extended this classic definition to reflect evolutionary changes in clinical practice.[6, 7] Such changes have included a mounting emphasis on the use of the outpatient setting for diagnostic investigations, an increasing number of immunocompromised patients (especially those with neutropenia), a proliferation of increasingly complex surgical and intensive care protocols, and the advent of the acquired immunodeficiency syndrome. In deference to this new practice environment, cases of FUO are currently codified into four distinct subclasses of the disorder: classic FUO, nosocomial FUO, immune-deficient FUO, and human immunodeficiency virus (HIV)-associated FUO (Table 44–1).

CLASSIC FEVER OF UNKNOWN ORIGIN

Classic FUO refers to the type of FUO defined by Petersdorf and Beeson in 1961.[3] The only alteration to their definition required to conform to modern medical practice is an emphasis on the outpatient setting, which has become the preferred venue for evaluation and treatment. Most patients with classic FUO, in fact, have subacute or chronic symptoms and, therefore, can be safely managed as outpatients. In a series of 53 such patients, for example, the median duration of fever before diagnosis was 40 days.[1] Even though the tempo and accuracy of clinical investigation has increased in recent years, many cases of classic FUO continue to elude diagnosis for extended periods, as reflected in the findings of a Japanese survey from 1982 to 1992, in which an average of 49 days (range 8 to 217 days) was required to complete the diagnostic evaluation.[8]

Of the many publications concerned with the etiology of FUO,[3, 9–15] most have dealt with classic FUO, rather than the other subclasses listed previously. In these investigations, a recurrent theme has emerged—of the myriad of disorders causing FUO, almost all belong to one of five general categories of diseases: infections, neoplasms, connective tissue diseases, miscellaneous disorders, and undiagnosed conditions. The relative frequencies of disorders within these five categories vary from series to series, depending on the geographic region, age of the patient, type of hospital, and other factors (Fig. 44–1). In most series, infection has been the commonest cause of FUO overall, accounting for 25 to 50% of cases. However, in patients older than 65 years, infections have been reported to be the second or even third most common cause of FUO.[8, 9]

In a series of 47 patients 65 years of age and older, Knockaert and associates identified infection as the cause of FUO in only 25% of cases.[9] Temporal arteritis and various connective tissue diseases accounted for 31% of cases and tumors for 12%. Only 8% of cases went undiagnosed—a percentage substantially lower than that reported in surveys involving younger adults, in which as many as 30% of cases remained undiagnosed (Fig. 44–2).[16] The longer the duration of fever before medical consultation, the less likely that a diagnosis will be reached.[17]

Among the infections responsible for classic FUO, abscesses, endocarditis, tuberculosis, and complicated urinary tract infections have consistently been some of the most important. These tend to vary in incidence according to locale. Visceral leishmaniasis, for example, although absent from most series of classic FUO, accounted for 8% of cases in a study reported in 1997 from Spain.[18] Other examples of causes of classic FUO with distinctive geographic distributions include melioidosis (Southeast Asia and northern Australia),[19] Kikuchi-Fujimoto disease (an unusual form of necrotizing

TABLE 44–1 Summary of Definitions and Major Features of the Four Subtypes of Fever of Unknown Origin (FUO)

	Classic FUO	Nosocomial FUO	Immune-Deficient FUO	HIV-Related FUO
Definition	>38.0°C, >3 wk, >2 visits or 3 d in hospital	>38.0°C, 3 d, not present or incubating on admission	>38.0°C, >3 d, negative cultures after 48 h	38.0°C, >3 w for outpatients, >3 d for inpatients, HIV infection confirmed
Patient location	Community, clinic, or hospital	Acute care hospital	Hospital or clinic	Community, clinic, or hospital
Leading causes	Cancer, infections, inflammatory conditions, undiagnosed, habitual hyperthermia	Nosocomial infections, postoperative complications, drug fever	Majority due to infections, but cause documented in only 40–60%	HIV (primary infection), typical and atypical mycobacteria, CMV, lymphomas, toxoplasmosis, cryptococcosis
History emphasis	Travel, contacts, animal and insect exposure, medications, immunizations, family history, cardiac valve disorder	Operations and procedures, devices, anatomic considerations, drug treatment	Stage of chemotherapy, drugs administered, underlying immunosuppressive disorder	Drugs, exposures, risk factors, travel, contacts, stage of HIV infection
Examination emphasis	Fundi, oropharynx, temporal artery, abdomen, lymph nodes, spleen, joints, skin, nails, genitalia, rectum or prostate, lower limb deep veins	Wounds, drains, devices, sinuses, urine	Skin folds, IV sites, lungs, perianal area	Mouth, sinuses, skin, lymph nodes, eyes, lungs, perianal area
Investigation emphasis	Imaging, biopsies, sedimentation rate, skin tests	Imaging, bacterial cultures	CXR, bacterial cultures	Blood and lymphocyte count; serologic tests; CXR; stool examination; biopsies of lung, bone marrow, and liver for cultures and cytologic tests; brain imaging
Management	Observation, outpatient temperature chart, investigations, avoidance of empirical drug treatments	Depends on situation	Antimicrobial treatment protocols	Antiviral and antimicrobial protocols, vaccines, revision of treatment regimens, good nutrition
Time course of disease	Months	Weeks	Days	Weeks to months
Tempo of investigation	Weeks	Days	Hours	Days to weeks

Abbreviations: CMV, Cytomegalovirus; CXR, chest radiograph; HIV, human immunodeficiency virus; IV, intravenous.
Adapted from Durack DT. Fever of unknown origin. In: Mackowiak PA, ed. Fever. Basic Mechanisms and Management. 2nd ed. Philadelphia: Lippincott-Raven; 1997:237–249.

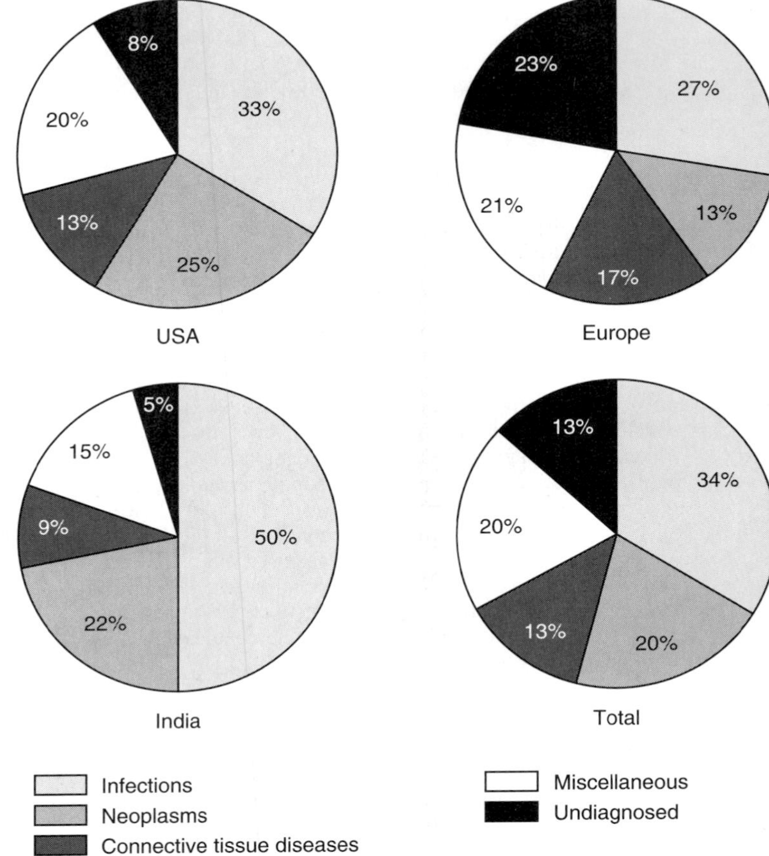

FIGURE 44–1. The five main etiologic categories of fever of unknown origin, comparing their frequency in series from three geographic regions. (Redrawn from Durack DT. Fever of unknown origin. In: Mackowiak PA, ed. Fever. Basic Mechanisms and Management. 2nd ed. Philadelphia: Lippincott-Raven; 1997:237–249.)

lymphadentitis seen primarily in Japan),[20] and familial Hibernian fever (an inherited periodic fever syndrome described only in Ireland).[21] The miscellaneous category contains both varied and individually rare causes of classical FUO (Table 44–2).

Of the connective tissue diseases responsible for classical FUO, Still's disease, systemic lupus erythematosus, and variants of rheumatoid arthritis predominate in younger patients, whereas temporal arteritis and polymyalgia rheumatica syndromes are more common in elderly patients. Malignant neoplasms, another important cause of FUO, can induce fever directly through the production and release of pyrogenic cytokines, as in the case of certain lymphomas. They can also generate fevers indirectly by undergoing spontaneous or induced necrosis or by creating conditions conducive to secondary infections, such as postobstructive pneumonia.[22] Although traditionally touted as an important cause of FUO,[3, 23] in reality, hypernephromas rarely present with fever.[24]

The relative frequency with which the major diagnostic categories are represented in series of classic FUO has varied according to both the era in which the series was published[6, 13] and its country of origin (see Fig. 44–1).[8, 15, 25, 26] Since the mid-1900s, the frequency with which infections and malignant neoplasms have been identified as causes of classic FUO has fallen steadily, whereas that of miscellaneous causes and undiagnosed conditions has risen.[25] However, in developing countries, the frequency with which infections are diagnosed has changed little.[15] Consequently, in these countries, malignant neoplasms and connective tissue disorders are comparatively less important as causes of classic FUO than in developed countries (see Fig. 44–1).[15]

TABLE 44–2 Examples of Rare Miscellaneous Causes of Fever

Alcoholic hepatitis	Immunoblastic lymphadenopathy
Allergic alveolitis	Inflammatory bowel disease
Aortitis	Kikuchi-Fujimoto disease
Aortic dissection	Lymphomatoid granulomatosis
Atrial myxoma	Metal fume fever
Behçet's syndrome	Myeloproliferative syndromes
Castleman's disease	Pancreatitis
Chronic meningitis	Paroxysmal hemoglobinurias
Cirrhotic fever	Pericarditis
Carcinomatous meningitis	Periodic fever
Cyclic neutropenia	Pheochromocytoma
Drug fever and other hypersensitivities	Pulmonary emboli
Erythema multiforme	Postpericardiotomy syndrome
Fabry's disease	Retroperitoneal fibrosis
Factitious fever	Sarcoidosis
Familial Hibernian fever	Schnitzler's syndrome
Familial Mediterranean fever	Serum sickness
Granulomatous hepatitis	Sjögren's syndrome
Granulomatous peritonitis	Subacute necrotizing lymphadenitis
Hemoglobinopathies	Thrombotic thrombocytopenic purpura
Hemolytic anemias	Thyroiditis and thyrotoxicosis
Histiocytosis X	Veno-occlusive disease
Hypereosinophilic syndrome	Wegener's granulomatosis
	Whipple's disease

Adapted from Durack DT. Fever of unknown origin. In: Mackowiak PA, ed. Fever. Basic Mechanisms and Management. 2nd ed. Philadelphia: Lippincott-Raven; 1997:237–249.

Infants and Children

The diseases responsible for classic FUO in infants differ from those in older children and adults. Respiratory infections cause classic FUO in infants more often than in children older than 12 months or adults.[10] The relative frequency of infections as a cause of FUO in infants is high, owing to the fact that connective tissue diseases and

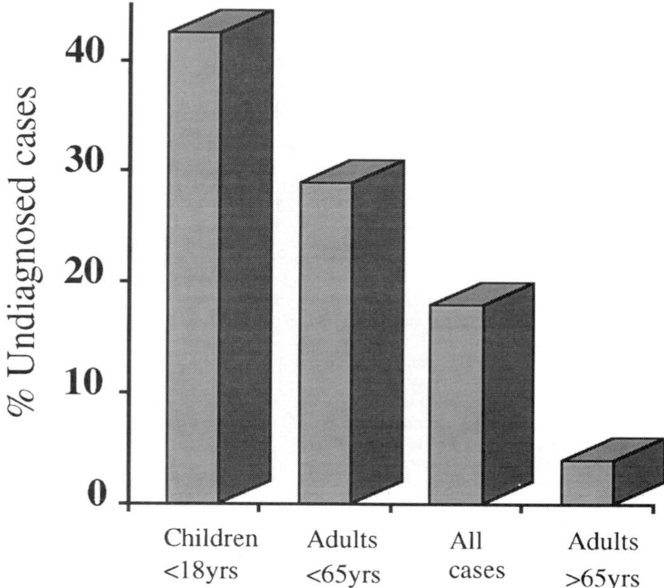

FIGURE 44–2. Frequency of undiagnosed causes of fever of unknown origin by age. (Adapted from Durack DT. Fever of unknown origin. In: Mackowiak PA, ed. Fever. Basic Mechanisms and Management. 2nd ed. Philadelphia: Lippincott-Raven; 1997;237–249.)

cancers are relatively rare in this age group. Kawasaki disease is predominantly a problem of children younger than 5 years, less so of older children. Whereas connective tissue diseases are rarely seen in children younger than 12 months, Still's disease is a leading cause of FUO in older children and young adults. Joint involvement in children with FUO usually signifies a serious underlying disorder, such as a connective tissue disease, endocarditis, or leukemia.[10]

In a series of 146 pediatric cases of FUO, Jacobs and Schutze established a diagnosis in only 84 (57.5%).[27] Of these, 64 (43.8%) had infections, 11 (7.5%) autoimmune disorders, 4 (2.7%) malignant neoplasms, and 5 (3.4%) a variety of other disorders, such as drug-induced fever, sarcoidosis, and mercury poisoning. The most common infectious diseases diagnosed in their series were Epstein-Barr virus infection (15%), osteomyelitis (10%), bartonellosis (5%), and urinary tract infections (4%).

Elderly Persons

One of the most striking features of classic FUO in patients older than 65 years is the relatively high frequency with which connective tissue diseases are identified as the cause of the illness (Table 44–3).[28, 29] In developed countries, connective tissue diseases surpass even infections as the leading cause of classic FUO in elderly patients.[8, 9] This is because the temporal arteritis and polymyalgia rheumatica syndromes are common in this setting.[8, 30] Unfortunately, these diagnoses are frequently missed or delayed because associated symptoms are subacute and nonspecific. In elderly patients in whom infections are identified as the cause of FUO, intra-abdominal abscesses, complicated urinary tract infections, tuberculosis, and endocarditis have predominated.[9, 14] For unclear reasons, factitious fever rarely causes FUO in older patients. Relatively few cases of FUO go undiagnosed in elderly patients (Table 44–3), and yet, elderly FUO patients have a distinctly poorer prognosis than their younger counterparts, because of a relatively high incidence of cancer.

NOSOCOMIAL FEVER OF UNKNOWN ORIGIN

Nosocomial FUO, as the name implies, is a hospital-associated disorder in which patients first manifest fever after having been hospitalized for at least 24 hours. Such FUO cases, as might be expected, are all-too-frequently attributable to risk factors encountered in the hospital environment—including surgical procedures, urinary and respiratory tract instrumentation, intravascular devices, drug therapy, and immobilization. Because acute febrile disorders are well recognized consequences of exposure to such risk factors, it has been assumed that these same acute disorders also occasionally manifest as FUOs. Examples of such disorders commonly offered, but not yet verified in actual surveys of nosocomial FUO, include septic thrombophlebitis, recurrent pulmonary emboli, *Clostridium difficile* colitis, and drug fever.[7, 31] Sinusitis has been better documented as a cause of FUO in intensive care unit patients, especially those with nasotracheal and nasogastric tubes.[32] However, our overall knowledge of nosocomial FUO is limited due to the lack of a published series specifically devoted to this category of FUO.

IMMUNE-DEFICIENT FEVER OF UNKNOWN ORIGIN

The number of patients with neutropenia or impaired cell-mediated immunity, or both, resulting from cytotoxic therapy or hematologic malignant neoplasms is rising, even as the average duration of neutropenia in such patients is falling, because of the increasing clinical application of colony-stimulating factors. Many episodes of fever in immune-deficient patients are short-lived, because they either respond quickly to treatment or are rapidly fatal infections. For this reason, the diagnostic evaluation of febrile episodes must be completed quickly, so that appropriate therapy can be administered without delay. Because of the impaired immune response of such patients, signs of inflammation other than fever are notoriously modest, leading in many cases to atypical clinical presentations of what otherwise would be readily apparent infectious diseases.

In series of patients with immune-deficient FUO, infection has been identified as the cause of the fever in 60% or more of cases.[33] In at least some cases, however, the diagnosis has been presumptive, based on a favorable clinical response to antimicrobial therapy, rather than on the result of definitive tests. Although Steinmetz and colleagues have reported that in neutropenic patients a raised serum concentration of interleukin-6 is a useful marker for septic episodes,[34] de Kleijn and associates did not find circulating levels of pyrogenic cytokines to be diagnostically useful in 123 patients with classic FUO.[35]

Infections caused by pyogenic bacteria are the most common cause of fever during episodes of neutropenia. These generally respond well to antibiotic therapy, whether or not the etiologic microorganism is isolated. In patients with impaired cell-mediated immunity,

TABLE 44–3 Final Diagnosis in Elderly Compared with Younger Patients with Fever of Unknown Origin

Diagnosis	<65 Years n = 152 (%)	>65 Years n = 201 (%)
Infections	33 (21%)	72 (35%)
Abscess	6	25
Endocarditis	2	14
Tuberculosis	4	20
Viral infections	8	1
Other	13	12
Tumors	8 (5%)	37 (19%)
Hematologic	3	19
Solid	5	18
Multisystem diseases*	27 (17%)	57 (28%)
Miscellaneous†	39 (26%)	17 (8%)
No diagnosis	45 (29%)	18 (9%)

*Rheumatic diseases, connective tissue disorders, vasculitis (including temporal arteritis), polymyalgia rheumatica, and sarcoidosis.

†Includes factitious fever (seven cases), habitual hyperthermia (five cases) and drug-induced fever (three cases).

Adapted from Iikuni Y, Okada J, Kondo H, et al. Current fever of unknown origin 1982–1992. Intern Med. 1994; 33:67–73; and Knockaert DC, Vanneste LJ, Bobbaers HJ. Fever of unknown origin in elderly patients. J Am Geriatr Soc. 1993; 41:1187–1192.

FUO is more often due to conditions other than pyogenic bacterial infections, as illustrated in a recent survey of transplant recipients by Chang and coworkers.[36] In their series, infections were the cause of 7 of the 12 (58%) episodes of fever in which a diagnosis could not be established during 3 days of intensive investigation; these included five cases of human herpes virus 6 infection, one of varicella zoster virus infection with atypical skin lesions, and one of pneumonia due to *Serratia marcescens* (in which the pulmonary infiltrate was initially inapparent radiographically). Three (25%) cases were due to noninfectious conditions (one malignant neoplasm, one drug-induced fever, and one case of adrenal insufficiency). In two (17%) cases, the cause of the fever could not be determined.

HUMAN IMMUNODEFICIENCY VIRUS–ASSOCIATED FEVER OF UNKNOWN ORIGIN

Episodes of fever are commonplace in patients infected with HIV—a special subgroup of immune-deficient patients.[37–39] The primary phase of the HIV infection itself is characterized by a mononucleosis-like illness in which fever is a prominent feature. All too often, primary HIV infection eludes diagnosis, because the illness is nonspecific and precedes seroconversion. For this reason, it represents an important cause of HIV-associated FUO. Once symptoms of the primary phase of the HIV infection resolve, HIV-infected patients exhibit only trivial elevations in oral temperature as a result of their persistent retroviral infection.[40] Consequently, in the later phases of the HIV infection, fever invariably signifies some superimposed illness. Because many of these are potentially devastating opportunistic infections (Table 44–4), febrile episodes in patients with advanced HIV infections must be diagnosed and treated as promptly as possible. Unfortunately, in acquired immunodeficiency syndrome patients, infections tend to present in atypical fashion, owing to the capacity both of the disordered immune response and of prior prophylactic antimicrobial therapy[41] to distort their clinical manifestations.

The salient features of HIV-associated FUO are amply illustrated in a survey by Bissuel and colleagues, wherein 57 cases of FUO were identified among 270 hospitalized HIV-infected patients.[39] The cause of FUO was determined in most cases (86%). In 23 (40%), mycobacterial infections were responsible for the FUO. Twelve were infected with mycobacteria other than *Mycobacterium tuberculosis,* 10 had tuberculosis, and one was diagnosed with a Calmette-Guérin bacillus infection.[39] Cytomegalovirus was identified as the cause of the FUO in 9% of the cases. Other diagnoses included disseminated leishmaniasis (illustrating the importance of the travel history in diagnosing FUO), *Pneumocystis carinii* pneumonia, and toxoplasmosis. Fourteen percent of the cases had noninfectious causes of FUO, including lymphomas and other miscellaneous diagnoses. Only 14% of the cases of FUO remained undiagnosed.

In a survey of 580 HIV-infected patients in Spain, 8% of the patients developed HIV-associated FUO.[38] Among these, a diagnosis was established in 88%—the majority of which were infections. More than half the infections involved mycobacteria, with the incidence of tuberculosis exceeding that of other mycobacterioses by a ratio of 3:1. Because of the frequency with which disseminated mycobacterial infections (and in some locales, visceral leishmaniasis[42]) have been identified as the cause of FUO in HIV-infected patients, several investigators have suggested that a bone marrow biopsy should be routinely examined during the evaluation of HIV-associated FUO.[18, 43] However, Kilby and colleagues have reported that in cases in which mycobacterial infections are diagnosed, bone marrow results seldom provide more immediate or specific information than centrifugation blood cultures.[44] Therefore, these investigators recommend that in HIV-infected patients in whom disseminated mycobacterial infections are suspected, a single lysis centrifugation blood culture should be obtained early in the routine evaluation.

TABLE 44–4 Causes of Fever of Unknown Origin in Human Immunodeficiency Virus–Infected Patients*

Cause	Percentage
Tuberculosis (pulmonary and extrapulmonary)	35.5
Mycobacterium avium complex (MAC) infection	11.5
Visceral leishmaniasis	9.9
Pneumocystis carinii pneumonia	5.6
Mycobacteria other than tuberculosis and MAC	4.5
Non-Hodgkin's lymphoma	4.2
Bacterial infections	3.9
Cytomegalovirus infection	2.5
Toxoplasmosis	2.4
Cryptococcosis	1.5
Fever due to human immunodeficiency virus	1.3
Histoplasmosis	0.5
Drug-induced fever	0.5
Other causes	2.2
Unknown	6.7
Nonspecified	7.2

*Data from a total of 594 episodes.
From Mayo J, Collazos J, Martinez E. Fever of unknown origin in the HIV-infected patient: New scenario for an old problem. Scand J Infect Dis. 1997; 29:327–336.

TABLE 44–5 General Diagnostic Evaluation of Patients with Fever of Unknown Origin

- Comprehensive history
- Repeated physical examinations
- Complete blood count
- Routine blood chemistry determinations
- Urinalysis, including microscopic examination
- Chest radiograph
- Erythrocyte sedimentation rate
- Antinuclear antibodies
- Rheumatoid factor
- Blood cultures: three or more separate specimens obtained in absence of antimicrobial therapy
- Cytomegalovirus IgM antibodies or viral detection in blood
- Heterophile antibody test in children and young adults
- Tuberculin skin test
- Computed tomography of abdomen, pelvis, or other sites
- Radionuclide scans
- Human immunodeficiency virus antibodies or viral detection assay
- Further evaluation of any abnormality detected by above tests
- Venous duplex imaging of lower limbs

Adapted from Arnow PM, Flaherty JP. Fever of unknown origin. Lancet. 1997;350:575–580.

EVALUATION

The initial evaluation of the patient with FUO typically includes a comprehensive history, repeated physical examinations, and a host of laboratory investigations (Table 44–5).

History and Physical Examination

The first step in the evaluation of the patient with FUO is to verify the presence of fever. The importance of this step is self-evident and yet all too often overlooked. In fact, in a series of 347 patients admitted to the National Institutes of Health for prolonged fever, 35% were ultimately determined either not to have fever or to have fever of factitious origin.[45]

Although fever patterns are rarely diagnostic, they may contain diagnostically useful information[46] and should, therefore, be examined carefully. In pediatric populations, for example, the height of a fever correlates roughly with the likelihood of bacteremia. McCarthy has reported that in young children with febrile illnesses, the likelihood of bacteremia is 7% in children with temperatures of 40°C or less, 13% with temperatures of 40.5°C to 41°C, and 26% with temperatures of 41.1°C or greater.[47, 48] Although there is a general perception that a similar relationship exists between the height of a fever and the likelihood of bacteremia in adults, this belief has not been substantiated. Unfortunately, the relationship is at best a relatively loose one even in children, with numerous examples of bacteremia in which there is little or no fever and nonbacteremic conditions, such as drug-induced fever, thrombophlebitis, and recurrent pulmonary emboli, in which extremely high fevers are encountered. Thus, although the height of fever might be useful in predicting bacteremia in febrile populations, the relationship should be invoked with caution in individual patients.

Clinicians have endeavored to diagnose particular diseases by analyzing fever patterns since the earliest days of clinical thermometry.[49] These efforts have given rise to a vast and frequently arcane terminology, including descriptors such as *remittent, intermittent, hectic, quotidian, picket fence, sustained, quartan,* and *saddleback.* Such terms have been used to codify fever patterns into general categories in an attempt to enhance their diagnostic utility. A few, such as the Pel-Ebstein pattern of Hodgkin's disease, the typhus inversus (i.e., reversal of the normal diurnal pattern) of disseminated tuberculosis, the pulse-temperature disassociation of typhoid fever, and the sustained fever of gram-negative bacterial pneumonia and central nervous system damage have been posited as having especially high specificity for particular diseases. Unfortunately, with the possible exception of the tertian and quartan patterns of malaria, these fever patterns are neither sensitive nor specific enough to be considered diagnostic of any disease.

This is not to say, however, that time spent scrutinizing fever patterns is necessarily unproductive or misleading. In the context of other signs and symptoms and laboratory data, distinctive patterns can suggest specific diagnoses to the alert clinician. Likewise, as noted later, the resolution of fever after the institution of disease-specific therapy is occasionally the most compelling, if not the only, evidence of the cause of a febrile illness.

Although it is axiomatic that a comprehensive history and careful physical examination are the cornerstones of the evaluation of any illness, they are especially important in determining the focus of the initial laboratory investigation in FUO. In the history, particular attention should be given to recent travel, exposure to pets and other animals, the work environment, and recent contact with persons exhibiting similar symptoms. The family history should be carefully scrutinized for hereditary causes of fever, as, for example, familial Mediterranean fever. Likewise, the past medical history must be examined for previously diagnosed conditions (e.g., lymphoma, rheumatic fever, or prior abdominal disorder) the reactivation of which might account for the source of fever. Finally, a complete list of the patient's medications must be obtained, so that each can be evaluated as a potential source of drug-induced fever.

In the investigation of FUO, several aspects of the physical examination should be accorded closer scrutiny than generally given to the evaluation of other illnesses (Table 44–6). All too frequently, key physical abnormalities in patients with FUO are so subtle as to require repeated examinations to be appreciated. The nodular or weakly pulsatile temporal artery of temporal arteritis, the telltale oral ulcer of disseminated histoplasmosis, and the vague rectal fluctuance of the perirectal abscess are but a few important examples. The diagnostic yield of the physical examination in the evaluation of FUO has not been studied directly. Nevertheless, in two pediatric series, abnormal physical findings were reported to have contributed to the diagnosis in 60% of cases of FUO.[50, 51] In half of these, the abnormalities were detected only after repeated examinations. Although a vigorous search for lymphadenopathy is generally recommended in patients with FUO, enlarged lymph nodes have not consistently correlated with specific diseases and when examined histopathologically, have not consistently yielded a correct diagnosis.[50, 52]

Laboratory Investigation

The literature is replete with algorithms for evaluating FUO.[53–59] Although useful as general guides to establishing a diagnosis, such algorithms tend to promote the use of large and frequently expensive batteries of clinical tests unless judiciously applied using clues to diagnosis gleaned from the history and physical examination. Moreover, when formulating a diagnostic plan for such patients, the clinician does well to remember that most often the cause of FUO is a common disorder presenting in atypical fashion rather than an exotic disease presenting in its typical form.

In most series, noninvasive laboratory tests have yielded the diagnosis in approximately a quarter of the cases of FUO studied.[9, 25, 26] The most useful of these have been serologic tests for microbial pathogens and for various rheumatologic diseases. Paradoxically, the advent of enhanced microbial culture systems has had less of an impact on the diagnosis of FUO than might have been anticipated. This is because such systems are so proficient at recovering fastidious bacteria, mycobacteria, and fungi that they now tend to provide the diagnosis in otherwise obscure febrile illnesses before conditions defining FUO are met.

Imaging studies have been used primarily to localize abnormalities as a preamble to more definitive (invasive) testing (Fig. 44–3). Computed tomography (CT) of the abdomen has been especially effective in this regard.[60] Structures appearing abnormal on CT are almost always confirmed as such on laparotomy or biopsy.[61] As a result, abdominal CT and, to a lesser extent, ultrasound imaging of the gallbladder and hepatobiliary system have been used extensively to evaluate cases of FUO. In fact, in one series, more than three CT or ultrasound examinations, or both, were performed for each FUO patient evaluated.[62] Unfortunately, the diagnostic yield per test performed has been little better than 10%. False-negative CT studies

TABLE 44–6 Examples of Subtle Physical Findings Having Special Significance in Patients with Fever of Unknown Origin

Body Site	Physical Finding	Diagnosis
Head	Sinus tenderness	Sinusitis
Temporal artery	Nodules, reduced pulsations	Temporal arteritis
Oropharynx	Ulceration	Disseminated histoplasmosis
	Tender tooth	Periapical abscess
Fundi or conjunctivae	Choroid tubercle	Disseminated granulomatosis*
	Petechiae, Roth's spot	Endocarditis
Thyroid	Enlargement, tenderness	Thyroiditis
Heart	Murmur	Infective or marantic endocarditis
Abdomen	Enlarged iliac crest lymph nodes, splenomegaly	Lymphoma,† endocarditis, disseminated granulomatosis*
Rectum	Perirectal fluctuance, tenderness	Abscess
	Prostatic tenderness, fluctuance	Abscess
Genitalia	Testicular nodule	Periarteritis nodosa
	Epididymal nodule	Disseminated granulomatosis
Lower extremities	Deep venous tenderness	Thrombosis or thrombophlebitis
Skin and nails	Petechiae, splinter hemorrhages, subcutaneous nodules, clubbing	Vasculitis, endocarditis

*Includes tuberculosis, histoplasmosis, coccidioidomycosis, sarcoidosis, and syphilis.
†See text for note on the nonspecificity of lymphadenopathy identified on physical examination.

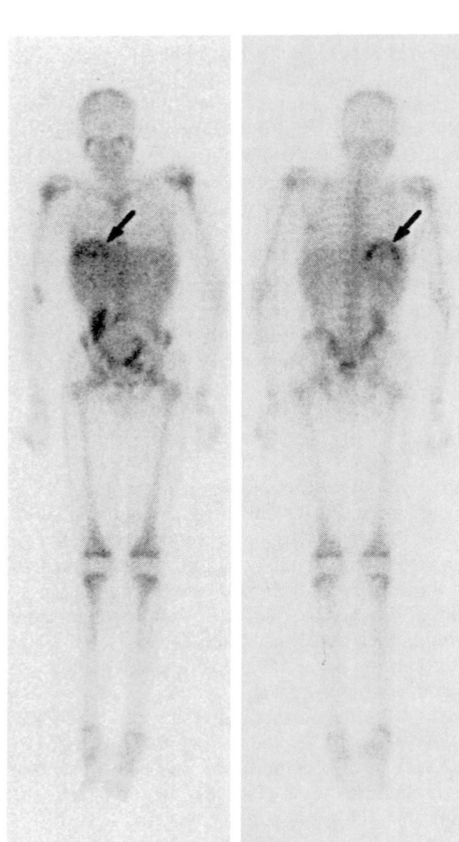

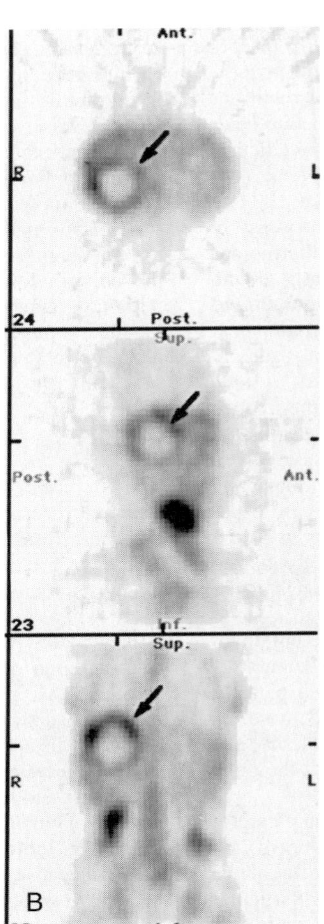

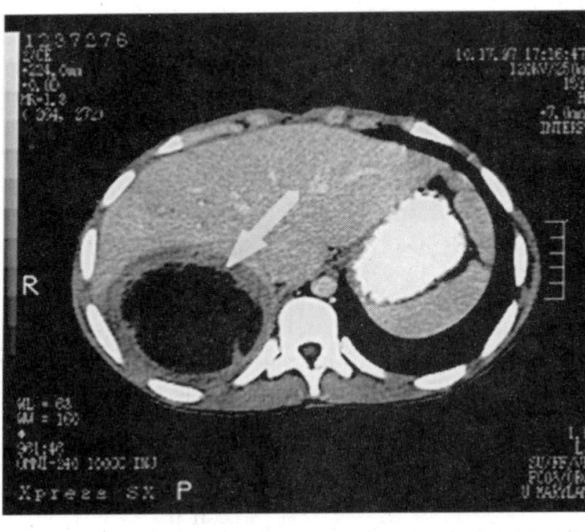

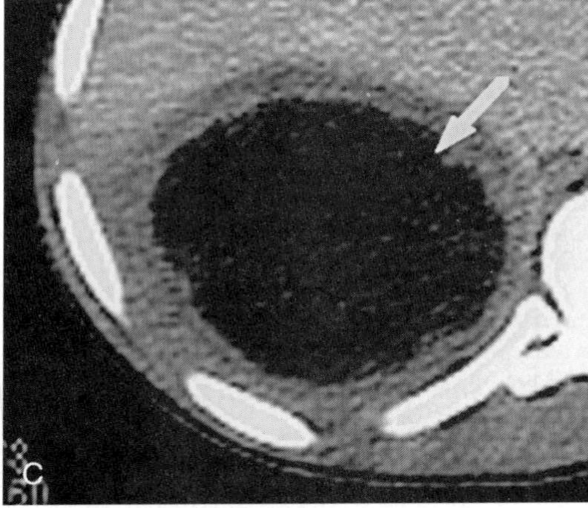

FIGURE 44–3. Anterior and posterior whole body ^{111}In white blood cell scan (*A*), transaxial, saggital and coronal multiplanar SPECT scan (*B*), and CT scan (*C*) performed during the initial evaluation of a 15-year-old boy with classic fever of unknown origin resulting from a large liver abscess (*arrow*). (Images provided courtesy of L. E. Holder, M.D., Department of Radiology, University of Maryland School of Medicine.)

have occasionally been encountered, even in cases of abscesses in solid organs, as a result of distortions of normal anatomy, small abscess size, or failure to use both oral and intravenous contrast agents.[63]

Scanning with labeled autologous leukocytes is a useful test for evaluating cases in which infections and malignant neoplasms are the cause of FUO. In such patients, labeled leukocyte scans have generally provided a higher yield overall than that obtained by either CT or ultrasound scanning.[64, 65] When contemplating the use of such scans in the investigation of undiagnosed fever, one must choose between ^{111}In-labeled mixed leukocytes, ^{111}In-labeled pure granulocytes, and ^{99m}Tc-labeled leukocytes.[66] The choice of one versus another depends on both local conditions and theoretical considerations. Although one might expect pure granulocytes to perform better than mixed leukocytes in patients with FUO, because a greater fraction of the injected label associates with migrating cells, the literature suggests that both preparations perform equally well.[66]

On theoretical grounds, ^{99m}Tc-labeled leukocytes should be less effective in the evaluation of FUO than ^{111}In-labeled leukocytes, even though they provide better photon flux and image resolution. This is because the infections responsible for FUO are frequently chronic and therefore involve mononuclear infiltrates. As a result, their visualization is critically dependent on 24-hour imaging. In both labeled cells and targeted inflammatory tissue, ^{99m}Tc is less stable than ^{111}In and has a shorter physical half-life.[67] Consequently, one might expect it to be less effective in visualizing infectious causes of FUO than ^{111}In. However, clinical experience has yet to show ^{111}In to be superior to ^{99m}Tc in the evaluation of FUO.[66]

Another useful technique for evaluating undiagnosed fever, especially FUO, is ^{67}Ga scanning. Its ability to image inflammation was first described by Lavender and colleagues.[68] Shortly thereafter, Hilson and Maisey reported positive results by ^{67}Ga scanning in 50 of 67 patients with FUO, of which 32 had abscesses.[69] The ^{67}Ga appears to be particularly effective in visualizing chronic infections. In a study by Sfakianakis and coworkers, five false-negative ^{67}Ga scans and seven false-negative ^{111}In-leukocyte scans were recorded in 32 febrile patients with 26 sites of proven infection.[70] The former studies were obtained in patients with fever of less than 1 week's duration, whereas the latter came from patients who had been febrile for longer than 2 weeks. These findings suggest that if fever due to infection has been present for longer than 2 weeks, ^{67}Ga scanning is the imaging technique most likely to visualize the infectious focus.

When labeled human polyclonal immunoglobulin G (IgG) was introduced as an inflammation imaging agent, hopes were raised that it would be both sensitive and specific for infection on the basis of binding of the Fc portion of the IgG molecule to local Fc receptors at sites of inflammation.[71, 72] Although this turned out not to be the case, interest in human polyclonal IgG has persisted, owing to the publication of several articles showing human polyclonal IgG and ^{111}In-leukocyte scanning to be equally effective in visualizing infectious foci.[73, 74]

The role of venous duplex imaging of the lower extremities in the evaluation of FUO is uncertain. In a survey of 89 patients with FUO, AbuRahma and colleagues used venous duplex imaging to identify lower extremity venous thrombosis as the probable cause of fever in 6% of the cases studied.[75] Their findings, which need to be corroborated by other investigators, suggest that in a small percentage of FUO patients, venous duplex imaging can establish the correct diagnosis.

Invasive Procedures

Excisional biopsy, needle biopsy, or laparotomy has been the definitive diagnostic procedure in less than half of the cases of FUO in most published series.[63] The majority of patients with FUO undergo at least one such procedure, even though the diagnostic yield of the procedures is only fair, with an average of 2.8 to 4.6 biopsies required per case to establish a final diagnosis.[13, 76] The diagnostic yield of operative and CT-guided biopsies is higher than that of bedside biopsy procedures.[13] For this reason, bedside biopsies should rarely be performed unless guided by additional localizing information. An important exception to the injunction against blind biopsies concerns the temporal artery, which may merit biopsy in an elderly FUO patient with an erythrocyte sedimentation rate above 50 mm/hour, even in the absence of localizing signs.[9]

Exploratory laparotomy is rarely performed today unless localized findings are present. This is because few anatomic abnormalities are currently missed by CT scanning, leaving only rare cases of vasculitis, polyarteritis nodosa, granulomatous disease, and chronic cholecystitis to be diagnosed by laparotomy.[61] Laparoscopy, including laparoscopic liver biopsy, has helped further obviate the need for laparotomy.[77] Blind liver biopsy, even in patients with liver abnormalities, is less accurate than laparoscopic liver biopsy.[78]

Therapeutic Trials

In the past, empirical trials of therapy with anti-inflammatory agents such as aspirin or corticosteroids or with antimicrobial agents have been employed as diagnostic tests in patients with FUO.[1] In some cases, antineoplastic drugs have even been used for this purpose. Today such trials are seldom indicated. However, in appropriate clinical settings, therapeutic trials employing agents with limited spectrums of activity (e.g., antimycobacterial drugs) continue to be an acceptable means of diagnosing FUO.

The limitations and risks of empirical therapeutic trials are obvious. Underlying diseases may remit spontaneously during the course of inappropriate therapy, giving the false impression of a successful therapeutic trial. Furthermore, empirical treatment is rarely specific. Rifampin, for example, although frequently included in empirical therapeutic regimens for tuberculosis, is active against numerous pyogenic bacteria as well as *M. tuberculosis.* Similarly, although fevers caused by malignant neoplasms have been reported to respond better to nonsteroidal anti-inflammatory agents, such as naproxen, than fevers of infectious origin,[79] the diagnostic accuracy of the so-called naproxen test in differentiating malignant from nonmalignant causes of FUO remains to be determined. For these reasons, therapeutic trials, even when successful in reducing fever, may delay both the diagnosis and appropriate treatment of FUO. Therefore, empirical therapeutic trials are probably best reserved for those few patients in whom all other approaches have failed, and for the occasional patient who is too ill for therapy to be withheld pending further observation.

MANAGEMENT

A fundamental principle in the management of classic FUO is that therapy should be delayed until the cause of the fever has been determined, so that the therapy can be tailored to a specific diagnosis.[1] This approach is based upon the oft-repeated observation that nonspecific treatment is rarely curative and has the potential to delay diagnosis. This ideal is, however, frequently ignored in clinical practice because, by definition, the road to diagnosis in FUO is long and tortuous. As a result, clinicians may feel compelled to treat symptoms empirically, even though the agents used may obscure the very signs and symptoms on which the diagnosis depends. This approach may be difficult to resist, for example, in the patient with suspected temporal arteritis, who is treated empirically with corticosteroids to prevent vascular complications such as cortical blindness. Primary care physicians, who have learned from experience that the most cost-effective approach to febrile illnesses is to attempt to eradicate them using empirical therapy before undertaking expensive diagnostic exercises, must recognize that this approach is less likely to succeed with FUO than with more mundane fevers.

In neutropenic FUO, the principles of treatment are different. Because of the relatively high prevalence of serious bacterial infections responsible for these fevers, febrile neutropenic patients should generally receive broad-spectrum antimicrobial therapy immediately after samples for appropriate cultures have been obtained.[33] Treatment regimens can be adjusted later, according to the results of cultures and the clinical response. Prompt antibiotic treatment is also frequently indicated in patients with nosocomial FUO, especially when such patients have severe underlying diseases or appear toxic.

PROGNOSIS

The prognosis of FUO is determined by both the cause of the fever and the underlying disease or diseases on which the disorder is superimposed. The time required to establish the diagnosis is less important. Elderly patients and those with malignant neoplasms have the poorest prognosis.[1] Diagnostic delay adversely affects the prognosis in intra-abdominal infections, miliary tuberculosis, disseminated fungal infections, and recurrent pulmonary emboli.[63]

Patients in whom FUO remains undiagnosed after extensive evaluation generally have a favorable outcome, characteristically with resolution of their fever in 4 or more weeks without sequelae.[3, 8, 76, 80] In a study of 61 patients followed long term for undiagnosed FUO, Knockaert and associates were largely unsuccessful in identifying specific diseases as the cause of undiagnosed FUO.[80] Most cases resolved spontaneously, generally obviating the need for corticosteroid therapy. Some patients, however, required nonsteroidal anti-inflammatory drugs for symptomatic relief. In this series, the 5-year mortality rate for undiagnosed FUO was only 3.2%.

SELECTED CAUSES

The following diseases are examples of some of the more important causes of FUO.

Disseminated Granulomatoses

Tuberculosis, histoplasmosis, coccidioidomycosis, blastomycosis, and sarcoidosis are all potential causes of FUO, especially when disseminated and lacking the classic miliary pattern on chest radiographs. An epididymal nodule or an oral mucosal ulcer in patients with FUO may be the only clues to disseminated tuberculosis and disseminated histoplasmosis, respectively, and should be diligently sought when performing the physical examination in FUO patients.

The disseminated granulomatoses are some of the most readily treatable causes of potentially fatal FUO and, therefore, merit close diagnostic attention.[63] Serial chest radiographs may demonstrate subtle infiltrates that increase gradually over time. The erythrocyte sedimentation rate is usually raised, and anemia is common. The tuberculin skin test has been reported to be nonreactive in as many as one half of patients with disseminated tuberculosis, and sputum smears reveal acid-fast bacilli in only one fourth to one half of cases. Biopsies of the lung and liver each demonstrate granulomas in 80 to 90% of cases of miliary tuberculosis. Bone marrow biopsy demonstrates granulomas in only half of the patients, unless anemia, leukopenia, or monocytosis is present, in which case the likelihood of finding granulomas increases above 80%. Bronchoalveolar lavage fluid is often culture positive but rarely reveals acid-fast bacilli on microscopic examination. Rapid diagnostic tests, such as polymerase chain reaction, permit earlier detection of *M. tuberculosis* and may be helpful in diagnosing selected cases of FUO.

Lymphoma

Fever is a well-recognized manifestation of malignant neoplasms, especially those originating in the hematopoietic system or with metastases to the liver.[3, 14, 79, 81] A number of different mechanisms have been postulated to cause such fevers, including tumor necrosis, inflammation, and increased heat production by the tumor cells themselves.[79] Current evidence, however, indicates that tumor-associated fever most often results from the production of pyrogenic cytokines, such as tumor necrosis factor-α and interleukin-1, either by the tumor cells themselves or by mononuclear cells that have infiltrated the tumors.[82–84]

Numerous studies have identified lymphomas as the neoplasms most commonly causing FUO in adults.[3, 13, 14, 29, 85] Periodic (Pel-Ebstein) fevers have been reported to be characteristic of fever associated with lymphomas, especially Hodgkin's disease.[86] However, such periodic fevers are rarely reported in current reviews of FUO.

Thromboembolic Disease

Thromboembolic disease has only occasionally been reported as a cause of FUO. However, a series by AbuRahma and coworkers suggests that in contrast to the findings of earlier surveys, lower extremity venous thrombosis and recurrent occult pulmonary embolism may be responsible for as many as 6% of today's cases of FUO.[75] The importance of thromboembolic disease as a cause of FUO belies its relatively low incidence, because it is potentially fatal and can be effectively treated. It is a diagnosis most likely to be overlooked as the cause of FUO when emboli are unaccompanied by pulmonary abnormalities and when the attending physician fails to recognize that thrombophlebitis (even in the absence of focal signs of inflammation) and pulmonary emboli (even in the absence of radiologically apparent pulmonary infiltrates) are capable of inducing high fevers of long duration.

Endocarditis

Microorganisms causing endocarditis are generally easily identified, because they circulate continuously in the blood stream, and because today's blood culture techniques are highly efficient in isolating the bacterial species most often responsible for the infection. For these reasons, endocarditis is a less common cause of FUO today than in earlier times. Those few cases that remain as causes of FUO belong to the special category of *culture-negative endocarditis.*

The incidence of culture-negative endocarditis has been reported to vary between 2.5 and 31% of cases of endocarditis.[87] The high rates of negative blood cultures reported in some of the early series most likely reflect the use of less effective culture techniques and less rigidly defined criteria for the diagnosis of endocarditis than those employed in more recent series. Today, unless blood cultures are obtained after the initiation of antimicrobial therapy (the most common cause of culture-negative endocarditis overall), less than 5% of cases of infective endocarditis exhibit negative blood cultures.[88]

Some species of microorganisms that cause endocarditis are difficult to isolate using standard blood-culture techniques.[87, 89, 90] Most, including the HACEK group of fastidious gram-negative bacilli (*Haemophilus* spp., *Actinobacillus actinomycetemcomitans, Cardiobacterium* spp., *Eikenella* spp., and *Kingella* spp.), *Brucella, Francisella,* and strains of nutritionally variant streptococci, can be isolated within 5 to 7 days using modern blood-culture media.[91] However, a few species, for example, *Bartonella* spp., may require prolonged incubation for 2 to 3 weeks, or special culture media. If blood cultures remain sterile after 5 to 7 days in cases in which a diagnosis of endocarditis seems likely, blind subculture from liquid onto solid media may shorten the time required to isolate the etiologic microorganism. Bacteria with deficient cell walls (L-forms) are no longer believed to be a cause of culture-negative endocarditis. Therefore, special hypertonic culture media, which in the past were recommended for the isolation of L-forms, are not currently indicated in the evaluation of culture-negative endocarditis.

Blood cultures are frequently sterile in cases of fungal endocarditis. This diagnosis should be considered as a cause of FUO in intravenous drug users, patients with prosthetic heart valves, and patients who have received prolonged intravenous antibiotic therapy.[92] In some cases of fungal endocarditis, the yield from blood cultures can be increased by using the lysis-centrifugation culture method.[87] *Aspergillus* spp., however, are seldom isolated from blood cultures, even during active endocarditis. Serologic studies may be helpful in diagnosing rare cases of endocarditis due to *Coxiella, Bartonella,* and *Legionella,* which should be considered in patients with suspected prosthetic valve endocarditis in whom standard blood cultures are sterile.[93]

Temporal Arteritis

Temporal arteritis (also known as giant cell arteritis) is a disease of protean manifestations.[94] No single clinical symptom, sign, or noninvasive laboratory test can be relied on to establish the diagnosis. More often than not, physical findings indicative of active arteritis are absent, and a history consistent with arteritis is obtained only after careful questioning by a clinician fully versed in the varied symptoms and signs of the disorder.[94] In geriatric patients, temporal arteritis may manifest as little more than unexplained fever, or prolonged malaise, depression, or anemia.

The erythrocyte sedimentation rate is usually markedly elevated (above 50 mm/hour) during active arteritis and is thus both useful as an aid to diagnosis and a clinical marker of disease activity. Occasionally, the erythrocyte sedimentation rate is normal during active arteritis. For this reason, symptoms or signs, or both, consistent with the disease should be pursued, even if the sedimentation rate is normal.

Nodules or diminished temporal artery pulsations need not be present for an arterial biopsy to reveal active arteritis. Because pathologic abnormalities may be confined to short segments of the artery, extensive (bilateral) segments of the temporal artery may need to be examined to establish the diagnosis. Blindness, the most feared complication of temporal arteritis, can generally be averted through the use of corticosteroid therapy.

Adult Still's Disease

Still's disease is a diagnosis based solely on clinical findings, because serologic markers and other diagnostic tests for the disorder do not exist.[95] Its clinical features include high spiking fever, arthralgias or arthritis, a transient maculopapular rash, lymphadenopathy, hepatosplenomegaly, serositis, and sore throat. Leukocytosis is generally marked, and rheumatoid factor and antinuclear antibody tests are negative.

The fever of Still's disease is characteristically high and spiking, with temperatures reaching levels of as high as 41.6°C. The fever pattern may be either intermittent (quotidian) or remittent. Although most patients seek medical attention within 2 weeks of the onset of symptoms, some 25% suffer for more than 4 weeks before doing so. A distinctive, evanescent, salmon-pink, macular or maculopapular rash is typically present during the course of the illness.

Hepatomegaly or abnormal liver function tests, or both, are common. Severe liver failure, however, is seen almost exclusively in conjunction with aspirin or other nonsteroidal anti-inflammatory drug therapy. In a third of patients, the disease has a self-limited course, in a quarter an intermittent course, and in a third a chronic course. In occasional patients, Still's disease has a fatal outcome.[95] Three predictors of an unfavorable outcome include root joint (shoulder and hip) arthritis on presentation, polyarthritis, and rash. No other clinical or laboratory manifestations, including human leukocyte antigen (HLA) tests, predict the outcome.[95]

Intra-abdominal Abscess

The particular site at which an intra-abdominal abscess develops to a large extent dictates its clinical manifestations.[63] Localizing symptoms, such as abdominal pain, nausea, vomiting, or diarrhea, are common in liver and intraperitoneal abscesses, and in chronic cholecystitis. Tenderness on examination is also characteristic of most cases of liver, splenic, and intraperitoneal abscess. Elderly patients, however, often have a subacute course with few signs and symptoms referrable to their abscess.[96] Certain antecedent conditions predispose to specific intra-abdominal abscesses. Crohn's disease, for example, has a propensity for causing intraperitoneal and retroperitoneal abscesses, whereas infective endocarditis, biliary tract disease, and pancreatitis are associated with abscesses in the spleen, liver, and pancreas, respectively.[63]

Drug Fever

Fever may be the sole or the most prominent feature of an adverse drug reaction.[97] In contrast to characterizations of drug-induced fever found in numerous textbooks and review articles, the disorder is generally not accompanied by other signs of drug allergy. Although occasionally present, neither rash nor eosinophilia is common. Relative bradycardia is, likewise, uncommon. Several authors have suggested that there might be a characteristic drug-induced fever pattern. However, no such pattern has yet emerged, perhaps because antipyretics and external cooling measures are so frequently used to treat drug-induced fever. Considerable variability has been reported in the length of time between the initiation of a drug therapy and the onset of fever due to the drug. Therefore, clinicians must not assume that because a patient has been taking a certain medication for an extended time, it is not likely the cause of FUO. Contrary to some early reports, there does not appear to be an association between drug fever and either systemic lupus erythematosus, atopy, female sex, or advanced age.[97]

Factitious Fever

Although in most series factitious fever has been a rare cause of FUO, in one report, it was identified as the cause of 9% of cases of prolonged FUO, suggesting that it might be a more common cause of the disorder than generally appreciated.[98] It has two forms—a fraudulent form and a self-induced form.[99] In the former instance, deceit is used to create the appearance of fever, whereas in the latter, genuine fever is induced by the injection or ingestion of pyrogenic materials. Fraudulent fever is most commonly created by means of thermometer manipulation involving the use of external heat sources, or substitute thermometers. Data falsification has also been used to create fraudulent fever in one instance.[100] Fraudulent fever by proxy, although rare in adults, has been reported in children.[101] Rumans and Vosti[102] reported two such cases in children, in whom the mother was believed to have manipulated thermometer readings to create the impression of fever in her children. She had previously been suspected of having orchestrated her own fraudulent fever. Patients with factitious fever may also induce fever through the self-administration of pyrogenic agents. Agents injected for this purpose have most often consisted of bacterial suspensions.

Patients with factitious fever are generally young women, approximately 50% of whom have had training in some aspect of health care, often as nurses. Physicians have rarely been diagnosed with the disorder. In the rare male patient who manifests factitious fever, the fraudulent variety is the one most likely to be diagnosed. In women, the self-induced variety predominates. In fact, all 12 cases of self-induced infection reported by Reich and Gottfried occurred among women.[103] Factitious fever (especially the fraudulent variety) appears to be increasing in frequency among geriatric patients.[104, 105]

Although retrospective analyses have suggested that underlying psychiatric illnesses are common in such patients, a survey of 41 cases of factitious disorders by Reich and Gottfried found no evidence of major psychiatric disorders among patients with either self-induced infection or simulated illnesses.[103] Nor did these investigators find evidence of psychosis on projective testing among the few patients who underwent detailed psychological analysis.

Patients with fraudulent fever are characteristically healthy in appearance and exhibit relative bradycardia during "febrile" episodes. They have unusual fever patterns (e.g., lack of diurnal rhythmicity) that are unresponsive to antipyretics. Laboratory studies are typically normal. In such patients, the diagnosis is usually confirmed by close observation and careful attention to temperature-monitoring procedures.

The classic presentation of self-induced fever is one involving recurrent polymicrobial abscesses or bacteremia, or both, without an apparent source. Such patients usually have complex medical histories. Many have been employed in the medical field.

Confrontation is the key to effective management. During the confrontation process, the clinician must be supportive and nonpunitive and should seek the assistance of a psychiatrist experienced in managing such disorders. In Reich and Gottfried's series, of 33 patients confronted, 12 admitted and 21 denied having had a role in the origin of their disorder.[102] After confrontation, symptoms resolved in many, including at least some of those denying complicity in their disorder.

Although data are scarce, the prognosis of factitious fever appears to be good. Once the diagnosis has been established, even some of the most chronic fevers have been reported to respond favorably to combined medical and psychiatric therapy.[104]

REFERENCES

1. Durack DT. Fever of unknown origin. In: Mackowiak PA, ed. Fever. Basic Mechanisms and Management. 2nd ed. Philadelphia: Lippincott-Raven; 1997:237–249.
2. Keefer CS, Leard SE. Prolonged and Perplexing Fevers. Boston: Little Brown; 1955:1–248.
3. Petersdorf RG, Beeson PB. Fever of unexplained origin: Report on 100 cases. Medicine. 1961;40:1–30.
4. Alt HL, Barker MH. Fever of unknown origin. JAMA. 1930;94:1457–1461.
5. Wong S, Lam M. Pyrexia of unknown origin—approach to management. Singapore Med J. 1995;36:204–208.
6. Smith JW. Fever of undetermined origin: Not what it used to be. Am J Med Sci. 1986;292:56–64.
7. Durack DT, Street AC. Fever of unknown origin reexamined and redefined. Curr Clin Top Infect Dis. 1991;11:35–51.
8. Iikuni Y, Okada J, Kondo H, et al. Current fever of unknown origin 1982–1992. Intern Med. 1994;33:67–73.
9. Knockaert DC, Vanneste LJ, Bobbaers HJ. Fever of unknown origin in elderly patients. J Am Geriatric Soc. 1993;41:1187–1192.
10. Chantada G, Casak S, Daza Plata J, et al. Children with fever of unknown origin in Argentina: An analysis of 113 cases. Pediatr Infect Dis J. 1994;13:260–263.
11. Knockaert DC, Vanneste LJ, Laurent J, et al. Recurrent or episodic fever of unknown origin: Review of 45 cases and survey of the literature. Medicine. 1993;72:184–196.
12. Knockaert DC. Diagnostic strategy for fever of unknown origin in the ultrasonography and computed tomography era. Acta Clin Belg. 1992;47.2:100–116.
13. Kazanjian PH. Fever of unknown origin: Review of 86 patients treated in community hospitals. Clin Infect Dis. 1992;15:968–973.
14. Larson EB, Featherstone HJ, Petersdorf RG. Fever of undetermined origin: Diagnosis and follow-up of 105 cases, 1970–1980. Medicine. 1982;61:269–292.
15. Sharma BK, Kumari S, Varma SC, et al. Prolonged undiagnosed fever in Northern India. Trop Geogr Med. 1992;44:32–36.
16. De Kleijn EMHA, Vandenbroucke JP, van der Meer, et al. Fever of unknown origin (FUO). I. A prospective multicenter study of 167 patients with FUO, using fixed epidemiologic entry criteria. Medicine. 1997;76:392–400.
17. Barbado FJ, Vazquez JJ, Pena JM, et al. Fever of unknown origin: A survey on 133 patients. J Med. 1984;15:185–192.

18. Benito N, Nunez A, de Gorgolas M, et al. Bone marrow biopsy in the diagnosis of fever of unknown origin in patients with acquired immunodeficiency syndrome. Arch Intern Med. 1997;157:1577–1580.
19. Handa R, Bhatia S, Wali JP. Meliodosis: A rare but not forgotten cause of fever of unknown origin. Br J Clin Pathol. 1996;50:116–117.
20. Norris AH, Krasinskas AM, Salhany KE, Glickman SJ. Kikuchi-Fujimoto disease: A benign cause of fever and lymphadenopathy. Am J Med. 1996;101:401–405.
21. McDermott EM, Smillie DM, Powell RJ. Clinical spectrum of familial Hibernian fever: A 14-year follow-up study of the index case and extended family. Mayo Clin Proc. 1997;72:806–817.
22. Klastersky J, Weerts D, Hensgens C, et al. Fever of unexplained origin in patients with cancer. Eur J Cancer. 1973;9:649–656.
23. Hamman L, Wainwright CW. The diagnosis of obscure fever. II. The diagnosis of unexplained high fever. Johns Hopkins Hosp Bull. 1936;58:307–331.
24. Berger L, Sinkoff MW. Systemic manifestations of hypernephroma: A review of 273 cases. Am J Med. 1957;22:791–796.
25. Shoji S, Imamura A, Imai Y, et al. Fever of unknown origin: A review of 80 patients from the Shin'etsu area of Japan from 1986–1992. Intern Med. 1994;33:74–76.
26. Saxe SE, Gardner P. The returning traveler with fever. Infect Dis Clin North Am. 1992;6:427–439.
27. Jacobs RF, Schutze GE: *Bartonella henselae* as a cause of prolonged fever and fever of unknown origin in children. Clin Infect Dis. 1998;26:80–84.
28. Gleckman RA, Esposito AL. Fever of unknown origin in the elderly: Diagnosis and treatment. Geriatrics. 1986;41:45–52.
29. Kauffman CA, Jones PG. Diagnosing fever of unknown origin in older patients. Geriatrics. 1984;39:46–51.
30. Ghose MK, Shensa S, Lerner PI. Arteritis of the aged (giant cell arteritis) and fever of unexplained origin. Am J Med. 1976;60:429–436.
31. Konecny P, Davidson RN. Pyrexia of unknown origin in the 1990s: Time to redefine. Br J Hosp Med. 1996;56:21–24.
32. Kountakis SE, Burke L, Rafie J-J, et al. Sinusitis in the intensive care unit patient. Otolaryngol Head Neck Surg. 1997;117:362–366.
33. Hughes WT, Armstrong D, Bodey GP, et al. Guidelines for the use of antimicrobial agents in neutropenic patients with unexplained fever. J Infect Dis. 1990;161:381–396.
34. Steinmetz H, Herbertz A, Bertram M, et al. Increase in interleukin-6 serum level preceding fever in granulocytopenia and correlation with death from sepsis. J Infect Dis. 1995;171:225–228.
35. De Kleijn EMHA, Dreuth JPH, Presman GJ, et al. Circulating and ex vivo production of pyrogenic cytokines and interleukin-1 receptor antagonist in 123 patients with fever of unknown origin. J Infect Dis. 1997;175:191–195.
36. Chang FY, Singh N, Gayowski T, et al. Fever in liver transplant recipients: Changing spectrum of etiologic agents. Clin Infect Dis. 1998;26:59–65.
37. Regnery RL, Anderson BE, Clarridge JE III, et al. Characterization of a novel *Rochalimaea* species, *R. henselae* sp nov, isolated from blood of a febrile, human immunodeficiency virus positive patient. J Clin Microbiol. 1992;30:265–274.
38. Miralles P, Moreno S, Perez-Tascon M, et al. Fever of uncertain origin in patients infected with the human immunodeficiency virus. Clin Infect Dis. 1995;20:872–875.
39. Bissuel F, Leport C, Perrone C, et al. Fever of unknown origin in HIV-infected patients: A critical analysis of a retrospective series of 57 cases. J Intern Med. 1994;236:529–535.
40. Wheeler DA, Call SC, Wasserman SS, et al. Relationship between basal body temperature and stage of disease in asymptomatic HIV-infected men. Infect Dis Clin Pract. 1997;6:47–50.
41. Sepkowitz KA. Effect of prophylaxis on the clinical manifestations of AIDS-related opportunistic infections. Clin Infect Dis. 1998;26:806–810.
42. Mayo J, Collazos J, Martinez E. Fever of unknown origin in the HIV-infected patient: New scenario for an old problem. Scand J Infect Dis. 1997;29:327–336.
43. Engels E, Marks PW, Kazanjian P. Usefulness of bone marrow evaluation of unexplained fever in patients infected with human immunodeficiency virus. Clin Infect Dis. 1995;21:427–428.
44. Kilby JM, Margues MB, Jaye DL, et al. The yield of bone marrow biopsy and culture compared with blood culture in the evaluation of HIV-infected patients for mycobacterial and fungal infections. Am J Med. 1998;104:123–128.
45. Aduan RP, Fauci AS, Dale DC, Wolff SM. Prolonged fever of unknown origin (FUO): A prospective study of 347 patients. Clin Res. 1978;26:558A.
46. Mackowiak PA. Commentary: Fever patterns. Infect Dis Clin Pract. 1997;6:308–309.
47. McCarthy PL, Dolan TF. Hyperpyrexia in children. Am J Dis Child. 1976;130:849–851.
48. McCarthy PL, Jekel JF, Dolan TF. Temperature greater than or equal to 40°C in children less than 24 months of age: A prospective study. Pediatrics. 1977;59:663–668.
49. Woodward TE. The fever pattern as diagnostic aid. In: Mackowiak PA, ed. Fever: Basic Mechanisms and Management, 2nd ed. Philadelphia: Lippincott-Raven; 1997;215–235.
50. Pizzo PA, Lovejoy FH, Smith DH: Prolonged fever in children: Review of 100 cases. Pediatrics. 1975;55:468–473.
51. Lohr JA, Hendley JO. Prolonged fever of unknown origin: A record of experiences with 54 childhood patients. Clin Pediatr. 1977;16:768–773.
52. Sheon RP, Van Ommeu RA. Fever of obscure origin: Diagnosis and treatment based on a series of sixty cases. Am J Med. 1963;34:486–499.
53. Vickery DM, Quinnell RK. Fever of unknown origin. An algorithmic approach. JAMA. 1977;238:2183–2188.
54. Esposito AL, Gleckman RA. A diagnostic approach to the adult with fever of unknown origin. Arch Intern Med. 1979;139:575–579.
55. Hurley DL. Fever in adults. What to do when the cause is not obvious? Postgrad Med. 1983;74:232–244.
56. Gries E, Hoensch H, Ohnhaus EE. Differential Diagnose bei bisher ungeklärtem Fieber: Bedeutung klinischer Begleir Symptome. Klin Wochenschr. 1986;64:307–313.
57. Nolan SM, Fitzgerald FT. Fever of unknown origin: The general internist's approach. Postgrad Med. 1987;81:190–205.
58. Koch H, Jenke V. Fieber unklarer Ursache—ein diagnostisches Basisprogramm. Z Gesamte Inn Med. 1990;1890:560–562.
59. Fischer JL, Henselmann L. Stufendiagnostik des Fieber unbekannter Ursache. Med Klin. 1987;82:229–235.
60. Rowland MD, Del Bene VE. Use of body computed tomography to evaluate fever of unknown origin. J Infect Dis. 1987;156:408–409.
61. Quinn MJ, Sheedy PF II, Stephen DH, Hattery RR. Computed tomography of the abdomen in evaluation of patients with fever of unknown origin. Radiology. 1980;136:407–411.
62. Knockaert DC, Vanneste LJ, Vanneste SB, Bobbaers HJ. Fever of unknown origin in the 1980s: An update of the diagnostic spectrum. Arch Intern Med. 1992;152:51–55.
63. Arnow PM, Flaherty JP. Fever of unknown origin. Lancet. 1997;350:575–580.
64. Knockaert DC, Mortelmans LA, De Roo MC, Bobbaers HJ. Clinical value of gallium-67 scintigraphy in evaluation of fever of unknown origin. Clin Infect Dis. 1994;18:601–605.
65. Syrjala MT, Valtonen V, Liewendahl K, Myllylä G. Diagnostic significance of indium-111 granulocyte scintigraphy in febrile patients. J Nucl Med. 1987;28:155–160.
66. Peters AM. Localizing the cause of undiagnosed fever. Eur J Nucl Med. 1996;23:239–242.
67. Peters AM, Roddie ME, Danpure HJ, et al. Tc-99m HMPAO labelled leucocytes: Comparison with In-111-tropolonate labelled granulocytes. Nucl Med Commun. 1988;9:449–463.
68. Lavender JP, Lowe J, Barker JR. Ga-67 citrate scanning in neoplastic and inflammatory lesions. Br J Radiol. 1971;44:361–366.
69. Hilson AJW, Maisey MN. Gallium-67 scanning in pyrexia of unknown origin. BMJ. 1979;II:1330–1331.
70. Sfakianakis GN, Al-Sheikh W, Heal A, et al. Comparison of scintigraphy with ^{111}In leukocytes and ^{67}Ga in the diagnosis of occult sepsis. J Nucl Med. 1982;23:618–626.
71. Rubin RH, Young LS, Hansen WP, et al. Specific and non-specific imaging of localized Fisher immunotype 1 *Pseudomonas aeruginosa* infection with radiolabeled monoclonal antibody. J Nucl Med. 1988;29:651–656.
72. Lind P, Langsteger W, Kotringer P, et al. Immunoscintigraphy of inflammatory processes with a technetium-99m–labeled monoclonal antigranulocyte antibody (Mab BW 250/183). J Nucl Med. 1990;31:417–423.
73. Oyen WJG, Claessens RAMJ, van der Meer JWM, et al. Detection of subacute infectious foci with In-111–labelled autologous leukocytes and In-111-labelled human nonspecific immunoglobulin G: A prospective comparative study. J Nucl Med. 1991;32:1854–1860.
74. Datz FL, Anderson CE, Ahluwalia R, et al. The efficacy of indium-111-polyclonal IgG for the detection of infection and inflammation. J Nucl Med. 1994;35:74–83.
75. AbuRahma AF, Saiedy S, Robinson PA, et al. Role of venous duplex imaging of the lower extremities in patients with fever of unknown origin. Surgery. 1997;121:366–371.
76. Larson EB, Featherstone HJ, Petersdorf RG. Fever of undetermined origin: Diagnosis and follow-up of 105 cases, 1970–1980. Medicine. 1982;61:269–292.
77. Solis-Herruzo JA, Benita V, Morillas JD. Laparoscopy in fever of unknown origin—study of seventy cases. Endoscopy. 1981;13:207–210.
78. Mitchell DP, Hanes TE, Hoyumpa AM Jr, Schenker S. Fever of unknown origin: Assessment of the value of percutaneous liver biopsy. Arch Intern Med. 1977;137:1001–1004.
79. Chang JC, Hawley BH. Neutropenic fever of undetermined origin (N-FUO): Why not use the naproxen test? Cancer Invest. 1995;13:448–450.
80. Knockaert DC, Dujardin KS, Bobbaers HJ. Long-term follow-up of patients with undiagnosed fever of unknown origin. Arch Intern Med. 1996;156:618–620.
81. Bodel P. Tumors and fever. Ann N Y Acad Sci. 1974;230:6–13.
82. Bodel P, Ralph P, Wenc K, Long JC. Endogenous pyrogen production by Hodgkin's disease and human histiocytic lymphoma cell lines *in vitro*. J Clin Invest. 1980;65:514–518.
83. Dinarello CA. Interleukin-1. Rev Infect Dis. 1984;6:51–95.
84. Lachman LB, Moore JO, Metzger RS. Preparation and characterization of LAF from acute monocytic and myelomonocytic leukemic cells. Cell Immunol. 1978;41:189–206.
85. Esposito AL, Gleckman R. Fever of unknown origin in the elderly. J Am Geriatr Soc. 1978;26:498–505.
86. Reimann HA. Periodic (Pel-Ebstein) fever of lymphomas. Ann Clin Lab Sci. 1977;7:1–5.
87. Cannady PB Jr, Sanford JP. Negative blood cultures in infective endocarditis: A review. South Med J. 1976;69:1420–1424.
88. Von Reyn CF, Levy BS, Arbeit RD, et al. Infective endocarditis: An analysis based on strict case definitions. Ann Intern Med. 1981;94:505–518.
89. Van Scoy RE. Culture-negative endocarditis. Mayo Clin Proc. 1982;57:149–154.

90. Washington JA II. The role of the microbiology laboratory in the diagnosis and antimicrobial treatment of infective endocarditis. Mayo Clin Proc. 1982;57:22–32.
91. O'Grady NP, Barie PS, Bartlett JC, et al. Practice guidelines for evaluating new fever in critically ill adult patients. Clin Infect Dis. 1998;26:1042–1059.
92. Rubinstein E, Noriega ER, Simberkoff MS, et al. Fungal endocarditis: Analysis of 24 cases and review of the literature. Medicine (Baltimore). 1975;54:331–334.
93. Tompkins LS, Roessler BJ, Redd SC, et al. Legionella prosthetic-value endocarditis. N Engl J Med. 1988;318:530–535.
94. Goodman BW. Temporal arteritis. Am J Med. 1979;67:839–852.
95. Pouchot J, Sampalis JS, Beaudet F, et al. Adult Still's disease: Manifestations, disease course, and outcome in 62 patients. Medicine. 1991;70:118–136.
96. Copper GS, Shlaes DM, Salata RA. Intraabdominal infection: Differences in presentation and outcome between younger patients and the elderly. Clin Infect Dis. 1994;19:146–148.
97. Mackowiak PA, LeMaistre CF. Drug fever: A critical appraisal of conventional concepts. Ann Intern Med. 1987;106:728–733.
98. Aduan RP, Fauci AS, Dale DC, et al. Factitious fever and self-induced infection, a report of 32 cases and review of the literature. Ann Intern Med. 1979;90:230–242.
99. Sarwari AR, Mackowiak PA. Factitious fever. Curr Clin Topics Infect Dis. 1997;17:88–94.
100. Petersdorf RG, Bennet IL. Factitious Fever. Ann Intern Med. 1957;46:1039–1062.
101. Rosenberg DA. Web of deceit: A literature review of Münchausen syndrome by proxy. Child Abuse Negl. 1987;11:547–563.
102. Rumans LW, Vosti KL. Factitious and fraudulent fever. Am J Med. 1978;65:745–755.
103. Reich D, Gottfried LA. Factitious disorders in a teaching hospital. Ann Intern Med. 1983;99:240–247.
104. Potin M, Regamey C, Glauser MP. Factitious fever as a cause of prolonged fevers (in French). J Suisse Med. 1983;113:1534–1539.
105. Marcus EL, Van Dijk JM. Fever of unknown origin (Letter). J Am Geriatr Soc. 1991;36:637–638.

Chapter 45

The Acutely Ill Patient with Fever and Rash

DAVID J. WEBER
MYRON S. COHEN
JO-DAVID FINE

A recognizable rash can lead to immediate diagnosis and appropriate therapy. Material isolated from involved skin, when properly handled, can confirm a specific diagnosis. Unfortunately, rashes often present a bewildering array of diagnostic possibilities. Dermatologists, who are generally more comfortable with evaluation of the skin, are not always available for immediate consultation. Furthermore, not infrequently, dermatologists and infectious disease specialists differ in their approach to the patient with a rash.

This chapter provides a framework for investigation of the cause of rash, with emphasis on the following: (1) a diagnostic approach to patients with fever and rash, (2) categories of skin lesions, and (3) brief descriptions of the most important febrile illnesses characterized by a rash.

APPROACH TO THE PATIENT

In the initial evaluation of patients with fever and rash, three concerns must be addressed immediately. First is whether the patient is well enough to provide further history, or whether cardiorespiratory support is urgently required. Second is whether the nature of the rash, in the context of presentation, demands institution of isolation precautions. Isolation is required primarily for patients whose illnesses allow droplet or airborne spread of the pathogen and includes both viral and bacterial disease. If deemed necessary, isolation practices should be scrupulously employed. Health care workers should exercise caution in all interactions with patients with undiagnosed infectious diseases, and they should use standard precautions including the avoidance of intimate contact with secretions.[1–6] Although the vast majority of skin eruptions are noninfectious in origin, gloves should always be worn during the examination of the skin whenever an infectious cause is being considered, because some infections (e.g., syphilis, herpes simplex) may be acquired by direct skin contact. In the event of potential exposure to a pathogen, health care workers should be evaluated by their occupational health service for postexposure prophylaxis or the need for work restrictions.[7] The third concern is whether the skin lesions are consistent with meningococcal disease (see later on); such cases require immediate institution of antibacterial therapy. Similar urgency may be warranted when lesions suggest bacterial septic shock or Rocky Mountain spotted fever, because appropriate use of antibiotics may improve survival.[8]

The history obtained from the patient should elicit the following information:

- Drug ingestion within the past 30 days
- Travel outside the local area
- Occupational exposure
- Sun exposure
- Immunizations
- Sexually transmitted disease exposure, including risk factors for infection with human immunodeficiency virus (HIV)
- Factors affecting immunologic status, including chemotherapy, steroid use, hematologic malignancy, solid organ or bone marrow transplantation, and functional or anatomic asplenia
- Valvular heart disease
- Prior illnesses, including a history of drug or antibiotic allergies
- Exposure to febrile or ill persons within the recent past
- Exposure to wild or rural habitats, insects, arthropods, and wild animals
- Pets and habits

The clinician should pay particular attention to the season of the year, which dramatically affects the epidemiology of febrile rashes of infectious origin.

Physical examination should focus on the following:

- Vital signs
- General appearance
- Signs of toxicity
- Presence and location of adenopathy
- Presence and morphology of genital, mucosal, or conjunctival lesions
- Detection of hepatosplenomegaly
- Presence of arthritis
- Signs of nuchal rigidity, meningismus, or neurologic dysfunction

Key ingredients in arriving at a correct diagnosis—or at least a useful, limited, "working" list of likely diagnoses—include determination of (1) the primary type(s) of skin lesions present, (2) the distribution of the eruption, (3) the pattern of progression of the rash, and (4) the timing of the onset of the rash relative to the onset of fever and other signs of systemic illness.[9–17] Whereas histologic findings from lesional skin biopsies may help to confirm some diagnoses,[18] the patterns observed are frequently not specific for a single organism, the presence of infectious agents may not always be detectable, and laboratory studies often require at least 24 hours to complete. Thus, the clinician must attempt to use other diagnostic skills during the early evaluation of a patient with fever and rash. As discussed elsewhere, specific types of primary skin lesions frequently suggest different infectious disorders in patients with fever and rash. For example, palpable purpura, the hallmark feature of leukoclastic vasculitis, is the prototypic early finding in meningococcemia and Rocky Mountain spotted fever, whereas rapidly enlarging but asymptomatic red dermal nodules instead suggest candidemia in the appropriate host. Skin nodules noted on very deep palpation are probably located within the subcutaneous fat, suggesting one of several types of panniculitis, including erythema nodosum, a disorder caused by many different types of inflammatory or infectious processes, and erythema induratum, which is a classic tuberculoid reaction.

Examples of differences in the types of primary skin lesions present in the setting of underlying systemic infectious diseases are summarized in Table 45–1, although it should be clear that such a classification, by itself, rarely ever suggests only a single diagnosis. On the other hand, the presence of other, more specific lesions, most notably "target" or "iris" lesions (as in erythema multiforme), may suggest a single diagnosis, implicating a limited group of underlying infectious diseases as possible causes. Similarly, the presence of some lesions in the setting of fever may immediately exclude an infectious disorder as the cause of rash. For example, high fever accompanying a paucity of tender, red to violaceous, peripherally mamillated plaques suggests Sweet's syndrome (a rare hypersensitivity reaction frequently associated with selected underlying malignancies) or, in the setting of chemotherapy, a rare drug-induced hypersensitivity phenomenon known as neutrophilic eccrine hidradenitis.[19]

Distribution or direction of spread of an eruption may be highly informative. The rash of Rocky Mountain spotted fever and acute meningococcal infection, for example, most often begins on the lower extremities and then spreads centrally (i.e., centripetally), whereas most drug- and viral infection–associated eruptions (with the exception of those caused by echoviruses and coxsackieviruses) begin on the face or trunk and spread outward (centrifugally). "Streaky" facial involvement, usually without other skin findings, is characteristic of infection due to parvovirus B19 (fifth disease, erythema infectiosum).

The number of lesions can also provide useful insight. For example, "rose spots" (see later on), the hallmark cutaneous feature of *Salmonella* infection, are characteristically present in much greater numbers in patients who have paratyphoid fever than in those who have typhoid fever. In contrast, brucellosis may be manifested by only one or a few clinically subtle skin lesions, as seen in a fixed drug eruption.

Finally, timing of the rash may be particularly helpful in allowing the clinician to exclude reactions due to certain drugs as the underlying cause. With the exception of urticarial eruptions, which usually occur within a few minutes to a few hours of the administration of a systemic agent, the more typical generalized maculopapular or morbilliform drug eruption typically occurs within the first 7 to 14 days of the first dose of the offending agent, suggesting the need for a very careful drug history (including start and stop dates for all medications taken within 30 days of the onset of eruption).

It must be emphasized that noninfectious processes often include skin rash and fever and should be among the diagnostic considerations in the initial evaluation.[20] As noted previously, the presence of some highly specific morphologic types or patterns of skin lesions may quickly suggest a noninfectious cause to the astute clinician, thereby obviating the need to pursue a more extensive clinical and laboratory evaluation.

About 5% of all patients to whom a drug is administered experience an adverse reaction. Adverse cutaneous reactions to drugs are frequent, affecting 2 to 3% of all hospitalized patients.[21–23] Therefore, a drug reaction must be considered in any patient with a generalized maculopapular rash, especially if associated with palmoplantar involvement. Severe cutaneous reactions often induced by drugs include Stevens-Johnson syndrome, toxic epidermal necrolysis, hypersensitivity syndrome, small-vessel vasculitis, serum sickness, anticoagulant-induced necrosis, and angioedema.[23]

Rashes associated with occupational exposures,[24, 25] athletics,[26] animal exposures,[27] and international travel[28, 29] have been reviewed elsewhere.

PATHOGENESIS OF SKIN RASH

Skin rash with fever can result from a local infectious process due to virtually any class of microbe that has been allowed to penetrate the stratum corneum and multiply locally. A typical example is streptococcal cellulitis. In rare cases, such localized inoculations result in more generalized eruptions, and the diagnosis is then relatively straightforward. However, eruptions that begin as generalized exanthems are the "rashes" that constitute the focus of this chapter.

An exanthem is a cutaneous eruption due to the systemic effects of a microorganism infecting the skin. An enanthem is an eruption caused in similar fashion but involving the mucous membranes. Microorganisms may produce eruptions by (1) multiplication in the skin (e.g., herpesviruses); (2) release of toxins that act on skin structures (e.g., in scarlet fever, infections due to *Pseudomonas aeruginosa*, toxic shock syndrome, staphylococcal scalded skin syndrome); (3) evoking an inflammatory response involving phagocytes and lymphocytes, in which the microbicidal/tumoricidal metabolism of host defense cells is directed at the skin; and (4) via effects on vasculature, including vaso-occlusion and necrosis or vasodilation with edema and hyperemia. Obviously, for many eruptions, several concurrent mechanisms can play a role.

DIFFERENTIAL DIAGNOSIS IN SKIN RASH

There are two ways to approach the investigation of infectious rash: either by the type of lesion visualized or by knowledge of individual pathogens and the rashes they produce (Table 45–2). Unfortunately, neither system alone serves both to generate a complete list of diagnostic possibilities to rule out disorders as appropriate. Accordingly, both approaches should be incorporated into evaluation of the patient with skin rash and fever.

Characteristics of the Lesion

Morphologic types of primary skin lesions include macules, papules, nodules, vesicles, bullae, pustules, and plaques. *Macules* are flat, nonpalpable lesions in the plane of the skin. *Papules* are small, solid, palpable lesions elevated above the plane of the skin. Large papules are referred to as *nodules. Vesicles* and *bullae* are small and large blisters, respectively, and *pustules* are usually small, palpable lesions filled with pus. *Plaques* are large, flat lesions, usually greater than 1 cm in diameter, that are palpable. In addition to morphology, lesions are characterized by their color and, particularly in the setting of a systemically ill-appearing patient, by the presence or absence of hemorrhage—hemorrhagic lesions being termed *purpura* or *petechiae*. Lesions may be skin-colored, hyperpigmented or hypopigmented, or any of several other colors of which red is the most common; the presence of such reddening is *erythema*. Blanching erythematous lesions are those in which erythema is due to vasodilatation, whereas nonblanching erythema may be due to extravasation of blood. As noted, purpuric lesions are those in which there is hemorrhage into the skin and may be small (petechial) or large (ecchymotic). For purposes of the following discussion, it is useful to divide eruptions into those that are maculopapular (characterized by both flat and elevated lesions), nodular, vesiculobullous, erythematous, and purpuric.

Maculopapular Rash

Maculopapular rashes are usually seen in viral illnesses, drug eruptions, and immune complex–mediated syndromes. Potentially responsible viral disorders include the classic childhood viral diseases such as measles, rubella, erythema infectiosum, and roseola.[30–32] Other viral agents that occasionally produce a maculopapular rash are coxsackieviruses, echoviruses, cytomegalovirus, and hepatitis B virus.

Erythema multiforme may be considered a special category of maculopapular rash. Usually, as the term *multiforme* signifies, this rash contains a wide range of different, concurrent morphologic types (including plaques, vesicles, and bullae), suggesting a much different diagnosis with a correspondingly different list of potential

TABLE 45–1 Systemic Infections with Prominent Cutaneous Manifestations

Organism/Disease	Macules, Papules	Vesicles, Bullae	Petechiae, Purpura
Viruses			
Human immunodeficiency virus type 1	X		
Echoviruses	X	X	X
Coxsackieviruses	X	X	X
Rubeola (measles)	X		
Atypical measles	X		X
Adenovirus	X		X
Lymphocytic choriomeningitis virus	X		
Dengue virus	X		X
Viral hemorrhagic fevers			X
Rubella (German measles)	X		X
Colorado tick fever	X		
Yellow fever			X
Varicella-zoster (disseminated)		X	
Herpes simplex (disseminated)		X	
Varicella (chickenpox)		X	
Vaccinia		X	
Cytomegalovirus	X		
Congenital cytomegalovirus			X
Epstein-Barr virus	X		X
Hepatitis B	X		X (as palpable purpura)
Parvovirus B19 (erythema infectiosum)	X		
Human herpesvirus 6	X		
Bacteria			
Chlamydia psittaci	X		
Mycoplasma pneumoniae	X	X	
Rickettsiae			
Rickettsia rickettsii (Rocky Mountiain spotted fever)	X		X
Rickettsia akari (rickettsialpox)	X	X	
Rickettsia prowazekii (epidemic/louse-borne typhus)	X		X
Rickettsia typhi (endemic/murine typhus)	X		
Rickettsia tsutsugamushi (scrub typhus)	X		
Bartonella henselae	X		
Bartonella quintana	X		
Salmonella typhi	X		
Francisella tularensis	X		
Streptobacillus moniliformis (rat-bite fever)	X		X
Treponema pallidum (secondary syphilis)	X		
Mycobacterium haemophilum	X		
Neisseria gonorrhoeae	X		X
Neisseria meningitidis			X
Leptospira spp.	X		
Listeria monocytogenes		X (rare)	
Bartonella bacilliformis	X		
Borrelia spp. (relapsing fever)	X		X
Borrelia burgdorferi (Lyme disease)	X (annular)		
Pseudomonas aeruginosa	X		
Spirillum minus (rat-bite fever)	X		
Staphylococcus aureus	X		X
Streptococci— group A (scarlet fever)	X		
Capnocytophaga canimorsus			X
Vibrio vulnificus		X	
Fungi (disseminated infection)			
Candida spp.	X		
Cryptococcus neoformans	X		
Histoplasma capsulatum	X		
Blastomyces dermatitidis	X		
Coccidioides immitis	X		
Fusarium spp. (agents of mucormycosis)	X		
Protozoa			
Plasmodium falciparum (malaria)			X

Data from refs. 11–15.

TABLE 45–2 Skin Lesions and Systemic Infections

Lesion	Common Pathogens	Histologic Findings	Smears Positive for Pathogens	Time to Appearance (after Onset of Illness)
Symmetric peripheral gangrene, purpura fulminans, acrocyanosis	Noninfectious or gram-negative bacteria, *Capnocytophaga canimorsus*	Bleeding in skin, vascular thrombosis, perivascular infiltration	No	12–36 h
Multiple purpuric lesions in severely ill patients	*Neisseria meningitidis, Capnocytophaga canimorsus, Rickettsia* spp., other gram-negative bacteria	Vascular thrombosis, perivascular hemorrhage	Yes*	12–36 h†
Echthyma gangrenosum, other bullous lesions	*Pseudomonas,* gram-negative bacteria, *Vibrio vulnificus*	Veins mainly involved, intima spared, inflammatory reaction	Yes	Several days
Macronodular lesions	*Candida, Cryptococcus neoformans, Histoplasma capsulatum, Fusarium*	Hyphae, mononuclear perivascular reaction	No	Several days
Delayed-onset rash with nonsymmetric, scattered, maculopapular or vesicular lesions	*Neisseria gonorrhoeae, Neisseria meningitidis* (chronic)	Perivascular mononuclear infiltrate, immune complex	Occasionally (few bacteria only)	3–10 d
Rose spots	*Salmonella* spp.	Perivascular mononuclear inflammation or leukocyoclastic vasculitis	No	5–10 d
"Toxic erythema"	*Staphylococcus aureus* (SSS)	Dilatation and perivascular edema	No	At presentation

*Except for Rocky Mountain spotted fever, in which biopsy and immunofluorescent staining are important for early diagnosis.
†In Rocky Mountain spotted fever, 1–7 days.
Adapted from Kingston ME, Mackey D. Skin clues in the diagnosis of life-threatening infections. Rev Infect Dis. 1986;8:1–11.

underlying infections and noninfectious causes to be excluded. Lesions of erythema multiforme usually begin as round to oval macules and papules that range in size from less than a centimeter up to 1 to 2 cm in diameter. The most characteristic lesions of erythema multiforme have central erythema surrounded by a narrow ring of normal-appearing skin that is in turn surrounded by another thin ring of erythema to form so-called target lesions (iris or "bull's-eye" lesions). The central area may be dark red, blue, or dusky gray in color and may develop into a blister. Lesions may be symmetrically or asymmetrically distributed on the trunk and extremities and may show a predilection for knees, elbows, palms, and soles. Mucosal involvement is usually present, accompanied by pain. The degree of mucosal involvement varies from oral blisters and erosions to a hemorrhagic conjunctivitis and stomatitis. When the latter are present with fever, the term *Stevens-Johnson syndrome* (erythema multiforme major) is applied.[21–23] In children and adults, infections constitute a leading cause (the most common being herpes simplex infection), but in adults, many cases are idiopathic or due to drug exposure. Infectious diseases linked to erythema multiforme are summarized in Table 45–3. More atypical rashes that may be initially suggestive of erythema multiforme may occur in chronic meningococcemia, bacterial endocarditis, secondary syphilis, staphylococcal scalded skin syndrome, Kawasaki disease, toxic shock syndrome, Rocky Mountain spotted fever, collagen vascular disease, and a variety of viral disorders. A clue useful in differentiating these disorders from erythema multiforme is the lack of target lesions.

Toxic epidermal necrolysis (TEN) constitutes a medical emergency, characterized by fever and generalized rash.[21, 22, 33] It may initially be confused with Stevens-Johnson syndrome (or, rarely, may even evolve from this condition). Untreated, TEN rapidly progresses to widespread full-thickness necrosis of the epidermis, resulting in separation of large sheets of epidermis from the underlying dermis either spontaneously or following the application of minimal lateral traction or pressure to the skin. TEN is almost always the result of a hypersensitivity reaction to a systemically administered drug. In some patients with early TEN (usually involving no more than 25% of the body surface area) in whom secondary infection was ruled out, remarkable reversal of this process was achieved after administration of high-dose corticosteroids, consistent with the inhibition of ongoing cellular immunologic reaction; this treatment remains controversial, however.[34] Both Stevens-Johnson syndrome and TEN are associated with significant morbidity and mortality, regardless of the underlying causative disorder. The causes of TEN are the same as those of Stevens-Johnson syndrome, but drugs are most frequently implicated. The mortality rate for Stevens-Johnson syndrome is 1 to 5%, and for TEN, 30 to 40%, with sepsis and gram-negative pneumonia the leading causes of death.

Human parvovirus B19 infection, the cause of erythema infectiosum (fifth disease), is manifested as a common exanthem in childhood and as a rheumatic syndrome in adults.[35, 36] Other disease manifestations include fever, anorexia, sore throat, abdominal pain, aplastic crisis in patients with hemoglobinopathies (e.g., sickle cell anemia), and hydrops fetalis with a risk of fetal death.[37–42] Erythema infectiosum is characterized by a three-stage rash. The initial stage is that of an erythematous, warm but nontender "slapped cheek" or streaked facial rash. Simultaneously or up to 4 days later, a more variable rash appears, most often on the upper extremities, that may have a morbilliform, confluent, lacelike ("reticulate"), or even annular appearance. Later the rash may remit, but it may recur with stress, exercise, exposure to sunlight, or bathing. The rash usually disappears within 1 to 2 weeks. Because by the time this rash has appeared in immunocompetent patients, viremia can no longer be detected, such patients are infective only prior to the appearance of the rash.[43] Rarely (approximately 25 cases reported), parvovirus B19 may cause the "papular-purpuric gloves and socks syndrome" (PPGSS), which is characterized by a rapidly progressive painful and highly pruritic, symmetric swelling and erythema of the distal hands and feet.[44] Confluent papular, purpuric lesions then develop that involve the dorsal and palmar surfaces of the hands and feet, with sharp margins at the wrists and ankles. Subsequently, most patients develop a polymorphous enanthem involving the hard and

TABLE 45-3 Known Causes of Erythema Multiforme

Noninfectious

Drugs (especially sulfonamides)
X-ray therapy

Infectious

Herpes simplex infections
Epstein-Barr virus (infectious mononucleosis)
Adenovirus type 7 (respiratory tract infection)
Coxsackieviruses A10, A16, B5 (enteroviral syndrome)
Echovirus type 6 (enteroviral syndrome)
Vaccinia virus (smallpox inoculation)
Variola virus (smallpox)
Varicella virus (chickenpox)
Orf (echthyma contagiosum)
Paravaccinia virus (milker's nodules)
Influenza A virus (influenza)
Mumps virus (mumps)
Hepatitis B virus (hepatitis)
Mycoplasma pneumoniae (respiratory infection)
Chlamydia psittaci (psittacosis)
Chlamydia trachomatis (lymphogranuloma venereum)
Bartonella henselae (cat-scratch disease)
Staphylococcus aureus (sepsis)
Streptococcus pyogenes (sepsis)
Neisseria gonorrhoeae (gonorrhea)
Corynebacterium diphtheriae (diphtheria)
Pseudomonas aeruginosa (sepsis)
Francisella tularensis (tularemia)
Salmonella typhi (typhoid fever)
Salmonella spp. (salmonellosis)
Yersinia spp. (gastroenteritis)
Vibrio parahaemolyticus (gastroenteritis)
Treponema pallidum (syphilis)
Mycobacterium tuberculosis (tuberculosis)
Mycobacterium leprae (leprosy)
Histoplasma capsulatum (histoplasmosis)
Coccidioides immitis (coccidioidomycosis)
Trichomonas vaginalis (vulvovaginitis)

soft palates, buccal mucosa, and lips. This syndrome generally clears spontaneously within 1 to 2 weeks.

In several life-threatening infections, the presenting manifestations may include blanching erythematous maculopapular lesions that later evolve into petechiae, making initial diagnosis difficult on the basis of lesion morphology alone. These infections include acute meningococcemia, Rocky Mountain spotted fever, and viral hemorrhagic fevers such dengue. Although a diagnostic feature of rheumatic fever is an annular or polycyclic, migrating (or expanding) erythema known as *erythema marginatum*, this disease may also be associated with the presence of a maculopapular eruption and subcutaneous nodules. Patients with enteric fever due to *Salmonella* may develop "rose spots," a transient scattering of rose-colored macules over the abdomen. Typically, the rose spots of typhoid fever are pale pink in color, oval or circular in shape, completely blanchable, few in number, moderately sized (up to 0.5 to 1.0 cm in diameter), and usually present on the abdomen or trunk.[45] In contrast, rose spots of paratyphoid fever are typically smaller in size and more numerous in number.

Physicians should be familiar with the cutaneous manifestations of syphilis, because primary and secondary syphilis and congenital syphilis continue to occur in the United States, especially in the South Atlantic states.[46, 47] The primary skin lesion (chancre) typically develops about 21 days after exposure. Secondary syphilis is often accompanied by a rash with highly variable morphology. Lesions may be macular, papular, maculopapular, papulosquamous, or pustular. Occasionally, all types of lesions may be present in the same patient. A characteristic presentation of secondary syphilis is that of a pityriasis rosea–like eruption, appearing as numerous, tan to reddish-brown, scaly macules, usually distributed along skin tension lines on the trunk and, to a lesser extent, other body sites. Typically, no herald patch (a hallmark feature of pityriasis rosea) is present when this eruption is caused by syphilis, and usually the patient with secondary syphilis lacks associated pruritus and may have concurrent "copper penny" macules or plaques on the palms or soles. Condylomata lata, which are grayish, raised, broad, flat-appearing papular lesions, may occur in skinfolds or apposed skin in moist areas, such as the anus, vulva, and scrotum.

Nodular Lesions

A nodule is a palpable, solid, round or ellipsoidal lesion, usually resulting from disease in the dermis. Nodules may contain various inflammatory cells (as part of a hypersensitivity phenomenon), organisms (most notably fungi, as in septic emboli), or tumor cells (from metastatic cancer, lymphoma, or leukemia cutis). In the appropriate clinical setting, sudden development of dermal nodules may suggest candidal sepsis (see later on), but other fungal diseases including blastomycosis, histoplasmosis, coccidioidomycosis, and sporotrichosis may produce skin nodules. Bacteria such as *Nocardia* and atypical mycobacteria (especially *Mycobacterium marinum*) may also cause nodular lesions (which typically later ulcerate).[48] Lesions consistent with echthyma gangrenosum, typified by the presence of deep, "punched-out" ulcerations with overlying black eschar and peripheral erythema, suggest *Pseudomonas* sepsis. A skin biopsy specimen with appropriate stains and cultures defines the diagnosis.

Subcutaneous nodules pose a real diagnostic challenge, because they may reflect the presence of a variety of underlying disorders, including hypersensitivity reactions to systemic infection. The lesions of erythema nodosum are characterized by tender, erythematous nodules that range in diameter from less than a centimeter to several centimeters. They are usually multiple and located on the anterior portions of the legs but may be solitary and occur on other parts of the body. They typically do not suppurate. These lesions often develop in crops and usually heal in days to a few weeks without scarring. Infectious agents are a prominent cause of this lesion (Table 45–4). In contrast, erythema induratum, a known tuberculoid reaction, typically presents as painful, red, subcutaneous nodules over the posterior ankles. These lesions tend to suppurate, distinguishing them morphologically from erythema nodosum and most

TABLE 45-4 Known Causes of Erythema Nodosum

Noninfectious

Systemic lupus erythematosus
Sarcoidosis
Ulcerative colitis
Crohn's colitis
Behçet's disease
Drugs (especially oral contraceptives)
Pregnancy

Infectious

Hepatitis C virus (hepatitis)
Herpes simplex virus
Streptococcus pyogenes (respiratory tract infection)
Chlamydia psittaci (psittacosis)
Chlamydia trachomatis (lymphogranuloma venereum)
Neisseria meningitidis (meningitis)
Bartonella henselae (cat-scratch disease)
Corynebacterium diphtheriae (diphtheria)
Campylobacter spp. (gastroenteritis)
Haemophilus ducreyi (chancroid)
Yersinia spp. (gastroenteritis)
Treponema pallidum (syphilis)
Mycobacterium tuberculosis (tuberculosis)
Mycobacterium leprae (leprosy)
Mycobacterium marinum (atypical mycobacteriosis)
Cryptococcus neoformans (cryptococcosis)
Blastomyces dermatitidis (blastomycosis)
Histoplasma capsulatum (histoplasmosis)
Coccidioides immitis (coccidioidomycosis)
Wuchereria bancrofti (filariasis)

other types of panniculitis. Furthermore, erythema induratum can usually be easily differentiated from erythema nodosum on histologic examination of a wedge biopsy specimen: inflammation can be seen within subcutaneous fat lobules in the former, rather than within septal connective tissue as classically seen in erythema nodosum. Acid-fast bacilli are rarely visible within the lesions of erythema induratum, because this condition typically represents reactivation of long-standing infection with, or hypersensitivity to, the tuberculosis bacilli that are present at distant sites.

Diffuse Erythema

Diffuse erythema, especially if desquamation or peeling is present, should lead to consideration of scarlet fever, toxic shock syndromes, mucocutaneous lymph node syndrome (Kawasaki disease), staphylococcal scalded skin syndrome, Stevens-Johnson syndrome, and TEN. Desquamation may occur late in all of these syndromes, and its absence early in the clinical course should not be considered a reason for excluding any disease process. Most of these disorders can be easily diagnosed on the basis of the patient's history and appropriate tests.

Vesiculobullous Eruptions

A vesicle is a circumscribed, elevated lesion containing free fluid. A vesicular lesion larger than 0.5 cm is termed a bulla. Most vesiculobullous eruptions are immunologic in origin; few are associated with infectious systemic infections. Infectious diseases to be considered include varicella, disseminated herpes simplex, eczema herpeticum (herpes simplex superinfection of atopic eczema), and infections due to echoviruses and coxsackieviruses (including coxsackievirus A16, the cause of hand-foot-and-mouth disease). Herpes simplex infection, the most common of these infections, is characterized by a grouped clustering of vesicles on an erythematous base that progresses to mucocutaneous ulceration.[49] Viral culture of a scraping from a blister may allow determination of a herpes infection. In addition, the demonstration of multinucleated giant cells in a scraping (Tzanck preparation) of the base of a vesicle indicates infection with herpes simplex or varicella-zoster virus. Older vesicles can be easily confused with pustules. A pustule is an elevation of the skin enclosing a purulent exudate. Vesicular lesions may at times become pustules, as can occur with herpes simplex or varicella-zoster lesions. Diffuse pustular diseases usually represent a noninfectious dermatologic illness (e.g., pustular psoriasis) or a cutaneous infection (e.g., pustular *Pseudomonas* lesions developing after the use of contaminated hot tubs or staphylococcal folliculitis).[50] Pustular skin lesions associated with arthralgias should lead to a consideration of gonococcemia, *Moraxella* bacteremia, chronic meningococcemia, subacute bacterial endocarditis, coxsackievirus infection, and Behçet's syndrome.

Bullous skin lesions with sepsis are suggestive of the following infections: group A streptococcal erysipelas with necrotizing fasciitis (gangrenous erysipelas), echthyma gangrenosum (due to *Pseudomonas aeruginosa* or *Aeromonas* spp.), *Vibrio* infections (especially those due to *Vibrio vulnificus*), staphyloccocal cellulitis or impetigo, and streptococcal cellulitis. Rarely, in immunocompromised patients the initial manifestation of gram-negative sepsis may be the appearance of a solitary hemorrhagic blister. *V. vulnificus* infection should be strongly considered in patients with preexisting liver disease, or other immunocompromising states, who have recently ingested raw seafood.[51, 52] Vesicopustular eruptions in the neonate may be due to both noninfectious and infectious causes. Potential infectious causes include congenital and neonatal candidiasis, staphylococcal infections, streptococcal infections, *Listeria monocytogenes* infection, herpes simplex, neonatal varicella, and bacterial sepsis (due to various organisms).[53]

Petechial and Purpuric Eruptions

Petechiae are lesions less than 3 mm in diameter containing extravasated red blood cells or hemoglobin. Larger lesions are termed ecchymoses or purpura. Diffuse petechial lesions should always prompt urgent investigation. In critically ill patients these lesions are often associated with symmetric peripheral gangrene (purpura fulminans), consumptive coagulopathy, and shock. The most common infectious agents include gram-negative organisms, especially *Neisseria meningitidis*, and rickettsiae. Less commonly, *L. monocytogenes* or staphylococci may be associated with a similar clinical picture. Asplenic patients are at an increased risk of overwhelming sepsis (lifetime risk of approximately 5%), which may be accompanied by symmetric peripheral gangrene.[54–62] About half of the latter infections are due to *Streptococcus pneumoniae*.[54, 55, 57, 62]

Viral illnesses associated with petechial rashes include infections due to coxsackievirus A9, echovirus 9, Epstein-Barr virus, or cytomegalovirus; atypical measles; and the viral hemorrhagic fevers (see Chapter 155). Although children with coxsackievirus and echovirus infections are usually nontoxic in appearance, some may appear very ill. In these patients, differential diagnosis from acute meningococcemia is difficult. However, in a series of children presenting with fever and petechiae, only 8% had meningococcal infections and 4% had bacterial sepsis secondary to other disorders.[63, 64]

Rashes are a prominent characteristic of all rickettsial diseases except for Q fever. Although Rocky Mountain spotted fever is the most common rickettsial disease in the United States, other rickettsial diseases may occur, including murine (endemic) typhus, rickettsialpox, and sylvatic typhus.[65] Lesions caused by rickettsiae are usually generalized and symmetric. An eschar *(tache noire)* characteristically develops at the site of inoculation in the following rickettsial infections: African tick typhus (caused by *Rickettsia conorii*), North Asian tick-borne rickettsiosis (due to *Rickettsia sibirica*), Queensland tick typhus (due to *Ricksettsia australis*), rickettsialpox (due to *Rickettsia akari*), and scrub- or chigger-borne typhus (due to *Ricksettsia tsutsugamushi*). New rickettsioses continue to be recognized worldwide that are characterized by generalized skin lesions, such as Japanese or Oriental spotted fever (caused by *Ricksettsia japonica*) and Flinders Island spotted fever (due to *Rickettsia honei*), or by a tache noire lesion, such as Astrakhan fever and African tick-bite fever (due to *Rickettsia africae*).[66]

In patients with an appropriate travel history, infection with *Plasmodium falciparum* must be considered.[67] In addition, clinicians should be aware that malaria may occasionally be acquired in the United States.[68] Heavy parasitization may lead to severe hemolysis, renal failure, central nervous system abnormalities, and petechiae secondary to thrombocytopenia (rash is present in about 5% of affected patients).

The most important causes of noninfectious petechiae are thrombocytopenia, large and small vessel necrotizing vasculitis (usually presenting as palpable purpura), and the pigmented purpuric eruptions (which usually represent capillaritis).

Enanthems

In attempting to classify the exanthem, it is essential that a thorough search of the mucous membranes (including the mouth, conjunctiva, and occasionally also the vagina, rectum, and glans penis) be made for the presence of enanthems. In many allergic reactions the mucous membranes are frequently involved. Koplick spots, diagnostic of rubeola, are tiny, white or blue-gray specks superimposed on an erythematous base, located on the buccal mucosa, most prominently on that adjacent to the molars. A "strawberry tongue" suggests the possibility of Kawasaki disease, toxic shock syndrome, or scarlet fever. Petechiae of the palate are common in scarlet fever and some vasculitides and with thrombocytopenia. In infectious mononucleosis, petechiae of both the hard palate and soft palate are common. Oral ulcers occur in a variety of noninfectious immunologic diseases and also with coxsackievirus A16 infection.

DERMATOLOGIC CONDITIONS ASSOCIATED WITH FEVER THAT ARE FREQUENTLY CONFUSED WITH INFECTIOUS PROCESSES

Sweet's Syndrome

Sweet's syndrome, also known as febrile neutrophilic dermatosis, is an unusual hypersensitivity phenomenon characterized by the development of one or more tender, red, edematous, urticarial plaques or large papules.[69, 70] Often the border of each plaque is studded with papules (or, infrequently, with vesicles or pustules), giving an irregularly contoured, mamillated appearance reminiscent of that of the aureoles of the breast. If solitary and large, such lesions may be confused with those caused by a variety of infectious processes including primary herpes simplex infection or streptococcal cellulitis. When solitary and present on the dorsum of the hand, a lesion of Sweet's syndrome may mimic erysipeloid or a severe reaction to an arthropod bite. Occasionally, these plaques become dusky in color and frankly hemorrhagic, suggesting instead erythema multiforme or leukocytoclastic vasculitis. Some lesions may also become bullous, suggesting bullous erythema multiforme or fixed drug eruption. Rare bullous lesions may erode or ulcerate, mimicking pyoderma gangrenosum. Mucosal surfaces may rarely be involved. Characteristically, patients with Sweet's syndrome have associated fever; other findings may include leukocytosis, malaise, arthralgias, myalgias, conjunctivitis, and episcleritis. The hallmark histologic feature of this disorder is the presence of numerous neutrophils within the dermis, especially in a perivascular array.

Sweet's syndrome responds rapidly to high-dose systemic corticosteroids, but relapse is frequent if tapering is too rapid. Although at times idiopathic, this disorder may be a marker for underlying leukemia (especially acute myelogenous leukemia), as well as other internal malignancies.

Dilantin Hypersensitivity Syndrome

The Dilantin (phenytoin) hypersensitivity syndrome is commonly confused with a variety of systemic infections, and the correct diagnosis is often realized only after exhaustive microbiologic cultures have proved negative and empirical antibiotics have been used without success. Patients with this unique hypersensitivity reaction typically manifest sudden fever, with temperatures often as high as 104°F (40°C), and a clinical appearance of toxicity, followed by the development of rash, generalized lymphadenopathy, and leukocytosis (sometimes with mild eosinophilia). In more protracted cases, hepatosplenomegaly may occur in association with elevated transaminase levels. Without treatment, small numbers of patients eventually die of either hepatic necrosis or renal failure.

This heterogeneous eruption is remarkably distinctive, allowing for its diagnosis at the bedside. The face is edematous and red. Lips may be similarly swollen and red. Confluent erythema is present on the central trunk, with a paucity of tiny sterile pustules studding the surface of the flanks. A more morbilliform maculopapular eruption is present acrally, and the palms and soles are also involved. In contrast to most drug eruptions, the Dilantin hypersensitivity syndrome typically occurs months or later into treatment with the drug and will recur if the patient receives any of several other anticonvulsants (most notably phenobarbital and carbamazepine [Tegretol]). Treatment involves discontinuation of the offending drug and administration of high-dose systemic corticosteroids; major flares can be expected if a very slow taper over several months is not used.

PATHOGENS OR INFECTIOUS CONDITIONS STRONGLY ASSOCIATED WITH RASH

As noted previously, the investigation of infectious rash requires consideration of not only the characteristics of the skin lesions but also the pathogens and infectious processes strongly associated with rash. The following discussion reviews the various skin manifestations of these pathologic processes.

Septicemia

Kingston and Mackey[18] have classified the skin lesions associated with septicemia into five pathogenic processes (major categories of infectious causes): (1) disseminated intravascular coagulation (DIC) and coagulopathy (due to *N. meningitidis,* streptococci, enteric gram-negative bacilli); (2) direct vascular invasion and occlusion by bacteria and fungi (*N. meningitidis, P. aeruginosa, Candida* spp., *Aspergillus* spp., *Rickettsia* spp.); (3) immune vasculitis and immune complex formation (associated with infection due to *N. meningitidis, Neisseria gonorrhoeae, Salmonella typhi*); (4) formation of emboli in endocarditis (due to *Staphylococcus aureus,* streptococci); and (5) vascular effects of toxins (in staphylococcal scalded skin syndrome, toxic shock syndrome, scarlet fever). Various systemic bacterial infections may spread to the skin, generally producing discrete lesions from which the organisms can be isolated or recognized on biopsy with special stains. Cutaneous manifestations of DIC include symmetric peripheral gangrene, purpura fulminans, localized gangrene, acrocyanosis, other types of purpura, ecchymoses, bleeding from wound and venipuncture sites, and subcutaneous hematomas.[20, 69] *Symmetric peripheral gangrene* is defined as ischemic necrosis simultaneously involving the distal portions of two or more extremities without proximal arterial obstruction.[70] Potential causative disorders include cardiogenic shock and other low-flow states, disorders that induce severe vasospasm such as ergot poisoning and Raynaud's syndrome, disorders that lead to obstruction of small blood vessels such as cold agglutinin disease/syndrome or primary polycythemia, snake bites, and infections.[70–72] *N. meningitidis* is the organism most commonly responsible for symmetric peripheral gangrene, but this disorder may also be due to *S. pneumoniae* and other streptococcal species, *S. aureus, Escherichia coli, Klebsiella* spp., *Proteus* spp., *Aeromonas hydrophila, Aspergillus*, and other gram-negative organisms.[69, 71, 73] Symmetric peripheral gangrene is preceded by bleeding into the skin, ecchymosis, purpura, and acrocyanosis (a grayish cyanosis that does not blanch on pressure and occurs on the lips, legs, nose, ear lobes, and genitalia). Subsequently, the ecchymotic lesions become confluent, blister, undergo necrosis and ulceration, and develop overlying eschars.[18] Histologic examination reveals a Shwartzman-like reaction in the skin characterized by diffuse and extensive hemorrhages, perivascular cuffing, and intravascular thrombosis. Bacteria are usually absent from smears of the lesions. Shock rather than DIC appears to be the major factor in the pathogenesis of symmetric peripheral gangrene.

The term *purpura fulminans* has been used synonymously with *symmetric peripheral gangrene* and in a more restricted sense to describe symmetric bleeding into the skin and subsequent necrosis after a benign infection.[20] This latter syndrome, although most commonly reported in children, may affect adults[74] as well and usually follows pharyngitis or a viral exanthem by several days.[71, 75, 76] Common preceding illnesses include scarlet fever, streptococcal pharyngitis, staphylococcal bacteremia, varicella, and measles. Histologically, it resembles an Arthus reaction or localized Shwartzman reaction[77] with deposition of antigen-antibody complexes in tissues. The pathogenesis of purpura fulminans appears to be related to an acquired or transient deficiency of protein C or protein S, or of both, because identical lesions have been seen in infants with homozygous protein C deficiency and in patients with heterozygous deficiency of protein C or S during the initial phase of warfarin sodium (Coumadin) therapy.[74]

Infections Due to *Neisseria* Species

Neisseria meningitidis *Infection*

Purpuric skin lesions have been noted in 50 to 90% of patients with fulminant meningococcemia.[78–80] The lesions characteristically are petechial but may be noted to blanch with pressure early in the course of infection, thus resembling a viral exanthem. The petechiae are irregular and small and are often accompanied by palpable purpuric lesions, some of which may have pale centers. Coalescing lesions, often macular, may have a characteristic gun metal–gray color centrally, consistent with epidermal necrosis. Lesions most commonly occur on the extremities and trunk but may also be found on the head, palms and soles, and mucous membranes. Symmetric peripheral gangrene may rapidly develop, often in association with DIC. Histologic examination reveals diffuse endothelial damage, fibrin thrombi, necrosis of the vessel walls, and perivascular hemorrhage in the involved skin.[79, 81] Gram staining of aspirates of the involved areas frequently reveals the presence of organisms.[78, 82]

Meningococcal endotoxin is a potent producer of the dermal Shwartzman reaction in mice and probably plays an important role in the frequency of hemorrhagic cutaneous manifestations in meningococcal infections.[83] Skin lesions and bacteremia are rarely findings in patients with meningococcal pneumonia.[84]

Chronic meningococcemia is a rare disease. The classic clinical constellation of symptoms includes intermittent or sustained fevers; recurring maculopapular, nodular, pustular, or petechial eruptions; and migratory arthritis or arthralgias with little systemic toxicity.[85, 86] In one large series comprising 148 patients, skin lesions were noted to occur in 93%.[86] A variety of skin lesions may occur in chronic meningococcemia, the most frequently reported being pale to pink-colored macules and papules, seen in over 40% of cases. Nodular lesions may occur, mostly on the lower extremities. Petechiae of variable size may be seen, with superimposed vesicules or pustules centrally. Small, irregularly round, subcutaneous hemorrhages with a bluish-gray center containing pus cells are a distinctive lesion of this syndrome. Ecchymotic areas or hemorrhagic, tender nodules that are located deep in the dermis may also occur. Lesions associated with chronic meningococcemia tend to appear in showers in association with the onset of fever. In contrast to the lesions associated with fulminant meningococcemia, those of chronic meningococcemia rarely include organisms demonstrable on Gram-stained smear or biopsy specimen.[87] In addition, purpura fulminans is not a typical finding in chronic meningococcemia.

Neisseria gonorrhoeae *Infection*

Disseminated gonococcal infection (DGI) follows untreated mucosal infection with *N. gonorrhoeae* in about 0.5 to 3% of patients.[88–91] Skin lesions are the most common manifestation of DGI and occur in 50 to 70% of patients.[92] The eruption typically appears during the first day of symptoms and may recur with each bout of fever.[93] The skin lesions associated with DGI begin as tiny red papules or petechiae 1 to 5 mm in diameter, many of which evolve rapidly through vesicular or pustular stages to develop a gray necrotic center, often on a hemorrhagic base.[93, 94] Papules, bullae, pustules, and hemorrhagic lesions all may be present simultaneously. The lesions tend to be scanty but widely distributed. The distal portions of the extremities are most commonly involved (at times associated with tenosynovitis), with sparing of the scalp, face, trunk, and oral mucous membranes. Histologic examination reveals leukocytoclastic vasculitis with fibrin thrombi.[95] Gram-stained smears of material from skin lesions infrequently contain organisms, although most smears are positive for gonococci when examined by immunofluorescence techniques. Circulating immune complexes may play a role in the pathogenesis of DGI-associated skin lesions and arthritis/tenosynovitis.[96]

Pseudomonas Infection

Superficial infection with *P. aeruginosa* (pseudomonal folliculitis) has followed bathing in contaminated whirlpools, hot tubs, and swimming pools.[97] The lesions appear as large, follicular-based, tender, red papules. They are present only in areas exposed to *Pseudomonas*-contaminated waters. Skin lesions have been reported to accompany *P. aeruginosa* sepsis in 13 to 39% of patients.[98–100] The dermatologic manifestations of *P. aeruginosa* sepsis include echthyma gangrenosum,[99–108] subcutaneous nodules,[99, 109–113] vesicular lesions,[99] gangrenous cellulitis, small papules sometimes resembling the macular rose spots of typhoid fever,[114] and grouped petechiae.[107] Echthyma gangrenosum, the most characteristic skin lesion caused by *P. aeruginosa*, has generally been reported to occur in 1.3 to 2.8% of septic patients,[98, 115, 116] but one report noted echthyma gangrenosum in 28% of patients with *Pseudomonas* bacteremia.[100]

Echthyma gangrenosum lesions begin as painless, round, erythematous macules, with or without adherent vesicles, that soon become indurated and progress to hemorrhagic bluish bullae. Later, the lesion sloughs to form a deep gangrenous ulcer with a gray-black eschar and a surrounding erythematous halo. The process evolves rapidly over a period of 12 to 24 hours. Lesions may be discrete or multiple and are usually found in the groin, axilla, or perianal areas but may occur anywhere on the body. Although most commonly associated with *P. aeruginosa* sepsis, echthyma gangrenosum–like lesions have also been reported in sepsis associated with other pseudomonal species,[117] *A. hydrophilia*,[118, 119] *Candida* spp.,[120] *Serratia marcescens*,[102] *S. aureus*,[102] *Aspergillus* spp.,[102] and *Mucor* spp.[101] It may also result from vasculitis or malignant infiltration.[121] Rarely, echthyma gangrenosum due to *P. aeruginosa* may occur in the absence of sepsis.[108, 122, 123]

Histologically, echthyma gangrenosum is characterized by three features: bacterial invasion of the media and adventitia of vein walls deep in the dermis, sparing of the intima and lumen, and minimal inflammation.[104, 106, 118, 121] Bacterial invasion results in marked fibrin exudation and frank hemorrhage, followed by bulla formation. Finally, necrosis of the dermis occurs. Bacteria are readily visible in biopsy samples and can be demonstrated in Gram-stained material scraped from the base of the lesion.[103]

Subcutaneous nodules may result from *P. aeruginosa* bacteremia. Characteristically, the nodules are erythematous and warm, may be either fluctuant or nonfluctuant, and may be tender. Despite prolonged antibiotic therapy, these lesions may contain viable bacteria weeks after the blood has been cleared of infection. The absence of fluctuance may be due to either the lack of pus in neutropenic patients or the deep location of the abscess, or both. Although successful treatment may require incision and drainage,[111, 112] prolonged antibiotic therapy without drainage may result in a cure.[109, 113]

Bacterial Endocarditis

Skin lesions have been reported to accompany bacterial endocarditis in 15 to 50% of cases.[124–127] Skin lesions include Osler's nodes, Janeway lesions, and petechiae. The prevalence of embolic and hypersensitivity lesions in skin and mucous membranes (50%) in heroin-associated infective endocarditis is similar to that described in patients with non–heroin-associated infective endocarditis.[128]

Osler's nodes occur in about 5 to 15% of patients with subacute bacterial endocarditis. These lesions are tender, indurated, erythematous nodules, with a pale center about 1.0 to 1.5 mm in diameter.[129, 130] Osler's nodes most commonly occur on the pads of the fingers or toes but may also occur on the thenar and hypothenar eminences and over the arms. Pain may be elicited by palpating the tips of the digits. Osler's nodes tend to occur in crops, are rarely numerous, and tend to be transient. The lesions usually resolve without necrosis or suppuration 1 to 3 days after antibiotic therapy is initiated. Histologically, Osler's nodes show microabscesses with microemboli in adjacent arterioles. Osler's nodes are most commonly associated with subacute bacterial endocarditis due to infection with streptococci but may occur in endocarditis due to infection with fungi or gram-negative bacilli[130] or in systemic lupus erythematosus, typhoid fever, and gonococcemia.[20] Osler's nodes probably represent the sequelae of vascular occlusion by microemboli leading to localized vasculitis.[131]

Janeway lesions consist of small erythematous macules or, less commonly, small nodular hemorrhages in the palms and soles. Although they may be seen in subacute bacterial endocarditis, they are more common in acute endocarditis, especially that due to *S. aureus*. Unlike Osler's nodes, Janeway lesions are painless. Histologically, they show microabscesses with neutrophil infiltration of capillaries.

Petechiae are the most common skin and mucous membrane lesions observed in endocarditis, occurring in about 50% of patients. The lesions are small, flat, reddish-brown lesions that do not blanch on pressure. Mucous membrane involvement is common. Petechiae frequently occur in small crops. Lesions usually are transient.

Infections Due to *Staphylococcus aureus* and *Streptococcus pyogenes*

Most commonly, *S. aureus* and *Streptococcus pyogenes* cause local skin infections including cellulitis and folliculitis (see Chapter 78). Both pathogens may produce serious local infection including abscesses, myositis, and fasciitis (see Chapter 79). *S. aureus* is responsible for a variety of infectious syndromes that may produce local or diffuse skin lesions.[132–138] Skin lesions arise from (1) production of toxins (as in staphylococcal scalded skin syndrome and toxic shock syndrome),[139, 140] (2) shock, and (3) vascular invasion, often in association with endocarditis.

Staphylococcal Scalded Skin Syndrome

S. aureus strains belonging to phage group II (types 3A, 3B, 3C, 55, 71) may produce exfoliative toxins. These toxins are capable of causing a clinical spectrum of disease that includes bullous impetigo, a generalized scarlatiniform eruption without exfoliation, and exfoliative disease—that is, staphylococcal scalded skin syndrome (SSSS).[134, 136, 141–144] Bullous impetigo, a disorder usually confined to children, which results from toxin-producing strains of *S. aureus*, is characterized by discrete, flaccid bullae containing clear or cloudy yellow fluid. Lesions are frequently localized to the umbilicus, groin, or axillae. The surrounding skin may appear normal or mildly erythematous. The bullae rapidly rupture, leaving raw, denuded erosions that reepithelialize in 5 to 7 days. Affected infants are usually afebrile and lack constitutional signs.

SSSS (Ritter's disease) usually occurs in neonates or young children but may affect older children or, rarely, adults. Most cases in adults occur in association with renal impairment, lymphoma, or immunosuppression.[144–149] A well-characterized animal model exists for SSSS. Unlike in bullous impetigo, in which the staphylococcal infection is in the skin at the site of the lesion, in SSSS the infection begins abruptly with a diffuse, blanchable erythema in association with marked skin tenderness, fever, and irritability. Light stroking of the ill-defined bullae causes rupture and separation of the upper portion of the epidermis (Nikolsky's sign). Generalized desquamation usually occurs. Unless secondary infection intervenes, the skin heals within 10 to 14 days. A skin biopsy specimen (or a frozen section of an induced peel for more rapid diagnosis) may be studied to distinguish between SSSS and TEN. In SSSS, the cleavage plane of the early intraepidermal bulla is just beneath the granular cell layer, whereas in TEN, the bulla is subepidermal and associated with full-thickness necrosis of the epidermis. Early distinction between these two diseases is important because the therapy for SSSS includes antistaphylococcal antibiotics, whereas in TEN discontinuation of treatment with the offending drug and initiation of aggressive burn unit intervention may be lifesaving.

A mild form of SSSS is characterized by a generalized scarlatiniform eruption with exfoliation ("staphylococcal scarlet fever"). The skin has a sandpaper roughness, and Pastia's lines are present, as in streptococcal scarlet fever, but the strawberry tongue and palatal enanthem of streptococcal scarlet fever are absent.

Staphylococcal Toxic Shock Syndrome

Toxic shock syndrome (TSS) is an acute febrile illness characterized by a generalized erythematous eruption that is due to in vivo production of a toxin at the site of localized, often relatively asymptomatic or unnoticed infection by *S. aureus* strains capable of toxin production.[134] The multisystem effects observed in TSS patients are induced by TSS toxin 1 (TSST-1), which has been shown to be identical[150] to enterotoxin F[151] and exotoxin C.[152] TSST-1 has been purified, cloned, and sequenced. It has been demonstrated to be a potent, nonspecific inducer of interleukin-1 (IL-1) and tumor necrosis factor; to be a potent, nonspecific T-cell mitogen; and to induce the suppression of a number of immune responses. Recent work has established that TSST-1 acts as a superantigen that stimulates T cells to proliferate nonspecifically through interaction with class II major histocompatibility complex products on antigen-presenting cells and then with variable regions on the Vβ-chain of the T-cell receptor complex.[153]

Bacterial superantigens include staphylococcal exotoxins, now designated as SEA, SEB, SEC, SED, SEE, TSST-1, and EXF-T, and group A streptococcal exotoxins SPeA, SPeB, SPeC, SPeF, and SSA.[153, 154] All of these toxins share the ability to cause symptoms via release of immune cytokines, leading to high fever and enhanced host susceptibility to lethal endotoxin shock.[153, 154]

TSST-1–producing coagulase-negative staphylococci have also been described.[155] In the early 1980s, most cases of TSS occurred in menstruating females, often in association with tampon use.[156, 157] At present, about 300 cases of TSS are reported each year, of which only half are associated with menstruation.[136] Nonmenstrual TSS has been associated with a variety of infections, including postoperative wounds, cutaneous infections, burn wounds, postpartum complications, and *S. aureus* respiratory infections, often after viral influenza.[159–165]

TSS may range in severity from a relatively mild disease, often misdiagnosed as a viral syndrome, to a severe life-threatening illness. The most common symptoms include a temperature greater than 104°F (40°C), hypotension, and diffuse erythroderma with desquamation 1 to 2 weeks after the onset of illness. Additional early features include conjunctival, oropharyngeal, and vaginal hyperemia; vomiting and diarrhea; and myalgias.[166–169] Most patients have abnormalities in three or more organ systems: (1) muscular—rhabdomyolysis; (2) central nervous system—toxic encephalopathy; (3) renal—azotemia; (4) liver—abnormal transaminases; and (5) hematologic—thrombocytopenia. The rash of TSS is almost always noted within the first 24 hours of illness. Desquamation occurs after 7 to 10 days, most prominently on the hands and feet. Histologically, the epidermis exhibits cleavage in the basilar layers, which differentiates TSS from SSSS and from viral and drug eruptions.[170] *S. aureus* septicemia may be associated with erythematous, petechial, or pustular lesions.[171] In addition, lesions associated with endocarditis such as Osler's nodes, Janeway lesions, and splinter hemorrhages may occur. Such skin lesions have been reported in 10 to 64% of patients with staphylococcal septicemia.[172] Purpuric lesions may in some cases be so extensive as to suggest meningococcemia or Rocky Mountain spotted fever.[173–176] Gram-stained smears of the material in these lesions usually demonstrate gram-positive cocci.

Streptococcal Infections

Group A streptococcal infections are associated with several cutaneous presentations, including impetigo (pyoderma), scarlet fever, erysipelas, cellulitis, lymphangitis, gangrene, and perianal cellulitis.[177] These manifestations of streptococcal infection occur via three distinct mechanisms:[178] (1) direct infection of the skin, (2) immunologically mediated disease, and (3) toxin-mediated disease. Rheumatic fever affects up to 3% of people with untreated group A hemolytic streptococcal infections of the nasopharynx. Cutaneous manifestations include erythema marginatum (occurring in 10 to 20% of cases), subcutaneous nodules (in up to 30%), and erythema papulatum (rare). Over the last decade the incidence of severe disease as a result of infection with *Streptococcus pyogenes* has increased dramatically.[179, 180] The term *streptococcal toxic shock syndrome* has been suggested to describe many of these patients with hypotension and multiorgan failure, as occurs in staphylococcal TSS (Table 45–5).[181] Many but not all patients have a rash at the time of presentation.[181–184] Skin manifestations include generalized erythroderma with desquamation and localized cellulitis with vesiculation or bulla formation.[182] Unlike in TSS, a focus of pyogenic inflammation is usually present, and a large proportion of the patients have documented bacteremia.[177] Rarely, Group G streptococci have been reported to cause myositis with toxic shock syndrome.[185]

Rickettsial Infections

Rickettsiae are obligate intracellular parasites whose primary target in humans appears to be the endothelial cell.[186] After parasitization of the endothelial cell, necrosis of the media and intima results in thrombosis, formation of microinfarcts, and extravasation of blood. The end result is increased vascular permeability and vasculitis.

Rash is a hallmark of Rocky Mountain spotted fever,[187–191] the most common rickettsial disease in the United States. Initially, a maculopapular rash develops. Subsequently, the rash becomes more petechial. Characteristically, the rash appears between the second and sixth days of illness (average 4 days). However, the rash may be absent in 5 to 17% of patients, and in up to 50% it may not appear within the first 3 days of illness.[187, 188, 190, 192, 193] Failure to initiate proper therapy within 5 days of onset of symptoms has been associated with an increased mortality.[194] Independent predictors of failure by the physician to initiate therapy the first time a patient was seen include absence of a rash, presentation between August 1 and April 30, and presentation within 3 days of illness. Most commonly, the rash begins on the extremities, often around the wrists and ankles, and spreads centripetally to the trunk, with relative sparing of the face. However, the rash may begin on the trunk (10%) and spread centrifugally or may have a diffuse distribution at the time of onset (10%). Characteristically, the rash involves the palms and/or soles in the later stages of infection. Over time, the rash, which begins as maculopapular lesions, may progress to become petechial or ecchymotic. Rarely, gangrene or skin necrosis that requires amputation may occur.[195] The rash may rarely be urticarial or pruritic. Because the mortality rate for infection may be decreased from 15% to 3%[196] with appropriate treatment, institution of antibiotic therapy should never be delayed in the absence of rash. Signs and symptoms similar to those of Rocky Mountain spotted fever may occur with ehrlichiosis (see later on).

Capnocytophaga canimorsus Infection

Capnocytophaga canimorsus (dysgonic fermenter-2 [DF-2]) is a fastidious, gram-negative, opportunistic pathogen that can cause serious multiorgan disease in humans. The organism is found worldwide. Studies suggest that it is part of the normal gingival flora of cats and dogs.

Over 50 cases of infection due to *C. canimorsus* have been described.[197–202] Although infected patients have ranged in age from 5 months to 77 years, most infections have been reported in adults over 40 years of age. Approximately 80% of patients described in the literature have a predisposing condition, most commonly surgical asplenia. Other predisposing factors have included Hodgkin's disease, trauma, idiopathic thrombocytopenic purpura, alcohol abuse, steroid therapy, and chronic lung disease.

Infection is strongly associated with dog bites, with more than 50% of patients reporting dog bites prior to clinical evidence of infection. Infections have also followed cat bites or scratches,[203] scratches from dogs, and contact with wild animals. An additional 20% of patients have reported exposure to dogs without a history of an actual bite or scratch. The clinical syndrome in humans is characterized by fever, DIC, cellular necrosis in certain organs such as kidneys and adrenal glands, thrombocytopenia, hypotension, and renal failure with oliguria and anuria. Dermatologic lesions occur in about 50% of patients and may include petechiae, a macular or papular eruption, eschar formation, or painful erythema. Patients frequently develop a hemorrhagic diathesis with purpuric skin lesions and petechiae that may progress to cutaneous gangrene.

The case-fatality rate is approximately 25%. Death has not been confined to immunocompromised patients. Infection with *C. canimorsus* should be considered in patients who have a compatible clinical syndrome coupled with a history of a dog bite or animal exposure. Definitive diagnosis requires isolation of the organism from blood or other body fluids or tissues. Empirical therapy based on the clinical presentation should be given. In patients who show high-grade bacteremia, the organism has been demonstrated in peripheral blood smears. Therefore, in all patients suspected of having *C. canimorsus* sepsis, especially splenectomized patients, Gram staining of the buffy coat should be performed.

Borrelia burgdorferi Infection

Lyme disease is a tick-borne borreliosis with broad distribution and myriad manifestations.[204] Skin lesions are prominent clinical manifestations of all stages of Lyme disease.[205–209] Approximately 50 to 75% of infected patients will develop the classic lesion of erythema chronicum migrans (ECM) at the site of the tick bite (stage 1). The initial macular lesion is usually homogeneous in its redness and may remain so until it heals. More commonly, the lesion partly or totally clears centrally, leaving an annular erythema that spreads centrifugally. ECM may develop anywhere, but the most frequently affected site is the lower leg. Although the lesion may last from a few days to about 1 year, it usually disappears within a few weeks to months. In about half of the patients, itching, dysesthesia/hyperesthesia, or sensations of heat may develop at the site of erythema.

TABLE 45–5 Staphylococcal Versus Streptococcal Toxic Shock Syndromes

Feature	Staphylococcal	Streptococcal
Age	Primarily 15–35 yr	Primarily 20–50 yr
Gender	Higher frequency in women	Men and women equally affected
Severe pain	Rare	Common
Hypotension	100%	100%
Erythroderma rash	Very common	Less common
Renal failure	Common	Common
Bacteremia	Low frequency	60%
Tissue necrosis	Rare	Common
Predisposing factors	Tampons, packing, nonsteroidal anti-inflammatory drug use?	Cuts, burns, bruises, varicella, nonsteroidal anti-inflammatory drug use?
Thrombocytopenia	Common	Common
Mortality rate	<3%	30–70%

Adapted from Stevens DL. The toxic shock syndromes. Infect Dis Clin North Am. 1996;10:727–746.

Many patients who develop disseminated infection (stage 2) will exhibit ECM-like lesions. The disseminated lesions are usually smaller than the primary lesion and often multiple. These lesions may be ring-shaped but are often homogeneous and nonmigrating. In Europe, borrelial lymphocytomas have been described during stage 2 illness.

Acrodermatitis chronica atrophicans (ACA) has been more commonly described in Europe but may occur in the United States and is a manifestation of chronic infection (i.e., stage 3). ACA begins with an inflammatory phase with a bluish-red erythema, usually on the distal lower leg or foot. The course is chronic, with persistence of inflammatory lesions for years and gradual conversion to markedly atrophic skin.

Candidiasis

The incidence and relative frequency of infections due to *Candida* as a nosocomial pathogen appear to be increasing.[210–216] Disseminated candidiasis is frequently fatal and is a major cause of death in immunocompromised patients.[217, 218] Predisposing factors are malignancy with cytotoxic therapy, neutropenia, antimicrobial therapy, hyperalimentation, severe burn injuries, very low birth weight, use of intravenous catheters, systemic administration of adrenocortical steroids, and gastrointestinal surgery.[217, 218]

Disseminated candidiasis may be accompanied by a characteristic macronodular skin rash in up to 13% of patients.[218] The lesions are discrete, firm, nontender, subcutaneous raised erythematous papules or nodules.[219–222] Nodules may sometimes have a pale center, and some may become hemorrhagic. Often the lesions are diffuse, but they may be localized to a small area. The face is usually spared. Histologically, the middle and lower portions of the dermis are involved and show vessels distended by fungal pseudohyphae, platelet aggregates, and fibrin. Scant lymphocytic perivenular infiltrate may be present.

The diagnosis of disseminated candidiasis may be established by biopsy and culture of the dermal lesions. However, the diagnosis may be missed unless multiple tissue sections are carefully examined.

Many other fungi produce nodular lesions identical to those caused by *Candida* and must be considered as possible pathogens in immunocompromised patients. In patients with acquired immunodeficiency syndrome (AIDS), cryptococci may cause umbilicated nodules that mimic the lesions of molluscum contagiosum.

NEW AND EMERGING INFECTIOUS DISEASES

The Institute of Medicine defines new and emerging diseases as "new, reemerging or drug-resistant infections whose incidence in humans has increased within the past two decades or whose incidence threatens to increase in the near future."[223] To this definition we suggest the addition of infections whose geographic range is increasing. The factors leading to the development of new and emerging diseases have been reviewed in the literature.[224, 225] It is important for infectious disease clinicians to realize that international travel has dramatically increased; accordingly, patients may present with diseases only rarely seen in the United States.[225] Many of these diseases may be associated with either local or generalized skin lesions, including dengue fever, yellow fever, viral hemorrhagic fevers, malaria, and leptospirosis.[225]

Infections Due to New Herpesviruses

In recent years, the number of human viruses in the herpesvirus family has increased from five to eight.[226] Human herpesvirus 6 (HHV-6) is now recognized as the cause of exanthem subitum in infants and other febrile diseases in children.[227] HHV-6 infection, a worldwide disease, is normally acquired at a very early age. Classically, patients with exanthem subitum present with a high fever that lasts from 3 to 5 days.[227] As the temperature normalizes, a macular or maculopapular rash develops, generally beginning on the trunk, with later spread to the extremities and often to the neck and face. Typical dermal lesions are 2 to 3 mm in diameter and blanch with pressure. In one study of Japanese children, about half had a morbilliform rash and half had a rubella-like rash.[228] However, a study of febrile children seen in an emergency department in the United States reported the following data on the frequency of rash in those children diagnosed as having HHV-6 infection: rash at presentation, 18% (described as macular or maculopapular); rash within 1 week of presentation, 18% (described as variable); and classic roseola-like rash after fever subsided, 9%.[229] In children, HHV-6 infection may be manifested as fever without a rash, rash without a fever, infectious mononucleosis–like illness, or, rarely, a vesicular rash.[230] Cases clinically identified as either measles or rubella can be due to primary HHV-6 infection.[230, 231] In adults, HHV-6 produces an infectious mononucleosis–like illness either occurring without a rash,[232] or associated with erythematous macules and papules[233] or erythroderma.[234] Human herpesvirus 7 (HHV-7) has not been firmly linked to human illness; it has been suggested as a cause of exanthem subitum,[235] but some investigators suggest that this association is related to the ability of HHV-7 to reactivate HHV-6 from latency.[236] Human herpesvirus 8 (HHV-8) has been linked to Kaposi's sarcoma.[226]

Viral Hemorrhagic Fever

Hemorrhagic fever may be caused by viruses belonging to several families including Arenaviridae (e.g., Argentine hemorrhagic fever, Lassa fever, Venezuelan hemorrhagic fever), Bunyaviridae (e.g., hantavirus pulmonary syndrome), Filoviridae (Ebola virus disease), and Flaviviridae (yellow fever, dengue fever, Omsk hemorrhagic fever).[237]

Hantaviruses are RNA viruses that belong to the family Bunyaviridae and include Hantaan, Seoul, Puumala, Dobrava, Sin Nombre, Bayou, Black Creek Canal, and New York viruses.[238] Hemorrhagic fever with renal syndrome (HFRS) may be caused by Hantaan, Seoul, Dobrava, and Puumala viruses. Severe forms of HFRS have characteristic phases that may not be seen with milder disease. After an incubation period of 2 to 3 weeks, patients present with abrupt onset of fever in association with malaise, headache, myalgias, back pain, abdominal pain, nausea, and vomiting. Conjunctival injection or hemorrhage with palatal and upper torso petechiae is commonly seen on physical examination.[238] During this phase, a characteristic erythematous flush that blanches with pressure may be observed, usually affecting the face, neck, and upper torso.[239] After the 3- to 7-day febrile phase, a period of hypotension and severe shock ensues that is characterized by hemorrhagic manifestations. Overall, about 20% of the patients manifest severe disease, with death from shock and renal failure in 5 to 10% of cases. The hantavirus pulmonary syndrome caused by the Sin Nombre virus is not associated with facial flushing, petechiae, or conjunctival injection.

Filoviruses include the agents that cause Marburg and Ebola hemorrhagic fever.[240–243] Ebola virus is more virulent than Marburg virus and causes more severe clinical disease, with an accelerated course and high morbidity and mortality. Patients present with an acute onset of fever, severe frontal headache, anorexia, malaise, and myalgias. These signs and symptoms are followed 2 to 3 days later by clinical deterioration heralded by pharyngitis, conjunctivitis, severe nausea and vomiting, abdominal pain, and watery diarrhea. Five days later, patients develop a maculopapular rash on the trunk and back that is followed by the appearance of petechiae, ecchymoses, subconjunctival hemorrhages, epistaxis, hemoptysis, hematemesis, and melena. Hemorrhagic shock may progress to death. Patients with Marburg virus infection may develop a scarlatiniform rash rather than a maculopapular rash. Considerations in the differential diagnosis of African hemorrhagic fevers also include yellow fever and Lassa fever, but these illnesses are not accompanied by a rash.

The etiologic agents of dengue fever are four serologically related RNA viruses belonging to the family Flaviviridae.[244, 245] Classic dengue fever begins after an incubation period of 3 to 15 days (average 5 to 8 days) with an abrupt onset of fever that may be accompanied by chills, headache, and general malaise. The fever usually lasts 3 to 7 days and may be biphasic. Erythema may appear shortly before the onset of fever, concurrently with fever onset, or 24 to 48 hours later. This rash may be noted as a flushing or erythematous mottling beginning on the trunk and spreading centrifugally to the face, neck, and extremities. Flushing may disappear after 1 or 2 days or may blend into an erythematous macular or maculopapular rash that develops anytime during the course of illness. Pruritus and desquamation, especially on the palms and soles, may follow termination of the eruption. Dengue hemorrhagic fever/dengue shock syndrome is a more severe disease whose skin manifestations may include petechiae, purpura, ecchymoses, epistaxis, and gum bleeding.

Bacterial Diseases Due to *Bartonella* Species

The genus *Bartonella* now contains four species demonstrated to be pathogenic in humans: *Bartonella bacilliformis, Bartonella henselae, Bartonella quintana*, and *Bartonella elizabethae*.[246–248] Disease syndromes caused by *Bartonella* spp. include cat-scratch disease *(B. quintana)*, trench fever *(B. quintana)*, and bartonellosis *(B. bacilliformis). B. henselae* is now considered the primary agent of cat-scratch disease (CSD). Infection with *Bartonella* spp. results in disease syndromes of variable severity, ranging from lymphadenopathy only (CSD) to systemic disease. As noted by Anderson and Neuman, the severity and presentation of disease are related to immune status.[247] In general (excluding *B. bacilliformis*), immunocompetent patients who are otherwise healthy tend to present with classic CSD when infected with *B. henselae*. Patients who are immunocompromised by having AIDS, chronic alcoholism, immunosuppression, or other serious health problems tend to have systemic disease. However, there have been rare reports of systemic disease, including bacillary angiomatosis, in immunocompetent persons.[249]

CSD occurs primarily in children and young adults. Characteristically, it presents as lymphadenopathy, usually preceded by an erythematous papule at the inoculation site. About 30% of the patients have low-grade fever and malaise. Less common clinical findings include rash, hepatosplenomegaly, lytic bone lesions, granulomatous conjunctivitis, pneumonitis, and central nervous system involvement.[250] Skin eruptions have included a papular or an urticarial rash, erythema nodosum, and a vesiculopapular eruption.[251] Uncomplicated CSD-mediated lymphadenopathy usually resolves spontaneously in 2 to 6 months. Manifestations of *Bartonella* infection in the immunocompromised patient include cutaneous bacillary angiomatosis (BA), extracutaneous lesions, bacillary peliosis hepatis, and fever with bacteremia.[250–260] BA is the most common clinical manifestation of *Bartonella* infection in the immunocompromised person. Several different skin lesions have been described in BA, including elevated, friable, firm, bright red papules (in approximately 67% of cases); subcutaneous nodules (in approximately 50%); and cellulitic plaques (in 5 to 10%). Lesions may be located anywhere on the body, and patients may have several forms of lesions at the same time or sequentially. The lesions of BA may be clinically and histologically similar to Kaposi's sarcoma; therefore, biopsy specimens and special stains may be required to confirm the diagnosis. Cutaneous BA may also have extracutaneous manifestations ranging from subclinical to life-threatening infection.[247] *Bartonella* infection may be associated with local or generalized complications[260, 261] or may manifest as overwhelming disseminated infection.[260] In addition to extracutaneous lesions, multiple cutaneous lesions may develop.[262] Visceral lesions may involve the respiratory or gastrointestinal mucosa, heart, liver, spleen, bone marrow, muscles, or lymph nodes. *B. quintana* and *B. henselae* have been successfully cultured from the blood or from cutaneous lesions of patients with BA.[263–265]

Arthropod-Borne Bacterial Diseases Due to *Ehrlichia* Species

Arthropod-borne diseases that occur in the United States include Rocky Mountain spotted fever, murine typhus, rickettsialpox, sylvatic typhus, Lyme disease, tick-borne relapsing fever, Colorado tick fever, and tularemia. Recently, *Ehrlichia* species have emerged as important and potentially life-threatening pathogens.[266–268] Two different illnesses have been described: human monocytic ehrlichiosis (HME), due to *Ehrlichia chaffeensis*, and human granulocytic ehrlichiosis (HGE) due to *Ehrlichia equi/phagocytophila*. The severity of HME and HGE ranges from subclinical to fatal. There are no clinical features that consistently distinguish HME from HGE. The onset of symptoms generally occurs about 1 week after tick exposure (range 0 to 34 days). Patients with ehrlichiosis characteristically present with abrupt onset of fever, headache, myalgia, and shaking chills. Less common signs and symptoms include nausea, vomiting, diarrhea, abdominal pain, cough, and confusion. A rash has been reported in about 30% of patients and may be more common in children.[268] Rashes may not develop until several days into the illness and are short-lived. Limited data suggest that rashes may be more common with HME than with HGE. The exanthems reported in patients with ehrlichiosis have been highly variable and have been described as macular, maculopapular, petechial, and even vesicular.

Involvement of the palms and soles is unusual, having been reported in less than 5% of patients. Several forms of rash may be present in the same patient. The clinical features of ehrlichiosis may mimic those of Rocky Mountain spotted fever, Kawasaki disease, meningococcemia, enterovirus and cytomegalovirus infections, infectious mononucleosis, leptospirosis, and babesiosis. The overall mortality rate has ranged from 2 to 5% for HME and from 7 to 10% for HGE, but these estimates are probably inflated, as severe cases are overrepresented in the literature.

Skin Lesions in Immunocompromised Patients

The diagnosis of skin lesions in the immunocompromised patient is complex because of the wide range of potential microbial pathogens that may cause disease in patients with abnormal immune responses (Table 45–6).[269–277] In addition, in immunocompromised persons, common infections may have unusual manifestations.[278] Cutaneous lesions of suspected infectious origin should undergo biopsy.[270] Biopsy samples should be processed by the most rapid and sensitive methods for detecting microbes both histologically and immunologically, and appropriate stains and cultures should be used to optimize the chance of identifying the pathogen. Biopsy samples should be divided into two portions. The first should be submitted for histologic evaluation by routine and special stains to detect fungi, mycobacteria, and bacteria. The second portion should be sent for microbiologic study including culture of aerobic and anaerobic bacteria, *Nocardia*, mycobacteria, and fungi. Direct fungal touch preparations should be made, and Gram, acid-fast, and modified acid-fast staining should be performed. Viral culture should be considered when herpesviruses are likely agents of infection.[276]

Solid organ transplant recipients are at high risk for disease due to opportunistic bacterial, viral, and fungal pathogens. The risk of infection and the most likely infecting pathogen depend on the type of transplant, type and dose of immunosuppressive medications, time since transplant, presence of coexisting diseases including viral infections, and epidemiologic exposures.

Kaye and colleagues[270] categorized cutaneous infections in immunocompromised persons into four groups based on pathophysiology: (1) infection originating in skin that is typical of those occurring in immunocompetent persons; (2) extensive cutaneous involvement with pathogens that normally produce trivial or well-localized disease in immunocompetent patients; (3) infection originating from a cutaneous source that is caused by opportunistic pathogens that rarely cause disease in immunocompetent patients but may cause either

TABLE 45-6 Cutaneous and Subcutaneous Lesions Caused by Opportunistic Organisms That Infect Immunocompromised Patients

Type of Lesion	Potentially Causative Organisms
Abscess	*Aspergillus* spp., *Chaetochonidium, Cryptococcus neoformans, Fusarium solani,* members of family Mucoraceae, *Mycobacterium avium-intracellulare, Mycobacterium fortuitum, Mycobacterium kansasii, Mycobacterium tuberculosis, Nocardia* spp., *Pseudomonas aeruginosa*
Cellulitis	*Aspergillus* spp., *Candida* spp., *C. neoformans, Histoplasma capsulatum,* members of family Mucoraceae, *M. kansasii, Nocardia* spp., *P. aeruginosa*
Ecthyma gangrenosum	*Candida* spp., members of family Mucoraceae, *P. aeruginosa,* other gram-negative bacilli
Erythematous macules	*Aspergillus* spp., members of family Mucoraceae, human immunodeficiency virus (acute infection)
Hemorrhagic lesions	*Aspergillus* spp., *Candida* spp., *C. neoformans, H. capsulatum*
Papules, nodules	*Aspergillus* spp., *Candida* spp., *C. neoformans, H. capsulatum,* members of family Mucoraceae, *M. tuberculosis* (miliary tuberculosis), *Mycobacterium chelonae, M. fortuitum, M. kansasii, Mycobacterium szulgai, Mycobacterium Trichosporon beigelii, Trichophyton rubrum, Pneumocystis carinii*
Plaques	*Alternaria alternata, Aspergillus* spp., *Candida* spp., *C. neoformans, M. kansasii, M. tuberculosis, Prototheca* spp., *Coccidioides immitis, H. capsulatum*
Pustules	*C. neoformans, Prototheca* spp., *Staphylococcus aureus*
Subcutaneous nodules, panniculitis	*Candida* spp., *Chaetoconidium, H. capsulatum,* members of family Mucoraceae, *M. fortuitum, M. intracellulare, M. kansasii, M. tuberculosis, Mycobacterium malmoense, Nocardia* spp., *Scytalidium hyalinum, F. solani, P. aeruginosa*
Vesicles, bullae	*Aspergillus* spp., *Alteraria* spp., *Candida* spp., *C. neoformans,* herpes simplex virus, herpes zoster virus, members of family Mucoraceae, *P. aeruginosa*
Ulcers	*Candida* spp., *Rhizopus* spp., *H. capsulatum*

Adapted from Wolfson JS, Sober AJ, Rubin RH. Dermatologic manifestations of infections in immunocompromised patients. Medicine (Baltimore). 1985;64:115–133.

localized or widespread disease in immunocompromised patients; (4) cutaneous or subcutaneous infection that represents metastatic spread from a noncutaneous site. Only life-threatening infections with cutaneous manifestations are discussed further here. In general, most cases of skin infection result from secondary dissemination after initial infection of the lungs or other organ systems. Primary cutaneous infection resulting from direct inoculation is less common. In transplant patients, infections with viruses and fungi are probably more common than skin infections caused by bacteria.

Immunocompromised patients are at increased risk for the development of cellulitis due to *S. pyogenes* and *S. aureus*. Neutropenic patients are also susceptible to more unusual pathogens such as members of the family Enterobacteriaceae and *Pseudomonas* spp. Patients with leukemia or impaired cell-mediated immunity may develop erysipelas-like lesions due to *Candida* spp. or *Cryptococcus neoformans*. Both local and diffuse skin infections with herpesviruses, especially herpes simplex and varicella-zoster, are very common.[272] Cutaneous cytomegalovirus infection has a highly variable appearance that may include nodules, ulcers, indurated plaques, maculopapular eruptions, vesicles, and petechiae.

Kaye and colleagues[270] noted that in immunocompromised patients, cutaneous lesions resulting from hematogenous spread of infection are caused by three classes of organisms: (1) *P. aeruginosa* and other bacteria; (2) the endemic systemic mycoses caused by *H. capsulatum, Coccidioides immitis*, and, rarely, *Blastomyces dermatitidis*; and (3) the opportunistic organisms *Aspergillus, Coccidiodes neoformans, Candida, Rhizopus*, and *Nocardia. P. aeruginosa* may cause either cellulitis or echthyma gangrenosum, which may develop in the absence of bacteremia. Patients with malignancy may develop sepsis associated with a variety of uncommon bacteria that are also associated with skin lesions (e.g., *A. hydrophila, C. canimorsus, Clostridium septicum*, mycobacteria, and *S. typhimurium*).[277] Of the three fungal pathogens, *H. capsulatum* appears to be the most likely to cause cutaneous lesions. Most commonly, *H. capsulatum* causes cellulitis, but it may also cause papules, nodules, pustules, and hemorrhagic lesions. Metastatic spread to the skin from noncutaneous sites of infection most commonly occurs with *Aspergillus* spp., *C. neoformans, Candida* spp., *Rhizopus* spp., and *Nocardia*. With the exception of *Candida*, the initial portal of entry is the respiratory tract. However, the respiratory tract infection may be asymptomatic, with the initial signs of illness seen in the skin. In neutropenic patients, cutaneous lesions due to *Aspergillus* spp. are often found in association with the sino-orbital form of disease.[274] Neutropenic patients may also develop disseminated infection with other fungi such as *Fusarium* spp. and *Trichosporon beigelii.*

Human Immunodeficiency Virus Infection

HIV infection commonly results in dermatologic disorders in both adults[279–295] and children.[296–301] Clinically, the skin lesions associated with HIV infection may be classified by morphologic appearance, stage of HIV infection, pathophysiology (infectious, neoplastic, vascular, miscellaneous), and, for infectious diseases, etiologic agent.

Skin disorders are clearly related to the stage of HIV infection. Initial infection with HIV may result in development of the acute retroviral syndrome, characterized by transient fever, myalgias, headache, urticaria, aseptic meningitis, and rash.[302–306] The rash is maculopapular and usually confined to the trunk.

The Centers for Disease Control and Prevention (CDC) uses several dermatologic disorders in its definition of symptomatic but not AIDS category of HIV infection.[307] These conditions may provide an early clue to unsuspected HIV infection and include bacillary angiomatosis (see later on); oropharyngeal candidiasis in a patient who has not recently received antibiotics, immunosuppressive medication, or chemotherapy; vulvovaginal candidiasis that is persistent, frequent, or poorly responsive to therapy; oral hairy leukoplakia; herpes zoster involving at least two distinct episodes or more than one dermatome; and idiopathic thrombocytopenic purpura. HIV infection should also be considered in persons with herpes simplex infection that is unusually prolonged or poorly responsive to acyclovir.

Several dermatologic conditions have been incorporated into the CDC's diagnostic criteria for AIDS. These include disseminated or extrapulmonary coccidioidomycosis, herpes simplex virus infection characterized by a mucocutaneous ulcer that persists longer than 1 month, extrapulmonary or disseminated histoplasmosis, Kaposi's sarcoma, and extrapulmonary or disseminated *Mycobacterium avium-intracellulare* or *Mycobacterium kansasii* infection.[307]

Like other immunocompromised patients, persons with AIDS develop infections with opportunistic pathogens that rarely if ever cause infection in immunocompetent people. Furthermore, infections due to common pathogens may have clinical manifestations that are unusual, more severe, more prolonged, or poorly responsive to therapy. Skin lesions often yield multiple pathogens.[308–310]

Several common pathogens may cause disease with unusual presenting manifestations. Severe, chronic herpes simplex lesions have been reported.[306] These ulcers are frequently perianal in homosexual men but may also involve the lips and perioral area. Severe herpetic whitlow may be confused with osteomyelitis or other chronic ulcerative conditions. Herpes zoster occurs with a higher than expected frequency in HIV-infected persons.[281] Chronic varicella-zoster infection has been reported[311–314] and may lead to severe scarring.[283] Molluscum contagiosum may involve both the genital area and the face. The number and size of the lesions and their response to therapy tend to correlate with the degree of immunosuppression.[284]

S. aureus is the most common cutaneous bacterial pathogen in HIV-infected persons. Infection usually presents as folliculitis of the face, trunk, or groin. Cutaneous staphylococcal infections may progress to botryomycosis, a rare condition characterized by aggregates of bacteria in skin. Syphilis is common in HIV-infected persons. Primary infection is manifested by a chancre. Secondary syphilis may manifest as a generalized maculopapular eruption with or without scaling; palmoplantar vesicles, papules, or macules; hypopigmented axillary macules; and oral lesions.[291] Unusual patterns of syphilis have been reported in the HIV-infected person, including coexistent lesions of secondary syphilis and tertiary gummas and nodulo-ulcerative lesions with lymphadenopathy in precocious tertiary syphilis. In patients with AIDS, typical serologic tests (i.e., Venereal Disease Research Laboratory [VDRL] and fluorescent treponemal antibody absorption test [FTA-ABS]) for syphilis may be unreliable, and a biopsy of the skin with silver staining to show the spirochetes may be required for diagnosis.[315] Scabies may be widespread and be manifested as an erythematous papulosquamous eruption in which numerous mites can easily be found in the skin scraping. Less commonly, classic Norwegian scabies with marked hyperkeratosis may occur.

Unusual pathogens that may involve the skin include cytomegalovirus,[307, 316] nontuberculous mycobacteria *(M. avium* complex, *Mycobacterium haemophilum, Mycobacterium fortuitum), Candida* spp. (disseminated candidiasis), *Acanthamoeba castellani, Pneumocystis carinii,* and *Toxoplasma gondii.* Dissemination to the skin may occur with histoplasmosis, cryptococcosis, and coccioidomycosis.[317] Cutaneous histoplasmosis may be manifested as slightly pinkish to red papules with little or no induration or inflammation, a cellulitis-like eruption, and ulcerations and acneiform papules and pustules.[283] The most common cutaneous presentation of cutaneous cryptococcosis is that of widespread dome-shaped papules with slight central umbilication and waxy translucence.[283] As these may mimic the papules of molluscum contagiosum, biopsy should be considered for diagnosis.[318]

Papulopustular lesions may be the presenting sign of disseminated coccidioidomycosis.[319] Gradon and colleagues[290] have classified the unusual skin and soft tissue manifestations of opportunistic infections in AIDS as follows: nodular lesions—*Sporothrix schenckii, M. tuberculosis, Corynebacterium jekeium, Demodex* mites, and *Sarcoptes scabiei*; ulcerating lesions—*M. haemophilum*, herpesviruses including herpes simplex virus and cytomegalovirus; scalded skin syndrome—*S. aureus*; and pyomyositis—*S. aureus* and group C streptococci. The treatment of infectious disorders of the skin in HIV-infected persons has been reviewed.[285]

Well-described primary dermatologic disorders not associated with fever but associated with HIV infection include psoriasis, seborrheic dermatitis,[283, 291] papular eruptions,[288] ichthyosis,[320, 321] infectious eczemoid dermatitis, yellow nail syndrome,[288] vitiligo,[288] telangiectasias of the anterior portion of the chest,[291, 319] and alopecia.[283, 291] Many of these diseases are more severe in patients with HIV infection, and their presence in undiagnosed patients should lead to consideration of HIV infection. Several patients have developed an eosinophilic pustular rash ("eosinophilic folliculitis"), responsive to ultraviolet therapy.[291]

Drug reactions are common in patients with AIDS.[288, 291] Up to 50% of HIV-infected patients who receive trimethoprim-sulfamethoxazole develop a rash, usually an erythematous, maculopapular rash involving the entire body that is commonly associated with fever. Stevens-Johnson syndrome may develop. Rash may also accompany pentamidine therapy or treatment with dapsone-trimethoprim.

REFERENCES

1. Garner JS. Guideline for isolation precautions in hospitals. Infect Control Hosp Epidemiol. 1996;17:53–80.
2. Centers for Disease Control and Prevention. Recommendations for prevention of HIV transmission in the health-care setting. MMWR Morb Mortal Wkly Rep. 1987;36(Suppl 2):3–18.
3. Centers for Disease Control and Prevention. Management of patients with suspected viral hemorrhagic fever. MMWR. 1988;37(Suppl 3):1–16.
4. Centers for Disease Control and Prevention. Risks associated with human parvovirus B19 infection. MMWR Morb Mortal Wkly Rep. 1989;38:8188, 8193–8197.
5. Centers for Disease Control and Prevention. Update: Universal precautions for prevention of transmission of human immunodeficiency virus: Hepatitis B virus, and other bloodborne pathogens in health-care settings. MMWR Morb Mortal Wkly Rep. 1988;37:377–388.
6. Centers for Disease Control and Prevention. Guidelines for prevention of transmission of human immunodeficiency virus and hepatitis B virus to health-care and public-safety workers. MMWR Morb Mortal Wkly Rep. 1989;38(Suppl 6):1–37.
7. Bolyard EA, Tablan OC, Williams WW, et al. Guideline for infection control in health care personnel, 1998. Am J Infect Control. 1998;26:289–354.
8. Kreger BE, Craven DE, McCabe WR. Gram-negative bacteremia. IV. Reevaluation of clinical features and treatment in 612 patients. Am J Med. 1980;68:344–355.
9. Valman HB. Common rashes. BMJ. 1981;283:970–971.
10. Fitzpatrick TB, Bernhard JD. The structure of skin lesions and fundamentals of diagnosis. In: Fitzpatrick TB, Eisen AZ, Wolff K, et al, eds. Dermatology in General Medicine. 4th ed. New York: McGraw-Hill; 1993:27–54.
11. Cropley TG, Fitzpatrick TB. Dermatologic diagnosis by recognition of clinical morphologic patterns and syndromes. In: Fitzpatrick TB, Eisen AZ, Wolff K, et al, eds. Dermatology in General Medicine. 4th ed. New York: McGraw-Hill; 1993:55–65.
12. Lazarus GS, Goldsmith LA, Tharp MD. Diagnosis of Skin Disease. Philadelphia: FA Davis; 1980.
13. Habif TP. Clinical Dermatology. St. Louis, Mosby, 1996.
14. Fitzpatrick TB, Johnson RA. Differential diagnosis of rashes in the actutely ill febrile patient and in life-threatening diseases. In: Jeffers JD, Scott E, White J, eds. Dermatology in General Medicine. Textbook and Atlas. 3rd ed. New York: McGraw-Hill; 1987:21–22.
15. Johnson M-L. Dermatologic problems. In: Samily AH, ed. Textbook of Diagnostic Medicine. Philadelphia: Lea & Febiger; 1987:768–789.
16. Corey L, Kirby P. Rash and fever. In: Braunwald E, Isselbacher KJ, Petersdorf RG, et al, eds. Harrison's Principles of Internal Medicine. 11th ed. New York: McGraw-Hill; 1987:240–244.
17. Kline PP. Fever and rash. Emerg Decisions. 1988;April:27–37.
18. Kingston ME, Mackey D. Skin clues in the diagnosis of life-threatening infections. Rev Infect Dis. 1986;8:1–11.
19. Harrist TJ, Fine JD, Berman RS, Murphy GF, Mihm MC. Neutrophilic eccrine hidradenitis: A distinctive type of neutrophilic dermatosis associated with myelogenous leukemia and chemotherapy. Arch Dermatol. 1982:118:263–266.
20. Lazar AP. Cutaneous manifestations of systemic diseases. Comprehensive Ther. 1992;18:5–9.
21. Manders SM. Serious and life-threatening drug eruptions. Am Fam Physician. 1995;51:1865–1872.
22. Roujeau JC, Sterm RS. Severe adverse cutaneous reactions to drugs. N Engl J Med. 1994;331:1272–1285.
23. Wolkenstein P, Revuz J. Drug-induced severe skin reactions. Drug Safety. 1995;13:56–68.
24. Veraldi S, Rizzitelli G, Schianchi-Veraldi R. Occupational cutaneous infections. Clin Dermatol. 1992;10:225–230.
25. Taylor JS. Occupational dermatoses. Dermatol Clin. 1994;12:461–610.
26. Conklin RJ. Common cutaneous disorders in athletes. Sports Med. 1990;9:100–119.
27. Thomsett L. Zoonotic skin diseases. Practitioner. 1990;234:52–55.
28. Lucchina LC, Wilson ME, Drake LA. Dermatology and the recently returned traveler: Infectious diseases with dermatologic manifestations. Int J Dermatol. 1997;36:167–181.
29. Wilson ME. Skin problems in the traveler. Infect Dis Clin North Am. 1998;12:471–488.
30. Resnick SD. New aspects of exanthematous diseases of childhood. Dermatol Clin. 1997;15:257–265.
31. Frieden IJ, Resnick SD. Childhood exanthems: Old and new. Pediatr Clin North Am. 1981;38:859–887.
32. Frieden IJ. Childhood exanthems. Curr Opin Pediatr. 1995;7:411–414.
33. Avakian R, Flowers FP, Araujo OE, Ramos-Caro FA. Toxic epidermal necrolysis: A review. J Am Acad Dermatol. 1991;25:69–79.
34. Fine JD. Management of acquired bullous skin diseases. N Engl J Med. 1995;333:1475–1484.

35. Anderson LJ. Human parvoviruses. J Infect Dis. 1990;161:603–608.
36. Thurn J. Human parvovirus B19: Historical and clinical review. Rev Infect Dis. 1988;10:1005–1011.
37. Kurtzman GJ, Ozawa K, Cohen B, et al. Chronic bone marrow failure due to persistent B19 parvovirus infection. N Engl J Med. 1987;317:287–294.
38. Frickhofen N, Abkowitz JL, Safford M, et al. Persistent B19 parvovirus infection in patients infected with human immunodeficiency virus type 1 (HIV-1): A treatable cause of anemia in AIDS. Ann Intern Med. 1990;113:926–933.
39. Faden H, Gary GW, Anderson LJ. Chronic parvovirus infection in a presumably immunologically healthy woman. Clin Infect Dis. 1992;15:595–597.
40. Levy R, Weissman A, Blomberg G, Hagay ZJ. Infection by parvovirus B19 during pregnancy: A review. Obstet Gynecol Surv. 1997;52:254–259.
41. Brown KE, Young NS. Parvovirus B19 in human disease. Annu Rev Med. 1997;48:59–67.
42. Alger LS. Toxoplasmosis and parvovirus B19. Infect Dis Clin North Am. 1997;11:55–75.
43. Anderson MJ, Higgins PG, Davis LR, et al. Experimental parvoviral infection in humans. J Infect Dis. 1985;152:257–264.
44. Smith PT, Landry ML, Carey H, et al. Papular-purpuric gloves and socks syndrome associated with acute parvovirus B19 infection: Case report and review. Clin Infect Dis. 1998;27:164–168.
45. Fine JD, Harris TJ. Cutaneous leukocytoclastic vasculitis in the rose spot of paratyphoid fever. Int J Dermatol. 1982;21:216–217.
46. Hook EW, Marra CM. Acquired syphilis in adults. N Engl J Med. 1992;326:1060–1069.
47. Centers for Disease Control and Prevention. Summary of notifiable diseases, United States, 1996. MMWR Morb Mortal Wkly Rep. 1996;45:1–88.
48. Street ML, Umbert-Millet IJ, Roberts GD, et al. Nontuberculous mycobacterial infections of the skin. J Am Acad Dermatol. 1991;24:208–215.
49. Arbesfeld DM, Thomas I. Cutaneous herpes simplex virus infections. Am Fam Physician. 1991;43:1655–1664.
50. Williams R. Pustular skin disease. Practitioner. 1991;235:332–339.
51. Koenig KL. *Vibrio vulnificus*: Hazard on the half shell. West J Med. 1991;155:400–403.
52. Lee CC, Tong KL, Howe HS, Lam MS. *Vibrio vulnificus* infections: Case reports and literature review. Ann Acad Med Singapore. 1997;26:705–712.
53. Esterly NB. Vesicopustular eruptions in the neonate. Australas J Dermatol. 1991;32:1–12.
54. Lynch AM, Kapila R. Overwhelming postsplenectomy infection. Infect Dis Clin North Am. 1996;10:693–707.
55. Baccarani M, Fiacchini M, Galieni P, et al. Meningitis and septicaemia in adults splenectomized for Hodgkin's disease. Scand J Haematol. 1986;36:492–498.
56. Scully RE, Mark EJ, McNeely BU, eds. Case records of the Massachusetts General Hospital. Case 29-1986. N Engl J Med. 1986;315:241–249.
57. Scully RE, Mark EJ, McNelly BU, eds. Case records of the Massachusetts General Hospital. Case 20-1983. N Engl J Med. 1983;308:1212–1218.
58. O'Neal BJ, McDonald JC. The risk of sepsis in the asplenic adult. Ann Surg. 1981;194:775–778.
59. Sekikawa T, Shatney CH. Septic sequelae after splenectomy for trauma in adults. Am J Surg. 1983;145:667–673.
60. Zarrabi MH, Rosner F. Serious infections in adults following splenectomy for trauma. Arch Intern Med. 1984;144:1421–1424.
61. Green JB, Shackford SR, Sise MJ, et al. Late septic complications in adults following splenectomy for trauma: A prospective analysis in 144 patients. J Trauma. 1986;26:999–1004.
62. Evans D. Postsplenectomy sepsis 10 years or more after operation. J Clin Pathol. 1985;38:309–311.
63. Baker RC, Seguin JH, Gilchrist MJ, Myers MG. Fever and petechiae in children. Pediatrics. 1989;84:1051–1055.
64. Van Nguyen Q, Nguyen EA, Weiner LB. Incidence of invasive bacterial disease in children with fever and petechiae. Pediatrics. 1984;74:77–80.
65. Myers SA, Sexton DJ. Dermatologic manifestations of arthropod-borne diseases. Infect Dis Clin North Am. 1994;8:689–712.
66. Raoult D, Roux V. Rickettsioses as paradigms of new or emerging infectious diseases. Clin Microbiol Rev. 1997;10:694–719.
67. Murphy GS, Oldfield EC. Falciparum malaria. Infect Dis Clin North Am. 1996;10:747–775.
68. Zucker JR. Changing patterns of autochthonous malaria transmission in the United States: A review of recent outbreaks. Emerging Infect Dis. 1996;2:37–43.
69. Sweet RD. Acute febrile neutrophic dermatosis—1978. Br J Dermatol. 1979;100:93–99.
70. Driesch PVD. Sweet's syndrome (acute febrile neutrophilis dermatosis). Am Acad Dermatol. 1994;31:535–556.
71. Conger LA, Grabski WJ. Dilantin hypersensitivity syndrome. Cutis. 1996;57:223–226.
72. Robboy SJ, Mihm MC, Colman RW, et al. The skin in disseminated intravascular coagulation. Prospective analysis of thirty-six cases. Br J Dermatol. 1973;88:221–229.
73. Goodwin JN, Berne TV. Symmetrical peripheral gangrene. Arch Surg. 1974;108:780–784.
74. Chu DZJ, Blaisdell FW. Purpura fulminans. Am J Surg. 1982;143:356–362.
75. Chasan PE, Hansbrough JF, Cooper ML. Management of cutaneous manifestations of extensive purpura fulminans in a burn unit. J Burn Care Rehabil. 1992;13:410–413.
76. Dudgeon DL, Kellogg DR, Gilchrist GS, et al. Purpura fulminans. Arch Surg. 1971;103:351–358.
77. Hjort PF, Rapaport SI, Jorgensen L. Purpura fulminans. Report of a case successfully treated with heparin and hydrocortisone. Review of 50 cases from the literature. Scand J Haematol. 1964;1:169–192.
78. Hjort PF, Rapaport SI. The Shwartzman reaction: Pathogenetic mechanisms and clinical manifestations. Annu Rev Med. 1965;16:135–169.
79. DeVoe IW. The meningococcus and mechanisms of pathogenicity. Microbiol Rev. 1982;46:162–190.
80. Salzman MB, Runin LG. Meningococcemia. Infect Dis Clin North Am. 1996;10:709–725.
81. Sotto MN, Langer B, Hoshimo-Shimizu S, et al. Pathogenesis of cutaneous lesions in acute meningococcemia in humans: Light, immunofluorescent, and electron microscopic studies of skin biopsy specimens. J Infect Dis. 1976;133:506–514.
82. Bernhard WG, Jordan AC. Purpuric lesions in meningococcic infections. J Lab Clin Med. 1944;29:273–281.
83. Davis CE, Arnold K. Role of meningococcal endotoxin in meningococcal purpura. J Exp Med. 1974;140:159–171.
84. Koppes GM, Ellenbogen C, Gebhart RJ. Group Y meningococcal disease in United States Air Force recruits. Am J Med. 1977;62:661–666.
85. Leibel RL, Fangman JJ. Chronic meningococcemia in childhood. Am J Dis Child. 1974;127:94–98.
86. Benoit FL. Chronic meningococcemia. Am J Med. 1963;35:103–112.
87. Ognibene AJ, Dito WR. Chronic meningococcemia. Arch Intern Med. 1964;114:29–32.
88. Barr J, Danielsson D. Septic gonococcal dermatitis. BMJ. 1971;1:482–485.
89. Holmes KK, Weisner PJ, Pederson AHB, et al. The gonococcal arthritis-dermatitis syndrome. Ann Intern Med. 1971;75:470–471.
90. Kerle K, Mascola JR, Miller TA. Disseminated gonococcal infection. Am Fam Physician. 1992;45:209–214.
91. Buntin DM, Rosen T, Lesher JL, et al. Sexually transmitted diseases: Bacterial infections. J Am Acad Dermatol. 1991;25:287–299.
92. Handsfield HH. Disseminated gonococcal infection. Clin Obstet Gynecol. 1975;18:131–142.
93. Abu-Nassar H, Hill N, Fred HL, et al. Cutaneous manifestations of gonococcemia. Arch Intern Med. 1963;112:731–737.
94. Holmes KK, Counts GW, Beaty HN. Disseminated gonococcal infection. Ann Intern Med. 1971;74:979–993.
95. Tronca E, Handsfield HH, Wiesner PJ, et al. Demonstration of *Neisseria gonorrhoeae* with fluorescent antibody in patients with disseminated gonococcal infection. J Infect Dis. 1974;129:583–586.
96. Walker LC, Ahlin TD, Tung KSK, et al. Circulating immune complexes in disseminated gonorrheal infection. Ann Intern Med. 1978;89:28–33.
97. Ratnam S, Hogan K, March SB, Butler RW. Whirlpool-associated folliculitis caused by *Pseudomonas aeruginosa*: Report of an outbreak and review. J Clin Microbiol. 1986;23:655–659.
98. Flick MR, Cluff LE. *Pseudomonas* bacteremia. Am J Med. 1976;60:501–508.
99. Forkner CE, Frei E, Edgcomb JH, et al. *Pseudomonas* septicemia. Am J Med. 1958;25:877–889.
100. Whitecar JP, Luna M, Bodey GP. *Pseudomonas* bacteremia in patients with malignant diseases. Am J Med Sci. 1970;260:216–223.
101. Anderson MG. *Pseudomonas* septicaemia and echthyma gangrenosum. S Afr Med J. 1979;55:504–509.
102. Bodey GP, Boliva R, Fainstein V, et al. Infections caused by *Pseudomonas aeruginosa*. Rev Infect Dis. 1983;5:279–313.
103. Curtin JA, Petersdorf RG, Bennett IL. *Pseudomonas* bacteremia: Review of ninety-one cases. Ann Intern Med. 1961;54:1077–1107.
104. Dorff GJ, Geimer NF, Rosenthal DR, et al. *Pseudomonas* septicemia. Arch Intern Med. 1971;128:591–595.
105. Fast M, Woerner S, Bowman W, et al. Ecthyma gangrenosum. Can Med Assoc J. 1979;120:332–334.
106. Greene SL, Su WPD, Muller SA. Ecthyma gangrenosum: Report of clinical, histopathologic, and bacteriologic aspects of eight cases. J Am Acad Dermatol. 1984;11:781–787.
107. Hall JH, Callaway JL, Tindall JP, et al. *Pseudomonas aeruginosa* in dermatology. Arch Dermatol. 1968;97:312–324.
108. van den Broek PJ, van der Meer JWM, Kunst MW. The pathogenesis of echthyma gangrenosum. J Infect. 1979;1:263–267.
109. Bagel J, Grossman ME. Subcutaneous nodules in *Pseudomonas* sepsis. Am J Med. 1986;80:528–529.
110. Llistosella E, Revella A, Moreno A, et al. Panniculitis in *Pseudomonas aeruginosa* septicemia. Acta Derm Venereol (Stockh). 1984;64:447–449.
111. Picou KA, Jarratt MT. Persistent subcutaneous abscesses following *Pseudomonas* sepsis. Arch Dermatol. 1979;115:459–460.
112. Reed RK, Larter WE, Sieber OF, et al. Peripheral nodular lesions in *Pseudomonas* sepsis: The importance of incisions and drainage. J Pediatr. 1976;88:977–979.
113. Schlossberg D. Multiple erythematous nodules as a manifestation of *Pseudomonas aeruginosa* septicemia. Arch Dermatol. 1980;116:446–447.
114. Stanley MM. *Bacillus pyocyaneus* infections. Am J Med. 1947;9:253–277.
115. Baltch AL, Griffin PE. *Pseudomonas aeruginosa* bacteremia: A clinical study of 75 patients. Am J Med Sci. 1977;274:119–129.
116. Bodey GP, Jadeja L, Elting L. *Pseudomonas* bacteremia. Arch Intern Med. 1985;145:1621–1629.
117. Mandell IN, Feiner HD, Price NM, et al. *Pseudomonas cepacia* endocarditis and echthyma gangrenosum. Arch Dermatol. 1977;113:199–202.

118. Ketover BP, Young LS, Armstrong D. Septicemia due to *Aeromonas hydrophila*: Clinical and immunologic aspects. J Infect Dis. 1973;127:284–290.
119. Shackelford PG, Ratzan SA, Shearer WT. Ecthyma gangrenosum produced by *Aeromonas hydrophila.* J Pediatr. 1973;83:100–101.
120. Fine JD, Miller JA, Harrist TJ, et al. Cutaneous lesions in disseminated candidiasis mimicking echthyma gangrenosum. Am J Med. 1981;70:1133–1135.
121. Musher DM. Cutaneous and soft-tissue manifestations of sepsis due to gram-negative enteric bacilli. Rev Infect Dis. 1980;2:854–866.
122. El Baze P, Ortonne J-P. Ecthyma gangrenosum. J Am Acad Dermatol. 1985;13:299–300.
123. Huminer D, Siegman-Igra Y, Morduchowicz G, et al. Ecthyma gangrenosum without bacteremia. Arch Intern Med. 1987;147:299–310.
124. Von Reyn CF, Levy BS, Arbeit RD, et al. Infective endocarditis: An analysis based on strict case definitions. Ann Intern Med. 1981;94:505–518.
125. Venezio FR, Westenfelder GO, Cook FV, et al. Infective endocarditis in a community hospital. Arch Intern Med. 1982;142:789–792.
126. Terpenning MS, Buggy BP, Kauffman CA. Infective endocarditis: Clinical features in young and elderly patients. Am J Med. 1987;83:626–634.
127. King K, Harnkess JL. Infective endocarditis in the 1980s. Part 1. Aetiology and diagnosis. Med J Aust. 1986;144:536–540.
128. Dreyer NP, Fields BN. Heroin-associated endocarditis. Ann Intern Med. 1973;78:699–702.
129. Alpert JS, Krous HF, Dalen JE, et al. Pathogenesis of Osler's nodes. Ann Intern Med. 1976;85:471–473.
130. Yee J, McAllister CK. Osler's nodes and the recognition of infective endocarditis: A lesion of diagnostic importance. South Med J. 1987;80:753–757.
131. Cardullo AC, Silvers DN, Grossman ME. Janeway lesions and Osler's nodes: A review of histopathologic findings. J Am Acad Dermatol. 1990;22:1088–1090.
132. Harvey D. Staphylococcal infections. J Antimicrob Chemother. 1979;5(Suppl A):21–26.
133. Sheagren JN. *Staphylococcus aureus.* The persistent pathogen (first of two parts). N Engl J Med. 1984;310:1368–1373.
134. Sheagren JN. *Staphylococcus aureus.* The persistent pathogen (second of two parts). N Engl J Med. 1984;310:1437–1442.
135. Sheagren JN. Staphylococcal infections of the skin and skin structures. Cutis. 1985;361:2–6.
136. Wickboldt LG, Fenske NA. Streptococcal and staphylococcal infections of the skin. Hosp Pract. 1986;21:41–47.
137. Williams RE, MacKie RM. The staphylococci. Dermatol Clin. 1993;11:201–206.
138. Aly R. The pathogenic staphylococci. Semin Dermatol. 1990;9:292–299.
139. Arbuthnott JP, Coleman DC, de Azavedo JS. Staphylococcal toxins in human diseases. Soc Appl Bacteriol Symp Ser 1990;19:101S–107S.
140. Ginsburg CM. Staphylococcal toxin syndromes. Pediatr Infect Dis J. 1991;10:319–321.
141. Dowsett EG. The staphylococcal scalded skin syndrome. J Hosp Infect. 1984;5:347–354.
142. Elias PM, Fritsch P, Epstein EH. Staphylococcal scalded skin syndrome. Arch Dermatol. 1977;113:207–219.
143. Hebert AA, Esterly NB. Bacterial and candidal cutaneous infections in the neonate. Dermatol Clin. 1986;4:3–21.
144. Melish ME, Glasggow LA. Staphylococcal scalded skin syndrome: The expanded clinical syndrome. J Pediatr. 1971;78:958–967.
145. Borchers SL, Gomez EC, Isseroff RR. Generalized staphylococcal scalded skin syndrome in anephric boy undergoing hemodialysis. Arch Dermatol. 1984;120:912–918.
146. O'Keefe R, Dagg JH, MacKie RM. The staphylococcal scalded skin syndrome in two elderly immunocompromised patients. BMJ. 1987;295:179–180.
147. Richard M, Mathieu-Serra A. Staphylococcal scalded skin syndrome in a homosexual adult. J Am Acad Dermatol. 1986;15:385–389.
148. Beers B, Wilson B. Adult staphylococcal scalded skin syndrome. Int J Dermatol. 1990;29:428–429.
149. Donohue D, Robinson B, Goldbert NS. Staphylococcal scalded skin syndrome in a woman with chronic renal failure exposed to human immunodeficiency virus. Cutis. 1991;47:317–318.
150. Igarashi H, Fujikawa H, Usami H, et al. Purification and characterization of *Staphylococcus aureus* FRI 1169 and 587 toxic shock syndrome exotoxins. Infect Immun. 1984;44:175–181.
151. Bergdoll MS, Crass BA, Reiser RF, et al. A new *Staphylococcus* enterotoxin, enterotoxin F, associated with toxic-shock syndrome *Staphylococcus aureus* isolates. Lancet. 1981;1:1017–1021.
152. Schlievert PM, Shands KN, Dan BB, et al. Identification and characteristics of an exotoxin from *Staphylococcus aureus* associated with toxic-shock syndrome. J Infect Dis. 1981;143:509–516.
153. Schlievert PM. Role of superantigens in human disease. J Infect Dis. 1993;167:997–1002.
154. Kotb M. Bacterial pyrogenic exotoxins as superantigens. Clin Microbiol Rev. 1995;8:411–426.
155. Crass BA, Bergdoll MS. Involvement of coagulase-negative staphylococci in toxic shock syndrome. J Clin Microbiol. 1986;23:43–45.
156. Davis JP, Chesney PJ, Wand PJ, et al. Toxic shock syndrome. Epidemiologic features, recurrence, risk factors, and prevention. N Engl J Med. 1980;303:1429–1435.
157. Fisher RF, Goodpasture HC, Peterie JD, et al. Toxic shock syndrome in menstruating women. Ann Intern Med. 1981;94:156–163.
158. Centers for Disease Control and Prevention. Summary of notifiable diseases, United States, 1990. MMWR Morb Mortal Wkly Rep. 1990;39:1–61.
159. Holt PA, Armstrong AM, Norfolk GA, et al. Toxic-shock syndrome due to staphylococcal infection of a burn. Br J Clin Pract. 1987;41:582–583.
160. Reingold AL, Dan BB, Shands KN, et al. Toxic-shock syndrome not associated with menstruation. Lancet. 1982;1:1–4.
161. Reingold AL, Hargrett NT, Dan BB, et al. Nonmenstrual toxic shock syndrome. A review of 130 cases. Ann Intern Med. 1982;96:871–874.
162. Bates I. Characteristic rash associated with staphylococcal pneumonia. Lancet. 1987;2:1026–1027.
163. Center for Disease Control and Prevention. Toxic shock syndrome associated with influenza—Minnesota. MMWR Morb Mortal Wkly Rep. 1986;35:143–144.
164. Center for Disease Control and Prevention. Toxic shock syndrome following influenza—Oregon; update on influenza activity—United States. MMWR Morb Mortal Wkly Rep. 1987;36:64–65.
165. Wilkins EGL, Ney F, Roberts C, et al. Probable toxic shock syndrome with primary staphylococcal pneumonia. J Infect. 1985;11:231–232.
166. Finch R, Whitby M: Toxic shock syndrome. J R Coll Physicians Lond. 1985;19:219–223.
167. Tofte RW, Williams DN. Clinical and laboratory manifestations of toxic shock syndrome. Ann Intern Med. 1982;96:843–847.
168. Tofte RW, Williams DN. Toxic shock syndrome: Clinical and laboratory features in 15 patients. Ann Intern Med. 1981;94:149–156.
169. Tofte RW, Williams DN. Toxic shock syndrome. Recognition and management of a diverse disease. Postgrad Med. 1983;73:275–288.
170. Todd J, Fishuat M, Kapral F, et al. Toxic-shock syndrome associated with phage-group-1 staphylococci. Lancet. 1978;2:1116–1117.
171. Plaut MD. Staphylococcal septicemia and pustular purpura. Arch Dermatol. 1969;99:82–85.
172. Musher DM, McKenzie SO. Infections due to *Staphylococcus aureus.* Medicine (Baltimore). 1977;56:383–409.
173. Aach R, Kissane J, eds. A thirty-eight year old woman with overwhelming sepsis. Am J Med. 1972;53:233–241.
174. Murray HW, Tuazon CU, Sheagren JN. Staphylococcal septicemia and disseminated intravascular coagulation. Arch Intern Med. 1977;137:844–847.
175. Milunski MR, Gallis HA, Fulkerson WJ. *Staphylococcus aureus* septicemia mimicking fulminant Rocky Mountain spotted fever. Am J Med. 1987;83:801–803.
176. Rahal JJ, MacMahon E, Weinstein L. Thrombocytopenia and symmetrical peripheral gangrene associated with staphylococcal and streptococcal bacteremia. Ann Intern Med. 1968;69:35–43.
177. Bisno AL. Group A staphylococcal infections and acute rheumatic fever. N Engl J Med. 1991;325:783–793.
178. Bryan BO, Frieden I. Streptococcal skin disease in children. Semin Dermatol. 1992;11:3–10.
179. Low DE, Schwartz B, McGeer A. The reemergence of severe group A streptococcal disease: An evolutionary perspective. In: Scheld WM, Armstrong D, Hughes JM, eds. Emerging Infections, V. 1. Washington, DC: ASM Press; 1998.
180. Musser JM, Krause RM. The revival of group A streptococcal diseases, with a commentary on staphylococcal toxic shock syndrome. In: Krause RM, ed. Emerging Infections. London: Academic Press; 1998.
181. Stevens DL. The toxic shock syndromes. Infect Dis Clin North Am. 1996;10:727–746.
182. Stevens DL, Tanner MH, Winship J, et al. Severe group A streptococcal infections associated with toxic shock–like syndrome and scarlet fever toxin A. N Engl J Med. 1989;321:1–7.
183. Drabick JL, Lennox JL. Group A streptococcal infections and toxic shock–like syndrome (Letter). N Engl J Med. 1989;321:1545.
184. Hess EV, Grant KD. Group A streptococcal infections and toxic shock–like syndrome (Letter). N Engl J Med. 1989;321:1545–1546.
185. Wagner JG, Schlievert PM, Assimacopoulos AP, et al. Acute group G streptococcal myositis associated with streptococcal toxic shock syndrome: Case report and review. Clin Infect Dis. 1996;23:1159–1161.
186. Walker DH. Rickettsial disease: An update. In: Majno G, Cotran RS, Kaufman N, eds. Current Topics in Inflammation and Infection. Baltimore: Williams & Wilkins; 1982;188–204.
187. Kirk JL, Fine DP, Sexton DJ, Muchmore HG. Rocky Mountain spotted fever: A clinical review based on 48 confirmed cases, 1943–1986. Medicine. 1990;69:35–45.
188. Helmick CG, Bernard KW, D'Angelo LJ. Rocky Mountain spotted fever: Clinical, laboratory, and epidemiological features of 262 cases. J Infect Dis. 1984;150:480–488.
189. Hazard GW, Ganz RN, Nevin RW, et al. Rocky Mountain spotted fever in the Eastern United States. N Engl J Med. 1969;280:57–62.
190. Kaplowitz LG, Fischer JJ, Sparling PF. Rocky Mountain spotted fever: A clinical dilemma. In: Remington JS, Swartz MN, eds. Current Clinical Topics in Infectious Diseases. New York: McGraw-Hill; 1981:89–108.
191. Sexton DJ, Burgdorder W. Clinical and epidemiologic features of Rocky Mountain spotted fever in Mississippi, 1933–1973. South Med J. 1975;68:1529–1535.
192. Cohen JI, Corson AP, Corey GR. Late appearance of skin rash in Rocky Mountain spotted fever. South Med J. 1983;76:1457–1458.
193. Ramsey PG, Press OW. Successful treatment of Rocky Mountain "spotless" fever. West J Med. 1984;140:94–96.
194. Kirkland KB, Wilkinson E, Sexton DJ. Therapeutic delay and mortality in cases of Rocky Mountain spotted fever. Clin Infect Dis. 1995;20:1118–1121.
195. Kirkland KB, Marcom PK, Sexton DJ, et al. Rocky Mountain spotted fever

complicated by gangrene: Report of six cases and review. Clin Infect Dis. 1993;16:629–634.
196. Harkess JR. Ehrlichiosis. Infect Dis Clin North Am. 1991;5:37–52.
197. Hicklin H, Verghese A, Alvarez S. Dysgonic fermenter 2 septicemia. Rev Infect Dis. 1987;9:884–890.
198. Zumla A, Lipscomb G, Corbett M, et al. Dysgonic fermenter—type 2: An emerging zoonosis: Report of two cases and review. Q J Med. 1988;257:741–752.
199. Job L, Horman JT, Grigor JK, Israel E. Dysgonic fermenter-2: A clinico-epidemiologic review. J Emerg Med. 1989;7:185–192.
200. Krol-van Staaten MJ, Landheer JE, de Maat CEM. *Capnocytophaga canimorsus* (formerly DF-2) infections: Review of the literature. Neth J Med. 1990;36:304–309.
201. Kullberg B-J, Westendorp RGJ, van't Wout JW, Meinders AE. Purpura fulminans and symmetrical peripheral gangrene caused by *Capnocytophaga canimorsus* (formerly DF-2) septicemia—a complication of dog bite. Medicine. 1991;70:287–292.
202. Bilgrama S, Bergstron SK, Peterson DE, et al. *Capnocytophaga* bacteremia in a patient with Hodgkin's disease following bone marrow transplantation: Case report and review. Clin Infect Dis. 1992;14:1045–1049.
203. Mahrer S, Raik E. *Capnocytophaga canimorsus* septicemia associated with cat scratch. Pathology. 1992;24:194–196.
204. Buchstein SR, Gardner P. Lyme disease. Infect Dis Clin North Am. 1991;5:103–116.
205. Trevisan G, Cinco M. Lyme disease. Int J Dermatol. 1990;29:1–8.
206. Thyresson N. Historical notes on skin manifestations of Lyme borreliosis. Scand J Infect Dis. 1991;77:9–13.
207. Hercogova J, Tomankova M, Bartak P. Contributions to the treatment of dermatologic manifestations of Lyme borreliosis. Cutis. 1992;49:409–411.
208. Asbrink E. Cutaneous manifestations of Lyme borreliosis. Scand J Infect Dis. 1991;77(Suppl):44–50.
209. Asbrink E, Hovmark A. Lyme borreliosis: Aspects of tick-borne *Borrelia burgdorferi* infection from a dermatologic viewpoint. Semin Dermatol. 1990;9:277–291.
210. Centers for Disease Control and Prevention. Nosocomial infection surveillance. MMWR Morb Mortal Wkly Rep. 1984;35(Suppl):17–29.
211. Drutz DJ, Jarvis WR, de Repentigny L, et al. Severe nosocomial yeast infections. Conservations Infect Control. 1985;6:1–12.
212. Morrison AJ, Freer CV, Searcy MA, et al. Nosocomial bloodstream infections: Secular trends in a statewide surveillance program in Virginia. Infect Control. 1986;7:550–553.
213. Weber DJ, Rutala WA. Epidemiology of nosocomial fungal infections. In: McGinnis MR, ed. Current Topics in Medical Mycology. v. 2. New York: Springer Publishing; 1988:305–337.
214. Schaberg DR, Culver D. Major trends in the microbial etiology of nosocomial infection. Am J Med. 1991;91(Suppl 3B):72–75.
215. Banerjee SN, Emori TG, Culver DH, et al. Secular trends in nosocomial primary bloodstream infections in the United States, 1980–1989. Am J Med. 1991;91(Suppl 3B):86–89.
216. Weber DJ, Rutala WA, Samsa GP, et al. Relative frequency of nosocomial pathogens at a university hospital during the decade 1980 to 1989. Am J Infect Control. 1992;20:192–197.
217. Bodey GP. Fungal infection and fever of unknown origin in neutropenic patients. Am J Med. 1986;80:112–119.
218. Maksymiuk AW, Thongprasert S, Hopfer R, et al. Systemic candidiasis in cancer patients. Am J Med. 1984;77(Suppl):20–27.
219. Bodey GP. Candidiasis in cancer patients. Am J Med. 1984;77(Suppl):13–19.
220. Balandran L, Rothschild H, Pugh N, et al. A cutaneous manifestation of systemic candidiasis. Ann Intern Med. 1973;78:400–403.
221. Jacobs MI, Magid MS, Jarowski CI. Disseminated candidiasis. Arch Dermatol. 1980;116:1277–1279.
222. Kirkpatrick CH. Host factors in defense against fungal infections. Am J Med. 1984;77(Suppl):1–12.
223. Lederberg J, Shope RE, Oaks SC. Emerging Infections: Microbial Threats to Health in the United States. Institute of Medicine. Washington, DC: National Academy Press; 1992.
224. Morse SS. Factors in the emergence of infectious diseases. Emerging Infect Dis. 1995;1:7–15.
225. Ostroff SM, Kozarsky P. Emerging infectious diseases and travel medicine. Infect Dis Clin North Am. 1998;12:231–241.
226. Levy JA. Three new human herpesviruses (HHV6, 7, and 8). Lancet. 1997;349:558–563.
227. Braun DK, Dominguez G, Pellett P. Human herpesvirus 6. Clin Microbiol Rev. 1997;10:521–567.
228. Asano Y, Nakashima T, Yoshikawa T, Suga S, Yazaki T. Severity of human herpesvirus-6 viremia and clinical findings in infants with exanthem subitum. J Pediatr. 1991;118:891–895.
229. Pruksananonda P, Hall CB, Insel R, et al. Primary human herpesvirus 6 infection in young children. N Engl J Med. 1992;326:1445–1450.
230. Black JB, Durigon E, Kite-Powell K, et al. Seroconversion to human herpesvirus 6 and human herpesvirus 7 among Brazilian children with clinical diagnoses of measles and rubella. Clin Infect Dis. 1996;23:1156–1158.
231. Tait DR, Ward KN, Brown DWG, Miller E. Measles and rubella misdiagnosed in infants as exanthem subitum (roseola infantum). BMJ. 1996;312:101–102.
232. Steeper TA, Horwitz CA, Ablashi D, et al. The spectrum of clinical and laboratory findings resulting from the human herpesvirus-6 (HHV-6) in patients with mononucleosis-like illnesses not resulting from Epstein-Barr virus or cytomegalovirus. Am J Clin Pathol. 1990;93:776–783.
233. Akashit K, Eizuru Y, Sumiyoshi Y, et al. Brief report: Severe infectious mononucleosis–like syndrome and primary herpesvirus 6 infection in an adult. N Engl J Med. 1993;329:168–171.
234. Sumiyoshi Y, Akashi K, Kikichi M. Detection of human herpes virus (HHV 6) in the skin of a patient with primary HHV 6 infection and erythroderma. J Clin Pathol. 1994;47:762–763.
235. Ablashi DV, Berneman ZN, Kramarsky B, et al. Human herpes virus-7 (HHV-7): Current status. Clin Diag Virol. 1995;4:1–13.
236. Katsafanas GC, Schirmer EC, Wyatt LS, Frenkel N. *In vitro* activation of human herpesviruses 6 and 7 from latency. Proc Natl Acad Sci U S A. 1996;93:9788–9792.
237. Melnick JL. Taxonomy of viruses. In: Murray PR, ed. Manual of Clinical Microbiology. 6th ed. Washington, DC: ASM Press; 1995.
238. Mertz GJ, Hjelle BL, Bryan RT. Hantavirus infection. Dis Mon. 1998;44:87–138.
239. Schmaljohn C, Hjelle B. Hantaviruses: A global disease problem. Emerging Infect Dis. 1997;3:95–103.
240. Gill MV, Cunha BA. Ebola hemorrhagic fever. Infect Dis Pract. 1995;19:37–41.
241. Klenk HD, Feldmann H. Marbug and Ebola viruses. Adv Virus Res. 1996;47:1–52.
242. Feldmann H, Slenczka W, Klenk HD. Emerging and reemerging of filoviruses. Arch Virol. 1996;11(Suppl):77–100.
243. Sodhi A. Ebola virus disease: Recognizing the face of a rare killer. Postgrad Med. 1996;99:75–76, 78.
244. Ramirez-Ronda CH, Garcia CD. Dengue in the Western Hemisphere. Infect Dis Clin North Am. 1994;8:107–125.
245. Rigau-Perez JG. Clinical manifestations of dengue hemorrhagic fever in Puerto Rico, 1990–1991. Rev Panam Salud Publica. 1997;1:381–387.
246. Spach DH, Koehler JE. *Bartonella*-associated infections. Infect Dis Clin North Am. 1998;12:137–155.
247. Anderson BE, Neuman MA. *Baronella* spp. as emerging human pathogens. Clin Microbiol Rev. 1997;10:203–219.
248. Maurin M, Raoult D. *Bartonella (Rochalimaea) quintana* infections. Clin Microbiol Rev. 1996;9:273–292.
249. Tappero JW, Koehler JE, Berger TM, et al. Bacillary angiomatosis and bacillary splenitis in immunocompetent adults. Ann Intern Med. 1993;118:363–365.
250. Margileth AM, Wear DJ, English CK. Systemic cat scratch disease: Report of 23 patients with prolonged or recurrent severe bacterial infection. J Infect Dis. 1987;155:390–402.
251. Jimenez-Acosta F, Pardo RJ, Cohen RJ, et al. Bacillary angiomatosis and acquired immunodeficiency syndrome: Case report and literature review. J Am Acad Dermatol. 1990;22:525–529.
252. Cockerell CJ. The clinicopathologic spectrum of bacillary (epithelioid) angiomatosis. Prog AIDS Pathol. 1990;2:111–126.
253. Cockerell CJ, LeBoit PE. Bacillary angiomatosis: A newly characterized, pseudoneoplastic, infectious, cutaneous vascular disorder. J Am Acad Dermatol. 1990;22:501–512.
254. Schwartzman WA, Marchevsky A, Meyer RD. Epithelioid angiomatosis or cat scratch disease with splenic and hepatic abnormalities in AIDS: Case report and review of the literature. Scand J Infect Dis. 1990;22:121–133.
255. LeBoit PE. Bacillary angiomatosis: A systemic opportunistic infection with prominant cutaneous manifestations. Semin Dermatol. 1991;10:194–198.
256. Schwartzman WA. Infections due to *Rochalimaea*: The expanding spectrum clinical spectrum. Clin Infect Dis. 1992;15:893–902.
257. LeBoit PE, Berger TG, Egbert BM, et al. Epithelioid haemangioma–like vascular proliferation in AIDS: Manifestation of cat scratch disease bacillus infection? Lancet. 1988;1:960–963.
258. Tompkins DC, Steigbigel RT. *Rochalimaea*'s role in cat scratch disease and bacillary angiomatosis. Ann Intern Med. 1993;118:388–389.
259. Kemper CA, Lombard CM, Deresinski SC, Tompkins LS. Visceral bacillary epithelioid angiomatosis: Possible manifestations of disseminated cat scratch disease in the immunocompromised host: A report of two cases. Am J Med. 1990;89:216–222.
260. Adal KA, Cockerell CJ, Petri WA. Cat scratch disease, bacillary angiomatosis, and other infections due to *Rochalimaea*. N Engl J Med. 1994;33:1509–1515.
261. Cockerell CJ, Whitlow MA, Webster GF, Friedman-Kien AE. Epithelioid angiomatosis: A distinct vascular disorder in patients with the acquired immunodeficiency syndrome or AIDS-related complex. Lancet. 1987:1:654–656.
262. Miam MW, Balerdi MJ, Toney JF, et al. Epithelioid angiomatosis secondary to disseminated cat scratch disease involving the bone marrow and skin in a patient with acquired immunodeficiency syndrome: A case report. Am J Med. 1990;88:180–183.
263. Koehler JE, Quinn FD, Berger TG, et al. Isolation of *Rochalimaea* species from cutaneous and osseous lesions of bacillary angiomatosis. N Engl J Med. 1992;327:1625–1631.
264. Welch DF, Pickett DA, Slater LN, et al. *Rochalimaea henselae* sp. nov., a cause of septicemia, bacillary angiomatosis, and parenchymal bacillary peliosis. J Clin Microbiol. 1992;30:275–280.
265. Slater LN, Welch DF, Hensel D, et al. A newly recognized fastidious gram-negative pathogen as a cause of fever and bacteremia. N Engl J Med. 1990;323:1578–1593.
266. Walker DH. Emerging human ehrlichiosis: Recently recognized, widely distributed, life-threatening tick-borne disease. In: Scheld WM, Armstrong D, Hughes JM, eds. Emerging Infections I. Washington, DC: ASM Press; 1998.
267. Walker DH, Dumler JS. Emergence of the ehrlichiosis as human health problems. Emerging Infect Dis. 1996;2:18–27.
268. Fritz CL, Glaser CA. Ehrlichiosis. Infect Dis Clin North Am. 1998;12:123–136.
269. Dreizen S, McCredie KB, Bodey GP, et al. Unusual mucocutaneous infections. Postgrad Med. 1986;79:287–294.

270. Kaye ET, Johnson RA, Wolfson JS, Sober AJ. Dermatologic manifestations of infection in the compromised host. In: Rubin RH, Young LS, eds. Clinical Approach to Infection in the Compromised Host. 3rd ed. New York: Plenum; 1994:105–119.
271. Parker C. Skin lesions in transplant patients. Dermatol Clin. 1990;8:313–325.
272. Koranda FC, Dehmel EM, Kahn G, Penn I. Cutaneous complications in immunocompromised renal homograph recipients. JAMA. 1974;229:419–424.
273. Wolfson JS, Sober AJ, Rubin RH. Dermatologic manifestations of infections in immunocompromised patients. Medicine. 1985;64:115–133.
274. Bodey GP. Dermatologic manifestations of infections in neutropenic patients. Infect Dis Clin North Am. 1994;8:655–675.
275. Gentry LO, Zeluff B, Kielhofner MA. Dermatologic manifestations of infectious diseases in cardiac transplant patients. Infect Dis Clin North Am. 1994;8:637–654.
276. LaRocco MT, Burgert SJ. Infection in the bone marrow transplant recipient and role of the microbiology laboratory in clinical transplantation. Clin Rev Microbiol. 1997;10:277–297.
277. Beebe JL, Koneman EW. Recovery of uncommon bacteria from blood: Association with neoplastic disease. Clin Rev Microbiol. 1995;8:336–356.
278. Hoppenjans WB, Bibler MR, Orme RL, Solinger AM. Prolonged cutaneous herpes zoster in acquired immunodeficiency syndrome. Arch Dermatol. 1990;126:1048–1050.
279. Valle S. Dermatologic findings related to human immunodeficiency virus infection in high-risk individuals. J Am Acad Dermatol. 1987;17:951–961.
280. Trianan AF, Shapiro RS, Polk BF, et al. Mucocutaneous findings in acquired immunodeficiency syndrome/AIDS-related complex patients. J Am Acad Dermatol. 1987;16:888–889.
281. Kaslow RA, Phair RP, Freidman HB, et al. Infection with the human immunodeficiency virus: Clinical manifestations and their relationship to immune deficiency. Ann Intern Med. 1987;107:474–480.
282. Matis WL, Triana A, Shapiro R, et al. Dermatologic findings associated with immunodeficiency virus infection. J Am Acad Dermatol. 1987;17:746–751.
283. Cockerell CJ. Cutaneous manifestations of HIV infection other than Kaposi's sarcoma: Clinical and histologic aspects. J Am Acad Dermatol. 1990;22:1260–1269.
284. Berger TG, Obuch ML, Goldschmidt RH. Dermatologic manifestations of HIV infection. Am Fam Physician. 1990;41:1729–1742.
285. Cockerell CJ. Human immunodeficiency virus infection and the skin. Arch Intern Med. 1991;151:1295–1303.
286. Berger TG, Greene I. Bacterial, viral, fungal, and parasitic infections in HIV disease and AIDS. Dermatol Clin. 1991;9:465–492.
287. Dover JS, Johnson RA. Cutaneous manifestations of human immunodeficiency virus syndrome. Part I. Arch Dermatol. 1991;127:1383–1391.
288. Dover JS, Johnson RA. Cutaneous manifestations of human immunodeficiency virus syndrome. Part II. Arch Dermatol. 1991;127:1549–1557.
289. LeBoit PE. Dermatopathologic findings in patients infected with HIV. Dermatol Clin. 1992;10:59–71.
290. Gradon JD, Timpone JG, Schnittman SM. Emergence of unusual opportunistic pathogens in AIDS: A review. Clin Infect Dis. 1992;15:134–157.
291. Zalla MJ, Su WPD, Fransway AF. Dermatologic manifestations of human immunodeficiency virus infection. Mayo Clin Proc. 1992;67:1089–1108.
292. Stratigos AJ, Johnson RA, Dover JS. Cutaneous manifestations of human immunodeficiency virus infection. Semin Neurol. 1992;12:299–311.
293. Kurgis BS. Skin manifestations of human immunodeficiency virus (HIV): Part 1. Infectious manifestations. J Am Osteopath Assoc. 1993;93:106–117.
294. McCrossin I, Wong D. HIV-related skin disease. Med J Aust. 1993;158:179–185.
295. Tappero JW, Perkins BA, Wenger JD, Berger TG. Cutaneous manifestations of opportunistic infections in patients infected with human immunodeficiency virus. Clin Microbiol Rev. 1995;8:440–450.
296. Prose NS. HIV infection in children. J Am Acad Dermatol. 1990;22:1223–1231.
297. Torre D, Zeroli C, Fiori GP, et al. Dermatologic manifestations of AIDS in children. Pediatrician. 1991;18:195–203.
298. Nance KV, Smith ML, Joshi VV. Cutaneous manifestations of acquired immunodeficiency syndrome in children. Int J Dermatol. 1991;30:531–539.
299. Prose NS. Mucocutaneous disease in pediatric human immunodeficiency virus infection. Pediatr Clin North Am. 1991;38:977–990.
300. Prose NS. Cutaneous manifestations of pediatric HIV infection. Pediatr Dermatol. 1992;9:326–328.
301. Lim W, Sadick N, Gupta A, et al. Skin diseases in children with HIV infection and their association with degree of immunosuppression. Int J Dermatol. 1990;29:24–30.
302. Calabrese LH, Proffitt MR, Levin KH, et al. Acute infection with the human immunodeficiency virus (HIV) associated with acute brachial neuritis and exanthematous rash. Ann Intern Med. 1987;107:849–851.
303. Denning DW, Amos A, Wall RA. Oral and cutaneous features of acute human immunodeficiency virus infection. Cutis. 1987;40:171–175.
304. Ho DD, Sarngadharan MG, Resnick L, et al. Primary human T-lymphotropic virus type III infection. Ann Intern Med. 1985;103:880–883.
305. Boyko WJ, Schechter MT, Craib KJP, et al. The Vancouver lymphadenopathy-AIDS study: 7. Clinical and laboratory features of 87 cases of primary HIV infection. Can Med Assoc J. 1987;137:109–113.
306. Goodman DS, Teplitz ED, Wishner A, et al. Prevalence of cutaneous disease in patients with acquired immunodeficiency syndrome (AIDS) or AIDS-related complex. J Am Acad Dermatol. 1987;17:210–220.
307. Centers for Disease Control and Prevention. 1993 revised classification system for HIV infection and expanded surveillance case definition for AIDS among adolescents and adults. MMWR Morb Mortal Wkly Rep. 1992;41(RR-17):1–19.
308. Pierard G, Pierard-Franchimont C, Estrada JA, et al. Cutaneous mixed infections in AIDS. Am J Dermatopathol. 1990;12:63–66.
309. Kwan TH, Kaufman HW. Acid-fast bacilli with cytomegalovirus and herpes inclusions in the skin of an AIDS patient. Am J Clin Pathol. 1986;85:236–238.
310. Gretzula J, Penneys NS. Complex viral and fungal skin lesions of patients with acquired immunodeficiency syndrome. J Am Acad Dermatol. 1987;16:1151–1154.
311. Gulick RM. Varicella-zoster virus disease in patients with human immunodeficiency virus infection. Arch Dermatol. 1990;126:1086–1088.
312. Janier M, Hillion B, Baccard M, et al. Chronic varicella zoster infection in acquired immunodeficiency syndrome. J Am Acad Dermatol. 1988;18:584–585.
313. Disler R, Dover JS. Chronic localized herpes zoster in the acquired immunodeficiency syndrome. Arch Dermatol. 1990;126:1101–1106.
314. Leibovitz E, Kaul A, Rigaud M, et al. Chronic varicella zoster in a child infected with human immunodeficiency virus: Case report and review of the literature. Cutis. 1992;49:27–31.
315. Hicks CB, Benson PM, Lupton GP, et al. Seronegative secondary syphilis in a patient infected with the human immunodeficiency virus (HIV) with Kaposi's sarcoma. Ann Intern Med. 1987;107:492–495.
316. Bournerias I, Boisnic S, Patey O, et al. Unusual cutaneous cytomegalovirus involvement in patients with immunodeficiency syndrome. Arch Dermatol. 1989;125:1234–1236.
317. Angeles AM. Fungal and mycobacterial skin infections. Clin Dermatol. 1991;9:65–69.
318. Manrique P, Mayo J, Alvarez JA, et al. Polymorphous cutaneous cryptococcosis: Nodular, herpes-like, and molluscum-like lesions in a patient with the acquired immunodeficiency syndrome. J Am Acad Dermatol. 1992;26:122–123.
319. Prichard JG, Sorotzkin RA, James RE. Cutaneous manifestations of disseminated coccidioidomycosis in the acquired immunodeficiency syndrome. Cutis. 1987;39:203–205.
320. Brenner S. Acquired ichthyosis in AIDS. Cutis. 1987;39:421–423.
321. Young LY, Steinman HK. Acquired ichthyosis in a patient with acquired immunodeficiency syndrome and Kaposi's sarcoma. Cutis. 1987;39:395–396.

SECTION B

UPPER RESPIRATORY TRACT INFECTIONS

Chapter 46

The Common Cold

JACK M. GWALTNEY, JR.

Common cold is the traditional term used by both physicians and laypersons for acute minor coryzal illness, although the existence of a single entity, as implied by the term, is incorrect. Instead, the "common cold" is a group of diseases caused, for the most part, by members of five families of viruses. The viruses in these families have distinctive biochemical properties that govern their differing pathogenic and epidemiologic behaviors. In addition, the immunotypes found in the various viral families have antigenic variations that are of biologic importance to the immune system of their human host. The problem of controlling acute respiratory disease presents a complex challenge that requires approaches suitable for the properties of the individual virus groups. Therefore, the hope for development of a single "cure" for the "common cold" is an unrealistic expectation that has led to the diversion of resources into attempts at simplistic and unrealistic solutions to the problem.

As a clinical entity, the common cold is a mild, self-limited, catarrhal syndrome that is the leading cause of acute morbidity and of visits to physicians in the United States. It is also a major cause of industrial and school absenteeism.[1] A small proportion of colds is complicated by bacterial infections of the paranasal sinuses and the middle ear, which require antimicrobial therapy.

Based on early observations of their contagious nature, colds have long been thought to be caused by infectious agents. However, it was not until the isolation of a number of new respiratory viruses in cell culture in the 1950s that the specific cause of colds was known. The first of these, a parainfluenza virus, was discovered in 1955.[2] In 1956, rhinoviruses were isolated from adults with common colds.[3, 4] The following year, respiratory syncytial virus (RSV) was associated with acute respiratory illness in infants,[5] and in 1958 one of the enteroviruses, coxsackievirus A21, was recovered from military recruits with mild respiratory disease.[6] The most recent group of common cold viruses to be discovered, the coronaviruses, was first reported in the 1960s.[7, 8] Since that time, no new cold viruses have been found, although the specific cause of some colds remains unknown. Other respiratory viruses, such as influenza virus and adenovirus, produce the common cold syndrome but are characteristically associated with a more severe illness, which often involves the lower respiratory tract.

ETIOLOGY

The major respiratory viruses causing colds and similar upper respiratory tract illnesses are found in the myxovirus, paramyxovirus, adenovirus, picornavirus, and coronavirus groups (Table 46–1).[9–12] Within three groups of viruses are many different antigenic types. The rhinovirus group, which accounts for approximately 40% of colds in adults, has 100 immunotypes. The percentage of colds caused by the coronavirus group and the number of immunotypes of this virus have not been fully determined, but it is believed that these viruses are an important cause of colds. The three parainfluenza viruses and the RSV each account for a proportion of colds on an annual basis. Influenza virus and adenovirus produce a spectrum of illness that overlaps the common cold syndrome. Some of the enteroviruses produce coryza,[13] as do some viruses that usually produce other characteristic findings, such as exanthems. Because mild streptococcal pharyngitis cannot be differentiated from viral pharyngitis on clinical grounds, it also is included as a cause of "colds." The cause of approximately one third to one fourth of colds in adults remains unknown. Some illnesses may be undiagnosed because of the insensitivity of methods currently used for detection of known viruses, and others may be caused by undiscovered agents. Colds in children are caused by the same viruses in roughly the same proportion, but the total number of colds that can be diagnosed in children is usually lower. In some studies, as many as 70% of acute respiratory illnesses in children cannot be assigned a cause.

Colds are frequent because of the large number of different causative viruses and also because reinfections may occur with the same virus type. Second infections probably occur with members of all the viral groups; with some, such as coronavirus, reinfections appear to be particularly common. Up to 80% of persons infected with coronavirus OC43 have prior neutralizing antibody to the virus.[14]

SEASONAL INCIDENCE

The respiratory viruses have a worldwide distribution. Annual epidemics of upper respiratory tract disease occur in the colder months in temperate areas and during the rainy season in the tropics. In the United States the respiratory disease season begins in late August to mid-September.[15, 16] Respiratory illness rates rise sharply for a few weeks and then remain elevated until spring. During March, April, and May, rates decline to the low summer level.

The events controlling the seasonal variation in attack rates of acute respiratory disease are not well understood. Adding to the complexity of the problem has been the discovery that some of the virus groups have their own seasonal pattern within the overall respiratory disease season. Rhinovirus outbreaks typically occur in the early fall and in middle to late spring,[16] and coronaviruses are most prominent in the winter.[14] Studies with a specific virus, rhinovirus type 15, showed that chilling of volunteers did not increase their susceptibility to infection and illness.[17] Therefore, the effect of ther-

TABLE 46–1 Viruses Associated with the Common Cold

Virus Group	Antigenic Types	Percentage of Cases*
Rhinoviruses	100 types and 1 subtype	30–40
Coronavirus	3 or more types	≥10
Parainfluenza virus	4 types	
Respiratory syncytial virus	2 types	
Influenza virus	3 types	10–15
Adenovirus	47 types	5
Other viruses (enteroviruses, rubeola, rubella, varicella)		5
Presumed undiscovered viruses		25–30
Group A β-hemolytic streptococci†		5–10

*Estimated percentage of colds annually.
†Included because differentiation of streptococcal and viral pharyngitis is not possible by clinical means.

mal cold per se on the host does not appear to explain the seasonal outbreaks of colds.

Undoubtedly, among the responsible variables for seasonal fluctuations in colds are the bringing together of children during school periods and the increased crowding indoors of populations during colder months.[18] Also, seasonal changes in relative humidity may be an important variable controlling prevalence of the different virus families because of the effect of relative humidity on virus survival. In general, enveloped viruses survive better under conditions of low relative humidity, as found in colder months of the year, and the converse is true for nonenveloped viruses.

ATTACK RATES

During peak months in the respiratory disease season in the United States, adults average 6 to 8 colds per 1000 persons per day.[16] In the summer, rates fall to 2 or 3 colds per 1000 per day. Overall, adults in the United States average two to four colds per year and children average six to eight.[15, 16] In one 10-year study of illness in families, young children in nursery school averaged up to nine colds for the period of September through May. Illness rates decline in older children and reach adult levels in adolescence. Boys have slightly more colds than girls until adolescence, but after that the incidence is slightly higher in women, perhaps reflecting their greater exposure to young children.[12] Adults with children in the home have more colds than those without this exposure.[15, 19] Tonsillectomy does not reduce the incidence of colds.[15] Cigarette smokers have the same incidence of colds as nonsmokers, but the severity of their illnesses is greater.[16, 20]

TRANSMISSION

The main reservoir of respiratory viruses is in the upper airway in young children. Spread of colds takes place most commonly in the home,[15, 19] in schools,[21] and in daycare centers.[22] Children acquire new viral strains from their schoolmates, which they then bring home and pass to other family members. Intervals of 1 to 5 days occur between cases. Secondary attack rates of family members vary depending on age, position in the family, and prior immunity to the virus. Age and immunity are related risk factors. Young children and mothers have high secondary attack rates as a result of close and prolonged exposure to schoolchildren in the family. The secondary attack rate of fathers is relatively low.

The natural mechanisms for the spread of cold viruses have not been well established. Possible means of transmission include (1) direct contact with infectious secretions on skin and environmental surfaces, (2) large particles of respiratory secretions that are briefly transported in air, (3) infectious droplet nuclei suspended in air, and (4) combinations of these methods.[23] For some viruses, such as rhinovirus, close physical contact appears to be necessary for efficient spread. Infectious rhinovirus is produced primarily in the nose and is shed in highest concentrations in nasal secretions. Peak viral titers in nasal mucus occur on the second to fourth days of experimental infection and coincide with the period of maximum communicability.[23] A high proportion of persons with natural and experimental rhinovirus colds have recoverable virus on their hands. With experimental rhinovirus infection, brief hand contact permits ready transfer of virus-contaminated nasal secretions from the hands of infected subjects to the hands of susceptible subjects. When the contaminated fingers of the susceptible subjects are then placed in contact with nasal and conjunctival mucosa, infection results in a high percentage of cases.[24] In one study conducted in the home setting, treatment of fingers with a virucidal solution reduced the rate of infection in mothers exposed to other family members with fresh colds.[25] This study provides direct evidence of the mechanisms of common cold transmission under natural conditions and suggests that a proportion of colds are spread by hand contamination and self-inoculation.

Another rhinovirus transmission model has been developed in which virus is reliably transmitted through the air in large-and/or small-particle aerosol.[26] This model demonstrates the feasibility of the aerosol route of spread but does not prove that it occurs under natural conditions. Studies conducted in the field with intervention techniques specific for aerosol transmission are needed to address that question. There is epidemiologic evidence that influenza and adenovirus may be spread, at least in part, by small airborne droplets. All respiratory viruses may not behave in the same way, and further studies are necessary to determine which routes of transmission are important in the natural dissemination of these viruses.

PATHOGENESIS

Viral invasion of the upper respiratory tract is the basic mechanism in the pathogenesis of colds, but the specific events leading to clinical illness have only recently been investigated. Infection with common cold viruses is characteristically of short duration and self-limited. For example, maximum rhinovirus shedding lasts 3 weeks or less in young adults with experimental colds,[27, 28] and coronavirus excretion has been detected for only 1 to 4 days.[14] Cold viruses are not usually present in asymptomatic persons,[29] although subclinical infections do occur and viral carriage may be somewhat prolonged in children.[30]

Characteristic changes have been described in sloughed columnar epithelial cells in nasal secretions of persons with natural colds of unknown cause.[31] Cells with persistent ciliary activity have been found in nasal secretions on days 1 through 3 of illness. Also, some exfoliated cells show degenerative changes characterized by progressive nuclear pyknosis and the formation of apparent inclusion bodies. Ciliated epithelial cells containing viral antigen have been found in the nasal mucus of volunteers with experimental rhinovirus colds.[32]

Attempts to demonstrate specific histopathologic changes in nasal biopsy specimens of volunteers with rhinovirus colds have not been successful.[33, 34] Examination by light and electron microscopy of nasal biopsy specimens from young adults with natural colds also confirmed the absence of destruction of the nasal epithelium.[35] In this study there was a significant increase in the number of neutrophils in the epithelium and in the lamina propria. The number of epithelial mast cells was not increased. The findings with rhinovirus contrast with the destructive changes to the respiratory epithelium that are seen with influenza virus and adenovirus infections.

With rhinovirus colds, the period of maximum viral excretion in nasal secretions coincides with the peak of clinical illness[36] and the appearance of ciliated epithelial cells in nasal mucus.[32] At that time, large quantities of protein, including immunoglobulins, are present in nasal secretions. In addition to any direct destructive effect that the virus may have on the respiratory mucous membrane, there is increasing evidence that chemical mediators and neurologic reflexes play a role in the pathogenesis of the common cold. Bradykinin,[37, 38] prostaglandin,[38, 39] histamine,[38, 40] interleukin-1,[41] interleukin-6,[42] and interleukin-8[43, 44] have been associated with rhinovirus pathogenesis and with parasympathetic[45] and α-adrenergic nerve pathways.[46] Pathogenic mechanisms for the various respiratory viruses are undoubtedly somewhat different.

A self-limited cold virus infection may lead to changes that affect the resident bacterial flora of the upper respiratory tract and result in secondary bacterial infection. Bacteria invade normally sterile areas such as the sinuses, middle ear, and perhaps the tracheobronchial tree. The events involved in triggering these secondary bacterial infections are unknown but probably include deposition of bacteria into the sinuses and middle ear, obstruction of outlet areas, and damage to mucociliary cleansing. Experimental and natural colds routinely lead to acute, reversible abnormalities of the ostiomeatal area and sinus cavities.[47, 48] It is unknown whether direct viral invasion of the sinus, middle ear, and tracheobronchial tree is necessary for subsequent bacterial infection to occur or whether the viral involvement can remain localized to the nasal and pharyngeal mucous membrane. However, respiratory viruses have been recovered from sinus[49] and middle ear[9, 50] aspirates obtained by direct puncture from patients with inflammation at these sites. Abnormalities in eustachian tube function and middle ear pressures have been consistently observed in volunteers with experimental rhinovirus infection.[51] During colds, increases have also been noted in titers of resident bacterial populations of the upper airways, but the significance of this is unknown.[52, 53]

CLINICAL CHARACTERISTICS

The incubation period of the common cold varies somewhat with the different viruses but is usually between 12 and 72 hours. The symptoms of experimental rhinovirus colds have an onset 8 to 16 hours after viral inoculation into the nose.[37, 54] The cardinal symptoms are nasal discharge, nasal obstruction, sneezing, sore or "scratchy" throat, and cough.[15, 20] Slight fever may be found, but temperature elevation of more than 1°F is distinctly uncommon in adults. Infants and young children may more frequently have temperature elevation. The early symptoms may be minimal, with only "scratchy" throat, mild malaise, and nasal complaints. With rhinovirus infection, sneezing, nasal discharge, and nasal obstruction usually begin simultaneously on the first day of illness and rapidly increase to maximum severity by the second or third day. Paralleling the nasal symptoms is a sore, dry, or "scratchy" throat. Cough and hoarseness may also begin early in the course of illness and, when present, tend to persist until the end of the first week of symptoms, by which time nasal and pharyngeal complaints have usually subsided. Limited information is available suggesting that symptom patterns are similar with coronavirus colds[14] (see Chapter 145).

The median duration of rhinovirus colds is 1 week, but in approximately one fourth of cases the illness lasts up to 2 weeks. In cigarette smokers with rhinovirus colds, cough is increased and prolonged. Other complaints may include mild burning of the eyes, but true conjunctivitis is not seen except in some adenovirus and enterovirus infections. There may also be loss of the senses of smell and taste and a feeling of facial pressure and fullness in the ears. The voice may have a nasal quality. Painful maceration of the skin around the nostrils is often bothersome when rhinorrhea has been profuse and persistent.

On physical examination, the findings are often minimal despite the subjective discomfort of the patient. A red nose and a dripping nasal discharge are the characteristic features of the patient with a cold, but many patients lack these outward manifestations of the infection. The nasal mucous membrane may have a glassy appearance owing to the exudation of serum proteins and increased mucus secretions. It is difficult to accurately detect the presence of increased erythema of the mucous membrane of the nose and throat because of normal variations in the color of these structures. Marked pharyngeal erythema and exudate are not seen with rhinovirus and coronavirus infections, but they do occur with pharyngoconjunctival fever of adenovirus infection and with primary herpes simplex pharyngitis. Examination of the chest may reveal the presence of rhonchi.

The clinical picture of the common cold is similar in children and in adults. However, in young children, parainfluenza virus and RSV infections may lead to viral pneumonia, croup, and bronchiolitis, whereas in adults these viruses usually cause only colds. In both adults and children, the upper airway manifestations of rhinovirus, coronavirus, parainfluenza virus, and RSV infections are indistinguishable in the individual patient.

DIAGNOSIS

The manifestations of the common cold are so typical and familiar that self-diagnosis by the patient is usually correct. Hay fever and vasomotor rhinitis may result in similar nasal symptoms, but the recurrent and chronic nature of these diseases is soon recognized by the patient and easily diagnosed by the physician from the patient's history. Diagnosis of the specific virus involved is usually not possible on the basis of clinical observation. Some acute respiratory infections, such as influenza and pharyngoconjunctival fever, when seen in a typical epidemiologic setting, can be recognized without benefit of viral culture or serologic tests. Knowledge of the characteristic seasonal patterns for the different virus groups may also suggest a particular virus.

The main challenge to the physician is to distinguish the uncomplicated cold from cases of secondary bacterial sinusitis (0.5 to 2% of colds)[15, 55] and otitis media (2%).[15] This is not easy because of the lack of inexpensive and noninvasive diagnostic tests for this purpose. A complete physical examination should be performed on the pharynx, nasal cavity, ears, and sinuses. In the pharynx, marked infection or exudate should raise suspicion of streptococcal or adenovirus infection, herpes simplex pharyningitis, Vincent's angina, mononucleosis, or diphtheria. Occasionally, patients have small vesicles on the palate as a result of coxsackievirus A infections. The presence of nasal polyps is suggestive of an underlying allergy problem. In children, a foreign body may lead to persistent nasal discharge. Examination of the ears is directed at finding changes in the appearance of the tympanum, indicating infection (see Chapter 50). The use of the pneumatic otoscope is helpful in determining whether fluid is present behind the ear drum. There may be sinus tenderness or swelling and erythema over the area of a sinus, but these findings are uncommon.

Sinus computed tomography scans are sensitive for detecting abnormalities in the sinuses of patients with cold symptoms.[48] The cost and inconvenience of computed tomography precludes its use in routine practice. More importantly, it is not an accurate way to distinguish between pure viral and secondary bacterial infections of the sinus. The most valuable laboratory test in patients with prominent pharyngeal complaints is rapid antigen detection for group A β-hemolytic streptococci, with throat culture when indicated. Many of the respiratory viruses can be isolated in cell culture, although specific virologic diagnosis is not usually available in clinical practice. Rhinoviruses grow in human embryonic lung cells, myxoviruses and paramyxoviruses in primary rhesus monkey kidney cells, and RSV in Hep2 cells. Isolation of coronavirus in cell culture has proved difficult with currently available techniques. The sensitivity of the tests for isolating viruses can vary widely owing to variations in the sensitivity of the cell cultures. Nucleic acid probes are being developed for detecting common cold viruses, but their utility in clinical practice has not been established.[56–58]

Serologic diagnostic analyses for influenza virus, parainfluenza virus, RSV, and adenovirus infection are available in some state health department laboratories. Serum specimens should be obtained in the acute phase of illness and again approximately 3 weeks later and tested simultaneously. A rise of fourfold or greater in antibody titer is indicative of infection. Serologic diagnosis of rhinovirus infection is not practical because of the many different antigenic types. Rapid techniques using fluorescent antibody or other immunodiagnostic procedures on respiratory secretions are being used in clinical laboratories for the diagnosis of influenza virus, parainfluenza virus, RSV, and adenovirus (see Chapters 14, 132, 146, 148, 153).

TREATMENT

Although a "cure" for the common cold remains elusive, some of the available commercial remedies provide good symptomatic relief. Leading the list of effective cold treatments are the first-generation antihistamines and the nonsteroidal anti-inflammatory drugs (NSAID). Antihistamines have only recently been tested in properly powered clinical trials in adults with colds.[59–61] Good relief was observed for sneezing, rhinorrhea, nasal mucus weights, and, with one of the drugs,[61] cough. The newer, nonsedating antihistamines do not appear to have the same effectiveness in treating cold symptoms.

NSAIDs sulindac,[62] indomethacin,[63] and naproxen[64] have shown effectiveness in reducing cough, presumably through blocking prostaglandin action.[38] These compounds also are useful for treating headaches, malaise, and other systemic complaints.

The combination of a first-generation antihistamine and an NSAID provides good relief of cold symptoms. In an unpublished trial I conducted in volunteers with experimental rhinovirus colds, I found that brompheniramine (12 mg, extended release) and naproxen sodium (275 mg) given on an every-12-hour schedule resulted in significant and clinically relevant reduction in sneezing, rhinorrhea, nasal mucus weights, nasal obstruction, cough, headache, and malaise. Treatment was begun 24 hours after viral challenge, during early symptomatic infection, and continued regularly for 5 days. This, or a similar combination of a first-generation antihistamine and an NSAID, is recommended for use at the first evidence of cold symptoms. First-generation antihistamines cause clinically important drowsiness in 10 to 15% percent of patients, and NSAIDs can result in gastric irritation.

Because this combined antihistamine-NSAID therapy relieves nasal obstruction, decongestant therapy may not be necessary. When required, oral decongestants are recommended to avoid the rebound nasal obstruction and pharyngeal irritation associated with topical preparations such as phenylephrine and oxymetazoline. Oral decongestants have been shown to be safe in patients with hypertension on therapy.[65] Dextromethorphan and codeine have been used successfully in practice for cough suppression, although their effectiveness has been difficult to demonstrate in controlled clinical trials in patients with colds.[66]

Sore throat can be relieved with warm saline gargles or lozenges containing a topical anesthetic. The regular application of an ointment containing a petrolatum base is useful in controlling painful maceration of the nares. The patient's activities should be restricted during the height of the illness, when the patient is most contagious to others. Regular hand washing and care to avoid contamination of the environment with nasal secretions may also help to prevent spread of infection.

Antibiotics have no place in the treatment of uncomplicated colds. Until specific treatment becomes available, there will continue to be fads in the use of "alternative" cold remedies. The ingestion of large doses of vitamin C has been widely used as a preventive or therapeutic measure for colds. Controlled studies have shown a modest therapeutic benefit of vitamin C for colds but have failed to show any usefulness in preventing cold.[67, 68] Vitamin C has mild anticholinergic activity.

Three properly designed clinical trials failed to show a beneficial effect of zinc for treatment of colds,[69–71] and positive studies probably reflected poor masking of subjects and other problems with experimental design.[72] Echinacea, an herbal medicine, has never received adequate testing for colds,[73] and has potentially serious side effects, involving T_4 lymphocyte suppression.[74, 75]

PROSPECTS FOR VACCINES, NEW TREATMENTS, AND INTERRUPTION OF TRANSMISSION

Vaccine development for the common cold has reached an impasse because of the discovery of the many different cold viruses, particularly the 100 different serotypes of rhinoviruses. Unless ways are found to combine large numbers of viral antigens effectively or to take advantage of minor antigenic cross-relationships that exist, prospects for common cold vaccines are not good. A number of chemical compounds have inhibitory activity against respiratory viruses in tissue culture systems, and attempts are being made to develop antiviral agents for clinical use. The activity of such compounds tends to be relatively group specific, but some have shown activity against most of the rhinoviruses.[76]

Intranasal recombinant human interferon alfa-2b has effective prophylactic activity against experimental rhinovirus infection.[77–79] When given therapeutically intranasally, interferon has reduced viral excretion, but its effect on illness has been of only minimal benefit.[80] In addition, chronic application of intranasal interferon is associated with local side effects such as nasal stuffiness, dryness, discomfort, and pinpoint areas of ulceration.[81, 82] Short-term contact prophylaxis with intranasal interferon by family members exposed to individuals with colds of recent onset reduced the incidence of total colds by 40% and virtually eliminated rhinovirus-specific infections.[83, 84] Side effects were avoided by the short duration of the course of interferon.

The therapeutic failure of potent antivirals such as interferon alfa-2b[80] and the capsid binders, which block viral attachment and uncoating,[85, 86] suggests that treatment with antiviral compounds alone may be insufficient to provide clinically useful benefits. This may be the result of the inflammatory events accompanying the infection, which would not be expected to respond to the antiviral. To test this hypothesis, an experimental treatment was developed that combined a compound with antiviral activity with other compounds that block selected pathways of inflammation. Promising results were obtained in a study in which volunteers with early rhinovirus colds were given interferon alfa-2b and ipratropium topically into the nose plus oral naproxen.[64] A new approach under investigation is the intranasal application of synthetic rhinovirus receptor (ICAM-I) to block viral attachment to cells in the nose. When this treatment was started 7 hours before or 12 hours after viral challenge, it reduced the severity of experimental rhinovirus colds.[87]

Another approach to control of colds is to interrupt the person-to-person transmission of the viruses. A virucidal hand treatment used in the home by mothers exposed to children with new colds reduced the mothers' incidence of total colds by 60% and eliminated laboratory-proven rhinovirus colds.[25] In another study, children trained to avoid self-inoculatory behavior had reduced cold-associated asthmatic attacks and laboratory-proven respiratory virus infections.[88] These studies suggest that spread of cold viruses occurs in part by direct hand contact and self-inoculation. Hand washing and avoidance of finger-nose and finger-eye contact should be practiced, particularly when there is exposure to someone with a cold. Also, covering of coughs and sneezes with disposable nasal tissues is recommended as a means of controlling aerosol transmission.

REFERENCES

1. Rice DP, Feldman JJ, White KL. The current burden of illness in the United States. Occasional Papers of the Institute of Medicine. Washington, DC: National Academy of Science; 1976:1.
2. Chanock RM. Association of a new type of cytopathogenic myxovirus with infantile croup. J Exp Med. 1956;104:55.
3. Pelon W, Mogabgab WJ, Phillips IA, et al. A cytopathogenic agent isolated from naval recruits with mild respiratory illness. Proc Soc Exp Biol Med. 1957;94:262.
4. Price WH. The isolation of a new virus associated with respiratory clinical disease in humans. Proc Natl Acad Sci U S A. 1956;43:892.
5. Chanock RM, Roizman B, Myers R. Recovery from infants with respiratory illness of a virus related to Chimpanzee Coryza Agent (CCA): I. Isolation, properties, and characterization. Am J Hyg. 1957;66:281.
6. Lennette EH, Fox VL, Schmidt NJ, et al. The COE virus: An apparently new virus recovered from patients with mild respiratory disease. Am J Hyg. 1958;68:272.
7. Tyrrell DAJ, Bynoe ML. Cultivation of a novel type of common-cold virus in organ cultures. BMJ. 1965;1:1467.
8. Hamre D, Procknow JJ. A new virus isolated from the human respiratory tract. Proc Soc Exp Biol Med. 1966;121:190.
9. Gwaltney JM Jr. Virology of middle ear. Ann Otol Rhinol Laryngol. 1971;80:365.
10. Stuart-Harris CH, Andrewes C, Andrews BE, et al. A collaborative study of the aetiology of acute respiratory infection in Britain 1961–4: A report of the Medical Research Council working party on acute respiratory virus infections. BMJ. 1965;2:319.
11. Hamre D, Connelly AP Jr, Procknow JJ. Virologic studies of acute respiratory disease in young adults: IV. Virus isolations during four years of surveillance. Am J Epidemiol. 1966;83:238.
12. Monto AS, Bryan ER, Ohmit S. Rhinovirus infections in Tecumseh, Michigan: Frequency of illness and number of serotypes. J Infect Dis. 1987;156:43–49.
13. Kepfer PD, Hable KA, Smith TF. Viral isolation rates during summer from children with acute upper respiratory tract disease and health children. AJCP. 1974;16:1–5.
14. Monto AS. Coronaviruses. In: Evans AS, ed. Viral Infections of Humans: Epidemiology and Control. 3rd ed. New York: Plenum; 1989:153–167.
15. Dingle JH, Badger GF, Jordan WS Jr. Illness in the Home: Study of 25,000 Illnesses

in a Group of Cleveland Families. Cleveland: The Press of Western Reserve University; 1964:1.
16. Gwaltney JM Jr, Hendley JO, Simon G, et al. Rhinovirus infections in an industrial population: I. The occurrence of illness. N Engl J Med. 1966;275:1261.
17. Douglas RG Jr, Lindgren KM, Couch RB. Exposure to cold environment and rhinovirus common cold: Failure to demonstrate effect. N Engl J Med. 1968;279:743.
18. Gwaltney JM Jr. The Jeremiah Metzger Lecture: Climatology and the common cold. Trans Am Clin Climatol Assoc. 1984;96:159.
19. Hendley JO, Gwaltney JM Jr, Jordan WS Jr. Rhinovirus infections in an industrial population: IV. Infections within families of employees during two fall peaks of respiratory illness. Am J Epidemiol. 1969;89:184.
20. Gwaltney JM Jr, Hendley JO, Simon G, et al. Rhinovirus infections in an industrial population: II. Characteristics of illness and antibody response. JAMA. 1967;202:494.
21. Beem MO. Acute respiratory illness in nursery school children: A longitudinal study of the occurrence of illness and respiratory viruses. Am J Epidemiol. 1969;90:30.
22. Frenck RW, Glezen WP. Respiratory tract infections in children in day care. Semin Pediatr Infect Dis. 1990;1:234–244.
23. Gwaltney JM Jr. Epidemiology of the common cold. Ann N Y Acad Sci. 1980;353:54.
24. Gwaltney JM Jr, Moskalski PB, Hendley JO. Hand-to-hand transmission of rhinovirus colds. Ann Intern Med. 1978;88:463.
25. Hendley JO, Gwaltney JM Jr. Mechanisms of transmission of rhinovirus infections. Epidemiol Rev. 1988;10:242.
26. Dick EC, Jennings LC, Mink KA, et al. Aerosol transmission of rhinovirus colds. J Infect Dis. 1987;156:442.
27. Cate TR, Couch RB, Johnson KM. Studies with rhinoviruses in volunteers: Production of illness, effect of naturally acquired antibody, and demonstration of a protective effect not associated with serum antibody. J Clin Invest. 1964;43:56.
28. Winther B, Gwaltney JM Jr, Mygind N, et al. Sites of rhinovirus recovery after point inoculation of the upper airway. JAMA. 1986;256:1763.
29. Hamre D, Rhinoviruses. In: Melnick JL, ed. Monographs in Virology 1. Basel: Karger; 1968;1.
30. Frank AL, Taber LH, Wells CR, et al. Patterns of shedding of myxoviruses in children. J Infect Dis. 1981;144:433.
31. Bryan WTK, Bryan MP, Smith CA. Human ciliated epithelial cells in nasal secretions. Transactions of the 85th Annual Meeting of the American Laryngological Association. 1964:145.
32. Turner RB, Hendley JO, Gwaltney JM Jr. Shedding of infected ciliated epithelial cells in rhinovirus colds. J Infect Dis. 1982;145:849.
33. Douglas RG Jr, Alford BR, Couch RB. Atraumatic nasal biopsy for studies of respiratory virus infection in volunteers. Antimicrob Agents Chemother. 1968;8:340.
34. Winther B, Farr B, Turner RB, et al. Histopathologic examination and enumeration of polymorphonuclear leukocytes in the nasal mucosa during experimental rhinovirus colds. Acta Otolaryngol (Stockh). 1984;413 (suppl):19–24.
35. Winther B, Brofeldt S, Christensen B, et al. Light and scanning electron microscopy of nasal biopsies from patients with naturally acquired common colds. Acta Otalaryngol. 1984;97:309.
36. Douglas RG Jr, Cate TR, Gerone PJ, et al. Quantitative rhinovirus shedding patterns in volunteers. Am Rev Respir Dis. 1966;94:159.
37. Naclerio RM, Proud D, Lichtenstein LM, et al. Kinins are generated during experimental rhinovirus colds. J Infect Dis. 1988;157:133.
38. Doyle WJ, Boehm S, Skoner DP. Physiologic responses to intranasal dose-response challenges with histamine, methacholine, bradykinin, and prostaglandin in adult volunteers with and without nasal allergy. J Allergy Clin Immunol. 1990;86:924–935.
39. Sperber SJ, Hendley JO, Hayden FG, et al. Effects of naproxen on experimental rhinovirus colds: A randomized, double-blind, controlled trial. Ann Intern Med. 1992;117:37–41.
40. Doyle WJ, McBride TP, Skoner DP, et al. A double-blind, placebo-controlled clinical trial of the effect of chlorpheniramine on the response of the nasal airway, middle ear and eustachian tube to provocative rhinovirus challenge. Pediatr Infect Dis J. 1988;7:229–238.
41. Proud D, Gwaltney JM Jr, Hendley JO, et al. Increased levels of interleukin-1 are detected in nasal secretions of volunteers during experimental rhinovirus colds. J Infect Dis. 1994;169:1007–1013.
42. Zhu Z, Tang W, Ray A, et al. Rhinovirus stimulation of interleukin-6 *in vivo* and *in vitro*: Evidence for NF-$_{\kappa}$B–dependent transcriptional activation. J Clin Invest. 1966;97:421–430.
43. Zhu A, Tang W, Gwaltney JM Jr, et al. Rhinovirus stimulation of interleukin-8 *in vivo* and *in vitro*: Role of NF-$_{\kappa}$B. Am J Physiol (Lung Cell Mol Physiol.) 1997;17:L814–L824.
44. Turner RB, Weingand K, Yeh CH, et al. Association between interleukin-8 concentration in nasal secretions and severity of symptoms of experimental rhinovirus colds. Clin Infect Dis. 1988;26:840–846.
45. Gaffey MJ, Hayden FG, Boyd JC, et al. Ipratropium bromide treatment of experimental rhinovirus infection. Antimicrob Agents Chemother. 1988;32:1644–1647.
46. Sperber SJ, Sorrentino JV, Riker DK, et al. Evaluation of an alpha agonist alone and in combination with a nonsteroidal anti-inflammatory agent in the treatment of experimental rhinovirus colds. Bull N Y Acad Med. 1989;65:145–160.
47. Turner BW, Cail WS, Hendley JO, et al. Physiologic abnormalities in the paranasal sinuses during experimental rhinovirus colds. J Allergy Clin Immunol. 1992;90:474–478.
48. Gwaltney JM Jr, Phillips CD, Miller RD, et al. Computed tomographic study of the common cold. N Engl J Med. 1994;330:25–30.
49. Evans FO Jr, Sydnor JB, Moore WEC, et al. Sinusitis of the maxillary antrum. N Engl J Med. 1975;293:735.
50. Arola M, Ruuskanen O, Ziegler T, et al. Clinical role of respiratory virus infection in acute otitis media. Pediatrics. 1990;86:848–855.
51. Doyle WJ, McBride TP, Skoner DP, et al. A double blind placebo-controlled clinical trial of the effect of chlorpheniramine on the response of the nasal airway, middle ear and eustachian tube to provocative rhinovirus challenge. Pediatr Infect Dis J. 1988;7:222.
52. Straker E, Hill AB, Lovell RA. A study of the nasopharyngeal bacterial flora of different groups of persons observed in London and south-east England during the years 1930 to 1937. Reports on Public Health and Medical Subjects, no. 90. London: His Majesty's Stationery Office; 1939;7.
53. Brimblecombe FSW, Cruickshank R, Master P, et al. Family studies of respiratory infections. BMJ. 1958;1:119.
54. Harris JM II, Gwaltney JM Jr. The incubation periods of experimental rhinovirus infection and illness. Clin Infect Dis. 1996;23:1286–1290.
55. Berg O, Carenfelt C, Rystedt G, et al. Occurrence of asymptomatic sinusitis in common cold and other acute ENT-infections. Rhinology. 1986; 24:223–225.
56. Myint S, Harmsen D, Raabe T, et al. Characterization of a nucleic acid probe for the diagnosis of human coronavirus 229E infections. J Med Virol. 1990; 31:165–172.
57. Johnston SL, Sanderson G, Pattemore PK, et al. Use of polymerase chain reaction for diagnosis of picornavirus infection in subjects with and without respiratory symptoms. J Clin Microbiol. 1993;31:111–117.
58. Arruda E, Hayden FG. Detection of human rhinovirus RNA in nasal washings by PCR. Mol Cell Probes. 1993;7:373–379.
59. Gwaltney JM Jr, Park J, Paul RA, et al. Randomized controlled trial of clemastine fumarate for treatment of experimental rhinovirus colds. Clin Infect Dis. 1996;22:656–662.
60. Turner RB, Sperber SJ, Sorrentino JV, et al. Effectiveness of clemastine fumarate for treatment of rhinorrhea and sneezing associated with the common cold. Clin Infect Dis. 1997;25:824–830.
61. Gwaltney JM Jr, Druce HM. Efficacy of brompheniramine maleate treatment for rhinovirus colds. Clin Infect Dis. 1997;25:1188–1194.
62. Nozhat JRM, Choudry B, Fuller RW. The effect of sulindac on the abnormal cough reflex associated with dry cough. J Pharmacol Exper Ther. 1990;255:161–164.
63. Fogari R, Zoppi A, Tettamanti F, et al. Effects of nifedipine and indomethacin on cough induced by angiotensin-converting enzyme inhibitors: A double-blind, randomized, cross-over study. J Cardiovas Pharmacol. 1992;19:670–673.
64. Gwaltney JM Jr. Combined antiviral and antimediator treatment of rhinovirus colds. J Infect Dis. 1992;166:776–782.
65. Coates ML, Rembold CM, Farr BM. Does pseudoephedrine increase blood pressure in patients with controlled hypertension? J Fam Pract. 1995;40:22–26.
66. Freestone C, Eccles R. Assessment of the antitussive efficacy of codeine in cough associated with common cold. J Pharm Pharmacol. 1997;49:1045–1049.
67. Walker GH, Bynoe ML, Tyrrell DAJ. Trial of ascorbic acid in prevention of colds. BMJ. 1967;1:603.
68. Schwartz AR, Togo Y, Hornick RB, et al. Evaluation of the efficacy of ascorbic acid in prophylaxis of induced rhinovirus 44 infection in man. J Infect Dis. 1973;128:500.
69. Farr BM, Gwaltney JM Jr. The problems of taste in placebo matching: An evaluation of zinc gluconate for the common cold. J Chronic Dis. 1987;40:875–879.
70. Farr BM, Conner EM, Betts FR, et al. Two randomized controlled trials of zinc gluconate lozenge therapy of experimentally induced rhinovirus colds. Antimicrob Agents Chemother. 1987;31:1183–1187.
71. Smith DS, Helzner EC, Nuttall CE Jr, et al. Failure of zinc gluconate in treatment of acute upper respiratory tract infections. Antimicrob Agents Chemother. 1989;33:646–648.
72. Farr BM, Hayden FG, Gwaltney J Jr. Zinc gluconated lozenges for treating the common cold (Letter). Ann Intern Med. 1997;126:738.
73. Bauer R, Wagner H. *Echinacea* species as potential immunostimulatory drugs. Economic and Medicinal Plants Research. 1991;5:253–321.
74. Gaisbauer M, Zimmermann W, Schleich T. Nat Med. 1986;3:6–10.
75. Coeugniet EG, Elek E. Immunomodulation with *Viscum album* and *Echinacea purpurea* extracts. Onkologie. 1987:10(suppl):27–33.
76. Sperber SJ, Hayden FG. Chemotherapy of rhinovirus colds. Antimicrob Agents Chemother. 1988;32:409–419.
77. Scott GM, Phillpotts RJ, Wallace J, et al. Purified interferon as protection against rhinovirus infections. BMJ. 1982;284:1822.
78. Hayden FG, Gwaltney JM Jr. Intranasal interferon-alpha$_2$ for prevention of rhinovirus infection and illness. J Infect Dis. 1983;148:543.
79. Samo T-C, Greenberg SB, Couch RB Jr, et al. Evaluations of efficacy and tolerance to intranasally applied recombinant leukocyte A interferon in normal volunteers. J Infect Dis. 1983;148:535.
80. Hayden FG, Gwaltney JM Jr. Intranasal interferon-α_2 treatment of experimental rhinoviral colds. J Infect Dis. 1984;150:174.
81. Douglas RM, ALbrecht JK, Miles HB, et al. Intranasal interferon-α_2 prophylaxis of natural respiratory virus infection. J Infect Dis. 1985;151:731.
82. Hayden FG, Gwaltney JM Jr, Johnson ME. Prophylactic efficacy and tolerance of low-dose intranasal interferon-alpha$_2$ in natural respiratory viral infections. Antiviral Res. 1985;5:11.
83. Hayden FG, Albrecht JK, Kaiser DL, et al. Prevention of natural colds by contact prophylaxis with intranasal alpha$_2$-interferon. N Engl J Med. 1986;314:71.
84. Douglas RM, Moore BW, Miles HB, et al. Prophylactic efficacy of intranasal

alpha$_2$-interferon against rhinovirus infections in the family setting. N Engl J Med. 1986;314:65.
85. Al-Nakib W, Higgins PG, Barrow GI, et al. Suppression of colds in human volunteers challenged with rhinovirus by a new synthetic drug (R61837). Antimicrob Agents Chemother. 1989;33:522–525.
86. Hayden FG, Andries K, Janssen PAJ. Safety and efficacy of intranasal pirodavir (R77975) in experimental rhinovirus infection. Antimicrob Agents Chemother. 1992;36:727–732.
87. Turner RB, Wecker MT, Pohl G, et al. Efficacy of soluble intercellular adhesion molecule-1 for prevention of experimental rhinovirus infection and illness in a randomized clinical trial. (In press).
88. Corley DL, Gevirtz R, Nideffer R, Cummins L. Prevention of postinfectious asthma in children by reducing self-inoculatory behavior. J Pediatr Psychol. 1987;12: 242–258.

Chapter 47

Pharyngitis

JACK M. GWALTNEY, JR.
ALAN L. BISNO

Acute pharyngitis is an inflammatory syndrome of the pharynx caused by several different groups of microorganisms. Most cases are of viral etiology and occur as part of common colds and influenzal syndromes. The most important of the bacterial infections is that due to group A β-hemolytic streptococci *(Streptococcus pyogenes).* It is important to differentiate streptococcal from viral pharyngitis because of the response of streptococcal infection to penicillin therapy and the ineffectiveness of antibiotic therapy in the viral infections. Also, streptococcal pharyngitis may be complicated by acute rheumatic fever and acute glomerulonephritis. There are other uncommon or rare types of pharyngitis, and for some of these treatment is also available. The list of microorganisms known to cause pharyngitis continues to grow as new etiologic associations are established.

ETIOLOGY

The known microbial causes of pharyngitis are listed in Table 47–1, which shows the syndromes of respiratory illness caused by the various agents[1–4] and their estimated contribution to all cases of pharyngitis.[5, 6] The relative importance of the different agents is not fully defined, and it is still not possible to determine the cause in a sizable proportion of cases. The results of epidemiologic investigations are influenced by the season of the year, the age of the population, the severity of illness, and the diagnostic methods used to detect cases. A large proportion of mild cases of pharyngitis is associated with rhinovirus and coronavirus colds. Adenovirus and herpes simplex virus pharyngitis, although less common, are important because of their clinical severity. Others of the known respiratory viruses each account for a small proportion of cases. The acute retroviral syndrome due to human immunodeficiency virus (HIV) has joined the list of viral infections associated with acute pharyngitis.[7]

Approximately 15% of all cases of pharyngitis are due to *S. pyogenes.* In children with sore throat, *S. pyogenes* may cause up to half of the cases during some periods. The importance of non–group A β-hemolytic streptococci as a cause of pharyngitis is not entirely clear. β-hemolytic streptococci of groups C and G have long been associated with foodborne outbreaks of pharyngitis.[8, 9, 9a, 10] Group C streptococci have also been associated with endemic pharyngitis in college students[11] and other adult populations.[12] There is also limited evidence to implicate group G streptococci in community outbreaks.[13] Other non–group A β-hemolytic streptococci have not been definitely implicated as a cause of endemic pharyngitis.[14–18] Mixed anaerobic bacterial infections (Vincent's angina) cause occasional cases of acute pharyngitis, as do *Corynebacterium diphtheriae, Arcanobacterium hemolyticum, Yersinia enterocolitica,* and *Neisseria gonorrhoeae. Mycoplasma pneumoniae* has been associated with pharyngitis since the late 1950s, but in epidemiologic studies of unselected patients, *M. pneumoniae* has not been an important cause of the disease.[5, 6, 14, 15, 19] The recognition of the role of *Chlamydia pneumoniae* (TWAR strain) in acute respiratory disease[20] has added another agent to the list of those causing pharyngitis, but its relative importance has yet to be determined.[21, 22]

EPIDEMIOLOGY

Most cases of pharyngitis occur during the colder months of the year, during the respiratory disease season. Viral agents such as rhinoviruses tend to have annual periods of peak prevalence in the fall and spring; coronaviruses have been found most often in the winter. Influenza appears in epidemics, which in the United States usually occur between December and April. In military recruits, adenoviruses cause the syndrome of acute respiratory disease (ARD) during the colder months. In civilians, wintertime ARD occurs, as do epidemics of pharyngoconjunctival fever in the summer. Streptococcal pharyngitis occurs during the respiratory disease season, with peak rates of infection in winter and early spring. Spread among family members in the home is a prominent feature of the epidemiologic behavior of most of these agents, with children being the major reservoir of infection. For details on the epidemiologic behavior of these organisms, the reader is referred to the chapters dealing with each.

PATHOGENESIS

Symptoms of sore or scratchy throat occur in approximately 50% of people with rhinovirus colds[23] and in 20 to 70% of people with respiratory illness due to coronavirus.[24, 25] Pharyngeal complaints are present in up to 80% of people with parainfluenza virus illness[26] and in approximately 50% of people with type A influenza and adenovirus illness.[26] Other viral respiratory illnesses with pharyngitis occur with coxsackievirus A21, echoviruses 6 and 20,[26] herpes simplex virus,[27] Epstein-Barr virus (EBV), and cytomegalovirus infections.

The pathogenic mechanisms are different for the various organisms. Nasal epithelial biopsies obtained from volunteers with experimental rhinovirus infections have shown little or no evidence of viral cytopathic effect.[28, 29] However, it has been noted that bradykinin and lysylbradykinin are generated in the nasal passages of persons with experimental and natural rhinovirus colds.[30, 31] These inflammatory mediators are potent stimulators of pain nerve endings. Also, volunteers given experimental intranasal challenge with bradykinin have developed symptoms of sore throat.[32] With other respiratory virus infections, such as those due to adenovirus and coxsackievirus, there is evidence that direct invasion of pharyngeal mucosa occurs.

The events leading to invasive streptococcal infection of the pharynx and tonsil are also not well understood. Pharyngeal carriage of *S. pyogenes* is commonly observed in asymptomatic people. Factors that influence the balance between colonization and invasive infection may include natural and acquired host immunity and interference among the bacteria present in the oropharynx. *S. pyogenes* elaborates a number of extracellular factors, including erythrogenic toxins, hemolysins, streptokinase, deoxyribonuclease, proteinase, and hyaluronidase, which are of known or possible pathogenic importance. Complications of acute streptococcal pharyngitis may include acute rheumatic fever, acute glomerulonephritis, and invasive infection. There is a general association of specific M serotypes with these complications.[33] It is likely, however, that strain-related virulence factors rather than M serotype per se are the major determinant of disease expression.

The usual pathologic changes occurring in viral pharyngitis are edema and hyperemia of the tonsils and the pharyngeal mucous

TABLE 47–1 Microbial Causes of Acute Pharyngitis

Pathogen	Syndrome/Disease	Estimated Importance*
Viral		
Rhinovirus (100 types and 1 subtype)	Common cold	20
Coronavirus (3 or more types)	Common cold	≥5
Adenovirus (types 3, 4, 7, 14, 21)	Pharyngoconjunctival fever, ARD	5
Herpes simplex virus (types 1 and 2)	Gingivitis, stomatitis, pharyngitis	4
Parainfluenza virus (types 1–4)	Common cold, croup	2
Influenza virus (types A and B)	Influenza	2
Coxsackievirus A (types 2, 4–6, 8, 10)	Herpangina	<1
Epstein-Barr virus	Infectious mononucleosis	<1
Cytomegalovirus	Infectious mononucleosis	<1
HIV-1	Primary HIV infection	<1
Bacterial		
Streptococcus pyogenes (group A β-hemolytic streptococci)	Pharyngitis/tonsillitis, scarlet fever	15–30
Group C β-hemolytic streptococci	Pharyngitis/tonsillitis	5–10
Mixed anaerobic infection	Gingivitis, pharyngitis (Vincent's angina)	<1
	Peritonsillitis/peritonsillar abscess (quinsy)	<1
Neisseria gonorrhoeae	Pharyngitis	<1
Corynebacterium diphtheriae	Diphtheria	≥1
Corynebacterium ulcerans	Pharyngitis, diphtheria	<1
Arcanobacterium haemolyticum (*Corynebacterium haemolyticum*)	Pharyngitis, scarlatiniform rash	<1
Yersinia enterocolitica	Pharyngitis, enterocolitis	<1
Treponema pallidum	Secondary syphilis	<1
Chlamydial		
Chlamydia pneumoniae	Pneumonia/bronchitis/pharyngitis	Unknown
Mycoplasmal		
Mycoplasma pneumoniae	Pneumonia/bronchitis/pharyngitis	<1
Mycoplasma hominis (type 1)	Pharyngitis in volunteers	Unknown
Unknown		30

*Estimated percentage of cases of pharyngitis due to indicated organism in persons of all ages.
Abbreviations: ARD, Acute respiratory disease; HIV, human immunodeficiency virus.
Data from refs. 1–6.

membrane. An inflammatory exudate may be present with adenovirus and EBV infections; with the latter, nasopharyngeal lymphoid hyperplasia also occurs. Vesiculation and mucosal ulceration may occur with herpes simplex virus and some coxsackievirus A infections. With streptococcal tonsillopharyngitis, there is an intense inflammatory response characterized by marked erythema and edema of the fauces and uvula, and frequently by a grayish-yellow tonsillar exudate. With diphtheria, a fibrous pseudomembrane containing necrotic epithelium, leukocytes, and bacterial colonies develops on the epithelial surface. For a more detailed discussion of the pathogenic events associated with infection by the wide variety of microorganisms that cause pharyngitis, the reader is referred to the chapters describing the individual agents.

CLINICAL PRESENTATION

Pharyngitis with the Common Cold

Mild to moderate pharyngeal discomfort is frequently present during a cold but is usually not the primary complaint. The symptom is characterized as soreness, scratchiness, or irritation. Severe pharyngeal pain and odynophagia are not characteristic of this type of pharyngitis. Nasal signs and symptoms and cough are also usually present. Systemic complaints of fever, chills, malaise, and myalgia are not prominent, and a temperature elevation is unusual in adults and older children. On examination, the pharynx may appear normal or show a mild amount of edema and erythema. Rhinorrhea and postnasal discharge are usually present. Pharyngeal and tonsillar exudates and painful lymphadenopathy are not seen. Pharyngeal complaints usually subside over 3 or 4 days, and most patients have recovered by the end of a week (see Chapter 46).

Human Immunodeficiency Virus Infection

Febrile pharyngitis is a characteristic feature of primary infection with HIV.[34, 35] Following an incubation period of 3 to 5 weeks, patients have developed fever and pharyngitis associated with varying amounts of myalgia, arthralgia, lethargy, and in some cases nonpruritic maculopapular rash. This has been followed in approximately 1 week by the development of lymphadenopathy. Pharyngeal hyperemia, sometimes marked, has been noted, as have mucosal ulcerations, but exudate has not been described (see Chapter 108).

Streptococcal Pharyngitis

The severity of illness associated with *S. pyogenes* infection of the pharynx varies greatly.[14] In severe cases, there is marked pharyngeal pain, odynophagia, and a temperature of 39.4°C or greater. Headache, chills, and abdominal pain may occur. The pharyngeal membrane is a fiery red, and a patchy, grayish-yellow exudate is present on the tonsils and at times may be seen on hypertrophied lymphoid nodules of the posterior pharynx. Edema of the uvula is often pronounced. Tender, enlarged cervical nodes and a leukocyte count of over 12,000/mm^3 complete the picture of an acute suppurative bacterial infection. Rhinorrhea and cough are more characteristic of viral infection but may occur.[23] At the other extreme are those streptococcal infections that are quite mild or may even go unrecognized by the patient. Infection with strains of *S. pyogenes* that produce erythrogenic toxin results in the characteristic erythematous rash of scarlet fever, which is followed by desquamation. The tongue is red, and the papillae are enlarged (strawberry tongue). It has recently been reported that noninvasive pharyngitis due to *S. pyogenes* may be the cause of streptococcal toxic shock syndrome[36, 37] (see Chapter 186).

The clinical features of pharyngeal infection with strains of group C and group G streptococci are similar to those of *S. pyogenes*, including the occurrence of purulent exudates, fever, and anterior cervical adenopathy.[11, 12] In group C–associated pharyngitis, the signs and symptoms on average are less severe than in group A pharyngitis but more so than in patients with negative bacterial cultures. Cases of group C and group G pharyngitis are often recognized in the setting of a common-source foodborne outbreak; milk, egg salad, and chicken salad have been recognized as vehicles.

Anaerobic Pharyngitis (Vincent's Angina)/Peritonsillitis/ Peritonsillar Abscess (Quinsy)

Pharyngeal and tonsillar infection with a mixture of anaerobic bacteria and spirochetes, while uncommon, still occurs. *S. pyogenes* and *Staphylococcus aureus* may play a role in some cases. With this infection, a purulent exudate coats the membrane, and there may be a foul odor to the breath. Postanginal septicemia (Lemierre's disease) is a specific form of the condition caused by *Fusobacterium necrophorum*.[38] It is associated with jugular vein septic thrombophlebitis and metastatic infection to the lung and other sites. The disease is most common in adolescents and young adults. Exudative tonsillitis or peritonsillar abscess may be present but in some cases will have subsided by the time the patient is seen. With jugular vein thrombophlebitis, there is pain, swelling, neck stiffness, and dysphagia.

With development of an abscess, pharyngeal pain is usually severe, and dysphagia and low-grade fever are common. On examination, there is inflammation and swelling of the peritonsillar area with medial displacement of the tonsil. The infection is usually limited to one side, but when the condition is bilateral, partial obstruction of the pharynx occurs. Rarely, there is extension of the infection along the carotid sheath and into the mediastinum[39] (see Chapter 53).

Gonococcal Pharyngitis

The incidence of gonococcal infections of the pharynx has increased in recent years. Most infections are asymptomatic, but gonorrheal infection may be responsible for an occasional case of mild pharyngitis[40] (see Chapter 200).

Pharyngitis with Influenza

Sore throat is a major complaint in some patients with influenza. It is usually associated with other manifestations of the disease, such as myalgia, headache, and cough.[14, 26] Coryzal symptoms and hoarseness may also be present. Temperature elevations are common in both adults and children, to levels of 38.3°C or higher. Edema and erythema of the pharyngeal mucosa may be present but are not marked. Pharyngeal exudates and painful cervical adenopathy are not part of influenzal pharyngitis. Defervescence occurs in 3 to 4 days on the average, but in some uncomplicated cases fever may last up to 1 week (see Chapter 153).

Pharyngoconjunctival Fever

The clinical presentation of adenoviral pharyngitis is usually more severe than pharyngitis associated with the common cold. Malaise, myalgia, headache, chills, and dizziness often accompany adenovirus infections. Temperature elevations persist for 5 to 6 days in studies of recognized cases. Sore throat is often marked. On examination, pharyngeal erythema and exudate may be present, mimicking streptococcal pharyngitis. A distinguishing feature of adenovirus pharyngitis, when present, is conjunctivitis, which occurs in one third to one half of cases. The conjunctivitis is of the follicular type and is bilateral in about one fourth of affected patients. Cough, hoarseness, and substernal pain occur in ARD in military recruits but are usually not prominent features of pharyngoconjunctival fever in civilian populations (see Chapter 132).

Acute Herpetic Pharyngitis

Primary infection with herpes simplex virus may present as an acute pharyngitis. Mild cases are indistinguishable from those caused by other respiratory viruses. In severe cases of herpetic pharyngitis, the presence of inflammation and exudate may mimic full-blown streptococcal pharyngitis. Vesicles and shallow ulcers of the palate are characteristic of herpetic infection and when present are helpful in the differential diagnosis. Tender cervical adenopathy and fever are noted in some cases. Vesicles or ulcers are present on the labial and buccal mucosa when there is an associated gingivostomatitis. Acute primary herpetic infection should be distinguished from chronic mucocutaneous infection of the oropharynx due to herpes simplex virus. The chronic form of the disease is seen exclusively in patients with impaired immunity and is characterized by large shallow, painful ulcers that slowly progress unless the patient's immune status improves or antiviral therapy is given (see Chapter 125).

Herpangina

Herpangina is an uncommon type of pharyngitis caused by coxsackieviruses and is distinguished by the presence of small vesicles (1 to 2 mm across) on the soft palate, uvula, and anterior tonsillar pillars. The lesions rupture to become small white ulcers. Herpangina has been recognized primarily in children, in whom it may be manifested as a severe febrile illness with marked sore throat and dysphagia. In some cases anorexia and abdominal pain mimic acute appendicitis (see Chapter 160).

Infectious Mononucleosis

Exudative tonsillitis or pharyngitis occurs in approximately one half of the cases of infectious mononucleosis due to EBV. Fever and cervical adenopathy are characteristically present. The pharyngeal complaints of mononucleosis are usually associated with other features of the disease, such as headache and persistent malaise and fatigue. Generalized adenopathy may be present, and there is enlargement of the spleen in approximately half the cases. The mononucleosis syndrome is also associated with cytomegalovirus infection. Some patients with cytomegalovirus mononucleosis have pharyngeal soreness, but on examination, the pharynx usually appears unremarkable (see Chapters 127 and 128).

Diphtheria

Although uncommon today, diphtheria still occurs in unvaccinated populations in the United States. The disease characteristically has a slow onset, and pharyngeal discomfort is usually not marked. Temperature elevation is present but is low grade. The characteristic tonsillar or pharyngeal membrane varies in color from light to dark gray and is firmly adherent to the tonsil and pharyngeal mucosa. Human infection with *Corynebacterium ulcerans* is a rare cause of human pharyngeal infection. It is associated with the consumption of raw milk and has presented as mild pharyngitis but in one case presented as serious diphtheria[41] (see Chapter 193).

Arcanobacterial Pharyngitis

A. haemolyticum has been increasingly identified as a cause of exudative pharyngitis, clinically similar to that caused by β-hemolytic streptococci.[42–45] Characteristically, the infection has been recognized in children, adolescents, and young adults and is associated with a diffuse, sometimes pruritic, erythematous maculopapular skin rash on the extremities and trunk. Cases of *A. haemolyticum* infection with membraneous pharyngitis that mimics diphtheria[46] and with peritonsillar abscess[47] have also been reported.

Yersinial Pharyngitis

Y. enterocolitica causes exudative pharyngitis, which is associated with ingestion of contaminated food and drink and in adults may occur without the typical enterocolitis seen in children. Fever, prominent cervical lymphadenopathy, and abdominal pain with or without diarrhea have been reported.[48, 49] A fulminant course with high mortality has been associated with reported cases of yersinial pharyngitis, making recognition important.

Chlamydial Pharyngitis

C. pneumoniae (strain TWAR) has been established as an etiologic agent of acute infections of the respiratory tract, some of which have pharyngeal manifestations.[22] Pharyngitis with or without fever has occurred as a separate illness and also in association with pneumonia or bronchitis.[21] Distinguishing clinical features of the pharyngitis have not been described, but chronicity of infection despite antimicrobial therapy has been noted.

Mycoplasmal Pharyngitis

Epidemiologic studies of pharyngitis have associated some cases with *M. pneumoniae* infection. The illnesses observed have been relatively mild and have had no distinguishing clinical features. *M. pneumoniae* characteristically causes bronchitis and primary atypical pneumonia (see Chapter 172).

Noninfectious Pharyngitis

Occasional cases presenting as an inflammatory pharyngitis may have noninfectious causes. These include conditions such as bullous pemphigoid, systemic lupus erythematosus, Behçet's disease, and paraquat ingestion. Kawasaki disease may manifest as a febrile sore throat without exudate. It occurs in children and is associated with characteristic lesions on the lips, tongue, and skin.

DIAGNOSIS

The primary objectives in the diagnosis of acute pharyngitis are to distinguish cases of common viral etiology from those due to *S. pyogenes* and to detect and identify the occasional case due to an unusual or rare cause for which treatment is available. In the majority of cases, an etiologic diagnosis is not possible on clinical grounds alone. The presence of pharyngeal or tonsillar exudates, tender adenopathy, skin rash, or conjunctivitis aids in the differential diagnosis, but these findings are not entirely specific and are not present with sufficient frequency to be helpful in most cases.

The list of etiologic agents associated with the presence of pharyngeal exudates includes group A, group C, and group G streptococci; the anaerobic bacteria; *C. diphtheriae; A. haemolyticum; Y. enterocolitica*; adenovirus; herpes simplex virus; and EBV. However, pharyngeal exudate is not always present with infections due to these infections so that its absence does not exclude them from consideration. On the other hand, exudate is rarely if ever seen in the large group of cases of pharyngitis due to the common cold viruses and influenza virus. The presence of skin rash suggests the possibility of infection with *S. pyogenes, A. haemolyticum,* HIV, and EBV. Toxic shock syndrome should also be considered. The presence of conjunctivitis suggests infection with adenovirus and some types of enterovirus.

The development of rapid antigen detection tests, using a specimen collected by throat swab, has made possible early microbiologic confirmation of the diagnosis of streptococcal pharyngitis.[50, 51] When such tests are used in clinical practice, the reported specificity has been over 90%, but the sensitivity has been lower (60 to 95%), depending in part on the sensitivity of the culture method used as a control.[52, 53]

The sensitivity of culture methods to detect *S. pyogenes* in pharyngeal secretions has been reviewed.[54] No single combination of medium and atmosphere was thought likely to detect all possible isolates of the bacterium, but four methods were judged capable of detecting 90 to 95% from symptomatic patients. These were sheep blood agar incubated anaerobically for 48 hours; sheep blood agar incubated aerobically (without CO_2 supplementation) for 48 hours, using a cover glass to reduce oxygen tension on the primary inoculum zone; and sheep blood agar containing sulfamethoxazole and trimethoprim incubated aerobically (5 to 10% CO_2) or anaerobically for 48 hours. The use of anaerobic conditions may improve recovery of group C streptococci.

The performance characteristics of the antigen detection tests have dictated a strategy in which a positive test result establishes the diagnosis of streptococcal pharyngitis, while a negative test result should be followed by a throat culture on sheep blood agar. Among the advantages of routinely performing an antigen detection test or culture in patients with pharyngitis are that test results may obviate unnecessary antimicrobial therapy in the patient and may influence the management of symptomatic family members.

The patient's history and a consideration of epidemiologic factors may be helpful in suggesting a specific etiologic diagnosis in cases in which results of throat culture or rapid antigen test are negative. Other family members frequently have common colds and influenzal illnesses. The season of the year and the occurrence of known epidemics may provide clues to diagnosis. Rhinovirus infections predominate in the fall and spring and coronavirus infections in the winter. The occurrence of an influenza epidemic in the community is usually known to the physician. Patients with pharyngoconjunctival fever, a summer illness, may give a history of swimming, and they or a family member may have conjunctivitis. The diagnosis of infectious mononucleosis, primary HIV infection, and diphtheria may be suggested by the nonpharyngeal manifestations of these infections.

Examination of the structures of the pharynx should be thorough and should include inspection of the nasopharynx and larynx when diphtheria is suspected. In children under the age of 3 years, the presence of an exudate is a less reliable indicator of streptococcal infection than it is in older children and adults. Diphtheria produces a pseudomembrane that may be mistaken for an exudate. The presence of small vesicles or ulcers suggests herpes simplex virus infection or herpangina. The mucosal lesions of herpangina are less numerous and more confined to the area of the palate than are those of herpes simplex virus, which may involve the entire oropharynx. Aphthous stomatitis, a benign condition of unknown cause, produces small painful mucosal ulcers that are sometimes confused with those of herpetic infection. Aphthosis tends to be recurrent, in contrast to acute herpetic pharyngitis, and with the usual case of aphthosis there are fewer lesions, which are usually located in the anterior part of the mouth.

Medial displacement of one or both tonsils is seen with peritonsillitis or peritonsillar abscess, and dysphagia may be present. Patients with postanginal septicemia with jugular vein thrombophlebitis have malaise, fever, and chills, suggestive of serious illness; also, pain, tenderness, and swelling at the angle of the jaw and stiff neck are characteristic, but these findings may be subtle. Patients with infectious mononucleosis usually have generalized adenopathy and may have enlargement of the spleen. Severe sore throat and odynophagia in an adult in the absence of findings in the pharynx should suggest epiglottitis (see Chapter 52).

Laboratory tests are available to help in the diagnosis of some of the aforementioned infections. *N. gonorrhoeae* may be detected on Thayer-Martin or other suitable media. Vincent's angina is diagnosed by a crystal violet–stained smear of the pharyngeal or tonsillar exudate showing the presence of numerous fusobacteria and spirochetes. Blood specimens for culture should be obtained in cases of suspected postanginal septicemia, and radiographic examination of the lungs, bones, and large joints may detect metastatic infection. A throat swab for culture using Löffler's medium should be obtained in all suspected cases of diphtheria (see Chapter 193). The hemolysis associated with *A. hemolyticum* becomes maximal at 48 to 72 hours and is more prominent on rabbit and human blood agar than sheep blood agar; thus, this organism may be missed on standard throat culture.[43, 45] The diagnosis of infectious mononucleosis can be confirmed by specific serologic tests (see Chapter 128). HIV antigen has been detected in the serum of patients with pharyngitis due to primary HIV infection.[30] Also, in suspected cases of this infection, follow-up to detect appearance of serum antibody to HIV is essential. Cultures and rapid diagnostic tests for influenza virus, adenovirus, herpes simplex virus, cytomegalovirus, and *M. pneumoniae* are now available in some laboratories. Acute and convalescent (3-week) serum specimens are necessary for serologic tests for these agents. Laboratory tests for the common cold viruses are not readily available. Diagnostic tests for *C. pneumoniae* are being developed[22] but are not commercially available at present.

Pharyngitis due to noninfectious causes may sometimes present a diagnostic problem. Pemphigus, bullous pemphigoid, and systemic lupus erythematosus are among the diseases that can cause pharyngeal inflammation and discomfort. Also, drug reactions are sometimes manifested by pharyngeal soreness, as is agranulocytosis. The presence of other manifestations of these diseases, particularly involvement of the skin, is helpful in leading to the diagnosis.

TREATMENT AND PREVENTION

Antimicrobial Therapy

Streptococcal Pharyngitis

Patients with pharyngitis due to *S. pyogenes* should receive a 10-day course of penicillin[50, 51, 55–58] or an equivalent antibiotic if they are allergic to penicillin (see Chapter 186, on *Streptococcus pyogenes,* for dosage schedule). An injection of long-acting benzathine penicillin is an excellent although painful form of therapy because it does not require patient compliance. The adult dose of benzathine penicillin is 1.2 million units. In patients who are allergic to penicillin, a 10-day course of erythromycin is recommended. In some areas of the world, erythromycin resistance among *S. pyogenes* strains is sufficiently prevalent to be a problem, but this has not occurred in the United States.[56] First-generation cephalosporins such as cephalexin and cefadroxil and a second-generation cephalosporin such as cefuroxime axetil are also suitable for treating streptococcal pharyngitis and have given clinical and microbiologic responses equivalent or superior to those achieved with penicillin G. Although a number of newer antimicrobial drugs have activity against *S. pyogenes,* they offer no advantage over penicillin or the first-generation cephalosporins and are more expensive.

The availability of rapid antigen detection tests for *S. pyogenes* has reduced but not eliminated the dilemma of when to begin antimicrobial therapy in the suspected case. In patients with a positive antigen test result, treatment should be started immediately, with the goals of providing maximal symptomatic relief for the acute illness, eradicating the infection to prevent transmission, and preventing suppurative and nonsuppurative complications.[56, 59–61] In patients in whom a rapid test is not performed or whose test result is negative and in whom the clinical diagnosis of streptococcal pharyngitis is still entertained, either of two strategies may be employed. It is generally preferable to await the results of throat culture before starting treatment when clinical suspicion of streptococcal infection is high and the clinical manifestations are severe. It is reasonable to begin therapy when the patient is originally seen and to discontinue treatment if the culture result is negative. Both of these approaches have advantages and disadvantages. Withholding treatment until culture results are known limits the immediate therapeutic benefit of antimicrobial therapy but reduces unnecessary drug use. Beginning treatment before the results of culture are known provides maximal therapeutic benefit but exposes many patients to an antimicrobial drug unnecessarily. Initiation of treatment within 1 week of the onset of streptococcal pharyngitis will prevent subsequent acute rheumatic fever,[62] and either of the two approaches will achieve this goal (see Chapter 187). Also, a 48-hour delay in the initiation of penicillin therapy for patients with *S. pyogenes* pharyngitis did not reduce the rate of recurrence with homologous serotypes compared with that in patients in whom treatment was started at the time of diagnosis.[63]

Reports of therapeutic failure with penicillin as manifested by recurrent symptomatic illness do not warrant the abandonment of penicillin as the drug of choice for streptococcal pharyngitis at the present time.[55–58] Penicillin is the only currently recommended drug that has been demonstrated to prevent rheumatic fever. There is no credible evidence that penicillin's efficacy in the treatment of acute streptococcal pharyngitis has diminished. Patients with recurrent pharyngitis associated with the documented presence of *S. pyogenes* in the pharynx require antimicrobial therapy. It is unavoidable that some "cases" of streptococcal pharyngitis, initial or recurrent, that are diagnosed by currently available means in reality represent persons with viral pharyngitis who are merely colonized with *S. pyogenes.*

Because the incidence of acute rheumatic fever had declined to a low level in the United States, the need for *any* antimicrobial treatment of streptococcal pharyngitis was questioned. However, the resurgence of rheumatic fever in some areas of the United States[64–66] and its continuing prevalence in other areas of the world are sufficient reasons not to abandon the general policy of using antimicrobials in the treatment of streptococcal pharyngitis. Discounting the benefit in rheumatic fever prevention and in reduction of acute morbidity, treatment is still important for limiting transmission to school and household contacts and for prevention of suppurative complications of streptococcal pharyngitis, which include sinusitis, otitis media, mastoiditis, lateral sinus thrombosis, bacteremia, and pneumonia.

Anaerobic Pharyngitis/Peritonsillitis/Peritonsillar Abscess

Oral penicillin is still recommended for the treatment of anaerobic pharyngitis and peritonsillitis, with clindamycin as an alternative. The use of early antimicrobial therapy has reduced but not eliminated the cases that require surgical drainage of an abscess. Suspected cases of postanginal septicemia require hospitalization and appropriate diagnostic evaluation.[38] Parenteral treatment with high doses of penicillin or another antimicrobial with activity against *F. necrophorum* should be given for a prolonged course.

Diphtheria

The treatment of diphtheria is described in Chapter 193.

Arcanobacterial Pharyngitis

A. haemolyticum pharyngitis has been reported not to respond to a standard 10-day course of penicillin V but did respond to one injection of benzathine penicillin or to a course of oral erythromycin.[42, 43, 45]

Yersinial Pharyngitis

Y. enterocolitica is usually susceptible to aminoglycosides, trimethoprim-sulfamethoxazole, and third-generation cephalosporins but resistant to penicillin (see Chapter 218).

Gonococcal Pharyngitis

The treatment of gonococcal infections is described in Chapter 200.

Mycoplasmal Pharyngitis

The treatment of *M. pneumoniae* infection is described in Chapter 172.

Viral Pharyngitis

Amantadine or rimantadine, if given early in the course of illness, has a therapeutic effect in type A influenza. It is recommended for cases of presumed influenzal pharyngitis occurring during a known influenza type A epidemic (see Chapter 153). Acyclovir and foscarnet are available for the treatment of ulcerative oropharyngeal herpes simplex virus infection in immunosuppressed patients (see Chapter 36).

Symptomatic Therapy

Treatment is directed at relieving pharyngeal discomfort and associated systemic or respiratory symptoms. Warm saline gargles and supportive measures such as rest, analgesics, and liquids are sufficient in most cases of viral pharyngitis. Ibuprofen was found to be superior to acetaminophen in relieving throat pain associated with tonsillitis and pharyngitis in 6- to 12-year-old children.[67] Symptomatic therapy is also helpful in relieving symptoms of streptococcal pharyngitis. Patients with severe streptococcal pharyngitis or peritonsillitis may be in extreme discomfort and require liberal use of analgesics during the early course of illness. Hospitalization is necessary with some types of pharyngitis that are associated with systemic illness or that have serious or life-threatening complications.

Prevention

Tonsillectomy has been shown to reduce the incidence of throat infections in children who were severely affected with recurrent pharyngitis.[68] However, it is not recommended as a routine practice.[69] Penicillin prophylaxis for *S. pyogenes* infection is required for patients at risk of recurrent rheumatic fever (see Chapter 187). Active immunization is available for type A and type B influenza and for diphtheria (see Chapters 153 and 312). The prophylactic administration of amantadine or rimantadine is also effective against type A influenza. Prophylactic intravenous and oral regimens of acyclovir are effective in preventing mucocutaneous herpes simplex virus infection in immunosuppressed patients (see Chapter 36). Live adenovirus vaccines have been used successfully in military populations but are not available for civilian use (see Chapter 132). There has been work on experimental vaccines for a number of the agents that cause pharyngitis, including *S. pyogenes,* but these vaccines are still in the experimental stage of development.

REFERENCES

1. Stuart-Harris CH, Andrewes C, Andrews BE, et al. A collaborative study of the aetiology of acute respiratory infection in Britain 1961–4. A report of the Medical Research Council working party on acute respiratory virus infections. BMJ. 1965;2:319.
2. Gwaltney JM Jr. Virology of middle ear. Am Otol Rhinol Laryngol. 1971;80:365.
3. Hamre D, Connelly AP Jr, Procknow JJ. Virologic studies of acute respiratory disease in young adults. IV. Virus isolations during four years of surveillance. Am J Epidemiol. 1966;83:238.
4. Monto AS, Ullman BM: Acute respiratory illness in an American community: The Tecumseh study. JAMA. 1974;227:164.
5. Evans AS, Dick EC. Acute pharyngitis and tonsillitis in University of Wisconsin students. JAMA. 1964;190:699.
6. Glezen WP, Clyde WA Jr, Senior RJ, et al. Group A streptococci, mycoplasmas, and viruses associated with acute pharyngitis. JAMA. 1967;202:455.
7. Valle S-L. Febrile pharyngitis as the primary sign of HIV infection in a cluster of cases linked by sexual contact. Scand J Infect Dis. 1987;19:13–17.
8. Stryker WS, Fraser DW, Facklam RR. Foodborne outbreak of group G streptococcal pharyngitis. Am J Epidemiol. 1982;116:533–540.
9. Cohen D, Ferne M, Rouach T, et al. Foodborne outbreak of group G streptococcal sore throat in an Israeli military base. Epidemiol Infect. 1987;99:249–255.

9a. Duca E, Teodorovici G, Radu C, et al. A new nephritogenic streptococcus. J Hyg (Lond). 1969;67:691–698.

10. Bisno AL. Acute pharyngitis: Etiology and diagnosis. Pediatrics. 1996; 97(Suppl):949–954.
11. Turner JC, Hayden GF, Kiselica D, et al. Association of group C β-hemolytic streptococci with endemic pharyngitis among college students. JAMA. 1990;264:2644–2647.
12. Meier FA, Centor RM, Graham L Jr, et al. Clinical and microbiological evidence for endemic pharyngitis among adults due to group C streptococci. Arch Intern Med. 1990;150:825–829.
13. Gerber MA, Randolph MF, Martin NJ, et al. Community-wide outbreak of group G streptococcal pharyngitis. Pediatrics. 1991;87:598–603.
14. McMillan JA, Sandstrom C, Weiner LB, et al. Viral and bacterial organisms associated with acute pharyngitis in a school-aged population. J Pediatr. 1986;109: 747–752.
15. Reed BD, Huck W, Lutz LJ, et al. Prevalence of *Chlamydia trachomatis* and *Mycoplasma pneumoniae* in children with and without pharyngitis. J Fam Pract. 1988;26:387–392.
16. Hofkosh D, Wald ER, Chiponis DM. Prevalence of non–group-A β-hemolytic streptococci in childhood pharyngitis. South Med J. 1988;81:329–331.
17. Hayden GF, Murphy TF, Hendley JO. Non–group A streptococci in the pharynx. Pathogens or innocent bystanders? Am J Dis Child. 1989;143:794–797.
18. Gaviria JM, Bisno AL. Group C and G streptococci. In: Stevens DL, Kaplan EL, eds. Streptococcal Infections. New York: Oxford University Press; 1999. In press.
19. Gwaltney JM Jr, Hendley JO, Simon G, et al. Rhinovirus infections in an industrial population. I. The occurrence of illness. N Engl J Med. 1966;275:1261.
20. Grayston JT, Kuo C-C, Wang S-P, et al. A new *Chlamydia psittaci* strain, TWAR, isolated in acute respiratory tract infections. N Engl J Med. 1986;315:161–168.
21. Hammerschlag MR, Chirgwin K, Roblin PM, et al. Persistent infection with *Chlamydia pneumoniae* following acute respiratory illness. Clin Infect Dis. 1992;14: 178–182.
22. Grayston JT. Infections caused by *Chlamydia pneumoniae* strain TWAR. Clin Infect Dis. 1992;15:757–563.
23. Gwaltney JM Jr. Rhinoviruses. In: Evans AS, ed. Viral Infections of Humans: Epidemiology and Control. 3rd ed. New York: Plenum; 1989:593–611.
24. Hendley JO, Fishburne HB, Gwaltney JM Jr. Coronavirus infections in working adults. Am Rev Respir Dis. 1972;105:805.
25. Wenzel RP, Hendley JO, Davies JA, et al. Coronavirus infections in military recruits. Three-year study with coronavirus strains OC43 and 229E. Am Rev Respir Dis. 1974;109:621.
26. Tyrrell DAJ: Common Colds and Related Diseases: Baltimore: Williams & Wilkins; 1965.
27. Glezen W, Fernald GW, Lohr JA. Acute respiratory disease of university students with special reference to the etiologic role of herpesvirus hominis. Am J Epidemiol. 1975;101:111.
28. Douglas RG Jr, Alford BR, Couch RB: Atraumatic nasal biopsy studies of respiratory virus infections in volunteers. Antimicrob Agents Chemother. 1968;8:340–342.
29. Winther B, Farr B, Turner RB, et al. Histopathologic examination and enumeration of polymorphonuclear leukocytes in the nasal mucosa during experimental rhinovirus colds. Acta Otolaryngol (Stockh) 1984;413(Suppl):19–24.
30. Naclerio RM, Proud D, Lichtenstein, et al. Kinins are generated during experimental rhinovirus colds. J Infect Dis. 1988;157:133–142.
31. Proud D, Naclerio RM, Gwaltney JM, et al. Kinins are generated in nasal secretions during natural rhinovirus colds. J Infect Dis. 1990;161:120–123.
32. Proud D, Reynolds CJ, Lacapra S, et al. Nasal provocation with bradykinin induces symptoms of rhinitis and a sore throat. Am Rev Respir Dis. 1988;137:613–616.
33. Johnson DR, Stevens DL, Kaplan EL. Epidemiologic analysis of group A streptococcal serotypes associated with severe systemic infections, rheumatic fever, or uncomplicated pharyngitis. J Infect Dis. 1992;166:374–382.
34. Kahn JO, Walker BD. Acute human immunodeficiency virus type 1 infection. N Engl J Med. 1998;339:33–39.
35. Kessler HA, Blaauw B, Spear J, et al. Diagnosis of human immunodeficiency virus infection in seronegative homosexuals presenting with an acute viral syndrome. JAMA. 1987;258:1196–1199.
36. Herold AH. Group A beta-hemolytic streptococcal toxic shock from a mild pharyngitis. J Fam Pract. 1990;31:549–551.
37. Chapnick EK, Gradon JD, Lutwick LI, et al. Streptococcal toxic syndrome due to noninvasive pharyngitis. Clin J Infect Dis. 1992;14:1074–1077.
38. Moreno S, Altozano JG, Pinilla B, et al. Lemierre's disease: Postanginal bacteremia and pulmonary involvement caused by *Fusobacterium necrophorum.* Rev Infect Dis. 1989;11:319–324.
39. Scully RE, Galdabini JJ, McNeely BU: Case records of the Massachusetts General Hospital. N Engl J Med. 1978;298:894.
40. Hutt DM, Judson FN. Epidemiology and treatment of oropharyngeal gonorrhea. Ann Intern Med. 1986;104:655.
41. Hart RJC. *Corynebacterium ulcerans* in humans and cattle in North Devon. J Hyg Camb. 1984;92:161–164.
42. Banck G, Nyman M. Tonsillitis and rash associated with *Corynebacterium haemolyticum.* J Infect Dis. 1986;154:1037–1040.
43. Miller RA, Brancato F, Holmes KK. *Corynebacterium haemolyticum* as a cause of pharyngitis and scarlatiniform rash in young adults. Ann Intern Med. 1986;105: 867–872.
44. Greenman JL. *Corynebacterium haemolyticum* and pharyngitis. Ann Intern Med. 1987;106:633.
45. Karpathios T, Drakonaki S, Zervoudaki, et al. *Arcanobacterium haemolyticum* in children with presumed streptococcal pharyngotonsillitis or scarlet fever. J Pediatr. 1992;12:735–737.
46. Green SL, LaPeter KS. Pseudodiphtheritic membranous pharyngitis caused by *Corynebacterium haemolyticum.* JAMA. 1981;245:2330.
47. Kovatch AL, Schuit KE, Michaels RH. *Corynebacterium haemolyticum* peritonsillar abscess mimicking diphtheria. JAMA. 1983;249:1757.
48. Rose FB, Camp CJ, Antes EJ. Family outbreak of fatal *Yersinia enterocolitica* pharyngitis. Am J Med. 1987;82:636–637.
49. Cover TL, Aber RC. *Yersinia enterocolitica.* N Engl J Med. 1989;321:16–24.

50. Dajani A, Taubert K, Ferrieri P, et al. Treatment of acute streptococcal pharyngitis and prevention of rheumatic fever: A statement for health professionals. Pediatrics. 1995;96:758–764.
51. Bisno AL, Gerber MA, Gwaltney JM Jr, et al. Group A streptococcal pharyngitis: Diagnosis and management. A practice guideline. Clin Infect Dis. 1977;25:574–583.
52. Rapid diagnostic tests for group A streptococcal pharyngitis. Med Lett. 1991;33: 40–41.
53. Wegner DL, White DL, Schrantz RD. Insensitivity of rapid antigen detection methods and single blood agar plate culture for diagnosing streptococcal pharyngitis. JAMA. 1992;267:695–697.
54. Kellog JA. Suitability of throat culture procedures for detection of group A streptococci and as reference standards for evaluation of streptococcal antigen detection kits. J Clin Microbiol. 1990;28:165–169.
55. Peter G. Streptococcal pharyngitis: Current therapy and criteria for evaluation of new agents. Clin Infect Dis. 1992;14(Suppl):S218–S223, S231–S232.
56. Denny FW. Current management of streptococcal pharyngitis. J Fam Pract. 1992;35:619–620.
57. Paradise JL. Etiology and management of pharyngitis and pharyngotonsillitis in children: A current review. Ann Otol Rhinol Laryngol. 1992;155:51–57.
58. Pichichero ME. The rising incidence of penicillin treatment failures in group A streptococcal tonsillopharyngitis: An emerging role for the cephalosporins? Pediatr Infect Dis J. 1991;10:S50–S55.
59. Nelson JD. The effect of penicillin therapy on the symptoms and signs of streptococcal pharyngitis. Pediatr Infect Dis. 1984;3:10.
60. Krober MS, Bass JW, Michels GN. Streptococcal pharyngitis. Placebo-controlled double-blind evaluation of clinical response to penicillin therapy. JAMA. 1985;253:1271.
61. Randolph MF, Gerber MA, DeMeo KK, et al. The effect of antibiotic therapy on the clinical course of streptococcal pharyngitis. J Pediatr. 1985;106:870.
62. Caranzaro FJ, Stetson CA, Morris AJ, et al: The role of the streptococcus in the pathogenesis of rheumatic fever. Am J Med. 1954;17:749.
63. Gerber MA, Randolph MF, DeMeo KK, et al. Lack of impact of early antibiotic therapy for streptococcal pharyngitis on recurrence rates. J Pediatr. 1990;117: 853–858.
64. Wald ER, Dashefsky B, Feidt C, et al. Acute rheumatic fever in western Pennsylvania and the tristate area. Pediatrics. 1987;80:371.
65. Veasy LG, Tani LY, Hill HR. Persistence of acute rheumatic fever in the intermountain area of the United States. J Pediatr. 1994;124:9–16.
66. Papadimos T, Escamilla J. Acute rheumatic fever at a Navy training center—San Diego, California. Leads from the MMWR. JAMA. 1988;259:1782.
67. Bertin L, Pons G, d'Athis P, et al. Randomized, double-blind, multicenter, controlled trial of ibuprofen versus acetaminophen (paracetamol) and placebo for treatment of symptoms of tonsillitis and pharyngitis in children. J Pediatr. 1991;119:811–814.
68. Paradise JL, Bluestone CD, Bachman RZ, et al. Efficacy of tonsillectomy for recurrent throat infection in severely affected children. Results of parallel randomized and nonrandomized clinical trials. N Engl J Med. 1984;310:674.
69. Hendley JO. Tonsillectomy: Justified but not mandated in special patients. N Engl J Med. 1984;310:717.

Chapter 48

Acute Laryngitis

MARY T. CASERTA

Acute laryngitis is a common clinical syndrome encountered by primary care physicians in patients of all ages. The symptoms are often described as the recent onset of hoarseness or a harsh voice with a deepened pitch.[1] There may be voice breaks or episodes of aphonia, which frequently occur in the context of an upper respiratory tract infection with rhinorrhea, cough, and sore throat.[2] The duration of symptoms is difficult to discern from the literature; however, in a study of 100 adults with the common cold, hoarseness was reported for a median of 3 days, with 8 days being the 75th percentile.[3] Although most literature describes acute laryngitis as a mild and self-limited syndrome, a survey of intercollegiate athletes found substantial morbidity associated with laryngitis.[4] Students reported laryngitis significantly more often as a cause of missing practice and as adversely affecting their athletic performance, compared with cough, nasal discharge, or myalgia.

The incidence of acute laryngitis reported in the literature is variable and highly dependent on the study methods used. In a report by Higgins of more than 3900 patients older than 5 years of age with acute respiratory infections, only 2% were given a primary diagnosis of laryngitis.[5] However, in other studies, 38% of patients with pneumonia reported hoarseness as a symptom, as did 33% of adults with colds.[6, 7] Laryngitis has also been noted in 24% of adolescents or school-aged children with sore throat and in 75% of toddlers with acute respiratory symptoms during a croup epidemic.[8, 9] Despite these studies demonstrating that laryngitis is a problem at all ages, a series of reports from Sweden of 235 patients seen in an ear, nose, and throat clinic showed that the majority of patients with acute laryngitis were young, nonsmoking women between 18 and 40 years of age.[2] In a smaller study from Japan, the mean age of the patients with laryngitis was 38 years.[10]

All of the major respiratory viruses have been etiologically associated with laryngitis. In the study by Higgins of patients older than 5 years of age with a primary diagnosis of laryngitis, 21% had infection with parainfluenza virus, 15% had rhinovirus, 3% had influenza virus, and 3% had adenovirus.[5] Only 18% of patients with laryngitis in this study had a viral pathogen recovered from the respiratory tract. Also, the pattern of infection was age dependent, with only parainfluenza virus identified in children 5 to 15 years of age. The risk of developing laryngitis with a particular type of respiratory infection is summarized in Table 48–1. McMillan and colleagues reported that laryngitis and cough were noted significantly more often among patients with influenza (29%) than among those with group A β-hemolytic streptococcal infection (2.3%).[8] In a retrospective review of an epidemic of influenza in the United Kingdom, the rate of laryngitis or tracheitis reported by general practitioners peaked at approximately 100 per 100,000 population, coincident with the peak of influenza illness.[11] Hoarseness has also been reported to be a prominent manifestation of infection with coronavirus and parainfluenza virus, identified in 63% and 90% of cases, respectively.[9, 12]

Bacterial respiratory infections have also been associated with acute laryngitis. Several authors have noted the presence of hoarseness in patients with acute streptococcal pharyngitis, as noted in Table 48–1. Laryngitis due to diphtheria has been virtually eliminated in the United States, although diphtheria continues to be an important cause of laryngeal disease worldwide. The possible etiologic role of *Moraxella* (*Branhamella*) *catarrhalis* in adults with acute laryngitis was investigated in several reports from Sweden. In an initial case-control study of 40 adults with hoarseness and symptoms of upper respiratory tract infection, 55% of the patients and 14% of controls had *M. catarrhalis* isolated from a nasopharyngeal culture.[13] This high rate of recovery of *M. catarrhalis* from adults with laryngitis was confirmed in two subsequent studies with 206 patients.[14, 15] *Haemophilus influenzae* was the second most frequently recovered bacterial pathogen from patients with laryngitis (8 to 20%), suggesting that it may also play a role in this condition. An in vitro study of 72 isolates of *M. catarrhalis* recovered from patients with laryngitis demonstrated that the majority of the strains were resistant to killing by complement, a characteristic associated with virulence.[16] However, treatment of patients with *M. catarrhalis* with oral penicillin or erythromycin for 5 days failed to show any objective clinical benefit over placebo, despite a significant rate of bacteriologic eradication, casting doubt on the significance of the association.[14, 15]

Unusual causes of acute laryngitis described in case reports include candida, *Coccidioides immitis*, *Cryptococcus neoformans*, and group G β-hemolytic streptococci in both normal and immunocompromised patients.[17–22] Laryngitis due to tuberculosis and blastomycosis is a complication of pulmonary infection, manifesting as hoarseness but accompanied by a brassy cough because of tracheobronchial lesions.[17, 23] Laryngeal tuberculosis is highly contagious owing to the large number of organisms in the sputum. Laryngeal histoplasmosis is a complication of disseminated infection and manifests as hoarseness of indolent onset without cough. Blastomycosis and histoplasmosis of the larynx can be mistaken for squamous carcinoma by the indolent onset, gross appearance on laryngoscopy,

TABLE 48–1 Frequency of Laryngitis Associated with Common Respiratory Pathogens

Pathogen	Frequency (%)	Study
Rhinovirus	29	Gwaltney, 1997[26]
Influenza	1–35	Gwaltney, 1997[26]; Bennett, 1973[27]; Chan et al., 1993[28]; Knott et al., 1994[29]
Parainfluenza	8.5–90	Hall et al., 1977[9]; Knott et al., 1994[29]
Adenovirus	22–35	McNamara et al., 1962[30]
Coronavirus	63	Wenzel et al., 1974[12]
Mycoplasma pneumoniae	3–37	Foy et al., 1970[6]; Thom et al., 1990[31]
Chlamydia pneumoniae	30–38	Thom et al., 1990[31]
Group A β-hemolytic streptococci	2.3–19	McMillan et al., 1986[8]; Gwaltney et al., 1997[26]

and pseudoepitheliomatous hyperplasia on biopsy. Fever is low grade or absent. Diagnosis depends on demonstration of the fungi in the submucosa. Hoarseness may also be noted as a component of other laryngeal infections, such as croup, acute epiglottitis or supraglottitis, and bacterial tracheitis. These conditions are discussed separately (in Chapters 49 and 52). Other noninfectious causes of acute laryngitis, including voice abuse, gastroesophageal reflux disease, and laryngeal malignancy, are beyond the scope of this chapter.

The diagnosis of acute laryngitis caused by an upper respiratory infection can often be made by history alone. Examination of the larynx reveals hyperemic vocal folds resulting from edema and vascular engorgement of the mucous membranes.[24, 25] Treatment needs to be directed at the underlying infectious cause of hoarseness but in general is symptomatic in nature, with voice rest and humidification.[25] As noted, studies evaluating the use of antibiotics for patients with acute laryngitis have not shown objective benefit, and they are not routinely recommended.

REFERENCES

1. Dettelbach M, Eibling DE, Johnson JT. Hoarseness: From viral laryngitis to glottic cancer. Postgrad Med. 1994;95:143.
2. Schalеæn L. Acute laryngitis in adults: Diagnosis, etiology, treatment. Acta Otolaryngol (Stockh). 1988;449:31.
3. Mossad SB, Macknin ML, Medendorp SV, et al. Zinc gluconate lozenges for treating the common cold: A randomized, double-blind, placebo-controlled study. Ann Intern Med. 1996;125:81.
4. Weidner TG. Reporting behaviors and activity levels of intercollegiate athletes with an URI. Med Sci Sports Exerc. 1994;26:22.
5. Higgins PG. Viruses associated with acute respiratory infections 1961–71. J Hyg Camb. 1974;72:425.
6. Foy HM, Kenney GE, McMahan R, et al. *Mycoplasma pneumoniae* pneumonia in an urban area: Five years of surveillance. JAMA. 1970;214:1666.
7. Tarlo S, Broder I, Spence L. A prospective study of respiratory infection in adult asthmatics and their normal spouses. Clin Allergy. 1979;9:293.
8. McMillan JA, Sandstrom C, Weiner LB, et al. Viral and bacterial organisms associated with acute pharyngitis in a school-aged population. J Pediatr. 1986;109:747.
9. Hall CB, Geiman JM, Breese BB, Douglas RG Jr. Parainfluenza viral infections in children: Correlation of shedding with clinical manifestations. J Pediatr. 1977;91:194.
10. Hashiguchi K, Ogawa H, Kazuyama Y. Seroprevalence of *Chlamydia pneumoniae* infections in otolaryngeal diseases. J Laryngol Otol. 1992;106:208.
11. Miller DL, Lee JA. Influenza in Britain 1967–68. J Hyg Camb. 1969;67:559.
12. Wenzel RP, Hendley JO, Davies JA, et al. Coronavirus infections in military recruits: Three-year study with coronavirus strains OC43 and 229E. Am Rev Respir Dis. 1974;109:621.
13. Schaleæn L, Christensen P, Kamme C, et al. High isolation rate of *Branhamella catarrhalis* from the nasopharynx in adults with acute laryngitis. Scand J Infect Dis. 1980;12:277.
14. Schaleæn L, Fex S, Christensen P, et al. Inefficacy of penicillin V in acute laryngitis in adults: Evaluation from results of double-blind study. Ann Otol Rhinol Laryngol. 1985;94:14.
15. Schaleæn L, Kamme C, Eliasson I, et al. Erythromycin in acute laryngitis in adults. Ann Otol Rhinol Laryngol. 1993;102:209.
16. Hol C, Schaleæn L, Verduin CM, et al. *Moraxella catarrhalis* in acute laryngitis: Infection or colonization? J Infect Dis. 1996;174:636.
17. Vrabec DP. Fungal infections of the larynx. Otolaryngol Clin North Am. 1993;26:1091.
18. Laing RBS, Wardrop PJC, Welsby PD, et al. Stridor in patients with HIV infection. J Laryngol Otol. 1995;109:1197.
19. Lawson R, Bodey G, Luna M. Case report: *Candida* infection presenting as laryngitis. Am J Med Sci. 1980;280:173.
20. Kobayashi RH, Rosenblatt HM, Carney JM, et al. *Candida* esophagitis and laryngitis in chronic mucocutaneous candidiasis. Pediatrics. 1980;66:380.
21. Browning DG, Schwartz DA, Jurado RL. Cryptococcosis of the larynx in a patient with AIDS: An unusual cause of fungal laryngitis. South Med J. 1992;85:762.
22. Nasri S, True LD, Abemayor E. Upper airway obstruction caused by Group G streptococcal laryngitis. Am J Otolaryngol. 1995;16:53.
23. Bachman AL, Zizmor J, Noyek AM. Tuberculosis of the larynx. Semin Roentgenol. 1979;14:325.
24. Lederer FJ, Soboroff BJ. Medical problems related to diseases of the larynx. Otolaryngol Clin North Am. 1970;Oct:599.
25. Vaughan CW. Current concepts in otolaryngology: Diagnosis and treatment of organic voice disorders. N Engl J Med. 1982;307:863.
26. Gwaltney JM Jr. Rhinoviruses. In: Evans AS, Kaslow RA, eds. Viral Infections of Humans, Epidemiology and Control. 4th ed. New York: Plenum Medical Book Company; 1997;815.
27. Bennett NM. Diagnosis of influenza. Med J Aust Suppl. 1973;1:19.
28. Chan L, Long CE, Hall CB. Influenza infections in the pediatric outpatient population. J Univ Rochester Med Ctr. 1993;5:12.
29. Knott AM, Long CE, Hall CB. Parainfluenza viral infections in pediatric outpatients: Seasonal patterns and clinical characteristics. Pediatr Infect Dis J. 1994;13:269.
30. McNamara MJ, Pierce WE, Crawford YE, et al. Patterns of adenovirus infection in the respiratory diseases of naval recruits: A longitudinal study of two companies of naval recruits. Am Rev Respir Dis. 1962;86:485.
31. Thom DH, Grayston JT, Wang S-P, et al. *Chlamydia pneumoniae* strain twar, *Mycoplasma pneumoniae*, and viral infections in acute respiratory disease in a university student health clinic population. Am J Epidemiol. 1990;132:248.
32. Grayston JT, Kuo C-C, Wang S-P, et al. A new *Chlamydia psittaci* strain, twar, isolated in acute respiratory tract infections. N Engl J Med. 1986;315:161.

Chapter 49

Acute Laryngotracheobronchitis (Croup)

CAROLINE BREESE HALL
JOHN T. McBRIDE

. . . the sharp stridulous voice which I can resemble to nothing more nearly than the crowing of a cock . . . is the true diagnostic sign of the disease.

Francis Home, 1765[1]

Croup, or acute laryngotracheobronchitis, is an age-specific viral infection of the upper and lower respiratory tract that produces inflammation in the subglottic area and results in a striking picture of dyspnea accompanied on inspiration by the characteristic stridulous notes of croup. Croup perhaps best demonstrates the piquant interaction of host and microorganism. Age, sex, an undefined predisposition of the child, and type of virus all appear to influence the susceptibility and severity of the infection.

Francis Home of Edinburgh first introduced the word *croup* in his treatise, "An Inquiry into the Nature, Causes and Cure of the

Croup," in which he describes 12 patients with croup.[1] The term *croup* has been traced to an Anglo-Saxon word *Kropan*[2] or the old Scottish term *roup*, which meant "to cry out in a shrill voice."

For the next century, the term *croup* was applied to a number of disease entities, including diphtheria. John Cheyne, however, appeared to describe not only diphtheria, "cynache trachealis," but also a croup that apparently was similar to the viral laryngotracheobronchitis of today.[3] Bretonneau, in 1859, argued that diphtheria was a separate and specific disease.[4] However, the confusion between "membranous" or "true" croup and "spasmodic" or "false" croup continued. Differentiation awaited Klebs' discovery of *Corynebacterium diphtheriae* in 1883. In 1948, Rabe[5] classified the forms of infectious croup according to etiology—bacterial or nonbacterial—and suggested that the latter, larger group was viral in origin. In only 15% of his 347 patients was he able to identify a pathogen, namely, *C. diphtheriae* or *Haemophilus influenzae* type b.

The term *croup* now generally refers to an acute laryngotracheitis or laryngotracheobronchitis caused by a viral infection. Many children develop croup only once during childhood despite multiple infections with the viruses that are the prime etiologic agents. In some children, however, such viral infections cause repeated episodes of croup in early childhood. In such children the illness is often called "spasmodic croup." An episode of the spasmodic croup cannot be differentiated from a single episode of the usual type of croup in its clinical manifestations, nor in its etiology, which is usually viral.

INCIDENCE

Croup is a relatively common illness in young children, accounting for about 10 to 15% of lower respiratory tract disease. In Hoekelman's prospective study[6] of infectious diseases occurring in the first year of life, 1.2% of the infants studied had croup. The peak occurrence is in the second year of life, with most cases occurring between 3 months and 3 years of age.[7–10] In a Seattle prepaid group practice, the annual incidence of croup per 1000 children younger than 6 years of age was seven episodes; in the first 6 months of life the rate was 5.2, and in the second 6 months it was 11.[7] The peak incidence was 14.9 in the second year of life and fell to half that rate in the third year. In a group practice in North Carolina, the incidence was three to five times higher, with a peak of 47 annual episodes per 1000 children in the second year of life.[10] Even in the first 6 months of life the incidence was 24, and after 6 years of age it was 4.6. In series of hospitalized or outpatient cases of croup, boys predominated, although the attack rates of upper respiratory tract illnesses by these same viral agents show no sex preference.[7, 9–13]

ETIOLOGY

Acute laryngotracheobronchitis may be caused by a variety of viral agents and occasionally by *Mycoplasma pneumoniae*.[7, 8, 10–16] Parainfluenza type 1 virus is the most common cause of croup in the United States and Great Britain (Table 49–1). Parainfluenza type 3 virus is usually the second most frequently associated agent. In infants this virus more commonly tends to cause bronchiolitis and pneumonia, but the more usual manifestation in children 2 to 3 years of age is croup, and in older children it is tracheobronchitis.[11, 17] Outbreaks with influenza A and B viruses, especially the former, may result in appreciable numbers of croup cases. Influenza, because of its unpredictable nature and fluctuating seasonal occurrence, may be a less common instigator of croup than the parainfluenza viruses, but some studies have reported it to be more severe,[18–20] although others have not.[10] Influenza A virus may produce croup in a broader age range of children and sometimes with a higher frequency of hospitalization. In Washington, D.C., between 1957 and 1976, 14.3% of the patients with croup had influenza A or B viral infection.[20] Influenza A virus more commonly caused croup than did influenza B virus, and the frequency of croup appeared to be related to the particular strain of influenza. Croup was more frequently observed in H3N2 than in H2N2 epidemics.[20]

Only a small proportion (approximately 5%) of respiratory syncytial viral infections result in croup, but 1 to 11% of reported croup cases have been associated with this virus (see Table 49–1). The mean age of croup cases associated with respiratory syncytial virus tends to be younger—less than 1 year, especially in hospitalized cases—and the course may be more severe and prolonged. Adenoviral infection infrequently results in croup, although laryngitis is a relatively common manifestation of adenoviral infection. In contrast, croup is the characteristic manifestation of parainfluenza type 2 viral infection. The total proportion of croup cases produced by parainfluenza type 2 virus is, however, less than that associated with types 1 and 3.[17] The seasonal pattern of parainfluenza type 2 virus also is less predictable, and sizable outbreaks of infection with parainfluenza type 2 virus are unusual in comparison to outbreaks with type 1.[9–11, 17] Rhinoviruses, enteroviruses, and *M. pneumoniae* all contribute to a small but variable percentage of cases.

The proportion of croup cases caused by the different agents varies somewhat according to age. The parainfluenza viruses remain

TABLE 49–1 Percentage of Croup Cases Associated with Various Agents

Agent	Reported Series								
	Cramblatt, 1977[14] (%)	Parrott et al, 1962[15] (%)	Loda et al, 1968[16] (%)	Glezen et al, 1971[11] (%)	Foy et al, 1973[7] (%)		Buchan et al, 1974[13] (%)	Downham et al, 1974[8] (%)	Denny et al, 1983[10] (%)
Parainfluenza virus									
Type 1	8	21	39	21	13*	6.4†	25	26	18
Type 2	6	8	1.6	4	1.4	7.3	1.7	6	3
Type 3	14	10	1.6	9	3	13	8	10	6.6
Influenza A virus	6	} 8	—	2	1	3.7	10	6	1.4
Influenza B virus	—		—	1	1	2	—	—	1.2
Respiratory syncytial virus	—	8	11.4	6	1	9	1.7	6	3.8
Adenovirus	4	9	3	1	4	4.6	1.7	3	—
Rhinovirus	—	—	—	0.6	2	—	1	6	—
Enterovirus	12	—	—	1	1	—	1	—	—
Other viruses	—	—	—	—	—	—	5	—	2
Mycoplasma pneumoniae	—	—	5	1.4	0.5	2	—	1	1.4
Total percentage of cases with identified agent	50	64	62	47	56		54	64	37.6

*Identified by isolation of agent.
†Identified by serology.

the major agents at all ages, but in the first few months of life respiratory syncytial virus ascends in importance, and the influenza viruses and *M. pneumoniae* predominantly cause croup in children older than 5 years of age.[10]

Of all these agents, only the parainfluenza viruses and influenza viruses occur in epidemics and have a predilection for causing croup great enough to produce during their season of activity an appreciable rise in the number of community croup cases.[7, 10, 13, 20, 21]

Outbreaks of measles in the United States or elsewhere serve as a reminder that rubeola in the prevaccine era often resulted in severe and complicated croup. During the 1989–1991 upsurge of measles cases in the United States, laryngotracheobronchitis complicated approximately 20% of the cases of measles in hospitalized patients in Los Angeles and Houston.[22, 23] Children with croup as a complication of their measles tended to be younger and had a more severe course, with 17 to 22% requiring intubation. In some the outcome was fatal.

EPIDEMIOLOGY

The epidemiologic patterns of croup reflect mainly the seasonal personalities of the major agents. The major peak of croup cases coincides with the height of activity of parainfluenza type 1 virus, which in recent years has been every other year in the fall.[9, 11, 13, 17] Parainfluenza type 2 virus also may contribute to outbreaks of croup occurring in the fall, whereas those in the winter to early spring are most apt to be related to influenza A and B viral activity and, to a lesser extent, to respiratory syncytial virus activity.[8–13, 17, 21] Sporadic cases of croup commonly are associated with parainfluenza type 3 virus. This virus previously tended to be present throughout much of the year, but more recently it has been observed to have swells of activity during the warmer months of late spring and summer.[8, 11, 13, 17] Sporadic cases of croup may also be caused by any of the less commonly associated agents, such as the adenoviruses, rhinoviruses, and *M. pneumoniae*, all of which may be prevalent through many months of the year. Croup caused by enteroviruses, although uncommon, tends to occur in the summer and early fall.

PATHOPHYSIOLOGY

The viral infection initially affects the upper respiratory tract, usually producing inflammation of the nasal passages and nasopharynx. Subsequently, the infection spreads downward to involve essentially all levels of the respiratory tract. The classic signs of croup—stridor, hoarseness, and cough—arise mostly from the inflammation that occurs in the larynx and trachea. Involvement of the lower respiratory tract is also present in most cases requiring hospitalization.[24] The inflammation and obstruction are greatest at the subglottic level. This is the least distensible part of the airway because it is encircled by the cricoid cartilage, with the narrow anterior ring and the larger posterior quadrangular lamina forming a "signet ring."

Inflammation at the subglottic level results in the characteristic obstruction observed in viral croup. The impeded flow of air through this narrowed area produces the classic high-pitched vibratory sounds, or *stridor*. This is most apparent on inspiration because the negative intraluminal pressure tends to narrow the extrathoracic airway further, much as sucking on a partially occluded paper straw causes it to collapse inwardly. This effect is enhanced in young children because their airway walls are relatively compliant.[25] In 1836, Ley[26] descriptively expressed the characteristic findings of croup as follows:

> *The shrill sonorous inspiration so characteristic of this complaint, marks very unequivocally its seat. . . . From some cause there is an unusual approximation of the sides of the glottis . . . the influence being very analogous to that produced by too strong compression of the reed against the mouthpiece of the clarionet by the lips of one who has made no great proficiency in that instrument, when a harsh, squeaking sound is produced abundantly discordant and grating to the ear.*

In histologic sections, inflammatory changes may be seen in the epithelium, the mucosa, and the submucosa of the larynx, in the trachea, and the linings of the bronchi, bronchioles, and even the alveoli.[27] Small areas of atelectasis may also be present.

Why children in the second year of life are particularly prone to develop croup is not entirely clear. Most of these children are experiencing primary infection with the viral agent, which is more likely to result in spread of the virus to involve the lower respiratory tract. The anatomy of the young child also may be important in the age predilection. The diameters of the larynx and glottis are relatively small in the young child, and inflammation of the membranes lining these passages causes an appreciably greater degree of obstruction. Airway resistance is highly sensitive to even small changes in the diameter of the airway, because the resistance to airflow is inversely related to the fourth power of the radius of the airway. The mucous membrane is also relatively looser and more vascular, and the cartilage ring is less rigid. Furthermore, nasal obstruction and crying can aggravate the dynamic narrowing of the child's airway.

Immunologic mechanisms also may be involved in the pathogenesis of croup. Urquhart and colleagues[28] suggested that the pathogenesis of croup may be different in children with abrupt instead of gradual onset. Noting a different serologic response in such children, they hypothesized that croup of sudden onset resulted from a hypersensitivity reaction to parainfluenza type 1 virus in children with previous infection with a closely related paramyxovirus, such as parainfluenza type 3. In children with a more gradual onset of prodromal upper respiratory tract symptoms (i.e., longer than 1 day), antibody to the parainfluenza viruses was less often present and was present in lower titers in acute phase sera, compared with sera from patients with a sudden onset of croup.

Greater concentrations of immunoglobulin E (IgE) antibody to parainfluenza viral antigen and histamine were detected in children with parainfluenza viral infections whose illness was manifested as croup, wheezing, or both, compared with those with only upper respiratory tract illness.[29] The lymphoproliferative responses of peripheral blood lymphocytes from children with parainfluenza viral croup were demonstrated to be significantly greater than those from children with upper respiratory tract illnesses, and their histamine-induced suppression of the lymphoproliferative response was diminished.[30] From these findings, Welliver and colleagues suggested that a defect in the regulation of the immune response, similar to that found in atopic subjects, contributes to the pathogenesis of croup.

Physiologic Correlations

When the infection produces obstruction at the subglottic level, the child's tidal volume initially declines. This is compensated by an increase in the respiratory rate to maintain adequate alveolar ventilation (Fig. 49–1). If the degree of obstruction worsens, the work of breathing may increase so much that the child tires and can no longer maintain the necessary compensatory respiratory effort. The tidal volume may then further decrease, and, as the respiratory rate declines, hypercarbia and secondary hypoxemia ensue.

The frequent occurrence of hypoxemia in children hospitalized with croup may not be suspected and may seem surprising because upper airway obstruction that does not disrupt the distribution of ventilation and perfusion in the lung should not cause hypoxemia. The inflammation in the lung parenchyma, however, results in areas of abnormally low ventilation-perfusion ratio and increased alveolar-to-arterial oxygen gradient (see Fig. 49–1). In some children, hypoxemia may result from transient airway hyperreactivity or from pulmonary edema caused by the marked negative intrathoracic pressures exerted during inspiration in an attempt to compensate for the obstruction of the upper airway. In those few patients who require intubation, the abrupt relief of the negative mean intrathoracic pressure can also be associated with acute onset of pulmonary edema.

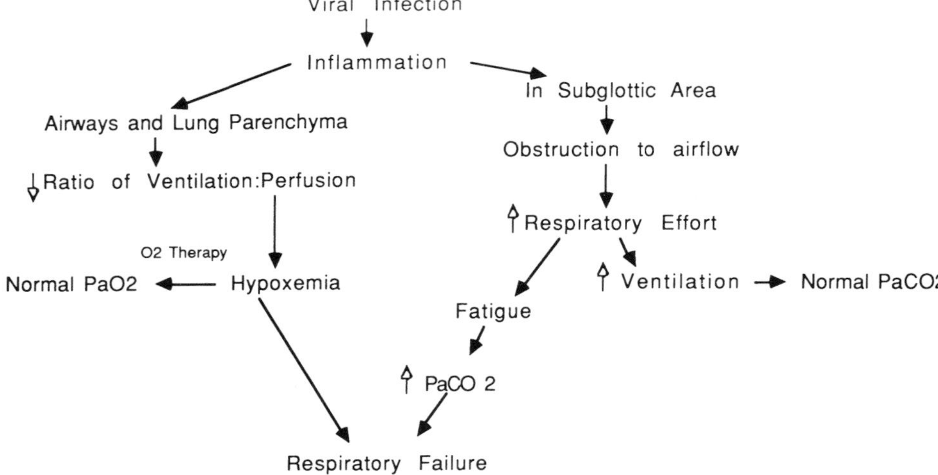

FIGURE 49–1. Physiologic abnormalities in croup.

CLINICAL MANIFESTATIONS

The disease generally comes on in the evening after the little patient has been exposed to the weather during the day and often after a slight catarrh of some days' standing. At first his voice is observed to be hoarse and pulling . . . he awakens with a most unusual cough, rough, and stridulous. And now his breathing is laborious, each inspiration being accompanied by a harsh, shrill noise.

—John Cheyne, 1814[2]

Most children with croup have a history of an upper respiratory tract infection for one to several days previously. Commonly the child has had rhinorrhea, a sore throat, and a mild cough. Most children have fever, either initially during the upper respiratory tract infection or at the onset of croup. Children with croup caused by influenza or parainfluenza viruses commonly have fevers with temperatures ranging from 38°C to 40°C.[31] Fever with respiratory syncytial viral infection tends not to be as high or may even be absent.

The onset of croup often is heralded by hoarseness and a deepening cough. The cough usually is not productive but has the striking brassy tone that has earned it the sobriquet "seal's bark." The child may awaken at night with this distinctive cough, tachypnea, and the characteristic inspiratory stridor. In 1836, Ley[26] described the stridor as "the crowing of a cock, the yelping of a fox, the barking of a dog, the braying of an ass, or a ringing sound, as if the voice came from a brazen tube." The child may sit forward in bed and appear apprehensive. Often accompanying the stridor are retractions of the chest wall, usually most marked in the supraclavicular and suprasternal areas.

In children who are more severely affected, auscultation of the chest may reveal not only the inspiratory stridor but also rales, rhonchi, or wheezing. Occasionally, a markedly distressed child has stridor on expiration as well as inspiration. The respiratory rate is commonly elevated to 35 to 45 per minute. Respiratory rates much above 50 per minute are unusual in children with croup, in contrast to the marked tachypnea that is often evident in bronchiolitis. With progression of the disease, auscultation of the chest may reveal poor exchange of air with diminished breath sounds.

One of the hallmarks of croup is its fluctuating course. A child may appear clinically to worsen or improve within an hour. In milder cases of croup, children commonly improve in the morning, only to worsen again at night. In most children the course of croup is 3 to 4 days, although the cough may persist for a longer period.

LABORATORY FINDINGS

In most cases of croup the leukocyte and differential counts are not particularly abnormal or helpful. In the more severely stressed child, the leukocyte count may be somewhat elevated, and an increase in the proportion of immature polymorphonuclear cells may be observed.

Hypoxemia occurs in most hospitalized children, and hypercapnea is present in more than half.[24] In the study of Newth and associates,[24] most children hospitalized with croup had arterial partial pressure of oxygen (PaO_2) values between 50 and 80 mmHg, and about half had $PaCO_2$ values in the normal range below 40 mmHg. The rest had $PaCO_2$ levels between 40 and 50 mmHg. Only 1 of the 35 children manifested hypercarbia greater than 50 mmHg. Few pulmonary function studies have been obtained in children with croup, but in five out of six children in one study the functional residual capacity was found to be increased.[32]

DIAGNOSIS

The diagnosis of croup is usually based on the characteristic clinical picture. Differentiation from noninfectious causes of stridor (e.g., foreign body aspiration, allergic reaction) and from bacterial epiglottitis usually may be made on the basis of both the history and the anterior-posterior and lateral roentgenograms of the neck.[33, 34]

Characteristically, the course of epiglottitis is much more rapidly progressive, and the children appear more toxic. The history of an upper respiratory tract infection with rhinorrhea and laryngitis usually is not present in epiglottitis. The absence of the distinctive cough or "seal's bark" and the presence of marked dysphagia with drooling are two of the more helpful differentiating clinical signs. In viral laryngotracheobronchitis the anteroposterior view of the neck (Fig. 49–2) shows the characteristic subglottic swelling, sometimes described as the "hourglass" or "steeple" sign. In epiglottitis, the lateral neck view may show the edematous epiglottis without subglottic narrowing (see Chapter 52). The roentgenographic picture may not, however, always be diagnostic for croup or epiglottitis, and controversy exists about its reliability and usefulness in the acute situation.[35–37]

Identification of the specific viral agent may be accomplished by isolation in tissue culture or by one of the newer techniques of rapid viral diagnosis.[38] In reported series, the cause was determined in approximately one third to two thirds of the patients with croup (see Table 49–1), which is higher than that generally reported for other respiratory tract syndromes. The time required for viral isolation may be shortened by the use of spin-enhanced cultures.[39] Rapid techniques may be used to identify the viral antigens in the respiratory secretions (e.g., immunofluorescence, other immunoassays) or to detect viral RNA (e.g., reverse transcriptase polymerase chain reaction, immunoassay).[40, 41] Serologic diagnosis generally may be made only retrospectively, and for some of the major agents of croup serologic rises are variable and unreliable. Heterotypic antibody rises are frequent among the various types of the parainfluenza viruses and related viruses such as mumps.[15, 42] Furthermore, during reinfection no measurable antibody responses may occur.[42]

COMPLICATIONS

The severity of croup appears to be influenced by both the virus and host factors. Some children appear predisposed to croup, with repetitive episodes from a variety of agents. John Cheyne[3] noted that ". . . the first attack establishes a predisposition to the disease. I have observed, that after the first attack, a slighter cause will produce Croup a second time than is required originally."

Children with repeated episodes of croup are sometimes diagnosed as having *spasmodic croup.*[43] An allergic diathesis or hyperreactivity of the airway may contribute to the illness in these children; positive intradermal skin tests and family members with allergy have been noted frequently in children with recurrent versus single episodes of croup.[44–48] A tendency toward lower serum IgA levels also has been noted in children with recurrent croup.[47] Nevertheless, a viral infection initiates croup even in these children, and the disease cannot be distinguished clinically.

Boys are particularly prone to develop croup, for reasons that are not entirely clear.[9–11, 13, 44–48] Taussig,[49] however, showed that young girls have significantly larger maximal air flow rates than do boys. This suggests that anatomic differences or differences in intrinsic airway resistance exist that are related to gender. This may in part explain why young boys tend to develop lower respiratory tract disease more frequently or more severely than do young girls.

Severe croup sometimes has been reported as being more common with influenza A viral infection than with the other viral agents.[18, 19] In the study of Howard and coworkers,[18] made during an outbreak of influenza A viral infection, 10 of 25 infants hospitalized with croup required tracheotomy. This complication was estimated to occur in about 5 to 12% of cases of croup.[48, 50, 51] The number of children requiring intubation has been reduced by newer modes of therapy, including nebulized racemic epinephrine and corticosteroids. The associated mortality rate in these series has ranged from 0 to 2.7%. Of the major acute complications, respiratory failure necessitating such airway intervention is the most common. Subglottic stenosis after intubation occasionally occurs in children with complicated and prolonged courses.[48, 50–53]

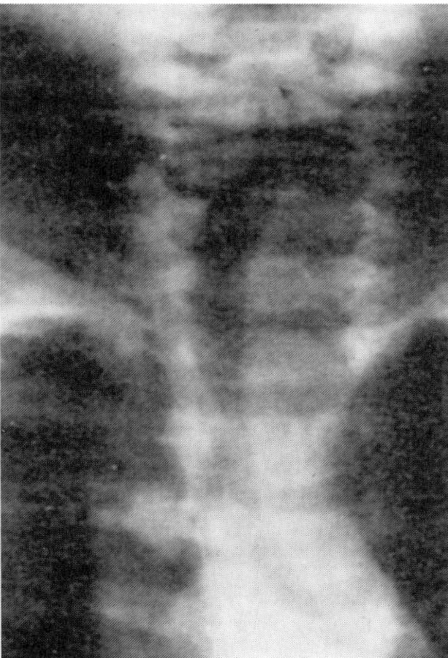

FIGURE 49–2. Roentgenogram of the neck of a child with viral croup that shows the characteristic narrowing of the air shadow of the trachea in the subglottic area.

Pneumonia cannot be considered a true complication of croup but should be thought of as a part of the disease. Parenchymal involvement, as evidenced by hypoxemia, is present in most hospitalized children, whether or not it is visible on the chest roentgenogram. Less common complications include pneumothorax, pulmonary edema, and aspiration pneumonia. Aspiration of gastric contents is most likely to occur during emergency intubation. Transient pulmonary edema without evidence of cardiac enlargement has been described in children with croup.[53–55] The mechanism leading to this complication is not completely understood, but it may arise from a neurogenic effect on the pulmonary vasculature, as a direct result of alveolar hypoxia, or possibly from an increased alveolar-capillary gradient causing a leakage of intravascular fluids.

Whether long-term complications can follow croup is speculative. The disease is self-limited, and recovery appears to be complete. Several follow-up studies of children with croup early in life, however, have shown an increased frequency of hyperreactivity of the airways and altered pulmonary function that may be clinically occult in some children.[32, 51, 56, 57] In one study of 12-year-old children who had a history of hospitalization for croup, elevated residual volumes and significant reduction in forced vital capacity (FVC), forced expiratory volume in 1 second (FEV_1), and maximal expiratory flow between 25 and 75% of vital capacity ($FEF_{25-75\%}$) were found.[57] The fact that hyperreactivity of the airways was observed in each of these follow-up studies could suggest that children who tend to develop croup are those who have an underlying predisposition to airway hyperreactivity. Detection of such abnormalities on follow-up examination therefore may reflect not the previous croup, but the predisposition of a selected population to acquire croup.[32, 51, 56, 57]

THERAPY

Despite a plethora of home therapies for croup, none has proved consistently effective. The natural fluctuations in the course of croup make evaluation of many therapies difficult. Vaporizers and other means of producing steam or mist in the home have long been advised. In the past century, steaming tea kettles were an integral, if not primary, mode of therapy.[58] Nevertheless, the beneficial effects of these devices have not been proved. These methods certainly provide humidification of the upper airway, but the droplet size produced is generally too large to reach the lower respiratory tract. The advantages of such home humidification devices must be balanced against the discomfort or fear they may produce in the child.[59] Crying and lack of rest may worsen the condition.

In hospitalized patients, the essence of successful management is close observation and good supportive care based on a thorough understanding of the physiologic changes associated with croup. Clinical estimation of the severity of croup is difficult. Cyanosis may not be present despite compromising degrees of hypoxemia.[60] Of the clinical signs, an increasing respiratory rate is often the best indication of hypoxemia. The severity of the stridor and retractions reflects the degree of subglottic obstruction and is not indicative of the arterial oxygen saturation. Oximetry offers a simple, noninvasive means of monitoring the child's arterial oxygen saturation.[61] In the more severely ill child, the PCO_2 also may need to be assessed. In most cases, however, blood drawing and other frightening procedures should be kept to a minimum to avoid compounding the dyspnea and respiratory obstruction. Inspirations that are rapid and shallow, such as commonly accompany anxiety and crying, aggravate the narrowing of the airway and further increase the metabolic demand for gas exchange. Most children with hypoxemia who are not hypercarbic respond to relatively low concentrations of supplemental oxygen, because the hypoxemia results primarily from areas of lung with an abnormal ratio of ventilation to perfusion[51, 62, 63] (see Fig. 49–1).

In the hospital, humidification of the airway may be administered by an ultrasonic nebulizer fitted to a mask or an oxygen tent.

Although humidification may aid the upper airway secretions, a beneficial effect on the subglottic swelling and on the lower parenchymal abnormalities has not been shown, and few controlled studies have examined this therapy. In one small, controlled trial of 16 children, humidification did not result in discernible improvement.[64] In another study, nebulized water administered to five children did not produce a change in the measured total respiratory resistance.[65]

In a dog model of croup, cold-dry, cold-moist, and dry air were more effective than warm-moist air in decreasing airway resistance.[66] All of these types of air contain little humidification compared with warm-moist air. These findings correlate with the clinical observation that many children with croup improve when taken out into cold night air, which would contain little moisture.

A variety of pharmacologic agents have been evaluated in the treatment of croup. Nebulized racemic epinephrine has appeared to provide clinical improvement to many children with marked stridor.[50, 67–70] L-Epinephrine, which contains only the active isomer, has been shown to be just as effective and may have fewer side effects.[71, 72] The α-adrenergic effect of racemic epinephrine—local vasoconstriction and diminished subglottic swelling—is probably the mechanism by which the stridor is ameliorated. The arterial oxygen saturation is not affected, and the clinical improvement is transient, lasting usually for a couple of hours.[68, 73] Children improving from such treatment should continue to be observed, since dyspnea and airway obstruction may recur in 1 to 3 hours. Despite the lack of benefit in terms of arterial oxygen saturation, nebulized racemic epinephrine has resulted in a less frequent need for intubation by alleviating the work of breathing and progression toward respiratory failure.[50, 67–70]

Corticosteroids have been added to the armamentarium for the treatment of croup. Although their use was long controversial,[69, 74–76] the majority of more recent studies have indicated significant clinical benefit in the hospitalized child with severe croup and even in children treated as outpatients.[77–82] Furthermore, significant clinical improvement has been reported in controlled studies to occur with varying routes of administration, including intramuscular, oral, and by nebulization, thus allowing the potential use of such therapy in outpatients.

Despite the general acknowledgment that viruses are the perpetrators of croup, antibiotics are frequently used.[69, 83] Bacterial infection superimposed or occurring after croup is uncommon, and administration of antibiotics to children with croup prophylactically or without evidence of concomitant bacterial infection is not warranted.[69, 83]

A few children, despite adequate supportive therapy, fatigue and develop respiratory failure, demonstrated by a climbing Pa_{CO_2} level. If a mechanical airway becomes necessary, nasotracheal intubation is the preferred method, provided personnel skilled in this technique are available.[51–53] In Schuller and Birck's[51] 8-year follow-up study of children receiving nasotracheal intubation for croup and epiglottitis, the rate of immediate and reversible complications was 7%, and that of delayed, irreversible complications was 1.6%. The average period of intubation for the children with croup was 88 hours, compared with 55 hours for those with epiglottitis.

BACTERIAL TRACHEITIS

An atypical form of croup with a clinical picture more similar to epiglottitis than to the usual case of laryngotracheobronchitis has been described and designated *bacterial tracheitis*.[84–89] Although this entity appears to have been described before 1940, it received little attention until it was rediscovered toward the end of the 1970s. This relatively uncommon disease tends to affect somewhat older children but may affect those of any age; it produces a dramatic, acute onset marked by high fever, stridor, and dyspnea with copious amounts of purulent sputum. The clinical picture may progress rapidly, requiring endotracheal intubation. The primary area of inflammation and obstruction is subglottic. The subglottis is covered with a thick exudate, but the epiglottis and supraglottic structures tend to be minimally inflamed. A lateral soft tissue roentgenogram of the neck characteristically reveals a normal epiglottis with subglottic narrowing within which a shaggy membrane may sometimes be visible.

The organisms most commonly recovered from this exudate are *Staphylococcus aureus*, group A β-hemolytic streptococci, and, at least before widespread immunization became available, *H. influenzae* type b.[84–89] The pathogenesis of this entity, nevertheless, is not clear. The syndrome appears to develop in children who are predisposed by previous conditions, especially those associated with injury to the trachea. Children who have been intubated recently and sometimes those with a preceding viral infection appear to be at greater risk, suggesting that mucosal damage or impairment of local immune mechanisms may predispose to invasive infections with common pyogenic organisms.

The rapidly progressive course of this disease demands its prompt diagnosis and differentiation from viral croup by its clinical and roentgenographic picture. Direct laryngoscopy can confirm the diagnosis and provide specimens of the localized exudate for culture. These children do not respond to nebulized racemic epinephrine. Initial antibiotic therapy should be broad enough to cover the associated major pathogens.

REFERENCES

1. Home F. An Inquiry into the Nature, Cause and Cure of Croup. Edinburgh: Printed for A. Kincaid & J. Bell; 1765.
2. Cherry JD. Croup. In: Kiple KF, ed. Cambridge History and Geography of Human Disease Project. Bowling Green, Ohio: University of Cambridge Press; 1990:654–657.
3. Cheyne J. Essays on the Diseases of Children, with Cases and Dissections: Philadelphia, 1802–1808. Philadelphia: Anthony Finley Merritt; 1814:20.
4. Semple RH. Memoirs on diphtheria. From the Writings of Bretonneau, Guersant, Trousseau, Bouchut, Empis, Daviot. London: New Sydenham Society Publication; 1859:5.
5. Rabe EF. Infectious croup: I. Etiology. Pediatrics. 1948;2:255–265.
6. Hoekelman RA. Infectious illness during the first year of life. Pediatrics. 1977:59:119–121.
7. Foy HM, Cooney MK, Maletzky AJ, et al. Incidence and etiology of pneumonia, croup and bronchiolitis in pre-school children belonging to a prepaid medical care group over a four year period. Am J Epidemiol. 1973;97:80–92.
8. Downham MAPS, McQuillan J, Gardner PS. Diagnosis and clinical significance of parainfluenza virus infections in children. Arch Dis Child. 1974;49:8–15.
9. Glezen WP, Denny FW. Epidemiology of acute lower respiratory disease in children. N Engl J Med. 1973;288:498–505.
10. Denny FW, Murphy TF, Clyde WA Jr, et al. Croup: An 11 year study in a pediatric practice. Pediatrics. 1983;71:871–876.
11. Glezen WP, Loda FA, Clyde WA Jr, et al. Epidemiological patterns of acute lower respiratory disease of children in a pediatric group practice. J Pediatr. 1971;78:397–406.
12. Loda FA, Glezen WP, Clyde WA Jr. Respiratory disease in group day care. Pediatrics. 1972;49:428–437.
13. Buchan KA, Marten KW, Kennedy DH. Aetiology and epidemiology of viral croup in Glasgow, 1966–72. J Hyg (Camb). 1974;73:143–150.
14. Cramblett HG. Croup (epiglottitis, laryngitis, laryngotracheobronchitis). In: Kendig EL Jr, Chernick V, eds. Disorders of the Respiratory Tract in Children. 3rd ed. Philadelphia: WB Saunders; 1977:353.
15. Parrott RH, Vargosko AJ, Kim HW, et al. Acute respiratory diseases of viral etiology: III. Myxoviruses: parainfluenza. Am J Public Health. 1962;52:907–917.
16. Loda FA, Clyde WA Jr, Glezen WP, et al. Studies of the role of viruses, bacteria, and *M. pneumoniae* as causes of lower respiratory tract infections in children. J Pediatr. 1968;72:161–176.
17. Knott A, Long CE, Hall CB. Parainfluenza viral infections in pediatric outpatients: Seasonal patterns and clinical characteristics. Pediatr Infect Dis J. 1993;13:269–273.
18. Howard JB, McCracken GH Jr, Luby JP. Influenza A 2 virus as a cause of croup requiring tracheotomy. J Pediatr. 1972;81:1148–1150.
19. Eller JJ, Fulginiti VA, Plunket DC, et al. Attack rates for hospitalized croup in children in a military population: Importance of A_2 influenza infection. Pediatr Res. 1972;6:126.
20. Kim HW, Brandt CD, Chanock RM, et al. Influenza A and B virus infection in infants and young children during the years 1957–1976. Am J Epidemiol. 1979;109:464–479.
21. Hall CB, Douglas RG Jr. Respiratory syncytial virus and influenza: Practical community surveillance. Am J Dis Child. 1976;130:615–620.
22. Ross LA, Mason WH, Lanson J, et al. Laryngotracheobronchitis as a complication of measles during an urban epidemic. J Pediatr. 1992;121:511–515.
23. Fortenberry JD, Mariscalco M, Louis PT, et al. Severe laryngotracheobronchitis complicating measles. Am J Dis Child. 1992;146:1040–1043.
24. Newth CJ, Levison H, Bryan AC. The respiratory status of children with croup. J Pediatr. 1972;81:1068–1073.

25. McBride JT. Stridor in childhood. J Fam Practice. 1984;19:782–790.
26. Ley H. An essay on the Laryngismus Stridulus or Croup-like Inspiration of Infants. London: Churchill; 1836:6.
27. Szpunar J, Glowacki J, Laskowski A, et al. Fibrinous laryngotracheobronchitis in children. Arch Otolaryngol. 1971;93:173–178.
28. Urquhart GED, Kennedy DH, Ariyawansa JP. Croup associated with parainfluenza type 1 virus: Two subpopulations. BMJ. 1979;1:1604.
29. Welliver RC, Wong DT, Middleton E Jr, et al. Role of parainfluenza virus-specific IgE in pathogenesis of croup and wheezing subsequent to infection. J Pediatr. 1982;101:889–896.
30. Welliver RC, Sun M, Rinaldo D. Defective regulation of immune responses in croup due to parainfluenza virus. Pediatr Res. 1985;19:716–720.
31. Hall CB, Geiman JM, Breese BB, et al. Parainfluenza viral infections in children: Correlation of shedding with clinical manifestations. J Pediatr. 1977;91:194–198.
32. Loughlin G, Taussig LM. Pulmonary function in children with a history of laryngotracheobronchitis. J Pediatr. 1979;94:365–369.
33. Rapkin RH. The diagnosis of epiglottitis: Simplicity and reliability of radiographs of the neck in the differential diagnosis of the croup syndrome. J Pediatr. 1972;80:96–98.
34. Wildin SR, Chonmaitree T, Swischuk LE. Roentgenographic features of common pediatric viral respiratory tract infections. Am J Dis Child. 1988;142:43–46.
35. Currarino G, Williams B. Lateral inspiration and expiration radiographs of the neck in children with laryngotracheobronchitis (croup). Radiology. 1982;195:365–366.
36. Jones JL. False positives in lateral neck radiographs used to diagnose epiglottitis (letter). Ann Emerg Med. 1983;12:797.
37. Stankiewicz JA, Bowes AK. Croup and epiglottitis: A radiologic study. Laryngoscope. 1985;95:1159–1160.
38. Miller MJ, Cherry JD. Use of diagnostic virology laboratory. In: Feigen RD, Cherry JD, eds. Textbook of Pediatric Infectious Diseases. 4th ed. Philadelphia: WB Saunders; 1998:2873–2891.
39. Olsen MA, Shuck KM, Sambol AR, et al. Isolation of seven respiratory viruses in shell vials: A practical and highly sensitive method. J Clin Microbiol. 1993;31: 422–425.
40. Karron RA, Froehlick JL, Bobo L, et al. Rapid detection of parainfluenza virus type 3 RNA in respiratory specimens: Use of reverse transcription-PCR-enzyme immunoassay. J Clin Microbiol. 1994;32:484–488.
41. Freymuth F, Vabret A, Galateau-Salle F, et al. Detection of respiratory syncytial virus, parainfluenzavirus 3, adenovirus and rhinovirus sequences in respiratory tract of infants by polymerase chain reaction and hybridization. Clin Diagn Virol. 1997;8:31–40.
42. Bloom HH, Johnson KM, Jacobsen R, et al. Recovery of parainfluenza viruses from adults with upper respiratory illness. Am J Hyg. 1961;74:50–59.
43. McLain LG. Croup syndrome. Am Fam Physician. 1987;36:207–214.
44. Hide DW, Guyer BM. Recurrent croup. Arch Dis Child. 1985;60:585–586.
45. Laufer P. The relationship of respiratory allergies to croup. J Asthma. 1986;23:9–10.
46. Zach M, Erban A, Olinsky A. Croup, recurrent croup, allergy, and airways hyperreactivity. Arch Dis Child. 1981;56:336–341.
47. Zach M. Serum IgA in recurrent croup. Am J Dis Child. 1983;137:184–185.
48. Postma DS, Jones RD, Pillsbury HC III. Severe hospitalized croup: Treatment trends and prognosis. Laryngoscope. 1984;94:1170–1175.
49. Taussig LM. Maximal expiratory flows at functional residual capacity: A test of lung function for young children. Am Rev Respir Dis. 1977;116:1031–1038.
50. Adair JC, Ring WH, Jordan WS, et al. Ten year experience with IPPB in the treatment of acute laryngotracheobronchitis. Anesth Analg. 1971;50:649–655.
51. Schuller DE, Birck HG. The safety of intubation in croup and epiglottitis: An eight-year follow-up. Laryngoscope. 1975;85:33–46.
52. Hen J Jr. Current management of upper airway obstruction. Pediatr Ann. 1986;15:274–294.
53. Kilham H, Gillies J, Benjamin B. Severe upper airway obstruction. Pediatr Clin North Am. 1987;34:1–14.
54. Broniatowski M. Croup. Ear Nose Throat J. 1985;64:12–21.
55. Travis KW, Todres ID, Shannon DC. Pulmonary edema associated with croup and epiglottitis. Pediatrics. 1977;59:695–698.
56. Zach MS, Schnall RP, Landau LI. Upper and lower airway hyperreactivity in recurrent croup. Am Rev Respir Dis. 1980;121:979–983.
57. Gurwitz D, Corey M, Levison H. Pulmonary function and bronchial reactivity in children after croup. Am Rev Respir Dis. 1980;122:95–99.
58. Baugh R, Gilmore BB Jr. Infectious croup: A critical review. Otolaryngol Head Neck Surg. 1986;95:40–46.
59. Henry R. Moist air in the treatment of laryngotracheitis. Arch Dis Child. 1983;58:577.
60. Hall CB, Hall WJ, Speers DM. Clinical and physiological manifestations of bronchiolitis and pneumonia: Outcome of respiratory syncytial virus. Am J Dis Child. 1979;133:798–802.
61. Gussack GS, Tacchi EJ. Pulse oximetry in the management of pediatric airway disorders. South Med J. 1987;80:1381–1384.
62. Barker GA. Current management of croup and epiglottitis. Pediatr Clin North Am. 1979;26:565–579.
63. Newth CJL, Levison H. Diagnosing and managing croup and epiglottitis. J Respir Dis. 1981;2:22–41.
64. Bourchier D, Dawson KP, Fergusson DM. Humidification in viral croup: A controlled trial. Aust Paediatr J. 1984;20:289–291.
65. Lenney W, Milner AD. Treatment of acute viral croup. Arch Dis Child. 1978;53:704–706.
66. Wolfsdorf J, Swift DL. An animal model simulating acute infective upper airway obstruction of childhood and its use in the investigation of croup therapy. Pediatr Res. 1978;12:1062–1065.
67. Westley CR, Cotton EK, Brooks JG. Nebulized racemic epinephrine by IPPB for the treatment of croup: A double-blind study. Am J Dis Child. 1978;132:484–487.
68. Taussig LM, Castro O, Beaudry PH, et al. Treatment of laryngotracheobronchitis (croup): Use of intermittent positive-pressure breathing and racemic epinephrine. Am J Dis Child. 1975;129:790–793.
69. Skolnik NS. Treatment of croup. Am J Dis Child. 1989;143:1045–1049.
70. Kuusela A-L, Vesikari T. A randomized double-blind, placebo-controlled trial of dexamethasone and racemic epinephrine in the treatment of croup. Acta Paediatr Scand. 1988;77:99–104.
71. Klassen TP. Managing croup: Racemic epinephrine versus L-epinephrine. J Respir Dis. 1995;16:245–246.
72. Waisman Y, Klein BL, Boenning DA, et al. Prospective randomized double-blind study comparing L-epinephrine and racemic epinephrine aerosols in the treatment of laryngotracheitis (croup). Pediatrics. 1992;89:302–306.
73. Fanconi S, Burger R, Maurer H, et al. Transcutaneous carbon dioxide pressure for monitoring patients with severe croup. J Pediatr. 1990;117:701–705.
74. Bass JW, Bruhn FW, Merrit WT. Corticosteroids and racemic epinephrine with IPPB in the treatment of croup. J Pediatr. 1980;96:173–174.
75. Tunnessen WW Jr, Feinstein AR. The steroid-croup controversy: An analytic review of methodologic problems. J Pediatr. 1980;96:751–756.
76. Kairys SW, Olmstead EM, O'Connor GT. Steroid treatment of laryngotracheitis: A meta-analysis of the evidence from randomized trials. Pediatrics. 1989;83:683–693.
77. Geelhoed GC, Macdonald WBG. Oral and inhaled steroids in croup: A randomized, placebo-controlled trial. Pediatr Pulmonol. 1995;20:355–361.
78. Geelhoed GC, Macdonald WBG. Oral dexamethasone in the treatment of croup: 0.15 mg/kg versus 0.3 mg/kg versus 0.6 mg/kg. Pediatr Pulmonol. 1995;20:362–368.
79. Geelhoed GC. Croup. Pediatr Pulmonol. 1997;23:370–374.
80. Klassen TP, Feldman ME, Watters, LK, et al. Nebulized budesonide for children with mild-to-moderate croup. N Engl J Med. 1994;331:285–289.
81. Klassen TP, Watters LK, Feldman ME, et al. The efficacy of nebulized budesonide in dexamethasone-treated outpatients with croup. Pediatrics. 1996;97:463–466.
82. Cruz MN, Stewart G, Rosenberg N. Use of dexamethasone in the outpatient management of acute laryngotracheitis. Pediatrics. 1995;96:220–223.
83. Pianosi P, Feldman W, Robson MG, et al. Inappropriate use of antibiotics in croup at three types of hospitals. Can Med Assoc J. 1986;134:357–359.
84. Jones R, Santos JI, Overall JC. Bacterial tracheitis. JAMA. 1979;242:721–726.
85. Liston SL, Gehrz RC, Jarvis CW. Bacterial tracheitis. Arch Otolaryngol. 1981;107:561–564.
86. Davidson S, Barzilay Z, Yahav J, et al. Bacterial tracheitis: A true entity? J Laryngol Otol. 1982;96:173–175.
87. Donnelly BW, McMillan JA, Weiner LB. Bacterial tracheitis: Report of eight new cases and review. Rev Infect Dis. 1990;12:729–735.
88. Dudin AA, Thalji A, Rambaud-Cousson A. Bacterial tracheitis among children hospitalized for severe obstructive dyspnea. Pediatr Infect Dis J. 1990;9:293–295.
89. Long SS. Bacterial tracheitis. Report on Pediatric Infectious Diseases. 1992;2:29–31.

Chapter 50

Otitis Externa, Otitis Media, and Mastoiditis

JEROME O. KLEIN

OTITIS EXTERNA

Infection of the external auditory canal (otitis externa) is similar to infection of skin and soft tissue elsewhere. Unique problems occur because the canal is narrow and tortuous; fluid and foreign objects enter, are trapped, and cause irritation and maceration of the superficial tissues. The pain and itching that results may be severe because of the limited space for expansion of the inflamed tissue. Infections of the external canal may be subdivided into four categories: acute localized otitis externa, acute diffuse otitis externa, chronic otitis externa, and malignant otitis externa. Reviews by Senturia and colleagues,[1] Hirsch,[2] and Rubin and Yu[3] provide more complete information.

Pathogenesis

The external auditory canal is approximately 2.5 cm long from the concha of the auricle to the tympanic membrane. The lateral half of the canal is cartilaginous; the medial half tunnels through the temporal bone. A constriction, the isthmus, present at the juncture of the osseous and cartilaginous portions, limits the entry of wax and foreign bodies to the area near the tympanic membrane. The skin of the canal is thicker in the cartilaginous portion and includes a well-developed dermis and subcutaneous layer. The skin lining the osseous portion is thinner and firmly attached to the periosteum and lacks a subcutaneous layer. Hair follicles are numerous in the outer third and sparse in the inner two thirds of the canal.

The microbial flora of the external canal is similar to the flora of skin elsewhere. There is a predominance of *Staphylococcus epidermidis, Staphylococcus aureus, Corynebacteria*, and, to a lesser extent, anaerobic bacteria such as *Propionibacterium acnes*.[4–6] Pathogens responsible for infection of the middle ear *(Streptococcus pneumoniae, Haemophilus influenzae*, or *Moraxella catarrhalis)* are uncommonly found in cultures of the external auditory canal when the tympanic membrane is intact.

The epithelium absorbs moisture from the environment. Desquamation and denuding of the superficial layers of the epithelium may follow. In this warm, moist environment, the organisms in the canal may flourish and invade the macerated skin. Inflammation and suppuration follow. Invasive organisms include those of the normal skin flora and gram-negative bacilli, particularly *Pseudomonas aeruginosa*. Invasive otitis media is a necrotizing infection frequently associated with *P. aeruginosa*. The organism gains access to the deeper tissues of the ear canal and causes a localized vasculitis, thrombosis, and necrosis of tissues. Diabetic microangiopathy of the skin overlying the temporal bone results in poor local perfusion and a milieu for invasion by *P. aeruginosa*.

Clinical Manifestations and Management

Acute localized *otitis externa* may occur as a pustule or furuncle associated with hair follicles; it is due to *S. aureus*. Erysipelas caused by group A *Streptococcus* may involve the concha and the canal. Pain may be severe. Bluish-red hemorrhagic bullae may be present on the osseous canal walls and also on the tympanic membrane. Adenopathy in the lymphatic drainage areas is often present. Local heat and systemic antibiotics are usually curative. Incision and drainage may be necessary to relieve severe pain.

Acute diffuse otitis externa (swimmer's ear) occurs mainly in hot, humid weather. The ear itches and becomes increasingly painful. The skin of the canal is edematous and red. Gram-negative bacilli, mainly *P. aeruginosa*, may play a significant role. A severe hemorrhagic external otitis due to *P. aeruginosa* was associated with mobile redwood hot tub systems.[7] Gentle cleansing to remove debris including irrigation with hypertonic saline (3%) and cleansing with mixtures of alcohol (70 to 95%) and acetic acid should be used initially. Hydrophilic solutions such as 50% Burrow's solutions may be used for 1 to 2 days to reduce inflammation. Ear drops of neomycin alone or with polymyxin combined with hydrocortisone or an oral quinolone, such as levofloxacin, ofloxacin, or ciprofloxacin plus topical hydrocortisone, diminish local inflammation and infection.

Chronic otitis externa is due to irritation from drainage through a perforated tympanic membrane. The underlying cause is chronic suppurative otitis media. Itching may be severe. Management is directed to treatment of the middle ear disorder. Rare causes of chronic otitis externa include tuberculosis, syphilis, yaws, leprosy, and sarcoidosis.

Invasive ("malignant") otitis externa is a severe, necrotizing infection that spreads from the squamous epithelium of the ear canal to adjacent areas of soft tissue, blood vessels, cartilage, and bone.[3, 8] Severe pain and tenderness of the tissues around the ear and mastoid are accompanied by the drainage of pus from the canal. Elderly, diabetic, immunocompromised, and debilitated patients are at particular risk. Life-threatening disease may result from spread to the temporal bone and then on to the sigmoid sinus, jugular bulb, base of the skull, meninges, and brain. Permanent facial paralysis is frequent, and cranial nerves 9, 10, and 12 may also be affected.[9] *Pseudomonas aeruginosa* is almost always the causative agent. The extent of damage to soft tissue and bone may be identified and monitored by the use of computed tomography and magnetic resonance imaging.[3] Diagnostic tests for underlying disease should be instituted. The canal should be cleansed, devitalized tissue removed, and ear drops with antipseudomonal antibiotics combined with steroid instilled into the external auditory canal. Systemic therapy with regimens including activity for *Pseudomonas* spp. should be used for 4 to 6 weeks. The combination of ceftazidime or an antipseudomonal penicillin (ticarcillin or piperacillin) with an aminoglycoside (gentamicin or tobramycin) should be considered. Oral quinolones with activity against *Pseudomonas* spp., such as ciprofloxacin, have been effective therapy early in the course of invasive external otitis.[10]

Fungal otitis may be part of a general or local fungal infection. *Aspergillus* spp. are responsible for most cases of fungal otitis.[11] *Candida albicans* is a frequent cause of external otitis in children with chronic mucocutaneous candidiasis.

OTITIS MEDIA

Otitis media, or inflammation of the middle ear, is defined by the presence of fluid in the middle ear accompanied by signs or symptoms of acute illness. In 1990, there were an estimated 24.5 million visits made to offices of physicians in the United States at which the principal diagnosis was otitis media. For children younger than 15 years, otitis media was the most frequent diagnosis in physicians' office practices. Office visits with a principal diagnosis of otitis media increased from 9.9 million visits in 1975 to 24.5 million visits in 1990.[12] The peak incidence occurs in the first 3 years of life. The disease is less common in the school-aged child, adolescents, and adults. Nevertheless, infection of the middle ear may be the cause of fever, significant pain, and impaired hearing in these age groups. In addition, adults suffer from the sequelae of otitis media of childhood: hearing loss, cholesteatoma, adhesive otitis media, and chronic perforation of the tympanic membrane. A comprehensive review of otitis media is included in the text *Otitis Media in Infants and Children*.[13]

Epidemiology

By 3 years of age, more than two thirds of children have had one or more episodes of acute otitis media, and one third have had three or more episodes.[14] The highest incidence of acute otitis media occurs between 6 and 24 months of age. Subsequently, the incidence declines with age except for a limited reversal of the downward trend between 5 and 6 years of age, the time of school entry. Otitis media is infrequent in adults, but the bacteriology and therapy are similar to those in children.[15, 16]

Longitudinal studies have provided information about the characteristics of children who have recurrent and severe episodes of acute otitis media. The vast majority of children have no obvious defect responsible for severe and recurrent otitis media, but a small number have anatomic changes (cleft palate, cleft uvula, submucous cleft), alteration of normal physiologic defenses (patulous eustachian tube), or congenital or acquired immunologic deficiencies. Children with acquired immunodeficiency syndrome have a higher age-specific incidence of otitis media, beginning at 6 months of age, than uninfected children or children who initially were positive for human immunodeficiency virus antibody but who seroreverted.[17]

As is true for most infectious diseases of childhood, acute otitis media occurs more often in males than in females. Correlation of the index child with severe or recurrent acute otitis media in a sibling or parent identifies a likely genetic susceptibility. The age at the time of the first episode of acute otitis media appears to be among the most powerful predictors of recurrent middle ear infections. Breast-feeding for 3 or more months is associated with a decreased risk of acute otitis media in the first year of life.[14] Race and ethnicity provide additional data suggesting a genetic basis for recurrent middle ear infections; Native Americans, Alaskan and Canadian Eskimos, and Australian aborigines have an extraordinary incidence and severity of otitis media.

The role of increased exposure to infectious agents and the importance of environmental pollutants are identified in studies of the incidence of infection in group day care and the effects of passive smoking on children. The introduction of infants into large day care groups increases the incidence of respiratory infections, including otitis media. The day care risk of infection is associated with the number of children in the facility. Almost one episode of respiratory tract infections a month occurs during the first year of life, and acute otitis media is a complication of about one third to one half of the respiratory tract infections.[18] Passive smoking documented by a biochemical marker, the serum nicotine level, increased the incidence of new episodes of otitis media with effusion and the duration of effusion.[19] Kim and colleagues identified an association of invasive pneumococcal disease and otitis media with atmospheric conditions, air pollution, and the isolation of respiratory viruses.[20] The study documented an association between pneumococcal infection and levels of sulfur dioxide as a marker for air pollution.

Pathogenesis

The middle ear is part of a continuous system that includes the nares, nasopharynx, and eustachian tube medially and anteriorly, and the mastoid air cells posteriorly. These structures are lined with a respiratory epithelium that contains ciliated cells, mucus-secreting goblet cells, and cells capable of secreting local immunoglobulins.

Anatomic or physiologic dysfunction of the eustachian tube appears to play a critical role in the development of otitis media. The eustachian tube has at least three physiologic functions with respect to the middle ear: protection of the ear from nasopharyngeal secretions, drainage into the nasopharynx of secretions produced within the middle ear, and ventilation of the middle ear to equilibrate air pressure with that in the external ear canal. When one or more of these functions is compromised, the results may be the development of fluid and infection in the middle ear. Congestion of the mucosa of the eustachian tube may result in obstruction. Secretions that are constantly formed by the mucosa of the middle ear accumulate behind the obstruction, and if a bacterial pathogen is present, a suppurative otitis media may result.

Microbiology

Bacteria

The bacteriology of otitis media has been documented by appropriate cultures of middle ear effusions obtained by needle aspiration. Many studies of the bacteriology of acute otitis media have been performed. The results are remarkably consistent in demonstrating the importance of *S. pneumoniae* and *H. influenzae* in all age groups (Table 50–1).[21, 22]

S. pneumoniae is the most important bacterial cause of otitis media. Relatively few types are responsible for most disease. The most common types in order of decreasing frequencies are 19, 23, 6, 14, 3, and 18.[23–25] All are included in the currently available 23-type pneumococcal polysaccharide vaccine. The greater immunogenicity of protein-conjugated pneumococcal vaccines now undergoing trial in young children should decrease the incidence of pneumococcal otitis media.

Otitis media due to *H. influenzae* is associated with nontypable strains in the vast majority of patients. In approximately 10%, the otitis is due to type B and should be preventable by immunization. Some of these patients appear to be in a very toxic state, and about one quarter have concomitant bacteremia or meningitis.[26] Nontypable strains of *H. influenzae* are a significant cause of otitis media in older children, adolescents, and adults.[15, 16]

TABLE 50–1 Bacterial Pathogens Isolated from Middle Ear Fluid in Children with Acute Otitis Media, 1980–1897*

Microorganism	Mean Percentage of Children with Pathogen
Streptococcus pneumoniae	39
Haemophilus influenzae	27
Streptococcus, group A	3
Staphylococcus aureus	2
Moraxella catarrhalis	10
Miscellaneous bacteria	8
None or nonpathogens	28

*Nine reports from centers in the United States and Canada.
Modified from Bluestone CD, Klein JO. Otitis media, atelectasis, and eustachian tube dysfunction. In: Bluestone CD, Stool SE, eds. Pediatric Otolaryngology. 3rd ed. Philadelphia: WB Saunders; 1996:388–582.

In 12 reports from the United States, Finland, and Canada, *M. catarrhalis* was isolated from a mean of 10% of children with acute otitis media (range 2 to 15%).[21, 27, 28] Before 1970, almost all strains of *M. catarrhalis* were sensitive to penicillin. Today most strains produce β-lactamase and are resistant to penicillin G, ampicillin, and amoxicillin.

Viruses

Virologic and epidemiologic data suggest that viral infection is frequently associated with acute otitis media.[29–31] In a study of children attending a day care program, isolation of viruses from the upper respiratory tract was correlated with a clinical diagnosis of otitis media. Virus outbreaks coincided with epidemics of otitis media. Recent studies identify respiratory viruses[29] or viral antigens[30] in approximately one quarter of middle ear fluids of children with acute otitis media. Respiratory syncytial virus, influenza virus, enteroviruses, and rhinoviruses were the most common viruses found in middle ear fluids. Many patients with virus in middle ear fluid have a mixed viral-bacterial infection. Respiratory signs may be prolonged in children with dual infection.[32, 33]

Mycoplasma, Chlamydia, and Unusual Organisms

Mycoplasma pneumoniae was responsible for hemorrhagic bullous myringitis in a study of nonimmune volunteers inoculated with the organism.[34] However, the middle ear fluid of a large number of patients (771) has been studied, and *M. pneumoniae* was isolated in only one case.[35, 36] Although mycoplasmas do not appear to play a significant role in acute otitis media, some patients with lower respiratory tract disease due to *M. pneumoniae* may have concomitant otitis media.

Chlamydia trachomatis is associated with acute respiratory infections in infants younger than 6 months and is a cause of acute infection of the middle ear in this age group. The organism has been isolated from middle ear fluid of infants with acute infection.[37]

Uncommon forms of otitis include diphtheritic otitis, tuberculous otitis, otogenous tetanus, otitis due to *Mycobacterium chelonae*,[38] and otitis due to *Ascaris lumbricoides* or Wegener's granulomatosis.

Immunology

The middle ear is the site of a secretory immune system similar to those of other areas of the respiratory tract. Local and systemic immune responses occur in patients with acute or chronic otitis media with effusion. In the middle ear, immunologically active antigen interacts with immunocompetent cells in the lamina propria to produce a local immune response. The middle ear effusion that results from acute or chronic infection contains all the major classes of immunoglobulins, complement, cells, immune complexes of antigen and antibody, and various chemical mediators of inflammation. The role of these substances in the course of otitis media is uncertain. The immune response to various antigens may prevent subsequent infection, assist in clearance of fluid during the acute episode, or contribute to the accumulation and persistence of fluid in the middle ear cavity, which becomes the culture medium for the next infection.

Diagnosis and Clinical Course

Acute otitis media is defined by the presence of fluid in the middle ear along with signs or symptoms of acute illness. Signs and symptoms may be specific, such as ear pain, ear drainage, or hearing loss, or may be nonspecific, such as fever, lethargy, or irritability. Vertigo, nystagmus, and tinnitus may occur. Redness of the tympanic membrane is an early sign of otitis media, but erythema alone is not diagnostic of middle ear infection since it may be caused by inflammation of the mucosa throughout the upper respiratory tract.

The presence of fluid in the middle ear is determined by the use of pneumatic otoscopy, a technique that permits an assessment of the mobility of the tympanic membrane. The motion of the tympanic membrane is proportional to the pressure applied by gently squeezing and then releasing the rubber bulb attached to the head of the otoscope. Normal mobility is apparent when positive pressure is applied and the tympanic membrane moves rapidly inward; with release of the bulb and the resulting negative pressure, the membrane moves outward. Fluid or high negative pressure in the middle ear dampens the mobility of the tympanic membrane. Adjunctive techniques are available to confirm the results of otoscopic examinations and assist in the accuracy of diagnosis. Tympanometry uses an electroacoustic impedance bridge to record compliance of the tympanic membrane and middle ear pressure. This technique presents objective evidence of the status of the middle ear and the presence or absence of fluid.[39] Acoustic reflectometry measures sound reflectivity from the middle ear and is able to distinguish an air- or fluid-filled space Spatial-gradient analysis is correlated with the probability of middle ear effusion in children.[40] In addition to a professional model, a consumer model (Becton-Dickinson) is available that permits home monitoring of the development or persistence of middle ear fluid.

Fluid persists in the middle ear for prolonged periods after the onset of acute otitis media even though symptoms usually resolve within a few days after the initiation of antimicrobial therapy. About 70% of children with otitis media have fluid in the middle ear 2 weeks after the onset of disease, 40% still have fluid 1 month after the onset, and 10% still have fluid 3 months after the first signs of middle ear infection.[13]

Patients with middle ear effusion suffer from hearing loss of variable severity. On average, a patient with fluid in the middle ear has a 25-dB (pure-tone average) loss.[41] Since development of speech, language, and cognitive skills is dynamic during infancy when the incidence of acute otitis media is highest, there is concern that any impediment to reception or interpretation of auditory stimuli might have an adverse effect. Recent studies suggest that children with histories of recurrent episodes of acute otitis media score lower in tests of speech, language, and cognitive abilities than do their disease-free peers.[42, 43]

The results of microbiologic studies of middle ear effusions in patients with acute otitis media are so consistent that the choice of antimicrobial agents may be based on knowledge of the bacteriologic characteristics of otitis media acquired from the many investigations rather than the results of cultures from other sites such as the throat or nasopharynx (Table 50–1). If the patient is toxic or has focal infection elsewhere, cultures of samples of the blood and of the focal infection are warranted. Needle aspiration of the middle ear effusion (tympanocentesis) to define the microbiological characteristics of the infection should be considered in selected patients: the patient who is critically ill at the onset, the patient who has not responded to initial antimicrobial therapy in 48 to 72 hours and is toxic, and the patient with altered host defenses (e.g., an immunologic defect, including the newborn infant).

Management

Acute Otitis Media

Antimicrobial Agents. The preferred antimicrobial agent for the patient with otitis media must be active against *S. pneumoniae, H. influenzae*, and *M. catarrhalis*. Group A streptococci and *S. aureus* are infrequent causes of acute otitis media and need not be considered in initial therapeutic decisions. Gram-negative enteric bacilli must be considered when otitis media occurs in the newborn infant, in the patient with a depressed immune response, and in the patient with suppurative complications of chronic otitis media. The antimicrobial agent should achieve concentrations in middle ear fluid above the expected minimal inhibitory concentration of the likely pathogens. Craig and Andes examined the relationship between bacteriologic cure in otitis media and serum and middle ear fluid concentrations for various antimicrobial agents.[44] They found that a bacteriologic cure required the presence of serum concentrations above the minimal inhibitory concentration for at least 70% of the dosing interval.

There are now 16 antimicrobial agents approved by the Food and Drug Administration for acute otitis media. Amoxicillin remains the drug of choice for initial treatment because of its 25-year record of clinical success, acceptability, limited side effects, and relatively low cost. The drug is ineffective against β-lactamase–producing strains of *H. influenzae* and *M. catarrhalis*. The current incidence of ampicillin-resistant *H. influenzae* and *M. catarrhalis* is not high enough to require a change in the initial therapy.

The rationale for the continued use of amoxicillin is as follows. *S. pneumoniae* is responsible for about 40% of cases of acute otitis media. Concentrations of amoxicillin can be achieved in the middle ear fluid sufficient to sterilize all but highly resistant strains. In recent years, less than 10% of pneumococci isolated from the nasopharynx of Boston children are resistant (minimal inhibitory concentrations ≥ 2 μg/ml) (S. I. Pelton, E. D. Barnett, and J. O. Klein, unpublished data), and treatment in about 4% of all children with acute otitis might fail if they are treated with regular doses of amoxicillin (40 mg/kg/day). The recent recommendation of doubling the dose of amoxicillin to 80 mg/kg/day will achieve higher concentrations in middle ear fluid and further reduce the number of children in whom amoxicillin therapy will fail because of resistant pneumococci. *H. influenzae* and *M. catarrhalis* are responsible for about 30 and 10% of acute otitis media cases, respectively. If 30% of the former and 75% of the latter are β-lactamase producing, then 16% of acute otitis media cases are caused by β-lactamase–producing organisms. If 50% improve spontaneously or despite β-lactamase activity, then less than 10% of the failures could be anticipated to be due to failure of amoxicillin to be active against β-lactamase–producing organisms. Although this incidence is not high enough to prompt abandonment of amoxicillin therapy, parents should be alerted to call the physician if a child does not respond to therapy.

Each of the other 15 drugs has documented clinical efficacy for acute otitis media. The drugs include amoxicillin-clavulanate, two sulfa-containing combinations (erythromycin plus sulfisoxazole and trimethoprim-sulfamethoxazole), two macrolides (azithromycin and clarithromycin), nine oral cephalosporins (cephalexin, cefaclor, cefixime, ceftibuten, cefprozil, cefpodoxime, cefuroxime axetil, cefprozil and cefdinir), and one parenteral cephalosporin (ceftriaxone). There is a paucity of data about the efficacy of the drugs in cases of acute otitis media due to resistant strains, and none of the drugs have approval for use in multidrug-resistant pneumococcal infections. All the drugs other than amoxicillin are unaffected by β-lactamase but have varied activity against strains of *H. influenzae*. Opinions vary about the optimal agent for acute otitis media that persists after the use of amoxicillin. An expert panel convened by the Centers for Disease Control and Prevention suggested regimens including an increased dosage schedule of amoxicillin clavulanate (90 mg/kg/day in two doses), cefuroxime axetil, or intramuscular ceftriaxone. For some children, the use of tympanocentesis to identify the bacterial pathogen and the susceptibility pattern may be necessary for choosing the most effective drug.[45]

Some children with acute otitis media due to a bacterial pathogen improve without the use of antimicrobial agents.[46, 47] Howie and Ploussard performed dual aspirates of middle ear fluid in children with acute otitis media 2 to 7 days apart with placebo given instead of an antibacterial drug: 19% of middle ear fluids infected initially with pneumococci became sterile; 48% of middle ear fluids infected initially with *H. influenzae* became sterile.[48] The discrepancy between the proportion of infections sterilized with the two bacterial species indicates that a simple mechanical effect (drainage of the infected fluid via a patent eustachian tube or a perforated tympanic membrane) was unlikely to be responsible for the microbiologic effect. A host mechanism (likely based on humoral or cellular immunity) acted preferentially to rid the ear of *H. influenzae* more frequently than of *S. pneumoniae*. The microbiologic results indicating that approximately one quarter of children have acute otitis media due to a viral pathogen and that some of the episodes of bacterial otitis media resolve without antibacterial drugs prompted some European physicians to withhold antibiotic therapy from children with ear infections.[49, 50] Because physicians cannot distinguish children who may benefit from antimicrobial therapy from those who respond without treatment, representatives of the Centers for Disease Control and Prevention and the American Academy of Pediatrics concluded that physicians should continue to treat all patients with a diagnosis of acute otitis media.[51]

With appropriate antimicrobial therapy, most children with acute otitis media are significantly improved within 48 to 72 hours. If there is no improvement, the patient should be reexamined. Toxicity with persistent or recurrent fever or otalgia should prompt reevaluation of the patient. The child may have developed a new focus of infection or have received inadequate therapy.

Decongestants, Antihistamines, and Corticosteroids. Nasal and oral decongestants, administered either alone or in combination with an antihistamine, are used extensively for the treatment of otitis media with effusion. The use of the drugs is based on the consideration that they reduce congestion of the respiratory mucosa and relieve the obstruction of the eustachian tube that results from inflammation caused by respiratory infection. The results of clinical trials, however, indicate no significant evidence of efficacy of any of these preparations, used alone or in combination, for relief of signs of disease or a decrease in the time spent with middle ear effusion.[52, 53] Although there are data suggesting efficacy of systemic corticosteroid therapy for the treatment of persistent middle ear effusion, particularly when combined with an antibiotic,[54] there are no studies of the use of corticosteroids alone or in combination with antimicrobial agents for amelioration or prevention of acute otitis media.

Chronic Otitis Media

The term *chronic otitis media* includes recurrent episodes of acute infection and a prolonged duration of middle ear effusion usually resulting from a previous episode of acute infection. For the prevention of recurrent episodes of acute otitis media, management includes the consideration of chemoprophylaxis (the use of antimicrobial agents) and immunoprophylaxis (the use of vaccines or immunoglobulin). For the management of persistent middle ear effusions, three surgical methods are considered: myringotomy, adenoidectomy, and the placement of tympanostomy tubes.

Chemoprophylaxis has been shown to be of value for the prevention of acute illness in children who have suffered from recurrences of middle ear infections. A reduction of episodes of acute febrile illnesses due to otitis media occurred.[55–57] On the basis of available information,[48] a protocol has been suggested that uses a once-a-day regimen of amoxicillin or sulfisoxazole during winter and spring, the periods of high incidence of infections of the respiratory tract. Children should be considered for prophylaxis if they have had two episodes of acute otitis media in the first 6 months of life or, in older children, three episodes in 6 months or four episodes in 1 year. Amoxicillin, 20 mg/kg, or sulfisoxazole, 50 mg/kg, may be administered once a day. Chemoprophylaxis may suppress symptoms of otitis media, but middle ear effusion may persist (though without apparent symptoms). The physician who chooses to use chemoprophylaxis to prevent acute recurrent disease must examine the patient at approximately 1-month intervals for middle ear effusion. The use of a modified course of antimicrobial drug may promote the selection of resistant bacteria in the nasopharynx and as the likely pathogens of episodes of acute otitis media. Because of concerns for the development of resistance, the physician should be certain that the episodes of acute otitis media are well documented and that the chemoprophylaxis is warranted.[51]

The concerns about antibiotic resistance have lead to innovative approaches to chemoprophylaxis including the use of oligosaccharides to prevent adhesion of bacterial pathogens to respiratory mucosa and the use of xylitol to inhibit bacterial colonization. Carbohydrates or homologues have been suggested as materials that might interfere with bacterial attachment to respiratory mucosa. Oligosaccharides interfere with the establishment and progression of experimental pneumococcal pneumonia[58] and human studies are now in progress to determine their efficacy when administered as a nasal spray for the prevention of acute otitis media. Xylitol is a polyol sugar alcohol produced from birch trees, strawberries, and other fruits that is effective in reducing dental caries, presumably because it inhibits the growth of *Streptococcus mutans*. Uhari and colleagues demonstrated in vitro reduction of growth of *S. pneumoniae* and a reduction in the number of episodes of acute otitis media in children who used daily xylitol chewing gum contrasted with those who used sucrose chewing gum.[59]

Pneumococcal vaccines have been evaluated for the prevention of recurrences of acute otitis media in children.[60–62] As in previous studies, children younger than 2 years had unsatisfactory responses to single-dose regimens. The vaccine reduced the number of episodes of acute otitis media due to types of *S. pneumoniae* present in the vaccine, but the reduction was not sufficient to alter the experience of the children with middle ear infections. The basis for failure of the vaccine was due to the poor immunologic response to the polysaccharide antigens in the young infants enrolled in the trials. The data suggested that the vaccine was likely to be more effective in children older than 2 years.[62] Vaccines composed of pneumococcal capsular polysaccharides conjugated to proteins increased immunogenicity in young infants and are currently undergoing clinical evaluation.

Because of the importance of respiratory viruses in the pathogenesis of acute otitis media, viral vaccines could be of preventive value. Influenza virus vaccine has been documented to decrease the incidence of acute otitis media in children in day care in Finland[63] and North Carolina.[64]

Surgical management of the persistent effusion of the middle ear includes the use of myringotomy, adenoidectomy, and the placement of tympanostomy tubes. Myringotomy, or incision of the tympanic membrane, is a method of draining middle ear fluid. Before the introduction of antimicrobial agents, myringotomy was the major method of managing suppurative otitis media. Today, the use of myringotomy is limited to the relief of intractable ear pain, hastening resolution of mastoid infection, and drainage of persistent middle ear effusion that is unresponsive to medical therapy.

Enlarged adenoids may obstruct the orifice of the eustachian tube in the posterior portion of the nasopharynx and interfere with adequate ventilation and drainage of the middle ear. Studies of the use of adenoidectomy in children with prolonged effusions in the middle

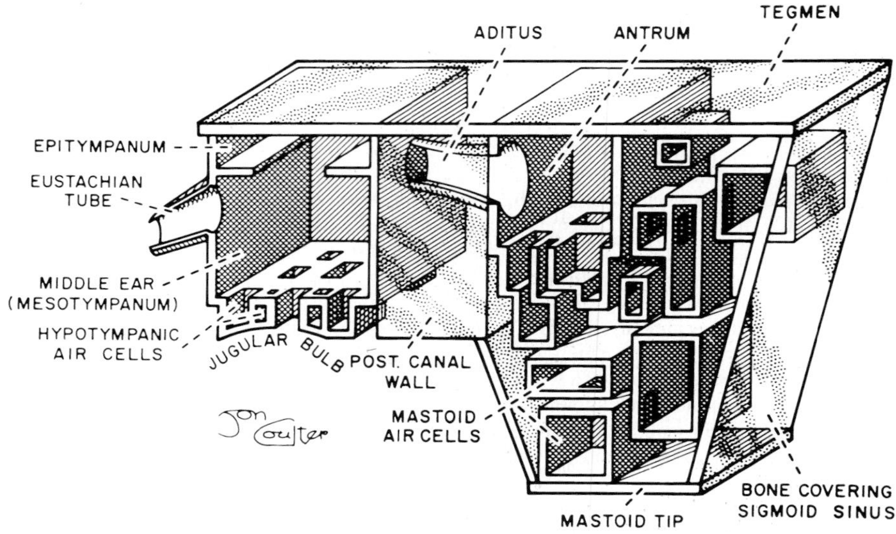

FIGURE 50–1. Diagrammatic representation of the anatomy of the middle and mastoid air cell system showing the narrow connection (aditus and antrum) between the two.

ear identify in selected children a beneficial effect in reducing the time spent with effusion.[65, 66]

Tympanostomy tubes resemble small collar buttons. They are placed through an incision in the tympanic membrane to provide drainage of fluid and ventilation of the middle ear. The placement of these tubes is now one of the most common surgical procedures in children. The criteria for the placement of tubes include persistent middle ear effusions unresponsive to adequate medical treatment over a period of 3 months and persistent negative pressure. Hearing improves dramatically after placement of the ventilating tubes. The tubes have also been of value in patients who have difficulty maintaining ambient pressure in the middle ear such as would occur due to barotrauma in airline personnel. The liabilities of the placement of tubes include those of anesthesia associated with the procedure, persistent perforation, scarring of the tympanic membrane, the development of cholesteatoma, and otitis media caused by swimming with ventilating tubes in place, but these occur infrequently.

MASTOIDITIS

The proximity of the mastoid to the middle ear cleft suggests that most cases of suppurative otitis media are associated with inflammation of the mastoid air cells (Fig. 50–1). The incidence of clinically significant mastoiditis, however, is low since the introduction of antimicrobial agents. Nevertheless, acute and chronic disease still occur and may be responsible for significant morbidity and life-threatening disease.

Pathogenesis

At birth, the mastoid consists of a single cell, the antrum, connected to the middle ear by a small channel. Pneumatization of the mastoid bone takes place soon after birth and is extensive by 2 years of age. The clinical importance of the mastoid is related to contiguous structures including the posterior cranial fossa, the middle cranial fossa, the sigmoid and lateral sinuses, the canal of the facial nerve, the semicircular canals, and the petrous tip of the temporal bone. The mastoid air cells are lined with modified respiratory mucosa, and all are connected with the antrum.

Infection in the mastoid follows middle ear infection. Initially, there is hyperemia and edema of the mucosal lining of the air cells. Serous, then purulent exudate collects in the cells. Necrosis of bone due to pressure of the purulent exudate on the thin bony septa follows. Coalescence of pus in contiguous areas results in abscess cavities.

Clinical Manifestations

Acute mastoiditis is usually accompanied by acute infection in the middle ear. During early stages, the signs are those of acute otitis media with hearing loss, otalgia, and fever. Subsequently, swelling, redness, and tenderness are present over the mastoid bone. The pinna is displaced outward and downward. A purulent discharge may emerge through a perforation in the tympanic membrane.

Chronic otitis media with mastoiditis can erode through the roof of the antrum, causing temporal lobe abscess, or extend posteriorly, causing septic thrombosis of the lateral sinus.

Diagnosis

Radiographs of the mastoid area may show a loss of sharpness of the shadows of cellular walls due to demineralization of bony septa and cloudiness of areas of pneumatization due to inflammatory swelling of the air cells. Computed tomography is very helpful in delineating the extent of disease.

Cultures for bacteria from ear drainage fluid must be taken with care to distinguish fresh drainage fluid from material in the external canal. The canal must be cleaned and fresh pus obtained as it exudes from the tympanic membrane. If the tympanic membrane is not perforated, tympanocentesis should be performed to obtain material from the middle ear.

Management

The antimicrobial drugs of choice for acute infection are similar to those for acute otitis media: antibiotics with activity against *S. pneumoniae* and *H. influenzae*. If the disease in the mastoid has had a prolonged course, coverage for *S. aureus* and gram-negative enteric bacilli may be considered for initial therapy until the results of cultures become available.

A mastoidectomy is performed when an abscess has formed in the mastoid bone. The procedure should be performed at a time when antimicrobial agents have controlled sepsis.

REFERENCES

1. Senturia BH, Marcus MD, Lucente FE. Diseases of the External Ear. An Otologic Dermatologic Manual. 2nd ed. New York: Grune & Stratton; 1980.
2. Hirsch BE. Disease of the external ear. In: Bluestone CD, Stool SE, eds. Pediatric Otolaryngology. 3rd ed. Philadelphia: WB Saunders; 1996:378–387.

3. Rubin J, Yu VL. Malignant external otitis: Insights into pathogenesis, clinical manifestations, diagnosis, and therapy. Am J Med. 1988;85:391–398.
4. Riding KH, Bluestone CD, Michaels RH, et al. Microbiology of recurrent and chronic otitis media with effusion. J Pediatr. 1978;93:739–743.
5. Pelton SI, Teele DW, Shurin PA, et al. Disparate cultures of middle ear fluids. Am J Dis Child. 1980;134:951–953.
6. Brook I, Schwartz R. Anaerobic bacteria in acute otitis media. Acta Otolaryngol. 1981;91:111–114.
7. Centers for Disease Control and Prevention. Otitis due to *Pseudomonas aeruginosa* serotype 0:10 associated with mobile redwood hot tub systems—North Carolina. MMWR Morb Mortal Wkly Rep. 1982;31:541–542.
8. Doroghazi RM, Nadol JB, Hyslop NE, et al. Invasive external otitis. Am J Med. 1981;71:603–613.
9. Johnson MP, Ramphal R. Malignant external otitis: Report on therapy with ceftazidime and review of therapy and prognosis. Rev Infect Dis. 1990;12:173–180.
10. Rapoport Y, Shalit I, Redianu C, Himmelfarb MZ. Oral ofloxacin therapy for invasive external otitis. Ann Otol Rhinol Laryngol. 1991;100:632–637.
11. Phillips P, Bryce G, Shepherd J. Invasive external otitis caused by *Aspergillus*. Rev Infect Dis. 1990;12:277–281.
12. Schappert SM. Office visits for otitis media: United States, 1975–90. In: Vital and Health Statistics of the Centers for Disease Control/National Centers for Health Statistics. Atlanta: Centers for Disease Control and Prevention, 1992;214:3–18.
13. Bluestone CD, Klein JO, eds. Otitis Media in Infants and Children. 2nd ed. Philadelphia: WB Saunders; 1995.
14. Teele DW, Klein JO, Rosner B. Epidemiology of otitis media during the first seven years of life in children in greater Boston: A prospective, cohort study. J Infect Dis. 1989;160:83–94.
15. Celin S, Bluestone C, Stephenson J, et al. Bacteriology of acute otitis media in adults. JAMA. 1991;266:2249–2252.
16. Schwartz LE, Brown RB. Purulent otitis media in adults. Arch Intern Med. 1992;152:2301–2304.
17. Barnett ED, Klein JO, Pelton SI, Luginbuhl LM. Otitis media in children born to human immunodeficiency virus–infected mothers. Pediatr Infect Dis J. 1992;11: 360–364.
18. Schwartz B, Giebink GS, Henderson GW, et al. Respiratory infections in day care. Pediatrics. 1994;94:1018–1020.
19. Etzel RA, Pattishall EN, Haley NJ, et al. Passive smoking and middle ear effusion among children in day care. Pediatrics. 1992;90:228–232.
20. Kim PE, Musher DM, Glezen WP, et al. Association of invasive pneumococcal disease with season, atmospheric condition, air pollution, and the isolation of respiratory viruses. Clin Infect Dis. 1996;22:100–106.
21. Bluestone CD, Klein JO. Otitis media, atelectasis, and eustachian tube dysfunction. In: Bluestone CD, Stool SE, eds. Pediatric Otolaryngology. 3rd ed. Philadelphia: WB Saunders; 1996;388–582.
22. Del Baccaro MA, Mendelman PM, Inglis AF, et al. Bacteriology of acute otitis media: A new perspective. J Pediatr. 1992;120:81–84.
23. Kamme C, Ageberg M, Lundgren K. Distribution of *Diplococcus pneumoniae* types in acute otitis media in children and influence of the types on the clinical course in penicillin V therapy. Scand J Infect Dis. 1970;2:183–190.
24. Austrian R, Howie VM, Ploussard JH. The bacteriology of pneumococcal otitis media. Johns Hopkins Med J. 1977;141:104–111.
25. Gray BM, Converse GM, Dillion HC. Serotypes of *Streptococcus pneumoniae* causing disease. J Infect Dis. 1979;140:979–983.
26. Harding AL, Anderson P, Howie VM, et al. *Haemophilus influenzae* isolated from children with otitis media. In: Sell SHW, Karzon DT,eds. *Haemophilus influenza*. Nashville: Vanderbilt University Press; 1973:21.
27. Van Hare GF, Shurin PA, Marchant CD, et al. Acute otitis media caused by *Branhamella catarrhalis*: Biology and therapy. Rev Infect Dis. 1987;9:16–27.
28. Kovatch AL, Wald ER, Michaels RH. β-Lactamase-producing *Branhamella catarrhalis* causing otitis media in children. J Pediatr. 1983;102:261–264.
29. Chonmaitree T, Howie VM, Truant AL. Presence of respiratory viruses in middle ear fluids and nasal wash specimens from children with acute otitis media. Pediatrics. 1986;77:698–702.
30. Klein BS, Dallette ER, Volken RH. The role of respiratory syncytial virus and other viral pathogens in acute otitis media. J Pediatr. 1982;101:16–20.
31. Henderson FW, Collier AM, Sanyal MA, et al. A longitudinal study of respiratory viruses and bacteria in the etiology of acute otitis media with effusion. N Engl J Med. 1982;306:1377.
32. Arola M, Ziegler T, Ruuskanen O. Respiratory virus infection as a cause of prolonged symptoms in acute otitis media. J Pediatr. 1990;116:697–701.
33. Chonmaitree T, Owen MJ, Patel JA, et al. Effect of viral respiratory tract infection on outcome of acute otitis media. J Pediatr. 1992;120:856–862.
34. Rifkind DR, Chanock RM, Kravetz H, et al. Ear involvement (myringitis) and primary atypical pneumonia following inoculation of volunteers with Eaton agent. Am Rev Respir Dis. 1962;85:479–489.
35. Klein JO, Teele DW. Isolation of viruses and mycoplasma from middle ear effusions: A review. Ann Otol Rhinol Laryngol. 1976;85:140–144.
36. Sobeslavsky O, Syrucek L, Bruckoya M, et al. The etiological role of *Mycoplasma pneumoniae* in otitis media in children. Pediatrics. 1965;35:652–657.
37. Tipple MA, Beem MO, Saxon EM. Clinical characteristics of the afebrile pneumonia associated with *Chlamydia trachomatis* infection in infants less than 6 months of age. Pediatrics. 1979;63:192–197.
38. Lowry PW, Jarvis WR, Oberle AD, et al. *Mycobacterium chelonae* causing otitis media in an ear-nose-and-throat practice. N Engl J Med. 1988;391:978–982.
39. Brookhouser PE. Use of tympanometry in office practice for diagnosis otitis media. Pediatr Infect Dis J. 1998;17:544–551.
40. Kimball S. Acoustic reflectometry: Spectral gradient analysis for improved detection of middle ear effusion in children. Pediatr Infect Dis J. 1998;17:522–555.
41. Fria TJ, Cantekin EI, Eichler JA. Hearing acuity of children with effusion. Arch Otolaryngol. 1985;111:10–16.
42. Holm VA, Kunze LH. Effects of chronic otitis media on language and speech development. Pediatrics. 1969;43:833–839.
43. Teele DW, Klein JO, Chase C, et al. Otitis media in infancy and intellectual ability, school achievement, speech and language at age 7 years. J Infect Dis. 1990;162:685–694.
44. Craig WA, Andes D. Pharmacokinetics and pharmacodynamics of antibiotics in otitis media. Pediatr Infect Dis J. 1996;15:255–259.
45. Dowell SF, Butler J, Giebink FS, et al. Acute otitis media: Management and surveillance in an era of pneumococcal resistance—a report from the drug-resistant *Streptococcus pneumoniae* therapeutic working group. Pediatr Infect Dis J. 1999;18:1–9.
46. Kaleida PH, Casselbrant ML, Rockette HE, et al. Amoxicillin or myringotomy or both for acute otitis media: Results of a randomized clinical trial. Pediatrics. 1991;87:466–474.
47. Marchant CD, Carlin SA, Johnson CE, Shurin PA. Measuring the comparative efficacy of antibacterial agents for acute otitis media: The "Pollyanna phenomenon." J Pediatr. 1992;120:72–77.
48. Howie VM, Ploussard JH. The "in-vivo sensitivity test": Bacteriology of middle ear exudate during antimicrobial therapy in otitis media. Pediatrics. 1969;44:940–944.
49. Van Buchem FL, Dunk JH, van't Hof MA. Therapy of acute otitis media: Myringotomy, antibiotics or neither? A double-blind study in children. Lancet. 1981:2:883–887.
50. Browning GG. Childhood otalgia: Acute otitis media. BMJ. 1990;300:1005–1007.
51. Dowell SF, Marcy SM, Phillips WR, et al. Otitis media: Principles of judicious use of antimicrobial agents. Pediatrics. 1998;101:165–171.
52. Cantekin EI, Mandel EM, Bluestone CD. Lack of efficacy of a decongestant-antihistamine combination for otitis media with effusion ("secretory" otitis media) in children. N Engl J Med. 1983;308:297–301.
53. Bluestone CD, Connell JT, Doyle WJ, et al. Symposium: Questioning the efficacy and safety of antihistamines in the treatment of upper respiratory infection. Pediatr Infect Dis J. 1988;7:15–42.
54. Berman S. Medical management of children with otitis media with effusion. The Report on Pediatric Infectious Diseases. New York: Churchill Livingstone; 1993: 37–38.
55. Perrin JM, Charney E, MacWhinney JB, et al. Sulfisoxazole as chemoprophylaxis for recurrent otitis media: A double-blind crossover study in pediatric practice. N Engl J Med. 1974;291:664–667.
56. Maynard JE, Fleshman JK, Tschopp CF. Otitis media in Alaskan Eskimo children: Prospective evaluation of chemoprophylaxis. JAMA. 1972;219:597–599.
57. Klein JO, Bluestone CD. Acute otitis media: Management of pediatric infectious diseases in office practice. Pediatr Infect Dis. 1982;1:66–73.
58. Idänpään-Heikkilä I, Simon PM, Zopf D, et al. Oligosaccharides interfere with the establishment and progression of experimental pneumococcal pneumonia. J Infect Dis. 1997;176:704–712.
59. Uhari M, Kontiokari T, Koskela M, Niemelä M. Xylitol chewing gum in prevention of acute otitis media: Double blind randomized trail. BMJ. 1996;313:1180–1184.
60. Teele DW, Klein JO, the Greater Boston Collaborative Study Group. Use of pneumococcal vaccine for prevention of recurrent acute otitis media in infants in Boston. Rev Infect Dis. 1981;3(Suppl):S113–118.
61. Sloyer JL, Ploussard JH, Howie VM. Efficacy of pneumococcal polysaccharide vaccine in preventing acute otitis media in infants in Huntsville, Alabama. Rev Infect Dis. 1981;3(Suppl):119.
62. Makela PH, Leinonen M, Pukander J, et al. A study of the pneumococcal vaccine in prevention of clinically acute attacks of recurrent otitis media. Rev Infect Dis. 1981;3(Suppl):124.
63. Heikkinen T, Ruuskanen O, Waris M, et al. Influenza vaccination in the prevention of acute otitis media in children. Am J Dis Child. 1991;145:445–448.
64. Clements DA, Langdon L, Bland C, et al. Influenza A vaccine decreases the incidence of otitis media in 6 to 30 month old children in day care. Arch Pediatr Adolesc Med. 1995;149:1113–1117.
65. Paradise JL, Bluestone CD, Rogers KD, et al. Efficacy of adenoidectomy in recurrent otitis media: Historical overview and preliminary results from a randomized, controlled trial. Ann Otol Rhinol Laryngol. 1980;89:319–321.
66. Gates GA, Avery CA, Prihoda TJ, et al. Effectiveness of adenoidectomy and tympanostomy tubes in the treatment of chronic otitis media with effusion. N Engl J Med. 1987;317:1444–1451.

Chapter 51

Sinusitis

JACK M. GWALTNEY, JR.

ACUTE

Classification

Sinusitis is a disease that usually results from an infection of one or more of the paranasal sinuses. Acute sinusitis can be classified into various categories on the basis of several characteristics including its occurrence in the community or hospital setting; the immune status of the patient; its infectious or noninfectious cause; and its viral, bacterial, or fungal cause (Table 51–1). Recognizing these categories and using precise terminology are of importance for understanding the pathogenesis and clinical expression of the disease and for optimizing approaches to diagnosis and treatment.

Diagnostic Challenges

Managing acute community-acquired sinusitis is a continuing challenge for physicians because of the difficulty of making an etiologic diagnosis with accuracy and evaluating the effectiveness of treatment with precision. These problems would not exist if the paranasal sinuses were accessible to direct examination and to noninvasive sampling for microbial culture. Because they are not, for diagnosis, physicians have to rely on clinical findings that are either insensitive or nonspecific.[1] It is now recognized that sinus disease is an inherent part of the common cold syndrome itself, and that a high proportion of patients with colds have sinus cavity disease.[2] Thus, the common cold is in reality a viral rhinosinusitis (VRS), not simply a rhinitis as traditionally held. Not appreciating this has led to confusion, because historically the term *acute sinusitis* has been used to identify acute community-acquired bacterial sinusitis (ACABS). Undoubtedly, this term has often been misapplied to cases with a viral or a combined viral-bacterial cause. Without the benefit of sinus puncture, these distinctions cannot be made with accuracy.

In cases of combined viral-bacterial infection, the clinical features of the illness reflect its dual nature. The viral component contributes to the overall severity and duration of the illness and, thus, complicates the diagnosis and confounds the assessment of antimicrobial effectiveness. Likewise, cases of pure VRS that are misdiagnosed as acute bacterial sinusitis are a cause of confusion in patient management and contaminate patient samples in clinical trials of antimicrobial therapy in which sinus aspirate culture is not used for diagnosis.

TABLE 51–1 Classification of Acute Sinusitis

Patient with Normal Immunity
Infectious
Community-Acquired
Viral
Viral-bacterial
Bacterial
Fungal (noninvasive)
Nonallergic
Allergic
Fungus ball
Nosocomial
Bacterial
Fungal
Noninfectious
Allergic
Toxic
Immunocompromised Patient
Viral
Bacterial
Fungal (invasive)

Anatomy and Physiology

Paranasal pneumaticity, the antorbital cavity, originated in animals somewhat earlier than the common ancestor of the dinosaurs.[3] A similar structure, the maxillary sinus, arose in the evolutionary line leading to humans. The ethmoid, frontal, and sphenoid sinuses are of more recent origin and have been described as characteristic of conventional mammals.[4] The function of the paranasal sinuses remains somewhat in doubt. It has been proposed that these structures reduce the bony mass and weight of the skull, participate in warming and humidification of inspired air, and add resonance to the voice.

The maxillary sinus has a pyramidal shape, with the base of the pyramid formed by the lateral wall of the nasal cavity, and the apex extending toward the zygomatic process (Fig. 51–1). In the adult, the maxillary sinus cavity has a volume of 15 to 30 ml. The sinus is lined with ciliated pseudostratified epithelium and is covered with a mucous blanket. The epithelium is well supplied with goblet cells (Table 51–2).[5,6] In contrast, seromucous gland densities in the sinus cavity are low compared with those in the nasal passages.[7]

The maxillary ostium is located on the highest part of the medial wall of the sinus cavity (see Fig. 51–1). It is connected to the nasal cavity by a small tubular passage, the infundibulum, which is encased in bone and lies directly under the lamina papyracea of the orbit. The infundibulum leads to the hiatus semilunaris of the middle meatus, which is posterolateral to the uncinate process in a shielded location. The anterior ethmoid and frontal sinuses also empty into the middle meatus. This area and the region of the anterior ethmoid are described together as the ostiomeatal complex.

The infundibulum is approximately 6 mm in length and has an average diameter of 3 mm, which is of adequate size to drain 30 ml (the maxillary sinus volume) of water by gravity in approximately

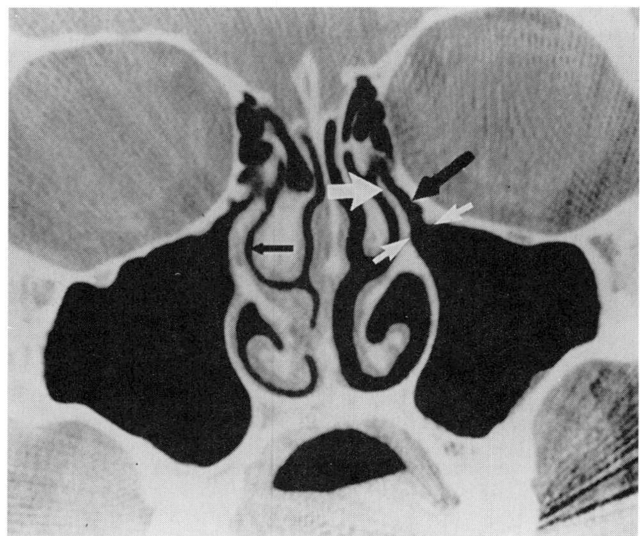

FIGURE 51–1. Selected features of the anatomy of the drainage system of the maxillary sinus shown on computed tomography scan. The ostium is located between the two *small white arrows.* The ostium opens into a tubular structure, the infundibulum, shown by the *large black arrow.* The *large white arrow* indicates the upper part of the uncinate process, which forms the inferior portion of the infundibulum. The infundibulum empties into the middle meatus. The *small black arrow* indicates the contralateral middle meatus, which is narrowed as a result of turbinal distention from the normal nasal cycle.

TABLE 51–2 Density (mm²) of Mucus-Producing Structures in the Nasal Passages and Paranasal Sinuses

	Goblet Cells*	Seromucous Glands†
Nasal passages	5700–11,000	8
Sinuses		
Maxillary	9700	0.2
Ethmoid	6500	0.5
Frontal	5900	0.08
Sphenoid	6200	0.05

*Data from Morgensen C, Tos M. Density of goblet cells in the normal adult human nasal septum. Anat Anz. 1977;141:237.
†Data from Morgensen C, Tos M. Quantitative histology of the maxillary sinus. Rhinology. 1977;55:129; and Morgensen C, Tos M. Quantitative histology of the normal sphenoid sinus. Rhinology. 1978;56:203.

11 seconds. Mucus and other fluids produced in the maxillary sinus cavity are transported by ciliary action in a spiral direction up to and through the infundibulum and delivered into the hiatus semilunaris of the middle meatus.[8, 9] Mucociliary transit times of 4.6 to 12.3 mm/minute have been measured in the nose[10] and are presumably similar in the sinus. The mucous blanket changes two to three times each hour,[11] and normally, mucus does not accumulate in the sinus cavity.

In 10 to 30% of adults, the maxillary sinus cavity is connected to the nasal passage by one or more accessory ostia that are located inferiorly to the infundibulum in the area of the anterior and posterior nasal fontanelles. The fontanelles are areas of very thin bone or membrane located in the lateral nasal wall at the level of the middle meatus and lying anteriorly and posteriorly to the uncinate process. Accessory ostia are created when they rupture.

The paranasal sinuses, although directly connected to the nasal passages, which are colonized with bacteria,[12] are themselves sterile under normal conditions.[13–16] Sterility is maintained in the sinus by mechanisms that are not fully understood but are believed to include mucociliary clearance, the immune system, and possibly antibacterial concentrations of nitric oxide gas in the sinus cavity.[17]

Epidemiology

In the United States, the incidence of VRS in children is six to eight and in adults two to three episodes per person per year.[18] VRS rates follow a well-established seasonal pattern with annual epidemics in the fall, winter, and spring and periods of relative inactivity during the summer. The periods of high prevalence for rhinovirus are early fall and late spring and for coronavirus, respiratory syncytial virus, and influenza, winter and early spring. A small proportion of VRS episodes are, in turn, complicated by an acute bacterial infection of the sinus. This has been reported to occur in 0.5 to 2% of cases.[19, 20] The seasonal trends in the incidence of presumed bacterial sinusitis have been shown to correlate with those of VRS.[21] In addition to VRS-related cases, ACABS occurs throughout the year associated with allergy, swimming, and nasal obstruction due to polyps, foreign bodies, and tumors. Other less common risk factors are immune deficiencies such as agammaglobulinemia and acquired immunodeficiency syndrome; abnormalities of white cell function as found in chronic granulomatous disease; structural defects, especially cleft palate; and disorders of mucociliary clearance including cilial dysfunction and cystic fibrosis.

Based on the epidemiologic findings described previously, approximately 1 billion cases of VRS can be expected to occur annually in the United States (260 million people [adults and children] × 4 acute respiratory illnesses = 1 billion cases or more of VRS annually), and these, in turn, can be expected to be complicated by 20 million cases of ACABS, assuming a 2% complication rate. Data from the National Ambulatory Medical Care Survey for 1991 show 11.57 million physician-patient contacts for acute upper respiratory illness and 2 million patient visits per year for presumed acute bacterial sinusitis.[22] Thus, in the United States, an estimated 1 in 100 VRS patients and 1 in 10 ACABS patients seek physician care for their illness.

Pathogenesis

Viral. A central feature of rhinovirus pathogenicity is the virus's ability to evade the host's protective defenses in the upper airway. The vulnerability of the nose to rhinovirus is shown by the fact that intranasal inoculation of virus in nonimmune volunteers routinely leads to a 90% or greater infection rate.[23] After infection, however, only three quarters of persons develop symptoms of a cold, the rest having an inapparent infection. Viral deposition in the nose is followed by transport to the posterior nasopharynx[24] and attachment to the rhinovirus receptor intercellular adhesion molecule 1 (ICAM-1).[25] In posterior pharyngeal biopsies, ICAM-1 has been located on M (membranous) cells present in the adenoid crypts but not on adjacent ciliated epithelial cells.[26, 27] Nucleic acid probe studies have shown only sparse and widely scattered foci of rhinovirus infection in biopsies of nasal turbinates of experimentally infected volunteers.[28] Infection leads to the activation of several inflammatory pathways and of the parasympathetic nervous system,[29] causing engorgement of the capacitance vessels in the venous erectile tissue of the nasal turbinates, intercellular leakage of plasma into the nose and presumably sinuses, discharge of seromucous glands and goblet cells, and stimulation of pain nerve and sneeze and cough reflexes.

In one study, sinus cavity abnormalities occurred in 87% of patients with early natural colds and included all the different sinuses (Table 51–3).[2] The presence of air bubbles in the material seen on computed tomography (CT) and the irregular distribution of the material on the walls of the sinus suggest that the exudate that is adherent to the floor, sides, and, in some cases, ceiling of the sinus cavity is highly viscous (Fig. 51–2). The material probably consists of excess amounts of goblet cell mucus and possibly plasma. The infundibulum was occluded in 77% of patients, and the ostiomeatal complex was also frequently congested. Also, observations from paired sinus CT scans in patients with VRS showed a failure of the cilia to move deposits of the material toward the ostium over a period of hours (Fig. 51–3).[30] Thus, acute sinus disease appears to be due to malfunction of mucociliary clearance as a result of increased amounts of viscous exudate as much as to infundibular occlusion. Viruses have been recovered from sinus cavity aspirates taken from patients with acute community-acquired sinusitis,[31] but it is not clear if viral invasion of the cavity is necessary to cause the disease. The erratic distribution of the abnormalities seen in different sinuses of the same patient seems more compatible with random viral invasion of a sinus than with a response to generalized activation of inflammatory mediators in the nasal passage.[2, 30]

Bacterial. The nasal passages and nasopharynx are colonized with the same bacterial species that cause ACABS,[12] and, undoubtedly, the bacteria in these areas serve as the reservoir for this infection. Sneezing, coughing, and nose blowing may create pressure differentials that deposit these bacteria into the sinuses. In a rabbit model, the introduction of *Streptococcus pneumoniae* or *Haemophilus in-*

TABLE 51–3 Frequency of Sinus Computed Tomographic Scan Abnormalities in Adults with Early Common Colds

	Percentage
Occlusion of infundibulum	77
Abnormality of sinus cavity	
Maxillary	87
Ethmoid	65
Frontal	32
Sphenoid	39

*Data from Gwaltney JM Jr, Phillips CD, Miller RD, Riker DK. Computed tomographic study of the common cold. N Engl J Med. 1994;330:25–30.

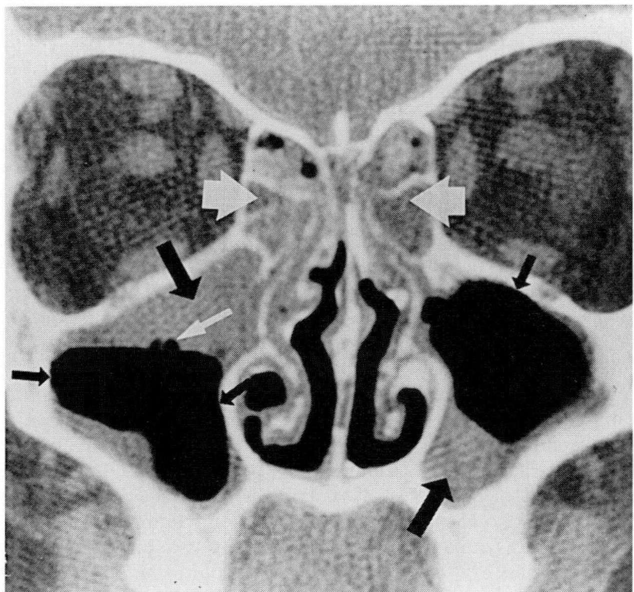

FIGURE 51–2. Sinus computed tomography scan from an adult with a common cold of 4 days' duration shows abnormalities of the roof and floor of the maxillary sinuses *(large black arrows)*. Gaseous bubbles in the material *(small white arrow)* and its irregular distribution along the walls of the sinus cavity suggest that it is thick exudate adherent to the sinus wall and not mucosal swelling. The *small black arrows* show portions of the air-bone interfaces of the sinus wall, which are normal. The uneven distribution of the abnormalities is not compatible with mucosal swelling, which would be expected to be more uniform. Bilateral disease of the ethmoid sinuses is also present *(large white arrows)*.

fluenzae into an acutely obstructed maxillary sinus led to infection and disease, whereas obstruction of the sinus ostium without bacterial instillation did not.[32, 33]

Once bacteria are deposited into the cavity of an obstructed sinus, growth conditions are favorable, as indicated by the high titers attained, which have been measured in sinus aspirates at concentrations of up to 10^7 colony-forming units per milliliter.[14] Cases of ACABS were also associated with a leukocytosis of 10,000 or more white blood cells per millimeter^3 in sinus aspirates. However, granulocyte phagocytosis may be impaired by the reduced oxygen tension present in an obstructed sinus.

In experimental sinus infections in rabbits, marked destruction of ciliated epithelial cells started on day 2 and day 4 (*Strep. pneumoniae*) and day 4 (*H. influenzae*).[33] By the fourth day, there was a 70 to 80% reduction in viable ciliated cells, and by the fifth day, the sinus was completely filled with a viscous material described as "mucopus." At this point, reversing the process involves more than simply relieving ostial obstruction. Regeneration of new ciliated epithelium is necessary to remove the considerable debris and bacteria that accumulate. Also, squamous cell metaplasia and increased numbers of goblet cells were observed in this model.[34, 35]

In humans, there is also evidence that acute bacterial sinusitis is a process of sufficient severity to require several weeks to heal. Studies using serial sinus imaging have shown resolving cavitary abnormalities that persist after clinical complaints have resolved.[14, 36, 37] In a study of 13 adults, serial sinus molecular resonance imaging studies showed a rapid increase in the mean aeration of the sinus cavity during the first 10 days of observation, but this was then followed by a slow resolution for up to day 56, the last day of observation.[37] The mean aeration had only approached 80% when observations were discontinued.

Microbial Cause

Specimen Collection. The method of specimen collection is critical in determining the accuracy of sinus culture results. Unless sinus cavity specimens are collected without contamination by nasal secretions, there is always the danger that the specimens will yield bacteria that are growing in the nose instead of the sinus. For this reason, sinus cavity culture obtained by puncture and aspiration has been the gold standard for microbial diagnosis (Table 51–4). Sinus puncture is a relatively painless and safe procedure when performed by an experienced operator, although it is not appropriate for routine clinical use. A spring-loaded device for performing sinus puncture has become commercially available. The bacteria recovered from sinus aspirates have shown pathogenic features including high titers, correlation with a simultaneous Gram stain, and association with leukocytosis in the aspirate.[14]

It is not possible to enter the sinus cavities with an endoscope by way of the natural ostia. With the maxillary sinus, the sheltered location of the hiatus semilunaris, behind the turbinate and uncinate process, and the small diameter of the infundibulum and its acute angle relative to the lower nasal passage make it physically impossible to pass an endoscope into the cavity (see Fig. 51–1).[38] It may be possible to enter the maxillary sinus cavity in some of the 10 to 30% of persons with accessory ostia, but to do so without contaminating the specimen with nasal secretions is difficult or impossible. Therefore, endoscopic sampling is actually directed at secretions in the middle meatus. It is not clear whether the middle meatus is normally sterile or is colonized or contaminated with nasopharyngeal bacteria. In rhinosinusitis patients who have excessive secretions, the possibility of contamination appears greater. In one unpublished study of 47 patients with ACABS, endoscopic sampling had a sensitivity of 65% and a specificity of 40% compared with sampling by sinus aspiration.[39] The sensitivity (79%) and specificity (85%) were improved when the data were analyzed for only *Strep. pneumoniae*, *H. influenzae*, and *Moraxella catarrhalis*. The limited amount of information from direct comparisons of aspiration and endoscopic sampling in the same patient does not permit replacement of aspirate cultures as the gold standard for microbiologic diagnosis at this time.

Viral. Only a limited number of sinus aspirates from patients with acute sinusitis have been tested for virus (Table 51–5). In one study, viruses were recovered from 11 (16%) of 70 positive aspirates.[31] Most of these specimens were collected after the first 3 days of illness when the chances of viral recovery declines. Rhinovirus, parainfluenza virus, and influenza virus were identified, which support the role of viruses in the pathogenesis of sinusitis.

Bacterial

Acute Community-Acquired. The etiology of ACABS has been well defined by puncture studies going back to the late 1940s and 1950s.[13, 14, 40–49] There has been good agreement among the results. *Streptococcus pneumoniae* and *H. influenzae* have been the most important pathogens, together accounting for more than 50% of cases (see Table 51–5). Other streptococcal species including *Streptococcus intermedius*, *Streptococcus pyogenes*, and other α-hemolytic streptococci; *M. catarrhalis*; *Staphylococcus aureus*; and anaerobic bacteria

TABLE 54–4 Method of Sinus Puncture and Aspiration for Specimen Collection

Disinfect the anterior nares and the area below the inferior turbinate (puncture site).
Anesthetize the puncture site with a topical anesthetic.
Puncture the medial wall of the antrum with a 12-gauge needle (or spring-loaded puncture device).
Aspirate the sinus contents into a syringe; if necessary, add 1–2 ml of sterile normal saline (without preservatives) to obtain a specimen.
Cap the syringe and transport the specimen in the syringe to the laboratory.
Obtain quantitative bacterial cultures if possible.

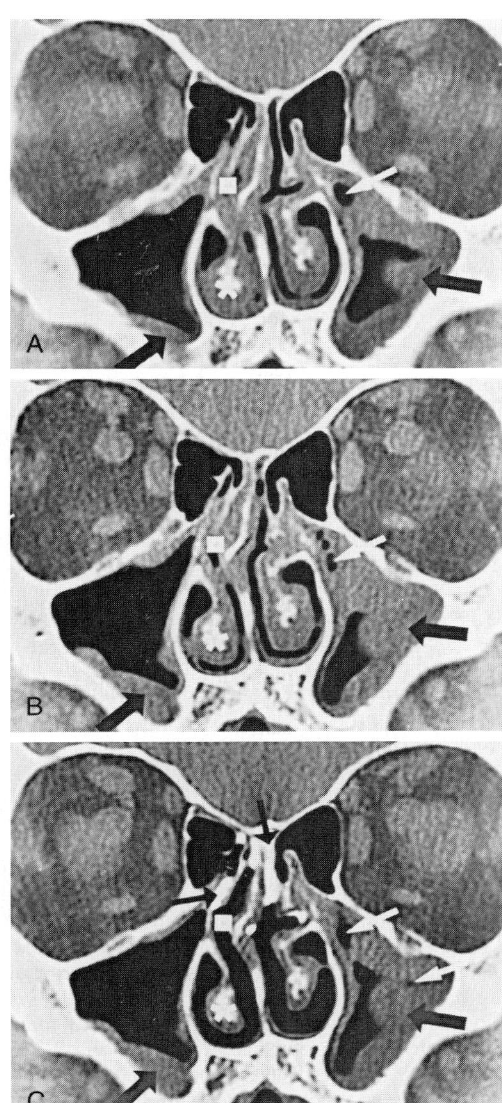

FIGURE 51–3. Serial sinus computed tomography scan from an adult with a common cold of 4 days' duration. *A,* Scan taken at 2:00 PM. There are abnormalities in both maxillary sinuses *(black arrows).* A gaseous bubble is present on the left *(white arrow),* indicating that the material causing the abnormality is thick fluid. The nasal turbinates are engorged *(asterisk),* and the middle meatus is congested *(square).* Immediately after the scan was obtained, the patient was given 60 mg of pseudoephedrine orally. *B,* Scan taken at 4:00 PM on the same day. The material in the maxillary sinuses *(black arrows)* has not moved, and the findings are essentially unchanged after treatment with pseudoephedrine. The turbinates remain engorged *(asterisk)* and the middle meatus congested *(square).* Immediately after the scan was obtained, the patient was given two intranasal sprays of .05% oxymetazoline. *C,* Scan taken 10 minutes after oxymetazoline administration, showing shrinkage of the turbinates *(asterisk)* and decongestion of the middle meatus *(square).* Omnipaque dye was given intranasally immediately before the scan with the patient supine and is present in the middle meatus and olfactory recess *(small black arrows).* The location of the material in the maxillary sinus cavities *(large black arrows)* has not changed.

each account for an additional proportion of cases. *M. catarrhalis* is more prevalent in children than in adults, whereas anaerobic infections are infrequent in children.[46] Most sinusitis due to anaerobic bacteria arises from infection of the roots of the premolar teeth, thus representing a pure bacterial infection. Some of the anaerobic infections have included up to six different species of microaerophilic and anaerobic bacteria. Viruses and bacteria have been recovered simultaneously from the same sinus aspirate, confirming the dual nature of the infection.

The relative importance of the different bacteria has not changed in the last half century, but there have been important changes in their antimicrobial susceptibilities. The appearance of penicillin resistance in *Staph. aureus* was followed by the emergence of β-lactam–resistant strains of *H. influenzae* and *M. catarrhalis.* The most recent and serious event has been the emergence of multiply resistant strains of *Strep. pneumoniae.*

Only approximately 60% of sinus aspirates in suspected cases of ACABS yield bacteria.[50] The cause of the culture-negative cases is not clear, but undoubtedly, many have a viral cause. *Chlamydia pneumoniae* has been identified in patients with respiratory illness that includes features of sinusitis.[51] However, until *C. pneumoniae* has been repeatedly identified in sinus aspirates, its role as a cause of sinusitis will remain unclear. Also, *M. pneumoniae* has been suggested as a cause of ACABS, but there are no reports of attempts to isolate it from sinus aspirates. Atypical pneumonia and bronchitis are the characteristic syndromes associated with *M. pneumoniae* infection. The clinical features of sinusitis have not been described with this infection.

Nosocomial. Nosocomial sinusitis has been most often associated with *Staph. aureus, Pseudomonas aeruginosa, Serratia marcescens, Klebsiella pneumoniae, Enterobacter* spp., and *Proteus mirabilis* and is often polymicrobic.[52–57] *Pseudomonas aeruginosa* is the most frequent isolate in sinus aspirates from patients with cystic fibrosis.[58] *Legionella pneumophila* was identified in sinus tissue from a patient with acquired immunodeficiency syndrome.[59]

Fungi. Fungi are a well-established cause of occasional cases of acute community-acquired sinusitis. Also, fungal infections occur in hospitalized patients and those with other diseases such as diabetes mellitus. In such patients, fungi may be the cause of serious life-threatening infections. An increasing number of fungal groups have been associated with sinus infection (Table 51–6).[14, 60–74]

TABLE 51–5 Viral and Bacterial Cause of Acute Community-Acquired Maxillary Sinusitis

	Mean Percentage of Cases (Range)	
	Adults	*Children*
Viruses*		
Rhinovirus	15	—
Influenza virus	5	—
Parainfluenza virus	3	2
Adenovirus	—	2
Bacteria†		
Streptococcus pneumoniae	31 (20–35)	36
Haemophilus influenzae (unencapsulated)	21 (6–26)	23
S. pneumoniae and *H. influenzae*	5 (1–9)	—
α-Streptococci	9 (3–19)	—
Moraxella catarrhalis	8 (2–10)	19
Anaerobic bacteria (*Bacteroides, Peptostreptococcus, Fusobacterium* spp., and so forth)	6 (0–10)	—
Staphylococcus aureus	4 (0–8)	—
Streptococcus pyogenes	2 (1–3)	2
Gram-negative bacteria‡	9 (0–24)	2

*Data from Hamory BH, Sande MA, Sydnor A Jr, et al. Etiology and antimicrobial therapy of acute maxillary sinusitis. J Infect Dis. 1979;139:197–202.
†Data from refs. 14, 40–49.
‡One study had 24% isolation of gram-negative bacteria, but in four other studies the recovery rate was not over 5%. Gram-negative bacteria recovered included *Pseudomonas aeruginosa, Klebsiella pneumoniae,* and *Escherichia coli.*

TABLE 51–6 Fungal Cause of Paranasal Sinusitis

	Community Acquired	Impaired Host
Aspergillus (*A. fumigatus*, *A. flavus*, *A. niger*, *A. oryzae*, *A. nidulans*)	Yes	Yes
Cryptococcus (*C. neoformans*)		Yes
Pseudallescheria (*P. boydii*)	Yes	Yes
Sporothrix (*S. schenckii*)	Yes	
Homobasidiomycetes (*Schizophyllum commune*)	Yes	Yes
Hyalohyphomycetes (*Penicillium melini*)	Yes	Yes
Phaeohyphomytes (*Bipolaris hawaiienis*, *B. spicifera*, *Exserohilum rostratum*, *E. mcginnisii*, *Alternaria alternata*, *Curvularia lunata*)	Yes	Yes
Zygomyces (*Mucor* spp., *Rhizopus* spp., *Cunninghamella bertholetiae*)	Yes	Yes

Clinical Features

Viral, Bacterial. ACABS is usually superimposed on preexisting VRS; therefore, the clinical features of the illness reflect the dual nature of the infection. In most cases, it is not possible to separate the clinical features of VRS from those of ACABS. Sneezing, nasal discharge, rhinorrhea, nasal obstruction, facial pressure, and headache commonly occur with both conditions. In addition, temperatures of 38°C or more, facial pain, and erythema occur in some cases of ACABS but are relatively uncommon. Purulence or a colored nasal discharge, which is commonly considered a sign of ACABS, also occurs in cases of VRS. Cough has been noted as a characteristic of ACABS in children[46] and is also a common complaint in adults with acute sinusitis. Hyposmia may also be present. When the sinusitis follows dental infection, molar pain and a foul odor to the breath are characteristic features.

Patients with bacterial infection of the sphenoid sinus have presented with severe frontal, temporal, or retroorbital headache that radiates to the occipital region and hypesthesia or hyperesthesia of the ophthalmic or maxillary dermatomes of the fifth cranial nerve.[75] Lethargy and the clinical findings of cavernous sinus or cortical vein thrombosis may also be present as well as signs of orbital cellulitis and abscess. With severe frontal sinusitis, pus may collect under the periosteum of the frontal bone causing swelling and edema of the forehead, which is known as *Pott puffy tumor*.[76]

Nosocomial. Nosocomial sinusitis of bacterial origin has features that are similar to those of ACABS, but because many patients with this condition are severely ill or unconscious, typical clinical features may not be obvious. Nosocomial sinusitis should be suspected when fever of undetermined origin occurs in patients with risk factors such as nasal intubation. Nosocomial sinusitis has been recognized as a risk factor for nosocomial pneumonia.

Fungal. Patients with community-acquired fungal sinusitis usually present with masses, proptosis, and bony erosion due to pressure effects. The invasive form of fungal sinusitis typically presents as a rapidly progressive infection.

Diagnosis

Viral, Bacterial. Diagnostic evaluation should include a history and an examination of the pharynx, nose, ears, sinuses, teeth, and chest. Information should be obtained about coryzal and influenzal illnesses, respiratory allergies, toothache, and other dental complaints. An initial distinction must be made between infectious and allergic or other noninfectious sinusitis syndromes. Differentiation must then be made between viral, combined viral-bacterial, or pure bacterial causes. It is desirable to determine the specific microbial cause, but this is not usually possible in the clinical setting. An allergic cause can usually be established by a history of paroxysmal sneezing, itching eyes, allergen exposure, and similar prior episodes. In one small study, adult patients were accurate in using self-diagnosis to make the distinction between allergy and infection.[77]

Separating viral from viral-bacterial or bacterial infections is a difficult problem. None of the signs and symptoms with which patients present are both sensitive and specific for this purpose (Table 51–7).[1] Another study examined adults with paranasal symptoms and pus observed coming from the middle meatus, using a purulent sinus aspirate (without bacterial culture) as the comparison standard.[78] The presence of two of the three findings of local pain with unilateral predominance, unilateral purulent rhinorrhea, and an erythrocyte sedimentation rate of more than 12 had a sensitivity of 79% and a specificity of 83%. In another study of adults in general practice using purulent maxillary sinus aspirate as the criterion standard, an elevated C-reactive protein concentration (>10 mg/liter) combined with an elevated erythrocyte sedimentation rate (10 mm/hour for men, 20 mm/hour for women) had a sensitivity of 82% and a specificity of 57%.[79] Other standard laboratory tests such as white blood cell and differential counts are not useful because of lack of sensitivity and specificity.

Because of its superior sensitivity, CT scanning of the sinuses has largely supplanted conventional radiography as the imaging method of choice. The cost of a CT scan limited to the sinuses is comparable to that of a plain sinus radiograph in many clinics and

TABLE 51–7 Sensitivity and Specificity of Clinical Findings in Adults with Acute Community-Acquired Sinusitis

Population	Criterion Standard	Finding	Sensitivity (%)	Specificity (%)
Males with nasal discharge*	Positive sinus radiologic examination	History of colored nasal discharge	72	52
		Cough	70	44
		Sneezing	70	34
		Poor response to decongestants	41	80
		Maxillary toothache	18	93
		Purulent secretion	51	76
		Sinus tenderness	48	65
		Temperature >38°C	16	85
Emergency ward patients with paranasal symptoms‡	Purulent sinus aspirate†	Purulent rhinorrhea, unilateral	48	—
		Pain, unilateral	37	—
		Purulent rhinorrhea, bilateral	35	—
		Sinus tenderness on percussion	43	—
		Pus in nasal cavity	41	—

*Data from Williams JW Jr, Simel DL, Roberts L, Samsa GP. Clinical evaluation for sinusitis. Making the diagnosis by history and physical examination. Ann Intern Med. 1992;117:705–710.
†Bacterial culture was not performed.
‡Data from Killingsworth SM, Wetmore SJ. *Curvularia/Drechslera* sinusitis. Laryngoscope. 1990;100:932–937.

TABLE 51–8 Categories of Severity and Management Plans for Suspected Acute Community-Acquired Bacterial Sinusitis*

Category	Features	Management Plan
Emergent	Signs and symptoms suggesting intracranial (meningitis, brain abscess) or orbital extension	Emergency diagnostic measures; head computed tomography, lumbar puncture, surgical consultation Intravenous antimicrobial therapy (vancomycin and a third-generation cephalosporin) while awaiting culture and susceptibility results
Urgent	Fever (temperature of ≥38°C), facial pain, edema, and erythema; maxillary toothache; classic air-fluid level	Oral antimicrobial therapy effective against sinus pathogenesis plus a decongestant, first-generation antihistamine, and mucoevacuant
Elective	Cold or "flu"-like illness that has persisted for 8–10 d or more with no improvement or with worsening	Antimicrobial and supportive treatment (as for urgent cases)

*In the setting of an illness beginning as a common cold, "flu"-like illness, or allergic rhinitis or associated with swimming or other risk factors.

hospitals. Imaging studies are not recommended for the routine diagnosis of community-acquired sinusitis because of their lack of specificity. Patients with VRS have sinus CT scan abnormalities that usually cannot be distinguished from those associated with ACABS.[2] However, the presence of a classic air-fluid level with a flat meniscus (indicating thin fluid in the cavity) correlates well with positive bacterial aspirate culture. In adults, an air-fluid level on a conventional sinus radiograph had a specificity of 89% when compared with positive aspirate culture, although the finding was present in only 37.5% of 48 positive examinations.[31]

As an aid to diagnosis, three categories of ACABS can be recognized (Table 51–8). The first presentation, which is rare, is that in which sinusitis has been complicated by meningitis, brain abscess, or orbital infection. In these cases, the clinical features of the sinus infection are overshadowed by the more serious illness. The second presentation is that in which the classic and relatively specific features of ACABS are present. These include fever of 38°C or higher and facial pain, marked tenderness, erythema, or swelling. Also in this category are patients with molar pain or other evidence of an odontogenic cause of the infection. The third presentation, which is most common, is that of a patient with VRS or an influenza-like illness in which symptoms have continued for 8 to 10 days or more and colored nasal discharge, nasal obstruction, facial pressure, and sometimes cough are no better or are worse. Uncomplicated rhinovirus colds have a median duration of 1 week.[80, 81] If still symptomatic, most cold patients are improved by the end of a week, so that worsening or continuing symptoms raise the suspicion of a complication. Also, sinus puncture studies have shown that approximately 60% of patients with an initial presentation of VRS who are no better after 1 week have a positive bacterial aspirate culture.[50]

Bacterial sinusitis associated with dental infection may go undiagnosed because the dental condition is unrecognized by the patient as a cause of the sinusitis. Previous or current toothache and dental care are important features of the history. A foul odor may be detected on examination of the pharynx.

Nosocomial. Nosocomial sinusitis resulting from indwelling nasal tubes has occurred most often during the second week of hospitalization. Fever and leukocytosis are common findings. Unexplained fever in patients with indwelling nasal tubes is an indication for obtaining a sinus CT scan. Sinus aspirate culture is recommended when possible.

Fungal. Acute fungal sinusitis can resemble bacterial sinusitis but occurs in patients with serious underlying diseases and has a marked propensity for invading through contiguous bone into the orbit, brain, and hard palate (see Chapters 248 and 249). Chronic fungal sinusitis has three forms: invasive sinusitis, fungus ball of the sinus, and allergic fungal sinusitis. Invasive infection resembles squamous carcinoma, Wegener's granulomatosis, midline granuloma, and rhinoscleroma. Fungus ball of the sinus is a benign mass of hyphae, usually *Aspergillus*. Allergic fungal sinusitis presents as chronic sinus pain and an expansile mass of inspissated mucus, eosinophils, and hyphae that can deform outward the bony wall between the ethmoid sinus and the orbit or between the maxillary sinus and the nasal cavity. Patients usually have a history of allergic rhinitis and nasal polyps.

Noninfectious. Noninfectious causes of sinus disease include chemical irritation, nasal and sinus tumors, foreign bodies, Wegener's granulomatosis, and midline granuloma. Rhinoscleroma, a chronic granulomatous disease of the mucosa of the upper airway caused by *Klebsiella rhinoscleromatis*, may also lead to bony invasion and obstruction of the nasal passages.

Complications

ACABS may lead to intracranial, orbital, and respiratory complications. The intracranial complications include meningitis, brain abscess, subdural empyema, and cavernous sinus and cortical vein thrombosis. Orbital complication are most common in young children and include orbital cellulitis, subperiosteal abscess, and orbital abscess. Sinusitis is also associated with the onset or exacerbation of asthma and bronchitis. Sinopulmonary disease is a well-recognized combination, especially when the condition has become chronic.

Whether the usual type of ACABS can lead to chronic sinus disease is unknown. Certain specific microorganisms might predispose to chronic sinus disease, or chronic sinus disease may be related more to problems with host immunity including allergy.

Therapy

Antimicrobial

General Considerations. The case for treating ACABS patients with antimicrobials is based on solid evidence of bacteriologic and clinical improvement.[82] Studies using pre- and post-treatment sinus aspirate cultures have shown that antimicrobials with appropriate spectra and given in adequate doses and with an adequate duration are effective in eradicating or substantially reducing bacterial titers in the sinus cavity compared with treatment in which the drug spectrum or the dose is inadequate (Table 51–9).[31, 44, 50, 83] Since the early 1970s, a number of antimicrobials have been tested in patients with ACABS using pre- and post-therapy aspirate cultures. With a 10-day course of an antimicrobial with an appropriate spectrum used at the correct dose, bacteriologic cure rates of 90% or higher have been routinely obtained.[50]

In clinical trials of antimicrobial therapy for ACABS, pretreatment bacterial aspirate culture is necessary to exclude cases of uncomplicated VRS, which invariably confound the patient sample if inclusion criteria are based solely on clinical and imaging parameters. Post-treatment aspirate culture is also necessary to determine the effectiveness of bacterial eradication. Currently, the Food and Drug Administration does not require post-treatment aspirate cultures for approval of a sinusitis treatment indication. In the literature, there are reports of "bacteriologic cures" in which post-therapy aspirate cultures were not performed and "bacteriologic cure" was based on clinical response and not on the results of aspirate cultures.

Evidence for clinical improvement after antimicrobial therapy in

TABLE 51–9 Comparative Bacteriologic Cure Rates (Determined by Sinus Puncture) in Patients with Acute Community-Acquired Bacterial Sinusitis

	No. Bacteriologic Cures/No. Cases
C Carenfelt et al[44]	
Antibiotic concentration ≥ MIC of causative bacteria*	19/21 (90%)
Antibiotic concentration < MIC of causative bacteria	15/33 (45%)
BH Hamory et al[31]	
Appropriate antimicrobial and dose	47/49 (96%)
Inappropriate antimicrobial†	0/6 (0)
C Carenfelt et al[83]	
Appropriate antimicrobial and dose	105/115 (91%)
Suboptimal dose‡	37/50 (74%)
JM Gwaltney Jr et al[50]	
Appropriate antimicrobial and dose	126/136 (93%)
Suboptimal dose‡	1/5 (20%)
Suboptimal dose§	15/21 (71%)

*Antibiotic concentration in sinus aspirate after 2–3 days of treatment.
†Clindamycin for *Haemophilus influenzae.*
‡Cefaclor 500 mg bid.
§Cefaclor 500 mg tid.
Abbreviations: MIC, Minimal inhibitory concentration.

ACABS may be found in a double-blind controlled trial of antimicrobial therapy in adults.[84] A significant difference in the duration of illness favoring antimicrobial therapy appeared by the third day of treatment and continued throughout the 30-day observation period (Fig. 51–4). By day 10, 86% of antimicrobial-treated patients were recovered or much better compared with 57% of those on placebo. By day 10, 86% of patients on treatment also showed sinus CT scan improvement compared with 66% on placebo. After 30 days, 25% of patients receiving placebo judged themselves to be still sick compared with 10% of those on antimicrobial treatment.

Recommendations for antimicrobial treatment have changed as the sensitivities of the causative bacteria have evolved. The emergence of penicillin- and methicillin-resistant *Staph. aureus* was not a major problem because of its relative infrequency as a cause of ACABS. The subsequent emergence of β-lactamase–producing strains of *H. influenzae* and *M. catarrhalis* reduced the usefulness of ampicillin, but a number of more expensive antimicrobials were still available.[50] The emergence of intermediate- and high-level resistant strains of *Strep. pneumoniae* is a much more serious problem. A number of antimicrobials that were previously useful in the treatment

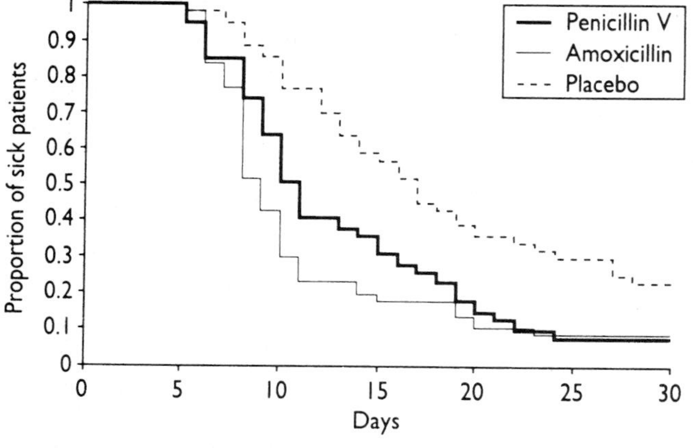

FIGURE 51–4. Duration of illness in adults with acute community-acquired sinusitis in a randomized double-blind clinical trial of antimicrobial treatment. (—— penicillin V, n = 39; —— amoxicillin, n = 44; ----- placebo, n = 44). (From Lindbaek M, Hjortdahl P, Johnsen U. Randomised, double-blind, placebo controlled trial of penicillin V and amoxycillin in treatment of acute sinus infections in adults. BMJ. 1996;313:325–329.)

of ACABS now have MIC_{90}s against intermediately resistant pneumococci that are not achievable.[85]

Current Recommendations. Antimicrobial therapy is usually selected on an empirical basis because sinus aspirate culture results are not available in the usual clinical setting. Treatment should be directed against the known sinus pathogens (see Table 51–5). The β-lactam antimicrobials that continue to show the best activity against intermediately resistant strains of pneumococci and are also effective against β-lactamase–producing *H. influenzae* and *M. catarrhalis* are amoxicillin-clavulanate, cefpodoxime, cefdinir, and cefuroxime. Also, the new quinolones provide excellent activity against pneumococci and other sinusitis pathogens. Of these drugs, amoxicillin-clavulanate, cefdinir, cefuroxime, and levofloxacin have been shown to be effective in pre- and post-therapy sinus puncture clinical trials in patients with ACABS.[48–50] A 10-day course of treatment with one of these antimicrobials is recommended for patients with ACABS (Table 51–10). There are no pre- and postsinus aspirate culture data on the effectiveness of longer or shorter courses of treatment for ACABS.

The symptoms of acute community-acquired sinusitis usually improve after 2 or 3 days of treatment and are generally resolved by 7 to 14 days.[37] *However, it is important to be aware that patients with acute sinusitis may have substantial symptomatic improvement despite the persistence in the sinus of purulent material containing high titers of bacteria.*[14] In one clinical trial, 38% of patients on placebo reported improvement by the third day of observation.[84] In patients with evidence of severe infection or in whom intracranial or orbital extension of infection is suspected, intravenous therapy should be started with vancomycin and ceftriaxone or cefotaxime until the results of culture and sensitivity testing are available for directing treatment. These patients should have emergency evaluations by CT or MRI, or both, and may also require diagnostic lumbar puncture or surgical decompression and drainage, or both. Antimicrobial treatment of patients with nosocomial sinusitis should be directed by culture and sensitivity information when available, or when empirical, should cover the usual pathogens responsible for these infections.

Fungal. Community-acquired fungal sinusitis in persons with normal immunity is usually effectively treated with surgical débridement of the affected sinus cavities. Complicated cases and patients with immunodeficiencies suspected of having invasive infection should be evaluated on an individual basis for appropriate surgical and antifungal therapy.

Ancillary. Most patients with ACABS are successfully treated as outpatients. Patients with severe infection, especially those in whom intracranial or orbital extension is suspected, require hospitalization. Ancillary treatment should be directed at drainage of the nasal passages and sinuses and the relief of sneezing, coughing, and systemic complaints.[86] Topical decongestants are rapidly effective in shrinking the erectile vascular tissue of the turbinates and, thus, helping relieve ostiomeatal and nasal obstruction (see Fig. 51–3).[30] However, sequential CT scans have shown that decongestants have no effect on opening the infundibulum and draining the sinus cavity itself. Also, the exudate in the sinus cavity is often too viscous to be moved by ciliary action. Decongestants do help to open and drain the nasal passages and ostiomeatal complex. Oral decongestants avoid rebound vasodilatation and pharyngeal irritation and are pre-

TABLE 51–10 Antimicrobial Treatment of Acute Community-Acquired Bacterial Sinusitis in Adults

Amoxicillin-clavulanate*	875-125 mg q12h
Cefdinir*	600 mg qd
Cefpodoxime proxetil	200 mg q12h
Cefuroxime axetil*	250 mg q12h
Levofloxacin*	500 mg qd
Trovafloxacin	200 mg qd

*Have been found effective in pre- and post-treatment sinus aspirate culture studies.

ferred over topical preparations. They have been shown to be safe in patients with stable hypertension on antihypertensive treatment.[87]

Topical steroids have not been rigorously evaluated in treating patients with ACABS,[86] add unnecessary expense, and are not recommended. The value of mucoevacuants, such as guaifenesin, is also not established, but they are used on theoretical grounds. Nonsteroidal anti-inflammatory drugs are useful in treating systemic complaints such as fever and malaise and may be helpful in reducing cough.[88, 89] Other cough suppressants such as dextromethorphan and codeine may be needed for cough control.

First-generation antihistamines have not been recommended in the past for treating VRS or ACABS because of their anticholinergic activity and the possibility of drying secretions. Although this is a reasonable theoretical consideration, actual testing under randomized controlled blinded conditions has shown an approximately 50% reduction in sneezing and a 30% reduction in rhinorrhea and nasal mucus weights in volunteers with experimental rhinovirus colds.[90, 91] Also, there was no evidence for worsening of other symptoms or prolongation of the overall illness. This indicates that the drying of secretions and the impairment of drainage were not problems. Also, by reducing sneezing and nose blowing, antihistamines may reduce the frequency of viral and bacterial dissemination in the nasal passages and into the sinus cavities. Experimental upper airway challenge with histamine in volunteers stimulates the release of secretions with an increased sulfate concentration characteristic of mucus, suggesting that histamine stimulates goblet cell exocytosis.[92] Thus, antihistamine therapy may reduce the amount of mucus that accumulates in the sinus cavity.

In patients with ACABS who do not respond to an initial course of therapy, sinus puncture and lavage, repeatedly if necessary, is highly recommended. This more invasive form of treatment is justified because once sinus disease has progressed to a chronic state, the prognosis for eventual recovery is reduced considerably.

Prevention

Preventing colds may be possible to some extent by avoiding contact with cold sufferers and by hygienic measures such as hand washing when contact occurs between infected and noninfected persons. Also, covering coughs and sneezes with disposable nasal tissues is desirable. Vaccine is effective in preventing influenza as is prophylactic amantadine or rimantadine during periods of epidemic influenza. There are no proven measures for preventing secondary bacterial infection of the sinuses, although avoiding vigorous nose blowing and the suppression of sneezes and coughs is of theoretical value. Also, the promotion of decongestion and drainage is possible in the lower nasal passages and ostiomeatal area but, as discussed previously, its value in clearing the sinus cavity is problematic. *Prophylactic antimicrobial administration to prevent recurrent ACABS is not recommended and, if used widely for such a common illness as VRS, would undoubtedly hasten the emergence of bacteria with new patterns of antibiotic resistance.* Better treatments for colds may be available in the future, and these, when given early in the course of the illness, may modify the viral sinusitis and, in turn, lower the incidence of secondary bacterial sinusitis.

Avoiding nasal intubation has been shown to be effective in reducing the incidence of nosocomial sinusitis.[57]

CHRONIC

Chronic sinus disease (CSD) remains a largely neglected area of study. Published sinus aspirate culture data on specimens obtained from intact sinuses of CSD patients is very limited. Understanding of the etiology and pathogenesis of CSD remains poor, and except for surgery, treatment modalities are inadequate. The disease is best classified into pre- and postsurgical categories because patients in these categories present somewhat different problems in management.

Presurgical Cases

Etiology and Pathogenesis

Approximately 5 to 10% of cases of ACABS fail to show bacteriologic cure after a course of antimicrobial therapy.[50] In a clinical trial of adults with acute community-acquired sinusitis, 25% of the patients who received placebo were still symptomatic after 1 month.[84] It is reasonable to speculate that most cases of CSD arise from patients with typical ACABS who are nonresponders to treatment or who have not received treatment, but good evidence for this view is lacking. Anecdotal evidence from clinical practice indicates that some cases of ACABS do not resolve despite repeated courses of more than adequate antimicrobial treatment. Post-therapy sinus aspirate cultures of these patients are often nonrevealing. This suggests that at least some or many cases of CSD do not evolve from typical ACABS but may represent a separate and distinct entity of undetermined cause. However, somewhat paradoxically, two small sinus puncture studies have recovered *Strep. pneumoniae*, *H. influenzae*, and other streptococcal species from aspirate cultures obtained from the intact sinuses of CSD patients.[93, 94]

It is well recognized that persistent sinus disease can result from certain conditions including obstruction of sinus drainage, abnormalities in mucociliary clearance, severe immunoglobulin deficiency, granulocyte dysfunction, and acquired immunodeficiency syndrome, but most CSD patients do not have these problems. Anecdotal evi-

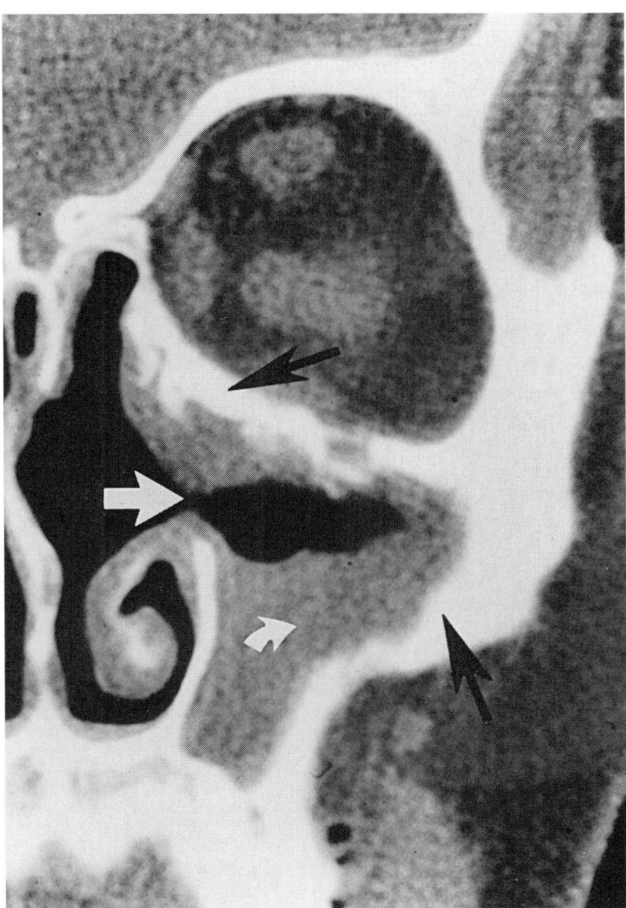

FIGURE 51–5. Bone remodeling *(black arrows)* in a 60-year-old diabetic with chronic sinus disease of 8 years' duration. Despite a widely patent surgical antrostomy *(large white arrow)*, exudate *(small curved arrow)* is present in the sinus cavity. A highly viscous exudate that grew a strain of *Pseudomonas aeruginosa* was removed by endoscopy.

dence may be accumulating that less severe immune problems such as deficiencies in immunoglobulin subtypes may play a role in the pathogenesis of CSD, but this is currently not well established. Also, there is a subset of patients with CSD associated with aspirin sensitivity, nasal polyposis, and asthma.

Management

A commonly used approach to the medical management of patients in whom an initial course of therapy for ACABS fails is to give additional courses of antimicrobials, sometimes guided by aspirate culture results; prescribe intranasal and sometimes oral steroids; and evaluate the patient for allergic and immune deficiency states. Sinus lavage was used in the preantibiotic era, and it still may be an effective form of treatment that is currently neglected or underused. When comprehensive medical management, including the previously mentioned therapies, has failed and there is sinus CT scan evidence of persistent disease, the patient should be evaluated as a candidate for sinus surgery.

Prolonged ineffective medical management is not recommended because of the theoretical risk that CSD may become so well established that the chances of success with sinus surgery may be lessened. Remodeling of the facial bones is often seen on CT scans of patients with prolonged CSD (Fig. 51–5), and evidence of osteomyelitis has been demonstrated in specimens from such patients (Fig. 51–6).[95] Also, there is the possibility that irreversible mucosal damage may occur.

Modern endoscopic surgery is reported to result in "marked" short-term improvement in approximately 85% of patients.[96] In the standard procedure, the ostiomeatal area is opened, antrostomies are created, and ethmoid partitions are removed. A portion of the anterior wall of the sphenoid sinus may be removed, but the frontal sinuses are usually not opened in the initial procedure.

Postsurgical Cases

Pathogenesis

Patients in whom sinus surgery fails continue to have chronic purulent nasal discharge, nasal crusting, anosmia, facial pain, headache, cough, and fatigue. When the condition is fully developed, it is the cause of serious morbidity and typically continues for years. Bacterial cultures obtained from the nasal passages and opened sinus cavities are usually positive but may be difficult to interpret (Table 51–11). Serial cultures are most often positive for *Staph. aureus*, *Pseudomonas* spp., *S. marcescens*, *Stenotrophomonas maltophilia*, and other gram-negative bacteria. These organisms appear to be the cause of the ongoing disease, although it is unlikely that they were responsible for the original problem. The reason that sinus surgery fails in some patients remains obscure, but as with presurgical CSD, host immune factors may play a role. As described previously, bony involvement is often identified.[95] Microbial factors such as the presence of small-colony bacterial variants may also have a role in the chronicity of the process.[97]

TABLE 51–11 Bacterial Culture Categories in Patients with Chronic Sinus Disease

Category 1: *Streptococcus pneumoniae, Haemophilus influenzae, Moraxella catarrhalis,* other species of *Streptococcus* (*intermedius,* etc.)
Setting: recovered in sinus aspirates; in high titers
Interpretation: cause of acute exacerbations or possibly of ongoing disease
Category 2: *Staphylococcus aureus* and/or *Pseudomonas aeruginosa* (and other *Pseudomonas* species)
Setting: recovered in sinus aspirates in cystic fibrosis; postoperative sinus cavity exudates; persistent infection
Interpretation: cause of disease (crusts, thick and/or "concretized" secretions)
Category 3: *Staphylococcus epidermidis* (other coagulase-negative staphylococci), *Corynebacterium* spp., anaerobes, gram-negative bacteria
Setting: recovered from tissue and swab specimens collected at time of surgery, in nasal and sinus swabs; low titers
Interpretation: role in pathogenesis unclear or suspect

Management

The management of CSD patients in whom surgery has failed is a difficult and frustrating challenge. Surgery is recommended on unopened areas that show continuing disease by CT scan examination. The most frequent targets for this are isolated ethmoid air cells and the sphenoid and frontal sinuses. Antimicrobial treatment should be based on serial culture and sensitivity results and coordinated with

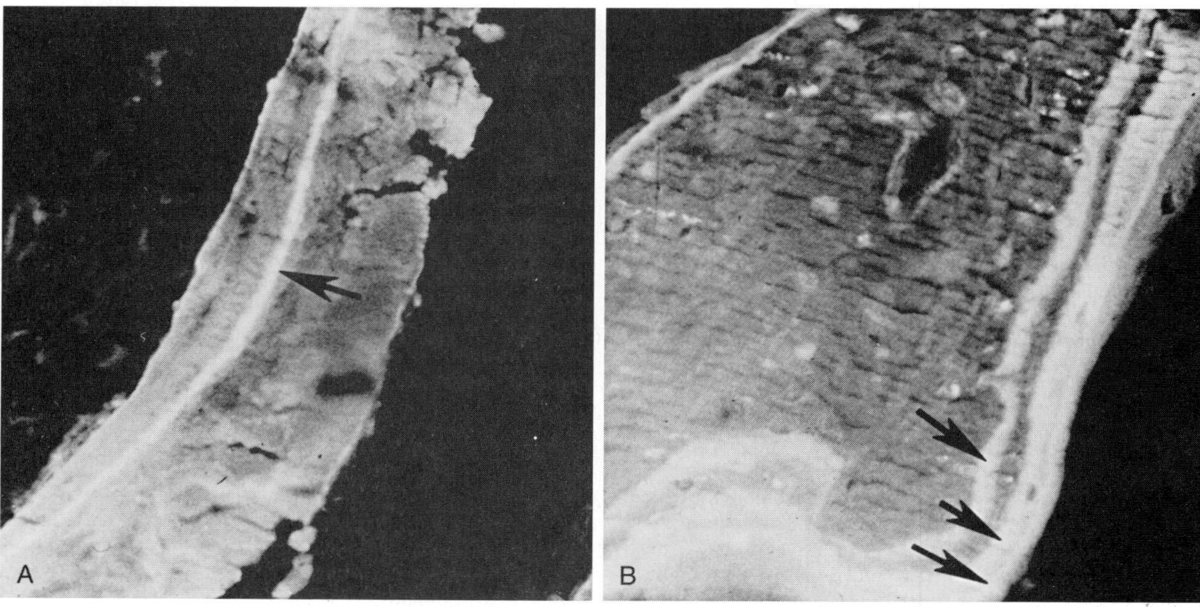

FIGURE 51–6. Tetracycline labeling of ethmoid bone removed from a normal control with a single area of neogenesis *(arrow) (A)* and a patient with chronic sinus disease with multiple areas of neogenesis *(arrows) (B).*

surgical drainage. Prolonged courses of therapy directed at bony involvement seem reasonable, but experience with this approach is limited and early results are not encouraging. Patients may have sustained improvement, but relapses are usually seen when antimicrobials are discontinued. Some physicians have observed sustained improvement with immunoglobulin replacement therapy, but evaluation of this form of treatment has not been subjected to controlled evaluation. Less aggressive management relies on short-term courses of antimicrobials during periods of unusually severe exacerbation combined with daily nasal irrigations and surgical removal of crusts when necessary. Irrigating fluids and devices should be maintained under sterile conditions, and unsterilized tap water lavages are not recommended.

REFERENCES

1. Williams JW Jr, Simel DL, Roberts L, Samsa GP. Clinical evaluation for sinusitis. Making the diagnosis by history and physical examination. Ann Intern Med. 1992;117:705–710.
2. Gwaltney JM Jr., Phillips CD, Miller RD, Riker DK. Computed tomographic study of the common cold. N Engl J Med. 1994;330:25–30.
3. Witmer LM. Homology of facial structures in extant archosaurs (birds and crocodilians), with special reference to paranasal pneumaticity and nasal conchae. J Morphol. 1995;225:269–327.
4. Rowe T. Definition, diagnosis, and the origin of Mammalia. J Vert Paleontol. 1988;8:241–264.
5. Morgensen C, Tos M. Quantitative histology of the maxillary sinus. Rhinology. 1977;55:129.
6. Morgensen C, Tos M. Quantitative histology of the normal sphenoid sinus. Rhinology. 1978;56:203.
7. Mogensen C, Tos M. Density of goblet cells in the normal adult human nasal septum. Anat Anz. 1977;141:237.
8. Hilding A. The physiology of drainage of nasal mucus. III. Experimental work on the accessory sinuses. Am J Rhinol. 1932;May:664–670.
9. Messerklinger W. Über die Drainage der menschlichen Nasennebenhöhlen unter normalen und pathologischen Bedingungen 1. Mitteilung Mschr Ohrenheillk Lar-Rhinol. 1966;100:56–58.
10. Deitmer T. Physiology and pathology of the mucociliary system. In: Pfaltz CR, ed. Advances in Oto-Rhino-Laryngology, v. 43. Basel: Karger; 1989;28.
11. Maran AGD, Lund VJ. Nasal physiology. In: Clinical Rhinology. New York, Thieme Medical; 1990;37.
12. Gwaltney JM Jr, Hayden FG. The nose and infection. In: Proctor DF and Andersen I, eds. The Nose. Upper Airway Physiology and the Atmospheric Environment. Amsterdam, Elsevier Biomedical; 1982;399–422.
13. Björkwall T. Bacteriological examinations in maxillary sinusitis: Bacterial flora of the maxillary antrum. Acta Otolaryngol Suppl (Stockh). 1950;83:33–58.
14. Evans FO Jr, Sydnor JB, Moore WEC, et al. Sinusitis of the maxillary antrum. N Engl J Med. 1975;293:735–739.
15. Bjuggren G, Kraepelien S, Lind J. Sinusitis in children at home and in day-nurseries. Ann Paediat. 1949;173:205–221.
16. Shapiero ED, Wald ER, Doyle WJ, Rohm DD. Bacteriology of maxillary sinuses of the rhesus monkey. Ann Otol Rhinol Laryngol. 1982; 91:150–151.
17. Runer T. Studies of Mucociliary Activity and Blood Flow in the Upper Airways, with Special Reference to Endothelins and Nitric Oxide. PhD thesis. Department of Oto-Rhino-Laryngology, Head and Neck Surgery, University of Lund, Sweden, 1996.
18. Gwaltney JM Jr. Rhinoviruses. In: Evans AS, Kaslow RA, eds. Viral Infections of Humans: Epidemiology and Control. 4th ed. New York, Plenum, 1997;815–838.
19. Dingle JH, Badger GF, Jordan WS Jr. Illness in the Home. A Study of 25,000 Illnesses in a Group of Cleveland Families. Cleveland, The Press of Western Reserve University, 1964;347.
20. Berg O, Carenfelt C, Rystedt G, Ånggåard A. Occurrence of asymptomatic sinusitis in common cold and other acute ENT-infections. Rhinology. 1986;24:223–225.
21. Gable CA, Jones JK, Floor M, et al. Chronic sinusitis: Relation to upper respiratory infections and allergic rhinitis. Pharmacoepidemiol Drug Safety. 1994;3:337–349.
22. Schappert SM. Vital and Health Statistics. National Ambulatory Medical Care Survey: 1991 Summary, Series 13: Data from the National Health Survey, No. 116. DHHS Publication No. (PHS) 94–1777. Atlanta: Centers for Disease Control and Prevention, National Center Health Statistics; 1994.
23. Gwaltney JM Jr, Hayden FG. Response to psychological stress and susceptibility to the common cold (Letter). N Engl J Med. 1992;326:644–645.
24. Winther B, Gwaltney JM Jr, Mygind N, et al. Sites of recovery after point inoculation of the upper airway. JAMA. 1986;256:1763–1767.
25. Greve JM, Davis G, Meyer AM, et al. The major human rhinovirus receptor is ICAM-1. Cell. 1989;56:839–847.
26. Winther B, Innes DJ. The human adenoid. A morphologic study. Arch Otolaryngol Head Neck Surg. 1994;120:144–149.
27. Winther B, Innes DJ, Hendley JO, et al. Distribution of the human rhinovirus receptor, ICAM-1, on epithelium of the upper airways. Abstract 100. J Jpn Rhinol Soc. 1991;100.
28. Arruda E, Boyle TR, Winther B, et al. Localization of human rhinovirus replication in the upper respiratory tract by in situ hybridization. J Infect Dis. 1995;171:1329–1333.
29. Gwaltney JM Jr, Ruckert RR. Rhinovirus. In: Richman DD, Whitley RJ, Hayden FG, eds. Clinical Virology. New York, Churchill Livingstone, 1997;1025–1047.
30. Gwaltney JM Jr. State-of-the-art. Acute community-acquired sinusitis. Clin Infect Dis. 1996;23:1209–1223.
31. Hamory BH, Sande MA, Sydnor A Jr, et al. Etiology and antimicrobial therapy of acute maxillary sinusitis. J Infect Dis. 1979;139:197–202.
32. Hinni ML, McCaffrey TV, Kasperbauer JL. Early mucosal changes in experimental sinusitis. Otolaryngol Head Neck Surg. 1992;107:537–548.
33. Fukami M, Norlander T, Stierna P, et al. Mucosal pathology of the nose and sinuses: A study in experimental maxillary sinusitis in rabbits induced by *Streptococcus pneumoniae, Bacteroides fragilis*, and *Staphylococcus aureus*. Am J Rhinol. 1993;7:125–132.
34. Westrin KM, Stierna P, Carlsöö B, Nord CE. Mucosubstance histochemistry of the maxillary sinus mucosa in experimental sinusitis: A model study on rabbits. ORL J Otolaryngol Relat Spec. 1991;53:508–513.
35. Fukami M, Norlander T, Stierna P, et al. Mucosal pathology of the nose and sinuses: A study in experimental maxillary sinusitis in rabbits induced by *Streptococcus pneumoniae, Bacteroides fragilis,* and *Staphylococcus aureus*. Am J Rhinol. 1993;7:125–132.
36. Axelsson A, Runze U. Comparison of subjective and radiological findings during the course of acute maxillary sinusitis. Ann Otol Rhinol Laryngol. 1983;92:75–77.
37. Lepold DA, Stafford CT, Sod EW, et al. Clinical course of acute maxillary sinusitis documented by sequential MRI scanning. Am J Rhinol. 1994;8:19–28.
38. Yanagisawa E, Yanagisawa K. Endoscopic view of maxillary sinus ostia. Ear Nose Throat J. 1993;72:518–519.
39. Talbot G, Kennedy D, Scheld M, et al. Utility of sinus endoscopy versus sinus aspiration for microbiologic documentation of acute maxillary sinusitis (AMS). Abstract D42. Presented at the Thirty-fifth Interscience Conference of Antimicrobial Agents and Chemotherapy, San Francisco, CA, September 17–20, 1995.
40. Urdal K, Berdal P. The microbial flora in 81 cases of maxillary sinusitis. Acta Otolaryngol (Stockh). 1949;37:20–25.
41. Lystad A, Berdal P, Lund-Iverson L. The bacterial flora of sinusitis with an in vitro study of the bacterial resistance to antibiotics. Acta Otolaryngol Suppl (Stockh). 1964;188:390–399.
42. Rantanen T, Arvilommi H. Double-blind trial of doxicycline in acute maxillary sinusitis: A clinical and bacteriological study. Acta Otolaryngol (Stockh). 1973;76:58–62.
43. Axelsson A, Brorson JE. The correlation between bacteriological findings in the nose and maxillary sinus in acute maxillary sinusitis. Laryngoscope. 1973;83:2003–2011.
44. Carenfelt C, Eneroth C-M, Lundberg C, Wretlind B. Evaluation of the antibiotic effect of treatment of maxillary sinusitis. Scand J Infect Dis. 1975;7:259–264.
45. Sydnor A Jr, Gwaltney JM Jr, Cocchetto DM, Scheld WM. Comparative evaluation of cefuroxime axetil and cefaclor for therapy of acute bacterial maxillary sinusitis. Arch Otolarngol Head Neck Surg. 1989;115:1054–1059.
46. Wald ER, Milmoe GJ, Bowen A, et al. Acute maxillary sinusitis in children. N Engl J Med. 1981;304:749–754.
47. Sydnor TA Jr, Scheld WM, Gwaltney J Jr, et al. Loracarbef (LY163892) vs amoxicillin/clavulanate in bacterial maxillary sinusitis. Ear Nose Throat J. 1992;71:225–232.
48. Gwaltney JM Jr, Savolainen S, Rivas P, et al. Comparative effectiveness and safety of cefdinir and amoxicillin-clavulanate in treatment of acute community-acquired bacterial sinusitis. Antimicrob Agents Chemother. 1997;41:1517–1520.
49. Sydnor A, Scheld WM, Gwaltney JM. A noncomparative study to evaluate the safety and efficacy of levofloxacin in the treatment of acute bacterial sinusitis in adults. Data on file. Raritan, NJ, The Robert Wood Johnson Pharmaceutical Institute/Ortho-McNeil Pharmaceutical, 1995.
50. Gwaltney JM Jr, Scheld WM, Sande MA, Sydnor A. The microbial etiology and antimicrobial therapy of adults with acute community-acquired sinusitis: A fifteen-year experience at the University of Virginia and review of other selected studies. J Allergy Clin Immunol. 1992;90:457–462.
51. Hahn DL, Dodge RW, Golubjantnikov R. Association of *Chlamydia pneumoniae* (strain TWAR) infection with wheezing, asthmatic bronchitis, and adult-onset asthma. JAMA. 1991;266:225–230.
52. Pope TL, Stelling CB, Leitner YB. Maxillary sinusitis after nasotracheal intubation. South Med J. 1981; 74:610–612.
53. Via-Reque E, Rattenborg CC. Prolonged oro- or nasotracheal intubation. Crit Care Med. 1981; 9:637–639.
54. Caplan ES, Hoyt NJ. Nosocomial sinusitis. JAMA. 1982;247:639–641.
55. Deutschman CS, Wilton PB, Sinow J, et al. Paranasal sinusitis: A common complication of nasotracheal intubation in neurosurgical patients. Neurosurgery. 1985;17:296–299.
56. Linden BE, Aguilar EA, Allen SJ. Sinusitis in the nasotracheally intubated patient. Arch Otolaryngol Head Neck Surg. 1988;114:860–861.
57. Rouby J-J, Laurent P, Gosnach M, et al. Risk factors and clinical relevance of nosocomial maxillary sinusitis in the critically ill. Am J Respir Crit Care Med. 1994;150:776–783.
58. Shapiro ED, Milmoe GJ, Wald ER, et al. Bacteriology of the maxillary sinuses in patients with cystic fibrosis. J Infect Dis. 1982;146–151.
59. Schlanger G, Lutwick LI, Kurzman M, et al. Sinusitis caused by *Legionella pneumophila* in a patient with the acquired immune deficiency syndrome. Am J Med. 1984;77:957–960.
60. Morriss FH Jr, Spock A. Intracranial aneurysm secondary to mycotic orbital and

sinus infection. Report of a case implicating *Penicillium* as an opportunistic fungus. Am J Dis Child. 1970; 119:357–362.
61. McGuirt WF, Harril JA. Paranasal sinus aspergillosis. Laryngoscope. 1979;89:1563–1570.
62. Stevens MH. Primary fungal infections of the paranasal sinuses. Am J Otolaryngol. 1981;2:348–357.
63. Romett J, Newman R. Aspergillosis of the nose and paranasal sinuses. Laryngoscope. 1982;92:764–766.
64. Rinaldi MG. Invasive aspergillosis. Rev Infect Dis. 1983;5:1061–1077.
65. Morgan MA, Wilson WR, Neel B III, Roberts GD. Fungal sinusitis in healthy and immunocompromised individuals. Am J Clin Pathol. 1984; 82:597–601.
66. Parfrey NA. Improved diagnosis and prognosis of mucormycosis. A clinico-pathologic of 33 cases. Medicine. 1986;65:113–120.
67. Kern ME, Uecker FA. Maxillary sinus infection caused by the homobasidio-mycetous fungus *Schizophyllum commune*. J Clin Microbiol. 1986;23:1001–1005.
68. MacMillan RH III, Cooper PH, Body BA, Mills AS. Allergic fungal sinusitis due to *Curvularia lunata*. Hum Pathol. 1987;18:960–964.
69. Washburn RG, Kennedy AW, Begley MG, et al. Chronic fungal sinusitis in apparently normal hosts. Medicine. 1988;67:231–247.
70. Killingsworth SM, Wetmore SJ. *Curvularia/Drechslera* sinusitis. Laryngoscope. 1990;100:932–937.
71. Zieske LA, Kipke RD, Hamill R. Dematiaceous fungal sinusitis. Otolaryngol Head Neck Surg. 1991;105:567–577.
72. Morrison VA, Weisdorf DJ. *Alternaria:* A sinonasal pathogen of immunocompromised hosts. Clin Infect Dis. 1993;16:265–270.
73. Fothergill AW. Identification of dematiaceous fungi and their role in human disease. Clin Infect Dis. 1996:22(Suppl 2):S179–S184.
74. Iwen PC, Rupp ME, Hinrichs SH. Invasive mold sinusitis: 17 cases in immunocompromised patients and review of the literature. Clin Infect Dis. 1997;1178–1184.
75. Lew D, Southwick FS, Montgomery WW, et al. Sphenoid sinusitis. A review of 30 cases. N Engl J Med. 1983;309:1149–1154.
76. Wells RC, Sty JR, Landers AD. Radiological evaluation of Pott puffy tumor. JAMA. 1986;255:1331–1333.
77. Williams RB, Gwaltney JM Jr. Allergic rhinitis or virus cold?: Nasal smear eosinophilia in differential diagnosis. Ann Allergy. 1972;80:189–194.
78. Berg O, Carenfelt C. Analysis of symptoms and clinical signs in the maxillary sinus empyema. Acta Otolaryngol (Stockh). 1988;105:343–349.
79. Hansen JG, Schmidt H, Rosborg J, Lund E. Predicting acute maxillary sinusitis in a general practice population. BMJ. 1995;311:233–236.
80. Gwaltney JM Jr, Hendley JO, Simon G, Jordan WS Jr. Rhinovirus infections in an industrial population. II. Characteristics of illness and antibody response. JAMA. 1967;202:494–500.
81. Gwaltney JM Jr, Buier RM, Rogers JL. The influence of signal variation, bias, noise, and effect size on statistical significance in treatment studies of the common cold. Antiviral Res. 1996;29:287–295.
82. Gwaltney JM Jr. Acute community-acquired bacterial sinusitis: To treat or not to treat. Can Respir J. In press.
83. Carenfelt C, Melen I, Ödkvist L, et al. Treatment of sinus empyema in adults. A coordinated Nordic multicenter trial of cefixime vs. cefaclor Acta Otolaryngol (Stockh). 1990;110:128–135.
84. Lindbæk M, Hjortdahl P, Johnsen U. Randomised, double-blind, placebo controlled trial of penicillin V and amoxycillin in treatment of acute sinus infections in adults. BMJ. 1996;313:325–329.
85. Doern GV, Brueggemann A, Holley HP Jr, Rauch AM. Antimicrobial resistance of *Streptococcus pneumoniae* recovered from outpatients in the United States during the winter months of 1994 to 1995: Results of a 30-center national surveillance study. Antimicrob Agents Chemother. 1996;40:1208–1213.
86. Zeiger RS. Prospects for ancillary treatment of sinusitis in the 1990s. J Allergy Clin Immunol. 1992;478–495.
87. Coates ML, Rembold CM, Farr BM. Does pseudoephedrine increase blood pressure in patients with controlled hypertension? J Fam Pract. 1995;40:22–26.
88. Sperber SJ, Hendley JO, Hayden FG, et al. Effects of naproxen on experimental rhinovirus colds. A randomized, double-blind, controlled trial. Ann Intern Med. 1992;117:37–41.
89. Gwaltney JM Jr. Combined antiviral and antimediator treatment of rhinovirus colds. J Infect Dis. 1992;166:776–782.
90. Gwaltney JM Jr, Park J, Paul RA, et al. A randomized controlled trial of clemastine fumarate in experimental rhinovirus colds. Clin Infect Dis. 1996;22:656–662.
91. Gwaltney JM Jr, Druce HM. Efficacy of brompheniramine maleate treatment for rhinovirus colds. Clin Infect Dis. 1997;25:1188–1194.
92. Brofeldt S, Mygind N, Srrensen GH, et al. Biochemical analysis of nasal secretions induced by methacholine, histamine, and allergen provocations. Am Rev Respir Dis. 1986; 133:1138–1142.
93. Wald E. Microbiology of acute and chronic sinusitis. In: Lusk RP, ed. Pediatric Sinusitis. New York, Raven, 1992:43–47.
94. Winther B, Vickery CL, Gross CW, Hendley JO. Microbiology of the maxillary sinus in adults with chronic sinus disease. Am J Rhinol. 1996;10:347–350.
95. Kennedy DW, Senior BA, Gannon FH, et al. Histology and histomorphometry of ethmoid bone in chronic rhinosinusitis. Laryngoscope. 1998;108:502–507.
96. Kennedy D. Prognostic factors, outcomes and staging in ethmoid sinus surgery. Laryngoscope. 1992;102:1–18.
97. Proctor RA, Balwit JM, Vesga O. Variant subpopulations of *Staphylococcus aureus* as cause of persistent and recurrent infections. Infect Agents Dis. 1994;3:302–312.

Chapter 52

Epiglottitis

JAMES E. BURNS
J. OWEN HENDLEY

Acute epiglottitis (supraglottitis) is a cellulitis of the epiglottis and adjacent structures that has the potential for causing abrupt, complete airway obstruction.

The typical patient has been a 2- to 4-year-old boy having a 6- to 12-hour history of fever, irritability, dysphonia, and dysphagia, which can occur at any time of the year. However, as the use of *Haemophilus influenzae* type B conjugated vaccine increases, the typical patient is becoming an adult with a sore throat. At the time medical attention is sought, varied degrees of respiratory distress may be evident. The pediatric patient usually prefers to sit leaning forward while drooling oral secretions. Respirations tend to be tentative and careful without marked tachypnea. Tachycardia is usually commensurate with fever but may be related to hypoxia and be out of proportion to fever.[1] Inspiratory stridor and hoarseness may occur, but the barking cough and aphonia typical in croup syndrome are rare. The diagnosis is established by visualizing an edematous "cherry-red" epiglottis (Figs. 52–1 and 52–2). The course of acute epiglottitis may be fulminating, as emphasized by the report of a patient who progressed from being completely asymptomatic to having complete airway obstruction in 30 minutes.[2]

Laboratory data may include moderate leukocytosis with a "shift to the left," positive cultures of blood and epiglottis, and evidence of pneumonia on chest radiographs in up to 25% of cases.[3] A radiograph of the lateral neck may show an enlarged epiglottis, ballooning of the hypopharynx, and normal subglottic structures.[4] However, the use of radiographs in the diagnosis of epiglottitis is questionable because of both the delay in securing an airway while the films are being obtained and the variable sensitivity (as low as 3%) and false-positive rates (as high as 30%) of this procedure.[1, 5, 6] Although careful analysis of the films may be able to improve their diagnostic efficiency, their clinical usefulness is limited.[7] The epiglottis should be visualized directly, even if the radiograph is negative, in those patients in whom there is a suspicion of epiglottitis. This examination should be performed only when one is prepared to immediately secure the airway. *H. influenzae* type B is isolated from

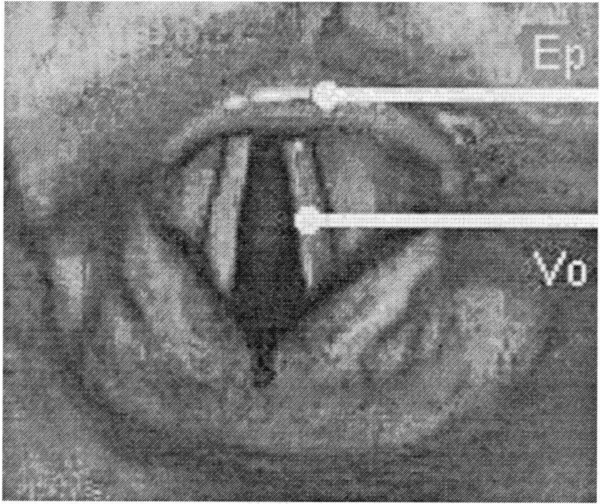

FIGURE 52–1. Normal epiglottis (Ep) and adjacent structures. *Abbreviation:* Vo, Vocal cords.

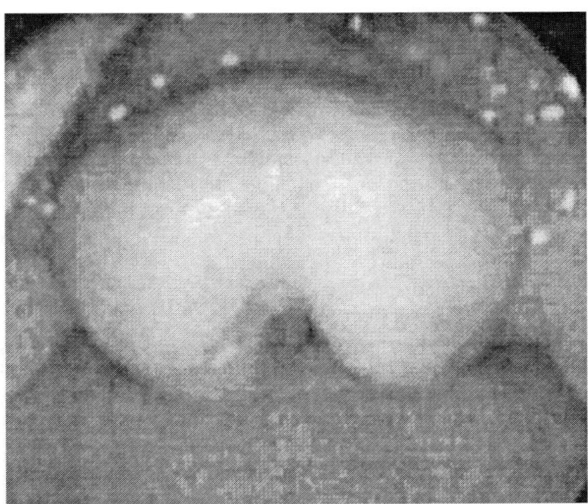

FIGURE 52–2. Epiglottitis showing a markedly enlarged epiglottis obscuring the adjacent structures. (Courtesy of Dr. Carlos Nunez, University of Miami, Miami, Fla.)

cultures of blood or epiglottis, or both, in most pediatric patients and in up to 26% of adult patients with epiglottitis.[8] Other agents occasionally implicated are pneumococci, staphylococci, and streptococci.[2, 8, 9] Establishing the etiologic role of rarer agents is difficult because of the small number of cases and the frequent lack of recovery of the same organism from both the epiglottis and the blood. Organisms can be incidentally cultured from the surface of the epiglottis or from blood without being etiologic. However, a large number of etiologic agents have been reported in association with epiglottitis (Table 52–1).[10] The role of viruses in epiglottitis, other than possible rare herpes simplex infections, has not been established.[10, 11] Patients with underlying diseases or immune system compromise appear more likely to have atypical causes.[10, 11]

H. influenzae bacteremia occurs in up to 100% of children with epiglottitis.[1] Significantly, this bacteremia has been associated with only a small number of metastatic infections such as meningitis and arthritis.[1, 2, 12]

EPIGLOTTITIS IN ADULTS

Epiglottitis in adults manifests as a sore throat with odynophagia. There is a 2:1 male predominance and variable seasonality. Most patients are in good health before the onset, but underlying conditions compromising immunity may be a factor in some patients. Up to 29% of adults at the time of diagnosis of epiglottitis had been previously seen for the same illness without the diagnosis being made, and 44% had an abnormal oropharyngeal examination without examination of the epiglottis. This emphasizes the need for a complete examination in adults with severe sore throats, which would include the epiglottis.[9] Predictors of airway compromise include sitting erect, stridor, high white blood cell counts, blood cultures positive for *H. influenzae,* and pneumonia on chest radiographs. Although the disease is generally milder in adults, Mayo-Smith and associates found the death rate for adults (3.2%) higher than that for children (2.2%).[13] In the same study, 3.7% of adults, compared with 4.5% of children, had airway obstruction on presentation. They speculated that there are two forms of disease in adults: a severe form caused by *H. influenzae* and a milder form caused by other organisms.

TABLE 52–1 Etiologic Agents That Have Been Associated with Epiglottitis

Infectious agents	*Propionibacterium*
Aspergillus	*Pseudomonas aeruginosa*
Bacteroides melaninogenicus	*Serratia marcescens*
β-Hemolytic streptococcus	*Staphylococcus aureus*
Branhamella catarrhalis	*Streptococcus milleri*
Candida albicans	*Streptococcus pneumoniae*
Citrobacter diversus	*Streptococcus pyogenes*
Cytomegalovirus	*Streptococcus viridans*
Enterobacter cloacae	Varicella-zoster virus
Epstein-Barr virus	*Vibrio vulnificus*
Escherichia coli	Chemical agents
Fusobacterium	Caustic ingestion
Haemophilus influenzae	Gastroesophageal reflux
Haemophilus parainfluenzae	Physical causes
Herpes simplex	Hot water ingestion or inhalation
Kingella kingae	Smoking illicit drugs
Klebsiella pneumoniae	Blind finger sweep
Mycobacterium tuberculosis	Laryngeal mask
Neisserria meningititis	Tonsillectomy complication
Pasteurella multocida	Other
Peptostreptococcus	Allergic reactions

DIFFERENTIAL DIAGNOSIS

The croup syndrome is the most frequent differential consideration in pediatric epiglottitis. Although the barking cough typical of croup is an infrequent feature of epiglottitis, differentiation from croup is sometimes difficult unless the epiglottis is visualized. In contrast to epiglottitis, croup is frequently preceded by an upper respiratory infection, has a more gradual onset, involves somewhat younger children (aged 3 months to 3 years), and may last up to a week. The cause is usually viral, and the area of obstruction is subglottic, whereas the epiglottis is normal. Children with croup are more likely to prefer to lie supine and do not have the dysphagia and drooling that are characteristic of epiglottitis. In croup, radiographs of the lateral neck may show the airway narrowed in the subglottic region and are likely to reveal a normal epiglottis.[4] However, such films may be falsely read as suggesting epiglottitis in up to 27% of patients.[5]

Diphtheria can be differentiated from epiglottitis by the presence of a pseudomembrane in the respiratory tract and the presence of typical organisms on direct smear and culture of the membrane. Allergic laryngeal edema (angioneurotic edema) and foreign body aspiration lack the toxic manifestations of epiglottitis and often have a history that is helpful in suspecting the correct diagnosis. Retropharyngeal abscess, peritonsillar abscess, bacterial tracheitis, epiglottic hemangioma, toxic epidermal necrolysis, and lingual tonsillitis are other rare causes of upper airway obstruction; these can usually be differentiated from epiglottitis on physical examination. Abcess formation may complicate epiglottitis.[14]

IMMUNE-COMPROMISED HOSTS

Epiglottitis may present a somewhat different clinical picture in patients with human immunodeficiency virus infection.[15] It may rarely be part of the initial presentation, the epiglottis may be "pale and floppy," the patients may demonstrate no leukocytosis, and the course may be more fulminant than in the immune-competent host.[16] Human immunodeficiency virus infection may also be associated with unique causes such as Kaposi's sarcoma[17] and organisms that are rare at this site such as *Candida.*[18]

Epiglottitis caused by rare organisms may be associated with other conditions that compromise immunity. Examples of these associations include single-case reports of polyarteritis nodosa and *Candida,* testicular cancer and *Kingella kingae,* thalassemia and *Vibrio vulnificus,* and various neoplasms and *Candida.* Necrotizing epiglottitis has been reported in leukemia with *Aspergillus* and in drug-induced neutropenia with *Escherichia coli.*[10, 17]

THERAPY

Maintenance of an adequate airway should be the primary concern as soon as the diagnosis of epiglottitis is even suspected in a child or an adult. Appropriate management of the pediatric patient with epiglottitis requires the immediate insertion of an endotracheal tube. Observation of a child with epiglottitis for signs of airway obstruction cannot be recommended, because the mortality is up to 25% in those observed and 80% in those in whom obstruction occurs.[2, 19]

Many more adults than children have been managed with observation and no artificial airway. There have been no reported cases of airway compromise precipitated by examination in adults, so all adults presenting with a severe sore throat and odynophagia should have their epiglottis examined by direct or indirect laryngoscopy.[3, 9, 13, 20] If laryngoscopy cannot be performed, a lateral neck radiograph may be obtained, but it will not always be positive in epiglottitis. Observation of an adult with epiglottitis can be dangerous.[3] Mayo-Smith and colleagues reported that only 7 of 220 adults managed with observation required an artificial airway, but 3 of these 7 died.[13] With careful observation and the ability to immediately secure an artificial airway, observation of adults without signs of airway compromise (stridor, dyspnea) may be relatively safe. Patients with higher temperatures and higher peripheral white blood cell counts warrant closer observation.

Pediatric patients even suspected of having acute epiglottitis should be handled as a medical emergency because of the potential for rapid deterioration to complete respiratory obstruction. Painful or anxiety-provoking procedures should be minimized until the airway is secured or the diagnosis has been eliminated. Patients should be allowed to maintain the posture that is most comfortable for them; separation from caregivers should be minimized. Patients being transported between medical facilities and within such facilities must be accompanied by personnel capable of securing the airway should obstruction occur.

The epiglottis can be visualized in many patients by inspection alone and in most patients by depressing the tongue with a depressor placed as far posteriorly as the tonsillar pillars. However, it may be unwise to examine the epiglottis of a pediatric patient suspected of having epiglottitis because of the possibility of precipitating complete airway obstruction or a vagally mediated cardiopulmonary arrest. This caution may, however, be more anecdotal than absolute.[3, 21] It is also unwise to restrain pediatric patients in the supine position as this may also lead to airway obstruction.[2] As a consequence, it is safer to transfer a pediatric patient thought to have epiglottitis to an operating room and to visualize the epiglottis with a laryngoscope or bronchoscope after the induction of anesthesia and after all is in readiness for the insertion of an artificial airway under controlled conditions. As soon as the diagnosis is made by visualization of the "cherry-red" epiglottis, an uncuffed endotracheal tube should be inserted. In spite of theoretical difficulties with the insertion of an endotracheal tube through the region of the inflammed epiglottis, this has generally not proved to be a problem. In rare circumstances in which difficulty is encountered, a bronchoscope may be used to secure and dilate the airway before insertion of the tube.[3, 22] If the epiglottis is normal, the patient may be managed in a manner appropriate for croup or laryngotracheobronchitis. If difficulty is encountered or if obstruction occurs while transporting the patient or while trying to establish the airway, the possibility of ventilating the apneic patient by bag and mask or mouth-to-mouth ventilation should not be overlooked.[23, 24] If these attempts are unsuccessful, a needle cricothyrotomy should be performed before a more stable airway is established.

Contrary to common belief, the sudden obstruction of the airway that can occur in epiglottitis is not due to the abrupt impaction of the edematous epiglottis into the laryngeal inlet. Instead, cellulitis of the supraglottic structures progressively narrows the airway. Airflow in the upper airways is turbulent,[25] and resistance is inversely proportional to the fifth power of the diameter.[26, 27] Therefore, reducing the airway diameter by half increases airflow resistance by 32 times. The potential abrupt airway obstruction in epiglottitis is a functional rather than a complete physical obstruction (although virtually complete physical obstruction can occur with severe edema). The airway resistance can simply exceed the patient's ability to overcome it, and this leads to respiratory failure.

After the establishment of an airway, blood and the surface of the epiglottis should be cultured, and the pediatric patient should be given intravenous antibiotic therapy directed at *H. influenzae.* In view of the risk of infection with ampicillin-resistant *H. influenzae,*[28] cefotaxime (50 to 180 mg/kg/day in four divided doses), ceftriaxone (80 to 100 mg/kg/day in two divided doses), or ampicillin-sulbactam (200 to 300 mg of ampicillin/kg/day in four divided doses) should be given as initial therapy. Adults should also receive a second- or third-generation cephalosporin.

Pediatric patients with acute epiglottitis usually improve 12 to 48 hours after the initiation of appropriate antibiotic therapy. Depending on the patient's progress, the artificial airway can usually be removed within this period.[3, 29] Before extubation the patient should be clinically improved, afebrile, and alert. The decision to extubate may be based on the clinical condition of the patient, evidence of resolution by direct visualization with a fiberoptic laryngoscope, or the presence of an air leak around the endotracheal tube. Antibiotics should be continued for 7 to 10 days. The clinical response and status of the patient should dictate the route by which the antibiotic is administered after extubation.

A small number of patients experiencing severe respiratory distress or arrest before intubation develop pulmonary edema. The cause of this complication is not known.[29, 30]

Nebulized epinephrine or steroids, or both, appear to be ineffective in epiglottitis.[9]

If the patient with *H. influenzae* epiglottitis has unvaccinated household contacts who are younger than 4 years, rifampin prophylaxis given once daily for 4 days in a dose of 20 mg/kg/day (maximum of 600 mg/day) is recommended for all household contacts, regardless of immunization status.[31] In addition, the patient should receive rifampin in the same dosage before discharge to eliminate carriage and to prevent reintroduction of the organism into the household (see Chapter 212).

IMMUNITY

An episode of *H. influenzae* epiglottis usually results in high levels of serum antibody to capsular polysaccharide.[32] This response appears to provide immunity, since second cases of epiglottitis are extremely rare. However, when epiglottitis occurs in children younger than 24 months, an age-appropriate immunization series should be completed, ignoring previously administered vaccine.[31] The presence of maternally derived serum antibody at birth explains the infrequent occurrence of *H. influenzae* infections in infants. After disappearance of this maternal antibody, there is an inverse relationship between rising naturally acquired antibody and the declining incidence of epiglottitis in unvaccinated populations.[33]

Widespread use of *H. influenzae* type B polysaccharide vaccine has dramatically decreased the incidence of invasive *H. influenzae* disease[34, 35] and epiglottitis.[36] The introduction of these vaccines began in the United States in 1985 with the polyribosyl-ribitol phosphate vaccine administered at 18 months of age. Conjugated vaccines, which were first licensed in 1987, are currently administered beginning at 2 months of age, a schedule started in 1990. Childhood vaccination will probably have little effect on the 2 in 100,000 incidence of disease in adults.[8, 9, 13] Vaccination will also not decrease *H. influenzae* disease due to serotypes other than B.

REFERENCES

1. Sendi K, Crysdale WS. Acute epiglottitis: Decade of change—a 10-year experience with 242 children. J Otolaryngol. 1987;16:196.
2. Bass JW, Steele RW, Wiebe RA. Acute epiglottitis: A surgical emergency. JAMA. 1974;229:671.
3. Andreassen UK, Baer S, Nielsen TG, et al. Acute epiglottitis—25 years experience

with nasotracheal intubation, current management policy, and future needs. J Laryngol Otol. 1992;106:1072.
4. Podgore JK, Bass JW. The "thumb sign" and "little finger sign" in acute epiglottitis. J Pediatr. 1976;88:154.
5. Stankiewicz JA, Bowes AK. Croup and epiglottitis: A radiologic study. Laryngoscope. 1985;95:1159.
6. Jones JL, Holland P. False positives in lateral neck radiographs used to diagnose epiglottitis. Ann Emerg Med. 1983;12:797.
7. Rothrock SG, Pignatiello GA, Howard RM. Radiologic diagnosis of epiglottitis: Objective criteria for all ages. Ann Emerg Med. 1990;19:978.
8. Trollfors B, Nylén O, Strangert K. Acute epiglottitis in children and adults in Sweden 1981–3. Arch Dis Child. 1990;65:491.
9. Frantz TD, Rasgon BM, Quesenberry CP. Acute epiglottitis in adults: Analysis of 129 cases. JAMA. 1994;272:1358.
10. Carey MJ. Epiglottitis in adults. Am J Emerg Med. 1996;14:421.
11. D'Angelo AJ Jr, Zweillenberg S, Oleskszyk JP, et al. Adult supraglottitis due to herpes simplex virus. J Otolaryngol. 1990;19:179.
12. Dajani AS, Asmar BI, Thirumoorthi MC. Systemic *Haemophilus influenzae* disease: An overview. J Pediatr. 1979;94:355.
13. Mayo-Smith MF, Spinale JW, Donskey CJ, et al. Acute epiglottitis: An 18-year experience in Rhode Island. Chest. 1995;108:1640.
14. Torkkeli T, Ruoppi P, Nuutinen J, Kari A. Changed clinical course and current treatment of acute epiglottitis in adults: A 12-year experience. Laryngoscope. 1994;104:1503.
15. Pedersen BK, Pedersen C. Epiglottitis as a manifestation of acute HIV infection. J Acquir Immune Defic Syndr. 1994;7:1210.
16. Rothstein SG, Persky MS, Edelman BA, et al: Epiglottitis in AIDS patients. Laryngoscope. 1989;99:389.
17. Laing RBS, Wadrop PJC, Welsby PD, Brettle RP. Stridor in patients with HIV infection. J Otolaryngol. 1995;109:1197.
18. Israel L, Sadigh M. *Candida* epiglottitis in an adult with acquired immunodeficiency syndrome treated with oral fluconazole. J Laryngol Otol. 1995;109:337.
19. Rapkin RH. Tracheostomy in epiglottitis. Pediatrics. 1973;52:426.
20. Dort JC, Frohlich AM, Tate RB. Acute epiglottitis in adults: Diagnosis and treatment in 43 patients. J Otolaryngol. 1994;23:281.
21. Mauro RD, Poole SR, Lockhart CH. Differentiation of epiglottitis from laryngotracheitis in the child with stridor. Am J Dis Child. 1988;142:679.
22. Walker P, Crysdale WS. Croup, epiglottitis, retropharyngeal abscess, and bacterial tracheitis: Evolving patterns of occurrence and care. Int Anesthesiol Clin. 1992;30:57.
23. Adair JC, Ring WH. Management of epiglottitis in children. Anesth Analg. 1975;54:622.
24. Blanc VF, Weber ML, Ludec C, et al. Acute epiglottitis in children: Management of 27 consecutive cases with nasotracheal intubation with special emphasis on anaesthetic considerations. Can Anaesth Soc J. 1977;24:1.
25. West JB. Respiratory Physiology—the Essentials. 5th ed. Baltimore: Williams & Wilkins; 1995:103.
26. Glauser SC, Glauser EM, Rusy BF. Influence of gas density and viscosity on the work of breathing. Arch Environ Health. 1969;19:654.
27. Watts AMI, McCallum MID. Acute airway obstruction following facial scalding: Differential diagnosis between a thermal and infective cause. Burns. 1996;22:570.
28. Kessler A, Wetmore RF, Marsh RR. Childhood epiglottitis in recent years. Int J Pediatr Otorhinolaryngol. 1993;25:155.
29. Butt W, Shann F, Walker C, et al. Acute epiglottitis: A different approach to management. Crit Care Med. 1988;16:43.
30. Bonadio WA, Losek JD. The characteristics of children with epiglottitis who develop the complication of pulmonary edema. Arch Otolaryngol Head Neck Surg. 1991;117:205.
31. Committee on Infectious Diseases, American Academy of Pediatrics. Report of the Committee on Infectious Diseases. 24th ed. Evanston, Ill. American Academy of Pediatrics; 1994.
32. Whisnant JK, Rogentine GN, Gralnick MA, et al. Host factors and antibody response in *Haemophilus influenzae* type b meningitis and epiglottitis. J Infect Dis. 1976;133:448.
33. Schneerson R, Rodrigues LP, Parke JC Jr, Robbins JB. Immunity to disease caused by *Hemophilus influenzae* type b. J Immunol. 1971;107:1081.
34. Centers for Disease Control and Prevention. Progress toward elimination of *Haemophilus influenzae* type b disease among infants and children—United States, 1987–1995. MMWR Morb Mortal Wkly Rep. 1996;45:901.
35. Adams WG, Deaver KA, Cochi SL, et al: Decline of childhood *Haemophilus influenzae* type b (Hib) disease in the Hib vaccine era. JAMA. 1993;269:221.
36. Takala AK, Petola H, Eskola J. Disappearance of epiglottitis during large-scale vaccination with *Haemophilus influenzae* type b conjugate vaccine among children in Finland. Laryngoscope. 1994;104:731.

Chapter 53

Infections of the Oral Cavity, Neck, and Head

ANTHONY W. CHOW

Infections of the oral cavity most commonly are odontogenic in origin and include dental caries, pulpitis, periapical abscess, gingivitis, and periodontal and deep fascial space infections. Although rare, such life-threatening complications as intracranial, retropharyngeal, or pleuropulmonary extension and hematogenous dissemination to heart valves, prosthetic devices, and other metastatic foci clearly indicate the potentially serious nature of these infections. Nonodontogenic infections of the oral cavity include ulcerative and gangrenous stomatitis and infection of the major salivary glands. Suppurative orofacial infections can also arise from the middle ear, oronasopharynx, and mastoids and paranasal sinuses; these have been discussed in Chapters 50 and 51, respectively.

Infections of the neck and head in the adult most commonly result from human or animal bites, trauma, irradiation, and surgical procedures. In children, cervical adenitis or thyroiditis due to bacterial or viral causes are more common. Rarely do embryologic cysts in the neck region become secondarily infected. These are considered separately from oral infections, since they frequently involve a different microflora and require alternative approaches to diagnosis and therapy.

OROFACIAL ODONTOGENIC INFECTIONS

Microbiologic Considerations

The microbiota associated with odontogenic infections is complex and generally reflects the indigenous oral flora. Despite this complexity, recent evidence strongly supports a causative role of specific microorganisms in different forms of odontogenic infections. This emerging concept of specific microbial cause has created a considerable dilemma in our traditional approach to the diagnosis and management of such infections. Since the microflora associated with these infections is typically polymicrobial, it does not necessarily follow that each component of this complex flora has equal pathogenic potential or that the numerically predominant cultivatable microflora are the most important. Furthermore, it may not be necessary to eradicate the complete microflora for effective therapy. An appreciation of the indigenous oral flora and the host factors that may modify its composition and knowledge of the specific microorganisms implicated in different odontogenic infections should therefore greatly assist in a more rational approach to such infections arising from the oral cavity.

Indigenous Oral Flora

The oral cavity cannot be regarded as a single, uniform environment. Although representative species of microorganisms can be isolated from most areas of the mouth, certain sites such as the tongue, tooth surface, gingival crevice, and saliva tend to favor colonization by specific organisms (Table 53–1).[1–3] Quantitative studies indicate that obligate anaerobes constitute a large and important part of the residential oral flora. In the gingival crevice of healthy adults, for example, the total microscopic counts averaged 2.7×10^{11} microorganisms/g wet weight.[4] The total cultivatable anaerobic bacteria averaged 1.8×10^{11} microorganisms/g, whereas facultative bacteria averaged 2.2×10^{10} microorganisms/g, an eightfold difference. Overall, *Streptococcus, Peptostreptococcus, Veillonella, Lacto-*

TABLE 53–1 Predominant Cultivatable Bacteria from Various Sites of the Oral Cavity

Type	Predominant Genus or Family	Total Viable Count (Mean %)			
		Gingival Crevice	*Dental Plaque*	*Tongue*	*Saliva*
Facultative					
Gram-positive cocci	*Streptococcus*	28.8	28.2	44.8	46.2
	S. mutans	(0–30)	(0–50)	(0–1)	(0–1)
	S. sanguis	(10–20)	(40–60)	(10–20)	(10–30)
	S. mitior	(10–30)	(20–40)	(10–30)	(30–50)
	S. salivarius	(0–1)	(0–1)	(40–60)	(40–60)
Gram-positive rods	*Lactobacillus*	15.3	23.8	13.0	11.8
	Corynebacterium				
Gram-negative cocci	*Moraxella*	0.4	0.4	3.4	1.2
Gram-negative rods	Enterobacteriaceae	1.2	ND	3.2	2.3
Anaerobic					
Gram-positive cocci	*Peptostreptococcus*	7.4	12.6	4.2	13.0
Gram-positive rods	*Actinomyces*				
	Eubacterium				
	Lactobacillus	20.2	18.4	8.2	4.8
	Leptotrichia				
Gram-negative cocci	*Veillonella*	10.7	6.4	16.0	15.9
		16.1	10.4	8.2	4.8
Gram-negative rods	*Fusobacterium*	1.9	4.1	0.7	0.3
	Prevotella or *Porphyromonas*	4.7	ND	0.2	ND
	Bacteroides	5.6	4.8	5.1	2.4
	Campylobacter	3.8	1.3	2.2	2.1
Spirochetes	*Treponema*	1.0	ND	ND	ND

Abbreviation: ND, Not detected.
Data from refs. 1–3.

bacillus, Corynebacterium, and *Actinomyces* account for more than 80% of the total cultivatable oral flora. Facultative gram-negative rods are uncommon in healthy adults but may be more prominent in seriously ill, hospitalized, and elderly patients.[5] Unique ecologic niches are observed. For example, *Streptococcus sanguis, Streptococcus mutans,* and *Streptococcus mitis* as well as *Actinomyces viscosus* preferentially colonize the tooth surface.[6] In contrast, *Streptococcus salivarius* and *Veillonella* spp. have a predilection for the tongue and buccal mucosa.[2] *Fusobacterium,* pigmented *Bacteroides* (*Porphyromonas* and *Prevotella*) and anaerobic spirochetes appear concentrated in the gingival crevice.[2] Factors that appear to govern these localization patterns include selective adherence characteristics of certain bacteria for various types of cells, local environmental conditions such as oxygen tension, oxidation-reduction potential (Eh) and pH, interbacterial coaggregation, and microbial inhibition.[2, 7, 8] Apart from anatomic considerations, numerous factors such as age, diet and nutrition, eruption of deciduous dentition, oral hygiene, smoking habits, the presence of dental caries or periodontal disease, antimicrobial therapy, hospitalization, pregnancy, and genetic and racial factors may influence the composition of the oral flora.[2, 6–8]

Microbial Specificity in Odontogenic Infections

Although it had been recognized for some time that odontogenic infections are initiated by microorganisms through the establishment of dental plaques, the microbial specificity of these infections was not fully appreciated until recently. This breakthrough was brought about by technologic advances in sampling and anaerobic culture of specimens as well as by improved methods for species identification and taxonomy.[9, 10] Important differences in bacterial compositions have been noted for dental caries, gingivitis, and different forms of periodontitis when compared with cultures from healthy tissues.[11, 12] An etiologic association of *S. mutans* in dental caries has been firmly established.[13, 14] *Streptococcus mutans* is the only organism consistently isolated from all decayed dental fissures and is the only organism consistently found in greater numbers in carious compared with noncarious teeth. The infectious and transmissible nature of this organism in dental caries has been demonstrated in both experimental animals and longitudinal studies in humans. Similarly, in gingivitis and periodontitis, a unique and specific bacterial composition of the subgingival plaque has been identified. In the healthy periodontium, the microflora is sparse and consists mainly of gram-positive organisms such as *Streptococcus oralis, S. sanguis,* and *Actinomyces* spp. In the presence of gingivitis, the predominant subgingival flora shifts to a greater proportion of anaerobic gram-negative rods, and *Prevotella intermedia* (formerly *Bacteroides intermedius*), *Capnocytophaga* spp., and *Peptostreptococcus* spp. are most commonly isolated.[11, 12, 15] With established periodontitis, the flora further increases in complexity, with a preponderance of anaerobic gram-negative and motile organisms and spirochetes (*Treponema denticola*).[11, 16] *Porphyromonas gingivalis* (formerly *Bacteroides gingivalis*), *Actinobacillus actinomycetemcomitans, Bacteroides forsythus, P. intermedia,* and *T. denticola* are most commonly isolated. In juvenile periodontitis, a clinical variant seen primarily in adolescents, the subgingival plaque mainly consists of saccharolytic organisms, with *A. actinomycetemcomitans* and *Capnocytophaga* spp. as the most common identifiable species. *P. gingivalis* is rarely found in this condition.[12, 17] In suppurative odontogenic infections such as periapical abscesses or deep fascial space infections, a polymicrobial flora is usually present, with *Fusobacterium nucleatum,* pigmented *Bacteroides, Peptostreptococcus, Actinomyces,* and *Streptococcus* as the most predominant isolates.[1, 17] Except in selected patients with serious underlying illnesses, facultative gram-negative bacilli and *Staphylococcus aureus* are uncommonly isolated.[18]

This microbial specificity demonstrated for different odontogenic infections probably reflects the acquisition of a unique microflora during the development of a supragingival dental plaque and its progression to a subgingival dental plaque.[19, 20] Plaques that accumulate above the gingival margin are composed mainly of gram-positive facultative and microaerophilic cocci and rods; plaques that accumulate below the gingival margin are composed mainly of gram-negative anaerobic rods and motile forms including spirochetes (Fig. 53–1). Microorganisms residing within the supragingival plaque are characterized by their ability to adhere to the tooth surface and by their saccharolytic activity. Microorganisms in the subgingival plaque are frequently asaccharolytic and need not be adherent.

Pathogenetic Mechanisms

Suppurative orofacial infections are usually preceded by dental caries or periodontal disease. The pathogenetic mechanisms of cariogenesis

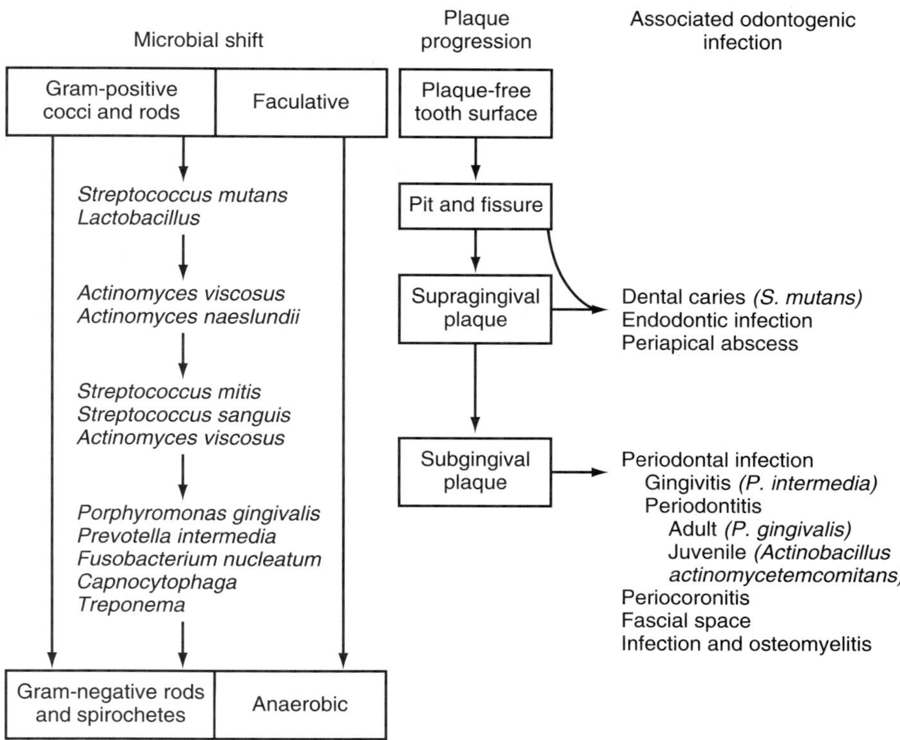

FIGURE 53–1. Microbial specificity in odontogenic infections. A unifying hypothesis demonstrating a microbial shift from a plaque-free tooth surface and progression to supragingival and subgingival plaque organisms. (Modified from Chow, AW. Odontogenic infections. In: Schlossberg D, ed. Infections of the Head and Neck. New York: Springer; 1987: 148.)

remain poorly defined. The most universally accepted theory is that originated by W. D. Miller in 1882, which proposes that bacterial action on carbohydrates produces acidic substances that cause demineralization and dissolution of the hard tissues of the tooth.[20, 21] In order for dental caries to develop three factors need to be present: (1) a susceptible tooth surface (host factors), (2) acidogenic (acid-producing) and aciduric (able to grow at low pH) bacteria within a dental plaque (microbial factors), and (3) simple sugars and other carbohydrates (dietary factors). In the healthy host, at least three mechanisms protect the tooth from carious decay: (1) the cleaning action of the tongue and buccal membranes, which removes any food particles from the proximity of the tooth; (2) the buffering effect of saliva, which has a neutral pH, washes away bacterial acids, and provides essential substrates for remineralization and repair of damaged tooth surfaces; and (3) the protective effect of an acellular bacteria-free coating of salivary origin on the tooth surface, known as the *acquired pellicle,* which acts as a surface barrier to most dietary and bacterial acids and other proteolytic substances. In the absence of tooth brushing and flossing, the acquired pellicle becomes rapidly colonized and is replaced by the bacterial plaque. It is not surprising, therefore, that carious lesions occur most often in areas inaccessible to the self-cleaning mechanisms of the mouth and on the occlusal surfaces and interproximal sites that are protected from the reaches of the toothbrush.

Unlike its effect on dental caries, diet does not appear to have a significant role in the pathogenesis of periodontal disease. The periodontal microflora associated with the subgingival plaque have the ability to penetrate the gingival epithelium and elicit an inflammatory host response that ultimately results in destruction of the periodontium.[11, 16, 19–22] Two major predisposing factors are poor oral hygiene and increasing age. Other factors include hormonal effects, with exacerbation of disease activity during puberty, menstruation, and pregnancy.[23, 24] Diabetes mellitus causes an increased incidence, particularly in juvenile diabetic patients. Finally, various genetic disorders are associated with an increased incidence of periodontal disease.[25] In particular, those with neutrophil defects (such as Chédiak-Higashi syndrome, agranulocytosis, cyclic neutropenia, and Down syndrome) have a higher incidence of periodontal disease.[26]

It is a tribute to the local defenses in the healthy host that infections within the oral cavity are not more common. The establishment of the normal resident flora appears to be particularly important in providing a strong mucosal defense against colonization and invasion by potential pathogens *(colonization resistance).*[27] Other nonspecific local defenses include the continuous cell shedding and turnover of the mucosal epithelium and the constant flow of saliva containing lysozyme, lactoferrin, β-lysin, lactoperoxidase, and other antimicrobial systems.[27] Various salivary glycoproteins and histidine-rich polypeptides have been reported to inhibit bacteria and fungi and may prevent infection by the inhibition of microbial attachment to oral epithelium by way of competition for cellular receptor sites or clumping of microorganisms. The epithelial barrier may be affected by radiation therapy, cancer chemotherapy, or trauma. A reduced turnover rate of the epithelial cells allows retention of adherent organisms. A reduction in saliva volume also has significant effects on the oral environment and predisposes to microbial invasion. In addition to nonspecific host defenses, specific humoral and cellular immune mechanisms are also important. Specific antibodies are present in saliva, with secretory immunoglobulin A (IgA) as the predominant immunoglobulin.[28] Salivary antibodies may affect the oral flora by the aggregation of organisms and the prevention of their attachment to mucosal epithelium. Cell-mediated immunity is important in oral defense against intracellular pathogens, including viruses, fungi, and bacteria. In the severely immunocompromised patient, a reactivation of viral infection involving the oral cavity is common, often with potentially life-threatening complications.[29] In addition to humoral and cellular immunity, various phagocytic cells in the oral mucosa also appear important. Phagocytic cells such as lymphocytes, granulocytes, and macrophages are abundant in the lamina propria and presumably contribute to the removal of foreign matter that has breached the epithelial barrier. Unique defects in host defenses have been identified in periodontal infections.[19] For example, impairment of neutrophil chemotaxis has been demonstrated in patients with juvenile periodontitis.[30] A number of oral anaerobes and streptococci implicated in periodontitis including *P. gingivalis, P. intermedia, Prevotella melaningogenica, Capnocytophaga* spp., *S. sanguis,* and *S. mitis* are found to secrete IgA proteases.[31] The pathogenic significance of this finding is uncertain at present; it has been suggested that cleavage of IgA by microbial IgA proteases may impair local mucosal immunity of the host. It remains to be seen if similar or other defects of host resistance can be identified in different forms of destructive odontogenic infections.

Anatomic Considerations

Soft tissue infections of odontogenic origin tend to spread along planes of least resistance from the supporting structures of the affected tooth to various potential spaces in the vicinity. Accumulated pus, therefore, must generally perforate bone at the site where it is thinnest and weakest before it extends into the periapical areas or deeper fascial spaces. In the mandible, this is usually in the region of the molar teeth on the lingual aspect and more anterior on the buccal aspect.[32] In the maxilla, the bone is weakest on the buccal aspect throughout and relatively thicker on the palatal aspect. If pus perforates through either the maxillary or the mandibular buccal plate, it presents intraorally if inside the attachment of the buccinator muscle to the maxilla or mandible and extraorally if outside this muscle attachment (Fig. 53–2). When a mandibular infection perforates lingually, it presents in the sublingual space if the apices of the involved teeth lie above the attachment of the mylohyoid muscle (e.g., mandibular incisor, canines, premolars, and first molars) and in the submandibular space if below the attachment of this muscle (e.g., second and third molars) (see Fig. 53–2). Thus, these local anatomic barriers of bone, muscle, and fascia predetermine the routes of spread, extent, and clinical manifestations of many orofacial infections of odontogenic origin. The clinically important "fascial spaces" most often involved are illustrated in Figures 53–3 and 53–4. These are potential spaces between layers of fascia normally bound together by loose connective tissue. The breakdown of these attachments by a spreading infective process results in a fascial space infection. These spaces intercommunicate with one another to varied degrees, and the potential pathways of extension from one space to another are illustrated in Figure 53–5. A thorough understanding of the potential *anatomic routes* of infection not only provides valuable information on the nature and extent of infection but also suggests the optimal surgical approach for effective drainage.

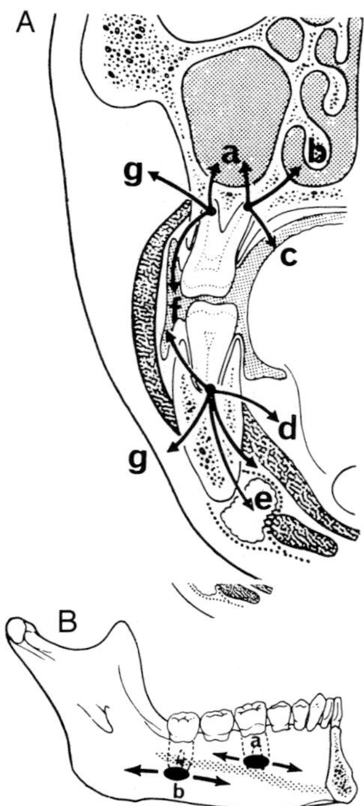

FIGURE 53–2. Routes of spread of odontogenic orofacial infections along planes of least resistance. *A,* Coronal section in the region of the first molar teeth: a, maxillary antrum; b, nasal cavity; c, palatal plate; d, sublingual space (above the mylohyoid muscle); e, submandibular space (below the mylohyoid muscle); f, intraoral presentation with infection spreading through the buccal plates inside the attachment of the buccinator muscle; g, extraoral presentation to buccal space with infection spreading through the buccal plates outside the attachment of the buccinator muscle. *B,* Lingual aspect of the mandible: a, apices of the involved tooth above the mylohyoid muscle, with spread of infection to the sublingual space; b, apices of involved tooth below the mylohyoid muscle, with spread of infection into the submandibular space. (From Chow AW, Roser SM, Brady FA. Orofacial odontogenic infections. Ann Intern Med. 1978; 88:392.)

Clinical Presentations

Odontogenic infections originate in either the dental pulp or the periodontium. The most common site is the dental pulp and results in dentoalveolar infections.

Dentoalveolar Infections

Pulpal infection most frequently results from carious exposure, rarely from physical or chemical injury. The carious process most frequently begins in pits and fissures on the occlusal surfaces of molars and premolars, which encourage food retention. Interproximal sites and the gingival margin are the next most common. Demineralization of the enamel results in discoloration, the first visible evidence of carious involvement. Destruction of the enamel and dentin and invasion of the pulp produce either a localized or a generalized pulpitis. If drainage from the pulp is obstructed, a rapid progression with pulpal necrosis and proliferation of endodontic microorganisms leads to invasion of the periapical areas (periapical abscess) and alveolar bone (acute alveolar abscess).

Clinically, the tooth is sensitive to percussion and to both heat and cold during early or reversible pulpitis, although the painful response stops abruptly when the stimulus is withdrawn. During late or irreversible pulpitis, the tooth is exquisitely painful to a hot stimulus, with prompt relief by the application of cold. If drainage is established through the tooth before extension into the periapical region, chronic irritation from the necrotic pulp may result in periapical granuloma or cyst formation that may be relatively asymptomatic. Dental radiographs are particularly helpful for the detection of silent lesions, particularly those caused by interproximal caries, which are difficult to detect clinically.

The principles of treatment in dentoalveolar infections include prompt elimination of the infected pulp, deep periodontal scaling, or extraction of the affected tooth. Dentoalveolar abscess should be surgically drained at the same time. Other supportive measures include hydration, a soft diet, analgesics, and oral hygiene. Antibiotic therapy is indicated primarily if drainage cannot be adequately established or when infection has perforated the cortex and spread into surrounding soft tissue.

Gingivitis and Periodontal Infections

Periodontal disease is a general term that refers to all diseases involving the supporting structures of the teeth (periodontium), which include the gingiva, periodontal ligament, alveolar bone, and cementum. In the early phase of periodontal disease, infection is confined to the gingiva (gingivitis). Later, the underlying supporting tissues are affected (periodontitis), ultimately leading to complete

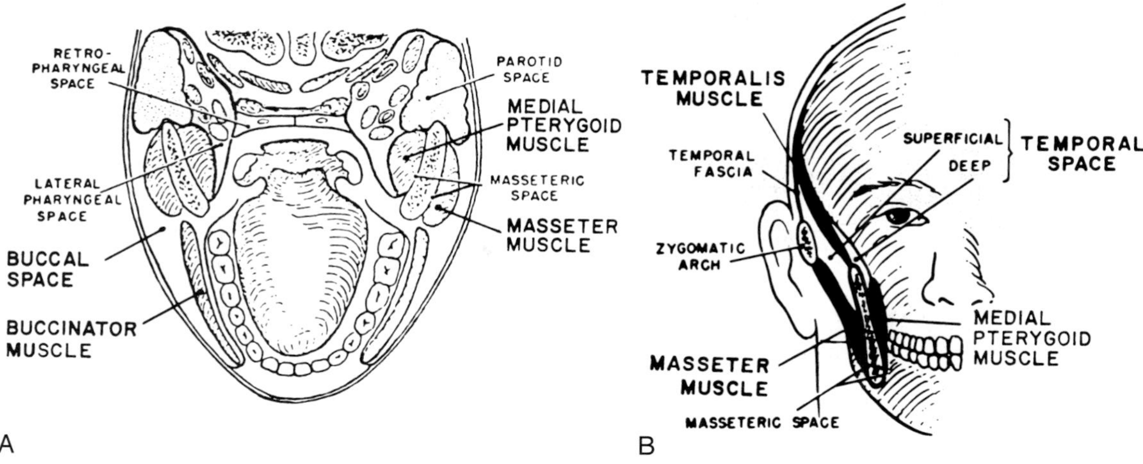

FIGURE 53–3. Fascial spaces around the mouth and face. *A,* Horizontal section at the level of the occlusal surface of the mandibular teeth. *B,* Frontal view of the face. (From Chow AW, Roser SM, Brady FA. Orofacial odontogenic infections. Ann Intern Med. 1978; 88:392.)

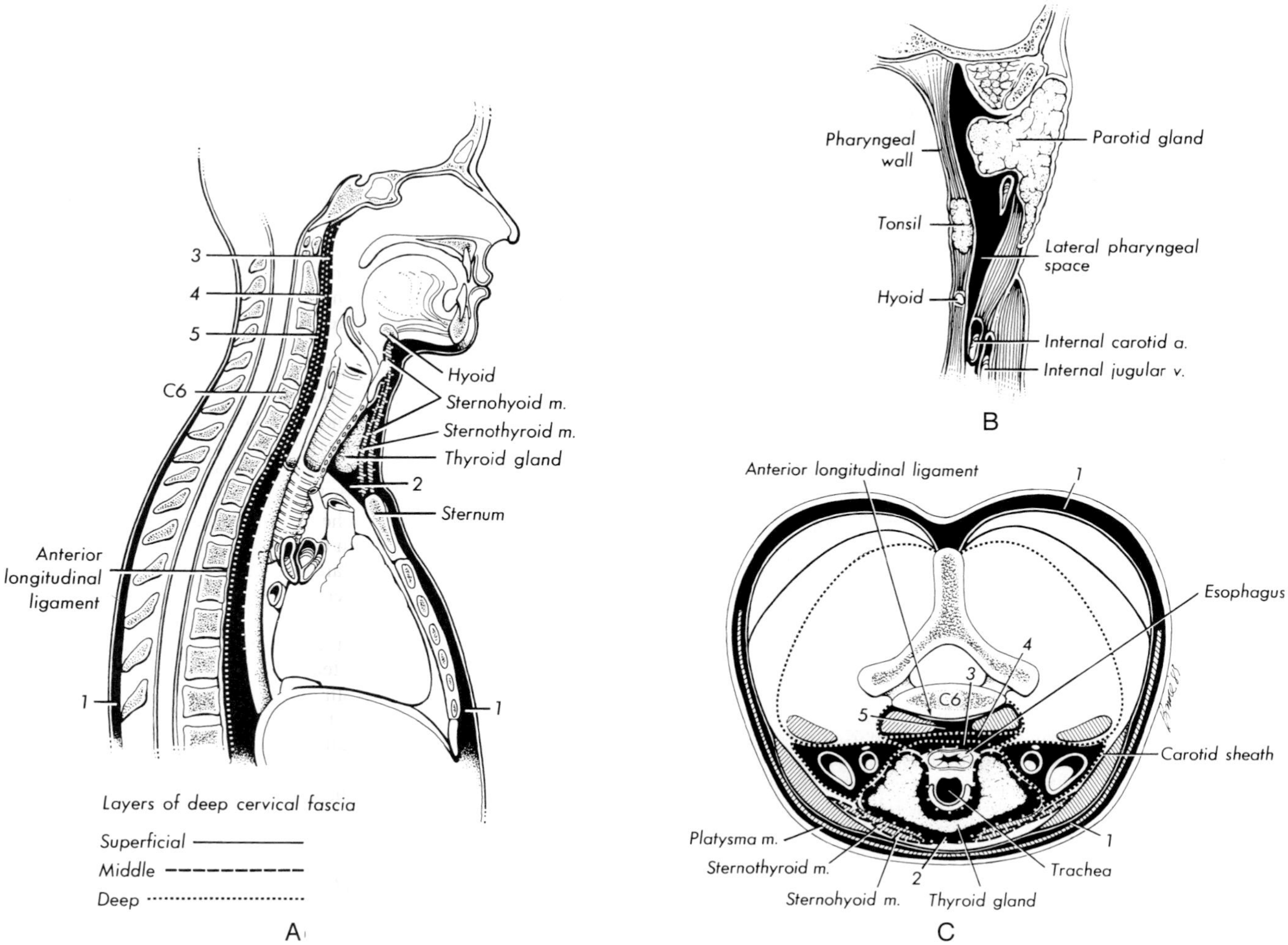

FIGURE 53–4. Relation of lateral pharyngeal, retropharyngeal, and prevertebral spaces to the posterior and anterior layers of the deep cervical fascia. 1: Superficial space; 2: pretracheal space; 3: retropharyngeal space; 4: "danger" space; 5: prevertebral space. *A,* Midsagittal section of the head and neck. *B,* Coronal section in the suprahyoid region of the neck. *C,* Cross-section of the neck at the level of the thyroid isthmus.

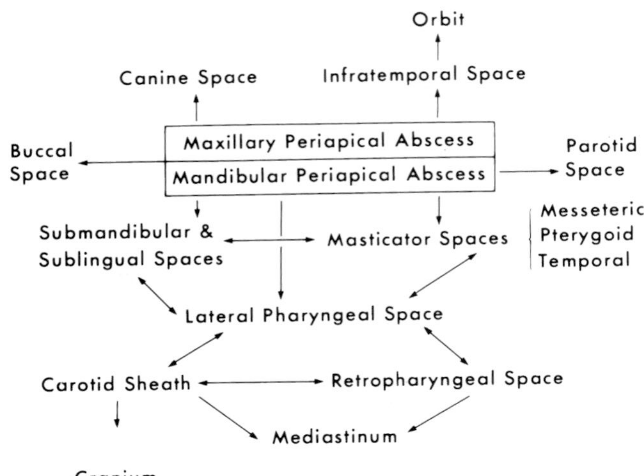

FIGURE 53–5. Potential pathways of extension in deep fascial space infections.

destruction of the periodontium and a permanent loss of teeth. Periodontal infections tend to localize in intraoral soft tissues and seldom spread into deeper structures of the face or neck.

Gingivitis. Acute and chronic inflammation of the gingiva is initiated by local irritation and microbial invasion.[11, 16, 26] Subgingival plaque is always present. In simple gingivitis, there is a bluish-red discoloration, with swelling and thickening of the free gingival margin. A tendency for bleeding of the gums after eating or toothbrushing may be one of the earliest findings. There is usually no pain, but a mild fetor oris may be noticed. In acute necrotizing ulcerative gingivitis (Vincent's disease, or trench mouth), the patient typically experiences a sudden onset of pain in the gingiva that interferes with normal mastication. Necrosis of the gingiva occurs mainly in the interdental papilla and results in a marginated, punched-out, and eroded appearance. A superficial grayish pseudomembrane is formed, and a characteristic halitosis with altered taste sensation is present. There is usually associated fever, malaise, and regional lymphadenopathy. Treatment includes local débridement and lavage with oxidizing agents, which usually brings relief from pain within 24 hours. Antibiotic therapy with penicillin or metronidazole is indicated and is highly effective.[33, 34]

Periodontitis. Chronic inflammation of the periodontium is the major cause of tooth loss in adults. The destructive process proceeds insidiously, usually beginning in early adulthood. Subgingival plaque is always present, and both supragingival and subgingival calculi are usually abundant. Unlike pulpal infection in which drainage is frequently obstructed, periodontal infections drain freely, and patients experience little or no discomfort. Associated sensations include pressure and an itchy feeling in the gums and between the teeth, a bad taste in the mouth, hot and cold sensitivity, and vague pains in the jaws. The gingiva is inflamed and discolored, bleeds readily, and presents as periodontal pockets around the affected teeth. Frank pus can be readily expressed by digital pressure or may exude freely from the pockets. As periodontitis advances, the supporting tissues are destroyed, ultimately leading to loosening and exfoliation of teeth. Localized juvenile periodontitis is a particularly destructive form of periodontitis seen in adolescents and is characterized by rapid vertical bone loss affecting the first molar and incisor teeth. Plaque is usually minimal, and calculus is absent. A specific defect with impaired neutrophil chemotaxis has been demonstrated in this condition. Recent experience suggests excellent therapeutic results with systemic tetracycline or metronidazole therapy combined with local periodontal treatment involving root débridement and surgical resection of inflamed periodontal tissues.[19, 35–37]

Periodontal Abscess. Periodontal abscesses may be focal or diffuse and present as red, fluctuant swelling of the gingiva, which is extremely tender to palpation. These abscesses are always in communication with a periodontal pocket from which pus can be readily expressed after probing. Treatment is surgical and aimed at drainage of loculated pus.

Pericoronitis. Pericoronitis is an acute localized infection associated with gum flaps overlying a partially erupted or impacted wisdom tooth. Food debris and microorganisms become entrapped under the affected gingival tissues. If drainage is interrupted due to sudden swelling or trauma, infection extends along fascial planes of least resistance into adjacent soft tissues. The underlying alveolar bone is usually not involved. Clinically, the pericoronal tissues are erythematous and swollen. Digital pressure produces a small amount of exudate from under the infected flap. Since the masticator spaces are often involved, marked trismus secondary to irritation of the masseter or medial pterygoid muscle is a prominent presenting feature. Treatment of pericoronitis includes gentle débridement and irrigation under the tissue flap. The use of antibiotics and incision and drainage may be necessary if cellulitis of fascial planes occurs. Excision of the operculum or extraction of the involved tooth may also be considered.

Deep Fascial Space Infections

Infections of either odontogenic or oropharyngeal origin may extend to potential fascial spaces of the lower part of the head and upper portion of the neck. These "space infections" can be conveniently divided into those around the face (masticator, buccal, canine, and parotid spaces), those in the suprahyoid region (submandibular, sublingual, and lateral pharyngeal spaces), and those involving the infrahyoid region or the total neck (retropharyngeal, "danger," and pretracheal spaces).[18, 32]

Masticator Spaces. Masticator spaces consist of the masseteric, pterygoid, and temporal spaces, all of which are well differentiated but intercommunicate with each other as well as with the buccal, submandibular, and lateral pharyngeal spaces (see Fig. 53–3). Infection of the masticator spaces occurs most frequently from molar teeth, particularly the third molars (wisdom teeth). Clinically, the hallmark of masticator space infection is trismus and pain in the area of the body or ramus of the mandible. Swelling may not be a prominent finding, especially in the masseteric compartment, since infection exists deep in large muscle masses, which obscures or prevents clinically apparent swelling. When present, swelling tends to be brawny and indurated, which suggests the possibility of cervicofacial actinomycosis or mandibular osteomyelitis. If infection extends internally, it can involve an area close to the lateral pharyngeal wall and result in dysphagia. A true lateral pharyngeal space infection, however, is accompanied by displacement of the lateral pharyngeal wall toward the midline and is a finding not present in masticator space infections. Infection of the deep temporal space usually originates from involvement of the posterior maxillary molar teeth. Very little external swelling is observed early in the course; if present, it usually affects the preauricular region and an area over the zygomatic arch. As infection progresses, the cheek, eyelids, and whole side of the face may be involved (Fig. 53–6). Infection may extend directly into the orbit via the inferior orbital fissure and produce proptosis, optic neuritis, and abducens nerve palsy.

Buccal, Canine, and Parotid Spaces. As noted previously, infections arising from mandibular or maxillary bicuspid and molar teeth tend to extend in a lateral or buccal direction. The relation of the root apices to the origins of the buccinator muscle determines whether infection will exit intraorally into the buccal vestibule or extraorally into the buccal space (see Fig. 52–2). Infection of the buccal space is readily diagnosed because of marked cheek swelling with minimal trismus and systemic symptoms. There is a great tendency to resolu-

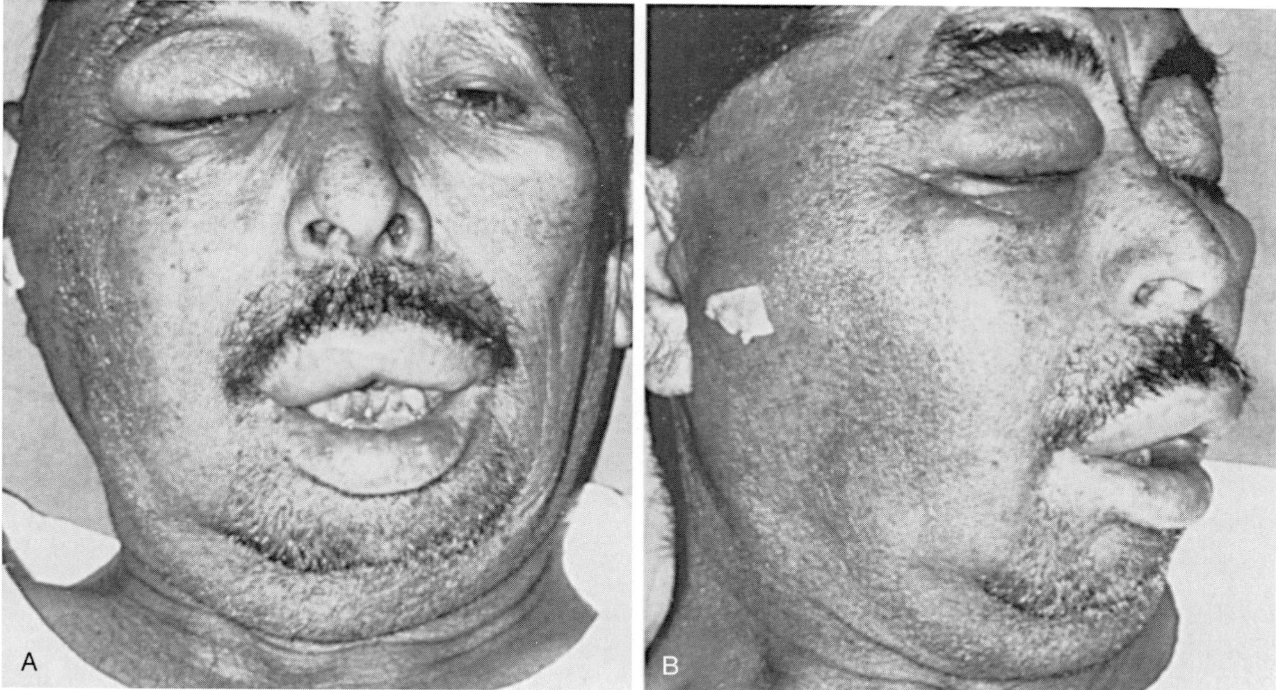

FIGURE 53–6. Deep temporal space infection with spread to the right parotid space and the orbit. This patient developed right optic neuritis with permanent loss of vision in that eye. *A,* Frontal view. *B,* Lateral view. (From Chow AW, Roser SM, Brady FA. Orofacial odontogenic infections. Ann Intern Med. 1978; 88:392.)

tion with antibiotic therapy alone. Drainage, if required, is superficial and should be performed extraorally. Involvement of the maxillary incisors and canines may result in a canine space infection, which presents as dramatic swelling of the upper lip, canine fossa, and frequently the periorbital tissues. Pain is usually moderate, and systemic signs are minimal. Occasionally, a purulent maxillary sinusitis may result due to direct extension of infection into the adjoining antrum. Treatment consists of antibiotics and drainage, which can be accomplished intraorally. Parotid space infection from an odontogenic cause generally represents secondary spread from a masseteric space infection in the area of the ramus of the mandible (see Fig. 53–3). There is marked swelling of the angle of the jaw without associated trismus. Pain may be intense and accompanied by high fever and chills. Because of its close relationship with the posterior aspect of the lateral pharyngeal space, a parotid space infection carries the potential risk of direct extension into the danger and visceral spaces and hence to the posterior mediastinum (see Fig. 53–4).

Submandibular and Sublingual Spaces. These two spaces are separated by the mylohyoid muscle (see Fig. 53–2), and the submandibular space is further divided into the submaxillary and submental spaces. Infection in these spaces usually arises from the second and third mandibular molar teeth since their root apices lie inferior to the mylohyoid muscle. There is typical swelling, although much less trismus in contradistinction to masseteric space infection, since the major muscles of mastication are usually not involved. Submandibular odontogenic infection should be distinguished from submandibular sialadenitis and lymphadenitis that are due to other causes. Therapy includes antibiotics, dental extraction, and extraoral surgical drainage. Infection of the sublingual space generally arises from mandibular incisors, since their root apices lie above the mylohyoid muscle. Clinically, this space infection presents as a brawny, erythematous, tender swelling of the floor of the mouth that begins close to the mandible and spreads toward the midline or beyond. Some elevation of the tongue may be noted in late states. Surgical drainage of the sublingual space should be performed intraorally by an incision through the mucosa parallel to Wharton's duct. If the submandibular space is also to be drained, both spaces can be reached through a submandibular approach.

The term *Ludwig's angina* has been loosely applied to a heterogenous array of infections involving the sublingual, submaxillary, and submandibular spaces.[38] However, for therapeutic and prognostic purposes, it is desirable to restrict this diagnosis to cases that conform to the following classic description: (1) the infection is always bilateral, (2) both the submandibular and sublingual spaces are involved, (3) the infection is a rapidly spreading indurated cellulitis without abscess formation or lymphatic involvement, and (4) the infection begins in the floor of the mouth. A dental source of infection has been found in 50 to 90% of reported cases. The second and third mandibular molars are most commonly involved. Clinically, patients present with a brawny boardlike swelling in the submandibular spaces that does not pit on pressure (Fig. 53–7). The mouth is usually held open and the floor elevated, which pushes the tongue to the roof of the mouth. Eating and swallowing are difficult, and respiration may be impaired by obstruction from the tongue. A rapid progression of the infection results in edema of the neck and glottis and may precipitate asphyxiation. Fever and systemic toxicity are usually present and may be severe. Treatment requires high doses of parenteral antibiotics, airway monitoring, early intubation or tracheostomy when required, soft tissue decompression, and surgical drainage.

Lateral Pharyngeal Space. The lateral pharyngeal space (also known as the pharyngomaxillary space) in the lateral aspect of the neck is shaped like an inverted cone, with its base at the skull and its apex at the hyoid bone (see Fig. 53–4). Its medial wall is contiguous with the carotid sheath, and it lies deep to the pharyngeal constrictor muscle. Infection of the lateral pharyngeal space may result from pharyngitis, tonsillitis, parotitis, otitis, or mastoiditis, as well as odontogenic infection, especially if the masticator spaces are primarily involved. If the anterior compartment is infected, the patient

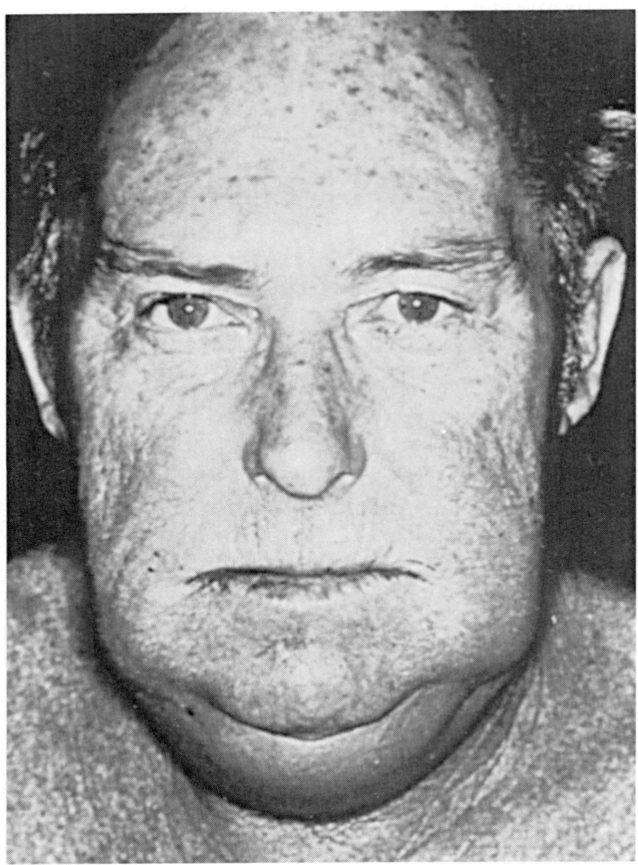

FIGURE 53–7. Early appearance of a patient with Ludwig's angina with a brawny, boardlike swelling in the submandibular spaces. (From Chow AW, Roser SM, Brady FA. Orofacial odontogenic infections. Ann Intern Med. 1978; 88:392.)

exhibits fever, chills, marked pain, trismus, swelling below the angle of the mandible, dysphagia, and medial displacement of the lateral pharyngeal wall. Although not prominent, dyspnea can occur. Posterior compartment infection is characterized by septicemia with little pain or trismus. Swelling is usually internal and deep and can often be missed because it is behind the palatopharyngeal arch. Complications, particularly if the posterior compartment is involved, include respiratory obstruction from edema of the larynx, thrombosis of the internal jugular vein, and erosion of the internal carotid artery. Because respiratory obstruction from laryngeal edema can occur suddenly, the patient must be closely observed, and prophylactic tracheostomy may be required. Treatment includes high levels of antibiotics and surgical drainage. It is usually prudent to wait for the infection to localize before drainage is attempted unless respiratory obstruction or hemorrhage necessitates early surgical intervention.

Retropharyngeal, Danger, and Pretracheal Spaces. The retropharyngeal space comprises the posterior part of the visceral compartment in which the esophagus, trachea, and thyroid glands are enclosed by the middle layer of deep cervical fascia (see Fig. 53–4). It lies behind the hypopharynx and the esophagus and extends inferiorly into the superior mediastinum to about the level from T1 to T2. Posterior to this compartment lies the danger space, which descends directly into the posterior mediastinum to the level of the diaphragm. Infection of the retropharyngeal space may result from contiguous infection of the lateral pharyngeal space or from lymphatic spread from more distant sites to involve the retropharyngeal lymph nodes. Dysphagia, dyspnea, nuchal rigidity, and esophageal regurgitation, as well as high fever and chills, may be present. Bulging of the posterior pharyngeal wall may be observed. Lateral soft tissue radiographs of the neck may reveal marked widening of the retropharyngeal space. Infection of the retropharyngeal space is potentially life-threatening and requires prompt surgical drainage. Complications include hemorrhage and spontaneous rupture into the airway with asphyxiation, laryngeal spasm, bronchial erosion, and thrombosis of the jugular vein. The pretracheal space comprises the anterior portion of the visceral compartment and completely surrounds the trachea. Most commonly, infections reach this space through perforations of the anterior esophageal wall, occasionally through contiguous extension from a retropharyngeal space infection. The clinical presentation is characterized by severe dyspnea, but hoarseness may be the first complaint. Swallowing is difficult, and regurgitation of fluids through the nose may occur. A pretracheal space infection is always serious because of possible extension into the mediastinum, and prompt surgical drainage is critically important.

Complications of Odontogenic Infections

Complications of odontogenic infections can occur either by hematogenous spread or by direct extension. Transient bacteremia is common during or after various dental procedures, especially the extraction of infected teeth.[39] The temporal relationship between these procedures and subsequent bacterial endocarditis and cardiovascular prosthetic infections is well documented.[40] Reports of infected total hip replacements after dental procedures add further concern.[26, 41] Prophylactic antibiotic treatment during dental procedures, although frequently used, remains a controversial issue, especially in the absence of preexisting valvular heart disease.[40] Complications of odontogenic infections secondary to direct extension include mediastinal spread,[42] intracranial suppuration (especially cavernous sinus thrombosis),[43] suppurative jugular thrombophlebitis, carotid artery erosion,[44] maxillary sinusitis,[1] and osteomyelitis.[45] Acute mediastinitis and intracranial suppuration secondary to odontogenic infections are relatively uncommon in the postantibiotic era.

Suppurative Jugular Thrombophlebitis and Carotid Artery Erosion

These are uncommon complications of oropharyngeal or odontogenic infections in the postantibiotic era. Extension of infection to the carotid sheath, which encloses both the internal jugular vein and the internal carotid artery, usually arises from the lateral pharyngeal space.[44] Since the carotid sheath space in this area is relatively compact with little areolar connective tissue, there is little tendency of spread up and down this vascular sheath, with the exception of possible retrograde thrombophlebitis and intracranial extension. The major concern is protracted septicemia and erosion of the carotid artery or one of its branches.

The onset of suppurative jugular thrombophlebitis is acute, with shaking chills, spiking fevers, and profound prostration. Localizing signs of pain and swelling at the angle of the jaw, tenderness and induration along the sternocleidomastoid muscle, and swelling of the lateral pharyngeal wall with dysphagia and neck ridigity are usually present. However, these findings may be subtle, and their clinical significance may not be fully recognized until postmortem examination. Systemic evidence of infection such as septic pulmonary emboli and metastatic abscesses to the brain, lungs, kidneys, and joints is not infrequent. The usual recommended treatment consists of external drainage of the lateral pharyngeal space and ligation of the internal jugular vein. *Fusobacterium necrophorum* has been the organism most frequently isolated from blood cultures, and mortality remains high. Important warning signals that may herald major hemorrhage due to erosion of the carotid artery include multiple episodes of minor bleeding from the oral cavity or ear and ecchymosis of oral and cervical tissue. With the onset of major hemorrhage, primary considerations are maintenance and protection of the airway because death may occur more rapidly from asphyxiation than from hemorrhagic shock. Appropriate treatment consists of emergency carotid ligation after the restoration of blood volume and pressure. Hemorrhage is controlled by local compression until ligation can be attempted. The mortality for emergency ligation ranges from 30 to 50%. Cerebrovascular accident is a significant complication in survivors.

Septic Cavernous Sinus Thrombosis

This dreaded complication is fortunately rare in the postantibiotic era. Facial furuncles and purulent paranasal sinusitis were the major predisposing conditions. Infection of the maxillary teeth was the most common dental cause. Eagleton described six criteria for the diagnosis of septic cavernous sinus thrombosis to help distinguish it from other less lethal infections, particularly those of the ethmoid sinus and the orbit: (1) a known site of infection; (2) evidence of blood stream invasion; (3) early signs of venous obstruction in the retina, conjunctiva, and eyelid; (4) paresis of the third, fourth, and sixth cranial nerves resulting from inflammatory edema; (5) abscess formation in neighboring soft tissue; and (6) evidence of meningeal irritation.[47] Before the antibiotic era, septic cavernous sinus thrombosis was virtually always fatal. Mortality since 1970 has been markedly reduced to 15 to 30%.[44, 48, 49] Treatment requires early recognition, high-dose intravenous antibiotics, and surgical decompression of the underlying predisposing infection. Anticoagulation and steroids therapy are not indicated.

Maxillary Sinusitis

In many people, the roots of the maxillary molars lie proximate to the maxillary antrum. At times, congenital bony defects occur, with the root adjacent to the sinus membrane. In these cases, sinusitis can result from direct extension of an odontogenic infection or from perforation of the sinus floor during extraction of a maxillary tooth.[49, 50] The clinical presentation of secondary sinus involvement is similar to that of primary sinus disease.

Osteomyelitis of the Jaws

The mandible is much more susceptible to osteomyelitis than is the maxilla, mainly because the cortical plates of the latter are thin and its medullary tissues are relatively poor in vascular supply.[45] In view of the large number of odontogenic infections and the intimate relationship of teeth to the medullary cavity, it is surprising that osteomyelitis of the jaws is not more frequent. When osteomyelitis occurs, there is usually a predisposing condition that affects host resistance such as a compound fracture, previous irradiation, osteopetrosis, Paget's disease, diabetes mellitus, or steroid therapy. With the initiation of infection, the intramedullary pressure markedly increases, further compromising blood supply and leading to bone necrosis. Pus travels through the haversian and perforating canals, accumulates beneath the periosteum, and elevates it from the cortex. If pus continues to accumulate, the periosteum is eventually penetrated, and mucosal and cutaneous abscesses and fistulas may develop. As the inflammatory process becomes more chronic, granulation tissue is formed. Spicules of necrotic and nonviable bone may become either totally isolated (sequestrum) or encased in a sheath of new bone (involucrum). Severe mandibular pain is a common symptom and may be accompanied by anesthesia or hypoesthesia on the affected side. In protracted cases, mandibular trismus may develop. A clinical variant is chronic sclerosing osteomyelitis associated with a proliferative periostitis. Clinically, it is characterized by a localized, hard, nontender swelling over the mandible. Actinomycosis and radiation necrosis are two common causes of this form of osteomyelitis of the jaws.

Diagnostic Approaches

Specimen Collection and Processing

For closed-space infections, it is imperative that the normal resident oral flora be excluded during specimen collection in order that the culture results be appropriately interpreted. Needle aspiration of loculated pus by an extraoral approach is desirable, and specimens should be transported immediately to the laboratory under anaerobic conditions. For intraoral lesions, direct microscopic examination of stained smears often provides more useful information than do culture results from surface swabs. Gram and acid-fast stains for bacteria and potassium hydroxide preparations for fungi should be routinely performed. Tissue biopsy specimens should be routinely examined for histopathologic evidence of acute or chronic inflammation and infection. The presence of specific microbial agents can be detected by immunofluorescence or polymerase chain reaction for certain suspected bacterial, mycobacterial, fungal, and viral infections. In chronic osteomyelitis, soft tissue swelling and draining fistulas are frequently present. Aspirates from the adjacent soft tissue swellings may be valuable, but cultures from the sinus tracts may be misleading, since these sinus tracts are often colonized by organisms that do not reflect what is actually occurring within the infected bone.[51] Bone biopsies for histopathologic examination and culture are often required for a definitive diagnosis.

Imaging Techniques for the Localization of Infection

Pantomography (orthopantomograph) may reveal the true extent of advanced periodontitis or the presence of periapical abscess. Ultrasonography, radionuclide scanning, computed tomography, and magnetic resonance imaging are particularly useful for the localization of deep fascial space infections of the head and neck.[52, 53] A lateral radiograph of the neck may demonstrate compression or deviation of the tracheal air column or the presence of gas within necrotic soft tissues.[54] In retropharyngeal infections, lateral radiographs of the cervical spine or computed tomographic scanning can help determine whether the infection is in the retropharyngeal space or the prevertebral space.[55] The former suggests an odontogenic source, whereas the latter suggests involvement of the cervical spine. Technetium bone scanning used in combination with gallium- or indium-labeled white blood cells is particularly useful for the diagnosis of acute or chronic osteomyelitis and for the differentiation of infection or trauma from malignancy. In acute osteomyelitis, both the bone scan and the gallium scan are likely to have positive findings. In chronic osteomyelitis, the gallium or indium scans may be negative, but the technetium scan may be positive. Similarly, both scans may be positive during infection and trauma, whereas neoplasms in the bone may be associated only with a positive bone scan but negative gallium or indium scan results.

Therapeutic Considerations

Dental Caries and Periodontitis

For both caries prevention and the treatment of periodontitis, the most important strategy is the effective control of the supragingival and subgingival plaques through active promotion of and meticulous attention to oral hygiene. The diet should be scrutinized to eliminate or discourage frequent snacking on carbohydrate-rich foods or the intake of sugar-containing beverages. Fluoride-containing dentifrices and rinses (e.g., sodium fluoride 1.1% or stannous fluoride 0.4%) and dentral flossing should be encouraged after each meal. Fluoride forms a complex with the apatite crystals in dentin by replacing the hydroxyl group, thereby lending strength to the entire structure. Further, fluoride promotes remineralization of the carious lesions and also exerts a bacteriostatic effect. Oral antimicrobial rinses with 0.12% chlorhexidine are also effective for the control of dental plaque bacteria that lead to gingivitis and periodontitis. Chlorhexidine acts as a cationic detergent killing a wide range of bacteria and is retained on the oral surfaces for prolonged periods to prevent plaque advancement.[26] Unfortunately, it has a bitter taste and stains the enamel and tongue. Prolonged application may also promote the emergence of resistant microorganisms. Among topical antibiotics, although both penicillin and tetracycline have cariostatic effects in animal models, only the topical application of vancomycin has been shown to reduce dental caries with some degree of success in humans. With the development of improved restorative dental care and dental restorative materials, such as bonding and fluoride-releasing agents, the need for dental extractions has become much less frequent than in the past.[56]

Acute necrotizing ulcerative gingivitis should be treated with systemic antimicrobials such as metronidazole or penicillin.[37] Certain types of severe periodontitis are amenable to systemic antimicrobial therapy in conjunction with mechanical débridement (scaling and root planing).[35] In localized juvenile periodontitis, systemic tetracycline therapy directed against *A. actinomycetemcomitans* and combined with local periodontal treatment has yielded excellent results.[35, 37] Unfortunately, the administration of tetracycline to children younger than 9 years can cause staining of the permanent dentition and is not generally recommended. Furthermore, tetracycline resistance among periodontal pathogens has been increasingly recognized.[57] In double-blind clinical studies of advanced periodontitis, systemic metronidazole (500 mg three times daily orally) or doxycycline (200 mg twice daily orally) for 1 or 2 weeks in conjunction with rigorous mechanical débridement of the root surfaces was found to reduce the need for radical surgery by 80% compared with débridement plus placebo control.[37] The routine use of systemic antimicrobial therapy prophylactically during oral or periodontal surgery, or both, in a healthy host is unwarranted since the risk of postoperative infections after periodontal surgery is less than 1%.[37]

Other important approaches to caries and periodontitis prevention include the active promotion of improved oral hygiene through more effective educational programs,[13] and behavioral modification of co-risk factors, such as tobacco smoking and reluctance to visit dental care professionals regularly.[23] The prospect of an effective and safe vaccine against dental caries, such as the use of various immunogens derived from *S. mutans*,[58, 59] remains remote and unlikely to be available for clinical application in the near future.[60]

Suppurative Odontogenic Infections

The most important therapeutic modality for pyogenic odontogenic infections is surgical drainage and the removal of necrotic tissue. Needle aspiration by the extraoral route can be particularly helpful both for microbiologic sampling and for evacuation of pus. The need for definitive restoration or extraction of the infected tooth, the primary source of infection, is readily apparent. Deep periodontal scaling and endodontic treatments with root filling may be required in most instances. Effective surgical management requires a thorough understanding of the most likely anatomic routes of spread. The neighboring potential fascial spaces should be carefully and systematically surveyed. The optimal timing for incision and drainage is equally important. Premature incision into an unlocalized cellulitis in an ill-conceived search for pus can disrupt the normal physiologic barriers and cause further diffusion and extension of infection.

Antibiotic therapy is important in halting the local spread of infection and in preventing hematogenous dissemination. Antimicrobial agents are generally indicated if fever and regional lymphadenitis are present or when infection has perforated the bony cortex and spread into surrounding soft tissue. Severely immunocompromised patients are particularly at risk for unhalted and spreading orofacial infections, and empirical broad-spectrum antimicrobial therapy in these patients is usually warranted.[61, 62] The initial choice of antibiotic regimens for the treatment of odontogenic infections requires not so much the results of bacterial culture and sensitivity as knowledge of the indigenous organisms that colonize the teeth, gums, and mucous membranes. By far most of these organisms, including both anaerobes and aerobes, are sensitive to penicillin.[61, 62] Thus, penicillin monotherapy in doses appropriate for the severity of infection remains a good choice. However, the problem of β-lactamase production and penicillin resistance among certain oral anaerobes, particularly pigmented *Prevotella* spp. and *F. nucleatum,* has been increasingly recognized, and treatment failure with penicillin in odontogenic infections because of such β-lactamase–producing strains has been well documented.[63, 64] Thus, in patients with life-threatening deep fascial space infections and in patients who have had an unfavorable or delayed response to penicillin, alternative therapy with a broader spectrum against anaerobes as well as facultative gram-negative bacilli may be considered.[62, 65] Ambulatory patients with less serious odontogenic infections may be treated with amoxicillin with or without a β-lactamase inhibitor, or with either penicillin or a fluoroquinolone in combination with metronidazole. Penicillin-allergic patients may be treated with clindamycin, cefoxitin, cefotetan, or ceftizoxime. Erythromycin and tetracycline are not recommended because of increasing resistance among some strains of streptococci.[57, 62] Metronidazole, although highly active against anaerobic gram-negative bacilli and spirochetes, is only moderately active against anaerobic cocci and is not active against aerobes, including streptococci.[1, 61, 66] Except in acute necrotizing gingivitis and in advanced periodontitis,[33, 34, 37] it should not be used as a single agent in odontogenic infections. In the compromised host such as the patient with leukemia and severe neutropenia after chemotherapy, it is prudent to cover for facultative gram-negative bacilli as well, and agents with broad-spectrum activity against both aerobes and anaerobes are desirable (Table 53–2).

TABLE 53–2 Empirical Antibiotic Regimens for Odontogenic Soft Tissue Infections

Normal host
Penicillin G, 1–4 MU IV q4–6h
Ampicillin-sulbactam, 1.5–3 g IV q6h
Clindamycin, 450 mg PO or 600 mg IV q6–8h
Metronidazole, 500 mg PO or IV q8h*
Doxycycline, 200 mg PO or IV q12h
Cefoxitin, 1–2 g IV q6h
Cefotetan, 2 g IV q12h
Ceftizoxime, 1–2 g IV q8–12h
Compromised host (one of following ± aminoglycoside)
Ceftizoxime, 4 g IV q8h
Cefotaxime, 2 g IV q6h
Piperacillin-tazobactam, 3 g IV q4h
Imipenem-cilastatin, 500 mg IV q6h

*Usually in combination with antibiotics active against aerobic organisms.

Osteomyelitis

Treatment of osteomyelitis of the jaws is complicated by the presence of teeth and persistent exposure to the oral environment. Antibiotic therapy needs to be prolonged, often for weeks to months. Adjuvant therapy with hyperbaric oxygen may prove beneficial in hastening the healing process.[45] Surgical management, including sequestrectomy, saucerization, decortication, and closed-wound suction irrigation, may occasionally be necessary. Rarely, in advanced cases, the entire segment of the infected jaw may have to be resected.

OROFACIAL NONODONTOGENIC INFECTIONS

Nonodontogenic infections of the oral cavity most frequently occur secondary to chemical, thermal, or traumatic injury. Virtually all infectious microorganisms can present with intraoral manifestations, particularly sexually transmitted agents and childhood viral enanthems. Cancer patients with mucositis from cytotoxic drugs are especially prone to acute and chronic opportunistic infections of the oral cavity, particularly candidiasis, aspergillosis, mucormycosis, herpetic gingivostomatitis, and mixed gram-negative infections.[67, 68] In this section, some of the conditions affecting primarily the oral mucosa and salivary glands in which an infectious cause is either proved or suspected are briefly discussed.

Infections of the Oral Mucosa

Noma, or Gangrenous Stomatitis

Noma, or gangrenous stomatitis, also known as cancrum oris, is an acute, fulminating, and gangrenous infection of the oral and facial tissues. It usually occurs in the presence of severe debilitation and malnutrition, and children are most often affected.[69] The earliest lesion is a small, painful, red spot or vesicle on the attached gingiva in the premolar or molar region of the mandible. A necrotic ulcer rapidly develops and undermines the deeper tissue. Painful cellulitis of the lips and cheeks is observed as the lesion extends outward in a conelike fashion. Within a short period, sloughing of necrotic soft tissues occurs and exposes underlying bone, teeth, and deeper tissues.

Fusospirochetal organisms such as *Borrelia vincentii* and *F. nucleatum* are consistently cultured from noma lesions. *Prevotella melaninogenica* may also be present. Biopsy specimens of tissue from the advancing lesion show a mat of predominantly gram-negative threadlike bacteria that cannot be positively identified.[70] Thus, this lesion bears a similarity to acute necrotizing ulcerative gingivitis in several respects but appears to be more focal and destructive, involving deeper tissues beyond the gingiva. Treatment of noma requires high doses of intravenous penicillin. Every effort should be directed to correct the dehydration and underlying malnutrition and debility. Loose teeth and sequestra may be removed, but saucerization should be avoided. Healing is by secondary intention. Serious multilation and facial deformity may require subsequent cosmetic surgery.

Aphthous Stomatitis

Aphthous ulcers are the most common cause of recurrent oral lesions. This entity must be distinguished from oral ulceration due to herpes simplex, coxsackievirus, agranulocytosis, and Behçet's and other diseases. Three major clinical variants are recognized: (1) minor aphthous ulcers, (2) major aphthous ulcers, and (3) herpetiform aphthous ulcers.[71] The true cause of aphthous ulcerations is not known, although a number of infectious agents including viruses have been implicated. The most prevailing hypothesis suggests that the mechanism causing the ulceration is autoimmune. Circulating humoral antibodies and sensitized T lymphocytes active against oral mucosa have been demonstrated in patients with aphthous ulcers.[71] Furthermore, the active T lymphocytes undergo a phase of rapid proliferation just before the onset of ulceration. The origin of the autoantibodies is not clear, and no common antigenic factor between oral epithelium and the indigenous microflora has been demonstrated.

In their most characteristic form, minor aphthous ulcers appear as a number of small ulcers on the buccal and labial mucosa, the floor of the mouth, or the tongue. The palatal soft tissues are rarely involved. Moreover, the ulcers are concentrated in the anterior part of the oral cavity, whereas the pharynx and tonsillar fauces are rarely implicated. A prodromal stage is usually present. The ulcers appear gray-yellow, often with a raised and erythematous margin, and are exquisitely painful. Lymph node enlargement is seen only with secondary bacterial infection. The course of ulceration varies from a few days to a little over 2 weeks and is followed by spontaneous healing. Major aphthous ulcers are more protracted and last up to several months. All areas of the oral cavity including the soft palate and tonsillar areas may be involved. Long periods of remission may be followed by intervals of intense ulcer activity. Herpetiform aphthous ulcers are small and multiple and characteristically affect the lateral margins and tip of the tongue. The ulcers are gray, without a delineating erythematous border, and are extremely painful, which makes eating and speaking difficult. Despite its name, there is little clinical resemblance to an acute herpetic gingivostomatitis. Although intranuclear inclusions have been demonstrated in herpetiform aphthous ulcers, there is no evidence to suggest that these inclusions bear any relationship to the presence of viruses.

The treatment of aphthous ulcers is primarily symptomatic. Strict oral hygiene should be maintained, and the use of antiseptic mouthwashes may be helpful in temporarily reducing secondary infection. Local anesthetic lozenges or gels may be used as a last resort for brief periods of pain relief. Topical or systemic steroids may be beneficial in selected people with extensive disease, but caution must be exercised in their administration. Thalidomide (100 to 200 mg/day orally for 2 to 6 weeks) has been reported to be effective for treatment of large aphthory lesions in patients with acquired immunodeficiency syndrome.[72]

Mucositis and Stomatitis in the Severely Immunocompromised Person

Much of what is known about the management of oromucosal infections has been studied in cancer patients being treated with radiotherapy, chemotherapy, and bone marrow transplantation.[67, 73] Other patient groups that develop oromucosal complications include those undergoing solid organ transplantation, patients with acquired immunodeficiency syndrome,[74] and those with autoimmune diseases associated with xerostomia and systemic immunosuppression. The underlying mechanism appears to be a breakdown of the mucosal epithelium that leads to mucositis, secondary bacterial or fungal infection, or reactivation of latent viral infection. Oral candidiasis, herpes simplex, varicella-zoster, and cytomegalovirus infections are the most common manifestations. Mucositis that complicates radiation or chemotherapy most commonly involves the nonkeratinized oral epithelium, including the buccal and labial mucosa, soft palate, oropharynx, floor of the mouth, and ventral and lateral surfaces of the tongue. Ulceration and pseudomembrane formation are evident usually between 4 and 7 days after the initiation of chemotherapy when the rate of destruction of the basal epithelium exceeds that of proliferation of new cells. The clinical manifestations may be quite variable. The lesions are often protracted in duration and may not be associated with an inflammatory reaction, thereby masking the usual signs and symptoms. Pain or tenderness may be the only abnormal finding. Since the etiologic agents of infection cannot be readily predicted on clinical grounds alone in such patients, specific microbiologic diagnosis by culture, histopathologic examination, or antigen detection techniques is critical for appropriate treatment. Topical as well as systemic antimicrobial agents may be indicated along with antiseptic (e.g., chlorhexidine) and anesthetic (e.g., benzydamine, viscous lidocaine) applications.[74] Frequent saline rinses may reduce mucosal irritation, remove thickened secretions or debris, and increase moisture in the mouth.[67] Coating agents such as milk of magnesia or aluminum hydroxide gel (Amphojel) have been useful for the symptomatic relief of painful oral lesions. Topical or oral cytoprotective agents (e.g., sucralfate) or nonsteroidal anti-inflammatory analgesics (e.g., benzydamine, salicylates) may provide additional benefit.[75, 76] Meticulous oral and dental hygiene, effective management of xerostomia, selective suppression of oropharyngeal microbial colonization, and early control of reactivation by latent viral infections appear to be the critical steps to prevent and reduce the overall morbidity of oromucosal infections in the severely immunocompromised person.[29, 77]

Infections of the Salivary Gland

Sialadenitis, or infection of salivary tissue, is a relatively common disease. Sialolithiasis in elderly patients leads to ductal obstruction and secondarily to suppuration of the salivary gland and appears to be a major predisposing condition. In this regard, stones of Wharton's duct are much more common than are those of Stensen's duct, and obstructive sialadenitis is much more frequent with the submandibular than the parotid gland.[78] Other predisposing factors for sialadenitis include dehydration, general debility, sialogogic drugs, and trauma.

Suppurative Parotitis

Acute bacterial parotitis is a specific clinical entity primarily affecting the elderly, malnourished, dehydrated, or postoperative patient. Clinically, there is a sudden onset of firm, erythematous swelling of the pre- and postauricular areas that extends to the angle of the mandible. This is associated with exquisite local pain and tenderness. Systemic findings of high fevers, chills, and marked toxicity are generally present. Progression of the infection may lead to massive swelling of the neck, respiratory obstruction, septicemia, and osteomyelitis of the adjacent facial bones. Staphylococci have been the predominant isolates, and antibiotic therapy should include an antistaphylococcal agent. Enterobacteriaceae, other gram-negative bacilli, and anaerobes have also been reported to cause parotitis.[79, 80] Early surgical drainage and decompression of the gland are generally required since spontaneous drainage is uncommon.

Chronic Bacterial Parotitis

In this condition, parotitis is recurrent with intermittent acute exacerbations. There is chronic, low-grade, bacterial infection resulting in functional destruction of the salivary gland. Pus, when obtained directly from the gland, usually reveals the growth of staphylococci or mixed oral aerobes and anaerobes. Sialography during remission may reveal a sialectatic pattern of pooling of contrast medium that suggests multiple cystic cavities in place of the normal acinar pattern. Chronic parotitis may be confused with Sjögren syndrome, a noninfectious illness characterized by the triad of xerostomia, keratoconjunctivitis, and systemic autoimmune disease such as rheumatoid arthritis, lupus erythematosus, scleroderma, periarteritis nodosa, and polymyositis. The presence of associated temporomandibular arthritis or arthralgia should strongly suggest Sjögren syndrome rather than chronic bacterial parotitis.

Therapy for chronic parotitis should initially be conservative and consists of systemic antibiotics and ductal saline or antibiotic irrigations. Parotidectomy may eventually be required for people with long-standing infection.

Viral Parotitis

Mumps parotitis is characterized by the rapid, painful swelling of one or both parotid glands within 2 to 3 weeks after exposure. A prodromal phase of preauricular pain, fever, chills, and headache may be present. Other viral causes of parotitis include influenza and enteroviruses, and virus cultures or serologic examinations may be required for distinguishing these from true mumps. Mumps parotitis usually resolves spontaneously in 5 to 10 days. Symptomatic relief of pain and fever is necessary, and prevention of dehydration and secondary bacterial infection is essential.

MISCELLANEOUS INFECTIONS OF THE NECK AND HEAD

In the antibiotic era, dental causes have surpassed oropharyngeal and tonsillar sources of deep neck infections.[49, 65] Other miscellaneous infections of the neck and head include suppurative cervical adenitis, infected embryologic cysts of the neck, various infections secondary to human and animal bites, maxillofacial trauma, irradiation, and surgical procedures of the head and neck.

Cervical Adenitis

Cervical adenitis, which presents unilaterally in association with warm, tender, enlarged, and fluctuant lymph nodes, is usually due to pyogenic infections. Its anatomic location in relationship to major cervical landmarks provides the clinical clues to the primary source of infection.[81, 82] Bilateral acute cervical adenitis generally suggests a nonspecific or viral cause, toxoplasmosis, or group A streptococcal infection. A more chronic or recurrent cervical adenitis should suggest the possibility of typical or atypical mycobacteriosis, human immunodeficiency virus infection, Epstein-Barr virus or cytomegalovirus mononucleosis, cat-scratch fever, actinomycosis, sarcoidosis, or lymphoproliferative and neoplastic disorders.

Infected Embryologic Cysts

Three distinct embryologic abnormalities can present with infection in the neck. They are (1) cystic hygroma or lymphangioma, (2) pharyngeal and bronchial cleft cysts, and (3) thyroglossal duct cysts. Cystic hygroma is associated with a diffuse tumor mass usually evident within the first 2 years of life. It commonly involves the lower aspect of the neck, but it can appear anywhere in the cervical region. It is probably an abnormal development of lymphatic vessels from the jugular lymphatic sacs. Sudden enlargement by infection or hemorrhage into a lymphangioma may cause obstruction of the upper airways. Pharyngeal cleft cysts can develop from the first, second, or third pharyngeal clefts, although the second is most common. They usually present in childhood as fistulas or masses just posterior to the angle of the mandible along the anterior border of the sternocleidomastoid muscle. The mass can fluctuate in size, and enlargement can be associated with upper respiratory infection. Thyroglossal duct cysts originate from the foramen cecum of the tongue and descend through the body of the hyoid bone into the anterior portion of the neck. Any residual secretory lining may give rise to a thyroglossal duct cyst that is midline. It can cause respiratory obstruction or fistula formation if secondarily infected. Treatment of these congenital abnormalities during secondary bacterial infection requires broad-spectrum antibiotics such as a cephalosporin. Definitive surgical excision to prevent recurrence should be performed after complete resolution of the acute process.

Suppurative Thyroiditis

Although infections of the thyroid gland are rare, they are potentially life-threatening. Such infections may arise by a variety of pathways, including hematogenous dissemination, direct spread from an adjacent deep fascial space infection, an infected thyroglossal fistula, or anterior perforation of the esophagus. Preexisting diseases of the thyroid gland such as a goiter or adenoma are frequently present.[83, 84] Acute suppurative thyroiditis is characterized by fever, local pain, tenderness, warmth, erythema, and symptoms of dysphagia, dysphonia, hoarseness, or pharyngitis. The infection may involve single or both lobes, and fluctuance may not be apparent until late in the course. Subacute thyroiditis may have similar local findings, but systemic manifestations are not as severe and tend to be more self-limiting. Laboratory investigation of thyroid infections should include ultrasonography, radionuclide scanning, and lateral radiographs or computed tomographic scanning of the neck for evidence of peritracheal extension; thyroid function tests; and diagnostic needle aspiration for microbiologic diagnosis. *Staphylococcus aureus, Streptococcus pyogenes,* and *Streptococcus pneumoniae* are most frequently isolated. Other pathogens include *Haemophilus influenzae,* viridans streptococci, *Eikenella corrodens,* and *Bacteroides, Peptostreptococcus,* and *Actinomyces* spp. Treatment requires specific antimicrobial agents and appropriate surgical drainage.

Infections from Bites, Maxillofacial Trauma, Irradiation, and Surgical Wounds

Human and Animal Bites

Human and animal bite wounds to the head and neck are relatively common. Although they may look innocuous initially, serious complications can occur. For this reason, empirical antibiotic therapy is recommended when the bite wound involves the face, head, or neck. Recent studies that used adequate anaerobic culture techniques indicate indigenous oral flora rather than the skin flora to be the major source of bite wound infections.[85] Streptococci, *E. corrodens,* and *S. aureus* are the most prevalent facultative organisms, and *Bacteroides* and *Peptostreptococcus* are the most common anaerobic isolates. Penicillin-resistant gram-negative rods are infrequent. *Eikenella corrodens* is unique in that it is susceptible to penicillin and ampicillin but resistant to oxacillin, methicillin, nafcillin, and clindamycin.[86] In animal bite wounds, *Pasteurella multocida* has been a common cause of infection.[87] It is susceptible to penicillin and cefoxitin, but resistant to clindamycin and erythromycin. In view of these findings, penicillin remains the antibiotic of choice for initial therapy for both human and animal bite wounds.

Maxillofacial Trauma

Automobile and motorcycle accidents cause the most severe maxillofacial trauma. Particular attention should be paid to fractures that may traverse sinus cavities and tooth-bearing areas of the maxilla or mandible, since secondary infection rates at these sites are particularly high. Treatment is aimed not only at correcting the fracture but also at the prevention of infection and subsequent osteomyelitis. Early stabilization of the fracture and the jaws is generally required to protect the airway. Tracheostomy with the use of inflated, cuffed endotracheal tubes may prevent aspiration of blood and other foreign materials. The occurrence of otorrhea or rhinorrhea with a persistent cerebrospinal fluid leak should be carefully observed.

Irradiation and Postsurgical Wounds

Malignancies of the head and neck are frequently treated with a combination of irradiation, chemotherapeutic agents, and surgical resection. Infectious complications are particularly common after such procedures. Pharyngocutaneous fistulas, osteonecrosis of the mandible, or radionecrosis of the laryngeal cartilage may occur. *Staphylococcus aureus* and *Pseudomonas aeruginosa* are frequent pathogens.[88] Prolonged courses of intravenous antibiotics selected according to culture and sensitivity data as well as frequent wound débridement and cleansing are indicated. Although some controversy still exists, immunocompromised patients undergoing oropharyngeal surgery for cancer should receive perioperative antibiotics since they are at particular high risk for infection. A broad-spectrum antibiotic such as cefazolin, cefuroxime, cefoxitin, or ceftizoxime appears appropriate in this setting.[89, 90]

REFERENCES

1. Chow AW, Roser SM, Brady FA. Orofacial odontogenic infections. Ann Intern Med. 1978;88:392.
2. Hardie J. Microbial flora of the oral cavity. In: Schuster GS, ed. Oral Microbiology and Infectious Disease, 2nd ed. Baltimore: Williams & Wilkins, 1983:162.
3. Hamada S, Slade HD. Biology, immunology and cariogenicity of *Streptococcus mutans.* Microbiol Rev. 1980;44:331.
4. Gordon DF, Stutman M, Loesche WJ. Improved isolation of anaerobic bacteria from the gingival crevice area of man. Appl Microbiol. 1971;21:1046.
5. Valenti WM, Trudell RB, Bentley DW. Factors predisposing to oropharyngeal colonization with gram-negative bacilli in the aged. N Engl J Med. 1978;298:1108.
6. Schuster GS. The microbiology of oral and maxillofacial infections. In: Topazian RG, Goldberg MH, eds. Oral and Maxillofacial Infections. 2nd ed. Philadelphia: WB Saunders; 1987:33.
7. Geddes DAM, Jenkins GN. Intrinsic and extrinsic factors influencing the flora of the mouth. In: Skinner FA, Carr JG, eds. The Normal Microbial Flora of the Mouth. London: Academic 1974:85.
8. Yao ES, Lamont RJ, Leu SP, et al. Interbacterial binding among strains of pathogenic and commensal oral bacterial species. Oral Microbiol Immunol. 1996;11:35.
9. Maiden MFJ, Macuch PJ, Murray L, et al. "Checkerboard" DNA-probe analysis and anaerobic culture of initial periodontal lesions. Clin Infect Dis. 1997;25(Suppl 2):S230.
10. Moore WEC, Moore LVH. The bacteria of periodontal diseases. Periodontol 2000. 1994;5:66.
11. Darveau RP, Tanner A, Page RC. The microbial challenge in periodontitis. Periodontol 2000. 1997;14:12.
12. Tanner A, Stillman N. Oral and dental infections with anaerobic bacteria: Clinical features, predominant pathogens, and treatment. Clin Infect Dis. 1993;16(Suppl 4):S304.
13. Shaw JH. Causes and control of dental caries. N Engl J Med. 1987;317:996.
14. Loesche WJ. Role of *Streptococcus mutans* in human dental decay. Microbiol Rev. 1986;50:353.
15. Johnson TC, Reinhardt RA, Payne JB, et al. Experimental gingivitis in periodontitis-susceptible subjects. J Clin Periodontol. 1997;24:618.
16. Rams TE, Flynn MJ, Slots J. Subgingival microbial associations in severe human periodontitis. Clin Infect Dis. 1997;25(Suppl 2):S224.
17. Matto J, Asikainen S, Vaisanen ML, et al. Role of *Porphyromonas gingivalis, Prevotella intermedia,* and *Prevotella nigrescens* in extraoral and some odontogenic infections. Clin Infect Dis. 1997;25(Suppl 2):S194.
18. Baker AS, Montgomery WW. Oropharyngeal space infections. Curr Clin Top Infect Dis. 1987;8:227.
19. Newman MG. Anaerobic oral and dental infection. Rev Infect Dis. 1984;6:107.
20. Chow AW. Odontogenic infections. In: Schlossberg D, ed. Infections of the Head and Neck. New York: Springer 1987:148.
21. Ishikawa I, Nakashima K, Koseki T, et al. Induction of the immune response to periodontopathic bacteria and its role in the pathogenesis of periodontitis. Periodontol 2000. 1997;14:79.
22. Offenbacher S. Periodontal diseases: Pathogenesis. Ann Periodontol. 1996;1:821.
23. Salvi SE, Lawrence HP, Offenbacher S, et al. Influence of risk factors in the pathogenesis of periodontitis. Periodontol 2000. 1997;14:173.
24. Genco RJ. Current view of risk factors for periodontal diseases. J Periodontol. 1996;67(Suppl 10):1041.
25. Hart TC, Korman KS. Genetic factors in the pathogenesis of periodontitis. Periodontol 2000. 1997;14:202.
26. Kureishi K, Chow AW. The tender tooth—dentoalveolar, pericoronal, and periodontal infections. Infect Dis Clin North Am. 1988;2:163.
27. Roscoe DL, Chow AW. Normal flora and mucosal immunity of the head and neck. Infect Dis Clin North Am. 1988;2:1.
28. McGhee JR, Michalek SM. Immunobiology of dental caries—microbial aspects and local immunity. Annu Rev Microbiol. 1981;35:595.
29. Epstein JB. Infection prevention in bone marrow transplantation and radiation. NCI Monogr. 1990;9:73.
30. Van Dyke TE, Horoszewicz HU, Cianciola LJ, et al. Neutrophil chemotaxis dysfunction in human periodontitis. Infect Immun. 1980;27:124.
31. Kilian M. Degradation of immunoglobulins A1, A2, and G by suspected principal periodontal pathogens. Infect Immun. 1981;34:757.
32. Thadepalli H, Mandal AK. Anatomic basis of head and neck infections. Infect Dis Clin North Am. 1988;2:21.
33. Shinn DLS, Squires S, McFadzean JA. The treatment of Vincent's disease with metronidazole. Dent Pract. 1965;15:275.
34. Stephen KW, McLatchie MF, Mason DK, et al. Treatment of acute ulcerative gingivitis (Vincent's type). Br Dent J. 1966;121:313.
35. Loesche WJ, Giordano J, Soehren S, et al. Nonsurgical treatment of patients with periodontal disease. Oral Surg Oral Med Oral Pathol Oral Radiol Endod. 1996;81:533.
36. Slots J, Reynolds HS, Genco RJ. *Actinobacillus actinomycetemcomitans* in human periodontal disease: A cross-sectional microbiological investigation. Infect Immun. 1980;29:1013.
37. Loesche WJ. Antimicrobials in dentistry: With knowledge comes responsibility. J Dent Res. 1996;75:1432.
38. Finch RG, Snider GE, Sprinkle PM. Ludwig's angina. JAMA. 1980;243:1171.
39. Crawford JJ, Sconyers JR, Moriarty JD, et al. Bacteremia after tooth extractions studied with the aid of prereduced anaerobically sterilized culture media. Appl Microbiol. 1974;27:927.
40. Hall G, Hedstrom SA, Heimdahl A, et al. Prophylactic administration of penicillins for endocarditis does not reduce the incidence of postextraction bacteremia. Clin Infect Dis. 1993;17:188.
41. Bartzokas CA, Johnson R, Jane M, et al. Relation between mouth and haematogenous infection in total joint replacements. BMJ. 1994;309:506.
42. McCurdy JA, MacInnis EL, Hays LL. Fatal mediastinitis after a dental infection. J Oral Surg. 1977;35:726.
43. Yoshikawa TT, Quinn W. The aching head—intracranial suppuration due to head and neck infections. Infect Dis Clin North Am. 1988;2:265.
44. Blomquist IK, Bayer AS. Life-threatening deep fascial space infections of the head and neck. Infect Dis Clin North Am. 1988;2:237.
45. Topazian RG. Osteomyelitis of the jaws. In: Topazian RG, Goldberg MH, eds. Oral and Maxillofacial Infections. 2nd ed. Philadelphia: WB Saunders; 1987;204.
46. Sinave CP, Hardy GJ, Fardy PW. The Lemierre syndrome: Suppurative thrombophlebitis of the internal jugular vein secondary to oropharyngeal infection. Medicine (Baltimore). 1989;68:85.
47. Eagleton WP. Cavernous Sinus Thrombophlebitis and Allied Septic and Traumatic Lesions of the Basal Venous Sinuses. A Clinical Study of Blood Stream Infection. New York: Macmillan; 1926.
48. Harbour RC, Trobe JD, Ballinger WE. Septic cavernous sinus thrombosis associated with gingivitis and parapharyngeal abscess. Arch Ophthalmol. 1984;102:94.
49. Chow AW. Life-threatening infections of the head and neck. Clin Infect Dis. 1992;14:991.

50. Chow AW. Infections of the sinuses and parameningeal structures. In: Gorbach SL, Barlett JC, Blacklow NR, eds. Infectious Diseases, 2nd ed. Philadelphia: WB Saunders; 1998:517.
51. Mackowiak PA, Jones SR, Smith JW. Diagnostic value of sinus-tract cultures in chronic osteomyelitis. JAMA. 1978;239:2772.
52. Salit IE. Diagnostic approaches to head and neck infections. Infect Dis Clin North Am. 1988;2:35.
53. Holt GR, McManus K, Newman RK, et al. Computed tomography in the diagnosis of deep-neck infections. Arch Otolaryngol. 1982;108:693.
54. Wholey MH, Bruwer AJ, Baker HL. The lateral roentgenogram of the neck. Radiology. 1958;71:350.
55. Bryan CS, King BG Jr, Bryant RE. Retropharyngeal infection in adults. Arch Intern Med. 1974;134:127.
56. Chow AW. Odontogenic infections in the elderly. Infect Dis Clin Pract. 1998;6:587.
57. Olsvik B, Tenover FC. Tetracycline resistance in periodontal pathogens. Clin Infect Dis. 1993;16(Suppl 4):S310.
58. Gregory RL, Filler SJ. Protective secretory immunoglobulin A antibodies in humans following oral immunization with *Streptococcus mutans*. Infect Immun. 1987;55:2409.
59. Taubman MA, Holmberg CJ, Smith DJ. Immunization of rats with synthetic peptide constructs from the glucan-binding or catalytic region of mutans streptococcal glucosyltransferase protects against dental caries. Infect Immun. 1995;63:3088.
60. Bowen WH. Vaccine against dental caries—a personal view. J Dent Res. 1996;75:1530.
61. Hill MK, Sanders CV. Principles of antimicrobial therapy for head and neck infections. Infect Dis Clin North Am. 1988;2:57.
62. Peterson LJ. Contemporary management of deep infections of the neck. J Oral Maxillofac Surg. 1993;51:226.
63. Lewis MA, Parkhurst CL, Douglas CW, et al. Prevalence of penicillin resistant bacteria in acute suppurative oral infection. J Antimicrob Chemother. 1995;35:785.
64. Heimdahl A, von Konow L, Nord CE. Isolation of β-lactamase producing *Bacteroides* strains associated with clinical failures with penicillin treatment of human orofacial infections. Arch Oral Biol. 1980;25:687.
65. Chow AW. Life-threatening infections of the head, neck, and upper respiratory tract. In: Hall JB, Schmidt GA, Wood LDH, eds. Principles of Critical Care, 2nd ed. New York: McGraw-Hill; 1998:887.
66. Hood FJC. The place of metronidazole in the treatment of acute orofacial infection. Antimicrob Agents Chemother. 1978;15:71.
67. Epstein JB. The painful mouth—mucositis, gingivitis and stomatitis. Infect Dis Clin North Am. 1988;2:183.
68. Barrett AP. A long-term prospective clinical study of oral complications during conventional chemotherapy for acute leukemia. Oral Surg. 1987;63:313.
69. Enwonwu CO. Noma: A neglected scourge of children in sub-Saharan Africa. Bull World Health Organ. 1995;73:541.
70. Topazian RG. Uncommon infections of the oral and maxillofacial regions. In: Topazian RG, Goldberg MH, eds. Oral and Maxillofacial Infections. 2nd ed. Philadelphia: WB Saunders; 1987:317.
71. Tyldesley WR. Recurrent oral ulcerations. In: Tyldesley WR, ed. Oral Medicine. Oxford: Oxford University Press; 1981:49.
72. Jacobson JM, Greenspan JS, Spritzler J, et al: Thalidomide for the treatment of oral aphthous ulcers in patients with human immunodeficiency virus infection: National Institute of Allergy and Infectious Diseases AIDS Clinical Trials Group. N Engl J Med 1997;336:1487.
73. Epstein JB, Gangbar SJ. Oral mucosal lesions in patients undergoing treatment for leukemia. J Oral Med. 1987;42:132.
74. Lee PL, Kiviat N, Truelove EL, et al. Oral manifestations in patients with AIDS or AIDS-related disorders. J Dent Res. 1987;66:183.
75. Epstein JB, Stevenson-Moore P. Benzydamine hydrochloride in prevention and management of pain in oral mucositis associated with radiation therapy. Oral Surg. 1986;62:145.
76. Adams S, Toth B, Dudley BS. Evaluation of sucralfate as a compounded oral suspension for the treatment of stomatitis. Clin Pharmacol Ther. 1985;2:178.
77. Epstein JB, Schubert MM. Synergistic effects of sialogogues in management of xerostomia following radiation therapy. Oral Surg. 1987;64:179.
78. Goldberg MH. Infections of the salivary glands. In: Topazian RG, Goldberg MH, eds. Oral and Maxillary Infections. 2nd ed. Philadelphia: WB Saunders; 1987:239.
79. Brook I, Finegold SM. Acute suppurative parotitis caused by anaerobic bacteria: Report of two cases. Pediatrics. 1978;62:1019.
80. Pruett TL, Simmons RL. Nosocomial gram-negative bacillary parotitis. JAMA. 1984;251:252.
81. Zeitoun IM, Dhanarajani PJ. Cervical cellulitis and mediastinitis caused by odontogenic infections. Report of two cases and review of literature. J Oral Maxillofac Surg. 1995;53:203.
82. Brook I. The swollen neck—cervical lymphadenitis, parotitis, thyroiditis and infected cysts. Infect Dis Clin North Am. 1988;2:221.
83. Berger SA, Zonszein J, Villanema P, et al. Infectious diseases of the thyroid gland. Rev Infect Dis. 1983;5:108.
84. Freidig EE, McClure SP, Wilson WR, et al. Clinical-histologic-microbiologic analysis of 419 lymph node biopsy specimens. Rev Infect Dis. 1986;8:322.
85. Goldstein EJC, Citron DW, Wield B, et al. Bacteriology of human and animal bite wounds. J Clin Microbiol. 1978;8:667.
86. Tami TA, Parker GS. *Eikenella corrodens*—an emerging pathogen in head and neck infections. Arch Otolaryngol. 1984;110:752.
87. Weber DJ, Hansen AR. Infections resulting from animal bites. Infect Dis Clin North Am. 1991;5:663.
88. Brook I, Hirokawa R. Microbiology of wound infection after head and neck cancer surgery. Ann Otol Rhinol Laryngol. 1989;98:323.
89. Gerard M, Meunier F, Dor P, et al. Antimicrobial prophylaxis for major head and neck surgery in cancer patients. Antimicrob Agents Chemother. 1988;32:1557.
90. Aldridge KE, Weeks LS, Stratton CW, et al. Differences in the in vitro inhibitory and bactericidal activity of ceftizoxime, cefoxitin, cefotetan, and penicillin G against *Bacteroides fragilis* group isolates. Comparison of time-kill kinetic studies with MIC values. Diagn Microbiol Infect Dis. 1990;13:311.

SECTION C

PLEUROPULMONARY AND BRONCHIAL INFECTIONS

Chapter 54

Acute Bronchitis

JACK M. GWALTNEY, JR.

Acute bronchitis is an inflammatory condition of the tracheobronchial tree that is usually associated with a generalized respiratory infection. It occurs most commonly during the winter months when acute respiratory tract infections are prevalent. Patients seen in general practices in Great Britain had annual attack rates of acute bronchitis that varied between 40 and 54 per 100,000.[1] Weekly attack rates peaked (117 to 171 per 100,000) in January and February and fell to trough levels (26 to 42 per 100,000) in August. The diagnosis was made most often in children younger than 5 years.

The syndrome of acute bronchitis is most often associated with respiratory viruses, both common cold viruses, such as rhinovirus and coronavirus, and those more invasive of the lower respiratory tract such as influenza and adenovirus. Nonviral causes of acute bronchitis also exist and include *Bordetella pertussis, Mycoplasma pneumoniae,* and *Chlamydia pneumoniae.* Secondary invasion with the common respiratory bacteria such as *Streptococcus pneumoniae* and *Haemophilus influenzae* may play a role in acute bronchitis, but this is uncertain.

ETIOLOGY

Cough occurs in approximately 50% of the cases of common respiratory illness in persons of all ages.[2] Cough is the localizing symptom in the respiratory tract that is most frequently associated with fever and is also highly associated with the occurrence of hoarseness. Infection with members of all the major respiratory virus groups causes cough (Table 54–1).[2–9] Cases of acute bronchitis are particularly common during influenza epidemics. Although rhinovirus infections do not produce as severe an involvement of the tracheobronchial tree as influenza, rhinovirus infections, because of their frequency, are an important cause of acute bronchitis. In populations of military recruits, adenovirus infections are a major cause of acute bronchitis. Among the other respiratory viruses that cause acute bronchitis, measles virus has been recognized as causing a particularly severe form of the disease.

TABLE 54–1 Cough Associated with Acute Viral Infections of the Respiratory Tract

Virus	Percentage of Cases with Cough (References)
Influenza virus	75–93 (2, 3)
Adenovirus	45–90 (4, 6)
Rhinovirus	32–60 (3, 5)
Coronavirus	10–50 (7, 8)
Parainfluenza virus	2–45 (5)
Respiratory syncytial virus	61 (9)
Coxsackievirus A21	26 (5)
Miscellaneous (rubeola, rubella, and so forth)	—

A small proportion of cases have a nonviral cause. *Mycoplasma pneumoniae* and *B. pertussis* are among the nonviral causes of acute bronchitis. The *C. pneumoniae* strain TWAR[10] has been associated with acute respiratory tract infections that have included cases with the clinical features of acute bronchitis.[11–15]

The etiologic role of *S. pneumoniae* and *H. influenzae* in acute bronchitis is not clear. Since these bacteria are carried in the resident flora of the upper respiratory tract of normal persons, it is difficult to evaluate studies in which expectorated sputum specimens have been cultured. To examine the role of secondary bacterial infection in the pathogenesis of acute bronchitis, it is necessary to conduct studies in which samples are collected from the tracheobronchial tree without contamination by nasopharyngeal flora.

PATHOGENESIS

The pathogenesis of acute bronchitis has not been well investigated for the viruses. One of the basic questions is whether the virus invades the lower airway and causes damage to the bronchial epithelium or whether cough results from more indirect mechanisms. Some viruses, such as influenza, routinely invade the lower airway. This may not be the case with a common cold virus such as rhinovirus; in such infections, various inflammatory mediators may play an important role in pathogenesis. During acute bronchial infection, the mucous membrane of the tracheobronchial tree is hyperemic and edematous, and there are increased bronchial secretions. Destruction of respiratory epithelium may be extensive in some infections, such as influenza[16, 17] but appears to be minimal in others, such as rhinovirus colds.[18, 19] Bronchial mucociliary function may be diminished in infections in which overt mucosal damage is limited.[20] With *M. pneumoniae* infection, the pathogenesis is similar to that of *B. pertussis* in that the organism attaches to the bronchial mucosa between the cilia of the epithelial cells.[21]

It is also possible that the severity of attacks of acute bronchitis may be increased by exposure to cigarette smoke and air pollutants. These substances, in association with recurrent acute bronchial infection, may result in permanent injury to the bronchial tree. Epidemiologic studies support the idea that acute respiratory infections play a role in the pathogenesis of chronic obstructive lung disease.[22, 23] Also, studies of pulmonary function in adults with acute bronchitis have shown abnormalities in airway resistance and reactivity.[24, 25]

The relationship between acute bronchitis and heightened airway reactivity has been investigated. Mild bronchial asthma was found to be increased in patients with a history of recurrent acute bronchitis over that seen in the general population.[26] Also, in a case-control study, patients with acute bronchitis were more likely to have a previous history of asthma and a history or diagnosis of atopic disease.[27] These findings have raised the question of the possible role of bronchospasm in some cases of prolonged cough associated with acute respiratory infection.

CLINICAL PRESENTATION

Cough begins early in the course of many acute respiratory infections and tends to become more prominent as the illness progresses. Of

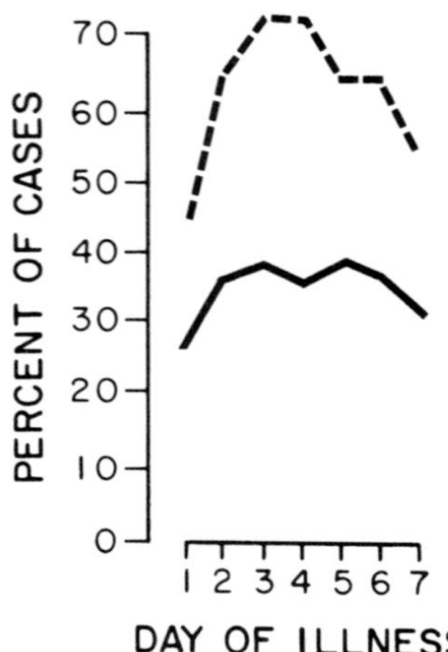

FIGURE 54–1. Occurrence of cough in rhinovirus colds (139 cases) *(solid line)* and type A_2 influenza (33 cases) *(broken line)* in young adults. (Modified from Gwaltney JM Jr. Rhinoviruses. In: Evans AS, ed. Viral Infections of Humans: Epidemiology and Control. 3rd ed. New York: Plenum; 1989:593–615.)

the different respiratory viruses, influenza virus, which routinely invades the lower airway, is the most important cause of cough. In a 6-year study of a group of young adults in which daily records of respiratory symptoms including cough were kept, the highest incidence of cough occurred in patients with influenza, reaching 70% on day 3 of the illness (Fig. 54–1).[28] In patients with rhinovirus colds, the incidence of cough remained at approximately 35% over the 7-day period of illness. Two syndromes, the common cold and what is called here *acute infectious bronchitis,* account for the overwhelming majority of cases of self-limited cough.[21] Although often caused by the same agents and showing overlap in clinical characteristics, the common cold and acute infectious bronchitis represent two distinct clinical syndromes (Table 54–2). In the typical common cold, cough is only one of several symptoms, is not unusually severe or predominant, and subsides along with the other complaints, although often lasting a few days longer. In the usual cold and influenzal illness, nasal and pharyngeal complaints subside after 3 or 4 days, whereas the cough tends to persist and to achieve greater prominence.[3]

With acute infectious bronchitis, cough is, or becomes, the predominant symptom and may last for several weeks. Patients with acute infectious bronchitis often present in the second or third week of their illness and represent a subset of all patients with acute respiratory infection. The episode may last up to a month or longer before eventually subsiding. Some cases with this syndrome progress into adult-onset asthma. In one prospective study of acute respiratory disease, 45% of patients were still coughing 2 weeks after presentation and 25% were still coughing after 3 weeks.[28] With a variety of different respiratory virus infections, sputum production was reported in approximately one-half of the cases in which cough occurred.[4, 5] Initially the cough of a cold results in mucoid sputum, which may develop a more purulent character in the later stages of illness. A study of natural rhinovirus infections in young adults has shown that the frequency and duration of cough is prolonged in cigarette smokers.[28] The prolonged cough of infectious bronchitis is typically nonproductive.

With severe tracheal involvement, there may be burning substernal pain associated with respiration and coughing. Dyspnea and cyanosis are not seen in adults unless the patient has underlying chronic obstructive pulmonary disease or other conditions that impair lung function. Rhonchi and coarse rales may be heard on examination of the chest. Signs of consolidation and alveolar involvement are not present in uncomplicated bronchitis. The frequency with which fever occurs depends on the specific infectious agent involved and the age of the patient. In adults, influenza virus, adenovirus, and *M. pneumoniae* infections are commonly associated with temperature elevations. Fever is unusual in adults with bronchitis associated with cold viruses, such as rhinovirus and coronavirus.

DIAGNOSIS

Bronchitis may be suspected in the patient with an acute respiratory infection with cough, but because a large number of more serious diseases of the lower respiratory tract cause cough, bronchitis must be considered to be a diagnosis of exclusion. A complete history should be obtained, including information on exposure to toxic substances and cigarette use. Complaints involving other organ systems should be sought. Epidemiologic considerations and a vaccination history may aid in the diagnosis of specific causes of bronchitis, such as influenza, *M. pneumoniae* infection, and whooping cough.

After every influenza epidemic, there is a small percentage of patients with influenza who, for unknown reasons, develop persistent bronchitis. Another important cause of persistent bronchitis that is receiving increasing attention is pertussis infection (whooping cough). The epidemiology of pertussis has changed due to widespread pertussis vaccination of children. A major reservoir of *B. pertussis* is now adults who were immunized as children but no longer have solid immunity. These individuals present with a severe bronchitis that is clinically indistinguishable from that of other infectious causes. Pertussis is often unrecognized; recent studies have shown that 20 to 25% of adults with episodes of acute, severe persistent cough have pertussis.

Included in a complete physical examination should be a careful evaluation of the chest for evidence of pneumonia and signs of cardiovascular and thromboembolic diseases. Radiologic examination of the chest may be required in the occasional patient in whom the question of parenchymal disease of the lung remains after the physical examination. Cultures of respiratory secretions for influenza virus, *M. pneumoniae,* and *B. pertussis* should be obtained when these diseases are suspected. Cultures and other diagnostic tests for the other respiratory viruses are available in some clinical microbiology laboratories. Culture methods and a microimmunofluorescence

TABLE 54–2 The Two Major Syndromes of Acute Self-Limited Cough

Syndrome	Clinical Features	Cause
Common cold	Cough is one of several symptoms Cough is not usually predominant symptom Cough usually subsides in 7–10 d	Rhinovirus Coronavirus Parainfluenza virus Respiratory syncytial virus Influenza virus
Acute infectious bronchitis	May begin as severe cold or "flulike" illness Cough is severe and becomes predominant complaint Cough persists for up to a month or longer May progress into adult-onset asthma	Influenza virus Adenovirus *Bordetella pertussis* *Mycoplasma pneumoniae* *Chlamydia pneumoniae*

test have been developed for the laboratory diagnosis of *C. pneumoniae*.[10] The use of an immunoglobulin M (IGM)–specific conjugate helps detect current infections. Routine bacterial cultures of expectorated sputum are not helpful because of the sampling problem of avoiding nasopharyngeal flora and because of the unknown importance of bacterial infection as the cause of acute bronchitis. Patients in whom cough persists beyond the expected duration of the acute illness should have further diagnostic examinations, including chest radiographs, sputum cytologic examination, and bronchoscopy to exclude foreign body aspiration, tuberculosis, tumors, and other chronic diseases of the tracheobronchial tree and lungs.

TREATMENT

Treatment of most cases of acute bronchitis is symptomatic and is directed primarily at the control of cough. Otherwise, healthy patients do not require hospitalization except in cases of unusual severity. Patients with underlying chronic cardiopulmonary diseases who contract influenzal or other severe forms of bronchitis may develop serious ventilatory abnormalities that require hospitalization with ventilatory assistance and oxygen therapy. Narcotic cough suppressants such as codeine and dextromethorphan have been the mainstay of treatment for cough associated with colds. Although clinical experience suggests that these drugs are useful, the results of placebo-controlled clinical trials have not supported their effectiveness in patients with upper respiratory tract infection.[29]

Placebo-controlled clinical trials have suggested that nonsteroidal anti-inflammatory drugs are effective in cough suppression. In two studies, naproxen at doses of 250 to 500 mg three times daily reduced cough severity in volunteers with experimental rhinovirus colds.[21] Also, ibuprofen 400 mg every 12 hours has shown promise as a cough suppressant in clinical practice. In a large placebo-controlled clinical trial, the first-generation antihistamine brompheniramine (12 mg every 12 hours) also reduced cough severity in volunteers with experimental rhinovirus colds.[30] Regular administration every 12 hours of combined therapy with a first-generation antihistamine such as brompheniramine and nonsteroidal anti-inflammatory drug is recommended for treating cough associated with the typical common cold. For patients with the prolonged cough of infectious bronchitis, short courses of oral or inhaled steroids are being used in clinical practice, but this treatment has not received adequate evaluation in controlled clinical trials. In one small controlled trial of oral dexamethasone in children with whooping cough, the results were not impressive.[31]

The value of expectorants is not well established,[32] and in patients with a good cough reflex, maintaining hydration is probably the most effective way to prevent the drying of bronchial secretions. Aspirin or acetaminophen and bed rest are beneficial in influenzal syndromes in which malaise and fever are prominent. Because of the apparent bronchospastic component in some cases of persistent cough, there has been an interest in treatment with β_2-adrenergic bronchodilators but results have not been impressive.[33–35]

Antibiotics are not recommended in the treatment of otherwise healthy patients with acute bronchitis of presumed viral cause. Controlled trials comparing antibiotic treatment to placebo in acute bronchitis have given conflicting results,[36–41] which could result from a number of variables, including the season of the year (reflecting the prevalence of different pathogens), and the adequacy of subject blinding related to drug side effects. With a self-limited disease such as acute bronchitis, therapeutic trials that compare one antibiotic with another but do not have a placebo group are difficult to interpret.

Mycoplasma pneumoniae infection should be treated with erythromycin or tetracycline (see Chapter 172), *B. pertussis* infection with erythromycin (see Chapter 219), and *C. pneumoniae* infection with tetracycline, erythromycin, or one of the newer macrolide or azalide antibiotics (see Chapter 27). During epidemics caused by influenza A virus, treatment with amantadine or rimantadine (100 mg orally twice daily) should be considered for patients with suspected influenza if the illness is less than 48 hours in duration. Also, annual immunization with influenza vaccine with consideration of prophylaxis with amantadine or rimantadine is recommended for patients with chronic cardiopulmonary problems (see Chapter 153). Children should receive pertussis vaccine as part of their routine immunizations. It is particularly important to discourage cigarette smoking in patients in whom acute respiratory tract infections are associated with protracted cough and sputum production.

REFERENCES

1. Ayres JG. Seasonal pattern of acute bronchitis in general practice in the United Kingdom 1976–83. Thorax. 1986;41:107–110.
2. Dingle JH, Badger GF, Jordon WS Jr. Illness in the Home: A Study of 25,000 Illnesses in a Group of Cleveland Families. Cleveland, Ohio: The Press of Western Reserve University; 1964:68.
3. Gwaltney JM Jr. Rhinoviruses. In: Evans AS, ed. Viral Infections of Humans: Epidemiology and Control. 3rd ed. New York: Plenum; 1989:593–615.
4. Dascomb HE, Hilleman MR. Clinical laboratory studies in patients with respiratory disease caused by adenovirus (RI-APC-ARD agents). Am J Med. 1956;21:161.
5. Tyrrell DAJ. Common Colds and Related Diseases. Baltimore: Williams & Wilkins; 1965.
6. Bloom HH, Forsyth BR, Johnson KM, et al. Patterns of adenovirus infections in Marine Corps personnel. I. A 42-month survey in recruit and nonrecruit populations. Am J Hyg. 1964;80:328.
7. Kaye HS, Marsh HB, Dowdle WR. Seroepidemiologic survey of coronavirus (strain OC43) related infections in a children's population. Am J Epidemiol. 1971;94:43.
8. Hendley JO, Fishburne HB, Gwaltney JM Jr. Coronavirus infections in working adults. Eight-year study with 229E and OC43. Am Rev Respir Dis. 1972;105:805.
9. Knight V, Kapikian AZ, Kravetz MH, et al. Ecology of a newly recognized common respiratory agent RS-virus. Ann Intern Med. 1961;55:507.
10. Grayston JT. Infections caused by *Chlamydia pneumoniae* strain TWAR. Clin Infect Dis. 1992;16:757–763.
11. Grayston JT, Kuo C-C, Wang S-P, et al. A new *Chlamydia psittaci* strain, TWAR, isolated in acute respiratory tract infections. N Engl J Med. 1986;315:161–168.
12. Grayston JT, Kuo C-C, Wang S-P, et al. Clinical findings in TWAR respiratory tract infections. In: Oriel JD, Ridgway G, Schacter J, et al, eds. Chlamydial Infections. Cambridge: Cambridge University Press; 1986:337–340.
13. Hahn DL, Dodge RW, Golubjatnikov R. Association of *Chlamydia pneumoniae* (strain TWAR) infection with wheezing, asthmatic bronchitis, and adult-onset asthma. JAMA. 1991;266:225–230.
14. Hammerschlag MR, Chirgwin K, Roblin PM, et al. Persistent infection with *Chlamydia pneumoniae* following acute respiratory illness. Clin Infect Dis. 1992;14:178–182.
15. Falck G. Heyman L, Gnarpe J, Gnarpe H. *Chlamydia pneumoniae* (TWAR): A common agent in acute bronchitis. Scand J Infect Dis. 1994;26:179–187.
16. Loosli CG, Stinson SF, Ryan DP, et al. The destruction of type 2 pneumocytes by airborne influenza PR8-A virus: Its effect on surfactant and lecithin content of the pneumonic lesions of mice. Chest. 1975;67(Suppl):7S.
17. Mulder J, Hers JFPh. Influenza. Groningen: Wolters-Noordhoff; 1972;1–300.
18. Douglas RG Jr, Alford BR, Cough RB: Atraumatic nasal biopsy for studies of respiratory virus infection in volunteers. Antimicrob Agents Chemother. 1968;8:340.
19. Winther B, Farr B, Turner RB, et al. Histopathologic examination and enumeration of polymorphonuclear leukocytes in the nasal mucosa during experimental rhinovirus colds. Acta Otolaryngol Suppl (Stockh). 1984;413:19–24.
20. Sasaki Y, Togo Y, Wagner NH Jr, et al. Mucociliary function during experimentally induced rhinovirus infection in man. Ann Otol. 1973;82:203.
21. Gwaltney J Jr. Clinical and mechanistic perspectives on acute self-limited cough. Symposium Report from the World Congress of Pharmacy and Pharmaceutical Sciences. Int Pharm J. 1997;11:5–7.
22. Lebowitz MD, Burrows B. The relationship of acute respiratory illness history to the prevalence and incidence of obstructive lung disorders. Am J Epidemiol. 1977;105:544.
23. Monto AS, Ross HW. The Tecumseh study of respiratory illness. X. Relation of acute infections to smoking, lung function and chronic symptoms. Am J Epidemiol. 1978;107:57.
24. Hall WJ, Hall CB, Speers DM. Respiratory syncytial virus infection in adults. Clinical, virologic, and serial pulmonary function studies. Ann Intern Med. 1978;88:203.
25. Boldy DAR, Skidmore SJ, Ayres JG. Acute bronchitis in the community: Clinical features, infective factors, changes in pulmonary function and bronchial reactivity to histamine. Respir Med. 1990;84:377–385.
26. Hallett JS, Jacobs RL. Recurrent acute bronchitis: The association with undiagnosed bronchial asthma. Ann Allergy. 1985;55:568–570.
27. Williamson HA, Jr, Schultz P. An association between acute bronchitis and asthma. J Fam Pract. 1987;24:35–38.
28. Gwaltney JM Jr, Hendley JO, Simon G, et al. Rhinovirus infections in an industrial population. II. Characteristics of illness and antibody response. JAMA. 1967;202:494.
29. Freestone C, Eccles R. Assessment of the antitussive efficacy of codeine in cough associated with common cold. J Pharm Pharmacol. 1997;49:1045–1049.

30. Gwaltney JM Jr, Druce HM. Efficacy of brompheniramine maleate treatment for rhinovirus colds. Clin Infect Dis. 1997;25:1188–1194.
31. Roberts I, Gavin R, Lennon D. Randomized controlled trial of steroids in pertussis (Letter). Pediatr Infect Dis J. 1992;11:982–983.
32. Kuhn JJ, Hendley JO, Adams KF. Antitussive effect of guaifenesin in young adults with natural colds. Objective and subjective assessment. Chest. 1982;82:713.
33. Melbye H, Aasebo U, Straume B. Symptomatic effect of inhaled fenoterol in acute bronchitis: A placebo-controlled double-blind study. Fam Pract. 1991;8:216–222.
34. Hueston WJ. A comparison of albuterol and erythromycin for the treatment of acute bronchitis. J Fam Pract. 1991;33:476–480.
35. Littenberg B, Wheeler M, Smith DS. A randomized controlled trial of oral albuterol in acute cough. J Fam Pract. 1996;42:49–53.
36. Stott NC, West RR. Randomized controlled trial of antibiotics in patients with cough and purulent sputum. BMJ. 1976;2:556.
37. Franks P, Gleiner JA. The treatment of acute bronchitis with trimethoprim and sulfamethoxazole. J Fam Pract. 1984;19:185–190.
38. Williamson HA Jr. A randomized, controlled trial of doxycycline in the treatment of acute bronchitis. J Fam Pract. 1984;19:481–486.
39. Brickfield FX, Carter WH, Johnson RE. Erythromycin in the treatment of acute bronchitis in a community practice. J Fam Pract. 1986;23:119–122.
40. Dunlay J, Reinhardt R, Roi LD. A placebo-controlled, double-blind trial of erythromycin in adults with acute bronchitis. J Fam Pract. 1987;25:137–141.
41. MacKay DN. Review: Antibiotics are ineffective for acute bronchitis. ACP J Club. 1997;March/April:39.

Chapter 55

Chronic Bronchitis and Acute Infectious Exacerbations

HERBERT Y. REYNOLDS

Chronic bronchitis features cough and excessive secretion of mucus from the tracheobronchial airways that is not attributed to other specific diseases such as bronchiectasis, asthma, or tuberculosis. The label *chronic bronchitic* is often applied loosely to patients and is very much a clinical diagnosis. The diagnosis is defined by having a productive cough on most days during at least 3 months in each of two successive years.[1, 2] Often, an element of airflow obstruction is present, in which case the designation of *chronic obstructive pulmonary disease* (COPD) is added.[1, 3] If wheezing and bronchospasm exist with chronic bronchitis or occur with exacerbations, the term *asthmatic bronchitis* (also *hyperactive airways disease*) may be used. Emphysema often coexists with COPD, although the precise diagnosis of emphysema is an anatomic one. Recognition that there are subsets of patients[2, 4] who have chronic bronchitis can be useful, as factors that cause acute exacerbations of chronic bronchitis may differ and therapy must be individualized. Three subsets can be identified, although there are overlapping features: simple chronic bronchitis, chronic or recurrent mucopurulent bronchitis, and chronic obstructive bronchitis.[2, 4]

ETIOLOGY AND PATHOLOGY

Several important factors contribute to chronic bronchitis: cigarette smoking, infection (viral and bacterial), inhalation of environmental pollutants (dust or fumes), and allergens causing allergic responses. Chronic bronchitis is common and may affect 10 to 25% of the adult population. It is estimated that over 12 million people in the United States have chronic bronchitis.[1] Bronchitis is more common in men than in women and more common in persons older than 40 years than in younger persons. Although cigarette smoking is most often associated with the disease, other factors must be important because only about 15% of tobacco smokers clinically develop chronic bronchitis.[5] Other diseases that can impair mucociliary transport in the lung should be suspected in appropriate patients. Recurrent respiratory infections and persistent chronic bronchitis could represent a defect in pulmonary host defenses[6, 7] or an immunodeficiency syndrome. This association may first become evident in teenagers or young adults and not just in young children as generally expected. Evaluation for cystic fibrosis, caused by a gene defect in the transmembrane conductance regulator of epithelial cells[8]; an immunoglobulin deficiency involving immunoglobulin A (IgA) or selective IgG subclasses, or both[9, 10]; a structural or acquired defect in cilia on epithelial cells impairing clearance of mucosal secretions[11]; and rarely abnormal polymorphonuclear (PMN) granulocyte function should be considered. Long-term, low-dose corticosteroid therapy in patients with asthma or with chronic bronchitis-emphysema has been reported to cause serum deficiencies in levels of IgG subclasses, particularly IgG_1.[12]

Although cigarette smoking is a significant airway irritant for most patients with chronic bronchitis,[13, 14] about 6 to 10% of nonsmoking men have persistent cough and phlegm production. Reports from the analysis of bronchoalveolar lavage fluid to obtain respiratory cells from human lungs have found a tremendous increase in the recovery of alveolar macrophages from cigarette smokers compared with nonsmokers.[15, 16] "Normal" smokers usually yield a small percentage of PMN inflammatory cells as well. A modest degree of smoking (2 to 5 pack-years) induces cellular and bronchoalveolar lavage fluid immunoglobulin changes similar to those found in heavy smokers. Postmortem examination of lungs obtained from young accident victims showed evidence of inflammation involving respiratory bronchioles in smokers but not in nonsmokers.[17] The lesion consisted of clusters of pigmented macrophages in association with edema, fibrosis, and epithelial hyperplasia of the bronchiolar and alveolar walls.[17] Thus, cigarette users, even those who smoke minimally, initiate irritation that may insidiously culminate years later as chronic bronchitis and possibly other forms of degenerative lung disease. The realization that cigarette smoke can inactivate the antiprotease function of α_1-antitrypsin in lung secretions further supports this sequence of destructive lung disease.[18, 19]

Several changes are found in the lungs of patients with chronic bronchitis. There is an increase in the number of goblet (mucus-secreting) cells in the surface epithelium of major and smaller bronchi,[3] such that the epithelium may consist almost entirely of such cells. In addition, mucus glands in the walls of the larger bronchi undergo hypertrophy, producing a high relative ratio of the mucous gland layer compared with the bronchial wall thickness—the Reid index.[20] Besides mucous gland enlargement, irritation of the airway mucosa occurs and more mucus is present in peripheral airways. The irritated airways respond by producing extra secretions, exposing sensitive stretch receptors (this aggravates cough), and making more neuropeptides that can promote bronchospasm. Inflammation of the mucosa causes swelling and edema and reflects the infiltration of PMN granulocytes in response to chemokines, such as interleukin-8 produced by epithelial cells.[21] Inflammation represents a complex interplay between irritants, such as microbes or environmental pollutants, reaching the airways; the generation of chemokines by epithelial cells that attract PMNs or eosinophils; and airway macrophages that may stimulate excessive mucus production.[22] Together these promote mucosal edema, more secretions, and clinical symptoms.[23–25]

CLINICAL PRESENTATION

Frequent coughing interrupts the life of most patients with advanced bronchitis, causing them to clear their throats frequently and expectorate sputum throughout the day. Many cough up the largest amount in the morning on arising. Sputum may be tenacious and sticky and vary in appearance from mucoid or whitish to yellowish-green and obviously purulent. Nasal or sinus congestion and a postnasal drip are often associated. Many patients with chronic bronchitis are not especially incapacitated unless an acute infection or some other illness occurs. However, some degree of expiratory airflow limitation is usually present that defines the physiology of COPD.[1, 2]

The clinical manifestations of COPD reflect a dynamic interplay between chronic bronchitis, emphysema, and often asthma; the relative proportion of each entity can vary for a particular patient, creating subsets of COPD patients with different symptoms and physiology.[1] Initial descriptions of COPD patients with American *emphysema* versus British *bronchitis*[26] defined radiographic groups of emphysematous, inflammatory, and unclassified patients who also had distinguishing symptoms and cardiopulmonary physiology. The major groups, types A and B, descriptively evolved as "pink puffers" and "blue bloaters," respectively. Clinically, this is an oversimplification because of type X, or indeterminate patients with a mixture of features. Nevertheless, for patients with COPD, separating the extreme forms as predominantly emphysema or predominantly bronchitis, based on clinical and physiologic criteria, remains very helpful[27] in assessing the impact of infection and planning therapy for acute exacerbations of chronic bronchitis (AECB).[2] Briefly, the emphysema-predominant patient typically has more dyspnea, less sputum, and fewer respiratory infections. The patient is more likely to be of thin habitus with a "barrel" chest, has diminished breath sounds but clear lungs on auscultation, maintains reasonably normal arterial blood gas levels, and has a hyperexpanded appearance of the lung fields on chest films. In contrast, the bronchitis-predominant patient has more productive coughing, is prone to infections, maintains body weight or is obese, and has lung crackles and wheezing, right heart failure, and pedal edema. Lethargy or somnolence can develop. Also, acrocyanosis, polycythemia, and arterial blood gas levels that feature hypoxemia, carbon dioxide retention, and acidemia are often present. Digital clubbing is not a finding in the uncomplicated bronchitic patient.

Previously, three distinctions among patients with chronic bronchitis were proposed that might be helpful for clinical and epidemiologic purposes[4]: (1) simple chronic bronchitis, based on a chronic or recurrent increase in the volume of mucoid bronchial secretions produced, which would help distinguish when an exacerbation from infection would create purulent sputum; (2) chronic or recurrent mucopurulent bronchitis in which the sputum was usually mucopurulent but was not attributed to localized disease (bronchiectasis, as an example) or to asthma unless infection had supervened; and (3) chronic obstructive bronchitis in which the chronic bronchitis was complicated by expiratory airflow obstruction. Overlap between these groups often existed.[4] However, a more recent approach seems more helpful[2] for separating subsets of patients with an AECB potentially from multiple causes so that an infection-related episode could be identified more accurately. Although the precise role of infection in causing AECB remains somewhat debatable and controversial,[5, 28–32] certain patients with more severe illness and worse dyspnea benefit slightly from antibiotic treatment.[33, 34] A first step is to establish the underlying severity of the patient's chronic bronchitis with a scoring system[2] that includes baseline lung function, age, smoking status, comorbid conditions, and the number of exacerbations within the past year. This would define patients with severe enough disease that antibiotic trials (with newer antibiotics) might be targeted toward them. In a similar fashion, Dr. Grossman[35] offered a stratification of patients according to risk factors related to the baseline clinical status that would allow the selection of patients for whom antibiotic therapy would be indicated to prevent treatment failures. Both of these reports[2, 35] stress that future appropriately designed clinical trials are required.

Evidence of an Acute Infectious Exacerbation

Objective signs that bronchitis has worsened because of an infection are not always evident. Reliance is placed on the patient's observation that the sputum has changed in color and consistency or has increased in amount. Patients may note increasing cough and dyspnea, but during an acute illness most do not have symptoms suggesting systemic toxicity such as chills and fever, nor do they develop a blood leukocytosis. Patients often experience chest tightness and increased fatigue. Because a precise definition of an AECB does not exist, it remains difficult to determine just when one has occurred or ended.

Sputum Analysis

Cellular analysis[36] of a fresh sputum specimen (early-morning sample) is helpful for evaluating patients with chronic bronchitis. Continual bronchial irritation is indicated by the presence of many PMN granulocytes, even during quiescent periods. Determining the number of eosinophils is important.[37] Ciliated epithelial cells can be recognized, and their number correlates reasonably well with the degree of vigorous coughing that was needed to produce the sputum specimen. A few alveolar macrophages may be identified that in the cigarette smoker characteristically contain yellowish-brown cytoplasmic inclusions. A Gram-stain smear often shows a mixture of gram-positive and gram-negative bacteria representing normal mouth flora or tracheal colonization by such species as *Haemophilus influenzae, Streptococcus pneumoniae,* and *Moraxella catarrhalis.*

The mucus secreted in chronic bronchitis contains various glycoproteins, mucopolysaccharide acids, transferrin, and albumin. Small amounts of immunoglobulin species are present, including secretory IgA, IgG, occasionally IgM and IgE, or proteolytic fragments derived from them because of the action of lysosomal enzymes and other degradative substances in sputum.[7, 38] Immunologic analysis of IgA in sputum may help in diagnosing the presence of infection in patients with a flare-up of chronic bronchitis. With active infection, the content of 7-S IgA is increased and free secretory component is all used; without infection, the 11-S IgA level is increased and excess secretory component exists.[39]

Radiologic Evidence

Standard chest radiographic films do not provide a definitive diagnosis of chronic bronchitis, but they are essential for excluding other diseases that may complicate the condition. The chest film can appear normal and not change during infectious exacerbations; therefore, it is not a very sensitive way of following most patients. However, chest computed tomography, especially high-resolution scans,[40] can identify parenchymal infections earlier or delineate other conditions such as bronchiectasis better.

RELATIONSHIP OF INFECTION TO ACUTE EXACERBATIONS

The role and evidence of bacterial infection in AECB have been discussed extensively.[28–32] Bacterial infection does not appear to initiate bronchitis except possibly in an adult patient with a history of frequent childhood respiratory infections.[29] However, bacteria are probably significant in perpetuating the overproduction of mucus[3] and account for some of the characteristic exacerbations. As the importance of infection as the cause of many exacerbations of chronic bronchitis is debated, a role for the nonspecific inflammatory response may be given more prominence.[41]

The lower airways of nonbronchitic patients who are free of other lung diseases are reasonably sterile,[42–44] although methods for culturing are not perfect and may not exclude some oral flora.[44] Pathogenic bacteria can be cultured from the bronchi of most patients with chronic bronchitis and from those with other conditions such as carcinoma of the lung or tuberculosis or after irradiation to the lung. A variety of damage to the lung may predispose to bacterial colonization. Routine sputum cultures from patients with chronic bronchitis commonly yield nonencapsulated *H. influenzae, S. pneumoniae,* and other oropharyngeal commensal flora. As one or both of these species is recovered from approximately 30 to 50% of the sputum specimens in most clinical series of chronic bronchitis, they represent the baseline microbial flora of many patients. *Moraxella*

TABLE 55–1 General Medical Measures

Have patient discontinue cigarette smoking, using cessation course and/or nicotine medication; if unsuccessful, at least attempt to reduce amount of daily smoking.
Assess for any concomitant allergic disease—rhinitis, asthma, sulfite sensitivity.
Judge involvement of sinus disease and/or nasal obstruction with baseline sinus CT scan; obtain otolaryngology consultation to evaluate possible obstruction from polyps or septal deviation.
Review for any potential host factor or hereditary illness causing recurrent sinopulmonary infections (e.g., immunoglobulin deficiency, cystic fibrosis, ciliary defect).
Have patient obtain nutritional counseling to reduce weight if obese, or use dietary supplementation if patient is malnourished or experiencing early satiety. Maintenance of stable weight is important but difficult in end-stage COPD.
Have patient minimize contact with environmental irritants.
Arrange for periodic cancer screening, as risk of lung cancer is usually increased.
Obtain pulmonary spirometry tests and oximetry for oxygen saturation on room air (baseline arterial blood gas levels are advised).
Have patient record daily peak-flow-meter readings (patient log).
Encourage pulmonary rehabilitation program or daily exercise routine. Use supplemental oxygen as dictated by oxygen desaturation with exercise, arterial blood gas values, and degree of pulmonary hypertension.
If fiberoptic bronchoscopy is required, consider a bronchitis index that gives a semiquantitative visual scale for airway inflammation (based on presence of mucosal edema, erythema, secretions, and friability).[14]
Give preventive immunization—pneumococcal vaccine and yearly influenza vaccine.
Have postural drainage done if sputum production is copious.

Abbreviation: COPD, Chronic obstructive pulmonary disease; CT, computed tomography.

catarrhalis is also considered a potential pathogen and can be recovered in sputum as well.[28] Anaerobic bacteria could be recovered in only 17% of transtracheal aspirate specimens.[45] *Haemophilus influenzae* and pneumococci tend to persist in sputum during quiescent intervals, and their frequency of recovery is not greatly increased during infectious episodes.[30] The development of purulent sputum is not correlated specifically with the presence of one or the other of these bacteria. However, evidence suggests that purulence is associated with a quantitative increase in the number of pneumococci cultured from sputum.[30] *Mycoplasma pneumoniae* does not seem to be of great importance, for some studies attribute only 1 to 10% of acute infections to this organism.[30, 31] Respiratory illness produced by *Chlamydia pneumoniae* (TWAR) may be associated with a subacute form of bronchitis in which symptoms, especially cough and reactive airway disease, last for days or weeks.[46–49] Also, infection with *Bordetella pertussis* has reemerged, especially when chronic cough develops.[50, 51] Bacteria heretofore considered part of the normal oropharyngeal flora and nonpathogens may be isolated from patients with bronchitis and be attributed to infection. This has been reported for *Corynebacterium pseudodiphtheriticum*.[52, 53]

The following statements broadly summarize the relationship between causative agents[28, 54, 55] and acute flare-ups of infection in chronic bronchitis: (1) Chronic colonization of the airways and sputum with unencapsulated strains of *H. influenzae* and with *S. pneumoniae* occurs in at least one half of the affected patients. Although it is difficult to incriminate one or both of these bacteria microbiologically, antibiotic selection is based on this probability. As noted, *M. catarrhalis,* perhaps *B. pertussis,* and newly recognized pathogens such as *C. pseudodiphtheriticum* should be included in antibiotic coverage for certain patients. (2) Other bacteria such as hemolytic species of streptococci, *Staphylococcus aureus,* and gram-negative enteric bacilli are infrequent causes of acute infection in chronic bronchitis. Only 5 to 10% of the sputum specimens contain significant numbers of these other bacteria. As sputum can be contaminated by oropharyngeal flora, these bacteria may not originate in the lower airways. (3) *Mycoplasma pneumoniae* infections can be sporadic and are infrequently responsible for acute exacerbations.[30, 31] (4) Viruses are frequent causes of acute infection, although many infections may remain asymptomatic.[30] About one third of acute exacerbations are related to these agents, including influenza virus, parainfluenza virus, respiratory syncytial virus, rhinovirus, and coronavirus. Viral infections are seasonal and occur more frequently in winter. (5) It is difficult to document the microbial cause of many respiratory infections even with optimal methods of culture and conscientious diagnostic evaluation.[47, 55] As an example, for only 50% of the acute pneumonia episodes in hospitalized patients was a specific cause found.[56]

MANAGEMENT

Overall Management

For patients with COPD and bronchitis and a propensity for acute flare-ups, overall management should address four areas: (1) maintenance therapy during quiescent intervals designed to optimize daily activity, enhance exercise tolerance, and keep secretions, cough, and wheezing minimal (Tables 55–1 and 55–2); (2) prevention of respiratory infections; (3) more intensive treatment when symptomatic bronchitis flares; and (4) selection of antibiotic therapy (Table 55–3). Recommendations reflect suggestions from several general sources that can be consulted for more details.[57–60]

Included among general measures (see Table 55–1) are suggestions that should be reviewed occasionally for any patient having risk factors contributing to other illnesses or in whom risk modification is needed to improve health. Therefore, smoking cessation, weight reduction or nutritional advice, screening for malignancy, and using preventive strategies are obvious considerations. A maintenance regimen (see Table 55–2) to improve symptoms from airflow obstruction for a COPD patient is usually required. A medication schedule must be designed that encourages compliance. The regular use of inhalers is advocated, rather than on an "as needed basis," including some objective monitoring such as of daily peak-flow expiratory volume. The patient with COPD and bronchitis who has daily expectoration of sputum, cough, wheezing on occasion, and dyspnea likely has a medication regimen similar to that as outlined in Table 55–2.[57] Metered-dose inhalers would include a β_2-agonist, an anticholinergic agent, and topical corticosteroids. The use of a combination inhaler of albuterol and ipratropium seems effective for these patients.[60–62] In addition to inhaled corticosteroids, a small oral dose of prednisone in the range of 5 to 10 mg/day can enhance the effectiveness of the inhaler regimen. The addition of theophylline may help some patients, but its excitatory effects have to be balanced. Finally, newer medications to inhibit leukotrienes[63] or to promote sputum removal[64] are being introduced that attack different mechanisms of the disease.

TABLE 55–2 Maintenance Therapy—Bronchodilator and Anti-inflammatory Medications*

Albuterol 2 puffs qid (or salmeterol 2 puffs bid—may decrease awakening during night with symptoms)
Ipratropium 2 puffs qid
Combination inhaler of albuterol-ipratropium, 2 puffs qid
Oral theophylline (for patients with suboptimal response to above bronchodilators); for example, Theo-Dur 200 or 300 mg bid or tid (dose of theophylline must be individualized based on peak serum concentration)
Inhaled triamcinolone, 2 or 4 puffs, given qid or bid, respectively (dose can be increased to 16 inhalations/day or 1600 μg)
Oral prednisone, dose 20–30 mg/day initially, with a tapering schedule and switching to alternate-day regimen of about 5–10 mg/day, if possible
Cough suppressant (example, benzonatate 100 mg bid)
For more severe asthma or to spare amount of corticosteroids, use inhibitor of cysteinyl leukotrienes (example—montelukast 10-mg tablet/day or zafirlukast 20-mg tablet bid
Aerosolized surfactant (palmitoylphosphadidylcholine) to improve sputum transport
Prophylactic antibiotic—rotating schedule with oral, broad-spectrum antibiotic is suggested (see text); requirement for continuous antibiotic is unusual

*Use of a spacer with an inhaler is recommended if patient has difficulty coordinating use.

TABLE 55–3 Oral Antibiotics for Common Agents Associated with an Exacerbation of Chronic Bronchitis

Antibiotic	Usual Oral Dosage	*Streptococcus pneumoniae**	*Haemophilus pneumoniae**	*Moraxella catarrhalis*	*Mycoplasma pneumoniae*	*Chlamydia pneumoniae*
Ampicillin	250 mg qid	±	–	–	–	–
Amoxicillin	250–500 mg tid	±	±	–	–	–
Amoxicillin-clavulanate	250-mg tablet tid	+	+	+	–	–
Doxycycline	200 mg first day, then 100 mg/day	–	±	–	+	+
Azithromycin	500 mg/day, then 250 mg/day	±	±	+	+	+
Trimethoprim-sulfamethoxazole (Bactrim DS)	160-800 mg (1 DS/day)	±	+	+	–	–
Cefuroxime axetil	250–500 mg bid	±	+	+	–	–
Levofloxacin†	500 mg/day	+	+	+	+	+

*Antibiotic resistance can occur with some strains, designated as ±. Antibiotic susceptibility testing is required.
†Selected as a representative of fluoroquinolones with enhanced activity for *S. pneumoniae*.
Modified from Reynolds HY. Antibiotic treatment of bronchitis and chronic lung disease. In: Cherniack NS, ed. Chronic Obstructive Disease. Philadelphia: WB Saunders; 1991:450–461.

Prophylactic antibiotic therapy may have some usefulness in highly selected patients who experience frequent exacerbations (four or more per year). A number of oral antibiotics suffice based on considerations of microbial sensitivity, the patient's tolerance, the dosing interval, and the cost. Several strategies appear to be effective. Patients may receive antibiotics daily during winter months, or 4 days per week during the winter, or a 7-day course at the first sign of a "chest cold."

Flare-ups of bronchitis, usually described as exacerbations of COPD in most patients, may occur at a rate of about 2.7 per patient per year,[65] although many are not reported or easily detected, so the rate is often reported as lower.[33] Factors predicting that a patient will have more exacerbations include having daily cough and sputum, daily wheezing, frequent flare-ups in the previous year, and comorbid illness.[66] Clues to document the exacerbations can be subtle and subjective, but usually some decrement in airflow (peak-flow meter values usually decrease), fatigue or not feeling well, and more secretions occur. Before automatically increasing therapy, it is important to estimate the severity of the exacerbation. If a scoring system has been used to determine the baseline severity of disease,[2] then subsets of patients can be identified who have disease of sufficient severity to justify inclusion in clinical trials of antibiotics.[2, 35, 66] With a symptomatic flare-up, all respiratory therapy is usually intensified, perhaps changing metered-dose inhalers to aerosolized nebulizer therapy and often boosting, or initiating, oral corticosteroids. A burst and taper regimen over 5 to 7 days is usually tried if the patient is not already on oral corticosteroids. If the patient is on a daily maintenance dose, it is increased to a 40 to 60 mg/day equivalent of prednisone for several days until symptoms stabilize, after which tapering of the dose can begin.

Antimicrobial Therapy

Antibiotic therapy is usually begun, although the effectiveness of the short-term use of antibiotics for acute exacerbations is difficult to assess. However, infection can cause acute decompensation, and it is the most common identifiable cause of death in these patients. On balance, an antibiotic does hasten recovery and improve clinical outcome.[34, 66] The usual strategy is to institute a course of antimicrobial therapy for a 7- to 10-day period and hope that the acute flare-up subsides; an objective end point for success is usually lacking. Oral administration of antibiotics is sufficient for most patients.

There are many considerations in selecting an appropriate antibiotic, as outlined by Schentag and Tillotson[67]; these include the spectrum of activity, mode of action, tissue penetration, tolerance of the drug by the patient, frequency of administration, modification of dose-based mechanism of excretion or inactivation, and cost. The array of acceptable antibiotics is large, and new agents are constantly being introduced. Only a limited number are listed, but these cover most of the microorganisms likely to be involved in AECB (see Table 55–3). Several references[67–69] discuss antimicrobial choices in relation to present antibiotic-resistant patterns, which are continuing to change.

REFERENCES

1. Celli BR, Snider GL, Heffner J, et al. American Thoracic Society Statement—Standards for the diagnosis and care of patients with chronic obstructive pulmonary disease. Am J Respir Crit Care Med. 1995;152:S77–S120.
2. Wilson R, Wilson CB. Defining subsets of patients with chronic bronchitis. Chest. 1997;112:303S–309S.
3. Rennard SI. COPD: Overview of definitions, epidemiology, and factors influencing its development. Chest. 1998;113:235S–241S.
4. Stuart-Harris CH, Crofton J, Gilson JC, et al. (Committee for the Medical Research Council). Definition and classification of chronic bronchitis for clinical and epidemiological purposes. Lancet. 1965;1:775–779.
5. Sethi S. Is chronic bronchitis an infectious disease? In: Nelson S, ed. Mediguide® to Pulmonary Medicine, v. 5, no. 1. New York: Lawrence DellaCorte; 1997:1–7.
6. Reynolds HY. Immunologic system in the respiratory tract. Physiol Rev. 1991;71:1117–1133.
7. Reynolds HY. Integrated host defense against infections. In: Crystal RG, West JB, Weibel ER, Barnes PJ, eds. The Lung: Scientific Foundations, v. 2. Philadelphia: Lippincott-Raven; 1997:2353–2365.
8. Welsh MJ, Ramsey BW. Research on cystic fibrosis—a journey from the Heart House. Am J Respir Crit Care Med. 1998;157:S148–S154.
9. Beck GS, Heiner DC. Selective immunoglobulin G4 deficiency and recurrent infections of the respiratory tract. Am Rev Respir Dis. 1981;124:94–96.
10. Reynolds HY. Immunoglobulin G and its function in the human respiratory tract. Mayo Clin Proc. 1988;63:161–174.
11. Afzelius BA. "Immotile-cilia" syndrome and ciliary abnormalities induced by infection and injury (Editorial). Am Rev Respir Dis. 1981;124:107–109.
12. Klaustermeyer WB, Gianos ME, Kurohara ML, et al. IgG subclass deficiency associated with corticosteroids in obstructive lung disease. Chest. 1992;102:1137–1142.
13. Linden M, Rasmussen JB, Piitulainen E, et al. Airway inflammation in smokers with nonobstructive and obstructive chronic bronchitis. Am Rev Respir Dis. 1993;148:1226–1232.
14. Thompson AB, Huerta G, Robbins RA, et al. The bronchitis index. A semiquantitative visual scale for the assessment of airways inflammation. Chest. 1993;103:1482–1488.
15. Reynolds HY, Merrill WW. Airway changes in young smokers that may antedate chronic obstructive lung disease. Med Clin North Am. 1981;65:667–689.
16. Sibille Y, Reynolds HY. Macrophages and polymorphonuclear neutrophils in lung defense and injury—state of the art. Am Rev Respir Dis. 1990;141:471–501.
17. Niewoehner DE, Kleinerman J, Rice DB. Pathologic changes in the peripheral airways of young cigarette smokers. N Engl J Med. 1974;291:755–788.
18. Gadek JE, Fells GA, Crystal RG. Cigarette smoking induces functional antiprotease deficiency in the lower respiratory tract of humans. Science. 1979;206:1315–1316.
19. Mason RJ, Crystal RG. Pulmonary cell biology. Am J Respir Crit Care Med. 1998;157:S72–S81.
20. Reid L. Measurement of the bronchial mucous gland layer: A diagnostic yardstick in chronic bronchitis. Thorax. 1960;15:132–141.
21. McElvaney NG, Nakamura H, Birrer P, et al. Modulation of airway inflammation in cystic fibrosis—in vivo suppression of interleukin-8 levels on the respiratory epithelial surface by aerosolization of recombinant secretory leukoprotease inhibitor. J Clin Invest. 1992;90:1296–1301.
22. Marom Z, Shelhamer JH, Kaliner M. Human pulmonary macrophage-derived mucus secretagogue. J Exp Med. 1984;159:884–860.
23. Rankin JA, Marcy T, Rochester CL, et al. Human airway macrophages—a technique for their retrieval and a descriptive comparison with alveolar macrophages. Am Rev Respir Dis. 1992;145:928–933.
24. Reynolds HY. Cytokines: Role in respiratory illnesses and potential control with immunomodulatory therapy. Focus and Opinion: Internal Medicine 1994;1(6):1–10.

25. Standiford TJ, Huffnagle JB. Cytokines in host defense against pneumonia. J Invest Med. 1997;45:335–345.
26. Burrows B, Niden AH, Fletcher CM, et al. Clinical types of chronic obstructive lung disease in London and Chicago. Am Rev Respir Dis. 1964;90:14–27.
27. Honig EG, Ingram RH Jr. Chronic bronchitis, emphysema, and airways obstruction. In: Fauci AS, Braunwald E, Isselbacher KJ, et al, eds. Harrison's Principles of Internal Medicine, 14th ed. New York: McGraw-Hill; 1998:1451–1460.
28. Murphy TF, Sethi S. Bacterial infection in chronic obstructive pulmonary disease—state of the art. Am Rev Respir Dis. 1992;146:1067–1083.
29. Leeder SR. Role of infection in the cause and course of chronic bronchitis and emphysema. J Infect Dis. 1975;131:731–742.
30. Gump DW, Phillips CA, Forsyth BR, et al. Role of infection in chronic bronchitis. Am Rev Respir Dis. 1976;113:465–474.
31. Tager I, Speizer FE. Role of infection in chronic bronchitis. N Engl J Med. 1975;292:563–571.
32. Wilson R. The role of infection in COPD. Chest. 1998;113:243S–248S.
33. Anthonisen NR, Manfreda J, Warren CPW, et al. Antibiotic therapy in acute exacerbations of chronic obstructive pulmonary disease. Ann Intern Med. 1987;106:196–204.
34. Saint S, Bent S, Vittinghoff E, et al. Antibiotics in chronic obstructive pulmonary disease exacerbations: A meta-analysis. JAMA. 1995;273:957–960.
35. Grossman RF. Guidelines for the treatment of acute exacerbations of chronic bronchitis. Chest. 1997;112:310S–313S.
36. Baigelman W, Chodosh S. Sputum "wet preps": Window on the airways. J Respir Dis. 1984;59–70.
37. Rothenberg ME. Eosinophilia—mechanisms of disease (Review). N Engl J Med. 1998;338:1592–1600.
38. Niederman MS, Merrill WW, Polomski LM, et al. Influence of sputum IgA and elastase on tracheal cell bacterial adherence. Am Rev Respir Dis. 1986;133:255–260.
39. Stockley RA, Afford SC, Burnett D. Assessment of 7S and 11S immunoglobulin A in sputum. Am Rev Respir Dis. 1980;122:959–964.
40. Wheeler JH, Fishman EK. Computed tomography in the management of chest infections: Current status. Clin Infect Dis. 1996;23:232–240.
41. Natsch S, vanderMeer JWM. Dosing of amoxicillin/clavulanate for treatment of lower respiratory tract infection. Clin Infect Dis. 1998;26:529–530.
42. Laurenzi GG, Potter RT, Kass EH. Bacterial flora of the lower respiratory tract. N Engl J Med. 1961;265:1273–1278.
43. Potter RT, Rotman F, Fernandez F, et al. The bacteriology of the lower respiratory tract. Bronchoscopic study of 100 clinical cases. Am Rev Respir Dis. 1968;97:1051–1061.
44. Halperin SA, Suratt PM, Gwaltney JM Jr, et al. Bacterial cultures of the lower respiratory tract in normal volunteers with and without experimental rhinovirus infection using a plugged double catheter system. Am Rev Respir Dis. 1982;125:678–680.
45. Hass H, Morris JF, Samson S, et al. Bacterial flora of the respiratory tract in chronic bronchitis. Comparison of transtracheal, fiber-bronchoscopic and oropharyngeal sampling methods. Am Rev Respir Dis. 1977;116:41–47.
46. Grayston JT. Infections caused by *Chlamydia pneumoniae* strain TWAR—state of the art (Clinical Article). Clin Infect Dis. 1992;15:757–763.
47. Reimer LG, Carroll KC. Role of the microbiology laboratory in the diagnosis of lower respiratory tract infections. Clin Infect Dis. 1998;26:742–748.
48. Emre U, Sokolovskaya N, Roblin PM, et al. Detection of anti-*Chlamydia pneumoniae* IgE in children with reactive airway disease. J Infect Dis. 1995;172:265–267.
49. Kutlin A, Roblin PM, Hammerschlag MR. Antibody response to *Chlamydia pneumoniae* infection in children with respiratory illness. J Infect Dis. 1998;177:720–724.
50. Nenning ME, Shinefield HR, Edwards KM, et al. Prevalence and incidence of adult pertussis in an urban population. JAMA. 1996;275:1672–1674.
51. Jansen DL, Gray GC, Putnam SD, et al. Evaluation of pertussis in US Marine Corps trainees. Clin Infect Dis. 1997;25:1099–1107.
52. Manzella JP, Kellogg JA, Parsey KS. *Corynebacterium pseudodiphtheriticum*: A respiratory tract pathogen in adults. Clin Infect Dis. 1995;20:37–40.
53. Ahmed K, Kawakami K, Watanabe K, et al. *Corynebacterium pseudodiphtheriticum*: A respiratory tract pathogen. Clin Infect Dis. 1995;20:41–46
54. Reynolds HY. Bacterial adherence to respiratory tract mucosa—A dynamic interaction leading to colonization. Semin Respir Infect. 1987;2:8–19.
55. Reynolds HY. Respiratory infections—community acquired pneumonia and newer microbes. Lung. 1996;174:207–224.
56. Bates JH, Campbell GD, Barron AL, et al. Microbial etiology of acute pneumonia in hospitalized patients. Chest. 1992;101:1005–1012.
57. Reynolds HY, Swisher JW. Preoperative management of chronic bronchitis. Infect Med. 1993;10:21–29.
58. Petty TL. Supportive therapy in COPD. Chest. 1998;113:256S–262S.
59. Mahler DA. Pulmonary rehabilitation. Chest. 1998;113:263S–268S.
60. Tolep K, Lando Y, D'Alonzo GE. Rethinking inhalative therapy for outpatients with chronic obstructive pulmonary disease. Clin Pulm Med. 1997;4:93–100.
61. Bone R, Boyars M, Braun SR, et al (Combivent Inhalation Aerosol Study Group). In chronic obstructive pulmonary disease, a combination of ipratropium and albuterol is more effective than either agent alone—an 85-day multi-center trial. Chest. 1994;105:1411–1419.
62. Wilson JD, Serby CW, Menjoge SS, Witek TJ Jr. The efficacy and safety of combination bronchodilator therapy. Eur Respir Rev. 1996;6:286–289.
63. O'Byrne PM, Israel E, Drazen JM. Antileukotrienes in the treatment of asthma—review. Ann Intern Med. 1997;127:472–480.
64. Anzueto A, Jubran A, Ohar JA, et al. Effects of aerosolized surfactant in patients with stable chronic bronchitis—a prospective randomized controlled trial. JAMA. 1997;278:1426–1431.
65. Seemungal TAR, Donaldson GC, Paul EA, et al. Effect of exacerbation on quality of life in patients with chronic obstructive pulmonary disease. Am J Respir Crit Care Med. 1998;157:1418–1422.
66. Grossman RF. The value of antibiotics and the outcomes of antibiotic therapy in exacerbations of COPD. Chest. 1998;113:249S–255S.
67. Schentag JJ, Tillotson GS. Antibiotic selection and dosing for the treatment of acute exacerbations of COPD. Chest. 1997;112:314S–319S.
68. Bartlett JG, Breiman RF, Mandell LA, et al. Community-acquired pneumonia in adults: Guidelines for management. Clin Infect Dis. 1998;26:811–838.
69. Jones RN, Jacobs MR, Washington JA, et al. A 1994–95 survey of *Haemophilus influenzae* susceptibility to ten orally administered agents—a 187 clinical laboratory center sample in the United States. Diagn Microbiol Infect Dis. 1997;27:75–83.

Chapter 56

Bronchiolitis

CAROLINE BREESE HALL
JOHN T. McBRIDE

In bronchiolitis we must now contend
with both the disease of the "now" and the "then";
For many such infants a mold has been cast,
perhaps by their unborn and unknown past,
which destines that they shall in time wheeze again.
For them this disease
is the distant, boding knell
Of vulnerable lungs
to a microbe's mystic spell.
C.B.H.

Bronchiolitis is an acute viral lower respiratory tract illness occurring during the first 2 years of life. The illness also has been called "wheezy bronchitis" and "asthmatic bronchitis." Whatever term is applied, the syndrome is caused by a viral infection. The characteristic clinical manifestations include an acute onset of wheezing and hyperinflation, most commonly associated with cough, rhinorrhea, tachypnea, and respiratory distress. The term *bronchiolitis* appears to have been born from a long lineage of confusing sobriquets, including "acute catarrhal bronchitis," "interstitial bronchopneumonia," "spastic bronchopneumonia," "capillary or obstructive bronchiolitis," and "asthmatic bronchiolitis."[1] Bronchiolitis, however, did not become recognized as a distinct entity until the 1940s.[2]

ETIOLOGY

Although bronchiolitis was initially thought to be caused by bacteria, viruses and occasionally *Mycoplasma pneumoniae* are now known to be the instigators of bronchiolitis. Respiratory syncytial virus (RSV) is clearly the major pathogen, and parainfluenza viruses are the second most commonly isolated agents (Table 56–1; Fig. 56–1).[3–12] A long-term study of respiratory illnesses associated with wheezing in children from a private practice in Chapel Hill, North Carolina, showed that RSV, parainfluenza 1 and 3 viruses, adenoviruses, rhinoviruses, and *M. pneumoniae* make up 87% of the isolates obtained from children of all ages.[3] Within the first 2 years of life, RSV accounted for 44% of the isolates, with parainfluenza 1 and 3

TABLE 56–1 Agents Causing Bronchiolitis

Agent	Percent of Cases	Epidemiologic Occurrence
Respiratory syncytial virus	45–75	Yearly epidemics, winter to spring
Parainfluenza viruses		
Type 3	8–15	Predominantly spring to fall
Type 1	5–12	Epidemics in fall every other year
Type 2	1–5	Fall
Rhinoviruses	3–8	Endemic, all seasons
Adenoviruses	3–10	Endemic, all seasons
Influenza viruses	5–8	Epidemic, winter to spring
Mycoplasma pneumoniae	1–7	Endemic, all seasons
Enteroviruses	1–5	Summer to fall

viruses and adenoviruses each accounting for about 13%. Similarly, RSV constituted 60% of the isolates obtained from children with bronchiolitis from two group practices in Rochester, New York, over an 11-year period.[13] The second most frequently identified agent was parainfluenza 3 virus, accounting for 12% of the cases. The relative proportions of these agents may change depending on the population and whether the cases occur as part of an epidemic. In hospitalized cases, the contribution of RSV is even higher, as demonstrated by studies from Newcastle-upon-Tyne, England, in which 74% of the infants hospitalized with bronchiolitis had infection with this agent.[10]

EPIDEMIOLOGY

Bronchiolitis shows a definite seasonal pattern in temperate climates, with a yearly upsurge in number of cases during winter to early spring.[3, 7–10, 13, 14] This pattern mirrors that of its prime agent, RSV. Lesser swells of activity are seen during fall and spring, when parainfluenza viruses are active.

Bronchiolitis is a common illness during the first year of life, the peak attack rate occurring between 2 and 10 months of age.[3, 5, 9, 10, 12, 14–17] In the Chapel Hill studies, the incidence of bronchiolitis was about 11 cases per 100 children for both the first and second 6 months of life.[3, 14] In the second year of life the incidence fell to approximately one-half that. A much higher incidence, however, has been reported in long-term studies of children in a daycare center who were examined regularly.[17] Because even the mildest cases were detected, the rate was much higher: 115 cases per 100 children aged 6 months or less per year. By the second year of life, this rate had declined to 32 cases per 100 children per year. Among children in the first year of life enrolled in a health maintenance organization in

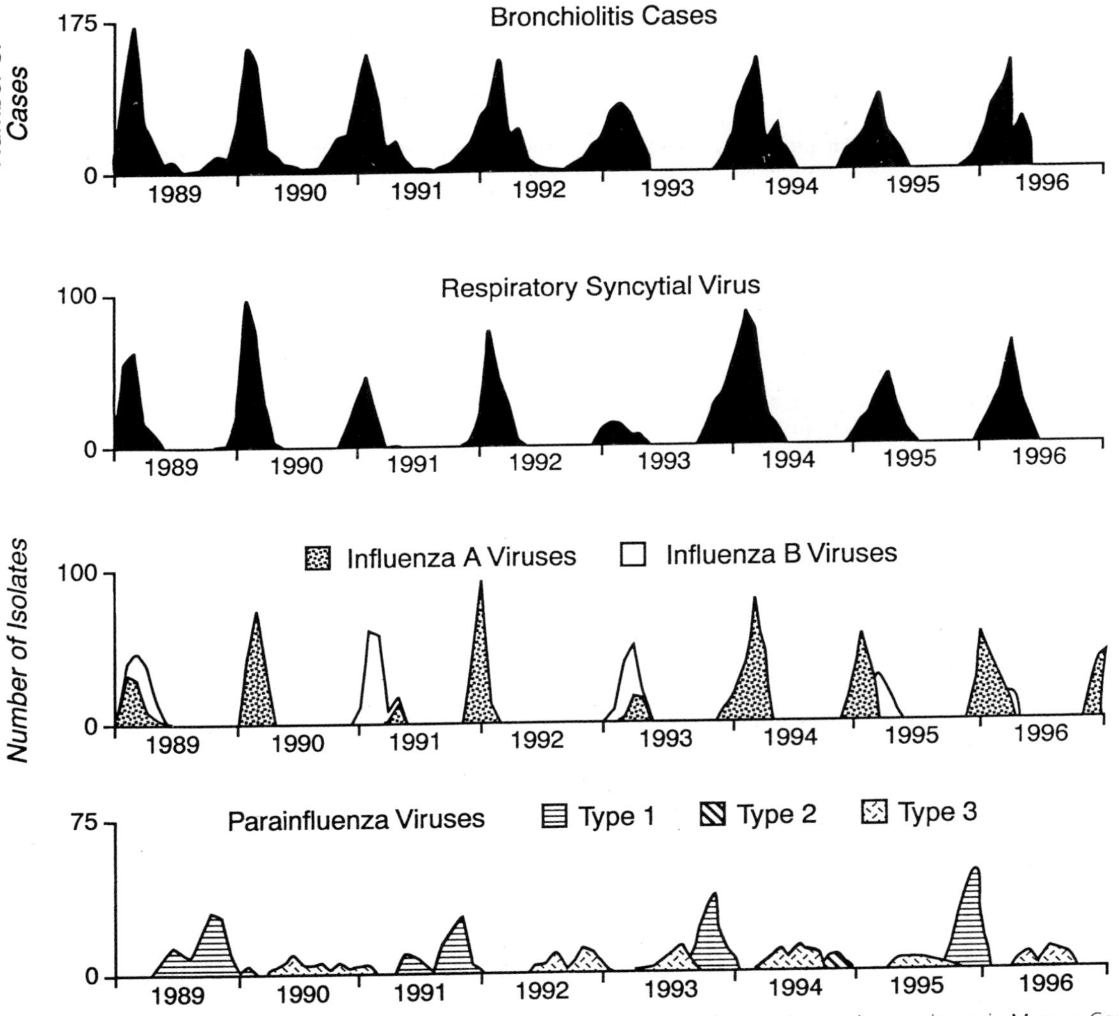

FIGURE 56–1. Patterns of reported cases of bronchiolitis shown in relation to the activity of the major respiratory viruses in Monroe County, New York. Data are obtained from a weekly community surveillance program for infectious diseases.

Tucson, Arizona, the rate of occurrence of lower respiratory tract illness was 32.9 cases per 100 children, of which 60% were bronchiolitis.[9]

An appreciable proportion of hospital admissions for infants within the first year of life is due to bronchiolitis, especially those cases resulting from RSV. In the review by Breese and colleagues of their group practice, bronchiolitis was the reason for admission in 4% of their patients of all ages who required hospitalization for medical illnesses.[18] In a Seattle prepaid medical care group, the rate of hospitalization among infants with bronchiolitis during the first 6 months of life was 6 per 1000 children per year.[5] Bronchiolitis is more common in boys, especially in those requiring hospitalization, with a gender ratio of about 1.5 to 1.[3, 16, 19]

Other factors described as increasing the chances that hospitalization will be required in otherwise normal children include young age, especially the first several months of life, as well as young maternal age, living in crowded and polluted surroundings, a greater number of siblings, lack of breast-feeding, a predisposition to atopy or hyperreactivity of the airway, and illness caused by RSV.[3, 12, 16, 17, 20–24]

PATHOPHYSIOLOGY

The term *bronchiolitis* was first used by Engle and Newns[2] in 1940 for the lower respiratory tract disease they observed in young infants that tended to be severe and often fatal and was probably viral in origin. They carefully described the pathologic findings in these infants dying of bronchiolitis, which over the subsequent half-century have been confirmed and expanded.[1, 25–29]

The pathologic findings in bronchiolitis are characteristically focused on the respiratory epithelium. The virus initially replicates in the epithelium of the upper respiratory tract but in the young infant tends to spread rapidly to the lower tract airways. Early inflammation of the bronchial and bronchiolar epithelium progresses rapidly to necrosis. Subsequently, the epithelium may proliferate and demonstrate cuboidal cells without cilia. Peribronchiolar infiltration, mostly with mononuclear cells, and edema of the submucosa and adventitia are observed. Necrosis of the bronchiolar epithelium and sloughing result (Figs. 56–2 and 56–3).

The pathologic findings in viral bronchiolitis are also characteristically generalized. Inflammatory changes, of variable severity, are observed in most small bronchi and bronchioles. Because resistance to the flow of air is related inversely to the cube of the radius of the airway, this inflammation and edema make the small-lumen airways in infants particularly vulnerable to obstruction. Plugs of necrotic material and fibrin may completely or partially obstruct the small airways.

Smooth muscle constriction does not appear to be important in the obstruction.[28] In areas peripheral to sites of partial obstruction, air becomes trapped by a process similar to a "ball-valve" mechanism. The negative intrapleural pressure exerted during inspiration allows air to flow beyond the point of partial obstruction. However, on expiration, the size of the lumen decreases with the positive pressure, thereby resulting in increased obstruction and hyperinflation. Thus, although airflow is impeded during both inspiration and expiration, the latter is more affected and prolonged. In areas peripheral to complete obstruction, the trapped air eventually becomes absorbed, which results in multiple areas of atelectasis. The degree of atelectasis or hyperinflation that develops may be greater in infants because collateral channels that maintain alveolar expansion in the presence of airway obstruction are not well developed early in life.

The physiologic correlates of this resistance to airflow are dyspnea, tachypnea, and a diminished tidal volume. The distribution of ventilation within the infant's lung also is altered markedly. Significant areas of lung parenchyma in which the ratio of ventilation to perfusion is low produces arterial hypoxemia. When an infant is no longer able to compensate for disordered gas exchange by increasing ventilation, hypercarbia may ensue. The pathologic process may progress to involve the alveolar walls and spaces, producing an interstitial pneumonitis. Recovery tends to be slow, requiring several weeks.

Experimental and clinical studies have suggested that the development of wheezing and the pathogenesis of bronchiolitis in some children and their risk for subsequent wheezing and pulmonary function abnormality are related to the type of inflammatory response initiated by RSV or other viruses and to a predisposition of the host. The presence and levels of immunoglobulin E (IgE) antibody to RSV and histamine, as well as leukotriene C_4 and eosinophilic cationic protein (ECP), have been related to the development of wheezing in infants with RSV infection.[30–39] The detection of a number of other cell-specific mediators in respiratory secretions of children with bronchiolitis, such as some of the chemokines (chemotactic cytokines), suggests that RSV and other viruses initiate the local migration and activation of eosinophils and basophils, resulting in an enhanced inflammatory response.[40–41]

Infection with RSV also elicits the release of certain neutrophilic chemotactic factors, interleukins IL-6 and IL-8. Accordingly, neutro-

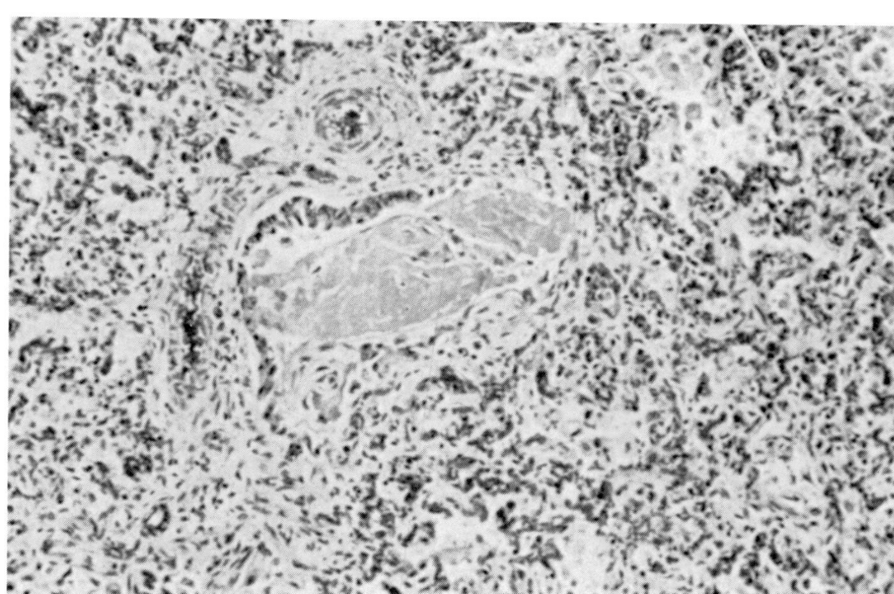

FIGURE 56–2. Inflammation and necrosis in bronchiolitis, resulting in obliteration of the bronchiolar lumen.

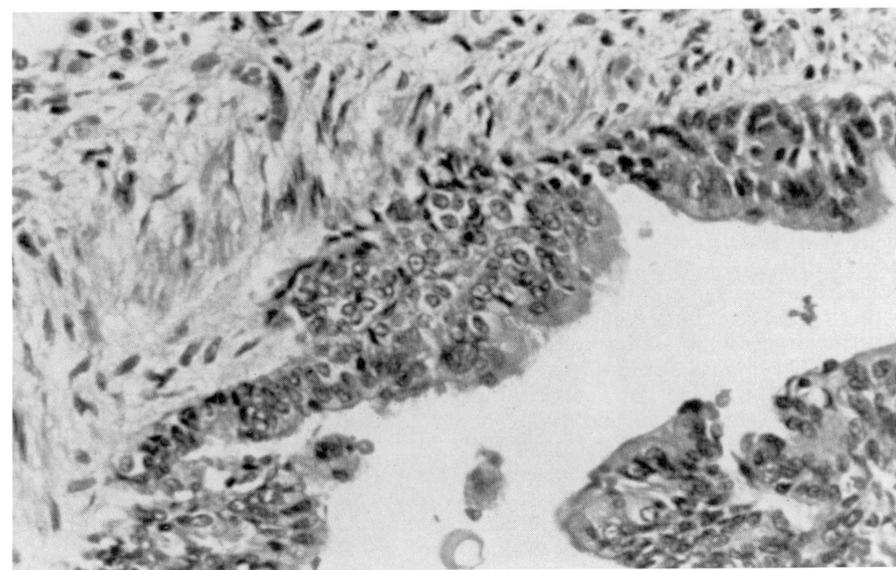

FIGURE 56–3. Inflammation of the bronchiole with regenerating epithelium.

phils are found in the bronchoalveolar lavage fluid of children with RSV infection.[42–44]

Evidence is lacking, however, that this inflammatory response that may elicit the acute syndrome of wheezing is related to subsequent hyperreactivity and abnormalities in subsequent lung function. The IgE response during the acute RSV infection appears possibly to be predictive of the IgE response to other viruses, but not to environmental allergens and to the development of asthma. This is suggested by the observation that RSV elicits a different pattern of mediator response (elevated interferon-γ and diminished IL-4) from that associated with atopy.[45] Some investigators, however, have characterized the immediate inflammatory response to RSV as involving both "atopic" (Th2) and "nonatopic" (Th1) cytokine profiles.[46]

Infants who develop bronchiolitis or wheezing early in life were previously thought to be at high risk for subsequent hyperreactivity of the airways and abnormalities in lung function because of modulation of or alteration in airway development and immune response induced by viral infection, but this concept has been modified. Recent studies suggest these early wheezers constitute two major groups of infants with different predisposing factors but who can be differentiated only by their subsequent clinical course and outcome.[47–52] Infants who are most likely to develop asthma and recurrent wheezing in later childhood constitute a minority of these early wheezers. They usually have evidence of atopy and a family history of atopy and of maternal smoking; typically, lung function is normal at birth, but recurrent episodes of bronchospasm tend to occur by 5 to 10 years. In the preschool years these children tend to wheeze only in association with colds and with attacks of shortness of breath.[51] Despite their propensity for asthma and recurrent wheezing, they are not at increased risk for chronic pulmonary function abnormalities in later life.

The larger group of infants who wheeze early are those who have no personal or family history of atopy but who have diminished lung function at birth. Although some may be premature, many are normal, healthy-appearing infants, and the anatomic basis of lower lung dysfunction in these infants is not clear. They may have a transitory tendency to wheeze with early episodes of viral respiratory infection, which are not associated with airway hyperreactivity, and they are often asymptomatic during their preschool years.[48, 49] Nevertheless, these infants appear to be at greater risk of developing chronic obstructive pulmonary disease as older adults than are the atopic children who wheeze when they reach school age.

Bronchiolitis and wheezing in early life are clearly instigated by RSV and other viral infections, but the role of viruses in causing an increased risk for subsequent pulmonary disease and asthma is unclear and unconfirmed. However, infants who develop wheezing and bronchiolitis with their initial infection with RSV or other respiratory viral infections early in life are those most likely to have some form of recurrent lower respiratory tract disease.

CLINICAL MANIFESTATIONS

Upper respiratory tract signs, especially coryza and cough, usually herald the onset of bronchiolitis. A prodromal period of 1 to 7 days marked by fever, usually mild, is common. Manifestations of lower respiratory tract involvement most frequently appear 2 to 3 days from the onset of the illness. The progression of the disease may be reflected initially in the development of a prominent cough and subsequently by an increase in the respiratory rate and in nonspecific systemic symptoms such as irritability, lethargy, and anorexia. With progression, tachypnea and tachycardia may be marked, although fever may no longer be present. Retractions of the chest wall, flaring of the nasal alae, and grunting are evidence of the increased work of breathing. Cyanosis rarely is evident even though moderate to severe hypoxemia may be present.[28, 53] Auscultatory findings, which may vary from hour to hour, include wheezing with or without crackles. Increasing dyspnea with decreasing lung sounds on auscultation and diminished movement of air may indicate progressive obstruction and impending respiratory failure.

A recent study of 21 infants with acute bronchiolitis, caused by RSV in 18 and parainfluenza virus in 3, demonstrated that bronchiolitis may result in significant cardiovascular effects in infants with no underlying cardiac or pulmonary disease.[54] During the acute phase of the illness, the 21 infants were evaluated by cross-sectional and Doppler echocardiography; 11 were demonstrated to have tricuspid valve regurgitation, usually accompanied by increased pulmonary artery systolic pressure. The presence of these abnormalities correlated with the clinical severity of the bronchiolitis. Subsequent serial evaluation studies indicated that these abnormalities disappeared as the infants recovered.

Dehydration is a common accompaniment of bronchiolitis, resulting from paroxysms of coughing, which may trigger vomiting, and from a poor oral intake related to the respiratory distress and lethargy. The tachypnea further increases the fluid requirement. Otitis media, occurring in 10 to 30% of infants, as well as mild conjunctivitis and occasionally diarrhea may also be present.

The acute course typically lasts 3 to 7 days. Most infants show improvement within 3 to 4 days, with a gradual recovery period of 1 to 2 weeks, which may be prolonged in some.[53, 55]

LABORATORY FINDINGS

The total white blood cell count is usually within the normal range or slightly elevated.[55, 56] In hospitalized infants, however, who are more seriously ill and hypoxemic, the white blood cell count may be elevated, and the differential count may show a leftward shift.[53, 56] Most hospitalized infants with bronchiolitis are hypoxemic, but the degree of hypoxemia is difficult to assess clinically.[53] The degree of wheezing and retractions cannot be assumed to be indicative of the level of oxygenation. An inverse correlation, however, appears to exist between the respiratory rate and the arterial oxygen saturation.[53, 57] Only the most severely ill children develop hypercarbia, as most are able to compensate for the increased work of breathing with an elevated respiratory rate.[53, 57, 58]

The hallmark of the chest roentgenogram in acute bronchiolitis is the characteristic hyperinflation with associated depressed diaphragms, hyperlucency of the parenchyma, and decreased costophrenic angle.[59–66] The bronchovascular markings are usually prominent, with linear densities seen radiating out from the hila. Multiple areas of atelectasis of variable degree also are commonly present and difficult to differentiate from the infiltrates of pneumonia. Indeed, both bronchiolitis and pneumonia frequently are present, especially with RSV infection.

In most cases of bronchiolitis, obtaining a chest roentgenogram is not necessary for diagnosis or management. The abnormalities observed on the chest roentgenogram in acute bronchiolitis often do not correlate with the degree of clinical illness; the child may be severely ill despite minimal findings on the chest roentgenogram. Furthermore, a recent study indicates that considerable intraobserver and interobserver variation occurs among radiologists in their assessment of radiographic findings for the diagnosis of lower respiratory tract disease in infants, especially those with bronchiolitis.[66]

DIAGNOSIS

The diagnosis of bronchiolitis is made most frequently on the basis of the characteristic clinical and epidemiologic findings. However, considerable confusion exists over the exact definition of bronchiolitis.[29, 67] A variety of entities may cause a similar picture of dyspnea and wheezing in the infant. Asthma is not easily differentiated, particularly if it is the infant's first episode. Furthermore, the two diseases may be combined. An appreciable proportion of wheezing episodes occurring in a child with an atopic diathesis may arise from viral infections.[68–70] RSV in particular has a propensity to induce wheezing in young children. Even in adults with acute RSV infection clinically manifested as upper respiratory tract infection, hyperreactivity of the airways may be detected by pulmonary function testing and may last for 1 or 2 months.[71]

The differential diagnosis of wheezing in an infant is broad and requires a careful history and examination.[67] Gastric reflux and aspiration may produce a picture that is indistinguishable clinically from acute bronchiolitis. Other considerations include obstruction of the airway from a foreign body, vascular rings, retropharyngeal abscess, and even enlarged adenoids. Wheezing may also be associated with cystic fibrosis, immunodeficiency, and congestive heart failure in young infants.

Identification of the specific agent of acute bronchiolitis can be made in an appreciable proportion of infants by viral isolation from respiratory secretions, preferably from a nasal wash.[3, 5–10, 72] In most cases the viruses associated with bronchiolitis may be identified in tissue culture within 3 to 7 days. Rapid viral diagnostic techniques are available, especially for RSV, that allow identification of the viral antigen in the respiratory secretions within hours[73, 74] (see Chapter 148). The sensitivity of these assays is variable, and the positive predictive value significantly diminishes if they are used when RSV infection is not epidemic in the community. The use of culture in addition to the rapid screening test may be of particular benefit when the suspected viral agent is not highly prevalent in the community and when results of rapid-technique tests are negative. Viral isolation procedures offer the advantage of detecting other agents that may be the cause of the illness or that are concurrently present. Serologic tests to determine the etiologic agent are rarely helpful. Antibody determinations in convalescent serum specimens provide information too late to be of help in clinical management. Also, maternally acquired antibody to many of the viral agents of bronchiolitis will be present in the sera of infants and will confound interpretation of most antibody tests.

THERAPY

More than 2 decades ago, Reynolds and Cook noted that "oxygen is vitally important in bronchiolitis, and there is little convincing evidence that any other therapy is consistently or even occasionally useful."[75] Today the mainstay of therapy for the hospitalized child remains oxygen administration to maintain the oxygen saturation level at 92% or greater, with careful supportive care.[1] Although mist therapy also is commonly employed, its use has not been proved beneficial, and chest physiotherapy has been shown to be of no help.[76, 77]

A variable but sometimes high proportion of infants with bronchiolitis, especially those with RSV infection who are admitted to the hospital, may require mechanical ventilation.[78, 79] High tidal volumes with high peak inspiratory pressures and low respiratory rates are often required to achieve an adequate minute ventilation. Even though infants with bronchiolitis generally have hyperexpanded lungs, most benefit from positive end-expiratory pressure.

The only specific therapy currently available for bronchiolitis caused by RSV is ribavirin (1-β-D-ribofuranosyl-1,2,4-triazole-3-carboxamide), a synthetic nucleoside[80] (see Chapter 36). This broad-spectrum antiviral agent has been approved only for infants hospitalized with RSV infections and is administered as a small-particle aerosol for 8 to 12 hours each day, usually for 2 to 5 days.[80–83] Shorter or intermittent periods of administration may be as beneficial, especially because very high levels of drug are achieved in the respiratory secretions by aerosol administration.[84, 85] Infants who should be considered for therapy with ribavirin are those who have or are at risk of developing severe or complicated RSV infection, such as those with underlying predisposing conditions, especially prematurity and cardiopulmonary disease.[83] Although in a number of relatively small placebo-controlled studies, clinical benefit and more rapid improvement in oxygen saturation levels have been demonstrated with ribavirin therapy, shortening of the duration of hospitalization has not been shown consistently. Further considerations in whether ribavirin should be used include the technical difficulty of preventing clogging of the circuits when the drug is administered via a mechanical ventilator and its considerable cost, which makes it of questionable benefit, especially in children without severe illness.

Bronchodilator therapy is perhaps the most frequently used therapy for bronchiolitis, despite lack of evidence supporting the efficacy of these agents in most children with bronchiolitis.[86–91] Bronchodilators are generally used in over 80% of hospitalized infants with bronchiolitis, and in a 1995 poll of members of the European Society for Paediatric Infectious Diseases, bronchodilators were used universally.[86–88] In most young infants, the major cause of the airway obstruction is the inflammation caused by the viral infection, rather than smooth muscle contraction, but hyperreactive airways may compound the obstruction.[92] Studies evaluating bronchodilators administered by a variety of routes have given conflicting results. The majority of studies have shown little or no significant benefit with regard to clinical status and pulmonary function.[88–94] Some studies have indicated modest clinical benefit, especially for treatment with epinephrine aerosols as opposed to albuterol.[95–100] Adverse effects of bronchodilator use may occur in some infants, including paradoxical airway obstruction and cardiovascular effects.[101–104]

Corticosteroids have been reported to be used in over 80% of children with bronchiolitis,[87] but their efficacy has been a matter of controversy. Some controlled studies have indicated these agents provide no appreciable clinical benefit in the hospitalized child whether given parenterally or orally with or without bronchodilators,[105–113] whereas others have shown a benefit.[114] In one controlled study of 54 patients, oral prednisolone was associated with a greater but modest decrease in the symptom score in the first 3 days, but the duration of hospitalization was not shortened.[115] A recent placebo-controlled study in 144 children with moderately severe croup reported beneficial effects with use of either intramuscular dexamethasone or nebulized budesonide, with the greatest benefit associated with dexamethasone.[116]

Other therapies evaluated in limited small studies for RSV-caused lower respiratory tract disease have included the use of interferon alfa-2A and vitamin A, but with little success.[117–119]

Antibacterial antibiotics should not be administered routinely to infants with bronchiolitis, because bacteria have no role in the etiopathogenesis. Furthermore, secondary bacterial infection is rarely observed after bronchiolitis.[120]

COMPLICATIONS

Almost all children recover from bronchiolitis without difficulty. Complications from bronchiolitis are relatively rare, especially in normal children. A number of studies have attempted to predict by epidemiologic and clinical characteristics which children with acute bronchiolitis are most likely to have complicated or severe courses. Infants with underlying diseases, especially cardiac, pulmonary, and immunodeficiency diseases, and those who were premature are most at risk for prolonged or complicated illness.[21, 22, 28, 66, 78, 83, 105, 106, 121, 122] Clinical characteristics at the onset of the acute illness, such as respiratory rate or lung sounds on auscultation have not been of consistent prognostic value, but diminished arterial oxygen saturation has been associated with complicated illness.[122, 123] With currently available technical and pharmacologic methods of management, the mortality from bronchiolitis is very low. Respiratory failure and prolonged hypoxemia are most likely to occur in infants with compromising underlying conditions and in very young infants.[53, 124] Apnea is a relatively common complication in reported series of hospitalized patients, especially very young infants with RSV infection.[53, 125–127]

Among potential complications following bronchiolitis, the major concern—which has been noted for decades—is the tendency for many children who had bronchiolitis early in life to experience recurrent episodes of wheezing or lower respiratory tract disease.[128–136] Some studies have shown that as many as 75% of infants hospitalized with acute bronchiolitis will have recurrent episodes of bronchospasm within the first 2 years after discharge. However, over subsequent years, the number of children with continued clinical episodes of bronchospasm tends to diminish.[130, 136, 137] Children who had milder bronchiolitis not requiring hospitalization may not have the same degree of risk.[130, 138, 139] More recent studies suggest that the infants who subsequently wheeze constitute two major groups of children: those without evidence of atopy, but who have diminished lung function at birth, and a smaller group of children who have an atopic predisposition (see Pathophysiology section).[47–52] Despite these differing predisposing factors, determining the prognosis for an individual child at the time of the initial episode of bronchiolitis is not possible at present.

Bronchiolitis Obliterans

A rare, chronic type of bronchiolitis termed *bronchiolitis obliterans* has been reported in both adults and children.[140–146] In adults, bronchiolitis obliterans recently has been reported most often as a complication, often severe, of heart-lung and bone marrow transplantation.[140–142, 144, 146] This unusual disease has also been noted in association with collagen vascular diseases.[145, 147] In infants and young children, bronchiolitis obliterans may also complicate transplantation, but it primarily occurs as a rare, frequently devastating sequela of acute viral bronchiolitis. The major association has been with adenovirus infection in infants with a certain undefined genetic predisposition.[140, 148–150] The disease has appeared to be particularly prevalent in Native American populations in central Canada and among Polynesians in New Zealand.[140, 148–150] Affected infants commonly have bronchopneumonia along with signs of bronchiolitis that continue for weeks to months with fluctuating severity. Approximately 60% of these children develop chronic disease with atelectasis, bronchiectasis, intermittent pneumonia, and hyperinflation. These sequelae are accompanied by severe pathologic abnormalities involving the occlusion and destruction of the bronchi and bronchioles.

REFERENCES

1. Wohl MEB. Bronchiolitis. In: Chernick V, Kendig EL Jr, eds. Kendig's Disorders of the Respiratory Tract in Children. 5th ed. Philadelphia: WB Saunders; 1990: 360–370.
2. Engle S, Newns GH. Proliferative mural bronchiolitis. Arch Dis Child. 1940;15:219–229.
3. Henderson FW, Clyde WA Jr, Collier AM, Denny FW. The etiologic and epidemiologic spectrum of bronchiolitis in pediatric practice. J Pediatr. 1979;95:183–190.
4. Chanock R, Chambon L, Chang W, et al. WHO respiratory disease survey in children. A serologic study. Bull World Health Organ. 1967;37:363–369.
5. Foy HM, Cooney MK, Maletzky AJ, et al. Incidence and etiology of pneumonia, croup and bronchiolitis in preschool children belonging to a prepaid medical care group over a four year period. Am J Epidemiol. 1973;97:80–92.
6. Glezen WP, Loda FA, Clyde WA Jr, et al. Epidemiologic patterns of acute lower respiratory tract disease of children in a pediatric group practice. J Pediatr. 1971;78:397–406.
7. Kim HW, Arrobio JO, Brandt CD, et al. Epidemiology of respiratory syncytial virus infection in Washington, D.C. I. Importance of the virus in different respiratory disease syndromes and temporal distribution of infection. Am J Epidemiol. 1973;98:216–225.
8. Loda FA, Glezen WP, Clyde WA Jr. Respiratory disease in group day care. Pediatrics. 1972;49:428–437.
9. Wright AL, Taussig LM, Ray CG, et al. The Tucson Children's Respiratory Study II. Lower respiratory illness in the first year of life. Am J Epidemiol. 1989;129:1232–1246.
10. Gardner PS. How etiologic, pathologic, and clinical diagnosis can be made in a correlated fashion. Pediatr Res. 1977;11:254–261.
11. Chang TC, Wang CL, Han HL. Etiologic and clinical investigation of bronchiolitis. Chinese Med J. 1978;4:135–141.
12. Everard ML, Milner AD. The respiratory syncytial virus and its role in acute bronchiolitis. Eur J Pediatr. 1992;151:638–651.
13. Hall CB. Infect Dis Newslett Commun Surveill. 1982–93;29–51:1.
14. Denny FW, Clyde WA Jr. Acute lower respiratory tract infections in non-hospitalized children. J Pediatr. 1986;108:635–646.
15. Glezen WP. Pathogenesis of bronchiolitis: Epidemiologic considerations. Pediatr Res. 1977;11:239–243.
16. Parrott RH, Kim HW, Arrobio JO, et al. Epidemiology of respiratory syncytial virus infection in Washington, D.C. II. Infection and disease with respect to age, immunologic status, race and sex. Am J Epidemiol. 1973;98:289–300.
17. Denny FW, Collier AM, Henderson FW, Clyde WA Jr. The epidemiology of bronchiolitis. Pediatr Res. 1977;11:234–236.
18. Breese BB, Disney FA, Talpey W. The nature of a small pediatric group practice. Part I. Pediatrics. 1966;38:264–277.
19. Kravits H. Sex distribution of hospitalized children with acute respiratory diseases, gastroenteritis and meningitis. Clin Pediatr (Phila). 1965;4:484–491.
20. Report to the Medical Research Council Subcommittee on Respiratory Syncytial Virus. Respiratory syncytial virus infection: Admission to hospital in industrial urban and rural areas. BMJ. 1978;2:796–798.
21. Carlsen K-H, Larsen S, Bjerve O, Leegaard J. Acute bronchiolitis: Predisposing factors and characterization of infants at risk. Pediatr Pulmonol. 1987;3:153–160.
22. Holberg CJ, Wright AL, Martinez FD, et al. Risk factors for respiratory syncytial virus–associated lower respiratory illnesses in the first year of life. Am J Epidemiol. 1991;133:1135–1151.
23. Simpson H, Matthew DJ, Inglis JM, George EL. Virological findings and blood gas tensions in acute lower respiratory tract infections in children. BMJ. 1974;2:629–632.
24. Martinez FD, Wright AL, Holberg CJ, et al. Maternal age as a risk factor for wheezing lower respiratory illnesses in the first year of life. Am J Epidemiol. 1992;136:1258–1268.

25. Aherne W, Bird T, Court SDM, et al. Pathological changes in virus infections of the lower respiratory tract in children. J Clin Pathol. 1970;23:7–18.
26. McLean KH. The pathology of bronchiolitis. A study of its evolution. I. The exudative phase. Aust Ann Med. 1956;5:254.
27. McLean KH. The pathology of bronchiolitis. A study of its evolution. II. The repair phase. Aust Ann Med. 1957;6:29.
28. Wohl MEB. Bronchiolitis. Pediatr Ann. 1986;15:307–313.
29. Price JF. Acute and long-term effects of viral bronchiolitis in infancy. Lung. 1990;168(Suppl):414–421.
30. Welliver RC, Wong DT, Sun M, et al. The development of respiratory syncytial virus specific IgE and the release of histamine in nasopharyngeal secretions after infection. N Engl J Med. 1981;305:841–846.
31. Welliver RC, Kaul TN, Sun M, et al. Defective regulation of immune responses in respiratory syncytial virus infection. J Immunol. 1984;133:1925–1930.
32. Welliver RC, Kaul A, Ogra PL. Cell-mediated immune response to respiratory syncytial virus infection: Relationship to the development of reactive airway disease. J Pediatr. 1979;94:370–375.
33. Welliver RC, Wong DT, Sun M, McCarthy N. Parainfluenza virus bronchiolitis: Epidemiology and pathogenesis. Am J Dis Child. 1986;14:34–40.
34. Welliver RC, Sun M, Rinaldo D, Ogra PL. Predictive value of respiratory syncytial virus specific IgE responses for recurrent wheezing following bronchiolitis. J Pediatr. 1986;109:776–780.
35. Volovitz B, Faden H, Ogra PL. Release of leukotriene C_4 in respiratory tract during acute viral infection. J Pediatr. 1988;112:218–222.
36. Volovitz B, Welliver RC, de Castro G, et al. The release of leukotrienes in the respiratory tract during infection with respiratory syncytial virus: Role in obstructive airway disease. Pediatr Res. 1988;24:504–507.
37. Garofalo R, Dorris A, Ahlstedt S, Welliver RC. Peripheral blood eosinophil counts and eosinophil cationic protein content of respiratory secretions in bronchiolitis: Relationship to severity of disease. Pediatr Allergy Immunol. 1994;5:111–117.
38. Reijonen TM, Korppi M, Kuikka L, et al. Serum eosinophil cationic protein as a predictor of wheezing after bronchiolitis. Pediatr Pulmonol. 1997;23:397–403.
39. Skoner D, Fireman P, Caliguiri L, Davis H. Plasma elevations of histamine and a prostaglandin metabolite in acute bronchiolitis. Am Rev Respir Dis. 1990;142:359.
40. Becker S, Reed W, Henderson FW, Noah TL. RSV infection of human airway epithelial cells causes production of the β-chemokine RANTES. Am J Physiol. 1997;272 (3 Pt 1:)L512–L520.
41. Berkman NA, Robichaeid A, Krishnan VL, et al. Expression of RANTES in human airway epithelial cells: Effect of corticosteroids and interleukin-4, -10, and -13. Immunology. 1996;87:599.
42. Everard ML, Swarbrick A, Wrightham J, et al. Analysis of cells obtained by bronchial lavage of infants with respiratory syncytial virus infection. Arch Dis Child. 1994;71:428–432.
43. Mastronarde JG, Monick MM, Cross TJ, Hunninghake GW. Amiloride inhibits cytokine production in epithelium infected with respiratory syncytial virus. Am J Physiol. 1996;271(2 Pt 1):L201–L207.
44. Noah TL, Becker S. Respiratory syncytial virus–induced cytokine production by a human epithelial cell line. Am J Physiol. 1993;265(5 Pt 1):L472–L478.
45. Welliver RC, Duffy L. The relationship of RSV-specific immunoglobulin E antibody responses in infancy, recurrent wheezing, and pulmonary function at age 7–8 years. Pediatr Pulmonol. 1993;15:19–27.
46. Khan MA, Kemeny MD, Milner AD. Cytokine Controlling Allergic Responses to Nasal Secretions of Infants with Respiratory Syncytial Virus Induced Bronchiolitis (Abstract). Washington, DC: American Pediatric Society/Society for Pediatric Research; April 1997;41(4):11a.
47. Martinez FD, Morgan WJ, Wright AL, et al. Diminished lung function as a predisposing factor for wheezing respiratory illness in infants. N Engl J Med. 1988;319:1112–1117.
48. Martinez FD, Stern DA, Wright AL, et al. Association of non-wheezing lower respiratory tract illnesses in early life with persistently diminished serum IgE levels. Thorax. 1995;50:1067–1072.
49. Martinez FD. Viral infections and the development of asthma. Am J Respir Crit Care. 1995;151:1644–1647.
50. Martinez FD, Wright AL, Taussig LM, et al. Asthma and wheezing in the first six years of life. N Engl J Med. 1995;332:133–138.
51. Dodge R, Martinez FD, Cline MG, et al. Early childhood respiratory symptoms and the subsequent diagnosis of asthma. J Allergy Clin Immunol. 1996;98:48–54.
52. Wilson N. The significance of early wheezing. Clin Exp Allergy. 1994;24:522–529.
53. Hall CB, Hall WJ, Speers DM. Clinical and physiologic manifestations of bronchiolitis and pneumonia. Am J Dis Child. 1979;133:798–802.
54. Sreeram N, Watson JG, Hunter S. Cardiovascular effects of acute bronchiolitis. Acta Paediatr Scand. 1991;80:133–136.
55. Ackerman BD. Acute bronchiolitis: A study of 207 cases. Clin Pediatr (Phila). 1962;1:75–81.
56. Portnoy B, Haynes B, Salvatore MA, et al. The peripheral white blood count in respirovirus infection. J Pediatr. 1966;68:181–188.
57. Reynolds EOR. Arterial blood gas tensions of babies with bronchiolitis. BMJ. 1963;1:1192–1195.
58. Downes JJ, Wood DW, Striker TW, et al. Acute respiratory failure in infants with bronchiolitis. Anesthesiology. 1968;29:426–434.
59. Simpson W, Hacking PM, Court SDM, Gardner PS. The radiological findings in respiratory syncytial virus infection in children. Pediatr Radiol. 1974;2:97–100.
60. Simpson W, Hacking PM, Court SDM, Gardner PS. The radiological findings in respiratory syncytial virus infection in children. Part II. The correlation of radiological categories with clinical and virological findings. Pediatr Radiol. 1974;2: 155–160.
61. Rice RP, Loda F. A roentgenographic analysis of respiratory syncytial virus pneumonia in infants. Radiology. 1966;87:1021–1027.
62. Koch DA. Roentgenologic considerations of capillary bronchiolitis. Am J Roentgenol Rad Ther Nucl Med. 1959;82:433–436.
63. Khamapirad T, Glezen WP. Clinical and radiographic assessment of acute lower respiratory tract disease in infants and children. Semin Respir Infect. 1987;2: 130–144.
64. Wildin SR, Chonmaitree T, Swischuk LE. Roentgenographic features of common pediatric viral respiratory tract infections. Am J Dis Child. 1988;142:43–46.
65. Friis B, Eiken M, Hornsleth A, Jensen A. Chest x-ray appearances in pneumonia and bronchiolitis. Acta Paediatr Scand. 1990;79:219–225.
66. Davies HD, Wang EE, Manson D, et al. Reliability of the chest radiograph in the diagnosis of lower respiratory infections in young children. Pediatr Infect Dis J. 1996;15:600–604.
67. Mahesh VK, Taussig LM. When an infant wheezes: Clues to the differential. J Respir Dis. 1990;11:739–750.
68. McIntosh K, Ellis EF, Hoffman LS, et al. The association of viral and bacterial respiratory infections with exacerbations of wheezing in young asthmatic children. J Pediatr. 1973;82:578–590.
69. Johnston SL, Pattemore PK, Sanderson G, et al. Community study of role of viral infections in exacerbations of asthma in 9–11 year old children. BMJ. 1995;310:1225–1228.
70. Heymann PW, Zambrano JC, Rakes GP. Virus-induced wheezing in children: Respiratory syncytial virus (RSV) and rhinovirus. Immunol Allergy Clin North Am. 1998;18:35–47.
71. Hall WJ, Hall CB, Speers DM. Respiratory syncytial virus infections in adults: Clinical, virologic and serial pulmonary function studies. Ann Intern Med. 1978;88:203–205.
72. Hall CB, Douglas RG Jr. Clinically useful method for the isolation of respiratory syncytial virus. J Infect Dis. 1975;131:1–5.
73. Kellogg JA. Culture vs. direct antigen assays for detection of microbial pathogens from lower respiratory tract specimens suspected of containing the respiratory syncytial virus. Arch Pathol Lab Med. 1991;115:451–458.
74. Tristram DA, Welliver RC. Respiratory syncytial virus. In: Murray PR, Baron EJ, Pfaller MA, et al, eds. Manual of Clinical Microbiology. 6th ed. Washington, DC: ASM Press; 1995;2–9.
75. Reynolds EOR, Cook CD. The treatment of bronchiolitis. J Pediatr. 1963;63:1205–1207.
76. Taussig LM: Mists and aerosols: New studies, new thoughts (Editorial). J Pediatr. 1974;84:619–622.
77. Webb MSC, Martin GA, Cartlidge PHT, et al. Chest physiotherapy in acute bronchiolitis. Arch Dis Child. 1985;60:1078–1079.
78. Frankel LR, Lewiston NJ, Smith DW, Stevenson DK. Clinical observations on mechanical ventilation for respiratory failure in bronchiolitis. Pediatr Pulmonol. 1986;2:307–311.
79. Outwater KM, Crone RK. Management of respiratory failure in infants with acute viral bronchiolitis. Am J Dis Child. 1984;138:1071–1075.
80. Knight V, Gilbert BE. Chemotherapy of respiratory viruses. Adv Intern Med. 1986;31:95–118.
81. Hall CB, McBride JT, Walsh EE, et al. Aerosolized ribavirin treatment of infants with respiratory syncytial virus infection: A randomized double-blind study. N Engl J Med. 1983;308:1443–1447.
82. Smith DW, Frankel LR, Mathers LH, et al. A controlled trial of aerosolized ribavirin in infants receiving mechanical ventilation for severe respiratory syncytial virus infection. N Engl J Med. 1991;325:24–29.
83. Report of the Committee of Infectious Diseases. Respiratory syncytial virus. In: Peter G, ed. Redbook. 24th ed. Elk Grove Village, Ill: American Association of Pediatrics; 1997:443–447.
84. Englund JA, Piedra PA, Jefferson LS, et al. High-dose, short-duration ribavirin aerosol therapy in children with suspected respiratory syncytial virus infection. J Pediatr. 1990;117:313–320.
85. Connor J. Ribavirin pharmacokinetics. Pediatr Infect Dis J. 1990;9:S91–S92.
86. Nahata MC, Schad PA. Pattern of drug usage in bronchiolitis. J Clin Pharm Ther. 1994;19:117–118.
87. Kimpen JL, Schaad UB. Treatment of respiratory syncytial virus bronchiolitis: 1995 poll of members of the European Society for Paediatric Infectious Diseases. Pediatr Infect Dis J. 1997;16:479–481.
88. Dobson JV, Stephens-Groff SM, McMahon SR, et al. The use of albuterol in hospitalized infants with bronchiolitis. Pediatrics. 1998;101:361–368.
89. Flores G, Horwitz RI. Efficacy of β_2-agonists in bronchiolitis: A reappraisal and meta-analysis. Pediatrics. 1997;100:233–239.
90. Kellner JD, Ohlsson A, Gadomski AM, Wang EEL. Efficacy of bronchodilator therapy in bronchiolitis. Arch Pediatr Adolesc Med. 1996;150:1166–1172.
91. Gadomski AM, Sawy BE, Khallaf N, Black RE. Oral virus nebulized albuterol in management of bronchiolitis in Egypt. Pediatrics. 1994;24:131–138.
92. Mahesh VK, Taussig LM. The wheezing infant: Acute and long-term management. J Respir Dis. 1990;11:799–810.
93. Sly PD, Lanteri CJ, Raven JM. Do wheezy infants recovering from bronchiolitis respond to inhaled salbutamol? Pediatr Pulmonol. 1991;10:36–39.
94. Hughes DM, Lesouef PN, Landau LI. Effect of salbutamol on respiratory mechanics in bronchiolitis. Pediatr Res. 1987;22:83–86.
95. Schuh S, Canny G, Reisman JJ, et al. Nebulized albuterol in acute bronchiolitis. J Pediatr. 1990;117:633–637.

96. Klassen TP, Rowe PC, Sutcliffe T, et al. Randomized trial of salbutamol in acute bronchiolitis. J Pediatr. 1991;118:807–811.
97. Sanchez I, DeKoster J, Powell RE, et al. Effect of racemic epinephrine and salbutamol on clinical score and pulmonary mechanics in infants with bronchiolitis. J Pediatr. 1993;122:145–151.
98. Menon K, Sutcliffe T, Klassen TP. A randomized trial comparing the efficacy of epinephrine with salbutamol in the treatment of acute bronchiolitis. J Pediatr. 1995;126:1004–1007.
99. Hickey RW, Gochman RF, Chande V, David HW. Albuterol delivered via metered-dose inhaler with spacer for outpatient treatment of young children with wheezing. Arch Pediatr Adolesc Med. 1994;148:189–194.
100. Kristjansson S, Lodrup Carlsen KC, Wennergren G, et al. Nebulised racemic adrenaline in the treatment of acute bronchiolitis in infants and toddlers. Arch Dis Child. 1993;69:650–654.
101. O'Callaghan C, Milner AD, Swarbrick A. Paradoxical deterioration in lung function after nebulized salbutamol in wheezy infants. Lancet. 1986;2:1424–1425.
102. Prendiville A, Green S, Silverman M. Paradoxical response to nebulized salbutamol in wheezy infants, assessed by partial expiratory flow-volume curves. Thorax. 1987;42:86–91.
103. Keller KA, Bhisitkul DM. Supraventricular tachycardia: A complication of nebulized albuterol. Pediatr Emerg Care. 1995;11:98–99.
104. Nelson HS. β-Adrenergic bronchodilators. Drug Therapy. 1995;333:499–506.
105. Connelly JH, Field CMB, Glasgow JFT, et al. A double blind trial of prednisolone in epidemic bronchiolitis due to respiratory syncytial virus. Acta Paediatr Scand. 1969;58:116.
106. Leer JA, Green JL, Heimlich EM, et al. Corticosteroid treatment in bronchiolitis. A controlled collaborative study in 297 infants and children. Am J Dis Child. 1969;117:495–503.
107. Yaffe SJ, Weiss CF, Cann HM, et al. Should steroids be used in treating bronchiolitis? Pediatrics. 1970;46:640–642.
108. Springer C, Bar-Yishay E, Uwayyed K, et al. Corticosteroids do not affect the clinical or physiological status of infants with bronchiolitis. Pediatr Pulmonol. 1990;9:181–185.
109. Maayan C, Itzhaki T, Bar-Yishay E, et al: The functional response of infants with persistent wheezing to nebulized beclomethasone dipropionate. Pediatr Pulmonol. 1986;2:9–14.
110. Carlsen K-H, Leegaard J, Larsen S, Orstavik I. Nebulized beclomethasone dipropionate in recurrent obstructive episodes after acute bronchiolitis. Arch Dis Child. 1988;63:1428–1433.
111. Klassen TP. Recent advances in the treatment of bronchiolitis and laryngitis. Pediatr Clin North Am. 1997;44:249–261.
112. Roosevelt G, Sheehan K, Grupp-Phelan J, et al. Dexamethasone in bronchiolitis: A randomized controlled trial. Lancet. 1996;348:292–295.
113. De Benedictis FM, Canny GJ, Levison H. The role of corticosteroids in respiratory diseases of children. Pediatr Pulmonol. 1996;22:44–57.
114. Jaffe DM: Treatment of croup with glucocorticoids. N Engl J Med. 1998;339: 553–554.
115. Van Woensel JBM, Wolfs TFW, van Aalderen WMC, et al. Randomised double blind placebo controlled trial of prednisolone in children admitted to hospital with respiratory syncytial virus bronchiolitis. Thorax. 1997;52:634–637.
116. Johnson DW, Jacobson S, Edney PC, et al. A comparison of nebulized budesonide, intramuscular dexamethasone and placebo for moderately severe croup. N Engl J Med. 1998;339:498–503.
117. Chipps BE, Sullivan WF, Portnoy JM. Alpha-2A-interferon for treatment of bronchiolitis caused by respiratory syncytial virus. Pediatr Infect Dis J. 1993;12: 653–658.
118. Neuzil KM, Gruber WC, Chytil F, et al. Safety and pharmacokinetics of vitamin A therapy for infants with respiratory syncytial virus infections. Antimicrob Agents Chemother. 1995;39:1191–1193.
119. Quinlan KP, Hayani KC. Vitamin A and respiratory syncytial virus infection, serum levels and supplementation trial. Arch Pediatr Adolesc Med. 1996;150:25–30.
120. Hall CB, Powell KR, Schnabel KC, et al. The risk of secondary bacterial infection in infants hospitalized with respiratory syncytial viral infection. J Pediatr. 1988;113:266–271.
121. Milner AD, Murray M. Acute bronchiolitis in infancy: Treatment and prognosis. Thorax. 1989;44:1–5.
122. Shaw KN, Bell LM, Sherman NH. Outpatient assessment of infants with bronchiolitis. Am J Dis Child. 1991;145:151–155.
123. Mulholland EK, Olinsky A, Shann FA. Clinical findings and severity of acute bronchiolitis. Lancet. 1990;335:1259–1261.
124. Wohl MEB, Stigol LC, Mead J. Resistance of the total respiratory system in healthy infants and infants with bronchiolitis. Pediatrics. 1969;43:495–509.
125. Bruhn FW, Mokrohisky ST, McIntosh K. Apnea associated with respiratory syncytial virus infection in young infants. J Pediatr. 1977;90:382–386.
126. Anas N, Boettrich C, Hall CB, Brooks JG. The association of apnea and respiratory syncytial virus in infants. J Pediatr. 1982;101:65–68.
127. Church NR, Anas NG, Hall CB, Brooks JG. Respiratory syncytial virus related apnea in infants: Demographics and outcome. Am J Dis Child. 1984;138:247–250.
128. Workshop on Bronchiolitis, sponsored by the National Heart, Blood and Lung Institute, Division of Lung Diseases, National Institutes of Health. Pediatr Res. 1977;11:209–270.
129. Twiggs JT, Larson LA, O'Connell EJ, Illstrup DM. Respiratory syncytial virus infection: Ten-year follow up. Clin Pediatr. 1981;20:187–190.
130. Hall CB, Hall WJ, Gala CL, et al. A long term prospective study of children following respiratory syncytial virus infection. J Pediatr. 1984;105:358–364.
131. Kattan M, Keens TG, Lapierre JG, et al. Pulmonary function abnormalities in symptom free children after bronchiolitis. Pediatrics. 1977;59:683–688.
132. Sims DG, Gardner PS, Weightman D, et al. Atopy does not predispose to RSV bronchiolitis or postbronchiolitic wheezing. BMJ. 1981;282:2086–2088.
133. McConnochie KM, Roughman KJ. Bronchiolitis as a possible cause of wheezing in childhood: New evidence. Pediatrics. 1984;74:1–10.
134. Duiverman EJ, Neijens HJ, van Strik R, et al. Lung function and bronchial responsiveness in children who had infantile bronchiolitis. Pediatr Pulmonol. 1987;3:38–44.
135. Webb MSC, Henry RL, Milner AD, et al. Continuing respiratory problems three and a half years after acute viral bronchiolitis. Arch Dis Child. 1985;60:1064–1067.
136. Mok JY, Simpson H. Outcome of acute lower respiratory tract infection in infants: Preliminary report of seven-year follow-up study. BMJ. 1982;285:333–337.
137. Pullan CR, Hey EN. Wheezing, asthma, and pulmonary dysfunction 10 years after infection with respiratory syncytial virus in infancy. BMJ. 1982;284:1665–1669.
138. McConnochie KM, Mark JD, McBride JT, et al. Normal pulmonary function measurements and airway reactivity in childhood after mild bronchiolitis. J Pediatr. 1985;107:54–58.
139. Morgan WJ. Viral respiratory infection in infancy: Provocation or propagation? Semin Respir Med. 1990;11:306–313.
140. Ralph DD, Springmeyer SC, Sullivan KM, et al. Rapidly progressive airflow obstruction in marrow transplant recipients. Am Rev Respir Dis. 1984;129: 641–644.
141. Chan CK, Hyland RH, Hutcheon MA, et al. Small-airways disease in recipients of allogeneic bone marrow transplants. Medicine. 1987;66:327–340.
142. McGregor CG, Jamieson SW, Baldwin JC, et al. Combined heart-lung transplantation for end-stage Eisenmenger's syndrome. J Thorac Cardiovasc Surg. 1986;91:443–450.
143. Garg K, Lunch DA, Newell JD, King TE Jr. Proliferative and constrictive bronchiolitis: Classification and radiologic features (Review). Am J Roentgenol. 1994;162:803–808.
144. Penn CC, Liu C. Bronchiolitis following infection in adults and children. Clin Chest Med. 1993;14:645–654.
145. Wells AU, du Bois RM. Bronchiolitis in association with connective tissue disorders. Clin Chest Med. 1993;14:655–666.
146. Crawford SW, Clark JG. Bronchiolitis associated with bone marrow transplantation. Clin Chest Med. 1993;14:741–749.
147. Nadorra RL, Landing BH. Pulmonary lesions in childhood onset systemic lupus erthematosus: Analysis of 26 cases, and summary of literature. Pediatr Pathol. 1987;7:1–18.
148. Gold R, Wilt JC, Adhikari PK, Macpherson RI. Adenoviral pneumonia and its complications in infancy and childhood. J Can Assoc Radiol 1969;20:218–224.
149. Lang WR, Howden CW, Lars J, Burton JF. Bronchopneumonia with serious sequelae in children with evidence of adenovirus type 21 infections. BMJ. 1969;1:73–79.
150. Chernick V, Macpherson RI. Respiratory syncytial and adenovirus infections of the lower respiratory tract in infancy. Clin Notes Respir Dis. 1971;10:3.

Chapter 57

Acute Pneumonia

GERALD R. DONOWITZ
GERALD L. MANDELL

In 1901, Sir William Osler noted in the fourth edition of his book *The Principles and Practice of Medicine* that "the most widespread and fatal of all acute diseases, pneumonia, is now Captain of the Men of Death."[1] A century later, the prominence of pneumonia as a clinical entity remains. It is the sixth most common cause of death in the United States and the most common cause of infection-related mortality.[2] The challenge confronting most clinicians is not in detecting the presence of the disease but rather in identifying its cause. It is now recognized that a wide array of microbial agents may cause acute pneumonia (Table 57–1), and no single antimicrobial regimen can be expected to cover all the possibilities. A specific etiologic diagnosis is often not possible, and empirical therapy is usually necessary. An understanding of the pathogenesis of the disease, evaluation of relevant data from a careful history and physical examination, recognition of common clinical patterns of infection, and information from the microbiology laboratory all aid in nar-

TABLE 57–1 Etiology Agents of Acute Pneumonia

- Bacterial
  - Common
    - *Streptococcus pneumoniae*
    - *Staphylococcus aureus*
    - *Haemophilus influenzae*
    - Mixed anaerobic bacteria (aspiration)
      - *Bacteroides* spp.
      - *Fusobacterium* spp.
      - *Peptostreptococcus* spp.
      - *Peptococcus* spp.
      - *Prevotella* spp.
    - Enterobacteriaceae
      - *Escherichia coli*
      - *Klebsiella pneumoniae*
      - *Enterobacter* spp.
      - *Serratia* spp.
    - *Pseudomonas aeruginosa*
    - *Legionella* spp. (including *L. pneumophila* and *L. micdadei*)
  - Uncommon
    - *Acinetobacter* var. *anitratus*
    - *Actinomyces* and *Arachnia* spp.
    - *Aeromonas hydrophilia*
    - *Bacillus* spp.
    - *Moraxella catarrhalis*
    - *Campylobacter fetus*
    - *Eikenella corrodens*
    - *Francisella tularensis*
    - *Neisseria meningitidis*
    - *Nocardia* spp.
    - *Pasteurella multocida*
    - *Proteus* spp.
    - *Pseudomonas pseudomallei*
    - *Salmonella* spp.
    - *Enterococcus faecalis*
    - *Streptococcus pyogenes*
    - *Yersinia pestis*
- Fungal
  - *Aspergillus* spp.
  - *Candida* spp.
  - *Coccidioides immitis*
  - *Cryptococcus neoformans*
  - *Histoplasma capsulatum*
  - Agents of mucormycosis
    - *Rhizopus* spp.
    - *Absidia* spp.
    - *Mucor* spp.
    - *Cunninghamella* spp.
- Rickettsial
  - *Coxiella burnetii*
  - *Rickettsia rickettsiae*
- Mycoplasma and chlamydia
  - *Mycoplasma pneumoniae*
    - *Chlamydia psittaci*
    - *Chlamydia trachomatis*
    - *Chlamydia pneumoniae* (TWAR)
  - Mycobacterial
    - *Mycobacterium tuberculosis*
    - Nontuberculous mycobacteria
- Parasitic
  - *Ascaris lumbricoides*
  - *Pneumocystis carinii*
  - *Strongyloides stercoralis*
  - *Toxoplasma gondii*
  - *Paragonimus westermani*
- Viral
  - Children
    - Common
      - Respiratory syncytial virus
      - Parainfluenza virus types 1, 2, 3
      - Influenza A virus
    - Uncommon
      - Adenovirus types 1, 2, 3, 5
      - Influenza B virus
      - Rhinovirus
      - Coxsackievirus
      - Echovirus
      - Measles virus
      - Hantavirus
  - Adults
    - Common
      - Influenza A virus
      - Influenza B virus
      - Adenovirus types 4 and 7 (in military recruits)
    - Uncommon
      - Rhinovirus
      - Adenovirus types 1, 2, 3, 5
      - Enteroviruses
        - Echovirus
        - Coxsackievirus
        - Poliovirus
      - Epstein-Barr virus
      - Cytomegalovirus
      - Respiratory syncytial virus
      - Varicella-zoster virus
      - Parainfluenza virus
      - Measles virus
      - Herpes simplex virus
      - Hantavirus
      - Human herpesvirus 6

rowing down the possible etiologic agents of pneumonia, thereby allowing reasonable empirical therapy to be selected.

HOST DEFENSES AND PATHOGENESIS

The lung is constantly exposed to a mixture of gases, particulate material, and microbes that constitute inspired air. In addition, organisms from oral secretions are frequently seeping down from the upper airways as a consequence of microaspiration. Yet, the lower airways usually remain sterile because of the defense mechanisms at work throughout the respiratory tract. The development of acute pulmonary infection indicates either a defect in host defenses, exposure to a particularly virulent microorganism, or an overwhelming inoculum. Infectious agents gain entry to the lower respiratory tract through aspiration of upper airway resident flora, inhalation of aerosolized material, and, less frequently, metastatic seeding of the lung from blood.

The pulmonary host defense system includes anatomic and mechanical barriers, humoral immunity, cell-mediated immunity, and phagocyte activity (Table 57–2).[3–12] The upper airways, including the nasopharynx, oropharynx, and larynx, are the sites first exposed to inhaled microorganisms. Particles greater than 10 μm are efficiently filtered by the hair in the anterior nares or impact onto mucosal surfaces because of the configuration of the upper airways and the nasal turbinates. The nasal mucosa contains ciliated epithelium and mucus-producing cells. Mechanical clearance of entrapped organisms occurs through the nasopharynx via expulsion or swallowing. In the oropharynx, the flow of saliva, sloughing of epithelial cells, local production of complement, and bacterial interference from resident flora serve as important factors in local host defense. Secretory immunoglobulin A (IgA) is the major immunoglobulin produced in the upper airways and accounts for 10% of the total protein of nasal secretions.[9] It possesses antibacterial and antiviral activity despite being a relatively poor opsonin. Low IgA levels have been associated with increased bacterial adherence.[13] IgG and IgM enter the airways predominantly via transudation from the blood. Their roles in bacterial opsonization, complement activation, agglutination, and neutralization activity are similar to those noted in serum.

Adherence of microorganisms to epithelial surfaces of the upper airways is a critical initial step in colonization and subsequent infection. Changes in fibronectin secretion and in binding characteristics

TABLE 57–2 Pulmonary Host Defenses

Location	Host Defense Mechanism
Upper airways	
Nasopharynx	Nasal hair
	Turbinates
	Anatomy of upper airways
	Mucocilliary apparatus
	IgA secretion
Oropharynx	Saliva
	Sloughing of epithelial cells
	Bacterial interference
	Complement production
Conducting airways	
Trachea, bronchi	Cough, epiglottic reflexes
	Sharp angled branching of airways
	Mucocilliary apparatus
	Immunoglobulin production (IgG, IgM, IgA)
Lower respiratory tract	
Terminal airways, alveoli	Alveolar lining fluid (surfactant, fibronectin, immunoglobulin, complement, free fatty acid, iron-binding proteins)
	Cytokines (TNF, IL-1, IL-8, and others)
	Alveolar macrophages
	Polymorphonuclear leukocytes
	Cell-mediated immunity

Abbreviations: IL, Interleukin; TNF, tumor necrosis factor.

of epithelium for various lectins occur as a response to underlying diseases. This may help to explain why colonization occurs in some clinical settings and not in others.[14, 15] Microbes possess surface adhesions, pili, exotoxins, and proteolytic enzymes that can degrade IgA, which serves to overcome host defenses and allow colonization.[10]

The cough and epiglottic reflexes keep most large particulate matter from reaching the central airways. The trachea and conducting airways are usually effective in entrapping particles from 2 to 10 μm. The sharp angles at which the central airways branch cause particles to impact on mucosal surfaces, where they are entrapped by endobronchial mucus. Once entrapped, particles are removed by ciliated epithelium to the oropharynx.

Particles in the range of 0.5 to 1 μm may reach the terminal airways and alveoli. No mucociliary apparatus exists at this level, yet a variety of humoral and cell-mediated host defenses function here. The alveolar lining fluid contains surfactant, fibronectin, IgG, and complement, all of which are effective opsonins. Free fatty acids, lysozyme, and iron-binding proteins are also present and may be directly microbicidal.

Four distinct populations of macrophages exist in the lung and vary in their location and function.[16] The alveolar macrophage is located in the alveolar lining fluid at the interphase between air and lung tissue. It serves as the resident phagocytic cell in the lower airway and is the first phagocyte encountered by inert particles and potential pathogens entering the lung via inspired air. Alveolar macrophages play several critical roles.[5] As phagocytic cells, they can eliminate certain organisms. If the numbers of organisms increase beyond the macrophages' capability to handle them or if the organisms involved are particularly virulent (i.e., *Pseudomonas aeruginosa*), the macrophage becomes a mediator of an inflammatory response by producing cytokines that recruit neutrophils into the lung.[8, 12, 17, 18]

Interstitial macrophages are located in the lung connective tissue and serve both as phagocytic cells and antigen-processing cells. Animal models suggest that interstitial cells, although equal to alveolar macrophages in Fc-receptor–dependent phagocytosis, are less active in demonstrating Fc-receptor–independent phagocytosis, cytokine production, and oxygen radical production. On the other hand, their class II antigen expression is superior to that of the alveolar macrophage.[16, 19, 20]

Dendritic cells develop from monocytes and have an enhanced capacity for class II antigen processing and expression.

The intravascular macrophage is located in the capillary endothelial cells. These cells are actively phagocytic and remove foreign or damaged material entering the lungs via the blood stream.

Neutrophil recruitment is central to the inflammatory response in the lung and is mediated by a variety of cytokines.[21, 22] These mediators are involved in both attracting and maintaining adequate numbers of neutrophils in areas of lung damage as well as in regulating the extent of inflammation. Interleukin-1 (IL-1), tumor necrosis factor-α (TNF-α), colony-stimulating factors, interferon-α, IL-10, IL-12, and the CXC, CC, and C chemokines are important mediators in this regard. Although TNF-α and IL-1 are not thought to have direct chemotactic activity, they induce the production of IL-8, which is a potent chemoattractant. In addition, the fifth component of complement (C5), leukotriene B_4, and formyl methionyl peptides of bacterial cell walls may be present in the lower airways and help recruit neutrophils into areas of inflammation as well.

Lung parenchymal cells may also help regulate the inflammatory response.[23, 24] Epithelial cells, endothelial cells, smooth muscle cells, dendritic cells, interstitial macrophages, and fibroblasts produce both proinflammatory (i.e., colony-stimulating factors, chemokines) and anti-inflammatory cytokines (IL-10).

A pathogen arriving in the lower airways is coated with alveolar lining fluid, and here it may interact with complement (C_3b), IgG, and nonspecific opsonins like fibronectin.[7, 9, 12] These molecules may opsonize the organism or demonstrate direct antibacterial activity especially against *Staphylococcus aureus* and some gram-negative bacilli.[25] Alveolar lining fluid also contains free fatty acids, lysozyme, and iron-binding proteins that have antibacterial activity. The complement cascade is activated by the alternate pathway or, if specific IgG is present, by the classic pathway with the generation of C5a. Phagocytosis by alveolar macrophages occurs and, depending on the nature and number of the organisms, cytokines such as IL-1 and TNF are released that mediate the inflammatory response. IL-8 is produced, and, in coordination with other cytokines and chemoattractants, neutrophils are recruited into the lung and ingest and kill the infecting organisms.

Cell-mediated immunity also plays a role in pulmonary host defenses and is especially important against certain pathogens including viruses and intracellular parasites that can survive within pulmonary macrophages (i.e., *Mycobacterium* spp., *Legionella* spp.). The lung has lymphoid tissue where homing and differentiation of previously uncommitted cells to memory T and B cells occur.[26] Most of the organized lymphoid tissue in the lung is located in follicles along the bronchial tree in bronchus-associated lymphoid tissues (BALT). The lymphoid centers are morphologically similar to Peyer's patches in the intestine and are similarly associated with mucosal epithelium. Inhaled antigens therefore are able to cross the epithelial surface and immediately encounter cells involved with antigen processing. Once these antigens are processed and presented, it is in the BALT that B and T lymphocytes localize and are stimulated to become memory cells and effector cells.

Normal lung parenchyma usually contains few lymphoid cells, representing only 5 to 10% of the total cell population. The lymphocytes present are memory cells located in the submucosa and lamina propria; effector cells located between epithelial cells and in the interstitium; and cells thought to be "preactivated," awaiting stimulation by inhaled antigens in the alveolus. The majority of lymphocytes are T cells, with 35 to 45% representing a CD_4 (helper, inducer) phenotype, and 18 to 32% representing a CD_8 (suppressor) phenotype.[27]

Antigens inhaled into the alveolus are processed and subsequently activate intra-alveolar lymphoid cells. These cells can stimulate the migration of memory lymphocytes into the area, leading to a localized accumulation of antigen-specific T and B lymphocytes, many of which possess effector cell function. As is true in other anatomic areas, binding of T cells to endothelium is a critical first step in the inflammatory process and is mediated by the interaction of leukocyte function–associated antigen-1 (LFA-1) integrins on the lymphocyte cell surface with ligands exposed by endothelium in areas of inflammation (intercellular adhesion molecules 1 and 2 and VCAM-1). Expression of these ligands on pulmonary endothelium is upregulated by inflammatory mediators such as IL-1, interferon-γ, and TNF-α as well as bacterial lipopolysaccharides.

Pulmonary lymphocytes are thought to shuttle between two functionally distinct lymphoid areas, the BALT, which can be viewed as the afferent limb where antigens first stimulate an immune response, and the lung parenchyma, where differentiated T and B cells participate in the inflammatory response, which can be viewed as the efferent limb. The increase in numbers of memory T cells after antigenic stimulation may occur as a result of local proliferation or via migration of cells from BALT.

Lymphocytes in the lung have three major roles;[28] (1) the production of antibody, (2) cytotoxic activity, and (3) production of inflammatory mediators. The lung contains a variety of cytotoxic T cells including natural killer cells (antigen nonrestricted), antibody-dependent cytotoxic cells, and antigen-restricted cytotoxic cells. Pulmonary T cells produce a large number of cytokines. Mouse models suggest that unstimulated T cells produce mainly IL-2. After stimulation and conversion to memory T cells, two distinct groupings of cytokines are produced. The Th1 and Th2 pattern of cytokine production noted in murine models occurs in humans, though it appears to be less restrictive. Th1 cells produce interferon-α, IL-2, and IL-10, whereas Th2 cells produce IL-4, IL-5, and IL-10. Further, IL-3,

TNF-α, granulocyte-macrophage colony-stimulating factor, and members of the chemokine family of proteins are secreted by both Th1 and Th2 phenotypes. Th1 cells are involved in cell-mediated inflammatory reactions, whereas Th2 cells stimulate antibody production, especially IgE, and stimulate eosinophil activity.

A number of factors are known to interfere with normal host defenses and to predispose to infection.[3] Alterations in the level of consciousness from any cause (stroke, seizures, drug intoxication, anesthesia, alcohol abuse, and even normal sleep) can compromise epiglottic closure and lead to aspiration of oropharyngeal flora into the lower respiratory tract.[29, 30] Cigarette smoke, perhaps the most common agent involved in compromising natural pulmonary defense mechanisms, disrupts both mucociliary function and macrophage activity.[31]

Infections with *Mycoplasma pneumoniae* or *Haemophilus influenzae* may interfere with normal ciliary function.[32] Viruses may also inhibit important host defenses.[11, 33] Viruses may actually destroy respiratory epithelium and may disrupt normal ciliary activity. Neutrophil function, including chemotaxis, phagocytosis, and stimulation of oxidative metabolism, may be inhibited by certain viral infections. Similarly, alveolar macrophage function may be inhibited.[33] Sepsis associated with extrapulmonary infections may also undermine lung defense mechanisms. In animal models, exposure to lipopolysaccharide or endotoxin decreases lung clearance of a bacterial challenge.[34, 35] Alcohol not only impairs the cough and epiglottic reflexes leading to an increased risk of aspiration but also has been associated with increased colonization of the oropharynx with aerobic gram-negative bacilli.[36] Alcohol has also been associated with decreased mobilization of neutrophils,[37] abnormal phagocyte oxidative metabolism, and abnormal chemotaxis.[38] Alcohol in animal models effectively blocks the TNF response to endotoxin.[39] The associated findings of decreased recruitment of neutrophils to the lung after endotoxin challenge suggests that endotoxin-induced stimulation of TNF is important in neutrophil mobilization of the lung and that alcohol may inhibit this component of the inflammatory response. Iatrogenic manipulations that bypass the usual host defenses of the upper airways (endotracheal tubes, nasogastric tubes, and respiratory therapy machinery) all predispose to infection.[40] A variety of commonly prescribed drugs have been shown to inhibit host defenses in vitro or in models, but the clinical significance of this is uncertain. These agents include aspirin,[41] erythromycin,[42] and aminophylline.[43] Other factors that impair pulmonary host defenses include hypoxemia,[44] acidosis, toxic inhalations,[45, 46] pulmonary edema,[47] uremia, malnutrition, immunosuppressive agents,[36, 48] and viral and mechanical obstruction.[4]

The effect of infection with the human immunodeficiency virus (HIV) on pulmonary host defenses remains incompletely understood.[49] Although specific defects have been defined, these data at times have been contradictory and have not fully explained the susceptibility of HIV-infected patients to pulmonary infections. Antigen presentation and expression by alveolar macrophages is diminished in HIV-infected patients, though phagocytic cell function and cytokine production appear intact. In BALT, destruction of dendritic cells and degeneration of lymphoid follicles have been noted in patients with acquired immunodeficiency syndrome (AIDS). Defective antigen presentation by dendritic cells has also been observed. Abnormal chemotaxis, phagocytosis, and oxidative metabolism have been noted in neutrophils from patients with AIDS.

Elderly persons are at increased risk for the development of pneumonia (see Chapter 306). Although a variety of factors play an important role in this regard, including an increased number and increased severity of underlying diseases and an increased number of hospitalizations, there are age-related impairments in host defenses.[50–52] Less effective mucociliary clearance and abnormal elastic recoil may lead to less effective coughing and clearing of the upper airways. Changes in humoral immunity and cell-mediated immune function have been documented in elderly persons.

Recurrent episodes of bacterial pneumonia suggest the presence of specific predisposing factors.[53–56] In children and young adults, recurrent pneumonia is associated with defects in host defenses, including leukocyte function[57] and immunoglobulin production.[57–60] Congenital defects in ciliary activity including the immotile-cilia syndrome,[61] Kartagener's syndrome (ciliary dysfunction, situs inversus, sinusitis, bronchiectasis),[62] Young's syndrome (azospermia, sinusitis, pneumonia),[63] and cystic fibrosis are other clinical entities associated with recurrent pneumonia in young persons. Structural lung abnormalities such as bronchiectasis and pulmonary sequestration[64] are also important predisposing factors for both younger and older patient populations.

Although most congenital defects in host defenses present in childhood, common variable hypogammaglobulinemia may first present in adulthood with recurrent pneumonia. Acquired host defense defects are more varied and include malignancies (lymphoma, chronic lymphocytic leukemia, myeloma), infection (AIDS), and iatrogenic causes (immune suppression associated with solid organ or marrow transplantation or cancer chemotherapy). Underlying respiratory tract disorders such as chronic obstructive pulmonary disease, bronchiectasis, adult-onset cystic fibrosis, bronchopulmonary sequestration, and tracheobronchiomegaly may present with pneumonia. Bronchial obstruction due to intrinsic compression (adenocarcinoma) or extrinsic compression (lymphadenopathy due to sarcoid or malignancy) has also been associated with recurrent episodes of pneumonia. Underlying diseases that predispose to aspiration lead to an increased incidence of pneumonia. These may be associated with gastrointestinal diseases (tracheoesophageal fistula, esophageal diverticula, esophageal reflux, esophageal stricture[65]), neuromuscular disorders (myasthenia gravis, dementia, amyotrophic lateral sclerosis), and cancer of the head and neck. Some systemic illnesses, including Weber-Christian disease, chronic renal failure, diabetes, and sickle cell disease, have been associated with pneumonia.[56]

CLINICAL EVALUATION

History

The history should attempt to define (1) signs and symptoms consistent with the diagnosis of pneumonia, (2) the clinical setting in which the pneumonia takes place, (3) defects in host resistance that could predispose to the development of pneumonia, and (4) possible exposures to specific pathogens.

Respiratory signs and symptoms are commonly encountered in primary care practices. In 1994, over 10 million visits were associated with a chief complaint of cough. Only 4% of the visits involved pneumonia.[66] Therefore, a serious effort should be made to differentiate pneumonia from other diagnostic possibilities with which it may be confused. Although the clinical findings of pneumonia related to the respiratory tract should be sought, including cough, sputum production, dyspnea, and fever, it should be recognized that nonrespiratory symptoms are commonly present. These include fatigue, sweats, headache, nausea, and myalgia.[67] With increasing age, both respiratory and nonrespiratory symptoms of pneumonia become less frequent.

Mycoplasmal pneumonia occurs more often in younger people[68, 69] but may be a cause of pneumonia requiring hospitalization in older age groups.[70] Gram-negative pneumonia tends to occur in elderly persons,[71] and tuberculosis has reemerged as an important cause of pulmonary disease and should be suspected in homeless persons, in those infected with HIV, and in those who come from developing countries where tuberculosis is prevalent.[72, 73]

Pneumonia has been noted to occur with increased frequency in patients with a variety of underlying disorders such as congestive heart failure, diabetes, alcoholism, and chronic obstructive pulmonary disease (COPD).[71, 74, 75, 76] In one series of 292 patients with pneumonia, only 18% were found to have no underlying disease.[71] A history of antecedent upper respiratory tract infection has been elicited in 36 to 50% of patients with acute pneumonia, especially in those with pneumococcal disease.[74, 77] Recent dental manipulations, sedative overdoses, seizures, alcoholism, or loss of consciousness for any reason should raise the suspicion of anaerobic infection due to aspiration of oral contents.[29, 30]

Specific etiologic agents of pneumonia have been associated with certain underlying diseases. An increased incidence of staphylococcal pneumonia has been noted during epidemics of influenza.[78]

Special note needs to be made of the relationship between pneumonia and patients with COPD.[79, 80] Although well-controlled studies are lacking, it does appear that patients with COPD have an increased incidence of pneumonia. However, since the tracheobronchial tree is often colonized with *Streptococcus pneumoniae* and *H. influenzae,* it has been difficult to distinguish clearly between colonization and infection in many studies. Although these organisms play an important role as etiologic agents of pneumonia in this patient population, most of the clinical studies were carried out before it was recognized that other less common pathogens also play a significant role in causing disease. The roles of *Moraxella catarrhalis, Legionella* spp., *Chlamydia pneumoniae*, and aerobic gram-negative rods including *P. aeruginosa* have recently been acknowledged.[80–83] Cystic fibrosis is associated with *Pseudomonas* and staphylococcal pulmonary infections.[84] Pulmonary alveolar proteinosis is associated with *Nocardia* infection.[85]

Patients infected with HIV are at high risk for the development of pulmonary infections.[86, 87] Although *Pneumocystis carinii* pneumonia remains an important clinical entity in this patient population, prophylaxis has reduced its incidence and importance as a cause of death.[88, 89] In considering the nature of pulmonary infection in patients infected with HIV, geographic exposures, demographic characteristics of the patient, and the degree of immune suppression need to be considered.[86, 87] *P. carinii* infection is relatively uncommon in Africa, but more frequent in Europe and the United States. *Mycobacterium tuberculosis* is more common in the northeastern United States than in other parts of the country.[90] Since fungal infections play a major role in this patient population, exposure in endemic areas of histoplasmosis, blastomycosis, and coccidioidomycosis needs to be considered. The overall incidence of bacterial pneumonia in patients with HIV is five times higher than in non–HIV-infected populations, and the greatest risk appears to be associated with intravenous and inhaled drug use.[86, 91, 92] Common pulmonary pathogens such as *S. pneumoniae, H. influenzae,* and *S. aureus* play an important role.[87] The incidence of pneumococcal pneumonia, including bacteremic disease, is 7 to 10 times higher in HIV-infected patients,[93] whereas the incidence of *H. influenzae* infection may be up to 100-fold higher than in the non–HIV-infected population.[94] *P. aeruginosa* pneumonia is often associated with bacteremia or cavitary lung disease and is a later complication of HIV infection occurring with CD_4 counts less than 25/μl. The infection is associated with the presence of central venous catheters, urinary catheters, and the use of steroids.[95, 96] Bacterial agents such as *Legionella* spp., *Nocardia* spp., aerobic gram-negative bacilli, and *Rhodococcus equi* are important causes of pneumonia.[97]

In patients infected with HIV, the relationship between the degree of immune suppression using the CD_4 count as a marker and the specific etiology of pneumonia deserves emphasis. Bacterial pneumonia and tuberculosis usually occur when the CD_4 count is less than 400/μl.[92, 98] *P. carinii* and disseminated tuberculosis are associated with CD_4 counts below 200/μl, and disseminated nontuberculosis mycobacterial infections and disseminated fungal infection occur with CD_4 counts less than 100/μl.[98] Pulmonary infections in HIV-infected patients are discussed in more detail in Chapter 109.

Pneumonia developing in hospitalized patients often involves Enterobacteriaceae, *P. aeruginosa,* and *S. aureus,* organisms that are unusual in community-acquired disease.[99] Similarly, pneumonia in elderly persons, especially those living in nursing homes or extended care facilities, is more often associated with gram-negative bacilli than is pneumonia in younger populations.[93–100]

An occupational history, a history of exposure to animals, a travel history, and a sexual history are all important in suggesting specific potential infectious agents (Table 57–3). The presence of noninfectious pulmonary disease such as tumors or pulmonary emboli, which may masquerade as pneumonia, may also be suggested by a careful history.

Physical Examination

Fever is usually present and may be sustained, remittent, or at times hectic. Fever patterns per se, however, are not useful for establishing a specific diagnosis. The temperature should be taken rectally to reduce error due to rapid mouth breathing. Recording of postural changes in blood pressure and pulse rate is useful in assessing hydration and intravascular fluid volume. The pulse usually increases by 10 beats/minute for every degree (C) of temperature elevation. A pulse temperature deficit (i.e., a relative bradycardia for the amount of fever) should suggest viral infection, mycoplasmal infection, chlamydial infection, tularemia, or infection with *Legionella* spp. Cyanosis, a rapid respiratory rate, the use of accessory muscles of respiration, sternal retraction, and nasal flaring suggest serious respiratory compromise.

Furuncles are rarely secondary to staphylococcal pneumonia acquired by the respiratory route but may signal a source of bacteremia with subsequent pneumonia via hematogenous spread. Herpes labialis is seen in up to 40% of patients with pneumococcal pneumonia.[101] Bullous myringitis is an infrequent although significant finding in mycoplasmal pneumonia.[69] The presence of poor dentition should suggest a mixed infection due to aspiration of anaerobes and aerobes that colonize the oropharynx. Although edentulous people may develop anaerobic pneumonia due to aspiration, it is uncommon.[102]

Examination of the thorax may reveal "splinting" or an inspiratory lag on the side of the lesion that is suggestive of bacterial pneumonia. Early in the disease process, definite signs of pulmonary involvement may be lacking or may be manifest only as fine rales. Chest examination may reveal these early signs of pneumonia even though the chest film is normal. Thin section computed tomographic scans can show infiltrates in patients with normal chest radiographs.

TABLE 57–3 Important Environmental Factors in Pneumonia

Pneumonia Associated with	Environmental History
Anthrax	Exposure to cattle, swine, horses, goat hair, raw wool, animal hides
Brucellosis	Exposure to cattle, goats, pigs; ingestion of unpasteurized dairy products; employment as abattoir worker or veterinarian
Melioidosis	Travel to W. Indies, Australia, Guam, S.E. Asia, South and Central America
Plague	Exposure to ground squirrels, chipmunks, rabbits, prairie dogs, rats
Tularemia	Exposure to tissue or body fluids of infected animals during trapping, hunting, or skinning (rabbits, hares, foxes, squirrels) or to bites of an infected arthropod (flies, ticks)
	Handling or ingesting poorly cooked meat from an infected animal
Psittacosis	Exposure to birds (parrots, budgerigars, cockatoos, pigeons, turkeys)
Leptospirosis	Exposure to wild rodents, dogs, cats, pigs, cattle, horses, or exposure to water contaminated with animal urine
Coccidioidomycosis	Reside in or travel to San Joaquin Valley, S. California, S.W. Texas, S. Arizona, New Mexico
Histoplasmosis	Exposure to bat droppings or dust from soil enriched with bird droppings
Q fever	Exposure to infected goats, cattle, sheep, domestic animals and their secretions (milk, amniotic fluid, placenta, feces)
Legionnaires' disease	Exposure to contaminated aerosols (e.g., air coolers, hospital water supply)
Pasteurella multocida	Exposure to infected dogs and cats
Hantavirus	Exposure to rodent droppings, urine, and saliva

Evidence of consolidation (dullness on percussion, bronchial breath sounds, and E to A changes) is highly suggestive of bacterial infection but may be absent in two thirds of patients ill enough to be hospitalized and may be absent more often in patients treated as outpatients.[103] Patients with mycoplasmal or viral infection may exhibit few abnormalities on physical examination despite the presence of impressive infiltrates on the chest film.

The usefulness of the history and physical examination to detect the presence of pneumonia has been studied.[104] A great deal of intraobserver variation exists in detecting the signs and symptoms of pneumonia. Rare findings such as egobronchophony and asymmetric chest movements have a high predictive value for pneumonia. Other findings are usually not helpful. An absence of any vital sign abnormalities (i.e., respiratory rate <30 breaths/minute, heart rate <100 beats/minute, and temperature <37.8°C) has been associated with a less than 1% chance of a patient's having pneumonia assuming a pneumonia prevalence of 5% in the population under study.[105]

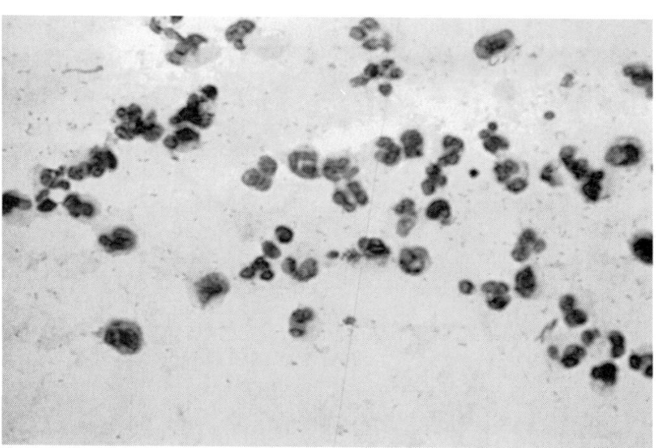

FIGURE 57–2. Expectorated sputum with gram-negative coccobacillary forms from a patient with *Haemophilus influenzae* pneumonia.

SPUTUM EXAMINATION

Microscopic examination and culture of expectorated sputum remain the mainstays of the laboratory evaluation of pneumonia despite ongoing controversy concerning their sensitivity and specificity.[106–115]

In the guidelines for the management of community-acquired pneumonia developed by the Infectious Disease Society of America, the sputum Gram stain is viewed as a simple, quick, inexpensive procedure that may serve as a guide to initial antibiotic therapy.[110] The overall helpfulness of the procedure for aiding in the etiologic diagnosis of pneumonia is unclear.[111] This is due in part to lack of a gold standard for the "true" cause of pneumonia, intraobserver variability, and the fact that 30 to 40% of patients fail to produce sputum.[111, 112] Increased accuracy appears to be associated with experience, with laboratory technicians having greater accuracy than house staff.[116] However, despite the pitfalls, the procurement of expectorated sputum is a noninvasive technique that can be carried out at no risk to the patient, and may allow the clinician to make a presumptive diagnosis.

Examination of the sputum should include observation of the color, amount, consistency, and odor of the specimen. Mucopurulent sputum is most commonly found with bacterial pneumonia or bronchitis. Sputum of a similar nature has been described in one third to one half of patients with mycoplasma[69] or adenovirus infections.[117, 118] However, scant or watery sputum is more often noted with these and other atypical pneumonias. "Rusty" sputum suggests alveolar involvement and has been most commonly (although not solely) associated with pneumococcal pneumonia.[119] Dark red, mucoid sputum (currant-jelly sputum) suggests Friedlander's pneumonia caused by encapsulated *Klebsiella pneumoniae.*[120] Foul-smelling sputum is associated with mixed anaerobic infections most commonly seen with aspiration.[102]

Where possible, frankly purulent material should be selected for microscopic examination and Gram stain. To maximize the diagnostic yield of the sputum examination, only samples with minimal oropharyngeal contamination should be reviewed. As a guide, the number of neutrophils and epithelial cells should be quantitated under low power (× 100), with further examination reserved for samples containing 25 or more neutrophils and 10 or fewer epithelial cells.[121] Samples with more epithelial cells and fewer neutrophils are usually nondiagnostic and should be discarded. The morphologic and staining characteristics of any bacteria seen should be recorded and an estimate made of the predominant organisms (Figs. 57–1 through 57–4). Where no bacterial predominance exists, this should be noted as well.

In the appropriate clinical setting, a predominance of gram-positive, lancet-shaped diplococci should suggest pneumococcal infection (Fig. 57–1). When strict criteria for Gram stain positivity are used (predominant flora or more than 10 gram-positive, lancet-shaped diplococci per oil immersion field [× 1000], or both), the specificity of the Gram stain for identifying pneumococci has been shown to be 85%, with a sensitivity of 62%.[122] The diagnostic yield of the

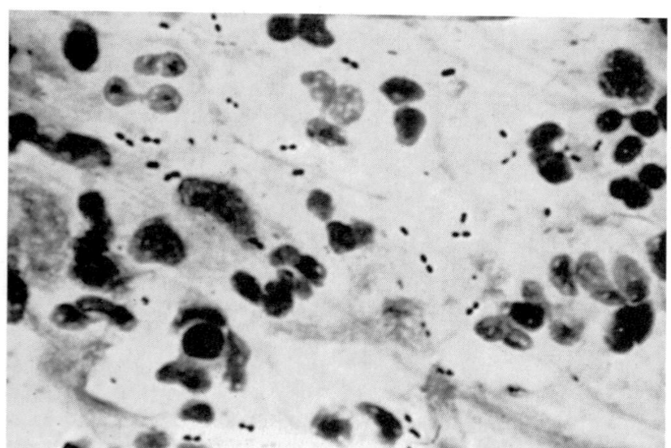

FIGURE 57–1. Expectorated sputum with gram-positive, lancet-shaped diplococci from a patient with pneumococcal pneumonia.

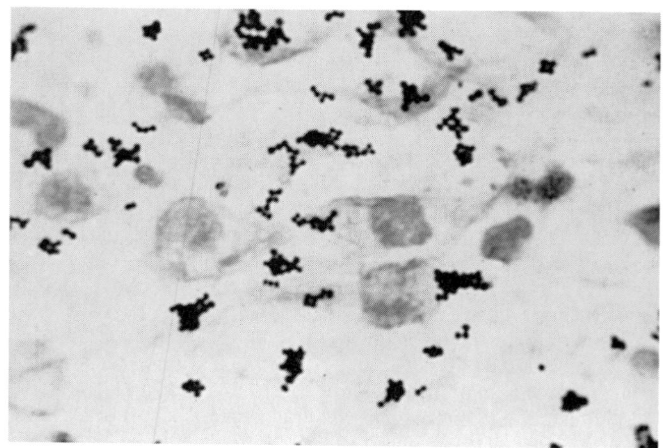

FIGURE 57–3. Expectorated sputum with gram-positive cocci in clumps from a patient with staphylococcal pneumonia.

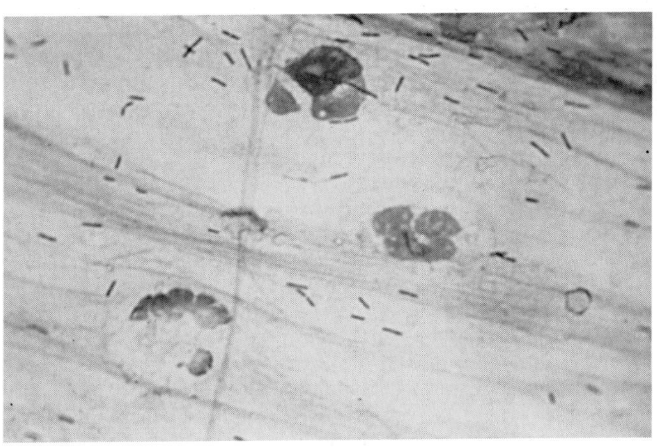

FIGURE 57–4. Expectorated sputum with gram-negative rods in a patient with *Escherichi coli* pneumonia.

sputum examination for pneumococci can be maximized by the use of the quellung reaction. Anticapsular antiserum reacts with capsular polysaccharide, and this may be seen as a distinctly outlined capsule. Rare false-positive results may occur with α-hemolytic streptococci. Occasional false-negative results may occur as well. An 89% correlation between pneumococcal isolation by culture and a positive sputum quellung test has been demonstrated.[107]

Since pneumococci may be part of the nasopharyngeal flora in up to 50% of healthy adults and may colonize the lower airways in patients with chronic bronchitis, identification of the organism does not mean that it is the cause of disease.[123–125] However, it is our experience that the large number of pneumococci necessary to produce a positive Gram stain or quellung reaction is unusual in carriers. Gram stain may reveal large numbers of organisms in patients with bronchitis.

The sputum Gram stain is helpful to identify organisms other than pneumococci. Small gram-negative coccobacillary organisms are characteristic of *H. influenzae* (Fig. 57–2). However, the sensitivity of sputum Gram stain for detecting *H. influenzae* is usually less than that for *S. pneumoniae* and has been reported to be 40 to 80%.[114, 116, 126] Staphylococci appear as gram-positive cocci in tetrads and grapelike clusters (Fig. 57–3). Organisms of mixed morphology are characteristic of anaerobic infection. Few bacteria are seen with legionnaires' disease, mycoplasma pneumonia, and viral pneumonia. When the criteria of more than 25 neutrophils and fewer than 10 squamous epithelial cells per low-power (× 100) magnification are met, and when a predominant morphology is observed, the sensitivity of sputum Gram stain in detecting organisms found in the blood was reported as 85% in patients with community-acquired pneumonia.[126] In contrast, sputum cultures positive for pneumococci are found in only 50 to 60% of patients with pneumonia and pneumococcal bacteremia.[127, 128] Sputum examination has been a useful means of diagnosing *P. carinii* pneumonia in patients with AIDS. The use of commercially available monoclonal antibodies or Giemsa's, Gomori's methanamine silver, or toluidine blue O stain has led to a diagnosis in more than 50% of cases, making more aggressive diagnostic procedures unnecessary.[129–131]

Antigen detection in respiratory secretions has been used for over 2 decades to try to maximize the diagnostic yield of sputum especially for infections caused by *S. pneumoniae, P. carinii, Legionella pneumophila,* and a variety of respiratory viruses.[132] In addition to the quelling reaction, counterimmunoelectrophoresis (CIE) and coagglutination have been used to detect pneumococcal polysaccharide with 70 to 90% sensitivity and a specificity of 80%. However, with these assays, colonization may be confused with infection, cross-reactivity with oral streptococci may occur, and prior therapy with antibiotics may lower overall sensitivity. Direct fluorescent antibody assays may detect *L. pneumophila* with a specificity of over 90%. Sensitivity ranges from 25 to 75% and non-*pneumophilia* strains of *Legionella* may be missed.[133, 134] Lipopolysaccharide detection with enzyme immunoassay has been used to detect both *Chlamydia trachomatis* and *C. pneumoniae* in respiratory tract secretions.[135] However, cross-reactivity with normal oral flora, relatively low amounts of lipopolysaccharide in respiratory secretions, and the inability to determine one species of chlamydia from another are persistent problems. Although direct fluorescent antibody tests have been used to detect *C. trachomatis,* the assay is insensitive in detecting *C. pneumoniae* and has a varied sensitivity of 20 to 60%.[132] The least problematic of the antigen detection assays is that used for the detection of *P. carinii.* Direct fluorescent antibody assays are over 80% sensitive and 90% specific.[136, 137]

Detection of microbial nucleic acid in clinical samples including respiratory tract secretions remains an area of ongoing interest. Initially, nucleic acid hybridization techniques were used to detect herpes simplex virus, cytomegalovirus, *M. pneumoniae, Legionella* spp., and mycobacteria. DNA probes for some organisms *(Legionella, Mycoplasma)* are no longer available, and others remain of unproven applicability.[132, 138–141] Nucleic acid amplification using the polymerase chain reaction (PCR) has received the most recent attention. The technique represents a rapid and relatively simple means of identifying organisms with potentially high specificity and sensitivity. The technique has been applied to organisms that are otherwise cumbersome to identify using usual microbiologic techniques including *L. pneumophila, M. pneumoniae, C. pneumoniae,* cytomegalovirus, and *P. carinii* as well as more common bacterial pathogens.[142–148] Although the majority of studies have involved sputum, PCR of throat swabs has been shown to be an effective way of diagnosing *L. pneumophila, M. pneumoniae,* and *C. pneumoniae* infections in small numbers of patients.[143] PCR offers the advantage of high sensitivity even early in the course of infection with no loss of sensitivity due to prior antibiotic usage. Further, the assay does not depend on a normal host response to infection. However, problems with the technique are numerous. Its high sensitivity makes laboratory contamination a real concern. Differentiation between infection and colonization and between active infection, latent infection, and past infection may be difficult. False-negative results may occur because of the presence of natural inhibitors. The technique has not yet been standardized and in most cases remains experimental.

Antibody coating of bacteria in respiratory secretions has been used as a means of differentiating infection from colonization in intubated patients.[149] Although the assay has been reported as specific for the presence of lower respiratory infection, the sensitivity is only 46%, and it cannot clearly differentiate purulent bronchitis from pneumonia.

The utility of the sputum culture as a means of diagnosing pneumonia has been questioned. First, only 60% of patients with pneumonia may produce sputum. As noted previously, patients with bacteremic pneumococcal pneumonia have been reported to have negative sputum cultures in 45 to 50% of cases, even when large numbers of organisms have been noted on Gram stain.[127, 128] Similarly, 34 to 47% of sputum cultures are negative with proven *H. influenzae* pneumonia.[150, 151] Furthermore, sputum cultures have frequently been shown to yield more bacterial species than more invasive methods of obtaining respiratory tract secretions.[152, 153] Contamination with gram-negative bacilli from the oropharynx has been noted in 32% of sputum cultures.[154] A lack of correlation of sputum culture findings and those from blood cultures and serologic studies has been observed.[112]

Several key parameters have been identified in efforts to maximize the diagnostic yield from sputum culture. Procurement of adequate sputum samples is an essential first step. When fewer than 10 epithelial cells and more than 25 neutrophils per low-power field are noted, oropharyngeal contamination is minimal and sputum samples are comparable to transtracheal aspirates in terms of the number of bacterial species isolated.[121] With increasing numbers of epithelial cells and decreasing numbers of neutrophils, an increased amount of oropharyngeal contamination is present, as indicated by the isolation of more bacterial species.

The presence of alveolar macrophages does not alter the bacteriologic findings when substantial numbers of epithelial cells are present, indicating that otherwise adequate samples of sputum can be contaminated with oropharyngeal contents and thereby rendered nondiagnostic. This type of initial screening has proved helpful in differentiating adequate sputum samples from saliva, thereby increasing the diagnostic yield of sputum culture. When organisms such as *M. tuberculosis, Legionella* spp., and *P. carinii* are found in sputum, this indicates clinical infection independent of the sputum quality because these organisms are not normal flora.[155]

When culture of sputum is delayed, the isolation of pneumococci is less likely due to overgrowth by oropharyngeal flora. Rapid processing of samples is therefore another important factor leading to higher diagnostic yields.

Laboratory techniques for maximizing the useful information from sputum cultures have included quantitative cultures, washing of samples to remove contaminating mouth flora, and the use of mucolytic agents. The varied results noted have not warranted the increased efforts required. Furthermore, washing samples does not guarantee that adequate samples of lower respiratory tract secretions are present.[156] Some reports suggest that with adequate sputum samples and prompt culture of specimens, the diagnostic yield of the sputum culture may be improved.[106, 157, 158]

TRANSTRACHEAL ASPIRATION

Although the sputum examination should always be included in the initial evaluation of patients with pneumonia, it may be inadequate for a presumptive diagnosis. In cases in which (1) no sputum is produced, (2) no clear predominance of a potential pathogen exists on sputum Gram stain or culture, (3) there has been a poor response to antibiotics chosen on the basis of expectorated sputum, (4) gram-negative rods or yeast forms are found in the sputum, or (5) the possibility of superinfection exists, a more direct method of obtaining lower respiratory tract secretions may be necessary.

In the past, transtracheal aspiration has been used as a means of obtaining lower respiratory tract secretions with minimal oropharyngeal contamination. However, because of the fear of adverse reactions, most clinicians now use other methods of obtaining lower respiratory tract secretions.

FIBEROPTIC BRONCHOSCOPY

Initial studies concerning the usefulness of fiberoptic bronchoscopy for the diagnosis of bacterial pneumonia demonstrated that the procedure was limited by contamination of specimens by oropharyngeal flora. Cultures obtained via the bronchoscope averaged two to three more bacterial isolates than samples from paired transtracheal aspirates.[159] In patients without lower respiratory tract infections, cultures of aspirates obtained at bronchoscopy produced an average of five different bacterial species.[160] The development of the protected brush catheter (a brush within two catheters sealed at the end with a polyethylene glycol plug) decreased but has not eliminated this problem.[161, 162] Quantitative culturing has been used to differentiate contaminants from true infecting agents.[161, 163, 164]

Approximately 10^6 to 10^8 organisms/ml are present in areas of pneumonia.[109] Accounting for dilution of samples, bacterial growth of more than 10^3 to 10^4 has been used as a breakpoint for determining the clinical significance of an isolate.

Studies employing the protected brush catheter have proved experimentally and clinically to be both sensitive (70 to 97%) and specific (95 to 100%) for the diagnosis of bacterial pneumonia.[163–166] However, not all series using this technique have produced impressive results,[167–169] and in some patient groups this technique is not useful. These include patients receiving prior antibiotics, patients with purulent bronchitis in whom bacterial counts above 10^3 are noted, and patients with underlying structural disease in whom over 50% of bronchoscopic specimens yield significant numbers of organisms even in the absence of pneumonia.[161, 166, 170] Detection of the antibody coating of organisms found at bronchoscopy has been used in an attempt to differentiate colonization from true infection. Experience has been limited and results have been mixed, with a high false-positive rate noted in patients with chronic bronchitis.[171, 172] Gram stain of specimens obtained from fiberoptic bronchoscopy has been used as a guide to empirical therapy while cultures are pending.[170, 173] A positive Gram stain predicts growth of more than 10^3 colony-forming units (CFU)/ml with up to 78% sensitivity.

In practice, however, fiberoptic bronchoscopy is usually not performed on patients with community-acquired pneumonia unless severe pneumonia, unresolving pneumonia, or a clear failure of antibiotic therapy is encountered.[174, 175] The procedure may be useful in defining the cause of ventilator-associated pneumonia. Bronchoscopy with a protected specimen brush has been shown to have a sensitivity of 82 to 100%, a specificity of 60 to 77%, a positive predictive value of 43 to 74%, and a negative predictive value of 85 to 100% when compared with quantitative cultures of infected lung.[176–181] Not all studies have shown such good results; sensitivity of 36%, specificity of 50%, and positive and negative predictive values of 43% have also been reported.[182, 183] Differences in exclusion and inclusion criteria, differing definitions of pneumonia, and the acceptance or rejection of patients with recent antibiotic changes may explain the different results. The use of antibiotics markedly diminishes the diagnostic yield of the procedure.[184–186] Most bacterial species initially found by a protected specimen brush are undetectable after 72 hours of antibiotic therapy, and the majority of organisms found are resistant to the antibiotics given. These may have no role in the infection. However, in a patient with ongoing pneumonia despite antibiotic therapy, bronchoscopy with a protected specimen brush should pick up resistant organisms that may be playing a role in infection.[177]

False-negative findings are seen in up to 30 to 40% of patients, which may reflect the fact that bacterial counts may differ 50-fold in areas of infected lung versus noninfected adjacent areas, making the sampling site an important consideration.[167, 179] Other possible explanations include prior antibiotic use, technique problems, and in some cases an early stage of pneumonia where bacterial numbers are not yet high enough to reach the breakpoint of the procedure.[187]

Broncheolar Lavage

Bronchoalveolar lavage (BAL) in which a segment of the lung is washed with sterile fluid has been used for determining the cause of pneumonia. Approximately 100 million alveolae are sampled, and consequently a larger area of lung is evaluated than with the protected specimen brush.[188] A diagnostic threshold of 10^4 CFU/ml is utilized with lavage since the procedure recovers 5 to 10 times more organisms than brushing. The most consistent results have been seen in the diagnosis of *P. carinii* pneumonia in patients with AIDS. Diagnostic yields of 89 to 98% have been reported.[189, 190] Excellent yields have been noted in detecting cytomegalovirus in patients with AIDS as well as in bone marrow transplant and solid organ transplant recipients.[191–193] The isolation of the organism does not prove that it is the cause of the pneumonia. By using immunofluorescent monoclonal antibodies to viral antigens or centrifuging lavage material into tissue culture preparations, the identification of cytomegalovirus may be made within hours rather than weeks.[194, 195]

BAL has proved especially useful for diagnosing pneumonia caused by *M. tuberculosis.*[196–198] Culture of BAL material has a sensitivity of 85%, even in the presence of negative cultures of expectorated sputum and gastric aspirate. In patients with miliary tuberculosis in whom sputum culture yields are low (25%), culture of BAL fluid approximates 100%. In addition to culture and staining, adenosine deaminase levels and enzyme-linked immunosorbent assay (ELISA) assays for antibodies to *M. tuberculosis* have been studied.[199–202] BAL has also been used for the diagnosis of atypical pneumonias, including those caused by *Legionella* spp. and *M. pneumoniae*.[199]

BAL has been used as a means of diagnosing ventilator-associated pneumonia. When compared with quantitative cultures of infected lung, sensitivities of up to 91%, specificities of 78 to 100%, positive predictive values of 83%, and negative predictive values of 87% have been noted.[177] Microscopic examination of cells from lavage have also been used to diagnose pneumonia. When greater than 5% of cells from bronchoalveolar lavage contain bacteria, pneumonia has been diagnosed with sensitivities of up to 90% and specificities of 89 to 100%.[177, 203] Similar values have been noted when more than 2%, or more than 7% of cells with intracellular bacteria have been used as the threshold for diagnosing pneumonia.[204, 205] The procedure appears to be repeatable and may yield results even if antibiotics are present, especially if no recent changes in antibiotics have occurred.[171, 185, 206] Studies vary as to threshold levels of bacteria, patient selection, and standards for determining the presence of pneumonia. Consequently, sensitivity, specificity, and predictive values vary. Overall, however, despite the inconsistencies of study design, bronchoalveolar lavage appears similar in efficacy to the protected specimen brush as a means of diagnosing the cause of ventilator-associated pneumonia.[207]

The use of BAL for the diagnosis of pneumonia in other clinical settings and with other pathogens is less well defined.[208, 209] By using cytologic screening, quantitative cultures of BAL fluid, or Gram stain criteria, bacterial pneumonia has been identified in non–AIDS-related immunosuppressed patients, patients with severe community-acquired pneumonia, and patients with nonresolving pneumonia.[175, 208, 209] In addition to quantitative culture and Gram stain of BAL fluid, quantitation of endotoxin has been used to detect the presence of gram-negative pneumonia.[210]

Although the risks of bronchoscopy are relatively small, hypoxia occurs in 13 to 28% of patients on ventilators undergoing BAL.[173, 211] In patients with gram-negative pneumonia, the procedure may be followed by a sepsis-like picture with increased temperature and decreased mean arterial pressure.[212]

OTHER TECHNIQUES

A variety of less invasive techniques have been used in attempts to determine the cause of pneumonia without resorting to bronchoscopy. Blind endotracheal suctioning with quantitative cultures has compared favorably with bronchoscopic procedures in some studies.[213, 214] With a threshold of greater than 10^5 CFU/ml, the sensitivity for predicting ventilator-associated pneumonia was comparable to that of lavage or protected brush procedures, although the specificity was somewhat lower.[214] Further, no differences in mortality, the length of stay in the intensive care unit, or the duration of mechanical ventilation were noted when quantitative endotracheal cultures were used as the sole means of diagnosis compared with its use with bronchioalveolar lavage and a protected specimen brush.[215] Others have reported false-negative rates of over 30% and many more organisms isolated by endotracheal suctioning than by brushing.[216] At present, this procedure is best used when bronchoscopy cannot be done.

The blind protected specimen brush has compared favorably with bronchoscopically guided procedures with 86% agreement.[215, 217] Nonbronchoscopic bronchioloalveolar lavage has been examined in some cases by a protected catheter to minimize contamination. Sensitivities of 70 to 80% and a specificity of 66 to 96% have been noted.[218–222] Mortality from ventilator-associated pneumonia is unchanged independent of whether bronchoscopic or nonbronchoscopic procedures are used for diagnosis.[223]

LUNG BIOPSY

Direct means of obtaining diagnostic material in patients with pneumonia include percutaneous lung aspiration, transbronchial lung biopsy, thoracoscopy, and open lung biopsy.[224] These procedures are usually reserved for cases of pneumonia in impaired hosts and in pediatric populations, in whom sputum is not routinely available.[225]

Biopsy procedures are rarely indicated in the normal person with acute pneumonia. The indications and usefulness of these invasive procedures remain controversial. Lung aspiration has provided a diagnostic yield of 30 to 82% in adults and children, though false-negative rates of up to 18% have been reported.[226–230] Bleeding and pneumothorax have been reported as major complications in 5 to 39% of procedures.[229–232] The use of transbronchial biopsy in the diagnosis of pneumonia has been reviewed, revealing similar diagnostic yields though somewhat lower complication rates.[233]

Thoracoscopy, in which the pleura and underlying lung are visualized before biopsy, has been used in several series of children and adults with pneumonia. Despite a diagnostic yield of over 90% and low complication rates,[234, 235] there has not been extensive experience with this procedure.

Open lung biopsy remains the definitive invasive procedure for making an etiologic diagnosis of pneumonia in immunosuppressed patients, with diagnostic yields of 60 to 100%.[232, 233, 236] The incidence of pneumothorax and bleeding is usually less than 10%, even in patients who are thrombocytopenic.[233] Some have questioned whether open lung biopsy provides meaningful information that significantly affects patients' clinical outcome.[237, 238]

EXAMINATION OF PLEURAL EFFUSIONS

The characteristics of pleural effusions and their importance in the differential diagnosis of pulmonary disease are discussed in Chapter 58. It should be noted that the incidence of pleural effusions associated with pneumonia varies with the etiologic agent, from approximately 10% with pneumococci to 50 to 70% with gram-negative bacilli to up to 95% with group A streptococci.[119, 239, 240] Pleural fluid cultures, when positive, are specific for the organism causing the underlying pneumonia. Furthermore, analysis of pleural fluid may play a major role in differentiating other causes of pulmonary infiltrates that may mimic pneumonia, including tuberculosis, tumors, pulmonary emboli, and collagen vascular diseases.[241] Pleural biopsy specimens from patients with acute bacterial pneumonia are nonspecific and are therefore of little use in the differential diagnosis. Analysis of pleural fluid may be of prognostic significance. A pleural fluid pH of less than 7.3 has been associated with the presence of a complicated parapneumonic effusion and the need for a tube thoracostomy.[242] Although the determination of glucose and lactate dehydrogerase levels has been suggested by some to discriminate between complicated and uncomplicated parapneumonic effusions, they do not appear to be as accurate as pH in this regard.

BLOOD CULTURE, SEROLOGIC STUDIES, ANTIGEN DETECTION, AND DNA AMPLIFICATION

Blood cultures are positive in only 1 to 16% of patients hospitalized with community-acquired pneumonia, and their usefulness and cost effectiveness have been questioned.[243, 244] However, the presence of positive blood cultures is highly specific, helps identify a patient population with a greater mortality rate, and may be of use in narrowing antibiotic coverage.[244, 245] In addition, patients with HIV infection, those with underlying malignancy, those receiving immunosuppressives, and those residing in nursing homes have an increased risk of bacteremia. Finally, unusual organisms may be identified that may not be adequately treated by routine empirical coverage.[246] Therefore, blood cultures should be obtained from all patients suspected of having bacterial pneumonia who are ill enough to be hospitalized.

S. pneumoniae produces a variety of antigens and surface markers that are type- or species-specific.[247] Since the demonstration by Dorff and associates that pneumococcal-related antigens could be detected by CIE,[248] a variety of techniques have been used to identify pneumococci in urine, serum, sputum, and pleural fluid. Most recent assays have involved recognition of one of two pneumococcal polysaccharides. Pneumococcal C polysaccharide is a teichoic acid constituent of the bacterial cell wall that is species- but not type-specific. Pneumococcal capsular polysaccharide antigens are constituents of the outer surface of the pneumocci that are type-specific. Three immunoassays have been used for antigen identification, including CIE, agglutination, and ELISA. ELISA has proved to be the most sensitive but is the most expensive and time-consuming. Latex agglutination, although easy to perform, is less sensitive for detecting urinary antigen. CIE may miss positively charged capsular polysaccharide antigen. Yields have been highest for antigen detection in sputum, with sensitivities of 72 to 94%.[249–253] Antigen detection in urine has been consistently less sensitive, with yields of 40 to 60%. The U.S. Food and Drug Administration approved a rapid test for urinary pneumococcal C-polysaccharide in August 1999. The manufacturer (Binax, Inc.) reports sensitivity of 86 to 90% in bacteremic pneumococcal pneumonia. Antigen detection in serum is unacceptably low, with sensitivities of 3 to 9%. Antigen may persist long after the onset of pneumonia, even in patients who are adequately treated and in whom cultures are no longer positive. Specificity of pneumococcal antigen in sputum remains a problem.[252, 254] False-positive rates of 18 to 20% are reported.[247, 255] Distinguishing colonization and oropharyngeal contamination from infection remains an unresolved problem with the technique.

Serologic assays have been used to detect antibodies against four pneumococcal antigens: pneumococcal C polysaccharide, capsular polysaccharide, phosphorylcholine, and the protein toxin pneumolysin. Antibody detection against the capsular polysaccharide and C polysaccharide have reported sensitivities of 89 and 97%, respectively.[254]

CIE and latex agglutination techniques have been used for the detection of *H. influenzae* and *Pseudomonas* antigens in patients with pneumonia, though clinical experience has been limited and the results inconsistent.[256]

A variety of assays have been utilized to detect pathogens that have been difficult to isolate using routine culture techniques. Serologic assays have been used to diagnose infections caused by *Legionella* spp., *M. pneumoniae, Chlamydia* spp., and *Coxiella burnetii*.[257] The sensitivity and specificity of the assays vary, and, since they are not available routinely, their usefulness in making a rapid diagnosis is limited. Soluble *L. pneumophila* antigen can be detected in urine using a radioimmunoassay, though it is useful for detecting only *L. pneumophila* serogroup 1.[258] This assay offers the advantage of being noninvasive, and has a sensitivity of 80 to 95% and a specificity estimated to be 99%. An ELISA test is also available. Although test results may be available on the day of testing, antigenuria may persist for weeks to months after therapy.[144]

Detection of microbial DNA using PCR techniques has been used to detect the cause of pneumonia. *S. pneumoniae* may be detected in the blood of bacteremic patients with a sensitivity as high as 100% and a specificity of 94%.[259] The highest diagnostic yields have been associated with phenol extraction of DNA to remove serum inhibitors, a technique that is labor-intensive and therefore not suited to most clinical labs. Moreover, only pneumonia associated with bacteremia would be expected to be detected. PCR has also been used to detect DNA from *P. carinii* in blood of patients with AIDS[260] and from BAL fluid.[145] Diagnostic efficacy has essentially been equal to that of immunofluoresence staining.

PCR techniques have been used to identify DNA from *M. tuberculosis* in both sputum and lavage fluid. Although sensitivity and specificity have been high even in patients who were smear-negative but culture-positive, PCR may be positive in 70% of people with prior exposure to tuberculosis but no active disease. This problem of false-positives remains.

Recent evidence suggests that cytokine responses may be a useful adjunct in diagnosing pneumonia.[261–264] C-reactive protein is an acute-phase reactant produced in the liver as a response to a variety of stimuli, including infection. Elevated C-reactive protein levels have been observed in patients with community-acquired pneumonia and appear to be a potential means of distinguishing pneumonia from purulent bronchitis and noninfectious conditions. Persistent elevations of C-reactive protein may suggest antibiotic failure or the development of other infectious complications. Other cytokines have also been studied including IL-6 and TNF-α. Correlations with pneumonia appear less consistent.

RADIOLOGIC EXAMINATION

The chest radiograph plays a critical role in the diagnosis of pneumonia. The differential diagnosis of respiratory complaints and abnormal physical findings includes upper respiratory as well as lower respiratory tract infection as well as an array of noninfectious entities.[265] Demonstration of an abnormal chest radiograph consistent with pneumonia differentiates a patient population that may benefit from antibiotic therapy from patient populations that will not. Overuse of antibiotics for therapy of upper respiratory infections has been documented and may contribute to the growing problem of antibiotic resistance. Identifying patients who really should be receiving antibiotic therapy is of obvious importance. The chest radiograph is readily available, is reasonably reliable as far as interobserver variability,[266] and should be obtained in most patients suspected of having pneumonia.[266, 267] The extent and nature of radiographic abnormalities may define patients who are more seriously ill and may need closer monitoring.[268] The chest film most frequently shows a pattern of infiltrates that is not very helpful in making a specific etiologic diagnosis (Fig. 57–5). However, certain features may be of some diagnostic aid. Lobar consolidation, cavitation, and large pleural effusions support a bacterial cause (Fig. 57–6). Most lobar pneumonias are pneumococcal, whereas most pneumococcal pneumonias are not lobar. In cases in which bilateral diffuse involvement is noted, *P. carinii* pneumonia, *Legionella* pneumonia, or a primary viral pneumonia should be suspected. Staphyloccal pneumonia may result from infection metastasizing from a primary focus unrelated to the lung. In these cases, multiple nodular infiltrates throughout the lung may be seen. Staphylococci may cause marked necrosis of lung tissue with ill-defined thin-walled cavities (pneumatoceles), bronchopleural fistulas, and empyema, especially in children (Fig. 57–7).[269–271] Although pneumatoceles are diagnostically significant findings in staphylococcal pneumonia, they may be seen in pneumonias with other causes, including *K. pneumoniae, H. influenzae, S. pneu-*

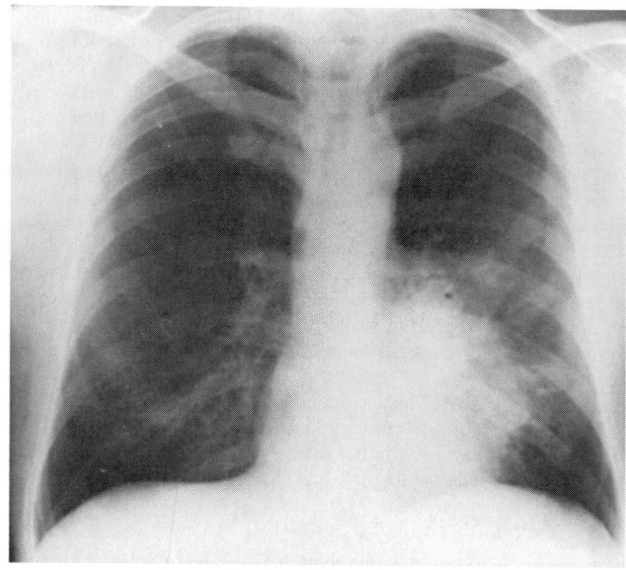

FIGURE 57–5. Patchy infiltrate representing bronchopneumonia in a patient with *Streptococcus pneumoniae* infection.

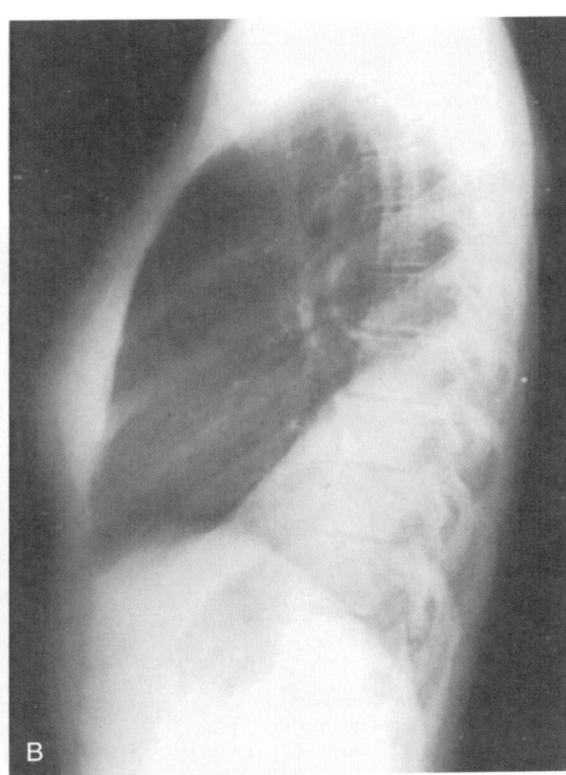

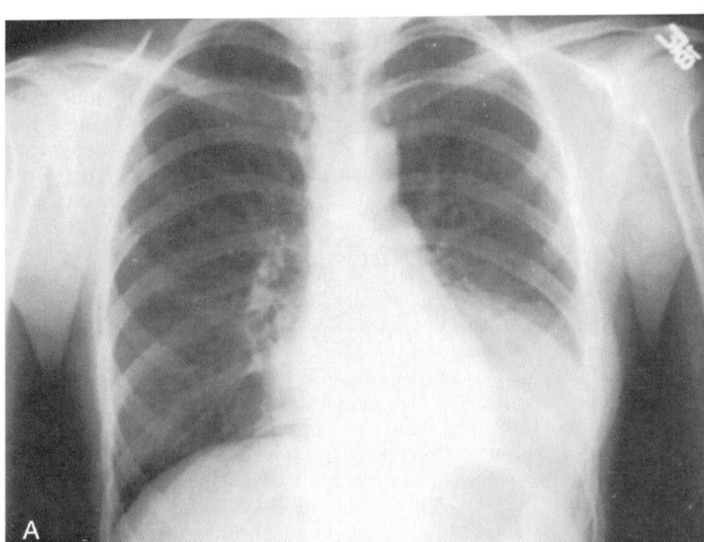

FIGURE 57–6. *A*, Posteroanterior film showing dense left lower consolidation consistent with bacterial pneumonia, in this case caused by *S. pneumoniae*. *B*, Lateral film of a patient with left lower lobe pneumococcal pneumonia.

moniae, and, more rarely, *P. carinii*.[272–274] Pulmonary infections due to *Pseudomonas* may cavitate. *Pseudomonas* and other gram-negative bacilli most commonly cause lower lobe pneumonia.[275]

Aspiration pneumonia should be considered along with gram-negative and staphyloccal pneumonias as a source of necrotizing pneumonia, cavitation, and empyema. Aspiration pneumonia commonly involves either the superior segment or the basilar segment of either lower lobe or the posterior segment of the upper lobes, depending on whether aspiration occurred in the dependent or the upright position.[276] Chronic aspiration most commonly results in a bilateral lower lobe pneumonia, although it may involve one side more than the other.[275]

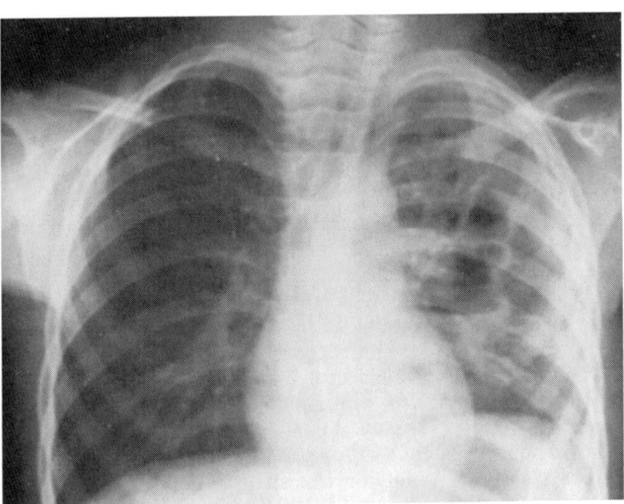

FIGURE 57–7. Pneumatocele formation in the left upper lobe of a patient with staphylococcal pneumonia.

Many viral pneumonias involve generalized destruction of ciliated epithelium with little radiologic distinction between the various viral causes. Initially, ciliated epithelial cells, goblet cells, and bronchial mucous gland cells are destroyed. Subsequent involvement may include terminal bronchioles and alveoli. Diffuse hemorrhagic congestion of alveolar septa with red blood cells and inflammatory edema fluid may be seen, especially with primary influenza pneumonia.[277] The radiographic concomitants of these pathologic findings are varied and may be confusing if a secondary bacterial infection complicates the initial process. Diffuse and localized involvement with both interstitial and alveolar patterns have been noted (Fig. 57–8).[278] Peribronchial involvement with nodular infiltrates is a pattern often seen with varicella.

Mycoplasmal pneumonia often manifests with an interstitial pattern in a peribronchial distribution. As more edema fluid is elaborated, there may be rapid progression to lobar or sublobar consolidation. Once this consolidation stage is reached, radiologic differentiation between bacterial and mycoplasmal pneumonia is difficult. *Mycoplasma* is usually associated with lower lobe disease. Cavitation is rare, although pleural effusion may be seen in 20% of the cases.[279]

Legionnaires' disease may initially present with a radiographic picture similar to that of mycoplasmal pneumonia. A patchy interstitial or finely nodular pattern is seen in the lower lobe.[280] However, unlike the situation with mycoplasmal pneumonia, pneumonia with more than two-lobe involvement is commonly seen. Rapid progression and pleural effusions are also common.[281] Pneumonia caused by *Legionella micdadei* may present with pulmonary nodules, either single or multiple, as well as with segmental infiltrates. As in pneumonia caused by *L. pneumophila*, rapid radiologic progression of the disease is characteristic.[282]

It must be recognized that chest radiographs are most helpful in

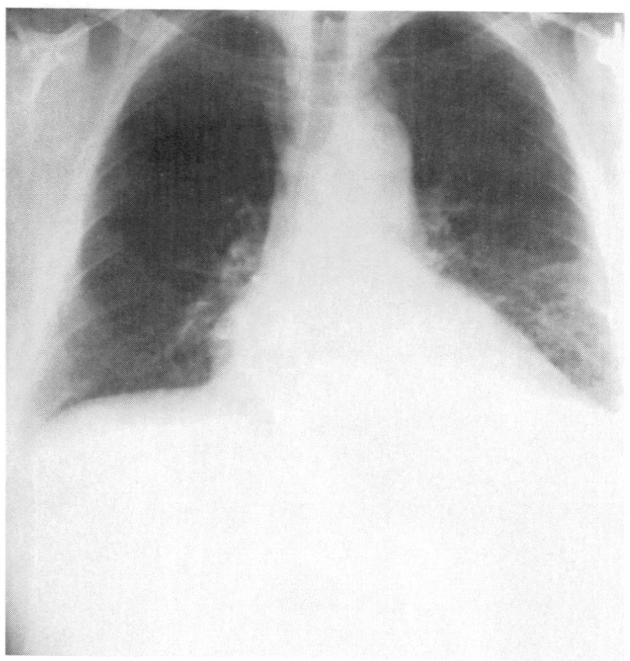

FIGURE 57–8. Bilateral involvement with a mixed interstitial-alveolar pattern in a patient with viral pneumonia.

conjunction with the clinical history and physical examination but are often not helpful in making a specific etiologic diagnosis. This point was clearly shown by Tew and associates, who evaluated readings of radiographs of patients with pneumonia made without clinical information.[283] Pneumonia was correctly identified as bacterial only 67% of the time and as viral only 65% of the time. Mycoplasmal pneumonia was incorrectly identified as bacterial 81% of the time.

The usefulness of computed tomography (CT) in managing chest infections, including pneumonia, has been reviewed.[284–286] In the immunocompetent host, chest CT is most helpful in evaluating recurrent pneumonia or infections unresponsive to therapy. Pneumonia developing behind an obstruction due to tumors or other masses and lung abscess may also be better defined by CT than by routine chest radiographs. High-resolution CT has been shown to improve radiographic characterization of lung infection.[284, 286] Compared with a routine chest radiograph, high-resolution CT detects the presence of pneumonia more often and does a better job in defining disease in the upper and lower lobes, and lingula.[285] However, exposure to more radiation (the radiation from one CT scan equals that from six to seven chest radiographs) and the increased expense (approximately seven times the cost of a chest radiograph) has limited its use as the initial radiographic procedure. In the immunocompromised host in whom infection is only one of the possible causes of abnormal chest radiographs, chest CT or one of its variations, such as spiral CT or high-resolution CT, may aid in better defining a "questionable" chest radiograph and may be helpful in localizing involved areas of lung as a guide to biopsy procedures.[285] Further, certain infections, such as those caused by *Aspergillus, M. tuberculosis*, and *P. carinii*, have characteristic appearances on CT that in the correct clinical setting may make invasive procedures unnecessary.

Nuclear medicine procedures have been used to detect pneumonia. These procedures include ^{67}Ga-citrate scans, ^{111}In-labeled granulocytes, and ^{99m}Tc-diethylenetriaminepenta-acetic acid aerosol clearance.[287] In general, these procedures have been used in patients with AIDS to define the presence of lung infection in the absence of abnormal chest radiographs. In patients with AIDS, diffuse uptake of gallium is usually seen with *P. carinii* infection but may also be seen with infection caused by *Mycobacterium avium* complex, cytomegalovirus, and *Cryptococcus neoformans*, and in patients with lymphoma. Localized uptake may be associated with bacterial disease. Focal uptake corresponding to lymph node areas has been associated with *M. avium* complex, *M. tuberculosis*, and lymphoma.

PNEUMONIA SYNDROMES

Acute Community-Acquired Pneumonia

As discussed previously, a long list of bacterial, fungal, viral, and protozoal agents may cause pneumonia. Since initial evaluation rarely results in a specific etiologic diagnosis, antibiotic therapy is usually begun empirically. Defining pneumonia syndromes based on clinical, epidemiologic, radiographic, and laboratory parameters with a limited number of organisms commonly associated with each syndrome has helped the clinician to select rational empirical therapy for the most likely organisms involved. One cannot determine the cause based on any specific clinical, radiographic, or laboratory parameter. In fact, many of the syndromes have overlapping signs and symptoms, which at times makes clear identification of a specific syndrome in an individual impossible.[288–290] Further, the characteristics of the syndrome of acute community-acquired pneumonia as defined almost 30 years ago[71, 74, 75] are changing.[290–304] The patient population is aging and includes more patients with significant coexistent diseases and more patients who are immunosuppressed. Microbial agents now recognized as potential causes of community-acquired pneumonia that were not previously recognized.[290, 299]

In 1993, the American Lung Association developed four subgroupings of community-acquired pneumonia based on the age of the patient, the need for hospitalization, the severity of illness, and the presence of coexisting disease.[303] This "splitting" of the syndrome of acute community-acquired pneumonia recognized the diversity of the patient population and of the organisms potentially involved. It grouped together bacterial causes usually involved in acute community-acquired pneumonia and those involved in atypical pneumonia syndromes including *M. pneumoniae, Chlamydia* spp., respiratory viruses, and *Legionella* spp. Treatment recommendations are made for each subgroup (see later).

In 1998, the Infectious Disease Society of America developed similar guidelines with the major criteria for antibiotic selection based on the severity of illness, comorbidity, exposure, and the epidemiologic setting.[110] The distinction of acute bacterial community-acquired pneumonia versus atypical pneumonia became blurred even further. However, attempts to define pneumonia syndromes as they have classically been described is a reasonable first step in dealing with clinical decision making.

Patients with acute community-acquired pneumonia are usually in their mid-fifties to late sixties.[243, 245, 295–298] Although peak incidences of disease in midwinter and early spring have been described, work has suggested that there is no "pneumonia season," and that disease takes place throughout the year.[299] Most patients (58 to 89%) have one or more chronic underlying diseases, including COPD, cardiovascular disease, neurologic disease, diabetes, or alcohol abuse.[243, 245, 290, 297, 301, 302, 305, 306] Immunosuppression including the presence of malignancy, neutropenia, the chronic use of steroids or myelosuppresive agents, or the presence of HIV infection may be present in up to 57% of patients.[114, 290, 307]

"Classically" community-acquired pneumonia presents with a sudden onset of a chill followed by fever, pleuritic chest pain, and cough productive of mucopurulent sputum. The presence of various signs and symptoms and physical findings varies according to the age of the patient, therapy with antibiotics before presentation, and the severity of illness. These classic findings in some combination are present in approximately 81% of patients with community-acquired pneumonia. Patients usually present after having been ill for a mean of 6 days.[300] Cough is noted in over 80% of patients and is productive in 60 to 80%.[290, 299, 302–306] Chest pain is present in 30 to 46% of cases, chills in 40 to 70%, and true rigors in 15%.[67, 297, 290, 299]

A variety of nonrespiratory symptoms are frequently associated with pneumonia, including fatigue (91%), anorexia (71%), sweats (69%), and nausea (41%).[67] Both respiratory and nonrespiratory findings occur less frequently in older age groups.[67]

Physical examination reveals fever in 68 to 78% of patients but may be seen less commonly in older populations. Tachypnea (respiratory rate greater than 24 to 30 breaths/minute) is noted in 45 to 69% of patients and may be more frequently seen in older age groups.[67] Tachycardia (pulse rate greater than 100 beats/minute) is noted in 45%. Rales are noted in 78% of patients, but signs of consolidation are noted in 29%.

Most commonly, the white blood cell count is in the range of 15,000 to 35,000/mm^3, and the differential cell count reveals an increased number of juvenile forms.[308] Leukopenia may be noted and is a poor prognostic sign.[309] The hematocrit and the red blood cell indices are usually normal. Sputum is thick and purulent and may be rust colored. The sputum Gram stain reveals numerous neutrophils and bacteria, often with a single organism predominating. Chest films show areas of parenchymal involvement, usually with an alveolar-filling process. There is moderate hypoxemia due to ventilation perfusion abnormalities. Even with rigorous laboratory evaluation and using definitions of *definite, probable*, and *possible* causes, a microbiologic diagnosis may be made in only 20 to 70% of cases of community-acquired pneumonia.[70, 114, 243, 268, 290, 293, 299, 305, 306, 308]

In the past, 50 to 90% of the cases of acute community-acquired pneumonia were caused by *S. pneumoniae*.[74, 75, 310] More recently, the relative importance of the pneumococcus has varied greatly in published reports from 16 to 60% of the cases of acute community-acquired pneumonia.[114, 290, 291, 293–302, 311–313] The pneumococcus remains the leading cause of the syndrome of acute community-acquired pneumonia in virtually all series.

Advanced age, cigarette smoking, institutionalization, dementia, seizures, malnutrition, and the presence of chronic illnesses such as COPD, chronic liver and kidney disease, congestive heart failure, and cerebrovascular disease have been identified as significant risk factors for the development of pneumococcal pneumonia.[314] Severe pneumococcal infections, including pneumonia, have been associated with prior splenectomy due to trauma or staging for Hodgkin's disease,[315, 316] abnormal immunoglobulin responses (myeloma, lymphoma, HIV infection),[317] and functional asplenia due to systemic lupus erythematosus or marrow transplant.

An estimated 3 to 15% of the cases of acute community-acquired pneumonia are caused by *H. influenzae*.[71, 75, 114, 243, 293, 311–313, 318, 319] The true incidence of this organism is obscured by the difficulty in isolating it from sputum and identifying it in sputum Gram stain, and by the difficulty in distinguishing colonization from infection. The age of patients, presence of underlying disease, and presentation are all similar to those of pneumococcal disease.

S. aureus accounts for 2 to 5% of acute community-acquired pneumonia cases[114, 320] and takes on increased importance as a cause of pneumonia in elderly patients, and in those with influenza.[321, 322] Patients developing postinfluenza pneumonia are usually younger and have less underlying disease than most other patients with community-acquired pneumonia. Clinical signs and symptoms of influenza are present but appear to resolve over several days. After a variable period of time ranging from 2 to 14 days, symptoms suddenly reappear, with the onset of shaking chills, pleuritic chest pain, and cough productive of purulent sputum. An elevated white blood cell count with a shift to the left, physical signs of pulmonary consolidation, and radiographic evidence of focal parenchymal disease appear. The sputum Gram stain is consistent with bacterial pneumonia. Although the pneumococcus still represents the most common etiologic agent, staphylococcal disease occurs with a higher frequency than that noted in noninfluenza-related, community-acquired pneumonia.[321, 322]

Aerobic gram-negative bacteria, exclusive of *H. influenzae*, and mixed aerobic and anaerobic infections cause most of the remaining cases of acute community-acquired pneumonia. Gram-negative rods may cause 7 to 18% of pneumonia cases[114, 311–313] and are particularly important pathogens in elderly persons.

The importance of *Legionella* spp. in causing pneumonia varies greatly in different geographic areas. Although incidences as high as 17 to 30% have been reported,[310, 323] some centers report significantly lower rates of 2 to 8%.[114, 290, 298, 299] No clinical features reliably distinguish *Legionella* spp. pneumonia from that caused by other bacteria. However, the presence of a high fever (>40°C), multilobar involvement, rapid progression of radiographic abnormalities, a need for intensive care, gastrointestinal and neurologic abnormalities, elevated liver enzyme levels, and increased creatinine levels have all been associated with *Legionella* pneumonia.[290, 323, 324]

Moraxella catarrhalis has also been identified as a cause of pneumonia.[325–327] The overall incidence of disease due to this bacterium is low, but it is an important pathogen in elderly patients with COPD and various forms of immunosuppression.

In contrast to disease patterns in adults, viruses are the most important cause of pneumonia in young children. Respiratory syncytial virus and parainfluenza virus type 3 are the major pathogens. Other parainfluenza viruses and low-numbered adenovirus serotypes are also important.

Mild Community-Acquired Pneumonia

Most of the information concerning the cause of community-acquired pneumonia has been gathered from series of hospitalized patients. Approximately 50 to 80% of episodes of community-acquired pneumonia are treated in the outpatient setting. The relative importance of various etiologic agents has not been well characterized in this patient population. *S. pneumoniae* has been implicated in 9 to 36% of outpatient community-acquired pneumonias. Although the relative importance of *H. influenzae* appears similar to that noted in inpatients, the percentage of *S. aureus* pneumonia appears lower (zero to 1%) and that of *M. pneumoniae* higher (up to 37%). Approximately 8 to 14% of mild pneumonias are viral in origin. Influenzae A and B, parainfluenza virus, adenovirus, and respiratory syncytial virus are the important agents involved.[328]

Community-Acquired Pneumonia in the Elderly Population

Pneumonia in the elderly population is a major cause of morbidity and mortality and in some series represents the leading cause of death (see Chapter 306).[329] The clinical presentation may be more subtle than in younger populations, with more gradual onset, less frequent complaints of chills and rigors, and less fever.[67, 290, 330–333]

The classic findings of cough, fever, and dyspnea may be absent in over half of elderly patients.[330, 334] Patients may present with a decline in functional status, weakness, subtle changes in mental status, anorexia, or abdominal pain.

The incidence of fever may decline with age, and the degree of fever appears lower in older populations.[67, 290, 299] Tachypnea (respiratory rate greater than 24 to 30 breaths/minute) is noted more frequently in up to 69% of patients. Although rales are common and are noted in 78% of patients, signs of true consolidation are found in only 29%. Bacteremia, metastatic foci of infection, and death are more frequent in older populations.[71, 100, 309]

Specific etiologic diagnoses are made less frequently in elderly patients, with approximately 20 to 40% of patients having an etiologic agent defined.[330, 335, 336] The absence of productive cough and prior use of antibiotics help to explain this observation. Causes have varied in different series according to the means of diagnosis, the patient population studied (outpatient versus institutionalized elderly patients), and the geographic location.[330] In general, the cause of community-acquired pneumonia in the elderly population follows the general trend of infection in younger populations. *S. pneumoniae* remains the predominant organism, accounting for 20 to 60% of cases.[330, 336, 337, 338] *Haemophilus influenzae*, usually a nontypable strain, is frequently the second most common agent, accounting for 7 to 11% of episodes. Other aerobic gram-negative bacilli, especially *K. pneumoniae* and *S. aureus*, play important roles as well, especially in elderly patients in nursing homes or extended care facilities.[330–333, 339] Although increased oropharyngeal colonization with aerobic gram-negative bacilli has been documented in the elderly population and is thought to explain the increased incidence of pneumonia caused by these organisms, colonization appears to be related to debility of the patient rather than age.[340] Other factors associated with increasing colonization with gram-negative organisms include prior use of antibiotics, decreased activity, diabetes, alcoholism, and incontinence.[331, 340–342] Elderly persons are at greater risk for infection with group B streptococci, *M. catarrhalis*, and *Legionella* spp., though their overall incidence among the elderly population is relatively low.[325–327] Polymicrobial infections and pneumonia due to aspiration have both been noted to occur more frequently in elderly patients.[100, 343, 344]

The role of agents causing atypical pneumonia in the elderly population is unclear. Most series suggest that *M. pneumoniae* pneumonia is unusual, though it has been documented by others to be a significant cause of pneumonia leading to hospitalization in elderly patients.[70, 336, 345] Chlamydial infections appear commonly in the elderly population and may cause pneumonia in up to 21%, though the incidence varies.[336, 346]

Viral agents may also play an important role in causing pneumonia in the elderly population. In one series, both respiratory syncytial virus and influenza A caused infection in 10 to 11% of the patients studied. Forty-eight percent of those infected with respiratory syncytial virus and 30% of those infected with influenza virus had pneumonia.[347] As in younger populations, dyspnea, wheezing, and sputum production are hallmarks of disease with those agents, with bronchospasm appearing more frequently with respiratory syncytial virus.[348] Coinfection with bacteria was noted in over 17% of cases, making interpretation of the actual role of viruses in the presenting symptoms of pneumonia somewhat unclear. Rhinovirus also appears to be an important cause of respiratory infection in elderly persons, with 24% of some populations infected. Although about two thirds of those infected have lower respiratory tract symptoms, the role of rhinovirus as a cause of pneumonia is unclear.[349]

Community-Acquired Pneumonia in Patients with Acquired Immunodeficiency Syndrome

The cause of community-acquired pneumonia in patients with AIDS has changed significantly since the beginning of the epidemic. Before the development of effective prophylactic regimens, *P. carinii* pneumonia occurred in approximately 85 percent of patients at some time during their course, with a mortality rate in 1987 of 32.5%.[350, 351] The incidence of *Pneumocystis* disease was halved and mortality rates dropped to 13.8% in 1992.[89, 352] In patients who refuse prophylaxis or who have advanced untreated HIV infection, *Pneumocystis* infection remains a significant problem. Further, even with prophylaxis, *Pneumocystis* infection may develop in the setting of severe immune deficiency.[89, 353] A multicenter prospective study of respiratory tract infection in 1353 HIV-infected patients has yielded valuable information concerning the number of pulmonary infections in this patient population.[354] The number of community-acquired pneumonia cases was five to eight times that of non–HIV-infected controls and *S. pneumoniae, H. influenzae*, and *S. aureus* were the predominant pathogens.[92, 352, 355] A variety of other bacteria have been implicated, including *R. equi* and *P. aeruginosa*, the latter being associated with late stages of disease, the presence of central venous catheters, the presence of urinary catheters, and the use of steroids.[356] *Mycobacterium tuberculosis*, nontuberculous mycobacteria, *Cryptococcus neoformans*, and cytomegalovirus also play important roles as etiologic agents (see Chapters 253 and 127).[355]

Severe Community-Acquired Pneumonia

Approximately 10% of community-acquired pneumonia cases are severe enough to require intensive care or mechanical ventilation, or both. These cases of "severe community-acquired pneumonia" have been reviewed.[297, 357–359] *S. pneumoniae* and *L. pneumophila* are the organisms most commonly involved in causing severe community-acquired pneumonia. Gram-negative bacilli, especially *Klebsiella* spp., must be considered in patients who have significant underlying disease such as COPD, diabetes, and alcohol abuse.[357, 360] In some series, *M. pneumoniae*, one of the agents causing atypical pneumonia, is involved in up to 11% of community-acquired pneumonia patients requiring intensive care.

A series of criteria have been developed that aid in identifying patients who may have severe community-acquired pneumonia and may require intensive care.[297, 361–363] These include

1. Respiratory rate above 30 breaths/minute
2. Pa_{O_2}/F_{IO_2} less than 250 or P_{O_2} less than 50 to 60 mmHg breathing room air
3. Chest radiographs showing bilateral involvement, multilobar involvement, or significant progression of disease in the first 48 hours of admission, or all of these
4. Hypotension (systolic blood pressure <90 mmHg or diastolic blood pressure <60 mmHg)
5. Requirement for vasopressors
6. Urine output less than 20 ml/hour or less than 80 ml over a 4-hour period
7. Abnormal mental status

Mortality rates in patients with severe pneumonia have ranged from 20 to 53%, which is higher than the 2 to 30% noted in all community-acquired pneumonias.[70, 114, 245, 297, 357–360, 364, 365] Tachypnea (>30 breaths/minute), diastolic blood pressure less than 60 mmHg, and blood urea nitrogen levels above 7 mmol/liter have been shown to be independently associated with death from pneumonia.[361–363] Other parameters identified with increased mortality include severe underlying disease, underlying neoplastic disease, age above 60 years, or absence of pleuritic chest pain, a change in mental status, acute respiratory failure requiring ventilatory support, bilateral involvement, bacteremia, a neutrophil count under 3500, a total serum protein level less than 45 g/liter, a serum creatinine level greater than 15 mg/liter, the presence of shock, inadequate initial antibiotic therapy, radiographic evidence of spreading disease, and pneumonia caused by *S. aureus* or gram-negative bacilli.[363, 366]

Slowly Resolving Community-Acquired Pneumonia

The natural history of adequately treated community-acquired pneumonia is usually that of prompt resolution.[367] In healthy young military personnel recovering from pneumococcal pneumonia, fever resolved after 2.5 days, cough after 7.9 days, and "crackles" on physical examination of the chest by 8 days.[368] Normalization of the white blood cell count occurred by day 4. Patients who are older or who have significant coexisting underlying disease have more gradual resolution of signs and symptoms. Radiographic abnormalities may take 4 to 10 weeks to normalize, with younger (<50 years of age) patients resolving more quickly.[369–371] Patients who fail to resolve their radiographic abnormalities by day 30, despite clearing of signs and symptoms, usually have significant underlying pulmonary disease such as emphysema, chronic bronchitis, pneumoconiosis, or asthma.

Slowly resolving pneumonia has been defined as less than 50% clearing of radiographic abnormalities at 2 weeks and less than complete clearing of abnormalities by 4 weeks.[370, 371] Host factors such as age above 50 years, a history of alcoholism, and the presence of significant underlying diseases (COPD, diabetes, congestive heart failure, asthma, malignancy) have been found to be associated with slow resolution of pneumonia. *S. pneumoniae* and *Legionella* spp.

are the organisms most often associated with slowly resolving pneumonia.[371, 372]

Atypical Pneumonia Syndrome

By the late 1930s most of the main bacterial causes of pneumonia had been defined. In 1938, Hobart Reiman described a small number of patients with a clinical picture that was "atypical" in that episodes began as a mild respiratory tract illness that was followed by an atypical pneumonia with dyspnea and cough without sputum.[373, 374] *M. pneumoniae, C. pneumoniae*, and *L. pneumophila* are the most significant causes of atypical pneumonia. Other agents such as *Chlamydia psittaci, C. burnetii*, and a variety of respiratory viruses may also cause atypical pneumonia but do so much less commonly. Although some series report that almost 50% of patients with community-acquired pneumonia demonstrate serologic evidence of mycoplasmal or chlamydial pneumonia, or both, other series suggest an incidence of 7 to 28%.[70, 112, 289, 375] The overall frequency of atypical pneumonia varies based on the means of diagnosis. A single IgG elevation that is commonly used as a means of diagnosis may not be as specific as a fourfold rise in antibody, thereby falsely increasing the incidence of disease. Other variables that play a role in the incidence of infection include the geographic location, the age of the patients, and the presence or absence of an epidemic during the study period.[375, 376] Further, dual infections, usually with a "typical" bacterial pathogen, may occur in up to two thirds of patients with suspected mycoplasmal or chlamydial infection, which raises the question as to the true role of atypical agents.[377, 378]

In the past, the epidemiology and clinical features of the atypical pneumonias were thought to be distinct enough to clearly differentiate them from other causes of community-acquired pneumonia. Although with their "classic" presentation this may be true, the overlap of demographic features, presenting signs and symptoms, and laboratory and radiographic characteristics make the clear differentiation between atypical agents and typical bacterial causes of community-acquired pneumonia problematic.[290, 300, 379] Despite these constraints, until rapid microbiologic assays are developed for the atypical agents, it is still instructive to use epidemiologic, clinical, laboratory, and radiographic findings to at least attempt to differentiate atypical pathogens from typical bacterial pathogens of community-acquired pneumonia, recognizing that it may not always be possible to do so.

The older child (older than 5 years), the adolescent, and the young adult are at greatest risk for developing infection with *M. pneumoniae*. Recent data suggest that *M. pneumoniae* is an etiologic agent of pneumonia leading to hospitalization in older patients as well, though the incidence of mycoplasma in the elderly population varies from less than 1 to 5%.[70, 345, 380] This agent accounts for 1 to 20% of cases of community-acquired pneumonia, with the highest percentages noted in patients who remain ambulatory.[70, 110, 114, 289] The majority of cases are in patients younger than 40 years. An increased incidence of disease and true epidemics have been documented in relatively enclosed populations of young adults at military bases, colleges, and boarding schools.[381–383] Mycoplasmal infection occurs throughout the year, although a relative increase in incidence is noted in the late summer and fall. In contrast, adenovirus infection, another cause of atypical pneumonia, most commonly occurs between January and April, outbreaks occurring primarily in military recruit camps.[381, 383, 384]

The course of the atypical pneumonias is characterized by up to 10 days of symptoms before presentation.[300]

In its classic form, mycoplasma infection presents with constitutional symptoms and a progression from the upper to lower respiratory tract. Sore throat is often the initial finding. Bullous myringitis is seen in only about 5% of cases but when present is suggestive of mycoplasmal infection. Fever, malaise, coryza, headache, and cough represent the major clinical findings. Pleuritic chest pain, splinting, and respiratory distress are not usually seen. Moist or crepitant rales may be heard. Sputum production is variable, and although it is purulent in one third to one half of the cases, Gram stain and culture of sputum usually reveal mouth flora. White blood cell counts greater than 10,000/mm^3 are uncommon, occurring in approximately 20% of the patients.[118] An elevated sedimentation rate is noted in about 25% of the cases.[300] Pulmonary involvement seen on radiographs is commonly more extensive than the physical examination would indicate. Unilateral or bilateral patchy infiltrates in one or more segments, usually in the lower lobes, are noted in a bronchial or peribronchial distribution. Upper lobe involvement and pleural effusions are rare. Progression of the radiographic picture, despite a stable clinical picture, may be seen. The overall clinical course in most cases is benign. Disappearance of constitutional symptoms is usually noted in the first and second weeks, although cough and radiographic changes may persist for several weeks. Occasionally, *M. pneumoniae* infection may present as severe community-acquired pneumonia requiring intensive care.[297] A large number of extrapulmonary manifestations may occur with *M. pneumoniae*, including involvement of skin, central nervous system, blood, and kidneys. These are reviewed in Chapter 172.

Other etiologic agents involved in the atypical pneumonia syndrome include *C. burnetii* (Q fever), *C. psittaci* (psittacosis), *C. trachomatis*, and *C. pneumoniae* (TWAR).

Chlamydia pneumoniae (TWAR) has emerged as an important cause of atypical pneumonia and may account for approximately 6 to 12% of community-acquired pneumonia cases.[70, 110, 114, 289, 385–388] Though disease is uncommon in those younger than 5 years, serologic evidence of infection has been noted in over 50% of adults.[389] Disease usually occurs sporadically, though several epidemics have been well documented. The majority of infections are either asymptomatic or produce mild symptoms.[392] In older age groups, most severe pneumonia with chlamydia occurs with reinfection rather than with primary infection.[391] As with mycoplasmal infection, sore throat and hoarseness herald the onset of pneumonia, though the progression of symptoms appears slower than that noted with mycoplasma or viral pneumonia.[389, 392] Cough may begin after several days to weeks, suggesting a biphasic illness. Hoarseness and sinus tenderness appear more commonly than in patients infected with mycoplasma or viruses.[389] The white blood cell count is rarely elevated. Pneumonia with *C. pneumoniae* is usually mild, though complete recovery may be slow. Cough and malaise may persist for weeks to months. Reinfection occurs and appears to be more mild than primary infection and is usually not associated with pneumonia. Chronic and latent infection have also been described. Infection with *C. pneumoniae* has been associated with exacerbations of COPD and asthma.[390, 393] In general, few features distinguish chlamydial pneumonia from infection caused by other atypical agents or other bacteria.[391, 394, 395] *Chlamydia pneumoniae* infections have been associated with extrapulmonary manifestations, including bronchitis, otitis, sinusitis, pericarditis, myocarditis, and endocarditis.[396] Chlamydial infection has been associated with coronary artery disease, and organisms have been demonstrated in atheromatous plaques.[397–399] Antibiotic therapy directed against *C. pneumoniae* has been associated with a decrease in the incidence of subsequent coronary events.[400, 401] Despite these interesting findings, the definite relationship between chlamydia and coronary artery disease remains unclear. (see Chapter 170).

C. trachomatis may be a pulmonary pathogen in immunocompromised as well as healthy hosts.[402–404] Productive cough, myalgias, and fever associated with diffuse nonsegmental infiltrates appear most commonly. The agent has also been associated with chronic pneumonia in neonates and infants. Onset occurs at 2 to 3 weeks of age and is associated with tachypnea, a staccato cough with periods of cyanosis and emesis, a lack of fever, and diffuse interstitial and patchy alveolar infiltrates on chest radiographs. Elevated IgG and IgM levels and absolute eosinophilia have also been noted.

Of the viral agents associated with atypical pneumonia in adults, influenza A and B, adenovirus types 3, 4, and 7 (especially in military recruits), parainfluenza virus,[405] and respiratory syncytial virus (especially in elderly and immune-suppressed patients) are the most common.[406–408] Data suggest that respiratory syncytial virus may cause pneumonia in 1 to 5% of immune-competent adults in whom wheezing by history and rhonchi on physical examination are characteristic.[409] Reports of other viral agents causing pneumonia are scant but have included rhinovirus,[254] enterovirus, coronavirus,[410] the herpesviruses,[411] and hantavirus.[412, 413]

Legionella spp. are now recognized as an important cause of community-acquired pneumonia, accounting for 2 to 8% of cases involving hospitalization.[70, 110, 112] Further, *Legionella* spp. are among the top three to four organisms causing pneumonia requiring intensive care unit monitoring.[365, 414, 415] Although approximately 40 different species of *Legionella* have been identified, fewer than half cause disease in humans. *Legionella pneumophila* causes over 90% of cases of *Legionella* pneumonia, with 70 to 80% of cases caused by serogroup 1.[375]

Inhalation of aerosolized organisms after exposure to environmental reservoirs, such as fresh water and moist soil, has been the accepted means of acquisition of the organism, although aspiration has been thought to be an alternate route of infection.[416] An increased incidence during summer months has been observed.[417]

Cigarette smoking, chronic lung disease, and immunosuppression are consistently noted risk factors for the development of disease. *Legionella* pneumonia may present as either a "typical" acute community-acquired pneumonia or as an atypical pneumonia. Although early symptoms of malaise, muscle aches, headaches, and nonproductive cough resemble the onset of a "viral syndrome," the rapid progression of pulmonary symptoms and relatively high fever, often exceeding 40°C, is noteworthy.[416, 418] *Legionella pneumophila* pneumonia is associated with a variety of extrapulmonary findings and laboratory abnormalities including mental status changes, abdominal complaints (loose stools or diarrhea), elevation of hepatic enzyme levels, hypophosphatemia, hyponatremia, elevated serum lactate dehydrogenase levels, headache, bradycardia, and elevated serum creatinine levels. Although no single finding or laboratory test can distinguish *L. pneumophila* pneumonia from pneumonias of other causes, with the use of groupings of symptoms and laboratory findings, scoring systems have been developed that may help identify *Legionella*. The systems have not been validated in large prospective series.[324, 419] Extrapulmonary infection is unusual, but when it does occur, it usually involves the heart with myocarditis, pericarditis, and postcardiotomy-like syndrome.[416] Unfortunately, none of these findings can distinguish between *L. pneumophila* pneumonia, pneumonia caused by other atypical agents, and pneumonia caused by more typical bacterial pathogens.[420] Similarly, radiographic manifestations do not distinguish *Legionella* infections from those of other causes. Patchy interstitial infiltrates, or nodular infiltrates that may progress rapidly even with adequate therapy, are characteristic. Pleural effusions may be noted in up to one third of patients.

Pneumonia in the Setting of Aspiration

The clinical setting in which aspiration occurs involves any disease state in which consciousness is altered and the normal gag and swallowing reflexes are abnormal. Elderly patients; patients in chronic care facilities, especially those who are neurologically impaired; patients during the acute phase of stroke; and patients with dementia fit into the category of individuals susceptible to aspiration.[343, 344]

The pathogenesis of lung injury due to acid aspiration has been delineated.[421] The presence of acidic contents in the lung induces the release of proinflammatory cytokines including TNF-α and IL-8. These and other cytokines recruit neutrophils into the lung. Activated neutrophils appear to be the key mediators of acute lung injury after acid aspiration, though a role for complement has also been demonstrated.[422] Bacterial aspiration pneumonia occurs in more than 60% of cases of chemical aspiration.[343]

Three major syndromes are recognized as a consequence of aspiration: chemical pneumonitis, bronchial obstruction secondary to aspiration of particulate matter, and bacterial aspiration pneumonia.[423, 424] Aspiration may be associated with acute respiratory distress syndrome atelectasis, bronchial hyperreactivity, and fibrosis. Although chemical pneumonitis and mechanical obstruction usually cause acute symptoms, aspiration pneumonia is more insidious, with symptoms usually occurring gradually several days after the initial episode of aspiration. Pneumonitis, necrotizing pneumonia, abscess, and empyema are common. Symptoms often include fever, weight loss, and productive cough. Putrid sputum is produced in 50% of the cases.[102, 276] Anemia and an elevated white blood cell count are frequently associated findings. The bacteriologic findings in aspiration pneumonia reflect the flora of the oropharynx, and the importance of periodontal disease in this regard has been noted. Anaerobic bacteria, alone (45 to 58% of the cases) or in combination with aerobes (22 to 46%), are most commonly seen when adequate culture techniques are used.[29, 102, 425]

Bacteroides spp., *Porphyromonas* spp., *Prevotella melaninogenica, Fusobacterium* spp., and anaerobic gram-positive cocci are the predominant anaerobes isolated. In community-acquired aspiration pneumonia, *Streptococcus* spp. are the most common aerobic isolates.[29, 424, 426, 427] *Moraxella catarrhalis* and *Eikenella corrodens* may also be involved.[428] In contrast, gram-negative bacilli and *S. aureus* are the most commonly isolated aerobes from nosocomial aspiration pneumonia.[424, 427]

Pulmonary Infiltrates with Eosinophilia

Pulmonary infiltrates with eosinophilia (PIE) is a syndrome associated with a variety of clinical entities, only some of which have an infectious cause.[429–432] Pulmonary eosinophilia with transient, peripheral pulmonary infiltrates and minimal symptoms has been associated with *Ascaris* and *Strongyloides* infections. Prolonged pulmonary eosinophilia associated with weight loss, fever, cough, and dyspnea may be due to tuberculosis, brucellosis, psittacosis, coccidioidomycosis, histoplasmosis, and parasitic infections including ascariasis, strongyloidiasis, paragonimiasis, echinococcosis, visceral larva migrans, cutaneous larva migrans, and infections with *Schistosoma, Dirofilaria immitis*, and *Ancylostoma* spp. Noninfectious causes include drug allergy, sarcoidosis, eosinophilic leukemia, Hodgkin's disease, and hypersensitivity pneumonitis (i.e., pigeon breeders' disease).[433] A PIE syndrome has been associated with *P. carinii* pneumonia in AIDS patients.[434, 435]

Acute eosinophilic pneumonia represents a distinct clinical entity occurring in younger (20 to 30 years old) otherwise healthy individuals. It is marked by the acute onset of dyspnea, nonproductive cough, fever, hypoxia, and chest pain.[436–438] Although leukocytosis is common, peripheral eosinophilia is usually absent. Bilateral, diffuse pulmonary infiltrates are commonly seen. Radiographic abnormalities usually begin as interstitial infiltrates that progress to alveolar infiltrates. Chest CT reveals a "ground glass" opacification with interlobular septal thickening.[436, 437] BAL yields marked (25 to 62%) eosinophilia, which is the diagnostic feature of the disease. Although most patients have received antibiotics, rapid stabilization occurs with steroid use.

It has been suggested that chronic eosinophilic pneumonia may represent a unique clinical entity that is a form of collagen-vascular disease or an infection in a hyperimmune patient.[439–442] A subacute onset of cough, dyspnea, fever, and weight loss associated with peripheral eosinophilia are the common features at presentation. Unlike the situation in acute eosinophilic pneumonia, respiratory failure is rare. Peripheral infiltrates are usually seen on radiographs. Focal interstitial fibrosis, bronchiolitis obliterans, microabscesses, and sarcoid-like granulomas are characteristic pathologic features. A rapid response to steroids has been reported.[441]

Tropical eosinophilia consists of myalgia, fatigue, weight loss, and anorexia associated with cough, frequently with nocturnal exacerbations, wheezing, dyspnea, and marked peripheral eosinophilia in patients who have lived in or visited the tropics.[443] Radiographic changes are distinctive and include increased interstitial markings with 2- to 4-mm nodules throughout the lungs with preferential involvement of the bases. Most cases are thought to represent immunologic hyperresponsiveness to microfilarial infection and can be treated with diethylcarbamazine.

Other causes of PIE syndrome include bronchopulmonary *Aspergillus*, which should be suspected when PIE presents with asthma and pulmonary vasculitis. Patients with the Churg-Strauss syndrome[431] frequently have eosinophilia along with allergic angiitis and granulomatosis and present with asthma, diffuse pulmonary infiltrates, and multiorgan involvement.[444]

Nosocomial Pneumonia and Pneumonia in the Immunosuppressed Host

Nosocomial pneumonia is the second leading type of nosocomial infection and accounts for 13 to 18% of all such infections. It is the leading cause of infection-related deaths in hospitalized patients with an attributable mortality of 27 to 33%.[445–450] Higher mortality rates have been observed when patients are bacteremic or have pneumonia caused by *P. aeruginosa* or *Acinetobacter* spp. The morbidity associated with nosocomial pneumonia includes longer hospital stays (an average of 7 to 9 days) and higher costs of health care (an estimated $2 billion annually).[451]

Risk factors for the development of nosocomial pneumonia have been categorized as patient related, infection-control related, or intervention related.[452] Patient-related risk factors include age greater than 70 years, severe underlying disease, malnutrition, coma, metabolic acidosis, and the presence of any of a number of comorbid illnesses (COPD, alcoholism, azotemia, central nervous system dysfunction). An association has been made between the presence of sinusitis and the subsequent development of pneumonia, though it remains unclear if the relationship is causal.[453] Infection-control–related risk factors include a lack of hand-washing and glove-use practices and the use of contaminated respiratory equipment. Intervention-related risk factors involve those procedures and therapies that undermine normal host defenses or allow the host to be exposed to large inocula of bacteria. Sedatives and narcotics may lead to aspiration; corticosteroids and cytotoxic agents blunt the normal host response to infection; and the prolonged use of antibiotics engenders resistance. The use of ventilatory support is perhaps the greatest risk factor for the development of nosocomial pneumonia, presenting a risk over 20 times that of unventilated patients.[454, 455] Data suggest that there is a 1 to 3%/day risk of developing pneumonia while on a ventilator.[454] Because of this preeminence as a risk factor, the term *ventilator-associated pneumonia* (VAP) has been introduced.

The use of antacids and histamine type 2 blockers that raise the gastric pH has been shown to increase stomach colonization with aerobic gram-negative rods. Whether this leads to an increase in nosocomial pneumonia remains controversial.[456–461] Demonstrating that gastric colonization precedes tracheal colonization has been inconsistent and has been noted in only 9 to 32% of patients observed. Further, the percentage of patients with VAP caused by organisms initially found in the stomach ranges from zero to 55%.[462]

Approximately 60% of cases of nosocomial pneumonia are caused by aerobic gram-negative bacilli, with members of the family Enterobacteriaceae (*K. pneumoniae, E. coli, Serratia marcescens, Enterobacter* spp.) and *Pseudomonas* spp. accounting for the majority of these. *S. aureus* causes 13 to 40% of nosocomial pneumonia and appears to be more common in burn units, in patients with wound infections, and in patients recently ventilated after neurosurgery or head trauma.[455, 463, 464] In contrast to its prominent role in community-acquired pneumonia, *S. pneumoniae* causes 3 to 20% of nosocomial pneumonias in most studies and is associated with infection developing early in the hospital course.[99, 465] Anaerobic bacteria have been isolated in up to 35% of cases of nosocomial pneumonia, though usually less than 5% of infections are thought to be due to these organisms.[466, 467] They play a role when aspiration is likely. Pneumonia caused by *Legionella* spp. may occur sporadically or as part of outbreaks.[468] As many as 60% of patients with nosocomial *Legionella* pneumonia are immunosuppressed. Inhalation of organisms from environmental sources has been suspected as the primary source of entry, though aspiration has been suspected as well.[469] Twenty-five to 46% of VAP may be polymicrobial.[454] Nosocomial viral infections have been recognized in children and adults. Respiratory syncytial virus, influenza, and parainfluenza make up the majority of viral causes.[470, 471]

Nosocomial pneumonia has been characterized as early, occurring within the first 4 days of hospitalization, or late, occurring after this time. Early-onset pneumonia usually involves organisms associated with community-acquired pneumonia including the pneumococcus, *Haemophilus influenzae*, and *M. catarrhalis*. Late-onset pneumonia is more often associated with enteric gram-negative bacilli (*E. coli, Enterobacter* spp., *Serratia* spp.), *P. aeruginosa*, and *S. aureus*.

The clinical features of nosocomial pneumonia are nonspecific, and a variety of noninfectious diseases may be responsible for fever, changing chest radiographs, purulent sputum, and an elevated white blood cell count in a critically ill patient. Using clinical criteria alone, the presence of nosocomial pneumonia may be missed 20 to 30% of the time and therapeutic decisions may be ineffective in two thirds of patients.[472] The role of invasive procedures in diagnosing nosocomial pneumonia, especially VAP, remains controversial.[473, 474] Although both bronchoscopic and nonbronchoscopic sampling of lower respiratory tract secretions have been used to successfully diagnose VAP, differences in patient populations examined differing results from different centers, a lack of agreement on quantitative breakpoints for a positive study, and lack of a clear "gold standard" have prevented meaningful comparisons of procedures. An in-depth discussion of nosocomial pneumonia can be found in Chapter 293.

Clinical Evaluation of and Therapy for Pneumonia

The first decision confronting the clinician is whether the patient presenting with respiratory symptoms in fact has pneumonia. The difficulties in establishing a diagnosis on clinical grounds and the potential problem of overprescribing empirical antibiotics for all patients with respiratory findings have been reviewed. A chest radiograph is usually necessary to establish a diagnosis of pneumonia.

The next decision confronting the clinician is whether the patient is to be hospitalized, as will be the case in approximately 18 to 30% of patients.[70, 475–477] A number of investigators have examined prognostic features and predictors of the clinical outcome for patients with community-acquired pneumonia that are useful to address this issue. Most use a combination of clinical, epidemiologic, laboratory, and radiographic parameters.[475–479]

One of the most extensive reviews derived a prediction system by analyzing over 14,000 hospitalized patients and applied it to over 40,000 patients in both an inpatient and outpatient setting.[480] In non–HIV-positive patients, the 30-day mortality was lowest (0.1%) in patients younger than 50 years with no coexisting condition (neoplasia, heart failure, cerebral vascular disease, renal disease, or liver disease) and normal physical findings (including normal mental status, pulse <125 beats/minute, respiratory rate <30/minute, systolic blood pressure >90 mmHg, and temperature >35°C and <40°C). For patients demonstrating some abnormalities, these and seven further laboratory and radiographic parameters were used to develop a severity index. In general, the older the patient, the greater the physiologic impairment, the greater the severity index, and the higher the associated mortality.[480] Those with the lowest scores and risk for death can be treated as outpatients.

In the absence of a formal severity index, practitioners have noted that normal respiratory status, normal mental status, and generally a "not very sick" appearance were important elements in deciding to treat patients outside the hospital. The reliability of the patient and adequate home care support were also important criteria for outpatient therapy.[477] In general, those subjective evaluations tended to overestimate the possible death of patients who were hospitalized and presumably led to more admissions. With the use of a highly select population, the use of a pneumonia severity index during the early decision-making process led to increased numbers of patients treated as outpatients.[481] It is important to note that indices serve only as guidelines and are not meant to be substituted for clinical judgment. Strict reliance on severity indices has failed to predict complex outcomes in up to 39% of patients thought to be well enough to be treated as outpatients.[482]

The next problem is determining the most likely cause of the pneumonia. If diagnostic studies, as described previously, yield a likely cause, then specific therapy should be initiated. However, most patients will fall into a group in which a specific diagnosis cannot be established with certainty.

The next step in managing the patient with pneumonia is selecting an empirical antibiotic regimen. The choice of antibiotic has been complicated by the increasing incidence of drug resistance in many strains of pneumococci, the ambiguous effect of this resistance on practical antibiotic selection, and the potential need to cover both typical and atypical pathogens in certain patient populations.

Although it was known that penicillin resistance could be induced in the pneumococcus in 1943,[483] it was not until the late 1960s and 1970s that penicillin nonsusceptibility was encountered clinically in Australia, Papua New Guinea, and South Africa.[484] In the United States, the incidence of penicillin nonsusceptibility has increased dramatically since the 1970s. Surveillance studies between 1979 and 1987 showed a 4 to 5% incidence of penicillin nonsusceptibility among pneumococci.[485] By the early 1990s, the incidence had increased to 20%, by the mid-1990s the incidence had increased 23.6%,[486–488] and by 1996–1997, the overall incidence was 33.5%, with 13.6% of strains demonstrating high-level (minimal inhibitory concentration >1 μg/ml) resistance.[488]

The real effect of this resistance pattern on the response to therapy remains unclear. From data presently available, it appears that penicillin and other β-lactam antibiotics still remain effective therapies for most penicillin-susceptible and nonsusceptible strains of *S. pneumoniae*. Few failures in the therapy of pneumococcal pneumonia have been associated with resistance.[489] Outcomes of penicillin therapy in patients with susceptible versus nonsusceptible strains of *S. pneumoniae* are similar.[490] An explanation for these observations comes from animal data that suggest that in vitro susceptibility data are not as predictive of clinical success or failure as is the amount of time serum antibiotic levels remain above the minimal inhibitory concentration of the infecting organism.[491] Maximal efficiency is achieved when drug levels are above the minimal inhibitory concentration for at least 40% of the dosing interval. Using higher doses of antibiotic or shorter dosing intervals may provide effective therapy for relatively resistant organisms. Oral penicillins such as amoxicillin and amoxicillin-clavulanic acid can provide this degree of activity. Among the oral cephalosporins, cefuroxime appears to be the most potentially useful, though only for penicillin-intermediate strains of pneumococci.[492] High-dose parenteral penicillin and third-generation cephalosporins like ceftriaxone and cefotaxime provide consistent coverage even for resistant strains. Other agents, such as ceftazidime and ceftizoxime, appear less potent.[493–496] Several "respiratory tract quinolones" (levofloxacin, trovafloxacin, grepafloxacin, sparfloxacin) have been licensed for use as therapy of respiratory infections. These agents not only possess activity against the majority of bacterial and atypical agents involved in lower respiratory infections but their potency is not significantly affected by the presence of penicillin resistance.

Pneumococcal resistance to penicillin has been paralleled by resistance to other agents frequently used in the therapy of pneumonia. Up to 25.5% of pneumococci resistant to penicillin are resistant to other antibiotics.[487, 497] Resistance patterns of penicillin-resistant pneumococci to other clinically important antibiotics are shown in Table 57–4.[491, 492, 496, 498, 499] Not enough data have been gathered to reasonably predict what level of resistance will yield clinical failures.

The new respiratory tract quinolones have demonstrated in vitro potency against penicillin-susceptible and nonsusceptible strains of *S. pneumoniae* as well as agents of atypical pneumonia, including *M. pneumoniae, Chlamydia* spp., and *Legionella* spp. Interestingly, when these agents are compared clinically with β-lactam antibiotics with varied activity against nonsusceptible strains of pneumococci and no real activity against atypical agents, the overall outcomes have, in general, been equivalent with those of rare studies showing superiority of the newer, broader-spectrum agents.[500–503] Although the numbers of patients studied may still be too small to detect a difference, the results underscore the fact that the definitive diagnosis of atypical pneumonia remains elusive and that some episodes of mycoplasmal and chlamydial pneumonia may improve independent of the antibiotic therapy chosen.

Even with these ambiguities and persistent questions noted, empirical regimens may still be selected that are broad enough and potent enough to treat the most significant causes of pneumonia. Several guidelines have been published and involve stratifying patients according to age, the severity of illness, comorbidity, and the prevalence of drug resistance.[110, 115]

For a patient who does not require hospitalization and who is relatively young (younger than 60 years) and for whom no clear distinction between typical (e.g., pneumococcal) and atypical (mycoplasmal, chlamydial) pneumonia can be made, both types of organisms can be covered (Table 57–5). Antibacterial therapy should address the possibility of infection with nonsusceptible strains of *S. pneumoniae* and β-lactamase–producing strains of *H. influenzae*. In this setting the choices include (1) an oral β-lactam plus erythromycin (examples of appropriate β-lactams include the second-generation cephalosporin cefuroxime axetil or the β-lactam–β-lactamase inhibitor combination amoxicillin-clavulanic acid); (2) azalides-macrolides (azithromycin, clarithromycin, or erythromycin); (3) one of the respiratory tract quinolones (examples include levofloxacin, trovafloxacin, grepafloxacin, sparfloxacin). Previously used agents like doxycycline and trimethoprim-sulfamethoxazole are less favored because of decreased activity against resistant strains of pneumococci.

Overall, no clear "best choice" emerges. In some centers erythromycin (despite poor activity against *H. influenzae*) is the most commonly used agent in this setting.[504] Decreased activity against penicillin-resistant strains of pneumococci and gastrointestinal intolerance have made this a less attractive choice than the newer azalides-

TABLE 57–4 Percentage of Penicillin-Sensitive, -Intermediate, and -Resistant Strains of *Streptococcus pneumoniae* That Show Resistance to Other Antibiotics*

	PCN^S	PCN^I	PCN^R
Amoxicillin-clavulanic acid	0.2	8–21	66–93
Cefuroxime	<1	21–50	100
Trimethoprim-sulfamethoxazole	1.8	40.6	91.6
Erythromycin-azithromycin-clarithromycin†	1.6	9.8	19.4–60
Ceftriaxone	0	0–1	22.2
Cefotaxime	0	1	14–27
Chloramphenicol	<1	5.4	10–19.4
Tetracycline	1.6	20.8	21–25
Imipenem	0	0	2.7
Respiratory tract quinolones† (levofloxacin, trovafloxacin, sparfloxacin, grepafloxacin)	0–0.4	0.4–1.2	1.1

*Data are presented as percentage of strains showing resistance based on MIC breakpoint data. Not all drugs were compared in all studies. The percentage of resistance varies between studies. Values of MICs may not predict clinical outcomes.

†Averages for the group.

Abbreviations: MIC, Minimal inhibitory concentration; PCN^S, penicillin-sensitive *S. pneumoniae* (MIC ≤ 0.06 μg/ml); PCN^I, penicillin-intermediate *S. pneumoniae* (MIC = 0.12–1 μg/ml); PCN^R, penicillin-resistant *S. pneumoniae* (MIC ≥ 2 μg/ml).

Data from refs 487, 488, 492, 496–499, 514.

TABLE 57–5 Strategy for Empirical Therapy of Pneumonia: Outpatient Therapy (Oral Therapy)

Patient population	<60 yr old, no significant comorbidity or underlying risk factor	>60 yr old, no significant comorbidity or underlying risk factor
Organisms of concern	*Streptococcus pneumoniae* *Haemophilus influenzae* *Legionella pneumophila* *Mycoplasma pneumoniae* *Chlamydia pneumoniae*	*Streptococcus pneumoniae* *Haemophilus influenzae* *Legionella pneumophila* *Mycoplasma pneumoniae* *Chlamydia pneumoniae*
Regimen	1. Respiratory tract quinolone (i.e., levofloxacin, trovafloxacin, grepafloxacin, sparfloxacin) *or* 2. β-Lactam (e.g., cefuroxime axetil,* amoxicillin-clavulanic acid) + erythromycin *or* 3. azalide-macrolide (i.e., azithromycin, clarithromycin)	1. Respiratory tract quinolone (i.e., levofloxacin, trovafloxacin, grepafloxacin, sparfloxacin) *or* 2. β-Lactam (e.g., cefuroxime axetil,* amoxicillin-clavulanic acid) + erythromycin *or* 3. azalide-macrolide (i.e., azithromycin, clarithromycin)

*Other agents within the same class may be used.

macrolides. Azithromycin or clarithromycin has been favored by some because of a spectrum of activity more directed toward the major respiratory tract pathogens and a satisfactory safety profile. However, increased resistance in strains of pneumococci is a concern. Although the newer quinolones maintain their potency against resistant strains of pneumococci, their spectrum of activity seems broader than is usually needed to treat most community-acquired pneumonias. Most of these agents cover a variety of gram-negative bacilli including *Pseudomonas* spp. and, in the case of trovafloxacin, anaerobes.

In older patients (older than 60 years) in whom atypical pneumonia is less likely and who are not ill enough to be hospitalized, a second-generation oral cephalosporin or a β-lactam–β-lactamase inhibitor combination with or without erythromycin represents reasonable therapy. The respiratory tract quinolones may be used as single agents, or the newer azalides-macrolides could be used.

In patients who are ill enough to be hospitalized, and in whom early evaluation is not diagnostic, empirical therapy should be aimed at covering *S. pneumoniae* including penicillin-resistant strains, *H. influenzae* (including β-lactamase–producing strains), *S. aureus*, and atypical agents including *Legionella* spp., *Chlamydia* spp., and *M. pneumoniae*. Parenteral therapy is indicated. A second-generation cephalosporin (such as cefuroxime) or a third-generation cephalosporin (such as cefotaxime or ceftriaxone) or a β-lactam–β lactamase inhibitor combination (such as ampicillin-sulbactam) could be utilized in combination with erythromycin. Parenteral levofloxacin or trovafloxacin are also acceptable choices and may be preferred when penicillin-resistant pneumococci are a particular problem (Table 57–6).

Elderly or debilitated patients with significant underlying disease, patients who are immunosuppressed, and patients admitted from extended care facilities may have infections caused by aerobic gram-negative rods as well as to the organisms already mentioned. Therapy with a third-generation cephalosporin, such as cefotaxime, ceftriaxone (ceftazidime or cefepime if *P. aeruginosa* is suspected) *or* an extended-spectrum penicillin (ticarcillin, piperacillin) or a β-lactam-β-lactamase inhibitor combination (ticarcillin-clavulanic acid, piperacillin-tazobactam) or a carbapenem (imipenem, meropenem) are reasonable choices.[505] The addition of a fluoroquinolone, a macrolide, or an azalide is warranted if *Legionella, mycoplasma*, or *Chlamydia* is suspected. Although debate exists as to whether agents such as aminoglycosides or quinolones need to be added to β-lactam therapy of gram-negative pneumonia, and although data exist to support both sides of the controversy, we favor a two-drug approach, at least initially, while cultures of sputum and blood are pending.[506, 507]

In the patient admitted to an intensive care unit, therapy should be directed against *S. pneumoniae* including penicillin-resistant strains, *Legionella* spp., gram-negative rods, and *M. pneumoniae*. We favor combination therapy as described in the preceding paragraph at least initially while cultures are pending and the patient is being stabilized. A fluoroquinolone, an azalide, or a macrolide should be used to treat the possibility of *Legionella* spp. and *M. pneumoniae*.

Studies suggest that parenteral therapy, once begun, need not be continued for the duration of therapy. Most patients outside an intensive care unit normalize previously abnormal findings, such as temperature elevation, tachycardia, tachypnea, and changes in mental status, within 3 to 7 days. Once clinical stability is reached, significant clinical deterioration is unusual.[508] Changing to oral therapy at this time provides comparable efficacy to parenteral therapy and is associated with shorter hospital stays, and a lower cost of care.[509–513]

Aspiration pneumonia and lung abscess are discussed in Chapter 59. Therapy for nosocomial pneumonia is discussed in Chapter 293.

TABLE 57–6 Strategy for Empirical Therapy of Pneumonia: Inpatient Therapy (Parenteral Therapy)

Patient population	Moderately ill patients	Elderly, debilitated patients with significant comorbid diseases, immune-suppressed, patients from extended care facilities, intensive care unit patients
Organisms of concern	*Streptococcus pneumoniae* *Haemophilus influenzae* *Staphylococcus aureus* *Mycoplasma pneumoniae* *Chlamydia pneumoniae* *Legionella* spp.	*Streptococcus pneumoniae* *Haemophilus influenzae* *Staphylococcus aureus* *Legionella* spp. *Chlamydia pneumoniae* Aerobic gram-negative bacilli *Pseudomonas aeruginosa*
Regimen	1. Second-generation cephalosporin (e.g., cefuroxime) *or* 2. Third-generation cephalosporin (e.g., cefotaxime, ceftriaxone) *or* 3. β-Lactam–β-lactamase inhibitor combination (e.g., ampicillin-sulbactam) *For all of the above*, consider adding erythromycin 4. Respiratory tract quinolone (e.g., levofloxacin, trovafloxacin)	1. Third-generation cephalosporin (e.g., cefotaxime, ceftriaxone; ceftazidime or cefepime if *Pseudomonas aeruginosa* is suspected) *or* 2. Extended spectrum penicillin (e.g., ticarcillin, piperacillin) *or* 3. β-Lactam–β-lactamase inhibitor combination (e.g., ticarcillin-clavulanic acid, piperacillin-tazobactam) *or* 4. Carbapenem (e.g., imipenem, meropenem) *For all of the above*, consider adding an aminoglycoside* and/or a respiratory tract quinolone†

*If *Pseudomonas aeruginosa* or *Enterobacter* spp. are suspected.
†If atypicals (*Mycoplasma, Chlamydia*, or *Legionella*) and/or penicillin-resistant *S. pneumoniae* are suspected.

REFERENCES

1. Osler W. The Principles and Practice of Medicine. 4th ed. New York: D Appleton; 1901:108.
2. Advanced Report of Final Mortality Statistics, v. 42. Hyattsville, Md: National Center for Health Statistics; 1992.
3. Johanson WG Jr, Gould KG Jr. Lung defense mechanisms. Basics RD. 1977;6:1–6.
4. Green G. In defense of the lung. Am Rev Respir Dis. 1970;102:691–703.
5. Sibille Y, Reynolds HY. Macrophage and polymorphonuclear neutrophils in lung defense and injury. Am Rev Respir Dis. 1990;141:471–501.
6. Shelhamer JH (moderator), Toews GB, Masur H, et al. Respiratory disease in the immunosuppressed patient. Ann Intern Med. 1992;117:415–431.
7. Reynolds HY. Pulmonary host defenses. Chest. 1989;95(Suppl):223S–230S.
8. Mason CM, Nelson S. Normal host defenses and impairments associated with the delayed resolution of pneumonia. Semin Respir Infect. 1992;7:243–255.
9. Reynolds H. Normal and defective respiratory host defense. In: Pennington JE, ed. Respiratory Infections: Diagnosis and Management. 2nd ed. New York: Raven; 1988:1–33.
10. Coonrod J. The role of extracellular bactericidal factors in pulmonary host defense. Semin Respir Infect. 1986;1:118–129.
11. Busse WW. Pathogenesis and sequelae of respiratory infections. Rev Infect Dis. 1991;13(Suppl 6):S477–S485.
12. Reynolds HY. Lung inflammation: Normal host defense or a complication of some diseases. Annu Rev Med. 1987;38:295–323.
13. Niederman MS, Merrill WW, Polonski LM, et al. Influence of sputum IgA and elastase on tracheal cell bacterial adherence. Am Rev Respir Dis. 1981;133: 255–260.
14. Niederman MS, Merrill WW, Ferrante RD, et al. Nutritional status and bacterial binding in the lower respiratory tract in patients with chronic tracheostomy. Ann Intern Med. 1984;100:795–800.
15. Palmer LB, Merrill WW, Neiderman MS, et al. Bacterial adherence to respiratory tract cells—relationship between in vivo and in vitro pH and bacterial attachment. Am Rev Respir Dis. 1986;133:784–788.
16. Lohmann-Matthes ML, Steinmüller C, Franke-Ullman G. Pulmonary macrophages. Eur Respir J. 1994;7:1678–1689.
17. Lipscomb MF, Onofrio JM, Nash EJ, et al. A morphological study of the role of phagocytes in the clearance of *Staphylococcus aureus* from the lung. J Reticuloendothel Soc. 1983;33:429–442.
18. MacNee W, Selby C. Neutrophil kinetics in the lung. Clin Sci. 1990;79:97–107.
19. Lavnikova N, Prokhorova S, Heylar L, Laskin DL. Isolation and partial characterization of subpopulations of alveolar macrophages granulocytes and highly enriched interstitial macrophages from rat lung. Am J Respir Cell Mol Biol. 1993;8:384–392.
20. Crowell RE, Heaphy E, Valdez Y, et al. Alveolar and interstitial macrophages in the murine lung. Exp Lung Res. 1992;18:435–446.
21. Strieter RM, Standiford TJ, Huffnagle GB, et al. The good, the bad, and the ugly: The role of chemokines in models of human disease. J Immunol. 1996;196:3583–3586.
22. Standiford TJ, Huffnagle GB. Cytokines in host defense against pneumonia. J Investig Med. 1997;45:335–343.
23. Standiford TJ, Kunkel SL, Basha MA, et al. Interleukin-8 gene expression by a pulmonary epithelial cell line—a model for cytokine networks in the lung. J Clin Invest. 1990;86:1945–1953.
24. Strieter RM, Kunkel S, Showell H, et al. Endothelial cell gene expression of a neutrophil chemotactic factor by TNF-α, LPS, and IL-β. Science. 1989;243:1467–1469.
25. Pikaar JC, Voorhout WF, Van Golde LMG, et al. Opsonic activities of surfactant proteins A and D in phagocytosis of gram-negative bacteria by alveolar macrophages. J Infect Dis. 1995;172:481–489.
26. Agostini C, Chilosi M, Zambello R, et al. Pulmonary immune cells in health and disease: Lymphocytes. 1993;6:1378–1401.
27. Fishman AP, Reynolds HY, Elias JA, et al. Pulmonary defense mechanisms against infection. In: Fishman AP, ed. Fishman's Pulmonary Diseases and Disorders. 3rd ed. New York: McGraw Hill; 1998;265–274.
28. Mosmann TR, Sad S. The expanding universe of T-cell subsets: Th1, Th2 and more. Immunol Today. 1995;17:138–146.
29. Bartlett J, Gorbach S, Finegold S. The bacteriology of aspiration pneumonia. Am J Med. 1974;56:202–207.
30. Huxley EJ, Viroslav J, Gray WR, et al. Pharyngeal aspiration in normal adults and patients with depressed consciousness. Am J Med. 1978;64:564–568.
31. Green GM, Carolin D. The depressant effect of cigarette smoke on the in vitro antibacterial activity of alveolar macrophages. N Engl J Med. 1967;276:421–427.
32. Nelson S, Mason LM, Kolls J, Summer WR. Pathophysiology of pneumonia. Clin Chest Med. 1995;16:1–12.
33. Warshauer D, Goldstein E, Akers T, et al. Effect of influenza viral infection on the ingestion and killing of bacteria by alveolar macrophages. Am Rev Respir Dis. 1977;115:269–277.
34. Harris SE, Nelson S, Astry CL, et al. Endotoxin-induced suppression of pulmonary antibacterial defenses against *Staphylococcus aureus*. Am Rev Respir Dis. 1988;138:1439–1443.
35. Nelson S, Chidiac C, Bagby G, et al. Endotoxin-induced suppression of lung host defenses. J Med. 1990;21:85–103.
36. Green GM, Kass EH. The role of the alveolar macrophage in the clearance of bacteria from the lung. J Exp Med. 1964;119:167–176.
37. MacGregor RR. Alcohol and immune defense. JAMA. 1986;256:1474–1479.
38. Schopf RE, Trompter M, Bork K, et al. Effects of ethanol and acetaldehyde on phagocytic function. Arch Dermatol Rev. 1985;277:131–137.
39. Nelson S, Bagby GJ, Bainton BG, et al. The effects of acute and chronic alcoholism on tumor necrosis factor and the inflammatory response. J Infect Dis. 1989;160:422–429.
40. Mason CM. The pathogenesis and presentation of nosocomial pneumonia. Crit Care Rev. 1991;2:145–155.
41. Espesito AL. Aspirin impairs antibacterial mechanisms in experimental pneumococcal pneumonia. Am Rev Respir Dis. 1984;130:857–862.
42. Nelson S, Summer WR, Terry PB, et al. Erythromycin-induced suppression of pulmonary antibacterial defenses: A potential mechanism of superinfection in the lung. Am Rev Respir Dis. 1987;136:1207–1212.
43. Nelson S, Summer WR, Jakab EJ. Aminophylline-induced suppression of pulmonary antibacterial defenses. Am Rev Respir Dis. 1985;131:923–927.
44. Green GM, Kass EH. The influence of bacterial species on pulmonary resistance to infection in mice subjected to hypoxia, cold stress and ethanolic intoxication. Br J Exp Pathol. 1965;46:360–366.
45. Coffin DL, Gardner DE, Holzman RS, et al. Influence of ozone on pulmonary cells. Arch Environ Health. 1968;16:633–636.
46. Ehrlich R, Henry MC. Chronic toxicity of nitrogen dioxide. 1. Effect on resistance to bacterial pneumonia. Arch Environ Health. 1968;17:860–865.
47. LaForce FM, Mullane JF, Boehme RF, et al. The effect of pulmonary edema on antibacterial defenses of the lung. J Lab Clin Med. 1973;82:634–648.
48. Huber GL, LaForce FM, Mason RJ, et al. Impairment of pulmonary bacterial defense mechanisms by immunosuppressive agents. Surg Forum. 1970;21:285–286.
49. Davis L, Beck JM, Shellito J. Update: HIV infection and pulmonary host defenses. Semin Respir Infect. 1993;8:75–85.
50. Gyetko MR, Toews GB. Immunology of the aging lung. Clin Chest Med. 1993;14:379–391.
51. Simons RJ, Reynolds HY. Altered immune status in the elderly. Semin Respir Infect. 1990;5:251–259.
52. Granton JT, Grossman RF. Community-acquired pneumonia in the elderly patient. Clin Chest Med. 1993;14:537–553.
53. Winterbauer RH, Bedon GA, Bal WC Jr. Recurrent pneumonia: Predisposing illness and clinical patterns in 158 patients. Ann Intern Med. 1969;70:689–700.
54. Roth RM, Gleckman RA. Recurrent bacterial pneumonia: A contemporary perspective. South Med J. 1985;78:573–579.
55. Ekdahl K, Braconier JH, Rollof J. Recurrent pneumonia: A review of 90 adult patients. Scand J Infect Dis. 1992;24:71–76.
56. Geppert EF. Chronic recurrent pneumonia. Semin Respir Infect. 1992;7:282–288.
57. Donowitz GR, Mandell GL. Clinical presentation and unusual infections. In: Gallin JI, Fauci AS, eds. Advances in Host Defense Mechanisms, v. 3. New York: Raven; 1983:55–75.
58. Donabedian H, Gallin JI. The hyperimmunoglobulin E recurrent infection (Jobs) syndrome. Medicine. 1983;62:195–208.
59. Beck S, Heiner DC. Selective immunoglobulin G_4 deficiency and recurrent infections of the respiratory tract. Am Rev Respir Dis. 1981;124:94–96.
60. Ammann AJ, Hong R. Selective IgA deficiency: Presentation of 30 cases and a review of the literature. Medicine. 1971;50:223–236.
61. Eliasson R, Mossberg B, Camner P, et al. The immotile-cilia syndrome. N Engl J Med. 1977;297:1–6.
62. Kartagener M. Zur Pathologie der Bronchiektasien: Bronkiectasien bei Situs Inversus. Beitr Klin Tuberk. 1933;83:489–501.
63. Handelsman DJ, Conway AJ, Boylan LM, et al. Young's syndrome: Obstructive azospermia and chronic sinopulmonary infections. N Engl J Med. 1984;310:3–9.
64. Savic B, Birtel FJ, Tholen W, et al. Lung sequestation: Report of seven cases and review of 540 published cases. Thorax. 1979;34:96–101.
65. Iverson LIG, May IA, Samson PC. Pulmonary complications in benign esophageal disease. Am J Surg. 1973;126:223–228.
66. Metlay JP, Stafford RS, Singer DE. National trends in the use of antibiotics by primary care physicians for adult patients with cough. Arch Intern Med. 1998;158:1813–1818.
67. Metlay JP, Schulz R, Li YH, et al. Influence of age on symptoms at presentation in patients with community-acquired pneumonia. Arch Intern Med. 1997;157:1453–1459.
68. Grayston JT, Alexander ER, Kenny GE, et al. *Mycoplasma pneumoniae* infections: Clinical and epidemiological studies. JAMA. 1965;191:369–374.
69. Murray HW, Masur H, Senterfit L, et al. The protean manifestations of *Mycoplasma pneumoniae* infection in adults. Am J Med. 1975;58:229–242.
70. Marston BJ, Plouffe JF, File TM, et al. Incidence of community-acquired pneumonia requiring hospitalization: Results of a population-based active surveillance study in Ohio. Arch Int Med. 1997;157:1709–1718.
71. Dorff GJ, Rytel MW, Farmer SG, et al. Etiologies and characteristic features of pneumonias in a municipal hospital. Am J Med Sci. 1973;266:349–358.
72. Bloch AB, Rieder HL, Kelly CD, et al. The epidemiology of tuberculosis in the United States. Semin Respir Infect. 1989;4:157–170.
73. Braun MM, Coté TR, Rabkin CS. Trends in death with tuberculosis during the AIDS era. JAMA. 1993;269:2865–2868.
74. Fekety FR, Caldwell J, Grump D, et al. Bacteria, viruses, and mycoplasmas in acute pneumonia in adults. Am Rev Respir Dis. 1971;104:499–507.
75. Sullivan RJ, Dowdle WR, Marine WM, et al. Adult pneumonia in a general hospital: Etiology and host risk factors. Arch Intern Med. 1972;129:935–942.
76. Fernandez-Solá J, Junque A, Estruch R, et al. High alcohol intake as a risk and prognostic factor for community-acquired pneumonia. Arch Intern Med. 1995;155:1649–1654.

77. Lepow ML, Balassanian N, Emmerich J, et al. Interrelationships of viral, mycoplasmal and bacterial agents in uncomplicated pneumonia. Am Rev Respir Dis. 1968;97:533–545.
78. Martin CM, Kunin CM, Gottlieb LS, et al. Asian influenza A in Boston, 1957–1958. II. Severe staphylococcal pneumonia complicating influenza. Arch Intern Med. 1959;103:532–542.
79. Sprunt K. Infection in chronic lung disease. Bull N Y Acad Med. 1972;48:698–703.
80. Griffith DE, Mazurek GH. Pneumonia in chronic obstructive lung disease. Infect Dis Clin North Am. 1991;5:467–484.
81. Davies BI. *Moraxella catarrhalis*: Clinical significant therapeutic problems. Infect Dis Newslett. 1991;10:73–77.
82. Wright PW, Wallace RJ, Shepard JR. A descriptive study of 42 cases of *Branhamella catarrhalis* pneumonia. Am J Med. 1990;88(Suppl 5A):SA25–SA75.
83. Torres A, Dorca J, Zalacain R, et al. Community-acquired pneumonia in chronic obstructive pulmonary disease: A Spanish multicenter study. Am J Respir Crit Care Med. 1996;154:1456–1461.
84. Hoiby N. Epidemiological investigations of the respiratory tract bacteriology in patients with cystic fibrosis. Acta Pathol Microbiol Scand B. 1974;82:541–550.
85. Burbank B, Marrione TG, Cutler SS. Pulmonary alveolar proteinosis and nocardiosis. Am J Med. 1960;28:1002–1007.
86. Wallace JM, Rao AV, Glassroth J, et al. Respiratory illness in person with acquired immunodeficiency virus infection. Am Rev Respir Dis. 1993;148:1523.
87. Rosen MJ. Overview of pulmonary complication. Clin Chest Med. 1996;17:621.
88. Hoover DR, Saah AJ, Bacellar H, Phair J. Clinical manifestations of AIDS in the era of pneumoscystis prophylaxis. N Engl J Med. 1993;329:1922.
89. Selik RM, Chu Sy, Ward JW. Trends in infectious diseases and cancers among persons dying of HIV infection in the United States from 1987–1992. Ann Intern Med. 1995;123:933.
90. Chan ISF, Neaton JD, Sarvolatz LD, et al. Frequencies of opportunistic diseases prior to death among HIV-infected persons. AIDS. 1995;98:1145–1151.
91. Caiaffa WT, Vlahov D, Graham NMH, et al. Drug smoking, *Pneumocystis carinii* pneumonia, and immune suppression, increase risk of bacterial pneumonia in human immunodeficiency virus-seropositive infection drug users. Am J Respir Crit Care Med. 1994;150:1493–1498.
92. Hirschtick RE, Glassroth J, Jordan MC, et al. Bacterial pneumonia in persons infected with the human immunodeficiency virus. N Engl J Med. 1995;333:845–851.
93. Garcia-Leoni ME, Moreno S, Rodeñó P, et al. Pneumococcal pneumonia: Adult hospitalized patients infected with the human immunodeficiency virus. Arch Intern Med. 1992;152:1808–1812.
94. Steinhart R, Reingold AL, Taylor F, et al. Invasive *Haemophilus influenzae* infection in men with HIV infection. JAMA. 1992;268:3350–3352.
95. Baron AD, Hollander H. *Pseudomonas aeruginosa* bronchopulmonary infection in late human immunodeficiency virus disease. Am Rev Respir Dis. 1993;148:992–996.
96. Dropulic LK, Leslie JM, Eldred LJ, et al. Clinical manifestations and risk factors of *Pseudomonas aeruginosa* infection in patients with AIDS. J Infect Dis. 1995;171:930–937.
97. Daley CL. Bacterial pneumonia in HIV-infected patients. Semin Respir Infect. 1993;8:104–115.
98. Hanson DL, Chusy SY, Farizo KM, et al. Distribution of CD_4 T lymphocytes at diagnosis of acquired immunodeficiency syndrome—defining and other human immunodeficiency virus-related illness. Arch Intern Med. 1995;155:1537.
99. Gross PA. Epidemiology of hospital-acquired pneumonia. Semin Respir Infect. 1987;2:2–7.
100. Marrie TJ, Haldane EV, Faulkner RS, et al. Community acquired pneumonia requiring hospitalization: Is it different in the elderly? J Am Geriatr Soc. 1985;33:671–680.
101. Heffron R. Pneumonia. New York: Commonwealth Fund; 1939:505.
102. Bartlett JG, Finegold SM. Anaerobic infections of the lung and pleural space. Am Rev Respir Dis. 1974;110:56–77.
103. Woodhead M. Management of pneumonia in the outpatient setting. Semin Respir Infect. 1998;13:848.
104. Metlay JP, Kapoor WN, Fine MJ. Does this patient have community-acquired pneumonia. JAMA. 1997;278:1440.
105. Gennis P, Gallagher J, Falvo C, et al. Clinical criteria for the detection of pneumonia in adults: Guidelines for ordering chest roentgenograms in the emergency department. J Emerg Med. 1989;7:263–268.
106. Thorsteinsson SB, Musher DM, Fagan T. The diagnostic value of sputum culture in acute pneumonia. JAMA. 1975;233:894–895.
107. Merrill C, Gwaltney JM, Hendley JO, et al. Rapid identification of pneumococci. N Engl J Med. 1973;288:510–512.
108. Drew WL. Value of sputum culture in diagnosis of pneumococcal pneumonia. J Clin Microbiol. 1977;6:62–5.0.
109. Bartlett RC, Melnick A. Usefulness of Gram stain and routing and quantitative culture of sputum in patients with and without acute respiratory infection. Conn Med. 1970;34:347–351.
110. Bartlett JG, Breiman RF, Mandell LA, File TM Jr. Community-acquired pneumonia in adults: Guidelines for management. Clin Infect Dis. 1998;26:811–838.
111. Reed WW, Byrd GS, Gates RH Jr, et al. Sputum Gram's stain in community-acquired pneumococcal pneumonia: A meta analysis. West J Med. 1996;165:197–204.
112. Ewig S, Bauer T, Hasper E, et al. Value of routine microbial investigation in community-acquired pneumonia treated in a tertiary care center. Respiration. 1996;63:164–169.
113. Marrie TJ. Community-acquired pneumonia. Clin Infect Dis. 1994;18:501–515.
114. Bartlett JG, Mundy LM. Community-acquired pneumonia. N Engl J Med. 1995;333:1618–1624.
115. Niederman MS, Bass JB Jr, Campbell GD, et al. Guidelines for the initial management of adults with community-acquired pneumonia: Diagnosis, assessment of severity and initial antimicrobial therapy. Am Rev Respir Dis. 1993;148:1418–1426.
116. Fine MJ, Orloff JJ, Rihs JD, et al. Evaluation of housestaff physician's preparation and interpretation of sputum Gram's stain for community-acquired pneumonia. J Gen Intern Med. 1991;6:189–198.
117. Bryant RE, Rhoades ER. Clinical features of adenoviral pneumonia in Air Force recruits. Am Rev Respir Dis. 1967;96(4):717–723.
118. Goerge RB, Ziskind MM, Rasch JR, et al. Mycoplasma and adenovirus pneumonias—comparison with other atypical pneumonias in a military population. Ann Intern Med. 1966;65:931–942.
119. Reimann H. The Pneumonias. Philadelphia: WB Saunders; 1938:67.
120. Solomon S. Primary Friedlander pneumonia. JAMA. 1937;108:937–947.
121. Murray PR, Washington JA III. Microscopic and bacteriologic analysis of expectorated sputum. Mayo Clin Proc. 1975;50:339–344.
122. Rein MF, Gwaltney JM, O'Brien WM, et al. Accuracy of the Gram's stain in identifying pneumococci in sputum. JAMA. 1978;239:2671–2673.
123. Hendley JO, Sande MA, Stewart PM, et al. Spread of *Streptococcus pneumoniae* in families. I. Carriage rates and distribution of types. J Infect Dis. 1975;132:55–61.
124. Finland M. Recent advances in the epidemiology of pneumococcal infections. Medicine. 1942;21:307–344.
125. Lees AW, McNaught W. Bacteriology of lower-respiratory tract secretions, sputum and upper-respiratory tract secretions in "normals" and "chronic bronchitis." Lancet. 1959;2:1112–1115.
126. Gleckman R, DeVita J, Hibert D, et al. Sputum Gram's stain assessment in community-acquired bacteremic pneumonia. J Clin Microbiol. 1988;26:846–849.
127. Barrett-Connor E. The non-value of sputum culture in the diagnosis of pneumococcal pneumonia. Am Rev Respir Dis. 1971;103:845–848.
128. Rathburn HK, Govani I. Mouse inoculation as means of identifying pneumococci in the sputum. Johns Hopkins Med J. 1967;120:46–48.
129. Zaman MK, Wooten OH, Suprahmonya B, et al. Rapid non-invasive diagnosing of *Pneumocystis carinii* from induced liquified sputum. Ann Intern Med. 1988;109:7–10.
130. Bigby TD, Margolskee D, Curtis JL, et al. The usefulness of induced sputum in the diagnosis of *Pneumocystis carinii* pneumonia in patients with the acquired immunodeficiency syndrome. Am Rev Respir Dis. 1986;133:515–518.
131. Pitchenik AE, Ganjei P, Torres A, et al. Sputum examination for the diagnosis of *Pneumocystis carinii* pneumonia in the acquired immunodeficiency syndrome. Am Rev Respir Dis. 1986;133:226–229.
132. Skerrett SJ. Diagnostic testing to establish a microbial cause is helpful in the management of community-acquired pneumonia. Semin Respir Infect. 1997;12:308–321.
133. Edelstein PH. Legionnaire's Disease. Clin Infect Dis. 1993;16:741–749.
134. Roig J, Domingo C, Morera J. Legionnaire's disease. Chest. 1994;105:1817–1825.
135. Kauppinen M, Saikku P. Pneumonia due to *Chlamydia pneumoniae*: prevalence, clinical features, diagnosis and treatment. Clin Infect Dis. 1995;21:S244–S252.
136. Ng VL, Virani NA, Chaisson RE, et al. Rapid detection of *Pneumocystis carinii* using a direct fluorescent monoclonal antibody stain. J Clin Microbiol. 1990;28:2228–2233.
137. Willocks L, Burns S, Cossor R, Breltte R. Diagnosis of *Pneumocystis carinii* pneumonia in a population of HIV-positive drug users with particular reference to sputum inductional fluorescent antibody techniques. J Infect Dis. 1993;26:257–264.
138. Peterson LR, Shanholtzer CJ. Using the microbiology laboratory in the diagnosis of pneumonia. Semin Respir Infect. 1988;3:106–112.
139. Sullivan CJ, Joran ML. Diagnosis of viral pneumonia. Semin Respir Infect. 1988;3:148–161.
140. Oldach DW, Gaydos CA, Mundy LM, et al. Rapid diagnosis of *Chlamydia psittaci* pneumonia. Clin Infect Dis. 1993;17:338–343.
141. Sills M, White P. Rapid identification of *Chlamydia psittaci* and TWAR *(C. pneumoniae)* in sputum samples using an amplified enzyme immunoassay (Letter). J Clin Pathol. 1990;43:260.
142. Van Kuppeveld FJ, Johansson KE, Galoma JM, et al. 16S mRNA based polymerase chain reaction compared with culture and serologic methods for diagnosis of *Mycoplasma pneumoniae* infection. Eur J Clin Microbiol Infect Dis. 1994;13:401–405.
143. Ramirez JA, Ahkee S, Tolentino A, et al. Diagnosis of *Legionella pneumophila, Mycoplasma pneumoniae* or *Chlamydia pneumoniae* lower respiratory infection using the polymerase chain reaction on a single throat swab specimen. Diagn Microbiol Infect Dis. 1996;24:7–14.
144. Shelhamer JH, Gill VJ, Quinn TC, et al. The laboratory evaluation of opportunistic pulmonary infections. Ann Intern Med. 1996;124:585–599.
145. Schluger NW, Rom WN. The polymerase chain reaction in the diagnosis and evaluation of pulmonary infections. Am J Respir Crit Care Med. 1995;152:11–16.
146. Gaydos CA, Roblin PM, Hammerschlag MR, et al. Diagnostic Utility of PCR-enzyme immunoassay, culture, and serology for detection of *Chlamydia pneumoniae* in symptomatic and asymptomatic patients. J Clin Microbiol. 1994;32:903–905.
147. Cartwright CP, Nelson NA, Gill VJ. Development and evaluation of a rapid and simple procedure for detection of *Pneumocystis carinii* by PCR. J Clin Microbiol. 1994;32:1634–1638.
148. Rudolph KM, Parkinson AJ, Black CM, Mayer LW. Evaluation of polymerase

chain reaction for diagnosis of pneumococcal pneumonia. J Clin Microbiol. 1993;31:2661–2666.
149. Wonderink RG, Russell GB, Mezger E, et al. The diagnostic utility of the antibody-coated bacteria test in intubated patients. Chest. 1991;99:84–88.
150. Wallace RJ, Musher DM, Martin RR. *Haemophilus influenzae* pneumonia in adults. Am J Med. 1978;64:87–93.
151. Levin D, Schwarz M, Matthay R, et al. Bacteremic *Haemophilus influenzae* pneumonia in adults. A report of 24 cases and a review of the literature. Am J Med. 1977;62:219–224.
152. Davidson M, Tempest B, Palmer DL. Bacteriologic diagnosis of acute pneumonia, comparison of sputum, transtracheal aspirates, and lung aspirates. JAMA. 1976;235:158–163.
153. Geckeler RW, Gremillion DH, McAllister CK, et al. Microscopic and bacteriological comparison of paired sputa and transtracheal aspirates. J Clin Microbiol. 1977;6:396–399.
154. Kalinske RW, Parker RH, Brandt D, et al. Diagnostic usefulness and safety of transtracheal aspiration. N Engl J Med. 1967;276:604–608.
155. Wilson ML. Assessing the quality of sputum specimens submitted for mycobacterial culture, old lessons, new lessons and the future. Am J Clin Pathol. 1996;105:625–666.
156. Hoeprich PD. Etiologic diagnosis of lower respiratory tract infections. Calif Med. 1970;112:1.
157. Tillotson JR, Lerner AM. Pneumonias caused by gram negative bacilli. Medicine. 1966;45:65–76.
158. Saadah HA, Nasr FL, Shagoury ME. Washed sputum Gram stain and culture in pneumonia. J Okla State Med Assoc. 1980;73:354–359.
159. Jordan GW, Wong GA, Hoeprich PD. Bacteriology of the lower respiratory tract as determined by fiber-optic bronchoscopy and transtracheal aspiration. J Infect Dis. 1976;134:428–435.
160. Bartlett JG, Alexander J, Mayhew J, et al. Should fiberoptic bronchoscopy aspirates be cultured? Am Rev Respir Dis. 1976;114:73–78.
161. Wimberly N, Faling LJ, Bartlett JG. A fiberoptic bronchoscopy technique to obtain uncontaminated lower airway secretions for bacterial cultures. Am Rev Respir Dis. 1979;119:337–342.
162. Meden G, Hall GS, Ahmad M. Retrieval of microbiological specimens through the fiberoptic bronchoscope. Cleve Clin Q. 1985;52:495–502.
163. Wimberly NW, Bass JB, Boyd BW, et al. Use of a bronchoscopic protected catheter brush for the diagnosis of pulmonary infections. Chest. 1982;81:556–582.
164. Hays DA, McCarthy LC, Friedman M. Evaluation of two bronchofiberscopic methods of culturing the lower respiratory tract. Am Rev Respir Dis. 1980;122:319–323.
165. Higuchi JH, Coalson JJ, Johanson WG. Bacteriologic diagnosis of nosocomial pneumonia in primates. Ann Rev Respir Dis. 1982;125:53–57.
166. Pollock HM, Hawkins EL, Bonner JR, et al. Diagnosis of bacterial pulmonary infections with quantitative protected catheter cultures obtained during bronchoscopy. J Clin Microbiol. 1983;17:255–259.
167. Halperin SA, Suratt PM, Gwaltney JM, et al. Bacterial cultures of the lower respiratory tract in normal volunteers with and without experimental rhinovirus infection using a plugged double catheter system. Am Rev Respir Dis. 1982;125:678–680.
168. Bordelon JY Jr, Legrand P, Gewin WL, et al. The telescoping plugged catheter in suspected anaerobic infections: A controlled series. Am Rev Respir Dis. 1983;128:465–468.
169. Wimberly NW, Bass JR Jr, Boyd DW, et al. Bronchial brush specimens from patients with stable chronic bronchitis. Chest. 1986;90:534–536.
170. Bass JB, Hawkins EL, Bonner JR, et al. Use of bronchoscopy protected catheter technique in the clinical evaluation of a new antibiotic. Diagn Microbiol Infect Dis. 1983;1:95–106.
171. Winterbauer RH, Hutchinson JF, Reinhardt GN, et al. The use of quantitative culture and antibody coating of bacteria to diagnose bacterial pneumonia by fiberoptic bronchoscopy. Am Rev Respir Dis. 1983;128:98–103.
172. Vereen L, Smart LM, George RB. Antibody coating and quantitative cultures of bacteria in sputum and bronchial brush specimens from patients with stable chronic bronchitis. Chest. 1986;90:534–536.
173. Guerra LF, Baughman RP. Use of bronchoalveolar lavage to diagnose bacterial pneumonia in mechanically ventilated patients. Crit Care Med. 1990;18:169–173.
174. Ortquist A, Kalin M, Lejdeborn L, et al. Diagnostic fiberoptic bronchoscopy and protected brush culture in patients with community-acquired pneumonia. Chest. 1990;97:576–582.
175. Feinsilver SH, Fein AM, Niederman MS, et al. Utility of fiberoptic bronchoscopy in nonresolving pneumonia. Chest. 1990;98:1322–1326.
176. Chastre J, Viau F, Brun P, et al. Prospective evaluation of the protected specimen brush for the diagnosis of pulmonary infections in ventilated patients. Am Rev Respir Dis. 1994;130:924–925.
177. Chastre J, Fagon J, Barnet-Lesco M, et al. Evaluation of bronchoscopic techniques for the diagnosis of nosocomial pneumonia. Am J Respir Crit Care Med. 1995;152:231–240.
178. Chastre J, Fagon JY, Soler P, et al. Diagnosis of nosocomial bacterial pneumonia in intubated patients undergoing ventilation: Comparison of the usefulness of bronchoalveolar lavage and the protected specimen brush. Am J Med. 1988;85:499.
179. Johanson WG, Seidenfeld JJ, Gomez P, et al. Bacteriologic diagnosis of nosocomial pneumonia following prolonged mechanical ventilation. Am Rev Respir Dis. 1988;137:259–269.
180. Mortos JA, Ferrer M, Torres A, et al. Specificity of quantitative cultures of protected specimen brush and bronchoalveolar lavage in mechanically ventilated patients. Am Rev Respir Dis. 1990;161:A276.
181. Broughton WA, Middleton RM, Kirkpatrick MB, et al. Bronchoscopic protected specimen brush and bronchoalveolar lavage in the diagnosis of bacterial pneumonia. Infect Dis Clin North Am. 1991;5:432–452.
182. Torres A, El-Ebiary M, Padro L, et al. Validation of different techniques for the diagnosis of ventilator-associated pneumonia: Comparison with immediate postmortem pulmonary biopsy. Am J Respir Crit Care Med. 1994;149:324–331.
183. Marquette CH, Copin M, Wallet F, et al. Diagnostic tests for pneumonia in ventilated patients: Prospective evaluation of diagnostic accuracy using histology as a diagnostic gold standard. Am J Respir Crit Care Med. 1995;151:1878–1888.
184. Montravers P, Fagon J, Chastre J, et al. Follow-up protected specimen brushes to assess treatment in nosocomial pneumonia. Am Rev Respir Dis. 1993;147:38–44.
185. Timsit J, Misset B, Renard B, et al. Effect of previous antimicrobial therapy on the accuracy of the main procedure used to diagnose nosocomial pneumonia in patients who are using ventilation. Chest. 1995;108:1036–1040.
186. DeCastro FR, Violan JS, Capuz BL, et al. Reliability of the bronchoscopic protected catheter brush in the diagnosis of pneumonia in the mechanically ventilated patient. Crit Care Med. 1991;19:171.
187. Torres A, El-Ebiary M. Invasive diagnostic techniques for pneumonia: Protected specimen brush, bronchoalveolar lavage and lung biopsy methods. Infect Dis Clin North Am. 1998;12:701–722.
188. Mayhall CG. Nosocomial pneumonia diagnosis and prevention. Infect Dis Clin North Am. 1997;11:427–457.
189. Broaddus C, Dake MD, Stulburg MS, et al. Bronchoalveolar lavage and transbronchial biopsy for the diagnosis of pulmonary infections in the acquired immunodeficiency syndrome. Ann Intern Med. 1986;102:747–752.
190. Jules-Elysee KM, Stover DE, Zaman MB, et al. Aerosolized pentamadine: Effect on diagnosis and presentation of *Pneumocystis carinii* pneumonia. Ann Intern Med. 1990;112:750–787.
191. Crawford SW, Bowden RA, Hackman RC, et al. Rapid detection of cytomegalovirus pulmonary infection by bronchoalveolar lavage and centrifugation culture. Ann Intern Med. 1988;108:180–185.
192. Spector SA. Diagnosis of cytomegalovirus infection. Semin Hematol. 1990;27: 11–16.
193. Pisani RJ, Wright AJ. Clinical utility of bronchoalveolar lavage in immunocompromised hosts. Mayo Clin Proc. 1992;67:221–227.
194. Crawford SW, Bowden RA, Hackman RC, et al. Rapid detection of cytomegalovirus pulmonary infection by bronchoalveolar lavage and centrifugation culture. Ann Intern Med. 1988;108:180–185.
195. Emmanuel D, Peppard J, Stover D, et al. Rapid diagnosis of cytomegalovirus pneumonia by bronchoalveolar lavage using human and murine monoclonal antibodies. Ann Intern Med. 1986;104:476–481.
196. Xavier R, Henn L, Costa R. Bronchoalveolar lavage in pulmonary tuberculosis. Chest. 1990;98:975.
197. DeGracia J, Curull V, Vidal R, et al. Diagnostic value of bronchoalveolar lavage in suspected pulmonary tuberculosis. Chest. 1988;93:329–332.
198. Baughman RP, Dohn MN, Loudon RG, et al. Bronchoscopy with bronchoalveolar lavage in tuberculosis and fungal infection. Chest. 1991;99:92–97.
199. Meduri GH, Baselski V. The role of bronchoalveolar lavage in diagnosing nonopportunistic bacterial pneumonia. Chest. 1991;100:179–190.
200. Bovornkittz S, Pushpakom R. Adenosine deaminase in bronchoalveolar lavage fluid. Chest. 1988;94:1113.
201. Levy H, Wadee AA, Feldman C, et al. Enzyme-linked immunosorbent assay for detection of antibodies against *Mycobacterium tuberculosis* in bronchial washings and serum. Chest. 1988;93:762–766.
202. Raja A, Baughman RP, Daniel TM. The detection by immune assay of antibody to mycobacterial antigens in bronchoalveolar lavage fluid from patients with tuberculosis and control subjects. Chest. 1988;94:133–137.
203. Torres A, El-Ebiary M, Fabregos N, et al. Value of intracellular bacteria detection in the diagnosis of ventilator associated pneumonia. Thorax. 1996;51:378–384.
204. Chastre J, Fagon JY, Soler P, et al. Quantification of BAL cells containing intracellular bacteria rapidly identifies ventilated patients with nosocomial pneumonia. Chest. 1989;15:190s–192s.
205. Allaouchiche B, Jaumain H, Dumontet C, et al. Early diagnosis of ventilator associated pneumonia: Is it possible to define a cutoff value of infected cells in BAL fluid? Chest. 1996;110:1558–1565.
206. Gerbeaux P, Ledoray V, Boussuges A, et al. Diagnosis of nosocomial pneumonia in mechanically ventilated patients. Am J Respir Crit Care Med. 1998;157:76–80.
207. Jourdain B, Joly-Guillou ML, Dombret MC, et al. Usefulness of quantitative cultures of BAL fluid for diagnosing nosocomial pneumonia in ventilated patients. Chest. 1997;111:411–418.
208. Stover DE, Zaman MB, Hajdu SI, et al. Bronchoalveolar lavage in the diagnosis of diffuse pulmonary infiltrates in the immunosuppressed host. Ann Intern Med. 1984;101:1–7.
209. Martin WJ, Smith TF, Sanderson DR, et al. Role of bronchoalveolar lavage in the assessment of opportunistic pulmonary infections: Utility and complications. Mayo Clin Proc. 1987;62:549–557.
210. Pugin J, Auckenthaler R, Delaspre O, et al. Rapid diagnosis of gram-negative pneumonia by assay of endotoxin in bronchoalveolar lavage fluid. Thorax. 1992;47:547–549.
211. Trouillet JL, Guiguet M, Gibert L, et al. Fiberoptic bronchoscopy in ventilated patients: Evaluation of cardiopulmonary risk under midazolam sedation. Chest. 1990;97:927–933.

212. Pugin J, Suter PM. Diagnostic bronchoalveolar lavage in patients with pneumonia produces sepsis-like systemic effects. Intensive Care Med. 1992;18:6–10.
213. Prokop A, Gawenda M, Krüger I, Pichlmaier H. Value of bronchoscopic pneumonia diagnosis: Prospective study. World J Surg. 1996;29:22–26.
214. El-Ebiary M, Torres A, Gonzalez J, et al. Quantitative cultures of endotracheal aspirates for the diagnosis of ventilator-associated pneumonia. Am Rev Respir Dis. 1993;148:1552–1557.
215. Sanchez-Nieto JM, Torres A, Garcia-Cordoba F, et al. Impact of invasive and non-invasive quantitative culture sampling on outcome of ventilator-associated pneumonia: A pilot study. Am J Respir Crit Care Med. 1998;157:371–376.
216. Jourdain B, Novora A, Joly-Guillou ML, et al. Role of quantitative values of endotracheal aspirate in the diagnosis of nosocomial pneumonia. Am J Respir Crit Care Med. 1995;152:241–246.
217. Marik PE, Brown WJ. A comparison of bronchoscopic vs blind protected specimen brush sampling in patients with suspected ventilator-associated pneumonia. Chest. 1995;108:203–207.
218. Gaussorgues P, Piperno D, Bachman P, et al. Comparison of non-bronchoscopic bronchoalveolar lavage to open lung biopsy for bacteriology diagnosis of pulmonary infection in mechanically ventilated patients. Intensive Care Med. 1989;15:94.
219. Rouby J, Rossignon MD, Nicholas MH, et al. A prospective study of protected bronchoalveolar lavage in the diagnosis of nosocomial pneumonia. Anesthesiology. 1989;71:679–685.
220. Meduri GU, Beals D, Maijub G, et al. Protected bronchoalveolar lavage, a new bronchoscopic technique to retrieve uncontaminated distal airway secretion. Am Rev Respir Dis. 1991;143:855–864.
221. Pugin J, Auckenthaler R, Mili N, et al. Diagnosis of ventilator-associated pneumonia by bacteriologic analysis of bronchoscopic and non-bronchoscopic "blind" bronchoalveolar lavage fluid. Am Rev Respir Dis. 1991;143:1121–1129.
222. Kollef MH, Bock KR, Richards RD, Hearns ML. The safety and diagnostic accuracy of minibronchoalveolar lavage in patients with suspected ventilator-associated pneumonia. Ann Intern Med. 1995;122:743–748.
223. Bregeon F, Papazian L, Visconti A, Gregoire R, et al. Relationship of microbiologic diagnostic criteria to morbidity and mortality in patients with ventilator-associated pneumonia. JAMA. 1997;277:655–662.
224. Busk MF, Rosenow EC III, Wilson WR. Invasive procedures in the diagnosis of pneumonia. Semin Respir Infect. 1988;3:113–122.
225. Manresa F, Dorca J. Needle aspiration techniques in the diagnosis of pneumonia. Thorax. 1991;46:601–603.
226. Mimica I, Donoso E, Howard JE, et al. Lung puncture in the etiological diagnosis of pneumonia. Am J Dis Child. 1971;122:278–282.
227. Klein JO. Diagnostic lung puncture in the pneumonias of infants and children. Pediatrics. 1969;44:486–492.
228. Bartlett JG. Invasive diagnostic techniques in respiratory infections. In: Pennington JE, ed. Respiratory Infections: Diagnosis and Management. New York: Raven; 1983:55–77.
229. Palmer DL, Davidson M, Lusk R. Needle aspiration of the lung in complex pneumonias. Chest. 1980;78:16–21.
230. Torres A, Jimenez P, de la Bellacasa JP, et al. Diagnostic value of nonfluoroscopic percutaneous lung needle aspiration in patients with pneumonia. Chest. 1990;98:840–844.
231. Bandt PD, Blank N, Castellino RA. Needle diagnosis of pneumonitis, value in high risk patients. JAMA. 1972;220:1578–1580.
232. Greenman RL, Goodall PT, King D. Lung biopsy in immune compromised hosts. Am J Med. 1975;59:488–496.
233. Cockerill FR III, Wilson WR, Carpenter HA, et al. Open lung biopsy in immunocompromised patients. Arch Intern Med. 1985;145:1398–1404.
234. Dijkman JH, van der Meer JWM, Bakker W, et al. Transpleural lung biopsy by the thoracoscopic route in patients with diffuse interstitial pulmonary disease. Chest. 1982;82:76–83.
235. Rodgers BM. Thoracoscopy in children. Poumon-Coeur. 1981;37:301–306.
236. Springmeyer SC, Silvestri RC, Sale GE, et al. The role of transbronchial biopsy for the diagnosis of diffuse pneumonias in immunocompromised marrow transplant recipients. Am Rev Respir Dis. 1982;116:763–765.
237. McCabe RE, Brooks RG, Mark JBD, et al. Open lung biopsy in patients with acute leukemia. Am J Med. 1985;78:609–616.
238. McKenna RJ, Mountain CF, McMurtrey MJ. Open lung biopsy in immunocompromised patients. Chest. 1984;86:671–674.
239. Lowell JR. Pleural Effusions—A Comprehensive Review. Baltimore: University Park Press; 1977:96.
240. Unger JD, Rose HD, Unger GF. Gram-negative pneumonia. Diagn Radiol. 1973;107:283–291.
241. Light RW. Pleural diseases. Dis Mo. 1992;38:266–331.
242. Heffner JE, Brown LK, Barbieri L, DeLeo JM. Pleural fluid chemical analysis in para-pneumonia effusions: A meta analysis. Am J Respir Crit Care Med. 1995;151:1700–1708.
243. Bothe R, van Furth R, van den Broeks PJ. A etiology of community-acquired pneumonia: A prospective study among adults requiring admission to hospital. Thorax. 1995;50:543–547.
244. Chalasani NP, Valdecanas MAL, Gopal AK, et al. Clinical utility of blood cultures in adult patients with community-acquired pneumonia without defined underlying risks. Chest. 1995;108:932–936.
245. Fine MJ, Smith MA, Carson LA, et al. Prognosis and outcomes of patients with community-acquired pneumonia: A meta-analysis. JAMA. 1996;275:134–141.
246. Berk SL. Justifying the use of blood cultures when diagnosing community-acquired pneumonia. Chest. 1995;108:891–892.
247. Venkatesan P, MacFarlane JT. Role of pneumococcal antigen in the diagnosis of pneumococcal pneumonia (Editorial). Thorax. 1992;47:329–331.
248. Dorff GJ, Coonrod JD, Rytel MW. Detection of immunoelectrophoresis of antigen in sera of patients with pneumococcal bacteremia. Lancet. 1971;1:578–579.
249. Örtquist A, Jonsson I, Kalin M, et al. Comparison of three methods for detection of pneumococcal antigen in sputum of patients with community-acquired pneumonia. Eur J Clin Microbiol Infect Dis. 1989;8:956–961.
250. Woodhead MA, MacFarlane JT, Finch RG, et al. A comparison of counter-current immunoelectrophoresis and latex agglutination for the detection of pneumococcal antigen in community based pneumonia study. Serodiagn Immunother Infect Dis. 1990;4:159–165.
251. Lenthe-Ebua S, Brighouse G, Auckenthaler R, et al. Comparison of immunological methods for diagnosis of pneumococcal pneumonia in biological fluids. Eur J Clin Microbiol. 1987;6:28–34.
252. Boermsa WG, Lowenberg A, Holloway Y, et al. Pneumococcal capsular antigen detection and pneumococcal serology in patients with community-acquired pneumonia. Thorax. 1991;46:902–906.
253. Tugwell P, Greenwood BM. Pneumococcal antigen in lobar pneumonia. J Clin Pathol. 1975;28:118–123.
254. Burman LA, Trollfors B, Andersson B, et al. Diagnosis of pneumonia by cultures, bacterial and viral antigen detective tests and serology with special reference to antibodies against pneumococcal antigens. J Infect Dis. 1991;163:1087–1095.
255. Boermsa WG, Lowenberg A, Holloway Y, et al. Pneumococcal antigen persistence in sputum from patients with community-acquired pneumonia. Chest. 1992;102:422–427.
256. Martin SJ, Hogansan DA, Thomas ET. Detection of *Streptococcus pneumoniae* and *Haemophilus influenzae* type B antigens in acute nonbacteremic pneumonia. J Clin Microbiol. 1987;25:248–250.
257. Campbell JF, Spika JS. The serodiagnosis of nonpneumococcal bacterial pneumonia. Semin Respir Infect. 1988;3:123–130.
258. Ruf B, Schurmann D, Horbach I, et al. Frequency and diagnosis of *Legionella pneumophila*: A 3 year prospective study with emphasis on application of urinary antigen detection. J Infect Dis. 1990;162:1341–1347.
259. Salo P, Örtquist Ä, Leinonen M. Diagnosis of bacteremic pneumococcal pneumonia by amplification of pneumolysia gene fragments in serum. J Infect Dis. 1995;171:479–482.
260. Schlager N, Godwin K, Sepkowitz D, et al. Application of the polymerase chain reaction in *Pneumocystis carinii* and frequent detection of *Pneumocystis carinii* in serum of patients with pneumocystis pneumonia. J Exp Med. 1992;176:1327–1333.
261. Smith RP, Lipworth BJ, Cree IA, et al. C-reactive protein: A clinical marker in community-acquired pneumonia. Chest. 1995;108:1288–1291.
262. Örtquist Ä, Hedlund J, Wretlind B, et al. Diagnostic and prognostic value of interleukin 6 and C-reactive protein in community-acquired pneumonia. Scan J Infect Dis. 1995;27:457–462.
263. Smith RP, Lipworth BJ. C-reactive protein in simple community-acquired pneumonia. Chest. 1995;107:1028–1031.
264. Puren AJ, Feldman C, Savage N, et al. Patterns of cytokine expression in community-acquired pneumonia. Chest. 1995;107:1342–1349.
265. Woodhead M. Management of pneumonia in the outpatient setting. Semin Respir Infect. 1998;13:8–16.
266. Albaum MN, Hill LC, Murphy M, et al. Interobserver reliability of the chest radiograph in community-acquired pneumonia. Chest. 1996;110:343–350.
267. Gonzales R, Steiner JF, Sande MA. Antibiotic prescribing for adults with colds, upper respiratory tract infections and bronchitis by ambulatory care physicians. JAMA. 1997;278:901–904.
268. Hasley PB, Albaum MN, Li Y-H, et al. Do pulmonary radiographic findings at presentation predict mortality in patients with community-acquired pneumonia? Ann Intern Med. 1996;156:2206–2212.
269. Lerner AM, Jankauskas K. The classic bacterial pneumonias. Dis Mon. Feb 1975:1–46.
270. Willman VL, Lewis JE, Hanlon CR. Staphylococcal pneumonia—Surgical considerations in cases in infants and children. Arch Surg. 1961;83:93–97.
271. Highman JH. Staphylococcal pneumonia and empyema in childhood. Am J Roentgenol. 1969;106:103–108.
272. Dines DE. Diagnostic significance of pneumatocoeles of the lung. JAMA. 1968;204:1169–1172.
273. Warner JO, Gordon I. Pneumatocoeles following *Haemophilus influenzae* pneumonia. Clin Radiol. 1981;32:99–105.
274. Luddy RE, Champion LA, Schwartz AD. *Pneumocystis carinii* pneumonia with pneumatocele formation. Am J Dis Child. 1977;131:470.
275. Scanlon GT, Unger JD. The radiology of bacterial and viral pneumonias. Radiol Clin North Am. 1973;11:317–338.
276. Bartlett JG, Finegold SM. Anaerobic pleuropulmonary infections. Medicine. 1972;51:413–450.
277. Lindsay MI, Morrow GW. Primary influenzal pneumonia. Postgrad Med. 1971;49:173–178.
278. Conte P, Heitzman ER, Markarian B. Viral pneumonia. Roentgen pathological correlations. Radiology. 1970;95:267–272.
279. Fine NL, Smith LR, Sheedy PF. Frequency of pleural effusions of mycoplasma and viral pneumonias. N Engl J Med. 1970;283:790–793.
280. Fraser DW, Tsai TR, Orenstein W, et al. Legionnaire's disease. Description of an epidemic of pneumonia. N Engl J Med. 1977;297:1189–1197.
281. Kirby BD, Snyder KM, Meyer RD, et al. Legionnaire's disease—a cluster of cases (Abstract). Clin Res. 1978;26:A399.

282. Pope TL, Armstrong P, Thompson R, et al. Pittsburgh pneumonia agent chest film manifestations. AJR. 1982;138:237–241.
283. Tew J, Calenoff L, Berlin BS. Bacterial or nonbacterial pneumonia: Accuracy of radiographic diagnosis. Radiology. 1977;124:607–612.
284. Wheeler JH, Fishman EK. Computed tomography in the management of chest infections: Current status. Clin Infect Dis. 1996;23:232–240.
285. Primack SL, Müller NL. High resolution computed tomography in acute diffuse lung disease in the immunocompromised patient. Radiol Clin North Am. 1994;32:731–744.
286. Syrjälä H, Broas M, Suramo I, et al. High resolution computed tomography for the diagnosis of community-acquired pneumonia. Clin Infect Dis. 1998;27:358–363.
287. Kramer EL, Chaitanya RD. Pulmonary applications of nuclear medicine. Clin Chest Med. 1991;12:55–75.
288. Sapira JD, Cochran J. Community-acquired pneumonia versus hospital-acquired pneumonia: What are we talking about? A skeptics review. Infect Dis Newslett. 1993;12:57–61.
289. Marrie TJ, Peeling RW, Fine MJ, et al. Ambulatory patients with community-acquired pneumonia: The frequency of atypical agents and clinical course. Am J Med. 1996;101:508–515.
290. Fang GD, Fine M, Orloff J, et al. New and emerging etiologies for community-acquired pneumonia with implications for therapy: A prospective multicenter study of 359 cases. Medicine. 1990;69:307–316.
291. Pennington JE. Community-Acquired Pneumonia and Acute Bronchitis in Respiratory Infections: Diagnosis and Management. New York: Raven; 1994.
292. Garibaldi RA. Epidemiology of community acquired respiratory tract infections in adults: Incidence, etiology, and impact. Am J Med. 1985;78(Suppl 6B):32–37.
293. Kerttula Y, Leinonen M, Koskela M, et al. The aetiology of pneumonia. Application of bacterial serology and basic laboratory methods. J Infect. 1987;14:21–30.
294. Gleckman R, DeVita J, Hibert D, et al. Sputum Gram's stain assessment in community-acquired bacteremic pneumonia. J Clin Microbiol. 1988;26:846–849.
295. Woodhead MA, Arrowsmith J, Chamberlain-Webber R, et al. The value of routine microbial investigation in community-acquired pneumonia. Respir Med. 1991;85:313–317.
296. Holmberg H, Bodin L, Jönsson I, et al. Rapid aetiological diagnosis of pneumonia based on routine laboratory features. Scand J Infect Dis. 1990;22:537–545.
297. The British Thoracic Society Research Committee and the Public Health Laboratory Service. The aetiology, management and outcome of severe community-acquired pneumonia on the intensive care unit. Respir Med. 1992;86:7–13.
298. Holmberg H. Aetiology of community-acquired pneumonia in hospital-treated patients. Scand J Infect Dis. 1987;19:491–501.
299. Marrie TJ, Durant H, Yates L. Community-acquired pneumonia requiring hospitalization: Five year prospective study. Rev Infect Dis. 1989;11:586–599.
300. Farr BM, Kaiser DL, Harrison BDW, et al. Prediction of microbial aetiology at admission to hospital for pneumonia from the presenting clinical features. Thorax. 1989;44:1031–1035.
301. Fine MJ, Orloff JJ, Arisumi D, et al. Prognosis of patients hospitalized with community-acquired pneumonia. Am J Med. 1990;88(5N):1N–8N.
302. Fine M, Smith D, Singer DE. Hospitalization decision in patients with community-acquired pneumonia: A prospective chart review. Am J Med. 1990;89:713–714.
303. American Thoracic Society. Guidelines for the initial management of adults with community-acquired pneumonia: Diagnosis, assessment of severity, and initial antimicrobial therapy. Am Rev Respir Dis. 1993;148:1418–1426.
304. Marrie TJ. Community-acquired pneumonia. Clin Infect Dis. 1994;18:501–515.
305. Bates JH, Campbell GD, Barron AI, et al. Etiology of acute pneumonia in hospitalized patients. Chest. 1992;101:1005–1012.
306. Karalus NC, Cursons RT, Leng RA, et al. Community-acquired pneumonia: Aetiology and prognostic index evaluation. Thorax. 1991;46:413–418.
307. Mundy LM, Auwaerter PG, Oldach D, et al. Community-acquired pneumonia: Impact of immune status. Am J Respir Crit Care Med. 1995;152:1309–1315.
308. Chatard JA. The leukocytes in acute lobar pneumonia. Johns Hopkins Hosp Rep. 1910;15:89–98.
309. Austrian R, Gold J. Pneumococcal bacteremia with especial reference to bacteremic pneumococcal pneumonia. Ann Intern Med. 1964;60:759–776.
310. MacFarlane JT, Finch RG, Ward MJ, et al. Hospital study of adult community acquired pneumonia. Lancet. 1982;2:255–258.
311. Klimek JJ, Ajemian E, Fontecchio S, et al. Community acquired bacterial pneumonia requiring admission to hospital. Am J Infect Control. 1983;11:79–82.
312. Levy M, Dromer F, Brion N, et al. Community-acquired pneumonia: Importance of initial non-invasive bacteriologic and radiographic investigations. Chest. 1988;92:43–48.
313. Stratton CW. Bacterial pneumonia. An overview with emphasis on pathogenesis, diagnosis and treatment. Heart Lung. 1986;15:226–244.
314. Lipsky BA, Boyko EJ, Inui TS, et al. Risk factors for acquiring pneumococcal infections. Arch Intern Med. 1986;146:2179–2185.
315. Rosner F, Zarrabi MH. Late infections following splenectomy in Hodgkin's disease. Cancer Invest. 1983;1:57–65.
316. Zarrabi MH, Rosner F. Serious infections in adults following splenectomy for trauma. Arch Intern Med. 1984;144:1421–1424.
317. Musher DM. Infections caused by *Streptococcus pneumoniae*: Clinical spectrum, pathogenesis, immunity and treatment. Clin Infect Dis. 1992;14:801–809.
318. Crofton J. The chemotherapy of bacterial respiratory infections. Am Rev Respir Dis. 1970;101:841–859.
319. Hirschmann JV, Everett ED. *Haemophilus influenzae* infections in adults: Report of nine cases and a review of literature. Medicine. 1979;58:80–94.
320. Hausmann W, Karlish AJ. Staphylococcal pneumonia in adults. BMJ. 1956;2:845–847.
321. Schwarzmann SW, Adler JL, Sullivan RJ, et al. Bacterial pneumonia during the Hong Kong influenza epidemic of 1968–1969. Experience in a city-county hospital. Arch Intern Med. 1971;127:1037–1041.
322. Louria DB, Blumenfeld HL, Ellis JT, et al. Studies on influenza. J Clin Invest. 1959;38:213–265.
323. Yu VL, Kroboth FJ, Shonnard J, et al. Legionnaire's disease: New clinical perspective from a prospective pneumonia study. Am J Med. 1982;73:357–361.
324. Cunha BA. Clinical features of legionnaires' disease. Semin Respir Infect. 1998;13:116–127.
325. Nicotra B, Rivera M, Luman I, et al. *Branhamella catarrhalis* as a lower respiratory tract pathogen in patients with chronic lung disease. Arch Intern Med. 1986;146:890–893.
326. Slevin NJ, Aitken J, Thornleg PE. Clinical and microbiological features of *Branhamella catarrhalis* bronchopulmonary infections. Lancet. 1987;1:782–783.
327. Wallace RJ Jr, Musher DM. In honor of Dr. Sarah Branham. A star is born: The realization of *Branhamella catarrhalis* as a respiratory pathogen. Chest. 1986;90:447–450.
328. Marrie TJ. Epidemiology of mild pneumonia. Semin Respir Infect. 1998;13:3–7.
329. Gross JS, Neufeld RR, Libon LS, et al. Autopsy study of the elderly institutionalized patients: Review of 234 autopsies. Arch Intern Med. 1988;148:173–176.
330. Granton JT, Grossman RF. Community-acquired pneumonia in the elderly patient. Clin Chest Med. 1993;14:537–553.
331. Musgrave T, Verghese A. Clinical features of pneumonia in the elderly. Semin Respir Infect. 1990;5:269–275.
332. Harper C, Newton P. Clinical aspects of pneumonia in the elderly veteran. J Am Geriatr Soc. 1989;37:867–872.
333. Venkatesan P, Gladman J, MacFarlane JT. A hospital study of community-acquired pneumonia in the elderly. Thorax. 1990;45:254–258.
334. Houston MS, Silverstein MD, Suman VJ. Community-acquired lower respiratory tract infection in the elderly: A community-based study of incidence and outcome. J Am Board Fam Pract. 1995;8:347–356.
335. Janssens JP, Gauthey L, Herrmann F, Thatch L, et al. Community-acquired pneumonia in older patients. JAGS. 1996;44:539–544.
336. Riquelme R, Torres A, El-Ebiary M, et al. Community-acquired pneumonia in the elderly: A multivariate analysis of risk and prognostic factors. Am J Respir Crit Care Med. 1996;154:1450–1455.
337. File TM Jr. Etiology and incidence of community-acquired pneumonia. Infect Dis Clin Pract. 1996;5(Suppl4):5127–5135.
338. Rello J, Rodriguez R, Jubert P, et al. Severe community-acquired pneumonia in the elderly. Clin Infect Dis. 1996;23:723–728.
339. Berk KC, Holtsdan SA, Wiener SL, et al. Nontypeable *Haemophilus influenzae* in the elderly. Arch Intern Med. 1982;142:532–539.
340. Valenti WM, Trudell RG, Bentley DW. Factors predisposing to oropharyngeal colonization with gram-negative bacilli in the aged. N Engl J Med. 1978;298:1108–1111.
341. Mackowiak PA, Martin RM, Jones SR, et al. Pharyngeal colonization by gram-negative bacilli in aspiration-prone persons. Arch Intern Med. 1978;138:1224–1247.
342. Nicolle L, McLeod J, McIntyre M, et al. Significance of pharyngeal colonization with aerobic gram-negative bacilli in elderly institutionalized men. Aging. 1986;15:47–52.
343. Kidd D, Lawson J, Nesbitt R, MacMahon J. The national history and clinical consequences of aspiration in acute stroke. Q J Med. 1995;88:409–413.
344. Pick N, McDonald A, Bennett N, et al. Pulmonary aspiration in a long-term care setting: Clinical and laboratory observation and an analysis of risk factors. JAGS. 1996;44:763–768.
345. Marrie TJ. *Mycoplasma pneumoniae* requiring hospitalization with emphasis on infection in the elderly. Arch Intern Med. 1993;153:488–494.
346. Orr PH, Peeling RW, Fast M, et al. Serologic study of responses to selected pathogens causing respiratory tract infection in the institutionalized elderly. Clin Infect Dis. 1996;23:1240–1245.
347. Falsey AR, Cunningham CK, Barber WH, et al. Respiratory syncytial virus and influenza A, infections in the hospitalized elderly. J Infect Dis. 1995;172:389–394.
348. Dowell SF, Anderson LJ, Gary HE Jr, et al. Respiratory syncytial virus is an important cause of community-acquired lower respiratory infection among hospitalized adults. J Infect Dis. 1996;174:456–462.
349. Nicholson KG, Kent J, Hammersley V, Cancio E. Risk factors for lower respiratory complications of rhinovirus infections in elderly people living in the community: Prospective cohort study. BMJ. 1996;313:1119–1123.
350. Murray JF, Felton CP, Garay SM, et al. Pulmonary complications of the acquired immunodeficiency syndrome. Report of a National Heart, Lung and Blood Institute Workshop. N Engl J Med. 1984;310:1682–1688.
351. Stover DE, White DA, Romano PA, et al. Spectrum of pulmonary diseases associated with the acquired immune deficiency syndrome. Am J Med. 1985;78:429–437.
352. Murray JF. Pulmonary complications of HIV infection. Annu Rev Med. 1996;47:117–126.
353. Saah AJ, Hoover DR, Pengy Phair JP, et al. Predictors for failure of *Pneumocystis carinii* pneumonia prophylaxis multicenter AIDS cohort study. JAMA. 1995;273:1197–1202.
354. Pulmonary Complications of HIV Infection Study Group: Design of a prospective study of the pulmonary complications of human immunodeficiency virus infection. J Clin Epidemiol. 1993;46:497.

355. Rosen MJ. Overview of pulmonary complications. Clin Chest Med. 1996;17: 621–631.
356. Dropulic LK, Leslie JM, Eldred LJ, et al. Clinical manifestation and risk factors of *Pseudomonas aeruginosa* in patients with AIDS. J Infect Dis. 1995;171:930–937.
357. Pachon J, Prados D, Capote F, et al. Severe community-acquired pneumonia: Etiology, prognosis, treatment. Am Rev Respir Dis. 1990;142:369–373.
358. Potgieter PD, Hammond JMJ. Etiology and diagnosis of pneumonia requiring ICU admission: A discussion. Chest. 1992;101:199–203.
359. Leroy O, Santre C, Beuscart C, et al. A five year study of severe community-acquired pneumonia with emphasis on prognosis in patients admitted to an intensive care unit. Intensive Care Med. 1995;21:44–51.
360. Torres A, Serra-Batlles J, Ferrer A, et al. Severe community-acquired pneumonia: Epidemiology and prognostic factors. Am Rev Respir Dis. 1991;144:312–318.
361. Farr BM, Sloman AJ, Fisch MJ. Predicting death in patients hospitalized for community-acquired pneumonia. Ann Intern Med. 1991;115:428–436.
362. The British Thoracic Society Research Committee and the Public Health Laboratory Service. Community-acquired pneumonia in adults in British hospitals in 1982–1983: A survey of aetiology, mortality, prognostic factors and outcome. Q J Med. 1987;62:195–220.
363. Fine MJ, Orloff JJ, Arisumi D, et al. Prognosis of patients hospitalized with community-acquired pneumonia. Am J Med. 1990;88:S-1N–S-8N.
364. Leeper KV Jr, Torres A. Community-acquired pneumonia in the intensive care unit. Clin Chest Med. 1995;16:155–178.
365. Leeper KV Jr. Severe community-acquired pneumonia. Semin Respir Infect. 1996;11:96–108.
366. Leroy O, Santre L, Beuscart L. A five-year old study of severe community-acquired pneumonia with emphasis on prognosis in patients admitted to an intensive care unit. Intensive Care Med. 1995;21:24–31.
367. Marrie TJ. Normal resolution of community-acquired pneumonia. Semin Respir Infect. 1992;7:256–270.
368. Lehtomaki K. Clinical diagnosis of pneumococcal adenoviral, mycoplasmal and viral pneumonia in young men. Eur Respir J. 1988;1:324–329.
369. Jay SJ, Johnson WG Jr, Pierce WK. The radiographic resolution of *Streptococcus pneumoniae* pneumonia. N Engl J Med. 1991;293:798–801.
370. Winterbauer RH, Bedon GA, Ball WC Jr. Recurrent pneumonia: Predisposing of illness and clinical patterns in 158 patients. Ann Intern Med. 1989;70:689–700.
371. Corley DE, Winterbauer RH. Infectious diseases that result in slowly resolving and chronic pneumonia. Semin Respir Med. 1993;8:3–13.
372. Feinsilver SH, Fein AM, Niederman MS, et al. Utility of fiberoptic bronchoscopy in nonresolving pneumonia. Chest. 1990;98:1322–1326.
373. Reiman HA. An acute infection of the respiratory tract with atypical pneumonia. JAMA. 1938;111:2377–2384.
374. Luby JP. Pneumonia caused by *Mycoplasma pneumoniae* infection. Clin Chest Med. 1991;12:237–244.
375. File TM, Tan JS, Plouffe JF. The role of atypical pathogens: *Mycoplasma pneumoniae, Chlamydia pneumoniae* and *Legionella pneumophila* in respiratory infection. Infect Dis Clin North Am. 1998;12:509–592.
376. File TM Jr, Tan JS, Plouffe TF. Community-acquired pneumonia: What's needed for accurate diagnosis. Postgrad Med J. 1996;99:95–107.
377. Gaydos CA, Eiden JJ, Oldach D, et al. Diagnosis of *Chlamydia pneumoniae* infection in patients with community-acquired pneumonia by polymerase chain reaction enzyme immunoassay. Clin Infect Dis. 1994;19:157–160.
378. Lieberman D, Schlaeffer F, Lieberman D, et al. *Mycoplasma pneumoniae* community-acquired pneumonia: A review of 101 hospitalized adult patients. Respiration. 1996;63:261–266.
379. Woodhead MA, MacFarlane JT. Comparative clinical and laboratory features of *Legionella* with pneumococcal and *Mycoplasma* pneumonias. Br J Dis Chest. 1987;81:133–139.
380. Riquelme R, Torres A, El-Ebiary M, et al. Community-acquired pneumonia in the elderly: A multivariate analysis of risk and prognostic factors. Am J Respir Crit Care Med. 1996;154:1450–1455.
381. Mogabgab WJ. *Mycoplasma pneumoniae* and adenovirus respiratory illness in military and university personnel 1959–1966. Am Rev Respir Dis. 1968;97: 345–358.
382. Forsyth BR, Bloom HH, Johnson KM, et al. Etiology of primary atypical pneumonia in a military population. JAMA. 1965;191:364–368.
383. Wenzel RP, McCormick DP, Smith EP, et al. Acute respiratory disease: Clinical and epidemiologic observations of military trainees. Mil Med. 1971;136:873–880.
384. Grayston JT, Kenny GE, Foy HM, et al. Epidemiological studies of *Mycoplasma pneumoniae* infections in civilians. Ann N Y Acad Sci. 1967;143:436–446.
385. Grayston JT, Diwan VK, Cooney M, et al. Community and hospital acquired pneumonia associated with chlamydia TWAR infection demonstrated serologically. Arch Intern Med. 1989;149:169–173.
386. Grayston JT, Kuo CC, Wang SP, et al. A new *Chlamydia psittaci* strain, TWAR, isolated in acute respiratory tract infection. N Engl J Med. 1986;315:161–169.
387. Marrie TJ, Grayston JT, Wang SP, et al. Pneumonia associated with the TWAR strain of *Chlamydia.* Ann Intern Med. 1987;106:507–511.
388. Thorn DH, Grayston JT. Infections with *Chlamydia pneumoniae* strain TWAR. Clin Chest Med. 1991;12:245–256.
389. Grayston JT, Campbell LA, Kuo CC, et al. A new respiratory tract pathogen: *Chlamydia pneumoniae* strain TWAR. J Infect Dis. 1990;161:618–625.
390. Von Hurtzen L, Alakarppa H, Koskinen R, et al. *Chlamydia pneumoniae* infection in patients with chronic obstructive pulmonary disease. Epidemiol Infect. 1997;118:155–164.
391. Kauppinen MT, Saikku P. Pneumonia due to *Chlamydia pneumoniae*: Prevalence, clinical features, diagnosis and treatment. Clin Infect Dis. 1995;21:5244–5252.
392. Kleemola M, Saikku P, Viskorpi R, et al. Epidemics of pneumonia caused by TWAR, a new *Chlamydia* organism in military trainees in Finland. J Infect Dis. 1988;157:230–236.
393. Weiss S, Quist J, Roblin P, et al. The relationship between *Chlamydia pneumoniae* (cp) and bronchospasm in adults. Abstract K39. Presented at 35th Interscience Conference on Antimicrobial Agents and Chemotherapy. San Francisco, September 1995.
394. Kauppinen MT, Saikku P, Kujala P, et al. Clinical picture of community-acquired *Chlamydia pneumoniae* pneumonia requiring hospital treatment. A comparison between chlamydial and pneumococcal pneumonia. Thorax. 1996;51:185–190.
395. Dalhoff K, Maass M. *Chlamydia pneumoniae* pneumonia in hospitalized patients. Chest. 1996;110:351–356.
396. Grayston JT. Infection caused by *Chlamydia pneumoniae* strain TWAR. Clin Infect Dis. 1992;15:757–763.
397. Kuo CL, Shor A, Campbell LA, et al. Demonstration of *Chlamydia pneumoniae* in atherosclerotic lesions of coronary arteries. J Infect Dis. 1993;167:841–849.
398. Thorn DH, Grayston JT, Siscovick DS, et al. Association of prior infection with *Chlamydia pneumoniae* and angiographically demonstrated coronary artery disease. JAMA. 1992;268:68–72.
399. Campbell LA, O'Brien ER, Cappuccio AL, et al. Detection of *Chlamydia pneumoniae* (TWAR) in human coronary atherectomy tissues. J Infect Dis. 1995;172:585–588.
400. Gupta S, Leatham EW, Carrington D, et al. Elevated *Chlamydia pneumoniae* antibodies, cardiovascular events and azithromycin in male survivors of myocardial infarction. Circulation. 1997;96:404–407.
401. Gurfinkel E, Bozovich G, Daroca A, et al. for the Roxis study group. Randomized trial of roxithromycin in non-Q-wave coronary syndromes: Roxis pilot study. Lancet. 1997;350:404–407.
402. Sawyer LA, Fishbein DB, McDale JE. Q fever: Current concepts. Rev Infect Dis. 1987;9:935–946.
403. Tack KJ, Peterson PK, Rasp FL, et al. Isolation of *Chlamydia trachomatis* from the lower respiratory tracts of adults. Lancet. 1980;1:116–120.
404. Komaroff AL, Aronson MD, Schachter J. *Chlamydia trachomatis* infections in adults with community acquired pneumonia. JAMA. 1981;245:1319–1322.
405. Wenzel RP, McCormick DP, Beam WE Jr. Parainfluenza pneumonia in adults. JAMA. 1972;221:294–295.
406. Falsey AR, Cunningham CK, Baber WH, et al. Respiratory syncytial virus and influenza A infections in the hospitalized elderly. J Infect Dis. 1995;172:389–394.
407. Englund JA, Sullivan CJ, Jordan MC, et al. Respiratory syncytial virus infections in immunocompromised adults. Ann Intern Med. 1988;109:203–208.
408. Harrington RD, Hooton TM, Hackman RC, et al. An outbreak of respiratory syncytial virus in a bone marrow transplant center. J Infect Dis. 1992;165:987–993.
409. Dowell SF, Anderson LJ, Gary HE Jr, et al. Respiratory syncytial virus is an important cause of community-acquired lower respiratory infection among hospitalized adults. J Infect Dis. 1996;174:456–462.
410. Greenberg SH. Viral pneumonia. Infect Dis Clin North Am. 1991;5:603–621.
411. Ruben FL, Nguyen MLT. Viral pneumonitis. Clin Chest Med. 1991;12:223–235.
412. Duchin JS, Koster FT, Peters CJ, et al. Hantavirus pulmonary syndrome: A clinical description of 17 patients with a newly recognized disease. N Engl J Med. 1994;330(14):949–955.
413. Jenison S, Hjelle BM, Simpson S, et al. Hantavirus pulmonary syndrome: Clinical, diagnostic and virologic aspects. Semin Respir Infect. 1995;10:259–269.
414. Rello J, Quintana E, Ausiner V, et al. A three-year study of severe community-acquired pneumonia with emphasis on outcome. Chest. 1993;103:232–235.
415. Leeper KV Jr, Torres A. Community-acquired pneumonia in the intensive care unit. Clin Chest Med. 1995;16:155–171.
416. Stout JE, Yu VL. Legionellosis. N Engl J Med. 1997;337:682–687.
417. Marston BJ, Lipman HB, Breiman RF. Surveillance for legionnaire's disease. Risk factors for morbidity and mortality. Arch Intern Med. 1994;154:2417–2422.
418. Cunha BA, Ortega AM. Atypical pneumonia. Postgrad Med. 1996;99:123–132.
419. Keller DW, Lipman HB, Marston BJ, et al. Clinical diagnosis of legionnaires disease (LD) using a multivariable model. Abstract K55. Presented at 35th Interscience Conference on Antimicrobial Agents and Chemotherapy. San Francisco, September 1995.
420. Sopena N, Sabria-Leal M, Pedro-Botet ML, et al. Comparative study of the clinical presentation of legionella pneumonia and other community-acquired pneumonias. Chest. 1998;113:1195–1200.
421. Matthay MA, Rosen GD. Acid aspiration induced lung injury: New insights and therapeutic options. Am J Respir Crit Care Med. 1996;154:277–278.
422. Robinovici R, Neville LF, Abdullah F, et al. Aspiration-induced lung injury: Role of complement. Crit Care Med. 1995;23:1405–1411.
423. Bartlett JG, Gorbach SL. The triple threat of aspiration pneumonia. Chest. 1979;68:560–566.
424. Wynne JW, Modell JH. Respiratory aspiration of stomach contents. Ann Intern Med. 1977;87:466–474.
425. Hammond JMJ, Potgieter PD, Hanslo D, et al. The etiology and antimicrobial susceptibility patterns of microorganisms in acute community-acquired lung abscess. Chest. 1995;108:937–941.
426. Finegold SM. Aspiration pneumonia. Rev Infect Dis. 1991;13(Suppl 9):S737–S742.
427. Lorber B, Swenson RM. Bacteriology of aspiration pneumonia: A prospective study of community and hospital-acquired cases. Ann Intern Med. 1974;81: 329–331.
428. Finegold SM. Aspiration pneumonia. Rev Infect Dis. 1991;13(Suppl 9):S737–S742.

429. Ludmerer KM, Kissare JM. Pulmonary infiltrates and eosinophilia in a young man. Am J Med. 1986;81:533–540.
430. Chemopathologic conference. Respiratory failure and eosinophilia in a young man. Am J Med. 1993;94:533–542.
431. Lanham JG, Elkon KB, Pusey CD, et al. A clinical approach to the Churg-Strauss syndrome. Medicine. 1984;63:65–81.
432. Allen JN, Davis WB. What is eosinophilic pneumonia. Arch Intern Med. 1992;152:1765–1766.
433. Schatz M, Wasserman S, Patterson R. Eosinophils and immunologic lung disease. Med Clin North Am. 1981;65:1055–1071.
434. Weber RW. Adverse drug effects and the spectrum of eosinophilic pulmonary disorders. Ann Allergy Asthma Immunol. 1995;74:451–453.
435. Fleury-Feith J, Van Nhieu JT, Picard L, et al. Bronchoalveolar lavage eosinophilia associated with *Pneumocystis carinii* pneumoritis in AIDS patients. Chest. 1989;95:1198–1201.
436. Pope-Harman AL, Davis WB, Allen ED. Acute eosinophilic pneumonia: A summary of 15 cases and a review of the literature. Medicine. 1996;75:334–342.
437. Cheon JE, Soo Lee K, Sik Jung G. Acute eosinophilic pneumonia: Radiographic and CT findings in six patients. AJR. 1996;167:1195–1199.
438. King MA, Pope-Harman AL, Allen JN. Acute eosinophilic pneumonia: Radiologic and clinical features. Radiology. 1997;203:715–719.
439. Citro LA, Gordon ME, Miller WT. Eosinophilic lung disease (or how to slice P.I.E.). AJR. 1973;117:787–797.
440. Liebow AA, Carrington CB. The eosinophilic pneumonias. Medicine. 1969;48:251–285.
441. Jederlinic PJ, Sicilian L, Graensler EA. Chronic eosinophilic pneumonia. Medicine. 1988;67:154–162.
442. Marchand E, Reynand-Gaubert M, Lauque D, et al. Idiopathic chronic eosinophilic pneumonia. Medicine. 1998;77:299–312.
443. Marshall BG, Wilkinson RJ, Davidson RN. Pathogenesis of tropical pulmonary eosinophilia, parasitic alveolitis, and parallels with asthma. Respir Med. 1998;92:1–3.
444. Kim Y, Soo Lee K, Choi DL, et al. The spectrum of eosinophilic lung disease: Radiographic findings. J Comput Assist Tomogr. 1997;21:920–930.
445. Haley RW, Culver DH, White JW, et al. The nationwide nosocomial infection rate: A new need for vital statistics. Am J Epidemiol. 1985;121:159–167.
446. Simmons BP, Wong ES. CDC guidelines for the prevention and control of nosocomial infections: Guideline for prevention of nosocomial pneumonia. Am J Infect Control. 1983;11:230–233.
447. Scheld WM, Mandell GL. Nosocomial pneumonia: Pathogenesis and recent advances in diagnosis and therapy. Rev Infect Dis. 1991;13(Suppl 9):S743–S751.
448. Torres A, Aznar R, Gatell JM, et al. Incidence of risk and prognosis of nosocomial pneumonia in mechanically ventilated patients. Am Rev Respir Dis. 1990;142: 523–528.
449. McEachern R, Campbell GD Jr. Hospital-acquired pneumonia: Epidemiology, etiology, and treatment. Infect Dis Clin North Am. 1998;12:761–779.
450. Fagon JY, Chastre J, Hance AJ, et al. Nosocomial pneumonia in ventilated patients: A cohort study evaluating attributable mortality and hospital stay. Am J Med. 1993;94:281–288.
451. Wenzel RP. Hospital-acquired pneumonia: An overview of the current state of the art for prevention and control. Eur J Clin Microbiol Infect Dis. 1989;8:56–60.
452. American Thoracic Society. Hospital-acquired pneumonia in adults: Diagnosis, assessment of severity, initial antimicrobial therapy, and prevention strategies. Am J Respir Crit Care Med. 1996;153:1711–1725.
453. Rouby JL, Laurent P, Gosnach M, et al. Risk factors and clinical relevance of nosocomial maxillary sinusitis in the critically ill. Am J Respir Crit Care Med. 1994;150:776–783.
454. George DL. Epidemiology of nosocomial pneumonia in intensive care unit patients. Clin Chest Med. 1995;16:29–44.
455. Craven DE, Steger KA. Epidemiology of nosocomial pneumonia: New perspectives on an old disease. Chest. 1995;108(2 Suppl):1S–16S.
456. Donowitz LG, Page MC, Mileur BL, et al. Alteration of normal gastric flora in critical care patients receiving antacid and cimetidine therapy. Infect Control. 1986;7:23–26.
457. Snepar R, Poporad GA, Romano JM, et al. Effect of cimetidine and antacid on gastric microbial flora. Infect Immun. 1982;36:518–524.
458. Driks MR, Craven DE, Celli BR, et al. Nosocomial pneumonia in intubated patients given sucralfate as compared with antacids or histamine type-2 blockers. The role of gastric colonization. N Engl J Med. 1987;317:1376–1382.
459. Cook DJ, Laine LA, Guyatt GH, et al. Nosocomial pneumonia and the role of gastric pH: A beta analysis. Chest. 1991;100:7–13.
460. Craven DE, Steger KA, Barber TW. Preventing nosocomial pneumonia: State of the art and perspective for the 1990s. Am J Med. 1991:91(Suppl 3B):44S–53S.
461. Simms HH, DeMoria E, McDonald L, et al. Role of gastric colonization in the development of pneumonia in critically ill trauma patients: Results of a prospective randomized trail. J Trauma. 1991;31:531–537.
462. Bonten MJM, Gaillard CA, deLeeuw PW, Stobberingh EE. Role of colonization of the upper intestinal tract in the pathogenesis of ventilator-associated pneumonia. Clin Infect Dis. 1997;24:309–319.
463. Rello J, Quintana E, Ausina V, et al. Risk factors for *Staphylococcus aureus* nosocomial pneumonia in critically ill patients. Am Rev Respir Dis. 1990;142:1320–1324.
464. Rello J, Ausina V, Castella J, et al. Incidence, etiology and outcome of nosocomial pneumonia in mechanically ventilated patients. Chest. 1991;100:439–444.
465. Septimus EJ. Nosocomial bacterial pneumonia. Semin Respir Infect. 1989;4: 245–252.
466. A'Court C, Garrard CS. Nosocomial pneumonia in the intensive care unit: Mechanism and significance. Thorax. 1992;47:465–473.
467. Bartlett JG, O'Keefe P, Tally FP, et al. Bacteriology of hospital-acquired pneumonia. Arch Intern Med. 1986;146:868–871.
468. Nguyen MH, Stout JE, Yu VL. Legionellosis. Infect Dis Clin North Am. 1991;5:561–584.
469. Carratala J, Guidol F, Pallares J, et al. Risk factors for nosocomial *Legionella pneumophila* pneumonia. Am J Respir Crit Care Med. 1994;149:625–629.
470. Graman PS, Hall CB. Nosocomial viral respiratory infections. Semin Respir Infect. 1989;4:253–260.
471. Holladay RC, Campbell GD Jr. Nosocomial viral pneumonia in the intensive care unit. Clin Chest Med. 1995;16:121–133.
472. Fagen JY, Chastre JY, Hance AJ, et al. Evaluation of clinical judgement in the identification and treatment of nosocomial pneumonia in ventilated patients. Chest. 1993;103:547–553.
473. Chastre J, Fagen JY. Invasive diagnostic testing should be routinely used to manage ventilated patients with suspected pneumonia. Am J Respir Crit Care Med. 1994;150:570–574.
474. Niederman MS, Torres A, Sumner W. Invasive diagnostic testing is not needed routinely to manage suspected ventilator-associated pneumonia. Am J Respir Crit Care Med. 1994;150:565–569.
475. Niederman MS, Peters SP. Update in pulmonary medicine. Ann Intern Med. 1998;128:208–215.
476. National Center for Health Statistics National Hospital Discharge Survey Annual Summary. 1990 Vital Health Stat. 1992;13:1–225.
477. Fine MJ, Hough LJ, Medsger AR, et al. The hospital admission decision for patients with community-acquired pneumonia: Results from the pneumonia patient outcomes research team cohort study. Arch Intern Med. 1997;157:36–44.
478. Black ER, Mushlin AI, Griner PF, et al. Predicting the need for hospitalization of ambulatory patients with pneumonia. J Gen Intern Med. 1991;6:394–400.
479. Fine MJ, Smith DN, Singer DE. Hospitalization decision on patients with community-acquired pneumonia: A prospective cohort study. Am J Med. 1990;89: 713–721.
480. Fine MJ, Auble TE, Yealy DM, et al. A prediction rule to identify low risk patients with community-acquired pneumonia. N Engl J Med. 1997;336:1248–1250.
481. Atlas SJ, Benzer TI, Borowsky LH, et al. Safely increasing the proportion of patients with community-acquired pneumonia treated as outpatients: An interventional trial. Arch Intern Med. 1998;158:1350–1356.
482. Porath A, Schlaeffer F, Lieberman D. Appropriateness of hospitalization of patients with community-acquired pneumonia. Ann Emerg Med. 1996;27:176–183.
483. Schmidt LN, Sesler CL. Development of resistance to penicillin by pneumococci. Proc Soc Exp Biol Med. 1943;52:353–357.
484. Klugman PK. Pneumococcal resistance to antibiotics. Clin Microbiol Rev. 1990;3:171–176.
485. Spika JS, Facklam RR, Rlikaytis BD, et al. Antimicrobial resistance to *Streptococcus pneumoniae* in the United States. 1979–1987. J Infect Dis. 1991;163:1273–1278.
486. Thornsberry C, Brown SD, Yee YC, et al. Increasing penicillin resistance in *Streptococcus pneumoniae* in the U.S. Effect on susceptibility to oral cephalosporins. Infect Med. 1993;10(Suppl D):15–24.
487. Doern GV, Brueggemann A, Holley HP Jr, et al. Antimicrobial resistance to *Streptococcus pneumoniae* recovered from outpatients in the United States during the winter months of 1994–1995: Results of a 30-center national surveillance study. Antimicob Agents Chemother. 1996;40:1208–1213.
488. Thornsberry C, Ogilvie P, Kahn J, et al. Surveillance of antimicrobial resistance in *Streptococcus pneumoniae, Haemophilus influenzae* and *Moraxella catarrhalis* in the United States in 1996–1997 Respiratory Season. Diagn Microbial Infect Dis. 1997;29:249–257.
489. Klugman KP, Feldman C. The clinical relevance of antibiotic resistance in the management of pneumococcal pneumonia. Infect Dis Clin Pract. 1998;7:180–184.
490. Pallares R, Liñares J, Vadillo M, et al. Resistance to penicillin and cephalosporin and mortality from severe pneumococcal pneumonia in Barcelona Spain. N Engl J Med. 1995;333:474–480.
491. Craig WA. Antimicrobial resistance issues of the future. Diagn Microbiol Infect Dis. 1996;25:213–217.
492. Low DE. Resistance issues and treatment implications: Pneumococcus, *Staphylococcus aureus,* and gram-negative rods. Infect Dis Clin North Am. 1998;12: 613–630.
493. Strachan SA, Friedland IR. Therapy for penicillin-resistant *Streptococcus pneumoniae.* J Med Microbiol. 1995;43:237–238.
494. Liñares J, Alonso T, Perez JL. Decreased susceptibility of penicillin-resistant pneumococci to twenty-four β-lactam antibiotics. J Antimicrob Chemother. 1992;30:279–288.
495. Haas DW, Stratton CW, Griffin JP, et al. Diminished activity of ceftizoxime in comparison to cefotaxime and ceftriaxone agents.
496. Barry AL, Brown SD, Novick WJ. In vitro activities of cefotaxime, ceftriaxone, ceftazidime, cefpirome, and penicillin against *Streptococcus pneumoniae* isolates. Antimicrob Agents Chemother. 1995;39:2193–2196.
497. Butler JC, Hofmann J, Cetron MS, et al. The continued emergence of drug-resistant *Streptococcus pneumoniae* in the United States: An update from the Centers for Disease Control and Prevention's Pneumococcal Sentinel Surveillance System. J Infect Dis. 1996;174:986–993.
498. Simor AE, Louie M, Low DE. The Canadian Bacterial Surveillance Network.

Canadian national survey of prevalence of antimicrobial resistance among clinical isolates of *Streptococcus pneumoniae.* Antimicrob Agents Chemother. 1996;40:2190–2193.

499. Thornburn CE, Knott SJ, Edwards DI. In vitro activities of oral β-lactams at concentrations achieved in humans against penicillin-susceptible and resistant pneumococci and potential to select resistance. Antimicrob Agents Chemother. 1998;42:1973–1979.
500. Donowitz GR, Brandon ML, Salisbury JP, et al. Sparfloxacin versus cefaclor in the treatment of patients with community-acquired pneumonia: A randomized, double-masked comparative multicenter study. Clin Thera. 1997;19:936–953.
501. File TM Jr, Segreti J, Dunbor L, et al. A multicenter, randomized study comparing the efficacy and safety of intravenous and/or oral levofloxacin versus ceftriaxone and/or cefuroxime treatment of adults with community-acquired pneumonia. Antimicrob Agents Chemther. 1997;41:1965–1972.
502. Adams M, Sullivan J, Henry D, et al. Comparison of grepafloxacin with cefaclor in the treatment of community-acquired pneumonia. Abstract LM-68. In: 37th ICAAC Toronto, Ontario, Canada. Sept 26-Oct 1, 1997.
503. Aubier M, Verster R, Regamy C, et al. Once-daily Sparfloxacin versus high-dosage amoxicillin in the treatment of community-acquired suspected pneumococcal pneumonia in adults. Clin Infect Dis. 1998;26:1312–1320.
504. Gleason PP, Kapoor WN, Stone RA, et al. Medical outcomes and antimicrobial costs with the use of the American Thoracic Society guidelines for outpatients with community-acquired pneumonia. JAMA. 1997;278:32–39.
505. Donowitz GR, Mandell GL. Beta-lactam antibiotics (parts 1 and 2). N Engl J Med. 1988;318:419–426, 490–500.
506. Craig WA, Andes D. Aminoglycosides are useful for severe respiratory tract infections. Semin Respir Infect. 1997;12:271–277.
507. Schentag JJ, Birmingham MC, Paladins JA, et al. Nosocomial pneumonia, optimizing antibiotics other than aminoglycosides is a more important determinant of successful clinical outcome and a better means of avoiding resistance. Semin Respir Infect. 1997;12:278–293.
508. Halm EA, Fine MJ, Marrie TJ, et al. Time to clinical stability in patients hospitalized with community-acquired pneumonia: Implication for practice guidelines. JAMA. 1998;279:1452–1457.
509. Hitt CM, Nightingale CH, Quintiianc R, Nicolau DP. Streamlining antimicrobial therapy for lower respiratory tract infections. Clin Infect Dis. 1997;24(Suppl 2):5231–5237.
510. Ramirez JA, Srinath L, Ahkee S, et al. Early switch from intravenous to oral cephalosporins in the treatment of hospitalized patients with community-acquired pneumonia. Arch Intern Med. 1995;155:1273–1276.
511. Ramirez JA. Switch therapy in community-acquired pneumonia. Diagn Microbiol Infect Dis. 1995;22:219–223.
512. Siegel RE, Halpern NA, Almenoff PL, et al. A prospective randomized study of inpatient IV antibiotics for community-acquired pneumonia: The optimal duration of therapy. Chest. 1996;110:965–971.
513. Chan R, Hemeryck L, O'Regan M, et al. Oral versus intravenous antibiotics for community-acquired lower respiratory tract infection in a general hospital, open, randomized controlled trial. BMJ. 1995;310:1360–1362.
514. Thornsberry C, Hickey ML, Diakun DR, et al. Sequential surveillance of antimicrobial resistance in the United States: *Streptococcus pneumoniae, Haemophilus influenzae,* and *Moraxella catarrhalis* (1997–1998 US 1996–1997) Abstract 22. Presented at 38th Interscience Conference in Antimicrobial Agents and Chemotherapy. September 24–27, 1998, San Diego, Calif.

Chapter 58

Pleural Effusion and Empyema

RICHARD E. BRYANT
CHRISTOPHER J. SALMON

Pleural empyema is a complex disease with a poor prognosis if the diagnosis is missed or if antimicrobial therapy or drainage is inadequate.[1–3] Recent developments in diagnostic imaging have greatly facilitated the recognition and management of this disease,[4–8] and scientific and technical advances have enhanced our understanding of its pathophysiology and appropriate therapy.[9–16] Microbial infection of the pleural space is usually secondary to pneumonia (56%) but may arise from extrapulmonic infection and follow surgery (22%), trauma (4%), esophageal perforation (4%), thoracentesis or chest tube placement (4%), subdiaphragmatic infection (3%), septicemia (1%), or, less commonly, other procedures or diseases.[17–22] The mode of presentation is modified by the origin of the infection, the infecting microorganisms, and the patient's underlying disease or diseases.

ETIOLOGY

Medical and societal changes have modified the types of organisms causing empyema.[1–3] In otherwise healthy adults with pneumonia, the most common bacteria causing pleural empyema are *Staphylococcus aureus, Streptococcus pneumoniae,* or *Streptococcus pyogenes.*[1, 7] Empyema caused by *Staph. aureus, Strep. pneumoniae,* or *Haemophilus influenzae* has been common in children.[23] The new conjugate vaccine has dramatically reduced the frequency of suppurative complications of *H. influenzae* infection in children.

The increased recognition of anaerobic empyema reflects improved microbiologic techniques and recognition of anaerobic infection associated with aspiration pneumonia, putrid lung abscess, and pleural infection arising from oropharyngeal or gastrointestinal sites.[24, 25] Bartlett and Finegold found that pleural empyema was caused by aerobic bacteria in 24%, anaerobic bacteria in 35%, and both aerobic and anaerobic bacteria in 41% of 83 medical service patients without prior antibiotic therapy or surgical procedures.[24] Ferguson and coworkers found malodorous empyema fluid in 62% of patients but grew anaerobes from only half of those specimens.[26] Recent studies suggest that anaerobic infection may occur in 25 to 33% of children with empyema.[27] Pleural infection secondary to subdiaphragmatic disease is often polymicrobial and anaerobic in origin.[28]

There is a high frequency of *Staph. aureus* and aerobic gram-negative bacillary infection in patients with empyema following trauma or surgery.[29, 30] Empyema complicating hemothorax is often staphylococcal, whereas that associated with pneumothorax or serous effusion is often caused by gram-negative aerobic bacilli. Microorganisms gain access to the pleura by direct extension from the lung or from blood or lymphatics; by extension from subdiaphragmatic, mediastinal, pericardial, or cervical infection; and by transthoracic entry from trauma, surgery, or manipulative procedures. Patients with trauma to the esophagus, mediastinum, or heart or those who have had surgery in those areas are at increased risk of infection extending to the pleura. Similarly, patients with retropharyngeal, vertebral, or paravertebral suppurative disease may present with pleural empyema. As the efficiency of trauma rescue programs increases, the frequency of empyema associated with chest and head trauma will increase. Immunocompromised patients have a higher frequency of empyema caused by fungi and gram-negative bacilli.[17, 21, 30] Organ transplant recipients and patients with the acquired immunodeficiency syndrome may reactivate pleural foci of mycobacterial or fungal infection but rarely present with empyema without disseminated disease. Unsuccessful resection of cavitary coccidioidomycosis may be complicated by empyema from that organism. The association of fistulous tracts from the pleura suggests the possibility of actinomycosis, nocardiosis, or tuberculosis. Less common causes of empyema include extension of subdiaphragmatic infections caused by *Salmonella, Clostridia,* or *Entamoeba histolytica.*

Inflammatory exudates may become loculated in a relatively small area or may extend to involve virtually the entire hemithorax, leading to ventilatory dysfunction and to the signs and symptoms of overwhelming sepsis and multiple organ failure. The exuberant inflammatory response can occasionally erode the chest wall, causing spontaneous drainage of the empyema (empyema necessitatis).

By convention, the phases of empyema formation are divided into the *exudative phase,* during which leukocyte accumulation causes the formation of pus; the *fibropurulent phase,* during which fibrin formation begins to limit expansion of the lung; and the *organizing phase,* during which fibroblast formation and scarring produce a thick, leathery encasement that traps the lung.[31] Early diagnosis and prompt intervention can prevent the development of more advanced disease but require a high index of suspicion for the presence of empyema and an appreciation of the subtleties of its presentation.

PATHOPHYSIOLOGY

Pleural effusions may be caused by altered oncotic or capillary pressure from renal, cardiac, hepatic, or metabolic diseases. Pleural effusions may occur in 40 to 50% of patients with pneumonia.[32] However, only 5% or less of parapneumonic effusions develop features of empyema.[1] Pleural fluid is readily infected. Neutrophils are dysfunctional in early phases of pleural infection because empyema fluid is deficient in the opsonins and complement needed for optimal phagocytic function and ultimately develops extremes of hypoxia and acidity that further impair local neutrophil activity.[33, 34] In addition, surface phagocytosis is impaired in pleural fluid.[35] Likewise, neutrophil lysozomal substances such as defensins, bactericidal permeability-increasing protein, lysozyme, cationic proteins, and high concentrations of zinc-binding proteins in pus may suppress bacterial growth and thereby suppress bacterial susceptibility to antibiotics. Endotoxins and other toxic factors elaborated by bacteria impair host defenses and permit the growth of microbes to concentrations of 10^8 bacteria per milliliter of empyema fluid.[36] Despite the elegance and complexity of the cytokine cascade and leukocyte host defense functions, the purulent environment becomes maladaptive and contributes to the refractory nature of pleural suppurative infection by inhibiting antimicrobial efficacy. The abscess environment suppresses the bacterial growth rate and secondarily suppresses antibiotic uptake and bactericidal activity in pleural fluid. Bacterial growth in suppurative environments may be slowed by 24- to 72-fold with a proportional reduction in the bacterial death rate after exposure to antibiotics.[37] The mechanisms by which this occurs are poorly understood but may reflect a downregulation of penicillin-binding proteins as organisms enter a stagnant phase of growth.[38] This may partially explain the requirements for prolonged antibiotic therapy of inadequately drained suppurative infections. Likewise, it explains the universally appreciated benefits of abscess or empyema drainage wherein the noxious inflammatory products and antibiotic-refractory bacteria are removed expeditiously.

The acid pH of abscess fluid adversely affects aminoglycoside activity because aminoglycoside uptake by bacteria is inhibited by acidic environments. Similarly, the increased concentration of magnesium, binding of aminoglycosides to the DNA in pus, and suppressive effect of hypoxia on membrane transport of aminoglycosides inhibit the activity of aminoglycosides in pus.[39, 40] β-Lactamase from microorganisms can degrade β-lactamase–susceptible β-lactam antibiotics, and chloramphenicol may be degraded by microbial enzymes in pus.[36]

EXPERIMENTAL EMPYEMA

Microbe-specific factors affect the pathophysiology of pleural space infection but are not easily identified experimentally because animal models lack many of the features of human disease. The induction of experimental empyema in guinea pigs requires the inoculation of more than 10^6 *Escherichia coli,* or *Staph. aureus* plus *Bacteriodes fragilis,* in order to infect more than 50% of animals.[41] The use of umbilical tape as a foreign body does not increase lethality, but the addition of blood greatly enhances the lethality of challenge with *E. coli* and *B. fragilis* mixtures.[41]

Rabbit models of pleural infection produced by inoculating *Strep. pneumoniae* or *Klebsiella pneumoniae* into a turpentine-induced chemical pleuritis heal spontaneously.[42] Streptokinase injection reduced the incidence of pleural adhesion in that model but increased the volume of pleural effusion that accumulated.[43] Studies with turpentine-induced *K. pneumoniae* empyema showed 60% cure rates of animals treated with gentamicin but 100% cure rates when gentamicin was used in conjunction with hyperbaric oxygen.[44] Those studies validate both the adverse effect of pus on gentamicin activity and the suboptimal performance of gentamicin as single drug therapy for empyema.

A rabbit model of *Pasteurella multocida* empyema was used to assess the effect of delayed pleural drainage on the course of pleural infection.[45] As anticipated, there was a significant reduction in the amount of pleural peel and pleural pus in animals with chest tubes placed within 24 to 48 hours when compared with animals with chest tubes placed after 72 hours.[45]

PRESENTATION OF EMPYEMA

Clinical Features

The clinical presentation of empyema is largely nonspecific and reflects the findings of pleural fluid accumulation and uncontrolled infection. Patients may have chest pain, dyspnea, weight loss, chills, fever, or night sweats.[1–3] The development or persistence of fever and leukocytosis, despite appropriate antibiotic therapy in a patient at risk of empyema, is a common clue to its presence. Physical examination often reveals only signs of an effusion with altered vital signs. It is unusual to demonstrate loculated pleural fluid on physical examination. A high index of suspicion and recognition of factors that predispose patients to the development of pleural empyema

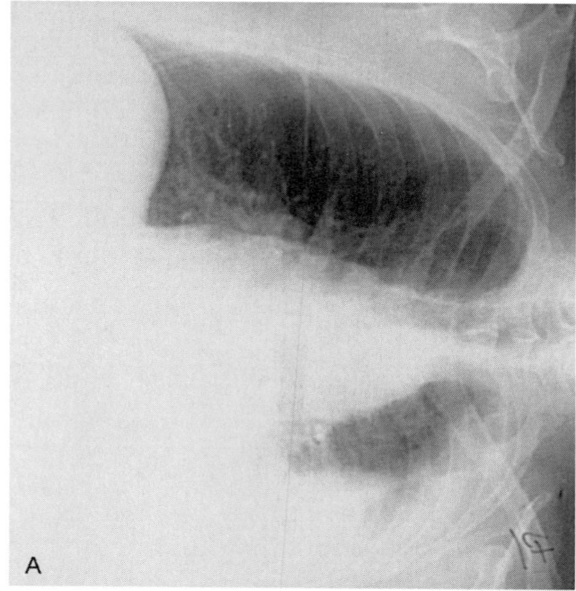

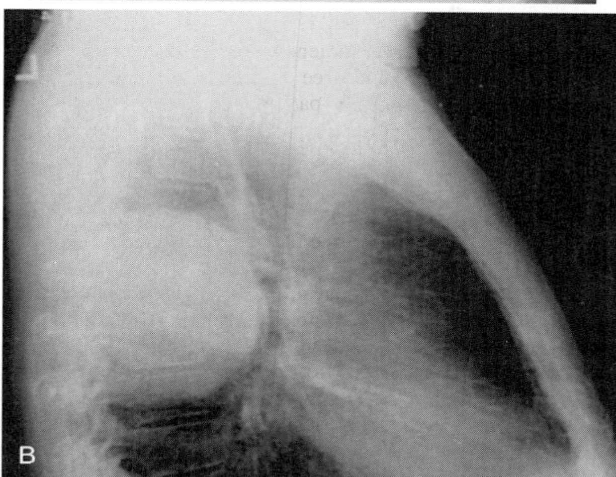

FIGURE 58–1. *A,* Empyema fluid is shown layering out along the dependent chest wall of a patient with left lower lobe pneumonia. *B,* D-shaped mass representing a loculated empyema at the site of a former right upper lobectomy.

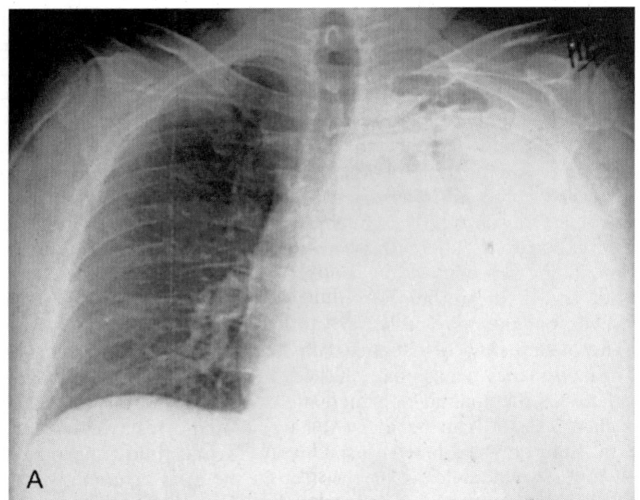

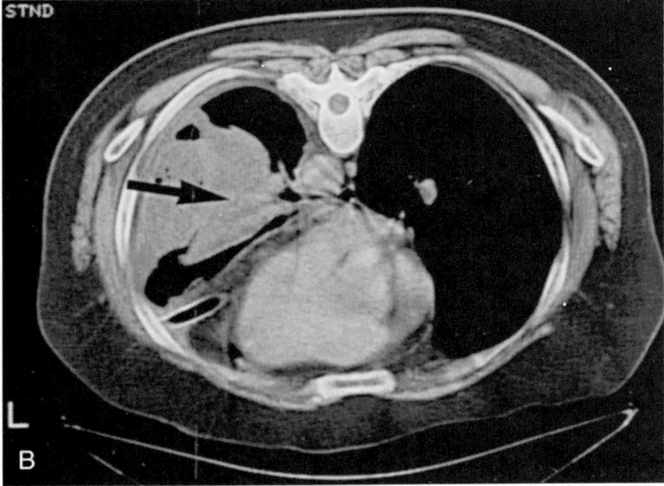

FIGURE 58–2. *A,* The patient's empyema progressed despite percutaneous drainage and appropriate antibiotic therapy. *B,* Computed tomography showed malposition of chest tubes, but all attempts at tube drainage failed. The *arrow* indicates the loculated empyema. The patient responded promptly to surgical decortication.

facilitate its recognition. The urgency of treatment is linked to the severity of infection and the degree of host defense deficits, because the sickest and most susceptible patients have the greatest need for rapid definitive therapy.[22, 46, 47]

Radiologic Features

The chest radiograph is usually the first imaging study demonstrating pleural disease (Fig. 58–1). As little as 25 ml of pleural fluid may alter the hemidiaphragm on a chest radiograph, but posterior costophrenic angle blunting requires effusion of at least 200 ml. Dependent, decubitus views of the chest with the affected side down may demonstrate layering of 5 to 10 ml of freely flowing fluid.[48] The disease-side-up decubitus view may facilitate better recognition of the extent of pulmonary disease. With extensive adjacent pulmonary consolidation and intrapleural loculations, the radiographic assessment of pleural collections becomes more difficult.

Ultrasonography provides a convenient method for thoracentesis or drainage catheter placement that can be transported to the bedside of critically ill patients. Its use decreases the incidence of pneumothorax after thoracentesis.[49, 50] Pleural collections vary in appearance from echo-free to very echogenic. Highly echogenic empyemas may mimic consolidated lung or pulmonary abscess.[51] Ultrasonography can distinguish solid from liquid pleural abnormalities with 92% accuracy, compared with 68% accuracy of chest radiography. When ultrasonography and the chest radiograph are used together, their combined accuracy rises to 98%.[52] Unlike consolidated lung or abscess, pleural fluid varies in sonographic configuration during the respiratory cycle. Ultrasonography may reveal fluid bronchograms in areas of consolidated lung to allow differentiation from empyema.[53]

Septations can be found by ultrasonography in up to 74% of intrapleural exudates,[54] even when they are invisible by computed tomography (CT). The presence of these septations has prognostic significance because loculated pleural collections require drainage and are usually larger than unloculated collections.[55]

CT has greatly improved the assessment of empyemas that appear round, ovoid, or crescent-shaped and are smoothly marginated (Fig. 58–2). The margins are formed by the inflamed and thickened visceral and parietal layers that enhance with intravenous contrast material and are separated by the interposed empyema fluid, giving rise to the *split pleura sign* of empyema.[56] The extrapleural or subcostal fat between the inflamed parietal pleura and internal surface of the ribs is shown by CT to increase in size in both acute and chronic empyema (Fig. 58–3). Plain radiography cannot distinguish this fatty hyperplasia from pleural thickening or effusion.

Lung abscess may mimic empyema, or empyema may coexist with adjacent pneumonia or lung abscess, which may be impossible to distinguish by clinical and radiographic means.[51] Fortunately, contrast-enhanced CT usually allows definitive diagnosis. Lung abscesses tend to be poorly defined, roughly spherical, and surrounded by irregularly consolidated lung. They often contain one or more cavities with shaggy margins. Because they are nearly spherical, peripheral lung abscesses usually form acute angles with the adjacent chest wall. Since they arise within and occupy consolidated lung, they rarely appear to displace pulmonary airways and vessels the way empyemas do. Empyemas may form acute or obtuse angles with the adjacent chest wall, but they have other distinguishing features on the CT examinations cited previously.[57]

Laboratory Diagnosis

Empyema is documented by finding pus or high concentrations of microorganisms, or both, in exudative pleural fluid obtained by thoracentesis. The character of the fluid depends on the type and duration of the infection and the associated trauma, surgery, malignancy, or other underlying disease. Initially, the fluid is thin and serous but becomes thick and purulent as neutrophil accumulation

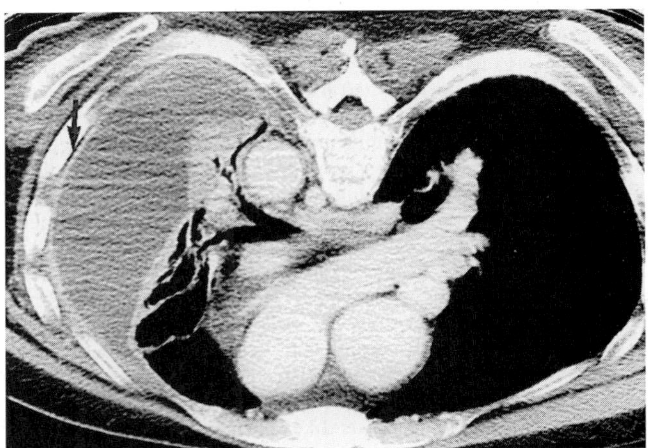

FIGURE 58–3. The *arrow* points to the "clear" area of fat hypertrophy between the pleural peel and inner margin of the rib.

occurs. The poor correlation between the white blood cell counts in empyema fluid and the clinical features of infection may reflect the lysis of neutrophils in pus. Frankly purulent specimens require only smear, culture, and drainage after demonstration by Gram's stain that bacteria are present. Less overtly purulent specimens should be assessed for pH, glucose levels, and lactic dehydrogenase levels in addition to appropriate smears and cultures.[1–3, 32] Empyema fluid characteristically has a pH of less than 7.2, glucose level less than 40 mg/dl, and lactic dehydrogenase activity of at least 1000 IU/liter. Demonstration of these features or the presence of large numbers of bacteria on Gram's stain indicates that drainage procedures are probably necessary. The pH of empyema fluid has the best correlation with the extent of the inflammatory process. Acid pH is primarily metabolic in origin but affected by local CO_2 retention. It is important to keep pleural fluid specimens tightly capped and on ice to prevent spurious changes in pH or glucose levels.[32] The mean lactic acid concentration of pus from human abscesses is 30 mg/dl, and pH values may be as low as 5.5. Empyema fluid pH values of 6 to 6.7 or lower may be associated with esophageal rupture—a condition with a mortality of at least 50% when treatment is delayed more than 24 hours.[32] Urgent intervention with the measurement of empyema fluid amylase levels, CT, a barium swallow, or endoscopic procedures may be required to direct therapy. Chronic abscesses or empyema may have comparably low pH values, but acute infection should not. Systemic acidosis may secondarily lower pleural fluid pH. Pleural fluid pH levels of at least 0.30 below arterial pH levels support the need for chest tube drainage.[32] At the other extreme, frankly purulent empyema fluid can have a disproportionately high pH when infection is caused by urea-splitting *Proteus* strains.[58] Empyema caused by anaerobic bacteria is malodorous in approximately 60% of instances.[59] Less specific findings of empyema fluid include a protein concentration of greater than 3.0 mg/dl and a specific gravity of greater than 1.018.

Microorganisms in empyema fluid can usually be seen on Gram's stain and grown in culture unless patients have received antibiotic therapy. Occasionally, smears are positive and cultures are negative. In some instances, the bacterial origin is clarified by cultures of blood, polymerase chain reaction testing, or the demonstration of *Legionella* antigen in urine. When the diagnosis is in question, pleural fluid can be tested for *Legionella* by direct fluorescent antibody stains and culture, because that organism will not be seen on conventional Gram's stains. Disseminated histoplasmosis can be diagnosed by antigen detection in serum or urine.[60] Empyema fluid devoid of microorganisms should also be examined for anaerobes, fungi, mycobacteria, or amoebae when appropriate. Approximately 98% of patients with pleural of pulmonary amebiasis have positive serologic tests for *E. histolytica*.[61] Those patients should have careful assessment for hepatic abscesses, which are almost always present. Pleural pus from patients at risk of developing nocardiosis should have modified acid-fast stains. Acridine orange may permit the visualization of organisms in abscess fluid that is smear-negative by Gram's stain. It should be noted that chylous pleural effusions may resemble purulent material but lack white cells or microorganisms and remain opaque after centrifugation. Empyema associated with systemic and pleural fluid eosinophilia is a rare condition that is highly suggestive of paragonimiasis. It can be confirmed serologically or by demonstrating eggs in stool, sputum, or, rarely, pleural fluid.[62]

Potts and coworkers found no bacteria on microscopic examination of 4 of 10 empyema fluids.[9] Two were sterile by culture. Smear-negative sterile empyema fluid has been reported in 6 to 15% of patients, and culture-negative empyema has been described in up to 33% of patients.[19] Although improper culture technique, fastidious microorganisms, and prior antibiotic therapy may account for many cases of sterile empyema, it is likely that certain organisms are killed in pus. However, frankly purulent empyemas must be drained, whether sterile or not.

Pleural tuberculosis may be diagnosed by pleural fluid stains in 18 to 23% of patients or by cultures and stains of pleural fluid or by histologic examination of pleural biopsy specimens in up to 95% of patients.[63] Liquid culture media are preferable to solid culture media.[64] It is rarely necessary to culture more than a single biopsy specimen. Radiometric culture detection and polymerase chain reaction methods may increase the speed and specificity of diagnosis in patients with pleural tuberculosis. Elevated levels of adenosine deaminase or tuberculostearic acid are indicative of tuberculous pleuritis but are not currently available in the United States. Increased risk of exposure to tuberculosis, host defense defects favoring reactivation, skin test conversion, or symptoms of weight loss, night sweats, and fever are helpful clues to the diagnosis of tuberculosis. However, patients may be both afebrile and anergic.

The pleural fluid of patients with rheumatoid arthritis, pancreatitis, or malignancy occasionally has features suggestive of empyema.[1] Exudates of rheumatoid or pancreatic origin only rarely have a pH less than 7.2 and can be identified by serologic tests or increased pleural fluid amylase levels, respectively. Pleural fluid from patients with lupus erythematosus or rheumatoid pleuritis characteristically have titers of antinuclear antibody of at least 1:160 or rheumatoid factor of at least 1:320, respectively, with values exceeding those found in serum.[65, 66] The rare malignant effusion with a pH of less than 7 is readily diagnosed by cytologic examination and is associated with a worse prognosis than that of alkaline malignant effusion.[67]

TREATMENT (Table 58–1)

Drainage

The goals of treatment for pleural empyema are the eradication of infection, drainage of pus, and expansion of the lung. The primary treatment of empyema is drainage, and this is necessary for patients with pleural fluid containing gross pus, which is usually characterized by a heavy growth of organisms visible by microscopy, a pH less than 7.2, glucose levels less than 40 mg/dl, and lactic dehydrogenase levels greater than 1000 IU/liter.[1–3] Those with smear-negative serous pleural fluid and a pH of at least 7.2 and intermediate lactic dehydrogenase and glucose levels may be treated with antibiotics and repeat thoracentesis in 12 to 18 hours to reassess the need for drainage procedures.[32] Those with improving pleural fluid parameters may be followed and reassessed. However, pleural fluid loculation indicates the presence of a complex parapneumonic process usually requiring more aggressive intervention with CT-guided tube drainage or thoracoscopy.[1, 32]

Light has described useful criteria for approaching parapneumonic effusions and empyema.[1] Effusions are categorized by the extent of purulence and the degree of complexity. Parapneumonic collections that move freely and are less than 1 cm in width, as measured on a lateral decubitus chest radiograph, can usually be managed medically and do not require fluid aspiration if the patient is doing well and there is radiographic improvement.[15, 22, 23] Patients with greater evidence of suppuration require more aggressive intervention. The pleural fluid character and location need to be documented promptly. Tube drainage is reserved for smear-positive collections or those with overt purulence or loculation indicating the need for thrombolytic therapy.

Repeated thoracentesis is rarely adequate unless the empyema fluid is quite thin and present in a small volume. Percutaneous drainage of thin or serous fluid with small-bore catheters early in the course of empyema has been successful. Closed chest tube drainage without thrombolytic therapy is successful in two thirds of patients, and the system can be placed by the surgeon, the radiologist, or the pulmonologist.[68, 69] Ferguson and associates found that medical therapy was successful in 80% of patients whose empyema occupied 20% or less of their hemithorax but in only 24% of those with empyema occupying 40% or more of their hemithorax.[26] Several reports support an expanded role for the interventional radiologist in

TABLE 58-1 Classification and Treatment of Suspected Empyema

Classification	Indices of Pleural Infection							Therapy and Procedures					
	pH	*Glucose (mg/dl)*	*LDH (IU/l)*	*Gram Stain +*	*Culture Growth*	*Frank Pus*	*Loculated Fluid*	*Antibiotics*	*Needle Aspiration*	*Tube Drainage*	*Urokinase Thrombolysis*	*VATS*	*Full Decortication*
Parapneumonic effusion	>7.2	>40	<1000	−	−	−	−	+	+[R]				
Parapneumonic exudate													
Minimally complex	≥7.2	>40	<1000	−	−	−	−	+	+[R]				
Moderately complex	≤7.2	<40	>1000	±	±	−	−	+	+	+	±[R]		
Extremely complex	≤7.0	<40	>1000	±	±	−	+	+	+	+	±[R*]	±*	
Empyema													
Not complex	NN	NN	NN	±	±	+	±	+	+	+	±[R*]	±*	
Complex	NN	NN	NN	±	±	+	+	+	+				

Free-flowing effusions less than 1 cm in width on lateral decubitus radiographs may not require aspiration.

Diagnostic and therapeutic interventions are based on the extent and severity of the inflammatory response and on the measures required to adequately drain pleural pus and to expand the lung.

*More aggressive intervention is required for extensive or complex disease that fails to respond to therapy.

Abbreviations: Gram stain +, Bacteria seen on Gram stain; LDH, lactic (acid) dehydrogenase; NN, not necessary to test; R, repeat as needed; VATS, video-assisted thoracoscopy; +, yes; −, no; ±, possibly.

Approach modified from Light RW. Parapneumonic effusions and empyema. In: Light RW, ed. Pleural Disease. 3rd ed. Baltimore: Williams & Wilkins; 1995;129–153.

the management of thoracic empyema.[70–74] Imaging guidance allows the precise placement of smaller-bore catheters (usually 15- to 16-French) into small pockets of unusual configuration previously considered inaccessible by tube thoracostomy alone. These tubes can be placed safely, with much less patient discomfort and morbidity and, with proper management, are at least as efficacious as 28-French or larger surgical tubes.[73–75] They do require periodic flushing and daily bedside assessment by the physician to maintain optimal patency and function.[71] For the occasional collection of very viscous pus, a catheter up to 24-French can be placed by a modified Seldinger technique.[8] The more traditional blind, bedside drainage of empyema by tube thoracostomy done only with reference to the chest radiograph is often unsuccessful, with a substantial proportion of patients needing further invasive treatment.[17, 26, 76] Relatively high morbidity, and mortality as high as 5%, have been reported.[22]

CT is the modality of choice for pleural empyema diagnosis and management, facilitating catheter placement and monitoring of the response to therapy. Percutaneous catheter placement can be done by direct trocar puncture or a modified Seldinger technique.[70, 74, 75] After tube placement and pus aspiration, the space is irrigated with sterile saline and the tube attached to a standard underwater-seal drainage system for continuous suction.

Pleural loculations form during the development of either complex parapneumonic effusions or empyemas,[1] indicating that the effusion has progressed to the fibropurulent stage with deposition of detectable quantities of fibrin on the pleural surfaces. Fibroblast ingrowth and fibrosis ensue rapidly unless the collections are evacuated and appropriate antibiotics given. Fibrin deposition enhances the development of subsequent fibrosis by creating a diffusional barrier to oxygen, since pleural fluid hypoxia and lactic acidosis have been shown to promote fibroblast collagen production.[43] These findings support the urgency of empyema drainage to prevent intrapleural fibrosis, which often requires surgical extirpation, and provide a rationale for therapies directed at the prevention of deposition and the removal of intrapleural fibrin early in the course of an empyema. The act of placing a catheter over a guide wire helps to break down at least some loculations, but additional measures may be required to achieve complete drainage. Repeated guide wire manipulations may be attempted or multiple catheters employed if urokinase therapy fails.[4, 70, 74, 75]

Enzymatic Therapy

Patients failing to respond to tube drainage within 24 hours should receive intrapleural urokinase therapy. Urokinase is nonantigenic and nonpyrogenic.[12–14, 77] Although "purified" forms of streptokinase are now available,[78] these may cause fever due to an antibody response, and this may falsely suggest the persistence of infection.

We favor intrapleural urokinase instillation by methods similar to those described.[13, 14] Each dose consists of 125,000 units given in 50 to 100 ml of 0.9% sterile saline solution. This is left in place for at least 2 hours. The patient may be moved into different positions to fully distribute the enzyme throughout the collection. The catheter or chest tube is then "unclamped" and suction restored. This process can be repeated as needed. Unused portions of the urokinase solution should be refrigerated. Although it is possible to give urokinase by transmural injection into an indwelling large surgical chest tube, it is more efficiently introduced by stopcock through a radiologically placed pleural drainage catheter. Catheter use ensures that the agent reaches and stays within the pleural collection.

Interval assessment of the response to urokinase therapy is usually best achieved by CT scans, which can be performed quickly and without contrast media for comparison with previous studies.[79] Pleural space manipulation with a soft guide wire may be done through the catheter and be repositioned as needed. Urokinase therapy usually obviates the need for multiple chest tubes. Some empyemas may require three instillations per day for 2 or more days to achieve complete drainage.

Thrombolytic therapy of empyema is reported to be successful in 69 to 92% of patients but is more likely to fail when used to treat advanced disease.[26, 79–81] Its successful use in 19 patients with human immunodeficiency virus infection was attributed to the early initiation of thrombolysis, which obviated the need for surgery despite a high frequency of virulent pathogens and a 31% incidence of bronchopleural fistula.[82]

The use of urokinase in the pleural space is safe. The total dose in the pleural space is only about one tenth that given intravascularly to lyse clots, and urokinase has an average serum half-life of about 20 minutes. The presence of a bronchopleural fistula is considered by some authors to be an absolute contraindication to intrapleural urokinase use.[12, 13]

The need for continued vacuum or water-sealed drainage is assessed by measuring the volume of fluid drained daily and by the size of the residual pleural cavity. Tubes can usually be withdrawn when the drainage is less than 50 ml/day and the cavity is less than 50 ml.[68]

Other Surgical Procedures

Empyema that fails to respond to chest tube drainage and thrombolytic therapy is largely the province of the chest surgeon, who should be involved early in the course of disease.[68] Immunocompromised patients may require more extensive drainage procedures, including early rib resection and open drainage.[10, 83–85] The management of open drainage tubes with daily irrigation and convalescence for 3 to 4 months is a tedious and time-consuming but time-honored method. In young adults who are otherwise healthy and are good operative candidates, video-assisted thoracoscopy (VATS) or decortication may be preferable.[86]

VATS is a significant new alternative for the treatment of multiloculated empyema refractory to urokinase therapy.[86–88] It is a less invasive procedure that permits the lysis of adhesion under direct thoracoscopic control and clear assessment of the need for a more extensive procedure, that is, decortication.[86–89] The efficacy and cost effectiveness of VATS has been shown by a number of reports with one randomized trial documenting shorter hospitalization associated with its use.[87] VATS also offers a better cosmetic alternative and lower morbidity than full thoracotomy.

Decortication may provide more rapid recovery and more complete restoration of pulmonary function in adults with complex empyema but is needed less frequently in children.[1, 85, 89] The control of infection is a primary indication for early VATS or decortication. Thoracotomy and decortication is traditionally advocated during the second or third week or after the sixth week of the disease in order to minimize the risk of tearing the poorly demarcated pleural peel during the 3 to 6 weeks of illness. The importance of surgical timing for the thoracotomy decortication has been questioned.[90]

Although small bronchopleural fistulas may close spontaneously, many are difficult to treat and require surgical closure. There is considerable variation in the frequency with which surgeons at different centers use rib resection, decortication, or empyectomy to manage empyema.[89, 91] Similarly, several methods are used to treat chronic empyema or empyema that occurs after pneumonectomy. These operative approaches are selected on the basis of expected benefits and risks. Tube drainage has the fewest side effects, is tried first, and is rarely successful in that setting. Alternatives include permanent drainage, obliteration of the empyema space by muscle flaps, sterilization by the instillation of antibiotics, and thoracoplasty.[92] The open window thoracostomy procedure devised by Eloesser was adapted to manage postpneumonectomy empyema. It can be used as permanent therapy for patients unable to undergo more extensive surgery.[89, 92] Patients with bronchopleural fistulas that do not close with tube drainage are often treated successfully with muscle flap transposition by suturing the muscle directly to the bronchus or adjacent to the closed bronchial stump and using the muscle mass to obliterate the empyema cavity.[92] Patients with empyema and residual lung after partial resection who do not have bronchopleural fistulas may respond to decortication or, if that fails, to myoplasty. Thoracoplasty is usually the procedure of last resort.[92]

Antimicrobial Therapy

Tuberculous pleural effusions rarely require more than antibiotic therapy unless a bronchopleural fistula is present. Special care should be taken not to introduce a secondary bacterial infection while performing a diagnostic or therapeutic thoracentesis of a tuberculous pleural effusion.

The guidelines for optimal antibiotic therapy of bacterial empyema differ little from the recommendations for the treatment of suppurative disease at other sites. Antibiotics are selected on the basis of their activity against microorganisms causing infection. It is unnecessary to administer antibiotics directly into the pleural space. Adequate levels of antibiotics are easily achieved in empyema fluid. β-Lactam antibiotics should be used in adequate doses 2 to 4 weeks for nontuberculous bacterial infections. A 2-week course is most appropriate for patients with good drainage and rapid clinical response. Patients with nocardiosis, actinomycosis, tuberculosis, or fungal empyema require even more prolonged therapy. In addition, patients with long-standing bacterial empyema may require prolonged therapy. Aminoglycosides should not be used as single-drug therapy of bacterial empyemas because they are toxic drugs with poor activity in the abscess milieu.[34] However, aminoglycosides may be combined with β-lactam antibiotics to achieve a synergistic activity against empyema caused by *Pseudomonas aeruginosa, Enterobacter cloacae, Acinetobacter calcoaceticus,* or *Serratia marcescens.*[40] Until more information is available, empyema caused by these multiresistant organisms should be treated initially with at least two effective antibiotics. Fluoroquinolones provide a less nephrotoxic alternative for concomitant or protracted therapy of empyema caused by those organisms.

Anaerobic pleural empyema can be treated adequately with clindamycin, carbapenems like imipenem or meropenem, or combinations of β-lactams and β-lactamase inhibitors. Although metronidazole is an excellent agent for anaerobic infection, it may be ineffective in anaerobic lung abscesses or partially drained empyemas because the drug is not reduced to its active metabolite in a partially oxygenated environment. Furthermore, it has poor activity against streptococci and actinomycetes. Chloramphenicol or tetracyclines are not sufficiently effective to be used to treat empyema caused by anaerobes.

PROGNOSIS

The mortality rate of pleural empyema is affected by the type and severity of infection, the patient's health or associated underlying diseases, and the adequacy of antibiotic therapy and drainage. Although mortality rates of 8 to 15% have been reported in otherwise healthy young patients,[82, 86] rates of 40 to 70% have been reported in elderly persons and in groups with severe underlying disease.[85, 91] Mortality is increased in patients with nosocomial infection or empyema caused by polymicrobial or resistant gram-negative bacteria.[32] Patients with inadequately drained empyemas often die.[24] There are no criteria validating the superiority of a single technique, but in general, the more fragile or compromised patient may need more rapid achievement of adequate drainage by whatever means. If tube drainage and urokinase infusion are unsuccessful, VAT drainage may prove to be a better-tolerated, efficacious alternative than the more traditional decortication. Adequate drainage early in the illness of patients who are vulnerable to the serious sequelae of malnutrition or chronic sepsis may avoid multiple organ failure associated with the delayed drainage of pus.[91] The adverse effect of delayed diagnosis and treatment is suggested by the report that the average duration of illness before admission was 4.8 days for children with empyema cured with antibiotics alone, 5.8 days for those requiring chest tubes, and 8 days for those requiring decortication.[93] None of the children with scoliosis due to empyema were cured medically, and 63% required decortication.[93]

Post-traumatic empyema has a worse prognosis and should be considered for early decortication if (1) sepsis is not contained despite adequate antibiotic therapy, (2) fluid levels persist, (3) ventilatory function is compromised by inadequate lung expansion, or (4) pleural drainage is inadequate after 2 weeks of therapy.[29, 91] An infected hemothorax rarely responds to tube drainage alone because clots obstruct the tube but may respond to urokinase infusion.[80] Polymicrobial or nosocomial infection carries a worse prognosis because such patients have multiple underlying diseases and poor host defenses.[30, 85] In addition, these patients have an increased frequency of colonization and infection with multiply resistant gram-negative bacilli.[30] Thus, the sickest and most infirm patients often have pus that is hard to drain and organisms that are difficult to treat.

REFERENCES

1. Light RW. Parapneumonic effusions and empyema. In: Light RW, ed. Pleural Diseases. 3rd ed. Baltimore: Williams & Wilkins; 1995:129–153.
2. Sahn SA. Management of complicated parapneumonic effusions. Rev Respir Dis. 1993;148:813–817.
3. Bryant RE, Salmon CJ. Pleural empyema. Clin Infect Dis. 1996;22:747–764.
4. O'Moore PV, Mueller PR, Simeone F. Sonographic guidance in diagnostic and therapeutic interventions in the pleural space. AJR. 1987;149:1–5.
5. Mirvis SE, Tobin KD, Kostrubiak I, et al. Thoracic CT in detecting occult disease in critically ill patients. AJR. 1987;148:685–689.
6. Van Sonnenberg E, Nakamoto SK, Mueller PR, et al. CT and ultrasound guided catheter drainage of empyemas after chest-tube failure. Radiology. 1984;151:349–353.
7. Yang PC, Luh KT, Chang DB, et al. Value of sonography in determining the nature of pleural effusion: Analysis of 320 cases. AJR. 1992;159:29–33.
8. Boland GW, Lee Mj, Silverman S, Mueller PR. Interventional radiology of the pleural space. Clin Radiol. 1995;50:205–214.
9. Potts DE, Levin DC, Sahn SA. Pleural fluid pH in parapneumonic effusions. Chest. 1976;70:328–331.
10. Houston MC. Pleural fluid pH: Diagnostic, therapeutic, and prognostic value. Am J Surg. 1987;154:333–337.
11. Poe RH, Marin MG, Israel RH, et al. Utility of pleural fluid analysis in predicting tube thoracostomy/decortication in parapneumonic effusions. Chest. 1991;100: 963–967.
12. Lee KS, Im J-G, Kim YH, et al. Treatment of thoracic multiloculated empyemas with intracavitary urokinase: A prospective study. Radiology. 1991;179:771–775.
13. Moulton JS, Moore PT, Mencini RA. Treatment of loculated pleural effusions with transcatheter intracavitary urokinase. AJR. 1989;153:941–945.
14. Robinson LA, Moulton AL, Fleming WH, et al. Intrapleural fibrinolytic treatment of multiloculated thoracic empyemas. Ann Thorac Surg. 1994;57:803–814.
15. Kaiser LR, Shrager JB. Video-assisted thoracic surgery: The current state of the art. AJR. 1995;165:1111–1117.
16. O'Brien J, Cohen M, Solit R, et al. Thoracoscopic drainage and decortication as definitive treatment for empyema thoracis following penetrating chest injury. J Trauma. 1994;36:536–540.
17. Varkey B, Rose HD, Kutty CPK, Politis J. Empyema thoracis during a ten-year period: Analysis of 72 cases and comparison to a previous study (1952 to 1967). Arch Intern Med. 1981;141:1771–1776.
18. Weese WC, Shindler ER, Smith IM, et al. Empyema of the thorax then and now. Arch Intern Med. 1973;131:516–520.
19. Yeh TJ, Hall DP, Ellison RG. Empyema thoracis: A review. Am Rev Respir Dis. 1963;88:785–790.
20. Snider GL, Saleh SS. Empyema of the thorax in adults; Review of 105 cases. Dis Chest. 1968;54:410–415.
21. Smith JA, Mullerworth MH, Westlake GW, Tatoulis J. Empyema thoracis: A 14-year experience in a teaching center. Ann Thorac Surg. 1991;51:39–42.
22. Sherman MM, Subramanian V, Berger RL. Management of thoracic empyema. Am J Surg. 1977;133:474–479.
23. Freij BJ, Kusmiesz H, Nelson JD, McCracken GH. Parapneumonic effusions and empyema in hospitalized children. A retrospective review of 227 cases. Pediatr Infect Dis. 1984;3:578–591.
24. Bartlett JG, Finegold SM. Anaerobic infections of the lung and pleural space. Am Rev Respir Dis. 1974;110:56–77.
25. Bartlett JG, Gorbach SL, Thadepalli H, Finegold SM. Bacteriology of empyema. Lancet. 1974;1:338–340.
26. Ferguson AD, Prescott RJ, Selkon JB, et al. The clinical course and management of thorasic empyema. Q J Med. 1996;89:285–289.
27. Brook I. Microbiology of empyema in children. Pediatrics. 1990;85:722–726.
28. Ballantyne KC, Sethia B, Reece IJ, et al. Empyema following intra-abdominal sepsis. Br J Surg. 1984;71:723–725.

29. Caplan ES, Hoyt NJ, Rodriguez A, et al. Empyema occurring in the multiply traumatized patient. J Trauma. 1984;24:785–798.
30. Vianna NJ. Nontuberculous bacterial empyema in patients with and without underlying disease. JAMA. 1971;215:69–71.
31. Andrews NC, Parker EF, Shaw RP, et al. Management of nontuberculous empyema. Am Rev Respir Dis. 1962;85:935–936.
32. Light RW. Management of empyema. Semin Respir Med. 1992;13:167–176.
33. Lew P, Zubler R, Vaudauz P. Decreased heat-labile opsonic activity and complement levels associated with evidence of C3 breakdown products in infected pleural effusions. J Clin Invest. 1979;63:326–334.
34. Bryant RE. Pus: Friend or foe? In: Root RK, Trunkey DD, Sande MA, eds. Contemporary Issues in Infectious Diseases, v. 6. New Surgical and Medical Approaches. New York: Churchill Livingstone; 1987:31–48.
35. Wood WB Jr, Smith MR, Watson B. Studies on the mechanism of recovery in pneumonoccal pneumonia. IV. The mechanism of phagocytosis in the absence of antibody. J Exp Med. 1946;84:387–402.
36. Bryant RE. Effect of the suppurative environment on antibiotic activity. In: Root RK, Sand MD, eds. Contemporary Issues in Infectious Diseases, v. 1: New Dimensions in Antimicrobial Therapy. New York: Churchill Livingstone; 1984;313–337.
37. Zak O, Sande MA. Correlation of the in vitro antimicrobial activity of antibiotics with results of treatment in experimental animal models and human infection. In: Sabath LD, ed. Action of Antibiotics in Patients. Bern, Switzerland: Hans Huber; 1992:55–67.
38. Stevens DL, Yan S, Bryant AE. Penicillin-bind protein expression at different growth stages determines penicillin-binding protein efficacy in vitro and in vivo: An explanation of the inoculum effect. J Infect Dis. 1993;167:1401–1405.
39. Vaudau P, Waldvogel RA. Gentamicin inactivation in purulent exudates: Role of cell lysis. J Infect Dis. 1980;142:586–593.
40. Bryant RE, Fox KE, Oh G, Morthland VH. β-Lactam enhancement of aminoglycoside activity under conditions of reduced pH and oxygen tension that may exist in infected tissues. J Infect Dis. 1992;165:676–682.
41. Mavroudis C, Ganzel BL, Cox SK, Polk HC Jr. Experimental aerobic-anaerobic thoracic empyema in the guinea pig. Ann Thorac Surg. 1987;43:298–302.
42. Sahn SA, Taryle DA, Good JT Jr. Experimental empyema: Time course and pathogenesis of pleural fluid acidosis and low pleural fluid glucose. Am Rev Respir. 1979;120:355–361.
43. Strange C, Tomlinson JR, Wilson C, et al. The histology of experimental pleural injury with teracycline, empyema, and carrageenan. Exp Mol Pathol. 1989;51: 205–219.
44. Shohet I, Yellin A, Meyerovitch J, et al. Pharmacokinetics and therapeutic efficacy of gentamicin in an experimental pleural empyema rabbit model. Antimicrob Agents Chemother. 1987;31:982–985.
45. Sasse S, Nguygen TK, Mulligan M, et al. The effect of early chest tube placement on empyema resolution. Chest. 1997;111:1679–1683.
46. Pothula V, Krellenstein DJ. Early aggressive surgical management of parapneumonic empyemas. Chest. 1994;105:832–836.
47. Cham CW, Haq SM, Rahamim J. Empyema thoracis: A problem with late referral? Thorax. 1993;48:925–927.
48. Moskowitz H, Platt RT, Schachar R, Mellins H. Roentgen visualization of minute pleural effusion: An experimental study to determine the minimum amount of pleural fluid visible on a radiograph. Radiology. 1973;109:33–35.
49. Seneff MG, Corwin RW, Gold LH, Irwin RS. Complications associated with thoracentesis. Chest. 1986;90:97–110.
50. Harnsberger HR, Lee TG, Mukono DH. Rapid, inexpensive real-time directed thoracentesis. Radiology. 1983;146:545–546.
51. Landay MJ, Conrad MR. Lung abscess mimicking empyema on ultrasonography. AJR. 1979;133:731–734.
52. Lipscombe DJ, Flower CDR, Hadfield JW. Ultrasound of the pleura: An assessment of its clinical value. Clin Radiol. 1981;32:289–290.
53. Doren HL. Differentiation of pulmonary parenchymal consolidation from pleural disease using the sonographic fluid bronchogram. Radiology. 1986;158:41–42.
54. Hirsch JH, Rogers JV, Mack LA. Real-time sonography of pleural opacities. AJR. 1981;136:297–301.
55. Lee MJ, Saini S. Brink JA, et al. Interventional radiology of the pleural space: Management of thoracic empyema with image-guided catheter drainage. Semin Intervent Radiol. 1991;8:29–35.
56. Stark DD, Federle MP, Goodman PC, Podrasky AE, Webb WR. Differentiating lung abscess and empyema: Radiography and computed tomography. AJR. 1983;141:163–167.
57. Salmon CJ, Bryant RE. Pleural effusion and empyema. In: Mandell GL, Simberkoff, eds. Atlas of Infectious Diseases, v. VI: Pleuropulmonary and Bronchial Infections. Philadelphia: Churchill Livingstone; 1996;9.1–9.20.
58. Pine JR, Hollman JL. Elevated pleural fluid pH in *Proteus mirabilis* empyema. Chest. 1983;84:109–111.
59. Sullivan KM, O'Toole RD, Fisher RH, Sullivan KN. Anaerobic empyema thoracis: The role of anaerobes in 226 cases of culture-proven empyemas. Arch Intern Med. 1973;131:521–527.
60. Wheat LJ, Connolly-Stringfield PA, Baker RL, et al. Disseminated histoplasmosis in the acquired immune deficiency syndrome: Clinical findings, diagnosis, and treatment, and review of the literature. Medicine (Baltimore). 1990;69:361–374.
61. Adams EB, MacLeod IN. Invasive amebiasis. I. Amebic dysentery and its complications. Medicine (Baltimore). 1977;56:315–323.
62. Skerrett SJ, Plorde JJ. Parasitic infections of the pleural space. Semin Respir Med. 1992;13:242–258.
63. Levine H, Metzger W, Lacera D, et al. Diagnosis of tuberculous pleurisy by culture of pleural biopsy specimen. Arch Intern Med. 1970;126:269–271.
64. Wichelhausen RH, McLean RL, Lowrey FB. Reinforcement of diagnostic value of pleural biopsy by culture in liquid medium. Am Rev Respir Dis. 1996;92:288–290.
65. Halla JT, Schrohenloher RE, Valanakis JE, et al. Immune complexes and other features of pleural effusions. Ann Intern Med. 1980;92:748–752.
66. Good JT Jr, King TE, Antony VB, et al. Lupus pleuritis: Clinical features and pleural fluid characteristics with special reference to pleural fluid antinuclear antibodies. Chest. 1983;84:714–718.
67. Good JA, Taryle DA, Maulitz RM, et al. The diagnostic value of pleural fluid pH. Chest. 1980;78:55–59.
68. Miller KS, Sahn SA. Chest tubes. Chest. 1987;91:258–264.
69. Hutter JA, Harari D, Braimbridge MV. The management of empyema thoracis by thoracoscopy and irrigation. Ann Thorac Surg. 1985;39:517–520.
70. Merriam MA, Cronan JJ, Dorgman GS, et al. Radiographically guided percutaneous catheter drainage of pleural fluid collections. AJR. 1988;151:1113–1116.
71. Goldberg MA, Mueller PR, Saini S, et al. Importance of daily rounds by the radiologist after interventional procedures of the abdomen and chest. Radiology. 1991;180:767–770.
72. Stavas J, van Sonneberg E, Casola G, Wittich GR. Percutaneous drainage of infected and noninfected thoracic fluid collections. J Thorac Imaging. 1987;2:80–87.
73. Kerr A, Vasudevan VP, Powell S, Ligenza C. Percutaneous catheter drainage for acute empyema: Improved cure rate using CAT scan, fluoroscopy, and pigtail drainage catheters. N Y State J Med. 1991;91:4–7.
74. Silverman SG, Mueller PR, Saini S, et al. Thoracic empyema: Management with image-guided catheter drainage. Radiology. 1988;169:5–9.
75. Hunnam GR, Flower CDR. Radiologically-guided percutaneous catheter drainage of empyemas. Clin Radiol. 1998;39:121–126.
76. Light RW. Parapneumonic effusions and empyema. Clin Chest Med 1985;6:55–62.
77. Lahorra JM, Haaga JR, Stellato T, et al. Safety of intracavitary urokinase with percutaneous abscess drainage. AJR. 1993;160:171–174.
78. Taylor RFH, Rubens MB, Pearson MC, Barnes NC. Intrapleural streptokinase in the management of empyema. Thorax. 1994;49:856–859.
79. Roupie E, Bouabdallah K, Delclaux C, et al. Intrapleural administration of streptokinase in complicated purulent pleural effusion: A CT-guided strategy. Intensive Care Med. 1996;22:1351–1353.
80. Jerjes-Sanchez C, Ramirez-Rivera A, Elizalde JJ, et al. Intrapleural fibrinolytics with streptokinase as an adjunctive treatment in hemothorax and empyema. Chest. 1996;109:1514–1519.
81. Temes RT, Folles F, Kessler RM, et al. Intrapleural fibrinolytics in management of empyema thoracis. Chest. 1996;110:102–106.
82. Borge JH, Michavila IA, Mendez JM, et al. Thoracic empyema in HIV infected patients. Chest. 1998;113:732–738.
83. Himelman RB, Callen PW. The prognostic value of loculations in parapneumonic pleural effusions. Chest. 1986;90:852–856.
84. Storm HKR, Krasnik M, Bang K, Fridmodt-Moller N. Treatment of pleural empyema secondary to pneumonia: Thoracentesis regimen versus tube drainage. Thorax. 1992;47:821–824.
85. Mandal AK, Thadepalli H. Treatment of spontaneous bacterial empyema thoracis. J Thorac Cardiovasc Surg. 1987;94:414–418.
86. Landreneau RJ, Keenan RJ, Hazelrigg SR, et al. Thoracoscopy for empyema and hemothorax. Chest. 1995;1995:18–24.
87. Wait MA, Sharma S, Hohn J, Nogare AD. A randomized trial of empyema. Chest. 1997;111:1548–1551.
88. Lawrence DR, Ohri SK, Moxon RE, et al. Thoracoscopic debridement of empyema thoracis. Ann Thorac Surg. 1997;64:1448–1450.
89. Mayo P. Early thoracotomy and decortication for nontuberculous empyema in adults with and without underlying diseases. Am Surg. 1985;4:230–236.
90. Hoover EL, Hsu H-K, Ross MJ, et al. Reappraisal of empyema thoracis. Chest. 1986;90:511–515.
91. Lemmer JH, Botham MJ, Orringer MD. Modern management of adult thoracic empyema. J Thorac Cardiovasc Surg. 1985;90:849–855.
92. Le Roux BT, Mohlala ML, Odell JA, et al. Suppurative diseases of the lung and pleural space. Part 1. Empyema thoracis and lung abscess. Curr Probl Surg. 1986;23:4–38.
93. Hoff SJ, Neblett WW, Edwards KM, et al. Parapneumonic empyema in children: Decortication hastens recovery in patients with severe pleural infections. Pediatr Infect Dis J. 1991;10:194–199.

Chapter 59

Lung Abscess

SYDNEY M. FINEGOLD

Lung abscess is a suppurative pulmonary infection involving the destruction of lung parenchyma to produce one or more large cavities with an air-fluid level. A similar process with multiple small cavitations (less than 2 cm in diameter) has been designated *necrotizing pneumonia* by some clinicians. The distinction is arbitrary since lung abscess and necrotizing pneumonia are different expressions of the same fundamental pathologic process. The earliest manifestation of this type of problem is pneumonia without excavation or abscess formation. In the absence of effective therapy, the disease may progress to lung abscess or to necrotizing pneumonia, with or without pleural empyema. Generally, the specific infecting organisms and the predisposing conditions do not influence the type of clinical disease that results as much as the size of the inoculum of organisms and the defense mechanisms of the host. Most often lung abscess follows aspiration, and anaerobic bacteria have been the major organisms involved. The spectrum of organisms causing lung abscess has widened, however, as patients present with more complex medical and surgical conditions.

PREDISPOSING CAUSES

By far the most important background factor for abscess of the lung is aspiration,[1] usually related to altered consciousness. Common causes of altered consciousness in such patients are alcoholism, cerebral vascular accident, general anesthesia, drug overdose or addiction, seizure disorder, diabetic coma, shock, and other serious illness. Other factors in aspiration include dysphagia due to either esophageal disease or neurologic disease, intestinal obstruction, tonsillectomy or tooth extraction, mechanical interference with the cardiac sphincter caused by nasogastric tubes, and endotracheal intubation. A study by Huxley and associates using a sensitive radioactive tracer technique determined that 70% of patients with depressed consciousness and 45% of healthy subjects in deep sleep aspirated.[2] Aspiration occurred more frequently and extensively in patients with depressed consciousness. Impairment of normal clearance mechanisms or the overwhelming of such mechanisms by large volumes of aspirated secretions may result in pulmonary infection. Alcoholic patients and patients who are acutely or chronically ill (whether or not they are hospitalized or in a nursing home) often demonstrate oropharyngeal colonization with gram-negative bacilli, particularly if they undergo endotracheal intubation and especially if they also receive histamine type 2 blockers or antacids.[3, 4]

Next to aspiration, the most important factor predisposing to lung abscess or to necrotizing pneumonia is periodontal disease or gingivitis. Lung abscess is rare in an edentulous person and suggests the possibility of an associated bronchogenic carcinoma.[5] Other underlying processes include bronchiectasis, secondary infection of a bland pulmonary embolus with infarction, septic embolization, bacteremia, inhalation of bacteria-containing aerosols, and intra-abdominal infection. Suppurative inflammation behind an obstruction in a bronchus is another important mechanism. Other conditions that may play a role include diabetes mellitus, malignancy, acquired immunodeficiency disease, and other immunocompromising conditions. Patients receiving immunosuppressive therapy may develop multiple lung abscesses due to *Nocardia* or other organisms.

PATHOGENESIS AND PATHOLOGIC CHARACTERISTICS

Lung abscess is primarily of endogenous origin. Most of the bacteria involved are elements of the normal flora of the upper respiratory tract. Infections involving *Staphylococcus aureus, Klebsiella,* and other organisms may be of nosocomial origin.

The primary site of lung abscess is the posterior segment of the right upper lobe, with the same segment on the left less commonly affected. Next in frequency of involvement are the apical segments of the lower lobes. These segments are dependent when the subject is in a horizontal position, and the localization relates to the fact that aspiration or inhalation is the primary background factor. Normally, aspirated material is handled effectively by ciliary action, cough, and alveolar macrophages. If the protective mechanisms are not effective, as with ethanol ingestion or viral disease, infection may result. Endotracheal tubes impair coughing, impede pulmonary clearance mechanisms, and allow leakage of oropharyngeal secretions into the tracheobronchial tree. Thick or particulate matter and foreign bodies are not easily removed and thus may lead to bronchial obstruction and atelectasis. With aspiration, gastric acid and enzymes may be the primary offending agents.

Subdiaphragmatic infection may extend to the lung or to the pleural space by way of lymphatics, directly through the diaphragm or defects in it, or by way of the blood stream. Most amebic lung abscesses are located in the right lower lobe adjacent to the diaphragm since they typically arise by direct extension of hepatic abscesses through the diaphragm.

Infection may arise in or behind an obstruction (neoplasm, foreign body, or enlarged mediastinal lymph node). Septic emboli from bacterial endocarditis of the right side of the heart or from pelvic or other deep vein thrombophlebitis may result in a metastatic lung abscess.

Although the virulence of the infecting organism or organisms may be a factor determining the nature and extent of the infectious process, this is not usually important in the case of the anaerobes except for *Fusobacterium necrophorum.* Certain other anaerobes, especially *Fusobacterium nucleatum,* the *Bacteroides fragilis* group, and *Clostridium perfringens,* are more likely to be present as the sole infecting organism, an indication of virulence. The number of organisms aspirated is probably an important factor. Anaerobic counts in oral flora are lower than usual in edentulous subjects and higher in patients with periodontal disease. With certain of the nonanaerobes such as *Klebsiella, Staphylococcus,* and group A streptococci, virulence may play an important role.

The pathologic characteristic is essentially that of necrosis supervened on inflammation with cavitation and abscess formation. The abscess cavity may become partially lined with regenerated epithelium, and localized bronchiectasis and emphysema may develop. There is usually no significant vascular involvement in lung abscess. However, a septic or bland pulmonary embolus may be the initial event. Once under way, the infection itself may give rise to pulmonary arteritis as in infection caused by *Pseudomonas aeruginosa.*

CLINICAL MANIFESTATIONS

Anaerobic Lung Abscess

In patients with lung abscess admitted to a hospital, symptoms have generally been present for at least 2 weeks. At times, the patient has had several weeks or even months of malaise, low-grade fever, and productive cough before seeking medical attention. Weight loss and anemia are common and confirm that the infection is indolent. Often the patient runs a low-grade fever, that is, a temperature about 101 to 102°F. Sputum production is usually copious. Foul-smelling sputum or empyema fluid occurs in only about one half of the patients.[1, 5, 6]

In patients in whom the course of the infection has been followed radiologically, pneumonia appears first and cavitation subsequently. The earliest time of appearance of a cavity is about 7 days after aspiration; the average is about 12 days. Mediastinal adenopathy occasionally accompanies the parenchymal disease in patients with lung abscess or with other types of anaerobic pulmonary infection.[6]

There may be a history of a period of unconsciousness, evidence of alcoholism, diseased gums, an absence of the gag reflex, or other indications of the predisposing condition.

The physical findings are those of a pneumonia, with or without pleural effusion, early in the course of the illness. Later there may be amphoric or cavernous breath sounds. Clubbing of the fingers is noted on occasion.

Anaerobic Necrotizing Pneumonia

Usually anaerobic necrotizing pneumonia is confined primarily to one pulmonary segment or lobe. However, it may extend to involve an entire lung or even both lungs (Fig. 59–1). This type of anaerobic pulmonary infection is the most severe of all. There may be an associated empyema. The disease often spreads rapidly and produces destruction that is characterized by ragged, greenish discoloration of the lung and large putrid sloughs of tissue. This process culminates in "pulmonary gangrene."[5–7]

The patients are generally quite ill, with a temperature of 102 to 103°F. Leukocytosis is usually pronounced, for example, more than 20,000/mm^3. Most of these patients have putrid sputum or empyema fluid when first seen.

Pulmonary actinomycosis may be manifested as a necrotizing pneumonia; a number of cases are complicated by extension of the process to the pleural space and to the chest wall.

Nonanaerobic Lung Abscess and Necrotizing Pneumonia

In primary infections due to organisms such as *S. aureus, Streptococcus pyogenes, Nocardia,* or *Klebsiella pneumoniae,* the symptoms are those of a severe pneumonia.

Secondary Lung Abscess and Necrotizing Pneumonia

In cases of secondary lung abscess, the basic process (bacteremia, endocarditis, septic thrombophlebitis, subphrenic infection, and so forth) are usually evident in addition to the pulmonary process. The most characteristic hematogenous lung abscess is seen in staphylococcal bacteremia, especially in children. These abscesses are commonly multiple and peripheral. There may be repeated episodes of pleuritic pain and hemoptysis. Empyema is frequently seen in this situation (Fig. 59–2). Repeated septic emboli should be suspected when multiple lesions appear over an extended period.

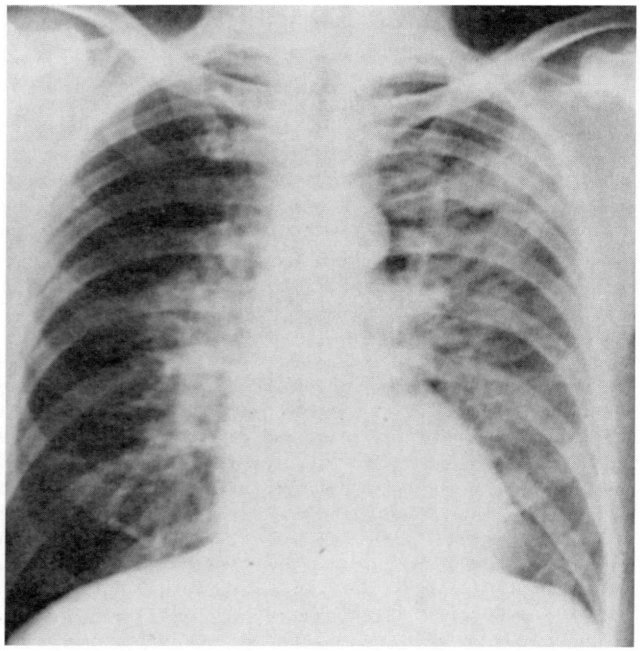

FIGURE 59–1. Posteroanterior (PA) chest film: anaerobic necrotizing pneumonia, and empyema. There is major involvement of the left lung, less involvement of the right. Note the multiple small excavations and one larger cavity in the left lung and blunting of the left costophrenic angle.

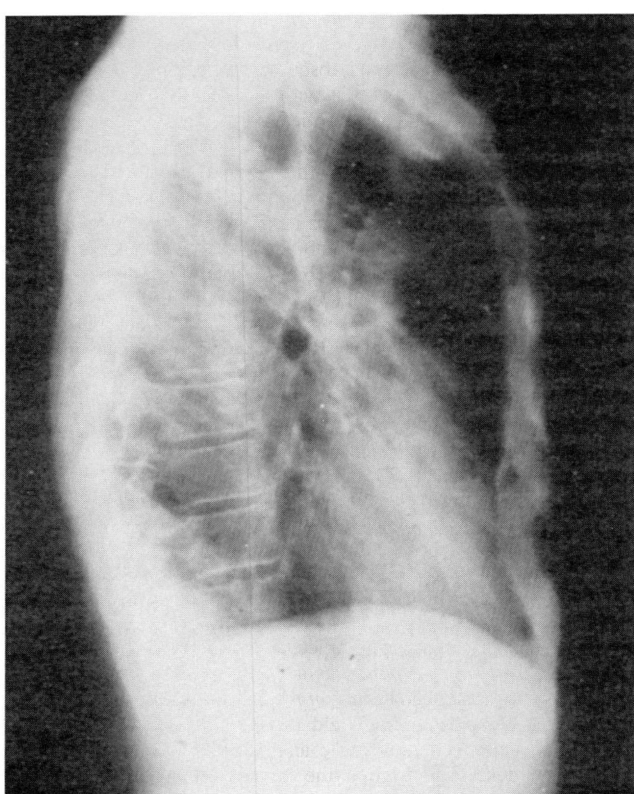

FIGURE 59–2. Lateral chest film: Hematogenous staphylococcal lung abscesses and empyema. Note the air-fluid levels.

Less than 5% of bland pulmonary infarcts become secondarily infected. Secondary infection of infarcts should be suspected if fever is persistent, if the temperature rises above 103°F for more than 48 hours, or if the white blood cell count rises to more than 20,000 cells/mm^3. Abscess formation may occur within a necrotic pulmonary tumor or behind an obstructing tumor.

The syndrome of tonsillitis or pharyngitis (Vincent's angina) with septicemia due to *F. necrophorum,* followed by widespread metastatic disease involving the lungs and other organs, is not commonly seen any longer, probably as a result of early antibiotic therapy for upper respiratory tract infections. However, it is important to be aware of this serious illness that occurs in children and young adults.

Amebic Lung Abscess

In patients with amebic lung abscess, the symptoms of the associated liver abscess often have been present before the rupture through the diaphragm. After perforation of the liver abscess into the lung, there is a gradually developing cough and expectoration of a peculiar chocolate– or anchovy sauce–like sputum. There is no odor to the sputum. The development of a pulmonary amebic abscess varies from a very insidious phenomenon to a dramatic onset with a sudden attack of severe cough productive of a large amount of brownish red sputum.[8] There may be a history of diarrhea, and an appropriate travel history may be elicited.

Complications

Approximately one third of lung abscesses are complicated by empyema. This may be seen with or without a bronchopleural fistula. Brain abscess may also be a complication in patients not receiving appropriate therapy early. A brain abscess is typically solitary. There is virtually never dissemination to other organs. Localized bronchiectasis may occur. Amyloidosis is no longer seen.

Complications of amebic abscess include spontaneous perforation creating a cutaneous sinus, hepatobronchial fistula, empyema, secondary bacterial infection, and amebic abscess of the brain.[9]

MICROBIOLOGIC CHARACTERISTICS

In a prospective study of 26 patients with lung abscesses by Bartlett and associates, anaerobic bacteria were recovered in 24 of the 26 transtracheal aspirate specimens.[1] Only anaerobes (including microaerophilic streptococci) were recovered from 16 of the 24 patients, whereas aerobic or facultative bacteria were recovered along with anaerobes in the other 8. Four patients had a single anaerobe recovered in pure culture, whereas 20 patients had multiple isolates, averaging 3.1 bacteria (2.6 anaerobes) per patient. The most commonly encountered anaerobes were gram-negative rods and gram-positive cocci.

Among 28 cases of anaerobic necrotizing pneumonia, 20 yielded only anaerobes.[5] Overall, there was an average of 2.3 anaerobes and 0.4 aerobes per case. *Fusobacterium nucleatum,* pigmented and other *Bacteroides* (some of which would now be classified as *Prevotella* or *Porphyromonas*), and anaerobic and microaerophilic streptococci and cocci predominated among the anaerobes. Another distinctive cause of necrotizing pneumonia is actinomycosis.

A retrospective study of anaerobic or mixed anaerobic empyema yielded an average of 3.5 anaerobes and 1.1 aerobic or facultative bacteria per specimen.[10] Of the 46 specimens studied, 19 yielded only anaerobes. The predominant nonanaerobes were α-hemolytic streptococci. The predominant anaerobes were pigmented and nonpigmented *Prevotella, Bacteroides* (including the *B. fragilis* group, *F. nucleatum,* and *Peptostreptococcus* spp.

The anaerobes most commonly encountered in anaerobic pleuropulmonary infection are listed in Table 59–1. Although clostridia, including *Clostridium perfringens,* may be recovered from patients with necrotizing pneumonia and empyema or other anaerobic pulmonary infections, there is usually nothing distinctive about the clinical picture in such cases.

TABLE 59–1 Anaerobes Most Commonly Encountered in Pleuropulmonary Infection

Gram-negative bacilli
- Pigmented *Prevotella*
- *Prevotella oralis* group
- *Prevotella oris*
- *Prevotella buccae*
- *Prevotella bivia*
- *Sutterella wadsworthensis*
- *Bacteroides fragilis* group
- *Fusobacterium nucleatum*
- *Fusobacterium necrophorum*
- *Fusobacterium naviforme*
- *Fusobacterium gonidiaformans*

Gram-positive cocci
- *Peptostreptococcus* (especially *Peptostreptococcus micros, Peptostreptococcus anaerobius, Peptostreptococcus magnus, Peptostreptococcus asaccharolyticus, Peptostreptococcus prevotii, Peptostreptococcus intermedius**)
- Microaerophilic streptococci

Gram-positive spore-forming bacilli
- *Clostridium perfringens, Clostridium ramosum*

Gram-positive non–spore-forming bacilli
- *Actinomyces* spp.
- *Propionibacterium propionicum*
- *Bifidobacterium dentium*

*This organism officially belongs in the genus *Streptococcus.* (Data from refs. 10–12, 22.)

There is an important difference in bacterial cause in terms of whether the patient aspirates in the community or in the hospital setting.[6, 13] Community-acquired aspiration pneumonia is primarily an anaerobic process, with 35 of 38 patients studied yielding anaerobes and 25 yielding only this type of organism.[13] On the other hand, cultures from patients aspirating in the hospital setting yielded anaerobes in 26 of 32 cases (in pure culture in only 7 cases) and, most importantly, as part of the other infecting flora yielded important nosocomial pathogens such as *S. aureus* and various aerobic and facultative gram-negative bacilli such as *Klebsiella, Pseudomonas,* and *Proteus.*

Nichols and Smith have shown that patients with bleeding or obstructing duodenal ulcers or with gastric ulcers or malignancy commonly have a much more profuse microflora in the stomach than do people without such pathologic conditions.[14] This flora includes various organisms from the oral flora such as streptococci and anaerobes of various types but also coliform bacilli and, on occasion, *B. fragilis.* Thus, aspiration of gastric contents in people with the aforementioned pathologic conditions would carry with it a greater risk of bacterial infection, and the infecting flora might be different from what would ordinarily be expected. Histamine type 2 blockers or antacids have commonly been used to prevent upper gastrointestinal bleeding due to stress ulcers in critically ill patients. This leads to an elevated gastric pH and gastric and pharyngeal (by the retrograde route) colonization with gram-negative bacilli. This may be avoided by the use of sucralfate.[3]

There are also several major aerobic causes of necrotizing pneumonia: *S. aureus, S. pyogenes, K. pneumoniae,* and *P. aeruginosa.* It is said that, on rare occasion, pneumococci (type 3) may cause a lung abscess. Infrequently, other gram-negative bacilli such as *Escherichia coli, Legionella pneumophila,* and perhaps *Proteus* spp. may cause pulmonary necrosis. Uncommon but important causes of cavitating pneumonia are *Nocardia* infection, *Rhodococcus,*[15] *Salmonella, Burkholderia, Paragonimus,* melioidosis, and glanders. In acute Friedländer's (*Klebsiella*) pneumonia, 25 to 50% of the patients develop one or more lung abscesses. Lung abscess due to *Pseudomonas cepacia* was reported by Poe and coworkers.[16] The source of the organism was determined to be the reservoir of an ultrasonic nebulizer. Such nebulizers have been implicated in gram-negative bacillary pneumonia by several groups of investigators. However, although necrotizing pneumonia is seen in a proportion of these groups, a solitary lung abscess is uncommon. In infants with staphylococcal pneumonia, pneumatoceles occur as frequently as abscesses, whereas in adults the radiolucencies almost always represent abscess formation. Mycobacteria may also cause necrotizing pneumonia, and fungal infection (particularly histoplasmosis, coccidioidomycosis, and aspergillosis) sometimes produces this lesion.

Three major groups of bacteria are involved in hematogenous spread to the lungs: gram-positive cocci, notably staphylococci; gram-negative enteric bacilli; and anaerobic bacteria. Multiple abscesses are likely to be of hematogenous origin, either as a result of bacteremia or of septic embolization. The most characteristic hematogenous lung abscess is seen in staphylococcal bacteremia. Hematogenous pulmonary infection with gram-negative enteric bacilli occurs in association with urinary tract infection or manipulation, after bowel surgery, after septic abortion, or as a nosocomial infection (usually in relation to vascular or urinary tract catheterization). Anaerobic or microaerophilic streptococci and gram-negative anaerobic bacilli may also produce hematogenous necrotizing pulmonary infection secondary to intra-abdominal or pelvic infections. In all these anaerobic infections, there may be only bacteremia or else a septic thrombophlebitis that results in septic embolization. Uncommon hematogenous necrotizing pulmonary processes are those seen with anthrax, plague, and *Salmonella choleraesuis* infection.

Metastatic lung abscess may occur as a result of septic emboli from bacterial endocarditis of the right side of the heart (*S. aureus* is the major pathogen in this setting) or from pelvic or other deep vein thrombophlebitis. Various anaerobic bacteria and also pyogenic cocci such as *S. aureus* and streptococci not infrequently cause septic thrombophlebitis. As noted earlier, the anaerobes may be involved in this type of process in association with pelvic or intra-abdominal infection or, uncommonly now, with jugular vein thrombophlebitis in association with tonsillopharyngeal infections. Thrombophlebitis of the cavernous sinus most often involves *S. aureus* or streptococci. *S. aureus* may also produce septic thrombophlebitis in association with superficial skin or soft tissue infections or in relation to intravenous catheters. The latter setting also may lead to septic thrombophlebitis involving gram-negative bacilli. Various organisms may be involved in secondary infection of bland pulmonary infarcts, including staphylococci, streptococci, pneumococci, gram-negative enteric bacilli, and anaerobes of various types. Infection within a necrotic pulmonary tumor or behind an obstructing tumor may lead to abscess formation. Anaerobic bacteria of various types are commonly involved in such infections, but various other infecting organisms including *Mycobacterium tuberculosis* and fungi, as well as a variety of other bacteria, may also be involved.

DIAGNOSIS

The typical lung abscess can be suspected on clinical grounds. Most diagnoses are made from the chest radiograph, specifically from the presence of a cavity with an air-fluid level or pneumonitis with multiple small excavations located in a dependent segment. CT scanning may be needed to detect cavities, and may give evidence of obstructing endobronchial lesions. Diagnosis of the specific cause as well as differentiation from similar lesions depends on definitive bacteriologic studies. Because of the presence of large numbers of anaerobes as indigenous flora in the mouth and the common presence in hospitalized people of potential pathogens such as *S. aureus* and *K. pneumoniae* as colonizers in the mouth or the upper respiratory tract, it is necessary to obtain a specimen other than expectorated sputum for bacteriologic diagnosis. Empyema fluid, if available, provides an excellent specimen. On occasion, particularly with a metastatic lung abscess, blood cultures may be positive; however, blood cultures may reveal only part of the infecting flora. In the absence of the aforementioned sources of specimens for diagnosis, percutaneous transtracheal aspiration may be performed to establish the specific cause of the lung abscess or necrotizing pneumonia in patients who are able to cooperate.[17] This procedure should not be used in people with a significant bleeding tendency or in those in whom it is difficult to provide adequate oxygenation. Percutaneous transthoracic aspiration may be useful, particularly in children, but provides a smaller, less satisfactory specimen. Obtaining specimens during fiberoptic bronchoscopy by means of a bronchial brush within a plugged double-lumen catheter[18] is much more widely used now than transtracheal aspiration. It is absolutely essential that the techniques as outlined in detail by Broughton and colleagues be used exactly as described[19] and that cultures be done quantitatively. Growth at a 10^{-3} dilution is considered significant. The amount of the secretions collected by the brush is 0.001 to 0.01 ml, so the 10^{-3} dilution represents 10^5 to 10^6 organisms/ml of lower respiratory tract secretions. The small volume of material obtained and the difficulty one would encounter to arrange for anaerobic transport are a concern; nevertheless, good results appear to have been obtained in a small number of cases of anaerobic pulmonary infection. Quantitative culture of fluid obtained by bronchoalveolar lavage (during bronchoscopy) has provided reliable results in bacterial pneumonia[20] and is rather widely used. There is little information available on the recovery of anaerobes from such specimens so far, but limited studies are promising.[21] It is likely that quantitative culture of other respiratory tract specimens (e.g., aspirates from tracheostomies or endotracheal tubes) would provide reliable information.

It is essential that material obtained for culture be placed under anaerobic conditions promptly before transport to the laboratory. It is usually desirable to aspirate the material to be cultured into a syringe, to expel all bubbles of air or gas from the syringe and needle, and then to transfer the specimen to a tube that has been gassed out with oxygen-free gas for transport to the laboratory.[22]

Demonstration of the usual underlying liver abscess is basic to the diagnosis of amebic lung abscess, but one may be able to demonstrate *Entamoeba histolytica* in the patient's sputum. Charcot-Leyden crystals in the sputum are suggestive of amebic infection. The usual procedures for the diagnosis of intestinal or hepatic amebiasis should be undertaken. The vast majority of patients with extraintestinal amebiasis have high titers of hemagglutinating or complement-fixing antibodies.

Differential Diagnosis

Factors that would suggest a cavitating carcinoma rather than lung abscess include the absence of predisposing factors for an aspiration abscess (including an edentulous patient), location of an abscess in a nondependent segment, an irregular abscess wall, and failure to respond to antibacterial therapy. Tuberculosis may also simulate a lung abscess or necrotizing pneumonia. Patients with infected lung cysts or bullae typically lack the systemic symptoms that may be seen in a lung abscess, the cavity wall is thin, and there is no surrounding pneumonitis.

THERAPY AND PROGNOSIS

The primary mode of therapy is the administration of antimicrobial agents. Treatment may need to be continued for 2 to 4 months to achieve cure without relapse. Features to be monitored include fever, sputum production, and the radiographic appearance of the abscess.

The anaerobes involved in lung abscess or in necrotizing pneumonia are increasingly resistant to penicillin G. Reports have appeared of a less than optimal response or even frank failure to cure anaerobic lung abscesses or necrotizing pneumonia with penicillin therapy,[23–25] primarily because of β-lactamase–producing, gram-negative anaerobic rods. Metronidazole, or clindamycin, supplemented with penicillin G, represents one of the treatments of choice for serious anaerobic pulmonary infections. Since some of the anaerobic cocci may require 8 units/ml or more of penicillin G for inhibition, one should use large doses of this agent (10 to 20 million units/day intravenously in adults). Thus, penicillin G (or penicillin V, ampicillin, or amoxicillin) should no longer be used as the sole initial therapy for patients with a suspected or proven anaerobic lung abscess or necrotizing pneumonia who are moderately or seriously ill. Patients who are not very ill may be treated satisfactorily with penicillin, at times even with an oral penicillin (or cephalosporin). Other penicillins are often considerably less active than is penicillin G.

A significant percentage of strains of most anaerobes are resistant to tetracyclines. Accordingly, these compounds should not be used. Clindamycin is active against most anaerobes with the exception of some strains of *Peptostreptococcus, Sutterella wadsworthensis, Fusobacterium varium,* and some strains of clostridia other than *C. perfringens*; 20% or more of the *B. fragilis* group are resistant in some centers. The addition of penicillin G would increase the spectrum of coverage except for the *B. fragilis* group and *Sutterella.* Metronidazole is active against all gram-negative anaerobes including the *B. fragilis* group and other β-lactamase producers except for some *S. wadsworthensis* strains. It is also essentially always active against all clostridia. Some anaerobic cocci and most microaerophilic streptococci, *Actinomyces,* and *Propionibacterium propionicum* strains are resistant. For this reason, metronidazole should ordinarily be used together with penicillin G (or erythromycin) in the treatment of anaerobic pulmonary infections. Certain β-lactam agents are quite active against the *B. fragilis* group and other β-lactamase–producing *Bacteroides* and most other anaerobes, although increasing resistance has been encountered in some centers. Included are cefoxitin, the carboxy penicillins (carbenicillin and ticarcillin), and piperacillin. Cefoxitin is inactive against one third of clostridia other than *C. perfringens* and against 15 to 20% of strains of the *B. fragilis* group in some centers. These agents, especially the broad-spectrum penicillins and cefoxitin, also have significant activity against various Enterobacteriaceae. Cefoxitin is also active against *S. aureus* and piperacillin has good activity against *P. aeruginosa.* The third-generation cephalosporins and related new compounds all have less activity against anaerobes, especially the *B. fragilis* group, than do cefoxitin and the broad-spectrum penicillins just discussed. Exceptions are imipenem and meropenem, which are active against virtually all anaerobes. Combinations of β-lactam drugs and β-lactamase inhibitors such as ticarcillin plus clavulanic acid and ampicillin plus sulbactam are active against essentially all anaerobes and have good activity against *S. aureus* and many gram-negative bacilli. Chloramphenicol is active against essentially all anaerobes and represents another option in a seriously ill patient with necrotizing pneumonia or lung abscess in whom β-lactamase–producing anaerobes may be present. The new quinolone trovafloxacin has excellent activity against anaerobes and many other organisms that may be involved in lung abscess.

For staphylococcal infections, a penicillinase-resistant penicillin is preferable, but one of the parenteral cephalosporins or vancomycin may be used in the event of significant allergy. Vancomycin is the drug of choice for methicillin-resistant *S. aureus.* Penicillin G is the drug of choice for group A streptococcal infection. For infections due to *K. pneumoniae* or other facultative or aerobic gram-negative bacilli that may be involved in the type of pulmonary infection under discussion, one of the aminoglycosides would represent a good choice, but the extended-spectrum penicillins, certain newer cephalosporins and aztreonam, and combinations of β-lactam drugs and β-lactamase inhibitors have very good activity against some of these organisms. This is also true of imipenem and meropenem. Trimethoprim-sulfamethoxazole and the newer quinolones have good activity against many nonanaerobic gram-negative rods and may be useful in combination regimens. Gentamicin is ordinarily suitable, but in certain hospitals significant numbers of gram-negative bacilli are resistant to gentamicin; amikacin would then be the aminoglycoside of choice. In seriously ill patients, particularly those who may be immunosuppressed, the use of appropriate β-lactam agents along with the aminoglycoside is desirable.

Postural drainage is an important aspect of the therapy for a lung abscess. Bronchoscopy may be helpful in effecting drainage and for the removal of foreign bodies and biopsy diagnosis of tumors. Surgical resection of lung abscesses is seldom required unless there is a coexisting malignant process. Indeed, surgery may be contraindicated because of the hazard of the spread of infection or asphyxiation from spillage of abscess contents. Surgical or percutaneous catheter drainage[26] of a lung abscess through the chest wall is also seldom indicated. Complicating empyemas do require drainage.

Prognosis

The prognosis varies with the type of underlying or predisposing pathologic process, if any, and, in the case of acute severe necrotizing pneumonias, the speed with which appropriate therapy is instituted. The mortality in anaerobic lung abscess is 15% or less. In anaerobic necrotizing pneumonia it is 25%. The mortality may be significantly higher in acute pneumonias caused by *S. aureus, K. pneumoniae,* and other facultative or aerobic gram-negative bacilli. The prognosis in amebic lung abscess is good when the diagnosis and treatment are prompt. Nocardiosis often has a relatively poor prognosis, especially when it complicates a serious underlying disease.

REFERENCES

1. Bartlett JG, Gorbach SL, Tally FP, et al. Bacteriology and treatment of primary lung abscess. Am Rev Respir Dis. 1974;109:510–518.
2. Huxley EJ, Viroslav J, Gray WR, et al. Pharyngeal aspiration in normal adults and patients with depressed consciousness. Am J Med. 1978;64:564–568.
3. Driks MR, Craven DE, Celli BR, et al. Nosocomial pneumonia in intubated patients given sucralfate as compared with antacids or histamine type 2 blockers. N Engl J Med. 1987;317:1376–1382.
4. Tryba M. Risk of acute stress bleeding and nosocomial pneumonia in ventilated intensive care unit patients: Sucralfate versus antacids. Am J Med. 1987;83(Suppl 3B):117–124.
5. Bartlett JG, Finegold SM. Anaerobic infections of the lung and pleural space. Am Rev Respir Dis. 1974;110:56–77.
6. Finegold SM. Anaerobic Bacteria in Human Disease. New York: Academic Press; 1977.
7. Bartlett JG, Finegold SM. Anaerobic pleuropulmonary infections. Medicine (Baltimore). 1972;51:413–450.
8. Craig DF. The Etiology, Diagnosis and Treatment of Amebiasis. Baltimore: Williams & Wilkins; 1944.
9. Ochsner A, DeBakey ME. Pleuropulmonary complications of amebiasis: An analysis of 153 collected and 15 personal cases. J Thorac Surg. 1936;5:225–258.
10. Civen R, Jousimies-Somer H, Marina M, et al. A retrospective review of cases of anaerobic empyema and update of bacteriology. Clin Infect Dis. 1995;20(Suppl 2):S224–S229.
11. Kirby BD, George WL, Sutter VL, et al. Gram-negative anaerobic bacilli: Their role in infection and patterns of susceptibility to antimicrobial agents. I. Little-known *Bacteroides* species. Rev Infect Dis. 1980;2:914–951.
12. George WL, Kirby BD, Sutter VL, et al. Gram-negative anaerobic bacilli: Their role in infection and patterns of susceptibility to antimicrobial agents. II. Little-known *Fusobacterium* species and miscellaneous genera. Rev Infect Dis. 1981;3:599–626.
13. Bartlett JG, Gorbach SL, Finegold SM. The bacteriology of aspiration pneumonia. Am J Med. 1974;56:202–207.
14. Nichols RL, Smith JW. Intragastric microbial colonization in common disease states of the stomach and duodenum. Ann Surg. 1975;182:557–561.
15. Savdie E, Pigott P, Jennis F. Lung abscess due to *Corynebacterium equi* in a renal transplant recipient. Med J Aust. 1977;1:817–819.
16. Poe RH, Marcus HR, Emerson GL. Lung abscess due to *Pseudomonas cepacia.* Am Rev Respir Dis. 1977;115:861–865.
17. Bartlett JG, Rosenblatt JE, Finegold SM. Percutaneous transtracheal aspiration in the diagnosis of anaerobic pulmonary infection. Ann Intern Med. 1973;79:535–540.
18. Wimberly NW, Bass JB Jr, Boyd BW, et al. Use of a bronchoscopic protected catheter brush for the diagnosis of pulmonary infections. Chest. 1982;81:556–562.
19. Broughton WA, Bass JB, Kirkpatrick MB. The technique of protected brush catheter bronchoscopy. J Crit Ill. 1987;2:63–70.
20. Kahn FW, Jones JM. Diagnosing bacterial respiratory infection by bronchoalveolar lavage. J Infect Dis. 1987;155:862–869.
21. Henriquez AH, Mendoza J, Gonzalez PC. Quantitative culture of bronchoalveolar lavage from patients with anaerobic lung abscesses. J Infect Dis. 1991;164:414–417.
22. Summanen P, Baron EJ, Citron DM, et al. Wadsworth Anaerobic Bacteriology Manual. 5th ed. Belmont, CA: Star Publishing; 1993.
23. Levison ME, Mangura CT, Lorber B, et al. Clindamycin compared with penicillin for the treatment of anaerobic lung abscess. Ann Intern Med. 1983;98:466–471.
24. Gudiol F, Manresa F, Pallares R, et al. Clindamycin vs penicillin for anaerobic lung infections. High rate of penicillin failures associated with penicillin-resistant *Bacteroides melaninogenicus.* Arch Intern Med. 1990;150:2525–2529.
25. Panwalker AP. Failure of penicillin in anaerobic necrotizing pneumonia. Chest. 1982;82:500–501.
26. Klein JS, Schultz S, Heffner JE. Interventional radiology of the chest: Image-guided percutaneous drainage of pleural effusions, lung abscess, and pneumothorax. Am J Radiol. 1995;164:581–588.

Chapter 60

Chronic Pneumonia

WILLIAM E. DISMUKES

For purposes of this chapter, *chronic pneumonia syndrome* is defined as a pulmonary parenchymal process that is caused by an infectious or a noninfectious agent, has been present for weeks to months rather than for days, and is manifested by abnormal chest radiographic findings and by chronic or progressive pulmonary symptoms. The abnormal chest radiograph, which may reveal any of several radiologic patterns, is probably the most important criterion. In many patients, the diagnosis of chronic pneumonia is based more on the pulmonary radiographic findings than on the pulmonary symptoms. However, asymptomatic patients who have abnormal findings, such as a solitary nodule, on routine evaluation should not be considered to have chronic pneumonia.

The emphasis in this chapter is on the chronic pneumonias caused by infectious agents; however, it is important to keep in mind that there are noninfectious causes of chronic pneumonia, including vasculitides,[1–4] neoplasia,[5–7] drugs,[8] radiation, amyloidosis,[9] sarcoidosis,[10] alveolar phospholipoproteinosis,[11] bronchiolitis obliterans organizing pneumonia,[12, 13] and other idiopathic causes.[14, 15]

ETIOLOGY

The infectious causes of chronic pneumonia can be divided into two main groups: (1) infectious agents that typically cause acute pneumonia and uncommonly cause chronic pneumonia and (2) infectious agents that typically cause chronic pneumonia. Among the agents that typically cause acute pneumonia—the anaerobes, *Staphylococcus* spp., *Haemophilus influenzae,* the Enterobacteriaceae, and *Pseudomonas aeruginosa*—are the organisms most likely to produce a persistent chronic pneumonia. This is usually a necrotizing process that most commonly occurs in patients with underlying disease such as alcoholism, diabetes mellitus, intrathoracic malignancy, or chronic obstructive lung disease or in patients who are hospitalized.[16–18] Acute pneumonias caused by most viruses or by *Streptococcus pneumoniae, Mycoplasma pneumoniae, Legionella* spp., *Coxiella burnetii,* or *Chlamydia pneumoniae*[19–21] rarely progress to a chronic pulmonary illness.

Table 60–1 shows the various causes of chronic pneumonia. In the normal host, tuberculosis,[22] other mycobacterial infections,[23–24] histoplasmosis,[25] coccidioidomycosis (in the appropriate geographic area),[26] mixed aerobic-anaerobic bacterial infection,[16–18] actinomycosis,[27] blastomycosis,[28] cryptococcosis,[29] paracoccidioidomycosis,[30] and sporotrichosis[31] are the infections deserving prime consideration. Adiaspiromycosis (caused by *Emmonsia*)[32] and pseudallescheriasis[33] are rare occurrences. In the immunocompromised host,[34, 35] chronic pneumonia should raise the possibility of tuberculosis,[22] nocardiosis, cryptococcosis,[29] aspergillosis,[36] and, in the appropriate geographic areas, coccidioidomycosis and histoplasmosis.[25, 26] In persons with acquired immunodeficiency syndrome (AIDS), a special immunocompromised population, the same infections are frequently seen.[26, 36–41] In addition, in these patients, chronic pneumonia may be caused by *Blastomyces dermatitidis,* atypical mycobacteria, *Rhodococcus equi, Penicillium marneffei, Pneumocystis carinii,* or cytomegalovirus, or by noninfectious disorders such as Kaposi's sarcoma, lymphoma, x-ray therapy, and nonspecific interstitial pneumonitis.[28, 42–46] The protozoa and worms listed in Table 60–1 are uncommon causes of chronic pneumonia syndrome among U.S. residents, but they are important considerations for patients who live in or have traveled in areas in which these agents are endemic.

No studies have been done to determine the approximate frequency of the various causes of chronic pneumonia in a large series of patients. This lack of perspective on the incidence of the various causes of chronic pneumonia contrasts with our better understanding of the *acute* pneumonia syndrome. In addition, since the introduction of antibiotics in the 1940s, the overall spectrum of pneumonia has changed; new pathogens have emerged, organisms that were previously considered to be harmless commensals now cause disease, and powerful immunosuppressive therapies render some patients more susceptible to certain microorganisms. Consequently, in considering the differential diagnosis in an individual patient, emphasis on specific entities usually must be based less on statistical likelihood and more on a thorough and methodic analysis of all available clinical, epidemiologic, and laboratory data.

TABLE 60–1 Etiology of Chronic Pneumonia Syndrome

Infectious Agents That Typically Cause Chronic Pneumonia
Bacteria and actinomycetes
Mixed aerobic-anaerobic bacteria
Actinomyces spp.
Propionibacterium propionicus
Nocardia spp.
Rhodococcus equi
Burkholderia pseudomallei
Mycobacteria
Mycobacterium tuberculosis
Mycobacterium kansasii
Mycobacterium avium complex
Fungi
Aspergillus spp.
Blastomyces dermatitidis
Coccidioides immitis
Cryptococcus neoformans
Emmonsia
Histoplasma capsulatum
Sporothrix schenckii
Paracoccidioides brasiliensis
Protozoa
Entamoeba histolytica
Worms
Echinococcus granulosus
Schistosomes: *Schistosoma hematobium, Schistosoma japonicum, Schistosoma mansoni*
Paragonimus westermani
Noninfectious Causes
Neoplasia
Carcinoma (primary or metastatic)
Lymphoma
Sarcoidosis
Amyloidosis
Vasculitis (autoimmune diseases)
Systemic lupus erythematosus
Polyarteritis nodosa
Allergic angiitis and granulomatosis (Churg-Strauss syndrome)
Progressive systemic sclerosis
Rheumatoid arthritis
Mixed connective tissue syndrome (overlap syndrome)
Wegener's granulomatosis
Lymphomatoid granulomatosis
Chemicals, drugs, or inhalation
Radiation
Recurrent pulmonary emboli
Bronchial obstruction with atelectasis (e.g., tumor, foreign body)
Pulmonary infiltration with eosinophilia syndrome
Löffler syndrome—usually transient
Tropical eosinophilia
Pneumonia plus asthma (e.g., allergic bronchopulmonary aspergillosis)
Bronchocentric granulomatosis
Vasculitis
Eosinophilic pneumonia—chronic
Pneumoconiosis
Chronic form of extrinsic allergic alveolitis (hypersensitivity pneumonitis)
Other lung disease—unknown cause
Bronchiolitis obliterans organizing pneumonia
Chronic interstitial pneumonia (fibrosing alveolitis, idiopathic pulmonary fibrosis)
Usual interstitial pneumonia (UIP)
Desquamative interstitial pneumonia (DIP)
Lymphocytic interstitial pneumonia (LIP)
Giant cell interstitial pneumonia (GIP)
Eosinophilic granuloma (histiocytosis X)
Lymphangioleiomyomatosis
Goodpasture's syndrome
Pulmonary alevolar proteinosis (phospholipoproteinosis)
Pulmonary alveolar microlithiasis
Idiopathic pulmonary hemosiderosis
Angiocentric immunoproliferative lesions

EPIDEMIOLOGY

Age, Gender, Race

In the United States over the past 2 decades, pulmonary tuberculosis has become a disease of the homeless, alcoholic, elderly, AIDS, and immigrant population groups. The significance of age and gender for patients with chronic pneumonia from other causes also usually relates, in an indirect manner, to associated epidemiologic factors. For example, an elderly patient is at higher risk of having a cerebrovascular accident, which in turn might predispose the patient to an aspiration episode and subsequent pneumonia and abscess. Likewise, older, debilitated patients are at higher risk for development of chronic gram-negative necrotizing pneumonia. In a similar manner, the gender of a given patient is likely to affect or determine occupation or avocation and therefore the likelihood of exposure to certain infectious agents or other etiologic vehicles. An exception is pulmonary lymphangioleiomyomatosis, which occurs exclusively in teenaged to middle-aged women.[47] The race of the patient may be a more important factor. For example, pulmonary tuberculosis should be the presumptive diagnosis in an African American with bilateral upper lobe cavitary disease; coccidioidomycosis is more likely to be severe in dark-skinned persons, including African Americans and Filipinos, who have lived or have traveled in the southwestern United States, the endemic area for the disease;[26] and chronic cavitary histoplasmosis is more likely to occur in the white male population.[25]

Occupation and Avocation

Certain occupations or hobbies should arouse suspicion of particular diseases. Despite the presence of *Cryptococcus neoformans* in pigeon droppings, most patients with pulmonary cryptococcosis have had no unusual exposure to pigeons. Occupational exposure to plant materials predisposes an individual to cutaneous and, according to some authorities, to pulmonary sporotrichosis. Other examples of occupationally or avocationally related conditions include the following: tuberculosis among health care workers; coccidioidomycosis among rock collectors, archeologists conducting excavations, construction workers, and others exposed to desert dust in the endemic area; histoplasmosis among persons who are exposed to pigeon or starling roosts, who clean out old chicken houses with dirt floors, who cut and clear hollow trees, or who explore old buildings or caves inhabited by bats; echinocococcosis among those who tend sheep; berylliosis among workers in the aircraft, electronics, and nuclear industries; the pneumoconioses (e.g., silicosis, asbestosis) among sandblasters and shipyard workers; and both chronic and acute pulmonary disease from repeated occupational or environmental exposure to organic antigen agents of extrinsic allergic alveolitis (hypersensitivity pneumonitis)[48] or to irritant gases such as phosgene, ammonia, ozone, and nitrogen dioxide.

Travel

Because the initial exposure to the microbiologic agents of many chronic or indolent infectious diseases may have occurred months or years before disease appears, it is necessary to inquire whether a patient has lived in or has traveled to another part of the United States or the world at any time. For example, a patient with bilateral upper lobe infiltrates with or without cavitation who has never traveled or lived in Central America, Mexico, South America, or west of the Mississippi River is unlikely to have coccidioidomycosis. On the other hand, if the patient has lived in the eastern half of the United States, especially the midcentral area, chronic pulmonary histoplasmosis should be considered, because histoplasmosis is endemic in that area. Paracoccidioidomycosis is acquired only during residence in Mexico, Central America, or parts of South America.

In addition to identifying a state or country visited, there may be a need for detailed questioning about rural or urban exposure, type of lodging, source of drinking water, exposure to native foods, and so forth. For example, if a person who has lived or traveled extensively in Southeast Asia, particularly in low-lying or rice-growing areas, subsequently manifests chronic pneumonia with pulmonary roentgenographic abnormalities resembling those of tuberculosis or a respiratory mycosis, melioidosis should be suspected.[49] Similarly, pulmonary paragonimiasis should be suspected in a businessperson who makes frequent trips to Japan and the Philippines; who eats raw or partly cooked crayfish, crabs or shrimp; and who has chronic pulmonary symptoms plus dense, nodular lung opacities and ring shadows.[50]

Contacts, Habits, and Drugs

In patients and health care workers in whom tuberculosis is suspected, contacts among companions, relatives, or patients with tuberculosis should be sought. In addition, tuberculosis should be suspected in persons living or working in closed environments such as jails and prisons, schools, daycare centers, and nursing homes. Inquiry should be made into the patient's smoking and drinking history and other personal habits. The likelihood of cancer of the lung in a patient with coal worker's pneumoconiosis is greater in a smoker than in a nonsmoker. Aspiration pneumonia, chronic gram-negative bacillary pneumonia, tuberculosis, and pulmonary sporotrichosis are more likely to occur in an alcoholic than in a nondrinker. Intravenous drug users who inject heroin or similar agents are at risk not only for infection with human immunodeficiency virus (HIV) and subsequent AIDS but also for septic pulmonary emboli followed by necrotizing pneumonia and single or multiple abscesses or an interstitial granulomatous reaction with pulmonary hypertension. Similarly, frequent use of free-base cocaine has been reported to cause bronchiolitis obliterans organizing pneumonia, eosinophilic lung disease, interstitial pneumonitis, and pulmonary hemorrhage and/or infarction.[51]

More than 100 different drugs have been reported to cause acute and chronic pulmonary symptoms with radiographic abnormalities.[8] Early in the course of drug-induced pulmonary disease, the chest roentgenogram findings may be normal; later, an interstitial, nodular, or alveolar pattern (or a combination of these) may be present. Still later, the chest radiograph may reveal only a fibrotic pulmonary process. The drugs that are most likely to cause chronic pulmonary disease include cytotoxic agents such as bleomycin, busulfan, cyclophosphamide, methotrexate, and nitrosoureas and noncytotoxic agents such as amiodarone, gold salts, nitrofurantoin, and penicillamine. Because drug-induced pulmonary disease may develop after drug therapy has been discontinued, the physician should inquire not only about all drugs the patient is presently taking but also about those taken in the recent past.

Important questions arise in regard to any previous or current antimicrobial therapy. Did the antimicrobial therapy result in roentgenographic or clinical improvement? If not, was the antimicrobial drug used in sufficient quantity to cure the suspected process or alter its course? Was the appropriate agent used? What effect did the antimicrobial agent have on the results of cultures? Is the report of "normal flora" on the sputum culture the result of elimination of a specific pathogen by antimicrobial therapy?

Underlying Disease

Pulmonary complications, including both acute and chronic or refractory pneumonia, are especially common among persons with AIDS[26, 28, 36–46] (see Chapter 116) or other immunocompromising conditions such as high-dose corticosteroid therapy, cytotoxic therapy, or organ transplantation.[34, 35] Patients with diabetes mellitus or preexisting chronic obstructive pulmonary disease are at high risk for development of chronic or persistent bacterial pneumonia. Similarly, chronic obstructive lung disease commonly precedes fibrocavitary histoplasmosis or *Mycobacterium avium* complex infection. Recurrent or persistent pneumonia in the same area of the lung raises the suspicion of a local endobronchial lesion that may not be apparent on routine chest radiographs. Because aspiration may predispose to chronic pneumonia, inquiry should be made into any history of recent dental problems or manipulation, sinusitis with chronic postnasal drip, disorders of swallowing resulting from neurologic or esophageal disease, seizure disorders, recent anesthesia, quantity and effect of alcohol, or any illness leading to an unconscious state. Finally, it should be determined whether the chronic pneumonia is community or hospital acquired.

CLINICAL FEATURES

Symptoms

There are many causes of chronic pneumonia, and no single symptom complex is common to all causes. Often, constitutional symptoms including fever, chills, and malaise are present initially. A history of progressive anorexia and weight loss usually indicates chronic illness. Pulmonary symptoms may be present early but frequently appear later in the course of the illness. Any patient with a prolonged illness and nonspecific constitutional complaints plus pulmonary symptoms—including a new or persistent cough, sputum production, hemoptysis, chest pain (especially pleuritic pain), or dyspnea—deserves medical evaluation, including a chest roentgenogram and, in some cases, a computed tomographic examination of the chest (chest CT).

Inquiries should be made to determine whether there is involvement of extrapulmonary organs. For example, skin lesions might suggest coccidioidomycosis, cryptococcosis, blastomycosis, nocardiosis, sporotrichosis, sarcoidosis, or Kaposi's sarcoma, whereas mucous membrane lesions would suggest histoplasmosis, paracoccidioidomycosis, Wegener's granulomatosis, or Kaposi's sarcoma. Monoarticular or polyarticular arthritis, polyarthralgias, or localized bone tenderness or pain might indicate a vasculitis. A history of persistent headache together with documentation of abnormal cerebrospinal fluid should raise the suspicion of tuberculosis, cryptococcosis, or coccidioidomycosis involving both the lungs and central nervous system. The presence of focal neurologic symptoms and signs argues strongly for a space-occupying lesion in the central nervous system; such findings in a patient with a cavitary infiltrate seen on a chest radiograph suggest the possibility of a brain abscess associated with chronic suppurative lung disease or pulmonary nocardiosis. Similarly, the triad of skin nodules, pulmonary nodules, and central nervous system abnormalities suggests lymphomatoid granulomatosis.[4]

Signs

Although the findings on physical examination of the chest usually are not helpful in differentiating specific causes of chronic pneumonia, the presence of generalized wheezing or other signs of bronchospasm, in the absence of underlying lung disease, indicates an asthmatic component to the pulmonary illness and raises the possibility of a disorder causing both pneumonia and asthma, such as extrinsic allergic alveolitis, allergic bronchopulmonary aspergillosis, or allergic angiitis and granulomatosis (Churg-Strauss syndrome).[3] Similarly, localized wheezing suggests the presence of an endobronchial obstructing lesion. The findings of tachycardia, cardiomegaly, gallop rhythm, and ankle edema provide evidence of cardiac disease and suggest that the pulmonary symptoms and signs result at least in part from cardiovascular causes. The presence of skin lesions, clubbing, cyanosis, or phlebitis is not specific for any single pulmonary disorder but may help to narrow the differential diagnosis, especially when considered along with other clinical and epidemiologic information. Similarly, the finding of jaundice, adenopathy, hepatomegaly, splenomegaly, or ascites suggests that a systemic disorder involving multiple organs is the cause.

DIAGNOSTIC PROCEDURES

Initial Laboratory Studies

Routine laboratory studies may provide some important clues to diagnosis. Pancytopenia may suggest miliary tuberculosis, disseminated histoplasmosis, or metastatic tumor in the bone marrow. Anemia alone is consistent with too many disorders to suggest a specific cause. A normal leukocyte count does not exclude infection. In particular, mycotic chronic pneumonia is usually associated with a normal or minimally elevated leukocyte count. Leukopenia or lymphopenia should raise the suspicion of infection with HIV. In addition, leukopenia should suggest sarcoidosis, systemic lupus erythematosus, tuberculosis, histoplasmosis, or tumor. A leukemoid reaction may be seen in disseminated mycobacteriosis. Leukocytosis is suggestive of but not specific for a bacterial cause.

Laboratory tests that measure the function of other organs may provide more helpful information. Liver function studies, including bilirubin, alkaline phosphatase, and serum aspartate aminotransferase determinations and prothrombin time, should be obtained for most patients. Urinalysis, with particular attention to the urinary sediment, plus tests of renal function including measurement of blood urea nitrogen and creatinine, should also be done. Abnormalities of liver function (especially elevated enzyme levels), kidney function, or both should raise the suspicion of disorders that are not limited to the lung but are known to involve multiple organs, including lung, liver, and kidney. Such disorders include disseminated histoplasmosis and disseminated mycobacteriosis as well as the vasculitides, sarcoidosis, and certain neoplastic diseases, especially the lymphoproliferative types.

In a patient with an abnormally low serum globulin level, a quantitative serum immunoglobulin determination should be obtained to evaluate the patient for hypogammaglobulinemia. Studies that should be performed in patients with suspected vasculitis include serologic tests for antinuclear antibodies, rheumatoid factor, antineutrophil cytoplasmic autoantibodies, and erythrocyte sedimentation rate. In addition, serum angiotensin-converting enzyme levels are increased in 30 to 80% of patients with sarcoidosis.[10]

Studies to Establish a Cause

A basic core of studies should usually be performed on all patients with chronic pneumonia, regardless of the suspected cause, but there should be flexibility in choosing additional tests or procedures to confirm a specific diagnosis. The orderly sequence of diagnostic studies described in the following sections necessarily results in oversimplification and consequently overlooks the unique aspects of a given patient's illness.

Chest Radiographic Studies. The chest radiographs, including a posteroanterior and a lateral film, and the chest CT are important diagnostic studies. Newer imaging techniques, including high-resolution thin-section chest CT[52, 53] and fluorodeoxyglucose positron emission tomography,[54] are being increasingly used, especially in the evaluation of the noninfectious causes of chronic pneumonia. Because of the singular importance of these various imaging studies, Table 60–2 is provided to emphasize the major radiologic patterns that may be seen. In Table 60–2, the disorders are grouped according to the type of radiologic abnormality that is characteristic of the disease. In some disorders there is a spectrum of radiologic manifestations, and these disorders appear more than once in the table. Typical radiographic findings may provide clues to specific diagnoses. For example, documentation of anterior mediastinal involvement argues strongly in favor of neoplasia, including lymphoma and metastatic carcinoma, as the cause of chronic pneumonia syndrome and argues against an infectious cause.

Tuberculosis and nontuberculous mycobacterial diseases, histoplasmosis, coccidioidomycosis, sporotrichosis, melioidosis, paragonimiasis, and the pneumoconioses, especially silicosis, characteristically produce fibrocavitary disease—a contracted area of lung with linear fibrosis, nodular or rounded densities, and cavitation. In addition, mycobacterial diseases, histoplasmosis, and silicosis characteristically involve the upper lobes. A thin-walled cavity is suggestive of coccidioidomycosis, sporotrichosis, or paragonimiasis, whereas a thick-walled cavity surrounded by an area of pneumonitis is more typical of tuberculosis, nontuberculous mycobacterial diseases, histoplasmosis, aspergillosis, melioidosis, nocardiosis, actinomycosis, pyogenic lung abscess, and lung disease caused by *R. equi.* Cavitation is less common in blastomycosis and cryptococcosis. Calcification is typical of tuberculosis, histoplasmosis, and coccidioidomycosis but is rare in actinomycosis, nocardiosis, blastomycosis, and cryptococcosis. Abscess of the chest wall or osteomyelitis of a rib adjacent to the pneumonia or pleural effusion may be seen in actinomycosis and nocardiosis. Although these radiographic manifes-

TABLE 60-2 Radiologic Patterns of Diseases That Commonly Cause Chronic Pneumonia Syndrome

Disease	Radiologic Characteristics
Diseases That Cause Patchy Infiltrates and/or Bronchopneumonia or Lobar Consolidation	
Infectious	
Aspiration pneumonia secondary to mixed aerobic and anaerobic infection	Usually dependent portions: superior or basilar segments of lower lobes or posterior segments of upper lobes; pleural involvement with empyema common
Necrotizing pneumonia secondary to infection by Enterobacteriaceae, *Pseudomonas aeruginosa,* or *Staphylococcus aureus*	Any lobe or segment Chronic *Klebsiella* pneumonia commonly involves upper lobes; may be multiple sites of pulmonary infection secondary to septic embolization
Actinomycosis	Commonly involves lower lobes; cavitation frequently present; pleural involvement with empyema common
Nocardiosis	No distinctive pattern; may involve single or multiple lobes; cavitation may be present; pleural involvement may occur
Tuberculous exudative pneumonia	Not restricted to upper lobes; often bilateral with perihilar distribution
Blastomycosis	Often a dense area of lobar or segmental consolidation; cavitation infrequent
Cryptococcosis	Single or multiple patchy infiltrates; less commonly, lobar consolidation; occasionally, single or diffuse nodular lesions
Paracoccidioidomycosis	Asymptomatic bilateral fluffy infiltrates; may be extremely indolent
Noninfectious	
Chronic eosinophilic pneumonia	Rapidly progressive, dense infiltrates; usually peripheral (reverse pattern of pulmonary edema)
Bronchiolitis obliterans organizing pneumonia	Patchy nonsegmental areas of consolidation, often subpleural and bilateral; large irregular nodules
Diseases That Cause Pulmonary Cavitation	
Infectious	
Pyogenic lung abscess	
Complicating aspiration pneumonia	Usually single cavity; location same as aspiration pneumonia; air-fluid level common
Complicating necrotizing pneumonia	May involve any lobe; often multiple and bilateral, depending on route of acquisition of pneumonia
Tuberculosis-reactivation or adult type	Usually upper lobes; often bilateral; may be multiple; fibrosis and calcification common
Atypical mycobacterial disease	Radiologically indistinguishable from tuberculosis, except that cavitation may be more frequent
Melioidosis	Simulates tuberculosis, but may involve any lobe
Rhodococcal lung disease	Simulates tuberculosis or nocardiosis; cavitation common
Histoplasmosis, chronic cavitary	Mimics tuberculosis; upper lobes frequently involved but can involve any lobe; unilateral or bilateral
Coccidioidomycosis	Usually single, thin-walled cavity with minimum involvement of surrounding lung; occasionally thick-walled cavity surrounded by extensive parenchymal disease
Sporotrichosis	May mimic tuberculosis but can involve any lobe; cavitation is frequent; thin-walled cavity more likely than thick-walled cavity
Aspergillosis	Single or multiple areas of pneumonia with or without central cavitation; not to be confused with intracavitary fungus ball
Paragonimiasis	Cystlike lesions as well as cavities, usually associated with linear or patchy infiltrates, fibrosis, and/or calcification
Echinococcosis	Single or multiple discrete, sharply defined, round lesions (cysts) with little surrounding inflammatory response; cavitation and/or calcification may occur
Noninfectious	
Wegener's granulomatosis and lymphomatoid granulomatosis	Often multiple nodules with cavitation; may be unilateral or bilateral
Silicosis	Associated with conglomerate nodular densities, frequently in upper lobes; usually superimposed on background of diffuse nodulation; rarely, eggshell calcification of hilar nodes
Bronchogenic carcinoma	Eccentric cavitation more common in squamous cell type
Lymphoma, especially Hodgkin's disease	Cavitation may occur in peripheral parenchymal nodules
Kaposi's sarcoma	Small or large nodules associated with peribronchial cuffing and tram track opacities
Infectious and Noninfectious Diseases That Cause Chronic Diffuse Pulmonary Infiltration and Fibrosis	
Bronchioloalveolar carcinoma Intrapulmonary bleeding (e.g., Goodpasture's syndrome) Pulmonary alveolar proteinosis	Alveolar pattern
Sarcoidosis Early asbestosis or berylliosis Bronchiolitis obliterans organizing pneumonia	Ground-glass interstitial pattern
Granulomatous infectious diseases (e.g., miliary tuberculosis, disseminated histoplasmosis) Sarcoidosis Lymphangitic carcinomatosis Wegener's granulomatosis Lymphomatoid granulomatosis Allergic angiitis and granulomatosis Rheumatoid lung disease Pneumoconiosis (including asbestosis, silicosis, and berylliosis)	Nodular interstitial pattern, including miliary spherical nodules
Chronic form of hypersensitivity pneumonitis Idiopathic pulmonary hemosiderosis Radiation injury—chronic Progressive systemic sclerosis Sarcoidosis	Linear interstitial pattern, including fine reticular markings and dense fibrosis
Advanced form of fibrosing alveolitis Bronchiectasis Eosinophilic granuloma (histiocytosis X) Sarcoidosis	Honeycombing (coarse reticular pattern with cystic airspaces)

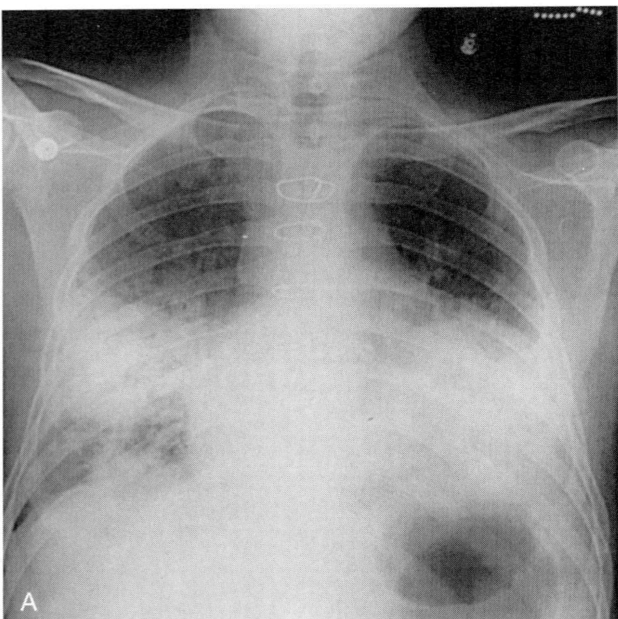

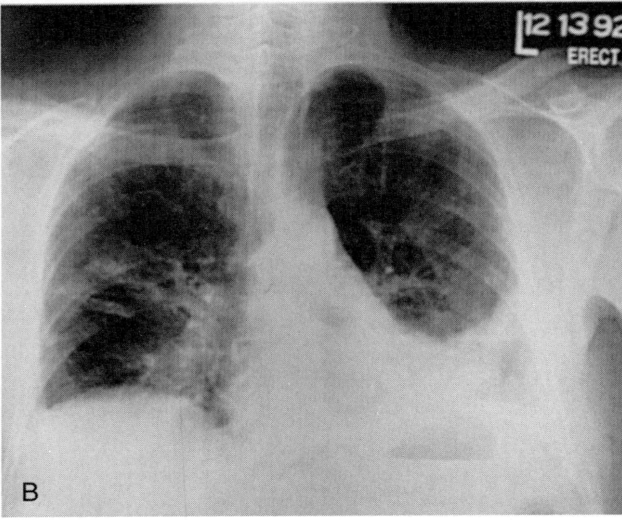

FIGURE 60–1. *A*, Bronchiolitis obliterans organizing pneumonia (BOOP) in a 32-year-old man who developed progressive chronic pneumonia several weeks after an open pericardiectomy to relieve cardiac tamponade associated with renal failure. Note the bilateral airspace consolidation. Bronchoscopy with transbronchial biopsy was nondiagnostic. The diagnosis of BOOP was established from tissue obtained at open lung biopsy. Corticosteroid therapy was dramatically beneficial. *B*, BOOP in a 60-year-old man with a 1-month illness manifested by fever, malaise, weight loss, nonproductive cough, dyspnea, and bilateral subpleural nodular opacities. Both symptoms and radiographic abnormalities progressed during antibiotic therapy. A bronchoscopy with transthoracic biopsy was nondiagnostic. The diagnosis of BOOP was made from tissue obtained at open lung biopsy. Corticosteroid therapy was beneficial.

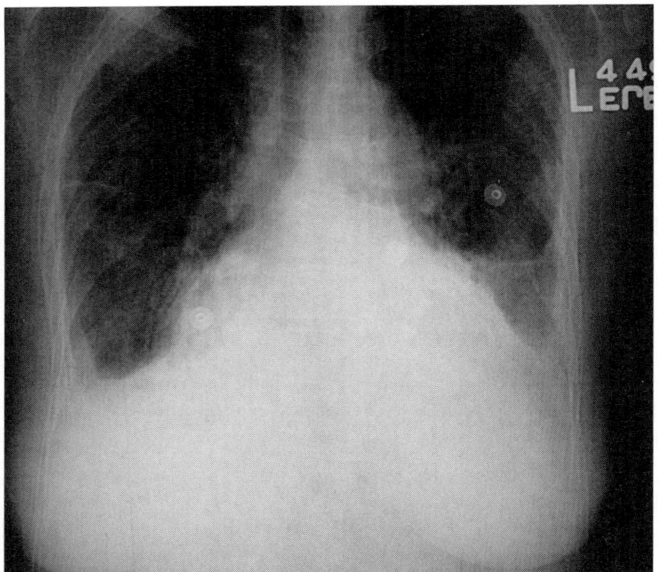

FIGURE 60–2. Systemic lupus erythematous in a previously healthy 66-year-old woman with a 5-month illness characterized by fever, nonproductive cough, shortness of breath, pleuritic chest pain, polyarthralgias, weakness, and proteinuria. Note the cardiomegaly, bilateral pleural effusions, and lower lobe pneumonitis. Cardiac echocardiogram showed a large pericardial effusion. Test results for antinuclear antibody and antibodies to double-stranded DNA were positive.

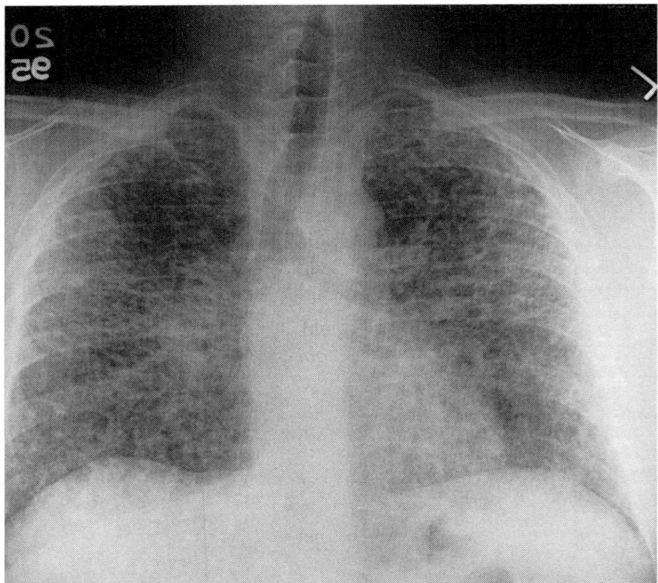

FIGURE 60–3. Pulmonary sarcoidosis in a 42-year-old man with a 6-month illness characterized by low-grade fever, intermittent night sweats, nonproductive cough, and progressive dyspnea. Note the bilateral panlobar reticulonodular pattern. A pathologic diagnosis was from lung tissue obtained by transbronchial biopsy.

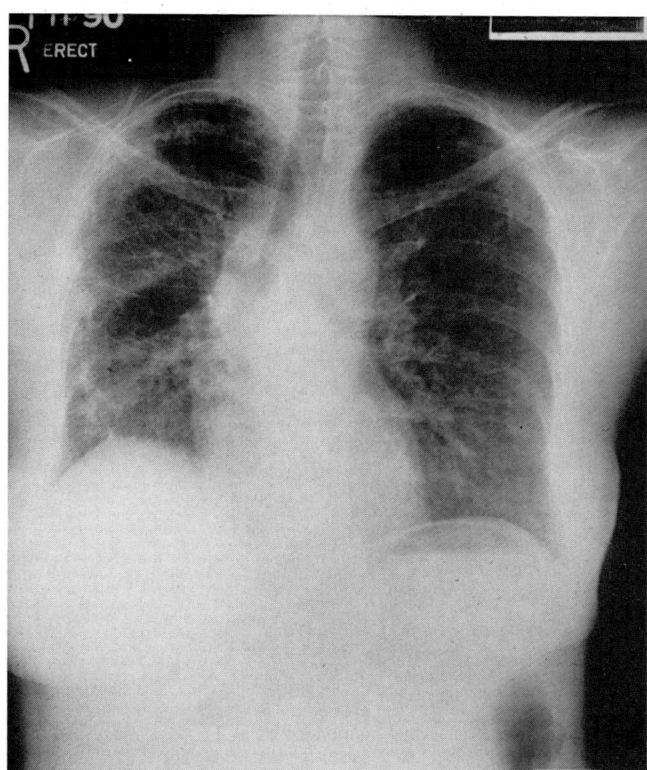

FIGURE 60–4. Drug-induced lung disease secondary to bleomycin in a 50-year-old woman receiving chemotherapy for Hodgkin's disease. She had noted fever, dyspnea, and nonproductive cough over the preceding 5-week period. Note the bilateral reticulonodular infiltrates, most prominent in the right middle and lower lung fields.

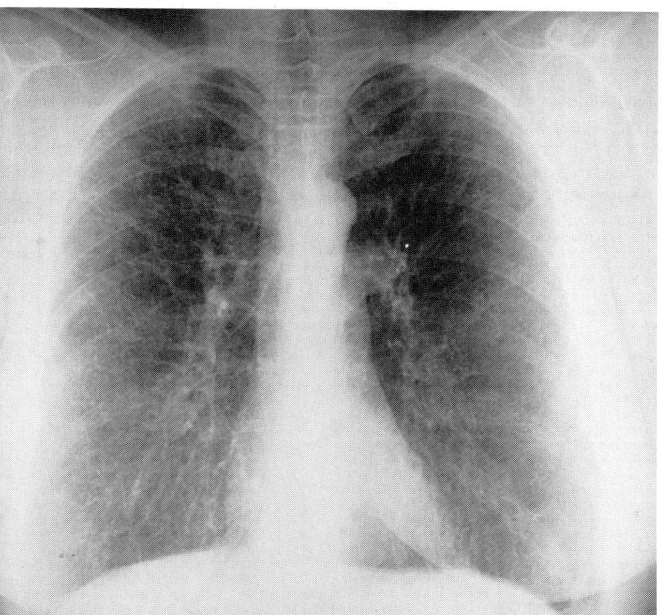

FIGURE 60–5. Lymphangioleiomyomatosis in a 42-year-old woman with a 6-month history of progressive dyspnea and intermittent blood-streaked sputum. She denied fever or history of pneumothorax. Note the diffuse reticular pattern with areas of cystic dilation and enlarged lung volumes. A pathologic diagnosis was made from lung tissue obtained by transbronchial biopsy.

tations of selected pulmonary diseases are typical in the majority of patients, experience during the AIDS epidemic has shown that pulmonary diseases in these patients may be highly atypical in radiographic appearance and clinical course.[26, 28, 36–46] Representative radiographs are shown in Figures 60–1 through 60–14.

Studies in Patients with Radiographic Evidence of Localized Infiltrates or Cavitation. In all patients with radiographic evidence of localized infiltrates or cavitation, examination of the sputum is essential. The specimen of sputum must be a representative sample. If the expectorated sputum is a deep, coughed specimen, of adequate volume and is acceptable after cytologic screening, other procedures to obtain sputum may not be necessary. Microscopic examination of sputum should include the following:

1. Gram staining for bacteria and actinomyces
2. Acid-fast staining for *Mycobacteria* and modified acid-fast staining for *Nocardia*
3. Wet mounts for fungi and eggs of *Paragonimus* (calcofluor white–potassium hydroxide preparation with phase contrast may enhance detection of fungi)
4. Gomori methenamine silver stain or the periodic acid–Schiff stain for fungi
5. Cytologic preparations for neoplastic cells, eosinophils, and fungi.

Generous volumes of expectorated sputum should also be sent to the microbiology laboratory for culture of bacteria, fungi, and mycobacteria. In addition, it is often diagnostically rewarding for the clinician to speak directly with the personnel in the microbiology laboratory to alert them to specific etiologic considerations. In this way, specimens can be inoculated on the most appropriate media, the microbi-

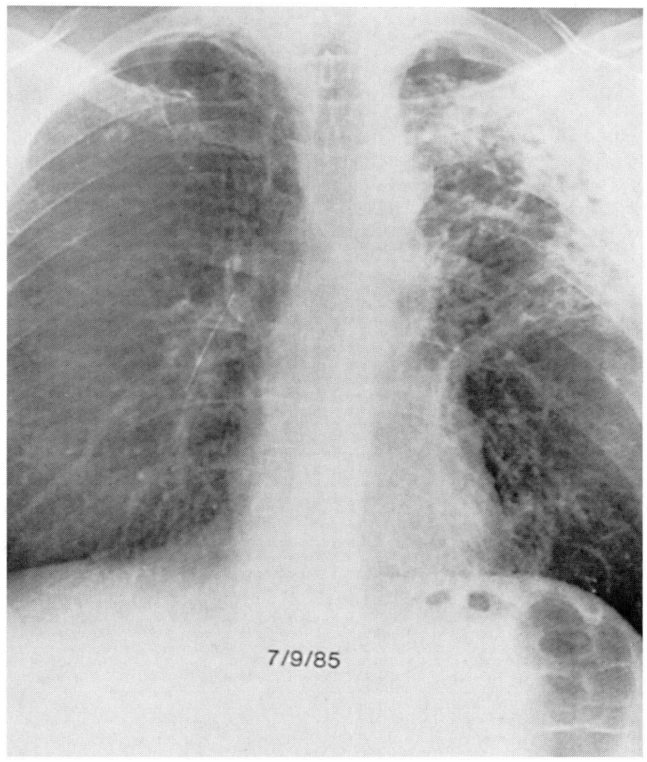

FIGURE 60–6. Chronic cavitary pulmonary histoplasmosis in a 53-year-old man with chronic obstructive pulmonary disease and a 3-month history of low-grade fever, night sweats, cough, progressive dyspnea, and weight loss. Note the bilateral fibrocavitary disease with prominent involvement of the left upper lobe.

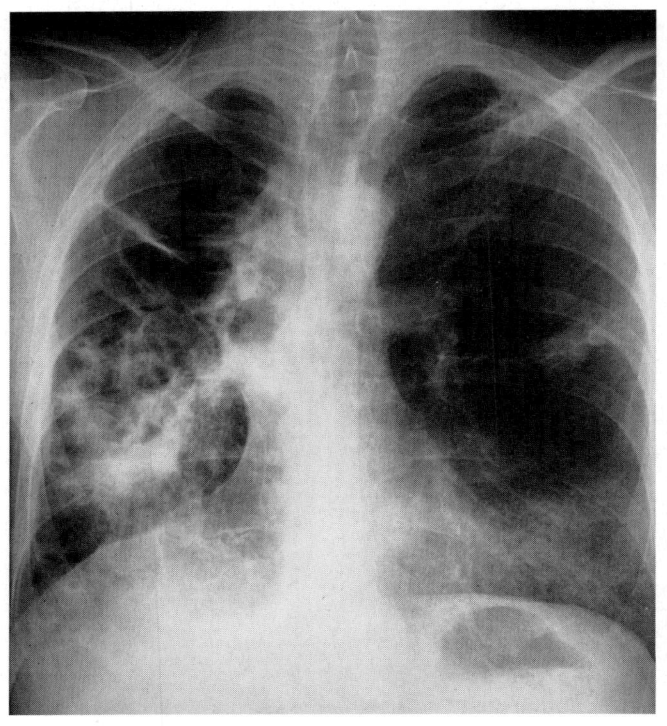

FIGURE 60–7. Atypical tuberculosis caused by *Mycobacterium avium* complex in a 52-year-old man with chronic obstructive pulmonary disease and an 18-month history of fever, weight loss, cough, intermittent hemoptysis, and progressive dyspnea associated with persistently positive acid-fast smears and cultures of expectorated sputum and worsening chest films despite appropriate antimycobacterial therapy. Note the bilateral lower lobe fibronodular disease, worse in the right lung, associated with cavitation.

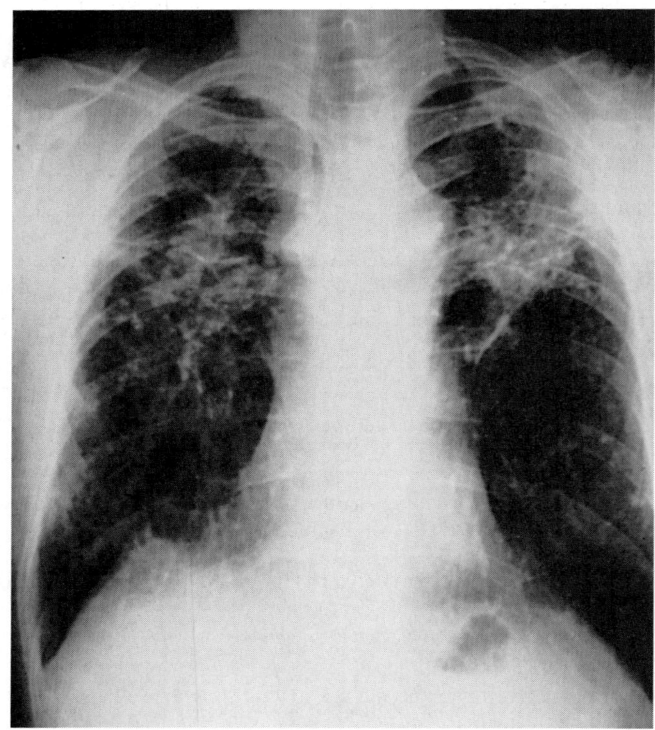

FIGURE 60–8. Chronic cavitary pulmonary coccidioidomycosis in a 55-year-old rancher from west Texas who had a history of an abnormal chest film result for the preceding 20 years. He had experienced a single episode of self-limited hemoptysis about 10 years earlier. At the time of this film, the patient noted subcutaneous nodules on his anterior chest. Histopathology of tissue obtained by skin biopsy revealed large, endospore-containing spherules, consistent with *Coccidioides immitis* infection. Note the bilateral fibrocavitary disease primarily involving the upper lobes.

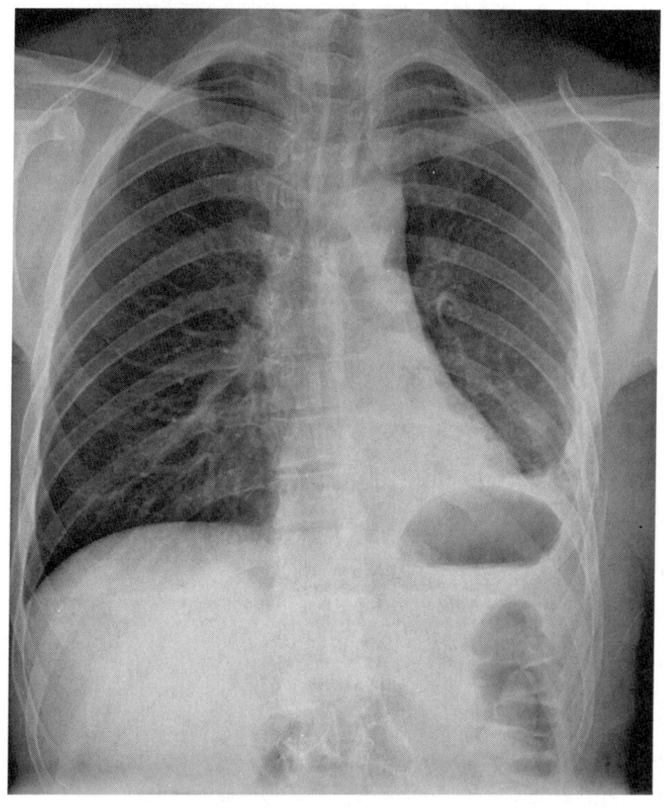

FIGURE 60–9. Pulmonary actinomycosis in a 53-year-old man with a 4-month history of malaise, low-grade fever, cough, and progressive left chest wall pain. He had severe dental caries and abused both alcohol and tobacco. Note the left lower lobe opacity, left pleural effusion, and left rib fracture. Microbiologic diagnosis was made by stains and culture of a biopsy specimen from a left chest wall draining mass lesion.

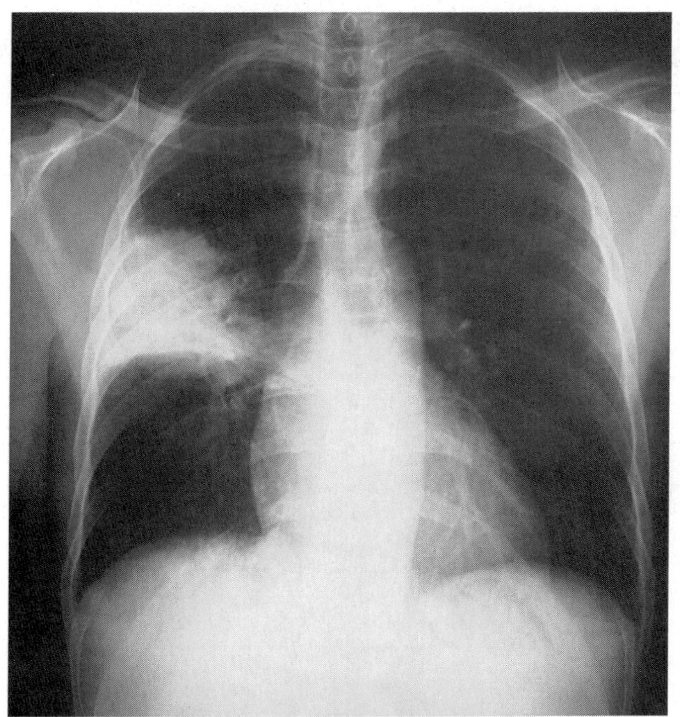

FIGURE 60–10. Pulmonary nocardiosis in a 40-year-old man with advanced acquired immunodeficiency syndrome ($CD4^+$ cell count 51/mm^3 and plasma human immunodeficiency virus RNA 72,000 copies/ml) and a 6-week illness consisting of fever, cough, pleuritic chest pain, shortness of breath, and nonresponsiveness to two courses of oral antibiotics. Note the pleural-based right upper lobe segmental bronchopneumonia. Microbiologic diagnosis was made from stains and cultures of bronchial washings obtained at bronchoscopy.

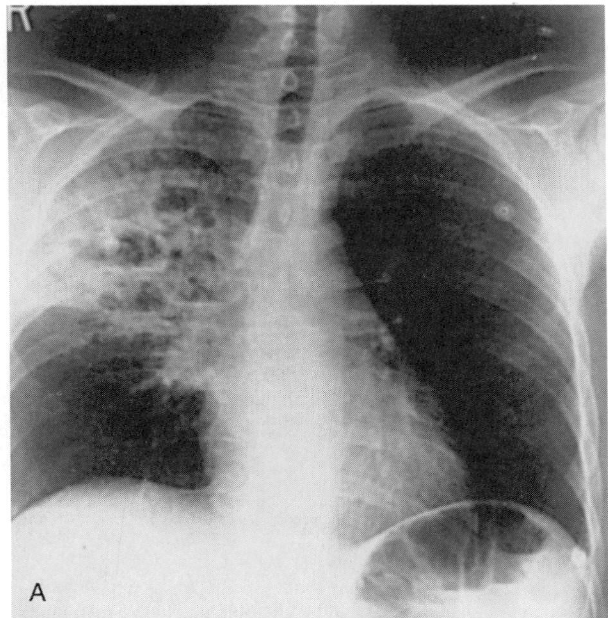

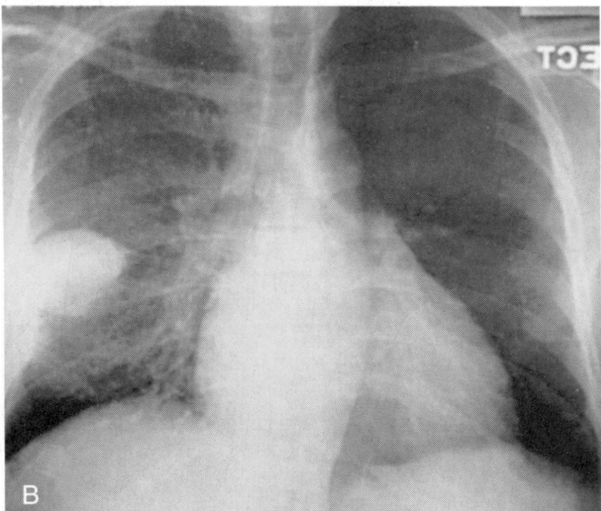

FIGURE 60–11. *A, Rhodococcus equi* pneumonia in a patient with acquired immunodeficiency syndrome (AIDS) who had a 2-month progressive illness characterized by fever, night sweats, weight loss, and nonproductive cough. Note the necrotizing, cavitary infiltrate involving the right upper lobe. The microbiologic diagnosis was made from washings and tissue obtained at bronchoscopy. *B, R. equi* pneumonia in an AIDS patient with a 6-week history of fever, weight loss, and right-sided pleuritic pain. Note the pleural-based, well-circumscribed mass lesion. The microbiologic diagnosis was made from tissue obtained at open lung biopsy.

ologists can be made more aware of the suspected pathogens, and recent microbiologic advances (e.g., rapid culture techniques, molecular probes) can be used to facilitate laboratory diagnosis.[55]

For all patients in whom an infectious cause is considered, cultures from sources other than sputum should be obtained. These sources might include blood, urine, pleural fluid in all patients with pleural effusion (pleural tissue should also be obtained for culture), cerebrospinal fluid in all patients with central nervous system symptoms or signs, synovial fluid in all patients with joint effusion, and samples of skin, mucous membrane, or any tissue obtained at biopsy.

To obtain sputum, if adequate sputum cannot be readily produced via spontaneous expectoration by the patient, consider the following: (1) sputum induction by hypertonic aerosol and ultrasonic nebulization, hydration, chest physiotherapy, or postural drainage and (2) bronchoscopy for bronchial brushing, transbronchial biopsy, bronchoalveolar lavage, or protected specimen brush sampling of lower respiratory tract secretions.[34, 56–58]

Skin tests should be made in all cases in which an infectious cause is considered. The tuberculin skin test with purified protein derivative (PPD) is the single most important test. Skin test antigens for the detection of infection with atypical mycobacteria are not commercially available. Skin tests of the tuberculin type are available for patients with suspected fungal disease. However, these are most valuable when they are used for epidemiologic studies to determine the prevalence of infection in a given population or in a certain geographic area; they are of little diagnostic value in the individual patient.

Serologic tests for HIV should be performed for all patients with unexplained chronic pneumonia. In addition, serologic tests may be helpful when other infectious causes, especially fungi, are considered. However, there are problems with these tests, including long delays in obtaining results, false-positive results because of cross-reactions to other antigens, and false-negative results. Serologic tests are most helpful when pulmonary mycoses, including coccidioidomycosis, cryptococcosis, histoplasmosis, and paracoccidioidomycosis, are suspected. Similarly, if hypersensitivity pneumonitis is suspected, serum should be examined for precipitating antibodies to various inhalant antigens, and, if allergic bronchopulmonary aspergillosis is suspected, total serum immunoglobulin E and serum anti-*Aspergillus* antibody should be measured. Finally, serologic tests for rarer causes of chronic pneumonia, such as *Legionella* species, *C. pneumoniae,* and *C. burnetii,* should be considered in selected patients.

Invasive Procedures. Certain clinical situations dictate a more aggressive diagnostic approach. In patients who are unable to raise sputum spontaneously and in whom attempts to induce sputum pro-

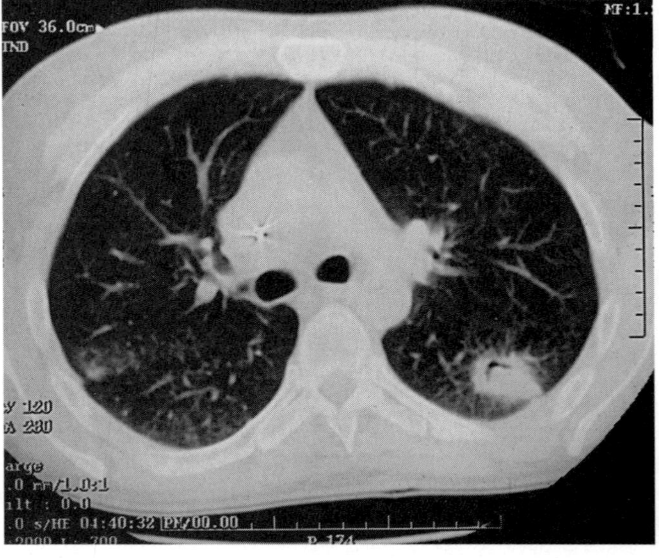

FIGURE 60–12. Invasive pulmonary aspergillosis in a 43-year-old man with prolonged granulocytopenia secondary to chemotherapy for acute myelocytic leukemia. For several weeks, the patient noted daily fevers, malaise, and left pleuritic chest pain, but no cough or shortness of breath. His symptoms persisted despite repeated courses of broad-spectrum antibiotics. Chest CT shows a pleural-based irregular rounded mass in the left lower lung and a smaller nodule in the right lower lung. Note the crescentric "halo" in the left lung mass. Stains and culture of lung tissue obtained by transthoracic needle aspiration confirmed the suspicion of *Aspergillus* as the causative fungus.

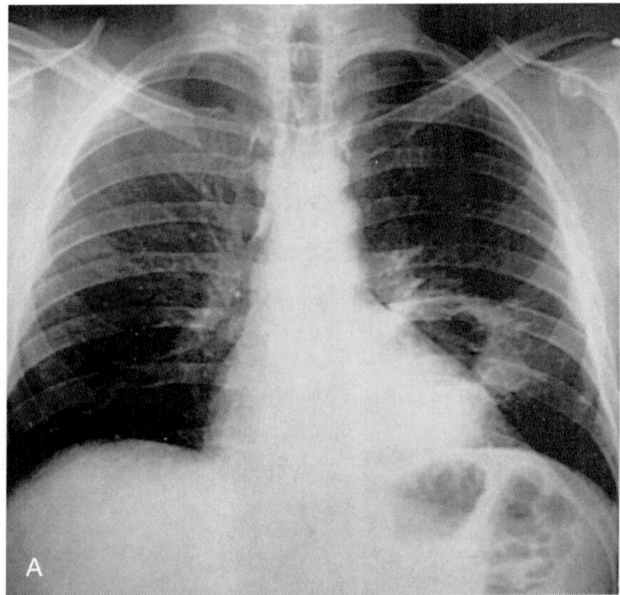

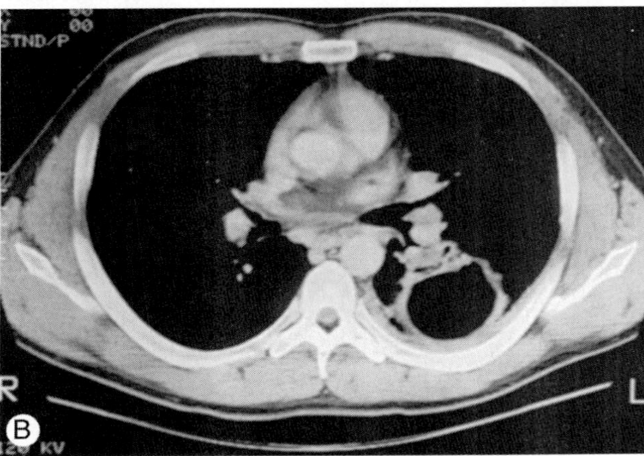

FIGURE 60–13. *A*, Wegener's granulomatosis in a 35-year-old cattle farmer with a 2-month illness manifested by fever, malaise, weight loss, pleurisy, polyarthralgias, and palpable purpura of the lower extremities. Laboratory studies included a markedly elevated erythrocyte sedimentation rate, a positive test result for antineutrophil cytoplasmic autoantibody, and an abnormal urine sediment. Note the large cavitary mass lesion of the left lower lobe. *B*, A chest computed tomography scan demonstrates the lower lobe cavitary lesion and a small pleural effusion but no other pulmonary parenchymal abnormalities.

duction are unsuccessful, invasive procedures may be necessary. Fiberoptic bronchoscopy usually is the initial procedure. It is diagnostically helpful when it is accompanied by bronchial washings and transbronchial biopsy with appropriate microbiologic and histologic studies.[34, 56–57] Analysis of bronchoalveolar lavage fluid may increase the diagnostic yield of bronchoscopy, especially in immunocompromised persons such as AIDS patients with suspected opportunistic infections or patients with suspected noninfectious causes of chronic pneumonia.[15, 34, 58] In a patient with extensive pleural involvement, thoracentesis and pleural biopsy, or rigid thoracoscopy in selected situations, may be more helpful diagnostically than bronchoscopy.[59] In some institutions, open lung biopsy is the procedure of choice for patients with interstitial lung disease and for many immunosuppressed patients with pulmonary disease because of the relatively large piece of tissue obtained, the expediency of diagnosis, and the safety of the procedure.[15, 60–61] By contrast, in other institutions with seasoned operators, transthoracic needle aspiration of the lung[62–63] or video-assisted thoracoscopy[59, 64] is preferred to open lung biopsy and is associated with low risk of complications and high sensitivity.

All specimens, regardless of source, should be submitted for microscopic examination and culture, as already described. Any lung or pleural tissue should also be submitted for histopathologic studies, including special stains. In any patient in whom there is extrapulmonary disease that probably results from the same cause as the chronic pneumonia, tissue or fluid from the extrapulmonary sites should be obtained for culture and histologic studies. In such patients, consider the following procedures: arthrocentesis, abdominal paracentesis, lumbar puncture, bone marrow biopsy, liver biopsy, lymph node biopsy, and skin and muscle biopsy.

Studies in Patients with Radiographic Evidence of Diffuse Pulmonary Infiltration and Fibrosis. In patients whose chest radiographs show a predominantly diffuse infiltrative pattern of either the alveolar or the interstitial type (see Table 60–2), pulmonary function studies

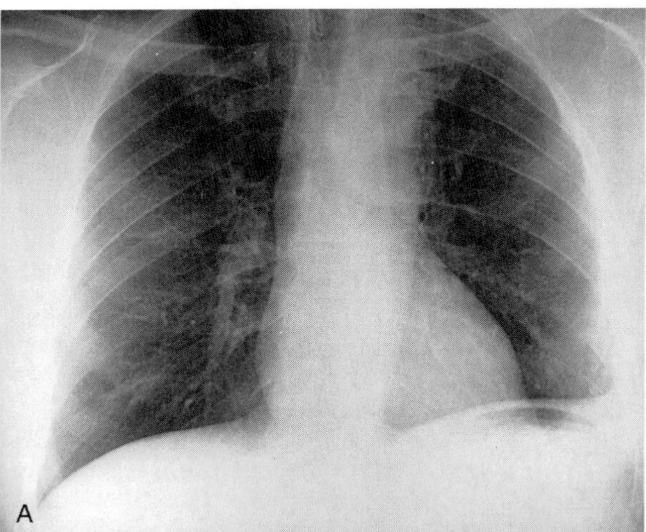

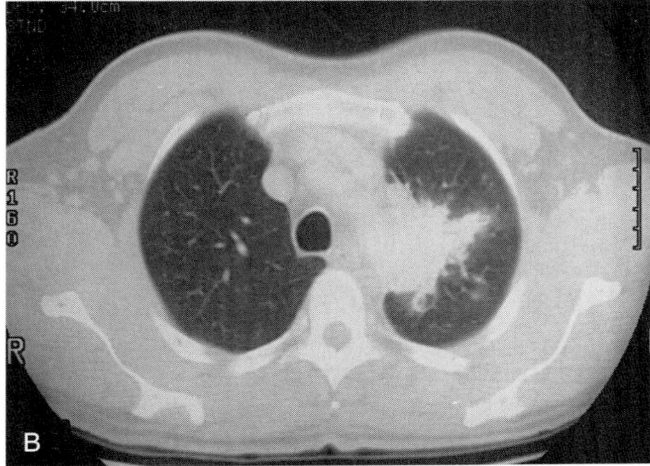

FIGURE 60–14. *A*, Pulmonary blastomycosis in a 49-year-old male logger with an illness consisting of low-grade fever, night sweats, and malaise for 8 months and, more recently, nonproductive cough and mild dyspnea but no hemoptysis, pleuritic chest pain, or skin lesions. Note the left upper lobe opacity, left-to-right shift of the trachea, and small left pleural effusion. *B*, Chest computed tomography scan shows a stellate irregular mass lesion without cavitation, interpreted as most consistent with malignancy. Specimens obtained at bronchoscopy with bronchial washings yielded both microbiologic and histopathologic evidence of blastomycosis.

may be of greater importance. These studies not only quantify the degree of pulmonary insufficiency but may help delineate the disease processes by virtue of the patterns of pulmonary function impairment. Accordingly, these tests are particularly useful in characterizing those diseases that impair gas transfer and predispose to ventilation-perfusion inequalities, such as sarcoidosis or other interstitial lung diseases.

Studies that may be especially useful in this group of patients include the following:

1. Arterial blood gas studies and exercise oximetry
2. Tests of pulmonary function, including spirometric measurements, measurements of lung volume, and measurement of pulmonary diffusing capacity
3. Studies on sputum as previously outlined (cytologic examination is especially important)
4. Lung biopsy to make an accurate morphologic diagnosis (transbronchial biopsy via the fiberoptic bronchoscope, open lung biopsy, or video-assisted thoracoscopy) is the procedure of choice.[15, 59, 64]

THERAPY

Antimicrobial Agents

If a specific infectious agent is readily identified as the cause of the chronic pneumonia, the appropriate antimicrobial agent or agents should be administered. In many patients, no etiologic agent is identified on the basis of the initial stains and cultures, and a definitive diagnosis must await the completion of serologic, histologic, and bacteriologic studies as well as other diagnostic tests. In such situations, if immediate empirical therapy is advisable, the choice of antimicrobial agents must be based on the available epidemiologic, clinical, and microbiologic data.

For example, if an otherwise healthy young patient has been ill for a relatively short period (2 to 3 weeks), the chest radiograph shows a lobar or patchy pneumonia, especially in the lower lobes; Gram stain of the sputum reveals few to moderate polymorphonuclear leukocytes and organisms resembling normal flora; and the patient acquired the infection outside the hospital, the patient may have persistent or chronic pneumonia as a complication of one or more common acute pneumonia syndromes, namely, pneumococcal pneumonia, *Mycoplasma* pneumonia, *Chlamydia* pneumonia, or legionnaires' disease. Reasonable empirical therapy in such a patient is a macrolide antibiotic (erythromycin, clarithromycin, or azithromycin) or one of the newer fluoroquinolones (levofloxacin or trovafloxacin), because these drugs in general provide effective treatment of these four pneumonias. If, on the other hand, a patient has chronic pneumonia after thoracotomy or has been chronically intubated in an intensive care unit, initial antimicrobial therapy should provide broad-spectrum coverage against hospital-acquired flora, including anaerobes, *Staphylococcus aureus,* and aerobic gram-negative bacteria. In both of the cases described, once the pathogen or pathogens have been identified and sensitivity testing has been completed, appropriate changes in the antibiotic regimen should be made.

If a patient has a more chronic indolent illness, is stable, and does not require immediate empirical therapy, a methodic and thorough diagnostic evaluation is the initial priority. In a patient with bilateral upper lobe cavitary disease in whom the initial microscopic examinations are nonrevealing, the leading considerations include tuberculosis, histoplasmosis, and coccidioidomycosis. If such a patient has a positive tuberculin skin response, tuberculosis should be presumed to be the diagnosis until proved otherwise, and antituberculosis therapy should be initiated and continued for at least 6 weeks, pending the final results of the mycobacterial cultures. Disseminated tuberculosis should be strongly suspected in any patient with unexplained fever and a chest radiograph showing a nodular interstitial pattern; prompt institution of antituberculosis therapy may be lifesaving in this otherwise fatal condition. Similarly, empirical antifungal therapy, usually with amphotericin B, may be indicated in an AIDS patient or other immunocompromised host with chronic pneumonia, because fungal pulmonary diseases in this setting can be severe and rapidly progressive.

Corticosteroids

The question of when to use corticosteroids in the treatment of a patient with chronic pneumonia frequently arises. If the cause of the illness is an infectious agent, particularly a bacterium or a fungus, steroids usually are not indicated. In contrast, corticosteroids may be beneficial in chronic pneumonia from noninfectious causes, such as the vasculitides,[1–4] sarcoidosis,[10] chronic eosinophilic pneumonia,[65] radiation injury, bronchiolitis obliterans organizing pneumonia,[12, 13] and many of the fibrotic lung diseases including chronic hypersensitivity pneumonitis (along with avoidance of exposure to the offending antigen).[48] Other immunosuppressive drugs, such as cyclophosphamide and azathioprine, may also be effective in some patients, especially those with a vasculitis.

Bronchoscopy and Surgery

Bronchoscopy may be used as a therapeutic adjunct, especially for patients who have thick, tenacious secretions that cannot be raised by noninvasive techniques. In other patients, mucus plugs or foreign bodies may predispose to atelectasis and chronic pneumonia; therapeutic bronchoscopy may be necessary to expand the collapsed lung.

Lobectomy or pneumonectomy should be considered in a patient with chronic destructive pneumonia, multiple macroabscesses or microabscesses involving an entire lobe or lung, and a ventilation-perfusion scan indicating nonfunction of the involved lung (pulmonary gangrene[66]). Thoracotomy may also be indicated for purposes of decortication of the pleura in patients whose chronic pneumonia has involved the pleura with resulting restrictive lung disease.

REFERENCES

1. Fauci AS, Haynes BF, Katz P, et al. Wegener's granulomatosis: Prospective clinical and therapeutic experience with 85 patients for 21 years. Ann Intern Med. 1983;98:76–85.
2. Hoffman GS, Kerr GS, Leavitt RY, et al. Wegener granulomatosis: An analysis of 158 patients. Ann Intern Med. 1992;116:488–498.
3. Lanham JC, Elkon KB, Pusey CD, et al. Systemic vasculitis with asthma and eosinophilia: A clinical approach to the Churg-Strauss syndrome. Medicine (Baltimore). 1984;63:65–80.
4. Fauci AS, Haynes BF, Costa J, et al. Lymphomatoid granulomatosis: Prospective clinical and therapeutic experience over 10 years. N Engl J Med. 1982;306:69–74.
5. Hill CA. Bronchioloalveolar carcinoma: A review. Radiology. 1984;150:15–20.
6. Cordier JF, Chailleux E, Lauque D, et al. Primary pulmonary lymphomas: A clinical study of 70 cases in nonimmunocompromised patients. Chest. 1993;103:201–208.
7. Casey KR. Neoplastic mimics of pneumonia. Semin Respir Infect. 1995;10:131–142.
8. Cooper JA Jr. Drug-induced lung disease. Adv Intern Med. 1997;42:231–268.
9. Cordier JF, Loire R, Brune J. Amyloidosis of the lower respiratory tract: Clinical and pathologic features in a series of 21 patients. Chest. 1986;90:827–831.
10. Lynch JP, Kazerooni EA, Gay SE. Pulmonary sarcoidosis. Clin Chest Med. 1997;18:755–785.
11. Prakash UB, Barham SS, Carpenter HA, et al. Pulmonary alveolar phospholipoproteinosis: Experience with 34 cases and a review. Mayo Clin Proc. 1987;62:499–518.
12. Epler GR. Bronchiolitis obliterans organizing pneumonia. Semin Respir Infect. 1995;10:65–77.
13. Lohr RH, Boland BJ, Douglas WW, et al. Organizing pneumonia: Features and prognosis of cryptogenic, secondary and focal variants. Arch Intern Med. 1997;157:1323–1329.
14. Crystal RG, Bitterman PB, Rennard SI, et al. Interstitial lung diseases of unknown cause: Disorders characterized by chronic inflammation of the lower respiratory tract. Parts 1 and 2. N Engl J Med. 1984;310:154–166, 235–244.
15. Schwartz MI. Clinical overview of interstitial lung disease. In: Schwarz MI, King TE Jr, eds. Interstitial Lung Disease. 2nd ed. St. Louis: Mosby–Yearbook; 1994:1–22.
16. Bartlett JG. Anaerobic bacterial infections of the lung. Chest. 1987;91:901–909.
17. Eisenstadt J, Crane LR. Gram-negative bacillary pneumonias. In: Pennington JE, ed. Respiratory Infections: Diagnosis and Management. 3rd ed. New York: Raven Press; 1994:369–406.
18. Kirtland SH, Winterbauer RH, Dreis DF, et al. A clinical profile of chronic bacterial pneumonia: Report of 115 cases. Chest. 1994;106:15–22.

19. Bartlett JG, Breiman RF, Mandel LA, et al. Community acquired pneumonia in adults: Guidelines for management. Clin Infect Dis. 1998;26:811–838.
20. Case records of the Massachusetts General Hospital. Case 8–1994. N Engl J Med. 1994;330:557–564.
21. Case records of the Massachusetts General Hospital. Case 48–1990. N Engl J Med. 1990;323:1546–1555.
22. Khan MA, Kovnat DM, Bachus B, et al. Clinical and roentgenographic spectrum of pulmonary tuberculosis in the adult. Am J Med. 1977;62:31–38.
23. Prince DS, Peterson DD, Steiner RM, et al. Infection with *Mycobacterium avium* complex in patients without predisposing conditions. N Engl J Med. 1989;321: 863–868.
24. Patz EF Jr, Swensen SJ, Erasmus J. Pulmonary manifestations of nontuberculous *Mycobacterium*. Radiol Clin North Am. 1995;33:719–729.
25. Goodwin RA, Owens FT, Snell JD, et al. Chronic cavitary histoplasmosis. Medicine (Baltimore). 1976;55:413–452.
26. Galgiani JN. Coccidioidomycosis. West J Med. 1993;159:153–171.
27. Hsieh MI, Liu HP, Chang JP, et al. Thoracic actinomycosis. Chest. 1993;104: 366–370.
28. Davies SF, Sarosi GA. Epidemiological and clinical features of pulmonary blastomycosis. Semin Respir Infect. 1997;12:206–218.
29. Balmes JR, Hawkins JG. Pulmonary cryptococcosis. Semin Respir Med. 1987;9:180–186.
30. Restreppo A, Robledo M, Giraldo H, et al. The gamut of paracoccidioidomycosis. Am J Med. 1976;61:33–42.
31. Plus JL, Opal SM. Pulmonary sporotrichosis: Review of treatment and outcome. Medicine (Baltimore). 1986;65:143–153.
32. Watts JC, Callaway CS, Chandler FW, et al. Human pulmonary adiospiromycosis. Arch Pathol. 1975;99:11–15.
33. Saadah HA, Dixon T. *Petriellidium boydii (Allescheria boydii)* necrotizing pneumonia in a normal host. JAMA. 1981;245:605–606.
34. Shelhamer JH, Toews GB, Masur H, et al. Respiratory disease in the immunosuppressed patient. Ann Intern Med. 1992;117:415–431.
35. Rivera MP, Jules-Elysee KM, Stover DE. Immunocompromised patients: nontransplant chemotherapy immunosuppression. In: Niederman MS, Sarosi GA, Glassroth J, eds. Respiratory Infections. Philadelphia: WB Saunders; 1994:163–181.
36. Denning DW. Invasive aspergillosis. Clin Infect Dis. 1998;26:781–805.
37. Barnes PF, Block AB, Davidson PT, et al. Tuberculosis in patients with human immunodeficiency virus infection. N Engl J Med. 1991;324:1644–1650.
38. Murray JF. Pulmonary complications of HIV infection. Ann Rev Med. 1996;47: 117–126.
39. Cameron ML, Bartlett JA, Gallis HA, et al. Manifestations of pulmonary cryptococcosis in patients with acquired immunodeficiency syndrome. Rev Infect Dis. 1991;13:64–67.
40. Wheat LJ, Connolly-Stringfield PA, Baker RL, et al. Disseminated histoplasmosis in the acquired immunodeficiency syndrome: Clinical findings, diagnosis and treatment, and review of literature. Medicine (Baltimore). 1990;69:361–374.
41. Gallant JE, Ko AH. Cavitary pulmonary lesions in patients infected with human immunodeficiency virus. Clin Infect Dis. 1996;22:671–682.
42. Kalavjiian RC, Toossi Z, Tomashefski JR Jr, et al. Pulmonary disease due to infection by *Mycobacterium avium* complex in patients with AIDS. Clin Infect Dis. 1995;20:1186–1194.
43. Mutaner L, Leyes M, Payeras A, et al. Radiologic features of *Rhodococcus equi* pneumonia in AIDS. Eur J Radiol. 1997;24:66–70.
44. Supparatpinyo K, Chiewchanvir S, Hirunsri P, et al. *Penicillium marneffei* infection in patients with human immunodeficiency virus. Clin Infect Dis. 1992;14:871–874.
45. Gruden JF, Huang L, Webb WR, et al. AIDS-related Kaposi sarcoma of the lung: Radiographic findings and staging system with bronchoscopic correlation. Radiology. 1995;195:545–552.
46. Suffredini AF, Ognibene FP, Lack EE, et al. Nonspecific interstitial pneumonitis: A common cause of pulmonary disease in the acquired immunodeficiency syndrome. Ann Intern Med. 1987;107:7–13.
47. Kitaichi M, Nishimura K, Itoh H, et al. Pulmonary lymphangioleiomyomatosis: A report of 46 patients including a clinicopthologic study of prognostic factors. Am J Respir Crit Care Med. 1995;151:527–533.
48. Sharma OP, Fujimura N. Hypersensitivity pneumonitis: A noninfectious granulomatosis. Semin Respir Infect. 1995;10:96–106.
49. Leelarasamee A, Bovornkitti S. Melioidosis: Review and update. Rev Infect Dis. 1989;11:413–425.
50. Im IG, Whang HY, Kim WS, et al. Pleuropulmonary paragonimiasis: Radiologic findings in 71 patients. AM J Roentgenol. 1992;159:39–43.
51. Haim DY, Lippman ML, Goldberg SK, et al. The pulmonary complications of crack cocaine: A comprehensive review. Chest. 1995;107:233–240.
52. Grenier P, Valeyre D, Cluzel P, et al. Chronic diffuse interstitial disease: Diagnostic value of chest radiography and high-resolution CT. Radiology. 1991;179:123–132.
53. Lynch DA, Gamsu G. Newer imaging techniques in the assessment of interstitial lung disease. In: Schwarz MI, King TE Jr, eds. Interstitial Lung Disease. 2nd ed. St. Louis: Mosby–Year Book; 1993:91–118.
54. Bury T, Dowlati A, Paulus P, et al. Evaluation of the solitary pulmonary nodule by positron emission tomography imaging. Eur Respir J. 1996;9:410–414.
55. Shelhamer JH, Gill VJ, Quinn TC, et al. The laboratory evaluation of opportunistic pulmonary infections. Ann Intern Med. 1996;124:585–589.
56. Feinsilver SH, Fein AM, Niederman MS, et al. Utility of fiberoptic bronchoscopy in non-resolving pneumonia. Chest. 1990;98:1322–1326.
57. Cazzadori A, DiPein G, Todeschini G, et al. Transbronchial biopsy in the diagnosis of pulmonary infiltrates in immunocompromised patients. Chest. 1995;107:96–100.
58. Pisani RJ, Wright AJ. Clinical utility of bronchoalveolar lavage in immunocompromised hosts. Mayo Clin Proc. 1992;67:221–227.
59. Harris RJ, Kavuru MS, Rice TW, et al. The diagnostic and therapeutic utility of thoracoscopy: A review. Chest. 1995;108:828–841.
60. Cockerill FR III, Wilson WR, Carpenter HA, et al. Open lung biopsy in immunocompromised patients. Arch Intern Med. 1985;145:1398–1404.
61. Cheson BD, Samlowski WE, Tang TT, et al. Value of open-lung biopsy in 87 immunocompromised patients with pulmonary infiltrates. Cancer. 1985;55:543–549.
62. Sokolowski JW Jr, Burgher LW, Jones FL Jr, et al. Guidelines for percutaneous transthoracic needle biopsy. Position paper of the American Thoracic Society. Am Rev Respir Dis. 1989;140:255–256.
63. Zalacain R, Llorente JL, Gazfelurrutia L, et al. Influence of three factors on the diagnostic effectiveness of transthoracic needle aspiration in pneumonia. Chest. 1995;107:96–100.
64. Bensard DD, McIntyre RC Jr, Waring BJ, et al. Comparison of video thorascopic lung biopsy to open lung biopsy in the diagnosis of interstitial lung diseases. Chest. 1993;103:765–770.
65. Jederline PJ, Sicilian L, Gaensler EA. Chronic eosinophilic pneumonia: A report of 19 cases and a review of the literature. Medicine (Baltimore). 1988;67:154–162.
66. Penner C, Maycher B, Long R. Pulmonary gangrene: A complication of bacterial pneumonia. Chest. 1994;105:567–573.

Chapter 61

Cystic Fibrosis

M. R. KNOWLES
P. H. GILLIGAN
R. C. BOUCHER

A clearer understanding of the recessive genetic disorder cystic fibrosis (CF) has evolved since identification of the CF gene in 1989,[1] but the molecular and organ-level pathogenesis is complex and the clinical syndrome is variable.[2–4] Currently, one third of identified CF patients are adults. Clinical manifestations include chronic obstructive lung disease and pancreatic exocrine insufficiency, with characteristic microbiologic flora, i.e., *Staphylococcus aureus* and mucoid *Pseudomonas aeruginosa,* in the sputum. The clinical diagnosis is usually supported by the hallmark laboratory abnormality, an elevated sweat chloride concentration. The upper limit of normal for sweat chloride concentrations measured by pilocarpine iontophoresis is higher in adults than in children; measured concentrations must be less than 40 mEq/liter to be clearly normal in children, whereas healthy adults may have concentrations of up to 70 mEq/liter.[2] The genetic diagnosis can be established by identification of a CF mutation on each allele of the CF gene.[5, 6]

CLINICAL MANIFESTATIONS

The clinical manifestations of CF reflect obstruction of organs by viscous secretions and the presence of chronic bacterial infection in the lung. Although multiple organ systems are involved, chronic suppurative airway disease is present in more than 98% of adults who have CF, and 95% of CF deaths are related to progressive pulmonary insufficiency. Most respiratory infections in affected adults are caused by *S. aureus, P. aeruginosa,* and *Haemophilus influenzae,* whereas the incidence of infections with most other infectious agents (e.g., *Mycoplasma pneumoniae,* viruses) is believed to be similar to that in the general population.[7] It has been recently noted that up to 20% of adults in some CF centers may harbor nontuberculous mycobacteria (NTM) in respiratory secretions[8, 9]; the general prevalence and pathogenic role of these organisms are not clearly defined.[10]

The clinical picture of CF is dominated by a chronic cough punctuated by episodes of clinical deterioration characterized by an increased volume and purulence of sputum, dyspnea, and sometimes anorexia and weight loss.[3, 11] Although adults with CF may exhibit low-grade fever with these exacerbations, high fever is unusual, and sepsis or bacteremia is uncommon despite the large number of bacteria in the airways (10^8 organisms per ml of sputum). Clinical exacerbations are associated with modest elevations in the white blood cell count and worsening spirometric values. The chest radiograph typically shows diffuse shadowing that reflects airway wall thickening and retained secretions and also cystic bronchiectatic changes. In many adult CF patients, these roentgenographic abnormalities are seen predominantly in upper lung zones, which may initially suggest tuberculosis. Significant gas exchange abnormalities usually occur only in the terminal stages of the disease, and hypoxemia and carbon dioxide retention are uncommon in adults with CF during acute exacerbations until the forced expiratory volume in 1 second (FEV_1) is less than 40% of the predicted value.[3, 11]

Adults with CF have frequent complications of hemoptysis and pneumothorax.[12] Minor hemoptysis is common, and massive hemoptysis occurs in about 1% of adult CF patients each year. Fortunately, medical (nonsurgical) intervention is usually sufficient for the treatment of pulmonary hemorrhage.[12, 13] Epithelial dysfunction in the nasal sinuses of CF patients and the frequent occurrence of nasal polyps make subacute or chronic sinusitis a major problem in many adult patients.[14] The microbiology of sinusitis is not always reflected by the flora identified in expectorated sputum.[15]

Because most CF patients have progressive pancreatic destruction and loss of function, the prevalence of diabetes mellitus in adult CF populations may be as high as 15%.[16, 17] The presence of glucose intolerance may add further difficulty to the treatment of pulmonary infection.

PATHOGENESIS

The clinical syndrome of CF reflects a genetic disorder inherited in autosomal recessive fashion. The CF gene was identified in 1989 and is located on the long arm of chromosome 7.[1] It is a relatively large gene consisting of 27 exons and codes for a 1480-amino-acid polypeptide known as cystic fibrosis transmembrane regulator (CFTR). Eight hundred different mutations have been identified in the CF gene. The most common mutation is a 3-base-pair deletion that leads to the absence of a phenylalanine from the CFTR protein at position 508 (ΔF508).[18]

The molecular pathogenesis of CF is complex and varies with the type of CF gene mutation. The CFTR protein appears to reside in the plasma membrane. Molecular modeling predicts that the polypeptide contains, in sequence, a six-transmembrane–spanning region, a nucleotide (adenosine triphosphate [ATP])-binding fold that is the site of the ΔF508 mutation, a large hydrophilic domain that is the site of kinase-phosphatase regulation (the R domain), another six-transmembrane–spanning region, and another nucleotide-binding fold.[1] The full spectrum of functions of CFTR protein is still not known. CFTR appears able to function as the cyclic adenosine monophosphate (cAMP)–regulated Cl^- channel in the plasma membrane[19, 20] but probably regulates other ion channels in the plasma membrane as well.[21, 22] The common CF mutation ΔF508 leads to abnormal folding of the CFTR polypeptide in the endoplasmic reticulum and degradation of the protein by intracellular "editing."[23] Thus, the cellular pathogenesis of the ΔF508 mutation reflects the absence of protein at the relevant cellular site, e.g., the plasma membrane. Other, less common CFTR mutations appear to allow the targeting of CFTR to the plasma membrane but lead to abnormal Cl^- channel regulation or abnormal Cl^- ion permeation, or both.

Two general features characterize the pathogenesis of CF at the cellular level: (1) the affected cells in target organs are epithelial cells; and (2) the abnormality in epithelial cells involves regulation of ion transport. The most prevalent defect is abnormal function of the cAMP-dependent plasma membrane Cl^- (CFTR) channels. Defective CFTR Cl^- channel function has been detected in the airways,[24] sweat ducts,[25] and small intestine[26] of CF patients. A second major defect in ion transport has been detected in CF airway epithelia; the rate of absorption of Na^+ ions from the airway lumen to the interstitium is raised threefold over that in non-CF epithelia.[27, 28] The molecular mechanisms that confer regulation of Na^+ transport by CFTR are not yet known but probably involve a cascade of protein-protein interactions.

The precise linkage between CF-specific ion transport defects and the pathogenesis of CF lung disease is not yet clear. The ion transport abnormalities that characterize CF may affect the volume or composition, or both, of the secretions that line the airway surfaces. One theory emphasizes the role of high salt content of CF secretions, perhaps via inactivation of defensin-like peptides in airway secretions, in the pathogenesis of CF airways infection.[29] A second theory emphasizes the roles of accelerated Na^+ absorption and reduced Cl^- secretion in decreasing the salt and water content of secretions.[30] The concomitant reduction in volume of secretions lining airway surfaces may deplete the layer in which cilia beat (the periciliary liquid layer), concentrate mucins on airway surfaces, and derange their viscoelastic properties, all of which lead to reductions in cilia-dependent and cough-effected mucus clearance. Whether reduced clearance of thickened secretions from airways is sufficient alone to lead to persistence of staphylococcal and pseudomonal infection is not yet clear. The activity of antimicrobial substances and neutrophils in thickened mucus has not yet been studied. A role for increased bacterial adherence to epithelia, particularly after the epithelium has been injured by the initial infection, has recently been postulated to contribute to disease pathogenesis.[31–34]

The development of persistent bacterial infection generates a complex series of events that lead to airway wall damage and ultimately to destroyed or bronchiectatic airways. Bacterial exoproducts from both *S. aureus* and *P. aeruginosa* have been implicated in airway destruction. In adults, lipopolysaccharides, exotoxin A, and a cell wall–associated rhamnolipid from *P. aeruginosa* have been implicated as important bacterial toxins.[35] The host inflammatory response appears intact in CF, and the vigorous host response contributes to airway damage.[36–38] Chemotactic agents, both bacterial and locally derived (e.g., arachidonic acid metabolites from airway epithelia), attract inflammatory cells into the airway lumen. Polymorphonuclear cell–derived enzymes (e.g., elastase) damage airway wall structures, and cleave immune receptors on neutrophils and bacteria,[39] thereby impairing immune function. In addition, the chronic antigenic stimulus of persistent airway infections generates immunologically mediated airway wall destruction.[37] Large amounts of neutrophil-derived DNA further thicken and impair clearance of airway secretions.[36] Eventually, the combination of retained secretions and airway damage deranges gas exchange, perturbs cardiac function, and leads to death.

MICROBIOLOGY

S. aureus and *P. aeruginosa* are the primary etiologic agents of pulmonary infection in patients with CF.[40] *S. aureus* often colonizes the respiratory tract in the first 2 years of life and can be found in approximately 30% of patients with CF in the United States. Before the advent of effective antistaphylococcal therapy, lung infection due to this organism was the leading cause of death. Antistaphylococcal penicillins such as oxacillin and nafcillin control infections with this organism. Ominously, resistance to these agents is increasing in CF patients; in some centers, 10 to 20% of CF patients are infected with methicillin-resistant *S. aureus* (MRSA). Person-to-person spread of MRSA has been documented in CF patients, with transmission from both CF and non-CF persons.[41, 42] In patients receiving long-term (for >3 months) prophylactic trimethoprim-sulfamethoxazole therapy, approximately 50% of *S. aureus* isolates are thymidine-dependent.[43] Thymidine-dependent *S. aureus* organisms give rise to small-colony variants.[44] It is speculated that these small-colony variants play a role in the persistence of *S. aureus* in CF patients who have received trimethoprim-sulfamethoxazole, much as they do in patients with chronic osteomyelitis due to this organism.[45] Because thymidine-dependent organisms grow poorly on most commonly used isolation media, and because mucoid *P. aeruginosa* may obscure recognition of its growth, mannitol salts agar must be used to ensure reliable recovery of *S. aureus.*

In childhood or early adolescence, patients with CF become chronically infected with *P. aeruginosa.* Up to 80% of adolescent and adult patients with CF are infected with this organism.[40] As this chronic infective state evolves, isolates of *P. aeruginosa* from these patients may produce large amounts of an extracellular mucoid polysaccharide called alginate.[46] Molecular studies suggest that biochemical factors in the airways of CF patients (high salt concentration and dehydration) switch on a series of genes that regulate production of this virulence factor.[46] Molecular studies also indicate that a large number of different *P. aeruginosa* strains are capable of producing alginate.[47, 48] Mucoid colonies that result from alginate production are predominant in infected CF patients but are rarely seen in other patients with chronic airway disease.[49] This mucoid variant is responsible for the formation of microcolonies that are believed to be resistant to both mechanical and immunologic clearance from the airways. The exuberant immune response to these microcolonies is believed to be responsible, in part, for the chronic deterioration in pulmonary function that is the hallmark of this disease.[50]

When first isolated, *P. aeruginosa* is usually susceptible to all antipseudomonal β-lactams, imipenem, quinolones, and aminoglycosides. With increasing antimicrobial pressure due to repeated antimicrobial treatment of pulmonary exacerbations, resistance to these agents may develop, especially if each one is used alone. Recent studies have suggested that mucoid variants when grown in biofilms are much more resistant to antimicrobials than nonmucoid variants of the same strain, further complicating antimicrobial therapy.[51] In patients who repeatedly require treatment for *P. aeruginosa* infection, the organism may remain susceptible only to polymixin B and colistin.[52]

As life expectancy has increased in CF patients, a third organism, *Burkholderia cepacia,* has emerged as an important pathogen in at least some CF centers. Some CF patients infected with *B. cepacia* develop what has been characterized as the "*cepacia* syndrome."[53] In this syndrome, adolescent and young adult CF patients with relatively mild pulmonary disease become infected, have rapid deterioration in pulmonary function, may develop bacteremia, and die within 6 months. Other CF patients may be infected with *B. cepacia* without a corresponding decline in clinical status.

Recent taxonomic and molecular studies of *B. cepacia* have begun to unravel some of the mystery surrounding this organism. On the basis of highly sophisticated molecular and cellular analysis, it is now accepted that *B. cepacia* can be divided into five different genomovars.[54] Most of the isolates recovered from CF patients belong to genomovars II and III. Genomovar II has recently been given the species designation *Burkholderia multivorans.*[55] Molecular analysis using pulsed-field gel electrophoresis has shown that a strain of genomovar III is highly transmissible and that it has been spread from North America to Europe.[56] Intimate social contact appears to be the major mode of spread.[57] This highly transmissible strain possesses an unusual adhesin called a cable pilin, which is speculated to have a role in this strain's transmissibility.[58] Segregation of *B. cepacia*–infected patients has been used successfully in some CF centers to prevent spread of *B. cepacia* to noninfected CF patients.[59] It is unclear whether all CF patients infected with a genomovar II or III strain should be segregated or just those with genomovar III isolates possessing the cable pilin.

B. cepacia is also a cause of concern in CF patients who undergo double lung transplantation. The transplanted lungs of CF patients frequently become reinfected with organisms that infected the native lungs and are still present in the sinuses or trachea of the recipient. At one center, where the highly transmissible genomovar III clone was first recognized, all 10 patients who had *B. cepacia* lung infections before transplantation became infected with *B. cepacia* after transplantation. Five additional CF patients developed noscomial *B. cepacia* pulmonary infections after transplantation, with an 80% mortality rate.[60] In a second center, three of six CF patients receiving lung transplants who were *B. cepacia*–positive died in the first year after transplantation, compared with a 1-year survival rate of 90% for CF patients infected with either susceptible or multidrug-resistant *P. aeruginosa.*[61] Because of the significant mortality associated with *B. cepacia* after transplantation, infection with *B. cepacia* is a contraindication to transplantation in some but not all centers performing CF lung transplantation.[60]

One of the major problems in managing *B. cepacia*–infected patients is the organism's resistance to antimicrobials. *B. cepacia* is intrinsically resistant to aminoglycosides and the polymixins. On initial isolation, the organism may be susceptible to trimethoprim-sulfamethoxazole and antipseudomonal β-lactams. However, under antimicrobial pressure, resistance quickly develops, and the clinician is frequently faced with the challenge of managing a patient infected with an organism resistant to all available antimicrobials.[53]

Another problem is detecting *B. cepacia* in the complex microbiologic milieu of CF respiratory secretions and then accurately identifying it. Unless specific isolation media are used, the organism, which grows comparatively slowly,[53] may be obscured, particularly by mucoid *P. aeruginosa.* Once the organism is isolated, the commercial identification systems used in many microbiology laboratories may not accurately identify it.[62] Referral of suspected *B. cepacia* isolates to reference laboratories that can use molecular identification techniques for confirmation is necessary for accurate identification of this organism.[54]

The role of mycobacteria in the lung disease of cystic fibrosis patients has recently come under scrutiny. Studies have shown that NTM, usually *M. avium intracellulare* complex organisms, can be isolated from the respiratory secretions of up to 20% of adult CF patients.[8, 9] CF patients colonized with these organisms are excluded as transplant candidates at some centers because of the difficulties in treating NTM infections. As with *B. cepacia,* special culture techniques are required to reliably prevent overgrowth of mucoid *P. aeruginosa* and allow recovery of NTM from CF respiratory secretions.[63] Although in most cases the presence of NTM is either transient or associated with asymptomatic infection, patients with persistently positive smears for acid-fast bacilli may have active infection with NTM.[64] On the other hand, *M. tuberculosis* is rarely recovered in this patient population.[64]

Other bacteria such as *H. influenzae, Moraxella catarrhalis, Stenotrophomonas maltophilia, Alcaligenes xylosoxidans, Burkholderia gladioli,* and members of the family Enterobacteriaceae are recovered from the respiratory tract of CF patients and may play a role in their pulmonary disease. As CF life expectancy increases and more CF patients survive into adulthood, the multidrug-resistant organisms *S. maltophilia* and *A. xylosoxidans* are being seen with increasing frequency. This is due to the selective pressure of repeated courses of antipseudomonal antimicrobials given to these patients.[65] The role of these organisms in CF lung disease is currently undefined.[66]

Aspergillus fumigatus may be cultured from specimens from CF patients.[53] However, the clinical diagnosis of allergic bronchopulmonary aspergillosis (ABPA) should be based on rigorous criteria, because many CF patients have positive results on immediate hypersensitivity skin testing and an assay for serum-precipitating antibodies to *Aspergillus* without the clinical syndrome of ABPA.[67, 68]

The role of viruses in the chronic lung disease of CF patients has not been determined. Acute respiratory infections due to respiratory syncytial virus, influenza A virus, and parainfluenza viruses have all been documented.[69–71] The rate of occurrence and severity of these viral respiratory infections in CF children are similar to those seen in their non-CF siblings.[70]

TREATMENT

The goal of therapy is to retard progressive lung damage by removing viscous and purulent airway secretions, by controlling bacterial infection with antibiotics, and by providing proper nutrition for host defense.[3, 11, 72, 73]

The presence of a large bacterial burden in the bronchiectatic airways of patients dictates that airway clearance techniques be combined with antibacterial therapy to achieve optimal results. Chest percussion with postural drainage is the time-honored method, but deep breathing and voluntary coughing, exercise, and other maneuvers are also effective.[11, 73] Aerosolized recombinant human DNAse I improves clearance of purulent airway secretions and offers another modality for treatment in some patients with DNA-laden secretions.[74] Anti-inflammatory agents may be useful in reducing the severity of mucosal edema and assisting in airway clearance. Oral administration of high-dose ibuprofen retards the decline in lung function in children with mild to moderate disease, but benefit has not been demonstrated in adults.[73, 75] The indications for systemic steroids are poorly defined,[11] and long-term usage of systemic steroids is associated with adverse side effects.[17, 76] The use of topical (inhaled) steroids is common, but benefit has not been established in clinical trials.[77, 78] Bronchodilators may assist in clearing retained secretions in some patients, but the finding of a paradoxical reduction in airflow in some patients,[79] coupled with potential acceleration of abnormal Na^+ transport,[27] suggests that these agents should be used intermittently and with caution in adult CF patients. There is little role for the use of inhaled mucolytic agents or bronchial lavage.[11]

Antibiotics have played a key role in improved survival.[80] Broad-spectrum oral antibiotics (amoxicillin, cephalexin, dicloxacillin, tetracycline, trimethoprim-sulfamethoxazole) can provide useful therapy for acute pulmonary exacerbations, despite the presence of *P. aeruginosa* organisms resistant to these agents. The clinical benefit may reflect antibiotic activity against pathogens that are difficult to culture in the presence of mucoid *P. aeruginosa (S. aureus, H. influenzae),* or in airway infection with high concentrations of bacteria ($>10^5$ organisms per ml) that are not typical pathogens,[81] or it may be due to inhibition of release of toxic bacterial exoproducts in the absence of bacterial killing.[53, 82] High doses and prolonged therapy (3 to 4 weeks) with oral agents are recommended for treatment of acute illnesses (exacerbations). Oral antibiotics are also of benefit in chronic bacterial sinusitis, which results from pathogens that are frequently sensitive to broad-spectrum antimicrobials.[14, 15] The use of oral antibiotics for prophylactic (maintenance) therapy is controversial but appears to have a useful role in some patients.

Quinolones are oral antipseudomonal drugs that are useful for intermittent therapy. The emergence of bacterial resistance during monotherapy with these drugs limits usefulness for long-term treatment, and the duration of periodic treatment should be limited to 2 to 4 weeks.[83, 84]

Aggressive parenteral therapy is indicated for clinical exacerbations that do not respond to oral antimicrobials.[3, 11, 73] Although sterilization of airway secretions rarely occurs and is not the goal of parenteral therapy, the bacterial burden in conducting airways can be reduced[85] and irreversible lung damage presumably retarded. Parenteral therapy should be guided by results of sputum bacteriologic and drug sensitivity studies, although treatment in adult CF patients is usually directed at *P. aeruginosa.* A combination of antibiotics is indicated to treat infection due to *P. aeruginosa* because thickened airway secretions prevent drug penetration, aminoglycoside activity is reduced by suppurative secretions, and a combination protects against the emergence of resistant strains.[86] The pharmacologic regimen usually includes an aminoglycoside (gentamicin, tobramycin, amikacin) plus another agent effective against *P. aeruginosa,* such as a cephalosporin (e.g., ceftazidime[87]), an antipseudomonal penicillin, or imipenem. If *S. aureus* is clinically suspected or cultured from sputum, addition of a specific antistaphylococcal agent should be considered if the antipseudomonal drug regimen is not adequate for treatment of *S. aureus* infection. Increased plasma clearance of almost all effective antibiotics in CF patients dictates the use of large, frequent doses of antimicrobials.[88, 89] For example, CF adults require 6 to 15 mg/kg/day of gentamicin to achieve desired peak serum levels of 10 μg/ml in an every-8-hour dosing regimen. Aminoglycoside toxicity is uncommon in CF patients, but trough serum levels should be monitored. Parenteral therapy should be continued for a minimum of 10 to 14 days or longer, if necessary, to achieve a full clinical and pulmonary functional response. Effective parenteral antibiotic therapy can be administered on an outpatient basis.[90, 91]

Aerosolized antibiotics can be used for subacute pulmonary exacerbations and to assist in the maintenance of stable clinical status.[92] A recent study demonstrated improved lung function and reduced episodes of respiratory illness with aerosolized tobramycin (TOBI) in clinically stable patients.[73, 93] Colistin is a useful alternative agent for inhalation therapy, because the rare development of bacterial resistance during prolonged aerosol therapy with colistin does not change the bacterial sensitivity to parenteral aminoglycosides.[94–96]

Of interest, despite intensive antibiotic exposure, symptomatic disease due to *Clostridium difficile* is uncommon in CF patients despite the presence of the organism in fecal samples.[97, 98] The asymptomatic carriage of *C. difficile* may reflect the inability of the CF intestinal epithelium to respond to *C. difficile*–derived secretory toxins.[26, 99]

Chronic malabsorption, coupled with increased caloric requirements due to chronic infection and increased respiratory activity, can induce malnutrition and impaired host defense mechanisms in CF patients. High caloric intake with supplemental pancreatic digestive enzymes and appropriate fat-soluble vitamins is standard treatment in these patients.[100]

Although *Aspergillus* organisms are frequently cultured from the sputum of CF adults, treatment is usually not indicated, unless the syndrome of ABPA is established.[67, 68] Treatment with systemic corticosteroids is usually sufficient, but antifungal agents may be useful for adjunctive therapy in some patients.[101] The increasing number of adults in the CF patient population is associated with increasing recovery of NTM from sputum cultures.[8, 9] Although as many as 20% of adult CF patients have NTM in respiratory secretions, the pathogenesis is not clearly defined, and clinical and radiologic studies should be monitored for evidence of pathogenic mycobacterial activity.[10]

Annual influenza vaccinations are recommended, but pneumococcal vaccine is not routinely indicated because of the relative absence of *Streptococcus pneumoniae* as a pathogen.

Heart-lung transplantation is a viable therapeutic option for patients with end-stage lung disease. In experienced lung transplant centers, the 1-year survival rate is 80 to 90%, and the 5-year survival rate may be as high as 50%.[102]

Recent progress in defining the organ-level and molecular pathogenesis of CF has led to the development of new therapeutic approaches.[103] Aerosolized and oral antiproteases are being tested as agents for treatment of secondary manifestations of the lung disease. Correction of abnormal airway epithelial ion transport, targeting defective Cl^- secretion with $P2Y_2$ receptor agonists,[104] offers the possibility of long-term "preventive" therapy that might impede the development of airway disease; these agents are being tested in clinical studies. Studies of other pharmacotherapies to enhance the cellular processing or function of CFTR are also under way.[103] Finally, gene transfer of a normal CFTR cDNA to airway cells offers the promise of treatment at the molecular level. Although this technique is some distance from clinical practice, several pilot studies of gene transfer with adenoviral and adeno-associated virus vectors and liposome-DNA complexes are under way.[103]

REFERENCES

1. Riordan JR, Rommens JM, Kerem B, et al. Identification of the cystic fibrosis gene: Cloning and characterization of complementary DNA. Science. 1989;245:1066.
2. Welsh MJ, Tsui L, Boat TF, Beaudet AL. Cystic fibrosis. In: Scriver CR, Beaudet AL, Sly WS, et al, ed. The Metabolic and Molecular Bases of Inherited Disease. 7th ed. New York: McGraw-Hill; 1995:3799.

3. Davis PB, Drumm M, Konstan MW. Cystic fibrosis. Am J Respir Crit Care Med. 1996;154:1229.
4. Stutts MJ, Boucher RC. Cystic fibrosis gene and functions of CFTR: Implications of dysfunctional ion transport for pulmonary pathogenesis. In: Yankaskas JR, Knowles MR, eds. Cystic Fibrosis in Adults. Philadelphia: Lippincott-Raven; 1998:3.
5. Rosenstein BJ, Cutting GR. The diagnosis of CF: A consensus statement. Cystic Fibrosis Foundation Consensus Panel. J Pediatr. 1998;132:589.
6. Stern RC. The diagnosis of cystic fibrosis. N Engl J Med. 1997;336:487.
7. Gilligan PH. Microbiology of cystic fibrosis lung disease. In: Yankaskas JR, Knowles MR, eds. Cystic Fibrosis in Adults. Philadelphia: Lippincott-Raven; 1998:93.
8. Kilby JM, Gilligan PH, Yankaskas JR, et al. Nontuberculous mycobacteria in adult patients with cystic fibrosis. Chest. 1992;102:70.
9. Aitken ML, Burke W, McDonald G, et al. Nontuberculous mycobacterial disease in adult cystic fibrosis patients. Chest. 1993;103:1096.
10. Olivier KN, Yankaskas JR, Knowles MR. Nontuberculous mycobacterial pulmonary disease in cystic fibrosis. Semin Respir Infect. 1996;11:272.
11. Turpin SV, Knowles MR. Treatment of pulmonary disease in cystic fibrosis. In: Davis PB, ed. Cystic Fibrosis. (Lung Biology in Health and Disease, v 64.) New York: Marcel Dekker; 1993:277.
12. Schidlow DV, Taussig LM, Knowles MR. Cystic Fibrosis Foundation Consensus Conference Report on pulmonary complications of cystic fibrosis. Pediatr Pulmonol. 1993;15:187.
13. Brinson GM, Noone PG, Mauro MA, et al. Bronchial artery embolization for the treatment of hemoptysis in patients with cystic fibrosis. Am J Respir Crit Care Med. 1998;157:1951.
14. Stern RC, Jones K. Nasal and sinus disease. In: Yankaskas JR, Knowles MR, eds. Cystic Fibrosis in Adults. Philadelphia: Lippincott-Raven; 1998:221.
15. Shapiro ED, Milmoe GJ, Wald ER, et al. Bacteriology of the maxillary sinuses in patients with cystic fibrosis. J Infect Dis. 1982;146:589.
16. Diagnosis, screening, and management of cystic fibrosis related diabetes mellitus: A Consensus Conference report. Consensus Conference: Concepts in Care CF Foundation V. 9, sec. 2. Bethesda, Md; 1999.
17. Robbins MK, Ontjes DA. Endocrine and renal disorders in cystic fibrosis. In: Yankaskas JR, Knowles MR, eds. Cystic Fibrosis in Adults. Philadelphia: Lippincott-Raven; 1998:383.
18. Collins FS. Cystic fibrosis: Molecular biology and therapeutic implications. Science. 1992;256:774.
19. Anderson MP, Rich DP, Gregory RJ, et al. Generation of cAMP-activated chloride currents by expression of CFTR. Science. 1991;251:679.
20. Kartner N, Hanrahan JW, Jensen TJ, et al. Expression of the cystic fibrosis gene in non-epithelial invertebrate cells produces a regulated anion conductance. Cell. 1991;64:681.
21. Gabriel SE, Clarke LL, Boucher RC, Stutts MJ. CFTR and outward rectifying chloride channels are distinct proteins with a regulatory relationship. Nature. 1993;363:263.
22. Stutts MJ, Canessa CM, Olsen JC, et al. CFTR as a cAMP-dependent regulator of sodium channels. Science. 1995;269:847.
23. Cheng SH, Gregory RJ, Marshall J, et al. Defective intracellular transport and processing of CFTR is the molecular basis of most cystic fibrosis. Cell. 1990;63:827.
24. Knowles MR, Stutts MJ, Spock A, et al. Abnormal ion permeation through cystic fibrosis respiratory epithelium. Science. 1983;221:1067.
25. Quinton PM. Chloride impermeability in cystic fibrosis. Nature. 1983;301:421.
26. Berschneider HM, Knowles MR, Azizkhan RG, et al. Altered intestinal chloride transport in cystic fibrosis. FASEB J. 1988;2:2625.
27. Boucher RC, Stutts MJ, Knowles MR, et al. Na^+ transport in cystic fibrosis respiratory epithelia. Abnormal basal rate and response to adenylate cyclase activation. J Clin Invest. 1986;78:1245.
28. Knowles M, Gatzy J, Boucher R. Increased bioelectric potential difference across respiratory epithelia in cystic fibrosis. N Engl J Med. 1981;305:1489.
29. Smith JJ, Travis SM, Greenberg EP, Welsh MJ. Cystic fibrosis airway epithelia fail to kill bacteria because of abnormal airway surface fluid. Cell. 1996;85:229.
30. Matsui H, Grubb BR, Tarran R, et al. Evidence for periciliary liquid layer depletion, not abnormal ion composition, in the pathogenesis of cystic fibrosis airways disease. Cell. 1998;95:1005–1015.
31. de Bentzmann S, Plotkowski C, Puchelle E. Receptors in the *Pseudomonas aeruginosa* adherence to injured and repairing airway epithelium. Am J Respir Crit Care Med. 1996;154:S155.
32. de Bentzmann S, Roger P, Dupuit F, et al. Asialo GM1 is a receptor for *Pseudomonas aeruginosa* adherence to regenerating respiratory epithelial cells. Infect Immun. 1996;64:1582.
33. de Bentzmann S, Roger P, Puchelle E. *Pseudomonas aeruginosa* adherence to remodelling respiratory epithelium. Eur Respir J. 1996;9:2145.
34. Imundo L, Barasch J, Prince A, Al-Awqati Q. Cystic fibrosis epithelial cells have a receptor for pathogenic bacteria on their apical surface. Proc Natl Acad Sci U S A 1995;92:3019.
35. Stutts MJ, Schwab JH, Chen MG, et al. Effects of *Pseudomonas aeruginosa* on bronchial epithelial ion transport. Am Rev Respir Dis. 1986;134:17.
36. Davis PB. Pathophysiology of the lung disease in cystic fibrosis. In: Davis PB, ed. Cystic Fibrosis. (Lung Biology in Health and Disease, v. 64.) New York: Marcel Dekker; 1993:193.
37. Konstan MW, Berger M. Infection and inflammation of the lung in cystic fibrosis. In: Davis PB, ed. Cystic Fibrosis. (Lung Biology in Health and Disease, v. 64.) New York: Marcel Dekker; 1993:219.
38. Noah TL, Black HR, Cheng P, et al. Nasal and bronchoalveolar lavage fluid cytokines in early cystic fibrosis. J Infect Dis. 1997;175:638.
39. Tosi MF, Zakem H, Berger M. Neutrophil elastase cleaves C3bi on opsonized *Pseudomonas* as well as CR1 on neutrophils to create a functionally important opsonin receptor mismatch. J Clin Invest. 1990;86:300.
40. FitzSimmons SC. The changing epidemiology of cystic fibrosis. J Pediatr. 1993;122:1.
41. Gilligan P, Jordan M, Wait K, et al. Oxacillin resistant *Staphylococcus aureus* in patients with cystic fibrosis (CF) (Abstract). Pediatr Pulmonol. 1996;13(Suppl):297.
42. Givney R, Vickery A, Pegler M, Benn R. Methicillin-resistant *Staphylococcus aureus* in a cystic fibrosis unit. J Hosp Infect. 1997;35:27.
43. Gilligan PH, Gage PA, Welch DF, et al. Prevalence of thymidine-dependent *Staphylococcus aureus* in patients with cystic fibrosis. J Clin Microbiol. 1987;25:1258.
44. Kahl B, Herrmann M, Everding AS, et al. Persistent infection with small colony variant strains of *Staphylococcus aureus* in patients with cystic fibrosis. J Infect Dis. 1998;177:1023.
45. Proctor RA, van Langevelde P, Kristjansson M, et al. Persistent and relapsing infections associated with small-colony variants of *Staphylococcus aureus.* Clin Infect Dis. 1995;20:95.
46. Govan JRW, Deretic V. Microbial pathogenesis in cystic fibrosis: Mucoid *Pseudomonas aeruginosa* and *Burkholderia cepacia.* Microbiol Rev. 1996;60:539.
47. Boukadida J, De Montalembert M, Lenoir G, et al. Molecular epidemiology of chronic colonisation by *Pseudomonas aeruginosa* in cystic fibrosis. J Med Microbiol. 1993;38:29.
48. Romling U, Grothues D, Koopmann U, et al. Pulsed-field gel electrophoresis analysis of a *Pseudomonas aeruginosa* pathovar. Electrophoresis. 1992;13:646.
49. McCarthy VP, Rosenberg G, Rosenstein BJ, Hubbard VS: Mucoid *Pseudomonas aeruginosa* from a patient without cystic fibrosis: Implications and review of the literature. Pediatr Infect Dis. 1986;5:256.
50. Konstan MW, Berger M. Current understanding of the inflammatory process in cystic fibrosis: Onset and etiology. Pediatr Pulmonol. 1997;24:137.
51. Parkins MD, Storey DG, Ceri H. The MBEC system, an *in vitro* model of biofilm growth for the study of antibiotic sensitivity and gene expression of *Pseudomonas aeruginosa* in cystic fibrosis (Abstract). Pediatr Pulmonol. 1998;17(Suppl):319.
52. Saiman L, Mehar F, Niu WW, et al. Antibiotic susceptibility of multiply resistant *Pseudomonas aeruginosa* isolated from patients with cystic fibrosis, including candidates for transplantation. Clin Infect Dis. 1996;23:532.
53. Gilligan PH. Microbiology of airway disease in patients with cystic fibrosis. Clin Microbiol Rev. 1991;4:35.
54. LiPuma JJ. *Burkholderia cepacia:* Management issues and new insights. Clin Chest Med. 1998;19:473.
55. Vandamme P, Holmes B, Vancanneyt M, et al. Occurrence of multiple genomovars of *Burkholderia cepacia* in cystic fibrosis patients and proposal of *Burkholderia multivorans* sp. nov. Int J Syst Bacteriol. 1997;47:1188.
56. Sun L, Jiang RZ, Steinbach S, et al. The emergence of a highly transmissible lineage of *cbl+ Pseudomonas (Burkholderia) cepacia* causing CF centre epidemics in North America and Britain. Nat Med. 1995;1:661.
57. Govan JRW, Brown PH, Maddison J, et al. Evidence for transmission of *Pseudomonas cepacia* by social contact in cystic fibrosis. Lancet. 1993;342:15.
58. Goldstein R, Sun L, Jiang RZ, et al. Structurally variant classes of pilus appendage fibers coexpressed from *Burkholderia (Pseudomonas) cepacia.* J Bacteriol. 1995;177:1039.
59. Smith DL, Smith EG, Gumery LB, Stableforth DE. *Pseudomonas cepacia* infection in cystic fibrosis. Lancet. 1992;339:252.
60. Snell GI, de Hoyos A, Krajden M, et al. *Pseudomonas cepacia* in lung transplant recipients recipients with cystic fibrosis. Chest. 1993;103:466.
61. Aris RM, Gilligan PH, Neuringer IP, et al. The effects of panresistant bacteria in cystic fibrosis patients on lung transplant outcome. Am J Respir Crit Care Med. 1997;155:1699.
62. Kiska DL, Kerr A, Jones MC, et al. Accuracy of four commercial systems for the identification of *Burkholderia cepacia* and other gram-negative nonfermenting bacilli recovered from patients with cystic fibrosis. J Clin Microbiol. 1996;34:886.
63. Whittier S, Hopfer RL, Knowles MR, Gilligan PH. Improved recovery of mycobacteria from respiratory secretions of patients with cystic fibrosis. J Clin Microbiol. 1993;31:861.
64. Torrens JK, Dawkins P, Conway SP, Moya E. Non-tuberculous mycobacteria in cystic fibrosis. Thorax. 1998;53:182.
65. Denton M, Todd NJ, Littlewood JM. Role of anti-pseudomonal antibiotics in the emergence of *Stenotrophomonas maltophilia* in cystic fibrosis patients. Eur J Clin Microbiol Infect Dis. 1996;15:402.
66. Gilligan PH: *Stenotrophomonas maltophilia, Burkholderia gladioli,* and related organisms: Are they emerging pathogens in CF? (Abstract). Pediatr Pulmonol. 1998;17(Suppl):117.
67. Hutcheson PS, Rejent AJ, Slavin RG. Variability in parameters of allergic bronchopulmonary aspergillosis in patients with cystic fibrosis. J Allergy Clin Immunol. 1991;88:390.
68. Knutsen AP, Slavin RG. Allergic bronchopulmonary mycosis complicating cystic fibrosis. Semin Respir Infect. 1992;7:179.
69. Abman SH, Ogle JW, Butler-Simon N, et al. Role of respiratory syncytial virus in early hospitalizations for respiratory distress of young infants with cystic fibrosis. J Pediatr. 1988;113:826.
70. Ramsey BW, Gore EJ, Smith AL, et al. The effect of respiratory viral infections on patients with cystic fibrosis. Am J Dis Child. 1989;143:662.

71. Conway SP, Simmonds EJ, Littlewood JM. Acute severe deterioration in cystic fibrosis associated with influenza A virus infection. Thorax. 1992;47:112.
72. Ramsey BW. Management of pulmonary disease in patients with cystic fibrosis. N Engl J Med. 1996;335:179.
73. Noone PG, Knowles MR. Standard therapy of cystic fibrosis lung disease. In: Yankaskas JR, Knowles MR, eds. Cystic Fibrosis in Adults. Philadelphia: Lippincott-Raven; 1998:145.
74. Fuchs HJ, Borowitz DS, Christiansen DH, et al. Effect of aerosolized recombinant DNase on exacerbations of respiratory symptoms and on pulmonary function in patients with cystic fibrosis. The Pulmoenzyme Study Group. N Engl J Med. 1994;331:637.
75. Konstan MW, Byard PJ, Hoppel CL, Davis PB. Effect of high-dose ibuprofen in patients with cystic fibrosis. N Engl J Med. 1995;332:848.
76. Rosenstein BJ, Eigen H. Risks of alternate-day prednisone in patients with cystic fibrosis. Pediatrics. 1991;87:245.
77. Bisgaard H, Pedersen SS, Nielsen KG, et al. Controlled trial of inhaled budesonide in patients with cystic fibrosis and chronic bronchopulmonary *Pseudomonas aeruginosa* infection. Am J Respir Crit Care Med. 1997;156:1190.
78. Nikolaizik WH, Schoni MH. Pilot study to assess the effect of inhaled corticosteroids on lung function in patients with cystic fibrosis. J Pediatr. 1996;128:271.
79. Shapiro GG, Bamman J, Kanerek P, Bierman CW. The paradoxical effect of adrenergic and methylxanthine drugs in cystic fibrosis. Pediatrics. 1976;58:740.
80. Michel BC. Antibacterial therapy in cystic fibrosis: A review of the literature published between 1980 and 1987. Chest. 1988;94:129S.
81. Myers MG, Koontz FP, Weinberger M. Lower respiratory infections in patients with cystic fibrosis. In: Lloyd-Still JD, ed. Textbook of Cystic Fibrosis. Boston: John Wright. PSG; 1983:91.
82. Grimwood K, To M, Rabin HR, Woods DE. Subinhibitory antibiotics reduce *Pseudomonas aeruginosa* tissue injury in the rat lung model. J Antimicrob Chemother. 1989;24:937.
83. Goldfarb J, Stern RC, Reed MD, et al. Ciprofloxacin monotherapy for acute pulmonary exacerbations of cystic fibrosis. Am J Med. 1987;82 (suppl 4A):174.
84. Schaad UB, Wedgwood J, Ruedeberg A, et al. Ciprofloxacin as antipseudomonal treatment in patients with cystic fibrosis. Pediatr Infect Dis J. 1997;16:106.
85. Smith AL, Redding G, Doershuk C, et al. Sputum changes associated with therapy for endobronchial exacerbation in cystic fibrosis. J Pediatr. 1988;112:547.
86. Mendelman PM, Smith AL, Levy J, et al. Aminoglycoside penetration, inactivation, and efficacy in cystic fibrosis sputum. Am Rev Respir Dis. 1985;132:761.
87. Reed MD, Stern RC, O'Brien CA, et al. Randomized double-blind evaluation of ceftazidime dose ranging in hospitalized patients with cystic fibrosis. Antimicrob Agents Chemother. 1987;31:698.
88. Kavanaugh RE, Unadkat JD, Smith AL. Drug disposition in cystic fibrosis. In: Davis PB, ed. Cystic Fibrosis. New York: Marcel Dekker; 1993:91.
89. Smith A, Cohen M, Ramsey B. Pharmacotherapy. In: Yankaskas JR, Knowles MR, eds. Cystic Fibrosis in Adults. Philadelphia: Lippincott-Raven; 1998:345.
90. Donati MA, Guenette G, Auerbach H. Prospective controlled study of home and hospital therapy of cystic fibrosis pulmonary disease. J Pediatr. 1987;111:28.
91. Strandvik B, Hjelte L, Malmborg AS, Widen B. Home intravenous antibiotic treatment of patients with cystic fibrosis. Acta Paediatr. 1992;81:340.
92. Ramsey BW, Dorkin HL, Eisenberg JD, et al. Efficacy of aerosolized tobramycin in patients with cystic fibrosis. N Engl J Med. 1993;328:1740.
93. Ramsey B, Burns J, Smith A. Safety and efficacy of tobramycin solution for inhalation in patients with cystic fibrosis: The results of two Phase III placebo controlled clinical trials. Pediatr Pulmonol Suppl. 1997;14:137.
94. Jensen T, Pedersen SS, Garne S, et al. Colistin inhalation therapy in cystic fibrosis patients with chronic *Pseudomonas aeruginosa* lung infection. J Antimicrob Chemother. 1987;19:831.
95. Dodd ME, Abbott J, Maddison J, et al. Effect of tonicity of nebulised colistin on chest tightness and pulmonary function in adults with cystic fibrosis. Thorax. 1997;52:656.
96. Diot P, Gagnadoux F, Martin C, et al. Nebulization and anti–*Pseudomonas aeruginosa* activity of colistin. Eur Respir J. 1997;10:1995.
97. Welkon CJ, Long SS, Thompson CM Jr, Gilligan PH. *Clostridium difficile* in patients with cystic fibrosis. Am J Dis Child. 1987;139:805.
98. Peach SL, Borriello SP, Gaya H, et al. Asymptomatic carriage of *Clostridium difficile* in patients with cystic fibrosis. J Clin Pathol. 1986;39:1013.
99. Gabriel SE, Brigman KN, Koller BH, et al. Cystic fibrosis heterozygote resistance to cholera toxin in the cystic fibrosis mouse model. Science. 1994;266:107.
100. Kalnins D, Stewart C, Tullis E, Pencharz PB: Nutrition. In: Yankaskas JR, Knowles MR, eds. Cystic Fibrosis in Adults. Philadelphia: Lippincott-Raven; 1998:289.
101. Denning DW, Van Wye JE, Lewiston NJ, Stevens DA. Adjunctive therapy of allergic bronchopulmonary aspergillosis with itraconazole. Chest. 1991;100:813.
102. Egan TM. Lung transplantation in cystic fibrosis. Semin Respir Crit Care Med. 1996;17:137.
103. Johnson LG, Knowles MR. New therapeutic strategies for cystic fibrosis lung disease. In: Yankaskas JR, Knowles MR, eds. Cystic Fibrosis in Adults. Philadelphia: Lippincott-Raven; 1998:233.
104. Bennett WD, Olivier KN, Zeman KL, et al. Effect of uridine 5′-triphosphate plus amiloride on mucociliary clearance in adult cystic fibrosis. Am J Respir Crit Care Med. 1996;153:1796.

SECTION D

Chapter 62

Urinary Tract Infections

JACK D. SOBEL
DONALD KAYE

Bacteriuria is a frequently used term and literally means "bacteria in the urine." The probability of the presence of infected urine in the bladder can be ascertained by means of quantifying numbers of bacteria in voided urine or in urine obtained via urethral catheterization. *Significant bacteriuria* is a term that has been used to describe the numbers of bacteria in voided urine that exceed the numbers usually due to contamination from the anterior urethra (i.e., $\geq 10^5$ bacteria/ml). The implication is that in the presence of at least 10^5 bacteria/ml of urine, infection must be seriously considered. *Asymptomatic bacteriuria* refers to significant bacteriuria in a patient without symptoms.

Urinary tract infection may involve only the lower urinary tract or may involve both the upper and the lower tracts. The term *cystitis* has been used to describe the syndrome involving dysuria, frequency, urgency, and occasionally suprapubic tenderness. However, these symptoms may be related to lower tract inflammation without bacterial infection and can be caused by urethritis (for example, gonorrhea or chlamydial urethritis). Furthermore, the presence of symptoms of lower tract infection without upper tract symptoms by no means excludes upper tract infection, which is also often present.

Acute pyelonephritis describes the clinical syndrome characterized by flank pain or tenderness, or both, and fever, often associated with dysuria, urgency, and frequency. However, these symptoms can occur in the absence of infection (for example, in renal infarction or renal calculus). A more rigorous definition of acute pyelonephritis is the previously described syndrome accompanied by significant bacteriuria and acute infection in the kidney.

Uncomplicated urinary tract infection refers to infection in a structurally and neurologically normal urinary tract. *Complicated urinary tract infection* refers to infection in a urinary tract with abnormalities. In general, infection in men, pregnant women, and children may be considered complicated. Some consider upper tract infection as complicated.[1–3]

Urinary tract infection may occur de novo or may be a recurrent infection. Recurrences may be either *relapses* or *reinfections.* Relapse of bacteriuria refers to a recurrence of bacteriuria with the same infecting microorganism that was present before therapy was started. This is due to persistence of the organism in the urinary tract. Reinfection is a recurrence of bacteriuria with a microorganism different from the original infecting bacterium. It is a new infection. Reinfection may occur with the same microorganism, which may have persisted in the vagina or feces. This can be mistaken for a relapse.

The term *chronic urinary tract infection* has little meaning in many patients. True chronic infection should really mean persistence of the same organism for months or years with relapses after treatment. Reinfections do not mean chronicity any more than repeated episodes of pneumonia indicate chronic pneumonia. Some authorities have inappropriately grouped patients with relapsing infections and frequent reinfections together as having "chronic infection."

The term *chronic pyelonephritis* is difficult to define and means different things to different authors. To some, chronic pyelonephritis refers to pathologic changes in the kidney due to infection only. However, identical pathologic alterations are found in several other entities such as chronic urinary tract obstruction, analgesic nephropathy, hypokalemic nephropathy, vascular disease, and uric acid nephropathy. Pathologic descriptions do not (and cannot) differentiate between the changes produced by infection versus those produced by these other entities.

Papillary necrosis from infection is an acute complication of pyelonephritis usually in the presence of diabetes mellitus, urinary tract obstruction, sickle cell disease, or analgesic abuse. Papillary necrosis can occur in the absence of infection in some of these conditions. The necrotic renal papillae may slough and cause unilateral or bilateral ureteral obstruction. *Intrarenal abscess* may result from bacteremia or may be a complication of severe pyelonephritis. *Perinephric abscess* occurs when microorganisms from either the renal parenchyma or blood are deposited in the soft tissues surrounding the kidneys.

PATHOLOGIC CHARACTERISTICS[4, 5]

Acute Pyelonephritis

In severe pyelonephritis the kidney is somewhat enlarged, and discrete, yellowish, raised abscesses are apparent on the surface. The pathognomonic histologic feature is suppurative necrosis or abscess formation within the renal substance.

Chronic Pyelonephritis (Chronic Interstitial Nephritis)

In chronic pyelonephritis, one or both kidneys contain gross scars, but even when involvement is bilateral, the kidneys are not equally damaged. This uneven scarring is useful in differentiating chronic pyelonephritis from diseases that cause symmetric contracted kidneys, for example, chronic glomerulonephritis. There are inflammatory changes in the pelvic wall with papillary atrophy and blunting. The parenchyma shows interstitial fibrosis with an inflammatory infiltrate of lymphocytes, plasma cells, and occasionally neutrophils (Fig. 62–1). The tubules are dilatated or contracted with atrophy of the lining epithelium. Many of the dilatated tubules contain colloid casts, which suggest the appearance of thyroid tissue ("thyroidization" of the kidney). There is also concentric fibrosis about the parietal layer of Bowman's capsule (termed *periglomerular fibrosis*) and vascular changes similar to those of benign or malignant arteriolar sclerosis.

Several studies have found little correlation between these pathologic findings and evidence for past or present urinary tract infection.[6–8] Clearly a better term for this pathologic entity would be *chronic interstitial nephritis* to encompass all the clinical states that can cause these changes. To incriminate infection as the sole cause of chronic interstitial nephritis, one needs evidence of past or present urinary tract infection and the absence of any other condition that can cause the pathologic picture of chronic interstitial nephritis. These criteria are seldom met, and even if they are, it is frequently impossible to establish whether infection is complicating interstitial nephritis of some unrecognized cause.

Papillary Necrosis Caused by Infection

Frequently both kidneys are affected, and one or more pyramids may be involved (Fig. 62–2). The pyramids are replaced by wedge-

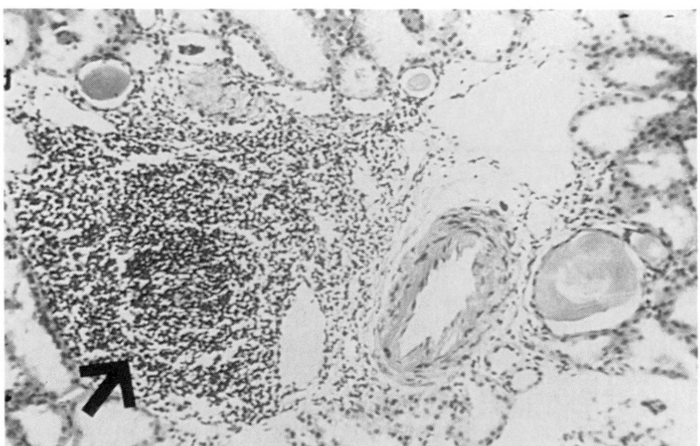

FIGURE 62–1. Chronic pyelonephritis. Tubules are filled with eosinophilic casts and surrounded by a dense infiltrate of lymphocytes and plasma cells *(arrow).*

shaped areas of yellow necrotic tissue with the base located at the corticomedullary junction. As the lesion progresses, a portion of the necrotic papilla may break off, producing a calyceal deformity that results in a recognizable radiologic filling defect. The sloughed portion may be voided and in some instances can be recovered from the urine. Microscopically, edema is initially seen in the interstitium. Eventually the lesion resembles an infarct with coagulation necrosis involving the entire pyramid. The collecting tubules are filled with bacteria and polymorphonuclear leukocytes.

PATHOGENESIS OF URINARY TRACT INFECTION

Urinary infections occur as a result of the interaction of bacterial virulence, and host biologic and behavioral factors as opposed to highly efficient host defense mechanisms. There are three possible routes by which bacteria can invade and spread within the urinary tract: the ascending, hematogenous, and lymphatic pathways.

Ascending Route

The urethra is usually colonized with bacteria. Studies using suprapubic puncture techniques have revealed the occasional presence of small numbers of microorganisms in the urine of uninfected persons.[9] Massage of the urethra in women[10] and sexual intercourse[11–16] can force bacteria into the female bladder. Condom use may heighten the traumatic effects.[17] Furthermore, just one catheterization of the bladder results in urinary tract infection in about 1% of ambulatory patients,[18] and infection develops within 3 or 4 days in essentially all patients with indwelling catheters with open drainage systems.[19] Both the diaphragm with nonoxynol 9 contraceptive jelly in women and the condom catheter in men have been shown to predispose to infection.[14, 16, 20–24] Studies have implicated the spermicide rather than the diaphragm. Spermicides increase colonization of the vagina with uropathogens.[25] Although the dominant *Lactobacillus* vaginal flora are more sensitive to nonoxynol 9 than *Escherichia coli,* it has not been proved that the high coliform presence in nonoxynol-9 users is due to a loss of lactobacilli. Spermicide use also increases adherence of *E. coli* to vaginal epithelial cells.[24]

The fact that urinary tract infection is much more common in women than in men gives support to the importance of the ascending route of infection. The female urethra is short and is in proximity to the warm moist vulvar and perianal areas, making contamination likely. It has been shown that the organisms that cause urinary tract infection in women colonize the vaginal introitus and the periurethral area before urinary infection results.[26] Once within the bladder, bacteria may multiply and then pass up the ureters, especially if vesicoureteral reflux is present, to the renal pelvis and parenchyma. Animal studies have also confirmed the importance of ascending infection.[27] If bladder bacteriuria is established after unilateral ureteral ligation, only the unligated kidney develops pyelonephritis. Finally, studies have correlated intestinal carriage of urovirulent *E. coli* and susceptibility to urinary tract infections in children.[28]

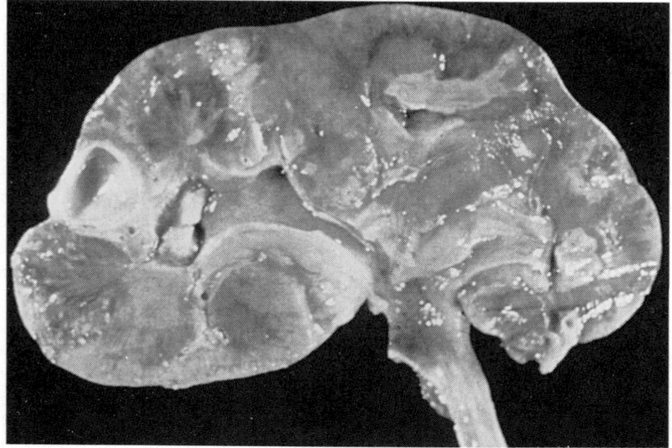

FIGURE 62–2. Necrotizing papillitis (papillary necrosis) complicating acute pyelonephritis in a diabetic patient. The pelvis is hemorrhagic. Note large and irregular defects. (Courtesy of M. Bergeron, M.D.)

Hematogenous Route

Infection of the renal parenchyma by blood-borne organisms clearly occurs in humans. The kidney is frequently the site of abscesses in patients with staphylococcal bacteremia or endocarditis, or both. Experimental pyelonephritis can be produced by the intravenous injection of several species of bacteria and *Candida.*[29] However, the production of experimental pyelonephritis by the intravenous route with gram-negative enteric bacilli, the common pathogens in urinary tract infection, is difficult. Additional manipulations such as the creation of ureteral obstruction are often necessary.[29] It would appear that in humans, infection of the kidney with gram-negative bacilli rarely occurs by the hematogenous route.

Lymphatic Route

Evidence for a significant role for renal lymphatics in the pathogenesis of pyelonephritis is unimpressive and consists of the demonstration of lymphatic connections between the ureters and kidneys in animals and the fact that increased pressure in the bladder can cause lymphatic flow to be directed toward the kidney.[30] Thus, it would seem that the ascending pathway of infection is the most important.

Host-Parasite Interaction

Organism

Although urinary tract infections are caused by many species of microorganisms, most are due to *E. coli.* However, only a few serogroups of *E. coli,* 01, 02, 04, 06, 07, 075, 0150, cause a high proportion of infections.[31] This has led to the concept of uropathogenic *E. coli* clones, or lineages, to differentiate pathogenic populations from commensals. Certain OKH serotypes also correlate with clinical severity, especially pyelonephritis. Accordingly, certain strains of *E. coli* are selected from the fecal flora by the presence of virulence factors that enhance both colonization and invasion of the urinary tract and the capacity to produce disease.[32] Johnson and colleagues confirmed that certain OKH serotypes are associated with urovirulence, and with the presence and expression of multiple chromosomal virulence factor determinants.[33] Recognized virulence factors include increased adherence to vaginal and uroepithelial cells,[34] resistance to serum bactericidal activity,[35] a higher quantity of K antigen,[35] the presence of aerobactin,[36] cytotoxic necrotizing factor type 1, and hemolysin production.[36] Genes for the various urovirulence factors are often duplicated in uropathogens and also frequently linked as large multigene chromosomal segments called *pathogenicity islands* and are absent in coliforms found in normal fecal flora. All uropathogens are able to use urine as a growth medium. Urine is, however, an incomplete growth medium; hence, the synthesis of one or more nutritional factors by uropathogenic *E. coli* is essential. Bacterial synthesis of guanine, arginine, and glutamine is required for optimal growth in urine.[37]

In particular, adhesive properties of the organism are involved in the selection of bacteria capable of colonizing the colon[28] and reaching and colonizing the normal urinary tract, and they influence the anatomic level of infection in the urinary tract (Table 62–1).[32, 38] Accordingly, bacteria with enhanced adherence to vaginal and periurethral cells would be selected to colonize the anatomic regions adjacent to the urethral orifice. Human studies and the mouse model of nonobstructive ascending pyelonephritis have confirmed the significance of the adhesive capacity of the urinary pathogen in causing lower and upper tract infection.[39–41] *Escherichia coli* pyelonephritis isolates adhere better than *E. coli* cystitis isolates, and urinary isolates tend to adhere more strongly to uroepithelial cells than random fecal *E. coli* isolates. The adhesins of uropathogenic *E. coli* exist either as filamentous surface organelles termed *pili* or *fimbriae* or as nonfilamentous proteins in the outer membrane. The fimbrial structure consists of helically arranged protein units. Genes encoding the expression of fimbriae on uropathogenic *E. coli* have been found on the chromosomes as opposed to the plasmid-encoded adhesins of enterotoxigenic *E. coli.* Methods such as electron microscopy, as well as erythrocyte agglutination, have been used to characterize fimbriae, and several specific morphologic and functional types have been identified. Numerous uropathogenic strains adhere in the absence of fimbriae. The binding of *E. coli* to epithelial cell receptors containing globoseries glycolipid accounts for the attachment of most strains causing kidney infection and is not inhibited by mannose (this binding is called MR for "mannose-resistant").[42, 43] Fimbriae attaching to globoseries receptors are termed *P fimbriae* since the receptor is a constituent of the P blood group antigen complex present in human erythrocytes and uroepithelial cells.[43] The globoseries glycolipid receptors (gal-gal) are distributed throughout the urinary tract, particularly in the kidney.[43]

P fimbriae are frequently present in uropathogens. They consist of the main subunit Pap A, which gives rise in its polymerized form to fibrillin, the structural protein of the fimbriae, and the carrier molecule for the adhesin (Pap G) on the tip of the fibrillin. A chromosomal gene cluster (genes *pap* A, B, C, D, E, F, G, H, I) code for different Pap proteins and for expression of the highly specific complex adhesion molecule.[44] P fimbriae reveal considerable antigenic variation, giving rise to multiple subgroups. Pap G tip adhesin of P fimbriae is essential in the pathogenesis of pyelonephritis.[45] The *pap* gene EFG sequences encode the adhesin complex. Three molecular variants of Pap G adhesin, encoded by Pap G alleles I through IV, exhibit subtle receptor-binding preferences influencing the clinical outcome. Allele II predominates among strains causing pyelonephritis and bacteremia, and class III allele is more commonly found in children and women with cystitis.[46] P fimbriae also appear to confer enhanced ability of *E. coli* uropathogenic clones to colonize the colon and spread to the perineum.[28] Although relatively resistant to phagocytosis by neutrophils, *E. coli* with P fimbriae paradoxically enhance the host inflammatory response by inducing the elaboration of proinflammatory cytokines.[47, 48] Neutrophils, however, lack receptors for P fimbriae. P-fimbriated *E. coli* dominate as a cause of pyelonephritis and urosepsis, and they especially dominate among blood isolates[44]; nevertheless, downregulation of P-fimbriae expression may occur in the bacteria when they are within the kidney, and this would facilitate parenchymal persistence. There are limited studies that indicate that there is a potential for the development of P-fimbriae–containing vaccines. In the mouse model of pyelonephritis, antibodies directed against P fimbriae that block bacterial adherence to uroepithelial cells in vitro prevent upper tract infection in vivo.[49] With the same model, a vaccine utilizing P fimbriae has shown some encouraging results.

Binding of *E. coli* to mannose-containing receptors occurs with most uropathogenic strains. In fact, strains from cystitis patients are more likely to bind than those from pyelonephritis patients.[41] Fimbriae attaching to mannosides are the common type 1 fimbriae (pili), and attachment is inhibited in the presence of mannose (MS for "mannose-sensitive"). Type 1 fimbriae bind mannose epitopes on secreted glycoproteins such as secretory IgA and Tamm-Horsfall protein (THP). Urinary mucus (THP), or slime, is rich in mannose residues, and hence *E. coli* possessing MS adhesins adheres avidly to urinary slime as well as to fibronectin.[50] The biologic significance of this phenomenon is unclear. Type 1 fimbriae are encoded by the *pil* or *fim* gene cluster including nine genes that encode structural and regulatory proteins.[34, 51] The gene *fim* A encodes the fimbrial subunit protein, which can be expressed independently of the *fim* H–encoded adhesin protein. The *fim* DNA sequences encoding type 1 fimbriae occur in most clinical isolates; consequently, epidemiologic evidence of an association between type 1 fimbriae and the site or severity of infection is more difficult to obtain. Expression of type 1 fimbriae is not especially evident among pyelonephritogenic strains. Nevertheless, experimental animal studies have correlated type 1 fimbriae with persistence of *E. coli* in the urinary tract, and the use of a *fim* H null mutant of a type 1–positive *E. coli* isolate resulted in rapid elimination of the mutant from the urinary tract.[51] Similarly, clinical

TABLE 62–1 Uropathogenic *Escherichia coli* Adhesins and Corresponding Epithelial Receptors

Adhesin	Genetic Sequence	Receptor	Comments
Type 1 fimbriae (MS)	*pil, fim*	D-mannose on epithelial cells and PMNs	Bind to THP and sIgA
P fimbriae (MR)*	*pap* G_{J96} (class I)	Gal (α1→4) Gal (P blood group antigen)	Rare (class I)
	pap GAP (class II)		Strongly associated with pyelonephritis (class II)
	prs (class III)		Associated with cystitis (class III)
S fimbriae (MR)*	*sfa*	Sialyl-(α2→3)-galactoside	Adherence inhibited by THP
Type 1c (MR)	*fac*	Undetermined	Possibly associated with pyelonephritis
G fimbriae (MR)		Terminal *N*-acetyl-D-glucosamine	
M fimbriae (MR)		Galactose-*N*-acetylgalactosamine	
		Blood group M (glycophoren A)	
Dr family (fimbriated and nonfimbriated)	*drb* operon adhesin (E gene)	Dr blood group antigen component of DAF	16% of first-time cystitis isolates
	afa E1-5		
	afa F		

*Associated with pyelonephritis.
Abbreviations: DAF, Decay-accelerating factor; MS, mannose sensitive; MR, mannose resistant; PMNs, polymorphonuclear leukocytes; sIgA, secretory IgA; THP, Tamm-Horsfall protein.

correlations in childhood urinary infections[51] suggest that type 1 fimbriae contribute to virulence in the urinary tract when expressed in the background of a fully virulent uropathogen. Paradoxically, *fim* H also promotes adhesion to phagocytic cells that should presumably result in early bacterial clearance due to enhanced intracellular killing. In fact antibody-opsonized and internalized type 1 fimbriae–bearing *E. coli* are rapidly killed. This is likely to occur within renal parenchyma, and hence type 1–fimbriated *E. coli* are programmed to shed their fimbriae upon reaching the renal pelvis. In contrast, *E. coli* internalized only by a type 1–fimbrial mechanism survive intracellularly within the phagocyte because the organism can attenuate, resulting in parasitism. Once inside the macrophage, the bacterium is safe from antibiotic assault, only to emerge later and possibly contribute to the relapse of bacteriuria.[52] Bacterial adherence to urinary catheters is also type 1 fimbria–dependent.

In addition to type 1 and P fimbriae, a variety of adhesins, including S (7% of uropathogenic strains); type 1c; G; and Dr fimbriae and M and X adhesins,[53, 54] with differing molecular binding specificities and serologic properties, have been identified on uropathogenic strains of *E. coli* and are expressed in vivo in urine (see Table 62–1). The Dr hemagglutinin family includes both fimbrial and nonfimbrial adhesins. Four genes (*dra* A, B, C, D) encoding the structural proteins and adhesins of the fimbriae have been identified. The adhesins bind to the Dr blood group antigen component of decay-accelerating factor, which is widely distributed along the urinary tract. Dr-expressing uropathogens are of relatively low invasive potential and demonstrate low multiplication rates; however, Dr-positive *E. coli* persist in renal infections and may play a role in chronic pyelonephritis and interstitial nephritis.[17, 55] Adherent bacteria not only persist within the urinary tract but have growth advantages and enhanced toxicity.[56] A possible correlation exists between the presence of bacterial adhesin and the difficulty in eradicating organisms with short-course antibiotic therapy.

Studies with other species of bacterial uropathogens, for example, *Proteus mirabilis and Klebsiella* spp., have similarly demonstrated the significance of adherence in the pathogenesis of urinary infections.[57] *Staphylococcus aureus* uncommonly causes cystitis and ascending pyelonephritis; in contrast, *Staphylococcus saprophyticus* is a frequent cause of lower urinary tract infections. *S. saprophyticus* adheres significantly better to uroepithelial cells than *S. aureus* or *Staphylococcus epidermidis.*[58] Trimethoprim-sulfamethoxazole, extensively used to prevent urinary infection, reduces the synthesis, expression, and adhesive function of type 1 fimbriae at concentrations well below the minimal inhibitory concentration.[59]

Evaluation of urinary isolates for virulence characteristics in the presence of underlying structural abnormalities (e.g., severe reflux) frequently fails to demonstrate the typical bacterial virulence factors. Therefore, in complicated urinary tract infections, virulence factors are often absent, and a natural selection of uropathogens is not apparent.[38, 44] Similarly, *E. coli* blood isolates obtained from patients with urosepsis after bladder instrumentation lack virulence factors.[60] Virulence determinants are more frequently expressed by urinary isolates of *E. coli* obtained from women with cystitis compared with fecal isolates from healthy women.[17, 61] No difference in the prevalence of *E. coli* virulence determinants was found between the subjects with first-time cystitis and those with recurrent cystitis, suggesting that host rather than bacterial factors determine the risk for recurrent infection. Stapleton and associates observed that *E. coli* isolates that caused cystitis in women using diaphragms with spermicides had fewer virulence determinants than those of nonusers,[61] suggesting that the use of diaphragms with spermicides may allow infection with less virulent *E. coli.*

The importance of adherence as a virulence factor is not complete without consideration of the role of the host. A difference in receptor density linked to a difference in genetic susceptibility to infection has been proposed. In women and children with recurrent urinary tract infection, an increased avidity of bacterial attachment to vaginal,[62] periurethral,[63] and uroepithelial[64, 65] cells has been found. However, some authors have failed to corroborate these findings.[66]

Certain other characteristics of bacteria may be important in the production of upper tract infection. Motile bacteria can ascend in the ureter against the flow of urine,[67] and the endotoxins of gram-negative bacilli have been shown to decrease ureteral peristalsis[68] and possibly contribute to the renal parenchymal inflammatory response by phagocytic cell activation.[69] In *Proteus* spp., the production of urease by infecting microorganisms has been correlated with the ability to cause pyelonephritis.[70] The presence of K capsular antigen protects bacteria from leukocyte phagocytosis. Most uropathogenic strains produce hemolysin, which facilitates tissue invasion and causes renal tubular epithelial and parenchymal cell damage,[71] possibly making iron available to invading *E. coli.* The hemolysin gene is frequently located adjacent to genes encoding for serious resistance and sialic acid–specific (S) fimbriae, but the pathogenic role of hemolysis in pyelonephritis remains controversial.[72] Aerobactin, an iron-scavenging protein or siderophore, is present with increased frequency in uropathogenic strains of *E. coli.*[34]

The greater the number of organisms delivered to the kidneys, the greater the chance of producing infection.[73] The kidney itself is not uniformly susceptible to infection, since very few organisms are needed to infect the medulla, whereas 10,000 times as many are needed to infect the cortex.[74] The greater susceptibility of the medulla may be due to the high concentration of ammonia, which may inactivate complement,[75] and to poor chemotaxis of polymorphonuclear neutrophils (PMNs) into an area of high osmolality, low pH, and low blood flow.[76]

Host

With the exception of urethral mucosa, the normal urinary tract is resistant to colonization by bacteria and for the most part efficiently and rapidly eliminates both pathogenic and nonpathogenic microorganisms that gain access to the bladder. This is achieved by the presence of several lower urinary tract antibacterial defense mechanisms (Table 62–2).

Uropathogenic clones elicit an inflammatory response at all levels in the urinary tract by stimulating uroepithelial and other cells to produce cytokines and other proinflammatory factors.[47, 48] Systemic elaboration of interleukin 1-β (IL-1β) and IL-6 may lead to fever and activation of the acute-phase response. The chemotactic cytokine IL-8 is released at the mucosal site recruiting PMNs, resulting in pyuria, and contributes to the eradication of bacteriuria. Cytokine elaboration is a consequence of bacterial adherence to epithelial cells and to a lesser extent a consequence of bacterial lipopolysaccharide.[77]

Mannhardt and coworkers have shown that direct contact between

TABLE 62–2 Antibacterial Host Defenses in the Urinary Tract

Urine (osmolality, pH, organic acids)
Urine flow and micturition
Urinary tract mucosa (bactericidal activity, cytokines)
Urinary inhibitors of bacterial adherence
Tamm-Horsfall protein
Bladder mucopolysaccharide
Low-molecular-weight oligosaccharides
sIgA
Lactoferrin
Inflammatory response
PMNs
Cytokines
Immune system
Humoral
Cell-mediated immunity
Miscellaneous
Prostatic secretions

Abbreviations: PMNs, Polymorphonuclear neutrophils; sIgA, secretory immunoglobulin A.

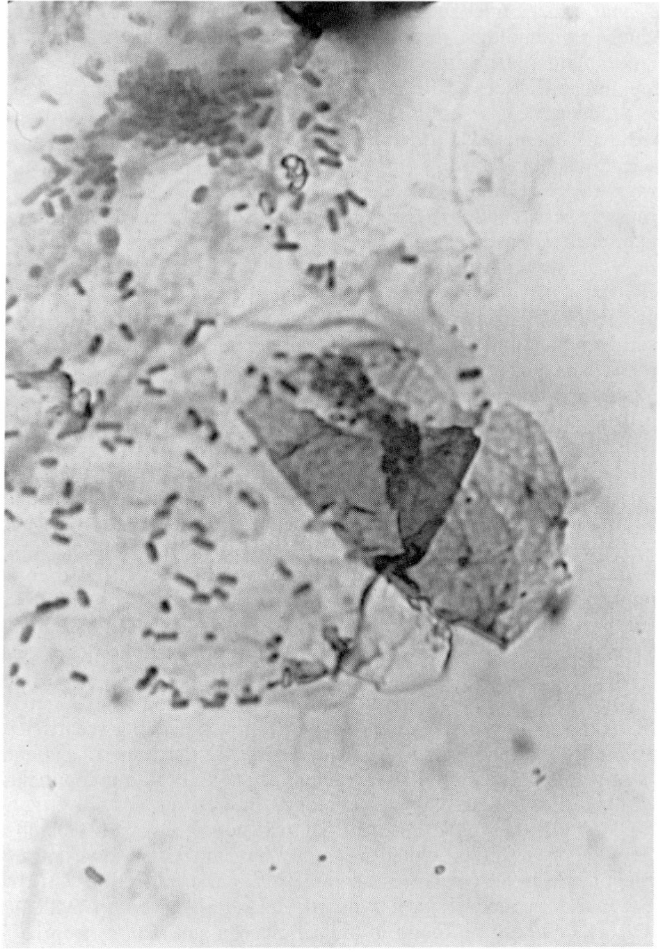

FIGURE 62–3. Light-microscopic specimen of urine showing uromucoid (Tamm-Horsfall protein) with large numbers of adherent uropathogenic bacteria.

adherent bacteria and uroepithelial cells may also result in bacterial growth suppression.[78] This antibacterial epithelial defense function is activated by transmembranous signals from bacteria attached to the host cell surface and involves adenylate cyclase activity.

Although urine is generally considered to be a good culture medium for most bacteria, it does possess antibacterial activity. Anaerobic bacteria and other fastidious organisms that make up most of the urethral flora generally do not multiply in urine. It has been shown that extremes of osmolality, a high urea concentration, and low pH levels are inhibitory for the growth of some of the bacteria that cause urinary tract infection.[79] Furthermore, the pH and osmolality of urine from pregnant women tend to be more suitable for bacterial growth than those of nonpregnant women, which in turn are more suitable for bacterial growth than those of urine from men.[80] The presence of glucose makes urine a better culture medium, whereas the addition of prostatic fluid to urine inhibits bacterial growth.[80, 81] Furthermore, urine has been shown to inhibit the migrating, adhering, aggregating, and killing functions of PMNs.[82]

By means of its mannose-containing side chains, THP, secreted by cells of the ascending loop of Henle, binds strongly to *E. coli* expressing type I and S fimbriae.[83] THP is the most abundant protein of renal origin in urine and may function as a urinary antibacterial defense mechanism by binding to MS strains of *E. coli,* preventing them from attaching to epithelial cell receptors (Fig. 62–3).[50] Clinical studies in adults have failed to show a relationship between urinary THP concentrations and the risk for urinary tract infection, although significantly reduced levels of THP in elderly persons occur during episodes of urinary tract infection.[84]

The flushing mechanism of the bladder exerts a major protective effect. When bacteria are introduced into the bladders of humans, there is a tendency for spontaneous clearance.[85] Since flushing alone would probably not completely clear the bacteria, there must be additional protective factors. Host factors including bladder catheterization influence the susceptibility of uroepithelial cells to attachment by uropathogens, and this in turn increases the susceptibility to bacteriuria.[86]

In a study of bladder defense mechanisms in dogs, Parsons and colleagues demonstrated an active antiadherence mechanism of bladder mucosa.[87] Pretreatment of the bladder with acid was shown to increase bacterial adherence 20- to 50-fold. The increased adherence was independent of the bacterial species employed. Histochemical studies revealed that bacterial adherence was increased by the removal of a surface mucopolysaccharide, glycosaminoglycan, which seems to be responsible for the natural resistance to adherence.[88] Thus, normally small inocula of bacteria are probably unable to adhere, remain suspended in urine, and are removed by voiding. In the presence of a larger bladder inoculum of bacteria, especially with good adhesive qualities, the primary defense of antiadherence may be overcome, colonization can occur, and subsequent bladder infection may result.[89] With the occurrence of bladder infection, secondary defense mechanisms such as mobilization of leukocytes, phagocytosis, and bacterial destruction are called on to remove bacteria.[89, 90] Bacteria stimulate PMNs to secrete IL-8, IL-1β, and tumor necrosis factor and stimulate lymphocytes to elaborate immunoregulatory cytokines ultimately resulting in immunoglobulin synthesis and modifying epithelial cell responses to bacteria. Epithelial cells participate in PMN recruitment by secreting neutrophil chemoattractants (e.g., IL-8) and by the expression of adhesion molecules involved in PMN transmigration (intercellular adhesion molecule 1).[91]

In women, colonization of the vaginal introitus and periurethral region by Enterobacteriaceae is critical in the pathogenesis of urinary tract infections.[26] Several authors have shown that periurethral colonization with the same organism almost invariably precedes episodes of significant bacteriuria.[26, 92, 93] Microbiologic studies have demonstrated that the urethra, periurethral region, and vaginal vestibule of women with recurrent urinary tract infections tend to be more commonly colonized with coliform bacteria.[62, 63, 92] Stamey has postulated that such colonization is often the prelude to new infection and that women with recurrent urinary tract infection have a biologic predisposition to infection.[92] The hypothesis is that some women have defective local perineal and vaginal defense mechanisms that result in increased susceptibility to introital and perineal colonization with urinary pathogens such as coliform bacteria.[92] In a series of studies, the effects of several factors in vaginal secretions on colonization were examined[62, 94–99] A low vaginal pH level was the most important factor related to a lack of colonization. Furthermore, serogroups of uropathogenic *E. coli* were more resistant to low pH levels. It was also found in these studies that *E. coli* was less susceptible to the inhibitory effects of vaginal fluid than *P. mirabilis* or *Pseudomonas aeruginosa.* Finally, it was noted that *E. coli* adhered more avidly to vaginal epithelial cells of women with recurrent urinary tract infection, and this was initially attributed to a reduced local production of antibodies in vaginal secretions.[62] Kallenius and Winberg however, showed that the periurethral cells of young girls prone to recurrent urinary tract infections were more susceptible to bacterial attachment,[63] and other authors found enhanced attachment of *E. coli* to uroepithelial cells of patients with recurrent urinary tract infections.[64, 65] These observations suggest a genetic cellular predisposition of some women to urinary tract infection. This hypothesis is further supported by the fact that women who are epithelial antigen and receptor nonsecretors may have an increased risk of urinary tract infection, and their uroepithelial cells bind *E. coli* more avidly than do cells from secretors.[100] In studying women prone to recurrent lower urinary tract infection, investigators found that these patients did not differ from control subjects with regard to the distribution of blood groups A, B, O, or P phenotypes but demonstrated an increased frequency of the Lewis blood group nonsecretor and recessive phenotype.[101, 102] Recently investigators failed to confirm that the nonsecretor phenotype was independently associated with an increased overall risk of sporadic urinary infection but the nonsecretor phenotype may still predispose to recurrent infection.[24, 103] Other endogenous factors, such as estrogenic hormones, may influence bacterial attachment to uroepithelial cells and affect the risk of urinary tract infection.[104] From an acquired or behavioral point of view, both colonization of the vaginal introitus and bacteriuria due to *E. coli* have been strongly associated with diaphragm and spermicide use, which may account for the increased risk of urinary tract infection associated with sexual activity.[14, 16] The dominant pathogenic mechanism is probably related to the differential antibacterial effect of nonoxynol 9, whereby more susceptible lactobacilli are replaced by coliform uropathogens.[105]

Not all authors agree that periurethral colonization is the most important factor in the pathogenesis of recurrent urinary tract infection.[93, 106–109] They point out that vestibular colonization with Enterobacteriaceae is as common in women not prone to infection. Furthermore, Parsons and Schmidt found no enhanced bacterial adherence to vaginal epithelial cells in women with recurrent urinary tract infection,[66] and Kurdydyk and coworkers studied immunoglobulin (IgG) and IgA levels in cervicovaginal washings and found no difference between washings from women prone to infection and those from women with no past history of urinary tract infection.[110] Kunin and associates stated that all women who do not have a structural or neurologic problem in the voiding mechanism are approximately at the same risk of having a first urinary tract infection.[93] In their view, once established, each infection sets the stage for the next episode, since infection and antibiotic treatment thereof may lead to colonization unless periurethral colonization is eradicated by therapy. Smith and colleagues reported that recent antimicrobial use increases a woman's risk of urinary infection by altering the indigenous urogenital flora, predisposing to vaginal colonization with uropathogens.[111] Antibiotics, especially β-lactams, promote vestibular colonization with *E. coli*.[112] The longer the interval between infections, the less likelihood there is for recurrences. The antagonists to Stamey's hypothesis have concluded that the decisive factor is not the colonization of the periurethral area per se but rather host factors and the ability of these organisms to ascend the urethra, including the ability of infecting organisms to adhere to mucosal cells and withstand normal host defense mechanisms.

The role of humoral immunity in the host's defense against infection of the urinary tract, although extensively studied, is poorly understood, as shown in several studies.[113–120] During acute pyelonephritis, there is a systemic antibody response. Antibodies against the O antigen and occasionally the K antigen of the infecting strain have been found, and antibodies to type 1 and P fimbriae were described.[115, 121] IgM antibodies dominate in the response to the first upper tract infection but not to subsequent episodes. Of note is the observation that high levels of IgG antibodies to lipid A correlate with the severity of renal infection and the progression of renal parenchymal destruction.[116] An antibody response consisting of IgG and secretory IgA antibodies can be detected in the urine. In contrast to upper tract infection, lower urinary infection is usually associated with a reduced or nondetectable serologic response, reflecting the superficial nature of the infection. Macrophages are well distributed in the submucosa throughout the urinary tract, and Ia-expressing cells, analogous to Langerhans cells, have been identified in the urinary mucosa, including among renal tubular cells.[122] IgA-producing lymphocytes are found in the submucosa of infected rat bladders. Similarly, Christmas observed high numbers of IgA-producing plasma cells in the bladder submucosa of patients with bacterial cystitis in comparison with healthy controls.[123] Finally, in animal models, antibody-secreting cells and B lymphocytes migrate to kidney and urinary tract submucosa during urinary tract infections. The reduced immunologic response to the infecting organism in cystitis may explain the phenomenon of reinfection with the same strain. Hopkins and associates, however, using a monkey model, reported the production of systemic and urinary IgG and IgA that accompanied experimental cystitis.[124]

In particular, antifimbrial antibodies are absent in the urine in lower tract infection.[124] At least one third of females with a second urinary tract infection have an identical strain isolated, indicating incomplete or inadequate immunity with a single episode of infection.[125] A systemic serologic response has been used to distinguish between upper and lower urinary tract infection but is not practical because of too many false-negative and false-positive results. However, local coating of bacteria with antibodies within the kidney (and prostate) has formed the basis of localization techniques that clarified modern approaches to therapy.

In spite of the impressive systemic and local urinary antibody production that follows acute pyelonephritis, the protective role of these antibodies is unclear. When bacteria persist in the kidney for several months, antigenic drift may occur.[117] Nevertheless, antibodies against several bacterial structures, including O and K antigen and more recently fimbrial antigens, have been found to protect against hematogenous or ascending pyelonephritis in experimental animals.[114, 115] Animal recipients of vaccines based on Pap A fimbriae were protected against experimental pyelonephritis caused by homologous and heterologous Gal-Gal–binding uropathogenic *E. coli* strains.[126]

Antibodies may be of value in limiting the damage incurred within the kidney or preventing colonization preceding recurrence. Svanborg-Eden and Svennerholm reported that the urine of patients with pyelonephritis inhibited the adherence of *E. coli* to uroepithelial cells and that this activity was removed by absorption with O antigen.[118] Antibodies have not been shown to protect against bladder infection.[119, 120] Cell-mediated immunity has not been shown to play a major role in host defenses against urinary tract infection. Urinary tract mucosa contains few T lymphocytes, although both $CD4^+$ and $CD8^+$ T cells can be found in the submucosa and lamina propria[123]; however, they generally lack γδ T cells.[127] Experimental studies in athymic mice showed similar resistance to intravesical infections when compared with normal controls.[128] Similarly, clinical experience in humans with severe defects in cell-mediated immunity does not indicate increased susceptibility to or severity of urinary infection. Nevertheless, a useful role for cell-mediated immunity may still exist in that T-cell–derived proinflammatory cytokines (e.g., interferon-γ) stimulate epithelial cells to produce IL-6[129] as do Th2 lymphocyte responses involving IL-4, IL-5, IL-10, and IL-13.[48] Thus, urinary tract T cells producing immunoregulatory cytokines may influence the mucosal epithelial cell response to bacterial adherence and invasion. The IL-6 secreted by renal tubular epithelial cells[47, 48, 129] may contribute to mucosal antibacterial activity by increasing IgA secretion by committed B cells.

During pyelonephritis, an acute inflammatory exudate consisting predominantly of PMNs is present. Although the inflammatory reaction is directed at limiting bacterial spread and persistence within the kidney, it has been suggested that the infiltrating phagocytic cells may contribute to tissue damage and renal scarring, as evidenced by reduced parenchymal kidney destruction in experimental neutropenia.[130] It has been suggested that chronic pyelonephritis and persistent renal damage may develop after successful eradication of bacterial pyelonephritis with antimicrobial therapy. According to these concepts, bacterial remnants or antigen persistence induces a chronic humoral immunologic response resulting in cryptogenic renal scarring.[131] Another theory suggests that during acute pyelonephritis, THP, normally present within intact renal tubules only, gains access to the renal interstitial space and induces a chronic autoimmune process leading to renal cortical scarring.[132] Neither of these theories has been substantiated or influences clinical management.

There are several abnormalities of the urinary tract that interfere with its natural resistance to infection. Obstruction to urine flow is the most important of these. Extrarenal obstruction can result from congenital anomalies of the ureter or urethra, such as valves, stenosis, or bands; calculi; extrinsic ureteral compression from a variety of causes; and benign prostatic hypertrophy. Intrarenal obstruction may be produced by entities such as nephrocalcinosis, uric acid nephropathy, analgesic nephropathy, polycystic kidney disease, hypokalemic nephropathy, and the renal lesions of sickle cell trait or disease.[133] Obstruction inhibits the normal flow of urine, and the resulting stasis is important in increasing susceptibility to infection.

In animals, obstruction of a ureter markedly increases susceptibility to hematogenous infection.[133] Intrarenal obstruction, experimentally produced by scars in a variety of ways, also increases the susceptibility of the kidney to infection. Medullary scars, which produce greater amounts of obstruction than cortical scars, increase the susceptibility of animals to infection more than cortical scars.[134] Furthermore, the intravenous injection of *E. coli* in animals with renal scars from prior staphylococcal pyelonephritis produces pyelonephritis in the regions of intrarenal hydronephrosis caused by the old scars.[135] Men of any age and pregnant women are the most prone to lesions that result in obstruction to the free flow of urine.

Calculi may increase susceptibility to urinary tract infection by producing obstruction (Fig. 62–4). However, not all stones obstruct, and local irritative phenomena may also be important. Furthermore, calculi may develop secondary to infection. It has been observed clinically and experimentally that *Proteus* spp. and other urea-splitting organisms (e.g., *Klebsiella*) are most likely to produce calculi.[136] Furthermore, bacteria survive deep within the calculi and are extremely difficult to eradicate even by artificial means such as by incubating in solutions containing antibiotics or iodine and alcohol.[137] This may account for the well-known difficulties encountered clinically in trying to cure urinary tract infection in the presence of stones.

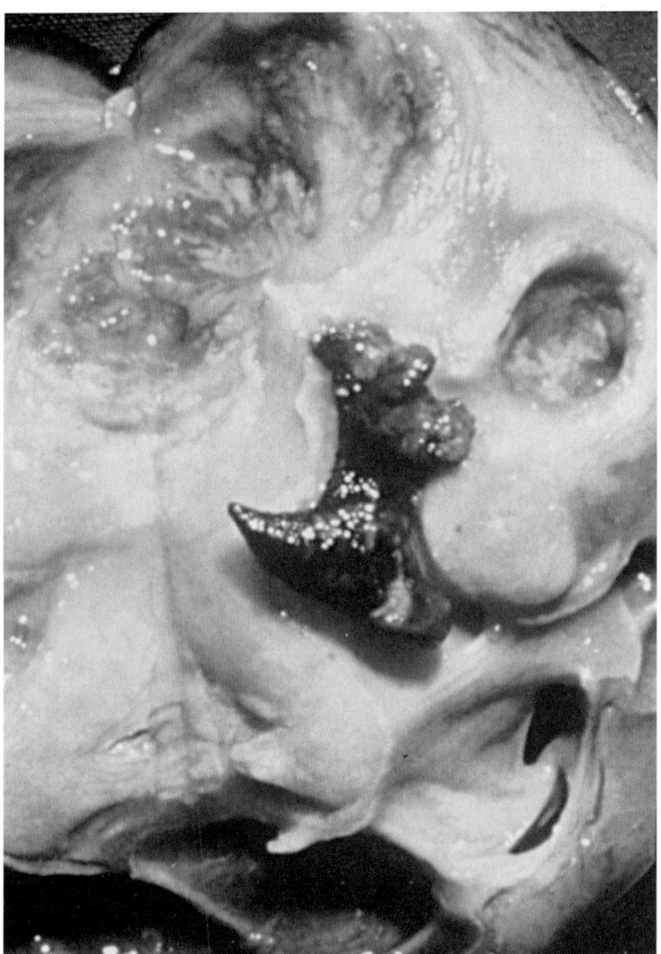

FIGURE 62–4. Staghorn calculus visible in the dilated pelvis of a hydronephrotic kidney. (Courtesy of M. Bergeron, M.D.)

Vesicoureteral reflux and urinary tract infection are also intricately related. Reflux due to a congenital abnormality, bladder overdistention, or unknown causes probably contributes to upper tract infection via the ascending route. On the other hand, clinical observations have demonstrated that infection may, in fact, produce reflux, especially in children.[138] Reflux tends to perpetuate infection by maintaining a residual pool of infected urine in the bladder after voiding. It is probable that reflux, especially in young children, plays an important role in the production of upper tract infection and subsequent scarring.[139] Patients with incomplete emptying of the bladder for either mechanical reasons (bladder neck obstruction, urethral valves, urethral strictures, prostatic hypertrophy) or neurogenic malfunctions (poliomyelitis, tabes dorsalis, diabetic neuropathy, cord injuries) are prone to frequent urinary tract infections. These patients are subject to bladder overdistention, which may interfere with local defense mechanisms, and, most importantly, frequent instrumentation of the urinary tract.

EPIDEMIOLOGY OF URINARY TRACT INFECTION

Infecting Organisms

More than 95% of urinary tract infections are caused by a single bacterial species. There is a great difference between the bacterial flora of the urine in patients with an initial episode of urinary tract infection compared with the flora from those with frequent recurrences of infection. *Escherichia coli* is by far the most frequent infecting organism in acute infection.[140, 141] In recurrent urinary tract infections, especially in the presence of structural abnormalities of the urinary tract (such as obstructive uropathy, congenital anomalies, neurogenic bladder, and fistulous communication involving the urinary tract), the relative frequency of infection caused by *Proteus, Pseudomonas, Klebsiella,* and *Enterobacter* spp. and by enterococci and staphylococci increases greatly. In the presence of structural abnormalities, it is also relatively common to isolate multiple organisms from the urine. Since instrumentation and repeated courses of antimicrobial therapy are common in these patients, antibiotic-resistant isolates might be expected.

The hospital environment is an important determinant of the nature of the bacterial flora in urinary tract infection. *Proteus, Klebsiella, Enterobacter,* and *Pseudomonas* spp. and staphylococci and enterococci are more often isolated from inpatients, compared with a greater preponderance of *E. coli* in an outpatient population.[142, 143] Cross-infections are important in the pathogenesis of hospital-related urinary tract infections, especially with indwelling catheters.[144, 145] *Corynebacterium* group D2 has been recognized as an important nosocomial pathogen. This gram-positive, urea-splitting, slow-growing bacillus may cause acute or chronic cystitis and pyelonephritis and is highly resistant to antimicrobials, although usually sensitive to vancomycin.[145] It should be considered in the presence of high urine pH, urologic problems, previous urinary tract infection, and recent antibiotic treatment.

Anaerobic organisms are rarely pathogens in the urinary tract. A variety of bacteria may be found in the urine of specific clinical settings. Fungi (particularly *Candida* spp.) occur in patients with indwelling catheters who are receiving antimicrobial therapy.[146] Coagulase-negative staphylococci are a common cause of urinary tract infection in some reports.[147] *Staphylococcus saprophyticus* tends to cause infection in young, sexually active females,[148–150] accounting for 5 to 15% of acute cystitis episodes in the United States. Coagulase-positive staphylococci most often invade the kidney from the hematogenous route, resulting in intrarenal or perinephric abscesses.

DNA typing of *E. coli* has substantially aided in the epidemiologic study of urinary tract infection.

Adenoviruses (particularly type 11) have been strongly implicated as causative agents in hemorrhagic cystitis in pediatric patients, especially boys, and in allogenic bone marrow transplant recipients.[151] Cell wall–deficient bacteria have been demonstrated in urine from patients with pyelonephritis, particularly in association with therapy using cell wall–active antibiotics.[152] However, these forms have not been consistently isolated from either urine or renal tissue despite the use of adequate techniques and are probably not of major importance.

Although Maskell and coworkers, using special media, have isolated fastidious microaerophilic organisms from women with lower tract symptoms,[153] the causal role of these organisms is controversial. Similarly *Gardnerella vaginalis* is frequently isolated from the urine of women with and without urinary tract symptoms, but its pathogenic role is unclear. *Ureaplasma urealyticum* and *Mycoplasma hominis* are possible but unproven causes of pyelonephritis and cystourethritis.[154, 155]

A report describes nanobacteria as tiny (0.05 to 0.5 mm) cell wall–possessing bacteria that are associated with renal stones.[156] In vitro, the organisms produce carbonate apatite that can fix calcium. In clinical material, all 30 kidney stones were positive for a nanobacteria-specific protein epitope, and organisms were seen in all 30 specimens examined by immunofluorescence microscopy.

Bacteriuria in Children

The problem of urinary tract infection spans all age-groups, beginning with neonates.[157–162] The frequency of urinary tract infection in infants is about 1 to 2%. It is much more common in boys during the first 3 months and thereafter occurs more often in girls. Bacteremia is common in association with urinary tract infection in male newborns. Autopsy series of infants with pyelonephritis have revealed a predominance of infant boys with pyelonephritis.[157] A lack of circumcision predisposes to urinary tract infection in infants and young boys.[161, 163]

During the preschool years, urinary tract infection is more common in girls than in boys. When infection occurs in preschool boys, it is frequently associated with serious congenital abnormalities. With repeated study over a period of 1 year, the period prevalence of significant bacteriuria in this age-group is 4.5% for girls and about 0.5% for boys. Infections during this period often are symptomatic, and it is believed that much of the renal damage that occurs from urinary tract infection takes place at this time (Fig. 62–5).[158, 164, 165]

Much information on the natural history and epidemiology of urinary tract infection has been gleaned from the studies of Kunin[166, 167] and associates[168] with schoolchildren from central Virginia. It was found that bacteriuria is common in girls in this population, is often asymptomatic, and frequently recurs. For example, the prevalence of bacteriuria among schoolgirls was about 1.2%, and about 5% of the girls had significant bacteriuria at some time before leaving high school. About one third of these patients had some symptom referable to the urinary tract when the bacteriuria was first detected. It was shown that each year about 0.3 to 0.4% of the female population (25% of those infected) was cured either spontaneously or with antimicrobial agents, and an equal number of girls developed new cases of bacteriuria. Bacteriuria was rare in schoolboys (prevalence, 0.03%).

These studies also provided an opportunity to treat the patients and follow their clinical course. Patients were initially treated for 10 days to 2 weeks. Girls with frequent infections were given longer courses of therapy (1 to 3 months). White girls tended to have frequent reinfections, whereas black girls became reinfected less frequently. With each course of therapy, about 20% of white girls went into long-term remission. However, when many of these girls were married or became pregnant, bacteriuria recurred at a rate far above that expected for the general population. Over 50% developed bacteriuria within 3 months after marriage. Thus, the presence of bacteriuria in childhood defines a population at higher risk for the development of bacteriuria in adulthood.

Bacteriuria in Adults

Once adulthood is reached, the prevalence of bacteriuria increases in the female population. The prevalence of bacteriuria in young nonpregnant women is about 1 to 3%.[169] Each year, about 25% of bacteriuric women clear their bacteriuria, and an equal number become infected (often women who have had urinary infection previously). At least 10 to 20% of the female population experience a symptomatic urinary tract infection at some time during their life.[169] Frequent sexual intercourse, diaphragm use, the use of a spermicide, a lack of urination after intercourse, and a history of recurrent infections are risk factors for urinary infection in women.[14, 16, 20–22, 24, 170, 171] The diaphragm can cause urinary obstruction in some women, but its main effect is probably a change in vaginal flora due to the spermicide.[22, 25] The risk of a second urinary tract infection in young women is greater than that of the first, with at least 20% developing a recurrent infection within 6 months of follow-up,[172, 173] *Escherichia coli* causing urinary tract infection may be transmitted between sexual partners, as the same strains have been found in the urine of men who are sexual partners of women with urinary tract infection.[174]

The prevalence of bacteriuria in adult men is low (0.1% or less) until the later years, when it rises. The increase in bacteriuria in older men is probably mainly related to prostatic disease and the resultant instrumentation. Men with bacteriuria frequently have anatomic abnormalities of the urinary tract. In young men, a lack of circumcision increases the risk of urinary tract infection caused by uropathogenic strains of *E. coli,* including the development of symptomatic urethritis.[175]

Bacteriuria in the Elderly Population

At least 10% of men and 20% of women older than 65 years have bacteriuria. In contrast to young adults, in whom bacteriuria is 30 times more frequent in women than in men, in those older than 65 years the ratio alters dramatically, with a progressive decrease in the female/male ratio.[176–178] In both sexes, the prevalence of bacteriuria rises substantially. Possible reasons for the high frequency of urinary tract infections in elderly patients include obstructive uropathy from the prostate and loss of the bactericidal activity of prostatic secretions in men, poor emptying of the bladder due to prolapse in women, soiling of the perineum from fecal incontinence in demented women, and neuromuscular diseases and increased instrumentation and bladder catheter usage in both sexes.[177] There is a high rate of spontaneous cure and reinfection in both women and men.[177] The spectrum of microorganisms is unaltered in the elderly population.

Bacteriuria in Patients with Other Conditions

There is a higher prevalence of bacteriuria in hospitalized patients than in outpatients.[179] The general ill health of hospitalized patients as well as the higher probability of urinary tract instrumentation are probably the major contributors to these differences.

A single catheterization causes urinary tract infection in only about 1% of ambulatory persons.[18] However, after catheterization of hospitalized patients, infection occurs in at least 10%. Race apparently does not appreciably affect the prevalence of bacteriuria. However, socioeconomic status is important, with pregnant women from lower socioeconomic groups having a higher prevalence of bacteriuria.[180–182]

Various underlying diseases have also been associated with an increased frequency of urinary tract infection. Diabetic women but not men have been found to have a higher prevalence of bacteriuria than nondiabetic patients.[183, 184]

Black women with sickle cell trait have a higher prevalence of

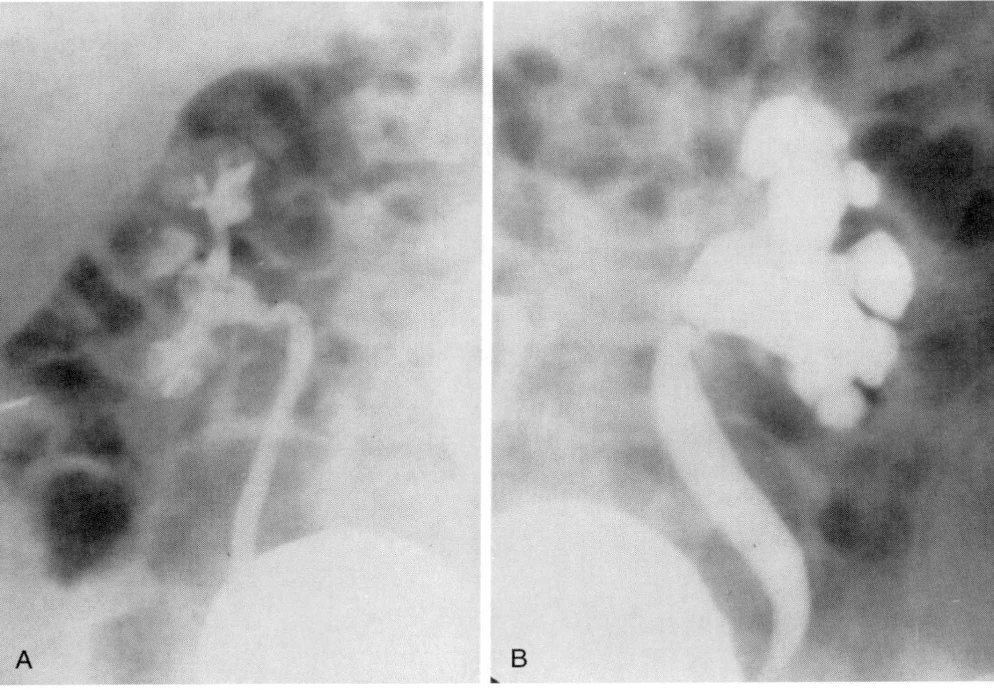

FIGURE 62–5. Vesicoureteral reflux in a young girl with recurrent urinary tract infections. *A,* Right kidney demonstrates grade II reflux. *B,* Left kidney shows dilatation of the ureter, grade III reflux, and calyceal clubbing. (Courtesy of T. Slovis, M.D.)

bacteriuria during pregnancy than black women without the sickle trait.[182, 184, 185] Other conditions stated to be associated with urinary tract infection (but without documentation) include chronic potassium deficiency, gout, hypertension, and other conditions causing interstitial renal disease. There is an increased frequency and severity (more sepsis) of urinary tract infection in renal transplant patients and men with acquired immunodeficiency disease.[186, 187] Evidence for an increase in the frequency or severity of infection in women with acquired immunodeficiency disease is lacking.

CLINICAL MANIFESTATIONS

Symptoms

Urinary tract infection in children tends to manifest with different symptoms depending on the age of the child. Symptoms in neonates and children younger than 2 years are nonspecific.[158–160, 162] Failure to thrive, vomiting, and fever seem to be the major manifestations. When children older than 2 years (and more consistently, older than 5 years) develop infection, they are more likely to display localizing symptoms such as frequency, dysuria, and abdominal or flank pain.

The manifestations of urinary tract infection in adults are usually easy to recognize. The lower tract symptoms result from bacteria producing irritation of urethral and vesical mucosa, causing frequent and painful urination of small amounts of turbid urine. Patients sometimes complain of suprapubic heaviness or pain. Occasionally the urine is grossly bloody or shows a bloody tinge at the end of micturition. Fever tends to be absent in infection limited to the lower tract.

The classic clinical manifestation of upper urinary tract infection includes fever (sometimes with chills), flank pain, and frequently lower tract symptoms (e.g., frequency, urgency, and dysuria). At times, the lower tract symptoms antedate the appearance of fever and upper tract symptoms by 1 or 2 days. It should be recognized that the symptoms described, although classic, may vary greatly. In fact, pyelonephritis may show protean clinical manifestations in adults as well as in children. Flank tenderness or discomfort is frequent in upper tract infection in adults and is more intense when there is obstructive disease. Severe pain with radiation into the groin is rare in acute pyelonephritis per se and suggests the presence of a renal calculus. The pain from the kidney is occasionally felt in or near the epigastrium and may radiate to one of the lower quadrants. These manifestations may offer difficulties in differential diagnosis and suggest gallbladder disease or appendicitis.

The vast majority of elderly patients with urinary infection are asymptomatic.[176–178] Symptoms, when present, are often not diagnostic, since noninfected elderly patients often experience frequency, dysuria, hesitancy, and incontinence. Nevertheless, typical symptoms may occur, and less frequently acute pyelonephritis develops, usually necessitating hospitalization. Gleckman and associates found a much higher frequency of bacteremia (61%) associated with pyelonephritis in elderly patients than is found in young patients, and shock commonly supervened.[188] Most of the patients had significant urologic abnormalities. The effect of asymptomatic bacteriuria on the general sense of well-being, appetite, and urinary continence has been studied, and no association could be demonstrated.[189, 190]

The clinical manifestations of recurrent or persistent urinary tract infection are more difficult to define. Patients with lower urinary tract involvement tend to have repeated bouts of transient symptomatic or asymptomatic infection. Patients with upper tract infection may have episodes of fever, pain in the renal regions, and dysuria during acute exacerbations or new bouts of infection. However, upper tract infection may result in only lower tract symptoms or no symptoms at all. Patients with urinary tract infection in the presence of an indwelling urinary catheter usually have no lower tract symptoms, but flank pain or fever may occur. Urinary tract infection is the most common source of bacteremia produced by gram-negative bacilli. Bacteremia may occur with no urinary symptoms, especially in the presence of an indwelling catheter.

Alterations in Renal Function

In experimentally produced pyelonephritis, the only consistent abnormality of renal function is the inability to concentrate the urine maximally.[191, 192] The mechanism of the concentrating defect is not clear but seems to be related in experimental animals to inflammation and perhaps to the increased production of prostaglandins.[192, 193] The concentrating defect occurs early in the course of experimental infection and is rapidly reversible with antimicrobial therapy and after the administration of prostaglandin inhibitors.[191, 192] The same phenomenon occurs in humans.[194]

Progressive destruction of the kidney (particularly in the presence of obstruction) may occur and give rise to clinical manifestations of renal insufficiency. Bilateral papillary necrosis occasionally can lead to rapidly progressive renal failure.[195]

DIAGNOSIS

Presumptive Diagnosis of Urinary Tract Infection

Microscopic examination of the urine is the first step in the laboratory diagnosis of urinary tract infection. A clean-catch midstream urine specimen is centrifuged for 5 minutes at 2000 rpm, and then the sediment is examined under high power. Each leukocyte seen represents about 5 to 10 cells/mm^3 of urine; 10 to 50 white cells/mm^3 are considered the upper limit of normal.[196] With this criterion, 5 to 10 leukocytes per high-power field in the sediment from a clean-catch midstream urine specimen is the upper limit of normal, as they represent 50 to 100 cells/mm^3. Although more elaborate and precise methods for determining the urinary concentration of leukocytes have been evaluated, it is generally not necessary to use these clinically.[196] It should be emphasized that the finding of pyuria is nonspecific, and patients with and without pyuria may or may not have infection.[197] However, the vast majority of patients with symptomatic infection have pyuria.[198] Using a broader definition of pyuria (at least 10 leukocytes/mm^3 of midstream urine by counting chamber), the vast majority of patients with either symptomatic or asymptomatic bacteriuria have pyuria. In fact, most have hundreds of leukocytes per cubic millimeter. However, pyuria without infection remains common.[199]

The dipstick leukocyte esterase test is a rapid screening test for detecting pyuria. It is both sensitive (75 to 96%) and specific (94 to 98%) for detecting more than 10 white blood cells/mm^3 of urine.[200–203] However, the leukocyte esterase test may not be reliable in daily practice. Hence, patients with a negative leukocyte esterase test and urinary tract infection symptoms should have a urine microscopic examination for pyuria or a urine culture.[202]

Microscopic or sometimes gross hematuria is occasionally seen in patients with urinary tract infection (i.e., hemorrhagic cystitis). However, red blood cells may be indicative of other disorders such as calculi, tumor, vasculitis, glomerulonephritis, and renal tuberculosis. White cell casts in the presence of an acute infectious process are strong evidence for pyelonephritis, but the absence of white cell casts does not rule out upper tract infection. White cell casts can also be seen in renal disease in the absence of infection.

Proteinuria is a common although not universal finding in urinary tract infection. Most patients with urinary tract infection excrete less than 2 g of protein in 24 hours; excretion of 3 g or more suggests glomerular disease.

One of the most useful tests for the presumptive diagnosis of urinary tract infection is the microscopic examination of a specimen for bacteria. The ability to identify bacteria in the urine depends on whether the specimen has been centrifuged and on whether it has been stained with Gram or methylene blue stain (Table 62–3).[200, 204] Smaller numbers of bacteria can be detected microscopically in a stained than in an unstained specimen, and smaller numbers can be detected in centrifuged than in uncentrifuged urine. The presence of at least one bacterium per oil-immersion field in a midstream, clean-catch, Gram-stained, uncentrifuged urine correlates with 10^5 bacteria or more per milliliter of urine. As this titer is regarded to represent significant bacteriuria, Gram staining of an uncentrifuged specimen is an easy, rapid, and relatively reliable way to detect significant numbers of organisms. The absence of bacteria in several fields in a stained sedimented specimen indicates the probability of fewer than 10^4 bacteria/ml.

TABLE 62–3 Correlation of Methods of Direct Examination of Urine for Bacteria with Quantitative Cultures

	Unstained	Stained
Uncentrifuged	$\geq 10^6$ ($\times 400$)	$\geq 10^5$ ($\times 1000$)
Centrifuged	$\geq 10^5$ ($\times 400$)	$\geq 10^4$ ($\times 1000$)

A number of rapid indirect methods have been devised to detect bacteriuria for presumptive diagnosis. Most common are tests that detect the presence of urine nitrite that is formed when bacteria reduce the nitrate that is normally present.[200–203] False-negative tests are common, especially in the detection of low-count bacteriuria (10^2 to 10^3/ml and with certain bacterial species) but false-positive results are unusual. Automated rapid screening tests have become available that may be cost-effective for processing large numbers of samples.[200]

Diagnosis of Urinary Tract Infection by Culture

General

Urine in the bladder is normally sterile. Since the urethra and periurethral areas are very difficult to sterilize, even the most carefully collected specimens (including those obtained by catheterization) are frequently contaminated. By quantitating bacteria in midstream, clean-voided urine, it is possible statistically to separate contamination from urinary tract infection. Patients with infection usually have at least 10^5 bacteria/ml in urine in the bladder, and therefore voided urine usually contains at least 10^5 bacteria/ml.[19] Patients without infection have sterile bladder urine, and with proper collection, voided urine usually contains less than 10^4 bacteria/ml. However, it is important to remember that about one third of young women with symptomatic lower tract infection have fewer than 10^5 bacteria/ml of urine (see "Urinary Tract Infection with Low Numbers of Organisms"). It is likely that a significant proportion of other patients with both symptomatic and asymptomatic infection have fewer than 10^5 bacteria/ml of urine. The Infectious Diseases Society of America consensus definition of cystitis for use in antibiotic treatment studies is 10^3 CFU/ml or more (sensitivity 80% and specificity 90%) and for pyelonephritis 10^4 CFU/ml or more (sensitivity 90% and specificity 95%).[205] These concentrations of microorganisms can be identified by standard microbiologic techniques in most clinical laboratories.

Calibrated loops serve as a simple inexpensive way to examine quantitatively the bacteriologic characteristics of urine specimens.[168] Platinum loops that deliver 0.01 ml and 0.001 ml are used to streak urine onto agar plates. After incubation at 37°C for 24 hours, the number of colony-forming units is counted, and the total number of organisms originally present in the specimen is estimated by multiplying the colony count by 10^2 or 10^3, respectively. A further refinement of the technique involves the use of differential agars to allow isolation from mixed cultures and more rapid identification.

The dip inoculum method in which an agar-coated glass slide is dipped into urine has an excellent correlation with calibrated-loop techniques and is available for office use at inexpensive prices.[206]

Acceptable methods for urine collection include (1) midstream clean catch, (2) catheterization, and (3) suprapubic aspiration. The clean-catch method is preferred for the routine collection of urine for culture. It avoids the risk of infection inherent in catheterization. The patient must be instructed in the proper technique of obtaining the urine; this is especially important in women. The woman should wash her hands, straddle the commode (facing the back of the commode), wash the vulva from front to back four times with four different sterile gauze pads soaked in green soap or another appropriate cleansing agent, and then rinse with two more sponges soaked in sterile distilled water. She should then spread the labia and void, discarding the first portion of urine and collecting the second. The urine should be processed immediately, or if refrigerated at 4°C, it can be cultured within 24 hours. In men the prepuce should be retracted, and thereafter the technique is similar. In infants and small children, sterile bags have been used for the collection of urine, but contamination is common.[159, 206]

In patients unable to cooperate, such as those with an altered sensorium, or those who are unable to void for neurologic or urologic reasons, catheterization may be necessary. When catheterization is performed, scrupulous aseptic technique should be observed.

The suprapubic aspiration method has been established as a safe technique in premature infants, neonates, children, adults, and even pregnant patients[9, 159, 185, 206] but is rarely used. With this method the bladder must be full. The patient refrains from voiding until the bladder can be percussed above the symphysis pubis, and suprapubic pressure causes the urge to void. After preparation of the skin, the bladder is then punctured above the symphysis pubis with a 22-gauge needle on a syringe (local anesthesia is not required). After the procedure, self-limited hematuria may be observed. Suprapubic aspiration may be indicated in special clinical situations such as in pediatric practice when urine is difficult to obtain. Another situation is the rare adult in whom infection is suspected, results obtained from more routine procedures have been confusing or equivocal, and diagnosis is critical.

If there are more than 10^5 bacteria/ml in a clean-catch urine specimen from an asymptomatic woman, there is an 80% probability that this represents true bacteriuria. If two different specimens demonstrate at least 10^5 of the same bacterium per milliliter, the probability increases to 95%. Thus two clean-catch specimens should be obtained in an asymptomatic woman to confirm the diagnosis. When the number of bacteria per milliliter is between 10^4 and 10^5 in an asymptomatic woman, a confirmatory second specimen will contain 10^5 or more bacteria/ml in only 5% of instances. Thus in asymptomatic women, 95% of the time 10^4 to 10^5 bacteria/ml represents contamination, with occasional infection manifested by fewer than 10^5 bacteria/ml of urine. In men, in whom contamination is less likely, 10^3 or more organisms/ml is suggestive of infection.[207] False-positive cultures are caused by contamination or incubation of urine before processing. False-negative cultures may be due to the use of antimicrobial agents, soap from the preparation falling into the urine, total obstruction below the infection, infection with a fastidious organism, renal tuberculosis, and diuresis.

These criteria apply only to the Enterobacteriaceae. Gram-positive organisms, fungi, and bacteria with fastidious growth requirements may not reach titers of 10^5/ml in patients with infection and may be in the 10^4 to 10^5/ml range. The organism recovered often helps to distinguish contamination from true bacteriuria. Samples with counts of less than 10^4 organisms/ml often contain saprophytic skin organisms such as diphtheroids, *Neisseria,* and staphylococci. Pure growth of Enterobacteriaceae is uncommonly found in low-titer specimens but is present in over 90% of the urine samples containing more than 10^5 bacteria/ml. High colony counts containing more than one species of bacteria from urine of asymptomatic persons often represent contamination but may be more significant in the presence of symptoms. Mixed infection occurs in about 5% of cases.

In patients with symptoms of urinary tract infection, one titer of 10^5 or more bacteria/ml of urine carries a 95% probability of true bacteriuria. With titers below 10^5/ml but in the presence of frequency, urgency, and dysuria, women have a 33% chance of having bacterial infection (see "Urinary Tract Infection with Low Numbers of Organisms"). The presence of low numbers of Enterobacteriaceae (i.e., 10^2 to 10^5/ml) in such women correlates highly with infection. The presence of fewer than 10^2/ml Enterobacteriaceae is evidence against urinary tract infection.

Samples obtained by catheterization from noninfected patients are less likely to become contaminated enough to demonstrate 10^5 bacteria/ml. For example, in an asymptomatic patient, one catheterized specimen that contains 10^5 or more organisms/ml has a 95% chance of indicating infection, and counts between 10^4 and 10^5/ml (which are uncommon) are significant at least 50% of the time. The contamination is presumably from the urethra. Bladder urine obtained by suprapubic aspiration is either sterile or contains significant growth even if bacterial numbers are below 10^5/ml. The practice of forcing fluids before the procedure tends to reduce numbers of organisms.[208] In fact, almost 50% of suprapubic aspirates from infected patients contain fewer than 10^5 organisms/ml. However, small numbers of bacteria may be found in aspirated urine from presumably noninfected persons.[7] This suggests that bladder urine may be occasionally contaminated from the urethra.

Urinary Tract Infection with Low Numbers of Organisms

Most women with an acute onset of frequency, urgency, or dysuria, or all of these, have urinary tract infection with 10^5 or more bacteria/ml of urine (Fig. 62–6). However, up to half are found to have fewer than 10^5 bacteria/ml of urine, and the term *urethral syndrome* has been used to refer to this entity. Stamm and associates have demonstrated that many of these women have urinary tract infection but with low numbers of organisms.[209–212] Using suprapubic bladder aspirates compared with voided midstream urine in acutely dysuric women, they found that 10^2 or more coliforms/ml in midstream urine had a sensitivity and specificity of 95 and 85%, respectively for urinary tract infection. These women have urinary infections mainly restricted to the lower tract. Furthermore, about one fourth of young women with symptomatic infection localized to the lower urinary tract have fewer than 10^5/ml bacteria in urine. Pyuria (defined as eight or more leukocytes/mm^3 of uncentrifuged urine) is found in these patients, with bacteria in the bladder but fewer than 10^5/ml in voided urine.

Kunin and colleagues, in a study of women coming to a university health clinic for any reason, demonstrated that stepwise increases in bacterial counts from 10^2 to 10^5 CFU/ml were significantly associated with an increased incidence of symptoms and pyuria. They postulated that low-count bacteriuria represents an early phase of urinary infection.[213] This hypothesis appears to have been supported in a clinical study in which 21 women with low-count bacteriuria (10^2 to less than 10^5 CFU/ml) had therapy delayed for 2 days, and reculture showed that 10 of 21 (48%) developed concentrations of or more 10^5 CFU/ml.[214]

The remaining patients with the urethral syndrome (after excluding those with bacteria in the bladder and those with genital herpes infection or vaginitis) can be divided into two groups: (1) those with sterile pyuria from urethritis due to *Chlamydia trachomatis* and less frequently *Neisseria gonorrhoeae* infection and (2) those without pyuria in whom all cultures are negative. The pathogenesis of this symptom complex is unknown, but *U. urealyticum* as well as noninfectious factors (traumatic, psychologic, allergic, and chemical) have been suggested as causes. Patients with *C. trachomatis* and *N. gonorrhoeae* urethritis respond to antimicrobial therapy. Komaroff and coworkers reported that vaginitis is a common cause of dysuria, and, accordingly, patients should be questioned regarding vaginal symptoms, particularly if the complaint of burning is external, such as pain felt in the inflamed labia during micturition.[215] If vaginitis is suspected, a pelvic examination should be performed. Dysuria has also been described in 10% of women with initial genital herpes infection.[216]

Although symptoms and the clinical settings cannot reliably distinguish between causes of frequency, urgency, and dysuria, they can be suggestive. Bacterial urinary tract infections tend to have a sudden onset of symptoms; suprapubic pain and hematuria may be present. Clinical clues to chlamydial infection include a patient with a gradual onset of internal dysuria; a sexually active patient with a recent new sexual partner; and a patient with no hematuria. The diagnosis of urethral chlamydial infection is confirmed by ligase chain reaction in the urine.[217] The findings of pyuria, fewer than 10^5/ml bacteria in urine, a negative gonococcal culture, and a negative pelvic examination in a sexually active woman with frequency and dysuria should suggest consideration of azithromycin or doxycycline therapy for *C. trachomatis* urethritis. Doxycycline would also constitute adequate therapy for the other major possibility—urinary tract infection with fewer than 10^5/ml bacteria in urine.

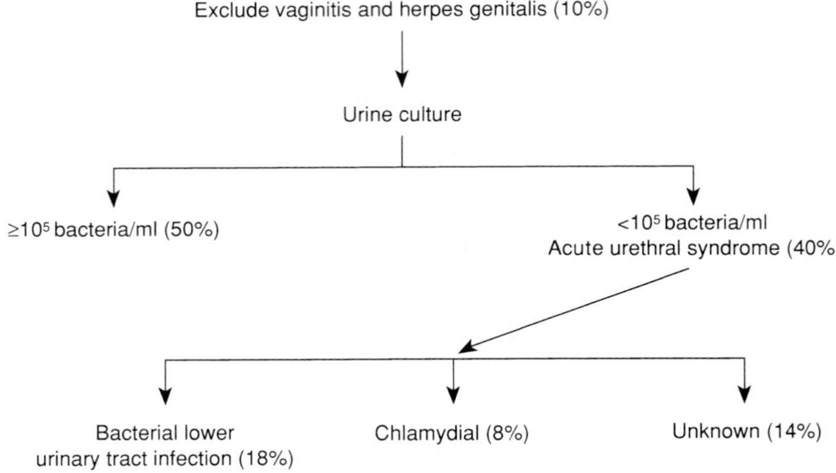

FIGURE 62–6. Relative frequencies of causes of acute onset of frequency or dysuria or both, in young women. (Adapted from data published in Stamm WE, Wagner KF, Amsel R, et al. Causes of acute urethral syndrome in women. N Engl J Med. 1980;303:409–415.)

Localization of Site of Infection

Localization of the site of infection to the kidney versus the bladder is not important in any given patient but has been useful in understanding the epidemiology and response to therapy of urinary tract infection.

Direct ureteral catheterization with quantitative cultures is an accurate but invasive method of localization.[218] The Fairley bladder-washout technique, which involves bladder catheterization,[219] is less invasive and less accurate.[220] Many other techniques such as measuring the urinary concentrating ability, urinary levels of various enzymes, urinary β_2-microglobulin levels, and serum antibody levels have been evaluated but are not reliable.[203, 221–225]

The antibody-coated bacteria test, which has been used for years to localize infection in treatment studies, has fallen out of favor because of concerns about its reliability.[226–233]

The outcome of therapy can also be used in a crude but useful manner to separate those with upper and lower tract infection. Virtually all patients with infection restricted to the lower tract can be cured with a short course of antimicrobial therapy.[234] However, the relapse rate with upper tract infection is appreciable, even with 7 to 10 days of therapy.

NATURAL HISTORY OF URINARY TRACT INFECTION

Children

In general, children with urinary tract infections without obstruction or vesicoureteral reflux have a very good prognosis.[158, 161, 162, 164, 235] In the presence of obstruction (e.g., urethral valves), severe destruction of renal parenchyma can occur.

Reflux is found in 30 to 50% of the children with asymptomatic or symptomatic bacteriuria (see Fig. 62–5).[158, 161, 164] Reflux can be caused by obstruction with increased pressure in the bladder, delayed development of the ureterovesical junction, a short intravesical ureter, or inflammation of the vesicoureteral junction, or all of these. Reflux in the presence of infection is associated with the development of scarring detected by intravenous pyelography.[164, 165, 206] Infants and young children (preschool age group) are at the highest risk for the development of progressive renal scarring.[158, 164, 165] These children frequently have severe degrees of reflux with repeated infections, and some develop end-stage renal disease and hypertension. Obstruction (most commonly in infant boys with congenital anomalies) is likely to be associated with marked reflux.

It should be emphasized that the contribution of reflux alone compared with reflux plus infection in the progression of renal scarring has not been clearly delineated. Reflux alone can apparently lead to renal damage and insufficiency.[236–238] Studies in uninfected animals[239] have demonstrated that reflux alone and in particular *intrarenal reflux* can produce "pyelonephritic" scars. It has also been shown that the immature kidneys of infants are more prone to intrarenal reflux.[240] The term *reflux nephropathy,* infected or uninfected, has been suggested to emphasize the primary role of reflux in scarring. However, it is probable that reflux is more likely to lead to severe damage and scarring when infection is also present.[239] It is also clear that infection tends to produce reflux or at least to make it more severe.

After the age of 5 years, children (predominantly girls) with bacteriuria frequently have renal scars presumably acquired during the preschool years. Many of these children also have reflux. Reflux tends to decrease with the elimination of bacteriuria. In addition, mild to moderate degrees of reflux are likely to disappear with the passage of time, probably in relation to maturation of the vesicoureteral junction.[241] Progression of scar already present or the development of new ones is uncommon after the age of 5 years.[241, 242] In fact, some investigators have questioned the need for detecting and treating bacteriuria in school-aged children (or, for that matter, in any asymptomatic children including infants).[162, 243] Furthermore, screening of children for asymptomatic bacteriuria is not cost-effective.[243] However, it is clear that progression does occur in some of these children, especially in the presence of severe reflux.[241]

Adults

Urinary tract infections are much more common in women than in men. Many of these patients previously had urinary tract infections as children and continue to have infections as adults.[162, 242] Once a woman develops infection, she is more likely to develop subsequent infections than a patient who has had no previous infections.

The courses of women with symptomatic recurrent urinary tract infections were described by Kraft and Stamey.[244] However, it was not defined whether these recurrences were reinfections or relapses. Twenty-three patients were followed over a total of 800 months, and each episode of urinary tract infection was treated. The overall attack rate was about 0.2 infections per month. Even in these women (i.e., those with recurrent urinary tract infections), significant bacteriuria (i.e., 10^5 or greater bacteria/ml urine) was present in only 70% of symptomatic episodes. Infections tended to occur in clusters with an increased attack rate of 0.5% per month. These periods of more frequent infection were followed by a remission or infection-free interval that averaged about 13 months. However, most remissions were followed by further clusters of infection. Thus, in many women it is more correct to use the term *remission* rather than *cure* of urinary tract infection. It may be a simple matter to cure an individual episode, but recurrence, most often reinfection, is common.

It is clear that urinary tract infection in adults can lead to progressive renal damage in the presence of obstruction. However, recurrent infection in adults in the absence of obstruction rarely, if ever, leads to renal failure.[169]

Autopsy studies have shown that it is difficult to implicate infection per se (i.e., in the absence of other renal abnormalities) as an important pathogenic factor in the production of severe renal disease in adults.[242] One exception might be severe papillary necrosis secondary to infection. In fact, one group of investigators was unable to find any case of uncomplicated pyelonephritis that progressed to end-stage renal disease among 173 patients admitted to dialysis programs.[245] In prospective studies, hundreds of patients with persistent or recurrent infections have been followed for years without documenting the progression of renal disease from infection alone.[162, 168, 246–250]

The role of infection in the progression of clinically or radiographically diagnosed interstitial renal disease has also been examined.[169, 251, 252] In general, these studies indicate that infection is rarely, if ever, the major factor leading to further renal decompensation. However, infection may occasionally accelerate the progression of the primary underlying disease process.[251] In summary, except for perhaps rare instances, there is no evidence to indicate that uncomplicated urinary tract infection alone produces renal failure in adults.

Some studies had demonstrated decreased survival among elderly people with bacteriuria.[253, 254] However, more recent studies have not confirmed this association.[254, 255] At present, it seems unlikely that asymptomatic bacteriuria in elderly persons has any deleterious effects. Furthermore, there is no evidence to suggest that treatment of asymptomatic bacteriuria in elderly patients has any beneficial effects.[256] Therefore, routine treatment of asymptomatic bacteriuria in elderly patients is not advocated by most experts.

Hypertension

It is clear that severe renal disease may cause hypertension. The entity of chronic interstitial renal disease (not necessarily related to infection) has also been related to hypertension.[252] It has been suggested that patients with bacteriuria in the absence of other renal disease are more likely to have hypertension, but the data have not shown a clear-cut relationship. No definite cause-and-effect relationships have been documented.

MANAGEMENT OF URINARY TRACT INFECTION

General Considerations

Ideally, antimicrobial agents should only be administered when there is reasonable evidence of infection in the urinary tract. Symptoms are not a reliable indication of infection. The diagnosis of infection in the asymptomatic patient should be made on no fewer than two cultures of clean-voided, midstream urine in which the same microorganism is present in significant titers. If the patient is symptomatic, one specimen suffices, and therapy should be started.

There has been much controversy about how vigorously chemotherapy should be pursued. A rational approach to the treatment of urinary tract infection depends on an appreciation of the prognosis of the untreated infection and the long-term results to be expected from therapy. The side effects, cost, and inconvenience of different therapeutic regimens must also be considered. As the prognosis of urinary tract infection in nonpregnant adult women seems to be quite good and reinfection is common, therapy probably makes little contribution to the patient's well-being other than eradicating symptoms.

Although bacteriuria in the elderly population is associated with degenerative and debilitating diseases and in some reports with mortality, there is no convincing evidence for a cause-and-effect relationship.[177, 254, 256, 257] There certainly is no evidence that treatment of the urinary tract infection alters the patient's course. Urinary tract infection serves as a marker for debilitating diseases, which in turn may contribute to mortality. In addition, urinary tract infection is very common in the elderly population, and many of these patients become reinfected or relapse after antimicrobial therapy. Furthermore, a higher frequency of side effects from chemotherapy would be expected in an older age group because of preexisting renal, auditory, and other diseases. Considering the large numbers of patients involved, intensive antimicrobial therapy may lead to an unwarranted financial burden and the danger of drug toxicity and thus may do more harm than good in elderly patients.

In contrast, bacteriuria in preschool children with vesicoureteral reflux (especially if congenital anomalies are present) can result in stunted growth of the kidney, scar formation, and, rarely, renal failure. Bacteriuria in pregnancy may also have serious implications. Treatment of children and pregnant women is most likely to be beneficial. Furthermore, it is feasible to treat all these patients since the prevalence of bacteriuria is relatively low in these groups.

Hospitalized patients with bacteriuria have higher mortality rates than those without bacteriuria.[258, 259] This observation may be related to deaths from bacteremia in patients with indwelling urinary catheters.

It is usually necessary to treat all symptomatic patients regardless of age, even when infection is likely to recur. Some patients have such frequent symptomatic episodes (either relapses or reinfections) that they are almost chronically incapacitated. In these patients, it may be necessary to give prolonged therapy or prophylaxis to prevent recurrent symptoms.

Nonspecific Therapy

Hydration

Forcing fluids has been advocated in the therapy of urinary tract infection. There is some theoretical support for this method of treatment. Hydration produces rapid dilution of the bacteria and removal of infected urine by frequent bladder emptying, which in the presence of minimal residual volume may offset the logarithmic growth of gram-negative bacilli. Forcing fluids usually results in a rapid reduction of bacterial counts. Permanent loss of bacteriuria has been reported in a few patients with rapid hydration, but in most patients bacterial counts return to the original levels when hydration is stopped (e.g., overnight when the urine flow rate and frequency of micturition are reduced).[260]

Medullary hypertonicity tends to inhibit leukocyte migration into the renal medulla, and the high concentration of ammonia tends to inactivate complement.[75, 76] Abolition of medullary hypertonicity by diuresis would be expected to reverse these effects. In addition, a reduction in bacterial counts in the urine by hydration would enhance the effect of factors otherwise overwhelmed by large numbers of bacteria (e.g., bladder mucosal defenses or the effect of relatively low concentrations of antimicrobial drugs).

Hydration may also have some disadvantages. Increased fluid intake could theoretically result in increased vesicoureteral reflux and possibly cause acute urinary retention in the partially obstructed bladder. The larger urine output results in dilution of antibacterial substances normally present in the urine as well as lower urinary concentrations of antimicrobial agents. Water diuresis also decreases urinary acidification, which enhances the antibacterial activity of urine and certain antimicrobial agents.

As there is no evidence that hydration improves the results of appropriate antimicrobial therapy, and because continuous hydration is inconvenient, we are not in favor of this approach.

Urinary pH

The antibacterial activity of urine results mainly from a high urea concentration and osmolality and is pH-dependent, being greater at a lower pH.[79] The pH-dependent activity may be related to a high concentration of various weakly ionizable organic acids, such as hippuric and β-hydroxybutyric acids.[261] The antibacterial activity of these organic acids is related to the concentration of the undissociated molecule, which probably penetrates better than the ionized form into the bacterial cell. As these organic acids have a relatively low pK_a (the pH at which 50% of the molecules are undissociated), the lower the urinary pH, the greater the concentration of undissociated molecules and the greater the antibacterial activity of the organic acid.

Hippuric acid is a common constituent of urine, being the glycine conjugate of dietary benzoic acid, and is bacteriostatic in proportion to the concentration of undissociated molecules. The production of antibacterial activity in urine by the ingestion of large volumes of cranberry juice (if the urinary pH level is kept low) results from the appearance in the urine of high concentrations of hippuric acid derived from precursors in the berry. The successful use of mandelic acid, another organic acid, is also dependent on the maintenance of a low urinary pH level.

The urinary pH level affects the antibacterial activity of many chemotherapeutic agents used in the treatment of urinary tract infections. The activity of methenamine results from the release of formaldehyde as the urinary pH level is decreased below 5.5. Clinically, methenamine is used in the form of its mandelic acid salt (methenamine mandelate) or its hippuric acid salt (methenamine hippurate). The antibacterial activity of these salts is related to the formation of the un-ionized organic acid and formaldehyde, which is highly dependent on the maintenance of a urinary pH of 5.5 or less. The effectiveness of nitrofurantoin (pK_a 7.2) is also greater at a low urinary pH level. In contrast, the aminoglycoside antibiotics such as gentamicin, tobramycin, and amikacin are more effective in alkaline urine.

Although different antimicrobial agents have maximal effectiveness at different pH levels, most agents exhibit adequate antibacterial activity at usual urinary pH levels. The maintenance of urine at the low pH level required for effective antibacterial activity of organic acids and methenamine can be accomplished by the administration of ascorbic acid or methionine. Acidification of the urine can result in precipitation of urate stones, and, since oxalate is a metabolite of ascorbic acid, large doses of ascorbic acid can cause the formation of oxalate stones.

To acidify the urine, it is often necessary to modify the diet by restriction of agents that tend to alkalinize the urine, for example, milk, fruit juices (except cranberry juice), and sodium bicarbonate. Another major problem with acidification is that patients with renal insufficiency are unable to excrete an acid load and may become systemically acidotic when urinary acidification is attempted. It may be impossible to acidify urine infected with urea-splitting organisms such as *Proteus* spp. because of the production of ammonia from urea. Acidification for long-term antimicrobial therapy should only be used with the concomitant use of organic acids or methenamine. Urinary acidification is frequently difficult to achieve[262] and is rarely if ever necessary.

Analgesics

Urinary analgesics such as phenazopyridine hydrochloride (Pyridium) have little place in the routine management of symptomatic infections. The dysuria of urinary tract infection usually responds rapidly to antibacterial therapy and requires no local analgesia. If flank pain or dysuria is severe, systemic analgesics can be used. Analgesics such as phenazopyridine hydrochloride may be useful in the management of certain patients with dysuria but without infection.

Principles of Antimicrobial Therapy

The selection of an appropriate antimicrobial agent has become complex because of the increasing number of compounds available, each with its characteristic spectrum and toxic properties. However, in most cases, any of many available agents are perfectly satisfactory. Given two or more drugs with equivalent activity against the infecting microorganism, the agent with the least toxicity should be chosen.

There is no evidence to support any superiority of bactericidal drugs over bacteriostatic agents in urinary tract infection. However, there may be theoretical reasons for using bactericidal drugs in the treatment of relapsing urinary tract infection.

Serum, Tissue, and Urine Concentrations of Antimicrobial Agents

A poor correlation exists between the response of bacteriuria and blood levels of antimicrobial agents.[263–265] In the dosages commonly used for urinary tract infection, many oral antimicrobial agents do not achieve serum levels above the minimal inhibitory concentration for most urinary pathogens.

The disappearance of bacteriuria is closely correlated with the sensitivity of the microorganism to the concentration of the antimicrobial agent achieved in the urine.[263–265] Inhibitory urinary concentrations are achieved after oral administration of essentially all commonly used antimicrobial agents. Although blood levels do not seem to be important in the treatment of urinary tract infection, they may be critical in patients with bacteremia and may be important in the cure of patients with renal parenchymal infection who relapse.

In patients with renal insufficiency, dosage modifications are necessary for agents that are excreted primarily by the kidneys and cannot be cleared by any other mechanism. In renal failure, the kidney may not be able to concentrate an antimicrobial agent in the urine, and difficulty in eradicating bacteriuria may occur. This may be an important factor in the failure of therapy for urinary tract infection with aminoglycosides.

In addition, high concentrations of magnesium and calcium as well as a low pH level can raise the minimal inhibitory concentration of aminoglycosides for gram-negative bacilli to levels above those achievable in the urine of patients with renal failure.[266] In general, the penicillins and cephalosporins attain adequate urine concentrations despite severely impaired renal function and are the agents of choice in renal insufficiency.[267]

Response to Therapy

The objective of antimicrobial therapy is to eliminate bacteria from the urinary tract. Symptoms usually abate spontaneously without chemotherapy, even though bacteriuria may persist. Therefore, the results of therapy can only be determined by follow-up urine cultures.

There are four patterns of response of bacteriuria to antimicrobial therapy: cure, persistence, relapse, and reinfection. Quantitative bacterial counts in urine should decrease within 48 hours after the initiation of an antimicrobial agent to which the microorganism is sensitive in vitro. If titers do not decrease within this time, the therapy being given will almost invariably be unsuccessful.

Cure is defined as negative urine cultures on chemotherapy and during the follow-up period (usually 1 to 2 weeks). However, it must be understood that many of these patients will develop reinfection at a later time.

Persistence has been used in two ways to describe a response to therapy: (1) persistence of significant bacteriuria after 48 hours of treatment and (2) persistence of the infecting organism in low numbers in urine after 48 hours. Significant bacteriuria usually persists only if the urinary levels of the antimicrobial agent are below the concentration of the drug needed to inhibit the microorganism. This can occur when the infecting strain is resistant to the urinary levels usually attained (i.e., a resistant organism) or because the urinary levels of the drug are inordinately low (i.e., from not taking the agent, insufficient dosage, poor intestinal absorption, or poor renal excretion as in renal insufficiency). Persistence of the infecting microorganism in low titers in voided urine may mean persistence in the urinary tract or contamination from the urethra or vagina. Bladder-puncture cultures would be needed to evaluate the significance of low titers of bacteria obtained when the patient is receiving therapy, and this procedure is rarely indicated. Bacteria may persist within the urinary tract during therapy without excretion of organisms in the urine. Sites of persistence within the urinary tract are the renal parenchyma, the renal calculi, and the prostate. The simplest way of determining the significance of persistence of the organism in low titers in the urine is to obtain follow-up urine cultures after therapy has been stopped. Prompt relapse of significant bacteriuria usually follows persistence of the organism in the urinary tract.

Relapse usually occurs within 1 to 2 weeks after the cessation of chemotherapy and is often associated with renal infection, with structural abnormalities of the urinary tract, or with chronic bacterial prostatitis. Relapse indicates that the infecting microorganism has persisted in the urinary tract during therapy. However, an apparent relapse can be related to reinfection (new infection) with the same microorganism. In spite of eradication from the urinary tract, the original infecting organism may still be present in the intestine, vagina, or external urethra and then may cause a new infection. Markedly delayed relapses (more than 1 month after stopping therapy) are much more likely due to this phenomenon or to chronic bacterial prostatitis than to true relapse. Relapses occurring within 1 to 2 weeks are usually true relapses. Cell wall–deficient forms of bacteria have been postulated to play a role in relapse, but there is little evidence to support this theory.[153]

After initial sterilization of the urine, *reinfection* may occur during the administration of chemotherapy (also called *superinfection*) or at any time thereafter. Reinfection is easy to identify when there is a change in bacterial species. However, there may be reinfection with a different serotype of the same species (usually *E. coli*) or even the same serotype.

Classification and Antimicrobial Therapy for Different Groups

Acute Pyelonephritis

Patients who are severely ill with pyelonephritis should be hospitalized. Although mild to moderate illness responds well to orally administered antimicrobial agents, nausea and vomiting may preclude oral treatment, necessitating parenteral therapy. The patient who is reliable, compliant, and tolerates oral therapy may be treated with a variety of oral antimicrobial agents. At the time of antibiotic selection, a Gram stain of the urine should have indicated the morphology of the infecting organism (e.g., gram-negative bacillus, gram-positive coccus), but the precise identity and antimicrobial susceptibility are usually unknown. Therefore, the selection of antimicrobial therapy is usually empirical. When gram-positive cocci in chains are seen on Gram stain, ampicillin or amoxicillin is probably the agent of choice. When staphylococci are implicated on Gram stain, cephalosporins (such as cephalexin) are appropriate agents.

Although ampicillin and amoxicillin have been mainstays of oral therapy for gram-negative bacillus infection for many years, these agents can no longer be recommended as reliable agents, since 25 to 35% of *E. coli* are now resistant.[268, 269] Accordingly, oral antimicrobial agents currently advocated for gram-negative bacillus urinary infection include trimethoprim, trimethoprim-sulfamethoxazole, cephalexin, amoxicillin-clavulanic acid, and the fluoroquinolones (e.g., norfloxacin and ciprofloxacin). The doses are listed under "Lower Urinary Tract Infection." A caveat is that resistance of *E. coli* to first-generation cephalosporins is increasing and approaching that of amoxicillin, and resistance to trimethoprim-sulfamethoxazole is approaching 20%, and if resistance continues to rise trimethoprim-sulfamethoxazole will no longer be the agent of choice as initial empirical therapy for acute pyelonephritis.[269, 270] There is increasing evidence that cell wall–active agents (e.g., penicillins and cephalosporins) are not as effective in eradicating infection in the kidneys, or for that matter anywhere in the urinary tract, as trimethoprim-sulfamethoxazole, quinolones, or aminoglycosides.[269–271] In all patients with symptoms of upper tract infection, therapy should be preceded by culture of a clean-catch midstream urine sample.

In hospitalized patients, particularly those with suspected gram-negative bacillary bacteremia complicating pyelonephritis (high fever, shaking chills, hypotension), parenteral therapy should be used and is directed at the life-threatening bacteremia. In these seriously ill patients, the spectrum of antibacterial activity of the initial agents should include all potential pathogens. In seriously ill patients with community-acquired acute pyelonephritis, when the Gram stain reveals gram-negative bacilli, empirical therapy includes a wide selection of antimicrobial agents: aminoglycosides (such as gentamicin, 3 to 5 mg/kg/day); aztreonam, 3 to 6 g/day; ureidopenicillins (mezlocillin or piperacillin, 18 g/day); the ampicillin-sulbactam combination (as 12 g of ampicillin/day); the ticarcillin-clavulanic acid combination (as 18 g of ticarcillin/day); third-generation cephalosporins (e.g., cefotaxime or ceftriaxone); or a parenteral fluoroquinolone. In patients with hospital-acquired gram-negative bacillary infection, particularly in those seriously ill, the initial selection of antibiotics should not leave any hiatus in the spectrum of activity and should anticipate the possibility of resistant microorganisms. Under these circumstances ceftazidime (3 to 6 g/day), cefepime (2 to 4 g/day), ticarcillin-clavulanic acid (as 18 g of ticarcillin/day), aztreonam (3 to 6 g/day), imipenem (2 g/day), or meropenem (1.5 to 3 g/day), often used in combination with aminoglycosides or a parenteral fluoroquinolone, can be recommended. When the susceptibility pattern of the infecting organism is known, therapy can be altered to less expensive single-agent therapy, and oral treatment can be used once a response has occurred.

Effective therapy results in a marked decrease in bacterial titers in the urine within 48 hours after the onset of treatment. Antimicrobial agents are sometimes effective in vivo even when disk sensitivity tests indicate drug resistance, because most antimicrobials are excreted in the urine in concentrations much higher than those tested for by disk sensitivity testing.

If a bacteriologic response does not occur by 48 hours, there is no point in continuing the same regimen. Therapy is then changed to an alternative drug on the basis of susceptibility tests (e.g., from the initial isolate). The finding of continuing positive blood cultures or persistent high fever and toxicity past the first 3 days suggests the need for investigation to exclude urinary obstruction or intrarenal or perinephric abscess formation. Investigation should include renal ultrasonography, a computed tomography (CT) or magnetic resonance imaging scan, and, according to the findings, perhaps an intravenous pyelography (IVP) examination. The availability of sensitive noninvasive studies has resulted in early diagnosis of intrarenal or perinephric abscess formation that may respond to antibiotic therapy alone. In uncomplicated pyelonephritis after a clinical response and defervesence occur, oral therapy is initiated and should be continued to complete a course of 14 days of antimicrobial therapy.[272] When upper tract infection is complicated by abscesses, more prolonged therapy and perhaps drainage is indicated (see the later sections "Perinephric Abscess" and "Intrarenal Abscess"). Routine imaging studies are not indicated in women with acute uncomplicated pyelonephritis.[273] Follow-up urine cultures are mandatory within 1 to 2 weeks of completion of therapy in pregnant women, children, and patients with recurrent symptomatic pyelonephritis in whom suppressive maintenance therapy is being contemplated. In the majority of nonpregnant adults who remain asymptomatic, follow-up cultures are optional.

Renal infection is a special problem in adults with hereditary polycystic disease. Although parenchymal infections respond well to appropriate antibiotics, cyst infections frequently fail to improve and may require antibiotics that diffuse into these closed sites (e.g., trimethoprim-sulfamethoxazole[274] or a fluoroquinolone[269]) or surgical aspiration or drainage. Emphysematous pyelonephritis is most often seen in elderly female diabetic patients with chronic urinary infections and renal vascular disease (Fig. 62–7). Because of the extraordinarily high mortality rate of 70% in spite of appropriate antibiotics and supportive therapy, immediate nephrectomy is almost always indicated for this condition.[275–277]

Lower Urinary Tract Infection

Conventional Therapy. In the past, 7 to 10 days of therapy were routinely recommended for patients with lower tract symptoms. However, in recent years it has become apparent that most women with lower tract infection have only a superficial mucosal infection and can be cured with much shorter courses of therapy and in fact with only a single dose of an antimicrobial agent.

Short-Course Therapy. Single-dose therapy with certain agents achieves high urinary concentrations that are prolonged for at least 12 to 24 hours and eliminates infection when presumably confined to the bladder. The most widely used regimens have been oral doses of 3 g of amoxicillin or one to two double-strength tablets of trimethoprim-sulfamethoxazole.[278] Other regimens have included sulfonamides (e.g., 2 g of sulfisoxazole orally), aminoglycosides (e.g., 150 mg of netilmicin intramuscularly), 2 g of tetracycline orally, 400 mg of trimethoprim orally, 200 mg of nitrofurantoin orally, cephalosporins (e.g., 0.5 g of ceftriaxone intramuscularly), and fluoroquinolones (e.g., 800 mg of norfloxacin orally).[278–282] Cure rates have ranged from 65 to 100%.

The advantages of single-dose therapy include a lesser expense, assured compliance, fewer side effects, and perhaps less intensive selective pressure for the emergence of resistant organisms in gut, urinary, or vaginal flora. Possible deleterious effects include a poorer outcome of infections that are actually in the upper tract. Finally, it should not be assumed that every antibiotic administered as a single dose will be effective even with regard to susceptible organisms. Results depend on high sustained urinary concentrations of the antimicrobial agent. For example, a 2-g oral dose of cefaclor resulted in a 57% failure rate.[283] Before using single-dose therapy, certain factors should be evaluated, including the frequency of attacks, a poor response to single-dose therapy in the past, known structural abnormalities, a history of childhood infection, symptoms longer than 7 days, pyelonephritis during the past year, and diabetes mellitus. Any of these factors increases the likelihood of upper tract infection and might mitigate against using single-dose therapy.

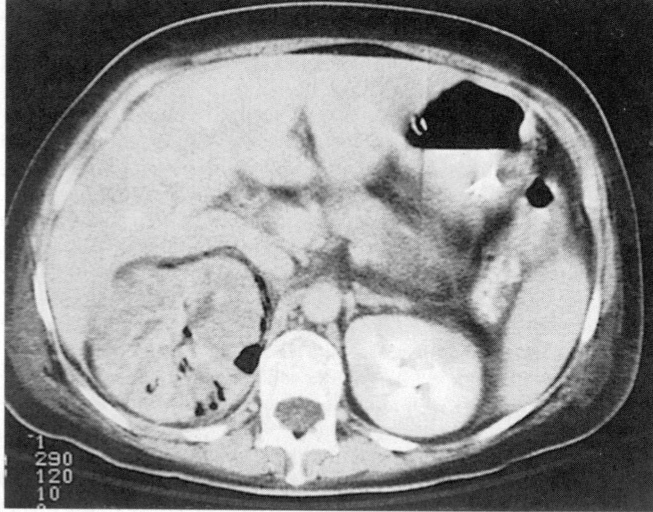

FIGURE 62–7. Emphysematous pyelonephritis in a patient with diabetes. The computed tomographic scan shows an enlarged, inflamed right kidney with air within the parenchyma and subcapsular space. (Courtesy of M. Bergeron, M.D.)

A by-product of single-dose therapy is that a failure to eradicate a urinary tract infection after a single dose of an agent may indicate a patient in whom further investigation should be considered. Response to single-dose therapy appears comparable with the antibody-coated bacteria test in localizing the site of infection.[234, 284]

Single-dose therapy gives basically 1 day of therapy with regard to antimicrobial activity in the urine. The same results should be achievable with 1 day of standard-dose antimicrobial therapy; however, the data to support this do not exist. Three reviews concluded that 3 days of therapy are superior to single-dose therapy.[278, 285, 286] It is our preference to use 3 days of therapy with standard doses. It seems clear that with either a single dose or 3 days of therapy, trimethoprim-sulfamethoxazole (and probably fluoroquinolones) are superior to β-lactam antibiotics in terms of both early (i.e., <2 weeks) and late (i.e., >2 weeks) follow-up.[268, 278, 279] Some of the preferred agents for 3 days of therapy are trimethoprim-sulfamethoxazole (one double-strength tablet twice a day), trimethoprim (100 mg twice a day), norfloxacin (400 mg twice a day), ciprofloxacin (500 mg twice a day), and other fluoroquinolones. Because of increased resistance of *E. coli* to trimethoprim-sulfamethoxazole, it may become less useful for this purpose.

We do not advocate the use of sulfonamides, ampicillin, or amoxicillin because of the relatively high frequency of *E. coli* resistant to these agents among community-acquired urinary tract infections.[268, 269]

The approach to the management of lower urinary tract infection has evolved to the point where short-course therapy should become the standard for most female patients with suspected lower tract infection. Some studies in pediatric populations have shown similarly good results, but others have not.[159] Short-course therapy has not been adequately evaluated in men and is not recommended at present. Short-course therapy is not appropriate for women who have a history of previous urinary infection caused by antibiotic-resistant organisms or more than 7 days of symptoms.[287] In these patients (who have an increased likelihood of upper tract infection) and in males, 7 to 10 days of therapy are recommended.

If symptoms do not respond or if they recur, a urine culture should be obtained. In pregnant women, children, and patients at high risk for renal damage who remain asymptomatic, follow-up cultures should be obtained 1 to 2 weeks after discontinuation of therapy to detect relapses.

Office Strategy for Frequency, Urgency, and Dysuria Syndrome

When a sexually active woman is first seen with frequency, urgency, and dysuria, urine culture is not mandatory, and the therapeutic decision is based on the clinical presentation and the presence or absence of pyuria. If pyuria (defined as at least 10 leukocytes/mm^3) is present, antimicrobial therapy is warranted for urinary tract infection. Dipstick methods of measuring pyuria are sufficiently accurate to be used. Short-course therapy is a reasonable first approach in women except in settings in which occult pyelonephritis is more likely, as described previously. An agent likely to be effective against most pathogens (e.g., trimethoprim, trimethoprim-sulfamethoxazole, amoxicillin-clavulanic acid, norfloxacin, ciprofloxacin) should be used. If a clinical response does not occur, a culture should be obtained (for the possibility of a resistant organism), and therapy should be changed and directed at *Chlamydia,* 100 mg of doxycycline twice a day for 7 days or azithromycin 1.0 g orally as a single dose.

In the nonsexually active female with symptoms of lower tract infection and pyuria, there is a high probability of urinary tract infection. A lack of response to therapy probably indicates a resistant organism and mandates a urine culture.

A symptomatic response followed by recurrence after therapy is discontinued indicates the probability of upper tract infection and the need for a culture and at least 2 weeks of therapy. Men and children should have a urine culture, and males should receive 7 to 10 days of treatment.

Asymptomatic Bacteriuria

Most patients with asymptomatic bacteriuria are women and are in the older age groups. Although cure may result after treatment, relapse and especially reinfection are common. The approach to asymptomatic bacteriuria depends on the age of the patient. In children, therapy should be given as described for symptomatic infection. A trial of short-course therapy is reasonable. In contrast, therapy for asymptomatic bacteriuria in the adult is by no means mandatory in the absence of obstruction except during pregnancy. Nonpregnant women can be treated providing that a nontoxic antimicrobial agent is used. If the infecting microorganism is resistant to all but toxic agents, then treatment should not be instituted in the nonobstructed patient.

Asymptomatic bacteriuria in elderly persons is a benign disease and need not be treated, especially since with vigorous treatment a great many people will be exposed to drug toxicity.

When dealing with asymptomatic bacteriuria, there is no urgency in treating. Therapy should be delayed until two cultures have been obtained for confirmation of the presence of bacteriuria. By that time, the identity and antimicrobial susceptibility pattern of the infecting organism will have been determined.

Relapsing Urinary Tract Infection

If the patient relapses after therapy for symptomatic urinary tract infection or for asymptomatic bacteriuria, the most likely possibilities are that the patient has (1) renal involvement, (2) a structural abnormality of the urinary tract (e.g., calculi), or (3) chronic bacterial prostatitis.

Relapses, especially in the absence of structural abnormalities, may be related to renal infection that may require a longer duration of therapy. Patients who relapse after a short course or 7 to 10 days of therapy should be considered for a 2-week course. Turck and colleagues[288] demonstrated that a 6-week course of therapy resulted in a higher cure rate than a 2-week course in patients who relapsed after 2 weeks of therapy.[288]

Structural abnormalities of the urinary tract predispose to relapse. Urinary tract infection in the presence of obstruction is likely to be associated with renal involvement, a tendency for renal functional impairment, and bacteremia. Obstructive lesions can be corrected surgically and should be sought in the evaluation of patients with relapsing infection. Calculi may be a cause of relapse of urinary tract infection. The ultimate success of chemotherapy is dependent on the removal of stones.

Some patients continue to relapse despite surgical correction of urologic abnormalities. In others, surgical correction may not be indicated or feasible, or no abnormalities may be found. In these patients who relapse after 2 weeks of chemotherapy, a repeat course of 2 weeks should be considered. After another relapse, a 4- to 6-week course should be considered. In men, chronic bacterial prostatitis should first be ruled out.

If relapse occurs after a 6-week course, therapy lasting 6 months or even longer may be considered. Only carefully selected patients, such as children, adults who have continuous symptoms, or adults who are at high risk of developing progressive renal damage (e.g., those with obstruction not amenable to surgery), should be considered for 4-week or longer courses of therapy. Asymptomatic adults without obstruction should not receive these longer courses. Some of the agents that can be used for long-term therapy are amoxicillin (250 mg three times a day), cephalexin, trimethoprim-sulfamethoxazole, trimethoprim, norfloxacin, and ciprofloxacin, in usual doses and nitrofurantoin in full dosage for 1 week and then half the usual dosage.

An antimicrobial agent being used for long-term therapy is continued only as long as significant bacteriuria is absent. If bacteriuria persists or relapses during chemotherapy (indicating that the infecting organism is now resistant to that agent), the agent is altered. The aim is to achieve continuous suppression of bacteriuria for the entire course of therapy. If relapse occurs after discontinuation of the antimicrobial agent, therapy is reinstituted with the same or another drug. If deemed necessary, this agent is administered for an additional 6 to 12 months (if bacteriuria remains suppressed). All patients are followed with urine cultures at least monthly while on therapy.

A creatinine clearance determination and imaging studies of the kidneys initially and yearly (or at least every 2 years) should be obtained on patients receiving long-term therapy to determine the glomerular filtration rate and structural changes in the kidneys. Blood counts, urinalyses, and liver chemistry tests (when indicated) are also obtained periodically as tests for drug toxicity.

Reinfection of the Urinary Tract

Patients with reinfection can generally be divided into two groups: (1) those who have relatively infrequent reinfections, perhaps only once every 2 or 3 years to several times a year; and (2) those who develop frequent reinfections. An extreme example of the latter group is patients who become reinfected during or shortly after each course of antimicrobial therapy. With infrequent reinfections, each episode can be approached with therapy as if it were a new episode of either symptomatic or asymptomatic infection. Short-course therapy should be used in women with lower tract symptoms. Women with reinfections associated with lower tract symptoms can be managed with self-administration of short-course therapy with the onset of symptoms.[289]

Many patients with frequent reinfections after therapy are middle-aged or elderly women in whom infection is limited to the lower urinary tract. Most asymptomatic reinfections in this group should not be treated, because the frequent use of antimicrobial agents in this group is apt to result in toxic side effects and because progressive destruction of the kidneys is rare. If, however, the episodes are symptomatic or if the likelihood of renal damage is increased, these patients should be treated.

Occasionally, patients of any age develop symptomatic reinfection so frequently that they can be incapacitated. In some women, these symptomatic reinfections are associated with sexual activity. Voiding immediately after intercourse may help prevent reinfection. However, single-dose prophylactic chemotherapy taken after sexual intercourse (e.g., a single-strength trimethoprim-sulfamethoxazole tablet or 100 mg of ciprofloxacin) is a more effective method of decreasing these episodes.[290–292]

In other patients with frequent symptomatic reinfections, no precipitating event is apparent; in these patients, when symptoms are severe, long-term chemoprophylaxis may be instituted. Although these courses seem to decrease the frequency of reinfections and symptoms in most patients, it is impossible to completely prevent reinfection in many patients. When reinfection occurs when the patient is receiving therapy, the prophylactic agent must be changed.

Long-term chemoprophylaxis should be considered for asymptomatic patients who reinfect frequently and are at risk of developing renal parenchymal damage with each reinfection (e.g., young children with vesicoureteral reflux and children and adults with obstructive uropathy). In these groups, keeping the patient abacteriuric helps to protect the kidneys. Several studies in patients with frequent reinfections indicate that such prolonged chemotherapy reduces the frequency of reinfections.

Long-term prophylactic antimicrobial agents have reduced the frequency of symptomatic infections of the urinary tract in older men, women, and children.[293–297] Before prophylaxis is initiated, the patient should receive a course of therapy with an appropriate antimicrobial agent. Trimethoprim-sulfamethoxazole, nitrofurantoin, or trimethoprim alone are particularly useful for long-term prophylaxis, because these drugs are inexpensive and are unlikely to allow the emergence of antimicrobial-resistant bacteria with prolonged use.[294–297]

Full antimicrobial dosage is not necessary for successful prophylaxis. One 50-mg capsule of nitrofurantoin or one half tablet of trimethoprim-sulfamethoxazole (40 mg of trimethoprim, 200 mg of sulfamethoxazole) nightly suffices. Fluoroquinolones and other agents have been used with good results.[268, 291, 298]

Patients receiving long-term prophylaxis should be followed with urine cultures monthly or more often if interim symptomatic episodes develop. Therapy is continued with the same agent as long as the patient remains abacteriuric. If bacteriuria persists or recurs during the administration of an antimicrobial agent, therapy is altered using the response of bacteriuria as a parameter of the adequacy of therapy. Long-term prophylaxis can be undertaken only if urine cultures are obtained periodically and therapy altered if bacteriuria recurs.

Another recent approach to preventing reinfections in postmenopausal women with frequent recurrent urinary tract infections is the use of oral or intravaginal estrogens. The use of estrogens in these women has resulted in a decrease in the number of episodes of urinary tract infection, probably by decreasing the vaginal pH, increasing colonization of the vagina with lactobacilli, and decreasing colonization with Enterobacteriaceae.[299, 300]

An investigational approach is to use vaginal mucosal immunization with a mixture of uropathogens.[301]

Fungal Infections

Most *Candida* urinary tract infections occur in patients with indwelling catheters. Although removal of the catheter may result in cure of candiduria, continuous amphotericin B bladder irrigation or oral fluconazole 100 mg per day for 7 days may also be necessary in association with removing (if possible) or replacing the catheter.[1, 146] However, there is no demonstrated benefit in the treatment of asymptomatic infection. Exceptions include renal transplant patients and patients who are to undergo elective urinary tract surgery.

URINARY TRACT INFECTION IN PREGNANCY

Physiologic Alterations in the Urinary Tract

During pregnancy, there is dilatation of the ureters and renal pelves with markedly decreased ureteral peristalsis. These changes begin as early as the seventh week of gestation and progress to term.[182] The bladder also decreases in tone so that late in gestation it can contain twice its normal contents without causing discomfort. These changes vary from patient to patient. They are more marked on the right side and are more likely to occur during the first pregnancy or when pregnancies occur in rapid succession. The urinary tract tends to revert to normal by the second month after delivery.[182, 302]

Changes similar to those of pregnancy have been described in the urinary tracts of women taking oral contraceptives.[303] Because of this observation, it has been suggested that the urinary tract alterations may be at least in part related to hyperestrogenism.[182] Other possible explanations for the alterations are obstruction of the ureters by the gravid uterus and hypertrophy of muscle bundles at the lower end of the ureter.[182] To investigate the effects of estrogens on these changes, Andriole and Cohn[304] treated nonpregnant female and male rats with estrogens and obtained intravenous pyelograms before and during treatment. Hydroureter and a markedly increased susceptibility to *E. coli* pyelonephritis were observed in both male and female animals.

Epidemiology

The microbiologic picture of bacteriuria during gestation is similar to that seen in nonpregnant women. The prevalence of asymptomatic bacteriuria in pregnancy ranges from 4 to 7%.[305, 306] However, recurrent episodes are more common in pregnant women who had bacteriuria documented at their initial prenatal visit. It is unclear if *U. urealyticum* and *G. vaginalis,* reported by some to be in bladder urine of an additional 10 to 15% of pregnant women, play a significant pathogenic role.[182] Pregnant women of higher socioeconomic status have a lower frequency of bacteriuria of pregnancy than women of lower socioeconomic status.[180] The prevalence of bacteriuria also rises with parity, age, and sexual activity, in diabetes mellitus, in women with sickle cell trait, and in women with a past history of urinary tract infection.[307, 308] For example, in low-income populations, the prevalence of bacteriuria is about 2% in primiparas younger than 21 years, compared with 8 to 10% in grandmultiparas older than 35 years.[306] Most women who develop bacteriuria during pregnancy have infection at the first prenatal visit. However, 1 to 1.5% of pregnant women or about 25% of those with bacteriuria of pregnancy develop infection in the later trimesters.[182, 305] The development of symptomatic pyelonephritis late in pregnancy is usually an expression of asymptomatic bacteriuria that was present early in parturition. The marked dilatation of the ureters during the later stages apparently allows bacteria in the bladder to reach the upper tract and to produce symptomatic pyelonephritis.

About 20 to 40% of the patients with untreated bacteriuria early in gestation develop acute symptomatic pyelonephritis later in pregnancy.[182, 306, 307, 309] In contrast, less than 1% of patients whose urine is uninfected early in gestation develop acute infection. Therefore, most of the cases of acute pyelonephritis can be prevented by eliminating asymptomatic bacteriuria in the early stages of pregnancy.[182, 306, 310] It has also been noted that those whose bacteriuria fails to respond to treatment are at the highest risk of developing symptomatic infection.[311] A lack of cure is probably an indication of upper versus lower tract infection.

An association between acute pyelonephritis of pregnancy and premature delivery was well known in the preantibiotic era.[182] The rate of prematurity can be as high as 20 to 50%. In 1959, Kass reported that there was an association between asymptomatic bacteriuria and prematurity and that the eradication of bacteriuria significantly reduced the rate of premature delivery.[307] Since then, there have been conflicting studies both supporting and denying these observations.[182, 306, 311, 312] It seems that prematurity and low birth weight[313] are increased in patients with asymptomatic bacteriuria, primarily in those women with renal involvement. McKenzie and associates reported a correlation between the acquisition of urinary antibodies to uropathogens in pregnancy and preterm delivery.[314] However, it does not necessarily follow that asymptomatic bacteriuria is a cause of prematurity. It is possible that certain patients are predisposed both to bacteriuria and to delivering premature infants. Some investigators have reported that the elimination of bacteriuria decreases the frequency of prematurity.[182, 306, 311] However, other studies have failed to show a decrease in prematurity or fetal wastage with the elimination of asymptomatic bacteriuria.[182, 315] Neonates of patients refractory to multiple courses of therapy have been reported to have a significantly lower birth weight than infants of those who respond; this phenomenon may be related to the presence of upper tract infection in these patients.[316, 317] There have been several studies that have attempted to relate asymptomatic bacteriuria to the development of hypertension in pregnancy, but the results have been unclear.[306]

Even though the data relating bacteriuria of pregnancy to prematurity are not clear-cut, the relationship of asymptomatic bacteriuria to the later development of acute pyelonephritis is indisputable. Acute pyelonephritis has possible serious consequence for both the mother and the fetus. Accordingly, screening for and treatment of bacteriuria of pregnancy seem justified. Quantitative urine cultures should be obtained in all pregnant patients at the initial prenatal visit because treatment given at that time would provide the greatest number of bacteriuria-free gestational weeks.[315] Unfortunately, semiquantitative tests and dipstick methods are of low predictive value.[318, 319]

Postpartum studies of patients with bacteriuria of pregnancy demonstrate a high frequency of bacteriuria even with treatment during the pregnancy.[320] Postpartum intravenous pyelography of these patients has shown that 10 to 30% have radiologic changes of "chronic pyelonephritis" and other abnormalities.[320] These abnormalities are most common in patients in whom renal bacteriuria has been demonstrated or in whom bacteriuria during pregnancy was difficult to eradicate with antimicrobial therapy.[182] However, pyelographic abnormalities should not necessarily be attributed to the infection that occurred during the pregnancy. In fact, these abnormalities probably antedate the pregnancy and in most cases are related to childhood infection. Treatment of bacteriuria of pregnancy has little effect on the long-term course of the patient. When patients who had bacteriuria of pregnancy were studied 10 to 14 years later, there were no differences between those who were treated and those who were not. About 25% of the women in each group had bacteriuria at the time of follow-up.[182]

Management of Bacteriuria of Pregnancy

Since screening and treatment of asymptomatic bacteriuria has been shown to prevent pyelonephritis,[310] treatment with an appropriate antimicrobial agent is recommended for all pregnant patients found to have significant bacteriuria.[182, 306, 321, 322] The goal of therapy is to maintain sterile urine throughout gestation and thereby to avoid the complications associated with urinary tract infection during pregnancy. The administration of a relatively nontoxic drug for 7 days (e.g., a sulfonamide, amoxicillin, amoxicillin-clavulanate, cephalexin, nitrofurantoin) eradicates bacteriuria in 70 to 80% of patients.[182, 306] Failure of treatment is most commonly seen in patients with renal infection or radiologic abnormalities of the urinary tract.[182, 306] Sulfonamides should not be administered in the last few weeks of gestation because they may contribute to hyperbilirubinemia and kernicterus in the newborn. Tetracyclines and quinolones should be avoided during pregnancy.

There are relatively few studies evaluating the efficacy of single-dose or 3-day antimicrobial therapy for asymptomatic bacteriuria during pregnancy. In general, results of single-dose therapy appear to be inferior to those of conventional therapy.[182, 323] However, 3 days of therapy has now emerged as the first option in both symptomatic and asymptomatic infection in an attempt to decrease drug administration in pregnancy. Acute pyelonephritis in pregnancy is treated vigorously with parenteral antibiotics as in the nongravid state, but mild episodes may respond to outpatient management.[324]

Urine cultures should be obtained 1 to 2 weeks after discontinuing therapy and at regular intervals (e.g., monthly) for the remainder of gestation. If bacteriuria recurs, therapy should be given for relapse or reinfection, as already discussed. Catheterization should be avoided at the time of delivery. If relapses or multiple reinfections occurred during pregnancy, radiologic evaluation should be considered postpartum. Effective prophylaxis for recurrent urinary infection in pregnancy can be achieved by postcoital prophylaxis consisting of a single oral dose of either cephalexin (250 mg) or nitrofurantoin macrocrystals (50 mg).[325]

PROSTATITIS

Bacterial prostatitis can manifest as either an acute or a chronic disease. Although the manner by which bacteria reach the prostate is unknown,[326, 327] possibilities include the hematogenous route, ascending infection from the urethra, and lymphatic spread from the rectum. Reflux of infected urine may also play a role in the pathogenesis of bacterial prostatitis.[328] Urethral instrumentation and prostatic surgery are known causes of prostatitis, but many patients have no history of a precipitating event.

Stamey has noted that male sex partners of women with vaginal colonization by gram-negative bacilli may develop transient urethral colonization with the same organisms.[329] He postulated that sexual intercourse might play an important role in infection of the prostate. Prostatic fluid constituents, notably zinc, normally have substantial antibacterial properties.[81, 330] However, the prostatic secretions of some patients with chronic bacterial prostatitis have been shown to lack such activity.[330] Bacterial prostatitis infrequently develops after transurethral prostatectomy in men who have infected urine.[326]

The syndromes of acute and chronic bacterial prostatitis are distinctly different. Acute prostatitis does not usually result in chronic prostatitis, and chronic bacterial prostatitis is not usually antedated by acute prostatitis. Acute prostatitis is similar to an acute localized infection in any other organ, producing local heat, tenderness, and fever. In contrast, chronic bacterial prostatitis often produces few or no symptoms related to the prostate, which just serves as a nidus of low-grade infection. Symptoms of acute cystitis or pyelonephritis occur when bacteria, which are repeatedly invading the bladder, overcome the defense mechanisms of the bladder.

Bacteria originating in the prostate may be coated with antibody and, therefore, are a cause of a false-positive antibody-coated bacteria test.[229] After acute bacterial prostatitis, a serum and local immune response is elicited, with the presence of IgA and IgG bacteria-specific immunoglobulins being detected in prostatic secretions. More prolonged prostatic secretion of antigen-specific IgG and IgA is observed in chronic bacterial prostatitis.[331]

Acute Prostatitis

Most cases of acute bacterial prostatitis in the preantibiotic era were caused by *N. gonorrhoeae*. Gram-negative enteric organisms, most commonly *E. coli*, are now the most frequent pathogens.[326, 327] *Neisseria gonorrhoeae* is currently an unusual cause.

Pathologically, acute bacterial prostatitis is characterized by inflammation of part or all of the gland with marked cellular infiltrate (predominantly PMNs), diffuse edema, and hyperemia of the stroma. Microabscesses may occur and may be followed by large, clinically apparent collections of pus. Transrectal ultrasonography is the study of choice to demonstrate the presence of an abscess. If ultrasonography is not available, a CT scan or magnetic resonance imaging of the pelvis may be useful.[332]

Acute bacterial prostatitis is characterized by high fever, chills, perineal and back pain, and symptoms of urinary tract infection such as frequency, urgency, and dysuria.[326] The patient may have urinary retention due to bladder outlet obstruction. The prostate gland is warm, swollen, and extremely tender on rectal examination. Expressed prostatic fluid contains many PMNs, and the infecting organism can frequently be seen on Gram stain. However, massage of the acutely infected prostate gland can precipitate bacteremia and should be discouraged. Since most patients also have bacteriuria, the infecting organism can usually be isolated by midstream urine culture. Many antibiotics diffuse well into the acutely inflamed prostate, and acute bacterial prostatitis responds well to appropriate antimicrobial therapy. Complications such as bacteremia, prostatic abscess, (Fig. 62–8), epididymitis, seminal vesiculitis, and pyelonephritis may occur.

Chronic Bacterial Prostatitis

Chronic bacterial prostatitis is most commonly caused by *E. coli* (80%), but *Klebsiella, Enterobacter, P. mirabilis,* and enterococci are also common causes.[326] Although *S. epidermidis, S. aureus,* and diphtheroids have been frequent isolates in some series,[333] there is considerable doubt as to their real pathogenic role, and most gram-positive bacteria cultured in association with prostatitis represent urethral commensals.[326] Reported rare causes of prostatitis include *Candida* spp., *Blastomyces dermatitidis, Histoplasma capsulatum,*

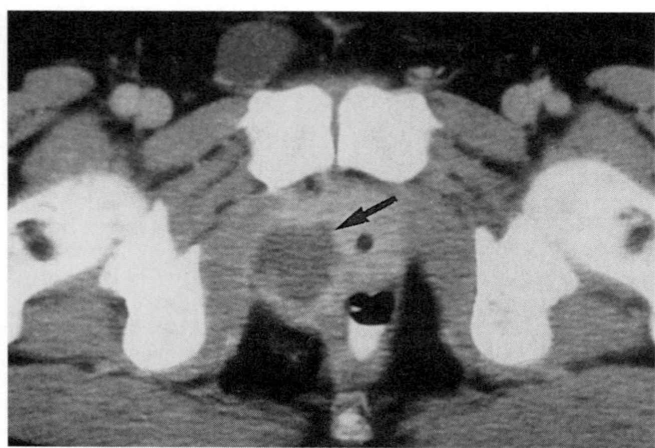

FIGURE 62–8. Computed tomogram demonstrating a large prostatic abscess *(arrow)* adjacent and lateral to the urethra. The rectum contains contrast material.

Mycobacterium tuberculosis, and nontuberculous *Mycobacteria.* The prostate gland has been identified as an important subclinical focus of *Cryptococcus neoformans* infection. Occasionally, histologic specimens of prostatic tissue reveal granulomatous prostatitis of unknown cause.

The histologic findings of chronic bacterial prostatitis are focal, nonacute inflammation. Similar findings may be noted in patients without evidence of bacterial infection and are therefore not diagnostic of bacterial prostatitis.

Many men with chronic infection of the prostate are totally asymptomatic. However, some have perineal discomfort, low back pain, or dysuria. Symptoms of acute urinary tract infection may appear periodically. In fact, chronic bacterial prostatitis is probably the most common cause of relapsing urinary tract infection in men. Fever, if present, tends to be low grade unless pyelonephritis occurs. The results of rectal examination and IVP are unremarkable unless the patient also has an enlarged prostate gland from benign prostatic hypertrophy or carcinoma.

Because of the focal nature of chronic bacterial prostatitis, needle biopsy of the prostate gland for culture of tissue is unreliable.[334] Demonstration of leukocytes in prostatic fluid is not specific for bacterial prostatitis. Most clinicians agree that more than 15 leukocytes per high-power field represents an abnormal number of leukocytes in prostatic fluid.[326] Provided that simultaneous urethral and midstream specimens show insignificant pyuria, this finding would indicate prostatic inflammation irrespective of the cause. Meares and Stamey have described a quantitative localization technique for making the bacteriologic diagnosis.[335] Because bacteria present in the urethra can contaminate prostatic secretions obtained by prostatic massage, accurate diagnosis requires simultaneous quantitative cultures of (1) urethral urine (VB_1), (2) midstream urine (VB_2), (3) prostatic secretions expressed by massage (EPS), and (4) the urine voided after massage (VB_3).

The specimens must be cultured immediately after collection, and methods of quantitating small numbers of bacteria must be used. The study should be done at a time the patient does not have significant bacteriuria. If bacteriuria is present, ampicillin, cephalexin, or nitrofurantoin should be given for 2 to 3 days to sterilize the urine; these agents will not affect bacterial counts in the prostate in chronic bacterial prostatitis. If chronic bacterial prostatitis is present, the number of bacteria in EPS or ejaculate will exceed those in VB_1 or VB_2 urine by at least 10-fold. If no EPS or ejaculate can be obtained, the bacterial counts in the VB_3 specimen should be at least 10-fold higher than the VB_1 or VB_2 samples.

Chronic bacterial prostatitis is very difficult to cure since few antimicrobial agents penetrate well into the noninflamed prostate. Furthermore, the nidus of infection in some patients may be small prostatic calculi or abscesses that presumably are difficult to sterilize. Transrectal ultrasonography will demonstrate prostatic calculi in many patients with chronic bacterial prostatitis.[327, 336] Chronic bacterial prostatitis is therefore likely to persist and cause relapsing urinary tract infection. Unlike classic urinary tract infection, relapses may occur after long periods without bacteriuria (e.g., months). Management may be difficult (see "Therapy").

Nonbacterial Prostatitis

Nonbacterial prostatitis is the most common type of prostatitis and represents an inflammatory condition of unknown cause.[326] The symptoms are perineal pressure, dysuria, urgency, or low back pain, or all of these, symptoms that can also be caused by chronic bacterial prostatitis. However, bacterial pathogens cannot be demonstrated using sequential quantitative cultures. Urinary tract infection does not occur, although prostatic secretions contain excessive numbers of leukocytes and fat-laden macrophages. Although *Chlamydia* and *Ureaplasma* have been implicated as causes of nonbacterial prostatitis, supporting evidence is not convincing.[326, 327, 332, 336–338] The term *prostadynia* or *prostatosis* refers to a similar clinical syndrome in the absence of any objective signs of prostatic inflammation. Some feel that the symptoms may be caused by spasm of the pelvic floor musculature.[327, 332, 336, 339] Others feel that there may be a major psychological component. Because the cause of both entities is unknown, therapy is difficult (see "Therapy").

Therapy

A dog model has been used to measure the diffusion of antimicrobial agents into the noninflamed prostate.[340] In this system, antimicrobial agents are infused, giving high and constant plasma levels, and prostatic secretions are simultaneously collected. Although the basic macrolides such as erythromycin penetrated well into prostatic secretions, penicillins, cephalosporins, tetracyclines, nitrofurantoin, and vancomycin did not. The explanation given was that only lipid-soluble and basic compounds are capable of entering the acid milieu of the prostate gland. Trimethroprim[341] and probably the fluoroquinolones diffuse into prostatic fluid in high concentrations.[327, 332, 336]

Acute bacterial prostatitis frequently responds dramatically to antibacterial therapy. It is thought that the intense diffuse inflammatory reaction of acute bacterial prostatitis allows the passage of antimicrobial agents from plasma into the prostate.[326] Therefore, in the management of acute prostatitis, antimicrobial agents should be given to the patient in doses that achieve therapeutic concentrations in the blood. Appropriate treatment of coliform infections includes trimethoprim-sulfamethoxazole, cephalosporins, amoxicillin, or any of the fluoroquinolones. Ciprofloxacin, 500 mg twice daily, is suitable for the occasional episodes caused by *P. aeruginosa.* Rarely, parenteral antibiotics are required. After a favorable clinical response, antimicrobial therapy should be continued for a minimum of 4 weeks to prevent the development of chronic bacterial prostatitis. Measures such as hydration, analgesics, bed rest, and stool softeners may be helpful. Urethral instrumentation should be avoided. If acute urinary retention occurs, suprapubic drainage of urine through a suprapubic catheter is required. Prostatic abscess is rarely cured by antimicrobial agents alone and requires surgical drainage. Drainage can often be achieved by an ultrasound-guided needle.

Chronic bacterial prostatitis is very difficult to cure. Partial transurethral prostatectomy is curative only if all the infected tissue is removed; about one third of the patients are cured by this procedure.[326] However, a higher percentage are cured if a radical transurethral prostatectomy is performed.[326] Complete prostatectomy is contraindicated because of the complications of sexual impotence and incontinence.

The primary approach to chronic bacterial prostatitis is an attempt at cure with antimicrobial therapy. Although occasional cures have been achieved with penicillins, cephalosporins, tetracyclines, or aminoglycosides, the focus of infection in the prostate has usually persisted, resulting in relapse after therapy was discontinued. Better results have been reported in limited trials with trimethoprim-sulfamethoxazole (one double-strength tablet twice a day). Cure rates have varied from one third to most of the patients treated for several months. The sulfonamide component of trimethoprim-sulfamethoxazole probably contributes little, and rifampin may be more suitable than sulfamethoxazole as a partner for trimethroprim.[342] Although prospective comparative studies are needed, clinical series indicate that fluoroquinolones—ciprofloxacin, 500 mg twice a day; norfloxacin, 400 mg twice a day; ofloxacin, 300 mg twice a day; and lomefloxacin, 400 mg once daily for 30 days—achieve comparable if not superior results to trimethoprim-sulfamethoxazole.[326, 327, 332, 336, 343–345] At present, the initial regimen of choice is trimethoprim-sulfamethoxazole or a quinolone. If therapy fails with these regimens, the patient should be managed either with treatment of acute exacerbations of urinary tract infection or with chronic suppressive therapy to prevent urinary tract infections using low daily doses (e.g., half-normal doses) of an antimicrobial agent. Although it is not widely accepted, some urologists recommend transurethral resection to unroof and remove calculi.[345]

Nonbacterial prostatitis can be treated empirically with erythromycin or a tetracycline, relying on the clinical response to justify a further trial of therapy. Reassurance is important.

PERINEPHRIC ABSCESS AND INTRARENAL ABSCESS

Perinephric Abscess

Perinephric abscess is an uncommon complication of urinary tract infection.[346] The most common predisposing factors are urinary tract calculi and diabetes mellitus. It usually occurs secondary to obstruction of an infected kidney or calyx or occasionally secondary to bacteremia. It may occur insidiously, and up to one third of cases may not be diagnosed until autopsy. The infecting bacteria are usually gram-negative enteric bacilli and occasionally gram-positive cocci when the infection is of hematogenous origin. Multiple bacterial species are present in about 25% of cases and occasionally fungi, especially *Candida* spp., can be cultured from the abscess. The abscess is usually confined by Gerota's fascia to the perinephric space but may extend throughout the retroperitoneum to affect adjacent structures.[347]

The patients have a syndrome suggestive of acute pyelonephritis, with fever, abdominal and flank pain (usually unilateral), and often symptoms of lower tract infection. However, presenting symptoms are often nonspecific. The patient has often been ill for 2 or more weeks. The diagnosis should be strongly considered in any patient with a febrile illness and unilateral flank pain who does not respond to therapy for acute pyelonephritis. A palpable mass may or may not be present. About one half of the patients have an abnormal plain film of the abdomen (e.g., an abdominal mass, an enlarged kidney with indistinct outlines, a loss of the psoas margin, a calculus, a poorly defined renal shadow). Pyuria and proteinuria are frequently found, but about 30% of patients have a normal urinalysis, and about 40% have sterile urine cultures.[347]

Intrarenal Abscess

Intrarenal abscess may occur as a consequence of bacteremia (often caused by coagulase-positive staphylococci). Hematogenous lesions are usually unilateral, single, and located in the cortex. However, these focal suppurative lesions are being recognized with increasing frequency as a complication of classic acute pyelonephritis and are located in the cortex, medulla, or both. The clinical setting is usually that of acute pyelonephritis with high fever, severe flank pain, and tenderness, but with no response or very slow response to appropriate antimicrobial therapy. Contrast-enhanced CT may detect intense parenchymatous inflammation and necrosis in a lobe of the kidney, termed *lobar nephronia* or *acute focal bacterial nephritis*. Although antibiotics may arrest progression at this stage, coalescence of microabscesses (multifocal bacterial nephritis) can lead to intrarenal abscess. Emphysematous pyelonephritis is an uncommon, severe, necrotizing form of acute multifocal bacterial nephritis in which retroperitoneal, extraluminal gas is seen in the renal parenchyma and perirenal space on an abdominal radiograph. The presence of gas suggests a gas-forming, gram-negative facultative anaerobic uropathogen. *Escherichia coli* is the most common organism associated with this complication, but *Klebsiella* spp., *P. mirabilis,* and *Citrobacter* spp. may be involved. This condition occurs most commonly in diabetic patients with or without urinary obstruction.[348] The mortality rate is 70% in spite of antibiotic therapy, and immediate nephrectomy is almost always necessary.[275–277]

Xanthogranulomatous pyelonephritis is an uncommon but severe focal or diffuse chronic infection of the renal parenchyma. Destroyed tissue is replaced by granulomatous tissue containing lipid-laden macrophages (foam cells). Predisposing factors include renal calculi, urinary obstruction, lymphatic obstruction, partially treated chronic urosepsis, renal ischemia and secondary metabolic alterations in lipid metabolism, an abnormal host immune response, and diabetes mellitus.[349]

Diagnosis and Therapy

Urinalysis is abnormal in 70% of patients with a corticomedullary abscess, whereas it is usually normal in the patient with a hematogenous cortical or perinephric abscess. Confirmation of the diagnosis requires radiographic techniques.

The introduction of renal ultrasonography and in particular CT scans has added a new dimension of sensitivity and specificity permitting the early diagnosis of intrarenal and perinephric abscesses (Figs. 62–9 through 62–11).[302, 350–352] The most common CT findings include thickening of Gerota's fascia, renal enlargement, focal parenchymal decreased attenuation, and fluid or gas, or both, in and around the kidney.[302, 353]

In patients with a clinical or radiographic suspicion of perinephric

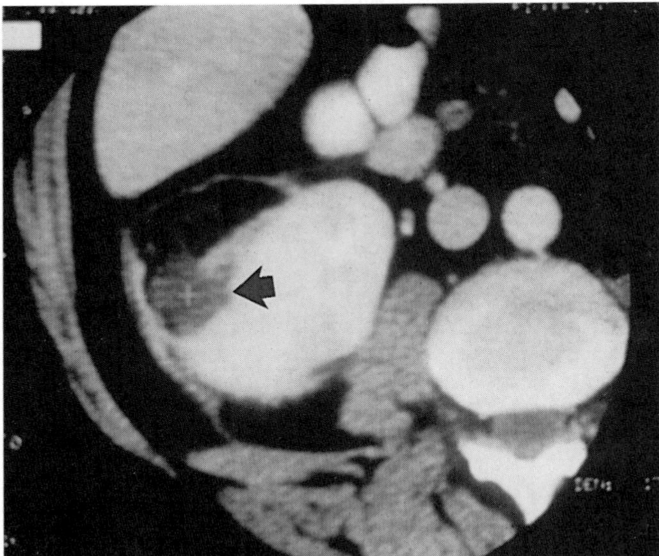

FIGURE 62–9. On computed tomography, an intrarenal abscess, evident as a well-delineated hypodense lesion *(arrow),* is seen extending into the intrarenal space. (Courtesy of M. Bergeron, M.D.)

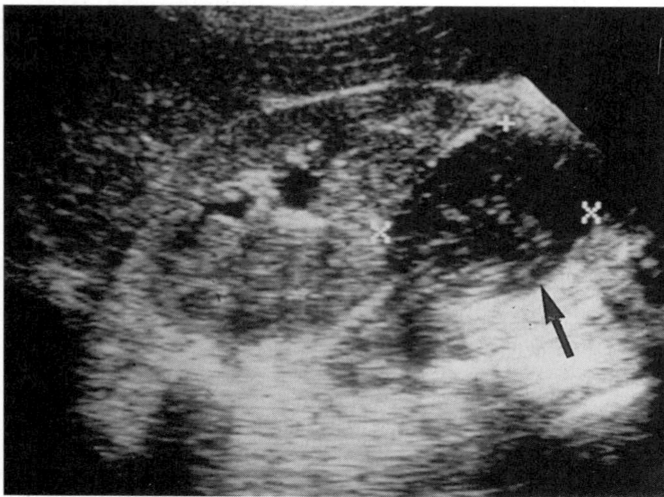

FIGURE 62–10. Ultrasound examination revealing a perinephric abscess *(arrow)*. (Courtesy of M. Bergeron, M.D.)

abscess, diagnostic needle aspiration can be safely performed by using ultrasonography or CT-scan guidance. When an abscess is confirmed, small catheters can be introduced percutaneously to provide immediate decompression as well as continuous and definitive drainage without the need for surgery.[350, 352] Advantages to guided percutaneous drainage compared with open surgical drainage include earlier diagnosis and treatment, the avoidance of general anesthesia and surgery, less expensive therapy, easier nursing care, and greater patient acceptance of closed drainage. Accordingly, it is now recommended that after antimicrobial therapy directed against the most likely pathogens is started, a trial of percutaneous drainage should be the initial mode of therapy for perinephric abscess. Surgical intervention should be undertaken only when percutaneous drainage fails or is contraindicated. Although parenteral antimicrobial therapy directed against the infecting organism isolated from blood or urine should be initiated before drainage, if additional organisms are isolated at the time of surgery, treatment directed against these organisms must be added. Therapy must also be used for the underlying disease (e.g., obstructive uropathy).

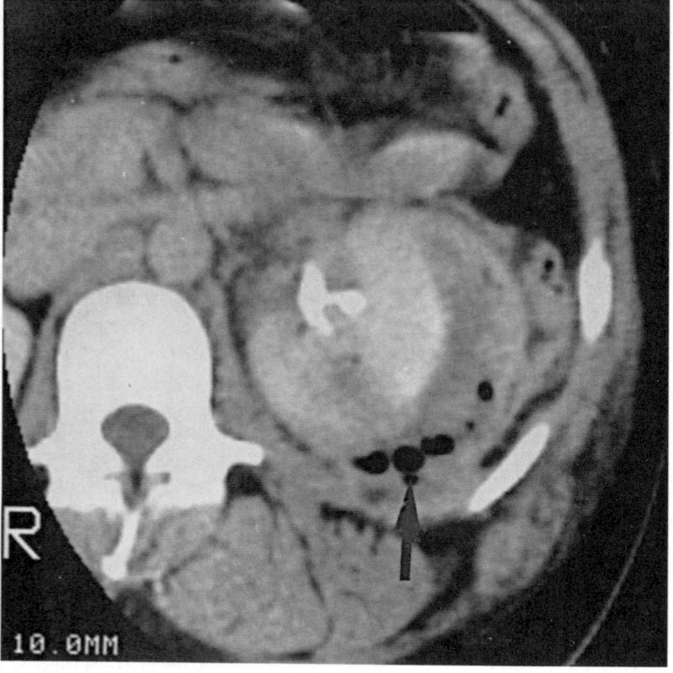

FIGURE 62–11. Computed tomography with contrast material demonstrating a large left perinephric abscess containing gas *(arrow)*.

When antimicrobial therapy with appropriate agents fails with infected renal cysts or abscesses, percutaneous drainage should be tried. Agents that diffuse into these closed sites such as trimethoprim-sulfamethoxazole and fluoroquinolones may have an advantage.[269, 274] Percutaneous drainage often avoids the previous approach of open surgical drainage or nephrectomy.[350, 352, 354, 355]

Successful percutaneous treatment has been reported in 90% of patients with renal or perinephric abscess formation.[352] In the past, delay and missed diagnosis resulted in mortality rates of 20 to 50% with approximately one third of cases diagnosed only postmortem. Today, with early recognition utilizing modern imaging techniques, together with prompt drainage and antibiotic therapy, the mortality is extremely low.[347] Most patients with intrarenal abscess respond, although slowly, to antimicrobial therapy, but fever and severe flank pain may persist for days. Siegel and coworkers reported that virtually all intrarenal abscesses less than 3 cm in diameter resolved on antibiotic therapy alone, as did 92% of those 3 to 5 cm in diameter, whereas larger abscesses (>5 cm) often required percutaneous (33%) or open surgical drainage (37%).[356] Nephrectomy is reserved for emphysematous pyelonephritis, patients with diffusely damaged renal parenchyma, or elderly septic patients requiring urgent intervention for survival.

RADIOLOGIC EVALUATION OF PATIENTS WITH URINARY TRACT INFECTION

Radiologic procedures play an important role in the management of patients with urinary tract infection,[302, 352] both in the control of complicated episodes of acute pyelonephritis and in the investigation of patients of all ages in whom the clinician suspects the presence of underlying structural abnormalities that may be surgically correctable. In adults, uncomplicated acute renal infections do not require radiologic workup. Studies are useful when the diagnosis is in doubt, in severely ill or immunocompromised patients, in those who fail to improve on antibiotic therapy, or when complications are suspected.

Radiologic assessment should commence with a plain film of the abdomen for the detection of urinary tract calculi, calcification, soft tissue masses, and abnormal gas collections. In the past, excretory urography in the form of IVP was the initial and definitive investigatory study but has been largely replaced by both ultrasonography and CT scans (Figs. 62–12 and 62–13). In general, sonography serves as a rapid, noninvasive, and relatively inexpensive means of evaluating the renal collecting system, parenchyma, and surrounding retroperitoneum.[351, 352] Ultrasonography is more sensitive than IVP for detecting parenchymal changes associated with renal infection.

Johnson and associates confirmed that ultrasonographically demonstrable renal swelling characteristically occurs in almost all women with acute pyelonephritis.[273] Enlargement may be unilateral or bilateral and correlates with protracted pretreatment symptoms, leukocytosis, high fever, focal suppurative complications, and prolonged hospitalization. The study also indicated that the frequency of underlying abnormalities and focal complications is low.[273] Several large studies have now confirmed that ultrasonography, especially when combined with a plain film of the abdomen, has become the radiologic investigation of choice in young women with urinary tract infection,[357, 358] replacing excretory urography.

CT is the most sensitive technique of all, and some radiologists consider contrast-enhanced CT as the study of choice.[302] Nevertheless, compared with CT, sonography offers several advantages, including no irradiation, portability, and relative accessibility.[357] The increased sensitivity of contrast-enhanced CT, especially helical CT, is particularly apparent in identifying renal parenchyma abnormalities

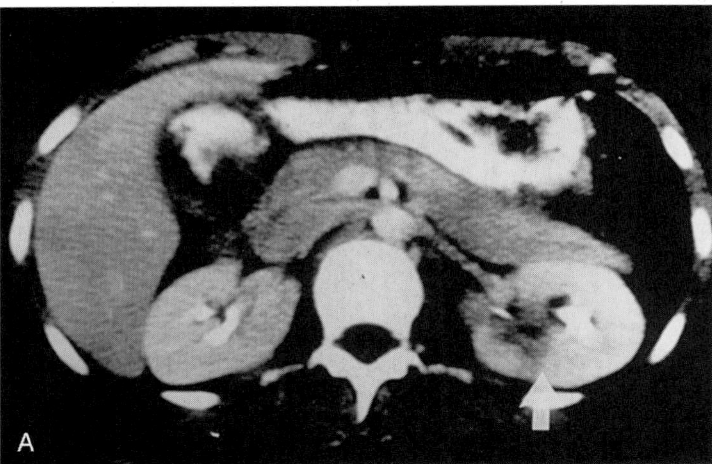

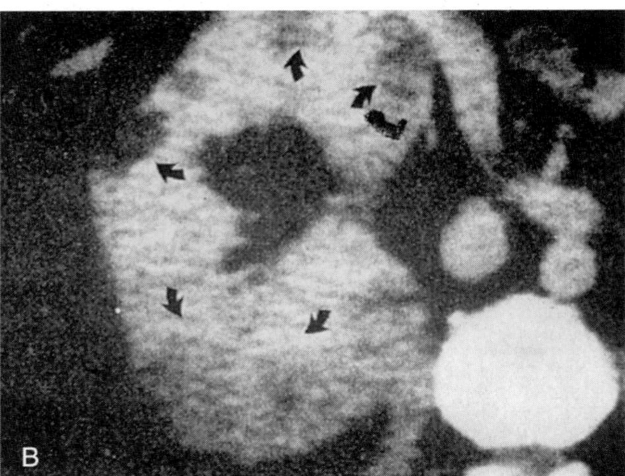

FIGURE 62–12. Computed tomography in acute pyelonephritis. The masslike lesion of pyelonephritis is often well defined, because it is less dense than the cortex. *A,* It can be irregular with a nonhomogeneous center *(arrow),* as seen in the left kidney. The contralateral kidney is normal. *B,* Acute pyelonephritis can appear as multifocal and diffuse masslike lesions *(arrows).* (Courtesy of Huang, M.D.)

in all but the mildest cases of acute pyelonephritis. Sonography is normal in most uncomplicated cases. A common CT finding is decreased opacification of the affected renal parenchyma, usually in a patchy, wedge-shaped, or linear pattern. Different patterns may coexist, and abnormalities vary in size. Non–contrast-enhanced CT is often normal but may show focal areas of decreased attenuation. Areas of markedly decreased attenuation should raise a suspicion of abscess formation, and then contrast material should, if possible, be administered. Other CT findings in pyelonephritis include diffuse or focal kidney enlargement, perinephric stranding, and mild collecting system dilatation. In moderate and severe cases of acute pyelonephritis, CT-scan abnormalities usually persist for several weeks, well after clinical symptoms and laboratory findings have returned to normal.[359] After adequate therapy, most cases eventually demonstrate complete resolution of imaging abnormalities. In recurrent infection associated with chronic reflux, the affected renal lobes develop changes of reflux nephropathy. Recurrent infection results in deformity and dilatation of calyces and focal cortical loss, with upper and lower poles severely affected.

Both CT and ultrasonography are sensitive in diagnosing intrarenal and perirenal suppuration. On contrast-enhanced CT, the hallmark of an abscess is a focal area that fails to enhance, indicating an avascular state. Abscesses are typically sharply demarcated and round or ovoid and contain a low-density center. The abscess wall enhances after contrast injection, resulting in the "rind sign" owing to the presence of inflamed dilated vessels.[350] When detected, gas within a low-density mass is pathognomonic for abscess formation. In contradistinction to pyelonephritis, intrarenal abscesses reaching 2 to 3 cm are well evaluated by ultrasonography, showing sharp demarcation and the presence of liquefaction.[348] Ultrasonography demonstrates a well-marginated, hypoechoic mass with good through transmission, an irregular interior wall margin, and scattered echogenic foci within the mass representing debris. Gas formation is highly echogenic. Both these procedures may be used for the guidance of percutaneous needle aspiration.

Neither CT scans nor ultrasonography reliably distinguish an uninfected obstructed renal collection system (hydronephrosis) from pyonephrosis. Suggestive findings on CT scan include an increased thickness of the renal pelvis wall and the presence of increased density within the renal pelvis indicative of pus or debris. The strongest indication of pyonephrosis on CT is the presence of gas within the collecting system, but this is uncommon. Sonography may identify echogenic contents or debris (Fig. 62–14).[302]

Gas formation within the renal parenchyma as a consequence of severe infection by facultative anaerobes and *Candida* spp. is termed *emphysematous pyelonephritis.* Although gas may be seen on plain radiographs, it is often mistaken for bowel gas. CT is exquisitely sensitive in the detection of gas, the latter appearing as small bubbles or as linear streaks. Gas often collects in a subcapsular location forming a sharp line around the margin of the kidney or may be seen within the renal collecting system.

IVP remains useful for detecting lesions of the collecting system and ureters. Contrast-enhanced CT provides physiologic information similar to that obtained with IVP, with much better parenchymal delineation but less optimal delineation of the collecting system.[353] For cases in which renal calculi may be present, the CT study should also include noncontrast images through the kidney. Helical CT without contrast material is a highly effective means to confirm or exclude the presence of obstructing ureteral calculi.[360]

All studies requiring the parenteral administration of contrast material are associated with some risk of allergy or contrast-induced renal insufficiency. Predisposing factors for renal insufficiency include myeloma, diabetes mellitus, preexisting renal failure, severe intravascular volume depletion, and the recent administration of large doses of iodinated contrast material. Magnetic resonance imaging offers no advantage over CT in the diagnosis of intrarenal or perinephric abscess but may be considered as an alternative to contrast-enhanced CT in patients with a contraindication to iodinated contrast administration.

Radioisotope studies play only a small role, if any, in the investigation of the urinary tract. Gallium-67 citrate scanning and indium-111–labeled white blood cell studies occasionally prove useful in localizing inflammation or infection to the kidneys in patients with fever of unknown origin (Fig. 62–15). Radionuclide scanning may be of value, after ultrasonography or CT scans have identified a solid renal mass, in suggesting the inflammatory nature of the lesion. Neither of these radionuclide studies distinguishes pyelonephritis from abscess.

Another important contribution provided by these radiologic modalities is the detection of surgically correctable abnormalities of the urinary tract. Investigation should be considered in patients at the greatest risk of having surgically correctable abnormalities. Persons with urinary tract infection included in this higher-risk category are all children, men of any age, patients who relapse after therapy, and patients whose infection has been complicated by bacteremia. In the past, excretory urography was indicated for all these categories and for adult women only after multiple episodes of urinary tract infection. As mentioned previously, given the value of ultrasonography,

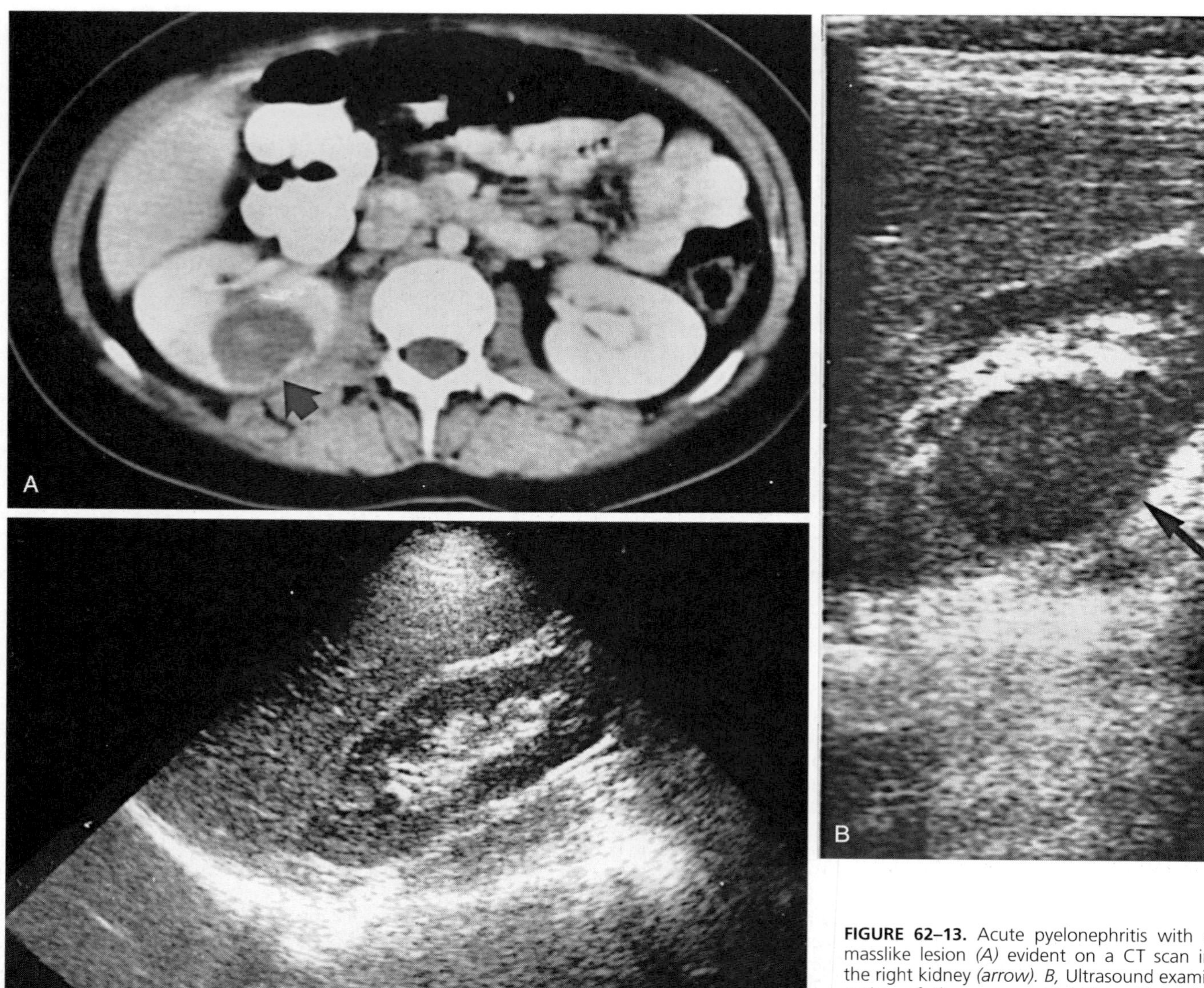

FIGURE 62–13. Acute pyelonephritis with a masslike lesion *(A)* evident on a CT scan in the right kidney *(arrow)*. *B,* Ultrasound examination of the same right kidney. Note the mass *(arrow),* which has resolved on the follow-up ultrasound study *(C)* performed 2 months later. (Courtesy of T. Slovis, M.D.)

its availability, and its safety, it might be reasonable to study all patients with upper tract infection by this method.[358] However, as indicated by Johnson and coworkers, even the routine use of noninvasive renal ultrasonography in women with acute uncomplicated pyelonephritis appears excessive since focal complications are rare and underlying structural abnormalities occur in only about 5% of cases.[273] Women with bacteriuria of pregnancy in whom eradication of infection is difficult should be evaluated. Whereas ultrasonography can be safely performed during pregnancy, accurate delineation of the urinary tract should be delayed until at least 2 months after delivery, by which time the physiologic alterations to the urinary tract that occur during pregnancy should be reversed.[184] Ultrasound examination is also useful in diagnosing lower urinary tract obstruction and detecting residual urine in the bladder. A radionuclide DPTA scan with furosemide to increase urine flow is useful in determining if there is structural as opposed to functional ureteropelvic junction obstruction.

In addition to delineating lesions amenable to surgical correction, urography frequently provides information previously unknown to the patient or physician. For example, unsuspected renal scarring may be seen, suggesting the presence of undiagnosed urinary tract infection in childhood. Occasionally, an unusual or unsuspected type of renal infection such as tuberculosis, papillary necrosis, or xanthogranulomatous pyelonephritis may be discovered.[302, 361] Two major radiologic patterns of xanthogranulomatous pyelonephritis are seen: that of a localized mass and that of diffuse nodularity (Fig. 62–16). When a mass lesion is present, differentiation from pyogenic abscess, tuberculous abscess, or avascular carcinoma may not be possible. Additional findings include nephromegaly, thickening of Gerota's fascia, and infiltration into perinephric space and surrounding retroperitoneal tissues.

Children with urinary tract infection are evaluated radiologically to identify those who may be at risk of chronic renal damage and in identifying children who require corrective surgery (Fig. 62–17).

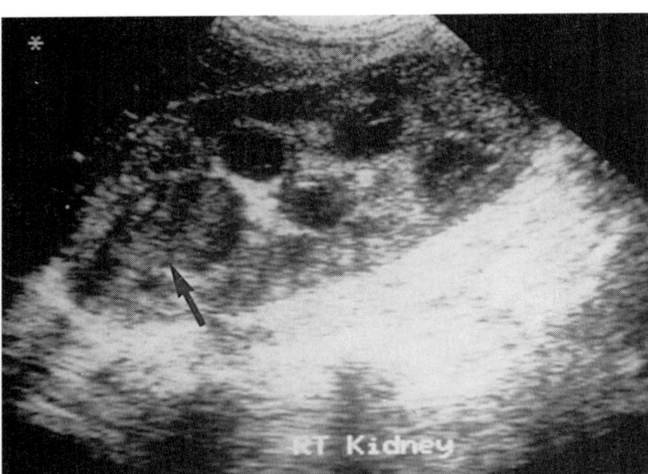

FIGURE 62–14. Ultrasound study demonstrating pyonephrosis (i.e., hydronephrosis) and echogenic content of the collecting system *(arrow)*.

Although controversial, ultrasonography and voiding cystourethrography are recommended in all boys after the first episode of urinary infection and in preschool girls at least after the second infection.[362–364] Investigation is indicated since the incidence of vesicoureteral reflux in this population has been reported to be 20 to 50% and obstruction is not uncommon in boys. Reflux is associated

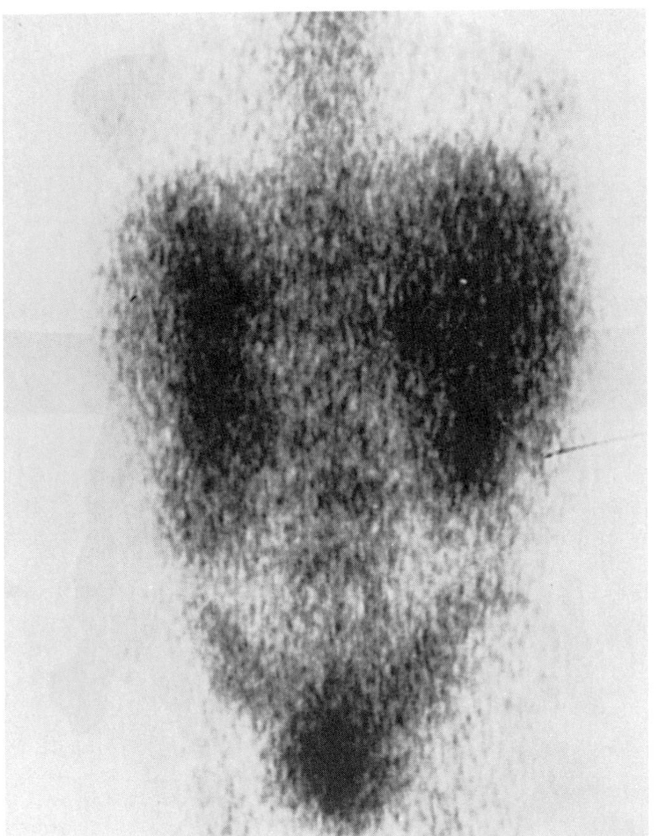

FIGURE 62–15. Renal gallium-67 scan in a young girl with bilateral acute pyelonephritis and increased uptake in both kidneys due to inflammation. (Courtesy of M. Bergeron, M.D.)

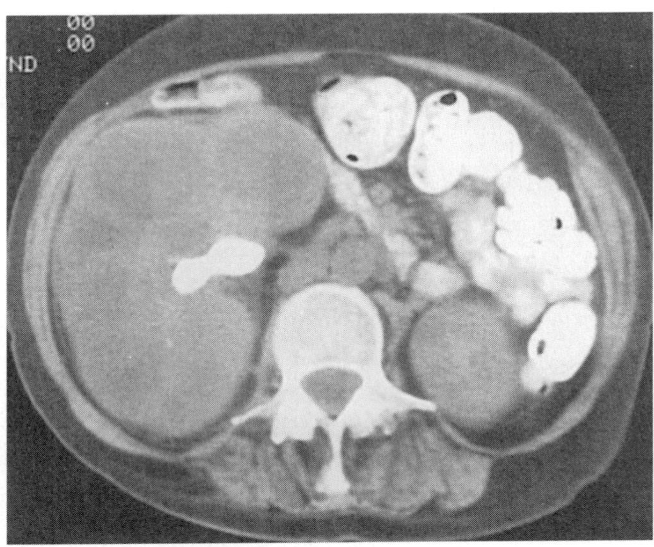

FIGURE 62–16. Computed tomography scan of a patient with right-sided xanthogranulomatous pyelonephritis. A huge multilobulated inflammatory mass replaces the right kidney. *Proteus mirabilis* was grown from the urine. (Courtesy of L. E. Nicolle, M.D.)

with renal scar formation, and surgery may be indicated in some of these children and infants. Several investigators consider that renal cortical scintigraphy is superior to renal ultrasonography and IVP in detecting evidence of both acute pyelonephritis and renal scarring.[365, 366] Performing both renal cortical scintigraphy and ultrasonography appears unnecessary, and both have largely eliminated the need for IVP in children.[367–369] Radionuclide scanning with either ^{99m}Tc-glucoheptonate or dimercaptosuccinic acid (DMSA) technetium have been shown to be sensitive means of identifying not only renal scars but acute and chronic renal infection and upper urinary tract involvement (Fig. 62–18). These scans are effective in screening to identify those children in whom lower urinary tract investigation is indicated to detect reflux, obstruction, or other congenital anomalies. DMSA abnormalities tend to resolve with time; however, an abnormal DMSA study at the time of urinary tract infection identifies most children with significant reflux.[370] As an elective procedure for the detection and evaluation of vesicoureteral reflux, conventional cystourethrography or high-resolution radionuclide voiding cystography are still required, especially since reflux with urinary tract dilatation is frequently undetected by ultrasonography and IVP (Fig. 62–19). The use of radionuclide cystography involves less irradiation and is better tolerated than conventional contrast material introduced by bladder catheterization.[367] Cystourethrography should be avoided in older children unless renal imaging shows evidence of renal scars. However, even with scars, if serial urographic evaluation demonstrates stability of upper tract lesions, the need for studying the lower tract is questionable unless the child experiences recurrent symptomatic infections. When reflux is found, it should be graded as minimal (grade I) to severe (grade IV), so progression or improvement can be quantitated and decisions on surgery can be made.[165, 371]

SURGICAL MANAGEMENT

Surgical therapy in the management of urinary tract infection consists of the elimination of obstructive lesions or calculi and the reimplantation of ureters in the bladder for reflux. An obstruction may be intrinsic (such as renal cysts), or it may be extrinsic anywhere along the urinary conduit from the ureteropelvic junction to the external urethral meatus. Surgical therapy should be directed toward eliminating the obstruction and preserving renal function. After the obstruc-

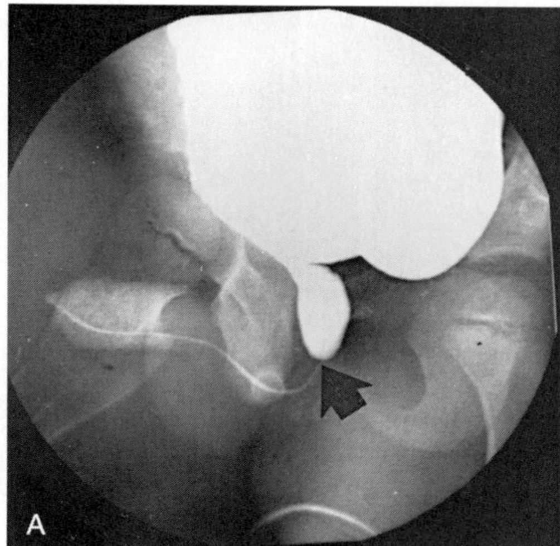

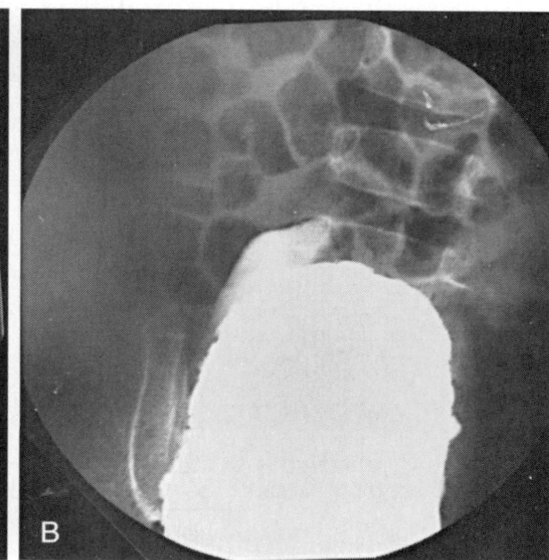

FIGURE 62–17. *A,* Voiding cystourethrogram. Posterior urethral valve on computed tomography scan. Note the discrepancy in size of the anterior *(arrow)* and the posterior urethra. *B,* There is irregular trabeculation of the bladder with right ureteric reflux. (Courtesy of T. Slovis, M.D.)

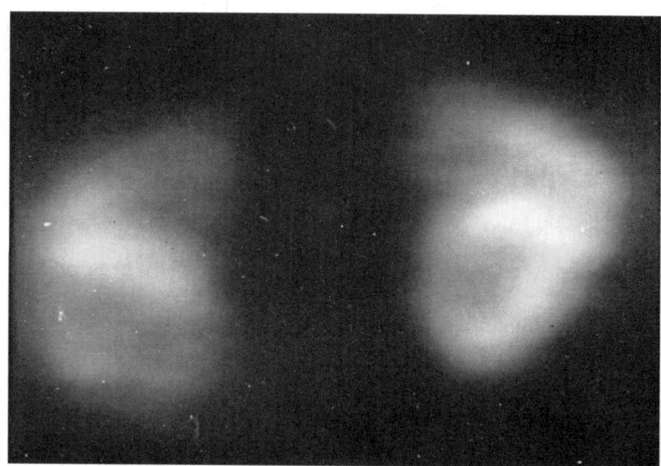

FIGURE 62–18. Acute pylonephritis. A ^{99m}Tc-glucoheptonate single photon emission CT scan with markedly decreased visualization of the upper and lower poles of the right kidney. The midportions are normal. (Courtesy of T. Slovis, M.D.)

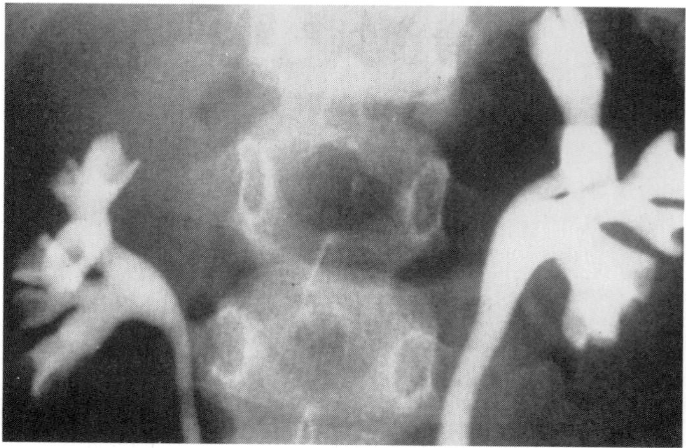

FIGURE 62–19. Grades II and III reflux in a voiding cystourethrograph study from a young boy presenting with recurrent urinary tract infection. Note early clubbing of the calyces and dilatation of the ureter on the left side. (Courtesy of L. E. Nicolle, M.D.)

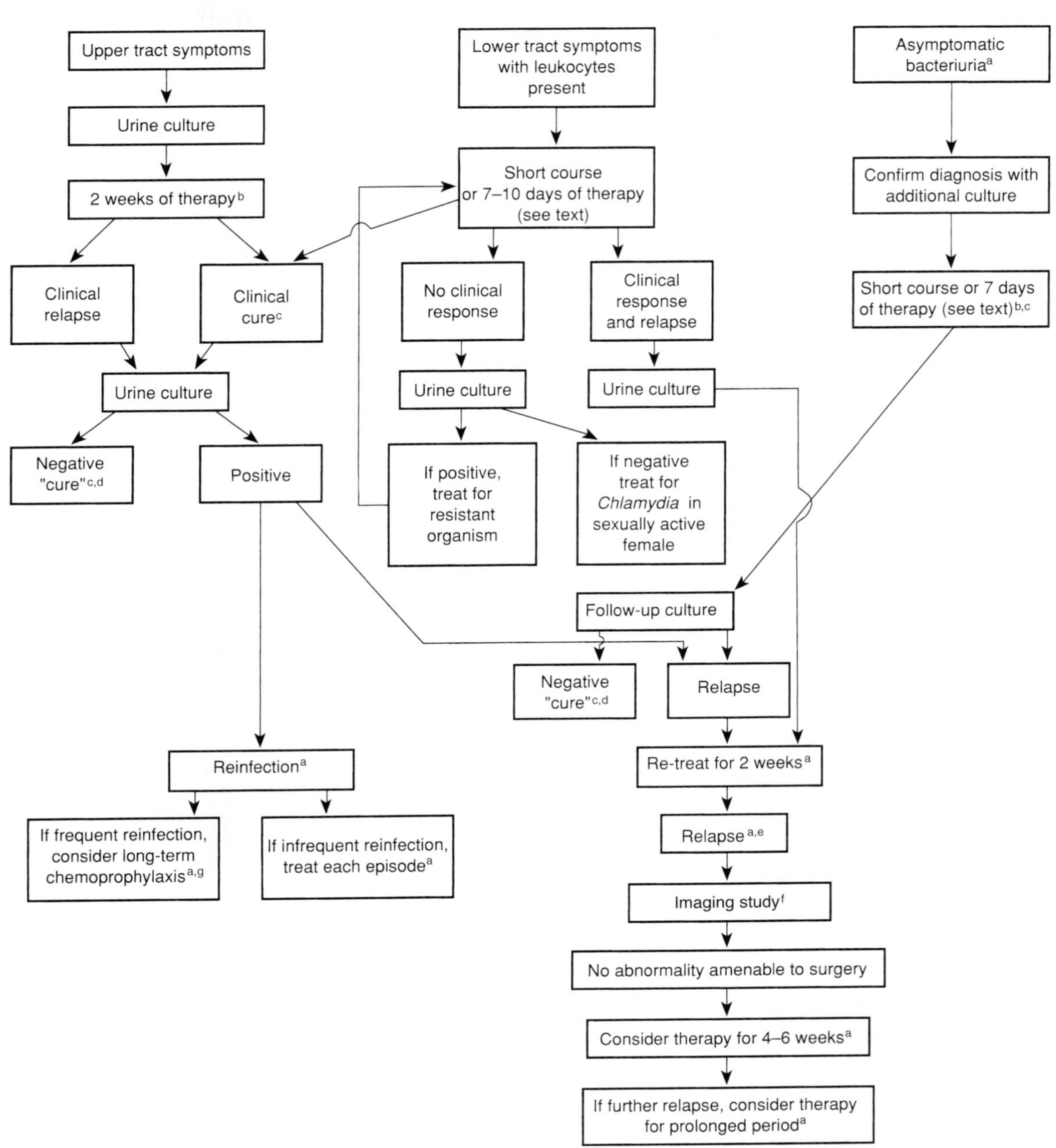

FIGURE 62–20. Approach to the management of urinary tract infection.
[a]Consider no therapy in nonpregnant adults without obstructive uropathy or symptoms of urinary tract infection.
[b]Consider imaging studies in all children and men with correction of significant lesions.
[c]Follow-up culture is required only in pregnancy, in children, and in adults with obstructive uropathy.
[d]Obtain follow-up cultures monthly in pregnant women and at 6 weeks and 6 months in children.
[e]Evaluate men for chronic bacterial prostatitis.
[f]Delay 2 months postpartum in pregnant women.
[g]Consider imaging studies after three to four reinfections in women.

tion is eliminated, the patient should be followed with urine cultures. Urinary tract infection should be treated before surgery to render the urine sterile at the time of surgery; this decreases the possibility of bacteremia occurring in association with the surgery. For management of perinephric or intrarenal abscess see "Perinephric Abscess" and "Intrarenal Abscess."

CATHETER-ASSOCIATED URINARY TRACT INFECTION

For a discussion of catheter-associated urinary tract infection, see Chapters 294 and 305.

SUMMARY FLOW SHEET

Figure 62–20 summarizes the approach to the management of urinary tract infection.

REFERENCES

1. Bacheller CD, Bernstein JM. Urinary tract infections. Med Clin North Am. 1997;81:719–730.
2. Hooton TM, Stamm WE. Diagnosis and treatment of uncomplicated urinary tract infection. Infect Dis Clin North Am. 1997;11:551–581.
3. Ronald AR, Harding GKM. Complicated urinary tract infections. Infect Dis Clin North Am. 1997;11:583–592.
4. Heptinstall RH. Urinary tract infection and clinical features of pyelonephritis. In: Pathology of the Kidney. 4th ed, v. 3. Boston: Little, Brown; 1992:1433–1488.
5. Heptinstall RH. Pyelonephritis: Pathologic features. In: Pathology of the Kidney. 4th ed, v. 3. Boston: Little, Brown; 1992:1489–1561.
6. Freedman L. Chronic pyelonephritis at autopsy. Ann Intern Med. 1967;66:697–710.
7. Huland H, Busch R. Chronic pyelonephritis as a cause of end stage renal disease. J Urol. 1982;127:642–643.
8. Kunin CM. Natural history of lower urinary tract infections. Infection. 1990;18(Suppl 2):S44–S49.
9. Monzon OT, Ory EM, Dobson HL, et al. A comparison of bacterial counts of the urine obtained by needle aspiration of the bladder, catheterization and midstream-voided methods. N Engl J Med. 1958;259:764–767.
10. Bran JL, Levison ME, Kaye D. Entrance of bacteria into the female urinary bladder. N Engl J Med. 1972;286:626–629.
11. Buckley RM, McGuckin M, MacGregor RR. Urine bacterial counts following sexual intercourse. N Engl J Med. 1978;298:321–324.
12. Kelsey MC, Mead MG, Gruneberg RN, et al. Relationship between sexual intercourse and urinary tract infection in women attending a clinic for sexually transmitted diseases. J Med Microbiol. 1979;12:511–512.
13. Nicolle LE, Harding GKM, Preiksaitis J, et al. The association of urinary tract infection with sexual intercourse. J Infect Dis. 1982;116:579–583.
14. Foxman B, Frerichs RR. Epidemiology of urinary tract infection. I. Diaphragm use and sexual intercourse. Am J Public Health. 1985;75:1308–1313.
15. Leibovici L, Alpert G, Laor A, et al. Urinary tract infections and sexual activity in young women. Arch Intern Med. 1987;147:345–347.
16. Strom BL, Collins M, West SL, et al. Sexual activity, contraceptive use, and other risk factors for symptomatic and asymptomatic bacteremia. Ann Intern Med. 1987;107:816–823.
17. Foxman B, Geiger A, Pali K, et al. First time urinary tract infection and sexual behavior. Epidemiology. 1995;6:162–168.
18. Turck M, Goffe B, Petersdorf RG. The urethral catheter and urinary tract infection. J Urol. 1962;88:834–837.
19. Kass EH. Asymptomatic infections of the urinary tract. Trans Assoc Am Physicians. 1956;69:56–64.
20. Gillespie L. The diaphragm an accomplice in recurrent urinary tract infections. Urology. 1984;24:25–30.
21. Fihn SD, Latham RH, Roberts P, et al. Association between diaphragm use and urinary tract infection. JAMA. 1985;254:240–245.
22. Fihn SD, Johnson C, Pinkstaff C, et al. Diaphragm use and urinary tract infections: Analysis of aerodynamic and microbiological factors. J Urol. 1986;136:853–856.
23. Johnson ET. The condom catheter: Urinary tract infection and other complications. South Med J. 1983;76:579–582.
24. Hooton TM, Scholes D, Hughes JP, et al. A prospective of risk factors for symptomatic urinary tract infections in young women. N Engl J Med. 1996;335:468–474.
25. Hooton TM, Hillier S, Johnson C, et al. *Escherichia coli* bacteriuria and contraceptive method. JAMA. 1991;265:64–69.
26. Stamey TA, Timothy M, Millar M, et al. Recurrent urinary infections in adult women. The role of introital enterobacteria. Calif Med. 1971;115:1–19.
27. Vivaldi E, Cotran R, Zangwill DP, et al. Ascending infection as a mechanism in pathogenesis of experimental non-obstructive pyelonephritis. Proc Soc Exp Biol Med. 1959;102:242–244.
28. Plos K, Connell H, Jodal U, et al. Intestinal carriage of P-fimbriated *Escherichia coli* and susceptibility to urinary tract infections in young children. J Infect Dis. 1995;171:625–631.
29. Measley RE, Levison ME. Host defense mechanisms in the pathogenesis of urinary tract infection. Med Clin North Am. 1991;75:275–286.
30. Murphy JJ, Schoenberg HW, Rattner WH, et al. The role of the lymphatic system in pyelonephritis. Surg Forum. 1960;10:880–883.
31. Roberts AP, Phillips R. Bacteria causing symptomatic urinary tract infection or bacteriuria. J Clin Pathol. 1979;32:492–496.
32. Svanborg-Eden C, Hagberg L, Hanson LA, et al. Adhesion of *Escherichia coli* in urinary tract infection. Ciba Found Symp. 1981;80:161–187.
33. Johnson JR, Orskov I, Orskov F, et al. O, K, and H antigens predict virulence factors, carboxylesterase B pattern, antimicrobial resistance and host compromise among *Escherichia coli* strains causing urosepsis. J Infect Dis. 1994;169:119–126.
34. Dennenberg MS, Welsh RA. Virulence determinants of uropathogenic *Escherichia coli*. In: Urinary tract Infections: Molecular Pathogenesis and Clinical Management. Washington DC: American Society for Microbiology, 1996;4:80–128.
35. Bjorksten B, Kaijser B. Interaction of human serum and neutrophils with *Escherichia coli* strains: Differences between strains isolated from urine of patients with pyelonephritis or asymptomatic bacteriuria. Infect Immun. 1978;22:308–311.
36. Johnson JR, Moseley SL, Roberts PL, et al. Aerobactin and other virulence factor genes among strains of *E. coli*. Infect Immun. 1983;40:265–272.
37. Hull R, Hull SI. Nutritional requirements for growth of uropathogenic *Escherichia coli* in human urine. Infect Immun. 1997;65:1960–1961.
38. Svanborg-Eden C, Gotschlich EC, Korhonen TK, et al. Aspects of structure and function of pili of uropathogenic *E. coli*. Prog Allergy. 1983;33:189–202.
39. Iwahi T, Abe Y, Nakao M, et al. Role of type 1 fimbriae in the pathogenesis of ascending urinary tract infection induced by *Escherichia coli* in mice. Infect Immun. 1983;40:265–315.
40. Hagberg L, Hull S, et al. Contribution of adhesin to bacterial persistence in the mouse urinary tract. Infect Immun. 1983;40:265–272.
41. Svanborg-Eden C, Eriksson B, Hanson LA. Adhesion of *Escherichia coli* to human uroepithelial cells in vitro. Infect Immun. 1977;18:767–774.
42. Kallenius G, Molby R, Svensson SB, et al. Occurrence of P-fimbriated *Escherichia coli* in urinary tract infections. Lancet. 1981;2:1369–1372.
43. Leffler H, Savnborg-Eden C. Glycolipid receptors for uropathogenic *Escherichia coli* binding to human erythrocytes and uroepithelial cells. Infect Immun. 1981;34:920–929.
44. Johnson JR. Virulence factors in *Escherichia coli* urinary tract infection. Clin Microbiol Rev. 1991;4:80–128.
45. Roberts JA, Marklund B-I, Ilver D, et al. The Gal (α1-4) Gal-specific tip adhesin of *Escherichia coli* P-fimbriae is needed for pyelonephritis to occur in the normal urinary tract. Proc Natl Acad Sci U S A. 1994;91:11,889–11,893.
46. Johnson JR, Russo TA, Brown JJ, Stapleton A. Pap G alleles of *Escherichia coli* strains causing first-episode or recurrent acute cystitis in adult women. J Infect Dis. 1998;177:97–101.
47. Agace W, Hedges S, Andersson U, et al. Selective cytokine production by epithelial cells following exposure to *Escherichia coli*. Infect Immun. 1993;61:602–609.
48. Hedges S, Agace W, Svanborg C. Epithelial cytokine responses and mucosal cytokine networks. Trends Microbiol. 1995;3:266–270.
49. Moayeri N, Collins M, O'Hanley P. Efficacy of a *Proteus mirabilis* outer membrane protein vaccine in preventing experimental *Proteus* pyelonephritis in a BALB/c mouse model. Infect Immun. 1991;59:3778–3786.
50. Orskov I, Ferencz A, Orskov F. Tamm-Horsfall protein or uromucoid is the normal urinary slime that traps type 1 fimbriated *Escherichia coli*. Lancet. 1980;1:887.
51. Connell H, Agace W, Klemm P, et al. Type 1 fimbrial expression enhances *Escherichia coli* virulence for the urinary tract. Proc Nat Acad Sci U S A. 1996;93:9827–9832.
52. Baorto DM, Gao Z, Malaviya R, et al. Survival of *fim H*–expressing enterobacteria in macrophages relies on glycolipid traffic. Nature. 1997;389:636–639.
53. Pere A, Nowicki B, Saxen H, et al. Expression of P_1 type-1 and type 1_c fimbriae of *Escherichia coli* in the urine of patients with acute urinary tract infection. J Infect Dis. 1987;156:567–574.
54. Nowicki B, Labigne A, Moseley S, et al. The Dr hemagglutinin, afimbrial adhesins AFA-1 and AFA-III, and F1845 fimbriae of uropathogenic and diarrhea-associated *Escherichia coli* belong to a family of hemagglutinins with Dr receptor recognition. Infect Immun. 1990;58:279–281.
55. Goluszka P, Popov V, Selvarangan R. Dr Fimbriae operon of uropathogenic *Escherichia coli* mediate microtublule dependent invasion to the HeLa epithelial cell line. J Infect Dis. 1997;176:158–167.
56. Zafriri D, Gron Y, Eisenstein BI, et al. Growth advantages and enhanced toxicity of *Escherichia coli* adherent to tissue culture cells due to restricted diffusion of products secreted by the cells. J Clin Invest. 1987;79:1210–1216.
57. Mobley HLT, Belas R, Lockatell V, et al. Construction of a flagellum-negative mutant of *Proteus mirabilis:* Effect of internalization by human renal epithelial cells and virulence in a mouse model of ascending UTI. Infect Immun. 1996;64:5332–5340.
58. Mardh PA, Colleen S, Hovelius B. Attachment of bacteria to exfoliated cells from the urogenital tract. Invest Urol. 1979;16:322–326.
59. Schifferli DM, Abraham SN, Beachey EH. Influence of trimethoprim and sulfamethoxazole on the synthesis, expression and function of type 1 fimbriae of *Escherichia coli*. J Infect Dis. 1986;154:490–496.
60. Johnson JR, Roberts PL, Stamm WE. P fimbriae and other virulence factors in *Escherichia coli* urosepsis: Association with patient's characteristics. J Infect Dis. 1987;156:225–229.
61. Stapleton A, Mosely S, Stamm WE. Urovirulence determined in *Escherichia*

coli isolates causing first-episode and recurrent cystitis in women. J Infect Dis. 1991;163:773–779.
62. Fowler JE Jr, Stamey TA. Studies of introital colonization in women with recurrent infections. VII. The role of bacterial adherence. J Urol. 1977;117:472–476.
63. Kallenius G, Winberg J. Bacterial adherence to periurethral epithelial cells in girls prone to urinary tract infection. Lancet. 1978;2:540–543.
64. Svanborg-Eden C, Jodal U. Attachment of *Escherichia coli* to urinary sediment epithelial cells from urinary tract infection prone and healthy children. Infect Immun. 1979;26:837–840.
65. Jacobson S, Carstensen A, Kallenius G, et al. Fluorescence-activated cell analyses of P-fimbriae receptor accessibility on uroepithelial cells of patients with renal scarring. Eur J Clin Microbiol. 1986;5:649–654.
66. Parsons CL, Schmidt JD. In vitro bacterial adherence to vaginal cells of normal and cystitis prone women. J Urol. 1980;123:184–187.
67. Weyrauch HM, Bassett JB. Ascending infection in an artificial urinary tract. An experimental study. Stanford Med Bull. 1951;9:25–29.
68. Boyarsky S, Labay P. Ureteral motility. Annu Rev Med. 1969;20:383–394.
69. Svanborg-Eden C, Hagberg L, Hull R, et al. Bacterial virulence versus host resistance in the urinary tracts of mice. Infect Immun. 1987;55:1224–1232.
70. Musher DM, Griffith DP, Yawn D, et al. Role of urease in pyelonephritis resulting from urinary tract infection with *Proteus.* J Infect Dis. 1975;131:177–181.
71. Mobley HLT, Green DM, Triffilis AL, et al. Pyelonephritogenic *Escherichia coli* and killing of cultured humans renal proximal tubular epithelial cells: Role of hemolysin in some strains. Infect Immun. 1990;58:1281–1289.
72. Connell H, de Man P, Jodal U, et al. Lack of association between hemolysin production and acute inflammation in human urinary tract infection. Microb Pathog. 1993;14:463–472.
73. Guze LB, Goldner BH, Kalmanson GM. Pyelonephritis. I. Observation on the course of chronic non-obstructed enterococcal infection in the kidney of the rat. Yale J Biol Med. 1961;33:372–385.
74. Freedman LR, Beeson PB. Experimental pyelonephritis. IV. Observations on infections resulting from direct inoculation of bacteria in different zones of the kidney. Yale J Biol Med. 1958;30:406–414.
75. Beeson PB, Rowley D. The anticomplementary effect of kidney tissue. Its association with ammonia production. J Exp Med. 1959;110:685–697.
76. Rocha H, Fekety FR. Acute inflammation in the renal cortex and medulla following thermal injury. J Exp Med. 1964;119:131–138.
77. Svensson M, Lindstedt R, Radin N, et al. Epithelial glycosphingo lipid expression as a determinant of bacterial adherence and cytokine production. Infect Immun. 1994;62:4404–4410.
78. Mannhardt W, Becker A, Putzer M, et al. Host defense within the urinary tract. Bacterial adhesion initiates uroepithelial defense mechanisms. Pediatr Nephrol. 1996;10:568–572.
79. Kaye D. Antibacterial activity of human urine. J Clin Invest. 1968;47:2374–2390.
80. Asscher AW, Sussman M, Weiser R. Bacterial growth in human urine. In: O'Grady F, Brumfitt W, eds. Urinary Tract Infection. London: Oxford University Press; 1968:3–13.
81. Stamey TA, Fair WR, Timothy MM, et al. Antibacterial nature of prostatic fluid. Nature. 1968;218:444–447.
82. Bryant RE, Sutcliffe MC, McGee FA. Human polymorphonuclear leukocyte function in urine. Yale J Biol Med. 1973;46:113–124.
83. Reinhart H, Obedeanu N, Sobel JD. Quantitation of Tamm-Horsfall protein binding to uropathogenic *Escherichia coli* and lectins. J Infect Immun. 1990;162:1335.
84. Reinhart H, Obedeanu N, Kaye D, et al. Urinary excretion of Tamm-Horsfall protein in elderly women. J Urol. 1991;146:806–808.
85. Cox CE, Hinman F Jr. Experiments with induced bacteriuria, vesical emptying and bacterial growth on the mechanism of bladder defense to infection. J Urol. 1961;86:739–748.
86. Daifuku R, Stamm WE. Bacterial adherence to bladder uroepithelial cell in catheter associated urinary tract infections. N Engl J Med. 1986;314:72–76.
87. Parsons CL, Greenspan C, Mulholland SG. The primary antibacterial defense mechanism of the bladder. Invest Urol. 1975;13:72–76.
88. Parsons CL, Mulholland SG, Anwar H. Antibacterial activity of bladder surface mucin duplicated by exogenous glycosaminoglycan (heparin). Infect Immun. 1979;24:552–557.
89. Mulholland SG. Lower urinary tract antibacterial defense mechanisms. Invest Urol. 1979;17:93–97.
90. Cobbs CG, Kaye D. Antibacterial mechanisms in the urinary bladder. Yale J Biol Med. 1967;40:93–108.
91. Agace W, Patarroyo M, Svensson M, et al. *Escherichia coli* induce transuroepithelial neutrophil migration by an ICAM-1 dependent mechanism. Infect Immun. 1995;63:4045–4062.
92. Stamey TA. The role of introital enterobactereria in recurrent urinary infections. J Urol. 1973;109:467–472.
93. Kunin CM, Polyak F, Postel E. Periurethral bacterial flora in women. Prolonged intermittent colonization with *Escherichia coli.* JAMA. 1980;243:134–139.
94. Stamey TA, Timothy MM. Studies of introital colonization in women with recurrent urinary infections. I. The role of vaginal pH. J Urol. 1975;114:261–263.
95. Stamey TA, Kaufman MF. Studies of introital colonization in women with recurrent urinary infections. II. A comparison of growth in normal vaginal fluid of common versus uncommon serogroups of *E. coli.* J Urol. 1975;114:264–267.
96. Stamey TA, Timothy MM. Studies of introital colonization in women with recurrent urinary infections. III. Vaginal glycogen concentrations. J Urol. 1975;114:268–270.
97. Stamey TA, Howell JJ. Studies of introital colonization in women with recurrent urinary infections. IV. The role of local vaginal antibodies. J Urol. 1976;115:413–415.
98. Stamey TA, Mihara G. Studies of introital colonization in women with recurrent urinary infections. V. The inhibitory activity of normal vaginal fluid on *Proteus mirabilis* and *Pseudomonas aeruginosa.* J Urol. 1976;115:416–417.
99. Stamey TA, Mihara G. Studies of introital colonization in women with recurrent urinary infections. VI. Analysis of segmented leukocytes on the vaginal vestibule in relation to enterobacterial colonization. J Urol. 1976;116:72–73.
100. Kinane DF, Blackwell CC, Brettle RP, et al. ABO blood group, secretor state, and susceptibility to recurrent urinary tract infection in women. BMJ. 1982;285:7.
101. Sheinfeld J, Schaeffer AJ, Cordon-Cardo C, et al. Association of the Lewis blood group phenotype with recurrent urinary tract infections in women. N Engl J Med. 1989;320:773–777.
102. Jantousch BA, Criss VR, O'Donnell, et al. Association of Lewis blood group phenotypes with urinary tract infection in children. J Pediatr. 1994;124:863–868.
103. Navas EL, Venegas MF, Duncan JL, et al. Blood group antigen expression on vaginal cells and mucus in women with and without a history of urinary tract infections. J Urol. 1994;152:345–349.
104. Reid G, Brooks HJK, Bacon DF. In vitro attachment of *E. coli* to human epithelial cells: Variations in receptivity during the menstrual cycle and pregnancy. J Infect Dis. 1983;148:412.
105. McGroarty FA, Chong S, Reid G, et al. Influence of the spermicidal compound nonoxynol-9 on the growth and adhesion of urogenital bacteria in vitro. Curr Microbiol. 1990;21:219–223.
106. Marsh FP, Murray M, Panchamia P. The relationship between bacterial cultures of the vaginal introitus and urinary infection. Br J Urol. 1972;44:368–375.
107. Elkins IB, Cox CE. Vaginal and urethral bacteriology of young women. I. Incidence of gram negative colonization. J Urol. 1974;111:88–92.
108. Cattell WR, McSherry MA, Northeast A, et al. Periurethral enterobacterial carriage in pathogenesis of recurrent urinary infection. BMJ. 1974;4:136–139.
109. Brumfitt W, Gargan RA, Hamilton-Miller JMT. Periurethral enterobacterial carriage preceding urinary infection. Lancet. 1987;1:824–826.
110. Kurdydyk LM, Kelly K, Harding GMK, et al. Role of cervicovaginal antibody in the pathogenesis of recurrent urinary tract infection in women. Infect Immun. 1980;29:76–82.
111. Smith HS, Hughes JP, Hooton TM, et al. Antecedent antimicrobial use increases the risk of uncomplicated cystitis in young women. Clin Infect Dis. 1997;25:63–68.
112. Hovelius BM, Hedstrom KG, Mollby R, et al. Pathogenesis of urinary tract infections—amoxicillin induces genital *E. coli* colonization. Infection. 1988;5:263.
113. Hanson LA, Ahlstedt S, Fasth A, et al. Antigens of *Escherichia coli,* human immune response, and the pathogenesis of urinary tract infections. J Infect Dis. 19797;136:S144–S149.
114. Kaijser B, Larson P, Olling S, et al. Protection against acute pyelonephritis caused by *Escherichia coli* in rats, using isolated capsular antigen conjugated to bovine serum albumin. Infect Immun. 1983;39:142–146.
115. Hanson LA, Fasth A, Jodal U, et al. Biology and pathology of urinary tract infection. J Clin Pathol. 1981;34:695–700.
116. Mattsby-Baltzer I, Claesson I, Hanson LA, et al. Antibodies to lipid A during urinary tract infection. J Infect Dis. 1981;144:319–328.
117. Mattsby-Baltzer I, Hanson LA, Kaijser B, et al. Experimental *Escherichia coli* ascending pyelonephritis in rats: Changes in bacterial properties and the immune response to surface antigens. Infect Immun. 1982;35:639–646.
118. Svanborg-Eden, Svennerholm AM. Secretory immunoglobulin A and G antibodies prevent adhesion of *Escherichia coli* to human urinary tract epithelial cells. Infect Immun. 1978;22:790–797.
119. Rene P, Dinolfo M, Silverblatt FJ. Serum and urogenital antibody response to *Escherichia coli* pili in cystitis. Infect Immun. 1982;38:542–547.
120. Rene P, Silverblatt FJ. Serological response to *Escherichia coli* pili in pyelonephritis. Infect Immun. 1982;37:749–753.
121. DeRee JM, Van DenBosch JF. Serological response to the P fimbriae of uropathogenic *Escherichia coli* in pyelonephritis. Infect Immun. 1987;55:2204–2207.
122. Kantele A, Papunes R, Virtahen E, et al. Antibody secreting cells in acute urinary tract infection as indicators of local immunoresponse. J Infect Dis. 1994;169:1023–1027.
123. Christmas T. Lymphocyte populations in the bladder wall in normal bladder, bacterial cystitis and interstitial cystitis. Br J Urol. 1994;73:508–512.
124. Hopkins WJ, Uehling DT, Balish E. Local and systemic antibody responses accompany spontaneous resolution of experimental cystitis in cynomolgus monkeys. Infect Immun. 1987;55:1951–1956.
125. Foxman B, Gillespie B, Koopman J, et al. Epidemiology of urinary tract infection: Risk factors for second infection. (in press 1999)
126. Denich K, Blyn LB, Craiu A, et al. DNA sequences of three *pap A* genes from uropathogenic *Escherichia coli* strains: Evidence of structural and serological conservation. Infect Immun. 1991;59:3849–3858.
127. Vroom TM, Scholte G, Osserdorp F, et al. Tissue distribution of human γ/δ T-cells: No evidence for general epithelial tropism. J Clin Pathol. 1991;44:1012–1017.
128. Svanborg-Eden C, Briles D, Hagberg L, et al. Genetic factors in host resistance to urinary tract infection. Infection. 1984;12:118–126.
129. Hedges S, Anderson P, Liden-Janson G, et al. Interlocking response to deliberate colonization of the human urinary tract with gram negative bacteria. Infect Immun. 1991;59:421–427.
130. Bille J, Glauser MP. Protection against chronic pyelonephritis in rats by suppression of acute suppuration. Effect of colchicine and neutropenia. J Infect Dis. 1982;146:220–226.

131. Aoki S, Imamura S, Aoki M, et al. Abacterial and bacterial pyelonephritis. Immunofluorescent localization of bacterial antigen. N Engl J Med. 1969;281:1375–1382.
132. Hanson LA, Fasth A, Jodal U. Autoantibodies to Tamm-Horsfall protein, a tool for diagnosing the level of urinary-tract infection. Lancet. 1976;1:226–228.
133. Rocha H. Pathogenesis and clinical manifestations of urinary tract infection. In: Kaye D, ed. Urinary Tract Infection and Its Management. St Louis: CV Mosby; 1972:6–27.
134. Rocha H, Guze LB, Freedman LR, et al. Experimental pyelonephritis. III. The influence of localized injury in different parts of the kidney on susceptibility to bacillary infection. Yale J Biol Med. 1958;30:341–354.
135. DeNavasquez SJ. Further studies in experimental pyelonephritis produced by various bacteria, with special reference to renal scarring as a factor in pathogenesis. J Pathol Bacteriol. 1956;71:27–32.
136. Cotran TS, Vivaldi E, Zangwill DP, et al. Retrograde pyelonephritis in rats. Am J Pathol. 1963;43:1–31.
137. Rocha H, Santos LCS. Relapse of urinary infection in the presence of urinary tract calculi: The role of bacteria within the calculi. J Med Microbiol. 1969;2:372–376.
138. Smellie JM, Normand ICS. Experience of follow-up of children with urinary tract infection. In: O'Grady F, Brumfitt W, eds. Urinary Tract Infection. London: Oxford University Press; 1968:123–138.
139. Smellie JM, Normand ICS. Bacteriuria, reflux, and renal scarring. Arch Dis Child. 1975;50:581–585.
140. Gould JC. The comparative bacteriology of acute and chronic urinary tract infection. In: O'Grady F, Brumfitt W, eds. Urinary Tract Infection. London: Oxford University Press; 1968:43–50.
141. Jellheden B, Norrby RS, Sanberg T. Symptomatic urinary tract infection in women in primary health care; bacteriological clinical and diagnostic aspects in relation to host response to infection. Scand J Prim Health Care. 1996;14:122–128.
142. Turck M, Stamm WE. Nosocomial infection of the urinary tract. Am J Med. 1981;70:651–654.
143. Bronsema DA, Adams JR, Pallares R, et al. Secular trends in rates and etiology of nosocomial urinary tract infections at a university hospital. J Urol. 1993;150:414–416.
144. Kippax PW. A study of *Proteus* infections in a male urological ward. J Clin Pathol. 1957;10:211–214.
145. Soriano F, Aguado JM, Ponto C, et al. Urinary tract infection caused by *Corynebacterium* group D2: Report of 82 cases and review. Rev Infect Dis. 1990;12:1019–1028.
146. Jacobs LG. Fungal urinary tract infections in the elderly. Drugs Aging. 1996;8:89–96.
147. Paed L, Crump J, Maskell R. Staphylococci as urinary pathogens. J Clin Pathol. 1977;30:427–431.
148. Jordan PA, Iravani A, Richard GA, et al. Urinary tract infection caused by *Staphylococcus saprophyticus*. J Infect Dis. 1980;142:510–515.
149. Hovelius B, Mardh P. *Staphylococcus saprophyticus* as a common cause of urinary tract infections. Rev Infect Dis. 1984;6:328–337.
150. Schneider PF, Riley TV. *Staphylococcus saprophyticus* urinary tract infections: Epidemiological data from Western Australia. Eur J Epidemiol. 1996;12:51–54.
151. Numazaki YN, Kumasaka T, Yana N, et al. Further study on acute hemorrhagic cystitis due to adenovirus 11. N Engl J Med. 1973;289:344–347.
152. Gutman LT, Turck M, Petersdorf RG, et al. Significance of bacterial variants in urine of patients with chronic bacteriuria. J Clin Invest. 1965;44:1945–1952.
153. Maskell R, Pead L, Sanderson RA. Fastidious bacteria and the urethral syndrome. Lancet. 1983;2:1277.
154. Thomsen AC. Mycoplasmas in human pyelonephritis. Demonstration of antibodies in serum and urine. J Clin Microbiol. 1978;8:197.
155. Pickering WJ, Birch DF, Kincaid-Smith P. Biochemical and histologic findings in experimental pyelonephritis due to *Ureaplasma urealyticum*. Infect Immun. 1990;58:3401–3406.
156. Kajander EO, Ciftcioglu N. Nanobacteria: An alternative mechanism for pathogenic intra- and extracellular calcification and stone formation. Proc Natl Acad Sci U S A. 1998;95:8274–8279.
157. Neumann CG, Pryles CV. Pyelonephritis in infants and children. Autopsy experience at the Boston City Hospital, 1933–1960. Am J Dis Child. 1962;104:215–229.
158. McCracken GH. Diagnosis and management of acute urinary tract infections in infants and children. Pediatr Infect Dis J. 1987;6:107–112.
159. Sherbotie JR, Cornfeld D. Management of urinary tract infections in children. Med Clin North Am. 1991;75:327–338.
160. Jones KV. Urinary tract infections in childhood. Practitioner. 1991;235:135–143.
161. Stull TL, LiPuma JJ. Epidemiology and natural history of urinary tract infections in children. Med Clin North Am. 1991;75:287–297.
162. Hansson S, Martinell J, Stokland E, Jodal U. The natural history of bacteriuria in childhood. Infect Dis Clin North Am. 1997;11:499–512.
163. Sureshkumar P, Craig C, Knight JF, et al. Effect of circumcision on incidence of urinary tract infection in preschool boys. J Pediatr. 1996;128:23–27.
164. Huland H, Bush R. Pyelonephritis scarring in 213 patients with upper and lower urinary tract infections: Long-term follow-up. J Urol. 1984;132:936–939.
165. Smellie JM. Reflections on 30 years of treating children with urinary tract infections. J Urol. 1991;146:665–668.
166. Kunin CM. The natural history of recurrent bacteriuria in school girls. N Engl J Med. 1970;282:1443–1448.
167. Kunin CM. Urinary tract infections in children. Hosp Pract. 1976;11:91–98.
168. Gillenwater JY, Harrison RB, Kunin CM. Natural history of bacteriuria in school girls. A long-term case-control study. N Engl J Med. 1979;301:396–399.
169. Ronald AR, Patrillo ALS. The natural history of urinary infection in adults. Med Clin North Am. 1991;75:299–312.
170. Fihn SD, Boyko EJ, Normand EH, et al. Association between use of spermicide-coated condoms and *Escherichia coli* urinary tract infection in young women. Am J Epidemiol. 1996;144:512–520.
171. Fihn SD, Boyko EJ, Chen CL, et al. Use of spermicide-coated condoms and other risk factors for urinary tract infection caused by *Staphylococcus saprophyticus*. Arch Intern Med. 1998;158:281–287.
172. Foxman B. Recurrent urinary tract infection: Incidence and risk factors. Am J Public Health. 1990;80:331–333.
173. Ikaheimo R, Siitonen A, Heiskanen T. Recurrence of urinary tract infection in a primary care setting: Analysis of a 1-year follow-up of 179 women. Clin Infect Dis. 1996;22:91–99.
174. Foxman B, Zhang L, Tallman P, et al. Transmission of uropathogens between sex partners. J Infect Dis. 1997;175:989–992.
175. Spach DH, Stapleton AE, Stamm WE. Lack of circumcision increases the risk of urinary tract infection in young men. JAMA. 1992;267:679–681.
176. Nordenstam G, Sundh V, Lincoln K, et al. Bacteriuria in representative population samples of persons aged 72–79 years. Am J Epidemiol. 1989;130:1176–1186.
177. Baldassarre JS, Kaye D. Special problems of urinary tract infection in the elderly. Med Clin North Am. 1991;75:375–390.
178. Nicolle LE. Asymptomatic bacteriuria in the elderly. Infect Dis Clin North Am. 1997;11:647–662.
179. Kaitz AL, Williams EJ. Bacteriuria and urinary tract infections in hospitalized patients. N Engl J Med. 1960;262:425–430.
180. Turck M, Goffe B, Petersdorf RG. Bacteriuria of pregnancy. N Engl J Med. 1962;266:857–860.
181. Lucas MJ, Cunningham FG. Urinary infection in pregnancy. Clin Obstet Gynecol. 1993;36:855–868.
182. Patterson FT, Andriole VT. Detection, significance, and therapy of bacteriuria in pregnancy. Infect Dis Clin North Am. 1997;11:593–608.
183. Zhanel GG, Harding GKM, Nicolle LE. Asymptomatic bacteriuria in patients with diabetes mellitus. Rev Infect Dis. 1991;13:150–154.
184. Patterson JE, Andriole VT. Bacterial urinary tract infections in diabetics. Infect Dis Clin North Am. 1997;11:735–750.
185. Andriole VT, Patterson TF. Epidemiology, natural history, and management of urinary tract infections in pregnancy. Med Clin North Am. 1991;25:359–373.
186. De Pinho AM, Lopes GS, Ramos-Filho CF, et al. Urinary tract infection in men with AIDS. Genitourin Med. 1994;70:30–34.
187. Tolkoff-Rubin NE, Rubin RH. Urinary tract infection in the immunocompromised host. Infect Dis Clin North Am. 1997;11:707–717.
188. Gleckman R, Blagg N, Hilbert D, et al. Acute pyelonephritis in the elderly. South Med J. 1982;75:551–554.
189. Boscia JA, Kobasa WB, Abrutyn E, et al. Lack of association between bacteriuria and symptoms in the elderly. Am J Med. 1986;81:979–982.
190. Ouslander JG, Schapira M, Schnelle JF, et al. Does eradicating bacteriuria affect the severity of chronic urinary incontinence in nursing home residents? Ann Intern Med. 1995;122:749–754.
191. Kaye D, Rocha H. Urinary concentrating ability in early experimental pyelonephritis. J Clin Invest. 1970;49:1427–1437.
192. Levison SP, Levison ME. The effect of indomethacin and sodium meclofenamate on the renal concentrating defect in experimental enterococcal pyelonephritis in rats. J Lab Clin Med. 1976;88:958–964.
193. Levison SP, Pitsakis PG, Levison ME. Free water reabsorption during saline diuresis in experimental enterococcal pyelonephritis in rats. J Lab Clin Med. 1982;99:474–480.
194. Norden CW, Tuttle EP. Impairment of urinary concentrating ability in pregnant women with asymptomatic bacteriuria. In: Kass EH, ed. Progress in Pyelonephritis. Philadelphia: FA Davis; 1965:73–80.
195. Hellebusch AA. Renal papillary necrosis. A urological emergency. JAMA. 1969;210:1098–1100.
196. Brumfitt W. Urinary cell counts and their value. J Clin Pathol. 1965;18:550–555.
197. Thysell H. Evaluation of chemical and microscopical methods for mass detection of bacteriuria. Acta Med Scand. 1969;185:393–400.
198. Brumfitt W, Percival A. Pathogenesis and laboratory diagnosis of non-tuberculous urinary tract infection: A review. J Clin Pathol. 1964;17:482–491.
199. Boscia JA, Levison ME, Abrutyn E, et al. Correlation of pyuria and bacteriuria in elderly ambulatory women. Ann Intern Med. 1989;110:404–405.
200. Pezzlo M. Detection of urinary tract infections by rapid methods. Clin Microbiol Rev. 1988;1:268–288.
201. Pels RJ, Bor D, Woolhandler S, et al. Dipstick urinalysis screening of asymptomatic adults for urinary tract disorders. JAMA. 1989;262:1221–1224.
202. Winkens RAG, Leffers P, Trienekens TAM, et al. The validity of urine examination for urinary tract infections in daily practice. Fam Pract. 1995;11:290–297.
203. Pappas PG. Laboratory in the diagnosis and management of urinary tract infections. Med Clin North Am. 1991;75:313–325.
204. Cobbs CG. Presumptive tests for urinary tract infections. In: Kaye D, ed. Urinary Tract Infection and Its Management. St Louis: CV Mosby; 1972:43–51.
205. Rubin RH, Shapiro ED, Andriole VT, et al. Evaluation of new anti-infective drugs for the treatment of urinary tract infections. Clin Infect Dis 1992;15:S216–S220.
206. Leung AKC, Robson WLM. Urinary tract infection in infancy and childhood. Adv Pediatr. 1991;38:257–285.
207. Lipsky BA. Urinary tract infections in men. Ann Intern Med. 1989;110:138–150.
208. Goldberg LM, Vosti KL, Rantz LA. Microflora of the urinary tract examined by

voided and aspirated urine culture. In: Kass EH, ed. Progress in Pyelonephritis. Philadelphia: FA Davis; 1965:545.
209. Stamm WE, Wagner KF, Amsel R, et al. Causes of the acute urethral syndrome in women. N Engl J Med. 1980;303:409–415.
210. Stamm WE, Running K, McKuvitt M, et al. Treatment of the acute urethral syndrome. N Engl J Med. 1981;304:956–958.
211. Stamm WE. Quantitative urine cultures revisited. Eur J Clin Microbiol. 1984;3:279–281.
212. Stamm WE, Counts GW, Running R, et al. Diagnosis of coliform infection in acutely dysuric women. N Engl J Med. 1982;307:463–468.
213. Kunin CM, White LVA, Hua TH. A reassessment of the importance of "low count" bacteriuria in young women with acute urinary symptoms. Ann Intern Med. 1993;119:454–460.
214. Arav-Boger R, Leibovici L, Danon YL. Urinary tract infections with low and high colony counts in young women. Arch Intern Med. 1994;154:300–304.
215. Komaroff AL, Pass TM, McCue JD, et al. Management strategies for urinary and vaginal infections. Arch Intern Med. 1978;138:1069–1073.
216. Stamm WE. Management of the acute urethral syndrome. Drug Ther. 1982;12:155–159.
217. Lee HH, Chernesky MA, Schachter J, et al. Diagnosis of *Chlamydia trachomatis* genitourinary infection in women by ligase chain reaction assay of urine. Lancet. 1995;345:213–215.
218. Stamey TA, Govan DE, Palmer JM. The localization and treatment of urinary tract infections: The role of bactericidal urine levels as opposed to serum levels. Medicine. 1965;44:1–36.
219. Fairley KF, Bond AG, Brown RB, et al. Simple test to determine the site of urinary tract infection. Lancet. 1967;2:427–428.
220. Fairley KF, Carson NE, Gutch RC, et al. Site of infection in acute urinary tract infection in general practice. Lancet. 1971;2:615–618.
221. Clark H, Ronald AR, Cutler RE, et al. The correlation between site of infection and maximal concentrating ability in bacteriuria. J Infect Dis. 1969;120:47–53.
222. Ronald AR, Cutler RE, Turck M. Effect of bacteriuria on renal concentrating mechanisms. Ann Intern Med. 1969;70:723–730.
223. Reeves DS, Brumfitt W. Localization of urinary tract infection. In: O'Grady F, Brumfitt W, eds. Urinary Tract Infection. London: Oxford University Press; 1968:53–67.
224. Andriole VT. Advances in the treatment of urinary infections. J Antimicrob Chemother. 1982;9(Suppl A):163–172.
225. Sheldon CA, Gonzalez RD. Differentiation of upper and lower urinary tract infections: How and when? Med Clin North Am. 1984;68:321–333.
226. Thomas V, Shelokov A, Forland M. Antibody-coated bacteria in the urine and the site of urinary tract infection. N Engl J Med. 1974;290:588–590.
227. Jones SR, Smith JW, Sanford JP. Localization of urinary tract infections by detection of antibody-coated bacteria in urine sediment. N Engl J Med. 1974;290:591–593.
228. Thomas VL, Forland M. Antibody coated bacteria in urinary tract infections. Kidney Int. 1982;21:1–7.
229. Jones SR. The current status of urinary tract infection localization by the detection of antibody-coated bacteria in the urinary sediment. In: Gilbert DN, Sanford JP, eds. Infectious Diseases. Current Topics, v. 1. New York: Grune & Stratton; 1979:97–106.
230. Merritt JL, Keys TF. Limitations of the antibody-coated bacteria test in patients with neurogenic bladders. JAMA. 1982;247:1723–1725.
231. Riedash G, Ritz E, Dreikorn K, et al. Antibody-coating of urinary bacteria in transplanted patients. Nephron. 1978;20:267–272.
232. Montplaisir S, Cote P, Martinelli B, et al. Localization du site de l'infection urinaire chez l'enfant par la recherche des bactéries recouvretes d'anticorps. Can Med Assoc J. 1976;115:1096–1099.
233. Hellerstein S, Kennedy E, Nussbaum L, et al. Localization of the site of urinary tract infections by means of antibody-coated bacteria in the urinary sediment. J Pediatr. 1978;92:188–193.
234. Ronald AR, Conway B, Zhanel GG. The value of single-dose therapy to diagnose the site of urinary infection. Chemotherapy. 1990;36(Suppl 1):2–9.
235. Martinell J, Lidin-Janson G, Jagenburg R, et al. Girls prone to urinary infections followed into adulthood: Indices of renal disease. Pediatr Nephrol. 1996;10:139–142.
236. Andriole VT. Advances in the treatment of urinary infections: J Antimicrob Chemother. 1982;9(Suppl A):163–172.
237. Bakshandeh K, Lynne C, Carrion H. Vesicoureteral reflux and end stage renal disease. J Urol. 1976;557:8.
238. Salfatierra O, Tangaho E. Reflux as a cause of end stage kidney disease. Report of 32 cases. J Urol. 1977;117:441–443.
239. Hodson J, Maling TMJ, McManamon PS, et al. Reflux nephropathy. Kidney Int. 1975;8:S50–S58.
240. Rolleston GI, Maling TMJ, Hodson CJ. Intrarenal reflux and the scarred kidney. Arch Dis Child. 1974;49:531–539.
241. Edwards D, Normand ICS, Prescod N, et al. Disappearance of vesicoureteric reflux during long-term prophylaxis of urinary tract infection in children. BMJ. 1977;2:285–288.
242. Kunin CM. Natural history of "lower" urinary tract infections. Infection. 1990;18(Suppl 2):S44–S49.
243. Kemper KJ. The case against screening urinalyses for asymptomatic bacteriuria in children. Am J Dis Child. 1992;146:343–346.
244. Kraft JK, Stamey TA. The natural history of symptomatic recurrent bacteriuria in women. Medicine (Baltimore). 1977;56:55–60.
245. Schechter H, Leonard CD, Cribner BH. Chronic pyelonephritis as a cause of renal failure in dialysis candidates. JAMA. 1971;216:514–517.
246. Bullen M, Kincaid-Smith P. Asymptomatic pregnancy bacteriuria: A followup study 4–7 years after delivery. In: Kinkaid-Smith PK, Fairley KF, eds. Renal Infection and Renal Scarring. 2nd ed. Melbourne: Mercedes; 1970:33.
247. Gower PE, Haswell B, Sidaway ME, et al. Follow-up of 164 patients with bacteriuria of pregnancy. Lancet. 1968;1:990–994.
248. Asscher AW, Chick S, Radford N, et al. Natural history of asymptomatic bacteriuria in non-pregnant women. In: Brumfitt W, Asscher AW, eds. Urinary Tract Infection. London: Oxford University Press; 1973:51–61.
249. Gaches CGC, Miller KW, Roberts BM, et al. The Bristol pyelonephritis registry: 10 years on. Br J Urol. 1976;47:721–725.
250. Zinner S, Kass EH. Long term (10 to 14 years) follow-up of bacteriuria of pregnancy. N Engl J Med. 1971;285:820–824.
251. Gower PE. A long-term study of renal function in patients with radiological pyelonephritis and other allied radiological lesions. In: Brumfit W, Asscher AW, eds. Urinary Tract Infection. London: Oxford University Press; 1973:74–80.
252. Murray T, Goldberg MD. Etiologies of chronic interstitial nephritis. Ann Intern Med. 1975;82:453–459.
253. Dontas AS, Kasviki-Charvati P, Panayiotis CL, et al. Bacteriuria and survival in old age. N Engl J Med. 1981;304:939–943.
254. Boscia JA, Abrutyn E, Kaye D. Asymptomatic bacteriuria in elderly persons. Treat or do not treat? Ann Intern Med. 1987;106:764–766.
255. Nordenstam GR, Brandberg CA, Oden AS, et al. Bacteriuria and mortality in an elderly population. N Engl J Med. 1986;314:1152–1156.
256. Abrutyn E, Mossey J, Berlin JA, et al. Does asymptomatic bacteriuria predict mortality and does antimicrobial treatment reduce mortality in elderly ambulatory women. Ann Intern Med. 1994;120:827–833.
257. Boscia JA, Kaye D. Asymptomatic bacteriuria in the elderly. Infect Dis Clin North Am. 1987:1893–1905.
258. Platt R, Polk BF, Murdock B, et al. Reduction of mortality associated with nosocomial urinary tract infection. Lancet. 1983;1:893–897.
259. Platt R. Adverse consequences of asymptomatic urinary tract infections in adults. Am J Med. 1987;82(Suppl 6B):47–52.
260. O'Grady F, Gauci CL, Watson BW, et al. In vitro models simulating conditions of bacterial growth in the urinary tract. In: O'Grady F, Brumfitt W, eds. Urinary Tract Infection. London: Oxford University Press; 1968:80–92.
261. Kass EH, Zangwill DP. Principles in the long-term management of chronic infection of the urinary tract. In: Quinn EL, Kass EH, eds. Biology of Pyelonephritis. Boston: Little, Brown; 1960:663–672.
262. Vainrub B, Musher DM. Lack of effect of methenamine in suppression of or prophylaxis against, chronic urinary infection. Antimicrob Agents Chemother. 1977;12:625–629.
263. McCabe WR, Jackson GG. Treatment of pyelonephritis: Bacterial, drug and host factors in success or failure among 252 patients. N Engl J Med. 1965;272:1037–1044.
264. Stamey TA, Fair WR, Timothy MM, et al. Serum versus urinary antimicrobial concentrations in case of urinary tract infections. N Engl J Med. 1974;291:1159–1163.
265. Stamey TA, Govan DE, Palmer JM. The localization and treatment of urinary tract infections: The role of bactericidal urine levels as opposed to serum levels. Medicine. 1965;44:1–36.
266. Minuth JN, Masher DM, Thorsteinsonn SB. Inhibition of the antibacterial activity of gentamicin by urine. J Infect Dis. 1976;133:14–21.
267. Kunin CM, Finkelberg Z. Oral cephalexin and ampicillin: Antimicrobial activity, recovery in urine, and persistence in blood of uremic patients. Ann Intern Med. 1970;72:349–356.
268. Hooton TM, Stamm WE. Management of acute uncomplicated urinary tract infection in adults. Med Clin North Am. 1991;75:339–357.
269. Bergeron MG. Treatment of pyelonephritis in adults. Med Clin North Am. 1995;79:619–649.
270. Hooton TM, Stamm W. Diagnosis and treatment of uncomplicated urinary tract infection. Med Clin North Am. 1997;11:551–581.
271. Nicolle LE. A practical guide to the management of complicated urinary tract infection. Drugs. 1997;53:583–592.
272. Stamm WE, McKevitt M, Counts GW. Acute renal infection in women: Treatment with trimethoprim-sulfamethoxazole or ampicillin for two or six weeks. A randomized trial. Ann Intern Med. 1987;106:341–345.
273. Johnson JR, Vincent LM, Wang K, et al. Renal ultrasonographic correlates of acute pyelonephritis. Clin Infect Dis. 1992;14:15–22.
274. Schwab SJ, Bander S, Klahr S. Renal infection in autosomal dominant polycystic kidney disease. Am J Med. 1987;82:714–718.
275. Michaeli J, Mogle D, Perlberg S, et al. Emphysematous pyelonephritis. J Urol. 1984;131:203–208.
276. Stein JP, Spitz A, Elmajian DA, et al. Bilateral emphysematous pyelonephritis. Urology. 1996;47:129–134.
277. Shokeir AA, El-Azab M, Mohsen T, et al. Emphysematous pyelonephritis. Urology. 1997;49:343–346.
278. Norrby SR. Short-term treatment of uncomplicated lower urinary tract infections in women. Rev Infect Dis. 1990;12:458–467.
279. Saginur R, Nicolle LE. Single-dose compared with 3-day norfloxacin treatment of uncomplicated urinary tract infection in women. Arch Intern Med. 1992;152:1233–1237.
280. Rosenstock J, Smith LP, Gurney M, et al. Comparison of single-dose tetracycline

hydrochloride to conventional therapy of urinary tract infection. Antimicrob Agents Chemother. 1985;27:652–654.

281. Harbord RB, Gruneberg RN. Treatment of urinary tract infection with a single dose of amoxycillin, cotrimoxazole or trimethoprim. BMJ. 1981;283:1301–1302.
282. Grossius G. Single dose nitrofurantoin therapy for urinary tract infections in women. Curr Ther Res. 1984;35:925–931.
283. Greenberg RN, Sanders CV, Lewis AC. Single-dose therapy for urinary tract infection with cefaclor. Am J Med. 1981;71:841–845.
284. Stamm WE. Single-dose treatment of cystitis. JAMA. 1980;244:591–592.
285. Philbrick JT, Bracikowski JP. Single-dose antibiotic treatment for uncomplicated urinary infections. Less for less? Arch Intern Med. 1985;145:1672–1678.
286. Stamey TA. Recurrent urinary tract infections in female patients: An overview of management and treatment. Rev Infect Dis. 1987;9(Suppl 2):S195–S208.
287. Johnson J, Stamm W. Diagnosis and treatment of acute urinary tract infection. Infect Dis Clin North Am. 1987;1:773–791.
288. Turck M, Ronald AR, Peterdorf RG. Relapse and reinfection in chronic bacteriuria. II. The correlation between site of infection and pattern of recurrence in chronic bacteriuria. N Engl J Med. 1968;278:422–427.
289. Wong ES, McKevitt M, Running K, et al. Management of recurrent urinary tract infections with patient-administered single-dose therapy. Ann Intern Med. 1985;102:302–307.
290. Vosti K. Recurrent urinary tract infection: Prevention by prophylactic antibiotics after sexual intercourse. JAMA. 1975;231:934–940.
291. Melekos MD, Asbach HW, Gerharz E, et al. Post-intercourse versus daily ciprofloxacin prophylaxis for recurrent urinary tract infections in premenopausal women. J Urol. 1997;157:935–939.
292. Pfau A, Sacks TG. Effective postcoital quinolone prophylaxis of recurrent urinary tract infections in women. J Urol. 1994;152:136–138.
293. Nicolle LE, Ronald AR. Recurrent urinary tract infection in adult women: Diagnosis and treatment. Infect Dis Clin North Am. 1987;1:793–806.
294. Stamey TA, Condy M, Mihara G. Prophylactic efficacy of nitrofurantoin macrocrystals and trimethoprim-sulfamethoxazole in urinary infection. N Engl J Med. 1977;296:780–783.
295. Light RB, Ronald AR, Harding GKM, et al. Trimethoprim alone in the treatment and prophylaxis of urinary tract infection. Arch Intern Med. 1981;141:1807–1810.
296. Gruneberg RN, Smellie JM, Leaky A, et al. Long-term low-dose, co-trimoxazole in prophylaxis of childhood urinary tract infection. Bacteriologic aspects. BMJ. 1976;2:206–208.
297. Brumfitt W, Smith GW, Hamilton-Miller JMT, et al. A clinical comparison between macrodantin and trimethoprim for prophylaxis in women with recurrent urinary infections. J Antimicrob Chemother. 1985;16:111–120.
298. Brumfitt W, Hamilton-Miller JMT. A comparative trial of low dose cefaclor and macrocrystalline nitrofurantoin in the prevention of recurrent urinary tract infection. Infection. 1995;23:98–102.
299. Raz R, Stamm WE. A controlled trial of intravaginal estriol in postmenopausal women with recurrent urinary tract infections. N Eng J Med. 1993;329:753–756.
300. Griebling TL, Nygaard TE. The role of estrogen replacement therapy in the management of urinary incontinence and urinary tract infection in post menopausal women. Endocrinol Metab Clin North Am. 1997;26:347–360.
301. Uehling DT, Hopkins WJ, Balish E, et al. Vaginal mucosal immunization for recurrent urinary tract infection: Phase II Clinical Trial. J Urol. 1997;157:2049–2052.
302. Kaplan DM, Rosenfeld AT, Smith RC. Advances in the imaging of renal infection: Helical CT and modern coordinated imaging. Infect Dis Clin North Am. 1997;11:681–706.
303. Guyer PB, Delaney D. Urinary tract dilatation and oral contraceptives. BMJ. 1970;4:588–590.
304. Andriole VT, Cohn GL. The effect of diethystilbestrol on the susceptibility of rats to hematogenous pyelonephritis. J Clin Invest. 1973;43:1136–1145.
305. Norden CW, Kass EH. Bacteriuria of pregnancy: A critical appraisal. Annu Rev Med. 1968;19:431–470.
306. Miller LK, Cox SM. Urinary tract infections complicating pregnancy. Infect Dis Clin North Am. 1997;11:13–26.
307. Kass E. Bacteriuria and pyelonephritis of pregnancy. Trans Assoc Am Physicians. 1959;72:257–264.
308. Golan A, Wexler S, Amit A, et al. Asymptomatic bacteriuria in normal and high risk pregnancy. Eur J Obstet Gynecol Reprod Biol. 1989;33:101–108.
309. Kincaid-Smith P, Bullen M. Bacteriuria in pregnancy. Lancet. 1965;1:395–399.
310. Gratacos E, Torres PJ, Vila J, et al. Screening and treatment of asymptomatic bacteriuria in pregnancy prevent pyelonephritis. J Infect Dis. 1994;169:1390–1392.
311. Condie AP, Williams JD, Reeves DS, et al. Complications of bacteriuria in pregnancy. In: O'Grady F, Brumfitt W, eds. Urinary Tract Infection. London: Oxford University Press; 1968:148–159.
312. Meis PJ, Michielutte R, Peters TJ, et al. Factors associated with preterm birth in Cardiff, Wales. Am J Obstet Gynecol. 1995;173:597–602.
313. Shieve LA, Handler A, Hershaw R, et al. Urinary tract infection during pregnancy, its association with maternal moridity and perinatal outcome. Am J Publ Health 1992;84:405–410.
314. McKenzie H, Donnet ML, Howie PW, et al. Risk of preterm delivery in pregnant women with group B streptococcal urinary infections or urinary antibodies to group B streptococcal and *E. coli* antigens. Br J Obstet Gynaecol. 1994;101:107–113.
315. Stenquist K, Dahlen-Nilsson I, Lidin-Janson G, et al. Bacteriuria in pregnancy. Am J Epidemiol. 1989;129:372–376.
316. Schultz R, Read AW, Straton JA, et al. Genitourinary tract infections in pregnancy and low birth weight: Case-control study in Australian aboriginal women. BMJ. 1991;303:1369–1373.
317. Gruneberg R, Leigh D, Brumfitt W. Relation of bacteriuria to acute pyelonephritis, prematurity and fetal mortality. Lancet. 1969;2:1–3.
318. Bhana MC, Hoosen AA, Moodley J, et al. Screening for bacteriuria using reagent strips in an indigent pregnant population. S Afr J Epidemiol Infect. 1994;9:48–50.
319. Bint AJ, Hill D. Bacteriuria in pregnancy, an update of significance and management. J Antimicrob Chemother. 1994;33(Suppl A):93–97.
320. Leigh D, Gruneberg R, Brumfitt W. Long term followup of bacteriuria in pregnancy. Lancet. 1968;1:603–605.
321. Vercaigne LM, Zhanel GC. Recommended treatment of urinary tract infection in pregnancy. Ann Pharmacol. 1994;28:248–251.
322. Loughlin KR. Management of urological problems in pregnancy. Urology. 1994;44:159–169.
323. Adelson MD, Graves WL, Osborne NG. Treatment of urinary infections in pregnancy using single versus 10-day dosing. J Natl Med Assoc. 1992;84:73–75.
324. Brooks AM, Garite TJ. Clinical trial of the outpatient management of pyelonephritis in pregnancy. Infect Dis Obstet Gynecol. 1995;3:50–55.
325. Pfau A, Sacks TG. Effective prophylaxis for recurrent urinary tract infections during pregnancy. Clin Infect Dis. 1992;14:810–814.
326. Meares EM Jr. Prostatitis. Med Clin North Am. 1991;75:405–424.
327. Roberts RO, Lieber MM, Bostwick DG, et al. A review of clinical and pathological prostatitis syndromes. Urology. 1997;49:809–821.
328. Kirby RS, Lowe ED, Bultitude MI, et al. Intraprostatic urinary reflux: An aetiological factor in abacterial prostatitis. Br J Urol. 1982;54:729–731.
329. Stamey TA. Urinary infections in males. In: Stamey TA, ed. Pathogenesis and Treatment of Urinary Tract Infections. Baltimore: Williams & Wilkins; 1980:342–429.
330. Fair WR, Cough J, Wehner N. The purification and assay of the prostatic antibacterial factor (PAF). Biochem Med. 1973;8:329–339.
331. Shortliffe LM, Wehner N. The characterization of bacterial and nonbacterial prostatitis by prostatic immunoglobulins. Medicine. 1986;65:399–414.
332. Luzzi G. The prostatitis syndromes. Int J STD AIDS. 1997;7:471–478.
333. Drach GW. Prostatitis: Man's hidden infection. Urol Clin North Am. 1975;2:499–520.
334. Kohnen PW, Drach GW. Patterns of inflammation in prostatic hyperplasia: A histologic and bacteriologic study. J Urol. 1979;121:755–760.
335. Meares EM, Stamey TA. Bacteriologic localization patterns in bacterial prostatitis and urethritis. Invest Urol. 1968;5:492–518.
336. Moul JW. Prostatitis. Postgrad Med. 1993;94:191–194.
337. Weidner W, Brunner H, Krause W. Quantitative culture of *Ureaplasma urealyticum* in patients with chronic prostatitis. J Urol. 1980;124:62–67.
338. Abdelatif OM, Chandler FW, McGuire BS Jr. Chlamydia trachomatis in chronic abacterial prostatitis: Demonstration by colorimetric in situ hybridzation. Hum Pathol. 1991;22:41–44.
339. Segura JW, Opitz J, Green LF. Prostatosis, prostatitis, or pelvic floor tension myalgia? J Urol. 1979;122:168–169.
340. Winningham DF, Nemoy NJ, Stamey TA. Diffusion of antibiotics from plasma into prostatic fluid. Nature. 1968;219:139–143.
341. Stamey TA, Bushby SRM, Bragonse J. The concentration of trimethoprim in prostatic fluid: nonionic diffusion or active transport. J Infect Dis. 1973;128 (Suppl):S686–S690.
342. Giamarellou H, Kosmidis J, Leonidas M, et al. A study of the effectiveness of rifampin in chronic prostatitis caused mainly by *Staphylococcus aureus*. J Urol. 1982;128:321–324.
343. Naber KG. The role of quinolones in the treatment of chronic bacterial prostatitis. Infection. 1991;19(S3):S170–S177.
344. Weidner W, Schiefer HG, Brahler E. Refractory chronic bacterial prostatitis: A re-evaluation of ciprofloxacin treatment after a median followup of 30 months. J Urol. 1991;146:350–352.
345. Pfau A. The treatment of chronic bacterial prostatitis. Infection. 1991;19(Suppl 3):S160–S164.
346. Thorley JD, Jones SR, Sanford JP. Perinephric abscess. Medicine (Baltimore). 1974;53:441–451.
347. Steinfeld J, Erturk E, Spataro Rd, et al. Perinephric abscess: Current concepts. J Urol. 1987;137:191–204.
348. Patel NP, Lavengood RW, Fernandes M, et al. Gas-forming infections in genitourinary tract. Urology. 1992;39:341–349.
349. Brown BS, Dodson M, Wemtraub PS. Xanthogranulomatous pyelonephritis: Report of nonsurgical management of a case and review of the literature. Clin Infect Dis. 1996;22:308–314.
350. Gerzof SG, Gale ME. Computed tomography and ultrasonography for diagnosis and treatment of renal and retroperitoneal abscesses. Urol Clin North Am. 1982;9:185–193.
351. Hoddick W, Jeffery RB, Goldberg HI. CT and sonography of severe renal and perirenal infections. AJR Am J Roentgenol. 1983;140:517–520.
352. Huligowska E, Newman B, White S, et al. Interventional ultrasound in detection and treatment of renal inflammatory disease. Radiology. 1983;147:521–526.
353. Bova JG, Potter JL, et al. Renal and perirenal infection. The role of computerized tomography. J Urol. 1985;133:375–378.
354. Costello AJ, Blandy JP, Hately W. Percutaneous aspiration of renal cortical abscess. Urology. 1983;21:201–204.
355. Finn DJ, Palestrant AM, DeWolf WC. Successful percutaneous management of renal abscess. J Urol. 1982;127:425–426.
356. Siegel JF, Smith A, Moldwin R. Minimally invasive treatment of renal abscess. J Urol. 1996;155:52–55.

357. McNicholas MM, Griffin JF, Cantwell DF. Ultrasound of the pelvis and renal tract combined with a plain film of the abdomen in young women with urinary tract infection: Can it replace intravenous urography? A prospective study. Br J Radiol. 1991;64:221–224.
358. Spencer J, Lindsell D, Mastorakou I. Ultrasonography compared with intravenous urography in investigation of urinary tract infection in adults. BMJ. 1990;301:221–224.
359. Papanicolaou N, Pfister RC. Acute renal infections. Radiol Clin North Am. 1996;34:965–995.
360. Smith RC, Verga M, McCarthy S, et al. Acute flank pain: Value of unenhanced helical CT. Am J Roentgenol. 1996;166:97–101.
361. Grainger RG, Longstaff AJ. Xanthogranulomatous pyelonephritis: A reappraisal. Lancet. 1982;1:1398–1401.
362. Hellerstein S, Wald ER, Winberg J, et al. Consensus: Roentgenographic evaluation of children with urinary tract infections. Pediatr Infect Dis. 1984;3:291–293.
363. Koff SA. A practical approach to evaluating urinary tract infection in children. Pediatr Nephrol. 1991;5:398–400.
364. Hanbury DC, Whitaker RH, Sherwood T, et al. Ultrasound and plain x-ray screening in childhood in urinary tract infection. Br J Urol. 1989;64:638–640.
365. Sreenarastmhaiah V, Alon US. Uroradiologic evaluation of children with urinary tract infection: Are both ultrasonography and renal cortical scintigraphy necessary? J Pediatr. 1995;127:373–377.
366. Preston AA. Imaging strategies and discussion of vesicoureteric reflux as a risk factor in the evaluation of urinary tract infection in children. Curr Opin Pediatr. 1994;6:178–182.
367. Honkinen O, Ruuskanen O, Rikalairen H, et al. Ultrasonography as a screening procedure in children with urinary tract infection. Pediatr Infect Dis. 1986;5:633–635.
368. Leonidas JC, McCauley RG, Klauber G, et al. Sonography as substitute for excretory urography in children with urinary tract infection. Am J Roentgenol. 1985;144:815–819.
369. Kangarloo H, Gold RH, Fine RN, et al. Urinary tract infection in infants and children evaluated by ultrasound. Radiology. 1985;154:367–373.
370. Rosenberg AR, Rossleigh MA, Brydon MP, et al. Evaluation of acute urinary tract infection in children by dimercaptosuccinic acid scintigraphy: A prospective study. J Urol. 1992;148:1746–1749.
371. Gordon I. Vesico-ureteric reflux, urinary tract infections, and renal damage in children. Lancet. 1995;346:489–490.

SECTION E

Chapter 63

Sepsis Syndrome

LOWELL S. YOUNG

Sepsis syndrome has been defined as the earliest stage during an infectious process at which evidence of altered organ perfusion can be detected.[1, 2] However, this concept is controversial because clinicians, intensivists, and infectious disease specialists have employed different terminologies for similar but overlapping clinical conditions. Additional difficulties relate to the challenge of establishing the cause and extent of an apparent infection. Some noninfectious clinical states (e.g., pancreatitis) may mimic an acute infectious process and be equally catastrophic.[2] Although infectious disease specialists have focused on bacterial infections (both gram positive and gram negative) for much of the last 4 decades, it is well recognized that fulminant parasitic infections, miliary tuberculosis, and systemic fungal disease can cause the same manifestations as gram-negative septicemia. One of the major gains of clinical research has been the identification of mediators or cytokines that appear to be responsible for the pathophysiologic changes associated with the systemic manifestations of infection.[3] These cytokines are produced when host cells such as monocytes and macrophages interact with microorganisms or their products, which may or may not be present in the peripheral circulation. Not surprisingly, as in the case of tumor necrosis factor-α (TNF-α), a specific molecule has been associated with the pathophysiologic changes observed in such diverse states as gram-negative bacillary septicemia, meningococcemia, staphylococcal toxic shock syndrome, pulmonary tuberculosis, and cerebral malaria.[4] In this sense, the sepsis syndrome may be considered a constellation of signs and symptoms that represents the host's response to infection, whereby the effects of cytokines (or substances triggered by cytokines) are responsible for most of the clinical manifestations.

With respect to the issue of definitions, Table 63–1 is an attempt to reconcile some of the concepts advanced by a committee of the American College of Chest Physicians/Society of Critical Care Medicine.[2] *Infection*, as defined by the presence of organisms in a normally sterile site, can be symptomatic but may also be inapparent or subclinical. *Bacteremia*—the presence of organisms that can be cultured from the blood—is probably a transient phenomenon for virtually every bacterial infection except endocarditis or severe intravascular infection. *Septicemia* is a term that traditionally has been used interchangeably with *bacteremia*, but many clinicians feel that it implies greater severity. To confuse matters further, the term *sepsis* has often been used in a manner synonymous with the term *infection* but without specifying culture positivity of the blood or body fluids. Increasingly, *septic* refers to individuals who are thought to have systemic infection or who have clinical and laboratory changes consistent with a systemic infection but who do not have positive blood cultures. Therefore, the term *sepsis* is used for a clinical situation in which there is evidence of infection plus a systemic response as manifested by an elevated temperature, tachycardia, increased respirations, leukocytosis or an impaired peripheral leukocyte response, and/or the presence of immature band forms in the peripheral circulation. Emphasizing a degree of increased severity, the term *sepsis syndrome* is defined as sepsis with evidence of altered organ perfusion and at least one of the following: hypoxemia, elevated lactate concentration, oliguria, and altered mentation. All of these conditions imply some degree of organ dysfunction. *Severe sepsis* clearly represents a more advanced degree of organ compromise. Tissue hypoperfusion in severe sepsis may include, among other manifestations, lactic acidosis, oliguria, or changes in mental status.

Clinically, one of the most frequently obtained bedside measurements is that of blood pressure. Often, the normal blood pressure of a person who is admitted to a hospital through an emergency room or to a critical care unit is unknown. A widely used breakpoint for *hypotension* is a systolic blood pressure of less than 90 mmHg or a reduction of more than 40 mmHg from baseline in the absence of other causes of hypotension. Blood pressure is a fluctuating variable, and some patients may have significant changes over a period of hours. Hypotension can readily be corrected by a fluid challenge, and therefore the term *septic shock* should be reserved for patients who have sepsis syndrome and hypotension despite fluid resuscitation of at least 500 ml of saline solution. Some patients who are receiving inotropic or vasopressor agents may not be hypotensive at

TABLE 63–1 Some Definitions of Sepsis, Sepsis Syndrome, Bacteremia, and Related Disorders

Disorder	Definition
Infection	Presence of organisms in a normally sterile site that is usually, but not necessarily, accompanied by an inflammatory host response
Bacteremia	Bacteria present in blood, as confirmed by culture; may be transient
Septicemia	Same as bacteremia, but implies greater severity
Sepsis	Clinical evidence of infection, plus evidence of a systemic response to infection. This systemic response is manifested by two or more of the following conditions: Temperature >38°C or <36°C Heart rate >90 beats/min Respiratory rate >20 breaths/min or Pa_{CO_2} <32 mmHg (<4.3 kPa) WBC >12,000 cells/mm³, <4000 cells/mm³, or >10% immature (band) forms
Sepsis syndrome	Sepsis plus evidence of altered organ perfusion with at least one of the following: hypoxemia, elevated lactate, oliguria, altered mentation
Hypotension	A systolic blood pressure of <90 mmHg or a reduction of >40 mmHg from baseline in the absence of other causes of hypotension
Severe sepsis	Sepsis associated with organ dysfunction, hypoperfusion, or hypotension. Hypoperfusion and perfusion abnormalities may include, but are not limited to, lactic acidosis, oliguria, or an acute alteration in mental status
Septic shock	Sepsis with hypotension despite adequate fluid resuscitation along with the presence of perfusion abnormalities that may include, but are not limited to, lactic acidosis, oliguria, or an acute alteration in mental status. Patients who are on inotropic or vasopressor agents may not be hypotensive at the time that perfusion abnormalities are measured
Refractory septic shock	Septic shock that lasts for more than 1 hour and does not respond to fluid administration or pharmacologic intervention
Systemic inflammatory response syndrome	Response to a wide variety of clinical insults, which can be infectious, as in sepsis, but can be noninfectious in etiology (e.g., burns, pancreatitis)

Data from refs. 1 and 2.

the time that perfusion abnormalities are measured but may yet have evidence for septic shock.

Refractory septic shock refers to septic shock that lasts for longer than 1 hour and does not respond to fluid administration or pharmacologic intervention with pressor agents. The 1-hour dividing point is admittedly arbitrary.

Finally, a term that is being increasingly used by intensivists is *systemic inflammatory response syndrome* (SIRS).[5] This is perhaps the broadest category of all; it includes a wide variety of clinical conditions that are essentially infectious in nature, such as the sepsis syndrome, but also encompasses noninfectious entities such as burns and pancreatitis when fever and organ hypoperfusion are present.[2] The sepsis syndrome can be considered a subset of patients with SIRS.

In an era of increasingly widespread use of antibiotics in the outpatient or home care setting, culture negativity in febrile patients with many of the hallmarks of bacterial infection is very common by the time such patients reach an acute treatment facility. The rationale for not requiring that bacteremia be present in the definition of the sepsis syndrome derives from a prospective study of sepsis and septic shock.[5] Prospective studies have validated the risk of progression and increasing mortality with SIRS, severe sepsis, and septic shock.[6, 7] Nonmicrobiologic terms such as *sepsis*, *sepsis syndrome*, and *SIRS*, although confusing, represent common clinical situations that prompt diagnostic measures and usually result in the initiation of antimicrobial therapy, depending on the severity of disease.

EPIDEMIOLOGIC CONSIDERATIONS

Terms such as *sepsis* and *sepsis syndrome* are clinical definitions and have no direct relation to microbiologic information. However, voluntary surveillance networks such as the National Nosocomial Infection System (NNIS) provide data from selected American hospitals on the relative occurrence of blood stream infections.[8] Before the institution of this voluntary (and therefore selective) surveillance system, information on important blood stream infections was inferred from the experience of teaching hospitals. A population-based estimate of aerobic gram-negative bacteremia in one U.S. county was 42 cases per 100,000 persons per year.[9] Data from the National Hospital Discharge survey collected from a stratified sample of U.S. acute care hospitals and weighted to reflect national distribution demonstrated a dramatic increase in the rate of septicemia, from 73.6 per 100,000 population (164,000 cases) in 1979 to 176 per 100,000 (425,000 cases) in 1987.[10] The total number of septicemia discharges was 2,570,000 for the 9-year period. Over the same period, the percentage of all hospital discharges that included septicemia as a diagnosis increased from 0.5 to 1.3%. For the United States in 1996, septicemia was the 10th leading cause of death[11]; however, cancer and pneumonia were independently listed as categories of mortality and were far more common.

Data from NNIS and from intrainstitutional surveys indicate an upsurge in gram-positive infections during the past 2 decades.[8, 12] Hospital-wide surveillance performed by NNIS indicates that the highest rates for hospital-acquired blood stream infection—1.0, 1.4, and 3.9 per 100 discharges—were observed for oncology, burn/trauma, and high-risk nursery services, respectively.[13] In the summary of the 1986–1997 period, coagulase-negative staphylococci and *Staphylococcus aureus* were the leading causes of nosocomial blood stream infection, followed by *Enterococcus* spp., *Candida albicans*, and *Enterobacter* spp.[8]

CLINICAL MANIFESTATIONS

Table 63–1 represents an attempt to categorize a set of overlapping clinical states and includes clinical conditions that may evolve from one stage to another. The clinician faces the task of determining the likely cause of the clinical state so that appropriate therapy can be instituted. Table 63–2 summarizes some of the common signs and symptoms seen in bacterial infections with either gram-positive or gram-negative organisms, recognizing that such findings are by no means restricted to bacterial processes. Such findings should prompt careful culture of blood, cultures of likely sources of infection, and prompt consideration of initiation of antimicrobial therapy. The distinction between primary manifestations and complications is arbitrary; indeed, onset of hypotension, bleeding, hypoxia, acidosis, and jaundice may be the major clues that first suggest sepsis. Although fever and chills are typical, some patients who develop systemic bacterial infections are debilitated and do not exhibit striking changes (e.g., rigors) early during the course of infection. Paradoxically, hypothermia rather than hyperthermia can occasionally be the manifestation of a systemic infection, and this is associated with a poor prognosis. Although neutropenia definitely predisposes to systemic infection, a precipitous decline in the neutrophil count from a normal or an already depressed level may be seen in immunosuppressed patients. The clinician should be alert to the possibility that hypotension, a fall in urine output, a decrease in circulating platelet levels, and evidence for bleeding even in the absence of fever and chills could be manifestations of a systemic infectious process or the result of the systemic absorption of microbial toxins from a focal infectious process.

Even before elevation of temperature or the onset of chills, bacteremic patients may begin to hyperventilate. Continuous monitoring of patients in intensive care units has indicated that the earliest clinical finding is apprehension and hyperventilation; therefore, the earliest metabolic change in the sepsis syndrome, and in gram-negative bacillary infections in particular, is a resultant respiratory alkalosis.[14] In the critically ill patient, a sudden change of status manifested by hyperventilation should lead to obtaining blood cultures and to a careful evaluation for the possibility of infection. Change in mental status can also be an important clinical clue: although the most common pattern is lethargy or obtundation, some patients become excited, agitated, or combative or display bizarre behavior.[15]

Cutaneous manifestations of the septic process can be seen with bacterial, viral, fungal, and even parasitic processes. In bacterial infections, it has long been recognized that staphylococcal or streptococcal disease can result in metastatic infection of the skin and thereby provide an opportunity for early diagnosis and initiation of specific antimicrobial treatment. In addition to causing cellulitis, the gram-positive pathogens can cause a diffuse erythroderma that is the result of the pathophysiologic action of pyrogenic or erythrogenic toxins.[16] As with the gram-negative endotoxins, these substances can cause multiorgan damage. From the viewpoint of clinical manifestations, erythroderma can be striking, and it may not be possible to distinguish between the advancing edge of a cellulitic process and the manifestations of one of these erythrogenic toxins. Aspiration of the leading edge of an advancing erythematous process may be clinically useful and may provide material for an early diagnosis.

Cutaneous manifestations of gram-negative bacillary bacteremia, usually colorful skin lesions, were described as early as the previous

TABLE 63–2 Signs and Symptoms Suggesting a Systemic Bacterial Infection as the Cause of Sepsis Syndrome

Primary	Complications
Fever	Hypotension
Chills	Bleeding
Hyperventilation	Leukopenia
Hypothermia	Thrombocytopenia
Skin lesions	Organ failure
Change in mental status	Lung: cyanosis, acidosis
	Kidney: oliguria, anuria, acidosis
	Liver: jaundice
	Heart: congestive failure

century.[17] Skin lesions have been most commonly associated with *Pseudomonas aeruginosa* bacteremia. The so-called pathognomonic skin lesion of *P. aeruginosa* bacteremia was described and given the name *ecthyma gangrenosum*.[17] Ecthyma gangrenosum lesions are round or oval, vary from 1 to 5 cm, and have a raised halo or rim of erythema and induration that surrounds a central area that may begin as a vesicle but usually evolves into a necrotic ulcer (Fig. 63–1). The appearance of these "bull's-eye"–type lesions strongly suggests *P. aeruginosa* infection and has been observed in 5 to 25% of all *Pseudomonas* bacteremias. In the thrombocytopenic patient, the periphery of these lesions may become ecchymotic. Biopsy of the lesions indicates that the underlying process is infectious, with direct vascular invasion by bacilli and thrombosis on the venous side of the capillary bed. It seems likely that extracellular products of bacteria such as proteases (elastases) and/or exotoxins are responsible for tissue damage. Nonetheless, there are some reports attributing this phenomenon to local manifestations of Shwartzman reactions in the skin, that is, a localized area of consumption coagulopathy where venous thrombosis, triggered perhaps by endotoxin, is the initiator of tissue injury. Most of these ecthyma lesions appear to be infectious, because organisms can be directly aspirated or cultured from these lesions and histopathologic sections reveal organisms invading blood vessel walls. Therefore, the presence of ecthyma lesions can be considered indicative of bacteremia.

Although ecthyma-type lesions are strongly suggestive of *P. aeruginosa* infection these are not the only organisms that can cause this characteristic lesion. *Aeromonas hydrophila* can produce a clinical picture similar to that of *P. aeruginosa* infection, and a large proportion of bacteremic patients have had ecthyma-like skin lesions.[18] Additionally, cutaneous lesions have been observed in septicemia caused by *Escherichia coli*,[19] *Klebsiella*, *Enterobacter*, and *Serratia*. Besides ecthyma lesions, colorful vesicular or bullous lesions, cellulitis, diffuse erythematous reactions (similar to scarlet fever), or showers of petechial lesions (not unlike meningococcemia) can be cutaneous manifestations of gram-negative bacteremia.[20] Therefore, cutaneous lesions should not lead the clinician to make a specific etiologic diagnosis (although ecthyma-type lesions in the neutropenic patient are most often caused by *P. aeruginosa*) but to alert medical personnel to the possibility of a systemic gram-negative bacillary infection and the need for diagnostic measures and therapeutic intervention. The availability of a lesion from which a biopsy specimen can be obtained and that is easily aspirated, cultured, and processed with Gram stain may provide the basis for an initial microbiologic diagnosis before the isolation and characterization of organisms from blood cultures.

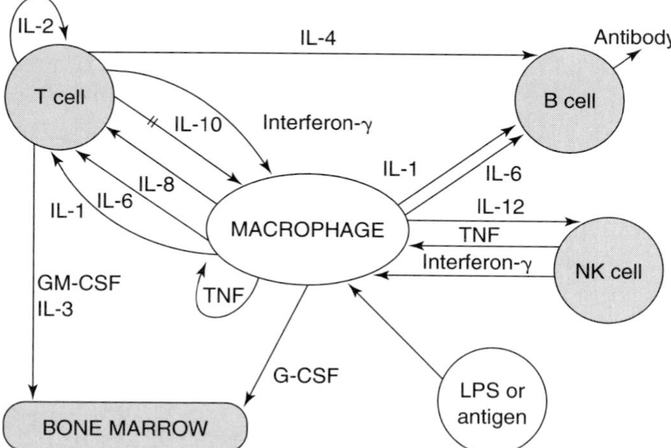

FIGURE 63–1. The interaction between an antigen such as bacterial lipopolysaccharide (LPS or endotoxin) and host mononuclear cells triggers an inflammatory cascade of cytokines that include two potent pyrogenic peptides that can induce hypotension and shock: tumor necrosis factor (TNF)-α and interleukin (IL)-1 (see text). Other peptides with proinflammatory effects include IL-2 (which stimulates T-cell growth), IL-6, IL-8, and interferon (IFN)-γ. Hematopoietic colony-stimulating activity is manifested by IL-3, granulocyte colony-stimulating factor (G-CSF), and granulocyte-macrophage colony-stimulating factor (GM-CSF). IL-4 and IL-10 (and to some degree IL-6) have downregulating effects on inflammation, and IL-12 activates natural killer (NK) cells.

Some patients may have a fulminating bacteremia manifested by shock or rapidly progressing to the stage of shock in a matter of hours. The latter course may be indistinguishable from that of meningococcemia and may be caused by *P. aeruginosa* or *Aeromonas* infection. More typically, however, the onset of shock is slower and follows a period of several hours of hemodynamic instability.

Oliguria, defined as hourly urine outputs of less that 20 ml, often follows the onset of hypotension. The hallmark of shock is tissue hypoperfusion resulting from a decrease in intravascular fluid volume, diminished vascular resistance, or both. Both vasodilatation and increased vascular permeability of some compartments of the circulation may be an initial manifestation of certain pathophysiologic processes (see Pathophysiology), and the net effect is a reduction in circulating blood volume.

Many patients have transient hypotension or oliguria that is quickly ameliorated by prompt corrective measures such as fluid administration. Others progress from an initial phase of hypotension, tachycardia, and peripheral vasodilatation ("warm shock") to a moribund phase of deep pallor, intense vasoconstriction, and anuria ("cold shock"). The latter state clearly reflects the inability of compensatory mechanisms to maintain perfusion even to vital organs. The onset of shock is seen in perhaps 20 to 35% of patients with gram-negative bacillary bacteremia and increases the mortality rate to perhaps twice that figure.

Although clinical findings are likely to reflect the severity and stage of shock rather than a specific microbial cause, hemodynamic differences in shock complicating gram-positive bacteremia compared with gram-negative bacillemia have been reported. Gunnar and colleagues[14] reported prospective hemodynamic studies in patients in shock associated with gram-positive cocci and gram-negative rods. Patients were hospitalized in the intensive care unit of a large municipal hospital, and most had procedures involving urinary tract instrumentation. A number of variables were monitored, including heart rate, cardiac index, left ventricular end-diastolic pressure, systemic vascular resistance, and mean arterial pressure (Table 63–3). Of these parameters, the cardiac rate and cardiac index (which parallels the cardiac rate) were significantly lower in patients with shock secondary to gram-negative bacillary infection. These findings were consistent with release of a vasodilator substance early during the course of gram-negative bacteremia, but ultimately vasoconstriction was more common in patients with gram-negative infections. Myocardial function was also depressed. Although changes in both cardiac rate and cardiac index reflect decreased tissue perfusion, the differences were small, with considerable overlap between the two groups. In the individual patient, a single measurement of either heart rate or cardiac index is likely to be of limited value in distinguishing whether the patient has gram-negative or gram-positive infection. For this reason, it still seems prudent in the critically ill patient with septic shock to initiate empirical antimicrobial therapy aimed at both gram-positive and gram-negative agents until the results of cultures are known.

A minority of patients have bacteremia originating from the lung. They may develop infection secondary to aspiration (bronchial embolism), whereby material containing organisms from the upper respiratory tract is aspirated into the lung parenchyma and pneumonitis and bacteremia develop subsequently. More commonly, diffuse pneumonitis develops secondary to bacteremia and is often of overwhelming severity. The attention of pulmonary physiologists and clinicians has been focused on this complication, which is often referred to as the adult respiratory distress syndrome (ARDS) or "shock lung."[21] ARDS probably reflects a wide variety of pathophys-

TABLE 63–3 Comparison between Hemodynamic Values during Septic Shock in 19 Patients with Gram-Positive Organisms and 31 Patients with Gram-Negative Organisms Cultured from Blood (Mean ± SE)

Organism	MAP (mmHg)	CVP (mmHg)	HR (per min)	CI (liter/min/m²)	SVR (mmHg/liter/min)	LVEDP (mmHg)
Gram-positive	57 ± 2	3.5 ± 0.06	119 ± 4	3.8 ± 0.3	8.5 ± 1.1	6.7 ± 1.3
Gram-negative	57 ± 3	5.1 ± 0.7	100 ± 4	2.9 ± 0.2	11.5 ± 0.9	9.8 ± 1.6
p (unpaired)	NS	NS	<.01	<.05	NS	NS

Abbreviations: CI, Cardiac index; CVP, central venous pressure; HR, heart rate; LVEDP, left ventricular end-diastolic pressure; MAP, mean arterial pressure; NS, not significant; SVR, systemic vascular resistance.
From Gunnar RM, Loeb HS, Winslow EJ, et al. Hemodynamic measurements in bacteremic and septic shock in man. J Infect Dis. 1973;128:287.

iologic mechanisms and clearly has no single cause; it can be caused by either gram-negative or gram-positive pathogens. The mechanism for the diffuse infiltrates may entail direct involvement of the lung by a bacteremic necrotizing pneumonitis or a combination of pulmonary edema (diffuse alveolar/capillary leak) associated with evidence for macroembolization and microembolization to the lung (consumption coagulopathy). That bacterial products can trigger intrinsic clotting and (pari passu) that the body has mechanisms for resorption of thrombi (activation of the fibrinolytic system) is well known. The complexity of the clinical situation probably relates to multiple events that are triggered by bacterial invasion of the blood stream and the ensuing host responses that are described in the following section. The characteristic clinical findings include hypoxia, evidence for a right-to-left shunt, and diffuse pulmonary infiltrates. The most important finding is the relatively normal pulmonary wedge pressure (left ventricular end-diastolic pressure) in the face of a high pulmonary arterial pressure and marked hypoxia (arterial partial pressure of oxygen <60 mmHg). This indicates that the diffuse pulmonary capillary leak syndrome and mechanical alterations in lung function are not secondary to left-sided cardiac failure but actually represent "noncardiogenic" pulmonary edema.

PATHOPHYSIOLOGY

Bacterial invasion of the host is a common setting for the sepsis syndrome. The best studied situation, both in experimental animal systems and in humans, involves systemic disease caused by gram-negative bacteria. The most consistent virulence factor of these gram-negative organisms is bacterial endotoxin or lipopolysaccharide (LPS).

It has become clear with intensive research that LPS triggers humoral enzymatic mechanisms involving the complement, clotting, fibrinolytic, and kinin pathways.[22, 23] Fever and inflammation are mediated by cytokines (peptide hormones acting on cells) that are released in response to the lipid A moiety of LPS (see Fig. 63–1). Some cytokines, such as TNF-α, interleukin-1 (IL-1), interferon-γ (IFN-γ), and various colony-stimulating factors, are produced within minutes to hours of contact between LPS and host defense cells such as monocytes and macrophages.[4, 22–30] IL-1 is the so-called classic endogenous pyrogen and in some animals can induce shock,[30] but TNF-α has potent fever-inducing properties as well.

Of all of the cytokines identified thus far, TNF-α appears to be the most potent mediator of the pathophysiology of the gram-negative sepsis syndrome. LPS in turn is a potent inducer of TNF-α, as are staphylococcal exotoxins, mycobacterial glycolipids, and yeast cell wall mannans.[4] The biologic properties of TNF-α, which are described as "proinflammatory," are summarized in Table 63–4. Evidence for the pivotal role of TNF-α in the pathophysiology of the gram-negative sepsis syndrome is derived from studies showing that (1) mice that are genetically unresponsive to endotoxin lack the capacity to produce murine TNF-α from their macrophages[31]; (2) the administration of endotoxin to human volunteers results in the liberation of free TNF-α in plasma accompanied by many symptoms typical of gram-negative infection[32] (IL-1 and IFN-γ were not detected at challenge doses of 4 ng/kg); (3) high levels of free TNF-α in plasma have been associated with morbidity and increased mortality in human meningococcemia[33] and human gram-negative bacteremia accompanied by shock[4]; (4) the administration of purified recombinant TNF-α to humans[32, 34, 35] and animals[36, 37] mimics most of the clinical, laboratory, and histopathologic findings seen in the gram-negative sepsis syndrome and shock; and (5) antibodies directed against TNF-α, particularly when given before endotoxin challenge, significantly increased the survival of experimental animals.[38, 39] Infusion of anti–TNF-α murine monoclonal antibodies into primates who were bacteremic abrogated the development of signs of endotoxicity. TNF-α can also act directly on cellular components of blood and vascular epithelium,[40] and TNF-α appears to trigger the release of prostaglandins that can act as "second messengers" of systemic toxicity.[41]

Although TNF-α is a potent pyrogen,[42] when used alone it may be insufficient to induce lethality in experimental animals.[43] However, TNF-α plus bacterial products or whole bacteria induce hemorrhagic necrosis of tissues and murine lethality.[4, 24] TNF-α plus IL-1, when given in doses that by themselves are not lethal for the host, rapidly induce animal lethality.[30, 44] Similarly, IFN-γ can be measured during the course of human and experimental disease but does not appear to induce shock by itself.[45] However, markedly enhanced lethality is observed experimentally when IFN-γ and TNF-α are administered together. Therefore, cytokines at concentrations that are not lethal per se can exert a lethal effect in combination. The inhibition of one or more of these cytokines could abrogate the inflammatory response that leads to the sepsis syndrome.

The effects of cytokines are certainly pleiotropic and sometimes paradoxical. In low doses cytokines such as IL-1 and TNF-α prime for host defense, but in larger quantities, such as might result from a massive invasion of the host, these cytokines appear to be lethal.[4, 46]

TABLE 63–4 Effects of the Proinflammatory Cytokine Tumor Necrosis Factor-α

- Inflammation
  - Fever
  - Leukocyte mobilization
- Cardiovascular
  - Tachycardia
  - Hypotension
  - Myocardial depression
  - Capillary leak
  - Endothelial changes
- Central nervous system
  - Anorexia
  - Fever
  - Headache
- Metabolic-hormonal
  - Acidosis
  - Bone resorption
  - Catabolic state leading to cachexia
  - Increased pituitary and stress hormone production
- Hematologic
  - Inhibition of erythropoiesis and inhibition of myelopoiesis
  - Leukopenia
  - Disseminated intravascular coagulation
- Renal
  - Oliguric renal failure
  - Renal cortical necrosis

Data from refs. 4, 52.

The pathophysiology of the sepsis syndrome involves an inflammatory cascade of reactions, with TNF-α as the principal mediator working synergistically with other biologically active products released by host cells. Clearly, other infectious processes such as parasitic or gram-positive infections can lead to TNF-α release, so its detection is not specific for gram-negative infection.[47] Therefore, the identification of TNF-α as an important mediator of septic shock suggests that the sepsis syndrome is an example of immune system "overresponsiveness" to invading pathogens[48, 49] or to large doses of provocative antigens (e.g., LPS) in a manner analogous to anaphylaxis.

IL-6 and IL-8 can also be measured during the course of gram-negative infection and may have diagnostic, prognostic, or therapeutic importance. IL-6 is a mild endogenous pyrogen but is relatively nontoxic per se.[50] It may function to downregulate TNF-α production.[51] IL-8 is primarily a chemotactic and activating factor for neutrophils.[52] IL-10 is a cytokine that acts on macrophages to downregulate TNF-α release.[53] Table 63–5 compares some of the biologic activities of these cytokines.

Cytokine release by itself is not the final pathway leading to host injury. Effects on tissue metabolism, cardiac function, and vascular tone are three major mechanisms for the damage exerted by TNF-α.[28] It has been shown that the combination of TNF-α with other cytokines such as IFN-γ and IL-1 can induce the enzyme nitric oxide synthase (iNOS) in many cells and tissues.[54, 55] The labile but toxic nitric oxide (NO) molecule (known previously as *endothelial relaxing factor*) is a potent vasodilator.[54, 56] The production of NO by iNOS appears to be responsible for hypotension after administration of LPS or TNF-α.[57, 58] NO has a half-life in the circulation of seconds, has potent antimicrobial activity, and has been shown in human and animal test systems to be responsible, in part, for the microbicidal activity of macrophages.[59, 60] Because NO has been detected in the circulation and cerebrospinal fluid (CSF) of septic patients, it has become the target of therapeutic strategies aimed at inhibiting iNOS[61] or scavenging NO radicals with chemical moieties.[60]

There are some provocative experiments that indicate that pretreatment of animal hosts with IL-1 or TNF-α actually induces protection against a bacterial challenge applied hours later.[46, 62] The apparent mechanism for this effect is that the host responds by the production of antagonists (IL-1-Ra) or soluble receptors of TNF-α and IL-1 or is capable of downregulating receptors for these proinflammatory cytokines.[29, 63, 64]

COAGULOPATHY IN THE SEPSIS SYNDROME

Disseminated intravascular coagulation (DIC) may become evident in several ways. Systemic activation of coagulation generates the deposition of fibrin in small blood vessels and microvascular thrombosis in critical target organs, leading to organ failure. Consumption of clotting proteins may lead to bleeding, so both clotting and bleeding can occur simultaneously in the same patient. The most convenient laboratory measurements include a decline in the platelet count and serum fibrinogen levels with an increase in measurable components of fibrin (fibrin "split" or degradation products, D-dimers). Studies carried out in humans or in nonhuman primates have identified the mechanisms involved in infection-triggered coagulopathy. Previously published experiments in rodents and in rabbits have their limitations because of intraspecies differences in the production of mediators or mediator-induced byproducts, and cogent reservations have been expressed about applying animal data to humans. LPS infusions into human volunteers have resulted in the sequential appearance of TNF-α, IL-1, IL-6, and IL-8.[65] The appearance of these cytokines was then followed by markers for the generation of thrombin, as illustrated in Figure 63–2. Other markers of fibrinogen to fibrin conversion, such as fibrinopeptide A, have also been documented. The use of recombinant TNF-α in cancer patients and healthy volunteers has shown a parallel activation of coagulation, and inhibition of endotoxin-induced TNF release in chimpanzees results in inhibition of the activation of coagulation.[66, 67] Taken together, these studies confirm the central role of TNF-α in endotoxin-triggered coagulopathy. Understanding of the roles of other cytokines such as IL-1, IL-6, and IL-8 is incomplete, but studies indicate that cytokines other than TNF significantly affect blood coagulation in vitro. IL-6 is a potent stimulus for platelet production.[52]

The well-established compartmentalization of clotting pathways into the intrinsic (contact activation–dependent) pathway and the extrinsic (tissue factor–dependent) pathway is summarized in Figure 63–2. Studies using large concentrations of LPS showed that factor XII (Hageman's factor) can be activated in vitro; this is an initial important event in the contact activation of the intrinsic clotting system. Additionally, clinical studies showed that low levels of factor XII are present in bacteremic patients, thereby supporting the role of the intrinsic pathway for activation. However, in experimental endotoxemia or after cytokine administration with TNF-α, highly sensitive assays have shown that the initial activation of coagulation in septic states appears to depend primarily on activation of the extrinsic pathway.[66, 67] The lines of evidence supporting this conclusion are as follows: (1) After endotoxin administration to healthy human volunteers or chimpanzees, or the administration of TNF-α to volunteers or cancer patients, substantial factor X–mediated generation of thrombin is observed. At the same time, plasma markers for intrinsic pathway clotting factor activation remain normal. (2) In vitro studies show that TNF-α induces the expression of tissue factor on monocytes, and tissue factor binds and activates factor VII, thereby forming a complex that can convert factor X and activate it. (3) Children with meningococcemia have increased tissue factor expression on circulating monocytes. (4) Studies of experimental bacteremia or endotoxemia in nonhuman primates in which the extrinsic clotting system was blocked by the simultaneous infusion of monoclonal antibodies directed either against tissue factor or against factor VII showed that LPS-induced thrombin and fibrin

TABLE 63–5 Biologic Activities of Cytokines That May Contribute to Septic Shock

Activity	IL-1	IL-2	GM-CSF	IL-4	IL-5	IL-8	TNF	IFN-γ
In vivo								
Hypotension	+	+					+	+
Fever	+	+	+		+		+	
Edema	+	+				+	+	
Leukocytosis	+		+		+			
Wasting	+						+	
In vitro								
Direct cytotoxicity	+	+	+				+	
Cell-mediated cytotoxicity	+		+	+			+	+
Proteases, O_2 radicals				+		+	+	
Chemotaxis			+	+		+		
Vascular adhesion	+			+			+	

Adapted from Cannon, JG. Cytokines and shock. In: Kimball ES, ed. Cytokines and Inflammation. Boca Raton, Fla: CRC Press; 1991:307–329.

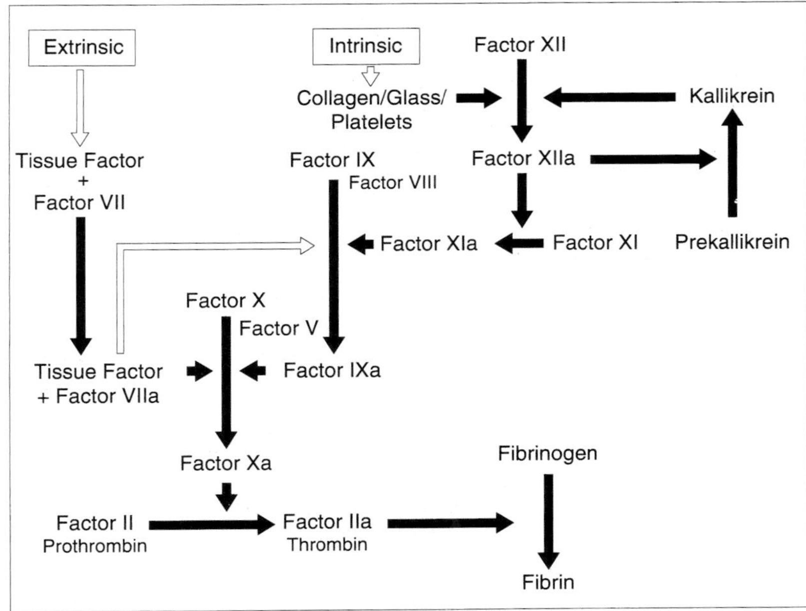

FIGURE 63–2. The coagulation system. Activation of the intrinsic or the extrinsic pathway results in the generation of thrombin and ultimately in fibrinogen-to-fibrin conversion. The tissue factor–factor VIIa complex is also able to directly activate Factor IX, which may be an important connecting link between both pathways. (From Levi M, ten Cate H, van der Poll T, et al. Pathogenesis of disseminated intravascular coagulation in sepsis. JAMA. 1993;27:975–979, with permission.)

conversion was completely blocked. Therefore, current evidence favors the concept that LPS-induced activation of coagulation is mediated in large part by TNF-α and is initially dependent on activation of the extrinsic pathway of coagulation.

Low levels of factor XII and prekallikrein and high plasma levels of complexes between kallikrein and C1 inhibitor and between factor XII and C1 inhibitor are measurable in septic patients. However, experimental studies indicate that activation of the contact system does not necessarily contribute to activation of the coagulation system in sepsis.[68] In experimental studies of *E. coli* bacteremia in baboons, blockade of the contact system by the simultaneous administration of anti–factor XII or anti–Hageman factor antibodies had no effect on the development of DIC.[65] However, inhibition of the contact activation system resulted in a reduction of *E. coli*–induced lethal hypotension. Therefore, the contact activation system of hemodynamic effects still appears to be important, and it is probably mediated by the generation of kinins, such as bradykinin, during activation of the contact system. Kinins have hypotension-inducing effects and have long been suspected of playing a role in septic shock.[69]

As might be anticipated, activation of the contact system can affect the fibrinolytic system. Activation of the contact system triggers plasminogen activator activity, initiating fibrinolysis. Activation of the contact system in septic patients does not appear truly to trigger coagulation but does seem to play an important role in the development of hypotension, which ultimately brings about activation of the fibrinolytic system.

With respect to fibrinolysis, low plasma levels of fibrinolytic proteins and inhibitors and increased plasma levels of fibrin degradation products indicate extensive activation of this system.[65] In response to coagulation, the fibrinolytic system initially becomes activated and subsequently inhibited. Healthy human volunteers given LPS or TNF-α show an increase in plasminogen activator activity.[66, 67] Both tissue-type plasminogen activator and urokinase-type plasminogen activator have been demonstrated.

The temporal relation between the appearance of TNF-α and the increase in fibrinolytic activity suggests that TNF-α is a mediator of this effect, but IL-1 may also contribute. In studies of chimpanzees given LPS in which endotoxin-induced TNF-α release was blocked, there was no activation of the fibrinolytic system after endotoxemia. In experiments in which the endotoxin-induced activation of coagulation was blocked by monoclonal antibodies inhibiting the extrinsic pathway, endotoxin-induced effects on fibrinolysis were unaffected. This supports the concept that fibrinolytic responses to endotoxin can be separated from activation of coagulation. Therefore, endotoxemia results in rapid activation and subsequent inhibition of fibrinolysis, and the response of the fibrinolytic system to endotoxin is mediated by TNF-α, resulting in inadequate removal of intravascular fibrin deposition.

PULMONARY VASCULAR ENDOTHELIAL INJURY AND THE ADULT RESPIRATORY DISTRESS SYNDROME

Various clinical settings, including infection, shock, and trauma, can trigger injury to the pulmonary vascular endothelium leading to ARDS. Models of acute lung injury leading to the development of ARDS use provocative stimuli such as endotoxin, thrombin, complement, platelet-activating factor (PAF), and arachidonate metabolites.[70] TNF-α and IL-1 appear to be central to the diverse processes leading to endothelial injury. Both LPS and thrombin induce IL-1 production at the endothelial surface.[71] IL-1 in turn induces endothelial biosynthesis of both arachidonate metabolites and PAF.[72] LPS activates complement, and complement cleavage products can induce TNF-α production, which in turn triggers the synthesis of arachidonate metabolites and PAF, which have the ability to initiate lung injury.

Both IL-1 and TNF-α have direct effects on granulocytes and endothelial cells.[73] Exposure of granulocytes to IL-1 in vitro does not facilitate adherence to cultured endothelial monolayers, but TNF-α increases granulocyte adherence within minutes. TNF-α rapidly induces surface expression of the adhesion molecule, CDW18, which is a complement receptor for CR3. Cytokine effects on granulocyte adherence to endothelial surfaces may explain the rapid margination phenomenon and granulocytopenia that follow infusion of substances such as LPS or cytokines.

Cytokines induce surface expression of an antigen, the endothelial leukocyte adhesion molecule, or ELAM-1.[70] This molecule also augments endothelial surface procoagulant activity.[71] Therefore, both IL-1 and TNF-α interact with endothelial receptors to stimulate synthesis and expression of surface proteins that recognize granulocyte surface adhesion molecules and enhance the endothelial "stickiness" for granulocytes. This stimulation is energy dependent, but once the antigen is expressed on the endothelial cell surface, endothelial metabolism is not required. In addition to direct effects on granulocyte-endothelial interactions, cytokine administration can recruit granulocytes. Pulmonary vascular endothelial injury appears to be facilitated by leukostasis and sequestration of granulocytes within the pulmonary vasculature. Coadministration of both recombinant IL-1 and TNF-α synergistically enhances pulmonary leukostasis in rabbits. Neutrophil release from the bone marrow is further facilitated and results in the release of mature neutrophils into the circulation. However, the presence of granulocytes adherent to pulmonary endothelium or in sequestered vascular channels is not essential for the development of noncardiogenic pulmonary edema. Even in neutropenic patients, complications such as ARDS occur, probably as a result of the direct effect of endotoxin-induced cytokines on endothelial surface integrity.[74]

The effects of cytokines on endothelium involve direct activities because they bind to specific endothelial cell receptors and cause morphologic changes. TNF-α also stimulates angiogenesis and neovascularization. IL-1 can enhance superoxide anion release from cultured endothelial cells. Therefore, endothelial cell–generated toxic oxygen radicals and granulocyte-derived oxygen intermediates can add to endothelial injury.

ROLE OF CYTOKINE-INDUCED PLATELET-ACTIVATING-FACTOR SYNTHESIS

Cytokines act by triggering other peptide molecules that can act on host tissues, and PAF can be produced after induction of phospholipase A_2 activity by antigens such as LPS.[73] Both IL-1 and TNF-α stimulate biosynthesis of PAF, and TNF-α–induced systemic hypotension and bowel necrosis can be prevented by PAF receptor antagonism. Because TNF-α can induce hypotension, acute lung injury or "shock lung" can contribute to hypotension and further damage to pulmonary cells. This damage, resulting in sustained hypotension as well as decreased systemic vascular resistance, can lead to increased hydrostatic pressures in the lung and increased noncardiogenic pulmonary edema.[73] Increased circulating or local levels of cytokines have been demonstrated in both experimental models of lung injury and clinical antecedents of ARDS. Furthermore, increased levels of cytokines have been demonstrated in lung parenchyma, bronchoalveolar lavage fluid, and during experimental lung injury, as well as in patients with ARDS.

An additional cytokine that induces the pulmonary vascular leak syndrome is IL-2 (although its effects might be related to TNF triggering). IL-2 recruits lymphoid elements to lung tissue and promotes growth of lymphocytes, and these cells can adhere to the microvascular endothelial surface.[52] Therefore, both IL-2 and lymphokine-activated killer cells have the potential to mediate pulmonary vascular endothelial injury as well.

CLINICAL APPROACH TO THE PATIENT

The sepsis syndrome usually is manifested by fever, but occasionally patients are hypothermic. The initial evaluation of the patient must begin with a carefully taken history. Special attention should be devoted to assessment of any underlying or predisposing disorder such as surgery, transplantation, chemotherapy, or trauma. Assessment of the treatment given to the underlying disorder and its clinical stage should also be carried out. A history of previous infections and antimicrobial treatment along with any microbiologic data that may be available from studies performed in the antecedent few weeks may often be particularly useful. In addition, symptoms or signs such as pain, erythema, swelling, or headache can all be important clues to the source and extent of an infectious process. An accurate dietary history, travel history, and exposure history, with special attention to infectious agents in contacts or in the environment, can be extremely valuable to the clinician in identification of an infectious process. Knowledge of the complications of previous treatment, such as drug reactions, can also be useful in the selection of therapy.

It is likely that a systemic infectious process, such as bacteremia or the sepsis syndrome with fever and other manifestations of systemic disease, has an initial focal source. However, a number of bacteremic infections have no known or easily identified source and are classified by the Centers for Disease Control and Prevention as "primary bacteremias." In many immunosuppressed patients, these primary bacteremias probably originate in the gastrointestinal tract. The sepsis syndrome can emanate from a localized focus of infection before bacteremia develops, and, if blood cultures are drawn early in the course of the infectious process, the bacteremia may not be documented. The administration of antimicrobial therapy can paradoxically exacerbate fever secondary to a bacteriolytic effect, which leads to endotoxin release or pyrogen release.[75]

The bedside approach to the patient involves not only an integration of the history with physical findings but a search for the clues to infection even though the patient may not have any localizing signs. A vigorous attempt should be made to obtain infected secretions or body fluids or to aspirate an area that is suspicious for infection, such as the advancing edge of cellulitis. Microbiologic studies should include not only blood cultures but study of any potential source of a systemic infection. If the patient has diarrhea, examination of the stool for fecal leukocytes and stool cultures may be appropriate, as may studies to detect *Clostridium difficile* toxin.

A complete physical examination should be undertaken as expeditiously as possible. Immunosuppressed and neutropenic patients may have a blunted inflammatory response, and typical signs of infection, such as induration, fluctuance, local heat, reactive lymphadenopathy, and exudation of pus, may not be present. Immunosuppressed patients may also have suppressed cough mechanisms and not produce purulent sputum or other exudates. Even with urinary tract infection, neutropenic or immunosuppressed patients may not have classic localizing symptoms or pyuria. In immunosuppressed patients with meningitis, the signs of nuchal rigidity may be absent, but two important clues remain: headache and impaired mental status. Erythema is a reliable clue to the presence of infection irrespective of the absolute leukocyte count and, along with pain, erythema may be more useful in the detection of a localized infectious process than swelling and warmth in immunosuppressed patients.

The selection of laboratory studies should be based on the physical findings and the overall clinical manifestations. Because the sepsis syndrome implies systemic disease, at least two sets of blood cultures taken at different sites should be obtained to detect bacteremia. In addition to sampling any potential focus of infection, a lumbar puncture should be performed for the patient who has an altered mental status or more specific signs of central nervous system infection, provided there is no evidence of increased intracranial pressure or of a focal supratentorial lesion.

If the clinical situation is deteriorating and the patient appears to be seriously ill, it is wise to obtain as many diagnostic studies as possible expeditiously and to initiate empirical antimicrobial therapy. Treatment can subsequently be modified if necessary for those patients with positive blood cultures. In practice, much of the therapy given in hospitals today is empirical, based on history, intuition, and bedside suspicion of the most likely infecting pathogens. The presence of sepsis syndrome, with the potential for shock and other severe complications, usually mandates prompt treatment.

Clearly, the status of host defense mechanisms and the ability to maintain function of vital organs are the factors that determine the outcome of any blood stream infection. Table 63–6 summarizes, in order of estimated importance, some of the factors that affect prognosis. In addition to underlying diseases and complications, several other factors have significant effects. Although quantitative blood cultures are now infrequently performed, several studies indicate that mortality is greater with high-grade bacteremia and with polymicrobial bacteremia.[76] The absence of a discernible focus of infection

TABLE 63-6 Factors Affecting the Outcome of Systemic Bacterial Infection

Underlying conditions
Neutropenia
Hypogammaglobulinemia
Diabetes
Alcoholism ± cirrhosis
Renal failure
Respiratory failure
Complications of the infectious event at the onset of treatment (e.g., shock, anuria)
Antimicrobial chemotherapy
Grade (severity) of bacteremia (polymicrobial bacteremia)
Source of infection
Interval after initiation of treatment
Age

may also be associated with a poorer prognosis. Age may have an impact on outcome, because a poorer survival rate is seen in the very young and in the older age groups. The selection of antimicrobial therapy and the rapidity with which it is administered can also affect outcome.[77] Detectable cytokine levels may be ephemeral, but sustained elevations of serum TNF-α (as well as LPS) have been linked to decreased survival in meningococcemia and gram-negative bacteremia.[78, 79]

ANTIMICROBIAL THERAPY FOR THE SEPSIS SYNDROME

Early clinical suspicion, rigorous diagnostic measures, aggressive initiation of appropriate antimicrobial therapy, comprehensive supportive care, and measures aimed at reversing predisposing causes are the cornerstones of successful management. It is obvious that clinical suspicion of the bacterial sepsis syndrome should promptly be confirmed by rapid identification and antimicrobial susceptibility testing of disease-causing organisms. Diagnostic microbiologic techniques are covered in more detail in Chapter 14.

Antimicrobial therapy remains the mainstay of treatment of the sepsis syndrome, but approaches aimed at correcting the predisposition to this complication have a critical bearing on the outcome of the infection. Amelioration of an underlying disease, such as achievement of remission in leukemia, is usually the major factor determining recovery, regardless of the choice of antimicrobial agents. The removal of foreign bodies that predispose to or potentiate infection, such as intravascular or urinary catheters, may alone cause resolution of symptoms and lead to a cure. Transient bacteremia is a well-documented event, particularly with urinary tract manipulation, and the latter accounts for a number of instances in which bacteremic patients have been cured either with inappropriate antibiotics or with no antimicrobial therapy at all.[77, 80] A major corollary of this observation is that attempts to drain abscesses or to remove obvious sources of infection such as obstructed abdominal viscera are of paramount importance in determining recovery. Antimicrobial sterilization of large abscesses seems futile, although it is possible that small foci of infection could be sterilized by aggressive antimicrobial therapy alone.

Analyses of the status of host factors, the severity of underlying disease, and the outcome of gram-negative bacillary bacteremia have consistently demonstrated increasing mortality in patients with "nonfatal," "ultimately fatal," and "rapidly fatal" disease. The classification of underlying disease, as proposed by McCabe and Jackson[81] and by others,[82] assumes critical importance when treatment results are compared, because of the heterogeneity of predisposing or underlying conditions. It is clearly unfair and unscientific to compare therapeutic results in patients with transient bacteremia secondary to a kidney stone (usually these are patients with nonfatal underlying disease) with results in patients who develop bacteremia during chemotherapy for acute unremitting leukemia (the usual example of a rapidly fatal disease). Classification of patients with postsurgical or post-traumatic conditions is more difficult, but for the most part intra-abdominal infections complicating surgical procedures or traumatic injury occur in nonimmunosuppressed patients without obvious derangement in host defense mechanisms.

During the 1960s, several major published reports indicated that appropriate antimicrobial therapy for gram-negative bacillary bacteremia (as defined by antimicrobials that inhibited the infecting strain) significantly reduced mortality in patients with nonfatal or ultimately fatal disease.[81, 82] Studies carried out since 1968 in patients with cancer and neutropenia have shown a general overall improvement in clinical response rates. Most of the studies of patients with neutropenia reported since 1985 showed survival rates ranging from 40 to 85%, especially with some of the most potent modern treatment regimens.[83, 84] These clinical trials have enrolled neutropenic patients because of their increased risk for sepsis and the relative ease in organizing evaluations of drug treatments in this patient population.

Many factors besides the introduction of new antimicrobial agents could account for the improved therapeutic results observed even in immunosuppressed patients. These factors include more aggressive approaches to diagnosis and the initiation of treatment, overall improvements in supportive care, and many of the adjunctive measures detailed in subsequent sections of this chapter.

One attitude that has become widely accepted in approaches to suspected infection in the critically ill has been the willingness to begin empirical broad-spectrum therapy before the results of cultures are obtained.[85] This approach has inherent dangers, such as the selection for antimicrobial resistance and the risk of drug toxicity. There are some patients with apparently intact host defenses in whom empirical therapy may not be indicated because there is adequate time to obtain material for culture and sensitivity testing (e.g., subacute bacterial endocarditis in a patient without congestive heart failure or emboli).

It is only logical that clinicians have used combinations of antimicrobial agents for serious infections, particularly for those patients with the most adverse prognostic factors. The supporting arguments for combination therapy are multiple and not mutually exclusive. (1) Combination therapy makes it possible to cover a broad range of diagnostic possibilities including both gram-positive and gram-negative infection, which may be difficult to distinguish clinically. (2) Because polymicrobial bacteremia may be present, the use of two agents, rather than being duplicative, may give appropriate therapy for dual infections. (3) The use of two agents may prevent the emergence of resistance by eliminating small subpopulations that are resistant to one of the components of the combination. (4) Two antimicrobials may interact either additively or synergistically, thereby enhancing the sum of antimicrobial activity or (in the case of synergy) permitting a reduction in dosage of one component of the combination, such as the agent that is potentially more toxic. Although there is no universally accepted definition of antimicrobial synergy and in practice dosage reduction is not usually carried out, there has been considerable investigative interest in determining whether the use of so-called synergistic combinations is associated with improved clinical results in humans. Experimental studies in animals with normal circulating granulocyte counts and in those rendered neutropenic have shown that use of synergistic combinations leads to a more favorable outcome in *P. aeruginosa* infections.[86] Several human studies have shown an association between the use of combinations that interact synergistically against infecting strains and improved clinical results.[87, 88]

Because multiple agents are usually given on different dosage schedules, it has been difficult to ensure that the drug concentrations that are achieved in vivo reflect test concentrations used in in vitro studies. The finding by one group of serum inhibitory titers equal to or exceeding 1:8 was associated with a favorable clinical outcome.[89] Still, it is possible that good clinical results obtained when using combinations of antimicrobial agents may not be related to synergistic interactions. For instance, with such commonly used agents as aminoglycosides and penicillins, which often interact synergistically in vitro, "peak" blood levels that are used to gauge in vitro susceptibility are actually maintained for rather short periods, followed by periods of rapid "decay." The use of a broad-spectrum penicillin with an aminoglycoside may merely ensure a more sustained interval of serum inhibitory or bactericidal activity or avoid too low "trough" levels of such activity. For critically ill patients with septicemia, it is implicit that all pharmacologic agents should be administered via the intravenous route.

A principle of empirical therapy is to provide broad initial coverage. Table 63–7 summarizes recommendations for initial empirical therapy for presumed gram-negative infection as the cause of the sepsis syndrome, but these regimens also provide coverage for *S. aureus* and streptococci (except enterococci). First- and second-generation cephalosporins alone may be justified for community-acquired bacteremia secondary to urinary tract infection in the non-neutropenic host where *E. coli* and *Klebsiella* are the main concerns. For the patient with nosocomial infection, initial therapy should consist of an aminoglycoside initially paired with a β-lactam agent. Preference is expressed for a cephalosporin as the β-lactam agent in the non-neutropenic patient because of the greater likelihood of *Klebsiella* and *Staphylococcus*. The regimen of an aminoglycoside paired with a penicillin or cephalosporin having antipseudomonal activity is preferred for the neutropenic patient, the patient receiving assisted ventilation, and the patient with an extensive burn injury.

The third-generation cephalosporins, related β-lactam agents, carbapenems such as imipenem, and monobactam agents such as aztreonam have markedly augmented activity against enteric bacteria but variable bactericidal effect against *P. aeruginosa*. The potency of cefotaxime, ceftizoxime, and ceftriaxone against *E. coli* and *Klebsiella* (minimal inhibitory concentrations often 0.5 μg/ml or less with achievable blood levels 100-fold or more higher) suggests that single-agent therapy directed against those bacteria may be successful even in severely compromised hosts. In contrast, resistance among *Pseudomonas*, *Serratia*, and *Enterobacter* species may emerge rapidly with monotherapy. Ceftazidime, cefepime, imipenem, and meropenem appear most active against *P. aeruginosa*. Monotherapeutic regimens (e.g., ceftazidime, imipenem, or a fluoroquinolone with good activity against gram-positive organisms, such as levofloxacin) may be effective for fevers of undetermined origin in neutropenic patients and for documented infections caused by highly susceptible gram-negative bacteria.[90] Cefepime appears to be an alternative to ceftazidime, as meropenem is an alternative to imipenem. Guidelines for initial use of antimicrobial agents in febrile neutropenic patients have been updated by the Infectious Diseases Society of America.[91]

Clinicians should not assume that the administration of apparently adequate doses of antimicrobial agents consistently ensures therapeutic levels. Aminoglycosides have a narrow therapeutic ratio, and there is marked variability in the individual peak blood levels of gentamicin.[92] Studies of patients with recurrent or breakthrough bacteremia have indicated an association with subinhibitory blood levels of agents such as gentamicin.[93] In view of the variations in blood pharmacokinetics of aminoglycosides, it would seem prudent in the critically ill patient to monitor blood levels frequently. There is some evidence that such monitoring may also avert potentially toxic complications.[94] The measurement of aminoglycoside blood levels usually is not indicated in patients with bacteremia from the genitourinary tract, inasmuch as the levels of many agents excreted in the urine are high. The average duration of treatment in normal hosts experiencing gram-negative sepsis is 10 to 14 days, but this may be longer if the patient has persistent infection at the source of bacteremia. Treatment of the neutropenic or immunocompromised patient may require an even longer duration. Patients in the latter group should be afebrile for a minimum of 4 to 7 days and have evidence of resolving infection at the source of bacteremia, and the neutrophil count should be rising and higher than 500/μl before drug therapy is stopped. The exception to this guideline would be patients with marrow failure syndromes, who are unlikely to generate leukocyte counts as high as 500/μl; in these subjects clinical defervescence alone should suffice.

Oral therapy is ill advised for the bacteremic patient with fever, hemodynamic instability, and factors that might limit absorption of antimicrobial agents from the gut. On the other hand, a change to an effective oral agent (as determined by in vitro testing) is often justified after defervescence if the patient's overall condition is improving. Potentially useful agents include the quinolones and some oral β-lactam agents.

TABLE 63–7 Recommended Antimicrobial Regimens for Initial (Presumptive) Therapy for the Sepsis Syndrome*

1. Community-acquired infection in the non-neutropenic patient (neutrophil count ≥1000/mm³)
    a. Suspected urinary tract source: a third-generation cephalosporin; a quinolone; or piperacillin, mezlocillin, ticarcillin ± an aminoglycoside
    b. Nonurinary tract source: a third-generation cephalosporin (+ metronidazole); or ticarcillin-clavulanate or ampicillin-sulbactam or piperacillin-tazobactam ± an aminoglycoside
2. Hospital-acquired infection, non-neutropenic patient: cefepime, a third-generation cephalosporin ± metronidazole, or ticarcillin-clavulanate or ampicillin-sulbactam or piperacillin-tazobactam, or imipenem; all + an aminoglycoside
3. Hospital-acquired infection, neutropenic patient: ticarcillin-clavulanate, or piperacillin-tazobactam + an aminoglycoside; or imipenem/meropenem ± an aminoglycoside or ceftazidime + an aminoglycoside
4. Thermal injury to at least 20% of the body surface area: ceftriaxone (ceftazidime) + an aminoglycoside; or vancomycin + antipseudomonal penicillin + an aminoglycoside
5. Established or suspected gentamicin resistance: use amikacin as the aminoglycoside
6. Evidence of indwelling vascular catheter infection: add vancomycin

* Regimens are choices for initial therapy and should be modified on the basis of culture results.

ADJUNCTIVE MEASURES IN THE TREATMENT OF THE SEPSIS SYNDROME

Maintenance of Adequate Tissue Perfusion with Volume Replacement

Management of fluid and electrolyte balance is a crucial aspect of the care of the patient with the sepsis syndrome, particularly if the course is complicated by shock. Perfusion of vital organs such as the brain and kidney must be maintained. It is clear that the body has an order of priorities that results in distribution of blood preferentially to vital organs; this causes splanchnic vasoconstriction as well as a marked reduction of circulation to the skin. When these compensatory changes are inadequate to maintain perfusion, central arterial pressure falls. The first goal of management of the patient with severe sepsis, particularly in the incipient stages of shock, is adequate monitoring of vital signs so that any hemodynamic changes can be readily counteracted. Insertion of a central venous pressure monitoring device, an arterial catheter, and Swan-Ganz catheters to determine the left atrial end-diastolic pressure are widely used measures in the critically ill, although it is clear that they present certain infection hazards. These monitoring devices are not used to determine optimal therapy but rather the limits of therapy. In other words, normal or low central venous pressure and left atrial end-diastolic pressures (pulmonary wedge pressures) in the presence of a declining systemic arterial blood pressure are an indication for further volume replacement. On the other hand, these parameters may rise to dangerous levels without being able to restore adequate arterial perfusion, and cautious use of inotropic agents should be considered in that setting (see later discussion).

There are a number of solutions that can be used to expand intravascular fluid volume and colloid oncotic pressure, including normal saline solution, fresh frozen plasma, albumin of the regular type or salt depleted, and various dextran preparations. If the patient is anemic as well as hypotensive, the transfusion of whole blood in the face of a low central venous pressure is justified. If there is no need for erythrocytes, one of the plasma fractions will suffice. With evidence for bleeding and consumption coagulopathy, the use of fresh frozen plasma may be indicated. There has been a tendency to avoid dextran preparations because of an association with hemorrhagic incidents. Other authorities have used crystalloid solutions in preference to colloid.[95] There is no evidence that exchange transfusions or plasmapheresis is beneficial for patients in septic shock.

Use of Sympathomimetic Amines

Sympathomimetic amines have been widely used to treat the hemodynamic complications of shock, but there have been no controlled or comparative studies of the efficacy of different compounds. For many years, norepinephrine and epinephrine were the principal agents available. Norepinephrine has intense peripheral vasoconstricting activity; the extravasation around intravenous infusion sites has led to ischemic necrosis of tissues. There is justifiable concern that its use compromises the perfusion of vital organs. Both norepinephrine and epinephrine increase myocardial irritability. Alternative agents such as isoproterenol, dopamine, and dobutamine have largely supplanted norepinephrine. They have an inotropic effect on myocardial function but because of β-adrenergic activity are capable of enhancing peripheral tissue perfusion. Isoproterenol increases the cardiac index but has little effect on mean arterial pressure.[96] Dopamine causes vasodilatation of renal, coronary, and cerebral blood flow while causing an increase in systolic blood pressure and heart rate and an effective reduction in the blood supplied to skeletal muscle. Dobutamine has little chronotropic activity and is otherwise similar to dopamine. Norepinephrine should be reserved only for those patients in whom it is not possible to support systemic blood pressure and vascular perfusion with dopamine or isoproterenol. Table 63–8 is a summary of recommended doses and techniques for administering sympathomimetic amines.

Sympathomimetic agents have important side effects, particularly on pulmonary airway passages and blood sugar. None of these considerations is as important as perfusion of vital organs during septic shock. Perhaps the critical factor that is often neglected in the management of patients with sympathomimetic amines is the relation between fluid therapy and the use of these agents. It is inappropriate to use dopamine and isoproterenol before aggressive volume replacement. If they are used in the presence of a reduced intravascular fluid volume, the vasodilatation secondary to β-adrenergic stimulation can cause a paradoxical decline in blood pressure and decreased tissue perfusion because of the sudden drop in effective intravascular volume. Because of this danger, monitoring of central venous pressure and pulmonary wedge pressure is indicated; some authors advocate fluid replacement to the point that either or both of the latter begin to rise to the upper limits of normal. At that juncture it would be appropriate to use an agent such as dopamine, dobutamine, or isoproterenol if the patient remains hypotensive.

Even with volume replacement and sympathomimetic amine administration, significant metabolic acidosis may ensue. Although primary efforts should still be aimed at enhancing tissue perfusion, temporary correction of acidosis may be achieved with infusions of sodium bicarbonate.

TABLE 63–8 Sympathomimetic Amines for Support of the Circulation in Septic Shock*

1. Dopamine, 2–25 μg/kg/min: increase the rate of infusion (D_5W or saline) q15–20 min until systolic blood pressure exceeds 90 mmHg and the urine output exceeds 30 ml/hr
2. Dobutamine, 2–25 μg/kg/min: titrate as with dopamine
3. Isoproterenol, 5 μg/ml/min: observe the effect within 15–25 min and double the rate of infusion if necessary
4. Norepinephrine: give a test dose of 0.1–0.2 μ/kg and observe the response (usually in minutes). The normal maintenance dose is 0.05 μg/kg/min delivered via a plastic catheter into a large peripheral or central vein

*Listed in order of preference, to be used after volume replacement and with careful monitoring of ECG, CVP, and BP.
Abbreviations: BP, Blood pressure; CVP, central venous pressure; D_5W, 5% dextrose in water; ECG, electrocardiogram.

Role of Corticosteroids in the Treatment of Gram-Negative Rod Septicemia and Its Complications

There have been decades of controversy over the effectiveness of corticosteroids as adjunctive therapy in the management of infection. Corticosteroids have a variety of metabolic, anti-inflammatory, and immunosuppressive effects. It is commonly observed that their short-term administration often results in defervescence, leading to a clinical impression of improvement. Weitzman and Berger emphasized the lack of convincing evidence from controlled studies that corticosteroids accelerate the rate of recovery or lower mortality from sepsis.[97] Much of the belief that steroids are useful in septic shock was derived from animal studies wherein healthy experimental subjects of varying susceptibility to the effects of bacterial endotoxin were given large doses of these substances to induce shock.

A major issue related to the efficacy of corticosteroids in human septic shock is dosage. Because relatively low doses (up to 1 mg/kg of betamethasone, or roughly 25–30 mg/kg equivalent of hydrocortisone) were used in one well-controlled, prospective study and showed no beneficial effect,[98] advocates of corticosteroid therapy have escalated their recommendations. One study reported a beneficial effect of corticosteroids in doses of 30 mg/kg of methylprednisolone or 2 mg/kg of dexamethasone.[99] Doses in this range were found to improve survival in one controlled clinical trial in patients with typhoid fever.[100] Another comparative study found that large doses of corticosteroids (2 g of methylprednisolone for the 70-kg patient) actually reversed septic shock in a significant number of patients. Although a transient, "early" effect in increased survival was noted, mortality at the conclusion of the study was similar in both groups, and steroid recipients had a higher incidence of superinfection.[101] Despite these results, however, the largest and most comprehensive controlled clinical trials in the United States have failed to confirm the beneficial effect of corticosteroids in septic shock. This conclusion was reached in the final report of a multicenter collaborative trial involving the Veterans Affairs Hospitals[102] and a multihospital collaborative group.[103] Two additional controlled human trials employed similar doses of corticosteroids for ARDS patients and obtained negative results.[104, 105] In view of these findings, large doses of prednisone, prednisolone, or dexamethasone cannot be recommended as adjunctive therapy for sepsis or shock. Replacement doses of corticosteroids are clearly justified in suspected adrenal insufficiency.

Anticoagulation

The use of anticoagulation, particularly heparinization, to treat septicemic states associated with DIC is logical because there is strong experimental and human clinical evidence that coagulopathy can be terminated by heparinization. At present, however, it is unclear whether anticoagulation has any effect in prolonging survival, however desirable it may be to abolish the sequence of events leading to clotting, consumption of clotting factors, and the onset or aggravation of bleeding. In both human and experimental animals, the use of agents such as heparin has failed to decrease significantly the mortality from bacteremic gram-negative infections.[106, 107] In human infection, the failure to show a difference may be related to the overall poor prognosis of the underlying disease that is complicated by bacteremia. Until a consistent reduction in mortality can be shown, the use of routine anticoagulation in the management of patients with DIC should be avoided especially in normotensive patients. If bleeding in such patients is associated with depressed levels of platelets or a specific factor, replacement therapy may be required to control the hemorrhage.

For hypotensive septicemic patients, measures aimed at controlling the infection and correcting hemodynamic alterations (volume replacement and sympathomimetic amines) are of primary importance. If the blood pressure responds to such measures (an effect is usually observed within 4 hours), consumption coagulopathy usually ceases. If the patient has bleeding because of the coagulopathy and not from another cause such as an associated gastrointestinal ulcer, replacement therapy is indicated. This should consist of platelet transfusions for thrombocytopenia, cryoprecipitate preparations for hypofibrinogenemia, and fresh-frozen plasma for depleted coagulation factors. Although this approach theoretically could aggravate coagulopathy by providing additional substrate for clotting, this complication is not commonly observed when replacement therapy is used in conjunction with measures aimed at controlling shock and infection.[108]

For patients with refractory shock and coagulopathy despite the preceding measures, heparin therapy may be beneficial in terminating DIC (without evidence that this prolongs life). Other patients who should be considered for anticoagulation are those who appear to have pulmonary embolic phenomena. This includes patients with pelvic thrombophlebitis. Heparin may be given by either intermittent or continuous infusion. The dose for intermittent infusion is 50 to 100 U/kg of aqueous heparin given by bolus infusion every 4 hours. For continuous infusion, the recommended dose of heparin in adult therapy is 10,000 U made up in 500 ml of 5% dextrose in water (D_5W) delivered over a period of approximately 4 to 6 hours. Because reversal of coagulation tendencies has an immediate effect, it would appear judicious to terminate therapy as soon as possible after the subsidence of fever.

Therapeutic Role of Granulocyte Transfusion and Colony-Stimulating Factors

Granulocyte transfusions were once popular for treatment of infections in neutropenic subjects, and their use was supported by the results of clinical trials.[109, 110] Subsequently, a much larger study that randomly assigned patients with documented gram-negative bacteremia to receive or not to receive neutrophil transfusions showed no difference in recovery rates or survival, even in the subset of patients without evidence of bone marrow recovery.[111] Correction of neutropenia is a desirable, although sometimes unattainable, goal in treatment of shock in the neutropenic patient. Use of granulocyte transfusions is discussed in Chapter 298. Guidelines for use of colony-stimulating factors (CSFs) are given in Chapters 37, 298, and 299.

Diuretics

Diuretics are commonly used in the management of the early oliguric or anuric phases of bacteremic shock. The use of agents such as furosemide is controversial, however, because there is no controlled study demonstrating that acute renal failure may be avoided by the aggressive use of such agents. The action of potent loop diuretics such as furosemide usually results in a significant increase in the output of dilute urine, but it is unclear whether the aggressive use of diuretics in the early oliguric phases of shock makes the ensuing renal failure less severe. What has been observed is that some agents such as furosemide may cause deafness, and there may be enhanced toxicity when these agents are simultaneously used with agents that can damage eighth-nerve or renal function, such as aminoglycoside antibiotics.

THERAPEUTIC ANTISERUM AND CYTOKINE INHIBITION IN SEPSIS

The use of antiserum to treat bacterial infections antedates the antimicrobial era, but was all but abandoned 5 decades ago. Resurgent interest in the therapeutic applications of antibody stems from the persistently high mortality rate associated with the gram-negative sepsis syndrome complicated by shock despite the use of appropriate antimicrobials.[112] There have been anecdotal reports of the successful use of antiserum for *P. aeruginosa* infection.[112] Ziegler and associates[113] reported the results of a large multicenter, double-blind, controlled trial of therapeutic antiserum prepared by immunizing donors with the J5 mutant of *E. coli* O111, a "rough mutant" with an LPS "core" structure. Mortality was 22% in 103 bacteremic recipients of antiserum and 39% in 109 similar subjects who received control serum therapy.[113] An even more significant difference was noted in the ability of antiserum to reverse profound shock. Therapeutic antiserum did not, however, significantly affect survival rates in patients with cancer and/or neutropenia, and no protective antibody titer or level could be inferred. A clinical trial of intravenous immunoglobulin G (IgG) was unsuccessful, possibly because of low titer or because IgG antibodies are not protective.[114]

The first large-scale, double-blind human trials aimed at reducing mortality in gram-negative sepsis syndrome used humanized[115] or murine[116] IgM antibodies directed against the "core" region (lipid A) or LPS. Although the initial results with these antibodies were considered positive and showed benefit in selected subgroups, subsequent reexamination of the original monoclonal data[117, 118] and the completion of subsequent human trials with the same intervention failed to confirm the original results.[119, 120] A similar disappointing pattern of clinical trial results has been observed with the use of recombinant IL-receptor antagonist (IL-1Ra),[121] monoclonal antibodies to TNF-α,[122, 123] and TNF-α receptors (p75 and p55) fused with IgG.[124, 125] In fact, trials of TNF-p75 receptor construct attempting to dampen the cytokine response suggested a deleterious effect in a subset of patients with gram-positive infections.[124] Similarly, clinical trials of pharmacologic agents in septic shock such as PAF antagonists,[126] bradykinin inhibitors,[127] and inhibitors of iNOS[61] have been disappointingly negative. These results provoked considerable discussion about the discordance between experimental data in animals and human trial results and prompted efforts to improve clinical trial design.[118, 128, 129] Major factors underlying the failure of these interventions include the timeliness of the intervention and the severity of underlying disease in the patients studied. The latter would make it difficult for any intervention to affect mortality end points. Because TNF-α and NO have beneficial effects on host defense, it remains a challenge to modulate their toxic effects during sepsis precisely.[130, 131]

PROPHYLAXIS OF SEPSIS

Measures to prevent sepsis have included meticulous efforts aimed at limiting the spread of infection within the hospital, the use of prophylactic antimicrobial agents of a topical or systemic form, management of high-risk patients in so-called protective environments, active or passive immunoprophylaxis with type-specific or cross-reactive antibodies, augmentation of the host granulocyte pool with prophylactic granulocyte transfusions, and stimulation of bone marrow with CSFs. It seems reasonable that the simplest and most cost-effective measures for the prophylaxis of gram-negative bacillary infections would involve minimizing the infection hazard associated with such procedures as Foley catheterization and prolonged intravascular catheterization. Logical applications of antimicrobial prophylaxis include topical application to the skin, the use of an oropharyngeal spray, and orally ingested nonabsorbable antibiotics to suppress the fecal flora. The application of topical agents such as silver nitrate, silver sulfadiazine, or sulfamylon to burned skin appears to have reduced significantly the incidence of burn wound sepsis caused by organisms such as *P. aeruginosa*.[132] The application of a polymyxin spray to the posterior portion of the pharynx appears to limit gram-negative bacillary colonization of the oropharynx and to prevent some cases of nosocomial gram-negative pneumonia.[133] However, such efforts offer the potential hazard of selecting for the emergence of organisms resistant to the prophylactic agent, as has been amply documented with the use of polymyxin sprays.[134]

Because the gastrointestinal tract is a vast reservoir of gram-negative bacilli, an essentially topical approach to prophylaxis is the use of oral nonabsorbable antimicrobial agents. Sterilization of bowel contents is unrealistic, but suppression of the aerobic fecal flora has been achieved to varying degrees with regimens that use polymyxin[135] or gentamicin[136] orally with vancomycin and nystatin. Randomized studies have shown a significant reduction in bacterial sepsis in neutropenic subjects given a polymyxin-containing regimen, compared with placebo.[135] The efficacy of gentamicin-vancomycin-nystatin has been assessed in a three-arm study with management of neutropenic patients in "protected environments" with laminar airflow and under regular ward care.[136] The reduction in infection was similar for both groups receiving oral antimicrobials and was not significantly greater for those additionally managed in laminar airflow rooms.

Regimens containing oral nonabsorbable agents are unpalatable, and patient compliance has been variable. Better-tolerated alternatives include trimethoprim-sulfamethoxazole[137] and the newer quinolones. Trimethoprim-sulfamethoxazole has been used to prevent both *Pneumocystis carinii* pneumonia and bacterial infection. It has no effect against *P. aeruginosa* and may predispose to superinfection with fungi and resistant bacilli. Some studies suggested a significant reduction in gram-negative infections occurring in neutropenic patients given quinolones but without any overall survival benefit.[91] Even more aggressive approaches have included both orally and systemically administered antibodies to achieve "gut decontamination." These approaches are controversial because no consistent benefit has been demonstrated, and there is concern about selection of resistant organisms.

AUGMENTATION OF HOST DEFENSES: GRANULOCYTE TRANSFUSIONS, COLONY-STIMULATING FACTORS, AND IMMUNOPROPHYLAXIS

In patients who are neutropenic or likely to become so, use of prophylactic granulocyte transfusions has been replaced by prophylactic CSFs. Benefit has been variable, but some studies show a decreased incidence of fevers, diminished use of systemic antibodies, and shortened hospitalizations.[138, 139]

With respect to the feasibility of immunoprophylaxis in the prevention of gram-negative bacteremia, the impetus for this approach is the convincing evidence that some bacterial infections can be prevented by active or passive immunization with either cell wall components of certain bacteria or toxoid preparations of extracellular toxins. Particularly with toxoid immunization (e.g., tetanus), immunity appears to be lifelong. Gram-positive infections, such as pneumococcal disease or group B streptococcal disease, may be prevented to some degree in selected populations by immunization or antimicrobial prophylaxis (see Chapters 188 and 190). Immunization of experimental animals or healthy people with a *Pseudomonas* LPS vaccine led to some augmentation of circulating antibody levels against these seven LPS antigens.[140] Some evidence exists from studies of patients with burn injuries that this vaccine is protective, but definitive double-blind controlled studies are lacking.[141] Other *Pseudomonas* LPS antigens have been used in controlled studies in burn patients, and the results have been significantly in favor of immunization.[142] A randomized, prospective study of *Pseudomonas* immunization in cancer patients showed some overall reduction in *Pseudomonas* infections as well as *Pseudomonas*-associated mortality but no significant reduction in bacteremic *P. aeruginosa* infections.[140]

Therefore, it appears that immunization alone is not likely to be successful in the prevention of gram-negative bacteremia in markedly immunosuppressed patients, particularly those who are neutropenic. Passive immunization with transfused antibodies is an alternative. Transfused immunoglobulins appear to be appropriate for hypogammaglobulinemic patients, but convincing evidence of prophylactic efficacy in preventing sepsis and related disorders in normal subjects is lacking.[143]

REFERENCES

1. Bone RC, Balk RA, Cerra FB, et al. Definitions for sepsis and organ failure and guidelines for the use of innovative therapies in sepsis. Chest. 1992;101:1644–1655.
2. American College of Chest Physicians/Society of Critical Care Medicine Consensus Conference Committee. Definitions for sepsis and organ failure and guidelines for the use of innovative therapies in sepsis. Crit Care Med. 1992;20:864–874.
3. Billiau A, Vandekerckhove F. Cytokines and their interactions with other inflammatory mediators in the pathogenesis of sepsis and septic shock. Eur J Clin Invest. 1991;21:559–573.
4. Beutler B, ed. Tumor Necrosis Factors: The Molecules and Their Emerging Role in Medicine. New York: Raven; 1992.
5. Bone RC. Toward an epidemiology and natural history of SIRS (systemic inflammatory response syndrome). JAMA. 1992;268:3452–3455.
6. Rangel-Frausto S, Pittet D, Costigan M, et al. The natural history of the systemic inflammatory response syndrome (SIRS): A prospective study. JAMA. 1995;273:117–123.
7. Rangel-Frausto S, Pittet D, Hwang T, et al. The dynamics of disease progression in sepsis: Markov modeling describing the natural history and the likely impact of effective antisepsis agents. Clin Infect Dis. 1988;27:185–190.
8. U.S. Department of Health and Human Services, Public Health Services: National nosocomial infectious surveillance (NNIS) report: Data summary for October 1986–April 1997. Am J Infect Control. 1997;25:477–487.
9. Martin MA. Epidemiology and clinical impact of gram-negative sepsis. Infect Dis Clin North Am. 1991;5:739–752.
10. Centers for Disease Control and Prevention. Increase in national hospital discharge survey rates for septicemia—United States, 1979–1987. MMWR Morb Mortal Wkly Rep. 1990;39:31–34.
11. National Center for Health Statistics. Health, United States, 1998 with Socioeconomic Status and Health Chartbook. DHHS Publication No. (PHS) 98-1232. Hyattsville, Md: NCHS; 1998:217 (Table 4).
12. Schaberg DR, Culver DH, Gaines KP. Major trends in the microbial etiology of nosocomial infection. Am J Med. 1991;90:725–735.
13. National Nosocomial Infections Surveillance (NNIS) System. Nosocomial infection rates for interhospital comparison: Limitations and possible solutions. Infect Control Hosp Epidemiol. 1991;12:609–621.
14. Gunnar RM, Loeb HS, Winslow EJ, et al. Hemodynamic measurements in bacteremic and septic shock in man. J Infect Dis. 1973;128:287.
15. Sprung CL, Peduzzi PN, Shatney CH, et al. Impact of encephalopathy on mortality in the sepsis syndrome. Crit Care Med. 1990;18:801–806.
16. Stevens DL, Tanner MH, Winship J, et al. Reappearance of scarlet fever toxin among streptococci in the Rocky Mountain West: Severe group A streptococcal infections associated with a toxic shock–like syndrome. N Engl J Med. 1989;321:1–7.
17. Dorff GJ, Geimer NF, Rosenthal DR, et al. *Pseudomonas* septicemia. Arch Intern Med. 1971;128:591.
18. Davis WA II, Kane JG, Garagusi VF. Human *Aeromonas* infections: A review of the literature and a case report of endocarditis. Medicine (Baltimore). 1978;57:267.
19. Fisher KW, Berger B, Keusch GT. Subepidermal bullae due to *E. coli*. Arch Dermatol. 1974;110:105.
20. Forkner CE, Frei E III, Edgcomb JH, et al. *Pseudomonas* septicemia. Observations on twenty-three cases. Am J Med. 1958;25:877.
21. Hopewell PC, Murray JS. The adult respiratory distress syndrome. Annu Rev Med. 1976;181:343.
22. Young LS, Proctor RA, Beutler B, et al. University of California/Davis Interdepartmental Conference on Gram-Negative Septicemia. Rev Infect Dis. 1991;13:666–687.
23. Wenzel RP, Pinsky MR, Ulevitch RJ, Young L. Current understanding of sepsis. Clin Infect Dis. 1996;22:407–413.
24. Rothstein JL, Schreiber H. Synergy between tumor necrosis factor and bacterial products causes hemorrhagic necrosis and lethal shock in normal mice. Proc Natl Acad Sci U S A. 1988;85:607–611.
25. Cannon JG, Tompkins RG, Gelfand JA, et al. Circulating interleukin-1 and tumor necrosis factor in septic shock and experimental endotoxin fever. J Infect Dis. 1990;161:79–97.
26. Heremans H, Van Damme J, Dillen C, et al. Interferon-γ, a mediator of lethal lipopolysaccharide-induced Shwartzman-like shock reactions in mice. J Exp Med. 1990;171:1853–1869.
27. Martich GD, Danner RL, Ceska M, et al. Detection of interleukin 8 and tumor necrosis factor in normal humans after intravenous endotoxin: The effect of anti-inflammatory agents. J Exp Med. 1991;173:1021–1024.
28. Parrillo JE. Pathogenetic mechanisms of septic shock. N Engl J Med. 1993;328:1471–1477.
29. van Deuren M, van der Ven-Jongekrijg J, Demacker PNM, et al. Differential expression of proinflammatory cytokines and their inhibitors during the course of meningococcal infections. J Infect Dis. 1994;169:157–161.
30. Okusawa S, Gelfland JA, Ikejima T, et al. Interleukin 1 induces a shock-like state in rabbits: Synergism with tumor necrosis factor and the effect of cyclooxygenase inhibition. J Clin Invest. 1988;81:1162–1172.
31. Beutler B, Krochin N, Milsark IW, et al. Control of cachectin (tumor necrosis factor) synthesis: Mechanisms of endotoxin resistance. Science. 1986;232:977–980.
32. Michie HR, Manogue KR, Spriggs DR, et al. Detection of circulating tumor necrosis factor after endotoxin administration. N Engl J Med. 1988;318:1481–1486.
33. Waage A, Halstensen A, Espevik T. Association between tumor necrosis factor in

serum and fatal outcome in patients with meningococcal disease. Lancet. 1987;1:355–357.
34. Tracey KJ, Lowry SF, Cerami A. Cachectin/TNF mediates the pathophysiological effects of bacterial endotoxin/lipopolysaccharide (LPS). In: Levin J, Buller HR, tenCate JW, et al, eds. Bacterial Endotoxins: Pathophysiological Effects, Clinical Significance, and Pharmacological Control. New York: Alan R. Liss; 1988:77–88.
35. Blick M, Sherwin SA, Rosenblum M, et al. Phase I study of recombinant tumor necrosis factor in cancer patients. Cancer Res. 1987;47:2986–2989.
36. Mathison JC, Wolfson E, Ulevitch RJ. Participation of tumor necrosis factor in the mediation of gram-negative bacterial lipopolysaccharide-induced injury in rabbits. J Clin Invest. 1988;81:1925–1937.
37. Stephens KE, Ishizaka A, Larrick JW, et al. Tumor necrosis factor causes increased pulmonary permeability and edema. Am Rev Respir Dis. 1988;137:1364–1370.
38. Beutler B, Milsark IW, Cerami A. Passive immunization with cachectin/tumor necrosis factor (TNF) protects mice from the lethal effects of endotoxin. Nature. 1985;229:869–871.
39. Tracey KJ, Fong Y, Hesse DG, et al. Anti-cachectin/TNF monoclonal antibodies prevent septic shock during lethal bacteremia. Nature. 1987;330:662–664.
40. Nawroth PP, Bank I, Handley D, et al. Tumor necrosis factor/cachectin interacts with endothelial cell receptors to induce release of interleukin-1. J Exp Med. 1986;163:1363–1375.
41. Kettelhut IC, Fiers W, Goldberg AL. The toxic effects of tumor necrosis factor in vivo and their prevention by cyclooxygenase inhibitors. Proc Natl Acad Sci U S A. 1987;84:4273–4277.
42. Dinarello CA, Cannon JG, Solff SM, et al. Tumor necrosis factor (cachectin) is an endogenous pyrogen and induces production of interleukin 1. J Exp Med. 1986;163:1433–1450.
43. Neilson IR, Neilson KA, Yunis EJ, et al. Failure of tumor necrosis factor to produce hypotensive shock in the absence of endotoxin. Surgery. 1989;106:439–443.
44. Waage A, Espevik T: Interleukin 1 potentiates the lethal effect of tumor necrosis factor α/cachectin in mice. J Exp Med. 1988;167:1987–1992.
45. Talmadge JE, Bowersox O, Tribble H, et al. Toxicity of tumor necrosis factor is synergistic with gamma-interferon and can be reduced with cyclooxygenase inhibitors. Am J Pathol. 1987;128:410–425.
46. Ozaki Y, Ohashi T, Minami A, et al. Enhanced resistance of mice to bacterial infection induced by recombinant human interleukin-1α. Infect Immun. 1987;55:1436–1440.
47. Scuderi P, Sterling KE, Lam KS, et al. Raised serum levels of tumor necrosis factor in parasitic infections. Lancet. 1986;2:1364–1365.
48. Tracey KJ, Beutler B, Lowry SF, et al. Shock and tissue injury induced by recombinant human cachectin. Science. 1986;234:470–474.
49. Ulich TR, Kaizhi G, del Castillo J. Rapid communication: Endotoxin-induced cytokine gene expression in vivo. I: Expression of tumor necrosis factor mRNA in visceral organs under physiologic conditions and during endotoxemia. Am J Pathol. 1989;134:11–14.
50. Papanicolaou DA, Wilder RL, Manolagas SC, Chrousos GP. NIH Conference: The pathophysiologic roles of interleukin-6 in human disease. Ann Intern Med. 1998;128:127–137.
51. Aderka D, Le J, Vilcek J. IL-6 inhibits lipopolysaccharide-induced TNF production in cultured human monocytes, U937 cells, and in mice. J Immunol. 1989;143:3517–3523.
52. Cannon JG. Cytokines and shock. In: Kimball ES, ed. Cytokines and Inflammation. Boca Raton, Fla: CRC Press; 1991:307–329.
53. De Waal MR, Abrams J, Bennet B, et al. Interleukin 10 (IL-10) inhibits cytokine synthesis by human monocytes: An autoregulatory role of IL-10 produced by monocytes. J Exp Med. 1991;174:1209–1220.
54. Moncada S, Higgs A. The L-arginine-nitric oxide pathway. N Engl J Med. 1993;329:2002–2012.
55. Nathan C. Inducible nitric oxide synthase: What difference does it make? J Clin Invest. 1997;100:2417–2423.
56. Pepke-Zaba J, Higenbottam TW, Dinh-Xuan AT, et al. Inhaled nitric oxide as a cause of selective pulmonary vasodilatation in pulmonary hypertension. Lancet. 1991;338:1173–1174.
57. Petros A, Bennett D, Vallance P. Effect of nitric oxide synthase inhibitors on hypotension in patients with septic shock. Lancet. 1991;338:1557–1558.
58. Kilbourn RG, Gross SS, Jubran A, et al. N^G-methyl-L-arginine inhibits tumor necrosis factor-induced hypotension: Implications for the involvement of nitric oxide. Proc Natl Acad Sci U S A. 1990;87:3629–3632.
59. Fang FC. Mechanisms of nitric oxide-related antimicrobial activity. J Clin Invest. 1997;99:2818–2825.
60. Shenep JL, Tuomanen E. Perspective: Targeting nitric oxide in the adjuvant therapy of sepsis and meningitis. J Infect Dis. 1998;177:776–779.
61. Watson D, Beerahee M, Holzapfel L, et al. Multicentre, placebo-controlled, double-blind study of the nitric oxide synthase inhibitor 546C88 in patients with septic shock: Effect on plasma nitrate profile. Abstract G-40. American Society for Microbiology: Abstracts of the 37th Interscience Conference on Antimicrobial Agents and Chemotherapy, Washington, DC, 1997.
62. Wallach D, Holtmann H, Engelmann H, et al. Sensitization and desensitization to lethal effects of tumor necrosis factor and IL-1. J Immunol. 1988;140:2994.
63. Van Zee KJ, Kohno T, Fischer E, et al. Tumor necrosis factor soluble receptors circulate during experimental and clinical inflammation and can protect against excessive tumor necrosis factor α in vitro and in vivo. Proc Natl Acad Sci U S A. 1992;89:4845–4849.
64. Alexander RH, Doherty GM, Buresh CM, et al. A recombinant human receptor antagonist to interleukin 1 improves survival after lethal endotoxemia in mice. J Exp Med. 1991;173:1029–1032.
65. Levi M, ten Cate H, van der Poll T, et al. Pathogenesis of disseminated intravascular coagulation in sepsis. JAMA. 1993;270:975–979.
66. van der Poll T, Buller HR, ten Cate H, et al. Activation of coagulation after administration of tumor necrosis factor to normal subjects. N Engl J Med. 1990;322:1622–1627.
67. van Deventer SJ, Buller HR, ten Cate JW, et al. Experimental endotoxemia in humans: Analysis of cytokine release and coagulation, fibrinolytic and complement pathways. Blood. 1990;76:2520–2526.
68. Warr TA, Mohan-Rao LV, Rapaport SI. Disseminated intravascular coagulation in rabbit induced by administration of endotoxin or tissue factor: Effect of anti-tissue factor antibodies and measurement of plasma extrinsic pathway inhibitor activity. Blood. 1990;75:1481–1489.
69. O'Donnell TF, Clowes GHA, Talamo RC, et al. Kinin activation in the blood of patients with sepsis. Surg Gynecol Obstet. 1976;143:539.
70. Bevilacqua MP. Endothelial-leukocyte adhesion molecules. Annu Rev Immunol. 1993;11:767–804.
71. Bevilacqua MP, Pober JS, Majeau GR, et al. Recombinant tumor necrosis factor induces procoagulant activity in cultures of vascular endothelium: Characterization and comparison with the actions of interleukin 1. Proc Natl Acad Sci U S A. 1986;83:4533–4537.
72. Dinarello CA, Wolff SM. The role of interleukin-1 in disease. N Engl J Med. 1993;328:106.
73. Goldblum SE. The role of cytokines in acute pulmonary vascular endothelial injury. In: Kimball ES, ed. Cytokines and Inflammation. Boca Raton, Fla: CRC Press; 1991:191–234.
74. Parsons PE, Worthen GS, Moore EE, et al. The association of circulating endotoxin with the development of the adult respiratory distress syndrome. Am Rev Respir Dis. 1989;140:294–301.
75. Maury E, Barakett V, Blanchard H, et al. Circulating endotoxin during initial antibiotic treatment of severe gram-negative bacteremic infections. J Infect Dis. 1998;178:270–273.
76. DuPont HL, Spink WW. Infections due to gram-negative organisms: An analysis of 860 patients with bacteremia at the University of Minnesota Medical Center, 1958–1966. Medicine (Baltimore). 1969;48:307.
77. Kreger BE, Craven DE, Carling P, et al. Gram-negative bacteremia: III. Reassessment of etiology, epidemiology, and ecology in 612 patients. Am J Med. 1980;68:332.
78. Brandtzaeg P, Kierulf P, Gaustad P, et al. Plasma endotoxin as a predictor of multiple organ failure and death in systemic meningococcal disease. J Infect Dis. 1989;159:195–204.
79. Calandra T, Baumgartner JD, Grau GE, et al. Prognostic values of tumor necrosis factor/cachectin, interleukin-1, alpha interferon and gamma interferon in the serum of patients with septic shock. J Infect Dis. 1990;149:982–987.
80. Anderson ET, Young LS, Hewitt WL. Antimicrobial synergism in the therapy of gram-negative bacteremia. Chemotherapy. 1978;24:45.
81. McCabe WR, Jackson GG. Gram-negative bacteremia: II. Clinical, laboratory and therapeutic observations. Arch Intern Med. 1962;110:856.
82. Bryant RE, Hood AF, Hood CE, et al. Factors affecting mortality of gram-negative rod bacteremia. Arch Intern Med. 1971;127:120.
83. Young LS. Treatment of infections due to gram-negative bacilli: A perspective of past, present and future. Rev Infect Dis. 1985;7(Suppl 4):572.
84. Calandra T, Cometta A. Antibiotic therapy for gram-negative bacteremia. Infect Dis Clin North Am. 1991;5:817–834.
85. Young LS. Empirical antimicrobial therapy in the neutropenic host. N Engl J Med. 1986;315:580.
86. Robson HG. Synergistic activity of carbenicillin and gentamicin in experimental *Pseudomonas* bacteremia in neutropenic rats. Antimicrob Agents Chemother. 1976;10:646.
87. Young LS. Review of clinical significance of synergy in gram-negative bacteremic infections at the UCLA hospital. Infection. 1978;10:247–254.
88. Klastersky J, Meunier-Carpentier F, Prevost JM. Significance of antimicrobial synergism for the outcome of gram-negative sepsis. Am J Med Sci. 1977;273:157.
89. Sculier JP, Klastersky J. Significance of serum bactericidal activity in gram-negative bacillary bacteremia in patients with and without granulocytopenia. Am J Med. 1984;76:429–435.
90. Rolston KVI, Berkey P, Bodey GP, et al. A comparison of imipenem to ceftazidime with or without amikacin as empiric therapy in febrile neutropenic patients. Arch Intern Med. 1992;152:283–291.
91. Hughes WT, Armstrong D, Bodey GP, et al. 1997 guidelines for the use of antimicrobial agents in neutropenic patients with unexplained fever. Clin Infect Dis. 1997;25:551–573.
92. Kaye D, Levison ME, Labovitz ED. The unpredictability of serum concentrations of gentamicin: Pharmacokinetics of gentamicin in patients with normal and abnormal renal function. J Infect Dis. 1974;130:150.
93. Anderson ET, Young LS, Hewitt WL. Simultaneous antibiotic levels in "breakthrough" gram-negative bacteremia. Am J Med. 1976;61:493.
94. Smith CR, Maxwell RR, Edwards CQ, et al. Nephrotoxicity induced by gentamicin and amikacin. Johns Hopkins Med J. 1978;142:85.
95. Shine K, Silver M, Young LS, et al. Aspects of the management of shock. Ann Intern Med. 1980;93:723–734.
96. Winslow EJ, Loeb HS, Pahimtoola SH, et al. Hemodynamic studies and results of therapy in 50 patients with bacteremic shock. Am J Med. 1973;54:421.

97. Weitzman S, Berger S. Clinical trial design in studies of corticosteroids for bacterial infections. Ann Intern Med. 1974;81:36.
98. Klastersky J, Cappel R, Debusscher L. Effectiveness of betamethasone in management of severe infections. N Engl J Med. 1971;284:1248.
99. Schumer W. Steroids in the treatment of clinical septic shock. Ann Surg. 1976;184:333.
100. Hoffman SL, Punjabi NH, Kumala S, et al. Reduction of mortality in chloramphenicol-treated severe typhoid fever by high-dose dexamethasone. N Engl J Med. 1981;301:456–457.
101. Sprung CL, Caralis PV, Marcial EH, et al. The effects of high-dose corticosteroids in patients with septic shock: A prospective controlled study. N Engl J Med. 1984;311:1137–1143.
102. Veterans Administration Systemic Sepsis Cooperative Study Group. Effect of high dose glucocorticoid therapy on mortality in patients with clinical signs of systemic sepsis. N Engl J Med. 1987;317:659–665.
103. Bone RC, Fisher CJ, Clemmer TP, et al. A controlled clinical trial of high-dose methylprednisolone in the treatment of severe sepsis and septic shock. N Engl J Med. 1987;317:653–658.
104. Bernard GR, Luce JM, Sprungs CL, et al. High-dose corticosteroids in patients with the adult respiratory distress syndrome. N Engl J Med. 1987;317:1565–1570.
105. Luce JM, Montgomery AB, Marks JD, et al. Ineffectiveness of high-dose methylprednisolone in preventing parenchymal lung injury and improving mortality in patients with septic shock. Am Rev Respir Dis. 1988;138:62–68.
106. Corrigan JJ Jr, Ray WL, May N. Change in blood coagulation system associated with septicemia. N Engl J Med. 1968;279:851.
107. Corrigan JC, Kiernat JF. Effect of heparin in experimental gram-negative septicemia. J Infect Dis. 1975;131:138.
108. Corrigan JJ. Heparin therapy in bacterial septicemia. J Pediatr. 1977;91:695.
109. Alavi JB, Root RK, Djerassi I, et al. A randomized clinical trial of granulocyte transfusions for infection in acute leukemia. N Engl J Med. 1977;296:706.
110. Vogler WR, Winton EF. A controlled study of the efficacy of granulocyte transfusions in patients with neutropenia. Am J Med. 1977;63:548.
111. Winston DJ, Ho WG, Gale RP. Therapeutic granulocyte transfusions for documented infections. Ann Intern Med. 1982;97:509.
112. Young LS. Immunoprophylaxis and serotherapy of bacterial infections. Am J Med. 1984;76:664–671.
113. Ziegler EJ, McCutchan JA, Fierer J, et al. Treatment of gram-negative bacteremia and shock with human antiserum to a mutant *Escherichia coli*. N Engl J Med. 1982;307:1225.
114. Calandra T, Glauser MP, Schellekens J, et al. Treatment of gram-negative septic shock with human IgG antibody to *Escherichia coli* J5: A prospective double-blind, randomized trial. J Infect Dis. 1988;158:312–319.
115. Ziegler EFJ, Fisher CJ Jr, Sprung CL, et al. Treatment of gram-negative bacteremia and septic shock with HA-1A human monoclonal antibody against endotoxin. N Engl J Med. 1991;324:429–436.
116. Greenman RL, Schein RMH, Martin MA, et al. A controlled clinical trial of E5 murine monoclonal IgM antibody to endotoxin in the treatment of gram-negative sepsis. JAMA. 1991;266:1097–1102.
117. Warren HS, Danner RL, Munford RS. Antiendotoxin monoclonal antibodies. N Engl J Med 1992:326:1153–1157.
118. Young LS, Wenzel RP: New immunotherapies for sepsis. Proc Assoc Am Physicians. 1995;79:361–369.
119. McCloskey RV, Straube RC, Sanders C, et al. Treatment of septic shock with human monoclonal antibody HA-1A. Ann Intern Med. 1994;121:1–5.
120. Bone RC, Balk RA, Fein AM, et al. A second large controlled clinical study of E5, a monoclonal antibody to endotoxin: Results of a prospective, multicenter, randomized, clinical trial. Crit Care Med. 1995;23:994–1006.
121. Fisher CJ Jr, Dhainaut FJ, Opal SM, et al. Recombinant human interleukin-1 receptor antagonist in the treatment of patients with sepsis syndrome: Results from a randomized, double-blind, placebo-controlled trial. JAMA. 1994;271:1836–1844.
122. Abraham E, Wunderink R, Silverman H, et al. Efficacy and safety of monoclonal antibody to human necrosis factor-alpha in patients with sepsis syndrome: A randomized, controlled, double-blind, multicenter clinical trial. JAMA. 1995;273:934–941.
123. Abraham E, for the Norsept II Study Group. Double-blind, randomized, controlled trial of monoclonal antibody to human tumor necrosis factor in treatment of septic shock. Lancet. 1998;351:929–933.
124. Fisher CJ Jr, Agosti JM, Opal SM, et al. Treatment of septic shock with the tumor necrosis factor: Fc fusion protein. N Engl J Med. 1996;334:1697–1702.
125. Abraham E, Glauser MP, Butler T, et al. Tumor necrosis factor receptor fusion protein in the treatment of patients with severe sepsis and septic shock. JAMA. 1997;277:1531–1538.
126. Dhainaut JR, Tenaillon A, LeTulzo Y, et al. Platelet-activating factor receptor antagonist BN 52021 in the treatment of severe sepsis: A randomized, double-blind, placebo-controlled, multicenter clinical trial. Crit Care Med. 1994;22:1720–1728.
127. Fein AM, Bernard GR, Criner GJ, et al. Treatment of severe systemic inflammatory response and sepsis with a novel bradykinin antagonist, delbitant (CP-0127). JAMA. 1997;277:482–487.
128. Bernard GR. Issues in the design of clinical trials for sepsis. In: Cytokines and Pulmonary Infections: Part II. American Thoracic Society. Am J Respir Crit Care Med. 1997;156(6 Suppl):1–6.
129. Natanson C. Re-evaluation of anti-inflammatory trials in sepsis: A metanalysis. In: Cytokines and Pulmonary Infections: Part II. American Thoracic Society. Am J Respir Crit Care Med. 1997;156(6 Suppl):7–18.
130. Grau GE, Maennel DN. TNF inhibition and sepsis: Sounding a cautionary note. Nat Med. 1997;3:1193–1195.
131. Cobb JP, Natanson C, Hoffman WD, et al. N^{Δ}-amino-L-arginine, an inhibitor of nitric oxide synthase, raises vascular resistance but increases mortality rates in awake canines challenged with endotoxin. J Exp Med. 1992;176:1175–1182.
132. Lindberg RB, Moncrief JA, Mason AD Jr. Control of experimental and clinical burn wound sepsis by topical application of sulfamylon compounds. Ann N Y Acad Sci. 1968;50:950.
133. Greenfield S, Teres D, Bushnell LS, et al. Prevention of gram-negative bacillary pneumonia using aerosol polymixin as prophylaxis. J Clin Invest. 1973;52:2935.
134. Feeley TW, du Moulin GC, Hedley-Whyte J, et al. Aerosol polymixin and pneumonia. N Engl J Med. 1975;293:471.
135. Storring RA, McElwain TJ, Jameson B, et al. Oral non-absorbed antibiotics prevent infection in acute non-lymphoblastic leukaemia. Lancet. 1977;2:837.
136. Schimpff SC, Greene WH, Young VM, et al. Infection prevention in acute non-lymphocytic leukemia: Laminar air flow room reverse isolation with oral, nonabsorbable antibiotic prophylaxis. Ann Intern Med. 1975;82:351.
137. Young LS. Trimethoprim-sulfamethoxazole and bacterial infections during leukemic therapy. Ann Intern Med. 1981;95:508.
138. Pizzo PA. Drug therapy: Management of fever in patients with cancer and treatment-induced neutropenia. N Engl J Med. 1993;328:1323–1332.
139. Rowe JM. Treatment of acute myeloid leukemia with cytokines: Effect on duration of neutropenia and response to infections. Clin Infect Dis. 1998;26:1290–1294.
140. Young LS, Meyer RD, Armstrong D. *Pseudomonas aeruginosa* vaccine in cancer patients. Ann Intern Med. 1973;79:518.
141. Alexander JW, Fisher MW, MacMillan BG. Immunological control of *Pseudomonas* infection in burn patients. A clinical evaluation. Arch Surg. 1971;102:31.
142. Jones RJ, Roe EA, Gupta JL. Low mortality in burned patients in a *Pseudomonas* vaccine trial. Lancet. 1978;2:401.
143. Dwyer JM. Manipulating the immune system with immune globulin. N Engl J Med. 1992;326:106–116.

SECTION F

Chapter 64

Peritonitis and Other Intra-abdominal Infections

MATTHEW E. LEVISON
LARRY M. BUSH

Intra-abdominal infection can take several forms. Infection may be in the retroperitoneal space or within the peritoneal cavity. Intraperitoneal infection may be diffuse or localized into one or more abscesses. Intraperitoneal abscesses may form in dependent recesses such as the pelvic space or Morison's pouch, in the various perihepatic spaces, within the lesser sac, or along the major routes of communication between intraperitoneal recesses, such as the right paracolic gutter. In addition, infection may be contained within the intra-abdominal viscera, as in hepatic, pancreatic, splenic, tuboovarian, or renal abscesses. Abscesses also frequently form about diseased viscera (pericholecystic, periappendiceal, pericolic, and tuboovarian) and between adjacent loops of bowel (i.e., interloop abscesses).

ANATOMY

The anatomic relationships within the abdomen are important in determining possible sources and routes of spread of infection. The peritoneal cavity extends from the undersurface of the diaphragm to the floor of the pelvis. In men, the peritoneal cavity is a closed space. In women, it is perforated by the free ends of the fallopian tubes. The stomach, jejunum, ileum, cecum, appendix, transverse and sigmoid colons, liver, gallbladder, and spleen lie within the peritoneal cavity, some being suspended by a mesentery.

The peritoneal reflections and mesenteric attachments compartmentalize the intraperitoneal space and route, spreading exudate to sites that are often distant from the source (Fig. 64–1). The transverse mesocolon divides the peritoneal cavity horizontally into an upper and a lower space. The greater omentum, extending from the transverse mesocolon and lower border of the stomach, covers the lower peritoneal cavity and further separates the upper from the lower peritoneal cavity (Fig. 64–2). The small bowel mesentery divides the lower peritoneal space.

The peritoneal cavity has several recesses into which exudate may become loculated. The most dependent recess of the peritoneal cavity in the supine position is in the pelvis. Between the rectum and bladder in men is a pouch of peritoneal cavity that extends slightly below the level of the seminal vesicles. In women, the uterus and fallopian tubes project into the pelvic recess. Between the rectum and the body of the uterus is the pouch of Douglas, which lies above the posterior fornix of the vagina. On either side of the rectum and bladder are the pararectal and paravesical fossae. The pelvic recess is continuous with both the right and left paracolic gutters.

The phrenicocolic ligament, which fixes the splenic flexure of the colon to the diaphragm, partially bridges the junction between the left paracolic gutter and the left perihepatic space. In contrast, the right paracolic gutter is continuous with the right subhepatic space and the right subphrenic space. A posterior superior extension of the right subhepatic space, Morison's pouch, is the most dependent portion in the supine position of the right paravertebral groove and lies just above the beginning of the transverse mesocolon. The horizontal posterior reflection of the serosal surface of the liver onto the diaphragm (the right triangular and coronary ligaments) and the vertical reflection (falciform ligament) divide the right perihepatic space into right subphrenic and right subhepatic spaces (see Figs. 64–1 and 64–2*A*). The left subphrenic and subhepatic spaces communicate freely around the smaller left lobe of the liver and its more superiorly placed left triangular ligament[1, 2] (see Figs. 64–1 and 64–2*B*). The right and left subphrenic spaces are separated by the falciform ligament, which probably prevents the spread of pus to the opposite side and explains why only about 5 to 15% of subphrenic abscesses are bilateral.[2] The left subhepatic space is divided by the gastrohepatic omentum into an anterior space and the lesser sac (see Fig. 64–2*B*). Abscesses within the perihepatic spaces become localized by pyogenic membranes. In the right subphrenic space, they lie anteriorly or posteriorly and in the subhepatic space superiorly or

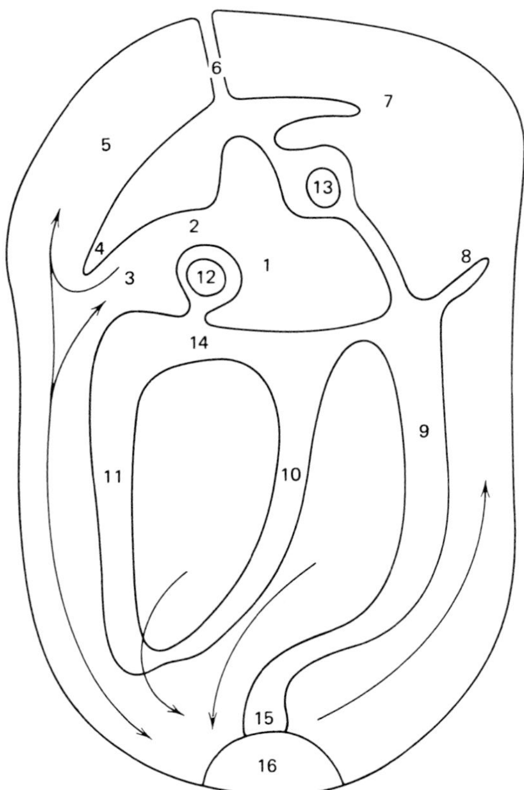

FIGURE 64–1. Schema of the posterior peritoneal reflections and recesses of the peritoneal cavity. 1, Lesser sac; 2, foramen of Winslow; 3, Morison's pouch; 4, right triangular ligament; 5, right subphrenic spaces; 6, falciform ligament; 7, left subphrenic space; 8, phrenocolic ligament; 9, bare area of the descending colon; 10, root of the small bowel mesentery; 11, bare area of the ascending colon; 12, duodenum; 13, esophagus; 14, root of the transverse mesocolon; 15, bare area of rectum; 16, bladder.

FIGURE 64–2. Schema of a sagittal section of the peritoneal cavity. *A*, Right upper quadrant. 1, Subphrenic space; 2, liver; 3, subhepatic space; 4, right kidney; 5, transverse colon. *B*, Left upper quadrant. 1, Subphrenic space; 2, liver, left lobe; 3, subhepatic space; 4; stomach; 5; transverse colon; 6, lesser sac; 7, pancreas; 8, duodenum; 9, transverse mesocolon; 10, omemtum; 11, left kidney.

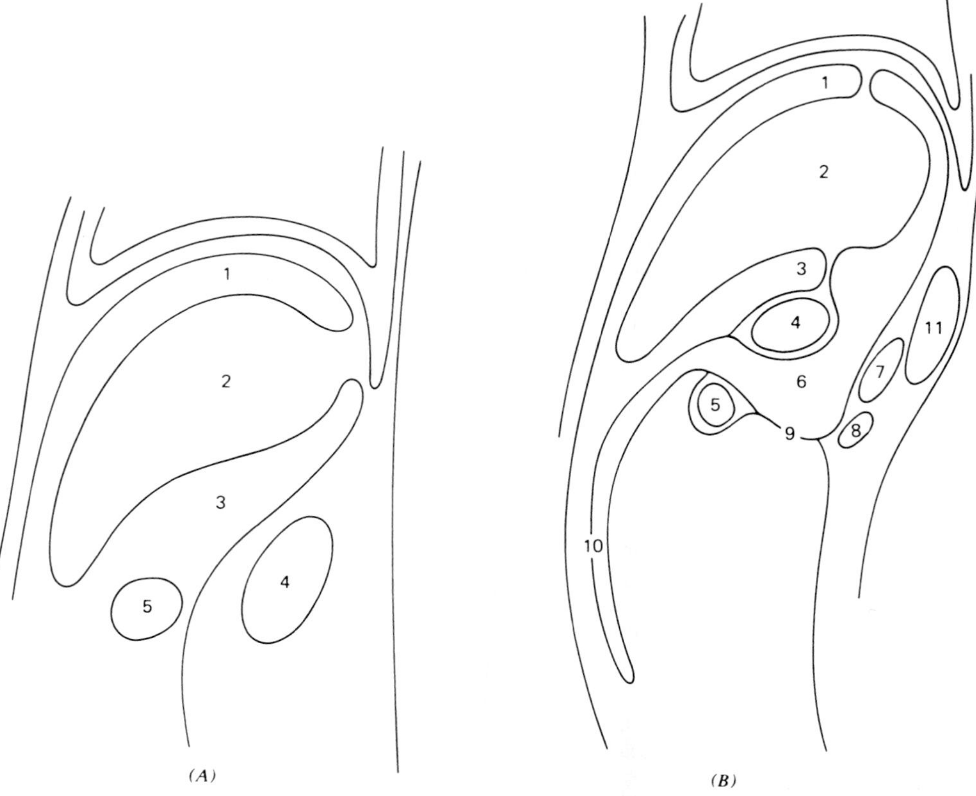

inferiorly.[1, 2] Abscesses of the left perihepatic space are either in the single left subphrenic space or in the lesser sac.[1, 2]

The lesser sac, the largest recess of the peritoneal cavity, is connected to the main peritoneal space by the foramen of Winslow, an opening situated between the free border of the gastrohepatic omentum and the posterior parietal peritoneum. The lesser sac is surrounded posteriorly by the pancreas and kidneys, anteriorly by the stomach, and laterally by the liver and spleen. It may also extend to a variable extent between the folds of the greater omentum. Because of the limited communication from the lesser sac to the major cavity via the foramen of Winslow, suppuration in the lesser sac may exist with little or no involvement of the major cavity. Abscesses in the lesser sac lie between the stomach and pancreas but may spread to the right and lie anterior to the right kidney and inferior to the liver.

After intraperitoneal injection of water-soluble contrast material selectively into various intraperitoneal spaces, Myers[3] demonstrated that the right paracolic gutter is the main communication between the upper and lower peritoneal cavities. Fluid introduced into the right upper peritoneal space gravitates toward Morison's pouch and then into the right subphrenic space and along the right paracolic gutter into the pelvic recess (Fig. 64–3). Flow of fluid in the left upper peritoneal space is mainly into the left subphrenic space. The phrenicocolic ligament limits flow inferiorly into the left paracolic gutter. Fluid introduced into the lower peritoneal cavity first gravitates to the pelvic recess and then ascends, whether in the supine or erect position, along the right paracolic gutter into the right subhepatic space, especially into Morison's pouch, and into the right subphrenic space. Ascension of fluid from the pelvic space along the left paracolic gutter is minimal and is limited by the phrenicocolic ligament. Although gravity would account for the pooling of fluid in the dependent peritoneal recesses, such as the pelvic recess and Morison's pouch, ascension of fluid from the pelvis to the subphrenic space is probably caused by hydrostatic pressure differences between the upper and lower peritoneal cavities created by diaphragmatic motion. Normal intestinal and abdominal wall motion would also account for some spread of intraperitoneal fluid.

The retroperitoneal space lies between the posterior peritoneal membrane and the transversalis fascia, extending from the diaphragm to the pelvic brim. In the anterior retroperitoneal space between the peritoneum and anterior renal fascia lie the ascending and descending colons, duodenum, and pancreas. The kidneys and ureters lie within the posterior retroperitoneal (perinephric) space, between the anterior and posterior renal fasciae. The renal fascia encloses the kidneys and adrenals superiorly and laterally, but not inferiorly, favoring spread of infection in this space inferiorly.[4]

The parietal peritoneum, mainly the anterior portion, is well supplied by somatic afferent nerves and is sensitive to all forms of stimuli. The ability of the anterior parietal peritoneum to sense sharp, well-localized pain in response to local inflammation is of primary importance in diagnosing abdominal infection and may be associated with involuntary abdominal muscle contraction, tenderness, and rebound tenderness. Irritation of the peripheral diaphragmatic peritoneum is felt as pain near the adjacent body wall, and irritation of the central portion is felt as pain referred to the shoulder. Stimulation of the visceral peritoneum, usually by distention of an organ, causes poorly localized, somewhat dull pain.

The peritoneal cavity is lined by a serous membrane. The surface area of this membrane approximates that of the skin. The membrane consists of a monolayer of flat polygonal cells beneath which are lymphatics, blood vessels, and nerve endings. Normally, the peritoneal space contains only sufficient fluid to maintain moistness of the surface, facilitating movements of the viscera. Noninflamed serous fluid is clear yellow with a low specific gravity ($<$1.016) and low protein content (usually $<$3 g/dl). The protein is predominantly albumin. Fibrinogen is not present, and serous fluid will not clot. Solute concentrations are almost identical to those in plasma. A few leukocytes ($<$300/mm^3), mostly mononuclear cells, and desquamated serosal cells may be found.

The peritoneal membrane is highly permeable. Bidirectional transfer of substances across this membrane is rapid and, because of the large surface area involved, potentially great in quality. In fact, the peritoneal surface has been used extensively as a dialyzing membrane for the treatment of uremia and has also been used for the administration of fluid, electrolytes, antibiotics, and even blood. The effective serum oncotic pressure and the hydrostatic pressure in the portal veins and lymphatics are major determinants of the rate and direction of fluid movement. The rate of movement of water and solutes between blood and peritoneal fluid also depends on concentration gradients between these compartments and has been studied in detail.[5, 6] Water and solutes diffuse via blood capillaries and to a lesser extent through the lymphatics. Lymphatics are primarily involved in removal of nonirritating colloids and particles into the blood stream. Absorption into lymphatics of particulate matter us thought to take place mostly from the diaphragmatic surface and is aided by the pumping action of diaphragmatic motion.[7] After infusion of ^{51}Cr-labeled red blood cells into the peritoneal cavity of dogs, Rochlin and associates[8] reported absorption of about 70% of the labeled cells by 48 to 96 hours. This absorption occurred mostly through the lymphatics. In humans, two thirds of intraperitoneally injected red blood cells in anticoagulated blood have been found in the circulation 8 to 12 days after infusion.[9] The quantity of resorbed cells was less when no anticoagulant was used with the transfused cells, presumably because of trapping of red blood cells in intraperitoneal clots.[9] Transport of other particulate matter, such as intraperitoneal bacteria, may be similarly impeded because of trapping in fibrinous intraperitoneal exudate.[10]

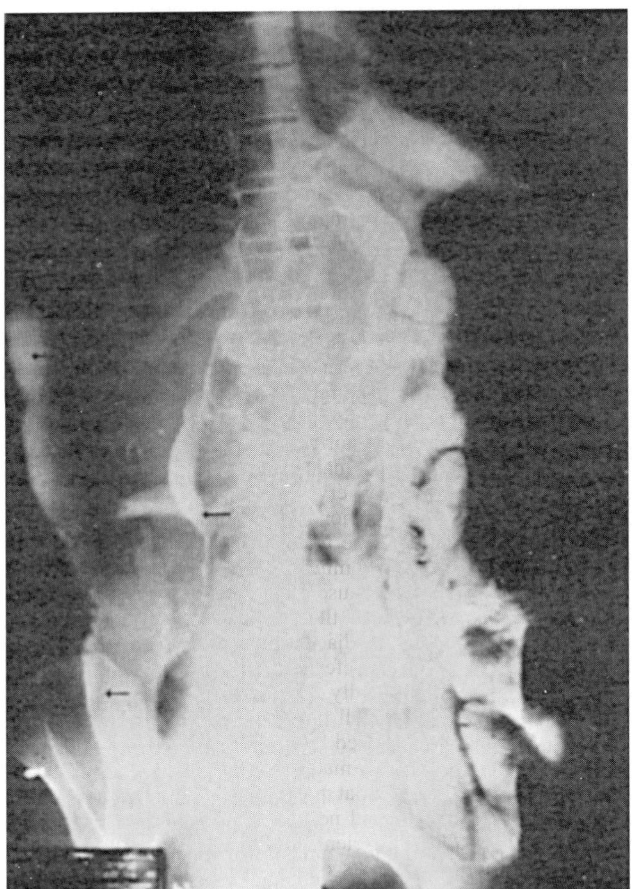

FIGURE 64–3. Abdominal radiograph (right decubitus) after oral administration of Gastrografin to a patient with dehiscence of an esophageal-gastric anastomosis. Radiopaque Gastrografin *(arrows)* can be seen in the subhepatic space, right paracolic gutter, and right subphrenic space, as well as within the lumen of the intestinal tract.

In addition, there are communications between the peritoneal and pleural cavities that are independent of the blood stream. In patients with Meigs' syndrome, for example, radioactive colloidal gold instilled into the peritoneal cavity appears in the pleural space, probably as a result of transdiaphragmatic lymphatic transport.[11]

PERITONITIS

Inflammation of the peritoneum may be the result of contamination of the peritoneal cavity with microorganisms, irritating chemicals, or both. Infective peritonitis has been categorized as either primary, secondary, or tertiary. Peritonitis complicating peritoneal dialysis can be considered as an additional category. In the primary variety, the peritoneal infection is not directly related to other intra-abdominal abnormalities. In the secondary variety, an intra-abdominal process, such as a ruptured appendix or a perforated peptic ulcer, is evident. Tertiary peritonitis has been conceived as a later stage of the disease, when clinical peritonitis and signs of sepsis persist after treatment for secondary peritonitis, and no pathogens or only low-grade pathogens are isolated from the peritoneal exudate.

Primary Peritonitis

Etiology

Primary peritonitis, sometimes referred to as spontaneous bacterial peritonitis (SBP), is probably not a specific entity with a common cause but represents a group of diseases with different causes having in common only infection of the peritoneal cavity without an evident source. Primary peritonitis occurs at all ages. The prevalence of primary peritonitis in children apparently has been decreasing.[12] In the preantibiotic era, primary peritonitis occurred in about 10% of all pediatric abdominal emergencies; it now accounts for less than 1 to 2%.[13, 14] The decline has been attributed to widespread use of antibiotics for minor upper respiratory tract illness. Although primary peritonitis may occur in children without predisposing disease,[12] it is known to occur particularly in children with postnecrotic cirrhosis[13, 15] and in 2% of children with the nephrotic syndrome.[12, 16] In one study, it was also frequently associated with urinary tract infections.[13] In some nephrotic children, repeated episodes of peritonitis occur, and peritonitis may precede other manifestations of nephrosis.[12]

In adults, primary peritonitis usually has been reported in patients with alcoholic cirrhosis and ascites. In 1971, Conn and Fessel[17] summarized their experience with 32 episodes in 28 patients and, in addition, reviewed 46 episodes in 42 patients reported in the literature. Subsequent reports have confirmed and extended their initial findings.[18–24] Primary peritonitis was found to occur in about 10% of the patients with alcoholic cirrhosis studied retrospectively.[17, 18] Among 63 consecutive patients with cirrhosis and ascites studied prospectively using optimal aerobic and anaerobic bacteriologic techniques, primary peritonitis was found in 5.[21] Primary peritonitis has also been reported in adults with postnecrotic cirrhosis,[15] chronic active hepatitis,[25] acute viral hepatitis,[26] congestive heart failure,[27] metastatic malignant disease,[28] systemic lupus erythematosus,[29] or lymphedema,[30] and, rarely, in those with no underlying disease.[31] The presence of ascites appears to be the common link among these various conditions.

Bacteriologic Characteristics

Several decades ago, the organisms reported to cause primary peritonitis in children were *Streptococcus pneumoniae* and group A streptococci.[12–14] By the 1970s the number of nephrotic children with streptococcal peritonitis had declined, and the relative frequency of peritonitis caused by gram-negative enteric bacilli[13, 14, 16] and by staphylococci[12, 14] apparently had increased.

In cirrhotic patients, microorganisms presumably of enteric origin account for up to 69% of the pathogens.[32] *Escherichia coli* is the most frequently recovered pathogen, followed by *Klebsiella pneumoniae*, *S. pneumoniae*, and other streptococcal species, including enterococci.[17, 20, 32–34] *Staphylococcus aureus* is an unusual isolate in primary peritonitis, accounting for 2 to 4% of the cases in most series, and it has been noted to occur in patients with an erosion of an umbilical hernia.[33] Anaerobes and microaerophilic organisms are infrequently reported.[20, 24] Possible explanations include the intrinsic bacteriostatic activity of ascites against *Bacteroides* spp.,[35] the relatively high partial pressure of oxygen of ascitic fluid,[36] and the lack of optimal anaerobic bacteriologic techniques to study patients with primary peritonitis in the past. In a review of 126 cases of primary peritonitis in cirrhotic patients recorded in the literature, only eight patients (6%) had disease caused by anaerobic or microaerophilic bacteria, including *Bacteroides* spp., *Bacteroides fragilis*, *Clostridium perfringens*, *Peptostreptococcus* spp., *Peptococcus* spp., and *Campylobacter fetus*.[20] Polymicrobial infection was present in four of these eight cirrhotic patients with peritonitis caused by anaerobes, in contrast to the relatively low frequency of polymicrobial infection (only 10 of 118 cases of peritonitis) when aerobes alone were involved.

Ascitic fluid with positive cultures but few leukocytes in patients without clinical findings of peritonitis has been noted.[34] This may represent early colonization before a host response.[24] However, patients with a low leukocyte response have the same mortality rate as those with a greater response.[23] Conversely, several series have identified cases of primary peritonitis with negative ascitic fluid cultures.[17, 24] In one series, sterile cultures occurred in 35% of patients with clinical findings consistent with primary peritonitis, ascitic fluid leukocyte counts greater than 500/mm^3, and no evident source of intra-abdominal infection.[37] Blood cultures were positive in one third of these patients.[37] The frequency of culture-negative ascitic fluid may be decreased by inoculating blood-cultured bottles with ascitic fluid at the bedside.[38]

Bacteremia is present in up to 75% of patients with primary peritonitis caused by aerobic bacteria,[32] but it is rarely found in those with peritonitis caused by anaerobes.[20] Usually the same organisms isolated from the peritoneal fluid are recovered from the blood.[17, 20]

Occasionally, peritonitis may result from infection with *Mycobacterium tuberculosis*, *Neisseriae gonorrhoeae*, *Chlamydia trachomatis*, or *Coccidioides immitis*, but this is usually the result of disseminated infection or sometimes spread from adjacent foci of infection (see "Pathogenesis").

Pathogenesis

The route of infection in primary peritonitis is usually not apparent, and often it is presumed to be hematogenous, lymphogenous, or transmural migration through an intact gut wall from the intestinal lumen, or, in women, from the vagina via the fallopian tubes. Conn and Fessel[17] postulated that the hematogenous route is most likely in cirrhotic patients: either (1) organisms removed from circulation by the liver contaminate hepatic lymph and pass through the permeable lymphatic walls into the ascitic fluid or (2) portosystemic shunting greatly diminishes hepatic clearance of bacteremia in the portal circulation, which would tend to perpetuate bacteremia and increase the opportunity to cause metastic infection at susceptible sites such as the ascitic collection. The infrequency of primary peritonitis in ascites (except that caused by liver disease) emphasizes the importance of intrahepatic shunting in the pathogenesis of this disease. The hepatic reticuloendothelial system is known to be a major site for removal of bacteria from blood,[39] and animal studies have suggested that destruction of blood-borne bacteria by the reticuloendothelial system is impaired in experimental cirrhosis[40] and in alcoholic liver disease.[41] The decrease in phagocytic activity seen in alcoholic cirrhosis is proportional to the severity of the liver disease.[42] Additionally, alcohol abuse and cirrhosis have been reported to be associated with impaired intracellular killing by monocytes and neutrophils[43] and with impaired opsonization[44] and low levels of serum complement.[45] The characteristics of ascitic fluid in nephrosis and cirrhosis predispose to infection. Opsonic activity, as reflected by low levels of complement and immunoglobulins, is reduced in the ascitic fluid of patients with the nephrotic syndrome and cirrhosis.[46, 47] Primary bacteremia, usually caused by coliforms, is a common complication in cirrhosis,[48] and metastatic infection in the pleural space has also been reported in cirrhotic patients.[49] An increased frequency of gram-negative endocarditis has also been noted in cirrhotics.[50]

Enteric bacteria may also gain access to the peritoneal cavity by directly traversing the intact intestinal wall. This has been demonstrated in animals: Schweinburg and coworkers[51] demonstrated in dogs that ^{14}C-labeled *E. coli* passed from the bowel into the peritoneal cavity after the introduction of hypertonic solutions into the peritoneum. A similar mechanism may explain the enteric bacterial peritonitis that frequently complicates peritoneal dialysis.[52] The infrequent occurrence of bacteremia and the multiplicity of species in peritoneal fluid when anaerobic bacteria are involved suggest that transmural migration of bacteria is the probable route of infection of ascitic fluid in the majority of these patients.[20] In addition, the occurrence of polymicrobial anaerobic perinotitis in two patients after infusion of vasopressin into the superior mesenteric or gastroduodenal arteries suggests that arterial vasoconstriction decreased the intestinal mucosal barrier and permitted transmural migration of enteric organisms.[19] Colonic microorganisms have been reported to colonize the upper small bowel in cirrhotic patients.[53]

The simultaneous presence of pneumococci in vaginal secretions and peritoneal fluid in prepubertal girls[54] makes an ascending infection of genital origin likely in these patients. The alkaline vaginal secretions of prepubertal girls may be less inhibitory to bacterial growth than the acidic secretions of postpubertal women. Transfallopian spread is also suggested by the development of peritonitis in women with intrauterine devices (IUDs).[55, 56] The route of spread in women with gonococcal or chlamydial perihepatitis (Fitz-Hugh-Curtis syndrome) is presumbly from the fallopian tubes and paracolic gutters to the subphrenic space, but it may also be hematogenous. In the one man with this syndrome, *N. gonorrhoeae* was recovered from a liver biopsy specimen, and the route of spread was presumably via bacteremia.[57]

Although tuberculous peritonitis may result from direct entry into the peritoneal cavity of tubercle bacilli (from the lymph nodes, intestine, or genital tract in patients with active disease of these organs), it is more likely to result from hematogenous dissemination from remote foci of tuberculosis, most commonly in the lung. Tuberculous peritonitis can become clinically evident after the initial focus has completely healed.

Clinical Manifestations

Primary peritonitis is an acute febrile illness often confused with acute appendicitis in children. Fever, abdominal pain, nausea, vomiting, and diarrhea are usually present with diffuse abdominal tenderness, rebound tenderness, and hypoactive or absent bowel sounds. In cirrhotic patients with primary peritonitis, preexisting ascites is present. In some patients, the clinical manifestations are atypical. For example, the onset may be insidious, and findings of peritoneal irritation may be absent in an abdomen distended with ascites. Fever (>37.8°C [100°F]) is the most common presenting sign, occurring in 50 to 80% of cases,[17, 23] and may be present without abdominal signs or symptoms, or the process may be completely silent. Primary peritonitis in cirrhotic patients is generally associated with other features of end-stage liver disease (hepatorenal syndrome, progressive encephalopathy, and variceal bleeding). Primary peritonitis should always be considered in the differential diagnosis of decompensation of previously stable chronic liver disease.

Fluid obtained by paracentesis should be examined for cell count, differential count, and protein concentration, and a Gram stain and culture of the fluid should be obtained.[67] The ascitic fluid protein concentration may be low[17] in abdominal inflammation because of (1) hypoalbuminemia[58] and (2) dilution of ascitic fluid with transudate from the portal system when there is cirrhosis or the portal vein is obstructed.[59] The leukocyte count in peritoneal fluid usually is greater than 300 cells/mm³ (in 85% of cases, >1000/mm³), with granulocytes predominating in more than 80% of cases.[22] However, the total leukocyte count of some patients with ascites uncomplicated by infection may be similarly elevated.[21] Indeed, an increase in ascites leukocyte counts has been noted during diuresis in patients with chronic liver disease.[60] Some studies of other parameters of ascitic fluid that might help in diagnosing primary bacterial peritonitis have found lactate concentration and pH to be useful.[61–63] Ascitic fluid pH less than 7.35 and a lactate concentration higher than 25 mg/dl were more specific but less sensitive than a leukocyte count greater than 500 cells/mm³, and using all three parameters together increased the diagnostic accuracy.[62, 63] Gram staining of the sediment, when positive, is diagnostic, but it is negative in 60 to 80% of patients with cirrhosis and ascites.[17, 22]

Gonococcal perihepatitis (Fitz-Hugh-Curtis syndrome) most often occurs in women. It manifests with sudden onset of pain in the right upper quandrant of the abdomen, at times referred to the right shoulder. There may be low-grade fever, right upper quadrant tenderness, guarding, and a friction rub over the liver.[64] Gonococcal cervicitis or salpingitis may or may not be clinically evident. Chlamydial and gonococcal perihepatitis are clinically indistinguishable.

Primary tuberculous peritonitis usually is gradual in onset, with fever, weight loss, malaise, night sweats, and abdominal distention. The abdomen may not be rigid and is often characterized as being "doughy" on palpation. The findings at operation or laparoscopy consist of multiple nodules scattered over the peritoneal surface and omentum. Adhesions and a variable amount of peritoneal fluid are usually present. Ascitic fluid may have an elevated protein concentration (>3 g/dl) and a lymphocytic pleocytosis, but neither may be present, especially in cirrhotic patients.[65] Similarly, *C. immitis* can cause a granulomatous peritonitis with a variable clinical manifestation.[66]

Diagnosis

The diagnosis of primary peritonitis is one of exclusion of a primary intra-abdominal source of infection. Oral and intravenous contrast with computed tomographic (CT) scanning has greatly enhanced detection of intra-abdominal sources of peritonitis. Surgery can often be directed toward an identified potential source of infection, rather than the approach of a full exploratory laparotomy, which was more commonly used before the availability of CT scans in this setting and was associated with high mortality in certain groups of patients, such as cirrhotics.[68] Patients with primary peritonitis usually respond within 48 to 72 hours to appropriate antimicrobial therapy.[69] The observation of an exponential rate of decline in the number of ascitic fluid leukocytes after the initiation of antimicrobial therapy for primary peritonitis has also been found to help differentiate primary from secondary bacterial peritonitis.[70]

Recovery of pneumococci from peritoneal fluid may not indicate primary peritonitis, as illustrated by a case report of appendicitis and secondary peritonitis due to pneumococci.[71] For this reason, some surgeons have considered the differential diagnosis in children between appendicitis and primary peritonitis too difficult to make without operative examination, even when gram-positive bacteria are identified in peritoneal fluid.[14] Paracentesis for smear and culture is indicated in all cirrhotic patients with ascites and in children with gross proteinuria and abdominal pain, whether or not the diagnosis of nephrotic syndrome has been established. However, paracentesis is not without hazard, especially in patients with hemorrhagic tendencies of bowel distention. In a retrospective analysis of 242 consecutive diagnostic abdominal paracenteses in patients with liver disease and ascites, major complications were reported in 7, including perforation of the bowel with generalized peritonitis or abdominal wall abscess and serious hemorrhage.[72]

The diagnosis of tuberculous peritonitis can usually be made at operation or laparoscopy and confirmed by the histologic characteristics of the peritoneal biopsy specimen[73] and by bacteriologic examination of the peritoneal biopsy specimen and fluid.[74] The diagnosis of *C. immitis* peritonitis is best made by culture of ascitic fluid.[66] The laboratory should be apprised of this diagnostic possibility because the fungus is a biohazard.

Prognosis

The treatment of primary peritonitis has been reported to be successful in more than one half of the cirrhotic patients, but, because of the frequency of accompanying end-state cirrhosis, the overall mortality rate in cirrhotic adults has been as high as 95%.[17] However, more recent studies have reported lower mortality rates of 70 and 57% with 28 and 40% dying from the primary peritonitis, respectively.[22, 23] Those patients with the poorest prognosis were found to have renal insufficiency, hypothermia, hyperbilirubinemia, and hypoalbuminemia. The lower mortality rates in these later series can perhaps be explained by the less frequent occurrence of hepatic encephalopathy. The lowest hospitalization mortality and infection-related mortality rates (37.8 and 2.2%, respectively), reported even more recently, were attributed to early diagnosis and treatment.[69] Treatment of peritonitis caused by gram-positive organisms and of early infections has been more frequently successful than treatment of gram-negative or late infections. In nephrotic patients with gram-positive infections and patients who do not have a preterminal underlying illness, the survival rate is greater than 90%.[12]

Treatment

Because the gram stain is frequently negative in primary bacterial peritonitis, the initial choice of antimicrobial drug is often empirical, based on the most likely pathogens. The antimicrobial regimen can be modified once the results of the culture and susceptibility tests are available.

Some of the third-generation cephalosporin antibiotics have been demonstrated to be as efficacious as the combination of ampicillin plus an aminoglycoside for empirical therapy in primary bacterial peritonitis.[75] They also avoid the risk of nephrotoxicity, which is sufficiently common in this group of patients to warrant the avoidance of aminoglycosides if an equally effective alternative antimicrobial regimen can be used.[23, 76] Other antimicrobial agents such as the broad-spectrum penicillins (e.g., mezlocillin, ticarcillin, piperacillin), carbapenems (e.g., imipenem or meropenem), β-lactam/β-lactamase combinations (e.g., piperacillin-tazobactam, ticarcillin-clavulanate, ampicillin-sulbactam), and the newer fluoroquinolones, levofloxacin or trovafloxacin, are potential alternatives.

Primary bacterial peritonitis caused by either *S. pneumoniae* or group A streptococci is best treated with high-dose penicillin, ceftriaxone, or cefotaxime. If the pneumococcal strain is highly resistant to these drugs, vancomycin would be the preferred drug. Peritonitis suspected of being caused by methicillin-sensitive *S. aureus* should be treated with a penicillinase-resistant penicillin (e.g., nafcillin) or with a first-generation cephalosporin (e.g., cefazolin); if the strain is methicillin resistant or the patient is allergic to penicillin, vancomycin can be used. If *Pseudomonas aeruginosa* is isolated, an aminoglycoside antibiotic combined with an antipseudomonal penicillin or ceftazidime, cefepime, aztreonam or a carbapenem (e.g., imipenem, meropenem), or a fluoroquinolone with good antipseudomonal activity (e.g., ciprofloxacin) combined with another antipseudomonal antibiotic[77] should be used. For those situations in which the gram stain is suggestive of *Bacteroides* or polymicrobial peritonitis is evident, antimicrobials with activity against *B. fragilis* and other anaerobic organisms (e.g., metronidazole, clindamycin) should be added, or a single agent with both aerobic and anaerobic antimicrobial activity, such as one of the β-lactam/β-lactamase-inhibitor combinations, one of the carbapenems, or trovafloxacin, should be used.

In those cases in which there is a strong clinical suspicion of primary bacterial peritonitis but all cultures are sterile, antimicrobial therapy should be continued. Clinical improvement together with a significant decline in the ascitic fluid leukocyte count should occur after 24 to 48 hours of antimicrobial therapy if the diagnosis is correct.[69, 70, 78] Lack of the expected clinical response or persistence of an elevated ascitic fluid leukocyte count should make other diagnoses a consideration. Antimicrobial therapy should be continued for 10 to 14 days if improvement is noted; however, shorter-course (5-day) therapy has been shown to be as efficacious.[69] The administration of intraperitoneal antimicrobials is not necessary.

Prevention

Selective decontamination of the bowel with oral norfloxacin (400 mg daily) or trimethoprim/sulfamethoxazole (one double-strength dose given once daily for 5 days each week) has been shown to decrease the frequency of spontaneous bacterial peritonitis and may be an option in patients awaiting liver transplantation, but it has not been shown to confer a survival advantage otherwise.[79]

Secondary Peritonitis

Etiology

Secondary intra-abdominal infection usually is caused by spillage of gastrointestinal or genitourinary microorganisms into the peritoneal cavity owing to loss of the integrity of the mucosal barrier. The primary intra-abdominal processes that can give rise to secondary peritonitis are numerous. They include diseases or injuries of the gastrointestinal or genitourinary tracts (e.g., perforation of a peptic ulcer, traumatic perforation of the uterus, urinary bladder, stomach, or small or large bowel; spontaneous perforation associated with typhoid, tuberculous,[80] amebic, *Strongyloides*, or cytomegalovirus [CMV] ulcers in immunocompromised persons; appendicitis, diverticulitis, or intestinal neoplasms; gangrene of the bowel from strangulation, bowel obstruction, or mesenteric vascular obstruction; suppurative cholecystitis; bile peritonitis; pancreatitis; operative contamination of the peritoneum or disruption of a surgical anastomosis site; septic abortion, puerperal sepsis, postoperative uterine infection, or endometritis complicating an IUD[81] and gonococcal salpingitis or gonococcal vulvovaginitis in children; suppurative prostatitis; and rupture of an intraperitoneal or visceral abscess (such as renal or perinephric, tuboovarian, liver, splenic, pancreatic abscess). Peritonitis is a major hazard of chronic ambulatory peritoneal dialysis (CAPD) used in the management of renal failure, fluid and electrolytic imbalance, and certain intoxications.[52] Not uncommonly, bacterial peritonitis occurs secondary to the use of peritoneovenous and ventriculoperitoneal shunts.[82, 83]

Microbiologic Characteristics

Infrequently, secondary peritonitis is caused by exogenous microorganisms such as *S. aureus*, *N. gonorrhoeae*, or *M. tuberculosis*, which cause infection in intra-abdominal or adjacent viscera and spread to involve the peritoneum. Most cases of secondary peritonitis, however, are endogenous in orgin and are caused by the large number and variety of microorganisms that normally colonize mucous membranes lining certain viscera within the abdominal cavity. Although forming a continuous surface, the mucous membranes of the stomach, upper small bowel, lower small bowel, and large bowel each have a characteristic microflora in terms of type of microbial species, total number of different species, and microbial density. The vagina also has a distinct microflora. Normally, invasive activities of indigenous bacteria are controlled by the intact mucosa of the gastrointestinal tract and vagina. Disturbances in this mucosal barrier can occur as a result of spontaneous disease, trauma, or surgical operations that permit escape of indigenous bacteria and cause an infection of the peritoneum, the abdominal viscera, or the retroperitoneal space. The frequency with which various indigenous organisms are recovered from intra-abdominal infections varies according to the site of the primary process and whether the primary process is associated with an alteration of the indigenous microflora.[84]

The stomach normally contains up to 10^3 colony-forming units (cfu) of microorganisms per milliliter in the fasting state. If bacteria are present, they are mostly facultative, gram-positive, salivary microorganisms such as candida, lactobacilli, and streptococci. The numbers of these organisms in stomach contents transiently increase after a meal.[85] Gastric flora is more numerous and may be composed of different organisms when there is achlorhydria (e.g., from cimetidine) or blood in the stomach.[85, 86] The flora of the upper small intestine is normally sparse and consists of salivary microorganisms.[87] But in the presence of achlorhydria,[85] intestinal obstruction, or other processes affecting intestinal motility or absorption, the flora of the small intestine is more profuse and varied. Conditions that favor small bowel stasis include scleroderma, regional enteritis, small bowel strictures, nontropical sprue, tropical sprue, duodenal and jejunal diverticula, presence of an afferent loop of the Billroth II gastrojejunostomy, and intestinal pseudo-obstruction.[88] Large bowel flora has been found in the proximal small bowel of cirrhotic patients.[53] The ileum normally contains *E. coli*, enterococci, and an equal number of microorganisms that are obligately anaerobic, such as *B. fragilis*.[87] It is the colon, however, in which a profuse microflora exists in concentrations of about 10^{11} bacteria per milliliter of feces, a wet sludge of practically pure bacteria.[89] The colonic flora is predominantly composed of the obligate anaerobes *B. fragilis* and *Bifidobacterium* spp., which outnumber facultative microorganisms, primarily *E. coli*, by 10^3: to 10^4:1. Other colonic bacteria are viridans streptococci, enterococci, *Eubacterium* spp., *Klebsiella* spp., *Proteus* spp., *Enterobacter* spp., and *C. perfringens*. The large bowel flora is relatively stable[89] but may be significantly altered by antibiotic therapy.[90]

With loss of the integrity of the mucosal barrier at some point along the gastrointestinal tract a variable number of bacteria (in terms of bacterial density and number of different species) is found in the peritoneal cavity, depending on the level of the mucosal defect and comorbid conditions. For example, with perforation of the colon, initially a total of more than 10^{11} cfu/ml of hundreds of different species spills into the peritoneal cavity. A simplification of the microflora then occurs, so that once peritoneal infection is established only about five species are isolated from peritoneal exudate, usually three anaerobic and two aerobic species, even when care is exercised to ensure recovery of the obligate anaerobes. The obligate anaerobes isolated from clinical specimens have been found to be more oxygen-tolerant and to have identifiable virulence factors, compared with the rest of the anaerobic microflora in the gut. The facultative anaerobes isolated also have virulence factors. *B. fragilis* is the most frequently isolated obligate anaerobe after colonic perforation, and *E. coli* is the most freqently isolated facultative anaerobe.

As would be anticipated from the nature of the gastrointestinal flora, Altemeier[91] reported anaerobes in 96% of 100 cases of peritonitis secondary to acute appendicitis with perforation. *Prevotella melaninogenica* and anaerobic gram-positive cocci were the most frequent isolates. Studies of the bacteriologic characteristics of intra-abdominal infections,[92–94] using modern bacteriologic techniques that provide an anaerobic environment during collection, transport, and incubation, have confirmed the findings of Altemeier that anaerobes play a major role. Finegold[92] reported that in a series of 73 intra-abdominal infections, including 16 cases of peritonitis, there were an average of 4.5 isolates per case (range, 1 to 12 organisms), with 2.5 anaerobes and 2 aerobes or facultative organisms. The most common isolate was *E. coli*, followed by *B. fragilis* (the most common anaerobic isolate), enterococci, other *Bacteroides* spp., *Fusobacterium*, *C. perfringens*, other clostridia, *Peptococcus*, *Peptostreptococcus*, and *Eubacterium*. Similar findings were reported by Gorbach and coworkers[93] in a series of 43 patients, including 10 with peritonitis, in 93% of whom anaerobes or a mixture of anaerobes and facultative organisms were recovered, and by Swenson and colleagues[95] in a series of 64 patients, including 26 with peritonitis, in 81% of whom anaerobes were recovered. In these series, bacteremia was reported in 20 to 30% of patients. Organisms recovered from blood frequently included *B. fragilis* or *E. coli*. In series of patients with *Bacteroides* bacteremia, 14 to 62% had a gastrointestinal source.[96–99]

In a study of perforated appendicitis in which careful anaerobic culture techniques were used, an average of 9.4 species of anaerobes were isolated from each patient.[100] *Biliophila wadsworthia*, a recently recognized anaerobic gram-negative bacillus, was the fourth most common obligate anaerobe recovered and was found in one third of patients with gangrenous appendicitis and one half of patients with perforated appendicitis.[101]

Relatively antibiotic-resistant organisms such as candida, enterococci, *Enterobacter*, *Serratia*, *Acinetobacter*, and *P. aeruginosa* are isolated more frequently from patients whose intra-abdominal infection developed while they were in the hospital, after they received broad-spectrum antimicrobial agents.[102, 103] However, several studies have found that *P. aeruginosa* makes up a more significant portion of the aerobic isolates in community-acquired intra-abdominal infections[104–107] than had been noted previously.[108] Monomicrobial infection with microorganisms that have relatively low pathogenicity, such as candida, enterococci, or coagulase-negative staphylococci, have also been observed in what was thought to be new-onset peritonitis in patients with severely impaired defenses.[109]

Penetrating injuries to the liver and spleen are rarely followed by infection because of the usual sterility of these organs.[110]

Quantitative studies[111–113] of sexually active women during the childbearing period have revealed that the predominant vaginal microflora is composed of five to seven different microorganisms and that anaerobes are approximately 10 times more numerous than facultative organisms. There are about 10^8 to 10^9 cfu of anaerobes and about 10^7 to 10^8 cfu of facultatives per milliliter of vaginal secretions. The most frequent isolates in titers of 10^5 per milliliter or more are obligate or facultative anaerobic lactobacilli, nonenterococcal streptococci, anaerobic gram-positive cocci, Bacteroidaceae other than *B. fragilis* (e.g., *Prevotella melaninogenica*, *Prevotella bivia*, *Prevotella ruminicola*), and a group of unidentified catalase-negative facultative bacilli. Diphtheroids and *S. epidermidis* have also been reported to be frequent vaginal isolates.[113] When specifically looked for, *Gardnerella vaginalis* in high counts has also been found to be only slightly less common than lactobacilli in the vaginal secretions of normal women.[111, 112]

Colonic organisms, such as *B. fragilis*, Enterobacteriaceae, and enterococci, are rarely found as predominant components of the normal vaginal flora and probably proliferate at this site only under exceptional circumstances. For example, these organisms have been reported to appear in vaginal secretions in the immediate postoperative period after vaginal operations,[114] and *C. perfringens* has been reported more frequently in vaginal secretions after difficult labor or abortion.[115] Hite and colleagues[116] noted the relative infrequency of *Bacteroides* and anaerobic gram-positive cocci in the vagina of normal prenatal women, whereas during the puerperium, in both women with postpartum endometritis and noninfected women, these organisms were found to be more prevalent.[116, 117] Factors favoring colonization by these anaerobes after surgery and in the puerperium are unknown but are possibly related to blood or necrotic tissue that provides the reduced, enriched environment required by these anaerobes.

Sequential sampling of vaginal secretions during the menstrual cycle has been reported to show constant levels of anaerobes, although recovery of specific organisms varied from specimen to specimen in each woman.[113] In contrast, levels of facultative organisms decrease 100-fold in the premenstrual week.[113] This variation in microflora may reflect cyclic fluctuation in the vaginal environment caused by changes in hormonal activity during the menstrual cycle. Because the vaginal flora varies under certain conditions and members of this flora have differing pathogenicity, the frequency of endogenous intra-abdominal infections of gynecologic origin and the types of pathogens involved vary accordingly. For example, the frequency of vaginal colonization with group B streptococci increases during pregnancy, and infections caused by these organisms are relatively common in the postpartum period.[118] In addition, in women with trichomoniasis, *Bacteroides* spp. may be found more often in vaginal secretions.[112, 116] Postpartum infection, presumably caused by anaerobes, has been reported to be more common in women who have trichomoniasis during pregnancy.[119]

The bacteriologic characteristics of intra-abdominal infections that complicate female genital tract infections are similar to those of secondary peritonitis from a gastrointestinal source, except for the occurrence of *N. gonorrhoeae* in cul-de-sac aspirates.[120] Data compiled by Swenson,[121] Thadepalli,[122] and Chow[123] and their colleagues indicate that anaerobes were found in 72% of 200 gynecologic infections. Anaerobes were especially frequent (92%) in closed-space infections such as tuboovarian and pelvic abscesses. *Bacteroides* spp., in particular *B. fragilis*, *P. melaninogenica*, and anaerobic gram-positive cocci were the most frequently isolated anaerobes. *E. coli* and streptococci were the most prevalent facultative organisms. Bacteriologic studies have demonstrated in the majority of patients, even those with acute salpingitis, the presence of anaerobes, usually gram-positive cocci in cul-de-sac aspirates, despite the recovery of gonococci from the endocervix.[124–126] The data are interpreted as supporting the concept of superinfection with anaerobes late in the course of this disease, after initial infection with *N. gonorrhoeae*.[127] In children, gonococcal peritonitis has been reported rarely with gonococcal vulvovaginitis.[128, 129]

Intraperitoneal rupture has been reported in 10% of the cases of amebic liver abscess, and it may cause acute generalized peritonitis or, less commonly, a localized intraperitoneal abscess, with a mortality rate of about 18%.[130] Perforation of the colon with bacterial peritonitis due to fulminant amebic colitis is also unusual but often fatal.[131] Similarly, *Strongyloides stercoralis* infestation of the small bowel may rarely cause fatal peritonitis, with or without concurrent bacterial contamination.[132] Intestinal perforation complicating penetrating CMV enterocolitis has been described as a cause of acute abdomen in these patients. *Candida* has been isolated from the abdominal fluid of patients undergoing peritoneal dialysis, as has *S. aureus*, Enterobacteriaceae, and *P. aeruginosa*.[133] *Candida* peritonitis has also been observed as a complication of gastrointestinal surgery or in perforation of a viscus,[134, 135] and its occurrence is related to numerous factors that increase the rate of *Candida* colonization in the gastrointestinal tract. These include immunosuppression, prolonged hospitalization, and antimicrobial or antacid therapy. *Candida* is most commonly isolated from the peritoneum after perforation of a gastric or duodenal peptic ulcer, or after spillage of colonic contents into the peritoneum as a result of trauma, mesenteric artery occlusion, or dehiscence of a surgical anastomosis.

Pathogenesis

The virulence of the bacteria that cause peritonitis is enhanced when certain microorganisms either are combined intraperitoneally with substances such as mucus, enzymes, or hemoglobin or are combined with certain other microorganisms.

Chemical peritonitis can be produced by escape of bile or of gastric or pancreatic secretions into the peritoneal cavity. When gastric acid escapes into the peritoneal cavity, there is an outpouring of serum protein and electrolytes from the blood into the peritoneal cavity. The acidity is quickly neutralized by these buffers and by diffusion of hydrogen ions into the body fluids.[136, 137] Widespread necrosis may result from enzymatic digestion after intraperitoneal spillage of potent pancreatic enzymes. Escape of bile into the peritoneal cavity is generally considered to be a very grave, often fatal situation.[138, 139] The severity of peritonitis after escape of these intestinal secretions results in part to subsequent bacterial peritonitis. Indeed, in the dog with experimentally produced partial biliary diversion into the peritoneal cavity, fatal effects were reduced by oral nonabsorbable or parenteral antibiotics.[140] Bacteria may enter the peritoneal cavity with contaminated intestinal secretions through perforations in the gastrointestinal wall, or by migration through the wall of the intact gastrointestinal tract, in response to the irritation of bile and possibly other intestinal tract secretions on the serosal surface.[51]

Nemir and associates[141, 142] demonstrated that after experimental strangulation obstruction of a loop of bowel in the dog, the animal usually died within 36 hours, and the peritoneal fluid at first was light pink and eventually became black. When this black fluid was removed and injected into the peritoneal cavity of a normal animal, the recipient also developed a similar fatal peritonitis, but the early peritoneal fluid was nontoxic.[141–143] The toxicity could be largely counteracted by instilling antibiotics into the obstructed loop of intestine or by giving antibiotics simultaneously when the fluid was injected into normal animals.[144, 145] Many workers in the past have shown that intraperitoneal injection of large numbers of organisms in pure culture is incapable of producing peritonitis unless some additional factor is present, such as gum tragacanth, talc, mucin, turpentine, or another irritant. It seemed unlikely, therefore, that the toxicity of strangulation obstruction fluid was caused by its bacterial content alone. Evidence has been reported that viable bacteria in addition to the presence of free hemoglobin in the peritoneal fluid are necessary to account for the lethality both of bowel strangulation and of the fluid that collects in the peritoneal cavity after bowel strangulation.[146–148] The mechanism by which free hemoglobin enhances peritoneal infection is unknown but perhaps is related to free iron. Iron is required for bacterial metabolism and, in amounts that leave an excess of free iron after having saturated transferrin, may greatly enhance infections caused by certain microorganisms, such as Enterobacteriaceae and *C. perfringens*.[149] Hau and colleagues[150] demonstrated that intraperitoneal hemoglobin depresses the influx of granulocytes into the peritoneal cavity in response to intraperitoneal bacteria, and hemoglobin depresses in vitro the chemotactic response of granulocytes and monocytes.

Intraperitoneal fluid and fibrin that enter the peritoneal cavity as a result of the increased vascular permeability caused by local trauma or bacterial infection are important components of the inflammatory response and play adjuvant roles. Low numbers of *E. coli* in small volumes of saline infused intraperitoneally are innocuous, but these numbers can become lethal in direct proportion to the increase in the volume of saline infused; this is thought to be related to dilution of opsonic proteins.[151] Trapping of bacteria beneath layers of fibrin may limit their spread but may also lead to abscess formation and isolation of bacteria from host defense mechanisms.[152–154]

A number of other substances, such as hog gastric mucin, bile salts,[155] and barium sulfate,[156, 157] have been used as adjuvants in producing lethal intraperitoneal infections. The mechanisms of their respective effects have been the subject of numerous studies. It has been postulated that hog gastric mucin coats bacteria, thereby protecting them from intraperitoneal phagocytosis.[158]

Cuevas and Fine[159] attributed the lethality of bowel strangulation and infectious or chemical irritation of the serosal surface of the bowel to endotoxemia. Endotoxin was thought to escape from the gut lumen, cross the intact bowel wall into the peritoneal cavity, and become absorbed into the systemic circulation. Within minutes after experimental superior mesenteric artery occlusion, endotoxin was detected in the systemic circulation before its appearance in the portal vein.[159] Similarly, endotoxin levels were reported to be increased in plasma or peritoneal fluid of patients with severe intra-abdominal infection, but this parameter was not of prognostic significance.[160]

Secondary peritonitis is usually a mixed infection involving predominantly obligate and facultative anaerobes. Obligate anaerobes are sensitive to oxygen in the molecular form and also to bound oxygen, as in organic peroxides. Survival and growth of anaerobes also depends on the oxidation-reduction potential, that is, the oxidizing capacity of their environment. Most pathogenic anaerobes require a negative potential of at least -150 mV. Low oxidation-reduction potentials are thought to occur in many abscesses,[161] and oxidation-reduction potentials of -150 mV or less are measured in abscesses from which anaerobes are recovered.[162] Some anaerobic organisms have additional requriements, such as vitamin K, arginine, serum, blood pigments, or bile, before growth is obtained. Therefore, establishment of an anaerobic infection requires an environment in which the oxygen tension is very low, the oxidation-reduction potential is low, and abundant nutrients are available to support anaerobic metabolism. These requirements usually are met by devitalized tissue as a consequence of ischemia, trauma, or neoplastic growth. Once proper conditions are obtained, anaerobic organisms can achieve doubling rates equivalent to those seen with aerobic enteric bacilli. In vivo, the rapidly expanding bacterial and inflammatory cell mass, fequently accompanied by gas production, can interrupt the blood supply to the immediately surrounding tissue and cause further tissue necrosis.

Gram-negative anaerobic cocci and bacilli (including *B. fragilis* and *P. melaninogenica*) possess endotoxins with much weaker biologic activity in comparison with those extracted from their aerobic counterparts, and they have low or absent 2-keto-3-deoxyoctanoate content.[163] In addition, certain anaerobes elaborate collagenase,[164] other proteolytic enzymes, and deoxyribonuclease.[165] Certain Bacteroidaceae are capable of degrading heparin,[166] an ability that may be responsible for the suppurative thrombophlebitis frequently seen in infections caused by these microorganisms.[167] These factors tend to provide more areas well adapted to the growth requirements of the anaerobe, with the result that the infection progresses.

In addition, anaerobes may be resistant to host defenses. For example, although leukocytes have been shown to have bactericidal activity under both aerobic and anaerobic conditions against several anaerobic species, including *B. fragilis*, presumably by mechanisms other than those dependent on the superoxide anion O_2^- or H_2O_2,[168] Keusch and Douglas[169] found that granulocytic killing of *C. perfringens* was impaired under anaerobic conditions. Also, a capsule has been demonstrated on *B. fragilis*[170] and *Porphyromonas asaccharolytica* (formerly *B. melaninogenicus* ssp. *asaccharolyticus*)[171] that might protect the organisms from phagocytosis and favor abscess formation.[172–174] Some anaerobes, especially *B. fragilis*, may be resistant to the normal bactericidal activity of serum.[168]

Many anaerobic infections appear to be synergistic. Although it is probable that the majority of bacteria isolated in mixed infections are nonpathogenic by themselves, their presence may nevertheless be essential for the pathogenicity of the bacterial mixture. Such examples of bacterial synergism in infection were demonstrated in periodontal infection by Socransky and Gibbons[175] and in peritonitis by Altemeier.[176]

Facultative organisms in mixed infections may be essential by providing a sufficiently reduced environment for the growth of obligate anaerobic organisms. Another mechanism of bacterial synergy is the generation of a substance by one organism that is essential for the growth of another, for example, the production of vitamin K (a required growth factor for *P. melaninogenica*) by diphtheroids. Anaerobes such as *Bacteroides* spp. have also demonstrated the ability to protect aerobic bacteria from phagocytic killing[177, 178] and from otherwise effective antibiotic therapy (e.g., via β-lactamase production).[179]

In addition, each component of the pathogenic mixture may contribute in different ways to the clinical picture. In a series of experiments, Weinstein and coworkers[180] clarified the sequence of events that occurs after contamination of the peritoneum with fecal flora. In this model, after implantation of fecal contents intraperitoneally into rats, Onderdonk and associates[181] observed that *E. coli* initially predominated in the peritoneal exudate. Bacteremia, caused by *E. coli* during this phase, was uniformly present and frequently fatal. In rats that survived, indolent intra-abdominal abscesses developed in which *B. fragilis* predominated. Elimination of *E. coli* by early administration of gentamicin reduced early mortality but did not prevent late intra-abdominal abscess caused by obligate anaerobes; on the other hand, elimination of obligate anaerobes with clindamycin did not prevent early mortaliy from *E. coli* bacteremia but reduced late abscess formation in survivors. These findings indicate that, although *E. coli* is responsible for early mortality, *B. fragilis*, in concert with *E. coli* and perhaps other microorganisms (e.g., enterococci,[182, 183]) is responsible for late intraperitoneal abscess formation. Such synergy between obligate and facultative anaerobes has long been recognized in mixed infections.[184]

Pathophysiologic Responses

Whatever the initiating cause of peritonitis, a similar series of reactions takes place, both locally and systemically.

Local Response. The local inflammatory response of the peritoneum is similar to that in other tissues, but the peritoneal lining presents a large exudative and absorptive surface. At sites of irritation there is an outpouring of fluid into the peritoneal cavity that, in contrast to normal serous fluid, has a high protein content (>3 g/dl) and many cells, primarily granulocytes, that phagocytose and kill organisms. The exudate contains fibrinogen that polymerizes, and plaques of fibrinous exudate form on the inflamed peritoneal surfaces. This exudate glues together adjacent bowel, mesentery, and particularly omentum. Localization is further aided by inhibition of motility in involved intestinal loops. Experimentally, radiopaque medium injected intraperitoneally at one locus can be demonstrated to have spread over much of the greater peritoneal sac within a short time. The extent and rate of intraperitoneal spread of contamination undoubtedly depend on the volume and nature of the exudate[10] and on the effectiveness of the localizing processes.

If peritoneal defenses aided by appropriate supportive measures control the inflammatory process, the disease may resolve spontaneously. A second possible outcome is a confined abscess. A third course results when the peritoneal and systemic defense mechanisms are unable to localize the inflammation, which then progresses to spreading diffuse peritonitis. Some of the factors favoring spread of the inflammatory process are (1) greater virulence of bacteria, (2) greater extent and duration of contamination, and (3) impaired host defenses.

The cytokine response in peritonitis has been subject of an excellent review.[185] Undoubtedly, many of the local abdominal and systemic manifestations of peritonitis are mediated by cytokines, including tumor necrosis factor (TNF), interleukin-1 (IL-1), IL-6, and interferon-γ (INF-γ). Cytokines appear in the peritoneal exudate to a much greater extent than in systemic circulation of patients with peritonitis.[186] These cytokines are produced by macrophages and other host cells in response to bacteria or bacterial products, such as endotoxin,[187] and by tissues traumatized during abdominal operative procedures.[188]

Cytokine responses have been studied in the peritoneal exudate in experimental animal models of peritonitis,[189–192] in patients with spontaneous bacterial peritonitis,[193, 194] in patients undergoing CAPD,[195–197] and in patients with severe secondary bacterial peritonitis who were undergoing planned relaparotomy.[198] Anti-TNF antibody failed to afford protection against death[199] and failed to reduce serum levels of IL-1 and IL-6 in an experimental model of peritonitis.[189, 192, 200] In contrast, in this model anti-endotoxin antibodies were found to prevent death[201] and to reduce bacterial numbers in the peritoneal exudate, as well as serum levels of TNF, IL-1 and IL-6. Anti-INF-γ antibodies also afforded a protective effect both in this model of experimental peritonitis and after intravenous injection of endotoxin.[202]

Systemic Response. Peritonitis leads to changes not only locally in the peritoneal cavity but throughout the body.

Gastrointestinal. Initially in peritonitis there is hypermotility, followed by paralysis of the bowel. Accumulation of fluid and electrolytes in the lumen of the adynamic bowel continues until distention is sufficient to inhibit capillary inflow and secretion ceases.

Cardiovascular. Because of the large surface area of the peritoneum, shifts of fluid into the peritoneal cavity, combined with fluid shifts into the bowel lumen, can produce a profound fall in circulating blood volume and elevation of the hematocrit.[203, 204] Fluid and electrolyte loss is further exaggerated by coexistent fever, vomiting, diarrhea, and loss of aspirated gastrointestinal fluid. As the process continues, the decreased venous return to the right side of the heart results in a drop in cardiac output, with resulting hypotension.[204] Usually there is evidence of increased adrenergic activity: sweating, tachycardia, and cutaneous vasoconstriction (i.e., cold moist skin, mottled and cyanotic extremities).

With adequate replacement of blood volume, cardiac output may be maintained above normal.[204] Cardiac output of two or even three times normal may be required to satisfy the increased metabolic needs of the body in the presence of infection. Failure to sustain increased cardiac output results in progressive lactic acidosis, oliguria, hypotension, and ultimately death if the infection cannot be controlled.

Respiratory. The intraperitoneal inflammation results in relatively high and fixed diaphragms and considerable pain on respiration. This results in basilar atelectasis with intrapulmonary shunting of blood. Satisfactory compensation is possible only if the increase in energy demands does not exceed the respiratory reserve. Heavy cigarette smoking, chronic bronchitis emphysema, and obesity compound the problem. With decompensation in respiratory function, hypoxemia is accompanied first by hypocapnia (respiratory alkalosis) and later by hypercapnia (respiratory acidosis). In some patients, pulmonary edema develops, not because of left ventricular failure but perhaps because of increased pulmonary capillary leakage as a consequence of hypoalbuminemia or direct effects of bacterial toxins (adult respiratory distress syndrome). In these patients, progressive hypoxemia develops with decreasing pulmonary compliance. This requires volume-cycled ventilatory assistance with increasingly higher concentrations of inspired oxygen and positive end-expiratory pressure.

Renal. Low renal perfusion may be followed by acute tubular necrosis and progressive azotemia.

Metabolic. The excretion of cortisol is increased during the first few days and subsequently returns to normal.[205] The increased energy demands of infection rapidly deplete body stores of glycogen; this leads to catabolism of protein (muscle) and fat, accounting for the rapid weight loss of severely infected patients. Prolonged intra-abdominal infection is associated with extreme wasting. Heat production may eventually fail, and body temperature then falls. Exhaustion and death may ensue.

Clinical Manifestations

Symptoms. The early manifestations of peritonitis that results from disease of abdominal viscera are frequently those of the primary disease process. Moderately severe abdominal pain is almost always the predominant symptom. The pain is aggravated by any motion, even respiration. The progression of abdominal pain is a function of the rate of dissemination of the material producing the pain stimulus. Rupture of a peptic ulcer with massive spillage of gastric contents produces severe epigastric pain that, within minutes, may spread to involve the entire abdomen. In contrast, the spread of pain from a lesion such as a ruptured appendix is much more gradual. Decreased intensity and extent of pain with time usually suggest localization of the inflammatory process.

Anorexia, nausea, and vomiting commonly accompany abdominal pain. Patients may also complain of feverishness, sometimes with chill, thirst, scanty urination, inability to pass feces or flatus, and abdominal distention.

The formation and progression of an intraperitoneal abscess is often gradual: The patient who seemed to be recovering from peritonitis or an abdominal operation stops improving; fever returns, and localizing symptoms may develop.

Physical Findings. Patients with peritonitis characteristically lie quietly in bed, supine, with the knees flexed and with frequent limited intercostal respirations, since any motion intensifies the abdominal pain. The patient is alert, restless, and irritable early in the course but later may become apathetic or delirious.

Body temperatures may reach 42°C. Subnormal temperatures in the range of 35°C are often seen in the early stages of chemical peritonitis; they are a grave sign late in the course in patients with continuing intra-abdominal sepsis or septic shock.

Increasing tachycardia with weak, thready peripheral pulses reflects decreased effective blood volume. The blood pressure is maintained within normal limits early in the disease process. As peritonitis progresses, the blood pressure lowers to shock levels. Respiration is increasingly rapid and shallow.

Marked abdominal tenderness to palpation is present, usually maximally over the organ in which the process originated. Rebound tenderness, both direct and referred, signifies parietal peritoneal irritation. This finding is sometimes more accurate than direct palpation in locating the point of maximal tenderness and delineating the extent of peritoneal irritation.

Muscular rigidity of the abdominal wall is produced both by voluntary guarding and reflex muscular spasm. Hyperresonance due to gaseous intestinal distention can usually be demonstrated by percussion. Pneumoperitoneum from a ruptured hollow viscus may produce decreased liver dullness to percussion. Bowel sounds, initially hypoactive, later disappear. Rectal and vaginal examination may reveal tenderness and the presence of a pelvic abscess and may indicate a primary focus in the female pelvic organs.

Abdominal pain and muscle spasm may be deceptively absent in some patients. Those with lax abdominal musculature (e.g., patients in the postpartum period, patients with ascites due to cirrhosis, patients with marked cachexia) may not have abdominal rigidity. Similarly, patients who are in shock, who are receiving glucocorticosteroid therapy, or in whom loculated intra-abdominal abscesses are not in contact with the anterior abdominal wall (e.g., subphrenic, lesser sac, pelvic) may not exhibit marked abdominal pain and spasm. Absent bowel sounds may be the only manifestation of peritonitis in such patients, and a high index of suspicion is necessary.

Diagnostic Studies

The differential diagnosis in patients with symptoms and signs of peritonitis includes pneumonia, sickle cell anemia, herpes zoster, diabetic ketoacidosis, tabes dorsalis, porphyria, familial Mediterranean fever, plumbism, lupus erythematosus, and uremia.

A peripheral blood leukocyte count of 17,000 to 25,000 cells/mm^3 is usual in acute peritonitis, the differential count showing polymorphonuclear predominance and a moderate to marked shift to the left. However, reliance on the significance of the total leukocyte count may be misleading. Massive peritoneal inflammation can mobilize leukocytes into the diseased area; for example, there may be fewer than 5000 leukocytes per milliliter in the circulating blood, but the differential smear in this situation may show an extreme shift to immature polymorphonuclear forms.

Hemoconcentration and dehydration are reflected by increased hematocrit and blood urea nitrogen values. Hyperglycemia and glycosuria usually are not present in peritonitis but may be seen in diabetic acidosis and acute pancreatitis, which can manifest with signs suggesting peritonitis. Hematuria and pyuria without bacteriuria may reflect intra-abdominal inflammatory disease such as appendicitis adjacent to the urinary tract. Elevated serum amylase levels may be seen in peritonitis from almost any cause, but very high levels are seen only in acute pancreatitis. Hyponatremia may be seen in patients given water to replace isotonic fluid losses, but it is also characteristic of porphyria. Acidosis, both metabolic and respiratory, is present in severe and late peritonitis.

Supine, upright, and lateral decubitus radiographs of the abdomen may reveal distention of both the small intestine and the colon, with adynamic loops of bowel or features of mechanical intestinal obstruction, volvulus, intussusception, or vascular occlusion. Inflammatory exudate and edema of the intestinal wall produces a widening of the space between adjacent loops. Peritoneal fat lines and psoas shadows may be obliterated. Free air may be visible if there is a ruptured viscus. Chest radiographs should always be taken to rule out a pulmonary or thoracic problem as the cause of the abdominal distress. The presence of air beneath the diaphragm may be best defined in these pictures. Trapped gas with a fluid level or mottling due to gas may also be visible in intraperitoneal or visceral abscesses. Calcification in the gallbladder or other organs may also be noted on radiographs.

Ultrasonography is frequently the initial step in evaluating intra-abdominal sepsis, especially for detecting processes in the right upper quadrant, retroperitoneum, and pelvis. However, dilated, air-filled loops of bowel, obesity, overlying lungs, bandages, wounds, drains, and ostomies can interfere with the quality of ultrasound images. CT scanning of the entire abdomen and pelvis with oral and intravenous contrast has become invaluable for evaluating patients with a suspected intra-abdominal infection. CT has frequently replaced exploratory laparotomy for this purpose. CT can facilitate detection of lesions outside the suspected area on the basis of clinical findings and guidance of percutaneous drainage of peritoneal fluid or abscesses. Although CT is more costly than ultrasound, it is the preferred initial study, except when the lesion is suspected to be in the right upper quadrant, retroperitoneum, or pelvis.[206–208] Ultrasound is also more operator-dependent than CT, and abdominal tenderness may preclude the use of the desired amount of external pressure to visualize the intra-abdominal contents adequately.

Needle aspiration of the peritoneal cavity is often helpful. If no fluid can be aspirated, peritoneal lavage with Ringer's lactate solution should be done to obtain fluid for examination. In performing a tap, the region of abdominal scars, where bowel may be adherent to the underside of the scar, should be avoided. The aspirate is examined grossly for content of blood, pus, bile, or digested fat; chemically for amylase content; and microscopically, with gram staining, for bacteria. A positive tap is meaningful; a dry or negative tap is of little significance. Guidance for the tap may be obtained by ultrasound or CT.

Prognosis

Survival of a patient with secondary peritonitis depends on many factors, including the age of the patient, comorbid conditions, the duration of peritoneal contamination, the presence of foreign material (bile or pancreatic secretions, barium), the primary intra-abdominal process, and the microorganisms involved.[209, 210] Altemeier[91] showed that the more organisms present in peritoneal exudate, the worse the prognosis, although there was no correlation between severity of infection and the presence of any particular organism. Mortality increases with more distal gastrointestinal sources of contamination.[211] In the very young patient, because of the relatively small omentum, the walling-off process is less effective and diffuse peritonitis occurs more frequently than in the adult. In the elderly, preexisting conditions such as emphysema, diabetes, or cardiovascular disease reduce the capacity of the patient to meet the demands on the cardiovascular, respiratory, and renal systems during this period of intense metabolic activity.[209] Mortality rates range from 3.5% in those with early infection caused by penetrating abdominal trauma to more than 60% in patients with established intra-abdominal infection and secondary organ failure.[212] Persistent peritoneal contamination, leakage of pancreatic enzymes, septicemia, fluid and electrolyte abnormalities, pneumonia,[213] and cardiovascular, renal, and respiratory failure[214] are the principal causes of death.

With a disease process that has widely varying mortality rates, the ability to predict outcome and stratify severity of disease is important for clinical decision-making and for ensuring comparability in trials that evaluate different management strategies with surgical protocols or antimicrobial agents.[215] Outcome has been found to be related mainly to host related factors (e.g., preoperative nutritional status, organ impairment, severity of the patient's systemic response, and the patient's premorbid physiologic reserves, as predicted by the Acute Physiologic and Chronic Health Evaluation II (APACHE II) scoring system,[216] rather than type and source of the infection.[217, 218]

Death from intra-abdominal infection, especially when the tertiary phase is reached, is thought to result from an exaggerated, uncontrolled cytokine release that is unresponsive to all therapeutic attempts.[219] This has led to the use of endotoxin and cytokine levels in circulation to predict outcome. However, the magnitude of levels of TNF-α and IL-6 in circulation in patients with peritonitis have not been invariably related to prognosis.[220–224] Determination of cytokine levels in the peritoneal exudate, rather than in blood, has been suggested to better reflect the severity of the compartmentalized peritoneal infection and predict outcome.[198]

Treatment

Antimicrobial Therapy. Medical management includes use of antimicrobial therapy and supportive measures to maintain vital functions (e.g., improve or maintain circulation, nutrition, and oxygenation to vital organs). As yet the clinical efficacy of "immunomodulators" such as anti-TNF antibodies, anti-endotoxin antibodies, and IL-1 receptor antagonists, is unproven.

Secondary peritonitis is typically polymicrobial, and the pathogens in most cases are derived from the gastrointestinal tract, even in patients with a primary gynecologic process. Typically, the facultative microorganisms are *E. coli*, *Klebsiella/Enterobacter* spp., *Proteus* spp., and enterococci, and the obligate anaerobes are *B. fragilis*, *P. melaninogenica*, *Peptococcus*, *Peptostreptococcus*, *Fusobacterium*, *Eubacterium lentum*, and *Clostridium*. Other less commonly isolated pathogens include *S. aureus*, *P. aeruginosa*, and *Candida*.

The role of antimicrobial therapy in the outcome of infection caused by anaerobes or by a mixture of anaerobes and facultative microorganisms is extremely difficult to assess. Often dramatic response to surgical drainage and débridement alone occurs when there is localized infection. Nevertheless, appropriate antimicrobial therapy has been shown to reduce significantly mortality among patients with bacteremic infections caused by Bacteroidaceae or Enterobacteriaceae.[99, 225, 226] Antimicrobial drugs are expected to control bacteremia and early metastatic foci of infection, to reduce suppurative complications if given early, and to prevent local spread of existing infection. Once suppuration has occurred, it may be difficult to cure the infection if antimicrobial drugs are used without drainage; also, antimicrobial drugs used alone may mask some of the clinical manifestations of abscess formation. However, some intra-abdominal abscesses can be treated successfully with antibiotics alone.[227, 228]

Antimicrobial agents must penetrate to the site of infection in concentrations that are sufficient to overcome the effects of a high bacterial density, the metabolic inactivity and slow growth rate of probably more than 90% of the bacterial inoculum, low pH, low redox potential, necrotic tissue, and bacterial products that may lower the drug's activity. For example, aminoglycosides and clindamycin are less active at acid pH, aminoglycosides are less active at low redox potentials, and β-lactams are less active against high bacterial densities.

Although the results of many antimicrobial trials for the treatment of intra-abdominal infections have been published, caution must be exercised when interpreting these studies because of the possibility of inadequate study design and analysis of data.[229] Some of the variables that must be considered are differences in patient populations, types and severity of underlying illnesses, community-versus hospital-acquired infection, and the pathogens isolated. Table 64–1 lists many of the antimicrobial regimens that have been found to be efficacious for the treatment of intra-abdominal infections in clinical trials.

Antimicrobial therapy should be started immediately after appropriate specimens (blood and, if possible, peritoneal fluid) are obtained for culture. This means that antimicrobial therapy is often started before the completion of in vitro antimicrobial sensitivity testing of the specific facultative pathogens. In addition, rapid isolation, identification, and in vitro sensitivity testing of anaerobes, in contrast to testing of facultative bacteria, are not possible in many community hospitals. Several factors account for the delay in obtaining anaerobic bacteriologic results. Infections caused by anaerobes frequently involve mixtures of five or more microorganisms, and cultures require long periods for growth and isolation. In addition, in vitro sensitivity testing by the conventional disk diffusion technique has not been standardized for anaerobes.[162] Such tests are influenced to a large extent by the growth rate of the bacteria, inoculum size, pH and type of medium, duration of incubation, and carbon dioxide concentration in the atmosphere.[241, 242] In vitro studies of the stability of the β-lactam antibiotics when exposed to reducing agents such as mercaptoamines (cysteine), which are frequently incorporated in media used for the growth of anaerobes, have shown that these compounds are able to open the β-lactam ring and to inactivate penicillins.[243] However, susceptibility of anaerobic organisms can be reliably determined by the broth or agar dilution technique with the use of appropriate media.[244] Because these tests are generally performed by research laboratories, knowledge of the antimicrobial susceptibility of anaerobes is gained from periodically published reports on anaerobic isolates by centers that specialize in performing these tests. Therefore, initial chemotherapy is usually empirical, based on the most reliable and least toxic antimicrobial agents for the most probable anaerobic and facultative pathogens. In vitro sensitivity reports (usually reliable only for the facultative or aerobic organisms) allow subsequent adjustment of the initial regimen to more specific therapy.

Because these infections are commonly polymicrobial, a broad spectrum of antimicrobial activity is required. Data suggest that survival in patients with intra-abdominal infection is diminished if

TABLE 64–1 Comparative Antimicrobial Trials for Treatment of Intra-abdominal Infections

Regimen	Reference
Cefoxitin ± aminoglycoside vs. clindamycin + aminoglycoside	230–232
Ticarcillin + aminoglycoside vs. clindamycin + aminoglycoside	233
Piperacillin vs. cefoxitin	234
Ampicillin-sulbactam vs. clindamycin + aminoglycoside	235
Imipenem vs. clindamycin + aminoglycoside	236–239
Aztreonam + clindamycin vs. clindamycin + aminoglycoside	240
Trovafloxacin vs. imipenem	240a

initial therapy is inadequate, regardless of the adequacy of subsequent treatment.[245] The ideal regimen remains controversial. The animal model of intra-abdominal sepsis demonstrated the necessity of treating both the facultative enteric gram-negative bacilli, namely *E. coli*, and the anaerobic gram-negative bacilli, namely *B. fragilis*. Empirical use of an antimicrobial regimen active against *E. coli* and *B. fragilis* has been well established. Indeed, the need for intraoperative cultures to document the etiologic microorganisms and their antimicrobial susceptibilities has been questioned because the results are rarely available to influence clinical decision-making.[246, 247]

Drugs active against anaerobic bacteria may be inactive against the accompanying aerobic or facultative pathogens in the mixed infections, and vice versa. For this reason, combinations of usually two or three drugs are used. These combinations of antimicrobial agents are selected for their activity against most of the more virulent pathogens in the infective mixture (e.g., the Enterobacteriaceae, *B. fragilis*), although monotherapy for polymicrobial intra-abdominal infection is now possible because of the availability of broad-spectrum agents with activity against both aerobes and anaerobes.[236]

Antibiotics need not be active against every pathogen isolated. It is apparent that if only some of the organisms can be eliminated, the synergistic effect may be removed and the patient's defenses may be able to eradicate the remaining organisms. For example, clindamycin alone (which has no activity against Enterobacteriaceae or enterococci) has been reported to be sufficient treatment for some patients with infections resulting from a mixture of Enterobacteriaceae, enterococci, and anaerobes.[248]

Although enterococci are found in about 20% of intra-abdominal infections, the exact role they play in polymicrobial intra-abdominal infection and the need for an antimicrobial regimen specific for these organisms is controversial.[249] In several studies, patients were treated successfully with clindamycin and gentamicin despite absence of activity of this therapeutic regimen against enterococci.[250, 251] Selective therapy against *E. coli* and *B. fragilis* that has no or borderline in vitro antimicrobial activity against enterococci has been found to be sufficient to reduce enterococcal counts.[252] Nevertheless, in animal models of experimental polymicrobial intra-abdominal infection, enterococci have been found to be a significant component of the inoculum; as such, they enhance abscess formation, weight loss, bacteremia with *B. fragilis* and *E. coli*, and mortality.[252, 253] Similarly, clinical reports have emphasized the importance of enterococci in intra-abdominal infection [254] and noted the emergence of enterococcal abscesses and bacteremia supervening after treatment of intra-abdominal sepsis with antimicrobial agents that lack significant in vitro enterococcal activity.[255–265] Enterococci have emerged as major nosocomial pathogens, undoubtedly as a result of their inherent resistance to many commonly used antimicrobial agents and their recent acquisition of resistance to previous standard therapy (i.e., ampicillin, aminoglycosides, and the glycopeptides, vancomycin and teicoplanin).[266–269] Only clinically unproven agents to which the strains are sensitive (e.g., doxycycline, novobiocin, chloramphenicol) and a new combination of two streptogramin antibiotics (Synercid), used alone or in combination to prevent emergence of resistance, are available as potential therapy for infections caused by these multiple-drug–resistant strains of enterococci. The efficacy of agents with anti-enterococcal activity for primary empirical therapy to prevent emergence of enterococcal superinfection is unknown. A multicenter study of intra-abdominal infection[270, 271] found that the presence of enterococci in the initial culture, independently from the APACHE II score, predicted treatment failure with broad-spectrum antimicrobial regimens that lacked specific enterococcal activity. APACHE II score, age, length of preinfection hospital stay, and postoperative infections predicted the presence of enterococci. It is unknown whether inclusion of antienterococcal therapy improves outcome in these high-risk patients.

Treatment for *Candida* in polymicrobial infections is also controversial.[272, 273] Isolation of this microorganism from blood cultures or as the sole organism within residual or recurrent intra-abdominal infection, or as the predominant organism on Gram staining of peritoneal exudate, represents an indication for specific antimicrobial therapy plus drainage of abscesses, if present.[134, 274, 275] Amphotericin B is standard therapy for invasive *Candida* infection, although lipid-associated amphotericin may be an efficacious, less nephrotoxic, but more expensive alternative. Fluconazole is also less toxic, although no comparative trials in *Candida* peritonitis exist. *Candida krusei* and *Torulopsis glabrata* are inherently more resistant to azoles, and resistance to azoles among previously sensitive *Candida* species is increasing.

When combinations of antibiotics are used, synergism or antagonism may occur. Chloramphenicol has been shown to impair early bactericidal activity of gentamicin in vitro, and antagonism was demonstrated in mice with experimental *Proteus mirabilis* infection when phagocytic function was impaired (i.e., in neutropenic mice).[276] Two studies suggest that clindamycin inhibits early in vitro killing of *E. coli* and *K. pneumoniae* by gentamicin.[277] However, in an in vivo study of aminoglycoside therapy of *E. coli* peritonitis and bacteremia in normal and neutropenic mice, prior or simultaneous administration of clindamycin with the aminoglycoside did not inhibit the therapeutic effect of the aminoglycoside.[278] Clindamycin combined in vitro with gentamicin has been reported to have indifferent or synergistic activity against Enterobacteriaceae after 18 hours of incubation.[279]

The activities of various antimicrobial agents against the usual peritoneal pathogens and the results of clinical trials are discussed in the sections that follow.

Chloramphenicol. At a concentration of 16 μg/ml, chloramphenicol has activity against more than 99% of the anaerobic pathogens involved in intra-abdominal infections, especially *B. fragilis*.[280] However, the availability of equally effective and potentially less toxic antimicrobial agents to treat anaerobic infections (e.g., clindamycin, metronidazole, imipenem) has all but eliminated the need for chloramphenicol,[281] except perhaps for significant infection caused by strains of enterococci that are resistant to all other antimicrobial agents.

Clindamycin. Clindamycin has been reported to inhibit more than 95% of the anaerobes, including *B. fragilis*, at a concentration of 8 μg/ml,[280] and early clinical trials established the efficacy of clindamycin plus aminoglycoside.[282, 283] About 15% of the strains of *Clostridium* spp. other than *C. perfringens*, *Peptococcus* spp., and rare strains of *Fusobacterium* spp. have been reported to be resistant to clindamycin. Most strains of *B. fragilis* have remained highly susceptible to clindamycin during the past decade.[284, 285] Plasmid-mediated, transferable clindamycin resistance in *B. fragilis* has been demonstrated,[284] and clindamycin resistance among *B. fragilis* has become a problem at certain medical centers. Clindamycin is active against only certain facultative gram-positive cocci, such as *S. aureus* and *Streptococcus pyogenes*, but not enterococci, and it has virtually no activity against Enterobacteriaceae.

Diarrhea is reported to be the most common side effect of clindamycin therapy, occurring at an incidence of 2 to 20%.[286] The severity of the diarrhea varies, but it may be associated with pseudomembranous colitis in up to one half of the patients with diarrhea, as reported in one study.[287] Toxic megacolon, colonic perforation, and death on rare occasions have been reported and attributed to an exotoxin produced by clindamycin-resistant strains of *C. difficile*.[286]

Metronidazole. Metronidazole is active against strict anaerobes, inhibits most *B. fragilis* strains, *Fusobacterium* spp., and *Clostridium* spp., and has a unique bactericidal action against *B. fragilis* and *C. perfringens*.[288] Resistance among *B. fragilis* to metronidazole is rare. However, the in vitro activity of metronidazole is poor against aerobes, microaerophiles, and anaerobes that may become somewhat aerotolerant on subculture (i.e., certain anaerobic gram-positive cocci and sporeless gram-positive rods),[280, 289] although there is some in vivo evidence in animal models and humans that metronidazole has activity against *E. coli* and other aerobes in mixed aerobic-anaerobic infections.[290, 291] The mechanism for this is poorly understood but may be related to the conversion by *B. fragilis* of metronidazole into active metabolites with activity against *E. coli* and other aerobes.[290] Nonetheless, because facultative gram-negative bacilli and microaerophilic gram-positive cocci, which are frequent copathogens in polymicrobial anaerobic infection, are resistant to metronidazole, the drug should be used in combination with another agent that is active against these pathogens to compensate for these defects in its spectrum.

The relative incidence of *C. difficile*–associated diarrhea and colonization was found to be less after use of metronidazole than after clindamycin in a retrospective study.[292] Metronidazole is the drug of choice for treatment of this disease.

Tetracyclines. The large number of resistant anaerobes, especially *B. fragilis*, precludes the use of these drugs,[293, 294] except perhaps for infection caused by strains of enterococci that are resistant to all other antimicrobial agents.

Cephalosporins. *B. fragilis* and other *Bacteroides* spp. usually are resistant to the so-called first-generation cephalosporins (e.g., cefazolin) and to some second-generation cephalosporins (e.g., cefuroxime). Cefoxitin is distinctly more active than any of the other second-generation cephalosporins against *Bacteroides* spp.,[280, 295, 296] but cefoxitin resistance has become a problem at certain medical centers.[285] Cefotetan has activity similar to that of cefoxitin except that it is ess active against the *B. fragilis* group (not including *B. fragilis*).[295, 296] These first- and second-generation cephalosporins are also active against most strains of *E. coli*, *P. mirabilis*, and *K. pneumoniae*. The third-generation cephalosporins (cefotaxime, ceftizoxime, cefoperazone, ceftriaxone, and ceftazidime) and cefepime have demonstrated significantly better activity against the Enterobacteriaceae. Only ceftazidime and cefepime, and to a lesser extent cefoperazone, have activity against *P. aeruginosa*. With a few exceptions, the third-generation cephalosporins have relatively poor activity against *B. fragilis* and other *Bacteroides* spp.[297] Ceftizoxime was reported to have good in vitro activity against *B. fragilis* and other *Bacteroides* spp. in some studies,[296, 298] but was inadequate against *Bacteroides* species, including *B. fragilis*, in other in vitro studies.[295, 299] Because the activity of ceftizoxime is greatly affected by the inoculum of *Bacteroides* in in vitro studies,[280] this antibiotic would most likely be inadequate to treat severe intra-abdominal infections in which the inoculum of organisms is great.[300, 301]

Regimens in which a third-generation cephalosporin is substituted for the aminoglycoside compare favorably to clindamycin plus aminoglycoside. However, resistance emerges readily under selective pressure of antimicrobial therapy with third-generation cephalosporins among certain gram-negative bacilli that produce chromosomal-encoded inducible β-lactamases, such as *Enterobacter*, *Serratia*, *Citrobacter*, *Morganella*, *Acinetobacter*, and *P. aeruginosa*. These organisms have a high spontaneous mutation rate for constitutive production of large amounts of these β-lactamases, which confer resistance to all β-lactams except imipenem, meropenem, and cefepime and are poorly antagonized by the clinically available β-lactamase inhibitors, sulbactam, clavulanic acid, and tazobactam. Patients who are likely to be infected with these organisms (those with prolonged hospital stays, prior antibiotic treatment, postoperative peritonitis, or tertiary peritonitis) are best treated with imipenem, meropenem, cefepime, a fluoroquinolone, or an aminoglycoside.

Strains of *K. pneumoniae* and, to a lesser extent, *E. coli*, have acquired plasmid-encoded, extended-spectrum β-lactamases that inactivate all third-generation cephalosporins, especially ceftazidime. These strains are also resistant to aztreonam, the monobactam, and frequently to the fluoroquinolones. These β-lactamases may be inactivated by sulbactam, clavulanic acid, and tazobactam, which confer activity to the β-lactam/β-lactamase inhibitor combinations containing these agents. Imipenem, meropenem, and, to a lesser degree, cefepime are reliably also likely to be active against these strains.

Penicillins. Penicillin G and ampicillin have excellent activity against all anaerobes, with the exception of *Bacteroides* spp. (especially *B. fragilis*) and *Fusobacterium* spp. other than *Fusobacterium nucleatum*. Ampicillin also is active against 70 to 80% of the strains of *E. coli* and almost all *P. mirabilis*. There is some evidence to suggest that penicillin G may fail to achieve inhibitory concentrations at sites of *B. fragilis* infection, because of both a reduction in penetration of penicillin into infected sites and inactivation of the drug by *B. fragilis*.[302] Therapeutic failures despite high doses of penicillin for *B. fragilis* bacteremia have been well documented.[96] Resistance of *B. fragilis* to penicillins is frequently caused by production of β-lactamase.[303]

About 80 to 90% of strains of *B. fragilis* may be sensitive to high concentrations (minimal inhibitory concentration [MIC], ≤125 μg/ml) of the extended-spectrum penicillins, piperacillin, ticarcillin, mezlocillin, and azlocillin,[304–306] and the clinical experience with these drugs in polymicrobial anaerobic infections has been favorable.[307–309] The spectrum of these penicillins also includes the majority of aerobic enteric gram-negative bacilli and *P. aeruginosa*, but is not likely to include *K. pneumoniae* and some strains of *E. coli* as a consequence of β-lactamase production. The combination of ticarcillin or piperacillin with the β-lactamase inhibitors clavulanic acid or tazobactam, respectively, confers activity against almost all β-lactamase–producing strains of *B. fragilis*, *E. coli*, and *K. pneumoniae*,[310–312] but does not confer activity against the chromosomal-encoded, inducible, β-lactamase-producing strains of *Serratia*, *Enterobacter*, *P. aeruginosa*, *Citrobacter*, *Acinetobacter*, and *Morganella*.[313] In addition, ticarcillin is inherently much less active against enterococci than piperacillin is. Ampicillin/sulbactam is active against many community-acquired, β-lactamase–producing bacteria that are resistant to ampicillin, including *E. coli*, *Klebsiella*, and *Bacteroides*,[314, 315] but it is inactive against nosocomial pathogens such as *Enterobacter*, *Serratia*, and *P. aeruginosa*. Monotherapy for polymicrobial anaerobic intra-abdominal infection is possible with these β-lactam/β-lactamase combinations, such as ampicillin/sulbactam, ticarcillin/clavulanate, and pipercillin/tazobactam, because of their broad spectrum of activity against both aerobes and anaerobes.

Other β-Lactams. The carbapenem antibiotics, imipenem and meropenem, have a very broad antimicrobial spectrum,[316] with activity against almost all aerobic and anaerobic pathogens. They are resistant to most β-lactamases, including chromosomal, inducible β-lactamases of bacteria, such as *Enterobacter*, *Serratia*, and *P. aeruginosa*,[317] except those produced by rare strains of *B. fragilis*[318] and *Stenotrophomonas maltophilia*. Monotherapy for polymicrobial anaerobic intra-abdominal infection is possible with meropenem or imipenem, because of their broad spectrum of activity against both aerobes and anaerobes.

Aztreonam, a monobactam antibiotic, has a spectrum of activity limited to aerobic gram-negative bacilli.[319] It would be necessary to use an antibiotic with activity against both anaerobes and microaerophilic and aerobic gram-positive cocci (i.e., clindamycin[320–322]) rather than metronidazole, which has poor activity against these common pathogens, along with aztreonam in the treatment of secondary intra-abdominal infections.

Aminoglycosides. Aminoglycosides, except for their excellent spectrum of activity against Enterobacteriaceae and *P. aeruginosa*, do not have much advantage over penicillins or cephalosporins against sensitive strains of these organisms for many reasons. The serum concentrations of gentamicin are unpredictable after a dose based on the body weight, so peak and trough serum levels must be confirmed by any of the various assay methods available.[323] In addition, the therapeutic range of peak serum concentrations of 4 to 8 μg/ml is narrow: Levels below 4 μg/ml may be below the MIC for the pathogen, and levels greater than 10 to 12 μg/ml may be toxic with an 8-hour dosing interval. Therefore, the peak serum levels are either equal to or only slightly greater than the MIC for the aminoglycoside in vitro.

Aminoglycosides are frequently underdosed because of fear of nephrotoxicity or ototoxicity, or because of underestimation of the expanded volume of distribution in critically ill patients with intra-abdominal sepsis. Once-daily aminoglycoside therapy, in which the total daily dose is given as a single dose every 24 hours rather than in multiple smaller, divided doses, obviates these problems, because both the bactericidal activity and the duration of the post antibiotic effect of aminoglycosides are concentration-dependent, whereas its nephrotoxicity is probably time-dependent. However, too limited numbers of severely ill patients with intra-abdominal sepsis have been studied to recommend general use of single daily dosing of these drugs. The use of aminoglycosides may be reduced by the availability of new alternative agents.

Aminoglycosides are inactive against obligate anaerobes, and their activity against sensitive pathogens is antagonized by an anaerobic environment[324] and by reducing substances such as sulfhydryl compounds. Aminoglycosides also are not active in acidic conditions. Both anaerobic and acidic conditions are frequently present in intra-abdominal abscesses. The β-lactams, in contrast, are relatively non-toxic, can be used in concentrations that are many times higher than the MIC for the pathogen, and are active under anaerobic or acidic conditions. For these reasons, the efficacy of aminoglycosides in intra-abdominal infection has been questioned.[325] The β-lactams are probably more reliable antibiotics than the aminoglycosides against sensitive pathogens. Therefore, if indicated on the basis of in vitro sensitivity testing, β-lactams should be used in preference to aminoglycosides. An aminoglycoside is usually included with a β-lactam antibiotic in the initial antimicrobial regimen for patients who are critically ill or in whom a resistant pathogen (e.g., *P. aeruginosa*) is suspected.

Quinolones. The fluoroquinolones (norfloxacin, ciprofloxacin, enoxacin, ofloxacin, lomefloxacin, levofloxacin, sparfloxacin, grepafloxacin, and trovafloxacin) are a class of antimicrobial agents related to nalidixic acid.[326] They are active against almost all aerobic gram-negative bacilli. Ciprofloxacin remains the most potent fluoroquinolone against *P. aeruginosa*. Levofloxacin, sparfloxacin, grepafloxacin, and especially trovafloxacin, in contrast to the older fluoroquinolones,[327] have activity against gram-positive cocci, although enterococci and methicillin-resistant *S. aureus* tend to be less susceptible than other gram-positive cocci. In addition, trovafloxacin has excellent potency against obligate anaerobes (comparable to metronidazole), unlike other fluoroquinolones.[328, 329] Their ability to kill bacteria in both the exponential and the stationary phases of growth, along with the lack of development of plasmid-mediated resistance, make the fluoroquinolones potentially valuable antimicrobial agents for the treatment of intra-abdominal infections, including abscesses.

Currently, four fluoroquinolones (ciprofloxacin, ofloxacin, levofloxacin, and trovafloxacin) are available for parenteral administration. These four, as well as sparfloxacin and grepafloxacin, are well absorbed after oral administration and are concentrated in tissues so that tissue levels are well in excess of the MICs of many sensitive pathogens. However, with current fluoroquinolone dosing regimens, these tissue levels may be inadequate to treat susceptible pathogens with relatively high MICs (e.g., >0.5 μg/ml of ciprofloxacin), which include some strains of *P. aeruginosa*, enterococci, and *S. aureus*, especially the methicillin-resistant strains.[330] If such organisms can be anticipated (e.g., in nosocomial infections), additional antimicrobial agents may be necessary to broaden the spectrum of an empirical regimen. The addition of an antimicrobial agent active against anaerobic bacteria and aerobic or microaerophilic gram-positive cocci (e.g., clindamycin, ampicillin-sulbactam, amoxicillin-clavulanic acid) would be required if the use of ciprofloxacin were considered for secondary intra-abdominal infection. However, monotherapy for polymicrobial intra-abdominal infection is possible with trovafloxacin because of its broad-spectrum activity against both aerobes and anaerobes.

Duration of Antimicrobial Therapy. Antibiotic therapy should be given before, during, and after surgery to ensure tissue and blood levels of the antibiotic that can combat local and metastatic spread of the infection. The duration of antimicrobial therapy after adequate surgery is usually 5 to 7 days and depends on severity of infection, clinical response, and normalization of the leukocyte count.[282, 331, 332] Only a short course of antimicrobial therapy (24 hours) is required for sterile peritonitis that occurs in the peritoneal space about an infected, but resectable intra-abdominal organ, such as appendix or gall bladder, after resection of the organ. Similarly, contamination of the peritoneum with bacteria from a defect in the intestinal wall, for example immediately following penetrating abdominal trauma, may also require only operative intervention to remove the diseased organ and to stop continued peritoneal contamination and a brief course of antimicrobial therapy.[282, 331, 332] Persistent sepsis suggests formation of an intra-abdominal abscess requiring drainage, continued contamination of the peritoneum from an inadequately controlled source, superimposed nosocomial infection with a resistant pathogen, or tertiary peritonitis.

The antibiotic regimen should be adjusted to include the most efficacious, least toxic, and least expensive agents, once cultures have been finalized, with the proviso that therapy must have activity against anaerobes even when they are not isolated, because anaerobic bacteriologic techniques are frequently inadequate.

In patients able to tolerate oral intake, conversion to oral therapy after an initial response to intravenous therapy is possible.[271] Oral therapy allows earlier discharge in some patients and reduces costs and risks of infusion-related complications. Once ileus no longer prohibits oral intake, efficacy of oral therapy depends on the adequacy of absorption after oral administration of the antimicrobial agents, the availability of potent oral agents against the significant pathogens, namely *E. coli* and *B. fragilis*, and the effects of oral versus intravenous administration of these agents on bowel flora. Potential oral agents include clindamycin, metronidazole, amoxicillin/clavulanic acid, trimethoprim-sulfamethoxazole, trovafloxacin, and ciprofloxacin.

The additon of antibiotics or antiseptics to intraperitoneal lavage fluid continues to be debated,[333–336] and its efficacy intraoperatively,[282] or by continuous peritoneal lavage postoperatively,[336] remains unclear. One study showed that irrigation of the peritoneal cavity with povidone-iodine decreased the frequency of intra-abdominal abscess formation, compared with saline irrigation.[337] However, povidone-iodine has been shown to be a potent inactivator of such neutrophil functions as chemotaxis and phagocytosis and therefore may have a detrimental effect.[338]

Hyperbaric Oxygen. The increased oxygen tension attainable with hyperbaric oxygen therapy inhibits and kills *C. perfringens*[339] and reduces the production of *C. perfringens* α-toxin. Hyperbaric oxygenation has been used clinically and experimentally for clostridial myonecrosis, with some reported success.[340] *C. perfringens* is a relatively oxygen-tolerant pathogen compared with other obligate anaerobes, and it is reasonable to assume that hyperbaric oxygen therapy would be at least equally efficacious with anaerobic infections caused by these more oxygen-sensitive anaerobes. However, except for a few reports,[341] almost no clinical or experimental data are available. Hill[342] reported suppression of experimental liver abscesses due to anaerobes in mice after treatment with hyperbaric oxygen therapy alone. In one study, it appeared that the use of hyperbaric oxygen therapy favorably affected the outcome of experimental sepsis in a rat model, perhaps by enhancing host defense mechanisms.[343] Consideration should also be given to the hazards of hyperbaric oxygen therapy. See Chapter 38 for a more detailed discussion.

Gastrointestinal Drainage. In the presence of peritonitis, the patient should receive nothing by mouth. If no distention is present when treatment is instituted, continuous gastric suction usually is sufficient. For those patients who are distended when treatment is started and for those who become distended despite gastric drainage, intubation of the small intestine should be instituted.

Water and Electrolyte Administration. The type of fluid replacement is determined in large part by the chemical abnormalities found. In general, hypovolemia, dehydration, and metabolic acidosis predominate, so plasma or albumin, Ringer's lactate solution, and 5% dextrose in water usually suffice. The amount to be given in the 2- to 4-hour period before anticipated surgery is determined by watching vital signs, hematocrit values, hourly urinary output, and central venous pressure.

Blood and Plasma Transfusion. Although many patients recover from an illness satisfactorily with a hemoglobin of 8 or 10 g/dl, some surgeons recommend that the patient be transfused to maintain levels as high as 12 to 13 g/dl, so as to provide a margin of safety should some complication such as septic shock or upper gastrointestinal hemorrhage supervene.

Respiratory Support. Fluid sequestered in the abdomen and loops of bowel distended by gas may elevate the diaphragm. Inflammation of the parietal peritoneum, including the diaphragmatic surface, leads to guarding and splinting of the muscular wall, which interferes with deep breathing and coughing. A subphrenic abscess may be responsible for splinting of the diaphragm. Retained bronchial secretions may lead to atelectasis and subsequent pneumonitis. These factors impair the ability to augment respiratory exchange in the face of the increased expenditure of energy required by the inflammatory process and produce hypoxemia and respiratory alkalosis. When the patient tires, the combination of metabolic and respiratory acidosis may develop and prove fatal.

Arterial blood gas studies are necessary to detect and quantitate respiratory decompensation. Measures aimed primarily at gastrointestinal decompression, elevation of the head of the bed, and control of the inflammation may sufficiently improve respiration. Administration of oxygen may improve arterial oxygen saturation. If these measures are inadequate, endotracheal intubation or tracheostomy should be done without delay. A volume-cycled respirator should be used and adjusted to give a partial pressure of oxygen of 80 to 100 mmHg and a normal pH. If the partial pressure of carbon dioxide is not then normal, metabolic acidosis or alkalosis may need to be treated. As the intra-abdominal process subsides, the patient may be able to breathe spontaneously again and may be weaned from the ventilator. In certain severe cases, positive end-expiratory pressure may also be necessary.

Operative Approach. Optimal management includes the following: (1) bowel decompression (e.g., by proximal colostomy for perforation, diverticulitis, or colonic carcinoma); (2) closure of traumatic perforations and resection of a diseased, perforated viscus to stop continued peritoneal contamination with bacteria and adjuvants; and (3) drainage of any purulent collections, which reduces the bacterial inoculum, removes excessive levels of proinflammatory cytokines and adjuvants (e.g., fecal matter, food, blood, bile, barium) that would enhance the virulence of peritoneal infection, and eliminates anaerobic conditions. In the absence of perforation, when the disease process (e.g., acute appendicitis, necrotic bowel) is anticipated to progress, the involved organ is resected. Operative intervention is generally not indicated for primary peritonitis, in patients in whom the disease process subsides and localizes while the patient is being prepared for surgery, in moribund patients, or in patients with pelvic peritonitis caused by pelvic inflammatory disease, which usually responds to medical management.

Intraoperative peritoneal lavage with saline, after drainage of purulent peritoneal exudates, fecal matter, food, and other foreign debris, is standard procedure during laparotomy for peritonitis. However, continuous postoperative peritoneal lavage for 48 to 72 hours or until the fluid is clear, using large volumes of fluid to ensure dispersion of the fluid and to prevent loculations, has failed to prove effective.[336, 344, 345] Radical peritoneal débridement of all fibrinous deposits on peritoneal surfaces is likewise no longer thought to be effective.[346, 347]

Initial reports were favorable for planned reexplorations in which a commitment is made at the first operation to perform laparotomies at frequent intervals until the abdomen is macroscopically clean, regardless of the patient's condition, with additional surgical procedures (e.g., resections) performed as necessary.[348, 349] The abdominal fascia is left open between laparotomies, with the abdominal wall defect bridged by saline-soaked gauze or by a temporary abdominal closure device such as mesh. On resolution of the septic process and establishment of granulation, the mesh is removed and a skin graft is applied to the granulating bed. These demanding and costly procedures have been complicated by multiple fistulas, wound contamination, incisional hernias, and secondary peritonitis with organisms such as entercocci or candida.[349–352] Indeed, repeated entry into the inflamed peritoneum may further escalate the cascade. A review concluded that, in the absence of randomized controlled prospective trials with appropriate stratification of patients by severity of illness, insufficient evidence now exists to determine whether these procedures improve outcome in severe diffuse peritonitis.[352]

In localized infection local drainage alone is adequate, because the risk of disseminating infection outweighs any possible benefit of removing foreign material that may have escaped mechanical removal.

Use of multiple drains for drainage of the general peritoneal cavity is physically impossible, because exudate and adhesions rapidly isolate and occlude the drains and may increase secondary infections.[353] However, drains are often placed in a dependent point to which fluid can be expected to gravitate or in an area of devitalized tissue that cannot be removed.

Prevention

Prevention of postoperative peritonitis requires avoiding contamination of the peritoneum with gastrointestinal or vaginal secretions. In addition to using good surgical technique, this can be accomplished by early treatment of an intra-abdominal infection. For example, Leigh and coworkers[354] noted that the rate of wound infection in patients with perforated appendix was greater than 50% if no antimicrobial therapy was used but only 15% in the group given appropriate therapy. Similarly, two studies demonstrated the efficacy of early use of antibiotics in penetrating wounds of the abdomen, especially those involving the colon.[355, 356] Surgeons have also used various means to reduce the complex gastrointestinal or vaginal flora before performing clean, contaminated surgery. Mechanical cleansing of the bowel with a low-residue diet and then a liquid diet, cathartics, and enemas can reduce the total fecal mass and coliform count in the colon, although not necessarily the predominant anaerobic flora.[357] The use of oral antibiotics preoperatively to reduce bowel flora is well accepted. *E. coli* in the colonic flora is sensitive to either oral neomycin or kanamycin, whereas *B. fragilis* frequently is sensitive to erythromycin or metronidazole. Therefore, combinations such as neomycin-erythromycin base have been shown to be effective in reducing total bowel flora preoperatively and decreasing the incidence of postoperative infection.[358]

Parenteral antibiotics have also been used in gastrointestinal and vaginal surgery prophylactically when there is a chance of contamination with normal microflora at the operative site (clean, contaminated surgery). Up to 30% of these types of operations may be complicated by infections. These procedures involve cutting through the large bowel without significant spillage; compromising the blood supply of the large bowel; cutting through the stomach or small bowel when there is anticipated intraluminal bacterial overgrowth; appendectomy for appendicitis without rupture; penetrating wounds of the abdomen; gallbladder surgery in the elderly; cesarean section after rupture of the membranes and labor; vaginal hysterectomy in the premenopausal woman; and radical pelvic surgery for gynecologic malignancy.[359] Several studies have shown significant reduction in the frequency of postoperative infection, from about 20 to 30% to about 4 to 8% after prophylactic antibiotic use in clean, contaminated surgery.[360, 361] The basic principle of antibiotic prophylaxis is to provide adequate tissue levels at the site of contamination and adequate blood levels during the procedure and for up to 24 hours after the procedure.

Peritonitis during Peritoneal Dialysis

Chronic Peritoneal Dialysis

Peritoneal dialysis has been used successfully to treat uremia in patients with end-stage renal disease since the mid-1940s. Peritonitis was a frequently associated side effect that hindered the acceptance of chronic peritoneal dialysis until an improved access catheter was developed by Tenckhoff in 1968. This catheter significantly decreased the incidence of peritonitis, but initial reports of patients undergoing CAPD with this catheter indicated peritonitis rates of more than six episodes per patient-year.[362, 363] This rate has appeared to decline with the introduction of collapsible plastic bags, improved adapters, and better techniques. However, peritonitis remains the major complication of CAPD today.[364] It occurs at a rate of about one episode per patient-year, with a range from less than 0.5 to 3 or more. Forty-five percent of patients experience peritonitis at least once during their initial 6 months of CAPD treatment. This rate increases to 60 to 70% during the first year.[365–367] Recurrent peritonitis occurs in 20 to 30% of patients and is one of the most common reasons for discontinuation of CAPD.[368] A small proportion of patients seem to have an unusually high frequency of peritonitis.[369] This disparity has been attributed, at least in part, to faulty sterile technique on the part of patients during self-administration of CAPD.

The origin of infection in most cases appears to be contamination of the catheter by common skin organisms.[363] Alterations of skin flora in CAPD patients[370] may lead to peritoneal contamination with enteric pathogens. A higher incidence of peritonitis has been reported in dialysis patients who are nasal carriers of *S. aureus*.[371] Pathogens may also contaminate the peritoneum from exit-site and subcutaneous-tunnel infections, transient bacteremia, and contamination of the dialysate delivery system during bag exchanges. As mentioned previously, enteric bacteria may also gain access to the peritoneal cavity by transmural migration through an intact intestinal wall after the introduction of hypertonic solutions into the peritoneum.[51] This mechanism may account for enteric bacterial peritonitis in dialysis patients.[52] Polymicrobial infection with fecal organisms suggests perforation of the bowel as a complication of catheter placement.

Alterations in peritoneal defenses may increase the risk of peritonitis in CAPD patients. The antimicrobial function of peritoneal macrophages and polymorphonuclear cells generally requires the presence of opsonins. A reduction in the levels of immunoglobutin G (IgG) and third component of complement (C3) has been noted in peritoneal dialysis effluents compared with serum, and the concentrations of these crucial opsonizing agents are inversely related to the frequency of peritonitis.[372] The addition of IgG to peritoneal dialysis fluid has been found to have a prophylactic effect.[373] Other important factors that impair host defense mechanisms are the low pH and high osmolality of peritoneal dialysis fluid, both of which can impair polymorphonuclear function and antibiotic efficacy.[374]

Gram-positive organisms comprise 60 to 80% of isolates, most commonly *S. epidermidis*, followed by *S. aureus*, *Streptococcus* spp., and diphtheroids. Staphylococcal isolates have been noted to grow on polymer surfaces and frequently produce an extracellular slime substance or biofilm that may protect these bacteria from host defenses.[375] Gram-negative organisms are obtained from 15 to 30% of isolates. *E. coli* is the most common, followed by *Klebsiella/Enterobacter*, *Proteus*, and *Pseudomonas* spp. Less common pathogens include *Acinetobacter* spp., *Candida albicans*, and anaerobic bacteria. Rare isolates include atypical mycobacteria (usually *Mycobacterium chelonei* or *Mycobacterium fortuitum*) *Mycobacterium tuberculosis*, *Candida parapsilosis*, *Aspergillus fumigatus*, *Nocardia asteroides*, and *Fusarium* spp.[369, 376–378]

Diagnosis of peritonitis is made when microorganisms and an increased number of leukocytes are present in the dialysate combined with a constellation of clinical findings that include abdominal pain and tenderness (found in 60 to 80% of patients), nausea and vomiting (in 30%), fever (in 10 to 20%), and diarrhea (in 10%).[363, 369, 377, 378] However, not all these criteria need to be met to fulfill the diagnosis.

The dialysate is almost always cloudy, and microscopic examination reveals a leukocyte count greater than 100 cells/mm^3, approximately 85% being more than 500/mm^3, with neutrophils predominating.[369] A preponderance of eosinophils in the peritoneal fluid is seen in a self-limited condition, known as eosinophilic peritonitis, that often follows placement of the Tenckhoff catheter and may represent allergy to the tubing.[379, 380] Peritoneal esosinophilia is also seen in fungal peritonitis. Gram staining of the fluid reveals organisms in 9 to 50% of cases.[363, 369] Peripheral leukocytosis has been reported to be a poor indicator for peritonitis in this group of patients.[377] Blood cultures are rarely positive, in contrast to the 30 to 50% positive rate in other types of intra-abdominal infection.

Peritonitis with negative cultures occurs in 5 to 10% of cases. Constant flow of dialysis fluid into and out of the peritoneal cavity dilutes the microbial density and may falsely lower the rate of positive dialysate culture results. Negative cultures may also result from infection with fastidious organisms, previous antimicrobial treatment, or inadequate culture techniques. One method that has been used to improve the yield of dialysate cultures is the filtration method. A 100-ml aliquot of peritoneal fluid is filtered through a 0.45-μm filter. The filter is then washed with sterile saline and incubated in thioglycolate broth.[377] Rubin and colleagues[363] compared the filtration method with direct inoculation of blood culture bottles and found no significant difference in positive culture rates. Still others found the inoculation of 2 to 3 ml of dialysate into thioglycolate broth to be the most sensitive culture technique.[377] A study comparing direct inoculation of dialysate into a biphasic blood culture system, direct inoculation of dialysate into routine blood culture bottles, and centrifugation of 50 ml of dialysate and culture of the sediment failed to demonstrate a significant difference among these methods in the recovery of a pathogen.[381] All cultures should be performed aerobically. Fungal, mycobacterial, and anaerobic cultures should be performed if clinically indicated (e.g., negative aerobic cultures).

The prognosis of peritonitis in dialysis patients is generally favorable. For example, one large series reported less than 1% mortality attributed directly to infection.[369] The duration of illness and positive peritoneal fluid cultures after institution of antimicrobial therapy is usually 1 to 4 days. However, some infections, especially those caused by *S. aureus*, *Pseudomonas*, or fungus, resolve more slowly and may cause relapse more frequently.[377]

Adequate levels of antimicrobial agents necessary to treat peritonitis successfully can be obtained in the peritoneal fluid by either the systemic or the intraperitoneal route.[369, 376, 377, 382] However, because CAPD peritonitis is a localized infection, the intraperitoneal route is preferred, because no therapeutic advantage of intravenously administered antibiotic has been demonstrated.[383] The increased use of intraperitoneal antibiotic therapy for peritonitis has allowed most patients to be treated on an ambulatory basis. Hospitalization is indicated for those who are severely ill or who are unable to manage the administration of intraperitoneal antibiotics at home. Although a variety of doses can be found in the literature, the initial doses recommended in Table 64–2 for intraperitoneal administration result in effective peritoneal fluid drug concentrations. Subsequent dosing is used to maintain these levels. The aim of the dosing regimen is to maintain a concentration of the drug in the peritoneal cavity fluid greater than the MIC of the offending pathogen for most if not all of the dosing interval. Caution must be exercised when reviewing the MIC and minimum bactericidal concentration (MBC) data, because these concentrations have been demonstrated to be markedly increased when peritoneal dialysis effluent is used as the in vitro growth medium.[384]

Because of the lack of comparative, prospective clinical trials, no one antimicrobial regimen can be called superior to another. After cultures are obtained, initial antimicrobial therapy should be based on the results of Gram staining or on the most likely pathogens if the Gram stain is not helpful. A reasonable initial empirical regimen would be vancomycin in combination with an aminoglycoside. Vancomycin is preferable to a cephalosporin because of the frequency of β-lactam resistance (i.e., methicillin resistance) in staphylococci, which predicts resistance to cephalosporins as well. Initial antibiotic choices should be modified, if necessary, after culture results are obtained. Because *P. aeruginosa* peritonitis is associated with high

TABLE 64–2 Antibiotic Dosage for Peritonitis during Peritoneal Dialysis

Drug	Initial Intraperitoneal Dosage (milligrams per liter dialysate)*	Intraperitoneal Maintenance Dosage (milligrams per liter dialysate)*
Amphotericin B	NA	1.5
Ampicillin	500	125
Cefazolin	500	125
Ceftazidime	250	125
Clindamycin	300	150
Gentamicin†	8	4–8
Piperacillin	4 g IV	250
Trimethoprim-sulfamethoxazole	320/1600	80/400
Vancomycin	1000	25

*Unless otherwise specified.
†Another option is single daily dosing of 0.6 mg/kg body weight in only one exchange per day.
Adapted from Keane WF, Alexander SR, Bailie GR, et al. Peritoneal dialysis–related peritonitis treatment recommendations: 1996 update. Perit Dial Intern. 1996;16:557–573.

failure rates and relapses, it is best treated with a combination of agents active against the infecting strain, in addition to catheter removal. The minimum length of therapy needed for dialysis-related peritonitis has not been determined, but the usual duration ranges from 10 days to 3 weeks. Most patients with CAPD peritonitis show clinical improvement within 48 to 96 hours after initiation of antimicrobial therapy. If the signs and symptoms of peritonitis persist after 96 hours of therapy, reevaluation is warranted, with consideration given to the possibilities of resistant pathogens, unusual organisms (e.g., mycobacterial, fungal), and other intra-abdominal processes, as recommended by Keane and colleagues.[383]

Fungal peritonitis, usually caused by *C. albicans*, should be treated with amphotericin B.[385–387] However, some molds including *Fusarium* spp. may be resistant to amphotericin. If CAPD is continued, amphotericin B should be given intraperitoneally, but it can cause appreciable abdominal pain when given by this route. However, most patients with fungal CAPD infection fail to respond unless the catheter is removed, after which amphotericin B should be given intravenously (about 30mg/day for a total dose of 250 to 500 mg). Flucytosine has also been recommended. However, this drug may be difficult to use in end-stage renal disease because of dose-dependent bone marrow toxicity. If this drug is used, serum levels should be monitored closely to prevent the development of toxic levels (>100 μg/ml). Experience is limited with the use of miconazole and ketoconazole in treating fungal peritonitis.[387a–c]

Removal of the catheter is necessary in 10 to 20% of patients. The indications for removal of the catheter include persistent skin exit-site or tunnel infection; fungal, fecal, or mycobacterial peritonitis; *P. aeruginosa* peritonitis; persistent peritonitis; recurrent peritonitis with the same organism; and catheter malfunction (e.g., poor flow). The catheter should also be removed in patients with intraperitoneal abscess. Use of oral or intraperitoneal antibiotics has not been shown to be effective in preventing peritonitis during peritoneal dialysis.[51, 388] In addition, topical mupirocin has been used to eliminate nasal carriage with *S. aureus* but has yet to be shown to significantly reduce the incidence of CAPD-related peritonitis.[389] Advances in CAPD instrumentation, such as titanium adapters, connector systems with disinfectant, and in-line filters, may decrease the frequency of peritonitis but will add to the overall cost of CAPD.

Acute Peritoneal Dialysis

The incidence of peritonitis during acute peritoneal dialysis has remained stable during the past 20 years. Innovations in technique, which began during the 1960s, reduced the rate of peritonitis from as high as 50% to acceptably low levels. These innovations included closed-drainage systems, small-bore catheters, limitation of dialysis to no longer than 48 to 72 hours, incorporation of a millipore filter into the tubing, and development of closed automatic systems. Also, the use of dry-heat incubators to warm the dialysate decreases the risk of contamination that may occur when water baths are used for this purpose.[390]

Some authorities have recommended that cultures of dialysate be obtained every 8 to 24 hours during acute peritoneal dialysis and at its termination. Culture of dialysate from the last exchange is more useful than culture of the catheter tip at the end of dialysis because of the frequent contamination of the catheter tip at the time of its removal. However, results of such routine cultures, in the absence of symptoms or cloudy fluid, provide a guide of doubtful value for initiation of therapy. More importantly, dialysate samples should be cultured and examined microscopically (cell count, Gram stain) if the dialysate becomes cloudy or the patient develops signs or symptoms of peritonitis (e.g., fever, abdominal pain). Cultures are best obtained by syringe from the port closest to the catheter.

Peritonitis during acute peritoneal dialysis is frequently caused by antibiotic-resistant, hospital-acquired, gram-negative bacilli and staphylococci. Therefore, it is recommended that therapy be initiated with intraperitoneal vancomycin and gentamicin (or tobramycin), with or without concurrent or subsequent addition of the same antibiotics parenterally, depending on the severity of the illness and the response to initial therapy (see Table 64–2 for dosages). Modification of the antibiotic regimen should be made when the culture results become available.

The clinical manifestations, prognosis, and response to therapy are similar to those described previously for peritonitis associated with chronic peritoneal dialysis.

INTRAPERITONEAL ABSCESSES

Etiology

Intraperitoneal abscess can complicate either primary or secondary peritonitis.[391, 392] Diseases causing secondary intraperitoneal abscesses include appendicitis, diverticulitis, biliary tract lesions, pancreatitis, perforated peptic ulcers, inflammatory bowel disease, trauma, and abdominal surgery. The relative frequency of abscess formation associated with appendicitis may be declining, and those of trauma and diverticulitis may be increasing.[392, 393] The location of an abscess is generally related to the site of primary disease and the direction of dependent peritoneal drainage. For example, appendicitis has been reported to be most commonly associated with right lower quadrant and pelvic abscesses; colonic diverticulitis with left lower quadrant and pelvic abscesses; and pancreatitis with lesser sac abscesses.[391] In one large series[391] of 194 intraperitoneal abscesses, about 44% were in the right lower quadrant, 14% in the left lower quadrant, and 14% in the pelvis, whereas 20% were perihepatic. In a series reported by Saini and associates,[392] the frequency of various abscess locations had changed somewhat, perhaps reflecting the change in the relative frequency of the various etiologic diseases.

Of the various perihepatic (right subphrenic, right subhepatic, left perihepatic, and lesser sac) abscesses, the most common continues to be in the right subphrenic space, but the difference in numbers between the right and left sides has been falling. In fact, in one large series of 267 cases of intra-abdominal abscesses, about one half were in the subphrenic space, 60% of which were noted in the left perihepatic space.[394] This increased frequency of left perihepatic space abscess was also noted by Ozeran,[395] Sherman and associates,[396] and Sanders.[397] This is in contrast to the series of Ochsner and DeBakey in 1938[398] when right subphrenic abscesses were most common, owing to the numerous ruptured appendices.

In children, appendicitis is still responsible for more than 50% of the cases of subphrenic abscess.[399] In adults, perihepatic abscesses currently are seen mainly as postoperative complications,[395–397, 400] rather than in neglected primary intra-abdominal infections such as appendicitis or perforated peptic ulcer. This may explain the increasing frequency of subphrenic abscess, especially on the left, compared with other intraperitoneal sites.[394] Usually, the surgery has been in the gastroduodenal and biliary tracts. One group of investigators[401] noted that abscesses that occurred after gastric operations were left subphrenic if incidental splenectomy had been performed but right subhepatic if splenectomy had not been done. The subhepatic space is less frequently involved than the subphrenic spaces. Lesser sac abscesses usually follow pancreatitis or perforation of the stomach or duodenum. Multiple perihepatic space abscesses have been reported in 5 to 26% of the patients.[395–397, 400, 401]

Bacteriologic Findings

These infections are typically polymicrobial. In studies in which bacteriologic techniques permitted isolation of anaerobes, anaerobes were found in 60 to 70% of cases.[391, 392, 400, 402] In one study,[400] anaerobes were recovered in 20 of 24 subphrenic abscesses, and *B. fragilis* was the most common pathogen, with anaerobic cocci and clostridia found in 50% of the patients. Other bacteria frequently recovered are *E. coli*, *Klebsiella/Enterobacter* group, *Proteus* spp., *P. aeruginosa*, *S. aureus*, and enterococci.[391, 395, 396, 400]

Pathogenesis

Intraperitoneal abscesses develop as a result of localizaton of diffuse peritonitis, usually in the pelvis, perihepatic spaces, and paracolic gutters. In addition, abscess may develop about diseased organs (e.g., periappendiceal or pericholecystic abscesses) or after a penetrating wound (stab, gunshot, auto accident, or other trauma) or surgical procedure. These abscesses are termed *secondary* and account for the majority of these cases. In contrast, the pathogenesis of primary abscesses is unknown and is presumably similar to that of primary peritonitis.

Clinical Manifestations

An acute course, with a high intermittent fever, shaking chills, abdominal pain, and tenderness over the involved area, is characteristic. The clinical pattern may be that of an acute secondary illness occurring after surgery for primary abdominal disease or prolonged recuperative course in a patient who has been receiving antibiotics after abdominal surgery. Various authors[396–401] have emphasized the occasional chronicity of subphrenic abscesses and have speculated that the course is often modified by antibiotics. Subphrenic abscesses have been described with 6 months or more of an indolent illness.[403]

Local symptoms and signs vary widely with the location and source of the abscess. Subphrenic abscesses are usually accompanied by chest findings with costal tenderness and pleural or pulmonary involvement, whereas subhepatic abscesses have more dominant signs of upper abdominal or subcostal involvement and fewer pulmonary changes.

Diagnosis

Noninvasive diagnostic procedures, including ultrasonography and CT, have provided greater sensitivity and specificity than routine radiography and radionuclide scanning.[404, 405] However, these latter techniques may be useful, on occasion, and sometimes a combination of diagnostic tests is the optimal approach to confirm the diagnosis of intra-abdominal abscess.[406]

Plain radiographs of the abdomen can suggest the location of abscesses in as many as 50% of patients.[407] Radiologic findings associated with a subphrenic abscess may include pleural effusion, elevation of the hemidiaphragm, and/or loss of diaphragmatic movement on fluoroscopy. Routine radiography may also reveal displacement of viscera by an abscess. These findings can be enhanced by contrast radiology. The stomach, for example, may be outlined with barium or air to indicate displacement caused by a left perihepatic or lesser sac abscess. The presence of gas, either as a single air-fluid level or as mottling within the abscess, may aid localization on routine abdominal radiography.

Leukocytes tagged with gallium-67 and indium-111 are used in radionuclide scans that at times may be helpful in detecting intra-abdominal abscesses, although they have been largely supplanted by the use of CT scans and magnetic resonance imaging (MRI). Unlike the technetium-93m sulfur colloid liver-spleen scan, which visualizes the entire organ and delineates abnormal areas as "cold" spots caused by decreased uptake of the isotope, ^{67}Ga- and ^{111}In-tagged leukocytes accumulate in areas of inflammation, such as abscesses, and appear as areas of increased radioactivity or "hot" spots[408–411] (Fig. 64–4). Gallium is excreted into the intestinal tract and can accumulate in any inflammatory process and in certain neoplasms. For these reasons, false-positive scan readings can occur when radioactivity within the lumen of the bowel, within the wall of an inflamed bowel, or within a noninfected operative site in the process of healing is misinterpreted as an intra-abdominal abscess.

^{111}In-tagged leukocyte scans are as sensitive as but more specific than ^{67}Ga scans: The labeled leukocytes tend to concentrate only in areas of inflammation, because, unlike ^{67}Ga, ^{111}In is not secreted into the bowel.[412, 413] Abscesses in the liver and spleen may be difficult to detect solely on ^{67}Ga- or ^{111}In-tagged leukocyte images, because normal accumulation of activity in these organs may mask an adjacent inflammatory focus. This problem can be overcome by comparing ^{67}Ga or ^{111}In images with ^{99m}Tc scans.

Ultrasonography is a noninvasive technique that is helpful in the determination of the size, shape, consistency, and anatomic relationships of an intra-abdominal mass.[414, 415] A pulsed, focused beam of high-frequency sound is directed into the suspect area of the patient's

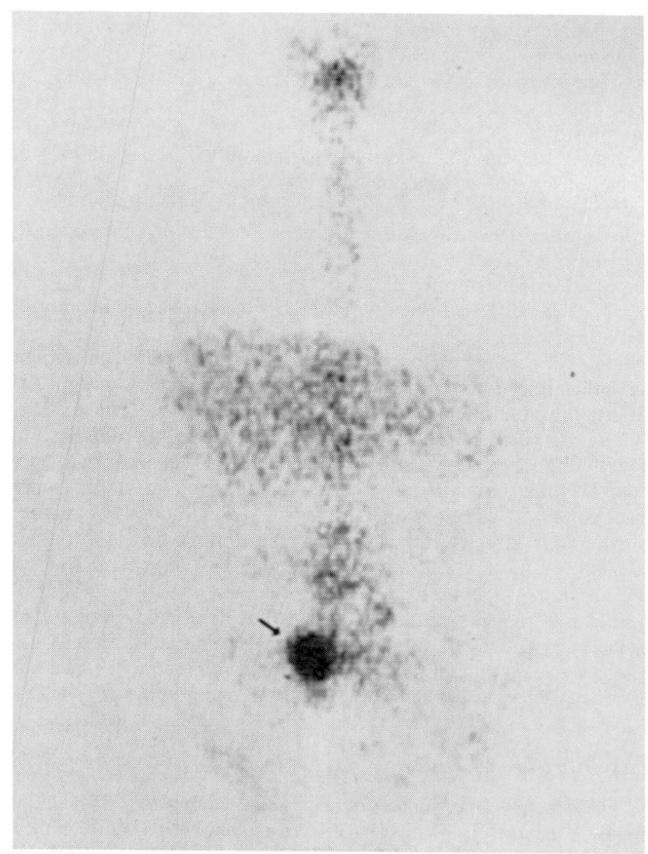

FIGURE 64–4. ^{67}Ga scan in a patient with regional enteritis and signs of an intra-abdominal abscess. Note the area of increased radioactivity in the right lower quadrant *(arrow)*.

body by means of a transducer. Echoes are received by the same transducer from skin and tissue planes. The echo pattern is displayed on an oscilloscope as the transducer is moved along the surface of the body. The appearance of abscesses may vary widely from echo-free lesions to highly echogenic masses, but they typically appear as a fluid collection with an irregular wall and the presence of a few internal echoes. Ultrasound images may be obscured by overlying gas-filled viscera and by postoperative wounds and drains.

CT has proven especially well suited for the diagnosis of intra-abdominal abscess.[416–421] Definition is unimpeded by intraluminal gas and postoperative changes, except in the presence of surgical metallic clips or residual barium that may disrupt the image. Observed findings consistent with abscess include a low-density tissue mass and a definable capsule. CT can detect extraluminal gas, a finding highly suggestive of abscess.[405] Contrast material is commonly administered orally and intravenously when attempting to diagnose intra-abdominal abscess. The intraluminal contrast material helps to distinguish loops of bowel from abscess cavities, and the parenteral contrast material may enhance a surrounding capsule, allowing for easier identification.

MRI has the potential to display normal anatomy and to show abnormal conditions in many of the body's organ systems and anatomic regions.[422, 423] However, only a few trials have compared MRI with older radiologic procedures. In one study, MRI demonstrated a clearer delineation of the extent of inflammatory changes than did CT, and it better distinguished the abscess from the surrounding structures.[424] In addition, the use of MRI does not require the administration of contrast medium and eliminates exposure to radiation, but it may be more costly than radiologic techniques.

Arteriographic localization has also been helpful. However, overreliance on any one of these techniques is dangerous, and results should be confirmed by other methods and by the clinical findings.

Prognosis

The period of morbidity is unusually prolonged in patients with intraperitoneal abscesses. Altemeier and colleagues[391] reported average hospital stays of 21 to 47 days. The presence of residual recurrent infection due to inadequate surgical drainage, more common in patients with multiple or bilateral abscesses, is associated with significantly greater mortality.

Treatment

The main therapy for any intraperitoneal abscess is drainage. Effective management depends on accurate localization of the abscess, discrimination between single and multiple abscesses, and early and adequate drainage. Conventional therapy for intraperitoneal abscesses has usually included surgical drainage. However, in recent years, successful therapy has been accomplished using percutaneous catheter drainage as an alternative to surgery.[425–427] This method has become possible with the use of refined imaging techniques, especially ultrasonography and CT.[428–430]

The general requirements for CT– or ultrasound–guided percutaneous catheter drainage include (1) an abscess that can be adequately approached via a safe percutaneous route; (2) an abscess that is unilocular; (3) an abscess that is not vascular and the patient has no coagulopathy; (4) joint radiologic and surgical evaluation, with surgical backup for any complication or failure; and (5) the possibility of dependent drainage via the percutaneously placed catheter. CT also allows detection of an unsuspected additional intra-abdominal problem that would otherwise require surgical intervention. Percutaneous catheter drainage can be used as an initial approach in a patient too unstable to withstand immediate surgery. Definitive surgery can be postponed until the patient is in better condition. Percutaneous drainage of periventricular or appendiceal abscesses may permit a subsequent one-stage procedure of primary resection and immediate anastomosis, rather than the more costly and complicated multistage procedure.[431] After percutaneous placement of the catheter with CT or ultrasound guidance and aspiration of the abscess cavity, the catheter is placed for drainage by gravity or low suction until the daily drainage volume is minimal. Clinical response and collapse of the abscess cavity on repeat scanning should follow successful drainage. Some patients with percutaneous catheter drainage can be managed at home with their catheters in place. Of the patients who fit these criteria, percutaneous drainage has been successful in 80 to 90%.[427, 432] Attempts at drainage of loculated, poorly organized, multiple, or extensive collections are less successful. In most series, the frequency of complications ranges from 5 to 15%,[425, 433] including septicemia, hemorrhage, peritoneal spillage, and fistula formation. In addition, failure may occur because of undrained abscesses or pus too viscid to drain via the catheter. Reports indicate that the morbidity and mortality associated with percutaneous drainage may be less than with surgical treatment.[426, 434]

Antimicrobial therapy should be started immediately after appropriate specimens (e.g., blood) are obtained for culture; usually this occurs before drainage. Because the pathogens usually are similar to those involved in secondary peritonitis, initial antibiotic therapy is similarly directed at the anaerobes, especially *B. fragilis* and the Enterobacteriaceae. The antimicrobial regimens discussed in the section on treatment of secondary peritonitis should be appropriate initial therapy. This antibiotic regimen should be adjusted to conform to results of in vitro testing of the infecting organisms isolated from blood or from purulent material obtained at surgery or catheter drainage. During the course of a prolonged illness, repeated cultures of blood and purulent collections, when clinically indicated, should provide a basis for change in antimicrobial therapy.

VISCERAL ABSCESS

Pancreatic Abscess

Etiology

Most pancreatic abscesses develop as a complication of pancreatitis, which may be biliary, alcoholic, postsurgical, or posttraumatic in origin. More recently, pancreatitis has been found to be a complication of endoscopic retrograde cholangiopancreatography (ERCP).[435] Pancreatic abscess occurs in about 1 to 9% of patients after acute pancreatitis.[436–440] The preceding attack of acute pancreatitis has been noted to be frequently severe.[441, 442] Occasionally, penetration of a peptic ulcer or secondary infection of a pancreatic pseudocyst may be the cause of a pancreatic abscess.

Bacteriologic Findings

About one third to one half of pancreatic abscesses have been reported to be polymicrobial, mainly with enteric facultative microorganisms such as *E. coli* and other Enterobacteriaceae, enterococci, viridans streptococci, and occasionally *S. aureus*.[438–441] However, because most studies have not used modern anaerobic bacteriologic techniques, it is unknown how frequently anaerobes are involved. More recent series have documented the presence of anaerobic bacteria in pancreatic abscesses.[437, 438, 443, 444] *M. tuberculosis* has also been cultured from pancreatic abscesses,[445] including from a patient with acquired immunodeficiency syndrome (Joseph F. John, Jr., M.D., personal communication).

Pathogenesis

The release of enzymes from an acutely damaged pancreas results in pancreatic necrosis. Infection of pancreatic necrosis is most likely a secondary event.[446, 447] The mixed enteric bacterial content of many pancreatic abscesses suggests that bacteria may reach the pancreas by reflux of contaminated bile. The frequency of bactobilia increases with biliary obstruction and with the patient's age, occurring in approximately 50% of those older than 70 years of age.[448] The hematogenous route may account for some of the monomicrobial infections, especially those caused by *S. aureus*.

Clinical Manifestations

The clinical manifestations are varied. The patient may fail to respond to therapy for pancreatitis, or 1 to 3 weeks after the onset of pancreatitis the patient may suddenly deteriorate after an initial response.[438–441] Abdominal pain, often radiating to the back, nausea, and vomiting are present in more than 80 to 90% of patients. Temperature higher than 38.3°C (101°F) and abdominal tenderness are usually present, although fever may be absent. Less frequently, jaundice, abdominal distention, or an abdominal mass may be present, or the patient may have generalized peritonitis. The serum amylase concentration is elevated in 21 to 66% of cases and may remain elevated.

Diagnosis

Radiologic, ultrasonic, radionuclide, and CT studies reveal the lesion in 80 to 90% of the cases. Plain films may show diaphragmatic elevation, pleural effusion, presence of a retrogastric mass, forward displacement of the gastric air shadow on cross-table lateral views of the abdomen, widening of the gastrocolic omentum as seen by an increase in the distance between gastric and colon gas, or mottling and the presence of gas bubbles in the gastrocolic or retrogastric region. Barium studies may show the visceral displacement (e.g., pressure effects in the posterior gastric wall or displacement and enlargement of the duodenal sweep). Ultrasonography and CT are also useful in the diagnosis of pancreatic abscess.[449, 450] CT appears to be superior to ultrasonography because the images are unaffected by overlying bowel gas and can better demonstrate pancreatic gas collections. It is, however, difficult to discern infected from noninfected pseudocysts by either method, and diagnostic needle aspiration under ultrasound or CT guidance is often helpful.[449] ^{67}Ga and ^{111}In radionuclide scans have not been found to be very helpful in differentiating pancreatitis or a pseudocyst from an abscess.[451, 452] To date, MRI also has not been a very helpful modality in imaging pancreatic abscesses.[453] Spleen scans, angiography, and retrograde duodenoscopic pancreatography may also be useful.[454]

Prognosis

The presence of proteolytic enzymes within the abscess may cause erosion of major blood vessels with intra-abdominal hemorrhage.[440, 441] Spread of infection may occur in the retroperitoneum, along the roots of the transverse mesocolon and small bowel mesentery, and may involve suppuration in the lesser sac with extension into the perihepatic spaces. Fistulas may form between the abscess cavity and the stomach, duodenum, or transverse colon. Patients with undrained abscesses seen in surgical practice have a 100% mortality rate.[439] About 53 to 86% of those operated on survive. Survival has depended on early surgical drainage.[438, 441, 443] Higher mortality has occurred in those with infected pancreatic necrosis[455] or biliary tract disease and in those who developed pancreatic abscess postoperatively. These were usually older patients who had ultimately fatal underlying disease. Death may result from septicemia, peritonitis, pleuropulmonary complications, or hepatic or renal failure.

Treatment

Early surgical drainage is most important.[456] Percutaneous drainage alone appears to be inadequate for the majority of pancreatic abscesses.[457, 458] However, it may do until the patient can be stabilized for surgical drainage,[459–461] and it can be definitive therapy in selected patients.[462, 463] Optimal treatment appears to require effective surgical débridement and drainage,[464, 465] although retroperitoneal laparoscopy has been reported to afford direct access to the pancreas and peripancreatic spaces for exploration and removal of necrotic infected material without the risk of peritoneal contamination.[466] Also, prompt reoperation is often necessary for persistent infection. The prophylactic use of antibiotics early in the course of pancreatitis has been shown to be ineffective in preventing the subsequent development of pancreatic abscess.[467] Initial antibiotic therapy should have adequate activity against *E. coli*, other Enterobacteriaceae, and anaerobic gram-negative bacilli. The regimens discussed in the section on treatment of secondary peritonitis would be appropriate choices. Antibiotic therapy should be adjusted according to the results of in vitro sensitivity testing. Routine therapy for pancreatitis should also be used.

Hepatic Abscess

Etiology

Bacterial abscesses of the liver are relatively uncommon lesions, despite the frequency of cholecystitis, appendicitis, diverticulitis, and peritonitis, which often are the sources of bacterial infections in the liver. More recently, pyogenic liver abscess has been noted to be one of the infectious complications occurring after liver transplantation,[468] and there is a high frequency of liver abscesses in patients with chronic granulomatous disease.[468] Bacterial abscesses have been reported to be more common than amebic liver abscess, especially in the northern United States.[469–472]

Liver abscesses caused by *Entamoeba histolytica* complicate 3 to 9% of the cases of amebic colitis.[469] Although there is no sex predominance in bacterial liver abscesses, more than 90% of amebic liver abscesses occur in men, and patients with amebic liver abscesses are generally younger than those with bacterial abscesses.[469, 472] Pyogenic abscesses have been reported in patients with sickle cell anemia.[473] Liver abscesses occur at all ages but are especially rare in children; they have been noted to follow umbilical vein catheterization in neonates.[474]

Bacteriologic Findings

Pyogenic hepatic abscess is frequently polymicrobial.[472, 475–477] Enteric gram-negative bacilli, usually *E. coli*, have been cultured from the majority of pyogenic hepatic abscesses.[472, 477, 478] The high frequency of "sterile" abscesses, reported in some series to be about 50%, is probably a result of inadequate anaerobic cultivation.[477, 479, 480] As a result of modern anaerobic bacteriologic techniques, anaerobic bacteria have become recognized as a major cause of hepatic abscesses. In reports in which modern anaerobic techniques were used, about 50% of all pyogenic liver abscesses were caused by anaerobes, and blood cultures were positive for anaerobes in up to 54% of these cases.[479, 481] These anaerobes included anaerobic gram-positive cocci, *Bacteroides* spp., *Fusobacterium* spp., and *Actinomyces* spp. Although the frequency of recovery of *S. aureus* or group A streptococci from liver abscesses varies among reports, these organisms occur in 20% or less of the cases.[469, 477, 480] *S. aureus* is more frequently isolated in children, primarily in those younger than 5 years of age,[477, 482] and is presumably of hematogenous origin.

S. aureus microabscesses in the liver may be associated with microabscesses in other organs as part of generalized hematogenous dissemination in children with impaired host defenses (e.g., acute leukemia, chronic granulomatous disease).[483]

On rare occasions, *Y. enterocolitica* has been isolated from liver abscesses.[484] It most commonly produces an acute gastroenteritis, especially in children, and a right iliac fossa syndrome resulting from inflammation of the terminal ileum or mesenteric lymphadenitis, or both.

Candida may invade the liver as part of a systemic infection.[485, 486]

Most of these patients have acute leukemia, usually granulocytic, and the microabscesses in the liver are probably secondary to intestinal *Candida* colonization and portal fungemia.[275] The diagnosis is most often delayed because of a nonspecific clinical presentation while the patient is neutropenic. Fever is usually the only sign of disseminated candidiasis. During this phase of the illness, ultrasound and CT are not helpful, and blood cultures are often negative. When the patient's neutropenia resolves, fever persists. After neutropenia resolves, ultrasonography or CT may reveal numerous abscesses in liver, spleen, and kidney.[486] The response to amphotericin therapy is slow, sometimes requiring 2 or 3 months for defervescence. Fluconazole can be used to extend the antifungal regimen provided that neutropenia does not return.[487–489]

The specific types of microorganisms that cause hepatic abscess probably vary with the underlying disease. For example, anaerobic abscesses are more frequently cryptogenic or portal in origin, whereas gallbladder disease was noted in one series in only 2 of 25 patients with anaerobic liver abscesses.[479] Group A streptococcal and *S. aureus* abscesses probably result from bacteremia due to these organisms. In the past, it was believed that 10 to 20% of amebic liver abscesses were secondarily infected with bacteria, usually of enteric origin.[471] However, in more recent series, superinfection was found to have occurred in up to 4% of cases.[472] Echinococcal hepatic cysts may also become secondarily infected.

Pathogenesis

The source of infection in the liver may be (1) biliary, in which disease of the extrahepatic biliary tract is caused by a calculus, stricture, or malignancy and results in ascending cholangitis; (2) portal, in which a pathologic process such as appendicitis, diverticulitis,[490] or inflammatory bowel disease[491] is in the bed of the portal venous circulation and may be associated with pyelophlebitis (acute suppurative thrombophlebitis in the portal venous system; (3) infection in a contiguous structure, such as the gallbladder, which spreads directly to the liver; (4) infected foci anywhere in the body via the hepatic artery; (5) infection secondary to penetrating wounds and even nonpenetrating trauma to the liver; or (6) cryptogenic, in which no source is evident. About one fourth of the liver abscesses are cryptogenic and are thought to be caused by infection of infarcted portions of the liver.[492] Although a portal venous source, mainly appendicitis, was a common cause of liver diseases in the past, biliary disease is now the most common source.[477, 493]

Pyogenic abscesses can be single or multiple. Multiple abscesses are more apt to be caused by biliary tract disease,[480] whereas abscesses arising via the portal vein are usually solitary[480]; the right lobe is more commonly involved than the left. Amebic abscesses are predominantly solitary in the right lobe.

Clinical Manifestations

The predominant symptoms of pyogenic hepatic abscess include fever and chills of several days' to several weeks' duration. Characteristically, multiple abscesses associated with ascending cholangitis give rise to spiking temperatures. Right upper quadrant pain may be dull, and abscesses high in the right lobe may cause respiratory symptoms such as cough and pleuritic pain with radiation to the right shoulder and an associated pleural rub. Tender hepatomegaly is present in 50 to 70% of the patients. Jaundice is not often present unless ascending choloangitis is a cause of the abscesses or there is extensive hepatic involvement, usually associated with multiple abscesses.[469, 477, 479] Either the indolence of the illness in some patients or the minimal physical findings (no hepatomegaly or abdominal tenderness) may account for some of these patients havings a "fever of unknown origin."[477]

Clinical differentiation of an amebic from a pyogenic abscess is greatly assisted by amebic serology. A history of diarrhea, the presence of chest findings, or the lack of spiking temperatures has been reported in some series to be more common in patients with amebic abscess, but these characteristics have not been especially frequent in other series of patients with amebic abscesses. Pain in the left upper quadrant of the abdomen in patients with amebic abscess is uncommon but may indicate a left lobe abscess that can extend into the pericardium.[130] Swelling may occur over the right chest wall, or there may be point tenderness that localizes abscesses caused by amebas.[130]

Alkaline phosphatase is the serum liver enzyme that is most frequently elevated. Blood cultures have been reported to be positive in about one half of the patients with pyogenic abscesses.[479, 480] The presence of viridans streptococcus in several blood cultures in patients with an indolent clinical course and elevated hepatic enzymes without evidence of endocarditis may be an important clue to the diagnosis of liver abscess.[494] Persistent recovery of viridans streptococci from liver also has been reported in the absence of bacteremia in a patient with an indolent clinical course and persistent serum alkaline phosphatase elevation.[495]

Diagnosis

Elevation and limitation of motion of the right diaphragm, basilar atelectasis, right pleural effusion, or gas within the abscess cavity may be noted on plain films of the abdomen or chest.[496] Scintigraph with ^{99m}Tc, ultrasonography, CT, and MRI are highly sensitive techniques for the detection of liver abscesses.[497]

The hepatic angiographic findings in liver abscess are the mass effect with stretching or displacement of blood vessels and an avascular area surrounded by a blush of contrast seen during the capillary-venous phase of the angiogram.[498]

The effectiveness of ultrasonography for the detection of liver abscess is now well documented.[478, 493, 499] It has proved especially useful for the evaluation of right upper quadrant structures, primarily because of the absence of the air-filled viscera that often impede visualization in other areas of the abdomen. As mentioned previously, the appearance of abscesses can vary from echo-free lesions to highly echogenic masses within the liver. Sonography, as opposed to ^{99m}Tc scintigraphy, can often distinguish an abscess from a tumor or other solid focal lesion. CT is also a highly sensitive technique for the diagnosis of liver abscess.[478, 500, 501] Abscesses produce areas of decreased attenuation on CT (Fig. 64–5).

Both ultrasound and CT can be used to guide needle aspiration for diagnostic and therapeutic purposes.[426, 501, 502] The aspirated mate-

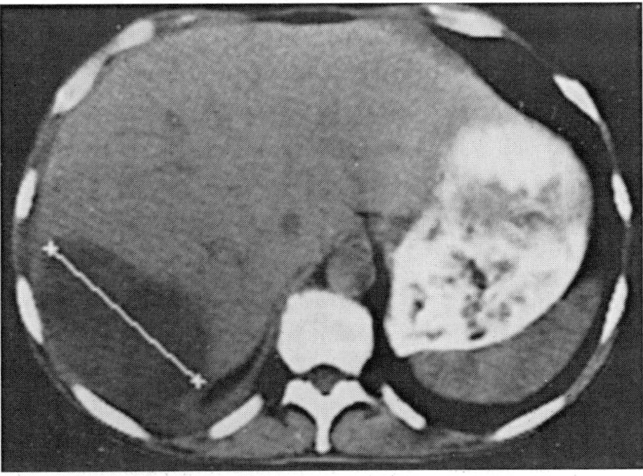

FIGURE 64–5. Abdominal computed tomography scan reveals a liver abscess *(arrow)* due to a mixture of anaerobic and aerobic pathogens. The abscess developed following drainage of an appendiceal abscess.

rial should be cultured aerobically and anaerobically. Ultrasound- or CT-guided percutaneous aspiration in patients with suspected amebic abscess has been recommended to rapidly rule out a pyogenic cause. Aspiration of sterile fluid that is brownish and without a foul odor is characteristic of an amebic abscess. However, fluid in amebic abscesses is frequently yellow or green and can be secondarily infected with enteric bacteria. Diagnosis is confirmed by finding *E. histolytica* on direct microscopy or culture of the aspirate or wall of the abscess. In endemic areas, aspiration usually is not performed if amebic abscess is suspected clinically because of the favorable response to drug therapy. Serologic tests indicative of past or present amebiasis are positive in more than 90% of amebic liver abscesses but may be misleading in endemic areas.[472]

Prognosis

The prognosis of pyogenic liver abscesses depends on the rapidity with which the diagnosis is made and treatment started. High mortality is also associated with advanced age and serious underlying disease. In the past, the mortality rate from pyogenic abscess ranged from 24 to 79%,[477, 479, 480] and undrained abscesses had a reported rate of up to 100%.[503, 504] More recent series have shown an improvement in prognosis, with cure rates of 88 to 100%.[227, 228, 502] Traditional therapy for pyogenic liver abscesses has been surgical drainage and antibiotics; however, the high success rates have occurred in patients treated with either antibiotics plus percutaneous drainage or antibiotics alone. The older series reporting high mortality rates for undrained abscesses may have included patients who were not candidates for surgical drainage because of poor clinical condition or extensive infection. (i.e., multiple small abscesses). The apparent improvement in prognosis in more recent years may be related to earlier diagnosis afforded by the use of ultrasonography and CT. The mortality rate in uncomplicated amebic abscesses is reported to be less than 1% in more recent series.[130, 472] However, amebic abscesses that rupture into the peritoneal or into pericardial cavity carry mortality rates of 18 or 30%, respectively, and amebic abscesses that rupture into the bronchi or pleura carry a 6% mortality rate.[130]

Treatment

The treatment of pyogenic liver abscesses has changed as the use of ultrasonography and CT has become common for diagnosis and therapy.[505] These imaging procedures offer the ability to follow closely the resolution of the abscess during therapy and allow precise placement of percutaneous catheters for single or continuous drainage. Some series have reported high cure rates after antibiotic treatment without concomitant percutaneous drainage.[227, 228] However, most other reports have emphasized the necessity of some drainage procedure to ensure a good outcome.[502, 503, 506, 507] Most patients defervesce within 2 weeks of the start of medical therapy and drainage.[472] Some patients who are cured by medical and drainage therapy may still take up to 4 weeks to experience defervescence.[472] It has been recommended that surgery be considered for patients whose fever persists for longer than 2 weeks despite percutaneous catheter drainage and appropriate antimicrobial therapy.[472]

The abscess should decrease in size after percutaneous catheter drainage. Should the patient's condition not improve and fever not resolve within 48 hours after catheter drainage, repeat ultrasound or CT scanning should be performed to assess for undrained loculations of pus. Surgery is required for hepatic abscesses resulting from biliary obstruction. Loculated or highly viscous abscesses also usually require surgical incision and drainage.

Antibiotic therapy should be started as soon as the diagnosis is suspected and should be directed at the expected pathogens. Because the pathogens usually are similar to those involved in secondary peritonitis, initial antibiotic therapy is similarly directed at the anaerobes (especially *B. fragilis*) and the Enterobacteriaceae. The antimicrobial regimens outlined in the section on treatment of secondary peritonitis would be appropriate initial therapy. At the time of drainage, cultures are taken of the abscess for aerobic and anaerobic incubation, and specific antibiotic therapy is instituted on the basis of the culture results. Therapy should be prolonged, usually for more than 1 month. Up to 4 months of antibiotic therapy for multiple pyogenic abscesses has been recommended to prevent relapses.[479]

Amebic abscess is usually treated with a tissue amebicide, such as metronidazole or parenteral dehydroemetine.[508] Metronidazole has cure rates similar to those of dehydroemetine and has the advantage of being active for both the hepatic and intestinal phases of the disease and of being less toxic. Aspiration of the cavity has been recommended not only for diagnosis but also for therapeutic drainage by some authors.[130] However, others have found aspiration to be unnecessary, except in the occasional patient who responds poorly to medical therapy or in patients with large left lobe abscesses that may rupture into the pericardium and cause death.[472] Aspiration may also be indicated to evacuate an expanding abscess in an attempt to prevent imminent rupture. Repeated aspiration has been recommended if more than 250 ml is obtained initially.[130] If a solitary right lobe abscess occurs in a man, despite the finding of bacteria in the aspirate, additional antiamebic therapy has been recommended initially because of the likelihood of a secondarily infected amebic abscess.

Splenic Abscess

Etiology

Splenic abscesses are uncommon lesions that may occur in patients with sickle hemoglobinopathies, trauma, or bacteremia or in intravenous drug abusers.[509] Usually multiple small abscesses develop as a complication of hematogenous dissemination. One fourth of these abscesses have been reported to be solitary.[510]

Bacteriologic Characteristics

Splenic abscesses that develop during the course of bacterial endocarditis are usually caused by *S. aureus* or streptococcus. Enterobacteriaceae (e.g., *Salmonella*) and anaerobic microorganisms have also been recovered.[509–511] In one series, the bacteriology of the abscess was polymicrobial in 25% and included anaerobes.[509] The proportion of splenic abscesses reported to have sterile cultures has declined as anaerobic culture techniques have improved. Fungi (mostly *Candida* spp.) have been isolated from splenic abscesses with greater frequency during the past decade as the population with conditions predisposing to infections with *Candida* has increased (e.g., patients receiving high-dose corticosteroids or cancer chemotherapy). Fungal splenic abscesses are often part of the syndrome of chronic disseminated candidiasis.[485, 490] Blood cultures have been reported to be positive in 70% of patients with multiple splenic abscesses but in only 14% of those with solitary abscesses.[509]

Pathogenesis

Splenic abscesses probably develop as a metastatic process, for example, as a complication of bacterial endocarditis,[512] disseminated tuberculosis,[513] or *Salmonella* bacteremia in patients infected with the human immunodeficiency virus (HIV).[514, 515] Some are related to infection in contiguous organs and others to infected traumatic hematomas or infarcts, (e.g., in patients with sickle hemoglobinopathies).

Manifestations

Left upper quadrant abdominal pain is usual. Irritation of the adjacent diaphragm may result in pain referred to the left shoulder. Splenic enlargement and tenderness are often present, with high, spiking temperatures and perhaps a splenic rub. No clinical findings to suggest splenic involvement may occur in some patients with multiple small splenic abscesses.[509, 510]

Diagnosis

Radiographic examination may reveal an elevated left hemidiaphragm, basilar pulmonary infiltrates, atelectasis, or left pleural effusion. Shift of the colon and stomach down and to the right and extraintestinal gas, either diffusely mottled or producing an air-fluid level in the left upper quadrant, may also be seen.[509, 510] Ultrasonography, CT, and MRI are the preferred diagnostic techniques for the evaluation of suspected splenic abscess.[516, 517] CT appears to be somewhat superior to ultrasound for visualization of the spleen because of the adjacent gas-filled viscera and the inconstant position in the left upper quadrant.[518]

Treatment

In untreated cases, the mortality rate with splenic abscess is 100%.[518] Initial antibiotic therapy should have a broad spectrum of activity. A combination of antibiotics that has activity against streptococci and both aerobic and anaerobic gram-negative bacilli would be appropriate initial antimicrobial therapy. Subsequent modifications of antibiotic therapy may be based on results of blood cultures or cultures of material obtained at the time of surgery. With multiple, small abscesses, and with some large solitary abscesses when feasible, splenectomy is the treatment of choice; otherwise, when the spleen is surrounded by extensive adhesions, incision and drainage may be preferred.[509–511, 519] Percutaneous drainage was successful in some patients,[509, 520] but its indications, efficacy, and safety remain to be determined.[521, 522]

SPECIFIC SOURCES OF INTRA-ABDOMINAL INFECTION

Acute Appendicitis

Appendicitis manifests as right lower quadrant abdominal pain accompanied by anorexia, nausea, and vomiting. When the inflamed appendix lies in the anterior position, tenderness is often maximal at or near McBurney's point, with low-grade fever, rebound tenderness, voluntary guarding at first, and then abdominal rigidity. Variations in the anatomic location of the appendix may result in variations in the location of the pain and physical findings. For example, a retrocecal appendix can cause principally flank or back pain and tenderness; a pelvic appendix can cause suprapubic pain; and on rectal examination pain may be felt locally and suprapubically. Because the clinical findings are frequently nonspecific, 50% of patients with suspected appendicitis are hospitalized and found to have another diagnosis, and at least 20% of patients with appendicitis are misdiagnosed. In this situation, appendiceal CT after instillation of contrast material into the colon has been shown to be a useful, cost-saving diagnostic procedure in the initial assessment of patients with suspected appendicitis for clinical decision-making.[523]

Persistent obstruction of the appendiceal lumen, usually caused by a fecalith, leads to gangrene and rupture of the pus-filled organ. During the several hours between onset of acute appendicitis and rupture, adjacent viscera and omentum may wall off and confine the subsequent spill to the periappendiceal area, with development of an inflammatory mass felt in the right lower quadrant. If the walling-off process is incomplete, spreading diffuse peritonitis occurs. The two sites for loculation of intraperitoneal spread are the pelvic recess and the right subhepatic space. Pyelophlebitis and liver abscess may complicate the picture. Colonic microflora, namely, a mixture of *B. fragilis*, *P. melaninogenica*, *Bilophila wadsworthia*, anaerobic gram-positive cocci, and Enterobacteriaceae, are the primary pathogens in appendicitis and its complications.[100, 101]

The therapy for appendicitis without rupture and for ruptured appendicitis with local or diffuse peritonitis is surgery. Periappendiceal abscess may be drained percutaneously with the aid of ultrasound- or CT-guidance, followed by appendectomy. Laparoscopic appendectomy has been recommended for acute appendicitis, with the option for conversion to open appendectomy if complications (i.e., perforation or an inflammatory mass) are found. If perforation is suspected to have occurred, antibiotic therapy is initiated while the patient is being prepared for surgery. For recommendation of specific antimicrobial agents, see the section on therapy for secondary peritonitis. The severity of appendicitis is related to the development of rupture of the appendix, which is more common in children and the elderly. Meckel's diverticulitis may manifest in a manner identical to that of acute appendicitis, and the therapeutic approach is similar.

Although not a source of intra-abdominal infection, nonspecific mesenteric lymphadenitis is often confused with appendicitis in children and may account for symptoms suggestive of appendicitis in up to 20% of these patients. In childhood it is a self-limited, sometimes recurrent illness of unknown cause that primarily involves mesenteric nodes in the right iliac fossa. The nodes are enlarged and discrete. The adjacent bowel and peritoneum are at most mildly inflamed, and a small amount of clear serous peritoneal fluid is frequently present. The patient has fever, poorly localized right lower quadrant tenderness, rebound tenderness, and voluntary guarding, but rarely abdominal rigidity. On occasion, leukocytosis is present.

Because the clinical manifestation of nonspecific mesenteric lymphadenitis is so similar to that of acute appendicitis, the therapeutic approach is surgical to rule out appendicitis. Even though the appendix may appear normal, an appendectomy should be done, because a recurrent episode of mesenteric adenitis may again lead to misinterpretation. An identical clinical picture can be caused by rubeola, infectious mononucleosis, and infection with *Yersinia* spp.

Diverticulitis

Diverticula of the colon are herniations of the mucosa and submucosa through the circular muscular layer. Diverticula are usually located in the sigmoid and descending colons. Inflammation is the most frequent complication of diverticulosis. Diverticulosis is extremely common and affects 5 to 10% of the population older than 45 years of age and almost 80% of those older than 85; but diverticulitis develops in only 20% of these patients.[524] The pathogenesis is similar to that of appendicitis.[524] Diverticulitis is more common in patients with widespread diverticulosis, and the frequency of the complication increases with age (more than 80% of patients with diverticulitis are older than 50 years of age) and perhaps with use of nonsteroidal anti-inflammatory drugs.[525] The inflammation may remain localized to the bowel wall as a simple diverticulitis. Complications such as confined perforation with pericolic abscess to which adjacent viscera and omentum are adherent,[526] fistula formation, or perforation with spreading peritonitis[527] may occur. Less commonly, rupture of an uninflamed and unobstructed diverticulum into the peritoneal cavity with gross fecal peritonitis can occur. Rupture of a localized peridiverticular abscess into the peritoneal cavity does not result in gross fecal peritonitis, presumably because the diverticular neck is obstructed by a fecalith.[524]

The clinical picture of uncomplicated sigmoid diverticulitis resembles that of appendicitis, but with findings on the left side of the abdomen. Urinary symptoms are sometimes present as a result of inflammation close to the bladder or ureter and may be followed by fistulization. Pneumaturia and fecaluria, often accompanied by chills and fever, indicate fistulization between the colon and urinary tract. Passage of flatus and feces through the vagina indicates fistulas into the uterus or vagina. With uncomplicated diverticulitis, low-grade fever and mild leukocytosis are usually found, with tenderness, some rigidity in the left lower quadrant and/or suprapubic area, and normal bowel sounds. Perforation produces clinical findings of an intraperitoneal abscess or of diffuse peritonitis.

It is advisable to defer the barium enema until acute diverticulitis has abated with conservative therapy. In fact, because the use of insufflation can result in a perforation, CT has replaced contrast enema in the investigation of patients with suspected diverticulitis.[524] Tomographic evidence of diverticulitis includes inflammation of the pericolic fat, the presence of diverticula, thickening of the bowel wall, or the presence of a peridiverticular abscess. CT also may facilitate percutaneous drainage of peridiverticular abscesses. Sigmoidoscopy is used to diagnose colon cancer or Crohn's disease as a possible cause of the patient's problem, and not to diagnose diverticulitis, which is almost always extraluminal. Nonoperative therapy on an outpatient basis should be tried for the first few attacks of acute uncomplicated diverticulitis and for well-localized, small (≤5 cm in diameter) peridiverticular abscesses provided the patient can tolerate oral therapy, which consists of a liquid diet and 7 to 10 days of oral broad-spectrum antimicrobial therapy. Drugs must have an antimicrobial spectrum that includes the aerobic and anaerobic colonic flora (e.g., amoxicillin/clavulanic acid, ciprofloxacin/metronidazole, trovafloxacin); otherwise, hospitalization with parenteral antimicrobial therapy is indicated. CT-guided percutaneous catheter drainage may be attempted for abscesses larger than 5 cm,[524, 528–531] but if the abscess cavity contains gross fecal material, surgery is indicated. Initial inpatient treatment consists of parenteral fluids, broad-spectrum antibiotics, and nasogastric suction. Antibiotic recommendations are similar to those discussed in the section on therapy for secondary peritonitis.

There are several procedures advocated for surgical management of perforated diverticulitis. The optimal procedure has not been clearly defined[532] because of the absence of properly controlled studies and the variety of complications of diverticulitis and patient characteristics that may influence outcome. Surgical management for infectious complications of diverticulitis consists of either (1) a three-stage procedure, which involves initial drainage and a proximal colostomy to decompress the bowel and divert the fecal stream, followed by resection of the diseased bowel and finally, several months later, by anastomosis to restore bowel continuity; (2) a two-stage procedure, which involves initial resection and temporary proximal colostomy, with either a mucous fistula or blind pouch (Hartmann's procedure), followed by anastomosis; or (3) a one-stage procedure of primary resection and immediate anastomosis.[524] The three-stage procedure, a prolonged and costly course of events, has been reserved traditionally for the critically ill, high-risk patient with uncontrolled sepsis, colonic obstruction, or fecal peritonitis. However, more recently the two-stage procedure has been advocated as safe and effective for these high-risk patients, because the first stage of the three-stage procedures fails to eliminate the source of continued peritoneal infection.[532, 533] The one-stage procedure traditionally has been questioned in the patient with colonic perforation, because the lumen of the bowel is not cleansed preoperatively and because of the assumed risk of breakdown of the anastomosis in the presence of peritonitis. In its favor, the one-stage primary resection and immediate anastomosis eliminates the need for further hospitalization and shortens colostomy-related disability. In recent studies, the one-stage procedure has been reported to be safe and efficacious in the moderate-risk patient with colonic perforation (APACHE II score, ≤15) even in an emergency situation when the bowel has not been cleansed or peritonitis is present.[533, 534] Operative intervention is also indicated if the patient with acute diverticulitis fails to respond promptly to conservative management in 48 to 72 hours, if there is a colonic fistula or persistent colonic obstruction, or if carcinoma is suspected.

Regional Enteritis

The onset of regional enteritis may be acute, especially in the young, and it may mimic acute appendicitis. The correct diagnosis of early regional enteritis may be made only at operation, which reveals a thickened bowel wall and mesenteric lymph node involvement. Usually, however, the diagnosis is established by contrast radiography.

Perforation as the result of an ulcer burrowing through the entire thickness of the bowel wall may occur.[535] Usually the perforation is confined and results in abscesses or internal fistulas; rarely does the ulcer perforate freely into the peritoneal cavity. Perianal or perirectal abscesses and fistulas are also common manifestations of regional enteritis.

Systemic antibiotics are often of value in the management of suppurative complications (see the section on antimicrobial therapy for secondary peritonitis). Surgery is indicated to drain abdominal abscesses, to correct fistulas, and for free perforation. The principal complications of surgery are enterocutaneous fistula, intraperitoneal or wound sepsis, and prolonged postoperative ileus.

Typhlitis

Typhlitis, or inflammation of the cecum, may occur in immunocompromised patients, such as patients with HIV infection.[536, 537] and those who are severely neutropenic from any cause, including acute leukemia, aplastic anemia, cyclic neutropenia, Felty's syndrome, and myelosuppressive chemotherapy.[538–540]

In neutropenic patients, pathologically, the bowel is edematous, with marked thickening of the wall. The luminal surface has discrete areas of punctate ulceration, which at times may coalesce. There is also transmural inflammation with hemorrhagic necrosis and degeneration of the muscularis mucosae. The inflammatory cells found in histologic specimens are almost always mononuclear. It is thought that bacteria found in the normal gut flora opportunistically invade the ulcerations in the bowel during periods of profound neutropenia. Because of the lack of granulocytes, these organisms proliferate and cause local destruction by elaboration of exotoxins.[538]

Initially, the signs and symptoms are similar to those of acute appendicitis. These patients present with a new fever, abdominal pain, rebound tenderness in the right lower quadrant (because of the predominance of cecal involvement), and diarrhea. Rapid progression to the development of an acute abdomen is not uncommon.

Plain radiographs of the abdomen may demonstrate a thickened cecum and possibly the presence of gas within the wall of the colon.[541]

The mortality rate with neutropenic enterocolitis is greater than 50%.[542] Although the management of this disease is somewhat controversial,[543, 544] antimicrobial therapy with activity against the aerobic and anaerobic gut bacteria, together with surgical resection of the necrotic bowel, is generally recommended.

Actinomycosis

Actinomycosis is an uncommon suppurative infection produced by the anaerobe *Actinomyces israelii* or one of several closely related species. The cecal area is the most common site of abdominal actinomycosis. Typically, the history begins with an attack of acute appendicitis or with recurrent bouts of right lower quadrant pain and fever that prompt surgery for a presumptive diagnosis of appendicitis. At surgery an indurated pericecal mass is found with sinus tracts. After appendectomy, persistent draining sinuses form. The diagnosis of actinomycosis is made by demonstration of "sulfur granules" in the purulent sinus discharge and by histologic examination of the tissues. Treatment is discussed in Chapter 245.

Acute Cholecystitis

Pathogenesis

In more than 90% of patients with acute cholecystitis, gallstones are impacted in the cystic duct.[545] It is generally assumed that a change in the degree of obstruction leads to a sudden increase in intraductal

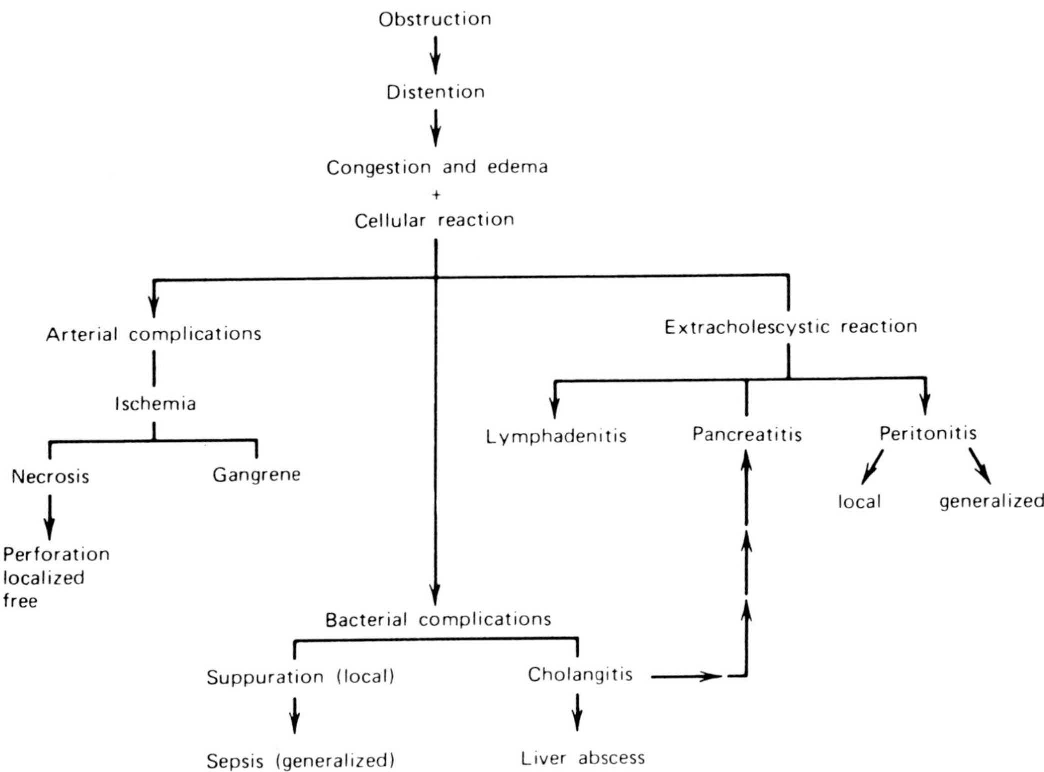

FIGURE 64–6. Pathogenesis of acute cholecystitis.

pressures, which produces distention of the gallbladder, compromising the blood supply and lymphatic drainage. This is followed by tissue necrosis and proliferation of bacteria present in calculous gallbladders. Although infection may not be a primary cause of acute cholecystitis, it develops in more than half of the cases. Infective complications include empyema or gangrene of the gallbladder, emphysematous cholecystitis, pericholecystic abscess, intraperitoneal abscess, peritonitis, cholangitis, liver abscess, and bacteremia. A detailed schema for the proposed pathogenesis of acute cholecystitis is shown in Figure 64–6.

Pathologic Findings

Acute cholecystitis is usually superimposed on a histologic picture of chronic cholecystitis. Ninety-five percent of the gallbladders removed for acute cholecystitis exhibit fibrosis, flattening of the mucosa, and clusters of chronic inflammatory cells as sequelae of previous disease. Rokitansky-Aschoff sinuses are present in 56% of the cases. These sinuses represent mucosal herniations, presumably related to increased hydrostatic pressure during previous episodes of cystic duct obstruction. The early acute changes may be only edema and venous congestion. These are followed by focal necrosis and an influx of neutrophils as secondary bacterial proliferation occurs. This may then be followed by actual gangrene or perforation (Table 64–3).

TABLE 64–3 Pathologic Classification of Acute Cholecystitis

Edema	Gangrene
Edema and congestion	Perforation
Focal necrosis	Localized
Suppuration	Free
Intramural	
Intraluminal	
Pericholecystic	

Symptoms and Signs

Initial obstruction of the cystic duct may be accompanied by only mild epigastric pain followed by reflex nausea and vomiting. If the obstruction is transient, these symptoms subside within 1 to 2 hours. With persistent obstruction, the findings of acute cholecystitis evolve. Pain shifts to the right upper quadrant and becomes increasingly severe. Signs of peritoneal irritation may be present, and in a small number of patients the pain may radiate to the right shoulder or scapula. The gallbladder is palpable in 30 to 40% of the cases.[546] Moderate temperature elevations are common, and minimal icterus may occur. However, repeated chills and fever, jaundice, or hypotension suggests suppurative cholangitis as a consequence of common duct obstruction (see "Bacteriologic Findings"). Most patients with acute cholecystitis have a complete remission within 1 to 4 days. However, 25 to 30% of patients require surgery or develop some complication.

Laboratory Findings

The laboratory data obtained rarely are required to make the diagnosis of acute obstructive cholecystitis, but they may be indicative of further complications (see "Bacteriologic Findings"). The leukocyte count is usually moderately elevated, with a slight increase in early segmented forms. About 50% of the patients have mild hyperbilirubinemia; 40% have a mild elevation of serum aspartate aminotransferase; 25% have increased alkaline phosphatase levels; and only 10% have mild elevations of serum amylase.[547]

Bacteriologic Findings

In the presence of cholecystitis and cholelithiasis, appreciable numbers of various bacteria may be found in the bile and walls of the gallbladder, even in the absence of symptoms. The frequency of bactobilia is higher with longer duration and severity of symptoms, in elderly patients (>60 to 70 years of age), in jaundiced patients, with acute (up to 94% of patients) versus chronic cholecystitis, and especially when the common duct is obstructed.[448, 548]

The organisms found in the biliary tract are commonly the same as the normal intestinal flora, namely, the enteric gram-negative bacilli, including *E. coli*, *Klebsiella/Enterobacter*, and *Proteus* spp., as well as the enterococci.[448, 549] In addition, studies have demonstrated the frequent recovery of anaerobic organisms, including *Bacteroides*, *Clostridia*, and *Fusobacterium* spp.[549] When present, these anaerobes are often involved in polymicrobic infections, mixed with other anaerobes and aerobic gram-negative bacilli.[550]

Patients from whom anaerobes were recovered were more likely to have had previous multiple, complex, biliary tract surgical procedures, especially biliary-intestinal anastomoses and common duct manipulations. These patients often had severe symptoms and a high incidence of postoperative infectious complications, especially wound infections.[551]

The source of bactobilia is unknown but has been assumed to be the duodenum, and spread is assumed to occur via an ascending route.[550] Although the duodenum normally has a sparse flora in the fasting state, higher counts occur transiently after meals and in conditions that allow bacterial overgrowth in the stomach (achlorhydria or gastric obstruction) or in the small bowel (obstruction, diverticula, or blind loops).

Radiographic and Related Studies

An upright chest radiograph is of limited value. In two thirds of cases the right hemidiaphragm is elevated. Because subdiaphragmatic free air cannot originate in the biliary tract, if it is present, it indicates another disease process. In only about 10 to 15% of cases are calcified gallstones seen on plain films of the abdomen, but this finding in any case indicates only cholelithiasis. Occasionally, a diffusely calcified gallbladder ("porcelainized gallbladder") may be seen. Because this condition rarely, if ever, causes acute cholecystitis, its presence should strongly suggest another diagnosis. The demonstration of gas limited to the gallbladder wall or lumen is diagnostic of emphysematous cholecystitis.

Oral cholecystography is of little value in diagnosing acute cholecystitis, because it requires too long a preparation time and is not applicable in jaundiced or vomiting patients. Intravenous cholangiography has been replaced by more sensitive and specific techniques. Advances in ultrasonography and nuclear medicine have made these modalities the diagnostic studies of choice for acute cholecystitis. Both are noninvasive, carry little reported morbidity, and have sensitivity and specificity values greater than 90%. Sonographic findings consistent with acute cholecystitis include the presence of stones, thickened gallbladder wall, dilated lumen of the gallbladder, or a pericholecystic collection.[552, 553] Hepatobiliary scanning with one of the ^{99m}Tc-labeled acetanilide iminodiacetic acid (IDA) derivatives is also a sensitive and rapid study for the diagnosis of acute cholecystitis.[552–554] Even in the presence of moderately severe liver dysfunction,[554] the IDA nuclide is concentrated in the liver and excreted into the bile, resulting in visualization of the functioning hepatobiliary system, including the gallbladder and duodenum, within the first hour. In acute cholecystitis, the cystic duct is occluded by a stone or mucosal inflammation, so the gallbladder is not visualized despite common duct and small bowel visualization. In patients with chronic cholecystitis, the cholescintigram may be either normal, or, in more than 50% of these patients, the gallbladder is only seen in delayed images obtained 4 hours after IDA administration.

Findings consistent with acute cholecystitis may also be demonstrated with CT, but this technique should not be used for initial screening.[555] MRI provides both functional and anatomic information and is sensitive in detecting gallbladder disease in patients with suspected cholecystitis.[556]

Complications

Perforation occurs in 10 to 15% of the cases. A small percentage of these are acute free perforations into the peritoneal cavity. These cases are readily recognizable because they produce the catastrophic symptoms and signs of diffuse peritonitis. More frequently, the omentum and serosa of contiguous viscera localize the perforation early. In such cases, there is persistent fever, often with a palpable mass that may be in a somewhat atypical location, and occasionally with a friction rub. Acute emphysematous cholecystitis is seen most commonly in elderly diabetic men. Systemic symptoms are more severe, and the classic radiographic picture of the abdomen reveals gas within the gallbladder lumen, frequently with a gas-fluid level, and gas in a ring along the contours of the gallbladder wall.[557] Cholangitis is described in detail in a later section. Pancreatitis can also complicate cholecystitis. Here the pain is more midline and may radiate to the back. Urine and serum amylase are often elevated.

Differential Diagnosis

In addition to the complications noted, the differential diagnosis should include myocardial infarction, perforating ulcer, right lower lobe pneumonia, intestinal obstruction, hepatitis, perihepatitis, and acute disease involving the right kidney. Radiographs of the chest and abdomen, electrocardiograms, and urinalysis can exclude these in most cases.

Antimicrobial Therapy in Acute Obstructive Cholecystitis

Severely ill or elderly patients and patients with infectious complications such as emphysematous cholecystitis, perforation with peritonitis or a pericholecystic collection and cholangitis should be treated early for infection possibly caused by enteric gram-negative bacilli and anaerobic bacteria, including *B. fragilis*.[439, 548, 549] An appropriate initial antibiotic regimen includes an aminoglycoside (gentamicin or tobramycin) and ampicillin or piperacillin, in addition to an agent such as clindamycin or metronidazole, to treat for *B. fragilis*. The antimicrobial regimens discussed in the section on treatment of secondary peritonitis would be appropriate alternatives. A more specific antibiotic regimen should be substituted when the results of antimicrobial sensitivity testing of the isolated pathogens become available.

The role of antibiotics for the treatment of uncomplicated acute cholecystitis remains unclear. In a large retrospective study, routine antibiotic therapy for acute cholecystitis did not appear to affect the outcome of the attack or to decrease the incidence of local infectious complications such as empyema or pericholecystic abscess formation.[558] These findings could occur because, although high concentrations of antibiotics may be present in blood, tissues, and common duct bile, these levels do not appear in the gallbladder bile, which is almost always blocked by cystic duct obstruction in acute cholecystitis, and therefore are unable to eradicate bactobilia.

Available evidence suggests that perioperative antibiotics are a helpful adjunct to surgery to prevent postoperative infectious complications.[559] Because wound infection is thought to be caused by contamination of the incision with infected bile at the time of operation, prophylactic antibiotics should be given in a manner that will achieve high blood and tissue concentrations at the time of surgery.

Perioperative antibiotics have been recommended in situations in which the frequency of bactobilia is high, for example in elderly patients and in those with a history of jaundice or jaundice at operation, common duct obstruction from stones, chills and fever, or previous biliary tract surgery. Also, it has been recommended that prophylactic antibiotics be administered according to the results of an intraoperative Gram stain of bile.[448] Although ineffective against enterococci and some anaerobes, a cephem antibiotic appears to be a reasonable choice,[559] but antibiotics such as ampicillin-sulbactam would have a broader spectrum of activity.

Surgery

Immediate surgery is indicated for gangrenous (emphysematous) cholecystitis, perforation with peritonitis, and suspected pericholecystic abscess. In these patients, cholecystectomy with intraoperative cholangiography is the procedure of choice. In patients with severe clinical deterioration, a cholecystostomy and removal of cystic duct stones may prove to be a temporizing life-saving measure until a second definitive procedure can be performed,[560, 561] provided there is no evidence of suppurative cholangitis (i.e., repeated chills, fever, jaundice, and hypotension), which would require immediate decompression of the common bile duct. Cholecystostomy is not an adequate operation for acute suppurative cholangitis unless the common duct is clearly decompressed through a large patent cystic duct. Laparoscopic cholecystectomy is an option for acute uncomplicated cholecystitis with conversion to an open procedure when technical difficulties are encountered.

The timing of surgery in patients with uncomplicated acute cholecystitis has been controversial. Supporters of delayed surgery after the acute attack has subsided with conservative management, believe that morbidity is decreased and that the delay lowers the frequency of unnecessary surgery when the diagnosis is unclear.[562] However, many series have supported early surgery, indicating that a deceptively benign presentation, especially in an elderly patient, can mask the presence of complications and prompt an inappropriate delay in surgery. Also, no difference in morbidity has been reported between early and delayed surgery, and advances in diagnostic studies have markedly decreased the incidence of misdiagnosis.[563, 564] The disadvantages of delayed surgery include prolonged hospitalization and a significant incidence of recurrent symptoms that may precipitate urgent surgery under less favorable conditions.

Cholangitis

Cholangitis may be defined as varying degrees of inflammation and/or infection involving hepatic and common bile ducts. Because the mucosa of the gallbladder is continuous with that of the common bile duct via the cystic duct, it is not surprising that varying degrees of choledochitis should occur as a limited cholangitis with cholecystitis. In fact, specimens of the common duct taken at the time of cholecystectomy for acute cholecystitis usually show localized edema and inflammation. However, this disease is indistinguishable from uncomplicated acute cholecystitis. This section focuses on the more severe entities of ascending cholangitis and acute obstructive suppurative cholangitis.

Pathogenesis

In a manner similar to that described for cholecystitis, obstruction of the common duct results in increased pressure, edema, congestion, and necrosis of the walls of the biliary tree, followed by rapid proliferation of bacteria within the biliary tree. In most instances, obstruction is caused by gallstones.[565] However, obstruction may result from previous biliary tract surgery, tumor, chronic calcific pancreatitis, and parasitic infections. Fulminant cholangitis has also been reported as a complication of endoscopic retrograde cholangiopancreatography.[566]

Pathogenic Findings

Microscopic examination of the common duct reveals marked fibrous thickening and focal areas of chronic inflammation. Superimposed on this picture is necrosis of the mucosa and dense infiltration of acute inflammatory cells. In the liver, portal inflammation is uniformly seen. Usually, this is a dense neutrophilic infiltrate. In 40% of cases, numerous microabscesses are present. Bile duct dilatation and cholestasis are also present.

Symptoms and Signs

Patients usually have an antecedent history compatible with gallbladder disease. The onset is usually acute, with high fever, chills, and diffuse pain and tenderness over the liver. Jaundice is usually prominent. In some cases, shock and other findings of gram-negative bacteremia may be present; altogether, 85% of the patients fulfill Charcot's triad of fever, chills, and jaundice.[567]

Laboratory Findings

There is usually marked leukocytosis with an increase in immature forms. The serum bilirubin concentration is often higher than 4 mg/dl, and the serum alkaline phosphatase level is significantly higher than that encountered in acute cholecystitis. Serum aspartate aminotransferase is modestly elevated. Biochemical and even clinical evidence of disseminated intravascular coagulation may be present.

Bacteriologic Findings

Adequate data are unavailable on the bacteriologic findings in cholangitis. Studies using detailed aerobic and anaerobic culture techniques suggest that the bacteriologic findings in cholangitis are similar to those in acute obstructive cholecystitis. Gram-negative enteric bacilli and anaerobic bacteria are the most common isolates. Those patients with a stent in their bile duct may harbor resistant flora such as *P. aeruginosa*. In contrast to uncomplicated cholecystitis, bacteremia occurs in approximately 50% of patients with cholangitis. *E. coli* (52% of the isolates), *B. fragilis* (22%), and *C. perfringens* (16%) are the organisms most frequently isolated from blood cultures.

Radiographic and Related Studies

An upright chest film is of limited value. The right hemidiaphragm is frequently elevated. Other findings are similar to those described for acute cholecystitis and are nonspecific. Oral cholecystography is of no value. Intravenous cholangiography usually is not helpful, because the serum bilirubin concentration frequently is higher than 4.0 mg/dl, and the technique has been replaced by less morbid and more sensitive techniques. Ultrasonography can easily be used to evaluate gallbladder size, the presence of stones, and the degree of bile duct dilatation. Marked bile duct dilatation in a patient with the appropriate clinical picture corroborates this diagnosis. It is important to note that not all patients with obstructive cholangitis have a grossly dilated biliary tree because of chronic inflammation of the biliary tract, and ultrasonography is unlikely to be helpful in these cases. Obstruction of the common bile duct can be diagnosed by hepatobiliary scanning with one of the ^{99m}Tc-labeled derivatives of IDA. In this case, no component of the biliary system or small bowel is visualized, despite adequate hepatic uptake. In obstructive cholangitis, however, ultrasonography is the preferred study because of its ability to visualize dilated ducts and the decreased dependability of IDA scintigraphy in the presence of severe jaundice.[568] Percutaneous transhepatic cholangiography and endoscopic retrograde cholangiography are extremely valuable in evaluating bile duct obstruction. However, it is seldom feasible to use these techniques in the patient who is acutely ill with cholangitis.

Complications

Bacteremia and shock occur commonly and perhaps are best included as part of the clinical picture of obstructive cholangitis. Perforation of the gallbladder may occur and is described in the section on complications of acute cholecystitis. In some less acute cases, macroscopic hepatic abscesses develop. This clinical picture may be similar to cholangitis alone, but ultrasonography, CT, or technetium or gallium scans may visualize multiple defects in the hepatic parenchyma. Finally, pancreatitis can occur as a complication.

Differential Diagnosis

Acute cholecystitis and its complications—hepatic abscess, perforating ulcer, pancreatitis, intestinal obstruction, right lower lobe pneumonia, acute disease involving the right kidney, and bacteremic shock related to another focus of infection—should all be considered in the differential diagnosis. In acute cholecystitis the patient is usually less ill; in addition, the serum bilirubin concentration is usually less than 4.0 mg/dl, serum alkaline phosphatase is not markedly elevated, and ultrasonography or cholescintigraphy usually demonstrates a patent, nondilated hepatic and common duct. Patients with hepatic abscesses not caused by obstructive cholangitis usually are not as acutely ill; hepatic tenderness, when present, is also not as severe, and liver function tests may be only minimally abnormal. Diagnostic studies usually detect a macroscopic parenchymal defect. In pancreatitis, the pain and tenderness are more midline and may radiate to the back. Serum and urine amylase levels are significantly elevated, but liver function tests are not markedly abnormal. Radiographs of the chest and abdomen and urinalysis exclude the majority of other possibilities.

Antimicrobial Therapy in Cholangitis

Prompt institution of appropriate antibiotic therapy is mandatory, because these severe infections are frequently complicated by bacteremia and shock. Based on the bacteriologic findings described and on the known in vitro susceptibilities of these organisms, the antimicrobial regimens discussed in the section on treatment of secondary peritonitis would be appropriate choices. This antibiotic regimen is directed primarily at the complicating bacteremia, because antibiotics alone cannot sterilize the biliary tract in the face of obstruction.[549]

Surgery

Prompt operative intervention with decompression of the common duct is mandatory in all but those few patients who respond promptly to antibiotics.[569] In all patients who undergo surgery, regardless of the procedure, operative cholangiography should be performed. The simplest but least satisfactory procedure is simple cholecystostomy if patency of the cystic duct is assured. However, if at all possible, a cholecystectomy should be performed, followed by common duct exploration and T-tube drainage. In more complicated cases, choledochoduodenostomy or cholecystoduodenostomy may have to be performed.

REFERENCES

1. Whalen JP, Bierny JP. Classification of perihepatic abscesses. Radiology. 1969;92:1427–1437.
2. Sanders RC, James AE Jr, Fischer K. Correlation of liver scans and images with abdominal radiographs in perihepatic sepsis. Am J Surg. 1972;124:346–352.
3. Myers MA. The spread and localization of acute intraperitoneal effusions. Radiology. 1970;95:547–554.
4. Altemeier WA, Culbertson WR, Fullen WD, et al. Intra-abdominal abscesses. Am J Surg. 1973;125:70–79.
5. Shear L, Swartz C, Shinaberger JA, et al. Kinetics of peritoneal fluid absorption in adult men. N Engl J Med. 1965;272:123–127.
6. Boen ST. Kinetics of peritoneal dialysis: A comparison with artificial kidney. Medicine (Baltimore). 1961;40:243–287.
7. Tsilibury EC, Wissig SL. Absorption from the peritoneal cavity: SEM study of the mesothelium covering the peritoneal surface of the muscular portion of the diaphragm. Am J Anat. 1977;149:127–133.
8. Rochlin DB, Zill H, Blakemore WS. Studies of the resorption of chromium-51 tagged erythrocytes from the peritoneal cavity: The absorption of fluids and particulate matter from the peritoneal cavity. Int Abstr Surg. 1958;107:1–14.
9. Pritchard JA, Adams RH. The fate of blood in the peritoneal cavity. Surg Gynecol Obstet. 1957;105:621–629.
10. Zinsser HH, Pryde AW. Experimental study of physical factors, including fibrin formation, influencing the spread of fluids and small particles within and from the peritoneal cavity of the dog. Ann Surg. 1952;136:818–827.
11. Macbeth RA, Mackenzie WC. The abdominal wall, umbilicus, peritoneum, mesenteries, and retroperitoneum. In: Sabiston DC Jr, ed. Davis-Christopher Textbook of Surgery. 10th ed. Philadelphia: WB Saunders; 1972:773–795.
12. Nohr CW, Marshall DG. Primary peritonitis in children. Can J Surg. 1984;27:179–181.
13. McDougal WS, Izant RJ, Zollinger RM Jr. Primary peritonitis in infancy and childhood. Ann Surg. 1975;181:310–313.
14. Golden GT, Shaw A. Primary peritonitis. Surg Gynecol Obstet. 1972;135:513–516.
15. Epstein M, Calia FM, Gabuzda GJ. Pneumococcal peritonitis in patients with postnecrotic cirrhosis. N Engl J Med. 1968;278:69–71.
16. Speck WT, Dresdale SS, McMillan RW. Primary peritonitis and the nephrotic syndrome. Am J Surg. 1974;127:267–269.
17. Conn HO, Fessel JM. Spontaneous bacterial peritonitis in cirrhosis: Variations on a theme. Medicine (Baltimore). 1971;50:161–197.
18. Conn HO. Spontaneous bacterial peritonitis, multiple revisitations. Gastroenterology. 1976;70:455–457.
19. Bar-Meir S, Conn HO. Spontaneous bacterial peritonitis induced by intra-arterial vasopressin therapy. Gastroenterology. 1976;70:418–421.
20. Targan SR, Chow AW, Guze LB. Role of anaerobic bacteria in spontaneous peritonitis of cirrhosis: Report of two cases and review of the literature. Am J Med. 1977;62:397–403.
21. Kline MM, McCallum RW, Guth PH. The clinical value of ascitic fluid culture and leukocyte count studies in alcoholic cirrhosis. Gastroenterology. 1976;70:408–412.
22. Weinstein MP, Iannini PB, Stratton CW, et al. Spontaneous bacterial peritonitis: A review of 28 cases with emphasis on improved survival and factors influencing prognosis. Am J Med. 1978;64:592–598.
23. Hoefs JC, Canawati HN, Sapico FL, et al. Spontaneous bacterial peritonitis. Hepatology. 1982;2:399–407.
24. Pinzello G, Simonetti R, Craxi A, et al. Spontaneous bacterial peritonitis: A prospective investigation in predominantly nonalcoholic cirrhotic patients. Hepatology. 1983;3:545–549.
25. Conn HO, Cirrhosis. In: Schiff L, Schiff ER, eds. Diseases of the Liver. 5th ed. Philadelphia: JB Lippincott; 1982:847–977.
26. Thomas FB, Fromkes JJ. Spontaneous bacterial peritonitis associated with acute viral hepatitis. J Clin Gastroenterol. 1982;4:259–262.
27. Runyon BA. Spontaneous bacterial peritonitis with cardiac ascites. Am J Gastroenterol. 1984;79:796.
28. Isner J, MacDonald JS, Schein PS. Spontaneous *Streptococcus pneumoniae* peritonitis in a patient with metastatic gastric cancer. Cancer. 1979;39:2306–2309.
29. Shesol BF, Rosato EF, Rosato FE. Concomitant acute lupus erythematosus and primary pneumococcal peritonitis. Am J Gastroenterol. 1975;63:324–326.
30. Friedland JA, Harris MN. Primary pneumococcal peritonitis in a young adult. Am J Surg. 1970;119:737–739.
31. Golden GT, Stevenson TR, Ritchie WP Jr. Primary peritonitis in adults. South Med J. 1975;68:413–414.
32. Wilcox CM, Dismukes WE. Spontaneous bacterial peritonitis: A review of pathogenesis, diagnosis and treatment. Medicine (Baltimore). 1987;66:447–456.
33. Correia JP, Conn HO. Spontaneous bacterial peritonitis in cirrhosis: Endemic or epidemic? Med Clin North Am. 1975;59:963–981.
34. Hoefs JC, Runyon BA. Spontaneous bacterial peritonitis. Dis Mon. 1985;31:1–48.
35. Fromkes JJ, Thomas FB, Mekhjian HS, et al. Antimicrobial activity of human ascitic fluid. Gastroenterology. 1977;73:668–672.
36. Scheckman P, Onderdonk AB, Bartlett JG, Anaerobes in spontaneous peritonitis. Lancet. 1977;2:1223.
37. Runyon BA, Hoefs JC. Culture-negative neutrocytic ascites: A variant of spontaneous peritonitis. Hepatology. 1984;4:1209–1211.
38. Runyon BA, Umland ET, Merlin T. Inoculation of blood culture bottles with ascitic fluid: Improved detection of spontaneous bacterial peritonitis. Arch Intern Med. 1987;147:73–75.
39. Beeson PB, Brannon ES, Warren JU. Observations on the sites of removal of bacteria from the blood in patients with bacterial endocarditis. J Exp Med. 1945;81:9–23.
40. Rutenburg AM, Sonnenblick F, Koven I, et al. Comparative response of normal and cirrhotic rats to intravenously injected bacteria. Proc Soc Exp Biol Med. 1959;101:279–281.
41. Lahnborg G, Friman L, Berghem L. Reticuloendothelial function in patients with alcoholic liver disease. Scand J Gastroenterol. 1981;16:481–489.
42. Rimola A, Soto R, Bory F, et al. Reticuloendothelial system phagocytic activity in cirrhosis and its relation to bacterial infections and prognosis. Hepatology. 1984;4:53–58.
43. Rajkovic IA, Williams R. Abnormalities of neutrophilic phagocytosis, intracellular killing and metabolic activity in alcoholic cirrhosis and hepatitis. Hepatology. 1986;6:252–262.
44. Wyke RJ, Rajkovic IA, Eddleston WF, et al. Defective serum opsonization in patients with chronic liver disease (Abstract). Gut. 1979;20:A931.
45. Yousif-Kadura AGM, Rajkovic IA, Wyke RJ, et al. Defects in serum attractant activity in different types of chronic liver disease. Gut. 1984;25:79–84.

46. Simberkoff MS, Moldover NH, Weiss G. Bactericidal and opsonic activity of cirrhotic ascites and nonascitic peritoneal fluid. J Lab Clin Med. 1978;91:831–839.
47. Runyon BA, Hoefs JC. Ascitic fluid analyis in the differentiation of spontaneous bacterial peritonitis from gastrointestinal performation into ascitic fluid. Hepatology. 1984;4:447–450.
48. Whipple RL Jr, Harris JF. *E. coli* septicemia in Laennec's cirrhosis of the liver. Ann Intern Med. 1950;33:462–469.
49. Murray HW, Marks SJ. Spontaneous bacterial empyema, pericarditis and peritonitis in cirrhosis. Gastroenterology. 1977;72:772–773.
50. Snyder N, Atterbury CE, Correia JP, et al. Increased concurrence of cirrhosis and bacterial endocarditis. Gastroenterology. 1977;73:1107–1113.
51. Schweinburg FB, Seligman AM, Fine J. Transmural migration of intestinal bacteria: A study based on the use of radioactive *Escherichia coli*. N Engl J Med. 1950;242:747–751.
52. Schwartz FD, Kallmeyer J, Durea G, et al. Prevention of infection during peritoneal dialysis. JAMA. 1967;199:79–81.
53. Gorbach SL, Lai D, Levitan R. Intestinal microflora in Laennec's cirrhosis (Abstract). J Clin Invest. 1970;49:36A.
54. McCartney JE, Fraser J. Pneumococcal peritonitis. Br J Surg. 1922;9:479–489.
55. Herbert TJ, Mortimer PP. Recurrent pneumococcal peritonitis associated with an intrauterine contraceptive device. Br J Surg. 1974;61:901–902.
56. Brinson RR, Kolts BE, Monif GRG. Spontaneous bacterial peritonitis associated with an intrauterine device. J Clin Gastroenterol. 1986;8:82–84.
57. Kimball MW, Knee S. Gonococcal perihepatitis in a male. The Fitz-Hugh-Curtis syndrome. N Engl J Med. 1970;282:1082–1084.
58. Luetscher JA Jr. Electrophoretic analysis of the proteins of plasma and serous effusions. J Clin Invest. 1941;20:99–106.
59. Witte MH, Witte CL, Davis WM, et al. Peritoneal transudate: A diagnostic clue to portal system obstruction in patients with intra-abdominal neoplasms or peritonitis. JAMA. 1972;221:1380–1383.
60. Hoefs JC. Increase in ascites white blood cell and protein concentrations during diuresis in patients with chronic liver disease. Hepatology. 1981;1:249–254.
61. Stassen WN, McCullough AJ, Bacon BR, et al. Immediate diagnostic criteria for bacterial infection of ascitic fluid: Evaluation of ascitic fluid polymorphonuclear leukocyte count, pH, and lactate concentration, alone and in combination. Gastroenterology. 1986;90:1247–1254.
62. Garcia-Tsao G, Conn HO, Lerner E. The diagnosis of bacterial peritonitis: Comparison of pH, lactate concentration and leukocyte count. Hepatology. 1985;5:91–96.
63. Yang C-Y, Liaw F, Chu E-M, et al. White count, pH and lactate in ascites in the diagnosis of spontaneous bacterial peritonitis. Hepatology. 1985;5:85–90.
64. Vickers FN, Maloney PJ. Gonococcal perihepatitis: Reports of three cases with comments on diagnosis and treatment. Arch Intern Med. 1964;114:120–123.
65. Burack WR, Hollister RM. Tuberculous peritonitis: A study of forty-seven proved cases encountered by a general medical unit in twenty-five years. Am J Med. 1960;28:510–523.
66. Saw EC, Shields SJ, Comer TP, et al. Granulomatous peritonitis due to *Coccidioides immitis*. Arch Surg. 1974;108:369–371.
67. Hoefs JC, Diagnostic paracentesis: A potent clinical tool. Gastroenterology. 1990;98:230–236.
68. Harrison RN, Cryer HM, Howard DA, et al. Clarification of risk factors for abdominal operations in patients with hepatic cirrhosis. Ann Surg. 1984;199:648–665.
69. Runyon BA, McHutchison JG, Antillon MR, et al. Short-course versus long-course antibiotic treatment of spontaneous bacterial peritonitis: A randomized controlled study of 108 patients. Gastroenterology. 1991;100:1737–1742.
70. Runyon BA, Hoefs JC. Spontaneous vs. secondary bacterial peritonitis: Differentiation by response of ascitic fluid neutrophil count to antimicrobial therapy. Arch Intern Med. 1986;146:1563–1565.
71. Dimond M, Proctor HJ. Concomitant pneumococcal appendicitis, peritonitis and meningitis. Arch Surg. 1976;111:888–889.
72. Mallory A, Schaefer JW. Complications of diagnostic paracentesis in patients with liver disease. JAMA. 1978;239:628–630.
73. Levine H. Needle biopsy of peritoneum in exudative ascites. Arch Intern Med. 1967;120:542–545.
74. Dineen P, Homan WP, Grafe WR. Tuberculous peritonitis: 43 years experience in diagnosis and treatment. Ann Surg. 1976;184:717–722.
75. Felisart J, Rimona A, Arroyo V, et al. Cefotaxime is more effective than is ampicillin-tobramycin in cirrhotics with severe infections. Hepatology. 1985;5:457–462.
76. Cabrera J, Arroyo V, Ballesta AM, et al. Aminoglycoside nephrotoxicity in cirrhosis: Value of urinary β_2-microglobulin to discriminate functional renal failure from acute tubular damage. Gastroenterology. 1982;82:97–105.
77. Forrest A, Nix DE, Ballow CH, et al. Phamacodynamics of intravenous ciprofloxacin in seriously ill patients. Antimicrob Agents Chemother. 1993;37:1073–1081.
78. Runyon BA, Hoefs JC. Ascitic fluid chemical analysis before, during and after spontaneous bacterial peritonitis. Hepatology. 1985;5:257–259.
79. Singh N, Gayowski T, Yu VL. Trimethoprim/sulfamethoxazole for the prevention of spontaneous bacterial peritonitis in cirrhosis: A randomized trial. Ann Intern Med. 1995;122:595–598.
80. Porter JM, Snowe RJ, Silver D. Tuberculous enteritis with perforation and abscess formation in childhood. Surgery. 1972;71:254–257.
81. Rowland TC Jr. Severe peritonitis complicating an intrauterine contraceptive device. Am J Obstet Gynecol. 1971;110:786–787.
82. Prokesch RC, Rimland D. Infectious complications of the peritoneovenous shunt. Am J Gastroenterol. 1983;78:235–240.
83. Reynold M, Sherman JO, Mclone DG. Ventriculoperitoneal shunt infections masquerading as an acute abdomen. J Pediatr Surg. 1983;18:951–954.
84. Nichols RL. Intra-abdominal infections: An overview. Rev Infect Dis. 1985;7(Suppl 4):S709–S715.
85. Drasar BS, Shiner M, McLeod GM. Studies on the intestinal flora: I. The bacterial flora of the gastrointestinal tract in healthy and achlorhydric persons. Gastroenterology. 1969;56:71–79.
86. Nichols RL, Smith JW. Intragastric microbial colonization in common disease states of the stomach and duodenum. Ann Surg. 1975;182:557–561.
87. Gorbach SL, Plaut AG, Nahas L, et al. Studies of intestinal microflora: II. Microorganisms of the small intestine and their relations to oral and fecal flora. Gastroenterology. 1967;53:856–867.
88. Drasar BS, Shiner M. Studies on the intestinal flora: Part II. Bacterial flora of the small intestine in patients with gastrointestinal disorders. Gut. 1969;10:812–819.
89. Gorbach SL, Nahas L, Lerner PI, et al. Studies of intestinal microflora: I. Effects of diet, age, and periodic sampling of numbers of fecal microorganisms in man. Gastroenterology. 1967;53:845–855.
90. Finegold SM. Interaction of antimicrobial therapy and intestinal flora. Am J Clin Nutr. 1970;23:1466–1471.
91. Altemeier WA. The bacterial flora of acute perforated appendicitis with peritonitis. Ann Surg. 1938;107:517–528.
92. Finegold SM. Abdominal and perineal infections. In: Finegold SM, ed. Anaerobic Bacteria in Human Disease. New York: Academic Press; 1977:257–313.
93. Gorbach SL, Thadepalli H, Norsen J, Anaerobic microorganisms in intra-abdominal infections. In: Balows A, de Haan RM, Dowell VR Jr, et al, eds. Anaerobic Bacteria: Role in Disease. Springfield, IL: Charles C Thomas; 1974:399–407.
94. Lorber B, Swenson RM. The bacteriology of intra-abdominal infections. Surg Clin North Am. 1975;55:1349–1354.
95. Swenson RM, Lorber B, Michaelson TC, et al. The bacteriology of intra-abdominal infections. Arch Surg. 1974;109:398–389.
96. Bodner SJ, Koenig MG, Goodman JS. Bacteremic *Bacteroides* infections. Ann Intern Med. 1970;73:537–544.
97. Gelb EF, Seligman SJ. Bacteroidaceae bacteremia: Effect of age and focus of infection upon clinical course. JAMA. 1970;212:1038–1041.
98. Fry DE, Garrison RN, Polk HC Jr. Clinical implications in *Bacteroides* bacteremia. Surg Gynecol Obstet. 1979;149:189–192.
99. Chow AW, Guze LB. Bacteroidaceae bacteremia: Clinical experience with 112 patients. Medicine (Baltimore). 1974;53:93–126.
100. Bennion RS, Thompson JL, Baron EL, et al. Gangrenous and perforated appendicitis with peritonitis: Treatment and bacteriology. Clin Ther. 1990;12(Suppl C):31–44.
101. Bennion RS, Thompson JL, Baron EL, et al. The bacteriology of gangrenous and perforated appendicitis—revisited. Ann Surg. 1990;211:165–167.
102. Tally FP, McGowan K, Kellum JM, et al. A randomized comparison of cefoxitin with or without amikacin and clindamycin plus amikacin in surgical sepsis. Ann Surg. 1981;193:318–323.
103. Rotstein OD, Pruett TL, Simmons RL. Microbiologic features and treatment of persistent peritonitis in patients in the intensive care unit, Can J Surg. 1986;29:247–250.
104. Aronoff SC, Olson MM, Gaudierer MWL, et al. *Pseudomonas aeruginosa* as a primary pathogen in children with bacterial peritonitis. J Pediatr Surg. 1987;22:861–864.
105. Heseltine PNR, Yellin AE, Applebaum MD, et al. Perforated and gangrenous appendicitis: An analysis of antibiotic failures. J Infect Dis.1983;148:322–329.
106. Bower RJ, Bell MJ, Ternberg JL. Controversial aspects of appendicitis management in children. Arch Surg. 1981;116:885–887.
107. Yellin AE, Heseltine PNR, Berne TV, et al. The role of *Pseudomonas* species in patients treated with ampicillin and sulbactam for gangrenous and perforated appendicitis. Surg Obstet Gynecol.1985;161:303–307.
108. Dunn DL, Simmons RL. The role of anaerobic bacteria in intra-abdominal infections. Rev Infect Dis. 1984; 6(Suppl 1):S139–S146.
109. Sawyer RG, Rosenlof LK, Adams RB, et al. Peritonitis in the 1990's: Changing pathogens and changing strategies in the critically ill. Am Surg. 1992;58:82–87.
110. Nichols RL, Smith JW, Klein DB, et al. Risk of infection after penetrating abdominal trauma. N Engl J Med. 1984;311:1065–1070.
111. Levison ME, Korman LC, Carrington ER, et al. Quantitative microflora of the vagina. Am J Obstet Gynecol. 1977;127:80–85.
112. Levison ME, Trestman I, Quach R, et al. Quantitative bacteriology of the vaginal flora in vaginitis. Am J Obstet Gynecol. 1979;133:139–144.
113. Bartlett JG, Onderdonk AB, Drude E, et al. Quantitative bacteriology of the vaginal flora. J Infect Dis. 1977;136:271–277.
114. Ohm M, Galask RP. The effect of antibiotic prophylaxis on patients undergoing vaginal operations: II. Alteration of microbial flora. Am J Obstet Gynecol. 1975;123:597–604.
115. Ramsay AM. The significance of *C. welchii* in the cervical swab and blood serum in postpartum and postabortum sepsis. J Obstet Gynecol. 1949;56:247–258.
116. Hite KE, Hesseltine HC, Goldstein L. A study of the bacterial flora of the normal and pathologic vagina and uterus. Am J Obstet Gynecol. 1947;53:233–240.
117. Gibbs RS, O' Dell TN, MacGregor RR, et al. Puerperal endometritis: A prospective microbiologic study. Am J Obstet Gynecol. 1975;121:919–925.
118. Baker CJ, Barrett FF, Yow MD. The influence of advancing gestation on group B streptococcal colonization in pregnant women. Am J Obstet Gynecol. 1975; 122:820–823.
119. Penza JF. Moniliasis and trichomoniasis. In: Charles D, Finland M, eds. Obstetric and Perinatal Infections. Philadelphia: Lea & Febiger; 1973:209.

120. Finegold SM. Female genital tract infections. In: Finegold SM, ed. Anaerobic Bacteria in Human Disease. New York: Academic Press; 1977:350–385.
121. Swenson RM, Michaelson TC, Daly MJ, et al. Anaerobic bacterial infections of the female genital tract. Obstet Gynecol. 1973;42:538–541.
122. Thadepalli H, Gorbach SL, Keith L. Anaerobic infections of the female genital tract: Bacteriologic and therapeutic aspects. Am J Obstet Gynecol. 1973;117:1034–1040.
123. Chow AW, Marshall JR, Guze LB. Anaerobic infections of the female genital tract: Prospects and perspectives. Obstet Gynecol Surg. 1975;30:477–494.
124. Chow AW, Malkasian KI, Marshall JR, et al. The bacteriology of acute pelvic inflammatory disease: Value of cul-de-sac cultures and relative importance of gonococcal and other aerobic and anaerobic bacteria. Am J Obstet Gynecol. 1975;122:876–879.
125. Eschenbach DA, Buchanon TM, Pollock HM, et al. Polymicrobial etiology of acute pelvic inflammatory disease. N Engl J Med. 1975;293:166–171.
126. Wasserheit JN, Bell TA, Kiviat NB, et al. Microbial causes of proven pelvic inflammatory disease and efficacy of clindamycin and tobramycin. Ann Intern Med. 1986;104:187–193.
127. Monif GRG, Welkos SI, Baer H, et al. Cul-de-sac isolates from patients with endometritis-salpingitis-peritonitis and gonococcal endocervicitis. Am J Obstet Gynecol. 1976;126:158–161.
128. Burry VF. Gonococcal vulvovaginitis and possible peritonitis in prepubertal girls. Am J Dis Child. 1971;121:536–537.
129. Fuld GL. Gonococcal peritonitis in a prepubertal child. Am J Dis Child. 1968;115:621–622.
130. Adams EB, MacLeod IN. Invasive amebiasis: II. Amebic liver abscess and its complications. Medicine (Baltimore). 1977;56:325–334.
131. Turner GR, Millikan M, Carter R, et al. Surgical significance of fulminating amebic colitis: Report of perforation of the colon with peritonitis. Am Surg. 1965;31:759–763.
132. Lintermans JP. Fatal peritonitis, an unusual complication of *Strongyloides stercoralis* infestation. Clin Pediatr. 1975;14:974–975.
133. Eisenberg ES, Leviton I, Soeiro R. Fungal peritonitis in patients receiving peritoneal dialysis: Experience with 11 patients and review of the literature. Rev Infect Dis. 1986;3:309–321.
134. Bayer AS, Blumenkrantz MJ, Montgomerie JZ, et al. Candida peritonitis: Report of 22 cases and review of the English literature. Am J Med. 1976;61:832–840.
135. Solomkin JS, Flohr AB, Quie PG, et al. The role of *Candida* in intraperitoneal infections. Surgery. 1980;88:524–530.
136. Howard JM, Singh LM. Peritoneal fluid pH after perforation of peptic ulcers. Arch Surg. 1963;87:483–484.
137. Mortez WH, Erickson WG. Neutralization of hydrochloric acid in the peritoneal cavity. Arch Surg. 1957;75:834–837.
138. Santschi DR, Huizenga KA, Scudamore HH, et al. Bile ascites. Arch Surg. 1963; 87:851–856.
139. Diamonon JS, Barnes JP. Choleperitoneum. Am Surg. 1964;30:331–334.
140. Cohn I, Coltar AM, Atik M, et al. Bile peritonitis. Ann Surg. 1960;152:827–835.
141. Nemir P Jr, Hawthorne HR, Cohn I, et al. I: The cause of death in strangulation obstruction. An experimental study. Ann Surg. 1949;130:857–873.
142. Nemir P Jr, Hawthorne HR, Cohn I, et al. II: The lethal action of the peritoneal fluid. Ann Surg. 1949;130:874–875.
143. Barnett WO, Hardy JD. Observations concerning the peritoneal fluid in experimental strangulated intestinal obstruction: The effects of removal from the peritoneal cavity. Surgery. 1958;43:440–444.
144. Barnett WO, Doyle RS. The effects of neomycin upon the toxicity of peritoneal fluid resulting from strangulation obstruction. Surgery. 1958;44:442–446.
145. Barnett WO, Messina AJ. The influence of massive antibiotics in experimental strangulation obstruction. Gastroenterology. 1959;36:534–536.
146. Davis JH, Yull AB. A possible toxic factor in abdominal surgery. J Trauma. 1962;2:291–300.
147. Filler RM, Sleeman HK, Hendry WS, et al. Lethal factors in experimental peritonitis. Surgery. 1966;60:671–678.
148. Lee JT, Ahrenholz DN, Nelson RD, et al. Mechanisms of the adjuvant effect of hemoglobin in experimental peritonitis: V. The significance of the coordinated iron component. Surgery. 1979;86:41–48.
149. Weingerg ED. Roles of iron in host-parasite interactions. J Infect Dis. 1971;124:401–410.
150. Hau T, Nelson RD, Fiegel VD, et al. Mechanisms of the adjuvant action of hemoglobin in experimental peritonitis-2: Influence of hemoglobin on human leukocyte chemotaxis in vitro. J Surg Res. 1977;22:174–180.
151. Dunn DL, Barke RA, Ahrenholz DH, et al. The adjuvant effect of peritoneal fluid in experimental peritonitis. Ann Surg. 1984;199:37–43.
152. Rotstein OD, Pruett TL, Simmons RD. Fibrin in peritonitis: V. Fibrin inhibits phagocytic killing of *Escherichia coli* by human polymorphonuclear leukocytes. Ann Surg. 1986;203:413–419.
153. McRitchie DI, Girotti MJ, Glynn MF, et al. Effect of systemic fibrinogen depletion on intraabdominal abscess formation. J Lab Clin Med. 1991;118:48–55.
154. Dubrow T, Schwartz RJ, Kissock J, et al. Effect of aerosolized fibrin solution in intraperitoneal contamination. Arch Surg. 1991;126:80–83.
155. Schneierson SS, Amsterdam D, Perlman E. Enhancement of intraperitoneal staphylococcal virulence for mice with different bile salts. Nature. 1961;190:829–830.
156. Sisel RJ, Donovan AJ, Yellin AE. Experimental fecal peritonitis: Influence of barium sulfate or water-soluble radiographic contrast material on survival. Arch Surg. 1972;104:765–768.
157. Westfall RH, Nelson RH, Musselman MM. Barium peritonitis. Am J Surg. 1966;112:760–763.
158. Olitzki L. Mucin as a resistance-lowering substance. Bacteriol Rev. 1948;12:149–172.
159. Cuevas P, Fine J. Role of intraintestinal endotoxin in death from peritonitis. Surg Gynecol Obstet. 1972;134:953–957.
160. Fugger R, Hamilton G, Rogy M, et al. Prognostic significance of endotoxin determination in patients with severe intraabdominal infection. J Infect Dis. 1990;161:1314–1315.
161. Bieluch VM, Tally FP. Pathophysiology of abscess formation. Clin Obstet Gynecol. 1983;10:93–103.
162. Gorbach SL, Bartlett JG. Anaerobic infections (third of three parts). N Engl J Med. 1974;290:1289–1294.
163. Hofstad T. Endotoxins of anaerobic gram-negative microorganisms. In: Balows A, de Haan RM, Dowell VR Jr, et al., eds. Anaerobic Bacteria: Role in Disease. Springfield, IL: Charles C Thomas; 1974:295.
164. Gibbons RJ, MacDonald JB. Degradation of collagenous substrates by *Bacteroides melaninogenicus*. J Bacteriol. 1961;81:614–621.
165. Bjornson HS. Enzymes associated with the survival and virulence of gram–negative anaerobes. Rev Infect Dis. 1984;6(Suppl 1):S21–S24.
166. Gesner BM, Jenkin CR. Production of heparinase by bacteroides. J Bacteriol. 1961;81:595–604.
167. Bjornson H, Hill EO. Bacteroidaceae in thromboembolic disease: Effects of cell wall components on blood coagulation in vivo and in vitro. Infect Immun. 1974;9:337–341.
168. Casciato DA, Rosenblatt JE, Goldberg LS, et al. In vitro interaction of *Bacteroides fragilis* with polymorphonuclear leukocytes and serum factors. Infect Immun. 1975;11:337–342.
169. Keusch GT, Douglas SD. Intraleukocytic survival of anaerobic bacteria. Clin Res. 1974;22:445A.
170. Kasper DL. The polysaccharide capsule of *Bacteroides fragilis* subspecies fragilis: Immunochemical and morphologic definition. J Infect Dis. 1976;133:79–87.
171. Mansheim BJ, Orderdonk AB, Kasper DL. Immunochemical characterization of surface antigens of *Bacteroides melaninogenicus*. Rev Infect Dis. 1979;1:263–277.
172. Onderdonk AB, Kasper DL, Cisneros RL, et al. The capsular polysaccharide of *Bacteroides fragilis* as a virulence factor: Comparison of the pathogenic potential of encapsulated and unencapsulated strains. J Infect Dis. 1977;136:82–89.
173. Ingham HR, Tharagonnet D, Sisson PR, et al. Inhibition of phagocytosis in vitro by obligate anaerobes. Lancet. 1977;2:1252–1254.
174. Simon GL, Klempner MS, Kasper DL, et al. Alterations in opsonophagocytic killing by neutrophils of *Bacteroides fragilis* associated with animal and laboratory passage: Effect of capsular polysaccharide. J Infect Dis. 1982;145:72–77.
175. Socransky SS, Gibbons RJ. Required role of *Bacteroides melaninogenicus* in mixed anaerobic infections. J Infect Dis. 1965;115:247–253.
176. Altemeier WA. The pathogenicity of the bacteria of appendicitis peritonitis. Surgery. 1942;11:374–384.
177. Namavar FA, Verweij MJ, Bal M, et al. Effects of anaerobic bacteria on killing of *Proteus mirabilis* by human polymorphonuclear leukocytes. Infect Immun. 1983;40:930–935.
178. Rotstein OD, Nasmith PE, Grinstein S. The bacteroides by-product succinic acid inhibits neutrophil respiratory burst by reducing intracellular pH. Infect Immun. 1987;55:864–870.
179. Brook I. Anaerobic infections in childhood. Rev Infect Dis. 1984;6(Suppl 1):S187–S192.
180. Weinstein WN, Onderdonk AB, Bartlett JG, et al. Experimental intra-abdominal abscesses in rats: Development of an experimental model. Infect Immun. 1974;10:1250–1255.
181. Onderdonk AB, Weinstein WN, Sullivan NM, et al. Experimental intra-abdominal abscess in rats: Quantitative bacteriology of infected animals. Infect Immun. 1974;10:1256–1259.
182. Weinstein WM, Onderdonk AB, Bartlett JG, et al. Antimicrobial therapy of experimental intraabdominal sepsis. J Infect Dis. 1975;132:282–286.
183. Onderdonk AB, Bartlett JG, Louie T, et al. Microbial synergy in experimental intra-abdominal abscess. Infect Immun. 1976;13:22–26.
184. Rotstein OD, Pruett TL, Simmons RL. Mechanisms of microbial synergy in polymicrobial surgical infections. Rev Infect Dis. 1985; 7:151–170.
185. Schein M, Wittmann DH, Holzheimer R, et al. Hypothesis: Compartmentalization of cytokines in intraabdominal infection. Surgery. 1996;119:694–700.
186. Holzheimer R, Schein M, Wittmann DH. Inflammatory response in peritoneal exudate and plasma of patients undergoing planned relaparotomy for severe secondary peritonitis. Arch Surg. 1995;130:1314–1319.
187. Giroir BP, Mediators of septic shock: New approaches for interrupting the endogenous inflammatory cascade. Crit Care Med. 1993;21:780–789.
188. Baigrie RJ, Lamont PM, Kwiatowski D, et al. Systemic cytokine response after major surgery. Br J Surg. 1992;79:757–760.
189. Bagby GJ, Plessala KJ, Wilson LA, et al. Divergent efficacy of antibody to tumor necrosis factor-δ in intravascular and peritonitis models of sepsis. J Infect Dis. 1991;163:83–88.
190. Asitz ME, Saha DC, Carpati CM, et al. Induction of endotoxin tolerance with monophosphoryl lipid A in peritonitis: Importance of localized therapy. J Lab Clin Med. 1994;123:89–93.
191. McMaster KM, Cheadle WG. Regulation of macrophage TNF-alpha, IL-1 beta and 1a (1a-alpha) mRNA expression during peritonitis is site dependent. J Surg Res. 1993;54:426–430.

192. Zannetti G, Heumann D, Gerain J, et al. Cytokine production after intravenous or peritoneal gram-negative bacterial challenge in mice. J Immunol. 1992;148:1890–1897.
193. Propst T, Propst A, Herold M, et al. Spontaneous bacterial peritonitis is associated with high levels of interleukin-6 and its secondary mediators in ascitic fluid. Eur J Clin Invest. 1993;23:823–836.
194. Zeni F, Tardy B, Vindimian M, et al. High levels of tumor necrosis factor-alpha and interleukin-6 in the ascitic fluid of cirrhotic patients with spontaneous bacterial peritonitis. Clin Infect Dis. 1993;17:218–223.
195. Nakahama H, Tanaka Y, Shirai D, et al. Plasma interleukin-6 levels in continuous ambulatory peritoneal dialysis and hemodialysis patients. Nephron. 1992;61:132–134.
196. Zemel D, Krediet RT, Koomen GC, et al. Interleukin-8 during peritonitis in patients treated with CAPD: An in-vivo model of acute inflammation. Nephrol Dial Transplant. 1994;9:169–176.
197. Zemel D, Koomen GC, Hart AA, et al. Relationship of TNF-alpha, interleukin-6, and prostaglandins to peritoneal permeability for macromolecules during longitudinal follow-up of peritonitis in continuous ambulatory peritoneal dialysis. J Lab Clin Med. 1993;22:686–696.
198. Holzheimer R, Schein M, Wittmann DH. Inflammatory response in peritoneal exudate and plasma of patients undergoing planned relaparotomy for severe secondary peritonitis. Arch Surg. 1995;130:1314–1320.
199. Slack AM, Saladino RA, Thompson C, et al. Failure of prophylactic and therapeutic use of murine anti-tumor necrosis factor monoclonal antibody in *Escherichia coli* sepsis in the rabbit. Crit Care Med. 1995;23:1512–1518.
200. Echtenacher B, Falk W, Mannel DN, et al. Requirement of endogenous tumor necrosis factor/cachectin for recovery from experimental peritonitis. J Immunol. 1990;145:3762.
201. Battafarano RJ, Burd RS, Kurrelmeyer KM, et al. Inhibition of splenic macrophage tumor necrosis factor alpha secretion in vivo by antilipopolysaccharide monoclonal antibodies. Arch Surg. 1994;129:179–181.
202. Kohler J, Heumann D, Garotta G, et al. IFN-gamma involvement in the severity of gram-negative infections in mice. J Immunol. 1993;151:916–921.
203. Rosoff L, Weil M, Bradely EC, et al. Hemodynamic and metabolic changes associated with bacterial peritonitis. Am J Surg. 1967;114:180–189.
204. MacLean LD, Mulugan WG, McLean APH, et al. Patterns of septic shock in man: A detailed study of 56 patients. Ann Surg. 1967;166:543–562.
205. Davis JH. Current concepts of peritonitis. Am Surg. 1967;33:673–681.
206. Debrin PB, Gully PH, Greenlee HB, et al. Radiographic diagnosis of an intra-abdominal abscess: Do multiple tests help? Arch Surg. 1986;121:41–46.
207. Gerzof SG, Johnson WC. Radiologic aspects of diagnosis and treatment of abdominal abscesses. Surg Clin North Am. 1984;54:53–65.
208. Haaga JR. Imaging intraabdominal abscesses and non-operative drainage procedures. World J Surg. 1990;14:204–209.
209. Pine RW, Wertz MJ, Lennard ES, et al. Determinants of organ malfunction or death in patients with intra-abdominal sepsis. Arch Surg. 1983;118:242–249.
210. Nystrom PO, Bax R, Dellinger EP, et al. Proposed definitions for diagnosis, severity scoring, stratification, and outcome for trials on intraabdominal infection: Joint Working Party of SIS North America and Europe. World J Surg. 1990;14:148–158.
211. Dellinger EP, Wertz MJ, Meakins JL, et al. Surgical infection stratification system for intra-abdominal infection. Arch Surg. 1985;120:21–29.
212. Meakins JL, Solomkin JS, Allo MD, et al. A proposed classification of intra-abdominal infections: Stratification of etiology and risk for future therapeutic trials. Arch Surg. 1984;119:1372–1378.
213. Mustard RA, Bohnen JM, Rosati C, et al. Pneumonia complicating abdominal sepsis: An independent risk factor for mortality. Arch Surg. 1991;126:170–175.
214. Runcie C, Ramsey G. Intra-abdominal infection: Pulmonary failure. World J Surg. 1990;14:196–203.
215. Nystrom PO, Bax R, Dellinger EP, et al. Proposed definitions for diagnosis, severity scoring, stratification, and outcome for trials on intra-abdominal infection. World J Surg. 1990;14:148–158.
216. Knaus WA, Draper EA, Wagner DP, et al. APACHE II: A severity of disease classification. Crit Care Med. 1985;13:818–829.
217. Pacelli F, Doglietto GB, Alfiere S, et al. Prognosis in intraabdominal infections: Multivariate analysis on 604 patients. Arch Surg. 1996;131:641–645, 665.
218. Christon NV, Barie PS, Dellinger EP, et al. Intra-abdominal study. Arch Surg. 1993;128:193–199.
219. Goris RJA, teBoekhorst, TPA, Nuytinck JKS, et al. Multiple-organ failure: Generalized autodestructive inflammation? Arch Surg. 1985;120:1109–1115.
220. Damas P, Ledoux D, Nys M, et al. Cytokine serum level severe sepsis in human: IL-6 as a marker of severity. Ann Surg. 1992;215:356–362.
221. Fugger R, Zadrobilek E, Gotzinger P, et al. Perioperative TNF-alpha and IL-6 concentrations correlate with septic state, organ dysfunction, and APACHE II scores in intra-abdominal infection. Eur J Surg. 1993;159:525–529.
222. Patel RT, Deen KI, Youngs J, et al. Interleukin 6 is a prognostic indicator of outcome in severe intra-abdominal sepsis. Br J Surg. 1994;81:1306–1308.
223. Hamilton G, Hofbauer S, Hamilton B. Endotoxin, TNF-alpha, interleukin-6 and parameters of cellular immune system in patients with intraabdominal sepsis. Scand J Infect Dis. 1992;24:361–368.
224. Barriere SL. An overview of mortality risk prediction in sepsis. Crit Care Med. 1995;23:376–393.
225. Nobles ER Jr. Bacteroides infections. Ann Surg. 1973;177:601–606.
226. Young LS, Martin WJ, Meyer RD, et al. Gram-negative rod bacteremia: Microbiologic, immunologic and therapeutic considerations. Ann Intern Med. 1977;86:456–471.
227. Maler JA Jr, Reynolds TB, Yellin AE. Successful medical treatment of pyogenic liver abscess. Gastroenterology. 1979;77:618–622.
228. Herbert DA, Fogel DA, Rothman J, et al. Pyogenic liver abscesses: Successful nonsurgical therapy. Lancet. 1982;1:134–136.
229. Solomkin JS, Meakins JC, Allo MD, et al. Antibiotic trials in intra-abdominal infections: A critical evaluation of study design and outcome reporting. Ann Surg. 1984;200:29–39.
230. Drusano GL, Warren WJ, Saah AJ, et al. A prospective randomized controlled trial of cefoxitin versus clindamycin-aminoglycoside in mixed aerobic-anaerobic infections. Surg Gynecol Obstet. 1982;154:715–720.
231. Tally FP, McGowan K, Kellum JM, et al. A randomized comparison of cefoxitin with or without amikacin and clindamycin plus amikacin in surgical sepsis. Ann Surg. 1981;193:318–323.
232. Nichols RL, Smith JW, Klein DB, et al. Risk of infection after penetrating abdominal trauma. N Engl J Med. 1984;311:1065–1070.
233. Tally FP, Kellum JM, Ho TF, et al. Randomized prospective study comparing moxalactam and cefoxitin with or without tobramycin for treatment of serious surgical infections. Antimicrob Agents Chemother. 1986;29:244–2249.
234. Najem AZ, Kaminski CR, Spiller CR, et al. Comparative study of parenteral piperacillin and cefoxitin in the treatment of surgical infections of the abdomen. Surgery. 1983;157:423–425.
235. Study Group of Intra-Abdominal Infections. A randomized controlled trial of ampicillin plus sulbactam vs gentamicin plus clindamycin in the treatment of intra-abdominal infections. Rev Infect Dis. 1986;8(Suppl 5):S533–S588.
236. Solomkin JS, Dellinger EP, Christou NV, et al. Results of a multicenter trial comparing imipenem cilastatin to tobramycin-clindamycin for intra-abdominal infections. Ann Surg. 1990;212:581–591.
237. Scandinavian Study Group. Imipenem-cilastatin versus gentamicin-clindamycin for treatment of serious bacterial infections. Lancet. 1983;1:868–871.
238. Solomkin JS, Fant WK, Rivera JO, et al. Randomized trial of imipenem-cilastatin versus gentamicin and clindamycin in mixed flora infections. Am J Med. 1985;78 (Suppl 6A):85–91.
239. Guerra JG, Casaline GE, Plomina JC, et al. Imipenem-cilastatin versus gentamicin-clindamycin for treatment of moderate to severe infections in hospitalized patients. Rev Infect Dis. 1985;7(Suppl 3):463–470.
240. Birolini D, Moraes MF, Soare de Souza O. Aztreonam plus clindamycin vs tobramycin plus clindamycin for the treatment of intra-abdominal infections. Rev Infect Dis. 1985;7(Suppl 4):S724–S728.
240a. Donahue PE, Smith DL, Yellin AE, et al. Trovafloxacin in the treatment of intra-abdominal infections: Results of a double-blind, multicenter comparison with imipenem/cilastatin. Am J Surg. 1998;176(Suppl 6A):53S–61S.
241. Stalons DR, Thonsberry C, Dawell VR. Effect of culture medium and carbon dioxide concentration of growth of anaerobic bacteria commonly encountered in clinical specimens. Appl Microbiol. 1974;27:1098–1104.
242. Rosenblatt JE, Schoenknecht F. Effect of several components of anaerobic incubation on antibiotic susceptibility test results. Antimicrob Agents Chemother. 1972;1:4337–440.
243. Wagoner ES, Gorman M. The reaction of cysteine and related compounds with penicillins and cephalosporins. J Antibiot (Tokyo). 1971;24:647–658.
244. Wilkins TD, Chalgren S. Medium for use in antibiotic susceptibility testing of anaerobic bacteria. Antimicrob Agents Chemother. 1976;10:926–928.
245. Mosdell DM, Morris DM, Voltura A, et al. Antibiotic treatment for surgical peritonitis. Ann Surg. 1991;214:543–549.
246. Wittmann DH, Bergstein JM, Franzides CT. Calculated empiric antimicrobial therapy for mixed surgical infections. Infection. 1991;19(Suppl 6):345–350.
247. Finegold SM, Wexler HM. Therapeutic implications of bacteriologic findings in mixed aerobic-anaerobic infections. Antimicrob Agents Chemother. 1988;32:611–616.
248. Gorbach SL, Thadepalli H. Clindamycin in pure and mixed anaerobic infections. Arch Intern Med. 1974;134:87–92.
249. Bartlett JG, Louie TJ, Gorbach SL, et al. Therapeutic efficacy of 29 antimicrobial regimens in experimental intraabdominal sepsis. Rev Infect Dis. 1981;3:535–542.
250. Fass RJ, Scholand JF, Hodges GR, et al. Clindamycin in the treatment of serious anaerobic infections. Ann Intern Med. 1973;78:853–859.
251. Levison ME, Santoro J, Bran JL, et al. In vitro activity and clinical efficacy of clindamycin in the treatment of infections due to anaerobic bacteria. J Infect Dis. 1977;135:S49–S53.
252. Montravers P, Andremont A, Massias L, et al. Investigation of the potential role of *Enterococcus faecalis* in the pathophysiology of experimental peritonitis. J Infect Dis. 1994;169:821–830.
253. Matlow AG, Bohnen JMA, Nohr C, et al. Pathogenicity of entercocci in a rat model of fecal peritonitis. J Infect Dis. 1989;160:142–145.
254. Doughtery SH. Role of enterococcus in intra-abdominal sepsis. Am J Surg. 1984;148:303–312.
255. Weinstein MP, Reller LB, Murphy J, et al. The clinical significance of positive blood cultures: A comprehensive analysis of 500 episodes of bacteremia and fungemia in adults. I: Laboratory and epidemiologic observations. Rev Infect Dis. 1983;5:35–53.
256. Shlaes DM, Levy J, Wolinksy E. Enterococcal bacteremia without endocarditis. Arch Intern Med. 1981;141:578–581.

257. Doughtery SH, Flohr AB, Simmons RL. Breakthrough enterococcal septicemia in surgical patients. Arch Surg. 1983;118:232–237.
258. Salzer W, Pegram PS, McCan CE. Clinical evaluation of moxalactam: Evidence of decreased efficacy in gram-positive aerobic infection. Antimicrob Agents Chemother. 1983;23:565–570.
259. Doughtery SH, Flohr AB, Simmons RL. "Breakthrough" entercoccal septicemia in surgical patients. Arch Surg.1983;118:232–238.
260. Murphy TF, Barza M, Treatment of intraabdominal infection with moxalactam. Rev Infect Dis. 1982;4:670–675.
261. Stellato TA, Danziger LH, Hau T, et al. Moxalactam vs. tobramycin-clindamycin: A randomized trial in secondary peritonitis. Arch Surg. 198;123:714–717.
262. Yu VL. Enterococcal superinfection and colonization after therapy with moxalactam, a new broad-spectrum antibiotic. Ann Intern Med. 1981;94:784–785.
263. Jones RN. Gram-positive superinfection following beta-lactam chemotherapy: The significance of the enterococcus. Infection. 1985;13(Suppl 1):S81–S88.
264. Barrall DT, Kenney PR, Slotman GJ, et al. Enterococcal bacteremia in surgical patients. Arch Surg. 1985;120:57–63.
265. Weigelt JA, Easley SM, Thal ER, et al. Abdominal surgical wound infection is lowered with improved enterococcus and bacteroides therapy. J Trauma. 1993;34:579–585.
266. Livornese LL Jr, Dias S, Samel C, et al. Hospital-acquired infection with vancomycin-resistant *Enterococcus faecium* transmitted by electronic thermometers. Ann Intern Med. 1992;117:112–116.
267. Murray BE. The life and times of the enterococci. Clin Microbiol Rev. 1990;3:46–65.
268. Courvalin P. Resistance of enterococci to glycopeptides. Antimicrob Agents Chemother. 1990;34;2291–2296.
269. Moellering RC. Emergence of enterococci as a significant pathogen. Clin Infect Dis. 1992;14:1173–1178.
270. Burnett RJ, Haverstock DC, Dellinger EP, et al. Definition of the role of enterococcus in intraabdominal infection: Analysis of a prospective randomized trial. Surgery. 1995;188:716–721.
271. Solomkin JS, Reinhart HH, Dellinger EP, et al. Results of a randomized trial comparing sequential intravenous/oral treatment with ciprofloxacin plus metronidazole to imipenem/cilastatin for intra-abdominal infections. Ann Surg. 1996;223:303–313.
272. Peoples JB. *Candida* and perforated peptic ulcers. Surgery. 1986;100:758–764.
273. Rutledge R, Mandel SR, Wilde RE. *Candida* species: Insignificant contaminant or pathogenic species? Am Surg. 1986;52:299–302.
274. Marsh PK, Tally FP, Kellum J, et al. *Candida* infections in surgical patients. Ann Surg. 1983;198:42–47.
275. Sobel JD. *Candida* infections in the intensive care unit. Crit Care Clin North Am. 1988;4:325–344.
276. Sande MA, Overton JW. In vivo antagonism between gentamicin and chloramphenicol in neutropenic mice. J Infect Dis. 1973;128;247–250.
277. Zinner SH, Provonchee RB, Elias KS. Effect of clindamycin on the in vitro activity of amikacin and gentamicin against gram negative bacilli. Antimicrob Agents Chemother. 1976;9:661–666.
278. Ekwo E, Peter G. Effect of clindamycin on aminoglycoside activity in murine model of *Escherichia coli* infection. Antimicrob Agents Chemother. 1976;10:893–898.
279. Fass RJ, Rotilie CA, Prior RB. Interaction of clindamycin and gentamicin in vitro. Antimicrob Agents Chemother. 1974;6:582–587.
280. Cuchural GJ Jr, Tally FB, Jacobus NV, et al. Susceptibility of the *Bactroides fragilis* group in the United States: Analysis by site of isolation. Antimicrob Agents Chemother. 1988;32:717–722.
281. Van Scoy RE, Wilkowske CJ, O'Fallon WM, et al. Clindamycin versus chloramphenicol in treatment of anaerobic infections: A prospective, randomized double-blind study. Mayo Clin Proc. 1984; 59:842–846.
282. Bohnen JMA, Solomkin JS, Dellinger EP, et al. Guidelines for clinical care: Anti-infective agents for intra-abdominal infection. A Surgical Infection Society policy statement. Arch Surg. 1992;127:83–89.
283. Shands JW Jr. Empiric antibiotic therapy of abdominal sepsis and serious perioperative infections. Surg Clin North Am. 1993;73:291–306.
284. Tally FB, Sosa A, Jacobus NV, et al. Clindamycin resistance in *Bacteroides fragilis*. J Antimicrob Chemother. 1981;8(Suppl):43–48.
285. Tally FP, Cuchural GH Jr, Jacobus NV, et al. Nationwide study of the susceptibility of the *Bacteroides fragilis* group in the United States. Antimicrob Agents Chemother. 1985;28:675–677.
286. Wilson WR, Cockerhill FR III. Tetracyclines, chloramphenicol, erythromycin and clindamycin. Mayo Clin Proc. 1987;62:906–915.
287. Tedesco FJ, Barton RW, Alpers DH. Clindamycin associated colitis: A prospective study. Ann Intern Med. 1974;81:429–433.
288. Ralph ED, Kirby WMM, Unique bactericidal action against *Bacteroides fragilis* and *Clostridium perfringens*. Antimicrob Agents Chemother. 1975;8:409–414.
289. Chow AW, Patten V, Guze LB. Susceptibility of anaerobic bacteria to metronidazole: Relative resistance of non-spore-forming gram-positive bacilli. J Infect Dis. 1975;131:182–185.
290. Onderdonk AB, Louie TJ, Tally FP, et al. Activity of metronidazole against *Escherichia coli* in experimental intra-abdominal sepsis. J Antimicrob Chemother. 1979;5:201–210.
291. Bartlett JG, Louie TJ, Gorbach SL, et al. Therapeutic efficacy of 29 antimicrobial regimens in experimental intra-abdominal sepsis. Rev Infect Dis. 1981;3:535–542.
292. Gerding DN, Olson MM, Johnson S, et al. *Clostridium difficile* diarrhea and colonization after treatment with abdominal infection regimens containing clindamycin or metronidazole. Am J Surg. 1990;159:212.
293. Sutter VL, Kwoh Y-Y, Finegold SM. Standardized antimicrobial disc susceptibility testing of anaerobic bacteria: I. Susceptibility of *Bacteroides fragilis* to tetracyclines. Appl Microbiol. 1972;23:268–275.
294. Sutter VL, Finegold SM. Susceptibility of anaerobic bacteria to 23 antimicrobial agents. Antimicrob Agents Chemother. 1976;10:736–752.
295. Wexler HM, Finegold SM. In vitro activity of cefotetan compared with that of other antimicrobial agents against anaerobic bacteria. Antimicrob Agents Chemother. 1988;32:601–604.
296. O'Keefe JP, Vlenezio FR, Divincenzo CA, et al. Activity of newer beta-lactam agents against clinical isolates of *Bacteroides fragilis* and other *Bacteroides* species. Antimicrob Agents Chemother. 1987;31:2002–2004.
297. Rolfe RD, Finegold SM. Comparative in vitro activity of new beta-lactam antibiotics against anaerobic bacteria. Antimicrob Agents Chemother. 1981;200:600–609.
298. Aldridge KE. Comparison of the activities of penicillin G and new beta-lactam antibiotics against clinical isolates of *Bacteroides* species. Antimicrob Agents Chemother. 1984;26:410–413.
299. Chow AW, Finegold SM. In vitro activity of ceftizoxime against anaerobic bacteria and comparison with other cephalosporins. J Antimicrob Chemother. 1982;10 (Suppl C):45–50.
300. Harding GJ, Vincelette A, Rachlis I, et al. A preliminary report on the use of ceftizoxime vs clindamycin/tobramycin for the therapy of intra-abdominal and pelvic infections. J Antimicrob Chemother. 1982;10(Suppl C):191–192.
301. Lou MA, Chen DF, Bansal M, et al. Evaluation of ceftizoxime in acute peritonitis. J Antimicrob Chemother. 1982;10(Suppl C):183–189.
302. O'Keefe JP, Tally FP, Barza M, et al. Inactivation of penicillin G during experimental infection with *Bacteroides fragilis*. J Infect Dis. 1978;137:437–442.
303. Sykes RB, Squibb Institute for Medical Research. The classification and terminology of enzymes that hydrolyze beta-lactam antibiotics. J Infect Dis. 1982;145:762–765.
304. Schoutens E, Yourassowsky E. Speed of bactericidal action of penicillin G, ampicillin and carbenicillin on *Bacteroides fragilis*. Antimicrob Agents Chemother. 1974;6:227–231.
305. Trestman I, Kaye D, Levison ME. Activity of semisynthetic penicillins and synergism with mecillinam against *Bacteroides* species. Antimicrob Agents Chemother. 1979;16:283–286.
306. Levison ME, Trestman I, Egert J, et al. Evaluation of ticarcillin in anaerobic infections (Abstract 176). 17th Interscience Conference on Antimicrobial Agents and Chemotherapy, New York; October 12–14, 1977.
307. Swenson RM, Lorber B. Clindamycin and carbenicillin in treatment of patients with intra-abdominal and female genital tract infections. J Infect Dis. 1977;135:S40–S45.
308. Winston DJ, Murphy W, Young LS, et al. Piperacillin therapy for serious bacterial infections. Am J Med. 1980;69:255–261.
309. Harding GKM, Buckwalk FJ, Ronald AR, et al. Prospective, randomized comparative study of clindamycin, chloramphenicol, and ticarcillin, each in combination with gentamicin, for therapy of intra-abdominal and female genital tract sepsis. J Infect Dis. 1980;142:384–393.
310. Gould IM, Wise R. Beta-lactamase inhibitors. In: Peterson PK, Verhoef J, eds. The Antimicrobial Agents Annual. 2nd ed. New York: Elsevier; 1987:58–69.
311. Wise R, Andrews JM, Bedford KA. Clavulanic acid and CP-45, 899: A comparison of their in vitro activity in combination with penicillins. J Antimicrob Chemother. 1980;6:197–206.
312. Donowitz GR, Mandell GL. Beta-lactam antibiotics (first of two parts). N Engl J Med. 1988;313:419–426.
313. Bansal MB, Chuah SK, Thadepalli H. In vitro activity and in vivo evaluation of ticarcillin plus clavulanic acid against aerobic and anaerobic bacteria. Am J Med. 1985;79(Suppl 5B):33–38.
314. Retsema JA, English AR, Girard A, et al. Sulbactam/ampicillin: In vitro spectrum, potency and activity in models of acute infection. Rev Infect Dis. 1986;8(Suppl 5):S528–S542.
315. Reinhardt JF, Johnston L, Ruane P, et al. A randomized double blind comparison of sulbactam/ampicillin and clindamycin for the treatment of aerobic–anaerobic infections.Rev Infect Dis. 1986;8(Suppl 5):S569–S575.
316. Jones RN. Review of the in vitro spectrum of activity of imipenem. Am J Med. 1985;78(Suppl 6A):22–32.
317. Sanders CC, Sanders WE Jr. Clinical significance of inducible beta-lactamase in gram-negative bacteria. Eur J Clin Microbiol. 1987;6:435.
318. Yotsuji A, Minami S, Inoue M, et al. Properties of a novel beta-lactamase produced by *Bacteroides fragilis*. Antimicrob Agents Chemother. 1983;24:925–929.
319. Jacobus NV, Ferreira MC, Barza M. In vitro activity of aztreonam, a monobactam antibiotic. Antimicrob Agents Chemother. 1982;22:832–838.
320. Williams RR, Hotchkin D. Aztreonam plus clindamycin versus tobramycin plus clindamycin in the treatment of intraabdominal infections. Rev Infect Dis. 1991;13(Suppl 7): S629–S633.
321. Berne TV, Yellin AE, Appleman MD, et al. Surgically treated gangrenous or perforated appendicitis: A comparison of aztreonam and clindamycin versus gentamicin and clindamycin. Ann Surg. 1987;205:133–137.
322. Birolini D, Morales MF, deSouza OS. Aztreonam plus clindamycin vs. tobramycin plus clindamycin for the treatment of intraabdominal infections. Rev Infect Dis. 1985;7(Suppl 4):S724–S729.

323. Kaye D, Levison ME, Labovitz ED. The unpredictability of serum concentrations of gentamicin: Pharmacokinetics of gentamicin in patients with normal and abnormal renal function. J Infect Dis. 1974;130:150–154.
324. Verklin RM Jr, Mandell GL. Alteration of effectiveness of antibiotics by anaerobiosis. J Lab Clin Med. 1977;89:65–71.
325. Ho JL, Barza M. Minireview. Role of aminoglycoside antibiotics in the treatment of intra-abdominal infection. Antimicrob Agents Chemother. 1987;31:485–491.
326. Wolfson JS, Hooper DC. The fluoroquinolones: Structures, mechanisms of action and resistance, and spectra of activity in vitro. Antimicrob Agents Chemother. 1985;28: 581–586.
327. Neu HE. New antibiotics: Areas of appropriate use. J Infect Dis. 1987;155:403–417.
328. Wexler HM, Molitoris E, Molitoris D, et al. In vitro activities of trovafloxacin against 557 strains of anaerobic bacteria. Antimicrob Agents Chemother. 1996;40:2232–2235.
329. Citron DM, Appleman MA. Comparative activities of trovafloxacin (CP-99, 219) against 221 aerobic and 217 anaerobic bacteria isolated from patients with intra-abdominal infections. Antimicrob Agents Chemother. 1997;41:2312–2316.
330. Forrest A, Nix DE, Ballow CH, et al. Phamacodynamics of intravenous ciprofloxacin in seriously ill patients. Antimicro Agents Chemother. 1993;37:1073–1081.
331. Lennard ES, Derllinger EP, Wertz MJ, et al. Implications of leukocytosis and fever at the conclusion of antibiotic therapy for intra-abdominal sepsis. Ann Surg. 1982;195:19–24.
332. Stone HH, Bourneuf AA, Stinson LD. Reliability of criteria for predicting persistent or recurrent sepsis. Arch Surg. 1985;120:17–20.
333. Hau T, Nishilawa R, Phuangsab A. Irrigation of the peritoneal cavity and antibiotics in the treatment of peritonitis. Surg Gynecol Obstet. 1983;156:25–30.
334. Rambo WM. Irrigation of the peritoneal cavity with cephalothin. Am J Surg. 1972;123:192–195.
335. Nichols RL. Management of intra-abdominal sepsis. Am J Med. 1985;80 (Suppl 6B):204–209.
336. Leiboff AR, Soroff HS. The treatment of generalized peritonitis by closed postoperative peritoneal lavage: A critical review of the literature. Arch Surg. 1987;122:1005–1010.
337. Sindelar WF, Mason GR. Intraperitoneal irrigation with povidone–iodine solution for the prevention of intra-abdominal abscess in the bacterially contaminated abdomen. Surg Gynecol Obstet. 1979;148:409–411.
338. Ahrenholz DH, Simmons RL. Povidone–iodine in peritonitis: I. Adverse effects of local instillation in experimental *E. coli* peritonitis. J Surg Res. 1979;26:458–463.
339. Hill GB, Osterhout S. Experimental effects of hyperbaric oxygen on selected clostridial species. In vitro studies. J Infect Dis. 1972;125:17–25.
340. Holland JA, Hill GB, Wolfe WG, et al. Experimental and clinical experience with hyperbaric oxygen in the treatment of clostridial myonecrosis. Surgery. 1975;77:75–85.
341. Schreiner A, Tonjum S. Digranes A. Hyperbaric oxygen therapy in bacteroides infections. Acta Chir Scand. 1974;140:73–76.
342. Hill GB. Hyperbaric oxygen exposures for intrahepatic abscesses produced in mice by non–spore-forming anaerobic bacteria. Antimicrob Agents Chemother. 1976;9:312–317.
343. Thom SR, Lavermann MW, Hart GB. Intermittent hyperbaric oxygen therapy for reduction of mortality in experimental polymicrobial sepsis. J Infect Dis. 1986;154:504–510.
344. Bhushan C, Mital VK, Elhence IP. Continuous postoperative peritoneal lavage in diffuse peritonitis using balanced saline antibiotic solution. Int Surg. 1975;60:526–528.
345. Hallerback B, Anderson C, Englund N, et al. A prospective randomized study of continuous peritoneal lavage postoperatively in the treatment of purulent peritonitis. Surg Gynecol Obstet. 1986;163:433–436.
346. Hudspeth AS. Radical surgical debridement in the treatment of advanced generalized bacterial peritonitis. Arch Surg. 1975;110:1233–1236.
347. Polk HC, Fry DE. Radical peritoneal debridement for established peritonitis: The result of a prospective randomized clinical trial. Ann Surg. 1980;192:350–355.
348. Aprahamian C, Wittman DH. Operative management of intraabdominal infection. Infection. 1991;19:453–455.
349. Wittman D, Aprahamian C, Bergstein J. Etappenlavage: Advance diffuse peritonitis managed by planned multiple laparotomies utilizing zippers, slide fastener, and Velcro analogue for temporary abdominal closure. World J Surg. 1990;14:218–226.
350. Teichmann W, Wittman DH, Andreone PA. Scheduled reoperations (etappenlavage) for diffuse peritonitis. Arch Surg. 1986;121:147–152.
351. Cuesta MA, Doblas M, Castaneda L, et al. Sequential abdominal reexploration with the zipper technique. World J Surg. 1991;15:74–80.
352. Schein M, Hirshberg A, Hashmonai M. Current surgical management of severe intraabdominal infection. Surgery. 1992;112:489.
353. Haller JA Jr. Shaker IJ, Donahoo JS, et al. Peritoneal drainage versus non-drainage for generalized peritonitis from ruptured appendicitis in children: A prospective study. Ann Surg. 1973;177:595–600.
354. Leigh DA, Simmons K, Norman E. Bacterial flora of the appendix fossa in appendicitis and postoperative wound infection. J Clin Pathol. 1974;27:997–1000.
355. Follen WD, Hunt J, Altemeier WA. Prophylactic antibiotics in penetrating wounds of the abdomen. J Trauma. 1972;12:282–288.
356. Fabian TC, Boldreghini SJ. Antibiotics in penetrating abdominal trauma: Comparison of ticarcillin plus clavulanic acid with gentamicin plus clindamycin. Am J Med. 1985;79(Suppl 5B):157–160.
357. Nichols RL, Gorbach SL, Condon RE. Alteration of intestinal microflora following preoperative mechanical preparation of the colon. Dis Colon Rectum. 1971;14:123–127.
358. Condon RE, Bartlett JG, Greenlee H, et al. Efficacy of oral and systemic antibiotic prophylaxis in colorectal operations. Arch Surg. 1983;118:496–502.
359. Kaiser AB. Antibiotic prophylaxis in surgery. N Engl J Med. 1986;315:1129–1138.
360. Baum ML, Anish DS, Chalmers TC, et al. A survey of clinical trials of antibiotic prophylaxis in colon surgery: Evidence against further use of nontreatment controls. N Engl J Med. 1981;305:795–799.
361. Guglielmo BJ, Hohn DC, Koo PJ, et al. Antibiotic prophylaxis in surgical procedures: A critical analysis of the literature. Arch Surg. 1983;118:943–955.
362. Holph KD, Sorkin M, Rubin J, et al. Continuous ambulatory peritoneal dialysis. Three-year experience at one center. Ann Intern Med. 1980;92:609–613.
363. Rubin J, Rogers WA, Taylor HM, et al. Peritonitis during continuous ambulatory peritoneal dialysis. Ann Intern Med. 1980;92:7–13.
364. Fenton SSA, Pei Y, Delmore T, et al. The CAPD peritonitis rate is not improving with time. Trans Am Soc Artif Intern Organs. 1986;32:546–549.
365. Vas SL. 2: Peritonitis of peritoneal dialysis patients: Pathogenesis and treatment. Med Microbiol. 1986;5:21–63.
366. Peterson PK, Matzke GR, Keane WF. Current concepts in the management of peritonitis in continuous ambulatory peritoneal dialysis patients. Rev Infect Dis. 1987;9:604–612.
367. Everett ED. Diagnosis, prevention and treatment of peritonitis. Perit Dial Bull. 1984;4(Suppl):139–142.
368. Steinberg SM, Cutler SJ, Novak JK, et al. Report of the National CAPD Registry of the National Institutes of Health: Characteristics of participants and selected outcome measures for the period January 1, 1981 through August 31, 1984. In: National CAPD Registry of the National Institute of Arthritis, Diabetes, and Digestive and Kidney Diseases. Washington, DC: US Public Health Services; 1985.
369. Kraus ES, Spector DA. Characteristics and sequelae of peritonitis in diabetics and non-diabetics receiving chronic intermittent peritoneal dialysis. Medicine (Baltimore). 1983;62:52–57.
370. Fenton S, Wu G, Cattran D, et al. Clinical aspects of peritonitis in patients on CAPD. Perit Dial Bull. 1981;1(Suppl):4–8.
371. Sewell CM, Clarridge J, Lacke C, et al. Staphylococcal nasal carriage and subsequent infection in peritoneal dialysis patients. JAMA 1982;248:1493–1495.
372. Keane WJ, Comty CM, Verbrugh HA, et al. Opsonic deficiency of peritoneal dialysis effluent in CAPD. Kidney Int. 1984;25:539–543.
373. Lamperi S, Carozzi S, Nasini MG. Intraperitoneal immunoglobulin treatment in prophylaxis of bacterial peritonitis in CAPD. In: Khanna R, Nolph KD, Provant B, et al., eds. Advances in CAPD. Toronto: University of Toronto Press; 1986:110.
374. Duwe AK, Vas SI, Weatherhead IW. Effects of composition of peritoneal dialysis fluid on chemiluminescence, phagocytosis and bacterial activity in vitro. Infect Immun. 1981;33:130–135.
375. Marrie TJ, Noble MA, Costerton JW. Examination of the morphology of bacteria adhering to peritoneal dialysis catheters by scanning and transmission electron microscopy. J Clin Microbiol. 1983;18:1388–1398.
376. Arfania D, Everett ED, Nolph KD, et al. Uncommon causes of peritonitis in patients undergoing peritoneal dialysis. Arch Intern Med. 1981;141:61–64.
377. Vas SI. Microbiologic aspects of chronic ambulatory dialysis. Kidney Int. 1983;23:83–92.
378. Peterson PK, Keane WF. Infections in chronic peritoneal dialysis patients. In: Remington JS, Swartz MN, eds. Current Clinical Topics in Infectious Diseases. New York: McGraw-Hill; 1985:239–260.
379. Digenis GE, Khanna K, Panatlony D. Eosinophilia after implantation of the peritoneal catheter. Peri Dial Bull. 1982;2:98–99.
380. Gokal R, Ramos JM, Ward MK, et al. "Eosinophilic" peritonitis in continuous ambulatory peritoneal dialysis (CAPD). Clin Nephrol. 1981;15:328–330.
381. Woods GL, Washington JA II. Comparison of methods for processing dialysate in suspected continuous ambulatory peritoneal dialysis–associated peritonitis. Diagn Microbiol Infect Dis. 1987;7:155–157.
382. Gokal R, Ramos JM, Francis DM, et al. Peritonitis in continuous ambulatory peritoneal dialysis: Laboratory and clinical studies. Lancet. 1982;2:1388–1391.
383. Keane WF, Alexander SR, Bailie GR, et al. Peritoneal dialysis–related peritonitis treatment recommendations: 1996 update. Perit Dial Intern. 1996;16:557–573.
384. Verbrogh HA, Keane WF, Conroy WE, et al. Bacterial growth and killing in chronic ambulatory peritoneal dialysis fluids. J Clin Microbiol. 1984;20:199–203.
385. Eisenberg ES, Leviton I, Soeiro R. Fungal peritonitis in patients receiving peritoneal dialysis: Experience with 11 patients and review of the literature. Rev Infect Dis. 1986;8:309–321.
386. Rubin J, Kirchner K, Walsh D, et al. Fungal peritonitis during continuous ambulatory peritoneal dialysis: A report of 12 cases. Am J Kidney Dis. 1987;10:361–368.
387. Vargemezis V, Papadopoulov ZL, Llamos H, et al. Management of fungal peritonitis during continuous ambulatory peritoneal dialysis (CAPD). Perit Dial Bull. 1986;6:17–20.
387a. McNeely DJ, Vas SI, Dambros N, et al. *Fusarium* peritonitis: An uncommon complication of continuous ambulatory peritoneal dialysis. Perit Dialy Bull. 1981;1:94–96.
387b. Chapman JR, Warnock DW. Ketoconazole and fungal CAPD peritonitis. Lancet. 1983;2:510–511.
387c. McGuire NM, Port FK, Kauffman CA. Ketoconazole pharmacokinetics in continuous peritoneal dialysis. Perit Dialy Bull. 1984;4:199–201.
388. Axelrod J, Meyers BR, Hirschman SZ, et al. Prophylaxis with cephalothin in peritoneal dialysis. Arch Intern Med. 1973;132:368–371.

389. Perez-Fontan M, Rosales M, Rodriguez-Carmona A, et al. Treatment of *Staphylococcus aureus* nasal carriers in CAPD with mupirocin. Adv Perit Dial. 1992;8:242–245.
390. Abrutyn E, Goodhart GL, Ries K, et al. *Acinetobacter calcoaeticus* outbreak associated with peritoneal dialysis. Am J Epidemiol. 1978;107:328–335.
391. Altemeir WA, Culbertson WR, Fullen WD, et al. Intra-abdominal abscesses. Am J Surg. 1973;125:70–79.
392. Saini S, Kellum JM, O'Leary MP, et al. Improved localization and survival in patients with intra-abdominal abscesses. Am J Surg. 1983;145:136–142.
393. Gibson DM, Feliciano DV, Mattox KL, et al. Intra-abdominal abscess after penetrating abdominal trauma. Am J Surg. 1981;142:699–703.
394. Patterson HC. Left subphrenic abscess. Am Surg. 1977;43:430–433.
395. Ozeran RS. Subdiaphragmatic abscess. Diagnosis and treatment. Am Surg. 1967;33:64–67.
396. Sherman NJ, Davis JR, Jesseph JE. Subphrenic abscess: A continuing hazard. Am J Surg. 1969;117:117–123.
397. Sanders RC. The changing epidemiology of subphrenic abscess and its clinical and radiological consequences. Br J Surg. 1970;57:449–455.
398. Ochsner A, DeBakey M. Subphrenic abscess. Collective review of 3608 collected and personal cases. Surg Gynecol Obstet. 1939;66:426.
399. Mackenzie M, Fordyle J, Young DG. Subphrenic abscess in children. Br J Surg. 1975;62:305–308.
400. Wang SMS, Wilson SE. Subphrenic abscess. The new epidemiology. Arch Surg. 1977;112:934–936.
401. DeCosse JJ, Poulin TL, Fox PS, et al. Subphrenic abscess. Surg Gynecol Obstet. 1974;138:841–846.
402. Gorbach SL. Treatment of intra-abdominal infection. Am J Med. 1984;76(Suppl 5A):107–110.
403. Milne GAC, Geere IW. Chronic subphrenic abscess: The missed diagnosis. Can J Surg. 1977;20:162–165.
404. Mueller PR, Simeone JF. Intra-abdominal abscesses: Diagnosis by sonography and computed tomography. Radiol Clin North Am. 1983;21:425–443.
405. Ferrucci JT Jr, Van Sonnenberg E. Role of ultrasound and computed tomography in the diagnosis and treatment of intraabdominal abscess. In: Remington JS, Swartz MN, eds. Current Clinical Topics in Infectious Diseases. New York: McGraw-Hill; 1982:136–159.
406. Kerlan RK Jr, Pogany AC, Jeffrey RB, et al. Radiologic management of abdominal abscesses. AJR Am J Roentgenol. 1985;144:145–149.
407. Connell TR, Stephens DH, Carlson HC, et al. Upper abdominal abscess: A continuing and deadly problem. AJR Am J Roentgenol. 1980;134:759–765.
408. Caffee HH, Watts G, Mena I. Gallium 67 citrate scanning in the diagnosis of intraabdominal abscess. Am J Surg. 1977;133:665–669.
409. Tsan M. Mechanism of gallium 67 accumulation in inflammatory lesions. J Nucl Med. 1985;26:88–92.
410. Disbro M, Datz F, Cook P, et al. Indium-111 labeled leukocytes: Clinical utility and accuracy. Clin Nucl Med. 1982;7:44–46.
411. Froelich JW, Krasicky GA. Radionuclide imaging of abdominal infections. Curr Concepts Diagn Nucl Med. 1985;2:12–16.
412. Coleman RE, Brack RE, Welch DM, et al. Indium-111 labeled leukocytes in the evaluation of suspected abdominal abscess. Am J Surg. 1980;139:99–104.
413. Sfakianakis GN, A-Shietch W, Heal A, et al. Comparisons of scintigraphy with In-111 Leukocytes and Ga^{67} in the diagnosis of occult sepsis. J Nucl Med. 1982;23:618–626.
414. Hill BA, Yamaguchi K, Flynn JJ, et al. Diagnostic sonography in general surgery. Arch Surg. 1975;110:1089–1094.
415. Goudie E, Andrew WK. The role of diagnostic ultrasound in the assessment of masses in the left upper quadrant of the abdomen. S Afr Med J. 1976;50:1391–1394.
416. Knochel JQ, Koehler PR, Lee TG, et al. Diagnosis of abdominal abscesses with computed tomography, ultrasound and ^{111}In leukocyte scans. Radiology. 1980;137:425–432.
417. Koehler PR, Moss AA. Diagnosis of intraabdominal and pelvic abscesses by computerized tomography. JAMA. 1980;224:49–52.
418. Gisi P, Graham DB. Splenic abscess: Two case reports. S D J Med. 1992;45:37–40.
419. Ooi LL, Nambiar R, Rauff A, et al. Splenic abscess. Aust N Z J Surg. 1992;62:780–784.
420. Balthazar EJ, Robinson DL, Megibow AJ, et al. Acute pancreatitis: Value of CT in establishing diagnosis. Radiology. 1990;174:331–336.
421. Brock JS, Pachter HL, Schreiber J, et al. Surgical diseases of the falciform ligament. Am J Gastroenterol. 1992;87:757–758.
422. Baker HL Jr, Berquist TN, Kispert DB, et al. Magnetic resonance imaging in a routine clinical setting. Mayo Clin Proc. 1985;60:75–90.
423. Cammoun D, Hendee WR, Davis KA. Clinical applications of magnetic resonance imaging: Current status. West J Med. 1985;143:793–803.
424. Wall SD, Fisher MR, Amparo EG, et al. Magnetic resonance imaging in the evaluation of abscesses. AJR Am J Roentgenol. 1985;144:1217–1221.
425. Gerzof SG, Robbins AH, Johnson WC, et al. Percutaneous catheter drainage of abdominal abscesses. N Engl J Med. 1981;305:653–657.
426. Mandel SR, Boyd D, Jaques PF, et al. Drainage of hepatic, intra-abdominal and mediastinal abscesses guided by computerized axial tomography: Successful alternative to open drainage. Am J Surg. 1983;145:120–125.
427. Pruett TL, Simmons RL. Status of percutaneous catheter drainage of abscesses. Surg Clin North Am. 1988;68:89–105.
428. Jaques P, Mauro M, Safrit H, et al. CT features of intraabdominal abscesses: Prediction of successful percutaneous drainage. Am J Radiol. 1986;146:1041–1045.
429. Malangioni MA. Pathogenesis and treatment of intraabdominal infection. Surg Gynecol Obstet. 1990;171:31–34.
430. Fornari F, Buscarini L. Ultrasonically guided fine-needle biopsy of gastrointestinal organs. Indications, results and complications. Dig Dis. 1992;10:121–133.
431. Flancbaum L, Nosh JL, Brolin RE, Percutaneous catheter drainage of abdominal abscesses associated with perforated viscus. Am J Surg. 1990;56:52–56.
432. Brolin RE, Nosher JL, Leiman S, et al. Percutaneous catheter versus open surgical drainage in the treatment of abdominal abscesses. Am Surg. 1984;50:102–108.
433. Van Sonnenberg E, Ferruci JT Jr, Mueller PR, et al. Percutaneous drainage of abscesses and fluid collections: Technique, results and applications. Radiology. 1982;142:1–10.
434. Olak J, Christov NV, Stein LA, et al. Operative vs percutaneous drainage of intraabdominal abscesses. Arch Surg. 1986;121:141–146.
435. Hurley JE, Vargish T. Early diagnosis and outcome of pancreatic abscesses in pancreatitis. Am Surg. 1987;53:29–33.
436. Kodesch R, DuPont HL. Infectious complications of acute pancreatitis. Surg Gynecol Obstet. 1973;136:763–768.
437. Becker JM, Pemberton JH, Diamgno EP, et al. Prognostic factors in pancreatic abscess. Surgery. 1984;96:455–460.
438. Shi ECP, Yeo BW, Ham JM. Pancreatic abscesses. Br J Surg. 1984;71:689–691.
439. Altemeier WA, Alexander JW. Pancreatic abscess: A study of 32 cases. Arch Surg. 1963;87:80–89.
440. Holden JL, Berne TV, Rosoff LSR, Pancreatic abscess following acute pancreatitis. Arch Surg. 1976;111:858–861.
441. Miller TA, Lindenauer SM, Frey CF, et al. Pancreatic abscess. Arch Surg. 1974;l08:545–551.
442. Ransom JHC, Balthazar E, Caccavale R, et al. Computed tomography and the prediction of pancreatic abscess in acute pancreatitis. Ann Surg. 1985;201:656–663.
443. Aranha GU, Prinz RA, Greenlee HB. Pancreatic abscess: An unresolved surgical problem. Am J Surg. 1982;144:534–538.
444. Bradley EL, Fulenwider JT. Open treatment of pancreatic abscess. Surg Gynecol Obstet. 1984;159:509–513.
445. Stambler JB, Klibaner MI. Tuberculous abscess of the pancreas. Gastroenterology. 1982;83:922–925.
446. Sostre CF, Flournoy JG, Bova P, et al: Pancreatic phlegmon: Clinical features and course. Dig Dis Sci. 1985;30:918–927.
447. Berger HG, Krautzberger W, Bittner R, et al. Results of surgical treatment of necrotizing pancreatitis. World J Surg. 1985;9:972–979.
448. Keighley MRB, Drysdale RB, Quoraiski AH, et al. Antibiotic treatment of biliary sepsis. Surg Clin North Am. 1975;55:1379–1390.
449. Crass RA, Meyer AA, Jeffrey RB, et al. Pancreatic abscess: Impact of computerized tomography on early diagnois and surgery. Am J Surg. 1985;150:127–131.
450. Williford ME, Foster WL Jr, Halversen RA, et al. Pancreatic pseudocyst: Comparative evaluation of sonography and computed tomography. AJR Am J Roentgenol. 1983;140:53–57.
451. Bicknell TA, Kohatsu S, Goodwin DA. Use of indium-111 labeled autologous leukocytes in differentiating pancreatic abscess from pseudocyst. Am J Surg. 1981;142:312–316.
452. Tanaka T, Miskin FS, Buozas DJ, et al. Pancreatic uptake of gallium-67 citrate in acute pancreatitis. Appl Radiol. 1978;1:163–165.
453. Paushter DM, Modic MT, Borkowski GP, et al. Magnetic resonance: Principles and applications. Med Clin North Am. 1984;68:1393–1421.
454. Weiss HD, Anacker H, Kramann B, et al. The diagnosis of necrotizing pancreatic lesions by means of duodenoscopic pancreatography: Its value for the surgical procedure. Am J Gastroenterol. 1975;64:26–33.
455. Fedorak IJ, Ko TC, Djuricin G, et al. Secondary pancreatic infections: Are they distinct clinical entities? Surgery. 1992;112:824–830.
456. D' Egidio A, Schein M. Surgical strategies in the treatment of pancreatic necrosis and infection. Br J Surg. 1991;78:133–137.
457. Rotman N, Mathieu D, Anglade MC, et al. Failure of percutaneous drainage of pancreatic abscesses complicating severe acute pancreatitis. Surg Gynecol Obstet. 1992;174:141–144.
458. Brolin RE, Flancbaum L, Ercoli FR, et al. Limitations of percutaneous catheter drainage of abdominal abscesses. Surg Gynecol Obstet. 1991;173:203–210.
459. Karlson KB, Martia EC, Fankochen EL, et al. Percutaneous drainage of pancreatic pseudocysts and abscesses. Radiology. 1982;142:619–624.
460. Pruett TC, Rotstein OD, Crass J, et al. Percutaneous aspiration and drainage for selected abdominal infections. Surgery. 1984;96:731–737.
461. Lang EK, Paolini RM, Pottmeyer A. The efficacy of palliative and definitive percutaneous versus surgical drainage of pancreatic abscesses and pseudocysts. A prospective study of 85 patients. South Med J. 1991;84:55–64.
462. Adams DB, Harvey TS, Anderson MC. Percutaneous catheter drainage of infected pancreatic and peripancreatic fluid collections. Arch Surg. 1990;125:1554–1557.
463. Lumsden A, Bradley EL 3rd. Secondary pancreatic infections. Surg Gynecol Obstet. 1990;170:459–467.
464. Ranson JH, Spencer FC. Prevention, diagnosis and treatment of pancreatic abscess. Surgery. 1977;82:99–106.
465. Warshaw AL, Jin G. Improved survival in 45 patients with pancreatic abscess. Ann Surg. 1985;202:408–415.
466. Van Vyve EL, Reynaert MS, Lengele BG, et al. Retroperitoneal laparostomy: Surgical treatment of pancreatic abscesses after acute necrotizing pancreatitis. Surgery. 1992;111:369–375.
467. Finch WT, Sawyers JL, Schenker S. A prospective study to determine the efficacy of antibiotics in acute pancreatitis. Ann Surg. 1976;183:667–671.

468. Kusne S, Dummer JS, Singh N, et al. Infections after liver transplantation: An analysis of 101 consecutive cases. Medicine (Baltimore). 1988;67:132–143.
469. Barbour GL, Juniper K Jr. A clinical comparison of amebic and pyogenic abscesses of the liver in sixty-six patients. Am J Med. 1972;53:323–334.
470. Dietrich RB. Experience with liver abscess. Am J Surg. 1984;147:288–291.
471. Ribaudo JM, Ochsner A. Intrahepatic abscesses: Amebic and pyogenic. Am J Surg. 1973;125:570–574.
472. Barnes PF, DeLock KM, Reynolds TN, et al. A comparison of amebic and pyogenic abscess of the liver. Medicine (Baltimore). 1987;66:472–483.
473. Shulman ST, Beem MO. A unique presentation of sickle cell disease: Pyogenic hepatic abscess. Pediatrics. 1971;47:1019–1022.
474. Williams JW, Rittenberry A, Dillard R, et al. Liver abscess in newborn: Complications of umbilical vein catheterization. Am J Dis Child. 1973;125:111–113.
475. Gyorffy EJ, Frey CF, Silva J Jr, et al. Pyogenic liver abscess: Diagnostic and therapeutic strategies. Ann Surg. 1987;206:699–705.
476. Sabbaj J. Anaerobes in liver abscess. Rev Infect Dis. 1984;6(Suppl 1):152–155.
477. Rubin RH, Swartz MN, Malt R. Hepatic abscess. Changes in clinical, bacteriologic and therapeutic aspects. Am J Med. 1974;57:601–610.
478. McDonald MI, Corey GR, Gallis HA, et al. Single and multiple pyogenic liver abscesses. Medicine (Baltimore). 1984;63:291–302.
479. Sabbaj J, Sutter VL, Finegold SM. Anaerobic pyogenic liver abscess. Ann Intern Med. 1972;77:629–638.
480. Lazarchick J, de Souza E, Silva NA, et al. Pyogenic liver abscess. Mayo Clin Proc. 1973;48:349–355.
481. Perera MR, Kirk A, Noone P. Presentation, diagnosis and management of liver abscess. Lancet. 1980;2:629–632.
482. Loh R, Wallace G, Thong Y. Successful non-surgical management of pyogenic liver abscess. Scand J Infect Dis. 1987;19:137–140.
483. Kaplan SL. Pyogenic liver abscess. In: Feigin RD, Cherry JD, eds. Textbook of Pediatric Infectious Disease. Philadelphia: WB Saunders; 1981:537–540.
484. Rabson AR, Koornhof HJ, Notman J, et al. Hepatosplenic abscesses due to *Yersinia Enterocolitica*. BMJ. 1972;4:341.
485. Haron E, Feld R, Tuffnell P, et al. Hepatitic candidiasis: An increasing problem in immunocompromised patients. Am J Med. 1987;83:17–26.
486. Thaler M, Pastakia B, Shawker T, et al. Hepatic candidiasis in cancer patients: The evolving picture of the syndrome. Ann Intern Med. 1988;108:88–100.
487. Flannery MT, Simmons DB, Saba H, et al. Fluconazole in the treatment of hepatosplenic candidiasis. Arch Intern Med. 1992;152:406–408.
488. Anaissie E, Bodey GP, Kantarjian H, et al. Fluconazole therapy for chronic disseminated candidiasis in patients with leukemia and prior amphotericin B therapy. Am J Med. 1991;91:142–150.
489. Kauffman CA, Bradley SF, Ross SC, et al. Hepatosplenic candidiasis: Successful treatment with fluconazole. Am J Med. 1991;91:137–141.
490. Wallack MK, Brown AS, Austrian R, et al. Pyogenic liver abscess secondary to asymptomatic sigmoid diverticulitis. Ann Surg. 1976;184:241–243.
491. Sparberg M, Gottschalk A, Kirsner JB. Liver abscess complicating regional enteritis: Report of two cases. Gastroenterology. 1965;49:548–551.
492. Lee JF, Block GE. The changing clinical pattern of hepatic abscesses. Arch Surg. 1972;104:465–470.
493. Miedema BW, Dineen P. The diagnosis and treatment of pyogenic liver abscesses. Ann Surg. 1984;200:328–335.
494. Williams RA, Finegold SM. Pyogenic and amebic liver abscess and splenic abscess. In: Wilson SE, Finegold SM, Williams RA, eds. Intra-Abdominal Infection. New York: McGraw-Hill; 1982:139–156.
495. Weinstein L. Bacterial hepatitis: A case report on an unrecognized cause of fever of unknown origin. N Engl J Med. 1978;299:1052–1054.
496. Foster SC, Schneider B, Seaman WB. Gas-containing pyogenic intra-hepatic abscesses. Radiology. 1970;94:613–618.
497. Stenson WF, Eckert T. Pyogenic liver abscess. Arch Intern Med. 1983;143:126–128.
498. Madayag MA, LeFleur RS, Braunstein P, et al. Radiology of hepatic abscesses. N Y State J Med. 1975;75:1417–1423.
499. Reynolds TB. Medical treatment of pyogenic liver abscesses. Ann Intern Med. 1982;96:373–374.
500. Callen PW. Computed tomographic evaluation of abdominal and pelvic abscesses. Radiology. 1979;131:171–175.
501. Koehler PR, Moss AA, Diagnosis of intraabdominal and pelvic abscesses by computerized tomography. JAMA. 1980;244:49–52.
502. Gerzof SG, Johnson WC, Robbins AH, et al. Intrahepatic pyogenic abscesses: Treatment by percutaneous drainage. Am J Surg. 1985;149:487–494.
503. Altemeier WA, Schowenserdt CG, Whiteby DH. Abscesses of the liver: Surgical consideration. Arch Surg. 1970;101:258–266.
504. DeBakey ME, Jordan GL Jr. Hepatic abscesses, both intra- and extra-hepatic. Surg Clin North Am. 1977;57:325–337.
505. Do H, Lambiase RE, Deyoe L, et al. Percutaneous drainage of hepatic abscesses: Comparison of results in abscesses with and without intrahepatic biliary communication. AJR Am J Roentgenol. 1991;157:1209–1212.
506. Attar B, Levendoglu H, Cuasay N. CT-guided percutaneous aspiration and catheter drainage of pyogenic liver abscesses. Am J Gastroenterol. 1986;81:550–555.
507. McCorkell SJ, Niles NC. Pyogenic liver abscess: Another look at medical management. Lancet. 1985;1:803–806.
508. Abramowicz M, ed. Drugs for parasitic infections. Med Lett. 1988;30:15–24.
509. Nelken N, Isnatius J, Skinner M, et al. Changing clinical spectrum of splenic abscess: A multicenter study and review of the literature. Am J Surg. 1987;154:27–34.
510. Gadacz T, Way LW, Dunphy JE. Changing clinical spectrum of splenic abscess. Am J Surg. 1974;128:182–187.
511. Chun CH, Raff MJ, Contreras L, et al. Splenic abscess. Medicine (Baltimore). 1980;59:50–63.
512. Robinson SL, Saxe JM, Lucas CE, et al. Splenic diseases associated with endocarditis. Surgery. 1992;112:781–786.
513. Khalil T, Uzoaru I, Nadimpalli V, et al. Splenic tuberculous abscess in patients positive for human immunodeficiency virus: Report of two cases and review. Clin Infect Dis. 1992;14:1265–1266.
514. Torres JR, Rodriquez Casas J, Balda E, et al. Multifocal *Salmonella* splenic abscess in an HIV-infected patient. Trop Geogr Med. 1992;44:66–68.
515. Drugas D, Duarte B, Barrett J. *Salmonella typhi* splenic abscess in an intravenous drug abuser following splenorrhaphy: Case report. J Trauma. 1992;33:143–144.
516. Grant E, Mertens MA, Mascatello VJ. Splenic abscess: Comparison of four imaging methods. AJR Am J Roentgenol. 1979;132:465–466.
517. Pawar S, Kay CJ, Gonzalez R, et al. Sonography of splenic abscess. AJR Am J Roentgenol. 1982;138:259–262.
518. Linos DA, Nagorney DM, McIlrath DC. Splenic abscess: The importance of early diagnosis. Mayo Clin Proc. 1983;58:261–264.
519. Sarr MG, Zuidema GD. Splenic abscess: Presentation, diagnosis and treatment. Surgery. 1982;92:480–485.
520. Chou YH, Hsu CC, Tiu CM, et al. Splenic abscess: Sonographic diagnosis and percutaneous drainage or aspiration. Gastrointest Radiol. 1992;17:262–266.
521. Quinn SF, von Sonnenberg E, Casola G, et al. Interventional radiology in the spleen. Radiology. 1986;161:289–291.
522. Levison MA, Percutaneous versus open operative drainage of intra-abdominal abscesses. Infect Dis Clin North Am. 1992;6:525–544.
523. Rao PN, Rhea JT, Novelline RA, et al. Effect of computed tomography of the appendix on treatment of patients and use of hospital resources. N Engl J Med. 1998;338:141–146.
524. Ferzoco LB, Paptopoulos V, Silen W. Acute diverticulitis. N Engl J Med. 1998;338:1521–1526.
525. Campbell K, Steele RJ. Non-steroidal anti-inflammatory drugs and complicated diverticular disease: A case-control study. Br J Surg. 1991;78:190–191.
526. Byrne RV. Localized perforated diverticulitis. Arch Surg. 1964;88:552–555.
527. Lozon AA, Duff JH. Acute perforation of the colon. Can J Surg. 1976;19:48–51.
528. Rodkey GV, Welch CE. Colonic diverticular disease with surgical treatment: A study of 338 cases. Surg Clin North Am. 1974;54:655–674.
529. Elfrink RJ, Miedema BW. Colonic diverticula: When complications require surgery and when they don't. Postgrad Med. 1992;92:97–98, 101–102.
530. Hemming A, Davis NL, Robbins RE. Surgical versus percutaneous drainage of intra-abdominal abscesses. Am J Surg. 1991;161:593–595.
531. Stabile BE, Puccio E, von Sonnenberg E, et al. Preoperative percutaneous catheter drainage of diverticular abscesses. Am J Surg. 1990;159:99–104.
532. Peoples JB, Vilk DR, Maguire JP, et al. Reassessment of primary resection of the perforated segment for severe colonic diverticulitis. Am J Surg. 1990;159:291–293.
533. Nespoli A, Razizzini C, Trivella M, et al. The choice of surgical procedure for peritonitis due to colonic perforation. Arch Surg. 1993;128:814–818.
534. Moreaux J, Vons C. Elective resection for diverticular disease of the sigmoid colon. Br J Surg. 1990;77:1036–1038.
535. Tugwell P, Southcott D, Walmesley P. Free perforation of the colon in Crohn's disease. Br J Clin Pract. 1972;26:44–45.
536. Till M, Lee N, Soper WD, et al. Typhlitis in patients with HIV-1 infection. Ann Intern Med. 1992;116:998–1000.
537. Wilson SE, Robinson G, Williams RA, et al. Acquired immune deficiency syndrome (AIDS) indications for abdominal surgery, pathology and outcome. Ann Surg. 1989; 210:428–434.
538. Prolla JC, Kirsner JB. The gastrointestinal lesions and complications of the leukemias. Ann Intern Med. 1964;61:1084–1103.
539. Pokorney BH, Jones JM, Skaikh BS, et al. Typhlitis: A treatable cause of recurrent septicemia. JAMA. 1980;243:682–683.
540. Mulholland MW, Delaney JP. Neutropenic colitis and aplastic anemia: A new association. Ann Surg. 1983;197:84–90.
541. Archibald RG. Nelson JA. Necrotizing enterocolitis in acute leukemia: Radiographic findings. Gastrointest Radiol. 1987;3:63–65.
542. Alt B, Glass NR, Sallinger H. Neutropenic enterocolitis in adults: Review of the literature and assessment of surgical intervention. Am J Surg. 1985;149:405–408.
543. Shaked A, Shinar E, Freund H. Neutropenic typhlitis: A plea for conservatism. Dis Colon Rectum. 1983;26:351–352.
544. Varki AP, Armitage JO, Feagler JR. Typhlitis in acute leukemias: Successful treatment by early surgical intervention. Cancer. 1979;43:695–697.
545. Berk JE, Zinbers SS. Acute cholecystitis: Medical aspects. In: Berk JE, Haubrich WS, Kalser MH, et al., eds. Gastroenterology. 4th ed. Philadelphia: WB Saunders; 1985;6:3597–3616.
546. Bailey HA, Thrush LB. Consideration of acute cholecystitis: An analysis of seventy-six cases. Am J Surg. 1951;82:328–333.
547. Schein CJ. Acute Cholecystitis. New York: Harper & Row; 1972:63–65.
548. Truedson H, Elmros T, Holm S. The incidence of bacteria in gallbladder bile at acute and elective cholecystectomy. Acta Chir Scand. 1983;149:307–313.
549. Pitt HA, Postier RG, Cameron JC. Biliary bacteria: Significance and alteration after antibiotic therapy. Arch Surg. 1982;117:445–449.
550. Finegold S. Anaerobes in biliary tract infection. Arch Intern Med. 1979;139:1338–1339.
551. Bourgalt AM, England DM, Rosenblatt JE, et al. Clinical characteristics on anaerobic bactobilia. Arch Intern Med. 1979;139:1346–1349.

552. Samuels BI, Freitas JE, Bree RL, et al. A comparison of radionuclide hepatobiliary imaging and real-time ultrasound for the detection of acute cholecystitis. Radiology. 1983;147:207–210.
553. Gill PT, Dillon E, Leahy AL, et al. Ultrasonography, HIDA scintigraphy or both in the diagnosis of acute cholecystitis? Br J Surg. 1985;72:267–268.
554. Johnson DG, Coleman RE. New techniques in radionuclide imaging of the alimentary system. Radiol Clin North Am. 1982;20:635–651.
555. Kane RA, Costello P, Duszlak E. Computed tomography in acute cholecystitis: New observations. AJR Am J Roentgenol. 1983;141:697–701.
556. McCarthy S, Hricak H, Cohen M, et al. Cholecystitis: Detection with MR imaging. Radiology. 1986;158:333–336.
557. Mentzer RM, Golden CT, Chandler JG, et al. A comparative appraisal of emphysematous cholecystitis. Am J Surg. 1975;125:10–15.
558. Kune GA, Burdon JGW. Are antibiotics necessary in acute cholecystitis? Med J Aust. 1975;2:627–630.
559. Hirschmann JV, Inui TS. Antimicrobial prophylaxis: A critique of recent trials. Rev Infect Dis. 1980;2:1–23.
560. Bulow S, Dronberg O, Lung-Kristenson K. Reappraisal of surgery for suppurative cholecystitis. Arch Surg. 1977;112:282–284.
561. Moore EE, Kelly GL, Driver T, et al. Reassessment of simple cholecystostomy. Arch Surg. 1979;114:515–518.
562. Naitove A. When cholecystectomy? Hosp Pract. 1978;13:121–128.
563. Jarvinen HJ, Hastbacka J. Early cholecystectomy for acute cholecystitis: A prospective randomized study. Ann Surg. 1980;191:501–505.
564. Morrow DJ, Thompson J, Wilson SE. Acute cholecystitis in the elderly: A surgical emergency. Arch Surg. 1979;113:1149–1152.
565. Thompson JE Jr, Tompkins RK, Longmire WP Jr. Factors in the management of acute cholangitis. Ann Surg. 1982;117:437–444.
566. Bilboa MK, Dotter CT, Lee TG, et al. Complications of endoscopic retrograde cholangiopancreatography: A study of 10,000 cases. Gastroenterology. 1976; 70:314–320.
567. Hinshaw DB. Acute obstructive cholangitis. Surg Clin North Am. 1973;53:1089–1094.
568. Ralls PW, Colletti PM, Halls JM, et al. Prospective evaluation of ^{99m}TC-IDA cholescintigraphy and gray-scale ultrasound in the diagnosis of acute cholecystitis. Radiology. 1982;144:369–371.
569. Welch JP, Donaldson G. The urgency of diagnosis and surgical treatment of suppurative cholangitis. Am J Surg. 1976;131:527–532.

S E C T I O N G

CARDIOVASCULAR INFECTIONS

Chapter 65

Endocarditis and Intravascular Infections

ARNOLD S. BAYER
W. MICHAEL SCHELD

INFECTIVE ENDOCARDITIS

The term *infective endocarditis* (IE) denotes infection of the endocardial surface of the heart and implies the physical presence of microorganisms in the lesion. Although the heart valves are most commonly affected, the disease may also occur within septal defects or on the mural endocardium. Infections of arteriovenous shunts and of arterioarterial shunts (patent ductus arteriosus), as well as infection related to coarctation of the aorta, are also included in the following discussion because the clinical manifestations are similar. The term *infective endocarditis,* first used by Thayer and later popularized by Lerner and Weinstein,[1, 2] is preferable to the old term *bacterial endocarditis* because chlamydiae, rickettsiae, mycoplasmas, fungi, and perhaps even viruses may be responsible for the syndrome.

In the past, the disease has been classified as "acute" or "subacute." This distinction was based on the usual progression of the untreated disease and is mainly of historical interest. The acute form follows a fulminant course, usually with high fever, systemic toxicity, and leukocytosis; death occurs in several days to less than 6 weeks. It is classically associated with infection caused by *Staphylococcus aureus, Streptococcus pyogenes, Streptococcus pneumoniae*, or *Neisseria gonorrhoeae.* The subacute (death occurring in 6 weeks to 3 months) and "chronic" (death occurring later than 3 months) forms are usually considered together. They commonly occur in the setting of prior valvular disease and are characterized by a slow, indolent course with low-grade fever, night sweats, weight loss, and vague systemic complaints. These two forms of the disease are classically caused by the viridans streptococci. Although useful conceptually, this classification ignores the nonbacterial forms of IE and the frequent overlap in manifestations of infection by specific organisms such as the enterococci. A classification based on the etiologic agent responsible is preferable, because it has implications for the course usually followed, the likelihood of preexisting heart disease, and the appropriate antimicrobial agent(s) to employ.

Although relatively uncommon, IE has received considerable attention by both clinicians and scientists for the past century. The clinical manifestations of the disease are so varied that they may be encountered in any of the medical subspecialties. Successful management is dependent on the close cooperation of medical and surgical disciplines. Indeed, endocarditis services have been created at several tertiary care centers in the United States. This collaboration has markedly improved the outcome of a disease that was universally fatal in the preantibiotic era. The disease has attracted considerable investigative interest. Although the factors that influence its development are now more clearly identified, many questions remain about the unique aspects of this infection, in particular:

1. Why do organisms lodge specifically on the cardiac valves rather than elsewhere in the vascular tree?
2. What enables the microorganisms to survive on the valve surface after colonization?
3. What are the primary host defenses against induction and progression of the infection?
4. Why do only a relatively small number of strains of bacteria produce the vast majority of cases of endocarditis, whereas many others produce only bacteremia?
5. What factors are responsible for the marked variation in the manifestations of the disease?
6. Why is the infection so difficult to eradicate with antibiotics even though the infecting organisms are often exquisitely sensitive to the drugs in vitro?

These questions are discussed in detail in the following sections.

Epidemiology

The incidence of IE is difficult to determine because the criteria for diagnosis and the methods of reporting vary with different series.[3, 4] An analysis based on strict case definitions often reveals that only a small proportion (≈20%) of clinically diagnosed cases are categorized as definite. Nevertheless, IE accounted for approximately 1 case per 1000 hospital admissions, with a range of 0.16 to 5.4 cases per 1000 admissions, in a review of 10 large surveys.[3, 5] This incidence has not changed in the past 30 years.[6] The mean annual incidence was 3.8 per 100,000 person-years in Olmstead County, Minnesota, from 1950 to 1981, with no significant change during this interval.[7] A similar figure of 1.7 per 100,000 person-years was reported from a prospective survey in Louisiana[8] and is analogous to results from the United Kingdom.[9] A series of 210 episodes of IE seen at a large community hospital in Youngstown, Ohio, from 1980 through 1990 documented annual rates of 0.32 to 1.30 (mean 0.75) episodes per 1000 admissions per year.[10] In an autopsy study[11] there was no change in the yearly number of cases of IE in the United Kingdom from 1939 to 1967. The proportion of acute cases has increased from approximately 20% in the preantibiotic era to 33%.[5, 6] Despite these changes in the disease spectrum, IE remains a prevalent disease with a significant mortality in the antibiotic era.[10, 12, 13] Estimates from the American Heart Association (AHA) place the annual incidence of IE at 10,000 to 20,000 new cases.

The mean age of patients with IE has gradually increased in the antibiotic era. In 1926, the median age was less than 30 years[14]; this had increased to 39 years by 1943, and currently over 50% of the patients are older than 50 years.[6, 10, 15, 16] At the present time, approximately 54% (range, 41 to 69%) of the cases occur in patients aged 31 to 60, 26% (range, 12 to 40%) in patients less than 30 years of age, and 21% (range, 8 to 38%) in people older than 60 years.[2] The mean age of patients with IE caused by group D streptococci is even higher: 61 to 67 years.[17] The disease remains uncommon in children, in whom it is associated primarily with (1) underlying structural congenital heart disease, particularly septal defects or complex lesions involving septal defects; (2) surgical repair of these defects; or (3) nosocomial catheter-related bacteremia, especially in infants.[18, 19] The mean age for men is 6 to 7 years older than that for women, and men are more commonly affected (54 to 69% of the cases; the mean male to female ratio is 1.7:1, with a range of 1.0 to 3.0:1 in 18 large series).[5] In patients under the age of 35 years, more cases occur in women. A number of factors may relate to this shift in age distribution. First, there has been a change in the nature of the underlying heart disease owing to a decline in the incidence of acute rheumatic fever and rheumatic heart disease countered by the increasing importance of degenerative heart disease in elderly patients. Second, the age of the population has been steadily increasing, and people with rheumatic or congenital heart disease are surviving longer. In addition, such patients are increasingly being subjected to prosthetic valve surgery, an important etiologic factor in the pathogenesis of IE. A new form of the disease—nosocomial endocarditis—secondary to new therapeutic modalities (intravenous catheters, hyperalimentation lines, pacemakers, dialysis shunts, and so forth) has emerged.[3] Of 125 cases of endocarditis reviewed in Seattle, 35 were nosocomial in origin (28%).[20] Although nosocomial endocarditis accounted for only 14.3% of cases in another recent study, 64% of patients were over 60 years of age, and mortality was high.[21] It is interesting, however, that the age-adjusted incidence for the most common causative organisms (viridans streptococci) has not appreciably changed.[22]

The heart valve involved by the infection varies considerably with the proportion of acute cases reported in each series. The distribution ranges from 28 to 45% of cases for the mitral valve alone, 5 to 36% for the aortic valve alone, and 0 to 35% for the aortic and mitral valves combined. The tricuspid valve is rarely involved (0 to 6% of the cases), and the pulmonary valve even less often (<1%).[15, 17, 20, 23] Both right- and left-sided disease are present in 0 to 4%.[2] Involvement of the aortic valve alone is increasing in frequency and correlates with the increase in acute cases; the incidence was 5% in 1938 and rose to 39% by 1978.[15] The aortic valve is involved in 61% of the male cases but in only 31% of the female cases.[20]

Almost any type of structural heart disease may predispose to IE, especially when the defect results in turbulence of blood flow. Rheumatic heart disease has been the underlying lesion in 37 to 76% of the infections in the past, and the mitral valve is involved in more than 85% of these cases.[5] If the mitral valve alone is involved, women outnumber men by 2 to 1. The aortic valve is affected in approximately 50% of these cases, and, if it alone is involved, men outnumber women by 4 to 1. Right-sided endocarditis is rare (except in intravenous drug users and patients with indwelling transvenous pacemakers) and accounts for less than 10% of all cases occurring in patients with rheumatic heart disease. The proportion of cases related to rheumatic heart disease has continued to decline to 25% or less in the past two decades.[24]

Congenital heart disease (especially patent ductus arteriosus, ventricular septal defect, coarctation of the aorta, bicuspid aortic valve, tetralogy of Fallot, and rarely, pulmonic stenosis) is responsible in 6 to 24% of the cases.[5] Endocarditis is uncommon in the secundum atrial septal defects, probably because this lesion results in a low-pressure shunt with little turbulence. The congenitally bicuspid aortic valve, erroneously attributed to rheumatic carditis in the past,[25] is now recognized as an important condition in elderly patients (especially men), and is the underlying lesion in over 20% of the cases occurring past the age of 60, and is associated with a poor prognosis despite rapid valve replacement.[26] Marfan's syndrome, when associated with aortic insufficiency, has also been associated with IE. Surgical closure of a ventricular septal defect lowers the risk of IE.[27]

The "degenerative" cardiac lesions (calcified mitral annulus, calcific nodular lesions secondary to arteriosclerotic cardiovascular disease, post–myocardial infarction thrombus, and so forth) assume the greatest importance in the 30 to 40% of the patients without any demonstrable underlying valvular disease. The actual contribution made by these lesions is unknown, but they occur with an increased incidence in the elderly. In one series, degenerative lesions were present in 50% of patients over 60 years old with native valve IE.[28] The contribution of these degenerative cardiac lesions to the development of IE is apparent in an analysis of 148 patients receiving treatment in London since 1970.[29, 30] The underlying structural cardiac defects were as follows: rheumatic heart disease, present in 39 of the patients; congenital defects, in 13; and normal or degenerate valves, in 65. Similarly, only 31% of patients with IE in another series[31] had known cardiac disease. Although a calcified mitral annulus is fairly frequent in elderly women, this lesion is rarely complicated by IE (only 3 of 80 in one report).[32] When acute cases of IE are considered separately, over 50% have no recognized underlying cardiac disease.[10]

Many other conditions such as luetic heart disease, arterioarterial fistulas, hemodialysis shunts or fistulas, intracardiac pacemaker wires, and intracardiac prostheses may predispose to endocarditis. Prosthetic valve endocarditis is rising in incidence in proportion to other forms of endocarditis and is discussed in Chapter 66. Infective endocarditis also occurs more frequently in seriously ill hospitalized patients who are compromised hosts and who are subjected to invasive intravascular access procedures (intravenous catheters, including central venous pressure monitoring lines, hyperalimentation lines, intracardiac pacemaker wires, and so on).[15] As noted previously, another group with an increased risk of IE comprises intravenous ("mainlining") drug users. (This group is considered in detail in a later section.) In this population, there is the added problem of a rapidly rising prevalence of IE in persons with human immunodeficiency virus (HIV) infection. In addition, intravenous drug users are also the group at greatest risk for recurrent as well as polymicrobial IE.[5, 33] Although the contribution of invasive procedures (e.g., sigmoidoscopy or colonoscopy) has been debated, native valve IE appears to be more frequent in patients with active inflammatory bowel disease (6 of 213 patients in one recent report[34]).

Although idiopathic hypertrophic subaortic stenosis (IHSS) or asymmetric hypertrophy of the interventricular septum has not classically been recognized as a condition leading to bacterial endocarditis, by 1982, 32 such cases had been reported in the literature.[35–37] In seven cases examined histologically, the infection was found on the aortic valve in three cases, mitral valve in two, both valves in one, and the subaortic endocardium in one. This distribution is probably related to the associated mitral regurgitation due to the displacement of the anterior leaflet by the abnormal ventricular architecture and by the turbulence of the jet stream affecting the aortic valve distal to the intraventricular obstruction. The age of patients developing endocarditis ranged from 20 to 66 years, and in most cases (70%) the disease was produced by viridans streptococci. Approximately 5% of patients with IHSS develop IE.[37] Infective endocarditis is more common in the subset of patients with IHSS who have hemodynamically severe forms of the disease manifested by a higher peak systolic pressure gradient and a high prevalence of symptoms. New murmurs develop in 36% of patients with IHSS complicated by IE, and this new physical finding correlates with a higher mortality rate.[37]

The association of the mitral prolapse syndrome and endocarditis has also been recognized. Of 87 consecutive cases of IE reported from Stanford University, 10 (11%) occurred in patients with well-documented mitral valve prolapse.[38] These 10 cases represented over one third of the 28 cases in which isolated mitral regurgitation was the predisposing condition. Four additional cases occurred in patients who were not studied by echocardiography or angiography but who had clinical evidence of the mitral prolapse syndrome. Thus, 40 to 50% of the cases of IE associated with isolated insufficient mitral valves probably occurred in patients with the mitral prolapse syndrome. In one series[23] of 63 cases of native valve endocarditis diagnosed in Memphis from 1980 to 1984, mitral valve prolapse was the most common underlying lesion (29%). In another study,[39] 5 of 58 patients with mitral valve prolapse followed prospectively for 9 to 22 years developed endocarditis. This syndrome should be suspected in patients with midsystolic clicks with or without a late systolic murmur. The condition is common and has been recognized in 0.5 to 20% of otherwise healthy people, especially young women. It has become apparent that mitral valve prolapse is only one component of a developmental syndrome. This lesion is often associated with a distinct habitus in women,[40] von Willebrand's disease, or ophthalmoplegia. Some of these characteristics may be useful in identifying patients at high risk for IE. It is important to emphasize that all 25 patients who developed IE on a prolapsing mitral valve had a holosystolic murmur, and none had the isolated click without a murmur.[38] The risk of IE appears to be increased in the subset of patients with mitral valve prolapse who exhibit thickened leaflets with valvular redundancy.[28] In addition, males older than 45 years who have mitral valve prolapse represent a group at increased risk for IE.[41] Nevertheless, the risk of IE is clearly higher in patients with mitral valve prolapse. In a careful retrospective epidemiologic matched case control analysis, the calculated odds ratio (8.2; 95% confidence interval, 2.4 to 28.4) indicates a substantially higher risk for the development of IE in these patients than in controls.[42] It appears that once IE develops in people with mitral valve prolapse, the symptoms and signs are more subtle and the mortality rate is less than in left-sided IE of other types.[43]

Pathogenesis and Pathophysiology

In vitro observations and studies in experimental animals have demonstrated that the development of IE probably requires the simultaneous occurrence of several independent events, each of which may be influenced by a host of separate factors. The valve surface must first be altered to produce a suitable site for bacterial attachment and colonization. Surface changes may be produced by various local and systemic stresses, including blood turbulence. These alterations result in the deposition of platelets and fibrin and in the formation of so-called sterile vegetation—the lesions of nonbacterial thrombotic endocarditis (NBTE). Bacteria must then reach this site and adhere to the involved tissue to produce colonization. Certain strains appear to have a selective advantage in adhering to platelets and/or fibrin and thus produce the disease with a lower inoculum. After colonization, the surface is rapidly covered with a protective sheath of fibrin and platelets to produce an environment conducive to further bacterial multiplication and vegetation growth. The interaction of these events is depicted in Figure 65–1. In the following sections, these factors are considered independently (see refs. 44 to 47 for in-depth discussions).

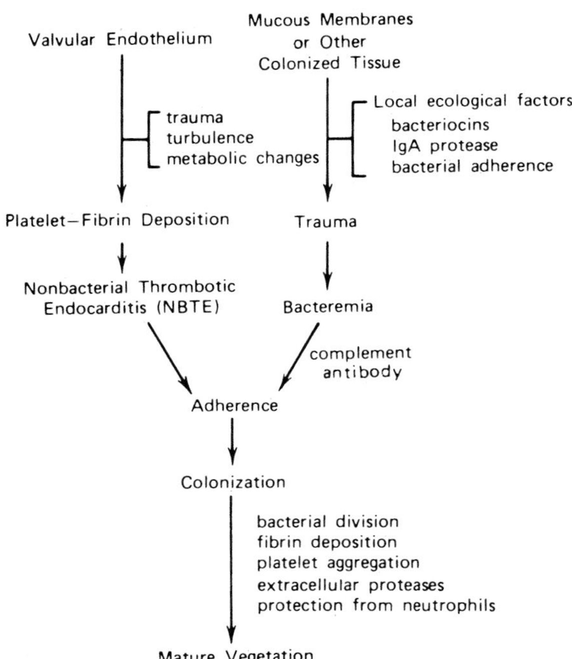

FIGURE 65–1. Proposed scheme for the pathogenesis of infective endocarditis.

Nonbacterial Thrombotic Endocarditis

Luschka, in 1852, first suggested that endocarditis resulted when septic coronary emboli lodged in the vessels of the cardiac valve.[48] This hypothesis was discarded because cardiac valves are poorly vascularized.[46, 49, 50] It is now clear that the initial colonization occurs on the endothelial surface of the valve. In experimental animals it is nearly impossible to produce IE with intravenous injections of bacteria unless the valvular surface is first damaged or otherwise altered. When a polyethylene catheter is passed across the aortic valve of a rabbit, endocarditis is readily produced with intravenously injected bacteria or fungi.[51, 52] Microscopic examination of this early lesion demonstrates the organisms intimately adherent to fibrin-platelet deposits overlying interstitial edema and mild cellular distortion that have formed in areas of valvular trauma.[53] Scanning electron micrographs of the damaged valvular surface confirm the adhesion of microorganisms to these areas of fibrin-platelet deposition early in the disease course.[54] The organisms are rapidly covered by fibrin.[55] Opossums and pigs are the only animals known to develop endocarditis readily without experimentally induced valvular alteration.[47, 56] The stress of captivity is apparently sufficient in these animals to produce subtle valvular changes that lead to both spontaneous endocarditis and a markedly increased susceptibility to the disease after the intravenous injection of bacteria. In other animals and probably in humans, alteration of the valve surface is a prerequisite for bacterial colonization. Angrist and Oka first recognized the importance of these deposits as the critical factor in allowing bacterial colonization of valve surfaces and suggested the term *nonbacterial thrombotic endocarditis.* Many forms of exogenous stress produce these lesions experimentally, including infection, hypersensitivity states, cold exposure, simulated high altitude, high cardiac output states, cardiac lymphatic obstruction, and hormonal manipulations.[47] These procedures all increase the susceptibility of the animals to IE.

Nonbacterial thrombotic endocarditis has been found in patients with malignancy (particularly pancreatic, gastric, or lung carcinoma) or other chronic wasting diseases, rheumatic or congenital heart disease,[49] uremia, or connective tissue diseases such as systemic lupus erythematosus, and after the placement of intracardiac catheters (e.g., Swan-Ganz), and even after a self-limited acute illness, and it generally reflects one of two pathogenic mechanisms: hypercoagulability or endothelial damage. In a careful analysis performed in Japan, NBTE was found in 2.4% of 3404 autopsies, especially in elderly people with chronic wasting disease.[57] NBTE was most frequent on the low-pressure side of the cardiac valves along the line of closure, precisely the site most often involved in IE. Whether this lesion is always essential for the development of endocarditis in humans is unknown.

Hemodynamic Factors

Infective endocarditis characteristically occurs on the atrial surface of the mitral valve and the ventricular surface of the aortic valve when associated with valvular insufficiency. Rodbard[58] showed that this localization is related to a decrease in lateral pressure (presumably with decreased perfusion of the intima) immediately "downstream" from the regurgitant flow. Lesions with high degrees of turbulence (small ventricular septal defect with a jet lesion, valvular stenosis resulting from insufficient valves) readily create conditions that lead to bacterial colonization, whereas defects with a large surface area (large ventricular septal defect), low flow (ostium secundum atrial septal defect), or attenuation of turbulence (chronic congestive heart failure with atrial fibrillation) are rarely implicated in IE. Cures of IE achieved with ligation alone of an arteriovenous fistula or patent ductus arteriosus also highlight the importance of hemodynamic factors. A hyperdynamic circulation itself, such as that developing after experimentally induced arteriovenous fistulas in dogs or after creation of fistulas and shunts in hemodialysis patients, indirectly may lead to IE by producing NBTE.[46, 47]

The degree of mechanical stress exerted on the valve also affects the location of the endocarditis.[59] In 1024 autopsy cases of IE reviewed through 1952, the incidence of valvular lesions was as follows: mitral, 86%; aortic, 55%; tricuspid, 19.6%; and pulmonic, 1.1%. This correlates with the pressure resting on the closed valve: 116, 72, 24, and 5 mmHg, respectively.

Transient Bacteremia

In the setting of preexistent NBTE, transient bacteremia may result in the colonization of these lesions and may lead to the development of IE.[60] Transient bacteremia occurs whenever a mucosal surface heavily colonized with bacteria is traumatized, such as with dental extractions and other dental procedures and gastrointestinal, urologic, and gynecologic procedures (Table 65–1).[60, 61] The degree of bacteremia is proportional to the trauma produced by the procedure and to the number of organisms inhabiting the surface, and the organisms isolated reflect the resident microbial flora. The bacteremia is usually low-grade—with 10 or fewer colony-forming units (cfu)/ml—and transient; the blood stream is usually sterile in less than 15 to 30 minutes. It is noteworthy that in two studies in which blood cultures were drawn from patients with severe gingival disease before the dental procedure, spontaneous bacteremia was identified in 9 to 11%. Other studies have demonstrated an even higher frequency of spontaneous bacteremia. Of the blood cultured from healthy people, 60 to 80% of specimens were positive when filters and anaerobic techniques were used.[62] The degree of bacteremia, however, was low, with only 2 to 10 cfu/5 ml of blood isolated. "Nonpathogenic" organisms such as *Propionibacterium acnes, Actinomyces viscosus, Staphylococcus epidermidis,* and other *Actinomyces* or streptococal species were responsible. Frequent episodes of silent bacteremia are also suggested by the identification of circulating humoral antibodies to the resident oral flora and by the noted increase in sensitized peripheral T cells to the flora of dental plaque.

Another factor of critical importance during the transient bacteremia stage is susceptibility of the potential pathogen to complement-mediated bactericidal activity. Only "serum-resistant" gram-negative aerobic bacilli—e.g., *Escherichia coli, Pseudomonas aeruginosa, Serratia marcescens*—reliably produce experimental IE in

TABLE 65–1 Incidence of Bacteremia after Various Procedures

Procedure/Manipulation	Percentage of Positive Blood Cultures
Dental	
Dental extraction	18–85
Periodontal surgery	32–88
Chewing candy or paraffin	17–51
Tooth brushing	0–26
Oral irrigation device	27–50
Upper airway	
Bronchoscopy (rigid scope)	15
Tonsillectomy	28–38
Nasotracheal suctioning/intubation	16
Gastrointestinal	
Upper GI endoscopy	8–12
Sigmoidoscopy/colonoscopy	0–9.5
Barium enema	11
Percutaneous needle biopsy of liver	3–13
Urologic	
Urethral dilation	18–33
Urethral catheterization	8
Cytoscopy	0–17
Transurethral prostatic resection	12–46
Obstetric/gynecologic	
Normal vaginal delivery	0–11
Punch biopsy of the cervix	0
Removal/insertion of an HUD	0

Abbreviations: GI, gastrointestinal; IUD, intrauterine (contraceptive) device.
From Everett ED, Hirschmann JV. Transient bacteremia and endocarditis prophylaxis: A review. Medicine (Baltimore). 1977;56:61.

rabbits,[63, 64] and this property is found in all isolates from human cases of IE. Although experimental IE can be induced in rats with "serum-sensitive" *E. coli,* the organisms are eliminated rapidly upon catheter removal.[64]

Microorganism–Nonbacterial Thrombotic Endocarditis Interaction

The ability of certain organisms to adhere to NBTE lesions is a crucial early step in the development of endocarditis. Gould and associates[65] showed that organisms frequently associated with IE (enterococci, viridans streptococci, *S. aureus, S. epidermidis, P. aeruginosa*) adhered more avidly to normal canine aortic leaflets in vitro than did organisms uncommon in IE (*Klebsiella pneumoniae, E. coli*). In addition, *S. aureus* and the viridans streptococci produce IE more readily than does *E. coli* in the rabbit model of IE.[66] This observation correlates with the relative frequency with which these organisms produce the disease in humans. The rarity of IE due to gram-negative aerobic bacilli may also be related to their "serum sensitivity," as noted previously.

Differences in the propensity to cause endocarditis are apparent even within a single species. Eleven capsular serotypes of *S. aureus* have been described to date; highly mucoid strains (e.g., serotypes 1 and 2) are rarely recovered from clinical isolates, whereas types 5 and 8 account for approximately 75% of isolates. Nevertheless, mutant strains devoid of microencapsulation had significantly lower median infective dose (ID_{50}) values in a rat (catheter-induced NBTE) endocarditis model[67] than wild-type parent strains. Thus, microcapsule expression may attenuate *S. aureus* endocarditis production by blocking bacterial cell surface adhesins, but this hypothesis requires confirmation.

Other studies using an elegant experimental model of IE after dental extraction in rats with periodontitis, which closely resembles the presumed pathogenetic sequence in humans, also suggest an important role for bacterial adhesion to NBTE in the early events. Although viridans streptococci were much more commonly isolated than were group G streptococci in blood cultures obtained 1 minute after extraction, the latter strains caused 83% of the IE episodes in this rat model.[68, 69] This propensity to cause IE was associated with an increased adhesion of group G streptococci to fibrin-platelet matrices in vitro.[69]

The adherence of oral streptococci to NBTE may depend on the production of a complex extracellular polysaccharide, dextran. This polymer plays an essential role in the pathogenesis of dental caries by *Streptococcus mutans.*[70] It allows the organism to adhere tightly to the surface of dental enamel. The enhanced ability to adhere to inert surfaces may also be important in IE. In an analysis of 719 cases of streptococcal infections in the United Kingdom, 317 cases of IE were found.[71] The most common etiologic agents were *Streptococcus sanguis* (16.4% of the cases), previously called "*Streptococcus* subacute bacterial endocarditis (SBE)," and *S. mutans* (14.2%). When a ratio denoting endocarditis to nonendocarditis bacteremia was derived (Table 65–2), the relative propensity for a particular organism to cause endocarditis could be predicted. The ratios range from 14.2:1 for *S. mutans* to a reversed ratio of 1:32 for *S. pyogenes.* Only the first four organisms listed in Table 65–2 (all with ratios greater than 3:1) produce extracellular dextran. This suggests that dextran production may also be a virulence factor in the pathogenesis of IE.

The role of dextran in the adherence of oral streptococci to NBTE has also been studied in vitro by using artificial fibrin-platelet matrices (simulating NBTE). The amount of dextran produced by the organism in broth correlated with adherence and was increased by incubating the organism in sucrose (which stimulates dextran production) and was decreased by the addition of dextranase (which removes the dextran from the cell surface). The addition of exogenous dextran to *S. sanguis* grown in sucrose-free media increased adherence. Dextran production also correlated directly with the abil-

TABLE 65-2 Ratio of Infective Endocarditis Cases to Nonendocarditis Bacteremia Cases for Various Streptococci and Enterococci

Organism	Endocarditis: Nonendocarditis
Streptococcus mutans	14.2:1
Streptococcus bovis I	5.9:1
DX+ *S. mitior**	3.3:1
Streptococcus sanguis	3.0:1
Streptococcus mitior	1.8:1
Unclassified "viridans" streptococci	1.4:1
Enterococcus faecalis	1:1.2
Miscellaneous streptococci	1:1.3
Streptococcus bovis II	1:1.7
Streptococcus anginosus	1:2.6
Group G streptococci	1:2.9
Group B streptococci	1:7.4
Group A streptococci	1:32.0

*DX+: dextran-positive.
Modified from Parker MT, Ball LC. Streptococci and aerococci associated with systemic infection in man. J Med Microbiol. 1976;9:275.

ity of these organisms to produce endocarditis in vivo in the rabbit model.[72] The strain of *S. sanguis* produced endocarditis less readily when incubated in dextranase than did control strains, and a strain that produced large quantities of dextran produced endocarditis more easily than did a strain that produced relatively small quantities of dextran. Dextran production also increases the adherence of *S. mutans* to traumatized canine aortic valves in vitro,[73] an effect dependent on polymers of higher molecular weight.[74] Thus, dextran formation (or, more properly, exopolysaccharide or glycocalyx production) by oral streptococci may be a virulence factor for the production of IE by these organisms.[75] Furthermore, continued in vivo synthesis of exopolysaccharide during experimental IE correlates with vegetation size and resistance to antimicrobial therapy.[76, 77] Measurement of cell-adherent glycocalyx by a quantitative spectrophotometric tryptophan assay among viridans streptococci isolated from blood cultures has potential value as an independent predictor of the likelihood of endocarditis.[78] It is clear, however, that non–dextran-producing streptococci may produce endocarditis in humans and adhere to artificial fibrin-platelet surfaces in vitro,[79] which suggests that other microbial surface characteristics are instrumental for this early event. Whatever the role of the extracellular glycocalyx in microbial adhesion, its presence may retard antimicrobial therapy for streptococcal endocarditis (see below).[76, 77, 80]

FimA is a surface adhesin expressed by viridans streptococci that serves as an important colonization factor in IE.[81] This 36-kDa protein is located at the tips of the fimbriae and has been shown to mediate the attachment of such organisms to platelet-fibrin matrices in vitro and to experimental NBTE lesions in the animal model of IE.[82] Of note, homologues of the *fimA* gene have been found widely distributed among clinical strains of viridans streptococci and enterococci, suggesting its importance in IE.[83] Several lines of experimental evidence have further confirmed the key role of FimA in the pathogenesis of IE. Inactivation of the *fimA* gene has yielded viridans streptococcal mutants exhibiting a significant decrease in virulence in experimental IE as compared with the parental strain having intact FimA expression.[82] In addition, animals either passively immunized with anti-FimA antibody or actively immunized with a FimA vaccine were significantly less susceptible to experimental IE than nonimmunized controls.[83]

A similar important role of adhesion to NBTE in the pathogenesis of IE has also been shown for yeasts. *Candida albicans* adheres readily to NBTE in vitro and produces IE in rabbits more readily than does *Candida krusei,* a nonadherent yeast rarely implicated in IE in humans.[84] Although microbial adhesion is a crucial early event in the pathogenesis of IE, the precise intracardiac loci are unknown and may differ among organisms. Most organisms probably adhere initially to a constituent of NBTE; some evidence implicates fibronectin as the host receptor within NBTE.[85] Recent studies[86, 87] support this concept. Low-fibronectin-binding mutants of *S. aureus* and *S. sanguis* had decreased ability to produce endocarditis in rats compared with high-fibronectin-binding parent strains. Other normal constituents of damaged endothelium or NBTE (e.g., fibrinogen, laminin, type 4 collagen[88]) may also serve to bind circulating bacteria. For example, *Streptococcus defectivus*—the major species isolated in cases of endocarditis due to "nutritionally variant streptococci" (NVS), discussed subsequently—bound the extracellular matrix of both fibroblasts and endothelial cells in a saturable specific manner, whereas *Streptococcus adjacens* and serotype III NVS strains did not bind.[89] A study also documented binding of *S. mutans, Streptococcus mitis, S. sanguis,* and *Enterococcus faecalis* to this extracellular matrix. Laminin-binding proteins (e.g., a 145-kD protein found in *Streptococcus gordonii* [formerly *S. sanguis I*]) have been found on the cell walls of organisms recovered from patients with endocarditis,[90] and the level of protein expression appeared to be regulated by the presence of extracellular matrix proteins. Other organisms may bind directly to, or become ingested by, endothelial cells as the initial event[91–94]; this sequence appears important in the initiation of IE by *S. aureus* on "normal" cardiac valves. A number of recent studies in experimental IE, utilizing *S. aureus* as the study organism, have shed additional light on the importance of microbial binding to specific matrix proteins found within the NBTE lesion upon the development of IE. It appears that the key adhesin possessed by the organism for induction of IE is one or more of its several fibrinogen-binding proteins (e.g., clumping factor, coagulase[95, 96]). Adhesins for other matrix molecules (e.g., fibronectin, collagen, thrombospondin[97–99]) are not pivotally involved in initial attachment of the organism to damaged endothelium but are crucial in the persistence of the microbe at this site. Moreover, additional virulence factors produced by this organism (α-toxin[100]) have also been identified in the experimental IE model as important for the persistence and proliferation of the organism within maturing vegetations in the post–valvular colonization stage of infection. Although the specific microbial surface–host receptor ligand relationship remains incompletely defined for all the major IE pethogens, this is an active area of investigation, because inhibition of these events may provide novel prophylactic strategies.

The importance of adherence characteristics in the development of endocarditis has also been examined by using preincubation of organisms with antibiotics. Many classes of drugs, after incubation even at subinhibitory concentrations, decrease the adhesion of streptococcal species to fibrin-platelet matrices and damaged canine valves in vitro.[101] Several elegant studies in animal models have verified the significance of this in vitro observation, because preincubation of the organism in subinhibitory antibiotic concentrations prevents the development of endocarditis in vivo.[102, 103] This has direct relevance to the chemoprophylactic prevention of IE (see Chapter 67). In one study, subinhibitory concentrations of penicillin were found to result in a loss of streptococcal lipoteichoic acid with reduced adhesion to NBTE-involved tissue and an impaired ability to produce IE in vivo.[104] Thus, antibiotics may prevent IE by at least two mechanisms: (1) bacterial killing and (2) inhibition of adhesion to NBTE-involved tissue.[105]

Because platelets are (with fibrin) the major constituents of NBTE, the role of the platelet in the pathogenesis of endocarditis has also been studied. Some strains of bacteria have been found to be potent stimulators of platelet aggregation and the release reaction.[106] In general, endocarditis-producing strains of staphylococci and streptococci more actively aggregate platelets than do other bacteria that less frequently produce IE. Bacterial-platelet aggregates have been found in the peripheral blood in patients with bacteremia. The importance of these bacterial-platelet aggregates in the formation of the vegetation or, conversely, in the effect of the aggregation on the rate of removal of organisms from the circulation is unknown. In one study, even small numbers of platelets greatly increased the adherence of oral streptococci to fibrin in vitro.[71] Other studies[107] have shown that *S. sanguis,* an important cause of IE, aggregates platelets and adheres to these blood components by protease-sensitive components, not dextrans. A platelet receptor for ligands on certain strains of *S. sanguis* was suggested. This platelet aggregation by viridans streptococci, however, requires both direct platelet binding and plasma components.[108] Other experiments implicate IgG in this specific streptococcal-platelet interaction and suggest that platelet activation is mediated through the platelet surface, Fc receptor, with a molecular weight of 40,000.[109]

Once the colonization of the valve occurs and a critical mass of adherent bacteria develops, the vegetation enlarges by further platelet-fibrin deposition and continued bacterial proliferation. The complex interplay among factors responsible for bacterial-platelet adhesion and aggregation has only been recently recognized. The ability of *S. sanguis* to induce platelet aggregation in vitro is conferred by two bacterial cell surface antigens: (1) class I antigen, which promotes adhesion of *S. sanguis* to platelets (adh$^+$), and (2) coexpression of class II antigen, which promotes platelet adhesion or platelet aggregation (agg$^+$). At least nine adh/agg phenotypes have been identified among naturally occurring variants, reflecting a range of platelet interactivity. Furthermore, intravenous inoculation of agg$^+$ *S. sanguis* strains into rabbits with catheter-induced aortic valve trauma leads to larger vegetations, a more severe clinical course, more gross lesions in major organs, and greater mortality than inoculation with a agg$^-$ strain or the agg$^+$ strains pretreated with Fab fragments specific for the platelet interactivity phenotype.[110] Platelet aggregation induced by *S. sanguis* in vivo appears to be an important virulence determinant of vegetation development and disease progression. Furthermore, streptococcal exopolysaccharide production inversely correlates with platelet adhesion while inhibiting aggregation,[111] indicating that these surface molecules may enhance endocarditis at some pathogenic steps but not others.

The manner in which *S. aureus* interacts with platelets in the pathogenesis of IE differs substantially with the viridans streptococci. This interaction does not require the presence of specific antistaphylococcal antibody and is thus not amplified by the platelet Fc receptor.[112] Moreover, platelet–*S. aureus* interactions for executing aggregation require fibrinogen as a bridging molecule but are independent of the primary platelet fibrinogen-binding site, the GpIIb/IIIa integrin receptor. In addition, it appears that *S. aureus* can bind to platelets via platelet-derived von Willebrand factor or directly to the von Willebrand factor receptor, at the von Willebrand factor–binding domain.[113, 114] In experimental IE, transposon inactivation of the putative *S. aureus* platelet-binding adhesin gene results in mutants with diminished capacity to adhere to platelets in vitro in either suspension or surface-bound monolayers.[115] In experimental IE due to such low-platelet-binding mutants, the induction rates of IE were equivalent to those of the parental strain, presumably because of the microbe's ability to attach to damaged endothelium by multiple adhesive mechanisms. However, the capacity of the mutant to persist and proliferate within experimental vegetations, as well as to hematogenously disseminate to the kidneys, was markedly impaired in the mutant strain.[115]

Platelets may also play a role in host defense within the cardiac vegetation during IE. Following specific exposure to thrombin, release of α-granule–derived platelet microbicidal proteins (PMPs, or thrombocidins) with bactericidal activity against some gram-positive cocci has been shown.[116] Although the ability of *S. aureus* to adhere to and aggregate platelets is a related property, the resistance to PMPs is an independent phenotypic characteristic and a potential virulence factor.[117] PMPs are low-molecular-weight (approximately 8 to 10 kD) cationic proteins and may act primarily on the bacterial cell membrane or cell wall synergistically with antibiotics to kill bacteria. PMPs may also demonstrate fungicidal activity against some yeasts in vitro.[118] Microbial resistance to the cidal activity of PMPs may contribute to the pathogenesis of IE. This hypothesis is supported by a reduction in vegetation weight and bacterial concentration in rabbits with experimental aortic valve *S. aureus* endocarditis after treatment with aspirin.[119] In addition, three recent studies in experimental IE as well as a clinical study have confirmed the importance of the relationship of PMP resistance and the pathogenesis of IE. In experimental viridans streptococcal IE and *S. aureus* IE, PMP-resistant strains exhibit an enhanced capacity to persist at sites of valvular damage.[120, 121] In addition, *S. aureus* strains exhibiting the PMP resistance phenotype in vitro are able to proliferate within the vegetation and hematogenously seeded extracardiac foci (kidneys, spleen) to a significantly greater extent than their isogenic counterparts that are PMP-susceptible in vitro.[122, 123] Furthermore, in a clinical study of bacteremic strains from patients with or without IE, viridans streptococcal and staphylococcal strains isolated from patients with IE tended to be substantially more resistant to PMPs in vitro.[121]

The bacterial colonies are found beneath the surface of the vegetation (at variable depth, depending on the intracardiac location[124]), and infiltration by phagocyte cells is minimal; thus the vegetation creates an environment of impaired host resistance. These conditions allow for relatively unbridled bacterial growth, resulting in extremely high colony counts of 10^9 to 10^{11} bacteria per gram of tissue. Bacteria deep within the fibrin matrix have been shown by autoradiography to reach a state of reduced metabolic activity.[125] Studies by Freedman and others suggest that impairment of host defenses (e.g., neutropenia, corticosteroids) potentiates progression of the disease when the tricuspid but not the aortic valve is involved[126, 127] but is largely dependent on the intracardiac location of the vegetation.[128] The role of granulocytes within the vegetation is unsettled. When vegetation formation is retarded with anticoagulants in experimental animals with IE, the organisms appear to divide on the surface, total bacterial titers are lower, and the clinical disease is more explosive.[129, 130] In addition, it has been suggested that phagocytosis of microorganisms by monocytes on or within the vegetation generates tissue thromboplastin formation; thromboplastin then acts as a stimulant to fibrin deposition and growth of the vegetation.[131] The best evidence, however, suggests that coagulation activation initiated by tissue factor,[132] with subsequent local thrombus formation, is responsible for the initiation of vegetation growth and persistence on the cardiac valve. It appears that some organisms (e.g., *S. aureus*) induce tissue factor production by endothelium without the necessity for host cytokines.[133]

Over the past several years, a number of important studies have elucidated the interaction between the invading microbe, the endothelium, the monocyte, and the pathogenesis of IE. Following internalization by endothelial cells in vitro, microbes such as *S. aureus* evoke a potent proinflammatory chemokine response (e.g., increase in expression of interleukin IL-6 or IL-8 or of monocyte chemotactic peptide).[134, 135] This event is also associated with increased expression upon the endothelial cell surface of several key adhesion molecules, especially intercellular adhesion molecule 1 (ICAM-1) and vascular cell adhesion molecule 1 (VCAM-1).[94, 134, 135] Among other cells, monocytes are drawn into this endothelial cell microenvironment; via their appropriate counterreceptors, monocytes can then bind avidly to such microbe-activated endothelial cells.[135] Extracellular bacteria circulating in the vascular system will then bind directly to the monocyte surface, inducing the release of tissue thromboplastin (tissue factor).[136, 137] This latter molecule participates in the catalytic conversion of prothrombin to thrombin, amplifying the procoagulant cascade at the site of endothelial cell colonization and leading to progressive evolution of the vegetative lesion in IE.

Immunopathologic Factors

Infective endocarditis causes the stimulation of both humoral and cellular immunity as manifested by hypergammaglobulinemia, splenomegaly, and the presence of macrophages in the peripheral blood. The possibility that preformed antibody can increase the likelihood of the development of IE was suggested by the spontaneous occurrence of IE in horses receiving repeated immunizations with live pneumococci.[138] It was suggested that these antibodies produced bacterial agglutination in vivo that increased the chances of valvular colonization. Studies in animals have suggested a protective role for circulating antibody. Rabbits preimmunized with heat-killed streptococci plus Freund's adjuvant had a significantly higher ID_{50} than that noted for nonimmunized controls after aortic valve trauma.[139] Other studies have yielded similar results with *S. sanguis, S. mutans,* and *S. pneumoniae.*[140, 141] In other experiments, antibody directed against cell surface components (including mannan) reduced the adhesion of *C. albicans* to fibrin and platelets in vitro and endocarditis production in vivo.[142] This effect may be dependent on the infecting organism, however, because antibody to *S. epidermidis* and *S. aureus* does not prevent the development of endocarditis in immunized animals or result in reduced bacterial concentrations in infected vegetations or kidneys,[143] perhaps because of the inability of immune sera to enhance opsonophagocytosis of staphylococci. Therefore, the role of preformed antibody in the pathogenesis of IE remains unclear. Intravascular agglutination of bacteria may, in fact, decrease the frequency of endocarditis by reducing the actual number of circulating organisms, but cross-protection is not achieved by passive transfer of high-titer immune globulin from *S. defectivus*–immunized rabbits to control animals.[141] Furthermore, nitrogen mustard–treated immunized rabbits lose their ability to efficiently clear *S. defectivus* from the circulation, a process partially restored by neutrophil transfusion.[144]

The role of the glycocalyx of *S. aureus,* and of antibodies directed against this exopolysaccharide, in the pathogenesis of IE remains controversial. Most experimental studies suggest that microencapsulation of strains by the common capsular types (5 and 8) may actually mitigate virulence of the organism in IE by obscuring key surface-expressed adhesins involved in colonization or persistence at endovascular damage sites.[145] Of interest, several recent studies have suggested a salutary effect of active or passive immunization strategies against this glycocalyx, in diminishing either the induction, progression, or metastatic infection phases of experimental IE.[146, 147]

Rheumatoid factor (anti-IgG IgM antibody) develops in about 50% of patients with IE of greater than 6 weeks' duration.[148] Rheumatoid factors have been found at the time of admission in 24% of the patients with acute staphylococcal endocarditis (less than 6 weeks' duration), and the frequency increased to 40% if fever persisted for 2 weeks after the initiation of antibiotic therapy.[149] Over two thirds of the patients became seronegative after 6 weeks of therapy, and two patients with a second episode of acute IE promptly redeveloped positive rheumatoid factors. The titers correlate with the level of hypergammaglobulinemia and decrease with therapy. Rheumatoid factor may play a role in the disease process by blocking IgG opsonic activity (by reacting with the Fc fragment), stimulating phagocytosis, or accelerating microvascular damage. Rheumatoid factor (IgM) has not been eluted from the immune complex glomerulonephritis associated with IE.[150] Antinuclear antibodies also occur in IE and may contribute to the musculoskeletal manifestations, low-grade fever, or pleuritic pain.[151]

Infective endocarditis, like malaria, schistosomiasis, syphilis, kala-azar, and leprosy, is associated with a constant intravascular antigenic challenge; therefore, the development of several classes of circulating antibody is not unexpected. Opsonic (IgG), agglutinating (IgG, IgM), and complement-fixing (IgG, IgM) antibodies and cryoglobulins (IgG, IgM, IgA, C3, fibrinogen), various antibodies to bacterial heat-shock proteins, and macroglobulins all have been described in IE.[152–154] Using the sensitive Raji cell or one C1q deviation techniques, circulating immune complexes have been found in high titers in virtually all patients with IE.[155] Circulating immune complexes are found with increased frequency in connection with a long duration of illness, extravalvular manifestations, hypocomplementemia, and right-sided IE. Levels fall and become undetectable with successful therapy. Patients with IE and circulating immune complexes may develop a diffuse glomerulonephritis that is analogous to the nephritis seen with infected ventriculoatrial shunts.[156] Immune complexes plus complement are deposited subepithelially along the glomerular basement membrane to form a "lumpy-bumpy" pattern. Immunoglobulin eluted from these lesions has been shown to cross react with bacterial antigens.[157] In addition, bacterial antigens have actually been demonstrated within circulating immune complexes.[158] Some of the peripheral manifestations of IE, such as Osler nodes, may also result from a deposition of circulating immune complexes. Pathologically these lesions resemble an acute Arthus reaction. However, the finding of positive culture aspirates in Osler nodes[159] suggests that they may in fact be due to septic emboli rather than immune complex deposition. In some diffuse purpuric lesions in IE, immune complex deposits (IgG, IgM, and complement) have been demonstrated in the dermal blood vessels by immunofluorescence.[160] Quantitative determinations of serum immune complex concentrations are useful in gauging the response to therapy. Effective treatment leads to a prompt decrease, with eventual disappearance of circulating immune complexes.[161] Conversely, therapeutic failures or relapses are characterized by rising titers or a reappearance of circulating immune complexes.[162]

Pathologic Changes

Heart. The classic vegetation of IE is usually located along the line of closure of a valve leaflet on the atrial surface for atrioventricular valves or the ventricular surface for semilunar valves. Vegetations may be single or multiple, are a few millimeters to several centimeters in size, and vary in color, consistency, and gross appearance. Microscopically, the lesion consists primarily of fibrin, platelet aggregates, and bacterial masses; neutrophils and red blood cells are rare. Destruction of the underlying valve may coexist. With treatment, healing occurs by fibrosis and occasionally calcification. The vegetation in acute cases is larger, softer, and more friable and may be associated with suppuration, more necrosis, and less healing than in subacute cases.[48, 163] This infection may lead to perforation of the valve leaflet, rupture of the chordae tendinae, interventricular septum, or papillary muscle. Staphylococcal endocarditis frequently results in valve ring abscesses[164] with fistula formation into areas of the myocardium or pericardial sac. Aneurysms of the valve leaflet or sinus of Valsalva are also common. Valvular stenosis may result from large vegetations. Myocarditis, myocardial infarction, and pericarditis[163, 164] are frequently found at autopsy. Myocardial abscesses are found in 20% of the autopsy cases and are associated primarily with acute staphylococcal endocarditis with hectic fever, a rapid onset of congestive heart failure, and conduction disturbances. Myocardial infarcts are found in as many as 40 to 60% of the autopsied cases, often without diagnostic changes in the electrocardiogram. Pericarditis is much more common in acute IE.

Although echocardiographic abnormalities are common in patients with AIDS, pericardial disease (pericarditis, effusions), myocardial disease leading to heart failure or arrhythmias, NBTE, and Kaposi sarcoma are all more frequent than IE.[165] AIDS patients with IE are usually intravenous drug users with right-sided involvement, with an increase in the prevalence of cases due to *S. aureus* or fungi.[165, 166] The clinical course in AIDS patients is often more fulminant than IE in intravenous drug users without AIDS; pneumonia and sepsis are common. IE has also been described in the transplanted heart.

Embolic phenomena are common in IE. In the preantibiotic era, 70 to 95% of the patients had clinically demonstrable embolic events, but this has decreased to 15 to 35% today. Pathologic evidence of embolization is still detected in 45 to 65% of autopsies, most frequently involving the renal, splenic, coronary, or cerebral circulation. Emboli and immune complex deposition contribute to the extracardiac manifestations of IE and may involve virtually any organ system. When large emboli occlude major vessels, fungal endocarditis, marantic endocarditis, or an intracardiac myxoma should be suspected.

Kidney. Three pathologic processes may be found in the kidney in IE: abscess, infarction, or glomerulonephritis. Abscesses are infrequent, but infarctions have been seen in 56% of the autopsy cases.[1] The kidney is usually normal in size but may be slightly swollen, and petechiae may be found in the capsule. When renal biopsies are done during active IE, the renal architecture is abnormal in *all* cases,[167] even in the absence of clinical or biochemical evidence of renal disease. "Focal" glomerulonephritis is found in 48 to 88% of the cases but is rare in acute IE. It is a focal, local, and segmental process characterized by endothelial and mesangial proliferation, hemorrhage, neutrophilic infiltration, fibrinoid necrosis, crescent formation, and healing by fibrosis. Diffuse glomerulonephritis is found in 17 to 80% of the cases and consists of generalized cellular hyperplasia in all glomerular tufts. A less common condition called *membranoproliferative glomerulonephritis* is associated with endocarditis due to *S. epidermidis* and characterized by marked mesangial proliferation and by splitting of the glomerular basement membrane. Renal interstitial cellular infiltration is common.[167]

Of the patients with IE, 10 to 15% will exhibit an immune complex glomerulonephritis similar to that seen in lupus erythematosus.[156, 157, 161, 162] The evidence for immune complex deposition rather than recurrent embolic phenomenon as the primary pathogenic mechanism includes the following:

1. Bacteria are rarely if ever seen in the lesions.
2. Glomerulonephritis can occur with right-sided IE.
3. Glomerulonephritis is rare in acute IE even though large, friable vegetations result in widespread metastatic abscess formation.
4. Immunofluorescent staining with anti-immunoglobulin antibody reveals the typical lumpy-bumpy distribution seen in other forms of immune complex nephritis.
5. In diffuse glomerulonephritis, subepithelial electron-dense deposits are seen by electron microscopy, with IgG, IgM, IgA, or complement demonstrated in these deposits by immunofluorescence.
6. Specific antibacterial antibody can be eluted from the lesions.[157]
7. Anti–glomerular basement membrane antibody has been found in a single case of IE with nephritis.
8. The glomerulonephritis is often accompanied by hypocomplementemia, with a positive result on serum assay for rheumatoid factor.
9. All these abnormalities usually resolve with successful antimicrobial therapy as the concentration of circulating immune complexes declines.

Mycotic Aneurysms. Mycotic aneurysms usually develop during active IE but are occasionally detected months or years after successful treatment. They are more common with viridans streptococcal infections and are found in 10 to 15% of autopsied cases. They may arise by any of the following mechanisms: (1) direct bacterial invasion of the arterial wall with subsequent abscess formation or rupture, (2) septic or bland embolic occlusion of the vasa vasorum, or (3) immune complex deposition with resultant injury to the arterial wall. The aneurysms tend to occur at bifurcation points. They are found most commonly in the cerebral vessels (primarily the peripheral branches of the middle cerebral artery), but they also occur in the abdominal aorta, sinus of Valsalva, a ligated patent ductus arteriosus, and the splenic, coronary, pulmonary, and superior mesenteric arteries. Myoctic aneurysms are usually clinically silent until rupture occurs; consequently, their true incidence in active IE is unknown.[168]

Central Nervous System. Cerebral emboli occur in at least one third of all cases[48] and most commonly affect the middle cerebral artery and its branches. Three percent of the cerebral emboli from all causes are secondary to IE. Cerebral infarction, arteritis, abscesses, mycotic aneurysms, intracerebral or subarachnoid hemorrhage, encephalomalacia, cerebritis, and meningitis all have been reported.[169] Hemorrhagic transformation of an ischemic infarct due to septic emboli is the most frequent mechanism leading to fatal intracerebral hemorrhage during IE.[170] True acute purulent meningitis is rare except in pneumococcal endocarditis, but multiple microabscesses (cerebritis) due to *S. aureus* are relatively common in acute staphylococcal endocarditis.

Spleen. Splenic infarctions have been reported in 44% of the autopsy cases but are often clinically silent.[48] Abscess formation and rupture have been described but are uncommon. Splenic enlargement is common, and virtually all cases are associated with hyperplasia of the lymphoid follicles, an increase in secondary follicles, proliferation of reticuloendothelial cells, and scattered focal necrosis.[163] Occasional cases of spontaneous rupture of the spleen have been observed.

Lung. When right-sided IE is present, pulmonary embolism with or without infarction, acute pneumonia, pleural effusion, or empyema is common; the emboli may be septic or bland in type.

Skin. Petechiae are found in 20 to 40% of the cases (Fig. 65–2) (see below). Osler nodes consist microscopically of arteriolar intimal proliferation with extension to venules and capillaries and may be accompanied by thrombosis and necrosis. A diffuse perivascular infiltrate consisting of neutrophils and monocytes surrounds the dermal vessels. Immune complexes have been demonstrated in the dermal vessels. Janeway lesions consist of bacteria, neutrophilic infiltration, necrosis, and subcutaneous hemorrhage (Fig. 65–3). Janeway lesions are due to septic emboli and reveal subcutaneous abscesses on histologic examination.[171]

Eye. "Roth spots" consist microscopically of lymphocytes surrounded by edema and hemorrhage in the nerve fiber layer of the retina (Fig. 65–4).[172]

Clinical Manifestations

The interval between an event likely to produce high-grade bacteremia (e.g., dental extraction) and the onset of symptoms of IE, contrary to older estimates, is actually quite short. The so-called

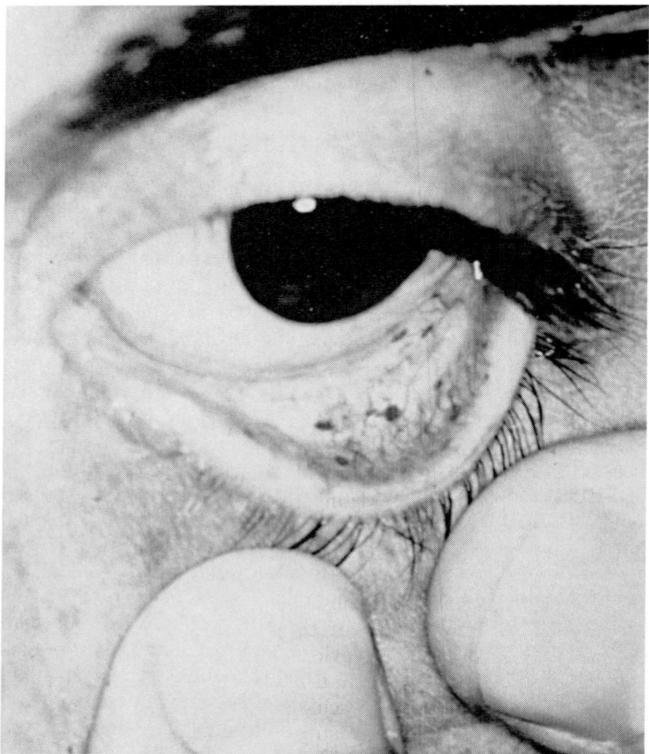

FIGURE 65–2. Conjunctival petechiae in a patient with bacterial endocarditis.

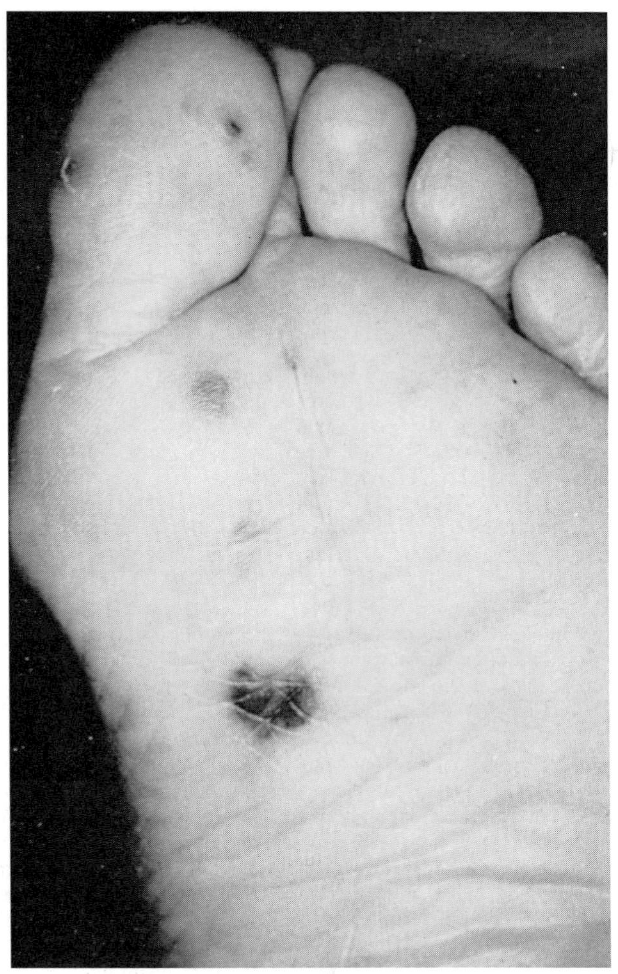

FIGURE 65–3. Janeway lesions in a patient with *Staphylococcus aureus* endocarditis. (From Sande MA, Strausbaugh LJ. Infective endocarditis. In: Hook EW, Mandell GL, Gwaltney JM Jr, et al, eds. Current Concepts of Infectious Diseases. New York: Wiley Press; 1977.)

"incubation period" in 84% of 76 cases of streptococcal endocarditis was less than 2 weeks.[173] However, the time from the onset of symptoms to diagnosis in the subacute form of IE is quite long, with a median interval of approximately 5 weeks. Symptom duration of cases managed in community hospitals is often shorter than in patients referred to a tertiary care center, reflecting "referral bias."[4]

The symptoms and signs (Table 65–3) are protean, and essentially any organ system may be involved. Four processes contribute to the clinical picture[48]: (1) the infectious process on the valve, including the local intracardiac complications; (2) bland or septic embolization to virtually any organ; (3) constant bacteremia, often with metastatic foci of infection; and (4) circulating immune complexes and other immunopathologic factors.[44–48, 174, 175] As a result, the clinical presentation of patients with IE is highly variable and the differential diagnosis often broad.[176]

Fever is common but may be absent (5% of the cases), especially in the setting of congestive heart failure (CHF), renal failure, a terminal disease, old age,[177] or previous antibiotic therapy. The fever pattern is usually remittent, and the patient's temperature rarely exceeds 40°C (103°F) except in acute IE.[174] Persistent fever during antimicrobial therapy of IE is relatively infrequent but may be an ominous sign. In a review[178] of 123 patients with IE managed in Cleveland from 1972 to 1984, approximately one half became afebrile within 3 days of the initiation of antibiotics; approximately 75% and approximately 90% had defervesced after 1 and 2 weeks of treatment, respectively. Prolonged fever (of ≥2 weeks' duration) is associated with specific etiologic agents (i.e., *S. aureus*, gram-negative bacilli, fungi, culture-negative endocarditis) but, perhaps more important, microvascular phenomena, embolization of major vessels, intracardiac (e.g., myocardial abscess) or peripheral complications, tissue infarction, a need for cardiac surgery, and a higher mortality rate.[178, 179] Pulmonary emboli (bland), drug reactions, and nosocomial infection unrelated to IE are also causes of prolonged fever in this patient population.

Nonspecific symptoms such as anorexia, weight loss, malaise, fatigue, chills, weakness, nausea, vomiting, and night sweats are common, especially in subacute cases.[20] These nonspecific symptoms often result in an incorrect diagnosis of malignancy, collagen vascular disease, tuberculosis, or other chronic diseases.

Audible heart murmurs occur in over 85% of the cases but may be absent with right-sided or mural infection. The classic "changing murmur" and the development of a new regurgitant murmur (usually aortic insufficiency) are uncommon and occur in 5 to 10% and in 3 to 5% of the cases, respectively. When present, these are diagnostically useful signs and usually complicate acute staphylococcal disease. New or changing murmurs are less common in the elderly and often lead to diagnositc confusion.[177, 180] Over 90% of patients who demonstrate a new regurgitant murmur will develop CHF. The incidence of CHF appears to be increasing (approximately 25% in 1966 and 67% in 1972)[20] and is now the leading cause of death in IE. Pericarditis is rare but, when present, is usually accompanied by myocardial abscess formation as a complication of staphylococcal infection. Although valvular regurgitation is the most important hemodynamic complication of IE, hemodynamically significant valvular obstruction requiring surgery may occur rarely, even without a prior history of valvular stenosis.[181]

The classic peripheral manifestations are found in up to one half of the cases, but the prevalence has decreased in recent years. Clubbing is present in 10 to 20%, especially if the disease is of long duration, and may recede with therapy. The complete syndrome of hypertrophic osteoarthropathy is rare. Splinter hemorrhages are linear red to brown streaks in the fingernails or toenails and are commonly found in IE. They are a nonspecific finding and are often seen in the elderly or in people experiencing occupation-related trauma. These

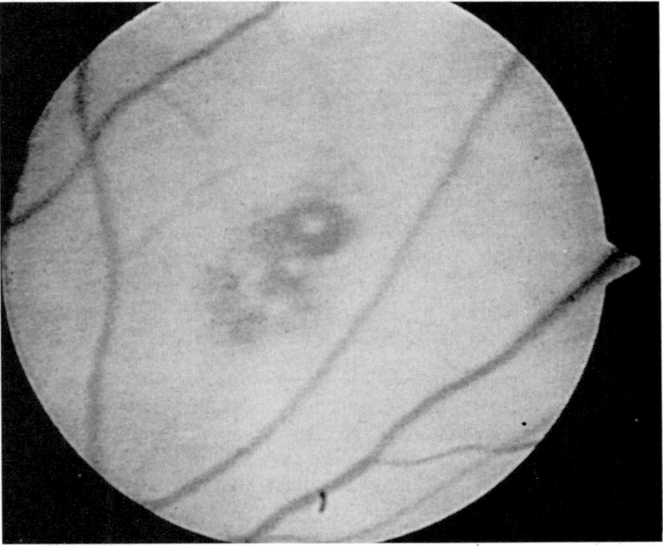

FIGURE 65–4. Retina from a patient with viridans streptococcal endocarditis showing Roth spots. (From Sande MA, Strausbaugh LJ. Infective endocarditis. In: Hook EW, Mandell GL, Gwaltney JM Jr, et al, eds. Current Concepts of Infectious Diseases. New York: Wiley Press; 1977.)

TABLE 65–3 Clinical Manifestations of Infective Endocarditis

Symptoms	% of Patients Affected	Signs	% of Patients Affected
Fever	80	Fever	90
Chills	40	Heart murmur	85
Weakness	40	Changing murmur	5–10
Dyspnea	40	New murmur	3–5
Sweats	25	Embolic phenomenon	>50
Anorexia	25	Skin manifestations	18–50
Weight loss	25	Osler nodes	10–23
Malaise	25	Splinter hemorrhages	15
Cough	25	Petechiae	20–40
Skin lesions	20	Janeway lesion	<10
Stroke	20	Splenomegaly	20–57
Nausea/vomiting	20	Septic complications (pneumonia, meningitis, etc.)	20
Headache	20	Mycotic aneurysms	20
Myalgia/arthralgia	15	Clubbing	12–52
Edema	15	Retinal lesion	2–10
Chest pain	15	Signs of renal failure	10–5
Abdominal pain	15		
Delirium/coma	10–15		
Hemoptysis	10		
Back pain	10		

Data from refs. 1, 20, 31, 174.

lesions are most suggestive of IE when located proximally in the nailbed. Petechiae are found in 20 to 40% of the cases, particularly after a prolonged course, and usually appear in crops on the conjunctivae (see Fig. 65–2), buccal mucosa, palate, and extremities. These lesions are initially red and nonblanching but become brown and barely visible in 2 to 3 days. Petechiae may result from either local vasculitis or emboli. Osler nodes are small, painful, nodular lesions usually found in the pads of fingers or toes and occasionally in the thenar eminence. They are 2 to 15 mm in size and are frequently multiple and evanescent, disappearing in hours to days. Osler nodes are rare in acute cases of IE but occur in 10 to 25% of all the cases. They are not specific for IE because they may be seen in systemic lupus erythematosus, marantic endocarditis, hemolytic anemia, and gonococcal infections and in extremities with cannulated radial arteries. Janeway lesions (see Fig. 65–3) are hemorrhagic, macular, painless plaques with a predilection for the palms or soles. They persist for several days and are thought to be embolic in origin and occur with greater frequency in staphylococcal endocarditis. Roth spots (see Fig. 65–4) are oval, pale, retinal lesions surrounded by hemorrhage and are usually located near the optic disk. They occur in less than 5% of the cases of IE and may also be found in anemia, leukemia, and connective tissue disorders such as systemic lupus erythematosus.

Splenomegaly has been reported in 25 to 60% of all the cases and is more common in patients with IE of prolonged duration. The incidence of splenomegaly appears to be progressively decreasing since the advent of antibiotics. Splenic septic emboli are common during IE, but localized signs and symptoms may be absent in approximately 90% of patients with this complication.[182] Abdominal computed tomography (CT) is highly sensitive and should be employed in cases with prolonged fever or sepsis. Serial CT studies can usually distinguish between bland septic emboli and splenic abscess.[183]

Musculoskeletal manifestations are common in IE. In a review of 192 cases,[184] 44% of the patients had musculoskeletal symptoms. These symptoms usually occurred early in the disease and were the only initial complaint in 15% of the cases. They included proximal oligo- or monoarticular arthralgias (38%), lower extremity mono- or oligoarticular arthritis (31%), low back pain (23%), and diffuse myalgias (19%). The back pain may be severe, limiting movement, and the initial complaint in 5 to 10% of cases.[10] These findings may mimic those in rheumatic disease, resulting in a diagnostic delay.

Major embolic episodes, as a group, are second only to CHF as a complication of IE and occur in at least one third of cases. Splenic artery emboli (as noted previously) with infarction may result in left upper quadrant abdominal pain with radiation to the left shoulder, a splenic or pleural rub, or a left pleural effusion. Renal infarctions may be associated with microscopic or gross hematuria, but renal failure, hypertension, and edema are uncommon. Retinal artery emboli are rare (occurring in fewer than 2% of the cases) and may be manifested by a sudden complete loss of vision. A panophthalmitis has been reported with pneumococcal IE. Pulmonary emboli secondary to right-sided IE constitute a common feature in narcotic addicts (see further on). Coronary artery emboli usually arise from the aortic valve and may cause myocarditis with arrythmias or myocardial infarction. This finding may be overlooked, especially given the time constraints of interventions such as thrombolytic therapy or angioplasty during acute myocardial infarction resulting in serious complications in patients with IE presenting as an acute myocardial infarction.[185] Major vessel emboli (affecting the femoral, brachial, popliteal, or radial artery) are more frequent in fungal endocarditis.

Neurologic manifestations occur in 20 to 40% of the cases and may dominate the clinical picture, especially in staphylococcal endocarditis. A sudden neurologic event in a young person should suggest IE. Major cerebral emboli afflict 10 to 30% of the patients and may result in hemiplegia, sensory loss, ataxia, aphasia, or an alteration in mental status.[169, 186] Of those patients with neurologic complications, up to 50% present with these signs and symptoms as the heralding features of their illness.[187, 188] The development of clinical neurologic deterioration during IE is associated with a two- to fourfold increase in mortality for the implicated etiologic microbe.[161] Mycotic aneurysms of the cerebral circulation occur in 2 to 10% of the cases. They are usually single, small, and peripheral and may lead to devastating subarachnoid hemorrhage. Other features include seizures, severe headache, visual changes (particularly homonymous hemianopsias), choreoathetoid movements, mononeuropathy, and cranial nerve palsies. A toxic encephalopathy with symptoms ranging from a mild change in personality to frank psychosis may occur, especially in elderly patients.

Patients with IE may have symptoms of uremia. In the preantibiotic era, renal failure developed in 25 to 35% of the patients, but presently fewer than 10% are affected. When uremia does develop, diffuse glomerulonephritis with hypocomplementemia is usually found, but focal glomerulonephritis has also been implicated. Renal failure is more common with long-standing disease but is usually reversible with appropriate antimicrobial treatment alone. IE may be confused with thrombotic thrombocytopenic purpura when neurologic signs, fever, renal failure, anemia, and thrombocytopenia are present.[189]

Infective Endocarditis in Drug Addicts

Acute infection accounts for approximately 60% of hospital admissions among intravenous drug users; IE is implicated in 5 to 15% of these episodes.[190] It has proved difficult to predict accurately the presence of IE in the febrile drug addict,[191] especially from history and physical examination findings alone,[192] although cocaine use by the intravenous drug user should heighten the suspicion of IE.[193] Cocaine was strongly associated with the presence of IE in 102 intravenous drug users in San Francisco when findings were analyzed by logistic regression analysis, but no such correlation was found among febrile addicts who did not use cocaine. The most reliable predictors of IE in febrile parenteral drug users are visualization of vegetations by echocardiography and the presence of embolic phenomena.[192] Although many of the aforementioned clinical manifestations are seen in addicts with IE, several distinctions are worthy of emphasis. In this group of patients, two thirds have no clinical evidence of underlying heart disease, and there is a predilection for the infection to affect the tricuspid valve. Only 35% of addicts ultimately proved to have IE demonstrate heart murmurs on admission.[190] The frequency of valvular involvement is as follows: tricuspid alone or in combination with others, 52.2%; aortic alone, 18.5%; mitral alone, 10.8%; and aortic plus mitral, 12.5%.[2] However, left-sided involvement has been more frequent in some series.[194]

Of those patients with tricuspid valve infection, 30% have pleuritic chest pain; pulmonary findings may dominate the clinical picture, and the chest roentgenogram will document abnormalities (infiltrates, effusion, and so forth) in 75 to 85%.[195] Roentgenographic evidence of septic pulmonary emboli is eventually present in 87% of cases.[196] Signs of tricuspid insufficiency (gallop rhythm, systolic regurgitant murmur louder with inspiration, large V waves, or a pulsatile liver) are present in only one third of the cases. Most of these patients are 20 to 40 years old (80%), and men predominate in a ratio of 4 to 6:1. Almost two thirds of these patients have extravalvular sites of infection, which are helpful in the diagnosis.[195–197] The course of acute staphylococcal endocarditis in the addict tends to be less severe than in nonaddicts,[195] although this may not be true in AIDS patients. HIV-seropositive patients acquire IE by one of two mechanisms: through intravenous drug abuse (IVDA) or as a complication of long-term central venous catheterization for administration of medications (e.g., for cytomegalovirus retinitis). In either situation, *S. aureus* is the most common etiologic organism. In the absence of IVDA, HIV-seropositive patients develop left-sided and right-sided IE with equal frequencies.[198] In contrast, in the setting of IVDA, HIV-seropositive patients develop predominantly right-sided IE. The IE-related morbidity and mortality rates in HIV-seropositive patients who do not have an AIDS-defining illness or criteria are similar to those in HIV-seronegative counterparts.[198]

Laboratory Findings

Hematologic parameters are often abnormal in IE, but none is diagnostic. Anemia is nearly always present (70 to 90% of the cases), especially in subacute cases, and has the characteristics of the anemia of chronic disease, with normochromic, normocytic indices, a low serum iron concentration, and a low iron-binding capacity. The anemia tends to worsen with the duration of the illness. Thrombocytopenia occurs in 5 to 15% of the cases but is common in neonatal IE. Leukocytosis is present in 20 to 30% of cases but is rare in the subacute variety, whereas counts of 15,000 to 25,000/mm^3 are not uncommon in acute IE. The differential count is usually normal, but there may be a slight shift to the left. Leukopenia is uncommon (5 to 15%) and, when present, is usually associated with splenomegaly. Large mononuclear cells (histiocytes) can be detected in the peripheral blood in approximately 25% of the patients, but the yield is higher in blood obtained by earlobe puncture. This finding is nonspecific, because similar cells have been found in malaria, typhus, typhoid fever, and tuberculosis.

The erythrocyte sedimentation rate (ESR) is nearly always (in 90 to 100% of cases) elevated, with a mean value of 57 mm/hr found in one large series.[20] In the absence of renal failure, CHF, or disseminated intravascular coagulation, a normal ESR is evidence against a diagnosis of IE. Hypergammaglobulinemia is detected in 20 to 30% of the cases and may be accompanied by a plasmacytosis in the bone marrow aspirate. A positive result on assay for rheumatoid factor is found in 40 to 50% of the cases, especially when the duration of the illness is greater than 6 weeks.[148] Hypocomplementemia (seen in 5 to 15% of cases) parallels the incidence of abnormal renal function test results (elevated creatinine level in 5 to 15%). A false-positive result on Venereal Disease Research Laboratory (VDRL) testing is uncommon (0.2%). Lyme serologic tests may be positive in patients with IE living in areas endemic for Lyme disease, which may lead to diagnostic confusion and delay.[199]

The urinalysis is frequently abnormal; proteinuria occurs in 50 to 65% of the cases, and microscopic hematuria in 30 to 60%. Red cell casts may be seen in as many as 12% of the cases[20]; gross hematuria, pyuria, white cell casts, and bacteriuria may also be found.

Circulating immune complexes can be detected in most cases of IE but are also found in 32% of the patients with septicemia but without endocarditis, in 10% of healthy persons, and in 40% of noninfected narcotic addicts.[148] However, levels of aggregated human γ-globulin equivalent greater than 100 μg/ml were found only in IE (35% of the cases). Detection of high levels of immune complexes may be useful in the diagnosis of right-sided IE in narcotic addicts or in culture-negative cases. In addition, because the levels fall with appropriate treatment, serial measurement of immune complexes may assist in management of the disease.[161, 162] Mixed-type cryoglobulins are detectable in 84 to 95% of the patients with IE but also constitute a nonspecific finding. Serial determination of the serum C-reactive protein concentration, although nonspecific and virtually always elevated in IE, may be useful to monitor therapy and detect intercurrent complications or infections.[200]

The detection of vegetations by gallium 67 (^{67}Ga) myocardial imaging initially appeared to be a useful diagnostic tool. Of 11 patients in one study,[201] 7 had infected vegetations localized by scans including one culture-negative case that was confirmed at autopsy. Further studies are needed to determine the potential value of noninvasive imaging of cardiac vegetations by using a radiolabeled compound, for example, technetium 99m (^{99m}Tc)–labeled antibacterial antibody[202] or indium 111 (^{111}In)–labeled platelets,[203] because both have shown promise in experimental endocarditis. At present, these techniques must be considered investigational. Radiographic techniques are occasionally useful in the diagnosis or in decisions regarding surgical intervention. For example, computed tomography (CT) of the abdomen detected splenic infarcts in 6 of 25 (24%) consecutive patients with IE in one series[204]: 2 of these 6 were asymptomatic.

The blood culture is the single most important laboratory test performed in a diagnostic workup for IE. The bacteremia is usually continuous and low-grade (80% of the cases have less than 100 cfu/ml of blood).[205] In approximately two thirds of the cases, all the blood specimens drawn will yield positive results on culture.[20] When bacteremia is present, the first two blood cultures will yield the etiologic agent more than 90% of the time. In a review of 206 cases of IE seen over a 15-year period at The New York Hospital,[206] 95% of the blood cultures were positive. In streptococcal endocarditis, the first blood culture was positive in 96% of cases, and one of the first two cultures was positive in 98%. When antibiotics had been administered in the previous 2 weeks, the rate of positive cultures declined from 97% to 91% ($p < .02$). The influence of outpatient antibiotic administration on blood culture positivity was more significant in another retrospective analysis[207]; 64% of 88 cultures were positive in 17 patients receiving antibiotics before hospitalization versus 100% in 15 patients without antibiotic exposure. In nonstreptococcal endocarditis, the first blood culture was positive in 86% of the cases and when two cultures were taken, in 100%. Most blood cultures contained only a few organisms; over 50% of the cultures contained 1 to 30 bacteria/ml. Only 17% of the cultures yielded more than 100 bacteria/ml. The bacteremia was also constant, with little variation in quantitative culture determinations in any individual patient. The sensitivity of blood cultures for the detection of streptococci is particularly susceptible to prior antibiotic therapy and is also affected by the media employed.[208]

On the basis of these studies, the following procedures for culturing blood are recommended. At least three blood culture sets (no more than two bottles per venipuncture) should be obtained in the first 24 hours. More specimens may be necessary if the patient has received antibiotics in the preceding 2 weeks. At least 10 ml of blood (when feasible) should be injected into both trypticase soy (or brain-heart infusion) and thioglycolate broth.[209, 210] Supplementation with 15% sucrose (in an attempt to isolate cell wall–deficient forms) or the use of prereduced anaerobic media is unrewarding.[211] The newer commercial media are also effective, but comparative data are few. In general, culture of arterial blood offers no advantage over use of venous blood. Inspection for macroscopic growth should be performed daily and routine subcultures done on days 1 and 3. The cultures should be held for at least 3 weeks. When gram-positive cocci grow on the initial isolation but fail to grow on subculture, nutritionally variant (thiol-dependent) streptococci should be suspected.[212] In this event, subculture inoculation should be onto media supplemented with either 0.05 to 0.1% L-cysteine or 0.001% pyridoxal phosphate.

Intraleukocytic bacteria have been visualized in peripheral blood in approximately 50% of the cases[213] by a simple "monolayer" technique. This may be helpful in culture-negative cases or when patients have been receiving antibiotics.[214]

Ribitol teichoic acids are major constituents of the cell wall of staphylococci. Gel diffusion and counterimmunoelectrophoresis techniques have been used to detect teichoic acid antibodies in the serum of patients suspected of having *S. aureus* endocarditis. Teichoic acid antibodies can be detected by counterimmunoelectrophoresis in over 95% of the patients,[215] but the rate of false-positive tests may exceed 10%. Serial titrations of serum with the double-agar diffusion technique can be used to detect the low titers found in some healthy people. Antibody titers of 1:4 or more are indicative of disseminated staphylococcal disease (endocarditis, multiple metastatic abscesses, or hematogenous osteomyelitis). Because these conditions all require prolonged antimicrobial therapy, this test may be of practical value if the results are positive. The value of a negative result is controversial; some authorities suggest that a short course of antimicrobial therapy is justified in this instance,[216] whereas others find a negative test response helpful only if all clinical signs are indicative of "benign" (i.e., superficial) staphylococcal bacteremia.[217] This issue is unresolved; we view this test as confirmatory of clinical suspicions only.

Special Diagnostic Tests. Special diagnostic tests are not routinely used (with the exception of echocardiography) in all cases of IE but may be useful in two situations: (1) in the diagnostic approach to culture-negative IE and (2) in decisions about surgical intervention during active infection.

The incidence of so-called blood culture–negative endocarditis has ranged from 2.5% to 31% in published series.[218, 219] If the patient has not received previous antibiotic therapy and the blood cultures are obtained as outlined, these cases should represent fewer than 5% of the total.[3] Some of the aforementioned tests (assays for rheumatoid factor and teichoic acid antibodies, examination of earlobe blood specimens for histiocytes, monolayer technique for detection of intraleukocytic bacteria) may be helpful in identifying such cases, but other procedures are often necessary. If the patient has received antibiotics, blood cultures in hypertonic media may allow detection of cell wall–defective organisms. Supplementation of media with vitamin B_6 or with cysteine may assist in the recovery of nutritionally variant streptococci (NVS). The lysis-centrifugation blood culture technique assists in the detection of staphylocci[220] and fungi, but NVS (now classified as *Abiotrophia* spp.) do not survive this procedure, and yields of pneumococci and anaerobes are decreased.[221] Routine use of this technique is not indicated, but it may be helpful in suspected culture-negative cases of IE. Because some anaerobes, *Brucella* spp., and members of the HACEK group (see "Unusual Gram-Negative Bacteria") are slow-growing organisms, holding cultures for 4 weeks may increase the recovery rate. Special efforts to neutralize or inactivate antimicrobial agents present in blood, such as the addition of penicillinase or of antibiotic-removal resins, do not substantially enhance the yield of positive blood cultures in IE and also increase the incidence of laboratory contamination of the blood culture. Thus, such maneuvers are not routinely recommended.[222, 223] Moreover, most automated blood culture detection systems use blood collection vials with antibiotic-binding resins. Cultures of bone marrow or urine may rarely be positive when blood cultures are negative. Serologic studies are necessary for the diagnosis of Q fever or murine typhus.[224] Psittacosis endocarditis is usually diagnosed with serologic methods but one recent case[225] yielded positive blood and pharyngeal cultures. Special culture techniques (e.g., for *Legionella* spp.[226]) are indicated in patients with suspected prosthetic valve endocarditis when initial cultures are "negative" (see Chapter 66). *Bartonella*, recently recognized as an important cause of apparent blood culture–negative IE (especially in homeless alcoholic patients), can also be isolated by prolonged incubation and subculture of the aerobic broth media.[227–231] Subculture on endothelial cell tissue may isolate *Bartonella* in certain cases.[227] Serologic strategies may also assist in the diagnosis of *Bartonella* IE.[228] In addition to blood culture and serodiagnostic strategies, as outlined previously, culture of valvular tissue or vegetations that have embolized to peripheral arteries, and which have been removed surgically, may yield the causative organism. Moreover, microscopy of such tissues, including direct fluorescence antibody techniques as well as electron microscopy, may also assist in making the etiologic diagnosis, particularly in cases caused by intracellular pathogens such as *Chlamydia, Coxiella*, and *Legionella*.[232] Furthermore, molecular techniques to recover specific DNA or 16S ribosomal RNA from tissue samples have been useful diagnostically in selected cases,[233] and polymerase chain reaction (PCR) studies performed on blood may be useful for the diagnosis of IE caused by difficult-to-grow pathogens such as *Bartonella*.[234] Other tests to exclude collagen vascular diseases are usually necessary in patients undergoing evaluation for culture-negative, native valve IE.[235]

Blood cultures are negative in over 50% of the cases of fungal endocarditis.[236] The lysis-centrifugation method of blood culture is also useful in detecting fungi. This form of the disease is increasing in frequency and usually affects narcotic addicts, patients with prosthetic valves, or hospitalized patients receiving antibiotics or hyperalimentation or both. Low-birth-weight neonates seem particularly prone to *Candida* IE, predominantly on the tricuspid valve or right atrial mural endocardium.[237] The Castaneda principle (a culture of blood in a bottle containing both agar and liquid broth) has been shown to increase the yield of fungal cultures.[211] Blastospores and pseudohyphae have been found in Wright-stained peripheral blood in at least one case of *Candida*-induced endocarditis.[238] Various serologic procedures have been used in an attempt to substantiate a diagnosis of fungal endocarditis. Tests for the determination of anti-*Candida* antibody are poorly standardized, variably sensitive, often nonspecific, and difficult to interpret.[239] In a rabbit model of *Candida*-induced endocarditis, both precipitating and agglutinating antibodies were detected after 12 days of active infection, and titers rose progressively until death of the animals.[240] In contrast, animals without endocarditis developed only a transient rise in antibody titers after a single intravenous injection of viable *C. albicans*. Tests for mannan antigenemia (a constituent of the cell wall of *Candida*) or enolase by hemagglutination inhibition or by the enzyme-linked immunosorbent assay (ELISA) method[241, 242] have been reported as helpful in the diagnosis of disseminated candidiasis. In addition, a reliable radioimmunoassay for the detection of *Aspergillus* antigenemia is currently under investigation. When embolism to major vessels occurs, an embolectomy should be performed, and the material should be examined by both special fungal stains and culture. Identification of the fungus by either technique is diagnostic of fungal endocarditis even when blood cultures are sterile.

The use of echocardiography in the diagnosis of IE was first reported in 1973.[243] Echocardiograms have correctly identified vegetations on all valves. Most reports have focused on left-sided disease. The sensitivity and the specificity of this technique are uncertain; however, two studies correctly identified 33 of 52 vegetations documented surgically or at autopsy with transthoracic methods.[244, 245] The characteristic finding is a shaggy dense band of irregular echoes in a nonuniform distribution on one or more leaflets, with full unrestricted motion of the valve. The smallest vegetation detected was approximately 2 mm, but the acoustic impedance of the mass relative to the surrounding structures is a more important factor than size in identifying the vegetation. The use of two-dimensional cross-sectional real-time techniques improves the diagnostic accuracy over M-mode methods.[246] If the vegetation is calcified (which may occur early and independent of the healing process), the sensitivity of echocardiography may be increased. Echocardiography has correctly localized vegetations in culture-negative cases. Echocardiography may be of special value in the detection of the large friable vegetations characteristic of fungal endocarditis. However, use of M-mode or two-dimensional transthoracic techniques with prosthetic heart valves has been disappointing because of the difficulty in resolution around the prosthetic device. Many reports[247] have evaluated the role of transthoracic echocardiography (TTE) in the diagnosis and management of suspected IE and have been summarized in cogent analyses.[248, 249] It appears from most analyses that TTE should be performed in all patients in whom IE appears to be a reasonable diagnosis. In contrast, TTE is not an appropriate screening test in the evaluation of febrile patients in whom IE is unlikely on clinical grounds, or in bacteremic patients with organisms that rarely cause IE (e.g., *E. coli*), particularly if there is another obvious focus to explain the clinical syndrome. TTE may be technically inadequate in up to 20% of adult patients owing to obesity, chronic obstructive pulmonary disease (COPD) or chest wall deformities. These studies also suggest the following: (1) TTE has variable sensitivity for the detection of vegetations (<50% to >90% positive), indicating that a negative study does not exclude IE; (2) the sensitivity of TTE for detecting vegetations is highest in right-sided IE, because the tricuspid and pulmonic valves lie relatively close to the chest wall; (3) false-positive results are extremely rare; (4) only technically adequate studies are of value, a characteristic heavily dependent on the experience of the person performing the examination; (5) echocardiography is extremely valuable in assessing local complications of IE, especially surrounding the aortic valve (however, the sensitivity for detecting such complications is relatively low for TTE [see further on]) and (6) patients with a "vegetation" identified by echocardiography are at an increased risk for subsequent systemic emboli, CHF, the need for emergency surgery, and death, especially with aortic valve involvement. This apparent influence on prognosis has hastened earlier surgery in some cases,[250] but this point remains controversial.[249, 251] Positive findings on the echocardiogram in a patient with IE should serve as adjunctive evidence, together with clinical parameters, in indicating surgical intervention. In one analysis from the Mayo Clinic,[252] emboli were not statistically more common in patients with left-sided native valve IE and echocardiographically documented vegetations within 72 hours of beginning antimicrobial therapy when compared with those without vegetations visualized by transthoracic techniques. The occurrence of emboli was positively correlated with the infecting microorganism, being more common in IE due to viridans streptococci than in *S. aureus* disease. Most studies suggest that mitral valve vegetations (particularly those attached to the anterior leaflet), regardless of size, are associated with higher rates of embolization (25%) than are noted with aortic valve vegetations (10%). This implicates the mechanical effects of abrupt mitral valve leaflet excursions, occurring twice per heart beat, in enhancing the embolic potential of vegetations.[253] Visualization of vegetations by echocardiography is not sufficient to prompt early surgery.[249, 254] Serial echocardiograms often reveal the persistence of vegetations after successful therapy, but sequential studies may be useful in the timing of surgical intervention. Short-term changes in vegetation size during therapy do not correlate well with clinical outcome.[255] However, a new technique, digital image processing of two-dimensional echocardiograms, may differentiate active from healed lesions.[256] If substantiated, this method may be useful in culture-negative cases (particularly with suspected recurrent IE) or when the response to therapy is suboptimal or inconclusive. One study suggested that an increase in vegetation size as seen by echocardiography during therapy of IE may well identify a subset of patients with a higher rate of complications, independent of the presence of persistent bacteremia or overt clinical stigmata of IE.[257] Some studies have suggested that highly mobile vegetations constitute an independent increase in risk for complications in IE.[258] However, in other studies, vegetation mobility on echocardiography has not been an important independent risk factor for embolic events in IE, because it is, in turn, strongly correlated with vegetation size (reviewed in ref. 259).[250]

Transesophageal echocardiography (TEE) has altered the diagnostic approach to some patients with suspected IE.[259–264] It utilizes a 5-mHz phased array transducer with Doppler and color flow-encoding capabilities mounted on the tip of a flexible endoscope. Biplane (horizontal and longitudinal) or omniplane imaging is preferred over TTE imaging because of (1) better spatial resolution with a higher frequency transducer; (2) lack of acoustic interference from the lungs, chest wall, and so forth; and (3) proximity to posterior structures (e.g., mitral valve, left atrium, interatrial septum, descending aorta).[261] TEE has proved useful in a wide variety of clinical situations, including detection of possible sources of emboli, diagnosis of thoracic aortic dissection, detection of prosthetic valve dysfunction, and evaluation of IE.[249, 259–261]

TEE is more sensitive than conventional TTE in the detection of intracardiac vegetations (approximately 95% and 60 to 65%, respectively), particularly in the setting of prosthetic valves (see Chapter 66). For example,[262] in one report of 96 patients with IE, the sensitivity of TEE was 100%, versus 63% for the transthoracic approach, with identical specificity values (98%). The advantage of TEE was particularly evident for vegetations less than 10 mm in diameter. In another study,[263] vegetations were detected by TEE in 82%, versus 69% for transthoracic echocardiography. Although negative results on TEE do not exclude IE,[259–261, 264] the procedure should be considered in patients with suspected IE and negative results on transthoracic study. Potential sources of false-negative TEE studies include very small vegetations and previous embolization of vegetations. When the clinical suspicion of IE is high and results of an initial TEE examination are negative, another TEE study is warranted within 7 to 10 days later.[204] TEE has also become the procedure of choice for the detection of perivalvular extension of infection in patients with IE.[265, 266] For example, Daniel and colleagues[266] reported diagnostic sensitivity and specificity of 87% and 95% for TEE for detection of IE-related abscess versus 28% and 99% for TTE. TEE should be performed (unless contraindicated, e.g., by significant esophageal disease) in all IE patients with a complicated course when perivalvular extension is suspected. Magnetic resonance imaging (MRI) also appears promising for the detection of these complications,[265] but clinical experience is limited. TEE is not a screening or noninvasive procedure but is generally safe[267] in experienced hands, and it may alter management in selected patients with proven or suspected IE. Furthermore, intraoperative TEE imaging has become a valuable new tool, often providing real-time feedback to the surgical team during the procedure.

In conjunction with the physical examination, phonocardiography, and electrocardiography, the echocardiogram may play an important role in assessing the severity of acute aortic insufficiency in cases of active IE.[268] In this setting, classic signs such as a wide pulse pressure and bounding pulses are often absent; however, there is usually a reduction in intensity of the first heart sound, and Austin Flint murmurs may be audible. Findings on the chest roentgenogram and electrocardiogram may be normal. The degree of mitral valve preclosure (as determined by echocardiography) correlates with the acute elevation in left ventricular end-diastolic pressure. If this event occurs before the Q wave on the electrocardiogram, urgent surgical intervention is recommended.

Cardiac catheterization with quantitative blood cultures obtained proximal and distal to suspected sites of infection has been useful in selected cases in the localization of vegetations in both right-sided and left-sided IE.[269] Multiple specimens from identical sites are necessary, because minor fluctuations in bacteremia do occur. Cardiac catheterization does provide valuable hemodynamic and anatomic information in patients with IE when surgical intervention is being considered.[197] Properly performed, the procedure is safe, as demonstrated by the lack of postcatheterization emboli or hemodynamic deterioration in 35 consecutive patients in one series.[270]

Previous diagnostic criteria for IE were published in 1982 by von Reyn and colleagues,[3] (Beth Israel criteria) but did not use echocardiographic findings in the case definitions, despite major improvements in echocardiographic technology (see previous discussion). In addition, the isolation of a "typical" IE pathogen from blood cultures was not considered in the Beth Israel definitions. Thus, many presumptive cases of IE were classified as not "definite" but "probable." With improved methodology *and* recognition of the central role of echocardiography in the evaluation of suspected IE, new case definitions and diagnostic criteria (the Duke criteria) proposed in 1994, are now widely used and have been accepted by most clinicians (Tables 65–4 and 65–5).[271] The new definitions retain, in slightly modified form, the pathologic parameters of the Beth Israel criteria[3] (see Table 65–4). The Duke criteria (modeled somewhat after the Jones criteria for diagnosing rheumatic fever[272]) build upon the Beth Israel criteria by including echocardiographic demonstration of vegetations or paravalvular complications of IE, as well as the isolation of typical IE pathogens from blood clutures, as "major criteria" for the clinically definite categorization of IE. In addition, the presence of recent IVDA is included in the Duke criteria as a "minor criterion" for diagnosing IE, recognizing the increased risk of IE in this patient population (see Table 65–5). Direct comparisons of the Duke and Beth Israel criteria have now been carried out in 11 major studies, including nearly 1400 patients. Patient populations from diverse geographic areas with presumed IE that have been studied include young, middle-aged, and geriatric adults; pediatric patients; patients with native or prosthetic valve involvement; and both IVDA and non-IVDA patients. These studies confirmed the increased sensitivity of the Duke criteria in clinically diagnosing IE and the diagnostic utility of echocardiography in identifying clinically definite cases (reviewed in detail by Bayer and associates[273]).

TABLE 64–4 Proposed Criteria for Diagnosis of Infective Endocarditis

Definite infective endocarditis
- Pathologic criteria
  - Microorganisms: demonstrated by culture *or* histology in a vegetation, or in a vegetation that has embolized, or in an intracardiac abscess, *or*
  - Pathologic lesions: vegetation or intracardiac abscess present, confirmed by histology showing active endocarditis
- Clinical criteria (using specific definitions for these terms as listed in Table 65–5)
  - 2 major criteria, *or*
  - 1 major and 3 minor criteria, *or*
  - 5 minor criteria

Possible infective endocarditis: findings consistent with infective endocarditis that fall short of *Definite*, but not *Rejected*

Rejected
- Firm alternate diagnosis explaining evidence of infective endocarditis, *or*
- Resolution of endocarditis syndrome, with antibiotic therapy for 4 days or less, *or*
- No pathologic evidence of infective endocarditis at surgery or autopsy, after antibiotic therapy for 4 days or less

Adapted from Durack DT, Lukes AS, Bright DK, et al. New criteria for diagnosis of infective endocarditis. Am J Med. 1994;96:200–209.

TABLE 65–5 Terminology Used in the Proposed Criteria for Infective Endocarditis

Major criteria

Positive blood culture for infective endocarditis
- Typical microorganism for infective endocarditis from 2 separate blood cultures
  - Viridans streptococci, *Streptococcus bovis*, HACEK group,* *or*
  - Community-acquired *Staphylococcus aureus* or enterococci, in the absence of a primary focus, *or*

Persistently positive blood cultures for any microorganism (i.e., from blood cultures drawn more than 12 hours apart), *or*

All of 3, or majority of 4 or more separate blood cultures, with first and last specimens drawn at least 1 hour apart

Evidence of endocardial involvement
- Findings on echocardiogram positive for infective endocarditis
  - Oscillating intracardiac mass on valve or supporting structures or in the path of regurgitant jets, or on iatrogenic devices, in the absence of an alternative anatomic explanation, *or*
  - Abscess, *or*
  - New partial dehiscence of prosthetic valve, *or*
- New valvular regurgitation (increase or change in preexisting murmur *not* sufficient)

Minor criteria

Predisposition: predisposing heart condition *or* intravenous drug use

Fever: ≥38.0°C (100.4°F)

Vascular phenomena: arterial embolism, septic pulmonary infarcts, mycotic aneurysm, intracranial hemorrhage, Janeway lesions

Immunologic phenomena: glomerulonephritis, Osler nodes, Roth spots, rheumatoid factor

Echocardiogram: findings consistent with infective endocarditis but not meeting major criterion above

Microbiologic evidence: positive blood culture but not meeting major criterion above, *or* serologic evidence of active infection with organism consistent with infective endocarditis

*As discussed in the text later on, the HACEK organisms are *Haemophilus*, *Actinobacillus*, *Cardiobacterium*, *Eikenella*, and *Kingella*.

Adapted from Durack DT, Lukes AS, Bright DK, et al. New criteria for diagnosis of infective endocarditis. Am J Med. 1994;96:200–209.

Etiologic Agents

Streptococci

A plethora of microorganisms have been implicated in IE, but streptococci and staphylococci account for 80 to 90% of the cases in which identification is made. The most common etiologic agents are outlined in Table 65–6. The streptococci still cause most cases of IE.[31] Although many community hospitals still report viridans streptococci as the most common isolates among patients with IE,[274, 275] and series from large tertiary care centers still represent these organisms among the major pathogens, staphylococci have assumed increasing importance among isolates in community hospitals in recent years (see farther on).[10, 275] Viridans streptococci remain the major

TABLE 65–6 Etiologic Agents in Infective Endocarditis

Agent	% of Cases
Streptococci	60–80
Viridans streptococci	30–40
Enterococci	5–18
Other streptococci	15–25
Staphylococci	20–35
Coagulase-positive	10–27
Coagulase-negative	1–3
Gram-negative aerobic bacilli	1.5–13
Fungi	2–4
Miscellaneous bacteria	<5
Mixed infections	1–2
Culture-negative	<5–24

cause of IE in children. The disease usually runs a subacute course with multiple nonspecific symptoms as outlined in Table 65–3. Over 80% of these patients have underlying heart disease. IE in young women with isolated mitral valve involvement is almost universally caused by viridans streptococci. Approximately 20% of the cases are seen because of embolic phenomena. With modern medical and surgical management, the cure rate should exceed 90% in nonenterococcal streptococcal endocarditis, although complications may ensue in more than 30% of cases.[274]

The nomenclature of the streptococci is confusing, and various authors differ in terminology used. As detailed in Chapters 191 and 192, current names for the α-hemolytic streptococci other than *S. pneumoniae* (i.e., "viridans streptococci") causing endocarditis are *S. mitis, S. sanguis, S. mutans, Streptococcus salivarius*, the "nutritionally variant streptococci" (now classified as *Abiotrophia* spp.), and some isolates of the "*S. intermedius* group" (*Streptococcus intermedius* and *Streptococcus anginosus*). *Streptococcus morbillorum* is now classified as *Gemella morbillorum; Streptococcus mitior* is now considered to be a "genospecies" of *S. mitis*. However, the name *S. mitior* is so deeply embeded in the endocarditis literature that it is retained in the discussion that follows. Group D streptococci are sometimes α-hemolytic, depending on the conditions and the isolate, but are not included among the viridans streptococci. Streptococci of the viridans group (not a true species) are α-hemolytic and usually nontypeable by the Lancefield system.

The most common streptococci isolated from cases of endocarditis are *S. sanguis, S. bovis, S. mutans,* and *S. mitior.*[71] In a series of 317 cases of streptococcal endocarditis, the breakdown was as follows: α-hemolytic, 45%; nonhemolytic, non–group D, 21%; group D, 25%; pyogenic (groups A, B, C, G), 5%; miscellaneous, 3%; and aerococci, 1.3%. The α-hemolytic strains included *S. sanguis* (16.4% of all cases of IE), nondextran-producing *S. mitior* (13.2%), dextran-positive *S. mitior* (7.3%), and an unclassified group (7.9%). Some isolates of *S. sanguis*, formerly called "*Streptococcus* SBE," are in Lancefield group H; however, most are nontypeable. *S. mutans* (14.2%), *S. anginosus* (5.4%), and *S. salivarius* (1.3%) comprised the nonhemolytic, non–group D strains. Group D organisms included the enterococci (8%) and *S. bovis* (17%). In another analysis,[276] viridans streptococci caused 58% of cases of IE at The New York Hospital from 1970 to 1978. The various responsible species were as follows: *S. mitior,* 31%; *S. bovis,* 27%; *S. sanguis,* 24%; *S. mutans,* 7%; vitamin B_6–dependent *S. mitior,* 5%; *S. anginosus,* 4%; and others, 2%—all of which are slightly different from those reported from the United Kingdom. A similar species distribution was observed in 48 patients (with 51 episodes of IE) reported from Washington, D.C.[277] There appears to be no correlation, however, between the clinical outcome and the species involved,[274, 277] with the exception of nutritionally deficient strains (see further on). Viridans streptococci remain the most commonly isolated pathogens in IE cases associated with mitral valve prolapse.[278] The relative role of each species overall is problematic, however, because species designations of identical strains among laboratories are often disparate,[274] and most blood and cerebrospinal fluid isolates of viridans or nonhemolytic streptococci are not from patients with IE.[279]

S. mutans, the etiologic agent in 14.2% of the cases in the review by Parker and Ball,[71] is microaerophilic, pleomorphic, and fastidious. Two thirds of strains will hydrolyze bile-esculin,[280] a test used to identify group D organisms, and thus may be confused with enterococci. Other characteristics of *S. mutans* include the absence of group D antigen (some strains are positive for group E), production of acid from mannitol, a failure to hydrolyze hippurate, and the formation of gelatinous deposits (dextran) in media containing 5% sucrose. This organism may be difficult to isolate and to identify. It often requires over 3 days for primary isolation, grows best on horse blood agar in 5 to 10% CO_2 on subculture, and is very pleomorphic, resulting in confusion with diphtheroids. *S. mutans* was first isolated in 1924 by Clark from dental caries lesions of humans and was first reported in 1928 to cause IE. The central importance of this organism in dental caries has been amply documented.

S. bovis is a normal inhabitant of the gastrointestinal tract of humans and many animal species. It is important to separate this organism from the other members of group D (the enterococci), because the respective therapeutic approaches to infection by these organisms are different (see further on). Group D organisms are presumptively identified by bile-esculin hydrolysis.[281, 282] However, only the enterococci (*E. faecalis* and its varieties *zymogenes* and *liquifaciens, Enterococcus faecium,* and *Enterococcus durans*) grow in 6.5% NaCl, whereas *S. bovis* and *Streptococcus equinus* (a very rare cause of IE) are salt-sensitive. Seventy-five percent of strains of *S. bovis* are heat-tolerant, and they may also grow and produce acid in "*E. faecalis* broth"; therefore, these methods are unreliable for separation.[283] Arginine hydrolysis by enterococci and starch hydrolysis by *S. bovis* are other means for reliable separation. The association of bacteremia due to *S. bovis* with carcinoma of the colon and other lesions of the gastrointestinal tract suggests that colonoscopy be performed when this organism is isolated from blood cultures.[284, 285]

Enterococci are normal inhabitants of the gastrointestinal tract and occasionally the anterior urethra. All enterococci are in Lancefield group D; are catalase-negative and nonmotile; and may exhibit α-, β-, or γ-hemolysis on blood agar. They grow well in sodium azide ("SF both"), 40% bile, 6.5% NaCl, and 0.1% methylene blue and can survive at 56°C for 30 minutes or at a pH of 9.6.[286] They should be separated from *S. bovis*. The *Enterococcus* group is responsible for 5 to 18% of the cases of IE, and the incidence appears to be increasing.[275, 287, 288] The disease usually runs a subacute course and affects older (mean age, 59 years) men after genitourinary manipulation or younger (mean age, 37 years) women after obstetric procedures. The mean duration of nonspecific symptoms such as malaise, fatigue, anorexia, and weight loss was 140 days in one review. Over 40% of the patients have no underlying heart disease, although more than 95% develop a heart murmur during the course of the illness. Classic peripheral manifestations are uncommon (fewer than 25% of the cases). Bacteriuria with enterococci is a helpful diagnostic clue and was found in 4 of 15 patients[286] in one study. Cure is difficult because of intrinsic resistance to many antibiotics, and a high mortality persists in this disease. With the increasing usage of third-generation cephalosporins, which are relatively inactive against enterococci in vitro, and other contributing factors (e.g., indwelling urinary catheters), some reports[288–290] emphasized an alarming increase in enterococcal bacteremias during the past 2 decades. Most enterococcal bacteremias are nosocomial in origin, often polymicrobial (42% in one large series[291]) and are associated with serious underlying disorders. Factors that suggest IE in patients with enterococcal bateremia include (1) community acquisition, (2) preexistent valvular heart disease, (3) a cryptogenic source, and (4) the absence of polymicrobial bacteremia.[291] Antibiotic usage patterns, the aging of the population, and more invasive procedures in hospitalized adults all portend a continued increase in serious enterococcal infections, including IE, in the future.

Before 1945, *S. pneumoniae* was responsible for approximately 10% of the cases of IE, but this has decreased to approximately 1 to 3% currently.[292] The course is usually fulminant and is often (in approximately one third of cases) associated with perivalvular abscess formation or pericarditis, or both. Left-sided involvement is the rule, and there is a predilection for the aortic valve (≈70% of cases). Many patients with pneumococcal endocarditis are alcoholic (≈40%), and concurrent meningitis is present in about 70% of cases.[292–294] The overall mortality rate remains at approximately 50% (≈60 to 65% in children[295]), with death usually due to rapid valvular destruction and hemodynamic compromise, although indolent presentations of pneumococcal endocarditis with a favorable outcome have been described.[296]

Nutritionally variant streptococci (NVS)—that is, *Abiotrophia* spp.—may cause difficulties in isolation and were implicated in 5.4% of the cases of streptococcal endocarditis at The New York Hospital.[297] The organisms do not grow on subculture unless L-cysteine or pyridoxal (vitamin B_6) is provided. IE due to nutritionally deficient streptococci is virtually always indolent in onset and associated with preexisting heart disease.[298] Therapy remains difficult because systemic embolization, relapse, and death are not infrequent (occurring in 17 to 27% of cases). A closely related species, *S. mitis,* although not nutritionally deficient, also causes serious infections, including IE, in adults[299] and has emerged as an important causative agent of IE among drug addicts in some areas (e.g., New York City[300]). Group B streptococci (*Streptococcus agalactiae*) are normal inhabitants of the mouth, vagina, and anterior urethra in 5 to 12% of the general population. In 149 patients with group B streptococcal infections, the serotypes isolated were Ia in 46%, II in 22%, and III in 11%.[301] Although long recognized as a cause of bacteremia and meningitis in neonates, serious *S. agalactiae* infections in adults have also been emphasized.[302] Risk factors for group B streptococcal sepsis and IE in adults include diabetes mellitus, carcinoma, alcoholism, hepatic failure, elective abortion, and intravenous drug use.[302–304] As with *S. bovis,* occasional cases occur in association with villous adenomas of the colon.[305] Over 90 cases of group B streptococcal IE have been reported.[303–307] Underlying heart disease is common, the male-to-female ratio is 1.4:1, the mean age is approximately 54 years, and left-sided involvement predominates. The overall mortality rate is nearly 50%. The organism does not produce fibrinolysin, which may be responsible for the large, friable vegetations and frequent major systemic emboli. A similar clinical picture with a destructive process, left-sided predominance, frequent complications, and high mortality (≈40%) has been observed in the 47 cases of group G streptococcal endocarditis reported in the literature.[308, 309] Most human infections with *Streptococcus suis* have presented as meningitis (with a striking predilection to cause deafness as a sequela) and sepsis with accompanying arthritis or endophthalmitis, but two cases of endocarditis due to serotype 2 have been described.[310] A history of pig or raw pork contact was a feature in both patients. Group A streptococci remain a very rare cause of IE in both adults and children.[311]

S. anginosus is a rare cause of IE (≈6 to 7% of cases) but is unusual among these streptococci in that it has a predilection to cause suppurative complications including brain, liver, perinephric, and other abscesses as well as cholangitis, peritonitis, and empyema.[312–314] Some of these complications occur during IE due to this organism and may require surgical attention. Approximately 50% of *S. anginosus* strains carry the group F antigen.[313] Infective endocarditis caused by *S. anginosus* may result in "virulent" intracardiac complications (e.g., myocardial abscess, purulent pericarditis) more typical of *S. aureus* infections.[315]

Infective endocarditis due to *Gemella haemolysans* has also been reported.[316] This organism is now placed in genus V of the family Streptococcaceae. *Gemella* should be suspected if blood cultures reveal a variable morphology (with some organisms resembling diphtheroids) and an indeterminate Gram stain. The antimicrobial susceptibility of *Gemella* spp. is similar to that of the viridans streptococci. Although misidentification in the microbiology laboratory is presumably common, six cases of IE due to *G. haemolysans* have been reported since 1982.[317]

Staphylococci

Staphylococci cause at least 20 to 30% of the cases of IE, and 80 to 90% of these are due to coagulase-positive *S. aureus*. This species is the causative agent in most cases of acute IE, but only a minority of patients with *S. aureus* bacteremia will have IE.[318, 319] The organism may attack "normal" (defined as no clinically detectable cardiac disease) heart valves in approximately one third of the patients. The course is frequently fulminant when it involves the mitral or aortic valve, with widespread metastatic infection, and results in death in approximately 40% of the patients.[320–323] As noted, the proportion of cases of IE due to *S. aureus* appears to be increasing at both community and university hospitals.[10, 274, 275, 324] It had been previously found that among cases of *S. aureus* IE, the vast majority were community-acquired.[325] However, recent experience from Duke University with 59 cases of definite *S. aureus* IE prospectively identified has suggested a demographic shift among patients with this infection.[326] In nearly half of the cases, the IE was acquired nosocomially, was frequently caused by methicillin-resistant *S. aureus* (MRSA) strains, and was often associated with intravascular device–related *S. aureus* infection. If this experience is confirmed in other centers, it would then appear that nosocomially-acquired *S. aureus* bacteremia should prompt a complete evaluation for underlying IE.

Myocardial abscesses (with conduction disturbances), purulent pericarditis, and valve ring abscesses are more common in staphylococcal endocarditis than in other forms of IE. Peripheral foci of suppuration (lung, brain, spleen, kidney, and so forth) are common and afflict over 40% of these patients.[320, 323, 324] These extravascular sites of involvement may offer clues to an early diagnosis, especially in addicts.[195, 196] This disease is often unsuspected and therefore not clinically recognized in older patients, and mortality rates often exceed 50% in patients over 50 years of age, especially when the infection is nosocomially acquired.[324, 327] The rare entity of neonatal endocarditis is also often caused by *S. aureus*[328]; survival is unusual.

Infective endocarditis in narcotic addicts is usually due to *S. aureus*, but the disease tends to be less severe, with mortality rates of 2 to 6%.[195, 196] This is directly related to the preponderance of cases affecting the tricuspid valve, a syndrome that usually responds to antimicrobial therapy in most cases.[325] The emergence of MRSA in addicts with staphylococcal IE, first documented in the Detroit area, is disturbing.[190, 329] Among 180 bacteremic addicts admitted to the Detroit Medical Center in 1 year, 24% grew MRSA, and 41% of the patients overall had IE. Previous hospitalizations, long-term addiction (particularly in males), and nonprescribed antibiotic use were predictive of MRSA acquisition (odds ratio, 8.6:1).[328]

S. epidermidis is an important agent in prosthetic valve endocarditis (see Chapter 66) and in infants with IE related to umbilical venous catheters in neonatal intensive care units.[330] Although such cases are still uncommon, some reports[331–333] have emphasized the importance of coagulase-negative staphylococci in native valve IE, particularly in patients with mitral valve prolapse.[331] Approximately two thirds of affected patients have preexistent valvular disease. Although the disease was indolent in onset, complications of IE were frequent; despite this, medical and/or surgical therapy was usually successful. Males predominate among the 85 patients reported, and the incidence of emboli, skin manifestations, and CHF is low.[334] Separation of IE from uncomplicated bacteremias due to *S. epidermidis* (implicated in ≈50% of cases of native valve coagulase-negative staphylococcal endocarditis) may be difficult, but a solid-phase radioimmunoassay for the detection of IgG antibodies is promising.[335] Extensive laboratory evaluation[336] reveals that most *S. epidermidis* endocarditis isolates are distinct and do not represent common-source outbreaks despite the frequent shift to a small-colony variant by many strains in vivo.[337] Rare cases of IE due to other coagulase-negative staphylococci (e.g., *Staphylococcus saprophyticus, Staphylococcus capitis*) have been reported.[338, 339] Over the past 5 years, a number of reports of IE caused by a coagulase-negative staphylococcus called *Staphylococcus lugdunensis* have been published.[340–343] This organism tends to cause a substantially more virulent form of IE than that due to other coagulase-negative staphylococci, with high morbidity rates despite nearly uniform in vitro susceptibilities to most antibiotics, including penicillins and cephalosporins.[340–343] These strains are frequently misidentified as *S. aureus* because they are often yellow-pigmented and yield complete hemolysis on blood agars. Their in vitro hemolytic capacities relate to the production of synergistic hemolysin. The differentiation of *S. lugdunensis* from *S. aureus* in the microbiology laboratory depends on the tube coagulase test and the ability of the former strains to cause ornithine decarboxylation. Distinguishing *S. lugdunensis* from other coagulase-negative staphylococci may be difficult using commercial identification schemata (e.g., API StaphIdent System[344]).

Gram-Negative Bacilli

Gram-negative aerobic bacilli have been reported to cause 1.3 to 4.8% of the cases of IE, but in two reports[345, 346] they accounted for over 10% of the cases. In the latter reports, approximately two thirds of the cases coexisted with or followed serious gram-positive infections. In spite of an increasing incidence of gram-negative bacillary septicemia, IE due to these organisms remains uncommon, but the incidence is increasing. Only 1.7% of 452 valvular infections reported in the 1960s were caused by gram-negative organisms, versus 7 to 15% in more recent series.[274, 347] A total of 56 cases of IE due to gram-negative bacteria were seen at the Mayo Clinic from 1958 to 1975, 35 from 1970 to 1975 alone.[348] Most cases were due to "fastidious" nonenteric organisms (see further on); this group caused 10% of the IE cases seen at this institution. Narcotic addicts, prosthetic valve recipients, and patients with cirrhosis[349] appear to be at an increased risk for the development of gram-negative bacillary endocarditis. The duration of illness is usually less than 6 weeks, most patients are aged 40 to 50 years, and males and females are affected equally.[350] In gram-negative septicemia, the blood stream is usually cleared readily with appropriate antimicrobial agents. In contrast, in gram-negative bacillary endocarditis, persistent bacteremia is common, even with high levels of antimicrobial activity. CHF is common, and the prognosis is poor. Most series report a mortality rate approaching 75 to 83%,[20, 350] but recent experience indicates a better prognosis,[348] with a cure rate of 62% in 21 patients infected with aerobic enteric bacilli. A heart murmur noted during an episode of gram-negative sepsis with unexplained anemia or the persistence of positive blood cultures despite adequate antibiotics may indicate endocarditis. In the early postoperative period after prosthetic valve replacement, sustained gram-negative bacillary bacteremia does not necessarily imply IE,[351] and other foci of infection (sternal wound, pneumonia, urinary tract, intravenous catheters, and so forth) should be carefully sought (see Chapter 66).

Among members of Enterobacteriaceae, *Salmonella* spp. were most common in early reports. These organisms have an affinity for abnormal cardiac valves, usually on the left side of the heart.[350, 352] Although many serotypes have been implicated, most cases are due to *Salmonella choleraesuis, Salmonella typhimurium*, and *Salmonella enteritidis*. Valvular perforation or destruction, atrial thrombi, myocarditis, and pericarditis are common, and the outlook is grave. Salmonellae may also produce endarteritis in aneurysms of major vessels (see further on).

In a review of 44 cases of Enterobacteriaceae endocarditis due to species other than *Salmonella* spp.[350] the following organisms were identified: *E. coli*, in 17 cases; *Citrobacter* sp., in 1 case; *Klebsiella-Enterobacter* spp., in 9; *S. marcescens*, in 13; *Proteus* spp. in 2; and *Providencia* spp., in 2. There were 19 additional cases of endocarditis due to *S. marcescens* reported from San Francisco[353]; 17 occurred in narcotic addicts. Two thirds of these patients had previously normal heart valves, and most of the infections occurred on the aortic and mitral valves. The cases are characterized by large vegetations with near-total occlusion of the valve orifice in the absence of significant underlying valvular destruction. The overall mortality rate ranges from 68 to 73%, because a cure of left-sided IE due to member of Enterobacteriaceae is uncommon with medical therapy alone. Since 1974, 17 more cases of IE due to *S. marcescens* have been observed in the San Francisco area; 15 occurred in intravenous drug abusers. As above, only 3 of 10 patients with left-sided involvement survived despite antimicrobial combination therapy and high serum bactericidal activity. Valve replacement after approximately 7 to 10 days of antibiotics was recommended for these difficult infections.[354] Approximately 12 cases of IE due to *Campylobacter fetus* have been reported since the first case in 1955.[355]

The first case of *Pseudomonas*-induced endocarditis was recognized in 1899; over 200 cases have subsequently been reported.[190, 329, 349, 356–359] Most (95%) of the patients have abused intravenous drugs.[329, 356–359] The male-to-female ratio is 2.5:1, and the mean age is 30 years. The organism affects normal valves in most cases. Major embolic phenomena, inability to sterilize valves, neurologic complications (53%), ring and annular abscesses, splenic abscesses, bacteremic relapses, and rapidly progressive CHF are common. Ecthyma gangrenosum, the necrotizing cutaneous lesion characteristic of *Pseudomonas* bacteremia, has occasionally been noted especially in cases of IE due to *Pseudomonas (Burkholdesia) cepacia*.[360] The disease carries the highest mortality in patients over 30 years of age (73%, versus 33%, in younger patients), when the duration of illness is less than 5 days (which raises the rate from 41% to 76%), and when there is left-sided cardiac involvement.[357, 359, 361] Owing to the gloomy outlook and frequent complications,[190] early surgery is recommended by many authorities for left-sided *Pseudomonas* endocarditis.[358, 359] In contrast, high-dose regimens of antipseudomonal penicillins combined with aminoglycosides have had a salutary effect in a majority of patents with isolated right-sided pseudomonal IE (see section on "Antimicrobial Therapy" later on). Nearly all addicts with *P. aeruginosa* endocarditis in recent reports[63, 329, 358, 359] have abused tripelennamine and pentazocine ("T's and blues").

Unusual Gram-Negative Bacteria

Endocarditis produced by several other gram-negative species has received recent attention. *N. gonorrhoeae* was responsible for at least 5 to 10% of the cases of IE before the introduction of penicillin but is now rarely implicated. In the older series, one half of the patients with gonococcal endocarditis had involvement of the right side of the heart and exhibited the characteristic double quotidian fever pattern. Of the cases of gonococcal endocarditis reported since 1949,[362–364] most occurred in young men. Skin manifestations consistent with the gonococcal arthritis-dermatitis syndrome or endocarditis are documented in only 20% of cases. Most of the cases of gonococcal endocarditis now follow an indolent course, in contrast to the often fulminant progression in the preantibiotic era. Aortic valve involvement, large vegetations seen on TTE, associated valve ring abscesses, CHF, and nephritis are quite common. Recently[364] a high frequency of late complement component deficiencies have been noted in patients with gonococcal endocarditis. Sudden hemodynamic deterioration despite appropriate therapy may occur,[362–364] and the mortality rate remains approximately 20%. Nonpathogenic *Neisseria* spp. (*Neisseria perflava, Neisseria flava, Neisseria pharyngis, Neisseria mucosa, Neisseria sicca, Neisseria flavesceus,* and especially *Moraxella [Neisseria] catarrhalis* and *Neisseria elongata* subsp. *nitroreducens* [CDC group M-6]) are now isolated more frequently in IE than are gonococci, but they usually produce infection on abnormal or prosthetic heart valves.[365–367] *Haemophilus* spp., predominantly *Haemophilus paraphrophilus, Haemophilus parainfluenzae*, and *Haemophilus aphrophilus*, account for 0.8 to 1.3% of all cases of IE.[368–371] This disease usually runs a subacute course and occurs in the setting of preexisting valvular disease. Emboli to major peripheral arteries were found in six of seven cases of *H. parainfluenzae* endocarditis,[368] and major central nervous system complications are relatively frequent.[371] *H. aphrophilus* produced a similar clinical pattern and has been transmitted from dogs to humans. Single cases of IE due to *Haemophilus segnis* and *Haemophilus aegyptius* have been reported from Denmark and Israel, respectively.[372, 373] A closely related organism, *Actinobacillus actinomycetemcomitans*, is a rare cause of subacute endocarditis (with approximately 35 cases reported), with a mortality of 34%.[374, 375] Infective endocarditis due to *Cardiobacterium hominis*[376] resembles the disease caused by *Haemophilus* spp.; 26 cases of IE due to this organism were reported by 1983. Only one extravascular infection due to *C. hominis* has been documented (meningitis during IE). At least 28 cases of *Kingella* endocarditis (*Kingella kingae*, 25; *Kingella denitrificans*, 2; *Kingella indologenes*, 1) have been reported.[377] Approximately 50% of patients develop complications, including acute stroke in approximately 25%. A dozen cases of IE due to *Eikenella corrodens* have been reported; intravenous drug use (especially amphetamines) was implicated in five patients.[378, 379] Dental infection or a history of dental procedures may be a feature, and drug users have often "cleaned" the injection site with saliva; *E. corrodens* is a usual habitant of the oropharynx. The disease generally has an indolent course but may present acutely.[379] All these organisms— the HACEK group: *Haemophilus, Actinobacillus, Cardiobacterium, Eikenella, Kingella*—are fastidious and may require 2 to 3 weeks for primary isolation. Routine subculturing onto supplemented chocolate agar or incubation in atmospheres of 5 to 10% CO_2 is necessary for the isolation of these organisms and should be performed in all culture-negative cases of IE. Granular growth in broth is characteristic and should suggest their presence. In addition, the clinical syndrome produced by this group is virtually identical with that in subacute IE: large friable vegetations, frequent emboli, and the development of CHF and often the eventual need for valve replacement.[380]

Gram-Positive Bacilli

Infective endocarditis due to various species of corynebacteria (diphtheroids) is uncommon and usually occurs on damaged or prosthetic valves,[381] although native valve infections (e.g., *Arcanobacterium* [Corynebacterium] haemolyticum in a drug addict) are rarely reported. About 19 cases of IE due to *Corynebacterium pseudodiphtheriticum* (previously *Corynebacterium hofmannii*) have been reported; native valves were involved in approximately 50% of these cases.[382] *Corynebacterium xerosis* is a very rare cause of native valve IE. Nontoxigenic *Conyebacterium diphtheriae* IE has been reported in more than 40 patients. A recent cluster of seven cases in 1 year from New South Wales, Australia,[383] emphasized the aggressive nature of the infection, including major vascular complications, the frequent occurrence of septic arthritis (in four of seven patients), and involvement of native valves. Intravenous drug use is also a predisposing factor. *Listeria monocytogenes* has been isolated in 44 cases of IE.[384, 385] Most cases of IE due to *Listeria* spp. have occurred in patients without any underlying defect in host defenses, although preexistent heart disease is present in approximately 50%. The mean age in the reported series was 51 years, and the overall mortality was 48%.[385] Lactobacilli have also been reported to cause a subacute form of IE, but such cases are rare, with only 41 reported.[386, 387] Despite an initial response to therapy, relapse of this infection is not unusual (≈60% of cases). Most cases occur on structurally abnormal native valves following dental manipulation.[387]

Therapy with single agents is often unsatisfactory, as lactobacilli, like enterococci, are tolerant to penicillins. Medical cure has been difficult to achieve in the past. These organisms also may take several weeks for isolation on blood culture. Over 90% of 49 serious infections caused by *Erysipelothrix rhusiopathiae* were characterized as endocarditis.[388] Occupational or vocational animal or fish exposure is a major risk factor, and approximately a third of patients are alcoholic. Most patients are male; a characteristic erysipeloid skin lesion is present in approximately 40% of cases, and the organism exhibits significant aortic valve tropism (involved in 70% of patients).[388] The overall mortality rate is 38%. Most cases of *Bacillus* endocarditis involve the tricuspid valve in addicts, but nonaddicts and prosthetic valve recipients have also been affected.[389] *Rothia dentocariosa* is a rare cause of IE (with six cases reported) but has led to significant central nervous system complications.[390, 391]

Anaerobic Bacteria

Nonstreptococcal anaerobic bacteria were responsible for 1.3% of all the cases of IE in 1970.[392] *Bacteroides fragilis* was the predominant pathogen in a review of 67 cases from the literature.[393] The following organisms were isolated: *B. fragilis*, 35.8%; *Bacteroides oralis*, 3.0%; *P. melaninogenica (Bacteroides melaninogenicus)*, 3.0%; *Fusobacterium necrophorum*, 13.4%; *Fusobacterium nucleatum*, 9.0%; *Clostridium* spp., 13.4%; *P. acnes*, 7.5%; *Dialister granuliformans*, 1.5%; and unidentified, 16.4%. Over one third of the unidentified cases were also thought by the authors to represent *B. fragilis*. Approximately 25% of these cases were polymicrobial, usually mixed with anaerobic or microaerophilic streptococci. The portal of entry for *B. fragilis* was probably the gastrointestinal tract, while *B. oralis, P. melaninogenica (B. melaninogenicus)*, or fusobacteria originated from the mouth or upper respiratory tract. Two thirds of the patients were over 40 years of age and had preexisting heart disease. The course is usually subacute except for that with infection due to *F. necrophorum*, which characteristically produces a more fulminant disease. These organisms usually cause extensive valve destruction, CHF, and major systemic emboli (in 60 to 70% of the cases). Thromboembolic episodes are especially common in infections caused by *B. fragilis*, a phenomenon that may be related to the heparinase produced by this organism. The mortality rate in cases of anaerobic endocarditis has ranged from 21 to 46%.[393] One series from California, however, noted no deaths in seven patients with anaerobic or microaerophilic endocarditis[394]; these cases constituted 10.6% of the IE cases seen. This is similar to a 7.7% incidence reported by other investigators[3] and suggests that anaerobic endocarditis may be more prevalent now than it was in 1970.[395] Isolation of these organisms may be improved by the newer anaerobic culture techniques currently in use.

Other Bacteria

Many other bacteria have been described in cases of IE; however, consideration of these organisms separately is beyond the scope of this chapter. These include *Acinetobacter* (approximately 20 reported cases; a maculopapular rash on the palms and soles may be present).[396] *Actinomyces,*[397] *Alcaligenes, Bordetella, Flavobacterium, Micrococcus, Moraxella, Paracolon, Stomatococcus mucilaginosus* (four cases of IE),[398] *Streptobacillus moniliformis* (16 cases; usually damaged native valves are involved),[399] *Vibrio*, and *Yersinia. Brucella* spp. continue as important etiologic agents in Spain and in Saudi Arabia, where these organisms are responsible for approximately 10% of IE cases.[400] Aggressive medical therapy with valve replacement is usually necessary for a cure of *Brucella* endocarditis.[401]

Etiology of Infective Endocarditis in Addicts

The organisms responsible for IE in narcotic addicts require separate consideration, because the distribution differs from that in other patients with IE. The frequencies of the etiologic agents isolated before 1977 in seven major series were as follows[2]: *S. aureus*, 38%; *P. aeruginosa*, 14.2%; *Candida* spp., 13.8%; enterococci, 8.2%; viridans streptococci, 6.0%; *S. epidermidis*, 1.7%; gram-negative aerobic bacilli, 1.7 to 15%; other bacteria, 2.2%; mixed infections, 1.3%; and culture-negative, 12.9%. In addition, there appears to be an unexplained geographic variation in the causal agents of narcotic-associated IE. *S. aureus* predominated in New York City, Washington, D.C., Chicago, and Cincinnati; *P. aeruginosa* was commonly isolated in Detroit, but methicillin-resistant *S. aureus* (MRSA) now predominates. The most recent compilation from Detroit indicates the distribution of causative agents in addicts with IE (n = 74) as follows: *S. aureus*, 60.8%; streptococci, 16.2%; *P. aeruginosa*, 13.5%; polymicrobial, 8.1%; and *Corynebacterium* JK, 1.4%. Polymicrobial endocarditis (as many as eight different pathogens have been recovered from blood cultures of an individual patient) is fairly common among drug addicts. Some authors have speculated that HIV infection predisposes intravenous drug users to IE due to unusual bacteria, including *Corynebacterium* or *Neisseria* spp.[402] Although *S. aureus* IE in this population was usually tricuspid, streptococci infected left-sided valves significantly more often than the other pathogens. Biventricular and multiple-valve infections occurred most commonly in *Pseudomonas* endocarditis; all of these patients abused "T's and blues." Left-sided IE due to *P. aeruginosa* is a devastating disease and usually presents as an acute illness refractory to seemingly optimal antimicrobial regimens. Complications including ring and annular abscesses, neurologic sequelae (≥253%), CHF, and splenic abscesses are frequent; surgery is often necessary for cure,[403] but the overall mortality rate still approaches 60%. There is an increased incidence of enterococcal endocarditis in Cleveland. *S. marcescens* was once an important pathogen in San Francisco,[354] but at present *S. aureus* is the most common (≅85%) etiologic agent (HF Chambers, personal communication). These differences do not correlate with contamination of "street" heroin.[404] The high incidence of staphylococcal endocarditis may be partially explained by an increase in nasal and oral carriage of this organism.[405] Heroin usage in the previous week was associated with an *S. aureus* isolation rate of 35% from skin, nose, or throat cultures; this rate declined to 11% (not significantly different from that in controls) if heroin has not been injected in the preceding 2 weeks. This suggests an endogenous source for the infecting organism, because *S. aureus* is infrequently (in < 5% of cases) isolated from street heroin or injection paraphernalia. The exact incidence of IE in narcotic addicts is unknown. A conservative estimate is 1.5 to 2 cases of IE per 1000 addicts at risk per year.[406] Moreover, intravenous drug use is the most common risk factor for the development of recurrent native valve IE; 43% of 281 patients surveyed from 1975 to 1986 with this syndrome were addicts[407] (see earlier).

Fungi

Most patients who have fungal endocarditis can be grouped into three categories: (1) narcotic addicts, (2) patients who have undergone reconstructive cardiovascular surgery, and (3) patients who have received prolonged intravenous or antibiotic therapy. In a review of 24 patients with fungal endocarditis seen at the New York University Medical Center from 1968 to 1973,[236] 11 were heroin addicts, 9 had undergone cardiac surgery, and 5 had other serious illnesses requiring antibiotics or hyperalimentation. Underlying heart disease and a tendency for major systemic embolization were noted in two thirds of these patients. *Candida parapsilosis* and *C. tropicalis* predominated in the addicts, whereas *C. albicans* and *Aspergillus* spp. caused most cases in nonaddicts. In a review of 23 addicts, *C. parapsilosis* was responsible in 12 patients (52%), and other *Candida* spp. (*Candida guillermondii, Candida stellatoidea, C. krusei, C. tropicalis*) caused most of the remaining cases. *C. albicans* was isolated in only 1 of the 23 addicts. In contrast, in 82 patients who developed fungal endocarditis after cardiac surgery, the reported distribution of causative organisms was different. *C. albicans* and *Aspergillus* spp. each accounted for approximately a third of the isolates. *C. parapsilosis* was found in fewer than 10%. Fungal endocarditis was documented in 29 patients after prolonged intravenous therapy, and in 17 it developed during the treatment of bacterial endocarditis. Half of these patients were infected with *C. albicans*.

The overall cure rate in cases of fungal endocarditis is poor (14.5% in cases treated since 1968). The poor prognosis may be due to (1) the large bulky vegetations, (2) the tendency for fungal invasion of the myocardium, (3) widespread systemic septic emboli, (4) the poor penetration of antifungal agents into the vegetation,[408] (5) the low toxic-therapeutic ratio of the available antifungal agents, and (6) the usual lack of fungicidal activity with these compounds. A cure is virtually impossible without surgical intervention (see further on).[409] Fatal endocarditis due to *Candida* spp. has also followed Swan-Ganz catheterization.

In a review of 25 cases of *Aspergillus*-induced endocarditis in which cultures were made,[410] the organisms isolated were as follows: *Aspergillus fumigatus*, 14; *Aspergillus flavus*, 4; *Aspergillus niger*, 3; and *Aspergillus ustus, Aspergillus sydowi, Aspergillus terreus,* and *Aspergillus glaucus,* 1 each. Only 5 of 34 patients in this series had positive blood cultures, and only 1 patient survived. A few cases, usually fatal, of *Aspergillus* endocarditis after coronary artery bypass surgery have been described. *Aspergillus clavatus* was isolated in one case. Other fungi that have caused IE include *Histoplasma, Blastomyces, Coccidioides, Cryptococcus, Hansenula, Fonsecaea* (*Hormodendrum*), *Scedosporium prolificans, Mucor, Paecilomyces,* and *Phialophora*. Of the eight reported cases of IE due to *Trichosporon beigelii*, six occurred on prosthetic valves; only two patients have survived a combined medical-surgical approach.[411] *Pseudallescheria boydii* has caused IE in approximately five reported patients; all were immunosuppressed (e.g., liver transplant, AIDS) or previous recipients of prosthetic heart valves.[412] Fungal endocarditis was unknown before 1945, and the incidence is increasing; at present, 1.2 to 2.6% of all cases of IE are due to fungi. Endocarditis has also been caused by higher bacteria such as *Actinomyces, Oerskoviai, Nocardia*, and *Mycobacterium* spp.

Other Microorganisms

Five cases of IE due to *Spirillum minor*, a spirochete, have been reported.[413] This organism is widely distributed in nature, especially in fresh or salt water with organic debris. *S. minor* is the etiologic agent of "rat-bite fever" (sodoku), but rodent transmission was not documented in the cases of endocarditis. Preexistent heart disease or severe underlying disease (e.g., aplastic anemia) is usually present, although one case occurred in an otherwise healthy person.

Infective endocarditis due to *Coxiella burnetii* (the cause of Q fever) is well documented in the United Kingdom, the United States, Canada, France, the Middle East, and Australia, with over 300 recognized cases.[414, 415] Ten cases of Q fever endocarditis were recognized in four Dublin teaching hospitals in only 3 years.[415] Q fever is usually a self-limited respiratory illness due to the inhalation of infected aerosols, especially from animal products. The first endocarditis cases were reported in 1959. Males outnumber females by 6 to 1, and 90% of the patients have preexisting heart disease. Most cases of IE are chronic, with a history of an influenza-like illness occurring 6 to 12 months previously. Risk factors may include exposure to parturient cats or rabbits. The aortic valve is involved in over 80% of the cases. Hematuria is uncommon, even though it is frequently observed in acute Q fever. Hepatosplenomegaly and hepatitis, common features in other types of Q fever, are usual in IE caused by this organism. Other important clues are thrombocytopenia (seen in 90% of cases) and hypergammaglobulinemia. Immune complex–mediated glomerulonephritis develops in approximately 25% of cases.[414–416] The rickettsiae were demonstrated histologically in the valve tissue in 62% of the cases, and the organism was isolated in 83%, although this poses a significant laboratory hazard.[414] The diagnosis is best made serologically; a positive titer of antibody to the phase I antigen as measured by complement fixation or ELISA is indicative of chronic infection, whereas a fourfold rise in titer of antibody to the phase II antigen is associated with active current infection. A phase I antibody titer (generally IgG and/or IgA) greater than 1:200 is considered virtually diagnostic of Q fever endocarditis and may be useful to follow the response to therapy.[414, 417] Isolation of *C. burnetii* by inoculation of valve suspensions into a human fetal diploid fibroblast cell line appears to be a promising technique.[418] DNA probes are under development. The prognosis with medical therapy alone is poor, and valve replacement is often necessary for a cure (see further on). This agent may also cause endarteritis. A single case of IE due to the causative agent of murine typhus has been reported.[224]

Chlamydia psittaci, the agent of psittacosis, has been implicated in at least 10 well-documented cases of IE.[419] This organism may also cause myocarditis or pericarditis. Most of the cases have been associated with psittacine bird exposure; in one case, chlamydiae were found in the liver of the suspected budgerigar. However, transmission from pet cats has also been proposed. The course is subacute, and the diagnosis is often made retrospectively. Most patients had preexisting heart disease, with a striking propensity for aortic valve involvement, and rapid valvular destruction leading to surgical intervention or death. A diagnosis can be established with the demonstration of complement-fixing antibodies. Cure usually requires valve replacement and prolonged antibiotic therapy. The mortality rate in this small group was 40%. Two well-documented cases of IE due to *Chlamydia trachomatis* have been reported.[420] Microimmunofluorescence tests are necessary for a diagnosis. Several cases of probable *Chlamydia pneumoniae* endocarditis have been reported.[421] IE due to *Mycoplasma pneumoniae* was proposed in one case report, but cultural confirmation was lacking.[422]

The role of viruses in IE is unknown. Experimentally, coxsackie B virus has been shown to produce valvular and mural endocarditis in mice and cynomolgus monkeys.[423] In these studies the viral antigen was demonstrated in the valvular tissue by immunofluorescence techniques. Although the enteroviruses are commonly implicated in cases of myocarditis or pericarditis in humans, there is no proof that viral infections produce IE in humans. Adenoviruses are also capable of producing IE in mice. Persand has described a case of "cytomegalovirus endocarditis," but bacteria were also cultured from a mural lesion.[424]

"Culture-Negative" Endocarditis

As discussed earlier, sterile blood cultures have been noted in 2.5 to 31% of the cases of IE.[425, 426] However, blood cultures are negative in only approximately 5% of patients with IE confirmed by strict diagnostic criteria.[427, 428] This may be due to several factors: (1) subacute right-sided endocarditis; (2) cultures taken toward the end of a chronic course (longer than 3 months); (3) uremia supervening in a chronic course; (4) mural endocarditis as in ventricular septal defects, post–myocardial infarction thrombi, or infection related to pacemaker wires; (5) slow growth of fastidious organisms such as anaerobes, *Haemophilus* spp., *Actinobacillus* spp., *Cardiobacterium* spp., NVS, or *Brucella* spp; (6) the prior administration of antibiotics[425, 426]; (7) fungal endocarditis; (8) endocarditis caused by obligate intracellular parasites such as rickettsiae, chlamydiae, and perhaps viruses; or (9) noninfective endocarditis or an incorrect diagnosis. Attention to the proper collection of blood culture specimens, care in the performance of serologic tests, and the use of newer diagnostic techniques may reduce the proportion of culture-negative cases.

Polymicrobial Endocarditis

The proportion of IE cases due to more than one pathogen may be increasing. In a literature review spanning the decade of the 1980s,[429] 101 cases of polymicrobial IE were found. The mean age was only 36.5 years, the male-to-female ratio was nearly 2:1, and 71 of the patients used intravenous drugs (as expected, tricuspid valve involvement with septic pulmonary emboli was frequent). Left-sided involvement, two organisms (versus three or more), and older age were associated with a higher mortality rate.

THERAPY FOR INFECTIVE ENDOCARDITIS

The response to antimicrobial therapy for IE is unique among bacterial infections. Although the organisms may exhibit exquisite susceptibility in vitro to the antibiotics used, complete eradication takes weeks to achieve, and relapse of the patient is not unusual. There are a few possible explanations for these phenomena: (1) the infection exists in an area of impaired host defense and is tightly encased in a fibrin meshwork in which the bacterial colonies are free to divide relatively free from interference from phagocytic cells, and (2) the bacteria in these vegetations reach tremendous population densities (often 10^9 to 10^{10} cfu/g). At these high populations, the organisms may exist in a state of reduced metabolic activity and cell division, as was suggested by Durack and Beeson[125] in studies of L-alanine incorporation into bacterial cell walls. A similar finding is observed in broth in vitro after 18 hours of incubation. In both situations the bacteria are less susceptible to the bactericidal action of penicillin or other drugs that require cell wall synthesis and division for maximum activity. The relative importance of antimicrobial penetration into vegetations and the response to therapy is unresolved. Although multiple studies have examined antibiotic concentrations in human cardiac valve tissue obtained during surgery,[430] usually in close agreement with concurrent serum concentrations, the relevance of these data to therapy for IE is unknown, so that current recommendations remain unaltered. Information on antimicrobial concentration in vegetations, either in experimental models or in humans with IE, is sparse. Recent experiments after a single dose of radiolabeled antimicrobial agents with autoradiographic analysis of drug dispersion within vegetations of animals with experimental IE revealed three patterns[431]: (1) concentration at the periphery of the vegetation without diffusion into the core (e.g., teicoplanin); (2) progressive diffusion but with a high gradient from periphery to core (e.g., ceftriaxone); or (3) homogeneous diffusion throughout the vegetation (e.g., several fluoroquinolones). The predictive value of these observations on therapeutic efficacy is unknown. However, the suboptimal clinical efficacy of teicoplanin in several clinical trials treating intravascular *S. aureus* infections may relate to the maldistribution of this agent within vegetations.[432] Analysis of pharmacodynamic variables (e.g., concentration-dependent bactericidal activity, postantibiotic effect) may also assist in the rational selection of regimens for the therapy of IE.[431] Studies in animals have confirmed that when vegetation formation is inhibited with anticoagulants, the organisms are eradicated more rapidly with penicillin treatment than in control animals with larger vegetations.[129] Furthermore, enzymatic modification of the glycocalyx in the vegetations of experimental streptococcal endocarditis by in vivo dextranase administration facilitates the bactericidal activity of penicillin by more rapid sterilization of the lesion.[433] In contrast, tissue-type plasminogen activator produced a concentration-dependent lysis of fibrin clots or vegetations infected with *S. epidermidis* or *S. sanguis* but did not enhance antimicrobial activity in in vitro models.[434, 435] Of interest, several recent studies in experimental IE have confirmed the utility of aspirin in reducing both the size of vegetations and the microbial densities within aortic vegetations.[436, 437] In addition, one clinical study in patients with established IE suggested that aspirin could mitigate the growth of vegetative lesions (as monitored echocardiographically) and prevent cerebral emboli.[438]

Certain general principles have been accepted that provide the framework for the current recommendations for treatment of endocarditis. Parenteral antibiotics are recommended over oral drugs in most circumstances because of the importance of sustained antibacterial activity. Erratic absorption with many classes of agents makes oral drugs less desirable. Short-term therapy has been associated with relapse, and most current recommendations emphasize extended drug administration. Early studies by the British Medical Research Council[439] first emphasized the necessity for prolonged treatment. Bacteriostatic antibiotics are generally ineffective in the treatment of bacterial endocarditis. Their use has been associated with frequent relapses or a failure to control the infection, or both. A symptomatic response to such agents as tetracycline, erythromycin, or, in some cases, clindamycin should not be accepted as indicative of successful treatment, because once treatment with these agents is discontinued, relapse is common. Likewise, antibiotic combinations should produce a rapid bactericidal effect. This is seen with synergistic combinations such as penicillin plus an aminoglycoside effective against most viridans streptococci or enterococci. In experimental animals, it has been shown that the rate of bactericidal action expressed by a drug or combination of drugs in broth is predictive of the relative rate at which the organisms will be eradicated from the cardiac vegetations in vivo. Antagonistic combinations such as penicillin plus chloramphenicol, which are less rapidly bactericidal, are less effective in experimental endocarditis than is the single bactericidal drug (penicillin) alone.[440] General guidelines for the evaluation of new antimicrobial agents for the therapy of IE were published recently.[441]

Patients with IE may have an associated myocarditis complicated by cardiac arrhythmias and CHF. Such patients (those with IE plus congestive heart failure) require close observation in an intensive care environment with electrocardiographic monitoring. As discussed subsequently, the selection of antibiotics should be based on antimicrobial susceptibility tests, and the treatment should be monitored clinically and with determination of antimicrobial blood levels when indicated. Blood cultures should be obtained during the early phase of therapy to ensure eradication of the bacteremia, and in patients with persistent or recurrent fever during therapy. The use of anticoagulants during therapy for native valve endocarditis has been associated with fatal subarachnoid hemorrhage and other bleeding complications. Most authorities agree that anticoagulant administration in this setting is contraindicated, but this area remains controversial. In cases of IE localized to mechanical prosthetic valves, many clinicians maintain anticoagulation within therapeutic range, provided that the patient has no evidence of major vascular emboli (e.g., central nervous system signs or symptoms).

Patients with left-sided IE should be managed at least initially in facilities with access to cardiothoracic surgery. Although persistent or recurrent fever despite appropriate antimicrobial therapy may be due to pulmonary or systemic emboli or drug hypersensitivity, the most common cause is extensive valve ring or adjacent structure infection or metastatic infection.[442] Approximately a third of patients with left-sided IE require surgery during the acute stages of infection for either valve replacement or metastatic infection.[271] Close monitoring and early surgical consultation of patients with IE, particularly those with signs of heart failure or persistent fever, are essential.

Tests Useful for Antimicrobial Treatment Monitoring

Management of IE demands careful consideration of the choice, dose, and duration of antimicrobial therapy. The following laboratory tests can help the physician to monitor treatment and can aid in rational therapeutic decisions. In every case of bacterial endocarditis, the etiologic agent must be isolated in pure culture, and the minimum inhibitory concentration (MIC) and the minimum bactericidal concentration (MBC) must be determined for the usual antibiotics used (see further on). Standard disk sensitivity testing is unreliable in the context of treating IE and results may be misleading without the quantitative information provided by determining the MIC and MBC. During therapy the serum can be monitored for bactericidal activity against the offending organism as originally described by Schlicter and Macllean.[443] The performance method for this test varies greatly, and consequently there are disagreements in interpretation. The inoculum size, composition of the broth, timing of samples ("peak" versus "trough"), methods of dilution and subculture, and criteria for determination of the bactericidal end point are among the important variables. Perhaps because of these problems and the frequent adverse events unrelated to bactericidal effects, the serum bactericidal titer (SBT) often correlates poorly with the clinical outcome in patients with IE. There is still intense disagreement regarding the value of this test in monitoring therapy for IE. A retrospective review[444] of 17 reports published between 1948 and 1980 failed to confirm any correlation between an SBT of 1:8 or greater and therapeutic success.[445] Controversy regarding the usefulness of peak versus trough SBT abounds.[446] When all of these variables are standardized,[447, 448] the SBT test may be useful in selected patients with IE. A recent prospective multicenter study[449] evaluated a standardized SBT method in 129 patients with bacterial endocarditis. Peak and trough SBT ratios of 1:64 or greater and 1:32, respectively, predicted bacteriologic cure in all patients, but specific levels could *not* be used to predict bacteriologic failure or clinical outcome accurately. Although there are problems with this study,[445] other data[449] support a role for the SBT when standardized and performed in the presence of 50% human serum: All patients with a peak SBT of 1:32 or greater were cured, whereas 7 of 21 (33%) with an SBT of 1:16 or less failed treatment.[450] Unless precluded by drug toxicity, it seems reasonable to attempt to achieve this level (1:8 to 1:16) of activity in patients, although this goal may be unattainable in some forms (e.g., gram-negative bacillary, enterococcal) of IE. Performance of the SBT test is usually unnecessary in patients with viridans streptococcal endocarditis and other antibiotic-susceptible forms of IE, but the SBT may be useful when (1) the organism is inherently resistant or tolerant to one of the drugs administered or (2) the response to therapy is suboptimal.

In some forms of IE, combinations of antibiotics are used routinely.[451] These regimens are based on synergy studies performed in vitro and on results obtained in experimental animal models of IE. In difficult cases with a slow therapeutic response or in those due to unusual organisms, a determination of synergistic combinations of antibiotics may be helpful. In these cases, tests for bactericidal synergism may be undertaken by standard techniques such as broth dilution, microtiter "checkerboards," or "time-kill" curves in broth. Proper attention to standardized techniques, especially inoculum size, is critically important for a meaningful interpretation of the results.

When aminoglycosides are used in therapy, the concentration of antibiotic in the serum should be periodically determined. These agents have a low toxic-therapeutic ratio, especially in elderly patients or in those with renal disease. Peak and trough concentrations should be measured, and the dose should be altered accordingly. This method is superior to reliance solely on nomograms for dosage changes. When synergy with another agent is demonstrable, serum concentrations of the aminoglycosides lower than those generally considered "therapeutic" may be adequate, thus lessening the potential for toxicity.

Antimicrobial Therapy

Recently, Wilson and colleagues and the AHA Committee on Endocarditis have reviewed the treatment of streptococcal, enterococcal, staphylococcal, nand HACEK IE in detail.[452]

"Penicillin-Sensitive" Streptococcal Endocarditis

Most strains of viridans streptococci, "other" streptococci (including *S. pyogenes*), and nonenterococcal group D streptococci (primarily *S. bovis*) are exquisitely sensitive to penicillins, with an MIC of less than 0.2 μg/ml. However, 15 to 20% of viridans streptococci are "resistant" to this arbitrary concentration of penicillin.[276, 297] In addition,[280] approximately 15% of the strains of *S. mutans* demonstrate a low MIC for penicillin (<0.1 μg/ml), but the MBC is considerably higher (1.25 to 50 μg/ml). These organisms should probably be considered "penicillin-tolerant" and should be treated accordingly. Although results are dependent on the in vitro methodology employed, studies suggest that tolerance to penicillin among viridans streptococci is more prevalent than previous reports suggested.[453] For example, 19% of viridans streptococci cultured from gingiva and blood after dental procedures were tolerant,[454] especially among *S. mutans* (27%) and *S. mitior* (20%) isolates. Almost identical figures were reported among blood culture isolates of viridans streptococci,[455] with tolerance defined as a penicillin MBC-to-MIC ratio exceeding 10:1. Nearly all strains of nutritionally dependent streptococci are tolerant to penicillin.[456, 457] The influence of the tolerance phenomenon on the response to penicillin therapy in experimental endocarditis is not known; two studies yielded conflicting results.[458, 459] Data on human infections with tolerant strains and the therapeutic results are unavailable. Except for NVS, we do not believe that the demonstration of tolerance by an isolate of viridans streptococci influences therapeutic decisions.

By broth dilution susceptibility tests, the usual MBC determinations for these so-called penicillin-sensitive streptococci are as follows: penicillin, 0.1 to 1.0 μg/ml; cephalothin, 0.15 to 1.25 μg/ml;

vancomycin, 0.15 to 0.4 μg/ml; streptomycin, 6.25 to 50 μg/ml; and gentamicin, 1.56 to 3.12 μg/ml.[460, 461] *S. bovis* is 10 to 5000 times more susceptible to penicillin than are the other group D species (enterococci). They are also relatively susceptible to oxacillin, methicillin, and lincomycin, whereas the enterococci are resistant.[282] Most streptococci in this group demonstrate synergism in vitro between penicillin or vancomycin and streptomycin, gentamicin, or kanamycin (see further on).[462, 463] The first strains of viridans streptococci with high-level streptomycin resistance (MIC of ≥1000 μg/ml) were reported in 1982 from Paris. Although these strains are rare (2 to 8% of isolates in some locales,[464] the documentation of aminoglycoside-modifying enzymes and the lack of penicillin-streptomycin synergy in vitro and in experimental animal models[464, 465] is alarming. These penicillin-susceptible strains are killed synergistically by penicillin-gentamicin combinations. Significant antibiotic antagonism has been shown with the combination of clindamycin and gentamicin for *S. mutans* IE. The in vitro synergism between penicillin and aminoglycosides has been found to correlate with a more rapid rate of eradication of bacteria from cardiac vegetations in vivo in the rabbit endocarditis model[466, 467] for the common viridans streptococci. All of these studies have been summarized in reviews.[468–470] Low-level penicillin resistance (MIC of 0.2 to 2.0 μg/ml) was found in 31% of viridans streptococci in Madrid in 1988 and 1989, and an additional 17% of strains demonstrated high-level resistance.[471] Perhaps most important, streptomycin and cefotaxime resistance was also "common."[470] The authors suggest a vancomycin-gentamicin regimen for IE due to viridans streptococci in Spain.

The combination of penicillin and streptomycin has been used in over 200 cases at the New York Hospital–Cornell Medical Center since 1959 without a documented relapse.[462] This clinical experience has been confirmed elsewhere,[2] but the overall reported relapse rate is 1.4%.[469] This regimen is as follows: aqueous penicillin G, 10 million to 20 million units intravenously (IV) daily, or procaine penicillin G, 1.2 million units intramuscularly (IM) every 6 hours for 4 weeks, combined with streptomycin, 0.5 g IM every 12 hours for the first 2 weeks. Studies by Wilson and colleagues at the Mayo Clinic[472, 473] demonstrated that a 2-week course of intramuscular procaine penicillin (1.2 million units every 6 hours) and streptomycin (0.5 g every 12 hours) cured at least 99% of patients with penicillin-sensitive streptococcal endocarditis. These results are similar to those obtained with therapy consisting of β-lactams alone for a total of 4 weeks[474, 475] but significantly better than those obtained with penicillin alone for 2 weeks; the latter regimen was associated with a 50% relapse rate when low doses of penicillin were used and improved to 17% with higher penicillin dosages. The 2-week penicillin-streptomycin regimen is the most cost-effective and had been preferred therapy among the three regimens in uncomplicated penicillin-sensitive (MIC of ≥ 0.1 μg/ml) streptococcal endocarditis in young patients. However, with the advent of ceftriaxone-based regimens (featuring 2 weeks of ceftriaxone + an aminoglycoside), many clinicians have opted for this approach[476, 477] (see later on). Four weeks of penicillin (or ceftriaxone; see later on) alone is recommended in patients with impaired renal function or those particularly susceptible to the low risk of streptomycin-induced ototoxicity (the elderly). The "Cornell regimen" of 4 weeks of penicillin plus an initial 2 weeks of streptomycin has been recommended in patients with a complicated course, a history of disease exceeding 3 months' duration, or prosthetic valve endocarditis due to these sensitive strains or when susceptibility testing reveals the rare penicillin-resistant streptococci.[478] The preferred regimen for IE due to "penicillin-tolerant" streptococci is unsettled. Most of the published clinical data with β-lactam-aminoglycoside regimens for the therapy of viridans streptococcal IE involves the use of penicillin or ampicillin plus streptomycin. However, on the basis of extensive in vitro and animal data, as well as a variety of other reasons, the AHA has deemed gentamicin as preferable to streptomycin in this context.[452] First, gentamicin is currently more widely available and used more often clinically than streptomycin in viridans streptococcal IE. Second, gentamicin (but not streptomycin) serum level determinations are routinely performed in most hospital laboratories. Third, gentamicin can be administered IV or IM, whereas streptomycin can be administered only IM. Because in vitro synergy against most viridans streptococci with penicillin or ampicillin in combination with gentamicin occurs at low gentamicin concentrations (1 to 3 μg/ml), most authorities recommend using gentamicin at a total daily dose of no more than 3 mg/day (IM or IV), split into either a twice-daily (every 12 hours) or thrice-daily (every 8 hours) dose regimen. However, a recent study, using ceftriaxone plus gentamicin given as a once-daily dose had excellent efficacy in the therapy of penicillin-susceptible streptococcal IE, with no increases in aminoglycoside-associated nephrotoxicity.[477] Despite the apparent safety of once-daily aminoglycoside dosing in this latter IE study, as well as in clinical trials involving patients with other infectious disorders,[479] it should be emphasized that the total number of patients receiving with such regimens for 2 weeks or more is relatively limited. Thus, as with any patients receiving aminoglycosides, appropriate clinical and blood level monitoring to mitigate ototoxicity and nephrotoxicity should be employed. Nomograms for prudent monitoring and adjustments of aminoglycoside dosages when once-daily regimens are employed have been published.[478]

Thus, we believe that gentamicin, at a total daily dosage of 3.0 mg/kg, should be substituted for streptomycin in the aforementioned regimens when combination therapy is deemed advisable. In addition, a penicillin-gentamicin regimen is indicated for viridans streptococcal endocarditis if high-level streptomycin resistance is present[464, 465] or for strains with a penicillin MIC more than 0.2 and less than 0.5 μg/ml.[452] Infections due to strains with a penicillin MIC above 0.5 μg/ml should be treated as for enterococcal endocarditis (see further on). Owing to the enhanced rate of bacterial killing in animal models[480, 481] and the high relapse rate of about 17%,[482] we also believe that the "Cornell regimen" (using gentamicin as the preferred aminoglycoside) should be employed for all patients with IE due to NVS. Although temafloxacin plus tobramycin was as effective as penicillin plus tobramycin in the therapy of experimental IE due to *S. adjacens* (an NVS species) in rabbits,[483] quinolones are best avoided for IE due to streptococci pending further data. In the penicillin-allergic patient when a cephalosporin is deemed safe, several regimens are acceptable for IE caused by penicillin-susceptible viridans streptococci: cefazolin, 1 to 2 g IM or IV every 8 hours for 4 weeks, combined with streptomycin, 0.5 g IM every 12 hours, or gentamicin (at the preceding dose regimens) for the initial 2 weeks or ceftriaxone 2 g IV or IM daily alone for 4 weeks. The latter regimen has proven efficacy for the therapy of penicillin-sensitive streptococcal endocarditis.[484, 485] For example, 55 of 59 patients in one uncontrolled trial in Europe completed treatment with 4 months to 5 years of follow-up. Treatment was completely uneventful in 71% of patients while valve replacement was eventually required in 10 patients. Ceftriaxone administered once daily may permit outpatient therapy in a majority of stable patients with this disease. In addition, ceftriaxone plus an aminoglycoside demonstrates in vivo synergy in experimental viridans streptococcal endocarditis.[486] Combination regimens of 2 weeks of once-daily ceftriaxone plus an aminoglycoside (netilmicin or gentamicin), which allows for shortened, predominantly outpatient, regimens has been recently studied in penicillin-susceptible viridans streptococcal IE.[476, 477] These trials performed in Europe and North and South America documented efficacy in this form of IE comparable to other two-week and four-week regimens.[476, 477] When treatment with β-lactams is contraindicated, the regimen of choice is vancomycin, 1 g IV every 12 hours for 4 weeks. A 4-week regimen of high-dose teicoplanin has been efficacious in a small number of patients with streptococcal endocarditis,[487] but the occurrence of drug fever and infection with teicoplanin-tolerant *S. bovis* are cause for concern.

"Penicillin-Resistant" Streptococcal and Enterococcal Endocarditis (e.g., MIC for Penicillin >1.0 μg/ml)[452]

IE due to enterococci is the third most common form of the disease and is the most resistant to therapy. The mortality rate still approximates 20%,[286] and relapses are not uncommon. By broth dilution susceptibility tests, the MIC determinations for many enterococci are as follows: penicillin, 0.4 to 12.5 μg/ml; ampicillin, less than 0.4 to 3.1 μg/ml; cephalothin, 12.5 to 25 μg/ml; vanomycin, 0.78 to 3.1 μg/ml; streptomycin, 3.1 to more than 50 μg/ml; and gentamicin, 6.25 to 25 μg/ml. Ampicillin is approximately twice as active as penicillin by weight. In contrast, the usual MBC determinations are as follows: penicillin, greater than 6.25 μg/ml (in 80% of cases, >100 μg/ml); cephalothin, more than 100 μg/ml; streptomycin, more than 25 μg/ml; vancomycin, more than 100 μg/ml; and gentamicin, 25 μg/ml or less.[488] *E. faecium* strains are more resistant to β-lactams than are *E. faecalis* strains.[489] Thus, in general these agents are bacteriostatic against the enterococci and should not be administered alone in this disease. This bacteriostatic action of agents known to inhibit cell wall synthesis is due to a defective bacterial autolytic enzyme system.[490, 491] As stated before, all β-lactams, including imipenem, are bacteriostatic against enterococci in vitro, and combination regimens are always employed in treating IE.[492] A new mechanism of penicillin resistance among *E. faecalis* strains was described in 1983: plasmid-mediated β-lactamase production. These strains remain relatively rare[493, 494]; *E. faecalis* predominates, but β-lactamase production was recently documented in *E. faecium*.[495] Ampicillin-sulbactam overcomes the β-lactamase production and appears equivalent to vancomycin[496, 497] (or teicoplanin[498]) in experimental IE due to these organisms and superior to therapy with ticarcillin-clavulanate.[497] Unfortunately, most β-lactamase–producing organisms also display high-level aminoglycoside resistance, thus further compromising and complicating the choice of available regimens (see further on). Still other enterococci, particularly *E. faecium* or *Enterococcus raffinosus,* may display high-level penicillin resistance in the absence of β-lactamase production related to perturbations in various penicilin-binding proteins; experimental IE due to these organisms responds to therapy with daptomycin or vancomycin.[499] To date, the number of reported cases of enterococcal IE caused by either β-lactamase–producing strains or those with high-level penicillin resistance on a nonenzymatic basis is very low. It should be noted that the traditional view of β-lactam tolerance among enterococci has been challenged[500] in that some strains demonstrate "paradoxical" tolerance (i.e., there is a higher percentage of survivors at higher antibiotic concentrations.) This phenomenon is more easily demonstrated in vitro at high bacterial densities in stationary growth phase, a situation presumably reflecting the in vivo conditions in the vegetation, and may be important in bacterial persistence or relapse during or following therapy of enterococcal endocarditis.

Cell wall–active antibiotics plus an aminoglycoside are synergistic and produce a bactericidal effect in vitro against most enterococcal strains. Successful treatment of enterococcal endocarditis requires such combinations. Studies in experimental models[501] suggest that "low-dose" streptomycin (peak serum concentrations of 9.1 μg/ml) in combination with penicillin is sufficient to treat streptomycin-susceptible enterococcal endocarditis. "High-level" streptomycin resistance (MIC of >2000 μg/ml) is demonstrable in at least 60% of current enterococcal strains. This resistance correlates with an inability to demonstrate in vitro synergism between penicillin and streptomycin.[502] These highly resistant strains demonstrate synergism between a penicillin and gentamicin in vitro[503, 504] at clinically achievable serum concentrations. Enhanced activity with the penicillin and gentamicin combination was seen in vivo for both streptomycin-resistant and streptomycin-sensitive enterococci in the rabbit model of IE. No differences in results were seen when penicillin was combined with low- versus high-dose gentamicin (peak serum levels of 3.06 and 8.05 μg/ml, respectively) in the treatment of experimental streptomycin-resistant enterococcal endocarditis.[505] Early reports[506, 507] revealed high-level gentamicin resistance among enterococci in up to 14% of isolates beginning in 1979. This phenomenon has become increasingly prevalent in many areas[508–510] beginning among *E. faecalis*, but now includes *E. faecium* as well.[510–512] High-level gentamicin resistance (MIC of ≥2000 μg/ml) now accounts for at least 35% of enterococcal blood isolates in many hospitals. The resistance is plasmid-mediated via the production of aminoglycoside-modifying enzymes and can be readily transferred among strains. A clonal dissemination is not the cause of the increased frequency of these resistant strains, because gentamicin resistance appears in a wide variety of different conjugative and nonconjugative plasmids among enterococci.[510] Although these strains seldom cause IE, they present major problems in nosocomial infections[510] and, because resistance to multiple aminoglycosides is common, represent a formidable therapeutic challenge.[513] In addition, penicillin- or vancomycin-aminoglycoside synergy is not apparent against these organisms in vitro.

The optimal therapy for IE due to these highly resistant strains has not been established. None of the currently recommended regimens is bactericidal against these isolates, and valve replacement[514] may be necessary for a cure. When these isolates are encountered, all available aminoglycosides must be tested separately because the organism may be susceptible to one but resistant to others. Some isolates are sensitive to quinolones or daptomycin, but these agents have received scant attention in human infections. At this time, we favor long-term therapy (8 to 12 weeks) with high dosages of penicillin (20 to 40 million units IV daily in divided doses) or ampicillin (2 to 3 g IV every 4 hours or by continuous infusion) for IE due to these multiply aminoglycoside-resistant enterococci, pending further data. Although results vary among experimental animal models of IE due to these strains,[513, 515] continuous infusion of high-dose ampicillin throughout the 24-hour period may be more effective than a divided-dose regimen and deserves a trial in recalcitrant cases. Even higher-dose aminoglycosides and trimethoprim-sulfamethoxazole were ineffective in animal models[516, 517] and cannot be recommended.

Vancomycin is also bacteriostatic against enterococci and exhibits synergy with the aminoglycosides in vitro. The vancomycin-streptomycin combination synergistically kills 40 to 80% of enterococcal strains, whereas the vancomycin-gentamicin combination demonstrates synergy against 93 to 98%.[518] In one study, vancomycin therapy alone was ineffective in eradicating enterococci from cardiac vegetations in the rabbit model of endocarditis, but the combination of vancomycin plus gentamicin rapidly achieved a bactericidal effect.[505] Vancomycin combined with rifampin has an indifferent effect against enterococci (43/48 strains) in vitro; antagonism is observed rarely.[519] Of some concern, outbreaks of infection due to vancomycin-resistant enterococci have been described.[520] Glycopeptide-resistant strains of enterococci were first isolated in France in 1986. Such strains have emerged rapidly in recent years in many geographic areas worldwide (e.g., New York City[521]) as an important cause of nosocomial infections. The genetics of vancomycin resistance[522] is described elsewhere (see Chapter 189), but multiple phenotypes exist that may confer cross-resistance to related agents (e.g., teicoplanin, daptomycin). Molecular analyses suggest that a highly mobile genetic element (i.e., a transposon) is responsible for the rapid spread of vancomycin-resistant enterococci.[521] The molecular basis for some forms of this resistance (substitutions of D-alanine–D-lactate for D-alanine–D-alanine in the terminal pentapeptide chain) has been defined. IE due to vancomycin-resistant enterococci has, so far fortunately, been unusual[523] but has occurred in transplanted hearts.[524]

The therapy of vancomycin-resistant enterococcal IE is unsettled. All suspected strains should be tested quantitatively (e.g., by determination of MIC or MBC) in vitro for susceptibility to glycopeptides, penicillins, and aminoglycosides. Teicoplanin—or, potentially, daptomycin—[525–527] may be useful, in combination with gentamicin, against some isolates with low-level vancomycin resistance that do not exhibit cross-resistance. Ramoplanin, a cyclic lipoglycopeptide, is active against more than 90% of strains of highly vancomycin-resistant enterococci in vitro,[528] but clinical experience with IE is virtually nonexistent. A triple combination of high-dose penicillin plus vancomycin plus gentamicin appears very promising in animal models of IE induced by such resistant enterococci[529, 530] and should be employed if in vitro susceptibility test results suggest multiply resistant isolates. The cephalosporins are relatively inactive against enterococci, even in combination with an aminoglycoside, and should not be used in this disease. The older-generation quinolones (e.g., ciprofloxacin) do not appear promising for the treatment of enterococcal endocarditis.[531] However, one recent study showed that a newer quinolone agent with an expanded in vitro spectrum against gram-positive cocci, trovafloxacin, had good in vivo activity against resistant enterococci in the experimental IE model.[532] This in vivo efficacy was noted for several resistant enterococcal strains, including a β-lactamase producer, as well as for strains exhibiting *vanA*- and *vanB*-mediated resistance (especially when trovafloxacin was combined with ampicillin-sulbactam). In addition, there are limited human treatment data supporting the efficacy of the fixed streptogram in combination of quinupristin-dalfopristin in the therapy of serious vancomycin-resistant enterococcal infections.[533] Among 115 patients with bacteremia due to such strains, including 5 who had IE, the overall frequency of clearance of bacteremia and clinical efficacy approached 70%.[534]

Although controlled trials are lacking, clinical experience would dictate that enterococcal endocarditis caused by strains with typical antibiotic susceptibility profiles be treated with combination antimicrobial therapy for at least 4 to 6 weeks.[468] The recommended regimen is as follows: aqueous penicillin G, 20 million units IV daily in divided doses (or ampicillin at doses as recommended for viridans streptococcal IE), combined with streptomycin, 0.5 g IM every 12 hours, or gentamicin, at the same regimen as that recommended for viridans stretococcal IE, for 4 to 6 weeks. It should be emphasized, however, that gentamicin should be given not once daily but at least twice daily for enterococcal IE. Experimental studies in enterococcal IE models show a greater reduction in vegetation bacterial densities when the aminoglycoside is administered in multidosing rather than once-daily regimens.[535, 536] If toxicity (vestibular, aural, or renal) occurs, the streptomycin dose is divided into an every-6-hour regimen. If the streptomycin MIC determined for the infecting strain is 2000 μg/ml or higher, gentamicin should be substituted for streptomycin, although relapses or therapeutic failures are unusual with penicillin plus streptomycin. We recommend penicillin plus gentamicin as the initial therapy. If the peak serum bactericidal titer is less than 1:8, the penicillin dose may be increased, or the aminoglycoside drug may be changed in accordance with in vitro tests results.

Wilson and associates[537] analyzed the experience at the Mayo Clinic with 56 patients who received treatment for 4 weeks with aqueous penicillin G (20 million units IV daily) combined with either streptomycin, 0.5 g IM every 12 hours, for enterococcal IE due to streptomycin-sensitive strains or gentamicin, 1 mg/kg IM every 8 hours, for IE due to streptomycin-resistant strains. Relapse rates were high (12.5%) for both regimens; however, all patients who relapsed had had symptoms suggestive of IE for longer than 3 months. Relapses also only occurred in patients with mitral valve involvement. All patients who received over 3 mg/kg daily of gentamicin developed reversible nephrotoxicity (defined as a twofold increase in serum creatinine concentration), and 19% of patients receiving streptomycin for 4 weeks developed irreversible vestibular toxicity. Although this was not a prospective randomized trial, we believe that in selected cases, enterococcal endocarditis may be treated with 4 weeks of combination therapy. The exceptions include mitral valve involvement, duration of symptomatic illness exceeding 3 months, enterococcal prosthetic valve endocarditis (PVE), and relapse(s) of enterococcal endocarditis.

The penicillin-allergic patient presents the clinician with a difficult therapeutic dilemma. Vancomycin as a single drug in a dose of 1 g IV every 12 hours has been used in the treatment of enterococcal endocarditis. However, experience is limited, and, because of its lack of bactericidal activity in vitro and poor performance in experimental endocarditis, vancomycin should be combined with gentamicin or streptomycin. Unfortunately, this combination is potentially more nephrotoxic, and clinical proof of the superiority of such regimens over vancomycin alone is not available. The other therapeutic option in the allergic patient is "penicillin desensitization" followed by the administration of penicillin and an aminoglycoside. The therapy of enterococcal IE due to highly aminoglycoside- or glycopeptide-resistant strains is discussed earlier.

Staphylococcal Endocarditis

The mortality rate in acute staphylococcal endocarditis still approximates 40%, and the preferred antibiotic regimen is controversial. Mortality is highest for men, patients over 50 years of age, and patients with left-sided involvement or central nervous system manifestations. In addition, narcotic addicts appear to have a lower mortality than do nonaddicts. Most *S. aureus* isolates, whether community- or hospital-acquired, are now resistant to penicillin G (MIC of >0.2 μg/ml). The current recommended regimen includes a penicillinase-resistant penicillin (nafcillin or oxacillin, 1.5 to 2 g IV every 4 hours) or a cephalosporin (cephalothin, 2 g IV every 4 hours, or cefazolin, 1 to 2 g IV or IM every 8 hours) given for 4 to 6 weeks.[452, 538] The addition of gentamicin produces a synergistic effect against *S. aureus* in vitro and in experimental staphylococcal endocarditis in rabbits.[539] However, the combination did not improve the survival rate (60%) over that observed with a penicillin derivative alone in a small group of patients.[323] Combination therapy did not improve the results of therapy for staphylococcal IE in addicts,[540] but the mortality rate is low in this subgroup of patients (≈2 to 8%) with this disease. Combination therapy may permit a shorter duration of therapy in addicts with *S. aureus* IE. Two weeks of nafcillin plus tobramycin (1 mg/kg IV every 8 hours) cured 47 of 50 (94%) intravenous drug users with right-sided endocarditis[541] without evidence of renal failure, extrapulmonary metastatic infectious complications, aortic or mitral involvement, meningitis, or infection by MRSA.

Since this original experience with "short-course" parenteral therapy for right-sided *S. aureus* IE in addicts,[541] there have been three recent randomized, prospective trials of such short-course regimens in this disease, comprising 121 patients (summarized by DiNubile.[542, 543] The combination regimens employed included intravenous cloxacillin with either gentamicin or amikacin.[544–546] The overall clinical and microbiologic cure rates exceeded 90% in these studies. Of note, in patients with HIV seropositivity (most having CD4$^+$ counts $>300 \times 10^6$ cells) and in those who had large tricuspid vegetations (≥10 mm in diameter), such regimens had excellent efficacy.[546] Of interest, in this latter study,[546] Ribera and coworkers showed an efficacy of intravenous cloxacillin equivalent to that of the cloxacillin-plus gentamicin regimen. Thus, it appears that for most addicted patients with uncomplicated right-sided *S. aureus* IE, such short-course parenteral regimens of an antistaphylococcal semisynthetic penicillin plus an aminoglycoside are interchangeable with longer-term (4 to 6 weeks) parenteral regimens. In addition, two studies have evaluated the use of predominantly oral 4-week antibiotic regimens (ciprofloxacin plus rifampin) for the therapy of uncomplicated right-sided *S. aureus* IE in addicts.[547, 548] In each study, including one in which more than 70% of patients were HIV-seropositive,[548] cure rates exceeded 90%.

Anecdotal case reports in nonaddicts with staphylococcal IE suggest that the addition of gentamicin may be of benefit in patients failing to respond to nafcillin therapy.[549] This issue was addressed in a multicenter prospective trial comparing nafcillin alone with nafcillin plus gentamicin (for the initial 2 weeks) in the treatment of endocarditis due to *S. aureus*.[550] Most of the patients in this study were nonaddicts who had left-sided IE. Although the combination resulted in a more rapid rate of eradication of the bacteremia, the incidence of nephrotoxicity was increased, and no improvement in mortality was achieved. Despite these results, many authorities still use combination therapy for short periods (e.g., 3 to 5 days) for left-sided *S. aureus* IE, especially in fulminant cases. If the organism is susceptible to penicillin (MIC of <0.1 μg/ml), then this agent in a dose of 20 million units IV daily should be used. The response to treatment may be slow, often with fever and positive blood cultures lasting up to 1 week.[320]

The therapy of staphylococcal endocarditis in penicillin-allergic patients, or when the isolate is methicillin-resistant (MRSA), is problematic. First-generation cephalosporins (as noted previously) are generally recommended in patients with non–life-threatening penicillin allergy, but nafcillin is more active in experimental methicillin-susceptible *S. aureus* endocarditis[551] and is preferred if results of skin tests for penicillin allergy are negative. With the exception of ceftazidime, the in vivo efficacy of cephalosporins in experimental *S. aureus* endocarditis has a positive correlation with in vitro activity (MIC) and the time (percentage) during the dosing interval in which the drug serum level exceeds the MIC.[551] Vancomycin is still recommended for the therapy of *S. aureus* endocarditis in patients with life-threatening penicillin allergy (e.g., anaphylaxis) or anaphylactoid reactions (e.g., giant urticaria), or when MRSA strains are involved; however, recent experience suggests caution, as suboptimal outcomes have been associated with the use of this agent in MRSA IE. Vancomycin is less rapidly bactericidal than nafcillin in vitro against *S. aureus*, especially at high inocula (approximately 10^7 cfu), mimicking intravegetation densities. Furthermore, failure rates of approximately 40% have been documented in patients with *S. aureus* endocarditis treated with vancomycin[552] despite right-sided involvement. In another study[553] utilizing vancomycin-based regimens (with or without rifampin), blood cultures were still positive after 7 days of therapy in approximately 50% of patients, again despite right-sided involvement and negative results in a large number of echocardiographic studies. Daptomycin and teicoplanin are unlikely to be acceptable substitutes, owing to unfavorable or unpredictable pharmacokinetics[554] or the development of resistance[555, 556] during therapy. For methicillin-susceptible *S. aureus* endocarditis in patients with anaphylactoid-type β-lactam allergy and suboptimal responses to vancomycin, the need for β-lactam desensitization should be considered.[557, 558]

Clindamycin has been used to treat over 60 cases of staphylococcal endocarditis but is associated with an unacceptable relapse rate, and its use is not recommended.[559] The optimal therapy for IE due to "tolerant" strains of *S. aureus* is controversial.[560, 561] One retrospective study[562] suggested that patients with IE due to these tolerant strains had a more complicated course; however, combination therapy did not appear to be of benefit. Tolerance does appear to influence the response to therapy in some experimental animal models of *S. aureus* endocarditis,[563] and the use of combination regimens appears prudent when these strains are recovered from patients, but this is not universally accepted. Another controversial area is the adjunctive role of rifampin, the most active antibiotic currently available against *S. aureus* in vitro in therapy for IE. Owing to the emergence of resistant strains, this drug is ineffective alone. Unfortunately, results of in vitro studies on rifampin combinations with either β-lactam agents or vancomycin are frequently contradictory, and clinical outcomes with experimental IE induced by *S. aureus* are dependent on which drug in the combination exerts the greatest bactericidal activity in vivo.[564] At present, rifampin should be reserved for patients demonstrating poor serum bactericidal activity during therapy with a β-lactam or vancomycin or in those with suppurative complications (e.g., valve-ring abscesses, hematogenous osteomyelitis, meningitis). Resistance to both clindamycin and rifampin has emerged during therapy of this condition, however.[565] The therapy of IE due to *S. aureus* displaying borderline susceptibility to antistaphylococcal penicillins, first described by McDougal and Thornsberry in 1986,[566] is also a matter of debate. Experimental models of IE induced with these isolates suggest, however, that nafcillin (or oxacillin) or ampicillin-sulbactam should be effective.[567, 568] Several newer agents, including teicoplanin, fosfomycin, and fluoroquinolones, are active against MRSA in vitro and are as rapidly bactericidal as vancomycin in experimental animal models of IE due to MRSA,[569, 570, 571] although resistance to the quinolones has emerged during therapy and frank failures have been recorded.[558, 572, 573] For patients with MRSA endocarditis not responding to vancomycin, several choices are available, including the addition of rifampin or gentamicin (or both), or other regimens including minocycline, trimethoprim-sulfamethoxazole, and ciprofloxacin-rifampin. Experience with these drugs in humans with *S. aureus* endocarditis is limited.[574] According to some authors,[575] when *S. aureus* bacteremia occurs in a patient with a removable focus of infection, the risk of concurrent IE is low, and treatment schedules may be shortened to 2 to 3 weeks. This approach avoids the high costs and risks of superinfection or antibiotic reactions associated with prolonged therapy. In one study, 8 of 21 patients with an infected intravenous catheter as the suspected source of *S. aureus* bacteremia developed endocarditis.[576] Bayer and associates[558, 577] identified four parameters predictive of the presence of IE in 72 patients with *S. aureus* bacteremia in a prospective study: (1) the absence of a primary site of infection; (2) community acquisition of infection; (3) metastatic sequelae; and (4) valvular vegetations detected by echocardiography. Therefore, short-term therapy should be used only if IE can be reasonably excluded by methods previously discussed. Other studies have suggested that occult IE in patients with nosocomial *S. aureus* bacteremia is uncommon.[557] Screening all patients with nosocomial *S. aureus* bacteremia by transthoracic echocardiography is not cost-effective and should be reserved for those with peripheral manifestations, known underlying valvular heart disease, persistent fever, bacteremia after removal of the presumed primary focus, or with new or significant heart murmurs.[557, 558] One recent study by Fowler and colleagues[326] has documented an apparent increase in the proportion of cases of IE complicating nosocomially acquired *S. aureus* bacteremia (mainly from infected intravascular catheters). In this group of 27 patients, classic manifestations of IE were infrequent, and TEE was useful in diagnosis of IE.

S. epidermidis is the most common etiologic agent in cases of prosthetic valve endocarditis. Most of these strains (87%) are methicillin-resistant when isolated within 1 year of valve implantation. One study[578] suggests that the optimal antimicrobial regimen for these infections is vancomycin plus rifampin, usually with the addition of an aminoglycoside. The emergence of vancomycin resistance among coagulase-negative staphylococci[579] is cause for concern. These concepts are discussed further in Chapter 66.

Endocarditis Due to Members of Enterobacteriaceae or Pseudomonas *Species*

Of 125 cases of IE reported from Seattle, 4.8% were due to gram-negative aerobic bacilli.[20] The mortality rate was 83%, and none of the patients in whom treatment did not include surgery survived. The prognosis is especially poor with left-sided cardiac involvement. Determinations of tube dilution MBC are necessary to guide therapy. Certain combinations of penicillins or cephalosporins and aminoglycosides have been shown to be synergistic against many of these strains and are usually recommended. For IE due to most strains of *E. coli* or *Proteus mirabilis*, a combination of a penicillin, either ampicillin (2 g IV every 4 hours) or penicillin (20 million units IV daily) with an aminoglycoside, usually gentamicin (1.7 mg/kg every 8 hours) or a broad-spectrum cephalosporin is suggested. Third-generation cephalosporins are extremely active against *E. coli* in vitro, and some (e.g., ceftriaxone) have proved effective in experimental animal models of *E. coli* endocarditis,[580] even when long dosing intervals were used. This group of agents deserves further evaluation in humans for IE due to susceptible gram-negative bacilli. A combination of a third-generation cephalosporin and an aminoglycoside (either gentamicin or amikacin) is recommended for *Klebsiella* endocarditis. Certain β-lactam/β-lactamase inhibitor combinations (e.g., piperacillin-tazobactam[581] but not ceftriaxone-sulbactam[582]) are active in vivo in experimental models of *Klebsiella* endocarditis in animals induced by TEM-3–producing isolates and deserve further evaluation in combination with an aminoglycoside in humans with this disease.

The specific aminoglycoside employed is a critical variable and cannot be totally predicted from MIC data alone, as pharmacodynamic characteristics differ markedly in animal models of IE due to gram-negative aerobic bacilli.[583, 584] Endovascular *Salmonella* infections, including IE, may also respond to third-generation cephalosporins (see further on).[585] Left-sided IE due to *S. marcescens* is refractory to medical therapy alone; valve replacement is invariably required to effect a cure.[354]

Pseudomonas aeruginosa remains an important pathogen in drug addicts with IE. Medical therapy may be successful in *P. aeruginosa* IE involving the right side of the heart in up to 50 to 75% of cases. If the disease is refractory to antibiotics, tricuspid valvulectomy or "vegetectomy"[586] without valve replacement is indicated.[587] Although valve replacement is often necessary for a cure of left-sided IE due to *P. aeruginosa*,[588] results[190] in a series of 10 patients (7 with left-sided involvement alone or in combination with tricuspid disease) suggest that medical therapy alone is occasionally curative. Studies in animals with experimental *Pseudomonas* endocarditis[589] offer a partial explanation for these disparate results: the penetration into vegetations and the time during which antibiotic concentrations exceeded the MBC were both significantly greater with tricuspid than with aortic vegetations for both ceftazidime and tobramycin.

The optimal antimicrobial regimen for *P. aeruginosa* IE is evolving; the most extensive experience has been at the Detroit Medical Center. Problems have emerged with all potential regimens in animal models of this disease: (1) therapy with β-lactams (e.g., ceftazidime) has failed, owing to the selection of clones within valve vegetations that exhibit constitutive hyperproduction of type Id β-lactamase[590]; (2) isolates demonstrating aminoglycoside resistance due to permeability defects emerge during therapy[591]; (3) no postantibiotic effect of β-lactams against *P. aeruginosa* is evident in vivo,[592] thus necessitating frequent (or continuous) drug administration; and (4) the alginate exopolysaccharide inhibits clearance of mucoid strains from the vegetation via cellular or antimicrobial mechanisms. This inhibition can be partially reversed by the coadministration of alginase in animal models of *Pseudomonas* endocarditis.[593]

Treatment failures of *Pseudomonas* endocarditis in humans have also been due to the selection of isolates with an enhanced production of type Id β-lactamase.[594] Based on clinical experience,[329, 356, 357] however, the preferred regimen for IE due to *P. aeruginosa* is high-dose tobramycin (8 mg/kg/day IV or IM in divided doses every 8 hours) with maintenance of peak and trough concentrations of 15 to 20 and 2 μg/ml or less, respectively, in combination with either an extended-spectrum penicillin (e.g., ticarcillin, piperacillin, azlocillin) or ceftazidime in full doses. The toxicity associated with this regimen is surprisingly low; combination treatment should be given for a minimum of 6 weeks. The use of quinolones (in combination with an aminoglycoside) appears promising for the treatment of *Pseudomonas* endocarditis on the basis of favorable results in animal models[590] and in humans,[595] but the development of stepwise resistance during therapy may limit the efficacy of this class of drugs in the future. Based on limited experimental data,[596] ceftazidime-tobramycin is preferred over aztreonam-tobramycin for this disease. Approximately seven cases of *P. aeruginosa* endocarditis have been successfully treated with imipenem plus an aminoglycoside,[597] but the potential for the development of resistance exists with any of these regimens.

In one study, IE due to *Haemophilus* spp. (and other members of the HACEK group) was usually responsive to ampicillin alone[348] administered for 3 weeks. Recently, however, β-lactamase–producing strains have been well documented. Because of difficulty in cultivating HACEK organisms in the laboratory, particularly for newer, automated susceptibility testing systems, such strains should be considered as ampicillin-resistant. The newer third-generation cephalosporins (e.g., ceftriaxone or cefotaxime) have excellent in vitro activity against HACEK organisms and also provide the potential for the avoidance of aminoglycoside-induced toxicity. Although clinical data are limited, the third-generation cephalosporins should be regarded as the drugs of choice for treatment of HACEK IE.[596] The place for quinolones (if any) in the therapy of these infections is not known.[599] Duration of treatment for HACEK IE should be 3 to 4 weeks for native valve infections and 6 weeks for prosthetic valve infections.[452, 598] We emphasize that the foregoing recommendations offer only a rough guide for initial treatment. However, it is imperative that each isolate be subjected to quantitative sensitivity testing in vitro to ensure the optimal selection of antibiotics.

Endocarditis Due to Anaerobic Bacilli

Although IE caused by anaerobic bacilli is uncommon, the mortality is high. *B. fragilis* is isolated in many of these cases and is responsible for most fatalities. Most strains of anaerobic bacilli, with the exception of *B. fragilis*, are sensitive to penicillin in vitro, and use of this agent, in a dose of 20 million units IV daily, is the recommended therapy.[392, 393] In addition, 33% of the strains of *B. fragilis* demonstrate an MIC for penicillin that is less than 0.25 μg/ml. However, penicillin is only bacteriostatic against these strains (the MBC is invariably greater than 100 μg/ml), and relapse is common. Although clindamycin, carbenicillin, and chloramphenicol readily inhibit most strains of *B. fragilis*, they lack bactericidal activity, and they are poor therapeutic choices even though several patients have been cured with either high-dose penicillin, chloramphenicol (1 g IV every 6 hours), clindamycin (600 mg IV every 6 hours), or carbenicillin (5 g IV every 3 hours). Owing to excellent bactericidal activity in vitro and the serum concentrations attained, metronidazole, ticarcillin plus clavulanic acid, or imipenem is a reasonable choice for therapy for anaerobic endocarditis.[394]

Pneumococcal, Gonococcal, and Meningococcal Endocarditis

IE caused by pneumococci, gonococci, or meningococci is now very rare. Pneumococcal endocarditis must be considered in any patient with pneumococcal bacteremia, especially if meningitis is present. This form of IE is most common in alcoholics; the organism generally attacks the aortic valve and results in valvular insufficiency, often with perivalvular abscess formation or pericarditis. Type 12 pneumococci cause over 20% of the cases of pneumococcal endocarditis but are a rare (5% of the cases) cause of pneumococcal pneumonia. Penicillin, 20 million units IV daily, or a third-generation cephalosporin for 4 weeks, is recommended for the treatment of pneumococcal endocarditis. In the rare circumstance of IE due to strains either moderately resistant or highly resistant to penicillin G, a third-generation cephalosporin or vancomycin would be the preferred choice.

The gonococci that cause systemic infection are usually susceptible to penicillin.[600] IE due to these organisms as well as the meningococci can be effectively treated with the same penicillin regimen recommended for pneumococcal endocarditis. Although endocarditis due to penicillin-resistant gonococci (on either a β-lactamase production basis or due to chromosomally mediated mechanisms) has not been reported, ceftriaxone has been used successfully to treat gonococcal endocarditis.[601]

Fungal Endocarditis

The incidence of IE caused by fungi has undergone a striking increase in the past decade. Fungal IE occurs principally in a setting of narcotic addiction, after cardiac surgery, after the prolonged intravenous administration of drugs (especially broad-spectrum antibiotics), and in the compromised host (including preterm neonates). The overall survival rate in patients treated since 1968 is only 14.5%.[236] The preferred mode of therapy has not been determined. The use of antifungal agents alone has been almost universally unsuccessful in achieving a cure of this disease. The addition of surgical measures to antifungal therapy may result in an improvement in prognosis, but to date there is insufficient clinical experience. When fungal IE is diagnosed, a combined medical-surgical approach is recommended.[409, 602]

The mainstay of antifungal drug therapy is amphotericin B. This agent is toxic and produces multiple side effects, including fever, chills, phlebitis, headache, anorexia, anemia, hypokalemia, renal tubular acidosis, nephrotoxicity, nausea, and vomiting. Drug toxicity is frequent and commonly necessitates alterations in the regimen. Dosages and the technique of administration are given in Chapter 35.

After 1 to 2 weeks of amphotericin B therapy at full dosages, surgery should probably be performed. If isolated tricuspid endocarditis is present, as in a narcotic addict, total tricuspid valvulectomy can usually be performed. Rarely, removal of the vegetation alone is curative. Most of the patients tolerate the valvulectomy without the development of significant right-sided heart failure for at least 3 to 5 years. Valve replacement is necessary for left-sided fungal endocarditis. The duration of antifungal therapy after surgery is empirical, but 6 to 8 weeks is usually recommended.

It is possible that combination antifungal therapy may improve the poor survival with fungal endocarditis. Some strains of *Candida* spp. and *Cryptococcus neoformans* are inhibited in vitro by concentrations of 5-fluorocytosine achieved with the oral administration of 150 mg/kg/day in six divided doses. Synergism between 5-fluorocytosine and amphotericin B has been documented for these yeasts in vitro and in the treatment of cryptococcal meningitis. This combination was fungicidal and perhaps instrumental in the cure of one case of *Aspergillus* endocarditis. However, in the rabbit model of endocarditis due to *C. albicans*[240] the addition of 5-fluorocytosine did not improve the rate of eradication of fungal organisms from the vegetation over that observed with amphotericin B alone. Potentiation of amphotericin B activity by rifampin has been noted for virtually all strains of *Candida* spp. tested and for a few isolates of *Histoplasma capsulatum.* The therapeutic advantage of the addition of 5-fluorocytosine or rifampin to amphotericin for fungal endocarditis requires further investigation, but initial results in animal models of disseminated candidiasis are not encouraging.[603] On the basis of animal model data,[604] high-dose intraconazole may be of value in the treatment of *Aspergillus* endocarditis, but valve replacement will probably remain imperative for a cure. Amphotericin B is more effective than fluconazole for the prophylaxis and treatment of experimental *Candida* IE[605] and remains the agent of choice. The use of fluconazole has apparently, however, led to long-term cures of *Candida* IE in a limited number of patients [409, 606–608] when valve replacement was considered to be contraindicated. This agent should be tried after an initial course of amphotericin B in this setting or used for long-term suppressive therapy. The role of amphotericin–lipid-liposomal complexes in the treatment of fungal endocarditis is unknown.

Q Fever Endocarditis

More than 300 well-documented cases of Q fever have been reported, and the mortality exceeds 65%.[414–417] Prolonged therapy with doxycycline and either trimethoprim-sulfamethoxazole or rifampin is considered to be the regimen of choice[414, 609–611] (see Chapter 177). A fluoroquinolone may be a useful addition to doxycycline.[414, 611] The acidic conditions of the phagolysosome, where the organism resides, may inhibit antibiotic activity.[611] Cure of the IE after treatment with a combination of doxycycline and hydroxychloroquine to alkalinize the phagolysosome for 1 year was reported in 20 patients.[414] Valve replacement is often required, and long-term prognosis is guarded. Careful follow-up to detect recrudescence of infection is essential. Most authorities recommend at least 3 to 4 years of therapy to eradicate both valvular and extravalvular Q fever (usually in the liver).

Infective Endocarditis Due to Chlamydiae

Albeit based on limited experience, a combination of valve replacement and prolonged (greater than 3 months) tetracycline therapy seems justified in these cases. Rifampin has cured at least one case of chlamydial IE after therapy with tetracyclines had failed, but exposure to this agent rapidly induces the emergence of drug resistance in *C. trachomatis* in tissue culture.[612] The role of combination regimens (e.g., rifampin plus erythromycin or tetracycline) deserves further study.

Culture-Negative Endocarditis

The therapy for culture-negative endocarditis in non–drug addicts is controversial, but the regimen usually used will "cover" enterococci, the HACEK group, and NVS. This consists of a combination of penicillin, 20 million units IV daily in divided doses, or ampicillin, 2 g IV every 4 hours, plus streptomycin, 0.5 g IM every 12 hours, or gentamicin, 1.7 mg/kg IM or IV every 8 hours, plus ceftriaxone, 2 g IV once daily. When staphylococcal endocarditis is likely (as in narcotic addicts), a penicillinase-resistant penicillin or a cephalosporin in full dosage should be added to the above regimen. If clinical improvement occurs, some authorities recommend discontinuation of treatment with the aminoglycoside after 2 weeks. The other agent(s) should be continued for a full 6 weeks of treatment. Continued surveillance for the causative agent and careful follow-up are mandatory. An analysis of any correlation between the response to empirical antimicrobial therapy and survival was performed in 52 patients with culture-negative endocarditis:[424] 92% of the patients who became afebrile within the first week of therapy survived, versus only 50% if fever persisted longer than 7 days. Most deaths were caused by major systemic emboli or uncontrollable CHF due to valvular insufficiency.

Surgical Therapy

Valve replacement has become an important adjunct to medical therapy in the management of IE and is now used in at least 25% of the cases. The generally accepted indications for surgical intervention during active IE are as follows: (1) refractory CHF; (2) more than one serious systemic embolic episode; (3) uncontrolled infection; (4) physiologically significant valve dysfunction as demonstrated by echocardiography; (5) ineffective antimicrobial therapy (e.g., as in fungal endocarditis); (6) resection of mycotic aneurysms; (7) most cases of prosthetic valve IE caused by more antibiotic-resistant pathogens e.g., staphylococci, enteric gram-negative bacilli; and (8) local suppurative complications including perivalvular or myocardial abscesses. The major indications in the past have been persistent infection and CHF[613–615] in both adults and children.[616] For example, CHF during active IE was the indication for surgery in 86% of 108 patients undergoing valve replacement at Stanford from 1963 to 1984.[615] Despite the widespread use of TTE and TEE at present in patients with IE, the indications for surgical intervention based on echocardiographic features remain controversial. The AHA Committee on IE, working from data reported in the recent literature, has identified the following echocardiographic features in IE as associated with a potential increased need for surgical intervention: (1) persistent vegetations after a major systemic embolic episode, (2) large (>1 cm in diameter) anterior mitral valve vegetations, (3) increase in vegetation size after 4 weeks of antibiotic therapy, (4) acute mitral insufficiency, (5) valve perforation or rupture, and (6) periannular extension of infection. (These data are reviewed in the article by Bayer and associates.[273])

The most frequent causes of death in IE, in approximate order, are neurologic and septic complications,[617] CHF, embolic phenomena, rupture of a mycotic aneurysm, complications of cardiac surgery, lack of response to antimicrobial therapy, and prosthetic valve endocarditis[2, 3, 6–9, 11, 12, 14–17, 20]

When acute aortic regurgitation complicated by CHF supervenes in IE, the mortality still exceeds 50%. The classic physical findings associated with chronic aortic regurgitation are often absent in these patients.[268] The current trend is to perform early surgery in this group of patients, because nothing is gained by delay. The merits of early valve replacement surgery were confirmed as early as 1972.[618] In a series of 28 patients from Birmingham, Alabama, with acute aortic regurgitation, 4 had no CHF and were managed medically, and all survived. In contrast, 7 of 11 patients with mild CHF and 7 of 8 with moderate to severe CHF died during medical therapy, often suddenly and with pathologic evidence of coronary emboli and myocardial infarction. Four of five patients with moderately severe CHF who underwent surgery survived. This suggests that early surgical intervention may improve survival in this setting. Valvular regurgitation on Doppler echocardiography is not predictive of death in the absence of CHF.[619]

The hemodynamic status of the patient, not the activity of the infection, is the critical determining factor in the timing of cardiac valve replacement (i.e., development of CHF in the setting of IE generally dictates valvular surgery irrespective of the acuity of infection or the amount of antibiotics already received by the patient).[620] The hemodynamic severity of the acute aortic regurgitation may be assessed by determining the degree of mitral valve preclosure by echocardiography. If premature closure of the mitral valve occurs before the Q wave of the electrocardiogram, then the left ventricular end-diastolic pressure is very high, and surgical intervention is urgently required. Nothing is gained by temporizing, even if only a few hours of antibiotics can be administered. When CHF persists despite digoxin, diuretics, and other therapeutic modalities (e.g., left ventricular afterload reduction), surgery is also indicated. In 80 patients subjected to aortic valve replacement for IE, the surgical cure rate was 72%. There were no instances of subsequent infection of the prosthesis, but 16% developed paravalvular regurgitation. This latter complication was usually easily controlled medically. Organisms visible on Gram stain, positive cultures, or annular abscesses at the time of surgery are associated with late complications.[617] Although not systematically studied, most authorities suggest that if there is evidence of active IE at the time of valve replacement surgery, antibiotic therapy should be continued postoperatively for at least several weeks. Such evidence includes vegetations that remain culture-positive or Gram stain–positive and those with significant polymorphonuclear inflammation.

In contrast to left-sided IE in which CHF is the usual indication for surgical intervention, persistent infection is the indication for surgery in over 70% of patients with right-sided IE. Most of the patients are narcotic addicts, with IE caused by organisms that are difficult to eradicate with antimicrobial therapy alone (e.g., fungi, gram-negative aerobic bacilli). Tricuspid valvulectomy or "vegetectomy" with valvuloplasty is now the procedure of choice for refractory right-sided IE.[621, 622] Valve replacement at a second operation is advised only when medical management fails to control the hemodynamic manifestations and the patient has ceased using illicit drugs. Combination antimicrobial therapy should be continued for 4 to 6 weeks postoperatively. These patients may develop mild to moderate right-sided heart failure, but this is easily tolerated, and the success rate with this approach is over 70%. However, eventual tricuspid valve replacement is usually required for progressive right heart failure. Persistent fever, recurrent pulmonary emboli, or vegetations demonstrable by echocardiography usually do not necessitate tricuspid valvulectomy in this setting.[623] In addition, many surgeons contend that a return to the use of illicit drugs and reinfection of the valve after initial cure is a contraindication to reoperation.[624]

Outstanding reviews on the indications for surgery during therapy for IE are available.[614, 625–628] The rationale for surgical intervention, including major and minor criteria for valve replacement, is discussed in detail. A point system weighting multiple factors has been devised by Alsip and colleagues to assist in decision making concerning sugery in patients with active IE.[625] The value of this system remains to be defined. It has become apparent that most patients with prosthetic valve endocarditis (except those with late disease caused by penicillin-sensitive viridans streptococci) require valve replacement for consistent cures (see Chapter 66). Valve replacement is also necessary in a significant proportion of patients with IE on native valves after a medical cure; aortic involvement is a predictor of the need for surgery.[629]

SUPPURATIVE THROMBOPHLEBITIS

Suppurative thrombophlebitis is an inflammation of the vein wall due to the presence of microorganisms and is frequently associated with thrombosis and bacteremia. In the following discussion, suppurative thrombophlebitis is differentiated from catheter-related sepsis. Suppuration of the vein wall is usually absent in intravenous catheter–related sepsis and bacteremia secondary to contaminated intravenous fluid but does occur. Suppurative thrombophlebitis may be classified into four forms: superficial, central (including pelvic), cavernous sinus, and infection of the portal vein (pyelophlebitis). The last two conditions have become rare since the introduction of antibiotics. Cavernous sinus thrombosis and thrombosis of the intracranial dural sinuses are discussed in Chapters 71 and 95. In contrast, superficial suppurative thrombophlebitis has been steadily increasing in incidence since the introduction of the plastic intravenous cannula. Superficial suppurative thrombophlebitis secondary to intravenous fluid therapy was first described in 1947,[630] when 93 cases were reported, 43 of which were amenable to surgical therapy.

Epidemiology

In 1973, approximately one of every four hospitalized patients received intravenous therapy, for a total of over 10 million patients annually in the United States.[631] It is estimated that more than half of the 40 million patients admitted to U.S. hospitals each year undergo intravascular catheterization.[632] Suppurative thrombophlebitis is a particular problem in burned patients, for whom it represents a common cause of death due to infection. In several large series of burned patients,[633–636] suppurative thrombophlebitis developed in 4 to 8% and increased in frequency if cutdowns were performed. Suppurative thrombophlebitis is also found in other hospitalized patients (especially those with cancer or those receiving steroid therapy).[637, 638] Seven such cases were recognized in an 18-month period in Charleston, South Carolina, and 35 cases were identified in 7 years in Louisville, Kentucky.[639] Eight cases were encountered during an 8-month period in Johannesburg; suppurative thrombophlebitis was estimated to represent a minimum incidence of 0.12% of all admissions.[640] In a study using strict diagnostic criteria, 29 episodes of suppurative thrombophlebitis in 27 patients were identified in a large Air Force hospital within 4 years.[641] Using data from the National Nosocomial Infection Study, Rhame and associates[642] estimated the overall incidence of suppurative thrombophlebitis as 88 per 100,000 discharges, but this disease is underreported. Suppurative thrombophlebitis is also common in drug addicts, particularly when injections are made in large, central veins (e.g., jugular or subclavian veins).[643] This condition is unusual during childhood[644] but may occur as a complication related to intravenous therapy. Catheter-related sepsis without suppurative thrombophlebitis is much more common and affects at least 50,000 to 100,000 patients per year in the United States.[645, 646] The risk of this complication is approximately 40 times higher with plastic cannulas (8%) than with steel or "scalp vein" cannulas (0.2%). Irritation to the vein wall with the subsequent development of suppurative thrombophlebitis is more common with polyethylene catheters than those constructed of Teflon or Silastic material. Central venous catheterization has been employed for more than 35 years for hemodynamic monitoring, total parenteral nutrition (TPN), and infusion of drugs. The exact incidence of suppurative thrombophlebitis of the central veins commonly cannulated (i.e., jugulars, subclavian, venae cavae) is unknown. Catheter-induced thrombosis is relatively common. Autopsy series have revealed central venous thrombosis in 37% of catheterized subjects, but this diagnosis is rarely recognized because most patients are asymptomatic. When examined by phlebography at the time of catheter withdrawal, 42% of catheters have sleeve thrombi, and another 8% reveal veno-occlusive thrombi.[647] In addition, sepsis has been reported in approximately 7% of patients receiving TPN and other medications by the central route. When thrombosis and bacterial or fungal contamination or sepsis coexist, suppurative thrombophlebitis may intervene. At least 50 cases of suppurative thrombophlebitis of the great thoracic veins have been reported in the literature,[648–650] but this is almost certainly a gross underestimate of the problem. Eight cases in 8 years due to *Candida* spp. alone were observed at the University of Wisconsin.[651] As another example, 53 cancer patients with catheter-related *S. aureus* bacteremia were identified over a 3-year period (1986 to 1989) at the M.D. Anderson Cancer Center; septic thrombosis was diagnosed in 12 (23%) and suspected in another 3 (6%) patients. Five of these 12 patients developed deep-seated complications, including septic pulmonary emboli and endocarditis, versus 2 of 38 without septic thrombosis ($p < .01$). Persistent fever despite appropriate antistaphylococcal agents was an early clue to the diagnosis.[652] Septic atrial thrombosis, occasionally with a coexistent Budd-Chiari syndrome, has complicated Broviac catheter insertion in infants.[653]

Superficial suppurative thrombophlebitis is a complication of either dermal infection or use of an indwelling intravenous catheter. Pelvic suppurative thrombophlebitis is associated with parturition, abortion, gynecologic surgery, or a pelvic abscess. Therefore, this is a disease of women of childbearing age, with most cases occurring between the ages of 15 and 40 years (mean, 20 years). In 123 cases in two reports,[654, 655] the predisposing conditions were as follows: vaginal delivery, 39 cases; cesarean section, 19 cases; abortion, 33 cases; and major gynecologic surgery, 32 cases. During a 9-year period in Atlanta, 27 cases of postpartum septic pelvic thrombophlebitis were identified in over 54,000 deliveries.[655] The relative risks for this condition were as follows: parturition, 1/2000 (highest in the inner-city population); septic abortion, 1/200; and major gynecologic surgery, 1/800. The incidence of suppurative thrombophlebitis rises proportionally with the degree of trauma to the pelvic tissues.

Pathogenesis

The pathogenesis of suppurative thrombophlebitis discussed in detail in reference 629, is poorly understood. A thrombus may act as a nidus for local entrapment and colonization of bacteria that gain access to the site from another focus. This is analogous to the proposed role of nonbacterial thrombotic endocarditis (NBTE) in the pathogenesis of IE. When superficial suppurative thrombophlebitis is associated with intravascular cannulas, the route of infection may be (1) migration from the skin between the catheter wall and perivascular tissue, (2) contamination of IV fluid, (3) contamination of the hub, (4) hematogenous dissemination from an infected focus elsewhere. The relative contributions of these four routes are unknown although most investigators believe that migration of organisms down the external surface of the catheter is the most important route of invasion.[632] However, the predominant organism in burn wounds, *P. aeruginosa*, is a rare cause of suppurative thrombophlebitis, and suppurative thrombophlebitis usually develops days to weeks after the cutdown incision is healed,[634, 635] arguing against a local cutaneous source in burn patients.

The venous system draining the pelvis includes the intervertebral venous plexus, the lumbar venous plexus, the superficial and deep veins of the abdominal wall, and the hemorrhoidal plexus. Any component of this system may be affected in pelvic suppurative thrombophlebitis, but the veins draining the uterus, including the ovarian veins and the inferior vena cava, are most often involved.[656] Thrombus formation may result from stasis of blood flow due to the gravid uterus or from the hypercoagulable state of parturition. Normal residents of the vaginal or perineal bacterial flora gain access to the thrombus via the blood stream regional lymphatics. There is often an associated endometritis or parametritis. Septic pulmonary emboli and metastatic abscess formation are common. Septic thrombosis of the portal vein is often associated with hepatic abscess (occurring in five of seven patients in one series[657]); an obvious extrahepatic source of intra-abdominal infection is usually absent.

Pathologic Changes

Regardless of the vein involved, the pathologic changes are similar. The vein is enlarged, tortuous, and thickened. There may be associated perivascular suppuration or hemorrhage, or both, and the vein lumen usually contains both pus and thrombus. Microscopically, endothelial damage, fibrinoid necrosis, and thickening of the vein wall are evident. Microabscesses may be present in the vein wall or in the surrounding tissue.[639, 658] Gross periphlebitic abscesses are not unusual and may be evident on physical examination. Thrombi frequently extend beyond the area of suppuration. In an autopsy series of peripheral suppurative thrombophlebitis in burned patients, extension of the clot into the great central veins was found in 18% of the cases.[634, 636] Metastatic abscess formation and septic pulmonary emboli with infarction are found in over 50% of the fatal cases. This may result from bacterial liquefaction and fragmentation of affected thrombi within the vein, because clot liquefaction is noted commonly in autopsy series.

Clinical Manifestations

Superficial suppurative thrombophlebitis is often difficult to identify because local findings of inflammation may be absent. The disease occurs more frequently when plastic catheters are inserted in the lower extremities, a common practice in burned patients. In 132 cases of superficial suppurative thrombophlebitis reported from the burn center at Fort Sam Houston, Texas, the distribution of affected vessels was as follows: lower extremity (predominantly saphenous system), 100; upper extremity (predominantly saphenous system), 100; upper extremity (predominantly antecubital fossa), 32; jugular vein, 7; and iliac vein, 4. The mean duration of preceding venous cannulation was 4.81 days, and the latent interval from removal of the catheter to the development of symptoms ranged from 2 to 10 days.[633, 635] Fever was present in over 70% of the cases, but rigors were rare. Local findings such as warmth, erythema, tenderness, swelling, or lymphangitis were present in only 32% of the patients; however, bacteremia with signs of systemic sepsis was found in 84%. Septic pulmonary emboli with secondary pneumonia—often the first diagnostic clue—occurred in 44%. Thus, pneumonia, sepsis, or metastatic abscess formation was the only manifestation of this disease in two thirds of the cases. The authors emphasize that the late onset of pneumonia or sepsis in a burned patient demands the careful inspection of all previously cannulated veins, because untreated suppurative thrombophlebitis is associated with a high mortality. In these series, fewer than 50% of the cases were diagnosed antemortem.[634]

In contrast to the experience with suppurative thrombophlebitis in burned patients, most medical and postoperative patients develop the disorder in the upper extremities, and signs of local inflammation are more commonly present (94% in one series).[643] Many of these patients are elderly (20/35 over 50 years old) with debilitating diseases and are often receiving antibiotics when superficial suppurative thrombophlebitis supervenes. As noted, the duration of intravenous catheterization is an important risk factor; 68% of implicated cannulas had been left in place for at least 5 days.[642, 643] The frequency of catheter manipulations has also been linked to catheter infections.[659]

Subperiosteal abscesses of adjacent long bones may complicate superficial suppurative thrombophlebitis in children.[660] The local findings in this condition, including bone tenderness, erythema, warmth, and limitation of motion with occasional extension into the joint space, may overshadow the suppurative thrombophlebitis itself. Septic deep vein thrombosis of the femoral vessels with swollen, tender, and inflamed inguinal areas has been described in intravenous users of heroin and cocaine. Contiguous pelvic bone osteomyelitis is unusual.

Suppurative thrombophlebitis of the thoracic central veins occurs in critically ill patients with central catheters in place, in those receiving TPN, or in patients after long-term cannulation with Broviac, Hickman, and other devices. The systemic findings associated with sepsis overshadow any local findings in venous occlusion (e.g., superior vena cava syndrome), which are rare in this setting. This syndrome should be suspected in any septic patient when bacteremia or fungemia fails to resolve upon removal of the central catheter and institution of appropriate antimicrobial therapy.

Pelvic suppurative thrombophlebitis usually develops 1 to 2 weeks postpartum or postoperatively and is associated with high fever, chills, anorexia, nausea, vomiting, abdominal pain, and a protracted course.[655] Flank pain may result from ureteral obstruction by enlarged veins. Abdominal tenderness, usually in the right lower quadrant, may be mild to severe. Approximately 80% of cases are unilateral on the right side, 14% are bilateral, and only 6% are unilateral and left-sided. This distribution is thought to result from compression of the right ovarian vein at the pelvic brim by the enlarged uterus with retrograde flow on the left and protection from ascending infection. However, the physical examination may be normal. A tender vein can be palpated in 30% of the cases on pelvic or abdominal examination.[654, 656] The uterus is usually freely movable. Spread of the process to the femoral vein with edema and tenderness of the lower extremity is unusual. Many of these patients are extremely ill, with an acute or chronic course characterized by little or no response to antibiotics and the development of multiple small septic pulmonary emboli. Since many of the manifestations are nonspecific, the differential diagnostic listing is broad and includes acute appendicitis, ureteral obstruction, torsion of an ovarian cyst, pyelonephritis, broad ligament hematoma, parametritis, endometritis, perinephric abscess, pelvic abscess, small bowel volvulus, pelvic inflammatory disease, sickle cell crisis, and ectopic pregnancy.

Laboratory Findings

Bacteremia occurs in 80 to 90% of the cases of superficial suppurative thrombophlebitis. Gross pus within the vein lumen is found in about half of the cases, and this finding establishes a diagnosis of suppurative phlebitis. When infection of a venous catheter is suspected, it should be removed and cultured. The results, however, may be misleading, because even though bacteria will be isolated in up to 60% of the cases, a positive culture does not correlate with inflammation.[661] The following semiquantitative culture technique has been developed in an attempt to differentiate catheter-related sepsis from suppurative thrombophlebitis. After preparing the skin with alcohol, the catheter is removed with sterile forceps (avoiding skin contact) and is placed in a sterile tube for transport. The catheter is then aseptically cut into 5.7-cm pieces, and each section is rolled across the surface of a 5% sheep blood agar plate. The growth of more than 15 colonies on the plate correlates well[661] with the presence of venous infection. In the few cases of suppurative thrombophlebitis studied by this technique, all catheters have yielded confluent growth. Because the standard 5.7-cm catheter retains approximately 0.7 to 1.5 mg of moisture on its surface and the plate growth has exceeded 1000 colonies in every case of suppurative thrombophlebitis, bacterial counts must exceed 10^6 organisms/g in the catheter wound. These titers are similar to those found with other types of infected wounds. This technique is simple, rapid, and inexpensive and may prove useful in establishing the need for exploratory venotomy. Simple needle aspiration of the suspected vein may also be diagnostic. ^{111}In-labeled leukocyte imaging studies have detected superficial suppurative thrombophlebitis, but experience is limited.

Other laboratory findings in patients with superficial suppurative thrombophlebitis, for example, leukocytosis, are nonspecific. The chest x-ray film may reveal multiple peripheral densities or a pleural effusion consistent with pulmonary emboli, infarction, abscess, or empyema. The diagnosis of an associated subperiosteal abscess is difficult: bone and gallium scans usually reveal hyperperfusion without definite osteomyelitis, routine x-ray films virtually always show no abnormalities, and CT scans often demonstrate only soft tissue swelling with obliteration of tissue planes. The use of high-resolution CT scans may improve these results.[660] The diagnosis of deep central vein suppurative thrombophlebitis in the thorax is established by venography, with the demonstration of thrombi in a patient with positive blood cultures, but CT with contrast enhancement is probably as sensitive and is noninvasive. CT scans are clearly useful in the diagnosis of suppurative phlebitis of the great central veins[662, 663] and the portal vein[645]; gas may be detected in the venular lumen, which is diagnostic of this condition. Experience with magnetic resonance imaging and ^{111}In-labeled leukocytes is meager.

In most cases of pelvic suppurative thrombophlebitis, there is a peripheral blood leukocytosis, and the urinalysis is usually normal. The chest x-ray film may reveal multiple septic pulmonary emboli. Intravenous pyelography can be useful in disclosing ureteral obstruction. Real-time ultrasonography is very helpful in delineating the location and extent of the thrombus, but the ileus that is often associated with this infection may render interpretation difficult. Ultrasonography may also demonstrate the presence of a periuterine, adnexal or tuboovarian mass. CT reveals low attenuation with contrast enhancement in suppurative venous thrombosis and is very sensitive in the diagnosis of pelvic suppurative thrombophlebitis.[664, 665] Magnetic resonance imaging may be even more sensitive and can differentiate fresh thrombus (≤ 1 week old) from organizing or subacute thrombus.[666] These sensitive and noninvasive techniques may lead to an increased recognition of pelvic suppurative thrombophlebitis, earlier diagnosis, and improved outcome. The role of newer diagnostic techniques such as pelvic venography, transuterine phlebography, ^{111}In-labeled leukocyte scanning, and laparoscopy is still undefined. Because bacteremia is demonstrated in only 20 to 30%[654, 655, 667] of cases of pelvic suppurative thrombophlebitis, negative blood cultures do not exclude the diagnosis.

Etiologic Agents

S. aureus was the causative agent of 65 to 78% of the cases of superficial suppurative thrombophlebitis reported before 1968. In recent years, most cases have been due to a member of Enterobacteriaceae, especially *Klebsiella-Enterobacter* spp.[637, 643] These agents are acquired nosocomially and are often resistant to multiple antibiotics. Nearly all patients with superficial suppurative thrombophlebitis due to gram-negative aerobic bacilli or fungi are receiving broad-spectrum antibiotics at the time the disease becomes manifested. In a review of 86 cases compiled from the literature reported since 1970, the organisms isolated were as follows: *Klebsiella-Enterobacter* spp., in 34 cases; *Providencia* spp., in 5 cases; *Proteus* spp., in 5; *Serratia* spp., in 3; *E. coli*, in 6; *P. aeruginosa*, in 3; *S. aureus*, in 15; *C. albicans*, in 9; *S. epidermidis*, in 4; and enterococci, in 2.[642, 643] Suppurative thrombophlebitis due to gram-negative pathogens and *E. faecalis* is more common (than *S. aureus*) in patients with significant intra-abdominal pathology.[641] *S. aureus*, other gram-positive cocci, and *Candida* spp. were more frequent when this risk factor was absent. Multiple organisms are isolated in up to 14% of cases. Anaerobic isolates are extremely rare. An increase in the incidence of superficial suppurative thrombophlebitis due to *Candida* spp. has been reported[668, 669]; all patients were receiving antibiotics without hyperalimentation. None were neutropenic or receiving corticosteroids. In one series of seven patients observed in a 15-month interval,[669] all had concomitant or preceding bacterial infections and had received multiple antibiotics; mean number 5 for at least 2 weeks. Preceding candidal colonization at other sites (e.g., sputum, urine) was often present.[669] *Malassezia furfur* is also seen as an opportunistic pathogen of deep vein catheters, especially in premature infants[670] and others in the pediatric age group receiving lipid emulsions, but this risk factor is not present in all patients. Septic thrombosis, endocarditis, and other metastatic complications are not uncommon in this setting of disseminated *Malassezia* infection.[670] Although not documented by culture, histopathologic evidence suggests that cytomegalovirus may cause suppurative thrombophlebitis in patients with AIDS despite therapy with ganciclovir.[671]

The responsible agents in pelvic suppurative thrombophlebitis are poorly defined, because blood cultures are often negative and most investigators did not use adequate anaerobic techniques. The organisms isolated in approximate order of frequency are *Bacteroides* spp., microaerophilic or anaerobic streptococci, *E. coli* and other coliforms, and β-hemolytic streptococci. The predominance of *Bacteroides* may be related to the heparinase produced by this organism. A prolonged latent period (up to 3 weeks) may occur before blood cultures become positive. The more extensive use of anaerobic isolation techniques and routine culturing of surgical specimens may serve to clarify the role of anaerobic bacteria in this entity.

Presumptive Therapy

Superficial suppurative thrombophlebitis is a lethal iatrogenic disease, and surgery is often necessary for cure. The first reported successful cure of suppurative thrombophlebitis followed surgical ligation of the vein by John Hunter in 1784.[672] All authorities strongly endorse surgical excision as an integral part of treatment. In a review of 24 patients,[634] 14 were managed medically alone, and all died either directly from suppurative thrombophlebitis with persistent bacteremia or secondary to metastatic complications. However, of 10 patients who underwent surgical exploration, 7 survived, and only 1 of the 3 deaths was attributable to suppurative thrombophlebitis. Antibiotics should also be used in the treatment of this disease; initial empirical treatment with a semisynthetic penicillin (e.g., nafcillin, 2 g IV every 4 to 6 hours) plus either an aminoglycoside (e.g., gentamicin, 1.0 to 1.7 mg/kg IV or IM every 8 hours) or a third-generation cephalosporin (e.g., cefotaxime) or a quinolone (e.g., ciprofloxacin) is recommended, because members of Enterobacteriaceae or staphylococci are the usual etiologic agents. The optimum duration of therapy is unknown and largely empirical. The role of antifungal therapy for superficial suppurative thrombophlebitis due to *C. albicans* is controversial.[668, 669] Most of these infections can be cured by vein excision. However, because of the propensity of this pathogen to hematogenously disseminate to visceral organs (e.g., kidney), a short course of amphotericin B (approximately 200 mg) or fluconazole (400 mg/d for 10 to 14 days) is advised postoperatively, pending further data. Antifungal therapy is mandatory in the immunosuppressed patient or if signs of metastatic complications (e.g., endophthalmitis) develop.

When superficial suppurative thrombophlebitis is a likely diagnosis, an exploratory venotomy may be necessary. This procedure should be performed proximal to the suspected site; the vein should be ligated and then "milked" in an attempt to express purulent material for inspection by Gram stain and culture. If no pus is apparent, further surgical exploration is necessary to establish the diagnosis. In older literature, simple ligation was thought to be sufficient, but the rate of relapse with ongoing sepsis was high. Therefore, the segment of vein and all its involved tributaries should be totally excised. Radical surgery from the ankle to the groin may be required in some burn patients. Nevertheless, local or regional anesthesia alone is often sufficient (approximately 90% of cases) for vein excision. Backbleeding, indicative of a patent lumen, should be evident at the point of vein transection. Vein excision is usually followed by prompt (≤24 hours) defervescence. If systemic symptoms, bacteremia, or marked local manifestations persist after vein excision, reexploration is necessary, with careful attention to total removal of all involved veins and drainage of contiguous (e.g., periphlebitic, subperiosteal) abscesses. We stress, however, that the role of less radical surgery in therapy for superficial suppurative thrombophlebitis has not been addressed adequately. Although the literature supports vein excision, this experience stems largely from burn centers. Despite infection with gram-negative bacilli or *Candida* spp., six of eight children with superficial suppurative thrombophlebitis were cured by local incision and drainage of the involved site plus parenteral antimicrobials.[641] Radical surgery with extensive excision can perhaps be reserved for patients in whom these measures fail. Delayed closure is preferred over primary wound closure. If osteomyelitis is documented in the adjacent long bones, antimicrobial therapy should be continued for at least 6 weeks. Resection of the involved vasculature in most patients with suppurative thrombophlebitis of the great central veins is technically impossible. Fortunately, medical therapy is usually sufficient.[648, 651, 673] The recommended approach is catheter removal, full-dose anticoagulation with heparin,[673, 674] and parenteral antibiotics. Although tissue plasminogen activator therapy has been used successfully in this setting,[675] experience is limited, and its use must be considered experimental. Septic thrombosis of the portal vein usually responds to systemic antimicrobial therapy directed at bowel flora with or without percutaneous drainage of any associated hepatic abscesses.[657]

The duration of therapy for septic phlebitis of deeper veins is unsettled; 2 to 3 weeks after catheter removal is suggested, with at least 4 weeks for *S. aureus* disease.[652] Experience with more potent agents (e.g., third-generation cephalosporins) for suppurative thrombophlebitis due to gram-negative bacilli is scant, but trials are indicated. Because heparin may precipitate vancomycin with a partial loss of antibacterial activity at concentrations present in intravenous lines,[674] these drugs should not be administered simultaneously by the same intravenous access line. Unlike *Candida* IE, suppurative thrombophlebitis of the great central veins due to *Candida* spp. is curable medically, but antifungal regimens must be continued longer than is usually adequate for superficial suppurative thrombophlebitis. Based on limited data,[651] amphotericin B at a daily dose of 0.7 mg/kg, to a total dosage of at least 22 mg/kg, plus 5-fluorocytosine (100 to 150 mg/kg/day in four divided doses, if tolerable) is recommended after catheter removal. Fluconazole (400 mg/day) for 4 to 6 weeks is an alternative in patients not able to tolerate amphotericin B. Surgery may, however, be essential in patients with suppurative thrombophlebitis of the thoracic or neck veins when perivascular collections are present.

The optimal therapy for pelvic suppurative thrombophlebitis is still controversial. Because anaerobic streptococci and *Bacteroides* spp. predominate, the initial antibiotics of choice are aqueous penicillin G, 20 million units IV daily, plus either clindamycin, 450 to 600 mg IV every 6 hours, or metronidazole, 500 to 750 mg IV every 8 hours. The use of heparin is debated. The addition of heparin after several days of unsuccessful treatment with antibiotics may itself produce an antipyretic effect.[667] In one series of 46 patients with pelvic suppurative thrombophlebitis,[655] including 7 with massive ovarian vein involvement and 15 with septic pulmonary emboli, 42 patients become afebrile within 7 days (mean, 2.5 days) while receiving penicillin, chloramphenicol, and heparin. Four patients required exploratory laparotomy, and pelvic abscesses were found in three. These results argue strongly that medical therapy alone is often effective, but no controlled studies on the use of heparin have been done. When medical therapy is unsatisfactory, surgery with drainage of abscesses and usually ligation of the implicated venous system must be performed. Some authorities[656] believe that ligation of the inferior vena cava or ovarian vein, or both, should be performed in all these cases, but the evidence for this approach is inconclusive.

Prevention

The incidence of superficial suppurative thrombophlebitis can be reduced by the same preventive procedures that are used for intravenous cannulas in general. These include the use of "scalp vein" cannulas whenever possible, the avoidance of lower extremity cannulations, insertion under aseptic conditions, secure anchoring of the cannula, and frequent replacement (at least every 48 to 72 hours) of intravenous fluid bottles, cannulas, and connecting tubing. Although neomycin–polymyxin B–bacitracin ointment is effective in reducing the incidence of cutdown infections,[676] use of this combination agent has not demonstrated consistent benefit with intravenous cannulas.[677]

A detailed discussion of prevention strategies for vascular catheters has been recently published by the Centers for Disease Control and Prevention.[678] When clinical signs of bacteremia occur in a patient receiving intravenous fluids, the following steps should be taken: (1) blood cultures specimens should be obtained, (2) intravenous administration should be discontinued and all cannulas removed, (3) the intravenous fluid itself should be cultured, (4) the cannula should be cultured semiquantitatively on blood agar as described by Maki and associates[661] and (5) appropriate antibiotic therapy should be instituted. If clinical signs of sepsis and bacteremia persist despite appropriate antibiotic therapy, then an intravascular focus (such as suppurative thrombophlebitis at a previously cannulated vein) should be sought as discussed previously.

INFECTIVE ENDARTERITIS AND "MYCOTIC ANEURYSMS"

The term *mycotic aneurysm* was coined by Osler in 1885 to describe a mushroom-shaped aneurysm that developed in a patient with subacute bacterial endocarditis. At that time *mycotic* was used to refer to all microorganisms. At present, the use of *mycotic* has been restricted specifically to fungal infections, but *mycotic aneurysm* is still used for all extra- (or intra-) cardiac aneurysms of infectious etiology except for syphilitic aortitis. Unfortunately, this term has also been used to describe preexisting aneurysyms secondarily infected from contiguous or distant foci or pseudoaneurysms arising from trauma or iatrogenic causes. *Endarteritis* refers to inflammation of the arterial wall, which may occur with or without coexistent aneurysmal dilatation. Unless an aneurysm or coarctation of the aorta is present, infective endarteritis is usually a postmortem diagnosis. Because infected aneurysms differ in their pathogenesis, the various classifications, given in Table 65–7, are examined separately in the following discussion.[679] Infections of arterial prosthetic devices are dealt with in detail in Chapter 66 and are not considered here.

Epidemiology

Although incidence figures are unavailable, a localized suppurative process of the arterial wall is rare. Estimates derived from autopsy series of aortic aneurysms are available but ignore infections at other locations in the arterial tree. In a review of over 22,000 autopsies performed at the Boston City Hospital from 1902 to 1951,[680] aortic aneurysms were found in 1.5%. However, mycotic aneurysms constituted only 2.6% of these lesions. In another review of 178 aneurysms found among more than 20,000 autopsies at the Mayo Clinic from 1925 to 1954,[681] only 6 were believed to be of infectious origin. Similarly, in a review[682] of 77 pure iliac artery aneurysms in 48 patients from a 21-year period, only 2 aneurysms (4.2%) were mycotic in origin. In the preantibiotic era, infected aneurysms were predominantly confined to patients with IE; in a series of 217 cases reported in 1923,[683] 86% were associated with IE. With the advent of antibiotics, mycotic aneurysms in IE have become less prevalent, and hematogenous seeding of a previously damaged arteriosclerotic vessel constitutes the most common mechanism.

TABLE 65–7 Classification of "Mycotic Aneurysms"

Preexistent Arterial Status	Source of Infection
Normal	Intravascular
Atherosclerotic	Embolism
Aneurysm	Bacteremia with "seeding"
Arterial prosthesis	Extension from adjacent endocardial focus on erosion
	Extravascular
	Contiguous site of infection
	Iatrogenic

Because most of these lesions arise in areas of severe atherosclerosis, males predominate over women by 3 to 1, and the average age has been 65 years. The mean age for mycotic aneurysms that occur with IE is younger (approximately 40 years), and men and women are affected approximately equally. Estimates of the incidence of mycotic aneurysms in patients with IE range up to 15%.[684–687] Approximately 2 to 4% of IE patients develop intracranial mycotic aneurysms,[687, 688] although a neurologic presentation is not uncommon in patients with IE (noted in approximately 16 to 23% of cases), and at least 30% of the patients develop neurologic manifestations.[689, 690] As discussed previously, the presence of such manifestations during IE has an adverse effect on the ultimate mortality rate. These lesions remain a significant cause of morbidity and mortality due to intracerebral and subarachnoid hemorrhage, especially in young people in developing countries where acute rheumatic fever, rheumatic heart disease, and resultant IE are still prevalent.[691] Nine intracranial mycotic aneurysms associated with IE were treated in one neurosurgical unit in South Africa in a recent 18-month period, with five deaths.[691] In addition, aortic root complications, including abscess or mycotic aneurysm, are associated with a poor outcome from IE. For example, in one review,[692] aortic root complications were documented in 23 of 50 cases of aortic valve IE (46%) over a 6-year period; prosthetic valve involvement was common, and the surgical mortality rate and the incidence of postoperative aortic regurgitation were higher in the group with root complications.

Mycotic aneurysms are extremely rare in childhood[693] and, when present, are usually associated with IE, cardiovascular malformations, or connective tissue disorders. However, a specific disease entity first described in 1970 is aneurysm associated with umbilical artery catheterization in newborn infants.[694] Such lesions are usually of staphylococcal etiology, and 34 cases had been reported in 1992, with the following distribution[694]: descending thoracic aorta, 14; abdominal aorta, 10; iliac arteries, 6; and multiple sites, 4.

Pathogenesis

Four different mechanisms have been postulated to produce infection of the arterial wall: (1) formation of mycotic aneurysms secondary to septic microemboli to the vasa vasorum ("embolomycotic aneurysms"), (2) extension from a contiguous infected focus, (3) hematogenous seeding of the intima during bacteremia originating from a distant infection, and (4) trauma to the arterial wall with direct contamination.[695] Embolomycotic aneurysms usually occur in patients with active IE, and the incidence of this type has declined in the antibiotic era. The source of infection is the cardiac vegetation, with production of arterial emboli that lodge in the vasa vasorum, often at points of bifurcation of the affected artery. Contiguous foci of infection (e.g., a caseous tuberculous lymph node or pyogenic vertebral osteomyelitis) may extend directly to major vessels, with subsequent aneurysm formation. The normal arterial intima is very resistant to infection. However, when this lining is altered by congenital malformations (e.g., coarctation of the aorta) or acquired disease (especially atherosclerotic plaques or ulcers), resistance to infection is lowered, and the surface may become colonized by blood-borne organisms. This hypothesis is analogous to the central role of NBTE in the pathogenesis of IE. An intraluminal thrombus associated with an atherosclerotic vessel may also serve as a nidus for colonization. Atherosclerosis accounts for over 74% of secondarily infected aneurysms. Luetic arteritis and cystic medial necrosis have also been associated with secondary infection.[684] Trauma to the arterial wall with subsequent infection has been documented in narcotic addicts, in whom it is due to needle trauma,[696] and has also been associated with gunshot wounds, vascular surgery, cardiac catheterization, percutaneous transluminal coronary angioplasty,[697, 698] and even puncture of a femoral artery for analysis of arterial blood gases.[679] These events, if associated with contamination, usually lead to pseudoaneurysm formation in a peripheral artery and a contiguous abscess in extravasated blood.

Pathologic Changes

Infection of the arterial tree has been recognized by pathologists for more than a century. Virchow first demonstrated local dilatation of the arterial wall at the site of a septic embolus in 1847. Infection superimposed on an atherosclerotic aorta was first reported by Koch in 1851. Stengel and Wolfroth[683] collected 217 cases of mycotic aneurysms in 1923. Because these lesions are probably underreported, pathologic material has been scant in recent years.

Most mycotic aneurysms that develop during the course of IE are situated in the sinus of Valsalva or in the supravalvular proximal thoracic aorta (>70% develop proximal to the aortic arch). Aneurysms are more frequent in the right or posterior sinus and may be complicated by acquired shunts (rupture into the right ventricle is the most common), tamponade, coronary artery occlusion, or an atrioventricular conduction block.[699] Less commonly, major visceral, intracranial, and peripheral arteries are involved. Intracranial mycotic aneurysms characteristically develop in the distribution of the middle cerebral artery at peripheral bifurcation points,[689, 690] versus a more proximal location for most congenital aneurysms. Multiple intracranial lesions may be present. Mycotic aneurysm of the extracranial carotid arteries is rare (26 case reports[700]), but most develop in association with IE, usually due to *S. aureus*. Less than 10% are found in the upper extremities, but these arteries are usually not examined adequately by pathologic or radiologic techniques. Infrafemoral aneurysms during IE or following its treatment[701] are also unusual. Multiple lesions are identified in many IE patients with mycotic aneurysms.[702] Saccular forms appear to be more common than fusiform ones.[680] The aneurysms vary in size from 1 mm to more than 10 cm. As mentioned before, many of these aneurysms arise from emboli to the vasa vasorum, and occasionally the embolus can be demonstrated grossly and microscopically. Acute and chronic inflammation is found diffusely through the arterial wall; necrosis, hemorrhage, abscess, and bacterial colonies may all be present in the sections. The elastica and muscularis layers are usually obliterated, but the intima is often intact. Rupture with surrounding hemorrhage and infection may be present.

Secondary infection of a preexisting aneurysm is most commonly found in the abdominal aorta (accounting for 70% of the cases), because this is the area most frequently and severely damaged by atherosclerosis. Ascending and descending aortic aneurysms each account for about 15% of the cases. The primary bacteremia most commonly originates from distal infections in soft tissue, lung, bone, or joint. The arterial infection usually begins in the distal abdominal aorta or iliac arteries as a focus of inflammation on an ulcerated atheromatous plaque. The wall of the aneurysm is thinned, and there is focal acute and chronic inflammation that may lead to arterial rupture. Even so-called bland aortic aneurysms commonly have some mild inflammation (characterized by a predominance of lymphocytes and mononuclear cells) in the wall; however, infected atherosclerotic aneurysms are characterized by acute inflammation with a predominance of polymorphonuclear leukocytes, necrosis, abscess formation, hemorrhage, and visible bacterial colonies. This lesion is probably underreported, because the focal suppuration may be limited in extent and overlooked unless routine culture and histologic sections are examined on every aortic aneurysm specimen. Erosion and rupture may be present without aneurysmal dilatation. Lumbar or thoracic osteomyelitis is present in up to a third of the cases[684] and may either precede the aneurysm or develop secondary to contiguous spread from the vascular infection.

When contamination accompanies arterial injury, an infected pseudoaneurysm may result. Such lesions are located in the extremities in over 80% of the cases and are characterized by more extensive local tissue inflammation than is seen with the two types mentioned previously. Infection as a cause of pseudoaneurysm formation is increasing; 17 of 57 (30%) such lesions seen in the 1980s[703] were infected. When endarteritis develops following angioplasty, it usually follows a second procedure or repuncture, and this scenario should suggest the diagnosis; all cases have been due to *S. aureus*.[694, 698] Distal emboli, pseudoaneurysm, and coexistent osteomyelitis are present in more than 50% of the cases. Infective aortic root aneurysm has also followed coronary artery bypass grafting, with disastrous results.[702, 704] Subclavian artery aneurysms may be present, with systemic findings plus unilateral upper extremity rash or splinter hemorrhages.[705] Nineteen cases of intracavernous carotid artery aneurysms have been reported,[706] usually occurring with meningitis with or without IE.

Of special interest are mycotic aneurysms in renal transplant patients. In 640 renal transplants performed at the University of Minnesota over a period of 8 years, perinephric infections developed in 28 patients, and 8 of these developed mycotic aneurysms.[707] These lesions were evident clinically 1.5 to 4 months after transplant. Six were located in the external iliac artery, with one each in the internal iliac artery and aorta. All these lesions were secondary to contiguous foci of infection in the deep tissues of the transplant wound.[708, 709]

Clinical Manifestations

When mycotic aneurysms occur during the course of IE, manifestations of the underlying disease may be evident. Peripheral middle cerebral artery aneurysms constitute 2.5 to 6.2% of all intracranial aneurysms[687–691, 709] and are usually secondary to infection. Intracranial mycotic aneurysms are usually clinically silent. When hemorrhage occurs, severe headache of sudden onset with rapid deterioration in the level of consciousness is noted. The time interval from the diagnosis of IE to the onset of hemorrhage is variable (0 to 35 days), with a mean of 18 days.[688] Some of these lesions produce premonitory or herald neurologic signs, including focal deficits and seizures. Unfortunately, such findings are relatively common in patients with IE without intracranial aneurysms, and the differential diagnosis as well as decisions regarding arteriography is difficult.[710] A sudden focal deficit consistent with embolism is seen in approximately 23% of patients and should prompt arteriography.[710] A high proportion of patients with intracranial mycotic aneurysm with severe, unremitting localized headache, often in association with homonymous hemianopsia (as a "herald" sign), has been reported in one series.[711] As noted, stroke syndromes may be seen and are manifested as focal neurologic deficits, headache, confusion, meningismus, seizures, or coma.[689, 690] Contrary to popular belief, the majority of intracranial hemorrhages associated with IE are due not to ruptured mycotic aneurysms but to septic necrotic arteritis.[689] Symptomatic intracranial hemorrhage was associated with a mortality rate of 60 to 90% in this study. Patients may present with bilateral cortical blindness as well. Unusual location or etiology of an intracranial mycotic aneurysm suggests a diagnosis other than IE.[712] Mycotic aneurysms tend to occur more commonly in females of a younger age than does IE in general. They must be differentiated from aneurysms secondary to tumor emboli (especially choriocarcinoma or atrial myxoma), trauma, arteritis, and moyamoya disease and from congenital aneurysms. Visceral artery aneurysms are uncommon but, when present, are almost uniformly due to infection[695] or polyarteritis nodosa. The most common location is in the superior mesenteric artery. Although superior mesenteric artery aneurysms account for only 8% of visceral artery aneurysms overall, most are of infectious etiology.[713] Symptoms include colicky abdominal pain of acute onset, but the presentation is variable. Hepatic artery aneurysms may produce colicky right upper quadrant pain, fever, jaundice, and gastrointestinal hemorrhage[714] or hemobilia.[715] Over 190 cases of this entity have been reported in the literature; 75% were extrahepatic and 25% intrahepatic. Ruptured mycotic aneurysm of the celiac artery may present as hemoptysis or hemothorax.[716] When the external iliac artery is involved, a triad of clinical signs may be present: pain in the lower extremity (especially the anterior aspect of the thigh) with quadriceps muscle wasting and a depressed knee jerk; arterial insufficiency of the extremity with coolness, pallor, and depressed pulses; and bacteremia.[717] Distal aneurysms (e.g., affecting the femora artery) occasionally have unusual presenting manifestations, including arthritis and purpura in the affected limb.

When more peripheral arteries are involved (usually with a pseudoaneurysm), a tender, diffusely indurated mass is present in 92% of cases. The mass is pulsatile, with an associated bruit, in 50 to 60% of patients, and approximately 20 to 30% have decreased peripheral pulses, skin changes, or even frank gangrene.[696] Local suppuration, petechiae, and purpura are often present, and the lesion may be confused with localized cellulitis or an abscess without consideration of vascular involvement. In users of illicit drugs, 80% of mycotic aneurysms occur in the lower extremity, with the remainder in the radial, brachial, or occasionally carotid artery. Only 50% of these patients are febrile on admission. A superimposed septic arthritis may also be present.[718]

Although most infected aortic atherosclerotic aneurysms occur in elderly men, no pathognomonic findings exist to separate these patients from those with bland uninfected aneurysms. Fever is a helpful differentiating sign (present in over 70% of the patients) because it is uncommon in patients with bland aneurysms. Back pain or abdominal pain each occur in about a third of the cases. A draining cutaneous sinus may be present. Separation of an infected aneurysm from the entity of inflammatory abdominal aortic aneurysm may be difficult. Inflammatory abdominal aortic aneurysms were first described in 1935 and account for 5 to 10% of abdominal aortic aneurysms; the lesions are usually infrarenal and often lead to ureteral obstruction owing to the densely adherent fibrotic mass surrounding the vessel.[719] In a large series of 2816 patients undergoing repair of abdominal aortic aneurysms, 127 (4.5%) had inflammatory abdominal aortic aneurysms.[720] Most patients (123/127) were men and heavy smokers. Inflammatory abdominal aortic aneurysms are associated with an elevated erythrocyte sedimentation rate (in 73% of the cases), weight loss, symptoms (back or abdominal pain in 30 to 50%), and a high operative mortality. Continuing bacteremia despite "appropriate" antimicrobial therapy in an elderly (especially diabetic) patient with no signs of IE is suggestive of an infected intravascular site. The aneurysm is palpable in 50 to 60% of the cases.[685, 695] In most cases, the onset is insidious, and a low-grade fever may be present for several months before diagnosis. The nonspecificity of the clinical manifestations is reflected by the 75% preoperative rupture rate for this entity. Rupture may occur into the retroperitoneal space or peritoneal cavity (56%), pleural cavity (9%), duodenum (12%), esophagus (6%), mediastinum (3%), or pericardium (3%). The most common site of aortoenteric fistula is between the aorta and the third portion of the duodenum. Short periods of "herald" bleeding are common warning signs before exsanguinating hemorrhage occurs.[721] Severe pain and the rapid onset of shock usually accompany rupture of the aneurysm.

Laboratory Findings

There are no characteristic laboratory abnormalities in this group of diseases. When mycotic aneurysms occur with IE, alterations suggesting the underlying disease may be present. CT is useful in patients with neurologic manifestations of IE, especially for the demonstration of intracranial hemorrhage. This modality is not sufficiently sensitive for the detection of intracranial mycotic aneurysms[689, 690]; however, these lesions are not likely when the appearance on CT scan is completely normal. Diagnosis of intracranial mycotic aneurysm is still best established by four-vessel cerebral arteriography, although magnetic resonance angiography[690] and the less dangerous and invasive procedure of intravenous digital subtraction angiography[722] are promising. Magnetic resonance angiography may detect aneurysms only 2 to 3 mm in diameter, but false-negative results occur (in 8 to 10% of such studies); therefore, this modality cannot substitute for selective angiography.

Patients with infected aortic aneurysms usually demonstrate a leukocytosis (65 to 83%), but this is nonspecific and may be present when the aneurysm is bland. Bacteremia is found in 53 to more than 90% of the cases, is continuous, and usually does not clear with antibiotic therapy alone. Evidence for a primary source of bacteremia (e.g., pneumonia, osteomyelitis) may be present but is absent in up to 46% of the cases.[684] The abdominal aorta is noted to be calcified on abdominal x-ray films in 47%,[686] and anterior vertebral body erosion has been demonstrated in 18%. A lack of calcification is suggestive of infection, because 70 to 80% of bland aneurysms demonstrate calcification on abdominal x-ray films. Certain procedures (e.g., intravenous pyelography, sonography, CT) may reveal the presence of an aneurysm but are often not satisfactory for preoperative detail. The absence of intimal calcification, an associated perianeurysmal fluid collection or osteomyelitis (usually shown by CT), and the sudden appearance of an aneurysm in a septic patient all are features suggestive of an infected abdominal aortic aneurysm.[723, 724] Gas in the aortic wall is diagnostic, but rare. Although the sensitivity is unknown, ^{67}Ga and ^{111}In leukocyte imaging have been used to localize intra-arterial infections.[725] Occult infected aneurysms have been identified in patients with fever of unknown origin and negative results on CT or magnetic resonance imaging studies with gallium[726] or leukocyte scintigraphy[727] and may separate seroma or hematoma from adjacent infection. Leukocyte imaging with ^{99}technetium-labeled cells also appears promising, but false-positive results have been noted.[728] Nevertheless, preoperative angiography is often preferred to delineate precisely the extent of aneurysmal involvement.[729] This information may alter the operative approach and may minimize the complications. Two-dimensional echocardiography (TTE or TEE) is a very useful noninvasive technique for documenting mycotic aneurysms in the vicinity of the aortic valve (e.g., sinus of Valsalva, supravalvular, subvalvular), and this technique is adjunctive to aortic root angiography preoperatively.[730] Infective endarteritis or mycotic aneurysm in the vicinity of a patent ductus arteriosus has also been successfully visualized with two-dimensional and Doppler echocardiography.[731, 732] Intraoperative epicardial echocardiography has also been used to facilitate the surgical approach. When a hepatic aneurysm is suspected, liver scanning and ultrasonography performed before angiography may be helpful.[714]

Etiologic Agents

Before the antibiotic era, mycotic aneurysms associated with IE were usually due to the more "virulent" organisms such as the β-hemolytic group A streptococci, pneumococci, or *Haemophilus influenzae*. With the decline of these organisms as causal agents in IE, most of these lesions are now due to streptococci or staphylococci (≥60% of cases) and follow the incidence patterns outlined in Table 65–4 for the underlying disease.

When bacteria "seed" a preexisting atherosclerotic vessel, the etiologic agents are markedly different from those found in mycotic aneurysms associated with IE. Gram-positive organisms cause approximately 60% of these lesions, but gram-negative bacilli (chiefly salmonellae) are isolated in 35%. Staphylococci are implicated in 40% of the cases and overall,[686] and over two thirds of these are *S. aureus*. Salmonellae cause 20% of the cases and involve, in order of frequency, the aorta and femoral and iliac arteries. Only 1 of 24 of such cases reported before 1974 was above the renal arteries.[733] Lumbar osteomyelitis due to *Salmonella* was present in one third of cases. The presumed portal of entry is the gastrointestinal tract. *Salmonella enteritidis* strains are isolated in 40% of cases, which is proportional to their overall rate of isolation in the United States. *Salmonella choleraesuis*, an uncommon clinical isolate, appears to be particularly pathogenic for this condition, because this species was isolated in 32% of the cases.[734] *Salmonella typhi* is rarely implicated in this disorder. *Salmonella* infections of aortic aneurysms were first reported in 1948. The predilection for involvement by this organism is not understood, but salmonellae tend to "seed" abnormal tissues during bacteremia (e.g., hematomas, malignant tumors, cysts, gallstones, bone infarcts, altered endothelium, aortic aneurysms). It has been estimated that 25% of patients over 50 years of age with *Salmonella* bacteremia have an intravascular focus of infection.[735, 736] *Arizona* species (especially *Arizona hinshawii*) are closely related to *Salmonella* spp., cause similar clinical syndromes, and also infect aortic aneurysms in elderly diabetic males.[737] The following organisms also produce infection in atherosclerotic aneurysms: *E. coli, P. aeruginosa, Proteus* spp., *Citrobacter freundii, Klebsiella-Enterobacter* spp., *Brucella* spp.,[738] *S. marcescens, C. fetus,*[739] *Listeria monocytogenes* (10 reported cases[740]), *B. fragilis*, gonococci, group A or C streptococci, corynebacteria, *Clostridium septicum,*[741] enterococci, and pneumococci.

Fungal mycotic aneurysms are rare in the intracranial compartment, with only 13 definite cases reported by 1981.[748] The most common etiologic agents are *Aspergillus* spp., agents of mucormycoses, and *Candida* spp. The first two agents may involve intracranial arteries by direct extension from foci of sinusitis. One case of multiple intracranial aneurysms due to *Coccidioides immitis* that occurred during therapy for basilar meningitis has been described. Fungal mycotic aneurysms tend to involve larger, more proximal vessels at the base of the brain (11/18 [61] carotid or basilar) than those involved in bacterial cases of IE[743] and may complicate intracranial surgery. *Aspergillus* mycotic aneurysms have followed transphenoidal resections. Fungi may also cause endarteritis in the aorta or on aortic grafts, including cases due to *Aspergillus* or *Bipolaris* spp.[744, 745] Mycotic aneurysms with subarachnoid bleeding may complicate the course of neurobrucellosis.[746] Tuberculous aneurysms are now uncommon and when present are due to contiguous foci of infection.

Pseudoaneurysms resulting from intra-arterial or perivascular injection of illicit street drugs, often in addicts with sclerosed veins due to repeated intravenous inoculation, are associated with contiguous abscesses. The causative agents are *S. aureus* (in 76% of cases), *P. aeruginosa* (in 18%), and many others.[696]

Therapy

No uniformly acceptable approach has been devised for the treatment of mycotic aneurysms in IE. The treatment of intracranial mycotic aneurysms is particularly controversial. Some of these lesions appear to resolve with antimicrobial therapy alone. In a review of 56 aneurysms occurring in 45 patients,[747] 3 of 20 patients died when treatment was limited to antibiotics alone. Mild to moderate neurologic deficits were observed in 8 of the 17 survivors. Likewise, 6 of 25 patients in whom treatment included both antibiotics and surgery died, and 9 of 19 survivors were left with mild to moderate neurologic deficits. In others studies, the investigators reported a different experience, with a higher mortality in the nonsurgical group,[688] but patients were selected only after subarachnoid hemorrhage had occurred. For example, in a review of 13 intracranial mycotic aneurysms,[688] 6 of 8 patients who received treatment with antibiotics alone died, and no deaths were observed in the surgical treatment group. In a review of 85 cases treated between 1954 and 1978, 20 of 38 patients managed solely with antibiotics died, versus 8 of 30 those operated upon.[687] The distal location of most intracranial mycotic aneurysms associated with IE may permit ligation and excision with fewer complications when compared with surgery for berry aneurysms in the circle of Willis. Of interest, the mortality rate was low in patients with multiple aneurysms (4/15) who received treatment with antibiotics alone. In one series, the mortality rate was 29% after rupture of an intracranial mycotic aneurysm.

Serial angiographic studies may be useful in following these patients, because the aneurysm(s) may change in size or new lesions may develop. In 21 patients studied by this modality, the mycotic aneurysm increased in size in 5, did not change in 1, became smaller in 6, and completely resolved in 11, and new aneurysms developed in 2. Therefore, over 50% of these peripheral intracranial aneurysms resolved with antibiotic therapy alone during the treatment of IE.[747] Surgery is indicated for aneurysms increasing in size on serial angiographic studies[748, 749] but may be deferred for 4 to 6 weeks for those remaining the same size (if the patient is an acceptable medical risk). The definitive treatment for aneurysms decreasing in size on subsequent serial angiographic studies repeated every 2 weeks is unclear. CT is not helpful in localizing the aneurysm but provides important information if hematomas, infarcts, or abscesses develop. The choice of antibiotics used is governed by the etiologic agent of the IE, but therapy for intracranial mycotic aneurysms, especially multiple lesions, must be individualized.[689, 690] (see earlier discussion). The AHA has recently reviewed this topic.[273] It was generally concluded that a single intracranial mycotic aneurysm distal to the first bifurcation of a major artery (e.g., middle cerebral artery) should be followed with frequent serial angiograms and promptly excised if the aneurysm enlarges or bleeds. Multiple aneurysms should be similarly monitored, and any enlarging one should be managed surgically. Aneurysms proximal to the first bifurcation are less amenable to surgical therapy, as they arise from major vessels and their ligation may result in severe neurologic deficits. These latter lesions should also be serially assessed, and surgery pursued should enlargement or leakage occur.

Peripheral vessels are usually involved when arterial trauma (narcotic addict, gunshot wound, iatrogenic) results in pseudoaneurysm formation with infection. Therapy with antibiotics, proximal ligation of the vessel, resection of the pseudoaneurysm, and appropriate drainage result in cures in 75% of the cases. Vascular reconstruction through uninfected tissue planes with autogenous grafts is necessary when limb viability is dependent on the affected vessel. This is encountered more frequently in the lower extremity. For example, severe ischemia developed in 9 to 28 patients after excision of mycotic aneurysms of the common femoral artery[696] in one series of 52 cases. Amputation was required in only 11% of a large series of 54 aneurysms among drug addicts recently seen at the Henry Ford Hospital; there were no deaths.[750]

The mortality rate in patients with infected atherosclerotic aneurysms often exceeds 90%; approximately 40 long-term survivors have been reported since 1962.[751–754] A high index of suspicion is necessary to allow surgical intervention before rupture occurs, because this complication is uniformly fatal and occurs in about 80% of the cases. When gram-negative bacilli are the cause of the infection, "early" (e.g., within 2 weeks after the first positive blood culture) rupture occurs much more frequently (84%) than if gram-positive bacteria are isolated (10%). Survival after surgery is also more common (75%) for patients with aneurysms infected with gram-positive cocci than for those with gram-negative bacilli (25 percent). Antibiotics should be used in this disease, however, even if the lesion is sterilized (reported in only three cases), the aneurysm may still continue to enlarge and rupture, and therefore surgery is required.

At surgery, the aneurysm and any intraluminal thrombus must be sectioned and Gram-stained, and specimens submitted for culture. If infection is present, all aneurysmal tissue and surrounding areas of inflammation must be resected before grafting. Basic principles of grafting in this situation include the use of autogenous rather than synthetic grafts and insertion only in clean noninfected tissue planes. If the graft is placed in the infected area, then continued infection, leakage, thrombus formation, abscess formation, or rupture usually results. Although some authorities have achieved a successful result by restoration of vascular continuity in situ after radical débridement,[751, 753] this approach is not recommended in most cases. Nevertheless, the type of reconstruction must be individualized, as results of in situ repair appear to be better when the aortic aneurysm is suprarenal[755–758] than when it is more distal in location if reconstruction is combined with prolonged courses of intravenous antimicrobial agents. Radical resection of intra-abdominal aortic aneurysms without prosthetic material has also been used in small numbers of cases.[759] In a review of 24 patients with abdominal aortic aneurysms infected with salmonellae, 10 died after rupture without surgery, and another 7 patients survived grafting only to succumb to continued leakage from the anastomosis (only 5 were long-term survivors). If a graft is inserted in situ and persistent fever with bacteremia or embolism in the lower extremities ensues, reoperation with extra-anatomic grafting is mandatory. Because the resected area is contaminated, special bypass techniques—especially thoracoiliac, transpubic, and axillofemoral—are usually required. When an axillofemoral approach is used, a single graft should be inserted for both lower extremities, because patency is prolonged under these circumstances.[752, 754] Bactericidal antibiotics should be continued for 6 to 8 weeks postoperatively. The choice of agents is dependent on the isolated organism (or the morphologic characteristics of the organisms in the surgical specimen) and on the results of in vitro susceptibility testing. Implantation of antibiotic-releasing carriers with in situ reconstruction has been used[760] but only in small numbers of patients without controlled trials; use of such carriers remains of unproven benefit in therapy for mycotic aneurysm.

REFERENCES

1. Lerner PI, Weinstein L. Infective endocarditis in the antibiotic era. N Engl J Med. 1966;274:199.
2. Watanakunakorn C. Changing epidemiology and newer aspects of infective endocarditis. Adv Intern Med. 1977;22:21.
3. von Reyn CF, Levy BS, Arbeit RD, et al. Infective endocarditis: An analysis based on strict case definitions. Ann Intern Med. 1982;94:505.
4. Steckelberg JM, Melton LJ III, Ilstrup DM, et al. Influence of referral bias on the apparent clinical spectrum of infective endocarditis. Am J Med. 1990;88:582.
5. Harris SL. Definitions and demographic characteristics. In: Kaye D, ed. Infective Endocarditis. New York: Raven Press; 1992:1.
6. Durack DT, Petersdorf RG. Changes in the epidemiology of endocarditis. In: Kaplan EL, Taranta AV, eds. Infective Endocarditis. An American Heart Association Symposium. Dallas: American Heart Association; 1977;3.
7. Griffin MR, Wilson WR, Edwards WD, et al. Infective endocarditis. Olmsted County, Minnesota, 1950 through 1981. JAMA. 1985;254:1199–1202.
8. King JW, Nguyen VQ, Conrad SA. Results of a prospective statewide reporting system for infective endocarditis. Am J Med Sci. 1988;295:517–527.
9. Shulman ST. Infective endocarditis:1986. Pediatr Infect Dis. 1986;5:691–694.
10. Watanakunakorn C, Burkert T. Infective endocarditis at a large community teaching hospital, 1980–1990. Medicine. 1993;72:90.
11. Hayward GW. Infective endocarditis: A changing disease. Br Med J. 1973;2:706.
12. Infective endocarditis (Editorial) Br Med J. 1981;1:677.
13. Gold MJ. Cure rates and long term prognosis. In: Kaye D, ed. Infective Endocarditis. New York: Raven Press; 1992:455.
14. Thayer WS. Studies on bacterial (infective) endocarditis. Johns Hopkins Hosp Rep. 1926;22:1.
15. Garvey GJ, Neu HC. Infective endocarditis: An evolving disease. Medicine (Baltimore). 1978;57:105.
16. Lien EA, Solberg CO, Kalager T. Infective endocarditis 1973–1984 at the Bergen University Hospital: Clinical features, treatment and prognosis. Scand J Infect Dis. 1988;20:239–246.
17. Come PC. Infective endocarditis: Current perspectives. Compr Ther. 1982;8:57.
18. Kaplan EL. Infective endocarditis in the pediatric age group: An overview. In: Kaplan EL, Taranta AV, eds. Infective Endocarditis. An American Heart Association Symposium. Dallas: American Heart Association; 1977:51.
19. Baltimore RS. Infective endocarditis in children. Pediatr Infect Dis J. 1992;11:907.
20. Pelletier LL, Petersdorf RG. Infective endocarditis: A review of 125 cases from the University of Washington Hospitals, 1963–72. Medicine (Baltimore). 1977;56:287.
21. Terpenning MS, Buggy BP, Kaufmann CA. Hospital-acquired infective endocarditis. Arch Intern Med. 1988;148:1601–1603.
22. Cherubin CE, Neu HC. Infective endocarditis at the Presbyterian Hospital in New York City from 1938–1967. Am J Med. 1971;51:83.
23. Roberts WC, Buchbinder NA. Right-sided valvular infective endocarditis. A clinicopathologic study of 12 necropsy patients. Am J Med. 1972;53:7.
24. Kaye D. Changing pattern of infective endocarditis. Am J Med. 1985;78(Suppl 6B):157–162.
25. Roberts WC, Perloff JK, Constantin T. Severe valvular aortic stenosis in patients over 65 years of age. Am J Cardiol. 1971;27:497.
26. Delahaye JP, Loire R, Milon H, et al. Infective endocarditis on stenotic aortic valves. Eur Heart J. 1988;9(Suppl E):S43–S49.
27. Gersony WM, Hayes CJ, Driscoll DJ, et al. Bacterial endocarditis in patients with aortic stenosis, pulmonary stenosis, or ventricular septal defect. Circulation. 1993;87(Suppl I):I-121.
28. McKinsey DS, Ratts TE, Bisno AL. Underlying cardiac lesions in adults with infective endocarditis. The changing spectrum. Am J Med. 1987;82:681–688.
29. Lowes JA, Hamer J, Williams G, et al. Ten years of infective endocarditis at St. Bartholomew's hospital: Analysis of clinical features and treatment in relation to prognosis and mortality. Lancet. 1980;1:133.
30. Moulsdale MT, Eykyn SJ, Phillips I. Infective endocarditis, 1970–1979. A study of culture-positive cases in St. Thomas' Hospital. Q J Med. 1980;49:315.
31. Venezio FR, Westenfelder GO, Cook FV, et al. Infective endocarditis in a community hospital. Arch Intern Med. 1982;142:789.
32. Fulkerson PK, Beaver BM, Aveson JC, et al. Calcification of the mitral annulus: Etiology, clinical associations, complications and therapy. Am J Med. 1979;66:967.
33. Welton DE, Young JB, Gentry LO, et al. Recurrent infective endocarditis: Analysis of predisposing factors and clinical features. Am J Med. 1979;66:932.
34. Kreuzpaintner G, Horstkotte D, Heyll A, et al. Increased risk of bacterial endocarditis in inflammatory bowel disease. Am J Med. 1992;92:391.
35. Cardelia JV, Befeler B, Hildner FJ, et al. Hypertrophic subaortic stenosis complicated by aortic insufficiency and subacute bacterial endocarditis. Am Heart J. 1971;81:543.
36. Wang K, Gobel FL, Gleason DF. Bacterial endocarditis in idiopathic hypertrophic subaortic stenosis, Am Heart J. 1975;89:359.
37. Chagnac A, Rudniki C, Loebel H, et al. Infectious endocarditis in idiopathic hypertrophic subaortic stenosis. Report of three cases and review of the literature. Chest. 1982;81:346.
38. Corrigan D, Bolen J, Hancock EW, et al. Mitral valve prolapse and infective endocarditis. Am J Med. 1977;63:215.
39. Jeresaty RM. Mitral valve prolapse—click syndrome. Prog Cardiovasc Dis. 1973;15:623.
40. Schutte JE, Gaffney FA, Blend L, et al. Distinctive anthropometric characteristics of women with mitral valve prolapse. Am J Med. 1981;71:533.
41. Devereux RB, Kramer-Fox R, Kligfield P. Mitral valve prolapse: Causes, clinical manifestations, and management. Ann Intern Med. 1989;111:305–317.
42. Clemens JD, Horwitz RI, Jaffe CC, et al. A controlled evaluation of the risk of bacterial endocarditis in persons with mitral-valve prolapse. N Engl J Med. 1982;307:776.
43. Nolan CM, Kane JJ, Grunow WA. Infective endocarditis and mitral prolapse. A comparison with other types of endocarditis. Arch Intern Med. 1981;141:447.
44. Scheld WM. Pathogenesis and pathophysiology of infective endocarditis. In: Sande MA, Kaye D, Root RK, eds. Endocarditis, v. 1. Contemporary Issues in Infectious Diseases. London: Churchill Livingstone; 1984:1–32.
45. Freedman LR. The pathogenesis of infective endocarditis. J Antimicrob Chemother. 1987;20(Suppl A):1–6.
46. Livornese LL Jr, Korzeniowski OM. Pathogenesis of infective endocarditis. In: Kaye D, ed. Infective Endocarditis. New York: Raven Press; 1992:19.
47. Tunkel AR. Scheld WM. Experimental models of endocarditis. In: Kaye D, ed. Infective Endocarditis. New York: Raven Press; 1992;37.
48. Weinstein L, Schlesinger JJ. Pathoanatomic, pathophysiologic, and clinical correlations in endocarditis (first of two parts). N Engl J Med. 1974;291:832.
49. Angrist AA, Oka M. Pathogenesis of bacterial endocarditis. JAMA. 1963;183:249.
50. Durack DT, Beeson PB. Pathogenesis of infective endocarditis. In: Rahimtoola SH, ed. Infective Endocarditis. New York: Grune & Stratton, 1978:1.
51. Durack DT, Beeson PB. Experimental bacterial endocarditis. I. Colonization of a sterile vegetation. Br J Exp Pathol. 1972;53:44.
52. Durack DT, Beeson PB, Petersdorf RG. Experimental endocarditis. III. Production and progress of the disease in rabbits. Br J Exp Pathol. 1973;54:142.
53. Durack DT. Experimental bacterial endocarditis. IV. Structure and function of very early lesions. J Pathol. 1975;115:81.
54. McGowan DA, Gillett R. Scanning electron microscopic observations of the surface of the initial lesion in experimental streptococcal endocarditis in the rabbit. Br J Exp Pathol. 1980;61:164.
55. Ferguson DJP, McColm AA, Ryan DM, et al. Experimental staphylococcal endocarditis and aortitis. Morphology of the initial colonization. Virchows Arch [A]. 1986;410:43–48.
56. Sherwood BF, Rowlands DT, Vakilzadeh J, et al. Experimental bacterial endocarditis in the opossum (*Didelphis virginiana*). Am J Pathol. 1971;64:513.
57. Chino F, Kodama A, Otake M, et al. Nonbacterial thrombotic endocarditis in a Japanese autopsy sample. A review of 80 cases. Am Heart J. 1975;90:190.
58. Rodbard S. Blood velocity and endocarditis. Circulation. 1963;27:18.
59. Lepeschkin E. On the relation between the site of valvular involvement in endocarditis and the blood pressure resting on the valve. Am J Med Sci. 1952;224:318.
60. Okell CC, Elliott SD. Bacteraemia and oral sepsis. With special reference to the aetiology of subacute endocarditis. Lancet. 1935;2:869.
61. Everett ED, Hirschmann JV. Transient bacteremia and endocarditis prophylaxis: A review. Medicine (Baltimore). 1977;56:61.
62. Loesche WJ. Indigenous human flora and bacteremia. In: Kaplan EL, Taranta AV, eds. Infective Endocarditis. An American Heart Association Symposium. Dallas: American Heart Association; 1977:40.
63. Durack DT, Beeson PB. Protective role of complement in experimental *Escherichia coli* endocarditis. Infect Immun. 1977;16:213.
64. Yersin B, Glauser M-P, Guze L, et al. Experimental *Escherichia coli* endocarditis in rats: Roles of serum bactericidal activity and duration of catheter placement. Infect Immun. 1988;56:1273–1280.
65. Gould K, Ramirez-Ronda CH, Holmes RK, et al. Adherence of bacteria to heart valves in vitro. J Clin Invest. 1975;56:1364.

66. Freedman LR, Valone J Jr. Experimental infective endocarditis. Prog Cardiovasc Dis. 1979;22:169.
67. Baddour LM, Lowrance C, Albus A, et al. *Staphylococcus aureus* microcapsule expression attenuates bacterial virulence in a rat model of experimental endocarditis. J Infect Dis. 1992;165:749.
68. Overholser CD, Moreillon P, Glauser MP. Experimental bacterial endocarditis after dental extractions in rats with periodontitis. J Infect Dis. 1987;155:107–112.
69. Moreillon P, Overholser CD, Malinverni R, et al. Predictors of endocarditis in isolates from cultures of blood following dental extractions in rats with periodontal disease. J Infect Dis. 1988;157:990–995.
70. Gibbons RJ, Nygaard M. Synthesis of insoluble dextran and its significance in the formation of gelatinous deposits by plaque-forming streptococci. Arch Oral Biol. 1968;13:1249.
71. Parker MT, Ball LC. Streptococci and aerococci associated with systemic infection in man. J Med Microbiol. 1976;9:275.
72. Scheld WM, Valone JA, Sande MA. Bacterial adherence in the pathogenesis of endocarditis. Interaction of bacterial dextran, platelets, and fibrin. J Clin Invest. 1978;61:1394.
73. Ramirez-Ronda CH. Adherence of glucan-positive and glucan-negative streptococcal strains to normal and damaged heart valves. J Clin Invest. 1978;62:805.
74. Ramirez-Ronda CH. Effects of molecular weight of dextran on the adherence of *Streptococcus sanguis* to damaged heart valves. Infect Immun. 1980;29:1.
75. Pelletier LL Jr, Coyle M, Petersdorf R. Dextran production as a possible virulence factor in streptococcal endocarditis. Proc Soc Exp Biol Med. 1978;158:415.
76. Pulliam L, Dall L, Inokuchi S, et al. Enzymatic modification of the glycocalyx in experimental endocarditis due to viridans streptococci. J Infect Dis. 1987;156:736.
77. Dall L, Barnes WG, Lane JW, et al. Enzymatic modification of glycocalyx in the treatment of experimental endocarditis due to viridans streptococci. J Infect Dis. 1987;156:736–740.
78. Dall LH, Herndon BL. Association of cell adherent glycocalyx and endocarditis production by viridans group streptococci. J Clin Microbiol. 1990;28:1698.
79. Crawford I, Russell C. Comparative adhesion of seven species of streptococci isolated from the blood of patients with subacute bacterial endocarditis to fibrin-platelet clots in vitro. J Appl Bacteriol. 1986;60:127-133.
80. Dall L, Keihofner M, Herndon B, et al. Clindamycin effect on glycocalyx production in experimental viridans streptococcal endocarditis. J Infect Dis. 1990;161:1221.
81. Fenno JC, LeBlanc DJ, Fives-Taylor P. Nucleotide sequence analysis of a type 1 fimbrial gene of *Streptococcus sanguis* FW213. Infect Immun. 1989;57:3527–3533.
82. Burnette-Curley D, Wells V, Viscount H, et al. FimA, a major virulence determinant associated with *Streptococus parasanguis* endocarditis. Infect Immun. 1995;63:4669–4674.
83. Viscount HB, Munro CL, Burnette-Curley D, et al. Immunization with FimA protects against *Streptococcus parasanguis* endocarditis in rats. Infect Immun. 1997;65:994–1002.
84. Scheld WM, Calderone RA, Alliegro GM, et al. Yeast adherence in the pathogenesis of *Candida* endocarditis. Proc Soc Exp Biol Med. 1981;168:208.
85. Scheld WM, Strunk RW, Balian G, et al. Microbial adhesion to fibronectin in vitro correlates with production of endocarditis in rabbits. Proc Soc Exp Biol Med. 1985;180:474–482.
86. Kuypers JM, Proctor RA. Reduced adherence to traumatized rat heart valves by a low-fibronectin-binding mutant of *Staphylococcus aureus*. Infect Immun. 1989;57:2306.
87. Lowrance JH, Baddour LM, Simpson WA. The role of fibronectin binding in the rat model of experimental endocarditis caused by *Streptococcus sanguis*. J Clin Invest. 1990;86:7.
88. Becker RC, DiBello PM, Lucas FV. Bacterial tissue tropism: An in vitro model for infective endocarditis. Cardiovasc Res. 1987;21:813–820.
89. Tart RC, van de Rijn I. Analysis of adherence of *Streptococcus defectivus* and endocarditis-associated streptococci to extracellular matrix. Infect Immun. 1991;59:857.
90. Sommer P, Gleyzal C, Guerret S, et al. Induction of a putative laminin-binding protein of *Streptococcus gordonii* in human infective endocarditis. Infect Immun. 1992;60:360.
91. Vercellotti G, Lussenhop D, Peterson PK, et al. Bacterial adherence to fibronectin and endothelial cells: A possible mechanism for bacterial tissue tropism. J Lab Clin Med. 1984;103:34–43.
92. Ogawa SK, Yurberg ER, Hather VB, et al. Bacterial adherence to human endothelial cells in vitro. Infect Immun. 1985;50:218–224.
93. Hamill RJ, Vann JM, Proctor RA. Phagocytosis of *Staphylococcus aureus* by cultured bovine aortic-endothelial cells: Model for post adherence events in endovascular infections. Infect Immun. 1986;54:833–836.
94. Yao L, Benjualid V, Lowy FB, et al. Internalization of *Staphylococcus aureus* by endothelial cells induces cytokine gene expression. Infect Immun. 1995;63:1835–1839.
95. Devitt D, Francois P, Vaudaux P, Foster TJ. Molecular characterization of the clumping factor (fibrinogen receptor) of *Staphylococcus aureus*. Mol Microbiol. 1994;11:237–248.
96. Moreillon P, Entenza JM, Francioli P, et al. Role of *Staphylococcus aureus* coagulase and clumping factor in pathogenesis of experimental endocarditis. Infect Immun. 1995;63:4738–4743.
97. Flock J-I, Hienz SA, Heimdahl A, Schennings T. Reconsideration of the role of fibronectin binding in endocarditis caused by *Staphylococcus aureus*. Infect Immun. 1996;64:1876–1878.
98. Heinz SA, Schennings T, Heimdahl A, Flock J-I. Collagen binding of *Staphylococcus aureus* is a virulence factor in experimental endocarditis. J Infect Dis. 1996;174:83–88.
99. Herrmann M, Suchard SJ, Boxer LA, et al. Thrombospondin binds to *Staphylococcus aureus* and promotes staphylococcal adherence to surfaces. Infect Immun. 1991;59:279–288.
100. Bayer AS, Ramos MD, Menzies BE, et al. Hyperproduction of α-toxin by *Staphylococcus aureus* results in paradoxically reduced virulence in experimental endocarditis—host defense role for platelet microbicidal proteins. Infect Immun. 1997;65:4652–4660.
101. Scheld WM, Zak O, Vosbeck K, et al. Bacterial adhesion in the pathogenesis of endocarditis. Effect of subinhibitory antibiotic concentrations on streptococcal adhesion in vitro and the development of endocarditis in rabbits. J Clin Invest. 1981;68:1381.
102. Bernard J-P, Francioli P, Glauser MP, et al. Vancomycin prophylaxis of experimental *Streptococcus sanguis* endocarditis: Inhibition of bacterial adherence rather than bacterial killing. J Clin Invest. 1981;68:1113.
103. Glauser MP, Francioli P. Successful prophylaxis against experimental streptococcal endocarditis with bacteriostatic antibiotics. J Infect Dis. 1982;146:806.
104. Lowry FD, Chang DS, Neuhaus EG, et al. Effect of penicillin on the adherence of *Streptococcus sanguis* in vitro and in the rabbit model of endocarditis. J Clin Invest. 1983;71:668.
105. Glauser MP, Bernard JP, Moreillon P, et al. Successful single-dose amoxicillin prophylaxis against experimental streptococcal endocarditis. Evidence for two mechanisms of protection. J Infect Dis. 1983;147:568.
106. Clawson CC, Rao Gunda HR, White JG. Platelet interaction with bacteria. IV. Stimulation of the release reaction. Am J Pathol. 1975;81:411.
107. Herzberg MC, Brintzenhofe KL, Clawson CC. Aggregation of human platelets and adhesion of *Streptococcus sanguis*. Infect Immun. 1983;39:1457.
108. Sullam PM, Valone FH, Mills J. Mechanisms of platelet aggregation by viridans group streptococci. Infect Immun. 1987;55:1743–1750.
109. Sullam PM, Jarvis GA, Valone FH. Role of immunoglobulin G in platelet aggregation by viridans group streptococci. Infect Immun. 1988;56:2907–2911.
110. Herzberg MC, MacFarlane GD, Gong K, et al. The platelet interactivity phenotype of *Streptococcus sanguis* influences the course of experimental endocarditis. Infect Immun. 1992;60:4809.
111. Sullam PM, Costerton JW, Yamasaki R, et al. Inhibition of platelet binding and aggregation by streptococcal exopolysaccharide. J Infect Dis. 1993;167:1123.
112. Bayer AS, Sullam PM, Ramos M, et al. *Staphylococcus aureus*–induced platelet aggregation—a fibrinogen-dependent mechanism that is integrin/RGD sequence-independent. Infect Immun. 1995;63:3634–3641.
113. Herrmann M, Hartleib J, Kehrel B, et al. Interaction of von Willebrand factor with *Staphylococcus aureus*. J Infect Dis. 1997;7:984–991.
114. Shenkman B, Varon D, Marinovitz U, et al. Mechanisms of *Staphylococcus aureus*–induced platelet aggregation: Involvement of glycoprotein Ib and glycoprotein IIb-IIIa. Abstract 50. Presented at the Annual Meeting of the Infectious Disease Society of America, San Francisco, Calif., September 1995.
115. Sullam PM, Bayer AS, Foss W, Cheung AL. Reduced platelet binding capacity of *Staphylococcus aureus* in vitro diminishes induction frequency and metastatic complications of experimental endocarditis. Infect Immun. 1996;64:4915–4921.
116. Yeaman MR, Puentes SM, Norman DC, et al. Partial characterization and staphylocidal activity of thrombin-induced platelet microbicidal protein. Infect Immun. 1992;60:1202.
117. Yeaman MR, Norman DC, Bayer AS. *Staphylococcus aureus* susceptibility to thrombin-induced platelet microbicidal protein is independent of platelet adherence and aggregation in vitro. Infect Immun. 1992;60:2368.
118. Yeaman MR, Ibrahim AS, Edwards JE Jr, et al. Thrombin-induced rabbit platelet microbicidal protein is fungicidal in vitro. Antimicrob Agents Chemother. 1993;37:546.
119. Nicolau DP, Freeman CD, Nightingale CH, et al. Reduction of bacterial titers by low-dose aspirin in experimental aortic valve endocarditis. Infect Immun. 1993;61:1593.
120. Dankert J, van der Werff J, Saat SAJ, et al. Involvement of bactericidal factors from thrombin-stimulated platelets in clearance of adherent viridans streptococci in experimental infective endocarditis. Infect Immun. 1995;63:633–671.
121. Wu T, Yeaman MR, Bayer AS. Resistance to platelet microbicidal protein in vitro among bacteremic staphylococcal and viridans streptococcal isolates correlates with an endocarditis source. Antimicrob Agents Chemother. 1994;38:729–732.
122. Dhawan V, Yeaman MR, Kim E, et al. Phenotypic resistance to thrombin-induced platelet microbicidal protein in vitro correlates with enhanced virulence in experimental endocarditis due to *Staphylococcus aureus*. Infect Immun. 1997;65:3293–3299.
123. Dhawan VK, Bayer AS, Yeaman MR. Influence of in vitro susceptibility to thrombin-induced platelet microbicidal protein on the progression of experimental *Staphylococcus aureus* endocarditis. Infect Immun. 1998;66:3476–3479.
124. Ferguson DJP, McColm AA, Ryan DM, et al. A morphological study of experimental staphylococcal endocarditis and aortitis II. Inter-relationship of bacteria, vegetation and cardiovasculature in established infections. Br J Exp Pathol. 1986;67 679–686.
125. Durack DT, Beeson PB. Experimental bacterial endocarditis. II. Survival of bacteria in endocardial vegetations. Br J Exp Pathol. 1972;53:50.
126. Yersin BR, Glauser MP, Freedman LR. Effect of nitrogen mustard on natural history of right-sided streptococcal endocarditis: Role of cellular host defenses. Infect Immun. 1982;35:320.
127. Meddens MJM, Thompson J, Eulderink F, et al. Role of granulocytes in experimental *Streptococcus sanguis* endocarditis. Infect Immun. 1982;36:325.

128. Meddens MJM, Thompson J, Mattie H, et al. Role of granulocytes in the prevention and therapy of experimental *Streptococcus sanguis* endocarditis in rabbits. Antimicrob Agents Chemother. 1984;25:263–267.
129. Hook EW III, Sande MA. Role of the vegetation in experimental *Streptococcus viridans* endocarditis. Infect Immun. 1974;10:1433.
130. Thorig L, Thompson J, Eulderink F, et al. Effects of monocytopenia and anticoagulation in experimental *Streptococcus sanguis* endocarditis. Br J Exp Pathol. 1980;61:108.
131. van Ginkel CJW, Thorig L, Thompson J, et al. Enhancement of generation of monocyte tissue thromboplastin by bacterial phagocytosis: Possible pathway for fibrin formation on infected vegetations in bacterial endocarditis. Infect Immun. 1979;25:388.
132. Drake TA, Rodgers GM, Sande MA. Tissue factor is a major stimulus for vegetation formation in enterococcal endocarditis in rabbits. J Clin Invest. 1984;73:1750–1753.
133. Drake TA, Pang M. *Staphylococcus aureus* induces tissue factor expression in cultured human cardiac valve endothelium. J Infect Dis. 1988;157:749–756.
134. Yao L, Berman JW, Factor SM, Lowy FD. Correlation of histopathologic and bacteriologic changes with cytokine gene expression in an experimental murine model of bacteremic *Staphylococcus aureus* infection. Infect Immun. 1997;65:3889–3995.
135. Beekhuizen H, van de Gevel JS, Veltrop MHAM, et al. Bacterial colonization of vascular endothelium in the pathogenesis of endocarditis. Abstract 145. Presented at the Fourth International Symposium on Modern Concepts in Endocarditis and Cardiovascular Infections, Yverdon, Switzerland, May 24–26, 1997.
136. Veltrop MHAM, Beekhuizen H, Thompson J. Procoagulant properties of endothelial cells after infection with bacteria. Abstract 148. Presented at the Fourth International Symposium on Modern Concepts in Endocarditis and Cardiovascular Infections, Yverdon, Switzerland, May 1997.
137. Bansci MJLFM, Veltrop MHAM, Bertina RM, Thompson J. Influence of monocytes and antibiotic treatment on tissue factor activity of endocardial vegetations in rabbits infected with *Streptococcus sanguis*. Infect Immun. 1996;64:448–451.
138. Mair W. Pneumococcal endocarditis in rabbits. J Pathol Bacteriol. 1923;26:426.
139. Scheld WM, Thomas JH, Sande MA. Influence of preformed antibody on experimental *Streptococcus sanguis* endocarditis. Infect Immun. 1979;25:781.
140. Durack DT, Gilliland BC, Petersdorf RG. Effect of immunization on susceptibility to experimental *Streptococcus mutans* and *Streptococcus sanguis* endocarditis. Infect Immun. 1978;22:52.
141. van de Rijn I. Analysis of cross-protection between serotypes and passively transferred immune globulin in experimental nutritionally variant streptococcal endocarditis. Infect Immun. 1988;56:117.
142. Scheld WM, Calderone RA, Brodeur JP, et al. Influence of preformed antibody on the pathogenesis of experimental *Candida albicans* endocarditis. Infect Immun. 1983;40:950.
143. Greenberg DP, Ward JI, Bayer AS. Influence of *Staphylococcus aureus* antibody on experimental endocarditis in rabbits. Infect Immun. 1987;55:3030–3034.
144. Sieling PJ, van de Rijn I. Evaluation of the immune response in protection against experimental *Streptococcus defectivus* endocarditis. J Lab Clin Med. 1991;117:402.
145. Albus A, Arbeit RD, Lee JC. Virulence of *Staphylococcus aureus* mutants altered in type 5 capsule production. Infect Immun. 1991;59:1008–1014.
146. Lee JC, Park J-S, Shepherd SE, Fattom A. Protective efficacy of antibodies to the *Staphylococcus aureus* type 5 capsular polysaccharide in a rat model of endocarditis. Infect Immun. 1997;65:4146–4151.
147. Bayer AS, Ing M, Kim E, et al. Role of anticapsular IgG in modifying the course of experimental *Staphylococcus aureus* endocarditis. Presented at the Thirty-sixth Interscience Conference on Antimicrobial Agents and Chemotherapy, Washington, D.C., 1996.
148. Williams RC, Kunkel HG. Rheumatoid factors and their disappearance following therapy in patients with SBE. Arthritis Rheum. 1962;5:126.
149. Sheagren JN, Tuazon CV, Griffin C, et al. Rheumatoid factor in acute bacterial endocarditis. Arthritis Rheum. 1976;19:887.
150. Phair JP, Clarke J. Immunology of infective endocarditis. Prog Cardiovasc Dis. 1979;22:137.
151. Bacon PA, Davidson C, Smith B. Antibodies to *Candida* and autoantibodies in subacute bacterial endocarditis. Q J Med. 1974;43:537.
152. Laxdal T, Messner RP, Williams RC. Opsonic, agglutinating, and complement-fixing antibodies in patients with subacute bacterial endocarditis. J Lab Clin Med. 1968;71:638.
153. Horwitz D, Quismorio FP, Friou GJ. Cryoglobulinemia in patients with infectious endocarditis. Clin Exp Immunol. 1975;19:131.
154. Qoronfleh MW, Weraarchakul W, Wilkinson BJ. Antibodies to a range of *Staphylococcus aureus* and *Escherichia coli* heat shock proteins in sera from patients with *S. aureus* endocarditis. Infect Immun. 1993;61:1567.
155. Bayer AS, Theofilopoulos AN, Eisenberg R, et al. Circulating immune complexes in infective endocarditis. N Engl J Med. 1976;295:1500.
156. Gutman RA, Striker GE, Gilliland BC, et al. The immune complex glomerulonephritis of bacterial endocarditis. Medicine (Baltimore). 1972;51:1.
157. Levy RL, Hong R. The immune nature of subacute bacterial endocarditis (SBE) nephritis. Am J Med. 1973;54:645.
158. Inman RD, Redecha PB, Knechtle SJ, et al. Identification of bacterial antigens in circulating immune complexes of infective endocarditis. J Clin Invest. 1982;70:271.
159. Alpert JS, Krous HF, Dalen JE, et al. Pathogenesis of Osler's nodes. Ann Intern Med. 1976;85:471.
160. Lowenstein MB, Urman JD, Abeles M, et al. Skin immunofluorescence in infective endocarditis. JAMA. 1977;238:1163.
161. Cabane J, Godeau P, Herreman G, et al. Fate of circulating immune complexes in infective endocarditis. Am J Med. 1979;66:277.
162. Kauffman RH, Thompson J, Valentijn RM, et al. The clinical implications and the pathogenetic significance of circulating immune complexes in infective endocarditis. Am J Med. 1981;71:17.
163. McFarland MM. Pathology of infective endocarditis. In: Kaye D, ed. Infective Endocarditis. New York: Raven Press; 1992:57.
164. Roberts WC. Characteristics and consequences of infective endocarditis (active or healed or both) learned from morphologic studies. In: Rahimtoola SH, ed. Infective Endocarditis. New York: Grune & Stratton; 1978:55.
165. Coplan NL, Bruno MS. Acquired immunodeficiency syndrome and heart disease: The present and future. Am Heart J. 1989;117:1175.
166. Francis CK. Cardiac involvement in AIDS. Curr Prob Cardiol. 1990;15:571.
167. Morel-Maroger L, Sraer JD, Herreman G, et al. Kidney in subacute endocarditis. Pathological and immunofluorescence findings. Arch Pathol. 1913;94:205.
168. Anderson CB, Butcher HR, Ballinger WF. Mycotic aneurysms. Arch Surg. 1974;109:712.
169. Greenlee JE, Mandell GL. Neurological manifestations of infective endocarditis: A review. Stroke. 1973;4:958.
170. Masuda J, Yutani C, Waki R, et al. Histopathologic analysis of the mechanisms of intracranial hemorrhage complicating infective endocarditis. Stroke. 1992;23:843.
171. Kerr A Jr, Tan JS. Biopsies of the Janeway lesion of infective endocarditis. J Cutan Pathol. 1979;6:124.
172. Silverberg HH. Roth spots. Mt Sinai J Med. 1970;37:77.
173. Starkebaum M, Durack D, Beeson P. The "incubation period" of subacute bacterial endocarditis. Yale J Biol Med. 1977;50:49.
174. Weinstein L, Rubin RH. infective endocarditis—1973. Prog Cardiovasc Dis. 1973;16:239.
175. Freedman LR. Infective endocarditis and other intravascular infections. In: Braude AI, David CE, Fierer J, eds. Medical Microbiology and Infectious Diseases. Philadelphia: WB Saunders; 1981:1511.
176. Hermans PE. The clinical manifestations of infective endocarditis. Mayo Clin Proc. 1982;57:15.
177. Terpenning MS, Buggy BP, Kauffman CA. Infective endocarditis: Clinical features in young and elderly patients. Am J Med. 1987;83:626–634.
178. Lederman MM, Sprague L, Wallis RS, et al. Duration of fever during treatment of infective endocarditis. Medicine (Baltimore). 1992;71:52.
179. Blumberg EA, Robbins N, Adimora A, et al. Persistent fever in association with infective endocarditis. Clin Infect Dis. 1992;15:983.
180. Espersen F, Frimodt-Moller N. *Staphylococcus aureus* endocarditis. A review of 119 cases. Arch Intern Med. 1986;146:1118–1121.
181. Charney R, Keltz TN, Attai L, et al. Acute vavular obstruction from streptococcal endocarditis. Am Heart J. 1993;125:544.
182. Ting W, Silverman NA, Arzaman DA, et al. Splenic septic emboli in endocarditis. Circulation. 1990;82(Suppl IV):IV-105.
183. Mansur AJ, Grinberg M, DaLuz PL, Bellotti G. The complications of infective endocarditis—a reappraisal in the 1980s. Arch Intern Med. 1992;152:2428–2432.
184. Churchill MA, Geraci JE, Hunder GG. Musculoskeletal manifestations of bacterial endocarditis. Ann Intern Med. 1977;87:754.
185. Herzog CA, Henry TD, Zimmer SD. Bacterial endocarditis presenting as acute myocardial infarction: A cautionary note for the era of reperfusion. Am J Med. 1991;90:392.
186. Lerner PI. Neurologic complications of infective endocarditis. Med Clin North Am. 1985;69:385–398.
187. Tunkel AR, Kaye D. Neurologic complications of infective endocarditis. Neurol Clin. 1993;11:419.
188. Selky AK, Roos KL. Neurologic complications of infective endocarditis. Semin Neurol. 1995;12:225.
189. Bayer AS, Theofilopulos AN, Eisenberg R, et al. Thrombotic thrombocytopenic purpura–like syndrome associated with infective endocarditis. A possible immune complex disorder. JAMA. 1977;238:408.
190. Levine DP, Crane LR, Zervos MJ. Bacteremia in narcotic addicts at the Detroit Medical Center II. Infectious endocarditis: A prospective comparative study. Rev Infect Dis. 1986;8:374–396.
191. Marantz PR, Linzer M, Feiner CJ, et al. Inability to predict diagnosis in febrile intravenous drug abusers. Ann Intern Med. 1987;106:823–828.
192. Weisse AB, Heller DR, Schimenti RJ, et al. The febrile parenteral drug user: A prospective study in 121 patients. Am J Med. 1993;94:274.
193. Chambers HF, Morris DL, Tauber MG, et al. Cocaine use and the risk for endocarditis in intravenous drug users. Ann Intern Med. 1987;106:833–836.
194. Graves MK, Soto L. Left-sided endocarditis in parenteral drug abusers: Recent experience at a large community hospital. South Med J. 1992;85:387.
195. Chambers HF, Korzeniowski OM, Sande MA, et al. *Staphylococcus aureus* endocarditis: Clinical manifestations in addicts and nonaddicts. Medicine (Baltimore). 1983;62:170.
196. Sklaver AR, Hoffman TA, Greenman RL. Staphylococcal endocarditis in addicts. South Med J. 1978;71:638.
197. Thadepalli H, Francis CK. Diagnostic clues in metastatic lesions of endocarditis in addicts. West J Med. 1978;128:1.
198. Nahass RG, Weinstein MP, Bartels J, Gocke BJ. Infectious endocarditis in intravenous drug users: A comparison of human immunodeficiency virus type-1-negative and -positive patients. J. Infect Dis. 1990;162:967–970.
199. Kaell AT, Volkman DJ, Gorevic PD, et al. Positive Lyme serology in subacute bacterial endocarditis. JAMA. 1990;264:2916.

200. McCartney AC, Orange GV, Pringle SD, et al. Serum C reactive protein in infective endocarditis. J Clin Pathol. 1988;41:44–48.
201. Wiseman J, Rouleau J, Rigo P, et al. Gallium-67 myocardial imaging for the detection of bacterial endocarditis. Radiology. 1976;120:135.
202. Wong DW, Dhawan VK, Tanaka T, et al. Imaging endocarditis with technetium 99m–labeled antibody—an experimental study: Concise communication. J Nucl Med. 1982;23:229.
203. Riba AL, Thakur ML, Gottschalk A, et al. Imaging experimental infective endocarditis with indium-111—labeled blood cellular components. Circulation. 1979;59:336.
204. Haft JI, Altieri J, Smight LG, et al. Computed tomography of the abdomen in the diagnosis of splenic emboli. Arch Intern Med. 1988;148:193–197.
205. Beeson PB, Brannon ES, Warren JV. Observations on the sites of removal of bacteria from the blood of patients with bacterial endocarditis. J Exp Med. 1945;81:9–23.
206. Werner AS, Cobbs CG, Kaye D, et al. Studies on the bacteremia of bacterial endocarditis. JAMA. 1967;202:199.
207. Pazin GJ, Saul S, Thompson ME. Blood culture positivity. Suppression by outpatient antibiotic therapy in patients with bacterial endocarditis. Arch Intern Med. 1982;142:263.
208. McKenzie R, Reimer LG. Effect of antimicrobials on blood cultures in endocarditis. Diagn Microbiol Infect Dis. 1987;8:165–172.
209. Aronson MD, Bos DH. Blood cultures. Ann Intern Med. 1987;106:246–253.
210. Washington JA II, Ilstrup DM. Blood cultures: Issues and controversies. Rev Infect Dis. 1986;8:792–802.
211. Washington JA II. The role of the microbiology laboratory in the diagnosis and antimicrobial treatment of infective endocarditis. Mayo Clin Proc. 1982;57:22.
212. Carey RB, Gross KC, Roberts RB. Vitamin-B_6–dependent *Streptococcus mitior (mitis)* isolated from patients with systemic infections. J Infect Dis. 1975;131:722.
213. Powers DL, Mandell GL. Intraleucocytic bacteria in endocarditis patients. JAMA. 1974;227:313.
214. Whitcomb DC. Bugs in the blood: Acute staphylococcal septicemia and endocarditis diagnosed by staining the buffy coat. N C Med J. 1986;47:293–295.
215. Tuazon CU, Sheagren JW. Teichoic acid antibodies in the diagnosis of serious infections with *Staphylococcus aureus*. Ann Intern Med. 1976;84:543.
216. Bayer AS, Tillman DB, Concepcion M, et al. Clinical value of teichoic acid antibody titers in the diagnosis and management of staphylococcemias. West J Med. 1980;132:294.
217. Kaplan JE, Palmer DL, Tung KSK. Teichoic acid antibody and circulating immune complexes in the management of *Staphylococcus aureus* bacteremia. Am J Med. 1981;70:769.
218. Cannady PB, Sanford JP. Negative blood cultures in infective endocarditis. A review. South Med J. 1976;69:1420.
219. Tunkel AR, Kaye D. Endocarditis with negative blood cultures. N Engl J Med. 1992;326:1215.
220. Walker RC, Henry NK, Washington JA II, et al. Lysis-centrifugation blood culture technique. Clinical impact in *Staphylococcus aureus* bacteremia. Arch Intern Med. 1986;146:2341–2343.
221. Washington JA II. The microbiological diagnosis of infective endocarditis. J Antimicrob Chemother. 1987;20(Suppl A):29–36.
222. Washington JA. The microbiologic diagnosis of infective endocarditis. J Antimicrob Chemother. 1987;20(Suppl A):29–36.
223. Tunkel AR, Kaye D. Endocarditis with negative blood cultures. N Engl J Med. 1992;326:1215–1217.
224. Austin SM, Smith SM, Co B, et al. Case report: Serologic evidence of acute murine typhus infection in a patient with culture-negative endocarditis. Am J Med Sci. 1987;293:320–323.
225. Shapiro DS, Kenney SC, Johnson M, et al. *Chlamydia psittaci* endocarditis diagnosed by blood culture. N Engl J Med. 1992;326:1192.
226. Tompkins LS, Roessler BJ, Redd SC, et al. *Legionella* prosthetic-valve endocarditis. N Engl J Med. 1988;318:530–535.
227. Spach DH, Kanter AS, Daniels NA, et al. *Bartonella (Rochalimaea)* species as a cause of apparent "culture-negative" endocarditis. Clin Infect Dis. 1995;20:1044–1047.
228. Larson AM, Cougherty MJ, Nowowiejski DJ, et al. Detection of *Bartonella (Rochalimaea)* by routine acridine orange staining of broth blood cultures. J Clin Microbiol. 1994;32:1492–1496.
229. Spach DH, Kanter AS, Dougherty MJ. et al. *Bartonella (Rochalimaea) quintana* bacteremia in inner-city patients with chronic alcoholism. N Engl J Med. 1995;332:419–423.
230. Drancourt M, Mainardi JL, Brouqui P, et al. *Bartonella (Rochalimaea) quintana* endocarditis in three homeless men. N Engl J Med. 1995;332:424–428.
231. Raoult D, Fournier PE, Drancourt M, et al. Diagnosis of 22 new cases of *Bartonella* endocarditis. Ann Intern Med. 1996;125:646–652.
232. Brouqui P, Dumler JS, Raoult D. Immunohistologic demonstration of *Coxiella burnetii* in the valves of patients with Q fever endocarditis. Am J Med. 1994; 451–458.
233. Hamed KA, Dormitzer PR, Su CK, Relman DA. *Haemophilus Parainfluenzae* endocarditis: Application of molecular approach for identification of pathogenetic bacterial species. Clin Infect Dis. 1994;19:677–683.
234. Goldenberger D, Kunzi A, Vogt P, et al. Molecular diagnosis of bacterial endocarditis by broad range PCR amplification and direct sequencing. J Cin Microbiol. 1997;35:2733–2739.
235. Walterspiel JN, Kaplan SL. Incidence and clinical characteristics of "culture-negative"infective endocarditis in a pediatric population. Pediatr Infect Dis. 1986;5:328–332.
236. Rubenstein E, Noriega ER, Simberkoff MS, et al. Fungal endocarditis: Analysis of 24 cases and review of the literature. Medicine (Baltimore). 1975–54:331.
237. Mayayo E, Moralejo J, Camps J, Guarro J. Fungal endocarditis in premature infants: Case report and review. Clin Infect Dis. 1996;22:366–368.
238. Kobza K, Steenblock U. Demonstration of candida in blood smears. Br Med J. 1977;1:1640.
239. Merz WG, Evans GL, Shadomy S, et al. Laboratory evaluation of serological tests for systemic candidiasis: A cooperative study. J Clin Microbiol. 1977;5:596.
240. Sande MA, Bowman CR, Calderone RA. Experimental *Candida albicans* endocarditis: Characterization of the disease and response to therapy. Infect Immun. 1977;17:140.
241. Warren RC, Bartlett A, Bidwell DE, et al. Diagnosis of invasive candidosis by enzyme immunoassay of serum antigen. Br Med J. 1977;1:1183.
242. Scheld WM, Borwn RS Jr, Harding SA, et al. Detection of circulating antigen in experimental *Candida albicans* endocarditis by an enzyme-linked immunosorbent assay. J Clin Microbiol. 1980;12:679.
243. Dillan JC, Feigenbaum H, Konecke LL, et al. Echocardiographic manifestations of valvular vegatations. AM Heart J. 1973;86:698.
244. Boucher CA, Fallion JT, Myers GS, et al. The value and limitations of echocardiography in recording mitral valve vegetations. Am Heart J. 1977;94:37.
245. Thomson KR, Nanda NC, Gramiak R. The reliability of echocardiography in the diagnosis of infective endocarditis. Radiology. 1977;125:473.
246. Melvin ET, Berger M, Lutzker LG, et al. Noninvasive methods for detection of valve vegetations in infective endocarditis. Am J Cardiol. 1981;47:271.
247. Mintz GS, Kotler MN. Clinical value and limitations of echocardiography. Its use in the study of patients with infectious endocarditis. Arch Intern Med. 1980;140:1022.
248. Popp RL. Echocardiography and infectious endocarditis. In: Remington JS, Swartz MN, eds. Current Clinical Topics in Infectious Diseases, v. 4. New York: McGraw-Hill; 1983:98.
249. Popp RL. Echocardiography. N Engl J Med. 1990;323:165.
250. Davis RS, Strom JA, Frishman W, et al. The demonstration of vegetations by echocardiography in bacterial endocarditis. An indication for early surgical intervention. Am J Med. 1980;57:69.
251. Martin RP, Mettzer RS, Chia EL, et al. Clinical utility of two-dimensional echocardiography in infective endocarditis. Am J Cardiol. 1980;46:379.
252. Steckelberg JM, Murphy JG, Ballard D, et al. Emboli in infective endocarditis; the prognostic value of echocardiography. Ann Intern Med. 1991;114:635.
253. Rohmann S, Erbel R, Gorge G, et al. Clinical relevance of vegetation localization by transesophageal echocardiography in infective endocarditis. Eur Heart J. 1992;13:446–452.
254. Bayer AS, Blomquist IK, Bello E, et al. Tricuspid valve endocarditis due to *Staphylococcus aureus*. Correlation of two-dimensional echocardiography with clinical outcome. Chest. 1988;93:247–53.
255. Manolis AS, Melita H. Echocardiographic and clinical correlates in drug addicts with infective endocarditis. Implication of vegetation size. Arch Intern Med. 1988;148:2461–2465.
256. Tak T, Rahimtoola SH, Kumar A, et al. Value of digital image processing of two-dimensional echocardiograms in differentiating active from chronic vegetations of infective endocarditis. Circulation. 1988;78:116–123.
257. Rohmann S, Erbel R, Darius H, et al. Prediction of rapid versus prolonged healing of infective endocarditis by monitoring vegetation size. J Am Soc Echocardiogr 1991;4:465–474.
258. SanFilippo AJ, Picard MH, Newell JB, et al. Echocardiographic assessment of patients with infective endocarditis. JACC. 1991;18:1191–1199.
259. Shapiro SM, Bayer AS. Transesophageal and Doppler echocardiography in the diagnosis and management of infective endocarditis. Chest. 1991;100:1125–1130.
260. Pearlman AS. Transesophageal echocardiography—sound diagnostic technique or two-edged sword? N Engl J Med. 1991;324:841.
261. Transesophageal echocardiography. Lancet. 1992;339:709.
262. Erbel R, Rohmann S, Drexler M, et al. Improved diagnostic value of echocardiography in patients with infective endocarditis by transesophageal approach: A prospective study. Eur Heart J. 1988;9:43.
263. Mügge A, Daniel WG, Frank G, et al. Echocardiography in infective endocarditis: Reassessment of prognostic implications of vegetation size determined by the transthoracic and transesophageal approach. J Am Coll Cardiol. 1989;14:631.
264. Sochowski RA, Chan K-L. Implication of negative results on a monoplane transesophageal echocardiographic study in patients with suspected infective endocarditis. J Am Coll Cardiol. 1993;21:216.
265. Carpenter JL. Perivalvular extension of infection in patients with infectious endocarditis. Rev Infect Dis. 1991;13:127.
266. Daniel WG, Mügge A, Martin RP, et al. Improvement in the diagnosis of abscesses associated with endocarditis by transesophageal echocardiography. N Engl J Med. 1991;324:795.
267. Daniel WG, Erbel R, Kasper W, et al. Safety of transesophageal echocardiography: A multicenter survey of 10419 examinations. Circulation. 1991;83:817.
268. Mann T, McLaurin L, Grossman W, et al. Assessing the hemodynamic severity of acute aortic regurgitation due to infective endocarditis. N Engl J Med. 1975;293:108.
269. Mills J, Abbott J, Utley JR, et al. Role of cardiac catheterization in infective endocarditis. Chest. 1977;72:576.
270. Welton DE, Young JB, Raizner AE, et al. Value and safety of cardiac catheterization during active infective endocarditis. Am J Cardiol. 1979;44:1306.

271. Durack DT, Lukes AS, Bright DK, et al. New criteria for diagnosis of infective endocarditis. Am J Med. 1994;96:200–209.
272. Dajani AS, Ayoub E, Bierman FZ, et al. Guidelines for the diagnosis of rheumatic fever: Jones criteria, 1992 update. JAMA. 1992;69:203–208.
273. Bayer AS, Bolger AF, Taubert KA, et al. Diagnosis and management of infective endocarditis and its complications. Circulation. 1998; 2936–2948.
274. Kim EL, Ching DL, Pien FD. Bacterial endocarditis at a small community hospital. Am J Med Sci. 1998;2936–2948.
275. Kazanjian PH. Infective endocarditis: Review of 60 cases treated in community hospitals. Infect Dis Clin Pract. 1993;2:41.
276. Roberts RB, Krieger AG, Schiller NL, et al. Viridans streptococcal endocarditis: The role of various species, including pyridoxal-dependent streptococci. Rev Infect Dis. 1979;1:955.
277. Tuazon CV, Gill V, Gill F. Streptococcal endocarditis: Single vs. combination antibiotic therapy and the role of various species. Rev Infect Dis. 1986; 8:54–60.
278. Baddour LM, Bisno AL. Infective endocarditis complicating mitral valve prolapse: Epidemiologic, clinical, and microbiologic aspects. Rev Infect Dis. 1986;8:117–37.
279. Hamoudi AC, Hribar MM, Marcon MJ, et al. Clinical relevance of viridans and nonhemolytic streptococci isolated from blood and cerebrospinal fluid in a pediatric population. Am J Clin Pathol. 1990;93:270.
280. Harder EJ, Wilkowske CJ, Washington JA, et al. *Streptococcus mutans* endocarditis. Ann Intern Med. 1974;80:364.
281. Watanakunakorn C. *Streptococcus bovis* endocarditis. Am J Med. 1974;56:256.
282. Moellering RC, Watson BK, Kunz LJ. Endocarditis due to group D streptococci. Comparison of disease caused by *Streptococcus bovis* with that produced by the enterococci. Am J Med. 1974;57:239.
283. Hoppes WL, Lerner PI. Nonenterococcal group D streptococcal endocarditis caused by *Streptococcus bovis*. Ann Intern Med. 1974;81:588.
284. Klein RS, Reuco RA, Catalano MT, et al. Association of *Streptococcus bovis* with carcinoma of the colon. N Engl J Med. 1977;297:800.
285. Steinberg D, Naggar CZ. *Streptococcus bovis* endocarditis with carcinoma of the colon. N Engl J Med. 1977;297:1354.
286. Mandell GL, Kaye D, Levison ME, et al. Enterococcal endocarditis: An analysis of 38 patients observed at the New York Hospital–Cornell Medical Center. Arch Intern Med. 1970;125:258.
287. Serra P, Brandimarte C, Martino P, et al. Synergistic treatment of enterococcal endocarditis. Arch Intern Med. 1977;137:1562.
288. Mergran DW. Enterococcal endocarditis. Clin Infect Dis. 1992;15:63.
289. Malone DA, Wagner RA, Myers JP, et al. Enterococcal bacteremia in two large community teaching hospitals. Am J Med. 1986;81:601–606.
290. Hoffmann SA, Moellering RC Jr. The enterococcus: "Putting the bug in our ears."Ann Intern Med. 1987;106:757–561.
291. Maki DG, Agger WA. Enterococcal bacteremia: Clinical features, the risk of endocarditis, and management. Medicine (Baltimore). 1988;67:248–269.
292. Ugolini V, Pacifico A, Smitherman TC, et al. Pneumococcal endocarditis update: Analysis of 10 cases diagnosed between 1974 and 1984. Am Heart J. 1986;112:813–819.
293. Powderly WG, Stanley SL Jr, Medoff G. Pneumococcal endocarditis: Report of a series and review of the literature. Rev Infect Dis. 1986;8:786–791.
294. Bruyn GAW, Thompson J, van der Meer JWM. Pneumococcal endocarditis in adult patients. A report of five cases and review of the literature. Q J Med. 1990;74:33.
295. Elward K, Hruby N, Christy C. Pneumococcal endocarditis in infants and children: Report of a case and review of the literature. Pediatr Infect Dis J. 1990;9:652.
296. Gelfand MS, Threlkeld MG. Subacute bacterial endocarditis secondary to *Streptococcus pneumoniae*. Am J Med. 1992;93:91.
297. Carey RB, Brause BD, Roberts RB: Antimicrobial therapy of vitamin B_6–dependent streptococcal endocarditis. Ann Intern Med. 1977;87:150.
298. Stein DS, Nelson KE. Endocarditis due to nutritionally deficient streptococci: Therapeutic dilemma. Rev Infect Dis. 1987;9:908–916.
299. Catto BA, Jacobs MR, Shlaes DM. *Streptococcus mitis*. A cause of serious infection in adults. Arch Intern Med. 1987;147:885–888.
300. Rapeport KB, Giron JA, Rosner F. *Streptococcus mitis* endocarditis. Report of 17 cases. Arch Intern Med. 1986;146:2361–2363.
301. Hager WD, Speck EL, Mathew PK, et al. Endocarditis with myocardial abscesses and pericarditis in an adult. Group B streptococcus as a cause. Arch Intern Med. 1977;137:1725.
302. Opal SM, Cross A, Palmer M, et al. Group B streptococcal sepsis in adults and infants. Contrasts and comparisons. Arch Intern Med. 1988;148:641–645.
303. Gallagher PG, Watanakunakorn C. Group B streptococcal endocarditis: Report of seven cases and review of the literature, 1962–1985. Rev Infect Dis. 1986;8:175–188.
304. Scully BE, Spriggs D, Neu HC. *Streptococcus agalactiae* (group B) endocarditis—a description of twelve cases and review of the literature. Infection. 1987;15:169–176.
305. Wiseman A, Rene P, Crelinsten GL. *Streptococcus agalactiae* endocarditis: An association with villous adenomas of the large intestine. Ann Intern Med. 1985;103:893–894.
306. Vartrian CV, Septimus EJ. Tricuspid valve group B streptococcal endocarditis following elective abortion. Rev Infect Dis. 1991;13:997.
307. Baddour LM. Infective endocarditis caused by β-hemolytic streptococci. Clin Infect Dis. 1998;26:66–71.
308. Venezio FR, Gullberg RM, Westenfelder GO, et al. Group G streptococcal endocarditis and bacteremia. Am J Med. 1986;81:29–34.
309. Smyth EG, Pallett AP, Davidson RN. Group G streptococcal endocarditis: Two case reports, a review of the literature and recommendations for treatment. J Infect. 1988;16:169–176.
310. Ho AKC, Woo KS, Tse KK, et al. Infective endocarditis caused by *Streptococcus suis* serotype 2. J Infect. 1990;21:209.
311. Liu VC, Stevenson JG, Smith AL. Group A *Streptococcus* mural endocarditis. Pediatr Infect Dis J. 1992;11:1060.
312. Murray HW, Gross KC, Masur H, et al. Serious infections caused by *Streptococcus milleri*. Am J Med. 1978;64:759.
313. Shlaes DM, Lerner PI, Wolinsky E, et al. Infections due to Lancefield group F and related streptococci *(S. milleri, S. anginosus)*. Medicine (Baltimore). 1981;60:197.
314. Gossling J. Occurence and pathogenicity of the *Streptococcus milleri* group. Rev Infect Dis. 1988;10:257–285.
315. Hosea SW: Virulent *Streptococcus viridans* bacterial endocarditis. Am Heart J. 1981;101:174.
316. Buu-Joi A, Sapoetra A, Branger C, et al. Antimicrobial susceptibility of *Gemella haemolysans* isolated from patients with subacute endocarditis. Eur J Clin Microbiol. 1982;1:102.
317. Frésard A, Michel VP, Rueda X, et al. *Gemella haemolysans* endocarditis. Clin Infect Dis. 1993;16:586.
318. Mylotte JM, McDermott C, Spooner JA. Prospective study of 114 consecutive episodes of *Staphylococcus aureus* bacteremia. Rev Infect Dis. 1987;9:891–908.
319. Eykyn SJ. Staphylococcal sepsis. The changing pattern of disease and therapy. Lancet. 1988;1:100–104.
320. Watanakunakorn C, Tan JS, Phair JP. Some salient features of *Staphylococcus aureus* endocarditis. Am J Med. 1973;54:473.
321. Musher DM, McKenzie SO. Infection due to *Staphylococcus aureus*. Medicine (Baltimore). 1977;56:383.
322. Bayer AS. Staphylococcal bacteremia and endocarditis. State of the art. Arch Intern Med. 1982;142:1169.
323. Thompson RL. Staphylococcal infective endocarditis. Mayo Clin Proc. 1982;57:106.
324. Sanabria TJ, Alpert JS, Goldberg R, et al. Increasing frequency of staphylococcal infective endocarditis. Experience at a university hospital, 1981 through 1988. Arch Intern Med. 1990;150:1305.
325. Ing MB, Baddour LM, Bayer AS. Bacteremia and infective endocarditis: Pathogenesis, diagnosis and complications. In: Crossley KB, Archer GL, eds. The Staphylococci in Human Disease. New York: Churchill Livingstone; 1997:331–354.
326. Fowler VG, Sanders LL, Kong L, et al. *Staphylococcus aureus* endocarditis: 59 prospectively identified cases with followup. Clin Infect Dis. 1998;28:106–114.
327. Julander I. Unfavourable prognostic factors in *Staphylococcus aureus* septicemia and endocarditis. Scand J Infect Dis. 1985;17:179–187.
328. O'Callaghan C, McDougall P. Infective endocarditis in neonates. Arch Dis Child. 1988;63:53–57.
329. Crane LR, Levine DP, Zervos MJ, et al. Bacteremia in narcotic addicts at the Detroit Medical Center. I. Microbiology, epidemiology, risk factors, and empiric therapy. Rev Infect Dis. 1986;8:364–373.
330. Noel GJ, O'Loughlin JE, Edelson PJ. Neonatal *Staphylococcus epidermidis* right-sided endocarditis: Description of five catheterized infants. Pediatrics. 1988;82:234–239.
331. Baddour LM, Phillips TN, Bisno AL. Coagulase-negative staphylococcal endocarditis. Occurrence in patients with mitral valve prolapse. Arch Intern Med. 1986;146:119–21.
332. Harris LF, O'Shields H. Coagulase-negative staphylococcal endocarditis: A view from the community hospital. South Med J. 1986;79:1379–1386.
333. Caputo GM, Archer GL, Calderwood SB, et al. Native valve endocarditis due to coagulase-negative staphylococci. Clinical and microbiologic features. Am J Med. 1987;83:619–625.
334. Arber N, Militano A, Ben-Yehuda A, et al. Native valve *Staphylococcus epidermidis* endocarditis: Report of seven cases and review of the literature. Am J Med. 1991;90:758.
335. Espersen F, Wheat LJ, Bemis AT, et al. Solid-phase radio-immunoassay for IgG antibodies to *Staphylococcus epidermidis:* Use in serious coagulase-negative staphylococcal infections. Arch Intern Med. 1987;147:689–693.
336. Etienne J, Brun Y, El Solh N, et al. Characterization of clinically significant isolates of *Staphylococcus epidermidis* from patients with endocarditis. J Clin Microbiol. 1988;26:613–617.
337. Baddour LM, Simpson WA, Weems JJ Jr, et al. Phenotypic selection of small-colony variant forms of *Staphylococcus epidermidis* in a rat model of endocarditis. J Infect Dis. 1988;157:757–763.
338. Singh VR, Radd I. Fatal *Staphylococcus saprophyticus* native valve endocarditis in an intravenous drug addict. J Infect Dis. 1990;162:783.
339. Lina B, Celard M, Vandenesch F, et al. Infective endocarditis due to *Staphylococcus capitis*. Clin Infect Dis. 1992;15:173.
340. DeHondt G, Leven M, Vandermersch C, Colaert J. Destructive endocarditis caused by *Staphylococcus lugdunensis*—case report and review of the literature. Acta Clin Belg. 1997;52:27–30.
341. Vandenesch F, Etienne J, Reverdy ME, Eykeyn SJ. Endocarditis due to *Staphylococcus lugdunensis:* Report of 11 cases and review. Clin Infect Dis. 1993;17: 871–876.
342. Celard M, Lelievre H, Obadia JF, et al. Long-standing bacteremia and endocarditis caused by *Staphylococcus lugdunensis* in a patient with an implantable cardioverter defibrillator. Clin Microbiol Infect. 1997;3:387–388.
343. Lessing MPA, Crook DWM, Bowler ICJ, Gribbin B. Native valve endocarditis caused by *Staphylococcus lugdunensis*. Q J Med. 1996;89:855–858.

344. Etienne J, Brun Y, Fleurette J. *Staphylococcus lugdunensis* endocarditis. J Clin Pathol. 1989;42:892–893.
345. Finland M, Barnes MW. Changing etiology of bacterial endocarditis in the antibacterial era. Experiences at Boston City Hospital 1933–1965. Ann Intern Med. 1970;72:341.
346. Pedersen FK, Petersen EA. Bacterial endocarditis of Blegdamshospitalet in Copenhagen 1944–1973. Scand J Infect Dis. 1976;8:99.
347. Cohen PS, Maquire JH, Weinstein L. Infective endocarditis caused by gram-negative bacteria: A review of the literature, 1945–1977. Prog Cardiovasc Dis. 1980;22:205.
348. Geraci JE, Wilson WR. Endocarditis due to gram-negative bacteria. Report of 56 cases. Mayo Clin Proc. 1982;57:145.
349. Snyder N, Atterbury CE, Correia JP, et al. Increased occurrence of cirrhosis and bacterial endocarditis. Gastroenterology. 1977;73:1107.
350. Carruthers M. Endocarditis due to enteric bacilli other than salmonellae: Case reports and literature review. Am J Med Sci. 1977;273:203.
351. Sande MA, Johnson WD, Hook EW, et al. Sustained bacteremia in patients with prosthetic cardiac valves. N Engl J Med. 1972;286:1067.
352. Schneider PJ, Nernoff J, Gold JA. Acute salmonella endocarditis. Report of a case and review. Arch Intern Med. 1967;120:478.
353. Mills J, Drew D. *Serratia marcescens* endocarditis. Ann Intern Med. 1976;85:397.
354. Cooper R, Mills J. *Serratia* endocarditis. A follow-up report. Arch Intern Med. 1980;140:199.
355. Caramelli B, Mansur AJ, Grinberg M, et al. *Campylobacter fetus* endocarditis on a prosthetic heart valve. South Med J. 1988;81:802–803.
356. Reyes MP, Brown WJ, Lerner AM. Treatment of patients with *Pseudomonas* endocarditis with high dose aminoglycoside and carbenicillin therapy. Medicine (Baltimore). 1978;57:57.
357. Reyes MP, Lerner AM. Current problems in the treatment of infective endocarditis due to *Pseudomonas aeruginosa*. Rev Infect Dis. 1983;5:314.
358. Wieland M, Lederman MM, Kline-King C, et al. Left-sided endocarditis due to *Pseudomonas aeruginosa*. A report of 10 cases and review of the literature. Medicine (Baltimore). 1986;65:180–189.
359. Komshian SV, Tablan OC, Palutke W, et al. Characteristics of left-sided endocarditis due to *Pseudomonas aeruginosa* in the Detroit Medical Center. Rev Infect Dis. 1990;12:693.
360. Noriega ER, Rubinstein E, Simberkoff M, et al. Subacute and acute endocarditis due to *Pseudomonas cepacia* in heroin addicts. Am J Med. 1975;59:29.
361. Reyes MP, Palutke WA, Wylin RF, et al. *Pseudomonas* endocarditis in the Detroit Medical Center 1969–1972. Medicine (Baltimore). 1973;52:173.
362. Jurica JV, Bomzer CA, England AC III. Gonococcal endocarditis: A case report and review of the literature. Sex Transm Dis. 1987;14:231–233.
363. Wall TC, Peyton RB, Corey GR. Gonococcal endocarditis: A new look at an old disease. Medicine. 1989;68:375.
364. Jackman JD Jr, Glamann DB. Gonococcal endocarditis: Twenty-five year experience. Am J Med Sci. 1991;301:221.
365. Wong JD, Janda JM. Association of an important *Neisseria* species, *Neisseria elongata* subsp. *nitroreducens,* with bacteremia, endocarditis, and osteomyelitis. J Clin Microbiol. 1992;30:719.
366. Ingram RJH, Cornere B, Ellis-Pegler RB. Endocarditis due to *Neisseria mucosa:* Two case reports and review. Clin Infect Dis. 1992;15:321.
367. Heiddal S, Sverrisson JT, Yngvason FE, et al. Native-valve endocarditis due to *Neisseria sicca:* Case report and review. Clin Infect Dis. 1993;16:667.
368. Chunn CJ, Jones SR, McCutchan JA, et al. *Haemophilus parainfluenzae* infective endocarditis. Medicine (Baltimore). 1977;56:99.
369. Lynn DJ, Kane JG, Parker RH. *Haemophilus parainfluenzae* and influenzae endocarditis: A review of forty cases. Medicine (Baltimore). 1977;56:115.
370. Geraci JE, Wilkowske CJ, Wilson WR, et al. *Haemophilus* endocarditis. Report of 14 cases. Mayo Clin Proc. 1977;52:209.
371. Parker SW, Apicella MA, Fuller CM. *Haemophilus* endocarditis. Two patients with complications. Arch Intern Med. 1983;143:48.
372. Bangsborg JM, Tuede M, Skinhoj P. *Haemophilus seguis* endocarditis. J Infect. 1988;16:81–85.
373. Porath A, Wanderman K, Simu A, et al. Case report: Endocarditis caused by *Haemophilus aegyptius*. Am J Med Sci. 1986;292:110–111.
374. Vandepitte J, DeGeest H, Jousten P. Subacute bacterial endocarditis due to *Actinobacillus actinomycetemcomitans*. Report of a case with a review of the literature. J Clin Pathol. 1977;30:842.
375. AhFat LNC, Patel BR, Pickens S. *Actinobacillus actinomycetemcomitans* endocarditis in hypertrophic obstructive cardiomyopathy. J Infect Dis. 1983;6:81.
376. Lane T, MacGregor RR, Wright D, et al. *Cardiobacterium hominis:* An elusive cause of endocarditis. J Infect. 1983;6:75.
377. Jenny DB, Letendre PW, Iverson G. Endocarditis due to *Kingella* species. Rev Infect Dis. 1988;10:1065–1066.
378. Decker MD, Graham BS, Hunter EB, et al. Endocarditis and infections of intravascular devices due to *Eikenella corrodens*. Am J Med Sci. 1986;292:209–12.
379. Patrick WD, Brown WD, Bowmer MI, et al. Infective endocarditis due to *Eikenella corrodens:* Case report and review of the literature. Can J Infect Dis. 1990;1:139.
380. Ellner JJ, Rosenthal MS, Lerner PI, et al. Infective endocarditis caused by slow-growing, fastidious, gram-negative bacteria. Medicine (Baltimore). 1979;58:145.
381. Gerry JL, Greenough WB. Diphtheroid endocarditis: Report of nine cases and review of the literature. Johns Hopkins Med J. 1976;139:61.
382. Morris A, Guild I. Endocarditis due to *Corynebacterium pseudodiphthericum:* Five case reports, review, and antibiotic susceptibilities of nine strains. Rev Infect Dis. 1991;13:887.
383. Tiley SM, Kociuba KR, Heron LG, et al. Infective endocarditis due to nontoxigenic *Corynebacterium diphtheriae:* Report of seven cases and review. Clin Infect Dis. 1993;16:271.
384. Bayer AS, Chow AW, Guze LB. *Listeria monocytogenes* endocarditis: Report of a case and review of the literature. Am J Med Sci. 1977;273:319.
385. Carvajal A, Frederiksen W. Fatal endocarditis due to *Listeria monocytogenes*. Rev Infect Dis. 1988;10:616–623.
386. Sussman JI, Baron EJ, Goldberg SM, et al. Clinical manifestations and therapy of *Lactobacillus* endocarditis: Report of a case and review of the literature. Rev Infect Dis. 1986;8:771–776.
387. Griffiths JK, Daly JS, Dodge RA. Two cases of endocarditis due to *Lactobacillus* species: Antimicrobial susceptibility, review, and discussion of therapy. Clin Infect Dis. 1992;15:250.
388. Gorby GL, Peacock JE Jr. *Erysipelothrix rhusiopathiae* endocarditis: Microbiologic, epidemiologic, and clinical features of an occupational disease. Rev Infect Dis. 1988;10:317–325.
389. Steen MK, Bruno-Murtha LA, Chaux G, et al. *Bacillus cereus* endocarditis: Report of a case and review. Clin Infect Dis. 1992;14:945.
390. Shands JW Jr. *Rothia dentocariosa* endocarditis. Am J Med. 1988;85:280–281.
391. Sudduth EJ, Rozich JD, Farrar WE. *Rothia dentocariosa* endocarditis complicated by perivalvular abscess. Clin Infect Dis. 1993;17:772.
392. Felner JM, Dowell UR. Anaerobic bacterial endocarditis. N Engl J Med. 1970;283:1188.
393. Nastro LJ, Finegold SM. Endocarditis due to anaerobic gram-negative bacilli. Am J Med. 1973;54:482.
394. Nastro FL, Sarma RJ. Infective endocarditis due to anaerobic and microaerophilic bacteria. West J Med. 1982;137:18.
395. Jackson RT, Dopp AC. *Bacteroides fragilis* endocarditis. South Med J. 1988; 81:781–782.
396. Gradon JD, Chapnick EK, Lutwick LI. Infective endocarditis of a native valve due to *Acinetobacter:* Case report and review. Clin Infect Dis. 1992;14:1145.
397. Lam S, Samraj J, Rahman S, et al. Primary actinomycotic endocarditis: Case report and review. Clin Infect Dis. 1993;16:481.
398. Ascher DP, Zbick C, White C, et al. Infections due to *Stomatococcus mucilaginosus:* 10 cases and review. Rev Infect Dis. 1991;13:1048.
399. Rupp ME. *Streptobacillus moniliformis* endocarditis: Case report and review. Clin Infect Dis. 1992;14:769.
400. Al-Kasab S, Fagih MR, Al-Yousef S, et al. *Brucella* infective endcarditis. Successful combined medical and surgical therapy. J Thorac Cardiovasc Surg. 1988;95:862–867.
401. Jacobs F, Abramowicz D, Vereerstrater P, et al. *Brucella* endocarditis. The role of combined medical and surgical treatment. Rev Infect Dis. 1990;12:740–743.
402. Szabo S, Lieberman JP, Lue YA. Unusual pathogens in narcotic-associated endocarditis. Rev Infect Dis. 1990;12:412.
403. Komshian SV, Tablan OC, Palutke W, et al. Characteristics of left sided endocarditis due to *Pseudomonas aeruginosa* in the Detroit Medical Center. Rev Infect Dis. 1990;12:693.
404. Tuazon CW, Hill R, Sheagren JW. Microbiologic study of street heroin and injection paraphernalia. J Infect Dis. 1974;129:327.
405. Tuazon CW, Sheagren JW. Increased rate of carriage of *Staphylococcus aureus* among narcotic addicts. J Infect Dis. 1974;129:725.
406. Reisberg BE. Infective endocarditis in the narcotic addict. Prog Cardiovasc Dis. 1979;22:193.
407. Baddour LM. Twelve-year review of recurrent native-valve infective endocarditis: A disease of the modern antibiotic era. Rev Infect Dis. 1988;10:1163–1170.
408. Rubenstein E, Noriega ER, Simberkoff MS, et al. Tissue penetration of amphotericin B in *Candida* endocarditis. Chest. 1974;66:376.
409. Moyer D, Edwards JE. Fungal endocarditis. In: Kaye D, ed. Infective Endocarditis. New York: Raven Press; 1992;299–312.
410. Carrizosa J, Levison ME, Lawrence T, et al. Cure of *Asperigillus ustus* endocarditis of prosthetic valve. Arch Intern Med. 1974;133:486.
411. Keay S, Denning DW, Stevens DA. Endocarditis due to *Trichosporon beigelii:* In vitro susceptibility of isolates and review. Rev Infect Dis. 1991;13:383.
412. Welty FK, McLeod GX, Ezratty C, et al. *Pseudallescheria boydii* endocarditis of the pulmonic valve in a liver transplant recipient. Clin Infect Dis. 1992;15:858.
413. McIntosh CS, Nickers PJ, Isaqacs AJ. *Spirillum* endocarditis. Postgrad Med J. 1975;51:645.
414. Marrie T, Raoult D. Q Fever. Clin Infect Dis. 1995; 20:489–495.
415. Applefield MM, Billingsley LJ, Tucker HJ, et al. Q fever endocarditis—a case occurring in the United States. Am Heart J. 1977;93:669.
416. Tobin MJ, Cahill N, Gearty G, et al. Q fever endocarditis. Am J Med. 1982;72:396.
417. Peter O, Flepp M, Bestetti G, et al. Q fever endocarditis: Diagnostic approaches and monitoring of therapeutic effects. Clin Invest. 1992;70:932.
418. Fernandez-Guerrero ML, Muelas JM, Aquado JM. Q fever endocarditis on porcine bioprosthetic valves. Ann Intern Med. 1988;108:209–213.
419. Jones RB, Priest JB, Kuo C-C. Subacute chlamydial endocarditis. JAMA. 1982;247:655.
420. Brearley BF, Hutchinson DN. Endocarditis associated with *Chlamydia trachomatis* infection. Br Heart J. 1981;46:220.
421. Marrie TJ, Harczy M, Mann OE, et al. Culture-negative endocarditis probably due to *Chlamydia pneumoniae*. J Infect Dis. 1990;161:127.
422. Popat K, Barnardo D, Webb-Peploe M. *Mycoplasma pneumoniae* endocarditis. Br Heart J. 1980;44:111.
423. Burch GE, Tsui CY. Evolution of coxsackie viral valvular and mural endocarditis in mice. Br J Exp Pathol. 1971;52:360.

424. Persand V. Two unusual cases of mural endocarditis with a review of the literature. Am J Clin Pathol. 1970;53:832.
425. Van Scoy RE. Culture-negative endocarditis. Mayo Clin Proc. 1982;57:149.
426. Pesanti EL, Smith IM. Infective endocarditis with negative blood cultures. An analysis of 52 cases. Am J Med. 1979;66:43.
427. Hoen B, Selton-Suty C, Lacassin F, et al. Infective endocarditis in patients with negative blood cultures—analysis of 88 cases from a one-year nationwide survey in France. Clin Infect Dis. 1995;20:501–506.
428. Tunkel BR, Kaye D. Endocarditis with negative blood cultures. N Engl J Med. 1992;326:1215–1217.
429. Baddour LM, Meyer J, Henry B. Polymicrobial infective endocarditis in the 1980's. Rev Infect Dis. 1991;13:963.
430. Daschner FD, Frank V. Antimicrobial drugs in human cardiac valves and endocarditis lesions. J Antimicrob Chemother. 1988;12:776–782.
431. Cremieux A-C, Carbon C. Pharmacokinetic and pharmacodynamic requirements for antibiotic therapy of experimental endocarditis. Antimicrob Agents Chemother. 1992;36:2069.
432. Gilbert DN, Wood CA, Kimbrough RC, et al. Failure of treatment with teicoplanin at 6 milligrams/kg/day in patients with *Staphylococcus aureus* intravascular infections. Chemotherapy. 1991;115:674–680.
433. Dall L, Barnes WG, Lane JW, et al. Enzymatic modification of glycocalyx in the treatment of experimental endocarditis due to viridans streptococci. J Infect Dis. 1987;156:736–740.
434. Buiting AGM, Thompson J, Emeis JJ, et al. Effects of tissue-type plasminogen activator on *Staphylococcus epidermidis*–infected plasma clots as a model of infected endocardial vegetations. J Antimicrob Chemother. 1987;19:771–780.
435. Buiting AG, Thompson J, Emeis JJ, et al. Effects of tissue-type plasminogen activator (t-PA) on *Streptococcus sanguis*–infected endocardial vegetations in vitro. J Antimicrob Chemother. 1988;21:609–620.
436. Nicolau DP, Marangos MN, Nightingale CH, Quinitiliani R. Influence of aspirin on development and treatment of experimental *Staphylococcus aureus* endocarditis. Antimicrob Agents Chemother. 1995;39:1748–1751.
437. Kupferwasser LI, Yeaman MR, Shapiro SM, et al. Beneficial effects of aspirin in experimental *Staphylococcus aureus* endocarditis: Microbiologic, echocardiographic and histopathologic analyses. Presented at the Ninety-eighth General Meeting of the American Society for Microbiology, Atlanta, Ga., May 17–21, 1998.
438. Taha TH, Durrant SS, Mazeika PK, et al. Aspirin to prevent growth of vegetations and cerebral emboli in infective endocarditis. J Intern Med. 1992;231:543–546.
439. Cates JE, Christie RV. Subacute bacterial endocarditis. Q J Med. 1951;20:93.
440. Carrizosa J, Kobasa WD, Kaye D. Antagonism between chloramphenicol and penicillin in streptococcal endocarditis in rabbits. J Lab Clin Med. 1975;85:307.
441. Wilson WR, Gilbert DN, Bisno AL, et al. Evaluation of new anti-infective drugs for the treatment of infective endocarditis. Clin Infect Dis. 1992;15(Suppl 1):S89.
442. Douglas A, Moore-Gillon J, Eykyn S. Fever during treatment of infective endocarditis. Lancet. 1986;1:1341–1343.
443. Schlicter JG, Macllean H. A method of determining the effective therapeutic level in the treatment of subacute bacterial endocarditis with penicillin. Am Heart J. 1947;34:209.
444. Coleman DL, Horwitz RI, Andriole VT. Association between serum inhibitory and bactericidal concentrations and therapeutic outcome in bacterial endocarditis. Am J Med. 1982;73:260.
445. Mellors JW, Coleman DL, Andriole VT. Value of serum bactericidal test in management of patients with bacterial endocarditis. Eur J Clin Microbiol. 1986;5:67–70.
446. Rahal JJ, Chan Y-K, Johnson G. Relationship of staphylococcal tolerance, teichoic acid antibody, and serum bactericidal activity to therapeutic outcome in *Staphylococcus aureus* bacteremia. Am J Med. 1986;81:43–52.
447. Wolfson JS, Swartz MN. Serum bactericidal activity as a monitor of antibiotic therapy. N Engl J Med. 1985;312:968–975.
448. Reller LB. The serum bactericidal test. Rev Infect Dis. 1986;8:803–808.
449. Weinstein MP, Stratton CW, Ackley A, et al. Multicenter collaborative evaluation of a standardized serum bactericidal test as a prognostic indicator in infective endocarditis. Am J Med. 1985;78:262–269.
450. Stratton CW. The role of the microbiology laboratory in the treatment of infective endocarditis. J Antimicrob Chemother. 1987;20(Suppl A):S41–S49.
451. Sande MA, Scheld WM. Combination antibiotic therapy of bacterial endocarditis. Ann Intern Med. 1980;92:390.
452. Wilson WR, Karchmer AW, Dajani AS, et al. Antibiotic treatment of adults with infective endocarditis due to streptococci, enterococci, staphylococci and HACEK microorganisms. JAMA. 1995;274:1706–1713.
453. Meylan PR, Francioloi P, Glauser MP. Discrepancies between MBC and actual killing by viridans group streptococci by cell-wall–active antibiotics. Antimicrob Agents Chemother. 1986;29:418–423.
454. Holloway Y, Pankert J, Hess J. Penicillin tolerance and bacterial endocarditis. Lancet. 1980;1:589.
455. Pulliam L, Inokuchi S, Hadley WK, et al. Penicillin tolerance in experimental streptococcal endocarditis. Lancet. 1979;2:957.
456. Gephart JF, Washington JA II. Antimicrobial susceptibilities of nutritionally variant streptococci. J Infect Dis. 1982;146:536.
457. Holloway Y, Dankert J. Penicillin tolerance in nutritionally variant streptococci. Antimicrob Agents Chemother. 1982;22:1073.
458. Lowry FD, Neuhas EG, Chang DS, et al. Penicillin therapy of experimental endocarditis caused by tolerant *Streptococcus sanguis* and nontolerant *Streptococcus mitis*. Antimicrob Agents Chemother. 1983;23:67.
459. Brennan RO, Durack DT. Therapeutic significance of penicillin tolerance in experimental streptococcal endocarditis. Antimicrob Agents Chemother. 1983;23:273.
460. Baker CW, Thornsberry C. Antimicrobial susceptibility of *Streptococcus mutans* isolated from patients with endocarditis. Antimicrob Agents Chemother. 1974;5:268.
461. Thornsberry C, Baker CN, Facklam RR. Antibiotic susceptibility of *Streptococcus bovis* and other group D streptococci causing endocarditis. Antimicrob Agents Chemother. 1974;5:228.
462. Wolfe JC, Johnson WD. Penicillin-sensitive steptococcal endocarditis. In vitro and clinical observations on penicillin-streptomycin therapy. Ann Intern Med. 1974;81:178.
463. Watanakunakorn C, Glotzbecker C. Synergism with aminoglycosides of penicillin, ampicillin, and vancomycin against nonenterococcal group D streptococci and viridans streptococci. J Med Microbiol. 1977;10:133.
464. Enzler MJ, Rouse MS, Henry NK, et al. In vitro and in vivo studies of streptomycin-resistant, penicillin-susceptible streptococci from patients with infective endocarditis. J Infect Dis. 1987;155:954–958.
465. Farber BF, Yee Y. High-level aminoglycoside resistance mediated by aminoglycoside-modifying enzymes among viridans streptococci: Implications for the therapy of endocarditis. J Infect Dis. 1987;155:948–953.
466. Sande MA, Irvin RG. Penicillin-aminoglycoside synergy in experimental *Streptococcus viridans* endocarditis. J Infect Dis. 1974;129:572.
467. Durack DT, Pelletier LL, Petersdorf RG. Chemotherapy of experimental streptococcal endocarditis. II. Synergism between penicillin and streptomycin against penicillin-sensitive streptococci. J Clin Invest. 1974;53:929.
468. Drake TA, Sande MA. Studies of the chemotherapy of endocarditis: Correlation of in vitro, animal model, and clinical studies. Rev Infect Dis. 1983;5(Suppl):S345.
469. Wilson WR, Geraci JE. Treatment of streptococcal infective endocarditis. Am J Med. 1985;78(Suppl 6B):S128–S137.
470. Scheld WM. Therapy of streptococcal endocarditis: Correlation of animal model and clinical studies. J Antimicrob Chemother. 1987;20(Suppl A):S71–S85.
471. Baquero F, Loza E. Penicillin resistance in Spain. Infect Dis Clin Pract. 1992;1:147.
472. Wilson WR, Geraci JE, Wilkowske CJ, et al. Short-term intramuscular therapy with procaine penicillin plus streptomycin for infective endocarditis due to viridans streptococci. Circulation. 1978;57:1158.
473. Wilson WR, Thompson RL, Wilkowske CJ, et al. Short-term therapy for streptococcal infective endocarditis. Combined intramuscular administration of penicillin and streptomycin. JAMA. 1981;245:360.
474. Karchmer AW, Mollering RC Jr, Maki DG, et al. Single antibiotic therapy for streptococcal endocarditis. JAMA. 1979;241:1801.
475. Malacoff RF, Frank E, Andriole VT. Streptococcal endocarditis (nonenterococcal, non–group A). Single vs. combination therapy. JAMA. 1979;241:1807.
476. Francioli P, Ruch W, Stamboulian D, et al. Treatment of staphylococcal endocarditis with a single daily dose of ceftriaxone and netilmicin for 14 days. Clin Infect Dis. 1998. In press.
477. Sexton DJ, Tenenbaum MJ, Wilson WR, et al. Ceftriaxone once daily for 4 weeks compared to ceftriaxone plus gentamicin once daily for 2 weeks for treatment of penicillin-susceptible streptococcal endocarditis. Clin Infect Dis. 1998;27:1470–1474.
478. Parillo JE, Borst GC, Mazur MH, et al. Endocarditis due to resistant viridans streptococci during oral penicillin chemoprophylaxis. N Engl J Med. 1979;300:296.
479. Nicolau DP, Freeman CD, Belliveau PP, et al. Experience with once-daily aminoglycoside program administered to 2,184 adult patients. Antimicrob Agents Chemother. 1995;39;650–655.
480. Bouvet A, Cremieux AC, Contrepois A, et al. Comparison of penicillin and vancomycin, individually and in combination with gentamicin and amikacin, in the treatment of experimental endocarditis induced by nutritionally variant streptococci. Antimicrob Agents Chemother. 1985;28:607–611.
481. Henry NK, Wilson WR, Roberts RB, et al. Antimicrobial therapy of experimental endocarditis caused by nutritionally variant viridans group streptococci. Antimicrob Agents Chemother. 1986;30:465–467.
482. Stein DS, Nelson KE. Endocarditis due to nutritionally deficient streptococci: Therapeutic dilemma. Rev Infect Dis. 1987;9:908–916.
483. Cremieux A-C, Saleh-Mghir A, Vallois J-M, et al. Efficacy of temafloxacin in experimental *Streptococcus adjacens* endocarditis and autoradiographic diffusion pattern of [^{14}C] temafloxacin in cardiac vegetations. Antimicrob Agents Chemother. 1992;36:2216.
484. Stramboulian D, Bonvehi P, Arevalo C, et al. Antibiotic management of outpatients with endocarditis due to penicillin-susceptible streptococci. Rev Infect Dis. 1991;13(Suppl 2):S160.
485. Francioli P, Etienne J, Hoigué R, et al. Treatment of streptococcal endocarditis with a single daily dose of ceftriaxone sodium for 4 weeks. Efficacy and outpatient treatment feasibility. JAMA. 1992;267:264.
486. Francioli PB, Glauser MP. Synergistic activity of ceftriaxone combined with netilmicin administered once daily for treatment of experimental streptococcal endocarditis. Antimicrob Agents Chemother. 1993;37:207.
487. Yenditti M, Gelfusa V, Serra P, et al. 4-week treatment of streptococcal native valve endocarditis with high-dose teicoplanin. Antimicrob Agents Chemother. 1992;36:723.
488. Watanakunakorn C. Penicillin combined with gentamicin or streptomycin: Synergism against enterococci. J Infect Dis. 1971;124:581.
489. Moellering RC Jr, Korzeniowski OM, Sande MA, et al. Species-specific resistance to antimicrobial synergism in *Streptococcus faecium* and *Streptococcus faecalis*. J Infect Dis. 1979;140:203.
490. Krogstad DJ, Parquette AR. Defective killing of enterococci: A common property

of antimicrobial agents acting on the cell wall. Antimicrob Agents Chemother. 1980;17:965.
491. Storch GA, Krogstad DA, Parquette AR. Antibiotic-induced lysis of enterococci. J Clin Invest. 1981;68:639.
492. Megran DW. Enterococcal endocarditis. Clin Infect Dis. 1992;15:63.
493. Murray BE, Church DA, Wanger A, et al. Comparison of two β-lactamase–producing strains of *Streptococcus faecalis*. Antimicrob Agents Chemother. 1986;30:861–864.
494. Ingerman M, Pitsakis PG, Rosenberg A, et al. β-Lactamase production in experimental endocarditis due to aminoglycoside-resistant *Streptococcus faecalis*. J Infect Dis. 1987;155:1226–1232.
495. Coudron PE, Markowitz SM, Wong ES. Isolation of a β-lactamase-producing, highly-gentamicin-resistant isolate of *Enterococcus faecalis*. Antimicrob Agents Chemother. 1992;36:1225.
496. Lavoie SR, Wong ES, Coudron PE, et al. Comparison of ampicillin-sulbactam with vancomycin for treatment of experimental endocarditis due to a β-lactamase-producing, highly-gentamicin-resistant isolate of *Enterococcus faecalis*. Antimicrob Agents Chemother. 1993;37:1447.
497. Thal LA, Vazquez J, Perri MB, et al. Activity of ampicillin plus sulbactam against β-lactamase-producing enterococci in experimental endocarditis. J Antimicrob Chemother. 1993;31:182.
498. Yao JDC, Thauvin-Eliopoulos C, Eliopoulos GM, et al. Efficacy of teicoplanin in two dosage regimens for experimental endocarditis caused by a β-lactamase-producing strain of *Enterococcus faecalis* with high level resistance to gentamicin. Antimicrob Agents Chemother. 1990;34:827.
499. Ramos MC, Grayson ML, Eliopoulos GM, et al. Comparison of daptomycin, vancomycin, and ampicillin-gentamicin for treatment of experimental endocarditis caused by penicillin-resistant enterococci. Antimicrob Agents Chemother. 1992;36:1864.
500. Fontana R, Grossato A, Ligozzi M, et al. In vitro response to bactericidal activity of cell wall–active antibiotics does not support the general opinion that enterococci are naturally tolerant to these antibiotics. Antimicrob Agents Chemother. 1990;34:1518.
501. Henry NK, Wilson WR, Geraci JE. Treatment of streptomycin-susceptible enterococcal experimental endocarditis with combinations of penicillin and low- or high-dose streptomycin. Antimicrob Agents Chemother. 1986;30:725–728.
502. Harwick HJ, Kalmanson GM, Guze LB. In vitro activity of ampicillin or vancomycin combined with gentamicin or streptomycin against enterococci. Antimicrob Agents Chemother. 1973;4:383.
503. Weinstein AJ, Moellering RC. Penicillin and gentamicin therapy for enterococcal infections. JAMA. 1973;223:1030.
504. Moellering RC, Wennersten C, Weinberg AW. Synergy of penicillin and gentamicin against enterococci. J Infect Dis. 1971;124(Suppl):S207.
505. Hook EW III, Roberts RB, Sande MA. Antimicrobial therapy of experimental enterococcal endocarditis. Antimicrob Agents Chemother. 1975;8:564.
506. Wright AJ, Wilson WR, Matsumoto JY, et al. Influence of gentamicin dose size on the efficacies of combinations of gentamicin and penicillin in experimental streptomycin-resistant enterococcal endocarditis. Antimicrob Agents Chemother. 1982;22:972.
507. Murray BE, Tsao J, Panida J. Enterococci from Bangkok, Thailand, with high-level resistance to currently available aminoglycosides. Antimicrob Agents Chemother. 1983;23:799.
508. Mederski-Samoraj BD, Murray BE. High-level resistance to gentamicin in clinical isolates of enterococci. J Infect Dis. 1983;147:751.
509. Zervos MJ, Dembinski S, Mikesell T, et al. High-level resistance to gentamicin in *Streptococcus faecalis:* Risk factors and evidence for exogenous acquisition of infection. J Infect Dis. 1986;153:1075–1083.
510. Patterson JE, Zervos MJ. High-level gentamicin resistance in *Enterococcus:* Microbiology, genetic basis, and epidemiology. Rev Infect Dis. 1990;12:644.
511. Zervos MJ, Terpenning MS, Schaberg DR, et al. High-level aminoglycoside-resistant enterococci. Arch Intern Med. 1987;147:1591–1594.
512. Eliopoulos GM, Wennersten C, Zighelboim-Daum S, et al. High-level resistance to gentamicin in clinical isolates of *Streptococcus (Enterococcus) faecium*. Antimicrob Agents Chemother. 1988;32:1528–1532.
513. Eliopoulos GM, Thauvin-Eliopoulos C, Moellering RC Jr. Contribution of animal models in the search for effective therapy for endocarditis due to enterococci with high-level resistance to gentamicin. Clin Infect Dis. 1992;15:58.
514. Fernandez-Guerrero ML, Barros C, Rodriquez Tudela JL, et al. Aortic endocarditis caused by gentamicin-resistant *Enterococcus faecalis*. Eur J Clin Microbiol. 1988;7:525–527.
515. Hellinger WC, Rouse MS, Robadan PM, et al. Continuous intravenous versus intermittent ampicillin therapy of experimental endocarditis caused by aminoglycoside-resistant enterococci. Antimicrob Agents Chemother. 1992;36:1272.
516. Fantin B, Carbon C. Importance of the aminoglycoside dosing regimen in the penicillin-netilmicin combination for treatment of *Enterococcus faecalis*–induced experimental endocarditis. Antimicrob Agents Chemother. 1990;34:2387.
517. Grayson ML, Thauvin-Eliopoulos C, Eliopoulos GM, et al. Failure of trimethoprim-sulfamethoxazole therapy in experimental enterococcal endocarditis. Antimicrob Agents Chemother. 1990;34:1792.
518. Watanakunakorn C, Bakie C. Synergism of vancomycin-gentamicin and vancomycin-streptomycin against enterococci. Antimicrob Agents Chemother. 1973;4:120.
519. Watanakunakorn C, Tisone JC. Effects of a vancomycin-rifampin combination on enterococci. Antimicrob Agents Chemother. 1982;22:915.
520. Uttley AH, Collins CH, Naidoo J, et al. Vancomycin-resistant enterococci. Lancet. 1988;1:57–58.
521. Frieden TR, Munsiff SS, Low DE, et al. Emergence of vancomycin-resistant enterococci in New York City. Lancet. 1993;342:76.
522. Courvalin P. Resistance of enterococci to glycopeptides. Antimicrob Agents Chemother. 1990;34:2291.
523. Murray BE. The life and times of the Enterococcus. Clin Microbiol Rev. 1990;3:46.
524. Venditti M, Biavasco F, Varaldo PE, et al. Catheter-related endocarditis due to glycopeptide-resistant *Enterococcus faecalis* in a transplanted heart. Clin Infect Dis. 1993;17:524.
525. Leclercq R, Derlot E, Dural J, et al. Plasmid-mediated resistance to vancomycin and teicoplanin in *Enterococcus faecium*. N Engl J Med. 1988;319:157–161.
526. Fantin B, Leclercq R, Arthur M, et al. Influence of low-level resistance to vancomycin on efficacy of teicoplanin and vancomycin for treatment of experimental endocarditis due to *Enterococcus faecium*. Antimicrob Agents Chemother. 1991;35:1570.
527. Caron F, Kitzis M-D, Gutmann L, et al. Daptomycin or teicoplanin in combination with gentamicin for treatment of experimental endocarditis due to a highly glycopeptide-resistant isolate of *Enterococcus faecium*. Antimicrob Agents Chemother. 1992;36:261.
528. Collins LA, Eliopoulos GM, Wennersten CB, et al. In vitro activity of ramoplanin against vancomycin-resistant gram-positive organisms. Antimicrob Agents Chemother. 1993;37:1364.
529. Caron F, Carbon C, Gutmann L. Triple-combination penicillin-vancomycin-gentamicin for experimental endocarditis caused by a moderately penicillin- and highly glycopeptide-resistant isolate of *Enterococcus faecium*. J Infect Dis. 1991;164:888.
530. Caron F, Lemeland J-F, Humbert G, et al. Triple combination penicillin-vancomycin-gentamicin for experimental endocarditis caused by a highly penicillin- and glycopeptide-resistant isolate of *Enterococcus faecium*. J Infect Dis. 1993;168:681.
531. Fernandez-Guerrero M, Rouse MS, Henry NK, et al. In vitro and in vivo activity of ciprofloxacin against enterococci isolated from patients with infective endocarditis. Antimicrob Agents Chemother. 1987;31:430–433.
532. Bayer AS, Li C, Kim E, Ing M. Efficacy of trovafloxacin (CP99219) in the therapy of experimental endocarditis due to drug-resistant enterococci. Abstract B257. Presented at the Thirty-sixth Interscience Conference on Antimicrobial Agents and Chemotherapy, New Orleans, La., September 1996.
533. Rubinstein E, Bompart F. Activity of quinupristin/dalfopristin against gram-positive bacteria: Clinical applications and therapeutic potential. J Antimicrob Ther. 1997;39(Suppl):S139–S143.
534. Moellering RC Jr. Early clinical results of RP59500 in bacteremia. Presented at the Third International Conference on the Macrolides, Azalides and Streptogramins, Lisbon, Portugal, 1996.
535. Fantin B, Carbon C. Importance of aminoglycoside dosing regimen in the penicillin-netilmicin combination for treatment of *Enterococcus faecalis*–induced experimental endocarditis. Antimicrob Agents Chemother. 1990;34:2387–2391.
536. Marangos MN, Nicolau DP, Nightingale CH, Quintiliani R. Influence of gentamicin dosing interval on the efficacy of penicillin-containing regimens in experimental *Enterococcus faecalis* endocarditis. Presented at the Thirty-sixth Interscience Conference on Antimicrobial Agents and Chemotherapy, New Orleans, La., September 15–18, 1996.
537. Wilson WR, Wilkowski CJ, Wright AJ, et al. Treatment of streptomycin-susceptible and streptomycin-resistant enterococcal endocarditis. Ann Intern Med. 1984;100:816–823.
538. Karchmer AW. Staphylococcal endocarditis. Laboratory and clinical basis for antibiotic therapy. Am J Med. 1985;78(Suppl B):S116–S127.
539. Sande MA, Courtney KB. Nafcillin-gentamicin synergism in experimental staphylococcal endocarditis. J Lab Clin Med. 1976;88:118.
540. Abrams B, Sklaver A, Hoffman T, et al. Single or combination therapy of staphylococcal endocarditis in intravenous drug abusers. Ann Intern Med. 1979;90:789.
541. Chambers HF, Miller RT, Newman MD. Right-sided *Staphylococcus aureus* endocarditis in intravenous drug abusers: Two week combination therapy. Ann Intern Med. 1988;109:619–624.
542. DiNubile MJ. Abbreviated therapy for right sided *Staphylococcus aureus* endocarditis in injecting drug users: The time has come? Eur J Clin Microbiol Infect Dis. 1994;13:533–534.
543. DiNubile MJ. Short-course antibiotic therapy for right sided *Staphylococcus aureus* endocarditis in injection drug users. Ann Intern Med. 1994;121:873–876.
544. Torres-Tortosa M, de Cueto M, Vergara A, et al. Prospective evaluation of a two-week course of intravenous antibiotics in intravenous drug addicts with infective endocarditis. Eur J Clin Microbiol Infect Dis. 1994;13:559–564.
545. Espinosa FJ, Valdes M, Martin-Luengo M, et al. Right sided endocarditis caused by *Staphylococcus aureus* in parenteral drug addicts: Evaluation of a combined therapeutic scheme for 2 weeks versus conventional treatment. Enferm Infecc Microbiol Clin. 1993;11:235–240.
546. Ribera E, Gomez-Jimenez J, Cortes E, et al. Effectiveness of cloxacillin with and without gentamicin in short-term therapy for right-sided *Staphylococcus aureus* endocarditis: A randomized, controlled trial. Ann Intern Med. 125:969–974.
547. Dworkin RJ, Lee BL, Sande MA, Chambers HF. Treatment of right-sided *Staphylococcus aureus* endocarditis in intravenous drug users with ciprofloxacin and rifampicin. Lancet. 1989;ii:1071–1073.
548. Heldman AW, Hartert TV, Ray SC, et al. Oral antibiotic treatment of right-sided staphylococcal endocarditis in injection drug users: Prospective randomized comparison with parenteral therapy. Am J Med. 1996;101:68–76.
549. Murray HW, Wigley FM, Mann JJ, et al. Combination antibiotic therapy in staphylococcal endocarditis: The use of methicillin sodium–gentamicin sulfate therapy. Arch Intern Med. 1976;136:480.
550. Korzeniowski OM, Sande MA, The National Collaborative Endocarditis Study

Group. Combination antimicrobial therapy for *Staphylococcus aureus* endocarditis in patients addicted to parenteral drugs and in nonaddicts. A prospective study. Ann Intern Med. 1982;97:496.
551. Steckelberg JM, Rouse MS, Tallan BM, et al. Relative efficacies of broad-spectrum cephalosporins for treatment of methicillin-susceptible *Staphylococcus aureus* experimental infective endocarditis. Antimicrob Agents Chemother. 1993;37:554.
552. Small PM, Chambers HF. Vancomycin for *Staphylococcus aureus* endocarditis in intravenous drug users. Antimicrob Agents Chemother. 1990;34:1227.
553. Levine DP, Fromm BS, Reddy BR. Slow response to vancomycin or vancomycin plus rifampin in methicillin-resistant *Staphylococcus aureus* endocarditis. Ann Intern Med. 1991;115:674.
554. Rybak MJ, Bailey EM, Lamp KC, et al. Pharmacokinetics and bactericidal rates of daptomycin and vancomycin in intravenous drug abusers being treated for gram-positive endocarditis and bacteremia. Antimicrob Agents Chemother. 1992;36:1109.
555. Kaatz GW, Seo SM, Reddy VN, et al. Daptomycin compared with teicoplanin and vancomycin for therapy of experimental *Staphylococcus aureus* endocarditis. Antimicrob Agents Chemother. 1990;34:2081.
556. Kaatz GW, Seo SM, Dorman NJ, et al. Emergence of teicoplanin resistance during therapy of *Staphylococcus aureus* endocarditis. J Infect Dis. 1990;162:103.
557. Mortara LA, Bayer AS. *Staphylococcus* bacteremia and endocarditis—New diagnostic and therapeutic concepts. Infect Dis Clin North Am. 1993;7:53.
558. Bayer AS. Infective endocarditis. Clin Infect Dis. 1993;17:313.
559. Watanakunakorn C. Clindamycin therapy of *Staphylococcus aureus* endocarditis. Clinical relapse and development of resistance to clindamycin, lincomycin, and erythromycin. Am J Med. 1976;60:419.
560. Kaye D. The clinical significance of tolerance of *Staphylococcus aureus*. Ann Intern Med. 1980;93:924.
561. Jackson MA, Hicks RA. Vancomycin failure in staphylococcal endocarditis. Pediatr Infect Dis J. 1987;6:750–752.
562. Rajashekaraiah KR, Rice T, Rao VS, et al. Clinical significance of tolerant strains of *Staphylococcus aureus* in patients with endocarditis. Ann Intern Med. 1980;93:796.
563. Voorn GP, Thompson J, Goessens WHF, et al. Role of tolerance in cloxacillin treatment of experimental *Staphylococcus aureus* endocarditis. J Infect Dis. 1991;163:640.
564. Zak O, Scheld WM, Sande MA. Rifampin in experimental endocarditis due to *Staphylococcus aureus* in rabbits. Rev Infect Dis. 1983;5(Suppl):481.
565. Tebas P, Martinez Ruiz R, Roman F, et al. Early resistance to rifampin and ciprofloxacin in the treatment of right-sided *Staphylococcus aureus* endocarditis. J Infect Dis. 1991;163:204.
566. McDougal LK, Thornsberry C. The role of β-lactamase in staphylococcal resistance to penicillinase-resistant penicillins and cephalosporins. J Clin Microbiol. 1986;23:832–839.
567. Hirano L, Bayer AS. β-Lactam–β-lactamase inhibitor combinations are active in experimental endocarditis caused by β-lactamase-producing oxacillin-resistant staphylococci. Antimicrob Agents Chemother. 1991;35:685.
568. Pefanis A, Thauvin-Eliopoulos C, Eliopoulos GM, et al. Activity of ampicillin-sulbactam and oxacillin in experimental endocarditis caused by β-lactamase–hyperproducing *Staphylococcus aureus*. Antimicrob Agents Chemother. 1993;37:507.
569. Fernandez-Guerrero M, Rouse M, Henry N, et al. Ciprofloxacin therapy of experimental endocarditis caused by methicillin-susceptible or methicillin-resistant *Staphylococcus aureus*. Antimicrob Agents Chemother. 1988;32:747–751.
570. Kaatz GW, Seo SM, Lamp KC, et al. CI-960, a new fluoroquinolone, for therapy of experimental ciprofloxacin-susceptible and -resistant *Staphylococcus aureus* endocarditis. Antimicrob Agents Chemother. 1992;36:1192.
571. Bayer AS, Li C, Ing M. Efficacy of trovafloxacin, a new quinolone antibiotic, in experimental staphylococcal endocarditis due to oxacillin-resistant strains. Antimicrob Agents Cheomother. 1998;42:1837–1841.
572. Kaatz GW, Seo SM, Barriere SL, et al. Development of resistance to fleroxacin during therapy of experimental methicillin-susceptible *Staphylococcus aureus* endocarditis. Antimicrob Agents Chemother. 1991;35:1547.
573. Munoz P, Berenguer J, Rodriguez-Creixems M, et al. Ciprofloxacin and infective endocarditis. Infect Dis Clin Pract. 1993;2:119.
574. Markowitz N, Quinn EL, Saravolatz LD. Trimethoprim-sulfamethoxazole compared with vancomycin for treatment of *Staphylococcus aureus* infection. Ann Intern Med. 1992;117:390–398.
575. Iannini PB, Crossley K. Therapy of *Staphylococcus aureus* bacteremia associated with a removable focus of infection. Ann Intern Med. 1976;84:558.
576. Watanakunakorn C, Baird IM. *Staphylococcus aureus* bacteremia and endocarditis associated with a removable infected intravenous device. Am J Med. 1977;63:253.
577. Bayer AS, Lam K, Ginzton L. *Staphylococcus aureus* bacteremia. Clinical, serologic, and echocardiographic findings in patients with and without endocarditis. Arch Intern Med. 1987;147:757–762.
578. Karchmer AW, Archer GL, Dismukes WE. *Staphylococcus epidermidis* causing prosthetic valve endocarditis: Microbiologic and clinical observations as guides to therapy. Ann Intern Med. 1983;98:447.
579. Schwalbe RS, Stapleton JT, Gilligan PH. Emergence of vancomycin resistance in coagulase-negative staphylococci. N Engl J Med. 1987;316:927–931.
580. Joly V, Parigon B, Vallois J-M, et al. Value of antibiotic levels in serum and cardiac vegetations for predicting antibacterial effect of ceftriaxone in experimental *Escherichia coli* endocarditis. Antimicrob Agents Chemother. 1987;31:1632–1639.
581. Caron F, Gutmann L, Bure A, et al. Ceftriaxone-sulbactam combination in rabbit endocarditis caused by a strain of *Klebsiella pneumoniae* producing extended-broad-spectrum TEM-3 β-lactamase. Antimicrob Agents Chemother. 1990;34:2070.
582. Mentec H, Vallois J-M, Bure A, et al. Piperacillin, tazobactam, and gentamicin alone or combined in an endocarditis model of infection by a TEM-3–producing strain of *Klebsiella pneumoniae* or its susceptible variant. Antimicrob Agents Chemother. 1992;36:1883.
583. Potel G, Caillon J, Fantin B, et al. Impact of dosage schedule on the efficacy of gentamicin, tobramycin, or amikacin in an experimental model of *Serratia marcescens* endocarditis: In vitro–in vivo correlation. Antimicrob Agents Chemother. 1991;35:111.
584. Potel G, Caillon J, LeGallou F, et al. Identification of factors affecting in vivo aminoglycoside activity in an experimental model of gram-negative endocarditis. Antimicrob Agents Chemother. 1992;36:774.
585. Rodriguez C, Olcoz MT, Izquierdo G, et al. Endocarditis due to ampicillin-resistant nontyphoid *Salmonella:* Cure with a third-generation cephalosporin. Rev Infect Dis. 1990;12:817.
586. Hughes CF, Noble N. Vegetectomy: An alternative surgical treatment for infective endocarditis of the atrioventricular valves in drug addicts. J Thorac Cardiovasc Surg. 1988;95:857–861.
587. Arbulu A, Thomas NW, Chiscano A, et al. Total tricuspid valvulectomy without replacement in the treatment of *Pseudomonas* endocarditis. Surg Forum. 1971;22:162.
588. Mammana RB, Levitsky S, Sernaque D, et al. Valve replacement for left-sided endocarditis in drug addicts. Ann Thorac Surg. 1983;35:436.
589. Bayer AS, Crowell DJ, Yih J, et al. Comparative pharmacokinetics and pharmacodynamics of amikacin and ceftazidine in tricuspid and aortic vegetations in experimental *Pseudomonas* endocarditis. J Infect Dis. 1988;158:355–359.
590. Bayer AS, Hirano L, Yih J. Development of β-lactam resistance and increased quinolone MIC's during therapy of experimental *Pseudomonas aeruginosa* endocarditis. Antimicrob Agents Chemother. 1988;32:231–235.
591. Parr TR Jr, Bayer AS. Mechanisms of aminoglycoside resistance in variants of *Pseudomonas aeruginosa* isolated during treatment of experimental endocarditis in rabbits. J Infect Dis. 1988;158:1003–1010.
592. Hessen MT, Pitsakis PG, Levison ME. Absence of a post-antibiotic effect in experimental *Pseudomonas* endocarditis treated with imipenem, with or without gentamicin. J Infect Dis. 1988;158:542–548.
593. Bayer AS, Park S, Ramos MC, et al. Effects of alginase on the natural history and antibiotic therapy of experimental endocarditis caused by mucoid *Pseudomonas aeruginosa*. Infect Immun. 1992;60:3979.
594. Jimenez-Lucho VE, Saravolatz LD, Medeiros AA, et al. Failure of therapy in *Pseudomonas* endocarditis: Selection of resistant mutants. J Infect Dis. 1986;154:64–68.
595. Daikos GL, Kathopalia SB, Lolans VT, et al. Long-term oral ciprofloxacin: Experience in the treatment of incurable infective endocarditis. Am J Med. 1988;84:786–790.
596. Pefanis A, Giamarellou H, Karayiannakos P, et al. Efficacy of ceftazidime and aztreonam alone or in combination with amikacin in experimental left-sided *Pseudomonas aeruginosa* endocarditis. Antimicrob Agents Chemother. 1993;37:308.
597. Fichtenbaum CH, Smith MJ. Treatment of endocarditis due to *Pseudomonas aeruginosa* with imipenem. Clin Infect Dis. 1992;14:353.
598. Francioli PB. Ceftriaxone and outpatient treatment of infective endocarditis. Infect Dis Clin North Am. 1993;17:313–322.
599. Pavicic MJAMP, van Winkelhoff AJ, de Graaff J. In vitro susceptibilities of *Actinobacillus actinomycetemcomitans* to a number of antimicrobial combinations. Antimicrob Agents Chemother. 1992;36:2634.
600. Weisner PJ, Handsfield HH, Holmes KK. Low antibiotic resistance of gonococci causing disseminated infection. N Engl J Med. 1973;288:1221.
601. Black JR, Brint JM, Reichart CA. Successful treatment of gonococcal endocarditis with ceftriaxone. J Infect Dis. 1988;157:1281–1282.
602. Melgar GR, Nasser RM, Gordon RM, et al. Fungal prosthetic valve endocarditis. An 11-year experience in a tertiary hospital. Medicine (Baltimore). 1997;76:94–103.
603. Ernst JD, Rusmak M, Sande MA. Combination antifungal chemotherapy for experimental disseminated candidiasis: Lack of correlation between in vitro and in vivo observations with amphotericin B and rifampin. Rev Infect Dis. 1983;5(Suppl):626.
604. Longman LP, Martin MV. A comparison of the efficacy of itraconazole, amphotericin B and 5-fluorocytosine in the treatment of *Aspergillus fumigatus* endocarditis in the rabbit. J Antimicrob Chemother. 1987;20:719–724.
605. Witt MD, Bayer AS. Comparison of fluconazole and amphotericin B for prevention and treatment of experimental *Candida* endocarditis. Antimicrob Agents Chemother. 1991;35:2481.
606. Venditti M, De Bernardis F, Micozzi A, et al. Fluconazole treatment of catheter-related right-sided endocarditis caused by *Candida albicans* and associated with endophthalmitis and folliculitis. Clin Infect Dis. 1992;14:422.
607. Czwerwiec FS, Bilsker MS, Kamerman ML, et al. Long-term survival after fluconazole therapy of candidal prosthetic valve endocarditis. Am J Med. 1993;94:545.
608. Nguyen MH, Nguyen ML, Yu VL, et al. *Candida* prosthetic valve endocarditis: Prospective study of six cases and review of the literature. Clin Infect Dis. 1996;22:262–267.
609. Haldane EV, Marrie TJ, Faulkner RS, et al. Endocarditis due to Q fever in Nova Scotia: Experience with five patients in 1981–1982. J Infect Dis. 1983;148:978–985.
610. Street AC, Durack DT. Experience with trimethoprim-sulfamethoxazole in treatment of infective endocarditis. Rev Infect Dis. 1988;10:915–922.
611. Levy PY, Drancourt M, Etienne J, et al. Comparison of different antibiotic regimens

for therapy of 32 cases of Q fever endocarditis. Antimicrob Agents Chemother. 1991;35:533.
612. Jones JB, Ridgeway GL, Boulding S, et al. In vitro activity of rifamycins alone and in combination with other antibiotics against *Chlamydia trachomatis*. Rev Infect Dis. 1983;5(Suppl):556.
613. McAnulty JH, Rahimtoola SH. Surgery for infective endocarditis. JAMA. 1979;242:77.
614. Dinubile MJ. Surgery in active endocarditis. Ann Intern Med. 1980;96:650.
615. D'Agostino RS, Miller DC, Stinson EB, et al. Valve replacement in patients with native valve endocarditis: What really determines operative outcome? Ann Thorac Surg. 1985;40:429–438.
616. Tolan RW Jr, Kleiman MB, Frank M, et al. Operative intervention in active endocarditis in children: Report of a series of cases and review. Clin Infect Dis. 1992;14:852.
617. Mansur AJ, Grinberg M, Lemosdaluz P, et al. The complications of infective endocarditis. Arch Intern Med. 1992;152:2428.
618. Griffin FM, Jones G, Cobb CG. Aortic insufficiency in bacterial endocarditis. Ann Intern Med. 1972;76:23–28.
619. Karalis DG, Blumberg AE, Vilaro JF, et al. Prognostic significance of valvular regurgitation in patients with infective endocarditis. Am J Med. 1991;90:193.
620. Wilson WR, Danielson GK, Giuliani ER, et al. Valve replacement in patients with active infective endocarditis. Circulation. 1978;58:585.
621. Arbulu A, Asfaw I. Tricuspid valvulectomy without prosthetic replacement. Ten years of clinical experience. J Thorac Cardiovasc Surg. 1981;82:684.
622. Straumann E, Stulz P, Jenzer HR. Tricuspid valve endocarditis in the drug addict: A reconstructive approach ("vegetectomy"). Thorac Cardiovasc Surg. 1990;38:291.
623. DiNubile M. Surgery for addiction-related tricuspid valve endocarditis: Caveat emptor. Am J Med. 1987;82:811–813.
624. Arbulu A, Asfaw I. Management of infective endocarditis: Seventeen years' experience. Ann Thorac Surg. 1987;43:144–149.
625. Alsip SG, Blackstone EH, Kirklin JW, et al. Indications for cardiac surgery in patients with active infective endocarditis. Am J Med. 1985;78(Suppl 6B): S38–S48.
626. Blumberg EA, Karalis DA, Chandrase Karan K, et al. Endocarditis-associated paravalvular abscesses—do clinical parameters predict the presence of abscess? Chest. 1995;107:898–903.
627. De Castro S, Magni G, Beni S, et al. Role of transthoracic echocardiography in predicting embolic events in patients with active endocarditis involving native cardiac valves. Am J Cardiol. 1997;57:329–343.
628. Moon MR, Stinson EB, Miller DC. Surgical treatment of endocarditis. Prog Cardiovasc Dis. 1997;40:239–264.
629. Tornos M-P, Permanyer-Miralda G, Olona M, et al. Long-term complications of native valve infective endocarditis in non-addicts. A 15-year follow-up study. Ann Intern Med. 1992;117:567.
630. Neuhof H, Seley GP. Acute suppurative phlebitis complicated by septicemia. Surgery. 1947;21:831.
631. Goldman DA, Maki DG, Rhame FS, et al. Guidelines for infection control in intravenous therapy. Ann Intern Med. 1973;79:848.
632. Rupp ME. Infections of intravascular catheters and vascular devices. In: Crossley KB, Archer GL, eds. The Staphylococci in Human Disease. New York: Churchill Livingstone; 1997;379–399.
633. O'Neill JA, Pruitt BA, Foley FD, et al. Suppurative thrombophlebitis—a lethal complication of intravenous therapy. J Trauma. 1968;8:256.
634. Stein JM, Pruitt BA. Suppurative thrombophlebitis: A lethal iatrogenic disease. N Engl J Med. 1970;282:1452.
635. Pruitt BA, Stein JM, Foley FD, et al. Intravenous therapy in burn patients. Suppurative thrombophlebitis and other life-threatening complications. Arch Surg. 1970;100:399.
636. Pruitt BA, McManus WF, Kim SH, et al. Diagnosis and treatment of cannula-related intravenous sepsis in burn patients. Ann Surg. 1980;191:546.
637. Garrison RN, Richardson JD, Fry DE. Catheter-associated septic thrombophlebitis. South Med J. 1982;75:917.
638. Sacks-Berg A, Strampfer MJ, Cunha BA. Suppurative thrombophlebitis caused by intravenous line sepsis. Heart Lung. 1987;16:318–320.
639. Munster AM. Septic thrombophlebitis. A surgical disorder. JAMA. 1974;230:1010.
640. Berkowitz FE, Argent AC, Baise T. Suppurative thrombophlebitis: A serious nosocomial infection. Pediatr Infect Dis J. 1987;6:64–67.
641. Johnson RA, Zajac RA, Evans ME. Suppurative thrombophlebitis: Correlation between pathogen and underlying disease. Infect Control. 1986;7:582–585.
642. Rhame FS, Maki DG, Bennett JV. Intravenous cannula–associated infections. In: Bennett JV, Brachman PS, eds. Hospital Infections. Boston: Little, Brown; 1979:433–442.
643. Baker CC, Peterson SR, Sheldon GF. Septic phlebitis: A neglected disease. Am J Surg. 1979;138:97.
644. Sears N, Grosfeld JL, Weber TR, et al. Suppurative thrombophlebitis in childhood. Pediatrics. 1981;68:630.
645. Zinner MJ, Zuidema GD, Lowery BD. Septic nonsuppurative thrombophlebitis. Arch Surg. 1976;111:122.
646. Maki DG. Infections due to infusion therapy. In: Bennet JV, Brachman PS, eds. Hospital Infections. Boston: Little, Brown; 1992:849.
647. Brismar B, Hardstedt C, Jacobson S. Diagnosis of thrombosis by catheter phlebography after prolonged central venous catheterization. Ann Surg. 1981;194:779–783.
648. Slagle DC, Gates RH Jr. Unusual case of central vein thrombosis and sepsis. Am J Med. 1986;81:351–354.
649. Kaufman J, Demas C, Stark K, et al. Catheter-related septic central venous thrombosis—current therapeutic options. West J Med. 1986;145:200–203.
650. Veghese A, Widrich WC, Arbeit RD. Central venous septic thrombophlebitis—the role of medical therapy. Medicine (Baltimore). 1985;64:394–400.
651. Strinden WD, Helgerson RB, Maki DG. *Candida* septic thrombosis of the great central veins associated with central catheters. Clinical features and management. Ann Surg. 1985;202:653–658.
652. Raad I, Narro J, Khan A, et al. Serious complications of vascular catheter–related *Staphylococcus aureus* bacteremia in cancer patients. Eur J Clin Microbiol Infect Dis. 1992;11:675.
653. Haddad W, Idowu J, Georgeson K, et al. Septic atrial thrombosis: A potentially lethal complication of Broviac catheters in infants. Am J Dis Child. 1986;140:778–780.
654. Collins CG, MacCallum EA, Nelson EW, et al. Suppurative pelvic thrombophlebitis. I. Incidence, pathology, and etiology. Surgery. 1951;30:298.
655. Josey WE, Staggers SR. Heparin therapy in septic pelvic thrombophlebitis: A study of 46 cases. Am J Obstet Gynecol. 1974;120:228.
656. Collins CG. Suppurative pelvic thrombophlebitis. A study of 202 cases in which the disease was treated by ligation of the vena cava and ovarian vein. Am J Obstet Gynecol. 1970;108:681.
657. Lim GM, Jeffrey RB Jr, Ralls PW, et al. Septic thrombosis of the portal vein: CT and clinical observations. J Comput Assist Tomogr. 1989;13:656.
658. Barenholtz L, Kaminsky NI, Palmer DL. Venous intramural microabscesses: A cause of protracted sepsis with intravenous cannulas. Am J Med Sci. 1973;265:335.
659. Syndman DR, Murray SA, Kornfeld SJ, et al. Total parenteral nutrition–related infections: Prospective epidemiologic study using semiquantitative methods. Am J Med. 1982;73:695.
660. Jupiter JB, Ehrlich MG, Novelline RA, et al. The association of septic thrombophlebitis with subperiosteal abscesses in children. J Pediatr. 1982;101:690.
661. Maki DG, Weise CE, Sarafin HW. A semiquantitative culture method for identifying intravenous-catheter-related infection. N Engl J Med. 1977;296:1305.
662. Ashkenazi S, Pickering LK, Robinson LH. Diagnosis and management of septic thrombosis of the inferior vena cava caused by *Candida tropicalis*. Pediatr Infect Dis J. 1990;9:446.
663. Mori H, Fukuda T, Isomoto I, et al. CT diagnosis of catheter-induced septic thrombosis of vena cava. J Comput Assist Tomogr. 1990;14:236.
664. Angel JL, Knuppel RA. Computed tomography in diagnosis of puerperal ovarian vein thrombosis. Obstet Gynecol. 1984;63:61–64.
665. Isada NB, Landy HJ, Larson JW Jr. Postabortal septic pelvic thrombophlebitis diagnosed with computed tomography. J Reprod Med. 1987;32:866–868.
666. Martin B, Molopulos GP, Bryan PJ. MRI of puerperal ovarian vein thrombosis. AJR. 1986;147:291–292.
667. Josey WE, Cook CC. Septic pelvic thrombophlebitis. Report of 17 patients treated with heparin. Obstet Gynecol. 1970;35:891.
668. Torres-Rojas JR, Stratton CW, Sanders CV, et al. Candidal suppurative peripheral thrombophlebitis. Ann Intern Med. 1982;96:431.
669. Walsh TJ, Bustamente CI, Valhov D, et al. Candidal suppurative peripheral thrombophlebitis: Recognition, prevention, and management. Infect Control. 1986;7:16–22.
670. Shek YH, Tucker MC, Viciana AL, et al. *Malassezia furfur*—disseminated infection in premature infants. Am J Clin Pathol. 1989;92:595.
671. Peterson P, Stahl-Bayliss CM. Cytomegalovirus thrombophlebitis after successful DHPG therapy. Ann Intern Med. 1987;106:632–633.
672. Miller CJ. Ligation and excision of pelvic veins in treatment of puerperal pyaemia. Surg Gynecol Obstet. 1917;25:431.
673. Topiel MS, Bryan RT, Kessler CM, et al. Treatment of Silastic catheter–induced central vein septic thrombophlebitis. Am J Med Sci. 1986;291:425–428.
674. Barg NL, Supena RB, Fekety R. Persistent staphylococcal bacteremia in an intravenous drug abuser. Antimicrob Agents Chemother. 1986;29:209–211.
675. Schranz D, Haugwitz D, Zimmer B, et al. Successful lysis of a septic thrombosis of the superior vena cava using recombinant tissue–plasminogen activator. Klin Padiatr. 1991;203:363.
676. Moran JM, Atwood RP, Rowe MI. A clinical and bacteriologic study of infections associated with venous cutdowns. N Engl J Med. 1965;272:554.
677. Norden CW. Application of antibiotic ointment to the site of venous catheterization—a controlled trial. J Infect Dis. 1969;120:611.
678. Centers for Disease Control and Prevention. Part 1. Intravascular device–related infection: An overview; and Part 2. Recommendations for prevention of intravascular device–related infections. Fed Register. 1995;60:49978.
679. Patel S, Johnston KW. Classification and management of mycotic aneurysms. Surg Gynecol Obstet. 1977;144:691.
680. Parkhurst GF, Decker JP. Bacterial aortitis and mycotic aneurysms of the aorta. A report of 12 cases. Am J Pathol. 1955;31:821.
681. Sommerville RL, Allen EV, Edwards JE. Bland and infected arteriosclerotic abdominal aortic aneurysms: A clinicopathologic study. Medicine (Baltimore). 1959;38:207.
682. Sekkal S, Cornu E, Cristides C, et al. Isolated iliac aneurysms. Seventy-seven cases in forty-eight patients. J Mal Vasc. 1993;18:13.
683. Stengel A, Wolfroth CC. Mycotic (bacterial) aneurysms of intravascular origin. Arch Intern Med. 1923;31:527.
684. Bennett DE, Cherry JK. Bacterial infection of aortic aneurysms. A clinicopathologic study. Am J Surg. 1967;113:321.
685. Cliff MM, Soulen RL, Firestone AJ. Mycotic aneurysms: A challenge and a clue. Arch Intern Med. 1970;126:977.

686. Jarrett F, Darling C, Mundth ED, et al. Experience with infected aneurysms of the abdominal aorta. Arch Surg. 1975;110:1281.
687. Bohmfalk GL, Story JL, Wissenger JP, et al. Bacterial intracranial aneurysm. J Neurosurg. 1978;48:369.
688. Frazee JG, Cahan LD, Winter J. Bacterial intracranial aneurysms. J Neurosurg. 1980;53:633.
689. Selky AK, Roos KL. Neurologic complications of infective endocarditis. Semin Neurol. 1992;12:225.
690. Tunkel AR, Kaye D. Neurologic complications of infective endocarditis. Neurol Clin. 1993;11:419.
691. Bullock R, Van Dellen JR, Van den Heever CM. Intracranial mycotic aneurysms. A review of 9 cases. S Afr Med J. 1981;60:970.
692. John RM, Pugsley W, Treasure T, et al. Aortic root complications of infective endocarditis—influence on surgical outcome. Eur Heart J. 1991;12:241.
693. Hollingworth J, Palmer KS, Simms MH. Ruptured mycotic aneurysm of the abdominal aorta in childhood. Eur J Vasc Surg. 1992;6:665.
694. Cribari C, Meadors FA, Crawford ES, et al. Thoraco-abdominal aortic aneurysm associated with umbilical artery catheterization: Case report and review of the literature. J Vasc Surg. 1992;16:75.
695. Jarrett F, Darling RC, Mundth ED, et al. The management of infected arterial aneurysms. J Cardiovasc Surg. 1977;18:361.
696. Johnson JR, Ledgerwood AM, Lucas CE. Mycotic aneurysm. New concepts in therapy. Arch Surg. 1983;118:577.
697. Brummitt CF, Kravitz GR, Granrud GA, et al. Femoral endarteritis due to *Staphylococcus aureus* complicating percutaneous transluminal coronary angioplasty. Am J Med. 1989;86:822.
698. Frazee BW, Flaherty JP. Septic endarteritis of the femoral artery following angioplasty. Rev Infect Dis. 1991;13:620.
699. Feigl D, Feigl A, Edwards JE. Mycotic aneurysms of the aortic root. A pathologic study of 20 cases. Chest. 1986;90:553–557.
700. Jebara VA, Dervanian P, Acar C, et al. Mycotic aneurysm of the carotid artery secondary to acute bacterial endocarditis. Arch Mal Coeur Vaiss. 1992;85:1615.
701. Akers DL Jr, Fowl RJ, Kempczinski RF, et al. Mycotic aneurysm of the tibioperoneal trunk: Case report and review of the literature. J Vasc Surg. 1992;16:71.
702. Dean RH, Mecham PW, Weaver FA, et al. Mycotic embolism and embolomycotic aneurysms. Neglected lessons of the past. Ann Surg. 1986;204:300–307.
703. Sedwitz MM, Hye RJ, Stabile BE. The changing epidemiology of pseudoaneurysm. Therapeutic implications. Arch Surg. 1988;123:473–476.
704. Morgan MB, Cintron G, Balis JV. Infective "mycotic" aortic root aneurysm following coronary artery bypass grafting. Am J Med. 1993;94:550.
705. Vyas SK, Law NW, Loehry CA. Mycotic aneurysm of the left subclavian artery. Br Heart J. 1993;69:455.
706. Hurst RW, Choi IS, Persky M, et al. Mycotic aneurysms of the intracavernous carotid artery: A case report and review of the literature. Surg Neurol. 1992;37:142.
707. Kyriakides GK, Simmons RL, Najarian JS. Mycotic aneurysms in transplant patients. Arch Surg. 1976;111:472.
708. Smith EJ, Milligan SL, Filo RS. *Salmonella* mycotic aneurysms after renal transplantation. South Med J. 1981;74:1399.
709. Olmsted WW, McGee TP. The pathogenesis of peripheral aneurysms of the central nervous system: A subject review from the AFIP. Radiology. 1977;123:661.
710. Salgado AV, Furlan AJ, Keys TF. Mycotic aneurysm, Subarachnoid hemorrhage, and indications for cerebral angiography in infective endocarditis. Stroke. 1987;18:1057–1060.
711. Wilson WR, Lie JT, Houser OW, et al. The management of patients with mycotic aneurysm. Curr Clin Top Infect Dis. 1981;2:151.
712. Barrow DL, Prats AR. Infectious intracranial aneurysms: Comparison of groups with and without endocarditis. Neurosurgery. 1990;27:562.
713. Friedman SG, Pogo GJ, Moccio CG. Mycotic aneurysm of the superior mesenteric artery. J Vasc Surg. 1987;6:87–90.
714. Sukerkar AN, Dulay CC, Anandappa E, et al. Mycotic aneurysm of the hepatic artery. Radiology. 1977;124:444.
715. Khoda J, Lantsberg L, Sebbag G. Hepatic artery mycotic aneurysm as a cause of hemobilia. J Hepatol. 1993;17:131.
716. Carrel D, Cohle SD, Chapman AJ. Fatal hemothorax from mycotic celiac artery aneurysm. Am J Med Pathol. 1992;13:233.
717. Feinsod FM, Norfleet RG, Hoehn JL. Mycotic aneurysm of the external iliac artery. A triad of clinical signs facilitating early diagnosis. JAMA. 1977;238:245.
718. Merry M, Dunn J, Weissmann R, et al. Popliteal mycotic aneurysm presenting as septic arthritis and purpura. JAMA. 1972;221:58.
719. Plate G, Forsley N, Stigsson L, et al. Management of inflammatory abdominal aortic aneurysm. Acta Chir Scand. 1988;154:19–24.
720. Pennell RC, Hollier LH, Lie JT, et al. Inflammatory abdominal aortic aneurysms: A thirty year review. J Vasc Surg. 1985;2:859–869.
721. Morrow C, Safi H, Beall AC Jr. Primary aortoduodenal fistula caused by *Salmonella* aortitis. J Vasc Surg. 1987;6:415–418.
722. Kimura I, Okumura R, Yamashita K, et al. Mycotic aneurysm. Radiat Med. 1989;7:121.
723. Vogelzang RL, Sohaey R. Infected aortic aneurysms: CT appearance. J Comput Assist Tomogr. 1988;12:109–112.
724. Blair RH, Resnik MD, Polga JP. CT appearance of mycotic abdominal aortic aneurysms. J Comput Assist Tomogr. 1989;13:101.
725. Rivera JV, Blanco G, Perez M, et al. Gallium-67 localization in a mycotic aneurysm of the thoracic aorta. Clin Nucl Med. 1985;10:814–816.
726. Zwas ST, Lorberboyin M, Schechter M. Occult aortic arch mycotic aneurysm diagnosed by radio gallium scintigraphy. Clin Nucl Med. 1992;17:797.
727. Ben-Haim S, Seabold JE, Hawes DR, et al. Leukocyte scintigraphy in the diagnosis of mycotic aneurysm. J Nucl Med. 1992;33:1486.
728. Ramo OJ, Vorne M, Lantto E, et al. Postoperative graft incorporation after aortic reconstruction—comparison between computerized tomography and Tc-99m-HMPAO labelled leukocyte imaging. Eur J Vasc Surg. 1993;7:122.
729. Brewster DC, Retana A, Waltman AC, et al. Angiography in the management of aneurysms of the abdominal aorta. N Engl J Med. 1972;292:822.
730. Griffiths BE, Petch MC, English TAH. Echocardiographic detection of subvalvular aortic root aneurysm extending to mitral valve annulus as complication of aortic valve endocarditis. Br Heart J. 1982;47:392.
731. Ozkutlu S, Ozbarlas N, Bilgi CA, et al. Mycotic aneurysm of the descending aorta diagnosed by echocardiography. Int J Cardiol. 1992;37:112.
732. Vargas-Barron J, Avila-Rosales L, Romero-Cardenas A, et al. Echocardiographic diagnosis of a mycotic aneurysm of the main pulmonary artery and patent ductus arteriosus. Am Heart J. 1992;123:1707.
733. Kanwar YS, Malhotra U, Anderson BR, et al. Salmonellosis associated with abdominal aortic aneurysm. Arch Intern Med. 1974;134:1095.
734. Cohen JI, Bartlett JA, Corey GR. Extra-intestinal manifestations of *Salmonella* infections. Medicine (Baltimore). 1987;66:349–388.
735. Cohen OS, O'Brien TF, Schoenbaum SC, et al. The risk of endothelial infection in adults with *Salmonella* bacteremia. Ann Intern Med. 1978;89:931.
736. Flamand F, Harris KA, DeRose G, et al. Arteritis due to *Salmonella* with aneurysm formation: Two cases. Can J Surg. 1992;35:248.
737. McIntyre KE Jr, Malone JM, Richards E. Mycotic aortic pseudoaneurysm with aortoenteric fistula caused by *Arizona hinshawii*. Surgery. 1982;91:173.
738. Kumar N, Prabhakar G, Kandeel M, et al. *Brucella* mycotic aneurysm of ascending aorta complicating discrete subaortic stenosis. Am Heart J. 1993;125:1780.
739. Anolik JR, Mildvan D, Winter JW, et al. Mycotic aortic aneurysm. A complication of *Campylobacter fetus* septicemia. Arch Intern Med. 1983;143:609.
740. Garto AR, Cone LA, Woodard DR, et al. Arterial infections due to *Listeria monocytogenes:* Report of four cases and review of world literature. Clin Infect Dis. 1992;14:23.
741. Hurley L, Howe K. Mycotic aortic aneurysm infected by *Clostridium septicum*—a case history. Angiology. 1991;42:585.
742. Mielke B, Weir B, Oldring D, et al. Fungal aneurysm: Case report and review of the literature. Neurosurgery. 1981;9:578.
743. Hadley MN, Martin NA, Spetzler RF, et al. Multiple intracranial aneurysms due to *Coccidioides immitis* infection. J Neurosurg. 1987;66:453–456.
744. Ogden PE, Hurley DL, Cain PT. Fatal fungal endarteritis caused by *Bipolaris spicifera* following replacement of the aortic valve. Clin Infect Dis. 1992;14:596.
745. Aguado JM, Valle R, Arjona R, et al. Aortic bypass graft infection due to *Aspergillus:* Report of a case and review. Clin Infect Dis. 1992;14:916.
746. McLean DR, Russell N, Khan MY. Neurobrucellosis: Clinical and therapeutic features. Clin Infect Dis. 1992;15:582.
747. Bingham WF: Treatment of mycotic intracranial aneurysms. J Neurosurg. 1977;46:428.
748. Leipzig MJ, Brown FD. Treatment of mycotic aneurysms. Surg Neurol. 1985;23:403–407.
749. Rodesch G, Noterman J, Thys JP, et al. Treatment of intracranial mycotic aneurysm: Surgery or not? Acta Neurochir. 1987;85:63–68.
750. Reddy DJ, Smith RF, Elliott JP Jr, et al. Infected femoral artery false aneurysms in drug addicts: Evolution of selective vascular reconstruction. J Vasc Surg. 1986;3:718–724.
751. Johansen K, Devin J. Mycotic aortic aneurysms. A reappraisal. Arch Surg. 1983;118:583.
752. Parsons R, Gregory J, Palmer DL. *Salmonella* infections of the abdominal aorta. Rev Infect Dis. 1983;5:227.
753. Bitseff EJ, Edwards WH, Mulherin JL Jr, et al. Infected abdominal aortic aneurysms. South Med J. 1987;80:309–312.
754. Taylor LM Jr, Deitz DM, McConnell DB, et al. Treatment of infected abdominal aneurysms by extra anatomic bypass, aneurysm excision, and drainage. Am J Surg. 1988;155:655–658.
755. Pasic M, Carrel T, von Segesser L, et al. In situ repair of mycotic aneurysm of the ascending aorta. J Thorac Cardiovasc Surg. 1993;105:321.
756. Cull DL, Winter RP, Wheeler JR, et al. Mycotic aneurysm of the suprarenal abdominal aorta. J Thorac Cardiovasc Surg. 1992;33:181.
757. Robinson JA, Johansen K. Aortic sepsis: Is there a role for in situ graft reconstruction? J Vasc Surg. 1991;13:677.
758. Pasic M, Carrel T, Vogt M, et al. Treatment of mycotic aneurysm of the aorta and its branches: The location determines the operative technique. Eur J Vasc Surg. 1992;6:419.
759. Viglione G, Younes GA, Coste P, et al. Mycotic aneurysm of the celiac trunk: Radical resection and reconstruction without prosthetic material. J Cardiovasc Surg. 1993;34:73.
760. Pasic M, von Segesser L, Turina M. Implantation of antibiotic-releasing carriers and in situ reconstruction for treatment of mycotic aneurysm. Arch Surg. 1992;127:745.

Chapter 66

Infections of Prosthetic Valves and Intravascular Devices

ADOLF W. KARCHMER

Implantable devices that assist in the maintenance of the hemodynamic capacity and electrical integrity of the heart and arterial blood supply enable the alleviation of cardiovascular and circulatory morbidity and mortality. The same devices, however, when infected cause extensive morbidity and mortality and constitute an important disease of medical progress. Because patient survival or anatomic integrity often requires that these devices be sustained in a functional capacity, their infection presents a major therapeutic challenge. That challenge is intensified by the fundamental difficulty associated with the eradication of infection that involves implanted foreign material.

PROSTHETIC VALVE ENDOCARDITIS

Prosthetic valve endocarditis (PVE) is a distinct and quantitatively important form of infective endocarditis. It accounts for 9.5 to 15% of all cases of endocarditis.[1, 2]

Epidemiology

Incidence. The frequency of PVE appears to have remained relatively stable over the past 4 decades. In reviews of large series the incidence of PVE among patients operated on before 1960, in the 1970s, and from 1970 to 1992 were 3.2, 2.1, and 3.3%, respectively.[3, 4] These rates, however, do not provide an accurate assessment of the risk of PVE, as they are primarily derived from series wherein there has not been comprehensive follow-up for either the occurrence of infection or the survival of the surgical cohort at risk. Studies utilizing active follow-up of all valve recipients and actuarial methods to estimate incidence of PVE suggest that between 3 and 5.7% develop valvular infection by 5 years after surgery (Table 66–1).[5–9] Furthermore, the risk of developing PVE is not uniform over time but it is increased during the initial 6 to 12 months after surgery. Estimates of the hazard function, that is, the risk of developing infection at a given point in time, indicate that the rate is greatest between the second and third month after valve surgery and that after 6 to 12 months have elapsed the rate falls to a low but constant rate of approximately 0.4% yearly.[4–6, 9] This rate appears to persist throughout prolonged follow-up, indicating the existence of a prolonged, if not lifelong, risk of PVE among valve recipients.[4, 5, 7]

Risks. Some studies have suggested that prostheses in the aortic position are more prone to infection than are mitral valve replacements.[3, 5, 8, 10] However, more recent studies have shown no difference in the rate of PVE at aortic and mitral sites.[5–7, 11] The data are also conflicting regarding whether replacing multiple valves increases the risk of PVE, especially during the initial postoperative months.[5–8, 11] Several studies, including randomized trials, have indicated that the overall risk of PVE is not associated with the type of valve implanted, that is, mechanical versus bioprosthetic devices with tissue leaflets.[5, 11–13] Ivert and associates found that the hazard of PVE was initially greater in mechanical valve recipients but that by the end of 6 months the risk of PVE in the two groups was indistinguishable.[6] Others have found similar differences in the risk of infection over time among recipients of different types of prostheses. Although there was no significant difference in the cumulative frequency of PVE among mechanical (5.0%) and bioprosthetic (6.3%) valve recipients 5 years after valve implantation, the frequency of infection for mechanical valves was significantly greater during the initial 3 months but that after 12 months the rate of infection was greater for bioprosthetic devices.[7] Other studies have found bioprosthetic valves at greater risk of infection than mechanical valves after the initial postoperative year.[8, 11] This temporal pattern, coupled with the leaflet localization of later-onset PVE involving bioprostheses, suggests that leaflet aging may result in local changes that increase valve vulnerability to infection.

Several studies have indicated, even after multivariate analyses, that patients undergoing valve replacement to correct structural damage due to endocarditis, whether active or healed, are at significantly increased risk to develop PVE.[6, 8, 9, 11] In some studies it was associated primarily with early-onset PVE, which, in combination with pathogen similarity between antecedent native valve endocarditis and subsequent PVE, suggests recrudescence of infection.[8, 9, 11] In other studies, however, the risk persisted years into the follow-up period, suggesting that patients with antecedent endocarditis were to a degree endocarditis prone.[8, 9]

TABLE 66–1 Cumulative Incidence of Prosthetic Valve Endocarditis

Study (Years) [Ref.]	Initial Cohort Size	Estimated Risk of Prosthetic Valve Endocarditis Months after Surgery			
		12	*24*	*48*	*60*
Rutledge et al. (1956–1981)[5]	1598	1.4			3.2
Ivert et al. (1975–1979)[6]	1465	3.0		4.1	
Calderwood et al. (1975–1982)[7]	2608	3.1		5.4	5.7
Arvay and Lengyel (1981–1985)[8]	912				4.9
Agnihotri et al. (1970–1992)[9]	2413*	1.0	1.5		3.0

*Aortic position only.

Pathogenesis

The biochemical and biophysical interactions between microorganisms and the cardiac endothelium, with or without a prostheses in place, result in adherence of organisms to specific sites and the initiation of infection. The interactions that give rise to PVE, are likely to be fundamentally the same as those that result in native valve endocarditis (see Chapter 65, "Endocarditis and Intravascular Infections"), although the site of these interactions can be altered markedly by the presence of the prosthesis. Early after valve implantation the prosthetic valve sewing ring and native valve annulus are not yet endothelialized and hence are a site of platelet fibrin thrombus formation and targets for adherence of microorganisms. Subsequently, with re-endothelialization, these areas may become less vulnerable to infection, whereas repetitive stress due to leaflet motion and aging may allow platelet fibrin aggregates to form on the leaflets of bioprostheses, thus establishing new sites for the adherence of organisms and development of PVE. This hypothesis is consistent with incidence over time of PVE involving mechanical and bioprosthetic valves as well as the pathology of PVE observed at various times after valve implantation.[14] The interaction of infecting organisms and foreign material, including the potential impairment of host defenses in the microenvironment of foreign material, is germane to both the initiation of PVE and its course as a result of the subsequent difficulties in eradicating infection with antimicrobial therapy alone.

The clinical events that contribute to the pathogenesis of PVE are related to the time of onset of infection. The microbiology of PVE that occurs during the initial 2 months after valve implantation (Table 66–2) strongly suggests a nosocomial origin for many of the episodes. The potential role of intraoperative contamination has been illustrated in several investigations. Kluge and colleagues, culturing intraoperatively, recovered microorganisms, especially *Staphylococcus epidermidis* and diphtheroids, from myocardial tissue surfaces and from the prostheses.[15] In another study the area over the opera-

TABLE 66–2 Microbiology of Prosthetic Valve Endocarditis (1975–1994)

Organism	Time of Onset after Cardiac Surgery		
	≤2 mos (N = 137)	>2–12 mos (N = 31)	>12 mos (N = 194)
Staphylococci			
Coagulase-negative	43 (31)	11 (35)	22 (11)
Staphylococcus aureus	32 (23)	4 (13)	34 (18)
Gram-negative bacilli	19 (14)	1 (3)	11 (6)
Streptococci	2 (1.5)	3 (10)	61 (31)
Enterococci	12 (9)	4 (13)	22 (11)
Diphtheroids	9 (7)	0	5 (3)
Fastidious gram-negative coccobacilli*	0	0	11 (6)
Fungi	12 (9)	2 (6)	3 (1)
Culture negative	4 (3)	4 (13)	16 (8)
Miscellaneous	4 (3)	2 (6)	9 (5)

**Haemophilus* species, *Cardiobacterium hominis, Actinobacillus actinomycetemcomitans.*
Data from refs. 7, 29–33.

tive site contained the greatest concentration of organisms and the bypass pump was also contaminated.[16] Several epidemiologic studies have linked intraoperative contamination to the subsequent development of PVE. Archer and associates epidemiologically linked cases of PVE caused by a unique clone of coagulase-negative staphylococci to intraoperative contamination by a single surgeon.[17] Of note, these patients presented clinically on average 5.3 months after surgery, with a delay of clinical onset in one case until 13 months after surgery. In three additional studies, 10 cases of coagulase-negative staphylococcal PVE were traced epidemiologically (and microbiologically in one report) to intraoperative contamination.[18–20] In 3 of 10 cases the clinical presentation of PVE was delayed from 84 days to 5.5 months.

The newly implanted prosthesis may be infected during bacteremia arising during the early postoperative period. Contamination of intravenous catheters and bacteremia as a consequence of thermodilution determination of cardiac output can seed the prosthesis.[21, 22] Additionally, in 31 to 92% of patients with PVE beginning within 2 months after surgery, the bacteria causing endocarditis were also implicated as causes of earlier or concurrent extracardiac nosocomial infections.[23–25] The association of postoperative wound infections and early-onset PVE was highly significant in one study and when associated there was a common responsible organism in 86% of patients.[9] Epidemiologic investigations, enhanced by molecular analysis of infecting organisms, have linked early postoperative exposure of wounds and chest or mediastinal tubes to *Legionella pneumophila* and *Legionella dumoffii* in tap water with subsequent development of PVE.[26] Lastly, the implantation of bioprostheses that had been contaminated during manufacturing with *Mycobacterium chelonae* has led to PVE.[27]

Fang and coworkers studied 171 patients with prosthetic valves who experienced bacteremia.[28] Among these patients, 56 had demonstrable PVE as a cause of the bacteremia. Among the remaining 115 patients, 18 (16%) were subsequently noted (median 28 days, range 7 to 170 days) to have new onset PVE. The frequency of new-onset PVE among patients experiencing staphylococcal and gram-negative bacillus bacteremia was 24 and 10%, respectively. Among the patients with PVE subsequent to the bacteremia, the portal of entry for bacteremia was either an intravascular catheter or skin/wound infection in 61%. Although some patients classified as having new-onset PVE might actually have had endocarditis causing the bacteremia and the attributable rate for endocarditis after bacteremia was not established from a non-bacteremic control group, this study illustrates the significant risk for developing PVE as a consequence of bacteremia from defined portals of entry and with diverse microorganisms (*Staphylococcus aureus, S. epidermidis, Pseudomonas aeruginosa, Proteus mirabilis,* other Enterobacteriaceae, *Enterococcus faecalis,* viridans streptococci, and *Candida albicans*). With the passage of time after valve implantation the events that result in bacteremia that in turn seeds the prosthesis are more likely community-acquired incidental infections or trauma to bacteria-laden mucosal surfaces than nosocomial events.[23, 24] At this point, the pathogenesis of PVE and community acquired native valve endocarditis become similar.

Microbiology

A wide spectrum of organisms has caused PVE. Nevertheless, when viewed in sequential time intervals after valve implantation the causes of PVE are relatively predictable (see Table 66–2). Among patients with PVE presenting within 2 months of valve implantation, coagulase-negative staphylococci are the predominant pathogen and account for at least 30% of cases.[7, 29–33] *S. aureus* causes the second largest proportion of cases occurring during this interval and is followed by gram-negative bacilli (primarily Enterobacteriaceae, *P. aeruginosa,* and occasional other nonfermentative species), enterococci, diphtheroids, and fungi, each of which contribute a roughly comparable proportion of cases.[7, 29–33] In the period encompassing month 3 through 12 after surgery the distribution of organisms is similar except that the proportions caused by gram-negative bacilli and diphtheroids are reduced and the frequency of streptococci is increased. Among the causes of PVE arising more than 12 months after surgery, coagulase-negative staphylococci, fungi, and diphtheroids are reduced whereas streptococci are increased further. Fastidious gram-negative coccobacilli, the so-called HACEK group (*Haemophilus aphrophilus, Actinobacillus actinomycetemcomitans, Cardiobacterium hominis, Eikenella* spp., and *Kingella* spp.), cause a small but significant proportion of these cases.[34] The microbiology of PVE during this last interval, with the exception of coagulase-negative staphylococci, resembles that of native valve endocarditis.

Reports of PVE have often referred to the causative coagulase-negative staphylococci as *S. epidermidis* without detailing careful speciation or have generally failed to report the antibiotic susceptibility of these organisms.[6, 10, 24, 33, 35–38] Careful study of coagulase-negative staphylococci reveals that from 84 to 87% of isolates causing PVE between 2 and 12 months after surgery are methicillin-resistant.[7, 39] In contrast, the frequency of methicillin-resistance among isolates causing PVE more than 12 months after valve surgery ranges from 22 to 30%.[7, 39] The mechanism whereby these organisms are resistant to methicillin is the same as that found in methicillin-resistant *S. aureus* and similarly mediates resistance to all currently available β-lactam antibiotics. Whereas the methicillin resistance genotype is present in all daughter cells of a resistant isolate, this phenotype is expressed in only 10^{-5} or 10^{-6} cells, a phenomenon called *heteroresistance,* which makes detection of this resistance difficult. Special tests are required to exclude methicillin resistance in coagulase-negative staphylococci causing PVE.[39] Of note, 53 of 55 coagulase-negative staphylococci causing PVE (primarily with onset within 12 months of surgery) were *S. epidermidis* (sensu stricto).[39] Among coagulase-negative staphylococci causing PVE with onset more than a year after valve surgery, almost half are non-*epidermidis* species.

PVE with onset within 2 months after valve surgery has been designated *early PVE,* whereas cases presenting later have been called *late PVE.* Early PVE, based on presumed pathogenesis and supported conceptually by the microbiology, has been considered nosocomial in contrast to late cases. The microbiology of cases occurring during the third through the twelfth month, particularly the characteristics of the coagulase-negative staphylococci, suggest that many of the cases occurring during this interval are nosocomial and relate to the surgical admission. This is corroborated by the delayed presentation of cases arising from intraoperative contamination.[17–19] Cases that are seen during this intermediate interval represent a mixture of nosocomial and community acquired episodes, whereas the cases arising more than 12 months after surgery are primarily community acquired.

Diphtheroids, corynebacteria other than *Corynebacterium diphtheriae,* although considered relatively avirulent, have been important causes of PVE. A variety of *Corynebacterium* species have caused PVE, and some of these strains have fastidious growth requirements and biochemical characteristics consistent with the highly antibiotic resistant JK group. Most diphtheroids are markedly susceptible to the bactericidal activity of vancomycin, and those strains that are not resistant to gentamicin are killed synergistically by the combination of penicillin and gentamicin.[40]

Fungi cause a small (4 to 6% overall) but important proportion of PVE.[14, 41] *C. albicans* is the most common fungal pathogen causing PVE and is followed in frequency by the non-*albicans Candida* species and *Aspergillus* spp.[14, 42, 43] Other pathogenic fungi have caused rare cases of PVE, including *Histoplasma capsulatum, Cryptococcus neoformans,* and the agents of mucormycosis. Fungi uncommonly pathogenic for humans are also rare causes of PVE, such as *Penicillium chrysogemum, Paecilomyces varioti, Trichosporon cutaneum, Curvularia geniculata,* and *Lecythophora (Phialophora) mutabilis.*[14, 43]

The diagnosis of fungal PVE is difficult. With the exception of infection due to *Candida* spp., and perhaps *C. neoformans,* blood cultures in patients with fungal PVE, even using lysis-centrifugation methods, are commonly negative. An etiologic diagnosis may require culture and microscopic examination of vegetative material from the heart or a peripheral embolus.

Pathology

Intracardiac Pathology. Infection involving mechanical prostheses often extends into the annulus and adjacent myocardium resulting in paravalvular abscess formation and partial dehiscence of the prosthetic valve with paravalvular regurgitation (Table 66–3).[23, 44–47] Large vegetations may encroach on the valve orifice, particularly that of prostheses in the mitral position, and cause functional obstruction.[44–46] Vegetations may also prevent valve closure and result in valve incompetence. Occasionally infection extends through the aortic annulus to cause pericarditis; extension into the membranous portion of the interventricular septum may disrupt the conduction system and cause various degrees of heart block.[44–46, 48] The frequency of invasive infection is more accurately derived from studies wherein pathologic findings from surgery and autopsy are expressed as a proportion of all patients encountered (Table 66–3). Among 85 patients with endocarditis involving a mechanical prosthesis, annulus invasion and myocardial abscess were noted in 42 and 14% of patients, respectively.[23, 47] Ismail and associates found annulus infection and valve dehiscence in 38 (82%) of 41 infected mechanical valves examined at surgery or autopsy.[24]

Initial studies of PVE involving bioprosthetic devices described infection largely confined to the leaflets and rarely invading the annulus. In a review of 47 patients, annular invasion was noted in only 4 patients while leaflet infection, often with invasion of the leaflet substance and tissue breakdown, was noted in the remainder. Stenosis caused by vegetations obstructing the orifice was noted in 13% of the cases.[49] In another report, among 10 infected bioprostheses, ring abscess was noted in 1 patient, cusp tears and valve perforations were noted in 3, and mitral valve stenosis was found in 2 patients.[50] However, it has subsequently been established that bioprosthetic valve infection is commonly associated with extension into the annulus.[33] Paravalvular abscesses were found in 14 of 39 patients treated surgically.[51] Fernicola and Roberts noted involvement of the annulus in 20 of 37 infected bioprosthetic valves examined at autopsy or surgery.[52] In 85 patients with PVE involving bioprosthetic valves treated between 1975 and 1983, annular or myocardial invasion occurred in 38 (45%); furthermore, invasive infection was more common among patients with PVE occurring during the initial postoperative year (59%) versus later onset cases (25%).[14] This same trend was noted among patients with bioprosthesis infection operated on between 1975 and 1992; 15 of 19 with infection in the first year after valve implantation and 22 of 71 with later-onset PVE had invasive disease.[53]

Invasive infection regardless of valve type has been correlated with the clinical findings of valvular dysfunction, persistent fever during appropriate antibiotic therapy (>9 days), new electrocardiographic conduction disturbances, and echocardiographic evidence of abscess formation.[54, 55] This clinical picture, which is suggestive of invasive disease, was noted in 64% of 116 patients and was significantly associated with infection involving aortic valve prostheses and onset of PVE within the initial year after valve surgery.[55]

Infection involving the leaflets of bioprosthetic valves can result in subtle tissue damage.[49–50] As a result, even if leaflets are not torn or perforated, late consequences may occur. Magilligan noted the delayed onset of leaflet stiffening and functional stenosis in 10 (37%) of 27 patients treated with antibiotics alone for PVE. As a result of this damage to valve leaflets, the period of effective bioprosthetic valve function may be reduced and late valve replacement required.

Clinical and Laboratory Manifestations

Clinical Features. The symptoms and signs of PVE are similar to those encountered in patients with native valve endocarditis (Table 66–4). Among patients developing PVE before discharge from the hospital after cardiac surgery, the manifestations of endocarditis are often overshadowed by findings related to postoperative complications. Hence, in evaluating the febrile valve recipient during the initial postoperative weeks, a high index of suspicions for PVE must be maintained. PVE may manifest as an exceptionally indolent illness with low-grade fever and immune-mediated manifestations, including glomerulonephritis. Alternatively, it can be a fulminant acute febrile illness with hypotension in 33% of patients with onset during the initial 2 months postoperatively and in patients who years after

TABLE 66–3 Intracardiac Pathology Associated with Infection of Mechanical Prosthetic Valves

Series [Ref.]	Total No. Patients	No. (%) with the Following Pathology			
		Annulus Invasion	*Myocardial Abscess*	*Valve Stenosis*	*Pericarditis*
Autopsy					
Arnett and Roberts[45]*	22	22	11	0	2
Anderson et al.[44]	22	11	4	0	2
Rose[46]†	30	30	9	2	2
TOTAL	74	63 (85)	24 (32)	14 (19)	4 (5)
Autopsy/Surgery					
Dismukes et al.[23]	38	8	3	2	2
Richardson et al.[47]	47	28	9	1	0
TOTAL	85	36 (42)	12 (14)	3 (4)	2 (2)

*Includes two homograft valves.
†Includes one bioprosthesis.
Adapted from Karchmer AW, Gibbons GW. Infections of prosthetic heart valves and vascular grafts. In: Bisno AL, Waldvogel FA, eds. Infections Associated with Indwelling Devices. 2nd ed. Washington, DC: American Society for Microbiology; 1994:213–249.

TABLE 66–4 Clinical Features of Prosthetic Valve Endocarditis

Symptom/Sign	Time of Onset after Surgery	
	≤ 2 Months (%)	> 2 Months (%)
Fever	95–100	95–100
New/changing murmur	50–70	40–60
Congestive heart failure	30–100	30
Shock	33	0–10
Conduction abnormality	15–20	5–10
Splenomegaly	20–30	15–40
Emboli	5–30	10–40
Petechiae	30–60	40–50
Osler's nodes, Janeway lesions, Roth's spots	5	15
Anemia	75	75
Leukocytosis	40	30–50
Hematuria		65

Adapted from Douglas JL, Cobbs CG. Prosthetic valve endocarditis. In: Kaye D, ed. Infective Endocarditis. 2nd ed. New York: Raven Press; 1992:375–396.

valve implantation develop acute endocarditis due to *S. aureus* and *Streptococcus pyogenes*.[32, 54, 56] PVE caused by *S. aureus* is very severe; central nervous system complications (stroke, hemorrhage, cerebritis, abscess, mycotic aneurysm) and intracardiac complications each occur in more than 40% of patients, and mortality rates range from 42 to 85%.[3, 32, 57] Although the true frequency of embolic complications is unknown (since many are asymptomatic), it is likely that they are common. At autopsy, 85% of patients had embolic complications and on routine abdominal computed tomography splenic infarcts were detected in 38% of cases.[44–58] The incidence of clinically detected emboli approaches 40%, and central nervous system complications, the majority of which are embolic infarcts or hemorrhagic events, are noted in 20 to 40% of patients.[10, 24, 30, 59]

Laboratory Findings. Anemia, leukocytosis, hematuria, and an elevated sedimentation rate, laboratory findings associated with native valve endocarditis, are found in patients with PVE as well (see Table 66–4). When PVE occurs in close proximity to cardiac surgery, these as well as other laboratory abnormalities must be interpreted with caution because they may relate more to the consequences and complications of surgery than to endocarditis. Increased concentrations of circulating immune complexes have been noted in patients with PVE, but a role in diagnosis or assessing response to therapy has not been defined. The laboratory findings of the greatest utility are those that provide insight into the etiology of the infection or the function of essential organs. Blood cultures, the primary method by which the etiology of PVE is established, will be positive in at least 90% of patients who have not received prior antibiotics. As in native valve endocarditis, bacteremia is continuous; hence, most blood cultures should be positive regardless of the relationship between the time at which they were obtained and body temperature. In fact, continuous bacteremia, noted as a high rate of positivity among cultures obtained over time, is strong evidence for intravascular infection. Occasionally, because of the confounding effect of antibiotics, infrequently obtained blood cultures, or perhaps paravalvular infection that does not communicate with the blood stream, only sporadic cultures are positive. If in this circumstance the isolate is a coagulase-negative staphylococcus or diphtheroid, it may be difficult to distinguish between recovery of a pathogen and a blood culture contaminant. Because in PVE the infecting organisms are generally from a single clone, molecular evaluation of the sporadic isolates to assess clonality may resolve this impasse.[60, 61]

It is unusual for patients with clinically evident PVE to have persistently negative blood cultures in the absence of prior antibiotic therapy. Nevertheless, such cases may be caused by microorganisms that are fastidious or otherwise difficult to recover from blood, for example, *Legionella* spp., *Bartonella* spp., *Coxiella burnetii, Mycoplasma hominis,* the HACEK group, and fungi other than *Candida* spp. Recovery of some of these organisms from blood can be enhanced by the use of lysis-centrifugation system including subculture on organism specific media, biphasic media, and incubation of blood cultures for 3 to 4 weeks. Also, some of these organisms may be implicated by serologic tests.[62] Occasionally the etiology of PVE is clarified by culture and histologic examination of a surgically removed embolic vegetation. Because of the exceptionally broad array of organisms that have caused PVE and the importance an etiologic diagnosis in designing therapy, cardiac surgery to recover vegetative material may be indicated.

Aside from an examination of vegetative material, no laboratory abnormality is diagnostic of PVE. Bacteremia with gram-negative bacilli (as opposed to gram-positive cocci) during the initial 85 days after valve surgery and in the presence of a peripheral source of septicemia was rarely associated with PVE.[63] Similarly, Fang and colleagues demonstrated that 57% of patients with prosthetic valves who had documented bacteremia neither had nor developed PVE.[28] Accordingly, if bacteremia and fever clear promptly with therapy, patients with bacteremia that is likely to have arisen peripherally and who have no other evidence of PVE can be treated with an antibiotic regimen designed for the peripheral source rather than PVE. If, however, the bacteremia fails to clear or there is evidence of valve dysfunction, the patient should be treated for PVE.

Special Studies. Evaluation of a prosthetic valve for infection requires thorough imaging by an experienced echocardiographer using both transthoracic echocardiography (TTE) and transesophageal echocardiography (TEE) using a high-resolution biplane or multiplane transducer capable of continuous-wave and pulse-wave Doppler and color flow imaging.[64, 65] The ventricular surfaces of prosthetic valves in the mitral, tricuspid, or aortic position are often more completely imaged using the TTE as compared with TEE. Alternatively, the atrial surface of prostheses in the mitral or tricuspid position is incompletely imaged with the TTE and better viewed using TEE. The aortic surface and outflow of an aortic valve prosthesis are better viewed using TEE. Doppler and color flow imaging allow full assessment of valve function, sites of dehiscence, fistulas, and sites where regurgitant jets impinge and initiate secondary infections. TEE is unquestionably superior to TTE when evaluating the anatomy and function of prosthetic valve in the mitral position and often the superior technique for interrogating a prosthetic aortic valve also. However, because the approaches are complementary, both TEE and TTE should be used to optimally assess a prosthesis.[65]

The diagnosis of PVE and assessment of prosthesis function have been markedly enhanced by TEE. Studies demonstrate that the sensitivity of TEE in the diagnosis of PVE ranges from 82 to 96% compared with 17 to 36% for TTE.[66–68] TEE overcomes technical difficulties in TTE acoustic access due to chest wall and pulmonary abnormalities and is able to detect smaller vegetations than TTE. TEE is superior to TTE for the diagnosis of PVE regardless of valve type or position[64–68] (Table 66–5). TEE substantially improved the preoperative detection of periprosthetic leaks, abscesses, and fistulas. In 16 patients with PVE involving a mitral or aortic valve, abscesses were detected in 14 (87%) by TEE compared with 5 (31%) by TTE.[69] The increased diagnostic sensitivity of TEE compared with TTE occurs without a significant decrease in specificity. Although the negative predictive value of a single TEE for PVE is 86 to 94%, to avoid missed diagnoses when PVE is strongly suspected a repeat examination several days later should be performed.[68, 70] By demonstrating that congestive heart failure is due to valvular dysfunction (as opposed to ventricular dysfunction) or that infection extends into myocardial tissues, echocardiography clarifies earlier the indications for surgical therapy as well as the pathology to be encountered at operation. Alternatively, the absence of intracardiac complications on echocardiography allows continued medical therapy.[71] Echocardiography has supplanted radioisotope cardiac imaging, cinefluoroscopy, and in very large measure cardiac catheterization (with the exception of defining coronary artery anatomy) in the assessment of PVE.

TABLE 66–5 Echocardiographic Diagnosis of Prosthetic Valve Endocarditis*

Prosthesis Position (Number Studied)	Number of Valves (%)			
	Transthoracic		*Transesophageal*	
	Nondiagnostic	*Diagnostic*	*Nondiagnostic*	*Diagnostic*
Aortic position (34)	16	18 (53)	5	29 (85)
Bioprosthesis (12)	6	6 (50)	1	11 (92)
Mechanical valve (22)	10	12 (55)	4	18 (82)
Mitral position (37)	32	5 (14)	4	33 (89)
Bioprosthesis (10)	8	2 (25)	2	8 (80)
Mechanical valve (27)	24	3 (11)	2	25 (93)

*Patients had pathoanatomic or clinically confirmed (Von Reyn criteria) PVE.
Data from refs. 67 and 68.

New or progressive conduction system abnormalities demonstrated by electrocardiography, especially in the setting of aortic PVE, provide indirect evidence of a septal abscess and demand intensive echocardiographic assessment.[48] Baumgartner and colleagues found myocardial abscesses at operation in 11 of 16 patients with PVE complicated by atrioventricular conduction abnormalities.[51]

Neurologic symptoms from presumed intracranial complications of PVE should be evaluated with contrast-enhanced magnetic resonance imaging or computed tomography, which will usually distinguish infarction, hemorrhage, and abscess formation.[72] If hemorrhage is detected, evaluation for a mycotic aneurysm should be undertaken using cerebral angiography.[73] The management of intracranial mycotic aneurysms complicating endocarditis is complex (see Chapters 65 and 77) and must be integrated with the treatment of PVE; this may include sequencing of neurosurgery and cardiac surgery based on the severity of the respective problems.[62] If PVE requires valve replacement, a bioprosthetic valve may be preferred if its use would obviate anticoagulation.

Diagnosis of Prosthetic Valve Endocarditis

PVE is a protean disease whose clinical presentation may be further confounded by the complications of recent cardiac surgery or other comorbidities. In the past the diagnosis has depended on a high index of suspicion, multiple positive blood cultures, a clinical appreciation of the range of the illness, and most recently an anatomic evaluation of the prosthesis by echocardiography. The Duke criteria for the diagnosis of endocarditis with its schema using major and minor criteria provide a systematic approach that can be applied to the diagnosis of PVE.[74] Classification of patients with suspected endocarditis by these criteria has correlated strongly with the diagnosis in pathologically confirmed cases and with the judgment of endocarditis experts who reviewed relevant medical records. Furthermore, the negative predictive value of these criteria has been 98 to 99%.[62] When these criteria were applied to 25 patients with pathologically confirmed PVE, the clinical categorizations were 76% definite, 24% possible, and none rejected.[75] Each case categorized as possible satisfied one major and either one or two minor criteria. TEE is essential for establishing the echocardiographic major criteria, if the schema is to be highly sensitive for PVE.[75] When the Duke criteria were used to categorize 17 patients with anatomically confirmed *S. aureus* PVE (treatment of some cases antedated TEE), 13 (76%) were classified clinically as definite and 4 (24%) as possible with these later cases manifesting a major and one or two minor criteria.[57] The Duke criteria can be used effectively to clinically diagnose PVE if applied longitudinally over the entire evaluation and if TEE is used to supplement nondiagnostic TTE evaluations. Blood cultures must be obtained optimally (multiple, over time, in the absence of antibiotic therapy) in order to correctly interpret organisms that are atypical for native valve endocarditis but common causes of PVE, for example, coagulase-negative staphylococci and diphtheroids. When these organisms are isolated sporadically, raising the question of blood culture contamination, molecular evaluations will be required to demonstrate that the isolates from different cultures are a single clone and thus unlikely to be contaminants.[60] Patients with prosthetic valves who, based on the Duke criteria, are judged to have definite or possible PVE must be treated for this infection. If these criteria are applied judiciously, rejection of bona-fide cases is unlikely.

Treatment of Prosthetic Valve Endocarditis

General Considerations. A single set of principles guide the treatment of both native valve endocarditis and PVE. To achieve optimal outcomes, these principles must be applied in concert with an understanding of the pathology of PVE, including considerations of the valve position, prosthesis type, and the time of onset after surgery. All patients should be hospitalized, at least during initial evaluation and treatment. To design optimal antimicrobial therapy it is essential that the etiologic agent be identified (not obscured by premature treatment). Accordingly, in hemodynamically stable patients presenting with indolent PVE antibiotics should be withheld initially, pending isolation of an organism from blood culture. If patients have received suboptimal antimicrobial therapy in the immediately preceding days, this brief delay (3 to 5 days) permits repeating blood cultures without the confounding effect of further antibiotic therapy. Patients presenting with PVE that is acute or that is complicated by hemodynamic instability should receive empirical antimicrobial therapy immediately after three to four sets of blood cultures have been obtained. All patients with PVE should undergo echocardiographic evaluation early in the course of treatment.

Antimicrobial Therapy. Antimicrobial therapy is based upon the in vitro susceptibility of the etiologic microorganism. A bactericidal antimicrobial or a combination of agents that together is bactericidal are necessary. The regimen should be administered parenterally for at least 6 weeks. Central venous catheters with their attendant risk of line-related septicemia should be avoided, if possible. The regimens advised for treatment of PVE (Table 66–6), although administered for a longer time, are similar to those used in the treatment of native valve endocarditis (see Chapter 65 for additional details about treatment of specific organisms).

For treatment of PVE caused by penicillin-susceptible (minimal inhibitory concentration [MIC] $\leq$0.1 μg/ml) streptococci, penicillin plus gentamicin given during the initial 2 weeks is recommended. Streptomycin can be used in lieu of gentamicin if the isolate is not resistant to streptomycin at 1000 μg/ml. If aminoglycoside therapy is relatively contraindicated, successful therapy has been provided with penicillin, a cephalosporin, or vancomycin alone.[14, 23] When treating PVE caused by streptococci that are relatively resistant to penicillin (MIC >0.1 μg/ml), the aminoglycoside component of therapy should be continued for 4 to 6 weeks.[76] Short-course (2 weeks) β-lactam plus aminoglycoside therapy as has been used in native valve streptococcal endocarditis is not effective for PVE, and

TABLE 66–6 Recommended Antibiotic Therapy for Prosthetic Valve Endocarditis

Infecting Organism	Antibiotic	Dose and Route*	Duration (wk)	Comments
1. Penicillin-susceptible viridans streptococci, *Streptococcus bovis*, and other streptococci (penicillin MIC ≤ 0.1 μg/ml)	A. Penicillin G plus gentamicin	18–24 million units IV daily in divided doses q4h 1 mg/kg IM or IV q8h	6 2	May omit aminoglycoside when potential for nephrotoxicity is increased.
	B. Ceftriaxone plus gentamicin	2 g IV or IM daily as single dose 1 mg/kg IM or IV q8h	6 2	Can be used in patients with nonimmediate penicillin allergy, intramuscular ceftriaxone is painful. Cephapirin 2 g IV q4h can be substituted for ceftriaxone.
	C. Vancomycin‡	15 mg/kg IV q12h	6	Use for patients with immediate or severe penicillin or cephalosporin allergy. Infuse doses over 1h to avoid histamine release reaction (redman syndrome).
2. Relatively penicillin-resistant streptococci (Penicillin MIC > 0.2 μg/ml)	A. Penicillin G plus gentamicin	24–30 million units IV daily in divided doses q4h 1 mg/kg IM or IV q8h	6 4	Preferred for the pyridoxal-requiring abiotrophia (formerly streptococci).
3. Enterococci (in vitro evaluation for MIC to penicillin and vancomycin, β-lactamase production, and high-level resistance to gentamicin and streptomycin required)	A. Penicillin G plus gentamicin	24–30 million units IV daily in divided doses q4h 1 mg/kg IV or IM q8h	6 6	Streptomycin can be used instead of gentamicin if streptomycin high-level resistance is not present. If high-level resistance to gentamicin but not to streptomycin is detected, streptomycin is preferred.
	B. Ampicillin plus gentamicin	2 g IV q4h Same dose as noted above	6 6	
	C. Vancomycin‡ plus gentamicin	15 mg/kg IV q12h Same dose as noted above	6 6	Use for patients with penicillin allergy. Do not use cephalosporins.
4. Staphylococci Methicillin-susceptible (assume penicillin-resistance)	A. Nafcillin or oxacillin plus gentamicin plus rifampin§	2 g IV q4h 1 mg/kg IV or IM q8h 300 mg PO q8h	6–8 2 6–8	Penicillin: 18–24 million units daily in divided doses q4h can be used instead of nafcillin or oxacillin if strains do not produce β-lactamase and penicillin MIC is ≤ 0.1 μg/ml. A first-generation cephalosporin can be used in lieu of nafcillin/oxacillin for patients with nonimmediate allergy to penicillins. Use gentamicin during initial 2 weeks. See text for alternates for gentamicin. For patients with immediate penicillin allergy, use regimen 5.
5. Staphylococci Methicillin-resistant	A. Vancomycin‡ plus gentamicin plus rifampin§	15 mg/kg IV q12h 1 mg/kg or IM q8h 300 mg PO q8h	6–8 2 6–8	Use gentamicin during the initial 2 weeks of therapy. See text for alternatives to gentamicin. Do not substitute a cephalosporin or imipenem for vancomycin.
6. HACEK organisms†	A. Ceftriaxone	2 g IV or IM daily as a single dose	6	Cefotaxime or other third-generation cephalosporin in comparable doses may be used.
	B. Ampicillin plus gentamicin	2 g IV daily in divided doses q4h 1 mg/kg IV or IM q8h	6 4	Test organism for β-lactamase production. Do not use this regimen if β-lactamase is produced.
7. Diphtheroids	A. Penicillin G plus gentamicin	18–24 million units IV daily in divided doses q4h 1 mg/kg IM or IV q8h	6	Bactericidal synergy results if isolate is not resistant to gentamicin (MIC ≥ 4 μg/ml).
	B. Vancomycin	15 mg/kg IV q12h	6	Use if organism resistant to gentamicin, highly resistant to penicillin, or patient is allergic to penicillin.

*Recommended doses are for adults with normal renal and hepatic function. Doses of gentamicin, streptomycin and vancomycin must be adjusted in patients with renal dysfunction. Use ideal body weight to calculate doses (men = 50 kg + 2.3 kg per inch over 5 feet; women = 45.5 kg plus 2.3 kg per inch over 5 feet). Do not use aminoglycosides as single daily doses.
†HACEK organisms include *Haemophilus parainfluenzae, Haemophilus aphrophilus, Actinobacillus actinomycetemcomitans, Cardiobacterium hominis, Eikenella corrodens, Kingella kingii.*
‡Peak levels obtained 1 h after completion of the infusion should be 30–45 μg/ml, trough level 10–20 μg/ml.
§Rifampin increases the dose of warfarin or dicumarol required for effective anticoagulation.
Abbreviation: MIC, Minimal inhibitory concentration.

once-daily dosing of aminoglycosides in the recommended regimens has not been studied in PVE and is not advised.[76] Vancomycin is recommended for treatment in patients with a history of immediate allergic reactions (urticarial and anaphylactic) to penicillins or cephalosporins. Cefotaxime or ceftriaxone may be used instead of penicillin in patients with other forms of penicillin allergy.

Combinations of penicillin or ampicillin (or vancomycin in penicillin-allergic patients) with an aminoglycoside have provided effective medical therapy for enterococcal PVE when the regimen has bactericidal synergistic activity against the implicated enterococcus.[76, 77] Antibiotic resistance among enterococci, however, is now sufficiently prevalent and complex that each isolate causing endocarditis must be studied in detail. Ideally, therapy combines a cell wall active agent (penicillin, ampicillin, vancomycin) with an aminoglycoside (gentamicin or streptomycin) to which the organism does not exhibit high-level resistance (growth in the face of streptomycin at 1000 μg/ml or gentamicin at 500 μg/ml). Resistance to each antibiotic is mediated by a unique gene that, although tending to congregate in strains, is acquired individually. Accordingly, in vitro screening of enterococci in search of a synergistic regimen should evaluate each potential component of a synergistic regimen.[78, 79] If because of high-level resistance to gentamicin and streptomycin a synergistic regimen is not feasible, prolonged therapy (8 to 12 weeks) with high doses of one of the cell wall active agents is recommended. Effective treatment of endocarditis due to vancomycin-resistant *Enterococcus faecium,* where coexistent resistance precluded penicillin plus aminoglycoside therapy, has not been defined. The efficacy of quinupristin-dalfopristin remains unclear. Patients with PVE caused by highly resistant strains of enterococci for which synergistic therapy is not available should be considered for surgical intervention during the course of suppressive bacteriostatic therapy.

Antibiotic therapy for PVE caused by staphylococci differs from that used when these organisms cause native valve endocarditis.[76] This difference is based on evidence from in vitro studies, animal model experiments, and clinical trials where treatment of infections associated with foreign material is enhanced by combination regimens, particularly ones including rifampin.[14, 39, 80–83] Rifampin is an essential element in the recommended regimens for staphylococcal PVE. Bacterial cells that are resistant to rifampin arise frequently from large populations of staphylococci like those found in PVE. Resistant strains are selected by ineffective rifampin-containing regimens and make subsequent therapy more complex.[14, 82] Accordingly, the rifampin component of therapy should not be started until treatment with two other antimicrobials known to be effective against the staphylococcus has been initiated. If two agents cannot be identified, therapy with a single effective agent should be given for a few days (3 to 5) before initiation of rifampin in an effort to reduce the staphylococcal population and the risk of subsequently selecting a rifampin-resistant subpopulation. Antibiotic treatment for staphylococcal PVE is based upon the susceptibility of the implicated isolate and not its production of coagulase. Thus, regimens do not distinguish between *S. aureus* and coagulase-negative staphylococci.[14, 76] For PVE caused by methicillin-resistant staphylococci, therapy is begun with vancomycin and gentamicin with rifampin added if the isolate is susceptible to both of the initial antimicrobials. The triple-drug regimen is continued for 2 weeks, after which time gentamicin is discontinued and vancomycin plus rifampin is continued to complete at least a 6-week course of therapy. If the strain is resistant to gentamicin, an alternate aminoglycoside to which it is susceptible in vitro should be sought. If an effective aminoglycoside cannot be identified, a fluoroquinolone to which the strain is highly susceptible should be used in lieu of an aminoglycoside. This recommendation is based on animal model experiments.[82–84] If the staphylococcus is susceptible to methicillin, a semisynthetic penicillinase-resistant penicillin should be substituted for vancomycin in the combination regimen. If the patient has a nonimmediate penicillin allergy, a first-generation cephalosporin can be used in place of the penicillin.

Occasional HACEK organisms have produced β-lactamase and thus are resistant to ampicillin. These strains, as well as those that are β-lactamase–negative, are highly susceptible to third-generation cephalosporins. As a result, ceftriaxone or a comparable third-generation cephalosporin is recommended for treatment of PVE caused by a HACEK organism. If a strain is β-lactamase–negative, treatment with ampicillin plus gentamicin can be used. In the absence of valvular dysfunction, HACEK PVE can generally be treated with antibiotics alone.[34]

Diphtheroids have variable susceptibility to penicillin; nevertheless, if strains are susceptible to gentamicin (MIC ≤ 4 μg/ml) the combination of penicillin and gentamicin will result in a synergistic bactericidal effect. If the strain is resistant to gentamicin, synergy will not be achieved.[85] Penicillin plus gentamicin is recommended for therapy when synergy is anticipated. Vancomycin is bactericidal for these organisms and provides alternative therapy for strains resistant to gentamicin. Vancomycin plus an aminoglycoside is not recommended because of the increased potential for nephrotoxicity.

Regimens for treating PVE caused by facultative gram-negative bacilli must be based on the in vitro susceptibility of the organism. Where possible, a synergistic bactericidal regimen is desirable. Most regimens will combine a potent β-lactam antibiotic with an aminoglycoside. The preferred antibiotic treatment for PVE caused by *P. aeruginosa* is an antipseudomonal penicillin (ticarcillin or piperacillin) plus high doses of tobramycin (8 mg/kg/day intravenously or intramuscularly in divided every-8-hour doses to achieve peak serum concentrations of 15 μg/ml).[86]

The consensus treatment of fungal PVE entails surgical therapy shortly after initiating antifungal antimicrobial therapy; a long course of antifungal therapy is given after surgery. Amphotericin B is the drug of choice for most fungi causing PVE; it is used in doses ranging from 0.7 to 1.0 mg/kg/day. The larger dose is used for PVE caused by *Aspergillus* spp. or *Mucor* spp., while smaller doses are used for PVE caused by *Candida* spp. Total doses of at least 2.0 g of amphotericin B are planned. In an effort to achieve a synergistic effect, 5-fluorocytosine (150 mg/kg/day in four divided doses with dose adjustments for renal dysfunction) is often used with amphotericin B.[42, 43] In one series using this approach to treat 15 patients (13 *Candida* spp., 1 *Histoplasma capsulatum* (although 5-fluorocytosine has no activity against *H. capsulatum*), and 1 *Saccharomyces cerevisiae*), 15 survived initial hospitalization; overall 10 patients (67%) survived with a mean follow-up of 4.5 years. Three patients experienced relapse late after treatment and were retreated in a similar fashion.[42] A review of *Candida* PVE reported since 1985 noted a 50% survival rate among 4 patients treated medically and a 46% survival rate among 13 patients treated with antifungal therapy and valve replacement surgery. All survivors had uncomplicated PVE (no evidence of invasive disease or valve dysfunction), and most patients remained on long-term suppressive fluconazole.[87] The clearly documented potential for *Candida* PVE to relapse long after initial therapy has lead many to place these patients on fluconazole 200 to 400 mg daily by mouth for long periods, possibly indefinitely.[42, 43, 87]

Empirical therapy for clinically apparent PVE wherein blood cultures are at present negative should include at least vancomycin and gentamicin. If there are clinical (peripheral site of infection) or epidemiologic clues, therapy should be expanded to cover the suggested microorganisms. If the onset of PVE is more than 12 months after valve surgery, coverage should be broadened to cover HACEK organisms by adding ceftriaxone or ampicillin.

Monitoring Therapy. Patients with PVE must be carefully monitored during therapy and for several months thereafter. Evaluations must determine the response to treatment (resolution of fever); development of intracardiac complications, valve dysfunction, and congestive heart failure; embolic complications; metastatic infection; or adverse events related to antimicrobial therapy. Occurrence of these events may indicate a need for a critical modification in antimicrobial therapy or surgical intervention for a threatening complication.

Measurement of the serum bactericidal titer (SBT)—the highest dilution of the patient's serum obtained at a given interdose time which in vitro kills 99.9% of an inoculum of the organism causing endocarditis—has been used to assess the efficacy of antimicrobial therapy. Studies have suggested that, when using a standardized SBT method with 50% human serum in the test, peak and trough titers of at least 1:64 or 1:32, and 1:32, respectively, have correlated with microbiologic cure (but not clinical outcome).[88, 89] The tests are used, however, are not standardized and are prone to exaggerated dilution effect when attempting to assess combination antibiotic therapy. Consequently, when using standard regimens that generate a predictably high SBT and that are considered clinically optimal, monitoring the SBT test is not recommended.[76] When treating PVE caused by unusual organisms for which optimal therapy is not established or when using unconventional regimens, the SBT test may be useful.

Some routine testing provides useful monitoring during the treatment of PVE. Serum concentrations of aminoglycosides and vancomycin should be measured to establish optimal dosing and avoid adverse events. Renal function should be followed when patients are treated with potentially nephrotoxic agents, and the complete blood count should be checked weekly when patients are treated with high-dose β-lactam agents. Blood cultures should be repeated during the initial days of therapy to confirm the eradication of bacteremia. Cure of PVE is often confirmed by obtaining blood cultures 2 to 8 weeks after completion of treatment. If there is recurrent fever after treatment, blood cultures must be obtained promptly to assess possible relapse.

Surgical Treatment. High mortality rates in patients with PVE have been associated with onset of infection within 2 months of surgery, nonstreptococcal etiologic agents, moderate to severe congestive heart failure, murmurs indicative of valve dysfunction, and fever persisting for 10 days or more in spite of appropriate antimicrobial therapy.[54, 55, 90, 91] Further analysis indicates that, with the exception of nonstreptococcal infection and onset early after surgery, these clinical observations are indicative of infection invasive into paravalvular tissue and valve dysfunction—pathology unlikely to be corrected with antimicrobial therapy alone.[54] Calderwood and colleagues defined invasive complicated disease as PVE with a new or increasing murmur of valve dysfunction, new or worsening congestive heart failure associated with dysfunction of the prosthesis, fever persisting for 10 or more days during appropriate antibiotic therapy, and new or progressive cardiac conduction abnormalities.[55] These investigators found that complicated disease was associated with prostheses in the aortic position and onset of infection within 1 year after surgery, that is, relatively early onset. In addition, complicated disease was strongly associated with mortality due to PVE. Recognition that these correlates of higher mortality, particularly congestive heart failure due to prosthesis dysfunction, were not amenable to antimicrobial therapy has resulted in increased and earlier surgical intervention. It has become clear that the mortality rate among patients with PVE who are treated surgically is no greater than that among those treated medically. In fact, several series indicate survival rates are higher among surgically treated patients than in those treated medically and that surgically treated patients have more favorable courses after discharge from the hospital than do PVE patients treated medically.[30, 55, 90, 91] Furthermore, the risk of recurrent endocarditis on the newly implanted prosthesis is not prohibitive.

Indications for cardiac surgical intervention as part of therapy for PVE have evolved (Table 66–7). Some of these indications are relative rather than absolute and require more integration of the entire clinical picture, including long-term morbidity, into the decision making process than are others. In some patients multiple indications will coexist, further strengthening the argument for surgical intervention.

Few, if any, patients with moderate to severe congestive heart failure due to prosthesis dysfunction survive beyond 6 months if treated medically.[47, 54] Outcome is improved in these patients when they are treated surgically.[92] For example, in a group of patients with PVE complicated by moderate to severe heart failure who were treated with antimicrobials plus valve replacement, 44 to 64% survived.[14, 47, 54] Paravalvular infection occurs in 45 to 60% of patients with PVE and is manifested by persistent fever during appropriate antimicrobial therapy, new and persistent conduction disturbances, valve instability, pericarditis in association with PVE at the aortic position, or echocardiographic evidence of abscess or fistula. In patients with invasive disease wherein survival was very unlikely, complex reconstructive procedures using homograft replacement of the aortic root and valve or reconstruction of the mitral or aortic valve using mechanical devices has led to 80% survival rates.[93, 94]

TABLE 66–7 Indications for Cardiac Surgery in Patients with Prosthetic Valve Endocarditis

Moderate to severe congestive heart failure due to valve dysfunction (regurgitant or stenotic)
Unstable prosthesis
Paravalvular extension of infection
Uncontrolled infection (persistent bacteremia) on optimal antimicrobial therapy
PVE caused by selected microorganisms
- Fungi
- *Pseudomonas aeruginosa*
- *Staphylococcus aureus*
- Enterococci in the absence of bactericidal therapy
- Other gram-negative bacilli and microorganisms that usually require surgery when infecting native valves, e.g., *Brucella* spp., *Coxiella burnetii*

Relapse after optimal therapy
Large (>10 mm) hypermobile vegetations
Culture negative prosthetic valve endocarditis with unexplained persistent (≥10 d) fever

Among PVE patients with relapsed endocarditis, cure rates are improved with combined antimicrobial and surgical treatment compared with antibiotics alone.[54, 55]

Demonstrating uncontrolled infection, that is, persistent bacteremia in the presence of maximal antimicrobial therapy, requires surgical intervention as a last resort. The outcome of medical therapy for PVE caused by some microorganisms has been so unfavorable that surgery is advocated because of the organism even in the absence of persistently positive blood cultures. The prototype of this scenario is PVE caused by *Candida* spp. or other fungi. Although reports suggest that chronic suppression of *Candida* PVE may be successful, this approach has been uniformly unsuccessful in patients with invasive *Candida* PVE and in general surgical intervention is preferred.[42, 43, 87]

The mortality attributed to *S. aureus* PVE when treated with antibiotics alone has been extraordinarily high (42 to 100%).[30, 32, 33, 91, 95, 96] Mortality has related to the severity of the cardiac infection or to central nervous system embolic complications.[30, 32] John and coworkers, in a multivariate analysis, noted that intracardiac complications were associated with a 13.7-fold increase in mortality and that mortality was reduced 20-fold among patients treated surgically during antibiotic therapy. This reduction in mortality occurred among both those with and without intracardiac complications.[57] This study further suggested that surgery remained appropriate for patients with early embolic CNS complications. Other investigators also have concluded that *S. aureus* PVE is best treated with early surgical intervention.[32, 33, 91, 95]

Patients with native valve endocarditis who have echocardiographically demonstrable vegetations that exceed 10 mm in greatest dimension experience more frequent systemic emboli than those with smaller vegetations.[97, 98] Although the same has not been demonstrated in patients with PVE, the overall frequency of embolic complications in those two forms of endocarditis is similar. In both groups the rate of embolic events decreases rapidly with duration of effective antibiotic therapy.[71, 99] Although it is clearly desirable to prevent central nervous system and coronary artery emboli, it has not been established that surgical intervention to prevent emboli enhances survival or reduces morbidity. Accordingly, most investigators do not consider vegetation size greater than 10 mm, increased vegetation motility, or a prior systemic embolus an absolute indication for surgical intervention. Rather, these findings are viewed as additional considerations that in concert with other clinical observations may prompt surgical intervention.

Patients with culture-negative endocarditis who continue to experience otherwise unexplained fever after 10 days of antibiotics should be considered for surgery. Surgery will provide access to vegetative material from which an etiologic agent can be sought and will allow débridement of invasive infection, if present. Surgery thus addresses the two major reasons for failure of empirical antibiotic therapy.

Not only is the decision to intervene surgically in the treatment of patients with PVE complex, but also the surgery itself can be unusually demanding as a consequence of the extent of infected cardiac tissue that requires débridement and the subsequent reconstruction. Elaborate reconstructions of the aortic and mitral valve apparatus and supporting structures have been accomplished using a valved conduit, cryopreserved homograft aortic root, or fresh autologous pericardium or glutaraldehyde fixed bovine pericardium in conjunction with prosthetic valves.[53, 93, 94, 100–102] Valve replacement and reconstructive surgery for highly invasive destructive PVE performed by experienced surgeons result in operative mortality rates (death before discharge) ranging from 10 to 30%; these rates are remarkably low considering the anticipated 100% mortality in the absence of surgery.[53, 93, 94, 100, 102] PVE recurs in only 6 to 15% of patients with active invasive PVE who are treated surgically.[51, 55, 93, 94, 103] In these surgically treated patients the need for further reoperation because of recurrent PVE or dehiscence of a sterile prosthesis with significant paravalvular leakage ranges from 18 to 26%.[51, 53,

[93, 103] The actuarial survival rate 5 years after surgical treatment for active PVE ranges from 54 to 82%.[51, 53, 93, 100]

The timing of surgical therapy for PVE must be individualized in an effort to perform surgery before the onset of severe end-stage heart failure and to minimize extravalvular tissue destruction. The hemodynamic state of the patient prior to surgery is the most important consideration in determining the time of surgical intervention. The operative mortality of patients with PVE, as is seen with surgically treated native valve endocarditis patients, is proportional to hemodynamic disability prior to surgery.[104] Renal failure, another indicator of cardiac decompensation, is associated with increased mortality as well.[51] Prolonging antimicrobial therapy in the face of deteriorating hemodynamics or persistent progressive infection does not correlate with sterilization of operative cultures or with increased survival rates.[51, 105] Accordingly, in patients with progressive infection or heart failure it is inappropriate to delay surgery solely to allow for the administration of additional antimicrobial therapy. On the other hand, there are occasional stable patients with mild heart failure due to paravalvular leak who have responded to antibiotic therapy in whom it is reasonable to delay surgery until antimicrobial therapy has been completed.

On careful evaluation, from 40 to 65% of patients with PVE may be candidates for surgical treatment.[55, 90] Alternatively, there are patients with PVE in whom medical therapy is as effective as antibiotics plus surgical intervention. This group of patients, for whom medical therapy is recommended, includes those with later-onset infection (>12 months after surgery) who are infected with less invasive organisms (viridans streptococci, HACEK organisms, and enterococci), and who do not have or develop invasive disease or other indications for surgery while being treated.[14]

Other Considerations Related to Surgery. To avoid neurologic deterioration and hemorrhagic intracranial complications in patients who have experienced a recent neurologic complication, it may be desirable to delay cardiac surgery and to consider a reconstruction that will not require long-term anticoagulation. If cardiac hemodynamics permit, surgery can be done safely 4 weeks after cerebral infarction. If surgery is performed 15 to 21 days after cerebral infarction, the frequency of neurologic deterioration is 10%, reduced from over 40% when surgery is performed within the week after infarction.[106] The risk of worsening neurologic status with cardiac surgery persists for at least 4 weeks after cerebral hemorrhage, unless the bleeding focus (mycotic aneurysm) can be repaired first.[72, 106]

The length of the antimicrobial treatment given after surgical intervention in patients with PVE should be based on the operative findings (including histopathologic and microbiologic information), the need for additional antimicrobial therapy for extracardiac focal infection, and the percentage of the standard antimicrobial regimen that had been administered preoperatively. A full course of the standard antimicrobial regimen should be given postoperatively to those patients wherein histopathology and cultures indicate continued inflammation or viable microorganisms. If there is no evidence of invasive infection (PVE is confined to the prosthesis) and the excised material is culture-negative, the sum of the preoperative and postoperative antibiotic treatment should be equal to at least the recommended therapy for PVE caused by the specific etiologic microorganism.

Anticoagulation. The optimal use of anticoagulant therapy in patients with active PVE, including warfarin versus heparin, remains controversial.[107, 108] Effective anticoagulation in patients with an infected mechanical valve reduces the frequency of strokes (16 events among 133 patients, 12%) when compared with no anticoagulant therapy (32 events in 76 patients, 42%) and does not increase the frequency of hemorrhagic complications (11% vs. 9%, respectively).[107] Accordingly, anticoagulation is recommended in patients with an infected mechanical valve. In patients with PVE involving a bioprosthetic valve that does not normally require anticoagulant therapy, the frequency of stroke during PVE, 2 events in 24 patients (8%), does not suggest a benefit from anticoagulant therapy. Bland infarcts can be converted to hemorrhagic infarcts with excessive anticoagulant therapy; hence, the intensity of anticoagulation must be monitored closely. I prefer coumadin anticoagulation (prothrombin time 1.5 times the control or International Normalized Ratio [INR] of 2.5 to 3.0), whereas others favor heparin.[4, 108] If extracardiac or nonendocarditis indications for anticoagulation arise, it is appropriate to judiciously anticoagulate the patient. If intracerebral bleeding occurs, anticoagulant effect should be reversed pending evaluation and resolution of the event. In general, mycotic aneurysms are a rare complication of endocarditis and rarely rupture after completion of effective antimicrobial therapy; hence anticoagulant therapy can be administered where indicated to patients with cured PVE.[108–110]

Prognosis

Although significantly improved from the early reports, the mortality associated with PVE remains high. In cases occurring before 1980, mortality rates in patients with PVE developing within 2 months of cardiac surgery and later were 77% (64/83) and 42% (62/147), respectively.[10, 23, 35, 36, 56] Among cases reported more recently, the mortality rate was 56% in 71 cases occurring within 2 months of surgery.[11, 32, 91] In 294 patients with PVE occurring later, the mortality rate was 32%.[11, 30, 32, 33, 91] Among 116 patients with PVE occurring between 1975 and 1982, Calderwood and associates reported that 77% survived initial treatment. In this series, mortality was significantly correlated with the presence of invasive infection but not with the time of onset relative to valve implantation.[55] Exceptionally high mortality rates continue among patients with *S. aureus* PVE. The improvements in the outcome of PVE noted in the past decade are likely the result of an increased awareness of the entity of PVE, early diagnosis and precise detection of intracardiac complications by TEE, the development of effective antimicrobial therapy for PVE caused by methicillin-resistant coagulase-negative staphylococci, and increased use of innovative surgical therapy early in the course of PVE to excise invasive infection and reconstruct damaged cardiac structures. Mortality rates ranging from 10 to 30% in series of surgically treated patients, whose anticipated mortality in the absence of surgery would have approached 100%, suggest that early aggressive surgical therapy may be the major contributor to improved outcome.[53, 94, 100, 102, 111] The favorable outcome in these reports also imply that patients with PVE, where feasible, should be treated in medical centers with specific expertise in management of this entity.

Prevention

Prophylactic antibiotics are routinely administered at the time of valve replacement surgery. Studies have compared first- and second-generation cephalosporin regimens for prophylaxis in cardiac surgery patients. Trials have not been significantly large to assess prevention of PVE but rather have focused on the prevention of surgical site wound infections. Cefazolin and cefuroxime appear to be among the most cost effective agents for perioperative prophylaxis. Vancomycin is used in patients with immediate type penicillin hypersensitivity and in institutions where methicillin-resistant *S. aureus* is an important cause of surgical wound infections. Medical problems that might predispose patients to PVE subsequently, for example, poor dental health, prostatic hypertrophy, and outflow obstruction, should be treated prior to valve replacement. Prosthetic valves remain vulnerable to infection during transient bacteremia indefinitely. Patients with prosthetic valves are considered at "high risk" for endocarditis according to the American Heart Association. These patients should be advised of their risk and strongly encouraged to seek prophylaxis before procedures that are likely to induce bacteremia.[112]

INFECTIONS OF PERMANENT PACEMAKERS

Pacemaker infections can be categorized from a clinical management perspective into two groups: infections that are restricted to the pulse generator pocket and/or the subcutaneous portion of the lead and infections that involve the transvenous intravascular electrode component with or without involvement of the generator unit. The latter category encompasses so-called pacemaker endocarditis. A 1 to 7% incidence of pacemaker infections, with an increased risk in association with generator unit reimplantation, is often cited.[113] Using careful follow-up and a precise definition of pacemaker endocarditis, a study of 8303 procedures noted pacemaker infections and endocarditis in 5.6 to 0.5% of patients, respectively.[114]

Clinical Manifestations

The most common pacemaker infection is that which is restricted to the generator unit and/or the lead wires in their subcutaneous position. These infections commonly arise in temporal proximity to pacemaker placement or generator exchange, although some will develop late after surgery as a consequence of the device eroding through chronically traumatized skin and subcutaneous tissue. Infection that complicates recent surgery on the generator pocket manifests as local swelling, erythema, pain, and possibly drainage through an incompletely healed incision or fistulous track. Clinical evidence of infection may be only local, or there may be systemic toxicity and bacteremia. Pacemaker infection, or perhaps more appropriately contamination, arising as a consequence of erosion may be asymptomatic aside from the erosion itself. These infections arise as a result of skin flora contamination of the surgical site. *S. aureus* and *S. epidermidis* account for 63 to 75% of the generator pocket infections.[113, 115] Streptococci, *Corynebacterium* spp., and *Proprionibacterium acnes,* that is, common skin flora, as well as Enterobacteriaceae and *Candida* spp., have been noted in these infections. The episodes arising during the initial 2 weeks after surgery are most likely caused by *S. aureus* and are more likely associated with bacteremia.[115]

Epicardial electrodes are occasionally infected by spread from the generator pocket or by direct contamination when placed. In addition to clinical findings of inflammation at the generator pocket, infection of these electrodes may be associated with pericarditis, mediastinitis, systemic toxicity, and bacteremia.

Infection of the intravascular portion of the transvenous electrode, which occurs primarily at an intracardiac site, most commonly arises from infection of the subcutaneous portion of the pacing apparatus that has tracked intravascularly.[114, 116, 117] Occasionally pacemaker endocarditis is due to bacteremic seeding from infection at a remote site.[118] Among patients with pacemaker endocarditis, from 27 to 36% present within 6 to 12 weeks after the last procedure at the implant site. The remainder of these infections manifests more than 6 to 12 weeks after the last procedure; among these patients there is a 25-month mean interval from the procedure to onset of symptoms.[116, 117] In the early presentations, the short time elapsed from pacemaker manipulation to acute pocket infection and evidence of systemic infection lead to prompt diagnosis. In contrast, mean intervals of 5 and 8 months from onset of symptoms to diagnosis emphasized the cryptic and often protean nature of this infection when presenting late.[116, 117] Fever (84 to 100%) and chills (75 to 84%) are the most common symptoms. Low-grade fever and failure to thrive may be the only symptoms in 25 to 35% of patients; however, patients occasionally present with sepsis and shock. Pouch infection, inflammation, or abnormalities resulting in multiple manipulations are reported in 25 to 55% of these patients. Pulmonary symptoms and findings consistent with pneumonia, bronchitis, lung abscess, or embolism are seen in 20 to 45% of patients and are more common among those with later onset infection. Overt pulmonary embolism is seen occasionally, and pulmonary scintigraphy may indicate embolism in 40% of the patients studied. New or changing heart murmurs and splenomegaly are uncommon. An elevated sedimentation rate (82 to 97%) and leukocytosis (50 to 66%) are common. TEE has demonstrated vegetations on the electrodes, tricuspid valve, or ventricular endocardium in 90 to 96% of patients studied.[116, 117] In contrast, TTE has been diagnostic or suggestive of endocarditis in only 22 to 54% of the patients examined.[114, 116, 117] The clinical constellation of symptoms, persistent bacteremia, and TEE findings allow definitive diagnosis in most episodes.

Microbiology

Although staphylococci are the predominant bacteria, a wide variety of organisms has caused pacemaker endocarditis. Among 129 episodes of precisely defined pacemaker endocarditis in three series, 14 patients had polymicrobial infection, 109 had a single organism isolated from blood or vegetation, and 6 were culture-negative.[114, 116, 117] Among the organisms recovered were *S. aureus* (27%), coagulase-negative staphylococci (56%), Enterobacteriaceae (6%), *P. aeruginosa* (3%), *C. albicans* (2%) and enterococci, *Corynebacteria, Listeria,* streptococci, and *Aspergillus* spp. (each causing $\leq$1%). The *S. aureus* and coagulase-negative staphylococci were distributed equally across early- and later-onset infections, and methicillin resistance was relatively common among both groups of staphylococci. Camus and colleagues demonstrated that *S. aureus* bacteremia apparently arising from sites other than the generator pocket in the early days after pacemaker placement is likely to infect the intravascular electrode.[118] In contrast, bacteremia with *S. aureus,* viridans streptococci, enterococci, and gram-negative bacilli arising from remote sites months and years after pacemaker placement does not uniformly seed the intravascular electrode.[118] These latter patients could be treated as having uncomplicated bacteremia rather than pacemaker endocarditis.

Treatment

In considering treatment of pacemaker infection, patients must be separated into those without bacteremia in whom infection is limited to the generator pocket or subcutaneous electrode and those with bacteremic pacemaker endocarditis with or without clinical involvement of the subcutaneous portion of the pacing system. When infection is limited to the subcutaneous elements, it is possible to perform a one-step direct exchange of the pacing system, if the pacemaker is truly required. While the patient is treated with antibiotics, a new pacemaker is inserted at a new site and immediately thereafter the infected device is removed. The infected subcutaneous pocket is left open and is treated with local wound care and abbreviated systemic antimicrobial therapy. In some instances, the removal of the infected device is separated from the insertion of the new pacer by a period of transvenous pacing using a temporary device.[115] Ideally, functionless electrodes, especially those contaminated in association with generator infection, should be extracted when the infected generators are removed.

Management of pacemaker endocarditis or bacteremia when pacemakers are in place remains somewhat controversial in the absence of prospective studies. The consensus approach to pacemaker endocarditis favors removing the generator and the electrode(s) as an integral part of treatment.[114, 116–118] Extraction of electrodes in place for less than 18 months can generally be accomplished with traction. Although it may be difficult, those in place for longer periods often can be removed with the Cook electrode extraction system. If the electrode cannot be safely removed transcutaneously, surgical removal by cardiotomy may be required. Additionally, in patients with large vegetations (>10 mm), surgical extraction may be advisable to prevent clinically significant pulmonary embolism.[116] For patients who continue to require a pacemaker, a new pacing unit can be inserted immediately using an epicardial lead or a temporary transvenous system can be used until systemic antibiotics have controlled endocardial infection, whereupon a new permanent transvenous unit can be placed.[113, 114, 116–118] A minimum of 2 weeks of antimicrobial therapy using an endocarditis regimen targeted to the causative organism (with clinical evidence that infection has been controlled) should be administered before reinsertion of a new permanent transvenous electrode. All patients with pacemaker endocarditis should receive a full course of parenteral antimicrobial therapy designed to treat endocarditis caused by the identified organism. Metastatic infection resulting from pacemaker endocarditis, for example, vertebral osteomyelitis, occasionally may require antibiotic therapy beyond that required for endocarditis.

Although electrode removal, especially if cardiotomy is required, is itself potentially associated with morbidity and mortality, the failure of antibiotic therapy alone, even when very prolonged, to eradicate pacemaker endocarditis supports removal of the entire system as the preferred therapy.[114, 116, 117] Camus and associates noted that initial therapy for staphylococcal pacemaker endocarditis was successful in 5 of 6 patients with electrode removal, whereas infection relapsed in all 7 patients from whom infected electrodes were not removed.[118] In the treatment of initial and relapse episodes of pacemaker endocarditis, these authors reported cure and survival in 10 of 11 patients from whom the electrodes were removed compared with documented cure in only 1 of 11 patients treated without extracting the infected electrode. Others have noted high failure rates with attempted salvage of infected electrodes by treatment with lengthy high-dose antibiotic therapy.[116, 117] In a review of nine retrospective series encompassing 190 cases of pacemaker endocarditis, the mortality rate of 29 patients treated with antibiotics alone was 41%, whereas the rate was only 19% among 161 patients treated with antibiotics plus removal of the entire pacing system.[117] These data, although potentially affected by selection bias, form the basis for the recommended early removal of the entire pacing system in the treatment of pacemaker endocarditis. In some patients, however, overall health status will not permit the procedures required to extract infected electrodes. In regard to this group, it is notable that a few patients with pacemaker endocarditis have been treated successfully with prolonged courses of parenteral therapy and that others have been managed using initial parenteral therapy followed by chronic suppressive oral antimicrobials.

INFECTION OF IMPLANTABLE CARDIOVERTER-DEFIBRILLATORS

The implantable cardioverter-defibrillator device (ICD), an important advance in the treatment of life-threatening ventricular arrhythmias, is a complex technology that continues to evolve. Originally, the ICD required surgical placement of not only the pulse generator but also extrapericardial or epicardial defibrillation patches, as well as a transvenous rate sensing electrode. Recently introduced systems use a transvenously implanted rate sensing lead and a superior vena caval coil electrode plus, as dictated by defibrillation threshold testing, additional subcutaneous or epicardial electrodes. All of the leads are ultimately connected to a subcutaneously or submuscularly placed pulse generator. The complexity of the systems and surgical implantation demands have often required coordinated two-staged placement procedures by cardiologists and thoracic surgeons. ICD infection rates have ranged from 2 to 11% among patients undergoing device placement by thoracotomy or sternotomy.[119, 120] Transvenous nonthoracotomy systems, the placement of which in many respects is similar to that for pacemakers, are less frequently complicated by infection, with rates ranging from 0.8 to 1.5%.[121–123] Although occasionally delayed-onset infections are noted, most ICD infections present clinically within 6 months, and usually with the initial 3 months, after placement. Pain, erythema, fluid collection, and drainage from around the generator, infraclavicular wound, or subcutaneous patch wound are the common presentations. If epicardial patches are infected, signs of deep infection and pericarditis may be present. Systemic symptoms, often with bacteremia, are noted in 50% of patients, particularly those with infection caused by *S. aureus.*[123] Patients occasionally present with septicemia and hypotension. The diagnosis of ICD infection is made clinically and confirmed by culture of sinus drainage or fluid aspirated from collections around the device. When an ICD is infected, cultures of the generator pocket are often positive even if that site does not manifest inflammatory changes.

Coagulase-negative staphylococci and *S. aureus* are the predominant pathogens causing ICD infection.[119, 123, 124] Nevertheless, a broad array of other microorganisms, including Enterobacteriaceae, *P. aeruginosa,* corynebacteria, *P. acnes, Candida* spp., streptococci, and atypical mycobacteria, have been noted to infect ICD. Polymicrobial infection of the generator pocket is not uncommon.[123, 124]

The management of ICD infection is complex. Most reports indicate that removal of the entire ICD system is required to eliminate infection, and this approach has been advocated, especially when infection has systemic features, is bacteremic, or is caused by *S. aureus.*[119, 123, 124] Infections restricted to the generator site have been managed by removing the generator, treating with parenteral antibiotics and wound care, and subsequently reimplanting a generator at a new site. If the patient's overall condition precludes removing the entire system, treatment of infection caused by low-virulence organisms with intravenous antimicrobials followed by continuous suppressive oral antibiotic therapy has been advocated.[123] The duration of parenteral therapy beyond that needed for soft tissue infection, regardless of whether the ICD is removed partially or entirely, should be determined by the potential for endocardial involvement and the implications of bacteremia, for example, sustained *S. aureus* bacteremia. The decision to replace the ICD after complete removal of the prior system and control of infection is difficult. The benefit of ICD reimplantation versus antiarrhythmic drug therapy is not resolved. If inducible arrhythmias persist and cannot be controlled or eradicated through other mechanisms, non-thoracotomy ICD systems can be reimplanted, when feasible. The timing of ICD replacement is determined to a significant degree by the perceived threat of the arrhythmia.

INFECTIONS OF VASCULAR GRAFTS

Incidence

The incidence of infection following arterial reconstruction using synthetic graft materials varies from less than 1 to 5%.[14] The frequency after reconstruction of the aorta and iliac arteries is 1%; infection complicates 2 to 5% of grafts that traverse the inguinal area (aortofemoral or femoropopliteal).

Pathogenesis

Although the mechanism initiating infection of an individual graft is not always evident, one of three mechanisms is thought responsible generally: (1) intraoperative contamination, (2) extension from adjacent infected or colonized tissue, or (3) hematogenous seeding.

The vulnerability of synthetic arterial grafts to hematogenous seeding has been established in animal models. In these models the incidence of graft infection after an intravenous challenge of *S. aureus* was universal initially and then declined with the time of challenge after graft placement and correlated inversely with the extent of neointimal development. In humans the inner surfaces of grafts develop a pseudointima and to a degree a true endothelium.[125] It is thought, however, that this coverage is incomplete, resulting in residual vulnerability to seeding during bacteremia. Although the frequency with which this mechanism leads to graft infection is difficult to ascertain, late infection of an aortic graft by *Pasteurella multocida* after a dog bite provides proof of principle.[126]

Intraoperative contamination is probably the most common mechanism of graft contamination and reflects a break, possibly unrecognized, in surgical technique. Additionally, investigators have found bacteria by culture in the wall of abdominal aortic aneurysms and in the aorta wall at repeat surgery.[127, 128] Patients with positive arterial wall cultures were at increased risk for graft infection; however, the incidence of graft infection was low and the significance of the positive arterial wall cultures is not known. Known or cryptic injury of the bowel may lead to graft contamination during aortic surgery.

Spread of bacteria from superficial and deep wound infections adjacent to grafts is a common mechanism of graft infection and accounts for many of the infections in areas such as the groin. Experimental studies suggest that lymphatics transport organisms from distally in the leg to proximal sites in contiguity with the graft. Protection can be obtained by ligation of the lymphatics.[129] Erosion of the aortic graft into the bowel wall and lumen results in direct contamination of the graft.

Microbiology

The most common microorganism causing graft infection is *S. aureus*. It is isolated in 24 to 36% of infected grafts. In addition, a broad range of bacteria cause these infections (Table 66–8). Graft infections beginning within days to weeks of surgery are caused by pyogenic organisms, particularly *S. aureus,* Enterobacteriaceae, and *P. aeruginosa.* Enterobacteriaceae are a common cause of intra-abdominal graft infection. Polymicrobial infections are noted in 12 to 37% of patients. Coagulase-negative staphylococci are often isolated from infections with delayed onset. Bandyk and associates have described indolent graft infections that present as anastomotic aneurysms very late (>14 months) after surgery and are commonly caused by *S. epidermidis.* Often these organisms are difficult to isolate, requiring sonication of the graft and culture in special media.[130, 131]

Clinical Presentation

The manifestations of graft infections vary with the anatomic site of the infected graft. Among infected grafts that cross the inguinal area, 50% will become apparent within 3 months of surgery or the most proximate graft manipulation.[132–135] These patients typically exhibit a localized inguinal mass with or without pain, erythema, and fever and may form a graft-cutaneous sinus track. A false aneurysm may be seen in some patients. This indicates infection at the artery-graft anastomosis, which may subsequently lead to hemorrhage, distal emboli, or graft thrombosis. Patients may complain of intermittent fever, malaise, anorexia, and weight loss as a reflection of indolent infection.

Graft infection arising in the abdominal cavity manifests subtly with low-grade fever, abdominal discomfort, retroperitoneal bleeding, or an abdominal mass due to a false aneurysm. There may be obstruction and hydronephrosis due to compression by a false aneurysm. Lower extremity emboli, and petechiae may be noted. Erosion of the graft into the gastrointestinal tract is another rare but notable form of infection. This occurs on average 5 to 6 years after graft replacement as a consequence of chronic pulsatile trauma to the intestinal wall overlying the graft. Erosion occurs most often into the distal duodenum but occasionally occurs into jejunum at the distal end of an aortoiliac graft. Fever (45 to 66%), distal emboli (33%), and positive blood culture with mixed enteric organisms (50 to 70%) may be seen. A cardinal finding is gastrointestinal bleeding, which may be quantitatively minor and due to mucosal injury if the erosion occurs over the shaft of the graft or massive exsanguination if the erosion occurs at the site of the graft to aorta anastomosis. An aortoenteric fistula should be suspected when a patient with an aortic graft develops hematemesis or melena.

Diagnosis

The approach to diagnosis is strongly influenced by the findings on physical examination. Clinical evidence of wound infection adjacent to a dysfunctional graft, for example, false aneurysm, recent thrombosis, or anastomotic bleeding, is virtually diagnostic, as is a sinus track to a graft or visible graft in an open wound. If the graft is not directly evaluable by physical examination, radiologic studies can be used to define anatomic abnormalities or perigraft inflammation. Computed tomography (CT) can reveal lack of incorporation by adjacent tissue, a false aneurysm, collections of fluid adjacent to the graft, perigraft tissue inflammation, or air adjacent to a graft, each of which can be suggestive of graft infection.[136] Oral contrast fluid can occasionally outline an aortic graft on CT when an aortoenteric fistula exists. Magnetic resonance imaging and angiography are also useful in evaluating graft anatomy, patency, tissue incorporation, perigraft fluid collections, and tissue inflammation.[137] In some instances, it may be difficult to distinguish changes due to surgery, that is, early lack of incorporation, from infection. Ultrasonography has had limited utility aside from demonstrating a false aneurysm, and radionuclide studies have foundered over issues of sensitivity and specificity. Establishing that a draining sinus extends to a graft by sinography is diagnostic. Stable patients with suspected aortoenteric fistula formation can be evaluated by endoscopy that extends to the fourth portion of the duodenum. Although a negative examination does not exclude a fistula, occasionally the graft will be visible or suspicious mucosal abnormalities noted. In the final analysis, diagnosis in some patients requires microbiologic examination of perigraft fluid or tissue or direct graft evaluation at surgery. If sufficient time has passed since graft placement, absence of incorporation of the graft into perigraft tissue as viewed by the surgeon correlates well with culture confirmation of infection and is sufficiently reliable to justify clinical management decisions.[138] Blood cultures, although

TABLE 66–8 Frequency of Bacteria Isolated from Infected Synthetic Arterial Grafts

	Percent Grafts Infected				
	Author (Ref.) [n = Number Patients]				
Organism	*Calligaro (135) [n = 42]*	*Cherry (140) [n = 39]*	*Mertens (132) [n = 59]*	*Edwards (133) [n = 24]*	*Lorentzen (134) [n = 62]*
S. aureus	24	24	30	29	36
Coagulase-negative staphylococci	11	8	10	4	21
Enterococci	11	10	6	—	11
Streptococci	7	4	12	—	—
Pseudomonas aeruginosa	12	6	12	4	1
Enterobacteriaceae	18	22	28	33	20
Bacteroides spp.	7	6	1	8	6
Corynebacterium	7		—		1
Culture-negative	—	8	2	21	4
Miscellaneous	3	12			
Number polymicrobial infections	[13]	[8]	[22]	[3]	[4]

sometimes positive, are often negative because infection does not extend to the graft lumen. Graft cultures themselves may be misleading either because of prior antibiotic exposure or because organisms are imbedded in a biofilm that must be disrupted if the culture effort is to be optimal.[130, 131]

Treatment

Although antibiotic therapy is an important component of treatment, the true burden of therapy falls on the vascular surgeon who must assess the risk of anastomotic disruption and death as well as the requirement for graft-provided arterial flow for vital organ or extremity survival. This assessment and the assessment of the extent of graft infection are combined to design surgery to remove the infected graft or a portion of it and to reperfuse the area by placing a new graft through an extra-anatomic uninfected route. The anatomic feasibility of the surgery as well as the morbidity and mortality risk of the proposed surgery must be considered. Staged procedures are required sometimes to accomplish the goal with acceptable operative risks. The guiding principles include complete resection of the infected graft, débridement of adjacent infected tissue, development of a healthy sterile arterial stump that can be securely closed, reperfusion through an uninfected pathway, and appropriate initial and long-term antibiotic therapy. Intensive antimicrobial therapy, as might be administered for endocarditis caused by the infecting organism or organisms, is recommended for the initial 4 to 6 weeks of therapy. Additionally, if the arterial wall at the site of stump closure has been culture-positive or is thought because of operative findings to be infected, 6 months of culture-specific suppressive antibiotics are advised to reduce the risk of stump disruption.[139]

Alternatives to the standard of extra-anatomic reperfusion through an uninfected route have been sought because of the surgical morbidity and mortality of the required procedures. Salvage of selected infected distal (outside the body cavities) grafts has been achieved when the anastomosis was not involved, the graft was patent, systemic sepsis was absent, and *P. aeruginosa* was not involved.[135, 140–142] In some instances salvage has been pursued when the anastomosis was intact but in the infected field.[143] Wounds have been managed by careful aggressive débridement and delayed secondary intention wound healing or by rotational muscle flaps. Culture-directed parenteral antibiotic therapy is given for at least 6 weeks. This approach has not, however, been subjected to randomized trials using graft excision and extra-anatomic reperfusion as the comparator. Some vascular surgeons do not consider this graft salvage approach optimal.[132] In Europe, cryopreserved arterial allografts have successfully been used for in situ replacement of infected synthetic aorta grafts. Although not studied in a randomized trial, this approach has been compared favorably with extra-anatomic reperfusion with a synthetic graft and resection of the infected graft.[144]

Outcome

The morbidity and mortality associated with infected arterial grafts and treatment vary with the position of the graft and the resultant treatment required. Mortality rates are higher and amputation rates lower when infections involve aortic grafts, for example, 37 and 21% at 1 year, respectively.[145] Infection of infrainguinal arterial grafts is associated with less mortality (18%) and with higher amputation rates (40%).[132]

REFERENCES

1. Wilson WR, Danielson GK, Giuliani ER, Geraci JE. Prosthetic valve endocarditis. Mayo Clin Proc. 1982;57:155–161.
2. Berlin JA, Abrutyn E, Strom BL, et al. Incidence of infective endocarditis in the Delaware Valley, 1988–1990. Am J Cardiol. 1995;76:933–936.
3. Mayer KH, Schoenbaum SC. Evaluation and management of prosthetic valve endocarditis. Prog Cardiovasc Dis. 1982;25:43–54.
4. Horskotte D, Piper C, Niehues R, Wiemer M, Schultheiss HP. Late prosthetic valve endocarditis. European Heart J. 1995;16(Suppl B):39–47.
5. Rutledge R, Kim J, Applebaum RE. Actuarial analysis of the risk of prosthetic valve endocarditis in 1,598 patients with mechanical and bioprosthetic valves. Arch Surg. 1985;120:469–472.
6. Ivert TSA, Dismukes WE, Cobbs CG, et al. Prosthetic valve endocarditis. Circulation. 1984;69:223–232.
7. Calderwood SB, Swinski LA, Waternaux CM, et al. Risk factors for the development of prosthetic valve endocarditis. Circulation. 1985;72:31–37.
8. Arvay A, Lengyel M. Incidence and risk factors of prosthetic valve endocarditis. Eur J Cardiothorac Surg. 1988;2:340–346.
9. Agnihotri AK, McGiffin DC, Galbraith AJ, O'Brien MF. The prevalence of infective endocarditis after aortic valve replacement. J Thorac Cardiovasc Surg. 1995;110:1708–1724.
10. Masur H, Johnson WD, Jr. Prosthetic valve endocarditis. J Thorac Cardiovasc Surg. 1980;80:31–37.
11. Grover FL, Cohen DJ, Oprian C, et al. Determinants of the occurrence of and survival from prosthetic valve endocarditis. J Thorac Cardiovasc Surg. 1994;108:207–214.
12. Hammermeister KE, Sethi GK, Henderson WG. A comparison of outcomes eleven years after heart valve replacement with a mechanical valve or prosthesis. N Engl J Med. 1993;328:1289–1296.
13. Bloomfield P, Wheatley DJ, Prescott RJ. Twelve-year comparison of a Björk-Shiley mechanical heart valve with procine bioprostheses. N Engl J Med. 1991;324:573–579.
14. Karchmer AW, Gibbons GW. Infections of prosthetic heart valves and vascular grafts. In: Bisno AL, Waldvogel FA, eds. Infections Associated with Indwelling Devices. 2nd ed. Washington, DC: American Society for Microbiology; 1994:213–249.
15. Kluge RM, Calia FM, McLaughlin JS, Hornick RB. Sources of contamination in open heart surgery. JAMA. 1974;230:1415–1418.
16. Blakemore WS, McGarrity GJ, Thurer RJ, et al. Infection by air-borne bacteria with cardiopulmonary bypass. Surgery. 1971;70:830–838.
17. Archer GL, Vishniavsky N, Stiver HG. Plasmid pattern analysis of *Staphylococcus epidermidis* isolates from patients with prosthetic valve endocarditis. Infect Immun. 1982;35:627–632.
18. Boyce JM, Potter-Bynoe G, Opal SM, et al. A common-source outbreak of *Staphylococcus epidermidis* infections among patients undergoing cardiac surgery. J Infect Dis. 1990;161:493–499.
19. Mickelsen PA, Plorde JJ, Gordon KP, et al. Instability of antibiotic resistance in a strain of *Staphylococcus epidermidis* isolated from an outbreak of prosthetic valve endocarditis. J Infect Dis. 1985;152:50–58.
20. van den Broek PJ, Lampe AS, Berbee GAM, et al. Epidemic of prosthetic valve endocarditis caused by *Staphylococcus epidermidis*. BMJ. 1985;291:949–950.
21. Freeman R, King D. Analysis of results of catheter tip cultures in open heart surgery patients. Thorax. 1975;30:26–30.
22. Stiles GM, Singh L, Imazaki G, Stiles QR. Thermodilution cardiac output studies as a cause of prosthetic valve bacterial endocarditis. J Thorac Cardiovasc Surg. 1984;88:1035–1037.
23. Dismukes WE, Karchmer AW, Buckley MJ, et al. Prosthetic valve endocarditis: Analysis of 38 cases. Circulation. 1973;48:365–377.
24. Ismail MB, Hannachi N, Abid F, et al. Prosthetic valve endocarditis: A survey. Br Heart J. 1987;58:72–77.
25. Wilson WR. Prosthetic valve endocarditis: Incidence, anatomic location, cause, morbidity, and mortality. In: Duma RJ, ed. Infections of Prosthetic Heart Valves and Vascular Grafts: Prevention, Diagnosis, and Treatment. Baltimore: University Park Press; 1977:3–16.
26. Tompkins LS, Roessler BJ, Redd SC, et al. Legionella prosthetic-valve endocarditis. N Engl J Med. 1988;318:530–535.
27. Rumisek JD, Albus RA, Clarke JS. Late *Mycobacterium chelonei* bioprosthetic valve endocarditis: Activation of implanted contaminant? Ann Thorac Surg. 1985;39:277–279.
28. Fang G, Keys TF, Gentry LO, et al. Prosthetic valve endocarditis resulting from nosocomial bacteremia: A prospective, multicenter study. Ann Intern Med. 1993;119:560–567.
29. Chen SC, Sorrell TC, Dwyer DE, et al. Endocarditis associated with prosthetic cardiac valves. Med J Aust. 1990;152:458–463.
30. Tornos P, Sanz E, Permanyer-Miralda G, et al. Late prosthetic valve endocarditis: Immediate and long-term prognosis. Chest. 1992;101:37–41.
31. Keys TF. Early-onset prosthetic valve endocarditis. Cleve Clin J Med. 1993;60:455–459.
32. Wolff M, Witchitz S, Chastang C, et al. Prosthetic valve endocarditis in the ICU: Prognosis factors of overall survival in a series of 122 cases and consequences for treatment decision. Chest. 1995;108:688–694.
33. Sett SS, Hudon MPJ, Jamieson WRE, Chow AW. Prosthetic valve endocarditis: Experience with porcine bioprostheses. J Thorac Cardiovasc Surg. 1993;105:428–434.
34. Meyer DJ, Gerding DN. Favorable prognosis of patients with prosthetic valve endocarditis caused by gram-negative bacilli of the HACEK group. Am J Med. 1988;85:104–107.
35. Rossiter SJ, Stinson EB, Oyer PE, et al. Prosthetic valve endocarditis: Comparison of heterograft tissue valves and mechanical valves. J Thorac Cardiovasc Surg. 1978;76:795–803.
36. Slaughter L, Morris JF, Starr A. Prosthetic valvular endocarditis: A 12 year review. Circulation. 1973;47:1319–1326.

37. Turina M. Prosthetic valve endocarditis. Thorac Cardiovasc Surgeon. 1982;30:350–353.
38. Paneth M. Native and prosthetic valve endocarditis. Thorac Cardiovasc Surgeon. 1982;30:362–364.
39. Karchmer AW, Archer GL, Dismukes WE. *Staphylococcus epidermidis* causing prosthetic valve endocarditis: Microbiologic and clinical observations as guides to therapy. Ann Intern Med. 1983;98:447–455.
40. Kazanjian P. Infective endocarditis: Review of 60 cases treated in community hospitals. Infect Dis Clin Pract. 1993;2:41–46.
41. Douglas JL, Cobbs CG. Prosthetic valve endocarditis. In: Kaye D, ed. Infective Endocarditis. 2nd ed. New York: Raven Press; 1992:375–396.
42. Melgar GR, Nasser RM, Gordon SM, et al. Fungal prosthetic valve endocarditis in 16 patients. An 11 year experience in a tertiary care hospital. Medicine. 1997;76:94–103.
43. Gilbert HM, Peters ED, Lang SJ, Hartman BJ. Successful treatment of fungal prosthetic valve endocarditis: Case report and review. Clin Infect Dis. 1996;22:348–354.
44. Anderson DJ, Bulkley BH, Hutchins GM. A clinicopathologic study of prosthetic valve endocarditis in 22 patients: Morphologic basis for diagnosis and therapy. Am Heart J. 1977;94:325–332.
45. Arnett EN, Roberts WC. Prosthetic valve endocarditis: Clinicopathologic analysis of 22 necropsy patients with comparison of observations in 74 necropsy patients with active infective endocarditis involving natural left-sided cardiac valves. Am J Cardiol. 1976;38:281–291.
46. Rose AG. Prosthetic valve endocarditis: A clinicopathological study of 31 cases. S Afr Med J. 1986;69:441–445.
47. Richardson JV, Karp RB, Kirklin JW, Dismukes WE. Treatment of infective endocarditis: A 10-year comparative analysis. Circulation. 1978;58:589–597.
48. Madison J, Wang K, Gobel FL. Prosthetic aortic valve endocarditis. Circulation. 1975;51:940–949.
49. Ferrans VJ, Boyce SW, Billingham ME, et al. Infection of glutaraldehyde-preserved porcine valve heterografts. Am J Cardiol. 1979;43:1123–1136.
50. Bortolotti U, Thiene G, Milano A, et al. Pathologic study of infective endocarditis on Hancock porcine bioprostheses. J Thorac Cardiovasc Surg. 1981;81:934–942.
51. Baumgartner WA, Miller DC, Reitz BA, et al. Surgical treatment of prosthetic valve endocarditis. Ann Thorac Surg. 1983;35:87–102.
52. Fernicola DJ, Roberts WC. Frequency of ring abscess and cuspal infection in active infective endocarditis involving bioprosthetic valves. Am J Cardiol. 1993;72:314–323.
53. Lytle BW, Priest BP, Taylor PC, et al. Surgery for acquired heart disease: Surgical treatment of prosthetic valve endocarditis. J Thorac Cardiovasc Surg. 1996;111:198–210.
54. Karchmer AW, Dismukes WE, Buckley MJ, Austen WG. Late prosthetic valve endocarditis: Clinical features influencing therapy. Am J Med. 1978;64:199–206.
55. Calderwood SB, Swinski LA, Karchmer AW, et al. Prosthetic valve endocarditis: Analysis of factors affecting outcome of therapy. J Thorac Cardiovasc Surg. 1986;92:776–783.
56. Wilson WR, Jaumin PM, Danielson GK, et al. Prosthetic valve endocarditis. Ann Intern Med. 1975;82:751–756.
57. John MVD, Hibberd PL, Karchmer AW, et al. *Staphylococcus aureus* prosthetic valve endocarditis: Optimal management and risk factors for death. Clin Infect Dis. 1998;26:1302–1309.
58. Ting W, Silverman NA, Arzouman DA. Splenic septic emboli in endocarditis. Circulation. 1990;82(Suppl IV):105–109.
59. Keyser DL, Biller J, Coffman TT, Adams HP, Jr. Neurologic complications of late prosthetic valve endocarditis. Stroke. 1990;21:472–475.
60. Archer GL, Karchmer AW, Vishniavsky N, Johnston JL. Plasmid-pattern analysis for the differentiation of infecting from noninfecting *Staphylococcus epidermidis*. J Infect Dis. 1984;149:913–920.
61. Breen JD, Karchmer AW. Usefulness of pulsed-field gel electrophoresis in confirming endocarditis due to *Staphylococcus lugdunensis*. Clin Infect Dis. 1994;19:985–986.
62. Bayer AS, Bolger AF, Taubert KA, et al. Diagnosis and management of infective endocarditis and its complications. Circulation. 1998;98:2936–2948.
63. Sande MA, Johnson WD, Hook EW, Kaye D. Sustained bacteremia in patients with prosthetic cardiac valves. N Engl J Med. 1972;286:1067–1070.
64. Khandheria BK. Transesophageal echocardiography in the evaluation of prosthetic valves. Am J Cardiac Imag. 1995;9:106–114.
65. Stewart WJ, Shan K. The diagnosis of prosthetic valve endocarditis by echocardiography. Sem Thorac Cardiovasc Surg. 1995;7:7–12.
66. Vered Z, Mossinson D, Peleg E, et al. Echocardiographic assessment of prosthetic valve endocarditis. Eur Heart J. 1995;16(Suppl B):63–67.
67. Daniel WG, Mugge A, Grote J, et al. Comparison of transthoracic and transesophageal echocardiography for detection of abnormalities of prosthetic and bioprosthetic valves in the mitral and aortic positions. Am J Cardiol. 1993;71:210–215.
68. Morguet AJ, Werner GS, Andreas S, Kreuzer H. Diagnostic value of transesophageal compared with transthoracic echocardiography in suspected prosthetic valve endocarditis. Herz. 1995;20:390–398.
69. Daniel WG, Mugge A, Martin RP, et al. Improvement in the diagnosis of abscesses associated with endocarditis by transesophageal echocardiography. N Engl J Med. 1991;324:795–800.
70. Sochowski RA, Chan KL. Implication of negative results on a monoplane transesophageal echocardiographic study in patients with suspected infective endocarditis. J Am Coll Cardiol. 1993;21:216–221.
71. Steckelberg JM, Murphy JG, Ballard D, et al. Emboli in infective endocarditis: The prognostic value of echocardiography. Ann Intern Med. 1991;114:635–640.
72. Gillinov AM, Shah RV, Curtis WE, et al. Valve replacement in patients with endocarditis and acute neurologic deficit. Ann Thorac Surg. 1996;61:1125–1130.
73. Huston JH, III, Nichols DA, Luetmer PH, et al. Blinded prospective evaluation of sensitivity of MR angiography to known intracranial aneurysms: Importance of aneurysm size. Am J Neuroradiol. 1994;15:1607–1614.
74. Durack DT, Lukes AS, Bright DK. New criteria for diagnosis of infective endocarditis: Utilization of specific echocardiographic findings. Am J Med. 1994;96:200–209.
75. Nettles RE, McCarty DE, Corey RG, et al. An evaluation of the Duke criteria in 25 pathologically confirmed cases of prosthetic valve endocarditis. Clin Infect Dis. 1997;25:1401–1403.
76. Wilson WR, Karchmer AW, Bisno AL, et al. Antibiotic treatment of adults with infective endocarditis due to viridans streptococci, enterococci, other streptococci, staphylococci, and HACEK microorganisms. JAMA. 1995;274:1706–1713.
77. Rice LB, Calderwood SB, Eliopoulos GM, et al. Enterococcal endocarditis: A comparison of prosthetic and native valve disease. Rev Infect Dis. 1991;13:1–7.
78. Eliopoulos GM. Enterococcal endocarditis. In: Kaye D, ed. Infective Endocarditis. 2nd ed. New York: Raven Press; 1992:209–223.
79. Eliopoulos GM. Aminoglycoside resistant enterococcal endocarditis. Infect Dis Clin North Am. 1993;7:117–133.
80. Archer GL, Johnston JL, Vazquez GJ, Haywood HB, III. Efficacy of antibiotic combinations including rifampin against methicillin-resistant *Staphylococcus epidermidis:* In vitro and in vivo studies. Rev Infect Dis. 1983;5(Suppl 3):S583–542.
81. Kobasa WD, Kaye KL, Shapiro T, Kaye D. Therapy for experimental endocarditis due to *Staphylococcus epidermidis*. Rev Infect Dis. 1983;5(Suppl 3):S533–537.
82. Chuard C, Herrmann M, Vaudaux P, et al. Successful therapy of experimental chronic foreign-body infection due to methicillin-resistant *Staphylococcus aureus* by antimicrobial combinations. Antimicrob Agents Chemother. 1991;35:2611–2616.
83. Lucet JC, Herrmann M, Rohner P, et al. Treatment of experimental foreign body infection caused by methicillin-resistant *Staphylococcus aureus*. Antimicrob Agents Chemother. 1990;34:2312–2317.
84. Rouse MS, Wilcox RM, Henry NK, et al. Ciprofloxacin therapy of experimental endocarditis caused by methicillin-resistant *Staphylococcus epidermidis*. Antimicrob Agents Chemother. 1990;34:273–276.
85. Murray BE, Karchmer AW, Moellering RC, Jr. Diphtheroid prosthetic valve endocarditis: A study of clinical features and infecting organisms. Am J Med. 1980;69:838–848.
86. Reyes MP, Lerner AM. Current problems in the treatment of infective endocarditis due to *Pseudomonas aeruginosa*. Rev Infect Dis. 1983;5:314–321.
87. Nguyen MH, Nguyen ML, Yu VL, et al. Candida prosthetic valve endocarditis: Prospective study of six cases and review of the literature. Clin Infect Dis. 1996;22:262–267.
88. Weinstein MP, Stratton CW, Ackley A, et al. Multicenter collaborative evaluation of a standardized serum bactericidal test as a prognostic indicator in infective endocarditis. Am J Med. 1985;78:262–269.
89. Stratton CW. The role of the microbiology laboratory in the treatment of infective endocarditis. J Antimicrob Chemother. 1987;20(Suppl A):41–49.
90. Saffle JR, Gardner P, Schoenbaum SC, Wild W. Prosthetic valve endocarditis: The case for prompt valve replacement. J Thorac Cardiovasc Surg. 1977;73:416–420.
91. Yu VL, Fang GD, Keys TF, et al. Prosthetic valve endocarditis: Superiority of surgical valve replacement versus medical therapy only. Ann Thorac Surg. 1994;58:1073–1077.
92. Horstkotte D, Bircks W, Loogen F. Infective endocarditis of native and prosthetic valves—the case for prompt surgical intervention? A retrospective analysis of factors affecting survival. Z Kardiol. 1986;75(Suppl 2):168–182.
93. Jault F, Gandjbakheh I, Chastre JC, et al. Prosthetic valve endocarditis with ring abscesses: Surgical management and long-term results. J Thorac Cardiovasc Surg. 1993;105:1106–1113.
94. Glazier JJ, Verwilghen J, Donaldson RM, Ross DN. Treatment of complicated prosthetic aortic valve endocarditis with annular abscess formation by homograft aortic root replacement. J Am Coll Cardiol. 1991;17:1177–1182.
95. Roder BL, Wandall DA, Espersen F, et al. A study of 47 bacteremic *Staphylococcus aureus* endocarditis cases: 23 with native valves treated surgically and 24 with prosthetic valves. Scand Cardiovasc J. 1997;31:305–309.
96. Kuyvenhoven JP, van Rijk-Zwickker GL, Hermans J, et al. Prosthetic valve endocarditis: Analysis of risk factors for mortality. Eur J Cardiothorac Surg. 1994;8:420–424.
97. Mugge A, Daniel WC, Frank G, Lichtlen PR. Echocardiography in infective endocarditis: Reassessment of prognostic implications of vegetation size determined by the transthoracic and transesophageal approach. J Am Coll Cardiol. 1989;14:631–638.
98. Aragam JR, Weyman AE. Echocardiographic findings in infective endocarditis. In: Weyman AE, ed. Principles and Practice of Echocardiography. 2nd ed. Philadelphia: Lea & Febiger; 1994;1178–1197.
99. Sanfilippo AJ, Picard MH, Newell JB, et al. Echocardiographic assessment of patients with infectious endocarditis: Prediction of risk for complications. J Am Coll Cardiol. 1991;18:1191–1199.
100. David TE. The surgical treatment of patients with prosthetic valve endocarditis. Sem Thorac Cardiovasc Surg. 1995;7:47–53.
101. Sande MA, Lee BL, Mills J, Chambers HF, III. Endocarditis in intravenous drug users. In: Kaye D, ed. Infective Endocarditis. 2nd ed. New York: Raven Press; 1992:345.

102. d'Udekem Y, David TE, Feindel CM, et al. Long-term results of operation for paravalvular abscess. Ann Thorac Surg. 1996;62:48–53.
103. Pansini S, di Summa M, Patane F, et al. Risk of recurrence after reoperation for prosthetic valve endocarditis. J Heart Valve Dis. 1997;6:84–87.
104. Reinhartz O, Herrmann M, Redling F, Zerkowski HR. Timing of surgery in patients with acute infective endocarditis. J Cardiovasc Surg. 1996;37:397–400.
105. Boyd AD, Spencer FC, Isom OW, et al. Infective endocarditis: An analysis of 54 surgically treated patients. J Thorac Cardiovasc Surg. 1977;73:23–30.
106. Eishi K, Kawazoe K, Kuriyama Y, et al. Surgical management of infective endocarditis associated with cerebral complications: Multicenter retrospective study in Japan. J Thorac Cardiovasc Surg. 1995;110:1745–1755.
107. Davenport J, Hart RG. Prosthetic valve endocarditis 1976–1987: Antibiotics, anticoagulation, and stroke. Stroke. 1990;21:993–999.
108. Delahaye JP, Poncet PH, Malquarti V, et al. Cerebrovascular accidents in infective endocarditis: Role of anticoagulation. Eur Heart J. 1990;11:1074–1078.
109. Hart RG, Kagan-Hallet K, Joerns SE. Mechanisms of intracranial hemorrhage in infective endocarditis. Stroke. 1987;18:1048–1056.
110. Salgado AV, Furlan AJ, Keys TF, et al. Neurologic complications of endocarditis: A 12-year experience. Neurology. 1989;39:173–178.
111. Kanter MC, Hart RG. Neurologic complications of infective endocarditis. Neurology. 1991;41:1015–1020.
112. Dajani AS, Taubert KA, Wilson W, et al. Prevention of bacterial endocarditis: Recommendations by the American Heart Association, from the Committee on Rheumatic Fever, Endocarditis, and Kawasaki Disease, Council on Cardiovascular Diseases in the Young. JAMA. 1997;277:1794–1801.
113. Waldvogel F. Pacemaker Infections. In: Bisno AL, Waldvogel FA, eds. Infections Associated with Indwelling Mechanical Devices. 2nd ed. Washington, DC: American Society for Microbiology; 1994;251–258.
114. Arber N, Pras E, Copperman Y, et al. Pacemaker endocarditis: Report of 44 cases and review of the literature. Medicine. 1994;73:299–305.
115. Lewis AB, Hayes DL, Holmes DR, Jr., et al. Update on infections involving permanent pacemakers: Characterization and management. J Thorac Cardiovasc Surg. 1985;89:758–763.
116. Klug D, Lacroix D, Savoye C, et al. Systemic infection related to endocarditis on pacemaker leads: Clinical presentation and management. Circulation. 1997;95:2098–2107.
117. Cacoub P, Leprince P, Nataf P, et al. Pacemaker infective endocarditis. Am J Cardiol. 1998;82:480–484.
118. Camus C, Leport C, Raffi F, et al. Sustained bacteremia in 26 patients with a permanent endocardial pacemaker: Assessment of wire removal. Clin Infect Dis. 1993;17:46–55.
119. Spinler SA, Nawarskas JJ, Foote EF, et al. Clinical presentation and analysis of risk factors for infectious complications of implantable cardioverter-defibrillator implantations at a university medical center. Clin Infect Dis. 1998;26:1111–1116.
120. Trappe HJ, Pfitzner P, Klein H. Infections after cardioverter-defibrillator implantation: Observations in 335 patients over 10 years. Br Heart J. 1995;73:20–24.
121. Smith PN, Vidaillet HJ, Hayes JJ. Infections with non-thoracotomy implantable cardioverter-defibrillators: Can these be prevented? Pacing Clin Electrophysiol. 1998;21:42–55.
122. Gold MR, Peters RW, Johnson JW. Complications associated with pectoral implantation of cardioverter defibrillators. Pacing Clin Electrophysiol. 1997;20:208–211.
123. O'Nunain S, Perez I, Roelke M, et al. The treatment of patients with infected implantable cardioverter-defibrillator systems. J Thorac Cardiovasc Surg. 1997;113:121–129.
124. Lai KK, Fontecchio SA. Infections associated with implantable cardioverter-defibrillators placed transvenously and via thoracotomies: Epidemiology, infection control, and management. Clin Infect Dis. 1998;27:265–269.
125. Wu MHD, Shi Q, Wechezak AR, et al. Definitive proof of endothelialization of a Dacron arterial prosthesis in a human being. J Vasc Surg. 1995;21:862–867.
126. Sanella NA, Tavano P, McGoldnak DM. Aortic graft sepsis caused by *Pasteurella multocida*. J Vasc Surg. 1987;5:887–888.
127. Schwartz JA, Powell TW, Burnham SJ. Culture of abdominal aortic aneurysm content: An additional series. Arch Surg. 1987;122:777–780.
128. Durham JR, Malone JM, Bernhard VM. The impact of multiple operations on the importance of arterial wall cultures. J Vasc Surg. 1987;5:160–169.
129. Rubin JR, Malone JM, Goldstone J. The role of lymphatic system in acute arterial prosthetic graft infections. J Vasc Surg. 1985;2:92–98.
130. Bandyk DF, Bergamini TM, Towne JB. *In situ* replacement of vascular prostheses infected by bacterial biofilms. J Vasc Surg. 1991;13:575–583.
131. Bergamini TM, Bandyk DF, Govostis D. Identification of *S. epidermidis* vascular graft infections: A comparison of culture techniques. J Vasc Surg. 1997;9:665–670.
132. Mertens RA, O'Hara PJ, Hertzer NR, et al. Surgical management of infrainguinal arterial prosthetic graft infections: Review of a thirty-five-year experience. J Vasc Surg. 1995;21:782–791.
133. Edwards WH, Jr., Martin RS, III, Jenkins JM, et al. Primary graft infections. J Vasc Surg. 1987;6:235–239.
134. Lorentzen JE, Nielsen OM, Arendrup H, et al. Vascular graft infection: An analysis of sixty-two graft infections in 2411 consecutively implanted synthetic vascular grafts. Surgery. 1985;98:81–86.
135. Calligaro KD, Veith FJ, Schwartz ML, et al. Are gram-negative bacteria a contraindication to selective preservation of infected prosthetic arterial grafts? J Vasc Surg. 1992;16:337–346.
136. Qvarfordt PG, Reilly LM, Marks AS. Computerized tomographic assessment of graft incorporation after aortic reconstruction. Am J Surg. 1985;150:227–231.
137. Hansen ME, Yucel EK, Waltman AC. STIR imaging of synthetic vascular graft infection. Radiology. 1993;16:30–36.
138. Padberg FT, Jr., Smith SM, Eng RHK. Accuracy of disincorporation for identification of vascular graft infection. Arch Surg. 1995;130:183–187.
139. Malone JM, Lalka SG, McIntyre KE, et al. The necessity for long-term antibiotic therapy with positive arterial wall cultures. J Vasc Surg. 1988;8:262–267.
140. Cherry JJ, Jr., Roland CF, Pairolero PC, et al. Infected femorodistal bypass: Is graft removal mandatory? J Vasc Surg. 1992;15:295–305.
141. Perler BA, Vander Kolk CA, Manson PM, Williams GM. Rotational muscle flaps to treat localized prosthetic graft infection: Long-term follow-up. J Vasc Surg. 1993;18:358–364.
142. Calligaro KD, Veith FJ, Sales CM, et al. Comparison of muscle flaps and delayed secondary intention wound healing for infected lower extremity arterial grafts. Ann Vasc Surg. 1994;8:32–37.
143. Calligaro KD, Veith FJ, Schwartz ML, et al. Selective preservation of infected prosthetic arterial grafts: Analysis of a 20-year experience with 120 extracavitary-infected grafts. Ann Surg. 1994;220:461–471.
144. Vogt PR, Brunner-LaRocca HP, Carrel T, et al. Surgery for adult cardiovascular disease: Cryopreserved arterial allografts in the treatment of major vascular infection: A comparison with conventional surgical techniques. J Thorac Cardiovasc Surg. 1998;116:965–972.
145. Quiñones-Baldrich WJ, Hernandez JJ, Moore WS. Long-term results following surgical management of aortic graft infection. Arch Surg. 1991;126:507–511.

Chapter 67

Prophylaxis of Infective Endocarditis

DAVID T. DURACK

Infective endocarditis continues to cause serious morbidity and mortality despite advances in diagnosis and treatment. The etiologic organisms usually can be eradicated by antibiotics, but microbiologic cure often does not prevent permanent cardiac valvular damage or other major sequelae. Only a minority of patients die during the active phase of endocardial infection, but many suffer later complications, including recurrent infective endocarditis, and have a shortened life span despite having been "cured" of the infection.[1, 2] The increasing prevalence of high-level antibiotic resistance among the common gram-positive cocci that cause most cases of endocarditis may further contribute to the risk of this disorder and its complications. For these reasons, prevention of IE remains an important objective.[3–9]

POTENTIAL INTERVENTIONS TO PREVENT ENDOCARDITIS

A variety of preventive measures could theoretically be used to interrupt the pathogenetic sequence that leads to endocarditis. These include alleviation of predisposing conditions, elimination of portals of entry for organisms, immunization against bacteria that cause endocarditis, inhibition of bacterial adherence to the endocardium, application of antiseptics in the mouth, and administration of antibiotics. Of these, administration of antibiotics has received the most attention.

Alleviation of Predisposing Conditions. Abnormalities that predispose to endocarditis can in some cases be corrected. For example, surgical repair of ventricular septal defect, patent ductus arteriosus (PDA), and coarctation of the aorta reduces or eliminates the significant risk for infective endocarditis associated with these conditions. In the past, the lifetime risk for infective endocarditis due to PDA was 25 to 40%, high enough to indicate surgical repair for this reason alone. In recent years, the lifetime risk has fallen to less than 5%, probably too low to justify surgery unless it is required for other indications.[10]

Elimination of Portals of Entry for Organisms. Most cases of infective endocarditis are caused by gram-positive cocci that originate from the mouth or the skin. Measures that prevent these organisms from entering and circulating in the blood stream should be effective in prevention of some cases of infective endocarditis. It is therefore desirable to maintain optimal oral health, especially healthy gums. Periodontal probing can cause bacteremias,[11] and periodontitis may be an exacerbating factor. Prevention and treatment of periodontal disease, and of other conditions associated with bacteremias such as dental abscesses, are strongly indicated in patients with cardiac conditions that predispose to infective endocarditis. Likewise, prevention and prompt treatment of skin diseases such as furuncles or cellulitis caused by staphylococci and streptococci should reduce the risk of infective endocarditis as a complication in predisposed patients. Catheter-related blood stream infections (CR-BSI) caused by gram-positive cocci and yeasts pose significant risk for development of nosocomial infective endocarditis, a risk that should be reduced by prevention or prompt treatment of these infections.

Immunization against Bacteria That Cause Endocarditis. Preexisting antibodies to bacteria that enter the blood potentially may either promote or prevent[12–19] development of endocarditis. Under defined conditions, prior immunization can prevent streptococcal infective endocarditis in rabbits.[15, 16, 19] A vaccine against FimA, a surface-associated protein found in about 80% of streptococci and enterococci that promotes adherence to fibrin, prevents experimental streptococcal endocarditis in rats.[12] Vaccines against various components of staphylococci that mediate adherence can prevent endocarditis,[17, 18, 20] catheter infection,[21] or septic death[22] in animal models, indicating that vaccines could possibly be developed to prevent staphylococcal bacteremias and hence infective endocarditis. Unfortunately, vaccination would be difficult to validate as a preventive strategy against this disorder, and to date it has not been attempted in humans.

Inhibition of Bacterial Adherence to the Endocardium. Adherence to the endocardium and local deposition of platelets and fibrin are essential early events in development of infective endocarditis. Inhibitors of these processes theoretically could prevent endocarditis. Anticoagulants have been tested in experimental animals but did not prevent infection.[23] As knowledge of the determinants of bacterial adherence progresses, new drugs that prevent attachment may be developed. A drug that prevented adherence of circulating bacteria might have advantages over antibiotics for the prevention of endocarditis because it would not be limited by antibiotic resistance.

Application of Antiseptics in the Mouth. The number of bacteria in the mouth and gingival crevices can be temporarily reduced by local irrigation with an antiseptic solution such as iodinated glycerol.[24] Some dental experts recommend routine use of this potentially useful de-germing measure before dental extractions.

Administration of Antibiotics. Development of recommendations for optimal use of antibiotics to prevent infective endocarditis has been hampered by a lack of quantitative information. Reliable data from human studies are not available to answer the following basic questions:

What is the risk of developing infective endocarditis after various procedures that cause bacteremia?

Is antibiotic prophylaxis effective? If so, which procedures and operations should be covered by antibiotics?

Which prophylactic antibiotic regimens are most effective?

Several case-control studies have been performed, but it is unlikely that sufficient epidemiologic data can be accumulated to answer these questions definitively.

Random, low-grade bacteremias with organisms originating from the mouth, the gut, or occasionally the skin occur commonly, probably daily.[25, 26] Thus, patients with underlying heart conditions that predispose to colonization are continually at some risk of developing infective endocarditis. In humans, it is usually impossible to determine with certainty what particular bacteremia (naturally occurring or induced by a medical or dental procedure) was responsible for an episode of endocarditis. Clinical studies on the prophylactic efficacy of antibiotics are also unlikely to provide the answers because an excessively large number of patients would be required to reach a significant conclusion, as the following example illustrates. To illustrate, let us make the following assumptions: that the risk of acquiring bacterial endocarditis after dental extraction is approximately 1 in 500;[27, 28] that approval for a randomized trial of antibiotic versus a placebo could be obtained from an ethics review committee; and that an antibiotic regimen is available that is 100% effective in preventing endocarditis. An imaginary clinical trial under these admittedly arbitrary conditions might yield the following figures:

Treatment Group	Number of Patients	Cases of Endocarditis
Placebo	3000	6
Antibiotic	3000	0
	Total 6000	$\chi^2 = 4.2$, $p < 0.05$

In this example, at least 6000 patients—all with preexisting valvular heart disease—would have to be studied during dental procedures for the results to reach statistical significance. Although these figures are based upon arbitrary and unproven assumptions, such a large study would probably be difficult or impossible to perform. However, it may be possible to demonstrate the efficacy of prophylaxis by selecting subgroups of patients at highest risk for endocarditis. Among patients with prosthetic heart valves undergoing various surgical procedures, no cases of endocarditis followed 287 procedures for which antibiotic prophylaxis was given, whereas 6 occurred after 390 procedures for which it was omitted.[28] This result, which needs to be independently confirmed by prospective studies, just reaches statistical significance.[28]

Attempted prevention of bacterial infections with antibiotics is most likely to be effective and cost-effective when a single antimicrobial drug is directed against a single pathogen and when the disease occurs with fairly high frequency in the absence of prophylaxis.[29] In the past, prevention of recurrent rheumatic fever in young patients met these conditions, and several studies proved that prevention of rheumatic fever was effective. Prevention of endocarditis does not meet these ideals, because a variety of antibiotics are used against a variety of organisms and because the disease occurs rarely even if prophylactic antibiotics are not given. Furthermore, only a small proportion (perhaps 1 to 5%, or 15% at the most) of all cases of infective endocarditis can be attributed to bacteremias caused by previous medical, surgical, or dental procedures.[9, 25, 30–32, 54] It follows that the proportion of potentially preventable cases is also small.

Because definitive data are lacking, prevention of infective endocarditis remains an empirical practice, characterized by uncertainty and controversy.[6, 31, 33, 34] Nevertheless, most authorities agree that prophylaxis should be offered to selected susceptible patients during certain procedures known to be associated with bacteremia.[3–5, 8, 25, 34] Controversy continues regarding the extent to which prophylaxis should be used and the specific risk factors for which antibiotic coverage should be provided.

ESTIMATES OF RISK FOR INFECTIVE ENDOCARDITIS

To determine whether antibiotic prophylaxis should be given to an individual patient, it is necessary to estimate that patient's relative risk of developing endocarditis. This can be done by evaluating the risks posed by the procedure versus those posed by the underlying cardiac condition.

Procedures Causing Bacteremia

The incidence of transient bacteremia after various manipulations has been extensively studied.[25, 26, 35–50] Much of the literature on infective endocarditis after dental procedures has emphasized tooth extraction, but bacteremias may occur after almost any form of dental manipulation.[25, 26] It should be noted that the reported incidence of bacteremia varies quite widely from study to study. Also, the presence in the blood of certain bacterial species associated with endocarditis, especially the viridans streptococci, may be more important than the overall frequency of bacteremia.[50] Some representative figures from selected studies are presented in Table 67–1.

Several hundred cases of endocarditis that were attributed to prior dental procedures have been recorded in the literature.[25, 51, 52] In many of these, the first symptoms of endocarditis appeared within less than 2 weeks.[52] Although the incubation period of endocarditis is not known precisely, the onset of symptoms soon after dental procedures in these cases makes a causal relationship seem likely. Similarly, more than 100 case reports provide reasonably good evidence that bacteremias originating from the genitourinary tract may cause endocarditis, especially when urologic or gynecologic procedures are carried out in the presence of bacterial infections of the urinary or reproductive system.[37] These uncontrolled case studies provide the basis for the belief that dental procedures often cause endocarditis—a belief that is widely but not universally accepted.[31, 32, 53–55]

The risk of developing infective endocarditis after a dental procedure certainly must be low, because such procedures are extremely common and they often cause bacteremias, yet endocarditis is a relatively rare disease. It has been variously estimated that the risk for a predisposed patient is 1 per 533,[27] 1 per 115,500,[56] or even zero.[55] The risk may be as high as 1.5 per 100 for patients with prosthetic valves.[57] Most authorities agree that dental operations do indeed pose some risk to susceptible patients, but it appears that the overall risk of acquiring infective endocarditis is less than 1% for each procedure, even if no antibiotic prophylaxis is given.

Evidence that other medical and surgical procedures cause infective endocarditis is sketchy. For example, only a handful of cases after miscellaneous operations such as drainage of soft tissue infections, abdominal surgery, diagnostic cardiac catheterization, and the use of oral irrigation devices have been recorded.[25, 58, 59] The frequency of bacteremia during normal delivery is very low,[60, 61] and few cases of endocarditis have been recorded in this setting.[61] Four cases following skin biopsy have been reported, two of which were due to *Staphylococcus aureus*.[62] Although bacteremias may occur during the performance of common diagnostic procedures such as endoscopy, barium enema, and liver biopsy, very few cases of endocarditis attributable to these procedures have been reported.[41, 47, 63–67] Table 67–2 presents listings of high-risk and lower-risk procedures that may cause bacteremias.

TABLE 67–1 Frequency of Bacteremia after Various Dental, Diagnostic, and Therapeutic Procedures

Procedure	% of Procedures Followed by Bacteremia	Range (if available)
None	0	0–3
Oral cavity		
Extraction of teeth	60	18–85
Periodontal surgery	88	60–90
Brushing teeth or irrigation	40	7–50
Tonsillectomy	35	33–38
Respiratory tract		
Tracheal intubation	<10	0–16
Nasotracheal suctioning	16	
Bronchoscopy: rigid bronchoscope	15	
Bronchoscopy: flexible bronchoscope	0	
Genitourinary tract		
Catheter insertion and removal	13	0–26
Prostatectomy: sterile urine	12	11–13
Prostatectomy: infected urine	60	58–82
Dilatation of strictures	28	19–86
Normal delivery	3	1–5
Intrauterine device insertion or removal	0	
Gastrointestinal tract		
Upper gastrointestinal endoscopy	4	0–8
Transesophageal echocardiography	1	0–17
Endoscopic retrograde cholangiopancreatography	5	0–6
Barium enema	10	5–11
Colonoscopy	5	0–5
Sigmoidoscopy: rigid sigmoidoscope	5	
Sigmoidoscopy: flexible sigmoidoscope	0	
Proctoscopy	2	
Hemorrhoidectomy	8	
Esophageal dilatation	45	
Vascular system		
Cardiac catheterization	2	0–5
Insufficient data		
Insertion and removal of tympanostomy tubes	?	
Cesarean section	?	

Data from studies reviewed by Everett and Hirschmann,[25] Shorvon et al.,[41] and Durack.[9, 123]

Underlying Cardiac Conditions

An assessment of risk of infective endocarditis in relation to the patient's underlying cardiac condition must also be made. The relative risks for various preexisting cardiac disorders are shown in Table 67–3. These estimates are based on the frequency with which such conditions are found in patients with infective endocarditis. Certain conditions clearly predispose to endocardial infection, including prosthetic valves, a previous episode of infective endocarditis, cyanotic congenital heart disease, congenital or acquired aortic valve disease, interventricular septal defects, and mitral stenosis or incompetence.[32, 58, 68, 69] In a case-control study, the odds ratio was 75:1 for patients with a prosthetic valve, 37:1 for patients with a previous history of infective endocarditis, and 17:1 for patients reporting any history of a cardiac valvular abnormality.[32] At the other end of the spectrum, uncomplicated secundum-type atrial septal defects carry such a low risk for infective endocarditis[58, 68] that prophylaxis is not recommended for patients with such defects.[9]

Mitral valve prolapse presents a special problem because it is common in the general population, being found in 4% or more according to the definition used.[70, 71] Mitral valve prolapse increases the risk of endocarditis by five- to eightfold[68, 70–72] and is present in 15 to 25% of the cases of subacute bacterial endocarditis.[73–75] The risk appears to be greater for those patients with a systolic murmur[72, 74] and for those with thickening and redundancy of the mitral leaflets on echocardiography.[71] Nevertheless, infective endocarditis is an uncommon disease; accordingly, mitral valve prolapse cannot be regarded as a high-risk lesion,[70] even when a murmur is present. At present, many authorities recommend prophylaxis for patients with prolapse and regurgitation.[76] A study of benefits versus costs by decision analysis indicated that prophylaxis for mitral valve prolapse could prevent some cases but probably would not be cost-effective.[77] Furthermore, because the incidence of endocarditis in patients with prolapse who undergo a dental procedure without prophylaxis is very low, the years of life lost from anaphylaxis due to parenteral penicillin could exceed the years of life saved by prevention of endocarditis.[77]

The American Heart Association (AHA) guidelines recommend that patients with mitral valve prolapse and regurgitation or thickening and redundancy of the leaflets on echocardiography should receive oral antibiotics before dental procedures because the costs and risks of taking one oral dose of amoxicillin are small, and because a serious disease may occasionally be prevented. However, the use of antibiotics could be considered optional rather than mandatory in this setting.[34] Parenteral prophylaxis should be avoided if possible.

TABLE 67–2 Risk of Infective Endocarditis with Various Procedures Associated with Potential Bacteremia

Relatively High-Risk Procedures	Lower-Risk Procedures
Dental extractions and gingival surgery, including implant placement	Other dental procedures, including orthodontia
Cystoscopy, urethral dilatation, urethral catheterization, urinary tract and prostatic surgery, if bacterial infection present	Injection of intraoral local anesthetic
Sclerotherapy for esophageal varices; esophageal dilatation	Genitourinary tract procedures or surgery in absence of bacterial infection
Incision, drainage, other surgical procedures in the presence of active bacterial infection at the site	Bronchoscopy with rigid bronchoscope
Vaginal delivery complicated by bacterial infection	Surgery involving gastrointestinal or upper respiratory mucosa in absence of bacterial infection
	Tonsillectomy or adenoidectomy
	Tympanostomy tube insertion
	Endotracheal tube insertion
	Bronchoscopy with flexible bronchoscope, with or without biopsy
	Gastrointestinal endoscopy, with or without biopsy
	Cardiac catheterization
	In the absence of bacterial infection: cesarean section, vaginal hysterectomy, urethral catheterization, dilatation and curettage, uncomplicated vaginal delivery, therapeutic abortion, insertion or removal of intrauterine devices, sterilization procedures, laparoscopy

Based on the reports by Dajani et al[76] and Durack.[34, 123]

INDIRECT EVIDENCE OF EFFICACY OF PROPHYLAXIS

In the absence of definitive data, recommendations for the prophylaxis of infective endocarditis must be based on secondary sources of information. These include anecdotal clinical experience, in vitro studies on the organisms that cause bacteremia and endocarditis, and evaluation of the prevention of infective endocarditis in experimental animals.

Uncontrolled Clinical Observations

Case reports describing patients who developed endocarditis after a procedure known to cause bacteremia despite the administration of antibiotics provide anecdotal evidence that attempts to prevent endocarditis are not uniformly successful.[75, 78] From 1979 to 1982, an AHA committee collected and recorded examples of apparent prevention failures.[75] Among 52 such cases, mitral valve prolapse was the single most common underlying cardiac lesion, present in 33%, followed by various congenital abnormalities in 29% and rheumatic heart disease in 21%; 19% had prosthetic valve endocarditis. Forty-eight cases (92%) followed a dental procedure, and 75% of cases were caused by viridans streptococci. Symptoms began fairly soon after the procedure suspected to have caused endocarditis: within 2 weeks in 50% and within 5 weeks in 79%. Most patients received oral penicillin as prophylaxis. Sixty percent of organisms for which antimicrobial susceptibility was known were sensitive to the antibiotics used for prophylaxis. This experience, although anecdotal, indicates that endocarditis prophylaxis failures may not be rare and that failures may occur even when the infecting organism is susceptible to the antibiotics used. It confirms that mitral valve prolapse is a common underlying lesion in patients with streptococcal endocarditis.

Case-Control Studies and Decision Analysis

Several case-control studies have been performed. One indicated that prophylaxis appeared to be effective,[79] but only eight cases were analyzed; in two of these, results of culture were negative. Two other large case-control studies concluded that attempted prevention with antibiotics in dental patients was of marginal or no value.[32, 53] Decision analysis led the authors of one study to doubt that prophylaxis would be cost-effective except in the highest-risk situations.[77] A cost-benefit analysis indicated that penicillin prophylaxis for dental patients would offer no net reduction in deaths.[80] These studies raise the possibility that the current practice of antibiotic prophylaxis for endocarditis is largely (or even entirely) ineffective.[34] It could even be counterproductive, by promoting antibiotic resistance and by diverting attention and resources from potentially more valuable interventions such as patient education and follow-up.

In Vitro Studies

A variety of organisms may be found in the blood stream after dental, surgical, and diagnostic procedures, including anaerobes and contaminants from the skin flora.[25, 27, 36, 81] However, only gram-positive cocci such as viridans streptococci, enterococci, and staphylococci commonly cause infective endocarditis in this setting. It is therefore appropriate to focus on the antibiotic susceptibilities of these organisms in attempting to formulate rational prophylactic programs. In the past, most of the bacteria in the oral flora that are

TABLE 67–3 Risk of Infective Endocarditis with Preexisting Cardiac Disorders

Relatively High Risk	Intermediate Risk	Very Low or Negligible Risk
Prosthetic heart valves	Mitral valve prolapse with regurgitation	Mitral valve prolapse without regurgitation
Previous infective endocarditis	Pure mitral stenosis	Trivial valvular regurgitation by echocardiography without structural abnormality
Cyanotic congenital heart disease	Tricuspid valve disease	Isolated atrial septal defect
Patent ductus arteriosus	Pulmonary stenosis	Arteriosclerotic plaques
Aortic regurgitation*	Asymmetric septal hypertrophy	Coronary artery disease
Aortic stenosis*	Bicuspid aortic valve or calcific aortic sclerosis with minimal hemodynamic abnormality	Cardiac pacemaker
Mitral regurgitation	Degenerative valvular disease in elderly patients	
Mitral stenosis and regurgitation		
Ventricular septal defect		
Coarctation of the aorta		
Surgically repaired intracardiac lesions with residual hemodynamic abnormality	Surgically repaired intracardiac lesions with minimal or no hemodynamic abnormality, less than 6 months after operation	Surgically repaired intracardiac lesions, with minimal or no hemodynamic abnormality, more than 6 months after operation

*Includes tricuspid, bicuspid, and unicuspid valves.

Adapted from Durack DT. Infective endocarditis. In: Alexander RW, Schlant RC, Fuster V, et al, eds. Hurst's The Heart, Arteries and Veins. 9th ed. New York: McGraw-Hill; 1998:2205–2239, with permission of The McGraw-Hill Companies.

likely to cause endocarditis were sensitive to penicillin G,[82] but some strains were partially resistant, with minimal bactericidal concentrations (MBCs) for penicillin G of 0.1 to 1.0 μg/ml or more.[83, 84] Ampicillin and amoxicillin possess good in vitro activity against many strains of streptococci associated with endocarditis[82] and provide good serum concentrations.[85] Unfortunately, penicillin resistance is increasing; a recent study in the United States documented strains with 43% intermediate and 13% high-level resistance among viridans streptococci.[86] Almost all strains of viridans streptococci, irrespective of their MBCs, are killed more rapidly and completely by a combination of a penicillin and an aminoglycoside than by a penicillin alone.[84, 87] Many strains of enterococci, although more likely to be resistant to both penicillins and aminoglycosides, are killed synergistically by these drugs in combination, both in vitro and in vivo.[84, 88, 89] Unfortunately, many strains of enterococci have now developed high-level resistance to penicillins, aminoglycosides, or glycopeptides, posing new problems for prophylaxis and treatment.[90]

Experimental Infective Endocarditis

Study of the prevention of experimental infective endocarditis in animal models has provided important information. In 1970 Garrison and Freedman[91] reported that placement of a polyethylene catheter in the rabbit heart led to the development of small sterile vegetations at points of contact between the catheter and endocardium. When staphylococci were placed in the lumen of the catheter, staphylococcal endocarditis resulted. Modification of this model by injecting organisms intravenously[92] provided a suitable in vivo system for examining the efficacy of various antibiotic regimens for the prophylaxis of endocarditis.[89, 93–96] A similar model in rats has also been used to investigate antibiotic prophylaxis.[97–102] Under experimental conditions, the time of onset of infective endocarditis is known exactly. Another important advantage is that the incidence of infection in untreated animals can be adjusted easily by altering the inoculum size; thus, the problem of very low infection rates in patients can be overcome by choosing an inoculum of the organism under investigation that is large enough to infect most of the animals. Significant differences among antibiotic regimens can then be demonstrated using manageable numbers of animals in each group.[89, 93, 95–101, 103, 104]

Early experiments comparing the success of various antibiotic regimens against viridans streptococci in this model system showed that bacteriostatic antibiotics were usually ineffective, that penicillin in low doses or in high doses of brief duration was often ineffective, that high penicillin concentrations in serum for 12 hours or more were more effective, that the combination of a penicillin plus an aminoglycoside was synergistic against viridans streptococci as well as enterococci, and that vancomycin provided an excellent alternative to regimens using penicillins.[89, 93, 94, 96, 103] Other antibiotics that have proved effective under controlled experimental conditions are ampicillin, amoxicillin,[95, 100, 101] ampicillin-sulbactam,[105] erythromycin,[101] clindamycin,[104] rifampin,[99] azithromycin, and clarithromycin.[106]

Further experiments have modified the view that bactericidal antibiotic activity is essential for prophylaxis. Streptomycin proved surprisingly effective in the prevention of experimental infection by some strains of enterococci, even though the serum concentrations of streptomycin were far too low to kill the organisms.[89] Subinhibitory concentrations of certain antibiotics, especially vancomycin, can inhibit the adherence of streptococci to fibrin surfaces in vitro.[107] Other experiments have demonstrated successful prophylaxis against various streptococci with sublethal doses of vancomycin, clindamycin, erythromycin, and even a tetracycline.[101, 103, 104] Penicillin was much less effective in the prevention of experimental streptococcal endocarditis if the infecting strain was tolerant to penicillin.[108] However, penicillin exhibited some prophylactic activity even if the strain was so tolerant that bactericidal concentrations of penicillin could not be achieved in serum.[108] All these findings suggest that prevention can sometimes be achieved by antibiotic effects that fall short of total bacterial killing, perhaps by an alteration of surface structures that mediate adherence to fibrin or by other unknown mechanisms. Bactericidal action may be sufficient but not necessary for prevention of endocarditis. The observation that successful prophylaxis with amoxicillin can be reversed by administration of penicillinase shortly *after* colonization of the vegetation shows that killing of organisms in the blood stream or prevention of their adherence to the endocardium is not essential for antibiotic prophylaxis in every situation.[97] The implications of these experimental findings for prophylaxis of infective endocarditis in humans are uncertain. At present, it still seems prudent to choose bactericidal drugs for the prophylaxis of infective endocarditis whenever possible.

To place these extensive experimental data into perspective, it should be emphasized that direct extrapolation of findings in animals to humans may not be meaningful. Although in vitro models provide a closer simulation of human endocarditis than any in vitro system could, there are at least two important differences. First, a foreign body was present throughout many of these experiments because the intracardiac catheter often was left in place. The presence of a foreign body in tissue lowers the inoculum required to initiate infection and then makes infection harder to eradicate. Therefore, the animal models probably simulate the situation in patients with prosthetic valves more closely than that in patients with congenital or rheumatic valvular disease. Second, in many of the experiments, a high inoculum was chosen deliberately, to make statistical comparisons possible with a relatively small number of animals. Because both the presence of a foreign body and the use of high inocula tend to make prevention harder to achieve, any regimen that proved effective under these rigorous experimental conditions is likely to provide a wide margin of safety in clinical use.

With these reservations in mind, what has been the real contribution of experimental studies of prevention? Animal models provide a convenient in vivo method for ranking prophylactic antibiotic regimens in order of efficacy, but they cannot be used to determine whether any particular antibiotic regimen will or will not prevent endocarditis in patients. For example, experimental findings do not exclude the possibility that tetracycline or other bacteriostatic drugs may prevent endocarditis in some patients. They do support the conclusion that one of the optimal bactericidal regimens such as one using vancomycin, or a β-lactam plus an aminoglycoside, should provide a much wider margin of safety than that conferred by a lower-ranking regimen such as one using erythromycin or tetracycline.[96]

PROPHYLAXIS FOR CARDIAC SURGERY

Most cardiovascular surgeons believe that the use of prophylactic antibiotics has reduced the incidence of postcardiotomy endocarditis.[69] Although this may be true, it should be noted that numerous technical improvements, introduced during the period when the incidence of postoperative endocarditis was falling, also may have contributed significantly. In fact, the efficacy of antibiotics for the prevention of postcardiotomy endocarditis has not yet been proved in any definitive controlled trial. However, the proven ability of antibiotics to prevent some other postoperative infections would make it difficult or impossible to obtain ethical approval to conduct a placebo-controlled trial.

Early-onset postcardiotomy endocarditis may be caused by a variety of organisms including staphylococci, gram-negative bacteria, and, rarely, fungi. No single antibiotic regimen is effective against all potential pathogens, and the use of broad-spectrum antibiotics may in itself predispose to superinfection with resistant organisms. Therefore, attempts to prevent endocarditis with antibiotics during open heart surgery should probably be limited to a short course of an antistaphylococcal agent such as a cephalosporin or vancomycin.[9] Some authorities recommend adding 1 to 3 doses of an aminoglycoside in the hope of taking advantage of possible synergism.

Diagnostic cardiac catheterizations (including Swan-Ganz catheters), insertion of pacemakers, coronary artery surgery, pericardial surgery, and the use of an intra-aortic balloon pump all appear to present little risk, and the administration of antibiotics specifically for the prevention of infective endocarditis is not usually recommended for these operations. Pulmonary artery catheters have been reported to predispose to both nonbacterial and bacterial endocarditis in patients with severe burns, who often develop bacteremias, but because these are often left in place over long periods, attempted antibiotic prophylaxis specifically for endocarditis is not indicated.[109]

Prosthetic Heart Valves

Extensive clinical experience has established that patients with prosthetic heart valves are at a relatively high risk for infective endocarditis.[28, 32, 68, 69, 110, 111] The high mortality and morbidity associated with prosthetic valve endocarditis and re-replacement of valves make its prevention a priority. Although the incidence of endocarditis after cardiac surgery has fallen steadily since these operations first became commonplace, the risk of early-onset endocarditis within 60 days of valve replacement remains in the region of 0.3 to 0.5% per year; thereafter, the risk approximates 0.5 to 1% per year.[69, 111] For comparison, the incidence of endocarditis is approximately 0.4% per year in patients with rheumatic heart disease.[112] It is important to recognize this risk and to take all possible steps to minimize it. Before elective valve replacement, the dental health of the patient must be evaluated and any necessary dental work completed under close medical observation and with appropriate antibiotic coverage. Healthy teeth should not be extracted, but if advanced dental or periodontal disease is present, extraction of all teeth should be considered. Thereafter, the patient should maintain good oral hygiene. Consultation between the patient's dentist and physician is important to ensure optimal antibiotic coverage during routine dental procedures. Some practitioners choose to administer antibiotic prophylaxis before diagnostic procedures such as colonoscopy that present negligible risk in patients without prosthetic valves (see Tables 67–1 and 67–2).

Late-onset prosthetic valve endocarditis (60 days after the operation) is more likely to be caused by organisms originating in the oral cavity and reaching the valve via the blood stream, just as for native valve endocarditis. Attempted prophylaxis for endocarditis in the setting of a dental procedure should be directed primarily against streptococci, not staphylococci or gram-negative bacilli, just as for patients without prosthetic valves.

Many cardiac patients receive anticoagulant therapy, which may alter the choice of prophylactic antibiotics. Intramuscular injections are contraindicated in patients receiving heparin and should be avoided if possible in patients receiving warfarin sodium. Usually an oral dose is used, but if parenteral antibiotic is given, the intravenous route should be used.

Timing of Prophylaxis

Antibiotics should be administered so as to provide peak serum levels at the time when the procedure that may cause bacteremia is performed. There is no rationale to support the common practice of beginning antibiotic therapy earlier than is necessary to meet this criterion. Indeed, if antibiotics are given more than a few hours before the procedure, penicillin-sensitive oral flora may be replaced by penicillin-resistant organisms, and endocarditis, should it occur, may be caused by resistant organisms.[78] For most regimens, the administration of antibiotics 30 to 60 minutes before the procedure is appropriate. If the operation is delayed for more than 1 to 2 hours, the dose should be repeated.

Duration of Prophylaxis

A single dose of antibiotic should suffice, as indicated by the success of single-dose regimens in animal models.[92–94, 96, 100] Many practitioners continue prophylaxis for longer than necessary.[75, 113, 114] This wastes antibiotic, may lead to the emergence of resistant organisms, and places the patient at an additional risk of adverse reactions. Moreover, a patient who is feeling perfectly well is unlikely to adhere to an unnecessarily prolonged regimen.

Prevention of Rheumatic Fever versus Prevention of Infective Endocarditis

Administration of low-dose penicillin orally or by monthly injection effectively prevents recurrences of rheumatic fever but is *inadequate* to prevent infective endocarditis. The incidence of infective endocarditis in children receiving penicillin for the prevention of rheumatic fever is no lower than in those with rheumatic heart disease who are not receiving prophylaxis.[112] Because patients taking low-dose oral penicillin for the prevention of rheumatic fever often carry moderately penicillin-resistant streptococci in the mouth, attempted prevention of infective endocarditis with an oral penicillin regimen in these patients is not advisable. They should receive clindamycin as an alternative (Table 67–4).

Prophylaxis for Children

Because bacteremia during dental procedures appears to be somewhat less common in children than in adults, it has been suggested that antibiotic prophylaxis for infective endocarditis is unnecessary in children.[116] However, careful studies indicate that bacteremia does indeed occur in a significant proportion of children after dental procedures,[117] and cases of endocarditis following soon after dental extraction have been reported.[117] The present consensus, therefore, is that children should receive antibiotic prophylaxis for infective endocarditis, with appropriate adjustment of dosages.

Compliance with Guidelines

Numerous studies and surveys have shown that most practitioners are aware of current recommendations, regarding them as authoritative. Nevertheless, physicians often do not follow these guidelines in practice.[118–120] The reasons for failure to comply with recommendations are not clear. However, compliance may be improving gradually over time.[115]

TABLE 67–4 Recommendations for Antibiotic Prophylaxis of Infective Endocarditis*

High-Risk vs. Lower-Risk Procedures†	Underlying Cardiac Risk Factors‡		
	Relatively High Risk	*Intermediate Risk*	*Very Low or Negligible Risk*
Relatively high-risk procedures	Prophylaxis recommended	Prophylaxis recommended	Prophylaxis not recommended
Lower-risk procedures	Optional—clinical judgment needed	Prophylaxis not recommended	Prophylaxis not recommended

*Note that antibiotics might be given in these settings for prevention of infections other than endocarditis, or for other indications.
†See Table 67–2.
‡See Table 67–3.

TABLE 67–5 Recommended Regimens for Prophylaxis of Endocarditis*

Indication	Regimen
Standard regimen	
For dental procedures; oral or upper respiratory tract surgery; minor GI or GU tract procedures	Amoxicillin, 2.0 g PO 1 h before†
Special regimens	
Oral regimen for penicillin-allergic patients (oral and respiratory tract only)	Clindamycin 600 mg PO 1 h before; then 300 mg 6 h later† *or* clarithromycin 0.5 g PO 1 h before
Parenteral regimen for high-risk patients; also for GI or GU tract procedures	Ampicillin 2.0 g IM or IV, *plus* gentamicin 1.5 mg/kg IM or IV, 0.5 h before
Parenteral regimen for penicillin-allergic patients	Vancomycin 1.0 g IV slowly over 1 h, starting 1 h before *Add* gentamicin, 1.5 mg/kg IM or IV, if GI or GU tract involved†
Cardiac surgery including implantation of prosthetic valves	Cefazolin 2.0 g IV at induction of anesthesia, repeated 8 and 16 h later†‡ *or* vancomycin 1.0 g IV slowly over 1 h starting at induction; then 0.5 g IV 12 h later†‡§

*__Note:__ No regimen has been proved effective for the prevention of endocarditis, and prevention failures may occur with any regimen. These guidelines do not define the standard of care and are not intended to cover all situations; the practitioner should use good clinical judgment on safety and cost-benefit issues in each case. One or two additional doses may be given if the period of risk for bacteremia is prolonged.
†Pediatric dosages: For ampicillin, 50 mg/kg; for cefazolin, 30 mg/kg; for clindamycin, in children who weigh more than 60 lb, use the same dose as for adults, and in children less than 60 lb, use half the adult dose; for gentamicin, 2.0 mg/kg; for amoxicillin, in children who weigh more than 60 lb, use the same dose as for adults, and in children less than 60 lb, use half the adult dose; and for vancomycin, 20 mg/kg.
‡Gentamicin 1.5 mg/kg IV may be given with each dose if postoperative gram-negative infections have occurred with significant frequency.
§This regimen is recommended for use in clinical units in which coagulase-negative staphylococcal prosthetic valve infections have occurred with significant frequency.
Abbreviations: GI, Gastrointestinal; GU, genitourinary.
Adapted from Dajani et al,[76] Durack,[9, 123] and Simmons.[122]

THE MALPRACTICE DILEMMA

The issue of professional liability in the prophylaxis of endocarditis often has led to allegations of negligence and malpractice claims.[121] Clearly, the lack of basic factual information, as noted previously, makes evaluation of such cases difficult. For example, it is hard to establish that any single procedure known to cause bacteremia was the "proximate cause" in a case of endocarditis. It is even harder to prove that the failure of a physician or a dentist to administer antibiotics was the direct cause of a patient's acquiring endocarditis. If strict demonstration of proximate cause were always required, it is doubtful that any claim based on the failure to administer prophylaxis could succeed, but juries are sometimes capricious in deciding liability in malpractice cases. Another common problem for the defense in claims based on failure to administer prophylaxis is our ignorance of the precise duration of the incubation period of infective endocarditis. Damages have been claimed when the first symptoms of endocarditis did not appear for months after a tooth extraction without antibiotic coverage. The likelihood of proximate cause in this circumstance is remote, because review of case reports indicates that the incubation period is 2 weeks or less in most instances.[52]

A reasonable standard of care requires that health care professionals be aware of the factors that may increase the risk of infective endocarditis. The practitioner should question the patient about underlying conditions that may predispose to endocarditis and should inform susceptible patients of the small risk that they may develop the disease. For the small subgroup of patients judged to be at relatively high risk, an antibiotic regimen should be administered before selected dental, surgical, and genitourinary tract manipulations that might cause bacteremia.[34, 76] Indications for prophylaxis outside these areas are less firmly established at present. A failure to use any recognized antibiotic regimen in preference to another should not be construed as negligence, because many different regimens have been published over the past 30 years. Although some authorities recognize evidence that certain antibiotic regimens probably provide a wider margin of efficacy than is conferred by others,[76, 122] this evidence is not yet firm enough to make the choice of any particular regimen mandatory.

The risks of toxicity from any prophylactic regimen must be considered carefully. Allergic reactions may occur even after low doses of penicillin; this risk is common to all regimens using a penicillin as the drug of choice. However, the risk of anaphylaxis to penicillin is much higher for parenteral than for oral administration. Other side effects such as ototoxicity and nephrotoxicity from aminoglycosides or vancomycin are extremely unlikely to occur after the very short courses (1 day or less) now used for the prophylaxis of infective endocarditis.

CURRENT RECOMMENDATIONS

An AHA committee[76] and various other authorities have published guidelines for the prophylaxis of infective endocarditis in the United States. Many groups in other countries have produced similar recommendations.[122] My recommendations are summarized in Tables 67–4 and 67–5.

REFERENCES

1. Tornos M-P, Permanyer-Miralda G, Olona M, et al. Long-term complications of native valve infective endocarditis in non-addicts. A 15-year follow-up study. Ann Intern Med. 1992;117:567–572.
2. Ormiston JA, Neutze JM, Agnew TM, et al. Infective endocarditis: A lethal disease. Aust N Z J Med. 1981;11:620–629.
3. Pallasch TJ. Antibiotic prophylaxis: The clinical significance of its recent evolution. J Calif Dent Assoc. 1997:25:619–632.
4. McGowan DA. A dental view of controversies in the prophylaxis of infective endocarditis. J Antimicrob Chemother. 1987;20(Suppl.A):105–109.
5. Kaye D. Prevention of bacterial endocarditis: 1991. Ann Intern Med. 1991;114:803–804.
6. Greenman RL, Bisno AL. Prevention of bacterial endocarditis. In: Kaye D, ed. Infective Endocarditis. 2nd ed. New York: Raven Press; 1992:465–481.
7. Finch R. Chemoprophylaxis of infective endocarditis. Scand J Infect Dis. 1990;70:102–110.
8. Durack DT. Current issues in prevention of infective endocarditis. Am J Med. 1985;78:149–156.
9. Durack DT. Prevention of infective endocarditis. N Engl J Med. 1995;332:38–44.
10. Thilen U, Astrom-Olsson K. Does the risk of infective endarteritis justify routine patent ductus arteriosus closure? Eur Heart J. 1997;18:503–506.
11. Daly C, Mitchell D, Grossberg D, et al. Bacteraemia caused by periodontal probing. Aust Dent J. 1997;42:77–80.
12. Viscount HB, Munro CL, Burnette-Curley D, et al. Immunization with FimA protects against *Streptococcus parasanguis* endocarditis in rats. Infect Immun. 1997;65:994–1002.
13. Adler SW, Selinger DS, Reed WP. Effect of immunization on the genesis of pneumococcal endocarditis in rabbits. Infect Immun. 1981;34:55–61.
14. Archer GL, Johnston JL. Effect of type-specific active immunization on the development and progression of experimental *Pseudomonas aeruginosa* endocarditis. Infect Immun. 1979;24:167–173.
15. Durack DT, Gilliland BC, Petersdorf RG. Effect of immunization on susceptibility to experimental *Streptococcus mutans* and *Streptococcus sanguis* endocarditis. Infect Immun. 1978;22:52–56.

16. Scheld WM, Thomas JH, Sande MA. Influence of preformed antibody on experimental *Streptococcus sanguis* endocarditis. Infect Immun. 1979;25:781–785.
17. Schennings T, Heimdahl A, Coster K, Flock JI. Immunization with fibronectin binding protein from *Staphylococcus aureus* protects against experimental endocarditis in rats. Microb Pathog. 1993;15:227–236.
18. Takeda S, Pier GB, Kojima Y, et al. Protection against endocarditis due to *Staphylococcus epidermidis* by immunization with capsular polysaccharide/adhesin. Circulation. 1991;84:2539–2546.
19. van de Rijn I. Role of culture conditions and immunization in experimental nutritionally variant streptococcal endocarditis. Infect Immun. 1985;50:641–646.
20. Lee JC, Park JS, Shepherd SE, et al. Protective efficacy of antibodies to the *Staphylococcus aureus* type 5 capsular polysaccharide in a modified model of endocarditis in rats. Infect Immun. 1997;65:4146–4151.
21. Kojima Y, Tojo M, Goldmann DA, et al. Antibody to the capsular polysaccharide/adhesin protects rabbits against catheter-related bacteremia due to coagulase-negative staphylococci. J Infect Dis. 1990;162:435–441.
22. Nilsson IM, Patti JM, Bremell T, et al. Vaccination with a recombinant fragment of collagen adhesin provides protection against *Staphylococcus aureus*–mediated septic death. J Clin Invest. 1998;101:2640–2649.
23. Hook EWI, Sande MA. Role of the vegetation in experimental *Streptococcus viridans* endocarditis. Infect Immun. 1974;10:1433–1438.
24. Bender IB, Naidorf IJ, Garvey GJ. Bacterial endocarditis: A consideration for physician and dentist. J Am Dent Assoc. 1984;109:415–450.
25. Everett ED, Hirschmann JV. Transient bacteremia and endocarditis prophylaxis. A review. Medicine. 1977;56:61–77.
26. Cobe HM. Transitory bacteremia. Oral Surg Oral Med Oral Pathol. 1954;7:609–615.
27. Kelson SR, White PD. Notes on 250 cases of subacute bacterial (streptococcal) endocarditis studied and treated between 1927 and 1939. Ann Intern Med. 1945;22:40–60.
28. Horstkotte D, Friedrichs W, Pippert H, et al. Nutzen der endokarditisprophylaxe bei patienten mit prothetischen herzklappen. Z Kardiol. 1986;75:8–11.
29. Sanford JP. Prophylactic use of antibiotics: Basic considerations. South Med J. 1977;70(Suppl 1):2–3.
30. Meyer GW. Antibiotic prophylaxis for gastrointestinal procedures: Who needs it? Gastrointest Endosc. 1994;40:645–646.
31. Guntheroth WG. How important are dental procedures as a cause of infective endocarditis? Am J Cardiol. 1984;54:797–801.
32. Strom BL, Abrutyn E, Berlin JA, et al. Dental and cardiac risk factors for infective endocarditis: A population-based case-control study. Ann Intern Med. 1998;129:761–769.
33. Chemoprophylaxis for infective endocarditis: Faith, hope, and charity challenged (Editorial). Lancet. 1992;339:525–526.
34. Durack DT. Antibiotics for prevention of endocarditis during dentistry: Time to scale back? Ann Intern Med. 1998;129:829–831.
35. Elliott SD. Bacteraemia and oral sepsis. Proc R Soc Med. 1939;32:747–754.
36. Rogosa M, Hampp EG, Nevin TA, et al. Blood sampling and cultural studies in the detection of postoperative bacteremias. J Am Dent Assoc. 1960;60:171–180.
37. Slade N. Bacteriaemia and septicaemia after urological operations. Proc R Soc Med. 1958;51:331–334.
38. LeFrock JL, Ellis CA, Turchik JB, Weinstein L. Transient bacteremia associated with sigmoidoscopy. N Engl J Med. 1973;289:467–469.
39. Le Frock J, Ellis CA, Klainer AS, Weinstein L. Transient bacteremia associated with barium enema. Arch Intern Med. 1975;135:835–837.
40. Hoffman BI, Kobasa W, Kaye D. Bacteremia after rectal examination. Ann Intern Med. 1978;88:658–659.
41. Shorvon PJ, Eykyn SJ, Cotton PB. Gastrointestinal instrumentation, bacteraemia, and endocarditis. Gut. 1983;24:1078–1093.
42. Baltch AL, Pressman HL, Schaffer C, et al. Bacteremia in patients undergoing oral procedures. Study following parenteral antimicrobial prophylaxis as recommended by the American Heart Association, 1977. Arch Intern Med. 1988;148:1084–1088.
43. Lamich R, Alonso C, Guma JR, et al. Prospective study of bacteremia during transesophageal echocardiography. Am Heart J. 1993;125:1454–1455.
44. Botoman VA, Surawicz CM. Bacteremia with gastrointestinal endoscopic procedures. Gastrointest Endosc. 1986;32:342–346.
45. Low DE, Shoenut JP, Kennedy JK, et al. Risk of bacteremia with endoscopic sphincterotomy. Can J Surg. 1987;30:421–423.
46. Ho H, Zuckerman MJ, Wassem C. A prospective controlled study of the risk of bacteremia in emergency sclerotherapy of esophageal varices. Gastroenterology. 1991;101:1642–1648.
47. Rodriguez W, Levine JS. Enterococcal endocarditis following flexible sigmoidoscopy. West J Med. 1984;140:951–953.
48. Low DE, Shoenut JP, Kennedy JK, et al. Prospective assessment of risk of bacteremia with colonoscopy and polypectomy. Dig Dis Sci. 1987;32:1239–1243.
49. Wolf D, Fleischer D, Sivak MV Jr. Incidence of bacteremia with elective upper gastrointestinal endoscopic laser therapy. Gastrointest Endosc. 1985;31:247–250.
50. Lockhart PB. An analysis of bacteremias during dental extractions. A double-blind, placebo-controlled study of chlorhexidine. Arch Intern Med. 1996;156:513–520.
51. Sale L. Some tragic results following extraction of teeth. II. J Am Dent Assoc. 1939;26:1647–1651.
52. Starkebaum MK, Durack DT, Beeson PB. The "incubation period" of subacute bacterial endocarditis. Yale J Biol Med. 1977;50:49–58.
53. van der Meer JTM, Van Wijk W, Thompson J, et al. Efficacy of antibiotic prophylaxis for prevention of native-valve endocarditis. Lancet. 1992;339:135–140.
54. van der Meer JTM, Thompson J, Valkenburg HA, Michel MF. Epidemiology of bacterial endocarditis in the Netherlands. II. Antecedent procedures and use of prophylaxis. Arch Intern Med. 1992;152:1869–1873.
55. Schwartz SP, Salman I. The effects of oral surgery on the course of patients with diseases of the heart. Am J Orthod. 1942;28:331–345.
56. Pogrel MA, Welsby PD. The dentist and prevention of infective endocarditis. Br Dent J. 1975;139:12–16.
57. Horstkotte D, Rosin H, Friedrichs W, Loogen F. Contribution for choosing the optimal prophylaxis of bacterial endocarditis. Eur Heart J. 1987;8:379–381.
58. Herrington DA, Hall RH, Losonsky G, et al. Toxin, toxin-coregulated pili, and the toxR regulon are essential for *Vibrio cholerae* pathogenesis in humans. J Exp Med. 1988;168:1487–1492.
59. Drapkin MS. Endocarditis after the use of an oral irrigation device. Ann Intern Med. 1977;87:455.
60. Sugrue D, Blake S, Troy P, MacDonald D. Antibiotic prophylaxis against infective endocarditis after normal delivery—is it necessary? Br Heart J. 1980;44:499–502.
61. Seaworth BJ, Durack DT. Infective endocarditis in obstetric and gynecologic practice. Am J Obstet Gynecol. 1986;154:180–188.
62. Spelman DW, Weinmann A, Spicer WJ. Endocarditis following skin procedures. J Infect. 1993;26:185–189.
63. Logan RF, Hastings JGM. Bacterial endocarditis: A complication of gastroscopy. BMJ. 1988;296:1107.
64. Pritchard TM, Foust RT, Cantey JR, Leman RB. Prosthetic valve endocarditis due to *Cardiobacterium hominis* occurring after upper gastrointestinal endoscopy. Am J Med. 1991;90:516–518.
65. Rigilino J, Mahapatra R, Barnhill J, Gutierrez J. Enterococcal endocarditis following sigmoidoscopy and mitral valve prolapse. Arch Intern Med. 1984;144:850–851.
66. Norfleet RG. Infectious endocarditis after fiberoptic sigmoidoscopy with a literature review. J Clin Gastroenterol. 1991;13:448–451.
67. Niv Y. Bacterial endocarditis after Hurst bougienage in a patient with a benign esophageal stricture and mitral valve prolapse. Gastrointest Endosc. 1985;31:265–267.
68. Steckelberg JM, Wilson WR. Risk factors for infective endocarditis. Infect Dis Clin North Am. 1993;7:9–19.
69. Braimbridge MV, Eykyn SJ. Prosthetic valve endocarditis. J Antimicrob Chemother. 1987;20:173–180.
70. Clemens JD, Horwitz RI, Jaffe CC, et al. A controlled evaluation of the risk of bacterial endocarditis in persons with mitral-valve prolapse. N Engl J Med. 1982;307:776–781.
71. Marks AR, Choong CY, Sanfilippo AJ, Weyman AE. Identification of high-risk and low-risk subgroups of patients with mitral-valve prolapse. N Engl J Med. 1989;320:1031–1036.
72. Danchin N, Briancon S, Mathiew P, et al. Mitral valve prolapse as a risk factor for infective endocarditis. Lancet. 1989;1:743–745.
73. Nolan CM, Kane JJ, Grunow WA. Infective endocarditis and mitral prolapse: A comparison with other types of endocarditis. Arch Intern Med. 1981;141:447–450.
74. MacMahon SW, Hickey AJ, Wilcken DEL, et al. Risk of infective endocarditis in mitral valve prolapse with and without precordial systolic murmurs. Am J Cardiol. 1986;58:105–108.
75. Durack DT, Kaplan EL, Bisno AL. Apparent failures of endocarditis prophylaxis: Analysis of 52 cases submitted to a national registry. JAMA. 1983;250:2318–2322.
76. Dajani AS, Taubert KA, Wilson W, et al. Prevention of bacterial endocarditis. Recommendations by the American Heart Association. Circulation. 1997;96:358–366.
77. Clemens JD, Ransohoff DF. A quantitative assessment of pre-dental antibiotic prophylaxis for patients with mitral-valve prolapse. J Chron Dis. 1984;37:531–544.
78. Garrod LP, Waterworth PM. The risks of dental extraction during penicillin treatment. Br Heart J. 1962;24:39–46.
79. Imperiale TF, Horwitz RI. Does prophylaxis prevent postdental infective endocarditis? A controlled evaluation of protective efficacy. Am J Med. 1990;88:131–136.
80. Bor DH, Himmelstein DU. Endocarditis prophylaxis for patients with mitral valve prolapse: A quantitative analysis. Am J Med. 1984;76:711–717.
81. Nikutta P, Mantey-Stiers F, Becht I, et al. Risk of bacteremia induced by transesophageal echocardiography: Analysis of 100 consecutive procedures. J Am Soc Echocardiogr. 1992;5:168–172.
82. Basker MJ, Sutherland R. Activity of amoxycillin, alone, and in combination with aminoglycoside antibiotics against streptococci associated with bacterial endocarditis. J Antimicrob Chemother. 1977;3:273–282.
83. Blount JG. Bacterial endocarditis. Am J Med. 1965;38:909–922.
84. Wilson WR, Geraci JE, Wilkowske CJ, Washington JA. Short-term intramuscular therapy with procaine penicillin plus streptomycin for infective endocarditis due to viridans streptococci. Circulation. 1978;57:1158–1161.
85. Shanson DC. The prophylaxis of infective endocarditis. J Antimicrob Chemother. 1978;4:2–4.
86. Doern GV, Ferraro MJ, Brueggmann AB, Ruoff KL. Emergence of high rates of antimicrobial resistance among viridans group streptococci in the United States. Antimicrob Agents Chemother. 1996;40:891–894.
87. Wolfe JC, Johnson WD. Penicillin-sensitive streptococcal endocarditis. In-vitro and clinical observations on penicillin-streptomycin therapy. Ann Intern Med. 1974;81:178–181.
88. Russell EJ, Sutherland R. Activity of amoxycillin against enterococci and synergism with aminoglycoside antibiotics. J Med Microbiol. 1973;8:1–10.
89. Durack DT, Starkebaum MK, Petersdorf RG. Chemotherapy of experimental streptococcal endocarditis. VI. Prevention of enterococcal endocarditis. J Lab Clin Med. 1977;90:171–179.

90. Murray BE. The life and times of the enterococcus. Clin Microbiol Rev. 1990;3:46–65.
91. Garrison PK, Freedman LR. Experimental endocarditis I. Staphylococcal endocarditis in rabbits resulting from placement of a polyethylene catheter in the right side of the heart. Yale J Biol Med. 1970;42:394–410.
92. Durack DT, Beeson PB, Petersdorf RG. Experimental bacterial endocarditis. III. Production and progress of the disease in rabbits. Br J Exp Pathol. 1973;54:142–151.
93. Durack DT, Petersdorf RG. Chemotherapy of experimental streptococcal endocarditis. I. Comparison of commonly recommended prophylactic regimens. J Clin Invest. 1973;52:592–598.
94. Pelletier LL Jr, Durack DT. Chemotherapy of experimental streptococcal endocarditis. J Clin Invest. 1975;56:319–330.
95. McGowan DA, Nair S, MacFarlane TW, MacKenzie D. Prophylaxis of experimental endocarditis in rabbits using one or two doses of amoxycillin. Br Dent J. 1983;155:88–90.
96. Durack DT. Experience with prevention of experimental endocarditis. In: Kaplan EL, Taranta AV, eds. Infective Endocarditis. An American Heart Association Symposium. American Heart Association Monograph Number 52. Dallas, Tex: American Heart Association, Inc; 1977:28–32.
97. Moreillon P, Francioli P, Overholser D, et al. Mechanisms of successful amoxicillin prophylaxis of experimental endocarditis due to *Streptococcus intermedius*. J Infect Dis. 1986;154:801–807.
98. Overholser CD, Moreillon P, Glauser MP. Experimental bacterial endocarditis after dental extractions in rats with periodontitis. J Infect Dis. 1987;155:107–112.
99. Malinverni R, Bille J, Glauser MP. Single-dose rifampin prophylaxis for experimental endocarditis induced by high bacterial inocula of viridans streptococci. J Infect Dis. 1987;156:151–157.
100. Malinverni R, Francioli PB, Glauser MP. Comparison of single and multiple doses of prophylactic antibiotics in experimental streptococcal endocarditis. Circulation. 1987;76:376–382.
101. Malinverni R, Overholser CD, Bille J, Glauser MP. Antibiotic prophylaxis of experimental endocarditis after dental extractions. Lab Invest. 1988;77:182–187.
102. Berney P, Francioli P. Successful prophylaxis of experimental streptococcal endocarditis with single-dose amoxicillin administered after bacterial challenge. J Infect Dis. 1990;161:281–285.
103. Bernard J, Francioli P, Glauser MP. Vancomycin prophylaxis of experimental *Streptococcus sanguis*; inhibition of bacterial adherence rather than bacterial killing. J Clin Invest. 1981;68:1113–1116.
104. Glauser MP, Francioli P. Successful prophylaxis against experimental streptococcal endocarditis with bacteriostatic antibiotics. J Infect Dis. 1982;146:806–810.
105. Ramos MC, Ing M, Kim E, et al. Ampicillin-sulbactam is effective in prevention and therapy of experimental endocarditis caused by beta-lactamase–producing coagulase-negative staphylococci. Antimicrob Agents Chemother. 1996;40:97–101.
106. Rouse MS, Steckelberg JM, Brandt CM, et al. Efficacy of azithromycin or clarithromycin for prophylaxis of viridans group streptococcus experimental endocarditis. Antimicrob Agents Chemother. 1997;41:1673–1676.
107. Scheld WM, Zak O, Vosbeck K, Sande MS. Bacterial adhesion in the pathogenesis of infective endocarditis. Effect of subinhibitory antibiotic concentrations on streptococcal adhesion in vitro and the development of endocarditis in rabbits. J Clin Invest. 1981;68:1381–1384.
108. Hess J, Dankert J, Durack DT. Significance of penicillin tolerance in endocarditis. Antimicrob Agents Chemother. 1983;11:555–564.
109. Ehrie M, Morgan AP, Moore FD, O'Connor NE. Endocarditis with the indwelling balloon-tipped pulmonary artery catheter in burn patients. J Trauma. 1978;18:665–666.
110. Ivert TSA, Dismukes WE, Cobbs CG, et al. Prosthetic valve endocarditis. Circulation. 1984;69:223–232.
111. Eliopoulos GM. Enterococcal endocarditis. In: Kaye D, ed. Infective Endocarditis. 2nd ed. New York: Raven Press; 1992:209–229.
112. Doyle EF, Spagnuolo M, Taranta A, et al. The risk of bacterial endocarditis during antirheumatic prophylaxis. JAMA. 1967;201:129–134.
113. Durack DT. Current practice in prevention of bacterial endocarditis. Br Heart J. 1975;37:478–481.
114. Brooks SL. Survey of compliance with American Heart Association guidelines for prevention of bacterial endocarditis. J Am Dent Assoc. 1980;101:41–43.
115. Brooks RG, Notario G, McCabe RE. Hospital survey of antimicrobial prophylaxis to prevent endocarditis in patients with prosthetic heart valves. Am J Med. 1988;84:617–621.
116. Hurwitz GA, Speck WT, Keller GB. Absence of bacteremia in children after prophylaxis. Oral Surg Oral Med Oral Pathol. 1971;32:891–894.
117. Johnson DH, Rosenthal A, Nadas AS. A forty-year review of bacterial endocarditis in infancy and childhood. Circulation. 1975;51:581–588.
118. Kunzel C, Sadowsky D. Knowledge acquisition processes: Dissemination of expert recommendations to general practice dentists. J Health Soc Behav. 1989;30:330–343.
119. Sadowsky D, Kunzel C. Recommendations for prevention of bacterial endocarditis: Compliance by dental general practitioners. Circulation. 1988;77:1316–1318.
120. van der Meer JTM, Van Wijk W, Thompson J, et al. Awareness of need and actual use of prophylaxis: Lack of patient compliance in the prevention of bacterial endocarditis. J Antimicrob Chemother. 1992;29:187–194.
121. Martin MV, Butterworth ML, Longman LP. Infective endocarditis and the dental practitioner: A review of 53 cases involving litigation. Br Dent J. 1997;182:465–468.
122. Simmons NA. Recommendations for endocarditis prophylaxis. J Antimicrob Chemother. 1993;31:437–453.
123. Durack DT. Prophylaxis of infective endocarditis. In: Mandell GL, Douglas RG Jr, Dolin R, eds. Principles and Practice of Infectious Diseases. 4th ed. New York: Churchill Livingstone; 1995:793–813.

Chapter 68

Myocarditis and Pericarditis

MARIA C. SAVOIA
MICHAEL N. OXMAN

Inflammatory processes affecting the heart frequently involve both the myocardium (myocarditis) and the pericardium (pericarditis). However, involvement of one or the other usually predominates, and the syndromes of myocarditis and pericarditis are sufficiently distinct in clinical presentation, etiology, and pathophysiology to warrant separate consideration.

MYOCARDITIS

Myocarditis, literally "inflammation of the myocardium," is a protean disease with a wide variety of infectious and noninfectious causes. Postmortem examinations reveal evidence of previously unsuspected myocarditis in 1 to 4% of unselected cases,[1, 2] with a higher incidence in young persons who have died suddenly.[3, 4] The diagnosis of infectious myocarditis usually is considered when unexplained heart failure or arrhythmias occur in the setting of a systemic febrile illness or after symptoms of an upper respiratory tract infection. In some cases, however, the antecedent systemic illness is mild or long forgotten. In addition, myocarditis has been found histologically in 10 to 20% of cases of idiopathic dilated cardiomyopathy.[5] In myocarditis, the inflammatory process may affect myocytes, vascular elements, the conducting system, autonomic nerves, or the interstitium. One or more of at least four mechanisms appear to be involved: (1) direct damage to cells by an infectious agent; (2) cytotoxicity caused by a circulating toxin; (3) cytotoxicity caused by infection-induced immune reactions; and (4) nonspecific damage to myocytes as a result of an adjacent inflammatory process. Damage to the vascular endothelium may also result in indirect myocardial injury.

Etiologic Agents

In most cases of myocarditis, no definite cause is ever established. Viruses are the most important infectious cause of myocarditis in the United States and western Europe, and many cases of idiopathic myocarditis are assumed to be viral in origin. Long before the era of modern virology, pericardial and myocardial involvement was recognized during outbreaks of mumps,[6] influenza,[7] measles,[8–10] poliomyelitis,[11] and enterovirus-associated pleurodynia.[12] In modern times, enteroviruses[13, 14] and especially group B coxsackieviruses[15, 16] have been the major agents implicated. These small, nonenveloped, single-stranded RNA viruses belonging to the picornavirus family attach to specific receptors on myocardial cells.[13] When sensitive techniques such as in situ hybridization or the polymerase chain reaction (PCR) are employed, enterovirus genome has been found in approximately 25% of persons with myocarditis and in 15% of samples of patients with dilated cardiomyopathy.[17] A study of 34 children with myocarditis using PCR found adenovirus genome in 15, enterovirus in 8, herpes simplex virus in 2, and cytomegalovirus in 1.[18] Symptomatic myocarditis or myopericarditis has also been reported in persons infected with many other viruses; additional viruses reported to cause myocarditis are listed in Table 68–1.

Myocardial involvement is the most common cause of death in diphtheria[60]; the toxin produced by *Corynebacterium diphtheriae* severely damages the myocardium and conduction system. The cardiac damage seen in patients with *Clostridium perfringens* may be the result of toxin, metastatic abscess formation, or both.[62, 63] The immunologically mediated carditis associated with acute rheumatic fever[64] is discussed in Chapter 187.

Invasion of the blood stream by any bacterial pathogen may result in metastatic foci in the myocardium, and myocarditis has been recognized in the course of meningococcemia,[66] salmonellosis,[67] brucellosis,[70] and streptococcal and staphylococcal bacteremia.[72] More commonly, bacteria invade the myocardium as a complication of endocarditis by contiguous spread from valvular tissue or via septic embolization of the coronary arteries.[115]

Myocarditis is a rare complication during *Legionella* infection.[76] Myocarditis has also been observed in the course of *Mycoplasma pneumoniae*,[77, 78] *Chlamydia psittaci*,[80] and *Chlamydia pneumoniae*[81, 82] infections and is commonly seen in rickettsial infections,[83] especially scrub typhus.[59, 84, 85] Approximately 10% of patients with Lyme disease develop cardiac abnormalities, most commonly conduction system disturbances; full recovery is the norm.[88, 89, 91] In South America, the principal agent responsible for myocarditis is *Trypanosoma cruzi*, the protozoan that causes Chagas disease. The initial infection is often asymptomatic, but it sometimes results in an acute illness complicated by myocarditis.[99] Myocarditis is the principal manifestation of chronic Chagas disease, which occurs in approximately 30% of infected individuals. These patients typically have cardiomegaly, congestive heart failure (often predominantly right-sided), and conduction disturbances.[100, 101] *Trypanosoma gambiense* and *Trypanosoma rhodesiense*, the agents of African trypanosomiasis, may also affect the heart with similar results, but central nervous system findings usually predominate.[105] Myocarditis is also observed in trichinosis[106–108] and is responsible for the occasional deaths that occur in severe infections.

In immunocompromised patients, myocarditis occurs as a consequence of a number of disseminated infections. Overt myocarditis is common in disseminated toxoplasmosis,[110–112] and systemic aspergillosis and candidiasis may also involve the heart.[93, 94] Cryptococcal, *Toxoplasma*, and *Aspergillus* myocarditis have been reported in patients with the acquired immunodeficiency syndrome (AIDS).[96–98, 109] Cardiac abnormalities in AIDS are common but are usually clinically silent.[119–121] A review of published autopsy series of AIDS cases by Kaul and associates suggested that the incidence of myocarditis in AIDS patients may be as high as 46%, although a strict definition of myocarditis requiring both myocardial inflammation and necrosis was not uniformly applied.[122] In a prospective study, DeCastro and colleagues reported the presence of echocardiographic abnormalities in 47 of 72 AIDS patients (65.2%), with cardiac involvement usually occurring late in the disease.[123] Cardiac dysfunction is appreciated clinically in approximately 20% of AIDS patients and frequently takes the form of dilated cardiomyopathy, which is associated with a poor prognosis. In a 1994 report, median survival time of patients at a similar stage of disease was reduced from 492 days to 101 days in those with cardiomyopathy.[124] A prospective study of 952 persons with human immunodeficiency virus (HIV) infection who did not use illicit drugs and had ratings of American Heart Association functional class I and US Centers for Disease Control and Prevention stage II showed that dilated cardiomyopathy developed in 76 (8%) during 5 years of follow-up.[125] A histologic diagnosis of myocarditis was made in 63 patients. HIV nucleic acid sequences were detected by in situ hybridization in biopsies of 36 (57%) of the patients with myocarditis. However, cultures were positive for group B coxsackievirus in four and for Epstein-Barr virus in four of those with myocarditis, and coinfection with HIV and other viruses was documented in nine.[125] In this study, as in others,[123, 126] cardiac dysfunction was highest in those with the most advanced disease. Although HIV has been cultured from endomyocardial biopsies[127, 128] and identified by Southern blot analysis[129] or in situ hybridization,[124, 130] in most AIDS patients with cardiac pathology HIV is found only rarely in myocytes,[124, 131] and, when it is, there is often no correlation with histopathologic or clinical evidence of heart muscle disease.[130] The isolation of known cardiotropic viruses from AIDS patients is not infrequently reported,[124, 128, 132] and a causal relation between HIV and myocarditis has yet to be firmly established. Malnutrition may also be a contributing factor to cardiac dysfunction in AIDS, and malnutrition and wasting are important independent predictors of cardiac morbidity and mortality.[133, 134] Antimyosin and anticardiac mitochondrial adenine nucleotide translocator antibodies have been identified in some AIDS patients with cardiac dysfunction.[135]

TABLE 68–1 Infectious Causes of Myocarditis

Viruses	Bacteria and rickettsia
Coxsackie A[13–15]	*Corynebacterium diphtheriae*[59–61]
Coxsackie B[13–16]	*Clostridium perfringens*[62, 63]
Echoviruses[19, 20]	*Streptococcus pyogenes*[57, 64, 65]
Polio[11, 21, 22]	*Neisseria meningitidis*[66]
Mumps[6, 23, 24]	*Salmonella*[67–69]
Rubeola[8–10]	*Brucella*[70, 71]
Influenza A and B[7, 25, 26]	*Staphylococcus aureus*[72]
Rabies[27]	*Listeria monocytogenes*[73–75]
Rubella[28, 29]	*Legionella pneumophila*[76]
Dengue[30, 31]	*Mycoplasma pneumoniae*[77–79]
Chikungunya[31]	*Chlamydia psittaci*[80]
Yellow fever[32]	*Chlamydia pneumoniae*[81, 82]
Argentinian hemorrhagic fever[33]	*Rickettsia rickettsii*[83]
Bolivian hemorrhagic fever[33]	*Rickettsia tsutsugamushi*[63, 84–86]
Lymphocytic choriomeningitis[34]	*Ehrlichia*[87]
Adenovirus[35, 36]	*Vibrio cholerae*[87a]
Varicella-zoster[37–40]	*Borrelia burgdorferi*[88–92]
Cytomegalovirus[41–46]	**Fungi**
Epstein-Barr[47, 48]	*Aspergillus*[93–96]
Vaccinia[49]	*Candida*[94]
Variola[50]	*Cryptococcus*[94, 96, 97]
Hepatitis B[51–53]	**Parasites**
Hepatitis C[54, 55]	*Trypanosoma cruzi*[99–104]
Respiratory syncytial virus[56]	*Trypanosoma gambiense*[105]
Parvovirus B19[57, 58]	*Trypanosoma rhodesiense*[105]
	Trichinella spiralis[106–108]
	Toxoplasma gondii[109–114]

Pathology and Pathogenesis

Myocardial pathology depends on the infecting agent, the mechanism of pathogenesis, and the duration of the process. The hallmarks of myocarditis are an inflammatory infiltrate and injury to adjacent myocardial cells. Pathologic changes may be acute or chronic and vary markedly in severity, depending on the nature of the disease and the point in its course at which tissue is obtained. Some agents, such as the coxsackie B viruses, infect the myocytes themselves, whereas agents such as varicella-zoster virus, cytomegalovirus, and hepatitis B virus appear to injure vascular endothelial cells. Although routine histology may help in the differential diagnosis, it rarely provides definitive information regarding an etiologic agent. Early in many viral infections, scattered hypereosinophilic myofibers, widespread edema, and only a few inflammatory cells may be present. Later, there is loss of striation, nuclear degeneration, and fragmentation of myofibers. The degenerating or partially necrotic myofibers are usually surrounded by lymphocytes, plasma cells, and macrophages.[15] The types of lymphocytes and macrophages that are present vary depending on the etiologic agent and the stage of infection.[131, 136–138] Polymorphonuclear cells are occasionally seen[3] (Fig. 68–1). Return to normal cardiac function usually precedes resolution of the histologic abnormalities.[139] The acute process may resolve completely; healing and chronicity are reflected by the development of interstitial fibrosis and loss of myofibers.[140]

The pathogenesis of human viral myocarditis is incompletely understood. Mouse models of myocarditis induced by infection with either coxsackievirus B3 or encephalomyocarditis virus have revealed several possible pathogenetic mechanisms. Susceptibility to

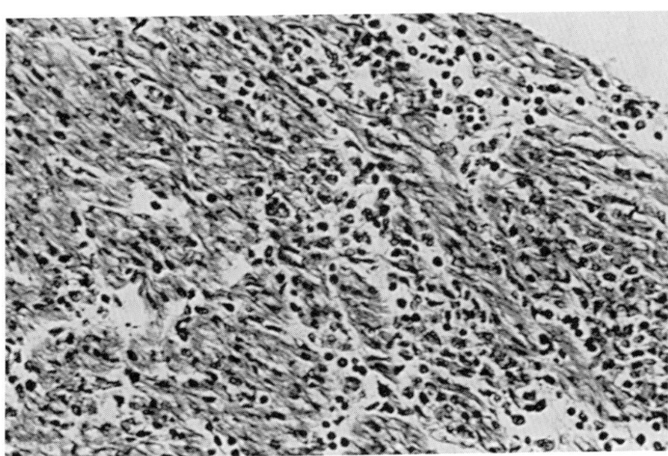

FIGURE 68–1. Coxsackievirus myocarditis with extensive infiltration of mononuclear cells, plasma cells, lymphocytes, and some eosinophils in the interstitial tissue (×250). (From Bloor CM. Pericarditis and myocarditis. In: Cardiac Pathology. Philadelphia: JB Lippincott; 1978:265–295.)

coxsackievirus B–induced myocarditis is age dependent and genetically determined.[141] Mechanisms of injury vary in different mouse strains.[142–145] In susceptible animals, acute myocarditis results from direct infection and cytolysis of myocytes.[3, 146, 147] In surviving animals, neutralizing antibody, perhaps in conjunction with macrophages[148, 149] and natural killer cells,[150] appears to terminate virus replication by 7 to 9 days after infection.[13, 151, 152] Exercise[3, 13, 153] and corticosteroids[154] markedly enhance mortality during the early stages of infection. Studies in mice also demonstrated increased virulence of coxsackie B3 virus in selenium-deficient mice, suggesting that "oxidative stress" may contribute to myocardial damage.[155] Nonsteroidal anti-inflammatory agents may also have deleterious effects,[156] perhaps through inhibition of interferon production.[157] Mice surviving the acute replicative phase of the virus infection may go on to develop severe myocarditis in the absence of recoverable virus. This second phase of virus-induced myocardial destruction depends on the presence of cytolytic T cells,[15, 158] which appear as productive virus replication ceases. Some of these cytolytic T cells recognize and lyse both infected and uninfected myocytes,[159] and their presence correlates with myocardial damage.[160, 161] The severity of myocardial damage caused by this immune mechanism is greatest in male mice and pregnant female mice.[162] In some strains of mice that are less prone to myocarditis, the cytolytic T-cell response appears to be inhibited by suppressor cells.[163] Variants of coxsackievirus B3 that do not evoke cytolytic T cells directed against both infected and uninfected myocytes fail to cause myocarditis, even though they are indistinguishable from myocarditic strains in their ability to replicate and stimulate neutralizing antibodies.[164] The foci responsible for the cardiovirulence of coxsackie B3 have been localized to two regions of the genome, the 5′ nontranslated region (NTR) and the capsid protein–encoding region.[165] Using two strains of coxsackievirus B3 that differ in their ability to produce autoimmunity, Weller and colleagues demonstrated that the viruses used different receptors for cell entry, indicating that the receptor used by a virus may be important in triggering autosensitization.[166] Interleukin-1, tumor necrosis factor, and bacterial lipopolysaccharide all enhance autoimmune injury and cause resistant mice to become susceptible.[167] Data demonstrating enhanced expression of intracellular adhesion molecule-1 in mice, and both type I and type II major histocompatibility complex (MHC) antigens in human myocarditis, also support the theory that autoimmunity plays a major role in the development of viral myocarditis.[168, 169]

In situ hybridization studies, however, suggest that the enterovirus genome can be found in all stages of acute and chronic infection and that virus persistence in the heart is characterized by restricted viral RNA and capsid protein synthesis. In one study, acute and chronic myocardial lesions were found consistently to be associated with infected myocardial cells, and mouse strains that cleared the virus after acute infection did not develop chronic disease.[170] Others have demonstrated the persistence of viral genome by PCR in mice after both culture and in situ hybridization techniques are negative.[171] However, in that study, there was no correlation between the occurrence of myocarditis and the presence of viral genome. A similar lack of correlation between the locations of heart inflammation and viral genome has been seen in humans,[172, 173] leading to the suggestion that this persistent viral genome does not have pathogenic or prognostic importance.[171, 172] Whether the persistence of viral genome plays any role in pathogenesis of myocarditis in humans has yet to be determined.

Mice and humans infected with coxsackievirus B3 also develop heart-reactive antibodies,[174–176] which may contribute to myocyte destruction.[143, 177–181] Zhang and colleagues demonstrated that a live attenuated variant of coxsackievirus B3 was able to protect mice against infection with the cardiovirulent wild-type strain. The attenuated virus was able to induce neutralizing antibodies but failed to induce significant levels of antibody against cardiac myosin, in contrast to wild-type virus.[182] In mice, susceptibility to damage from antimyosin antibodies is strain specific and appears to involve a genetically determined difference in target-organ sensitivity.[183] The role that autoantibodies play against structures such as the B adrenoreceptors, myosin heavy chains, cardiac mitochondrial adenosine diphosphate/triphosphate carrier proteins, and aminin has not been clearly elucidated, but, for example, some antisarcolemmal antibodies that cross-react with enteroviral epitopes lyse myocytes.[177, 179] Of note, Huber and associates also demonstrated three monoclonal antibodies to group A streptococcus that also bind to various heart antigens and neutralize a myocarditic strain of coxsackievirus B3.[184]

In human enteroviral infection, direct injury to myocytes appears to play a major role in neonatal infection and some cases of fulminant acute myocarditis in adults.[185] In situ hybridization studies also document the presence of enterovirus genome in 20 to 30% of cases of acute myocarditis and in some cases of dilated cardiomyopathy.[17] Patients with myocarditis also have been found to possess both cytotoxic lymphocytes that react with normal myocytes and high titers of antimyocyte antibodies.[185–187]

Another mechanism that may explain the myocardial dysfunction and myocyte necrosis observed in viral myocarditis is damage to coronary vasculature with luminal narrowing, spasm, and obstruction leading to myocyte ischemia. This has been demonstrated in murine coxsackievirus B3 myocarditis,[188] and a similar mechanism appears to underlie the development of dilated cardiomyopathy in some humans after viral or idiopathic myocarditis.

In mouse models of cytomegalovirus myocarditis, genes linked to the H-2 complex influence susceptibility.[189] Cardiac lesions develop in and around the small penetrating blood vessels of the heart. When infected mice are depleted of $CD4^+$ T lymphocytes, myocardial lesions fail to develop even though viral titers may be increased.[190] Cytomegalovirus also induces antibodies that cross-react with cardiac myosin.[191] In contrast, in reovirus-induced murine myocarditis, humoral immunity and cellular immunity protect against cardiac damage; myocarditis results from direct virus injury to myocytes.[192]

In acute Chagas' disease, pathologic examination often reveals parasites within cardiac myocytes. When rupture of the cysts occurs, there is a marked inflammatory infiltrate consisting of lymphocytes, plasma cells, macrophages, and some eosinophils.[99, 193] In chronic Chagas' disease, the heart is often enlarged and flabby. Aneurysm formation may be present at the apex. The conduction system is often involved, and this is reflected by a high frequency of rhythm disturbances. Microscopic examination reveals focal mononuclear cell infiltrates and fibrosis.[100, 193] In this stage, parasites can be identified only in 25% of patients.[100] Epitopes shared by *T. cruzi* and cardiac myocytes and recognized by cytotoxic T cells may play an important role in the progression of myocarditis late in disease.[194]

The heart, as well as the central nervous system, is often prominently involved in disseminated toxoplasmosis. *Toxoplasma* pseudocysts containing numerous organisms may be readily identified in cardiac tissue, and there is a striking absence of cellular response around them (Fig. 68–2). Rupture of parasitized fibers is followed by infiltration of neutrophils and eosinophils.[193]

Myocardial microabscesses, affecting both myocytes and the conducting system, may occur in the course of systemic bacterial infections with organisms such as *Staphylococcus aureus*, but heart failure is rarely a direct consequence of such lesions.[115] In experimental animals, *Borrelia burgdorferi* has a predilection for connective tissue in the heart base, and disease severity correlates with the number of spirochetes found.[195] Mouse models suggest that infection with *B. burgdorferi* has a different pathogenesis than enterovirus myocarditis, because injury is independent of class II MHC/T-cell interactions and results from the response of macrophages to the spirochetes.[196]

Rickettsia and most fungi produce vasculitic lesions with surrounding inflammation. Damage to myocytes may be caused by the adjacent inflammatory process or may reflect anoxia caused by occlusion of small blood vessels.

Diphtheria toxin inhibits cellular protein synthesis. This results in hyaline degeneration and necrosis of myocardial fibers, with a secondary inflammatory response.[3, 60]

Clinical Manifestations

Patients with myocarditis may be asymptomatic, or they may have a rapidly progressive fatal disease. The diagnosis of infectious myocarditis usually is considered when a young person develops unexplained heart failure or arrhythmias, or when cardiac abnormalities occur in the course of a recognized systemic infection. Fever, malaise, arthralgias, upper respiratory tract symptoms, and chest pain may precede or accompany coxsackievirus myocarditis,[185, 197] but these symptoms are not specific. Supraventricular tachycardia and ventricular extrasystoles are common.[198] Arrhythmias provide early evidence of involvement of the conduction system and are responsible for the occurrence of sudden death in patients with myocarditis. Myocarditis may mimic acute myocardial infarction,[199–203] but care should be taken not to mistake myocardial infarction occurring in a patient with infection for myocarditis.[204] In acute myocarditis, cardiac enzymes may be elevated and remain so for several days.[205] Symptomatic pericarditis may or may not be present.

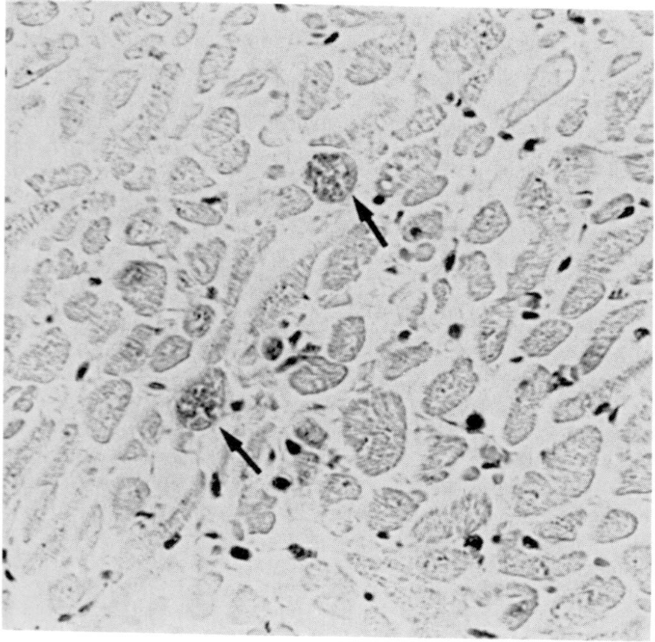

FIGURE 68–2. Cysts of *Toxoplasma gondii (arrows)* are easily visible in the heart of this immunosuppressed patient who died with disseminated toxoplasmosis.

Diagnosis

Diagnosis of myocarditis requires a high index of suspicion. In infants, myocarditis is often just one manifestation of a widespread fulminant systemic infection. Involvement of the lungs, liver, and central nervous system, disseminated intravascular coagulation, and circulatory collapse may obscure the clinical signs of cardiac disease.[35, 206] Recognition of myocarditis can also present difficulties in older children and adults when it occurs as part of an overwhelming systemic infection. When sought, however, signs of cardiac dysfunction usually are apparent. Even when cardiac signs and symptoms predominate, establishing a firm diagnosis may be difficult.

Nonspecific ST-segment and T-wave abnormalities on electrocardiography are frequently cited as presumptive evidence of myocarditis. Classically in myocarditis, there are sequential ST-segment elevations and T-wave inversions, which usually resolve in a month or two without the development of Q waves or R-wave depression.[207] The degree of ST-segment elevation and the extent and duration of later T-wave inversion have been reported to correlate with myocardial enzyme release and therefore with the amount of cell necrosis.[208] However, similar ST-segment and T-wave changes may also be seen with fever, hypoxia, tachycardia, and electrolyte disturbances, and they frequently occur during uncomplicated childhood viral infections.[209] Failure to reverse such ST-segment and T-wave changes with β-blockade is thought by some to be indicative of myocarditis,[210] but physicians should approach a diagnosis of myocarditis based solely on the presence of nonspecific ST-segment and T-wave abnormalities with skepticism.

Tachycardia out of proportion to the height of the fever, ventricular and supraventricular arrhythmias, and atrioventricular or intraventricular conduction disturbances may also be indicative of myocarditis. In a study of 45 patients with active myocarditis, the presence of Q waves in addition to ST-segment elevation frequently heralded a fulminant course, and abnormal QRS complexes and left bundle branch block were indicative of an increased risk of sudden cardiac death.[211]

The MB fraction of creatinine kinase (CK-MB) is frequently elevated in patients with acute myocarditis and significant ST-segment elevation.[207] Elevated serum levels of troponin T, a component of the myocyte contractile apparatus, persist in the serum for up to 14 days after myocyte injury.[207] Although elevations of cardiac troponin occur more frequently than do elevations of CK-MB, in one study only 34% (18/53) of those with biopsy-proven myocarditis had increased levels, as did 11% (4/35) of patients without myocarditis.[212] An increased troponin level reflects cardiac injury but is neither sensitive nor specific in the diagnosis of myocarditis. A variety of heart-reactive antibodies have been detected in patients with myocarditis, and their persistence at high titer appears to be a poor prognostic sign. However, the clinical utility of these assays remains to be demonstrated.

Echocardiography is useful in detecting and quantifying impaired systolic function. Inflammation and edema may cause local thickening of the myocardium, and regional wall motion abnormalities are often observed.[213–216] Repeated echocardiographic examinations may be used to monitor the resolution or progression of myocarditis. Persistent wall motion abnormalities and ventricular dilation suggest the development of chronic myocarditis or dilated cardiomyopathy.

Indium 111-labeled antimyosin antibody imaging detects myocardial necrosis rather than inflammation but appears to be more sensitive for diagnosing myocarditis than endomyocardial biopsy.[217–221]

Increased myocardial uptake is observed in almost all patients with myocarditis who have positive endomyocardial biopsies, but it is also observed in many comparable patients with negative biopsies.[217–221] A negative ^{111}In-antimyosin antibody scan is highly predictive of a negative endomyocardial biopsy.[220] However, scans may continue to be positive long after the active phase of myocarditis, and this may account for at least some of the positive scans observed in biopsy-negative patients. In one study, 15 of 21 patients with dilated cardiomyopathy had positive scans before cardiac transplantation, but careful examination of their explanted hearts revealed histologic evidence of myocarditis in only 7.[222] Indium 111 scanning has also been useful in distinguishing patients with acute myocarditis from those with acute myocardial infarction.[223]

Magnetic resonance imaging (MRI), which can detect small increases in the water content of tissues, has proved reliable in the diagnosis of cardiac allograft rejection.[224, 225] Limited experience indicates that MRI also provides a sensitive means of detecting acute viral or idiopathic myocarditis.[226] In one study, MRI detected focal myocardial edema in two patients that corresponded anatomically to segmental wall-motion abnormalities detected by echocardiography and that normalized after the acute phase.[227] In another study, abnormal myocardial signal intensities indicative of edema were detected in 6 of 6 children with acute myocarditis proven by endomyocardial biopsy, but in none of the 5 biopsy-negative controls.[226] Both MRI and ^{111}In-antimyosin antibody scans were reported to be positive in a patient with endomyocardial biopsy-proven Lyme myocarditis.[228] Friedrich and coworkers serially studied 19 patients who presented with symptoms of acute myocarditis using contrast media–enhanced MRI and concluded that acute myocarditis evolves from a focal to a disseminated process during the first 2 weeks after the onset of symptoms.[229]

The gold standard for the premortem diagnosis of myocarditis has traditionally been endomyocardial biopsy,[230–233] although some studies have questioned its value.[18, 234, 235] Biopsy confirmation of the clinical diagnosis of myocarditis is highly variable, ranging from 10 to 100% in different series.[233–241] Results of endomyocardial biopsy have also been highly variable in patients with unexplained congestive heart failure, with evidence of active myocarditis being found in 2 to 80% of these patients.[207, 230, 242–246] Several factors contribute to this variability and make interpretation of the literature difficult. These include lack of uniform clinical and histopathologic criteria for the diagnosis of myocarditis, a high degree of interobserver variability, sampling error, and marked variation in the timing of biopsies with respect to the onset of disease.[140, 207–231, 247–249] Agreement among pathologists on histopathologic criteria for the diagnosis of myocarditis (the *Dallas criteria*) has been a helpful development, but problems remain.[250] Scattered small collections of inflammatory cells with focal necrosis of myocytes may occur in response to stress or the administration of vasopressors,[250] and their presence in patients with heart failure may not be indicative of myocarditis. Conversely, a single small focus of myocarditis in the conducting system may be responsible for a fatal arrhythmia in someone without significant myocarditis elsewhere, and multiple endomyocardial biopsies are often necessary to establish this diagnosis.[234, 235] Timing of biopsy is also critical. Early in enteroviral myocarditis there is necrosis of myocytes but not the lymphocytic infiltration demanded by the Dallas criteria.[251, 252] Persistence of myocarditis is also highly variable; in some patients with acute enteroviral or idiopathic myocarditis, histopathologic abnormalities may resolve within a month or two after onset.[200, 232]

Dilated cardiomyopathy may represent, at least in some cases, the end stage of viral myocarditis.[5, 207, 244, 253, 254] This concept is supported by data from the mouse model, by serial biopsies demonstrating progression to dilated cardiomyopathy in some patients with acute myocarditis, by evidence of active myocarditis in many patients with idiopathic dilated cardiomyopathy who are biopsied soon after the onset of their symptoms, and by the detection of enterovirus RNA in biopsies and explanted hearts.[17, 230, 231, 236, 242, 253, 255–258]

Proof of causation requires isolation of virus from the myocardium or demonstration of viral proteins or nucleic acids in the myocardium. Except in neonatal myocarditis and myocarditis occurring in immunocompromised patients, virus has rarely been isolated from cardiac tissue.[17, 259] Detection of viral proteins has been difficult, primarily because lack of specificity has led to false-positive results, but the use of antiserum to purified coxsackievirus capsid proteins produced by recombinant DNA technology may overcome this difficulty. To date, diagnosis of viral myocarditis has generally been based on the isolation of virus from another site (e.g., stool), the demonstration of a fourfold or greater rise in antibody titer from acute to convalescent sera, or the demonstration of a high titer of virus-specific immunoglobulin M antibody in serum.[13, 15–17, 185] At best, such data provide only circumstantial evidence of causation of myocarditis and must be interpreted with caution because of the prevalence of asymptomatic infections by the same agents that cause myocarditis. In a typical prospective study, 26% of patients without myocarditis had serologic evidence of infection with agents known to cause myocarditis.[198] These traditional methods have failed to provide a specific diagnosis in most patients with myocarditis of presumed viral origin.

The use of newer techniques for the detection and amplification of viral nucleic acids and their application to cardiac tissue obtained by endomyocardial biopsy is now providing interesting but confusing data on the viral etiology of myocarditis and dilated cardiomyopathy.[17, 259–264] Cloned DNA fragments complementary to different regions of the enterovirus genome serve as type-specific or broadly cross-reactive hybridization probes or polymerase chain reaction (PCR) primers capable of detecting or amplifying nucleic acid sequences of a specific virus (e.g., coxsackievirus B3) or most of the enteroviruses. In situ hybridization, although somewhat less sensitive than PCR, has the advantage of identifying the specific cells that are infected, whereas PCR can increase the sensitivity of the assay to between 1 and 10 viral genomes per milligram of tissue. Overall, enteroviral RNA has been detected by these techniques in approximately 25% of specimens from patients with myocarditis and in 15 to 19% of patients with dilated cardiomyopathy.[17, 262]

Results from individual studies have varied markedly, however. A large proportion of cases in which coxsackieviruses were implicated serologically did not give positive results by in situ hybridization.[173, 265] Furthermore, the cells that contained enteroviral RNA were generally not in areas of myocarditis.[173] Moreover, enteroviral RNA was detected by PCR in cardiac tissue from control patients with a variety of other conditions, including those with normal hearts, although not from noncardiac control tissues.[258] These results raise a number of difficult questions, including the specificity of the assays, the sensitivity and validity of the histopathologic assessments, and the pathogenetic significance of enteroviral RNA in the absence of inflammation or necrosis. Interpretation of such results is even more problematic when the viruses in question are members of the herpesvirus family, which regularly persist in normal persons and which may even be present in the blood.[44] In some studies presence of enteroviral RNA in patients with myocarditis or dilated cardiomyopathy has been associated with a favorable[266] prognosis, but in other studies those with demonstrated enteroviral RNA have had a poor outcome.[267, 268]

The criteria for endomyocardial biopsy have evolved over time. At this time, myocardial biopsy is clearly indicated only in the monitoring of cardiac allograft rejection and anthracycline cardiotoxicity.[207] Many experts believe that endomyocardial biopsy is not warranted in most cases of myocarditis or dilated cardiomyopathy.[241, 269–272] However, the availability of PCR and in situ hybridization techniques and the development of antiviral drugs capable of inhibiting enteroviral replication may eventually justify endomyocardial biopsy during the acute phase of presumed infectious or idiopathic myocarditis in patients with positive ^{111}In -antimyosin antibody scans. Complications from right ventricular endomyocardial biopsy occur in approximately 6% of cases; serious adverse consequences (i.e., death, tamponade, perforation) occur in less than 1% if the operator is experienced.[273]

A wide variety of noninfectious diseases and agents may mimic infectious myocarditis and produce identical clinical syndromes (Table 68–2).

Treatment

Treatment of myocarditis should be directed at the specific etiologic agent involved whenever possible. Based on inferences from the murine model of coxsackievirus B3 myocarditis, bed rest remains an important part of therapy. Usual adjunctive care includes ensuring adequate oxygenation, avoiding and treating fluid overload if it develops, and monitoring for the development of ventricular arrhythmias. Some of the medications prescribed in the routine management of congestive heart failure may in the future play a more specific role in the treatment of myocarditis. In mice infected with either coxsackievirus B3 or encephalomyocarditis virus, treatment with captopril, an angiotensin-converting enzyme inhibitor used in the treatment of heart failure from a variety of causes, reduced inflammation and enhanced survival. Enalapril, however, did not reduce cardiac injury in a murine model of encephalomyocarditis,[291] suggesting that captopril's oxygen radical scavenging properties may be responsible for its beneficial effect.[292] Although verapamil and diltiazem are not useful agents in the treatment of human heart failure caused by ischemic disease,[293, 294] experimental data in animals suggest that they may be useful in the treatment of some forms of infectious myocarditis treatment.[295, 296] Amlodipine, a novel dihydropyridine calcium-channel blocker, both reduces myocardial injury in a murine myocarditis model (perhaps through an inhibition of nitric oxide)[297] and improved mortality in a double-blind, placebo-controlled study of patients with nonischemic dilated cardiomyopathy.[298] In severe cases of myocarditis, cardiac assist devices may be lifesaving.[299]

Most patients with viral myocarditis recover completely,[300, 301] and the factors that predispose certain patients to a poor outcome are not clear. Early in experimental coxsackievirus B3 infection in mouse models, indomethicin, salicylates, and ibuprofen all increase viral replication and mortality.[156, 302, 303] No controlled data about their use in patients with myocarditis are available. Administration of glucocorticoids during the acute phase of viral myocarditis has been associated with rapid clinical deterioration, and the deleterious effects of these drugs have been clearly demonstrated in the acute phase of coxsackievirus infection in mice.[154, 304] In some uncontrolled trials, patients with myocarditis proven by endomyocardial biopsy[305, 306] or with positive gallium scans[307] who were given immunosuppressive agents showed improvement; but controlled trials, with the exception of one trial in children[308] that had methodologic flaws,[268] have failed to show benefit from treatment with prednisone alone or with combinations of prednisone-azathioprine or prednisone-cyclosporine.[241, 268, 309] As knowledge of the pathogenesis of viral myocarditis increases and the ability to detect and identify the etiologic agents improves, subgroups that might benefit from immunosuppressive therapy may emerge. Data from mice and uncontrolled studies in humans suggest a beneficial role for immunoglobulins in the treatment of viral myocarditis and dilated cardiomyopathy. In a mouse model of coxsackievirus B3 myocarditis, immunoglobulin administration increased survival when given both simultaneously with virus inoculation and on day 14 after inoculation.[310] Marsch and colleagues demonstrated improvement of hemodynamic function and the eradication of virus after hyperimmunoglobulin treatment of patients with cytomegalovirus.[311] Immunoglobulin administration also led to significantly improved ejection fractions in 10 patients with new-onset dilated cardiomyopathy or myocarditis who had New York Heart Association class III/IV heart failure before therapy.[312] Controlled trials, however, are lacking. The role for interferon in the treatment of acute myocarditis also remains to be elucidated. Studies in mice[313, 314] and anecdotal reports[266] suggest potential benefit, although a small, single-center, matched-cohort trial demonstrated no significant difference in results between patients receiving interferon and controls.[315] Based on current understanding of the pathogenesis of acute viral myocarditis, cytokine manipulation or blockade may eventually prove to be useful therapy.[316, 317]

Ganciclovir has been used successfully in the treatment of severe cytomegalovirus infection, including myocarditis.[318] Although no antiviral drugs with efficacy against the enteroviruses are commercially available at this time, pleconaril (VP63843), an oral agent active against most of the picornavirus family, has shown promise in clinical trials (see Chapter 36). WIN54954, an earlier compound in the same family, had potent antiviral effects in mouse models of coxsackievirus B3 myocarditis,[319–322] but adverse effects limited its development. The clinical efficacy of pleconaril has been demonstrated in human respiratory tract infections with coxsackie A virus.[323] In a completed phase-II, double-blind, placebo-controlled study of naturally occurring enteroviral meningitis, those treated with pleconaril experienced significant reduction in symptoms and shortening of disease duration.[324] Documented adverse effects to date have been mild,[323] and pleconaril has been made available for compassionate use in serious enterovirus infection, including myocarditis. In cases of severe myocarditis with progressive or fulminant heart failure, transplantation may be required if less aggressive therapy fails.

TABLE 68–2 Noninfectious Causes of Myocarditis

Collagen vascular disease[274–280]	Drug-induced (hypersensitivity)[286]
Systemic lupus erythematosus	Methyldopa
Systemic sclerosis	Sulfonamides
Rheumatoid arthritis	Tetracycline
Dermatomyositis/polymyositis	Scorpion, wasp, and spider stings[282, 287]
Still's disease	Agents not yet identified
Thyrotoxicosis[274]	Kawasaki disease[288]
Thrombotic thrombocytopenic purpura[281]	Giant cell myocarditis[289]
Pheochromocytoma[282]	Sarcoid[290]
Peripartum[283]	
Radiation-induced[284]	
Drug-induced (direct toxic)[285]	
Cocaine	
Alcohol	
Emetine	
Catecholamines	
Arsenic	
Cyclophosphamide	
Daunorubicin	
Adriamycin	

PERICARDITIS

Pericarditis (inflammation of the pericardium) may be caused by any of a wide variety of infectious and noninfectious processes. It may be clinically silent or may result in severe hemodynamic compromise and death. In 1892, Sir William Osler called attention to the frequency with which pericarditis was overlooked by the practitioner,[325] and series indicate that this is still true today.[326–328] Advances in medicine, including antibiotic therapy, cardiac surgery, hemodialysis, cancer chemotherapy, and organ transplantation, have altered the etiologic spectrum of pericarditis over the course of the 20th century. Idiopathic and viral pericarditis now predominate and usually result in a benign, self-limited disease. Purulent bacterial pericarditis and tuberculous pericarditis are now less common, but they still cause significant morbidity and mortality and present a diagnostic challenge.

Etiologic Agents

Because of the difficulty in establishing a specific diagnosis, the cause of acute, self-limited pericarditis in most cases is never determined, and the disease is classified as idiopathic. In some series, idiopathic pericarditis accounted for 40 to 86% of patients hospitalized with acute pericarditis.[328–330] There are no clinical or epidemiologic features that distinguish idiopathic pericarditis from acute pericarditis of proven viral origin. Therefore, it is likely that viral infections are responsible for many, if not most, cases of acute pericarditis presently classified as idiopathic.

Most viruses infecting the heart affect both the myocardium and the pericardium (see previous discussion). Of the many viruses associated with heart disease, the enteroviruses, especially the coxsackieviruses, are most frequently implicated in pericarditis.[16, 331, 332] The association of myopericarditis with coxsackieviruses was first demonstrated in neonates with overwhelming, fatal systemic infections.[333] Pericarditis has also been recognized in the setting of epidemic coxsackievirus infection.[334, 335] A century ago, cases of acute benign pericarditis were recognized during epidemics of Bornholm disease (epidemic pleurodynia), and it was postulated that the etiologic agent of the two diseases was the same.[334] Subsequently, the group B coxsackieviruses were shown to be the principal cause of epidemic pleurodynia, and their etiologic role in the associated cases of pericarditis was well established.[334, 335]

Coxsackieviruses have only rarely been isolated from pericardial fluid,[336, 337] and, as with myocarditis, most diagnoses have been based on the isolation of virus from other body sites (e.g., stool) or the demonstration of a fourfold or greater rise in antibody titer after the acute illness, or both. A number of other viruses have also been shown to cause pericarditis, but symptomatic involvement of the pericardium is uncommon. When it occurs, it is often a manifestation of severe disseminated infection. Viruses known to cause pericarditis are listed in Table 68–3.

A wide variety of bacteria can cause pericarditis. In the preantibiotic era, purulent pericarditis occurred primarily as a complication of pneumonia in previously healthy children and adults.[327, 365, 366, 373] Of the 425 cases of purulent pericarditis reported in 1961 by Boyle and colleagues,[365] 43% were associated with pleuropulmonary infections. *Streptococcus pneumoniae* and *Staph. aureus* accounted for more than half of the cases. With the advent of antibiotics, the incidence of purulent pericarditis decreased markedly. Although staphylococci and streptococci are still etiologic in a substantial number of cases, the incidence of pneumococcal pericarditis has declined substantially, and gram-negative bacilli have assumed a much more important role.[326, 327, 366, 373] Patients with purulent pericarditis are now often older and have an underlying predisposing condition.[326, 327, 366, 373] A recent report emphasized the importance of anaerobic bacteria such as *Prevotella*, *Peptostreptococcus*, and *Propionibacterium* in pericarditis complicating esophageal perforation and mediastinitis from head and neck infections,[390] but anaerobes can also seed the pericardium via the blood stream.[391] Purulent pericarditis may occur as a complication of meningococcal meningitis or fulminant meningococcemia, but *Neisseria meningitidis*, especially serogroup C, also causes primary pericarditis.[376, 377] A reactive, culture-negative pericarditis, presumably of immune origin, may also occur after successful treatment of meningococcal infection at another site.[376, 377] *M. pneumoniae* can cause pericarditis; although it is uncommon, this manifestation has been observed in almost 1% of patients hospitalized with this infection.[395–399] *Legionella pneumophila* has been isolated from the pericardial fluid,[400–402] and pericarditis has occurred in association with pneumonia[400–404] and endocarditis.[405] Bacterial infections account for proportionately more pericarditis in children; after *S. aureus*, *Haemophilus influenzae*, and *N. meningitidis* are the most common etiologic agents.[380, 441] Childhood immunization with *H. influenzae* type B conjugate vaccine has markedly reduced the frequency of *H. influenzae* type B infection in children, and this should result in a comparable reduction in the incidence of *H. influenzae* type B pericarditis.

Acute or chronic pericarditis is reported to occur in approximately 1% of patients with pulmonary tuberculosis.[409] Before the AIDS epidemic, because of the declining incidence of primary tuberculosis and the use of effective chemotherapy, *Mycobacterium tuberculosis* accounted for fewer than 5% of cases of acute pericarditis in Europe and North America.[329, 410, 435] In contrast, tuberculous pericarditis is a major cause of heart disease in Africa[444, 445] and in patients with AIDS.[123, 446, 447] Diagnosis is difficult and mortality remains high.[411, 448] *M. tuberculosis* remains an important treatable cause of chronic pericardial effusion and constrictive pericarditis.[412, 444, 445, 449, 450] (see Chapter 240).

Fungi are infrequently recognized as a cause of pericarditis. However, in large outbreaks, pericarditis occurred in 6% of patients with acute symptomatic histoplasmosis.[416] In most, it appeared to represent a sterile inflammatory response to infection in adjacent mediastinal lymph nodes and resolved spontaneously without specific therapy. In disseminated histoplasmosis the pericardium itself may be infected with *Histoplasma capsulatum*.[418] Pericarditis is rarely recognized in acute coccidioidomycosis. Spontaneously resolving cases resembling those seen in acute histoplasmosis have been described,[419] but most reported cases have occurred in the setting of disseminated coccidioidomycosis and represent *Coccidioides immitis* infection of the heart.[420] Fungal pericarditis (resulting from direct inoculation or extension of mediastinal infection) is seen with increasing frequency as a complication of cardiothoracic surgery.[373] Pericarditis caused by *Candida* spp., *Aspergillus* spp., *Cryptococcus neoformans*, and other fungi occurs as a consequence of disseminated infection in severely debilitated and immunocompromised patients, especially those with prolonged neutropenia who are receiving multiple courses of antibiotics.[423–428] Pericardial effusions occur in 16 to 40% of patients with AIDS.[122, 123] Although they are generally idiopathic, a wide variety of viral, bacterial, and fungal agents have been isolated from the pericardial fluid, and malignant effusions have also been observed.[122, 447, 451] As with myocarditis, pericardial effusion in HIV-infected patients is associated with advanced stages of infection.[452] The rare parasitic causes of pericarditis are referenced in Table 68–3.

TABLE 68–3 Infectious Causes of Pericarditis

Viruses	Fungi
Coxsackie A[338–340]	*Histoplasma capsulatum*[416–418]
Coxsackie B[16, 331, 332, 334–337]	*Coccidioides immitis*[419–421]
Echovirus[330, 341–344]	*Blastomyces dermatitidis*[365, 422]
Adenovirus[330, 339, 345–347]	*Cryptococcus neoformans*[423]
Mumps[330, 348]	*Candida*[424–427]
Influenza[349–351]	*Aspergillus*[373, 428–431]
Epstein-Barr[352–354]	Parasites
Varicella-zoster[355]	*Toxoplasma gondii*[432–435]
Cytomegalovirus[356–361]	*Entamoeba histolytica*[436–440]
Herpes simplex[362, 363]	*Toxocara canis*[441]
Hepatitis B[364]	Schistosomes[442]
Bacteria	
Streptococcus pneumoniae[365–368]	
Other *Streptococcus* spp.[369–372]	
Staphylococcus aureus[365, 366, 373–375]	
Neisseria meningitidis[376, 377]	
Neisseria gonorrhoeae[378, 379]	
Haemophilus influenzae[365, 380–382]	
Enteric gram-negative rods[366, 383, 384]	
Salmonella[365, 385]	
Campylobacter[386]	
Brucella[387]	
Actinomyces[388, 389]	
Prevotella[390, 391]	
Peptostreptococcus[390, 391]	
Propionibacterium acnes[390, 391]	
Bacteroides[391, 392]	
Nocardia[393]	
Listeria monocytogenes[394]	
Mycoplasma[395–399]	
Legionella pneumophila[400–405]	
Chlamydia[406]	
Borrelia burgdorferi[88, 89, 219, 407, 408]	
Mycobacterium tuberculosis[409–414]	
Mycobacterium avium-intracellulare[415]	

Pathology, Pathogenesis, and Pathophysiology

The pericardium has two opposing mesothelial surfaces. The parietal pericardium forms a flask-shaped sac that encloses the heart and the origins of the great vessels. It consists of a 1-mm-thick layer of dense collagen lined by a single layer of mesothelial cells, which are covered by microvilli. The mesothelial cell layer is reflected onto the epicardial surface of the heart to form the visceral pericardium. The parietal pericardium has firm attachments to the sternum, the diaphragm, and the adventitia of the great vessels. The function of the normal pericardium has been a matter of considerable investigation and speculation.[453] It normally contains 15 to 50 ml of clear fluid, which may act as a lubricant. The pericardium reacts to acute injury by exuding fluid, fibrin, and cells in various combinations.[450] Acute pericarditis may resolve completely or progress to fibrous thickening, with or without constriction.

Cardiotropic viruses usually spread to the myocardium and pericardium hematogenously. Inflammation occurs in both visceral and parietal portions; effusion may develop and may be serous, serofibrinous, or serosanguineous. Concomitant myocarditis may or may not be evident. Although most patients with viral pericarditis recover completely, some have repeated disabling recurrences.[328, 454] The pathophysiology of these recurrences has not been established, but it probably involves immunologic mechanisms and not recurrent or persistent virus replication. Rarely, viral pericarditis leads to constriction as a late complication.[455]

Bacterial pericarditis results from (1) spread from a contiguous focus of infection within the chest, either de novo or after surgery or trauma; (2) spread from a focus of infection within the heart, most commonly from endocarditis; (3) hematogenous infection; or (4) direct inoculation as a result of penetrating injury or cardiothoracic surgery. The incidence of purulent pericarditis arising from a contiguous pneumonia has steadily decreased and now usually occurs only when there has been significant delay in antibiotic therapy.[327, 366, 367] Pericarditis after cardiothoracic or esophageal surgery often occurs in patients with sternal wound infections or mediastinitis[373] and may be overlooked. Mortality is high. Pericarditis not infrequently accompanies fatal endocarditis,[115] especially that caused by *S. aureus*.[72] It often results from extension of a perivalvular abscess into the pericardium.[115] However, pericardial effusions in endocarditis may also be hemorrhagic[456] or sympathetic and sterile.[457] The presence of preexisting nonbacterial pericardial effusion may predispose to the development of purulent pericarditis in bacteremic patients. Although the pericardial fluid may initially be clear,[365, 373] it is usually grossly purulent and may be loculated by the time the disease is clinically apparent. Subsequent organization with adhesions, obliteration of the pericardial space, and calcification may occur and result in constrictive pericarditis.

Tuberculous pericarditis may develop from a hematogenous focus present from the time of primary infection; as a result of lymphatic spread from peritracheal, peribronchial, or mediastinal lymph nodes; or by contiguous spread from a focus of infection in lung or pleura. Four pathologic stages in tuberculous pericarditis have been described.[450, 458] In the first stage, there is diffuse fibrin deposition, and granulomas with viable mycobacteria are present (Fig. 68–3). A serous or serosanguineous pericardial effusion then develops, usually quite slowly and often without symptoms. Lymphocytes, monocytes, and plasma cells replace the polymorphonuclear cells that are present early in infection. In the third stage, the effusion is absorbed, the pericardium thickens, granulomas proliferate, and a thick coat of fibrin is deposited on the parietal pericardium. Acid-fast bacilli become difficult to find as dense fibrous tissue and collagen are deposited. In stage 4, which is associated with constriction, the pericardial space is obliterated by dense adhesions, the parietal pericardium is markedly thickened, and many granulomas are replaced by fibrous tissue. This is often followed by the accumulation of cholesterol crystals and calcification. Constrictive pericarditis may develop in up to 50% of patients with tuberculous pericarditis despite the use of antituberculous chemotherapy.[414, 459] Although the incidence of

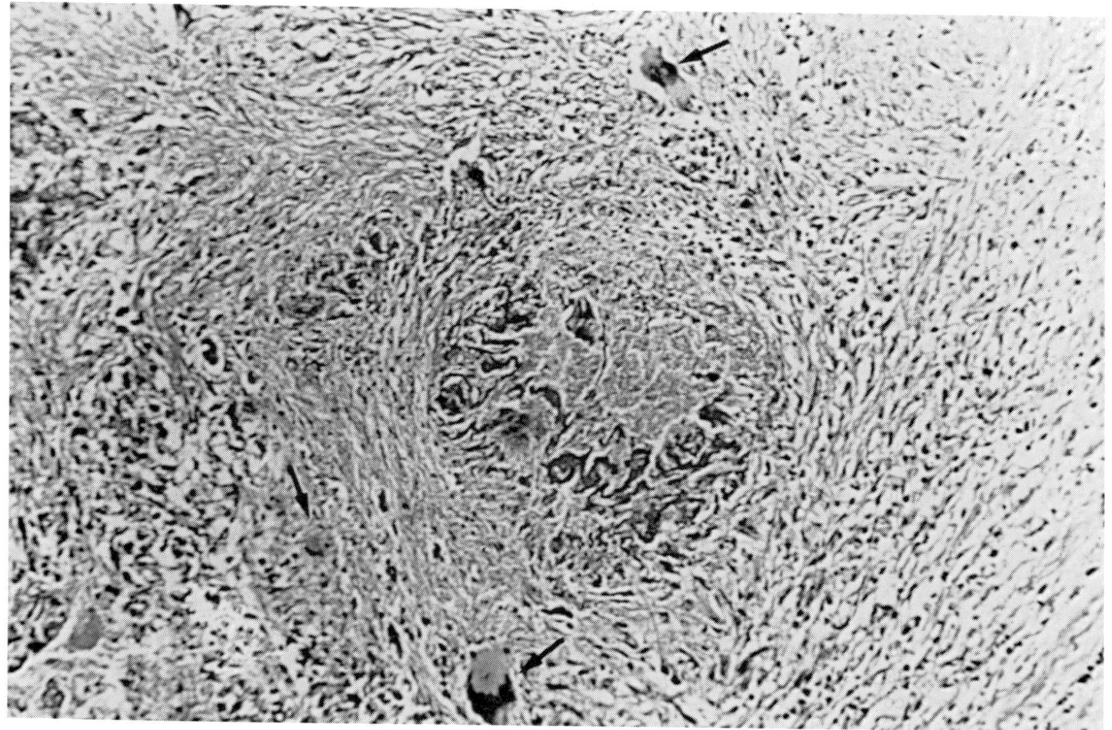

FIGURE 68–3. Tuberculous pericarditis, with a typical granuloma in the pericardium. There is central necrosis with aggregates of epithelioid cells at the periphery. Several multinucleated giant cells *(arrows)* are present (×40). (From Bloor CM. Pericarditis and myocarditis. In: Cardiac Pathology. Philadelphia: JB Lippincott; 1978:265–295.)

tuberculosis has declined, it remains an important cause of constrictive pericarditis, especially in underdeveloped countries.[444, 449, 450]

Regardless of the cause, if fluid accumulates rapidly in the pericardium and intrapericardial pressure rises, cardiac tamponade may result. Tamponade implies a progressive limitation of ventricular diastolic filling, with resultant reduction in stroke volume and cardiac output. In a series of medical patients with early cardiac tamponade, the cause was infectious in 12.5%, noninfectious in 74%, and undetermined in the remainder.[460]

Clinical Manifestations

The presentation of acute pericarditis varies depending on the cause. In viral or idiopathic pericarditis, chest pain is an important feature. This pain is often retrosternal, radiating to the shoulder and neck, and typically is aggravated by breathing, swallowing, and lying supine. In Smith's review of coxsackievirus B heart disease in adults,[332] 67% of patients had chest pain. Fever was present in 59%. A concurrent or prodromal flu-like illness with malaise, arthralgias, myalgias, and occasionally cough with sputum was present in 36%.

Bacterial pericarditis usually develops during the course of a severe systemic infection.[326, 327, 373] The patient is usually acutely ill; fever is almost always present, and dyspnea is common. However, chest pain is reported by only one third of patients with purulent pericarditis, and a pericardial friction rub, pathognomonic of pericarditis, is likewise present in only about one third.[326, 327] The symptoms and signs of pericarditis that are present (i.e., fever, dyspnea, and tachycardia), are often attributed to the underlying disease. Consequently, purulent pericarditis is recognized in many patients only at necropsy or after severe hemodynamic compromise has developed.[326, 327]

Tuberculous pericarditis most often has an insidious onset. Chest pain is present in 39 to 76%[414] but may be vague in nature. Weight loss, night sweats, cough, and dyspnea are common. Pericardial effusions in HIV-infected patients are usually asymptomatic or may be overlooked in those with severe intercurrent illness.[460a]

The classic physical finding in acute pericarditis is the three-component pericardial friction rub, which reflects cardiac motion during atrial systole, ventricular systole, and rapid ventricular filling in early diastole. This three-component rub was present in 50% of patients with acute pericarditis reported by Spodick.[461] The ventricular systolic component is often the loudest and most frequently appreciated. Rubs are often evanescent and may vary in quality; they are characteristically high-pitched, scratching, or grating. In the presence of significant pericardial effusion, there may be jugular venous distention, the most common physical finding in acute cardiac tamponade. Enlargement of the cardiac silhouette usually does not occur until at least 250 ml of fluid has accumulated in the pericardial space[462]; if fluid accumulates rapidly, tamponade may occur without detectable cardiomegaly. A pulsus paradoxus of more than 10 mmHg and a prominent x descent with loss of the y descent in the jugular venous pressure may be present. Dyspnea is common, but signs of left-sided heart failure usually are absent in cardiac tamponade, and clear lung fields may help to differentiate tamponade from cardiogenic shock.

Although the pericardium produces no electrical activity, the electrocardiogram is abnormal in 90% of patients with acute pericarditis,[462] reflecting diffuse subepicardial inflammation. Characteristic electrocardiographic changes are seen in approximately 50% of patients.[463, 464] Early in pericarditis, ST-segment elevation without change in QRS morphology typically occurs in multiple leads. Several days later, the ST segment returns to baseline, and there is T-wave flattening. During these early stages, there may also be depression of the PR segment. In contrast to myocardial infarction, the T-wave inversions in pericarditis usually do not occur until after the ST segment has returned to baseline. These T-wave inversions may last for weeks or months. Large pericardial effusions may be associated with reduced QRS voltage and electrical alternans. Sinus tachycardia is common, but the presence of other arrhythmias suggests preexisting underlying heart disease or significant myocardial involvement.[465]

Echocardiography has proved to be an extremely useful tool for diagnosis of pericardial effusion and should be performed if the situation is not immediately life-threatening. The size of the effusion can be roughly quantitated, and early hemodynamic compromise can often be detected.[462] Computed tomography has been useful in demonstrating pericardial thickening and, in some cases, in differentiating an uncomplicated transudate from a high-density exudate.[466, 467] MRI techniques also can easily detect pericardial fluid and thickening[468] but have no particular advantage over echocardiography.

Diagnosis

A wide variety of agents and diseases can cause pericarditis and pericardial effusion (Tables 68–3 and 68–4). Low-grade fever is common to many. A careful history, knowledge of the clinical setting in which the pericarditis occurs, and a search for clues outside the cardiovascular system are helpful in establishing a diagnosis. In a young person without underlying illness who presents with acute pericardial pain, the most likely diagnosis is viral or idiopathic pericarditis. However, establishing a specific viral diagnosis is difficult, costly, and often possible only in retrospect. Virus isolation can be attempted from throat and stool, and acute and convalescent sera can be tested for antibodies to potential pathogens (e.g., the coxsackie B viruses and any other enteroviruses prevalent locally at the time), but these approaches frequently fail to yield a specific diagnosis. Viruses are rarely isolated from pericardial fluid, even in patients in whom the diagnosis of viral myocarditis is highly probable.

If the clinical suspicion of viral or idiopathic pericarditis is strong in an otherwise healthy patient with uncomplicated pericarditis, pericardiocentesis or other invasive procedures add little diagnostically[435] and carry a small but definite risk.[489] After excluding patients with postpericardiotomy syndrome, myocardial infarction, renal failure, known neoplastic disease, trauma, and irradiation, Soler-Soler and colleagues prospectively evaluated 256 immunocompetent patients with primary acute pericardial disease.[329] After thorough diagnostic evaluation, 221 (86%) were thought to have acute idiopathic pericarditis. Unsuspected neoplastic pericarditis was found in 12 (5%), tuberculosis in 11 (4%), and collagen vascular disease in 4. Purulent pericarditis and viral pericarditis were each found in 3 patients, and *T. gondii* infection was found in 4. The diagnostic yield was substan-

TABLE 68–4 Major Noninfectious Causes of Acute Pericarditis

- Acute myocardial infarction[469–471]
- Uremia[472, 473]
- Neoplasia[462]
  - Primary
  - Metastatic
- Irradiation[474, 475]
- Cardiac injury[476]
  - Trauma (penetrating or blunt)[462]
  - Myocardial infarction (Dressler's) syndrome[477]
  - Postpericardiotomy[478]
- Dissecting aortic aneurysm[462, 479]
- Sarcoidosis[480]
- Collagen vascular diseases
  - Systemic lupus erythematosus[481]
  - Rheumatoid arthritis[482–484]
  - Scleroderma[485, 486]
  - Rheumatic fever[482]
- Inflammatory bowel disease[487]
- Drug-induced[462]
  - Procainamide
  - Hydralazine
  - Other
- Myxedema[488]

tial when pericardiocentesis or pericardiectomy with biopsy was done to relieve cardiac tamponade (28% and 54%, respectively), but led to a specific etiology only 5% and 4%, respectively, when these procedures were done solely for the purpose of diagnosis. The authors concluded that the presence of a pericardial effusion per se is not an indication for an invasive procedure; in patients with pericardial effusion that has persisted for longer than 3 weeks, an invasive procedure may be indicated. In a similar study of patients with large (>20 mm echo-free space in diastole) pericardial effusions without tamponade physiology or suspected purulent pericarditis, the diagnostic yield for pericardiocentesis or surgery was only 7%. Among those observed expectantly without a drainage procedure, no patient developed tamponade or died as a result of pericardial disease; moderate or large effusions persisted in only 2 of 45 patients.[490] Similarly, small, asymptomatic pericardial effusions in patients with HIV infection do not routinely require diagnostic evaluation. In a study of 13 AIDS patients who underwent surgical pericardial drainage, Kaposi's sarcoma was found in 3 (all with preexisting extracardiac lesions), but no other specific causes were identified.[491] However, in patients who are symptomatic, about two thirds of cases are caused by potentially treatable infection or neoplasm.[492]

When an invasive procedure is necessary, pericardiotomy with biopsy and drainage is preferable to pericardiocentesis because of greater diagnostic yield and fewer complications.[462] Pericardiocentesis alone establishes a specific etiologic diagnosis in 20 to 25% of cases; the availability of both fluid and tissue improves this yield to 54%.[435, 493] The technique of percutaneous pericardial biopsy is an alternative to surgery for obtaining tissue, and it appears to be safe and effective in patients with a thickened pericardium.[494–496] Noninfectious diseases predominate as causes of significant pericardial effusion and cardiac tamponade,[460] but bacterial and tuberculous effusions are more likely to have serious hemodynamic consequences.[489] Untreated purulent pericarditis usually is rapidly fatal.[373] In acutely ill patients in whom purulent pericarditis is suspected, the diagnosis should be pursued quickly and aggressively.

Treatment

Bed rest, symptomatic therapy for pain, and careful monitoring for the development of hemodynamic compromise are the mainstays of treatment for presumed viral or idiopathic pericarditis. Nonsteroidal anti-inflammatory agents are often successful in relieving symptoms but should be avoided in those with myocarditis based on data from animal models.[156, 302, 303] Because myocarditis often accompanies viral pericarditis and steroids enhance myocardial injury during active virus replication, we believe that steroids should be avoided during the acute illness. Viral or idiopathic pericarditis is generally benign and self-limited, but recurrences[454] and late constriction[455] do occur. Although prospective, double-blind clinical trials are lacking, several studies have suggested colchicine (1 mg/day) may be useful in limiting recurrences and may also be effective in the initial treatment of idiopathic pericarditis.[497–499] Steroids and other immunosuppressive agents have also been used to treat debilitating recurrences of idiopathic pericarditis, but controlled trials are lacking here also, and serious adverse effects with these regimens are more common.[500]

Surgical drainage of the pericardium, in addition to appropriate antibiotic therapy, is essential in almost all patients with purulent pericarditis.[365, 373, 380] Initial pericardiocentesis may be lifesaving, but fluid often reaccumulates, and constriction can develop rapidly.[373, 380] There is little rationale for irrigating the pericardium with antibiotics, because penetration of antibiotics from serum is excellent.[496] With early diagnosis and aggressive therapy, *H. influenzae* pericarditis in young patients has a good prognosis.[380] However, overall mortality in bacterial pericarditis remains high (30%), especially when it develops after surgery or occurs in the course of endocarditis.[373]

The treatment of tuberculous pericarditis remains controversial. Antituberculous therapy has reduced mortality substantially.[501] However, constrictive pericarditis may develop in 20 to 50% of patients despite appropriate treatment,[450, 459] and those with the clinical features of tamponade at presentation are at increased risk.[502] The addition of steroids to reduce inflammation and avoid late constriction is favored by many, including the authors.[445, 449, 503] The use of corticosteroids, in addition to antituberculous therapy, is supported by the results of two large, controlled trials in Transkei reported by Strang and associates.[445, 449] In patients with tuberculous pericardial effusions, the addition of prednisone to a four-drug antituberculosis regimen reduced the risk of death, the need for repeat pericardiocentesis, and the need for open surgical drainage because of rapid reaccumulation of pericardial fluid; constrictive pericarditis developed in 8% of steroid recipients and 12% of controls.[445] Prednisone was given in a dose of 60 mg daily for 4 weeks, followed by 30 mg daily for 4 weeks, 15 mg daily for 2 weeks, and 5 mg daily for 1 week. In a similar trial in patients with active tuberculous constrictive pericarditis, the addition of prednisone increased the rate of clinical improvement.[449] In 10 patients treated initially with 120 mg of prednisone daily, dramatic improvement occurred over a 1-week period, and the author suggested that higher initial doses might allow for shorter duration of treatment. Early surgical intervention is advocated in patients with hemodynamic compromise from recurrent effusion or progressive pericardial thickening.[459, 501, 504] In a retrospective study of children with tuberculous pericarditis reported from Africa, 5 (40%) of 12 patients with evidence of constriction at presentation required pericardiectomy.[505] These authors recommended observation for a period of 6 weeks to 3 months after the initiation of treatment, with pericardiectomy reserved for those who fail to improve or deteriorate. This procedure frequently results in striking hemodynamic improvement, but if diagnosis and therapy have been delayed, myocardial function may be affected, leading to less satisfactory results.[504] In some patients, resolution of venous congestion requires several months.[505] Patients with calcific tuberculous pericarditis have a poorer prognosis than those who undergo operation earlier in the course of disease.[505]

REFERENCES

1. Saphir O. Myocarditis: A general review with an analysis of two hundred and forty cases. Arch Pathol. 1941;32:1000-51 and 1942;33:88–137.
2. Gravanis MG, Sterby NH. Incidence of myocarditis. Arch Pathol Lab Med. 1991;115:390–392.
3. Bloor CM. Pericarditis and myocarditis. In: Cardiac Pathology. Philadelphia: JB Lippincott; 1978:265–295.
4. Bandt CM, Staley NA, Noren GR. Acute viral myocarditis: Clinical and histological changes. Minn Med. 1979;62:234–237.
5. Sole MJ, Lui P. Viral myocarditis: A paradigm for understanding the pathogenesis and treatment of dilated cardiomyopathy. J Am Coll Cardiol. 1992;22(Suppl A):99A–105A.
6. Bengtsson E, Orndahl G. Complications of mumps with special reference to the incidence of myocarditis. Acta Med Scand. 1954;149:381–388.
7. Lucke B, Wight T, Kime E. Pathologic anatomy and bacteriology of influenza: Epidemic of autumn 1918. Arch Intern Med. 1919;24:154–237.
8. Degen JA Jr. Visceral pathology in measles; clinicopathologic study of 100 fatal cases. Am J Med Sci. 1937;194:104–111.
9. Lucke B. Postmortem findings in measles bronchopneumonia and other acute infections. JAMA. 1918;70:2006–2011.
10. Frustaci A, Abdulla AK, Caldarulo M, et al. Fatal measles myocarditis. Cardiologia. 1990;35:347–349.
11. Saphir O, Wile SA. Myocarditis in poliomyelitis. Am J Med Sci. 1942;203:781–788.
12. Sylvest E. Epidemic Myalgia: Bornholm Disease. London: Oxford University Press; 1934.
13. Reyes MP, Lerner AM. Coxsackievirus myocarditis—with special reference to acute and chronic effects. Prog Cardiovasc Dis. 1985;27:373–394.
14. Hirschman SZ, Hammer GS. Coxsackie virus myopericarditis. A microbiological and clinical review. Am J Cardiol. 1974;34:224–232.
15. Woodruff JF. Viral myocarditis. Am J Pathol. 1980;101:427–478.
16. Grist NR, Bell EJ. A six-year study of coxsackievirus B infections in heart disease. J Hyg (Lond). 1974;73:165–172.
17. Hyypia T. Etiologic diagnosis of viral heart disease. Scand J Infect Dis. 1993;88(Suppl):25–31.
18. Martin AB, Webber S, Fricker FJ, et al. Acute myocarditis: Rapid diagnosis by PCR in children. Circulation. 1994;90:330–339.
19. Russell SJM, Bell EJ. Echoviruses and carditis. Lancet. 1970;1:784–785.

20. Bell EJ, Grist NR. ECHO viruses, carditis and acute pleurodynia. Am Heart J. 1971;82:133–138.
21. Jungeblut CW, Edwards JE. Isolation of poliomyelitis virus from the heart in fatal cases. Am J Clin Pathol. 1951;21:601–623.
22. Weinstein L, Shelokov A. Cardiovascular manifestations in acute poliomyelitis. N Engl J Med. 1951;244:281–285.
23. Roberts WC, Fox SM III. Mumps of the heart: Clinical and pathological features. Circulation. 1965;32:342–345.
24. Chaudary S, Jaski BE. Fulminant mumps myocarditis. Ann Intern Med. 1989;110:569–570.
25. Hamburger WW. The heart in influenza. Med Clin North Am. 1938;22:111–121.
26. Verel D, Warrack AJN, Potter CW, et al. Observations on the A2 England influenza epidemic. A clinicopathological study. Am Heart J. 1976;92:290–296.
27. Ross E, Armentrout SA. Myocarditis associated with rabies. Report of a case. N Engl J Med. 1962;266:1087–1089.
28. Ainger LE, Lawyer NG, Fitch CW. Neonatal rubella myocarditis. Br Heart J. 1966;28:691–697.
29. Kriseman T. Rubella myocarditis in a 9 year old patient. Clin Pediatr. 1984;23:240–241.
30. Chuah SK. Transient ventricular arrhythmia as a cardiac manifestation in dengue haemorrhagic fever—a case report. Singapore Med J. 1987;28:569–572.
31. Obeyesekere I, Hermon Y. Myocarditis and cardiomyopathy after arbovirus infections (dengue and chikungunya fever). Br Heart J. 1972;34:821–827.
32. Cannell DE. Myocardial degenerations in yellow fever. Am J Pathol. 1928;4:431–443.
33. Milei J, Bolomo NJ. Myocardial damage in viral hemorrhagic fevers. Am Heart J. 1982;104:1385–1391.
34. Thiede WH. Cardiac involvement in lymphocytic choriomeningitis. Arch Intern Med. 1962;109:50–54.
35. Henson D, Mufson MA. Myocarditis and pneumonitis with type 21 adenovirus infection: Association with fatal myocarditis and pneumonitis. Am J Dis Child. 1971;121:334–336.
36. Karjalainen J, Heikkila J, Nieminen MS, et al. Etiology of mild acute infectious myocarditis. Relation to clinical features. Acta Med Scand. 1983;213:65–73.
37. Waagner DC, Murphy TV. Varicella myocarditis. Pediatr Infect Dis J. 1990;9:360–363.
38. Woolf PK, Chung T-S, Stewart J, et al. Life-threatening dysrhythmias in varicella myocarditis. Clin Pediatr. 1987;26:480–482.
39. Coppack SW, Doshi R, Ghose AR. Fatal varicella in a healthy young adult. Postgrad Med J. 1985;61:529–531.
40. Tsintsof A, Delprado WJ, Keogh AM. Varicella zoster myocarditis progressing to cardiomyopathy and cardiac transplantation. Br Heart J. 1993;70:93–95.
41. Tiula E, Leinikki P. Fatal cytomegalovirus infection in a previously healthy boy with myocarditis and consumption coagulopathy as presenting signs. Scand J Infect Dis. 1972;4:57–60.
42. Maisch B, Schonian U, Crombach M, et al. Cytomegalovirus associated inflammatory heart muscle disease. Scand J Infect Dis. 1993;88:135–148.
43. Millett R, Tomita T, Marshall HE, et al. Cytomegalovirus endomyocarditis in a transplanted heart. A case report with in situ hybridization. Arch Pathol Lab Med. 1991;115:511–515.
44. Schonian U, Crombach M, Maisch B. Assessment of cytomegalovirus DNA and protein expression in patients with myocarditis. Clin Immunol Immunopathol. 1993;68:229–233.
45. Ando H, Shiramizu T, Hisanou R. Dilated cardiomyopathy caused by cytomegalovirus infection in a renal transplant recipient. Jpn Heart J. 1992;33:409–412.
46. Arbustini E, Grasso M, Diegoli M, et al. Histopathologic and molecular profile of human cytomegalovirus infections in patients with heart transplants. Am J Clin Pathol. 1992;98:205–213.
47. Webster BH. Cardiac complications of infectious mononucleosis: A review of the literature and report of five cases. Am J Med Sci. 1957;234:62–70.
48. Tyson AA Jr, Hackshaw BT, Kutcher MA. Acute Epstein-Barr virus myocarditis simulating myocardial infarction with cardiogenic shock. S Med J. 1989;82:1184–1187.
49. Matthews AW, Griffiths ID. Post vaccinal pericarditis and myocarditis. Br Heart J. 1974;36:1043–1045.
50. Anderson T, Foulis MA, Grist NR, et al. Clinical and laboratory observations in a smallpox outbreak. Lancet. 1951;1:1248–1252.
51. Mahapatra RK, Ellis GH. Myocarditis and hepatitis B virus. Angiology. 1985;36:116–119.
52. Bell H. Cardiac manifestations of viral hepatitis. JAMA. 1971;218:387–391.
53. Ursell PC, Habib A, Sharma P, et al. Hepatitis B virus and myocarditis. Hum Pathol. 1984;15:481–484.
54. Okabe M, Fukuda K, Arakawa K, et al. Chronic variant of myocarditis associated with hepatitis C virus infection. Circulation. 1997; 96(1):22–24.
55. Matsumori A, Maloba Y, Sasayama S. Dilated cardiomyopathy associated with hepatitis C virus infection. Circulation. 1995;92:2519–2525.
56. Thomas JA, Raroque, S, Scott WA, et al. Successful treatment of severe dysrhythmias in infants with respiratory syncytial virus infections: Two cases and a literature review. Crit Care Med. 1997;25(5):880–886.
57. Enders G, Deotsch J, Bauer J, et al. Life-threatening parvovirus B19–associated myocarditis and cardiac transplantation as possible therapy: Two case reports. Clin Infect Dis. 1998;26(2):355–358.
58. Schowengerdt KO, Ni J, Denfield SW, et al. Association of parvovirus B19 genome in children with myocarditis and cardiac allograft rejection: Diagnosis using the polymerase chain reaction. Circulation. 1997;96(10):3549–3554.
59. Gore I, Saphir O. Myocarditis. A classification of 1402 cases. Am Heart J. 1947;34:827–830.
60. Gore I. Myocardial changes in fatal diphtheria; summary of observations in 221 cases. Am J Med Sci. 1948;215:257–266.
61. Havaldar PV, Patil VD, Siddibhavi BM, et al. Fulminant diptheretic myocarditis. Indian Heart J. 1989;41:265–269.
62. Roberts WC, Berard CW. Gas gangrene of the heart in clostridial septicemia. Am Heart J. 1967;74:482–488.
63. Guneratne F. Gas gangrene (abscess) of heart. N Y State J Med. 1975;75:1766.
64. Joshi MK, Kandoth PW, Barve RJ, et al. Rheumatic fever: Clinical profile of 339 cases with long term follow up. Indian Pediatr. 1983;20:849–853.
65. Karjalainen J. Streptococcal tonsillitis and acute nonrheumatic myopericarditis. Chest. 1989;95:359–363.
66. Brasier AR, Macklis JD, Vaughan D, et al. Myopericarditis as an initial presentation of meningococcemia. Unusual manifestation of infection with serotype W135. Am J Med. 1987;82:641–644.
67. Cohen JI, Bartlett JA, Corey GR. Extra-intestinal manifestations of *Salmonella* infections. Medicine. 1987;66:349–388.
68. Wamder GS, Khurana SB, Puri S. *Salmonella* myopericarditis presenting with acute pulmonary oedema. Indian Heart J. 1992;44:55–56.
69. Baysal K, Sancak R, Ozturk F, et al. Cardiac involvement due to *Salmonella typhi* infections in children. Ann Trop Paediatr. 1998;188(1):23–25.
70. Lubani M, Sharda D, Helin I. Cardiac manifestations in brucellosis. Arch Dis Child. 1986;61:569–572.
71. Jubber AS, Gunawardana DR, Lulu AR. Acute pulmonary edema in *Brucella* myocarditis and interstitial pneumonitis. Chest. 1990;97:1008–1009.
72. Watanakunakorn C, Tan JS, Phair JP. Some salient features of *Staphylococcus aureus* endocarditis. Am J Med. 1973;54:473–481.
73. Tice AD, Nelson JS, Visconti EB. *Listeria monocytogenes* pericarditis and myocardial abscess. R I Med J. 1979;62:135–138.
74. McCue MJ, Moore EE. Myocarditis with microabscess formation caused by *Listeria monocytogenes* associated with myocardial infarct. Hum Pathol. 1979;10:469–472.
75. Stamm AM, Smith SH, Kirklin JK, et al. Listerial myocarditis in cardiac transplantation. Rev Infect Dis. 1990;12:820–823.
76. Armengol S, Domingo C, Mesalles E. Myocarditis: A rare complication during *Legionella* infection. Int J Cardiol. 1992;27:418–420.
77. Chen S-C, Tsai CC, Nouri S. Carditis associated with *Mycoplasma pneumoniae* infection. Am J Dis Child. 1986;140:471–472.
78. Lind K. Manifestation and complications of *Mycoplasma pneumoniae* disease: A review. Yale J Biol Med. 1983;56:461–468.
79. Karjalainen J. A loud third heart sound and asymptomatic myocarditis during *Mycoplasma pneumoniae* infection. Eur Heart J. 1990;11:960–963.
80. Dymock IW, Lawson JM, MacLennan WJ, et al. Myocarditis associated with psittacosis. Br J Clin Pract. 1971;25:240–242.
81. Gran JT, Hjetland R, Andreassen AH. Pneumonia, myocarditis and reactive arthritis due to *Chlamydia pneumoniae*. Scand J Rheumatol. 1993;22:43–44.
82. Wesslen LP, Pahlson C, Friman G, et al. Myocarditis caused by *Chlamydia pneumoniae* (TWAR) and sudden unexpected death in a Swedish elite orienteer (Letter). Lancet. 1992;340:427–428.
83. Marin-Garcia J, Mirvis DM. Myocardial disease in Rocky Mountain spotted fever: Clinical, functional, and pathologic findings. Pediatr Cardiol. 1984;5:149–154.
84. Brown GW, Shirai A, Jegathesan M, et al. Febrile illness in Malaysia—an analysis of 1629 hospitalized patients. Am J Trop Med Hyg. 1984;33:311–315.
85. Ognibene AJ, O'Leary DS, Czarnecki SW, et al. Myocarditis and disseminated intravascular coagulation in scrub typhus. Am J Med Sci. 1971;262:233–239.
86. Diab SM, Araj GF, Fenech FF. Cardiovascular and pulmonary complications of epidemic typhus. Trop Geog Med. 1989;41:76–79.
87. Williams JD, Snow RM, Arciniegas JG. Myocardial involvement in a patient with human ehrlichiosis. Am J Med. 1995;98:414–415.
87a. Leon F, Badui E, Campos A, et al. Cholera and mycarditis—a case report. Angiology. 1997; 48:545–549.
88. Steere AC, Batsford WP, Weinberg M, et al. Lyme carditis: Cardiac abnormalities of Lyme disease. Ann Intern Med. 1980;93:8–16.
89. McAlister HF, Klementowicz PT, Andrews C, et al. Lyme carditis: An important cause of reversible heart block. Ann Intern Med. 1989;110:339–345.
90. van der Linde MR. Lyme carditis: Clinical characteristics of 105 cases. Scand J Infect Dis. 1991;77:81–84.
91. Midttun M, Lebech AM, Hansen K, et al. Lyme carditis: A clinical presentation and long time follow-up. Scand J Infect Dis. 1997;29:153–157.
92. Segal LH. Early dissemenated Lyme disease: Cardiac manifestations. Am J Med. 1995; 98(Suppl 4A):258–285.
93. Williams AH. *Aspergillus* myocarditis. Am J Clin Pathol. 1974;61:247–256.
94. Atkinson JB, Connor DH, Robinowitz M, et al. Cardiac fungal infections: Review of autopsy findings in 60 patients. Hum Pathol. 1984;15:935–942.
95. Rogers JG, Windle JR, McManus BM, et al. *Aspergillus* myocarditis presenting as myocardial infarction with complete heart block. Am Heart J. 1990;120:430–432.
96. Cox JN, Di Dio F, Pizzolato G-P, et al. *Aspergillus* endocarditis and myocarditis in a patient with the acquired immunodeficiency syndrome (AIDS): A review of the literature. Virchows Arch. 1990;417:255–259.
97. Lewis W, Lipsick J, Cammarosano C. Cryptococcal myocarditis in acquired immune deficiency syndrome. Am J Cardiol. 1985;9:1240.
98. Lafont A, Wolff M, Marche C, et al. Overwhelming myocarditis due to *Cryptococcus neoformans* in an AIDS patient. Lancet. 1987;2:1145–1146.
99. Rosenbaum MB. Chagasic myocardiopathy. Prog Cardiovasc Dis. 1964;7:199–255.
100. Mott KE, Hagstrom JWC. The pathologic lesions of the cardiac autonomic nervous system in chronic Chagas' myocarditis. Circulation. 1965;31:273–286.

101. Mendoza I, Camardo J, Moleiro F, et al. Sustained ventricular tachycardia in chronic Chagasic myocarditis. Am J Cardiol. 1986;57:423–427.
102. Higuchi M de L. Chronic chagasic cardiopathy: The product of a turbulent host-parasite relationship. Rev Inst Med Trop Sao Paulo. 1997;39:53–60.
103. Fuenmayor AJ, Fuenmayor AM, Carrasco H, et al. Results of electrophysiologic studies in patients with acute chagasic myocarditis. Clin Cardiol. 1997;20:1021–1024.
104. de Carvalho VB, Sousa EF, Vila JH, et al. Heart transplantation in Chagas' disease. 10 years after the initial experience. Circulation. 1996;94:1815–1817.
105. Poltera AA, Owor R, Cox JN. Pathological aspects of human African trypanosomiasis in Uganda. Virchows Arch. 1977;373:249–265.
106. Barr R. Human trichinosis: Report of 4 cases with emphasis on central nervous system involvement and a survey of 500 consecutive autopsies at the Ottawa Civic Hospital. CMAJ. 1966;95:912–917.
107. Grey DF, Morse BS, Phillips WF. Trichinosis with neurologic and cardiac involvement. Review of the literature and report of three cases. Ann Intern Med. 1962;57:230–244.
108. Compton SJ, Celum CL, Lee C, et al. Trichinosis with ventilatory failure and persistent myocarditis. Clin Infect Dis. 1993;16:500–504.
109. Hofman P, Drici MD, Gibelin P, et al. Prevalence of toxoplasma myocarditis in patients with the acquired immunodeficiency syndrome. Br Heart J. 1993;70:376–381.
110. Yermakov V, Rashid RK, Vuletin JC, et al. Disseminated toxoplasmosis. Case report and review of the literature. Arch Pathol Lab Med. 1982;106:524–528.
111. Matturri L, Quattrone P, Varesi C, et al. Cardiac toxoplasmosis in pathology of acquired immunodeficiency syndrome. Panminerva Med. 1990;32:194–196.
112. Israelski DM, Remington JS. Toxoplasmosis in the non-AIDS immunocompromised host. Cur Clin Topics Infect Dis. 1993;13:322–356.
113. Duffield JS, Jacob AJ, Miller HC. Recurrent, life-threatening atrioventricular dissociation associated with toxoplasma myocarditis. Heart. 1996; 76:453–454.
114. Montoya JG, Jordan R, Lingamneni S, et al. Toxoplasmic myocarditis and polymyositis in patients with acute acquired toxoplasmosis diagnosed during life. Clin Infect Dis. 1997;24:676–683.
115. Buchbinder NA, Roberts WC. Left-sided valvular active infective endocarditis. A study of 45 necropsy patients. Am J Med. 1972;53:20–35.
116. Welch K, Finkbeiner W, Alpers CE, et al. Autopsy findings in the acquired immune deficiency syndrome. JAMA. 1984;252:1152–1159.
117. Baroldi G, Carallo S, Moroni M, et al. Focal lymphocytic myocarditis in acquired immunodeficiency syndrome (AIDS): A correlative morphologic and clinical study in 26 consecutive fatal cases. J Am Coll Cardiol. 1988;12:463–469.
118. Cammarosano C, Lewis W. Cardiac lesions in acquired immune deficiency syndrome (AIDS). J Am Coll Cardiol. 1985;5:703–706.
119. Fink L, Reichek N, St. John Sutton MG. Cardiac abnormalities in acquired immune deficiency syndrome. Am J Cardiol. 1984;54:1161–1163.
120. Milei J, Grana D, Fernández Alonso G, et al. Cardiac involvement in acquired immunodeficiency syndrome—a review to push action. The Committee for the Study of Cardiac Involvement in AIDS. Clin Cardiol. 1998;21:465–472.
121. Yunis NA, Stone VE. Cardiac manifestations of HIV/AIDS: A review of disease spectrum and clinical management. J Acq Immune Def Syndr Hum Retrovirol. 1998;18:145–154.
122. Kaul S, Fishbein MC, Siegel RJ. Cardiac manifestations of acquired immune deficiency syndrome: A 1991 update. Am Heart J. 1991;122:537–544.
123. De Castro S, Migliau G, Silvestri A, et al. Heart involvement in AIDS: A prospective study during various stages of the disease. Eur Heart J. 1992;13:1452–1459.
124. Currie PF, Jacob AJ, Foreman AR, et al. Heart muscle disease related to HIV infection: Prognostic implications. BMJ. 1994; 309:1605–1607.
125. Barbaro G, Di Lorenzo G, Grisorio B, et al. Incidence of dilated cardiomyopathy and detection of HIV in myocardial cells of HIV-positive patients. N Engl J Med. 1998;339:1093–1099.
126. Boller A-M, Al-Attar I, Orav EJ, Lipshultz SE. Cardiovascular morbidity and mortality in pediatric HIV infection. In: Lipshultz SE, ed. Cardiology in AIDS. New York: Chapman & Hall; 1998:77–94.
127. Calabrese LH, Proffitt MR, Yen-Lieberman B, et al. Congestive cardiomyopathy and illness related to the acquired immunodeficiency syndrome (AIDS) associated with isolation of retrovirus from myocardium. Ann Intern Med. 1987;107:691–692.
128. Dittrich H, Chow L, Denaro F, et al. Human immunodeficiency virus, coxsackievirus, and cardiomyopathy (Letter). Ann Intern Med. 1988;108:308–309.
129. Factor S, Flomenbaum M, Vdem S, et al. Proliferative membranopathy and human immunodeficiency virus in AIDS hearts (Abstract). Circulation. 1989;80(Suppl II):535.
130. Grody W, Cheng L, Pang M, et al. Direct infection of the heart by human immunodeficiency virus (HIV) (Abstract). Circulation. 1989;80(Suppl II):665.
131. Beschorner WE, Baughman K, Turnicky RP, et al. HIV-associated myocarditis: Pathology and immunopathology. Am J Pathol. 1990;137:1365–1371.
132. Wu TC, Pizzorno MC, Hayward GS, et al. In situ detection of human cytomegalovirus immediate-early gene transcripts within cardiac myocytes of patients with HIV-associated cardiomyopathy. AIDS. 1992;6:777–785.
133. Luginbuhl LM, Orav EJ, McIntosh K, Lipshultz SE. Cardiac morbidity and related mortality in children with HIV infection. JAMA. 1993;269:2869–2875.
134. Lipshultz SE. Dilated cardiomyopathy in HIV infected patients. N Engl J Med. 1998;339:1153–1154.
135. Herskowitz A, Ansori A, Neumann D, et al. Cardiomyopathy in acquired immunodeficiency syndrome: Evidence for autoimmunity. Circulation. 1989;80(Suppl II):322.
136. Parravicini C, Baroldi G, Gaiera G, et al. Phenotype of intramyocardial leukocytic infiltrates in acquired immunodeficiency syndrome (AIDS): A postmortem immunohistochemical study in 34 consecutive cases. Mod Pathol. 1991;4:559–565.
137. Mues B, Brisse E, Zwadlo G, et al. Phenotyping of macrophages with monoclonal antibodies in endomyocardial biopsies as a new approach to diagnosis of myocarditis. Eur Heart J. 1990;11:619–627.
138. Chow LH, Ye Y, Linder J, et al. Phenotypic analysis of infiltrating cells in human myocarditis. An immunohistological study in paraffin-embedded tissue. Arch Pathol Lab Med. 1989;113:1357–1362.
139. Keogh AM, Billingham ME, Schroeder JS. Rapid histological changes in endomyocardial biopsy specimens after myocarditis. Br Heart J. 1990;64:406–408.
140. Edwards WD. Myocarditis and endomyocardial biopsy. Cardiol Clin. 1984;2:647–656.
141. Lyden D, Olszewski J, Huber S. Variation in susceptibility of BALB/c mice to coxsackievirus group B type 3-induced myocarditis with age. Cell Immunol. 1987;105:332–339.
142. Herskowitz A, Wolfgram LJ, Rose NR, et al. Coxsackievirus B3, murine myocarditis: A pathologic spectrum of myocarditis in genetically defined inbred strains. J Am Coll Cardiol. 1987;9:1311–1319.
143. Huber SA, Lodge PA. Coxsackievirus B-3 myocarditis. Identification of different pathogenic mechanisms in DBA/2 and BALB/c mice. Am J Pathol. 1986;122:284–291.
144. Wolfgram LJ, Beisel KW, Herskowitz A, et al. Variations in the susceptibility to coxsackievirus B3-induced myocarditis among different strains of mice. J Immunol. 1986;136:1846–1852.
145. Khatib R, Probert A, Reyes MP, et al. Mouse strain–related variation as a factor in the pathogenesis of coxsackievirus B3 murine myocarditis. J Gen Virol. 1987;68:2981–2988.
146. Chow LH, Beisel KW, McManus BM. Enteroviral infection of mice with severe combined immunodeficiency. Evidence for direct viral pathogenesis of myocardial injury. Lab Invest. 1992;66:24–31.
147. McManus BM, Chow LH, Wilson JE, et al. Direct myocardial injury by enterovirus: A central role in the evolution of murine myocarditis. Clin Immunol Immunopathol. 1993;68:159–169.
148. Rager-Zisman B, Allison AC. The role of antibody and host cells in the resistance of mice against infection by coxsackie B-3 virus. J Gen Virol. 1973;19:329–338.
149. Woodruff JF. Lack of correlation between neutralizing antibody production and suppression of coxsackievirus B-3 replication in target organs: Evidence for involvement of mononuclear inflammatory cells in host defense. J Immunol. 1979;123:31–36.
150. Godeny EK, Gaunt CJ. In situ immune autoradiographic identification of cells in heart tissue of mice with coxsackievirus B3–induced myocarditis. Am J Pathol. 1987;129:267–276.
151. Godeny EK, Gaunt CJ. Murine natural killer cells limit coxsackievirus B3 replication. J Immunol. 1987;139:913–918.
152. Godeny EK, Gaunt CJ. Involvement of natural killer cells in coxsackievirus B3–induced murine myocarditis. J Immunol. 1986;137:1695–1702.
153. Keil RJ, Smith FE, Chason J, et al. Coxsackievirus B3 myocarditis in C3H/Hej mice: Description of an inbred model and the effect of exercise on virulence. Eur J Epidemiol. 1989;5:348–350.
154. Kilbourne ED, Wilson CB, Perrier D. The induction of gross myocardial lesions by a coxsackie (pleurodynia) virus and cortisone. J Clin Invest. 1956;35:362–370.
155. Beck MA, Kolbeck PC, Rohr LH, et al. Benign human enterovirus becomes virulent in selenium-deficient mice. J Med Virol. 1994;43:166–170.
156. Rezkalla S, Khatib G, Khatib R. Coxsackievirus B3 murine myocarditis: Deleterious effects of nonsteroidal anti-inflammatory agents. J Lab Clin Med. 1986;107:393–395.
157. Khatib R, Reyes MP, Smith F, et al. Enhancement of coxsackievirus B4 virulence by indomethacin. J Lab Clin Med. 1990;116:116–120.
158. Kishimoto C, Abekmann WH. In vivo significance of T cells in the development of coxsackievirus B3 myocarditis in mice. Immature but antigen-specific T cells aggravate cardiac injury. Circ Res. 1990;67:589–598.
159. Huber SA, Lodge PA. Coxsackievirus B-3 myocarditis in BALB/c mice. Evidence for autoimmunity to myocyte antigens. Am J Pathol. 1984;116:21–29.
160. Guthrie M, Lodge PA, Huber SA. Cardiac injury in myocarditis induced by coxsackievirus group B, type 3 in BALB/c mice is mediated by Lyt 2^+ cytolytic lymphocytes. Cell Immunol. 1984;88:558–567.
161. Kishimoto C, Kuribayashi K, Masuda T, et al. Immunologic behavior of lymphocytes in experimental viral myocarditis: Significance of T lymphocytes in the severity of myocarditis and silent myocarditis in BALB/c-nu/nu mice. Circulation. 1985;71:1247–1254.
162. Lyden DC, Huber SA. Aggravation of coxsackievirus, group B, type 3–induced myocarditis and increase in cellular immunity to myocyte antigens in pregnant BALB/c mice and animals treated with progesterone. Cell Immunol. 1984;87:462–472.
163. Job LP, Lyden DC, Huber SA. Demonstration of suppressor cells in coxsackievirus group B, type 3 infected female BALB/c mice which prevent myocarditis. Cell Immunol. 1986;98:104–113.
164. Huber SA, Job LP. Differences in cytolytic T cell response of BALB/c mice infected with myocarditic and non-myocarditic strains of coxsackievirus group B, type 3. Infect Immun. 1983;39:1419–1427.
165. Lee C, Maull E, Chapman N. Genomic regions of coxsackievirus B3–associated with cardiovirulence. J Med Virol. 1997;62:341–347.
166. Weller AH, Simpson K, Herzum M, et al. Coxsackievirus-B3–induced myocarditis: Virus receptor antibodies modulate myocarditis. J Immunol. 1989;143:1843–1850.

167. Lane JR, Neumann DA, Lafond-Walker A, et al. Role of IL-1 and tumor necrosis factor in coxsackievirus-induced autoimmune myocarditis. J Immunol. 1993;151:1682–1690.
168. Seko Y, Matsuda H, Kato K, et al. Expression of intercellular adhesion molecule-1 in murine hearts with acute myocarditis caused by coxsackievirus B3. J Clin Invest. 1993;91:1327–1336.
169. Herskowitz A, Admed-Ansari A, Neumann DA, et al. Induction of major histocompatibility complex antigens within the myocardium of patients with active myocarditis: A nonhistologic marker of myocarditis. J Am Col Cardiol. 1990;15:624–632.
170. Kandolf R, Klingel K, Zell R, et al. Molecular pathogenesis of enterovirus-induced myocarditis: Virus persistence and chronic inflammation. Intervirology. 1993;35:140–151.
171. Rabausch-Starz A, Schwaiger K, Grunewald H-K, et al. Persistence of virus and viral genome in myocardium after coxsackievirus B3–induced murine myocarditis. Clin Exp Immunol. 1994; 96:69–74.
172. Keeling PJ, Jeffrey S, Caforio AL, et al. Similar prevalence of enteroviral genome within the myocardium from patients with idiopathic dilated cardiomyopathy and controls by the polymerase chain reaction. Br Heart J. 1992; 68:554–559.
173. Easton AJ, Eglin RP. The detection of coxsackievirus RNA in cardiac tissue by in situ hybridization. J Gen Virol. 1988;69:285–291.
174. Wolfgram LJ, Beisel KW, Rose NR. Heart-specific autoantibodies following murine coxsackievirus B3 myocarditis. J Exp Med. 1985;161:1112–1121.
175. Neu N, Beisel KW, Traystman MD, et al. Autoantibodies specific for the cardiac myosin isoform are found in mice susceptible to coxsackievirus B3–induced myocarditis. J Immunol. 1987;138:2488–2492.
176. Gauntt C, Higdon A, Bowers D, et al. What lessions can be learned from animal model studies in viral heart disease? Scand J Infect Dis. 1993;88(Suppl):49–65.
177. Maisch B, Trostel-Soeder R, Stechemesser E, et al. Diagnostic relevance of humoral and cell-mediated immune reactions in patients with acute viral myocarditis. Clin Exp Immunol. 1982;48:533–545.
178. Shulze K, Becker B, Schauer R, Schultheib HP. Antibodies to the ADP-ATP carrier—an autoantigen in myocarditis and dilated cardiomyopathy—impair cardiac function. Circulation. 1990;81:959–969.
179. Maisch B, Deeg P, Liebau G, et al. Diagnostic relevance of humoral and cytotoxic immune reactions in primary and secondary dilated cardiomyopathy. Am J Cardiol. 1983;52:1072–1078.
180. Schultheib HP. The significance of autoantibodies against the ADP/ATP carrier for the pathogenesis of myocarditis and dilated cardiomyopathy—clinical and experimental data. Semin Immunopath. 1993;68:229–233.
181. Neu N, Rose NR, Beisel KW, et al. Cardiac myosin induces myocarditis in genetically predisposed mice. J Immunol. 1987;139:3630–3636.
182. Zhang H, Morgan-Capner P, Latif N, et al. Coxsackievirus B3–induced myocarditis. Characterization of stable attenuated variants that protect against infection with the cardiovirulent wild-type strain. Am J Pathol. 1997;150:2197–2207.
183. Liao L, Sindhwani R, Rojkind M, et al. Antibody-mediated autoimmune myocarditis depends on genetically determined target organ sensitivity. J Exp Med. 1995;181:1123–1131.
184. Huber S, Polgar J, Moraska A, et al. T-lymphocyte responses in CVR3-induced murine myocarditis. Scand J Infect Dis. 1993;88(Suppl):67–78.
185. See DM, Tilles JG. Viral myocarditis. Rev Infect Dis. 1991;13:951–956.
186. Maisch B, Bauer E, Cirsi M, et al. Cytolytic cross-reactive antibodies directed against the cardiac membrane and viral proteins in coxsackievirus B3 and B4 myocarditis. Characterization and pathogenetic relevance. Circulation. 1993;87(Suppl 5):IV49–65.
187. Herzum M, Maisch B. Humoral and cellular immune reactions to the myocardium in myocarditis. Herz. 1992;17:91–96.
188. Silver MA, Kowalczyk BS. Coronary microvascular narrowing in acute murine coxsackie B3 myocarditis. Am Heart J. 1989;118:173–174.
189. Lawson CM, O'Donoghue H, Bartholomaeus WN, et al. Genetic control of mouse cytomegalovirus–induced myocarditis. Immunology. 1990;69:20–26.
190. Craighead JE, Martin WB, Huber SA. Role of CD4+ (helper) T cells in the pathogenesis of murine cytomegalovirus myocarditis. Lab Invest. 1992;66:755–761.
191. Lawson CM, O'Donoghue HL, Reed WD. Mouse cytomegalovirus infection induces antibodies which cross-react with virus and cardiac myosin: A model for the study of molecular mimicry in the pathogenesis of viral myocarditis. Immunology. 1992;75:513–519.
192. Sherry B, Li XY, Tyler KL, et al. Lymphocytes protect against and are not required for reovirus-induced myocarditis. J Virol. 1993;67:6119–6124.
193. Bloor CM. Protozoal, helminthic and fungal heart disease. In: Cardiac Pathology. Philadelphia: JB Lippincott; 1978:335–366.
194. Felix JC, von Kreuter BF, Santos-Buch CA. Mimicry of heart cell surface epitopes in primary anti-*Trypanosoma cruzi* lyt 2+ T lymphocytes. Clin Immunol Immunopathol. 1993;68:141–146.
195. Armostrong AL, Barthold SW, Persing DH, et al. Carditis in Lyme disease: Susceptible and resistant strains of laboratory mice infected with *Borrelia burgdorferi*. Am J Trop Med Hyg. 1992;47:249–258.
196. Ruderman RM, Kerr JS, Telford SR III, et al. Early murine lyme carditis has a macrophage predominance and is independent of major histocompatibility complex class II–CD4+ T cell interactions. J Infect Dis. 1995;171:362–370.
197. Abelmann WH. Virus and the heart. Circulation. 1971;44:950–956.
198. Vikerfors T, Stjerna A, Olcen P, et al. Acute myocarditis. Serologic diagnosis, clinical findings and follow-up. Acta Med Scand. 1988;223:45–52.
199. Stratmann HG. Acute myocarditis versus myocardial infarction: Evaluation and management of the young patient with prolonged chest pain—case reports. Angiology. 1988;39:253–258.
200. Miklozek CL, Crumpacker CS, Royal HD, et al. Myocarditis presenting as acute myocardial infarction. Am Heart J. 1988;115:768–776.
201. Spodick DH. Infection and infarction. Acute viral (and other) infection in the onset, pathogenesis, and mimicry of acute myocardial infarction. Am J Med. 1986;81:661–668.
202. Beaufils P, Slama R. Myocarditis confirmed by biopsy presenting as acute myocardial infarction. Br Heart J. 1986;4:420.
203. Dec GW Jr, Waldman H, Southern J, et al. Viral myocarditis mimicking acute myocardial infarction (see comments). J Am Coll Cardiol. 1992;20:85–89.
204. Griffiths PD, Hannington G, Booth JC. Coxsackie B virus infections and myocardial infarction. Results from a prospective, epidemiologically controlled study. Lancet. 1980;1:1387–1389.
205. Heikkila J, Karjalainen J. Evaluation of mild acute infectious myocarditis. Br Heart J. 1982;47:381–391.
206. Kaplan MH, Kelin SW, McPhee J, et al. Group B coxsackievirus infection in infants younger than three months of age: A serious childhood illness. Rev Infect Dis. 1983;5:1019–1032.
207. Karjalainen J. Clinical diagnosis of myocarditis and dilated cardiomyopathy. Scand J Infect Dis. 1993;88(Suppl):33–43.
208. Karjalainen J, Heikkila J. Acute pericarditis: Myocardial enzyme release as evidence for myocarditis. Am Heart J. 1986;111:546.
209. Scott LP III, Gutelius MF, Parrott RH. Children with acute respiratory tract infections. An electrocardiographic survey. Am J Dis Child. 1970;119:111–113.
210. Karjalainen J. Functional and myocarditis-induced T-wave abnormalities: Effect of orthostasis, beta blockade, and epinephrine. Chest. 1983;83:868–872.
211. Morgera T, Di Lenarda A, Dreas L, et al. Electrocardiography of myocarditis revisited: Clinical and prognostic significance of electrocardiographic changes. Am Heart J. 1992;124:455–467.
212. Smith SC, Landenson JH, Mason JW, et al. Elevations of cardiac troponin I associated with myocarditis. Experimental and clinical correlates. Circulation. 1997;95:163–168.
213. Weinhouse E, Wanderman KL, Sofer S, et al. Viral myocarditis simulating dilated cardiomyopathy in early childhood: Evaluation by serial echocardiography. Br Heart J. 1986;56:94–97.
214. Nieminen MS, Heikkila J, Karjalainen J. Echocardiography in acute infectious myocarditis: Relation to clinical and electrocardiographic findings. Am J Cardiol. 1984;53:1331–1337.
215. Kondo M, Takahashi M, Shimono Y, et al. Reversible asymmetric septal hypertrophy in acute myocarditis. Serial findings of two-dimensional echocardiogram and thallium-201 scintigram. Jpn Circ J. 1985;49:589–593.
216. Pinamonti B, Alberti E, Cigalotto A, et al. Echocardiographic findings in myocarditis. Am J Cardiol. 1988;62:285–291.
217. Yasuda T, Palacios IF, Dec W, et al. Indium-111 monoclonal antimyosin antibody imaging in the diagnosis of acute myocarditis. Circulation. 1987;76:306–311.
218. Carrio I, Berna L, Ballester M, et al. Indium-111 antimyosin scintigraphy to assess myocardial damage in patients with suspected myocarditis and cardiac rejection. J Nucl Med. 1988;29:1893–1900.
219. Casans I, Villar A, Almenar V, et al. Lyme myocarditis diagnosed by indium-111 antimyosin scintigraphy. Eur J Nucl Med. 1989;15:330–331.
220. Dec W, Palacios I, Yasuda T, et al. Antimyosin antibody cardiac imaging: Its role in the diagnosis of myocarditis. J Am Coll Cardiol. 1990;16:97–104.
221. Nakata T, Gotoh M, Noto T, et al. Quantification of antimyosin uptake and infarct size at various stages of myocardial infarction. Int J Cardiol. 1992;34:85–95.
222. Obrador D, Ballester M, Carrio I, et al. Active myocardial damage without attending inflammatory response in dilated cardiomyopathy. J Am Coll Cardiol. 1993;21:1667–1671.
223. Narula J, Khaw BA, Dec GW Jr, et al. Brief report: recognition of acute myocarditis masquerading as acute myocardial infarction. N Engl J Med. 1993;328:100–104.
224. Aherne T, Tscholakoff D, Finkbeiner W, et al. Magnetic resonance imaging of cardiac transplants: The evaluation of rejection of cardiac allografts with and without immunosuppression. Circulation. 1986;74:145–156.
225. Sasaki H, Sada M, Nishimura T, et al. The expanded scope of effectiveness of nuclear magnetic resonance imaging to determine cardiac allograft rejection. Transplant Proc. 1987;19:1062–1064.
226. Gagliardi MG, Bevilacqua M, Di Renzi P, et al. Usefulness of magnetic resonance imaging for diagnosis of acute myocarditis in infants and children, and comparison with endomyocardial biopsy. Am J Cardiol. 1991;68:1089–1091.
227. Chandraratna AN, Nimalasuriya A, Reid CL, et al. Left ventricular asynergy in acute myocarditis. Simulation of acute myocardial infarction. JAMA. 1983;250:1428–1430.
228. Bergler-Klein J, Sochor H, Stanek G, et al. Indium 111-monoclonal antimyosin antibody and magnetic resonance imaging in the diagnosis of acute Lyme myopericarditis. Arch Intern Med. 1993;153:2696–2700.
229. Friedrich MG, Strohm O, Schulz-Menger J, et al. Contrast media–enhanced magnetic resonance imaging visualizes myocardial changes in the course of viral myocarditis. Circulation. 1998;97:1802–1809.
230. O'Connel JB, Mason JW. Diagnosing and treating active myocarditis. West J Med. 1989;150:431–435.
231. Peters NS, Poole-Wilson PA. Myocarditis—continuing clinical and pathologic confusion. Am Heart J. 1991;121:942–947.
232. Billingham ME. The safety and utility of endomyocardial biopsy in infants, children and adolescents. J Am Coll Cardiol. 1990;15:443–445.

233. Fowles RE, Mason JW. Endomyocardial biopsy. Ann Intern Med. 1982;97:885–894.
234. Hauch AJ, Kearney DL, Edwards WD. Evaluation of postmortem endomyocardial biopsy specimens from 38 patients with lymphocytic myocarditis: Implications for the role of sampling error. Mayo Clin Proc. 1989;64:1235–1245.
235. Chow LH, Radio SJ, Sears TD, et al. Insensitivity of right ventricular endomyocardial biopsy in the diagnosis of myocarditis. J Am Coll Cardiol. 1989;14:915–920.
236. Nippoldt TB, Edwards WD, Holmes DR, et al. Right ventricular endomyocardial biopsy. Clinicopathologic correlates in 100 consecutive patients. Mayo Clin Proc. 1982;57:407–418.
237. Parrillo JE, Aretz HT, Palacios I, et al. The results of transvenous endomyocardial biopsy can frequently be used to diagnose myocardial diseases in patients with idiopathic heart failure. Endomyocardial biopsies in 100 consecutive patients revealed a substantial incidence of myocarditis. Circulation. 1984;69:93–101.
238. Takahashi O, Kamiya T, Echigo S, et al. Myocarditis in children—clinical findings and myocardial biopsy findings. Jpn Circ J. 1983;47:1298–1303.
239. Vasiljevic JD, Kanjuh V, Seferovic P, et al. The incidence of myocarditis in endomyocardial biopsy samples from patients with congestive heart failure. Am Heart J. 1990;120:1370–1377.
240. Herskowitz A, Campbell S, Deckers J. Demographic features and prevalence of idiopathic myocarditis in patients undergoing endomyocardial biopsy. Am J Cardiol. 1993;71:982–986.
241. Mason JW, O'Connell JB, Herskowitz A, et al. A clinical trial of immunosuppressive therapy for myocarditis. N Engl J Med. 1995;333:269–275.
242. Dec GW, Palacios IF, Fallon JT, et al. Active myocarditis in the spectrum of acute dilated cardiomyopathies. Clinical features, histologic correlates, and clinical outcome. N Engl J Med. 1985;312:885–890.
243. Zee-Cheng C-S, Tsai CC, Palmer DC, et al. High incidence of myocarditis by endomyocardial biopsy in patients with idiopathic congestive cardiomyopathy. J Am Coll Cardiol. 1984;3:63–70.
244. Fenoglio JJ, Ursell PC, Kellogg CF, et al. Diagnosis and classification of myocarditis by endomyocardial biopsy. N Engl J Med. 1983;308:12–18.
245. Mason JW, Billingham ME, Ricci DR. Treatment of acute inflammatory myocarditis assisted by endomyocardial biopsy. Am J Cardiol. 1980;45:1037–1044.
246. Chow LC, Dittrich HC, Shabetai R. Endomyocardial biopsy in patients with unexplained congestive heart failure. Ann Intern Med. 1988;109:535.
247. Shanes JG, Ghali J, Billingham ME, et al. Interobserver variability in the pathologic interpretation of endomyocardial biopsy results. Circulation. 1987;75:401–405.
248. Billingham M. Acute myocarditis: A diagnostic dilemma. Br Heart J. 1987;58:6–8.
249. Kereiakes DJ, Parmley WW. Myocarditis and cardiomyopathy. Am Heart J. 1984;108:1318–1326.
250. Aretz HT, Billingham ME, Edwards WD, et al. Myocarditis, a histopathologic definition and classification. Am J Cardiovasc Pathol. 1987;1:3–14.
251. Morita H, Kitaura Y, Deguchi H, et al. Coxsackie B5 myopericarditis in a young adult. Clinical course and endomyocardial biopsy findings. Jpn Circ J. 1983;47:1077–1083.
252. Fukuhara T, Konoshita M, Bito K, et al. Myopericarditis associated with echovirus type 3 infection. A case report. Jpn Circ J. 1983;47:1274–1280.
253. Friman G, Fohlman J. The epidemiology of viral heart disease. Scand J Infect Dis. 1993;88(Suppl):7–10.
254. Kawai C, Matsumori A, Fujiwara H. Myocarditis and dilated cardiomyopathy. Annu Rev Med. 1987;38:221–239.
255. Kopecky SL, Gersh BJ. Dilated cardiomyopathy and myocarditis: Natural history, etiology, clinical manifestations, and management. In: O'Rourke RA, Crawford MH, eds. Current Problems in Cardiology. Chicago: Year Book Medical Publishers; 1987:569–647.
256. Lowry BS. Viruses and heart disease: A problem in pathogenesis. Ann Clin Lab Sci. 1986;16:358–364.
257. Weiss LM, Liu XF, Chang KL, et al. Detection of enteroviral RNA in idiopathic dilated cardiomyopathy and other human cardiac tissues. J Clin Invest. 1992;90:156–159.
258. Keeling PJ, Tracy S. Link between enteroviruses and dilated cardiomyopathy: Serological and molecular data. Br Heart J. 1994;72(Suppl):S25–29.
259. Weinstein C, Fenoglio JJ. Myocarditis. Hum Pathol. 1987; 18:613–618.
260. Rotbart HA, Eastman PS, Ruth JL, et al. Nonisotopic oligomeric probes for the human enteroviruses. J Clin Microbiol. 1988;26:2669–2671.
261. Erlich HA, Gelfand DH, Saiki RK. Specific DNA amplification. Nature. 1988;331:461–462.
262. Schwaiger A, Umlauft F, Weyrer K, et al. Detection of enteroviral ribonucleic acid in myocardial biopsies from patients with idiopathic dilated cardiomyopathy by polymerase chain reaction. Am Heart J. 1993;126:406–410.
263. Baboonian C, Treasure T. Meta-analysis of the association of enteroviruses with human heart disease. Heart. 1997;78:539–543.
264. Caforio AL, Baboonian C, McKenna WJ. Postviral autoimmune heart disease—fact or fiction? Eur Heart J. 1997;18:1051–1055.
265. Tracy S, Wiegand V, McManus B, et al. Molecular approaches to enteroviral diagnosis in idiopathic cardiomyopathy and myocarditis. J Am Coll Cardiol. 1990;15:1688–1694.
266. Figulla HR, Stille-Siegener M, Mall G, et al. Myocardial enterovirus infection with left ventricular dysfunction: A benign disease compared with idiopathic dilated cardiomyopathy. J Am Coll Cardiol. 1995;25:1170–1175.
267. Martino T, Liu P, Sole MJ. Viral infection and the pathogenesis of dilated cardiomyopathy. Circ Res. 1994;74:182–188.
268. Why HJ, Meany BT, Richardson PJ, et al. Clinical and prognostic significance of detection of enteroviral RNA in the myocardium of patients with myocarditis or dilated cardiomyopathy. Circulation. 1994;89:2582–2589.
269. McKenna WJ, Davies MJ. Immunosuppression for myocarditis. N Engl J Med. 1995;333:312–313.
270. Garg A, Shiau J, Guyatt G. The ineffectiveness of immunosuppressive therapy in lymphocytic myocarditis: An overview. Ann Intern Med. 1998;128:317–322.
271. Grogan M, Redfield MM, Bailey KR, et al. Long term outcomes of patients with biopsy-proven myocarditis: Comparison with idiopathic dilated cardiomyopathy. J Am Coll Cardiol. 1995;25:80–84.
272. Chow LC, Dittrich HC, Shabetai R. Endomyocardial biopsy in patients with unexplained congestive heart failure. Ann Intern Med. 1988;109:535–539.
273. Deckers JW, Hare JM, Baughman KL. Complications of transvenous right ventricular endomyocardial biopsy in adult patients with cardiomyopathy: A seven year survey of 516 consecutive diagnostic procedures in a tertiary referral center. J Am Coll Cardiol. 1992;19:43–47.
274. Fowler NO. The secondary cardiomyopathies. In: Fowler NO. Myocardial Disease. New York: Grune & Stratton; 1973:337–359.
275. Bank I, Marboe CC, Redberg RF, et al. Myocarditis in adult Still's disease. Arthritis Rheum. 1985;28:452–454.
276. Vintila M, Tanaseanu S, Luca R, et al. Is cardiac involvement in collagen diseases important? A clinical study in 917 patients. Med Int. 1990;28:219–227.
277. Goldenberg J, Ferraz MB, Pessoa AP, et al. Symptomatic cardiac involvement in juvenile rheumatoid arthritis. Int J Cardiol. 1992;34:57–62.
278. Askari AD, Huettner TL. Cardiac abnormalities in polymyositis/dermatomyositis. Sem Arthritis Rheum. 1982;12:208–219.
279. Tami LF, Bhasin S. Polymorphism of the cardiac manifestations in dermatomyositis. Clin Cardiol. 1993;16:260–264.
280. Clemson BS, Miller WR, Luck JC, et al. Acute myocarditis in fulminant systemic sclerosis. Chest. 1992;101:872–874.
281. Webb JG, Butany J, Langer G, et al. Myocarditis and myocardial hemorrhage associated with thrombotic thrombocytopenic purpura. Arch Intern Med. 1990;150:1535–1537.
282. Myocarditis. In: Braunwald E, ed. Heart Disease, a Textbook of Cardiovascular Medicine. 3rd ed. Philadelphia: WB Saunders; 1988:1440–1469.
283. Midei MG, DeMent SH, Feldman AM, et al. Peripartum myocarditis and cardiomyopathy. Circulation. 1990;81:922–928.
284. Ikaheimo MJ, Niemela KO, Linnaluoto MM, et al. Early cardiac changes related to radiation therapy. Am J Cardiol. 1988;56:943–946.
285. Isner JM, Chokshi SK. Cardiac complications of cocaine abuse. Ann Rev Med. 1991;42:133–138.
286. Taliercio CP, Olney BA, Lie JT. Myocarditis related to drug hypersensitivity. Mayo Clin Proc. 1985;60:463–468.
287. Brand A, Keren A, Kerem E, et al. Myocardial damage after a scorpion sting: Long-term echocardiographic follow-up. Pediatr Cardiol. 1988;9:59–61.
288. Matsuura H, Ishikita T, Yamamoto S, et al. Gallium-67 myocardial imaging for the detection of myocarditis in the acute phase of Kawasaki disease (mucocutaneous lymph node syndrome): The usefulness of single photon emission computed tomography. Br Heart J. 1987;58:385–392.
289. Humbert P, Faivre R, Fellman D, et al. Giant cell myocarditis: An autoimmune disease? Am Heart J. 1988;115:485–487.
290. Temple-Camp CR. Sarcoid myocarditis: A report of three cases. N Z Med J. 1989;102:501–502.
291. Suzuki H, Matsumori A, Kawai CH. Effects of angiotensin converting enzyme inhibitors on myocardial injury and congestive heart failure due to myocarditis in mice: Comparison with captopril and enalapril. Circulation. 1991;84(Suppl III):634.
292. Rezkalla SH, Raikar S, Kloner RA. Treatment of viral myocarditis with focus on captopril. Am J Cardiol. 1996;77:634–637.
293. Ferling J, Gallo CT. Responses of patients in heart failure to long term oval verapamil administration (Abstract). Circulation. 1984;70 (Suppl II):305.
294. Goldstein RE, Boccuzzi SJ, Cruess D, Nattel S. Diltiazem increases last-onset congestive heart failure in postinfarction patients with early reduction in ejection fraction. Circulation. 1991;83:52–60.
295. Factor SM, Minase T, Cho S, et al. Microvascular spasm in the cardiomyopathic Syrian hamster: A preventable cause of focal myocardial necroses. Circulation. 1982;66:342–354.
296. Morris SA, Weiss LM, Factor S, et al. Verapamil ameliorates clinical, pathologic and biochemical manifestations of experimental chagasic cardiomyopathy in mice. J Am Coll Cardiol. 1989;14:782–789.
297. Wang WZ, Matsumori A, Yamada T, et al. Beneficial effects of amlodipine in a murine model of congestive heart failure induced by viral myocarditis. Circulation. 1997;95:245–251.
298. Packer M, O'Connor CM, Ghali JK, et al. For the PRAISE study group. Effect of amlodipine on morbidity and mortality in severe chronic heart failure. N Engl J Med. 1996;335:1107–1114.
299. Moreno-Cabral CE, Moreno-Cabral RJ, McNamara JJ, et al. Prolonged extracorporeal circulation for acute myocarditis. Int J Artif Organs. 1992;15:475–480.
300. Hayakawa M, Inoh T, Yokota Y, et al. A long-term follow-up study of acute viral and idiopathic myocarditis. Jpn Circ J. 1983;47:1304–1309.
301. Remes J, Helin M, Vaino P, et al. Clinical outcome and left ventricular function 23 years after acute coxsackie virus myopericarditis. Eur Heart J. 1990;11:182–188.
302. Khatib R, Reyes MP, Smith F, et al. Enhancement of coxsackie B3 virulence by indomethacin. J Lab Clin Med. 1990;116:116–120.
303. Costanzo-Norden MR, Reap EA, O'Connell JB, et al. A nonsteroid anti-inflammatory drug exacerbates coxsackie B3 murine myocarditis. J Am Coll Cardiol. 1985;6:1078–1082.

304. Tomioka N, Kishimoto C, Matsumori A, et al. Effects of prednisolone on acute viral myocarditis in mice. J Am Coll Cardiol. 1986;7:868–872.
305. Ettinger J, Feucht H, Gartner R, et al. Cyclosporine A (CyA) for successful treatment of myocarditis (Letter). Eur Heart J. 1986;7:452.
306. Chan KY, Iwahara M, Benson LM, et al. Immunosuppressive therapy in the management of acute myocarditis in children: A clinical trial. J Am Coll Cardiol. 1991;17:458–460.
307. O'Connell JB, Robinson JA, Henkin RE, et al. Immunosuppressive therapy in patients with congestive cardiomyopathy and myocardial uptake of gallium-67. Circulation. 1981;64:780–786.
308. Camargo PR, Snitcowsky R, da Luz PL, et al. Favorable effects of immunosuppressive therapy in children with dilated cardiomyopathy and active myocarditis. Pediatr Cardiol. 1995;16:61–68.
309. Anandasabapathy S, Frishman WH. Innovative drug treatments for viral and autoimmune myocarditis. J Clin Pharm. 1998;35:295–308.
310. Takada H, Kishimoto C, Hiraoka Y. Therapy with immunoglobulin suppresses myocarditis in a murine coxsackie B3 model. Antiviral and antiinflammatory effects. Circulation. 1995;92:1604–1611.
311. Maisch B, Herzum M, Hufnagel G, Schonean U. Immunosuppressive and immunomodulatory treatment for myocarditis. Curr Opin Cardiol. 1996;11:310–324.
312. McNamara DM, Rosemblum WD, Janosko KM, et al. Intravenous immune globulin in the therapy of myocarditis and acute cardiomyopathy. Circulation. 1997;95:2476–2478.
313. Kishimoto C, Crumpacker CS, Abelmann WH. Prevention of murine coxsackie B3 viral myocarditis and associated lymphoid organ atrophy with recombinant human leukocyte interferon alpha A/D. Cardiovasc Res. 1988;22:732–738.
314. Hiraoka Y, Kishimoto C, Takada H, et al. Colony-stimulating factors and coxsackie B3 myocarditis in mice: Macrophage colony stimulating factor suppresses acute myocarditis with increasing interferon-alpha. Am Heart J. 1995;130:1259–1264.
315. Miric M, Vasilijevic J, Bojic M, et al. Long term follow up of patients with dilated heart muscle disease treated with human leucocytic interferon alpha or thymic hormones. Initial results. Heart. 1996;75:596–601.
316. Matsumori A. The use of cytokine inhibitors: A new therapeutic insight into heart failure. Int J Cardiol. 1997;62(suppl I):S3–S12.
317. Gebhard JR, Perry CM, Harkins S, et al. Coxsackievirus B3–induced myocarditis: Perforin exacerbates disease, but plays no detectable role in virus clearance. Am J Pathol. 1998;153:417–428.
318. McCormack JG, Bowler SD, Donnelly JE, Steadman C. Successful treatments of severe cytomegalovirus infection with ganciclovir in an immunocompetent host. Clin Infect Dis. 1998;26:1007–1008.
319. Woods MG, Diana GD, Rogge MC, et al. In vitro and in vivo activities of WIN 54954, a new broad-spectrum antipicornavirus drug. Antimicrob Agents Chemother. 1989;33:2069–2074.
320. Pauksen K, Ilback NG, Friman G, et al. Therapy of coxsackievirus B3–induced myocarditis with WIN 54954 in different formulations. Scand J Infect Dis. 1993;88(Suppl):125–130.
321. See DM, Tilles JG. Treatment of coxsackievirus A9 myocarditis in mice with WIN 54954. Antimicrob Agents Chemother. 1993;36:425–428.
322. Fohlman J, Pauksen K, Hyypia T, et al. Antiviral treatment with WIN 54954 reduces mortality in murine coxsackie B2 myocarditis. Circulation. 1996;94:2254–2259.
323. Schiff GM, McKinlay MA, Sherwood JR. Oral efficacy of VP63843 in coxsackie A21–infected volunteers. Abstracts of the 36th Interscience Conference and Antimicrobial Agents and Chemotherapy, New Orleans, La; 1996:171.
324. Rotbart HA, O'Connell JF, McKinlay MA. Treatment of human enterovirus infections. Antiviral Res. 1998;38:1–14.
325. Osler W. The Principles and Practice of Medicine. New York: D Appleton; 1892.
326. Sagrista-Sauleda J, Barrabes JA, Permanyer-Miralda G, et al. Purulent pericarditis: Review of a 20 year experience in a general hospital. J Am Coll Cardiol. 1993;22:1661–1665.
327. Park S, Bayer AS. Purulent pericarditis. Curr Clin Topics Infect Dis. 1992;12:56–82.
328. Ilan Y, Oren R, Ben-Chetrit E. Acute pericarditis: Etiology, treatment and prognosis. Jpn Heart J. 1991;32:315–321.
329. Soler-Soler J, Permanyer-Miralda G, Sagrista-Sauleda J. A systematic diagnostic approach to primary acute pericardial disease. The Barcelona experience. Cardiol Clin. 1990;8:609–620.
330. Johnson RT, Portnoy B, Rogers NG, et al. Acute benign pericarditis: Virologic study of 34 patients. Arch Intern Med. 1961;108:823.
331. Koontz CH, Ray CG. The role of coxsackie group B virus infections in sporadic myopericarditis. Am Heart J. 1971;82:750–758.
332. Smith WG. Coxsackie B myopericarditis in adults. Am Heart J. 1970;80:34–46.
333. Montgomery J, Gear JHS, Prinslou FR, et al. Myocarditis of the newborn. An outbreak in a maternity home in Southern Rhodesia associated with coxsackie group-B virus infection. S Afr Med J. 1955;29:608–612.
334. Bain HW, McLean DM, Walker SJ. Epidemic pleurodynia (Bornholm disease) due to coxsackie B5 virus. Pediatrics. 1961;27:889–902.
335. Helin M, Savola J, Lapinleimu K. Cardiac manifestations during a coxsackie B5 epidemic. BMJ. 1968;2:97–99.
336. Brodie HR, Marchessault V. Acute benign pericarditis caused by coxsackie virus group B. N Engl J Med. 1960;262:1278–1280.
337. Kagan H, Bernkopf H. Pericarditis caused by coxsackie virus B. Ann Pediatr. 1957;189:44–50.
338. Grist NR, Bell EJ. Coxsackie viruses and the heart. Am Heart J. 1969;77:295–300.
339. Van Reken D, Strauss A, Henandez A, et al. Infectious pericarditis in children. J Pediatr. 1974;85:165–169.
340. Movitt ER, Lenette EH, Mangum JF, et al. Acute benign pericarditis: Report of 2 cases associated with group A and group B coxsackie viruses. N Engl J Med. 1958;158:1082–1086.
341. Russell SJM, Bell EJ. Echoviruses and carditis. Lancet. 1970;1:784–785.
342. Celers J, Celers P, Bertocchi A. Non-polio enterovirus in France from 1974 to 1985. Pathol Biol. 1988;36:1221.
343. Grist NR, Beil EJ, Assaad F. Enteroviruses in human disease. Prog Med Virol. 1978;24:114–157.
344. Roberts R. Viral pericarditis. Med Serv J Can. 1961;17:588.
345. Canas JA, Balsam D, Leggiadro RJ. Adenovirus pericarditis. N Y State J Med. 1986;86:269–270.
346. Nahmias AJ, Griffith D, Snitzer J. Fatal pneumonia associated with adenovirus type 7. Am J Dis Child. 1967;114:36–41.
347. Odio C, McCracken GH Jr, Nelson JD. Disseminated adenovirus infection: A case report and review of the literature. Pediatr Infect Dis. 1984;3:46–49.
348. Kleinfeld M, Milles S, Lidsky M. Mumps pericarditis: Review of the literature and report of a case. Am Heart J. 1958;55:153–156.
349. Proby CM, Hacket D, Gupta S, et al. Acute myopericarditis in influenza A infection. QJM. 1986;60:887–892.
350. Adams CW. Postviral myopericarditis associated with the influenza virus: Report of 8 cases. Am J Cardiol. 1959;4:56–67.
351. Hildenbrandt HM, Maassab HF, Willis PW III. Influenza virus pericarditis: Report of a case with isolation of Asian influenza virus from the pericardial fluid. Am J Dis Child. 1962;104:579.
352. Cheng TC. Severe chest pain due to infectious mononucleosis. Postgrad Med. 1983;73:149–152.
353. Shugoll GI. Pericarditis associated with infectious mononucleosis. Arch Intern Med. 1957;100:630–634.
354. Satoh T, Kojima M, Ohshima K. Demonstration of the Epstein-Barr genome by the polymerase chain reaction and in situ hybridization in a patient with viral pericarditis. Br Heart J. 1993;69:563–564.
355. Williams AJ, Freemont AJ, Barnett DB. Pericarditis and arthritis complicating chickenpox. Br J Clin Pract. 1983;37:226–227.
356. Kassab A, Demoulin JC, Vanlancker MA, et al. Cytomegalovirus hemopericarditis. Report of 1 case with histologic confirmation. Acta Cardiol. 1987;42:69–72.
357. Martin V, Miranda ML, Stiefel P, et al. Acute pericarditis caused by cytomegalovirus in a normal host (Letter). Enferm Infec Microbiol Clin. 1989;7:515.
358. Nathan PE, Arsura EL, Zappi M. Pericarditis with tamponade due to cytomegalovirus in the acquired immunodeficiency syndrome. Chest. 1991;99:765–766.
359. Powell KF, Bellamy AR, Catton MG. Cytomegalovirus myocarditis in a heart transplant recipient: Sensitive monitoring of viral DNA by the polymerase chain reaction. J Heart Transplant. 1989;8:465–470.
360. Scott PJ, Conway SP, Da Costa P. Cardiac tamponade complicating cytomegalovirus pericarditis in a patient with AIDS. J Infect. 1990;20:92.
361. Campbell PT, Li JS, Wall TC, et al. Cytomegalovirus pericarditis: A case series and review of the literature. Am J Med Sci. 1995;309(4):229–234.
362. Freedberg RS, Gindea AJ, Dieterich DT, et al. Herpes simplex pericarditis in AIDS. N Y State J Med. 1987;87:304–306.
363. Toma E, Poisson M, Claessens MR, et al. Herpes simplex type 2 pericarditis and bilateral facial palsy in a patient with AIDS (Letter). J Infect Dis. 1989;160:553–554.
364. Adler R, Takahashi M, Wright HT Jr. Acute pericarditis associated with hepatitis B infection. Pediatrics. 1978;61:716–719.
365. Boyle JD, Pearce ML, Guze LB. Purulent pericarditis: Review of literature and report of eleven cases. Medicine. 1961;40:119–144.
366. Klacsmann PG, Bulkley BH, Hutchins GM. The changed spectrum of purulent pericarditis. An 86 year autopsy experience in 200 patients. Am J Med. 1977;63:666–673.
367. Kauffman CA, Watanakunakorn C, Phair JP. Purulent pneumococcal pericarditis. A continuing problem in the antibiotic era. Am J Med. 1973;54:743–750.
368. Saenz RE, Sanders CV, Aldridge KE, et al. Purulent pericarditis with associated cardiac tamponade caused by a *Streptococcus pneumoniae* strain highly resistant to penicillin, cefotaxime, and ceftriaxone. Clin Infect Dis. 1998;26(3):762–763.
369. Pruitt JL. Group A streptococcal pericarditis in a previously well child (Letter). Pediatr Infect Dis J. 1989;8:338.
370. Karikm MA, Bach RG, Dressler F, et al. Purulent pericarditis caused by group B streptococcus with pericardial tamponade. Am Heart J. 1993;126:727–730.
371. Halverson KC, Van Etta LL, Langager JH. Group G streptococcal purulent pericarditis. A case report. Minn Med. 1991;74:27–29.
372. Hirata K, Asato H, Maeshiro M. A case of effusive constrictive pericarditis caused by *Streptococcus milleri*. Jpn Circ J. 1991;55:154–158.
373. Rubin RH, Moellering RC. Clinical, microbiologic and therapeutic aspects of purulent pericarditis. Am J Med. 1975;59:68–78.
374. Kopec JS, Grifka RG, Karpawich PP. Isolated staphylococcal pericarditis following varicella in an adolescent: An unusual age-associated complication. Pediatr Emerg Care. 1990;6:38–39.
375. Demey HE, Eycken M, Vandermast M. Purulent pericarditis due to methicillin-resistant *Staphylococcus aureus*. A case report. Acta Cardiol. 1991;46:485–491.
376. Blaser MJ, Reingold AL, Alsever RN, et al. Primary meningococcal pericarditis: A disease of adults associated with serogroup C *Neisseria meningitidis*. Rev Infect Dis. 1984;6:625–632.
377. Finkelstein Y, Adler Y, Nussinovitch M, et al. A new classification for pericarditis associated with meningococcal infection. Eur J Pediatr. 1997;156:585–588.

378. Coe MD, Hamer DH, Levy CS, et al. Gonococcal pericarditis with tamponade in a patient with systemic lupus erythematosus. Arthritis Rheum. 1990;33:1438–1441.
379. Wilson J, Zaman AG, Simmons AV. Gonococcal arthritis complicated by acute pericarditis and pericardial effusion. Br Heart J. 1990;63:134–135.
380. Fyfe DA, Hagler DJ, Puga FJ, et al. Clinical and therapeutic aspects of *Haemophilus influenzae* pericarditis in pediatric patients. Mayo Clin Proc. 1984;59:415–422.
381. Schwartz KV, Guercio CA, Katz A. *Haemophilus influenza* pericarditis. Conn Med. 1987;51:423–424.
382. Welikovitch L, Knight JL, Burggraf GW, et al. Cardiac tamponade secondary to *Haemophilus* pericarditis: A case report. Can J Cardiol. 1992;8:303–305.
383. Corachan M, Poore P, Hadley GP, et al. Purulent pericarditis in Papua New Guinea: Report of 12 cases and review of the literature in a tropical environment. Trans R Soc Trop Med Hyg. 1983;77:341–343.
384. Lecomte F, Eustache M, Lemeland JF, et al. Purulent pericarditis due to *Yersinia enterocolitica* (Letter). J Infect Dis. 1989;159:363.
385. Sanchez-Guerrero J, Alarcon-Segovia D. *Salmonella* pericarditis with tamponade in systemic lupus erythematosus. Br J Rheumatol. 1990;29:69–71.
386. Morrison VA, Lloyd BK, Chia JK, et al. Cardiovascular and bacteremic manifestations of *Campylobacter fetus* infection: Case report and review. Rev Infect Dis. 1990;12:387–392.
387. Ugartemendia MC, Curos-Abadal A, Pujol-Rakosnik M, et al. *Brucella melitensis* pericarditis. Am Heart J. 1985;109:1108.
388. Ramsdale DR, Gautam PC, Perera B, et al. Cardiac tamponade due to actinomycosis. Thorax. 1984;39:473–474.
389. O'Sullivan RA, Armstrong JG, Rivers JT, et al. Pulmonary actinomycosis complicated by effusive constrictive pericarditis. Aust N Z J Med. 1991;21:879–880.
390. Brook E, Frazier EH. Microbiology of acute purulent pericarditis. A 12 year experience in a military hospital. Arch Int Med. 1996;156:1857–1860.
391. Skiest DJ, Steiner D, Werner M, et al. Anaerobic pericarditis: Case report and review. Clin Infect Dis. 1994;19:435–440.
392. Lam S, Greenberg R, Bank S. An unusual presentation of colon cancer: Purulent pericarditis and cardiac tamponade due to *Bacteroides fragilis*. Am J Gastroenterol. 1995;90:1518–1520.
393. Poland GA, Jorgensen CR, Sarosi GA. *Nocardia asteroides* pericarditis: Report of a case and review of the literature (see comments). Mayo Clin Proc. 1990;65:819–824.
394. Ferguson R, Yee S, Finkle H, et al. *Listeria*-associated pericarditis in an AIDS patient. J Natl Med Assoc. 1991;85:225–228.
395. Linz DH, Tolle SW, Elliott DL. *Mycoplasma pneumoniae* pneumonia. Experience at a referral center. West J Med. 1984;140:895–900.
396. Ponka A. The occurrence and clinical picture of serologically verified *Mycoplasma pneumoniae* infections with emphases on central nervous system, cardiac and joint manifestations. Ann Clin Res. 1979;24:1–60.
397. Sands MJ, Satz JE, Turner WE Jr, et al. Pericarditis and perimyocarditis associated with active *Mycoplasma pneumoniae* infection. Ann Intern Med. 1977;86:544–548.
398. Balaguer A, Boronat M, Carrascosa A. Successful treatment of pericarditis associated with *Mycoplasma pneumoniae* infection. Pediatr Infect Dis J. 1990;9:141–143.
399. Kenny RT, Li JS, Clyde WA, et al. Mycoplasmal pericarditis: Evidence of invasive disease. Clin Infect Dis. 1993;1(Suppl I) :S58–62.
400. Maycock R, Skale B, Kohler RB. *Legionella pneumophila* pericarditis proved by culture of pericardial fluid. Am J Med. 1983;75:534–536.
401. Reyes RR, Noble RC. Legionnaires' pericarditis. J Ky Med Assoc. 1983;81:757–758.
402. Luck PC, Helbig JH, Wunderlich E, et al. Isolation of *Legionella pneumophila* serogroup 3 from pericardial fluid in a case of pericarditis. Infection. 1989;17:388–390.
403. Svendsen JH, Jonsson V, Niebuhr U. Combined pericarditis and pneumonia caused by *Legionella* infection. Br Heart J 1987;58:663–664.
404. Puleo J, Matar FA, McKeown PP, et al. *Legionella* pericarditis diagnosed by direct fluorescent antibody staining. Ann Thoracic Surg. 1995;60:444–446.
405. Friedland L, Snydman DR, Weingarden AS, et al. Ocular and pericardial involvement in Legionnaires' disease. Am J Med 1984;77:1105–1107.
406. Odeh M, Oliven A. Chlamydial infections of the heart. Eur J Clin Microbiol Infect Dis. 1992;11:885–893.
407. Bruyn GW, DeKoning J, Reijsoo FJ, et al. Lyme pericarditis leading to tamponade. Br J Rheumatol. 1994;33:862–866.
408. Horowitz HW, Belkin RN. Acute myopericarditis resulting from Lyme disease. Am Heart J. 1995;130(1):176–178.
409. Larrieu AJ, Tyers GFO, Williams EH, et al. Recent experience with tuberculous pericarditis. Ann Thorac Surg. 1980;29:464–468.
410. Sagrista-Sauleda J, Permanyer-Miralda G, Soler-Soler J. Tuberculous pericarditis: Ten year experience with a prospective protocol for diagnosis and treatment. J Am Coll Cardiol. 1988;11:724–728.
411. Rooney JJ, Crocco JA, Lyons HA. Tuberculous pericarditis. Ann Intern Med. 1970;72:73–78.
412. Desai HN. Tuberculous pericarditis. A review of 100 cases. S Afr Med J. 1979;55:877–880.
413. Dalli E, Quesada A, Juan G, et al. Tuberculous pericarditis as the first manifestation of acquired immunodeficiency syndrome. Am Heart J. 1987;114:905–906.
414. Ortbals DW, Avioli LV. Tuberculous pericarditis. Arch Intern Med. 1979;139:231–234.
415. Woods GL, Goldsmith JC. Fatal pericarditis due to *Mycobacterium avium-intracellulare* in acquired immunodeficiency syndrome. Chest. 1989;95:1355–1357.
416. Wheat LJ, Stein L, Corya BC, et al. Pericarditis as a manifestation of histoplasmosis during two large urban outbreaks. Medicine. 1983;62:110–119.
417. Young EJ, Vainrub B, Musher DM. Pericarditis due to histoplasmosis. JAMA. 1978;240:1750.
418. Wheat J. Histoplasmosis. Experience during outbreaks in Indianapolis and review of the literature. Medicine. 1997;76(5):339–354.
419. Larson R, Scherb RI. Coccidioidal pericarditis. Circulation. 1953;7:211–217.
420. Chapman MG, Kaplan L. Cardiac involvement in coccidioidomycosis. Am J Med. 1957;23:87–98.
421. Amundson DE. Perplexing pericarditis caused by coccidioidomycosis. So Med J. 1993;86:694–696.
422. Witorsch P, Utz JP. North American blastomycosis: A study of 40 patients. Medicine (Balt). 1968;47:169–200.
423. Duvall CP, Carbone PP. *Cryptococcus neoformans* pericarditis associated with Hodgkin's disease. Ann Intern Med. 1966;64:850–856.
424. Kraus WE, Valenstein PN, Corey GR. Purulent pericarditis caused by *Candida*: Report of three cases and identification of high-risk populations as an aid to early diagnosis. Rev Infect Dis. 1988;10:34–41.
425. Eng RHK, Sen P, Browne K, et al. *Candida* pericarditis. Am J Med. 1981;70:867–869.
426. Kaufman LD, Seifert FC, Eilbott DJ, et al. *Candida* pericarditis and tamponade in a patient with systemic lupus erythematosus. Arch Intern Med. 1988;148:715–717.
427. Schrank JH, Dooley DP. Purulent pericarditis caused by *Candida* species: Case report and review. Clin Infect Dis. 1995;21:182–187.
428. Walsh TJ, Bulkley BH. *Aspergillus* pericarditis: Clinical and pathologic features in the immunocompromised patient. Cancer. 1982;49:48–54.
429. Cooper JAD, Weinbaum DL, Aldrich TK, et al. Invasive aspergillosis of the lung and pericardium in a nonimmunocompromised 33 year old man. Am J Med. 1981;71:903–907.
430. Ross EM, Macher AM, Roberts WC. *Aspergillus fumigatus* thrombi causing total occlusion of both coronary arterial ostia, all four major coronary arteries and coronary sinus and associated with purulent pericarditis. Am J Cardiol. 1985;56:499.
431. Le Moing V, Lortholary O, Timsit JF, et al. *Aspergillus* pericarditis with tamponade: Report of a successfully treated case and review. Clin Infect Dis. 1998;26(2):451–460.
432. Theologides A, Kennedy BJ. Toxoplasmic myocarditis and pericarditis (Editorial). Am J Med. 1969;47:169–174.
433. Sagrista-Sauleda J, Permanyer-Miralda G, Juste-Sanchez C, et al. Huge chronic pericardial effusion caused by *Toxoplasma gondii*. Circulation. 1982;66:895–897.
434. Lyngberg KK, Vennervald BJ, Bygbjerg IC, et al. *Toxoplasma* pericarditis mimicking systemic lupus erythematosus. Diagnostic and treatment difficulties in one patient. Ann Med. 1992;24:337–340.
435. Permanyer-Miralda G, Sagrista-Sauleda J, Soler-Soler J. Primary acute pericardial disease: A prospective series of 231 consecutive patients. Am J Cardiol. 1985;56:623–630.
436. Ibarra-Perez C, Green LS, Calvello-Juarez M, et al. Diagnosis and treatment of rupture of amebic abscess of the liver into the pericardium. J Thorac Cardiovasc Surg. 1972;64:11–17.
437. Rab SW, Alam N, Hoda AN, et al. Amoebic liver abscess. Some unique presentations. Am J Med. 1967;43:811–816.
438. Baid CS, Varma AR, Lakhotia M. A case of subacute effusive constrictive pericarditis with a probable amoebic aetiology. Br Heart J. 1987;58:296–298.
439. Strang JIG. Two-dimensional echocardiography in the diagnosis of amoebic pericarditis. A case report. S Afr Med J. 1987;71:328–329.
440. Chao TH, Li YH, Tsai LM, et al. Amoebic liver abscess complicated with cardiac tamponade and mediastinal abscess. J Formosan Med Assoc. 1998;97(3):214–216.
441. Herry I, Philippe B, Hennequin C. Acute life-threatening toxocaral tamponade. Chest. 1997;112(6):1692–1693.
442. Van der Horst R. Schistosomiasis of the pericardium. J R Soc Trop Med Hyg. 1979;73:243–244.
443. Dupuis C, Gronnier P, Kachaner J, et al. Bacterial pericarditis in infancy and childhood. Am J Cardiol. 1994;74:807–809.
444. Strang JIG. Tuberculous pericarditis in Transkei. Clin Cardiol. 1984;5:667.
445. Strang JI, Kakaza HH, Gibson DG, et al. Controlled clinical trial of complete open surgical drainage and of prednisone in treatment of tuberculous pericardial effusion in Transkei. Lancet. 1988;2:759–764.
446. D'Cruz IA, Sengupta EE, Abrahams C, et al. Cardiac involvement, including tuberculous pericardial effusion, complicating acquired immune deficiency syndrome. Am Heart J. 1986;5:1100.
447. Kwan T, Karve MM, Emerole O. Cardiac tamponade in patients infected with HIV. Chest. 1993;104:1059–1062.
448. Fowler NO. Tuberculous pericarditis (see comments). JAMA. 1991;266:99–103.
449. Strang JI, Kakaza HH, Gibson DG, et al. Controlled trial of prednisolone as adjuvant in the treatment of tuberculous constrictive pericarditis in Transkei. Lancet. 1987;2:1418.
450. Roberts WC, Spray TL. Clinical and morphologic spectrum of pericardial heart disease. Curr Probl Cardiol. 1977;2:1–71.
451. Moreno F, Sharkey-Mathis PK, Mokulis E, et al. *Mycobacterium kansasii* pericarditis in patients with AIDS. Clin Infect Dis. 1994;19:967–969.
452. Moreno R, Villacastin J, Bueno H, et al. Clinical and echocardiographic findings in HIV patients with pericardial effusion. Cardiology. 1997;88:397–400.
453. Shabetai R. Function of the pericardium. In: Fowler NO, ed. The Pericardium in Health and Disease. Mount Kisco, NY: Futura; 1985:19–50.
454. Fowler NO, Harbin AD. Recurrent acute pericarditis: Follow-up study of 31 patients. J Am Coll Cardiol. 1986;7:300–305.

455. Matthews JD, Cameron SJ, George M. Constrictive pericarditis following coxsackie virus infection. Thorax. 1970;25:624–626.
456. Utley JR, Mills J. Annular erosion and pericarditis. Complications of endocarditis of the aortic root. J Thorac Cardiovasc Surg. 1972;64:76–81.
457. Ribeiro P, Shapiro L, Nihoyannopoulos P, et al. Pericarditis in infective endocarditis. Eur Heart J. 1985;6:975–978.
458. Peel AAF. Tuberculous pericarditis. Br Heart J. 1948;10:195–207.
459. Carson TJ, Murray GF, Wilcox BR, et al. The role of surgery in tuberculous pericarditis. Ann Thorac Surg. 1974;17:163–167.
460. Guberman BA, Fowler NO, Engel PJ, et al. Cardiac tamponade in medical patients. Circulation. 1981;64:633–640.
460a. Heidenreich PA, Eisenberg MJ, Kee LL, et al. Pericardial effusion in AIDS. Incidence and survival. Circulation. 1995; 92:3229–3234.
461. Spodick DH. Pericardial rub: Prospective multiple observer investigation of pericardial friction rub in 100 patients. Am J Cardiol. 1975;35:357–362.
462. Lorell BH, Braunwald E. Pericardial disease. In: Braunwald E, ed: A Textbook of Cardiovascular Medicine. 4th ed. Philadelphia: WB Saunders; 1992:1465–1516.
463. Spodick DH. Electrocardiogram in acute pericarditis. Distributions of morphologic and axial changes by stages. Am J Cardiol. 1974;33:470–447.
464. Shabetai R. Acute pericarditis. Cardiol Clin. 1990;8:639–644.
465. Spodick DH. Frequency of arrhythmias in acute pericarditis determined by holter monitoring. Am J Cardiol. 1984;53:842–845.
466. Isner JM, Carter BL, Bankoff MS, et al. Computed tomography in the diagnosis of pericardial heart disease. Ann Intern Med. 1982;97:473–479.
467. Tomoda H, Hoshiai M, Furuya H, et al. Evaluation of pericardial effusion with computed tomography. Am Heart J. 1980;99:701–706.
468. Sechtem U, Tscholakoff D, Higgins CB. MRI of the abnormal pericardium. AJR. 1986;147:245–252.
469. Krainin FM, Flessas AP, Spodick DH. Infarction associated pericarditis. Rarity of diagnostic electrocardiogram. N Engl J Med. 1984;311:1211–1214.
470. Galve E, Garcia-del-Castillo H, Evangelista A, et al. Pericardial effusion in the course of myocardial infarction: Incidence, natural history, and clinical relevance. Circulation. 1986;73:294.
471. Gregoratos G. Pericardial involvement in acute myocardial infarction. Cardiol Clin. 1990;8:601–608.
472. Renfrew R, Buselmeier TJ, Kjeilstrand CM. Pericarditis and renal failure. Annu Rev Med. 1980;31:345–360.
473. Rutsky EA, Rostand SG. Treatment of uremic pericarditis and pericardial effusion. Am J Kidney Dis. 1987;10:2.
474. Brosius FC, Waller BF, Roberts WC. Radiation heart disease. Am J Med. 1981;70:519–530.
475. Stewart JR, Fajardo LF. Radiation-induced heart disease: An update. Prog Cardiovasc Dis. 1984;27:173.
476. Khan AH. The postcardiac injury syndromes. Clin Cardiol. 1992;15:67–72.
477. Dressler W. Post-myocardial infarction syndrome. JAMA. 1956;160:1379–1383.
478. Engle MA, Gay WA Jr, Zabriskie JB, et al. The post pericardiotomy syndrome: 25 years experience. J Cardiovasc Med. 1984;4:321–332.
479. Saner HE, Gobel FL, Nicoloff DM, et al. Aortic dissection presenting as pericarditis. Chest. 1987;91:71.
480. Silverman KJ, Hutchins GM, Bulkley BH. Cardiac sarcoid: A clinicopathologic study of 84 unselected cases with systemic sarcoidosis. Circulation. 1978;58:1204–1211.
481. Ansari A, Larson PH, Bates HD. Cardiovascular manifestations of systemic lupus erythematosis: Current perspective. Prog Cardiovasc Dis. 1985;27:421–434.
482. Lebowitz WB. The heart in rheumatoid arthritis (rheumatoid disease). A clinical and pathological study of sixty-two cases. Ann Intern Med. 1963;58:102–123.
483. Kelly CA, Bourke JP, Malcolm A, et al. Chronic pericardial disease in patients with rheumatoid arthritis: A longitudinal study. Q J Med. 1990;75:461–470.
484. Goldenberg J, Ferraz MB, Pessoa AP, et al. Symptomatic cardiac involvement in juvenile rheumatoid arthritis. Int J Cardiol. 1992;34:57–62.
485. McWhorter JE, LeRoy RC. Pericardial disease in scleroderma (systemic sclerosis). Am J Med. 1974;57:566–575.
486. Janosik DL, Osborn TG, Moore TL, et al. Heart disease in systemic sclerosis. Semin Arthritis Rheum. 1989;19:191.
487. Abid MA, Gitlin N. Pericarditis— an extraintestinal complication of inflammatory bowel disease. West J Med. 1990;153:314–315.
488. Zimmerman J, Yahalom J, Bar-On H. Clinical spectrum of pericardial effusion as the presenting feature of hypothyroidism. Am Heart J. 1983;106:770–771.
489. Krikorian JG, Hancock EW. Pericardiocentesis. Am J Med. 1978;65:808–814.
490. Mercé J, Sagristá-Sauleda J, Permanyer-Miralda G, et al. Should pericardial drainage be performed routinely in patients who have a large pericardial effusion without tamponade? Am J Med. 1998;105:106–109.
491. Gouny P, Lancelin C, Girard PM, et al. Pericardial effusion and AIDS: Benefits of surgical drainage. Eur J Cardiothorac Surg. 1998;13:165–169.
492. Estok L, Wallach F. Cardiac tamponade in a patient with AIDS. A review of pericardial disease in patients with HIV infection. Mt Sinai J Med. 1998;65:33–39.
493. Corey GR, Campbell PT, Van Trigt P, et al. Etiology of large pericardial effusions. Am J Med. 1993;95:209–213.
494. Uthaman B, Endrys J, Abushaban L, et al. Percutaneous pericardial biopsy: Technique, efficacy, safety, and value in the management of pericardial effusion in children and adolescents. Pediatr Cardiol. 1997;18:414–418.
495. Selig MB. Percutaneous pericardial biopsy under echocardiographic guidance. Am Heart J. 1991; 122:879–882.
496. Tan JS, Holmes JC, Fowler NO, et al. Antibiotic levels in pericardial fluid. J Clin Invest. 1974;53:7–12.
497. Adler Y, Finkelstein Y, Guindo J, et al. Colchicine treatment for recurrent pericarditis. A decade of experience. Circulation. 1998;97:2183–2185.
498. Guindo J, Adler Y, Spodick DH, et al. Colchicine for recurrent pericarditis: 51 patients followed up for 10 years. Circulation. 1997;96(Suppl I):1–29.
499. Millaire A, deGroote P, Docoulx E, et al. Treatment of recurrent pericarditis with colchicine. Eur Heart J. 1994;15:120–121.
500. Marcolongo R, Russo R, Laveder F, et al. Immunosuppressive therapy prevents recurrent pericarditis. J Amer Coll Card. 1995;26(5):1276–1279.
501. Quale JM, Lipschik GY, Heurich AE. Management of tuberculous pericarditis. Ann Thorac Surg. 1987;43:653–655.
502. Suwan PK, Potjalongslip S. Predictors of constructive pericarditis after tuberculous pericarditis. Br Heart J. 1995;73:187–189.
503. Alzeer AH, FitzGerald JM. Corticosteroids and tuberculosis: Risks and use as adjunct therapy. Tuber Lung Dis. 1993;74:6–11.
504. Arsan S, Mercan S, Sarigül A, et al. Long-term experience with pericardiectomy: Analysis of 105 consecutive patients. Thorac Cardiovasc Surg. 1994;42:340–344.
505. Fennell WM. Surgical treatment of constrictive tuberculous carditis. S Afr Med J. 1982;62:353.

Chapter 69

Mediastinitis

MARK E. RUPP

Acute mediastinitis is an uncommon, but potentially devastating, infection involving the structures of the mediastinum. Before the development of sophisticated techniques in cardiovascular and thoracic surgery, most cases resulted from esophageal perforation or contiguous spread from oropharyngeal foci. Mediastinitis now occurs most frequently as a postoperative infection following median sternotomy. Regardless of the pathogenesis of acute mediastinitis, a high index of clinical suspicion must be maintained for this serious infection in order to diagnose mediastinitis promptly and institute potentially life-saving medical and surgical therapy. Sclerosing mediastinitis, also known as *fibrosing* or *granulomatous mediastinitis*, often due to *Histoplasma capsulatum*, is also discussed.

ANATOMIC CONSIDERATIONS

The mediastinum is the region within the thorax between the pleural sacs (Fig. 69–1). It extends from the diaphragm inferiorly to the superior aperture of the thorax. The sternum and costal cartilages make up the anterior boundary, and the 12 thoracic vertebral bodies border the mediastinum posteriorly. The mediastinum is arbitrarily divided into four subdivisions: superior, posterior, anterior, and mid-

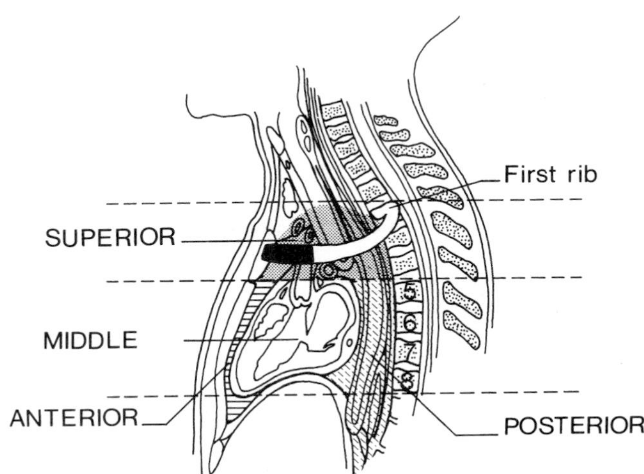

FIGURE 69–1. Anatomic boundaries and divisions of the mediastinum.

dle. Structures within the mediastinum include the heart and great vessels; the distal portion of the trachea and mainstem bronchi; the esophagus; the vagus nerves; the phrenic nerves; the remains of the thymus; and the thoracic duct. These structures are surrounded by adipose tissue, loose connective tissue, and lymph nodes. The mediastinum communicates with the structures of the head and neck via several fascial planes and potential spaces (see Fig. 53–4). Detailed descriptions of mediastinal anatomy are available,[1–4] and the major points are reviewed below. The three major routes by which infection spreads from the head and neck to the mediastinum are (1) the pretracheal space, (2) the long fascial planes of the posterior neck, and (3) the viscerovascular or lateral pharyngeal space. The long fascial planes of the posterior neck extend from the base of the skull to the diaphragm and are made up of the retropharyngeal or retrovisceral space, the prevertebral space, and the danger space. Pearse[1] attempted to delineate the relative importance of each route in the pathogenesis of mediastinitis and found the retropharyngeal space to be involved in 71% of cases, followed by the lateral pharyngeal space in 21% and the pretracheal space in 8%.

ACUTE MEDIASTINITIS

Epidemiology and Pathogenesis

Primary infection of the mediastinum is a rare event. Essentially all cases of mediastinitis are secondary to the spread of infection from other sites or direct inoculation due to trauma. The causes of mediastinitis are summarized in Table 69–1 and can be grouped into the following four categories: esophageal perforation, head and neck infection, infection originating at another site, and cardiothoracic surgery. The pathogenesis, clinical manifestations, and treatment vary according to the underlying cause of mediastinitis.

Mediastinitis Secondary to Infections of the Head and Neck and Other Contiguous Structures

Before the development of cardiac surgery, perforation of the esophagus was the leading cause of mediastinitis, followed by suppurative infections of the oropharynx.[1] In 1724, Herman Boerhaave described the first case of mediastinitis due to spontaneous rupture of the esophagus in a Dutch admiral who self-induced emesis.[111, 112] Subsequently, this entity has been known as *Boerhaave syndrome*. Currently, esophageal perforation is most frequently due to iatrogenic events.[6] Flexible fiber-optic endoscopy of the upper gastrointestinal tract is complicated by esophageal perforation in 0.074 to 0.4% of procedures.[4, 16, 113] This occurs more frequently when sclerotherapy or dilation procedures are performed.[6] Swallowed foreign bodies, esophageal carcinoma, and nonsurgical trauma may also result in perforation of the esophagus and mediastinitis.

Depending on where the esophageal perforation occurs, mediastinitis may result from direct spillage of esophageal contents into the posterior mediastinum or migration into the mediastinum via the fascial planes of the neck. A necrotizing chemical mediastinitis ensues that is followed by an aerobic and anaerobic bacterial mediastinitis. Often a synergistic necrotizing form of mediastinitis is observed.[33] Spread of infection from the neck into the mediastinum is influenced by respiratory dynamics in which the negative intrathoracic pressure generated during respiration tends to force the infection into the mediastinum.[24]

Before antibiotics were widely available, odontogenic and pharyngeal infections caused from 10 to 31% of cases of mediastinitis.[1, 2, 114] Fortunately, they are a rare cause of mediastinitis today. The prototypic odontogenic infection leading to mediastinitis is Ludwig's angina. This generally arises from an infection of the second or third mandibular molar to involve the sublingual and submandibular spaces. From there, the infection can spread via the lateral pharyngeal space to involve the retropharyngeal space or carotid sheath and thus track into the mediastinum. During the antibiotic era, approximately 3.5% of cases of Ludwig's angina have been complicated by mediastinitis.[41] Mediastinitis resulting from infections involving the lateral pharyngeal space may originate from a number of sources, including the teeth, parotid glands, tonsils, or, rarely, otitis or mastoiditis. Retropharyngeal space infections generally arise from perforation of the esophagus or extension from pharyngitis, epiglottitis, or tonsillitis. From the long fascial planes of the neck these infections easily spread into the superior mediastinum, or, if the danger space is involved, the posterior mediastinum.[33, 34] The pretracheal space descends into the anterior mediastinum and most often is involved in mediastinitis complicating surgery of the thyroid or trachea.[1]

TABLE 69–1 Causes of Acute Mediastinitis

Esophageal Perforation

Iatrogenic
- Esophagogastroduodenoscopy,[5–9] esophageal dilation,[5–9] esophageal variceal sclerotherapy,[10, 11] nasogastric tube,[6] Sengstaken-Blakemore tube,[12] endotracheal intubation,[13] esophageal surgery,[14] paraesophageal surgery[6, 15]

Swallowed foreign bodies
- Bones,[16] coins,[6] can pull tabs,[6] drug-filled condoms,[17] swords[6]

Trauma
- Penetrating
  - Gunshot wound,[18] knife wound[18]
- Blunt
  - Steering wheel injury,[19] seat-belt injury,[20] cardiopulmonary resuscitation,[21] whiplash injury,[22] barotrauma[23]

Spontaneous or other
- Emesis,[6, 24–26] cricoid pressure during anesthesia induction,[27] heavy lifting[28] defecation,[29, 30] parturition,[31] carcinoma[32]

Head and Neck Infections

Odontogenic,[1, 4, 33–40] Ludwig's angina,[1, 4, 41, 42] pharyngitis,[43–45] tonsillitis,[46] parotitis,[47] epiglottitis[48]

Infection Originating at Another Site

Pneumonia[49, 50]; pleural space infection or empyema[51]; subphrenic abscess[51]; pancreatitis[52]; cellulitis or soft-tissue infection of the chest wall[53–55]; osteomyelitis of sternum, clavicle, ribs, or vertebrae[2]; hematogenous spread from distant foci[56, 57]

Cardiothoracic Surgery

Coronary artery bypass grafting,[58–97] cardiac valve replacement,[65–97] repair of congenital heart defect,[98, 99] heart transplantation,[100–108] heart-lung transplantation, cardiac assist devices,[106–110] other types of cardiothoracic surgery

Mediastinitis Secondary to Cardiothoracic Surgery

Since the refinement of cardiothoracic surgery in the 1960s and 1970s, mediastinitis has become largely a postsurgical infection. Numerous studies have documented the incidence of mediastinitis following cardiothoracic surgery and the risk factors for development of this serious complication. In 1984, Sar and colleagues[77] reviewed the available literature and found the incidence of mediastinitis to be from 0.4 to 5% of patients undergoing median sternotomy. Since that time, studies documenting the experience in over 125,000 patients have been published, with incidence rates ranging from 0.4 to 2.4%.[58, 62–69, 71–74, 78, 79, 81, 84, 89, 90] The incidence of mediastinitis during outbreaks has been as high as 5 to 23.7%.[115–119] patients undergoing heart transplantation are at higher risk of developing mediastinitis, with incidences of 2.5 to 7.5%.[100–102] This increased risk of mediastinitis is particularly true if a mechanical device, such as a left ventricular assist device or a total artificial heart, is used to support a patient while awaiting a suitable donor heart. Incidences of mediastinitis in this situation range from 7.5 to 35.7%.[105–109]

A number of factors have been suggested to increase the risk of mediastinitis. The studies examining these risk factors are primarily retrospective case-control studies and, thus, are limited by the problems inherent in retrospective surveys. Risk factors can be divided into the following groups: preoperative, intraoperative, and postoperative. Risk factors that can be identified preoperatively include diabetes mellitus, obesity, previous sternotomy, chronic obstructive pulmonary disease, a history of endocarditis, cigarette smoking, low cardiac output states, remote infection, hair removal with razor versus removal with electric clippers, and prolonged preoperative hospitalization.[58, 61, 63–69, 72–77, 80, 84] Intraoperative and surgical factors include the complexity of surgery, the type of bone saw used, the type of sternal closure, the use of internal mammary arteries in coronary artery bypass grafting, the use of bone wax, a prolonged operative time, a prolonged time on cardiopulmonary bypass, blood transfusions, the indiscriminate use of electrocautery, tearing of the aortic or femoral artery, a prolonged aortic cross-clamp time, and antibiotic prophylaxis.[58–73, 77, 80–89, 92–95, 120] Postoperatively, patients at greater risk for mediastinitis have been found to have had reexploration to control bleeding, a prolonged length of stay in the intensive care unit, mechanical ventilation for greater than 24 to 48 hours, tracheostomy, cardiopulmonary resuscitation, temporary pacing wires, concurrent leg wound infection at the saphenous vein harvest site, and low cardiac-output states.[58, 63–70, 72, 73, 75, 77, 80–84, 92, 94, 97] There is not universal agreement regarding any of these factors. For instance, despite over 3 decades of surgical experience, it is unclear whether the use of internal mammary artery grafts in coronary artery bypass surgery predisposes patients to mediastinitis. In 1972, Arnold[121] suggested that, based on anatomic studies of sternal blood supply, the use of the internal mammary artery in coronary artery bypass procedures might lead to significant sternal ischemia and thus predispose patients to sternal osteomyelitis and mediastinitis. This has been supported by several laboratory and clinical studies.[59, 70, 84, 92, 122] However, other investigators have observed no significant increase in sternal wound infections in patients undergoing coronary artery bypass grafting when the internal mammary artery is used.[58, 60, 61, 69, 76, 123–125] More recently, Grover and colleagues[62] reviewed the data obtained from over 14,000 patients in the Department of Veterans Affairs Cardiac Surgery Database. Although operative mortality was significantly decreased in patients who received internal mammary artery grafts, there was an increased risk of mediastinitis, particularly when multiple internal mammary artery grafts were used.

It is generally believed that the pathogenesis of postcardiac surgery mediastinitis is related to the inoculation of organisms from the patient's endogenous bacterial flora or from the surgical field into the operative wound. Bacteria are able to propagate in the relatively protected avascular area of the surgical wound and cause infection. Thus, factors such as the length of time of surgery, the complexity of surgery, and the need for reexploration might be expected to increase the risk of mediastinitis. Outbreaks of mediastinitis that have been epidemiologically linked to sources such as bacteria from a surgeon's hands or nares lend support to this concept.[119–126] Ferrazzi and associates[88] observed a significant decrease in the incidence of gram-negative mediastinitis but no significant change in gram-positive infections with changes in the operating room environment, supporting the belief that many of these infections arise from a reservoir of gram-positive organisms resident on the patient's skin. Archer and Tenenbaum[127] and Archer and Amstrong[128] have demonstrated that patients are colonized by small numbers of antibiotic-resistant coagulase-negative staphylococci that become the predominant species when subjected to the selective pressure of prophylactic antibiotics. In addition, various postulated immunosuppressive effects of cardiopulmonary bypass may contribute to the pathogenesis of postcardiac surgery mediastinitis.[129, 130] Outbreaks of mediastinitis that have been linked to environmental sources and poor handwashing techniques have indicated the importance of postoperative factors.[115–118, 131–133] Controlled prospective studies are needed to define better the factors that influence postcardiac surgery mediastinitis.[134]

TABLE 69–2 Microbiology of Mediastinitis

Organisms Frequently Recovered in Mediastinitis Secondary to Infection of the Head and Neck or Esophageal Perforation*

- Anaerobic
  - Gram-positive cocci
    - *Peptostreptococcus* spp.
  - Gram-positive bacilli
    - *Actinomyces*
    - *Eubacterium*
    - *Lactobacillus*
  - Gram-negative cocci
    - *Veillonella*
  - Gram-negative bacilli
    - *Bacteroides* spp.
    - *Fusobacterium* spp.
    - *Prevotella* spp.
    - *Porphyromonas* spp.
- Aerobic or facultative
  - Gram-positive cocci
    - *Streptococcus* spp.
    - *Staphylococcus* spp.
  - Gram-positive bacilli
    - *Corynebacterium*
    - Gram-negative cocci
    - *Branhamella*
  - Gram-negative bacilli
    - Enterobacteriaceae
    - *Pseudomonas* spp.
    - *Eikenella corrodens*
  - Fungi
    - *Candida albicans*

Organisms Recovered in Mediastinitis Secondary to Cardiothoracic Surgery†

Organism	Range (%)	Representative Rate (%)
Gram-positive cocci		
Staphylococcus aureus	7.1–66.7	25
Staphylococcus epidermidis	6–45.5	30
Enterococcus spp.	8–18.8	10
Streptococcus spp.	0–18.2	2
Gram-negative bacilli		
Escherichia coli	0–12.5	5
Enterobacter spp.	4–21.4	10
Klebsiella spp.	0–21.1	3
Proteus spp.	0–7.1	2
Other Enterobacteriaceae	0–20	2
Pseudomonas spp.	0–54	2
Fungi		
Candida albicans	0–14.3	<2
Polymicrobial	0–40	10
Others occasionally reported		

Acinetobacter,[80] *Legionella* spp.,[141] *Bacteroides fragilis,*[142, 144] *Corynebacterium* spp.,[144] *Mycoplasma hominis,*[145] *Candida tropicalis,*[146] *Nocardia* spp.,[147] *Kluyvera,*[148] *Mycobacterium fortuitum,*[149] *Mycobacterium chelonei,*[149] *Rhodococcus bronchialsis*[150]

Other Unusual Causes of Mediastinitis

Anthrax,[151] brucellosis,[152] actinomycosis,[153] paragonimiasis,[154] *Streptococcus pneumoniae* infection[155]

*See references 3, 4, 13, 33, 34, 36, 38, 41, 50, 51, and 135 through 137.
†See references 58, 63, 65–70, 72, 74, 75, 77, 78, 80, 81, 83, 118, 132, and 138 through 140.

Bacteriology

The bacteriology of mediastinitis related to cardiovascular surgery and that secondary to odonotogenic or other head and neck infections is strikingly different, as summarized in Table 69–2. Mediastinitis secondary to cardiothoracic surgery is primarily due to gram-positive cocci with lesser contributions by gram-negative bacilli. *Candida* appears to be responsible for a growing number of cases of mediastinitis following cardiothoracic surgery.[139, 140] The bacteriology of mediastinitis secondary to extension from head and neck sources is largely polymicrobic. Often a synergistic infection made up of a number of oral anaerobes and gram-negative bacilli is present. The most frequently isolated organisms include viridans streptococci, peptococci, peptostreptococci, *Bacteroides* spp., and *Fusobacterium*. The relative frequency with which these organisms are isolated is uncertain.[135]

Clinical Manifestations and Diagnosis

The clinical manifestations of mediastinitis also differ according to the underlying cause of disease. Patients with mediastinitis from extension of odontogenic or pharyngeal infections generally have obvious primary infections with significant pain, fever, and swelling at the affected site. Esophageal perforation may be clinically obvious or inapparent. Early in the course of mediastinitis, signs and symptoms may be subtle, but, as the condition progresses, patients note increasing chest pain, respiratory distress, and dysphagia. Chest pain is often the most prominent symptom and may localize depending on which portion of the mediastinum is involved. In anterior mediastinitis, pain is often located in the cervical or substernal region. Pain due to posterior mediastinitis may localize to the epigastric area with radiation to the interscapular region.[16, 24, 50, 114] Pleuritic chest pain may also be experienced due to the relatively frequent complication of pleural effusion. Retroperitoneal extension may be accompanied by acute abdominal signs and may prompt unnecessary exploratory laparotomy.[33] Examination may reveal fever, tachycardia, crepitus, and edema of the chest or neck. Hamman's sign, a crunching rasping sound heard over the precordium synchronous with the cardiac rhythm, due to emphysema of the mediastinum, may be present in up to 50% of patients with pneumomediastinum.[156, 157] The heart sounds may appear distant and dull. In the later stages of disease, signs of bacteremia and sepsis may predominate. The early diagnosis of mediastinitis in the infant or neonate is particularly challenging. A peculiar, interrupted, staccato type of inspiration has been described in a number of cases.[158] The signs and symptoms of mediastinitis in older children are similar to those observed in adults.[159] Laboratory tests usually reveal a leukocytosis with a leftward shift evident on the differential. Radiographically, plain films of the chest may reveal mediastinal widening, air-fluid levels, and subcutaneous or mediastinal emphysema.[8, 9, 16, 34, 38, 160] The lateral chest radiograph may be useful in demonstrating superior mediastinal gas not evident on upright films. Approximately 50% of cases of pneumomediastinum are not evident without lateral views.[161] Complications of mediastinitis, such as pleural effusion or pneumoperitoneum, may also be evident on the chest radiograph. Esophageal perforation is best demonstrated by contrast esophagography, which reveals extravasation of dye in 59 to 100% of cases.[9, 16, 162, 166] It is recommended that a water-soluble contrast agent be used initially to avoid the inflammation and granuloma formation evoked by extravasated barium.[167] If extravasation is not observed, barium should be used to detect subtle defects, as it provides a better definition of the anatomy.[167] Computed tomography (CT) is often helpful in cases in which the diagnosis is not evident clinically or on plain films.[168, 169] Technetium-labeled white blood cell scans have been reported helpful in the diagnosis of mediastinitis in specialized circumstances when CT scan was not readily available.[170] The role of magnetic resonance imaging has not been well established.

Postcardiothoracic surgery mediastinitis usually presents within the first 2 weeks after surgery.[65–68, 74, 77–80] However, rare cases have been described occurring up to 416 days postoperatively.[75] Infections due to gram-negative organisms generally present earlier. One study found that all cases of mediastinitis presenting later than 2 weeks postoperatively were due to gram-positive organisms.[75] El Oakley and Wright[171] have proposed a classification system in which patients with postcardiothoracic surgery are divided into seven groups depending on the time to presentation, underlying risk factors, and prior therapeutic efforts. Mediastinitis may present fulminantly or subtly. Some cases may present as sepsis without localizing signs.[77] Patients may experience greater-than-normal postoperative pain, which may be pleuritic in nature. Dysphagia is a rare complaint. Fever and an abnormal appearance of the surgical wound, characterized by erythema, cellulitis, or purulent discharge, are the most frequent signs of mediastinitis.[59, 65–68, 75, 77, 79, 80, 90, 92] Sternal instability, dehiscence, or the observation of bubbles emanating from the sternal wound are less frequent findings. Occasionally chest wall emphysema is observed. Poststernotomy mediastinitis presenting as a deep neck abscess without abnormal findings on chest examination has been reported.[172] Laboratory tests usually show a moderate leukocytosis with a leftward shift on the white blood cell differential. Radiographically, mediastinal widening is a rare finding on plain chest films, and generally routine radiographs are of very little use in the diagnosis of mediastinitis following cardiothoracic surgery.[75, 77, 169] CT scanning has proved helpful in many cases of postoperative mediastinitis, particularly in differentiating superficial wound infections from deeper retrosternal processes.[168, 169, 173, 174] Characteristic findings include soft tissue swelling, pleural effusion, subcutaneous fluid collection, and sternal erosion.[168, 169, 173, 174] However, normal postoperative collections of fluid and gas are at times difficult to differentiate from early signs of mediastinitis.[168] The diagnostic value of nuclear scans has been espoused by several investigators.[175–177] Browdie and colleagues[178] studied the relative value of CT, ^{111}In-labeled leukocyte scanning, and epicardial pacer wire cultures in 24 patients being evaluated for possible mediastinitis. They found that CT had a sensitivity of 67% and a specificity of 71%. The ^{111}In-labeled leukocyte scan was 83% sensitive and 100% specific, and epicardial pacer wire cultures were reported to be 100% sensitive and 92% specific. Robicsek,[179] however, found epicardial pacer wire cultures to be associated with an unacceptably high false-positive rate, and in a study of 565 patients Maroto and associates[180] found epicardial wire cultures to be only 75% sensitive and 83.4% specific and to have a positive and negative predictive value of 11.6 and 99.1%, respectively. The role of magnetic resonance imaging is not well delineated, and it is contraindicated in instances in which ferromagnetic metals are used in sternal wires, artificial heart valves, cardiac pacemakers, or vascular clips. Several investigators have found mediastinal needle aspiration useful in the diagnosis of mediastinitis.[69, 70, 77, 90, 181] This method, which has been reported positive in 65.8% of patients, appears to be particularly useful in diagnosing mediastinitis before it becomes more clinically obvious.[69, 70, 181]

Treatment

Therapy that includes both medical and surgical techniques should be promptly initiated once the diagnosis of mediastinitis is made. Barrett[182] is credited with documenting the first successful treatment of mediastinitis due to esophageal perforation. Since then, most authorities recommend aggressive surgical drainage, débridement, and repair in cases of mediastinitis secondary to esophageal perforation.[7–9, 16, 162, 183–185] However, based on experience with eight patients, Cameron and colleagues[186] identified a subset of patients who could be treated without surgical intervention. These patients should have a well-contained disruption of the esophagus, the abscess should drain back into the esophagus, minimal symptoms should be present, and there should be minimal evidence of clinical toxicity. Shaffer and coworkers[163] expanded on these recommendations based on the recognition of patients with esophageal perforation due to instrumentation before major mediastinal contamination had occurred. Santos and Frator[187] have recommended transesophageal irrigation for patients in whom primary repair of the esophagus is not possible due to advanced local infection with extensive tissue necrosis.

As in cases of mediastinitis due to esophageal perforation, cases secondary to descending odontogenic or pharyngeal infection require prompt surgical intervention. Several authors have warned that a transthoracic approach is necessary and that transcervical drainage is often inadequate.[33, 40] Roberts and associates[188] have reported the successful management of a patient with descending necrotizing mediastinitis by thoracoscopic drainage.

Although the importance of supportive therapy and surgical intervention cannot be overemphasized, the administration of appropriate antibiotics is an essential component of therapy. Empirical regimens are based on the underlying cause and should cover the major pathogens listed in Table 69–2. Penicillin G has traditionally been the antibiotic of choice in the treatment of anaerobic infections arising above the diaphragm and continues to exhibit excellent activity against most oral anaerobic bacteria. However, oral anaerobes such as *Prevotella* and *Porphyromonas* spp. (formerly *Bacteroides* spp.) are often resistant to penicillin G, and, therefore, when infection with those organisms is suspected, treatment with metronidazole, clindamycin, or broad-spectrum β-lactam–β-lactamase combinations, imipenem, or meropenem, which have activity against penicillin-resistant anaerobes as well as other oropharyngeal anaerobes, may be indicated.[135] In addition, gram-negative enteric bacilli are often implicated in mediastinitis and should be covered in initial empirical therapy. Antibiotic therapy should then be more specifically tailored to the infecting organisms when definitive culture results are available, but therapy directed against anaerobic oropharyngeal organisms should probably be continued due to the difficulty in obtaining reliable anaerobic cultures.[135] The duration of therapy, which may range from weeks to months, is determined by the virulence of the bacteria, host factors, and the patient's response to therapy.

The treatment of postcardiac surgery mediastinitis generally requires aggressive surgical drainage and débridement. A small number of patients have been successfully treated via percutaneous catheter drainage.[189] Two approaches have been utilized in the surgical management of postcardiac surgery mediastinitis: an open technique and a closed technique. The open technique involves débridement of infected tissue and open packing of the wound with delayed closure.[58, 69, 70, 77, 89, 92, 190] Disadvantages of this technique include respiratory insufficiency due to a lack of mechanical support for the thorax, delayed healing and closure of the surgical wound, and hemorrhage from exposed vessels.[62, 77, 90, 92] The closed method involves débridement of affected tissues, closure of the sternum, and postoperative irrigation through drainage tubes within the mediastinum.[58, 69, 70, 77, 89, 92, 190, 191] Irrigants have included a variety of antimicrobial and antiseptic solutions, such as neomycin, gentamicin, bacitracin, polymyxin B, saline, and Dakin's solution. They have been associated with a variety of complications, including the emergence of resistant organisms, pericardial and tissue toxicity, and systemic absorption and toxicity.[91, 192–194] The most commonly employed irrigant is povidone-iodine. The use of povidone-iodine has been associated with iodine toxicity, renal failure, metabolic acidosis, and seizures.[195–197] Therefore, this agent must be used with caution, and it has been recommended that the serum iodide concentration be measured to ensure that toxic levels are not reached.[195–197] Durandy and coworkers[198] reported a closed technique successfully utilizing Redon drainage devices in 11 patients who did not require postoperative irrigation. A number of investigators have reported the successful use of muscle flaps and omental grafts, often at the time of initial débridement, to close mediastinal wounds with or without postoperative irrigation.[69, 92, 98, 190, 191, 199–203]

The use of parenteral antibiotics has remained a cornerstone of therapy. Generally, empirical therapy should be directed at staphylococci and gram-negative aerobic bacilli until definitive culture results are available. As with mediastinitis secondary to infection of the head and neck, the duration of therapy is determined by a number of factors and may be quite prolonged. Although controlled studies are lacking, in several cases of mediastinitis recalcitrant to more traditional therapy, packing the wound with granulated sugar or honey has been used successfully to eradicate infection.[204–207] It appears that the sugar lowers the water activity of the tissue substrate to a level at which bacterial growth is inhibited.[205]

Antibiotic Prophylaxis

Although cardiothoracic surgical procedures are classified as clean procedures and the risk of infection is low, the consequences of infection can be devastating. Therefore, despite the lack of placebo-controlled studies documenting its efficacy, antibiotic prophylaxis has become commonplace. Cefazolin or cefuroxime have generally been regarded as the drugs of choice for prophylaxis.[208] In a comparison among vancomycin, cefazolin, and cefamandole, Maki and associates[209] demonstrated a significant reduction in postoperative wound infection in patients receiving vancomycin prophylaxis. Vancomycin should be considered for prophylaxis in medical centers in which there is a high prevalence of infections due to methicillin-resistant staphylococci. However, the use of vancomycin for surgical prophylaxis must be tempered by the risk of development of vancomycin resistance in enterococci and staphylococci.

Complications and Prognosis

Complications of mediastinitis include extension of the infection into a number of contiguous structures and spaces, including the pericardial space, resulting in pericardial effusion and tamponade, the pleural space, and the peritoneum, resulting in peritonitis.[24, 33] A major complication of postcardiac surgery mediastinitis is sternal osteomyelitis. Before the development of modern surgery and antibiotics, mediastinitis, due primarily to esophageal perforation, was regarded as uniformly fatal. Unfortunately, since the time of Barrett's first successful surgical repair of the esophagus in 1946,[112] morbidity and mortality have remained high, with many studies recording mortality rates of 30 to 50%.[9, 33, 40, 58, 67, 75] However, recent studies have reported mortality rates of less than 10 to 15%.[63, 65, 66, 171, 190, 191] In examining the economic ramifications of mediastinitis, Loop and coworkers[58] found that the hospital charges for coronary artery bypass surgery patients who experience mediastinitis were 280% greater than those of patients with uncomplicated bypass surgery, and the median length of stay ranged from 38 to 51 days. Mossad and associates[68] found that patients with deep sternal wound infections due to coagulase-negative staphylococci required an excess hospital stay of 21.5 days at a cost of $20,000 per patient compared with patients without infection. The most important factor in determining outcome has been the length of time to diagnosis and the initiation of definitive therapy.[9, 40, 50, 69, 70, 162] Other prognostic indicators have included the blood urea nitrogen level, white blood cell count, culture positivity, type of surgical repair, and cytomegalovirus shedding[69, 210, 211]

SCLEROSING MEDIASTINITIS

Sclerosing, fibrosing, or *granulomatous mediastinitis* are terms for a chronic form of mediastinitis characterized by an invasive and compressive inflammatory infiltrate. The first report of this entity, which can cause up 10% of all primary mediastinal masses,[212] reportedly dates to a description by Ulmont in 1855.[213] Although the cause of up to 83% of cases of sclerosing mediastinitis remain obscure,[212] many authorities believe that most cases are secondary to infection with *H. capsulatum*.[214–218] Gryboski and associates[216] and Peabody and coworkers[217] found that up to 73% of cases previously characterized as nonspecific granulomatous mediastinitis could be reclassified as secondary to *H. capsulatum* infection by restaining the tissue with fungal stains and a thorough review of the pathologic sections. Other reported infectious causes of this condition include tuberculosis,[219, 220] actinomycosis,[221, 222] nocardiosis,[223] blastomycosis,[224] coccidioidomycosis,[225] aspergillosis,[225] *Rhizopus* spp. infection[226] and *Wucheria bancrofti* infection.[227] The older literature often lists syphilis as a prominent cause of this condition. However, this was erroneously based simply on seropositivity without other supporting evidence. Other conditions that closely mimic this entity include sarcoidosis,[212, 228] silicosis,[212] lymphoma,[228] mesothelioma,[229] and mediastinal fibrosis associated with idiopathic retroperitoneal fibrosis, Riedel's struma, or sclerosing cholangitis.

Approximately 40% of patients with sclerosing mediastinitis are asymptomatic and come to medical attention when a chest roentgenogram incidentally reveals a mediastinal mass.[215] Symptomatic patients usually note symptoms related to invasion or obstruction of structures within or adjacent to the mediastinum (Table 69–3). Sclerosing mediastinitis is the most common nonmalignant cause of

TABLE 69–3 Complications and Manifestations of Sclerosing Mediastinitis

Superior vena cava obstruction
Inferior vena cava obstruction
Esophageal obstruction
Esophagobronchial obstruction
Tracheobronchial obstruction
Pulmonary venous or arterial obstruction
Pulmonary hypertension
Pulmonary infarction
Cor pulmonale
Thoracic duct obstruction
Constructive pericarditis
Coronary artery stenosis
Mediastinal nerve entrapment
Recurrent laryngeal nerve palsy

superior vena cava syndrome, responsible for up to 23% of cases.[230] These patients generally present with plethora and edema of the face, neck, and upper torso; neck vein distention; headache; and visual disturbances. Patients presenting with obstruction of the pulmonary arteries often note cough, dyspnea, and symptoms consistent with right-sided heart failure. Pulmonary infarction, although rare, has been reported to occur in patients with fibrosing mediastinitis.[231] Pulmonary venous obstruction causes patients to experience cough, dyspnea, and hemoptysis. Patients with airway obstruction due to sclerosing mediastinitis usually present with wheezing, cough, hemoptysis, and recurrent episodes of bacterial bronchitis or pneumonia. Patients complaining of dysphagia may have esophageal obstruction due to posterior extension of the mediastinitis.

Radiographically, patients with fibrosing mediastinitis are often observed to have a mediastinal mass, most frequently located in the superior mediastinum at the level of the bifurcation of the trachea. Kerley B lines may be present.[232] CT often reveals calcification and delineates the extent of infection, whereas magnetic resonance imaging is superior in the assessment of the vascular integrity.[233] Ventilation-perfusion lung scans often reveal large perfusion deficits due to obstruction of the pulmonary vessels.

The diagnosis of fibrosing mediastinitis requires pathologic examination. There is a continuum of disease ranging from a predominantly granulomatous entity to an almost completely fibrosing process. Lesions described include caseating granuloma, dense hyalinized collagenous tissue, and infiltrations of lymphocytes, plasma cells, and giant cells. Specific stains for fungi often reveal organisms consistent with *Histoplasma*, but cultures are usually negative.[212, 224]

The pathologic features of this disease suggest a marked inflammatory reaction. Several different mechanisms have been proposed to explain the pathology of fibrosing mediastinitis. Some investigators believe that a caseous lymph node from primary infection with *Histoplasma* ruptures into the mediastinum, invoking an intense inflammatory reaction.[212, 224] A second hypothesis is the development of a delayed hypersensitivity reaction due to the spread of soluble *Histoplasma* antigens into the mediastinum.[234] An alternate explanation proposes that fibrosing mediastinitis represents an abnormality of collagen production and organization similar to that of idiopathic retroperitoneal fibrosis[234] or Riedel's struma.[234] Noguchi and coworkers[235] have incriminated the eosinophil in the pathogenesis of fibrosing mediastinitis by demonstrating eosinophils or major basic protein in tissue specimens from five of seven patients with fibrosing mediastinitis.[235]

No controlled trials of medical or surgical therapy in the treatment of fibrosing mediastinitis have been conducted. Although there is some anecdotal evidence of a beneficial effect of antifungal agents,[236] most authorities believe that at the time of presentation there is little evidence of an active infection, and the antifungal agents are not indicated.[214, 224, 232] Because the natural history of this disease is variable, with some patients progressing to compression of vital structures whereas others seem to have self-limited disease,[224] it is difficult to make recommendations regarding the timing of surgical intervention. It has been suggested that early surgical intervention and removal of granulomatous tissue may prevent the development of subsequent end-stage fibrosis and involvement of vital structures.[237] Clearly, patients experiencing obstruction or invasion of mediastinal structures require intervention, even though such surgery is often difficult and results are at times less than optimal.[224] Therapy with corticosteroids does not appear to have a role in the treatment of fibrosing mediastinitis.[238]

REFERENCES

1. Pearse HE, Jr. Mediastinitis following cervical suppuration. Ann Surg. 1938;108:588–611.
2. Neuhof H, Jemerin EE. Acute Infections of the Mediastinum. Baltimore: Williams & Wilkins; 1943.
3. De Marie S, Tjon A, Tham RTO, et al. Clinical infections and nonsurgical treatment of parapharyngeal infections complicating throat infection. Rev Infect Dis. 1989;11:975–982.
4. Chow AW. Life-threatening infections of the head and neck. Clin Infect Dis. 1992;14:991–1004.
5. Silvis SE, Nebel O, Rogers G, et al. Endoscopic complications: Results of the 1974 American gastrointestinal endoscopy survey. JAMA. 1976;235:928–930.
6. Michael L, Grillo HC, Malt RA. Esophageal perforation. Ann Thorac Surg. 1982;33:203–210.
7. Goldstein LA, Thompson WR. Esophageal perforations: A 15 year experience. Am J Surg. 1982;143:495–503.
8. Sarr MG, Pemberton JH, Payne WS. Management of instrumental perforations of the esophagus. J Thorac Cardiovasc Surg. 1982;84:211–218.
9. Moghissi K, Pender D. Instrumental perforations of the oesophagus and their management. Thorax. 1988;43:642–646.
10. Edling JE, Bacon BR. Pleuropulmonary complications of endoscopic variceal sclerotherapy. Chest. 1991;99:1252–1257.
11. Baydur A, Korula J. Cardiorespiratory effects of endoscopic esophageal variceal sclerotherapy. Am J Med. 1990;89:477–482.
12. Conn HO. Hazards attending the use of esophageal tamponade. N Engl J Med. 1958;259:701–707.
13. Uram J, Hauser MS. Deep neck and mediastinal necrotizing infection secondary to a traumatic intubation. J Oral Maxillofac Surg. 1988;46:788–791.
14. Aggerholm K, Illum P. Surgical treatment of Zenker's diverticulum. J Laryngology Otol. 1990;104:312–314.
15. Wang RC, Perlman PW, Parnes SM. Near-fatal complications of tracheotomy infections and their prevention. Head Neck. 1989;11:528–533.
16. Wychulis AR, Fontana RS, Payne WS. Noninstrumental perforations of the esophagus. Dis Chest. 1969;55:190–196.
17. Johnson JA, Landreneau RJ. Esophageal obstruction and mediastinitis: A hard pill to swallow for drug smugglers. Am Surgeon. 1991;57:723–726.
18. Miller RH, Duplechain JK. Penetrating wounds of the neck. Otolaryngol Clin North Am. 1991;24:15–29.
19. Gulbrandson RN, Gaspard DJ. Steering wheel rupture of the pharyngoesophagus: A solitary injury. J Trauma. 1977;17:74–77.
20. Micon L, Geis L, Siderys H, et al. Rupture of the distal thoracic esophagus following blunt trauma. J Trauma. 1990;30:214–217.
21. Rotstein OD, Rhame FS, Molina E, Simmons RL. Mediastinitis after whiplash injury. Can J Surg. 1986;29:54–56.
22. Mensah GA, Gold JP, Schreiber T, Isom OW. Acute purulent mediastinitis and sternal osteomyelitis after closed chest cardiopulmonary resuscitation: A case report and review of the literature. Ann Thorac Surg. 1988;46:353–355.
23. Ribet M, Pruvot FR. Barotraumatic rupture of the esophagus. J Chir Paris. 1986;123:164–168.
24. Payne WS, Larson RH. Acute mediastinitis. Surg Clin North Am. 1969;49:999–1009.
25. Bennett DJ, Deveridge RJ, Wright JS. Spontaneous rupture of the esophagus: A review with reports of six cases. Surgery. 1970;68:766–770.
26. Derbes VJ, Mitchell RE Jr. Rupture of the esophagus. Surgery. 1956;39:688–709,865–888.
27. Ralph SJ, Wareham CA. Rupture of the esophagus during cricoid pressure. Anaesthesia. 1991;46:40–41.
28. Mackler SA. Spontaneous rupture of the esophagus. Surg Gynecol Obstet. 1952;95:345–355.
29. Tidman MK, John HT. Spontaneous rupture of the esophagus. Br J Surg. 1967;54:286–292.
30. Beal JM. Spontaneous rupture of the esophagus. Ann Surg. 1949;512–516.
31. O'Connell ND. Spontaneous rupture of the esophagus. Am J Roentgenol.1967;99:186–203.
32. Kimose HH, Lund O, Hasenkam JM, et al. Independent predictors of operative mortality and postoperative complications in surgically treated carcinomas of the oesophagus and cardia—Is the aggressive surgical approach worthwhile? Acta Chir Scand. 1990;156:373–382.
33. Estrera AS, Landay MJ, Grishom JM, et al. Descending necrotizing mediastinitis. Surg Gynecol Obstet. 1983;157:545–552.

34. Levine TM, Wurster CF, Krespi YP. Mediastinitis occurring as a complication of odontogenic infections. Laryngoscope. 1986;96:747–750.
35. Moncada R, Warpeha R, Pickleman J, et al. Mediastinitis from odontogenic and deep cervical infection. Chest. 1978;73:497–500.
36. Steiner M, Grau MJ, Wilson DL, Snow NJ. Odontogenic infection leading to cervical emphysema and fatal mediastinitis. J Oral Maxillofac Surg. 1982;40:600–604.
37. Zachariades N, Mezitis M, Stavrinidis P, Agourdaki EK. Mediastinitis, thoracic empyema, and pericarditis as complications of a dental abscess. J Oral Maxillofac Surg. 1988;46:493–495.
38. Rubin MM, Cozzi GM. Fatal necrotizing mediastinitis as a complication of an odontogenic infection. J Oral Maxillofac Surg. 1987;45:529–533.
39. Masgrove BT, Malden NJ. Mediastinitis and pericarditis caused by dental infection. Br J Oral Maxillofac Surg. 1989;27:423–428.
40. Wheatley MJ, Stirling MC, Kirsh MM, et al. Descending necrotizing mediastinitis: Transcervical drainage is not enough. Ann Thorac Surg. 1990;49:780–484.
41. Moreland LW, Corey J, McKenzie R. Ludwig's angina: Report of a case and review of the literature. Arch Intern Med. 1988;148:461–466.
42. Van der Brempt X, Derue G, Severin F, et al. Ludwig's angina and mediastinitis due to *Streptococcus milleri*: Usefulness of computed tomography. Eur Respir J. 1990;3:728–731.
43. Baker AR, Moir AA, Donnelly PK. Life-threatening peripharyngeal sepsis with mediastinitis. Br J Clin Pract. 1990;44:640–641.
44. Zaltman M, Kallenbach J, Hockman M, et al. Fatal intrathoracic sepsis associated with neck space infection. Thorax. 1983;38:143–145.
45. Enquist RW, Blanck RR, Butler RH. Nontraumatic mediastinitis. JAMA. 1976;236:1048–1049.
46. Komatsu ES, Costa F, Marchese LT, Filho SV. Abscess of the mediastinum: A case report. J Pediatr Surg. 1989;24:1125.
47. Guardia SN, Cameron R, Phillips A. Fatal necrotizing mediastinitis secondary to acute suppurative parotitis. J Otolarngol. 1991;20:54–56.
48. Chong WH, Woodhead MA, Millard FJC. Mediastinitis and bilateral thoracic empyemas complicating adult epiglottitis. Thorax. 1990;45:491–492.
49. Pane GA, Hamilton GC, Call E. Nontraumatic suppurative mediastinitis presenting as acute mediastinal widening. Ann Emerg Med. 1983;12:777–779.
50. Freidman BC, Pickul DC. Acute mediastinitis: What to do when the cause is nonsurgical. Postgrad Med. 1990;87:273–285.
51. Hardy CC, Raza SN, Isalska B, Barber PV. Atraumatic suppurative mediastinitis and purulent pericarditis due to *Eikenella corrodens*. Thorax. 1988;43:494–495.
52. Iacono C, Procacci C, Frigo F, et al. Thoracic complications of pancreatitis. Pancreas. 1989;4:228–236.
53. Dreyfuss D, Djedaini K, Lapomme CB, Coste F. Nontraumatic acute anterior mediastinitis in two HIV-positive heroin addicts. Chest. 1992;101:583–585.
54. Duncan GW, Randall WE, Mulholland JH. *Hemophilus influenzae* type B, mediastinitis cellulitis, bacteremia, and meningitis in an adult. Am Rev Respir Dis. 1981;123:333–335.
55. Barradas MCR, Muscher DM, Hamill RJ, et al. Unusual manifestations of pneumococcal infection in human immunodeficiency virus-infected individuals: The past revisited. Clin Infect Dis. 1992;14:192–199.
56. Antreasian B. Mediastinal abscess: Two case reports. Indiana Med. 1988;81:528–532.
57. Smith A, Sinzobahamvya N. Anterior mediastinal abscess complicating septic arthritis. J Pediatr Surg. 1992;27:101–102.
58. Loop FD, Lytle BW, Cosgrove DM, et al. Sternal wound complications after isolated coronary artery bypass grafting: Early and late mortality, morbidity, and cost of care. Ann Thorac Surg. 1990;49:179–187.
59. Grossi EA, Esposito R, Harris LJ et al. Sternal wound infections and use of internal mammary artery grafts. J Thorac Cardiovasc Surg. 1991;102:342–347.
60. Sethi GK, Copeland JG, Moritz T, et al. Comparison of postoperative complications between saphenous vein and IMA grafts to left anterior descending coronary artery. Ann Thorac Surg. 1991;51:733–738.
61. Sutherland RD, Martinez HE, Guynes WA, Miller L. Postoperative chest wound infections in patients requiring coronary bypass. J Thorac Cardiovasc Surg. 1977;73:944–947.
62. Grover FL, Johnson RR, Marshall G, Hammermeister KE. Impact of mammary grafts on coronary bypass operative mortality and morbidity. Ann Thorac Surg. 1994;57:559–569.
63. El Oakley R, Paul E, Wong PS, et al. Mediastinitis in patients undergoing cardiopulmonary bypass: Risk analysis and midterm results. J Cardiovasc Surg. 1997;38:595–600.
64. Milano CA, Kesler K, Archibald N, et al. Mediastinitis after coronary artery bypass graft surgery. Circulation. 1995;92:2245–2251.
65. Munuz P, Menasalvas A, Bernaldo de Quiros JCL, et al. Postsurgical mediastinitis: A case-control study. Clin Infect Dis. 1997;25:1060–1064.
66. Bitkover CY, Garlund B. Mediastinitis after cardiovascular operations: A case-control study of risk factors. Ann Thorac Surg. 1998;65:36–40
67. Farinas MC, Paralta FG, Bernal JM, et al. Suppurative mediastinitis after open-heart surgery: A case-control study covering a seven-year period in Santander, Spain. Clin Infect Dis. 1995;20:272–279.
68. Mossad SB, Serkey JM, Longworth DL, et al. Coagulase-negative staphylococcal sternal wound infections after open heart operations. Ann Thorac Surg. 1997;63:395–401.
69. Grossi EU, Culliford AT, Kriegu KH, et al. A survey of 77 major infectious complications of median sternotomy: A review of 7949 consecutive operative procedures. Ann Thorac Surg. 1985;40:214–223.
70. Culliford AT, Cunningham JN, Zeff RH, et al. Sternal and costochondral infections following open-heart surgery. J Thorac Cardiovasc Surg. 1976;72: 714–726.
71. Hammermeister KE, Burchfiel C, Johnson R, Grover FL. Identification of patients at greatest risk for developing major complications at cardiac surgery. Circulation. 1990;82 (Suppl IV):380–389.
72. Ottino G, De Paulis R, Pansini S, et al. Major sternal wound infection after open-heart surgery: A multivariate analysis of risk factors in 2579 consecutive operative procedures. Ann Thorac Surg 1987;44:173–179.
73. Newman LS, Szczukowski LC, Bain RP, Perlino CA. Suppurative mediastinitis after open heart surgery. Chest. 1988;94:546–553.
74. Nagachinta T, Stephens M, Reitz B, Polk BF. Risk factors for surgical-wound infection following cardiac surgery. J Infect Dis. 1987;156:967–973.
75. Bor DH, Rose RM, Modlin JF, et al. Mediastinitis after cardiovascular surgery. Rev Infect Dis. 1983;5:885–897.
76. Engleman RM, Williams CD, Gouge TH, et al. Mediastinitis following open-heart surgery. Arch Surg. 1973;107:772–778.
77. Sarr MG, Gott VL, Townsend TR. Mediastinal infection after cardiac surgery. Ann Thorac Surg. 1984;38:415–423.
78. Verkkala K, Jarvinen A. Mediastinal infection following open-heart surgery. Scand J Thor Cardiovasc Surg. 1986;20:203–207.
79. Kutsal A, Ibrisim E, Catav Z, et al. Mediastinitis after open heart surgery. J Cardiovasc Surg. 1991;32:38–41.
80. Farrington M, Webster M, Fenn A, Phillips I. Study of cardiothoracic wound infection at St. Thomas's hospital. Br J Surg. 1985;72:759–762.
81. Miholic J, Hudec M, Domanig E, et al. Risk factors for severe bacterial infections after valve replacement and aortocoronary bypass operations: Analysis of 246 cases by logistic regression. Ann Thorac Surg. 1985;40:224–228.
82. Serry C, Bleck PC, Javid H, et al. Sternal wound complications. J Thorac Cardiavasc Surg. 1980;80:861–867.
83. Sanfelippo PM, Danielson GK. Complications associated with median sternotomy. J Thorac Cardiovasc Surg. 1972;63:419–423.
84. Kouchoukos NT, Wareing TH, Murphy SF, et al. Risks of bilateral internal mammary artery bypass grafting. Ann Thorac Surg. 1990;49:210–219.
85. Nishida H, Grooters RK, Soltanzadeh H, et al. Discriminate use of electrocautery on the median sternotomy incision. J Thorac Cardiovasc Surg. 1991;101:488–494.
86. Doebbeling BN, Pfaller MA, Kuhns KR, et al. Cardiovascular surgery prophylaxis. J Thorac Cardiovasc Surg. 1990;99:981–989.
87. Ko W, Lazenby D, Zelano JA, et al. Effects of shaving methods and intraoperative irrigation on suppurative mediastinitis after bypass operations. Ann Thorac Surg. 1992;53:301–305.
88. Ferrazzi P, Allen R, Crupi G, et al. Reduction of infection after cardiac surgery. Ann Thorac Surg. 1986;42:321–325.
89. Cheung EH, Craver JM, Jones EL, et al. Mediastinitis after cardiac valve operations. J Thorac Cardiovasc Surg. 1985;90:517–522.
90. Jimenez-Martinez M, Arguero-Sanchez R, Perez-Alvarez JJ, Mina-Casteneda P. Anterior mediastinitis as a complication of median sternotomy incisions. Surgery. 1970;67:929–934.
91. Thurur RJ, Bognolo D, Vargas A, et al. The management of mediastinal infection following cardiac surgery. J Thorac Cardiovasc Surg. 1974;68:962–968.
92. Grmoljez PF, Barner HK, Willman VL, Kaiser GC. Major complications of median sternotomy. Am J Surg. 1975;130:679–681.
93. Firor WB. Infection following open-heart surgery, with special reference to the role of prophylactic antibiotics. J Thorac Cardiovasc Surg. 1967;53:371–378.
94. Brown AH, Baimbridge MV, Panagopoulos P, Sabar EF. The complications of median sternotomy. J Thorac Cardiovasc Surg. 1969;58:189–197.
95. Ochsner JL, Mills NL, Woolverton WC. Disruption and infection of the median sternotomy incision. J Cardiovasc Surg. 1972;13:394–399.
96. Macmanus Q, Okies JE. Mediastinal wound infection and aortocoronary graft patency. Am J Surg. 1976;132:558–561.
97. Rutledge R, Applbaum RE, Kim BJ. Mediastinal infection after open heart surgery. Surgery. 1985;97:88–92.
98. Stiegel RM, Beasley ME, Sink JD, et al. Management of postoperative mediastinitis in infants and children by muscle flap rotation. Ann Thorac Surg. 1988;46:45–46.
99. Orringer MB, Murray GF, Haller JA, Gott VL. Median sternotomy and outflow patch infections in total repair of tetralogy of Fallot. J Thorac Cardiovasc Surg. 1972;63:442–448.
100. Miller R, Rudler J, Karwande SV, Burton NA. Treatment of mediastinitis after heart transplantation. J Heart Transplant 1986;5:477–479.
101. Trento A, Dummer GS, Hardesty RL, et al. Mediastinitis following heart transplantation: Incidence, treatment, results. Heart Transplantation. 1984;3:336–340.
102. Baldwin RT, Radovancevic B, Sweeney MS, et al. Bacterial mediastinitis after heart transplantation. J Heart Lung Transplant. 1992;11:545–549.
103. Pearl SN, Weiner MA, Dibbell DG. Sternal infection after cardiac transplantation. J Thorac Cardiovasc Surg. 1982;83:632–634.
104. Lonchyna VA, Pifarre R, Sullivan H, et al. Successful use of the total artificial heart as a bridge to transplantation with no mediastinitis. J Heart Lung Transplant. 1992;11:803–811.
105. Griffith BP, Kormos RK, Hardesty RL, et al. The artificial heart: Infection-related morbidity and its effect on transplantation. Ann Thorac Surg. 1988;45:409–414.
106. Pennington DG, McBride LR, Kanter KR, et al. Bridging to heart transplantation with circulatory support devices. J Heart Transplant. 1989;8:116–123.
107. Rooks JR, Burton NA, Lefrak EA, Macmanus Q. Mediastinitis complicating successful mechanical bridge to heart transplantation. J Heart Lung Transplant. 192;11:261–264.

108. Phillips WS, Burton NA, Macmanus Q, Lefrak EA. Surgical complications in bridging to transplantation: The thermo cardiosystems LVAD. Ann Thorac Surg. 1992;53:482–486.
109. Didsheim P, Olsen DB, Farrar DJ, et al. Infections and thromboembolism with implantable cardiovascular devices. Trans Am Soc Artif Intern Organs. 1989;35:54–70.
110. Hazelrigg SR, Auer JE, Seifert PE. Experience in 100 transthoracic balloon pumps. Ann Thorac Surg. 1992;54:528–532.
111. Boerhaave H. Artocis, nec descripti prius Morbi Historia. Secundem Artis Leges Conscripta. Lugdunis Batavorum Bouresteniana; 1724.
112. Barrett NR. Spontaneous perforation of the oesophagus. Thorax. 1946;1:48–70.
113. Katz D. Morbidity and mortality in standard and flexible gastrointestinal endoscopy. Gastrointest Endosc. 1969;15:134–141.
114. Keefer CS. Acute and chronic mediastinitis. Arch Intern Med. 1938;62:109–136.
115. DeSilva MI, Rissing JP. Postoperative wound infections following cardiac surgery: Significance of contaminated cases performed in the preceding 48 hours. Infect Control. 1984;5:371–377.
116. Dandalides PC, Rutala WA, Sarubbi FA Jr. Postoperative infections following cardiac surgery: Association with an environmental reservoir in a cardiothoracic intensive care unit. Infect Control. 1984;5:378–384.
117. Palmer DL, Kuritsky JN, Lapham SC, et al. *Enterobacter* mediastinitis following cardiac surgery. Infect Control. 1985;6:115–119.
118. Ehrenkranz NJ, Pfaff SJ. Mediastinitis complicating cardiac operations: Evidence of postoperative causation. Rev Infect Dis. 1991;13:803–814.
119. Boyce JM, Bynoe GP, Opal SM, et al. A common-source outbreak of *Staphylococcus epidermidis* infections among patients undergoing cardiac surgery. J Infect Dis. 1990;161:493–499.
120. Nelson DR, Buxton TB, Luu QN, Rissing JP. The promotional effect of bone wax on experimental *Staphylococcus aureus* osteomyelitis. J Thorac Cardiovasc Surg. 1990;99:977–980.
121. Arnold M. The surgical anatomy of sternal blood supply. J Thorac Cardiovasc Surg. 1972;64:596–610.
122. Lust RM, Sun YS, Chitwood WR Jr. Internal mammary artery use: Sternal revascularization and experimental infection patterns. Circulation. 1991;84(Suppl 3):285–289.
123. Kay EB, Naraghipour H, Beg RA, et al. Internal mammary artery bypass graft: Long-term patency rate and follow-up. Ann Thorac Surg. 1974;18:269–279.
124. Green GE. Internal mammary artery-to-coronary artery anastomosis: Three-year experience with 165 patients. Ann Thorac Surg. 1972;14:260–265.
125. Tector AJ, Davis L, Gabiel R, et al. Experience with internal artery grafts in 298 patients. Ann Thorac Surg. 1976;22:515–519.
126. Gaynes R, Marosok R, Hanley JM, et al. Mediastinitis following coronary artery bypass surgery: A 3-year review. J Infect Dis. 1991;163:117–121.
127. Archer GL, Tenenbaum MJ. Antibiotic-resistant *Staphylococcus epidermidis* in patients undergoing cardiac surgery. Antimicrob Agents Chemother. 1980;17:269–272.
128. Archer GL, Armstrong BC. Alteration of staphylococcal flora in cardiac surgery patients receiving antibiotic prophylaxis. J Infect Dis. 1983;147:642–649.
129. Chenoweth DE, Cooper SW, Hugli TE, et al. Complement activation during cardiopulmonary bypass. N Engl J Med. 1981;304:497–503.
130. Kirklin JK, Westaby S, Blackstone EH, et al. Complement and the damaging effects of cardiopulmonary bypass. J Thorac Cardiovasc Surg. 1983;86:845–857.
131. Weinstein RA, Jones EL, Schwarzmann SW, Hatcher CR Jr. Sternal osteomyelitis and mediastinitis after open-heart operation: Pathogenesis and prevention. Ann Thorac Surg. 1976;21:442–444.
132. Rosendorf LL, Daicoff G, Baer H. Sources of gram-negative infection after open-heart surgery. J Thorac Cardiovasc Surg. 1974;67:195–201.
133. Andersen BM, Sorlie D, Hotvedt R, et al. Multiply beta-lactam resistant *Enterobacter cloacae* infections linked to the environmental flora in a unit for cardiothoracic and vascular surgery. Scand J Infect Dis. 1989;21:181–191.
134. Kaiser AB. Risk factors for infection in cardiac surgery: Will the real culprit please stand up? Infect Control. 1984;5:369–370.
135. Murray M, Finegold SM. Anaerobic mediastinitis. Rev Infect Dis. 1984;6:S123–S127.
136. Howell HS, Prinz RA, Pickleman JR. Anaerobic mediastinitis. Surg Gynecol Obstet. 1976;143:353–359.
137. Weil RJ. Candidal mediastinitis after surgical repair of esophageal perforation. South Med J. 1991;84:1052–1053.
138. Yardena SI, Shafir R, Weiss J, et al. Serious infectious complications of midsternotomy: A review of bacteriology and antimicrobial therapy. Scand J Infect Dis. 1990;22:633–643.
139. Glower DD, Douglas JM, Gaynor JW, et al. *Candida* mediastinitis after a cardiac operation. Ann Thorac Surg. 1990;49:157–163.
140. Clancy CJ, Nguyen MH, Morris AJ. Candidal mediastinitis: An emerging clinical entity. Clin Infect Dis. 1997;25:608–613.
141. Lowry PW, Blankenship RJ, Gridley W, et al. A cluster of *Legionella* sternal wound infections due to postoperative topical exposure to contaminated tap water. N Engl J Med. 1991;324:109–113.
142. Czachor JS, Hawley HB. Anaerobic wound infection: *Bacteroides* mediastinitis after cardiovascular surgery. Heart Lung. 1988;17:335–338.
143. Cerat GA, McHenry MC, Loop FD. Median sternotomy wound infection and anterior mediastinitis caused by *Bacteroides fragilis*. Chest. 1976;69:231–232.
144. King CT. Sternal wound infection due to *Corynebacterium xerosis*. Clin Infect Dis. 1994;19:1171–1172.
145. Sielaff TD, Everett JE, Shumway SJ, et al. *Mycoplasma hominis* infections occurring in cardiovascular surgical patients. Ann Thorac Surg. 1996;61:99–103.
146. Isenberg HD, Tucci V, Cintron F, et al. Single-source outbreak of *Candida tropicalis* complicating coronary bypass surgery. J Clin Microbiol. 1989;27:2426–2428.
147. Thaler F, Gotainer B, Teodori G, et al. Mediastinitis due to *Nocardia asteroides* after cardiac transplantation. Intens Care Med. 1992;18:127–128.
148. Madero JS, Pratt K, Hall GS, et al. *Kluyvera* mediastinitis following open-heart surgery: A case report. J Clin Microbiol. 1990;28:2848–2849.
149. Hoffman PC, Fraser DW, Robicsek F, et al. Two outbreaks of sternal wound infections due to organisms of the *Mycobacteriun fortuitum* complex. J Infect Dis. 1981;143:533–542.
150. Richet HM, Craven PC, Brown JM, et al. A cluster of *Rhodococcus* (*Gordona*) *bronchialis* sternal wound infections after coronary artery bypass surgery. N Engl J Med. 1991;324:104–109.
151. Plotkin SA, Brachman PS, Utell M, et al. An epidemic of inhalation anthrax, the first in the twentieth century. Am J Med. 1960;29:992–1001.
152. Gelfand MS, Kaiser AR, Dale WA. Localized brucellosis: Popliteal artery aneurysm, mediastinitis, dementia, and pneumonia. Rev Infect Dis. 1989;11:783–788.
153. Morgan DE, Nath H, Sanders C, Hasson JH. Mediastinal actinomycosis. AJR. 1990;155:735–737.
154. Yokogawa S, Cort WW, Yokogawa M. *Paragonimus* and paragonimiasis. Exp Parasitol. 1960;10:139–205.
155. Maroto LC, Aguado JM, Carrascal AP, et al. Role of epicardial pacing wire cultures in the diagnosis of poststernotomy mediastinitis. Clin Infect Dis. 1997;24:419–421.
156. Hamman L. Spontaneous mediastinal emphysema. Bull Johns Hopkins Hosp. 1939;64:1–21.
157. Aragon SB, Dolwick F, Buckley S. Pneumomediastinum and subcutaneous cervical emphysema during third molar extraction under general anesthesia. J Oral Maxillofac Surg. 1986;44:141–144.
158. Feldman R, Gromisch DS. Acute suppurative mediastinitis. Am J Dis Child. 1971;121:79–81.
159. Meade RH. Laryngeal obstruction in children. Pediatr Clin North Am. 1962; 9:233–262.
160. Rossiter JL, Hendrix RA. Iatrogenic subcutaneous cervicofacial and mediastinal emphysema. J Otolaryngol. 1991;20:315–319.
161. Kirshner JA. Cervical mediastinal emphysema. Arch Otolaryngol. 1980;106:368–375.
162. Burnett CM, Rosemurgy AS, Pfeiffer EA. Life-threatening acute posterior mediastinal due to esophageal perforation. Ann Thorac Surg. 1990;49:979–983.
163. Shaffer HA, Valenzuela G, Mittal RK. Esophageal perforation. Arch Intern Med. 152:757–761.
164. Elleson DA, Rowley SD. Esophageal perforation: Its early diagnosis and treatment. Laryngoscope. 1982;92:678–680.
165. Appleton DS, Sandrasagra FA, Flower CDR. Perforated esophagus: Review of twenty-eight consecutive cases. Clin Radiol. 1979;30:493–497.
166. Berry BE, Ochsner JL. Perforation of the esophagus: A 30 year review. J Thorac Cardiovasc Surg. 1973;65:1–7.
167. Vessal K, Mantali RJ, Larson SM, et al. Evaluation of barium and Gastrografin as contrast media for the diagnosis of esophageal ruptures or perforations. AJR. 1975;123:307–319.
168. Carrol CL, Jeffrey B Jr, Federle MP, Vernacchia FS. CT evaluation of mediastinal infections. J Comput Assist Tomogr. 1987;11:449–454.
169. Breatnach E, Nath PH, Delany DJ. The role of computed tomography in acute and subacute mediastinitis. Clin Radiol. 1986;37:139–145.
170. Kao CH, Wang SJ. Spread of infectious complications of odontogenic abscess detected by technetium-99m–HMPAO-labeled WBC scan of occult sepsis in the intensive care unit. J Nucl Med. 1992;33:254–255.
171. El Oakley RM, Wright JE. Postoperative mediastinitis: Classification and management. Ann Thorac Surg. 1996;61:1030–1036.
172. Simpson LC, Peters GE. Poststernotomy infections presenting as deep neck abscess. Arch Otolaryngol Head Neck Surg. 1988;114:909–912.
173. Kay HR, Goodman LR, Teplick SK, Mundth ED. Use of computed tomography to assess mediastinal complications after median sternotomy. Ann Thorac Surg. 1983;36:706–714.
174. Misawa Y, Fuse K, Hasegwa T. Infectious mediastinitis after cardiac operations: Computed tomographic findings. Ann Thorac Surg. 1998;65:622–624.
175. Quirce R, Serano J, Arnal C, et al. Detection of mediastinitis after heart transplantation by gallium-67 scintigraphy. J Nucl Med. 1991;32:860–861.
176. Bahar RH, Shuhaiber HJ, Dayem HMA. The value of gallium-67 scintigraphy in localizing infection following cardiac surgery. Int J Cardiol. 1986;11:125–127.
177. Bitkover CY, Garlund B, Larsson SA, et al. Diagnosing sternal wound infections with ^{99m}Tc-labeled monoclonal granulocyte antibody scintigraphy. Ann Thorac Surg. 1996;62:1412–1417.
178. Browdie DA, Bernstein RW, Agnew R, et al. Diagnosis of poststernotomy infection: Comparison of three means of assessment. Ann Thorac Surg 1991;51:290–292.
179. Robicsek F. Posternotomy infections. Ann Thorac Surg. 1991;52:896–900.
180. Maroto LC, Aguado JM, Carrascal Y, et al. Fulminant mediastinitis due to *Streptococcus pneumoniae* following cardiac surgery; report of a case. Clin Infect Dis. 1996;22:594–595.
181. Sarr MG, Watkins L Jr, Stewart JR. Mediastinal tap as useful method for the early diagnosis of mediastinal infection. Surg Gynecol Obstet. 1984;159:79–82.
182. Barrett NR. Report of a case of spontaneous perforation of the oesophagus successfully treated by operation. Br J Surg. 1947;35:216–218.

183. Finley RJ, Pearson FG, Weisel RD, et al. The management of nonmalignant intrathoracic esophageal perforations. Ann Thorac Surg. 1980;30:575–583.
184. Trastek VF. Esophageal perforation: A reassessment of the criteria for choosing medical or surgical therapy. Arch Intern Med. 1992;152:693.
185. Kiernan PD, Conte JV Jr, Petri R, et al. Thoracic esophageal perforations at a Virginia hospital 1979–1990. V Med Q. 1992;119:102–104.
186. Cameron JL, Kieffer RF, Hendrix TR, et al. Selective nonoperative management of contained intrathoracic esophageal disruptions. Ann Thorac Surg. 1979;27:404–408.
187. Santos GH, Frater WM. Transesophageal irrigation for the treatment of mediastinitis produced by esophageal rupture. J Thorac Cardiovasc Surg. 1986;91:57–62.
188. Roberts JR, Smythe R, Weber RW, et al. Thoracoscopic management of descending necrotizing mediastinitis. Chest. 1997;112:850–854.
189. Gobien RP, Stanley JH, Gobien BS, et al. Percutaneous catheter aspiration and drainage of suspected mediastinal abscesses. Radiology. 1984;151:69–71.
190. Jones G, Jurkiewicz MJ, Bostwick J, et al. Management of the infected median sternotomy wound with muscle flaps. Ann Surg. 1997;225:766–778.
191. El Gamel A, Yonan NA, Hassan R, et al. Treatment of mediastinitis: Early modified Robicsek closure and pectoralis major advancement flaps. Ann Thorac Surg. 1998;65:41–47.
192. Gruhl VR. Renal failure, deafness, and brain lesions following irrigation of the mediastinum with neomycin. Ann Thorac Surg. 1971;11:376–379.
193. Kopel ME, Riemersma L, Finlayson DC, et al. Gentamicin solution for mediastinal irrigation: Systemic absorption, bactericidal activity, and toxicity. Ann Thorac Surg. 1989;48:228–231.
194. Kratz JM, Metcalf JS, Sade RM. Pericardial injury by antibacterial irrigants. J Thorac Cardiovasc Surg. 1983;86:785–787.
195. Zec N, Donovan JW, Kincaid RL, Demers LM. Seizures in a patient treated with continuous povidone-iodine mediastinal irrigation. N Engl J Med. 1992;326:1784.
196. Glick PL, Guglielmo BJ, Tranbaugh RF, Turley K. Iodine toxicity in a patient treated by continuous povidone-iodine mediastinal irrigation. Ann Thorac Surg. 1985;39:478–480.
197. Campistol JM, Abad C, Nogue S, Bertran A. Acute renal failure in a patient treated by continuous povidone-iodine mediastinal irrigation. J Cardiovasc Surg. 1988;29:410–412.
198. Durandy Y, Batisse A, Bourel P, et al. Mediastinal infection after cardiac operation: A simple closed technique. J Thorac Cardiovasc Surg. 1989;97:282–285.
199. Nahai F, Rand RP, Hester TR, et al. Primary treatment of the infected sternotomy wound with muscle flaps: A review of 211 consecutive cases. Plast Reconstr Surg. 1989;84:434–441.
200. Scully HE, Leclerc Y, Martin RD, et al. Comparison between antibiotic irrigation and mobilization of pectoral muscle flaps in treatment of deep sternal infections. J Thorac Cardiovasc Surg. 1985;90:523–231.
201. Majure JA, Albin RE, O'Donnell RS, Arganese TJ. Reconstruction of the infected median sternotomy wound. Ann Thorac Surg. 1986;42:9–12.
202. Miller JI, Nahai F. Repair of the dehisced median sternotomy incision. Surg Clin North Am. 1989;69:1091–1102.
203. Heath BJ, Bagnato VJ. Poststernotomy mediastinitis treated by omental transfer without postoperative irrigation or drainage. J Thorac Cardiovasc Surg. 1987;94:355–360.
204. Szerafin T, Vaszily M, Peterffy A. Granulated sugar treatment of severe mediastinitis after open-heart surgery. Scand J Thorac Cardiovasc Surg. 1991;25:77–80.
205. Chirfe J, Scarmato G, Herszage L. Scientific basis for use of granulated sugar in treatment of infected wounds. Lancet. 1982;1:560–561.
206. Efem SEE. Clinical observations on the wound healing properties of honey. Br J Surg. 1988;75:679–681.
207. Trouillet JL, Chastre J, Fagon JY, et al. Use of granulated sugar in treatment of open mediastinitis after cardiac surgery. Lancet. 1985;2:180–184.
208. Abramowicz M, ed. Antimicrobial prophylaxis in surgery. Med Lett. 1997;39:97–102.
209. Maki DG, Bohn MJ, Stolz SM, et al. Comparative study of cefazolin, cefamandole, and vancomycin for surgical prophylaxis in cardiac and vascular operations. J Thorac Cardiovasc Surg. 1992;104:1423–1434.
210. Hoen B, Gerard A, Berne C. Prognostic factors for mediastinitis following cardiac surgery. Abstract 1258. In: Abstracts of the 32nd Interscience Conference on Antimicrobial Agents and Chemotherapy. Washington, DC: American Society for Microbiology; 1992;320.
211. Domart Y, Trouillet JL, Fagon JY, et al. Incidence and morbidity of cytomegaloviral infection in patients with mediastinitis following cardiac surgery. Chest. 1990;97:18–22.
212. Schowengerdt CG, Suyemoto R, Main FB. Granulomatous and fibrous mediastinitis. J Thorac Cardiovasc Surg. 1969;57:365–379.
213. Hache L, Woolner LB, Bernatz PE. Idiopathic fibrous mediastinitis. Dis Chest. 1962;41:9–25.
214. Strimlan CV, Dines DE, Payne WS. Mediastinal granuloma. Mayo Clin Proc. 1975;50:702–705.
215. Dines DE, Payne WS, Bernatz PE, Pairolero PC. Mediastinal granuloma and fibrosing mediastinitis. Chest. 1979;75:320–324.
216. Gryboski WA, Crutcher RR, Holloway JB, et al. Surgical aspects of histoplasmosis. Arch Surg. 1963;87:590–599.
217. Peabody JW, Brown RB, Sullivan MB, Cannon A. Mediastinal granulomas. J Thorac Surg. 1958;35:384–396.
218. Goodwin RA, Loyd JE, Des Prez RM. Histoplasmosis in normal hosts. Medicine. 1981;60:231–266.
219. Ramakantan R, Shah P. Dysphagia due to mediastinal fibrosis in advanced pulmonary tuberculosis. AJR. 1990;154:61–63.
220. Shah P, Ramakantan R. Hoarseness of the voice due to left recurrent laryngeal nerve palsy in tuberculous mediastinitis. Arch Otolaryngol Head Neck Surg. 1990;116:108.
221. Weese WC, Smith IM. A study of 57 cases of actinomycosis over a 36-year period. Arch Intern Med. 1975;135:1562–1568.
222. Bennhoff DF. Actinomycosis: Diagnostic and therapeutic considerations and a review of 32 cases. Laryngoscope. 1984;94:1198–1217.
223. Poland GA, Jorgensen CR, Sarosi GA. *Nocardia asteroides* pericarditis: Report of a case and review of the literature. Mayo Clin Proc. 1990;65:819–824.
224. Dunn EJ, Ulicny KS Jr, Wright CB, Gottesman L. Surgical implications of sclerosing mediastinitis. Chest. 1990;97:338–346.
225. Ahmad M, Weinstein AJ, Hughes JA, Cosgrove DE. Granulomatous mediastinitis due to *Aspergillus flavus* in a nonimmunocompromised patient. Am J Med. 1981;70:887–890.
226. Leong ASY. Granulomatous mediastinitis due to *Rhizopus* species. Am J Clin Pathol. 1978;70:103–107.
227. Gilbert HM, Hartman BJ. Short report; a case of fibrosing mediastinitis caused by *Wuchereria bancrofti*. Am J Trop Med Hyg. 1996;54:596–599.
228. Case records of the Massachusetts General Hospital (case 6-1989). N Engl J Med. 1989;320:380–389.
229. Grotty TB, Colby TV, Gay PC, Pisani RJ. Desmoplastic malignant mesothelioma masquerading as sclerosing mediastinitis. Hum Pathol. 1992;23:79–82.
230. Loeb JM, Lombard CM. Idiopathic mediastinitis with superior vena cava obstruction, cardiac tamponade, and cutaneous vasculitis. West J Med. 1991;155:296–299.
231. Williamson WA, Tronic BS, Levitan N, et al. Pulmonary venous infarction. Chest. 1992;102:937–940.
232. Berry DF, Buccigrossi BS, Peabody J, et al. Pulmonary vascular occlusion and fibrosing mediastinitis. Chest. 1986;89:296–301.
233. Rholl KS, Levitt RG, Glaser HS. Magnetic resonance imaging of fibrosing mediastinitis. AJR. 1985;145:255–259.
234. Feigin DS, Eggleston JC, Siegelman SS. The multiple roentgen manifestations of solerosing mediastinitis. Johns Hopkins Med J. 1979;144:1–8.
235. Noguchi H, Kephart GM, Colby TV, Gleich GJ. Tissue eosinophilia and eosinophil degranulation in syndromes associated with fibrosis. Am J Pathol. 1992;140:521–528.
236. Urschel HC Jr, Razzuk MA, Netto GJ, et al. Sclerosing mediastinitis: Improved management with histoplasmosis titer and ketoconazole. Ann Thorac Surg. 1990;50:215–221.
237. Zajtchuk R, Strevey TE, Heydorn WH, Treasure RL: Mediastinal histoplasmosis: Surgical considerations. J Thorac Cardiovasc Surg. 1973;66:300–304.
238. Cardasco EM Jr, Ahmad N, Mehta A, Rubio F. The effects of steroid therapy on pulmonary hypertension secondary to fibrosing mediastinitis. Cleve Clin J Med. 1990;57:647–652.

SECTION H

CENTRAL NERVOUS SYSTEM INFECTIONS

Chapter 70

Approach to the Patient with Central Nervous System Infection

THOMAS P. BLECK
JOHN E. GREENLEE

Many infections of the central nervous system (CNS) can be rapidly progressive, producing death or permanent damage in a short period of time. In order to provide effective therapy in a timely manner, all clinicians need to have a basic understanding of the anatomic and physiologic determinants underlying the signs and symptoms of these infections. This chapter presents a discussion of the major manifestations of these conditions and then examines important anatomic and physiologic concepts in the greater detail needed by the infectious disease specialist.

COMMON CLINICAL MANIFESTATIONS SUGGESTING CENTRAL NERVOUS SYSTEM INFECTION

The major manifestations suggesting infection of the CNS include altered awareness, headache and other manifestations of elevated intracranial pressure (ICP), seizures, and focal neurologic signs and symptoms. A systematic approach to the patient suspected of having a CNS infection requires a basic understanding of the neuroanatomic and neurophysiologic principles that underlie these clinical phenomena.

Anatomy and Physiology of Altered Awareness

Consciousness depends upon the interaction of the cerebral hemispheres with the reticular system of the upper brain stem and thalamus. As a general rule, anatomic or physiologic disruption of *both* hemispheres *or* the reticular system is required for the alteration of consciousness, but there are a few acute focal cortical disorders that produce findings that may be confused with altered consciousness.[1] For example, right parietal lesions can cause apraxia of eye opening, making the person appear somnolent when the level of consciousness is normal. Other disorders may disturb memory or the patient's interaction with the environment, such as complex partial seizures.

The interaction of the midbrain reticular formation with the cerebral hemispheres is mediated through a set of pathways traversing the diencephalon for which the thalamic reticular nuclei are a crucial way station. Herniation syndromes that disturb transmission through this system can produce stupor or coma without anatomic lesions in either the midbrain or the cerebral hemispheres. Although the classic explanation of altered consciousness due to herniation stressed vertical (downward) displacement of the diencephalon,[2] research in the 1980s proves the importance of horizontal shift in disrupting these connections.[3] This work shows a stronger correlation between the distance of horizontal shift and the level of consciousness than with the degree of vertical displacement (Fig. 70–1).[4] A corollary observation is that early in the course of horizontal shift, lateral displacement of the diencephalon pulls the midbrain with it.

Thus, a right hemisphere mass pushes the diencephalon from right to left, initially resulting in (1) altered consciousness from disruption of reticular transmission through the diencephalon; (2) secondary movement of the midbrain, such that the perimesencephalic cistern is initially *larger* on the right; and (3) a right third–cranial nerve palsy resulting from stretching of the nerve between its origin from the midbrain and its attachment to the cavernous sinus (rather than resulting from compression of the third nerve by the herniating temporal lobe, as had previously been stressed; Fig. 70–2). Later in the course of herniation, the ipsilateral medial temporal lobe may cross the tentorial edge and compress both the third nerve and the posterior cerebral artery, but this is usually a preterminal condition. As the ICP increases, the pressure gradients across the tentorium and across the foramen magnum result in vertical herniation, commonly downward, but in the case of posterior fossa lesions, occasionally upward.

Although the third-nerve palsy associated with lateral cerebral masses was classically thought to begin with a dilated pupil without paresis of extraocular movement, these phenomena often occur simultaneously, or the eye movement disorder may precede the pupillary problem. Thus, the clinician must maintain a high index of suspicion of a mass lesion in any patient with acute third–cranial

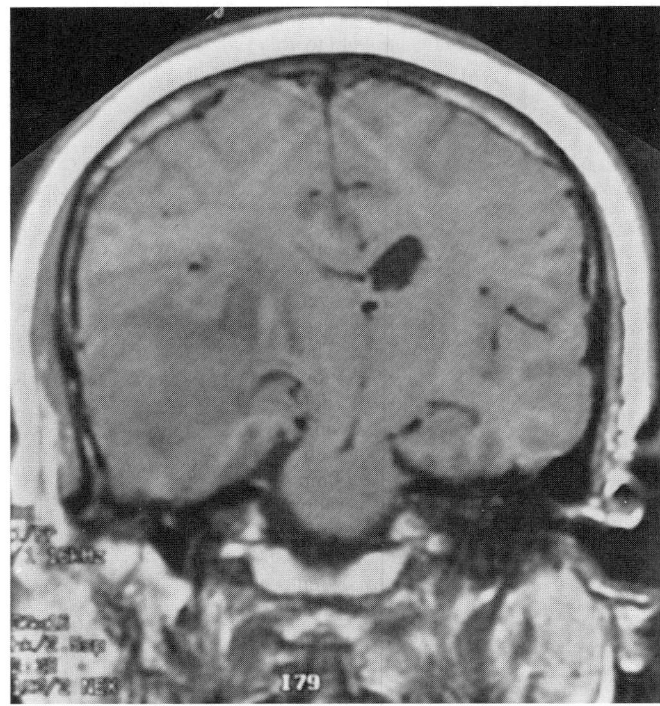

FIGURE 70–1. Coronal magnetic resonance image from a patient with a right hemisphere brain abscess. Note that the diencephalon is pushed to the left, and the midbrain is pulled to the left owing to its attachment to the diencephalon. The cistern adjacent to the midbrain on the right is enlarged by the shift, rather than being occupied by the medial temporal lobe as would have been predicted by older concepts of herniation.

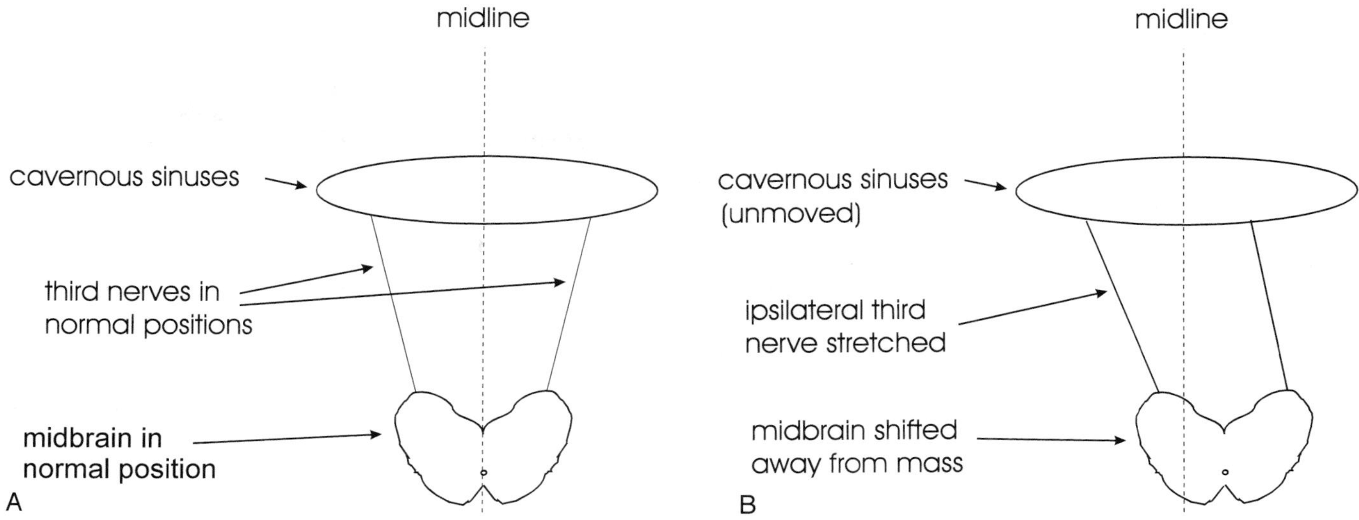

FIGURE 70–2. Production of an ipsilateral third cranial nerve palsy by a lateral mass lesion. *A,* The third cranial nerves are tethered posteriorly at the front of the midbrain and anteriorly where they enter the cavernous sinuses. *B,* When lateral movement of the diencephalon causes displacement of the midbrain out of its normal midline position, the ipsilateral third cranial nerve is stretched, producing a third nerve palsy.

nerve dysfunction. The clinical relevance of this newer anatomic understanding is the recognition that an acute third-nerve palsy may appear early in the development of a mass lesion, at a time when it is still quite amenable to treatment. The administration of mannitol when a herniation syndrome is suspected may be lifesaving while diagnostic studies are undertaken.

Headache and Other Manifestations of Elevated Intracranial Pressure

Three recognized mechanisms help to explain headache in the patient with a CNS infection: the infection may raise ICP by producing a mass effect, may raise ICP by producing hydrocephalus, or may cause meningeal irritation independent of an effect on ICP.

Headaches associated with intracranial pressure elevation are classically described as diffuse, and may be worse in the morning. This latter observation probably reflects the tendency to retain some carbon dioxide during the night, which causes cerebral vasodilation and thereby contributes to further elevation of the ICP. The normal ICP ranges up to 18 cm cerebrospinal fluid (CSF) (15 mmHg); headache may begin with sustained levels over about 24 cm CSF. The headache associated with a mass may also involve meningeal irritation if the mass is appropriately located. The other findings seen in patients with ICP elevation are probably more closely related to changes in cerebral perfusion pressure (CPP, defined as the mean arterial pressure [MAP] at the level of the brain minus the ICP; that is, CPP = MAP − ICP) than to the ICP itself. These include diminution or loss of consciousness, and the components of the Cushing reflex. The Cushing reflex represents a brain stem–mediated attempt to maintain CPP by raising MAP, followed by a reflex bradycardia, findings that are sometimes accompanied by respiratory irregularities.

Respiratory disturbances in patients with intracranial infections are usually manifestations of the elevation of ICP. Rarely, infection of the brain stem (e.g., *Listeria* rhombencephalitis) produces a primary disorder of respiration. As in other conditions causing respiratory failure, this problem can be divided conceptually into *oxygenation* failure and *ventilatory* failure. Most cases of oxygenation failure in CNS infections are a consequence of *neurogenic pulmonary edema,* which is itself a manifestation of elevated ICP. However, concurrent pneumonia, congestive heart failure, or pulmonary embolism must be considered.

Patients with elevated ICP from any cause occasionally demonstrate central neurogenic hyperventilation, in which the $Paco_2$ is low and the Pao_2 is normal. The other respiratory manifestations of elevated ICP are a consequence of the stepwise loss of higher centers, which allows anatomically more caudal systems to function without their usual control and integration. Bilateral cerebral hemispheral dysfunction, as may be seen in meningitis, results in Cheyne-Stokes respiration. Dysfunction affecting the lower midbrain–upper pontine region occasionally produces central neurogenic hyperventilation but more commonly causes neurogenic pulmonary edema. The patient is hyperpneic in both conditions, but in the case of neurogenic pulmonary edema the hyperpnea is a consequence of hypoxemia. The other classically described respiratory patterns associated with brain stem dysfunction (apneusis and ataxic respiration) are rare, occur in lower brain stem lesions, and are described elsewhere.[5]

Seizures

Seizures represent an excess of excitation over inhibition in the cerebral cortex. In most infectious diseases affecting the CNS, seizures reflect an area of cortical irritation. Brain abscesses, extra-axial suppurations (subdural empyema or epidural abscess), and focal encephalitides (e.g., herpes simplex encephalitis) typically produce seizures that arise in the adjacent cortex. More diffuse conditions such as bacterial meningitis may cause several areas of irritation in the cerebral cortex, presumably by producing microvascular disorders, any of which may give rise to seizures. Local mediators of inflammation may also be epileptogenic. One exception to this may be seizures associated with *Shigella* infection in children, which may directly lower the seizure threshold through a toxin not yet fully characterized.[6]

The major excitatory neurotransmitter in the cerebral cortex is glutamate, and the main inhibitory transmitter is γ-aminobutyric acid. The glutamate concentration in CSF is increased in patients with meningitis[7] and other CNS infections; excessive glutamate can produce seizures and is one of the major contributors to neuronal cell death by the process of *excitotoxicity.* Some penicillins and imipenem are potent γ-aminobutyric acid antagonists, explaining the propensity of these drugs to produce or exacerbate seizures, especially in patients with blood-brain barrier defects or renal failure.

Seizures induce a marked increase in cerebral blood flow and often cause further elevation of ICP.

Focal Neurologic Signs and Symptoms

A complete description of the focal findings that may be encountered in patients with CNS infection would constitute an entire textbook of neurologic diagnosis. The most important observation is that a rapid search for focal findings is important in the initial evaluation of the patient suspected of having acute bacterial meningitis, because the sequence of diagnostic studies and the decision to treat empirically differ if such findings are present. Localized infections, such as brain abscesses, are seldom confused with meningitis because the focal nature of the condition dominates the clinical picture. Subdural empyema, in contrast, may be more difficult to distinguish from meningitis, in part because the patient appears systemically ill more commonly than the patient with an intraparenchymal abscess, and in part because the inflammatory response renders a larger portion of the cortex dysfunctional.

There are some characteristic findings in infectious diseases that are important clues to diagnosis. For example, involvement of the temporal lobes of the brain is typical of herpes simplex encephalitis and of many brain abscesses of otic origin. The patient with such involvement may experience the intermittent behavioral alterations characteristic of complex partial seizures. There is nothing specific about seizures in these conditions that distinguish them from those due to other pathologic processes in the same brain region.

ANATOMIC RELATIONSHIPS OF THE BRAIN AND SPINAL CORD

Relationships of the Brain and Spinal Cord to the Meninges and Bony Structures

The brain and spinal cord are surrounded by three meningeal layers (Fig. 70–3). The pia mater is the direct investment of the CNS itself. The space between the pia and the arachnoid, the subarachnoid space, contains the CSF and the medium-caliber arteries that supply blood to the brain. During development, the arterial supply to the brain grows in from this space and carries the pia into the brain, where it forms the perivascular space of Virchow and Robin. This Virchow-Robin space is the site of accumulation of inflammatory cells in the brain and serves as a route of exit for these cells in a manner analogous to the lymphatic system in the rest of the body (the CNS lacks lymphatics).[8] Between the dura mater and the arachnoid lies the subdural space, through which course the veins bridging the distance from the brain surface to the large venous sinuses.

The subarachnoid space is unobstructed, allowing free movement of CSF (and blood, inflammatory material, or neoplastic cells) throughout the entire space. The subarachnoid space communicates with the ventricular system of the brain through the foramina of Luschka and Magendie. The bulk of the CSF is produced in the choroid plexus of the ventricles and exits through these foramina into the subarachnoid space surrounding the brain and spinal cord. The CSF is resorbed at the arachnoid granulations, which transport its contents into the sagittal sinus. Thus, meningitis frequently spreads into the ventricular system, producing ventriculitis, and may impede resorption of the CSF, resulting in communicating hydrocephalus.

Unless the subarachnoid space is compressed, or occluded by adhesions, the pressure in the lumbar subarachnoid space and that in the ventricular are equal (except for the hydrostatic differences imposed by the patient's position). Thus, with the patient in the lateral decubitus position, the pressure measured during a lumbar puncture should closely approximate ICP. However, with compression (as in the case of an epidural mass) or obstruction (e.g., within the ventricular system), a pressure gradient develops across the level of the lesion. In such a situation, lumbar puncture carries a risk of herniation that is not well quantitated but merits consideration. The greatest risk appears to be in the setting of complete occlusion of the subarachnoid space at the tentorial incisura, at the foramen magnum, or within the spinal canal. Some, but probably less, risk accompanies lesions that raise ICP but have not produced occlusion of the subarachnoid space.

In contrast, the spread of alien material through the subdural space is constrained by dural reflections at the falx cerebri, the falx cerebelli, the tentorium, and the diaphragma sellae. Subdural empyemas are usually limited to one of these spaces, such as that over one cerebral hemisphere. Because the spread of infectious material is unrestricted within the space, it tends to layer over the brain in a concave shape; and because it incites such a dramatic response in the underlying cortex, it is usually quite thin at the time of clinical presentation. Before magnetic resonance imaging, this thinness made the empyema difficult to recognize, but this is seldom a problem with modern imaging.

Between the skull and the dura mater is the epidural space. There are more limitations to the spread of alien material within the epidural space, as it adheres to the skull in the manner of a periosteum. Epidural abscesses, therefore, tend to assume a convex shape. Furthermore, the greater thickness and impermeability of the dura limits inflammation of the underlying brain, resulting in a clinical presentation more resembling a slowly growing mass lesion.

These same spaces exist around the spinal cord but are much smaller, with the result that extra-axial infections of the spinal cord tend to produce early and dramatic symptoms. The more rudimentary blood supply of the spinal cord means that the vasculitic complications of infection may have even more devastating consequences, as occurs with infarction of the distribution of the anterior spinal artery.

Relationship of the Brain and Meninges to Cranial Structures

The brain rests within divisions of the skull that constitute the anterior, middle, and posterior fossae. The poles of the frontal lobes are in contact with the frontal and ethmoid sinuses, from which infection may spread to surround or involve these lobes. The sella turcica forms the roof of the sphenoid sinus, which lies between the middle fossae containing the temporal lobes. Infection of the sphenoid sinus can spread into these adjacent structures.[9] Because of proximity to the optic nerves and the cavernous sinuses, sphenoid sinusitis can produce many ocular manifestations.[10] Infection may also spread from the middle ear or mastoid sinus to either the middle fossa or the posterior fossa.

Volume Relationships within the Skull (the Monro-Kellie Doctrine)

The intact skull can contain a fixed volume of brain, blood, and CSF. As fluids, these components are essentially incompressible. Introduction of alien tissue (such as tumor or abscess material), or an increase in the volume of the normal cranial contents, initially elicits a rise in ICP; this rise is proportional both to the volume of material added and to the rate of addition; slower rates allow more effective compensation. The early compensatory mechanisms involved include movement of CSF out of the skull through the foramen magnum and compression of veins, decreasing the venous blood volume. These initial changes produce little physiologic effect and correspond to the initial portion of the intracranial compliance curve where a given increase in volume produces only a small increase in pressure. Once these easily displaced components have exited the skull, however, further increases in volume produce large increases in pressure (poor compliance, corresponding to the rapidly rising portion of the compliance curve). As the ICP approaches MAP, brain perfusion suffers, and if the rise in ICP is unchecked, brain death eventually occurs.

In conditions characterized by diffuse brain swelling, as may occur in acute bacterial meningitis, or when communicating hydro-

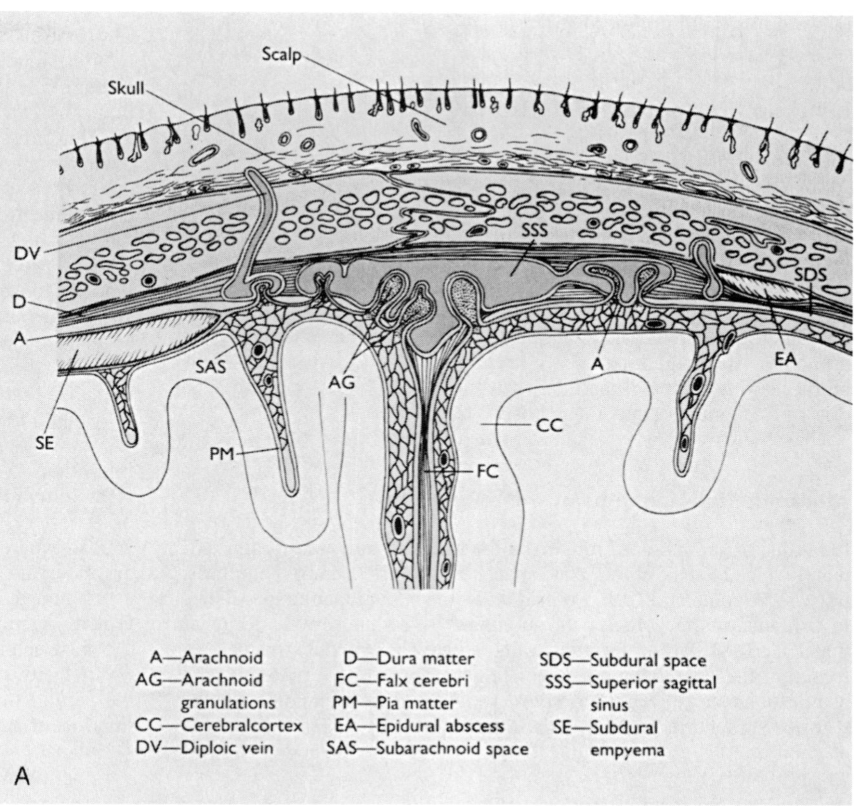

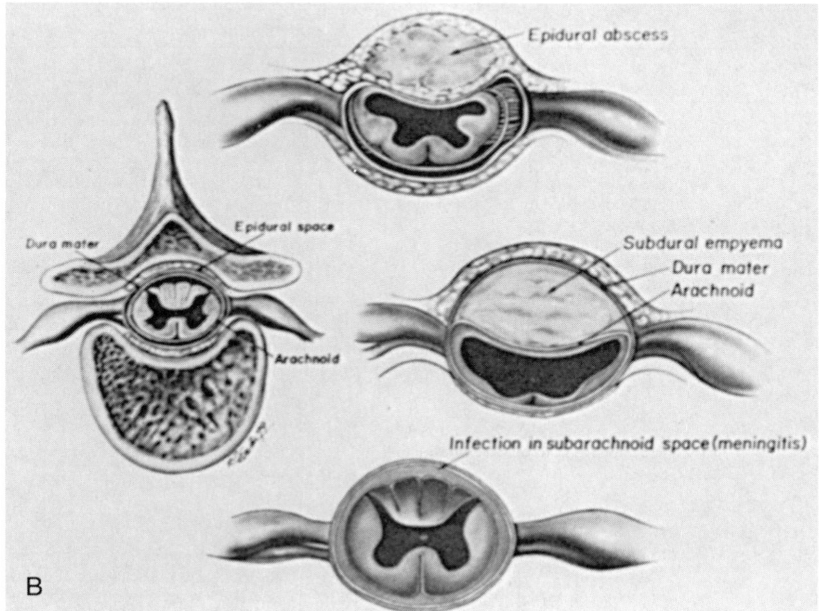

FIGURE 70–3. *A,* Anatomy of the intracranial dural spaces. Intracranial subdural empyema and epidural abscess are suppurative infections of the cerebral dural spaces and constitute neurologic emergencies. Intracranial subdural empyema may represent up to 23% of all intracranial infections, with intracranial epidural abscess being about half as common. A subdural empyema develops in the existing space between the dura and arachnoid, whereas cranial epidural abscess forms in the potential space between the dura and skull. The anatomy of the dural spaces helps explain the characteristic distribution of these infections. Intracranial epidural abscesses tend to be localized, limited by the dural attachment to the skull. Intracranial subdural empyemas are usually diffuse and occur most commonly over the cerebral hemispheres, where the subdural space is largest. Parafalcine, subtentorial, and multiple empyemas may be present in up to 20% of cases. (From Small M, Dale BA. Intracranial suppuration 1968–1982—a 15-year review. Clin Otolaryngol. 1984;9:315–321.) *B,* The spinal meninges and epidural space: normal anatomic relationships and alterations in epidural abscess, subdural empyema, and meningitis.

cephalus develops, there is minimal risk of brain displacement (although there eventually will be some downward displacement of the cerebellar tonsils). However, if a lateralized cerebral mass or a posterior fossa mass is present, there is the additional risk of a pressure gradient developing between the hemispheres or across the tentorium, resulting in herniation.

Injury to Cranial Nerves during Infections

The cranial nerves traverse the meninges after exiting the brain. They may be affected by the inflammatory response to infections involving the meningeal spaces they must traverse, by displacement or compression due to herniation of brain structures, or, at least in the case of the abducens nerve, potentially by the effect of increased ICP (Table 70–1). Cranial nerve palsies are particularly common in the chronic basilar meningitides (e.g., tuberculous meningitis). The oculomotor, trochlear, and abducens nerves, and at least the first branch of the trigeminal nerve, run through the cavernous sinus before exiting the skull, and their functions are typically impaired in cases of cavernous sinus thrombosis.

Anatomic Relationships of the Spinal Cord

In adults, the spinal cord runs from the foramen magnum to approximately the level of L1–2 disk space. Below the conus medullaris, only nerve roots and CSF are present in the subarachnoid space. The investment of the cord by the meninges is essentially the same as that described earlier for the brain. However, the dura mater surrounding the cord does not adhere to the vertebral periosteum, and in consequence the epidural space provides a freer conduit for the spread of infection (see Fig. 70–3*B*).

ROLE OF THE INTRACRANIAL CIRCULATION IN CENTRAL NERVOUS SYSTEM INFECTIONS

Vascular Anatomy

Arteries

The arterial supply of the brain derives from the internal carotid arteries and the vertebral arteries (Fig. 70–4). The carotid passes through the cavernous sinuses before giving off its small initial branches (which include the ophthalmic artery, the posterior communicating artery, and the anterior choroidal artery). It then gives rise to the anterior cerebral artery and terminates in the middle cerebral artery. The anterior cerebral arteries are connected by the anterior communicating artery. The vertebral arteries join to form the basilar artery, which gives off several branches before terminating in the posterior cerebral arteries. The posterior communicating arteries join with the posterior cerebral arteries to complete the circle of Willis. All these medium-sized arteries run in the subarachnoid space and branch several times after entering the brain substance itself. In addition, the components of the circle of Willis give off perforating branches that enter the brain directly.

Emboli to the brain (e.g., as a consequence of infective endocarditis) may lodge either in major or in branch arteries, producing infarction. A brain abscess may also occur as a consequence of septic embolism. Infectious material may lodge in the vasa vasorum of an artery, typically one that has already entered the brain substance, where it can produce a mycotic aneurysm. Rupture of such an aneurysm typically produces an intracerebral hemorrhage, often at an unusual location for such a hemorrhage; in comparison, the typical saccular aneurysm arises at a branch point of an artery within the subarachnoid space, resulting in a subarachnoid hemorrhage.

In contrast to infarction due to embolism, infarcts occurring in the setting of hypotension (e.g., as a consequence of septic shock) may occur in the "watershed" areas of blood supply at the borders

TABLE 70–1 Cranial Nerve Involvement in Central Nervous System Infections

Nerve or Nerves	Anatomic Features	Significance	Consequence
I	Traverses dura and ethmoid bone; surrounded by cuff of arachnoid; terminates in free nerve endings with nasal mucosa and nasopharynx	Only cranial nerve in direct contact with external environment	Potential route for viral entry
II	Embryologically part of brain; contained within subarachnoid space up to back of globe in over 90% of patients	Increased ICP can cause papilledema (except in rare patient in whom dural investment terminated before globe)	Papilledema not accompanied by remarkable change in visual acuity until late in course
	Myelin of optic nerve is formed by oligodendroglia rather than Schwann cells	May be target of immune response in CNS postinfectious syndromes (such as acute disseminated encephalomyelitis) but not peripheral nerve myelin disorders (such as Guillain-Barré syndrome)	Demyelinating lesions of optic nerve tend to produce early visual loss
III	Runs from anterior surface of midbrain through cavernous sinus	In most cases of elevated ICP, early CN III palsy represents stretching of nerve due to lateral displacement of midbrain; CN III compression by uncal herniation occurs later (see text)	Paresis of parasympathetic function causes pupillary dilation; loss of extraocular movement control leaves CN IV and VI unopposed, deviating eye laterally and slightly down
III, IV, V_1, VI	Travel together in wall of cavernous sinus	Commonly affected in cavernous sinus thrombosis	Complete external ophthalmoplegia, pupillary dilation and loss of light reflex; loss of sensation in distribution of ophthalmic division of trigeminal nerve (may involve maxillary division as well)
V, VI	Travel in close proximity to tip of petrous bone	May be damaged by osteomyelitis of petrous tip, usually as consequence of chronic otitis media	Abducens palsy and ipsilateral pain or sensory loss
VII	Sensory nerve cell bodies in geniculate ganglion	In facial nerve zoster (Ramsay-Hunt syndrome), facial palsy accompanied by vesicles in external auditory canal and skin near the meatus	Usually produces brain stem encephalitis of varied severity, often with auditory nerve involvement as well
IX, X, XI	Exit from skull through jugular foramen	May be affected by jugular vein thrombosis or osteomyelitis of skull base	Ipsilateral weakness of palate, trapezius, and sternocleidomastoid muscles
III–XII	Myelin sheaths of these nerves composed of peripheral nerve myelin distal to arachnoid membrane	May be affected in peripheral neuropathies (e.g., Guillain-Barré syndrome, Lyme disease)	Most commonly affects facial nerve

Abbreviations: CN, Cranial nerve; CNS, central nervous system; ICP, intracranial pressure.

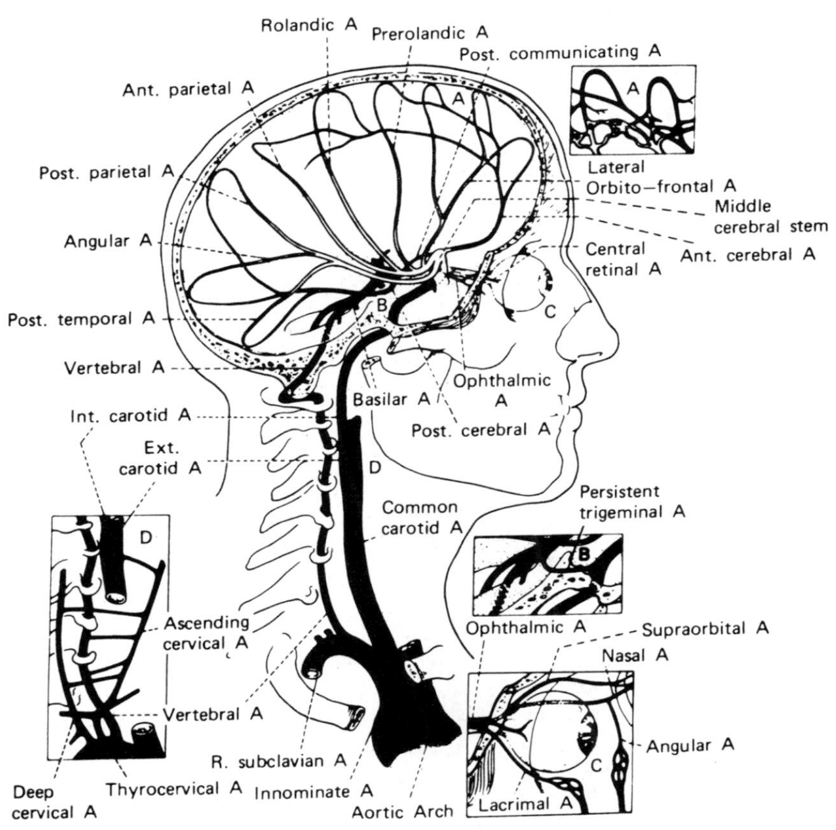

FIGURE 70–4. Arterial supply of central nervous system. (From Adams RD, Victor M. Principles of Neurology. 2nd ed. New York: McGraw-Hill; 1981:532.)

between vessels (e.g., at the border between the anterior and the middle cerebral arteries). The white matter also represents a watershed region, receiving blood from both the superficial and the deep arterial circulations. This presumably accounts for the tendency of hematogenously derived abscesses to form at the gray-white junction or in the white matter.[11]

Veins

Two groups of veins drain the brain: the superficial veins receive blood from the external portions of the cerebrum and brain stem, and the deep veins drain the white matter, basal ganglia, and thalamus. The blood then enters the venous sinuses, which are contained within the dura. The superficial veins above the sylvian fissure drain into the superior sagittal sinus, and those below the fissure drain into basilar venous sinuses. The bulk of venous blood leaves the skull via the internal jugular veins. Although there is communication between the superficial and deep venous systems at the torcula, the vast majority of blood from the superior sagittal sinus drains via the right internal jugular vein, whereas the deep veins drain predominantly through the left internal jugular vein. There are extensive interconnections between the superficial and deep venous systems, as well as anastomoses among the sinuses themselves. The superficial veins and the venous sinuses also connect with extracranial veins through emissary veins that traverse the meninges and the skull. There are no valves in the cerebral veins or sinuses, permitting reversal of flow if the jugular venous pressure begins to exceed the ICP (Fig. 70–5).

Thrombosis of cerebral veins may be asymptomatic or minimally symptomatic if it occurs in a region with good collateral drainage, or may produce devastating infarction. Such infarction is typically hemorrhagic and does not follow the expected distribution of arterial lesions. Thrombosis of the posterior portion of the superior sagittal sinus can induce cortical venous thrombosis of both hemispheres.

The venous sinuses resorb CSF through the arachnoid granulations, the majority of which drain into the anterior third of the superior sagittal sinus. Therefore, thrombosis of this sinus may produce communicating hydrocephalus. Occlusion of subsequent venous drainage via the lateral sinuses may have a similar effect.

Capillaries

Most of the capillaries of the brain and spinal cord are invested by astrocytic processes, which, in concert with the tight junctions of the endothelial cells, constitute the blood-brain barrier. There are actually separate barriers between the circulation and the parenchyma, the circulation and the CSF, and the CSF and the parenchyma. This distinction has some practical consequences, as seen in the tendency of clindamycin to accumulate in the brain but not in the CSF. The relative impermeability of the barrier to immunoglobulin, complement, and antimicrobial agents plays an important role in the pathogenesis of CNS infections and is a major consideration in the choice of therapy for them.

There are a few areas in which this barrier is different or lacking: the pituitary, the choroid plexus, the area postrema, and the circumventricular organs. These regions share the need to sample substances from the systemic circulation.

Vascular Supply of the Spinal Cord

The major arterial supply of the spinal cord comes from the anterior spinal artery. This artery arises from branches of the vertebral artery and receives contributions from radicular and aortic branches. In most patients, the anterior spinal artery receives a major aortic branch in the lower thoracic region known as the artery of Adamkiewicz. The posterior columns and horns of the cord receive arterial blood from the small, paired posterior spinal arteries. The venous drainage of the spinal cord follows a similar distribution to that of the arteries.

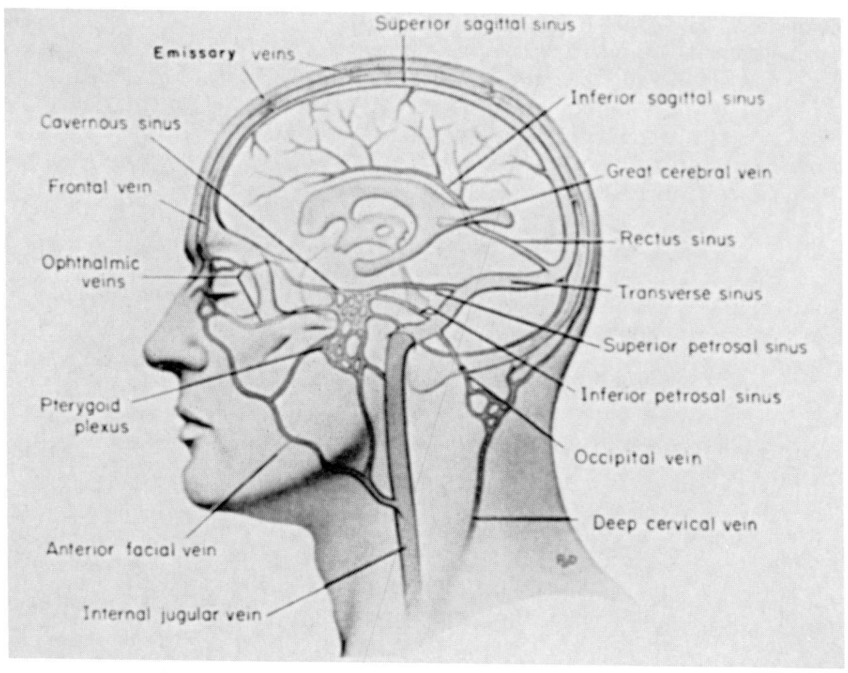

FIGURE 70–5. Venous supply of the central nervous system. (From Truax RC, Carpenter MB. Neuroanatomy. 6th ed. Baltimore: Williams & Wilkins; 1969:80.)

Role of Central Nervous System Vessels in Infection

The most common routes of infection of the brain are hematogenous, either to the choroid plexus (as in many cases of meningitis) or directly to the brain parenchyma (as in abscess consequent to septic embolism). Infection of the vessels themselves, or their occlusion by septic emboli, may also result in vascular compromise or hemorrhage. In some forms of meningitis, inflammation of the vessel wall leads to thrombosis. Multiplication of organisms within the arterial wall may produce occlusion (e.g., in Rocky Mountain spotted fever[12]). Vasculitis also plays a role in the syndrome of ipsilateral carotid arterial distribution infarction seen after ophthalmic division herpes zoster.

The veins of the CNS may also thrombose in response to inflammation and may be the source of sterile or septic emboli to other parts of the CNS or to the lungs.

Capillary injury plays a central role in the pathogenesis, diagnosis, and therapy of many CNS infections. Damage from septic emboli may allow organisms to enter areas of brain that have been rendered ischemic, providing the appropriate circumstances for abscess development. Cytokine release, triggered as a consequence of microbial products acting on astrocytes and macrophage-derived cells (including microglia),[13] can further disrupt the integrity of the blood-brain barrier.[14] Nitric oxide production by inflammatory cells can further disrupt the blood-brain barrier.[15]

Vasogenic cerebral edema, produced by the transudation of fluid across the damaged capillaries, can raise ICP and produce tissue shifts with secondary vascular compromise. This edema results in low-attenuation areas on computed tomographic scanning, and in areas of increased T_2 signal intensity on magnetic resonance images. Loss of the barrier function also permits radiographic and paramagnetic contrast agents to accumulate in the damaged areas of the brain and spinal cord.

The loss of barrier function allows antibiotics of limited lipophilicity, which are normally excluded from the CNS or kept at low concentrations, to penetrate the brain and the CSF. As the brain recovers, there may be a corresponding decrease in penetration.

The vessels supplying the spinal cord are much less frequently involved in infection than those supplying the brain. This probably reflects the much higher blood flow to the brain than the spinal cord, and the caliber of the vessels, rather than any intrinsic resistance to infection of the spinal vessels. On occasion, septic emboli may lodge in the anterior spinal artery, producing infarction. These vessels may also be involved in vasculitic disorders.

ROLE OF THE CEREBROSPINAL FLUID CIRCULATION IN CENTRAL NERVOUS SYSTEM INFECTIONS

About 85% of the CSF is produced by the choroid plexi, located within the ventricular system. The remainder arises from diffusion from the brain and spinal cord across the pia into the subarachnoid space. Under normal circumstances, the ventricular system and the cranial subarachnoid space contain about 70 ml of fluid, and the spinal subarachnoid space an equal amount. The CSF normally turns over three or more times per day (Fig. 70–6).

Chemical and cellular changes in the CSF provide important information about infection in the subarachnoid space. However, the lumbar CSF may not yield microbiologically useful information in circumstances in which the flow of fluid is obstructed, as may occur with chronic basilar meningitides (e.g., that due to *Mycobacterium tuberculosis*). Culturing large volumes of CSF from more than one lumbar puncture may be useful in this setting, as may cultures of fluid obtained from cisternal or lateral cervical taps. Parameningeal infections and unruptured brain abscesses may alter the composition of the CSF, often inducing a mild lymphocytosis and elevating the protein content without affecting the glucose concentration. If the flow of CSF is completely obstructed, as may occur with a lesion (e.g., an epidural abscess) that obliterates the subarachnoid space, the protein content in the lumbar fluid may reach 1 g/dl or greater (Froin's syndrome). However, CSF seldom provides useful information in patients with parameningeal infection or brain abscess, and in these conditions a lumbar puncture is usually inadvisable because of the risk of herniation.

Patients who have undergone ventriculoperitoneal or ventriculoatrial shunting may have two separate CSF spaces; the lumbar fluid may not reflect the ventricular fluid, and on occasion separate analyses of fluid from each space may be required. Many shunts are equipped with ports that allow sampling of ventricular CSF without disrupting the integrity of the shunt.

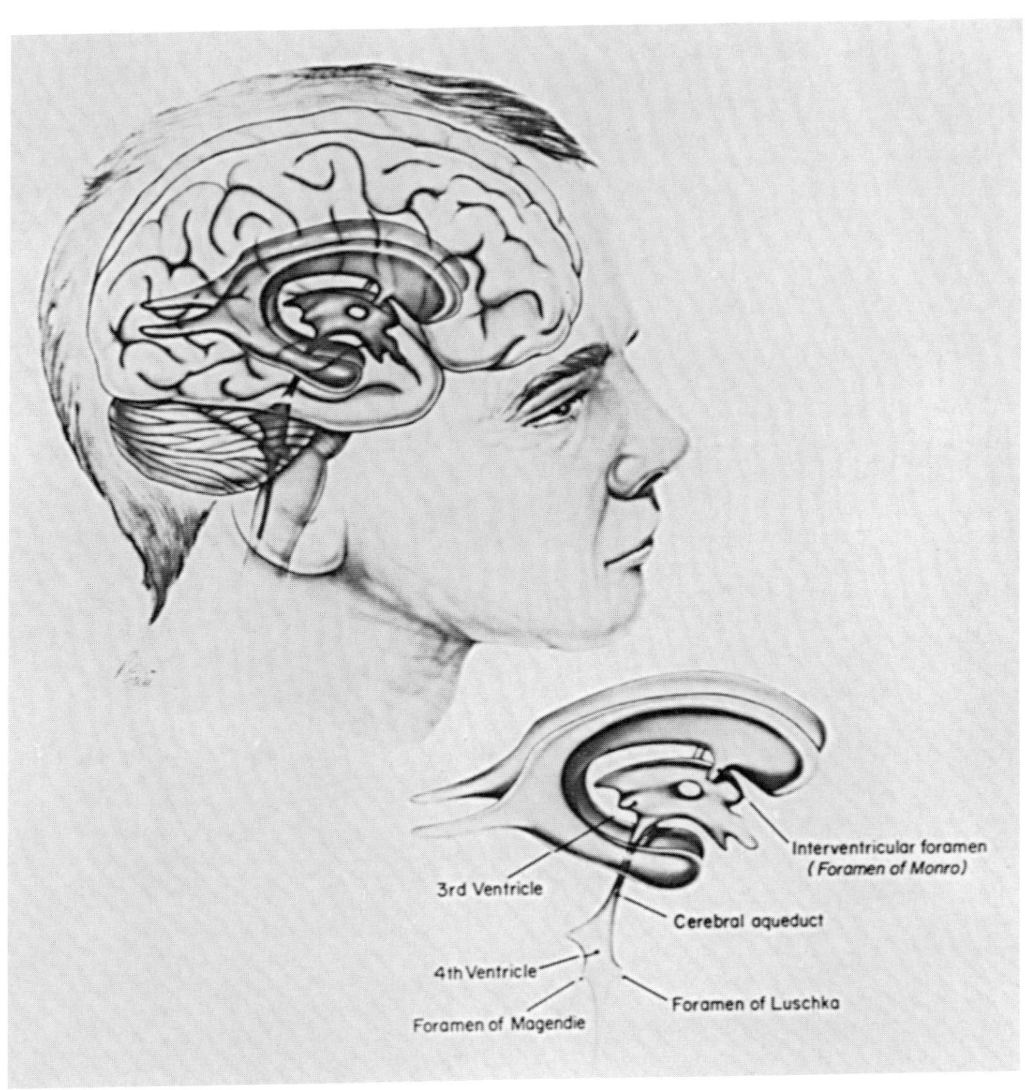

FIGURE 70–6. The cerebral ventricles. The ventricular system is narrowest and hence most easily obstructed at the foramen of Monro, the cerebral aqueduct (aqueduct of Sylvius), and the foramina of Luschka and Magendie.

In rare cases, patients may require the direct administration of antimicrobial agents into the CSF. Although this has traditionally been accomplished by repeated lumbar puncture, it is difficult to obtain useful concentrations of drugs in the ventricular system by this route. Placing an Ommaya reservoir allows direct access to the ventricular system for both fluid analysis and drug delivery.

ROUTES OF ENTRY INTO THE CENTRAL NERVOUS SYSTEM BY INFECTIOUS AGENTS

Most infectious agents reach the CNS via either (1) hematogenous dissemination from an extraneural site or (2) retrograde propagation of infected thrombi within emissary veins. Bacteria and viruses may enter through blood vessels of the choroid plexus, the meninges, or the parenchyma. Tuberculous meningitis typically develops from subependymal or submeningeal granulomata that seed the CSF. Cranial epidural abscess or subdural empyema may originate from infected veins or from spread of infection through the skull, usually from infected paranasal sinuses. In contrast, spinal epidural or subdural infections are commonly hematogenous in origin.[16] The organisms of intraparenchymal abscesses may arrive via either arteries or veins.

Most viruses infecting the CNS arrive via hematogenous spread. Prominent exceptions to this rule include herpesviruses (herpes simplex and zoster) and rabies virus.[17] The herpesviruses, after initial infection, produce latent infection of sensory ganglia. Some cases of herpes simplex encephalitis may result from reactivation of virus latent in the trigeminal ganglia; others appear to result from de novo infection, perhaps via the olfactory nerve. Rabies virus enters the CNS via retrograde movement within motor neurons.

RESPONSE OF THE CENTRAL NERVOUS SYSTEM TO INFECTION

Many viruses produce widespread infection of the brain and meninges; the term *aseptic meningitis* is usually a misnomer because of the associated brain involvement. Some viruses infect specific cell types. For example, poliomyelitis virus infects motor neurons. Progressive multifocal leukoencephalopathy, produced by a papovavirus, infects oligodendrocytes. Herpes simplex virus preferentially infects the temporal lobes, resulting in characteristic clinical findings.

Organisms producing acute infection, such as most forms of bacterial meningitis, elicit a polymorphonuclear neutrophil response. Subacute or chronic infections, such as those caused by *M. tuberculosis,* fungi, or viruses, often produce an initial polymorphonuclear neutrophil response, which is quickly followed by a lymphocytic

TABLE 70–2 Acute Medical Therapies for Elevated Intracranial Pressure

Therapy	Proposed Mechanisms of Action	Dosage or Therapeutic End Point	Comments
Hyperventilation	Cerebral vasoconstriction	Increase minute ventilation to reach initial Pa_{CO_2} of about 30 mmHg; further increases in minute ventilation should be in small increments	Important variable is change in CNS extracellular pH, which controls arterial caliber Lowers ICP very rapidly (seconds to minutes) Because mechanism of ICP reduction is vasoconstriction, may produce or worsen cerebral ischemia Bicarbonate clearance by choroid plexus brings CNS extracellular pH back toward normal over 6–12 h; ICP follows pH, not Pa_{CO_2} Further decreases in Pa_{CO_2} again decrease cerebral blood flow and lower ICP Increasing minute ventilation may raise intrathoracic pressure, impeding jugular venous drainage and paradoxically increasing ICP
Steroids	Decreasing fluid and electrolyte leakage across damaged or abnormal capillaries	Dexamethasone, 10 mg initially, then 4 mg q4–6h When required for chronic use, effect tends to increase with dose	Effective only in circumstances of vasogenic edema due to abnormal blood-brain barrier function (e.g., abscess, tumor) Ineffective in other forms of vasogenic edema (e.g., surrounding intracerebral hemorrhage) or cytotoxic edema (e.g., due to stroke)
Mannitol	Osmotic dehydration Improved microvascular flow due to increased RBC deformability Free-radical scavenging	0.25–1.0 gm/kg q4h	Actually mechanism(s) of action unknown Avoid systemic volume depletion due to osmotic diuretic effect, which may produce hypotension (resulting in cerebral ischemia) Excessive systemic hyperosmolality (e.g., exceeding 320 mOsm/L) may cause acute renal failure Potential for rebound brain swelling if systemic osmolality falls abruptly necessitates tapering over days after prolonged administration Hypertonic saline may be useful alternative
Barbiturates or propofol	Decreasing cerebral metabolism causes decrease in demand for cerebral blood flow without inducing ischemia	Pentobarbital, 5–12 mg/kg intravenous loading dose (infuse slowly), with infusion of 1–5 mg/kg/h titrated to ICP and CPP (not to exceed 50 mg/min) *or* Propofol, 1–3 mg/kg loading dose, with infusion of 20–100 μg/kg/min titrated to ICP and CPP	Initial hypotensive effect due to venodilation; can be treated with volume administration Subsequent myocardial depression at higher doses requiring inotropic agents (e.g., dopamine or dobutamine) and arterial dilatation requiring vasoconstrictors (e.g., norepinephrine or phenylephrine) and central venous or pulmonary capillary wedge pressure monitoring Immunosuppressive effects

Abbreviations: CNS, Central nervous system; CPP, cerebral perfusion pressure; ICP, intracranial pressure; RBC, red blood cell.

reaction. The same sequence is often found in brain abscesses. Plasma cells may be found within the inflammatory infiltrates, and there is local production of immunoglobulin. The inflammatory response within the brain and spinal cord is usually less intense than that seen in the peripheral tissues. In addition, microglial cells, which are probably derived from the monocyte-macrophage system, and astrocytes tend to proliferate within the area of infection. When abscesses develop within the brain, they are less likely to be surrounded by a fibrotic capsule but are instead surrounded by an area of gliosis. When the brain has suffered a previous ischemic injury, the inflammatory response may be minimal, and reactive gliosis may not occur.

In infections due to some viruses or *Mycoplasma,* or following immunization, the host may develop an immune response not only against the causative agent but also against myelin basic protein. Reaction against peripheral myelin produces segmental demyelination, and at times its total loss within nerve roots and peripheral nerves, causing the Guillain-Barré syndrome. Reaction against CNS myelin produces the condition known as acute disseminated encephalomyelitis.

Role of Edema and Brain Herniation in Central Nervous System Infections

The inflammatory response to infection produces not only local injury to the nervous system parenchyma, but also loss of capillary integrity with transudation of intravascular fluid into the brain and spinal cord.[18] The edema produced by this process is an invariable and potentially lethal consequence of CNS infection (see Chapter 71). Several factors contribute to the development of cerebral edema. Bacterial products, such as endotoxins produced by gram-negative organisms and the teichoic acid produced by *Staphylococcus aureus,* cause the release of tumor necrosis factor and many other cytokines and chemokines.[19–21] These inflammatory mediators produce a loss of capillary integrity, resulting in vasogenic cerebral edema. The effects of tumor necrosis factor are synergistic with the inflammatory effects of bacterial cell wall constituents.[22] The enhanced activity and CNS penetration of the third-generation cephalosporins can paradoxically worsen this problem by rapidly lysing large numbers of bacteria, increasing the signals for the generation of inflammatory mediators.

The development of vasogenic edema can be slowed or reversed by corticosteroids; these agents are very useful for ICP reduction in patients with brain abscesses. The controversial role of corticosteroids in treatment of bacterial meningitis is discussed in Chapter 71.

The primary therapy for ICP disorders associated with CNS infection is treatment of the underlying condition. This includes surgical extirpation of epidural abscess or subdural empyema. The timing of surgery for parenchymal brain abscess is discussed in Chapter 74. Critical elevations of ICP constitute an indication for craniotomy and aspiration or resection of an abscess regardless of its maturity. Posterior fossa mass lesions are especially dangerous, as they may rapidly compress the brain stem and may constitute a surgical emergency. Hydrocephalus can complicate the management of intracranial infections and require CSF drainage or shunting.

Medical therapies for ICP elevation (Table 70–2) may be lifesaving acutely but are only adjuncts to definitive treatment.[23] In the absence of a ventriculostomy as a site for pressure measurement, placement of an intraparenchymal ICP monitor should be considered in order to guide therapy. Patients requiring these therapies should usually be managed in critical care units.

REFERENCES

1. Bleck TP. Levels of consciousness and attention. In: Goetz CG, Pappert EJ, eds. Textbook of Clinical Neurology. Philadelphia: WB Saunders; 1998:2–29.
2. Plum F, Posner JB. The Diagnosis of Stupor and Coma. Philadelphia: FA Davis; 1980.
3. Ropper AH. A preliminary MRI study of the geometry of brain displacement and level of consciousness with acute intracranial masses. Neurology. 1989;39:622–627.
4. Ropper AH. Transtentorial herniation. In: Young GB, Ropper AH, Bolton CF, eds. Coma and Impaired Consciousness: A Clinical Perspective. New York: McGraw-Hill; 1998:119–130.
5. Brock DG, Bleck TP. Coma: A practical approach. In: Bone RC, Dantzker D, George R, et al, eds. Pulmonary and Critical Care Medicine, v. 3. Chicago: Mosby–Year Book; 1995:1–11.
6. Yuhas Y, Weizman A, Dinari G, Ashkenazi S. An animal model for the study of neurotoxicity of bacterial products and application of the model to demonstrate that Shiga toxin and lipopolysaccharide cooperate in inducing neurologic disorders. J Infect Dis. 1995;171:1244–1249.
7. Tucci S, Pinto C, Goyo J, et al. Measurement of glutamine and glutamate by capillary electrophoresis and laser induced fluorescence detection in cerebrospinal fluid of meningitis in sick children. Clin Biochem. 1998;31:143–150.
8. Esiri MM, Gay D. Immunological and neuropathological significance of the Virchow-Robin space. J Neurol Sci. 1990;100:3–8.
9. Brockbank MJ, Brookes GB. The sphenoiditis spectrum. Clin Otolaryngol. 1991;16:15–20.
10. Dale BA, Mackenzie IJ. The complications of sphenoid sinusitis. J Laryngol. 1983;97:661–670.
11. Wispelwey B, Dacey RG Jr, Scheld WM. Brain abscess. In: Scheld WM, Whitley RJ, Durack DT, eds. Infections of the Central Nervous System. 2nd ed. New York: Raven; 1997:463–493.
12. Miller JQ, Price TR. The nervous system in Rocky Mountain spotted fever. Neurology. 1972;22:561–566.
13. Gruol DL, Nelson TE. Physiological and pathological roles of interleukin-6 in the central nervous system. Mol Neurobiol. 1997;15:307–339.
14. Schwartz D, Engelhard D, Gallily R, et al. Glial cell production of inflammatory mediators induced by *Streptococcus pneumoniae:* Inhibition by pentoxifylline, low-molecular-weight heparin and dexamethasone. J Neurol Sci. 1998;155:13–22.
15. Buster BL, Weintrob AC, Townsend GC, Scheld WM. Potential role of nitric oxide in the pathophysiology of experimental bacterial meningitis in rats. Infect Immun. 1995;63:3835–3839.
16. Brock DG, Bleck TP. Extra-axial suppurations of the central nervous system. Semin Neurol. 1992;12:263–272.
17. Bleck TP, Rupprecht CE. Rabies. In: Richman DD, Whitley RJ, Hayden FG, eds. Clinical Virology. New York: Churchill Livingstone; 1997:879–897.
18. Wilson SL, Drevets DA. *Listeria monocytogenes* infection and activation of human brain microvascular endothelial cells. J Infect Dis. 1998;178:1658–1666.
19. Mastroianni CM, Lancella L, Mengoni F, et al. Chemokine profiles in the cerebrospinal fluid (CSF) during the course of pyogenic and tuberculous meningitis. Clin Exp Immunol. 1998;114:210–214.
20. Yokoyama T, Oda M, Seino Y. Interleukin-1 beta and interleukin-1 receptor antagonist levels in cerebrospinal fluid of aseptic meningitis patients. Pediatr Allergy Immunol. 1998;9:91–96.
21. Quagliarello VJ, Wispelwey B, Long WJ Jr, Scheld WM. Recombinant human interleukin-1 induces meningitis and blood-brain barrier injury in the rat. Characterization and comparison with tumor necrosis factor. J Clin Invest. 1991;87:1360–1366.
22. Angstwurm K, Freyer D, Dirnagl U, et al. Tumour necrosis factor alpha induces only minor inflammatory changes in the central nervous system, but augments experimental meningitis. Neuroscience. 1998;86:627–634.
23. Ford G, Bleck TP. Increased intracranial pressure. In: Parrillo JE, ed. Current Therapy in Critical Care Medicine. 3rd ed. Toronto: BC Decker; 1997:323–327.

Chapter 71

Acute Meningitis

ALLAN R. TUNKEL
W. MICHAEL SCHELD

Meningitis or inflammation of the meninges is identified by an abnormal number of white blood cells in cerebrospinal fluid (CSF). Acute meningitis is clinically defined as a syndrome characterized by the onset of meningeal symptoms over the course of hours up to several days. Headache is a prominent early symptom, often followed later by confusion or coma. Examination reveals few focal findings early during infection, although signs of meningeal irritation (e.g., Kernig's or Brudzinski's sign) are common. The acute meningitis syndrome blurs imperceptibly into the syndromes of chronic meningitis (see Chapter 72) and encephalitis (see Chapter 73). Chronic meningitis has an onset measured in weeks to months (but is generally defined when symptoms, signs, and the CSF remain abnormal for at least 4 weeks), whereas encephalitis is distinguished by the presence of decreased mentation (i.e., confusion or stupor) early in the course of disease and minimal meningeal signs. The distinction between these syndromes is clinically useful in guiding management but is obviously artificial in terms of etiology and pathology. For example, tuberculous meningitis may have a subacute or chronic onset.

The acute meningitis syndrome may be caused by a wide variety of infectious agents and may also be a manifestation of noninfectious diseases (Table 71–1). Diseases in which meningeal symptoms occur but are not predominant (e.g., measles) are excluded. Many of the causes of chronic meningitis, which can be manifested acutely, have been omitted but are listed in Chapter 72. Here, we review the common infectious causes of acute meningitis with particular emphasis on epidemiology and etiology, pathogenesis and pathophysiology, clinical features, diagnosis, treatment, and prevention.

EPIDEMIOLOGY AND ETIOLOGY

Viral Meningitis

Viruses are the major cause of the *acute aseptic meningitis syndrome*, a term used to define any meningitis (infectious or noninfectious), particularly one with a lymphocytic pleocytosis, for which a cause is not apparent after initial evaluation and routine stains and cultures of CSF.[1, 2] Over the years 1982 to 1988, from 8300 to 12,700 cases of aseptic meningitis were reported to the Centers for Disease Control and Prevention (CDC)[1] although these figures probably underestimate the importance of this syndrome because not all cases are reported and cases with a nonviral etiology are not reported as aseptic meningitis. In another large retrospective review of all cases of central nervous system (CNS) infection in Olmstead County, Minnesota, from 1950 to 1981,[3] 283 cases met the criteria for definite aseptic meningitis, for an adjusted incidence rate of 10.9/100,000 person-years. A specific viral etiology was only established in 33 (11%) of the cases, probably because of limitations of microbiologic techniques in the past and the low frequency of microbiologic searches for the virus in the patient population. More recent studies identify a specific viral pathogen in as many as 55 to 70% of cases when consistent diagnostic microbiologic principles are applied.[2, 4] Common viral etiologic agents that cause the acute aseptic meningitis syndrome are discussed in the following sections.

Enteroviruses. Enteroviruses, currently the leading recognizable cause of aseptic meningitis syndrome, account for 85 to 95% of all cases in which a pathogen is identified.[1, 2] Enteroviruses are worldwide in distribution. In temperate climates they appear with a marked summer/fall seasonality, although in tropical and subtropical areas a high year-round incidence is observed. Periods of warm weather and wearing sparse clothing may facilitate the fecal-oral spread of these organisms; enteroviruses may also be recovered from houseflies, wastewater, and sewage.[2] In the United States, the 15 most commonly occurring enteroviral serotypes account for more than 80% of isolates.[5] The predominant enteroviruses isolated from patients with meningitis during the years 1970 to 1983 were (in decreasing order)

TABLE 71–1 Differential Diagnosis of Acute Meningitis

Major infectious etiologies	Protozoa and helminths
Viruses	*Naegleria fowleri*
Nonpolio enteroviruses*	*Angiostrongylus cantonensis*
Mumps virus	*Strongyloides stercoralis* (hyperinfection syndrome)
Arboviruses†	Other infectious syndromes
Herpesviruses‡	Parameningeal foci of infection§
Lymphocytic choriomeningitis virus	Infective endocarditis
Human immunodeficiency virus	Viral postinfectious syndromes
Adenovirus	Postvaccination**
Parainfluenza virus types 2 and 3	Noninfectious causes and diseases of unknown etiology
Influenza virus	Intracranial tumors and cysts
Measles virus	Craniopharyngioma
Rickettsiae	Dermoid/epidermoid cyst
Rickettsia rickettsii (Rocky Mountain spotted fever)	Teratoma
Rickettsia conorii	Medications
Rickettsia prowazekii (epidemic or louse-borne typhus)	Antimicrobial agents††
Rickettsia typhi (endemic or murine typhus)	Nonsteroidal anti-inflammatory agents‡‡
Rickettsia tsutsugamushi (scrub typhus)	Muromonab-CD3 (OKT3)
Ehrlichia spp.	Azathioprine
Bacteria	Cytosine arabinoside (high dose)
Haemophilus influenzae	Carbamazepine§§
Neisseria meningitidis	Immune globulin
Streptococcus pneumoniae	Ranitidine
Listeria monocytogenes	Phenazopyridine
Streptococcus agalactiae	Systemic illnesses
Propionibacterium acnes	Systemic lupus erythematosus
Staphylococcus epidermidis	Vogt-Koyanagi-Harada syndrome
Enterococcus faecalis	Procedure related
Escherichia coli	Postneurosurgery
Klebsiella pneumoniae	Spinal anesthesia
Pseudomonas aeruginosa	Intrathecal injections***
Salmonella spp.	Chymopapain injection
Nocardia spp.	Miscellaneous
Mycobacterium tuberculosis	Seizures
Spirochetes	Migraine or migraine-like syndromes
Treponema pallidum (syphilis)	Mollaret's meningitis
Borrelia burgdorferi (Lyme disease)	
Leptospira spp.	

*Primarily echoviruses and coxsackieviruses.
†In the United States, the major etiologic agents are the mosquito-borne California, St. Louis, Eastern equine, Western equine, and Venezuelan equine encephalitis viruses and tick-borne Colorado tick fever.
‡Primarily herpes simplex virus type 2, but also herpes simplex virus type 1, varicella-zoster virus, cytomegalovirus, Epstein-Barr virus, and human herpesvirus 6.
§Brain abscess, sinusitis, otitis, mastoiditis, subdural abscess, epidural abscess, venous sinus thrombophlebitis, pituitary abscess, cranial osteomyelitis.
**Mumps, measles, polio, pertussis, rabies, vaccinia.
††Trimethoprim, sulfamethoxazole, trimethoprim-sulfamethoxazole, ciprofloxacin, penicillin, isoniazid.
‡‡Ibuprofen, sulindac, naproxen, tolmetin.
§§In patients with connective tissue diseases.
***Air, isotopes, antimicrobial agents, antineoplastic agents, steroids, radiographic contrast media.

echovirus 11; echovirus 9; coxsackievirus B5; echoviruses 30, 4, and 6; coxsackieviruses B2, B4, B3, and A9; echoviruses 3, 7, 5, and 21; and coxsackievirus B1.[5] In one epidemiologic investigation in New York state,[6] 20% of isolates were echovirus 30. In addition, the newly numbered enteroviruses 70 and 71 have been reported to commonly cause CNS disease.[2]

Infants and young children are the primary victims of enteroviral meningitis because they are the most susceptible host population (i.e., absence of previous exposure and immunity) within the community. In one large cohort study from Finland,[7] children younger than 1 year had an annual incidence of viral meningitis of 219 cases per 100,000 population versus an incidence of 19 cases per 100,000 population in children between the ages of 1 and 4 years; the incidence dropped even further with advancing age. The vast majority of these viral pathogens were enteroviruses. More than one episode of enteroviral meningitis may develop, although the same enteroviral serotype has not been implicated more than once in any immunocompetent patient.[2] Immunodeficiency and possibly physical exercise also predispose to enteroviral meningitis.

Arboviruses. The most common arthropod-transmitted cause of aseptic meningitis is St. Louis encephalitis virus, a flavivirus.[8] Aseptic meningitis accounts for about 15% of all symptomatic cases of St. Louis encephalitis and may be as high as 35 to 60% in children.[2] Patients older than 60 years rarely present with aseptic meningitis if infected with St. Louis encephalitis virus; encephalitis is the more common finding. These infections are more frequent in warmer months when contact with the insect vector is more likely. Vector exposure is more likely to occur indoors than outside because poorly sealed residences appear to be a risk factor.[9] Other arboviruses reported to cause aseptic meningitis include the California encephalitis group of viruses (e.g., La Crosse, Jamestown Canyon, and snowshoe hare viruses, which are bunyaviruses) and the agent of Colorado tick fever, a coltivirus seen in the mountainous and western regions of the United States and Canada.[10, 11]

Mumps Virus. In an unimmunized population, mumps is one of the most common causes of aseptic meningitis and encephalitis; symptomatic meningitis is estimated to occur in 10 to 30% of mumps patients overall.[12] CNS disease caused by mumps virus can occur in patients without evidence of parotitis[2, 12, 13] and 40 to 50% of patients with mumps meningitis have no evidence of salivary gland enlargement. Meningitis is the most common neurologic manifestation of infection with mumps virus[2, 12] and is usually a benign and self-limited process. Males are affected two to five times more often than females, and the peak incidence is in children aged 5 to 9 years.[12] Cases of vaccine-associated mumps meningitis have also been reported.[14]

Lymphocytic Choriomeningitis Virus. Lymphocytic choriomeningitis virus was one of the earliest and seemingly most significant viruses to be associated with human aseptic meningitis[1, 2]; this virus is now rarely reported as an etiologic agent. Lymphocytic choriomeningitis virus is transmitted to humans by contact with rodents (e.g., hamsters, rats, mice) or their excreta[15–17]; the greatest risk of infection is in laboratory workers, pet owners, and persons living in impoverished and nonhygienic situations. A recent outbreak was described in laboratory workers who were caring for nude mice that had been injected with lymphocytic choriomeningitis virus–infected tumor cell lines.[18] Presumed routes of transmission are ingestion of food contaminated with animal urine and exposure of open wounds to dirt. No evidence of human-to-human transmission has been reported.

Herpesviruses. Herpesviruses are DNA viruses and include herpes simplex virus types 1 and 2, varicella-zoster virus, cytomegalovirus, Epstein-Barr virus, and human herpesviruses 6, 7, and 8. Although neurologic complications are known to occur with some of these viruses,[19–25] complications associated with herpes simplex viruses are of the most significance. Overall, herpes simplex viruses account for approximately 0.5 to 3% of all cases of aseptic meningitis.[26] In patients beyond the neonatal period, it is critical to differentiate between herpes simplex encephalitis, a potentially fatal form of encephalitis, and herpes simplex meningitis, a self-limited syndrome. The syndrome of herpes simplex virus aseptic meningitis is most commonly associated with primary genital infection with herpes simplex virus type 2[19–21]; in one study, an aseptic meningitis syndrome developed in 36% of women and 13% of men concomitant with primary infection.[21] Meningitis is less likely with recurrences of genital herpes.[27] Primary genital infection with herpes simplex virus type 1 and nonprimary genital infection with herpes simplex virus of either type rarely result in meningitis.[21] Acute aseptic meningitis has also been associated with herpes zoster in patients with or without typical skin lesions,[22, 28, 29] the latter known as *zoster sine herpete*. Cases of Mollaret's recurrent meningitis have been associated with herpes simplex virus type 1,[30, 31] herpes simplex virus type 2,[32, 33] and Epstein-Barr virus.[34] Human herpesvirus 6 has also been associated with meningitis[35] in conjunction with roseola infantum; however, this virus can exhibit persistence in the CNS and has been demonstrated in the CSF of asymptomatic persons.[36] Cytomegalovirus and Epstein-Barr virus may cause aseptic meningitis in association with a mononucleosis syndrome,[24, 37] particularly in an immunocompromised host.

Human Immunodeficiency Virus. Human immunodeficiency virus (HIV) can infect the meninges early and persist in the CNS after initial infection.[38] Meningitis associated with HIV may occur as part of the primary infection or occur in an already infected patient[39]; HIV has been isolated from the CSF in some of these cases. However, acute meningitis does not occur in every individual who becomes infected and can be silent. Retrospective studies have noted that an acute meningoencephalitis is observed in 5 to 10% of HIV-infected patients during or after the mononucleosis-like syndrome that heralds the initial infection.[38, 40, 41]

Bacterial Meningitis

Bacterial meningitis remains a very important disease worldwide. Data defining the frequency of isolation of specific meningeal pathogens in cases of bacterial meningitis in the United States are shown in Table 71–2.[42–44] The overall annual attack rate for bacterial meningitis, as defined by a surveillance study of 27 states in the United States from 1978 through 1981, was approximately 3.0 cases per 100,000 population, although variability based on age, race, and sex was noted.[42] The three most common meningeal pathogens, *Haemophilus influenzae, Neisseria meningitidis*, and *Streptococcus pneumoniae*, accounted for more than 80% of cases. In a surveillance study conducted during 1995 in laboratories serving all the acute care hospitals in 22 counties of four states (>10 million population),[44] the incidence of bacterial meningitis decreased dramatically. This decrease was a result of a vaccine-related decline in meningitis caused by *H. influenzae* type B vaccine (from 2.9 cases per 100,000 population in 1986 to 0.2 cases per 100,000 population in 1995)[43, 44] such that in the United States, bacterial meningitis is now a disease predominantly of adults rather than infants and children.

TABLE 71–2 Etiology of Bacterial Meningitis in the United States

Organism	Percentage of Total Cases		
	United States (1978–1981)	*United States (1986)*	*United States (1995)*
Haemophilus influenzae	48	45	7
Neisseria meningitidis	20	14	25
Streptococcus pneumoniae	13	18	47
Streptococcus agalactiae	3	6	12
Listeria monocytogenes	2	3	8
Other	8	14	—
Unknown	6	—	—

Data from refs. 42–44.

TABLE 71–3 Etiology of Bacterial Meningitis in Patients 16 Years and Older

Organism	Percentage of Total Cases	
	United States (1962–1988)	Iceland (1975–1994)
Haemophilus influenzae	4	5
Neisseria meningitidis	14	56
Streptococcus pneumoniae	38	20
Listeria monocytogenes	11	6
Other*	20	—
Unknown	13	8

*Includes gram-negative bacilli, streptococci, enterococci, *Staphylococcus aureus*, anaerobes, and diphtheroids.

Data from Sigurdardottir B, Bjornsson OM, Jonsdottir KE, et al. Acute bacterial meningitis in adults. A 20-year overview. Arch Intern Med. 1997;157:425–430; and Durand ML, Calderwood SB, Weber DJ, et al. Acute bacterial meningitis in adults. A review of 493 episodes. N Engl J Med. 1993;328:21–28.

In patients 16 years or older the relative frequency of isolation of meningeal pathogens in patients with community-acquired bacterial meningitis is somewhat different[45, 46] (Table 71–3), with most cases caused by *S. pneumoniae, N. meningitidis*, and *Listeria monocytogenes*. Case-fatality rates for single episodes of community-acquired meningitis were 25% in one study.[46] Risk factors for death among patients with community-acquired meningitis included age 60 years or older, obtunded mental status on admission, and seizures within the first 24 hours.

Bacterial meningitis is also a significant problem in hospitalized patients. In a recent review of 493 episodes of bacterial meningitis in adults 16 years or older at the Massachusetts General Hospital from 1962 through 1988,[46] 40% of episodes were nosocomial in origin, with most cases (38%) caused by gram-negative bacilli. The overall case-fatality rate for patients with single episodes of nosocomial meningitis was 35% and did not vary significantly over the 27 years of the study.

In addition, bacterial meningitis is a major problem in other areas of the world[47–49] (Table 71–4). The largest review, approximately 4100 cases of bacterial meningitis at Hospital Couta Maia in Salvador, Brazil, from 1973 through 1982, revealed an attack rate of 45.8 cases per 100,000 population.[49] The overall case-fatality rate was 33% with 50% of deaths occurring within 48 hours of hospitalization. *H. influenzae, N. meningitidis*, and *S. pneumoniae* accounted for 62% of the cases and 70% of the deaths. The case-fatality rates for meningitis caused by the Enterobacteriaceae was 86%; more than half of these cases in children younger than 24 months were caused by *Salmonella* sp., an unusual meningeal pathogen in industrialized nations.

The likely etiologic agents of bacterial meningitis vary according to the age and underlying disease status of the patient (Table 71–5). The following sections review the epidemiology and etiology of specific meningeal pathogens.

Haemophilus influenzae. *H. influenzae* was previously isolated in 45 to 48% of all cases of bacterial meningitis in the United States[42, 43]; this organism is now isolated in only 7% of cases.[44] The overall mortality rate is 3 to 6%.[42–44] Most episodes of meningitis previously occurred in infants and children younger than 6 years (peak incidence of 6 to 12 months), with 90% of cases caused by capsular type B strains. Isolation of this organism in older children and adults should suggest the presence of certain underlying conditions, including sinusitis, otitis media, epiglottitis, pneumonia, diabetes mellitus, alcoholism, splenectomy or asplenic states, head trauma with CSF leak, and immune deficiency (e.g., hypogammaglobulinemia).[50–53] Recently, a profound reduction has been seen in the incidence of invasive infections (including bacterial meningitis) caused by *H. influenzae* type B in the United States and Western Europe.[54] This decrease in infection is attributed, in part, to the recent widespread use of conjugate vaccines against *H. influenzae* type B that have been licensed for routine use in all children beginning at 2 months of age. The number of cases of *H. influenzae* type B meningitis since the introduction of vaccination has decreased more than 90%.[55–58] However, in developing countries, because of vaccine expense, the results are not as dramatic.

TABLE 71–4 Etiology of Bacterial Meningitis in Three Selected Series outside the United States

Organism	Percentage of Total Cases		
	United Kingdom (1980–1984)	Dakar, Senegal (1970–1979)	Salvador, Brazil (1973–1982)
Haemophilus influenzae	29	20	23
Neisseria meningitidis	25	11	22
Streptococcus pneumoniae	20	29	17
Streptococcus agalactiae	7	4	—
Listeria monocytogenes	2	<0.5	—
Other	16	9	20
Unknown	—	26	18

Data from refs. 47–49.

TABLE 71–5 Common Bacterial Pathogens Based on Predisposing Factor in Patients with Meningitis

Predisposing Factor	Common Bacterial Pathogens
Age	
0–4 wk	*Streptococcus agalactiae, Escherichia coli, Listeria monocytogenes, Klebsiella pneumoniae, Enterococcus* spp., *Salmonella* spp.
4–12 wk	*S. agalactiae, E. coli, L. monocytogenes, Haemophilus influenzae, Streptococcus pneumoniae, Neisseria meningitidis*
3 mo to 18 yr	*H. influenzae, N. meningitidis, S. pneumoniae*
18–50 yr	*S. pneumoniae, N. meningitidis*
>50 yr	*S. pneumoniae, N. meningitidis, L. monocytogenes*, aerobic gram-negative bacilli
Immunocompromised state	*S. pneumoniae, N. meningitidis, L. monocytogenes*, aerobic gram-negative bacilli (including *Pseudomonas aeruginosa*)
Basilar skull fracture	*S. pneumoniae, H. influenzae*, group A β-hemolytic streptococci
Head trauma; postneurosurgery	*Staphylococcus aureus, Staphylococcus epidermidis*, aerobic gram-negative bacilli (including *P. aeruginosa*)
Cerebrospinal fluid shunt	*S. epidermidis, S. aureus*, aerobic gram-negative bacilli (including *P. aeruginosa*), *Propionibacterium acnes*

Neisseria meningitidis. *N. meningitidis* most commonly causes meningitis in children and young adults and is associated with an overall mortality rate of 3 to 13%.[42–44] Meningococci of serogroups B, C, and Y account for most of the endemic disease in the United States.[59] Disease caused by serogroups A and C may occur in epidemics; group Y strains may be associated with pneumonia. Several outbreaks of disease caused by serogroup C meningococci have been reported in the United States and Canada, with most caused by one strain of electrophoretic type 37 (ET-37) termed ET-15.[60, 61] Isolates of the ET-37 complex were also responsible for most cases of sporadic serogroup C meningococcal disease in another study.[62] Patients with deficiencies in the terminal complement components (C5, C6, C7, C8, and perhaps C9), the so-called membrane attack complex, have a markedly increased incidence of neisserial infection,[63–68] including that caused by *N. meningitidis*, although mortality rates in patients with meningococcal disease are lower than those in patients with an intact complement system (3 versus 19% in the general population). An increased risk of invasive meningococcal disease has also been described in a Dutch family with dysfunctional properdin,[69] which suggests a potential role for the alternative pathway in complement-mediated resistance against meningococci.

Streptococcus pneumoniae. *S. pneumoniae*, the most frequently observed etiologic agent of bacterial meningitis in the United States, now accounts for 47% of the total cases[44]; the mortality rate ranges from 19 to 26%.[42–44] Of the 83 known pneumococcal serotypes, 18 are responsible for 82% of the cases of bacteremic pneumococcal pneumonia, with a close correlation between bacteremic subtypes and those implicated in meningitis.[70–72] Patients often have contiguous or distant foci of pneumococcal infection such as pneumonia, otitis media, mastoiditis, sinusitis, and endocarditis. Serious infection may be observed in patients with various underlying conditions (e.g., splenectomy or asplenic states, multiple myeloma, hypogammaglobulinemia, alcoholism, malnutrition, chronic liver or renal disease, malignancy, and diabetes mellitus).[73–78] The pneumococcus is the most common etiologic agent of meningitis in patients who have suffered basilar skull fracture with CSF leak.[79]

Listeria monocytogenes. *L. monocytogenes* causes 8% of cases of bacterial meningitis in the United States and carries a mortality rate of 15 to 29%.[42–44] Serotypes 1/2b and 4b have been implicated in up to 80% of meningitis cases caused by this organism. *Listeria* has been isolated from dust, soil, water, sewage, and decaying vegetable matter (including animal feed and silage). Listerial infection is most common in infants younger than 1 month (up to 10% of cases), adults older than 60 years, alcoholics, cancer patients, those receiving corticosteroid therapy, and immunosuppressed adults (e.g., renal transplant recipients).[80–86] Other predisposing conditions include diabetes mellitus, liver disease, chronic renal disease, collagen-vascular diseases, and conditions associated with iron overload. Although colonization rates are low, pregnant women (who account for 25% of all cases of listeriosis) may harbor the organism asymptomatically in their genital tract and rectum and transmit the infection to their infants. *Listeria* meningitis is found infrequently in patients with HIV infection[87, 88] despite its increased incidence in patients with deficiencies in cell-mediated immunity. Meningitis can also occur in previously healthy adults.[89] Outbreaks of *Listeria* infection have been associated with the consumption of contaminated coleslaw, raw vegetables, milk, and cheese, with sporadic cases traced to contaminated cheese, turkey franks, and alfalfa tablets, thus pointing to the intestinal tract as the usual portal of entry.[81, 85, 90–93]

Streptococcus agalactiae. Group B streptococcus is a common cause of meningitis in neonates,[94] with 52% of all cases in the United States reported during the first month of life.[44] In the United States the overall mortality rate ranges from 7 to 27%.[42–44] Group B streptococcus has been isolated from the vaginal or rectal cultures of 15 to 35% of asymptomatic pregnant women[95, 96]; colonization rates do not vary during pregnancy, and carriage may be chronic (40%), transient, or intermittent. The risk of transmission from mother to infant is increased when the inoculum of organisms and the number of sites of maternal colonization are increased; the route of delivery does not influence transmission. Horizontal transmission has also been documented from the hands of nursery personnel to the infant. Most cases of neonatal meningitis are caused by subtype III organisms and occur after the first week of life. Group B streptococcus can also cause meningitis in adults.[97–101] Risk factors in adults include age older than 60 years, diabetes mellitus, pregnancy or the postpartum state, cardiac disease, collagen-vascular diseases, malignancy, alcoholism, hepatic failure, renal failure, previous stroke, neurogenic bladder, decubitus ulcers, and corticosteroid therapy; in one review of group B streptococcal meningitis in adults, no underlying illnesses were found in 43% of patients.[98]

Aerobic Gram-Negative Bacilli. Aerobic gram-negative bacilli (e.g., *Klebsiella* spp., *Escherichia coli*, *Serratia marcescens*, *Pseudomonas aeruginosa*, *Salmonella* spp.) have become increasingly important as etiologic agents in patients with bacterial meningitis.[102–109] These agents may be isolated from the CSF of patients after head trauma or neurosurgical procedures and may also be found in neonates, the elderly, immunosuppressed patients, and patients with gram-negative septicemia. Some cases have been associated with disseminated strongyloidiasis in the hyperinfection syndrome, a condition in which meningitis caused by enteric bacteria occurs secondary to seeding of the meninges during persistent or recurrent bacteremias associated with the migration of infective larvae.[110] Alternatively, the larvae may carry enteric organisms on their surfaces or within their own gastrointestinal tracts as they exit the intestine and subsequently invade the meninges. In patients with *E. coli* meningitis, 75% of cases are caused by strains possessing the K1 antigen.[94] Almost half of pregnant women have this organism isolated on rectal culture, and as many as 75% of their infants will be colonized during the first days of life; horizontal transmission from nursery staff members or other infants has also been reported.

Staphylococci. Meningitis caused by *Staphylococcus aureus* is usually found in early postneurosurgical or post-trauma patients and in those with CSF shunts; other underlying conditions include diabetes mellitus, alcoholism, chronic renal failure requiring hemodialysis, injection drug use, and malignancies.[111–114] Thirty-five percent of cases are observed in the setting of head trauma or after neurosurgery, and an additional 20% of patients have underlying infective endocarditis or paraspinal infection. Other sources of community-acquired *S. aureus* meningitis include patients with sinusitis, osteomyelitis, and pneumonia. Mortality rates have ranged from 14 to 77% in various series. *Staphylococcus epidermidis* is the most common cause of meningitis in patients with CSF shunts.[115, 116]

Other Bacteria. A review of 28 cases of nocardial meningitis revealed predisposing conditions in approximately 75% of patients,[117] including immunosuppressive drug therapy, malignancy, head trauma, CNS procedures, chronic granulomatous disease, and sarcoidosis. Anaerobic meningitis is unusual and is generally associated with contiguous foci of infection (e.g., otitis, sinusitis, pharyngitis, brain abscess, head and neck malignancy, recent head and neck surgery or wound infection, and CNS trauma and neurosurgery[118–122]; in many cases more than one organism may be recovered. Enterococci are unusual etiologic agents of bacterial meningitis; most adult patients have underlying illnesses, and disease is often associated with immunosuppressive therapy, CNS trauma or surgery, or an enterococcal infection outside the CNS.[123] Diphtheroids, particularly *Propionibacterium acnes*, have become important etiologic agents of meningitis in patients with CNS shunt infections.[115]

Spirochetal Meningitis

Treponema pallidum. *T. pallidum* disseminates to the CNS during early infection.[124] The organism can be isolated from the CSF of patients with primary syphilis, and CSF laboratory abnormalities are detected in 5 to 9% of patients with seronegative primary syphilis. The actual rate of invasion of the CNS during these early stages is likely to be considerably higher, however. Clinical neurosyphilis can be divided into four distinct syndromes[124]: syphilitic meningitis, meningovascular syphilis, parenchymatous neurosyphilis, and gummatous neurosyphilis. Some overlap may be seen in the clinical and laboratory findings of these syndromes. The incidence of syphilitic meningitis is greatest in the first 2 years after infection and is estimated to occur in only 0.3 to 2.4% of syphilis cases. In contrast, meningovascular syphilis is found in 10 to 12% of individuals with CNS involvement[124, 125] and occurs months to years after syphilis acquisition (peak incidence, approximately 7 years). Parenchymatous neurosyphilis has two variants, general paresis and tabes dorsalis. Both are relatively rare today and do not become apparent until 10 to 20 years after the acquisition of infection. Gummas are late manifestations of tertiary syphilis and may occur anywhere[124]; gummatous neurosyphilis is rare.

The overall incidence of neurosyphilis has recently increased, with many of the cases reported seen in patients with HIV infection.[126–128] In one report,[129] 44% of all patients with neurosyphilis had acquired immunodeficiency syndrome (AIDS); the remaining patients, who may have had HIV infection without AIDS, were not addressed in this report. The study also showed that 1.5% of patients with AIDS were found to have neurosyphilis at some point during the course of their disease. In a more recent review of neurosyphilis cases during the HIV era in San Francisco from 1985 to 1992, neurosyphilis was identified in young patients most often with HIV coinfection.[130]

Borrelia burgdorferi. The nervous system is eventually involved clinically in at least 10 to 15% of patients with Lyme disease, either while erythema migrans is still present or 1 to 6 months later.[131–133] A 1992 study used polymerase chain reaction (PCR) to detect spirochetal DNA in CSF samples from 8 of 12 patients with acute (<2 weeks) disseminated Lyme borreliosis,[134] which indicates that *B. burgdorferi* usually invades the CNS early in infection.

Protozoal and Helminthic Meningitis

Amebas. Despite the hundreds of species of free-living amebas that are known, only a few have been reported to infect humans.[135, 136] The most important are in the genera *Naegleria* and *Acanthamoeba*. *Naegleria fowleri*, the main protozoan causing primary amebic meningoencephalitis in humans, has been recovered from lakes, puddles, pools, ponds, rivers, sewage sludge, tap water, air conditioner drains, and soil. Sporadic cases of primary amebic meningoencephalitis occur when persons, usually children and young adults, swim or play in water containing the amebas or when swimming pools or water supplies have become contaminated, often through failure of chlorination. Asymptomatic carriage by humans can also occur. The incidence of infection is unknown, although a study of Florida lakes reported only 7 documented cases of primary amebic meningoencephalitis in over 1 billion swimming episodes.[137] Several cases have recently been reported in HIV-infected patients, all with advanced HIV disease at the time of amebic infection.[138–141]

Angiostrongylus cantonensis. Infection of humans by larvae of the nematode *A. cantonensis* can lead to the development of an eosinophilic meningitis.[110, 142] The larvae invade the brain either directly from the blood stream or after migrating through other organs before reaching the spinal cord and brain. Once in the CNS, the larvae mature into adult worms that migrate through the brain. *A. cantonensis* is widespread and human infection is fairly common and reported from many parts of the world (Thailand, India, Malaysia, Vietnam, Indonesia, Papua New Guinea, and the Pacific Islands, including Hawaii).[110, 142, 143] The parasites may spread to many countries by rats moving freely from port to port on ships.[142, 144] The rat infection rate in urban Bangkok has reached about 40%.[145]

PATHOGENESIS AND PATHOPHYSIOLOGY

Viral Meningitis

Initiation of Infection. After the colonization of mucosal surfaces throughout the body by various viruses, the host possesses numerous barriers to prevent viral entry.[146] For example, the respiratory tract contains a thin film of mucus and a mucociliary elevator that moves viral particles away from the lower respiratory tract; even if this barrier is crossed, alveolar macrophages are actively phagocytic for viral particles. Gastric acidity inactivates most swallowed viruses, and gastrointestinal enzymes and bile also disrupt viral envelopes, capsid proteins, and lipoprotein membranes; however, some nonenveloped, acid-resistant viruses (e.g., enteroviruses, adenoviruses, reoviruses, parvoviruses) are adapted for replication in the gastrointestinal tract. When the host has had previous contact with the viral agent, the mucosa of the gastrointestinal and respiratory tracts may be coated with secretory IgA, which neutralizes the virus and prevents attachment and subsequent cell penetration. If certain viruses are able to escape initial host defense mechanisms, they may replicate and disseminate with the potential for CNS invasion.

Viremia and Central Nervous System Invasion. After hematogenous dissemination of the virus, CNS infection may occur. Most neurotropic viruses first multiply at extraneural sites (initially at the portal of entry), establish viremia, and then cross the blood-brain barrier (BBB) to invade the CNS.[147, 148] For example, enteroviruses initially multiply in the peritonsillar lymphatics, Peyer's patches, lamina propria of the intestine, and vascular and endothelial cells, depending on the particular agent. M cells may mediate virus penetration from the gut lumen to lymphoid cells. From this initial site, the virus then disseminates to vascular tissue (e.g., liver, spleen, and muscle), where further multiplication augments the viremia.[149] After viremia, viral particles are normally cleared by the reticuloendothelial system, with the speed of removal directly related to virus size (i.e., large viruses are cleared more promptly from the blood stream). Viruses may also elude host clearance by associating with certain cells. Some viruses (e.g., measles, herpes, mumps) grow in human leukocytes, which protects them from phagocytosis by the reticuloendothelial system, neutralization by circulating antibody, and inactivation by nonspecific serum inhibitors.

CNS invasion by viruses may occur via several mechanisms. Most viruses invade directly across cerebral capillary endothelial cells, the major site of the BBB. Some viruses directly infect cerebral microvascular endothelial cells before infection of adjacent glia and neurons,[149] whereas others initially infect glia without evidence of endothelial cell infection. Still other viruses may be carried between cerebral endothelial cells in infected leukocytes after BBB disruption. Another site of virus entry is the choroid plexus epithelium. Studies of mumps virus in hamsters have shown a sequence of infection from the choroid plexus to the ependyma to parenchymal cells; viral nucleocapsids have been found in the choroid plexi and ependymal cells of humans with mumps meningitis.

Viruses may reach the CNS by spread along olfactory nerves.[146, 147, 149, 150] In an experimental hamster model,[146] intranasal inoculation of herpes simplex virus and togaviruses led to early infection of the olfactory bulb, which could be inhibited by cutting the olfactory tracts or chemical treatment of the olfactory mucosa. Peripheral nerve spread by viruses may also lead to CNS invasion. A recent study used a transgenic mouse model to demonstrate that after intramuscular inoculation of poliovirus in the limb, infectious poliovirus was first detected in the inferior segment of the spinal cord and then in the superior segment and the brain,[151] thus suggesting that poliovirus initially spreads to the CNS through peripheral nerve pathways.

Virus Spread within the Central Nervous System. Regardless of the mechanism of CNS invasion, the production of disease requires viral attachment to and penetration of susceptible cells, spread within the nervous system, and induction of cellular changes. Viral entry into the subarachnoid space via the choroid plexus leads to dispersion of virus within CSF in contact with meningeal and ependymal cells[146]; sequential spread of virus may then occur in a contiguous fashion to glia and neurons. Other viruses spread through extracellular gaps between cells and CNS processes (e.g., dendrites, axons, or glia), transit along the extensive axonal and dendritic ramifications of neurons by way of the glia, or are carried by mobile leukocytes in the inflammatory response. Experimental evidence supports each mode of transit, and all may be involved to various degrees in different viral infections.

Once viral infection of the CNS occurs, inflammatory cells usually accumulate although the mechanisms leading to inflammatory cell recruitment and their role in viral CNS infections are only partially understood.[146, 147] It appears that the initial inflammatory response is immunologically specific and consists of a population of lymphocytes sensitized by the virus. However, an inflammatory response may fail to develop in other viral CNS infections, a response that may be dependent on host age rather than the virus itself. Sensitized lymphocytes probably respond to a virus-specific protein that diffuses or is transported to the luminal surface of the endothe-

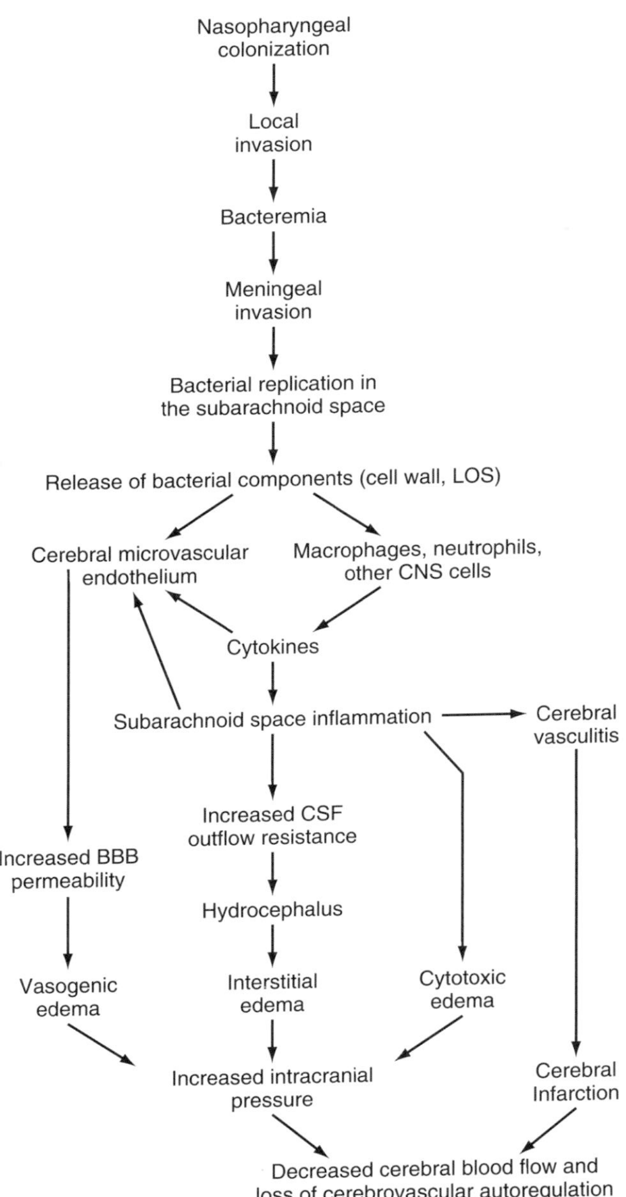

FIGURE 71–1. Pathogenesis and pathophysiology of bacterial meningitis. *Abbreviations*: BBB, Blood-brain barrier; CSF, cerebrospinal fluid; CNS, central nervous system; LOS, lipo-oligosaccharide. (From Tunkel AR, Scheld WM. Pathogenesis and pathophysiology of bacterial meningitis. Clin Microbiol Rev. 1993; 6:118–136.)

lium with subsequent passage through endothelial cells and release of inflammatory cytokines. In an experimental mouse model of meningitis caused by lymphocytic choriomeningitis virus,[152] elevated CSF concentrations of interleukin-6 (IL-6) and interferon-γ (IFN-γ) were demonstrated. CSF IL-6 concentrations began to rise 24 hours after intracerebral infection, followed by a rapid increase after day 4. IFN-γ was not detected in CSF until 5 to 6 days after infection, but then it markedly increased. CSF concentrations of these cytokines were only slightly and transiently elevated in athymic nude mice. In one review, IFN-γ was also detectable in the CSF in 75% of 16 patients with enteroviral meningitis,[153] with more consistent production and higher titers noted with coxsackievirus than with echovirus. Elevated CSF IL-6 concentrations were also detected in 12 of 15 samples from patients with acute aseptic meningitis.[152]

Other inflammatory cytokines have been measured in the CSF of patients with aseptic meningitis. In one study,[154] CSF concentrations of tumor necrosis factor-α (TNF-α) and IL-1β were measured in 36 patients with aseptic meningitis, 13 of whom had culture-proven enteroviral meningitis, and in 14 controls. None of the samples from the patients with aseptic meningitis or controls had detectable TNF-α activity, whereas 86% of patients with aseptic meningitis had detectable CSF IL-1β concentrations; only 2 of 14 control patients had elevated concentrations. The increased CSF IL-1β concentrations correlated with CSF white blood cell counts.

After development of a CSF inflammatory response, alterations in the BBB permit the traversal into CSF of serum proteins, including immunoglobulins. In addition, local CNS immunoglobulin synthesis occurs as B cells enter the CSF and differentiate into plasma cells. Intracerebral synthesis of immunoglobulins also occurs and is reflected by an increase in the CSF : serum ratios of specific immunoglobulins that persist for several weeks after infection.[146] The production of oligoclonal IgG proteins within the CNS has been demonstrated in patients with meningitis caused by mumps virus, varicella-zoster virus, and HIV.[13, 22, 155, 156] Furthermore, elevated CSF concentrations of oligoclonal IgG may persist for up to 1 year in patients with mumps meningitis,[13] which suggests the possibility of viral persistence and ongoing antigenic stimulation.

An intact host immune response appears to be important for clearance of virus from the CNS[146, 147]; T-cell responses appear to be more important than B-cell responses. Failure of an immune response to develop may be a result of immunologic tolerance, host immune defects, or the ability of the virus to escape immune surveillance. Chronic infections with varicella-zoster virus, cytomegalovirus, adenovirus, and measles virus have developed in patients with depressed cell-mediated immunity.

Bacterial Meningitis

Numerous investigations over the last 20 years have elucidated many of the pathogenic and pathophysiologic mechanisms operable in bacterial meningitis.[147, 157–161] Figure 71–1 shows a hypothetic scheme of these mechanisms, which are discussed in greater detail in the following sections.

Mucosal Colonization and Systemic Invasion

The early pathogenic events that result in bacterial meningitis depend on an interplay between specific virulence factors and host defense mechanisms (Table 71–6). The initiation of infection with meningeal pathogens usually begins with host acquisition of a new organism by nasopharyngeal colonization.[162] Many of the major meningeal pathogens possess surface characteristics that enhance mucosal colonization. For example, the fimbriae (or pili) of *N. meningitidis* mediate adherence of this organism to nasopharyngeal epithelial cells; these fimbriated strains accounted for 80% of primary meningococcal isolates from nasopharyngeal carriers and from the CSF of patients with meningococcal meningitis,[159] although all fimbriae were lost on

TABLE 71–6 Factors Involved in the Pathogenesis of Bacterial Meningitis

Pathogenic Event	Bacterial Factors	Host Factors
Mucosal colonization	Fimbriae, polysaccharide capsule, IgA protease production	Mucosal epithelium, secretory IgA, ciliary activity, anticapsular antibodies
Intravascular survival	Polysaccharide capsule	Complement
Meningeal invasion	Fimbriae, association with monocytes, the gene *ibe10*	Blood-brain barrier
Survival within the subarachnoid space	Polysaccharide capsule	Poor opsonic activity

serial subculture in the laboratory. The fimbriae appear morphologically as aggregated bundles or single filaments.[163] Aggregated bundles are found primarily among disease isolates exhibiting a low degree of adherence to human buccal epithelial cells, whereas the single filaments have medium to high adherence characteristics and are found predominantly among colonizing isolates. Once meningococci attach to nonciliated nasopharyngeal epithelial cells via a specific cell surface receptor, they are transported across these cells within a phagocytic vacuole[162]; this process appears to be essential for the subsequent development of invasive meningococcal disease.

Fimbriae have also been implicated in the attachment of *H. influenzae* to upper tract respiratory epithelial cells,[159] although fimbriae have not been found on isolates from the CSF or blood of patients with invasive disease. This observation suggests that although fimbriae play an initial role in adherence of *H. influenzae* within the nasopharynx, their presence is not necessary for the development of invasive disease, including meningitis. Furthermore, the type of fimbriae expressed by *H. influenzae* type B strains may facilitate adherence to select nasopharyngeal sites: α-fimbriae enhance adherence in the anterior of the nasopharynx, whereas β-fimbriae facilitate the process more posteriorly (A. L. Smith, personal communication). In addition, acquisition and colonization by *H. influenzae* type B may be promoted after respiratory tract infection by viral agents such as influenzae A Victoria and respiratory syncytial virus,[164] although the precise role of a preceding upper respiratory viral infection in the enhancement of nasopharyngeal colonization by *H. influenzae* type B is controversial. After nasopharyngeal colonization, invasion into the blood stream by *H. influenzae* appears to occur via a breakdown in the tight junctions between epithelial cells (in contrast to *N. meningitidis*, which invades via parasite-directed endocytosis), thereby leading to invasion by an intercellular mechanism.[162]

Surface encapsulation may also be an important virulence factor for nasopharyngeal colonization and systemic invasion of meningeal pathogens. Among the six encapsulated types of *H. influenzae* (A through F), type B strains constitute less than 5% of nasopharyngeal isolates but cause more than 95% of systemic and meningeal infections.[164] In an experimental infant rat model, it has been demonstrated that although all encapsulated strains of *H. influenzae* had the potential for systemic invasion after intraperitoneal inoculation, type B strains were the most virulent and were the only capsular types capable of systemic invasion after intranasal inoculation.[159, 164] Indeed, antibodies to type B capsule, which are almost uniformly detected in humans by the age of 4 years even in the absence of known exposure to *H. influenzae* type B, are protective against invasive disease. Polysaccharide capsule may also be an important virulence factor for the development of invasive disease by *S. pneumoniae*. In addition, in vivo capsular transformation events may equip pneumococcal strains with highly virulent blood invasive phenotypes, thereby increasing the seriousness of pneumococcal infection, especially that caused by multidrug-resistant strains.[165]

Adherence of microorganisms to mucosal surfaces may be inhibited by natural antibodies found in mucosal secretions, such as IgA. However, it appears that the presence of high concentrations of circulating IgA antibodies to *N. meningitidis* may permit the development or progression of invasive disease by preferentially binding to the organism and blocking the beneficial effects of IgG and IgM antibodies.[159] In addition, species of many pathogenic bacteria (e.g., *Neisseria, Haemophilus, Streptococcus*) produce IgA_1 proteases that cleave IgA in the hinge region and facilitate the adherence of bacterial strains to mucosal surfaces through local destruction of IgA. However, the exact role of IgA protease production in this pathogenic sequence remains unclear. The presence of anticapsular polysaccharide antibodies may also be effective in decreasing nasopharyngeal carriage of meningeal pathogens. In an intralitter transmission model in which infant rats were intranasally inoculated with *S. pneumoniae* and placed in a cage with other infant rats, pretreatment of uninoculated rats with systemic IgG antibodies to pneumococcal polysaccharide reduced the intralitter transmission of *S. pneumoniae*,[166] which suggests that IgG antibodies to pneumococcal polysaccharide may be sufficient to reduce pneumococcal nasopharyngeal carriage in humans.

Intravascular Survival

Once bacteria cross the mucosal barrier and gain access to the blood stream, they must overcome additional host defense mechanisms to survive. The presence of bacterial capsule, by effectively inhibiting neutrophil phagocytosis and resisting classic complement-mediated bactericidal activity, may enhance blood stream survival of the organism, thereby facilitating intravascular replication.[147, 159] The most common meningeal pathogens *(H. influenzae, N. meningitidis, S. pneumoniae, E. coli, S. agalactiae)* are all encapsulated. In addition, certain capsular types are disproportionately associated with the development of meningitis. For example, about 84% of cases of neonatal meningitis caused by *E. coli* are caused by strains bearing the K1 antigen[167]; in the absence of specific host antibody to the K1 capsule, these organisms are profoundly resistant to phagocytosis. Presence of the K1 capsule and a high degree of bacteremia are key determinants in the development of *E. coli* meningitis.[168]

The host possesses several defense mechanisms to counteract the antiphagocytic effects of bacterial capsule.[147, 159] For example, activation of the alternative complement pathway by the capsular polysaccharide of *S. pneumoniae* results in the cleavage of C3 with attachment of C3 to the bacterial surface. This series of events facilitates opsonization, phagocytosis, and intravascular clearance of the organism. Impairment of the alternative complement pathway (e.g., in patients with sickle cell anemia and those who have undergone splenectomy) predisposes to the development of pneumococcal meningitis. *H. influenzae* type B also activates the complement cascade. Experimental studies in a rat model have shown that after intravenous or intraperitoneal challenge with *H. influenzae* of varying serotypes (A, B, C, or D), a greater incidence and magnitude of bacteremia developed in rats depleted of C3. Although the incidence of bacteremia caused by type B organisms increased from 63 to 95% in complement-depleted rats, the incidence and severity of meningitis were unaffected by complement depletion.

Complement system activation is also an essential host defense mechanism against invasive disease caused by *N. meningitidis*. Patients with deficiencies in the membrane attack complex are particularly prone to neisserial infections, although usually with a more favorable outcome when appropriate therapy is instituted.[63] The reasons for the worse outcome in patients with an intact complement system are unclear, although a qualitative relationship can be shown among the concentration of circulating meningococcal lipo-oligosaccharide, a fatal outcome, and the degree of complement activation.[169]

Meningeal Invasion

The mechanism or mechanisms by which meningeal pathogens gain access to the CNS remain unknown. The development of a sustained, high-grade bacteremia has been suggested as one important factor.[170] In one study, culture-positive meningitis was produced in an experimental infant rat model only after an intense bacteremia had been present for at least 6 hours.[171] However, sustained bacteremia cannot be the sole factor responsible for meningeal invasion because many other organisms (e.g., viridans streptococci) that produce high-grade bacteremia during infective endocarditis rarely produce meningitis.

The site of CNS invasion by meningeal pathogens is also unclear. Early studies suggested that invasion from the blood stream was via the dural venous sinus system, whereas other experiments suggested that the site of invasion was above the cribriform plate or via the choroid plexi (because of their exceptionally high rate of blood flow of approximately 200 ml/g/minute).[170] Recent experimental studies, however, have demonstrated that receptors for some meningeal pathogens are present on cells of the choroid plexi and cerebral capillaries. In cryostat sections of infant rat brain cortical slices, *E. coli* strains possessing S fimbriae have been shown to bind specifically to the luminal surfaces of the vascular endothelium and the epithelium lining the choroid plexi and brain ventricles.[172] Phase variation to the nonfimbriated form may then be necessary for these bacteria to invade the CNS.[173] To understand the cellular mechanisms important for meningeal invasion, the invasion of *E. coli* into endothelial and epithelial cell cultures was studied. It appeared that microtubule-dependent and/or microfilament-dependent pathways, which rearrange the cell cytoskeleton, may be important for bacterial uptake and crossing of the BBB.[174] *N. meningitidis* was also shown to adhere in vivo to the endothelium of both the choroid plexus and meninges in a fatal case of meningococcemia[175]; isolates obtained from the CSF expressed significantly more PilC protein than did the blood isolates, which suggests that PilC plays an important role for this organism to cross the BBB. Despite these studies, the importance of adherence of meningeal pathogens to sites within the CNS requires further investigation.

To further assess the molecular mechanisms important in meningeal invasion, the ability of strains of *E. coli* to invade endothelial cells was determined. A gene (termed *ibe10*) has been cloned and found to encode an 8.2-kD protein that permits *E. coli* to invade brain microvascular endothelial cells both in vitro and in vivo.[176] The prevalence of *ibe10* was also increased in *E. coli* isolates from CSF versus feces or blood,[177] although further studies are needed to assess the role of this virulence determinant in meningeal invasion. In addition, the *aslA* gene product of *E. coli* K12 has been shown to have homology to the DNA adjacent to the Tn*phoA* insertion site, which potentially contributes to the invasion process of meningitic *E. coli* into the BBB.[178]

Another pathogenic mechanism postulated to promote CNS invasion by meningeal pathogens is association of the organism with circulating monocytes. Histologic and scanning microscopic techniques were used to examine the neuraxes of pigs inoculated with a strain of *Streptococcus suis* type 2,[179] and the only pathologic lesions detected were associated with the choroid plexus and were manifested as brush-border disruption, decrease in the number of Kolmer cells, and exudation of fibrin and inflammatory cells into the ventricles. Intracellular bacteria were demonstrated in the parenchyma of the choroid plexus, in ventricular monocytes, and within circulating peripheral blood monocytes, thus suggesting that bacteria may gain access to the CSF in association with monocytes migrating along normal pathways.

Transcytosis through microvascular endothelial cells has been investigated as another possible mechanism of meningeal invasion during bacterial meningitis. In an in vitro model using rat and human brain microvascular endothelial cells,[180] the transparent phase variants of pneumococci that gained access to an intracellular vesicle from the apical side of the microvascular endothelial cell monolayer were able to transcytose to the basal surface of these cells in a manner dependent on the platelet-activating factor (PAF) receptor and the presence of pneumococcal choline-binding protein A; the remaining transparent bacteria entering the cell underwent a previously unrecognized recycling to the apical surface. These data suggest that interaction of pneumococci with the PAF receptor results in sorting so that bacteria can be transcytosed across the cell, whereas non-PAF receptor entry shunts bacteria for exit and reentry on the apical surface. This bidirectional trafficking of pneumococci represents an important potential bioprobe to investigate transport across mammalian cells.

Bacterial Survival within the Subarachnoid Space

Once meningeal pathogens enter the subarachnoid space, host defense mechanisms are generally inadequate to control the infection.[147, 159] CSF concentrations of complement components are absent or minimal; meningeal inflammation leads to increased, although low CSF complement concentrations. This relative complement deficiency may be of critical importance because specific antibody, complement, or both are essential for opsonization of encapsulated meningeal pathogens and efficient phagocytosis. Observations in experimental animal models and in patients with meningitis have revealed absent or barely detectable opsonic and bactericidal activity. The explanation for this low level of complement components during bacterial meningitis is unclear. It has been suggested that degradation of complement components crossing the BBB by leukocyte proteases may result in inefficient opsonic activity at the site of infection. Indeed, in an experimental rabbit model of pneumococcal meningitis, the intracisternal inoculation of a nonspecific protease inhibitor (phenylmethylsulfonyl fluoride) led to a decline in pneumococcal concentrations in CSF when compared with saline-inoculated controls.

Immunoglobulin concentrations are also low in normal CSF (blood : CSF ratio of IgG of about 800:1), and although concentrations increase during bacterial meningitis, they remain low in comparison to simultaneous serum concentrations.[147, 159] In an experimental rabbit model, the intravenous administration of a bactericidal monoclonal antibody against the polyribosylribitol phosphate of *H. influenzae* type B produced high serum antibody concentrations, but BBB permeability was poor (5.5% or less), even in the presence of meningeal inflammation, which suggests that systemic administration of type-specific antibodies alone is likely to be suboptimal in therapy for bacterial meningitis.

Bacterial meningitis is characterized by the development of a neutrophilic pleocytosis within the CSF, although the precise mechanism of leukocyte traversal across the BBB is undefined.[159] The complement component C5a has been suggested as one chemotactic component, with chemotactic activity appearing 2 to 4 hours before neutrophil influx into CSF. In an experimental rabbit model, the intracisternal inoculation of C5a led to an influx of leukocytes into CSF 1 hour after inoculation,[181] a response that was attenuated by coadministration of prostaglandin E_2 (PGE_2) in a dose- and time-dependent manner, which suggests a direct anti-inflammatory action of PGE_2 on C5a-induced CSF pleocytosis during bacterial meningitis. Elevated CSF concentrations of two alternative-pathway complement activation proteins, C3 and factor B, have also been found in mice and in patients with bacterial meningitis.[182, 183] In the mouse model of *Listeria* meningitis,[182] intrathecal synthesis of C3 and factor B occurred during the course of the disease.

Recent studies have examined other chemotactic factors and their role in mediating CSF chemotactic activity. In an experimental mouse model of *Listeria* meningoencephalitis, the macrophage inflammatory proteins MIP-1α and MIP-2 were important in the recruitment of leukocytes into the CSF.[184] Elevated CSF concentrations of MIP-1α and MIP-1β, as well as other chemokines (IL-8, growth-related gene product-α, and monocyte chemotactic protein 1), have also been found to be increased in patients with bacterial meningitis.[185, 186] However, no significant correlation was found between CSF leukocyte counts and chemokine concentrations or chemotactic activity mediated by CSF, thus suggesting that other factors influence the extent of CSF pleocytosis in vivo. In another study, the significant correlation of elevated CSF concentrations of IL-8 and growth-related gene product-α with the number of granulocytes that immigrated into the CSF of patients with bacterial meningitis[187] suggested the importance of these chemokines in the recruitment of leukocytes into the subarachnoid space.

Despite this early influx of leukocytes in bacterial meningitis, host defense in CSF remains suboptimal because of the lack of functional opsonic and bactericidal activity. With inefficient phagocytosis, bacteria can multiply to huge concentrations in the CSF during meningitis.

The precise pathway of leukocyte traversal into the CSF is unknown, although adherence to vascular endothelial cells is a likely prerequisite. Pretreatment of noncerebral endothelial cells in culture with lipo-oligosaccharide or cytokines (IL-1 or TNF) has been shown to induce the formation of specific adhesion molecules such as endothelial leukocyte adhesion molecule 1 and intercellular adhesion molecule 1 (ICAM-1).[158] It is unclear whether similar adhesion mechanisms exist between neutrophils and cerebral vascular endothelium. In an infant mouse model of hematogenous bacterial meningitis,[188] mice genetically deficient in the gene coding for ICAM-1 production had a higher incidence of *H. influenzae* type B bacteremia than did wild-type mice, and more ICAM-1–deficient mice had positive CSF cultures for *H. influenzae* type B. In contrast, the incidence of *S. pneumoniae* bacteremia was equivalent in both groups of mice, and all were CSF culture positive, although mortality was higher for ICAM-1–deficient mice at 24 hours. These results suggested that ICAM-1 deficiency may be protective early in *H. influenzae* type B infection but detrimental in *S. pneumoniae* infection. In an experimental rat model, a monoclonal antibody (CD54) directed against ICAM-1 significantly reduced the accumulation of leukocytes in CSF during the early phase of bacterial meningitis,[189] which makes this adhesion molecule a promising target in the development of adjunctive strategies to treat bacterial meningitis.

Other families of leukocyte receptors have also been studied to determine their role in leukocyte-mediated damage in bacterial meningitis. In an experimental rabbit model, the intravenous inoculation of a monoclonal antibody (IB4) directed against the CD18 family of receptors on leukocytes (leukocyte integrins) blocked the accumulation of leukocytes in CSF despite the intracisternal inoculation of *H. influenzae* type B, *N. meningitidis*, pneumococcal cell wall, or lipo-oligosaccharide[190]; increased protein concentrations in CSF were also attenuated by IB4. In addition, the monoclonal antibody prevented the development of cerebral edema and death in animals challenged with lethal doses of *S. pneumoniae*. CSF penetration of antibiotics, CSF bactericidal concentrations, and the bactericidal response to ampicillin therapy were not affected by administration of the monoclonal antibody, although the onset of bacteremia was delayed and the CSF inflammatory response was attenuated after ampicillin-induced bacterial killing.

Selectins also play an important role in promoting the margination and reversible rolling of leukocytes at sites of tissue inflammation. After intravenous administration of prokaryotic peptides that mimic selectins (the S2 and S3 subunits of pertussis toxin) and competitively inhibit adherence of neutrophils to endothelial cells in vitro, recruitment of leukocytes into the CSF of rabbits with pneumococcal meningitis was disrupted, thus suggesting that these peptides have therapeutic anti-inflammatory potential.[191] An anti-CD11b monoclonal antibody (1B6) was studied in an infant rat model of *H. influenzae* sepsis and meningitis[192]; 1B6 played a role in inhibiting neutrophil emigration to sites of inflammation within the CNS but was not beneficial in decreasing mortality in this model. Furthermore, in an experimental cytokine-induced model of meningitis, mice deficient in P- and E-selectins displayed nearly complete inhibition in CSF leukocyte accumulation and BBB permeability versus only partial inhibition in P-selectin–deficient mice.[193] In additional studies, after intravenous treatment with the polysaccharide fucoidin, a homopolymer of sulfated L-fucose known to block the function of the leukocyte "rolling receptor" L-selectin,[194] leukocyte rolling was rapidly and profoundly reduced (confirmed by intravital microscopy in muscle), and the accumulation of both leukocytes and plasma proteins into the CSF of rabbits challenged intrathecally with pneumococcal antigen was profoundly reduced. These findings suggest that inhibition of selectin-mediated leukocyte rolling may be an effective therapeutic approach to the attenuation of leukocyte-mediated damage during bacterial meningitis.[195]

The dynamic aspects of these leukocyte–endothelial cell interactions were also examined in a meningitis model by means of confocal laser scanning microscopy, a new microscopic technique with much improved depth discrimination properties. In an experimental model of pneumococcal meningitis, the behavior of rhodamine 6G–labeled leukocytes in pial vessels was determined.[196] When compared with controls, the number of adherent leukocytes significantly increased within 1 hour after intracisternal challenge with *S. pneumoniae*, with further increases noted up to 6 hours after infection. Pretreatment with dexamethasone significantly attenuated the adherence and transendothelial passage of leukocytes. In another study using this technique, heparin was found to significantly attenuate leukocyte rolling, as well as leukocyte sticking, after the induction of pneumococcal meningitis.[197] Therefore, this technique has potential usefulness in investigation of the efficacy of anti-inflammatory agents that may interfere with leukocyte adherence.

Induction of Subarachnoid Space Inflammation

The induction of a marked subarachnoid space inflammatory response by meningeal pathogens contributes to many of the pathophysiologic consequences of bacterial meningitis and therefore to significant morbidity and mortality from this disorder. Recent experimental studies have focused on the virulence factors of meningeal pathogens and the specific inflammatory mediators that they induce (Table 71–7) to learn more about the mechanisms responsible for subarachnoid space inflammation.

Despite the importance of the polysaccharide capsule of bacteria in the survival of meningeal pathogens in the intravascular and subarachnoid space, capsular polysaccharides are remarkably noninflammatory even when inoculated in purified form into the CSF of animals. In contrast, the cell walls of *S. pneumoniae* are potent inducers of CSF inflammation,[198] and even independent intracisternal inoculation of the major components of the pneumococcal cell wall, teichoic acid and peptidoglycan, induces CSF inflammation.[199] These findings lend support to the concept that release of pneumococcal cell wall lytic products during antibiotic-induced autolysis in the treatment of bacterial meningitis contributes to an accentuated host inflammatory response in the subarachnoid space. Pneumolysin, an intracellular polypeptide toxin of *S. pneumoniae* that is released after bacterial cell lysis, does not appear to play a role in postantibiotic enhancement of meningeal inflammation.[200] Subarachnoid space inflammation is also induced by the intracisternal inoculation of purified *H. influenzae* type B lipo-oligosaccharide,[201, 202] a response blocked by pretreatment of lipo-oligosaccharide with polymyxin B or neutrophil acyloxyacyl hydrolase, thus supporting the importance of the lipid A region of the lipo-oligosaccharide molecule in the induction of inflammation.

Recently, however, experimental evidence has supported the concept that pneumococcal cell wall or lipo-oligosaccharide does not directly induce subarachnoid space inflammation, but does so through the local CNS release of inflammatory mediators such as IL-1, TNF, and prostaglandins. In an experimental rat model, the intracisternal inoculation of purified *H. influenzae* type B lipo-oligosaccharide led to elevated CSF concentrations of IL-1 and TNF within 30 to 120 minutes[159]; elevated CSF concentrations of TNF have also been found in an experimental rabbit model,[203] with peak activity at 2

TABLE 71–7 Potential Factors Contributing to Subarachnoid Space Inflammation

Bacterial factors
Cell wall components
Lipo-oligosaccharide
Outer-membrane vesicles
Peptidoglycan
Host factors
Prostaglandins (PGE_2, prostacyclin)
Interleukins (IL-1β, IL-6, IL-8, IL-12)
Interferon-γ
Growth-related gene product-α
Tumor necrosis factor-α
Platelet-activating factor
Macrophage inflammatory proteins 1 and 2
Leukocyte integrins (CD18)
Leukocyte selectins
Endothelial leukocyte adhesion molecule 1
Intercellular adhesion molecule 1

hours and persistence for about 5 hours. Similar results were observed after intracisternal challenge with live *H. influenzae* type B, although TNF activity persisted longer (about 14 hours). The TNF was produced principally within the CNS (i.e., no TNF activity was detected in serum samples) in this experimental animal model system, a finding that has also been observed in patients with bacterial meningitis.[204] In addition, the finding of increased CSF concentrations of TNF-α may be specific for bacterial meningitis. The presence of TNF-α in CSF appears to be indicative of a bacterial etiology,[204–208] although the absence of TNF-α does not exclude the diagnosis of bacterial meningitis. Furthermore, elevated CSF concentrations of PGE_2, prostacyclin, IL-1β, and TNF have been found in most infants and children with bacterial meningitis.[209]

Direct intracisternal inoculation of these inflammatory mediators can also induce CSF inflammation. In an experimental rabbit model, injection of purified rabbit TNF-α or human recombinant IL-1β produced significant CSF inflammation.[210] This effect was synergistic when lower doses of each cytokine were administered simultaneously, with more rapid and significantly increased leukocyte influx than when each cytokine was administered alone. In contrast, in an experimental rabbit model of pneumococcal meningitis, the parameters of CSF leukocytosis, BBB permeability, and brain edema were induced by intracisternal inoculation of human recombinant TNF-α, MIP-1 and MIP-2, and IL-α, but not by IL-1β.[211] Leukocytosis and brain edema were inhibited by antibodies homologous to each mediator, as well as in rabbits treated with a monoclonal antibody to CD18 to render neutrophil–endothelial cell interactions dysfunctional. PAF is also inflammatory in the CNS and causes significant BBB permeability and cerebral edema[212]; at higher doses these effects are accompanied by CSF leukocytosis, which can be inhibited by the administration of antibody to the CD18 family of leukocyte adhesion molecules. In an experimental rabbit model, treatment with a PAF receptor antagonist decreased CSF cytochemical values induced by intracisternal challenge with pneumococci but not *H. influenzae*,[212] thus suggesting a specific role for PAF in pneumococcal disease. In addition, another study using an experimental rat model found that PAF augmented the meningeal inflammation and BBB permeability elicited by *H. influenzae* type B lipo-oligosaccharide.[213] It would appear that these inflammatory mediators have multiple complex and interrelated activities in the CNS that contribute to inflammation and tissue damage during bacterial meningitis.

These findings have importance with regard to outcome in patients with bacterial meningitis. Outcome after gram-negative bacillary meningitis has been correlated with the persistence of organisms and higher concentrations of endotoxin (as measured by the *Limulus* lysate assay) in CSF.[214] In children with *H. influenzae* type B meningitis, CSF concentrations of free lipopolysaccharide correlated with the Herson-Todd severity score and the number of febrile hospital days.[215] In an experimental rabbit model of *E. coli* meningitis, a single intravenous dose of an antimicrobial agent (cefotaxime, cefpirome, meropenem, chloramphenicol, or gentamicin) caused a 2- to 10-fold increase in free CSF lipopolysaccharide concentrations within 2 hours, although free lipopolysaccharide concentrations increased almost 100-fold in untreated animals 4 hours later as bacteria continued to multiply.[216] The degree of elevated CSF concentrations of IL-1β also correlated with outcome after neonatal gram-negative bacillary meningitis.[217] Furthermore, in infants and children with predominantly *H. influenzae* type B meningitis, patients with CSF concentrations of IL-1β of 500 pg/ml or more were more likely to have neurologic sequelae[218]; elevated CSF concentrations of TNF were not associated with outcome. Elevated CSF concentrations of PAF have been demonstrated in children with *H. influenzae* meningitis[219] and correlate with bacterial density and with CSF concentrations of lipo-oligosaccharide and TNF-α; these increased concentrations of TNF-α and PAF were associated with severity of disease. This association was confirmed in more recent studies that demonstrated that elevated CSF concentrations of TNF-α and soluble TNF receptor, the natural homeostatic regulator of the actions of TNF-α, were important for predicting neurologic sequelae in bacterial meningitis.[220, 221] In an experimental rabbit model, intracisternal inoculation of rabbit recombinant IL-1β and TNF-α combined with IL-1 receptor antagonist and soluble TNF receptor produced less inflammation in rabbits than after inoculation of these cytokines alone.[222] However, IL-1 receptor antagonist and soluble TNF receptor did not reduce the meningeal inflammatory response associated with intracisternal inoculation of *H. influenzae* type B lipo-oligosaccharide, thus indicating that these cytokine inhibitors may not be effective in modulating inflammation induced by a broad inflammatory stimulus such as gram-negative bacteria or their products.

More recently, the role of other cytokines in the subarachnoid space inflammatory response in bacterial meningitis has been studied. Elevated CSF concentrations of IL-6 have been observed in the CSF of patients with bacterial meningitis[223–226]; these increased concentrations occurred after the release of TNF-α and before neutrophilic infiltration into CSF.[227] IL-8, a cytokine with potent chemoattractant and activating effects on neutrophils, has been detected in the CSF of patients with bacterial meningitis[228–230]; IL-8 may also have a role as a neutrophil chemotactic factor in nonbacterial meningitis. IL-10, an anti-inflammatory protein formed by T lymphocytes and monocytes, inhibits the production of proinflammatory cytokines such as TNF-α and has been detected in the CSF of animals and humans with bacterial meningitis.[231–234] In an experimental rabbit model, IL-10 modulated CSF TNF-α concentrations in experimental meningitis caused by *H. influenzae* type B lipo-oligosaccharide, *H. influenzae* type B, or *L. monocytogenes*, an effect that was maximal when IL-10 was combined with dexamethasone.[235] Finally, production of IFN-γ was induced by IL-12 (which is produced by phagocytic cells in response to infection and stimulates adaptive immunity), with TNF-α as a costimulator, and was inhibited by IL-10[236]; this IFN-γ production may contribute to the natural immunity against microorganisms in CSF during the acute phase of bacterial meningitis. Therefore, it appears that release of inflammatory mediators in the CNS is responsible for induction of a marked subarachnoid space inflammatory response and may correlate with morbidity and mortality in patients with bacterial meningitis.

Alterations of the Blood-Brain Barrier

Bacterial meningitis has been shown to increase permeability across the BBB, which is composed of the arachnoid membrane, choroid plexus epithelium, and cerebral microvascular endothelium; the cerebral microvascular endothelium has been the site of intensive study in bacterial meningitis. An adult experimental rat model was used to examine the propensity for meningeal pathogens to induce functional and morphologic alterations of the BBB.[237] After intracisternal inoculation of either *E. coli*, *S. pneumoniae*, or *H. influenzae* type B, alterations of the BBB were found with all three pathogens and were manifested morphologically by an early and sustained increase in pinocytotic vesicle formation and progressive separation of intercellular tight junctions; these morphologic changes correlated with the functional penetration of albumin, a molecule normally excluded by an intact BBB, into the CSF. Intracisternal inoculation of an unencapsulated strain of *H. influenzae* caused an increase in pinocytotic vesicle formation without separation of intercellular tight junctions, which suggests that encapsulation of *H. influenzae* was not essential for BBB injury but facilitated its progression by avoidance of host defense mechanisms. The increased BBB permeability was observed in both normal and leukopenic animals,[238] although permeability was augmented by the presence of leukocytes. The site of BBB injury was subsequently examined by in situ tracer perfusion and immunolabeling procedures to identify the topography and microvascular exit pathways of bovine serum albumin (BSA).[239] Exit of both perfused colloidal gold–BSA and immunodetectable BSA was through open intercellular junctions of venules in the pia-arachnoid, thus specifically and topographically localizing the BBB injury in bacterial meningitis to the meningeal venules.

Because surface encapsulation was not an essential virulence factor for the production of BBB injury, BBB permeability was examined after the intracisternal inoculation of purified *H. influenzae* type B lipo-oligosaccharide.[202] Purified lipo-oligosaccharide was shown to increase BBB permeability in an experimental rat model in both a dose- and time-dependent manner (maximum change at a dose of 20 ng 4 hours after intracisternal inoculation), with a close correlation between permeability and CSF pleocytosis 4 hours after intracisternal inoculation. Increased BBB permeability was also observed after the intracisternal inoculation of *H. influenzae* type B outer-membrane vesicles,[240] an effect that was blocked by preincubation with polymyxin B but not by a monoclonal antibody directed against the oligosaccharide side chain of the lipo-oligosaccharide; no change in permeability was observed in leukopenic animals. *H. influenzae* type B peptidoglycan has also been shown to induce meningeal inflammation and BBB permeability in an infant rat model.[241]

Further experiments demonstrated that lipo-oligosaccharide did not directly mediate the increased BBB permeability but did so by inducing the production of various inflammatory cytokines (e.g., IL-1 and TNF) within the CNS; intracisternal inoculation of purified lipo-oligosaccharide led to increased CSF concentrations of both IL-1 and TNF within 30 to 120 minutes.[159] Furthermore, the intracisternal inoculation of human recombinant IL-1β into rats led to a peak increase in BBB permeability about 3 hours after inoculation, earlier than the peak response obtained after inoculation with lipo-oligosaccharide (4 hours).[242] No permeability changes were induced after the intracisternal inoculation of human recombinant TNF-α, although all available evidence suggests that these cytokines act synergistically inasmuch as inoculation with submaximal doses of IL-1β plus TNF-α, at concentrations that produced no changes individually, enhanced BBB permeability. In contrast, in a study of patients with bacterial meningitis,[243] CSF concentrations of TNF-α, but not IL-1β correlated with BBB disruption (assessed by CSF protein concentrations); synergy between IL-1β and TNF-α was also noted in this study.

The effects of lipo-oligosaccharide on BBB permeability in the experimental rat model have also been examined in an in vitro model by growing purified preparations of cerebral microvascular endothelium on a semipermeable support.[244–246] Several investigators have demonstrated increased permeability across this monolayer after exposure to *H. influenzae* type B or purified lipo-oligosaccharide. The mechanism for this increased permeability is unclear, however. It may be related to a direct cytotoxic effect of lipo-oligosaccharide,[246] for instance, through effects of serum components such as lipo-oligosaccharide–binding protein on the cerebral microvascular endothelium,[247] or could be related to lipo-oligosaccharide–induced formation of various second messengers (e.g., cyclic adenosine or guanosine monophosphate) by endothelial cells.[159]

Increased Intracranial Pressure

Cerebral edema is the major element contributing to increased intracranial pressure during bacterial meningitis and may result in life-threatening cerebral herniation and other complications.[159] The origin of the cerebral edema may be vasogenic, cytotoxic, interstitial, or any combination; all three elements probably contribute to cerebral edema during bacterial meningitis. Vasogenic cerebral edema is primarily a consequence of increased BBB permeability; cytotoxic cerebral edema results from swelling of the cellular elements of the brain, most likely through release of toxic factors from neutrophils, bacteria, or both; and interstitial cerebral edema reflects obstruction of the flow of normal CSF as in hydrocephalus. The last factor has been examined in an experimental rabbit model of pneumococcal or *E. coli* meningitis in which the CSF outflow resistance (defined as factors that inhibit the flow of CSF from the subarachnoid space to the major dural sinuses) was markedly elevated and remained elevated for as long as 2 weeks despite rapid CSF sterilization with penicillin therapy.[248]

These concepts have been examined in greater detail in an experimental animal model of pneumococcal meningitis by measuring brain water content (indicative of cerebral edema if elevated), CSF lactate concentrations, and CSF pressure.[249] All three parameters were elevated in infected animals. Although treatment with ampicillin rapidly sterilized the CSF and normalized the brain water content and CSF pressure, the CSF lactate concentration remained elevated. The bacterial virulence factor responsible for the production of brain edema was subsequently examined in an experimental animal model of *E. coli* meningitis in which therapy with cefotaxime, but not chloramphenicol induced a marked rise in CSF endotoxin concentrations that was associated with increased brain water content.[250] The peptidoglycan of the *H. influenzae* cell wall also induced cerebral edema without perturbing the other parameters of inflammation (i.e., increased BBB permeability),[251] which suggests that peptidoglycan induces cytotoxic rather than vasogenic cerebral edema. Neutrophils appeared to contribute to the development of cerebral edema if adequately stimulated,[252] although the parameters of increased intracranial pressure and increased CSF concentrations of lactate and protein were unrelated to the presence of neutrophils. However, this area remains controversial because neutrophils are required for the increased BBB permeability seen in response to the intracisternal inoculation of bacterial virulence factors and inflammatory mediators.[202, 242]

Variability among bacterial strains may also be an important determinant in production of the subarachnoid space inflammatory response and brain edema in bacterial meningitis. Intracisternal inoculation of three different pneumococcal isolates resulted in pronounced differences in the pathophysiologic profiles 24 hours after challenge.[253] When pneumococcal cell wall fragments were inoculated intracisternally, the chemical composition of the fragments, specifically the degree of teichoication, influenced the induction of brain edema. In a subsequent study in an experimental rabbit model,[254] serotype-specific characteristics of pneumococci were found to play a major role in the subarachnoid space inflammatory process, although significant differences in brain water content were observed only with one of the serotypes tested. It is unclear, however, whether these differences affect the clinical expression of disease in patients with bacterial meningitis.

The infusion of hypertonic mannitol to treat increased intracranial pressure has been evaluated in a rabbit model of *H. influenzae* type B meningitis.[255] In all animals, mannitol consistently reduced intracisternal pressure, although the magnitude of reduction was greater in infected animals and brain water content was no different in mannitol-treated animals than in untreated ones. In contrast, in an experimental rat model of pneumococcal meningitis, mannitol modulated changes in cerebral blood flow, intracranial pressure, and brain water content,[256] perhaps by a mechanism of scavenging hydroxyl radicals, which have been shown to be involved in the pathogenesis and pathophysiology of cerebral ischemia and neuronal injury in bacterial meningitis (see later).

Alterations in Cerebral Blood Flow

Bacterial meningitis exerts profound effects on blood vessels coursing through the subarachnoid space,[159] and the resulting vasculitis leads to narrowing and/or thrombosis of cerebral blood vessels and the propensity for ischemia and/or infarction of underlying brain. In combination with increased intracranial pressure, these changes may result in altered cerebral blood flow in patients with bacterial meningitis. An infant rhesus monkey model of *H. influenzae* meningitis demonstrated that cerebral cortical hypoperfusion occurs during meningitis and causes relative cerebral anoxia.[170] Cerebrovascular autoregulation, in which cerebral blood flow increases when systemic pressure is increased and decreases when blood pressure is lowered, is also lost during experimental bacterial meningitis.[257] Furthermore, studies in an experimental rabbit model of pneumococcal meningitis have demonstrated that animals given a lower intravenous fluid regimen (50 ml/kg per 24 hours) of normal saline had a lower mean arterial pressure, lower cerebral blood flow, and a higher concentration of CSF lactate than did animals that received a higher fluid regimen (150 ml/kg per 24 hours).[258] In the first 4 to 6 hours of antibiotic administration, rabbits receiving lower fluid regimens had a significant decrease in mean arterial pressure and cerebral blood flow and a significant increase in CSF lactate concentrations when compared with rabbits receiving higher fluid regimens. These results, in combination with other experimental studies that have noted an increase in cerebral blood flow within the first few hours of intracisternal inoculation of either live pneumococci or pneumococcal cell wall fragments,[259] have suggested that maintenance of adequate intravascular volume and minimization of stimuli that increase systemic blood pressure may be important in the treatment of bacterial meningitis. These findings may also be of potential clinical relevance inasmuch as inadvertent increases in mean arterial pressure directly increase cerebral blood flow and intracranial pressure and depletion of intravascular volume with decreases in mean arterial pressure can cause parallel decreases in cerebral blood flow and a reduction in substrate delivery to the brain. Therefore, the brain is at risk from either hypoperfusion or hyperperfusion. As demonstrated by near-infrared spectroscopy in conjunction with measurement of cerebral blood flow in an experimental rabbit model of pneumococcal meningitis, infected animals had a relative increase in the deoxygenated hemoglobin fraction and a decrease in the oxygenated hemoglobin fraction,[260] thus supporting the possibility of cerebral venous engorgement in bacterial meningitis, which may contribute to intracranial hypertension in this disorder.

Additional studies have examined the importance of the subarachnoid space inflammatory response in alterations of cerebral blood flow during bacterial meningitis. In an experimental rabbit model of *H. influenzae* type B meningitis, CSF leukocytes were found to not be reponsible for the hyperemic response,[261] which suggests that cerebral hyperemia in bacterial meningitis is induced directly by bacterial components or indirectly by components of the inflammatory cascade. More recently, endothelin (which has been found to regulate vascular tone and integrity and act as a mediator of inflammation) has been investigated as a possible mediator of cerebrovascular complications in bacterial meningitis. In an experimental rat model of pneumococcal meningitis, endothelin contributed to the increased cerebral blood flow (as measured by laser Doppler flowmetry), intracranial pressure, brain water content, and CSF pleocytosis.[262] Elevated CSF concentrations of endothelin have also been found in patients during the acute stage of bacterial meningitis,[263] which suggests a potential role for endothelin in mediation of meningitis-induced cerebral hypoperfusion and brain infarction.

Cerebral blood flow has been measured in patients with bacterial meningitis. In an early study,[264] measurement of cerebral blood flow (by the xenon 133 intra-arterial injection method) revealed a 30 to 40% reduction in average total blood flow in five patients with pneumococcal meningitis (mean age of 54 years), but not in five patients with meningococcal meningitis (mean age of 20 years). An inverse relationship between cerebral blood flow and intracranial pressure has been observed in infants with bacterial meningitis[265]; among eight patients, alterations were noted only in the four older infants (age range of 3 to 10 months) and not in the four neonates (age range of 5 to 30 days) in whom no changes in cerebral blood flow velocity were detected. In another study of 17 children (aged 8 days to 6 years) with bacterial meningitis, transcranial Doppler ultrasound monitoring demonstrated an improvement in cerebral blood flow velocity with resolution of meningitis.[266] This observation suggests that in the early phase of bacterial meningitis, increased cerebrovascular resistance may contribute to a relative impairment in cerebral perfusion; transcranial Doppler ultrasound may be a useful technique for the early detection of deterioration in cerebral hemodynamics.

In a subsequent study in 20 children seriously ill with bacterial meningitis,[267] total and regional cerebral blood flow measured by stable xenon computed tomography (CT) revealed a global decrease in flow and even more regional variability. Although autoregulation of cerebral blood flow was preserved in the patients studied, hyperventilation reduced flow below the ischemic threshold, which raises important concerns about the routine use of hyperventilation in the management of increased intracranial pressure in patients with bacterial meningitis.[268] In another study of 86 adult patients with bacterial meningitis,[269] cerebral angiography was performed on 27 patients who had focal deficits (either clinically, on cranial CT, or both) and who had persistent coma without an explained cause despite 3 days of antimicrobial therapy. Thirteen of the patients who underwent angiography had alterations in their blood vessel system; the prognosis in these patients was poor. However, definitive changes in cerebral blood flow during bacterial meningitis are controversial and may vary with the stage of disease. These blood flow alterations may lead to regional hypoxia, increased lactate concentrations in the brain secondary to utilization of glucose by anaerobic glycolysis, and CSF acidosis, which may be a precursor to encephalopathy.[270]

Neuronal Injury

Recent data have suggested that oxygen radicals may contribute to the increased brain water content, intracranial pressure, and changes in regional blood flow (see later) in bacterial meningitis. In an experimental rat model of pneumococcal meningitis after intracisternal inoculation of live pneumococci or pneumococcal cell wall components,[271] the increases in brain water content and intracranial pressure were prevented, and the increase in regional blood flow was significantly attenuated by conjugated superoxide dismutase and deferoxamine. Catalase, which eliminates hydrogen peroxide, also significantly attenuated the increase in regional blood flow and brain water content, although only a trend toward a reduction in intracranial pressure was observed.[272] Furthermore, in a neonatal rat model of group B streptococcal meningitis, generation of reactive oxygen intermediates (localized to cells constituting the subarachnoid and ventricular inflammation and to the cerebral vasculature) was a major contributor to cerebral ischemia and necrotic and apoptotic neuronal injury[273]; the free radical scavenger α-phenyl-tert-butyl nitrone inhibited the biologic effect of the reactive oxygen intermediates, thereby improving cerebral cortical perfusion and reducing the extent of both necrotic and apoptotic neuronal injury. It also appeared that TNF-α plays a critical role in neuronal apoptosis in the hippocampus in rats with group B streptococcal meningitis,[274] although it was not essential for the development of inflammation and cortical injury in this model.

Evidence has suggested that reactive nitrogen intermediates may also play a role in the inflammatory process and other pathophysiologic events during bacterial meningitis.[275, 276] In an experimental rat model of pneumococcal meningitis utilizing treatment with the nitric oxide synthase inhibitor *N*-nitro-L-arginine, it was determined that nitric oxide accounted for the regional cerebral blood flow changes and pial arteriolar vasodilation in the early phase of meningitis and was involved as a mediator of brain edema and meningeal inflammation[277]; stimulation of cerebral endothelial cells with pneumococci released nitric oxide, presumably via inducible nitric oxide synthase. In addition, inhibition of the neuronal nitric oxide synthase pathway with 7-nitroindazole also prevented pneumococci-induced pial arteriolar vasodilation.[278] Similarly, in another rat model of meningitis, CSF concentrations of nitrite (a major metabolic product of nitric oxide in vivo) rose after challenge with live *H. influenzae* type B or *H. influenzae* type B lipo-oligosaccharide, in direct correlation with increased permeability of the BBB.[279] This result was confirmed by another study in an experimental rat model in which excessive nitric oxide production contributed to BBB disruption[280]; administration of aminoguanidine, an inhibitor of inducible nitric oxide synthase, during meningeal inflammation significantly diminished meningeal nitric oxide production, attenuated white blood cell migration into the CSF, and maintained normal BBB permeability.

A subsequent study also demonstrated that inhibition of nitric oxide production with aminoguanidine increased cortical hypoperfusion and ischemic neuronal injury,[281] which suggests that nitric oxide attenuates the development of cortical ischemia and neuronal injury in bacterial meningitis. Locally produced inflammatory mediators may also have effects on these processes in bacterial meningitis. Bradykinin has been shown to be involved as a mediator in the early phase of pneumococcal meningitis in the rat and contributes to the increase in regional blood flow, intracranial pressure, and brain water content[282]; administration of a bradykinin B_2 receptor antagonist may prevent nitric oxide release. In addition, systemic administration of IL-10 may interfere with the production of reactive nitrogen intermediates, thereby attenuating the pathophysiologic changes (increased regional cerebral blood flow, brain water content, intracranial pressure, and CSF white blood cell count) during the early phase of experimental pneumococcal meningitis.[283]

The role of nitric oxide has also been examined in patients with bacterial meningitis. It has been suggested that nitric oxide may contribute to anaerobic glycolysis and neurologic damage in children with bacterial meningitis.[284] The induction of nitric oxide synthase, and consequently the production of nitric oxide, may be induced by TNF in CSF,[285] which in turn mediates the increased BBB permeability in bacterial meningitis.

Finally, a potential role for excitatory amino acids in the pathogenesis of brain injury in bacterial meningitis has been proposed. In an experimental rabbit model, intracisternal inoculation of *S. pneumoniae* led to significant increases in CSF concentrations of glutamate, aspartate, glycine, taurine, and alanine[286]; elevated glutamate concentrations were also found in the brain extracellular space, which suggests that excitotoxic neuronal injury may play a role in bacterial meningitis. In an experimental rat model of group B streptococcal meningitis, administration of kynurenic acid attenuated the toxic effects of glutamate by inhibition of neuronal excitatory amino acid receptors, and treated animals showed significantly less neuronal injury in the cortex and hippocampus than did untreated controls,[287] thus demonstrating the important contribution of glutamate to neurotoxicity in bacterial meningitis. Excess CSF concentrations of glutamate have also been detected in patients with bacterial meningitis[288, 289]; a prolonged increase in CSF glutamate concentrations may predict a poor outcome in patients with bacterial meningitis, possibly because of the sustained neurotoxic effects of this excitatory neurotransmitter.

CLINICAL FEATURES

Viral Meningitis

Enteroviruses. The clinical manifestations of enteroviral meningitis depend on host age and immune status.[2] In neonates (2 weeks of age or younger) with proven enteroviral meningitis, fever is a ubiquitous finding and is usually accompanied by any combination of vomiting, anorexia, rash, and upper respiratory symptoms and signs. Neurologic involvement may be associated with nuchal rigidity and a bulging anterior fontanelle, although infants younger than 1 year are less likely to demonstrate meningeal signs. Mental status may be altered, but focal neurologic signs are uncommon. A more severe form of meningoencephalitis may be seen in neonates, who appear to be at greatest risk for morbidity and mortality (rates as high as 74 and 10% respectively),[290] particularly when symptoms and signs develop during the first day of life (after presumed transplacental transmission of the virus). With disease progression, hepatic necrosis, myocarditis, and necrotizing enterocolitis may develop. Findings in the CNS are of an encephalitis associated with seizures and focal neurologic findings. Lack of humoral antibody may contribute to the severity of neonatal infection.

The findings in neonates contrast with the clinical findings of enteroviral meningitis beyond the neonatal period (older than 2 weeks), in which severe disease and poor outcome are rare. In this patient population the onset of illness is usually sudden, with fever present in 76 to 100% of patients[291]; the fever may be biphasic, initially appearing with nonspecific constitutional symptoms, disappearing, and then reappearing with the onset of meningeal signs. More than half of patients have nuchal rigidity. Headache (often severe and frontal in location) is nearly always present in adults; photophobia is also common. Nonspecific symptoms and signs include vomiting, anorexia, rash, diarrhea, cough, upper respiratory findings (especially pharyngitis), and myalgias. Other clues to the presence of enteroviral disease, in addition to the time of year and known epidemic disease in the community, include the presence of exanthems, myopericarditis, conjunctivitis, and specifically recognizable enteroviral syndromes such as pleurodynia, herpangina, and hand-foot-and-mouth disease.[1] In addition, specific clinical stigmata may be associated with certain enteroviral serotypes.[2] For example, echovirus 9 is associated with scattered maculopapular rashes. Herpangina, in particular the finding of painful vesicles on the posterior of the oropharynx, is associated with coxsackievirus A; the presence of pericarditis or pleurisy may identify coxsackievirus B. The duration of illness in enteroviral meningitis is usually less than 1 week, with many patients reporting improvement after lumbar puncture,[292] presumably as a result of a reduction in intracranial pressure.

A unique clinical situation is seen in children and adults with absent or deficient humoral immunity that impairs clearance of enteroviruses. In persons who are agammaglobulinemic, a chronic enteroviral meningitis or meningoencephalitis may develop and last several years, often with a fatal outcome.[293] In about half of these patients a rheumatologic syndrome, usually dermatomyositis, also develops, probably as a direct result of enteroviral invasion of affected tissues.

Mumps Virus. In patients with mumps, CNS symptoms usually follow the onset of parotitis, when present, by about 5 days. The most frequent clinical manifestation of mumps CNS infection is the triad of fever, vomiting, and headache[12] (Table 71–8). The fever is usually high and lasts for 72 to 96 hours. Salivary gland enlargement is present in only about 50% of patients. Other findings include neck stiffness, lethargy or somnolence, and abdominal pain. Most patients have signs of meningitis, but no evidence of cortical dysfunction. Defervescence is usually accompanied by clinical recovery, and in uncomplicated cases, the total duration of illness is 7 to 10 days. Rarely, mumps may cause encephalitis, seizures, polyradiculitis, polyneuritis, cranial nerve palsies, myelitis, Guillain-Barré syndrome, and fatality.[12]

Lymphocytic Choriomeningitis Virus. Lymphocytic choriomeningitis virus infection begins with nonspecific viral symptoms. After a brief period of improvement, severe headache, photophobia, lightheadedness, lumbar myalgias, and pharyngitis develop in approximately 15% of patients.[1] Occasionally, orchitis, arthritis, myopericarditis, and alopecia are also seen, usually as late manifestations.

Herpesviruses. Meningitis associated with herpes simplex virus type 2 infection is usually characterized by stiff neck, headache, and fever.[21] In one review of 27 patients with herpes simplex virus type

TABLE 71–8 Initial Symptoms and Signs in Patients with Central Nervous System Mumps

Symptom or Sign	Relative Frequency (%)
Fever	88–100
Vomiting	68–94
Headache	47–88
Salivary gland swelling	47–62
Meningismus	43–93
Lethargy	28–69
Abdominal pain	14–23
Seizures	14–18

Adapted from Gnann JW Jr. Meningitis and encephalitis caused by mumps virus. In: Scheld WM, Whitley RJ, Durack DT, eds. Infections of the Central Nervous System. 2nd ed. Philadelphia: Lippincott-Raven; 1997:169–180.

2 meningitis,[27] neurologic complications were found in 37% of cases and consisted of urinary retention, dysesthesias, paresthesias, neuralgia, motor weakness, paraparesis, concentration difficulties of about 3 months' duration, and impaired hearing. All complications, however, subsided within 6 months in all patients. Recurrent meningitis was documented in five patients. Pharyngitis, lymphadenopathy, and splenomegaly should suggest Epstein-Barr virus infection. A diffuse vesiculopustular rash may be seen in meningitis caused by varicella-zoster virus.

Human Immunodeficiency Virus. HIV-infected patients may present with a typical aseptic meningitis syndrome associated with acute infection (i.e., the mononucleosis-like syndrome).[38, 39, 41] In addition, some patients may present with an atypical aseptic meningitis that is often chronic, tends to recur, and often includes cranial neuropathies (usually cranial nerves V, VII, and VIII) or long-tract findings.[294] The most common features are headache, fever, and meningeal signs. The illness is self-limited or recurrent rather than progressive.

Bacterial Meningitis

Patients with bacterial meningitis classically present with fever, headache, meningismus, and signs of cerebral dysfunction (i.e., confusion, delirium, or a declining level of consciousness ranging from lethargy to coma)[73, 295, 296] (Table 71–9). In a review of 493 cases of acute bacterial meningitis in adults,[46] the classic triad of fever, nuchal rigidity, and change in mental status was found only in two thirds of patients, but all had at least one of these findings. The meningismus may be subtle, marked, or acccompanied by Kernig's, Brudzinski's, or both signs.[297] Kernig's sign is elicited with the patient in the supine position, with the thigh flexed on the abdomen and the knee flexed. The leg is then passively extended, and in the presence of meningeal inflammation, the patient resists leg extension; this technique differs somewhat from the maneuver as first described by Kernig, in which the patient was initially placed in the seated position. Several signs were described by Brudzinski, although the best known is the nape-of-the-neck sign, in which passive flexion of the neck results in flexion of the hips and knees. However, these signs are elicited in only about 50% of adult patients with bacterial meningitis, and their absence does not rule out the diagnosis. Cranial nerve palsies (especially those involving cranial nerves III, IV, VI, and VII) and focal cerebral signs are seen in 10 to 20% of cases. Cranial nerve palsies probably develop as the nerve becomes enveloped by exudate in the arachnoid sheath surrounding the nerve, or they may be a sign of increased intracranial pressure. Seizures occur in about 30% of patients. Focal neurologic deficits and seizures arise from cortical and subcortical ischemia, which results from inflammation and thrombosis of blood vessels, often within the subarachnoid space. Hemiparesis may also result from the presence of a large subdural effusion and arises when infection in the adjacent subarachnoid space leads to increased permeability of the thin-walled capillaries and veins of the inner layer of the dura; this condition is usually self-limited, although an enlarging effusion can lead to a mass effect with resultant hemiparesis. Papilledema is seen in less than 1% of cases early in infection, and its presence should suggest an alternative diagnosis. With disease progression, signs of increased intracranial pressure may develop, including coma, hypertension, bradycardia, and palsy of cranial nerve III.

TABLE 71–9 Initial Symptoms and Signs in Patients with Bacterial Meningitis

Symptom or Sign	Relative Frequency (%)
Headache	≥90
Fever	≥90
Meningismus	≥85
Altered sensorium	>80
Kernig's sign	≥50
Brudzinski's sign	≥50
Vomiting	~35
Seizure	~30
Focal findings	10–20
Papilledema	<1

A specific etiologic diagnosis in patients with bacterial meningitis may be suggested by certain symptoms or signs. About 50% of patients with meningococcemia, with or without meningitis, present with a prominent rash located principally on the extremities.[296] Early in the course of illness, the rash is typically erythematous and macular, but it quickly evolves into a petechial phase with further coalescence into a purpuric form. The rash often matures rapidly, with new petechial lesions appearing during the physical examination. In one review of the clinical features of 255 patients with acute meningococcal meningitis,[298] a petechial rash was observed in three quarters of the patients; the rash was more commonly seen in children and adults younger than 30 years (81%) than in patients 30 years and older (62%). A similar rash may also be seen in splenectomized patients with rapidly overwhelming sepsis caused by *S. pneumoniae* or *H. influenzae* type B. In patients who have suffered a basilar skull fracture in which a dural fistula is produced between the subarachnoid space and nasal cavity, paranasal sinuses, or middle ear, a common finding is rhinorrhea or otorrhea secondary to a CSF leak[79]; in these patients, meningitis may be recurrent and is most commonly caused by *S. pneumoniae*. Patients with *L. monocytogenes* meningitis have an increased tendency to have seizures and focal deficits early in the course of infection, and some patients may present with ataxia, cranial nerve palsies, or nystagmus secondary to rhomboencephalitis[80, 81, 84, 85]; however, patients with *Listeria* meningitis may not present with any focal signs.

Some categories of patients may not manifest many of the classic symptoms and signs of bacterial meningitis.[299] For example, neonates with bacterial meningitis usually do not have meningismus.[94] Clinical clues to the presence of meningitis in neonates are temperature instability (hypothermia or hyperthermia), listlessness, high-pitched crying, fretfulness, lethargy, refusal to feed, weak suck, irritability, jaundice, vomiting, diarrhea, or respiratory distress. A change in the child's affect or state of alertness is one of the most important signs of meningitis. A bulging fontanelle (seen in one third of cases) usually occurs late during the course of illness; seizures are observed in 40% of neonates with bacterial meningitis. In children 1 to 4 years of age, fever (94%), vomiting (82%), and nuchal rigidity (77%) are the most common initial symptoms.[300] Elderly patients, especially those with underlying conditions (e.g., diabetes mellitus or cardiopulmonary disease), may present insidiously with lethargy or obtundation, no fever, and variable signs of meningeal inflammation. In one review,[301] confusion was very common in elderly patients on initial examination and occurred in 92 and 78% of those with pneumococcal and gram-negative bacillary meningitis, respectively. Elderly patients may also present with an antecedent or concurrent bronchitis, pneumonia, or paranasal sinusitis. The diagnosis of bacterial meningitis in neutropenic patients requires a high index of suspicion because symptoms and signs may initially be subtle because of the impaired ability of the patient to mount a subarachnoid space inflammatory response.[302] In patients with head trauma, the symptoms and signs of meningitis may be present as a result of the underlying injury and not meningitis.[79] In all of these subgroups of patients, altered or changed mental status should not be ascribed to other causes until bacterial meningitis has been excluded by CSF examination.

Cerebrospinal Fluid Shunt Infections

The clinical features of CSF shunt infection can be quite variable and depend on the pathogenesis of infection, organism virulence, and type of shunt.[303] The most frequent symptoms are headache, nausea, lethargy, and change in mental status; these symptoms occur as a result of shunt malfunction. Fever is reported in as few as 14% to as many as 92% of cases, so its absence cannot be interpreted as a factor against infection. Pain, often related to infection at the peritoneal or pleural endings of the shunt, may be absent in up to 60% of infections. Symptoms and signs of CSF shunt infection may be referable to either the proximal or distal portions of the shunt. Infection beginning in the proximal portion of the shunt (i.e., the catheter within the CSF space) results in meningitis or ventriculitis in about 30% of cases.[303, 304] However, meningeal symptoms should not be expected with infected ventricular shunts because communication between the infected ventricles and the CSF in contact with the meninges is usually absent. Infections with symptoms referable to the distal portion of the shunt are more specific to terminus location: infected vascular shunts lead to bacteremia, whereas shunts that terminate in the pleural or peritoneal space lead to an inflammatory response in the absorbing tissue (i.e., pleuritis or peritonitis). Furthermore, some shunt infections are insidious and cause few or no symptoms, perhaps only an intermittent low-grade fever or general malaise.

Spirochetal Meningitis

Treponema pallidum. The clinical features of neurosyphilis that have been described are based on studies compiled before the availability of penicillin, and it is not known whether the clinical findings of symptomatic neurosyphilis have been modified in the antibiotic era or by associated HIV infection.[124] Although the clinical features of neurosyphilis are numerous, only patients with acute meningitis and meningovascular syphilis are discussed here.

Patients with syphilitic meningitis usually present similarly to patients with other forms of aseptic meningitis and have complaints of headache, nausea, and vomiting; in one series, these complaints were present in 91% of patients.[305] Meningismus occurred in 59% and fever in less than half of the patients with syphilitic meningitis. Seizures occurred in 17% of patients, whereas cranial nerve palsies were found in 45% of cases (most commonly cranial nerves VII and VIII, followed by II, III, VI, and V). Focal abnormalities such as hemiplegia, aphasia, and mental status changes were seen less commonly. Syphilitic meningitis rarely affects the spinal cord.

Meningovascular syphilis is clinically distinguished from syphilitic meningitis temporally and on the basis of focal neurologic findings as a result of focal syphilitic arteritis, which almost always occurs in association with meningeal inflammation.[124, 125, 306] Most patients experience weeks to months of episodic prodromal symptoms and signs, including headache or vertiginous episodes, personality changes (e.g., apathy or inattention), behavioral changes (e.g., irritability or memory impairment), insomnia, or seizures. Focal deficits, which reflect episodes of ischemia in regions of the brain by involved blood vessels (usually in the distribution of the middle cerebral artery), may also occur; if untreated, these deficits may progress to a stroke syndrome with attendant irreversible neurologic deficits.

Coinfection with HIV may modify the clinical spectrum of syphilis. Case reports and small series have suggested that patients with HIV infection are more likely to progress to neurosyphilis and have accelerated disease courses.[126–129, 307] However, few clinical data currently support these hypotheses. In one study of HIV-infected and HIV-uninfected patients with syphilis at sexually transmitted disease clinics in Baltimore,[308] no significant differences were observed in clinical stage or in disease progression.

Borrelia burgdorferi. Meningitis is the most important neurologic abnormality of acute disseminated Lyme disease, usually following erythema migrans by 2 to 10 weeks[131]; however, only about 40% (range of 10 to 90%) of cases of Lyme meningitis are preceded by this characteristic rash.[133, 309] Headache is the single most common symptom (30 to 90% of patients) in Lyme meningitis, whereas neck stiffness is seen in only 10 to 20% of cases.[131] Photophobia, nausea, and vomiting are intermediate in frequency between headache and neck stiffness. About two thirds of patients have accompanying systemic symptoms, including malaise, fatigue, myalgias, fever, arthralgias, and involuntary weight loss. In untreated cases, the duration of symptoms ranges from 1 to 9 months. Patients typically experience recurrent attacks of meningeal symptoms lasting several weeks and alternating with similar periods of milder symptoms.[131–133, 309]

About half of patients with Lyme meningitis have mild cerebral symptoms consisting most commonly of somnolence, emotional lability, depression, impaired memory and concentration, and behavioral symptoms.[131–133, 309] These symptoms may fluctuate in severity in untreated patients before resolution. Transverse myelitis, spastic paraparesis or quadriparesis, disturbances of micturition, and Babinski's sign are also reported during this stage. Approximately 50% of patients also have cranial neuropathies. Facial nerve palsy is the most common (80 to 90%) of the cranial nerve palsies overall and occurs with rapid onset (often in 1 to 2 days), frequently accompanied by slight ipsilateral facial numbness or tingling or ipsilateral ear or jaw pain. The facial palsy is bilateral in 30 to 70% of cases, although the two sides are affected asynchronously in most cases. Other cranial nerves affected less commonly are cranial nerves II, III, the sensory portion of V, VI, and the acoustic portion of VIII. Recovery usually takes place within 2 months.

Protozoal and Helminthic Meningitis

Amebas. Primary amebic meningoencephalitis occurs in two forms.[135, 136] The acute form (incubation period of 3 to 8 days) is characterized by the sudden onset of high fever, photophobia, headache, and progression to stupor or coma and is usually indistinguishable from acute bacterial meningitis, although focal signs and seizures are more common in amebic meningoencephalitis. Because of early involvement of the olfactory area, early symptoms of abnormal smell or taste may be reported. Confusion, irritability, and restlessness progress to delirium, stupor, and finally, coma. Death in untreated patients generally occurs within 2 to 3 days from the onset of symptoms.

In contrast, the subacute or chronic form of primary amebic meningoencephalitis is manifested more insidiously by low-grade fever, headache, and focal signs (e.g., hemiparesis, aphasia, cranial nerve palsies, visual field disturbances, diplopia, ataxia, seizures)[135, 136]; the olfactory bulbs are usually spared. Deterioration occurs over a period of 2 to 4 weeks until death. However, longer durations of illness have also been reported (range of 5 to 18 months).

Angiostrongylus cantonensis. Symptoms of meningitis begin 6 to 30 days after the ingestion of raw mollusks or other sources of the parasite.[110, 310] Findings include severe headache (90%), stiff neck (56%), paresthesias (54%), and vomiting (56%). Moderate fever is present in about half of the cases.

DIAGNOSIS

Viral Meningitis

Cerebrospinal Fluid Examination. CSF pleocytosis is almost always present in patients with enteroviral meningitis, although some enteroviruses have been isolated from young infants with clinical evidence of meningitis but no CSF white blood cells.[1, 2] The cell count is usually 100 to 1000/mm^3, although counts in the several thousands have also been reported; higher CSF white blood cell counts have been associated with a greater likelihood of isolating the causative enterovirus.[311] Early in infection, neutrophils may dominate the CSF profile, although this situation quickly gives way to a lymphocytic predominance over the first 6 to 48 hours. Elevated CSF protein and decreased CSF glucose concentrations, if present, are usually mild, although extreme degrees of both have been reported. A specific virologic diagnosis of enteroviral meningitis depends on isolation of the virus from the CSF in tissue culture,[312, 313] although the sensitivity for enteroviral serotypes is only 65 to 75%, largely a result of the inability to grow many coxsackievirus A serotypes, which require suckling mouse inoculations.[2] The difficulty in isolation of enteroviruses from CSF may also relate to the low titers of enterovirus in CSF (as low as a median tissue culture infective dose of 10^1 to 10^3 per milliliter of CSF). The mean time for CSF enteroviruses to grow is 3.7 to 8.2 days. Although isolation of a nonpolio enterovirus from the throat or rectum of a patient with aseptic meningitis is suggestive of an etiologic diagnosis, the mean shedding periods from those sites after infection are 1 week and several weeks, respectively. In addition, viral shedding can occur in 7.5% of healthy controls during enterovirus epidemics.[1] Therefore, shedding from a past infection cannot be ruled out. Furthermore, a recent study found that non-CSF viral cultures were not helpful in predicting enteroviral CNS infection inasmuch as enteroviruses were isolated at the same frequency from non-CSF sites in infants in whom enteroviruses were cultured from CSF as in hospitalized infants with an acute illness whose CSF was negative.[314] Follow-up acute and convalescent serologic testing for the specific isolated strain may confirm the etiologic diagnosis.[1]

Rapid diagnosis of enterovirus infection by immunoassay techniques has been hampered by the lack of a common antigen among the various serotypes and the low concentrations of virus in body fluids.[1, 2] However, several recent studies have reported success with the use of polyclonal or monoclonal antibodies. Tests to detect specific IgM enteroviral antibodies have also been attempted,[315] although the specificity of some of the tests has been unsatisfactory. Complementary DNA nucleic acid probes have been prepared and can detect multiple enteroviral serotypes, but the clinical sensitivity was only 33% or less,[2] undoubtedly a result of low titers of enteroviruses in CSF specimens from patients with aseptic meningitis. PCR is the most promising alternative to viral culture for the diagnosis of enteroviral meningitis. All the primers are directed at highly conserved regions of the 5′ noncoding region of the viral genome and designed for reverse transcription combined with PCR. Enteroviral reverse transcription–PCR has been tested in clinical settings by numerous investigators and found to be more sensitive than culture and 94 to 100% specific for the diagnosis of enteroviral meningitis.[2, 316–319]

Patients with mumps meningitis almost always have CSF pleocytosis (usually less than 500/mm^3), primarily mononuclear cells (greater than 80% lymphocytes in 80 to 90% of patients)[13]; the pleocytosis may persist for weeks. CSF protein levels are reported in some series to be normal in more than half of patients with mumps meningitis.[12] The CSF glucose content is normal in most patients, but it may be depressed in up to 25% of cases.[12, 15] Complement fixation and hemagglutination inhibition on serum specimens are the most reliable serologic tests for the diagnosis of mumps. Testing of paired acute and convalescent sera should demonstrate a diagnostic fourfold rise in mumps antibody titer. Mumps virus can be grown from CSF in tissue culture for at least 1 week after the onset of disease, but the sensitivity of this technique is highly variable (30 to 50% if collected from CSF early during the course of mumps CNS infection).[12] Application of molecular diagnostic techniques such as PCR may make the diagnosis of mumps faster and more reliable in the future.

The CSF of patients with meningitis caused by lymphocytic choriomeningitis virus typically shows a lymphocytic pleocytosis (usually less than 750/mm^3, although counts up to several thousand may be seen).[1, 320] Hypoglycorrhachia is seen in up to 25% of cases. No rapid detection method is available. The virus may be cultured from blood and CSF early in infection and later from urine. The diagnosis is usually made by a fourfold rise between acute and convalescent sera.

Patients with herpes simplex virus type 2 meningitis also have a lymphocytic meningitis (less than 500/mm^3) and a normal glucose content.[1] The virus has been cultured from the CSF and buffy coat of some patients. PCR appears promising for the diagnosis of CNS infections caused by herpes simplex virus. With PCR, herpes simplex virus type 2 has been strongly associated with typical cases of Mollaret's meningitis in patients without symptoms or signs of genital infection.[32] PCR has also been used to confirm the presence of varicella-zoster viral DNA in the CSF of patients with herpes zoster meningitis.[321, 322] The CSF in HIV-infected patients during the acute retroviral syndrome typically shows a mild lymphocytic pleocytosis (<200/mm^3), mildly elevated protein concentrations, and a normal or slightly decreased glucose content[41, 294]; these CSF parameters improve and sometimes resolve within 2 weeks. HIV has been isolated from the CSF of some patients with neurologic disease,[41, 323] although it can be isolated from HIV-infected patients without neurologic symptoms or signs.[323, 324] HIV RNA has also been detected in the CSF of patients with meningitic disease.[325, 326] A few mononuclear cells and elevated protein concentrations in CSF are commonly documented in HIV-positive patients throughout the course of infection. The CSF findings in patients with arboviral meningitis are similar to those caused by enteroviruses.[1, 2] Virus has been cultured from blood and CSF, but the diagnosis is usually made by comparison of acute and convalescent sera.

Bacterial Meningitis

Cerebrospinal Fluid Examination. The diagnosis of bacterial meningitis rests on CSF examination by lumbar puncture[296, 327]; typical CSF findings in acute bacterial meningitis are shown in Table 71–10. In virtually all cases the opening pressure is elevated, with values over 600 mmH_2O suggesting the presence of cerebral edema, intracranial suppurative foci, or communicating hydrocephalus. The white blood cell count is elevated in untreated bacterial meningitis, usually 1000 to 5000/mm^3 (range of less than 100 to more than 10,000/mm^3). Neutrophils usually predominate, although approximately 10% of patients with acute bacterial meningitis present with a predominance of lymphocytes in spinal fluid; such predominance is more common in neonatal gram-negative bacillary meningitis and meningitis caused by *L. monocytogenes* (about 30% of cases). Patients with very low CSF white cell counts (0 to 20/mm^3) despite high CSF bacterial concentrations tend to have a poor prognosis. The absence of a CSF pleocytosis can characterize up to 4% of cases of bacterial meningitis overall,[328] most commonly in premature neonates (up to 15% of cases) and infants younger than 4 weeks (17% of cases). In addition, normal CSF white blood cell counts have been seen in patients with meningococcal meningitis[329, 330] and accounted for almost 10% of all cases of meningococcal meningitis in one study.[329] Therefore, a Gram stain and culture should be performed on all spinal fluid specimens even if the white blood cell count is normal. A CSF glucose concentration decreased to less than 40 mg/dl is found in about 60% of patients and a CSF : serum glucose ratio less than 0.31 in about 70% of patients.[331] CSF protein concentrations are elevated in virtually all patients, presumably because of disruption of the BBB. However, a normal CSF white blood cell count and protein concentration may be seen in specimens obtained at the onset

TABLE 71–10 Typical Cerebrospinal Fluid Findings in Patients with Bacterial Meningitis

Cerebrospinal Fluid Parameter	Typical Findings
Opening pressure	>180 mmH_2O
White blood cell count	1000–5000/mm^3 (range, <100 to >10,000)
Percentage of neutrophils	≥80%
Protein	100–500 mg/dl
Glucose	≤40 mg/dl
Lactate	≥35 mg/dl
Gram stain	Positive in 60–90%
Culture	Positive in 70–85%
Limulus lysate	Positive in gram-negative meningitis
Bacterial antigen detection	Positive in 50–100%
Polymerase chain reaction	Promising*

*See the text for details.

of meningitis, in some cases of neonatal meningitis, and in severely immunocompromised patients. A CSF glucose concentration less than 34 mg/dl, a CSF : blood glucose ratio less than 0.23, a CSF protein concentration more than 220 mg/dl, more than 2000 leukocytes per cubic millimeter of CSF and more than 1180 neutrophils per cubic millimeter of CSF were found to be individual predictors of bacterial rather than viral meningitis with 99% certainty or better.[332] This model was validated in one retrospective review of patients with meningitis,[333] although proof of the utility of this model will require a prospective application. Elevated CSF lactate concentrations (especially above 35 mg/dl) may also be useful in differentiating bacterial from nonbacterial meningitis in patients who have not received prior antimicrobial therapy.[334]

Gram-stain examination of CSF permits rapid, accurate identification of the causative microorganism in 60 to 90% of patients with bacterial meningitis and has a specificity of nearly 100%.[331] The likelihood of detecting the organism by Gram stain correlates with the concentration of bacteria in CSF; concentrations of 10^3 or fewer colony-forming units per milliliter are associated with positive Gram stains about 25% of the time, whereas CSF concentrations of bacteria of 10^5 or above lead to positive microscopy results in up to 97% of cases.[335] The clinical utility of the Gram stain also depends on the bacterial pathogen[336, 337]: bacteria have been observed in 90% of cases of meningitis caused by *S. pneumoniae*, 86% of cases caused by *H. influenzae*, 75% of cases caused by *N. meningitidis*, and 50% of cases caused by gram-negative bacilli; the CSF Gram stain is positive in less than 50% of patients with *L. monocytogenes* meningitis. In addition, the probability of identifying the organism may decrease in patients who have received prior antimicrobial therapy (40 to 60% and less than 50% positivity on Gram stain and culture, respectively).[338, 339] In studies of infants and children with bacterial meningitis, initially positive CSF cultures became sterile in 90 to 100% of patients within 24 to 36 hours of administration of "appropriate" antimicrobial therapy.[328] However, in most infants and children with bacterial meningitis who have received prior antimicrobial therapy, no significant differences in the CSF formula occur, although two studies revealed significantly lower CSF protein concentrations and rates of Gram-stain positivity.[338, 340]

Several rapid diagnostic tests have been developed to aid in the diagnosis of bacterial meningitis.[337] Counterimmunoelectrophoresis may detect specific antigens in CSF when the meningitis is caused by meningococci (serogroups A, C, Y, or W135), *H. influenzae* type B, pneumococci (83 serotypes), type III group B streptococci, and *E. coli* K1; the sensitivity ranges from 50 to 95%, although the test is highly specific. However, more recent tests that are more rapid (15 minutes or less) and 10-fold more sensitive than counterimmunoelectrophoresis are now available and include staphylococcal coagglutination and latex agglutination[337] (Table 71–11). Currently available latex agglutination techniques detect the antigens of *H. influenzae* type B, *S. pneumoniae*, *N. meningitidis*, *E. coli* K1, and the group B streptococci. However, many of the test kits do not include tests for group B meningococci, and other kits are probably poor because of the limited immunogenicity of group B meningococcal polysaccharide. Performance of one of these rapid diagnostic tests may be considered on CSF specimens from patients with presumed bacterial meningitis and a negative CSF Gram stain, although it must be emphasized that a negative test does not rule out infection caused by a specific meningeal pathogen. Lysate prepared from the amebocytes of the horseshoe crab *Limulus polyphemus* may be useful in suspected cases of gram-negative meningitis; a positive test indicates the presence of endotoxin.[337] A correctly performed *Limulus* lysate assay can detect about 10^3 gram-negative bacteria per milliliter of CSF; the sensitivity and specificity of this assay are 93 and 99.4%, respectively. However, this test does not distinguish between specific gram-negative organisms, and a negative test does not rule out the diagnosis of gram-negative meningitis. PCR has been used to amplify DNA from patients with meningitis caused by several meningeal pathogens.[341–347] In one study of CSF samples from patients with meningococcal meningitis,[342] the sensitivity and specificity of PCR were both 91%. Problems with false-positive results arise when using PCR, although further refinements in this technique may lead to its usefulness in the diagnosis of bacterial meningitis, particularly when CSF Gram stain, bacterial antigen tests, and cultures are negative.

TABLE 71–11 Sensitivity of Assays for Detection of Bacterial Antigens in Cerebrospinal Fluid from Patients with Bacterial Meningitis

Organism	Sensitivity (%)	
	Coagglutination	*Latex Agglutination*
Haemophilus influenzae type B	66–100	78–100
Neisseria meningitidis	50–78	50–93
Streptococcus pneumoniae	59–93	67–100
Streptococcus agalactiae	62–87	69–100

Adapted from Gray LD, Fedorko DP. Laboratory diagnosis of bacterial meningitis. Clin Microbiol Rev. 1992;5:130–145.

Radiography. Cranial CT or magnetic resonance imaging does not aid in the diagnosis of acute bacterial meningitis. However, one of these modalities should be considered during the course of illness in patients who have persistent or prolonged fever, clinical evidence of increased intracranial pressure, focal neurologic findings or seizures, enlarging head circumference (in neonates), persistent neurologic dysfunction, or persistently abnormal CSF parameters or cultures[94, 327] (Fig. 71–2). Cranial CT or magnetic resonance imaging has been recommended at the end of antimicrobial therapy in newborn infants to be certain that no intracranial complications have occurred.[94] In one review of 107 children with bacterial meningitis who underwent CT scanning,[348] one or more abnormalities were found in 52% of cases, although most findings did not require specific intervention. However, children with fever and subdural collections detected by CT may require a drainage procedure.

Radiographic studies may be useful in the subset of patients with meningitis as a result of a basilar skull fracture with CSF leak.[79, 115] CT scanning may detect air-fluid levels, opacification of the paranasal sinuses, or intracranial air; CT scanning with sagittal reconstruction can also be used to document or localize fracture sites. Radioisotope cisternography with cottonoid pledgets placed at the outlet of the sinuses within the nasal passage can be used to document a CSF leak, although high-resolution CT scanning with water-soluble contrast enhancement of the CSF (metrizamide cisternography) is the best test for defining the site of leakage.

Spirochetal Meningitis

Treponema pallidum. For the diagnosis of CNS involvement in patients with syphilis, no single routine laboratory test is definitive. CSF cellular and protein abnormalities have been reported to occur in 10 to 20% of patients with primary syphilis, 30 to 70% of patients with secondary syphilis, and 10 to 30% of patients with latent syphilis.[128] CSF abnormalities are common in patients with syphilitic meningitis, but they are nonspecific. Findings include a mononuclear pleocytosis (more than 10 cells/mm^3 in most patients), elevated CSF protein concentrations (78% of patients), and mild decreases in CSF glucose concentrations (less than 50 mg/dl in 55% of patients).[305] Oligoclonal bands and intrathecally produced antitreponemal antibodies are frequently present. Isolation of *T. pallidum* from CSF specimens is difficult, expensive, time consuming, and not routinely performed.[128]

Given the difficulties in the diagnosis of neurosyphilis, other CSF laboratory tests, particularly serologic testing (i.e., Venereal Disease Research Laboratory [VDRL] and fluorescent treponemal antibody tests) have been used.[128, 305, 349] However, serologic testing of CSF in patients with syphilis is problematic. For example, CSF collected by lumbar puncture is subject to blood contamination in about 10% of patients, which may lead to contamination of CSF and, therefore, a

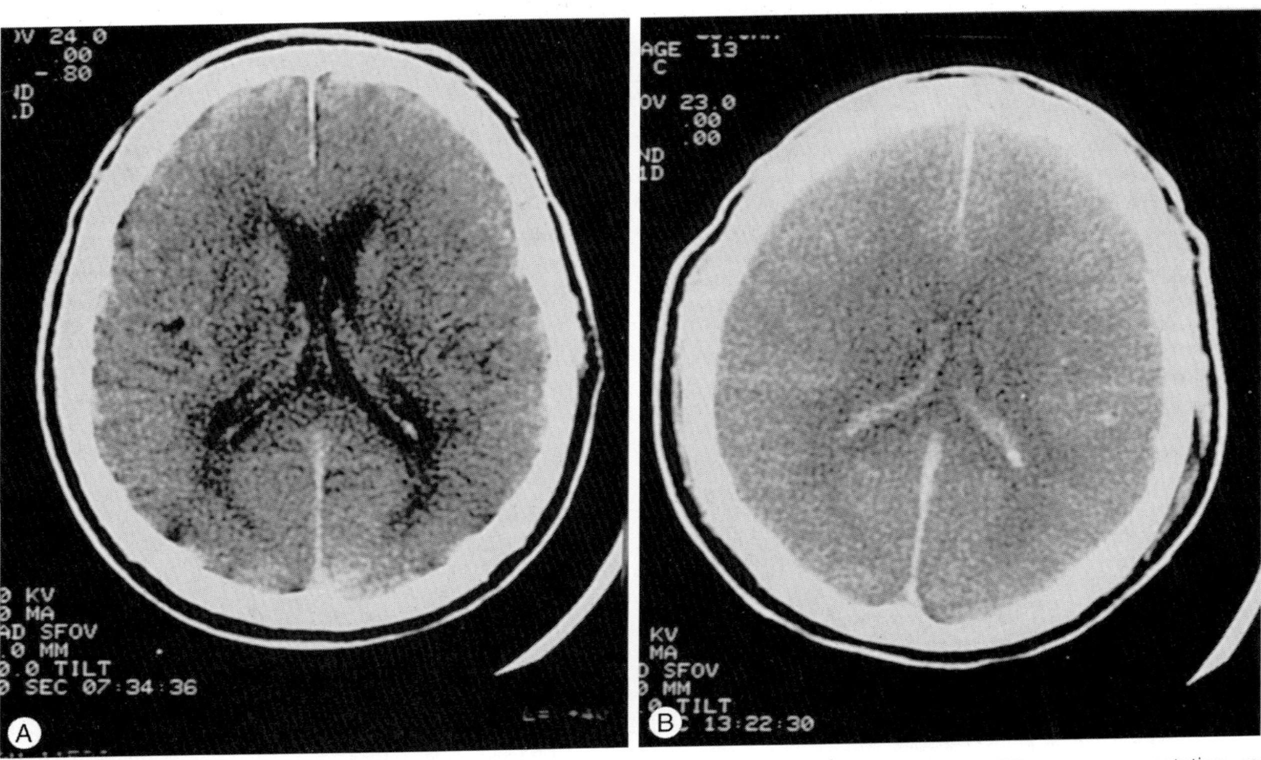

FIGURE 71–2. Computed tomography (CT) scans of the head in a patient with pneumococcal meningitis. *A*, CT scan on presentation, revealing moderate cortical atrophy; *B*, CT scan 3 days later, revealing diffuse swelling of the cerebral hemispheres bilaterally with effacement of the ventricular system.

false-positive serologic test result[124]; the likelihood of a false-positive test depends on the relative amount of contamination, the antibody titer in blood, and the sensitivity of the test. For patients with a serum VDRL value of 1:256 or less, sufficient blood contamination to be visible to the naked eye is required to cause false-positive CSF VDRL results. Although the specificity of the CSF VDRL test for the diagnosis of neurosyphilis is high, the sensitivity is low (reactive tests in only 30 to 70% of patients).[349] Therefore, a reactive CSF VDRL test in the absence of blood contamination is sufficient to diagnose neurosyphilis; a nonreactive result does not exclude the diagnosis. The CSF fluorescent treponemal antibody absorption (FTA-ABS) test has also been examined as a possible diagnostic test for neurosyphilis.[124, 349, 350] A nonreactive test effectively rules out the likelihood of neurosyphilis, but the specificity of the test is much less than the CSF VDRL test because of the possibility of leakage of small amounts of antibody from the serum into CSF. Furthermore, no compelling data confirm the significance of a reactive CSF FTA-ABS as being useful for the diagnosis of neurosyphilis.[124] PCR has been used to detect *T. pallidum* DNA in CSF samples in patients with acute symptomatic neurosyphilis.[351] Further large-scale studies are needed to determine the sensitivity and specificity of this technique. Based on the low sensitivity of the CSF VDRL test and until further studies demonstrate the usefulness of rapid diagnostic techniques, the diagnosis of neurosyphilis is based on elevated CSF concentrations of white blood cells, protein, or both in the appropriate clinical and serologic setting.

Borrelia burgdorferi. Typical CSF changes in patients with Lyme meningitis are a pleocytosis (usually fewer than 500 cells/mm^3, but up to 3500 cells/mm^3), with more than 90% lymphocytes in 75% of cases[131]; plasma cells may also be present. CSF protein concentrations are usually elevated (up to 620 mg/dl) and the CSF glucose concentration is usually normal, although glucose can be low in patients with illness of long duration. Oligoclonal banding may be present, with the bands reactive to *B. burgdorferi* antigens.

The best currently available laboratory test for the diagnosis of Lyme disease is demonstration of specific serum antibody to *B. burgdorferi*, in which a positive test in a patient with a compatible neurologic abnormality is strong evidence for the diagnosis.[131, 352] However, these tests are not standardized, and marked variability is seen between laboratories.[353] Most laboratories now use an enzyme-linked immunosorbent assay (ELISA) with sonicated *B. burgdorferi* as the antigen, although others still use the immunofluorescence technique. By the time that subacute disseminated (i.e., stage II) disease develops in most patients, they have elevated serum concentrations of IgG antibody to *B. burgdorferi*. False-positive reactions have been reported in patients with rheumatoid arthritis, Rocky Mountain spotted fever, infectious mononucleosis, tuberculous meningitis, leptospirosis, yaws, syphilis, and relapsing fever,[131] although high titers of cross-reacting IgG antibodies have been detected only in patients with syphilis or relapsing fever. False-negative results may be obtained from an unreliable assay, early infection, or early antibiotic use, which may blunt the normal humoral immune response. It is currently recommended that when the pretest probability of Lyme disease is 0.20 to 0.80, sequential testing with ELISA and Western blot is the most accurate method for ruling in or out the possibility of Lyme disease.[354, 355] Specific antibody against *B. burgdorferi* also appears in the CSF, and calculation of a specific antibody-IgG index for serum and CSF may indicate intrathecal antibody synthesis,[131] although demonstration of the usefulness of CSF antibody must await prospective studies with adequate sample size.[354] The technique of PCR on CSF samples has also been successfully used to identify *B. burgdorferi* DNA in patients with Lyme neuroborreliosis[356, 357] (see Chapter 231), although PCR must still be considered experimental in the diagnosis of CNS Lyme disease.

Radiologic studies may also be useful in patients with CNS manifestations of Lyme disease. CT has shown both enhancing and nonenhancing low-density lesions, mass effect, and cerebral demyelination. Magnetic resonance imaging may reveal punctate hyperresonant areas without mass effect within the cerebral white matter (Fig. 71–3).

Protozoal and Helminthic Meningitis

Amebas. The CSF formula in patients with the acute form of primary amebic meningoencephalitis reveals a neutrophilic pleocytosis, low glucose concentrations, an elevated protein concentration, and red blood cells.[135, 136] Gram stain is always negative. However, examination of fresh, warm specimens of CSF can reveal the ameboid movements of motile trophozoites.[358] After death, trophozoites can be demonstrated by light or electron microscopy of brain tissue.

Patients with the subacute or chronic form of the illness have a less florid CSF inflammatory response with a predominant mononuclear leukocytosis. The CSF protein concentration is elevated, and the glucose content is often normal or slightly reduced. Because amebas are not found in CSF, the diagnosis usually requires examination of a biopsy or necropsy specimen revealing the characteristic cysts. The value of serologic tests is variable.[135] Serum immunofluorescence, amebic immobilization titers, and complement-fixing antibodies support the diagnosis, although demonstration of rising titers is necessary to establish the diagnosis because some healthy persons have circulating antibodies.

Angiostrongylus cantonensis. The combination of a history of ingestion of suspected food, moderate to high peripheral eosinophilia, and CSF eosinophilia leads to the suspicion of angiostrongyloidiasis.[135] The CSF leukocytosis is moderate, with 16 to 72% eosinophils and an increased protein concentration; larvae are occasionally found in the CSF.

INITIAL MANAGEMENT OF PATIENTS WITH ACUTE MENINGITIS

The initial management of a patient with presumed bacterial meningitis includes performance of a lumbar puncture to determine whether the CSF formula is consistent with that diagnosis[359, 360] (Fig. 71–4). If purulent meningitis is present, institution of antimicrobial therapy should be based on the results of Gram staining or rapid bacterial antigen tests[360] (Table 71–12). However, if no etiologic agent can be identified by these means or if performance of the lumbar puncture is delayed (i.e., longer than 90 to 120 minutes), institution of empirical antimicrobial therapy should be based on the patient's age and underlying disease status (Table 71–13). Although no prospective data are available on the timing of administration of antimicrobial therapy in patients with bacterial meningitis, a recent retrospective cohort study in patients with community-acquired bacterial meningitis demonstrated that a delay in initiation of antimicrobial therapy after patient arrival in the emergency room was associated with an adverse clinical outcome when the patient's condition

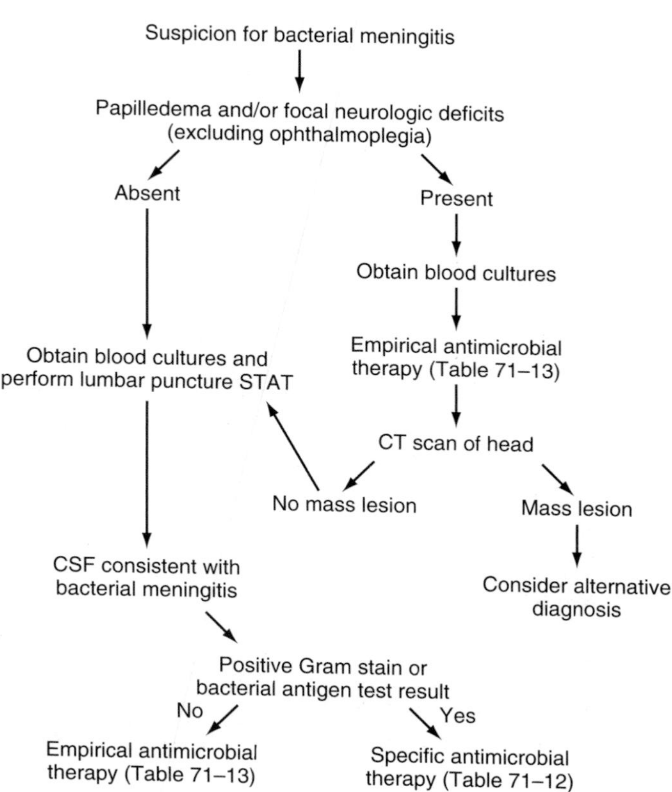

FIGURE 71–4. Algorithm for the initial management of the patient with meningitis. (From Tunkel AR, Scheld WM. Acute bacterial meningitis. Lancet. 1995;346:1675–1680. © by The Lancet Ltd., 1995.)

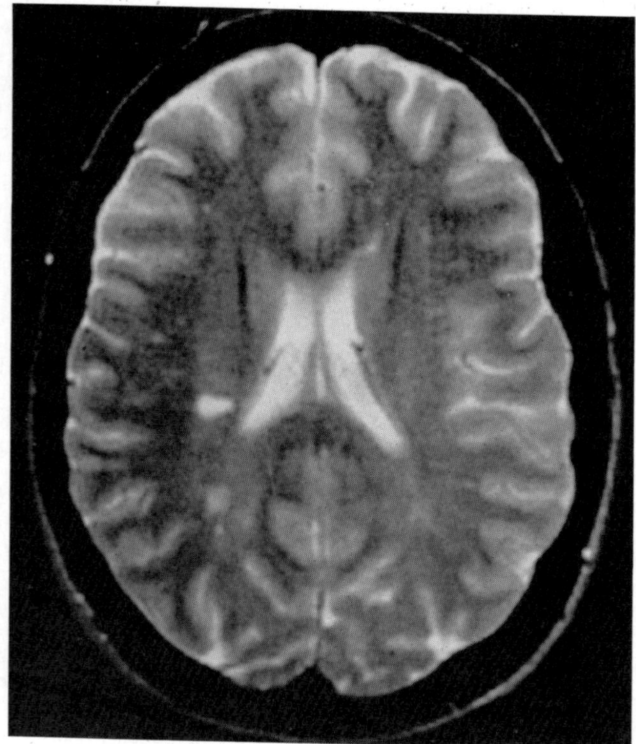

FIGURE 71–3. T_2-weighted magnetic resonance imaging scan in a patient with Lyme disease, revealing areas of increased signal intensity in the cerebral white matter.

TABLE 71–12 Recommended Antimicrobial Therapy for Acute Bacterial Meningitis Based on the Presumptive Pathogen Identified by Positive Gram Stain or Bacterial Antigen Test

Microorganism	Antimicrobial Therapy
Haemophilus influenzae type B	Third-generation cephalosporin*
Neisseria meningitidis	Penicillin G or ampicillin†
Streptococcus pneumoniae	Vancomycin plus a third-generation cephalosporin*
Listeria monocytogenes	Ampicillin or penicillin G‡
Streptococcus agalactiae	Ampicillin or penicillin G‡
Escherichia coli	Third-generation cephalosporin*

*Cefotaxime or ceftriaxone.
†Some authorities would prefer a third-generation cephalosporin if a resistant organism is suspected; the superiority of a third-generation cephalosporin over penicillin for these organisms has not been proved.
‡The addition of an aminoglycoside should be considered.
From Tunkel AR, Scheld WM. Acute bacterial meningitis. Lancet. 1995;346:1675–1680. © The Lancet Ltd., 1995.

TABLE 71–13 Empirical Therapy for Purulent Meningitis*

Predisposing Factor	Antimicrobial Therapy
Age	
0–4 wk	Ampicillin plus cefotaxime; or ampicillin plus an aminoglycoside
4–12 wk	Ampicillin plus a third-generation cephalosporin†
3 mo to 18 yr	Third-generation cephalosporin†; or ampicillin plus chloramphenicol
18–50 yr	Third-generation cephalosporin†‡
>50 yr	Ampicillin plus a third-generation cephalosporin†
Immunocompromised state	Vancomycin plus ampicillin plus ceftazidime
Basilar skull fracture	Third-generation cephalosporin†
Head trauma; postneurosurgery	Vancomycin plus ceftazidime
Cerebrospinal fluid shunt	Vancomycin plus ceftazidime

*Vancomycin should be added to empirical therapeutic regimens when highly penicillin- or cephalosporin-resistant strains of *Streptococcus pneumoniae* are suspected; see the text for details.
†Cefotaxime or ceftriaxone.
‡Add ampicillin if meningitis caused by *Listeria monocytogenes* is suspected.

advanced to a high stage of prognostic severity,[361] thus supporting the assumption that treatment of bacterial meningitis before it advances to a high level of clinical severity improves clinical outcome. In patients who present with focal neurologic findings or who have papilledema and bacterial meningitis is suspected, a CT scan of the head should be performed before lumbar puncture to rule out the presence of an intracranial mass lesion because of the potential risk of herniation[331]; the true incidence of this problem is unclear but has been suggested to be less than 1.2% in patients with papilledema and about 12% in patients without papilledema but with elevated intracranial pressure. However, the time involved in waiting for a CT scan significantly delays the initiation of antimicrobial therapy, with the potential for increased morbidity and mortality in patients with bacterial meningitis. Therefore, emergency empirical antimicrobial therapy, after obtaining blood cultures, should be initiated before sending the patient to the CT scanner. Although CSF cultures may be sterile after the initiation of antimicrobial therapy, pretreatment blood cultures and the CSF formula, Gram stain, or bacterial antigen tests will probably provide evidence for or against a diagnosis of bacterial meningitis. In one retrospective review of 177 patients (39 of whom had received prior antimicrobial therapy) with CSF culture–proven bacterial meningitis,[362] the combination of blood culture, CSF Gram strain, and/or latex agglutination identified the causative bacterium in 92% of patients. Once the infecting meningeal pathogen is isolated and susceptibility testing known, antimicrobial therapy can be modified for optimal treatment (Table 71–14). Recommended dosages of antimicrobial agents in adults for infections of the CNS are shown in Table 71–15, and those for neonates, infants, and children are presented in Table 71–16.

In addition, certain patients should receive adjunctive dexamethasone therapy when presenting with suspected or proven bacterial meningitis (see "Adjunctive Therapy," later, for complete details on adjunctive therapies in bacterial meningitis). Currently, data support the routine use of adjunctive dexamethasone therapy (0.15 mg/kg every 6 hours for 2 to 4 days) in infants and children with meningitis caused by *H. influenzae* type B.[360] In adults or in patients with meningitis caused by other bacteria, dexamethasone is not routinely recommended, although some authors recommend its use in all patients with presumed bacterial meningitis.[158] Rigorously controlled clinical data are not available to support this recommendation. Patients with severely impaired mental status, cerebral edema, or markedly elevated intracranial pressure may benefit most from adjunctive dexamethasone, but definitive data are lacking. When adjunctive dexamethasone is to be given, administration just before or concomitant with the first dose of an antimicrobial agent is optimal to obtain maximal attenuation of the subarachnoid space inflammatory response.

ANTIMICROBIAL THERAPY

Viral Meningitis

Specific antiviral chemotherapy for the enteroviruses is not currently available; treatment is supportive. A number of drugs have been

TABLE 71–14 Specific Antimicrobial Therapy for Acute Meningitis

Microorganism	Standard Therapy	Alternative Therapies
Bacteria		
Haemophilus influenzae		
β-Lactamase negative	Ampicillin	Third-generation cephalosporin,* cefepime, chloramphenicol, aztreonam
β-Lactamase positive	Third-generation cephalosporin*	Cefepime, chloramphenicol, aztreonam, fluoroquinolone
Neisseria meningitidis		
Penicillin MIC <0.1 μg/ml	Penicillin G or ampicillin	Third-generation cephalosporin,* chloramphenicol
Penicillin MIC 0.1–1.0 μg/ml	Third-generation cephalosporin*†	Chloramphenicol, fluoroquinolone
Streptococcus pneumoniae		
Penicillin MIC <0.1 μg/ml	Penicillin G or ampicillin	Third-generation cephalosporin,* chloramphenicol, vancomycin
Penicillin MIC 0.1–1.0 μg/ml	Third-generation cephalosporin*	Meropenem, vancomycin‡
Penicillin MIC ≥2.0 μg/ml	Vancomycin plus a third-generation cephalosporin*‡	Meropenem
Enterobacteriaceae	Third-generation cephalosporin*	Aztreonam, fluoroquinolone, trimethoprim-sulfamethoxazole, meropenem
Pseudomonas aeruginosa	Ceftazidime§	Aztreonam,§ fluoroquinolone,§ meropenem§
Listeria monocytogenes	Ampicillin or penicillin G§	Trimethoprim-sulfamethoxazole
Streptococcus agalactiae	Ampicillin or penicillin G§	Third-generation cephalosporin,* vancomycin
Staphylococcus aureus		
Methicillin sensitive	Nafcillin or oxacillin	Vancomycin
Methicillin resistant	Vancomycin	
Staphylococcus epidermidis	Vancomycin‡	
Spirochetes		
Treponema pallidum	Penicillin G	Doxycycline,** ceftriaxone**
Borrelia burgdorferi	Third-generation cephalosporin*	Penicillin G, doxycycline
Protozoa/helminths		
Naegleria fowleri	Amphotericin B†† plus rifampin plus doxycycline	

*Cefotaxime or ceftriaxone.
†Superiority of a third-generation cephalosporin over penicillin has not been established.
‡The addition of rifampin may be considered; see the text for indications.
§The addition of an aminoglycoside should be considered.
**The value of these antimicrobial agents has not been established.
††Intravenous and intraventricular administration.
Abbreviation: MIC, Minimal inhibitory concentration.

TABLE 71–15 Recommended Dosages of Antimicrobial Agents for Meningitis in Adults with Normal Renal and Hepatic Function*

Antimicrobial Agent	Total Daily Dose	Dosing Interval (h)
Amikacin†	15 mg/kg	8
Ampicillin	12 g	4
Aztreonam	6–8 g	6–8
Cefotaxime	8–12 g	4–6
Ceftazidime	6 g	8
Ceftriaxone	4 g	12–24
Chloramphenicol‡	4–6 g	6
Ciprofloxacin	800 mg	12
Doxycycline	200–400 mg	12
Gentamicin†	3–5 mg/kg	8
Meropenem	6 g	8
Nafcillin	9–12 g	4
Oxacillin	9–12 g	4
Penicillin G	24 million units	4
Rifampin§	600 mg	24
Tobramycin†	3–5 mg/kg	8
Trimethoprim-sulfamethoxazole**	10–20 mg/kg	6–12
Vancomycin† ††	2–3 g	8–12

*Unless indicated, therapy is administered intravenously.
†Need to monitor peak and trough serum concentrations.
‡Higher dose recommended for pneumococcal meningitis.
§Oral administration.
**Dosage based on trimethoprim component.
††May need to monitor cerebrospinal fluid concentrations in severely ill patients.

developed with efficacy in vitro and in animal models of enteroviral infection, but they have not yet reached clinical trials.[2] One of these drugs, disoxaril, protects mice from echoviral meningoencephalitis and has been shown to cure mice of chronic enteroviral meningitis; oral administration has also been shown to reduce the incidence of paralysis caused by echovirus 9. No specific antiviral therapy exists for the arboviruses, mumps virus, or lymphocytic choriomeningitis virus. Antiretroviral therapy for HIV-infected patients is discussed in Chapter 115.

Recovery of patients with herpes simplex virus type 2 meningitis is usually complete without neurologic sequelae. It is not clear whether antiviral treatment alters the course of mild meningitis. However, treatment with acyclovir is generally indicated for primary genital herpes infection[26] (see Chapter 125). Intravenous acyclovir is used if the meningitis is associated with genital herpes simplex infection.

Bacterial Meningitis

Principles of Therapy

Many factors influence the choice of an antimicrobial agent in the treatment of bacterial meningitis. Utilization of animal models of infection has permitted quantification of the relative penetration of drug into CSF, the effects of meningitis on this entry parameter, and the relative bactericidal efficacy (defined as the rate of bacterial eradication) within purulent CSF.[363]

The first factor relates to penetration of the antimicrobial agent into CSF, which depends, to a great extent, on the status of the BBB. For example, β-lactam antibiotics such as penicillin penetrate into CSF poorly (about 0.5 to 2.0% of peak serum concentrations) when the BBB is normal.[157, 359, 363] In the presence of meningeal inflammation, CSF penetration of the antibiotic is enhanced owing to increased permeability across the BBB, perhaps as a result of separation of intercellular light junctions and increased numbers of pinocytotic vesicles in cerebral microvascular endothelial cells.[237] Antimicrobial entry decreases as inflammation subsides, indicating that maximal parenteral doses of antimicrobial agents should be continued throughout the course of therapy to maintain adequate CSF concentrations. Antibiotic entry into CSF is also enhanced by drugs with a high lipid solubility, low molecular weight, low degree of protein binding in serum, and low degree of ionization at physiologic pH.

The second factor is the bactericidal activity of the antimicrobial agent within purulent CSF.[157, 359, 363] Because of the accumulation of lactate in CSF during bacterial meningitis, the pH of CSF is decreased, thereby inhibiting the bactericidal activity of the aminoglycosides; this has likely contributed to the poor response observed with the aminoglycosides in the therapy of meningitis in experimental animal models and in patients. Elevated CSF protein concentrations may decrease the efficacy of antimicrobial agents that are highly protein bound because free drug is needed for the antibacterial effect. Drug that penetrates the CSF may be removed by an active transport system that exists in the choroid plexus (as for the penicillins and cephalosporins), or it may be converted to an inactive metabolite. In addition, other drugs may influence antibiotic activity within purulent CSF. In experimental animal models of meningitis, antagonism has been shown when a bactericidal agent is coadministered with a bacteriostatic antibiotic (e.g., chloramphenicol plus gentamicin). However, in other instances the combination of antibiotics may be synergistic, as in the combination of penicillin or ampicillin with gentamicin in *L. monocytogenes* meningitis and ampicillin plus gentamicin against *S. agalactiae*.

A final factor concerns the importance of bactericidal activity in CSF for optimal therapy inasmuch as bacterial meningitis represents an infection in an area of impaired host defense. Multiple studies in experimental animal models have shown that rapid bacterial killing is observed in vivo only when CSF concentrations of β-lactams or aminoglycosides exceed the minimal bactericidal concentration by about 10- to 20-fold.[364] The importance of rapid bacterial killing has

TABLE 71–16 Recommended Dosages of Antimicrobial Agents for Meningitis in Neonates, Infants, and Children with Normal Renal and Hepatic Function*

Antimicrobial Agent	Total Daily Dose (Dosing Interval in Hours)		
	Neonates (0–7 d)†	*Neonates (8–28 d)†*	*Infants and Children*
Amikacin‡	15–20 mg/kg (12)	20–30 mg/kg (8)	20–30 mg/kg (8)
Ampicillin	100–150 mg/kg (8–12)	150–200 mg/kg (6–8)	200–300 mg/kg (6)
Cefepime	—	—	50 mg/kg (8)
Cefotaxime	100 mg/kg (12)	150–200 mg/kg (6–8)	200 mg/kg (6–8)
Ceftazidime	60 mg/kg (12)	90 mg/kg (8)	125–150 mg/kg (8)
Ceftriaxone	—	—	80–100 mg/kg (12–24)
Chloramphenicol	25 mg/kg (24)	50 mg/kg (12–24)	75–100 mg/kg (6)
Gentamicin‡	5 mg/kg (12)	7.5 mg/kg (8)	7.5 mg/kg (8)
Nafcillin	100–150 mg/kg (8–12)	150–200 mg/kg (6–8)	200 mg/kg (6)
Penicillin G	0.1–0.15 mU/kg (8–12)	0.15–0.2 mU/kg (6–8)	0.25 mU/kg (4–6)
Rifampin§**	—	—	10–20 mg/kg (12–24)
Tobramycin‡	5 mg/kg (12)	7.5 mg/kg (8)	7.5 mg/kg (8)
Trimethoprim-sulfamethoxazole††	—	—	10–20 mg/kg (6–12)
Vancomycin‡	20 mg/kg (12)	30–40 mg/kg (8)	50–60 mg/kg (6)

*Unless indicated, therapy is administered intravenously.
†Smaller dosages and longer intervals of administration may be advisable for very low birth weight neonates (<2000 g).
‡Need to monitor peak and trough serum concentrations.
§Oral administration.
**Maximum daily dosage of 600 mg.
††Dosage based on trimethoprim component.

also been examined in patients with bacterial meningitis. One study that compared outcomes in infants and children with bacterial meningitis who had negative or positive CSF cultures 18 to 36 hours after the initiation of antimicrobial therapy revealed an increased rate of neurologic complications (i.e., ataxia, hemiparesis, developmental delay, moderate to severe hearing impairment) in the group in whom the causative organism could still be recovered after this interval.[365]

Specific Antimicrobial Therapy

Haemophilus influenzae. Therapy for meningitis caused by *H. influenzae* type B has been markedly altered by the emergence of β-lactamase–producing strains. These strains accounted for approximately 24% of all CSF isolates in the United States based on a surveillance study of 27 states from 1978 through 1981.[42] A subsequent surveillance study of five states and Los Angeles County in 1986 found the incidence of these β-lactamase–producing strains to be 32%.[43] Resistance of *H. influenzae* to chloramphenicol has also been described, although more commonly from areas such as Spain[366, 367] (more than 50% of isolates) than the United States[368] (less than 1% of isolates). Even in patients with chloramphenicol-sensitive isolates, a recent prospective study found chloramphenicol to be bacteriologically and clinically inferior to ampicillin, ceftriaxone, or cefotaxime in the treatment of childhood bacterial meningitis caused predominantly by *H. influenzae* type B.[369] Furthermore, the use of chloramphenicol can be problematic because of its unpredictable metabolism in young infants and its pharmacologic interactions with other concomitantly administered drugs such as phenobarbital, rifampin, phenytoin, and acetaminophen, which increase the likelihood of toxicity.[370] Several studies have documented the efficacy of third-generation cephalosporins (particularly cefotaxime or ceftriaxone) to be similar to that of the combination of ampicillin plus chloramphenicol for bacterial meningitis.[371, 372] Based on these findings, the American Academy of Pediatrics has recommended the use of a third-generation cephalosporin as empirical antimicrobial therapy for children with bacterial meningitis.[373] Cefepime has been studied in the treatment of bacterial meningitis. Cefepime has in vitro activity similar to that of cefotaxime and ceftriaxone against *H. influenzae*, *N. meningitidis*, and *S. pneumoniae* and greater in vitro activity against *Enterobacter* spp. and *P. aeruginosa*. In a prospective randomized comparison of cefepime and cefotaxime for the treatment of bacterial meningitis in infants and children,[374] cefepime was found to be safe and therapeutically equivalent to cefotaxime and can be considered a suitable therapeutic alternative for the treatment of patients with this disease.

Despite initial studies suggesting that cefuroxime, a second-generation cephalosporin, was as efficacious as the combination of ampicillin plus chloramphenicol for childhood bacterial meningitis,[375] this finding has been questioned. In one study comparing cefuroxime with ceftriaxone, both regimens were efficacious in the treatment of bacterial meningitis, although some patients did not respond as satisfactorily to cefuroxime and had slower rates of CSF sterilization (0 versus 9% of CSF cultures positive at 24 hours in patients treated with cefuroxime, $p < .001$) and a higher incidence of hearing impairment (18 versus 11%).[376] Another prospective randomized study comparing ceftriaxone with cefuroxime for the treatment of childhood bacterial meningitis documented more rapid CSF sterilization (2 versus 12% of CSF cultures positive at 18 to 36 hours, $p = .11$) and a lower incidence of hearing impairment (4 versus 17%, $p = .05$) in the patients receiving ceftriaxone.[377] Furthermore, delayed CSF sterilization has been reported in patients receiving cefuroxime for *H. influenzae* meningitis,[375] as well as the development of *H. influenzae* meningitis in patients receiving cefuroxime for nonmeningeal *H. influenzae* disease.[378] Therefore, cefuroxime cannot be recommended as a first-line drug for the treatment of bacterial meningitis. In addition, single case reports of delayed CSF sterilization in patients with *H. influenzae* meningitis treated with ceftizoxime or ceftazidime have appeared.[379] However, resistance of *H. influenzae* to third-generation cephalosporins and fluoroquinolones in vitro has not been described to date.[380]

Neisseria meningitidis. Penicillin G and ampicillin are the antimicrobial agents of choice for meningitis caused by *N. meningitidis*. However, these recommendations may need to be modified in the future because of trends in the antimicrobial susceptibility of meningococci. Meningococcal strains that are relatively resistant to penicillin G and have a minimal inhibitory concentration (MIC) range of 0.1 to 1.0 μg/ml have recently been reported from several areas (particularly Spain).[381, 382] For example, of 3264 strains of *N. meningitidis* isolated from blood and CSF in Spain during 1978 to 1985,[383] only one resistant isolate was observed, whereas 9 of 168 (5%) invasive isolates relatively resistant to penicillin G were found in the first 6 months of 1986; this figure reached 20% in 1989. This resistance was reported to be mediated by a reduced affinity of the antibiotic for penicillin-binding proteins 2 and 3.[383, 384] High-level penicillin resistance resulting from β-lactamase production has also been reported, and the MICs for these strains may be as high as 256 μg/ml.[385] Furthermore, high-level chloramphenicol resistance (MIC of ≥64 μg/ml) has been described as resulting from the presence of the *catP* gene on a truncated transposon that has lost mobility because of internal deletions[386]; transmission of genetic material between strains of *N. meningitidis* probably played an important role in dissemination of the gene.

In the United States, meningococcal strains relatively resistant to penicillin have also been described.[387–389] In a population-based surveillance study of invasive meningococcal disease in selected areas of the United States, 3 of 100 isolates had penicillin MICs of 0.125 μg/ml.[387] These data indicate the importance of continued surveillance for these resistant strains.

The clinical significance of these isolates is unclear at present because many patients with meningitis caused by relatively penicillin-resistant meningococci have recovered with standard penicillin therapy. However, isolated reports of treatment failure have been described.[390, 391] Furthermore, in a study from Spain, reduced susceptibility of *N. meningitidis* to penicillin was seen in 34% of 213 children with meningococcal meningitis[392]; in this report, reduced penicillin susceptibility was more frequent in strains responsible for death or sequelae (60 versus 32%, $p = .04$). Based on these data, some authorities would treat patients with meningococcal meningitis with a third-generation cephalosporin (either cefotaxime or ceftriaxone). Susceptibility testing of the isolate should be performed for patients who fail to respond appropriately. Trovafloxacin was found to be equivalent to ceftriaxone in children with meningococcal meningitis in one report,[393] although further studies are needed before trovafloxacin can be recommended for the treatment of meningococcal meningitis.

Streptococcus pneumoniae. Therapy for meningitis caused by the pneumococcus has recently been modified according to current pneumococcal susceptibility patterns. In the past, pneumococci were uniformly susceptible to penicillin, with MICs of 0.06 μg/ml or less. Numerous reports from throughout the world have now documented strains of pneumococci that are relatively resistant to penicillin (MIC range of 0.1 to 1.0 μg/ml), as well as strains that are highly resistant to penicillin (MIC of 2.0 μg/ml or higher).[157, 360, 394–396] The mechanism of this resistance is an alteration in the structure and molecular size of penicillin-binding proteins. Resistance has been reported in several different pneumococcal serotypes, although the overwhelming majority of resistant strains are serotypes 6, 14, 19, and 23; most of the multiresistant strains isolated in the United States disseminated from a multiresistant serotype 23F clone of *S. pneumoniae* that was isolated in Spain as early as 1978.[397] In some areas of the United States, 25 to 30% of invasive pneumococcal isolates were found to have either relative or high-level resistance to penicillin.[398, 399] Factors reported to predispose to resistance include the patient's age (younger than 10 or older than 50 years), immunosuppression, prolonged hospital stay, children in daycare settings, infection by serotypes 14 and 23, and frequent, prolonged, or prophylactic use of antimicrobial therapy.[360, 393, 400–402]

Several alternative agents for the treatment of meningitis caused by penicillin-resistant pneumococci have been evaluated by in vitro susceptibility testing, in animal models, and in patients.[360, 396, 403] Here, we will restrict our discussion to agents that have been examined in clinical trials, unless animal model data have influenced treatment recommendations. Chloramphenicol is one agent that has been studied for the treatment of pneumococcal meningitis. However, clinical failures with chloramphenicol have been reported in patients with penicillin-resistant isolates, probably because of the poor bactericidal activity of chloramphenicol against these strains; 20 of 25 children had an unsatisfactory outcome (i.e., death, serious neurologic deficit, poor clinical response) in one study.[404] Despite susceptibility on disk testing, chloramphenicol minimal bactericidal concentrations of the penicillin-resistant pneumococcal isolates were significantly higher than those for the penicillin-sensitive isolates, with subsequent subtherapeutic bactericidal activity and treatment failure.

Third-generation cephalosporins have been considered the treatment of choice in relatively penicillin-resistant pneumococcal meningitis.[360, 403] Cefotaxime and ceftriaxone are the third-generation agents of choice; ceftizoxime is not recommended because its MIC to resistant pneumococci tends to be higher than that of either cefotaxime or ceftriaxone.[405, 406] However, some reports of meningitis treatment failure with the third-generation cephalosporins have appeared, and pneumococcal strains have emerged that are resistant to these agents (MIC $\geq$ 2 μg/ml).[407–414] When the MIC to the third-generation cephalosporin is 1 μg/ml or less, some patients have been treated successfully with either high-dose cefotaxime or ceftriaxone alone,[410, 415] although one study found that high-dose cefotaxime did not have reliably sufficient CSF bactericidal activity against cephalosporin-resistant pneumococci.[416]

Vancomycin has been evaluated in 11 adult patients with meningitis caused by relatively penicillin-resistant pneumococcal strains.[417] This therapy was associated with clinical failure in 4 patients; no failures occurred in 14 subsequent patients treated with ceftriaxone. In two of the failures, CSF vancomycin concentrations were undetectable at 48 hours, and in a third patient, symptoms recurred on the eighth day of antimicrobial therapy. The concomitant administration of dexamethasone and the subsequent decreased inflammation and poor entry of vancomycin into CSF may have contributed to this negative outcome; this explanation has been supported in an experimental rabbit model of pneumococcal meningitis.[418] These data support the concept that vancomycin should not be used alone for the treatment of pneumococcal meningitis.

In view of the aforementioned data, penicillin can never be recommended as empirical therapy in patients with suspected pneumococcal meningitis. As an empirical regimen, the combination of vancomycin plus a third-generation cephalosporin (either cefotaxime or ceftriaxone) is recommended.[360, 403] This combination was synergistic in a rabbit model of penicillin-resistant pneumococcal meningitis[419] and was synergistic, or at least additive, in the CSF of children with meningitis.[420, 421] The addition of rifampin to vancomycin with or without a third-generation cephalosporin has been recommended by some authorities, although clinical data are lacking; rifampin should be added only if the organism is demonstrated to be susceptible and the expected clinical or bacteriologic response is delayed.[403] In patients not responding, intrathecal or intraventricular vancomycin also remains a reasonable option.[422] Once susceptibility studies of the isolated pneumococcus are performed, antimicrobial therapy can be modified for optimal treatment (see Table 71–14).

With continued emergence of penicillin- and cephalosporin-resistant strains of *S. pneumoniae*, other antimicrobial agents have been evaluated for their efficacy in pneumococcal meningitis. Meropenem, a carbapenem with a broad spectrum of in vitro activity, including activity against penicillin-resistant pneumococci,[423, 424] has recently been approved by the Food and Drug Administration for the treatment of bacterial meningitis in children 3 months and older. Meropenem has been studied for the treatment of meningitis in both adults and children in several clinical trials,[425, 426] with microbiologic and clinical outcomes similar to those with either cefotaxime or ceftriaxone. Meropenem was also used successfully in one patient with multiply resistant pneumococcal meningitis.[427] However, further studies are needed to determine the efficacy of meropenem in pneumococcal meningitis caused by penicillin- and cephalosporin-resistant strains.

The fluoroquinolones have generally lacked sufficient in vitro activity against *S. pneumoniae* to warrant their investigation in the treatment of CNS infections. However, newer agents have shown excellent in vitro activity and have been evaluated in experimental animal models of infection. Trovafloxacin has excellent CSF penetration[428] and has demonstrated bactericidal activity in an experimental rabbit model of penicillin-resistant pneumococcal meningitis,[429] an effect that was not altered by the coadministration of dexamethasone. Another agent, moxifloxacin, was shown to be as effective as ceftriaxone in the rabbit model of meningitis caused by a penicillin-sensitive pneumococcal strain[430]; CSF penetration was only slightly reduced by the coadministration of dexamethasone. Moxifloxacin has also shown efficacy in the treatment of penicillin-resistant pneumococcal meningitis in rabbits.[431] Clinical trials are currently in progress to determine the usefulness of these agents in patients with bacterial meningitis.

Listeria monocytogenes. Despite their broad range of in vitro activity, third-generation cephalosporins are inactive in meningitis caused by *L. monocytogenes*. For patients with *Listeria* meningitis, therapy should consist of ampicillin or penicillin G[80, 81, 83–86]; the addition of an aminoglycoside should be considered in proven infection because of in vitro synergy and enhanced killing in vivo, as documented in a variety of animal models of *Listeria* infection. Nevertheless, it is important to emphasize that a controlled clinical trial comparing ampicillin with ampicillin plus gentamicin has never been performed in humans with listeriosis. An alternative agent in a penicillin-allergic patient is trimethoprim-sulfamethoxazole,[432] which is bactericidal against *Listeria* in vitro. Although chloramphenicol has varying activity against *Listeria* in vitro, its use has been associated with an unacceptably high failure rate in patients with *Listeria* meningitis. Vancomycin is also unsatisfactory for *Listeria* meningitis despite favorable in vitro susceptibility results. However, intraventricular administration of vancomycin was successful in one case of recurrent *L. monocytogenes* meningitis.[433] Rifampin is bacteriostatic against *L. monocytogenes* in vitro and was no better than penicillin alone when evaluated in the experimental rabbit model of meningitis.[434] Meropenem is active in vitro and in experimental animal models of *L. monocytogenes* meningitis[435] and may be a useful alternative if found to be clinically efficacious.

Streptococcus agalactiae. Standard therapy for neonatal meningitis caused by the group B streptococcus is the combination of ampicillin plus an aminoglycoside,[94] which is also recommended for adult patients with meningitis caused by this organism[98]; this combination is recommended because of documented in vitro synergy and recent reports detailing the presence of penicillin-tolerant strains. Alternative agents are the third-generation cephalosporins; vancomycin is reserved for patients who are allergic to penicillin.

Aerobic Gram-Negative Bacilli. Treatment of bacterial meningitis caused by enteric gram-negative bacilli has been revolutionized by the availability of third-generation cephalosporins.[436–439] Previous mortality rates with standard regimens (usually an aminoglycoside with or without chloramphenicol) ranged from 40 to 90% versus cure rates of 78 to 94% with the third-generation cephalosporins. Cefotaxime is preferred over ceftriaxone as the third-generation cephalosporin for use in neonates because it has been used more extensively and is not excreted in bile, which may have an inhibitory effect on the bacterial flora of the intestinal tract[327]; ceftriaxone also has increased protein binding. One particular third-generation cephalosporin, ceftazidime, has enhanced in vitro activity against *P. aeruginosa* and resulted in the cure of 19 of 24 patients in one study of *P. aeruginosa* meningitis when administered alone or in combination with an aminoglycoside.[440] In another study of 10 pediatric patients with *Pseudomonas* meningitis, 7 patients were cured clinically and 9 were cured bacteriologically when treated with ceftazidime-containing regimens.[441] Concomitant intrathecal or intraventricular aminoglycoside therapy should be considered in patients with gram-negative meningitis who are not responding to conventional parenteral therapy. However, this mode of administration is rarely needed at present and was associated with a higher mortality rate than was systemic therapy alone in infants with gram-negative meningitis and ventriculitis.[442]

Several other antimicrobial agents have been used in patients with meningitis caused by aerobic gram-negative bacilli. Aztreonam attains excellent CSF concentrations and has been shown to be efficacious in the treatment of gram-negative meningitis.[443] Imipenem was found to be efficacious in one case of *Acinetobacter* meningitis[444] and in bacterial eradication from CSF in a recent study of 21 children with bacterial meningitis (most cases caused by *H. influenzae* type B and *N. meningitidis*),[445] although a high rate of seizure activity (33%) limits its usefulness in the treatment of bacterial meningitis. High-dose meropenem (2 g every 8 hours) given for 18 weeks was successful in a lymphoma patient with *P. aeruginosa* meningitis who had failed therapy with ceftazidime plus gentamicin,[446] as well as in a patient with post-traumatic meningitis caused by *P. aeruginosa*.[447] Newer cephalosporins (e.g., cefepime, cefpirome) are being evaluated in clinical trials of patients with gram-negative meningitis. The fluoroquinolones (e.g., ciprofloxacin, pefloxacin) have been used successfully in some patients with gram-negative meningitis.[448–450] The limited published literature on use of the fluoroquinolones suggests that the primary area of usefulness of these agents is for the treatment of multidrug-resistant gram-negative organisms (e.g., *P. aeruginosa*) or when the response to conventional β-lactam therapy is slow (e.g., meningitis caused by *Salmonella* spp.). Data are insufficient to recommend any fluoroquinolone for empirical therapy in any patient with community-acquired bacterial meningitis.

Staphylococci. *S. aureus* should be treated with nafcillin or oxacillin,[112] with vancomycin reserved for patients allergic to penicillin or when methicillin-resistant organisms are suspected or isolated. The addition of rifampin should be considered in patients not responding to therapy. Meningitis caused by coagulase-negative staphylococci, the most commonly encountered organisms in CSF shunt infections, should be treated with vancomycin; rifampin should be added if the patient fails to improve.[115] Removal of the shunt is often necessary to optimize therapy (see the next section).

Cerebrospinal Fluid Shunt Infections. Numerous methods of treating CSF shunt infections have been reported, although no randomized, prospective studies have been performed.[115, 303] In suspected infection, CSF should be removed from the shunt via the reservoir and sent for cell count, glucose and protein determination, Gram stain, and culture. Antimicrobial therapy should be initiated before culture results if meningeal inflammation is present (see Table 71–13); therapy can then be modified according to culture results (see Table 71–14). Occasionally, direct instillation of antimicrobial agents into the ventricles (i.e., through an external ventriculostomy or shunt reservoir) is necessary in patients with infections that are difficult to eradicate or when the patient is unable to undergo the surgical components of therapy[303] (see later). Vancomycin has been directly instilled into the ventricles to overcome the relatively meager CSF penetration after intravenous administration; daily dosages have ranged from 4 to 10 mg. Gentamicin (1 to 2 mg daily for infants and children and 4 to 8 mg daily for adults) can be administered, always in combination with a parenteral agent (e.g., a β-lactam), for infections caused by susceptible gram-negative organisms. Teicoplanin, a glycopeptide antimicrobial agent, was also found to be successful after intraventricular administration in seven patients with staphylococcal neurosurgical shunt infections.[451] Empirical dosing should initially be used, with subsequent dosage adjustments based on CSF antimicrobial concentrations.

In addition, patients with CSF shunt infections should undergo removal of all components of the infected shunt at the beginning of antimicrobial therapy, with an external ventriculostomy placed to clear the ventriculitis and monitor CSF findings.[115, 303] The ability of many organisms to adhere to prostheses and survive antimicrobial therapy precludes optimal treatment in situ. Furthermore, the propensity for the entire shunt to become contaminated when one portion becomes infected argues against partial revisions. With externalization, treatment success is usually greater than 90%.

Duration of Therapy

The duration of therapy for bacterial meningitis has been based more on tradition than on scientific evidence. The duration of antimicrobial therapy in patients with bacterial meningitis has been 10 to 14 days for cases of nonmeningococcal meningitis.[452, 453] Several studies comparing 7 with 10 days of treatment in infants and children with *H. influenzae* type B meningitis, however, have documented that 7 days of therapy is safe and effective,[454, 455] although therapy must be individualized and some patients may require longer courses. Meningococcal meningitis can be treated for 7 days with intravenous penicillin, and some authors have also suggested that 4 days of therapy are adequate[456]; this study requires confirmation because only 50 patients were studied and no control group was included. A single dose, or even two to three doses, of long-acting penicillin or chloramphenicol has been used successfully in developing countries to treat meningococcal meningitis,[453] although this therapy is not considered standard. In adults with meningitis caused by enteric gram-negative bacilli, treatment regimens should be continued for 3 weeks because of the high rate of relapse in patients treated with shorter courses of therapy. Ten to 14 days is recommended for the treatment of meningitis caused by *S. pneumoniae* and 14 to 21 days for group B streptococci. *L. monocytogenes* meningitis should be treated for at least 21 days.[85, 86]

Spirochetal Meningitis

Treponema pallidum. In syphilis patients with CSF abnormalities but without clinically apparent disease, the goals of therapy are to prevent progression to symptomatic disease and ameliorate the laboratory abnormalities thought to indicate disease activity.[124] For patients with clinical neurosyphilis syndromes, the goal may be to reverse clinical symptoms and signs or to arrest disease progression. In patients with syphilitic meningitis whose clinical picture is that of meningeal inflammation as a result of the acute inflammatory response, clinical findings other than cranial nerve abnormalities usually resolve without therapy. In patients with meningovascular syphilis, the prognosis after therapy is quite good, except perhaps in patients with larger, clinically apparent neurologic deficits before therapy; therapy in this situation may halt progression and prevent further ischemic events caused by neurosyphilis.

The drug of choice for the treatment of neurosyphilis is penicillin G (see Table 71–14), although considerable controversy remains regarding the most appropriate total dose and the formulation and duration of therapy.[124, 128] Therapy with benzathine penicillin (2.4 million units intramuscularly) does not reliably produce CSF penicillin concentrations above 0.018 μg/ml and should not be used for the treatment of neurosyphilis. Furthermore, a small but poorly defined proportion of patients with syphilis treated with benzathine penicillin fail therapy, defined as persistent CSF abnormalities with clinically apparent neurosyphilis. However, many patients treated with benzathine penicillin resolve their CSF abnormalities and do not progress, which suggests that factors other than CSF concentrations of penicillin play a role in response to therapy.

The preferred antimicrobial regimen for the treatment of CNS syphilis is intravenous aqueous crystalline penicillin G at a dose of 12 to 24 million units daily in divided doses every 4 hours for 10 to 14 days.[124] Alternatively, procaine penicillin, 2.4 million units intramuscularly daily, plus probenecid, 500 mg orally four times daily, both for 10 to 14 days, can be used. Some experts also recommend follow-up therapy with one injection of benzathine penicillin G (2.4 million units intramuscularly), although no data support this recommendation. No large studies have been performed to evaluate alternative antimicrobial agents for neurosyphilis. The tetracyclines, chloramphenicol, and ceftriaxone have all been described to be of potential clinical utility in penicillin-allergic patients based on case reports, clinical experience, and extrapolations from experimental animal studies. One experimental study, however, suggested that ceftriaxone may not be adequate therapy for neurosyphilis.[457] Furthermore, a recent study of 43 HIV-infected patients with latent syphilis or neurosyphilis treated with ceftriaxone (1 or 2 g daily for 10 to 14 days) had a 23% failure rate,[458] similar to that seen in 13 HIV-infected patients with latent syphilis or neurosyphilis treated with benzathine penicillin (30%). Erythromycin is not recommended because of treatment failures in erythromycin-treated patients. In HIV-infected patients with neurosyphilis, careful monitoring for response to therapy is needed.[127, 459] Follow-up lumbar puncture should be performed every 6 months in all patients until the CSF changes have normalized. Several reports of failures in HIV-infected patients receiving standard therapy for neurosyphilis have appeared; these failures probably occurred because the patient's immunologic response has an important role in controlling the infection even in the presence of "adequate" antimicrobial therapy.

Borrelia burgdorferi. Parenteral antimicrobial therapy is usually needed to treat the neurologic manifestations of Lyme disease, including meningitis (see Table 71–14). Initial studies used high-dose (15 to 20 million units daily) intravenous penicillin G for 10 to 14 days,[131, 352] although one author found the benefits limited to patients treated within 5 weeks of the onset of neurologic symptoms. The meningeal and systemic reactions tend to improve within days, whereas radicular pain and motor deficits improve over many weeks. CNS abnormalities are arrested by treatment and may slowly improve, but some residual deficit is common. Some patients have also responded to treatment with oral or intravenous doxycycline, which has been found to be as efficacious as penicillin in several studies.[460, 461] Patients who have failed to respond to intravenous penicillin have responded to therapy with intravenous cefotaxime, ceftriaxone, or chloramphenicol.[131] In one prospective randomized trial,[462] ceftriaxone was superior to penicillin in therapy for late Lyme borreliosis. The current recommendation is to treat most patients with Lyme meningitis with intravenous ceftriaxone at a dosage of 2 g daily for 2 to 4 weeks[131, 352]; the literature contains no agreement on the duration of therapy or on the minimal adequate dose of the antimicrobial. No evidence supports treatment durations longer than 4 weeks. However, no regimen has proved to be universally effective. Although one report has indicated that high-dose oral doxycycline may produce inhibitory concentrations against *B. burgdorferi* in CSF,[463] parenteral regimens are generally necessary for CNS infection.

Protozoal and Helminthic Meningitis

Amebas. Many antimicrobial agents, including amphotericin B, the tetracyclines, the imidazoles, qinghaosu, and rifampin, have in vitro activity against free-living amebas[136]; phenothiazines are amebicidal only at high concentrations (100 μm). Amphotericin B is rapidly amebicidal against *N. fowleri* in vitro, but it is much less active against *Acanthamoeba*. Only four patients reported in the literature have survived after therapy for primary amebic meningoencephalitis.[135, 464, 465] All received amphotericin B along with various other antimicrobial agents. The best documented survivor received amphotericin B and miconazole intravenously and intrathecally, rifampin, sulfisoxazole, and dexamethasone. However, no effective regimen has been established. Therapy with parenteral and intracisternal amphotericin B combined with rifampin and tetracycline has been suggested[136]; the addition of experimental therapies such as one of the phenothiazines or qinghaosu may also be justified in view of the extremely poor outcome in patients with primary amebic meningoencephalitis. Therapy is continued for 2 to 3 weeks if the clinical response is good and no complications occur.

Angiostrongylus cantonensis. Treatment of symptoms such as headache, nausea, and vomiting is indicated for eosinophilic meningitis caused by *A. cantonensis*. Most patients recover within 1 to 2 weeks.[135] The benzimidazoles have been tried in humans without definite benefit; thiabendazole cleared *A. cantonensis* from rats in one study.[142] Thiabendazole has been used in the early stages of migration of the larvae of *A. cantonensis*, but the drug fails as soon as the worm reaches the CNS.

ADJUNCTIVE THERAPY

Viral Meningitis

As a result of the lack of effective antiviral therapy against the enteroviruses, other adjunctive measures have been used in seriously ill patients with enteroviral meningitis. Because enteroviral clearance from the host is antibody mediated, exogenously administered antibody has been examined.[2] Administration of immune globulin by multiple routes (including directly into the CNS) has led to stabilization or improvement of agammaglobulinemic patients with chronic enteroviral meningitis or meningoencephalitis. Neonates with overwhelming enteroviral sepsis and meningitis have received intravenous immune globulin, maternal plasma, and exchange transfusions with occasional success. A single randomized trial of intravenous immune globulin plus standard therapy versus standard therapy alone in neonates suspected of having enteroviral infection during the first 2 weeks of life enrolled too few patients for a definitive conclusion[466]; 75% of these patients had clinical or laboratory evidence of meningitis.

Specific hyperimmune globulin has been shown to reduce the incidence of orchitis in a single prospective controlled trial in patients with mumps,[2] but no benefit in neurologic syndromes has been proved. Anecdotal reports have appeared on the use of corticosteroids in patients with mumps encephalitis,[12] but no benefits have been documented.

Bacterial Meningitis

Anti-inflammatory Agents

Despite the availability of effective bactericidal antimicrobial agents in the treatment of bacterial meningitis, morbidity and mortality from this disorder remain unacceptably high. Because the subarachnoid space inflammatory response is a major factor contributing to morbidity and mortality, investigators have examined whether attenuation of this response would improve outcome in bacterial meningitis. As stated earlier (see "Pathogenesis and Pathophysiology"), generation of pneumococcal cell wall components in an experimental animal model of pneumococcal meningitis after treatment with bacteriolytic antibiotics may contribute to the inflammatory response in the subarachnoid space.[198, 199] The inflammatory response induced by either live pneumococci or pneumococcal cell wall was reduced by agents (e.g., methylprednisolone, oxindanac) that inhibit the cyclo-oxygenase pathway of arachidonic acid metabolism, and a correlation was noted between CSF concentrations of the arachidonic acid metabolite PGE_2 and CSF leukocytes.[467] In another study, administration of the anti-inflammatory agent indomethacin decreased both brain water content and CSF concentrations of PGE_2 during experimental pneumococcal meningitis, although intracranial pressure was not reduced.[468] In addition, the administration of either dexamethasone or oxindanac lessened the massive influx of serum albumin and other proteins of high and low molecular weight into the CSF during the early stages of experimental pneumococcal meningitis.[469]

Several corticosteroid agents have also been examined in experimental animal models of meningitis. Early studies revealed that methylprednisolone administration led to a significant reduction in the mass of leukocytes within the meninges of rabbits with pneumococcal meningitis.[470] Another study demonstrated that CSF outflow resistance was reduced by methylprednisolone therapy and to a greater extent than in untreated or penicillin-treated rabbits with pneumococcal meningitis.[248] In further studies that examined the effects of corticosteroids (methylprednisolone or dexamethasone) on brain water content, CSF pressure, and CSF lactate in rabbits with pneumococcal meningitis, it was found that both agents completely reversed the development of brain edema but that only dexamethasone led to a reduction in CSF pressure and lactate[249]; however, neither agent was superior to therapy with ampicillin alone in reducing cerebral edema or intracranial pressure, and no comparison was made between ampicillin alone and the combination of ampicillin plus corticosteroids, a comparison that would have been relevant to the potential clinical usefulness of adjunctive corticosteroid therapy in bacterial meningitis. A subsequent study did examine treatment with ceftriaxone versus ceftriaxone plus dexamethasone in an experimental rabbit model of *H. influenzae* meningitis.[471] Although combination therapy consistently reduced the brain water content, CSF pressure, and CSF lactate to a greater degree than ceftriaxone did alone, the differences were not statistically significant. The authors suggested, however, that adjunctive dexamethasone might be more beneficial if administered early or even before antibiotic-induced bacterial lysis and release of microbial products. In a subsequent analysis using the experimental rabbit model of *H. influenzae* type B meningitis,[472] ceftriaxone administration led to a significant increase in CSF endotoxin concentrations 2 hours after administration, which was followed by a rise in CSF TNF concentrations. Simultaneous administration of dexamethasone and ceftriaxone did not affect the release of endotoxin into CSF, but it markedly attenuated CSF concentrations of TNF measured 8 hours later. Adjunctive dexamethasone therapy also resulted in a significant decrease in CSF leukocytosis and a trend toward earlier improvement in CSF concentrations of glucose, lactate, and protein. These parameters improved without any apparent decrease in the rate of bacterial killing within the CSF in vivo.

On the basis of these observations, several clinical trials were undertaken to determine the effects of adjunctive dexamethasone on outcome in patients with bacterial meningitis[473–485] (Table 71–17). One meta-analysis of these clinical studies confirms the benefit of adjunctive dexamethasone (0.15 mg/kg every 6 hours for 2 to 4 days) for *H. influenzae* type B meningitis and, if commenced with or before parenteral antimicrobial therapy, suggests benefit for pneumococcal meningitis in childhood.[486] Evidence of clinical benefit was strongest for hearing outcomes. In contrast, a retrospective, nonrandomized study of children with pneumococcal meningitis published after the meta-analysis demonstrated that the use of adjunctive dexamethasone was not associated with a beneficial effect,[485] although the dexamethasone was administered before or within 1 hour of the first dose of antibiotic and the children in the dexamethasone group had a higher severity of illness. Dexamethasone therapy does not appear to be compromised by significant adverse effects if the duration of treatment is limited to 2 days, which is likely to be as effective as 4 days of therapy.[487]

When dexamethasone is used, the timing of administration is crucial. Administration before or concomitant with antimicrobial therapy is optimal for attenuating the subarachnoid space inflammatory response. In addition, patients should be carefully monitored for the possibility of gastrointestinal hemorrhage. In adults or in patients with meningitis caused by other bacterial organisms, the routine use of adjunctive dexamethasone cannot be recommended pending results of ongoing studies,[488] although some authors recommend its use in all cases of meningitis with a probable bacterial etiology (i.e., demonstrable bacteria on CSF Gram stain, which may predict the patients at greatest risk for bacteriolysis-induced exacerbation of inflammation)[158]; however, no rigorously controlled clinical data support this recommendation. Adults with severely impaired mental status (stupor or coma), documented cerebral edema (e.g., by CT scan), or markedly elevated intracranial pressure (i.e., high opening pressure on lumbar puncture, palsy of cranial nerve VI) may benefit from adjunctive dexamethasone, although data are lacking. The use of adjunctive dexamethasone is of particular concern in patients with pneumococcal meningitis caused by highly penicillin- and cephalosporin-resistant strains, in which case patients may require antimicrobial therapy with vancomycin. A diminished CSF inflammatory response after dexamethasone administration might significantly reduce vancomycin penetration into CSF and delay CSF sterilization, as shown in an experimental rabbit model of penicillin- and cephalosporin-resistant pneumococcal meningitis.[418] This result was confirmed in another rabbit model of pneumococcal meningitis in which significantly lower CSF vancomycin concentrations and differences in bacterial killing were found in the dexamethasone-treated rabbits.[489] However, CSF vancomycin penetration was not reduced by dexamethasone in a study in children.[420] Despite these conflicting reports, many experts have expressed concern regarding the use of adjunctive dexamethasone in treating pneumococcal meningitis caused by penicillin- and cephalosporin-resistant strains.[360, 490] CSF concentrations of ceftriaxone are not significantly altered in animals or patients treated with adjunctive dexamethasone.[418, 488, 491] For any patient receiving adjunctive dexamethasone who is not improving as expected or who has a pneumococcal isolate for which the cefotaxime or ceftriaxone MIC is 2.0 μg/ml or greater, a repeat lumbar puncture 36 to 48 hours after initiation of antimicrobial therapy is recommended to document the sterility of CSF.[492]

Other agents that reduce subarachnoid space inflammation have also been examined as possible adjuncts in the treatment of bacterial meningitis. Pentoxifylline, a phosphodiesterase inhibitor that decreases endotoxin-induced TNF-α production, attenuates the inflammatory action of IL-1 and TNF on leukocyte function, and blocks the lipo-oligosaccharide–induced release of TNF and IL-1 from microglial cell cultures, has been examined in an experimental rabbit model of *H. influenzae* type B meningitis.[493] Administration of pentoxifylline 20 minutes before intracisternal challenge with *H. influenzae* type B lipo-oligosaccharide significantly reduced CSF concentrations of leukocytes, protein, and lactate. However, dexamethasone was superior to pentoxifylline in modulation of these CSF inflammatory changes, and no appreciable synergism was observed when both agents were administered. Thalidomide, which also inhibits TNF-α production, was recently studied in an experimental rabbit model of meningitis. Thalidomide reduced TNF-α production after intracisternal challenge with either *H. influenzae* type B or *S. pneumoniae*, although it had a relatively greater effect on the inflammatory response to *S. pneumoniae*.[494]

Other studies have examined the effects of a monoclonal antibody (IB4) directed against the CD18 family of receptors on leukocytes to reduce CSF inflammation. Intravenous inoculation of IB4 blocked the accumulation of leukocytes in CSF despite intracisternal challenge with *H. influenzae* type B, *N. meningitidis*, pneumococcal cell wall, or lipo-oligosaccharide.[189] Furthermore, the monoclonal antibody was effective in preventing the development of cerebral edema and death in animals challenged with lethal doses of *S. pneumoniae*. In a second study using an experimental rabbit model of *H. influenzae* type B meningitis,[495] the concomitant administration of dexamethasone and IB4 led to a marked attenuation of all indices of meningeal inflammation and a reduction in brain water content when compared with the results obtained in untreated animals or when each agent was used alone. Clinical trials with this agent, perhaps in conjunction with dexamethasone, will be needed to determine whether outcome (i.e., morbidity or mortality) can be improved by the administration of IB4 in patients with bacterial meningitis.

Bactericidal/permeability-increasing protein, which is present in

TABLE 71–17 Outcome in Patients Receiving Adjunctive Dexamethasone Therapy for Bacterial Meningitis in Published Clinical Trials From 1988 to 1998

Study	Design	Antimicrobial Regimen	Results	Concerns
Lebel et al.[473]	Randomized, placebo controlled; 200 infants and children 2 mo to 16 yr old; 77% of cases caused by *Haemophilus influenzae* type B	Cefuroxime or ceftriaxone	More rapid normalization of CSF parameters (glucose, protein, lactate) and temperature; lower incidence of moderate to severe bilateral sensorineural hearing loss (15.5 vs 3.3%, $p < .01$)	Audiologic sequelae only significantly reduced in patients receiving cefuroxime; gastrointestinal hemorrhage developed in 4 patients receiving dexamethasone
Lebel et al.[474]	Randomized, placebo controlled; 60 infants and children 3 mo to 16 yr old; 75% of cases caused by *H. influenzae* type B	Cefuroxime	No significant differences in audiologic or neurologic sequelae	Small study size
Girgis et al.[475]	Randomized, not placebo controlled; 429 children and adults 3 mo to 60 yr old; 62% of cases caused by *Neisseria meningitidis,* 25% by *Streptococcus pneumoniae,* 13% by *H. influenzae* type B	Ampicillin plus chloramphenicol	Lower mortality rate in patients with pneumococcal meningitis (13.5 vs 40.7%, $p < .01$); lower incidence of sensorineural hearing loss in patients with pneumococcal meningitis (0 vs 12.5%, $p < .05$)	No differences in normalization of CSF parameters; no documentation of possible adverse effects; high percentage (>60%) of patients presented in a comatose state; most patients (370 of 429) received inadequate therapy for 3–5 d before hospitalization; antibiotics administered intramuscularly; no differences in outcome in patients with meningitis caused by *N. meningitidis* or *H. influenzae* type B
Odio et al.[476]	Randomized, placebo controlled; 101 infants and children 6 wk to 13 yr old; dexamethasone given 15–20 min before antibiotic; 78% of cases caused by *H. influenzae* type B	Cefotaxime	Significantly better clinical condition and mean prognostic score at 24 h ($p \leq .001$); by 12 h all indices of CSF inflammation improved with dexamethasone associated with a decrease in TNF-α and PAF; decreased incidence of one or more neurologic sequelae in patients monitored a mean of 15 mo (10 vs 31%, $p = .008$); trend in reduction of audiologic sequelae in patients monitored a mean of 15 mo (6 vs 16%, $p = .18$)	
Kennedy et al.[477]	Retrospective; 97 infants and children 2 mo to 15 yr old; 100% of cases caused by *S. pneumoniae*	Cefotaxime, ceftriaxone, cefuroxime, ampicillin, or penicillin	Significant reduction in total long-term neurologic outcome (11 vs 33%, $p = .033$); trend to reduction in neurologic (6 vs 16%, $p = .18$) and audiologic outcome (9 vs 21%, $p = .14$)	Retrospective review; no data on differences with regard to specific antibiotic used
Schaad et al[478]	Randomized, placebo controlled; 115 infants and children 3 mo to 16 yr old; dexamethasone given 10 min before antibiotic; 58% of cases caused by *H. influenzae* type B, 24% by *N. meningitidis*	Ceftriaxone	Reduction in one or more neurologic or audiologic sequelae 15 mo after discharge (5 vs 16%, $p = .066$); relative risk of sequelae of 3.27 in patients receiving placebo	Dexamethasone given every 12 h for 2 d
King et al.[479]	Randomized, placebo controlled; 101 children 1 mo to 18 yr old; 55% of cases caused by *H. influenzae* type B, 18% by *N. meningitidis,* 13% by *S. pneumoniae*	Ceftriaxone	No significant reduction in audiologic sequelae (10.4 vs 11.1% in placebo recipients); no significant reduction in neurologic sequelae (10.9 vs 8.6% in placebo recipients)	Dexamethasone given within 24 h of antibiotic (median of 11 h); only 8 of 50 patients received dexamethasone within 4 h; study stopped prematurely because standard of care became early administration of dexamethasone
Wald et al.[480]	Randomized, placebo controlled; 143 infants and children 8 wk to 12 yr old; 53% of cases caused by *H. influenzae* type B, 23% by *S. pneumoniae,* 16% by *N. meningitidis*	Ceftriaxone	No significant differences in neurologic sequelae or developmental outcome; no significant differences in unilateral (10.3 vs 13.5% in placebo recipients) or bilateral (4.4 vs 9.4% in placebo recipients, $p = .33$) deafness; of 22 children who were deaf at entry, no significant differences were noted in resolution of hearing impairment	Dexamethasone given within 4 h of first dose of antibiotic; lack of follow-up for 13% of study population and incomplete follow-up for an additional 18%
Kanra et al.[481]	Randomized, placebo controlled; 56 children 2–16 yr old; 100% of cases caused by *S. pneumoniae*	Ampicillin-sulbactam	No significant differences in moderate or severe unilateral or bilateral sensorineural hearing loss or neurologic sequelae at 6 wk (7.4 vs 23% in the placebo group, $p = .11$) or 1 yr (7.4 vs 26.9% in the placebo group, $p = .062$); significant reduction in hearing impairment at 3 mo (3.7 vs 23%, $p = .044$)	Did not use standard antibiotic therapy for bacterial meningitis; no data on antimicrobial resistance of pneumococcal isolates; Glasgow coma score significantly lower in the dexamethasone group ($p = .004$)
Kilpi et al.[482]	Randomized, not placebo controlled; 122 infants and children 3 mo to 15 yr old; 53% of cases caused by *H. influenzae* type B, 33% by *N. meningitidis,* 10% by *S. pneumoniae*	Ceftriaxone	Dexamethasone recipients showed only a tendency to less severe hearing impairment	Some patients in each group also received therapy with oral glycerol; small sample size

TABLE 71–17 Outcome in Patients Receiving Adjunctive Dexamethasone Therapy for Bacterial Meningitis in Published Clinical Trials From 1988 to 1998
Continued

Study	Design	Antimicrobial Regimen	Results	Concerns
Macaluso et al.[483]	Retrospective; 179 children 1 mo to 16 yr old; 37% of cases caused by *H. influenzae* type B, 22% by *N. meningitidis*, 9% by *S. pneumoniae*	Benzylpenicillin plus chloramphenicol	Rate of discharge without sequelae was higher in the dexamethasone group (70 vs. 56%, p = .07); in children aged 6–59 mo, those treated with dexamethasone had a significantly lower case-fatality rate (11 vs. 25%, p = .05) and a better rate of discharge without sequelae (73 vs 52%, p = .02)	Retrospective; benefits observed only for children aged 6–59 mo; no causative organism identified in 27% of cases; no follow-up to assess the incidence of permanent neurologic sequelae
Qazi et al.[484]	Randomized, placebo controlled; 89 children 2 mo to 12 yr old; 20% of cases caused by *H. influenzae* type B, 9% by *N. meningitidis*, 7% by *S. pneumoniae*	Ampicillin plus chloramphenicol	Higher mortality rate in patients treated with adjunctive dexamethasone (25 vs 12%); in the survivors who received dexamethasone, the frequency of neurologic sequelae was 26.5% (vs 24% in placebo recipients) and the frequency of hearing impairment was 42.3% (vs 30% in placebo recipients)	No causative organism identified in 55% of cases; differences in mortality were not statistically significant because of small sample size; no correlation of severity of illness with outcome; not all patients may have received appropriate intensive care
Arditi et al.[485]	Retrospective; children 3 to 16.5 yr old; 100% of cases caused by *S. pneumoniae*	Variable	The dexamethasone group had a higher incidence of any moderate or severe hearing loss (46 vs 23%, p = .016) or any neurologic deficits (55 vs 33%, p = .02); no significant differences in deafness (p = .06) or neurologic sequelae (p = .10) when data controlled for severity of disease	Retrospective; children in the dexamethasone group more frequently required intubation and mechanical ventilation and had a lower initial CSF glucose concentration; no data on use of specific antimicrobial agents in each group; no long-term follow-up of patients with hearing loss or neurologic deficits

Abbreviations: CSF, Cerebrospinal fluid; PAF, platelet-activating factor; TNF-α, tumor necrosis factor-α.

the azurophilic granules of neutrophils and binds to and neutralizes the biologic activity of the lipid A portion of lipo-oligosaccharide, has also been studied for its effects on CSF inflammation in bacterial meningitis. In an experimental rabbit model, the intracisternal inoculation of recombinant bactericidal/permeability-increasing protein significantly reduced CSF inflammation in response to meningococcal endotoxin[496]; this effect was not seen after systemic administration, probably because of failure of this protein to cross the BBB.

Reduction of Intracranial Pressure

Patients with bacterial meningitis who have signs of increased intracranial pressure (e.g., altered level of consciousness; dilated, poorly reactive or nonreactive pupils; ocular movement disorders) and who are stuporous or comatose may benefit from the insertion of an intracranial pressure monitoring device.[497] Intracranial pressures exceeding 20 mmHg are abnormal and should be treated. Furthermore, there is rationale for treating smaller pressure elevations (i.e., above 15 mmHg) to avoid larger elevations, so-called plateau waves, that can lead to cerebral herniation and irreversible brain stem injury.

Several methods are available to reduce intracranial pressure,[497] including elevation of the head of the bed to 30 degrees to maximize venous drainage with minimal compromise of cerebral perfusion; hyperventilation to maintain the Pa_{CO_2} between 27 and 30 mmHg, which causes cerebral vasoconstriction and a reduction in cerebral blood volume; use of hyperosmolar agents (e.g., mannitol) to make the intravascular space hyperosmolar to the brain and permit movement of water from brain tissue into the intravascular compartment; and corticosteroids. However, some experts have questioned the routine use of hyperventilation to reduce intracranial pressure in patients with bacterial meningitis.[267] In infants and children with bacterial meningitis who have initially normal CT scans of the head, hyperventilation can safely reduce elevated intracranial pressure because it is unlikely that cerebral blood flow would be reduced to ischemic thresholds. However, in children with cerebral edema on head CT, cerebral blood flow is more likely to be normal or reduced. Although hyperventilation might decrease intracranial pressure, it would do so at the cost of a significant reduction in cerebral blood flow, possibly approaching ischemic thresholds. These patients may benefit more from the early use of diuretics, osmotically dehydrating agents (provided that intravascular volume is protected), and corticosteroids; however, controlled trials exploring these issues have yet to be performed.

Glycerol, an osmotic dehydrating agent that can be given orally, has been evaluated in a trial of 122 infants and children with bacterial meningitis.[482] Patients in this study were randomized to receive adjunctive intravenous dexamethasone, oral glycerol, dexamethasone plus glycerol, or neither. Seven percent of the glycerol-treated patients and 19% of those not given glycerol had audiologic or neurologic sequelae (p = .052). However, further placebo-controlled, blinded studies are required before glycerol can be routinely recommended in patients with bacterial meningitis.

Patients who continue to have elevated intracranial pressures despite the aforementioned measures may be treated with high-dose barbiturate therapy,[296, 497] which decreases cerebral metabolic demands and cerebral blood flow. Barbiturates can also cause vasoconstriction in normal tissue, thereby shunting blood to ischemic tissue and protecting the brain from ischemic insult. During the administration of pentobarbital, the patient is monitored to measure decreases in intracranial pressure, or the dose can be titrated to the development of a burst suppression pattern on the electroencephalogram. Cardiac parameters also need to be monitored (by placement of a Swan-Ganz catheter) because of the risk of cardiac toxicity (e.g., decreased cardiac output, decreased contractile force, arrhythmias) with high-dose barbiturate therapy. This mode of treatment for meningitis and elevated intracranial pressure is of unproven benefit, however, and must be considered experimental.

Surgery

Surgical intervention may be required in some patients with bacterial meningitis. Patients who have suffered a basilar skull fracture with CSF leak may have persistent dural defects that can lead to recurrent episodes of bacterial meningitis.[79] Many leaks will cease spontaneously, but surgery is indicated for leaks that persist for several weeks or in patients who present with delayed or recurrent infection. Surgery is not indicated in the acute phase (before 7 days) of leakage; no difference in outcome is seen when patients with acutely repaired leaks are compared with those whose leaks stop spontaneously within 7 days. Surgical intervention may also be required in patients in whom recurrent meningitis develops from congenital or acquired cranial defects and dermal sinuses.[115]

PREVENTION

Viral Meningitis: Immunoprophylaxis

The cornerstone of prevention of mumps is active immunization with the live-attenuated mumps vaccine. Administration is in the second year of life, and protective serum antibody concentrations are seen in more than 97% of patients.[12] Widespread use of the mumps vaccine has greatly reduced the incidence of mumps and mumps meningoencephalitis. By the mid-1980s, mumps was the seventh most common cause of viral encephalitis in the United States (approximately 0.5% of cases), whereas it was the leading cause of viral encephalitis through the mid-1960s.[12] Mumps meningitis has been reported in children 11 days to 2 months after vaccine administration,[498, 499] although it is not clear whether these cases represented vaccine failure or meningitis from the vaccine strain of mumps virus.

Bacterial Meningitis

Haemophilus influenzae Chemoprophylaxis. It has become clear that the spread of several types of bacterial meningitis can be prevented by prophylaxis of contacts of cases with antimicrobial agents. Several studies have documented the transmission of *H. influenzae* type B from patients with meningitis to household contacts.[500, 501] The risk is markedly age dependent, highest for children younger than 2 years. Most secondary cases (75%) occur within 6 days of onset of the index case, although untreated household contacts remain at increased risk for *H. influenzae* type B disease for at least 1 month after onset in the index case. Daycare outside the home is considered another risk factor for transmission[42]; secondary disease is more likely to develop in children younger than 2 years. Controversy regarding the magnitude of the risk to children in daycare settings, however, has led to disagreement concerning the recommendation for chemoprophylaxis of children in these facilities.

The rationale for the use of chemoprophylaxis for prevention of secondary disease is eradication of nasopharyngeal colonization of *H. influenzae* type B, thereby preventing transmission to young, susceptible contacts and the development of invasive disease in those already colonized. The recommended chemoprophylactic agent of choice is rifampin (20 mg/kg daily for 4 days) for all individuals, including adults, in households with at least one unvaccinated or incompletely vaccinated child younger than 48 months[501, 502] (see Chapter 212). One study suggested that 2 days of rifampin therapy was equally efficacious to 4 days' treatment,[503] although further study is required before a recommendation to shorten the duration of prophylaxis can be made. The index patient may also need to receive rifampin prophylaxis. Ampicillin and chloramphenicol, unlike ceftriaxone and cefotaxime, do not effectively eliminate nasopharyngeal colonization. Rifampin is not recommended for pregnant women who are contacts of infected infants because the risk of rifampin to the fetus has not been established. Chemoprophylaxis is not currently recommended for daycare contacts 2 years or older unless two or more cases occur in the daycare center within a 60-day period. For children younger than 2 years, the CDC recommends prophylaxis for daycare contacts, whereas the American Academy of Pediatrics does not in most cases.[501] The question of whether to administer prophylaxis in this setting needs to be individualized and should be considered more strongly in daycare centers that resemble households where children have prolonged contact.

Neisseria meningitidis Chemoprophylaxis. Chemoprophylaxis is also necessary for close contacts of patients with invasive meningococcal disease; up to 10% of meningococcal meningitis cases have had contact with another known case. The estimated prevalence of meningococcal carriage in the United States is 5 to 10% under nonepidemic conditions. In closed populations such as military recruits, carriage rates can reach levels of 40 to 90%.[296] Household contacts exposed to a case of meningococcal disease have a 500- to 800-fold to 3000- to 4000-fold increased risk of invasive disease.[59] Secondary systemic meningococcal disease often develops within 5 days of recognition of the index case, with 70 to 80% of secondary cases occurring within 14 days of the primary case; in one report, 9 of 17 (53%) secondary cases occurred 5 to 39 weeks after the primary case.[504] Transmission of *N. meningitidis* has also been documented in a campus bar, dance club, and sports club.[505–507]

Chemoprophylaxis is recommended for close contacts of the index case, defined as household contacts, daycare center members, and anyone directly exposed to the patient's oral secretions (e.g., through kissing, mouth-to-mouth resuscitation, endotracheal intubation, or endotracheal tube management).[508] Chemoprophylaxis is not recommended for school, work, or transportation contacts. Chemoprophylaxis may also need to be administered to the index case before hospital discharge because certain antimicrobial agents (e.g., high-dose penicillin or chloramphenicol) do not reliably eradicate meningococci from the nasopharynx of colonized patients. Chemoprophylaxis should be administered as soon as possible (ideally within 24 hours) after the case is identified; administration 14 or more days after the onset of illness in the index patient is probably of limited value.

The optimal chemoprophylactic agent to prevent invasive meningococcal disease is controversial. The CDC currently recommends the administration of rifampin at 12-hour intervals for 2 days in the following dosages: adults, 600 mg; children 1 month or older, 10 mg/kg; and infants younger than 1 month, 5 mg/kg.[508] However, rifampin has several shortcomings, including nasopharyngeal eradication rates of only about 80%, adverse events, necessity for multiple doses over a 2-day period, and emergence of resistant organisms (up to 10 to 27% of isolates), which may then cause invasive disease. In the search for alternative agents, ceftriaxone (intramuscular administration of 250 mg in adults and 125 mg in children) eliminated the serogroup A carrier state in 97% of patients in one study for up to 2 weeks,[509] although parenteral administration is required. Additional studies have demonstrated a single dose of oral ciprofloxacin (500 mg in adults) to be very effective in elimination of the nasopharyngeal carriage of *N. meningitidis*.[448] Ciprofloxacin concentrations in nasal secretions have been shown to exceed the MIC_{90} for meningococci.[510] Ciprofloxacin may well supplant rifampin for chemoprophylaxis in adults. Ciprofloxacin is not recommended for use in children because of concern regarding cartilage damage. In pregnant patients, ceftriaxone is probably the safest alternative agent for chemoprophylaxis. Widespread chemoprophylaxis to low-risk contacts should be discouraged because of the concern over emergence of resistant organisms and possible future limitations on this approach.

Streptococcus pneumoniae Chemoprophylaxis. The risk of secondary pneumococcal disease in contacts of infected patients has not been defined, although outbreaks have been described in closed populations such as gold miners, military recruits, and jail inmates.[502] In one outbreak in a daycare center,[511] treatment of 97% of the daycare center children and staff with rifampin (10 mg/kg twice daily for 2 days) resulted in a 70% reduction (i.e., only partial eradication) of positive nasopharyngeal cultures for *S. pneumoniae* but did not prevent new acquisition of this organism by three children and one family member. Further studies are needed before chemoprophylaxis is recommended for contacts of patients with pneumococcal meningitis. Some authors do recommend prophylaxis with oral penicillin in patients with sickle cell disease; therapy in such patients has been shown to reduce the incidence of pneumococcal bacteremia by 84%.[512] The CDC has recommended daily penicillin prophylaxis for children with sickle cell hemoglobinopathy beginning before 4 months of age,[513] although consensus has not been reached regarding the age when prophylaxis should be discontinued.

Streptococcus agalactiae Chemoprophylaxis. Administration of ampicillin during labor to mothers with prenatal vaginal or rectal group B streptococcal colonization and obstetric risk factors (e.g., premature labor, prolonged rupture of membranes, or intrapartum fever) has been associated with reduced rates of colonization and early-onset streptococcal sepsis in the neonate.[514] The CDC has recently established guidelines for the prevention of group B streptococcal infection by chemoprophylaxis.[515] All pregnant women should be screened at 35 to 37 weeks' gestation for anogenital colonization with group B streptococci. Maternal group B streptococcal carriers, identified either antepartum or intrapartum, should receive chemoprophylaxis if one or more of the following risk factors are present: preterm labor at less than 37 weeks' gestation, fever (temperature of 38°C or higher) during labor, or after membranes have been ruptured 18 or more hours during any gestation. Furthermore, previous delivery of a sibling with invasive group B streptococcal disease warrants intrapartum maternal chemoprophylaxis in each subsequent pregnancy. Chemoprophylaxis should consist of intrapartum intravenous ampicillin (2 g initially and then 1 to 2 g every 4 hours) or penicillin G (5 million units initially and then 2.5 million units every 4 hours) until delivery; intravenous clindamycin or erythromycin should be used in penicillin-allergic patients.

Basilar Skull Fracture. A number of studies have used prophylactic antibiotics in patients with basilar skull fractures and CSF leak on the premise that in patients with a dural defect, the CSF is exposed to pathogenic organisms from the nasopharynx, nasal or mastoid sinuses, or external auditory canal.[79, 115] Interpretation and comparison of the various studies examining this question are confounded by multiple variables, including patient selection, choice of antimicrobial agents, and definition of infection. No prospective controlled trials have examined the efficacy of prophylactic antimicrobial agents in these patients, although a recent meta-analysis suggested that antibiotic prophylaxis did not prevent meningitis in patients with basilar skull fracture.[516] Antibiotic use does not appear to change the incidence of post-traumatic bacterial meningitis and may result in the selection and growth of resistant organisms.

Haemophilus influenzae Immunoprophylaxis. Vaccination to prevent infection with specific meningeal pathogens is a very useful measure for decreasing the incidence of bacterial meningitis. For *H. influenzae* type B, the availability of conjugate vaccines has decreased the number of cases of *H. influenzae* type B meningitis more than 90%.[44, 55–58] Three *H. influenzae* type B conjugate vaccines are now licensed for infant immunization. The American Academy of Pediatrics has recommended vaccine doses at 2, 4, and 6 months of age[517]; if PRP-OMP (PedvaxHIB) is administered at 2 and 4 months, a dose at 6 months is not required.

Neisseria meningitidis Immunoprophylaxis. Monovalent vaccines using purified serogroup capsular polysaccharide antigens of *N. meningitidis* have been shown to be immunogenic in humans,[518] although the serogroup C component is poorly immunogenic in recipients younger than 2 years. Serogroup A and C vaccines have demonstrated estimated clinical efficacies of 85 to 100% in older children and adults and are useful in controlling epidemics. The duration of efficacy, however, decreases markedly during the first 3 years after a single dose of vaccine, a decrease that occurs more rapidly in infants and children than in adults. Bactericidal antibody responses are also elicited in adults with the newly licensed quadrivalent vaccine (activity against serogroups A, C, Y, and W135). However, a major obstacle to the efficacy of meningococcal vaccine is the lack of a suitable vaccine against serogroup B. Vaccination with the quadrivalent meningococcal vaccine is currently recommended for patients in certain high-risk groups, including those with terminal complement component or properdin deficiency or dysfunction, patients with anatomic or functional asplenia, those who travel to areas with hyperendemic or epidemic meningococcal disease (e.g., Nigeria), military recruits, and those who are close contacts of the primary case, as an adjunct to chemoprophylaxis, although this use is controversial and of unproven efficacy.[518] Research, industrial, and clinical laboratory personnel who are routinely exposed to *N. meningitidis* in solutions that may be aerosolized should also be considered for vaccination. The vaccine is not recommended for routine use in the United States because of the overall low risk of infection, the inability to protect against serogroup B disease, and the inability to provide lasting immunity to young children.

Streptococcus pneumoniae Immunoprophylaxis. Use of the current 23-valent pneumococcal vaccine is currently recommended for prevention of bacteremic pneumococcal disease in certain high-risk groups[513]: persons 65 years and older; persons aged 2 to 64 years with chronic cardiovascular disease, chronic pulmonary disease, diabetes mellitus, alcoholism, chronic liver disease, CSF leaks, or functional or anatomic asplenia; and those living in special environments or social settings (including Alaskan natives and certain Native American populations). Immunocompromised persons 2 years or older with HIV infection, hematologic or generalized malignancies, chronic renal failure, or nephrotic syndrome, those receiving immunosuppressive chemotherapy (including corticosteroids), and those who have received an organ or bone marrow transplant should also be vaccinated. Efficacy of the vaccine in prevention of pneumococcal meningitis has never been proved, although it may be assumed that the overall efficacy of the vaccine is about 50% against pneumococcal meningitis (with a wide 95% confidence interval); in addition, no data have proved efficacy in infants and very young children.[518] One recent study examined the efficacy of a heptavalent conjugate pneumococcal vaccine in 37,000 infants and children and demonstrated an effectiveness of 100% in the prevention of invasive pneumococcal disease in fully vaccinated children.[519] Further studies may lead to the recommendation to include pneumococcal conjugate vaccines in routine childhood immunization programs.[520]

REFERENCES

1. Connolly KJ, Hammer SM. The acute aseptic meningitis syndrome. Infect Dis Clin North Am. 1990;4:599–622.
2. Rotbart HA. Viral meningitis and the aseptic meningitis syndrome. In: Scheld WM, Whitley RJ, Durack DT, eds. Infections of the Central Nervous System. 2nd ed. Philadelphia: Lippincott-Raven; 1997:23–46.
3. Nicolosi A, Hauser WA, Beghi E, et al. Epidemiology of central nervous system infections in Olmstead County, Minnesota, 1950–1981. J Infect Dis. 1986;154:399–408.
4. Berlin LE, Rorabaugh ML, Heldrich F, et al. Aseptic meningitis in infants <2 years of age: Diagnosis and etiology. J Infect Dis. 1993;168:888–892.
5. Strikas RA, Anderson LJ, Parker RA. Temporal and geographic patterns of isolates of nonpolio enterovirus in the United States, 1970–1983. J Infect Dis. 1986;153:346–351.
6. Centers for Disease Control and Prevention. Aseptic meningitis—New York state and United States, weeks 1–36, 1991. MMWR Morb Mortal Wkly Rep. 1991;40:773–775.
7. Rantakallio P, Leskinen M, von Wendt L. Incidence and prognosis of central nervous system infections in a birth cohort of 12,000 children. Scand J Infect Dis. 1986;18:287–294.
8. Monath TP, Heinz FX. Flaviviruses. In: Fields BN, Knipe DM, Howley PM, eds. Virology. Philadelphia: Lippincott-Raven; 1996:961–1034.
9. Tsai TF, Canfield MA, Reed CM, et al. Epidemiologic aspects of a St. Louis encephalitis outbreak in Harris County, Texas, 1986. J Infect Dis. 1988;157:351–356.
10. Emmons RW. Ecology of Colorado tick fever. Annu Rev Microbiol. 1988;42:49–64.
11. Goodpasture HC, Poland JD, Francy DB, et al. Colorado tick fever: Clinical, epidemiologic, and laboratory aspects of 228 cases in Colorado in 1973–1974. Ann Intern Med. 1978;88:303–310.
12. Gnann JW Jr. Meningitis and encephalitis caused by mumps virus. In: Scheld WM, Whitley RJ, Durack DT, eds. Infections of the Central Nervous System. 2nd ed. Philadelphia: Lippincott-Raven; 1997:169–180.
13. Levitt LP, Rich TA, Kinde SW, et al. Central nervous system mumps. Neurology. 1970;20:829–834.
14. Miller E, Goldacre M, Pugh S, et al. Risk of aseptic meningitis after measles, mumps, and rubella vaccine in UK children. Lancet. 1993;341:979–982.

15. Deibel R, Woodall JP, Decher WJ, et al. Lymphocytic choriomeningitis virus in man. Serologic evidence of association with pet hamsters. JAMA. 1975;232:501–504.
16. Vanzee BE, Douglas RG Jr, Betts RF, et al. Lymphocytic choriomeningitis in university hospital personnel. Clinical features. Am J Med. 1975;58:803–809.
17. Hirsch MS, Moellering RC Jr, Pope HG, et al. Lymphocytic-choriomeningitis–virus infection traced to a pet hamster. N Engl J Med. 1974;291:610–612.
18. Dykewicz CA, Dato VM, Fisher-Hoch SP, et al. Lymphocytic choriomeningitis outbreak associated with nude mice in a research institute. JAMA. 1992;267:1349–1353.
19. Olsen LC, Beuscher EL, Artenstein MS, et al. Herpesvirus infections of the human central nervous system. N Engl J Med. 1967;277:1271–1277.
20. Craig CP, Nahmias AJ. Different patterns of neurologic involvement with herpes simplex virus types 1 and 2: Isolation of herpes simplex virus type 2 from the buffy coat of two adults with meningitis. J Infect Dis. 1973;127:365–372.
21. Corey L, Adams HG, Brown ZA, et al. Genital herpes simplex virus infection: Clinical manifestations, course, and complications. Ann Intern Med. 1983;98:958–972.
22. Echevarria JM, Martinez-Martin P, Tellaz A, et al. Aseptic meningitis due to varicella-zoster virus: Serum antibody levels and local synthesis of specific IgG, IgM, and IgA. J Infect Dis. 1987;155:959–967.
23. Barnes DW, Whitley RJ. CNS diseases associated with varicella zoster virus and herpes simplex virus infection. Pathogenesis and current therapy. Neurol Clin. 1986;4:265–283.
24. Causey JQ. Spontaneous cytomegalovirus mononucleosis-like syndrome and aseptic meningitis. South Med J. 1976;69:1384–1387.
25. Duchowny M, Caplan L, Siber G. Cytomegalovirus infection of the adult nervous system. Ann Neurol. 1979;5:458–461.
26. Corey L, Spear PG. Infections with herpes simplex viruses (second of two parts). N Engl J Med. 1986;314:749–757.
27. Bergström T, Vahlne A, Alestig K, et al. Primary and recurrent herpes simplex virus type 2–induced meningitis. J Infect Dis. 1990;162:322–330.
28. Mayo DR, Booss J. Varicella zoster–associated neurologic disease without skin disease. Arch Neurol. 1989;46:313–315.
29. Karp SJ. Meningitis and cutaneous disseminated zoster complicating herpes zoster infection. J Neurol Neurosurg Psychiatry. 1983;46:582–590.
30. Steel JG, Dix RD, Baringer JR. Isolation of herpes simplex virus type 1 in recurrent (Mollaret) meningitis. Ann Neurol. 1982;11:17–21.
31. Yamamoto LJ, Tedder DG, Ashley R, et al. Herpes simplex virus type 1 DNA in cerebrospinal fluid of a patient with Mollaret's meningitis. N Engl J Med. 1991;325:1082–1085.
32. Tedder DG, Ashley R, Tyler KL, Levin MJ. Herpes simplex virus infection as a cause of benign recurrent lymphocytic meningitis. Ann Intern Med. 1994;121:334–338.
33. Picard FJ, Dekaban GA, Silva J, Rice GPA. Mollaret's meningitis associated with herpes simplex type 2 infection. Neurology. 1993;43:1722–1727.
34. Graman PS. Mollaret's meningitis associated with acute Epstein-Barr virus mononucleosis. Arch Neurol. 1987;44:1204–1205.
35. Huang LM, Lee CY, Lee PI, et al. Meningitis caused by human herpesvirus-6. Arch Dis Child. 1991;66:1443–1444.
36. Caserta MT, Hall CB, Schnabel K, et al. Neuroinvasion and persistence of human herpesvirus 6 in children. J Infect Dis. 1994;170:1586–1589.
37. Silverstein A, Steinberg G, Nathanson M. Nervous system involvement in infectious mononucleosis. Arch Neurol. 1972;26:353–358.
38. Berger JR, Simpson DM. Neurological complications of AIDS. In: Scheld WM, Whitley RJ, Durack DT, eds. Infections of the Central Nervous System. 2nd ed. Philadelphia: Lippincott-Raven; 1997;255–271.
39. McArthur JC. Neurologic manifestations of AIDS. Medicine (Baltimore). 1987;66:407–437.
40. Carne CA, Tedder RS, Smith A, et al. Acute encephalopathy coincident with seroconversion for anti-HTLV-III. Lancet. 1985;2:1206–1208.
41. Hollander H, Stringari S. Human immunodeficiency virus–associated meningitis. Clinical course and correlations. Am J Med. 1987;83:813–816.
42. Schlech WF III, Ward JI, Band JD, et al. Bacterial meningitis in the United States, 1978 through 1981. The National Bacterial Meningitis Surveillance Study. JAMA. 1985;253:1749–1754.
43. Wenger JD, Hightower AW, Facklam RR, et al. Bacterial meningitis in the United States, 1986: Report of a multistate surveillance study. J Infect Dis. 1990;162:1316–1323.
44. Schuchat A, Robinson K, Wenger JD, et al. Bacterial meningitis in the United States in 1995. N Engl J Med. 1997;337:970–976.
45. Sigurdardottir B, Bjornsson OM, Jonsdottir KE, et al. Acute bacterial meningitis in adults. A 20-year overview. Arch Intern Med. 1997;157:425–430.
46. Durand ML, Calderwood SB, Weber DJ, et al. Acute bacterial meningitis in adults. A review of 493 episodes. N Engl J Med. 1993;328:21–28.
47. Noah ND. Epidemiology of bacterial meningitis: UK and USA. In: Williams JD, Burnie J, eds. Bacterial Meningitis. London: Academic; 1987:93–115.
48. Greenwood BM. The epidemiology of acute bacterial meningitis in tropical Africa. In: Williams JD, Burnie J, eds. Bacterial Meningitis. London: Academic; 1987:61–91.
49. Bryan JP, de Silva HR, Tavares A, et al. Etiology and mortality of bacterial meningitis in northeastern Brazil. Rev Infect Dis. 1990;12:128–135.
50. Spagnuolo PJ, Ellner JJ, Lerner PI, et al. *Haemophilus influenzae* meningitis: The spectrum of disease in adults. Medicine (Baltimore). 1982;61:74–85.
51. Crowe HM, Levitz RE. Invasive *Haemophilus influenzae* disease in adults. Arch Intern Med. 1987;147:241–244.
52. Takala AK, Eskola J, van Alphen L. Spectrum of invasive *Haemophilus influenzae* type b disease in adults. Arch Intern Med. 1990;150:2573–2576.
53. Farley MM, Stephens DS, Brachman PS, et al. Invasive *Haemophilus influenzae* disease in adults. A prospective, population-based surveillance. Ann Intern Med. 1992;116:806–812.
54. Robbins JB, Schneerson R, Anderson P, Smith DH. Prevention of systemic infections, especially meningitis, caused by *Haemophilus influenzae* type b. JAMA. 1996;276:1181–1185.
55. Garpenholt O, Silfverdal SA, Hugosson S, et al. The impact of *Haemophilus influenzae* type b vaccination in Sweden. Scand J Infect Dis. 1996;28:165–169.
56. Van Alphen L, Spanjaard L, Van der Ende A, et al. Effect of nationwide vaccination of 3-month-old infants in The Netherlands with conjugate *Haemophilus influenzae* type b vaccine: High efficacy and lack of herd immunity. J Pediatr. 1997;131:869–873.
57. Mulholland K, Hilton S, Adegbola R, et al. Randomised trial of *Haemophilus influenzae* type-b tetanus protein conjugate for prevention of pneumonia and meningitis in Gambian infants. Lancet. 1997;349:1191–1197.
58. Steinhoff MC. *Haemophilus influenzae* type b infections are preventable everywhere. Lancet. 1997;349:1186–1187.
59. Riedo FX, Plikaytis BD, Broome CV. Epidemiology and prevention of meningococcal disease. Pediatr Infect Dis J. 1995;14:643–657.
60. Jackson LA, Schuchat A, Reeves MW, Wenger JD. Serogroup C meningococcal outbreaks in the United States. An emerging threat. JAMA. 1995;273:383–389.
61. Whalen CM, Hockin JC, Ryan A, Ashton R. The changing epidemiology of invasive meningococcal disease in Canada, 1985 through 1992. Emergence of a virulent clone of *Neisseria meningitidis*. JAMA. 1995;273:390–394.
62. Raymond NJ, Reeves M, Ajello G, et al. Molecular epidemiology of sporadic (endemic) serogroup C meningococcal disease. J Infect Dis. 1997;176:1277–1284.
63. Ross SC, Densen P. Complement deficiency states and infection: Epidemiology, pathogenesis and consequences of neisserial and other infections in an immune deficiency. Medicine (Baltimore). 1984;64:243–273.
64. Ellison RT III, Kohler PF, Curd JG, et al. Prevalence of congenital or acquired complement deficiency in patients with sporadic meningococcal disease. N Engl J Med. 1983;308:913–916.
65. Rosen MS, Lorber B, Myers AR. Chronic meningococcal meningitis. An association with C5 deficiency. Arch Intern Med. 1988;148:1441–1442.
66. Fijen CAP, Kuijper EJ, Hannema AJ, et al. Complement deficiencies in patients over ten years old with meningococcal disease due to uncommon serogroups. Lancet. 1989;2:585–588.
67. Zoppi M, Weiss M, Nydegger UE, et al. Recurrent meningitis in a patient with congenital deficiency of the C9 component of complement. First case of C9 deficiency in Europe. Arch Intern Med. 1990;150:2395–2399.
68. Fijen CAP, Kuijper EJ, Tjia HG, et al. Complement deficiency predisposes for meningitis due to nongroupable meningococci and *Neisseria*-related bacteria. Clin Infect Dis. 1994;18:780–784.
69. Sjöholm AG, Kuijper EJ, Tijssen CC, et al. Dysfunctional properdin in a Dutch family with meningococcal disease. N Engl J Med. 1988;319:33–37.
70. Fraser DW, Geil CC, Feldman RA. Bacterial meningitis in Bernalillo County, New Mexico: A comparison with three other American populations. Am J Epidemiol. 1974;100:29–34.
71. Gray BM, Converse GM III, Dillon HC Jr. Serotypes of *Streptococcus pneumoniae* causing invasive disease. J Infect Dis. 1979;140:979–983.
72. Broome CV, Facklam RR, Allen JR, et al. Epidemiology of pneumococcal serotypes in the United States. J Infect Dis. 1980;141:119–123.
73. Geiseler PJ, Nelson KE, Levin S, et al. Community-acquired purulent meningitis: A review of 1,316 cases during the antibiotic era, 1954–1976. Rev Infect Dis. 1980;2:725–745.
74. Burman LA, Norrby R, Trollfors B. Invasive pneumococcal infections: Incidence, predisposing factors, and prognosis. Rev Infect Dis. 1985;7:133–142.
75. Olopoenia L, Frederick W, Greaves W, et al. Pneumococcal sepsis and meningitis in adults with sickle cell disease. South Med J. 1990;83:1002–1004.
76. Godeau B, Bachir D, Schaeffer A, et al. Severe pneumococcal sepsis and meningitis in human immunodeficiency virus–infected adults with sickle cell disease. Clin Infect Dis. 1992;15:327–329.
77. Musher DM. Infections caused by *Streptococcus pneumoniae*: Clinical spectrum, pathogenesis, immunity, and treatment. Clin Infect Dis. 1992;14:801–809.
78. Kragsbjerg P, Kallman J, Olcen P. Pneumococcal meningitis in adults. Scand J Infect Dis. 1994;26:659–666.
79. Tunkel AR, Scheld WM. Acute infectious complications of head trauma. In: Braakman R, ed. Handbook of Clinical Neurology, Head Injury. Amsterdam: Elsevier; 1990:317–326.
80. Gellin BG, Broome CV. Listeriosis. JAMA. 1989;261:1313–1320.
81. Cherubin CE, Appleman MD, Heseltine PNR, et al. Epidemiological spectrum and current treatment of listeriosis. Rev Infect Dis. 1991;13:1108–1114.
82. Anaissie E, Kontoyiannis DP, Kantarjian H, et al. Listeriosis in patients with chronic lymphocytic leukemia who were treated with fludarabine and prednisone. Ann Intern Med. 1992;117:466–469.
83. Skogberg K, Syrjänen J, Jahkola M, et al. Clinical presentation and outcome of listeriosis in patients with and without immunosuppressive therapy. Clin Infect Dis. 1992;14:815–821.
84. Kessler SL, Dajani AS. *Listeria* meningitis in infants and children. Pediatr Infect Dis J. 1990;9:61–63.
85. Lorber B. Listeriosis. Clin Infect Dis. 1997;24:1–11.

86. Mylonakis E, Hohmann EL, Calderwood SB. Central nervous system infection with *Listeria monocytogenes*. 33 years' experience at a general hospital and review of 776 episodes from the literature. Medicine (Baltimore). 1998;77:313–336.
87. Decker CF, Simon GL, DiGioia RA, et al. *Listeria monocytogenes* infections in patients with AIDS: Report of five cases and review. Rev Infect Dis. 1991;13:413–417.
88. Berenguer J, Solera J, Diaz MD, et al. Listeriosis in patients infected with human immunodeficiency virus. Rev Infect Dis. 1991;13:115–119.
89. Zuniga M, Aguado JM, Vada J. *Listeria monocytogenes* meningitis in previously healthy adults: Long-term follow-up. Q J Med. 1992;85:911–915.
90. Schuchat A, Deaver KA, Wenger JD, et al. Role of foods in sporadic listeriosis. I. Case-control study of dietary risk factors. JAMA. 1992;267:2041–2045.
91. Pinner RW, Schuchat A, Swaminathan B, et al. Role of foods in sporadic listeriosis. II. Microbiologic and epidemiologic investigation. JAMA. 1992;267:2046–2050.
92. Bula CJ, Bille J, Glauser MP. An epidemic of food-borne listeriosis in western Switzerland: Description of 57 cases involving adults. Clin Infect Dis. 1995;20:66–72.
93. Calder JAM. *Listeria* meningitis in adults. Lancet. 1997;350:307–308.
94. Saez-Llorens X, McCracken GH Jr. Bacterial meningitis in neonates and children. Infect Dis Clin North Am. 1990;4:623–644.
95. Regan JA, Klebanoff MA, Nugent RP. The Vaginal Infections and Prematurity Study Group. The epidemiology of group B streptococcal colonization in pregnancy. Obstet Gynecol. 1991;77:604–610.
96. Schuchat A. Epidemiology of group B streptococcal disease in the United States: Shifting paradigms. Clin Microbiol Rev. 1998;11:497–513.
97. Farley MM, Harvey RC, Stull T, et al. A population-based assessment of invasive disease due to group B streptococci in nonpregnant adults. N Engl J Med. 1993;328:1807–1811.
98. Dunne DW, Quagliarello V. Group B streptococcal meningitis in adults. Medicine (Baltimore). 1993;72:1–10.
99. Jackson LA, Hilsdon R, Farley MM, et al. Risk factors for group B streptococcal disease in adults. Ann Intern Med. 1995;123:415–420.
100. Domingo P, Barquet N, Alvarez M, et al. Group B streptococcal meningitis in adults: Report of twelve cases and review. Clin Infect Dis. 1997;25:1180–1187.
101. Robibaro B, Vorbach H, Weigel G, et al. Group B streptococcal meningoencephalitis after colonization in a nonpregnant woman. Clin Infect Dis. 1998;26:1243–1244.
102. Mangi RJ, Quintiliani R, Andriole VT. Gram-negative bacillary meningitis. Am J Med. 1975;59:829–836.
103. Cherubin CE, Marr JS, Sierra MF, et al. *Listeria* and gram-negative bacillary meningitis in New York City, 1972–1979. Am J Med. 1981;71:199–209.
104. Gower DJ, Barrows AA, Kelly DL, et al. Gram-negative bacillary meningitis in the adult: Review of 39 cases. South Med J. 1986;79:1499–1502.
105. Campbell JR, Diacovo T, Baker CJ. *Serratia marcescens* meigitis in neonates. Pediatr Infect Dis J. 1992;11:881–886.
106. Unhanand M, Mustafa MM, McCracken GH Jr, et al. Gram-negative enteric bacillary meningitis: A twenty-one-year experience. J Pediatr. 1993;122:15–21.
107. Ventura G, Tumbarello M, Tacconelli E, et al. Gram-negative bacillary meningitis in adults. J Chemother. 1995;7(Suppl 4):S177–S179.
108. Tang LM, Chen ST. *Klebsiella oxytoca* meningitis: Frequent association with neurosurgical procedures. Infection. 1995;23:163–167.
109. Papadakis KA, Vartivarian SE, Vassilaki ME, Anaissie EJ. *Stenotrophomonas maltophilia* meningitis. Report of two cases and review of the literature. J Neurosurg. 1997;87:106–108.
110. Cameron ML, Durack DT. Helminthic infections of the central nervous system. In: Scheld WM, Whitley RJ, Durack DT, eds. Infections of the Central Nervous System. 2nd ed. Philadelphia: Lippincott-Raven; 1997:845–878.
111. Gordon JJ, Harter DH, Phair JP. Meningitis due to *Staphylococcus aureus*. Am J Med. 1985;78:965–970.
112. Schlesinger LS, Ross SC, Schaberg DR. *Staphylococcus aureus* meningitis: A broad-based epidemiologic study. Medicine (Baltimore). 1987;66:148–156.
113. Jensen AG, Espersen F, Skinhoj P, et al. *Staphylococcus aureus* meningitis. A review of 104 nationwide, consecutive cases. Arch Intern Med. 1993;153:1902–1908.
114. Lerche A, Rasmussen N, Wandall JH, Bohr VA. *Staphylococcus aureus* meningitis: A review of 28 consecutive community-acquired cases. Scand J Infect Dis. 1995;27:560–573.
115. Kaufman BA, Tunkel AR, Pryor JC, et al. Meningitis in the neurosurgical patient. Infect Dis Clin North Am. 1990;4:677–701.
116. Bayston R. Hydrocephalus shunt infections. J Antimicrob Chemother. 1994;34(Suppl A): S75–S84.
117. Bross JE, Gordon G. Nocardial meningitis: Case reports and review. Rev Infect Dis. 1991;13:160–165.
118. Heerema MS, Ein ME, Musher DM, et al. Anaerobic bacterial meningitis. Am J Med. 1979;67:219–227.
119. Feder HM Jr. *Bacteroides fragilis* meningitis. Rev Infect Dis. 1987;9:783–786.
120. Long JG, Preblud SR, Keyserling HL. *Clostridium perfringens* meningitis in an infant: Case report and literature review. Pediatr Infect Dis J. 1987;6:752–754.
121. Law DA, Aronoff SC. Anaerobic meningitis in children: Case report and review of the literature. Pediatr Infect Dis J. 1992;11:968–971.
122. Korman TM, Athan E, Spelman DW. Anaerobic meningitis due to *Peptostreptococcus* species: Case report and review. Clin Infect Dis. 1997;25:1462–1464.
123. Stevenson KB, Murray EW, Sarubbi FA. Enterococcal meningitis: Report of four cases and review. Clin Infect Dis. 1994;18:233–239.
124. Hook EW III. Central nervous system syphilis. In: Scheld WM, Whitley RJ, Durack DT, eds. Infections of the Central Nervous System. 2nd ed. Philadelphia: Lippincott-Raven; 1997:669–684.
125. Simon RP. Neurosyphilis. Arch Neurol. 1985;42:606–613.
126. Hook EW III. Syphilis and HIV infection. J Infect Dis. 1989;160:530–534.
127. Musher DM, Hamill RJ, Baughn RE. Effect of human immunodeficiency virus (HIV) infection on the course of syphilis and on the response to treatment. Ann Intern Med. 1990;113:872–881.
128. Hook EW III, Marra CM. Acquired syphilis in adults. N Engl J Med. 1992;326:1060–1069.
129. Katz DA, Berger JR. Neurosyphilis in acquired immunodeficiency syndrome. Arch Neurol. 1989;46:895–898.
130. Flood JM, Weinstock HS, Guroy ME, et al. Neurosyphilis during the AIDS epidemic, San Francisco, 1985–1992. J Infect Dis. 1998;177:931–940.
131. Reik L Jr. Lyme disease. In: Scheld WM, Whitley RJ, Durack DT, eds. Infections of the Central Nervous System. 2nd ed. Philadelphia: Lippincott-Raven; 1997;685–718.
132. Reik L, Steere AC, Bartenhagen NH, et al. Neurologic abnormalities of Lyme disease. Medicine (Baltimore). 1979;58:281–294.
133. Pachner AR, Steere AC. The triad of neurologic manifestations of Lyme disease: Meningitis, cranial neuritis and radiculoneuritis. Neurology. 1985;35:47–53.
134. Luft BJ, Steinman CR, Neimark HC, et al. Invasion of the central nervous system by *Borrelia burgdorferi* in acute disseminated infection. JAMA. 1992;267:1364–1367.
135. Niu MT, Duma RJ, Meningitis due to protozoa and helminths. Infect Dis Clin North Am. 1990;4:809–841.
136. Durack DT. Amebic infections. In: Scheld WM, Whitley RJ, Durack DT, eds. Infections of the Central Nervous System. 2nd ed. Philadelphia: Lippincott-Raven; 1997:831–844.
137. Wellings FM, Amuso PT, Chang SL, et al. Isolation and identification of pathogenic *Naegleria* from Florida lakes. Appl Environ Microbiol. 1977;34:661–667.
138. Gardner HAR, Martinez AJ, Visvesvara GS, et al. Granulomatous amebic encephalitis in an AIDS patient. Neurology. 1991;41:1993–1995.
139. Di Gregorio C, Rivasi R, Mongiardo N, et al. *Acanthamoeba* meningoencephalitis in a patient with acquired immunodeficiency syndrome. Arch Pathol Lab Med. 1992;116:1363–1365.
140. Gordon SM, Steinberg JP, DuPuis MH, et al. Culture isolation of *Acanthamoeba* species and leptomyxid amebas from patients with amebic meningoencephalitis, including two patients with AIDS. Clin Infect Dis. 1992;15:1024–1030.
141. Hawley HB, Czachor JS, Malhotra V, et al. *Acanthamoeba* encephalitis in patients with AIDS. AIDS Reader. 1997;7:137–142.
142. Koo J, Pien F, Kliks MM. *Angiostrongylus (Parastrongylus)* eosinophilic meningitis. Rev Infect Dis. 1988;10:1155–1162.
143. Kliks MM, Palumbo NE. Eosinophilic meningitis beyond the Pacific basin: The global dispersal of a peridomestic zoonosis caused by *Angiostrongylus cantonensis*, the nematode lungworm of rats. Soc Sci Med. 1992;34:199–212.
144. Campbell BG, Little MD. The finding of *Angiostrongylus cantonensis* in rats in New Orleans. Am J Trop Med Hyg. 1988;38:568–573.
145. Schmutzhard E, Boongird P, Vejjajiva A. Eosinophilic meningitis and radiculomyelitis in Thailand, caused by CNS invasion of *Gnathostoma spinigerum* and *Angiostrongylus cantonensis*. J Neurol Neurosurg Psychiatry. 1988;51:80–87.
146. Johnson RT. Pathogenesis of CNS infections. In: Viral Infections of the Central Nervous System. New York: Raven; 1982:37–60.
147. Tunkel AR, Wispelwey B, Scheld WM. Pathogenesis and pathophysiology of meningitis. Infect Dis Clin North Am. 1990;4:555–581.
148. Cassady KA, Whitley RJ. Pathogenesis and pathophysiology of viral infections of the central nervous system. In: Scheld WM, Whitley RJ, Durack DT, eds. Infections of the Central Nervous System. 2nd ed. Philadelphia: Lippincott-Raven; 1997:7–22.
149. Johnson RT, Mims CA. Pathogenesis of viral infections of the nervous system. N Engl J Med. 1968;278:23–30, 84–92.
150. Kristensson K, Ghetti B, Wisniewski HM. Study on the propagation of herpes simplex virus (type 2) into brain after intraocular injection. Brain Res. 1974;69:189–201.
151. Ren R, Racaniello VR. Poliovirus spreads from muscle to the central nervous system by neural pathways. J Infect Dis. 1992;166:747–752.
152. Frei K, Leist TP, Meager A, et al. Production of B cell stimulatory factor-2 and interferon γ in the central nervous system during viral meningitis and encephalitis: Evaluation in a murine model infection and in patients. J Exp Med. 1988;168:449–453.
153. Chonmaitree T, Baron S. Bacteria and viruses induce production of interferon in the cerebrospinal fluid of children with acute meningitis: A study of 57 cases and review. Rev Infect Dis. 1991;13:1061–1065.
154. Ramilo O, Mustafa MM, Porter J, et al. Detection of interleukin 1β but not tumor necrosis factor-α in cerebrospinal fluid of children with aseptic meningitis. Am J Dis Child. 1990;144:349–352.
155. Resnick L, diMarzo-Veronese F, Schüpbach J, et al. Intra–blood-brain-barrier synthesis of HTLV-III–specific IgG in patients with neurologic symptoms associated with AIDS or AIDS-related complex. N Engl J Med. 1985;313:1498–1504.
156. Gnann JW Jr, Whitley RJ. Neurologic manifestations of varicella and herpes zoster. In: Scheld WM, Whitley RJ, Durack DT, eds. Infections of the Central Nervous System. 2nd ed. Philadelphia: Lippincott-Raven; 1997:91–105.
157. Tunkel AR, Wispelwey B, Scheld WM. Bacterial meningitis: Recent advances in pathophysiology and treatment. Ann Intern Med. 1990;112:610–623.
158. Quagliarello V, Scheld WM. Bacterial meningitis: Pathogenesis, pathophysiology, and progress. N Engl J Med. 1992;327:864–872.

159. Tunkel AR, Scheld WM. Pathogenesis and pathophysiology of bacterial meningitis. Clin Microbiol Rev. 1993;6:118–136.
160. Pfister HW, Fontana A, Tauber MG, et al. Mechanisms of brain injury in bacterial meningitis: Workshop summary. Clin Infect Dis. 1994;19:463–479.
161. van Furth AM, Roord JJ, van Furth R. Roles of proinflammatory and anti-inflammatory cytokines in pathophysiology of bacterial meningitis and effect of adjunctive therapy. Infect Immun. 1996;64:4883–4890.
162. Stephens DS, Farley MM. Pathogenic events during infection of the human nasopharynx with *Neisseria meningitidis* and *Haemophilus influenzae*. Rev Infect Dis. 1991;13:22–33.
163. Greenblatt JJ, Floyd K, Philipps MW, et al. Morphologic differences in *Neisseria meningitidis* pili. Infect Immun. 1988;56:2356–2362.
164. Smith AL. Pathogenesis of *Haemophilus influenzae* meningitis. Pediatr Infect Dis J. 1987;6:783–786.
165. Nesin M, Ramirez M, Tomasz A. Capsular transformation of a multidrug-resistant *Streptococcus pneumoniae* in vitro. J Infect Dis. 1998;177:707–713.
166. Malley R, Stack AM, Ferretti ML, et al. Anticapsular polysaccharide antibodies and nasopharyngeal colonization with *Streptococcus pneumoniae* in infant rats. J Infect Dis. 1998;178:878–882.
167. Robbins JB, McCracken GH Jr, Gotschlich EL, et al. *Escherichia coli* K1 capsular polysaccharide associated with neonatal meningitis. N Engl J Med. 1974;290:1216–1220.
168. Kim KS, Itabashi H, Genski P, et al. The K1 capsule is the critical determinant in the development of *Escherichia coli* meningitis in the rat. J Clin Invest. 1992;90:897–905.
169. Brandtzaeg P, Mollnes TE, Kierulf P. Complement activation and endotoxin levels in systemic meningococcal disease. J Infect Dis. 1989;160:58–65.
170. Smith AL, Daum RS, Scheifele D, et al. Pathogenesis of *Haemophilus influenzae* meningitis. In: Sell SH, Wright PF, eds. *Haemophilus influenzae:* Epidemiology, Immunology, and Prevention of Disease. New York: Elsevier; 1982:89–109.
171. Ostrow PT, Moxon ER, Vernon N, et al. Pathogenesis of bacterial meningitis. Studies on the route of meningeal invasion following *Haemophilus influenzae* inoculation in infant rats. Lab Invest. 1979;40:678–685.
172. Parkkinen J, Korhonen TK, Pere A, et al. Binding sites in the rat brain for *Escherichia coli* S fimbriae associated with neonatal meningitis. J Clin Invest. 1988;81:860–865.
173. Saukkonen KM, Nowicki B, Leinonen M. Role of type 1 and S fimbriae in the pathogenesis of *Escherichia coli* O18:K1 bacteremia and meningitis in the infant rat. Infect Immun. 1988;56:892–897.
174. Meier C, Oelschlaeger TA, Merkert H, et al. Ability of *Escherichia coli* isolates that cause meningitis in newborns to invade epithelial and endothelial cells. Infect Immun. 1996;64:2391–2399.
175. Pron B, Taha MK, Rambaud C, et al. Interaction of *Neisseria meningitidis* with the components of the blood-brain barrier correlates with an increased expression of PilC. J Infect Dis. 1997;176:1285–1292.
176. Huang SH, Wass C, Fu Q, et al. *Escherichia coli* invasion of brain microvascular endothelial cells in vitro and in vivo: Molecular cloning and characterization of invasion gene *ibe10*. Infect Immun. 1995;63:4470–4475.
177. Bingen E, Bonacorsi S, Brahimi N, et al. Virulence patterns of *Escherichia coli* K1 strains associated with neonatal meningitis. J Clin Microbiol. 1997;35:2981–2982.
178. Hoffman JA, Zhang Y, Badger JL, Kim KS. Identification of a novel gene locus contributing to *E. coli* invasion of the blood-brain barrier. In: Program and Abstracts of the 37th Interscience Conference on Antimicrobial Agents and Chemotherapy. Washington, DC: American Society for Microbiology; 1998.
179. Williams AE, Blakemore WF. Pathogenesis of meningitis caused by *Streptococcus suis* type 2. J Infect Dis. 1990;162:474–481.
180. Ring A, Weiser JN, Tuomanen EI. Pneumococcal trafficking across the blood-brain barrier. Molecular analysis of a novel bidirectional pathway. J Clin Invest. 1998;102:347–360.
181. Kadurugamuwa JL, Hengstler B, Zak O. Inhibition of complement-factor-5a–induced inflammatory reactions by prostaglandin E_2 in experimental meningitis. J Infect Dis. 1989;160:715–719.
182. Stahel PF, Frei K, Fontana A, et al. Evidence for intrathecal synthesis of alternative pathway complement activation proteins in experimental meningitis. Am J Pathol. 1997;151:897–904.
183. Stahel PF, Nadal D, Pfister HW, et al. Complement C3 and factor B cerebrospinal fluid concentrations in bacterial and aseptic meningitis. Lancet. 1997;349:1886–1887.
184. Seebach J, Bartholdi D, Frei K, et al. Experimental *Listeria* meningoencephalitis. Macrophage inflammatory protein-1α and -2 are produced intrathecally and mediate chemotactic activity in cerebrospinal fluid of infected mice. J Immunol. 1995;155:4367–4375.
185. Inaba Y, Ishiguro A, Shimbo T. The production of macrophage inflammatory protein-1α in the cerebrospinal fluid at the initial stage of meningitis in children. Pediatr Res. 1997;42:788–793.
186. Spanaus KS, Nadal D, Pfister HW, et al. C-X-C and C-C chemokines are expressed in the cerebrospinal fluid in bacterial meningitis and mediate chemotactic activity on peripheral blood–derived polymorphonuclear and mononuclear cells in vitro. J Immunol. 1997;158:1956–1964.
187. Sprenger H, Rosler A, Tonn P, et al. Chemokines in the cerebrospinal fluid of patients with meningitis. Clin Immunol Immunopathol. 1996;80:155–161.
188. Tan TQ, Smith W, Hawkins EP, et al. Hematogenous bacterial meningitis in an intercellular adhesion molecule-1–deficient infant mouse model. J Infect Dis. 1995;171:342–349.
189. Weber JR, Angstwurm K, Burger W, et al. Anti ICAM (CD 54) monoclonal antibody reduces inflammatory changes in experimental bacterial meningitis. J Neuroimmunol. 1995;63:63–68.
190. Tuomanen EI, Saukkonen K, Sande S, et al. Reduction of inflammation, tissue damage, and mortality in bacterial meningitis in rabbits treated with monoclonal antibodies against adhesion-promoting receptors of leukocytes. J Exp Med. 1989;170:959–968.
191. Rozdzinski E, Jones T, Burnette WN, et al. Antiinflammatory effects in experimental meningitis of prokaryotic peptides that mimic selectins. J Infect Dis. 1993;168:1422–1428.
192. Tan TQ, Smith W, Hawkins EP, Kaplan SL. Anti-CD11b monoclonal antibody in an infant rat model of *Haemophilus influenzae* type b sepsis and meningitis. J Antimicrob Chemother. 1997;39:209–216.
193. Tang T, Frenette PS, Hynes RO, et al. Cytokine-induced meningitis is dramatically attenuated in mice deficient in endothelial selectins. J Clin Invest. 1996;97:2485–2490.
194. Granert C, Raud J, Xie I, et al. Inhibition of leukocyte rolling with polysaccharide fucoidin prevents pleocytosis in experimental meningitis in the rabbit. J Clin Invest. 1994;93:929–936.
195. Tuomanen E. A spoonful of sugar to control inflammation? J Clin Invest. 1994;93:917–918.
196. Lorenzl S, Loedel U, Dirnagl U, et al. Imaging of leukocyte-endothelium interaction using in vivo confocal laser scanning microscopy during the early phase of experimental pneumococcal meningitis. J Infect Dis. 1993;168:927–933.
197. Weber JR, Angstwurm K, Rosenkranz T, et al. Heparin inhibits leukocyte rolling in pial vessels and attenuates inflammatory changes in a rat model of experimental bacterial meningitis. J Cereb Blood Flow Metab. 1997;17:1221–1229.
198. Tuomanen E, Tomasz A, Hengstler B, et al. The relative role of bacterial cell wall and capsule in the induction of inflammation in pneumococcal meningitis. J Infect Dis. 1985;151:535–540.
199. Tuomanen E, Liu H, Hengstler B, et al. The induction of meningeal inflammation by components of the pneumococcal cell wall. J Infect Dis. 1985;151:859–868.
200. Friedland IR, Paris MM, Hickey S, et al. The limited role of pneumolysin in the pathogenesis of pneumococcal meningitis. J Infect Dis. 1995;172:805–809.
201. Syrogiannopoulos GA, Hansen EJ, Erwin AL, et al. *Haemophilus influenzae* type b lipooligosaccharide induces meningeal inflammation. J Infect Dis. 1988;157:237–244.
202. Wispelwey B, Lesse AJ, Hansen EJ, et al. *Haemophilus influenzae* lipopolysaccharide–induced blood brain barrier permeability during experimental meningitis in the rat. J Clin Invest. 1988;82:1339–1346.
203. Mustafa MM, Ramilo O, Olsen KD, et al. Tumor necrosis factor in mediating experimental *Haemophilus influenzae* type b meningitis. J Clin Invest. 1989;84:1253–1259.
204. Moller B, Mogensen SC, Wendelboe P, et al. Bioactive and inactive forms of tumor necrosis factor-α in spinal fluid from patients with meningitis. J Infect Dis. 1991;163:886–889.
205. Leist TP, Frei K, Kam-Hansen S, et al. Tumor necrosis factor α in cerebrospinal fluid during bacterial, but not viral, meningitis. Evaluation in murine model infections and in patients. J Exp Med. 1988;167:1743–1748.
206. Nadal D, Leppert D, Frei K, et al. Tumor necrosis factor-α in infectious meningitis. Arch Dis Child. 1989;64:1274–1279.
207. Glimaker M, Kragsbjerg P, Forsgren M, et al. Tumor necrosis factor-α (TNFα) in cerebrospinal fluid from patients with meningitis of different etiologies: High levels of TNFα indicate bacterial meningitis. J Infect Dis. 1993;167:882–889.
208. Lopez-Cortes LF, Cruz-Ruiz M, Gomez-Mateos J, et al. Measurement of levels of tumor necrosis factor-α and interleukin-1β in the CSF of patients with meningitis of different etiologies: Utility in the differential diagnosis. Clin Infect Dis. 1993;16:534–539.
209. Mustafa MM, Ramilo O, Saez-Llorens X, et al. Cerebrospinal fluid prostaglandins, interleukin 1β, and tumor necrosis factor in bacterial meningitis. Clinical and laboratory correlations in placebo-treated and dexamethasone-treated patients. Am J Dis Child. 1990;144:883–887.
210. Ramilo O, Saez-Llorens X, Mertsola J, et al. Tumor necrosis factor α/cachectin and interleukin 1β initiate meningeal inflammation. J Exp Med. 1990;172:497–507.
211. Saukkonen K, Sande S, Cioffe C, et al. The role of cytokines in the generation of inflammation and tissue damage in experimental gram-positive meningitis. J Exp Med. 1990;171:439–448.
212. Cabellos C, MacIntyre DE, Forrest M, et al. Differing roles for platelet-activating factor during inflammation of the lung and subarachnoid space. The special case of *Streptococcus pneumoniae*. J Clin Invest. 1992;90:612–618.
213. Townsend GC, Scheld WM. Platelet-activating factor augments meningeal inflammation elicited by *Haemophilus influenzae* lipooligosaccharide in an animal model of meningitis. Infect Immun. 1994;62:3739–3744.
214. McCracken GH Jr, Mustafa MM, Ramilo O, et al. Cerebrospinal fluid interleukin 1-beta and tumor necrosis factor concentrations and outcome from neonatal gram-negative enteric bacillary meningitis. Pediatr Infect Dis J. 1989;8:155–159.
215. Arditi M, Ables L, Yogev R. Cerebrospinal fluid endotoxin levels in children with *H. influenzae* meningitis before and after administration of intravenous ceftriaxone. J Infect Dis. 1989;160:1005–1011.
216. Friedland IR, Jafari H, Ehrett S, et al. Comparison of endotoxin release by different antimicrobial agents and the effect on inflammation in experimental *Escherichia coli* meningitis. J Infect Dis. 1993;168:657–662.
217. Mustafa MM, Mertsola J, Ramilo O, et al. Increased endotoxin and interleukin-1β concentrations in cerebrospinal fluid of infants with coliform meningitis and ventriculitis associated with intraventricular gentamicin therapy. J Infect Dis. 1989;160:891–895.

218. Mustafa MM, Lebel MH, Ramilo O, et al. Correlation of interleukin-1β and cachectin concentrations in cerebrospinal fluid and outcome from bacterial meningitis. J Pediatr. 1989;115:208–213.
219. Arditi M, Manogue KR, Caplan M, et al. Cerebrospinal fluid cachectin/tumor necrosis factor-α and platelet-activating factor concentrations and severity of bacterial meningitis in children. J Infect Dis. 1990;162:139–147.
220. Ossege LM, Sindern E, Voss B, Malin JP. Expression of tumor necrosis factor-α and transforming growth factor-β1 in cerebrospinal fluid cells in meningitis. J Neurol Sci. 1996;144:1–13.
221. Ichiyama T, Hayashi T, Furukawa S. Cerebrospinal fluid concentrations of soluble tumor necrosis factor receptor in bacterial and aseptic meningitis. Neurology. 1996;46:837–838.
222. Paris MM, Friedland IR, Ehrett S, et al. Effect of interleukin-1 receptor antagonist and soluble tumor necrosis factor receptor in animal models of infection. J Infect Dis. 1995;171:161–169.
223. Rusconi F, Parizzi F, Garlaschi L, et al. Interleukin 6 activity in infants and children with bacterial meningitis. Pediatr Infect Dis J. 1991;10:117–121.
224. Waage A, Halstensen A, Shalaby R, et al. Local production of tumor necrosis factor α, interleukin 1, and interleukin 6 in meningococcal meningitis. Relation to the inflammatory response. J Exp Med. 1989;170:1859–1867.
225. Chavanet P, Bonnotte B, Guiguet M, et al. High concentrations of intrathecal interleukin-6 in human bacterial and nonbacterial meningitis. J Infect Dis. 1992;166:428–431.
226. Azuma H, Tsuda N, Sasaki K, Okuno A. Clinical significance of cytokine measurements for detection of meningitis. J Pediatr. 1997;131:463–465.
227. Waage A, Brandtzaeg P, Halstensen A, et al. The complex pattern of cytokines in serum from patients with meningococcal septic shock. Association between interleukin 6, interleukin 1, and fatal outcome. J Exp Med. 1989;169:333–338.
228. Halstensen A, Ceska M, Brandtzaeg P, et al. Interleukin-8 in serum and cerebrospinal fluid from patients with meningococcal disease. J Infect Dis. 1993;167:471–475.
229. Lopez-Cortes LF, Cruz-Ruiz M, Gomez-Mateos J, et al. Interleukin-8 in cerebrospinal fluid from patients with meningitis of different etiologies: Its possible role as neutrophil chemotactic factor. J Infect Dis. 1995;172:581–584.
230. Ostergaard C, Benfield TL, Sellebjerg F, et al. Interleukin-8 in cerebrospinal fluid from patients with septic and aseptic meningitis. Eur J Clin Microbiol Infect Dis. 1996;15:166–169.
231. Frei K, Nadal D, Pfister HW, Fontana A. *Listeria* meningitis: Identification of a cerebrospinal fluid inhibitor of macrophage listericidal function as interleukin-10. J Exp Med. 1993;178:1255–1261.
232. van Furth AM, Seijmonsbergen EM, Langermans JAM, et al. High levels of interleukin-10 and tumor necrosis factor in cerebrospinal fluid during the onset of bacterial meningitis. Clin Infect Dis. 1995;21:220–222.
233. Diab A, Zhu J, Lindquist L, et al. Cytokine mRNA profiles during the course of experimental *Haemophilus influenzae* bacterial meningitis. Clin Immunol Immunopathol. 1997;85:236–245.
234. Kornelisse RF, Savelkoul HFJ, Mulder PHG, et al. Interleukin-10 and soluble tumor necrosis factor receptors in cerebrospinal fluid of children with bacterial meningitis. J Infect Dis. 1996;173:1498–1502.
235. Paris MM, Hickey SM, Trujillo M, et al. The effect of interleukin-10 on meningeal inflammation in experimental bacterial meningitis. J Infect Dis. 1997;176:1239–1246.
236. Kornelisse RF, Hack CE, Savelkoul HFJ, et al. Intrathecal production of interleukin-12 and gamma interferon in patients with bacterial meningitis. Infect Immun. 1997;65:877–881.
237. Quagliarello VJ, Long WJ Jr, Scheld WM. Morphologic alterations in the blood-brain barrier with experimental meningitis in the rat. Temporal sequence and role of encapsulation. J Clin Invest. 1986;77:1084–1095.
238. Lesse AJ, Moxon ER, Zwahlen A, et al. Role of cerebrospinal fluid pleocytosis and *Haemophilus influenzae* type b capsule on blood brain barrier permeability during experimental meningitis in the rat. J Clin Invest. 1988;82:102–109.
239. Quagliarello VJ, Ma A, Stukenbrok H, et al. Ultrastructural localization of albumin transport across the cerebral microvasculature during experimental meningitis in the rat. J Exp Med. 1991;174:657–672.
240. Wispelwey B, Hansen EJ, Scheld WM. *Haemophilus influenzae* outer membrane vesicle–induced blood-brain barrier permeability during experimental meningitis. Infect Immun. 1989;57:2559–2562.
241. Roord JJ, Apicella M, Scheld WM. The induction of meningeal inflammation and blood-brain barrier permeability by *Haemophilus influenzae* type b peptidoglycan. J Infect Dis. 1994;170:254–256.
242. Quagliarello VJ, Wispelwey B, Long WJ Jr, et al. Recombinant human interleukin-1 induces meningitis and blood-brain barrier injury in the rat. Characterization and comparison with tumor necrosis factor. J Clin Invest. 1991;87:1360–1366.
243. Sharief MK, Ciardi M, Thompson EJ. Blood-brain barrier damage in patients with bacterial meningitis: Association with tumor necrosis factor-α but not interleukin-1β. J Infect Dis. 1992;166:350–358.
244. Tunkel AR, Scheld WM. Alterations in the blood-brain barrier in bacterial meningitis: In vivo and in vitro models. Pediatr Infect Dis J. 1989;8:911–913.
245. Tunkel AR, Rosser SW, Hansen EJ, et al. Blood-brain barrier alterations in bacterial meningitis: Development of an in vitro model and observations on the effects of lipopolysaccharide. In Vitro Cell Dev Biol. 1991;27A:113–120.
246. Patrick D, Betts J, Frey EA, et al. *Haemophilus influenzae* lipopolysaccharide disrupts confluent monolayers of bovine brain endothelial cells via a serum-dependent cytotoxic pathway. J Infect Dis. 1992;165:865–872.
247. Tobias PS, Mathison JC, Ulevitch RJ. A family of lipopolysaccharide binding proteins involved in responses to gram-negative sepsis. J Biol Chem. 1988;263:13479–13481.
248. Scheld WM, Dacey RG, Winn HR, et al. Cerebrospinal fluid outflow resistance in rabbits with experimental meningitis. Alterations with penicillin and methylprednisolone. J Clin Invest. 1980;66:243–253.
249. Täuber MG, Khayam-Bashi H, Sande MA. Effects of ampicillin and corticosteroids on brain water content, cerebrospinal fluid pressure, and cerebrospinal fluid lactate levels in experimental pneumococcal meningitis. J Infect Dis. 1985;151:528–534.
250. Täuber MG, Shibl AM, Hackbarth CJ, et al. Antibiotic therapy, endotoxin concentrations in cerebrospinal fluid, and brain edema in experimental *Escherichia coli* meningitis in rabbits. J Infect Dis. 1987;156:456–462.
251. Burroughs M, Prasad S, Cabellos C, et al. The biologic activities of peptido-glycan in experimental *Haemophilus influenzae* meningitis. J Infect Dis. 1993;167:464–468.
252. Täuber MG, Borschberg U, Sande MA. Influence of granulocytes on brain edema, intracranial pressure, and cerebrospinal fluid concentrations of lactate and protein in experimental meningitis. J Infect Dis. 1988;157:456–464.
253. Täuber MG, Burroughs M, Neimoller UM, et al. Differences of pathophysiology in experimental meningitis caused by three strains of *Streptococcus pneumoniae*. J Infect Dis. 1991;163:806–811.
254. Engelhard D, Pomeranz S, Gallily R, et al. Serotype-related differences in inflammatory response to *Streptococcus pneumoniae* in experimental meningitis. J Infect Dis. 1997;175:979–982.
255. Syrogiannopoulos GA, Olsen KD, McCracken GH Jr. Mannitol treatment in experimental *Haemophilus influenzae* type b meningitis. Pediatr Res. 1987;22:118–122.
256. Lorenzl S, Koedel U, Pfister HW. Mannitol, but not allopurinol, modulates changes in cerebral blood flow, intracranial pressure, and brain water content during pneumococcal meningitis in the rat. Crit Care Med. 1996;24:1874–1880.
257. Tureen JH, Dworkin SL, Kennedy SL, et al. Loss of cerebrovascular autoregulation in experimental meningitis in rabbits. J Clin Invest. 1990;85:577–581.
258. Tureen JH, Täuber MG, Sande MA. Effect of hydration status on cerebral blood flow and cerebrospinal fluid lactic acidosis in rabbits with experimental meningitis. J Clin Invest. 1992;89:947–953.
259. Pfister HW, Koedel U, Haberl RL, et al. Microvascular changes during the early phase of experimental bacterial meningitis. J Cereb Blood Flow Metab. 1990;10:914–922.
260. Tureen J, Liu Q, Chow L. Near-infrared spectroscopy in experimental pneumococcal meningitis in the rabbit: Cerebral hemodynamics and metabolism. Pediatr Res. 1996;40:759–763.
261. Slater AJ, Berkowitz ID, Wilson DA, Traystman RJ. Role of leukocytes in cerebral autoregulation and hyperemia in bacterial meningitis in rabbits. Am J Physiol. 1997;42:H380–H386.
262. Koedel U, Lorenzl S, Gorriz C, et al. Endothelin B receptor–mediated increase of cerebral blood flow in experimental pneumococcal meningitis. J Cereb Blood Flow Metab. 1998;18:67–74.
263. Koedel U, Gorriz C, Lorenzl S, Pfister HW. Increased endothelin levels in cerebrospinal fluid samples from adults with bacterial meningitis. Clin Infect Dis. 1997;25:329–330.
264. Paulson OB, Brodersen P, Hansen EL, et al. Regional cerebral blood flow, cerebral metabolic rate of oxygen, and cerebrospinal fluid acid-base variables in patients with acute meningitis and with acute encephalitis. Acta Med Scand. 1974;196:191–205.
265. McMenamin JB, Volpe JJ. Bacterial meningitis in infancy: Effects on intracranial pressure and cerebral blood flow velocity. Neurology. 1984;34:500–504.
266. Goh D, Minns RA. Cerebral blood flow velocity monitoring in pyogenic meningitis. Arch Dis Child. 1993;68:111–119.
267. Ashwal S, Stringer W, Tomasi L, et al. Cerebral blood flow and carbon dioxide reactivity in children with bacterial meningitis. J Pediatr. 1990;117:523–530.
268. Ashwal S, Tomasi L, Schneider S, et al. Bacterial meningitis in children: Pathophysiology and treatment. Neurology. 1992;42:739–748.
269. Pfister HW, Borasio GD, Dirnagl U, et al. Cerebrovascular complications of bacterial meningitis in adults. Neurology. 1992;42:1497–1504.
270. Guerra-Romero L, Täuber MG, Fournier MA, et al. Lactate and glucose concentrations in brain interstitial fluid, cerebrospinal fluid, and serum during experimental pneumococcal meningitis. J Infect Dis. 1992;166:546–550.
271. Pfister HW, Koedel U, Lorenzl S, et al. Antioxidants attenuate microvascular changes in the early phase of experimental pneumococcal meningitis in rats. Stroke. 1992;23:1798–1804.
272. Pfister HW, Ködel U, Dirnagl U, et al. Effect of catalase on regional cerebral blood flow and brain edema during the early phase of experimental pneumococcal meningitis. J Infect Dis. 1992;166:1442–1445.
273. Leib SL, Kim YS, Chow LL, et al. Reactive oxygen intermediates contribute to necrotic and apoptotic neuronal injury in an infant rat model of bacterial meningitis due to group B streptococci. J Clin Invest. 1996;98:2632–2639.
274. Bogdan I, Leib SL, Bergeron M, et al. Tumor necrosis factor-α contributes to apoptosis in hippocampal neurons during experimental group B streptococcal meningitis. J Infect Dis. 1997;176:693–697.
275. Shenep JL, Tuomanen E. Perspective: Targeting nitric oxide in the adjuvant therapy of sepsis and meningitis. J Infect Dis. 1998;177:766–769.
276. Kortytko PJ, Boje KMK. Pharmacological characterization of nitric oxide production in a rat model of meningitis. Neuropharmacology. 1996;35:231–237.
277. Koedel U, Bernatowicz A, Paul R, et al. Experimental pneumococcal meningitis: Cerebrovascular alterations, brain edema, and meningeal inflammation are linked to the production of nitric oxide. Ann Neurol. 1995;37:313–323.

278. Paul R, Koedel U, Pfister HW. 7-Nitroindazole inhibits pial vasodilation in a rat model of pneumococcal meningitis. J Cereb Blood Flow Metab. 1997;17:985–991.
279. Buster BL, Weintrob AC, Townsend GC, Scheld WM. Potential role of nitric oxide in the pathophysiology of experimental bacterial meningitis in the rat. Infect Immun. 1995;63:3835–3839.
280. Boje KMK. Inhibition of nitric oxide synthase attenuates blood-brain barrier disruption during experimental meningitis. Brain Res. 1996;720:75–83.
281. Leib SL, Kim YS, Black SM, et al. Inducible nitric oxide synthase and the effect of aminoguanidine in experimental neonatal meningitis. J. Infect Dis. 1998;177:692–700.
282. Lorenzl S, Kodel U, Frei K, Pfister HW. Effect of the bradykinin B_2 receptor antagonist Hoe140 in experimental pneumococcal meningitis in the rat. Eur J Pharmacol. 1996;308:335–341.
283. Koedel U, Bernatowicz A, Frei K, et al. Systematically (but not intrathecally) administered IL-10 attenuates pathophysiologic alterations in experimental pneumococcal meningitis. J Immunol. 1996;157:5185–5191.
284. Kornelisse RF, Hoekman K, Visser JJ, et al. The role of nitric oxide in bacterial meningitis in children. J Infect Dis. 1996;174:120–126.
285. van Furth AM, Seijmonsbergen EM, Groeneveld PHP, et al. Levels of nitric oxide correlate with high levels of tumor necrosis factor α in cerebrospinal fluid samples from children with bacterial meningitis. Clin Infect Dis. 1996;22:876–878.
286. Guerra-Romero L, Tureen JH, Fournier MA, et al. Amino acids in cerebrospinal and brain interstitial fluid in experimental pneumococcal meningitis. Pediatr Res. 1993;33:510–513.
287. Leib SL, Kim YS, Ferriero DM, Täuber MG. Neuroprotective effect of excitatory amino acid antagonist kynurenic acid in experimental bacterial meningitis. J Infect Dis. 1996;173:166–171.
288. Spranger M, Krempien S, Schwab S, et al. Excess glutamate in the cerebrospinal fluid in bacterial meningitis. J Neurol Sci. 1996;143:126–131.
289. Spranger M, Schwab S, Krempien S, et al. Excess glutamate levels in the cerebrospinal fluid predict clinical outcome of bacterial meningitis. Arch Neurol. 1996;53:992–996.
290. Kaplan MH, Klein SW, McPhee J, et al. Group B coxsackievirus infections in infants younger than three months of age: A serious childhood illness. Rev Infect Dis. 1983;5:1019–1032.
291. Wilfert CM, Lehrman SN. Enteroviruses and meningitis. Pediatr Infect Dis. 1983;2:333–341.
292. Jaffe M, Srugo I, Tirosh E, et al. The ameliorating effect of lumbar puncture in viral meningitis. Am J Dis Child. 1989;143:682–685.
293. McKinney RE Jr, Katz SL, Wilfert CM. Chronic enteroviral meningoencephalitis in agammaglobulinemic patients. Rev Infect Dis. 1987;9:334–356.
294. Gaduzda DH, Hirsch MS. Neurologic manifestations of infection with human immunodeficiency virus. Clinical features and pathogenesis. Ann Intern Med. 1987;107:383–391.
295. Carpenter RR, Petersdorf RG. The clinical spectrum of bacterial meningitis. Am J Med. 1962;33:262–275.
296. Roos KL, Tunkel AR, Scheld WM. Acute bacterial meningitis in children and adults. In: Scheld WM, Whitley RJ, Durack DT, eds. Infections of the Central Nervous System. 2nd ed. Philadelphia: Lippincott-Raven; 1997:335–401.
297. Verghese A, Gallemore G. Kernig's and Brudzinski's signs revisited. Rev Infect Dis. 1987;9:1187–1192.
298. Anderson J, Backer V, Voldsgaard P, et al. Acute meningococcal meningitis: Analysis of features of the disease according to the age of 255 patients. J Infect. 1997;34:227–235.
299. Geiseler PJ, Nelson KE. Bacterial meningitis without clinical signs of meningeal irritation. South Med J. 1982;75:448–450.
300. Ashwal S, Perkin RM, Thompson JR, et al. Bacterial meningitis in children: Current concepts of neurologic management. Curr Probl Pediatr. 1994;24:267–284.
301. Gorse GJ, Thrupp LD, Nudleman KL, et al. Bacterial meningitis in the elderly. Arch Intern Med. 1989;149:1603–1606.
302. Tunkel AR, Scheld WM. Central nervous system infection in the compromised host. In: Rubin RH, Young LS, eds. Clinical Approach to Infection in the Compromised Host. 3rd ed. New York: Plenum; 1994:163–210.
303. Kaufman BA. Infections of cerebrospinal fluid shunts. In: Scheld WM, Whitley RJ, Durack DT, eds. Infections of the Central Nervous System. 2nd ed. Philadelphia: Lippincott-Raven; 1997:555–577.
304. Odio C, McCracken GH Jr, Nelson JD. CSF shunt infections in pediatrics. Am J Dis Child. 1984;138:1103–1108.
305. Merritt HH, Moore M. Acute syphilitic meningitis. Medicine (Baltimore). 1935;14:119–183.
306. Holmes MD, Zawadzki B, Simon RP. Clinical features of meningovascular syphilis. Neurology. 1984;34:553–555.
307. Johns DR, Tierney M, Felsenstein D. Alteration in the natural history of neurosyphilis by concurrent infection with the human immunodeficiency virus. N Engl J Med. 1987;316:1569–1572.
308. Hutchinson CM, Rompalo AM, Reichart CA, et al. Characteristics of patients with syphilis attending Baltimore STD clinics: Multiple, high-risk subgroups and interactions with human immunodeficiency virus infection. Arch Intern Med. 1991;151:511–516.
309. Reik L, Burgdorfer W, Donaldson JO. Neurologic abnormalities in Lyme disease without erythema chronicum migrans. Am J Med. 1986;81:73–78.
310. Kuberski T, Wallace GD. Clinical manifestations of eosinophilic meningitis due to *Angiostrongylus cantonensis*. Neurology. 1979;29:1566–1570.
311. Dagan R, Henista JA, Menegus MA. Association of clinical presentation, laboratory findings, and virus serotypes with the presence of meningitis in hospitalized infants with enterovirus infection. J Pediatr. 1988;113:975–978.
312. Wildin S, Chonmaitree T. The importance of the virology laboratory in the diagnosis and management of viral meningitis. Am J Dis Child. 1987;141:454–457.
313. Chonmaitree T, Baldwin CD, Lucia HL. Role of the virology laboratory in diagnosis and management of patients with central nervous system disease. Clin Microbiol Rev. 1989;2:1–14.
314. Johnson GM, McAbee GA, Seaton ED, et al. Suspect value of non-CSF viral cultures in the diagnosis of enteroviral CNS infections in young infants. Dev Med Child Neurol. 1992;34:876–884.
315. Glimaker M, Samuelson A, Magnius L, et al. Early diagnosis of enteroviral meningitis by detection of specific IgM antibodies with a solid-phase reverse immunosorbent test (SPRIST) and μ-capture EIA. J Med Virol. 1992;36:193–201.
316. Rotbart HA. Diagnosis of enteroviral meningitis with the polymerase chain reaction. J Pediatr. 1990;117:85–89.
317. Sawyer MH, Holland D, Aintablian N. Diagnosis of enteroviral central nervous system infection by polymerase chain reaction during a large community outbreak. Pediatr Infect Dis J. 1994;13:177–182.
318. Rotbart HA, Sawyer MH, Fast S, et al. Diagnosis of enteroviral meningitis using the polymerase chain reaction with a colorimetric microwell detection assay. J Clin Microbiol. 1994;32:2590–2592.
319. Ahmed A, Brito F, Goto C, et al. Clinical utility of polymerase chain reaction for diagnosis of enteroviral meningitis in infancy. J Pediatr. 1997;131:393–397.
320. Ratzan KR. Viral meningitis. Med Clin North Am. 1985;69:399–413.
321. Echevarria JM, Cases I, Tenoirio A, et al. Detection of varicella-zoster virus–specific DNA sequences in cerebrospinal fluid from patients with acute aseptic meningitis and no cutaneous lesions. J Med Virol. 1994;43:331–335.
322. Shoji H, Honda Y, Murai I, et al. Detection of varicella-zoster virus DNA by polymerase chain reaction in cerebrospinal fluid of patients with herpes zoster meningitis. J Neurol. 1992;239:69–70.
323. Hollander H, Levy JA. Neurologic abnormalities and recovery of human immunodeficiency virus from cerebrospinal fluid. Ann Intern Med. 1987;106:692–695.
324. Chalmers AC, Aprill BS, Shephard H. Cerebrospinal fluid and human immunodeficiency virus. Findings in healthy, asymptomatic, seropositive men. Arch Intern Med. 1990;150:1538–1540.
325. Pratt RD, Nichols S, McKinney N, et al. Virologic markers of human immunodeficiency virus type 1 in cerebrospinal fluid of infected children. J Infect Dis. 1996;174:288–293.
326. Conrad AJ, Schmid P, Syndulko K, et al. Quantifying HIV-1 RNA using the polymerase chain reaction on cerebrospinal fluid and serum of seropositive individuals with and without neurologic abnormalities. J Acquir Immune Defic Syndr. 1995;10:425–435.
327. Feigin RD, McCracken GH Jr, Klein JO. Diagnosis and management of meningitis. Pediatr Infect Dis J. 1992;11:785–814.
328. Bonadio WA. The cerebrospinal fluid: Physiologic aspects and alterations associated with bacterial meningitis. Pediatr Infect Dis J. 1992;11:423–432.
329. Coll MT, Uriz MS, Pineda V, et al. Meningococcal meningitis with 'normal' cerebrospinal fluid. J Infect. 1994;29:289–294.
330. Sivakmaran M. Meningococcal meningitis revisited: Normocellular CSF. Clin Pediatr (Phila). 1997;36:351–355.
331. Marton KI, Gean AD. The spinal tap: A new look at an old test. Ann Intern Med. 1986;104:840–848.
332. Spanos A, Harrell FE Jr, Durack DT. Differential diagnosis of acute meningitis. An analysis of the predictive value of initial observation. JAMA. 1989;262:2700–2707.
333. McKinney WP, Heudebert GR, Harper SA, et al. Validation of a clinical prediction rule for the differential diagnosis of acute meningitis. J Gen Intern Med. 1994;9:8–12.
334. Genton B, Berger JP. Cerebrospinal fluid lactate in 78 cases of adult meningitis. Intensive Care Med. 1990;16:196–200.
335. La Scolea LJ Jr, Dryja D. Quantitation of bacteria in cerebrospinal fluid and blood of children with meningitis and its diagnostic significance. J Clin Microbiol. 1984;19:187–190.
336. Greenlee JE. Approach to diagnosis of meningitis. Cerebrospinal fluid evaluation. Infect Dis Clin North Am. 1990;4:583–597.
337. Gray LD, Fedorko DP. Laboratory diagnosis of bacterial meningitis. Clin Microbiol Rev. 1992;5:130–145.
338. Kaplan SL, O'Brian Smith E, Wills C, et al. Association between preadmission oral antibiotic therapy and cerebrospinal fluid findings and sequelae caused by *Haemophilus influenzae* type b meningitis. Pediatr Infect Dis J. 1986;5:626–632.
339. Blazer S, Berant M, Alon U. Bacterial meningitis: Effect of antibiotic treatment on cerebrospinal fluid. Am J Clin Pathol. 1983;80:386–387.
340. Davis SD, Hill HR, Feigl P, et al. Partial antibiotic therapy in *Haemophilus influenzae* meningitis. Its effect on cerebrospinal fluid abnormalities. Am J Dis Child. 1975;129:802–807.
341. Kristiansen BE, Ask E, Jenkins A, et al. Rapid diagnosis of meningococcal meningitis by polymerase chain reaction. Lancet. 1991;337:1568–1569.
342. Ni H, Knight AI, Cartwright K, et al. Polymerase chain reaction for diagnosis of meningococcal meningitis. Lancet. 1992;340:1432–1434.
343. Jaton K, Sahli R, Bille J. Development of polymerase chain reaction assays for detection of *Listeria monocytogenes* in clinical cerebrospinal fluid samples. J Clin Microbiol. 1992;30:1931–1936.
344. Radstrom P, Backman A, Qian N, et al. Detection of bacterial DNA in cerebrospinal fluid by an assay for simultaneous detection of *Neisseria meningitidis, Haemophilus influenzae*, and streptococci using a seminested PCR strategy. J Clin Microbiol. 1994;32:2738–2744.

345. Hall LMC, Duke B, Urwin G. An approach to the identification of the pathogens of bacterial meningitis by polymerase chain reaction. Eur J Clin Microbiol Infect Dis. 1995;14:1090–1094.
346. Caugant DA, Hoiby EA, Froholm LO, Brandtzaeg P. Polymerase chain reaction for case ascertainment of meningococcal meningitis: Application to the cerebrospinal fluids collected in the course of the Norwegian meningococcal serogroup B protection trial. Scand J Infect Dis. 1996;28:149–153.
347. Saunders NB, Shoemaker DR, Brandt BL, Zollinger WD. Confirmation of suspicious cases of meningococcal meningitis by PCR and enzyme-linked immunosorbent assay. J Clin Microbiol. 1997;35:3215–3219.
348. Friedland IR, Paris MM, Rinderknecht S, et al. Cranial computed tomographic scans have little impact on management of bacterial meningitis. Am J Dis Child. 1992;146:1484–1487.
349. Hart G. Syphilis tests in diagnostic and therapeutic decision making. Ann Intern Med. 1986;104:368–376.
350. Davis LE, Schmitt JW. Clinical significance of cerebrospinal fluid tests for neurosyphilis. Ann Neurol. 1989;25:50–55.
351. Noordhoek GT, Wolters EC, de Jonge MEJ, van Embden JDA. Detection by polymerase chain reaction of *Treponema pallidum* DNA in cerebrospinal fluid from neurosyphilis patients before and after antibiotic treatment. J Clin Microbiol. 1991;29:1976–1984.
352. Steere AC. Lyme disease. N Engl J Med. 1989;321:586–596.
353. Corpuz M, Hilton E, Lardis MP, et al. Problems in the use of serologic tests for the diagnosis of Lyme disease. Arch Intern Med. 1991;151:1837–1840.
354. American College of Physicians. Guidelines for laboratory evaluation in the diagnosis of Lyme disease. Ann Intern Med. 1997;127:1106–1108.
355. Tugwell P, Dennis DT, Weinstein A, et al. Laboratory evaluation in the diagnosis of Lyme disease. Ann Intern Med. 1997;127:1109–1123.
356. Keller TL, Halperin JJ, Whitman M. PCR detection of *Borrelia burgdorferi* DNA in cerebrospinal fluid of Lyme neuroborreliosis patients. Neurology. 1992;42:32–42.
357. Lebech AM, Hansen K. Detection of *Borrelia burgdorferi* DNA in urine samples and cerebrospinal fluid samples from patients with early and late Lyme neuroborreliosis by polymerase chain reaction. J Clin Microbiol. 1992;30:1646–1653.
358. Martinez AJ, Visvesvara GS. Laboratory diagnosis of pathogenic free-living amoebas: *Naegleria, Acanthamoeba* and *Leptomyxid*. Clin Lab Med. 1991;11:861–872.
359. Tunkel AR, Scheld WM. Therapy of bacterial meningitis: Principles and practice. Infect Control Hosp Epidemiol. 1989;10:565–569.
360. Tunkel AR, Scheld WM. Acute bacterial meningitis. Lancet. 1995;346:1675–1680.
361. Aronin SI, Peduzzi P, Quagliarello VJ. Community-acquired bacterial meningitis: Risk stratification for adverse clinical outcome and effect of antibiotic timing. Ann Intern Med. 1998;129:862–869.
362. Coant PN, Kornberg AE, Duffy LC, et al. Blood culture results as determinants in the organism identification of bacterial meningitis. Pediatr Emerg Care. 1992;8:200–205.
363. Tunkel AR, Scheld WM. Applications of therapy in animal models to bacterial infection in human disease. Infect Dis Clin North Am. 1989;3:441–459.
364. Täuber MG, Sande MA. General principles of therapy of pyogenic meningitis. Infect Dis Clin North Am. 1990;4:661–676.
365. Lebel MH, McCracken GH Jr. Delayed cerebrospinal fluid sterilization and adverse outcome of bacterial meningitis in infants and children. Pediatrics. 1989;83:161–167.
366. Campos J, Garcia-Tornel S, Sanfeliu I. Susceptibility studies of multiply resistant *Haemophilus influenzae* isolated from pediatric patients and contacts. Antimicrob Agents Chemother. 1984;25:706–709.
367. Campos J, Garcia-Tornel S, Gairi JM, et al. Multiply resistant *Haemophilus influenzae* type b causing meningitis: Comparative clinical and laboratory study. J Pediatr. 1986;108:897–902.
368. Givner LB, Abramson JS, Wasilauskas B. Meningitis due to *Haemophilus influenzae* type b resistant to ampicillin and chloramphenicol. Rev Infect Dis. 1989;11:329–334.
369. Peltola J, Anttila M, Renkonen OV, The Finnish Study Group. Randomised comparison of chloramphenicol, ampicillin, cefotaxime, and ceftriaxone for childhood bacterial meningitis. Lancet. 1989;1:1281–1287.
370. McCracken GH Jr. Current management of bacterial meningitis in infants and children. Pediatr Infect Dis J. 1992;11:169–174.
371. del Rio M, Chrane D, Shelton S, et al. Ceftriaxone versus ampicillin and chloramphenicol for treatment of bacterial meningitis in children. Lancet. 1983;1:1241–1244.
372. Jacobs RF, Wells TG, Steele RW, et al. A prospective randomized comparison of cefotaxime vs ampicillin and chloramphenicol for bacterial meningitis in children. J Pediatr. 1985;107:129–133.
373. American Academy of Pediatrics Committee on Infectious Diseases. Treatment of bacterial meningitis. Pediatrics. 1988;81:904–907.
374. Saez-Llorens X, Castano E, Garcia R, et al. Prospective randomized comparison of cefepime and cefotaxime for treatment of bacterial meningitis in infants and children. Antimicrob Agents Chemother. 1995;39:937–940.
375. Marks WA, Stutman HR, Marks MI, et al. Cefuroxime versus ampicillin plus chloramphenicol in childhood bacterial meningitis: A multicenter randomized controlled trial. J Pediatr. 1986;109:123–130.
376. Lebel MH, Hoyt MJ, McCracken GH Jr. Comparative efficacy of ceftriaxone and cefuroxime for treatment of bacterial meningitis. J Pediatr. 1989;114:1049–1054.
377. Schaad UB, Suter S, Gianella-Borradori A, et al. A comparison of ceftriaxone and cefuroxime for the treatment of bacterial meningitis in children. N Engl J Med. 1990;322:141–147.
378. Arditi M, Herold BC, Yogev R. Cefuroxime treatment failure and *Haemophilus influenzae* meningitis: Case report and review of the literature. Pediatrics. 1989;84:132–135.
379. Hatch DL, Overturf GD. Delayed cerebrospinal fluid sterilization in infants with *Haemophilus influenzae* type b meningitis. J Infect Dis. 1989;160:711–715.
380. Jorgensen JH. Update on mechanisms and prevalence of antimicrobial resistance in *Haemophilus influenzae*. Clin Infect Dis. 1992;14:1119–1123.
381. Campos J, Mendelman PM, Sako MU, et al. Detection of relatively penicillin G–resistant *Neisseria meningitidis* by disk susceptibility testing. Antimicrob Agents Chemother. 1987;31:1478–1482.
382. Van Esso D, Fontanals D, Uriz S, et al. *Neisseria meningitidis* with decreased susceptibility to penicillin. Pediatr Infect Dis. 1987;6:438–439.
383. Saez-Nieto JA, Lujan R, Berron S, et al. Epidemiology and molecular basis of penicillin-resistant *Neisseria meningitidis* in Spain: A 5-year history (1985–1989). Clin Infect Dis. 1992;14:394–402.
384. Mendelman PM, Campos J, Chaffin DO, et al. Relative penicillin G resistance in *Neisseria meningitidis* and reduced affinity of penicillin-binding protein 3. Antimicrob Agents Chemother. 1988;32:706–709.
385. Oppenheim BA. Antibiotic resistance in *Neisseria meningitidis*. Clin Infect Dis. 1997;24(Suppl 1):S98–S101.
386. Galimand M, Gerbaud G, Guibourdenche M, et al. High-level chloramphenicol resistance in *Neisseria meningitidis*. N Engl J Med. 1998;339:868–874.
387. Jackson LA, Tenover FC, Baker C, et al. Prevalence of *Neisseria meningitidis* relatively resistant to penicillin in the United States, 1991. J Infect Dis. 1994;169:438–441.
388. Buck GE, Adams M. *Meningococcus* with reduced susceptibility to penicillin isolated in the United States. Pediatr Infect Dis J. 1994;13:156–157.
389. Woods CR, Smith AL, Wasilauskas BL, et al. Invasive disease caused by *Neisseria meningitidis* relatively resistant to penicillin in North Carolina. J Infect Dis. 1994;170:453–456.
390. Casado-Flores J, Osona B, Comingo P, Barquet N. Meningococcal meningitis during penicillin therapy for meningococcemia. Clin Infect Dis. 1997;25:1479.
391. Goldani LZ. Inducement of *Neisseria meningitidis* resistance to ampicillin and penicillin in a patient with meningococcemia treated with high doses of ampicillin. Clin Infect Dis. 1998;26:772.
392. Cubells CL, Garcia JJG, Martinez JR, Otin CL. Clinical data in children with meningococcal meningitis in a Spanish hospital. Acta Paediatr. 1997;86:26–29.
393. Hopkins S, Williams D, Dunne M, et al. A randomized, controlled trial of oral or IV trovafloxacin vs. ceftriaxone in the treatment of epidemic meningococcal meningitis. In: Program and Abstracts of the 36th Interscience Conference on Antimicrobial Agents and Chemotherapy. Washington, DC: American Society for Microbiology; 1996.
394. Appelbaum PC. Antimicrobial resistance in *Streptococcus pneumoniae*: An overview. Clin Infect Dis. 1992;15:77–83.
395. Austrian R. Confronting drug-resistant pneumococci. Ann Intern Med. 1994;121:807–809.
396. Paris MM, Ramilo O, McCracken GH Jr. Management of meningitis caused by penicillin-resistant *Streptococcus pneumoniae*. Antimicrob Agents Chemother. 1995;39:2171–2175.
397. McDougal LK, Facklam R, Reeves M, et al. Analysis of multiply antimicrobial-resistant isolates of *Streptococcus pneumoniae* from the United States. Antimicrob Agents Chemother. 1992;36:2176–2184.
398. Hofmann J, Cetron MS, Farley MM, et al. The prevalence of drug-resistant *Streptococcus pneumoniae* in Atlanta. N Engl J Med. 1995;333:481–486.
399. Jernigan DB, Cetron MS, Breiman RF. Minimizing the impact of drug-resistant *Streptococcus pneumoniae* (DRSP). A strategy from the DRSP working group. JAMA. 1996;275:206–209.
400. Clavo-Sanchez AJ, Giron-Gonzalez JA, Lopez-Prieto D, et al. Multivariate analysis of risk factors for infection due to penicillin-resistant and multidrug-resistant *Streptococcus pneumoniae*: A multicenter study. Clin Infect Dis. 1997;24:1052–1059.
401. Yagupsky P, Porat N, Fraser D, et al. Acquisition, carriage, and transmission of pneumococci with decreased antibiotic susceptibility in young children attending a day care facility in southern Israel. J Infect Dis. 1998;177:1003–1012.
402. Guillemot D, Carbon C, Balkau B, et al. Low dosage and long treatment duration of β-lactam. Risk factors for carriage of penicillin-resistant *Streptococcus pneumoniae*. JAMA. 1998; 279:365–370.
403. American Academy of Pediatrics, Committee on Infectious Diseases. Therapy for children with invasive pneumococcal infections. Pediatrics. 1997;99:289–299.
404. Friedland IR, Klugman KP. Failure of chloramphenicol therapy in penicillin-resistant pneumococcal meningitis. Lancet. 1992;339:405–408.
405. Haas DW, Stratton CW, Griffin JP, et al. Diminished activity of ceftizoxime in comparison to cefotaxime and ceftriaxone against *Streptococcus pneumoniae*. Clin Infect Dis. 1995;20:671–676.
406. Waites KB, Rivers T. Bactericidal activities of ceftizoxime and cefotaxime against *Streptococcus pneumoniae*. Antimicrob Agents Chemother. 1998;42:1869–1870.
407. Sloas MM, Barrett FF, Chesney PJ, et al. Cephalosporin treatment failure in penicillin- and cephalosporin-resistant *Streptococcus pneumoniae* meningitis. Pediatr Infect Dis J. 1992;11:622–626.
408. John CC. Treatment failure with use of a third-generation cephalosporin for penicillin-resistant pneumococcal meningitis: Case report and review. Clin Infect Dis. 1994;18:188–193.
409. Catalan MJ, Fernandez JM, Vazquez A, et al. Failure of cefotaxime in the treatment of meningitis due to relatively resistant *Streptococcus pneumoniae*. Clin Infect Dis. 1994;18:766–769.

410. Tan TQ, Schutze GE, Mason EO Jr, Kaplan SL. Antibiotic therapy and acute outcome of meningitis due to *Streptococcus pneumoniae* considered intermediately susceptible to broad-spectrum cephalosporins. Antimicrob Agents Chemother. 1994;38:918–923.
411. Guibert M, Chahime H, Petit J, et al. Failure of cefotaxime treatment in two children with meningitis caused by highly penicillin-resistant *Streptococcus pneumoniae*. Acta Paediatr. 1995;84:831–833.
412. Ruiz-Irastorza GR, Garea C, Alonso JJ, et al. Failure of cefotaxime treatment in a patient with penicillin-resistant pneumococcal meningitis and confirmation of nosocomial spread by random amplified polymorphic DNA analysis. Clin Infect Dis. 1995;21:234–235.
413. Florez C, Silva G, Martin E. Cefotaxime failure in pneumococcal meningitis caused by a susceptible isolate. Pediatr Infect Dis J. 1996;15:723–724.
414. Pacheco TR, Cooper CK, Hardy DJ, et al. Failure of cefotaxime in an adult with *Streptococcus pneumoniae* meningitis. Am J Med. 1997;102:303–305.
415. Viladrich PF, Cabellos C, Pallares R, et al. High doses of cefotaxime in treatment of adult meningitis due to *Streptococcus pneumoniae* with decreased susceptibilities to broad-spectrum cephalosporins. Antimicrob Agents Chemother. 1996;40:218–220.
416. Friedland IR, Klugman KP. Cerebrospinal fluid bactericidal activity against cephalosporin-resistant *Streptococcus pneumoniae* in children with meningitis treated with high-dose cefotaxime. Antimicrob Agents Chemother. 1997;41:1888–1891.
417. Viladrich PF, Gudiol F, Linares J, et al. Evaluation of vancomycin for therapy of adult pneumococcal meningitis. Antimicrob Agents Chemother. 1991;35:2467–2472.
418. Paris MM, Hickey SM, Uscher MI, et al. Effect of dexamethasone on therapy of experimental penicillin- and cephalosporin-resistant pneumococcal meningitis. Antimicrob Agents Chemother. 1994;38:1320–1324.
419. Friedland IR, Paris M, Ehrett S, et al. Evaluation of antimicrobial regimens for treatment of experimental penicillin- and cephalosporin-resistant pneumococcal meningitis. Antimicrob Agents Chemother. 1993;37:1630–1636.
420. Klugman KP, Friedland IR, Bradley JS. Bactericidal activity against cephalosporin-resistant *Streptococcus pneumoniae* in cerebrospinal fluid of children with acute bacterial meningitis. Antimicrob Agents Chemother. 1995;39:1988–1992.
421. Doit C, Barre J, Cohen R, et al. Bactericidal activity against intermediately cephalosporin-resistant *Streptococcus pneumoniae* in cerebrospinal fluid of children with bacterial meningitis treated with high doses of cefotaxime and vancomycin. Antimicrob Agents Chemother. 1997;41:2050–2052.
422. Ahmed A. A critical evaluation of vancomycin for treatment of bacterial meningitis. Pediatr Infect Dis J. 1997;16:895–903.
423. Bradley JS. Meropenem: A new, extremely broad spectrum beta-lactam antibiotic for serious infections in pediatrics. Pediatr Infect Dis J. 1997;16:263–268.
424. Fitoussi F, Doit C, Benali K, et al. Comparative in vitro killing activities of meropenem, imipenem, ceftriaxone, and ceftriaxone plus vancomycin at clinically achievable cerebrospinal fluid concentrations against penicillin-resistant *Streptococcus pneumoniae* isolates from children with meningitis. Antimicrob Agents Chemother. 1998;42:942–944.
425. Schmutzhard E, Williams KJ, Vukmirovits G, et al. A randomised comparison of meropenem with cefotaxime or ceftriaxone for the treatment of bacterial meningitis in adults. J Antimicrob Chemother. 1995;36(Suppl A):S85–S97.
426. Bradley JS, Scheld WM. The challenge of penicillin-resistant *Streptococcus pneumoniae* meningitis: Current antibiotic therapy in the 1990s. Clin Infect Dis. 1997;24(Suppl 2):S213–S221.
427. John CC, Aouad G, Berman B, Schreiber JR. Successful meropenem treatment of multiply resistant pneumococcal meningitis. Pediatr Infect Dis J. 1997;16:1009–1011.
428. Cutler NR, Vincent J, Jhee SS, et al. Penetration of trovafloxacin into cerebrospinal fluid in humans following intravenous infusion of alatrofloxacin. Antimicrob Agents Chemother. 1997;41:1298–1300.
429. Kim YS, Liu Q, Chow LL, Täuber MG. Trovafloxacin in treatment of rabbits with experimental meningitis caused by high-level penicillin-resistant *Streptococcus pneumoniae*. Antimicrob Agents Chemother. 1997;41:1186–1189.
430. Schmidt H, Dalhoff A, Stuertz K, et al. Moxifloxacin in the therapy of experimental pneumococcal meningitis. Antimicrob Agents Chemother. 1998;42:1397–1401.
431. Ostergaard C, Sorensen TK, Knudsen JD, Frimodt-Moller N. Evaluation of moxifloxacin, a new 8-methoxyquinolone, for treatment of meningitis caused by a penicillin-resistant *Pneumococcus* in rabbits. Antimicrob Agents Chemother. 1998;42:1706–1712.
432. Levitz RE, Quintiliani R. Trimethoprim-sulfamethoxazole for bacterial meningitis. Ann Intern Med. 1984;100:881–890.
433. Richards SJ, Lambert CM, Scott AC. Recurrent *Listeria monocytogenes* meningitis treated with intraventricular vancomycin. J Antimicrob Chemother. 1992;29:351–353.
434. Scheld WM. Evaluation of rifampin and other antibiotics against *Listeria monocytogenes* in vitro and in vivo. Rev Infect Dis. 1983;5(Suppl):S593–S599.
435. Nairn K, Shepard G, Edwards JR. Efficacy of meropenem in experimental meningitis. J Antimicrob Chemother. 1995;36(Suppl A):73–84.
436. Cherubin CE, Eng RHK, Norrby R, et al. Penetration of newer cephalosporins into cerebrospinal fluid. Rev Infect Dis. 1989;11:526–548.
437. Kaplan SL, Patrick CC. Cefotaxime and aminoglycoside treatment of meningitis caused by gram-negative enteric organisms. Pediatr Infect Dis J. 1990;9:810–814.
438. Cherubin CE, Corrado ML, Nair SR, et al. Treatment of gram-negative bacillary meningitis: Role of the new cephalosporin antibiotics. Rev Infect Dis. 1982;4(Suppl):S453–S464.
439. Landesman SH, Corrado ML, Shah PM, et al. Past and current roles of cephalosporin antibiotics in treatment of meningitis. Emphasis on use in gram-negative bacillary meningitis. Am J Med. 1981;71:693–703.
440. Fong IW, Tomkins KB. Review of *Pseudomonas aeruginosa* meningitis with special emphasis on treatment with ceftazidime. Rev Infect Dis. 1985;7:604–612.
441. Rodriguez WJ, Khan WN, Cocchetto DM, et al. Treatment of *Pseudomonas* meningitis with ceftazidime with or without concurrent therapy. Pediatr Infect Dis J. 1990;9:83–87.
442. McCracken GH Jr, Mize SG, Threlkeld N. Intraventricular gentamicin therapy in gram-negative bacillary meningitis of infancy: Report of the second neonatal meningitis cooperative study group. Lancet. 1980;1:787–791.
443. Kilpatrick M, Girgis N, Farid Z, et al. Aztreonam for treating meningitis caused by gram-negative rods. Scand J Infect Dis. 1991;23:125–126.
444. Rodriguez K, Dickinson GM, Greenman RL. Successful treatment of gram-negative bacillary meningitis with imipenem/cilastatin. South Med J. 1985;78:732–733.
445. Wong VK, Wright HT Jr, Ross LA, et al. Imipenem/cilastatin treatment of bacterial meningitis in children. Pediatr Infect Dis J. 1991;10:122–125.
446. Donnelly JP, Horrevorts AM, Sauerwein RW, et al. High-dose meropenem in meningitis due to *Pseudomonas aeruginosa*. Lancet. 1992;339:1117.
447. Chmelik V, Gutvirth J. Meropenem treatment of post-traumatic meningitis due to *Pseudomonas aeruginosa*. J Antimicrob Chemother. 1993;32:922–923.
448. Tunkel AR, Scheld WM. Treatment of bacterial meningitis. In: Wolfson JS, Hooper DC, eds. Quinolone Antimicrobial Agents. Washington, DC: American Society for Microbiology; 1993:481–495.
449. Wong-Beringer A, Beringer P, Lovett MA. Successful treatment of multidrug-resistant *Pseudomonas aeruginosa* meningitis with high-dose ciprofloxacin. Clin Infect Dis. 1997;25:936–937.
450. D'Antuono VS, Brown I. Successful treatment of *Enterobacter* meningitis with ciprofloxacin. Clin Infect Dis. 1998;26:206–207.
451. Cruciani M, Navarra A, Di Perri G, et al. Evaluation of intraventricular teicoplanin for the treatment of neurosurgical shunt infections. Clin Infect Dis. 1992;15:285–289.
452. Radetsky M. Duration of treatment in bacterial meningitis: A historical inquiry. Pediatr Infect Dis J. 1990;9:2–9.
453. O'Neill P. How long to treat bacterial meningitis. Lancet. 1993;341:530.
454. Jadavji T, Biggar WD, Gold R, et al. Sequelae of acute bacterial meningitis in children treated for seven days. Pediatrics. 1985;78:21–25.
455. Lin TY, Chrane DF, Nelson JD, et al. Seven days of ceftriaxone therapy is as effective as ten days' treatment for bacterial meningitis. JAMA. 1985;253:3559–3563.
456. Viladrich PF, Pallares R, Ariza J, et al. Four days of penicillin therapy for meningococcal meningitis. Arch Intern Med. 1986;146:2380–2382.
457. Marra CM, Slatter V, Tartaglione TA, et al. Evaluation of aqueous penicillin G and ceftriaxone for experimental neurosyphilis. J Infect Dis. 1991;165:396–397.
458. Dowell ME, Ross PG, Musher DM, et al. Response of latent syphilis or neurosyphilis to ceftriaxone therapy in persons infected with human immunodeficiency virus. Am J Med. 1992;93:481–488.
459. Hook EW III. Management of syphilis in human immunodeficiency virus–infected patients. Am J Med. 1992;93:477–479.
460. Kohlhepp W, Oschmann P, Mertens HG. Treatment of Lyme borreliosis: Randomized comparison of doxycycline and penicillin G. J Neurol. 1989;236:464–469.
461. Karlsson M, Hammers-Berggren S, Lindquist L, et al. Comparison of intravenous penicillin G and oral doxycycline for treatment of Lyme neuroborreliosis. Neurology. 1994;44:1203–1207.
462. Dattwyler RJ, Halperin JJ, Volkman DJ, et al. Treatment of late Lyme borreliosis—randomised comparison of ceftriaxone and penicillin. Lancet. 1988;1:1191–1194.
463. Dotevall L, Hagberg L. Penetration of doxycycline into cerebrospinal fluid in patients treated for suspected Lyme neuroborreliosis. Antimicrob Agents Chemother. 1989;33:1078–1080.
464. Sischel JS, Harmatz P, Visvesvara GS, et al. Successful treatment of primary amebic meningoencephalitis. N Engl J Med. 1982;306:346–348.
465. Brown RL. Successful treatment of primary amebic meningoencephalitis. Arch Intern Med. 1991;151:1201–1202.
466. Abzug MJ, Keyserling HL, Lee ML, et al. Neonatal enterovirus infection: Virology, serology, and effects of intravenous immune globulin. Clin Infect Dis. 1995;20:1201–1206.
467. Tuomanen E, Hengstler B, Rich R, et al. Nonsteroidal anti-inflammatory agents in the therapy for experimental pneumococcal meningitis. J Infect Dis. 1987;155:985–990.
468. Tureen JH, Täuber MG, Sande MA. Effect of indomethacin on the pathophysiology of experimental meningitis in rabbits. J Infect Dis. 1991;163:647–649.
469. Kadurugamuwa JL, Hengstler B, Zak O. Cerebrospinal fluid protein profile in experimental pneumococcal meningitis and its alteration by ampicillin and anti-inflammatory agents. J Infect Dis. 1989;159:26–34.
470. Nolan CM, McAllister CK, Walters E, et al. Experimental pneumococcal meningitis. IV. The effect of methylprednisolone on meningeal inflammation. J Lab Clin Invest. 1978;91:979–988.
471. Syrogiannopoulos GA, Olsen KD, Reisch JS, et al. Dexamethasone in the treatment of experimental *Haemophilus influenzae* type b meningitis. J Infect Dis. 1987;155:213–219.
472. Mustafa MM, Ramilo O, Mertsola J, et al. Modulation of inflammation and cachectin activity in relation to treatment of experimental *Haemophilus influenzae* type b meningitis. J Infect Dis. 1989;160:818–825.

473. Lebel MH, Freij BJ, Syrogiannopoulos GA, et al. Dexamethasone therapy for bacterial meningitis. Results of two double-blind, placebo-controlled trials. N Engl J Med. 1988;319:964–971.
474. Lebel MH, Hoyt MJ, Waagner DC, et al. Magnetic resonance imaging and dexamethasone therapy for bacterial meningitis. Am J Dis Child. 1989;143:301–306.
475. Girgis NI, Farid Z, Mikhail IA, et al. Dexamethasone treatment for bacterial meningitis in children and adults. Pediatr Infect Dis J. 1989;8:848–851.
476. Odio CM, Faingezicht I, Paris M, et al. The beneficial effects of early dexamethasone administration in infants and children with bacterial meningitis. N Engl J Med. 1991;324:1525–1531.
477. Kennedy WA, Hoyt MJ, McCracken GH Jr. The role of corticosteroid therapy in children with pneumococcal meningitis. Am J Dis Child. 1991;145:1374–1378.
478. Schaad UB, Lips U, Gnehm HE, et al. Dexamethasone therapy for bacterial meningitis in children. Lancet. 1993;342:457–461.
479. King SM, Law B, Langley JM, Heurter H. Dexamethasone therapy for bacterial meningitis: Better never than late? Can J Infect Dis. 1994;5:1–7.
480. Wald ER, Kaplan SL, Mason EO Jr, et al. Dexamethasone therapy for children with bacterial meningitis. Pediatrics. 1995;95:21–28.
481. Kanra GY, Ozen H, Secmeer G, et al. The beneficial effects of dexamethasone in children with pneumococcal meningitis. Pediatr Infect Dis J. 1995;14:490–494.
482. Kilpi T, Peltola H, Jauhiainen T, et al. Oral glycerol and intravenous dexamethasone in preventing neurologic and audiologic sequelae of childhood bacterial meningitis. Pediatr Infect Dis J. 1995;14:270–278.
483. Macaluso A, Pivetta S, Maggi RS, et al. Dexamethasone adjunctive therapy for bacterial meningitis in children: A retrospective study in Brazil. Ann Trop Paediatr. 1996;16:193–198.
484. Qazi SA, Khan MA, Mughal N, et al. Dexamethasone and bacterial meningitis in Pakistan. Arch Dis Child. 1996;75:482–488.
485. Arditi M, Mason EO Jr, Bradley JS, et al. Three-year multicenter surveillance of pneumococcal meningitis in children: Clinical characteristics, and outcome related to penicillin susceptibility and dexamethasone use. Pediatrics. 1998;102:1087–1097.
486. McIntyre PB, Berkey CS, King SM, et al. Dexamethasone as adjunctive therapy in bacterial meningitis. A meta-analysis of randomized clinical trials since 1988. JAMA. 1997;278:925–931.
487. Syrogiannopoulos GA, Lourida AN, Theodoridou MC, et al. Dexamethasone therapy for bacterial meningitis in children: 2- versus 4-day regimen. J Infect Dis. 1994;169:853–858.
488. Enting R, the Dutch Bacterial Meningitis Study Group. Dexamethasone for bacterial meningitis: We need the answer. Lancet. 1997;349:1179–1180.
489. Cabellos C, Martinez-Lacasa J, Martox A, et al. Influence of dexamethasone on efficacy of ceftriaxone and vancomycin therapy in experimental pneumococcal meningitis. Antimicrob Agents Chemother. 1995;39:2158–2160.
490. Prober CG. The role of steroids in the management of children with bacterial meningitis. Pediatrics. 1995;95:29–31.
491. Gaillard JL, Abadie V, Cheron G, et al. Concentrations of ceftriaxone in cerebrospinal fluid of children with meningitis receiving adjunctive dexamethasone therapy. Antimicrob Agents Chemother. 1994;38:1209–1210.
492. Kaplan SL, Mason EO Jr. Management of infections due to antibiotic-resistant *Streptococcus pneumoniae*. Clin Microbiol Rev. 1998;11:628–644.
493. Saez-Llorens X, Ramilo O, Mustafa MM, et al. Pentoxifylline modulates meningeal inflammation in experimental bacterial meningitis. Antimicrob Agents Chemother. 1990;34:837–843.
494. Burroughs MH, Tsenova-Berkova L, Sokol K, et al. Effect of thalidomide on the inflammatory response in cerebrospinal fluid in experimental bacterial meningitis. Microb Pathog. 1995;19:245–255.
495. Saez-Llorens X, Jafari HS, Severien C, et al. Enhanced attenuation of meningeal inflammation and brain edema by concomitant administration of anti-CD18 monoclonal antibodies and dexamethasone in experimental *Haemophilus* meningitis. J Clin Invest. 1991;88:2003–2011.
496. Kartalija M, Kim Y, White ML, et al. Effect of recombinant N-terminal fragment of bactericidal/permeability-increasing protein ($rBPI_{23}$) on cerebrospinal fluid inflammation induced by endotoxin. J Infect Dis. 1995;171:948–953.
497. Lyons MK, Meyer FB. Cerebrospinal fluid physiology and the management of increased intracranial pressure. Mayo Clin Proc. 1990;65:684–707.
498. Colville A, Pugh S. Mumps meningitis and measles, mumps, and rubella vaccine. Lancet. 1992;340:786.
499. Forsey T, Bentley ML, Minor PD, et al. Mumps vaccines and meningitis. Lancet. 1992;340:980.
500. Band JD. Chemoprophylaxis of *Haemophilus influenzae* type b disease: A strategy for preventing secondary cases. In: Sell SH, Wright PF, eds. *Haemophilus influenzae*: Epidemiology, Immunology, and Prevention of Disease. New York: Elsevier; 1982:309–315.
501. Peter G. Treatment and prevention of *Haemophilus influenzae* type b meningitis. Pediatr Infect Dis J. 1987;6:787–790.
502. Lieberman JM, Greenberg DP, Ward JI. Prevention of bacterial meningitis. Vaccines and chemoprophylaxis. Infect Dis Clin North Am. 1990;4:703–729.
503. Green M, Li KI, Wald ER, et al. Duration of rifampin chemoprophylaxis for contacts of patients infected with *Haemophilus influenzae* type b. Antimicrob Agents Chemother. 1992;36:545–547.
504. Cooke RPD, Riordan T, Jones DM, Painter MJ. Secondary cases of meningococcal infection among close family and household contacts in England and Wales, 1984–7. BMJ. 1989;298:555–558.
505. Imrey PB, Jackson LA, Ludwinski PH, et al. Meningococcal carriage, alcohol consumption, and campus bar patronage in a serogroup C meningococcal disease outbreak. Antimicrob Agents Chemother. 1995;33:3133–3137.
506. Cookson ST, Corrales JL, Lotero JO, et al. Disco fever: Epidemic meningococcal disease in northeastern Argentina associated with disco patronage. J Infect Dis. 1998;178:266–269.
507. Koh YM, Barnes GH, Kaczmarski E, Stuart JM. Outbreak of meningococcal disease linked to a sports club. Lancet. 1998;352:706–707.
508. Centers for Disease Control and Prevention. Control and prevention of meningococcal disease and control and prevention of serogroup C meningococcal disease: Evaluation and management of suspected outbreaks. MMWR Morb Mortal Wkly Rep. 1997;46(RR-5):1–11.
509. Schwartz B, Al-Tobaiqi A, Al-Ruwais A, et al. Comparative efficacy of ceftriaxone and rifampicin in eradicating pharyngeal carriage of group A *Neisseria meningitidis*. Lancet. 1988;1:1239–1242.
510. Darouiche R, Perkins B, Musher D, et al. Levels of rifampin and ciprofloxacin in nasal secretions: Correlation with MIC_{90} and eradication of nasopharyngeal carriage of bacteria. J Infect Dis. 1990;162:1124–1127.
511. Rauch AM, O'Ryan M, Van R, et al. Invasive disease due to multiply resistant *Streptococcus pneumoniae* in a Houston, Tex, day-care center. Am J Dis Child. 1990;144:923–927.
512. Gaston MH, Verter JI, Woods G, et al. Prophylaxis with oral penicillin in children with sickle cell anemia. A randomized trial. N Engl J Med. 1986;314:1593–1599.
513. Centers for Disease Control and Prevention. Prevention of pneumococcal disease: Recommendations of the Advisory Committee on Immunization Practices (ACIP). MMWR Morb Mortal Wkly Rep. 1997;46(RR-8):1–23.
514. Zangwill KM, Schuchat A, Wenger JD, Group B Streptococcal Disease Study Group. Group B streptococcal disease in the United States, 1990: Report from a multistate active surveillance system. MMWR Morb Mortal Wkly Rep. 1992;41:25–32.
515. Centers for Disease Control and Prevention. Prevention of perinatal group B streptococcal disease: A public health perspective. MMWR Morb Mortal Wkly Rep. 1996;45(RR-7):1–24.
516. Villalobos T, Arango C, Kubilis P, Rathore M. Antibiotic prophylaxis after basilar skull fracture. Clin Infect Dis. 1998;27:364–369.
517. American Academy of Pediatrics, Committee on Infectious Diseases. Recommended childhood immunization schedule—United States, January–December 1998. Pediatrics. 1998;101:154–157.
518. Peltola H. Vaccines against bacterial meningitis. In: Scheld WM, Whitley RJ, Durack DT, eds. Infections of the Central Nervous System. 2nd ed. Philadelphia: Lippincott-Raven; 1997:1013–1039.
519. Black S, Shinefield H, Ray P, et al. Efficacy of heptavalent conjugate pneumococcal vaccine (Wyeth Lederle) in 37,000 infants and children: Results of the Northern California Kaiser Permanente Efficacy Trial. In: Program and Abstracts of the 38th Interscience Conference on Antimicrobial Agents and Chemotherapy. Washington, DC: American Society for Microbiology; 1998.
520. Kayhty H, Eskola J. New vaccines for the prevention of pneumococcal infections. Emerg Infect Dis. 1996;2:289–298.

Chapter 72

Chronic Meningitis

BARBARA M. GRIPSHOVER
JERROLD J. ELLNER

A large number of infectious and noninfectious diseases can cause the clinical syndrome of chronic meningitis (Tables 72–1 and 72–2). The onset of symptoms in such cases typically is subacute to chronic with signs of meningoencephalitis such as fever, headache, lethargy, confusion, nausea, vomiting, and stiff neck. Cerebrospinal fluid (CSF) is abnormal with elevated protein concentrations, a pleocytosis that usually is predominantly lymphocytic, and sometimes a low glucose level. The major difficulty during initial evaluation is in distinguishing the rare patient with chronic meningitis from those patients with the more common syndromes of acute meningitis and encephalitis. If the neurologic symptoms and signs either persist or progress clinically and the CSF remains abnormal for at least 4 weeks, the diagnosis of chronic meningitis is appropriate.[1–9] The diagnosis of chronic meningitis has a number of implications; particularly important are those that relate to etiology, management, and prognosis. This duration of symptoms was derived empirically to

TABLE 72–1 Infectious Diseases That May Manifest as Chronic Meningitis: Usual Presentation in the Central Nervous System

Meningitis	Focal Lesions	Encephalitis
Acanthamoeba infection	Actinomycosis	African trypanosomiasis
Angiostrongylus cantonensis infection	Blastomycosis	Cytomegalovirus infection
Brucellosis	Coenurosis	Enterovirus (in patients with hypogammaglobulinemia)
Candidiasis	Cysticercosis	Measles (subacute sclerosing panencephalitis)
Coccidioidomycosis	Molds: aspergillosis, phaeohyphomycosis, pseudallescheriasis	Rabies
Cryptococcosis	Nocardiosis	Viral encephalitis (see Chapter 73)
Histoplasmosis	Schistosomiasis	
Lyme disease	Toxoplasmosis	
Sporotrichosis		
Syphilis		
Tuberculosis		

optimize the distinction between patients with chronic progressive disease and those with self-limited processes. In practice, patients frequently are seen by a physician within 1 to 4 weeks after the onset of symptoms. Prompt diagnosis and institution of appropriate treatment, therefore, may abort the neurologic process before the criteria for chronic meningitis are fulfilled.

Central nervous system (CNS) involvement by most diseases causing chronic meningitis has a high morbidity and mortality. Successful intervention requires the early administration of specific, often potentially toxic forms of therapy. Furthermore, drugs appropriate for treating one cause of chronic meningitis may be contraindicated in others. Therefore, a precise etiologic diagnosis is critical in modifying the course of this syndrome, and broad empirical therapeutic regimens are a poor and sometimes hazardous substitute. Whereas exact diagnosis may prove difficult (one third of cases in a retrospective series of 87 patients with chronic meningitis were undiagnosed[4]), certain aspects of the presentation can be helpful in determining causality or at least limiting the differential diagnosis.

HISTORY

The exposure history may be important in suggesting certain infectious diseases such as tuberculosis, coccidioidomycosis, histoplasmosis, brucellosis, cysticercosis, syphilis, Lyme disease, and, especially, acquired immunodeficiency syndrome (AIDS) with its distinctive spectrum of pathogens. The exposure history should direct the evaluation to include specific serologic studies and other diagnostic tests. Because the presence of human immunodeficiency virus (HIV) infection significantly alters the differential diagnosis, HIV testing should be done on all patients with chronic meningitis. This chapter discusses chronic meningitis in the HIV-seronegative patient, except where specifically noted.

The history also is of importance in distinguishing chronic meningitis from two superficially similar syndromes, acute meningitis (or encephalitis) with a protracted recovery period and recurrent meningitis. In chronic meningitis, onset is insidious and symptoms are chronic, although they may wax and wane. Episodes of acute neurologic deterioration sometimes punctuate the clinical course and may be caused by cerebral edema, hydrocephalus, cerebrovascular occlusions, or seizures. Even when symptoms temporarily regress, CSF abnormalities persist and reflect continued disease activity. In the protracted recovery period that sometimes follows pyogenic or aseptic meningitis and viral encephalitis, actual progression of disease is confined to the acute stages of the illness; clearing of the signs, symptoms, and CSF abnormalities, although gradual, may occur during observation. The second syndrome that must be differentiated from chronic meningitis is recurrent meningitis.[10] Patients with recurrent meningitis usually have repeated episodes of acute disease followed by periods during which signs and symptoms are absent and the CSF is normal (Table 72–3).

The history also is important in defining the cause of meningitis in those instances in which CNS extension occurs as a late manifestation of a previously diagnosed systemic disease. These conditions include acute leukemia, lymphoma, blastomycosis, and Behçet's disease.

PHYSICAL EXAMINATION

Diagnostic physical findings are rare. However, physical examination may delineate signs of an associated systemic disease that provide a potential source of rapid diagnosis. Skin lesions, although infrequent, are particularly important for their diagnostic value. Even benign-appearing superficial lesions, subcutaneous nodules and abscesses, or draining sinuses should be cultured and biopsy specimens obtained. Among the causes of chronic meningitis that are notable for manifesting with skin lesions are cryptococcosis (Fig. 72–1), sarcoidosis, *Acanthamoeba* infection, coccidioidomycosis, blastomycosis, and secondary syphilis; in addition, the subcutaneous nodules of cysticercosis and metastatic carcinoma (e.g., breast, melanoma) are important signs. The eye examination may be helpful if such lesions as choroidal tubercles, sarcoid granulomas, or uveitis are demonstrable. The finding of papilledema also is of significance, because it alters the course of the neurologic workup and contraindicates lumbar puncture. Hepatomegaly may reflect systemic disease involving the liver and increases the potential diagnostic yield of a liver biopsy.

Neurologic examination is of obvious importance in delineating the extent of CNS involvement. However, it is of limited use in differentiating among specific causes, because mental status changes, meningismus, oculomotor palsies, and, less frequently, focal findings, evidence of increased intracranial pressure, and spinal cord signs can be caused by most processes associated with chronic meningitis. Focal signs, however, often reflect a parenchymal mass such as an

TABLE 72–2 Noninfectious Causes of Chronic Meningitis

Behçet's disease
Chronic benign lymphocytic meningitis
Chronic meningitis of unknown cause
Granulomatous angiitis
Neoplasm
Sarcoidosis
Uveomeningoencephalitis

TABLE 72–3 Differential Diagnosis of Recurrent Meningitis

Drug-induced (with rechallenge)[11–14]
Parameningeal focus
Infection (sinusitis, mastoiditis, osteomyelitis, brain abscess)
Tumor (epidermoid cyst, craniopharyngioma)[15–18]
Posttraumatic (bacterial)
Mollaret's meningitis[19–22]
Systemic lupus erythematosus[23–26]
Herpes simplex virus

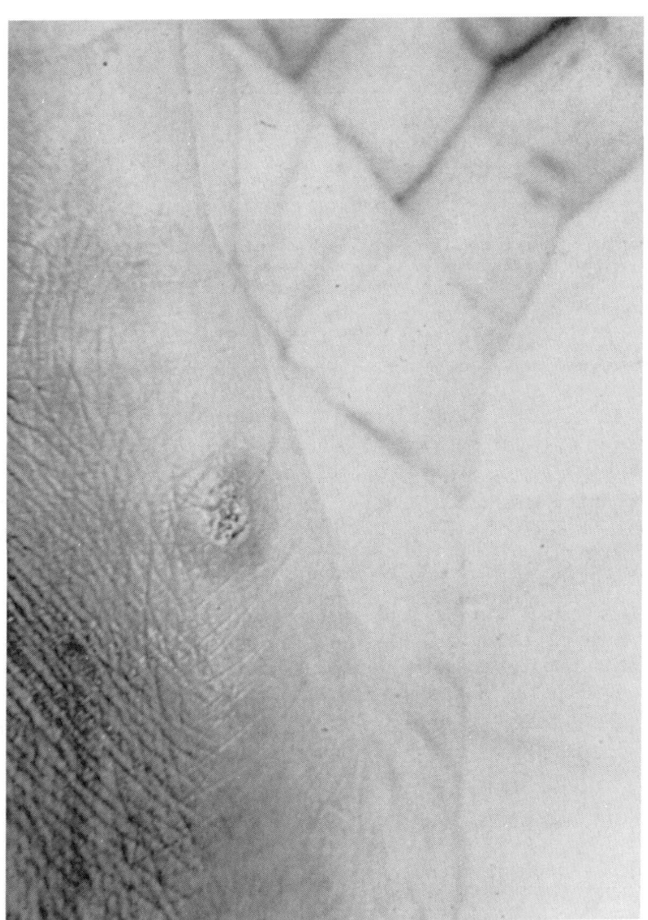

FIGURE 72–1. Skin lesion of a woman with chronic lymphocytic leukemia treated with corticosteroids and cytotoxic drugs, admitted with chronic meningitis. Material expressed from the lesion was positive on India ink preparation and culture for *Cryptococcus neoformans.*

abscess or granuloma that would dictate specific diagnostic and therapeutic maneuvers. Involvement of multiple levels of the neuraxis is suggestive of meningeal carcinomatosis. Hydrocephalus may complicate chronic meningitis, and appropriate neuroradiographic evaluation should be initiated when the constellation of headache, nausea, vomiting, mental changes, ataxia, incontinence, and papilledema is present. The finding of hydrocephalus, particularly with associated cranial neuropathies, is suggestive of an infectious cause with basilar leptomeningitis, although hydrocephalus also may complicate sarcoidosis, cysticercosis, and CNS tumor. Peripheral neuropathy is noted uncommonly in chronic meningitis and is suggestive of sarcoidosis or Lyme disease. In patients infected with HIV-1, radiculomyelitis should suggest cytomegalovirus infection.

LABORATORY EVALUATION

The cause of chronic meningitis ultimately must be established in the laboratory (Table 72–4). Abnormalities on chest radiographs may reflect systemic involvement by the underlying infectious process, carcinoma, or sarcoidosis. These findings should be pursued in an attempt to define the cause of the meningitis. In more enigmatic cases, biopsy of lung lesions may be indicated; this is associated with less morbidity and greater yield than is a brain biopsy.

The CSF formula is never itself diagnostic. However, certain abnormalities and patterns are more characteristic of a restricted group of causes of chronic meningitis (Table 72–5).

Lumbar puncture must be repeated periodically both for culture and to follow the course of meningeal inflammation. India ink preparations should be made from the sediment of 3 to 5 ml of CSF. The entire slide must be examined, because cryptococci may be present in small numbers. As opposed to artifacts that are seen commonly, encapsulated yeast has a regular, round, distinct capsule and a refractile central structure; budding yeast forms also may be found. The India ink preparation is more likely to be positive in patients with relatively acute presentations and in immunosuppressed patients with lymphoma or AIDS. In the latter setting, yeast organisms often far outnumber leukocytes in the CSF. CSF cytologic studies are indicated in all patients with chronic meningitis. Multiple specimens may be necessary for the diagnosis of CNS involvement by tumor, and negative cytologic studies do not preclude this possibility.[29] Demonstration of a clonal origin of CSF lymphocytes with the use of B- and T-cell immunologic markers also is helpful in the diagnosis of lymphomatous meningitis,[30, 31] as is polymerase chain reaction (PCR) detection of clonal immunoglobulin or T-cell receptor rearrangement.[32]

Serologic studies of serum and CSF are extremely important in evaluating the patient for coccidioidomycosis, cryptococcosis, and syphilis and should be performed routinely. In the case of cryptococcal meningitis, testing for cryptococcal polysaccharide antigen is helpful; testing for antibody is not useful. Serum antibodies to *Brucella* and *Toxoplasma* also may suggest these infections when they are present in high or increasing titers. Serum antibodies to *Histoplasma* are found in 60% of patients with *Histoplasma* meningitis.[33] Complement-fixing antibodies to *Histoplasma* are found in the CSF of most patients with CNS histoplasmosis, although they may also be detected in coccidioidal and cryptococcal infection.[34, 35] More specific is the detection of *Histoplasma capsulatum* antigen in serum, urine, or CSF by radioimmunoassay or enzyme-linked immunosorbent assay; however, this assay is less sensitive, with only 25% of patients with meningitis caused by this organism having detectable antigen in the CSF.[36] The antigen test is more likely to be positive in HIV-infected persons with *Histoplasma* meningitis.[33] The ELISA for antibody to *Sporothrix schenckii* in CSF has also been useful, although the disease rarely causes meningitis.[37] Identification of *Mycobacterium tuberculosis* DNA in CSF by PCR is more sensitive than culture, detecting 27 to 85% of cases of presumed tuberculous meningitis that responded to therapy.[38–43]

Skin testing should be limited to tuberculin purified protein derivative (PPD). The value of anergy testing is controversial. Repeated skin testing may be helpful when tuberculosis is a possibility. Fungal skin test antigens should not be used. They are of no value diagnostically and may cause confusion by altering the fungal serology results, particularly in the case of histoplasmosis.

Cultures are mandatory even when a specific diagnosis is suggested by serology or other studies. CSF should be cultured at least three times for bacteria, acid-fast bacilli, and fungi, and more numerous samples should be obtained and cultured in their entirety when the cause of the meningitis remains uncertain after the initial diagnostic evaluation is complete. The low density of fungi in the CSF and the difficulty in culturing certain organisms may delay the diagnosis of some mycotic infections. In such cases, the yield can be improved by inoculating Sabouraud's agar layered on the bottom of Erlenmeyer flasks with large volumes of CSF. The finding of even a single colony of an organism capable of causing chronic meningitis such as *S. schenckii* should never be disregarded as a contaminant (Fig. 72–2).[44] In fact, it may be useful to continue to examine fungal cultures for at least 4 to 6 weeks, because the growth of such organisms can be exceedingly slow. Ventricular CSF may have a higher cultural yield than lumbar CSF in certain infections.[45] Urine, sputum, and blood cultures should be obtained and processed routinely for mycobacteria and fungi even in the absence of clinical evidence of extraneural infection. These ancillary cultures frequently are positive in cases of cryptococcosis, tuberculosis, histoplasmosis, and blastomycosis. Special culture techniques such as anaerobiasis

TABLE 72–4 Evaluation of Patients with Chronic Meningitis

Initial Evaluation of All Patients

History: travel to southwestern United States, developing countries, or tropical Africa; new sexual partner, high-risk activity for HIV, household member with tuberculosis, brucellosis exposure such as meat packing, intravenous drug abuse, skin lesion resembling erythema migrans, childhood measles

Physical examination: complete examination, including search for skin lesions or subcutaneous nodules; ocular examination for retinal lesions, papilledema, uveitis, or iritis; lymphadenopathy; hepatosplenomegaly; neurologic examination

Laboratory tests: complete blood count with differential analysis and sedimentation rate; liver and renal function; PPD; chest radiograph; magnetic resonance imaging with gadolinium enhancement or computed tomography (with special attention for parameningeal foci in paranasal sinus or mastoids, intracerebral lesions, epidermoid cysts, and hydrocephalus); blood culture for fungi and mycobacteria by lysis centrifugation; urine culture for fungi and mycobacteria; serology for HIV, syphilis, cryptococcal antigen, and antinuclear antibody; lumbar puncture for opening pressure, leukocytes, protein, glucose (simultaneous blood glucose), cytospin cytology, VDRL, cryptococcal antigen, India ink, acid-fast stain, *Mycobacterium tuberculosis* PCR and large-volume (3 to 5 ml) cultures each for fungus, mycobacteria

Tests Indicated by Appropriate Exposure History

Serum serology for antibody to *Histoplasma, Coccidioides, Brucella,* and *Borrelia burgdorferi* (Lyme disease agent)

Cerebrospinal fluid antibody to *Histoplasma, Coccidioides, Blastomycosis, Taenia solium* (cysticercosis), *Brucella* and measles virus; *Histoplasma* antigen; stain CSF leukocytes for eosinophils; *Brucella* culture; blood smear for trypanosomes

Enigmatic Cases

Repeat PPD in 2 to 4 weeks; serum immunoglobulins and angiotensin-converting enzyme; CSF for antibody to *Sporothrix;* enteroviral culture and PCR (if low serum immunoglobulin G), repeat cytology and PCR for lymphocyte gene rearrangement. Consider brain biopsy for diffuse carcinomatosis or gliomatosis, *Acanthamoeba,* mold infections, or granulomatous angiitis.

Abbreviations: HIV, Human immunodeficiency virus; PCR, polymerase chain reaction; PPD, purified protein derivative of tuberculin; VDRL, Venereal Disease Research Laboratory test for syphilis.

or increased carbon dioxide tension also are appropriate in the search for certain pathogens such as *Actinomyces* species and *Brucella abortus,* respectively. Consultation with a clinical microbiologist may be helpful in difficult cases.

Biopsy of specific tissues should be directed by abnormal findings on physical examination. Skin, lymph node, and liver biopsy specimens may demonstrate granulomas, sometimes with caseation and occasionally with an organism demonstrable on special staining. Caseation is suggestive of tuberculosis, histoplasmosis, or coccidioidomycosis. Focal necrosis may be found in brucellosis. All biopsy specimens should be cultured for bacteria, fungi, and mycobacteria. Bone marrow biopsy and culture are particularly useful in tuberculosis and histoplasmosis. Liver biopsy is indicated when miliary tuberculosis is suspected, and it has a greater yield when liver function tests suggest an infiltrative process (increased alkaline phosphatase and glutamyltranspeptidase). Meningeal and brain biopsies should be performed and ventricular fluid should be sampled at the time of craniotomy for exploration of a mass or other focal lesion or for indicated ventricular shunting procedures. Brain and meningeal biopsy also should be considered in undiagnosed cases with a deteriorating course, recognizing that the yield of treatable causative organisms is low. In series reported from referral centers, the yield of a definitive diagnosis from leptomeningeal brain biopsy in chronic meningitis was 20 to 39%,[7, 8] and the most common diagnosis at biopsy was neoplastic meningitis. However, if the biopsy was in a site of gadolinium-enhanced meninges on a magnetic resonance imaging study, the diagnostic yield increased to 80%.[7] Despite the low yield, patients with hypoglycorrhachia and CSF pleocytosis greater than 50 cells/μl progressing on empirical antituberculosis therapy should be considered for biopsy. Earlier biopsy may be indicated, especially if the PPD skin test is negative and the clinical course is deteriorating without a diagnosis.

Radiographic Techniques

MRI or computed tomography (CT) should be performed for all patients with chronic meningitis to search for parameningeal lesions (especially paranasal sinus and mastoids), ependymona, glioma, and other parenchymal lesions. MRI provides a better evaluation of the meninges than CT; the high density of the bone of the skull on CT can obscure enhancement in the meninges, whereas bone on MRI is void of signal (and therefore black adjacent to the bright inflamed meninges).[46] However, all causes of chronic meningitis can result in meningeal enhancement, so this finding, although potentially useful in selecting patients and sites for brain biopsy, does not help to narrow the differential diagnosis. Hydrocephalus is also detected by imaging; the demonstration of hydrocephalus is not in itself a sufficient indication for ventricular shunting, because neurosurgical procedures have a high morbidity and failure rate in patients with chronic meningitis. Furthermore, hydrocephalus may clear spontaneously with treatment of the underlying condition. Nonetheless, if

TABLE 72–5 Cerebrospinal Fluid Characteristics of Various Causes of Chronic Meningitis

Pleocytosis <50 Cells/μl	Neutrophilic Pleocytosis[27]	Eosinophilic Pleocytosis[28]	Low Glucose
Behçet's disease	Bacteria	Chemical	Bacteria
Benign lymphocytic meningitis	*Actinomyces*	*Coccidioides*	*Actinomyces*
Carcinoma	*Nocardia*	Lymphoma	*Nocardia*
Cryptococcus in HIV-infected patients	Chemical	Parasites	Carcinoma
Sarcoidosis	Cytomegalovirus in HIV-infected patients	*Angiostrongylus*	*Cysticercus*
Vasculitis	Early *Mycobacterium tuberculosis* infection	*Cysticercus*	Fungi (all)
	Fungi	*Schistosoma*	*Mycobacterium tuberculosis*
	Aspergillus		Postsubarachnoid hemorrhage
	Candida		Sarcoidosis
	Systemic lupus erythematosus		Syphilis
			Toxoplasma
			Viral
			Chronic enterovirus
			Cytomegalovirus in HIV-infected patients

Abbreviation: HIV, Human immunodeficiency virus.

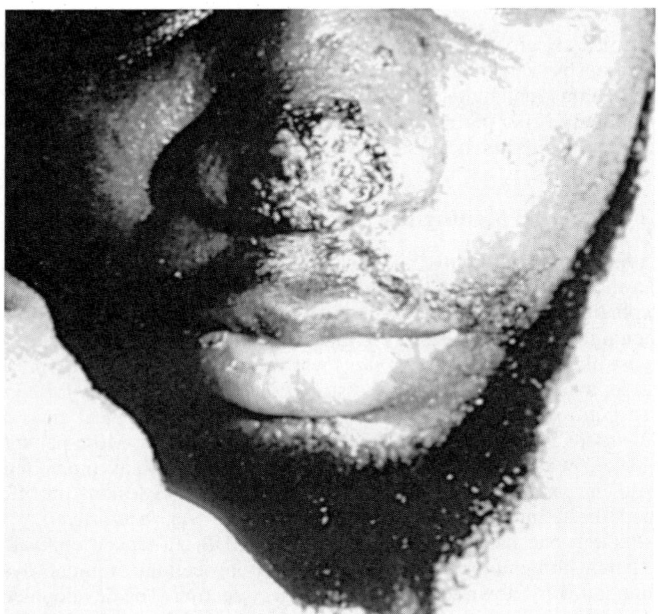

FIGURE 72–2. Skin lesions developed in this patient with enigmatic chronic meningitis after ventriculojugular shunting for hydrocephalus. A discarded cerebrospinal fluid culture from an earlier admission was found overgrown with mold, subsequently identified as *Sporothrix schenchii.*

clinical deterioration attributable to hydrocephalus occurs, a surgical approach must be considered.

Ancillary procedures such as mammography and gastrointestinal radiographic series may be appropriate in the search for a primary carcinoma when meningeal carcinomatosis is suspected.

THERAPEUTIC TRIALS

Therapeutic trials are indicated when the specific cause remains uncertain despite comprehensive evaluation. However, further attempts at establishing a diagnosis should be continued actively during such trials. Interpretation of the response to empirically administered drugs may be difficult, because clinical improvement is often slow, even when the agent selected is appropriate. When the patient is stable, sequential trials are indicated.

Tuberculous meningitis is the most common cause of chronic meningitis[4] where tuberculosis is endemic; therefore, an empirical trial of antituberculosis drugs clearly is appropriate when the presentation and CSF formula are consistent with tuberculosis and there is evidence of active or prior tuberculous infection. Studies suggest that initial tuberculin skin test results are negative in up to two thirds of patients with tuberculous meningitis.[47–50] Therefore, empirical antituberculosis therapy is indicated in many cases of undiagnosed chronic meningitis. Adequate cultures of CSF, urine, sputum, or gastric aspirates must be obtained before therapy is begun, and biopsy specimens of liver and bone marrow should be included if miliary disease is suspected. Repeat intermediate-strength PPD skin testing after 2 to 4 weeks also may be of value if the initial studies are negative.[50] Positive cultures or a clinical response to antituberculosis treatment despite negative cultures would be an indication to complete a full course of therapy.

Fluconazole is potentially useful as empirical therapy for chronic meningitis caused by *Cryptococcus neoformans, Coccidioides immitis,* and *Candida albicans.* No clinical trials have been published to guide empirical use. The diagnostic value of empirical fluconazole is limited by the slow response known to occur in documented cases. Improvement may not be obvious for several months, during which time meningitis resulting from other causes may irreversibly deteriorate. If such a trial is attempted, a dose of 400 mg/day is indicated, and repeated CSF examinations should be obtained to monitor the results of therapy. Should the patient respond but the condition remain undiagnosed, a minimum course would probably be at least 6 months.

Traditionally, empirical trials of corticosteroids have been avoided because of the potential catastrophic adverse effects in patients with unrecognized tuberculosis or fungal meningitis. However, chronic meningitis in areas where tuberculosis is not endemic usually is not infectious.[6, 7] Of 49 patients with chronic idiopathic meningitis at the Mayo Clinic from 1978 through 1990, 85% had a prolonged but benign course, with one half responding promptly to empirical corticosteroids. No patient responded to empirical tuberculosis therapy.[6] In selected patients in whom an infectious cause has been fairly excluded, serious consideration should be given to an empirical trial of corticosteroid therapy. Negative tests on serum and CSF should include cryptococcal antigen, *Histoplasma* antigen and antibody, and, depending on endemic area, *Coccidioides* and Lyme disease antibody. Normal chest radiograph and negative PPD skin test results, no history of exposure to tuberculosis, and CSF cell count below 20 leukocytes/mm^3 would also support this consideration.

DIFFERENTIAL DIAGNOSIS

A number of conditions can cause syndromes resembling chronic meningitis superficially but usually distinguishable from it on clinical grounds at presentation or during evaluation and observation of the patient (Table 72–6). In addition, a careful history is important to differentiate between recurrent and chronic meningitis, since the former syndrome connotes a different spectrum of diseases (see Table 72–3).

Those infections causing the syndrome of chronic meningitis (see Table 72–1) are discussed in detail in other chapters. Features that are important in establishing the cause of the chronic meningitis are reviewed here.

Mollaret's Meningitis

Mollaret's meningitis[51] is not a chronic meningitis; rather, it is a rare syndrome in which recurrent episodes of aseptic meningitis are characterized by acute onset of fever, headache, and nuchal rigidity.[10, 51] The symptoms resolve spontaneously within 2 to 5 days, and the patient returns to normal, only to undergo recurrent attacks weeks to months later.

This disease is most commonly seen in young adults, although the age range of reported cases is 5 to 57 years. There is no predisposition by sex. Lumbar puncture reveals a mixed lymphocytic and polymorphonuclear pleocytosis, with leukocytes ranging from hundreds to thousands per cubic millimeter. The protein concentra-

TABLE 72–6 Diseases That Sometimes Resemble Chronic Meningitis

Infectious diseases
Aseptic meningitis
Infective endocarditis
Parameningeal infections
Partially treated bacterial meningitis
Viral and nonviral encephalitis
Noninfectious diseases
Brain tumor
Giant cell arteriitis
Metabolic and other encephalopathies
Multiple sclerosis
Postinfectious encephalitis
Subarachnoid hemorrhage
Subdural hematoma
Systemic lupus erythematosus
Thrombotic thrombocytopenic purpura

tion is only mildly elevated, usually being less than 100 mg/ml, and the glucose concentration is usually normal. Early in an attack, large, fragile mononuclear cells are seen. Mollaret called these "endothelial" cells.[51] However, electron microscopy and monoclonal antibody techniques have demonstrated that these cells are monocytes.[52, 53] After 24 hours, the CSF pleocytosis has greatly decreased and is mainly lymphocytic; Mollaret's "endothelial" cells and PMN have disappeared. By 1 week, the CSF has completely normalized. Rarely, focal neurologic deficits have been associated with acute episodes, but they are self-limited and resolve during the episode without sequelae.

Studies have shown a probable link between herpes simplex virus (HSV) and at least some cases of Mollaret's meningitis.[19–22, 54] HSV-2 (and less commonly HSV-1) DNA has been detected in the CSF by PCR in patients with benign recurrent aseptic meningitis. In one report, the classic Mollaret cells were seen in the same CSF samples that contained the HSV-2 DNA.[20] CSF from patients between episodes or from control patients without a recurrent meningitis syndrome did not have the viral DNA. This association with HSV has potential therapeutic importance because acyclovir therapy might prevent further recurrences.

Tuberculous Meningitis

Tuberculous meningitis[47–50, 55–66] results from rupture of a superficial infective focus into the subarachnoid space. In younger patients, this event typically is associated with active, progressive systemic disease. Stigmata of miliary tuberculosis may be present on physical examination and on chest x-ray films. Tuberculin skin test results frequently are negative initially but convert on repeated testing. The diagnosis of tuberculosis usually is confirmed by smear, biopsy, and cultures obtained from extraneural specimens as well as CSF culture. In contrast, tuberculous meningitis in the adult more frequently results from the discharge of an old tuberculous focus into the subarachnoid space. As a result, physical examination, chest x-ray films, and extraneural cultures often are not helpful; despite presumably long-standing tuberculous infection, series indicate that the initial tuberculin skin test result is negative in 50 to 65% of patients.[47–50] The diagnosis rests on the outcome of CSF cultures. As a result of the frequent early use of antituberculous therapy empirically, more cases now are "unproved" microbiologically but with the diagnosis of tuberculosis suggested by an apparent response to treatment.

Overall there is nothing about the clinical syndrome of tuberculous meningitis that distinguishes it from other causes of chronic meningitis. About one half of the patients have had symptoms for longer than 2 weeks. Ocular palsies, particularly those caused by involvement of cranial nerve VI, are found in 30 to 70% of the cases. The typical CSF findings consist of a lymphocytic pleocytosis (usually of 100 to 500 cells/mm^3), increased protein concentration, and depressed glucose levels in two thirds of the patients on the initial lumbar puncture. This formula also is not specific for tuberculous meningitis. However, in unclear cases, progressive decrease in CSF glucose in the absence of specific treatment may be useful in distinguishing tuberculosis from aseptic meningitis and viral encephalitis. Cytologic examination of CSF often shows activated monocytoid cells and rarely Langhans' cells.[61] It should be noted that neutrophils may predominate, particularly during the first 10 days of symptoms.[47, 49] CSF smears contain acid-fast bacilli in 10 to 22% of the cases.[47–49, 65, 66] Proteinaceous spinal fluid contains fibrinogen and forms a clot or pellicle on standing; staining of the pellicle may increase the yield of the direct smear.[62] CSF cultures are positive in 38 to 88% of the cases, and sputum in about 14 to 50%.

CSF tests evaluated for the presumptive diagnosis of tuberculous meningitis include various antibody and antigen detection assays,[67] although currently detection of mycobacterial DNA by PCR shows the most promise. Sensitivity of PCR ranges from 27 to 85% in series, with specificity of 95 to 100%. The low amount of mycobacterial DNA in the CSF limits the sensitivity, but in all studies it is significantly greater than that of culture.[38–43] Adenosine deaminase is released by T lymphocytes, and increased CSF levels are found in tuberculous meningitis but not in viral or bacterial meningitides.[68–70] Specificity is not perfect, because elevations are seen also in lymphomatous meningitis, neurosarcoidosis, and brucellosis.

Cryptococcal Meningitis

Cryptococcal meningitis[47, 71–81] manifests in several different fashions, but the most characteristic, that of a subacute to chronic meningoencephalitis, is not at all distinctive among the causes of chronic meningitis. Exposure history is of little value clinically, because the yeast-like fungus *C. neoformans* var. *neoformans* is a widespread saprophyte with a worldwide distribution. However, *C. neoformans* var. *gattii* is most often found in the tropical and subtropical areas of Australia, Southeast Asia, Africa, and South America. More patients infected with the latter variety were previously normal, more have indolent onset, and they more often have focal CNS lesions on MRI than those infected with the *C. neoformans* var. *neoformans*.[82, 83] Although one half of patients in the pre-AIDS era lacked clinically apparent immunologic deficits, an underlying cellular immune dysfunction was known to predispose to this infection. The development of chronic meningitis in patients with Hodgkin's disease or lymphosarcoma, in persons receiving high-dose daily corticosteroid therapy, or in persons at risk for AIDS suggests cryptococcal meningitis.

In the previously healthy person, cryptococcal meningitis may cause an extremely indolent illness with gradual progression of dementia. The India ink preparation frequently is negative in such cases. More commonly, the onset of disease is subacute, at times mimicking a brain tumor, particularly when signs of increased intracranial pressure are present. In patients with hematologic malignancies or AIDS, the initial manifestation of cryptococcosis may be unexplained fever. However, CNS involvement often proceeds rapidly. CSF abnormalities include a lymphocytic pleocytosis (usually with 40 to 400 cells/mm^3) and a depressed glucose level in 55% of cases. In patients with AIDS, the CSF often shows little evidence of an inflammatory response.[75–78, 80] Overall, the India ink preparation suggests the diagnosis of cryptococcal meningitis in more than one half of cases. The yield is highest in patients with an acute syndrome. More than 85% of patients have cryptococcal polysaccharide antigen in the CSF. However, serum also should be processed for this antigen; the overlap between significant antigen titers in the serum and in the CSF allows a presumptive diagnosis of cryptococcosis in 94% of the cases.

Negative serology findings do not exclude a diagnosis of cryptococcal meningitis,[84, 85] and false-positive tests are not rare. Cultural confirmation of the diagnosis is mandatory. The initial CSF culture is positive in three quarters of patients; additional CSF cultures increase this yield and are indicated. Cultures of urine, sputum, and blood also should be obtained. They have both diagnostic and prognostic value and frequently are positive in the absence of overt signs of extraneural infection. CSF cultures and serologies also are indicated in all patients with extraneural cryptococcal infection, because they may have subclinical CNS disease; this is particularly likely in the immunocompromised host.

Coccidioidal Meningitis

Exposure history is important in the diagnosis of coccidioidal meningitis, because this infection is endemic in certain arid and semiarid areas of the Western Hemisphere.[86–95] CNS infection may be a part of generalized coccidioidomycosis, or it may represent the sole extrapulmonary site of active clinical disease. One third of patients with extrapulmonary coccidioidomycosis have meningeal involvement. Meningitis usually occurs within 6 months after the primary pulmonary infection; however, it has developed as long as 12 years after the initial infection.[92] Headache is the most prominent finding in patients with coccidioidal meningitis; the clinical syndrome is, however, in no way distinctive from the other causes of chronic meningitis. Skin tests with spherulin are positive in one third to one half of patients with meningitis.[91, 92] Complement-fixing antibody to the causative organism is found in the CSF of 55 to 95% of such patients. One study suggests that detection of CSF antibodies to a 33-kD antigen from the sperule by ELISA is more sensitive than detection of complement fixation antibodies.[96] Eosinophils are commonly seen in the CSF of patients with coccidioidal meningitis, with 30% of patients having more than 10 eosinophils/mm^3.[93] A presumptive diagnosis is possible when chronic meningitis occurs in the presence of demonstrated systemic coccidioidomycosis or a serum complement fixation titer to *C. immitis* of at least 1:16. CSF findings resemble those of cryptococcal meningitis; CSF cultures are positive in one third to one half of the cases, and spherules of *C. immitis* are sometimes present on a smear.

Histoplasma Meningitis

Histoplasma meningitis[33–36, 97–100] is a rare complication of infection with *Histoplasma capsulatum.* However, in one fourth of cases of *Histoplasma* meningitis, disease is limited to the CNS. Clinical presentation is not differentiable from that seen with other causes of chronic meningitis; fever is almost universally present.[33] Symptoms may have been present for weeks or many months. Oral mucosal lesions, although found in only 16% of patients with *Histoplasma* meningitis, can be diagnostic if present and are more common than skin lesions. CSF cultures are positive in only 27 to 65% of cases, making diagnosis problematic. Blood cultures should always be done; use of isolator tubes significantly increased the yield of blood cultures in a study of AIDS patients.[101] As discussed previously, detection of serum and CSF antibodies to the fungus is the most sensitive test for histoplasmosis; however, it is not specific, because the antibodies may cross-react with other fungi. Persons with positive *Histoplasma* serology should have their cryptococcal antigen level checked; if the patient is from an endemic area, coccidioidal serology should also be done to detect a false-positive test result. The serum antibody tests are negative in 10 to 40% of proven cases of *Histoplasma* meningitis. *Histoplasma* polysaccharide antigen may be detected in urine, blood, or CSF in 61% of patients with *Histoplasma* meningitis;[33] yields are even higher in HIV-infected persons.[101]

Lyme Disease

Infection with the spirochete *Borrelia burgdorferi* frequently involves the CNS.[102–107] The spirochete is introduced into its human host by an often unrecognized bite of the small deer tick, *Ixodes scapularis (dammini).* Early infection is characterized by a flulike syndrome and the pathognomonic rash of erythema chronicum migrans. Neurologic symptoms follow the rash by a median of 4 weeks; headache and lymphocytic pleocytosis are seen in almost all patients with neuroborreliosis. Cranial nerve palsies (especially facial nerve) and peripheral neuropathies may be prominent and help to differentiate Lyme disease from the other chronic meningitides except sarcoidosis, which can manifest similarly. Exposure history is key in guiding appropriate serologic testing; in the absence of exposure, a positive serology result is more likely to represent a false-positive test than to be diagnostic for Lyme disease.[108] False-positive tests have been associated with infectious mononucleosis, rheumatoid arthritis, systemic lupus erythematosus, other spirochetal disease such as syphilis and periodontal disease, and malignancy.[107] However, in endemic areas, up to 25% of healthy people are seropositive, so antibody detection in serum alone is not diagnostic. Persons in an endemic area who have an appropriate clinical presentation and positive serology results should be treated as having neuroborelliosis. Almost all persons with CNS Lyme disease have positive serologic evidence of Lyme disease and CSF pleocytosis.[108] The most specific test is the detection of synthesis of intrathecal antibody to *B. burgdorferi* in the CNS.[108–110] PCR detection of *Borrelia* DNA in the CSF is specific but has limited sensitivity for neuroborreliosis (38% in acute cases and 25% in chronic cases).[111]

Cysticercosis

Cysticercosis[112–119] is the most common parasitic disease of the CNS. Highly endemic areas include Mexico, central and upper South America, China, India, sub-Saharan Africa, and the Caribbean. In the United States, immigrants from Mexico are the largest infected population and can present with symptoms up to 25 years after leaving Mexico. The infection is acquired by eating food contaminated with stool containing the eggs of the tapeworm *Taenia solium*; these hatch in the small intestine, with the larvae invading the blood stream and infecting muscle, eye, and brain. In these sites the larvae mature into cysts and remain asymptomatic for an average of 4 to 5 years. The person develops symptoms as the larvae begin to die, inciting an increased inflammatory response. Symptoms vary depending on the part of the brain infected; intraparenchymal neurocysticercosis (the most common manifestation) results in seizures and focal neurologic deficits. Cysts in the subarachnoid space can collect in the basilar cisterns and induce a chronic basilar meningitis with hydrocephalus. CSF shows a lymphocytic pleocytosis, and hypoglycorrhachia occurs in up to one fourth of patients. Cysts can also occur in the ventricles, causing ventriculitis or internal hydrocephalus.

Diagnosis is suggested by characteristic multiple cystic or calcified lesions detected by head CT scan in a person who has been in an endemic area; early in infection the calcium may not be present. Subcutaneous cysts were present in one fourth of patients with neurocysticercosis in a large series; biopsy revealed the larval tapeworm.[115] Skeletal muscle calcification on plain film is also suggestive of cysticercosis; however, the yield was low (<10%) in a series from the United States.[116] Serologic studies of serum and particularly of CSF are helpful, but negative serology studies do not rule out neurocysticercosis, because serum antibodies are negative in up to 50% of cases. The yield in CSF is high (up to 84% positive serology findings) in patients with meningitis or hydrocephalus. Detection of antibodies in a patient from an endemic area with a typical history and characteristic head CT scan confirms the diagnosis.

Other Infectious Causes

Candida meningitis[5, 120–125] is rare and often is associated with widely disseminated disease. Risk factors for meningitis are similar to those for candidemia, including prolonged antimicrobial therapy, indwelling venous catheters, hyperalimentation, corticosteroid use, recent intra-abdominal surgery, and intravenous drug abuse. CSF shunts and ventricular catheters have also been associated specifically with meningitis. Neonates, and especially premature infants, seem to be at increased risk for candidal meningitis (11 of 17 patients in one series were younger than 1 year of age).[122] Presentation ranges from subacute to indolent, with the interval from onset of symptoms to diagnosis ranging from days to months. Most commonly the disease manifests acutely as a complication of disseminated *Candida* infection; the clinical presentation and CSF findings can mimic those of bacterial meningitis. However, *Candida* meningitis can manifest as chronic meningitis progressing over months, similar to the endemic fungi.[123] CSF shows pleocytosis with a predominance of neutrophils in one half of cases and hypoglycorrhachia in 60%. Gram staining reveals yeast in one third of smears, and CSF culture is usually diagnostic. However, culture of large volumes of CSF and filtering of CSF with culture of the filter contents may be necessary.[123]

Syphilitic meningitis[126–130] is a rare but easily diagnosed and treated form of secondary syphilis. The disease is usually subacute, with the symptoms persisting for longer than 1 month in about one quarter of the cases. Meningitis is the first overt sign of syphilis in 25% of meningitic patients. When extraneural manifestations occur, they generally precede CNS involvement by less than 2 years. The clinical presentation and CSF abnormalities resemble those of the other causes of chronic meningitis; however, cranial nerve palsies are seen in almost one half of cases, with a special predilection for nerves VII and VIII. Hypoglycorrhachia is present in 55% of the cases. The diagnosis of syphilitic meningitis is suggested by positive CSF and serum serology results for syphilis. Detection of *Treponema pallidum* DNA by PCR has been reported in neurosyphilis, but this test is not as sensitive as CSF-VDRL with conventional CSF analysis.[130] Transient dramatic deterioration of patients with meningitis after the initiation of penicillin therapy should suggest a Jarisch-Herxheimer reaction and the possibility of syphilis.

A meningoencephalomyelitis may follow the initial manifestations of brucellosis by 2 months to 2 years in fewer than 5% of cases.[131–135] Exposure to unpasteurized milk products or contact with cows, goats, sheep, swine, or their carcasses suggests the diagnosis. The patient also may have current or past symptoms and signs of systemic brucellosis, such as night sweats, unexplained fever, orchitis, and hepatosplenomegaly. The clinical manifestations of the meningitis and CSF abnormalities usually are nonspecific, with a lymphocytic pleocytosis in all and hypoglycorrhachia in one half of cases. However, transient episodes of hemianesthesia or paresthesia can be prominent in neurobrucellosis. In chronic cases, calcified foci may be noted in the liver and spleen on abdominal x-ray films. Cultures should be maintained in an increased carbon dioxide atmosphere for 3 weeks. CSF cultures are positive for *Brucella* in fewer than one half of the cases. Blood cultures occasionally are positive. The diagnosis is made by detection of *Brucella* antibodies in the serum and CSF.

S. schenckii has been described as a cause of chronic meningitis,[37, 44, 136] and the CSF may demonstrate *Sporothrix* antibody before the fungus is recovered by culture.[37] *Angiostrongylus cantonensis* is a nematode endemic to Southeast Asia and the Pacific Islands and is the most common cause worldwide of eosinophilic meningitis.[137] Symptoms develop approximately 1 week after ingestion of raw fish or snails and persist for 2 to 4 weeks, usually resolving spontaneously. Rarely, the living larvae may be found in the CSF or eye; however, the diagnosis is usually made clinically (eosinophilic meningitis with the correct exposure history).

CNS involvement in a large number of infections commonly is expressed as brain abscesses or other focal lesions occurring by hematogenous seeding or direct extension from clinically apparent extraneural sites. Rarely, the syndrome of chronic meningitis may be caused by these agents, sometimes without other stigmata of the infection. Infectious diseases belonging in this category include North American blastomycosis,[138–140] paracoccidioidomycosis,[141] cerebral phaeohyphomycosis,[142] actinomycosis,[143–145] nocardiosis,[146–149] and toxoplasmosis.[150–152] Several infectious agents have been documented to cause chronic meningitis in unique epidemiologic circumstances *(Coenurus cerebralis)*[1] or in isolated case reports (*Leptospira icterohaemorrhagiae,* mucormycosis)[1, 153] and are not discussed here. Other infections in which CNS involvement is a late manifestation with few related symptoms, or leptomeningitis is noted pathologically but not clinically, also are not reviewed.

Neoplastic Meningitis

The noninfectious diseases causing chronic meningitis may be difficult to diagnose and distinguish from occult infections (see Table 72–2). Primary and metastatic, hematologic, and solid tumors all may involve the meninges diffusely to cause a similar clinical syndrome. In the case of acute leukemia and lymphoma,[154–157] CNS involvement usually occurs in the setting of known underlying malignancy. The major diagnostic problem is to distinguish CNS involvement by the tumor from superimposed CNS infection and the uncommon paraneoplastic syndromes. Primary brain tumors, including gliomas, pinealomas, ependymomas, and choroid plexus tumors, may involve the meninges diffusely,[158] sometimes without gross parenchymal involvement. A diagnosis can be difficult in such cases. In metastatic "meningeal carcinomatosis,"[29, 159–167] the nature of the meningeal process also may be difficult to ascertain. In one large series, the primary tumor had not been diagnosed by the time of onset of neurologic symptoms in 75% of the patients,[161] although the figure was 8% in patients selected by admission to an oncology center.[29] Typically, the onset of symptoms is subacute, with intractable headache a prominent complaint along with mental changes. Cranial neuropathy occurs in 50% of the cases, and meningismus in about 20%. Fever usually is absent, or when it occurs it is associated with an intercurrent infection. Characteristically, neurologic signs far exceed symptoms and indicate widespread neurologic dysfunction; cerebral, cranial nerve, and spinal involvement are noted in one half of the patients on initial physical examination.

The CSF is abnormal; 72% of patients have a pleocytosis, often minimal, although some patients have a marked cellular response. The glucose content is depressed in 38% of the patients initially and in 72% during serial examinations. The finding of marked hypoglycorrhachia in the presence of minimal pleocytosis should suggest this diagnosis. In one series, CSF cytology results were diagnostic in 42% of patients in the first study and in 74% when multiple specimens were processed.[29] Of the ancillary neurodiagnostic tests, the myelogram was particularly helpful diagnostically and revealed multiple nodular deposits on nerve roots in 39% of the cases. MRI of the brain with gadolinium reveals enhancement and thickening in the meninges with better sensitivity than CT scan, but this finding is not specific.[168, 169] The finding of markedly elevated CSF levels of β-glucuronidase is suggestive of meningeal carcinomatosis.[170, 171] The most common primary sites of malignancy causing this syndrome are the breast, lung, stomach, pancreas, and skin (melanoma). Although neurologic signs may fluctuate and even partly regress, the course of meningeal carcinomatosis usually is rapidly progressive with involvement of all parts of the neuraxis. Because the primary tumor may be occult and extraneural metastatic sites lacking, cytologic examination of multiple CSF specimens is appropriate in all patients with undiagnosed chronic meningitis.

Sarcoid Meningitis

Neurologic involvement is seen in 5% of patients with sarcoidosis[172–180]; however, among these patients, almost one third present with neurologic signs as their initial indication of sarcoidosis and 17% have neurologic signs as the sole manifestation of the disease.[178] The clinical syndrome of sarcoid meningitis often includes cranial nerve palsies, long-tract and cerebellar abnormalities, and changes in mentation. Peripheral seventh cranial nerve paralysis is the most common manifestation of neurosarcoidosis.[181] The predilection for the basilar meninges with extension to the hypothalamus results in diabetes insipidus in 14 to 30% of cases; this is of diagnostic significance because it rarely occurs in other forms of chronic meningitis. In addition, peripheral neuropathies accompany CNS sarcoidosis in 14% of patients but generally are unusual in chronic meningitis except for Lyme disease. Seizures occur in 15% of patients and are associated with an acute, severe, progressive, and relapsing course.[182]

Characteristic CSF abnormalities consist of a minimal lymphocytic pleocytosis in 60% of patients and hypoglycorrhachia in 10 to 18%. The diagnosis of CNS sarcoidosis in patients with classic systemic manifestations of the disease is complicated by the necessity of excluding superimposed tuberculosis or cryptococcosis, both of which occur with increased frequency in patients with sarcoidosis and in patients receiving corticosteroid therapy. The diagnosis is more difficult when disease is limited to the CNS. Even the demonstration of granulomas in meningeal biopsy specimens is not specific. Serum and CSF concentrations of angiotensin-converting enzyme may be elevated in neurosarcoidosis,[183–185] although increased concentrations also are seen in malignant and bacterial meningitis.[184] More than two thirds of patients with neurosarcoid have evidence of thoracic disease; chest radiography and gallium scanning may be helpful in locating a site for diagnostic biopsy.[178, 180] Prolonged corticosteroid therapy is recommended for the treatment of CNS sarcoidosis; cytotoxic drug therapy may be required in some cases.[181, 186] Cyclosporine has also been used in refractory cases.[187] Low-dose irradiation of the CNS has been used with apparent advantage in several patients.[178, 188] Overall prognosis is good.[178]

Other Noninfectious Causes

Granulomatous angiitis is a necrotizing vasculitis of small leptomeningeal and perforating arteries and veins usually isolated to the CNS.[189–198] The process usually manifests as headache, confusion, focal neurologic findings, and CSF pleocytosis. Mean age of onset is the mid-forties. CSF findings include a lymphocytic pleocytosis and increased protein levels. Cerebral angiograms show a "string of beads" appearance in 27 to 65% of patients with primary angiitis of the CNS; however, a normal angiogram is seen in 13 to 44% of reported cases.[197] Biopsy is the gold standard for diagnosis; because of the focal nature of the disease, the sensitivity is only 71%.[195] Untreated, this disease is thought to be uniformly fatal. Successful long-term outcomes have been reported with a combination of corticosteroid and cytotoxic immunosuppressive therapy.[192] On clinical and pathologic grounds, this syndrome is distinct from sarcoidosis, giant cell arteritis, and Wegener's granulomatosis. An ipsilateral granulomatous angiitis of the middle cerebral artery may follow ophthalmic zoster; in some instances, varicella-zoster virus has been cultured from involved cerebral blood vessels.

A subacute meningoencephalitis usually occurs early in the course of the Vogt-Koyanagi-Harada syndrome (uveomeningoencephalitis).[199–203] The diagnosis is established by the development of severe, protracted, granulomatous uveitis; depigmentary skin changes such as poliosis (whitening of the eyebrows and eyelashes) and vitiligo; and dysacusia and tinnitis 3 months or more into the illness. The CSF shows predominantly lymphocytic pleocytosis. The CNS disease gradually resolves spontaneously. This syndrome is considered to be an autoimmune disease directed against melanocytes. It has a predilection for races with greater pigmentation: Asians, Hispanics, American Indians, and Asian Indians. Corticosteroids have been reported to preserve visual acuity.[202]

Of the patients with Behçet's disease (recurrent oral and genital ulcerations and uveitis), CNS involvement develops in 10 to 25%.[204–209] The neurologic manifestations include aseptic meningitis, meningoencephalitis, seizures, cranial nerve palsies, and hemiparesis. Occasionally, they precede other features of the syndrome. CSF abnormalities include a slight elevation of protein concentrations, normal glucose, and minimal pleocytosis (usually less than 60 cells/mm^3 with both lymphocytes and polymorphonuclear cells reported).

Other connective tissue diseases that may mimic chronic meningitis include systemic lupus erythematosus (SLE), Sjögren's syndrome, polyarteritis nodosa, and Wegener's granulomatosis. SLE can manifest as acute aseptic meningitis (less than 5% of patients with SLE),[210] but most SLE patients presenting with meningitis have an infectious cause.[211] Polyarteritis nodosa involves the CNS in 23 to 53% of cases, but almost all have evidence of systemic disease also (e.g., abdominal pain, renal dysfunction).[212] Although CNS involvement in Wegener's granulomatosis occurs in 25 to 50% of cases, meningitis is a rare manifestation, causing headache, cranial neuropathies, and a mild lymphocytic pleocytosis.[213] Sjögren's syndrome has been associated with a chronic inflammatory meningoencephalitis mimicking Alzheimer's dementia; the CSF is remarkably normal, but perivascular inflammation is seen on brain biopsy. This complication of Sjögren's syndrome responds dramatically to glucocorticoid therapy.[214]

A syndrome of benign chronic lymphocytic meningitis was first reported in 1973 from the National Hospitals for Nervous Diseases in London.[215] Over a 6-year period, observers identified 12 cases of idiopathic chronic meningitis. Five patients had very low CSF glucose or severe neurologic deficit, which distinguished them from the 7 other patients with chronic benign lymphocytic meningitis. The CSF of these patients had only mildly elevated protein, modest CSF pleocytosis (usually $<$50 cells/mm^3), and normal glucose. Three patients were treated with glucocorticoids, and two improved on this therapy. Patients observed for 1 to 9 years had persistent pleocytosis but no significant clinical deterioration.

Three more recent studies have confirmed the existence of a benign or steroid-responsive chronic meningitis.[4, 6, 7] In a retrospective review of chronic meningitis in a New Zealand hospital, 28 of 83 patients had idiopathic meningitis.[4] Of these, one half responded to empiric antituberculosis therapy, one third responded to steroids, and 14% improved on no therapy. A distinguishing feature of the steroid-responsive group was a normal CSF glucose concentration. Two patients died after withdrawal of glucocorticoid therapy. In a series of 37 patients who underwent brain biopsy for chronic meningitis at the Mayo Clinic between 1989 and 1993,[7] two thirds of patients ultimately were treated with glucocorticoids after the biopsy revealed chronic inflammation. Half of these patients improved, and none was reported to have deteriorated on corticosteroid therapy. A large series from the Mayo Clinic reported on 49 patients with chronic meningitis seen between 1978 and 1990.[6] Although only 10 of these patients ultimately had a definitive diagnosis, of whom 8 had neoplastic meningitis, the follow-up observations of the 39 idiopathic cases revealed that 85% had a good outcome despite a prolonged illness. Approximately one half of the patients received glucocorticoid therapy, often with prompt resolution of symptoms. No patient responded to empirical antituberculosis therapy.

In contrast to the patients with unexplained minimal, self-limited disease, an additional group of patients have an enigmatic chronic meningitis with significant neurologic involvement, a high CSF protein concentration, and sometimes a depressed glucose level.[1] The prognosis in this group is poor. Therapeutic trials may alter the course of the disease, the cultures, and the pathologic findings. A specific diagnosis may be apparent at autopsy, but this is not always the case. A temporal response to antifungal therapy in some cases has implicated an infectious cause; mycotic meningitis too often is associated with negative CSF cultures (as discussed previously) and only diagnosed after death. Therefore, a thorough diagnostic evaluation followed ultimately by meningeal and brain biopsy and, if appropriate, an empirical trial of amphotericin B with or without glucocorticoid therapy is indicated.

THE IMMUNOCOMPROMISED PATIENT

Chronic meningitis in the immunosuppressed patient with impaired cellular immunity requires special consideration because of the distinctive differential diagnosis. Among renal transplant recipients and patients with lymphoma or leukemia, *C. neoformans* is the most common cause of chronic meningitis.[216] *M. tuberculosis, Toxoplasma gondii, Nocardia, Histoplasma,* and *Coccidioides* also cause chronic meningitis more often in such patients. Progressive multifocal leukoencephalopathy (caused by papovaviruses) may produce profound focal neurologic deficits with minimal or no abnormalities in the CSF. JC virus DNA can be detected in the CSF by the PCR technique.[217] CT scans in such cases demonstrate low-density, nonenhancing, progressive lesions in the white matter without mass effect. Lesions are even better visualized by MRI. Hypogammaglobulinemic patients are susceptible to chronic meningoencephalitis secondary to enteroviral infections.[218] Symptoms include headache, seizures, lethargy, weakness, and ataxia; the CSF shows lymphocytic pleocytosis with hypoglycorrhachia.

Aseptic meningitis with fever, headache, and meningismus is common in primary HIV infection;[219] symptoms resolve rapidly, but CSF pleocytosis can be found in 10% of asymptomatic HIV-infected patients.[220] A mild elevation in protein is also seen, but glucose remains normal. *Cryptococcus*, the most common opportunistic pathogen to cause meningitis in patients with AIDS, occurs in about 1 to 2% of patients in the United States, the incidence having fallen since highly active antiretroviral therapy became available. There is often little inflammatory reaction in the CSF, but, in contrast to the situation in HIV-negative patients, this has not been a risk factor for poor outcome.[77, 78] Tuberculous meningitis is a more common complication of tuberculosis in HIV-infected persons, occurring in 10% of tuberculosis patients with HIV disease and only 2% of tuberculosis patients without HIV infection in Spain.[221] In one series of predominantly HIV-infected drug users from Madrid, tuberculous meningitis was more common than cryptococcal disease.[222] Clinical presentation, CSF findings, and mortality in HIV-infected patients were similar to those in HIV-negative patients with tuberculous meningitis. Risk factors for poor outcome were duration of symptoms greater than 2 weeks before admission and a CD4-positive T-lymphocyte count lower than 200 cells/cm^3.[221] Meningitis secondary to *Coccidioides*,[223] *Histoplasma*,[101] and *Blastomyces*[140] has also been reported with HIV. Reactivation of *T. gondii* is common in AIDS patients but usually causes ring-enhancing mass lesions rather than meningitis. CNS lymphoma similarly manifests more frequently as mass lesions; lymphocytic meningitis is much less common. PCR detection of Epstein-Barr viral DNA in the CSF suggests primary CNS lymphoma.[224] End-stage AIDS patients are at risk for cytomegalovirus ventriculoencephalitis;[225, 226] presenting symptoms include cranial nerve palsies, nystagmus, and confusion, usually in patients with previously diagnosed cytomegalovirus end-organ disease (e.g., retinitis). MRI scans show ependymal enhancement; the CSF has a neutrophilic pleocytosis with hypoglycorrachia. Cytomegalovirus DNA is detectable by PCR in the CSF.[224] An associated ascending radiculomyelitis with flaccid weakness and hyporeflexia is often seen. Prognosis is grim, with death occurring a median of 4 weeks after diagnosis despite antiviral chemotherapy. Progression of syphilis is accelerated in HIV-infected patients, with more syphilitic meningitis and uveitis seen;[128] usually, routine serologic tests confirm the diagnosis.[129, 227] Negative serology results in patients with frank syphilitic meningitis have been reported, but follow-up serologic studies were positive.[228, 229] Thirty percent of patients with advanced HIV infection and a documented previous history of syphilis have a negative fluorescent treponemal antibody absorption (FTA-ABC) test, calling into question the interpretation of negative serologic findings in AIDS patients.[230] When clinical suspicion for syphilis is high, serologic studies should be repeated in follow-up, looking for delayed seroconversion.

REFERENCES

1. Ellner JJ, Bennett JE. Chronic meningitis. Medicine (Baltimore). 1976;55:341–369.
2. Wilhelm C, Ellner JJ. Chronic meningitis. Neurol Clin. 1986;4:115–141.
3. Swartz M. Chronic meningitis: Many causes to consider. N Engl J Med. 1987;317:957–959.
4. Anderson NE, Willoughby EW. Chronic meningitis without predisposing illness: A review of 83 cases. Q J Med. 1987;63:283–295.
5. Salaki JS, Louria DB, Chmel H. Fungal and yeast infections of the central nervous system: A clinical review. Medicine (Baltimore). 1984;63:108–132.
6. Smith JE, Asamit AJ. Outcome of chronic idiopathic meningitis. Mayo Clin Proc. 1994;69:548–556.
7. Cheng TM, O'Neill BP, Scheithauer BW, et al. Chronic meningitis: The role of meningeal or cortical biopsy. Neurosurgery. 1994;34:590–596.
8. Anderson NE, Willoughby EW, Synek BJL. Leptomeningeal and brain biopsy in chronic meningitis. Aust N Z J Med. 1995;25:703–706.
9. Gripshover BM, Ellner JJ. Chronic meningitis syndrome and meningitis of noninfective or uncertain etiology. In: Scheld WM, Whitley RJ, Durak DT: Infections of the Central Nervous System. Philadelphia: Lippincott Raven; 1997:881–896.
10. Hermans PE, Goldstein NP, Wellman WE. Mollaret's meningitis and differential diagnosis of recurrent meningitis. Am J Med. 1972;52:128–140.
11. Joffle AM, Farley JD, Linden D, et al. Trimethoprim-sulfamethoxazole–associated aseptic meningitis: Case reports and review of the literature. Am J Med. 1989;87:332–338.
12. Marinac JS. Drug- and chemical-induced aseptic meningitis: A review of the literature. Ann Pharmacother. 1992;26:813–821.
13. Chez M, Sila CA, Ranshoff RM, et al. Ibuprofen-induced meningitis: Detection of intrathecal IgG synthesis and immune complexes. Neurology. 1989;39:1578–1580.
14. River Y, Averbuch-Heller L, Weinberger M, et al. Antibiotic induced meningitis. J Neurol Neurosurg Psychiatry. 1994;57:705–708.
15. Lunardi P, Missori P. Cranial and spinal tumors with meningitic onset. Ital J Neurol Sci. 1990;11:145–151.
16. Achard JM, Lallement PY, Veyssier P. Recurrent aseptic meningitis secondary to intracranial epidermoid cyst and Mollaret's meningitis: Two distinct entities or a single disease? A case report and a nosologic discussion. Am J Med. 1990;89:807–810.
17. Crossley GH, Dismukes WE. Central nervous system epidermoid cyst: A probable etiology of Mollaret's meningitis. Am J Med. 1990;89:805–806.
18. Kuroda Y, Abe M, Nagumo F, et al. Neuroepithelial cyst presenting as recurrent aseptic meningitis. Neurology. 1991;41:1834–1835.
19. Berger JR. Benign aseptic (Mollaret's) meningitis after genital herpes. Lancet. 1991;337:1360–1361.
20. Picard FJ, Dekaban GA, Silva J, et al. Mollaret's meningitis associated with herpes simplex type 2 infection. Neurology. 1993;43:1722–1727.
21. Tedder DG, Ashley R, Tyler KL, et al. Herpes simplex virus infection as a cause of benign recurrent lymphocytic meningitis. Ann Intern Med. 1994;121:334–338.
22. Monteyne P, Sindic CJM, Laterre EC. Recurrent meningitis and encephalitis associated with herpes simplex type 2: Demonstration by polymerase chain reaction. Eur Neurol. 1996;36:176–177.
23. Pasquale M, Finelli F, Yockey CC, et al. Recurrent aseptic meningitis in an elderly man: Unusual prodrome of systemic lupus erythematosus. JAMA. 1976;235:1142–1144.
24. Welsby P, Smith C. Recurrent sterile meningitis as a manifestation of systemic lupus erythematosus. Scand J Infect Dis. 1977;9:149–150.
25. Sands ML, Ryczak M, Brown RB. Recurrent aseptic meningitis followed by transverse myelitis as a presentation of systemic lupus erythematosus. J Rheumatol. 1988;15:862–864.
26. Kanekura T, Mizumoto J, Setoyama M. A case of lupus meningitis treated successfully with methylprednisone pulse therapy. J Dermatol. 1993;20:566–571.
27. Peacock JE Jr, McGinnis MR, Cohen MS. Persistent neutrophilic meningitis: Report of four cases and review of the literature. Medicine (Baltimore). 1984;63:379–395.
28. Weller PF. Eosinophilic meningitis. Am J Med. 1993;95:250–253.
29. Olson ME, Chernik NL, Posner JH. Infiltration of the leptomeninges by systemic cancer: A clinical and pathologic study. Arch Neurol. 1974;30:122–137.
30. Goodson JD, Strauss GM. Diagnosis of lymphomatous leptomeningitis by cerebrospinal fluid lymphocyte cell surface markers. Am J Med. 1979;66:1057–1059.
31. Kranz BR, Thiel E, Thierfelde R. Immunocytochemical identification of meningeal leukemia and lymphoma: Poly-L-lysine–coated slides permit multimarker analysis even with minute cerebrospinal fluid cell specimens. Blood. 1989;73:1942–1950.
32. Rhodes CH, Glantz MJ, Glantz L, et al. A comparison of polymerase chain reaction examination of cerebral spinal fluid and conventional cytology in the diagnosis of lymphomatous meningitis. Cancer. 1996;77:543–548.
33. Wheat LJ, Batteiger BE, Sathapatayarongs B. *Histoplasma capsulatum* infections of the central nervous system: A clinical review. Medicine (Baltimore). 1990;69:244–260.
34. Plouffe JF, Fass RJ. *Histoplasma* meningitis: Diagnostic value of cerebrospinal fluid serology. Ann Intern Med. 1980;92:189–191.
35. Wheat J, French M, Batteiger B, et al. Cerebrospinal fluid *Histoplasma* antibodies in central nervous system histoplasmosis. Arch Intern Med. 1985;145:1237–1240.
36. Wheat LJ, Kohler RB, Tewari RP, et al. Significance of *Histoplasma* antigen in the cerebrospinal fluid of patients with meningitis. Arch Intern Med. 1989;149:302–304.
37. Scott EN, Kaufman L, Brown AC, et al. Serologic studies in the diagnosis and management of meningitis due to *Sporothrix schenckii*. N Engl J Med. 1987;317:935–940.
38. Kox LFF, Kuijper S, Kolk AHJ. Early diagnosis of tuberculous meningitis by polymerase chain reaction. Neurology. 1995;45:2228–2232.
39. Lin JJ, Harn HJ, Hsu YD, et al. Rapid diagnosis of tuberculous meningitis by polymerase chain reaction assay of cerebrospinal fluid. J Neurol. 1995;242:147–152.
40. Miorner H, Sjobring U, Nayak P, et al. Diagnosis of tuberculous meningitis: A comparative analysis of 3 immunoassays, an immune complex assay and the polymerase chain reaction. Tuber Lung Dis. 1995;76:381–386.
41. Nguyen LN, Kox LFF, Pham LD, et al. The potential contribution of the polymerase chain reaction to the diagnosis of tuberculous meningitis. Arch Neurol. 1996;53:771–776.
42. Seth P, Ahuja K, Bhanu NV, et al. Evaluation of polymerase chain reaction for rapid diagnosis of clinically suspected tuberculous meningitis. Tuber Lung Dis. 1996;77:353–357.
43. Bonington A, Strang JIG, Klapper PE, et al. Use of Roche AMPLICOR *Mycobacterium tuberculosis* PCR in early diagnosis of tuberculous meningitis. J Clin Microbiol. 1998;36:1251–1254.
44. Ewing GE, Bose GJ, Petersen PK. *Sporothrix schenckii* meningitis in a farmer with Hodgkin's disease. Am J Med. 1980;68:455–457.
45. Kravitz GR, Davies SF, Eckman MR, et al. Chronic blastomycotic meningitis. Am J Med. 1981;71:501.
46. Sze G. Diseases of the intracranial meninges: MR imaging features. AJR Am J Roentgenol. 1993;160:727–733.
47. Stocksill MT, Kauffman CA. Comparison of cryptococcal and tuberculous meningitis. Arch Neurol. 1983;40:81–85.

48. Klein NC, Damsker B, Hirschman SZ. Mycobacterial meningitis: Retrospective analysis from 1970–1983. Am J Med. 1985;79:29–34.
49. Ogawa SH, Smith MA, Brennessel DJ, et al. Tuberculous meningitis in an urban medical center. Medicine (Baltimore). 1987;66:317–326.
50. Kent SJ, Crowe SM, Yung A, et al. Tuberculous meningitis: A thirty year review. Clin Infect Dis. 1993;17:987–994.
51. Mollaret MP. La meningite endothelio-leucotaire multirecurrent benigne: Syndrome nouveau ou maladie nouvelle? Rev Neurol. 1981;9:81–84.
52. Lowe E. Mollaret's meningitis: A case report. Acta Cytol. 1982;26:338–340.
53. Stoppe G, Stark E, Patzold U. Mollaret's meningitis: CSF immunohistological examinations. J Neurol. 1987;234:103–106.
54. Yamamoto LJ, Tedder DG, Ashley R, et al. Herpes simplex virus type 1 DNA in the cerebrospinal fluid of a patient with Mollaret's meningitis. N Engl J Med. 1991;325:1082–1085.
55. Rich AR, McCordock HA. The pathogenesis of tuberculous meningitis. Bull Johns Hopkins Hosp. 1933;52:5–38.
56. Merritt HH, Fremont-Smith F. Cerebrospinal fluid in tuberculous meningitis. Arch Neurol Psychol. 1935;33:516–536.
57. Lepper MH, Spies HW. The present status of the treatment of tuberculosis of the central nervous system. Ann N Y Acad Sci. 1963;106:106–123.
58. Weiss W, Flippin HF. The changing incidence and prognosis of tuberculous meningitis. Am J Med Sci. 1965;250:46–59.
59. Barrett-Connor EB. Tuberculous meningitis in adults. South Med J. 1967;60:1061–1067.
60. Kennedy DH, Fallon FJ. Tuberculous meningitis. JAMA. 1979;241:264–268.
61. Jeren T, Beus I. Characteristics of cerebrospinal fluid in tuberculous meningitis. Acta Cytol. 1982;26:678.
62. Johnson JL, Ellner JJ. Tuberculous meningitis. In: Evans RW, Baskin DS, Vatsu FM, eds. Prognosis in Neurological Disease. New York: Oxford University Press; 1991:209–225.
63. Yechoor VK, Shandera WX, Rodriguez P, et al. Tuberculous meningitis among adults with and without HIV infection. Arch Intern Med. 1996;156:1710–1716.
64. Girgis NI, Sultan Y, Farid Z, et al. Tuberculosis meningitis, Abbassia Fever Hospital Naval Medical Research Unit No. 3—Cairo, Egypt, from 1976 to 1996. Am J Trop Med Hyg. 1998;58:28–34.
65. Porkert MT, Sotir M, Parrott-Moore P, et al. Tuberculous meningitis at a large inner city medical center. Am J Med Sci. 1997;313:325–331.
66. Verdon R, Chevret S, Laissy JP, et al. Tuberculous meningitis in adults: A review of 48 cases. Clin Infect Dis. 1996;22:982–988.
67. Daniel TM. New approaches to the rapid diagnosis of tuberculous meningitis. J Infect Dis. 1987;155:599–602.
68. Ribera E, Martinez-Vazquez JM, Ocana I, et al. Activity of adenosine deaminase in cerebrospinal fluid for the diagnosis and follow up of tuberculous meningitis in adults. J Infect Dis. 1987;155:603–607.
69. Petterson T, Klockars M, Weber TH, et al. Diagnostic value of cerebrospinal fluid adenosine deaminase determination. Scand J Infect Dis. 1991;23:97–100.
70. Lopez-Cortez LF, Cruz-Ruiz M, Gomez-Mateous J, et al. Adenosine deaminase activity in the CSF of patients with aseptic meningitis: Utility in the diagnosis of tuberculous meningitis or neurobrucellosis. Clin Infect Dis. 1995;20:525–530.
71. Spickard A, Butler WT, Andriole V, et al. The improved prognosis of cryptococcal meningitis with amphotericin B therapy. Ann Intern Med. 1963;58:66–83.
72. Butler WT, Alling DW, Spickard A, et al. Diagnostic and prognostic value of clinical and laboratory findings in cryptococcal meningitis: A follow-up study of forty patients. N Engl J Med. 1964;270:59–66.
73. Littman ML, Walter JE. Cryptococcosis: Current status. Am J Med. 1968;45:922–932.
74. Diamond RD, Bennett JE. Prognostic factors in cryptococcal meningitis: A study of 111 cases. Ann Intern Med. 1974;80:176–181.
75. Kovacs JA, Kovacs AA, Polis M, et al. Cryptococcosis in the acquired immunodeficiency syndrome. Ann Intern Med. 1985;103:533–538.
76. Zuger A, Louie E, Holzman RS, et al. Cryptococcal disease in patients with the acquired immunodeficiency syndrome: Diagnostic features and outcome of treatment. Ann Intern Med. 1986;104:234–240.
77. Chuck SZ, Sande MA. Infections with *Cryptococcus neoformans* in the acquired immunodeficiency syndrome. N Engl J Med. 1989;321:794–799.
78. Clark RA, Greer D, Atkinson W, et al. Spectrum of *Cryptococcus neoformans* infection in 68 patients infected with human immunodeficiency virus. Rev Infect Dis. 1990;12:768–777.
79. Saag MS, Powderly WG, Cloud GA, et al. Comparison of amphotericin B with fluconazole in the treatment of acute AIDS-associated cryptococcal meningitis. N Engl J Med. 1992;326:83–89.
80. Darras-Joly C, Chevret S, Wolff M, et al. *Cryptococcus neoformans* infection in France: Epidemiologic features of and early prognostic parameters for 76 patients who were infected with human immunodeficiency virus. Clin Infect Dis. 1996;23:369–376.
81. Van der Horst CM, Saag MS, Cloud GA, et al. Treatment of cryptococcal meningitis associated with the acquired immunodeficiency syndrome. N Engl J Med. 1997;337:15–21.
82. Mitchell DH, Sorrell TC, Allworth AM, et al. Cryptococcal disease of the CNS in immunocompetent hosts: Influence of cryptococcal variety on clinical manifestations and outcome. Clin Infect Dis. 1995;20:611–616.
83. Speed B, Dunt D. Clinical and host differences between infections with the two varieties of *Cryptococcus neoformans*. Clin Infect Dis. 1995;21:28–34.
84. Currie BP, Freundlich LF, Soto MA, et al. False-negative cerebrospinal fluid cryptococcal latex agglutination tests for patients with culture-positive cryptococcal meningitis. J Clin Microbiol. 1993;31:2519–2522.
85. Agrawal JP, Tachibana H, Okuda B, et al. Latex agglutination test negative cryptococcal meningitis in an immuno-competent individual: A case report. Clin Neurol Neurosurg. 1994;96:250–253.
86. Smith CE, Saito MT, Simons SA. Pattern of 39,500 serologic tests in coccidioidomycosis. JAMA. 1956;160:546.
87. Winn WA. The treatment of coccidioidal meningitis: The use of amphotericin B in a group of 25 patients. Calif Med. 1964;101:75–89.
88. Winn WA. Coccidioidal meningitis: A follow-up report. In: Ajello L, ed. Coccidioidomycosis. Tucson: University of Arizona Press; 1967:55.
89. Candill RG, Smith CE, Reinarz JA. Coccidioidal meningitis: A diagnostic challenge. Am J Med. 1970;49:360.
90. Deresinski SC, Stevens DA. Coccidioidomycosis in compromised hosts. Medicine (Baltimore). 1974;54:377.
91. Bouza E, Dreyer JS, Hewitt WL, et al. Coccidioidal meningitis: An analysis of 31 cases and review of the literature. Medicine (Baltimore). 1981;60:139–171.
92. Vincent T, Galgiani JN, Huppert M, et al. The natural history of coccidioidal meningitis: VA-Armed Forces cooperative studies 1955–1958. Clin Infect Dis. 1993;16:247–254.
93. Ragland S, Arsura E, Ismail Y, et al. Eosinophilic pleocytosis in coccidioidal meningitis: Frequency and significance. Am J Med. 1993;95:254–257.
94. Galgiani JN, Cantanzaro A, Cloud GA, et al. Fluconazole therapy for coccidioidal meningitis. Ann Intern Med. 1993;119:28–35.
95. Tucker RM, Denning DW, Dupont B, et al. Itraconazole therapy for chronic coccidioidal meningitis. Ann Intern Med. 1990;112:108–112.
96. Galgiani JN, Peng T, Lewis ML, et al. Cerebrospinal fluid antibodies detected by ELISA against a 33-kDa antigen from spherules of *Coccidiodes immitis* in patients with coccidioidal meningitis. J Infect Dis. 1996;173:499–502.
97. Tynes BS, Crutcher JC, Utz JP. Histoplasma meningitis. Ann Intern Med. 1963;59:615–621.
98. Smith JW, Utz JP. Progressive disseminated histoplasmosis. Ann Intern Med. 1972;76:557.
99. Gilden DH, Miller EM, Johnson WG. Central nervous system histoplasmosis after rhinoplasty. Neurology (Minn). 1974;24:874–877.
100. Gelfand JA, Bennett JE. Active *Histoplasma* meningitis of 22 years duration. JAMA. 1975;233:1294–1295.
101. Wheat LJ, Connolly-Stringfield PA, Baker RJ, et al. Disseminated histoplasmosis in the acquired immunodeficiency syndrome: Review of the literature. Medicine (Baltimore). 1990;69:361–374.
102. Pachner AR, Steere AC. The triad of neurologic manifestations of Lyme disease: Meningitis, cranial neuritis, and radiculoneuritis. Neurology (NY). 1985;35:47–53.
103. Pachner AR. Neurologic manifestations of Lyme disease, the new "Great Imitator." Rev Infect Dis. 1989;11:S1482–S1486.
104. Halperin JJ, Volkeman DJ, Wu P. Central nervous system abnormalities in Lyme neuroborreliosis. Neurology. 1991;41:1571–1582.
105. Finkel MJ, Halperin JJ. Nervous system Lyme borreliosis revisited. Arch Neurol. 1992;49:102–107.
106. Rahn DW, Malawista SE. Lyme disease: Recommendations for diagnosis and treatment. Ann Intern Med. 1991;114:472–481.
107. Pachner AR. Early disseminated Lyme Disease: Lyme meningitis. Am J Med. 1995;98:4a30s–4a43s.
108. Tugwell P, Dennis DT, Weinstein A, et al. Laboratory evaluation in the diagnosis of Lyme Disease. Ann Intern Med. 1997;127:1109–1123.
109. Wilske B, Schierz G, Preac-Mursic V, et al. Intrathecal production of specific antibodies against *Borrellia burgdorferi* in patients with lymphocytic meningoradiculitis (Bannworth's syndrome). J Infect Dis. 1986;153:304–314.
110. Steere AC, Berrardi VP, Weeks KE, et al. Evaluation of the intrathecal antibody response to *Borrelia burgdorferi* as a diagnostic test for Lyme neuroborreliosis. J Infect Dis. 1990;761:1203–1209.
111. Nocton JJ, Bloom BJ, Rutledge BJ, et al. Detection of *Borrelia burgdorferi* DNA by polymerase chain reaction in cerebrospinal fluid in Lyme neuroborreliosis. J Infect Dis. 1996;174:623–627.
112. Denti JH. Cysticercosis cerebri-cestode infestation of the human brain. JAMA. 1957;164:401.
113. Lombardo LL, Mateos JH. Cerebral cysticercosis in Mexico. Neurology (Minn). 1961;11:824–826.
114. Loo L, Braude A. Cerebral cysticercosis in San Diego: A report of 23 cases and a review of the literature. Medicine (Baltimore). 1982;61:341–359.
115. Nash TE, Neva FA. Recent advances in the diagnosis and treatment of cerebral cysticercosis. N Engl J Med. 1984;311:1492–1496.
116. Earnest MP, Reller LD, Filley CM, et al. Neurocysticercosis in the United States: 35 cases and a review. Rev Infect Dis. 1987;9:961–979.
117. Del Brutto OH, Sotelo J. Neurocysticercosis: An update. Rev Infect Dis. 1988;10:1075–1087.
118. Bandres JC, White AC, Samo T, et al. Extraparenchymal neurocysticercosis: Report of five cases and review of management. Clin Infect Dis. 1992;15:799–811.
119. Shandera WX, White AC, Chen JC, et al. Neurocysticercosis in Houston, Texas: A report of 112 cases. Medicine (Baltimore). 1994;73:37–52.
120. DeVita VT, Utz JP, Williams T, et al. *Candida* meningitis. Arch Intern Med. 1966;117:527–535.
121. Bayer AS, Edwards JE Jr, Seidel JS, et al. *Candida* meningitis. Medicine (Baltimore). 1976;55:477–486.
122. Smego RA, Perfect JR, Durach DT. Combined therapy with amphotericin B and 5-fluorocytosine for candida meningitis. Rev Infect Dis. 1984;6:791–801.

123. Voice RA, Bradley SF, Sangeorzan JA, et al. Chronic candidal meningitis: An uncommon manifestation of candidiasis. Clin Infect Dis. 1994;19:60–66.
124. Nguyen MH, Yu VL. Meningitis caused by *Candida* species: An emerging problem in neurosurgical patients. Clin Infect Dis. 1995;21:323–327.
125. Casado JL, Quereda C, Oliva J, et al. Candidal meningitis in HIV-infected patients: Analysis of 14 cases. Clin Infect Dis. 1997;25:673–676.
126. Merritt HH, Adams RD, Solomon HC. Neurosyphilis. New York: Oxford University Press; 1946:24.
127. Hooshmand H, Escobar MR, Kopf SW. Neurosyphilis: A study of 241 patients. JAMA. 1972;219:726–729.
128. Katz DA, Berger JR, Duncan RC. Neurosyphilis: A comparative study of the effects of infection with human immunodeficiency virus. Arch Neurol. 1993;50:243–249.
129. Flood J, Weinstock HS, Guroy M, et al. Neurosyphilis during the AIDS epidemic, San Francisco, 1985–1992. J Infect Dis. 1998;177:931–940.
130. Marra CM, Gary DW, Kuypers J, et al. Diagnosis of neurosyphilis in patients infected with human immunodeficiency virus type 1. J Infect Dis. 1996;174:219–221.
131. Nichols E. Meningoencephalitis due to brucellosis. Ann Intern Med. 1951;35:673.
132. Fincham RW, Sahs AL, Joynt RJ. Protean manifestations of nervous system brucellosis. JAMA. 1963;184:97–103.
133. Mousa AR, Koshy TS, Araj GF, et al. Brucella meningitis: Presentation, diagnosis and treatment. A prospective study of ten cases. Q J Med. 1986;60:873–885.
134. Bouza E, Garcia de la Torre M, Parras F, et al. Brucella meningitis. Rev Infect Dis. 1987;9:810–822.
135. Mc Lean DR, Russell N, Khan MY. Neurobrucellosis: Clinical and therapeutic features. Clin Infect Dis. 1992;15:582–590.
136. Pollner JH, Khan A, Tuazon CU. *Sporothrix schenckii* meningitis in a patient with AIDS. Clin Infect Dis. 1992;15:741–743.
137. Koo J, Pien F, Kliks MM. *Angiostrongylus (Parastrongylus)* eosinophilic meningitis. Rev Infect Dis. 1988;10:1155–1162.
138. Wilhelmj CM. The primary meningeal form of systemic blastomycosis. Am J Med Sci. 1925;169:172.
139. Buechner HA, Clawson CM. Blastomycosis of the central nervous system: II. A report of nine cases from the Veterans Administration Cooperative Study. Am Rev Respir Dis. 1967;95:820.
140. Pappas PG, Pottage JC, Powderly WF, et al. Blastomycosis in patients with the acquired immunodeficiency syndrome. Ann Intern Med. 1992;116:847–853.
141. Pereira WC, Raphael A, Tehuto RA, et al. Localizacao encefalica da blastomicose sulAmericana: Consideracoes a proposito de 9 casos. Arq Neuropsiquiatr. 1965;23:113.
142. Bennett JE, Bonner H, Jennings AE, et al. Chronic meningitis caused by *Cladosporium trichoides*. Am J Clin Pathol. 1973;59:398–407.
143. Bolton CF, Ashenhurst EM. Actinomycosis of the brain: Case report and review of the literature. Can Med Assoc J. 1964;90:922–928.
144. Brown JR: Human actinomycosis. Hum Pathol. 1973;4:319–330.
145. Smego RA Jr. Actinomycosis of the central nervous system. Rev Infect Dis. 1987;9:855–865.
146. King RB, Stoops WL, Fitzgibbons J, et al. *Nocardia asteroides* meningitis. A case successfully treated with large doses of sulfadiazine and urea. J Neurosurg. 1966;24:749.
147. Richter RW, Silva M, Neu HC, et al. The neurological aspects of *Nocardia asteroides* infection. Infect Nerv Sys. 1968;44:424.
148. Bross JE, Gordon G. Nocardial meningitis: Case reports and review. Rev Infect Dis. 1991;13:160–165.
149. Mok CC, Lau CS, Poon SP. Primary nocardial meningitis in systemic lupus erythematosus. Br J Rheumatol. 1995;34:178–181.
150. Kramer W. Frontiers of neurological diagnosis in acquired toxoplasmosis. Psychiatr Neurol Neurochirg. 1966;69:43.
151. Townsend JJ, Wolinsky JS, Baringer JR, et al. Acquired toxoplasmosis: A neglected cause of treatable nervous system disease. Arch Neurol. 1975;32:335–343.
152. Grines C, Plouffe JF, Baird IM, et al. *Toxoplasma* meningoencephalitis with hypoglycorrhachia. Arch Intern Med. 1981;141:935.
153. Jones PG, Gilman RM, Medeiros AA, et al. Focal intracranial mucormycosis presenting as chronic meningitis. JAMA. 1981;24:2063.
154. Moore EW, Thomas LB, Shaw RK, et al. The central nervous system in acute leukemia. Arch Intern Med. 1960;105:451.
155. Hyman CB, Boyle JM, Brubaker CA, et al. Central nervous system involvement by leukemia in children. Blood. 1965;25:1.
156. Griffin JW, Thompson RW, Mitchinson MJ, et al. Lymphomatous leptomeningitis. Am J Med. 1971;51:200–208.
157. Hoffman MA, Valderrama E, Fuchs A, et al. Leukemic meningitis in B-cell prolymphocytic leukemia. Cancer. 1995;75:1100–1103.
158. Berg L. Hypoglycorrhachia of noninfectious origin: Diffuse meningeal neoplasia. Neurology (Minn). 1953;3:811–824.
159. Fischer-Williams M, Bosanquet FD, Daniel P. Carcinomatosis of the meninges. Brain. 1955;78:42–58.
160. Dinsdale HB, Taghavy A. Carcinomatosis of the meninges. Can Med Assoc J. 1964;90:505–512.
161. Vital C, Bruno-Martin F, Henry P, et al. La carcinomatose méningée. Bordeaux Med. 1970;12:2927–2944.
162. Gonzalez-Vitale JC, Garcia-Bunvel R. Meningeal carcinomatosis. Cancer. 1976;37:2906.
163. Little JR, Dale AJ, Okazaki H. Meningeal carcinomatosis. Arch Neurol. 1974;30:138–143.
164. Wasserstrom WR, Glass P, Posner JB. Diagnosis and treatment of leptomeningeal metastases from solid tumors. Cancer. 1982;49:759–772.
165. Rosen ST, Aisner J, Makuch RW. Carcinomatous leptomeningitis in small cell lung cancer. Medicine (Baltimore). 1982;61:45–53.
166. Jayson GC, Howell A, Harris M, et al. Carcinomatous meningitis in patients with breast cancer. Cancer. 1994;74:3135–3141.
167. Lyster MT, Kies MS, Kuzel TM. Neurologic complications of patients with small cell prostate carcinoma. Cancer. 1994;74:3159–3163.
168. Sze G, Soletsky S, Bronen R, et al. MR imaging of the cranial meninges with emphasis on contrast enhancement and meningeal carcinomatosis. AJNR Am J Neuroradiol. 1989;10:965–975.
169. Phillips ME, Ryals TJ, Kambhu SA, et al. Neoplastic vs. inflammatory meningeal enhancement with Gd-DTPA. J Comput Assist Tomogr. 1990;14:536–541.
170. Shuttleworth E, Allen N. CSF β-glucuronidase assay in the diagnosis of neoplastic meningitis. Arch Neurol. 1980;37:684–687.
171. Tallman RD, Kimbrough SM, O'Brien JF, et al. Assay for β-glucuronidase in cerebrospinal fluid: Usefulness for the detection of neoplastic meningitis. Mayo Clin Proc. 1985;60:293–298.
172. Wiederholt WC, Siekert RB. Neurological manifestations of sarcoidosis. Neurology (Minn). 1965;15:1147–1154.
173. Mathews WB. Sarcoidosis of the nervous system. J Neurol Neurosurg Psychiatry. 1965;28:23.
174. Gaines JD, Eckman PB, Remington JS. Low CSF glucose level in sarcoidosis involving the central nervous system. Arch Intern Med. 1970;125:333–336.
175. Douglas AC, Maloney AFJ. Sarcoidosis of the central nervous system. J Neurol Neurosurg Psychiatry. 1973;36:1024.
176. Delaney P. Neurological manifestations in sarcoidosis. Ann Intern Med. 1977;87:336–345.
177. Stern BJ, Knumholz A, Scott P, et al. Sarcoidosis and its neurological manifestations. Arch Neurol. 1985;42:909–917.
178. Chapelon C, Ziza JM, Piette JC, et al. Neurosarcoidosis: Signs, course and treatment in 35 confirmed cases. Medicine (Baltimore). 1990;69:261–276.
179. Oksanen V. Neurosarcoidosis: Clinical presentations and course in 50 patients. Acta Neurol Scand. 1986;73:283–290.
180. Sharma OP. Neurosarcoidosis: A personal perspective based on the study of 37 patients. Chest. 1997;112:220–228.
181. Lower EE, Broderick JP, Brott TG, et al. Diagnosis and management of neurological sarcoidosis. Arch Intern Med. 1997;157:1864–1868.
182. Krumholz A, Stern BJ, Stern EG. Clinical implications of seizures in neurosarcoidosis. Arch Neurol. 1991;48:842–844.
183. Chan Seu CP, Norfolk G, Spokes EG. CSF angiotensin-converting enzyme in neurosarcoidosis. Lancet. 1985;1:456–457.
184. Oksaner V, Fyhrquist F, Somer H, et al. Angiotensin converting enzyme in cerebrospinal fluid: A new assay. Neurology. 1985;35:1220–1223.
185. Jones DB, Mitchell D, Horn DB, et al. Cerebrospinal fluid angiotensin converting enzyme levels in the diagnosis of neurosarcoidosis. Scott Med J. 1991;36:144–145.
186. Agobogu BN, Stern BJ, Sewell C, et al. Therapeutic considerations in patients with refractory neurosarcoidosis. Arch Neurol. 1995;52:875–879.
187. Stern BJ, Schonfield SA, Sewell C, et al. The treatment of neurosarcoidosis with cyclosporine. Arch Neurol. 1992;49:1065–1072.
188. Grizzanti JN, Knapp AB, Schecter AJ, et al. Treatment of sarcoid meningitis with radiotherapy. Am J Med. 1982;73:605–608.
189. Kolodny EM, Rebeiz JJ, Caviness VS, et al. Granulomatous angiitis of the central nervous system. Arch Neurol. 1968;19:510–524.
190. Nurick S, Blackwood W, Mair WGP. Giant cell granulomatous angiitis of the central nervous system. Brain. 1972;95:133–142.
191. Mohr JP, Powell HC. Clinicopathologic conference: Headache and progressive mental deterioration in a 45-year-old man. N Engl J Med. 1976;295:944.
192. Cupps TR, Moore PM, Fauci AS. Isolated angiitis of the central nervous system: Prospective diagnostic and therapeutic experience. Am J Med. 1983;74:97–105.
193. Reik L, Grunnet ML, Spencer RP, et al. Granulomatous angiitis presenting as chronic meningitis and ventriculitis. Neurology (NY). 1983;33:1609–1612.
194. Stein RL, Martino CR, Weinert DM, et al. Cerebral angiography as a guide for therapy in isolated central nervous system vasculitis. JAMA. 1987;257:2193–2196.
195. Calabrese LH, Mallek JA. Primary angiitis of the central nervous system: Report of 8 new cases, review of the literature and proposal for new diagnostic criteria. Medicine (Baltimore). 1987;67:20–39.
196. Lie JT. Primary (granulomatous) angiitis of the central nervous system: A clinicopathologic analysis of 15 new cases and a review of the literature. Hum Pathol. 1992;23:164–171.
197. Vollmer TL, Guarnaccia J, Harrington W, et al. Idiopathic granulomatous angiitis of the central nervous system. Arch Neurol. 1993;50:925–930.
198. Parisi JE, Moore PM. The role of biopsy in vasculitis of the central nervous system. Semin Neurol. 1994;14:341–348.
199. Cowper AR. Harada's disease and Vogt-Koyanagi syndrome. Arch Ophthalmol. 1951;45:367.
200. Pattison EM. Uveomeningoencephalitis syndrome. Arch Neurol. 1965;12:197–205.
201. Riehl J-L, Andrews JM. The uveomeningoencephalitis syndrome. Neurology (Minn). 1966;16:603–609.
202. Rubasamen PE, Gass DM. Vogt-Koyanagi-Harrada syndrome: Clinical course, therapy and long-term visual outcome. Arch Opthalmol. 1991;109:682–687.
203. Moorthy RS, Inomata H, Rao NA. Vogt-Koyanagi-Harrada syndrome. Surv Opthalmol. 1995;39:265–292.
204. Schotland DL, Wolf SM, White HH, et al. Neurologic aspects of Behçet's disease. Am J Med. 1963;34:544–552.

205. Wolf SM. Involvement of nervous system in Behçet's syndrome. Arch Neurol. 1965;12:315–325.
206. O'Duffy JD, Goldstein NP. Neurologic involvement in seven patients with Behçet's disease. Am J Med. 1976;61:170–178.
207. Chajek T, Fainaru M. Behçet's disease: Report of 41 cases and a review of the literature. Medicine (Baltimore). 1975;54:179–196.
208. Kozin F, Haughton V, Bernhard GC. Neuro-Behçet disease: Two cases and neuroradiographic findings. Neurology. 1977;27:1148–1152.
209. Hersskovitz S, Lipton RB, Lantos G. Neuro-Behçet's disease: CT and clinical correlates. Neurology. 1988;38:1714–1720.
210. Sergent JS, Lockshin MD, Klempner MS, et al. Central nervous system disease in systemic lupus erythematosus: Therapy and prognosis. Am J Med. 1975;58:644–654.
211. Wong KL, Woo EK, Yu YL, et al. Neurological manifestations of systemic lupus erythematosus: A prospective study. Q J Med. 1991;81:857–870.
212. Sigal LH. The neurological presentation of vasculitic and rheumatologic syndromes. Medicine (Baltimore). 1987;66:157–179.
213. Jinnah HA, Dixon A, Brat DJ, et al. Chronic meningitis with cranial neuropathies in Wegener's granulomatosis. Arthritis Rheum. 1997;40:573–577.
214. Casselli RJ, Scheithauer BW, O'Duffy JD, et al. Chronic inflammatory meningoencephalitis should not be mistaken for Alzheimer's disease. Mayo Clin Proc. 1993;68:846–853.
215. Hopkins AP, Harvey PKP. Chronic benign lymphocytic meningitis. J Neurol Sci. 1973;18:443–453.
216. Hooper DC, Pruitt AA, Rubin RH. Central nervous system infection in the chronically immunosuppressed. Medicine (Baltimore). 1982;61:166–188.
217. Fong IW, Britton CB, Luinstra KE, et al. Diagnostic value of detecting JC virus DNA in cerebrospinal fluid of patients with progressive multifocal leukoencephalopathy. J Clin Microbiol. 1995;33:484–486.
218. McKinney RE, Katz SL, Wilfert CM. Chronic enteroviral meningoencephalitis in agammaglobulinemic patients. Rev Infect Dis. 1987;9:334–356.
219. Schacker T, Collier AC, Hughes J, et al. Clinical and epidemiologic features of primary HIV infection. Ann Intern Med. 1996;125:257–264.
220. Appleman ME, Marshall DW, Porey RL, et al. Cerebrospinal fluid abnormalities in patients without AIDS who are seropositive for the human immunodeficiency virus. J Infect Dis. 1988;158:193–199.
221. Berenguera J, Moreno S, Laguna F, et al. Tuberculous meningitis in patients infected with the human immunodeficiency virus. N Engl J Med. 1992;326:668–672.
222. Sanchez-Portocarrero J, Perez-Cecila E, Jimenez-Escrig A, et al. Tuberculous meningitis: Clinical characteristics and comparison with cryptococcal meningitis in patients with human immunodeficiency virus infection. Arch Neurol. 1996;53:671–676.
223. Fish DG, Ampel NM, Galgiani JN, et al. Coccidioidomycosis during human immunodeficiency virus infection: A review of 77 patients. Medicine (Baltimore). 1990;69:384–391.
224. Cinque P, Scarpellini P, Vago L, et al. Diagnosis of central nervous system complications in HIV-infected patients: Cerebrospinal fluid analysis by the polymerase chain reaction. AIDS. 1997;11:1–17.
225. Kalayjian RC, Cohen MC, Bonomo RA, et al. Cytomegalovirus ventriculoencephalitis in AIDS: A syndrome with distinct clinical and pathological features. Medicine (Baltimore). 1993;72:67–77.
226. McCutchan JA. Cytomegalovirus infections of the nervous system in patients with AIDS. Clin Infect Dis. 1995;20:747–754.
227. Matlow AG, Rachlis AR. Syphilis serology in human immunodeficiency virus-infected patients with symptomatic neurosyphilis: Case report and review. Rev Infect Dis. 1990;12:703–707.
228. Feraru ER, Aronow HA, Lipton RB. Neurosyphilis in AIDS patients: Initial CSF VDRL may be negative. Neurology. 1990;40:541–543.
229. Hicks CB, Benson PM, Lupton GP, et al. Seronegative secondary syphilis in a patient infected with the human immunodeficiency virus (HIV) with Kaposi's sarcoma. Ann Intern Med. 1987;107:492–495.
230. Haas JS, Bolan G, Larse SA, et al. Sensitivity of treponemal tests for detecting prior treated syphilis during human immunodeficiency virus infection. J Infect Dis. 1990;162:862–866.

Chapter 73

Encephalitis, Myelitis, and Neuritis

DIANE E. GRIFFIN

The terms *encephalitis, myelitis,* and *neuritis* refer to inflammations of brain, spinal cord, and peripheral nerves, respectively. If sensory or motor spinal roots are specifically involved, the term *radiculitis* may be used. Because meningeal inflammation often accompanies these inflammatory processes, compounded terms such as *meningoencephalitis* and *meningoencephalomyelitis* are sometimes used. None of these terms, however, differentiates between the inflammatory diseases caused by direct invasion of agents and the postinfectious or parainfectious demyelinating processes that may involve the brain, spinal cord, or peripheral nerves. Because of the diversity of clinical symptoms and signs that can occur with these inflammatory diseases, infectious or parainfectious causes must be entertained in the differential diagnosis of a great variety of neurologic diseases. As with all neurologic diseases, the differential diagnosis is determined by the temporal evolution of signs and symptoms and by the localization of the disease process to one or more anatomic sites by physical findings. Systemic involvement (skin, lung, salivary glands, liver, gastrointestinal tract) or fever may suggest an infectious cause, but these signs may also be absent.

ENCEPHALITIS AND MYELITIS

This section deals with infectious and postinfectious encephalitis and myelitis together because they are often considered in the same differential diagnosis and have considerable overlap in manifestation and causation. Peripheral neuropathies caused by infectious agents are considered, along with tetanus and botulism, in a separate section.

Pathogenesis and Pathologic Characteristics

Infectious agents can produce clinical symptoms and signs within the central nervous system (CNS) by either direct or indirect involvement of neural tissue. Infectious agents can invade the CNS by several pathways. The most common is via the blood. This is best documented for viral infections but probably is also important in rickettsial, bacterial, and fungal infections.[1-3] The initial site of entry of a pathogen and the primary site of replication may be the respiratory tract (e.g., measles, mumps, varicella-zoster viruses, *Mycobacterium tuberculosis, Cryptococcus neoformans*), the gastrointestinal tract (e.g., poliovirus, echovirus, *Listeria monocytogenes*), the genital tract (e.g., herpes simplex virus), or subcutaneous tissue (e.g., arthropod-borne viruses, *Rickettsia rickettsia, Rickettsia typhi,* trypanosomes). Involvement of the CNS is, for the most part, an infrequent consequence of common infections.

In certain viral infections, entry into the CNS occurs by way of the peripheral nerves. Transport systems within motor and sensory axons carry substances from the cell body to the periphery (anterograde transport) and from the periphery to the cell body (retrograde transport). The neural route of entry is important in viral infections such as rabies[4] and, occasionally, poliomyelitis.[5] Retrograde transport from the skin or mucous membranes moves herpes simplex and varicella-zoster viruses into sensory ganglia at the time of primary infection, and anterograde transport carries reactivated virus from the ganglia to the periphery during exacerbations.[6] On occasion, reactivated virus may also be carried retrograde to the CNS.

Entry of infectious agents into the CNS by way of the exposed olfactory nerves in the nasal mucosa has been demonstrated in experimental animals[7, 8] but is of proven clinical importance only for free-living amebas, which enter the olfactory and frontal lobes of the brain through the nasal mucosa and across the cribriform plate.[9]

Once the infective agent is within the CNS, only certain cells may be infected. This gives rise to variations in clinical manifestations. Neuronal infection may cause seizure activity, which, depending on the areas involved, may be focal or generalized. Infection of oligodendroglia may cause demyelination alone. Cortical infection or reactive parenchymal swelling may give rise to changes in the state of consciousness,[10] and infection of specific brain stem neurons can cause coma or respiratory failure.[11] Infection of microglia and macrophages may lead to neurologic dysfunction through indirect effects on neuronal function.[12, 13]

In fatal viral encephalitis, an inflammatory reaction is usually prominent in the meninges and in a perivascular distribution within the brain. Although the perivascular inflammatory reaction is composed predominantly of mononuclear cells, polymorphonuclear cells may be evident. Neural cells may show degenerative changes, and apparent phagocytosis of neurons by macrophages or microglial cells (neuronophagia) is often found. Multinucleated giant cells containing viral antigen are found in the brains of patients with encephalitis induced by human immunodeficiency virus (HIV).[14] CNS lesions in HIV infections may also include myelin pallor, vacuolar myelopathy, and gracile tract degeneration.[14, 15] Whether these pathologic changes are direct or indirect consequences of viral infection is not yet clear. Intranuclear inclusion bodies are seen in herpesvirus,[6] adenovirus,[16] and subacute and chronic forms of measles virus infections.[17] Cytomegalovirus infections produce characteristic pathologic changes with the induction of cytomegalic cells containing inclusion bodies.[18] Negri bodies are found in rabies virus encephalitis.[19]

Rickettsiae tend to invade and to multiply in vascular endothelial cells, resulting in widespread vasculitis of capillaries, arterioles, and small arteries,[20] including the retina.

Infectious agents can give rise to signs or symptoms suggesting encephalitis or myelitis without actually invading CNS parenchyma. One mechanism is the development of adhesive meningitis and vasculitis during the course of subacute or chronic leptomeningeal infection. In chronic tuberculous, fungal, or syphilitic meningitis, or untreated or partially treated bacterial meningitis, the chronic meningeal reaction may cause obstruction of cerebrospinal fluid (CSF) flow, resulting in hydrocephalus, cranial nerve palsies, or gliosis in the underlying cerebral cortex. In addition, vasculitis involving large vessels may lead to infarctions of brain and focal neurologic deficits. This sequence of events is frequently observed in tuberculosis,[21] aspergillosis,[22] and meningovascular neurosyphilis[23] and occasionally in coccidioidomycosis[24] and herpes zoster.[25] Syphilis of the meningovascular type appears relatively early in the course of this disease, and, in contrast to the parenchymatous manifestations (tabes dorsalis and paresis) that appear later, it is inflammatory and often reversible. *Cryptococcus* produces a chronic meningitis with little inflammatory reaction even in the immunologically normal host.[26] In chronic bacterial or fungal meningitis, organization of a subarachnoid exudate at the base of the brain may lead to communicating hydrocephalus and cranial nerve palsies.[3, 27]

When acute demyelinating disease complicates viral exanthems or respiratory or gastrointestinal infections, it is not known whether invasion of the virus into the CNS is a prerequisite to disease. The pathogenesis of this syndrome is thought to be related to induction of an immune response to CNS myelin.[28] This mechanism is analogous to neurologic complications of neural tissue–derived rabies vaccines.[29]

The pathologic changes of postinfectious and postvaccinal encephalomyelitis are characterized by perivascular infiltration of mononuclear inflammatory cells and perivenous demyelination. Acute hemorrhagic leukoencephalitis, characterized by fibrinoid necrosis of arterioles and hemorrhage in addition to the perivenular demyelination, represents a more severe form of postinfectious encephalomyelitis.[30]

On the other hand, Reye's syndrome is a distinct acute encephalopathy associated with mitochondrial dysfunction that usually follows a viral infection. This syndrome affects children and is characterized by acute fatty liver and noninflammatory cerebral edema. Reye's syndrome has been most commonly associated with varicella and influenza virus infections and is epidemiologically related to administration of salicylates during infection.[31]

Neurotoxins produced by bacteria infecting gastrointestinal and respiratory sites have been postulated to cause the acute CNS diseases seen occasionally with shigellosis[32] and melioidosis.[33] The role of the organism in the encephalopathy associated with cat-scratch disease is unknown.[34]

Clinical Findings

Infections limited to the leptomeninges manifest with signs and symptoms of meningeal irritation: headache, stiff neck, and pleocytosis. If the meningeal process is chronic, as in tuberculosis, manifesting symptoms and signs may be those of a communicating hydrocephalus (headache, nausea and vomiting, mental deterioration, or spastic paraparesis), a localized infarction secondary to vasculitis, or both.[35] The chronic form of cryptococcal meningitis may manifest as progressive mental deterioration rather than with headache, fever, and meningismus, as is seen in the more acute form.[27, 36]

Patients with viral encephalitis usually have signs and symptoms of meningeal inflammation, but, in addition to headache, fever, and nuchal rigidity, their encephalitis is characterized by alterations of consciousness: mild lethargy may progress to confusion, stupor, and coma. Focal neurologic signs usually develop, and seizures are common. Motor weakness, accentuated deep tendon reflexes, and extensor plantar responses may be observed. Abnormal movements are seen in some cases of encephalitis, and, rarely, a tremor characteristic of Parkinson's disease may develop. The hypothalamic pituitary axis may be involved, causing severe hyperthermia or poikilothermia, diabetes insipidus, and inappropriate antidiuretic hormone secretion. Involvement of the spinal cord can lead to flaccid paralysis, depression of tendon reflexes, and paralysis of bowel and bladder. Increased intracranial pressure can cause papilledema and third and sixth cranial nerve palsies.

In herpes simplex encephalitis, signs often include personality change, hallucinations, and aphasia, suggesting the temporal lobe localization typical of that infection.[6, 37] Rabies may begin with local paresthesia at the site of the bite.[38] A parkinsonian syndrome is common in Japanese encephalitis.[39] Acute contralateral hemiparesis may occur after herpes zoster ophthalmicus infection related to a localized cerebral angiitis, causing frontal lobe infarction.[25] With Lyme neuroborreliosis, both peripheral nervous system and CNS complications occur, ranging from severe meningoencephalitis to isolated cranial nerve palsies.[40, 41]

Myelitis can occur, with or without encephalitis. Transverse myelitis simulates acute transection of the cord, with rostral limb weakness, sensory level, and loss of bowel and bladder control. Ascending myelitis leads to an ascending flaccid paralysis and rising sensory deficit and is characterized by early bowel and bladder involvement. Poliomyelitis, in which anterior horn cells are involved primarily, typically causes flaccid paralysis and muscular pain without sensory loss or bladder dysfunction.

In postinfectious encephalomyelitis, the time lapse between manifestations of the primary infection and onset of symptoms referable to the nervous system ranges between 2 and 12 days. The onset is often abrupt, with depression of consciousness or seizure.[28, 30]

Systemic findings of particular importance are the rashes of Lyme disease, Rocky Mountain spotted fever (palms and soles), typhus, varicella, herpes B virus, and herpes zoster. An exanthem is also occasionally seen with *Mycoplasma,* coxsackievirus, and echovirus infections. A history of tick bite is often obtained in Rocky Mountain spotted fever, Lyme disease, ehrlichiosis, and Colorado tick fever. A history of animal or bat bite may be obtained in rabies, although most patients in the United States never give such a history.[42]

Mycobacterial and fungal infections often manifest as chronic and, on occasion, fluctuating disease, but in certain cases (including mucormycosis) they may progress very rapidly.

Bacterial infections usually manifest with an acute onset, but certain infections such as neurosyphilis, Lyme disease, relapsing fever, brain abscess, brucellosis, and Whipple's disease can have an insidious onset and an indolent, chronic, or even fluctuating course. The neurologic features of Whipple's disease, which may occur without significant manifestations of malabsorption, can include dementia, supranuclear ophthalmoplegia, myoclonus, spastic paresis, ataxia, and papilledema.[43] The rickettsial diseases are usually acute in onset, causing fever, headache, and myalgias. Rocky Mountain spotted fever and typhus are associated with a rash before or after neurologic disease,[44, 45] whereas a rash is rarely present in ehrlichiosis.[46]

Viral infections also may be acute, subacute, or chronic. Encephalitis due to adenovirus and enteroviruses has occurred both as acute disease in immunologically healthy persons and as subacute disease in immunologically compromised persons.[1, 16, 47] A number of CNS infections such as Creutzfeldt-Jakob disease, subacute sclerosing panencephalitis, rubella panencephalitis, HIV encephalopathy and myelopathy, tropical spastic paraparesis, and progressive multifocal leukoencephalopathy are slowly progressive diseases with an insidious onset and absence of fever.[1, 48–50]

Laboratory Findings

Peripheral blood counts are rarely helpful in this group of diseases, because they may be normal or may show a moderate leukocytosis or leukopenia. Peripheral blood smears may show atypical lymphocytes in Epstein-Barr virus infections, the diagnostic gametocytes of *Plasmodium falciparum* in malaria, the morulae of *Ehrlichia,* the borreliae in relapsing fever, or the trypanosomes in trypanosomiasis. The serum amylase concentration may be elevated in mumps virus infection. Pulmonary infiltrates may accompany lymphocytic choriomeningitis virus, typhus, *Legionella, Chlamydia,* and *Mycoplasma* infections.

CSF examination is essential. The pleocytosis of viral encephalomyelitis is variable (10 to 2000 cells/mm^3), and mononuclear cells usually predominate; however, early in any of these diseases there may be no cells, or polymorphonuclear cells may be present in considerable numbers. Repeat examination of the CSF in 24 hours is often useful.[51] Significant numbers of red blood cells may be found in herpes simplex encephalitis,[52] acute necrotizing hemorrhagic leukoencephalitis,[30] and *Naegleria* encephalitis.[53] In the chronic fungal and bacterial meningitides, a moderate mononuclear pleocytosis usually is found.[27] Meningoencephalitis caused by *Naegleria, Nocardia, Actinomyces, Candida,* or *Aspergillus* elicits a polymorphonuclear response.[53, 54]

The CSF protein level is usually increased in encephalomyelitis, and in chronic infections an increased proportion of this protein is immunoglobulin G (IgG) (normal is $<12\%$).[55] Under normal conditions, CSF IgG is derived primarily from the serum, and antibodies are present in the CSF at a ratio of about 1:200 with the serum concentration.[56] During acute inflammatory reactions a transudate of protein occurs, including serum immunoglobulins. During convalescence, plasma cells may produce pathogen-specific IgG within the CNS, as is seen after mumps,[57] herpes simplex,[52] and zoster[58] encephalitides. In chronic infection, examination of the CSF for specific antibody can be diagnostic in syphilis,[59] Lyme disease,[60] tropical spastic paraparesis,[49] subacute sclerosing panencephalitis,[61] progressive multifocal leukoencephalitis,[62] and rubella panencephalitis[63] and may be more useful than serum determinations, in the viral, rickettsial, fungal, and bacterial encephalitides for which antibody tests are available. If antibody to a particular pathogen is present at a comparable or higher amount in CSF than in serum and the CSF protein is only moderately elevated, it is indicative of CNS infection with the agent.

For diagnosis by serum antibodies, it is important to obtain serum early in the course (acute phase) for comparison with serum taken after 1 to 3 weeks of illness to demonstrate a significant antibody increase.[64] Tests for specific IgM in serum and CSF often allow for earlier diagnoses.[65, 66] This diagnosis is often of more than academic interest, because presumptive therapy begun early may then be discontinued if a diagnosis is established. Tests for cold agglutinins and heterophile antibody may yield false-negative results in the diagnosis of *Mycoplasma* and Epstein-Barr virus infections, respectively; therefore, organism-specific antibody tests are preferred.

The CSF glucose level is usually within the normal range during viral or rickettsial infections of the CNS, although a mild depression may be seen. The glucose level is usually low in tuberculous,[67] fungal,[27] bacterial, or amebic[53] infections.

Direct examination of the CSF by Gram stain for bacteria, by acid-fast stain for mycobacteria, and by India ink for *Cryptococcus* should be performed and may be diagnostic. Wet preparation of CSF may reveal free-living amebae, and Giemsa stain identifies trypanosomes. Bacteria, mycobacteria, fungi, amebae, and viruses may also be recovered from the CSF by appropriate culture techniques. Microbial antigen detection methods have proved particularly useful in cryptococcal disease.[36] Detection of nucleic acid in CSF by polymerase chain reaction is useful for a number of viral infections, particularly herpesviruses.[3]

The electroencephalogram is often abnormal in acute and chronic forms of herpes simplex encephalitis and may provide early localizing information in herpesvirus encephalitis. The computed tomographic scan is useful for ruling out space-occupying lesions but is often unrevealing in encephalitis and myelitis. Magnetic resonance imaging allows better visualization of the spinal cord, is a sensitive indicator of demyelination, and can detect the edematous changes that are often an early feature of encephalitis.

Etiology of Encephalomyelitis

Table 73–1 lists the viruses known to cause acute encephalitis or myelitis and those associated with postinfectious encephalomyelitis. Many of these infections have distinct seasonal variations that are helpful in narrowing the differential diagnosis (Fig. 73–1). The alphavirus, flavivirus, and bunyavirus encephalitides (except rubella) are arthropod-borne and therefore occur when their insect vectors are biting. The mosquito-borne encephalitides peak in late summer in temperate regions.[68] The tick-borne diseases occur most often in spring and early summer.[69–71] Enteroviruses are the most common

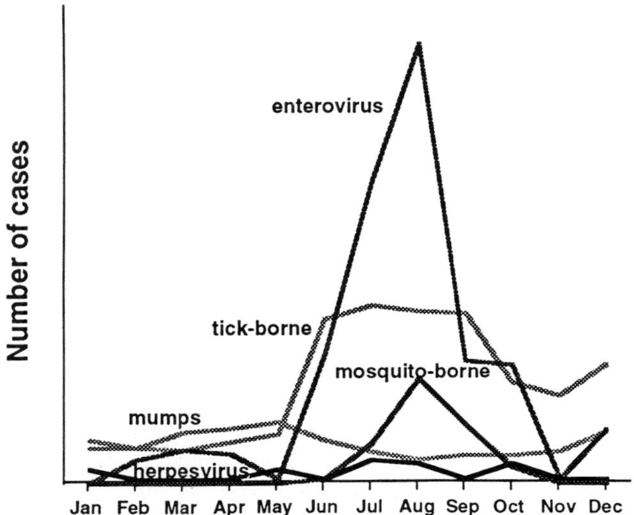

FIGURE 73–1. Seasonal variation in temperate zones of the Northern Hemisphere for the encephalitides caused by mosquito-borne viruses, enteroviruses, mumps virus, herpesvirus, and tick-borne diseases.

TABLE 73–1 Viral Causes of Acute Encephalomyelitis

Direct Infection	Postinfection
Togaviridae	Togaviridae
Alphaviruses	Rubivirus
Eastern equine	Rubella
Western equine	Orthomyxoviridae
Venezuelan equine	Influenza
Flaviviridae	Paramyxoviridae
St. Louis	Rubulavirus
Murray Valley	Mumps
West Nile	Morbillivirus
Japanese	Measles
Dengue	Poxviridae
Tick-borne complex	Orthopoxvirus
Bunyaviridae	Vaccinia
La Crosse	Herpesviridae
Rift Valley	Herpesvirus
Toscana	Varicella-zoster virus
Paramyxoviridae	Epstein-Barr virus
Paramyxovirus	
Mumps	
Morbillivirus	
Measles	
Hendra	
Nipah (Hendra-like)	
Arenaviridae	
Arenavirus	
Lymphocytic choriomeningitis	
Machupo	
Lassa	
Junin	
Picornaviridae	
Enterovirus	
Poliovirus	
Coxsackievirus	
Echovirus	
Hepatitis A	
Reoviridae	
Colorado tick fever	
Rhabdoviridae	
Lyssavirus	
Rabies	
Filoviridae	
Ebola	
Marburg	
Retroviridae	
Lentivirus	
Human immunodeficiency virus	
Herpesviridae	
Herpesvirus	
Herpes simplex virus types 1 and 2	
Varicella-zoster virus	
Herpes B virus	
Epstein-Barr virus	
Cytomegalovirus	
Human herpesvirus 6	
Adenoviridae	
Adenovirus	

cause of viral encephalitis and occur primarily in late summer and fall. In contrast, the herpesvirus encephalitides occur throughout the year. Lymphocytic choriomeningitis virus is most common in the winter, when rodents come indoors, and leptospirosis is more common in the warm months, when rodents and people are in contact with ponds and streams.[64]

In addition to the season, geographic and travel histories may be helpful in the diagnosis of vector-borne encephalitides. For instance, eastern equine encephalitis is most common in the Great Lakes region and along the Atlantic and Gulf coasts, whereas western equine encephalitis is most common in the western states. LaCrosse and St. Louis encephalitides are widespread in the United States.[1, 72] Lyme disease is endemic in the northeast and upper midwestern United States and in Europe.[73] Japanese encephalitis is found in most of Asia,[74] and tick-borne encephalitis occurs over a wide area of eastern Europe and northern Asia.[75]

Exposure to infected animals can transmit viral agents of encephalitis, even when the animals do not appear ill. Herpes B virus encephalitis may occur in monkey handlers who have been bitten or scratched by infected monkeys. Hendra virus, a member of the Paramyxoviridae family and formerly called equine morbillivirus, has caused encephalitis in a few Australian horse handlers. In 1999 an outbreak of encephalitis in Malaysia was caused by a Hendra-like virus, called Nipah virus, in persons in contact with swine.

Infections with eastern equine encephalitis virus produce clinically evident encephalitis with high frequency in all age groups,[76] in contrast to the other causes of viral encephalitis, in which a large majority of the infections are subclinical. Clinical disease with St. Louis and western equine encephalitis viruses occurs in about 1% of infections, and infants and adults older than 50 years of age are most likely to develop encephalitis.[72, 77] California virus infects persons of all ages but produces encephalitis predominantly in children.[78] Venezuelan equine encephalitis virus primarily causes a flulike illness in humans but can produce encephalitis in any age group.[79]

Nonviral causes of encephalomyelitis are listed in Table 73–2. Some of these diseases are of known and others of unknown cause, and the clinical presentations are often indistinguishable from those of viral encephalitis.[80–83] They include drug reactions such as the neuroleptic malignant syndrome[84] and chemotherapy-induced leukoencephalopathy,[85] which may be confused with infection. Many are treatable. One of the most important concerns in evaluating a patient with encephalomyelitis is consideration of treatable entities.

The cause of encephalitis is frequently different in immunodeficient patients. Patients with hypogammaglobulinemia may have chronic encephalitis with enterovirus.[47] Patients with defects in cell-mediated immunity have unusual forms of encephalitis or myelitis with herpesviruses,[18, 86, 87] a subacute inclusion body encephalitis with measles,[3, 17] meningoencephalitis with adenovirus,[16] and *Acanthamoeba.*[88] In acquired immunodeficiency syndrome (AIDS) a number of unusual agents, principally *Toxoplasma, Pneumocystis, Cryptococcus, Histoplasma,* cytomegalovirus, and papovavirus (progressive multifocal leukoencephalopathy), may cause CNS disease, either singly or in combination.[18, 36, 48, 88–90]

Transverse myelitis caused by a vasculitis of the anterior spinal artery has been seen in varicella-zoster virus infections, tuberculosis, syphilis, and schistosomiasis.[3, 91, 92] Postinfectious transverse myelitis has been associated with measles, rubella, mumps, and upper respiratory tract diseases.[93, 94] Direct infection of the spinal cord with varicella-zoster virus or Lyme borrelia may also produce a transverse myelitis.[3, 95] Infection with human T-lymphotropic virus type I causes disease primarily in the thoracic cord, leading to progressive spastic paraparesis.[49] Infection with HIV causes myelopathy manifested by spastic paraparesis and sensory ataxia.[48] An ascending myelitis may also occur in rabies.[96] The lower motor neuron variety of myelitis causing flaccid paralysis (poliomyelitis) may be produced by a number of enteroviruses, particularly poliovirus and enterovirus 71.[3, 97]

TABLE 73–2 Nonviral Causes of Encephalomyelitis

Rocky Mountain spotted fever	*Nocardia*
Typhus	Actinomycosis
Ehrlichia	Tuberculosis
Q fever	*Cryptococcus*
Chlamydia	*Histoplasma*
Mycoplasma	*Naegleria*
Legionella	*Acanthamoeba*
Brucellosis	*Ballamuthia mandrillaris*
Subacute bacterial endocarditis	*Toxoplasma*
Listeria	*Plasmodium falciparum*
Whipple's disease	Trypanosomiasis
Cat-scratch disease	Behçet's disease
Syphilis (meningovascular)	Vasculitis
Relapsing fever	Carcinoma
Lyme disease	Drug reactions
Leptospirosis	

Presumptive Treatment

Specific therapy is available for most of the diseases listed in Table 73–2 and should be instituted as soon as possible if a presumptive diagnosis can be made. In addition, effective therapy is available with acyclovir for herpes simplex, varicella-zoster, and herpes B[98–100] virus encephalitis. Cytomegalovirus encephalitis and radiculomyelitis can be treated with ganciclovir or foscarnet.[18, 101] HIV-associated neurologic disease may improve with antiretroviral treatment.[102] None of these treatments eliminates the latent state of these viruses in the nervous system.

Patients in coma caused by encephalitis or postinfectious encephalomyelitis may make remarkable recoveries even after prolonged periods of unconsciousness. For this reason vigorous supportive treatment is indicated, and the complications of ventilator therapy, catheters, intravenous lines, and so forth should be avoided if possible and should be treated vigorously if they occur. Blood glucose levels and electrolytes should be monitored closely, because the hypothalamic area may be involved in the encephalitic process. Seizures should be controlled, if they occur. Some fever may be beneficial, but extreme hyperthermia may aggravate seizures, as may hypoxia. Cerebral edema can be damaging in itself and should be controlled with steroids if necessary.

NEURITIS

Neuritis is an inflammatory disease involving the peripheral nerves. Leprosy, trypanosomes, microsporidia, and cytomegalovirus cause a direct infection of nerves leading to clinical signs of peripheral neuropathy. Neuroborreliosis frequently causes radiculoneuritis and cranial neuritis associated pathologically with inflammation.[3, 103] Herpes simplex virus and varicella-zoster virus infect sensory ganglia, and reactivation may be associated with radicular pain. Herpes zoster may also be complicated by a postherpetic pain syndrome in the distribution of nerves supplied by the affected ganglia. Three bacterial toxins affect peripheral nerves either directly (diphtheria) or indirectly (tetanus, botulism), each causing distinct syndromes. The Guillain-Barré syndrome is a postinfectious inflammatory process of peripheral nerves that can involve destruction of axons or myelin.

Pathologic Characteristics and Pathogenesis

In lepromatous leprosy the immunologic response does not effectively control the infection. There is a widespread distribution of *Mycobacterium leprae*. Nerves in the skin may exhibit only minor changes, but larger peripheral nerves contain many leprosy bacilli in Schwann cells. The organisms grow best in the cooler parts of the body, and nerves close to skin surface and distal nerves are affected preferentially. In late stages of the disease, extensive axonal degeneration may occur.[104]

Tuberculoid leprosy is characterized by a marked granulomatous reaction to the infection and few demonstrable bacilli. Cutaneous nerves beneath the depigmented skin macules are destroyed, producing anesthesia. The peripheral nerves are nodular and thickened, with destruction of the normal architecture. Segmental demyelination and axonal degeneration result in nerve destruction and severe fibrosis.

Trypanosoma cruzi, Trypanosoma gambiense, and *Trypanosoma rhodesiense* all can invade and replicate in tissue of the peripheral nervous system as well as the CNS. *T. cruzi* preferentially damages cells of the autonomic nervous system by replicating in the supporting Schwann cells, satellite cells, and capsular fibroblasts rather than in the neurons. In Africa, trypanosomiasis patients dying with encephalomyelitis often have evidence of neuritis.[105] The microsporidia *Nosema connori* can invade the nerve fibers of Auerbach's plexus, causing nerve dysfunction.[105]

Tetanus toxin, produced by *Clostridium tetani* under anaerobic conditions, is transported up the axon and binds to the presynaptic endings on motor neurons in the anterior horns of the spinal cord, where it cleaves synaptic vesicle components, blocking inhibitory input.[3, 106] This results in uncontrolled motor input to skeletal muscle and the spasms typical of this disease. Because of this transport mechanism for entry into the CNS, patients may have only localized disease in the area of the *Clostridium*-containing wound.

Botulinum toxin is produced during anaerobic metabolism of *Clostridium botulinum* and may be either ingested as preformed toxin (food botulism) or produced by organisms that are in the intestine (infant botulism) or are introduced into a wound (wound botulism). Botulinum toxin binds to the presynaptic axon terminal of the neuromuscular junction and cleaves components of exocytic synaptic vesicles, preventing release of acetylcholine and leading to flaccid paralysis.[3, 106] Little, if any, histologic abnormality is seen in either tetanus or botulism.

Diphtheria toxin is produced by *Corynebacterium diphtheriae* lysogenized by a phage coding for this toxin. The toxin is a protein with two subunits; subunit A inhibits protein synthesis by adenosine diphosphate ribosylation of elongation factor 2, and subunit B binds to cell membranes and enables the active subunit A to enter the cell.[107] The effect of this toxin on peripheral nerves is to cause a noninflammatory demyelination. Both cranial and peripheral nerves may be demyelinated, although cranial nerves are more frequently affected.

The Guillain-Barré syndrome usually follows within 4 weeks after a respiratory or gastrointestinal infection, immunization, trauma, or metabolic insult. Infections with *Campylobacter jejuni,* herpes viruses, *Mycoplasma pneumoniae,* and a few other organisms have been associated with this syndrome. *C. jejuni* is the most common preceding infection, particularly in patients with axonal degeneration and in children.[108, 109] Specific strains may be involved.[110] Two types of nerve pathology are recognized: mononuclear inflammation with demyelination,[109, 111] and axonal degeneration. The mechanisms by which these apparently autoimmune diseases are induced are not yet clear, but induction of antibody to gangliosides in the nervous system appears to be involved in some forms of the disease.[112]

Clinical Findings

Leprosy has two distinctive manifestations, depending on whether the disease is of the tuberculoid or the lepromatous type. Tuberculoid leprosy produces a mononeuropathy beneath the sharply demarcated, hypopigmented skin patches. Peripheral nerves may be palpably and visibly enlarged, and the neurologic involvement is a prominent part of the disease. In lepromatous leprosy, a distal hypesthesia with selective loss of pain and temperature is most common, although a mononeuropathy may be present. Cooler areas of the body are more strikingly affected, and the loss of pain sensation results in mutilation and eventual loss of digits.[104]

Tetanus usually manifests with rigidity of muscles, which may be painful. The initial manifestation may be "local tetanus," in which the rigidity affects only the limb or area of the body in which the *Clostridium*-containing wound is located. Stiffness of the jaw muscles causes trismus, and stiffness of the facial muscles may cause a change of expression. This mild picture can progress to generalized rigidity with reflex spasms and dysphagia. The history of a soil-contaminated puncture wound should be sought. The wound may have seemed insignificant at the time of the injury and may appear well healed at the time of the neurologic disease.[3, 113]

Botulism characteristically manifests 12 to 36 hours after ingestion of the toxin with weakness, dizziness, and dryness of the mouth. Neurologic symptoms follow within 12 to 72 hours with blurred vision, diplopia, dysphonia, dysphagia, and muscle weakness. On examination sensation is preserved, the tendon reflexes are depressed or absent, and the paralysis is flaccid.[3, 114] The same picture can develop more gradually in a patient with wound botulism. The original wound is usually of a rather severe traumatic nature and may appear to be healing well at the time of neurologic disease.[3, 114, 115]

The earliest sign of pharyngeal diphtheria (5 to 12 days) is paralysis of the palate, which produces a nasal quality of the voice and an increasing tendency to regurgitate fluids through the nose. Other cranial nerves (particularly the third, sixth, seventh, ninth, and tenth) may become involved, with blurring of vision and inability to accommodate as early symptoms. Later in the course of the disease, after the previous symptoms have subsided (4 to 8 weeks), a predominantly motor polyneuropathy involving initial symmetric weakness of distal extremities occurs and may appear similar to Guillain-Barré syndrome. There is a flaccid paralysis with loss of deep tendon reflexes that may be accompanied by the signs and symptoms of a diphtheritic myocarditis.[116]

Neuropathies associated with HIV infection include acute and chronic inflammatory demyelinating polyneuropathies, sensory ganglioneuritis, and polyradiculopathy early in infection and a distal, symmetric, primarily sensory neuropathy later, after AIDS has developed.[117]

In approximately 60% of cases, Guillain-Barré syndrome follows an infection or immunization.[108] Clinically it manifests with subjective paresthesias or weakness, or both, which may continue to progress for up to 4 weeks.[109, 118] Examination typically reveals a flaccid paralysis with loss of deep tendon reflexes. Involvement of the autonomic nervous system resulting in lability of blood pressure, inappropriate antidiuretic hormone secretion, and inability to compensate for volume changes occurs in approximately 20% of the cases.[119] These problems frequently necessitate the management of patients in an intensive care unit even though they may not require ventilatory assistance. The condition of an individual patient can change rapidly either during progression or during recovery. Improvement is often slow, however, and may continue for up to 12 months.[108, 109, 118]

Laboratory Findings

Routine blood chemistry analyses are not helpful in this group of diseases. If botulism is suspected, serum for mouse inoculation should be procured and CSF should also be obtained. In Guillain-Barré syndrome or diphtheritic polyneuritis, an increased protein level, with few cells (albuminocytologic dissociation) in the CSF, is the characteristic finding; however, some patients have a normal protein level, particularly early in the disease. Others, especially those with HIV infection, also have a moderate pleocytosis.[120, 121] The CSF findings are normal in tetanus, botulism, and leprosy. Neurometric tests that aid in localization of the pathologic changes and therefore the diagnosis, are *(1)* the measurement of nerve conduction times, to look for the slowed conduction found in the peripheral nerve lesions of Guillain-Barré syndrome and diphtheria (F-wave measurements may allow identification of abnormalities if lesions are very proximal), and *(2)* the recording from muscle during repetitive nerve stimulation, to look for the incremental response characteristic of botulism[114] and not found in Guillain-Barré syndrome. Nerve biopsies may be useful in identifying the granulomas and/or acid-fast bacilli of leprosy.

Presumptive Treatment

In this group of clinically distinctive diseases, it is important to recognize the disease and to treat it appropriately. Most patients with Guillain-Barré syndrome benefit from plasmapheresis or intravenous immunoglobulin therapy, especially when early in the disease.[120, 122] Patients must be closely monitored for vital capacity, electrolytes, blood pressure, temperature, and heart rate, and those with respiratory failure should be ventilated mechanically. Patients with autonomic nervous system dysfunction should be treated with short-acting drugs, because autonomic function in these patients can be very labile. A patient who is hypertensive in the morning may be distressingly hypotensive in the evening, and vice versa. Patients may not adjust to abrupt changes in intravascular volume, so intravenous fluids should be carefully controlled.

REFERENCES

1. Johnson RT. Viral Infections of the Nervous System, 2nd ed. Philadelphia: Lippincott-Raven; 1998.
2. Mims CA. The Pathogenesis of Infectious Diseases, 3rd ed. New York: Academic Press; 1987.
3. Scheld WM, Whitley RJ, Durack DT. Infections of the Central Nervous System, 2nd ed. Philadelphia: Lippincott-Raven; 1997.
4. Tsiang H. Pathophysiology of rabies virus infection of the nervous system. Adv Virus Res. 1993;42:375–412.
5. Wyatt HV. Incubation of poliomyelitis as calculated from the central nervous system via the peripheral nerve pathways. Rev Infect Dis. 1990;12:547–556.
6. Whitley RJ, Kimberlin DW, Roizman B. Herpes simplex viruses. Clin Infect Dis. 1998;26:541–555.
7. Monath TP, Cropp CP, Harrison AK. Mode of entry of a neurotropic arbovirus into the central nervous system: Reinvestigation of an old controversy. Lab Invest. 1983;48:399–410.
8. Barnett EM, Perlman S. The olfactory nerve and not the trigeminal nerve is the major site of CNS entry for mouse hepatitis virus, strain JHM. Virology. 1993;194:185–191.
9. Ma P, Visvesvara GS, Martinez AJ, et al. *Naegleria* and acanthamoeba infections: Review. Rev Infect Dis. 1990;12:490–513.
10. Johnson RT. Selective vulnerability of neural cells to viral infection. Brain. 1980;103:447–472.
11. Johnson RT, Burke DS, Elwell M, et al. Japanese encephalitis: Immunocytochemical studies of viral antigen and inflammatory cells in fatal cases. Ann Neurol. 1985;18:567–573.
12. Epstein LG, Gendelman HE. Human immunodeficiency virus type 1 infection of the nervous system: Pathogenetic mechanisms. Ann Neurol. 1993;33:429–436.
13. Tyor WR, Wesselingh SL, Griffin JW, et al. Unifying hypothesis for the pathogenesis of HIV-associated dementia complex, vacuolar myelopathy, and sensory neuropathy. J Acquir Immune Defic Syndr Hum Retrovirol. 1995;9:379–388.
14. Budka H. Neuropathology of human immunodeficiency virus infection. Brain Pathol. 1991;1:163–175.
15. Rance NE, McArthur JC, Cornblath DR, et al. Gracile tract degeneration in patients with sensory neuropathy and AIDS. Neurology. 1988;38:265–271.
16. Davis D, Henslee PJ, Markesbery WR. Fatal adenovirus meningoencephalitis in a bone marrow transplant patient. Ann Neurol. 1988;23:385–389.
17. Roos RP, Graves MC, Wollmann RL, et al. Immunologic and virologic studies of measles inclusion body encephalitis in an immunosuppressed host: The relationship to subacute sclerosing panencephalitis. Neurology. 1981;31:1263–1270.
18. McCutchan JA. Cytomegalovirus infections of the nervous system in patients with AIDS. Clin Infect Dis. 1995;20:747–754.
19. Dupont JR, Earle KM. Human rabies encephalitis: A study of forty-nine fatal cases with a review of the literature. Neurology. 1964;15:1023–1034.
20. Miller JQ, Price TR. The nervous system in Rocky Mountain spotted fever. Neurology. 1972;22:561–566.
21. Dastur DK, Lalitha VS, Udani PM, et al. The brain and meninges in tuberculous meningitis: Gross pathology in 100 cases and pathogenesis. Neurol India. 1970;18:86–100.
22. Walsh TJ, Hier DB, Caplan LR. Aspergillosis of the central nervous system: Clinicopathological analysis of 17 patients. Ann Neurol. 1985;18:574–582.
23. Greenfield JG. Infectious diseases of the central nervous system: Neurosyphilis. In: Blackwood W, McMenemey WH, Meyer A, et al, eds. Greenfield's Neuropathology. Baltimore: Williams & Wilkins; 1963:164.
24. Mischel PS, Vinters HV. Coccidiodomycosis of the central nervous system: Neuropathological and vasculopathic manifestations and clinical correlates. Clin Infect Dis. 1995;20:400–405.
25. Gray F, Belec L, Lescs MC, et al. Varicella-zoster virus infection of the central nervous system in the acquired immunodeficiency syndrome. Brain 1994;117:987–999.
26. Baker RD, Haugen RK. Tissue changes and tissue diagnosis in cryptococcosis: A study of 26 cases. J Clin Pathol. 1955;25:14.
27. Ellner JJ, Bennett JE. Chronic meningitis. Medicine (Baltimore). 1976;55:341–369.
28. Johnson RT, Griffin DE, Hirsch RL, et al. Measles encephalomyelitis: Clinical and immunologic studies. N Engl J Med. 1984;310:137–141.
29. Hemachudha T, Griffin DE, Giffels JJ, et al. Myelin basic protein as an encephalitogen in encephalomyelitis and polyneuritis following rabies vaccination. N Engl J Med. 1987;316:369–374.
30. Dangond F, Lacomis D, Schwartz RB, et al. Acute disseminated encephalomyelitis progressing to hemorrhagic encephalitis. Neurology. 1991;41:1697–1698.
31. Hardie RM, Newton LH, Bruce JC, et al. The changing clinical pattern of Reye's syndrome 1982–1990. Arch Dis Child. 1996;75:400–405.
32. Goren A, Freier S, Passwell JH. Lethal toxic encephalopathy due to childhood shigellosis in a developed country. Pediatrics. 1992;89:1189–1193.
33. Woods ML II, Currie BJ, Howard DM, et al. Neurological melioidosis: Seven cases from the Northern Territory of Australia. Clin Infect Dis. 1992;15:163–169.
34. Marra CM. Neurologic complications of *Bartonella henselae* infection. Curr Opin Neurol. 1995;8:164–169.
35. Osuntokun BO, Adeuja AOG, Familusi JB. Tuberculous meningitis in Nigerians: A study of 194 patients. Trop Geogr Med. 1971;23:225–231.
36. Moosa MYS, Coovadia YM. Cryptococcal meningitis in Durban, South Africa: A comparison of clinical features, laboratory findings, and outcome for human immunodeficiency virus (HIV)-positive and HIV-negative patients. Clin Infect Dis. 1997;24:131–141.

37. Dominques RB, Tsanaclis AMC, Pannuti CS, et al. Evaluation of the range of clinical presentations of herpes simplex encephalitis by using polymerase chain reaction assay of cerebrospinal fluid samples. Clin Infect Dis. 1997;25:86–91.
38. Hattwick MAW. Human rabies. Public Health Rep. 1981;96:580–584.
39. Dickerson RB, Newton JR, Hansen JE. Diagnosis and immediate prognosis of Japanese B encephalitis. Am J Med. 1952;12:277–288.
40. Halperin JJ, Volkman DJ, Wu P. Central nervous system abnormalities in Lyme neuroborreliosis. Neurology. 1991;41:1571–1582.
41. Halperin JJ, Golightly M, Andriola M, et al. Lyme borreliosis in Bell's palsy. Neurology. 1992;42:1268–1270.
42. Centers for Disease Control and Prevention. Human rabies—Montana, and Washington, 1997. MMWR Morb Mortal Wkly Rep. 1997;46:770–774.
43. Adams M, Rhyner PA, Day J, et al. Whipple's disease confined to the central nervous system. Ann Neurol. 1987;21:104–108.
44. Kirk JL, Fine DP, Sexton DJ, et al. Rocky Mountain spotted fever: A clinical review based on 48 confirmed cases, 1943–1986. Medicine (Baltimore). 1990;69:35–45.
45. Psi H, Sohn S, Seong Y, et al. Central nervous system involvement in patients with scrub typhus. Clin Infect Dis. 1997;24:436–440.
46. Ratnasamy N, Everett ED, Roland WE, et al. Central nervous system manifestations of human ehrlichiosis. Clin Infect Dis. 1996;23:314–319.
47. McKinney RE Jr, Katz SL, Wilfert CM. Chronic enteroviral meningoencephalitis in agammaglobulinemic patients. Rev Infect Dis. 1987;9:334–356.
48. McArthur JC. Neurologic manifestations of human immunodeficiency virus infection. Medicine (Baltimore). 1987;66:407–437.
49. Levin MC, Jacobson S. HTLV-1 associated myelopathy/tropical spastic paraparesis (HAM/TSP): A chronic progressive neurologic disease associated with immunologically mediated damage to the central nervous system. J Neurovirol. 1997;3:126–140.
50. Will RG, Ironside JW, Zeidler M, et al. A new variant of Creutzfeldt-Jakob disease in the UK. Lancet. 1996;347:921–925.
51. Feigin RD, Shackelford PG. Value of repeat lumbar puncture in the differential diagnosis of meningitis. N Engl J Med. 1973;289:571–574.
52. Koskiniemi M, Vaheri A, Taskinen E. Cerebrospinal fluid alterations in herpes simplex virus encephalitis. Rev Infect Dis. 1984;6:608–618.
53. Carter RF. Primary amoebic meningoencephalitis: An appraisal of present knowledge. Trans R Soc Trop Med Hyg. 1972;66:193–208.
54. Peacock JE Jr, McGinnis MR, Cohen MS. Persistent neutrophilic meningitis: Report of four cases and review of the literature. Medicine (Baltimore). 1984;63:379–395.
55. Link H, Muller R. Immunoglobulins in multiple sclerosis and infections of the nervous system. Arch Neurol. 1971;25:326–344.
56. Tourtellotte W. On cerebrospinal fluid immunoglobulin-G (IgG) quotients in multiple sclerosis and other diseases. J Neurol Sci. 1970;10:279–304.
57. Vandvik B, Nilsen RE, Vartdal F, et al. Mumps meningitis: Specific and nonspecific antibody responses in the central nervous system. Acta Neurol Scand. 1982;65:468–487.
58. Vartdal F, Vandvik B, Norrby E. Intrathecal synthesis of virus-specific oligoclonal IgG, IgA, and IgM antibodies in a case of varicella-zoster meningoencephalitis. J Neurol Sci. 1982;57:121–132.
59. Vartdal F, Vandvik B, Michaelson TE, et al. Neurosyphilis: Intrathecal synthesis of oligoclonal antibodies to *Treponema pallidum*. Ann Neurol. 1982;11:35–40.
60. Steere AC, Berardi VP, Weeks KE, et al. Evaluation of the intrathecal antibody response to *Borrelia burgdorferi* as a diagnostic test for Lyme neuroborreliosis. J Infect Dis. 1990;161:1203–1209.
61. Salmi AA, Norrby E, Panelius M. Identification of different measles virus-specific antibodies in the serum and cerebrospinal fluid from patients with subacute sclerosing panencephalitis and multiple sclerosis. Infect Immun. 1972;6:248–254.
62. Weber T, Trebst C, Frye S, et al. Analysis of the systemic and intrathecal humoral immune response in progressive multifocal leukoencephalopathy. J Infect Dis. 1997;176:250–254.
63. Townsend JJ, Baringer JR, Wolinsky JS, et al. Progressive rubella panencephalitis: Late onset after congenital rubella. N Engl J Med. 1975;292:990–993.
64. Meyer HM, Johnson RT, Crawford IP, et al. Central nervous system syndromes of "viral" etiology: A study of 713 cases. Am J Med. 1960;29:334–347.
65. Calisher CH, Berardi VP, Muth DJ, et al. Specificity of immunoglobulin M and G antibody responses in humans infected with eastern and western equine encephalitis viruses: Application to rapid serodiagnosis. J Clin Microbiol. 1986;23:369–372.
66. Burke DS, Nisalak A, Ussery MA, et al. Kinetics of IgM and IgG responses to Japanese encephalitis virus in human serum and cerebrospinal fluid. J Infect Dis. 1985;151:1093–1099.
67. Ogawa SK, Smith MA, Brennessel DJ, et al. Tuberculous meningitis in an urban medical center. Medicine (Baltimore). 1987;66:317–326.
68. Lennette EH, Longshore WA. Western equine and St. Louis encephalitis in man: California 1945–1950. Calif Med. 1951;75:189.
69. Spruance SL, Bailey A. Colorado tick fever: A review of 115 laboratory confirmed cases. Arch Intern Med. 1973;131:288–293.
70. Wilfert CM, MacCormack JN, Kleeman K, et al. Epidemiology of Rocky Mountain spotted fever as determined by active surveillance. J Infect Dis. 1984;150:469–479.
71. Ciesielski CA, Hightower AW, Horsley R, et al. The geographic distribution of Lyme disease in the United States. Ann N Y Acad Sci. 1989;539:283–288.
72. Calisher CH. Medically important arboviruses of the United States and Canada. Clin Microbiol Rev. 1994;7:89–116.
73. Schmid GP. The global distribution of Lyme disease. Rev Infect Dis. 1985;7:41–50.
74. Rosen L. The natural history of Japanese encephalitis virus. Annu Rev Microbiol. 1986;40:395–414.
75. Monath TP. Flaviviruses. In: Fields BN, Knipe DM, Howley PM, et al, eds. Virology, 3rd ed. New York: Lippincott-Raven; 1996;961–1034.
76. Przelomski MM, O'Rourke E, Grady GF, et al. Eastern equine encephalitis in Massachusetts: A report of 16 cases, 1970–1984. Neurology. 1988;38:736–739.
77. Southern PM, Smith JW, Luby JP, et al. Clinical and laboratory features of epidemic St. Louis encephalitis. Ann Intern Med. 1969;71:681.
78. Woodruff BA, Baron RC, Tsai TF. Symptomatic LaCrosse virus infections of the central nervous system: A study of risk factors in an endemic area. Am J Epidemiol. 1992;136:320–327.
79. Rivas F, Diaz LA, Cardena VM, et al. Epidemic Venezuelan equine encephalitis in La Guajira, Columbia, 1995. J Infect Dis. 1997;175:828–832.
80. Koskiniemi M, Rautonen J, Lahtokoski-Lehtiniemi E, et al. Epidemiology of encephalitis in children: A 20 year survey. Ann Neurol. 1991;29:492–497.
81. Kolski H, Ford-James EL, Richardson S, et al. Etiology of acute childhood encephalitis at the Hospital for Sick Children, Toronto 1994–1995. Clin Infect Dis. 1998;26:398–409.
82. Johnson JD, Raff MJ, Van Arsdall JA. Neurologic manifestations of Legionnaires' disease. Medicine (Baltimore). 1984;63:303–310.
83. Korman TM, Turnidge JD, Grayson ML. Neurological complications of chlamydial infections: Case report and review. Clin Infect Dis. 1997;25:847–851.
84. Bristow MF, Kohen D. Neuroleptic malignant syndrome. Br J Hosp Med. 1996;55:517–520.
85. Glass JP, Lee YY, Bruner J, et al. Treatment-related leukoencephalopathy: A study of three cases and literature review. Medicine (Baltimore). 1986;65:154–162.
86. Gray F, Belec L, Lescs MC, et al. Varicella-zoster virus infection of the central nervous system in the acquired immunodeficiency syndrome. Brain. 1994;117:987–999.
87. Chretien F, Belec L, Hilton DA, et al. Herpes simplex virus type 1 encephalitis in acquired immunodeficiency syndrome. Neuropathol Appl Neurobiol. 1996;22:394–404.
88. Gordon SM, Steinberg JP, DuPuis MH, et al. Culture isolation of *Acanthamoeba* species and leptomyxid amebas from patients with amebic meningoencephalitis, including two patients with AIDS. Clin Infect Dis. 1992;15:1024–1030.
89. Mariuz P, Bosler EM, Luft BJ. Toxoplasmosis in individuals with AIDS. Infect Dis Clin North Am. 1994;8:365–381.
90. Fong IW, Toma E, Canadian Study Group. The natural history of progressive multifocal leukoencephalopathy in patients with AIDS. Clin Infect Dis. 1995;20:1305–1310.
91. Cohen J, Capildeo R, Rose FC, et al. Schistosomal myelopathy. BMJ. 1977;1:1258.
92. Kenyon LC, Dulaney E, Montone KT, et al. Varicella-zoster ventriculoencephalitis and spinal cord infarction in a patient with AIDS. Acta Neuropathol. 1996;92:202–205.
93. Lipton HL, Teasdall RD. Acute transverse myelopathy in adults. Arch Neurol. 1973;28:252.
94. Christensen PB, Wermuth L, Hinge HH, et al. Clinical course and long-term prognosis of acute transverse myelopathy. Acta Neurol Scand. 1990;81:431–435.
95. Devinsky O, Cho E-S, Petito CK, et al. Herpes zoster myelitis. Brain. 1991;114:1181–1196.
96. Chopra JS, Banerjee AK, Murthy JMK, et al. Brain. 1989;103:789–802.
97. Melnick JL. Enterovirus type 71 infections: A varied clinical pattern sometimes mimicking paralytic poliomyelitis. Rev Infect Dis. 1984;6(Suppl 2):S387–S390.
98. Whitley RJ, Lakeman F. Herpes simplex virus infections of the central nervous system: Therapeutic and diagnostic considerations. Clin Infect Dis. 1995;20:414–420.
99. Weigler BJ. Biology of B virus in macaque and human hosts: A review. Clin Infect Dis. 1992;14:555–567.
100. Whitley RJ, Gnann JW Jr, Hinthorn D, et al. Disseminated herpes zoster in the immunocompromised host: A comparative trial of acyclovir and vidarabine. J Infect Dis. 1992;165:450–455.
101. Cinque P, Baldanti F, Vago L, et al. Ganciclovir therapy for cytomegalovirus (CMV) infection of the central nervous system in AIDS patients: Monitoring by CMV DNA detection in cerebrospinal fluid. J Infect Dis. 1995;171:1603–1606.
102. Sidtis JJ, Gatsonis C, Price RW, et al. Zidovudine treatment of the AIDS dementia complex: Results of a placebo-controlled trial. Ann Neurol. 1993;33:343–349.
103. Cadavid D, Barbour AG. Neuroborreliosis during relapsing fever: Review of the clinical manifestations, pathology, and treatment of infections in humans and experimental animals. Clin Infect Dis. 1998;26:151–164.
104. Sabin TD, Swift TR, Jacobson RR. Leprosy. In: Dyck PJ, Thomas PK, Griffin JW, et al, eds. Peripheral Neuropathy. Philadelphia: WB Saunders; 1993:1354–1379.
105. Connor DH, Manz HJ. Parasitic infections of the peripheral nervous system. In: Dyck PJ, Thomas PK, Griffin JW, et al, eds. Peripheral Neuropathy. Philadelphia: WB Saunders; 1993:1380–1400.
106. Montecucco C, Schiavo G. Mechanism of action of tetanus and botulinum neurotoxins. Mol Microbiol. 1994;13:1–8.
107. London E. Diphtheria toxin: Membrane interaction and membrane translocation. Biochim Biophys Acta. 1992;1113:25–51.
108. Winer JB, Hughes RAC, Osmond C. A prospective study of acute idiopathic neuropathy: 2. Antecedent events. J Neurol Neurosurg Psychiatry. 1988;51:613–618.
109. Hughes RA, Rees JH. Clinical and epidemiological features of Guillain-Barré syndrome. J Infect Dis. 1997;176(Suppl 2):592–598.
110. Nishimura M, Nukina M, Kuroki S, et al. Characterization of *Campylobacter jejuni* isolates from patients with Guillain-Barré syndrome. J Neurol Sci. 1997;153:91–99.

111. Asbury AK, Arnason BG, Adams RD. The inflammatory lesion in idiopathic polyneuritis: Its role in pathogenesis. Medicine (Baltimore). 1969;48:173–215.
112. Rees JH, Gregson NA, Hughes RA. Anti-ganglioside GM1 antibodies in Guillain-Barré syndrome and their relationship to *Campylobacter jejuni* infection. Ann Neurol. 1995;38:809–816.
113. Weinstein L. Tetanus. N Engl J Med. 1973;289:1293.
114. Cherington M. Clinical spectrum of botulism. Muscle Nerve. 1998;21:701–710.
115. Weber JT, Goodpasture HC, Alexander H, et al. Wound botulism in a patient with a tooth abscess: Case report and review. Clin Infect Dis. 1993;16:635–639.
116. McDonald WI, Kocen RS. Diphtheritic neuropathy. In: Dyck PJ, Thomas PK, Griffin JW, et al, eds. Peripheral Neuropathy. Philadelphia: WB Saunders; 1993:1412–1417.
117. Parry GJ. Peripheral neuropathies associated with human immunodeficiency virus infection. Ann Neurol. 1988;23(Suppl):S49–S53.
118. Barohn RJ, Saperstein DS. Guillain-Barré syndrome and chronic inflammatory demyelinating polyneuropathy. Semin Neurol. 1998;18:49–61.
119. Lichtenfeld P. Autonomic dysfunction in the Guillain-Barré syndrome. Am J Med. 1971;50:772–780.
120. Cornblath DR, McArthur JC, Kennedy PGE, et al. Inflammatory demyelinating peripheral neuropathies associated with human T cell lymphotropic virus type III infection. Ann Neurol. 1987;21:32–40.
121. Wiederholt WC, Mulder DW, Lambert EH. The Landry-Guillain-Barré-Strohl syndrome or polyradiculoneuropathy: Historical review, report on 97 patients, and present concepts. Mayo Clin Proc. 1964;39:427.
122. Hund EF, Bare ICO, Cornblath DR, et al. Intensive management and treatment of severe Guillain-Barré syndrome. Crit Care Med. 1993;21:433–446.

Chapter 74

Brain Abscess

ALLAN R. TUNKEL
BRIAN WISPELWEY
W. MICHAEL SCHELD

Brain abscess is a focal, intracerebral infection that begins as a localized area of cerebritis and develops into a collection of pus surrounded by a well-vascularized capsule.[1] Brain abscess was an almost uniformly fatal disease before the late 1800s, when surgical techniques (i.e., drainage) led to cure in selected patients.[2] Further advances in the management of brain abscess were made after the introduction of antimicrobial therapy and stereotactic brain biopsy and aspiration techniques. Here we review the common bacterial, fungal, and protozoal causes of brain abscess, highlighting the clinical presentation, diagnosis, and approach to management.

EPIDEMIOLOGY AND ETIOLOGY

Brain abscess is one of the most serious complications of head and neck infections. Before the advent of human immunodeficiency virus (HIV) infection, brain abscess accounted for about 1 in 10,000 general hospital admissions with 1500 to 2500 cases treated in the United States each year.[3] In most pediatric and adult series, a male predominance exists with a median age between 30 and 40 years, although the age distribution varies depending on the predisposing condition leading to the formation of brain abscess. When the abscess is related to a focus in the paranasal sinuses, most patients are 10 to 30 years of age; when the abscess is from an otitic focus, patients are younger than 20 or older than 40 years.[3,4] Overall, about 25% of brain abscess cases occur in children, most in the 4- to 7-year age group, usually in patients in whom they originate from an otitic focus or in patients with cyanotic congenital heart disease. Brain abscess is extremely rare in patients younger than 2 years.

Case-fatality rates in patients with brain abscess, even in the antibiotic era, have ranged from 30 to 60% (similar to the rates in the preantibiotic era) until the period since the late 1970s, when the overall mortality rate has ranged from zero to 24%.[3–5] This improvement has been attributed to the availability of more effective antimicrobial regimens (e.g., the addition of metronidazole), new surgical techniques, and, most importantly, the availability of computed tomography (CT) scanning. Data from the University of California in San Francisco demonstrated a decrease in the overall mortality rate from 44% during the 3 years before CT scanning to zero for the 3 years following the introduction of CT scanning in 1977.[6] This lower mortality rate was principally related to early diagnosis and an accurate method of postoperative follow-up with CT. The incidence of neurologic sequelae in patients who survive their brain abscess has ranged from 20 to 70%. In one study of factors influencing the outcome in 39 cases of bacterial brain abscess,[7] the prognosis was primarily determined by the rapidity of progression of the disease before hospitalization and the patient's mental status on admission. Therefore, early recognition of predisposing conditions is an important means of improving the outcome in this disorder.

When the microorganisms likely to be responsible for causing brain abscesses are evaluated, the isolation frequency depends on the predisposing condition (Table 74–1).[3] Improved microbiologic culture techniques, particularly for anaerobes, have had a significant impact on the awareness of microorganisms that are found in brain abscesses. The following sections review the common bacteria, fungi, protozoans, and helminths that can produce brain abscess.

Bacterial Brain Abscess

Streptococci (aerobic, anaerobic, and microaerophilic) are the bacteria most commonly (up to 70% of cases) cultured from patients with bacterial brain abscess, and are frequently isolated in mixed infections (30 to 60% of cases).[3] These bacteria, especially the *Streptococcus milleri* group (*Streptococcus anginosus*, *Streptococcus constellatus*, and *Streptococcus intermedius*), normally reside in the oral cavity, appendix, and female genital tract, and have a proclivity for abscess formation.[8,9] *Staphylococcus aureus* accounts for 10 to 15% of isolates, usually in patients with cranial trauma or infective endocarditis, and is often isolated in pure culture. The attention to proper culture techniques has increased the isolation of anaerobes from brain abscesses (40 to 100% of cases) with *Bacteroides* and *Prevotella* species isolated in 20 to 40% of patients, often in mixed culture.[10,11] Enteric gram-negative bacilli (e.g. *Proteus* spp., *Escherichia coli, Klebsiella* spp., and *Pseudomonas* spp.) are isolated in

TABLE 74–1 Predisposing Conditions and Microbiology of Brain Abscess

Predisposing Condition	Usual Microbial Isolates
Otitis media or mastoiditis	Streptococci (anaerobic or aerobic), *Bacteroides* and *Prevotella* spp., Enterobacteriaceae
Sinusitis (frontoethmoid or sphenoid)	Streptococci, *Bacteroides* spp., Enterobacteriaceae, *Staphylococcus aureus, Haemophilus* spp.
Dental sepsis	Mixed *Fusobacterium, Prevotella* and *Bacteroides* spp., streptococci
Penetrating trauma or postneurosurgical	*S. aureus,* streptococci, Enterobacteriaceae, *Clostridium* spp.
Lung abscess, empyema, bronchiectasis	*Fusobacterium, Actinomyces, Bacteroides* and *Prevotella* spp., streptococci, *Nocardia* spp.
Bacterial endocarditis	*S. aureus,* streptococci
Congenital heart disease	Streptococci, *Haemophilus* spp.
Neutropenia	Aerobic gram-negative bacilli, *Aspergillus* spp., Mucorales, *Candida* spp.
Transplantation	*Aspergillus* spp., *Candida* spp., Mucorales, Enterobacteriaceae, *Nocardia* spp., *Toxoplasma gondii*
HIV infection	*Toxoplasma gondii, Nocardia* spp., *Mycobacterium* spp., *Listeria monocytogenes, Cryptococcus neoformans*

Abbreviation: HIV, Human immunodeficiency virus.

23 to 33% of patients, often in patients with otitic foci of infection or in those who are immunocompromised. The incidence of negative cultures has ranged from zero to 43% in selected series,[3, 10, 12, 13] with the frequency often correlating with prior use of antimicrobial therapy.

Other bacterial pathogens may be isolated from brain abscesses in selected patients or from those who are immunocompromised. Although *Haemophilus influenzae, Streptococcus pneumoniae, and Listeria monocytogenes* are common etiologic agents of bacterial meningitis, they are rarely isolated from patients with pyogenic brain abscesses (<1% of cases).[14–18] In contrast, although meningitis caused by other facultative gram-negative organisms (e.g., *Citrobacter diversus*, *Proteus* spp., *Serratia marcescens*, or *Enterobacter* spp.) is infrequent, it is associated with concomitant brain abscess in more than 75% of cases[1, 19–22]; children with bacteremia or meningitis caused by these organisms should be evaluated for the possibility of brain abscess. Actinomycosis of the central nervous system (CNS) may present as brain abscess, usually secondary to hematogenous spread from a primary infection in the lung, abdomen, or pelvis, although contiguous spread from foci of infection in the ears, paranasal sinuses, or cervicofacial regions may occur.[23] Nocardial brain abscess may occur as an isolated CNS lesion or as part of a disseminated infection in association with pulmonary or cutaneous disease.[1] This organism is most often isolated in patients with defects in cell-mediated immunity (secondary to corticosteroid therapy; in organ transplant recipients; in patients infected with HIV; and in patients with neoplastic disease),[24–29] although up to 50% of patients with nocardiosis have no underlying conditions. Cases of nocardial brain abscess have also been seen in pregnant patients.[30] *Mycobacterium tuberculosis* and nontuberculous mycobacteria have been increasingly observed to cause focal CNS lesions,[1, 3] with several cases reported in patients with HIV infection.[31–33]

Fungal Brain Abscess

The incidence of fungal brain abscess has increased due to the prevalent administration of immunosuppressive agents, broad-spectrum antimicrobial therapy, and corticosteroids.[34–38] Unfortunately, the diagnosis of fungal brain abscess is often unexpected, and many cases are not discovered until autopsy. In autopsy studies, *Candida* spp. have emerged as the most prevalent etiologic agents[39, 40]; neuropathologic lesions include microabscesses, macroabscesses, noncaseating granulomas, and diffuse glial nodules. Risk factors for invasive *Candida* infection include the use of corticosteroids, broad-spectrum antimicrobial therapy, or hyperalimentation; disease is also seen in premature infants; in patients with malignancy, neutropenia, chronic granulomatous disease, diabetes mellitus, or thermal injuries; and in those with a central venous catheter in place.[35, 38, 41] However, several other pathogenic fungi should be considered in the differential diagnosis of fungal brain abscess, particularly in the immunosuppressed patient, and are described in detail.

Cases of intracranial infection caused by *Aspergillus* spp. have been reported worldwide, with most cases occurring in adults. Cerebral aspergillosis is reported in 10 to 20% of all cases of invasive aspergillosis, and only rarely is the brain the only site of infection.[42] The lungs are the usual site of primary infection, and intracranial seeding occurs during dissemination of the organism or by direct extension from an area anatomically adjacent to the brain (e.g., the paranasal sinuses).[38] Most cases of invasive aspergillosis are found in neutropenic patients who have an underlying hematologic malignancy.[43, 44] Other risk groups include patients with hepatic disease, Cushing's syndrome, diabetes mellitus, chronic granulomatous disease, or HIV infection; injection drug abusers; postcraniotomy patients; organ transplant recipients; and patients receiving chronic corticosteroid therapy.[34, 42, 45–49]

Mucormycosis (zygomycosis, phycomycosis) is one of the most acute, fulminant fungal infections known. Many predisposing conditions to mucormycosis have been described including diabetes mellitus (70% of cases), usually in association with acidosis, acidemia from profound systemic illnesses (e.g., sepsis, severe dehydration, severe diarrhea, chronic renal failure), hematologic neoplasms, renal transplantation, injection drug use, and the use of deferoxamine.[38, 50–55] Less than 5% of cases involve normal hosts. CNS disease may result from direct extension of the rhinocerebral form of mucormycosis, by open head trauma or by hematogenous dissemination. The order Mucorales includes many species that have caused brain lesions (see Chapter 249), with *Rhizopus oryzae* being one of the most common.[56]

Pseudallescheria boydii is a common mold readily isolated from soil that may cause CNS disease in both normal and immunocompromised hosts (e.g., those with neutropenia or cellular immunodeficiency).[38, 57–61] This organism is being increasingly referred to as *Scedosporium apiospermum*, the asexual form of *P. boydii*. *Pseudallescheria boydii* may enter the CNS by direct trauma, by hematogenous dissemination from a pulmonary route, by way of an intravenous catheter, or by direct extension from infected sinuses. Brain abscess is the usual CNS manifestation, although meningitis and ventriculitis have also been reported. There is an association between near-drowning and subsequent illness, due to the pathogen's presence in contaminated water and manure.

Many of the etiologic agents of fungal meningitis may also cause brain abscess (e.g., *Cryptococcus neoformans, Coccidioides immitis, Histoplasma capsulatum,* and *Blastomyces dermatitidis*); the epidemiologic and etiologic characteristics of these organisms are described in other chapters of this book. In addition, many of the dematiaceous fungi have also been reported to cause brain abscess; these include, in particular, *Cladophialophora bantiana, Bipolaris hawaiiensis, Bipolaris spicifera, Exophiala dermatitidis, Ochroconis gallopava, Ramichloridium mackenzei,* and *Curvularia pallescens.*

Protozoal and Helminthic Brain Abscess

Several protozoans and helminths have been reported to produce brain abscess.[1, 3, 62] These include *Trypanosoma cruzi*, *Entamoeba histolytica*, *Schistosoma* spp., and *Paragonimus* spp.[62–65] Neurocysticercosis, caused by the larval form of *Taenia solium*, is a major cause of brain lesions in the developing world.[66] The epidemiologic features and approach to diagnosis and management of these organisms are discussed in other chapters of this book.

Disease caused by *Toxoplasma gondii* is the most common protozoal cause of brain abscess. The incidence of human infection caused by *T. gondii* depends on dietary habits (especially the amount of meat consumed and whether eaten rare, raw, or well done), the number of stray cats living in close proximity to humans, climatic conditions (moderate temperatures and high humidity favor oocyst survival in soil), and the overall level of sanitation and hygiene.[67] *Toxoplasma gondii* can infect the CNS in a variety of syndromes but is usually associated with the development of intracerebral mass lesions or encephalitis in immunocompromised hosts. In the past, most cases of CNS toxoplasmosis occurred from reactivation of disease in patients with reticuloendothelial malignancies (either due to the malignancy itself or associated immunosuppressive or cytotoxic therapy), or in patients receiving immunosuppressive therapy after organ transplantation or for treatment of collagen vascular disorders.[67–73] Disease in organ transplant recipients not only occurs secondary to reactivation, but may occur after the transfer of infected cysts in the allograft, most commonly in heart transplant recipients.[71, 74, 75] The number of cases of CNS toxoplasmosis increased dramatically since 1981, specifically in patients with HIV infection.[76–79] The use of trimethoprim-sulfamethoxazole prophylaxis of *Pneumocystis carinii* pneumonia and highly active antiretroviral therapy has now decreased the incidence of *Toxoplasma* encephalitis substantially.

PATHOGENESIS AND PATHOPHYSIOLOGY

Pathogenesis

Microorganisms can reach the brain by several different mechanisms (see Table 74–1).[1, 3, 4, 5, 12, 14] The most common pathogenic mechanism of brain abscess formation is spread from a contiguous focus of infection, most often in the middle ear, mastoid cells, or paranasal sinuses. Brain abscess occurring secondary to otitis media is usually localized to the temporal lobe or cerebellum. Early studies reported that 40% of brain abscesses were associated with otitis media, but this number has been decreasing. However, if antimicrobial therapy of otitis is neglected, there is an increased risk of intracranial complications. Paranasal sinusitis continues to be an important condition predisposing to brain abscess. The frontal lobe is the predominant abscess site, although when brain abscess complicates sphenoid sinusitis, the temporal lobe or sella turcica is usually involved. Dental infections are a less common cause of brain abscess; infections of molar teeth seem most often to be the inciting factor. The frontal lobe is the usual site of the abscess after dental infection, but temporal lobe extension has also been reported.

A second mechanism of brain abscess formation is hematogenous dissemination to the brain from a distant focus of infection. These abscesses are usually multiple and multiloculated, and they have a higher mortality rate than abscesses that arise secondary to contiguous foci of infection.[3, 4] The most common sources of initial infection in adults are chronic pyogenic lung diseases, especially lung abscess, bronchiectasis, empyema, and cystic fibrosis. Brain abscess may also occur hematogenously from wound and skin infections, osteomyelitis, pelvic infection, cholecystitis, and other intra-abdominal infections. Another predisposing factor leading to hematogenously acquired brain abscess is cyanotic congenital heart disease,[80–82] accounting for about 5 to 15% of all brain abscess cases, with higher percentages in some pediatric series. These are most commonly seen in patients with tetralogy of Fallot or transposition of the great vessels. Brain abscess is rare after bacterial endocarditis (less than 5% of cases in most series),[83, 84] despite the presence of continuous bacteremia. Hereditary hemorrhagic telangiectasia is a predisposing factor for brain abscess and is almost always observed in those patients with coexisting pulmonary arteriovenous malformations, perhaps by allowing septic emboli to cross the pulmonary circulation without capillary filtration.[85–88] Brain abscesses have also developed after esophageal dilation or after sclerosing therapy for esophageal varices.[89, 90]

Trauma is a third pathogenic mechanism in the development of brain abscess, occurring secondary to an open cranial fracture with dural breach, following neurosurgery, or as a result of a foreign body injury.[91] The incidence of brain abscess formation after head trauma ranges from 3 to 17% in military populations, where it is usually secondary to retained bone fragments or contamination of initially "sterile" missile sites with bacteria from skin, clothes, and the environment.[92] Predisposing conditions in the civilian population include compound depressed skull fractures, dog bites, rooster pecking, and, especially in children, injury from lawn darts and pencil tips.[93, 94] Brain abscess is cryptogenic in about 20% of patients.

Initiation of Infection

There are few studies that have focused on the identification of the specific virulence factors of microorganisms that produce brain abscess. Contrary to common views, the brain may be more susceptible to infection than many other tissues. For example, compared with skin, the brain is significantly more susceptible to appropriate bacterial challenge. This was studied in a rat model of experimental brain abscess in which injections of 10^4 CFU of *S. aureus* or 10^6 CFU of *E. coli* failed to cause infection in the skin, whereas brain tissue was susceptible to as few as 10^2 CFU of either organism with resultant abscess formation.[95] The brain may also have differing susceptibility to infection by different organisms. In a rat model of experimental brain abscess, strains of *E. coli* were more virulent (i.e., leading to abscess formation at lower inocula) than either *Pseudomonas aeruginosa*, *S. aureus*, or *Streptococcus pyogenes*.[96] Furthermore, *E. coli* strains possessing the K1 antigen were more infective than K1-negative strains, indicating that certain encapsulated strains may be more virulent in the production of brain abscess. However, the role of capsule among other bacterial species in the pathogenesis of brain abscess has not been evaluated. The inoculation of *Bacteroides fragilis* or microaerophilic organisms such as *S. intermedius* into rat brain failed to produce infection and abscess formation, although these organisms account for a high percentage of isolates from brain abscess patients (see previous). This discrepancy may be explained because brain abscess is often a result of contiguous spread of chronic otitic or sinus infections, and the synergistic infectivity of mixed populations of anaerobes plus a facultative organism may be necessary to establish the disease.[97, 98] In an experimental dog model of brain abscess formation, the inoculation of *B. fragilis* in mixed culture with *Staphylococcus epidermidis* caused a virulent reaction,[99] although each organism was not tested separately.

The role of other bacterial virulence factors in brain abscess formation has not been evaluated. Despite extensive evidence implicating bacterial lipopolysaccharide in the pathogenesis of bacterial meningitis (see Chapter 71), similar studies on the effect, if any, of lipopolysaccharide on brain abscess formation and evolution are unavailable. *Bacteroides fragilis*, a major pathogen producing brain abscess, has a lipopolysaccharide that is chemically distinct from the lipopolysaccharide of aerobic gram-negative bacilli, but the biologic function of *B. fragilis* lipopolysaccharide is poorly defined and is unknown in the CNS.

An additional concern is the formation of brain abscesses in patients with bacterial meningitis. Brain abscess is a rare complication of bacterial meningitis with the exception of the high prevalence of abscess formation in neonates with *C. diversus* meningitis.[21, 22] In this disease, there is a propensity of contiguous inflammation in the cerebral white matter, which may reflect the effects of endotoxin on the small penetrating vessels in this area. This was examined in an infant rat model, in which infection was initiated with a high-grade bacteremia, followed by infiltration of the leptomeninges and the development of ventriculitis.[100] Brain abscesses in these animals were found exclusively in the periventricular white matter, apparently from disruption of the ventricular ependymal lining and direct extension of the infection into the parenchyma. The virulence factors responsible for the propensity of this organism to cause brain abscess are undefined, although a minor outer-membrane protein (32 kD) may be a marker for strains more likely to produce ventriculitis and brain abscess[101]; strains that lack the 32-kD outer-membrane protein cause more bacteremia, meningitis, and death. Other factors, such as fimbriation, biotype, and hemolysis did not correlate with CNS invasion.

Natural History of Infection

Several animal models have been used to examine the pathophysiologic consequences and temporal course of brain abscesses after the initiation of infection. A canine model was utilized to define the pathologic stages of brain abscess formation after the inoculation of α-hemolytic streptococci.[102] Based on detailed histologic evaluation, four stages of brain abscess evolution were defined: early cerebritis (days 1 to 3), late cerebritis (days 4 to 9), early capsule formation (days 10 to 13), and late capsule formation (day 14 and later after initial inoculation). Although these stages are somewhat arbitrary, they are useful in classification and comparisons of virulence between organisms in the production of brain abscess. The early cerebritis stage is characterized by an acute inflammatory infiltrate with visible bacteria on Gram stain and marked edema surrounding the lesion. The center of the lesion becomes necrotic during the late cerebritis stage, and macrophages and fibroblasts begin to invade the periphery. With early capsule formation, the necrotic center begins to decrease in size with simultaneous development of a collagenous capsule that is less prominent on the ventricular side of the lesion; cerebral edema also starts to regress during this stage. In this canine model, the collagen capsule was complete circumferentially by the end of the second week and then increased in density and thickness. Similar neuropathologic findings have been observed in a model of experimental anaerobic brain abscess,[99] although capsule formation could not be divided into early and late stages because of delayed encapsulation. A subsequent study revealed that *S. aureus* was more virulent than the α-hemolytic streptococci in brain abscess formation[103]; the amount of necrosis, the total area of involvement after staphylococcal challenge, the course of infection as it progressed toward resolution, the time for the abscess to reach a stable size, and the time to contain the necrotic region with a collagenous capsule were all longer after inoculation of *S. aureus*. Capsule formation was less prominent on the ventricular than on the cortical surface in these studies,[99, 102, 103] perhaps because differences in vascularity between cortical gray and white matter allowed greater fibroblast proliferation on the cortical side of the abscess. This may explain the tendency for brain abscesses to rupture into the ventricular system rather than into the subarachnoid space. An alternative hypothesis was supported in an experimental rat model after inoculation of *E. coli*.[104] It was suggested in this study that brain abscesses tended to rupture intraventricularly because the infectious process is directed along the major white matter tracts (areas of low tissue resistance) rather than as a result of asymmetric collagen deposition.

Host Defense Mechanisms

The brain is usually protected from infection by an intact blood-brain barrier. However, once brain infection is established, immune defenses are inadequate to control the infection. Because local opsonization is deficient, encapsulated bacteria such as *E. coli* and *B. fragilis* may escape efficient phagocytosis within the brain parenchyma. Several studies have shown that phagocytosis of *Bacteroides* spp. requires heat-labile serum factors (i.e., complement, lysozyme, or others),[105, 106] and these factors are likely absent, or at very low concentrations, even in the presence of CNS inflammation early in disease. In addition, an outer-membrane component of *Bacteroides* spp. may be important in the inhibition of neutrophil chemotaxis, thus reducing the host response to brain abscess associated with this organism.[107]

The host inflammatory response following the initiation of infection has been evaluated by serial pathologic analysis in several animal models of brain abscess formation.[99, 102, 103] During the early cerebritis stage, a border around the initial area of inoculation, composed of acute inflammatory cells, is observed and is accompanied by the rapid development of a perivascular infiltration consisting of neutrophils, plasma cells, and mononuclear cells. With progression to the late cerebritis stage, the acute inflammatory cells become mixed with macrophages and fibroblasts, and reticulin formation surrounds the necrotic center. As the capsule begins to form, increased numbers of fibroblasts and macrophages infiltrate the periphery, and mature collagen is deposited to form a capsule. With further encapsulation, the necrotic center continues to decrease in size while marked gliosis develops outside the capsule.

The importance of this host inflammatory response in containment of the brain abscess has been examined in immunosuppressed animals. Initial studies in the dog model of experimental brain abscess with *S. aureus* or *P. mirabilis* demonstrated that the administration of dexamethasone slowed, but did not fully impair, capsule formation.[108] In contrast, in another study no evidence of encapsulation was found when dexamethasone was given to rabbits at the same time as inoculation of either *S. pyogenes* or *S. aureus*.[109] In an experimental rat model of *E. coli* brain abscess, dexamethasone administration led to a reduction in the macrophage and glial response, collagen deposition, and host survival, with an increased number of viable bacteria in the brain abscess.[104] Coadministration of dexamethasone also impaired the lymphocytic and fibroblastic response in a rat model of experimental *S. aureus* brain abscess[110] but did not entirely halt the encapsulation or reduce the associated cerebral edema. Another study utilized dogs that were immunosuppressed with azathioprine and prednisone 7 days before the intracerebral inoculation of α-hemolytic streptococci.[111] The immunosuppressed animals manifested a decreased inflammatory response characterized by a reduction in neutrophils and macrophages in the lesion, a decrease and delay in collagen deposition, and persistence of viable organisms into the late capsule stage. Neutrophils, plasma cells, lymphocytes, and macrophages were markedly reduced in the areas surrounding the necrotic center of the abscess, and cerebritis was also decreased outside the developing capsule. Gliosis, however, was markedly increased in the area surrounding the collagen capsule in these immunosuppressed dogs. Although this decreased inflammatory response and edema formation resulted in less mass effect initially, the eventual size and area of the abscess may have become larger as a result of the diminished host response.

CLINICAL PRESENTATION

The clinical course of brain abscess may range from indolent to fulminant.[1, 3, 5, 7, 12, 14, 112] Most of the clinical manifestations (Table 74–2) are not due to the systemic signs of infection, but rather to the size and location of a space-occupying lesion within the brain and the virulence of the infecting microorganism. Headache is the most common presenting symptom and is observed in approximately 70% of patients. The headache may be moderate to severe and hemicranial or generalized in location but is without particularly distinguishing features, accounting for frequent delays in diagnosis. Sudden worsening of the headache, accompanied by a new onset of meningismus, may signify rupture of the abscess into the ventricular space[113]; this complication is often associated with a high mortality rate. Less than 50% of patients with brain abscess present with the classic triad of fever, headache, and focal neurologic deficit. In addition, the clinical presentation of brain abscess in the immunocompromised patient may be masked by the diminished inflammatory response.[34, 36]

The location of the brain abscess defines the clinical presentation.[3, 5, 12, 14] Patients with a frontal lobe abscess often present with headache, drowsiness, inattention, deterioration of mental status, hemiparesis with unilateral motor signs, and a motor speech disorder. The clinical presentation of cerebellar abscesses includes ataxia, nystagmus, vomiting, and dysmetria.[114] Temporal lobe abscesses may cause ipsilateral headache and aphasia if the lesion is in the dominant hemisphere; a visual field defect (e.g., an upper homonymous quadrantanopsia) may be the only presenting sign of a temporal lobe abscess. Abscesses of the brain stem usually present with facial weakness, fever, headache, hemiparesis, dysphagia, and vomiting.[115, 116] The classic findings of a well-defined brain stem syndrome may frequently be lacking in patients with brain stem abscesses because the abscess is likely to extend longitudinally along fiber tracts rather than expand transversely.[1]

TABLE 74–2 Common Symptoms and Signs in Brain Abscess

Symptom or Sign	Frequency (%)
Headache	~70
Mental status changes	≤70
Focal neurologic deficits	>60
Fever	45–50
Triad of headache, fever, and focal deficit	<50
Seizures	25–35
Nausea and vomiting	25–50
Nuchal rigidity	~25
Papilledema	~25

Certain pathogens may lead to the development of specific clinical characteristics after CNS infection. In patients with nocardial brain abscess, the presentation is generally nonspecific with fever, headache, and focal deficits determined by the site and size of the lesion.[24–30, 117] The clinical suspicion of nocardial brain abscess may be increased by the presence of pulmonary, skin, or muscle lesions, which are present concurrently in many, but not all, cases. All patients with pulmonary nocardiosis should undergo evaluation to exclude CNS disease.

Patients with *Aspergillus* brain abscess most commonly manifest signs of a stroke syndrome (secondary to ischemia or intracerebral hemorrhage, or both) referable to the involved area of brain.[38] Headache, encephalopathy, and seizures may also occur. Fever is not a consistent feature, and signs of meningeal irritation are rare. Patients who are severely immunocompromised usually present with nonspecific findings (i.e., alteration in mental status or seizures, or both) shortly before death, whereas those patients less immunocompromised are more likely to have headache and focal neurologic deficits.[42] Patients with *Aspergillus* brain abscess commonly have evidence of aspergillosis involving other organ systems.[44, 48, 118]

Rhinocerebral mucormycosis initially manifests with complaints referable to the eyes or sinuses including headache (often unilateral), facial pain, diplopia, lacrimation, and nasal stuffiness or epistaxis[38, 51, 52, 119]; fever is usual. As the infection spreads to contiguous structures, necrotic lesions appear in the turbinates, nose, paranasal skin or hard palate. Chemosis, proptosis, and external ophthalmoplegia may occur. Cranial nerve abnormalities are common (including cranial nerves II through VII, IX, and X), and blindness may occur as a result of invasion of the cavernous sinus, ophthalmic artery, and orbit. Thrombosis is a striking feature of this disease because the organism has a proclivity for blood vessel invasion. Focal neurologic deficits such as hemiparesis, seizures, or monocular blindness suggest far-advanced disease. With further progression, invasion of the internal carotid artery in the cavernous sinus can occur, accompanied by metastatic lesions in the frontoparietal cortex and deepening coma.[120] In patients with nonrhinocerebral brain abscess caused by the Mucorales, fever, headache, or focal neurologic deficits were present in more than half the patients. In one review of 22 cases,[53] 50% of the patients were injection drug users and the basal ganglia were the most commonly involved CNS site (83% of patients).

Brain abscess due to *P. boydii* tends to occur in immunocompromised patients or in patients 15 to 30 days after an episode of near-drowning.[59, 60] Brain abscesses can be located in the cerebrum, cerebellum, or brain stem; clinical presentations include seizures, altered consciousness, headache, meningeal irritation, focal neurologic deficits, abnormal behavior, and aphasia. The clinical manifestations of CNS disease caused by *Cryptococcus, Histoplasma, Coccidioides, Candida*, and other fungal pathogens depend on the intracranial location of the abscess. In one review, nearly one third of bone marrow transplant recipients with brain abscess caused by *Candida* spp. had no signs or symptoms[36]; these infections were commonly diagnosed postmortem.

The clinical manifestations of CNS toxoplasmosis in the immunocompromised patient may be variable, ranging from an insidious process evolving over several weeks to acute onset with a confusional state; the initial symptoms and signs may be focal, nonfocal, or both.[67] *Toxoplasma gondii* has a predilection to localize in the basal ganglia and brain stem, producing extrapyramidal symptoms resembling those of Parkinson's disease. Generally, patients who present with nonfocal abnormalities develop signs of focal neurologic disease as the infection progresses, although some patients develop a diffuse, rapidly fatal encephalopathic process. Nonfocal evidence of neurologic dysfunction may predominate and includes generalized weakness, headache, confusion, lethargy, alteration of mental status, personality changes, and coma. CNS toxoplasmosis may also present differently depending on the risk group. Infection in transplant recipients is often diffuse, disseminated disease.[69, 71, 72, 74, 75] Localizing neurologic signs tend to occur late in the course of infection in transplant recipients or not at all. In patients with underlying malignancies (e.g. Hodgkin's disease), the presentation of toxoplasmic encephalitis is evenly distributed between focal and nonfocal manifestations of encephalitis.[68–70] Patients with acquired immunodeficiency syndrome (AIDS) often present subacutely with nonspecific symptoms such as neuropsychiatric complaints, headache, disorientation, confusion, and lethargy progressing over 2 to 8 weeks; associated fever and weight loss are also common.[67, 76–79] Patients then develop clinical evidence of focal CNS mass lesions with ataxia, aphasia, hemiparesis, visual field loss, vomiting, or a more generalized encephalitis with increasing confusion, dementia, and stupor; seizures are common and may be the presenting clinical manifestation of CNS toxoplasmosis in patients with AIDS.

DIAGNOSIS

CT has revolutionized the diagnosis of brain abscess. Before the advent of CT, delays in diagnosis contributed significantly to the high morbidity and mortality in patients with brain abscess. CT has rendered diagnostic tests such as angiography, ventriculography, pneumoencephalography, and radionuclide brain scanning virtually obsolete[121]; therefore, these modalities will not be discussed here. CT is not only an excellent means of examination of the brain parenchyma but is superior to these standard radiographic procedures for examination of the paranasal sinuses, mastoids, and middle ear.[122, 123] The characteristic CT appearance of brain abscess is that of a hypodense center with a peripheral uniform ring enhancement following the injection of contrast material; this is surrounded by a variable hypodense area of brain edema (Fig. 74–1). Other CT findings include nodular enhancement and areas of low attenuation without enhancement, the latter of which is observed during the early cerebritis stage before abscess formation; as the abscess progresses, contrast enhancement is observed. Once the abscess becomes encapsulated in the later stages, contrast material no longer differentiates the lucent center and the CT appearance is similar to that of the early cerebritis stage. CT scanning is also useful for following the course of brain abscess, although after aspiration, improvement in the CT appearance may not be seen for up to 5 weeks or longer.

Magnetic resonance imaging (MRI) has been extensively evaluated in the diagnosis of brain abscess and is the first imaging choice in the evaluation of a patient suspected of having this disorder. MRI is more sensitive than CT and, therefore, offers significant advantages in the early detection of cerebritis, cerebral edema with greater contrast between edema and adjacent brain, more conspicuous spread of inflammation into the ventricles and subarachnoid space, and earlier detection of satellite lesions (Fig. 74–2).[124] On T_1-weighted images, the abscess capsule often appears as a discrete rim that is isointense to mildly hyperintense. Contrast enhancement with the paramagnetic agent gadolinium diethylenetriaminepentaacetic acid provides the added advantage of clearly differentiating the central abscess, surrounding enhancing rim, and cerebral edema surrounding the abscess. On T_1-weighted images, enhancement of the abscess capsule occurs. On T_2-weighted images, the zone of edema that surrounds the abscess is one of marked high signal intensity; the capsule now appears as a well-defined hypointense rim at the margin of the abscess. It is important to note that therapy with corticosteroids can decrease enhancement with both CT and MRI.

CT and MRI are also quite sensitive in defining the lesions in patients with fungal brain abscess; these modalities, however, are not specific, although some exceptions do exist. The finding of a cerebral infarct in a patient with risk factors for invasive aspergillosis should suggest that diagnosis.[38] The areas of infarction typically develop into either single or multiple abscesses involving the cerebrum (usually frontal or temporal lobes) or cerebellum. In patients with rhinocerebral mucormycosis, CT and MRI may show characteristic changes, including sinus opacification, erosion of bone, and obliteration of deep fascial planes.[125, 126] Frontal lobe involvement in mucormycosis may show little or no ring enhancement; the lack of contrast

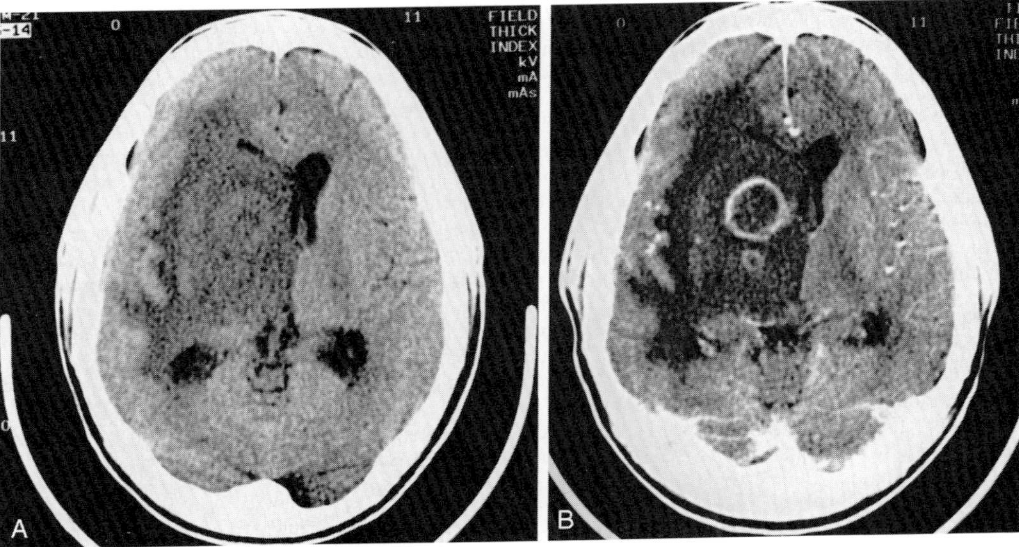

FIGURE 74–1. Computed tomography scan of the head revealing a large rounded area of low attenuation in the right lentiform nucleus with compression of the right horn of the right lateral ventricle and a shift to the left with vasogenic edema. *A*, Unenhanced scan reveals increased signal within the center of the area of low attenuation. *B*, Following the administration of intravenous contrast, there is ring enhancement of the abscess and evidence of a smaller satellite lesion.

enhancement is a poor prognostic sign as it indicates failure of host defense mechanisms to isolate or encapsulate the offending organism. Cavernous sinus involvement may be seen on MRI.

When CT or MRI is inconclusive in the diagnosis of brain abscess, radionuclide imaging may assist in clarifying the diagnosis. Leukocytes radiolabeled with ^{111}In will migrate to and accumulate in a focus of active inflammation and may assist in differentiating brain abscess from other mass lesions in the CNS. Two studies have demonstrated a diagnostic accuracy for brain abscess of 88 and 96% with the use of ^{111}In-labeled leukocytes,[127, 128] although it must be noted that necrotic tumors occasionally yield false-positive results and that the concomitant use of corticosteroids may produce false-negative scans in patients with abscesses. A second isotope, ^{99}Tc-hexamethylpropyleneamine oxime was evaluated in 23 patients with intracranial mass lesions and correctly identified all 10 confirmed cases of brain abscess[129]; no false-positive results were noted. Magnetic resonance spectroscopy, in combination with MRI, was useful in diagnosing two cases of bacterial brain abscess,[130] although further studies are needed to verify the diagnostic utility of this technique.

CT and MRI are both extremely useful in the diagnosis of CNS toxoplasmosis.[67, 77, 131, 132] The characteristic CT appearance (seen in 90% of patients) is that of rounded isodense or hypodense lesions with ring enhancement after the administration of contrast material; however, homogeneous enhancement or no enhancement can also be seen. There are multiple lesions in 70 to 80% of cases, often involving the corticomedullary junction and the basal ganglia, although any part of the CNS may be involved. Marked edema and a mass effect are also frequently observed. A double-dose delayed-contrast study may be a more sensitive method for delineating the true extent of disease.[133] Unfortunately, CT usually underestimates the number of lesions documented pathologically at autopsy.[76] MRI has a greater sensitivity than CT and has detected lesions in patients with active toxoplasmic encephalitis whose CT scans were normal. Therefore, MRI should be performed in AIDS patients with neurologic symp-

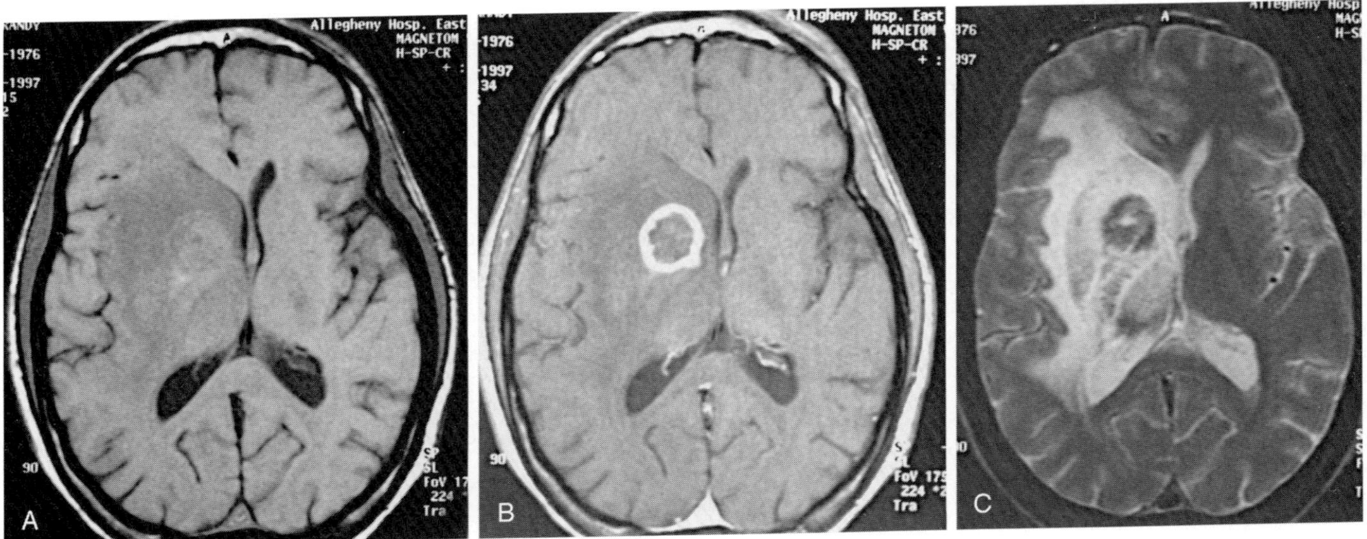

FIGURE 74–2. Magnetic resonance imagining of the brain (same patient as shown in Fig. 74–1) revealing a 2-cm, round ring-enhancing lesion in the right lentiform nucleus with associated vasogenic edema and midline shift to the left. *A*, T_1-weighted image reveals an ill-defined area of low attenuation. *B*, T_1-weighted image following administration of gadolinium, which reveals ring enhancement of the abscess. *C*, T_2-weighted image demonstrates hypointensity of the rim of the abscess with a large area of high signal intensity consistent with cerebral edema.

toms in whom CT shows no abnormality (or only cerebral atrophy). CT and MRI may also be useful in following the response to therapy, since most patients demonstrate radiographic evidence of improvement within 10 to 14 days of initiation of anti-*Toxoplasma* therapy.[79, 134]

In the immunosuppressed host with presumed toxoplasmic encephalitis, serologic testing is of value to aid in the diagnosis. For example, in AIDS patients, toxoplasmic encephalitis occurs as a result of a recrudescence of a latent infection.[76–79] In this situation, the presence of anti-*Toxoplasma* immunoglobulin G (IgG) antibody can almost uniformly be demonstrated before the development of the encephalitis. In AIDS patients, more than 97% of patients with toxoplasmic encephalitis have serum IgG antibody titers against *T. gondii* ranging from 1:8 to more than 1:1024[67]; the predictive value of a positive serologic result in patients with characteristic abnormalities on radiographic studies may be as high as 80% in the United States.[77, 135] In contrast, in a retrospective review of 115 patients with AIDS and CNS toxoplasmosis at San Francisco General Hospital between 1981 and 1990, 4 of 18 patients with pathologically confirmed disease had undetectable anti-*Toxoplasma* IgG antibody by an indirect immunofluorescence assay.[79] Despite these conflicting data, many physicians in the United States initiate a therapeutic trial of anti-*Toxoplasma* chemotherapy in an AIDS patient who is seropositive for *T. gondii* and has characteristic neuroradiographic abnormalities.[136] This is generally a valid approach in AIDS patients with presumed CNS toxoplasmosis (see Chapter 268).

A major advance in the use of CT scanning in patients with suspected brain abscess is the ability to perform stereotactic CT-guided aspiration to facilitate microbiologic diagnosis and guide antimicrobial therapy. Aspiration during the cerebritis stage, however, may be complicated by hemorrhage. At the time of aspiration, specimens should be sent for Gram stain, routine aerobic and anaerobic cultures, and cultures for mycobacteria and fungi. In addition, other special stains such as acid-fast stains for mycobacteria, modified acid-fast stains for *Nocardia,* and special stains (e.g., mucicarmine, methenamine silver) for fungi should be used to aid in making an etiologic diagnosis. For example, *Aspergillus* spp. manifest as septate hyphae in tissue sections with acute-angle, dichotomous branching. Biopsy of cerebral lesions in mucormycosis usually demonstrates irregular hyphae, right-angle branching, and a lack of septae. *Pseudallescheria boydii* hyphae cannot be distinguished reliably from *Aspergillus* spp.[59] In patients with CNS toxoplasmosis, diagnosis may require specialized immunohistochemical techniques (peroxidase-antiperoxidase) in order to detect the organisms or its antigens.[137] Pseudocysts and tachyzoites, which are easily identifiable by histopathologic stains, may not be found in the center of the necrotic lesion and are best identified at the periphery of the lesion or within normal brain tissue. A sensitive test for rapid diagnosis is the immunofluorescence technique, using monoclonal anti-*Toxoplasma* antibodies on brain touch preparations.[138]

INITIAL MANAGEMENT OF THE PATIENT WITH BRAIN ABSCESS

The initial approach to the patient with a suspected brain abscess is a multidisciplinary one and should include a neuroradiologist, neurosurgeon, and infectious diseases specialist. The following steps are a recommended approach to the patient with a suspected brain abscess[139]:

1. Contrast CT or MRI should be performed to verify the suspicion of brain abscess.
2. If single or multiple ring-enhancing lesions are found, the patient should be taken urgently to surgery. All lesions greater than 2.5 cm in diameter should be excised or stereotactically aspirated and specimens sent to the microbiology and pathology laboratories (see previous). For abscesses in the early cerebritis stage or when the abscesses are 2.5 cm in diameter or less, the largest lesion should be aspirated for diagnosis and organism identification.
3. Once abscess material has been obtained for microbiologic and histopathologic studies, empirical antimicrobial therapy should be initiated based on the patient's predisposing conditions and the presumed pathogenesis of abscess formation (Table 74–3). If a primary source of infection outside the CNS, which likely led to formation of the brain abscess, is identified, empirical antimicrobial therapy can be based on microbiologic studies from the other source (e.g., positive blood cultures in a patient with infective endocarditis).
4. Therapy with corticosteroids should be initiated in patients with significant edema and an associated mass effect causing increased intracranial pressure or a predisposition to transtentorial herniation. Phenytoin should be considered to prevent seizures during early stages of therapy.

The empirical approach to antimicrobial therapy for bacterial brain abscess should take into account the frequency of isolation of certain organisms.[3] Because of the high rate of isolation of streptococci (particularly the *S. intermedius [milleri]* group) from brain abscesses of various causes, high-dose intravenous penicillin G or another drug (e.g., a third-generation cephalosporin, either cefotaxime or ceftriaxone) active against this organism should be included in the initial therapeutic regimen. Penicillin G is also active against most anaerobic species with the notable exception of *B. fragilis,* which may be isolated in a high percentage of brain abscess cases; metronidazole should be included in the initial regimen when this organism is suspected. Metronidazole has bactericidal activity against *B. fragilis* and *Prevotella melaninogenica* and attains high concentrations in brain abscess pus, and its entry into cerebral abscesses is not affected by concomitant corticosteroid therapy.[140–142] When *S. aureus* is considered a likely pathogen (e.g., after cranial trauma or after neurosurgery), nafcillin should be used, with vancomyin reserved for patients allergic to penicillin or when methicillin-resistant organisms are suspected or isolated[143]; vancomycin should also be used in patients with abscesses after penetrating cranial trauma or recent neurosurgery. If *P. aeruginosa* is a likely infecting pathogen, ceftazidime is the agent of choice. In patients with a bacterial brain abscess of unclear pathogenesis, empirical therapy with vancomycin, metronidazole, and a third-generation cephalosporin (cefotaxime or ceftriaxone, or ceftazidime if *P. aeruginosa* is suspected) is recommended pending culture results.[144, 145]

In HIV-infected patients with CNS mass lesions, the initial approach to management is somewhat different because of the high likelihood of the diagnosis of toxoplasmic encephalitis.[77, 146] For patients with large lesions demonstrating a mass effect and threatening impending herniation, open biopsy with decompression is the standard. In HIV-infected patients with multiple ring-enhancing lesions on contrast CT or MRI and positive anti-*Toxoplasma* IgG serologic tests, empirical therapy for toxoplasmic encephalitis should

TABLE 74–3 Empirical Antimicrobial Therapy for Bacterial Brain Abscess

Predisposing Condition	Antimicrobial Regimen
Otitis media or mastoiditis	Metronidazole + a third-generation cephalosporin*
Sinusitis (frontoethmoid or sphenoid)	Metronidazole + a third-generation cephalosporin*,†
Dental sepsis	Penicillin + metronidazole
Penetrating trauma or postneurosurgical	Vancomycin + a third-generation cephalosporin*,‡
Lung abscess, empyema, bronchiectasis	Penicillin + metronidazole + a sulfonamide§
Bacterial endocarditis	Vancomycin + gentamicin or nafcillin + ampicillin + gentamicin
Congenital heart disease	Third-generation cephalosporin*
Unknown	Vancomycin + metronidazole + a third-generation cephalosporin*,‡

*Cefotaxime, ceftriaxone, or cefepime.
†Add vancomycin when infection caused by methicillin-resistant *Staphylococcus aureus* is suspected.
‡Use ceftazidime as the third-generation cephalosporin if *Pseudomonas aeruginosa* is suspected.
§Trimethoprim-sulfamethoxazole; include if a *Nocardia* spp. is suspected.

be initiated (Table 74–4); clinical and radiographic improvement should be observed within 10 to 14 days in patients with toxoplasmic encephalitis.[134] For patients with positive anti-*Toxoplasma* IgG serologic tests and a single lesion identified by MRI, consideration should be given to thallium-201 single photon emission computed tomography (^{201}Tl-SPECT) scanning. Although ^{201}T1-SPECT scans are not sensitive, positive scans are highly specific for the diagnosis of primary CNS lymphoma and would warrant stereotactic brain biopsy.[147–149] Similar results have been obtained with positron-emission tomography scanning employing ^{18}F-fluorodeoxyglucose (^{18}FDG-PET).[150, 151] In patients with mass lesions and negative anti-*Toxoplasma* IgG serologic tests, the diagnosis of toxoplasmic encephalitis is possible, but unlikely; scanning with ^{201}Tl-SPECT or ^{18}FDG-PET may also be helpful in this setting. Brain biopsy is optimal, although some experts have recommended an empirical trial of therapy for toxoplasmic encephalitis in patients with multiple ring-enhancing lesions even if the anti-*Toxoplasma* IgG serologic test is negative.[146] However, brain biopsy should be performed in patients who fail to respond. Patients with single lesions on MRI and negative serologic tests should undergo a stereotactic brain biopsy. A strategy for the management of suspected *Toxoplasma* CNS lesions in HIV-infected patients can be found in Chapter 268.

THERAPY

Once the infecting pathogen is isolated, antimicrobial therapy can be modified for optimal therapy. Our recommendations for standard therapy, with alternative agents, are shown in Table 74–4. Doses of these agents used for CNS infections are in Table 74–5. The following sections review the principles of use of antimicrobial and surgical therapy for bacterial and fungal brain abscesses. The therapeutic approach to toxoplasmic encephalitis is discussed in Chapter 268.

Bacterial Brain Abscess

Antimicrobial Therapy

Antimicrobial therapy for bacterial brain abscess should include agents that penetrate into the abscess cavity and have in vitro activity against the pathogens isolated.[1, 3–5, 152, 153] Few studies have addressed the penetration of antimicrobials into brain abscess fluid, and the published studies have included limited numbers of patients. Concentrations of penicillin G have been measured in brain abscess pus but were detected consistently only if the daily dosage in adults exceeded 24 million units; in some cases penicillin G may be inactivated in pus, and bacteria may still be cultured despite adequate penicillin concentrations.[154] Limited data are available on the penetration of the semisynthetic penicillins (e.g., nafcillin, oxacillin) into brain abscesses, although some studies suggest that concentrations of these drugs in brain abscess fluid are variable.[10] Metronidazole has excellent in vitro activity against strict anaerobes, making it an important agent for the therapy of patients with brain abscess.[140–142] Its excellent pharmacokinetic profile (i.e., good oral absorption and penetration into brain abscess cavities), has made metronidazole a more attractive antianaerobic agent than chloramphenicol for therapy of brain abscess. However, metronidazole must always be used in combination with an antimicrobial agent effective against streptococci, since polymicrobial infections are common in patients with brain abscesses. Vancomycin has also been shown to demonstrate excellent concentrations in brain abscess fluid (90% of serum concentrations) after prolonged therapy.[143]

The role of newer antimicrobial agents in the therapy of brain abscess is evolving. The third-generation cephalosporins are attractive agents for the therapy of brain abscess, given their good CNS penetration and excellent in vitro activity against many of the pathogens isolated from bacterial brain abscesses. When cefotaxime is

TABLE 74–4 Antimicrobial Therapy of Brain Abscess

Organism	Standard Therapy	Alternative Therapies
Bacteria		
Actinomyces spp.	Penicillin G	Clindamycin
Bacteroides fragilis	Metronidazole	Clindamycin
Enterobacteriaceae	Third-generation cephalosporin*	Aztreonam, trimethoprim-sulfamethoxazole, fluoroquinolone, meropenem
Fusobacterium spp.	Penicillin G	Metronidazole
Haemophilus spp.	Third-generation cephalosporin*	Aztreonam, trimethoprim-sulfamethoxazole
Listeria monocytogenes	Ampicillin or penicillin G†	Trimethoprim-sulfamethoxazole
Mycobacterium tuberculosis	Isoniazid + rifampin + pyrazinamide ± ethambutol	
Nocardia spp.	Trimethoprim-sulfamethoxazole or sulfadiazine	Minocycline, imipenem, a third-generation cephalosporin,* amikacin
Prevotella melaninogenica	Metronidazole	Clindamycin, cefotaxime
Pseudomonas aeruginosa	Ceftazidime†	Aztreonam,† fluoroquinolone,† meropenem†
Staphylococcus aureus		
Methicillin-sensitive	Nafcillin or oxacillin	Vancomycin
Methicillin-resistant	Vancomycin	
Streptococcus intermedius group (*milleri*), other streptococci	Penicillin G	Third-generation cephalosporin,* vancomycin
Fungi		
Aspergillus spp.	Amphotericin B‡	Itraconazole,§ amphotericin B lipid complex, liposomal amphotericin B
Candida spp.	Amphotericin B‡	Fluconazole, liposomal amphotericin B,§ amphotericin B lipid complex§
Cryptococcus neoformans	Amphotericin B‡	Fluconazole, liposomal amphotericin B,§ amphotericin B lipid complex§
Mucorales	Amphotericin B	Liposomal amphotericin B,§ amphotericin B lipid complex§
Pseudallescheria boydii	Miconazole	Itraconazole§
Protozoa		
Toxoplasma gondii	Pyrimethamine + sulfadiazine	Pyrimethamine + clindamycin; pyrimethamine + azithromycin, clarithromycin, atovaquone, or dapsone

*Cefotaxime, ceftriaxone, or cefepime.
†Addition of an aminoglycoside should be considered.
‡Addition of flucytosine should be considered.
§Efficacy not yet proved in brain abscess caused by this organism.

TABLE 74–5 Recommended Dosages of Antimicrobial Agents for Central Nervous System Infections in Adults*

Antimicrobial Agent	Total Daily Dosage	Dosing Interval (hs)
Amikacin†	15 mg/kg	8
Amphotericin B	0.6–1.0 mg/kg‡	24
Amphotericin B lipid complex	5 mg/kg	24
Ampicillin	12 g	4
Atovaquone	3000 mg	6
Azithromycin	1200–1500 mg	24
Aztreonam	6–8 g	6–8
Cefepime	4–6 g	8–12
Cefotaxime	8–12 g	4–6
Ceftazidime	6 g	8
Ceftriaxone	4 g	12
Chloramphenicol	4–6 g	6
Ciprofloxacin	800 mg	12
Clindamycin	1200–4800 mg§	6
Dapsone‖	100 mg	24
Ethambutol‖	15 mg/kg	24
Fluconazole	400–800 mg	24
Flucytosine‖	150 mg/kg	6
Gentamicin†	3–5 mg/kg	8
Imipenem	2 g	6
Isoniazid‖	300 mg	24
Itraconazole	800 mg	12
Liposomal amphotericin B (AmBisome)	3–5 mg/kg	24
Meropenem	6 g	8
Metronidazole	30 mg/kg	6
Miconazole	1.5–3 g	8
Nafcillin	9–12 g	4
Oxacillin	9–12 g	4
Penicillin	24 million units	4
Pyrazinamide‖	15–30 mg/kg	24
Pyrimethamine‖	50–75 mg§	24
Rifampin‖	600 mg	24
Sulfadiazine‖	4–6 g	6
Tobramycin‖	3–5 mg/kg	8
Trimethoprim-sulfamethoxazole	10–20 mg/kg¶	6–12
Vancomycin†	2–3 g	8–12

*Patients with normal renal and hepatic function. Unless indicated, the intravenous mode of administration is used.

†Need to monitor peak and trough serum concentrations.

‡Dosages up to 1.5 mg/kg/day may be used for aspergillosis or mucormycosis.

§Higher dosages utilized in acquired immunodeficiency syndrome patients with toxoplasmic encephalitis.

‖Dosage for oral administration.

¶Dosage based on trimethoprim component; higher dose utilized for *Nocardia* brain abscess.

given in high doses (3 g every 8 hours), brain abscess concentrations of cefotaxime and its active metabolite, desacetylcefotaxime, were above the minimal inhibitory concentrations of the majority of gram-positive and gram-negative organisms against which cefotaxime is used systemically.[145] When combined with metronidazole and used in conjunction with surgical excision, high doses of cefotaxime have also been effective clinically in the treatment of brain abscess.[155] Ceftriaxone, ceftizoxime, and ceftazidime have all been used in the treatment of brain abscess,[156, 157] although only a small number of patients have been studied. Moxalactam has been found to be efficacious in the treatment of brain abscess with good concentrations found in abscess fluid[158]; however, the potential for vitamin K–related bleeding disorders with the use of moxalactam limits the therapeutic usefulness of this agent. Ampicillin-sulbactam has also demonstrated therapeutic success in patients with brain abscesses[159]; intracavitary concentrations were variable, but adequate, in most cases.

Imipenem has been used successfully for the treatment of pyogenic and nocardial brain abscesses,[160, 161] although the use of imipenem has been associated with an increased risk of seizures, limiting its usefulness in patients with CNS mass lesions. Meropenem, a carbapenem antimicrobial agent similar to imipenem, was successful in one case of an *Enterobacter cloacae* brain abscess,[162] suggesting that this agent may be useful in brain abscess cases, especially when caused by resistant pathogens. The fluoroquinolones have good CNS penetration and have been used anecdotally in the treatment of brain abscess patients.[163] Data are inadequate to recommend any fluoroquinolone for the therapy of brain abscess.

Antimicrobial therapy with high-dose intravenous antibiotics has traditionally been administered for 6 to 8 weeks in patients with bacterial brain abscesses.[1] This is often followed by oral antibiotic therapy for 2 to 6 months if an appropriate agent or agents are available, although the efficacy and necessity of this approach has not been established. Shorter courses (3 to 4 weeks) of antimicrobial therapy may be adequate for patients who have undergone surgical excision of the abscess. Surgical therapy (i.e., excision or aspiration) is often required for the optimal management of brain abscess (see later), although certain subsets of patients may be treated with antimicrobial therapy alone.[116, 164–166] These are patients with medical conditions that increase the risk of surgery, multiple abscesses, abscesses in a deep or dominant location, concomitant meningitis or ependymitis, early abscess reduction with clinical improvement after antimicrobial therapy, and abscess size under 3 cm. However, in one series, no abscess larger than 2.5 cm resolved without surgical therapy.[164] Furthermore, patients treated with antimicrobial therapy alone may require prolonged (up to 12 weeks) courses of parenteral treatment, and must receive careful clinical and radiographic follow-up.

When a brain abscess due to *Nocardia* is suspected or proved, the sulfonamides, with or without trimethoprim, are recommended as first-line therapy,[167, 168] although treatment failures have been reported.[169] Alternative agents include minocycline, amikacin, imipenem, the third-generation cephalosporins, and the fluoroquinolones, which are among the most active agents against *Nocardia* in vitro.[170, 171] However, in vitro activity may not always correlate with clinical efficacy.[172] Combination therapies have been studied,[173–177] and combination regimens containing the third-generation cephalosporins or imipenem along with a sulfonamide should be considered for immunocompromised patients or those in whom therapy fails.[1] The duration of antimicrobial therapy for nocardial brain abscess has ranged from 3 to 12 months.[26, 178] However, therapy in immunosuppressed patients should probably be continued for up to 1 year,[117] with careful follow-up to monitor for relapse.

Surgical Therapy

Most patients with bacterial brain abscess require surgical management for optimal therapy. The two procedures available are aspiration of the abscess after burr hole placement and complete excision after craniotomy.[13, 14, 179] No prospective trial comparing the two procedures has ever been performed. Therefore, the choice of procedure must be individualized for each patient. Aspiration may be performed by a stereotactic procedure utilizing CT or MRI guidance, which affords the surgeon rapid, accurate, and safe access to virtually any intracranial point, including those areas located in deep critical regions of the CNS (e.g., brain stem, cerebellum, or diencephalic structures adjacent to the ventricles)[157, 180–187]; aspiration can also be used for swift relief of increased intracranial pressure.

Complete excision by craniotomy is now infrequently performed because of the development of the aspiration and closed drainage techniques described previously but may be required in patients with multiloculated abscesses (for whom aspiration techniques have failed) or for abscesses that fail to resolve. Craniotomy with total excision is difficult in cases of nocardial brain abscess, because these abscesses are usually multilocated.[117]

Fungal Brain Abscess

The optimal therapy of fungal brain abscesses usually requires a combined medical and surgical approach; surgery includes either excision or drainage of the abscess. However, therapy of fungal brain abscess in immunocompromised patients carries a high mortality rate despite surgery and antifungal therapy. Nevertheless, early recognition of this infection can lead to a successful outcome, especially if leukocyte counts return to normal or if the dosages of immunosuppressive agents can be reduced.[1] The mainstay of medical therapy for candidal brain abscess is amphotericin B plus 5-flucytosine. The efficacy of fluconazole in the therapy of *Candida* brain abscess has not been evaluated, although one case report in a premature infant with *C. albicans* brain abscess demonstrated a decrease in abscess size after the addition of fluconazole to amphotericin B plus 5-flucytosine.[188]

The antifungal therapy of choice for *Aspergillus* brain abscess is amphotericin B deoxycholate (0.8 to 1.25 mg/kg/day); doses up to 1.5 mg/kg/day can be used depending on the clinical response.[189] However, few instances of survival have been recorded in CNS aspergillosis despite the administration of this agent.[45, 46] Most patients have required a total of more than 3 g of amphotericin B for eradication of CNS disease. Concomitant therapy with 5-flucytosine or rifampin has been tried, although no controlled trials have been performed to examine the efficacy of this approach. A literature review suggested that success rates in CNS aspergillosis may be greater with the addition of 5-flucytosine to amphotericin B.[189] Itraconazole has in vitro activity against *Aspergillus*,[190] and high-dose therapy (800 mg daily for 5 months followed by 400 mg daily for 4.5 months) resulted in complete resolution of cerebral abscesses caused by *Aspergillus fumigatus* in an elderly asthmatic patient who was treated with corticosteroids.[191] Despite this and a few other case reports of the successful use of high-dose itraconazole, the unreliable absorption and very modest reported experience in *Aspergillus* brain abscess makes itraconazole more promising as an extension of successful therapy than as primary therapy. Excisional surgery or drainage was a key factor in the successful management of several cases of CNS aspergillosis.[47, 192–194] Mucormycosis should also be treated with amphotericin B, along with correction of underlying metabolic derangements and aggressive surgical débridement.[38, 51, 52, 195] The role of surgery in the treatment of cerebral mucormycosis cannot be overemphasized. Because of their propensity to invade blood vessels, the Mucorales cause extensive tissue infarction, thereby impairing the delivery of antifungal agents to the site of infection. This often leaves surgery as the only modality that may effectively eliminate the invading microorganisms. Hyperbaric oxygen therapy has been reported to be a useful adjunct in cerebral mucormycosis,[196, 197] although no prospective, controlled trials have been performed to adequately assess its efficacy.

For *P. boydii* brain abscess, surgical drainage is the cornerstone of effective therapy.[59] The organism demonstrates in vitro resistance to amphotericin B; the antifungal treatment of choice is intravenous miconazole.[59, 60, 198, 199] Failures and relapses are common, and few hospitals stock the drug.[38] Despite the report of partial response to fluconazole (600 to 800 mg/day), activity of this azole against molds has been modest or nonexistent.[200] Itraconazole has been used successfully to treat pulmonary infection,[201] but its efficacy in CNS disease is unknown. Itraconazole oral suspension has better absorption than the capsules and is probably the de facto drug of choice. Saperconazole, an investigational azole, resulted in failure when combined with surgical drainage and intensive methods to lower intracranial pressure in one case report.[202]

The addition of granulocyte or macrophage colony-stimulating factors, which enhanced neutrophil-mediated killing of fungi in vitro,[203, 204] may deserve study in fungal brain abscess. Administration of these agents may be considered in patients who fail conventional therapy.

REFERENCES

1. Mathisen GE, Johnson JP. Brain abscess. Clin Infect Dis. 1997;25:763–781.
2. Canale DJ. William Macewen and the treatment of brain abscesses: Revisited after one hundred years. J Neurosurg. 1996;84:133–142.
3. Wispelwey B, Dacey RG Jr, Scheld WM. Brain abscess. In: Scheld WM, Whitley RJ, Durack DT, eds. Infections of the Central Nervous System. 2nd ed. Philadelphia: Lippincott-Raven; 1997:463–493.
4. Heilpern KL, Lorber B. Focal intracranial infections. Infect Dis Clin North Am. 1996;10:879–898.
5. Kaplan K. Brain abscess. Med Clin North Am. 1985;69:345–360.
6. Rosenblum ML, Joff JT, Norman D, et al. Decreased mortality from brain abscesses since advent of computerized tomography. J Neurosurg. 1978;49:658–668.
7. Seydoux C, Francioli P. Bacterial brain abscess: Factors influencing mortality and sequelae. Clin Infect Dis. 1992;15:394–401.
8. Murray HW, Gross KC, Masur H, et al. Serious infections caused by *Streptococcus milleri*. Am J Med. 1978;64:759–764.
9. Shlaes DM, Lerner PI, Wolinsky E, et al. Infections due to Lancefield group F and related streptococci (*S. milleri, S. anginosus*). Medicine. 1981;60:197–207.
10. De Louvois J, Gortvai P, Hurley R. Bacteriology of abscesses of the central nervous system. A multicentre prospective study. BMJ. 1977;2:981–984.
11. De Louvois J: The bacteriology and chemotherapy of brain abscess. J Antimicrob Chemother. 1978;4:395–413.
12. Yang SY. Brain abscess: A review of 400 cases. J Neurosurg. 1981;55:794–799.
13. Mampalam TJ, Rosenblum ML. Trends in the management of bacterial brain abscesses: A review of 102 cases over 17 years. Neurosurgery. 1988;23:451–458.
14. Chun CH, Johnson JD, Hofstetter M, et al. Brain abscess. A study of 45 consecutive cases. Medicine. 1986;65:415–431.
15. Lechtenberg R, Sierra MF, Pringle GF, et al. *Listeria monocytogenes:* Brain abscess or meningoencephalitis? Neurology. 1979;29:86–90.
16. Nieman RE, Lorber B. Listeriosis in adults: A changing pattern. Report of eight cases and review of the literature. Rev Infect Dis. 1980;2:207–227.
17. Berenguer J, Solera J, Diaz MD, et al. Listeriosis in patients infected with human immunodeficiency virus. Rev Infect Dis. 1991;13:115–119.
18. Grigoriadis E, Gold WL. Pyogenic brain abscess caused by *Streptococcus pneumoniae*: Case report and review. Clin Infect Dis. 1997;25:1108–1112.
19. Renier D, Flandin C, Hirsch E, Hirsch JF. Brain abscesses in neonates: A study of 30 cases. J Neurosurg. 1988;69:877–882.
20. Ries M, Deeg KH, Heininger U, Stehr K. Brain abscess in neonates—report of three cases. Eur J Pediatr. 1993;152:745–746.
21. Kline MW. *Citrobacter* meningitis and brain abscess in infancy: Epidemiology, pathogenesis, and treatment. J Pediatr. 1988;113:430–434.
22. Morgan MG, Stuart C, Leonard AT, Enright M, Cole GF. *Citrobacter diversus* brain abscess: Case reports and molecular epidemiology. J Med Microbiol. 1992;36:273–278.
23. Smego RA Jr, Foglia G. Actinomycosis. Clin Infect Dis. 1998;26:1255–1263.
24. Curry WA. Human nocardiosis. A clinical review with selected case reports. Arch Intern Med. 1980;140:818–826.
25. Wilson JP, Turner HR, Kirchner KA, et al. Nocardial infections in renal transplant recipients. Medicine. 1989;68:38–57.
26. Berkey P, Bodey GP. Nocardial infection in patients with neoplastic disease. Rev Infect Dis. 1989;11:407–412.
27. Holtz HA, Lavery DP, Kapila R. Actinomycetales infection in the acquired immunodeficiency syndrome. Ann Intern Med. 1985;102:203–205.
28. Kim J, Minamoto GY, Grieco MH. Nocardial infection as a complication of AIDS: Report of six cases and review. Rev Infect Dis. 1991;13:624–629.
29. Lerner PI. Nocardiosis. Clin Infect Dis. 1996;22:891–905.
30. Braun TI, Kerson LA, Eisenberg FP. Nocardial brain abscesses in a pregnant woman. Rev Infect Dis. 1991;13:630–632.
31. Farrar DJ, Flanigan TP, Gordon NM, et al. Tuberculous brain abscess in a patient with HIV infection: Case report and review. Am J Med. 1997;102:297–301.
32. Gordon SM, Blumberg HM. *Mycobacterium kansasii* brain abscess in a patient with AIDS. Clin Infect Dis. 1992;14:789–790.
33. Monno L, Carbonara S, Costa D, et al. Cerebral lesions in two patients with AIDS: The possible role of *Mycobacterium kansasii*. Clin Infect Dis. 1996;22:1130–1131.
34. Salaki JS, Louria DB, Chmel H. Fungal and yeast infections of the central nervous system: A clinical review. Medicine. 1984;63:108–132.
35. Burgert SJ, Classen DC, Burke JP, Blatter DD. Candidal brain abscess associated with vascular invasion: A devastating complication of vascular catheter-related candidemia. Clin Infect Dis. 1995;21:202–205.
36. Hagensee ME, Bauwens JE, Kjos B, Bowden RA. Brain abscess following marrow transplantation: Experience at the Fred Hutchinson Cancer Center, 1984–1992. Clin Infect Dis. 1994;19:402–408.
37. Selby R, Ramirez CB, Singh R, et al. Brain abscess in solid organ transplant recipients receiving cyclosporine-based immunosuppression. Arch Surg. 1997;132:304–310.
38. Sepkowitz K, Armstrong D. Space-occupying fungal lesions. In: Scheld WM, Whitley RJ, Durack DT, eds. Infections of the Central Nervous System. 2nd ed. Philadelphia: Lippincott-Raven; 1997:741–762.
39. Parker JC Jr, McCloskey JJ, Lee RS. The emergence of candidosis: The dominant postmortem cerebral mycosis. Am J Clin Pathol. 1978;70:31–36.
40. Lipton SA, Hickey WF, Morris JH, et al. Candidal infection in the central nervous system. Am J Med. 1984;76:101–108.
41. Walsh TJ, Hier DB, Caplan LP. Fungal infections of the central nervous system: Comparative analysis of risk factors and clinical signs in 57 patients. Neurology. 1985;35:1654–1657.
42. Denning DW. Invasive aspergillosis. Clin Infect Dis. 1998;26:781–805.
43. Young RC, Bennett JE, Vogel CL, et al. Aspergillosis: The spectrum of the disease in 98 patients. Medicine. 1970;49:147–173.
44. Meyer RD, Young LS, Armstrong D, et al. Aspergillosis complicating neoplastic disease. Am J Med. 1973;54:6–15.
45. Weiland D, Ferguson RM, Peterson PK, et al. Aspergillosis in 25 renal transplant patients. Epidemiology, clinical presentation, diagnosis, and management. Ann Surg. 1983;198:622–629.

46. Britt RH, Enzmann DR, Remington JS. Intracranial infection in cardiac transplant recipients. Ann Neurol. 1981;9:107–119.
47. Green M, Wald ER, Tzakis A, et al. Aspergillosis of the CNS in a pediatric liver transplant recipient: Case report and review. Rev Infect Dis. 1991;13:653–657.
48. Beal MF, O'Carroll P, Kleinman GM, et al. Aspergillosis of the nervous system. Neurology. 1982;32:473–479.
49. Minamoto GY, Barlam TF, Vander Els NJ. Invasive aspergillosis in patients with AIDS. Clin Infect Dis. 1992;14:66–74.
50. McNulty JS. Rhinocerebral mucormycosis: Predisposing factors. Laryngoscope. 1982;92:1140–1143.
51. Parfrey NZ. Improved diagnosis and prognosis of mucormycosis. Medicine. 1986;65:113–123.
52. Morduchowicz G, Shmueli D, Shapira Z, et al. Rhinocerebral mucormycosis in renal transplant recipients. Rev Infect Dis. 1986;8:441–446.
53. Stave GM, Heimberger T, Kerkering TM. Zygomycosis of the basal ganglia in intravenous drug users. Am J Med. 1989;86:115–117.
54. Daly AL, Velazquez LA, Bradley SF, et al. Mucormycosis: Association with deferoxamine therapy. Am J Med. 1989;87:468–471.
55. Sugar AM. Mucormycosis. Clin Infect Dis. 1992;14:S126–S129.
56. Rinaldi MG. Zygomycosis. Infect Dis Clin North Am. 1989;3:19–41.
57. Fry VG, Young CN. A rare fungal brain abscess in an uncompromised host. Surg Neurol. 1981;15:446–448.
58. Travis LB, Roberts GD, Wilson WR. Clinical significance of *Pseudallescheria boydii:* A review of ten years' experience. Mayo Clin Proc. 1985;60:531–537.
59. Berenguer J, Diaz-Mediavilla J, Urra D, et al. Central nervous system infection caused by *Pseudallescheria boydii.* Rev Infect Dis. 1989;11:890–896.
60. Dworzack DL, Clark RB, Borkowski WJ, et al. *Pseudallescheria boydii* brain abscess: Association with near-drowning and efficacy of high-dose, prolonged miconazole therapy in patients with multiple abscesses. Medicine. 1989;68:218–224.
61. Kershaw P, Freeman R, Templeton D, et al. *Pseudallescheria boydii* infection of the central nervous system. Arch Neurol. 1990;47:468–472.
62. Bia FJ, Barry M. Parasitic infections of the central nervous system. Neurol Clin. 1986;4:171–206.
63. Solari A, Saavefra H, Sepulveda G, et al. Successful treatment of *Trypanosoma cruzi* encephalitis in a patient with hemophilia and AIDS. Clin Infect Dis. 1993;16:255–259.
64. Ohnishi K, Murata M, Kojima H, et al. Brain abscess due to infection with *Entamoeba histolytica.* Am J Trop Med Hyg. 1994;51:180–182.
65. Campbell S. Amebic brain abscess and meningoencephalitis. Semin Neurol. 1993;13:153–160.
66. White AC Jr. Neurocysticercosis: A major cause of neurological disease worldwide. Clin Infect Dis. 1997;24:101–115.
67. Dukes CS, Luft BJ, Durack DT. Toxoplasmosis of the central nervous system. In: Scheld WM, Whitley RJ, Durack DT, eds. Infections of the Central Nervous System. 2nd ed. Philadelphia: Lippincott-Raven; 1997:785–806.
68. Carey RM, Kimball AC, Armstrong D, et al. Toxoplasmosis. Clinical experiences in a cancer hospital. Am J Med. 1973;54:30–38.
69. Ruskin J, Remington JS. Toxoplasmosis in the compromised host. Ann Intern Med. 1976;84:193–199.
70. Hakes TB, Armstrong D. Toxoplasmosis. Problems in diagnosis and treatment. Cancer. 1983;52:1535–1540.
71. Hakim M, Esmore D, Wallwork J, et al. Toxoplasmosis in cardiac transplantation. BMJ. 1986;292:1108.
72. Reynolds ES, Walls KW, Pfeiffer RI. Generalized toxoplasmosis following renal transplantation. Arch Intern Med. 1966;118:401–405.
73. Deleze M, Mintz G, Carmen Majia MD. *Toxoplasma gondii* encephalitis in systemic lupus erythematosus, a neglected cause of treatable nervous system infection. J Rheumatol. 1985;12:994–996.
74. Luft BJ, Naot Y, Araujo FG, et al. Primary and reactivated *Toxoplasma* infection in patients with cardiac transplants. Ann Intern Med. 1983;99:27–31.
75. Nagington J, Martin AL. Toxoplasmosis and heart transplantation. Lancet. 1983;2:679.
76. Navia BA, Petito CK, Gold JWM, et al. Cerebral toxoplasmosis complicating the acquired immune deficiency syndrome: Clinical and neuropathological findings in 27 patients. Ann Neurol. 1986;19:224–238.
77. Luft BJ, Remington JS. Toxoplasmic encephalitis in AIDS. Clin Infect Dis. 1992;15:211–222.
78. Renold C, Sugar A, Chave JP, et al. *Toxoplasma* encephalitis in patients with acquired immunodeficiency syndrome. Medicine. 1992;71:224–239.
79. Porter SB, Sande MA. Toxoplasmosis of the central nervous system in the acquired immunodeficiency syndrome. N Engl J Med. 1992;327:1643–1648.
80. Yang SY. Brain abscess associated with congenital heart disease. Surg Neurol. 1989;31:129–132.
81. Park SC, Neeches WH. The neurologic complications of congenital heart disease. Neurol Clin. 1993;11:441–462.
82. Takeshita M, Kagawa M, Yato S, et al. Current treatment of brain abscess in patients with congenital cyanotic heart disease. Neurosurgery. 1997;41:1270–1279.
83. Pruitt AA, Rubin RHJ, Karchmer AW, Duncan GW. Neurologic complications of bacterial endocarditis. Medicine. 1978;57:329–343.
84. Tunkel AR, Kaye D. Neurologic complications of infective endocarditis. Neurol Clin. 1993;11:419–440.
85. Press OW, Ramsey PG. Central nervous system infections associated with hereditary hemorrhagic telangiectasia. Am J Med. 1984;77:86–92.
86. Gelfand MS, Stephens DS, Howell EI, et al. Brain abscess: Association with pulmonary arteriovenous fistula and hereditary hemorrhagic telangiectasia. Report of three cases. Am J Med. 1988;85:718–720.
87. Walder LA, Anastasia LF, Spodick DH. Pulmonary arteriovenous malformations with brain abscess. Am Heart J. 1994;127:227–232.
88. Thurnheer R, Vernazza PL, Galeazzi RL. Recurrent brain abscesses in an HIV-positive patient with hereditary hemorrhagic telangiectasia and arteriovenous malformation of the lung. Eur J Clin Microbiol Infect Dis. 1996;15:407–410.
89. Kuman P, Mehta SK, Deri BI, et al. Pyogenic meningitis and cerebral abscesses after endoscopic injection sclerotherapy. Am J Gastroenterol. 1991;86:1672–1674.
90. Algood L, Boon P, DeVos M, et al. Brain abscess after esophageal dilatation for stenosis. Clin Neurol Neurosurg. 1992;94:169–172.
91. Tunkel AR, Scheld WM. Acute infectious complications of head injury. In: Handbook of Clinical Neurology, v. 57: Head Injury. Amsterdam: Elsevier Science; 1990:317–326.
92. Rish BL, Careness WF, Dillon JD, et al. Analysis of brain abscess after penetrating craniocerebral injuries in Vietnam. Neurosurgery. 1981;9:535–541.
93. Foy P, Schair M. Cerebral abscesses in children after pencil tip injuries. Lancet. 1980;2:662–663.
94. Tay JS, Garland JS. Serious head injuries from lawn darts. Pediatrics. 1987;79:260–263.
95. Mendes M, Moore P, Wheeler CB, et al. Susceptibility of brain and skin to bacterial challenge. J Neurosurg. 1980;52:772–775.
96. Costello GT, Heppe R, Winn HR, et al. Susceptibility of brain to aerobic, anaerobic, and fungal organisms. Infect Immun. 1983;41:535–539.
97. Onderonk AB, Kasper DL, Cisneros RL, Bartlett JG. The capsular polysaccharide of *Bacteroides fragilis* as a virulence factor: Comparison of the pathogenic potential of encapsulated and unencapsulated strains. J Infect Dis. 1977;136:82–89.
98. Onderonk AB, Kasper DL, Mansheim BJ, et al. Experimental animal models for anaerobic infections. Rev Infect Dis. 1979;1:291–301.
99. Britt RH, Enzmann DR, Placone RC Jr, et al. Experimental anaerobic brain abscess. Computerized tomographic and neuropathological correlations. J Neurosurg. 1984;60:1148–1159.
100. Kline MW, Kaplan SL, Hawkins EP, Mason EO Jr. Pathogenesis of brain abscess formation in an infant rat model of *Citrobacter diversus* bacteremia and meningitis. J Infect Dis. 1988;157:106–112.
101. Kline MW, Mason EO Jr, Kaplan SL. Characterization of *Citrobacter diversus* strains causing neonatal meningitis. J Infect Dis. 1988;157:101–105.
102. Britt RH, Enzmann DR, Yeager AS. Neuropathological and computerized tomographic findings in experimental brain abscess. J Neurosurg. 1981;55:590–603.
103. Enzmann DR, Britt RR, Obana WG, et al. Experimental *Staphylococcus aureus* brain abscess. Am J Neuroradiol. 1986;7:395–402.
104. Neuwelt EA, Lawrence MS, Blank NK. Effect of gentamicin and dexamethasone on the natural history of the rat *Escherichia coli* brain abscess model with histopathological correlation. Neurosurgery. 1984;15:475–483.
105. Casciato DA, Rosenblatt JE, Goldberg LS, Bluestone R. In vitro interaction of *Bacteroides fragilis* with polymorphonuclear leukocytes and serum factors. Infect Immun. 1975;11:337–342.
106. Ingham HR, Sisson PR, Middleton RL, et al. Phagocytosis and killing of bacteria in aerobic and anaerobic conditions. Med Microbiol. 1981;14:391–399.
107. Adamu SA, Sperry JF. Polymorphonuclear neutrophil chemotaxis induced and inhibited by *Bacteroides* spp. Infect Immun. 1981;33:806–810.
108. Long WD, Meacham WF. Experimental method for producing brain abscess in dogs with evaluation of the effect of dexamethasone and antibiotic therapy on the pathogenesis of intracerebral abscesses. Surg Forum. 1968;19:437–438.
109. Quartey GRC, Johnston JA, Rozdilsky B. Decadron in the treatment of cerebral abscess. An experimental study. J Neurosurg. 1976;45:301–310.
110. Yildizhan A, Pasaoglu A, Kandemir B. Effect of dexamethasone on various stages of experimental brain abscess. Acta Neurochir. 1989;96:141–148.
111. Obana WG, Britt RH, Placone RC, et al. Experimental brain abscess development in the chronically immunosuppressed host. Computerized tomographic and neuropathologic correlations. J Neurosurg. 1986;65:382–391.
112. Brewer NS, MacCarty CS, Wellman WE. Brain abscess: A review of recent experience. Ann Intern Med. 1985;82:571–576.
113. Zeidman SM, Geisler FH, Olivi A. Intraventricular rupture of a purulent brain abscess: Case report. Neurosurgery. 1995;36:189–193.
114. Shaw MDM, Russell JA. Cerebellar abscesses—a review of 47 cases. J Neurol Neurosurg Psych. 1975;38:429–435.
115. Dake MD, McMurdo SK, Rosenblum ML, et al. Pyogenic abscess of the medulla oblongata. Neurosurgery. 1986;18:370–372.
116. Carpenter JL. Brain stem abscesses: Cure with medical therapy, case report, and review. Clin Infect Dis. 1994;18:219–226.
117. Mamelak AN, Obana WG, Flaherty JF, Rosenblum ML. Nocardial brain abscess: Treatment strategies and factors influencing outcome. Neurosurgery. 1994;35:622–631.
118. Walsh TJ, Hier DB, Caplan LR. Aspergillosis of the central nervous system: Clinicopathological analysis of 17 patients. Ann Neurol. 1985;18:574–582.
119. Rangel-Guerra R, Martinez HR, Saenz C. Mucormycosis. Report of 11 cases. Arch Neurol. 1985;42:578–581.
120. Anaissie EJ, Shikhani AH. Rhinocerebral mucormycosis with internal carotid occlusion: Report of two cases and review of the literature. Laryngoscope. 1985;95:1107–1113.
121. Osenbach RK, Loftus CM. Diagnosis and management of brain abscess. Neurosurg Clin North Am. 1992;3:403–420.
122. Miller ES, Psrilal SD, Uttley D. CT scanning in the management of intracranial abscess: A review of 100 cases. Br J Neurosurg. 1988;2:439–446.
123. Zimmerman RD, Weingarten K. Neuroimaging of cerebral abscesses. Neuroimaging Clin North Am. 1991;1:1–16.

124. Zimmerman RA, Girard NJ. Imaging of intracranial infections. In: Scheld WM, Whitley RJ, Durack DT, eds. Infections of the Central Nervous System. 2nd ed. Philadelphia: Lippincott-Raven; 1997:923–944.
125. Anderson D, Matick H, Naheedy MH, et al. Rhinocerebral mucormycosis with CT scan findings. Comput Radiol. 1984;8:113–117.
126. Press GA, Weindling SM, Hesselink JR, et al. Rhinocerebral mucormycosis: MR manifestations. J Comput Assist Tomogr. 1988;12:744–749.
127. Rehncrona S, Brismar J, Holtas S. Diagnosis of brain abscesses with indium-111 labeled leukocytes. Neurosurgery. 1985;16:23–36.
128. Bellotti C, Aragno MG, Medina M, et al. Differential diagnosis of CT-hypodense cranial lesions with indium-111-oxine–labeled leukocytes. J Neurosurg. 1986;64:750–753.
129. Grimstad IA, Hirschberg H, Rootwelt K. 99 Tc Hexamethylpropyleneamine oxime leukocyte scintigraphy and C-reactive protein levels in the differential diagnosis of brain abscess. J Neurosurg. 1992;77:732–736.
130. Martinez-Perez I, Moreno A, Alonso J, et al. Diagnosis of brain abscess by magnetic resonance spectroscopy. Report of two cases. J Neurosurg. 1997;86:708–713.
131. Elkin CM, Leon E, Grenell SL, et al. Intracranial lesions in the acquired immunodeficiency syndrome. Radiological (computed tomographic) features. JAMA. 1985;253:393–396.
132. Post MJD, Sheldon JJ, Hensley GT, et al. Central nervous system disease in acquired immunodeficiency syndrome: Prospective correlation using CT, MR imaging and pathologic studies. Radiology. 1986;158:141–148.
133. Post MJD, Kursunoglu SJ, Hensley GT, et al. Cranial CT in acquired immunodeficiency syndrome: Spectrum of diseases and optimal contrast enhancement technique. AJNR Am J Neuroradiol. 1985;6:743–754.
134. Luft BJ, Hafner R, Korzun AH, et al. Toxoplasmic encephalitis in patients with the acquired immunodeficiency syndrome. N Engl J Med. 1993;329:995–1000.
135. Cohn JA, McMeeking A, Cohen W, et al. Evaluation of the policy of empiric treatment of suspected *Toxoplasma* encephalitis in patients with the acquired immunodeficiency syndrome. Am J Med. 1989;86:521–527.
136. Cimino C, Lipton RB, Williams A, et al. The evaluation of patients with human immunodeficiency virus–related disorders and brain mass lesions. Arch Intern Med. 1991;151:1381–1384.
137. Conley FK, Jenkins KA, Remington JS. *Toxoplasma gondii* infection of the central nervous system. Use of the peroxidase-antiperoxidase method to demonstrate *Toxoplasma* in formalin fixed, paraffin embedded tissue sections. Hum Pathol. 1981;12:690–698.
138. Sun T, Greenspan J, Tenenbaum M, et al. Diagnosis of cerebral toxoplasmosis using fluorescein-labeled antitoxoplasma monoclonal antibodies. Am J Surg Pathol. 1986;10:312–316.
139. Mamelak AN, Mampalam TJ, Obana WG, Rosenblum ML. Improved management of multiple brain abscesses: A combined surgical and medical approach. Neurosurgery. 1995;36:76–86.
140. Ingram HR, Selkon JB, Roxby CM. Bacteriologic study of otogenic cerebral abscesses: Chemotherapeutic role of metronidazole. BMJ. 1977;2:991–993.
141. Holm S, Kourtopoulos H. Penetration of antibiotics into brain tissue and brain abscesses. An experimental study in steroid treated rats. Scand J Infect Dis Suppl. 1985;44:68–70.
142. Alderson D, Strong AJ, Ingham MR, et al. Fifteen year review of the mortality of brain abscess. Neurosurgery. 1981;8:1–6.
143. Levy RM, Gutin PH, Baskin DS, et al. Vancomycin penetration of a brain abscess: Case report and review of the literature. Neurosurgery. 1986;18:633–636.
144. Greene BM, Thomas FE Jr, Alford RH. Trimethoprim-sulfamethoxazole and brain abscess. Ann Intern Med. 1975;82:812–813.
145. Sjölin J, Eriksson N, Arneborn P, et al. Penetration of cefotaxime and desacetylcefotaxime into brain abscesses in humans. Antimicrob Agents Chemother. 1991;35:2606–2610.
146. Quality Standards Subcommittee of the American Academy of Neurology. Evaluation and management of intracranial mass lesions in AIDS. Neurology. 1998;50:21–26.
147. Ruiz A, Ganz WI, Post MJD, et al. Use of thallium-201 brain SPECT to differentiate cerebral lymphoma from *Toxoplasma* encephalitis in AIDS patients. AJNR Am J Neuroradiol. 1994;15:1885–1894.
148. Berry I, Gaillard JF, Guo Z, et al. Cerebral lesions in AIDS. What can be expected from scintigraphy? Cerebral tomographic scintigraphy using thallium-201: A contribution to the differential diagnosis of lymphomas and infectious lesions. J Neuroradiol. 1995;22:218–228.
149. O'Malley JP, Ziessman HA, Kumar PN, et al. Diagnosis of intracranial lymphoma in patients with AIDS: Value of 201 TL single-photon emission computed tomography. AJR Am J Roentgenol. 1994;163:417–421.
150. Hoffman JM, Waskin HA, Schifter T, et al. FDG-PET in differentiating lymphoma from nonmalignant central nervous system lesions in patients with AIDS. J Nucl Med. 1993;34:567–575.
151. Pierce MA, Johnson MD, Maciunas RJ, et al. Evaluating contrast-enhancing brain lesions in patients with AIDS by using positron emission tomography. Ann Intern Med. 1995;123:594–598.
152. De Louvois J. Antimicrobial chemotherapy in the treatment of brain abscess. J Antimicrob Chemother. 1983;11:205–207.
153. Black P, Graybill JR, Charache P. Penetration of brain abscess by systemically administered antibiotics. J Neurosurg. 1973;38:705–709.
154. De Louvois J, Gortvai P, Hurley R. Antibiotic treatment of abscesses of the central nervous system. BMJ. 1977;2:985–987.
155. Sjölin J, Lilja A, Eriksson N, et al. Treatment of brain abscess with cefotaxime and metronidazole: Prospective study on 15 consecutive patients. Clin Infect Dis. 1993;17:857–863.
156. Green HT, O'Donoghue MAT, Shaw MDM, Dowling C. Penetration of ceftazidime into intracranial abscesses. J Antimicrob Chemother. 1989;24:431–436.
157. Skrap M, Melatini A, Vassallo A, Sidoti C. Stereotactic aspiration and drainage of brain abscesses. Experience with 9 cases. Minim Invasive Neurosurg. 1996;39:108–112.
158. Yamamoto M, Jimbo M, Ide M, et al. Penetration of intravenous antibiotics into brain abscesses. Neurosurgery. 1993;33:44–49.
159. Adova M, Akalin HE, Korten V, et al. Treatment of intracranial abscesses: Experience with sulbactam/ampicillin. J Chemother. 1993;5:181–185.
160. Aseni V, Carton JA, Maradona JA, et al. Imipenem therapy of brain abscesses. Eur J Clin Microbiol Infect Dis. 1996;15:653–657.
161. Aseni V, Carton JA, Maradona JA, et al. Therapy of brain abscess with imipenem—a safe therapeutic choice? J Antimicrob Chemother. 1996;37:200–203.
162. Meis JFGM, Groot-Loonen J, Hoogkamp-Korstanje JAA. A brain abscess due to multiply-resistant *Enterobacter cloacae* successfully treated with meropenem. Clin Infect Dis. 1995;20:1567.
163. Wessalowksi R, Thomas L, Kivit J, Voit T. Multiple brain abscesses caused by *Salmonella enteritidis* in a neonate: Successful treatment with ciprofloxacin. Pediatr Infect Dis J. 1993;12:683–688.
164. Rosenblum ML, Hoff JT, Norman D, et al. Nonoperative treatment of brain abscesses in selected high-risk patients. J Neurosurg. 1980;52:217–225.
165. Boom WH, Tuazon CU. Successful treatment of multiple brain abscesses with antibiotics alone. Rev Infect Dis. 1985;7:189–199.
166. Fulgham JR, Wijdicks EFM, Wright AJ. Cure of a solitary brainstem abscess with antibiotic therapy: Case report. Neurology. 1996;46:1451–1454.
167. Wallace RJ Jr, Septimus EJ, Williams TW Jr, et al. Use of trimethoprim-sulfamethoxazole for treatment of infections due to *Nocardia*. Rev Infect Dis. 1982;4:315–325.
168. Smego RA Jr, Moeller MB, Gallis HA. Trimethoprim-sulfamethoxazole therapy for *Nocardia* infections. Arch Intern Med. 1983;143:711–718.
169. Overkamp D, Waldmann B, Lins T, et al. Successful treatment of brain abscess caused by *Nocardia* in an immunocompromised patient after failure of co-trimoxazole. Infection. 1992;20:365–366.
170. Wallace RJ Jr, Steele LC, Sumter G, et al. Antimicrobial susceptibility patterns of *Nocardia asteroides*. Antimicrob Agents Chemother. 1988;32:1776–1779.
171. Berkey P, Moore D, Rolston K. In vitro susceptibilities of *Nocardia* species to newer antimicrobial agents. Antimicrob Agents Chemother. 1988;32:1078–1079.
172. Fried J, Hinthorn D, Ralstin J, et al. Cure of brain abscess caused by *Nocardia asteroides* resistant to multiple antibiotics. South Med J. 1988;81:412–413.
173. Krone A, Schaal KP, Brawanski A, Schuknecht B. Nocardial cerebral abscess cured with imipenem/amikacin and enucleation. Neurosurg Rev. 1989;12:333–340.
174. Kim J, Minamoto GY, Hoy CD, et al. Presumptive cerebral *Nocardia asteroides* infection in AIDS: Treatment with ceftriaxone and minocycline. Am J Med. 1991;90:656–658.
175. Garlando F, Bodmer T, Lee C, et al. Successful treatment of disseminated nocardiosis complicated by cerebral abscess with ceftriaxone and amikacin: Case report. Clin Infect Dis. 1992;15:1039–1040.
176. Jansen C, Frenay HM, Vandertop WP, Visser MR. Intracerebral *Nocardia asteroides* abscess treated by neurosurgical aspiration and combined therapy with sulfadiazine and cefotaxime. Clin Neurol Neurosurg. 1991;93:253–255.
177. Gombert ME, du Bouchet L, Aulicino TM, Berkowitz LB. Antimicrobial synergism in the therapy of experimental cerebral nocardiosis. J Antimicrob Chemother. 1989;24:39–43.
178. Filice GA, Simpson GL. Management of *Nocardia* infections. In: Remington JS, Swartz MN, eds. Current Clinical Topics in Infectious Diseases. New York: McGraw-Hill; 1984:49–64.
179. Stephanov S. Surgical treatment of brain abscess. Neurosurgery. 1988;22:724–730.
180. Appuzzo MLJ, Sabshin JK. Computed tomographic guidance stereotaxis in the management of intracranial mass lesions. Neurosurgery. 1983;12:277–285.
181. Lunsford D, Martinez AJ. Stereotactic exploration of the brain in the era of computed tomography. Surg Neurol. 1984;22:222–230.
182. Dyste GN, Hitchon PW, Menezes AH, et al. Stereotaxic surgery in the treatment of multiple brain abscesses. J Neurosurg. 1988;69:188–194.
183. Rossitch E, Alexander E, Schiff SJ, et al. The use of computed tomography–guided stereotactic techniques in the treatment of brain stem abscesses. Clin Neurol Neurosurg. 1988;90:365–368.
184. Itakura T, Yokote H, Ozaki F, et al. Stereotactic operation for brain abscess. Surg Neurol. 1987;28:196–200.
185. Lunsford LD. Stereotactic drainage of brain abscesses. Neurol Res. 1987;9:270–274.
186. Shahzadi S, Lozano AM, Bernstein M, et al. Stereotactic management of bacterial brain abscesses. Can J Neurol Sci. 1996;23:34–39.
187. Laborde G, Klimek L, Harders A, Gilsbach J. Frameless stereotactic drainage of intracranial abscesses. Surg Neurol. 1993;40:16–21.
188. Kamitsuka MD, Nugent NA, Conrad PD, Swanson TN. *Candida albicans* brain abscesses in a premature infant treated with amphotericin B, flucytosine and fluconazole. Pediatr Infect Dis J. 1995;14:329–331.
189. Denning DW, Stevens DA. Antifungal and surgical treatment of invasive aspergillosis: Review of 2,121 published cases. Rev Infect Dis. 1990;12:1147–1201.
190. Zuckerman J, Tunkel AR. Itraconazole: A new triazole antifungal agent. Infect Cont Hosp Epidemiol. 1994;15:397–410.
191. Sanchez C, Mauri E, Dalmau D, et al. Treatment of cerebral aspergillosis with

itraconazole: Do high doses improve the prognosis? Clin Infect Dis. 1995;21:1485–1487.
192. Goodman ML, Coffey RJ. Sterotactic drainage of *Aspergillus* brain abscess with long-term survival: Case report and review. Neurosurgery. 1989;24:96–99.
193. Venugopal PV, Venugopal TV, Thiruneelakantan K, et al. Cerebral aspergillosis: Report of two cases. Sabouraudia. 1977;15:225–230.
194. Klein HJ, Richter HP, Schachenmayr W. Intracerebral *Aspergillus* abscess: Case report. Neurosurgery. 1983;13:306–309.
195. Ochi JW, Harris JP, Feldman JI, et al. Rhinocerebral mucormycosis: Results of aggressive surgical debridement and amphotericin B. Laryngoscope. 1988;98:1339–1342.
196. Couch L, Theilen F, Mader JT. Rhinocerebral mucormycosis with cerebral extension successfully treated with adjunctive hyperbaric oxygen therapy. Arch Otolaryngol Head Neck Surg. 1988;114:791–794.
197. Ferguson BJ, Mitchell TG, Moon R, et al. Adjunctive hyperbaric oxygen for treatment of rhinocerebral mucormycosis. Rev Infect Dis. 1988;10:551–559.
198. Fisher JF, Shadomy S, Teabeaut JR, et al. Near-drowning complicated by brain abscess due to *Petriellidium boydii.* Arch Neurol. 1982;39:511–513.
199. Perez RE, Smith M, McClendon J, et al. *Pseudallescheria boydii* brain abscess. Complication of an intravenous catheter. Am J Med. 1988;84:359–362.
200. Bailey T, Graham MB, Powderly W. Disseminated *Pseudallescheria boydii* infection treated with fluconazole. Abstract 71. In: Sixth International Symposium on Infections in the Immunocompromised Host, Peebles, Scotland, 1990.
201. Nomdedeu J, Brunet S, Martino R, et al. Successful treatment of pneumonia due to *Scedosporium apiospermum* with itraconazole: Case report. Clin Infect Dis. 1993;16:731–733.
202. Hachimi-Idrissi S, Willemsen M, Desprechins B, et al. *Pseudallescheria boydii* and brain abscess. Pediatr Infect Dis J. 1990;9:737–741.
203. Roilides E, Sein T, Holmes A, et al. Effects of macrophage colony-stimulating factor on antifungal activity of mononuclear phagocytes against *Aspergillus fumigatus*. J Infect Dis. 1995;172:1028–1034.
204. Dale DW, Liles C, Summer WR, Nelson S. Granulocyte colony-stimulating factor—role and relationships in infectious diseases. J Infect Dis. 1995;172:1061–1075.

Chapter 75

Subdural Empyema

THOMAS P. BLECK
JOHN E. GREENLEE

The two outer layers of the meninges, the dura mater and the arachnoid membrane, enclose a potential subdural space that is traversed by numerous small veins. Anatomic barriers to the extension of infection within the space exist only at the falx cerebri, the tentorium, the base of the brain, the foramen magnum, and the anterior spinal canal, where the arachnoid and dura are joined by penetrating nerves and vessels. These structures divide the subdural space into several large compartments, within each of which subdural infection can spread, but in which the infection will be confined. Cranial subdural empyemas, described by Sir Richard Bright in 1836,[1] account for 13 to 23% of localized intracranial bacterial infections.[2–5] These infections usually behave as rapidly expanding, space-occupying lesions.

ETIOLOGY AND PATHOGENESIS

In most cases, infection reaches the subdural space via emissary veins or by extension from the skull, with an accompanying epidural abscess.[6] In more than half the cases, the source of infection is the paranasal sinuses,[7] with the frontal and ethmoid sinuses involved in 50 to 80% of cases.[8] The percentage may be even higher in children.[9] The middle ear and mastoid are the source in 10 to 20%. In about 5% of cases, the infection is metastatic, principally from the lung. Subdural empyema may also follow trauma,[10] surgical procedures,[11] burns,[12] dental infections,[13] pharyngitis,[14] or infection of a pre-existing subdural hematoma.[15–17] In one report, intracranial procedures were more commonly the cause of subdural empyema (66%) than sinusitis or otitis (29%) in adults.[18]

In infants, subdural empyema may complicate acute bacterial meningitis. In one series, subdural empyema was the most common indication for neurosurgical intervention in meningitis patients younger than 9 months.[19] Bacterial meningitis and subdural empyema occasionally coexist in adults,[20] although it is not always certain which was present first.

MICROBIOLOGIC CHARACTERISTICS

Aerobic streptococci have been isolated in 35% of reported cases, and staphylococci in 17%. A variety of other organisms, including *Streptococcus pneumoniae, Haemophilus influenzae*, and gram-negative organisms, have been reported in 14% of cases.[15, 21–25] Enterococci may emerge as an important pathogen in this condition.[26] Anaerobic organisms including anaerobic and microaerophilic streptococci (in particular, the *Streptococcus intermedius* group[27]), *Clostridium perfringens*,[28] and *Bacteroides fragilis* have been recovered in up to 100% of cases in some series.[29, 30] Skin flora such as *Propionibacterium acnes* are occasionally encountered after neurosurgical procedures or trauma.[31] In immunocompromised hosts, especially those with human immunodeficiency virus infection, *Salmonella* and unusual pathogens should be considered.[32–36] Polymicrobial infections are common. *Mycobacterium tuberculosis* has been reported to produce a cranial subdural empyema.[37] Fungi such as *Candida* are occasionally responsible.[38]

PATHOLOGIC CHARACTERISTICS

The infection may involve one or both hemispheres and may occur at the base of the brain, over the cerebral convexity, or along the falx cerebri.[39] The posterior fossa is seldom involved.[40] The subdural space contains an inflammatory exudate that is largest over the frontal lobes if the empyema follows sinusitis, or over the temporal and occipital lobes if it follows otitis. The empyema may be multiloculated and may occur contralateral to the associated sinusitis. The focal, inflammatory reaction is frequently present within the subarachnoid space, but purulent meningitis occurs in only 14% of cases. Focal osteomyelitis or epidural abscesses are present in as many as 50% of cases. Septic thrombosis of veins within the empyema may extend into the venous sinuses or the cortical veins, causing hemorrhage infarction and superficial abscess formation. Arteries are less commonly affected.[41] Cerebral edema develops rapidly and contributes to the mass effect produced early in the course of infection. Herniation may occur unless there is prompt surgical evacuation of the empyema and may be precipitated by lumbar puncture.[42]

CLINICAL FEATURES

Subdural empyema may develop at any age but is most common in the second and third decades. Men are affected four times as commonly as women.[6] In 60 to 90% of cases, there is an accompanying, often asymptomatic, sinusitis or otitis. Extension of the infection into the subdural space produces fever, focal headache (which eventually becomes generalized), vomiting, and signs of meningeal irritation. Altered mental status may have an insidious onset and is present in 50% of the patients early in the infection. Within 24 to 48 hours, focal neurologic signs appear and progress rapidly to dysfunction of an entire cerebral hemisphere, with hemiparesis, hemisensory deficit, and hemianopia. Seizures, usually focal, occur in 50% of cases.[43] Aphasia is common when the dominant hemisphere is involved. Unless treatment is instituted, neurologic signs worsen progressively. Signs of increased intracranial pressure appear, leading to herniation and death. The course of the illness is sufficiently rapid that papilledema develops in less than half the patients.

Several exceptions to this clinical picture exist. Symptoms may be fulminant in onset or may develop over a period of several weeks. The development of symptoms after craniotomy may be extremely insidious. Prior antibiotic therapy may minimize systemic symptoms and may mask sinusitis or otitis. In this situation, clinical presentations resemble those of brain abscess. Rarely, cases of chronic subdural empyema, presumably made sterile by antibiotic treatment given for another diagnosis, are discovered at craniotomy performed for presumed meningiomas.[44] In infections metastatic to the subdural space, particularly in an alcoholic with an infected subdural hematoma, the patient often is seen late in the illness, and death is a frequent outcome.

DIAGNOSIS

Subdural empyema should be suspected in any patient with meningeal signs and a focal neurologic deficit, particularly when the deficit indicates extensive dysfunction of one cerebral hemisphere. Sinusitis followed by meningeal signs should also suggest the diagnosis, because bacterial meningitis per se is rarely due to sinusitis.

Magnetic resonance imaging with gadolinium enhancement is the diagnostic procedure of choice (Fig. 75–1)[45] and may detect empyema not seen on contrast-enhanced computed tomography.[39, 46] Sinusitis or otitis is present on skull radiographs or computed tomographic scans in over two thirds of patients. In infants, cranial ultrasonography is useful for detecting subdural empyemas and can aid in their distinction from sterile subdural effusions in cases of meningitis.[47] Spinal fluid changes are nonspecific, and the danger of transtentorial herniation represents a contraindication to lumbar puncture when subdural empyema is suspected.[48]

Other diseases, especially neoplasms, may rarely produce a radiographic picture that resembles subdural empyema.[49]

THERAPY

Aerobic and anaerobic cultures of blood and other material should be obtained, and antibiotics should be instituted as outlined in Table 75–1. Increased intracranial pressure should be managed as described in Chapter 70. Magnetic resonance imaging may detect subdural empyemas too small to be surgically drained. Early subdural empyema can sometimes be treated with antibiotics alone. In most instances, however, because of the rapidly progressive nature of the infection and the tendency for radiologic studies to understate the actual volume of the empyema, emergent surgical as well as medical intervention is necessary. Craniotomy is commonly believed to have a lower rate of complications than the use of bur holes alone and may be essential in posterior fossa lesions. However, the use of bur holes and irrigation of the subdural space can be effective,[50] particularly in early cases.[51] Empyema fluid should be submitted for Gram stain and culture, including anaerobic culture. Otitis or sinusitis may require simultaneous surgery. The possibility of multiloculated or parafalcine infection must be considered. Postoperative recurrence of the empyema may necessitate further surgery. Antibiotic therapy should be continued for at least 3 weeks.

PROGNOSIS

When treatment is prompt, there is a good likelihood of neurologic recovery, but a delay in therapy greatly increases the risk of permanent neurologic sequelae. Overall mortality ranges from 14 to 18% in published series. If the patient is alert on presentation, the mortality is 4 to 8%, but if the patient is comatose on presentation, this rises to 75%. The prognosis is poorer in aged persons, or when the infection is precipitous in onset. Late focal or generalized seizures develop in 42% of patients surviving subdural empyema and usually appear within 16 months. The likelihood of developing late seizures is not influenced by the presence of seizures during the acute illness.

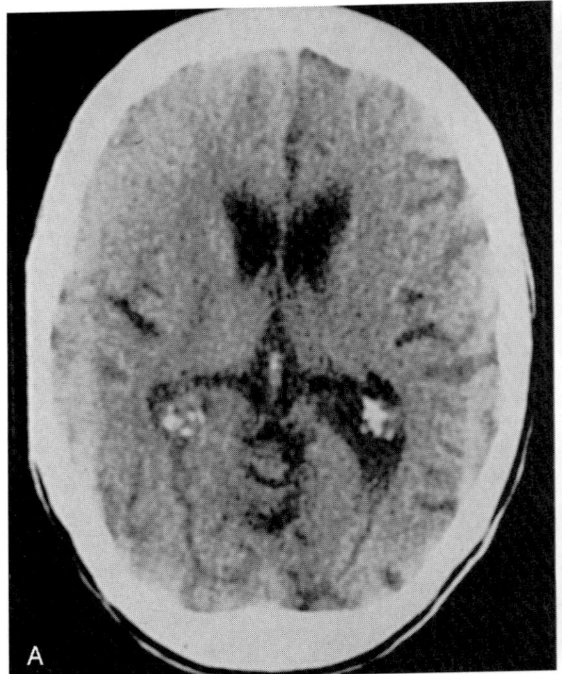

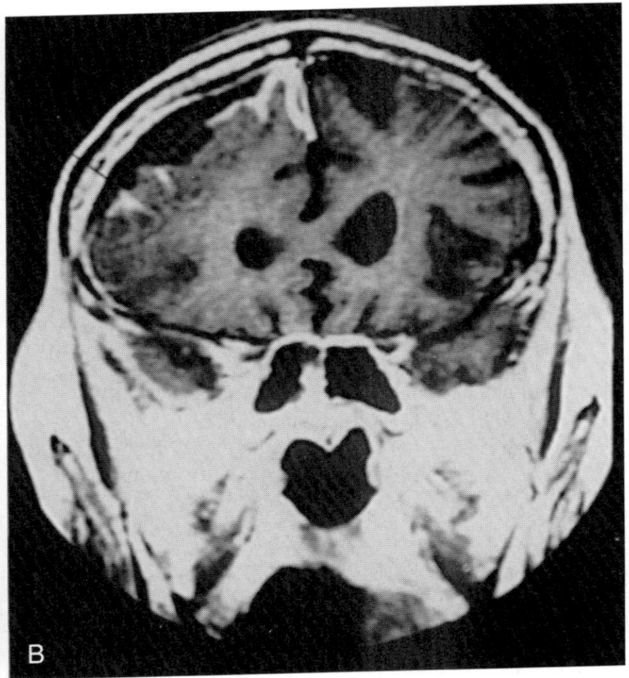

FIGURE 75–1. Computed tomography (CT) scan and gadolinium-enhanced magnetic resonance imaging (MRI) scan of patient with subdural empyema. *A*, CT scan. There is effacement of sulci over the right hemisphere, without obvious fluid collection or evidence of empyema. *B*, Gadolinium-enhanced coronal MRI obtained shortly after CT scan, showing a large subdural empyema. (Courtesy of Dr. Rick Harnsberger, University of Utah.)

TABLE 75–1 Bacterial Cause of and Initial Antibiotic Therapy for Subdural Empyema, Epidural Abscess, and Septic Intracranial Thrombophlebitis

Condition	Primary Infection	Probable Organisms	Suggested Initial Therapy
Subdural empyema, epidural abscess, or septic intracranial thrombophlebitis: older children or adults	Paranasal sinuses	Aerobic, microaerophilic, and anaerobic streptococci (especially *S. intermedius*); *Bacteroides fragilis* and other anaerobes; *Staphylococcus aureus;* Enterobacteriaceae; *Haemophilus* spp.	Metronidazole plus ceftriaxone, cefotaxime, or cefepime
	Otitis media or mastoiditis	Aerobic, microaerophilic, and anaerobic streptococci (especially *S. intermedius*); *Bacteroides fragilis* and other anaerobes; *S. aureus;* Enterobacteriaceae	Ceftriaxone, cefotaxime, or cefepime plus metronidazole
	After cranial surgery or trauma	*S. aureus;* coagulase-negative staphylococci; *Clostridium* spp.; Enterobacteriaceae	Vancomycin plus ceftriaxone (or cefepime or ceftazidime if *Pseudomonas aeruginosa* may be present)
	After dental sepsis	Mixed *Fusobacterium, Bacteroides,* and aerobic and anaerobic streptococci	Metronidazole plus either penicillin or ceftriaxone
Subdural empyema in neonates	Associated with meningitis	Enterobacteriaceae; group B streptococci	Ceftriaxone, cefotaxime, or cefepime
Subdural empyema in older infants and small children	Associated with meningitis	*Haemophilus influenzae, Streptococcus pneumoniae, Neisseria meningitidis*	Ceftriaxone, cefotaxime, or cefepime
Spinal epidural abscess or subdural empyema	Hematogenous or direct extension from bone	*S. aureus, Streptococcus* spp., Enterobacteriaceae	Nafcillin (or ceftriaxone if gram-negative infection suspected)

SUBDURAL EMPYEMA IN INFANTS AND YOUNG CHILDREN

In children younger than 5 years, intracranial subdural empyema almost invariably follows bacterial meningitis. The causative organism is that of the meningitis. Early signs of irritability, poor feeding, or an increase in head circumference occur but are nonspecific. By the time the child is seen by a physician, hemiparesis, seizures, and altered mental status are common, but fever may be absent. Examination may reveal an increased head circumference and a bulging fontanelle. Papilledema is unusual. The empyema fluid is often too turbid to allow transillumination. In infants, the diagnosis may be made by subdural taps, although this procedure will not detect a parafalcine empyema. Radiologic diagnosis and surgical therapy are as described previously for adults. The initial antibiotic therapy is that appropriate for the underlying meningitis (see Chapter 71).

SPINAL SUBDURAL EMPYEMA

Spinal subdural empyema is rare and usually metastatic. Occasional cases follow invasive procedures such as diskography.[52] Etiologic organisms are usually *Staphylococcus aureus*, and less commonly streptococci, gram-negative organisms, coagulase-negative staphylococci, or *Candida albicans*.[7] The empyema is usually posterior to the cord and involves the thoracic and lumbar regions more commonly than the cervical. Radicular pain and symptoms of cord compression may occur at multiple levels. Spinous process tenderness is often absent, and vertebral osteomyelitis rare. High-resolution computed tomography may detect the lesion at one level but cannot give accurate information regarding the extent of the empyema. Magnetic resonance imaging is the diagnostic procedure of choice.

Surgical decompression, usually emergent,[53] is the treatment of choice, preferably with a wide laminectomy,[6] although sometimes a less aggressive procedure has succeeded.[54] Intraoperative ultrasonography is useful for determining the extent of the lesion.[55] About half the reported patients have made good or full recoveries. The duration of antibiotic treatment has ranged from 2 to 6 weeks in published series. There does not appear to be a role for antibiotic therapy without surgery.

REFERENCES

1. Bleck TP. Richard Bright's 1836 description of subdural empyema. Neurology. 1992;42 (Suppl 1):394.
2. Harris LF, Haws FP, Triplett JN, Maccubbin DA. Subdural empyema and epidural abscess: Recent experience in a community hospital. South Med J. 1987;80:1254–1258.
3. Mauser HW, Tulleken CA. Subdural empyema. A review of 48 patients. Clin Neurol Neurosurg. 1984;86:255–263.
4. Weinmann D, Samarasinghe HHR. Subdural empyema. Aust N Z J Surg. 1972;41:324–330.
5. Gallagher RM, Gross CW, Phillips CD. Suppurative intracranial complications of sinusitis. Laryngoscope. 1998;108:1635–1642.
6. Brock DG, Bleck TP. Extra-axial suppurations of the central nervous system. Semin Neurol. 1992;12:263–272.
7. Dolan RW, Chowdhury K. Diagnosis and treatment of intracranial complications of paranasal sinus infections. J Oral Maxillofac Surg. 1995;53:1080–1087.
8. Maniglia AJ, Goodwin WJ, Arnold JE, Ganz E. Intracranial abscesses secondary to nasal, sinus, and orbital infections in adults and children. Arch Otolaryngol Head Neck Surg. 1989;115:1424–1429.
9. Giannoni C, Sulek M, Friedman EM. Intracranial complications of sinusitis: A pediatric series. Am J Rhinol 1998;12:173–178.
10. Dee KE, Newell DW, Cohen WA. Subdural empyema after depressed frontal sinus fracture. AJR Am J Roentgenol. 1998;170:790.
11. Gocer AI, Cetinalp E, Tuna M, Gezercan Y, Ildan F. Fatal complication of the percutaneous radiofrequency trigeminal rhizotomy. Acta Neurochir (Wien). 1997;139:373–374.
12. Sekaran MR, Sekaran VI, Gajendran R. Subdural empyema due to external burns. J Indian Med Assoc. 1997;95:84.
13. Woolley EJ, Patel M. Subdural empyema resulting from displacement of a root into the maxillary antrum. Br Dent J. 1997;182:430–432.
14. Gettler JF, el-Sadr W. Group C streptococcal subdural empyema in a healthy man: Possible complication of pharyngitis. Clin Infect Dis. 1993;16:726–727.
15. Levy I, Sood S. *Staphylococcus aureus* dissemination to a preexisting subdural hematoma. Pediatr Infect Dis J. 1996;15:1139–1140.
16. Aoki N, Sakai T, Oikawa A, et al. Infected subdural effusion associated with resolving subdural hematoma—case report. Neurol Med Chir (Tokyo). 1997;37:637–639.
17. Bakker S, Kluytmans J, den Hollander JC, Lie ST. Subdural empyema caused by *Escherichia coli*: Hematogenous dissemination to a preexisting chronic subdural hematoma. Clin Infect Dis. 1995;21:458–459.
18. Hlavin ML, Kaminski HJ, Fenstermaker RA, White RJ. Intracranial suppuration: A modern decade of postoperative subdural empyema and epidural abscess. Neurosurgery. 1994;34:974–980.
19. Chang YC, Huang CC, Wang ST, Chio CC. Risk factor of complications requiring neurosurgical intervention in infants with bacterial meningitis. Pediatr Neurol. 1997;17:144–149.
20. Pfister HW, Feiden W, Einhaupl KM. Spectrum of complications during bacterial meningitis in adults. Results of a prospective clinical study. Arch Neurol. 1993;50:575–581.
21. Silverberg AL, DiNubile MJ. Subdural empyema and cranial epidural abscess. Med Clin North Am. 1985;90:361–374.
22. Mauser HW, Van Houwelingen HC, Tulleken CA. Factors affecting the outcome in subdural empyema. J Neurol Neurosurg Psychiatry. 1987;50:1136–1141.
23. Yoshikawa TT, Chow AW, Guze LB. Role of anaerobic bacteria in subdural empyema: Report of four cases and review of 327 cases from the English literature. Am J Med. 1975;58:99–104.
24. Jain KC, Mahapatra AK. Subdural empyema due to salmonella infection. Pediatr Neurosurg. 1998;28:89–90.
25. Ellner PD, Correa-Londono A. *Pasteurella multocida* as a cause of subdural empyema. J Infect. 1981;3:79–81.
26. Jones BL, Wilcox MH. Subdural empyema due to *Enterococcus faecalis*. Scand J Infect Dis. 1997;29:627–628.

27. Skelton R, Maixner W, Isaacs D. Sinusitis-induced subdural empyema. Arch Dis Child. 1992;67:1478–1480.
28. Meschia JF, Bhat RK, Dwinnell B, et al. *Clostridium perfringens* subdural empyema and meningitis. Neurology. 1994;44:1357–1358.
29. Brook I. Aerobic and anaerobic bacteriology of intracranial abscesses. *Pediatr Neurol.* 1992;8:210–214.
30. Dill SR, Cobbs CG, McDonald CK. Subdural empyema: Analysis of 32 cases and review. Clin Infect Dis. 1995;20:372–386.
31. Critchley G, Strachan R. Postoperative subdural empyema caused by *Propionibacterium acnes*—a report of two cases. Br J Neurosurg. 1996;10:321–323.
32. Aliaga L, Mediavilla JD, Lopez de la Osa A, et al. Nontyphoidal salmonella intracranial infections in HIV-infected patients. Clin Infect Dis. 1997;25:1118–1120.
33. Balfour-Lynn IM, Ryley HC, Whitehead BF. Subdural empyema due to *Burkholderia cepacia*: An unusual complication after lung transplantation for cystic fibrosis. J R Soc Med. 1997;90(Suppl 31):59–64.
34. Shoshan Y, Maayan S, Gomori MJ, Israel Z. Chronic subdural empyema: A new presentation of neurobrucellosis. Clin Infect Dis. 1996;23:400–401.
35. Parkers PJ, Harland SP, Protheroe AS. Subdural empyema in an HIV positive patient. Br J Neurosurg. 1995;9:85–86.
36. Mussini C, Trenti F, Manicardi G, et al. Non-typhoid *Salmonella* subdural empyema in a patient with AIDS. Scand J Infect Dis. 1995;27:173–174.
37. Van Dellen A, Nadvi SS, Nathoo N, Ramdial PK. Intracranial tuberculous subdural empyema: Case report. Neurosurgery. 1998;43:370–373.
38. Duffner F, Brandner S, Opitz H, et al. Primary *Candida albicans* empyema associated with epidural hematomas in craniocervical junction. Clin Neuropathol. 1997;16:143–146.
39. Kubik CS, Adams RD. Subdural empyema. Brain. 1943;66:18–42.
40. Morikawa M, Rothman MI, Numaguchi Y. Infratentorial subdural empyema: MR findings. AJR Am J Roentgenol. 1994;163:1270.
41. Mitsuoka H, Tsunoda A, Mori K, et al. Hypertrophic anterior falx artery associated with interhemispheric subdural empyema—case report. Neurol Med Chir (Tokyo). 1995;35:830–832.
42. Coonrod JD, Dans PE. Subdural empyema. Am J Med. 1972;53:85–91.
43. Peter JC, Bok AP. Rhinogenic subdural empyema in older children and teenagers. S Afr Med J. 1994;84:847–849.
44. Kulali A, Erel C, Ozyilmaz F, Simsek P. Giant calcified subdural empyemas. Surg Neurol. 1994;42:442–447.
45. Campbell BG, Zimmerman RD. Emergency magnetic resonance of the brain. Top Magn Reson Imaging. 1998;9:208–227.
46. Conlon BJ, Curran A, Timon CV. Pitfalls in the determination of intracranial spread of complicated suppurative sinusitis. J Laryngol Otol. 1996;110:673–675.
47. Chen CY, Huang CC, Chang YC, et al. Subdural empyema in 10 infants: US characteristics and clinical correlates. Radiology. 1998;207:609–617.
48. Kaufman DM, Miller MH, Steigbigel NH. Subdural empyema: Analysis of 17 recent cases and review of the literature. Medicine (Baltimore). 1975;54:485–498.
49. Yokote H, Terada T, Nakai K, Itakura T. Subdural and meningeal involvement related to Wegener's granulomatosis: Case report. Neurosurgery. 1997;40:1071–1073.
50. De Falco R, Scarano E, Cigliano A, et al. Surgical treatment of subdural empyema: A critical review. J Neurosurg Sci. 1996;40:53–58.
51. Ak HE, Ozkan U, Devecioglu C, Kemaloglu MS. Treatment of subdural empyema by burr hole. Isr J Med Sci. 1996;32:542–544.
52. Zeidman SM, Thompson K, Ducker TB. Complications of cervical discography: Analysis of 4400 diagnostic disc injections. Neurosurgery. 1995;37:414–417.
53. Levy ML, Wieder BH, Schneider J, et al. Subdural empyema of the cervical spine: Clinicopathological correlates and magnetic resonance imaging. Report of three cases. J Neurosurg. 1993;79:929–935.
54. Sathi S, Schwartz M, Cortez S, Rossitch E Jr. Spinal subdural abscess: Successful treatment with limited drainage and antibiotics in a patient with AIDS. Surg Neurol. 1994;42:424–427.
55. Price DB, Gottesman MH, Adelman R, Schneider SJ. Spinal subdural empyema: Appearance on intraoperative sonography. J Ultrasound Med. 1993;12:493–495.

Chapter 76

Epidural Abscess

THOMAS P. BLECK
JOHN E. GREENLEE

An epidural abscess represents localized infection between the outermost layers of the meninges, the dura mater, and the overlying skull or vertebral column. Within the skull, the dura forms the inner layer of the cranial periosteum, and an epidural abscess must form by stripping the periosteum away from the bone. Such an abscess is almost always sharply confined and accompanied by focal osteomyelitis. Because of the ease with which infection can cross cranial dura along emissary veins, subdural empyema is often present as well. Within the spinal canal, however, the dura mater is separated from the vertebrae by an epidural space filled with fat and vascular areolar tissue. Although the spinal dura itself is only rarely breached by bacteria, the spinal epidural space offers low resistance to the longitudinal spread of infection. For this reason, a spinal epidural abscess often occupies several vertebral segments, and, within the narrow confines of the vertebral canal, may cause extensive cord compression and necrosis.

INTRACRANIAL EPIDURAL ABSCESS

The cause, pathogenesis, and bacteriology of intracranial epidural abscess are identical to those described for intracranial subdural empyema (see Chapter 75).[1] Virtually all cases follow frontal sinusitis, craniotomy, or mastoiditis.[2] In one large series, epidural abscesses accounted for 23% of intracranial infectious complications of sinusitis.[3] Rare cases may complicate nasopharyngeal malignancies.[4] *Staphylococcus aureus* is a frequent isolate in cases associated with surgical procedures or cranial trauma. Individual cases have been associated with *Eikenella*,[5] *Salmonella*,[6] *Pseudallescheria boydii*,[7] *Aspergillus*,[8, 9] and *Mucor (Rhizopus)*. An epidural tuberculoma has been reported in a patient with acquired immunodeficiency syndrome.[10]

Pathologic Characteristics

Epidural abscess most often arises adjacent to the frontal sinuses. In almost all cases, osteomyelitis is present within overlying bone, and there is septic thrombosis of veins bridging the skull and meninges. Subdural empyema is present in 81% of autopsy cases with epidural abscess, 38% of the cases also having meningitis and 17% having brain abscess.[11] Rarely, infection of the bridging veins may produce venous necrosis and epidural hemorrhage rather than abscess.[12]

Clinical Features

The onset of symptoms may be insidious and at first may be overshadowed by sinusitis or otitis. The abscess produces local pain followed by generalized headache, at times with alteration of mental status. Focal neurologic signs and focal or generalized seizures then appear. An epidural abscess near the petrous bone may involve cranial nerves V and VI, with unilateral facial pain and lateral rectus weakness (Gradenigo's syndrome). An occipital epidural abscess may obstruct the superior sagittal sinus.[13] As the abscess enlarges, papilledema and other signs of elevated intracranial pressure develop. Extension of the infection into the subdural space is accompanied by rapid neurologic deterioration.

Diagnosis

Persistent fever, lymphocytosis, an elevated erythrocyte sedimentation rate, and focal or generalized neurologic signs in the setting of sinusitis or otitis suggest the presence of intracranial infection. Edema or cellulitis of the face or scalp may be present. Gadolinium-enhanced magnetic resonance imaging (MRI) is the diagnostic procedure of choice (Fig. 76–1).[14] This imaging technique will identify pachymeningeal enhancement or epidural collections of pus not yet detectable by computed tomography and may also demonstrate the presence of sinusitis or otitis. Computed tomography may be used to image bone and as the major diagnostic study for the abscess itself if MRI is not available (Fig. 76–2). The spinal fluid is usually sterile, and the risk of herniation contraindicates the use of lumbar puncture.

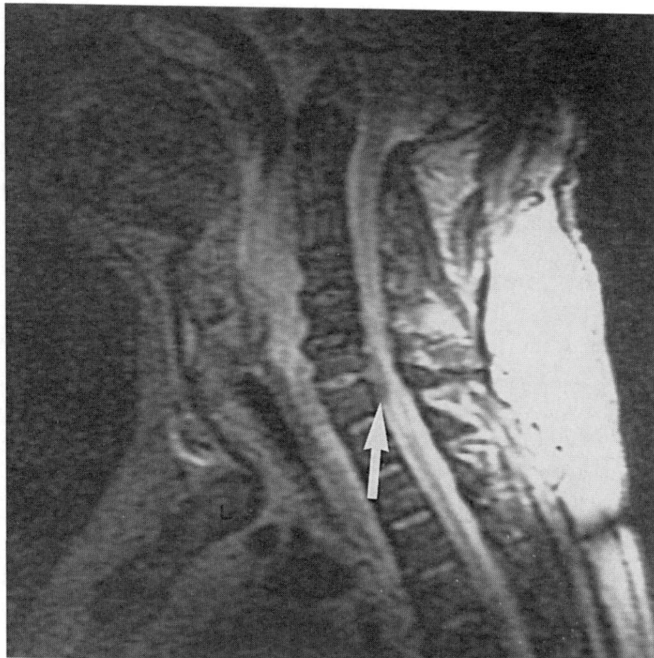

FIGURE 76–1. Magnetic resonance imaging scan of a patient with an anterior cervical epidural abscess. The abscess is seen as an area of diminished attenuation bulging into the spinal canal and compressing the spinal cord *(arrow)*. The infection also affects the adjacent disk space. (Courtesy of Dr. J. Richard Baringer, Salt Lake City, Utah.)

Therapy

In most cases, therapy of a cranial epidural abscess consists of antibiotic therapy and emergent surgical drainage to prevent the development of subdural empyema. Concomitant surgical therapy of sinusitis, otitis, or osteomyelitis may be required as well. Antibiotic therapy should be directed against aerobic and anaerobic streptococci, *S. aureus*, and gram-negative aerobic and anaerobic organisms. The ability of MRI to allow repeated noninvasive imaging of cranial epidural abscess has made it possible, in a small number of cases, to treat with antibiotics alone, using repeated imaging to ensure that the abscess is resolving. If surgery is deferred, MRI should be repeated frequently to confirm a reduction in abscess volume and to ensure that extension into the subdural space has not occurred.

SPINAL EPIDURAL ABSCESS

Etiology and Pathogenesis

The overall incidence of spinal epidural abscess may be as high as 1.96 patients per 10,000 hospital admissions.[15] Both acute and chronic spinal epidural abscesses follow infection elsewhere in the body. In most cases, infection reaches the epidural space by hematogenous spread, either by directly seeding the epidural space or by producing vertebral osteomyelitis with extension into the spinal epidural space. Intravenous drug abuse is increasingly recognized as an etiologic factor.[16] Infection of the epidural space may also be caused by penetrating injuries, or by extension of decubitus ulcers or paraspinal abscesses.

Epidural abscess has occurred after back surgery, lumbar puncture, and epidural anesthesia.[17] No abscesses were reported in a series of 1062 patients receiving epidural analgesia for up to 14 days.[18] In contrast, a series of 91 cancer patients receiving chronic epidural analgesia described 11 (12%) who developed spinal epidural abscesses.[19] Thus, the duration of catheter placement appears to influence the risk of abscess development, along with host factors. Epidural abscess is also being reported with increasing frequency as the use of epidural injections for the control of chronic pain becomes more prevalent.[20] Occasionally, epidural abscess arises as a complication of abdominal surgery. Rarely, the infection may spread along a persistent dermal sinus. In 10 to 30% of cases, there is a history of back trauma, and, less frequently, a history of diabetes mellitus or recent pregnancy.[16] Cases due to extension of a retropharyngeal abscess,[21] or to a colospinal fistula after radiation therapy,[22] point out the need for a high index of suspicion for the diagnosis of spinal epidural abscess.

Microbiology

S. aureus is the agent responsible in 60 to 90% of both the acute and the chronic cases and in some series is the only organism recovered.[16] Aerobic and anaerobic streptococci cause approximately 18% of cases, whereas gram-negative organisms, especially *Escherichia coli* and *Pseudomonas aeruginosa*, are responsible for 13%.[1, 23] Other organisms occasionally reported to be responsible for epidural abscess formation include coagulase-negative staphylococci, *Streptococcus pneumoniae, Haemophilus aphrophilus*,[24] *Nocardia asteroides*,[25] *Echinococcus*,[26] *Actinomyces israelii*,[1] and *Aspergillus*.[27] More than one organism is isolated in approximately 10% of cases.[16, 28] Combined infection with *S. aureus* and *Cryptococcus neoformans* has occurred in a patient infected with human immunodeficiency virus.[29] Chronic epidural infection may be caused by *Mycobacterium tuberculosis*, frequently without other detectable evidence of infection. *Candida* spp. are occasionally reported.[30]

Pathology

The abscess involves the thoracic spine in 50 to 80% of cases, the lumbar spine in 17 to 38%, and the cervical spine in 10 to 25%.[31] In

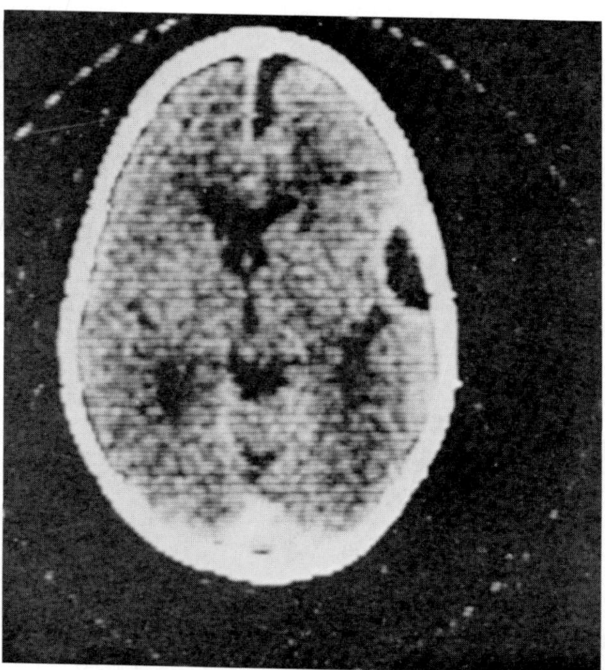

FIGURE 76–2. Computed tomography scan of a right-sided epidural abscess. A subdural empyema is also present between the falx cerebri and the medial aspect of the right frontal lobe. (Courtesy of Drs. D. M. Kaufman, N. E. Leeds, and I. Krichef. (From Kaufman DM, Leeds NE. Computed tomography [CT] in the diagnosis of intracranial abscess. Neurology. 1977; 27:1069–1073.)

children, the cervical and lumbar spine regions are more commonly involved. Abscesses may be posterior to the spinal cord, anterior to it, or circumferential. Anterior abscesses usually occur at cervical levels, except in tuberculosis, in which the anterior thoracic or lumbar epidural spaces may also be involved. Diskitis or vertebral osteomyelitis, detectable by MRI, may be present in 80 to 100% of cases. Acute abscesses consist of granulation tissue containing loculated pus; in chronic abscesses, there may be a prominent fibroblastic component. The abscess on average occupies about four vertebral segments[32] but may extend the entire length of the spinal cord. Enlargement of the abscess produces myelomalacia or cord necrosis, both by compression and by invasion of the spinal venous plexus.[23] Extension of infection into the subarachnoid space occurs in 12 to 25% of cases.[28]

Clinical Features

Spinal epidural abscess is significantly more common in men than in women and may occur at any age. The abscess may develop acutely within hours to days or may pursue a chronic course over months. Most abscesses, however, pass through four clinical stages, differing only in time course. Initially, there is focal vertebral pain; following this, pain radiates along the course of involved nerve roots.[28] This is followed by evidence of spinal cord compression (long-tract findings), which may progress to paralysis below the level of the lesion. Acute metastatic infection of the epidural space produces rapid progression with prominent systemic signs of infection, and severe or local pain. Such patients usually seek medical attention within the first few days of illness, when radicular signs are already present. When an epidural abscess arises from vertebral osteomyelitis, vertebral pain may develop over 2 to 3 weeks, but progression is rapid once radicular symptoms appear. Chronic epidural abscesses may manifest with a course indistinguishable from that of an epidural neoplasm, and without systemic signs of infection. Where the cervical spinal cord is involved, respiratory function may be impaired. A rapidly developing cervical epidural abscess may produce flaccid hyporeflexia, similar to that seen in the Guillain-Barré syndrome.[28]

Diagnosis

Epidural abscesses are a diagnostic consideration in any patient with localized back pain and radicular symptoms, especially when a source of infection is evident. Headache is a common additional complaint. Nuchal rigidity and focal tenderness to percussion are almost universally present.[23, 28] In acute cases, the white blood cell count and the erythrocyte sedimentation rate are elevated. Plain films of the spine may show osteomyelitis but are often normal. MRI is the procedure of choice for diagnosis (see Fig. 76–1).[14] When an epidural abscess is suspected, one should proceed immediately to MRI, rather than first obtaining plain films, since the MRI will be necessary regardless of the plain film findings. Time should not be wasted getting plain films first. Lumbar puncture should not be performed when an epidural abscess is suspected. Blood cultures and cultures of abscess material should be submitted for aerobic, anaerobic, mycobacterial, and fungal cultures.

Therapy

The danger of spinal cord necrosis requires surgical drainage, usually via laminectomy, as soon as the diagnosis of epidural abscess is made. Endoscopic surgical techniques represent a promising alternative to the open procedure[33] but remain in their infancy. Antibiotic coverage should be initiated before surgery. Minimally, coverage should be directed against *S. aureus*, usually with nafcillin or vancomycin. Gram-negative coverage, consisting of ceftriaxone and anaerobic coverage with metronidazole, should be added if there is any suspicion of the presence of such organisms. If the patient has recently been bacteremic, therapy directed against the offending organism should also be included. Since the epidural space lies outside the blood-brain barrier, the choice of other antibiotics need not be limited by this concern. Antibiotic therapy should be modified based on culture results. In some patients, needle aspiration guided by computed tomography may be used in place of laminectomy.

Antibiotic therapy alone, with meticulous frequent neurologic examinations and serial MRI studies, may be considered if the patient has localized pain or radicular symptoms without long-tract findings, worsening pain, increasing fever, or increasing leukocytosis.[34] If these latter findings develop, surgery is indicated.[35] Antimicrobial treatment should be continued for at least 3 to 4 weeks in uncomplicated spinal epidural abscess, and for 8 weeks or more if osteomyelitis is present. A recent study suggests that relapse may be less likely if antibiotic treatment is given for at least 8 weeks.[36] Severe destruction of bone may require surgery for stabilization once the infection is cured. The prognosis for neurologic recovery is excellent if therapy is begun before or during the stage of radicular symptoms but diminishes rapidly when evidence of cord damage appears. A multivariate analysis of factors influencing the outcome of patients operated for spinal epidural abscess found that the age of the patient and the degree of thecal sac compression were the only independent predictors.[37] The likelihood of neurologic improvement is dismal if surgery is delayed more than 24 hours after the onset of paralysis. Mortality of epidural abscess in recent series has been approximately 59%.

HYPERTROPHIC SPINAL PACHYMENINGITIS

Rarely, chronic inflammation or infection within the spinal canal involves the dura mater alone, producing a diffuse fibrosing pachymeningitis.[38] Cases have been associated with tuberculosis, syphilis, and infection with *Streptococcus intermedius, Aspergillus flavus*, or *P. boydii*, but in many cases no etiologic organism can be identified. The fibrosis compresses nerve roots and if extensive may injure the spinal cord. Early symptoms are pain, weakness, and muscle atrophy occurring in a radicular pattern. The spinal fluid protein level is elevated, but cells are not present. Electromyography may localize the process to nerve roots. In older cases, the diagnosis was made by myelography; more recently, MRI has been employed successfully. The treatment involves surgical removal of hypertrophied dura and antibiotic therapy of any diagnosed infection.

REFERENCES

1. Silverberg AL, DiNubile MJ. Subdural empyema and cranial epidural abscess. Med Clin North Am. 1985;69:361–374.
2. Dolan RW, Chowdhury K. Diagnosis and treatment of intracranial complications of paranasal sinus infections. J Oral Maxillofac Surg. 1995;53:1080–1087.
3. Gallagher RM, Gross CW, Phillips CD. Suppurative intracranial complications of sinusitis. Laryngoscope. 1998;108:1635–1642.
4. Kaplan RJ. Neurological complications of infections of the head and neck. Otolaryngol Clin North Am. 1976;9:729–749.
5. Akhtar MJ, Chandler JR. Periorbital, subgaleal, and epidural empyema secondary to *Eikenella* sinusitis. Ear Nose Throat J. 1979;58:358–361.
6. Aliaga L, Mediavilla JD, Lopez de la Osa A, et al. Nontyphoidal salmonella intracranial infections in HIV-infected patients. Clin Infect Dis. 1997;25:1118–1120.
7. Berenguer J, Diaz-Mediavilla J, Urra D, Munoz P. Central nervous system infection caused by *Pseudallescheria boydii*: Case report and review. Rev Infect Dis. 1989;11:890–896.
8. Hendrix WC, Arruda LK, Platts-Mills TA, et al. *Aspergillus* epidural abscess and cord compression in a patient with aspergilloma and empyema. Survival and response to high dose systemic amphotericin therapy. Am Rev Respir Dis. 1992;145:1483–1486.
9. Letscher V, Herbrecht R, Gaudias J, et al. Post-traumatic intracranial epidural *Aspergillus fumigatus* abscess. J Med Vet Mycol. 1997;35:279–282.
10. Gettler JF, el-Sadr W. Cranial epidural abscess due to *Mycobacterium tuberculosis* in a patient infected with the human immunodeficiency virus. Clin Infect Dis. 1993;17:289–290.
11. Slager UT. Infection and parainfectious inflammation. In: Slager UT, ed. Basic Neuropathology. Baltimore: Williams & Wilkins; 1970:89–125.

12. Rajput AJ, Rozdilsky B. Extradural hematoma following frontal sinusitis. Report of a case and review of the literature. Arch Otolaryngol. 1971;94:83–86.
13. Mineura K, Kamisato N, Miura S, et al. Occipital epidural abscess causing superior sagittal sinus obstruction. Clin Neurol Neurosurg. 1990;92:277–281.
14. Bleck TP. Imaging in the diagnosis of CNS infections. In: Mandell GM, Bennett JE, Dolin R, eds. Principles and Practice of Infectious Diseases Updates, v. 4, no. 1. New York: Churchill Livingstone; 1995:1–13.
15. Hlavin ML, Kaminski HJ, Ross JS, Ganz E. Spinal epidural abscess: A ten-year perspective. Neurosurgery. 1990;27:177–184.
16. Nussbaum ES, Rigamonti D, Standiford H, et al. Spinal epidural abscess: A report of 40 cases and review. Surg Neurol. 1992;38:225–231.
17. Shintani S, Tanaka H, Irifune A, et al. Iatrogenic acute spinal epidural abscess with septic meningitis: MR findings. Clin Neurol Neurosurg. 1992;94:253–255.
18. Burstal R, Wegener F, Hayes C, Lantry G. Epidural analgesia: Prospective audit of 1062 patients. Anaesth Intensive Care. 1998;26:165–172.
19. Smitt PS, Tsafka A, Teng-van de Zande F, et al. Outcome and complications of epidural analgesia in patients with chronic cancer pain. Cancer. 1998;83:2015–2022.
20. Knight JW, Cordingley JJ, Palazzo MG. Epidural abscess following epidural steroid and local anaesthetic injection. Anaesthesia. 1997;52:576–578.
21. Jang YJ, Rhee CK. Retropharyngeal abscess associated with vertebral osteomyelitis and spinal epidural abscess. Otolaryngol Head Neck Surg. 1998;119:705–708.
22. Wang WY, Hernandez JE, Denny B, et al. Postradiation colospinal fistula: A rare cause of spinal epidural abscess. AJNR Am J Neuroradiol. 1998;19:1959–1960.
23. Baker AS, Ojemann RG, Swartz MN, Richardson EP Jr. Spinal epidural abscess. N Engl J Med. 1975;293:463–468.
24. Hung CC, Hsueh PR, Chen YC, et al. *Haemophilus aphrophilus* bacteraemia complicated with vertebral osteomyelitis and spinal epidural abscess in a patient with liver cirrhosis. J Infect. 1997;35:304–308.
25. Harvey AL, Myslinski J, Ortiz L. A case of *Nocardia* epidural abscess. J Emerg Med. 1998;16:579–581.
26. Kaufman DM, Kaplan JG, Litman N. Infectious agents in spinal epidural abscesses. Neurology. 1980;30:844–850.
27. Witzig RS, Greer DL, Hyslop NE Jr. *Aspergillus flavus* mycetoma and epidural abscess successfully treated with itraconazole. J Med Vet Mycol. 1996;34(2):133–137.
28. Darouiche RO, Hamill RJ, Greenberg SB, et al. Bacterial spinal epidural abscess. Review of 43 cases and literature survey. Medicine (Baltimore). 1992;71:369–385.
29. Pirofski L, Casadevall A. Mixed staphylococcal and cryptococcal epidural abscess in a patient with AIDS. Rev Infect Dis. 1990;12:964–965.
30. Bonomo RA, Strauss M, Blinkhorn R, Salata RA. *Torulopsis (Candida) glabrata*: A new pathogen found in spinal epidural abscess. Clin Infect Dis. 1996;22:588–589.
31. Brock DG, Bleck TP. Extra-axial suppurations of the central nervous system. Semin Neurol. 1992;12:263–272.
32. Wong D, Raymond NJ. Spinal epidural abscess. N Z Med J. 1998;111:345–347.
33. Roselli R, Iacoangeli M, Pompucci A, et al. Anterior cervical epidural abscess treated by endoscopy-assisted minimally invasive microsurgery via posterior approach. Minim Invasive Neurosurg. 1998;41:161–165.
34. Nordberg G, Mark H. Epidural abscess after epidural analgesia treated successfully with antibiotics. Acta Anaesthesiol Scand. 1998;42:727–731.
35. Hanigan WC, Asner NG, Elwood PW. Magnetic resonance imaging and the nonoperative treatment of spinal epidural abscess. Surg Neurol. 1990;34:408–413.
36. Mackenzie AR, Laing RB, Smith CC, et al. Spinal epidural abscess: The importance of early diagnosis and treatment. J Neurol Neurosurg Psychiatry. 1998;65:209–212.
37. Khanna RK, Malik GM, Rock JP, Rosenblum ML. Spinal epidural abscess: Evaluation of factors influencing outcome. Neurosurgery. 1996;39:958–964.
38. Uemura K, Matsumura A, Kobayashi E. Idiopathic chronic hypertrophic craniocervical pachymeningitis: Case report. Neurosurgery. 1995;37:358.

Chapter 77

Suppurative Intracranial Phlebitis

THOMAS P. BLECK
JOHN E. GREENLEE

Septic intracranial thrombophlebitis most frequently follows infection of the paranasal sinuses, middle ear, mastoid, face, or oropharynx.[1] The infection spreads centrally along emissary veins. Septic thrombophlebitis may also occur in association with epidural abscess, subdural empyema, or meningitis. Occasionally, the infection is metastatic from lungs or other distant sites.[2] The likelihood of thrombosis is increased by states altering blood viscosity or coagulability, including dehydration, polycythemia, pregnancy, oral contraceptive use, sickle cell disease, malignancy, or trauma. *Staphylococcus aureus* is the most frequent isolate.[1] A minority of cases are due to *Staphylococcus epidermidis*, streptococci including *Streptococcus pneumoniae*, gram-negative bacilli, and anaerobic organisms. Craniofacial mucormycosis and human immunodeficiency virus and cytomegalovirus infections[3] may also be complicated by venous sinus thrombosis. Multiple infecting organisms may be present.[4]

PATHOLOGIC CHANGES

Septic intracranial thrombophlebitis may begin within veins or venous sinuses and may involve additional vessels by propagation or discontinuous spread.[5] The pathologic changes are those of both venous thrombosis and suppuration. Venous occlusion may produce no local injury, but, if collateral veins are compromised, edema and hemorrhagic infarction result. The most common sites of infarction are the area of venous watershed immediately above the Sylvian fissure and the medial surfaces of the cerebral hemispheres. Thrombosis of the anterior portion of the superior sagittal sinus or of the lateral sinuses may block reabsorption of cerebrospinal fluid with resultant communicating hydrocephalus. Local suppuration may produce venous necrosis and hemorrhage or may cause epidural abscess, subdural empyema, meningitis, or brain abscess. Septic embolization may produce pulmonary infarction, abscesses in lungs or other organs, or mycotic aneurysm.[6]

CLINICAL FEATURES

Cortical Vein Thrombosis

If collateral venous drainage is adequate, septic venous thrombosis may produce only transient neurologic findings or may be silent except for its metastatic consequences. If the thrombus outstrips collateral flow, however, a progressive neurologic deficit will result and may mimic brain abscess, with impairment of consciousness, focal or generalized seizures, and increased intracranial pressure. Focal neurologic findings include hemiparesis, which involves the face and hand if veins over the cerebral convexity are involved.[3] Thrombosis of veins along the falx cerebri may produce unilateral leg weakness, which becomes bilateral if propagation of the thrombus involves the veins of the contralateral hemisphere. Aphasia is common when the dominant hemisphere is involved. Transient hemodynamic variation in venous collateral flow may cause considerable fluctuation in neurologic signs.

Venous Sinus Thrombosis

The clinical findings vary with the sinus involved and are summarized in Table 77–1. The cavernous sinus, lateral sinus, and superior sagittal sinus are most often involved. Cavernous sinus thrombosis most commonly follows infections of the face or of the sphenoid and ethmoid sinuses.[7] The onset is abrupt, with diplopia, photophobia, orbital edema, and progressive exophthalmos.[8] Involvement of cranial nerves III, IV, V, and VI produces ophthalmoplegia, a midposition fixed pupil, a loss of the corneal reflex, and diminished sensation over the upper face. Obstruction of venous return from the retina results in papilledema, retinal hemorrhages, and visual loss. Similar findings appear in the opposite eye as the infection spreads to the contralateral cavernous sinus. Engorgement or thrombosis of facial veins may occur.

Thrombosis of the anterior third of the superior sagittal sinus may impair reabsorption of cerebrospinal fluid to produce intracranial hypertension without other signs.[9] A contemporary series found that 22% of cases of pseudotumor cerebri in children resulted from venous sinus thrombosis, and an additional 8% were attributable to other complications of otitis.[10] More extensive thrombosis of the

TABLE 77–1 Symptoms of Intracranial Venous Sinus Occlusion

Venous Sinus Involved	Associated Infection	Anatomic Structures Affected*	Clinical Findings*
Cavernous sinus	Paranasal sinusitis, especially of frontal, ethmoid or sphenoid sinuses, infection of face or mouth	Venous drainage from orbit and eye Cranial nerves III, IV, V, and VI within the cavernous sinus [venous supply of frontal lobe and pituitary]	Unilateral periorbital edema, exophthalmos, and chemosis Examination shows papilledema, ocular palsies, diminished pupillary reactivity, frequently diminished corneal reflex, and impaired sensation in first and second divisions of V Extension to contralateral sinus may duplicate these findings in opposite eye [seizures, frontal lobe deficits, hypopituitarism]
Lateral sinus	Otitis media or mastoiditis Rarely, pharyngitis	Cranial nerves V and VI Venous route of CSF reabsorption [venous supply of temporal lobe, jugular bulb, cranial nerves IX, X, XI at jugular foramen]	Lateral rectus weakness Facial pain and altered facial sensation Increased intracranial pressure with papilledema if other lateral sinus is also compromised [temporal lobe seizures] Jugular foramen syndrome with ipsilateral palatal weakness, diminished gag reflex, and weakness of trapezius and sternomastoid
Superior sagittal sinus	Infections of face, scalp, subdural or epidural spaces Meningitis	Venous drainage from medial portion of cerebral hemispheres CSF reabsorption	Bilateral leg weakness Intracranial hypertension
Superior petrosal sinus	Otitis media or mastoiditis	Trigeminal ganglion [venous drainage from temporal lobe]	Ipsilateral pain or sensory deficit [temporal lobe seizures]
Inferior petrosal sinus	Otitis media or mastoiditis	Cranial nerves V and VI at tip of petrous bone	"Gradenigo's syndrome" Ipsilateral facial pain and sensory deficit Ipsilateral lateral rectus palsy

*Brackets indicate structures affected or symptoms produced by extension of the sinus thrombus into cortical veins.
Abbreviation: CSF, Cerebrospinal fluid.

superior sagittal sinus, however, results in bilateral leg weakness followed by arm weakness and clouding of consciousness as cortical veins are affected. Occlusion of the lateral sinus produces pain over the ear and mastoid and may cause edema over the mastoid (Griesinger's sign). Impairment of veins supplying cranial nerves V and VI produces ipsilateral facial pain and lateral rectus weakness (Gradenigo's syndrome). Septic cortical vein or venous sinus occlusion may produce subdural empyema, meningitis, or brain abscess. The danger of septic pulmonary embolization is always present.[5]

DIAGNOSIS

Although infection accounts for less than 5% of cases of cranial venous thrombosis in some recent series,[11] in other series it accounts for the majority.[12] An infectious cause must be considered in the differential diagnosis of any patient with this condition. Septic intracranial thrombophlebitis may manifest as sepsis without neurologic signs or with stupor and focal neurologic signs in the presence of cranial infection. In the latter instance, septic thrombophlebitis may be indistinguishable from brain abscess or subdural empyema. Fever, leukocytosis, and an elevated erythrocyte sedimentation rate are usually present. Skull radiographs should be evaluated for the presence of sinusitis or mastoiditis. However, computed tomographic scanning or magnetic resonance imaging is much more sensitive and specific for the diagnosis of sinusitis. If a lumbar puncture is performed, it may reveal increased pressure, slight lymphocytic pleocytosis, and mild elevation of the protein level. Computed tomographic scanning with intravenous contrast material may reveal evidence of superior sagittal sinus or lateral sinus thrombosis, manifested as a filling defect in the vessel. However, computed tomography may yield a false-positive diagnosis of sagittal sinus thrombosis in up to 30% of cases.[13] Magnetic resonance imaging can distinguish between flowing blood and thrombus. Magnetic resonance angiography is the procedure of choice for the diagnosis of venous thrombosis (Fig. 77–1).[14] Computed tomography and magnetic resonance imaging can detect concomitant cerebral infection or infarction as well as infection in the epidural or subdural spaces. The role of conventional angiography in the diagnosis of venous thrombosis is diminishing.[15] Blood cultures may be diagnostically useful, as may cultures of any extracranial infected material.

TREATMENT

Appropriate antibiotic therapy, the reversal of elevated intracranial pressure, and control of seizures are the goals of therapy. Initial antibiotic therapy should be directed against *S. aureus*, aerobic streptococci, and anaerobes. Control of infection may require urgent surgery of infected cranial structures or drainage of intra- or extracranial abscess. Intracranial hypertension may require treatment (see Chapter 70). Communicating hydrocephalus may require serial lumbar punctures or ventricular drainage. The use of anticoagulants is controversial,[16] but the weight of opinion currently favors the use of heparin followed by warfarin. However, heparin-induced thrombocytopenia may complicate the use of heparin in septic venous thrombosis.[17] The role of thrombolytic therapy remains to be defined[18] but appears promising.[19] Internal jugular vein ligation has been used with lateral sinus thrombosis. In rare instances, thrombectomy has been successfully performed.

PROGNOSIS

Even when an apparently fixed neurologic deficit is present, intracranial venous infarction carries a better likelihood of functional recovery than does arterial infarction, but permanent deficits may occur. Overall mortality in suppurative intracranial thrombophlebitis is 34%.[20] Mortality in complete occlusion of the superior sinus, however, is 78%. Ominous prognostic signs are coma, progression of focal seizures to generalized ones, generalized seizures as an initial symptom, and bilateral signs, particularly bilateral flaccid hemiplegia.

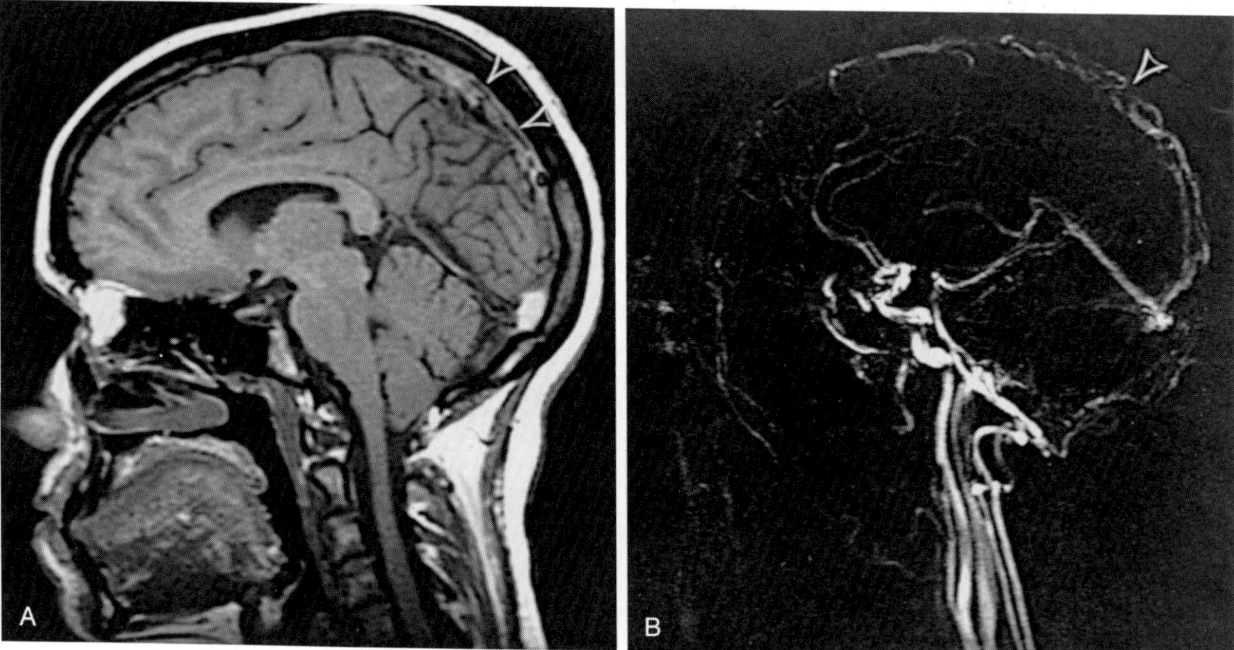

FIGURE 77–1. *A*, Magnetic resonance image of superior sagittal sinus thrombosis. There is increased signal within the vessel on T_2-weighted images *(arrows)*, indicating the presence of thrombus. *B*, Magnetic resonance angiogram of the same patient, showing nonfilling of the superior sagittal sinus. The sinus is surrounded by tortuous collateral vessels *(arrow)*. (Courtesy of Dr. Wayne Davis, University of Utah.)

REFERENCES

1. Southwick FS, Richardson EP, Swartz MN. Septic thrombosis of the dural venous sinuses. Medicine. 1986;65:82–106.
2. Stuart EA, O'Brien FH, McNally WJ. Cerebral venous thrombosis. Ann Otolaryngol. 1951;60:406–438.
3. Meyohas MC, Roullet E, Rouzioux C, et al. Cerebral venous thrombosis and dual primary infection with human immunodeficiency virus and cytomegalovirus. J Neurol Neurosurg Psychiatry. 1989;52:1010–1011.
4. Pallares R, Santamaria J, Ariza X, et al. Polymicrobial anaerobic septicemia due to lateral sinus thrombophlebitis. J Laryngol Otolaryngol. 1984;98:895–899.
5. Diaz JM, Schiffman JS, Urban ES, et al. Superior sagittal sinus thrombosis and pulmonary embolism: A syndrome rediscovered. Acta Neurol Scand. 1992;86:390–396.
6. Courville CB, Nielson JM. Fatal complications of otitis media. Arch Otolaryngol. 1934;19:451–459.
7. DiNubile MJ. Septic thrombosis of the cavernous sinuses. Arch Neurol. 1988;45:567–572.
8. Thatai D, Chandy L, Dhar KL. Septic cavernous sinus thrombophlebitis: A review of 35 cases. J Indian Med Assoc. 1992;90:290–292.
9. Johnston I, Hawke S, Halmagyi M, Teo C. The pseudotumor syndrome. Disorders of cerebrospinal fluid circulation causing intracranial hypertension without ventriculomegaly. Arch Neurol. 1991;48:740–747.
10. Dhiravibulya K, Ouvrier R, Johnston I, et al. Benign intracranial hypertension in childhood: A review of 23 patients. J Paediatr Child Health. 1991;27:304–307.
11. Daif A, Awada A, al-Rajeh S, et al. Cerebral venous thrombosis in adults. A study of 40 cases from Saudi Arabia. Stroke. 1995;26:1193–1195.
12. Gates PC. Cerebral venous thrombosis. A retrospective review. Aust N Z J Med. 1986;16:766–770.
13. Davies RP, Slavotinek JP. Incidence of the empty delta sign in computed tomography in the paediatric age group. Australas Radiol. 1994;38:17–19.
14. Medlock MD, Olivero WC, Hanigan WC, et al. Children with cerebral venous thrombosis diagnosed with magnetic resonance imaging and magnetic resonance angiography. Neurosurgery. 1992;31:870–876.
15. Perkins GD. Cerebral venous thrombosis: Developments in imaging and treatment. J Neurol Neurosurg Psychiatry. 1995;59:1–3.
16. Villringer A, Einhaupl KM. Dural sinus and cerebral venous thrombosis. New Horiz. 1997;5:332–341.
17. Kyritsis AP, Williams EC, Schutta HS. Cerebral venous thrombosis due to heparin-induced thrombocytopenia. Stroke. 1990;21:1503–1505.
18. Gerszten PC, Welch WC, Spearman MP, et al. Isolated deep cerebral venous thrombosis treated by direct endovascular thrombolysis. Surg Neurol. 1997;48:261–266.
19. Higashida RT, Halbach VV, Barnwell SL, et al. Thrombolytic therapy in acute stroke. J Endovasc Surg. 1994;1:4–15.
20. Kalbag RM, Woolf AL. Cerebral venous thrombosis. London: Oxford University Press; 1967:242–243.

SECTION I
SKIN AND SOFT TISSUE INFECTIONS

Chapter 78

Cellulitis and Subcutaneous Tissue Infections

MORTON N. SWARTZ

CELLULITIS AND SUPERFICIAL INFECTIONS

Major attention should be directed to determination of the specific microbial cause of any infection involving the skin. This chapter considers bacterial and mycotic infection, exclusive of that caused by the common dermatophytes. Classification of cutaneous infections on morphologic and clinical grounds can be most helpful in providing initial clues regarding the most likely responsible infectious agents (Table 78–1).

Primary Pyodermas

Impetigo

Impetigo is an initially vesicular, later crusted, superficial infection of the skin. Most cases occur in children. Previously, group A streptococcus was considered the principal cause of impetigo and was isolated from about 80% of cases, either alone or mixed with *Staphylococcus aureus*.[1] In the past 15 years group A streptococcus has been found less commonly (20 to 30%) in impetigo and appears to have been supplanted by *S. aureus* in frequency.[2–4] Occasional studies, however, continue to implicate group A streptococci as a major cause of impetigo.[5] These differences may well reflect geographic shifts in streptococcal hyperendemicity over time. As a cautionary note, the role of staphylococci may be overestimated inasmuch as they are common secondary invaders and some strains appear to produce bacteriocins that may make it more difficult to isolate group A streptococci in their presence.[6]

Pathologic Characteristics and Pathogenesis. Histopathologically, impetigo consists of a superficial, intraepidermal, unilocular vesicopustule. In epidemiologic studies, group A streptococcal acquisition on normal skin antedates the appearance of impetigo by about 10 days.[1] During that time, minor trauma (insect bites, abrasions) predisposes to the development of infected lesions. Impetigo is most common during hot, humid summer weather. Two to 3 weeks after skin acquisition of streptococci, pharyngeal colonization by the same organism occurs in about 30% of children with skin lesions. (The sporadic cases of facial impetigo occurring in cooler climates probably result from contiguous spread from an initial nasopharyngeal infection, and the serotypes involved are those commonly causing pharyngeal disease.) In contrast, in the cases of staphylococcal impetigo (where *S. aureus* is the only pathogen), nasal colonization precedes that of the normal skin; skin lesions then follow such colonization.[7, 8]

Evidence suggests that nonbullous impetigo caused by group A streptococcus *(Streptococcus pyogenes)* begins when the corneal layer of the epidermis is disrupted and the bacteria gain access to highly differentiated subcorneal keratinocytes. Adherence of impetigo strains, but not pharyngeal strains of *S. pyogenes* is furthered by keratinocyte differentiation.[9] M protein of *S. pyogenes* mediates binding of the bacteria to keratinocytes.[10] A second streptococcal surface protein, protein F, or fibronectin-binding protein, mediates adherence to antigen-presenting Langerhans' cells located along the basal layer of the epidermis.

Impetigo is a highly communicable infection. Spread in families (particularly among preschool children) is facilitated by crowding and poor hygiene.

Clinical Findings. Streptococcal impetigo begins as small vesicles, sometimes with narrow inflammatory halos, that rapidly pustulate and readily rupture. The purulent discharge dries and forms the characteristic thick, golden-yellow "stuck-on" crusts. Exposed areas are the most common sites for lesions. Pruritus is common, and scratching of lesions can spread infection. Occasionally, large crusts are produced by coalescence of smaller pustules. The lesions remain superfical and do not ulcerate or infiltrate the dermis, and mild regional lymphadenopathy is common. Healing occurs without scarring. The lesions are painless, and constitutional manifestations are minimal.

Laboratory Findings. Gram-stained smears of vesicles show gram-positive cocci. Culture of exudate beneath an unroofed crust reveals group A streptococci, *S. aureus*, or a mixture of streptococci and *S. aureus*. The anti–streptolysin O titer after streptococcal impetigo is scant, probably related to inhibition of streptolysin O by skin lipids at the infection site. In contrast, the anti–DNase B response readily occurs (elevated titers in 90% of patients with nephritis complicating streptococcal skin infections).[11]

Etiologic Agents. The group A streptococci responsible for impetigo usually belong to different M serotypes (e.g., 2, 49, 52, 55, 57, 59–61) than found in the strains producing pharyngitis (e.g., 1, 2, 4, 6, 25). Group C and G streptococci may rarely cause impetigo; group B streptococci have been associated with impetigo in the newborn.

Differential Diagnosis. Although the initial vesicular lesions may resemble early varicella, the crusts of the latter are darker brown and harder. The central clearing of a confluent cluster of lesions of impetigo may suggest tinea circinata but can be distinguished by the thick crusts that are not formed in the fungus infection. When the vesicles of herpes simplex become turbid, they may look like impetigo. Acute palmoplantar pustulosis, a sterile, idiopathic, self-limiting pustular eruption on the palms and soles, sometimes occurring after pharyngitis, may initially resemble impetigo.[12] Localized acute pustular psoriasis may also be mistaken for impetigo. Primary cutaneous listeriosis, an occupational disease of veterinarians and farmers involved in calving, is characterized by papulovesicular and pustular lesions on the forearms that may resemble those of impetigo.[13]

Presumptive Therapy. Penicillin in the past has been the drug of choice for the treatment of ordinary impetigo because of the then predominant role of group A streptococci and the possible occurrence of acute glomerulonephritis as a sequela. Whether penicillin therapy is effective (because of delay in seeking medical attention for such a mild infection) in reducing the incidence of streptococcal pyoderma-associated nephritis remains unclear. Penicillin is administered either as a single intramuscular injection of benzathine penicillin (300,000 to 600,000 units for children, 1,200,000 units for adults), as oral penicillin V (25,000 to 90,000 units/kg/day in divided doses every 6 hours for 10 days), or as amoxicillin. Erythromycin (30 to 50 mg/kg/day in divided doses every 6 hours for 10 days for children,

TABLE 78–1 Classification of Bacterial and Mycotic Infections of the Skin

Type of Lesion	Etiologic Agents
Primary pyodermas	
Impetigo	*Staphylococcus aureus,* group A streptococci
Folliculitis	*S. aureus, Candida, Pseudomonas aeruginosa, Pityrosporum ovale*
Furuncles and carbuncles	*S. aureus*
Paronychia	*S. aureus,* group A streptococci, *Candida, P. aeruginosa*
Ecthyma	Group A streptococci
Erysipelas	Group A streptococci
Chancriform lesions	*Treponema pallidum, Haemophilus ducreyi, Sporothrix, Bacillus anthracis, Francisella tularensis, Mycobacterium ulcerans, Mycobacterium marinum*
Membranous ulcers	*Corynebacterium diphtheriae*
Cellulitis	Group A streptococci, *S. aureus;* rarely, various other organisms
Infectious gangrene and gangrenous cellulitis	
Streptococcal gangrene and necrotizing fasciitis	Group A streptococci, mixed infections with Enterobacteriaceae and anaerobes
Progressive bacterial synergistic gangrene	Anaerobic streptococci plus a second organism (*S. aureus, Proteus*)
Gangrenous balanitis and perineal phlegmon	Group A streptococci, mixed infections with enteric bacteria (*Escherichia coli, Klebsiella,* etc.) and anaerobes
Gas gangrene, crepitant cellulitis	*Clostridium perfringens* and other clostridial species; *Bacteroides,* peptostreptococci, *Klebsiella, E. coli*
Gangrenous cellulitis in immunosuppressed patients	*Pseudomonas, Aspergillus,* agents of mucormycosis
Erythrasma	*Corynebacterium minutissimum*
Nodular lesions	*Candida, Sporothrix, S. aureus* (botryomycosis), *M. marinum, Nocardia brasiliensis, Leishmania brasiliensis*
Hyperplastic (pseudoepitheliomatous) and proliferative lesions (mycetomas, etc.)	*Nocardia, Pseudallescheria boydii, Blastomyces dermatitidis, Paracoccidioides brasiliensis, Phialophora, Cladosporium*
Vascular papules/nodules (bacillary angiomatosis, epithelioid angiomatosis)	*Bartonella (Rochalimaea) henselae, Bartonella (Rochalimaea) quintana*
Annular erythema (erythema chronicum migrans)	*Borrelia burgdorferi*
Secondary bacterial infections complicating preexisting skin lesions such as the following:	
Burns	*P. aeruginosa, Enterobacter,* various other gram-negative bacilli, various streptococci, *S. aureus, Candida, Aspergillus*
Eczematous dermatitis and exfoliative erythrodermas	*S. aureus,* group A streptococci
Chronic ulcers (varicose, decubitus)	Coliform bacteria, *P. aeruginosa,* peptostreptococci, enterococci, *Bacteroides, C. perfringens*
Dermatophytosis	*S. aureus,* group A streptococci
Traumatic lesions (abrasions, animal bites, insect bites, etc.)	*P. multocida, C. diphtheriae, S. aureus,* group A streptococci
Vesicular or bullous eruptions (varicella, pemphigus)	*S. aureus,* group A streptococci
Acne conglabata	Propionibacterium acnes
Hidradenitis suppurativa	*S. aureus, Proteus* and other coliforms, streptococci, peptostreptococci, *Bacteroides*
Intertrigo	*S. aureus,* coliforms, *Candida*
Pilonidal and sebaceous cysts	Peptostreptococci, *Bacteroides,* coliforms
Pyoderma gangrenosa	*S. aureus,* peptostreptococci, *Proteus* and other coliforms, *P. aeruginosa*
Cutaneous involvement in systemic bacterial and mycotic infections	
Bacteremias	*S. aureus,* group A streptococci (also other groups such as D), *Neisseria meningitidis, Neisseria gonorrhoeae, P. aeruginosa, Salmonella typhi; Haemophilus influenzae*
Endocarditis	Viridans streptococci, *S. aureus,* group D streptococci, etc.
Fungemias	*Candida, Cryptococcus, Blastomyces dermatitidis, Fusarium*
Listeriosis	*Listeria monocytogenes*
Leptospirosis (Weil's disease and pretibial fever)	*Leptospira interrogans* serotypes
Rat-bite fever	*Streptobacillus moniliformis, Spirillum minus*
Melioidosis	*Burkholderia pseudomallei*
Glanders	*Burkholderia mallei*
Carrión's disease (verruga peruana)	*Bartonella bacilliformis*
Scarlet fever syndromes	
Scarlet fever	Group A streptococci, rarely *S. aureus*
Scalded skin syndrome	*S. aureus* (phage group II)
Toxic shock syndrome	*S. aureus* (pyrogenic toxin–producing strains)
Para-infectious and postinfectious nonsuppurative complications	
Purpura fulminans	Group A streptococci, *S. aureus,* pneumococcus
Erythema nodosum	Group A streptococci, *Mycobacterium tuberculosis, Mycobacterium leprae, C. immitis, L. autumnalis, Yersinia enterocolitica, Legionella pneumophila*
Erythema multiforme–like lesions (rarely), guttate psoriasis	Group A streptococci

250 to 500 mg orally every 6 hours for adults) is an alternative for penicillin-allergic patients. Currently, it should be noted that the efficacy of erythromycin may be reduced in areas where erythromycin-resistant streptococci (and staphylococci) are prevalent. Local care (removal of crusts by soaking with soap and water) is helpful.

Mixed streptococcal-staphylococcal impetigo has the same crusted lesions and clinical course as streptococcal impetigo and may respond to treatment with penicillin G.[14] However, currently, because *S. aureus*, either alone or in concert with *S. pyogenes* as the etiology of impetigo commonly produces penicillinase, treatment with penicillin alone often fails. Penicillinase-resistant oral penicillins (e.g., dicloxacillin) or cephalosporins (e.g., cephalexin, cefadroxil) are very effective[2, 15] (see later).

A topical antibiotic, mupirocin ointment in a polyethylene glycol base, has been shown to be as effective as oral erythromycin in the treatment of impetigo[3] and more effective when erythromycin-resistant *S. aureus* strains were involved.[4] With the recent increased frequency of isolation of *S. aureus* from the lesions of patients with impetigo, some physicians favor alternative (but more expensive) approaches such as the use of cephalexin (25 to 50 mg/kg orally daily for children in two divided doses), cefadroxil (30 mg/kg orally daily for children in two divided doses), or dicloxacillin (12.5 mg/kg orally daily for children in four divided doses).[15] For most patients with nonbullous impetigo, erythromycin (or penicillin) or topical mupirocin is appropriate therapy unless problems in the community with erythromycin-resistant organisms are suspected.

Mupirocin has also been used topically to eradicate methicillin-resistant *S. aureus* from secondarily infected skin lesions and from colonized patients. However, because resistance in *S. aureus* strains has emerged sooner than anticipated after the introduction of mupirocin, particularly when long-term therapy has been used, prolonged administration should probably be avoided.

Bullous Impetigo

Clinical Findings. The bullous form of impetigo is due to *S. aureus* of phage group II (usually type 71), occurs principally in newborn and younger children, and represents about 10% of all cases of impetigo. The lesions begin as vesicles that turn into flaccid bullae initially containing clear yellow fluid. No erythematous areola is noted, and the Nikolsky sign is absent. The bullae quickly rupture, leave a moist red surface, and then form thin, "varnish-like," light brown crusts. Bullous impetigo, like the staphylococcal scalded skin syndrome (SSSS) and the staphylococcal scarlatiniform syndrome, represents a form of cutaneous response to the two extracellular exfoliative toxins produced by *S. aureus* of phage group II. The gene for one of the toxins (ETA) is chromosomal in origin and that of the other (ETB) is located on a plasmid[16]; ETA appears to have an amino acid sequence similar to that of an *S. aureus* serine protease. The toxin apparently acts extracellularly and causes subcorneal separation of cells of the epidermis.[16] Staphylococci are regularly isolated from the skin lesions of bullous impetigo. Streptococcal superinfection rarely complicates bullous impetigo, probably because type 71 strains of *S. aureus* produce a bacteriocin that inhibits streptococci. Fever and constitutional symptoms are uncommon, and healing occurs without scarring.

Presumptive Therapy. Extensive bullous impetigo responds to treatment with a penicillinase-resistant penicillin (e.g., in children, cloxacillin, 12.5 to 25 mg/kg, or dicloxacillin, 3.125 to 6.25 mg/kg in divided doses orally every 6 hours) or erythromycin in a penicillin-allergic patient.

Staphylococcal Scalded Skin Syndrome. SSSS is the most severe manifestation of infection with *S. aureus* strains producing an exfoliative exotoxin and is characterized by widespread bullae and exfoliation.[17–19] Pemphigus neonatorum (Ritter's disease) is SSSS in the newborn. The more general term *toxic epidermal necrolysis* is often used to encompass both SSSS and a morphologically identical syndrome of various etiologies (drug reactions, viral illnesses) (see Chapter 183).

Clinical Findings. SSSS usually occurs in younger children, but it can rarely develop in adults. Epidemics have occurred in neonatal nurseries.[20] SSSS begins abruptly (sometimes a few days after a recognized staphylococcal infection) with fever, skin tenderness, and a scarlatiniform rash. The Nikolsky sign can be demonstrated. Large, flaccid, clear bullae form, promptly rupture, and result in the separation of sheets of skin. New bullae appear over a period of 2 to 3 days. Exfoliation exposes large areas of bright red skin surface (Fig. 78–1). With appropriate fluid replacement and antimicrobial therapy, the skin lesions heal within 2 weeks, in contrast to drug-induced toxic epidermal necrolysis, in which recovery is more prolonged because the entire epidermis must be replaced and scarring is more frequent.

Presumptive Therapy. Intravenous use of a penicillinase-resistant penicillin (e.g., nafcillin, 50 to 100 mg/kg/day in newborns, 100 to 200 mg/kg/day for older children) is indicated in the initial treatment of SSSS because of the presence of active staphylococcal infection and rapid progression of the skin lesions. Topical treatment consists of cool saline compresses. Systemic corticosteroids alone should not be used in the treatment of SSSS, although they may be indicated in therapy for drug-induced toxic epidermal necrolysis.

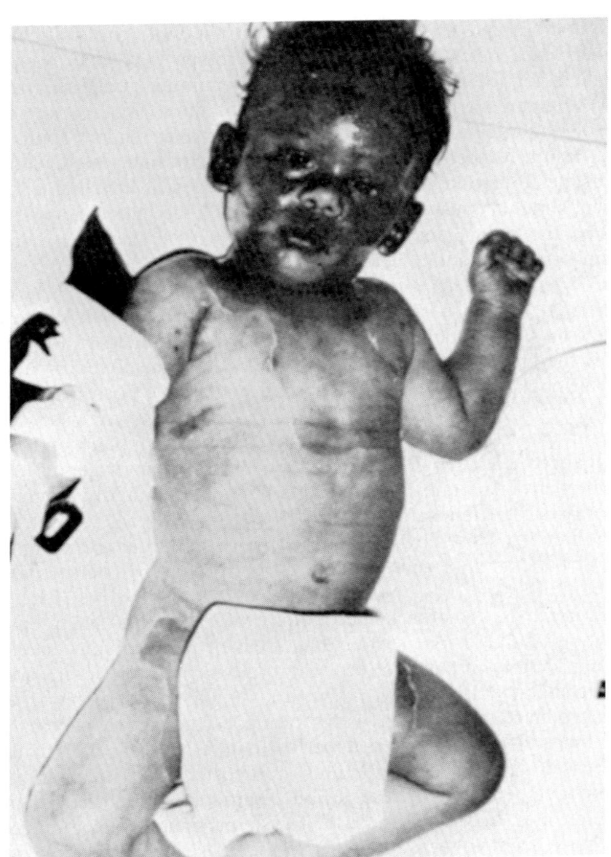

FIGURE 78–1. Staphylococcal scalded skin syndrome in a young infant. Exfoliation has occurred on the face, chest, and groin, exposing areas of bright red skin surface.

Staphylococcal Scarlet Fever

Staphylococcal scarlet fever is fundamentally a forme fruste of SSSS that does not progress beyond the initial stage of a generalized erythematous eruption. However, *S. aureus* enterotoxins (A to D) and toxic shock syndrome toxin 1 are more frequently associated with staphylococcal scarlet fever than are exfoliative toxins A and B.[21] The rash is indistinguishable from that of scarlet fever, and Pastia's lines can develop. However, pharyngitis is not usually present, and an enanthem does not develop. Desquamation, beginning on the face and involving most of the body, occurs 2 to 5 days after onset of the scarlatiniform rash. Antibiotic treatment with penicillinase-resistant penicillins is indicated.

Toxic Shock Syndrome

Toxic shock syndrome is another acute febrile illness with a generalized scarlatiniform eruption associated with *S. aureus* infection. Other elements of the syndrome include (1) hypotension (for shock), (2) functional abnormalities of three or more organ systems, and (3) desquamation in the evolution of the skin lesions[22–24] (see Chapter 183).

Folliculitis

Folliculitis is a pyoderma located within hair follicles and the apocrine regions. The lesions consist of small (2 to 5 mm) erythematous, sometimes pruritic papules often topped by a central pustule. Sycosis barbae is a distinctive form of deep folliculitis, often chronic, that occurs on bearded areas. *S. aureus* is the usual etiology of folliculitis. *Pseudomonas aeruginosa* (most often serotype 0-11) has been responsible for folliculitis acquired from swimming pools and whirlpools contaminated with large numbers of these organisms.[25] This type of skin infection produces pruritic, sometimes tender papulourticarial lesions (appearing within 48 hours of exposure) that eventuate in pustule formation. Lesions in different stages of development are present simultaneously. Preferred sites include the buttocks, hips, and axillae; the palms and soles are spared. Otitis externa is also a common manifestation. Healing occurs spontaneously within 5 days, either by drainage or regression. Scarring develops rarely when an occasional pustule has progressed to furuncle formation. When acquired in a whirlpool, the lesions are sharply limited to the trunk below the upper part of the chest or neck. Inadequate chlorine levels in whirlpools, hot tubs, and swimming pools have been responsible for many of the outbreaks reported. *P. aeruginosa* can also cause superinfection in acne. In granulocytopenic or immunosuppressed hospitalized patients, *P. aeruginosa* 0-11 from tap water used for washing has been implicated in folliculitis that has rapidly progressed to ecthyma gangrenosum.[26]

Folliculitis caused by Enterobacteriaceae can occur as a complication in patients with acne, usually during prolonged courses of oral antibiotic therapy.[27]

Candida is sometimes the etiology of folliculitis and produces pruritic satellite lesions surrounding areas of intertriginous candidiasis, particularly in patients receiving prolonged antibiotic or corticosteroid therapy. *Malassezia furfur*, a common skin saprophyte, may also produce a folliculitis with pruritic erythematous papules and papulopustules on the trunk, upper extremities, and face, particularly in the setting of diabetes mellitus, corticosteroid administration, or granulocytopenia.[28, 29] These lesions, particularly the early papular nodular ones, may suggest those of systemic candidiasis, a diagnosis that may seem to be supported by the presence of budding yeast forms on Gram-stained material from unroofed lesions. Unlike *Candida, M. furfur* requires lipid-supplemented media for primary isolation. Eosinophilic pustular folliculitis, a rare pruritic dermatosis characterized by recurrent crops of follicular papules and pustules with eosinophilic infiltration of perifollicular dermis, occurs particularly in the setting of acquired immunodeficiency syndrome (AIDS) and resembles bacterial or mycotic folliculitis but is a sterile process.[30]

Local measures (saline compresses and topical antibacterials or antifungals such as clotrimazole) are usually sufficient to control the infection.

Furuncles and Carbuncles

Definition and Pathologic Characteristics. A furuncle is a deep inflammatory nodule that usually develops from preceding folliculitis. A carbuncle is a more extensive process extending into the subcutaneous fat in areas covered by thick, inelastic skin. In the latter, multiple abscesses separated by connective tissue septa develop and drain to the surface along hair follicles. *S. aureus* is almost invariably the etiologic agent (see also Chapter 183).

Clinical Findings. Furuncles occur in skin areas that are subject to friction and perspiration and contain hair follicles (neck, face, axillae, buttocks). Predisposing factors include obesity, blood dyscrasias, treatment with corticosteroids, defects in neutrophil function, and probably diabetes mellitus. A furuncle begins as a firm, tender, red nodule that soon becomes painful and fluctuant. Spontaneous drainage of pus commonly occurs, and the lesion subsides. A carbuncle is a larger, deeper, indurated, more serious lesion, usually located at the nape of the neck, on the back, or on the thighs. Fever and malaise are frequent, and some patients are acutely ill. As the lesion progresses, drainage occurs externally along the course of multiple hair follicles. A leukocytosis occurs, particularly when the lesion contains a large amount of undrained pus or when a complicating cellulitis or bacteremia is present.

Blood stream invasion may occur unpredictably (but is sometimes precipitated by manipulation of the lesions) and result in osteomyelitis, endocarditis, or other metastatic foci. Lesions about the upper lip and nose present the special problem of spread of infection via the facial and angular emissary veins to the cavernous sinus.

Presumptive Therapy. Most furuncles are satisfactorily treated by the application of moist heat, which promotes localization and drainage of the process. A carbuncle or a furuncle with surrounding cellulitis or fever or one located about the midface should be treated with an antistaphylococcal antibiotic (e.g., cloxacillin, 0.5 to 1.0 g, or dicloxacillin, 0.125 to 0.25 g orally every 6 hours for an adult). In a penicillin-allergic adult, clindamycin (150 to 300 mg orally every 6 hours) or erythromycin (0.25 to 0.5 g orally every 6 hours) is an alternative. If the lesions are large and fluctuant, surgical drainage is indicated. Antibiotic treatment should be continued until evidence of acute inflammation has subsided.

Management of patients with recurrent furunculosis presents a troublesome problem. This disease does not appear to be due to specific staphylococcal strains with special biologic properties, and most patients do not have definable underlying defects in host defenses. Prophylaxis of recurrent episodes involves several measures:

1. *Antibiotic treatment*. Systemic antibiotic treatment, as described earlier, should be administered for the most recent episode. Prolonged treatment (2 months) is no more effective than a 10- to 14-day course in preventing recurrences.[31]
2. *General skin care*. Soap and water should be used to reduce the number of *S. aureus* organisms on the body surface, and careful hand washing should be performed after contact with lesions. A separate towel and washcloth (carefully washed in hot water before reuse) should be reserved for the patient. Chlorhexidine solution (4%), an antimicrobial skin cleanser, or hexachlorophene may be used to further decrease staphylococcal skin colonization.
3. *Care of clothing*. Sheets and underclothing should be laundered at high temperatures and changed daily for problem patients.
4. *Care of dressings*. Draining lesions should be covered at all times with sterile dressings to prevent autoinoculation, and the dressings should be wrapped and promptly disposed after removal.

Further measures aimed at elimination of nasal carriage and subsequent shedding of *S. aureus* (methicillin susceptible or methicillin resistant) onto the skin may be warranted in the management of refractory cases. Intranasal application of a 2% mupirocin calcium ointment in a white, soft paraffin base for 5 days can eliminate *S. aureus* carriage in healthy persons for up to 90 days[32] (bacitracin or neomycin ointments have been used previously for the same purpose). Similarly, prophylaxis with antibiotic ointment (fusidic acid) in the nares twice daily every fourth week (along with a peroral antistaphylococcal antimicrobial for 10 to 14 days for the patient) has been used with some success in patients and family members who are nasal carriers.[31] Oral antibiotics such as rifampin (600 mg daily for 10 days) have been effective in eradicating coagulase-positive staphylococci from most nasal carriers for periods up to 3 months.[33] Such use of rifampin to eliminate nasal carriage of *S. aureus* and interrupt a continuing cycle of recurrent furunculosis might be considered in patients for whom other measures have failed. However, such therapy can lead to rapid selection of rifampin-resistant strains. The addition of a second drug (cloxacillin if the *S. aureus* is methicillin susceptible; trimethoprim-sulfamethoxazole, ciprofloxacin, or minocycline if the strain is methicillin resistant) has been used to reduce the emergence of rifampin resistance.[34] In one very limited study, prophylaxis with oral clindamycin alone (150 mg daily for 3 months), without an accompanying intranasal antimicrobial agent, reduced the frequency of recurrent staphylococcal skin infection.[35] Various staphylococcal vaccines have not proved effective in preventing recurrent furunculosis.

Ecthyma

Clinical Findings. The lesions of ecthyma begin in a fashion similar to those of impetigo but penetrate through the epidermis. Group A streptococci either produce the lesions de novo or secondarily infect preexisting superficial lesions (insect bites, excoriations), with both mechanisms resulting in the same clinical picture.[36] It is important to note that lesions with the same ultimate appearance can be produced in the course of *Pseudomonas* bacteremia (see later). Ecthyma lesions most frequently occur on the lower extremities, particularly in children and the elderly. They consist of "punched-out" ulcers covered by greenish yellow crusts that extend deeply into the dermis and are surrounded by raised violaceous margins. Treatment is the same as for impetigo. Very extensive involvement with complicating bacteremia has occurred in a patient with AIDS.[37]

Chancriform Lesions

A variety of infections, often with systemic consequences, are characterized by an initial chancriform lesion (see Table 78–1). Of the nonvenereal infections, anthrax has one of the most prominent chancriform lesions.

Anthrax. See Chapter 196 for a detailed discussion.

Pathogenesis. Anthrax is a very rare disease in the United States. Infections are limited to persons working with raw imported wool and other animal products contaminated with highly resistant spores of *Bacillus anthracis*. Routine safety measures for employees in wool plants and so forth have virtually eliminated anthrax from this group; sporadic cases still occur in transient workers in factories (e.g., ventilation repairmen) and in persons directly importing wool for their own weaving. Most infections occur on the face, neck, or arms in an area with a minor abrasion. Rarely, pulmonary infection follows inhalation of *B. anthracis*, or intestinal anthrax results from ingestion of the organism.

Clinical Findings. After an incubation period of 1 to 3 days, a painless papule develops on an exposed area. The lesion enlarges, vesiculates ("malignant pustule"), and is surrounded by a wide zone of brawny, erythematous, gelatinous, nonpitting edema.[38, 39] Malaise and low-grade fever are present. As the lesion evolves, the vesicle becomes hemorrhagic, necrotic, and covered by an eschar of variable dimensions (Fig. 78–2). At all stages the lesion remains painless. Bacteremic dissemination of infection from a skin site may occur and be accompanied by high fever and hypotension. Meningitis may complicate such a bacteremic infection or primary pulmonary anthrax.

The epidemiologic background and the striking appearance of extensive gelatinous edema serve to distinguish anthrax from other types of chancriform lesions. A staphylococcal pustule or carbuncle with a necrotic eschar may be mistaken for early anthrax. However, the former is very painful and tender, and the etiologic agent can usually be demonstrated on a Gram-stained smear of material from the lesion.

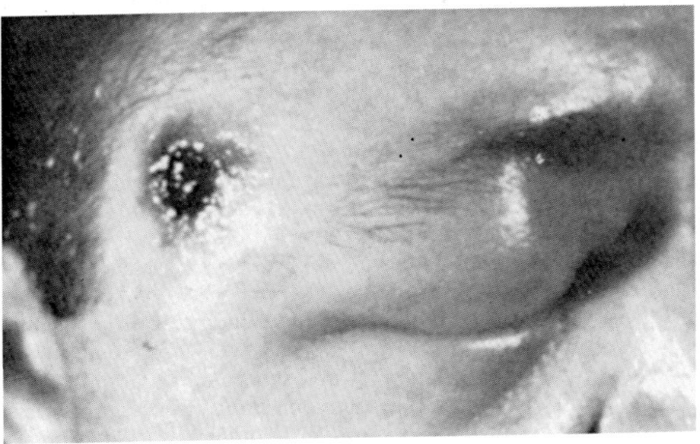

FIGURE 78–2. Chancriform lesion of anthrax on the forehead. There is a prominent surrounding zone of gelatinous edema that is most evident on the eyelids. (Courtesy of Dr. Louis Weinstein, Boston, Mass.)

Presumptive Treatment. Incision and débridement should be avoided because they increase the likelihood of bacteremia. Parenteral penicillin G (1 million units every 4 to 6 hours) is used. In a penicillin-allergic patient, tetracycline (1.0 to 2.0 g/day intravenously in an adult) is an alternative.

Erysipelas

Erysipelas is a distinctive type of superficial cellulitis of the skin with prominent lymphatic involvement. It is almost always due to group A streptococci (uncommonly, group C or G). Group B streptococci have produced erysipelas in the newborn. Evidence of streptococcal infection (groups A, G, and C) was found in 26 of 27 patients with clinical erysipelas by using the combination of direct immunofluorescence and cultures of punch biopsy specimens along with serologic titers.[40] Very rarely, a similar skin lesion is caused by *S. aureus*.

Clinical Findings. Erysipelas is more common in infants, young children, and older adults. Formerly, the face was most commonly involved, and an antecedent streptococcal respiratory tract infection preceded cutaneous involvement in about one third of patients even though streptococci might not be found on culture at the time that the skin lesion became evident. Now, the distribution of erysipelas has changed: 70 to 80% of the lesions are on the lower extremities and 5 to 20% are on the face.[41] Portals of entry are commonly skin ulcers, local trauma or abrasions, psoriatic or eczematous lesions, or fungal infections; in the neonate, erysipelas may develop from an infection of the umbilical stump. Predisposing factors include venous stasis, paraparesis, diabetes mellitus, and alcohol abuse. Patients with the nephrotic syndrome are particularly susceptible. Erysipelas tends to occur in areas of preexisting lymphatic obstruction or edema (e.g., after a radical mastectomy). Also, because erysipelas itself produces lymphatic obstruction, it tends to recur in an area of earlier infection. Over a 3-year period, the recurrence rate is about 30%,[41] predominantly in individuals with venous insufficiency or lymphedema.

Streptococcal bacteremia occurs in about 5% of patients with erysipelas; group A, C, or G streptococci can be isolated on throat culture from about 20% of cases.[41]

Erysipelas is a painful lesion with a bright red, edematous, indurated ("peau d'orange") appearance and an advancing, raised border that is sharply demarcated from the adjacent normal skin (Fig. 78–3). Fever is a feature. A common form of erysipelas involves the bridge of the nose and the cheeks. Uncomplicated erysipelas remains confined primarily to the lymphatics and the dermis. Occasionally, the infection extends more deeply and produces cellulitis, subcutaneous abscess, and necrotizing fasciitis.

Leukocytosis is common with erysipelas. Group A streptococci cannot usually be cultured from the surface of the skin lesion, and only rarely can they be isolated from tissue fluid aspirated from the advancing edge of the lesion. In cases of erysipelas complicating infected ulcers, group A streptococci have been isolated from the ulcerated area in 30% of patients.

Differential Diagnosis. The diagnosis is made on the basis of the appearance of the lesion and the clinical setting. Early herpes zoster involving the second division of the fifth cranial nerve may resemble unilateral facial erysipelas but can be distinguished by the pain and hyperesthesia preceding the skin lesions. Occasionally, contact dermatitis or giant urticaria may look like erysipelas but can be distinguished by the absence of fever and the presence of pruritus. Lesions closely resembling erysipelas, but apparently not caused by streptococcal infection may occur repeatedly in patients with familial Mediterranean fever. Diffuse inflammatory carcinoma of the breast may mimic low-grade erysipelas. Erythema chronicum migrans, the

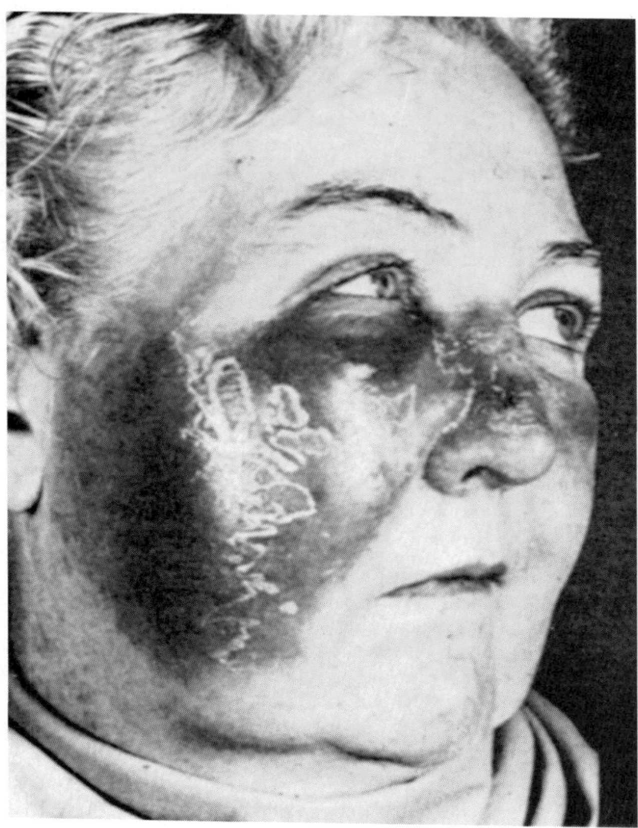

FIGURE 78–3. Facial erysipelas involving both cheeks and the bridge of the nose. The sharp demarcation between the bright red area of erythema and the normal surrounding skin is evident. (From Fitzpatrick TB, Eisen AZ, Wolff K, et al, eds. Dermatology in General Medicine. New York: McGraw-Hill; 1971.)

cutaneous lesion of Lyme disease, resembles erysipelas but is not painful and progresses much more slowly, and the associated fever is less marked. An erysipelas-like skin lesion has occurred in several patients with hypogammaglobulinemia and *Campylobacter jejuni* bacteremia.[42]

Presumptive Therapy. Mild early cases of erysipelas in an adult may be treated with intramuscular procaine penicillin (600,000 units once or twice daily) or oral penicillin V (250 to 500 mg every 6 hours). Erythromycin (250 to 500 mg orally every 6 hours) is a suitable alternative. For more extensive erysipelas, patients should be hospitalized and receive parenteral aqueous penicillin G (600,000 to 2,000,000 units every 6 hours). Although typical erysipelas can be readily distinguished from cellulitis (which can be of staphylococcal as well as streptococcal etiology), differentiation may not be clear cut in occasional circumstances. Under such conditions, particularly in an acutely ill patient, intravenous administration of a penicillinase-resistant penicillin (nafcillin or oxacillin) or a first-generation cephalosporin is warranted.

Cellulitis

Cellulitis is an acute spreading infection of the skin that extends deeper than erysipelas and involves the subcutaneous tissues. Group A streptococcus or *S. aureus* is most frequently the etiologic agent.

Clinical Findings. Previous trauma (laceration, puncture wound) or an underlying skin lesion (furuncle, ulcer) predisposes to the development of cellulitis; rarely, the latter may result from blood-borne spread of infection to the skin and subcutaneous tissues. Within several days of the inciting trauma, local tenderness, pain, and erythema develop and rapidly intensify. Malaise, fever, and chills develop. The involved area is often extensive and the lesion is very red, hot, and swollen. In contrast to erysipelas, the borders of an area of cellulitis are not elevated and sharply demarcated. Regional lymphadenopathy is common, and bacteremia can occur. Local abscesses may develop; small patches of overlying skin may subsequently undergo necrosis. Superinfection with gram-negative bacilli may supervene.

Cellulitis caused by group A streptococci may occur as a postoperative wound infection. Although uncommon today, it is particularly noteworthy because of the rapidity with which it can spread and invade the blood stream. Such infection may be manifested within 6 to 48 hours of surgery (comparable to the short incubation period of postoperative clostridial myonecrosis), earlier than the usual postoperative staphylococcal infection, which is not evident for at least several days after surgery. Hypotension, often caused by bacteremia, may be the initial sign of infection before significant erythema is evident about the incision. A thin serous discharge may be expressed on compression of the wound margins, and streptococci can be identified on a Gram-stained smear.

Cellulitis is a serious disease because of the propensity of infection to spread via the lymphatics and blood stream. Cellulitis of the lower extremities in older patients may be complicated by thrombophlebitis. In patients with chronic dependent edema, cellulitis may spread extremely rapidly.

A distinctive (by virtue of the clinical setting) form of cellulitis occurs in the lower extremities of patients whose saphenous veins have been removed for coronary artery bypass surgery.[43] Occasionally, an associated lymphangitis is present. In some patients, episodes of cellulitis are recurrent. Systemic manifestations such as chills, high fever, and toxicity are prominent. The area of cellulitis extends along the course of the saphenous venectomy. Edema, erythema, and tenderness are marked. Occasionally, the involved areas are somewhat similar to those of erysipelas ("pseudoerysipelas"). Although a bacterial etiology has not been defined in most cases, isolates available from involved skin or blood implicate non–group A β-hemolytic streptococci (groups C, G, B) as major causes.[44] The portal of entry of the infection is often an associated area of tinea pedis. The combination of compromised lymphatic drainage and minor venous insufficiency secondary to saphenous venectomy may result in lower leg edema, a favorable setting for cellulitis. The inflammation from an initial episode of cellulitis, erysipelas, or lymphangitis obstructs lymphatic drainage, thus enhancing the predisposition to further episodes of infection.

Similar recurrent episodes of cellulitis or pseudoerysipelas caused by group B and G streptococci have occurred in patients with lower extremity lymphedema secondary to radical pelvic surgery, radiation therapy, or neoplastic involvement of pelvic lymph nodes.[45] Typically, the cellulitis involves the vulva, inguinal areas, and both lower extremities. In this setting, recurrent episodes have occurred in association with recent coitus.[46]

An uncommon, but distinctive form of cellulitis, perianal streptococcal (group A) cellulitis, occurs principally in children.[47] The clinical features consist of intense perianal erythema, pain on defecation, blood-streaked stools from anal fissures, and chronicity (months) if not treated with penicillin.

A rare, but particularly troublesome, chronic, and progressive form of cellulitis, known as *dissecting cellulitis of the scalp* or *perifolliculitis capitis* is probably similar to hydradenitis suppurativa and acne conglobata in pathogenesis. The clinical features consist of recurrent painful, fluctuant dermal and subcutaneous nodules, purulent drainage from burrowing interconnecting abscesses, scarring, and alopecia. The pathogenesis, as in hydradenitis suppurativa, is probably related to follicular plugging, secondary infection, and deep dissecting inflammation. *S aureus* is most commonly isolated. Effective treatment has involved wide excision and skin grafting.[48]

A very similar, if not identical process, folliculitis decalvans is characterized by chronic perifollicular lesions, coalescence of pustules *(S. aureus)* and ulcers on the scalp, hair loss, and subsequent scarring.[49]

Lymphatic cutaneous metastases from neoplasms, particularly adenocarcinoma, may produce a localized, edematous, erythematous lesion resembling cellulitis. Inflammatory carcinoma of the breast, or carcinoma erysipeloides, involves the skin overlying the site of the primary tumor. Very rarely, lymphomatous involvement of subpectoral or retromammary nodes may produce an erythematous lymphedema of the breast suggesting subacute cellulitis or inflammatory carcinoma of the breast.

A polymorphonuclear leukocytosis is usually present regardless of the bacterial etiology.

Etiologic Agents. Group A streptococci and *S. aureus* are responsible for the overwhelming majority of cases of cellulitis, but other organisms may occasionally be involved. Streptococci belonging to other groups (group C, group G, and in neonates particularly, group B) are sometimes the etiologic agents.

Erysipelothrix rhusiopathiae is the etiologic agent of erysipeloid, a cellulitis occurring principally in persons handling saltwater fish, shellfish, poultry, meat, and hides (see Chapter 198). The infection, which usually occurs in the summer, is introduced through an abrasion on the hands. A painful violaceous area appears within 1 week of the injury. As the process spreads peripherally with distinct raised borders, the central portion of the lesion clears. Ulceration is not a feature. Occasionally, an adjacent joint is involved, and rarely, bacteremia and endocarditis may follow. The causative organism is not generally observed in Gram-stained drainage from the lesion but may be isolated on culture of a biopsy specimen taken from the advancing margin of the lesion. The development of a typical lesion in a person handling fish or meat products suggests the diagnosis. Other forms of bacterial cellulitis or erysipelas may resemble erysipeloid, particularly when the lesion is on the hand. A somewhat similar lesion of unknown etiology, "seal finger," occurs in aquarium workers and veterinarians secondary to seal bites or trauma sustained in caring for these animals. Whereas penicillin is the antibiotic of choice in the treatment of erysipeloid, it appears that seal finger responds to tetracycline.[50]

Rare cases of pneumococcal cellulitis acquired through the bacteremic route have been reported.[51] Soft tissue infections by the pneumococcus can bear a striking resemblance to streptococcal erysipelas. A variety of bacteria (*Serratia*, *Proteus*, and other Enterobacteriaceae) and fungi *(Cryptococcus neoformans)*[52] that are not the cause of cellulitis in healthy individuals may produce cellulitis in an immunocompromised or granulocytopenic patient. *Legionella* spp. have very rarely produced cellulitis: *Legionella pneumophila* in association with pneumonia[53] and *Legionella micdadei* in a renal transplant recipient.[54] Spontaneous *Escherichia coli* cellulitis occurs in children with the nephrotic syndrome in relapse.[55]

An environmental gram-negative bacillus found particularly in lakes, rivers, and soil, *Aeromonas hydrophila* may produce an acute cellulitis after introduction of the organism through a laceration acquired during swimming in fresh water.[56]

Cellulitis, bullous lesions, or necrotic ulcers may complicate infection of a traumatic wound sustained in salt water (or brackish inland waters) or exposed to drippings from raw seafood. Such infections, caused by *Vibrio* spp. (primarily *Vibrio vulnificus* but also occasionally *Vibrio alginolyticus*, non–serogroup 01 *Vibrio cholerae*, and *Vibrio parahaemolyticus*), can result in bacteremia and progress to necrosis, which requires extensive surgical débridement.[57, 58] A rapidly progressive primary septicemia caused by *V. vulnificus* may follow entry of the organism through the gastrointestinal tract (e.g., consumption of raw oysters) rather than through abraded skin. Cellulitis with hemorrhagic skin bullae often rapidly follows the bacteremia. Particularly at risk for the septicemic form of disease are patients with alcoholic cirrhosis, hemochromatosis, and thalassemia—presumably as a result of enhanced growth of *V. vulnificus* mediated by these processes with enhanced iron storage.[59] These vibrios are generally susceptible in vitro to tetracyclines, chloramphenicol, the aminoglycosides, and third-generation cephalosporins. Tetracyclines have been considered the treatment of *V. vulnificus* infections, although more recently, use of the combination of a third-generation cephalosporin plus an aminoglycoside has been advocated.[58]

Envenomation after puncture wounds by the spines of a stonefish (indigenous to shallow waters of the South Pacific) produces local edema and erythema that may suggest acute bacterial cellulitis acquired in seawater.[60] This reaction may be accompanied by serious systemic toxicity, including acute pulmonary edema.

Although needle aspiration of the lesion of erysipelas is commonly unsuccessful in providing a bacteriologic diagnosis (by Gram stain or culture), it is sometimes helpful in defining the pathogen in cases of cellulitis. Aspiration of material from the advancing edge of cellulitis, skin biopsy, and blood cultures are successful in isolating potential pathogens in only about 25% of patients.[61] Positive cultures can be obtained from 30% of closed lesions of cellulitis by the use of a fine-needle aspiration technique.[62] In view of the overall limited yield of pathogens on aspiration of areas of cellulitis, it is reasonable to use this technique primarily when unusual pathogens are suspected (e.g., in immunocompromised patients), when fluctuant areas are detected, or when initial antimicrobial therapy has been unsuccessful.[63] When a site of origin (abrasion, ulcer) for the infection is present, isolates of potential pathogens (*S. aureus*, group A streptococci) can be obtained in about one third of cases.

The appearance and clinical features of a noninfectious process, eosinophillc cellulitis, may suggest the appearance of bacterial cellulitis on the extremities or trunk.[64] The involved area is moderately erythematous and edematous. The lesion develops rapidly, is often accompanied by fever, and enlarges over several days. It can be distinguished from the usual bacterial cellulitis by its minimal tenderness, lack of local heat, and failure to respond to antibiotics. Biopsy of the early lesion shows marked infiltration of the dermis with eosinophils. The lesions resolve in several weeks but frequently recur.

Presumptive Therapy. If a mild early cellulitis is suspected to be of streptococcal etiology, it may be treated with an initial injection of aqueous penicillin G (600,000 units), followed by intramuscular procaine penicillin (600,000 units every 8 to 12 hours). When staphylococcal infection is suspected or when no initial clues to the etiology are present, a penicillinase-resistant penicillin (e.g., dicloxacillin, 0.25 to 0.5 g orally every 6 hours) should be used. In adults allergic to penicillin, erythromycin (0.5 g orally every 6 hours) is an alternative. For more severe infections in which both streptococcal and staphylococcal etiologies are possible, parenteral administration of a penicillinase-resistant penicillin (e.g., nafcillin, 1.0 to 1.5 g intravenously every 4 hours) should be used. Vancomycin (1.0 to 1.5 g/day intravenously) is an alternative for highly penicillin-allergic patients. If the clinical setting suggests a gram-negative bacillus as a possible etiology of a serious cellulitis, an aminoglycoside such as gentamicin may be added to the semisynthetic penicillin initially while awaiting definitive bacteriologic results. In the setting of diabetes mellitus and a diabetic leg ulcer, the development of cellulitis may warrant broader initial antimicrobial coverage such as with a parenteral cephalosporin (cefazolin or cefoxitin) plus an aminoglycoside or with a combination of clindamycin and an aminoglycoside. Gentamicin, along with a penicillinase-resistant penicillin, is probably indicated in the initial treatment of a rapidly progressive cellulitis developing after a freshwater injury. *A. hydrophila* is usually susceptible to gentamicin, chloramphenicol, trimethoprim-sulfamethoxazole, ciprofloxacin, and aztreonam (tetracycline to a slightly lesser degree).

Initial local care of cellulitis includes immobilization and elevation of the involved limb to reduce swelling and a cool sterile saline dressing to remove purulent exudate from any associated ulcer or infected abrasion and decrease local pain.

Patients who have cellulitis at the saphenous site after coronary bypass surgery and fungal infection in the interdigital spaces should be treated topically for the latter with miconazole or clotrimazole. The initial antibiotic (penicillin or nafcillin) should be given in high dosage by the intravenous route for 6 to 7 days to ensure prompt resolution before switching to other routes of therapy. Attention to the problem of tinea pedis before bypass surgery can prevent this form of cellulitis. Similar prompt attention to pedal epidermophytosis in patients who have had one such episode of cellulitis can obviate subsequent episodes.

Recurrent episodes of cellulitis usually occur in patients with peripheral edema. The use of support stockings and good skin hygiene can reduce its frequency or eliminate recurrences. In the occasional patient who continues to have frequent episodes of cellulitis or erysipelas despite such measures, prophylactic penicillin G (250 to 500 mg orally twice daily) or erythromycin (250 mg orally once or twice daily) if penicillin allergic may be indicated.[65]

Membranous Ulcers

Infected ulcers of varied or mixed bacterial etiology may be covered at their base by a layer of necrotic debris resembling a membrane. The latter is not usually strongly adherent and can be removed without much difficulty. In addition, such a lesion has abundant purulent drainage attributable to infection with pyogenic bacteria. Membrane-covered lesions (both superficial and deep ulcers) are also produced by cutaneous infection with *Corynebacterium diphtheriae*.

Cutaneous Diphtheria. Cutaneous diphtheria (see Chapter 193) is uncommon in developed countries; most cases occur in unimmunized persons in overcrowded, underdeveloped parts of the world, particularly in tropical areas, and are associated with skin trauma and poor hygiene. Recent increases in cutaneous diphtheria have been noted in the Pacific Northwest and the South.

Clinical Findings. Three types of cutaneous lesions have been described in cutaneous diphtheria: (1) *wound diphtheria*—secondary *C. diphtheriae* infection of a preexisting wound, which becomes partially covered by a membrane and encircled by a zone of erythema; (2) *primary cutaneous diphtheria*—a disease of the tropics that begins as a single or as several pustules, usually on a lower extremity, and progresses to form a punched-out ulcer covered by a gray-brown membrane; and (3) *superinfection of exzematized skin lesions*—a superficial membranous infection. *C. diphtheriae* has also been isolated from lesions resembling impetigo, ecthyma, and infected insect bites, where they may represent true infections or merely a cutaneous carrier state.[66] Chronic, nonhealing skin ulcers in intravenous drug users that are due to trauma and are infected with *S. aureus* or various types of streptococci have been found on occasion to be superinfected with nontoxigenic strains of *C. diphtheriae*.[67] Cutaneous diphtheria may be as contagious as the respiratory form of the disease among school children.

Occasionally, membranous pharyngitis may accompany cutaneous diphtheria. However, 20 to 40% of patients with cutaneous diphtheria carry *C. diphtheriae* in their upper respiratory tract.[66, 68] Myocarditis is extremely rare as a complication of cutaneous diphtheria, but cranial nerve palsies and Guillain-Barré syndrome occur in 3 to 5% of patients with membranous diphtheritic skin ulcers.

Laboratory Findings. Characteristic beaded, metachromatically staining bacilli can be found in methylene blue–stained smears of the edge of the membrane. However, the diagnosis can be established only by isolation of *C. diphtheriae* from a suggestive skin lesion. Selective media (Löffler's or tellurite agar) are necessary for isolation to inhibit other bacteria in skin ulcers. In addition to isolation of the organism, toxigenicity should be demonstrated by an Elek plate (agar diffusion precipitin reaction) or by guinea pig inoculation (dermonecrosis).

Differential Diagnosis. Pyogenic infection of ulcerated traumatic lesions is usually purulent, and the lesions are not covered by a membrane. Cutaneous fungal infections have more proliferative and irregular margins. The early stages of primary cutaneous diphtheria and secondary infection of insect bites and abrasions with *C. diphtheriae* may closely resemble impetigo.

Presumptive Therapy. If a presumptive diagnosis of ulcerative cutaneous diphtheria is made on clinical grounds and on the basis of preliminary bacteriologic findings, antitoxin is administered (20,000 to 40,000 units intramuscularly or intravenously) after testing for sensitivity to horse serum. Antibiotic administration (erythromycin, 2.0 g/day orally, or procaine penicillin, 1.2 to 2.4 million units/day intramuscularly in adults for 7 to 10 days) also assists in elimination of the convalescent carrier state. Removal of necrotic debris aids in healing of the lesions.

Infectious Gangrene (Gangrenous Cellulitis)

Infectious gangrene is a cellulitis that has rapidly progressed, with extensive necrosis of subcutaneous tissues and the overlying skin. Several different clinically distinguishable pictures may be produced, depending to varying extents on the specific causative organism, the anatomic location of the infection, and the predisposing conditions. Such clinical entities include (1) necrotizing fasciitis (type I, or polymicrobial, often including *Enterobacteriaceae* and anaerobes; type II, or streptococcal gangrene caused by *S. pyogenes*); (2) gas gangrene (clostridial myonecrosis) and anaerobic cellulitis; (3) progressive bacterial synergistic gangrene; (4) synergistic necrotizing cellulitis, perineal phlegmon, and gangrenous balanitis; (5) gangrenous cellulitis in an immunosuppressed patient; and (6) very localized areas of skin necrosis complicating conventional cellulitis.

Pathologic Characteristics and Pathogenesis. The pathologic changes of gangrenous cellulitis are those of necrosis and some hemorrhage in the skin and subcutaneous tissues. In most types of gangrenous cellulitis, an abundant polymorphonuclear leukocytic exudate is present, but in clostridial myonecrosis, the exudate is thin and consists of fluid, fibrin, and gas, but few leukocytes. In most types of gangrenous cellulitis (particularly streptococcal gangrene), fibrin thrombi are present in small arteries and veins of the dermis and subcutaneous fat.[69] In most instances, gangrenous cellulitis has developed secondary to introduction of the infecting organism at the infected site. It may also result from extension of infection from a deeper site to involve the subcutaneous tissues and skin (as in clostridial myonecrosis after intestinal surgery or in perineal phlegmon after dissection of infection from a perirectal abscess). Occasionally, gangrenous cellulitis may begin at a site of metastatic infection in the course of a bacteremia (clostridial myonecrosis caused by *Clostridium septicum* at a peripheral site secondary to spread from an associated colonic neoplasm; *Pseudomonas* gangrenous cellulitis).

Clinical Findings

Streptococcal Gangrene. Streptococcal gangrene is a rare form of gangrene caused by group A (or C or G) streptococci that usually develops at a site of trauma on an extremity but may occur in the absence of an obvious portal of entry (see "necrotizing fasciitis," type II, later). The lesion begins as a local painful area of erythema and edema. Over the next 1 to 3 days the skin becomes dusky. Bullae containing yellowish to red-black fluid develop and rupture.[70] The lesion evolves into a sharply demarcated area covered by necrotic eschar and surrounded by a border of erythema. The process at this point resembles a third-degree burn, for which it could be mistaken if a history were not available. Lymphangitis is rarely evident. Extensive necrotic sloughing can result because of deep penetration of the infection along fascial planes. Bacteremia, metastatic abscesses, and death may result from this life-threatening illness if appropriate antibiotic therapy is not initiated promptly.

Secondary thrombophlebitis may be a complication when the lower extremities are involved. Streptococci can usually be cultured from the early bullous lesions and frequently from blood.

Progressive Bacterial Synergistic Gangrene. This distinctive lesion usually follows infection at an abdominal operative wound site (frequently when wire sutures have been used), about an ileostomy or colostomy, at the exit of a fistulous tract, or in proximity to chronic ulceration on an extremity.[71, 72] It begins as a local tender area of swelling and erythema that subsequently ulcerates. The painful, shaggy ulcer gradually enlarges and is characteristically encircled by a margin of gangrenous skin (Fig. 78–4). Surrounding the latter is a violaceous zone that fades into an outer pink edematous border area. If untreated, the process extends slowly but relentlessly, ultimately producing an enormous ulceration. A related lesion, Meleney's ulcer, is essentially bacterial synergistic gangrene with the additional feature of burrowing necrotic tracts through tissue planes emerging at distant skin sites.

Microaerophilic or anaerobic streptococci can be recovered from aspirates of the advancing margin of the lesion, and *S. aureus* (or occasionally *Proteus* or other gram-negative bacilli) are present in the ulcerated area. Meleney has reproduced the same type of lesions by experimentally injecting both microaerophilic streptococci and *S. aureus* (but not either alone) into the skin of animals. The similarity between the appearance of Meleney's progressive bacterial synergistic gangrene and amebic *(Entamoeba histolytica)* skin gangrene, as well as the usual occurrence of both processes at abdominal or thoracic operative wound sites, has led to the suggestion that *E. histolytica* is the principal cause of Meleney's gangrene.[73] However, development of the latter after gynecologic surgery and its occurrence in countries where amebic infections are rare argue against this concept of pathogenesis. Nonetheless, the capacity of amebic infection to involve the skin of the abdominal wall in a gangrenous process after abdominal surgery should not be overlooked,[74] and appropriate measures (stool examination for amebas, serologic tests, periodic acid–Schiff stain of scrapings, or biopsy of the lesion) should be undertaken to exclude this diagnosis.

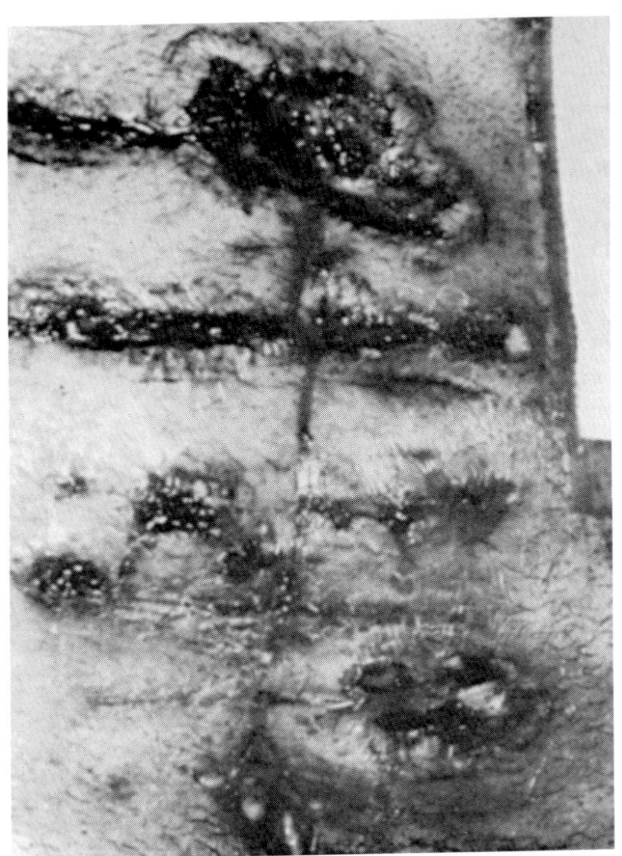

FIGURE 78–4. Progressive bacterial synergistic gangrene of the abdominal wall. Ulcerated areas had developed about wire stay sutures that have since been removed. (From Bornstein DL, Weinberg AN, Swartz MN, et al. Anaerobic infections. Review of current experience. Medicine [Baltimore]. 1964;43:207.)

Gas Gangrene, Anaerobic Cellulitis, and Other Forms of Crepitant Cellulitis. See Chapters 79 and 236 and the later section "Subcutaneous Infections and Abscesses."

Gangrenous Cellulitis in a Predisposed Host. The etiologic considerations in cellulitis occurring in a compromised host include agents that produce such infections in healthy persons, as well as a variety of other organisms not ordinarily regarded as causes of cellulitis. Mucormycotic gangrenous cellulitis may be engrafted on an extensive burn wound, or it may rarely develop in patients with diabetes mellitus or in those who are receiving immunosuppressive therapy. Local factors (open fracture sites, ileostomy stomas, fistulous tracts) also play a predisposing role in this type of infection. Spores of *Rhizopus* spp. (members of the Mucoraceae) contaminating Elastoplast tape used for occlusive dressings have resulted in progressive local and disseminated infection in immunosuppressed patients.[75] The infection may exhibit an indolent course with minimal fever and a slowly enlarging black ulcer, or it may follow a rapidly progressive febrile course. The characteristic lesion consists of a central anesthetic black necrotic area with a surrounding raised zone of violaceous cellulitis and edema.[76] Superficial vesicles and blistering may occur in the gangrenous area. Hematogenous dissemination is not ordinarily demonstrable, and the skin infection usually does not result from an initial pulmonary or rhinocerebral focus. Cultures of the necrotic skin or aspirates from the advancing margin usually do not reveal the fungus. Definition of the etiology is best obtained on biopsy specimens: fungal wet mount on a crushed tissue preparation, tissue sections stained with hematoxylin and eosin (showing tissue and vascular invasion by characteristic broad hyphae), and culture. Necrotizing angioinvasive cellulitis caused by the zygomycete *Apophysomyces elegans* has occurred in a small number of nonimmunocompromised patients after traumatic injury potentially contaminated with soil.[77]

Pseudomonas bacteremia may also produce a gangrenous cellulitis (see the section "Cutaneous Involvement in Systemic Bacterial and Mycotic Infections" later in this chapter) in immunocompromised hosts, patients with thermal burns, and so forth. In similar settings, gangrenous skin lesions may occur with disseminated aspergillosis.

Prominent necrosis of skin and subcutaneous fat occurs rarely in patients who have chronic renal failure (with secondary hyperparathyroidism), in those maintained by chronic dialysis, in patients with extensive calcification of small arteries of subcutaneous tissue, and in those in whom the calcium-phosphate product is markedly elevated.[78] The process that results in acute local calcification has been termed *calciphylaxis*.[79] Precipitating factors for the development of calciphylaxis are poorly defined but include local trauma and systemic infection. The skin lesions begin as dark red irregular areas resembling livido reticularis. They become plaquelike or nodular, are painful, and rapidly increase in size but remain well demarcated. They progress to gangrenous necrosis with eschar formation. Secondary infection of necrotic areas may follow. Histologically, involved areas show extensive vascular calcification, calcinosis cutis, and ischemic skin necrosis. Bacteremia originating elsewhere may contribute to the local ischemic process through further lesional thromboses mediated by disseminated intravascular coagulopathy. These necrotic skin ulcers in patients with chronic renal failure resemble those of infective gangrenous cellulitis, particularly if they become secondarily infected.

Differential Diagnosis. See Table 78–2. The bite of the brown recluse house spider can produce a necrotizing skin lesion that resembles infectious gangrenous cellulitis. The occurrence of fever and chills 24 to 48 hours after the bite enhances the mimicry.

Presumptive Therapy. Treatment of streptococcal gangrene consists of immediate surgical drainage with longitudinal incisions extending through the deep fascia and beyond the involved gangrenous and undermined areas.[70] Initial resuscitation measures with intravenous fluids are essential in the presence of hypotension caused by accompanying streptococcal bacteremia or the streptococcal toxic shock–like syndrome.[80] Areas of cutaneous necrosis are excised and nonviable fascia is débrided. Reexploration is commonly performed within 24 hours. Antibiotic therapy consists of parenteral aqueous penicillin G (600,000 to 2,000,000 units every 4 to 6 hours). If there is any question regarding the etiologic agent (e.g., possibly *S. aureus* rather than group A streptococcus), nafcillin (1.5 to 2.0 g intravenously every 4 to 6 hours) should be used. The etiology of necrotizing fasciitis resulting from mixed anaerobes and facultative organisms (synergistic necrotizing cellulitis) can usually be suspected at the outset from the foul odor and the appearance of the exudate on a Gram-stained smear. After surgery, the wound is treated with elevation and moist dressings. Skin grafting is usually required later.

Progressive bacterial synergistic gangrene is very difficult to treat. Local irrigation with bacitracin and systemic therapy with parenteral penicillin (4 to 6 million units/day intravenously) and a second drug (based on antibiotic susceptibility testing of bacteria other than microaerophilic streptococci isolated from the lesion) are sometimes helpful. However, wide excision of all necrotic tissue (extending well into normal tissue) combined with antibiotic treatment is usually required.

Erythrasma

Clinical Findings. Erythrasma is a common superficial bacterial infection of the skin characterized by slowly spreading, pruritic, reddish brown macular patches, usually located in the genitocrural area.[81] The lesions are finely scaled and finely wrinkled, and they are more common in men and in obese individuals with diabetes mellitus. The disease may be asymptomatic or may undergo periodic exacerbations. The etiology appears to be bacterial: *Corynebacterium minutissimum*, a species that can be grown aerobically. Gram-stained imprints of the skin surface show large numbers of small gram-positive bacilli. Examination of the lesions under Wood's lamp reveals a distinctive coral red fluorescence.

The principal superficial skin infections to be considered in the differential diagnosis are tinea versicolor lesions on the trunk and tinea cruris (a deeper, more inflammatory, and more rapidly progressive process).

Treatment with oral erythromycin (1.0 g/day orally for 5 to 7 days) is usually efficacious and clears the lesions within several weeks. Topical treatment with an aqueous solution of 2% clindamycin hydrochloride can also be effective.[82]

C. minutissimum is also the causative agent of pitted keratolysis, a superficial process consisting of crateriform pits up to 7 mm in width occurring on the pressure-bearing areas of the sole and on the ventral aspect of the toes.[83] The lesions are malodorous and associated with hyperhidrosis.

Secondary Bacterial Infections Complicating Preexisting Skin Lesions

A variety of skin lesions (burns, eczematous dermatitides, traumatic lesions, and so on) may become secondarily infected (see Table 78–1). Such infected lesions usually do not exhibit distinctive morphologic characteristics based on the infecting organism; rather, the appearance of the lesions is determined to a large measure by the nature of the preexisting injury or dermatosis, such as dermatophytosis and acne conglabata, which are often treated primarily by dermatologists. Several of the other secondarily infected dermatoses have some distinctive clinical and bacteriologic features and merit brief consideration.

Diabetic Foot and Other Chronic Superficial Skin Ulcers

A variety of aerobic and facultative organisms (*Pseudomonas*, *Proteus*, enterococci, and so on) colonize and secondarily infect decubitus ulcers. Only in recent years has the prominent role of anaerobic bacteria in such infections been recognized. The character of the ulcers (extensive undermining and necrosis of tissue) and their location, frequently in proximity to the anus, provide the opportunity for invasion by anaerobes. *Bacteroides fragilis* and other Bacteroidaceae and *Clostridium perfringens* have commonly been isolated from infected decubitus ulcers. Such lesions have been the source of symptomatic bacteremias caused by *B. fragilis*, *Peptostreptococcus* spp., *S. aureus*, *Enterococcus*, various streptococci, and a variety of facultative gram-negative bacilli.[84]

Chronic foot infections in patients with diabetes mellitus are common and difficult problems. They usually begin after minor trauma in patients with peripheral neuropathy, neuropathic ulcers, and arterial vascular insufficiency and take the form of cellulitis, soft tissue necrosis, or osteomyelitis with a draining sinus. For convenience, foot infections in diabetic patients are classified into two categories[85]: *non–limb-threatening infections* (superficial, lack systemic toxicity, minimal cellulitis extending less than 2 cm from the portal of entry, ulceration [if present] not fully extending through the skin, lacking significant ischemia) and *limb-threatening infections* (more extensive cellulitis, lymphangitis, ulcers penetrating through the skin into subcutaneous tissue, prominent ischemia). *S. aureus* is the major pathogen in the former. Facultative streptococci are isolated in about one third of patients. Facultative gram-negative bacilli and anaerobes are uncommonly isolated. In the limb-threatening category, in contrast, infection is commonly polymicrobial.[85–87] *S. aureus*, group B streptococci, *Enterococcus*, and facultative gram-negative bacilli are major pathogens in this situation, along with anaerobic gram-positive cocci and *Bacteroides* species.

Deep tissue cultures provide the most reliable bacteriologic information in diabetic foot infections. When not available, cultures and Gram-stained smears of material obtained from curettage of the base of the ulcer or from a purulent exudate may provide the information needed to guide antimicrobial therapy. Gas present in surrounding tissues on radiologic examination may represent air introduced through the ulcer or gas generated in soft tissues by the infecting anaerobic or coliform organisms.

Antibiotic treatment of infected diabetic foot ulcers is based on bacteriologic data if available and meaningful. Initial antimicrobial treatment in a previously untreated patient with a non–limb-threatening infection is focused primarily on staphylococci and streptococci. For mild infections that can be treated at home, oral clindamycin or cephalexin for 2 weeks has been satisfactory.[85] Similarly, cloxacillin or dicloxacillin might be effective. When superficial ulcers are complicated by cellulitis warranting parenteral antibiotics, cefazolin intravenously is effective.[85] Initial antimicrobial treatment of limb-threatening infections involves the use of broad-spectrum antibiotics aimed at its polymicrobial nature (group B streptococci, other streptococci, Enterobacteriaceae, anaerobic gram-positive cocci, and *Bacteroides* spp., including *B. fragilis*). In the past, the combination of clindamycin and an aminoglycoside has often been administered. In addition cefoxitin or ceftizoxime has been used. Although ciprofloxacin has been successful as monotherapy, potential problems are presented by the possible role of *Bacteroides* spp. in these infections and by the emerging resistance to this drug among *S. aureus* strains. Currently, a variety of regimens are advocated for initial empirical therapy for limb-threatening infections[85]: ampicillin-sulbactam or imipenem-cilastatin,[88] clindamycin plus a third-generation cephalosporin, ticarcillin-clavulanate, and clindamycin plus ciprofloxacin.

TABLE 78–2 Differential Diagnosis of Infectious Gangrene and Gangrenous Cellulitis

	Progressive Bacterial Synergistic Gangrene	Synergistic Necrotizing Cellulitis*	Streptococcal Gangrene†	Clostridial Myonecrosis (Gas Gangrene)	Necrotizing Cutaneous Mucormycosis	Bacteremic *Pseudomonas* Gangrenous Cellulitis	Pyoderma Gangrenosum
Predisposing conditions	Surgery, draining sinus	Diabetes common	Occasionally diabetes or myxedema, after abdominal surgery	Local trauma	Diabetes, corticosteroid therapy	Burns, immunosuppression	Ulcerative colitis, rheumatoid arthritis
Pain	Prominent	Prominent	Prominent	Prominent	Minimal	Mild	Moderate
Systemic toxicity	Minimal	Marked	Marked	Very marked	Variable	Marked	Minimal
Course	Slow	Rapid	Very rapid	Extremely rapid	Rapid	Rapid	Slow
Fever	Minimal or absent	Moderate	High	Moderate or high	Low grade	High	Low grade
Anesthesia of lesion	–	–	±	–	+	±	–
Crepitus	–	Often present	–	+	–	–	–
Appearance of the involved area	Central shaggy, necrotic ulcer surrounded by dusky margin and erythematous periphery	Crepitant cellulitis; thick, copious foul-smelling "dishwater" drainage from scattered areas of skin necrosis	Necrosis of subcutaneous tissue and fascia, black necrotic "burned" appearance of overlying skin	Marked swelling, yellow-bronze discoloration of skin, brown bullae, green-black patches of necrosis, serosaguineous discharge	Usually a central black necrotic area with a purple raised margin; may also appear as just a black ulcer	A sharply demarcated necrotic area with black eschar and surrounding erythema resembling a decubitus ulcer; may evolve from initial hemorrhagic bulla	Begin as bullae, pustules, or erythematous nodules that ulcerate deeply; often multiple, large and coalesce; usually on lower extremities or abdomen
Etiology	Microaerophilic streptococci plus *Staphylococcus aureus* (or *Proteus* sometimes)	Usually a mixture of organisms (e.g., *Bacteroides,* peptostreptococci, *Escherichia coli,* etc.)	Primarily group A streptococci; when develops secondary to abdominal surgery, enteric bacteria also involved	*Clostridium perfringens* (occasionally other clostridia)	*Rhizopus, Mucor, Absidia*	*Pseudomonas aeruginosa*	Not an infection primarily; may be confused with such resulting from secondary colonization by Enterobacteriaceae, microaerophilic streptococci, *P. aeruginosa, S. aureus*

*Similar to necrotizing fasciitis type I.
†Necrotizing fasciitis type II.
Modified from Wilson CB, Siber GR, O'Brien TF, et al. Phycomycotic gangrenous cellulitis. Arch Surg. 1976;111:531. Copyright 1976, American Medical Association.

Initial surgical management includes unroofing of encrusted areas and probing the wound to determine the extent of tissue destruction and possible bone involvement. Edema should be reduced by bed rest, elevation, and diuretic therapy as indicated. Control of diabetes is of considerable importance. Open ulcers should be gently packed three times daily with sterile gauze moistened with normal saline or one-quarter-strength povidone-iodine (Betadine). Surgical débridement and drainage should be carried out promptly in patients with deep ulcers extending to subcutaneous tissue or when deep tissue necrosis or suppuration is present.[85]

Occupationally related contaminated traumatic wounds often involve loss of skin and subcutaneous tissue, with ensuing cellulitis and deeper infections. Comparison of the bacteriology of initial wounds sustained in factories with those sustained on farms (associated with corn-harvesting machinery) indicates that gram-negative bacilli (particularly *Enterobacter* spp. and *Pseudomonas maltophilia*) are 10 times more common in the latter.[89]

A newly described, often occupationally related (fish farmers, fish cutters, cooks) form of cellulitis caused by *Streptococcus iniae* has occurred in individuals exposed to aquacultured fish, primarily tilapia.[90] *S. iniae* is a fish pathogen that has caused outbreaks of invasive disease with high mortality among tilapia in aquaculture farms or merely colonization of the surface of fish. Human infection occurs after a puncture wound of the hand by a fish bone or knife while handling or preparing fish. Cellulitis develops rapidly (within 6 to 24 hours of the injury). Fever, lymphangitis originating from the site of injury, and bacteremia are frequent. Metastatic infections such as septic arthritis, meningitis, and endocarditis may occur. Bulla formation and skin necrosis are not features. Penicillin G is the treatment of choice, but *S. iniae* is also susceptible in vitro to cefazolin and ceftriaxone.

Sport fishing in fresh water may result in puncture wounds or lacerations incurred from the venomous spines of catfish.[91] Such wounds may rapidly become secondarily infected, particularly by gram-negative bacilli found in ponds and lakes (e.g., *A. hydrophila*, *Klebsiella*, *E. coli*).

Post-traumatic Opportunistic Skin Infections in Immunocompromised Patients

A variety of unusual pathogens may invade the skin of immunocompromised patients after some local, often minor laceration or abrasion. Such pathogens include fungi *(Paecilomyces, Penicillium, Trichosporon, Fusarium, Alternaria)*, mycobacteria *(Mycobacterium marinum)*, and even algae *(Prototheca wickerhamii)*.[75] The lesions are usually ulcerative or nodular[92] but, in the case of *M. marinum*, may take the form of a nodular lymphangitis extending from the original focus. Cutaneous protothecosis *(P. wickerhamii)* occurs occasionally in patients with AIDS or other immunosuppressed states.[93] Protothecosis occurs rarely in nonimmunosuppressed patients who have been exposed to trauma, water, and local corticosteroid injections.[94] Excision therapy or the use of amphotericin B has been successful. A typical dermatophyte, *Trichophyton rubrum*, which ordinarily produces only superficial skin infections, may invade the deeper subcutaneous tissues of immunosuppressed hosts and produce multiple nodular or fluctuant masses.[95] Primary cutaneous *Bacillus cereus* infection can occur in neutropenic patients[96] and has occurred in a patient with severe immunodeficiency disease.[97] The lesions are vesicular or pustular and usually occur on the hand or an extremity during warm weather. Bacteremia is not a feature. Intravenous vancomycin is the preferred treatment.[96]

Rarely, scattered papular and nodular lesions in patients with AIDS show on biopsy an abscess containing a granule consisting of basophilic-staining cocci surrounded by eosinophilic material (Splendore-Hoeppli phenomenon). This particle superficially resembles a "sulfur granule" of actinomycosis or a mycetoma but is the lesion of botryomycosis and is caused by *S. aureus*.[98] Botryomycosis also occurs in immunocompetent patients; a foreign body may play a role in initiating or perpetuating the lesion, which has the gross appearance of a small infected sebaceous cyst or may resemble prurigo nodulans. Several cases of botryomycosis have occurred in patients with the hyperimmunoglobulin E syndrome associated with recurrent staphylococcal infections.

Bacillary Angiomatosis in Patients with Acquired Immunodeficiency Syndrome

Bacillary angiomatosis (epithelioid angiomatosis) is an infection that primarily involves the skin but also visceral organs in patients with AIDS. The lesions begin as tiny red papules that enlarge to become exophytic or pedunculated nodules, occasionally reaching several centimeters in diameter.[99] They are often dome-shaped vascular lesions with a collarette of scale.[100] Deeper nodules that may occur in the dermis or subcutaneous tissue are flesh colored and somewhat rubbery to firm in consistency and may be movable or fixed to underlying structures. The lesions bleed readily if incised. Only a few may be present, or they may number in the hundreds and cover the body. Oral, nasal, conjunctival, genital, and anal mucosal lesions occur. Visceral involvement takes the form of bacillary peliosis hepatis with hypodense lesions of the liver and spleen demonstrable on abdominal computed tomographic scans.

The lesions of bacillary angiomatosis grossly resemble those of Kaposi's sarcoma, pyogenic granuloma, hemangioma, subcutaneous tumors, or verruga peruana (eruptive phase of bartonellosis in Peru and Ecuador). Histologically, bacillary angiomatosis consists of a circumscribed lobular proliferation of capillaries lined with prominent large endothelial cells, an inflammatory infiltrate with neutrophils, and characteristically, aggregates of bacillary bodies that are demonstrable on Warthin-Starry stain.

The initially uncultivatable etiologic agent of bacillary angiomatosis was first defined in tissue samples as a rickettsia-like organism closely related to *Bartonella quintana* by using techniques for analysis of phylogenetic relatedness of eubacterial 16S ribosomal gene fragments.[101] A newly described species of *Bartonella, Bartonella henselae*, a fastidious gram-negative organism, has been isolated in blood cultures of immunocompromised and nonimmunocompromised patients with an abrupt febrile illness, as well as from cutaneous and osseous lesions of patients with bacillary angiomatosis.[100] *B. quintana* has been cultured from other patients with bacillary angiomatosis.

Based on results of a recently developed immunofluorescence assay for antibody to *B. henselae* and on isolation of this organism from the lymph nodes of several nonimmunosuppressed patients with clinical cat-scratch disease, *B. henselae* (or a closely related organism) appears to be the causative agent in most cases of cat-scratch disease. It is of interest that many patients with bacillary angiomatosis have a history of cat contact or cat scratches.

The diagnosis of bacillary angiomatosis is made by the clinical appearance of the lesions in a human immunodeficiency virus–infected patient and confirmed on biopsy (Warthin-Starry stain). Because the skin lesions are often extensive and systemic manifestations (fever, peliosis hepatis) can be features, antimicrobial treatment is indicated. Erythromycin (0.5 g orally four times daily for 2 to 8 weeks) or another macrolide is the drug of choice. Some patients have responded to doxycycline, and azithromycin (1.0 g orally once daily) has been used successfully in a patient with skin lesions, fever, and bacillary peliosis hepatis.

Hidradenitis Suppurativa

Hidradenitis suppurativa is an extremely troublesome, chronic, suppurative, ciccatricial disease of apocrine glands in the axillary, genital, and perianal areas. The primary lesion appears to be an unexplained keratinous plugging of the ducts of the apocrine glands that results in dilation and eventually rupture of the gland and surrounding tissue inflammation. The initial lesions are reddish purple nodules that slowly become fluctuant and drain. Irregular sinus tracts are formed with repeated crops of lesions; reparative processes are only partially successful. Ultimately, the involved areas show a mixture of burrowing, draining tracts and ciccatricial scarring. In some patients, hidradenitis suppurativa is associated with acne conglobata or dissecting cellulitis of the scalp. In such patients, a distinctive spondyloarthropathy may occur.[102]

Although not initially infected, the lesions frequently become infected secondarily.[103] Staphylococci, nonhemolytic streptococci, *Streptococcus milleri*, *E. coli*, *Proteus*, and *Pseudomonas* are often isolated from draining lesions. Anaerobic organisms (*Bacteroides*, anaerobic gram-positive cocci) have also been reported from such lesions. The foul odor of the discharge from such lesions would suggest the presence of anaerobes.

Treatment of hidradenitis suppurativa is difficult, particularly when the process is chronic and extensive, because of the multiple deep-seated sites of secondary infection that are inaccessible to antibiotics. Antimicrobial therapy (based on Gram-stained smears and culture results) and local moist heat to establish drainage are helpful in treatment of the initial phases of infection. Surgical drainage is required in the management of large abscesses. In very severe, resistant cases exhibiting chronicity and scarring, radical excision of most of the involved area followed by skin grafting may become necessary.

Infected Epidermal Cysts

Epidermal cysts are closed sacs lined with proliferating epidermal cells located about the head, trunk, extremities, and vulvovaginal and scrotal areas. Lacking communication with the skin surface, they can become infected and result in abscess formation. *S. aureus* (frequently present as the sole aerobic organism) and various streptococci are the principal aerobic/facultative isolates from these abscesses. *Peptostreptococcus* and *Bacteroides* spp., the primary anaerobic isolates, are often present in polymicrobial mixtures in cyst abscesses about the head, perineum, and vulvovaginal area.[104] Treatment consists principally of surgical drainage, and initial antimicrobial therapy (clindamycin, cefoxitin, or amoxicillin-clavulanate), if needed, is aimed at *S. aureus* and the probable anaerobes pending results of Gram-stained smears and cultures.

Self-Induced Skin Infections

Rarely, persisting unexplained skin ulcers are self-induced. Their colonization with a variety of gram-negative and gram-positive bacteria is inevitable. However, the continuing ulceration is the result of repeated, self-induced trauma rather than bacterial infection per se. Very rarely, unexplained continuing or recurrent polymicrobial (oral or intestinal flora) cellulitis or a subcutaneous abscess is the result of injection of foreign material containing saliva or contaminated fluids into subcutaneous tissue. Examination of biopsy specimens from the involved area by polarizing microscopy may reveal the presence of birefringent foreign bodies, which suggest the true diagnosis.

Cutaneous Involvement in Systemic Bacterial and Mycotic Infections

Cutaneous manifestations may be a feature of a variety of bacteremias, fungemias, and systemic bacterial infections[105] (see Table 78–1). In leptospirosis, rat-bite fever, and listeriosis, cutaneous manifestations are a small part of the total clinical picture and are considered elsewhere in chapters dealing with the responsible organisms. In some systemic infections, cutaneous manifestations are noninfectious complications of the illness (erythema nodosum, purpura fulminans).

Bacteremias

Staphylococcus aureus. The occurrence of skin lesions (pustules, subcutaneous abscesses, purulent purpura) in the course of bacteremia or endocarditis secondary to *S. aureus* can provide a clue to the nature of the infecting organism. The most distinctive of these lesions is purulent purpura, a small area of purpura with a white, purulent center. Aspiration of the contents of the central portion reveals staphylococci and polymorphonuclear leukocytes. Rarely, scattered tender subcutaneous nodules may develop during *S. aureus* bacteremia.

Pseudomonas aeruginosa. Five types of skin lesion have been described in the course of *Pseudomonas* septicemia:

1. *Vesicles and bullae.* These lesions occur as isolated bullae or occasionally in small clusters anywhere on the skin surface. They rapidly become hemorrhagic and have a narrow encircling zone of dusky erythema. Occasionally, in infants the lesions are surrounded by large, erythematous halos resembling insect bites or erythema multiforme.
2. *Ecthyma gangrenosum.* This lesion is a round, indurated, ulcerated, painless area with a central gray-black eschar and a surrounding narrow zone of erythema. These lesions may develop de novo or may evolve from an initial bullous lesion.
3. *Subcutaneous nodules.* Solitary or multiple, minimally fluctuant, subcutaneous nodules are uncommon features of *Pseudomonas* bacteremia, primarily in immunocompromised hosts.[106] Similar nodules in immunocompromised patients may have other infectious etiologies: *S. aureus* and botryomycosis, mycobacterial infections, candidiasis and other deep mycoses, protothecosis, *Acanthamoeba* infection, and bacillary angiomatosis.
4. *Gangrenous cellulitis.* Grangrenous cellulitis is either a superficial, sharply demarcated necrotic area that may resemble a decubitus ulcer or an area of cellulitis with edema and some necrosis of the overlying skin.
5. *Macular or maculopapular lesions.* These lesions are small, oval, erythematous macules located predominantly over the trunk that resemble the "rose spots" of typhoid fever. Such lesions have been reported, particularly in the tropics, in association with fever and diarrhea in the syndrome described as *Shanghai fever.*

The foregoing types of metastatic lesions contain numerous gram-negative bacilli but relatively few polymorphonuclear leukocytes. The development of such lesions in a febrile patient with leukemia who is undergoing induction chemotherapy or on uninvolved skin areas of a patient with extensive thermal burns should strongly suggest the presence of *Pseudomonas* bacteremia. Presumptive antibiotic management should be aimed at *P. aeruginosa* and includes a combination of ceftazidime or ticarcillin with tobramycin or a fluoroquinolone. Rarely, ecthyma gangrenosum occurs in the course of bacteremia caused by other gram-negative bacilli or in disseminated candidiasis, or it may occur in the absence of bacteremia as progression of *Pseudomonas* folliculitis in an immunocompromised patient.[107]

Neisseria meningitidis. The skin lesions of acute meningococcemia consist of erythematous macules (initially), petechiae, purpura, and ecchymoses located on the extremities and trunk. Extensive gun-metal gray, hemorrhagic, necrotic patches can develop by confluence of petechial and purpuric lesions in fulminant meningococcemia. Symmetric peripheral gangrene and purpura fulminans occur with prominent disseminated intravascular coagulation. Occasionally, gram-negative diplococci can be observed on smears of serum obtained from the skin lesions of patients with acute meningococcemia.

Skin lesions are an important feature of the unusual syndrome of chronic meningococcemia, which is characterized by recurrent cycles of fever, arthralgia, and rash over a period of 2 to 3 months.[108] The rash appears in crops, each consisting of a small number of individual lesions during febrile episodes. The lesions are generally located on the extremities, particularly about joints. They may consist of erythematous maculopapules, petechiae, petechiae with vesiculopustular centers, petechiae with small areolas of pale erythema, suggillations, or tender erythema nodosum–like nodules. Biopsy specimens of the lesions reveal the histologic picture of leukocytoclastic angiitis, a finding that may erroneously direct attention toward the diagnosis of a small vessel hypersensitivity vasculitis and away from that of vasculitis secondary to systemic infection.

Neisseria gonorrhoeae. The skin lesions of gonococcemia consist of a mixture of pustules surrounded by a thin zone of purpura, macules, papules, purpuric vesicles and bullae, and purpuric infarcts. The lesions are few, scattered over the distal ends of extremities in particular, and frequently painful. They are part of the gonococcemic dermatitis-arthritis syndrome.[109] *N. gonorrhoeae* is isolated from less than 5% of skin lesions, but in one study, gonococcal antigens were identified by immunofluorescent staining procedures in most lesions. In addition to arthralgias and frank arthritis, tenosynovitis may be a conspicuous feature.

Salmonella typhi. "Rose spots" frequently appear 7 to 10 days into the febrile course of untreated typhoid fever. The lesions are slightly raised, small (1 to 3 mm), pink papules that tend to occur in crops of 10 to 20 lesions. They are found most commonly on the upper part of the abdomen, lower part of the chest, and back. Rose spots are less frequently found in enteric fever caused by *Salmonella* spp. other than *S. typhi.* Early treatment with ciprofloxacin or chloramphenicol will prevent the appearance of these skin lesions. *S. typhi* can sometimes be found on Gram-stained preparations from the papules and isolated on culture.

Haemophilus influenzae. Cellulitis involving the face, neck, or upper extremities occasionally occurs with bacteremic *H. influenzae* type B infection in children, particularly those younger than 3 years. Although commonly described as having a peculiar purple-red or blue-red hue, the lesion most often is erythematous, indurated, and indistinguishable from cellulitis caused by streptococci or staphylococci. The site of primary infection is in the pharynx, the middle ear, or elsewhere in the upper respiratory tract. Direct invasion across traumatized buccal mucous membranes by *H. influenzae* type B colonizing the respiratory tract has been suggested as the pathogenesis of most cases of buccal cellulitis in children.[110] This infection is life threatening and acute, and bacteremia (sometimes complicated by meningitis) occurs in about 80% cases.[111] Until recently, this uncommon lesion had been described only in pediatric practice, but now a few cases have been reported in adults with epiglottitis and other forms of upper respiratory disease caused by *H. influenzae*.[112] *H. influenzae* type B cellulitis in children has almost disappeared in developed countries since widespread immunization with conjugate vaccines was introduced a decade ago. Although almost all cases of *H. influenzae* cellulitis in adults have involved cervical or thoracic areas, one case of bacteremic *H. influenzae* type B cellulitis has occurred on the foot of an otherwise healthy octogenarian.[113] In view of the increased incidence of ampicillin resistance in clinical strains of *H. influenzae* type B, provisional antibiotic therapy should use a third-generation cephalosporin or chloramphenicol (either alone or in combination with ampicillin) until the isolate can be tested for β-lactamase activity.

Helicobacter cinaedi Bacteremia. A syndrome of *H. cinaedi* febrile, indolent bacteremia with resultant recurrent multifocal cellulitis has been described.[114] Although *H. cinaedi* was originally described in homosexual men with gastroenteritis, gastroenteritis has not been a feature of patients with the bacteremia-cellulitis syndrome. The patients have been immunocompromised to a large extent, often with human immunodeficiency virus infection. In the latter group the infection may be sexually transmitted. The cellulitis in some patients is described as having an atypical appearance: red-brown or copper colored and lacking the expected local heat. *H. cinaedi* is susceptible to tetracyclines, aminoglycosides, rifampin, and often ciprofloxacin. Prolonged therapy (2 to 6 weeks) is usually required to ensure resolution of symptoms and prevent recurrence.[115]

Infective Endocarditis

The cutaneous lesions of subacute bacterial endocarditis consist of petechiae, subungual "splinter" hemorrhages, Osler's nodes, and Janeway lesions. Petechiae tend to occur in small crops, particularly in the conjunctivae, on the palate, and on the upper part of the chest and extremities, and are the most common skin lesions of endocarditis. Rarely, petechiae are extremely numerous, particularly on the lower extremities, and suggest a primary vasculitis. Osler's nodes are split pea–sized, erythematous, tender nodules located principally on the pads of the fingers and toes. They are few at any given time and occur in about 15% of patients with subacute bacterial endocarditis. The lesions are usually transient and clear in 1 to 2 days. Similar lesions may also occur in acute endocarditis (e.g., secondary to *S. aureus*). Histologic examination of such lesions in several cases of acute endocarditis has suggested septic embolization in their pathogenesis.[116] The genesis of Osler's nodes in subacute bacterial endocarditis may have a different basis, perhaps sterile embolization or an allergic vasculitis. Janeway lesions are painless, small erythematous macules or minimally nodular hemorrhages in the palms or soles occurring in either acute or subacute endocarditis (more commonly in the former, particularly when *S. aureus* is the etiology). Histologic findings in a case of *S. aureus* endocarditis indicate that Janeway lesions are caused by septic microembolization.[117]

Fungemias: Candida albicans

Systemic candidiasis developing in the setting of leukemia, immunosuppression, extensive antibiotic therapy, hyperalimentation, heroin addiction, cardiac surgery, and so on may be difficult to diagnose clinically until the organism is isolated from routine blood cultures—often not until after 5 to 7 days of incubation (more rapidly with lysis-centrifugation culture methods). The portal for disseminated candidiasis (or aspergillosis) may be an area of skin injured in the course of intravenous therapy (or trauma induced by adhesive tape or extravasation of intravenous fluid).[75] Examination of the optic fundi (for evidence of candidal ophthalmitis) and a search for *Candida* pseudohyphae and yeast forms on a smear of buffy coat of venous blood are sometimes helpful in making an early diagnosis of candidal fungemia while awaiting isolation of the organism from blood cultures. In occasional patients, the appearance of multiple discrete (2 to 5 mm) pink maculopapules (sometimes with pale centers) on the trunk or extremities can suggest the diagnosis.[118] In some of these patients, severe diffuse muscle tenderness has been present, and muscle biopsy specimens have shown necrosis with yeast and pseudohyphal forms.[119] Occasionally, subcutaneous abscesses caused by *Candida* may develop in the course of fungemia. Aspiration of such abscesses reveals the etiology on stained smear. Punch biopsy specimens of the maculopapular lesions provide a more accurate diagnosis than simple culture does because histologic sections can reveal *Candida* emboli in blood vessels and pseudohyphae in adjacent soft tissue. Isolation of *Candida* from an unroofed lesion may represent only surface colonization or may be consistent with *Candida* folliculitis rather than disseminated candidiasis.

SUBCUTANEOUS TISSUE INFECTIONS AND ABSCESSES

Exact categorization of some bacterial infections of the soft tissues (skin, subcutaneous tissue, fascia, and skeletal muscle) may be difficult. Although differences between a superficial pyoderma and a necrotizing myositis[120] such as gas gangrene are readily apparent, distinctions between many other types of soft tissue infection are sometimes blurred. Classification is usually based on features such as the anatomic structure involved, the infecting organism(s), and the clinical picture. Unfortunately, for convenience in categorization, some infections may involve several components of the soft tissue, and multiple bacterial species may produce infections with the same clinical appearance.

To further compound the problem of classification, a variety of designations have been given to closely related or virtually identical processes. For example, *streptococcal gangrene* has also been referred to as *necrotizing fasciitis*. Subsequent to the initial descriptions of this condition, it became apparent that it was sometimes caused by bacteria other than group A streptococci.[121] Thus, streptococcal gangrene can be considered the major subset of necrotizing fasciitis. For convenience, because a major feature of its manifestation is cutaneous gangrene, streptococcal gangrene has been considered in the preceding section with cellulitis and infectious cutaneous gangrene. Necrotizing fasciitis is reconsidered in this section on subcutaneous tissue infections, particularly in relation to its nonstreptococcal etiologies. Another example of the problems in nomenclature is that presented by infections that involve multiple soft tissue strata and that can be caused by a variety of bacterial species. Thus, the condition known as *synergistic necrotizing cellulitis* has also been described as *gram-negative anaerobic cutaneous gangrene* and *synergistic nonclostridial anaerobic myonecrosis*.[122, 123] Because of the prominence of subcutaneous tissue involvement in this condition, it is considered primarily in this part of the chapter, although it could be considered almost as readily in the first part ("Cellulitis and Superficial Infections") or in the chapter on myositis (see Chapter 79).

Clostridial Anaerobic Cellulitis

Clostridial anaerobic cellulitis is a necrotizing clostridial infection of devitalized subcutaneous tissue. Deep fascia is not appreciably involved, and ordinarily, no associated myositis is present. Gas formation is common and often extensive. Anaerobic cellulitis is several times more common than gas gangrene in war wounds.

Pathogenesis and Pathologic Characteristics. Clostridial species, usually *C. perfringens*, are introduced into subcutaneous tissue through a dirty or inadequately débrided traumatic wound, through contamination at surgery, or from a preexisting localized infection. The last is frequently located in the perineum, abdominal wall, buttocks, and lower extremities, areas that are readily contaminated with fecal flora. The presence of foreign debris and necrotic tissue in the depths of a wound provides a suitable anaerobic milieu for clostridial proliferation. Very rarely, clostridial anaerobic cellulitis develops not after primary cutaneous injury, but rather as a consequence of *C. septicum* bacteremia in the setting of leukemia and granulocytopenia.[124] Intestinal erosions are the presumed initial portals of entry. This type of *C. septicum* cellulitis should be distinguished from the even more life-threatening bacteremic *C. septicum* myonecrosis, which is often associated with a cryptic underlying colonic neoplasm (see Chapter 79).

Clinical Findings. The incubation period is several days, longer than the 1 to 2 days for clostridial myonecrosis. The onset is gradual, but the process may subsequently spread rapidly.[125] Local pain, tissue swelling, and systemic toxicity are not prominent features, and the relative mildness of the process helps distinguish it from true gas gangrene. The dark blebs and bronzing of the skin seen in gas gangrene are not usually features of clostridial cellulitis. Thin, dark, sometimes foul-smelling drainage (often containing fat globules) from the wound is characteristic, as is extensive tissue gas formation, more prominent than that observed in clostridial myonecrosis. Frank crepitus is present in the involved area and may extend very widely, even beyond the limits of the active infection.

Gram-stained smears of drainage material show numerous blunt-ended, thick, gram-positive bacilli and variable numbers of polymorphonuclear leukocytes. Soft tissue x-ray films show abundant gas, but not usually in the feathery linear pattern in muscles observed in clostridial myonecrosis.

Etiologic Agents. *C. perfringens* is the most common clostridial species responsible for this infection, but *C. septicum* and other species have been isolated. Sometimes, clostridia are present in mixed culture with facultative organisms.

Differential Diagnosis. When crepitus is observed with a wound, a variety of possibilities must be considered in the differential diagnosis (Table 78–3). The first is clostridial myonecrosis (gas gangrene) because of the fulminant nature of the infection and the requirement for emergency surgery. At the same time, distinguishing between clostridial gas gangrene and anaerobic cellulitis is essential to avoid performing unnecessarily extensive surgery. Ultimately, the two processes are differentiated in the operating room when the wound is laid open and the viability and appearance of the muscle are observed. The muscle is normal (pink) in clostridial cellulitis but distinctly abnormal (discolored, fails to contract on stimulation, does not bleed from a cut surface) in clostridial myonecrosis (see Chapter 79).

Presumptive Therapy. Surgical exploration is essential to determine the presence of any muscle involvement. If no myonecrosis is found, treatment should be limited to débridement of necrotic tissue and drainage of pus after the wound is opened widely. Initial antimicrobial management of clostridial cellulitis involves the use of several antibiotics because until surgical exploration has been carried out to distinguish between clostridial myonecrosis and anaerobic cellulitis and until Gram-stained smears of material from the lesion have been evaluated, gas gangrene or a potentially polymicrobial infection is an important consideration. Intravenous penicillin (1 to 2 million units every 3 hours) or ampicillin (1 to 1.5 g every 3 to 4 hours) plus intravenous clindamycin (0.6 g every 6 to 8 hours) or metronidazole (1 g loading dose followed by 0.5 g every 6 hours) provides a two-drug combination for treating anaerobic organisms likely to be involved. Use of an additional antimicrobial (an aminoglycoside, ciprofloxacin, or a third-generation cephalosporin) aimed at aerobic gram-negative bacilli would be based on evaluation of Gram-stained smears of exudate and tissue. Definitive antimicrobial selection is subsequently based on results of cultures and antimicrobial-susceptibility tests.

Nonclostridial Anaerobic Cellulitis

A clinical picture very similar to that of clostridial anaerobic cellulitis can be produced by infection with a variety of non–spore-forming anaerobic bacteria (various *Bacteroides* spp., peptostreptococci, peptococci—either alone or as mixed infections).[123] The anaerobic bacteria may be present along with facultative species (coliform bacilli, various streptococci, staphylococci) in a mixed infection. Gas-forming soft tissue infections have been produced by *E. coli*, *Klebsiella*, *Aeromonas*, and perhaps other facultative bacteria.[120, 126]

Because the clinical features and setting are very similar to those of clostridial anaerobic cellulitis, the same initial antimicrobial therapy (see earlier) would be appropriate to cover the mixed bacterial nature of the infection. In the past, the combination of penicillin or ampicillin (aimed at *Peptostreptococcus* spp., *Peptococcus* spp., *Clostridium* spp., and various streptococcal species) plus chloramphenicol (directed at *Bacteroides* spp. and facultative gram-negative bacilli) has been used as preliminary therapy and is still favored by some. Ampicillin-sulbactam can also be used as initial therapy. Evaluation of Gram-stained smears of exudate aspirated from the lesion supplies a more focused basis for initial antimicrobial therapy. Subsequent results of cultures and susceptibility testing of aspirates or tissue removed at surgical exploration provide the information needed for narrowing (or extending) antimicrobial therapy. The surgi-

TABLE 78–3 Differential Diagnosing of Crepitant Soft Tissue Wounds*

	Clostridial Cellulitis	Nonclostridial Anaerobic Cellulitis	Clostridial Myonecrosis (Gas Gangrene)	Anaerobic Streptococcal Myositis	Necrotizing Fasciitis†	Infected Vascular Gangrene	Synergistic Necrotizing Cellulitis‡	Noninfectious Causes of Gas in Tissues
Predisposing conditions	Local trauma or surgery	Diabetes mellitus, preexisting localized infection	Local trauma or surgery	Local trauma	Diabetes mellitus, abdominal surgery, perineal infection	Peripheral arterial insufficiency	Diabetes mellitus, cardiorenal disease, obesity, perirectal infection	Mechanical effects of penetrating trauma, injuries involving the use of compressed air, entrapment of air under loosely sutured wounds or under ulcers, irrigation of wounds with hydrogen peroxide, intravenous catheter placement, dissection of air from tracheostomy or spontaneous mediastinal emphysema
Incubation period	Usually over 3 d	Several days	1–2 d	3–4 d	1–4 d	>5 d	3–14 d	Less than an hour
Onset	Gradual	Gradual or rapid	Acute	Not as rapid as gas gangrene	Acute	Gradual	Acute	Usually present immediately after trauma or manipulation; may not be recognized until examined several hours later
Pain	Mild	Mild	Marked	Occurs late, marked	Moderate or severe	Variable	Severe	Mild
Swelling	Moderate	Moderate	Marked	Moderate	Marked	Moderate or marked	Moderate or marked	Slight or absent
Skin appearance	Minimal discoloration	Minimal discoloration	Yellow-bronze, dark bullae, green-black patches of necrosis	Erythema	Erythematous cellulitis, areas of skin necrosis	Discolored or black	Scattered areas of skin necrosis	Only those resulting from the initiating trauma
Exudate	Thin, dark	Dark pus	Serosanguineous	Abundant seropurulent	Seropurulent	0	"Dishwater" pus	0
Gas	+ + + +	+ + + +	+ +	±	+ +	+ + +	+ +	Variable but present; does not extend
Odor	Sometimes foul	Foul	Variable, slightly foul or peculiarly sweet	Slight; "sour"	Foul	Foul	Foul	0
Systemic toxicity	Minimal	Moderate	Marked	Only late in course	Moderate or marked	Minimal	Marked	0
Muscle involvement	0	0	+ + + +	+ + +	0	Dead	+ +	0

*In addition to the causes of crepitant infections listed in this table, *Aeromonas hydrophila* myositis may be associated with gas in soft tissues.
†The term *necrotizing fasciitis* is used here to designate forms of this syndrome other than streptococcal gangrene.
‡Synergistic necrotizing cellulitis is essentially the same process as type I necrotizing fasciitis. Because the former occasionally tends to involve muscle, it is given a separate designation here; however, the two processes are clinically indistinguishable in most instances.
Key: ±, Rarely present; + +, present to mild extent; + + +, present to moderate extent; + + + +, extensive.
Modified from Finegold SM. Anaerobic Bacteria in Human Disease. New York: Academic Press; 1977.

cal approach used is the same as in the treatment of clostridial anaerobic cellulitis.

Necrotizing Fasciitis

The term *necrotizing fasciitis* encompasses two bacteriologic entities.[127] In *type I*, the first entity, at least one anaerobic species (most commonly *Bacteroides* and *Peptostreptococcus* spp.) is isolated in combination with one or more facultative anaerobic species such as streptococci (other than group A) and members of the Enterobacteriaceae (e.g., *E. coli*, *Enterobacter*, *Klebsiella*, *Proteus*). An obligate aerobe such as *P. aeruginosa* is only rarely a component of such a mixed infection. Cases in which only anaerobes are present appear to be rare.

In *type II*, the second entity (corresponding to the entity also known as *hemolytic streptococcal gangrene*), group A streptococci are isolated either alone or in combination with other species, *S. aureus* most commonly. Streptococcal gangrene has been considered in the first part of this chapter as a form of gangrenous cellulitis. At this point, specific comments about streptococcal gangrene will be limited to the expanded setting in which the disease can appear and the changes in clinical features noted with the very recent apparent increase in bacteremic and severe invasive group A streptococcal infections and their association with the *streptococcal toxic shock–like syndrome*.[2, 128, 129] Hemolytic streptococcal gangrene occurs after minor trauma, stab wounds, or surgery, particularly in the background of diabetes and peripheral vascular disease, but cirrhosis and corticosteroid therapy have also been predisposing factors.[130] In outbreaks of streptococcal toxic shock–like syndrome, chills, fever (or profound hypothermia and shock), confusion, vomiting, diarrhea, tachycardia, hypotension, and multiorgan failure are prominent features. Necrotizing fasciitis is present in about half of cases of streptococcal toxic shock syndrome.[2] Streptococcal strains of M protein types 1, 3, 12, and 28 are most commonly involved and, in the United States, usually elaborate pyrogenic exotoxin A. The use of nonsteroidal anti-inflammatory agents may delay the diagnosis by reducing inflammatory features and thereby masking the diagnosis. Leukocytosis, thrombocytopenia, azotemia, and increased serum levels of creatine phosphokinase were commonly present. Rising creatine phosphokinase levels may serve as an indication of progression of streptococcal cellulitis to necrotizing fasciitis and myositis. Unlike many earlier studies of hemolytic streptococcal gangrene, which affected older individuals with underlying diseases, this recent outbreak of streptococcal toxic shock–like syndrome occurred primarily in young, previously healthy adults after minor trauma. In 70% of the patients, soft tissue findings progressed to hemolytic streptococcal gangrene with the development of vesicles, violaceous bullae, and necrosis of subcutaneous tissues typical of necrotizing fasciitis (or myositis) and requiring surgical débridement.[128] The mortality rate was about 30%. In young children the skin lesions of varicella can be superinfected with group A streptococci and become a risk factor for group A streptococcal necrotizing fasciitis.[131, 132]

In a study in Ontario, Canada, in the late 1980s, a primary site of infection could be defined in 38 of 50 (76%) cases of severe, invasive group A streptococcal infection.[133] Of these, skin and soft tissue infections numbered 26 (68%), and necrotizing fasciitis was present in 15 (57%) of these cases. The most common group A streptococci in recent outbreaks have been M1/T1 or M12/T12 types containing pyrogenic exotoxin A (spe A) or C (spe C) genes[133] and M1 or M3 types producing pyrogenic exotoxins A or B.[129] Recent examination of type M1 and M3 isolates from cases of streptococcal toxic shock–like syndrome suggests their possible clonal origin.[134] The finding of a characteristic restriction enzyme fragment profile of streptococcal DNA (hybridized with a spe A probe) from patients with serious streptococcal disease (mainly toxic shock–like syndrome) of several different serotypes further suggests that the invasive strains are not serotype specific but that a strain of a given serotype can acquire a new gene (toxin gene) and, with it, enhanced virulence.[135] The more general features of necrotizing fasciitis will now be considered.

Clinical Findings. Necrotizing fasciitis is an uncommon severe infection involving the subcutaneous soft tissues, particularly the superficial (and often the deep) fascia. It is usually an acute process but rarely may follow a subacute progressive course. Necrotizing fasciitis can affect any part of the body but is most common on the extremities, particularly the legs. Other sites of predilection are the abdominal wall, perianal and groin areas, and postoperative wounds.[136] The portal of entry is usually a site of trauma (laceration, abrasion, burn, insect bite), a laparotomy performed in the presence of peritoneal soiling (penetrating abdominal trauma or perforated viscus) or another surgical procedure (e.g., hemorrhoidectomy or vasectomy), perirectal abscess, decubitus ulcer, or an intestinal perforation. The last may be secondary to occult diverticulitis,[137, 138] rectosigmoid neoplasm, or a foreign body such as a chicken bone or toothpick. Necrotizing fasciitis from such intestinal sources may occur in the lower extremity (extension along the psoas muscle), as well as in the groin or abdominal wall (via a colocutaneous fistula). Particular clinical settings in which necrotizing fasciitis may develop include diabetes mellitus, alcoholism, and parenteral drug abuse.[139]

In the newborn, necrotizing fasciitis can be a serious complication of omphalitis. Initial swelling and erythema about the umbilicus can progress over several hours to several days and result in purplish discoloration and periumbilical necrosis.[140] Involvement of the anterior abdominal wall frequently extends to the flanks and even onto the chest wall.

The affected area is initially erythematous, swollen, without sharp margins, hot, shiny, exquisitely tender, and painful.[141] Lymphangitis and lymphadenitis are infrequent. The process progresses rapidly over several days, with sequential skin color changes from red-purple to patches of blue-gray. Within 3 to 5 days of onset can be seen skin breakdown with bullae (containing thick pink or purple fluid) and frank cutaneous gangrene (resembling a thermal burn). By this time, the involved area is no longer tender but has become anesthetic secondary to thrombosis of small blood vessels and destruction of superficial nerves located in the necrotic undermined subcutaneous tissue. The development of anesthesia may antedate the appearance of skin necrosis and provide a clue that the process is necrotizing fasciitis and not a simple cellulitis. Marked swelling and edema may produce a compartment syndrome with complicating extensive myonecrosis requiring prompt fasciotomy. Measurement of compartment pressure may be helpful during evaluation in early situations in which marked pain and swelling are present without concomitant skin changes that would indicate the diagnosis.[2] Subcutaneous gas is often present in the polymicrobial form of necrotizing fasciitis, particularly in patients with diabetes mellitus. Systemic toxicity is prominent, and the temperature is elevated in the 102°F to 105°F range. On probing of the lesion with a hemostat through a limited incision, the instrument easily passes along a plane just superficial to the deep fascia. Such easy passage would not occur with ordinary cellulitis.

Leukocytosis is commonly present. Gram-stained smears of exudate usually reveal a mixture of organisms or, in the case of streptococcal gangrene, chains of gram-positive cocci. In one instance, we observed numerous long gram-positive bacilli with subterminal spores (along with gram-negative bacilli) in the foul-smelling, purulent exudate of a patient with crepitant necrotizing fasciitis after a lower leg amputation for peripheral vascular disease. The presence of numerous spores in the wound exudate indicated that the gram-positive bacilli were unlikely to be *C. perfringens*. Before surgery the patient had *Clostridium difficile* enterocolitis, and *C. difficile* was isolated along with several members of the Enterobacteriaceae from the wound drainage material.

Blood cultures are frequently positive. Hypocalcemia (without tetany) may occur when necrosis of subcutaneous fat is extensive.

Fournier's Gangrene. A form of necrotizing fasciitis occurring about the male genitals is known as *Fournier's gangrene*[123, 127] *(idiopathic gangrene of the scrotum, streptococcal scrotal gangrene, perineal phlegmon).* It may be confined to the scrotum or may extend to involve the perineum, penis, and abdominal wall. Predisposing factors include diabetes mellitus, local trauma, paraphimosis, periurethral extravasation of urine, perirectal or perianal infections,[142] and surgery in the area (circumcision, herniorrhaphy). In cases originating in the genitalia, the infecting bacteria probably pass through Buck's fascia of the penis and spread along the dartos fascia of the scrotum and penis, Colles' fascia of the perineum, and Scarpa's fascia of the anterior abdominal wall. In view of the typical foul odor associated with this form of necrotizing fasciitis, a major role for anaerobic bacteria is likely. Mixed cultures containing facultative organisms (*E. coli*, *Klebsiella*, enterococci), along with anaerobes (*Bacteroides*, *Fusobacterium*, *Clostridium*, anaerobic or microaerophilic streptococci), have been obtained from the lesions in the limited number of cases studied. Group A streptococcal gangrene evolving from streptococcal balanitis can, on rare occasion, also involve the male genital area.

The infection commonly starts as cellulitis adjacent to the portal of entry. Early in the course of Fournier's gangrene, the involved area is swollen, erythematous, and tender as the infection begins to involve the deep fascia. Pain is prominent; fever and systemic toxicity are marked.[143] Swelling and crepitus of the scrotum quickly increase, and dark purple areas develop and progress to extensive scrotal gangrene. If the abdominal wall becomes involved in an obese patient with diabetes, the process can spread like wildfire.

Other Special Anatomic Forms of Necrotizing Fasciitis. Necrotizing fasciitis of the face and eyelids,[144] the neck,[145] and the lip[146] are uncommon but life-threatening forms of this disease. Although most often caused by group A streptococci, alone or with *S. aureus* and representing strepococcal gangrene, they occasionally represent mixed infections of group A streptococcus with Enterobacteriaceae or oral *Bacteroides* spp. Although necrotizing fasciitis of the head and neck is often considered a single entity, in fact it represents two conditions etiologically.[147] Craniofacial necrotizing fasciitis is commonly caused by group A streptococci, whereas cervical necrotizing fasciitis often represents a polymicrobial process (e.g., group A streptococci, various other streptococcal species, *Bacteroides* spp., *Peptostreptococcus* spp.). In mixed infections, crepitus may be a feature, as well as necrosis of the epidermis and superficial fascia. Trauma is the usual precipitating cause of necrotizing fasciitis of the periorbital areas and face; dental, oral, or pharyngeal infections predispose to cervical necrotizing fasciitis. Differentiation of the latter from cervical soft tissue infection of odontogenic origin may be difficult, but rapid spread of infection to other areas of the neck, severe pain, and systemic symptoms along with subcutaneous crepitus suggest the diagnosis of necrotizing fasciitis. When crepitus is not palpable, soft tissue radiographs may help in the diagnosis by demonstrating subcutaneous gas. The mortality associated with cervical necrotizing fasciitis is about four times as high as that from craniofacial necrotizing fasciitis.[147]

Other Microbial Etiologies of Necrotizing Fasciitis. Necrotizing fasciitis in neutropenic children receiving cancer chemotherapy may be due to *P. aeruginosa* or Enterobacteriaceae.[148] The acute cellulitis caused by *V. vulnificus* and other *Vibrio* species (described earlier) may extend to the superficial and deep fascia and produce necrotizing fasciitis. Very rare causes of necrotizing fasciitis include environmental species such as *Flavobacterium odoratum*,[149] *Serratia marcescens*,[150] and *Ochrobactrum anthropi*.[151]

Differential Diagnosis. See Table 78–3.

Presumptive Therapy. Prompt diagnosis is of paramount importance because of the rapidity with which the process can progress. The mortality rate of necrotizing fasciitis ranges from 20 to 47% overall (13 and 22% for Fournier's gangrene).[142, 143] Among patients (including those with either type I or type II necrotizing fasciitis) in whom the diagnosis is made within 4 days of appearance of the initial symptoms, the mortality rate is reduced to 12%.[152] Early clinical differentiation of necrotizing fasciitis from cellulitis may be difficult because the initial signs, including pain, edema, and erythema, are not distinctive. However, the presence of marked systemic toxicity out of proportion to the local findings should alert the physician. Computed tomography and magnetic resonance imaging can demonstrate subcutaneous and fascial edema, as well as tissue gas, in patients with necrotizing fasciitis and distinguish this process from cellulitis.[153, 154] However, in patients in whom the diagnosis is clearly suspected, the most expeditious route to diagnosis is through surgical exploration or biopsy without introducing delay for imaging studies. Where imaging studies can be most useful is early in the process when pain and swelling are evident but cutaneous changes are absent and the diagnosis is uncertain. Imaging studies may also be helpful in monitoring clinical progress after surgical débridement when further surgery may need to be considered. Imaging studies may also be helpful in the diagnosis and management of necrotizing fasciitis in areas of the body where the process may be more inaccessible (e.g., retroperitoneal involvement) or where the infection may readily spread to other tissue compartments (e.g., cervical fasciitis spreading to the mediastinum, pleura, and pericardium). Frozen section examination of biopsy specimens (including dermis, infected subcutaneous tissue, fascia, and underlying muscle) has been found to be helpful for early diagnosis.[153] Once the diagnosis is made, immediate surgical débridement is essential. In patients in whom the diagnosis is clearly suspected on clinical grounds—deep pain with patchy areas of surface hypoesthesia, crepitation, or bullae and skin necrosis—direct operative intervention is indicated. Extensive incisions should be made through the skin and subcutaneous tissues and go beyond the area of involvement until normal fascia is found. Necrotic fat and fascia should be excised, and the wound should be left open. A second-look procedure is frequently necessary 24 hours later to ensure adequacy of the initial débridement.[141] In the case of Fournier's gangrene, orchiectomy is almost never required because the testes have their own blood supply independent of the compromised fascial and cutaneous circulation of the scrotum. Initial antimicrobial therapy is based on the evidence for prominent roles of anaerobic bacteria, Enterobacteriaceae, and various streptococci in this process and on the specific findings on Gram-stained smears. Antibiotics used before obtaining bacteriologic data include combinations of ampicillin, gentamicin, and clindamycin; ampicillin, gentamicin, and metronidazole; ampicillin-sulbactam and gentamicin; or imipenem and metronidazole.

Several ancillary therapies, neither a substitute for prompt surgical débridement nor of proven efficacy, have been described. One is the use of intravenous immune globulin in the streptococcal toxic shock syndrome accompanying the treatment of group A streptococcal necrotizing fasciitis.[2] The other is the use of hyperbaric oxygen in the treatment of polymicrobial necrotizing fasciitis, particularly of the trunk.[127]

Synergistic Necrotizing Cellulitis

Clinical Findings. Synergistic necrotizing cellulitis (gram-negative anaerobic cutaneous gangrene, necrotizing cutaneous myositis, synergistic nonclostridial anaerobic myonecrosis) is a variant of necrotizing fasciitis, with prominent involvement of skin *and muscle*, as well as subcutaneous tissue and fascia. Some cases of Fournier's gangrene extending onto the abdominal wall are examples of this condition. Predisposing factors include diabetes mellitus, obesity, advanced age, and cardiorenal disease. Most infections are located on the lower extremities or near the perineum (e.g., originating in a perirectal abscess).[122]

The lesion may first be manifested as small skin ulcers draining foul-smelling reddish-brown ("dishwater") pus. Circumscribed areas of blue-gray gangrene surround these draining sites, but the intervening skin appears normal despite necrosis of underlying subcutaneous tissue, fascia, and muscle. Local pain and tenderness are marked. Tissue gas is noted in about a quarter of patients. Systemic toxicity is a feature; about half the patients have bacteremia.

Etiologic Agents. Cultures consistently show mixtures of anaerobic (anaerobic streptococci and/or *Bacteroides*) and facultative bacteria *(Klebsiella-Enterobacter, E. coli, Proteus)*.[122] *Bacteroides* has been reported as the major pathogen on occasion.[155]

Presumptive Therapy. Initial surgery involves incision and drainage, but radical débridement is often necessary because of extensive involvement of deep fascia and muscle.[122, 155] Amputation may be required. Antibiotic management is initially based on the results of Gram-stained smears of wound exudates, but it should include an antimicrobial effective against *Bacteroides* (see "Presumptive Therapy," earlier, for type I necrotizing fasciitis).

Miscellaneous Infections Secondary to Trauma

Bite Infections.[156] See Chapter 311.

Burn Infections. See Chapter 310.

Injection Site Abscesses. Subcutaneous and intramuscular abscesses infrequently occur after therapeutic injections. *S. aureus*, facultative gram-negative bacilli, and anaerobic bacteria are usually implicated. Hematomas may be the site of delayed infections. Gas gangrene has followed various injections, particularly epinephrine in oil.[120] Subcutaneous and intramuscular abscesses caused by a variety of oral anaerobes and streptococci have occurred after "skin popping" or attempted intravenous injections by narcotic addicts.[123] In the case of subcutaneous abscesses secondary to intravenous drug abuse, appropriate débridement and drainage should include excision of involved veins, which often contain pus or an infected thrombus.[157]

Factitial Disease (Self-Induced Abscesses). Occasionally, subcutaneous abscesses and cellulitis are produced when a patient deliberately injects or inserts contaminated substances into the skin.[158, 159] Such abscesses are often recurrent and may be of monomicrobial or polymicrobial etiology (often consisting of oral or fecal flora). Sterile abscesses may be induced by the introduction of foreign material without bacterial contamination. Such foreign material may be identified by examination of biopsy specimens with polarizing microscopy.

Subcutaneous Infections Originating in Contiguous Foci

Osteomyelitis. In an occasional patient, most commonly a child, acute hematogenous osteomyelitis may be manifested as subcutaneous abscess. Under these circumstances, a subperiosteal abscess has ruptured through intervening tissue into the subcutaneous tissue. *S. aureus* is the most common etiologic agent in such infections. It is important to recognize the nature of the process because of the different therapeutic programs required for osteomyelitis in contrast to a subcutaneous abscess of cutaneous origin. Involvement of subcutaneous tissue as a consequence of osteomyelitis may also occur in the form of a draining sinus associated with chronic osteomyelitis and sequestrum formation. Multiple draining sinuses may occur as a result of multiple foci of osteomyelitis in disseminated blastomycosis.

Actinomycosis. Subcutaneous abscesses frequently develop in the course of cervical, thoracic, or sometimes abdominal actinomycosis. Draining sinuses ultimately result (see Chapter 245).

Primary Pyodermas. On occasion, more superficial skin infections beginning as folliculitis, furunculosis, or cellulitis may progress into the deeper subcutaneous tissue and form a subcutaneous (sometimes "cold") abscess. *S. aureus* is commonly the etiology. Such progression repeatedly might suggest certain underlying phagocytic cell defects such as chronic granulomatous disease of childhood or hyperimmunoglobulin E syndrome (Job's syndrome).[160, 161]

In a cataloguing of the bacteriology of a large number of cutaneous abscesses (unspecified individual predisposing causes), *S. aureus* was the single most common aerobic/facultative isolate, followed in frequency by streptococci, groupable (A, B, C, D) and nongroupable.[162] Among anaerobic isolates, *Bacteroides* spp. (most commonly *B. fragilis* group) are most frequent, followed by *Peptostreptococcus* spp. and *Clostridium* spp. These abscesses are commonly polymicrobial (mixed aerobic-anaerobic). As might be predicted, *S. aureus* is the principal isolate in infections (both abscesses and wounds) of the extremities and trunk, whereas anaerobes are more numerous than aerobic/facultative species in such infections in the genital, perirectal, inguinal, and head and neck areas.

Subcutaneous Abscesses in the Course of Bacteremic Infections

Metastatic pyogenic infections can occur during the course of bacteremias or endocarditis caused by various common invasive organisms (e.g., *S. aureus*) in subcutaneous tissue, as well as a variety of other organs and tissues. These abscesses are tender and fluctuant. Rarely, multiple, firm, nodular subcutaneous lesions clinically resembling those of Weber-Christian disease occur in the course of a staphylococcal bacteremia. If promptly identified and treated, the process may be aborted before frank abscess formation occurs.

Less common bacterial pathogens, infrequently responsible for bacteremia (e.g., *Nocardia* spp.,[163] *Corynebacterium jeikeium*[164]) may also occasionally produce metastatic cutaneous abscesses in immunocompromised or debilitated individuals.

Mycetoma

See Chapter 252.

REFERENCES

1. Ferrieri P, Dajani AS, Wannamaker LW, et al. Natural history of impetigo. I. Site sequence of acquisition and familial patterns of spread of cutaneous streptococci. J Clin Invest. 1972;51:2851.
2. Bisno AL, Stevens DL. Streptococcal infections of skin and soft tissues. N Engl J Med. 1996;334:240.
3. Britton JW, Fajardo JE, Krafte-Jacobs B. Comparison of mupirocin and erythromycin in the treatment of impetigo. J Pediatr. 1990;117:827.
4. Dagan R, Bar-David Y. Double-blind study comparing erythromycin and mupirocin for treatment of impetigo in children: Implications of a high prevalence of erythromycin-resistant *Staphylococcus aureus* strains. Antimicrob Agents Chemother. 1992;36:287.
5. Esterly NB, Nelson DB, Dunne WM Jr. Impetigo. Am J Dis Child. 1991;145:125.
6. Dajani AS, Wannamaker LW. Experimental infection of the skin in the hamster simulating human impetigo. III. Interaction between staphylococci and group A streptocci. J Exp Med. 1971;134:588.
7. Dajani AS, Ferrieri P, Wannamaker LW. Natural history of impetigo. II. Etiologic agents and bacterial interactions. J Clin Invest. 1972;51:2863.
8. Dillon HC. Impetigo contagiosa: Suppurative and non-suppurative complications. I. Clinical bacteriologic, and epidemiologic characteristics of impetigo. Am J Dis Child. 1968;115:530.
9. Darmstadt GL, Fleckman P, Jonas M, et al. Differentiation of cultured keratinocytes promotes the adherence of *Streptococcus pyogenes*. J Clin Invest. 1998;101:128.
10. Okada N, Pentland AP, Falk P, et al. M protein and protein F act as important determinations of cell-specific tropism of *Streptococcus pyogenes* in skin tissue. J Clin Invest. 1994;94:965.
11. Dillon HC. Post-streptococcal glomerulonephritis following pyoderma. Rev Infect Dis. 1979;1:935.
12. Burge SM, Ryan TJ. Acute palmoplantar pustulosis. Br J Dermatol. 1985;113:77.
13. McLaughlin J, Low JC. Primary cutaneous listerosis in adults: An ocupational disease of veterinarions and farmers. Vet Rec. 1994;135:615.
14. Baltimore RS. Treatment of impetigo: A review. Pediatr Infect Dis. 1985;4:597.
15. Feder HM Jr, Abrahamian LM, Grant-Kels JM. Is penicillin still the drug of choice for non-bullous impetigo? Lancet. 1991;2:803.
16. Gemmell CG. Staphylococcal scalded skin syndrome. J Med Microbiol. 1995;43:318.

17. Dajani AS. The scalded-skin syndrome: Relation to phage group II staphylococci. J Infect Dis. 1972;125:548.
18. Melish ME, Glascow LA, Turner MD, et al. The staphylococcal epidermolytic toxin: Its isolation, characterization, and site of action. Ann N Y Acad Sci. 1974;236:317.
19. Elias PM, Fritsch P, Epstein EH Jr. Staphylococcal scalded skin syndrome: Clinical features, pathogenesis, and recent microbiological and biochemical developments. Arch Dermatol. 1977;113:207.
20. Curran JP, Al-Salihi FL. Neonatal staphylococcal scalded skin syndrome: Massive outbreak due to an unusual phage type. Pediatrics. 1980;66:285.
21. Lina G, Gillet Y, Vandenesch F, et al. Toxin involvement in staphylococcal scalded skin syndrome. Clin Infect Dis. 1997;25:1369.
22. Shands KN, Schmid GP, Dan BB, et al. Toxic-shock syndrome in menstruating women: Its association with tampon use and *Staphylococcus aureus* and the clinical features in 52 cases. N Engl J Med. 1980;303:1436.
23. Institute of Medicine, National Academy of Science. Conference on the Toxic Shock Syndrome. Ann Intern Med. 1978;96:835.
24. Todd JT, Fishaut M, Kapral F, et al. Toxic shock syndrome associated with phase-group-I staphylococci. Lancet. 1978;2:1116.
25. Gustafson LT, Band JD, Hutcheson RH, et al. *Pseudomonas* folliculitis: An outbreak and review. Rev Infect Dis. 1983;5:1.
26. El Baze P, Thyss A, Caldini C, et al. *Pseudomonas aeruginosa* 0-11 folliculitis: Development into ecthyma gangrenosum in immunosuppressed patients. Arch Dermatol. 1985;121:873.
27. Noble WC. Gram-negative bacterial skin infections. Semin Dermatol. 1993;12:336.
28. Klotz SA, Drutz DJ, Huppert M, et al. *Pityrosporum* folliculitis. Its potential for confusion with skin lesions of systemic candidiasis. Arch Intern Med. 1982;142:2126.
29. Bufill JA, Lum LG, Caya JG, et al. *Pityrosporum* folliculitis after bone marrow transplantation. Ann Intern Med. 1988;108:560.
30. Buchness MR, Lim HW, Hatcher VA, et al. Eosinophilic pustular folliculitis in the acquired immunodeficiency syndrome. N Engl J Med. 1988;318:1183.
31. Hedstrom SA. Treatment and prevention of recurrent staphylococcal furunculosis: Clinical and bacteriologic follow-up. Scand J Infect Dis. 1985;17:55.
32. Reagan DR, Doebbeling BN, Pfaller AM, et al. Elimination of coincident *Staphylococcus aureus* nasal and hand carriage with intranasal application of mupirocin calcium ointment. Ann Intern Med. 1991;114:101.
33. Wheat LJ, Kohler RB, Luft FC, et al. Long-term studies of the effect of rifampin on nasal carriage of coagulase-positive staphylococci. Rev Infect Dis. 1983;5(Suppl):S459.
34. Darouiche R, Wright C, Hammill R, et al. Eradication of colonization by methicillin-resistant *Staphylococcus aureus* using oral minocycline-rifampin and topical mupirocin. Antimicrob Agents Chemother. 1991;35:1612.
35. Klempner MS, Styrt B. Prevention of recurrent staphylococcal skin infections with low-dose oral clindamycin therapy. JAMA. 1988;260:2682.
36. Allen AM, Taplin D, Twigg L. Cutaneous streptococcal infections in Vietnam. Arch Dermatol. 1971;104:271.
37. Hewitt WD, Farrar WE. Case report: Bacteremia and ecthyma caused by *Streptococcus pyogenes* in a patient with acquired immunodeficiency syndrome. Am J Med Sci. 1988;295:52.
38. Smego RA, Gebrain B, Desmangels G. Cutaneous manifestations of anthrax in rural Haiti. Clin Infect Dis. 1998;26:97.
39. Aksaray N, Cinaz P, Coskum U, et al. Cutaneous anthrax. Trop Georg Med. 1990;42:168.
40. Bernard P, Bedame C, Mounier M, et al. Streptococcal cause of erysipelas and cellulitis in adults. Arch Dermatol. 1989;125:779.
41. Jorup-Ronstrom C. Epidemiological, bacteriological and complicating features of erysipelas. Scand J Infect Dis. 1986;18:519.
42. Kerstens PJ, Endtz HP, Meis JF, et al. Erysipelas-like lesions associated with *Campylobacter jejuni* septicemia in patients with hypogammaglobulinemia. Eur J Clin Microbiol Infect Dis. 1992;11:842.
43. Baddour LM, Bisno AL. Recurrent cellulitis after saphenous venectomy for coronary bypass surgery. Ann Intern Med. 1982;97:493.
44. Baddour LM, Bisno AL. Non–group A beta-hemolytic streptococcal cellulitis. Association with venous and lymphatic compromise. Am J Med. 1985;79:155.
45. Chmel H, Hamdy M. Recurrent streptococcal cellulitis complicating radical hysterectomy and radiation therapy. Obstet Gynecol. 1984;63:862.
46. Ellison RT III, McGregor JA. Recurrent postcoital lower extremity streptococcal erythroderma in women. Streptococcal-sex syndrome. JAMA. 1987;257:3260.
47. Spear RM, Rothbaum RJ, Keating JP, et al. Perianal streptococcal cellulitis. J Pediatr. 1985;107:557.
48. Williams CN, Cohen M, Ronan GS, et al. Dissecting cellulitis of the scalp. Plast Reconstr Surg. 1986;77:378.
49. Araújo A, Andrada-Serpa MJ, Paulo-Filho TA, et al. Folliculitis decalvans and human T cell lymphotropic virus type I–associated myelopathy/tropical spastic paraparesis. Clin Infect Dis. 1995;20:696.
50. Markham RB, Polk BF. Seal finger. Rev Infect Dis. 1979;1:567.
51. Patel M, Ahrens JC, Moyer DV, et al. Pneumococcal soft-tissue infections: A problem deserving more recognition. Clin Infect Dis. 1994;19:149.
52. Anderson DJ, Schmidt C, Goodman J, et al. Cryptococcal disease presenting as cellulitis. Clin Infect Dis. 1992;14:666.
53. Waldor MK, Wilson B, Swartz M. Cellulitis caused by *Legionella pneumophila*. Clin Infect Dis. 1993;16:51.
54. Kilborn JA, Manz LA, O'Brien M, et al. Necrotizing cellulitis caused by *Legionella micdadei*. Am J Med. 1992;92:104.
55. Asmar BI, Bashour BN, Fleischmann LE. *Escherichia coli* cellulitis in children with idiopathic nephrotic syndrome. Clin Pediatr (Phila). 1987;26:592.
56. Gold WL, Salit IE. *Aeromonas hydrophila* infections of skin and soft tissue: Report of 11 cases and review. Clin Infect Dis. 1993;16:69.
57. Bonner JR, Coker AS, Berryman CR, et al. Spectrum of *Vibrio* infections in a Gulf Coast community. Ann Intern Med. 1983;99:464.
58. Chuang Y-C, Yuan C-Y, Liu C-Y, et al. *Vibrio vulnificus* infection in Taiwan: Report of 28 cases and review of clinical manifestations and treatment. Clin Infect Dis. 1992;15:271.
59. Arnold M, Woo M-L, French GL. *Vibrio vulnificus* septicemia presenting as spontaneous necrotizing cellulitis in a woman with hepatic cirrhosis. Scand J Infect Dis. 1989;21:727.
60. Lehman DF, Hardy JC. Stonefish envenomation. N Engl J Med. 1993;329:510.
61. Hook EW III, Hooton TM, Horton CA, et al. Microbiologic evaluation of cutaneous cellulitis in adults. Arch Intern Med. 1986;146:295.
62. Sigurdsson AF, Gundmundsson S. The etiology of bacterial cellulitis as determined by fine-needle aspiration. Scand J Infect Dis. 1989;21:537.
63. Sachs MK. The optimum use of needle aspiration in the bacteriologic diagnosis for cellulitis in adults. Arch Intern Med. 1990;150:1907.
64. Saulsbury FT, Cooper PH, Bracikowski A, et al. Eosinophilic cellulitis in a child. J Pediatr. 1983;102:266.
65. Kremer M, Zuckerman R, Avraham Z, et al. Long-term antimicrobial therapy in the prevention of recurrent soft-tissue infections. J Infect. 1991;22:37.
66. Belsey MA, Sinclair M, Roder MR, et al. *Corynebacterium diphtheriae* skin infections in Alabama and Louisiana. A factor in the epidemiology of diphtheria. N Engl J Med. 1969;280:135.
67. Gruner E, Opravil M, Altwegg M, et al. Nontoxigenic *Corynebacterium diphtheriae* isolated from intravenous drug users. Clin Infect Dis. 1994;18:94.
68. Koopman JS, Campbell J. The role of cutaneous diphtheria infections in a diphtheria epidemic. J Infect Dis. 1975;131:239.
69. Barker FG, Leppard BJ, Seal DV. Streptococcal necrotizing fasciitis: Comparison between histological and clinical features. J Clin Pathol. 1987;40:335.
70. Strasberg SM, Silver MS. Hemolytic streptococcus gangrene. An uncommon but frequently fatal infection in the antibiotic era. Am J Surg. 1968;115:763.
71. Meleney FL. Bacterial synergism in disease processes with a confirmation of the synergistic bacterial etiology of a certain type of progressive gangrene of the abdominal wall. Ann Surg. 1931;94:961.
72. Husseinzadeh N, Nahas WA, Manders EK, et al. Spontaneous occurrence of synergistic bacterial gangrene following external pelvic irradiation. Obstet Gynecol. 1984;63:859.
73. Davson J, Jones DM, Turner L. Diagnosis of Meleney's synergistic gangrene. Br J Surg. 1988;75:267.
74. Turner L, Jones DM, Davson J. Cutaneous amoebiasis: Case report. BMJ. 1985;291:635.
75. Wolfson JS, Sober AJ, Rubin RH. Dermatologic manifestations in the compromised host. Annu Rev Med. 1983;14:205.
76. Wilson CB, Siber GR, O'Breín TF, et al. Phycomycotic gangrenous cellulitis. Arch Surg. 1976;111:532.
77. Weinberg WG, Wade BH, Cierny G III, et al. Invasive infection due to *Apophysomyces elegans* in immunocompetent hosts. Clin Infect Dis. 1993;17:881.
78. Richardson JA, Herron G, Reitz R, et al. Ischemic ulcerations of skin and necrosis of muscle in azotemic hyperparathyroidism. Ann Intern Med. 1969;71:129.
79. Khafif RA, DeLima C, Silverberg A, et al. Calciphylaxis and systemic calcinosis. Arch Intern Med. 1990;150:956.
80. Cone LA, Woodward DA, Schlievert PM, et al. Clinical and bacteriologic observations of a toxic-shock–like syndrome due to *Streptococcus pyogenes*. N Engl J Med. 1987;317:146.
81. Sarkany I, Taplin D, Blank H. The etiology and treatment of erythrasma. J Invest Dermatol. 1961;37:283.
82. Sindhuphak W, MacDonald E, Smith EB. Erythrasma: Overlooked or misdiagnosed. Int J Dermatol. 1985;24:95.
83. Takama H, Tamada Y, Yano K, et al. Pitted keratolysis: Clinical manifestations in 53 cases. Br J Dermatol. 1997;137:282.
84. Allman RM. Pressure ulcers among the elderly. N Engl J Med. 1989;320:850.
85. Karchmer AW, Gibbons GW. Foot infections in diabetes: Evaluation and management. In: Remington JS, Swartz MN, eds. Current Clinical Topics in Infectious Diseases, v. 14. Boston: Blackwell; 1994:7–10.
86. Gerding DM. Foot infections in diabetic patients: Role of anaerobes. Clin Infec Dis. 1995;20:5283.
87. Wheat LJ, Allen SD, Henry M, et al. Diabetic foot infections: Bacteriologic analysis. Arch Intern Med. 1986;146:1935.
88. Grayson ML, Gibbons GW, Habershaw GM, et al. Use of ampicillin/sulbactam versus imipenem/cilastatin in the treatment of limb-threatening foot infections in diabetic patients. Clin Infect Dis. 1994;18:683.
89. Agger WA, Cogbill TH, Busch H Jr, et al. Wounds caused by corn-harvesting machines: An unusual source of infection due to gram-negative bacilli. Rev Infect Dis. 1986;8:927.
90. Weinstein MR, Litt M, Kertess DA, et al. Invasive infections due to a fish pathogen. N Engl J Med. 1997;337:589.
91. Baack BR, Kucan JO, Zook EG, et al. Hand infections secondary to catfish spines: Case reports and literature review. J Trauma. 1991;31:1432.
92. Benedict LM, Kusne S, Torre-Cisneros J, et al. Primary cutaneous fungal infection after solid-organ transplantation: Report of five cases and review. Clin Infect Dis. 1992;15:17.
93. Carey WP, Kaykova Y, Bandres JC, et al. Cutaneous protothecosis in a patient

with AIDS and a severe functional neutrophil defect: Successful therapy with amphotericin B. Clin Infect Dis. 1997;25:1265.

94. Walsh SV, Johnson RA, Tahan SR. Protothecosis; an unusual cause of chronic subcutaneous and soft tissue infection. Am J Dermatopathol. 1998;20:379.
95. Novick NL, Tapia L, Bottone EJ. Invasive *Trichophyton rubrum* infection in an immunocompromised host. Am J Med. 1987;82:321.
96. Henrickson KJ, Flynn PM, Shenep JL, et al. Primary cutaneous *Bacillus cereus* infection in neutropenic children. Lancet. 1989;1:601.
97. Machado LS, Sleasman JW, Ford MJ. *Bacillus* species infection of the skin as a presentation of severe combined immunodeficiency disease. J Am Acad Dermatol. 1998;39:285.
98. Patterson JW, Kitces EN, Neafie RC. Cutaneous botryomycosis in a patient with acquired immunodeficiency syndrome. J Am Acad Dermatol. 1987;16:238.
99. Cockerell CJ, LeBoit PE. Bacillary angiomatosis: A newly characterized, pseudoneoplastic, infectious, cutaneous vascular disorder. J Am Acad Dermatol. 1990;22:501.
100. Schwartzman WA. Infections due to *Rochalimaea*: The expanding clinical spectrum. Clin Infect Dis. 1992;15:893.
101. Relman DA, Loutit JS, Schmidt TM, et al. The agent of bacillary angiomatosis. An approach to the identification of uncultured pathogens. N Engl J Med. 1990;323:1573.
102. Olafsson S, Khan MA. Musculoskeletal features of acne, hidradenitis suppurativa, and dissecting cellulitis of the scalp. Rheum Dis Clin North Am. 1992;18:215.
103. Jemec GBE, Faber M, Gutschik E, et al. The bacteriology of hydrodenitis suppurativa. Dermatology. 1996;193:203.
104. Brook I. Microbiology of infected epidermal cysts. Arch Dermatol. 1989;125:1658.
105. Kingston ME, Mackey D. Skin clues in the diagnosis of life-threatening infections. Rev Infect Dis. 1986;8:1.
106. Bourelly PE, Grossman ME. Subcutaneous nodule as a manifestation of *Pseudomonas* sepsis in an immunocompromised host. Clin Infect Dis. 1998;26:188.
107. Huminer D, Siegman-Igra Y, Morduchowicz G, et al. Ecthyma gangrenosum without bacteremia: Report of six cases and review of the literature. Arch Intern Med. 1987;147:299.
108. Benoit FL. Chronic meningococcemia. Am J Med. 1963;35:103.
109. O'Brien JP, Goldenberg DL, Rice PA. Disseminated gonococcal infection: A prospective analysis of 49 patients and a review of pathophysiology and immune mechanisms. Medicine (Baltimore). 1983;62:395.
110. Chartrand SA, Harrison CJ. Buccal cellulitis reevaluated. Am J Dis Child. 1986;140:891.
111. Walker JS, Corcoran KJ. Buccal cellulitis. Am J Emerg Med. 1990;8:542.
112. Drapkin MS, Wilson ME, Shrager SM, et al. Bacteremic *Hemophilus influenzae* type B cellulitis in the adult. Am J Med. 1977;63:449.
113. Bernard P, Mounier M, Acouturier P, et al. *Haemophilus influenzae* type B cellulitis of the lower extremity in a non-immunosuppressed elderly patient. Acta Dermatol Venereol (Stockh). 1990;70:359.
114. Kiehlbauch JA, Tauxe RV, Baker CM, et al. *Helicobacter cinaedi*–associated bacteremia and cellulitis in immunocompromised patients. Ann Intern Med. 1994;121:90.
115. Burman WJ, Cohn DL, Reves RR, et al. Multifocal cellulitis and monarticular arthritis as manifestations of *Helicobacter cinaedi* bacteremia. Clin Infect Dis. 1995;20:564.
116. Alpert JS, Krous HF, Dalen JE. Pathogenesis of Osler's nodes. Ann Intern Med. 1976;85:471.
117. Cardullo AC, Silvers DN, Grossman ME. Janeway lesions and Osler's nodes: A review of histopathologic findings. J Am Acad Dermatol. 1990;22:1088.
118. Balandral L, Rothschild H, Pugh N, et al. A cutaneous manifestation of systemic candidiasis. Ann Intern Med. 1973;78:400.
119. Jarowski CI, Fialk MA, Murray HW, et al. Fever, rash, and muscle tenderness. A distinctive clinical presentation of disseminated candidiasis. Arch Intern Med. 1978;138:544.
120. Bornstein DL, Weinberg AN, Swartz MN, et al. Anaerobic infections. Review of current experience. Medicine (Baltimore). 1964;43:207.
121. Wilson HD, Haltalin KC. Acute necrotizing fasciitis in childhood. Am J Dis Child. 1973;125:591.
122. Stone HH, Martin JJ Jr. Synergistic necrotizing cellulitis. Ann Surg. 1972;175:702.
123. George WL. Other infections of skin, soft tissue, and muscle. In: Finegold SM, George WL, eds. Anaerobic Infections in Humans. New York: Academic; 1989;492–504.
124. Moses AE, Hardan I, Simhon A, et al. *Clostridium septicum* bacteremia and diffuse spreading cellulitis of the head and neck in a leukemic patient. Rev Infect Dis. 1991;15:525.
125. MacLennan JD. The histotoxic clostridial infections of man. Bacteriol Rev. 1962;26:177.
126. Bessman AN, Wagner W. Nonclostridial gas gangrene. JAMA. 1975;233:958.
127. Green RJ, Dafoe DC, Raffin TA. Necrotizing fasciitis. Chest. 1996;110:219.
128. Stevens DL, Tanner MH, Winship J, et al. Severe group A streptococcal infections associated with a toxic shock–like syndrome and a scarlet fever toxin A. N Engl J Med. 1989;321:1.
129. Stevens SL. Invasive group A streptococcus infections. Clin Infect Dis. 1992;14:2.
130. Aitken DR, Mackett MC, Smith LL. The changing pattern of hemolytic streptococcal gangrene. Arch Surg. 1982;117:561.
131. Brogan TV, Nizet V, Waldhausen JHT, et al. Group A streptococcal necrotizing fasciitis complicating varicella: A series of fourteen patients. Pediatr Infect Dis J. 1995;14:588.
132. Wilson GJ, Talkington DF, Guber W, et al. Group A streptococcal necrotizing fasciitis following varicella in children: Case reports and review. Clin Infect Dis. 1995;20:1333.
133. Demers B, Simor AE, Vellend H, et al. Severe invasive group A streptococcal infections in Ontario, Canada: 1987–1991. Clin Infect Dis. 1993;16:792.
134. Musser JM, Hauser AR, Kim MH, et al. *Streptococcus pyogenes* causing toxic-shock–syndrome and other invasive diseases: Clonal diversity and pyrogenic exotoxin expression. Proc Natl Acad Sci U S A. 1991;88:2668.
135. Cleary PP, Kaplan EL, Handley JP, et al. Clonal basis for resurgence of serious *Streptococcus pyogenes* disease in the 1980s. Lancet. 1992;339:518.
136. Casali RE, Tucker WE, Petrino RA, et al. Postoperative necrotizing fasciitis of the abdominal wall. Am J Surg. 1980;140:787.
137. Galbut DL, Gerber DL, Belgraier AH. Spontaneous necrotizing fasciitis. Occurrence secondary to occult diverticulitis. JAMA. 1977;238:2302.
138. Barza MJ, Proppe KH. Case records of the Massachusetts General Hospital. N Engl J Med. 1979;301.370.
139. Schecter W, Meyer A, Schecter G, et al. Necrotizing fasciitis of the upper extremity. J Hand Surg. 1982;7:15.
140. Lally KP, Atkinson JB, Woolley MM, et al. Necrotizing fasciitis: A serious sequela of omphalitis in the newborn. Ann Surg. 1984;199;101.
141. Sudarsky LA, Laschinger JC, Coppa GF, et al. Improved results from a standardized approach in treating patients with necrotizing fasciitis. Ann Surg. 1987;206:661.
142. Iorianni P, Oliver GC. Synergistic soft tissue infections of the perineum. Dis Colon Rectum. 1992;35:640.
143. Nickel JC, Morales A. Necrotizing fasciitis of the male genitalia (Fournier's gangrene). Can Med Assoc J. 1983;129:445.
144. Kronish JW, McLeish WM. Eyelid necrosis and periorbital necrotizing fasciitis. Report of a case and review of the literature. Ophthalmology. 1991;98:92.
145. Rapoport Y, Himelfarb MZ, Zikk D, et al. Cervical necrotizing fasciitis of odontogenic origin. Oral surg Oral Med Oral Pathol. 1991;72:15.
146. Margolis RD, Cohen KR, Loftus MJ, et al. Nonodontogenic β-hemolytic necrotizing fasciitis of the face. J Oral Maxillofac Surg. 1989;47:1098.
147. Banerjee AR, Murty GE, Moir AA, et al. Cervical necrotizing fasciitis. A distinct clinocopathological entity? J Laryngol Otol. 1996;110:81.
148. Murphy JJ, Granger R, Blair GK, et al. Necrotizing fasciitis in childhood. J Pediatr Surg. 1995;30:1131.
149. Hsuch P-R, Wu J-J, Hsiue T-R, et al. Bacteremic necrotizing fasciitis due to *Flavobacterium odoratum*. Clin Infect Dis. 1995;21:1337.
150. Zipper RP, Bustamente MA, Khatib R. *Serratia marcescens*: A single pathogen in necrotizing fasciitis. Clin Infect Dis. 1996;23:648.
151. Brivet F, Guibert M, Kiredjian M, et al. Necrotizing fasciitis, bacteremia, and multiorgan failure caused by *Ochrobactrum anthropi*. Clin Infect Dis. 1993;17:516.
152. Stamenkovic I, Lew PD. Early recognition of potentially fatal necrotizing fasciitis: Use of frozen-section biopsy. N Engl Med. 1984;310:1689.
153. Walshaw CF, Deans H. CT findings in necrotizing fasciitis—a report of four cases. Clin Radiol. 1996;51:429.
154. Schmid MR, Kossman T, Duewell S. Differentiation of necrotizing fasciitis and cellulitis using MR imaging. Am J Roentgenol. 1998;170:615.
155. Baxter CR. Surgical management of soft tissue infections. Surg Clin North Am. 1972;52:1483.
156. Talan DA, Citron DM, Abrahamian FM, et al. Bacteriologic analysis of infected dog and cat bites. N Engl J Med. 1999;340:85.
157. Biderman P, Hiatt JR. Management of soft-tissue infections of the upper extremity in parenteral drug abusers. Am J Surg. 1987;154:526.
158. Aduan RP, Fauci AS, Dale DC, et al. Factitious fever and self-induced infection: A report of 32 cases and review of the literature. Ann Intern Med. 1979;90:230.
159. Reich P, Gottfried LA. Factitious disorders in a teaching hospital. Ann Intern Med. 1983;99:240.
160. Dreskin SC, Gallin JI. Evolution of the hyperimmunoglobulin E and recurrent infection (HIE, Job's) syndrome in a young girl. J Allergy Clin Immunol. 1987;80:746.
161. Curnutte JT, Boxer LA. Clinically significant phagocytic cell defects. In: Remington JS, Swartz MN, eds. Current Clinical Topics in Infectious Diseases, v. 6. New York: McGraw-Hill; 1985:103–156.
162. Brook I, Frazier EH. Aerobic and anaerobic bacteriology of wounds and cutaneous abscesses. Arch Surg. 1990;125:1990.
163. Curley RK, Hayward T, Holden CA. Cutaneous abscesses due to systemic nocardiosis. Clin Exp Dermatol. 1990;15:459.
164. Dan M, Somer I, Knobel B, et al. Cutaneous manifestations of infection with *Corynebacterium* group JK. Rev Infect Dis. 1988;10:1204.

Chapter 79

Myositis

MORTON N. SWARTZ

Infection of skeletal muscle (infectious myositis) is uncommon. When it occurs, a wide range of organisms may be responsible: bacteria, mycobacteria, fungi, viruses, and parasitic agents. Bacteria invade muscle either from contiguous sites of infection (skin and subcutaneous abscesses, penetrating wounds, decubitus ulcers, osteomyelitis) or by hematogenous spread from a distant focus. It is helpful to categorize infectious myositis on the basis of clinical manifestations. These may be very distinctive, as in clostridial gas gangrene, and suggest the specific etiologic agent; or they may be very nonspecific, as in the myalgias of viral infections and infective endocarditis (Table 79–1). In certain instances (e.g., psoas abscess), it is the anatomic location rather than the morphologic characteristics of the lesion or the nature of the infecting agent that distinguishes the particular type of muscle infection.

PYOMYOSITIS

Pyomyositis is an acute bacterial infection of skeletal muscle usually caused by *Staphylococcus aureus*. The accumulation of pus is always intramuscular initially and is not secondary to infection of adjacent skin, soft tissue, or bone. Clinically, it is characterized by fever, localized muscle pain and stiffness, swelling, and tenderness.

Pathogenesis and Pathologic Characteristics

Bacterial infections of muscle usually occur after a penetrating wound, prolonged vascular insufficiency in an extremity, or a contiguous infection. Bacteremic spread of infection to skeletal muscle is extremely uncommon. Of fatal cases of staphylococcal septicemia, abscesses in skeletal muscle are found in less than 1%.[1] Pyomyositis (primary muscle abscess) is a bacterial infection of muscle that occurs in the absence of a predisposing site of infection. *S. aureus* is the most common cause.[2] Blood cultures are positive in 5 to 35% of the cases at the time of clinical manifestation; metastatic infections in tissue other than muscle are rare.

Most cases of pyomyositis occur in the tropics; hence, the term *tropical pyomyositis*. It accounts for 1 to 4% of hospital admissions in some tropical areas.[2, 3] In the United States pyomyositis is very uncommon (only about 100 cases reported over the past 20 years in North America), occurring both in persons who have recently immigrated from the tropics and in those who have always resided in a temperate climate.[4, 5] It occurs at all ages, in the tropics more frequently among children, but in North America more often in adults and the elderly. As yet, no convincing evidence to relate pyomyositis causally to predisposing circumstances peculiar to the tropics (e.g., malaria, filariasis, arbovirus infection) has been developed. Migration of the guinea worm, *Dracunculus medinensis*, in the deep connective tissues of the lower extremities may be complicated by staphylococcal abscesses. However, these are located between muscle groups and are not the intramuscular abscesses typical of pyomyositis. About 40% of cases in temperate climates lack any relevant underlying disease, but the remainder have possible predisposing conditions: diabetes mellitus; alcoholic liver disease; corticosteroid therapy; immunosuppressive illnesses such as leukemia, lymphoma, or other hematologic processes (Felty syndrome, myelodysplasia, sickle cell disease); and human immunodeficiency virus (HIV) infection.[5] Pyomyositis has been reported in more than 25 patients with HIV infection, with or without acquired immunodeficiency syndrome (AIDS) (including one neonate); and in one quarter of these patients it was caused by *S. aureus*.[4, 6–11] The predisposition to pyomyositis in patients with AIDS probably stems from the combination of defective bactericidal activity of neutrophils,[12] the underlying cell-mediated immunodeficiency, and the potential for muscle injury (HIV myopathy, zidovudine-associated mitochondrial myopathy, myositis from parasitic disease, *Mycobacterium avium complex* infection) associated with this disease. Pyomyositis has been reported in 12 intravenous drug abusers; it was caused by *S. aureus*

TABLE 79–1 Classification of Infectious Myositis

Type of Process	Clinical Pattern	Principal Specific Causes
Pyogenic and predominantly localized (spreading by contiguity)	Pyomyositis	*Staphylococcus aureus;* group A streptococcus (rarely); gram-negative bacilli (very rarely)
	Gas gangrene	*Clostridium perfringens;* occasionally other histotoxic clostridial species
	Nonclostridial (crepitant) myositis	
	Anaerobic streptococcal gangrene	*Peptostreptococcus* (plus group A streptococci or *S. aureus*)
	Group A streptococcal necrotizing myositis	Group A streptococcus
	Synergistic nonclostridial anaerobic myonecrosis	Mixed infections: *Bacteroides* and other anaerobic non–spore-forming gram-negative bacilli; *Peptostreptococcus* and various streptococci; *Escherichia coli; Klebsiella; Enterobacter*
	Infected vascular gangrene	Same as for synergistic nonclostridial anaerobic myonecrosis
	Aeromonas hydrophila myonecrosis	*A. hydrophila*
	Psoas abscess	Gram-negative bacilli; *S. aureus;* mixed infections; *Mycobacterium tuberculosis*
Nonpyogenic and predominantly generalized	Myalgias	Viral infections (e.g., influenza, dengue); infective endocarditis; bacteremias (e.g., meningococcemia); rickettsioses (e.g., Rocky Mountain spotted fever); toxoplasmosis
	Pleurodynia	Coxsackievirus B
	Myalgias with eosinophilia	
	Trichinosis	*Trichinella spiralis*
	Cysticercosis (also subcutaneous nodules)	*Taenia solium*
	Muscle degeneration and destruction associated with infections elsewhere	
	Acute rhabdomyolysis	Viral influenza, echovirus, coxsackie and Epstein-Barr viruses, *Legionella*

in one half and by either gram-negative bacilli or multiple organisms (including anaerobes) in the remainder.[13] AIDS was a contributing factor in five of these patients.

The presumed pathogenesis of pyomyositis involves a prior bacteremia, commonly asymptomatic and transient. Because traumatizing muscle (locus minoris resistentiae) is necessary in order to produce pyomyositis in experimental animals after intravenous injection of *S. aureus*,[14] a role for local mechanical injury has been hypothesized.

Clinical Findings

In 20 to 50% of cases, there has been recent blunt trauma to or vigorous exercise of the involved area. The clinical picture often involves three stages. In the first or *invasive* stage, the onset is subacute with variable fever, local swelling with or without erythema, mild pain, and minimal tenderness. The area is indurated or has a wooden consistency. This stage is often overlooked. Because the initial swelling is firm and pain is not striking, attention is directed away from an infectious cause. Aspiration, if attempted, yields no pus. The second or *suppurative* stage occurs 10 to 21 or more days later, and this is the time when most patients are seen and diagnosed. Distinct muscle tenderness and swelling (tending to conform to the shape of the involved muscle) are present, and the patient is febrile. The overlying skin is intact and warm, and erythema is commonly absent. At this point, pus can be aspirated from the involved muscle. In the third stage, systemic manifestations of sepsis and local findings of erythema, exquisite tenderness, and fluctuance are striking. If untreated, the infection can progress to metastatic abscesses, shock, and renal failure.

In an occasional patient the onset is acute rather than subacute, with malaise, chills, and high fever. In a rare patient, the clinical picture is combined with that of toxic shock syndrome.[15] Because the muscle abscesses are contained by the overlying fascia, local erythema and heat may be minimal until the process extends through to the subcutaneous tissues some days to weeks later. Regional lymphadenitis is not a feature. Usually only a single muscle group is involved, but multiple muscle abscesses occur in up to 40% of the patients. The most frequent sites of involvement are the large muscles of the lower extremities (e.g., quadriceps femoris, gluteus group) and the trunk muscles. Involvement of the abdominal muscles is uncommon but noteworthy, because it may mimic an acute abdomen.[16]

A leukocytosis occurs. Eosinophilia is common in patients (even in the presence of a prominent leukocytosis) with tropical pyomyositis and appears to reflect the prevalence of parasitic infestation. Serum muscle enzyme levels may be elevated but frequently are normal despite gross muscle destruction. However, marked rhabdomyolysis with myoglobinuria and acute renal failure have developed in a patient with pyomyositis.[17]

Etiologic Agents

S. aureus is responsible for 95% of the cases in tropical areas. In North America, *S. aureus* is the cause of 66% of cases.[5] Group A streptococci account for 1 to 5% of the cases. Other gram-positive organisms uncommonly implicated in pyomyositis include various streptococci (groups B, C, and G), *Streptococcus pneumoniae*,[18] and *Streptococcus anginosus*. Other very rare causes include Enterobacteriaceae (*Escherichia coli, Klebsiella oxytoca, Serratia marcescens, Morganella morganii*,[9] *Citrobacter freundii, Salmonella* spp.), *Yersinia enterocolitica, Neisseria gonorrhoeae, Haemophilus influenzae*, and *Aeromonas hydrophila*.[4,5] Anaerobes *(Fusobacterium nucleatum, Clostridium septicum)* have been the cause in several cases. *Burkholderia mallei* and *Burkholderia pseudomallei* in the past have very rarely caused abscesses in muscle in the septicemic or chronic suppurative forms of the diseases they produce (glanders and melioidosis, respectively). *Aspergillus fumigatus* has caused a localized muscle abscess in rare patients with myelodysplasia or AIDS and in patients who have received corticosteroids. Hematogenously disseminated candidiasis in neutropenic patients can manifest with fever and muscle pain. The scattered *Candida* abscesses in the muscle are too small to localize by symptoms and physical examination, but myositis in these patients is often accompanied by small, tender, erythematous skin lesions. Punch biopsy of a skin lesion shows numerous *Candida* in the dermis. Tuberculous pyomyositis has occurred in a patient with disseminated tuberculosis,[19] and necrotizing pyomyositis due to *M. avium* complex has occurred in a patient with AIDS.[10] Extrapulmonary *Pneumocystis carinii* infection is relatively uncommon in patients with AIDS, but in one patient it manifested as an intramuscular, localized, painful thigh swelling with typical granulomatous histopathology.[20]

Differential Diagnosis

Early in the course of pyomyositis, other diagnoses may be suspected, particularly in nontropical areas: fever of obscure origin (in the early phase when localizing findings may be minimal or absent), osteomyelitis, septic arthritis, appendicitis or diverticulitis, muscle hematoma, muscle rupture, and thrombophlebitis. Iliopsoas myositis has mimicked appendicitis[21]; iliacus pyomyositis has mimicked septic arthritis of the hip[22]; and pyriformis muscle pyomyositis has simulated an epidural abscess because of severe back and radiating (sciatic) leg pain.[23] Muscle infarction is an uncommon condition that occurs most frequently in the quadriceps in poorly controlled diabetics with nephropathy, neuropathy, and hypertension. It may suggest pyomyositis because of the acute onset of pain and presence of tender local swelling, but, unlike pyomyositis, fever is absent.[24] The presence of a slowly enlarging, painful mass in an extremity of a patient with only low-grade fever may suggest the diagnosis of sarcoma. Pyomyositis of the pectoral muscle may pose a particular problem in diagnosis because it must be distinguished not only from muscle rupture, hematoma, and sarcoma but also from cryptic abscessed subpectoral nodes developing via lymphatic extension of an initiating infection on the thumb or index finger of the ipsilateral hand. Streptococcal necrotizing fasciitis, like gangrenous streptococcal myositis, produces localized swelling, tenderness, and erythema, but it is less common and produces necrosis of fascia and skin. Rapid frozen-section biopsy or surgical exploration may be needed to distinguish among these processes.

In the patient with multiple sites of muscle involvement and eosinophilia (from incidental parasitic infestation), the picture may suggest trichinosis. This resemblance ends when localized swellings become prominent and markedly tender. Rupture of the muscle abscess through the fascia into subcutaneous tissues may suggest the diagnosis of cellulitis. Radionuclide (^{67}Ga) scanning shows diffuse uptake in the involved area but does not distinguish an intramuscular abscess from necrotizing myositis or necrotizing fasciitis. It may be helpful when several areas of pyomyositis are present, or it may be helpful in the patient with diffuse myalgias in the early phase of the disease. Computed tomography can reveal low-density areas with loss of muscle planes, a central fluid collection, and a surrounding rim of contrast enhancement characteristic of pyomyositis.[25] Enlargement of the involved muscle is usually evident. CT findings of a superimposed cellulitis may sometimes be evident on CT, namely, skin thickening, stranding of subcutaneous fat with blurring of fat and fascial planes, and subcutaneous venous distention. Sonography may reveal an increase in muscle mass and a hypoechoic collection with internal echoes,[26] but it is less useful than computed tomography (CT) scanning or magnetic resonance imaging (MRI) for early diagnosis. MRI scanning can demonstrate enlargement of involved muscles and slight increase in signal intensity on T_1-weighted images in the involved area, with a hypointense central area and surrounding gadolinium-enhanced rim; and a diffuse increase in signal intensity on T_2-weighted images with a central high-signal-intensity fluid collection surrounded by a low-intensity rim.[25] Sonography or CT scanning can guide aspiration, which provides specific diagnosis of pyomyositis.

Presumptive Therapy

Surgical (open or ultrasound-guided percutaneous) drainage of all abscesses is essential. Initial antibiotic therapy should consist of intravenous administration of a β-lactamase-resistant penicillin because of the preponderance of penicillin-resistant *S. aureus* isolates from such abscesses. If a group A streptococcus is isolated, treatment should be changed to penicillin G. Early modification of initial antimicrobial therapy is based on interpretation of a Gram-stain smear of pus and subsequent results of cultures and susceptibility testing. Continued fever after surgical drainage of a muscle abscess while the patient is receiving appropriate antimicrobial therapy should suggest the presence of other undrained suppurative foci. Pyomyositis may be complicated by a compartment syndrome, particularly when it occurs in the anterior tibial compartment, and may require additional surgical drainage, fasciotomies, and débridement beyond simple percutaneous drainage.[27]

GROUP A STREPTOCOCCAL NECROTIZING MYOSITIS

In addition to producing an occasional case of typical pyomyositis with abscess formation, on rare occasions group A streptococci cause a fulminant form of myositis (peracute streptococcal pyomyositis, streptococcal necrotizing myositis, or spontaneous streptococcal gangrenous myositis).[28, 29] Reports such as that of one case of myositis and of three cases of myositis with necrotizing fasciitis among 20 patients in an outbreak of invasive group A streptococcal infections associated with a toxic shock-like syndrome suggest that this form of infection may be currently more frequent than in the past.[30] The entire clinical course may be telescoped to 2 to 3 days. The clinical features are usually intense pain, boardlike swelling of the affected muscle, and fever. The overlying skin may be uninvolved, or it may become erythematous and contain petechiae and vesicles.[31] Most cases involve the extremities and appear to develop spontaneously without antecedent pharyngitis or tonsillitis. Bacteremia and toxemia are prominent features and contribute to the very high mortality rate (80 to 100%).[30] The rapid spread of infection in a closed compartment of muscles can markedly raise intramuscular pressure, resulting in further necrosis of muscle.[31, 32] However, both processes may be simultaneously present in the same area. The compartment syndrome with group A streptococcal myositis (e.g., a tibial compartment syndrome may develop in the absence of fascial and muscle necrosis but be associated with muscle bulging secondary to edema and serosanguineous exudate.[33] Compartment pressures when measured are elevated. The clinical features of such a syndrome include weakness of the compartment muscles, which are swollen and tender, severe pain on movement of the lower leg, and overlying cutaneous hyperesthesia.

Streptococcal necrotizing fasciitis may resemble streptococcal myositis clinically, although the presence of tense bullae and areas of skin necrosis are more suggestive of the former. Sometimes both conditions are present together. MRI may disclose the structure involved predominantly, but surgical exploration should provide a clear answer. A rare case of acute streptococcal myositis with the toxic shock syndrome caused by group G streptococcus has been reported.[34]

Laboratory findings include a leukocytosis and elevated serum creatine phosphokinase levels.

This disease is a medical emergency requiring prompt clinical diagnosis with verification at surgery. Distinguishing group A streptococcal necrotizing myositis from streptococcal necrotizing fasciitis and spontaneous clostridial myonecrosis may be difficult clinically, but gas in the tissue would suggest the latter. Sonography, CT, or MRI scanning usually reveals muscle swelling and fluid collection in muscle compartments. Early, aggressive surgical intervention with fasciotomy and débridement of necrotic tissue is indicated; in some instances amputation is required. Antibiotic therapy involves high doses of penicillin G (2 million units intravenously every 3 to 4 hours) along with clindamycin[35] (600 mg intravenously every 6 to 8 hours) based on the Gram-stain smear.

GAS GANGRENE (CLOSTRIDIAL MYONECROSIS)

Gas gangrene is a rapidly progressive, life-threatening, toxemic infection of skeletal muscle caused by clostridia (principally *Clostridium perfringens*). It usually occurs after muscle injury and contamination, as in a dirty traumatic wound, or sometimes after surgery.

Pathogenesis and Pathologic Characteristics

Gas gangrene occurs in settings having in common muscle injury and contamination with soil or other foreign material containing spores of *C. perfringens* or other histotoxic clostridial species: (1) accidental traumatic civilian injuries such as compound fracture[36]; (2) penetrating war wounds[37]; (3) surgical wounds, particularly after bowel or biliary tract surgery[38]; and (4) arterial insufficiency in an extremity.[38] Rare cases of gas gangrene have occurred after parenteral injection of medication, particularly epinephrine in oil. A fulminant case was described beginning at the site of a simple venipuncture in a granulocytopenic patient.[38] *C. perfringens* are usually present in large numbers as normal flora in human feces and therefore can endogenously contaminate skin surfaces. Despite a high frequency (up to 88%) of clostridial contamination of major traumatic, open wounds, the incidence of gas gangrene in this setting is only 1 to 2%,[39] emphasizing the importance of devitalized tissue and the presence of foreign bodies in the pathogenesis of gas gangrene. The minimal dose of *C. perfringens* needed to produce fatal gas gangrene in the experimental animal is reduced by a factor of 10^6 when injected into devitalized muscle contaminated with sterile dirt rather than into normal muscle. The policy of prompt, thorough débridement and of leaving wounds open has decreased the incidence of gas gangrene in wartime injuries; only 22 cases among 139,000 combat casualties in Vietnam were reported.[40]

Gas gangrene may occasionally develop in the absence of an obvious external wound. This form of clostridial myonecrosis is designated *spontaneous, nontraumatic gas gangrene*. Its principal cause is *C. septicum*, a relatively aerotolerant species, which is spread by the bacteremic route and is apparently more capable of establishing infection without significant antecedent tissue injury than other clostridia. Intestinal tract abnormalities (colon cancer, diverticulitis, bowel infarction, necrotizing enterocolitis, volvulus) are the major predisposing conditions.[41] Colon cancer, often cryptic, is the most common of these, occurring in up to 88% of patients with *C. septicum* bacteremia. Other predisposing disorders include leukemia, other causes of neutropenia, and diabetes mellitus. The primary source of the organism is probably mucosal ulceration or perforation of the intestinal tract. The spread by the bacteremic route probably accounts for the occasional bilateral (but separated) involvement observed in a few patients with spontaneous gas gangrene. However, it may manifest in the buttocks or flanks as the consequence of an intra-abdominal catastrophe, with rapid extension of infection along the iliopsoas or other deep muscle groups. The progression of *C. septicum* spontaneous gas gangrene may be even more fulminant than that of traumatic *C. perfringens* gas gangrene; the mortality rate of the former is 67 to 100%, with most dying within 24 hours after onset.[41]

The involved muscle undergoes rapid disintegration. Initially, it may exhibit only pallor, edema, and loss of elasticity. When examined in the operating room, it fails to contract on stimulation and does not bleed from a cut surface. Later it becomes discolored (reddish purple, then greenish purple and gangrenous) and friable.

Histologically, the muscle fibers show coagulation necrosis, contain cavities caused by gas production, and have a destroyed supporting connective tissue; numerous gram-positive bacilli are present. Few if any inflammatory cells are present. Evidence suggests that the α and θ toxins of *C. perfringens* are major virulence factors that play important roles in myonecrosis and reduction of the inflammatory response at the site of infection.[42]

Clinical Findings

The usual incubation period between injury and the development of clostridial myonecrosis is 2 to 3 days, but it may be as short as 6 hours. The onset is acute. Pain is the earliest and most important symptom, although on occasion a sense of heaviness may be the only initial symptom. It rapidly increases in intensity, is more severe than the pain that is generally associated with the preceding injury or surgical procedure, and may become excruciating. The patient soon appears severely ill, pale, and sweaty. The pulse is rapid, the blood pressure falls, and shock and renal failure follow. The patient may be apathetic or may be apprehensive and restless but mentally clear. Delirium, stupor, and unconsciousness may supervene. Fever is frequently present, but often with a temperature of less than 38.3°C (101°F). Hypothermia is a poor prognostic sign and is usually associated with shock. Jaundice may become evident. The process may rapidly progress over a period of hours, with a fatal outcome if not properly treated.

Very early, tense edema and local tenderness may be the only findings of local lesions. If an open wound is present, swollen muscle may herniate through. A serosanguineous, dirty-appearing discharge, containing numerous organisms but few leukocytes, escapes from the wound. The wound has a peculiar foul odor. Gas bubbles may be visible in the discharge. Crepitus is usually present but not prominent; sometimes it is completely obscured by very marked edema. The skin adjacent to the wound is initially swollen and white but rapidly takes on a yellowish or bronze discoloration (Fig. 79–1). Tense blebs containing thin serosanguineous or dark fluid develop in the overlying skin, and areas of green-black cutaneous necrosis appear. In fulminant cases, progression of the changes occurs over 2 to 4 hours, as indicated by the advance of the area of edema and crepitation.

Laboratory Findings

The hematocrit level is usually reduced. *C. perfringens* bacteremia occurs in about 15% of the patients with gas gangrene.[43] Intense bacteremia (with associated intravascular hemolysis) is more likely to occur as a complication of uterine infection.[44] A leukocytosis is common.

A Gram-stain smear of the wound exudate or of an aspirate from one of the blebs reveals many large, gram-positive bacilli with blunt ends but few polymorphonuclear leukocytes (see Chapter 236). In almost all cases, spores are not evident. The presence of spores (subterminal) might suggest *C. septicum*.[45] Not infrequently, scattered gram-negative bacilli are also present, particularly in grossly contaminated wounds. The growth of *C. perfringens* in culture can be extraordinarily rapid (generation time, as little as 8 minutes), paralleling the rapidity of advance of the infection in devitalized tissue. Examination of liquid anaerobic cultures for gas production (and subsequent Gram-stain examination as little as 6 hours after inoculation may provide an early presumptive diagnosis of the infecting species.

X-ray films of the involved areas show extensive and progressive gaseous dissection of muscle and fascial planes.

Etiologic Agents

C. perfringens is most commonly isolated from the lesions of gas gangrene (80 to 95% of the cases).[36, 40] *Clostridium novyi* is involved in 10 to 40% of the cases, and *C. septicum* in 5 to 20%. Other clostridial species *(Clostridium bifermentans, Clostridium histolyticum, Clostridium fallax)* have been implicated on rare occasions. In addition to clostridia, other organisms (e.g., *E. coli, Enterobacter*, enterococci) are sometimes isolated from the lesions of gas gangrene, reflecting the contaminated character of the initiating trauma or lesion.[43]

Differential Diagnosis

The major considerations in differential diagnosis are gas-forming infections of the soft tissues (clostridial anaerobic cellulitis, nonclostridial crepitant myositis, nonclostridial crepitant cellulitis). Clostridial anaerobic cellulitis (see Chapter 78) is more gradual in onset and progression, and the systemic manifestations of illness are much milder than in gas gangrene. Local pain is relatively mild, and the skin lesions of gas gangrene (bronzing, dark blebs) do not develop. Gas formation is often much more extensive in clostridial cellulitis than in gas gangrene. Clinically, it is often difficult to distinguish between early clostridial cellulitis and myonecrosis. Definitive evaluation requires examination in the operating room for the characteristic changes of myonecrosis described earlier. The clinical picture of nonclostridial crepitant cellulitis is very similar to that of clostridial cellulitis. Although contamination of an operative or traumatic wound may be the source of infection in both types of cellulitis, nonclostridial crepitant cellulitis frequently develops in the setting of vascular insufficiency or perirectal infection. Bacteria isolated from nonclostridial crepitant cellulitis include facultative species (*E. coli, Klebsiella*, various streptococci) and anaerobic bacteria *(Bacteroides, Peptostreptococcus)*. Commonly, these are present in mixed culture and can be seen on the Gram-stain smear of a wound aspirate.

Presumptive Therapy

Treatment includes emergency surgical exploration both to define the nature of the process (gas gangrene versus crepitant cellulitis) by direct examination of muscles at the site of infection and to carry out appropriate débridement. Prompt and extensive surgery is the principal element in the treatment of gas gangrene. This includes excision of involved muscles (or amputation when necessary) and fasciotomies to decompress and drain the swollen fascial compartments. Antibiotic therapy is an important adjunct to surgical management. Penicillin G has been the antibiotic of choice in the past and is administered intravenously in a dosage for the adult of 1 to 2 million units every 2 to 3 hours. Currently, the combination of penicillin with clindamycin (600 mg intravenously every 6 to 8 hours) is widely used in treatment. The addition of clindamycin is based on results of experimental studies of fulminant clostridial myonecrosis in mice, in which clindamycin, metronidazole, and tetracycline were each more effective than penicillin.[46] In vitro, the addition of penicillin to metronidazole antagonizes the activity of the latter; in contrast, the combination of penicillin with clindamycin provides slightly greater efficacy than clindamycin alone but significantly enhanced efficacy over that of penicillin alone.[47]

An additional antimicrobial (e.g., ciprofloxacin, third-generation cephalosporin, chloramphenicol) may be employed initially when Gram-stain smears of the wound exudate show gram-negative bacilli as well as the predominant gram-positive bacilli. In addition to clindamycin, chloramphenicol is also a good alternative drug in the highly penicillin-allergic patient; it is preferable to tetracycline in view of the resistance of some clostridia to the latter. Although the majority of *C. perfringens* isolates are susceptible in vitro to first-, second-, and third-generation cephalosporins, the minimum inhibitory concentrations for at least 10% of isolates are above levels readily achievable in vivo.[40] The demonstration of plasmids mediating transferable drug resistance (tetracycline and chloramphenicol; perhaps erythromycin and clindamycin) in *C. perfringens*[49] suggests

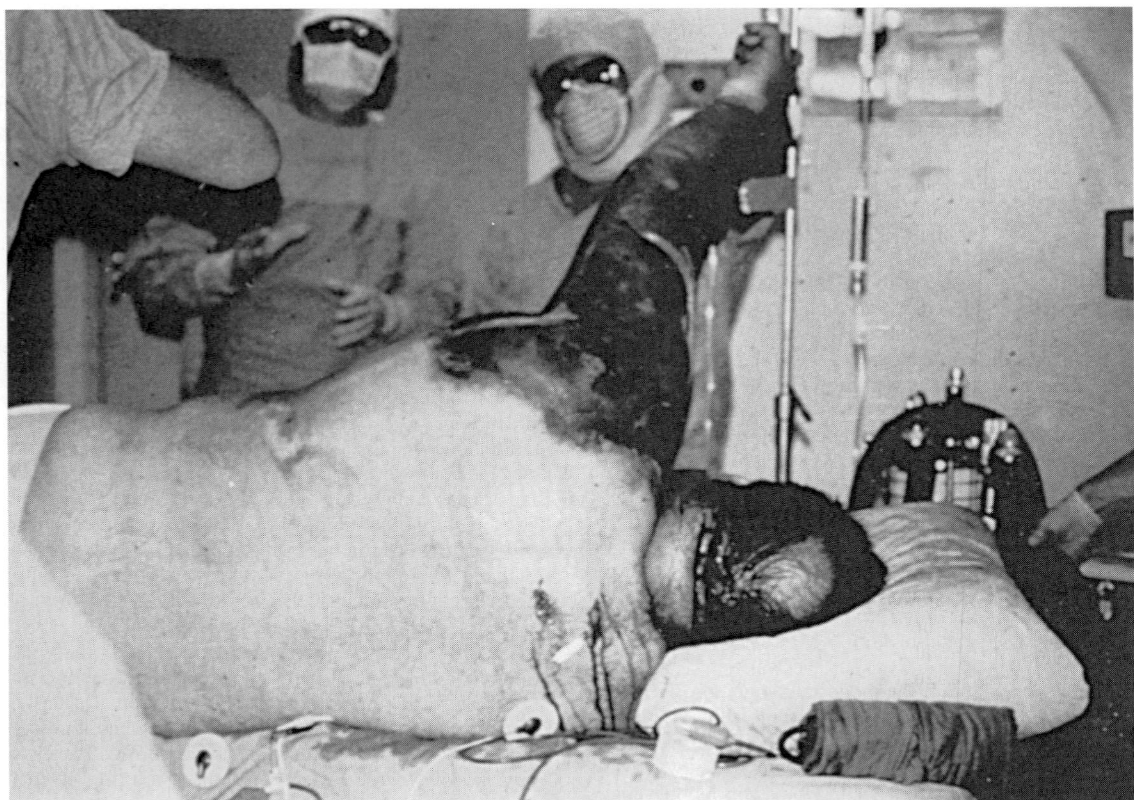

FIGURE 79–1. Clostridial gas gangrene of the left upper extremity. There is prominent characteristic bronze discoloration of the skin extending over the shoulder. Crepitus could be palpated beyond the area of discoloration onto the back.

the need for periodic monitoring of antibiotic susceptibilities of clinical isolates. Some strains of this organism may be showing somewhat less susceptibility in vitro to penicillin than was formerly the case.[48] *C. perfringens* are susceptible in vitro to metronidazole, but experience with the clinical use of this drug alone in clostridial myonecrosis is lacking.

The role of hyperbaric oxygen therapy is still under debate (see Chapter 38). Its use should never delay immediate surgical débridement when possible. Its most appropriate role at present would appear to be in the management of patients with extensive involvement of the trunk in whom surgical excision would be impossible (paraspinal sites) or mutilating.[50] In a murine model of *C. perfringens* myonecrosis initiated with a high inoculum, clindamycin therapy was more effective than hyperbaric oxygen, and the addition of the latter provided no further efficacy to use of clindamycin alone.[51] Initial hyperbaric oxygen therapy may reduce the extent of débridement necessary under these circumstances. The efficacy of intravenously administered polyvalent gas gangrene antitoxin has never been established clinically, and it is no longer available. Ancillary therapy is essential in the management of gas gangrene. This includes attention to fluid and electrolyte replacement and maintenance of adequate hematocrit levels by transfusions.

NONCLOSTRIDIAL (CREPITANT) MYOSITIS

Nonclostridial (crepitant) myositis includes four relatively distinct entities that differ from gas gangrene in their clinical picture and bacteriologic characteristics: (1) anaerobic streptococcal myonecrosis, (2) synergistic nonclostridial anaerobic myonecrosis, (3) infected vascular gangrene, and (4) *Aeromonas hydrophila* myonecrosis.

Anaerobic Streptococcal Myonecrosis

Anaerobic streptococcal myonecrosis is an acute interstitial myositis that clinically resembles subacute clostridial gas gangrene. The initial manifestations are swelling and a copious seropurulent exudate occurring 3 to 4 days after injury. Pain develops later, unlike the early occurrence of pain in gas gangrene. Tissue gas is present in muscle and fascial planes but is not extensive. The wound has an unpleasant, sour odor. The involved muscles are discolored but do react to stimulation. In contrast to gas gangrene, early cutaneous erythema is prominent. If it is not adequately treated, the infection progresses, with the development of toxemia, frank gangrene, and shock.

Numerous streptococci and polymorphonuclear leukocytes are present in the exudate. The infection is usually mixed (anaerobic streptococci with group A streptococci or *S. aureus*). A mixed infection of muscle with both peptostreptococci and *Bacillus subtilis* has been observed on several occasions in the setting of vascular injury. The clinical picture, along with the appearance of the Gram-stain smear, initially might suggest the diagnosis of clostridial myonecrosis.[52] Treatment involves the use of large doses of penicillin (and an antistaphylococcal agent, if indicated) and surgical débridement.

Synergistic Nonclostridial Anaerobic Myonecrosis

Synergistic nonclostridial anaerobic myonecrosis, a severe infection, is also known as *synergistic necrotizing cellulitis* (see Chapter 78); it involves skin, subcutaneous tissue, fascia, and muscle. The most extensive involvement is in the subcutaneous tissues and fascia; changes in the overlying skin and underlying muscle are usually secondary.

Very rarely crepitant myonecrosis may be caused by *Klebsiella pneumoniae*, unaccompanied by other organisms (aerobic or anaerobic), in a patient with diabetes mellitus.[53] The clinical course is rapidly progressive, with a fatal outcome.

Infected Vascular Gangrene

Infected vascular gangrene is a mixed infection developing in a group of muscles or in a limb devitalized as a result of arterial insufficiency, particularly in patients with diabetes mellitus. *Proteus, Bacteroides*, and anaerobic streptococci are among the bacteria found in such lesions. Gas formation and foul-smelling pus are prominent. The infection does not extend beyond the area of vascular gangrene to involve healthy muscle. *Bacillus cereus* infection has been associated with myonecrosis with slight crepitance after thrombosis of arterial grafts.[54]

Aeromonas hydrophila Myonecrosis

Rapidly progressive myonecrosis caused by *Aeromonas hydrophila*, a facultatively anaerobic, gram-negative bacillus, may occur after penetrating trauma in a freshwater environment or associated with fish or other aquatic animals.[55, 56] In a few instances, myonecrosis has been accompanied by gas spreading extensively in soft tissue planes. The rapid onset (24 to 48 hours) and rapid progression after trauma resemble those of clostridial gas gangrene. The prominence of pain, marked edema, serosanguineous bullae, and toxicity, in addition to the presence of gas in fascial planes, adds to the similarity of these conditions. Bacteremia is frequently present. Treatment consists of extensive surgical débridement and prompt initiation of antimicrobial therapy. Most isolates of *Aeromonas* are susceptible in vitro to gentamicin, tobramycin, trimethoprim-sulfamethoxazole, chloramphenicol, and ciprofloxacin.[57] Third-generation cephalosporins and aztreonam also appear to be active.

PSOAS ABSCESS

Infection of the psoas muscle takes the form of either an abscess or a phlegmon. It is usually the consequence of spread of infection from an adjacent structure. Rarely, it develops by the hematogenous route[58]; in children particularly, there may be no prior inciting event such as trauma or preceding infection, and *S. aureus* is the most common cause in this setting. Psoas abscess usually is confined within the psoas fascia, but occasionally, because of anatomic relations, infection extends to the buttock, hip, or upper thigh. Psoas abscess may complicate pyogenic or tuberculous vertebral osteomyelitis. The latter was formerly the principal cause of a psoas abscess; now psoas abscesses most commonly result from direct extension of intra-abdominal infections (e.g., diverticulitis, appendicitis, Crohn's disease).[59] Occasionally, a psoas abscess results from extension of a perinephric abscess or from secondary infection of a retroperitoneal hematoma. The organisms involved in spread of infection from an intestinal site are usually members of the aerobic and anaerobic bowel flora. *S. aureus* is the most common cause of psoas abscess secondary to vertebral osteomyelitis.

The iliacus muscle, applied to the ilium in the iliac fossa, forms a conjoined tendon with the lower portion of the psoas muscle. Osteomyelitis of the ilium or septic arthritis of the sacroiliac joint can penetrate the sheaths of either or both muscles in this location, producing an iliacus or psoas abscess.[60]

Clinical manifestations of a psoas abscess include fever, lower abdominal or back pain, or pain referred to the hip or knee. A limp may be evident, and flexion deformity of the hip may develop from reflex spasm, suggesting septic arthritis of the hip. The psoas sign is evident. Often a tender mass can be palpated in the groin.

Roentgenograms may show a bulge produced by a psoas muscle abscess or the presence of gas within the psoas sheath. Calcification in a psoas abscess strongly suggests a tuberculous cause.

Of the five noninvasive techniques currently available for visualization of the psoas (and iliacus) muscles, CT scanning is the most rapid and sensitive. Ultrasound is less reliable for detecting small lesions or a phlegmon. Gallium scanning does not provide as sharp a localization and takes up to 72 hours; indium-labeled leukocyte scanning may be preferable to the latter. CT scanning may show diffuse enlargement of the psoas (phlegmon) or sharply circumscribed, low-density fluid collections (abscess) within the muscle, or it may demonstrate the presence of gas within the muscle (indicative of abscess).[61] MRI scanning of the pelvis can show enlarged psoas and iliacus muscles displaying grossly abnormal signal intensities.

Pyogenic psoas abscesses are treated by surgical drainage and provisional initial antibiotic therapy based on knowledge of the origin of the infection. CT scanning may be of considerable value for guidance of direct needle aspiration of an abscess for culture or for drainage when the direct surgical approach is not preferable or warranted. When the process appears to be a phlegmon, repeated CT scanning during the course of antibiotic therapy can confirm resolution of the anatomic changes.

OTHER SPECIFIC SITES OF MUSCLE ABSCESSES

Infective myositis or pyomyositis may occasionally occur in unusual anatomic areas for these processes and mimic other more common infections. Iliacus pyomyositis[22] and pyomyositis of the adductor muscles may mimic septic arthritis of the hip; pyriformis pyomyositis may suggest a spinal epidural abscess[23]; iliopsoas myositis[21] may mimic appendicitis.

MYALGIAS

Myalgias are prominent features of a variety of infections such as dengue, influenza, and Rocky Mountain spotted fever. Little information is available on the presence of specific histologic findings indicative of myositis.

Influenza

Muscle aches are common early in the course of influenza. Occasionally, severe bilateral muscle pains in the lower limbs may develop in the recovery phase, particularly in young children.[62, 63] Muscle tenderness, principally in the gastrocnemius and soleus muscles, is demonstrable, and calf swelling may be present. Deep tendon reflexes and muscle strength are normal, but there is considerable difficulty in walking. The leg pains and muscle tenderness subside in less than a week. Mild elevations of serum concentrations of aldolase and creatine phosphokinase occur. The few biopsies performed have shown either nonspecific degenerative changes or muscle necrosis with polymorphonuclear leukocytic infiltration. Whether this "myositis" is caused by direct viral invasion or by some immunologic or other response is unknown. However, influenza A virus was isolated from the muscle biopsy specimen of an adult with generalized muscle weakness occurring during an influenza A outbreak.[64]

Infective Endocarditis

Prominent myalgias occur in about 15% of patients with infective endocarditis.[65] They may be either diffuse or localized. The pathogenesis is not known, but in one instance muscle biopsy specimens showed a small focus of muscle fiber destruction and leukocytic infiltration consistent with embolization to a small artery.[65]

Toxoplasmosis

The major features of acute acquired disseminated toxoplasmosis are those of meningoencephalitis, myocarditis, pneumonitis, skin rash, and occasionally hepatitis (see Chapter 268). In rare instances, polymyositis may be a prominent clinical manifestation. Marked myalgias, muscle weakness and swelling, and fasciculations occur in such patients. Muscle biopsy specimens show interstitial myositis with destruction of muscle fibers, and pseudocysts of *Toxoplasma gondii* can be found in areas of muscle free of inflammatory reaction. In several cases *Toxoplasma* have been isolated by animal inoculation.[66, 67]

Other Causes

Occasionally, the only clinical manifestations of initial infection with HIV-1 are those of polymyositis (myalgias, muscle weakness, and increased serum levels of muscle enzymes). HIV-1 viral antigens can be found in CD4 T cells in areas of muscle fiber inflammation and necrosis.[68] During the subsequent course of HIV-1 infection, various forms of muscular involvement may develop, including generalized or localized myalgias, HIV myopathy (polymyositis),[69] muscle atrophy secondary to the anorexia and cachexia of the "wasting syndrome" of AIDS,[70] and the mitochondrial myopathy related to prolonged zidovudine therapy.[71] The clinical presentation of HIV-1 myopathy (inflammatory polymyositis) is that of progressive proximal muscle weakness. Elevated serum creatine phosphokinase and electromyographic changes assist in diagnosis. Muscle biopsy material shows either of two histologic patterns alone or in combination: (1) an inflammatory myopathy with lymphocytic infiltration and muscle fiber necrosis or (2) abundant nemaline rod bodies and muscle fiber necrosis. In patients receiving prolonged zidovudine therapy in whom myopathy develops, muscle biopsy material shows a combination of endomyosial inflammatory infiltrate (CD8 T cells and macrophages) and a mitochondrial myopathy characterized by proliferation of large numbers of abnormal mitochondria ("ragged-red fibers") in the subsarcolemmal spaces.[72] The mitochondrial changes appear to represent toxic changes associated with zidovudine therapy, and clinical improvement in some patients may occur after discontinuance of the drug. The inflammatory myopathy may represent primarily an HIV-associated autoimmune process and may respond clinically to prednisone.

Inflammatory myositis with a lymphoplasmacytic cellular response was the major feature in a case of Lyme disease.[73] Spirochetes morphologically similar to *Borrelia burgdorferi* were present on Dieterle silver stain of biopsied muscle. Rarely, *Sarcocystis* (an intracellular sporozoan parasite) infection has been observed in histologic sections of muscle of individuals, mainly from abroad, with muscle pain or weakness.[74] Microsporidia myositis has been reported in a patient with AIDS.[75]

PLEURODYNIA SYNDROMES

Epidemic pleurodynia is an acute, febrile disease caused by group B coxsackieviruses that is characterized by the sudden onset of sharp chest pain over the lower ribs or sternum (see Chapter 160). Paroxysms of knifelike pain are precipitated by voluntary or respiratory movements. Muscle tenderness may be present. Abdominal pain may also be present in some patients; in others, abdominal pain may be the sole manifestation, simulating intraperitoneal processes.

Group B coxsackieviruses produce visceral lesions and also some focal myositis in experimental animals. Myositis has not been demonstrated as a feature pathologically either in fatal cases of severe neonatal coxsackievirus B infection or in the few biopsy specimens obtained from affected muscles of patients with epidemic pleurodynia.[76, 77]

MYALGIAS WITH EOSINOPHILIA (PARASITIC MYOSITIS)

Trichinosis

Trichinosis is acquired from ingestion of insufficiently cooked pork or, less commonly, from bear meat, wild boar, or walrus. The prominent clinical manifestations of trichinosis include fever, myositis, periorbital edema, and eosinophilia. An initial intestinal phase (nausea, vomiting, nonbloody diarrhea) during the first week is followed during the second week by larval invasion of skeletal muscle (see Chapter 277). Serious complications in the form of myocarditis, meningoencephalitis, and pneumonitis can occur.[78] Myalgias, frequently accompanied by muscle swelling and weakness and occasionally associated with fasciculations, are present in most patients with the disease. Muscles commonly involved include the extraocular muscles, flexor muscles of the extremities, back muscles, and the muscles used in chewing and swallowing. Periorbital edema, chemosis, and conjunctival hemorrhages are related to larval invasion of extraocular muscles. The inflammatory response in muscle produces increased serum levels of muscle enzymes.

Muscle biopsy specimens reveal encysted larval trichinae in necrotic muscle fibers surrounded by inflammatory cells (predominantly eosinophils and neutrophils, but also lymphocytes). Severe skeletal muscle involvement has been reported in a case of trichinosis in an immunosuppressed patient.[79] Although granulomatous reactions have been observed in the heart and lungs of fatal cases, larval encystment does not take place in organs other than skeletal muscle.

Trichinella spiralis is the most common cause of human trichinosis, but other species can infect humans. *Trichinella pseudospiralis* has caused a large outbreak of trichinosis in Thailand.[80] Because this species, unlike *T. spiralis*, does not undergo encystment in skeletal muscle, prolonged larval migration and clinical symptoms ensue.

Diagnosis of trichinosis is made on the basis of the clinical picture, eosinophilia, serology (enzyme-linked immunosorbent assay, bentonite flocculation), and, when needed, muscle biopsy.

Benzimadazole compounds (thiabendazole, mebendazole, albendazole) are the most effective therapies for acute symptomatic disease. Albendazole may have the advantage of being better tolerated.[80]

Trichinosis should be distinguished from the eosinophilia-myalgia syndrome resulting from the ingestion of certain tryptophan products and characterized by prominent myalgias, fatigue, and eosinophilia, followed, in some instances, by development of neurologic and scleroderma-like skin changes.[81]

Cysticercosis (Cysticercus Cellulosal Myositis)

Human cysticercosis is rare in the United States but is common in Latin America and Asia. It results from the ingestion and subsequent hatching of viable eggs of *Taenia solium* into the larval form of the parasite *Cysticercus cellulosae* (see Chapter 280). Eggs reach the upper intestinal tract from food contaminated by feces from a person parasitized by the adult worm. Autoinfection can occur through the fecal-oral route and possibly when reverse peristalsis introduces egg-laden proglottids back into the duodenum or stomach, where they hatch. From there they are distributed widely (skeletal muscle, subcutaneous tissues, heart, eye).

Symptomatic involvement of muscle is uncommon. Occasionally, the stage of invasion is characterized by fever, muscle tenderness, and eosinophilia. More characteristically, asymptomatic calcified cysts ("puffed rice" appearance) are detected in muscles on soft tissue x-ray films of patients with neurologic manifestations.

MUSCLE DEGENERATION ASSOCIATED WITH INFECTIONS AT OTHER SITES

Acute Rhabdomyolysis

Myoglobinuria occasionally follows an acute illness with symptoms suggesting an upper respiratory tract infection. Scattered cases have been shown to follow documented influenza A virus infections in children and adults,[82] legionnaires' disease, leptospirosis (Weil's disease),[83] pneumococcal sepsis,[84] meningococcal sepsis,[85] echovirus infection,[86] and infections caused by coxsackievirus, Epstein-Barr virus, and adenovirus.[87] Diffuse muscle pains (especially in the extremities), weakness, swelling, and tenderness are prominent features, along with myoglobinuria. Rhabdomyolysis has occurred in patients with no previous episodes and no family history of this condition. Like the myositis that occurs after influenza in children, it develops when respiratory symptoms are resolving.

Muscle Proteolysis and Mediators of Fever in Patients with Sepsis

Muscle involvement, in the form of myalgias and weakness, is common in the course of systemic infections. Accelerated catabolism of skeletal muscle contributes to the marked weakness and muscle wasting that can be observed in systemic infections. This appears to be part of a protective "acute phase" host response to sepsis and trauma. Important roles are played by interleukin-1 (IL-1), tumor necrosis factor, interferon-α, and IL-6. A polypeptide (possibly a breakdown product of IL-1) that produces a rapid increase in protein degradation in rat or human muscle preparations[88] has been observed in the plasma of patients with sepsis. Similar changes are produced by IL-1 itself.[89] This accelerated proteolysis is effected through increased synthesis in muscle of prostaglandin E_2, which in turn activates proteases in muscle-cell lysosomes. This catabolic activity is accompanied by IL-1–stimulated hepatic protein synthesis (using the newly generated source of amino acids) and other elements of the acute phase response and by fever (also generated by IL-1 and mediated by prostaglandin E_2). The important role of prostaglandin E_2 in the generation of the muscle aches and fever of infection is consistent with the amelioration of these symptoms produced by prostaglandin synthesis inhibitors such as aspirin.

REFERENCES

1. Smith IM, Vickers AB. Natural history of 338 treated and untreated patients with staphylococcal septicaemia. Lancet. 1960;1:1318.
2. Levin MJ, Gardner P, Waldvogel FA. "Tropical" pyomyositis: An unusual infection due to *Staphylococcus aureus*. N Engl J Med. 1971:284:196.
3. Horn CV, Master S. Pyomyositis tropicans in Uganda. E Afr Med J. 1968;45:463.
4. Christin L, Sarosi GA. Pyomyositis in North America: Case reports and review. Clin Infect Dis. 1992;15:668.
5. Harbarth SJ, Lew DP. Pyomyositis as a nontropical disease. In: Remington J, Swartz MN, eds. Current Clinical Topics in Infectious Diseases, v. 17. Malden, Mass: Blackwell Science Publishers; 1997:37–50.
6. Gardiner JS, Zauk AM, Minnefor AB, et al. Pyomyositis in an HIV-positive premature infant: Case report and review of the literature. J Pediatr Orthop. 1990;10:791.
7. Rodgers WB, Yodlowski ML, Mintzer CM. Pyomyositis in patients who have the human immunodeficiency virus: Case report and review of the literature. J Bone Joint Surg A. 1993;75:588.
8. Medina F, Fuentes M, Jara LJ, et al. Salmonella pyomyositis in patients with the human immunodeficiency virus. Br J Rheumatol. 1995;34:568.
9. Arranz-Caso JA, Cuadrado-Gomez LM, Romanik-Cabrera J, et al. Pyomyositis caused by *Morganella morganii* in a patient with AIDS. Clin Infect Dis. 1996;22:372.
10. Miralles GD, Bregman Z. Necrotizing pyomyositis caused by *Mycobacterium avium* complex in a patient with AIDS. Clin Infect Dis. 1994;18:833.
11. Mylonakis E, Rich JD, Flanigan T, et al. Muscle abscess due to *Aspergillus fumigatus* in a patient with AIDS. Clin Infect Dis. 1996;23:1323.
12. Murphy PM, Lane HC, Fauci AS, et al. Impairment of neutrophil bactericidal capacity in patients with AIDS. J Infect Dis. 1988;158:627.
13. Hsueh P-R, Hsiue TR, Hsieh W-C. Pyomyositis in intravenous drug abusers: Report of a unique case and review of the literature. Clin Infect Dis. 1996;22:858.
14. Miyake H. Beitrag zur Kenntniss des sogenannten Myositis infectiosa. Mitt Grenzgeb Med Chir. 1904;13:155.
15. Immerman RP, Greenman RL. Toxic shock syndrome associated with pyomyositis caused by a strain of *Staphylococcus aureus* that does not produce toxic-shock-syndrome toxin—1. Infect Dis. 1987;156:505.
16. Kennedy CA, Mathisen G, Goetz MB. Tropical pyomyositis of the abdominal wall musculature mimicking acute abdomen. West J Med. 1990;152:296.
17. Armstrong JH. Tropical pyomyositis and myoglobinuria. Arch Intern Med. 1978;138:1145.
18. Collazos J, Fernandez A, Martinez E, et al. Pneumococcal pyomyositis: Case report, review of the literature, and comparison with classic pyomyositis caused by other bacteria. Arch Intern Med. 1996;156:1470.
19. Bonomo RA, Graham R, Makley JT, et al. Tuberculous pyomyositis: An unusual presentation of disseminated *Mycobacterium tuberculosis* infection. Clin Infect Dis. 1995;20:1576.
20. Pearl GS, Sieger B. Granulomatous *Pneumocystis carinii* myositis presenting as an intramuscular mass. Clin Infect Dis. 1996;22:577.
21. Wysoki MG, Angeid-Backman, Izes BA. Iliopsoas myositis mimicking appendicitis: MRI diagnosis. Skeletal Radiol. 1997;26:316.
22. Chen W-S, Wan Y-L. Iliacus pyomyositis mimicking septic arthritis of the hip joint. Arch Orthop Trauma Surg. 1996;115:233.
23. Chusid MJ, Hill WC, Bevan JA, et al. Proteus pyomyositis of the pyriformis muscle in a swimmer. Clin Infect Dis. 1998;26:194.
24. Case Records of the Massachusetts General Hospital. Skeletal muscle infarction associated with diabetes mellitus. N Engl J Med. 1997;337:839.
25. Gordon BA, Martinez S, Collins AJ. Pyomyositis: Characteristics at CT and MRI imaging. Radiology. 1995;197:279.
26. Quillin SP, McAlister WH. Rapidly progressive pyomyositis: Diagnosis by repeat sonography. J Ultrasound Med. 1991;10:181.
27. Cone LA, Lamb RB, Graff-Radford A, et al. Pyomyositis of the anterior tibial compartment. Clin Infect Dis; 1997:25:146.
28. Svane S. Peracute spontaneous streptococcal myositis. Acta Chir Scand. 1971;137:155.
29. Moore DL, Delage G, Labelle H, et al. Peracute streptococcal pyomyositis: Report of two cases and review of the literature. J Pediatr Orthop. 1986;6:232.
30. Stevens DL, Tanner MH, Winship J, et al. Severe group A streptococcal infections associated with a toxic shock-like syndrome and scarlet fever toxin A. N Engl J Med. 1989;321:1.
31. Johnson L, Berggren L, Björsell-Östling E, et al. Streptococcal myositis. Scand J Infect Dis. 1992;24:661.
32. Yoder EL, Mendez J, Khatib R. Spontaneous gangrenous myositis induced by *Streptococcus pyogenes*: Case report and review of the literature. Rev Infect Dis. 1987;9:382.
33. Case Records of the Massachusetts General Hospital. Group A beta-hemolytic streptococcus infection, with the compartment and toxic shock syndrome. New Engl J Med. 1995;333:113.
34. Wagner JG, Schlievert PM, Assimacopoulos AP, et al. Acute Group G streptococcal myositis associated with streptococcal toxic shock syndrome: Case report and review. Clin Infect Dis. 1996;23:1159.
35. Stevens DL, Gibbons AE, Bergstrom R, et al. The Eagle effect revisited: Efficacy of clindamycin, erythromycin, and penicillin in the treatment of streptococcal myositis. J Infect Dis. 1988;158:23.
36. Altemeier WA, Fullen WD. Prevention and treatment of gas gangrene. JAMA. 1971;217:806.
37. MacLennan JD. The histotoxic clostridial infections of man. Bacteriol Rev. 1962;26:177.
38. Bornstein DL, Weinberg AN, Swartz MN, et al. Anaerobic infections: Review of current experience. Medicine (Baltimore). 1964;43:207.
39. Altemeier WA, Furste WL. Gas gangrene. Surg Gynecol Obstet. 1947;84:507.
40. Finegold SM. Anaerobic Bacteria in Human Disease. New York: Academic Press; 1977:424.
41. Stevens DL, Musher DM, Watson DA, et al. Spontaneous, nontraumatic gangrene due to *Clostridium septicum*. Rev Infect Dis. 1990;12:286.
42. Stevens DL, Tweten RK, Awad MM, et al. Clostridial gas gangrene: Evidence that α and θ toxins differentially modulate the immune response and induce acute tissue necrosis. J Infect Dis. 1997;176:189.
43. Caplan ES, Kluge RM. Gas gangrene: Review of 34 cases. Arch Intern Med. 1976;136:788.
44. Dyelewski J, Wiesenfeld H, Latour A. Postpartum uterine infection with *Clostridium perfringens*. Rev Infect Dis. 1989;11:470.
45. Case Records of the Massachusetts General Hospital. N Engl J Med. 1993; 328:340.
46. Stevens DL, Maier KA, Laine BM, et al. Comparison of clindamycin, rifampin, tetracycline, metronidazole, and penicillin for efficacy in prevention of experimental gas gangrene due to *Clostridium perfringens*. J Infect Dis. 1987;155:220.
47. Stevens DL, Laine BM, Mitten JE. Comparison of single and combination antimicrobial agents for prevention of experimental gas gangrene caused by *Clostridium perfringens*. Antimicrob Agents Chemother. 1987;31:312.
48. Marrie TJ, Haldane EV, Swantee CA, et al. Susceptibility of anaerobic bacteria to nine antimicrobial agents and demonstration of decreased susceptibility of *Clostridium perfringens* to penicillin. Antimicrob Agents Chemother. 1981;19:51.
49. Brefort G, Magot M, Ionesco H, et al. Characterization and transferability of *Clostridium perfringens* plasmids. Plasmid. 1977;1:52.
50. Shupak A, Halpern P, Ziser A, et al. Hyperbaric oxygen therapy for gas gangrene casualties in the Lebanon War, 1982. Isr J Med Sci. 1984;20:323.
51. Stevens DL, Bryant AE, Adams K, et al. Evaluation of therapy with hyperbaric oxygen for experimental infection with *Clostridium perfringens*. Clin Infect Dis. 1993;17:231.
52. Chambers CH, Bond GF, Morris JH. Synergistic necrotizing myositis complicating vascular injury. J Trauma. 1974;14:980.
53. Bruno-Murtha LA, Sedghivaziri MA, Arbeit RD. Crepitant myonecrosis caused by *Klebsiella pneumoniae* in an immunocompromised diabetic patient. J Infect Dis. 1990;162:1416.
54. Johnson DA, Aulicino PL, Newby JG. *Bacillus cereus*–induced myonecrosis. J Trauma. 1984;24:267.
55. Davis WA, Kane JG, Garagusi VF. Human *Aeromonas* infections: A review of the literature and case report of endocarditis. Medicine (Baltimore). 1978;57:267.
56. Heckerling PS, Stine TM, Pottage JC, et al. *Aeromonas hydrophila* myonecrosis and gas gangrene in a nonimmunocompromised host. Arch Intern Med. 1983;143:2005.
57. San Joaquin VH, Scribner RK, Picket DA, et al. Antimicrobial susceptibility of

Aeromonas species isolated from patients with diarrhea. Antimicrob Agents Chemother. 1986;30:794.
58. Steiner JL, Septimus EJ, Vartian CV. Infection of the psoas muscle secondary to *Streptococcus pneumoniae* infection. Clin Infect Dis. 1992;15:1047.
59. Kyle J. Psoas abscess in Crohn's disease. Gastroenterology. 1971;61:149.
60. Simons GW, Sty JR, Starshak RJ, et al. Retroperitoneal and retrofascial abscesses. J Bone Joint Surg A. 1983;65:1041.
61. Gordin F, Stamler C, Mills J. Pyogenic psoas abscesses: Noninvasive diagnostic techniques and review of the literature. Rev Infect Dis. 1983;5:1003.
62. Middleton PJ, Alexander RM, Szymanski MT. Severe myositis during recovery from influenza. Lancet. 1970;2:533.
63. Mejlszenkier JD, Safran AP, Healy JJ, et al. The myositis of influenza. Arch Neurol. 1973;29:441.
64. Kessler HA, Trenholme GM, Harris AA, et al. Acute myopathy associated with influenza A/Texas/1/77 infection. JAMA. 1980;243:461.
65. Churchill MA, Geraci JE, Hunder GG. Musculoskeletal manifestations of bacterial endocarditis. Ann Intern Med. 1977;87:754.
66. Greenlee JE, Johnson WD, Campa JF, et al. Adult toxoplasmosis presenting as polymyositis and cerebral ataxia. Ann Intern Med. 1975;82:367.
67. Kass EH, Andrus SB, Adams RD, et al. Toxoplasmosis in the human adult. Arch Intern Med. 1952;89:759.
68. Dalakas MC, Pezeshkpour GH, Gravell M, et al. Polymyositis associated with AIDS retrovirus. JAMA. 1986;256:2381.
69. Simpson DM, Bender AN. Human immunodeficiency virus-associated myopathy: Analysis of 11 patients. Ann Neurol. 1988;24:79.
70. Grunfeld C, Feingold KR. Metabolic disturbances and wasting in the acquired immunodeficiency syndrome. N Engl J Med. 1992;327:329.
71. Till M, MacDonell KB. Myopathy with human immunodeficiency virus type 1 (HIV-1) infection: HIV-1 or zidovudine? Ann Intern Med. 1990;113:492.
72. Dalakas MC, Illa I, Pezeshkpour GH, et al. Mitochondrial myopathy caused by long-term zidovudine therapy. N Engl J Med. 1990;322:1098.
73. Atlas E, Novak SN, Duray P, et al. Lyme myositis: Muscle invasion by *Borrelia burgdorferi*. Ann Intern Med. 1988;109:245.
74. Beaver PC, Gadgil RK, Morera P. Sarcocystis: A review and report of five cases. Am J Trop Med Hyg. 1979;28:819.
75. Ledford DK, Overman MD, Gonzalvo A, et al. Microsporidiosis myositis in a patient with the acquired immunodeficiency syndrome. Ann Intern Med. 1985;102:628.
76. Adams RD. Diseases of Muscle: A Study in Pathology. Hagerstown, Md.: Harper & Row; 1975:318.
77. Cherry JD. Enteroviruses. In: Remington JS, Klein JO, eds. Infectious Diseases of the Fetus and Newborn Infant. Philadelphia: WB Saunders; 1976:397.
78. Clausen MR, Meyer CN, Krantz T, et al. Trichinella infection and clinical disease. Q J Med. 1996;89:631.
79. Jacobson ES, Jacobson HG. Trichinosis in an immunosuppressed human host. Am J Clin Pathol. 1977;68:791.
80. Cabié A, Bouchard O, Houzé, et al. Albendazole versus thiabendazole as therapy for trichinosis: A retrospective study. Clin Infect Dis. 1996;22:1033.
81. Culpepper RC, Williams RG, Mease PJ, et al. Natural history of the eosinophilia-myalgia syndrome. Ann Intern Med. 1991;115:437.
82. Minow RA, Gorbach S, Johnson BL, et al. Myoglobinuria associated with influenza A infection. Ann Intern Med. 1974;80:359.
83. Solbrig MV, Sher JH, Kula RW. Rhabdomyolysis in leptospirosis (Weil's disease). J Infect Dis. 1987;156:692.
84. Naschitz JE, Yeshurun D, Shagrawi I. Rhabdomyolysis in pneumococcal sepsis. Am J Med. 1989;87:479.
85. Van Deuren M, Neeleman C, Assmann KJM, et al. Rhabdomyolysis during the subacute stage of meningococcal sepsis. Clin Infect Dis. 1998;26:214.
86. Josselson J, Pula T, Sadler JH. Acute rhabdomyolysis associated with an echovirus 9 infection. Arch Intern Med. 1980;140:1671.
87. Meshkinpour H, Vaziri ND. Acute rhabdomyolysis associated with adenovirus infection. J Infect Dis. 1981;143:133.
88. Clowes GHA Jr, George BC, Villee CA Jr, et al. Muscle proteolysis induced by a circulating peptide in patients with sepsis or trauma. N Engl J Med. 1983;308:545.
89. Baracos V, Rodemann HP, Dinarello CA, et al. Stimulation of muscle protein degradation and prostaglandin E_2 release by leukocytic pyrogen (interleukin-1): A mechanism for the increased degradation of muscle proteins during fever. N Engl J Med. 1983;308:553.

Chapter 80

Lymphadenitis and Lymphangitis

MORTON N. SWARTZ

LYMPHADENITIS

Lymphadenitis is an acute or chronic inflammation of lymph nodes. It may be restricted to a solitary node or to a localized group of nodes draining an anatomic area (regional lymphadenitis), or the involvement can be generalized during a systemic infection. The gross features may be those of nonsuppurative, suppurative, necrotizing, or caseous inflammation, depending on the nature of the infecting microorganism.

Pathogenesis and Pathologic Changes

Acute Lymphadenitis

Lymph nodes serve as filters, removing infectious agents from lymphatics draining areas of acute inflammation. The initial histologic response consists of swelling and hyperplasia of sinusoidal lining cells and the infiltration of leukocytes. Depending on the nature of the infecting organism, host defenses, and antimicrobial therapy, the process may or may not progress to abscess formation. With some microorganisms, a more distinctive pathologic picture may be seen: caseation necrosis with infections due to *Mycobacterium tuberculosis, Histoplasma capsulatum, Coccidioides immitis*, and various atypical mycobacteria; stellate abscesses surrounded by palisading epithelioid cells ("granulomatous abscess")[1] with lymphogranuloma venereum, cat-scratch disease, tularemia, yersiniosis, fungal lymphadenitis, and chronic granulomatous disease; or reactive follicular hyperplasia with scattered clusters of epithelioid histiocytes, located in cortical and paracortical zones and characteristically blurring the margins of germinal centers, along with focal distention of subcapsular and trabecular sinuses by monocytoid cells (monocytoid B cells), in toxoplasmosis.[2] The necrotizing granulomatous lymphadenitis that occurs in tularemia can resemble that occurring in cat-scratch disease but often exhibits more granulomatous inflammation. *Yersinia (Yersinia pseudotuberculosis* or *Yersinia enterocolitica)* infection in mesenteric lymph nodes can also cause a necrotizing lymphadenitis. Necrotizing nongranulomatous lymphadenitis may be a feature of processes to which an infectious cause has not yet been ascribed: Kikuchi's necrotizing lymphadenitis, Kawasaki syndrome, and systemic lupus erythematosus.[3]

Chronic Lymphadenitis

Histologically, the response is proliferative with hyperplasia of reticuloendothelial cells, prominent germinal centers, and dilated lymph sinuses filled with mononuclear cells. This picture is nonspecific, can be seen with a variety of infections, and may be observed initially on biopsy in a patient subsequently proven to have a lymphoproliferative disorder.

Dermatopathic lymphadenitis is a distinctive form of chronic lymphadenitis involving lymph nodes draining sites of chronic pruritic dermatitides. Histologically, the enlarged nodes show hyperplasia of reticulum cells in the germinal follicles and of sinusoidal lining cells, as well as the accumulation of lipid and melanin in macrophages (released from the inflammatory process in the skin). The latter feature is the basis for the pathologic designation *lipomelanotic reticuloendotheliosis*. The hyperplastic appearance of such nodes may be so prominent as to suggest erroneously the diagnosis of a lymphoproliferative disorder.

Clinical Findings

Acute Regional Lymphadenitis Due to Pyogenic Bacteria

Palpable lymph nodes do not always indicate serious or ongoing disease. Some degree of inguinal lymphadenopathy is relatively common, reflecting prior episodes of infection in the lower extremities (e.g., interdigital web infections secondary to epidermophytosis); similarly, minor enlargement of cervical nodes may be the residual from previous pharyngeal or dental infections. Lymphadenopathy in certain anatomic areas (preauricular, posterior auricular, supraclavicular, deltoidopectoral, and pectoral) should be viewed with greater suspicion because these nodes are not frequently enlarged as a result of local subclinical infections or minor trauma. Enlargement of superficial lymph nodes along the external jugular vein, as well as of nodes that drain the earlobe and the floor of the external acoustic meatus, is very infrequent but may be associated with superficial infection accompanying recent initial earring insertion. Rarely, a firm mass in the tail or lateral aspect of the breast, suggestive of carcinoma, proves to be an enlarged lymph node in an unusual location due to toxoplasmosis.[2]

Acute suppurative lymphadenitis is more common in children than in adults. In the past four decades, *Staphylococcus aureus* has superseded group A streptococci as the most frequent etiologic agent. The most common sites of involvement are, in descending order, submandibular (submaxillary), anterior and posterior cervical, inguinal, and axillary lymph nodes. The portal of entry for infection is frequently difficult to determine in children when cervical lymph nodes are involved.

On examination, the involved area is swollen, and the node(s) is usually at least 3 cm in diameter and tender. Fever is commonly present. The node(s) may be very firm or frankly fluctuant. The overlying skin is warm and often erythematous and edematous.

Syndromes Due to Suppurative Lymphadenitis at Specific Anatomic Sites

Cervical Lymphadenitis

Acute unilateral adenitis of pyogenic origin occurs most often in pre-school-aged children. The temperature is usually elevated (100°F to 101°F), and local swelling may have been present for some days before the patient is seen by a physician. In only a minority of the cases is there a history of sore throat. However, in the past, group A streptococci have been implicated in about 75% of the cases of untreated suppurative cervical lymphadenitis in children.[4, 5] *S. aureus*, or a combination of *S. aureus* and group A streptococci, is often the etiologic agent of suppurative cervical lymphadenitis associated with pyodermas of the face and scalp. Acute torticollis may result from cervical lymphadenitis, of either bacterial or viral (e.g., infectious mononucleosis) origin, and may be the initial symptom that brings the child to the physician.[6]

On examination, there is prominent swelling of the neck or face owing to the enlargement usually of a single node, which is often walnut-sized. The node is exquisitely tender and firm but may be fluctuant. The swelling may be sufficiently marked to interfere with opening of the mouth. A leukocytosis with a white blood cell count of 12,000 to 25,000/mm^3 is a common finding.

Acute bilateral cervical adenitis usually involves multiple nodes that are enlarged and somewhat tender in association with viral pharyngitis, infectious mononucleosis, streptococcal pharyngitis, or periodontal infection. Such lymphadenopathy does not oridinarily go on to suppuration unless the symptomatic streptococcal pharyngitis or periodontal infection is ignored.

Acute Axillary Lymphadenitis

This process, when due to *S. pyogenes*, is characterized by an abrupt onset with chills, fever, marked axillary pain, and prominent edema of the shoulder, arm, axilla, supraclavicular fossa, and pectoral areas.[7] The site of initiating infection is usually a pustule or traumatic lesion on the hand or arm. The involved area, although edematous, does not have features of cellulitis, lymphangitis, or erysipelas. Ipsilateral pleural effusion may develop owing to blockage of lymphatic vessels draining the parietal pleura into involved lymph nodes at the junction of the internal jugular and subclavian veins. Thrombosis of the axillary and subclavian veins may be a complication.

Subpectoral Lymphadenitis

An unusual course may be taken occasionally by infection (usually streptococcal but sometimes staphylococcal) of the thumb or of the interdigital web between the thumb and index finger. Lymphatics from this area do not pass through the epitrochlear nodes but drain directly into the axillary nodes, which in turn communicate with the subpectoral nodes. If infection is not contained in the axillary nodes, subpectoral lymphadenitis develops.[8] Suppuration of these subpectoral nodes can follow. Infection in this area may dissect downward and manifest as cellulitis over the lower chest and upper abdomen, suggesting an intra-abdominal infection. Occasionally, large subpectoral abscesses may suggest a tumor, because the overlying pectoralis major obscures the local warmth and erythema commonly associated with infection. Rarely, contraction of the pectoral muscle (as on elevating the arm) causes cephalic movement of the pectoral area swelling, suggesting avulsion of the inferior attachments of this muscle to sternum, sixth costal cartilage, and the aponeurosis of the external abdominal oblique muscle. The suppurating nodes may drain onto the chest wall. A pleural effusion may develop on the involved side.

Acute Suppurative Epitrochlear Lymphadenitis

The epitrochlear nodes receive lymphatic drainage from the middle, ring, and little fingers and from the medial portion of the hand and the ulnar aspect of the forearm. Acute suppurative epitrochlear lymphadenitis is uncommon. The site of the initiating infection in most patients is a primary pyoderma or secondarily infected skin lesion. Unilateral tender swelling, erythema, and induration of the epitrochlear area develop and may subsequently spread along the medial aspect of the arm and forearm. Pain on movement of the elbow is evident. There is often a moderate fever and leukocytosis. The diagnosis is apparent when a discrete, tender nodular swelling can be palpated; but when the area is diffusely swollen and movement at the elbow is limited, the picture may suggest septic arthritis or osteomyelitis.[9] Group A streptococci and *S. aureus* are implicated most commonly.

Suppurative Iliac Lymphadenitis

The iliac lymph nodes are located along the external and common iliac arteries in the anterior retroperitoneal space. They receive deep lymphatic drainage from the lower abdominal wall and afferents from the superficial and deep inguinal nodes. Iliac lymphadenitis may develop secondary to infection of the lower extremities, lower abdominal wall, perineum, and so forth, or rarely, it may result from hematogenous infection. After infection develops, it appears to break through fascial compartments in the iliac fossa, and abscess formation ensues. Formerly, most cases occurred in children and young adults, but more recently there appears to be no age predilection. The suppurative lymphadenitis progresses to abscess formation in the space between the posterior peritoneum and the psoas and iliacus fascia.[10] An unexplained limp may be the initial symptom; the acute onset with fever may not occur for some days or weeks. Back and hip pain becomes prominent; extension of the thigh is very painful, but abduction and adduction of the hip evoke minimal discomfort. The symptomatology and clinical findings direct attention to the diagnostic possibilities of septic arthritis and osteomyelitis. Only after some days or weeks does lower abdominal pain develop, and the patient becomes acutely ill with high fever and marked leukocytosis. Examination at this point reveals a tightly flexed hip, rectus muscle spasm on the affected side, possibly a tender posterolateral pelvic mass, or a tender inguinal mass suggesting an incarcerated inguinal hernia. By this stage, the abscess may be sizable and may produce elevation and medial displacement of the sigmoid colon and medial displacement of the lower third of the ureter. When the symptoms are on the right side, the diagnosis of *retrocecal* appendicitis with abscess may be suggested, but the antecedent limp is an important clinical clue. Other diagnoses that may be suggested by the clinical manifestations include tuberculosis of the spine with psoas abscess formation, pelvic inflammatory disease, and tumor of the thigh.[11] Body computed tomography (CT) scanning can be very helpful in defining an inflammatory collection abutting the psoas and iliacus muscles. *S. aureus* is the microorganism most commonly implicated, followed in frequency by streptococci.

Acute Regional Lymphadenitis Due to Infecting Agents Other than Pyogenic Bacteria

A variety of organisms other than the common pyogens may produce localized lymphadenitis (in some cases, going on to abscess and sinus tract formation). These infections resemble pyogenic lymphadenitis but are distinguishable by a prolonged and indolent course, the atypical anatomic areas involved, the lack of prior pyogenic infection, and clues in the history (e.g., scratch by a cat, previous tuberculosis, recent sexual exposure). Occasionally, the nature of the clinical setting broadens the spectrum of microorganisms to be considered as the cause of firm or fluctuant lymphadenitis. Mycotic (*Candida albicans, Aspergillus* spp.) cervical lymphadenitis has occurred after oral mucositis in neutropenic children with leukemia[12]; but a rare case of bilateral cervical lymphadenopathy due to *Aspergillus fumigatus* has been described in a young girl without underlying disease, neutropenia, or immunosuppression.[13] In patients with suppurative lymphadenitis complicating chronic granulomatous disease, the microbial etiology is usually a catalase-positive pathogen. In addition to the commonly involved *S. aureus*, these include members of the family Enterobacteriaceae *(Klebsiella, Serratia, Salmonella), Pseudomonas* (often *Pseudomonas cepacia*), *Aspergillus, Nocardia,* Calmette-Guérin bacillus (BCG), and *Chromobacterium violaceum.*[14–16]

A variety of opportunistic pathogens rarely may be responsible for peripheral lymphadenitis in patients with HIV infection. These include *Cryptococcus neoformans*,[17] *Pneumocystis carinii*,[18] and *Bartonella henselae*[19] (bacillary angiomatosis). In addition, unusual pathogens have been responsible for lymphadenitis on rare occasions in immunocompetent persons. Such microorganisms include *Rhodococcus equi*[20] and *Y. pseudotuberculosis*.[21]

Specific Types of Nonpyogenic Regional Lymphadenitis

Scrofula (Tuberculous Cervical Lymphadenitis)

Tuberculous cervical adenitis, formerly a common disease in children and young adults, has become infrequent. It is still occasionally seen in older adults who many years earlier had immigrated to this country from endemic areas (British Isles, Europe, and the Far East) or who lived in rural areas in this country. In this setting it represents breakdown of prior cervical node tuberculosis, acquired either by ingestion of infected milk (bovine tuberculosis) or by lymphohematogenous spread of infection from an initial pulmonary focus to this group of lymph nodes. *M. tuberculosis* is seen in this country as the etiologic agent of cervical adenitis also in adults of particular ethnic groups: Native Americans, Hispanics, and recent immigrants from Haiti and Asia. In this country, mycobacterial cervical lymphadenitis (scrofula) is four to five times more frequently due to atypical mycobacteria, commonly *Mycobacterium scrofulaceum* in children,[22] than to *M. tuberculosis*. In certain areas of the United States, *Mycobacterium avium-intracellulare* complex is the principal etiologic agent[23] in children and in adults. Recently, newly recognized, difficult-to-isolate and uncommon mycobacterial species have been reported as occasionally causing childhood cervical lymphadenitis[23]: *Mycobacterium interjectum, Mycobacterium malmoense, Mycobacterium haemophilum, Mycobacterium xenopi*, and *Mycobacterium szulgai*. Two additional newly described slowly growing mycobacterial species have been described very recently: one, *Mycobacterium lentiflavum*[24] is yellow-pigmented, and the other, *Mycobacterium heidelbergense*,[25] is nonphotochromogenic. *M. tuberculosis* infections, including cervical lymphadenitis, are frequent in the human immunodeficiency virus (HIV)–infected population. *M. tuberculosis* lymphadenitis in the HIV-infected patient differs in several respects from the infection in HIV-negative patients: higher frequency of fever, often negative results on purified protein derivative (PPD) skin testing, and higher frequency of positive smears for acid-fast bacilli (and greater numbers of organisms) on fine-needle aspirates of involved lymph nodes.[26] In parts of the world where BCG vaccination of infants is commonly practiced, subcutaneous abscesses and regional lymphadenitis are not uncommon complications, occurring 2 to 8 weeks after vaccination, but these usually resolve spontaneously. Occasionally, the regional (axillary, supraclavicular, or cervical) lymphadenitis progressively enlarges and goes on to caseating suppuration.[27] This has been reported to occur at a frequency of 0.1 to 4.3 cases per 100,000 doses administered to children younger than 2 years of age.[28]

The onset of scrofula is insidious, and fever and other systemic manifestations are absent. Several nodes are enlarged and matted together; the mass so formed may develop a swollen fluctuant area, and this brings the patient to medical attention. The process is usually painless. In most cases, clinical evidence of tuberculosis elsewhere is absent. Spontaneous drainage of caseous material onto the skin surface (scrofuloderma) may eventually occur.

Definition of the mycobacterial species involved is important. The atypical mycobacteria causing cervical lymphadenitis are frequently resistant to the usual antituberculous chemotherapy, and surgical excision of the involved fluctuant node(s) is indicated. Antituberculous therapy is usually not needed for BCG nonsuppurative lymphadenitis, but if suppurative lymphadenitis develops, complete excision[28] and antituberculous chemotherapy are indicated.

Granulomatous Lymphadenitis Caused by Nondiphtheria Corynebacteria

Subacute or chronic relapsing lymphadenitis has been reported occasionally to be due to *Corynebacterium pseudotuberculosis (Corynebacterium ovis)*.[29] Most patients have lived in Australia[30] and have had extensive contact with animals, particularly sheep in which *C. pseudotuberculosis* is a common cause of caseous lymphadenitis. The histologic picture is that of a suppurative or necrotizing granulomatous process. Treatment consists of prolonged antibiotic (erythromycin or penicillin) therapy combined with surgical drainage or excision of the involved nodes.

Oculoglandular (Parinaud's) Syndrome

Preauricular lymphadenopathy can occur secondary to granulomatous nodular conjunctival infection caused by the introduction of certain pathogens onto the external eye. Oculoglandular syndromes occur occasionally in tularemia, cat-scratch disease,[31] listeriosis, sporotrichosis, and lymphogranuloma venereum. Epidemic keratoconjunctivitis due to adenoviruses is often associated with an enlarged preauricular lymph node.

Cat-Scratch Disease[31]

Cat-scratch disease is a slowly progressive and sometimes chronic form of regional lymphadenitis caused by *B. henselae* (see Chapter 224). Although cat-scratch disease is usually a benign and ultimately self-limited process, it may be complicated by acute encephalitis, hepatitis, osteolysis, neuroretinitis, arthritis, pleuritis, atypical pneumonia, hilar adenopathy, and thrombocytopenia.

B. henselae bacilli are slow-growing, requiring 2 to 6 weeks' incubation in a moist environment (e.g., in a sealed, gas-permeable plastic bag) under 5% CO_2 for growth on blood agar plates (human blood is preferable to sheep or horse blood) (see Chapter 224).[32]

About 90% of patients with cat-scratch disease give a history of contact with cats (most often kittens), and most have been scratched. A primary lesion (small papule or vesicle resembling an insect bite) develops at the site of the scratch 7 to 14 days after contact with the animal. This primary lesion lasts for several weeks to months and may be helpful in diagnosis. Lymphadenopathy develops within 1 to 2 weeks of the appearance of the skin papule.[33] There is no lymphangitis. The lymphadenopathy progresses to suppuration in 10 to 50% of cases, but the course is slower than that of suppurative lymphadenitis due to pyogenic bacteria, and most patients are only mildly ill. Regional lymphadenitis is the sole manifestation of cat-scratch disease in half of the cases. Almost any peripheral lymph node may be involved, but the axillary nodes are most commonly affected. The nodes are tender, acutely so when there is frank suppuration. Fever is present in only about a third of patients and is low grade. About 10 to 15% of patients suffer features of a more systemic illness: anorexia, headache, weight loss, and splenomegaly. Unusual clinical presentations include Parinaud's oculoglandular syndrome (conjunctivitis from ocular inoculation associated with ipsilateral preauricular lymphadenopathy) in 4% of patients, neuroretinitis, and, rarely, acute encephalitis/encephalopathy, usually with a sudden seizure as the initial neurologic manifestation, occurring several weeks after the first symptoms of cat-scratch disease. In one patient with cervical lymphadenopathy and another patient with Parinaud's oculoglandular syndrome, *B. henselae* was isolated on blood culture after prolonged incubation (9 days in one case).[34]

Inguinal Buboes of Venereal Origin

Inguinal lymphadenopathy due to pyogenic infections or cat-scratch disease is usually unilateral. Prominent bilateral (or unilateral) adenopathy, particularly in men, is suggestive of several venereal diseases. The genital chancre of primary syphilis is usually accompanied by one or several discrete, firm, nonsuppurative, painless, enlarged nodes in one or both inguinal areas. Constitutional signs are lacking. The overlying skin is uninflamed. In secondary syphilis, the lymphadenopathy is generalized and painless and usually precedes the cutaneous eruption.

In lymphogranuloma venereum (LGV), the primary genital lesion (painless papule, vesicle, or erosion) is usually transient and asymptomatic. The initial manifestation of the disease is usually the characteristic inguinal bubo, occurring 10 to 30 days after sexual exposure and 1 to 2 weeks after the primary lesion. The adenopathy is more commonly unilateral. Initially the node is tender, discrete, hard, and movable, but subsequently the inflammatory process involves multiple nodes in the area. Chills, fever, and constitutional symptoms are common at this stage. As a result of periadenitis, the nodes become fixed and matted into an oval or lobulated mass. The mass is adherent to the overlying skin, which is purplish in color. Foci of suppuration develop, with multiple fistulous tracts. A central lengthwise linear depression (so-called groove sign of LGV) is produced by involvement of nodes above and below the inguinal ligament. Although characteristic of LGV, the groove sign may rarely be produced by suppurative bacterial lymphadenitis or by lymphomatous involvement of inguinal nodes.

Chancroid is usually accompanied by painful, tender inguinal adenopathy. The primary lesion is a papule or pustule that progresses to form an extremely painful and tender but nonindurated ulceration with undermined edges, quite in contrast to a syphilitic chancre. Autoinoculation is common with lesions on opposing or contiguous areas of the skin. The adenopathy of chancroid develops about 1 week after the primary lesion appears and, unlike in LGV, is present while the ulcer is still active. Systemic symptoms accompany chancroid only rarely. The chancroidal bubo is typically unilateral and made up of fused inguinal nodes and is more painful than that of LGV. Unilocular suppuration may develop. However, in most patients, the lymphadenitis subsides without suppuration.

Primary genital herpetic infection in men and women is often associated with tender inguinal adenopathy. Histologically, the nodes show paracortical hyperplasia (with a prominent admixture of immunoblasts, plasma cells, and macrophages), along with sinus histiocytosis, discrete foci of necrosis, and intranuclear inclusions within scattered mononuclear and giant cells. Similar, histologically proven, recurrent, localized as well as generalized herpetic lymphadenitis can occur in immunocompromised patients in the absence of overt mucocutaneous lesions.[35, 36] The "pseudobuboes" of granuloma inguinale are produced by subcutaneous granulomatous infection rather than by suppurative lymphadenitis.

Suppurative inguinal lymphadenitis due to group A streptococci has been superimposed on chronic lymphadenopathy in homosexual men.[37]

Inguinal Buboes of Nonvenereal Origin

Inguinal or femoral buboes occur in bubonic plague, because the flea bite initiating the infection is commonly on a lower extremity.[38] However, involvement of most other peripheral nodes can occur. The disease begins with fever, malaise, headache, and tender regional adenopathy after an incubation period of 2 to 6 days. Only rarely is a lesion (papule, pustule) at the site of the insect bite evident at the onset of clinical illness. A large, matted collection of lymph nodes with surrounding edema quickly develops and may go on to suppuration and spontaneous drainage. If not treated promptly, the infection rapidly progresses to a septicemic phase. The diagnosis should be suspected in a febrile, acutely ill patient with a large cluster of extremely tender lymph nodes and a history of exposure to fleas, rodents, or rabbits in the western United States. (Tularemia may mimic the epidemiologic and clinical features of bubonic plague but is more likely to produce an *ulceroglandular syndrome* [Table 80–1], with a primary lesion at the site of inoculation.[39]) Diagnostic procedures include blood cultures (which yield uniformly positive results in the septicemic phase of plague), as well as cultures and stained smears (see Chapter 216) of carefully obtained bubo aspirates. Appropriate treatment (see later on) should be instituted immediately, before results of cultures become available, if bubonic plague is suspected.

Generalized Lymphadenitis Associated with Systemic Infections

Widespread lymphadenitis is a feature of a variety of infections disseminated by the blood stream. In most instances, suppuration of the involved nodes does not occur. Generalized lymphadenopathy is a feature, for example, of secondary syphilis, HIV infection, infectious mononucleosis, leptospirosis, and miliary tuberculosis. Generalized lymphadenopathy associated with infections is commonly due to the presence of the invading microorganism in the nodes. Generalized lymph node enlargement is a feature of a variety of infectious diseases due to bacterial, rickettsial, chlamydial, spirochetal, viral, protozoal, and helminthic agents (see Table 80–1).

Etiologic Agents and Differential Diagnosis

It is helpful for purposes of the differential diagnosis to consider infective lymphadenitis in several categories (see Table 80–1): (1) regional lymphadenopathy, (2) regional lymphadenopathy with breakdown of nodes, (3) inguinal bubo formation, (4) ulceroglandular syndrome, (5) oculoglandular syndrome, and (6) generalized lymphadenopathy.

In distinguishing among the causes of fluctuant cervical lymphadenitis, the history may suggest a streptococcal (preceding tonsillitis), staphylococcal (recent facial or neck infection), or tuberculous (prior exposure to tuberculosis) disease or cat-scratch disease (exposure to cat) as the causative disorder. In a study of suppurative cervical adenitis, *S. aureus* was the etiologic agent more frequently than group A streptococci (36% versus 26%), and in another one quarter of the cases, a bacteriologic diagnosis could not be made.[40] A subacute clinical course with little fever and a normal leukocyte count would be more consistent with cat-scratch disease or tuberculous involvement. Sinus tract formation suggests infection due to *M.*

TABLE 80–1 Clinical Patterns and Microbial Agents of Infectious Lymphadenitis

		Form of Lymphadenitis					
Disease	**Infecting Organism**	***Regional***	***Regional with Suppuration (or Caseation)***	***Inguinal Bubo Formation***	***Ulceroglandular***	***Oculoglandular***	***Generalized***
Bacterial							
Pyogenic	Group A or B streptococci; *Staphylococcus aureus*	+	+				
Scarlet fever	Group A streptococci	+	+				+
Diphtheria	*Corynebacterium diphtheriae*	+					
Fusospirochetal angina	*Prevotella melaninogenica;* peptostreptococci, etc.	+					
Scrofula	*Mycobacterium tuberculosis*	+	+				
	Mycobacterium scrofulaceum; Mycobacterium avium-intracellulare	+	+				
Miliary tuberculosis	*M. tuberculosis*						+
Brucellosis	*Brucella*						+
Leptospirosis	*Leptospira*						+
Syphilis	*Treponema pallidum*	+					+
Chancroid	*Haemophilus ducreyi*			+			
Plague	*Yersinia pestis*	+	+	+			
Tularemia	*Francisella tularensis*		+		+	+	
Rat-bite fever	*Streptobacillus moniliformis; Spirillum minus*	+ +			+		
Anthrax	*Bacillus anthracis*	+			+		
Listeriosis	*Listeria monocytogenes*					+	
Melioidosis	*Burkholderia pseudomallei*	+	+				+
Glanders	*Burkholderia mallei*	+	+				+
Cat-scratch fever	*Bartonella henselae*	+	+		±	+	
Typhoid fever	*Salmonella typhi*						+
Mycotic							
Histoplasmosis	*Histoplasma capsulatum*						+
	H. capsulatum var. *duboisii*	+					
Coccidioidomycosis	*Coccidioides immitis*	+					
Paracoccidioidomycosis	*Paracoccidioides brasiliensis*	+					
Cryptococcosis	*Cryptococcus neoformans*	+					+
Rickettsial							
Boutonneuse fever, etc.	*Rickettsia conorii*				+		
Scrub typhus	*Rickettsia tsutsugamushi*	+					+
Rickettsialpox	*Rickettsia akari*	+					
Chlamydial							
Lymphogranuloma venereum	*Chlamydia trachomatis*			+		+	+
Viral							
Measles	Measles virus						+
Rubella	Rubella virus						+
Infectious mononucleosis	Epstein-Barr virus						+
Cytomegalovirus mononucleosis	Cytomegalovirus						+
Dengue fever	Dengue virus						+
West Nile fever	West Nile virus						+
Lassa fever	Lassa fever virus						+
Genital herpes infection	Herpes simplex virus type 2	+					
Pharyngoconjunctival fever	Adenovirus (types 3 and 7)	+				+	
Epidemic keratoconjunctivitis	Adenovirus (types 8 and 19)					+	
AIDS; AIDS-related complex	Human immunodeficiency virus						+
Protozoan							
Kala azar	*Leishmania donovani*						+
African trypanosomiasis	*Trypanosoma brucei*	+					+
Chagas disease	*Trypanosoma cruzi*					+	+
Toxoplasmosis	*Toxoplasma gondii*						+
Helminthic							
Filariasis	*Wucheria bancrofti*						+
	Brugia malayi						+
Loiasis	*Loa loa*			+			
Onchocerciasis	*Onchocerca volvulus*			+			

Abbreviation: AIDS, Acquired immunodeficiency syndrome.

tuberculosis or an atypical mycobacterium. Gram-stained and Ziehl-Neelsen smears and culture (including cultures for mycobacteria) of material aspirated or drained from suppurating nodes provides a diagnosis in about two thirds of such cases of cervical lymphadenitis. Further information may be provided by skin tests (PPD), serologic tests (antistreptolysin O antibody titer), and histologic examination (e.g., caseation necrosis suggesting mycobacterial infection or bimorphic appearance suggesting cat-scratch disease) of an excised node when culture of aspirated material is unrevealing.

A variety of noninfectious processes may resemble unilateral cervical lymphadenitis. Lymphoma may be suggested by the indolent course of cat-scratch disease. Acute febrile mucocutaneous lymph node syndrome (Kawasaki syndrome), a disease of infants and young children of unknown etiology, is characterized by nonsuppurative cervical lymphadenopathy.[41] The age of the patient, febrile course, conjunctival injection, erythematous rash, and subsequent desquamation suggest the diagnosis. In some patients, unilateral lymphadenitis may precede mucocutaneous manifestations and make diagnosis more difficult by initially suggesting bacterial involvement.[42] A more recently described benign disorder of lymph nodes, histiocytic necrotizing lymphadenitis or Kikuchi's disease, was first recognized in Japan and now has been observed in the United States.[43] Clinical features consist of localized, sometimes tender cervical lymphadenopathy, often with an upper respiratory prodrome and associated in some patients with fever. Most cases occur in women, commonly under 40 years of age. The involved nodes are usually rubbery or firm, discrete, and rarely greater than 2 cm in diameter.[44] Occasional patients present with generalized lymphadenopathy, and rarely, hepatosplenomegaly occurs.[45] Less frequent symptoms include nausea, vomiting, weight loss, and night sweats, suggesting the diagnosis of lymphoma. Mild leukopenia and lymphocytosis may suggest infectious mononucleosis. The illness does not respond to antibiotics, but it usually resolves spontaneously within 1 or 2 months. Occasionally, recurrences may be a feature. Histologically, surgical biopsy specimens may be erroneously interpreted as lymphoma, but the principal findings are those of focal or confluent nodules (made up of crescentic histiocytes, plasmacytoid monocytes, immunoblasts and karyorrhectic debris) combined with patchy areas of coagulative necrosis. Neutrophils are few or absent. Diagnosis has been made in some cases by fine-needle aspiration cytology.[46] Histologically, the lymph node appearance in systemic lupus erythematosus is very similar to that in Kikuchi's disease, but hematoxylin bodies are characteristic of the former. Serologic studies (e.g., antinuclear antibody or anti-DNA antibody assays) are warranted to help distinguish between the two processes. Although a viral origin is suspected on the basis of the clinical features, serologic and ultrastructural studies have failed to identify a specific agent. A case of parvovirus B19–associated hemophagocytic syndrome causing cervical lymphadenopathy with histologic features resembling those of Kikuchi's disease was recently described.[47]

Bronchial cleft cysts and cystic hygromas may be mistaken for cervical lymphadenitis, particularly if infected; thyroglossal duct cysts may suggest infected submental nodes. Lymphoepithelial cysts, indolent lesions of the salivary glands (usually the parotid) occurring in HIV-infected patients, may mimic preauricular lymphadenopathy or suggest Sjögren's syndrome.[48] Submaxillary sialadenitis or salivary gland tumors may mimic submandibular lymphadenitis. Bimanual (intraoral and submandibular) palpation can be helpful in distinguishing between these processes.

Isolated inguinal lymphadenitis or bubo formation in the adult suggests venereal disease (syphilis, LGV, chancroid). Distinctive associated primary lesions are usually features of syphilis and chancroid but not of LGV. The inguinal adenopathy of primary syphilis consists of painless, firm, discrete, movable nodes without erythema of the overlying skin. The nodes do not suppurate, whereas spontaneous rupture of the buboes of LGV and chancroid may occur. The groove sign is suggestive of LGV. The buboes of chancroid are characteristically painful. Axillary, cervical, and inguinal buboes may occur with plague and tularemia. In plague, an inguinal location is common. The geographic locale and a history of animal exposure are important clues to the diagnosis. Inguinal and femoral nodes can be involved in cat-scratch disease, although much less frequently than axillary or cervical nodes.

Generalized lymphadenopathy is frequently a manifestation of disseminated infection (see Table 80–1). Clues may be provided by the age of the patient and the presence of a characteristic rash (childhood exanthems, secondary syphilis), geographic factors (dengue, filariasis, localized *Leishmania* lymphadenitis,[49] histoplasmosis), occupation and dietary history (brucellosis, toxoplasmosis), exposure to animals (leptospirosis), and the presence of atypical lymphocytes (infectious mononucleosis, cytomegalovirus infection). Diagnosis of toxoplasmic lymphadenitis in the immunocompetent patient is based primarily on serologic testing, although sometimes a node biopsy is performed because of initial concern for lymphoma. A negative result on the Sabin-Feldman dye test or on a comparable test for *Toxoplasma* IgG antibody (indirect immunofluorescence [IIF], passive hemagglutination [PHA], or enzyme-linked immunosorbent assay [ELISA]) practically excludes the diagnosis. Between 3 and 6 months after clinical onset of *Toxoplasma* lymphadenitis, Sabin-Feldman dye titers are 1:1,024 or greater.[50] With toxoplasmosis the ELISA is positive for IgM antibodies within the first 3 months of infection in most patients. In the occasional patient with negative, low-positive, or equivocal titers of IgM antibodies, diagnosis may be made by detection of IgA or IgE antibodies or an acute pattern in the differential agglutination test (comparing titers obtained with formalin-fixed tachyzoites with those obtained with acetone-fixed or methanol-fixed tachyzoites—essentially differentiating between avidity of IgG antibodies in acute and nonacute infections). In a study of serodiagnosis in 40 consecutive patients with biopsy-confirmed toxoplasmic lymphadenitis, a serologic profile (dye test; IgM, IgG, and IgE antibody titers; and differential agglutination test) had a sensitivity of 100% with use of the first serum specimen drawn after clinical onset of lymphadenitis.[50]

Laboratory diagnosis of acute toxoplasmic lymphadenitis can also be made by seroconversion from a negative to a positive result on IgG antibody testing or by demonstration of a fourfold rise in titer over 3 weeks. In endemic areas, generalized nonsuppurative (and, very rarely, suppurative) lymphadenopathy occurs in typhoid fever.[51]

Widespread suppurative infections of lymph nodes occur as a result of the microbicidal defect characteristic of neutrophils and monocytes of patients with chronic granulomatous disease. Recurrent infections (involving skin, bones, lungs, and liver, as well as lymph nodes) beginning in childhood and due to *S. aureus* and certain gram-negative bacilli *(Escherichia coli*, salmonellae, *Serratia marcescens)* suggest the diagnosis.

Widespread lymphadenopathy may be a feature of many noninfectious diseases, particularly infiltrative processes such as lymphoma and reticuloendothelioses. Prominent peripheral lymphadenopathy may be a feature of rheumatoid arthritis. Lymphadenopathy may occur as an adverse effect of prolonged use of phenytoin. Widespread lymphadenopathy is a feature of the syndrome of immunoblastic lymphadenopathy, which is often accompanied by skin rash, polyclonal hypergammaglobulinemia, and immunosuppression. This disorder of immune regulation often eventuates in B-cell or T-cell lymphomas.[52]

Sinus histiocytosis with massive lymphadenopathy (Rosai-Dorfman disease) is another benign process that produces extensive, painless lymphadenopathy in the cervical areas in children and adolescents.[53] It is often accompanied by fever, neutrophilic leukocytosis, and polyclonal hypergammaglobulinemia. Histologically, there is extensive proliferation of histiocyte-like cells within the sinuses of the involved lymph nodes.[54] The etiology is unknown, and the prognosis is favorable. A very rare form of regional lymphadenopathy, showing sinus histiocytosis (with the cells seen to contain metal granules) histologically, can be the result of wear-induced debris from an adjacent metallic prosthesis.[55, 56] Similarly, enlarged regional lymph nodes (showing noncaseating granulomas containing silicone) have been described draining areas in which a silicone mammary prosthesis or a Silastic joint prosthesis[57] had been inserted previously.

Generalized Lymphadenopathy with the Acquired Immunodeficiency Syndrome

Patients with acquired immunodeficiency syndrome (AIDS) or with the AIDS-related complex may have generalized lymphadenopathy in which involvement with opportunistic infection or neoplastic disease (particularly Kaposi's sarcoma) is evident on histologic examination. The infections have included those due to cytomegalovirus and *M. avium-intracellulare*.[58] Those caused by the latter usually show a few poorly formed or no granulomas and a prominent histiocytic reaction. Large clusters ("globi") of acid-fast bacilli are present within the cytoplasm of histiocytes. Kaposi's sarcoma in patients with AIDS may follow the pattern of generalized lymph node involvement and a fulminant course with mucosal and visceral lesions.[59] In AIDS, other neoplasms can involve lymph nodes. These are primarily of the B-cell type and include B-cell immunoblastic sarcomas, small non–cleaved cell Burkitt-type lymphoma, and plasmacytoid lymphocytic lymphoma.[60]

Lymphadenopathy occurs in 50 to 75% of patients at risk for AIDS who develop an acute illness approximately 3 to 6 weeks after initial exposure to HIV.[61, 62] It often is one feature of a mononucleosis-like syndrome consisting of fever, malaise, myalgias, headaches, sore throat, diarrhea, leukopenia, thrombocytopenia, and a maculopapular rash. After the acute clinical illness subsides, lymphadenopathy may remain as persistent generalized lymphadenopathy, involving at least several extrainguinal sites, of at least 3 months' duration. This progressive lymphadenopathy early in the course of this infection may be the result of an active immune response against HIV in the affected lymph nodes[63] (see Chapter 107). The nodes are discrete and nontender; suppuration does not occur. HIV replication takes place in such lymph nodes, which histologically show follicular hyperplasia or mixed follicular and interfollicular hyperplasia.[64] Regression of the lymphadenopathy may occur after 8 to 19 months in some patients.

Presumptive Treatment

Initial treatment of infective lymphadenitis requires some narrowing of the diagnostic possibilities (see Table 80–1). Localized pyogenic lymphadenitis responds well to early antibiotic treatment. When cervical lymphadenitis has developed from a pharyngeal or periodontal portal, initial treatment with penicillin is appropriate (procaine penicillin G, 300,000 to 600,000 units intramuscularly every 12 to 24 hours initially to ensure receipt of the therapeutic agent when the patient may be nauseated; subsequently, 250 to 500 mg of penicillin V may be administered orally every 6 hours, or 250 to 500 mg of amoxicillin every 8 hours, for at least 20 days in older children and adults). In patients who are more acutely ill, larger doses of aqueous penicillin G parenterally are indicated. Erythromycin (20 to 40 mg/kg/day orally in divided doses every 6 hours) is an alternative for patients allergic to penicillin.

Pyogenic lymphadenitis complicating skin infections may be of staphylococcal or streptococcal etiology, and a penicillinase-resistant penicillin is the drug of choice (e.g., dicloxacillin, 0.25 to 0.5 g orally every 6 hours for the older child or an adult). In the more acutely ill patient, intravenous administration of a semisynthetic penicillinase-resistant penicillin (e.g., nafcillin) or a first-generation cephalosporin should be employed. Failure to show improvement, or progression to suppuration, is an indication for percutaneous needle aspiration (for bacteriologic diagnosis and treatment) or surgical drainage.

For cat-scratch disease, usually a self-limited process resolving in 2 to 4 months, treatment is principally symptomatic. If the nodes become fluctuant, aspiration is appropriate both for relief of pain and for bacteriologic diagnosis. The few strains of *B. henselae* from cases of cat-scratch disease that have been studied show in vitro susceptibility to a variety of antimicrobial agents, with the notable exception of first-generation cephalosporins.[32] In a retrospective review of antimicrobial treatment of several hundred patients with cat-scratch disease, clinical efficacy (58 to 87%) was attributed to four drugs (in increasing order): trimethoprim-sulfamethoxazole, gentamicin, ciprofloxacin, and rifampin.[65] Antimicrobial therapy may be reasonable in patients with more severe or extranodal cat-scratch disease. Bacillary angiomatosis and bacillary peliosis hepatitis, infections in patients with AIDS that are due to *B. henselae* or a closely related Bartonellaceae species, appear to respond to prolonged antimicrobial therapy with either erythromycin, doxycycline, or rifampin.[66]

If the diagnosis of bubonic plague is suspected, antibiotic treatment should be instituted promptly. Streptomycin (1.0 g intramuscularly every 12 hours in adults), alone or in combination with tetracycline (0.5 g orally every 6 hours in adults), are the preferred drugs, and treatment is continued for 10 days.

LYMPHANGITIS

Lymphangitis is an inflammation of lymphatic channels, usually in the subcutaneous tissues. It occurs either as an acute process of bacterial origin or as a chronic process of mycotic, mycobacterial, or filarial etiology.

Pathologic Changes and Pathogenesis

The visible red streaking in acute lymphangitis stems from the inflammatory process in the walls (and surrounding tissue spaces) of dilated lymphatic channels. Lymphatic obstruction often occurs on healing, resulting sometimes in persistent lymphedema. Cutaneous lymphatic sporotrichosis, a form of chronic lymphangitis, produces a combined suppurative and granulomatous response.

Clinical Findings

Acute Lymphangitis

Acute lymphangitis develops when an infection, commonly on an extremity, is not contained locally but spreads along lymphatic channels. Such infections are most often due to group A streptococci (and occasionally are due to streptococci of other groups and, very rarely, to *S. aureus*). Systemic manifestations may develop rapidly before evidence of infection becomes apparent at the site of inoculation of organisms, and they may be more prominent than might be anticipated on the basis of local pain and erythema. Red linear streaks, a few millimeters to several centimeters in width, extend from the initial site of infection toward the regional lymph nodes, which are enlarged and tender. Peripheral edema of the involved extremity often occurs. The time course of this type of infection can be accelerated from initial lesion to lymphangitis to complicating bacteremia in 24 to 48 hours. Occasionally, recurrent episodes of lymphangitis occur, with the initial episode causing some degree of chronic lymphedema, in turn predisposing to another episode. Rarely, elephantiasis nostras, a temporate-zone (nonfilarial) form of progressive lymphatic obstruction of a lower limb, can follow recurrent episodes of streptococcal lymphangitis. With each episode, further localized edema occurs, eventuating in grotesque enlargement of the extremity due to permanent solid edema, fibrosis of dermis and subcutaneous tissues, and verrucous pachyderma.[67]

The peripheral white blood cell count is commonly elevated. The etiologic agent often can be identified on Gram-stained smears and cultures obtained from the initial lesion. Blood cultures also may reveal the causative organism.

Acute lymphangitis or lymphadenitis, usually involving the lower extremities, is a feature of filariasis due to *Wuchereria bancrofti* (and sometimes to *Brugia malayi*).[68] These mosquito-borne diseases are endemic to Africa, Southeast Asia and the Pacific, and tropical South America. The acute form of disease is characterized by recurrent episodes of headache, backache, lymphangitis, lymphadenitis, epididymitis, and orchitis. Bancroftian lymphangitis may involve the breast, with a clinical appearance suggesting carcinoma.[69] Fever is uncommon. The adult filariae reside in lymphatics and lymph nodes and discharge microfilariae into the blood stream. With prolonged exposure in an endemic area, chronic lymphatic obstruction can develop with elephantiasis of the skin and scrotum.[70] In this setting, recurrent episodes of lymphangitis may be the result of both the parasitic infestation and superimposed streptococcal infections (to which the chronic lymphedema predisposes).[71] Serologic tests for filariasis may be helpful in diagnosis if microfilariae are not found, but results of such tests are positive in many other filarial infections. Lymph node or lymphatic vessel biopsy may be necessary for diagnosis.

Chronic Granulomatous Lymphangitis

Unlike acute lymphangitis, chronic granulomatous lymphangitis is an indolent process associated with little pain or systemic evidence of infection. Sporotrichosis is most commonly the underlying disease.[72] This infection frequently is introduced by minor trauma (e.g., from a thorn of a barberry or rose bush) into the skin of a gardener. An erythematous subcutaneous nodule (often becoming fluctuant) or a chancriform ulcer subsequently develops at the site of inoculation of *Sporothrix schenckii* (present on some plants and in sphagnum moss used in gardening) on the hand or finger. The lesion does not respond to local treatment or to administration of the common antibacterial agents. Slowly, multiple subcutaneous nodules appear and extend proximally along the course of regional lymphatics, which become thickened. Other infections producing a sporotrichoid pattern are characterized as nodular lymphangitis.[73]

Cutaneous infection (''swimming pool granuloma'') with *M. marinum*—an atypical mycobacterium that grows optimally at 25°C to 32°C and is found in swimming pools and fish tanks—produces a chronic nodular, verrucous or ulcerative lesion at the site of an abrasion, usually about the knees or elbows. The lesion is usually solitary, but in an occasional patient new lesions develop proximally, as in sporotrichosis. Multiple sporotrichoid lesions have occurred in occasional infections due to *Nocardia brasiliensis*[74] and in rare infections due to *Mycobacterium kansasii, Mycobacterium chelonae*, and *Nocardia asteroides*. Even rarer causes of nodular lymphangitis include leishmaniasis,[75] staphylococcal lymphangitis,[76] botryomycosis, and tularemia (reported earlier this century but not in the past 40 years).[73]

A very rare but most troublesome process is localized granulomatous lymphangitis of the penile and scrotal skin with resulting chronic edema of the genital area. It may be associated with lymphogranuloma venereum, granuloma inguinale, Milroy's disease, self-inflicted trauma, Melkersson-Rosenthal syndrome, or Chrohn's disease, or it may be idiopathic.[77] Penile edema either can be an initial manifestation of Crohn's disease or may develop as a late complication of well-established gastrointestinal disease.

Etiologic Agents

In the United States, acute lymphangitis is most commonly due to group A streptococci, and chronic lymphangitis is usually caused by *S. schenckii*. Other infectious agents occasionally produce lymphangitis (Table 80–2).

Differential Diagnosis

The combination of a peripheral infection or traumatic lesion and the acute onset of fever with proximal red linear streaks directed toward regional lymph nodes is diagnostic of acute lymphangitis. In the legs, thrombophlebitis may produce linear areas of tender erythema, but the absence of an initiating lesion and of tender regional adenopathy is helpful in distinguishing it from lymphangitis. A history of rat bite and the subsequent development of lymphangitis suggest *Spirillum minus* infection. Filariasis is a consideration when an appropriate geographic history is obtained. Sporotrichosis is considered when chronic ulcerative lymphangitis develops in a person working with plants, soil, or timbers. *M. marinum* is suggested as the etiologic agent when sporotrichoid lesions develop in a person who has been around swimming pools and fish tanks.

TABLE 80–2 Causes of Lymphangitis

Clinical Form	Etiologic Agent	Relative Frequency as Cause of Lymphangitis
Acute	Group A streptococci	Common
	Staphylococcus aureus	Occasional
	Pasteurella multocida	Occasional
	Spirillum minus (rat-bite fever)	Rare
	Wuchereria bancrofti; Brugia malayi (filariasis)	Rare (only in immigrants from endemic areas)
Chronic	*Sporothrix schenckii* (sporotrichosis)	Occasional
	Mycobacterium marinum (swimming pool granuloma)	Occasional
	Mycobacterium kansasii	Rare
	Nocardia brasiliensis	Rare
	Wuchereria bancrofti; B. malayi	Rare (only in immigrants from endemic areas)
	Nocardia asteroides	Very rare
	Mycobacterium chelonae	Very rare
	S. aureus (botryomycosis)	Very rare
	Leishmania brasiliensis or *Leishmania mexicana*	Very rare
	Francisella tularensis	Very rare

Presumptive Therapy

Penicillin therapy is the recommended initial treatment for acute lymphangitis. In a mildly ill adult, 600,000 units of procaine penicillin G once or twice daily is administered initially, with supplementary oral penicillin V. More acutely ill patients in whom bacteremia may have developed should be hospitalized and given parenteral aqueous penicillin G (600,000 to 2,000,000 units every 4 to 6 hours). If a staphylococcal etiology is suspected, a penicillinase-resistant penicillin is used.

The initial treatment of presumptive lymphocutaneous sporotrichosis is itraconazole, and saturated solution of potassium iodide is also effective[73] (see Chapter 250). If sporotrichoid *M. marinum* infection is suspected, the diagnosis should be confirmed by demonstration of acid-fast bacilli and by isolation of the organism at 30°C on appropriate media. Localized swimming pool granulomas are often treated by surgical excision. Chemotherapy is reserved for more extensive and sporotrichoid forms of infection. On the basis of limited data, the combination of choice would appear to be rifampin and ethambutol[73, 78] (see Chapter 243). Prolonged tetracycline or minocycline therapy has also been reported as successful in a small number of cases,[73, 79] but in vitro resistance to and treatment failure with doxycycline have been reported.[80] Trimethoprim-sulfamethoxazole has been reported as effective in several studies. However, in vitro activity requires drug concentrations greater than those usually achieved in serum and tissues.[81]

Chronic lymphedema, a complication of recurrent lymphangitis, has been treated primarily in the past with elevation and elastic hosiery. Newer and more successful methods to increase lymph drainage for problematic patients have recently been developed and include remedial exercises, manual massage, multilayered bandage wrapping, and intermittent pneumatic compression massage.[82]

REFERENCES

1. Case Records of the Massachusetts General Hospital. N Engl J Med. 1993;329:714.
2. McCabe RE, Brooks RG, Dorfman RF, et al. Clinical spectrum in 107 cases of toxoplasmic lymphadenopathy. Rev Infect Dis. 1987;9:754.
3. Strickler JG, Warnke RA, Weiss LM. Necrosis in lymph nodes. Pathol Annu. 1987;2:253.
4. Scobie WG. Acute suppurative adenitis in children. Scot Med J. 1969;14:352.
5. Dajani AS, Garcia RE, Wolinski E. Etiology of cervical lymphadenitis in children. N Engl J Med. 1963;268:1329.
6. Bredenkamp JK, Maceri DR. Inflammatory torticollis in children. Arch Otolaryngol Head Neck Surg. 1990;116:310.
7. Boyce JM. Severe streptococcal lymphadenitis. N Engl J Med. 1990;323:655.
8. Amren DP. Unusual forms of streptococcal disease. In: Wannamaker LW, Matsen JM, eds. Streptococci and Streptococcal Disease. New York: Academic Press; 1972:545.
9. Currarino G. Acute epitrochlear lymphadenitis. Pediatr Radiol. 1977;6:160.
10. Maull KI, Sachatello CII. Retroperitoneal iliac fossa abscess. A complication of suppurative iliac lymphadenitis. Am J Surg. 1974;127:270.
11. Oliff M, Chuang VP. Retroperitoneal iliac fossa pyogenic abscess. Radiology. 1978;126:647.
12. Shenep JL, Kalwinsky DK, Feldman S, et al. Mycotic cervical lymphadenitis following oral mucositis in children with leukemia. J Pediatr. 1985;106:243.
13. Mazzoni A, Ferrarese M, Manfredi R, et al. Primary lymph node invasive aspergillosis. Infection. 1996;24:39.
14. Curnutte JT, Boxer LA. Clinically significant phagocytic cell defects. In: Remington JS, Swartz MN, eds. Current Clinical Topics in Infectious Diseases. v. 4. New York: McGraw-Hill; 1985;103–155.
15. Sorensen RU, Jacobs MR, Shurin SB. *Chromobacterium violaceum* adenitis acquired in the northern United States as a complication of chronic granulomatous disease. Pediatr Infect Dis. 1985;4:701.
16. Kobayashi Y, Komazawa Y, Kobayashi M, et al. Presumed BCG infection in a boy with chronic granulomatous disease. A report of a case and review of the literature. Clin Pediatr. 1984;23:586.
17. Alfonso F, Gallo L, Winkler B, et al. Fine needle aspiration cytology of peripheral lymph node cryptococcosis. Acta Cytol. 1994;38:459.
18. Ramponi A, Angeli G, Rizzo GM, et al. Laterocervical lymphadenitis caused by *Pneumocystis carinii* in a patient with AIDS. Histopathology. 1994;24:91.
19. Haught WH, Steinbach J, Zander DS, et al. Case report: Bacillary angiomatosis with massive visceral lymphadenopathy. Am J Med Sci. 1993;306:236.
20. Lee-Chiong T, Sodigh M, Simms M, et al. Case reports: Pericarditis and lymphadenitis due to *Rhodococcus equi*. Am J Med Sci. 1995;310:31.
21. Pouchot J, Bortolotti V, Sterkers O, et al. Cervical suppurative lymphadenitis due to *Yersinia pseudotuberculosis*. Clin Infect Dis. 1995;21:1063.
22. Lincoln EM, Gilbert LA. Disease in children due to mycobacteria other than *Mycobacterium tuberculosis*. Am Rev Respir Dis. 1972;105:683.
23. Wolinsky E. Mycobacterial lymphadenitis in children; a prospective study of 105 nontuberculous cases with long-term follow-up. Clin Infect Dis. 1995;20:954.
24. Haase G, Kentrup H, Skopnik H, et al. *Mycobacterium lentiflavum*: An etiologic agent of cervical lymphadenitis. Clin Infect Dis. 1997;25:1245.
25. Haas WH, Butler WR, Kirschner P, et al. A new agent of mycobacterial lymphadenitis in children: *Mycobacterium heidelbergense* sp. nov. J Clin Microbiol. 1997;35:3203.
26. Shriner KA, Mathisen GE, Goetz MB. Comparison of mycobacterial lymphadenitis among persons infected with human immunodeficiency virus and seronegative controls. Clin Infect Dis. 1992;15:601.
27. Victoria MS, Shah BR. Bacillus Calmette-Guérin lymphadenitis: A case report and review of the literature. Pediatr Infect Dis. 1985;4:295.
28. Oguz F, Mujgan S, Alper G, et al. Treatment of bacillus Calmette-Guérin–associated lymphadenitis. Pediatr Infect Dis. J. 1992;11:887.
29. Lipsky BA, Goldberger AC, Tompkins LS, et al. Infections caused by non-diphtheria corynebacteria. Rev Infect Dis. 1982;4:1220.
30. Peel MM, Palmer GG, Stacpoole AM, et al. Human lymphadenitis due to *Corynebacterium pseudotuberculosis*: Report of ten cases from Australia and review. Clin Infect Dis. 1997;24:185.
31. Carithers HA, Carithers CM, Edwards RO Jr. Cat-scratch disease. Its natural history. JAMA. 1969;207:312.
32. Dolan MJ, Wong MT, Regnery RL, et al. Syndrome of *Rochalimaea henselae* adenitis suggesting cat scratch disease. Ann Intern Med. 1993;118:331.
33. Carithers HA. Cat-scratch disease. An overview based on a study of 1,200 patients. Am J Dis Child. 1985;139:1124.
34. Wong MT, Dolan MJ, Lattuada CP, et al. Neuroretinitis, aseptic meningitis, and lymphadenitis associated with *Bartonella (Rochalimaea) henselae* infection in immunocompetent patients and patients infected with human immunodeficiency virus type 1. Clin Infect Dis. 1995;21:352.
35. Epstein JI, Ambinder RF, Kuhajda, et al. Localized herpes simplex lymphadenitis. Am J Clin Pathol. 1986;86:444.
36. Miliauskas JR, Leong AS. Localized herpes simplex lymphadenitis: Report of three cases and review of the literature. Histopathology. 1991;19:355.
37. Ho DD, Murata GH. Streptococcal lymphadenitis in homosexual men with chronic lymphadenopathy. Am J Med. 1984;77:151.
38. Reed WB, Palmer DL, Williams RC, et al. Bubonic plague in southwestern United States. Medicine. 1970;49:465.
39. Young LS, Bicknell DS, Archer BG, et al. Tularemia epidemic: Vermont 1968. Forty-seven cases linked to contact with muskrats. N Engl J Med. 1969;280:1253.
40. Barton LL, Feigin RD. Childhood cervical lymphadenitis: A reappraisal. J Pediatr. 1974;84:846.
41. Feigin RD, Schleien CI. Kawasaki's disease. In: Remington J, Swartz MN, eds. Current Clinical Topics in Infectious Disease, v. 4. New York: McGraw-Hill; 1983;30.
42. Waggoner-Fountain LA, Hayden GF, Hendley JO. Kawasaki syndrome masquerading as bacterial lymphadenitis. Clin Pediatr. 1995;34:185.
43. Unger PD, Rappaport KM, Strauchen JA. Necrotizing lymphadenitis (Kikuchi's disease). Arch Pathol Lab Med. 1987;111:1031.
44. Tsang WYW, Chan JKC, Ng CS. Kikuchi's lymphadenitis: A morphologic analysis of 75 cases with special reference to unusual features. Am J Surg Pathol. 1994;18:219.
45. Dorfman RF. Histiocytic necrotizing lymphadenitis of Kikuchi and Fujimoto. Arch Pathol Lab Med. 1987;111:1026.
46. Tsang WYW, Chan JKC. Fine needle aspiration cytologic diagnosis of Kikuchi's lymphadenitis. A report of 27 cases. Am J Clin Pathol. 1994;102:454.
47. Yufu Y, Matsumoto M, Miyamura T, et al. Parvovirus B19–associated haemophagocytic syndrome with lymphadenopathy resembling histiocytic necrotizing lymphadenitis (Kikuchi's disease). Br J Haematol. 1997;96:868.
48. Maiorano E, Favia G, Viale G. Lymphoepithelial cysts of salivary glands: An immunohistochemical study of HIV-related and HIV-unrelated lesions. Hum Pathol. 1998;29:260.
49. Garcia-González R, Sanz I, Saus C, et al. Localized lymphadenitis due to leishmania. Diagnosis by fine needle aspiration cytology. Postgrad Med J. 1990;66:326.
50. Montoya JG, Remington JS. Studies on the serodiagnosis of toxoplasmic lymphadenitis. Clin Infect Dis. 1995;20:781.
51. Naqvi SH, Thobani S, Moazam F, et al. Generalized suppurative lymphadenitis with typhoidal salmonellosis. Pediatr Infect Dis J. 1988;7:882.
52. Abruzzo LV, Schmidt K, Weiss LM, et al. B-cell lymphoma after angioimmunoblastic lymphadenopathy: A case with oligoclonal gene rearrangements associated with Epstein-Barr virus. Blood. 1993;82:241.
53. Rosai J, Dorfman RF. Sinus histiocytosis with massive lymphadenopathy, a pseudolymphomatous benign disorder: Analysis of 34 cases. Cancer. 1972;30:1174.
54. Paulli M, Locatelli F, Kindl S, et al. Sinus histiocytosis with massive lymphadenopathy (Rosai-Dorfman disease). Clinico-pathological analysis of a paediatric case. Eur J Pediatr. 1992;151:672.
55. Shinto Y, Uchida A, Yoshikawa H, et al. Inguinal lymphadenopathy due to metal release from a prosthesis. J Bone Joint Surg. 1993;75B:266.
56. O'Connell JX, Rosenberg AE. Histiocytic lymphadenitis associated with a large joint prosthesis. Am J Clin Pathol. 1993;99:314.
57. Rogers LA, Longtine JA, Garnick MB, et al. Silicone lymphadenopathy in a long distance runner: Complication of a Silastic prosthesis. Hum Pathol. 1988;19:1237.
58. Fauci AS, Macher AM, Longo DL, et al. Acquired immunodeficiency syndrome: Epidemiologic, clinical, immunologic, and therapeutic considerations. Ann Intern Med. 1984;100:92.
59. Gottlieb MS, Groopman JE, Weinstein WM, et al. The acquired immunodeficiency syndrome. Ann Intern Med. 1983;99:208.
60. Levine AM, Meyer PR, Begandy MK, et al. Development of B-cell lymphoma in homosexual men: Clinical and immunological findings. Ann Intern Med. 1984;100:7.
61. Kinloch-de Loës S, deSaussure P, Saurat J-H, et al. Symptomatic primary infection due to human immunodeficiency virus type 1: Review of 31 cases. Clin Infect Dis. 1993;17:59.
62. Clark SJ, Saag MS, Decker WD, et al. High titers of cytopathic virus in plasma of patients with symptomatic primary HIV-1 infection. N Engl J Med. 1991;324:954.
63. Pantaleo G, Graziosi C, Fauci AS. The immunopathogenesis of human immunodeficiency virus infection. N Engl J Med. 1993;328:327.
64. Baroni CD, Uccini S. The lymphadenopathy of HIV infection. Am J Clin Pathol. 1993;99:397.
65. Margileth AM. Antibiotic therapy for cat-scratch disease: Clinical study of therapeutic outcome in 268 patients and a review of the literature. Pediatr Infect Dis J. 1992;11:474.
66. Koehler JE, Quinn FD, Berger TG. Isolation of *Rochalimaea* species from cutaneous and osseous lesions of bacillary angiomatosis. N Engl J Med. 1992;327:1625.
67. Sanders LJ, Slomsky JM, Burger-Caplan C. Elephantiasis nostras: An eight year observation of progressive nonfilarial elephantiasis of the lower extremity. Cutis. 1988;42:406.
68. Grove DI, Warren KS, Mahmoud AAF. Algorithms in the diagnosis and management of exotic diseases. VI. The filariases. J Infect Dis. 1975;132:340.
69. Jungmann P, Figueredo-Silva J, Dreyer G. Bancroftian lymphangitis in north-eastern Brazil: A histopathological study of 17 cases. J Trop Med Hyg. 1992;95:114.
70. Pani SP, Yuvaraj J, Vanamial P, et al. Episodic adenolymphangitis and lymphoedema in patients with bancroftian filariasis. Trans R Soc Trop Med Hyg. 1995;89:72.
71. Gyapong JO, Gyapong M, Adjel S. The epidemiology of acute adenolymphangitis due to lymphatic filariasis in northern Ghana. Am J Trop Med Hyg. 1996;54:591.
72. Orr ER, Riley HD Jr. Sporotrichosis in childhood: Report of ten cases. J Pediatr. 1971;78:951.
73. Heller HM, Swartz MN. Nodular lymphangitis: Clinical features, differential diagnosis and management. In: Remington JS, Swartz MN, eds. Current Clinical Topics in Infectious Diseases, v. 14. Boston: Blackwell Scientific; 1994:142–158.
74. Sachs MK. Lymphocutaneous *Nocardia brasiliensis* infection acquired from a cat scratch: Case report and review. Clin Infect Dis. 1992;15:710.

75. Graafar A, Ismail A, El Kadaro AY, et al. Necrotizing and suppurative lymphadenitis in *Leishmania major* infections. Trop Med Int Health. 1996;1:243.
76. Lieberman AA, Grossman ME, Bloomgarden D. Sporotrichoid lymphangitis due to *Staphylococcus aureus* in a diabetic patient. Clin Infect Dis. 1995;21:433.
77. Mors Y, Zaidi SZ, Rose DSC, et al. Granulomatous lymphangitis of the penile skin as a cause of penile swelling in children. J Urol. 1997;158:591.
78. Van Dyke JJ, Lake KB. Chemotherapy for aquarium granuloma. JAMA. 1975;233:1380.
79. Izumi AK, Hanke W, Higaki M. *Mycobacterium marinum* infections treated with tetracycline. Arch Dermatol. 1977;1313:1067.
80. Ljungberg B, Christensson B, Grubb R. Failure of doxycycline treatment in aquarium-associated *Mycobacterium marinum* infections. Scand J Infect Dis. 1987;19:539.
81. Sanders WJ, Wolinsky E. In vitro susceptibility of *Mycobacterium marinum* to eight antimicrobial agents. Antimicrob Agents Chemother. 1980;18:529.
82. Consensus Document of the International Society of Lymphology. The diagnosis and treatment of peripheral lymphedema. Lymphology. 1995;28:113.

SECTION J

GASTROINTESTINAL INFECTIONS AND FOOD POISONING

Chapter 81

Principles and Syndromes of Enteric Infection

RICHARD L. GUERRANT
THEODORE S. STEINER

Gastrointestinal infections encompass a wide variety of symptom complexes and recognized infectious agents. With the exception of *Helicobacter pylori* gastritis, the term *gastroenteritis* is applied to syndromes of diarrhea or vomiting that tend to involve noninflammatory infection in the upper small bowel or inflammatory infection in the colon. Other enteric infections and infestations cause predominantly systemic symptoms. Infections of the gastrointestinal tract, especially infectious diarrhea, are among the most common debilitating infectious diseases, afflicting people of all ages around the world. In many heavily populated areas, deaths from diarrheal illnesses exceed those from any other single cause.

In the absence of demonstrable causal forces, many descriptive terms have arisen through the years. Names such as Montezuma's revenge, Delhi belly, Aden gut, gyppi tummy, Aztec two-step, Greek gallop, Rome runs, Hong Kong dog, Turkey trots, La turista, Basra belly, and back door sprint illustrate the widespread occurrence of these infections. Although an etiologic agent is not found in many cases, the infectious nature of most acute diarrheal diseases is suggested by their epidemiologic behavior showing case clustering, spread in families and other groups, and occurrence among travelers. In the last two decades, much has been learned about bacterial and viral agents capable of causing acute gastrointestinal illnesses. These include *Escherichia coli* that produce enterotoxins, which cause fluid secretion, other *E. coli* capable of causing tissue destruction and inflammation, and pathogens such as *Yersinia, Campylobacter, Clostridium, Cryptosporidium, Cyclospora,* rotaviruses, and Norwalk-like viruses. With the development of new tools for diagnosis, important information has been gained in our understanding of the causes, pathogenesis, epidemiology, and control of acute gastrointestinal infections.

OCCURRENCE AND SCOPE OF GASTROINTESTINAL INFECTIONS

On a global scale, diarrheal diseases are second only to cardiovascular diseases as a cause of death[1]; they are the leading cause of childhood death, and, in some populous, developing areas, they are responsible for more years of potential life loss than all other causes combined.[2] Estimates are that 4,600,000 to 6,000,000 children die each year (>12,600/day) in Asia, Africa, and Latin America[3–6] and that more than 10,000 die from diarrhea each year in the United States.[7, 8] More than 13% of the children born in certain parts of Latin America die before their fifth birthday. In more than half, diarrhea is the major or associated cause of death.[2] Although the global mortality is decreasing (especially with oral rehydration therapy [ORT]),[9] in some areas diarrhea mortality is worsening[10] and prolonged diarrhea is emerging as the major cause of death.[11] Even greater than the mortality is the serious morbidity from diarrheal diseases, especially in association with malabsorption and malnutrition in tropical, developing areas. In areas such as Bangladesh, India, Guatemala, and Brazil, the attack rates often reach 7 to 19 cases per person per year among children younger than 2 years of age.[12–17] The attack rate is highest at the time of weaning.[15–18]

More than 60% of the children dying with diarrhea in Latin America also had nutritional deficiencies as associated causes of death, suggesting that diarrhea may precipitate malnutrition.[2] Acute infectious diarrhea exacerbates nutritional deficiencies in several ways. As with any acute infection, caloric demands are increased, and often catabolic steroids, glucagon, and adrenergic amines cause increased breakdown of structural proteins.[18] Through vicious cycles of transient malabsorption and anorexia, repeated bouts of acute diarrhea are major contributors to malnutrition.[19–25] The converse is also true; undernutrition appears to reduce resistance to acute infectious diarrhea. Increased attack rates and increased mortality from acute infectious diarrheal illnesses occur with progressive severity of malnutrition.[25–28] As a specific example, shigellae are shed longer and there is an increased relapse rate in children if they are malnourished.[26] In addition, malnutrition appears to predispose to more prolonged diarrheal illnesses.[28, 29]

More recent data suggest that there is also a complex interaction between poor nutritional status and persistent diarrheal illnesses, usually defined as diarrhea lasting longer than 14 days. These illnesses constituted a majority of total diarrheal burden in several cohorts of children living in impoverished areas.[16, 30, 31] A bidirectional interaction exists between malnutrition and persistent diarrhea. Malnutrition (as measured by growth shortfalls) predisposes to subsequent persistent diarrheal illness,[28] and each persistent diarrheal illness during the first 2 years of life may itself be associated with subsequent growth shortfalls.[32] Moreover, studies have demonstrated that carriage of the persistent diarrheal pathogens *Cryptosporidium parvum, Giardia lamblia,* and enteroaggregative *E. coli* is associated with poor growth even in the absence of diarrhea.[32–35] These early findings suggest that the overall global impact of childhood diarrheal illnesses may be even greater than previously suspected.

Military history indicates that acute diarrheal illnesses have played decisive roles in numerous campaigns. Diarrheal diseases and enteric infections were the major nontraumatic cause of hospitalization among U.S. troops in Vietnam and in Saudi Arabia, their number approaching the number of hospitalizations resulting from injuries due to hostile action.[36–38] Overall rates of gastrointestinal illness in the United States ranged from 1.5 to 5 illnesses per person per year in studies done in communities and in daycare centers, respectively.[5, 39–41] Rates are highest in young children but may sometimes increase during young adulthood (as with *Campylobacter jejuni* in the second weaning)[42] or in the elderly (as with *Clostridium difficile* and *Salmonella*).[5, 7, 43] Diarrhea remains the third most common syndrome in general practice.[37] In studies of community illness among urban and suburban families in Cleveland, Dingle and colleagues[39] identified "infectious gastroenteritis" as the second most common class of illness, after common respiratory diseases. In this community, 1.5 bouts of gastroenteritis occurred per person each year, accounting for 16% of all illnesses.

EPIDEMIOLOGIC AND ENVIRONMENTAL FACTORS

The frequency, type, and severity of enteric infections are determined by *who* you are, *where* you are, and *when* you are there.

Who is at risk of acquiring a gastrointestinal infection varies greatly with age, living conditions, personal and cultural habits, and group exposures. Although the infant who is being breast-fed is relatively protected from contaminated food and water and probably to some degree by maternal colostral antibodies and lactoferrin, at weaning there is a great increase in the risk of diarrheal illness. Adults, particularly if they live for many years in the same environment, may become asymptomatic reservoirs of microorganisms that cause diarrhea in the immunologically untutored child or visitor. Living conditions often reflect socioeconomic conditions; type of housing, population density, sanitation facilities, and water sources are major determinants of environmental exposure to enteric pathogens.[44] The impact of water quality and quantity cannot be overemphasized. As shown in Table 81–1, there are five basic ways in which a shortage of clean water can lead to transmission of enteric infections.[45] Personal hygienic habits determine how many organisms are ingested. Although the infectious dose varies with the organism, relatively small inocula of certain organisms may result in disease. Shigellae are acquired with an unusually low infectious dose and are often spread by direct contact among children in daycare centers. Conversely, *C. difficile* colitis occurs with increasing frequency with age. The majority of nonspecific diarrheal illnesses acquired in communities occur in family clusters, often with small children having the first illness. Of great importance whenever a patient has an enteric illness is a careful history of other illnesses in the family or community. Multiple illnesses and common exposure may be clues to a foodborne outbreak or to the causative agent.

The second epidemiologic determinant of risk for enteric infection is *where* you are. The pattern of illnesses and the etiologic agents vary greatly with climate. For example, *E. coli* that produce heat-labile (LT) or heat-stable (ST) enterotoxins cause disease primarily in the tropics, where the heaviest burden of parasites also occurs. Viral causes of common enteric illnesses have been found among young children in temperate and tropical climates. Despite their clustering, however, many community cases of diarrhea remain unexplained.

Finally, the third determinant of risk is *when* you are there. The majority of enteric illnesses in temperate climates occur during winter months. The opposite is true in tropical countries, where distinct summer peaks of illnesses are common. The role of rainfall is uncertain, and some adjacent areas with similar monsoon climates have opposite seasons of major diarrheal illnesses, as illustrated by the peak seasons for cholera in different parts of Bengal. In Dhaka, endemic cholera occurs during the winter dry months; less than 200 miles away, the peak cholera season in Calcutta occurs during the summer monsoon.

TABLE 81–1 Types of Water-Related Diseases

Waterborne	Diseases transmitted by ingestion of contaminated drinking water. Examples: cholera, typhoid fever, cryptosporidiosis.
Water-carried	Diseases acquired by accidental ingestion of, or exposure to, contaminated recreational water. Examples: cryptosporidiosis, giardiasis, *Pseudomonas* dermatitis.
Water-washed	Diseases transmitted person-to-person as a result of poor sanitation due to inadequate quantities of water for washing hands, utensils, and so on. Examples: shigellosis, hepatitis A, cryptosporidiosis.
Water-based	Diseases caused by pathogens with an obligatory life-cycle phase occurring in the water. Examples: schistosomiasis, dracunculiasis.
Water-vectored	Diseases transmitted by insects that breed or bite in or near water. Examples: malaria, yellow fever, dengue, African trypanosomiasis.

Table adapted from data published in Steiner TS, Theilman NM, Guerrant RL. Protozoal agents: What are the dangers for the public water supply? Annu Rev Med., 1997;48:329–340.

TABLE 81–2 Enteric Host Defenses

Host species, genotype, and age
Personal hygiene
Gastric acidity and other physical barriers
Intestinal motility
Enteric microflora
Specific immunity
- Phagocytic
- Humoral
- Cell-mediated

Nonspecific protective factors and human milk
Intestinal receptors

HOST FACTORS

Considering the ubiquity of potential enteric pathogens, it is surprising that enteric infections are not even more common. After exposure to infectious agents, several host factors determine who becomes ill. Several enteric host defenses provide substantial protection against many intestinal pathogens (Table 81–2).

Host Species, Genotype, and Age

Host species, genotype, and age are complex but major determinants of susceptibility to colonization and disease with enteric pathogens. Although a broad spectrum of animal hosts can be infected with pathogens such as *Salmonella enteritidis* and *C. jejuni,* only primates and humans are characteristically infected with *Salmonella typhi* or *Shigella* spp. In addition, the intestinal cell receptors for the K88, K99, and colonization factor antigen (CFA) attachment traits of enterotoxigenic *E. coli* (ETEC) are largely species specific.[46, 47] Interspecies variation and host genotype are also important. Persons with blood group O appear to be more susceptible to cholera, and possibly others with type A to giardiasis.[48, 49] Furthermore, Rutter and associates[50] have bred a strain of piglets that do not have the single-locus dominant allele for the intestinal receptor for *E. coli* K88 adherence antigen and consequently are resistant to diarrhea caused by these organisms. Such species or even genotype specificities play tremendously important roles in determining host susceptibility and the epidemiology of these infections. Genotypic differences in susceptibility to enteric infections may have far-reaching implications. For example, it has been suggested that the high prevalence of mutations in the cystic fibrosis transmembrane regulatory protein in Caucasians may have been maintained by a selective heterozygote advantage in susceptibility to *S. typhi.*[51]

The role of age in determining host susceptibility is complex. In animals a narrow "age window" of susceptibility to specific enteric infections is well recognized. In humans, the tendency of rotaviral and enteropathogenic *E. coli* (EPEC) infections to affect young children is impressive. The explanations probably reside in age-related changes in gut mucus, cell-surface factors, microbial flora, environmental exposure, and specific immune factors. In addition, specific receptors for microbial adhesins or toxins may be developmentally regulated, such as that for *Shigella,* Shiga-like, cholera, *E. coli,* and *C. difficile* enterotoxins.[52–55] This may explain in part the predisposition to hemolytic-uremic syndrome in children. Moreover, like certain strains of rotavirus, toxigenic strains of *C. difficile* are carried frequently by healthy young infants, in whom they seldom cause disease.

Specific receptor components or antagonists (e.g., mono-saccharides like *N*-acetylneuraminic acid) can be added exogenously and compete with intestinal binding sites for *E. coli.*[47, 56] Conversely, lectin-like substances that bind to the intestinal cell receptors may compete with the bacterial attachment factors. Positive chemotaxis of *Vibrio cholerae, E. coli,* and *Salmonella typhimurium* has been shown toward rabbit ileal mucosa, and a role of negative chemotactic factors as a new type of host defense has been postulated.[57]

Personal Hygiene

Whether a person acquires an enteric infection depends first on the number of pathogens ingested. Almost all agents of concern are acquired by the oral route. The majority of identified enteric pathogens have come from other mammalian intestinal tracts; often a human fecal-oral route can be traced. A plentiful, conveniently located supply of uncontaminated water, in conjunction with improved sanitary facilities, is critically important in reducing this mode of spread.[44, 58] Studies of presumptive viral agents that have not yet been defined strongly implicate the human fecal-oral route of infection.[59, 60] Usually in bacterial infections, a large number of organisms (100,000 to 100,000,000) must be ingested to overcome host defenses and cause disease[61] (Table 81–3). Such numbers may result from growth in food that is allowed to stand unrefrigerated for several hours after the initial contaminating inoculum. Exceptions to the large number of organisms usually required for an infecting dose are *Shigella* and cysts of certain parasites, which can be reproducibly transmitted with only 10 to 100 organisms. A mathematical model based on a large waterborne outbreak of cryptosporidiosis in Milwaukee, Wisconsin, in 1993 suggested that some people may have been infected after ingesting a single oocyst.[62] This small inoculum can readily be transmitted directly by person-to-person contact (as in daycare centers). This is an unusual route of spread for other bacterial enteric pathogens except in hosts with impaired defenses and newborn infants.

Gastric Acidity and Other Physical Barriers

Most bacterial pathogens that are ingested never reach the intestinal tract because of the normal gastric acid barrier. When this barrier is neutralized with antacids, both the susceptibility and the severity of several enteric bacterial and parasitic infections are increased. At the normal gastric pH (<4), more than 99.9% of ingested coliform bacteria are killed within 30 minutes. There is no reduction of an experimental bacterial inoculum in achlorhydric stomachs after 1 hour. Not surprisingly, then, the gastric coliform flora in fasting subjects (normally fewer than 10 organisms/ml) exceed 10,000/ml in the majority of achlorhydric patients.[63] Excessive numbers of normal bacterial flora in the upper small bowel may contribute to malabsorption and diarrheal syndromes.[64, 65]

The inoculum of *V. cholerae* required to cause disease can be reduced 10,000-fold (from 10^8 to 10^4 organisms) by neutralization of gastric acid with 2 g of sodium bicarbonate.[66] In an outbreak of cholera in Israel, 25% of the patients had had previous gastric resection, whereas none of a comparable control group had had gastric surgery.[67] A similar association of previous gastric surgery or achlorhydria with increased frequency and severity of *Salmonella* infections has also been noted in several studies.[68] Likewise, the frequency of enteric multiplication of a vaccine strain of *Shigella flexneri* increases threefold with sodium bicarbonate neutralization of gastric acid. With *C. jejuni,* a substantial range in infectious doses has been documented with different strains.[69] Although gastric acidity may enhance the process of excystation and infection by some parasites after ingestion of the ova, it may provide protection against other parasites. The fragile trophozoite of *G. lamblia* (requiring a pH of 6.4 to 7.1) causes more severe symptoms in association with hypochlorhydria or achlorhydria, perhaps because of increased survival of trophozoites refluxed to the stomach and proximal duodenum. The association of achlorhydria and hypochlorhydria with symptomatic strongyloidiasis has also been noted. Some have suggested that vitamin B_{12} deficiency occurs more often in association with fish tapeworm *(Diphyllobothrium latum)* in patients who are achlorhydric and who have high jeujunal infestations. Finally, certain parasitic, viral, or bacterial processes such as *H. pylori* infections may in themselves alter gastric acidity and thereby increase host susceptibility to other enteric pathogens.[70] The further importance of gastric acidity in preventing gastric, pharyngeal, and tracheal colonization by gram-negative bacilli and even nosocomial pneumonia has been shown by the increased risk of patients taking antacids or histamine (H_2) blockers compared with sucralfate, which preserves gastric acidity.[71]

Other physical barriers such as mucus and mucosal tissue integrity are important resistance factors in healthy hosts and work in concert with gastric acidity and intestinal motility to clear many bacteria from the upper small bowel.[72] Continuous removal and renewal of gastrointestinal mucus may bind organisms and toxins and further aid in protecting the intact mucosa from enzymatic and microbial attack.[73]

TABLE 81–3 Infectious Doses of Enteric Pathogens

Pathogen	Dose
Shigella	10 to 10^2
Campylobacter jejuni	10^2 to 10^6
Salmonella	10^5
Escherichia coli	10^8
Vibrio cholerae	10^8
Giardia lamblia	10 to 10^2 cysts
Entamoeba histolytica	10 to 10^2 cysts
Cryptosporidium parvum	1 to 10^3 oocysts

Intestinal Motility

Intestinal motility plays several important roles in normal intestinal physiology: (1) in the fluid absorptive process, (2) in maintaining the appropriate distribution of indigenous enteric microflora, and (3) in ridding the host of pathogenic microorganisms. The role of motility in aiding fluid absorption was demonstrated in a study done with human volunteers by Higgens and associates.[74] Using methantheline bromide (Banthīne), they showed that inhibition of normal intestinal motility resulted in impaired absorption of radiolabeled water and sodium. Whereas more than 90% of a labeled saline bolus was normally absorbed in less than 10 minutes, less than 70% was absorbed in 30 minutes after methantheline bromide administration. Intraluminal distribution of a barium bolus in small bowel before and after methantheline bromide administration suggested that a reasonable explanation for this impaired absorption was a reduction in the absorptive surface area exposed to the intraluminal fluid. In contrast to the distribution within 2 to 3 minutes of the bolus of barium throughout the small bowel of healthy persons, methantheline bromide caused a puddling of barium near the injection site in the upper small bowel, which often persisted for longer than 60 minutes.

Motility also helps to maintain normal distribution and flow of microflora. The risk of bowel stasis is evident in the bacterial overgrowth syndromes in the small bowel and in the added risk of "toxic megacolon" in inflammatory bowel disease after antimotility drugs are administered.

In addition, intestinal motility appears to play a role in providing protection from enteric pathogens. Experimental animals are much more easily infected with enteric pathogens after inhibition of gut motility with opiates.[75] *Salmonella* bacteremia may develop in patients after opiates are taken for relatively mild gastroenteritis.[76] A controlled study of adults with shigellosis treated with diphenoxylate hydrochloride with atropine (Lomotil) revealed that the antimotility drug abolished antibiotic effectiveness in reducing diarrhea and positive cultures and was associated with prolonged fever and shedding of the *Shigella* organisms.[77] Moreover, case reports suggest that complications of *Campylobacter* and *C. difficile* enteritis are more common in patients who have received antimotility agents.[78, 79] These drugs also predispose patients to hemolytic-uremic syndrome after infection with enterohemorrhagic *E. coli* (EHEC).[80] Gut motility and diarrhea that help rid the host of offending pathogens may therefore be analogous to the cough in pulmonary infections as a mechanism to expel pathogens.

Normal Enteric Microflora

There have been several developments in the understanding of the composition of intestinal microflora. With improved culture techniques,[81] it is now recognized that 99.9% of the normal enteric bacterial flora are anaerobes (approximately 10^{11} organisms per gram of normal feces). These organisms (*Bacteroides,* clostridia, peptostreptococci, peptococci, and others) far exceed the number of aerobes. *E. coli* number 10^8 per gram; *Klebsiella, Proteus,* enterococci, and other species number approximately 10^5 to 10^7 per gram. The role of normal flora as an extremely important and often overlooked host defense is beginning to be appreciated. In several situations normal bacterial flora can be shown to be highly effective in resisting colonization by potentially pathogenic invaders. The loss of normal flora or a shift in their balance caused by use of antibiotics often leads to their replacement by organisms such as *Pseudomonas, Klebsiella, Clostridium,* and *Candida.* When these organisms take up residence, they may cause serious systemic infections, especially in a nosocomial setting. There are numerous examples of increased susceptibility to infection in patients with reduced bacterial flora.[82, 83] Several enteric infections, such as infant botulism, nosocomial salmonellosis, and EPEC, occur with increased frequency in newborn infants who have not yet acquired a normal enteric flora. Diarrhea associated with the use of antibiotics is common and in many cases is probably related to an alteration in the balance of normal enteric microflora.

The basis for the resistance provided by normal bacterial flora in the intestinal tract was elucidated in an elegant series of studies by Bohnhoff and coworkers.[84] In experimental mice, they showed that the protective effect of normal flora is eradicated by a single injection of streptomycin. The infecting dose of *S. typhimurium* was reduced more than 100,000-fold by the administration of a single dose of streptomycin. This reduced resistance correlated with the reduction in the normal colonic flora and their toxic acidic products. Resistance was restored with the return of enteric flora (especially *Bacteroides*), either by inoculation or naturally. The importance of a reduced pH and volatile fatty acids from the anaerobic flora in colonization resistance was further shown by Van der Waaj and colleagues[85] and by Que and colleagues.[86]

Indigenous microbes such as *Lactobacillus, Bacteroides,* and *Clostridium* spp. attach to the intestinal epithelial surface and act synergistically with the host immunity to interfere with experimental *S. typhimurium* challenge.[87] Enteric bacteria, including *Proteus, Enterobacter,* and *E. coli,* also act synergistically in mice with vibriocidal immunity from vaccination to antagonize *V. cholerae.*[88] The protective role of normal enteric bacterial flora in humans was documented by the increased frequency of *Salmonella* infections among Swedish tourists who took a prophylactic antibiotic compared with those who took no antimicrobial agent.[83] In a huge outbreak of antimicrobial-resistant *S. typhimurium* enteritis involving almost 200,000 people in Illinois in the spring of 1985, there was a significant association of illness with a history of having taken antimicrobial drugs the month before the illness. There was a fivefold difference (6% versus 30%) between well controls and ill persons in the percentage who took antibiotics to which the outbreak strain was resistant.[89] Others have reported an increased risk of infection with antimicrobial-sensitive *Salmonella* after antimicrobial exposure.[90] Some have even used normal colonic or other competing bacterial flora to treat refractory *C. difficile* colitis.[91, 92] In addition, cytotoxic chemotherapy with agents such as methotrexate, cyclophosphamide, or fluorouracil may also suppress normal flora and predispose to *C. difficile* colitis.[92–96]

Intestinal Immunity

Enteric immunity is composed of phagocytic, humoral, and cell-mediated elements. Each component makes specific contributions to host resistance to enteric infections. The normal intestinal mucosa demonstrates a state of "physiologic inflammation" in the lamina propria, with numerous neutrophils, macrophages, plasma cells, and lymphocytes, that suggests a constant battle of the host with luminal challenges to maintain the integrity of the mucosa. The importance of intact phagocytic immunity becomes evident when neutrophils are absent in hosts, who then become particularly susceptible to gram-negative rod infections that often originate in the gastrointestinal tract.[97] In addition, neutropenic patients may develop stomatitis or necrotizing typhlitis (with fever, abdominal pain, cecal necrosis and edema, and sometimes bloody diarrhea).[98–101] The importance of immunity is also demonstrated by the potentially severe adenoviral, rotaviral, coxsackieviral, and *C. difficile* infections in patients undergoing bone marrow transplantation.[102]

Diarrhea in patients with the acquired immunodeficiency syndrome (AIDS) is common in those who are unable to receive highly active antiretroviral therapy and raises a special set of diagnostic and therapeutic questions. The growing range of severe, recurring enteric infections in immunocompromised patients,[101] especially those with AIDS, demonstrates the critical role of immunity in resisting a broad range of viral, bacterial, parasitic, and fungal enteric infections. The majority of AIDS patients with diarrhea have a documentable infectious cause such as cytomegalovirus, *Entamoeba histolytica, Cryptosporidium, Microsporidia, Salmonella, Giardia, C. jejuni, Shigella, Mycobacterium, Cyclospora,* enteroaggregative *E. coli* (EAggEC), or herpes simplex virus.[103–106] In Haiti and Africa, up to 95% of AIDS patients initially present with diarrhea; up to 50% have *Cryptosporidium* infections, and 15% have *Isospora belli.*[107–109]

The gut-associated lymphoid tissue comprises Peyer's patches, lamina propria lymphocytes, and intraepithelial lymphocytes.[110] Microfold (M) cells take up antigen and microbes such as *Yersinia, Shigella,* and *Cryptosporidium.*[111–113] Specific active humoral intestinal immunity (coproantibody) arises either from a leakage of serum immunoglobulin (predominantly IgG or IgM) or from the formation of IgA by plasma cells located predominantly in the lamina propria. Secretory IgA (an 11S dimer [Mr 390,000] with a secretory piece [Mr 60,000] from the mucosal epithelial cells) is found in the lumen.[114–116] Selective deficiency of secretory component has been associated with intestinal candidiasis.[116] Certain mucosal pathogens produce an IgA protease or degrade IgA.[117, 118] Both serum and secretory antibody responses have been demonstrated in response to parenteral and intraluminal challenge with cholera toxoid.[119] Secretory IgA is resistant to intraluminal degradation by enzymatic proteolysis and sulfhydryl reduction. The dynamics of local intestinal immunity have been elucidated in several experimental models. The most efficient method of eliciting a local antibody response is with a parenteral priming challenge followed by an intestinal booster antigen challenge. Studies of cholera toxoid immunity in rats suggest that the parenteral priming toxoid prepares a widespread distribution of precursor lymphocytes in areas such as the Peyer's patches.[120] These cells are then capable of responding to a booster challenge to produce many large IgA-bearing lymphocytes that appear in the thoracic duct before "homing" back to the lamina propria as specific IgA-secreting plasma cells at or distal to this site of booster toxoid. Passively acquired IgA probably accounts for part of the protection against enteric infections in infants who are breast-fed. Colostral antibody against rotaviruses and the enterotoxins of *V. cholerae* and *E. coli* have been demonstrated in breast milk.[121, 122]

Intestinal antibodies may be directed at any of a number of different bacterial antigens such as endotoxin, capsular material, or exotoxins and may have bactericidal, opsonic, or neutralizing effects. Although IgA can have hemagglutinating, precipitating, or virus-neutralizing properties, it does not appear capable of fixing complement so as to have the direct bactericidal effect that IgG and IgM may have. Selective IgA deficiency is often associated with a compensatory increase in IgM levels. Hereditary telangiectasia with IgA deficiency is associated with recurrent rhinopulmonary infection but is rarely associated with intestinal infection or dysfunction.[114] Although debated by others,[123] Zinneman and Kaplan[124] and Ament and associates[125] have suggested that patients with giardiasis have lower IgA levels and that hypogammaglobulinemic patients have more malabsorption and diarrhea with giardiasis. Patients with type 2 combined IgA and IgM deficiency and small intestinal lymphoid hyperplasia with a sparsity of plasma cells may have diarrhea, malabsorption, and giardiasis.[126] Crabbe and Heremans[127] described three patients with another type of selective IgA deficiency with spruelike intestinal symptoms and histopathologic changes. The role of cell-mediated immune processes in the intestine is suggested by adjuvant enhancement of vaccine efficacy against intracellular infections such as *S. typhi.*[128]

Other Protective Factors in Human Milk and Serum

The protection afforded by breast-feeding probably relates to several passively transmitted factors and to reduced exposure to a contaminated environment.[15–18, 129, 130] In addition to antibody, these factors include lactoferrin, lysozyme, phagocytes, high lactose, low protein, low phosphate, low pH (in part from bifidobacteria), and oligosaccharide fractions.[129–135] The role of lactoferrin in human milk is suggested by the abolition of milk's bacteriostatic properties against *V. cholerae* and EPEC by saturation with iron.[134] In addition, patients with chronic iron excess from hemolytic processes such as malaria, sickle cell anemia, and Oroya fever are at increased risk of infection with organisms such as *Salmonella*, and patients receiving the iron-chelating drug desferrioxamine may be at increased risk for infection with *Yersinia enterocolitica.*[135a] Some of the bacteriostatic properties of normal serum were abolished when iron-binding proteins were saturated with iron.[134]

MICROBIAL FACTORS

A number of bacterial virulence traits determine the pathogenic mechanisms responsible for diarrhea. This entire range of traits is demonstrated by the various types of *E. coli*, as summarized in Table 81–4. This versatile species may represent the predominant normal colonic flora or may be a urinary or enteric pathogen. Depending largely on the transmissible virulence traits encoded on plasmids or phage, *E. coli* may produce one of three families of enterotoxins (LT, STa, or STb), may be invasive (enteroinvasive *E. coli* [EIEC]), may cause hemorrhagic colitis (EHEC), or may exhibit three or four distinct types of adherence: class I and II EPEC, with or without the plasmid-encoded focal HEp-2 cell enteroadherence factor (EAF); aggregative adherence (EAggEC); and one of the recognized colonization traits (CFA-I, CFA-II, E8775, 260-1, and O159:H4). Study of *E. coli* with these varied pathogenic traits has greatly helped to unravel the mechanisms by which enteric pathogens alter normal intestinal absorptive function to cause diarrheal diseases.[136, 137]

Toxins

Toxic microbial components or products are implicated in the disease-producing capacity of several enteric pathogens. Culture filtrates

TABLE 81–4 Pathogenic Mechanisms of *Escherichia coli* Diarrhea*

Type	Mechanism	Model	Gene Code	Predominant Serogroups
I. Enterotoxigenic *E. coli* (ETEC)	Adherence via CFA-I through CFA-IV	Mannose-resistant hemagglutination (for most)	Plasmid	—
LT *E. coli*	Adenylate cyclase–like cholera toxin	Rabbit loops (18h) CHO, Y1 cell immunoassay	LT-I Plasmid, LT-II Chromosome	LT: O groups 1, 6, 7, 8, 9, 128 LT + ST: O groups 11, 15, 20, 25, 27, 60, 63, 75, 80, 85, 88, 89, 99, 101, 109, 114, 139, 153
STa *E. coli*	Guanylate cyclase	Suckling mice	Plasmid	ST: O groups 12, 78, 115, 148, 149, 153, 159, 166, 167
STb *E. coli*	Cyclic nucleotide–independent bicarbonate secretion	Piglet loops	Plasmid	—
II. Enterohemorrhagic *E. coli* (EHEC)	Attaching/effacing (analogous to EPEC), Shiga-like (Vero) toxin 1 or 2 inhibits protein synthesis	HeLa cell cytotoxicity Fluorescent actin–staining	Chromosome (pathogenicity island), phage	Predominantly O157:H7, O26:H11; O103:H2; O111:H^-; O113:H21+, some 50 others
III. Enteroinvasive *E. coli* (EIEC)	Local mucosal invasion, EIET	Sereny test, rabbit ileal loops, Ussing chambers	Plasmid, chromosome	O groups 11, 28ac, 29, 112ac, 115, 124, 136, 143, 144, 147, 152, 164, 167, 173
IV. Enteropathogenic *E. coli* (EPEC)				
Locally adherent	Adhere focally via bundle-forming pili	Localized HEp-2 cell adherence	Plasmid (60 MDa, pMAR2, with EAF and bfpA)	O18:H^-, 7, 14; O26:H^-, 11; O44:H18, 44; O55:H^-, 6, 7; O86:H34; 088; O111:H^-, 2, 12, 21; O114:H2; O119:H^-, 6; O125ac:H^-, 21; O126:H^-, 27; O127:H^-, 6†; O128ab:H2, 7; O142:H6; O145; O157:H8; O158:H23
Attaching and effacing *E. coli*	Attach to and efface brush border epithelium via injection and phosphorylation of Tir and subsequent intimin binding	Fluorescent actin staining	Chromosome locus of enterocyte effacement (LEE)	
V. Enteroaggregative *E. coli* (EAggEC)	Aggregative adherence to HEp-2 cells	Aggregative pattern of HEp-2 cell adherence	Plasmid	O3:H2; O44; O78:H33; O15:H11; O77:H18; O51:H11, O?:H10, among others (O78, 86, 91, 92)
EAST-1	Guanylate cyclase	Ussing chamber	Plasmid	
PET	Secretion, cytotoxicity	Ussing chamber	Plasmid	
VI. Diffusely adherent *E. coli* (DAEC)	Diffuse adherence	Diffuse adherence to HEp-2 cells	Chromosomal	(Strain F1845, 189, 57-1)
Normal enteric flora	?Adherence traits	—	—	O groups 1, 2, 4, 6, 7, 25, 45, 75, 81
Genitourinary, blood stream, or meningeal pathogens	?Capsular polysaccharide ± adherence pili, CNF-I and CNF-II; adenosine diphosphate-ribosylate Rho proteins	Several animals (mice, rabbits), cytotoxicity	Plasmid (CNF-II)	O groups 1, 2, 4, 6, 7, 11, 18, 22, 25, 45, 62, 75, 81 (K antigens 1, 2, 3, 5, 13)

*In addition, nontoxigenic *E. coli* with recognized or new colonization factor fimbriae can cause diarrhea, as documented in experimental animals and in human volunteers; several reviews comment on O and H serotypes.[396–400]

†O127:H6 is the focally HEp-2 cell adherent strain (E2348) from which the plasmid pMAR-2 was isolated.

Abbreviations: CFA, Colonization factor antigen; CHO, Chinese hamster ovary; CNF, colony necrotizing factor; EAF, enteroadherence factor; EAST, enteroaggregative STa-like toxin; LT, heat-labile; ST, heat-stable; PET, plasmid-encoded toxin.

of toxigenic microorganisms are capable of altering gastrointestinal structure or function in the absence of the organisms themselves. Toxins produced by enteric pathogens can be classified as *neurotoxins, enterotoxins*, or *cytotoxins* (Table 81–5).

Neurotoxins

Neurotoxins usually are ingested as preformed toxins that often cause enteric symptoms. These include staphylococcal, *Bacillus cereus*, and botulinum toxins. Although staphylococcal food poisoning is an abrupt upper gastrointestinal syndrome attributed to staphylococcal enterotoxin, the effect appears to be caused by the action of this toxin on the central autonomic nervous system rather than by destruction or fluid secretion in the intestine per se.[138, 139] An exotoxin related to enterotoxin A may cause fluid accumulation in rabbit ileal loops directly.[140, 141] A different staphylococcal α-toxin elicits hyperperistalsis. Certain strains of *B. cereus* isolated from patients with acute food poisoning also produce a highly heat-stable emetic toxin (especially when cultured with rice) that is a small (M_r<5000), nonantigenic polypeptide capable of causing vomiting in monkeys, much like staphylococcal enterotoxin.[142, 143] Botulinum toxin has a primary effect on the neuromuscular junction to prevent the release of acetylcholine from the presynaptic vesicle.[139]

Enterotoxins

True enterotoxins are defined as those having a direct effect on the intestinal mucosa to elicit net fluid secretion. The classic enterotoxin, cholera toxin, has been extensively studied and causes fluid secretion after the ganglioside-binding subunit releases the A2 toxin subunit, which activates basolateral epithelial adenylate cyclase via adenosine diphosphate–ribosylation of Gsα to increase concentrations of intestinal cyclic adenosine monophosphate (cAMP).[144, 145] In addition, prostaglandins, platelet-activating factor, and possibly neurohumoral mediators such as serotonin may be involved in the secretory or tissue culture responses to cholera toxin.[146–150] Antigenically and mechanistically similar toxins have been described for other closely related vibrios[151, 152] and *E. coli*.[153, 154]

Because there are no reliable markers such as serotype or biotype for enterotoxigenicity, demonstration of the toxin itself is necessary to identify which *E. coli* are enterotoxigenic. The genetic codes for enterotoxigenicity reside on transmissible plasmids that can be lost or transferred to other *E. coli* by conjugation[155, 156] or by phage transduction.[157] To recognize which *E. coli* are enterotoxigenic, enterotoxin activity must be identified in culture filtrates of the organisms in question. At one time this required inoculation into a ligated rabbit ileal segment[158] or into rabbit skin to test for toxin-associated "permeability factor."[159] The ability of the heat-labile enterotoxin of *E. coli* to activate adenylate cyclase has been used in the development of tissue culture bioassays.[160, 161] Its similar antigenicity to cholera toxin has provided immunoassay techniques as well.[162–164] Oligonucleotide gene probes for LT and STa are now available with nonradioactive enzyme markers and provide a simple, sensitive, and highly specific detection method for these enterotoxins.[165] The LT-producing *E. coli* are associated with watery diarrhea among adults in Asia,[166, 167] travelers to Central America,[168–170] and children in a number of areas.[171–173] In addition, *Klebsiella, Citrobacter, Salmonella*, and *C. jejuni* produce cholera-like heat-labile toxins that also activate adenylate cyclase, bind to ganglioside, and share some immunogenicity with *E. coli* LT.[174–180]

Another plasmid-mediated but smaller, less antigenic, heat-stable toxin can be produced by *E. coli*. The ST-producing *E. coli*, first described as a cause of diarrhea in piglets and calves,[46, 181] are capable of causing diarrhea in human volunteers as well.[182] It appears to be significantly associated with diarrhea among tourists to Central America,[183] in occasional newborn nursery outbreaks in this country,[184] and among adults with noninflammatory diarrhea on a Navajo reservation[185] and in Brazil.[16, 186] The mechanism of action of ST involves the specific activation of intestinal guanylate cyclase.[187–189] Like cAMP, cyclic guanosine monophosphate (cGMP) analogues (e.g., 8Br-GMP) can mimic the secretory effect of the enterotoxin.[187] *Yersinia*, non-O1 *V. cholerae*, and *Citrobacter freundii* also produce cross-reacting homologous ST of 17 to 19 amino acids with conservation of six cysteines (with three disulfide bonds) and a central Asp-Pro-Ala region that is required for ST-binding and activation of enterocyte guanylate cyclase.[190–195] Furthermore, endogenous ST-like compounds now being isolated from mammalian cells may play key roles in normal intestinal and renal physiology.[195–197]

Several other bacterial products induce intestinal secretion via electrogenic ion secretion. These include a chromosomally mediated 68- to 80-kD secretory toxin produced in iron-deprived conditions by EIEC called EIET,[198] a 2- to 5-kD heat-stable, plasmid-encoded STa-like toxin produced by many strains of EAggEC and EHEC called EAST-1,[199, 200] a 108-kD protein called PET from some isolates of EAggEC,[201] and the thermostable direct hemolysin of *Vibrio parahaemolyticus*.[202]

A protein neuroenterotoxin isolated from *Shigella dysenteriae* 1 (which may be responsible for the headache, meningismus, and seizures) also causes fluid secretion in rabbit ileal loops.[203] Although experimental findings have been contradictory, the activation of adenylate cyclase by this *Shigella* enterotoxin has been demonstrated in rabbit ileal loops.[204] Noninflammatory secretion also occurs in the small bowel of experimental monkeys infected with *S. flexneri* 2A,[205] and 80% of the patients infected with *S. flexneri* or *Shigella sonnei* develop neutralizing antibodies to the toxin.[206] However, the toxin alone does not appear to be sufficient to cause *Shigella* diarrhea, because toxigenic, noninvasive opaque colonial mutants of virulent *Shigella* are totally avirulent.[207, 208] Certain strains of *B. cereus* have also been reported to produce a heat-labile, adenylate cyclase–activating rabbit ileal loop–positive, dermonecrotic, and intestinonecrotic enterotoxin.[142, 143, 209, 210]

Another mechanism of several bacterial toxins is cytoskeletal disruption, which can lead to loss of tight junctions and perturbations in absorptive and barrier function of the intestinal epithelium. For example, a toxin identified from *Bacteroides fragilis* isolates from children and adults with diarrhea in Montana and Arizona has been cloned.[211, 212] This toxin disrupts tight junctions in intestinal epithelial

TABLE 81–5 Enteric Bacterial Toxins

Neurotoxin group
Clostridium botulinum
Staphylococcus aureus (enterotoxin b)
Bacillus cereus (emetic toxin)
Secretory enterotoxin group
Vibrio cholerae (cAMP)
Noncholera vibrios
Escherichia coli—LT (cAMP)
E. coli—STa (cGMP)
E. coli—STb
Salmonella
Klebsiella
Clostridium perfringens (A)
Shigella dysenteriae
B. cereus
Possible enterotoxins
E. coli: EIET, EAST, EALT, PET
V. cholerae: Ace, Zot
Bacteroides fragilis
Cytotoxin group
Shigella
C. perfringens (A)
Vibrio parahaemolyticus
S. aureus
Clostridium difficile (A and B)
E. coli (EHEC) (certain O groups: 26, 39, 128, 157); *Campylobacter jejuni; Helicobacter pylori*

Abbreviations: cAMP, Cyclic adenosine monophosphate; EALT, enteroaggregative *E. coli* heat labile toxin; EAST, enteroaggregative STa-like toxin; EHEC, enterohemorrhagic *E. coli;* EIET, enteroinvasive *E. coli* toxin; LT, heat-labile; PET, plasmid-encoded toxin; ST, heat-stable.

cells.[213, 214] The toxins of *C. difficile* disrupt epithelial integrity by performing an enzymatic monoglucosylation of the Thr-37 residue of small GTP-binding proteins of the Rho family, leading to their inactivation.[215, 216] The zonula occludens toxin of *V. cholerae*, which causes paracellular leak, may contribute to the diarrhea of cholera.[217] The plasmid-encoded cytotoxin (PET) from EAggEC isolates from children with diarrhea in Mexico City causes both fluid secretion and unique ultrastructural changes in the intestinal epithelium.[201]

Certain strains of *S. typhimurium* cause severe watery, cholera-like diarrhea[218, 219] that can be prevented in experimental models by indomethacin. As noted in Chapter 85, the products of an inflammatory response could act to cause mucosal secretion.[220, 221] Sandefur and Peterson[177] described a heat-labile enterotoxin-like effect in rabbit skin and Chinese hamster ovary cell models after separation from an inhibitor. A role of inflammatory mediators in *C. difficile* diarrhea is suggested by the prevention of hemorrhagic fluid accumulation in experimental animals by anti-inflammatory compounds, including receptor antagonists for platelet-activating factor or substance P, blocking antibodies against leukocyte adhesion molecules, ketotifen (which inhibits mast-cell activation), and indomethacin.[222–226] Others have described a heat-stable enterotoxin from *Salmonella*.[227] Other enteric organisms with which enterotoxin-like activity has been reported include *Klebsiella, Citrobacter, Aeromonas*, and *Enterobacter* spp.[175, 176, 228–230] Both heat-labile and heat-stable toxins have been reported. Although these enterotoxigenic organisms appear to be infrequent, much needs to be learned about the occurrence and the mechanism of action of enterotoxins from these organisms other than *E. coli*.

Cytotoxins

Cytotoxic products of several enteric pathogens are responsible for the mucosal destruction that often results in inflammatory colitis. Bacillary dysentery is a colonic mucosal destructive process in which a cytotoxin isolated from *S. dysenteriae* type 1 may play a role.[208, 231] Whether this cytotoxin is a component or a digestive product of the larger neuroenterotoxin mentioned previously is unknown.

EHEC that cause hemorrhagic colitis or the hemolytic-uremic syndrome (O groups 26, 39, 111, 113, 121, 128, and 157) produce one or two Shiga-like Vero-cell cytotoxins.[232–236] Two groups have recorded the transfer of Vero toxin production to recipient *E. coli* or its association with a large plasmid[234, 236]; others have associated the production of Shiga-like toxins (SLT) I and II with bacteriophages in *E. coli* O157:H7.[237] The heat-labile Vero cytotoxin, initially found in *E. coli* O26:H11, O128, and O39, has a slight secretory effect in 18-hour ligated rabbit ileal loops.[233] The multistate outbreak of hemorrhagic colitis with *E. coli* O157:H7 in 1982[235] was followed by studies showing the near-identity (one amino acid difference) of Vero cytotoxin to Shiga toxin (hence the term *Shiga-like toxin*) and the increasing association of these EHEC with numerous outbreaks and sporadic cases of hemorrhagic colitis or childhood hemolytic-uremic syndrome in schools, daycare centers, nursing homes, and communities, including more than 500 documented cases and four deaths in four western states associated with a single hamburger chain in 1993.[235, 238–242] A massive outbreak in 1996 involving more than 10,000 Japanese schoolchildren was presumptively traced to contaminated radish sprouts; there was a relatively low incidence of hemolytic-uremic syndrome in this population.[243, 244]

Like Shiga toxin, *E. coli* SLT has binding and active subunits, is neutralized by anti–Shiga toxin antibody, and binds to globotriaosylceramide (Gb3) via its B subunit, and the active A subunit (analogous to that of the plant toxin, ricin) enzymatically cleaves the *N*-glycoside bond of adenine at position 4324 in the 28SrRNA of the 60S ribosomal subunit to prevent elongation factor 1–dependent aminoacyl transfer RNA binding to the ribosome and thereby halt protein synthesis.[203, 238, 245–249] Subtle differences in the B-subunit specificities for Gb4 or Gb5 (globotetraosyl or globopentaosyl ceramide, respectively) as well as Gb3 may help explain differences in cell culture effects and in the disease manifestations of SLT-I and SLT-II, SLT-IIvh, and SLT-IIvp (to cause bloody diarrhea or hemolytic-uremic syndrome in patients or edema diseases in swine).[248–250] Shiga toxin causes limb paralysis and death in mice and rabbits, and axonal transport of toxin with vagal sensory neuron damage has been described.[251–254] Examination of histopathologic secretions, however, suggests that neuronal damage may be indirect, resulting from endothelial cell damage.[251, 252] In addition, a 110-kD heat- and trypsin-labile cytotoxin that is distinct from Shiga toxin has been implicated in patients with seizures or encephalopathy with shigellosis.[255]

C. perfringens enterotoxin also produces cytotoxicity similar to that of *S. dysenteriae* toxin in HeLa cells and in animal models.[256] Vero cells have been used to detect a cytotoxicity in fecal filtrates that is neutralized by specific antiserum or toxin fragments.[257–259] These methods have enabled studies that implicate enterocytotoxigenic *C. perfringens* in geriatric institutions and in cases of antibiotic-associated diarrhea.[260–261] *C. perfringens* type C produces a trypsin-sensitive β-toxin.[263] Another enteric pathogen that releases a cytotoxin is *V. parahaemolyticus*, an important cause of seafood-borne diarrheal illness outbreaks. There is a strong association between clinical disease and the presence of the gene for thermostable direct hemolysin,[264, 265] a toxin with both cytotoxic (believed to be a result of pore-forming ability)[266] and enterotoxic (via mobilization of intracellular calcium in rabbit loops) activities.[202] Others have noted the tendency of *V. parahaemolyticus* to penetrate and cause bacteremia in animal models[267] or an invasive colitis in patients.[268] *V. parahaemolyticus* typically causes explosive watery diarrhea in foodborne outbreaks in coastal areas of the United States.[269]

S. aureus produces a nonantigenic Δ-toxin that impairs water absorption and causes cytotoxic disruption of intestinal mucosa or cells in tissue culture.[270] The clindamycin-resistant *C. difficile* isolated from patients with antibiotic-associated pseudomembranous enterocolitis produces a potent cytotoxin that is capable of causing cytotoxicity in tissue culture and death in a hamster model[271–273]; it also produces an enterotoxic product that causes hemorrhagic fluid secretion in rabbit ileal loops.[273, 274] Finally, the pathogenesis of *C. jejuni, H. pylori*, and possibly even *V. cholerae* may also involve cytotoxic products.[275–283]

Attachment

The ability of many enteric pathogens to cause disease depends not only on the organism's ability to penetrate the mucosa or to produce enterotoxin or cytotoxin but also on its ability to adhere to and colonize the mucosa. This adherence capacity has been well described with ETEC, which, to cause disease, must first adhere to and colonize the upper small bowel of humans or animals. This adherence capacity for *E. coli* is variously called K88, K99, or CFA for strains affecting piglets, calves, and humans, respectively. As with enterotoxigenicity, the production of these adherence antigens appears to be genetically encoded by transmissible plasmids. These fimbriate bacterial surface adhesins are distinct from type 1 pili and from recognized urinary tract adhesins[284, 286] and usually cause hemagglutination that is mannose resistant.[287, 288] Although these adhesins hold great promise for immunization against colonization, there are now at least five different types of CFA, among human ETEC: CFA-I, CFA-II, E8775, 260-1, and O159:H4.[281, 287–291]

Analogous to ETEC adhesins, fimbriate or fibrillar adhesins may also aid in the initial colonization of EHEC O157, EPEC, and EAggEC. The Shiga-like toxin–producing EHEC O26 has been shown to adhere to the mucosa of human fetal small intestinal tissue in vitro in a mannose-resistant fashion, a trait that is transmissible by a colicinogenic conjugative plasmid.[292] In addition, EHEC strain O157:H7 has been shown to have a 60-MDa plasmid that encodes a new type of fimbria that appear to mediate attachment to Henle 407 cells in tissue culture.[293]

Classic EPEC exhibit a qualitatively different localized and attaching and effacing adherence and F-actin polymerization in intestinal brush border and in HEp-2 cells.[294–300] This localized EPEC adherence involves a complex array of plasmid-mediated adherence,[301, 302] followed by chromosomally mediated effacement, protein phosphorylation, and actin condensation in the host cell.[303] The 50- to 60-MDa plasmid in EPEC encodes inducible, bundle-forming pili that share amino-terminal sequence homology with the toxin-coregulated pili in *V. cholerae* and are responsible for efficient adherence to HEp-2 cells in "localized" colonies.[303–305] This is followed by injection of a 90-kD protein known as Tir (translocated intimin receptor) directly into the host cytosol via a type III secretion system. Tyrosine phosphorylation of Tir readies it to act as a receptor for the 94-kD bacterial chromosomally encoded protein intimin, which leads to intimate attachment to intestinal epithelial cells. Subsequent actin accumulation and effacement (encoded by genes in the *locus of enterocyte effacement [LEE]* on the EPEC chromosome) create the characteristic "pedestal" on which the bacterium sits.[306, 307] EHEC isolates may share a similar mechanism of attachment, although the ultrastructural appearance of the "pedestal" is qualitatively different.[308]

Distinct from the localized adherence of EPEC to HEp-2 cells are the "aggregative" and "diffuse" adherence patterns (AA and DA, respectively), for which gene probes have been developed that detect some, but not all, *E. coli* with these phenotypes.[309–313] EAggEC have been associated with persistent diarrhea in children in a number of developing areas, in adults with AIDS, in travelers from developed areas, and, more recently, in a large outbreak in Japanese schoolchildren.[314–317] Several potentially pathogenic products of EAggEC include EAST-1,[199] a 12-kD heat-labile hemolysin,[318] the 108-kD PET,[201] and a heat-stable protein factor that causes interleukin-8 release from intestinal epithelial cells.[35] The diffusely adherent *E. coli* (DAEC) represent several serotypes as identified by gene probes for strain 1845[319] and for a 100-kb plasmid-encoded 100-kD protein adhesin (AIDA-I) from strain 2787 (O126:H27).[320] Because DAEC have been variably seen in association with diarrhea and controls, a pathogenic role has not yet been established.[321, 322]

Finally, *E. coli* with the colonization traits mentioned previously, but without enterotoxin production, like an engineered, colonizing, multiply toxin–deleted *V. cholerae* vaccine strain (lacking ctxA, zot, ace, and hly), is capable of causing diarrhea in animals[323–328] and in human volunteers fed *E. coli* with the colonization trait as a potential vaccine. This diarrhea was associated with modest elevations in fecal lactoferrin, implying an inflammatory component.[329] Whether such colonizing *E. coli* are responsible, alone or in part, for naturally occurring acute or prolonged diarrhea remains to be determined.

Invasiveness

The capacity of organisms such as *Shigella* and certain invasive strains of *E. coli* to invade and destroy epithelial cells is responsible for the inflammatory or dysenteric diarrhea they cause. This capacity is demonstrated in the laboratory by the guinea pig conjunctivitis (Sereny) test.[330] There is cell destruction and superficial inflammatory invasion of the cornea similar to that noted in colonic mucosa. Modifications in the specific components of the O side chain of the cell wall lipopolysaccharide alter this invasive property in *Shigella*.[331, 332] There is also evidence that the invasiveness of certain *E. coli* may be reflected in their O antigens or serotype.[333, 334] Invasiveness is also associated with large, 120- to 140-MDa plasmids in *S. sonnei*,[204] *S. flexneri*,[335] and invasive *E. coli*.[336] HeLa cell, rabbit loop, and Sereny test invasiveness can be genetically constructed by the sequential transfer of defined chromosomal and plasmid genes for *S. flexneri* to *E. coli* K12.[337]

Cell invasion, unlike superficial colonization, may involve attachment to transmembrane glycoproteins (instead of carbohydrates and glycolipids) such as integrin bound by *Yersinia* invasin.[338] The expression of "invasiveness" is complex. In *Shigella* and EIEC, it appears to involve a series of plasmid-encoded invasion and adhesin proteins (ipaA through ipaD) that are regulated by key chromosomal codons (e.g., kcpA).[337–339] Once *Shigella* enters the host cell, a complex array of proteins induces condensation of host actin in a polar fashion, which allows the bacterium to propel itself through the cytoplasm to enhance its invasive properties.[340] In *Salmonella*, adherence and invasion appear to be closely linked and may require bacterial proteins that are induced by trypsin and neuraminidase-sensitive structures present on the epithelial cell surface.[341] The capacity of *Entamoeba histolytica* to adhere and "invade" relates, at least in part, to a GalNAc-inhibitable amebic lectin that leads to contact-dependent cytolysis of host cells, particularly attracted neutrophils.[342–344] As discussed previously, cytotoxic exotoxins may well play roles in the invasive and destructive properties of certain shigellae, *V. parahaemolyticus*, staphylococci, and clostridia.

Finally, many enteric pathogens include a vigorous host response which in and of itself can lead to diarrhea. For example, invasion by *Shigella* or *Salmonella* and adherence by *E. histolytica* lead to release of a wide array of proinflammatory cytokines from intestinal epithelial cells.[345] In addition, secreted or otherwise released culture products of several bacteria (including EAggEC, *H. pylori*, and *C. difficile*) have been shown to cause release of interleukin-8 from intestinal epithelial cells.[35, 346, 347] This leads to accumulation of neutrophils that can release 5′-AMP, which is cleaved to adenosine by an apical 5′-nucleotidase, causing electrogenic chloride secretion.[348] Even noninvasive, nontoxigenic organisms may induce fluid secretion by causing subepithelial cells to secrete prostaglandins or other secretory mediators. In the case of *C. parvum*, this host response is vigorous enough to create a secretory effect of stool from infected patients in the absence of any identifiable enterotoxin.[349] Whether induction of host inflammation is of itself a pathogenic feature of these organisms remains to be determined.

Other Virulence Factors

In addition to enterotoxin production and adherence, an orchestrated set of additional virulence traits appears to be critical to the ability of pathogens such as *V. cholerae* to succeed in colonizing the intestinal mucosa. These include motility,[350, 351] chemotaxis,[57, 352] and mucinase production,[353, 354] any one of which can be missing and lead to reduced virulence. The virulence of certain enteric pathogens such as *S. typhi* appears to be related to the Vi antigen[352] and to the polysaccharide composition of the O side chain of its lipopolysaccharide cell wall content,[355, 356] both of which have been used in vaccine production.[357–359] The virulence factors that enable enteric pathogens such as *Y. enterocolitica* to cause an enteric fever–like illness or mesenteric adenitis are less clear.

Another potential enteric pathogen that is increasingly recognized with improved culture techniques is *Campylobacter. C. jejuni* tends to cause more diarrhea than *Campylobacter fetus*; some *C. jejuni* have been reported to produce an LT-like enterotoxin,[360] or a cytotoxin,[277] and *C. fetus* causes more febrile systemic illness with bacteremia, perhaps related to the lipopolysaccharide and greater serum resistance of the organism.[361, 362] The mechanisms by which *Campylobacter* causes disease remain unclear.[361]

Still another way that organisms can cause diarrhea involves the selective destruction of absorptive cells (villus tip cells) in the mucosa, leaving secretory cells (crypt cells) intact.[362–365] Both the rotaviruses and the Norwalk-like viruses, which selectively infect and disrupt the villus tip cells, alter the normal absorptive fluid balance, and reduce the brush-border digestive enzymes present during active infection.[364, 365] Such an imbalanced disruption of the specialized absorptive surface may also be involved in other small bowel infections that are often associated with villus tip flattening or microvillus destruction, including bacterial overgrowth syndromes, EPEC infections, giardiasis, strongyloidiasis, and cryptosporidiosis.

MAJOR SYNDROMES OF DERANGED GASTROINTESTINAL PHYSIOLOGY

The elements of net fluid balance in the healthy adult intestinal tract are shown diagrammatically in Figure 81–1. With a daily oral intake

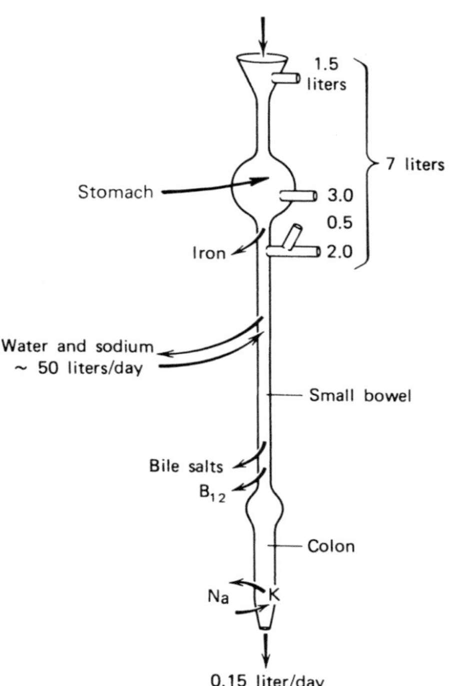

FIGURE 81–1. Diagram of fluid balance in the healthy adult gastrointestinal tract.

of 1.5 liters, salivary, gastric, biliary, and pancreatic secretions contribute a total of approximately 8.5 liters of fluid that enters the upper gastrointestinal tract each day. However, daily fecal fluid excretion is normally less than 150 ml, indicating a net absorption of more than 8 liters each day by the intestinal tract. More than 90% of this net absorption occurs in the small bowel, where there is a massive bidirectional flux that probably exceeds 50 liters/day. A relatively slight shift in the bidirectional flux can result in substantial overload of the colonic absorptive capacity, which rarely exceeds 2 to 3 liters/day. As in the kidney, there are hormonal, physical, and osmotic factors active in the intestinal tract. Aldosterone, for example, enhances intestinal sodium absorption at the expense of potassium.[366, 367] Excessive fluid volume results in a "third factor" effect that may elicit or prolong diarrhea,[368] and osmotic laxatives are as familiar as osmotic diuretics.

Enteric disease can be produced by microbe-host interactions that alter normal intestinal physiology in one of three ways: (1) a shift in the delicate balance of bidirectional water and electrolyte fluxes in the upper small bowel by intraluminal toxins or minimally invasive organisms (e.g., *Giardia, Cryptosporidium*), (2) inflammatory destruction of the ileal or colonic mucosa, or (3) penetration through an intact mucosa to the reticuloendothelial system. These three types of enteric infections are outlined in Table 81–6. They can often be distinguished by a quick, simple examination. Mucus from a fresh stool specimen is mixed with a drop of methylene blue on a slide and examined for the presence of fecal leukocytes.[369, 370] In most cases, no leukocytes are noted. This suggests a noninflammatory process in which diarrhea usually arises from the upper small bowel by the action of a true enterotoxin or agents such as *Giardia* or viruses. The secretory effects of certain enterotoxins share similar mechanisms with noninfectious endocrine causes of diarrhea such as non–β-cell islet tumors, medullary carcinoma of the thyroid, carcinoid tumors, and other benign or malignant neoplasms that are associated with increased serum prostaglandins, vasoactive intestinal polypeptide, or changes in cyclic nucleotide concentrations.[371] Impaired small bowel absorption is important in tropical sprue, enzyme deficiencies, and solute loads. Enhanced colonic secretion without an inflammatory response characteristic of microbial or ulcerative colitis may result from excessive bile salts or fatty acids or from malignancies such as villous adenomas.

The presence of numerous polymorphonuclear leukocytes documents an inflammatory or invasive process that usually arises from the colon or distal small bowel. Amebic colitis can often be distinguished from bacterial dysenteries by microscopic fecal examination. In addition to the amebic trophozoites or cysts, fecal neutrophils are usually pyknotic or absent with amebiasis, probably because of the cytopathic effect of virulent amebae on mammalian cells, including neutrophils.[372, 373] Impaired colonic absorption may contribute to the diarrhea in inflammatory colitis caused by shigellosis, pseudomembranous enterocolitis, amebic colitis, or idiopathic ulcerative colitis. In addition, evidence suggests that the products of the lipoxygenase and other pathways in neutrophils may also contribute to a secretory process.[220, 221] Agents that cause an inflammatory colitis may require specific antimicrobial intervention as well as supportive fluid therapy.[370]

The third type of enteric infection is caused by organisms that penetrate the intact intestinal mucosa, often in the distal small bowel, to multiply in the lymphatic or reticuloendothelial cells. This usually results in a febrile systemic illness with or without diarrhea. If diarrhea is present, mononuclear leukocytes may be found in the stools of these patients.[369] Cultural documentation of the pathogen is important, because a bacteremia that necessitates specific antimicrobial therapy may result in this setting.

The tripartite distinction among enteric infections is by no means absolute. For example, *C. difficile* colitis is pathophysiologically an inflammatory diarrhea, although there are often no visible fecal leukocytes. In addition, certain pathogens considered noninflammatory (e.g., *Cryptosporidium*, EPEC, EAggEC) actually are associated with varying degrees of villus destruction and inflammation, as measured both by histopathology and by more sensitive assays for fecal inflammatory markers such as lactoferrin, interleukin-1, and interleukin-8.[35, 374] As more of the pathophysiology of enteric infections is understood, these categories may require further revision.

DIAGNOSTIC APPROACH TO ENTERIC INFECTIONS

The appropriate diagnostic approach to diarrheal illness is determined by the patient's age, the severity of illness, the duration of illness, the type of illness, and the available facilities. Of greatest importance in patients with diarrhea are a careful history, physical examination, and examination of a fresh stool specimen for fecal leukocytes. A history of recent antibiotic use, weight loss, underlying diseases, other illnesses in the family or in other contacts, or travel outside the United States, to the seacoast, or to rural mountainous areas should elicit a more careful investigation of specific etiologic agents. A prompt evaluation of physical signs of fever, toxicity, or severe dehydration may result in lifesaving supportive fluid therapy. Particularly worrisome signs of severe dehydration, especially in children, include lethargy, postural hypotension and tachycardia, sunken fontanelles, and dry skin (with decreased turgor), dry eyes, or dry mucous membranes.

As noted in Figure 81–2, if the history or physical findings indicate anything more than a mild, isolated, afebrile illness, examination of a fresh stool specimen, preferably collected in a cup, is particularly valuable. First, it provides the physician with an objective determination of the patient's subjective complaints. Second, a gross description of the stool as either watery, mucoid, or bloody provides important clues about its cause and appropriate management. Third, a microscopic examination for fecal leukocytes, as described previously, may reveal heavy parasitic intestinal infestations or maldigested fat or meat fibers suggesting pancreatic insufficiency, or lipid droplets suggesting malabsorption with steatorrhea. If fever or fecal neutrophils are present, the physician should selectively take a culture for the most commonly recognized invasive

TABLE 81-6 Three Types of Enteric Infection

Characteristic	Type I	Type II	Type III
Mechanism	Noninflammatory (enterotoxin or adherence/superficial invasion)	Inflammatory (invasion, cytotoxin)	Penetrating
Location	Proximal small bowel	Colon	Distal small bowel
Illness	Watery diarrhea	Dysentery	Enteric fever
Stool examination	No fecal leukocytes Mild or no ↑ lactoferrin	Fecal polymorphonuclear leukocytes ↑ ↑ lactoferrin	Fecal mononuclear leukocytes
Examples	*Vibrio cholerae* *Escherichia coli* (ETEC, LT, ST) *Clostridium perfringens* *Bacillus cereus* *Staphylococcus aureus* Also†: *Giardia lamblia* Rotavirus Norwalk-like viruses *Cryptosporidium parvum* *E. coli* (EPEC, EAggEC) Microsporidia *Cyclospora cayetanensis*	*Shigella* *E. coli* (EIEC, EHEC) *Salmonella enteritidis* *Vibrio parahaemolyticus* *Clostridium difficile* *Campylobacter jejuni* *Entamoeba histolytica**	*Salmonella typhi* *Yersinia enterocolitica* *?Campylobacter fetus*

*Although amebic dysentery involves tissue inflammation, the leukocytes are characteristically pyknotic or absent, having been destroyed by the virulent amebae.[372]
†Although not typically enterotoxic, these pathogens alter bowel physiology via adherence, superficial cell entry, cytokine induction, or toxins that inhibit cell function.

pathogens—*C. jejuni, Salmonella*, and *Shigella*.[370] Cup specimens, when promptly examined for leukocytes, provide a highly sensitive screen for invasive processes such as shigellosis or *C. jejuni* enteritis.[374, 374a, 375] Swab or diaper specimens appear to be less sensitive.[375] A newer and simpler test for fecal lactoferrin provides a rapid, sensitive marker for fecal leukocytes that is effective even with swab or refrigerated samples.[376] Any grossly bloody stool specimen should also be examined for *E. coli* O157 by growth on sorbitol-McConkey agar and for other SLT-producing *E. coli* by a newer SLT assay. In the United States, EHEC is the most common cause of bloody diarrhea and should be suspected particularly if fever is absent.[80] Any patient with a history of recent antibiotic or antineoplastic drug use should have a stool assay for *C. difficile* toxins, regardless of the results of the microscopic stool examination. A history of recent antibiotic use, weight loss, and chronic diarrhea (>10 days); seacoast or other exposures; or immunocompromised states should prompt the physician to consider other agents as noted.

Other diagnostic studies that can be made on fecal specimens include special stains for fat or muscle and determinations of pH and reducing substances. A Sudan stain may reveal many large (10 to 75 μm), orange-stained globules of fat, suggesting malabsorption, or smaller (1 to 4 μm) globules or needle-like crystals of fatty acid that may be normal. Numerous undigested muscle fibers may be seen with an aqueous 2% eosin stain and suggest pancreatic insufficiency and maldigestion.

An acidic stool pH can be helpful in the identification of lactose intolerance, especially in children with diarrhea. Although breast-fed infants have a fecal pH ranging from 4.7 to 5.1, stool pH usually exceeds 7.0 if the infant is on a regular milk-containing diet. On a regular diet, a fecal pH less than 5.0 suggests the presence of lactic acid from the action of colonic bacterial flora on unabsorbed lactose. Stool-reducing substances may also be helpful in the detection of carbohydrate malabsorption. A simple test uses copper sulfate (Clinitest) tablets. Mix 1 ml stool with 2 ml water, add 15 drops of this mixture to a test tube, and then add one copper sulfate tablet. A reduction positive for "sugar" indicates reducing substances. Positive tests for blood may suggest an invasive process such as amebiasis or shigellosis. Although this is usually evident from a gross examination of the stool, tests for occult blood are much more sensitive but less specific. Tests for hemoglobin peroxidase use orthotolidine, benzidine, or guaiac reagents, in descending order of sensitivity. Some are so sensitive that they may be positive with ingested meat myoglobin. Twenty-four-hour determinations for fecal fat (normal <7.2 g/day fecal fat or <150 to 200 g/day total stool weight) may also be of value.

For culture of enteric pathogens, the specimen should be inoculated onto culture plates as promptly as possible.[377] The media used are selective and often contain indicator substances that aid in initial identification. Routine techniques must now include selective culture for *C. jejuni*, one of the most common causes of inflammatory diarrhea throughout the world.[378] For optimal results, this test requires a highly selective atmosphere of reduced oxygen (4 to 6%) and increased carbon dioxide (6 to 10%) and an increased incubator temperature (42°C). Selective media and means to obtain the proper atmosphere are now available.[378–381] When culturing stool from homosexual men with diarrhea, it should be kept in mind that *Helicobacter cinaedi* and *Campylobacter fenelliae* do not grow at 42°C. Routine stool culture also includes a medium, such as MacConkey's or eosin methylene blue (EMB) agar, that inhibits gram-positive organisms and selects predominantly for aerobic gram-negative rods. In addition, more selective media (e.g., xylose-lysine-deoxycholate, *Salmonella-Shigella* agar) and enrichment broths (e.g., gram-negative, selenite, tetrathionate) that inhibit most organisms except *Salmonella* and *Shigella* should be used. However, because highly selective media are also more inhibitory, the less selective MacConkey's and EMB agar should also be examined for non–lactose-fermenting (colorless) colonies that may be salmonellae or shigellae. Even the best techniques with fresh specimens may miss fragile organisms such as shigellae.[377, 380] Fecal cultures failed to yield shigellae in 40% of volunteers with inflammatory diarrhea from experimental *Shigella* infection.[369] When immediate culture is impossible, specimens may be transported to a laboratory in a non-nutrient holding medium, such as Cary-Blair soft agar, that prevents drying and overgrowth of normal flora.

Culture of vibrios (*V. cholerae, V. parahaemolyticus*, and others), which should be suspected after any exposure to coastal areas or seafood, requires the highly selective thiosulfate citrate bile salt sucrose agar.[6, 381] Selective culture for *C. difficile* and examination for fecal cytotoxin[268, 269, 382] may be indicated in patients with refractory antibiotic-associated diarrhea or colitis. Culture of *Y. enterocolitica* may require the selective process of "cold enrichment" on sheep blood agar or phosphate-buffered saline for 2 to 3 weeks[383] and should be considered for patients receiving desferrioxamine or with a history of raw pork consumption.

E. coli that grow readily as dry, lactose-fermenting (purple) colonies on EMB or MacConkey's agar are major aerobic constituents of normal fecal flora but should also be considered as potential pathogens. Certain serotypes have been associated with inflammatory diarrhea,[357] bloody diarrhea,[232–237] outbreaks of diarrhea in newborn nurseries, or even ST or LT production.[384] However, determination

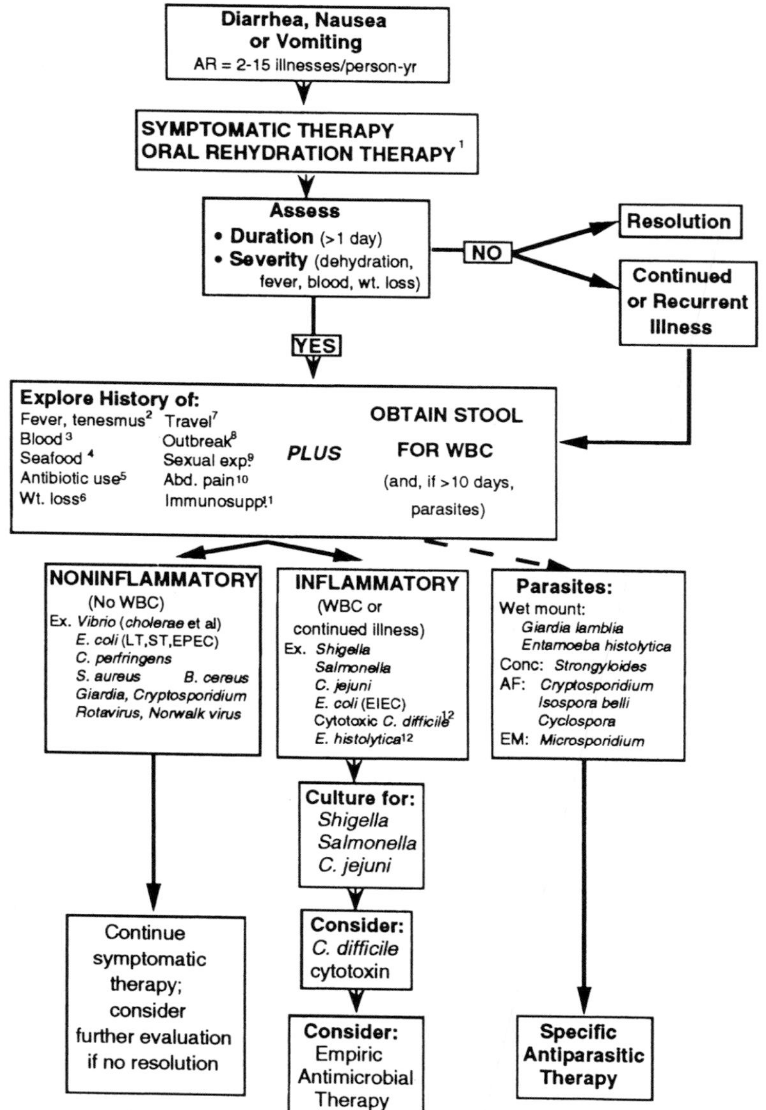

FIGURE 81–2. Approach to diagnosis and management of infectious diarrhea. Key to superscripts: *1.* Oral rehydration solution (ORS) can be prepared by adding 3.5 g NaCl, 2.5 g NaHCO3 (or 2.9 g Na citrate), 1.5 g KCl, and 20 g glucose or glucose polymer (e.g., 40 g sucrose; 4 tablespoons sugar; 50 to 60 g cereal flour such as rice, maize, sorghum, millet, wheat, or potato) to 1 liter (1.05 qt) of clean water. This makes approximately Na 90, K 20, Cl 80, HCO3 30, and glucose 111 mmol/liter. One level teaspoon table salt and 8 level teaspoons table sugar per liter makes about 86 mmol Na and 30 g sucrose/liter, to which one could add 1 cup orange juice or two bananas for potassium. *2.* Fever or tenesmus suggests an inflammatory proctocolitis. *3.* Diarrhea with blood, especially without fecal leukocytes, suggests enterohemorrhagic (Shiga-like toxin–producing) *Escherichia coli* or amebiasis (in which leukocytes are destroyed by the parasite). *4.* Ingestion of inadequately cooked seafood should prompt consideration of infections with *Vibrio* or Norwalk-like viruses. *5.* Antibiotics should be stopped if possible and cytotoxigenic *Clostridium difficile* considered. Antibiotics may also predispose to other infections such as salmonellosis. *6.* Persistence (>10 days) with weight loss should prompt consideration of giardiasis, cyclosporiasis, cryptosporidiosis. *7.* Travel to tropical areas increases the chance of developing enterotoxigenic *E. coli* (ETEC) as well as viral (Norwalk-like or rotaviral), parasitic *(Giardia, Entamoeba, Strongyloides, Cryptosporidium)*, and, if fecal leukocytes are present, invasive bacterial infections as noted in the algorithm. *8.* Outbreaks should prompt consideration of *Staphylococcus aureus, Bacillus cereus*, anisakiasis (incubation period <6 hours), *Clostridium perfringens, Cryptosporidium*, ETEC, *Vibrio, Salmonella, Campylobacter, Shigella*, or enteroinvasive *E. coli* (EIEC) infection. During spring and summer months, *Cyclospora* should also be considered. Consider saving *E. coli* for LT, ST, invasiveness, adherence testing, and serotyping; stool for rotavirus; and stool plus paired sera for Norwalk-like virus or toxin testing. *9.* Sigmoidoscopy in symptomatic homosexual men should distinguish proctitis in the distal 15 cm only (caused by herpesvirus, gonococcal, chlamydial, or syphilitic infection) from colitis (*Campylobacter, Shigella, C. difficile*, or chlamydial [LGV serotypes] infections) or noninflammatory diarrhea (giardiasis). *10.* If unexplained abdominal pain and fever persist or suggest an appendicitis-like syndrome, culture for *Yersinea enterocolitica* with cold enrichment. *11.* In immunocompromised hosts, a wide range of viral (cytomegalovirus, herpes simplex virus, coxsackievirus, rotavirus), bacterial (*Salmonella, Mycobacterium avium* complex), and parasitic *(Cryptosporidium, Isospora, Strongyloides, Entamoeba*, and *Giardia)* agents should be considered. *12.* If the fecal lactoferrin latex agglutination titer is 1:50 or higher, even if fecal leukocytes are absent, an inflammatory diarrhea should be considered, because some inflammatory colonic pathogens such as cytotoxigenic *C. difficile* or *Entamoeba histolytica* can destroy fecal leukocyte morphology. (Adapted from Guerrant RL, Bobak DA. Bacterial and protozoal gastroenteritis. N Engl J Med. 1991;325:327–340, with permission.)

of enterotoxigenicity depends not on serotypes but on detection of the toxin itself. Therefore, routine serotyping of *E. coli* in sporadic cases is of limited value and should be considered a special tool for investigating epidemic diarrhea in settings such as newborn nurseries or unexplained dysentery. Special tests for the cholera-like, heat-labile, adenylate cyclase–activating enterotoxin may use rabbit ileal loop,[158] rabbit skin permeability,[159] Chinese hamster ovary cell,[160] Y1 adrenal cell,[161] immunoassay,[162–164] or direct assay for the enterotoxin gene.[165, 385] The heat-stable enterotoxin acts through a different mechanism and currently requires the suckling mouse assay for its detection.[386, 387] EIEC may be identified by inoculation into the conjunctival sac of guinea pigs (Sereny test).[357]

When diarrhea persists unexplained, especially with blood or weight loss, examinations for protozoa and *Strongyloides stercoralis* are indicated, using specific techniques for the pathogens suspected. An acid-fast stain detects *Cryptosporidium* and *Cyclospora*; two newer tests for the former that require less technical experience are an enzyme immunoassay and a fluorescent-tagged antibody stain. A modified trichrome stain for microsporidia should also be considered for patients with AIDS. If *Giardia* or *E. histolytica* is suspected, specific enzyme immunassays, which offer an alternative to microscopic examination, are available.

Proctoscopic examination can be very helpful in the differential diagnosis, especially when inflammatory colitis is present. Although necrotic ulcers may be seen in acute shigellosis, discrete ulcers are more suggestive of amebiasis or Crohn's disease. Mucosal friability is more suggestive of inflammatory bowel disease (e.g., ulcerative colitis). The appearance of raised, plaque-like pseudomembranes is diagnostic of pseudomembranous colitis due to toxigenic *C. difficile*. Large amounts of mucus may be present in "mucous colitis" or with a villous adenoma; melanosis coli may suggest laxative abuse.

Rectal mucosal biopsy specimens, especially when ulcers are present, can be of great help for identification of the parasite *E. histolytica*, granulomata, amyloidosis (with Congo red stain), or Whipple's disease (with periodic acid–Schiff stain). Small bowel biopsy specimens may also be diagnostic in Whipple's disease, giardiasis, amyloidosis, a β-lipoproteinemia, lymphoma, cryptosporidiosis, giardiasis, microsporidiosis, or mast-cell disease. Characteristic but not necessarily diagnostic histopathologic changes may be seen in celiac disease, tropical sprue, eosinophilic gastroenteritis, dermatitis herpetiformis, and dysgammaglobulinemia. However, several conditions, including Crohn's disease, bacterial overgrowth syndrome, and pancreatic or bile salt insufficiency, may be associated with normal small bowel histologic findings or with nonspecific changes.

Radiologic studies of the intestinal tract may reveal toxic megacolon, pancreatic calcifications, or nodular adrenal calcifications suggestive of tuberculosis or histoplasmosis. Colonic mucosal edema with a "thumbprint" appearance has been reported on barium enema studies of patients with bloody diarrhea and *E. coli* O157 infection.[235] Although barium studies may reveal nonspecific changes in the small bowel (giardiasis) or colon (inflammatory colitis), they are less useful in diagnosing microbial diarrheas. Indeed, the barium contrast material renders a microscopic examination of stool virtually useless.

Bacterial overgrowth syndrome may result in deconjugation of bile salts that can be tested with a ^{14}C-glycocholic acid breath test. Carbon-14–labeled carbon dioxide in the breath represents the degradation product of bacterial deconjugation of bile salts.

PREVENTION, CONTROL, AND THERAPY

The public health measures of improved water supply and sanitation facilities are most important for the control of the majority of enteric infections. Another important area for intervention lies in the quality control of commercial products such as bottled water and beverages. These may have been responsible for outbreaks of significant enteric infections such as cholera in Portugal[388] and typhoid fever in Mexico.[389]

Nonspecific host factors should be appreciated to minimize their violation. Examples include careful personal hygiene and limited, judicious use of antacids, antimotility drugs, and antimicrobial agents.

Vaccines may be used to boost specific immune processes directed against the bacteria themselves, or against adherence appendages, cytotoxins, or enterotoxins. Perhaps the most useful are the live gal-epimerase mutant typhoid vaccine[355] and the Vi polysaccharide capsule vaccine against typhoid fever.[356, 358] A live, attenuated cholera vaccine (CVD-103HgR) is currently available in Europe. In addition, a tetravalent rotavirus vaccine has been approved for use in the United States.[390] To date, there are no effective vaccines against a parasitic enteric infection, and much new work is required to improve the understanding of host defenses against enteric parasitic processes.

New possibilities for pharmacologic antagonists to microbial adherence or to toxin action are on the horizon. New types of "antibiotics" may work by blocking the formation of bacterial adherence factors, binding bacterial adherence appendages, or acting as lectin-like competitors for the host cell receptors that enable microorganisms to colonize the gastrointestinal tract.[391] Finally, specific competitors for either the binding or the action of enterotoxins hold promise. For example, monosialoganglioside (G_{m1}) successfully binds cholera toxin or the heat-labile enterotoxin of *E. coli* in vitro and in animal experiments. Pharmacologic reversal of the cyclic nucleotide–associated secretory process may also be possible. Such a mechanism has been suggested for bismuth subsalicylate (Pepto-Bismol).[392]

Specific antimicrobial chemotherapy may be indicated, especially in inflammatory processes such as shigellosis or in parasitic diseases such as giardiasis or amebiasis.

Of greatest importance in the treatment of microbial diarrhea, regardless of the cause or category, is fluid replacement (ORT). The degree of volume depletion must first be assessed by examining the turgor of the skin and mucous membranes, by noting the amount of lacrimation, and by obtaining a history of urinary output. Postural lightheadedness with changes in pulse and blood pressure are helpful objective parameters of volume depletion. It has been documented that, despite the severest form of secretory derangement in cholera, glucose absorption and its coupled sodium and water absorption remain intact in the upper small bowel. Therefore, many patients can be completely rehydrated and maintained by a simple oral glucose–containing electrolyte solution. A controlled study of patients with cholera and other noninflammatory watery diarrheal diseases in Dacca, Bangladesh, documented the efficacy of both sucrose (table sugar) and glucose in the ORT solution.[393] Electrolyte losses in severe watery diarrhea are similar to the electrolyte composition of serum, and fluid replacement should contain approximately these concentrations of electrolytes.

A standard ORT regimen contains 3.5 g NaCl, 2.5 g $NaHCO_3$, 1.5 g KCl, and 20 g glucose per liter of boiled water. This corresponds to sodium 90, potassium 20, bicarbonate 30, chloride 80, and glucose 110 mmol/liter.[344] A similar solution may be prepared with 3 level tablespoons of sugar, ¾ teaspoon salt, ½ teaspoon sodium bicarbonate in 1 cup of orange juice to make up 1 liter (1.05 qt) in water. If there is concern about hypertonicity, particularly in children, the salt can be reduced in cases of milder diarrhea, and the solution should be given with ad libitum water. Still another alternative is 1 level teaspoon of salt and 8 level teaspoons of sugar per liter (or quart) of water, which makes approximately 86 mmol sodium and 30 g sucrose per liter, to which one could add 1 cup of orange juice or two bananas for potassium. A further improvement can be made by substituting 40 to 50 g cereal flour (rice, maize, sorghum, millet, wheat, or potato) for glucose.[395] The electrolyte contents of commonly available soft drinks are variable, although solutions of similar electrolyte composition to the ideal described here can be made in dilute solutions of bouillon or gelatin water. New developments in ORT include the use of rice powder or other glucose polymers and the use of amino acids such as glycine, alanine, and glutamine, which enhance sodium absorption independently of glucose. Glutamine-containing ORT solutions are of particular interest because of the importance of glutamine as the major enterocyte energy source; current studies examining whether these solutions offer an advantage over standard ORT appear promising.[32, 401–403]

REFERENCES

1. World Health Organization. Tropical disease 1990. ASM News. 1990;56:358–359.
2. Guerrant RL, McAuliffe JF. Special problems in developing countries. In: Gorbach SL, ed. Infectious Diarrhea. Boston: Blackwell Scientific; 1986:287–307.
3. Snyder JD, Merson MH. The magnitude of the global problem of acute diarrhoeal disease: A review of active surveillance data. Bull World Health Organ. 1982;60:604–613.
4. Warren KS. Tropical medicine or tropical health: The Heath Clark Lectures, 1988. Rev Infect Dis. 1990;12:142–156.
5. Guerrant RL, Hughes JM, Lima NL, et al. Diarrhea in developed and developing countries: Magnitude, special settings, and etiologies. Rev Infect Dis. 1990;12(Suppl 1):S41–S50.
6. Guerrant RL, Bobak DA. Bacterial and protozoal gastroenteritis. N Engl J Med. 1991;325:327–340.
7. Cohen ML. The epidemiology of diarrheal disease in the United States. Infect Dis Clin North Am. 1988;2:557–570.
8. Ho M-S, Glass RI, Pinsky PR, et al. Diarrheal deaths in American children: Are they preventable? JAMA. 1988;260:3281–3285.
9. Impact of oral rehydration therapy on hospital admission and case-fatality rates for diarrhoeal disease: Results from 11 countries. WHO Weekly Epidemiol Rec No. 8. 1988;49–52.
10. Yunes J. Evaluation of infant mortality and proportional infant mortality in Brazil. World Health Stats Q. 1981;34:200–219.
11. McAuliffe JF, Shields DS, de Souza MA, et al. Prolonged and recurring diarrhea in the northeast of Brazil: Examination of cases from a community-based study. J Pediatr Gastroenterol Nutr. 1986;5:902–906.
12. Schorling JB, Wanke CA, Schorling SK, et al. A prospective study of persistent diarrhea among children in an urban Brazilian slum. Am J Epidemiol. 1990;132:144–156.
13. Bhatnager S, Dosajh U. Diarrhoeal disease morbidity in children below 5 years in urban slums of Delhi. Indian J Med Res. 1986;84:53–58.
14. Black RE, Brown KH, Becker S, et al. Longitudinal studies of infectious diseases and physical growth of children in rural Bangladesh. Am J Epidemiol. 1982;115:315–324.
15. Mata LJ. The Children of Santa Maria Cauque: A Prospective Field Study of Health and Growth. Cambridge, MA: MIT Press; 1978.
16. Guerrant RL, Kirchhoff LV, Shields DS, et al. Prospective study of diarrheal illness in northeastern Brazil: Patterns of disease, nutritional impact, etiologies and risk factors. J Infect Dis. 1983;148:986.
17. Guerrant RL, Moore RA, Kirschenfeld PM, et al. Role of toxigenic and invasive bacteria in acute diarrhea in childhood. N Engl J Med. 1975;293:567–573.
18. Gordon JE, Chitkara ID, Wyon JB. Weanling diarrhea. Am J Med Sci. 1963;245:345.
19. Gordon JE, Scrimshaw NS. Infectious disease in the malnourished. Med Clin North Am. 1970;54:1495.
20. Lindenbaum J. Malabsorption during and after recovery from acute intestinal infection. BMJ 1965;2:326.
21. Hirschhorn N, Molla A. Reversible jejunal disaccharidase deficiency in cholera and other acute diarrheal diseases. J Hopkins Med J. 1969;125:291.
22. Lindenbaum J, Kent TH, Sprinz H. Malabsorption and jejunitis in American Peace Corps volunteers in Pakistan. Ann Intern Med. 1966;65:1201.
23. Chen LC, Scrimshaw NS, eds. Diarrhea and Malnutrition: Interactions, Mechanisms and Interventions. New York: Plenum Press; 1983.
24. Schorling JB, Guerrant RL. Diarrhea and catch-up growth. Lancet 1990;335:599–600.
25. Guerrant RL, Schorling JB, McAuliffe JF, et al. Diarrhea as a cause and effect of malnutrition: Diarrhea prevents catch-up growth and malnutrition increases diarrhea frequency and duration. Am J Trop Med Hyg. 1992;47:28–35.
26. Gordon JE, Guzman MA, Ascoli W, et al. Acute diarrhoeal disease in less developed countries: 2. Patterns of epidemiological behaviour in rural Guatemalan villages. Bull World Health Organ. 1964;31:9.
27. Bowie MD. Malnutrition and diarrhea. S Afr Med J. 1960;34:344.
28. Schorling JB, McAuliffe JF, de Souza MA, et al. Malnutrition is associated with increased diarrhoea incidence and duration among children in an urban Brazilian slum. Int J Epidemiol. 1990;19:728–735.
29. Black RE, Brown RH, Becker S. Malnutrition in determining factor in diarrheal duration, but not incidence, among young children in a longitudinal study in rural Bangledesh. Am J Clin Nutr. 1984;37:87–94.
30. McAuliffe JF, Shields DS, de Souza MA, et al. Prolonged and recurring diarrhea in the Northeast of Brazil: Examination of cases from a community-based study. J Pediatr Gastroenterol Nutr. 1986;5:902–906.
31. Schorling JB, Wanke CA, Schorling SK, et al. A prospective study of persistent diarrhea among children in an urban Brazilian slum. Am J Epidemiol. 1990;132:144–156.
32. Lima AAM, Barboza MS Jr, Melo AS, et al. Magnitude, impact and control of persistent diarrhea and malnutrition in a prospective cohort study of children in Northeast Brazil. Presented at International Centers for Tropical Disease Research meeting, National Institutes for Health, Bethesda, Md, May 2, 1998.
33. Checkley W, Gilman RH, Epstein LD, et al. Asymptomatic and symptomatic cryptosporidiosis: Their acute effect on weight gain in Peruvian children. Am J Epidemiol. 1997;145:156–163.
34. Agnew DG, Lima AAM, Newman RD, et al. Cryptosporidiosis in northeastern Brazilian children: Association with increased diarrheal morbidity. J Infect Dis. 1998;177:754–760.
35. Steiner T, Lima A, Nataro J, et al. Enteroaggregative *Escherichia coli* produce intestinal inflammation and growth impairment and cause interleukin-8 release from intestinal epithelial cells. J Infect Dis. 1998;177:88–96.
36. Sheehy TW. Digestive diseases as a national problem: VI. Enteric disease among United States troops in Vietnam. Gastroenterology. 1968;55:105.
37. Hodgkin K. Towards Earlier Diagnosis. A Family Doctor's Approach. Baltimore: Williams & Wilkins; 1963.
38. Hyams KC, Malone JD, Kapikian AZ, et al. Norwalk virus infection among Desert Storm troops. J Infect Dis. 1993;167:986–987.
39. Dingle JH, Badger GF, Jordan WS Jr. Illnesses in the Home: A Study of 25,000 Illnesses in a Group of Cleveland Families. Cleveland: The Press of Western Reserve University; 1964.
40. Bartlett AV, Moore M, Gary GW, et al. Diarrheal illness among infants and toddlers in daycare centers: II. Comparison with daycare home and households. J Pediatr. 1985;107:503–509.
41. Guerrant RL, Lohr JA, Williams EK. Acute infectious diarrhea: I. Epidemiology, etiology, and pathogenesis. Pediatr Infect Dis J. 1986;5:353–359.
42. Tauxe RV, Deming MS, Blake PA. *Campylobacter jejuni* infections on college campuses: A national survey. Am J Public Health. 1985;75:659–660.
43. Bartlett JG. *Clostridium difficile:* Clinical considerations. Rev Infect Dis. 1990;12(Suppl 2):S243–S251.
44. Hollister AC, Beck MD, Gittelsohn AM, et al. Influence of water availability on *Shigella* prevalence in children of farm labor families. Am J Public Health. 1955;45:354.
45. Steiner TS, Theilman NM, Guerrant RL. Protozoal agents: What are the dangers for the public water supply? Annu Rev Med. 1997;48:329–340.
46. Smith HW, Linggood MA. Observations of the pathogenic properties of the K88, Hly and Ent plasmids of *Escherichia coli* with particular reference to porcine diarrhea. J Med Microbiol. 1971;4:467.
47. Evans DG, Silver RP, Evans DJ, et al. Plasmid-controlled colonization factor associated with virulence in *Escherichia coli* enterotoxigenic for humans. Infect Immun. 1975;12:656.
48. Levine MM, Nalin DR, Rennels MB, et al. Genetic susceptibility to cholera. Ann Hum Biol. 1979;6:369–379.
49. Zisman M. Blood group A and giardiasis. Lancet. 1977;2:1285.
50. Rutter JM, Burrows MR, Sellwood R, et al. A genetic basis for resistance to enteric disease caused by *E. coli*. Nature. 1975;257:135.
51. Pier GB, Grout M, Zaidi T, et al. *Salmonella typhi* uses CFTR to enter intestinal epithelial cells. Nature. 1998;393:79–82.
52. Mobassaleh M, Koul O, Mishra K, et al. The developmental pattern of the regulatory enzymes involved in the synthesis and breakdown of the Shiga toxin receptor in rabbit small intestine. Gastroenterology. 1992;102:A567.
53. Chu SW, Walker WA. Bacterial toxin interaction with the developing intestine: A possible explanation for toxigenic diarrhea of infancy. Gastroenterology. 1993;104:916–925.
54. Cohen MB, Giannella RA. Jejunal toxin inactivation regulates susceptibility of the immature rat to STa. Gastroenterology. 1992;102:1988–1996.
55. Eglow R, Pothoulakis C, Itzkowitz S, et al. Diminished *Clostridium difficile* toxin A sensitivity in newborn rabbit ileum is associated with decreased toxin A receptor. J Clin Invest. 1992;90:822–829.
56. Bergman MJ, Evans DG, Sullivan JA, et al. Attachment of *E. coli* to human intestinal epithelial cells: A functional in vitro test for intestinal colonization factor. Trans Assoc Am Physicians. 1978;91:80.
57. Allweiss B, Dostal J, Carey KE, et al. The role of chemotaxis in the ecology of bacterial pathogens of mucosal surfaces. Nature. 1977;266:448.
58. Briscoe J. A role for water supply and sanitation in the child survival revolution. PAHO Bull. 1987;21:93–105.
59. Dolin R, Treanor JJ, Madore HP. Novel agents of viral enteritis in humans. J Infect Dis. 1987;55:365–375.
60. Blackow NR, Greenberg HB. Viral gastroenteritis. N Engl J Med. 1991;325:252–264.
61. Blacklow NR, Dolin R, Fedson DS, et al. Acute infectious nonbacterial gastroenteritis: Etiology and pathogenesis. Ann Intern Med. 1972;76:993.
62. Haas CN, Rose JB. Reconciliation of microbial risk models and outbreak epidemiology: The case of the Milwaukee outbreak. Proc Am Water Works Assoc 1994;517–523.
63. Giannella RA, Broitman SA, Zamcheck N. Gastric acid barrier to ingested microorganisms in man: Studies in vivo and in vitro. Gut. 1972;13:251.
64. Gorbach SL. Progress in gastroenterology: Intestinal microflora. Gastroenterology. 1971;60:1110.
65. Roberts SH, James O, Jarvis EH. Bacterial overgrowth syndrome without "blind loop": A cause for malnutrition in the elderly. Lancet. 1977;2:1193.
66. Hornick RB, Musik SI, Wenzel R, et al. The Broad Street pump revisited: Response of volunteers to ingested cholera vibrios. Bull N Y Acad Med. 1971;47:1181.
67. Gitelson S. Gastrectomy, achlorhydria and cholera. Isr J Med Sci. 1971;7:663.

68. Giannella RA, Broitman SA, Zamcheck N. Influence of gastric acidity on bacterial and parasitic enteric infections: A perspective. Ann Intern Med. 1973;78:271.
69. Black RE, Levine MM, Clements ML, et al. Experimental *Campylobacter jejuni* infection in humans. J Infect Dis. 1988;157:472–479.
70. Nurko SS, Garcia-Aranda JA, Consuelo A, et al. Is *Helicobacter pylori* a significant risk factor for persistent diarrhea in Mexican children? (Abstract). Gastroenterology. 1993;104:A160.
71. Driks MR, Craven DE, Celli BR, et al. Nosocomial pneumonia in intubated patients given sucralfate as compared with antacids or histamine type 2 blockers: The role of gastric colonization. N Engl J Med. 1987;317:1376.
72. Dixon JMS. The fate of bacteria in the small intestine. J Pathol Bacteriol. 1960;79:131.
73. Schrager J. The chemical composition and function of gastrointestinal mucus. Gut. 1970;11:450.
74. Higgens JA, Code CF, Orvis AL. The influence of motility on the rate of absorption of sodium and water from the small intestine of healthy persons. Gastroenterology. 1956;31:708.
75. Formal SB, Abrams GD, Schneider H, et al. Experimental *Shigella* infections: VI. Role of the small intestine in an experimental infection in guinea pigs. J Bacteriol. 1963;85:119.
76. Sprinz H. Pathogenesis of intestinal infections. Arch Pathol. 1969;87:556.
77. DuPont HL, Hornick RB. Adverse effect of Lomotil therapy in shigellosis. JAMA. 1973;226:1525.
78. Smith GS, Blaser MJ. Fatalities associated with *Campylobacter jejuni* infections. JAMA. 1985;253:2873–2875.
79. Feingold SM, George WL. Therapy directed against *Clostridium difficile* and its toxins: Complications of therapy. In: Rolfe RD, Feingold SM, eds. *Clostridium difficile*: Its role in intestinal disease. New York: Academic Press; 1988:342–357.
80. Slutsker L, Ries AA, Greene KD, et al. *Escherichia coli* O157:H7 diarrhea in the United States: Clinical and epidemiologic features. Ann Intern Med. 1997;126:505–513.
81. Holdeman LV, Cato EP, Moore WEC, eds. Anaerobe Laboratory Manual. Blacksburg, VA: Virginia Polytechnic and State University Anaerobe Laboratory; 1977.
82. Price DJE, Sleigh JD. Control of infection due to *Klebsiella* aerogenes in a neurosurgical unit by withdrawal of all antibiotics. Lancet. 1970;2:1213.
83. Mentzing LO, Ringertz O. *Salmonella* infection in tourists: 2. Prophylaxis against salmonellosis. Acta Pathol Microbiol Scand. 1968;74:405.
84. Bohnhoff M, Miller CP, Martin WR. Resistance of the mouse's intestinal track to experimental *Salmonella* infections. J Exp Med. 1964;120:805.
85. Van der Waaj D, Berguis JM, Lekkerkerk JEC. Colonization resistance of the digestive tract of mice during systemic antibiotic treatment. J Hyg. 1972;70:605–610.
86. Que JU, Casey SW, Hentges DJ. Factors responsible for increased susceptibility of mice to intestinal colonization after treatment with streptomycin. Infect Immun. 1986;53:116–123.
87. Tannock GW, Savage DC. Indigenous microorganisms prevent reduction in fecal size induced by *Salmonella typhimurium* in vaccinated gnotobiotic mice. Infect Immun. 1976;13:172.
88. Schrank GD, Verwey WF. Distribution of cholera organisms in experimental *Vibrio cholerae* infections: Proposed mechanisms of pathogenesis and antibacterial immunity. Infect Immun. 1976;13:195.
89. Ryan CA, Nickels MK, Hargrett-Bean NT, et al. Massive outbreak of antimicrobial-resistant salmonellosis traced to pasteurized milk. JAMA. 1987;258:3269–3274.
90. Pavia AT, Shipman LD, Wells JG, et al. Epidemiologic evidence that prior antimicrobial exposure decreases resistance to infection by antimicrobial-sensitive *Salmonella*. J Infect Dis. 1990;161:255–260.
91. Gorbach SL, Chang T-W, Goldin B. Successful treatment of relapsing *Clostridium difficile* colitis with lactobacillus GG. Lancet. 1987;2:1519.
92. Tvede M, Rask-Madsen J. Bacteriotherapy for chronic relapsing *Clostridium difficile* diarrhoea in six patients. Lancet. 1989;1:1156–1160.
93. Cuzzolin L, Zambreri D, Donini M, et al. Influence of radiotherapy on intestinal microflora in cancer patients. J Chemother. 1992;4:176–179.
94. Cudmore MA, Silva J Jr, Fekety R, et al. *Clostridium difficile* colitis associated with cancer chemotherapy. Arch Intern Med. 1982;142:333–335.
95. Silva J, Fekety R, Werk C, et al. Inciting and etiologic agents of colitis. Rev Infect Dis. 1984;6:S214.
96. Milligan DW, Kelly JK. Pseudomembranous colitis in a leukemia unit: Report of five fatal cases. J Clin Pathol. 1979;32:1237–1243.
97. Bodey GP, Buckley M, Sathe YS, et al. Quantitative relationships between circulating leukocytes and infection in patients with acute leukemia. Ann Intern Med. 1966;64:328.
98. Gandy W, Greenberg BR. Successful medical management of neutropenic enterocolitis. Cancer. 1983;51:1551–1555.
99. Dosik GM, Luna M, Valdivieso M, et al. Necrotizing colitis in patients with cancer. Am J Med. 1979;67:646–656.
100. Hopkins DG, Kushner JP. Clostridial species in the pathogenesis of necrotizing enterocolitis in patients with neutropenia. Am J Hematol. 1983;14:289–295.
101. Bodey GD, Fainstein V, Guerrant RL. Infections of the gastrointestinal tract in the immunocompromised patient. Annu Rev Med. 1986;37:271–281.
102. Yolken RH, Bishop CA, Townsend TR, et al. Infectious gastroenteritis in bone-marrow-transplant recipients. N Engl J Med. 1982;306:1009.
103. Smith PD, Lane C, Gill VJ, et al. Intestinal infections in patients with the acquired immunodeficiency syndrome (AIDS). Ann Intern Med. 1988;108:328–333.
104. Sperber SJ, Schleupner CJ. Salmonellosis during infection with human immunodeficiency virus. Rev Infect Dis. 1987;9:925–934.
105. Thielman NM, Guerrant RL. An algorithmic approach to the workup and management of HIV-related diarrhea. J Clin Outcomes Management. 1997;4:36–47.
106. Wanke CA, Mayer H, Weber R, et al. Enteroaggregative *Escherichia coli* as a potential cause of diarrheal disease in adults infected with human immunodeficiency virus. J Infect Dis. 1998;178:185–190.
107. Soave R, Johnson WD. *Cryptosporidium* and *Isospora belli* infections. J Infect Dis. 1988;157:225–229.
108. Colebunders R, Franastt, Mann J, et al. Persistent diarrhea, strongly associated with HIV infection in Kinshasa, Zaire. Am J Gastroenterol. 1987;82:859–864.
109. Sewankambo N, Mugerwa RD, Goodgame R, et al. Enteropathic AIDS in Uganda. An endoscopic, histological and microbiological study. AIDS. 1987;1:9–13.
110. Brandtzaeg P, Halstensen TS, Kett K, et al. Immunobiology and immunopathology of human gut mucosa: Humoral immunity and intraepithelial lymphocytes. Gastroenterology. 1989;97:1562–1584.
111. Grutzkau A, Hanski C, Hahn H, et al. Involvement of M cells in the bacterial invasion of Peyer's patches: A common mechanism shared by *Yersinia enterocolitica* and other enteroinvasive bacteria. Gut. 1990;31:1011–1015.
112. Wassef JS, Keren DF, Mailloux JL. Role of M cells in initial antigen uptake and in ulcer formation in the rabbit intestinal loop model of shigellosis. Infect Immun. 1989;57:858–863.
113. Marcial MM, Madara JL. *Cryptosporidium*: Cellular localization, structural analysis of absorptive cell-parasite membrane–membrane interactions in guinea pigs, and suggestion of protozoan transport by M cells. Gastroenterology. 1986;90:583–594.
114. Bull DM, Tomasi TB. Deficiency of immunoglobulin A in intestinal disease. Gastroenterology. 1968;54:313.
115. Hirschowitz B, Streeton D, Pollard M, et al. Role of gastric secretions in activation of peptic ulcers by corticotrophin (ACTH). JAMA. 1955;158:27–32.
116. Strober W, Krakauer R, Klaeveman HL, et al. Secretory component deficiency: A disorder of the IgA immune system. N Engl J Med. 1976;294:351–356.
117. Plaut AG. The IgAI proteases of pathogenic bacteria. Annu Rev Microbiol. 1983;37:603–622.
118. Kelsall BL, Ravdin JI. Degradation of human immunoglobulin by *Entamoeba histolytica*. 39th Meeting of the American Society for Microbiology, Nov. 4–8, 1990. Abstract No. 284:197.
119. Pierce NF, Reynolds HY: Immunity to experimental cholera: II. Secretory and humoral antitoxin response to local and systemic toxoid administration. J Infect Dis. 1975;131:383.
120. Pierce NF, Gowans JL. Cellular kinetics of the intestinal immune responses to cholera toxoid in rats. J Exp Med. 1975;142:1550.
121. Stoliar OA, Pelley RP, Kaniecki-Green E, et al. Secretory IgA against enterotoxins in breast-milk. Lancet. 1976;1:1258.
122. Brown SE III, Sauer KT, Nations-Shields M, et al. Comparison of paired whole milk and dried filter paper samples for antienterotoxin and anti-rotavirus activities. J Clin Microbiol. 1982;16:103.
123. Jones EG, Brown WR. Serum and intestinal fluid immunoglobulins in patients with giardiasis. Am J Dig Dis. 1974;19:791.
124. Zinneman HH, Kaplan AP. The associate of giardiasis with reduced intestinal secretory immunoglobulin A. Am J Dig Dis. 1972;17:793.
125. Ament ME, Ochs HD, Davis SD. Structure and function of the gastrointestinal tract in primary immunodeficiency syndromes: A study of 39 patients. Medicine. 1973;52:227.
126. Hermans PE, Huizenga KA, Hoffman HN, et al. Dysgammaglobulinemia associated with nodular lymphoid hyperplasia of the small intestine. Am J Med. 1966;40:78.
127. Crabbe PA, Heremans JF. Lack of gamma A-immunoglobulin in serum of patients with steatorrhea. Gut. 1966;7:119.
128. Collins FM, Carter PB. Cellular immunity in enteric disease. Am J Clin Nutr. 1974;27:1424.
129. Welsh JK, May JT. Anti-infective properties of breast milk. J Pediatr. 1979;94:1.
130. McClelland DBL, McGrath J, Samson RR. Antimicrobial factors in human milk: Studies of concentration and transfer to the infant during the early stages of lactation. Acta Paediatr Scand. 1978;27(Suppl):1.
131. Arnold RR, Cole MF, McGhee JR. A bactericidal effect for human lactoferrin. Science. 1977;197:263.
132. Griffiths E, Humphreys J. Bacteriostatic effect of human milk and bovine colostrum on *Escherichia coli*: Importance of bicarbonate. Infect Immun. 1977;15:396.
133. Bullen JJ, Rogers HJ, Leight L. Iron-binding proteins in milk and resistance to *Escherichia coli* infection in infants. BMJ 1975;1:69.
134. Hanson LA, Winberg J. Breast milk and defence against infection in the newborn. Arch Dis Child. 1972;47:845.
135. Cravioto A, Tello A, Villafán H, et al. Inhibition of localized adhesion of enteropathogenic *Escherichia coli* to HEp-2 cells by immunoglobulin and oligosaccharide fractions of human colostrum and breast milk. J Infect Dis. 1991;163:1247–1255.
135a. Robins-Browne RM, Prpic JK. Effects of iron and desferrioxamine on infections with *Yersinia enterocolitica*. Infect Immun. 1985;47:774–779.
136. Levine MM. *Escherichia coli* that cause diarrhea: Enterotoxigenic enteropathogenic, enteroinvasive, enterohemorrhagic, and enteroadherent. J Infect Dis. 1987;155:377–388.
137. Schlager TA, Guerrant RL. Seven possible pathogenic mechanisms for *Escherichia coli* diarrhea. Infect Dis Clin North Am. 1988;2:1–18.
138. Bobak DA, Guerrant RL. New developments in enteric bacterial toxins. Adv Pharmacol. 1992;23:85–108.
139. Lamanna C, Carr CJ. The botulinal, tetanal, and enterostaphylococcal toxins: A review. Clin Pharmacol Ther. 1967;8:286.

140. Koupal A, Deibel RH. Rabbit intestinal fluid accumulation by an enterotoxigenic factor of *Staphylococcus aureus*. Infect Immun. 1977;18:298–303.
141. Freer JH, Arbuthnott JP. Toxins of *Staphylococcus aureus*. In: Dorner F, Drews J, eds. Pharmacology of Bacterial Toxins. Oxford: Pergamon Press; 1986:581–633.
142. Terranova W, Blake PA. *Bacillus cereus* food poisoning. N Engl J Med. 1978;298:143.
143. Turnbull PCB. *Bacillus cereus* toxins. In: Dorner F, Drews J, eds. Pharmacology of Bacterial Toxins. Oxford: Pergamon Press; 1986:397–448.
144. Chen LC, Rohde JE, Sharp GWG. Intestinal adenyl-cyclase activity in human cholera. Lancet. 1971;1:939.
145. Guerrant RL, Chen LC, Sharp GWG. Intestinal adenyl-cyclase activity in canine cholera: Correlation with fluid accumulation. J Infect Dis. 1972;125:377.
146. Peterson JW, Ochoa G. Role of prostaglandins and cAMP in the secretory effects of cholera toxin. Science. 1989;245:857–859.
147. Peterson JW, Chopra AK, Prasad R. Fine mapping of the rrnE, purHD, and hydGH operons on the *Escherichia coli* chromosome. J Bacteriol. 1991;173:3274–3275.
148. Fang GD, Fonteles MC, Barrett LJ, et al. Inhibition by platelet activating factor (PAF) antagonists of the effects of choleratoxin on intestinal secretion and cytoskeleton of Chinese hamster ovary (CHO) cells (Abstract). Clin Res. 1993;41:222A.
149. Cassuto J, Jodal M, Tuttle R, et al. On the role of intramural nerves in the pathogenesis of cholera toxin-induced intestinal secretion. Scand J Gastroenterol. 1981;16:377–384.
150. Beubler E, Horina G. 5-HT_2 and 5-HT_3 receptor subtypes mediate cholera toxin-induced intestinal fluid secretion in the rat. Gastroenterology. 1990;99:1–7.
151. Honda T, Shimizu M, Takeda Y, et al. Isolation of a factor causing morphological changes of Chinese hamster ovary cells from the culture filtrates of *Vibrio parahemolyticus*. Infect Immun. 1976;14:1028.
152. Blake PA, Weaver RE, Hollis DG. Diseases of humans (other than cholera) caused by vibrios. Annu Rev Microbiol. 1980;34:341.
153. Evans DJ Jr., Chen LC, Curlin GT. Stimulation of adenyl cyclase by *Escherichia coli* enterotoxin. Nature. 1972;236:137.
154. Guerrant RL, Ganguly U, Casper AGT, et al. Effect of *Escherichia coli* on fluid transport across canine small bowel: Mechanism and time-course with enterotoxin and whole bacterial cell. J Clin Invest. 1973;52:1707.
155. Skerman FJ, Formal SB, Falkow S. Plasmid-associated enterotoxin production in a strain of *Escherichia coli* isolated from humans. Infect Immun. 1972;5:622.
156. Lathe R, Hirth P. Cell-free synthesis of enterotoxin of *E. coli* from a cloned gene. Nature. 1980;284:473.
157. Takeda Y, Murphy J. Bacteriophage conversion of heat-labile entertoxin in *Escherichia coli*. J Bacteriol. 1978;133:172.
158. Evans DG, Evans DJ Jr, Pierce NF. Differences in the response of rabbit small intestine to heat-labile and heat-stable enterotoxins of *Escherichia coli*. Infect Immun. 1973;7:873.
159. Craig JP. A permeability factor (toxin) found in cholera stools and culture filtrates and its neutralization by convalescent cholera sera. Nature. 1965;207:614.
160. Guerrant RL, Brunton LL, Schnaitman TC, et al. Cyclic adenosine monophosphate and alteration of Chinese hamster ovary cell morphology: A rapid, sensitive in vitro assay for the enterotoxins of *Vibrio cholerae* and *Escherichia coli*. Infect Immun. 1974;10:320.
161. Donta ST, Moon HW, Whipp SC. Detection of heat-labile *Escherichia coli* enterotoxins with the use of adrenal cells in tissue culture. Science. 1974;183:334.
162. Greenberg HB, Sack DA, Rodriguez W, et al. A microtiter solid-phase radioimmunoassay for detection of *Escherichia coli* heat-labile enterotoxin. Infect Immun. 1977;17:541.
163. Yoiken RH, Greenberg HB, Merson MH, et al. Enzyme-linked immunosorbent assay for detection of *Escherichia coli* heat-labile enterotoxin. J Clin Microbiol. 1977;6:439.
164. Honda T, Tage S, Takeda Y, et al. Modified Elek test for detection of heat-labile enterotoxin of enterotoxigenic *E. coli*. J Clin Microbiol. 1981;13:1.
165. Sommerfelt H, Svennerholm AM, Kalland KH, et al. Comparative study of colony hybridizations with synthetic oligonucleotide probes and enzyme-linked immunosorbent assay for identification of *Escherichia coli*. J Clin Microbiol. 1988;26:530–534.
166. Gorbach SL, Banwell JG, Chatterjee BD, et al. Acute undifferentiated human diarrhea in the tropics. I. Alterations in intestinal microflora. J Clin Invest. 1971;50:881.
167. Ryder RW, Sack DA, Kapikian AZ, et al. Enterotoxigenic *Escherichia coli* and reovirus-like agent in rural Bangladesh. Lancet. 1976;1:659.
168. Gorbach SL, Kean BH, Evans DG: Traveler's diarrhea and toxigenic *Escherichia coli*. N Engl J Med. 1975;292:933.
169. Merson MH, Morris GK, Sack DA, et al. Travelers' diarrhea in Mexico: A prospective study. Abstract 149. Presented at the 15th Interscience Conference on Antimicrobial Agents and Chemotherapy. September 1975.
170. Guerrant RL, Rouse JD, Hughes JM. Turista among members of the Yale Glee Club in Latin America. Am J Trop Med Hyg. 1980;29:895.
171. Gorbach SL, Khurana CM. Toxigenic *Escherichia coli*: A cause of infantile diarrhea in Chicago. N Engl J Med. 1972;287:791.
172. Sack RB, Hirschhorn N, Brownlee I, et al. Enterotoxigenic *Escherichia coli*–associated diarrheal disease in Apache children. N Engl J Med. 1975;292:1041.
173. Guerrant RL, Moore RA, Kirschenfeld PM, et al. Role of toxigenic and invasive bacteria in acute diarrhea of childhood. N Engl J Med. 1975;293:567.
174. Guerrant RL, Dickens MD, Wenzel RP, et al. Toxigenic bacterial diarrhea: Nursery outbreak involving multiple bacterial strains. J Pediatr. 1976;89:885–891.
175. Wachsmuth K, Wells J, Shipley P. Heat-labile enterotoxin production in isolates from a shipboard outbreak of human diarrheal illness. Infect Immun. 1979;24:793–797.
176. Honda T, Shimizu M, Takeda Y, et al. Isolation of a factor causing morphological changes of Chinese hamster ovary cells from the culture filtrates of *Vibrio parahemolyticus*. Infect Immun. 1976;14:1028–1033.
177. Sandefur PD, Peterson JW. Neutralization of *Salmonella* toxin-induced elongation of Chinese hamster ovary cells by cholera antitoxin. Infect Immun. 1977;15:988–992.
178. Ruiz-Palacios GM, Torres J, Torres NI, et al. Cholera-like enterotoxin produced by *Campylobacter jejuni*: Characterization and clinical significance. Lancet. 1983;2:250–253.
179. Ruiz-Palacios GM, Lopez-Vidal Y, Torres J, et al. Serum antibodies to heat-labile enterotoxin of *Campylobacter jejuni*. J Infect Dis. 1985;152:413–416.
180. Daikoku T, Kawagughi M, Takama K, et al. Partial purification and characterization of the enterotoxin produced by *Campylobacter jejuni*. Infect Immun. 1990;58:2414–2419.
181. Gyles CL. Heat-labile and heat-stable forms of the enterotoxin from *E. coli* strains enteropathogenic for pigs. Ann N Y Acad Sci. 1971;176:315.
182. Levine MM, Caplan ES, Waterman D, et al. Diarrhea caused by *Escherichia coli* that produce only heat-stable enterotoxins. Infect Immun. 1977;17:78.
183. Sack DA, Wells JG, Merson MH. Diarrhoea associated with heat-stable enterotoxin-producing strains of *Escherichia coli*. Lancet. 1975;2:239.
184. Ryder RW, Wachsmuth IK, Buxton AE, et al. Infantile diarrhea produced by heat-stable enterotoxin *Escherichia coli*. N Engl J Med. 1976;295:849.
185. Hughes JM, Rouse JD, Barada FA, et al. Etiology of summer diarrhea among the Navajo. Am J Trop Med Hyg. 1980;29:613.
186. Korzeniowski OM, Dantas W, Trabulsi LR, et al. A controlled study of endemic sporadic diarrhoea among adult residents of southern Brazil. Trans R Soc Trop Med Hyg. 1984;78:363–369.
187. Hughes JM, Murad F, Chang B, et al. Role of cyclic GMP in the action of heat-stable enterotoxin of *Escherichia coli*. Nature. 1978;271:755.
188. Field M, Graf LH Jr, Laird WJ, et al. Heat stable enterotoxin of *E. coli*: In vitro effects on guanylate cyclase activity, cyclic GMP concentration, and ion transport in small intestine. Proc Natl Acad Sci U S A. 1978;75:2800.
189. Guerrant RL, Hughes JM, Chang B, et al. Activation of intestinal guanylate cyclase by heat-stable enterotoxin of *E. coli*. Studies of tissue specificity, potential receptors and intermediates. J Infect Dis. 1980;142:220.
190. Aimoto S, Takao T, Shimonishi Y, et al. Amino-acid sequence of a heat stable enterotoxin produced by human enterotoxigenic *Escherichia coli*. Eur J Biochem. 1982;129:257–263.
191. Takao T, Hitouji T, Aimoto S, et al. Amino-acid sequence of a heat-stable enterotoxin isolated from enterotoxigenic *Escherichia coli* strain 18D. FEBS Lett. 1983;152:1–5.
192. Guarino A, Giannella R, Thompson MR. *Citrobacter freundii* produces an 18-amino-acid heat-stable enterotoxin identical to the 18-amino-acid *Escherichia coli* heat-stable enterotoxin (ST Ia). Infect Immun. 1989;57:649–652.
193. Takeda T, Balakrish Nair G, et al. Production of a monoclonal antibody to *Vibrio cholerae* non-O1 heat-stable enterotoxin (ST) which is cross-reactive with *Yersinia enterocolitica* ST. Infect Immun. 1990;58:2755–2759.
194. Guerrant RL, Fang G, Lima AAM, et al. Pathophysiology of enterotoxic diarrhea. 28th Joint Conference US-Japan Cooperative Medical Science Program on Cholera and Related Diarrheal Diseases Panel, Tokyo, July 1992. 20:31–36.
195. Fonteles MC, Lima AAM, Fang G, et al. Effect of STa and cholera toxin on renal electrolyte transport: Possible roles of an endogenous ST-like compound in the isolated kidney. 27th US Japan Cholera Meeting, Charlottesville, Va, 1991;100–105.
196. Currie MG, Fok KF, Kato J, et al. Guanylin: An endogenous activator of intestinal guanylate cyclase. Proc Natl Acad Sci U S A. 1992;89:947–951.
197. Fonteles MC, Villar-Palasi C, Fang G, et al. Partial characterization of an ANF/urodilatin-like substance released from perfused rabbit kidney under hypoxia. Brazilian J Med Biol Res. 1993;26:75–79.
198. Fasano A, Kay BA, Russell RG, et al. Enterotoxin and cytotoxin production by enteroinvasive *Escherichia coli*. Infect Immun. 1990;58:3717–3723.
199. Savarino S, Fasano A, Robertson D, et al. Enteroaggregative *Escherichia coli* elaborate a heat-stable enterotoxin demonstrable in an in vitro intestinal model. J Clin Invest. 1991;87:1450–1455.
200. Yamamoto T, Echeverria P. Detection of the enteroaggregative *Escherichia coli* heat-stable enterotoxin-1 gene sequences in enterotoxigenic *E. coli* strains pathogenic for humans. Infect Immun. 1996;64:1441–1445.
201. Navarro-Garcia F, Eslava C, Villaseca JM, et al. In vitro effects of a high-molecular-weight heat-labile enterotoxin from enteroaggregative *Escherichia coli*. Infect Immun. 1998;66:3149–3154.
202. Raimondi F, Kao JP, Kaper JB, et al. Calcium-dependent intestinal chloride secretion by *Vibrio parahaemolyticus* thermostable direct hemolysin in a rabbit model. Gastroenterology. 1995;109:381–386.
203. Keusch GT, Grady GF, Mata LJ, et al. The pathogenesis of *Shigella* diarrhea: I. Enterotoxin production by *Shigella dysenteriae* 1. J Clin Invest. 1972;51:1212.
204. Charney AN, Gots RE, Formal SB, et al. Activation of intestinal mucosal adenylate cyclase by *Shigella dysenteriae* I enterotoxin. Gastroenterology. 1976;70:1085.
205. Rout WR, Formal SB, Giannella RA, et al. Pathophysiology of *Shigella* diarrhea in the rhesus monkey: Intestinal transport, morphological and bacteriological studies. Gastroenterology. 1975;68:270.
206. Keusch FT, Jacewicz M. Serum enterotoxin neutralizing antibody in human shigellosis. Nature. 1973;241:31.

207. Kopecko DJ, Washington O, Formal SB. Genetic and physical evidence for plasmid control of *Shigella sonnei* form I cell surface antigen. Infect Immun. 1980;29:207.
208. Keusch GT. Invasive bacterial diarrhea. In: LC Chen, NS Scrimshaw, eds. Diarrhea and Malnutrition. New York: Plenum Press; 1983:45.
209. Turnbull PCB: Studies on the production of enterotoxins by *Bacillus cereus*. J Clin Pathol. 1976;29:941–949.
210. Gilbert RJ, Kramer JM. *Bacillus cereus* enterotoxins: Present status. Biochem Soc Trans. 1984;12:198–200.
211. Franco AA, Mundy LM, Trucksis M, et al. Cloning and characterization of the *Bacteroides fragilis* metalloprotease toxin gene. Infect Immun. 1997;65:1007–1013.
212. Moncrief JS, Obiso R Jr., Barroso LA, et al. The enterotoxin of *Bacteroides fragilis* is a metalloprotease. Infect Immun. 1995;63:175–181.
213. Chambers FG, Koshy SS, Saidi RF, et al. *Bacteroides fragilis* toxin exhibits polar activity on monolayers of human intestinal epithelial cells (T84 cells) in vitro. Infect Immun. 1997;65:3561–3570.
214. Saidi RF, Jaeger K, Montrose MH, et al. *Bacteroides fragilis* toxin rearranges the actin cytoskeleton of HT29/C1 cells without direct proteolysis of actin or decrease in F-actin. Cell Motil Cytoskeleton. 1997;37:159–165.
215. Just I, Wilm M, Selzer J, et al. The enterotoxin from *Clostridium difficile* (ToxA) monoglucosylates the Rho proteins. J Biol Chem. 1995;270:13932–13936.
216. Just I, Wilm M, Selzer J, et al. Glucosylation of Rho proteins by *Clostridium difficile* toxin B. Nature. 1995;375:500–503.
217. Fasano A, Uzzau S, Fiore C, et al. The enterotoxic effect of zonula occludens toxin on rabbit small intestine involves the paracellular pathway. Gastroenterology. 1997;112:839–846.
218. Giannella RA, Formal SB, Dammin GJ, et al. Pathogenesis of salmonellosis. Studies of fluid secretion, mucosal invasion, and morphologic reaction in the rabbit ileum. J Clin Invest. 1973;52:441.
219. Giannella RA, Gots RE, Charney AN, et al. Pathogenesis of *Salmonella*-mediated intestinal fluid secretion: Activation of adenylate cyclase and inhibition by indomethacin. Gastroenterology. 1975;69:1238.
220. Musch MW, Miller RJ, Field M, et al. Stimulation of colonic secretion by lipoxygenase metabolites of arachidonic acid. Science. 1982;217:1255.
221. Madara JL, Patapoff TW, Gillece-Castro B, et al. 5′-Adenosine monophosphate is the neutrophil-derived paracrine factor that elicits chloride secretion from T-84 intestinal epithelial cell monolayers. J Clin Invest. 1993;91:2320–2325.
222. Kelly CP, Becker S, Linevsky JK, et al. Neutrophil recruitment in *Clostridium difficile* toxin A enteritis in the rabbit. J Clin Invest. 1994;93:1257–1265.
223. Pothoulakis C, Casagliuolo I, LaMont JT, et al. CP-96,345, a substance P antagonist, inhibits rat intestinal responses to *Clostridium difficile* toxin A but not cholera toxin. Proc Natl Acad Sci U S A. 1994;91:947–951.
224. Fang GD, Lima AAM, Thielman NM, et al. Role of phospholipase A2 in the histologic, epithelial, and secretory responses to *Clostridium difficile* toxin A. Biomed J. 1994;1:71–76.
225. Fonteles M, Fang G, Thielman NM, et al. Role of platelet activating factor in the inflammatory and secretory effects of *Clostridium difficile* toxin A. J Lipid Mediat Cell Signal. 1995;11:133–143.
226. Pothoulakis C, Karmeli F, Kelly CP, et al. Ketotifen inhibits *Clostridium difficile* toxin A–induced enteritis in rat ileum. Gastroenterology. 1993;105:701–707.
227. Koupal LR, Deibel RH. Assay, characterization and localization of an enterotoxin produced by *Salmonella*. Infect Immun. 1975;11:14.
228. Klipstein FA, Holdeman LV, Corcino JJ. Enterotoxigenic intestinal bacteria in tropical sprue. Ann Intern Med. 1973;79:632.
229. Wasdtrom T, Aust-Kettis A, Habte D, et al. Enterotoxin-producing bacteria and parasites in stools of Ethiopian children with diarrhoeal disease. Arch Dis Child. 1976;51:865.
230. Ljungh A, Popoff M, Wadstrom T. *Aeromonas hydrophila* in acute diarrheal disease: Detection of enterotoxin and biotyping of strains. J Clin Microbiol. 1977;6:96.
231. Keusch GT, Jacewicz M. The pathogenesis of *Shigella* diarrhea: V. Relationship of Shiga enterotoxin, neurotoxin and cytotoxin. J Infect Dis. 1975;131S:S33.
232. Konowalchuk J, Speirs JI, Stavric S. Vero response to a cytotoxin of *Escherichia coli*. Infect Immun. 1977;18:775.
233. Konowalchuk J, Dickie N, Stavric S, et al. Properties of an *Escherichia coli* cytotoxin. Infect Immun. 1978;10:575.
234. Scotland SM, Day NP, Willshaw GA, et al. Cytotoxic enteropathogenic *Escherichia coli*. Lancet. 1980;1:90.
235. Riley LW, Remia RS, Helgerson SD, et al. Outbreaks of hemorrhagic colitis associated with a rare *Escherichia coli* serotype. N Engl J Med. 1983;308:681.
236. Johnson WM, Lior H, Bezanson GS. Cytotoxic *Escherichia coli* O157:H7 associated with hemorrhagic colitis in Canada. Lancet. 1983;1:76.
237. Strockbine NA, Marques LRM, Newland JW, et al. Two toxin-converting phages from *E. coli* O157:H7 strains 933 encode antigenically distinct toxins with similar biologic activities. Infect Immun. 1986;53:135–140.
238. Karmali MA, Petric M, Lim C, et al. The association between idiopathic hemolytic uremic syndrome and infection by verotoxin producing *E. coli*. J Infect Dis. 1985;151:775–782.
239. Pai CH, Gordon R, Sims HU, et al. Sporadic cases of hemorrhagic colitis associated with *E. coli* O157:H7. Ann Intern Med. 1984;101:738–742.
240. Carter AO, Borczyk AA, Carlson AK, et al. A severe outbreak of *E. coli* O157:H7 associated hemorrhagic colitis in a nursing home. N Engl J Med. 1987;317:1496–1500.
241. Griffin PM, Tauxe RV. The epidemiology of infections caused by *Escherichia coli* O157:H7, other enterohemorrhagic *E. coli*, and the associated hemolytic uremic syndrome. Epidemiol Rev. 1991;13:60–98.
242. Centers for Disease Control and Prevention. Update: Multistate outbreak of *E. coli* O157:H7 infections from hamburgers—W. U.S., 1992–1993. MMWR Morb Mortal Wkly Rep. 1993;42:258–263.
243. Watanabe H, Wada A, Inagaki Y, et al. Outbreaks of enterohaemorrhagic *Escherichia coli* O157:H7 infection by two different genotype strains in Japan. Lancet. 1996;348:831–832.
244. Watanabe H, Guerrant RL. Summary: Nagasaki enterohemorrhagic *Escherichia coli* meeting and workshop. J Infect Dis. 1997;176:247–249.
245. O'Brien AD, Holmes RK. Shiga and shiga-like toxins. Microbiol Rev. 1987;51:206–220.
246. Obrig TG, Moran RP, Colinas RJ. Ribonuclease activity associated with the 60-S ribosome inactivating proteins Ricin A, phytolaccin and shiga toxin. Biochem Biophys Res Commun. 1985;1300:8790–8840.
247. Reisbig R, Olsnes S, Eiklid K. The cytotoxic activity of *Shigella* toxin: Evidence for catalytic inactivation of the 60-S ribosomal subunit. J Biol Chem. 1981;2560:8739–8744.
248. Jackson MP. Structure-function analysis of Shiga toxin and the Shiga-like toxins. Microb Pathog. 1990;8:235–242.
249. Karmall MA. Infection by verocytotoxin-producing *Escherichia coli*. Clin Microbiol Rev. 1989;2:15–38.
250. Samuel JE, Perera LP, Ward S, et al. Comparison of the glycolipid receptor specificities of Shiga-like toxin type II and Shiga-like toxin type II variants. Infect Immun. 1990;58:611–618.
251. Bridgewater FAJ, Morgan RS, Rowson KEK, et al. The neurotoxin of *Shigella shigae*. Morphological and functional lesions produced in the central nervous system of rabbits. Br J Exp Pathol. 1955;36:447–453.
252. Cavanagh JB, Howard JG, Whitby JL. The neurotoxin of *Shigella shigae*: A comparative study of the effects produced in various laboratory animals. Br J Exp Med. 1956;370:272–278.
253. Howard JG. Observations on the intoxication produced in mice and rabbits by the neurotoxin of *Shigella shigae*. Br J Exp Pathol. 1955;36:439–446.
254. Wiley RG, Donohue-Rolfe A, Keusch GT. Axonally transported *Shigella* cytotoxin is neuronotoxic. J Neuropathol Exp Neurol. 1985;440:496–506.
255. Ashkenazi A, Cleary KR, Pickering LK, et al. The association of Shiga toxin and other cytotoxins with the neurologic manifestations of shigellosis. J Infect Dis. 1990;161:961–965.
256. McDonel JL, Duncan CL. Histopathological effect of *Clostridium perfringens* enterotoxin in the rabbit ileum. Infect Immun. 1975;12:1214.
257. Bartholomew BA, Stringer MF. Observations on the purification of *Clostridium perfringens* type A enterotoxin and the production of a specific antiserum. Fems Microbiol Lett. 1983;18:43–48.
258. Bartholomew BA, Stringer MF. *Clostridium perfringens* enterotoxin: A brief review. Biochem Soc Trans. 1984;12:195–197.
259. Horiguchi Y, Akai T, Sakaguchi G. Isolation and function of a *Clostridium perfringens* enterotoxin fragment. Infect Immun. 1987;55:2912–2915.
260. Borriello SP, Barclay F, Welch AR, et al. Epidemiology of diarrhea caused by enterotoxigenic *Clostridium perfringens*. J Med Microbiol. 1985;20:363–372.
261. Borriello SP, Welch AR, Larson HE, et al. Enterotoxigenic *Clostridium perfringens*: A possible cause of antibiotic associated diarrhea. Lancet. 1984;1:305–307.
262. Larson HE, Borriello SP. Infectious diarrhea due to *Clostridium perfringens*. J Infect Dis. 1988;157:390–392.
263. Lawrence GW, Lehmann D, Anian G, et al. Impact of active immunization against enteritis necroticans in Papua New Guinea. Lancet. 1990:336.
264. Sanyal SC, Sen PC. Human volunteer study on the pathogenicity of *Vibrio parahaemolyticus*. In: International symposium on *Vibrio parahaemolyticus*. Tokyo, Japan, Sept. 17–18, 1973. Tokyo:Saikon:227–230.
265. Shirai H, Ito H, Hirayama T, et al. Molecular epidemiologic evidence of association of thermostable direct hemolysin (TDH) and TDH-related hemolysin of *Vibrio parahaemolyticus*. Infect Immun. 1990;58:3568–3573.
266. Huntley JS, Hall AC. Nature of the cation leak induced in erythrocyte membranes by Kanagawa hemolysin of *Vibrio parahaemolyticus*. Biochem Biophys Acta. 1996;1281:220–226.
267. Calia FM, Johnson DE. Bacteremia in suckling rabbits after oral challenge with *Vibrio parahaemolyticus*. Infect Immun. 1975;11:1222.
268. Bolen JL, Zamiska SA, Grennough WB III. Clinical features in enteritis due to *Vibrio parahaemolyticus*. Am J Med. 1974;57:638.
269. Barker WH, MacKowiak PA, Fishbein M, et al. *Vibrio parahaemolyticus* gastroenteritis outbreak in Covington, Louisiana in August 1972. Am J Epidemiol. 1974;100:316.
270. Kapral FA, O'Brien AD, Ruff PD, et al. Inhibition of water absorption in the intestine by *Staphylococcus aureus* delta toxin. Infect Immun. 1976;13:140.
271. Bartlett JG, Chang TW, Gurwith M, et al. Antibiotic-associated pseudomembranous colitis due to toxin-producing clostridia. N Engl J Med. 1978;298:531.
272. Rifkin GD, Fekety FR, Silva J Jr, et al. Antibiotic-induced colitis: Implication of a toxin neutralized by *Clostridium sordelli* antitoxin. Lancet. 1977;2:1103.
273. Taylor NS, Thorne GM, Bartlett JG. Comparison of two toxins produced by *Clostridium difficile*. Infect Immun. 1981;34:1036.
274. Lima AAM, Lyerly DM, Wilkins TD, et al. Effects of *Clostridium difficile* toxins A and B in rabbit small and large intestine in vivo and on cultured cells in vitro. Infect Immun. 1988;56:582–588.
275. Johnson WM, Lior H. Toxins produced by *Campylobacter jejuni* and *Campylobacter coli*. Lancet. 1984;1:229–230.
276. Yeen WP, Pothocheary SD, Pang T. Demonstration of a cytotoxin from *Campylobacter jejuni*. J Clin Pathol. 1983;36:1237–1240.

277. Guerrant RL, Wanke CA, Pennie RA, et al. Production of a unique cytotoxin by *Campylobacter jejuni*. Infect Immun. 1987;55:2526–2530.
278. Perez-Perez GL, Cohn DL, Guerrant RL, et al. Clinical and immunologic significance of cholera-like toxin and cytotoxin production by *Campylobacter* species in patients with acute inflammatory diarrhea in the USA. J Infect Dis. 1989;160:460–467.
279. Leunk RD, Johnson PT, David BC, et al. Cytotoxic activity in broth-culture filtrates of *Campylobacter pylori*. J Med Microbiol. 1988;26:93–99.
280. Leunk RD, Ferguson MA, Morgan DR, et al. Antibody to cytotoxin in infection by *Helicobacter pylori*. J Clin Microbiol. 1990;28:1181–1184.
281. Guerrant RL, Lingwood CA. Glycoconjugate receptors for adhesins and toxins. In: Marshall BJ, McCallum RW, Guerrant RL, eds. *Helicobacter pylori* in Peptic Ulceration and Gastritis. Boston: Blackwell Scientific Publications; 1991:66–80.
282. Smoot DT, Mobley HLT, Chippendale GR, et al. *Helicobacter pylori* urease activity is toxic to human gastric epithelial cells. Infect Immun. 1990;58:1992–1994.
283. Fasano A, Baudry B, Pumplin DW, et al. *Vibrio cholerae* produces a second enterotoxin which affects intestinal tight junctions. Proc Natl Acad Sci U S A. 1991;88:5242–5246.
284. Salit IE, Gostchlich EC. Type I *Escherichia coli* pili: Characterization of binding to monkey kidney cells. J Exp Med. 1977;146:1182.
285. Silverblatt FJ. Host parasitic in the rat renal pelvis: A possible role for pili in the pathogenesis of pyelonephritis. J Exp Med. 1974;140:1696.
286. Eden CS, Hausson S, Jodal U, et al. Host-parasite interaction in the urinary tract. J Infect Dis. 1988;157:421–426.
287. Evans DG, Satterwhite TK, Evans DJ Jr, et al. Differences in serological responses and excretion patterns of volunteers challenged with enterotoxigenic *Escherichia coli* with and without the colonization factor antigen. Infect Immun. 1978;19:883.
288. Bergman MJ, Updike WS, Wood SJ, et al. Attachment factors among enterotoxigenic *Escherichia coli* from patients with acute diarrhea from diverse geographic areas. Infect Immun. 1981;32:881.
289. Thomas LV, Cravioto A, Scotland SM, et al. New fimbrial antigenic type E8775 that may represent a colonization factor in enterotoxigenic *E. coli* in humans. Infect Immun. 1982;35:1119–1124.
290. Honda T, Arita M, Miwatani T: Characterization of new hydrophobic pili of human enterotoxigenic *Escherichia coli*: A possible new colonization factor. Infect Immun. 1984;43:959–965.
291. Tacket CO, Maneval DR, Levine MM. Purification, morphology, and genetics of a new fimbrial putative colonization factor of enterotoxigenic *Escherichia coli* O159:H4. Infect Immun. 1987;55:1063–1069.
292. Williams PH, Sedgwick MI, Evans N, et al. Adherence of an enteropathogenic strain of *Escherichia coli* is mediated by a colicinogenic conjugative plasmid. Infect Immun. 1978;22:393.
293. Karch H, Heesemann J, Laufs R, et al. A plasmid of enterohemmorhagic *Escherichia coli* O157:H7 is required for expression of a new fimbrial antigen and for adhesion to epithelial cells. Infect Immun. 1987;55:455–461.
294. Levine MM, Nalin DR, Hornick RB, et al. *Escherichia coli* strains that cause diarrhea but do not produce heat-labile or heat-stable enterotoxins and are noninvasive. Lancet. 1978;1:1119.
295. Ulshen MH, Rollo JL. Pathogenesis of *Escherichia coli* gastroenteritis in man: Another mechanism. N Engl J Med. 1980;302:99.
296. Polotsky YE, Dragunskaya EM, Seliverstova VG, et al. Pathogenic effect of enterotoxigenic *Escherichia coli* and *Escherichia coli* causing infantile diarrhoea. Acta Microbiol Acad Sci Hung. 1977;24:221.
297. Guerrant RL. Yet another pathogenic mechanism for *Escherichia coli* diarrhea? N Engl J Med. 1980;302:113.
298. Rothbaum R, McAdams AJ, Giannella R, et al. A clinicopathologic study of enterocyte-adherent *Escherichia coli*: A cause of protracted diarrhea in infants. Gastroenterology. 1982;83:441.
299. Cravioto A, Gross RJ, Scotland S, et al. An adhesive factor found in strains of *Escherichia coli* belonging to the traditional infantile enteropathogenic serotypes. Curr Microbiol. 1979;3:95–99.
300. Knutton S, Baldwin T, Williams PH, et al. Actin accumulation at sites of bacterial adhesion to tissue culture cells: Basis of a new diagnostic test for enteropathogenic and enterohemorrhagic *Escherichia coli*. Infect Immun. 1989;57:1290–1298.
301. Baldini MM, Kaper JB, Levine MM, et al. Plasmid mediated adhesion of enteropathogenetic *Escherichia coli*. J Pediatr Gastroenterol Nutr. 1983;2:534–548.
302. Jerse AE, Martin WC, Galen JE, et al. Oligonucleotide probe for detection of the enteropathogenic *Escherichia coli* (EPEC) adherence factor of localized adherent EPEC. J Clin Microbiol. 1990;28:2842–2844.
303. Francis CL, Jerse AE, Kaper JB, et al. Characterization of interactions of enteropathogenic *Escherichia coli* O127:H6 with mammalian cells *in vitro*. J Infect Dis. 1991;164:693–703.
304. Vuopio-Varkila J, Schoolnik GK. Localized adherence by enteropathogenic *Escherichia coli* is an inducible phenotype associated with the expression of new outer membrane proteins. J Exp Med. 1991;174:1167–1177.
305. Girón JA, Ho ASY, Schoolnik GK. An inducible bundle-forming pilus of enteropathogenic *Escherichia coli*. Science. 1992;254:710.
306. Kenny B, DeVinney R, Stein M, et al. Enteropathogenic *E. coli* (EPEC) transfers its receptor for intimate adherence into mammalian cells. Cell. 1997;91:511–520.
307. Rosenshine I, Ruschkowski S, Stein M, et al. A pathogenic bacterium triggers epithelial signals to form a functional bacterial receptor that mediates actin pseudopod formation. EMBO J. 1996;15:2613–2624.
308. Yamamoto T. Distinct attaching and effacing phenomena observed with enterohemorrhagic *Escherichia coli* (EHEC) and enteropathogenic *E. coli* (EPEC). 33rd U.S.-Japan Cholera and Related Diarrheal Diseases Joint Panel Meeting. The United States-Japan Cooperative Medical Sciences Program: Clearwater Beach, Fla, Dec. 23–25, 1997:126–130.
309. Nataro JP, Kaper JB, Robins-Browne R, et al. Patterns of adherence of diarrheagenic *Escherichia coli* to HEp-2 cells. Pediatr Infect Dis J. 1987;6:829–831.
310. Mathewson JJ, Johnson PC, Dupont HL, et al. Pathogenicity of enteroadherent *Escherichia coli* in adult volunteers. J Infect Dis. 1986;154:524–527.
311. Scaletsky ICA, Silva MLM, Toledo MRF, et al. Correlation between adherence to HeLa cells and serogroups, serotypes, and bioserotypes of *Escherichia coli*. Infect Immun. 1985;49:528–532.
312. Mathewson JJ, Cravioto A. HEp-2 cell adherence as an assay for virulence among diarrheagenic *Escherichia coli*. J Infect Dis. 1989;159:1057–1060.
313. Baudry B, Savarino SJ, Vial P, et al. A sensitive and specific DNA probe to identify enteroaggregative *Escherichia coli*, a recently discovered diarrheal pathogen. J Infect Dis. 1990;161:1249–1251.
314. Bhan MK, Raj P, Levine MM, et al. Enteroaggregative *Escherichia coli* associated with persistent diarrhea in a cohort of rural children in India. J Infect Dis. 1989;159:1061–1064.
315. Bhan MK, Khoshoo V, Sommerfelt H, et al. Enteroaggregative *Escherichia coli* and *Salmonella* associated with nondysenteric persistent diarrhea. Pediatr Infect Dis J. 1989;8:499–502.
316. Wanke CA, Schorling JB, Barrett LJ, et al. Adherence traits of *Escherichia coli*, alone and in association with other stool pathogens: Potential role in pathogenesis of persistent diarrhea in an urban Brazilian slum. Pediatr J Infect Dis. 1991;10:746–751.
317. Itoh Y, Nagano I, Kunishima M, et al. Laboratory investigation of enteroaggregative *Escherichia coli* O untypable:H10 associated with a massive outbreak of gastrointestinal illness. J Clin Microbiol. 1997;35:2546–2550.
318. Baldwin TJ, Knutton S, Sellers L, et al. Enteroaggregative *Escherichia coli* strains secrete a heat-labile toxin antigenically related to *E. coli* hemolysin. Infect Immun. 1992;60:2092–2095.
319. Bilge SS, Clausen CR, Lau W, et al. Molecular characterization of a fimbrial adhesin, F1845, mediating diffuse adherence of diarrhea-associated *Escherichia coli* to HEp-2 cells. J Bacteriol. 1989;171:4281–4289.
320. Benz I, Schmidt MA. Isolation and serologic characterization of AIDA-I, the adhesin mediating the diffuse adherence phenotype of the diarrhea-associated *Escherichia coli* strain 2787 (O126:H27). Infect Immun. 1992;60:13–18.
321. Girón JA, Fry J, Frankel G, et al. Diffuse-adhering *Escherichia coli* (DAEC) as a putative cause of diarrhea in Mayan children in Mexico. J Infect Dis. 1991;163:507–513.
322. Baqui AH, Sack RB, Black RE, et al. Enteropathogens associated with acute and persistent diarrhea in Bangladeshi children <5 years of age. J Infect Dis. 1992;166:792–796.
323. Wanke C, Guerrant RL. Small-bowel colonization alone is a cause of diarrhea. Infect Immun. 1987;55:1924–1926.
324. Schlager TA, Wanke CA, Guerrant RL. Net fluid secretion and impaired villous function induced by colonization of the small intestine by nontoxigenic colonizing *Escherichia coli*. Infect Immun. 1990;58:1337–1343.
325. Tacket CO, Losonsky G, Nataro JP, et al. Safety, immunogenicity and transmissibility of live oral cholera vaccine candidate CVD110, a delta CTXA delta ZOT delta ace derivative of El Tor Ogawa *Vibrio cholerae*. J Infect Dis. 1993;168:1536–1540.
326. Trucksis M, Galen JE, Michalski J, et al. Accessory cholera enterotoxin (Ace) the third member of a *Vibrio cholerae* virulence cassette. Proc Natl Acad Sci U S A. 1993;90:5267–5271.
327. Madden JM, McCardell MBA, Shah DB. Cytotoxin production by members of genus *Vibrio*. Lancet. 1984;1:1217–1218.
328. Kandel G, Donohue-Rolfe A, Donowitz M, et al. Pathogenesis of *Shigella* diarrhea: XVI. Selective targeting of shigatoxin to villous cells of rabbit jejunum explains the effect of toxin on intestinal electrolyte transport. J Clin Invest. 1989;84:1509–1517.
329. Silva TM, Schleupner MA, Tacket CO, et al. New evidence for an inflammatory component in diarrhea caused by selected new, live attenuated cholera vaccines and by El Tor and O139 *Vibrio cholerae*. Infect Immun. 1996;64:2362–2364.
330. Sereny B. Experimental *Shigella* keratoconjunctivitis: A preliminary report. Acta Microbiol Acad Sci Hung. 1955;2:293.
331. Gemski P Jr, Sheahan DG, Washington O, et al. Virulence of *Shigella flexneri* hybrids expressing *Escherichia coli* somatic antigens. Infect Immun. 1972;6:104.
332. Keusch GT. *Shigella* infections. Clin Gastroenterol. 1979;8:645.
333. Trabulsi LR, Fernandes MFR. *Escherichia coli* serogroup O115 isolated from patients with enteritis: Biochemical characteristics and experimental pathogenicity. Rev Inst Med Trop Sao Paulo. 1969;11:358.
334. DuPont HL, Formal SB, Hornick RB, et al. Pathogenesis of *Escherichia coli* diarrhea. N Engl J Med. 1971;285:1.
335. Sansonetti PJ, Kopecko DJ, Formal SB. Involvement of a plasmid in the invasive ability of *Shigella flexneri*. Infect Immun. 1982;35:852.
336. Harris JR, Wachsmuth IK, Davis BR, et al. High-molecular-weight plasmid correlates with *Escherichia coli* invasiveness. Infect Immun. 1982;37:1295.
337. Sansonetti PJ, Hale TL, Oaks EV. Genetics of virulence in enteroinvasive *Escherichia coli*. Microbiology. 1985;74–77.
338. Isberg RR. Discrimination between intracellular uptake and surface adhesion of bacterial pathogens. Science. 1991;252:934–938.
339. Maurelli AT, Sansonetti P. Identification of a chromosomal gene controlling temperature-regulated expression of *Shigella* virulence. Proc Natl Acad Sci U S A. 1988;85:2820–2824.
340. Bernardini ML, Mounier J, D'Hauteville H, et al. Identification of *icsA*, a plasmid locus that governs intra- and intercellular spread through interaction with F-actin. Proc Natl Acad Sci U S A. 1989;86:3867–3871.

341. Finlay BB, Heffron F, Falkow S. Epithelial cell surfaces induce *Salmonella* proteins required for bacterial adherence and invasion. Science. 1989;243:940–943.
342. Ravdin JI, Guerrant RL. Role of adherence in cytopathogenic mechanisms of *Entamoeba histolytica.* J Clin Invest. 1981;68:1305–1313.
343. Guerrant RL, Brush JE, Ravdin JI, et al. Interaction between *Entamoeba histolytica* and human polymorphonuclear leukocytes. J Infect Dis. 1981;143:83–93.
344. Petri WA Jr, Chapman MD, Snodgrass T, et al. Subunit structure of the galactose and *N*-acetyl-D-galactosamine-inhibitable adherence lectin of *Entamoeba histolytica*. J Biol Chem. 1989;264:3007–3012.
345. Jung HC, Eckmann L, Yang SK, et al. A distinct array of proinflammatory cytokines is expressed in human colon epithelial cells in response to bacterial invasion. J Clin Invest. 1995;95:55–65.
346. Aihara M, Tsuchimoto D, Takizawa H, et al. Mechanisms involved in *Helicobacter pylori*–induced interleukin-8 production by a gastric cancer cell line, MKN45. Infect Immun. 1997;65:3218–3224.
347. Mahida YR, Makh S, Hyde S, et al. Effect of *Clostridium difficile* toxin A on human intestinal epithelial cells: Induction of interleukin-8 production and apoptosis after cell detachment. Gut. 1996;38:337–347.
348. Madara JL, Patapoff TW, Gillece-Castro B, et al. 5′-Adenosine monophosphate is the neutrophil-derived paracrine factor that elicits chloride secretion from T84 intestinal epithelial cells. J Clin Invest. 1993;91:2320–2325.
349. Guarino A, Canani RB, Pozio E, et al. Enterotoxic effect of stool supernatant of *Cryptosporidium*-infected calves on human jejunum. Gastroenterology. 1994;106:28.
350. Guentzel MN, Berry LJ. Motility as a virulence factor for *Vibrio cholerae*. Infect Immun. 1975;2:890–897.
351. Freter R, Allweiss B, O'Brien PCM, et al. Role of chemotaxis in the association of motile bacteria with intestinal mucosa: In vitro studies. Infect Immun. 1981;34:241–249.
352. Hornick RB, Greisman SE, Woodward TE, et al. Typhoid fever: Pathogenesis and immunologic control. N Engl J Med. 1970;283:686.
353. Schneider DR, Parker CD. Isolation and characterization of protease-deficient mutants of *Vibrio cholerae*. J Infect Dis. 1978;138:143–151.
354. Schneider DR, Parker CD. Purification and characterization of the mucinase of *Vibrio cholerae*. J Infect Dis. 1982;145:474–482.
355. Robbins PW, Uchida T. Determinants of specificity in *Salmonella*: Changes in antigenic structure mediated by bacteriophage. Immunochemistry. 1962;21:702.
356. Germanier R, Furer E. Isolation and characterization of Gal E Mutant Ty 21a of *Salmonella typhi*: A candidate strain for a live, oral typhoid vaccine. J Infect Dis. 1975;131:533.
357. Levine MM, Kaper JB, Black RE, et al. New knowledge on pathogenesis of bacterial enteric infections as applied to vaccine development. Microbiol. Rev. 1983;47:510–550.
358. Acharva IL, Lowe CU, Thapa R, et al. Prevention of typhoid fever in Nepal with the Vi capsular polysaccharide of *Salmonella typhi*. N Engl J Med. 1987;317:1102–1104.
359. Klugman KP, Koornhof H, Schneerson R, et al. Protective activity of Vi capsular polysaccharide vaccine against typhoid fever. Lancet. 1987;2:1165–1167.
360. Ruiz-Palacios GM, Torres J, Torres NI, et al. Cholera-like enterotoxin produced by *Campylobacter jejuni*: Characterization and clinical significance. Lancet. 1983;2:250.
361. Guerrant RL, Lahita RG, Winn WC Jr, et al. Campylobacteriosis in man: Pathogenic mechanisms and review of 91 bloodstream infections. Am J Med. 1978;65:584.
362. Perez-Perez GI, Hopkins JA, Blaser MJ. Antigenic heterogeneity of lipopolysaccarides from *Campylobacter jejuni* and *Campylobacter fetus*. Infect Immun. 1985;48:528–533.
363. Field M. Cholera toxin, adenylate cyclase, and the process of active secretion in the small intestine: The pathogenesis of diarrhea in cholera. In: Andreoli TE, Hoffman JF, Fauestil DD, eds. Physiology of Membrane Disorder. New York: Plenum Press; 1978.
364. Davidson GP, Barnes GL. Structural and functional abnormalities of the small intestine in infants and young children with rotavirus enteritis. Acta Paediatr Scand. 1979;68:181.
365. Agus SG, Dolin R, Wyatt RG, et al. Acute infectious nonbacterial gastroenteritis: Intestinal histopathology, histologic and enzymatic alterations during illness produced by Norwalk agent in man. Ann Intern Med. 1973;79:18.
366. Levitan R, Ingelfinger FJ. Effect of D-aldosterone on salt and water absorption from the intact human colon. J Clin Invest. 1965;44:801.
367. Guerrant RL, Chen LC, Rohde JE. Effect of spironolactone on stool electrolyte losses during human cholera. Gut. 1972;13:197.
368. Guerrant RL, Carpenter CCJ. Diarrheagenic effect of volume expansion: Intestinal fluid secretion without mucosal adenyl cyclase stimulation. Johns Hopkins Med J. 1975;136:209.
369. Harris JC, DuPont HL, Hornick RB. Fecal leukocytes in diarrheal illness. Ann Intern Med. 1972;76:697.
370. Guerrant RL, Shields DS, Thorson SM, et al. Evaluation and diagnosis of acute infectious diarrhea. Am J Med. 1985;78:91–98.
371. Said SI, Faloona GR. Elevated plasma and tissue levels of vasoactive intestinal polypeptide in the watery-diarrhea syndrome due to pancreatic, bronchogenic and other tumors. N Engl J Med. 1975;293:155.
372. Guerrant RL, Brush JE, Ravdin JI, et al. The interaction between *Entamoeba histolytica* and human polymorphonuclear leukocytes. J Infect Dis. 1981;143:83.
373. Ravdin JI, Guerrant RL. A review of the parasite cellular mechanisms involved in the pathogenesis of amebiasis. Rev Infect Dis. 1982;4:1185.
374. Seydel KB, Zhang T, Champion GA, et al. *Cryptosporidium parvum* infection of human intestinal xenografts in SCID mice induces production of human tumor necrosis factor and interleukin-8. Infect Immun. 1998;66:2379–2382.
374a. Guerrant RL. *Campylobacter* enteritis. In: Wyngaarden JB, Smith LH Jr, eds. Cecil Textbook of Medicine. Philadelphia: Saunders; 1988;1648–1651.
375. Korzeniowski OM, Basada FA, Rouse JD, et al. Value of examination for fecal leukocytes in the early diagnosis of shigellosis. Am J Trop Med Hyg. 1979;28:1031–1035.
376. Guerrant RL, Araujo V, Soares E, et al. Measurement of fecal lactoferrin as a marker of fecal leuckocytes. J Clin Microbiol. 1992;30:1238–1242.
377. Rahaman MM, Huq I, Dey CR: Superiority of MacConkey's agar over *Salmonella-Shigella* agar for isolation of *Shigella dysenteriae* type 1. J Infect Dis. 1975;131:700.
378. Blaser MJ, Reller LB. Campylobacter enteritis. N Engl J Med. 1981;305:1444.
379. Kaplan RL, Barrett JE. Monograph: *Campylobacter.* Kansas City, Mo: Marion Scientific, 1981.
380. Rahaman MM, Khan MM, Azi KMS, et al. An outbreak of dysentery caused by *Shigella dysenteriae* type I on a coral island in the Bay of Bengal. J Infect Dis. 1975;132:15.
381. Feeley JC, Balows A. *Vibrio*. In: Lennette EH, Spaulding EH, Truant JP, eds. Manual of Clinical Microbiology. Washington, DC: American Society for Microbiology; 1974:238.
382. Ryan RW, Kwasnik I, Tilton Rc. Rapid detection of *Clostridium difficile* in human feces. J Clin Microbiol. 1980;12:776.
383. Morris GK, Feeley JC, Martin WT, et al. Isolation and identification of *Yersinia enterocolitica*. Public Health Lab. 1977;35:217.
384. Merson MH, Black RE, Gross RJ, et al. Use of antisera for identification of enterotoxigenic *E. coli*. Lancet. 1980;2:222.
385. Moseley SL, Escheverria P, Seriwatana J, et al. Identification of enterotoxigenic *E. coli* by colony hybridization using three enterotoxin gene probes. J Infect Dis. 1982;145:863.
386. Dean AG, Ching Y-C, Williams RG, et al. Test for *Escherichia coli* using infant mice: Application in a study of diarrhea in children in Honolulu. J Infect Dis. 1972;125:407.
387. Giannella RA. Suckling mouse model for detection of heat-stable *Escherichia coli* enterotoxin: Characteristic of the model. Infect Immun. 1976;14:95.
388. Blake PA, Rosenberg ML, Florencia J, et al. Cholera in Portugal, 1974. Am J Epidemiol. 1977;105:344.
389. Lee JA, Kean BH. International Conference on the Diarrhea of Travelers. New Directions in Research: A summary. J Infect Dis. 1978;137:360.
390. Perez-Schael I, Guntinas MJ, Perez M, et al. Efficacy of the rhesus rotavirus-based quadrivalent vaccine in infants and young children in Venezuela. N Engl J Med. 1997;337:1181–1187.
391. Costerton JW, Geesey GG, Cheng K-J. How bacteria stick. Sci Am. 1977;1:86.
392. Ericsson CD, Evans DG, DuPont HL, et al. Bismuth subsalicylate inhibits activity of crude toxins of *Escherichia coli* and *Vibrio cholerae*. J Infect Dis. 1977;136:693.
393. Palmer DL, Koster FT, Islam AFRM, et al. A comparison of sucrose and glucose in oral electrolyte treatment of cholera and other severe diarrhea. N Engl J Med. 1977;297:1107.
394. Oral glucose/electrolyte therapy for acute diarrhea. (Editorial). Lancet. 1975;1:79.
395. Molla AM, Molla A, Nath SK, et al. Food-based oral rehydration salt solutions for acute childhood diarrhoea. Lancet. 1989;2:429–431.
396. Robbins-Browne RM. Traditional enteropathogenic *Escherichia coli* of infantile diarrhea. Rev Infect Dis. 1987;9:28–53.
397. Echeverria P, Orskov F, Orskov I, et al. Attaching and effacing enteropathogenic *Escherichia coli* as a cause of infantile diarrhea in Bangkok. J Infect Dis. 1991;164:550–554.
398. Levine MM, Edelman R. Enteropathogenic *Escherichia coli* of classic serotypes associated with infant diarrhea. Epidemiol Rev. 1984;6:31–51.
399. Whittam TS, Wolfe ML, Wachsmuth IK, et al. Clonal relationships among *Escherichia coli* strains that cause hemorrhagic colitis and infantile diarrhea. Infect Immun. 1993;61:1619–1629.
400. Scotland SM, Willshaw GA, Cheasty T, et al. Strains of *Escherichia coli* O157:H8 from human diarrhoea belong to attaching and effacing class of *E. coli*. J Clin Pathol. 1992;45:1075–1078.
401. Soares AM, Freire JE Jr, Lima AAM. Mathematical dose-response model in sodium intestinal cotransport with glutamine and glucose on isolated rabbit ileum mucosa. Braz J Med Biol Res. 1992;25:1141–1144.
402. Lima AAM, Soares AM, Freire JE Jr, et al. Cotransport of sodium with glutamine, alanine and glucose in the isolated rabbit ileal mucosa. Braz J Med Biol Res. 1992;25:637–640.
403. Silva AC, Santos-Neto MS, Soares AM, et al. Efficacy of a glutamine-based oral rehydration solution on the electrolyte and water absorption in a rabbit model of secretory diarrhea induced by cholera toxin. J Pediatr Gastroenterol Nutri. 1998;26:513–519.

Chapter 82

Esophagitis

PAUL S. GRAMAN

Esophagitis, or inflammation of the esophagus, is most often caused by noninfectious conditions, and gastroesophageal reflux disease is the most common. Esophageal infection occurs predominantly in patients with impaired immunity resulting from cancer chemotherapy, transplantation, or human immunodeficiency virus (HIV) infection and occasionally in persons who are otherwise healthy. *Candida albicans*, cytomegalovirus (CMV), and herpes simplex virus (HSV) are the leading etiologic agents of esophageal infection. Among patients with HIV infection, aphthous ulceration of the esophagus is a well-recognized entity. Acute HIV infection may also be a direct cause of esophageal ulceration.[1] A variety of other fungal, viral, mycobacterial, and parasitic agents have been shown to cause esophagitis on rare occasion. Pill-induced esophagitis resulting from local mucosal injury has been attributed to antimicrobial agents and many other drugs, particularly when these are ingested without water or in the supine position.[2, 3] Infectious and noninfectious etiologies of esophagitis are listed in Table 82–1. Multiple concomitant etiologies of esophagitis are not uncommon in patients who are significantly immunosuppressed or critically ill.[10]

CLINICAL MANIFESTATIONS

Most patients with esophagitis present with odynophagia (pain on swallowing) or dysphagia, described as difficulty swallowing or a sense of obstruction either substernal, epigastric, or in the throat. Liquids are often better tolerated than solids such as meats, which may worsen both odynophagia and dysphagia. Pain may be exacerbated by the ingestion of acidic liquids and by eructation. Ulcerative esophagitis is characterized primarily by odynophagia, which can be severe, at times to the point of limiting oral intake and resulting in weight loss and dehydration. Spontaneous substernal pain or burning may also occur intermittently, unrelated to swallowing. Gastrointestinal bleeding is rarely the initial manifestation of esophagitis, but it does occur.[22] Among patients evaluated for nausea and vomiting or abdominal pain, endoscopically proven esophagitis may be present in the absence of specific esophageal symptoms. In a recent review, odynophagia or dysphagia was absent in 21 to 41% of patients with documented esophagitis caused by *Candida*, HSV, CMV, or *Mycobacterium tuberculosis*.[23] Fever accompanied esophagitis in 20% of patients with CMV or mycobacterial infection, but it was less common among those with *Candida* or HSV. Nausea and vomiting were most common (42%) in patients with CMV esophagitis, possibly reflecting the fact that CMV infection is seldom confined to the esophagus. Oral lesions frequently provide clues to the diagnosis of esophagitis, particularly in patients with acquired immunodeficiency syndrome (AIDS). Oral thrush is seen in most patients with esophageal candidiasis and AIDS.[24] The finding of oropharyngeal candidiasis in a patient with esophageal symptoms and AIDS has a positive predictive value of 70% or higher for esophageal involvement.[8, 10, 25–27] Similarly, oropharyngeal vesicles or ulcerations may suggest, but do not prove concomitant esophageal HSV or aphthous ulceration in a symptomatic patient.

TABLE 82–1 Etiology of Esophagitis

Common	Uncommon
Infectious	
Candidiasis	Tuberculosis[4–7]
Cytomegalovirus	*Mycobacterium avium* complex[8, 9]
Herpes simplex virus	Cryptococcosis[10, 11]
HIV infection, acute	Histoplasmosis[12]
	Actinomycosis[13, 14]
	Cryptosporidiosis[15]
	Pneumocystosis[16]
	Varicella-zoster virus[17, 18]
	Epstein-Barr virus[19]
Noninfectious	
Gastroesophageal reflux	Ingestion of corrosives (e.g., lye)
Mucositis from cancer chemotherapy	Local mucositis from tablets or capsules[2, 3] (e.g., doxycycline, zidovudine,[20] ddC[21])
Mucositis from radiation therapy	
Aphthous ulcers	

Abbreviation: ddC, Dideoxycytidine (zalcitabine).
Adapted from Polis M. Esophagitis. In: Mandell GL, Bennett JE, Dolin R, eds. Principles and Practice of Infectious Diseases. 4th ed. New York: Churchill Livingstone; 1995:962–965.

SPECIFIC ETIOLOGIC AGENTS

Candida Esophagitis

C. albicans is the predominant pathogen of esophagitis (see Chapter 247). Non-*albicans* species of *Candida*, including *Candida tropicalis*, *Candida parapsilosis*, *Candida krusei*, and *Candida glabrata*, are implicated less often but may play a greater role as a result of selective pressure among patients who have received antifungal agents.[28] Small numbers of *C. albicans* are part of the normal oral flora, and esophageal colonization may be present in up to 20% of the population,[29] particularly in patients treated with H_2 blockers.[30] Colonization is the initial process whereby superficial adherence and proliferation of organisms remain confined to the superficial mucosa, without penetration or inflammation of the epithelium. Colonization progresses to infection when systemic and local defenses are inadequate to prevent invasion into deeper epithelial layers, with pseudohyphae seen at the advancing margin of tissue involvement. On endoscopic examination, the esophagus appears hyperemic with discrete, yellow-white mucosal plaques that are firmly adherent and, when removed, reveal an underlying rough and friable surface (Fig. 82–1). Lesions are most frequently located in the distal third of the esophagus. A scoring system for the severity of *Candida* esophagitis on endoscopy has been proposed: grade 1, few raised white plaques up to 2 mm in size, no ulceration; grade 2, multiple larger plaques, without ulceration; grade 3, confluent, linear, and nodular elevated plaques with ulceration; and grade 4, features of grade 3 with luminal narrowing.[2] Perforation of the esophagus is a rare complication.

Systemic host factors predisposing to esophageal candidiasis include acute[31] and advanced HIV infection, diabetes mellitus, leukemia and lymphoma, broad-spectrum antimicrobial therapy, antineoplastic therapy, corticosteroid therapy, and bone marrow or solid organ transplantation. In addition to immune dysfunction, contributing local factors are those that impair esophageal motility, such as systemic sclerosis, achalasia, esophageal webs or rings, or obstructing esophageal cancer, and conditions that result in mucosal injury, such as reflux esophagitis. Esophageal symptoms occur in up to half of all patients with AIDS,[8, 32] and *Candida* accounts for 50% or more of these cases.[10, 27] Porro and colleagues documented esophageal candidiasis in 48% of AIDS patients admitted to the hospital, although 40% of those infected reported no esophageal symptoms.[26] Transplant recipients, many of whom receive routine antifungal prophylaxis, appear less susceptible to *Candida* esophagitis, which developed in 5 (2.2%) of 224 renal transplant patients[33] and none of 304 cardiac transplant recipients.[34] Among symptomatic bone marrow transplant patients, esophageal infection was diagnosed in 21 of 46 endoscopic examinations, but *Candida* accounted for only 5 of the 21 infections, the remainder being caused by CMV, HSV, or both.[35]

Accurate diagnosis of esophageal candidiasis is established by endoscopy with directed brushings and biopsies. The characteristic gross appearance of candidiasis is suggestive, but occasionally misleading inasmuch as white exudative lesions may also be visualized with HSV or CMV infection or pill esophagitis. Brushings of exuda-

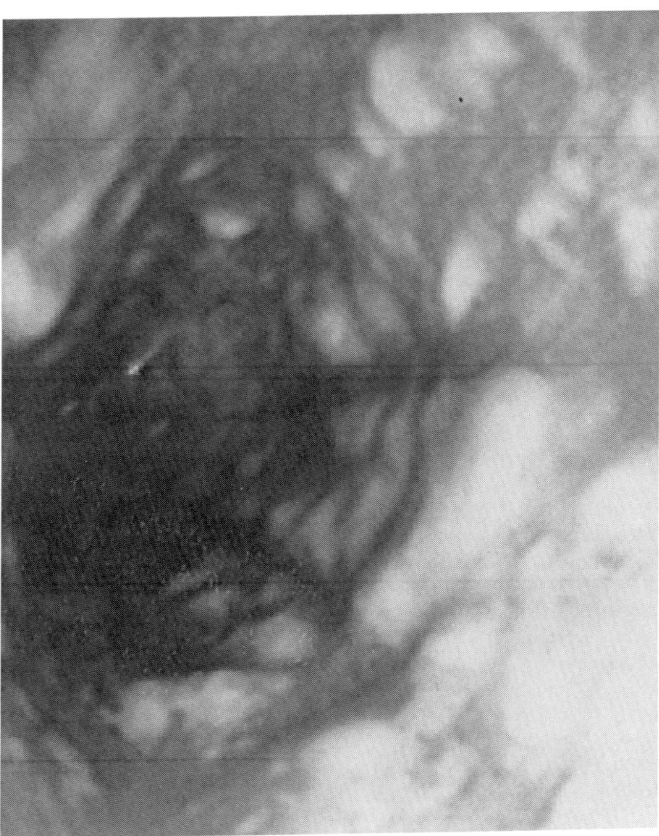

FIGURE 82–1. Endoscopic appearance of esophageal candidiasis, showing typical white plaques and nodules, in a patient with multiple myeloma. (Courtesy of Dr. Arthur DeCross, Rochester, NY.)

tive lesions and ulcer craters are obtained with a sheathed cytology brush, smeared onto slides, and submitted for periodic acid–Schiff, silver, or Gram stain. Biopsies of lesions and the edges of ulcers are submitted for histopathologic examination and for viral culture to identify CMV and HSV. Masses of yeast and pseudohyphae seen in tissue or brushings are diagnostic of *Candida* infection. Fungal cultures are not generally helpful, except to identify the pathogen in cases of fungal esophagitis that are refractory to treatment. Blind brushing of the esophagus via a nasogastric tube has been advocated as an alternative to endoscopy in patients with HIV infection and suspected esophagitis; this technique was 96% sensitive and 87% specific for the diagnosis of candidiasis.[25]

Radiologic contrast studies are of limited diagnostic value and seldom performed in patients with esophagitis. Although focal or confluent plaques or a diffuse "shaggy" appearance is characteristic of candidiasis on the esophagogram (Fig. 82–2), the examination result may be normal in some patients, and visualized abnormalities such as plaques, ulcerations, fistulas, or masses are often nonspecific; concurrent infections are likely to be missed.[22, 36] Radiographic studies may be useful if endoscopy is unavailable.

Cytomegalovirus Esophagitis

CMV esophagitis occurs most often in patients with AIDS or severe immunosuppression. CMV was an esophageal pathogen or copathogen in 33 (30%) of 110 patients with HIV infection and esophageal symptoms[10] and in 7 (33%) of 21 symptomatic recipients of bone marrow transplants.[35] Rare cases in immunocompetent hosts are reported.[37] Symptoms are indistinguishable from those associated with *Candida* or HSV esophagitis. The endoscopic appearance of CMV esophagitis is typified by large (>10 cm^2), shallow "punched-out" ulcers, solitary or multiple in number, located in the middle to distal part of the esophagus.[38] The ulcer margins are distinct and the intervening mucosa appears relatively normal. Isolation of CMV in culture is not diagnostic because virus harbored in blood or saliva may contaminate esophageal specimens. Conversely, culture is not positive in all cases. Histopathologic examination is the most reliable diagnostic method when mucosal and submucosal biopsies are obtained from the ulcer edge and ulcer base; routine hematoxylin and eosin staining demonstrates enlarged endothelial cells or fibroblasts containing large, dense intranuclear inclusions.[38] Immunohistochemical and direct fluorescent staining techniques, highly specific for CMV and HSV, may also help etablish these diagnoses. Coinfections of the esophagus are common in patients with CMV; concomitant candidiasis (73%) and HSV (12%) have been reported among these patients.[10]

Herpes Simplex Esophagitis

Herpes simplex esophagitis is usually identified in patients with AIDS or other significant immunosuppression, although cases in healthy adults are also seen. Among 23 patients with HSV esophagitis reported by McBane and associates, 7 (30%) had hematologic malignancies, 4 (17%) had received chemotherapy or irradiation for solid tumors, 8 (35%) had been treated with immunosuppressive agents for nonmalignant conditions, and 1 was otherwise healthy.[39] HSV esophagitis accounts for 6 to 16% of HIV-infected patients with esophageal symptoms.[32] In a series of 21 bone marrow transplant recipients with esophagitis, HSV was identified in 48%.[35] More than 35 cases of HSV esophagitis have been described in immunocompetent hosts, in whom the infection is self-limited.[40, 41] Odyno-

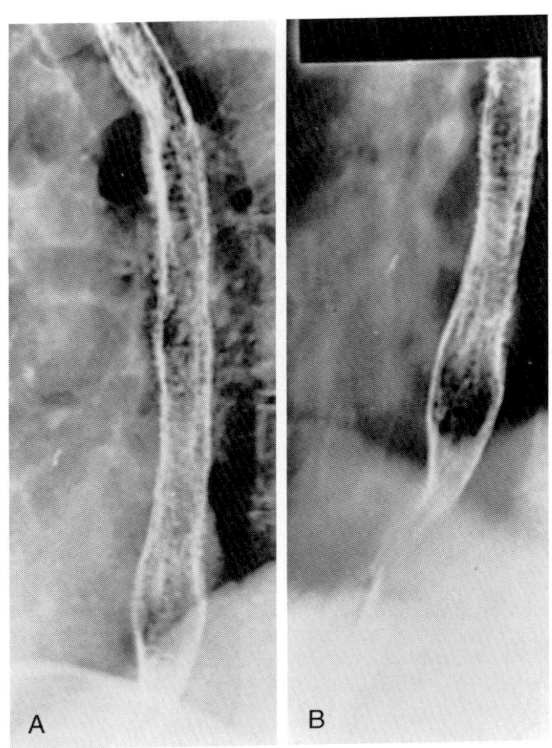

FIGURE 82–2. *A* and *B*, Barium contrast esophagograms of *Candida* esophagitis showing a markedly irregular esophagus due to multiple plaques in a patient with acquired immunodeficiency syndrome and severe odynophagia. (From Polis M. Esophagitis. In: Mandell GL, Bennett JE, Dolin R, eds. Principles and Practice of Infectious Diseases. 4th ed. New York: Churchill Livingstone; 1995:962–965.)

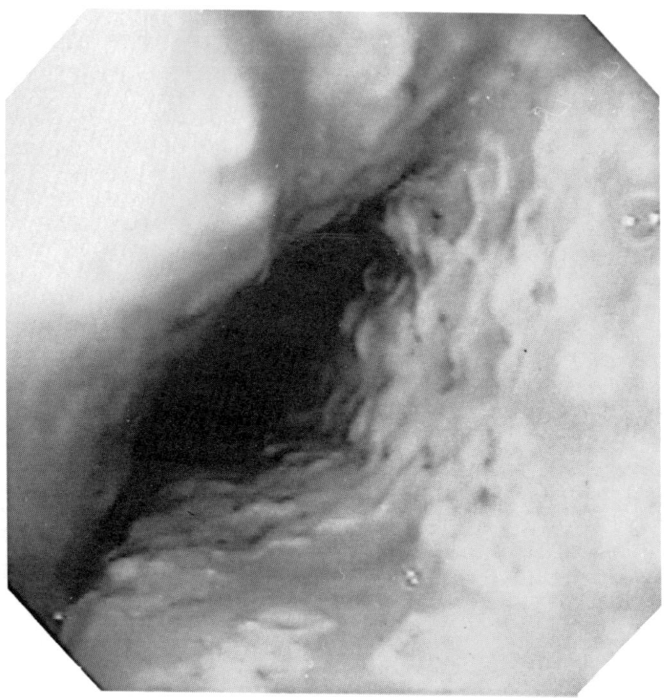

FIGURE 82–3. Herpes simplex esophagitis, characterized by numerous small ulcerations, in an immunocompetent adult with fever and odynophagia. (Courtesy of Dr. Charles Michalko, Rochester, NY.)

phagia, chest pain, fever, nausea, and vomiting are the most common initial symptoms; clinically significant gastrointestinal bleeding occurs in 15 to 25%.[39] Oral, labial, or cutaneous HSV is clinically evident in only 19 to 38% of cases.[40, 42] Typical lesions appear endoscopically as multiple, small superficial ulcers in the distal third of the esophagus; larger confluent ulcers, pseudomembranes, or diffusely denuded epithelium may be seen as the infection progresses (Fig. 82–3). "Volcano ulcers" may have raised margins around the central crater. Vesicles are rarely visualized. Double-contrast esophagography demonstrates ulcerative irregularities that are not specific or diagnostic. Viral culture of brushings or biopsies is the most sensitive diagnostic tool and is positive for HSV-1 in most, but not all cases; HSV-2 has rarely been implicated.[42] Histologic examination may show characteristic ballooning degeneration, multinucleated giant cells, and prominent intranuclear Cowdry type A inclusion bodies in 55 to 70% of biopsy specimens.

Aphthous (Idiopathic) Ulceration of the Esophagus

Aphthous or idiopathic ulceration, an important variant of esophagitis in patients with advanced HIV infection, accounts for approximately 5% of AIDS patients with esophagitis.[8, 10] No specific etiology is evident in 40% of AIDS patients with esophageal ulceration,[43] and painful ulcers are often present in the oropharynx as well.[44] Esophageal ulceration has also been described in patients with acute HIV infection presenting initially with odynophagia, and detection of HIV virions by electron microscopy in the margins of these ulcers has suggested to some a direct pathogenic role for HIV itself.[1] Others, having detected HIV nucleic acid by *in situ* hybridization or polymerase chain reaction in the esophageal mucosa of up to 80% of AIDS patients with idiopathic ulceration or with specific etiologic diagnoses (*Candida*, CMV, or HSV esophagitis), have concluded that HIV is not a primary pathogen in ulcerative disease.[27, 45] Other unrecognized infectious agents may contribute to the pathogenesis of these idiopathic ulcerations.

TABLE 82–3 Etiology of Esophagitis in Symptomatic Patients with Underlying Disease*

Etiology	AIDS† (n = 183)	Bone Marrow Transplant‡ (n = 39)	Solid Organ Transplant§ (n = 88)
Candida alone	38	10	3
Candida + other	22	3	
Cytomegalovirus	21	26	6
Herpes simplex virus	11	26	7
Aphthous ulceration	4		
Kaposi's sarcoma	7		

*Patients on whom upper endoscopy was performed to evaluate odynophagia, dysphagia, epigastric pain, nausea and vomiting, or gastrointestinal bleeding. Values are percentages of patients.
†Data from refs. 8, 10, and 27.
‡Data from ref. 35.
§Data from refs. 34 and 48.

MANAGEMENT OF ESOPHAGEAL INFECTION

General Considerations in Therapy

Specific therapies for infectious etiologies of esophagitis are listed in Table 82–2. The approach to diagnosis and therapy in a particular patient often depends on the presence of underlying disease and the severity of immunosuppression (Table 82–3).

Patients receiving cancer chemotherapy may experience severe mucositis with odynophagia that is clinically indistinguishable from fungal or viral esophagitis. Diagnostic endoscopy should be pursued whenever possible, but in practice the procedure is frequently deferred because of bleeding, severe pain, mucosal friability, or critical illness; empirical therapy for *Candida* and HSV is appropriate in the interim period, particularly if oral thrush or mucocutaneous HSV lesions are clinically evident or cultures are positive. Patients with fever and neutropenia (less than 100 neutrophils/mm^3) are usually treated empirically with amphotericin B in doses (0.5 to 1.0 mg/kg/day) sufficient to treat either esophageal or disseminated candidiasis. Intravenous acyclovir is often administered in this acute setting if HSV stomatitis or labialis is present or if esophageal symptoms are severe. Allogeneic bone marrow transplant recipients who are

TABLE 82–2 Treatment of Esophagitis

Etiology	Usual Therapy (Adult Dose)	Alternative Drugs
Candida	Fluconazole, 100–200 mg/d PO or IV for 14–21 d; maintenance suppressive therapy may be necessary in AIDS (fluconazole, 100–200 mg/d PO)	Itraconazole, 100 mg bid oral suspension PO Amphotericin B, 0.3 mg/kg/d IV for 7 d, or 500 mg qid oral suspension PO; used if refractory to other agents
Herpes simplex	Acyclovir, 5 mg/kg IV q8h for 7–14 d or 400 mg 5×/d PO for 14–21 d; maintenance suppressive therapy may be necessary in AIDS	Foscarnet, 90 mg/kg q12h IV for 7–14 d; used if acyclovir resistant Famciclovir, 500 mg bid PO (not for acyclovir resistant)
Cytomegalovirus	Ganciclovir, 5 mg/kg IV q12h for 14–21 d; maintenance suppressive therapy usually necessary in AIDS (ganciclovir, 5 mg/kg/d IV or 6 mg/kg/d IV 5×/wk)	Foscarnet, 90 mg/kg q12h for 14–21 d; suppression with foscarnet, 90–120 mg/kg/d IV
Aphthous (in AIDS)	Prednisone,[46] 40 mg/d PO for 14 d, then taper	Thalidomide,[47] 200 mg/d PO*

*Not approved by the Food and Drug Administration for this indication.

neutropenic commonly receive antiviral prophylaxis until engraftment occurs. Esophageal infections in bone marrow transplant patients usually begin more than 40 days after transplantation, and neutrophil counts are generally within the normal range at that time; CMV and HSV are at least as common as *Candida* in this group of patients, and treatment should be guided by the results of endoscopic diagnosis.[35] Similarly, treatment of esophagitis in solid organ transplant recipients or immunocompetent hosts should be guided by endoscopic appearance, culture data, and histopathology. Tacrolimus and cyclosporine levels may be elevated and should be monitored in transplant patients receiving concomitant fluconazole or itraconazole.

Esophagitis in Patients with Acquired Immunodeficiency Syndrome

Esophageal symptoms occur in 40 to 50% of patients with AIDS at some point in the course of their disease and may have a significant impact on nutritional status and overall morbidity.[8, 22, 32] The frequencies of various etiologies are shown in Table 82–3, and treatment regimens are listed in Table 82–2. *Candida* esophagitis is the most common and is treated empirically with fluconazole if oropharyngeal candidiasis is also observed in a symptomatic patient; oral thrush is predictive of esophageal involvement in more than 70% of such cases.[8, 10, 25–27] Ketoconazole is erratically absorbed and is less effective. Patients who fail to respond to empirical fluconazole therapy within 7 days should have endoscopy performed to establish a diagnosis.

A viral etiology is identified in approximately one third of cases, often in association with candidiasis. Empirical antiviral therapy for CMV or HSV is discouraged. Patients with CMV esophagitis confirmed by culture and histopathologic examination are treated with ganciclovir, 5 mg/kg intravenously every 12 hours. Cases refractory to ganciclovir may respond to foscarnet, 90 mg/kg intravenously every 12 hours. A partial or complete response to induction therapy is observed in 75 to 85% of patients treated with either ganciclovir or foscarnet,[49–51] but relapses are common with or without maintenance therapy. Documented HSV esophagitis is usually treated with intravenous acyclovir initially in severe cases; therapy may be continued with oral acyclovir or famciclovir. Complete resolution is reported in 70% of patients treated with acyclovir, but relapse occurs in 15% of patients within 4 months.[42] Patients who fail acyclovir therapy because of resistance are not expected to respond to ganciclovir and should receive foscarnet.

Patients with aphthous ulceration of the esophagus have improved on a regimen of prednisone, 40 mg daily for 2 weeks, in more than 90% of cases.[46] A placebo-controlled trial demonstrated complete healing of AIDS-associated oropharyngeal aphthous ulcers in 55% of 29 patients treated with thalidomide, 200 mg daily for 1 month, as compared with only 7% of patients in the placebo group.[47] In a series of 12 patients with idiopathic esophageal ulceration, 92% experienced complete resolution of symptoms with the same regimen.[52] Use of these therapies should be considered in patients with esophageal ulcerations not attributable to specific pathogens. Zidovudine and zalcitabine (ddC) capsules may also cause esophageal ulceration; patients should be advised to take these and all oral medications in the upright position with sufficient water.[20, 21]

Approximately 5% of patients with endoscopically proven *Candida* esophagitis are refractory to fluconazole therapy because of either acquisition of a resistant strain or gradual emergence of resistance over time. Refractory candidiasis is most common in patients with advanced AIDS and long-term exposure to antifungal agents. Patients unresponsive to fluconazole, 200 mg daily for 2 weeks, are not likely to respond to higher doses; 50 to 60% of refractory patients have responded to itraconazole oral solution, 200 to 400 mg daily.[53, 54] Itraconazole tablets are less efficacious.[55] Amphotericin B oral solution is an effective alternative for many patients; parenteral amphotericin is reserved for patients who fail other therapies. Relapse rates are higher with refractory candidiasis, and maintenance therapy is nearly always required. Antiretroviral therapy should also be optimized in such patients. To reduce the risk of refractory disease, continuous antifungal prophylaxis should be avoided in most AIDS patients with mucosal candidiasis unless recurrences are particularly frequent or severe.[53]

Various other pathogens have caused rare cases of esophagitis in patients with AIDS, including *Pneumocystis carinii*,[16] Epstein-Barr virus,[19] *Mycobacterium avium* complex,[8, 9] *Histoplasma capsulatum*,[12] *Cryptococcus neoformans*,[10] *Cryptosporidium*,[15] and *Actinomyces*.[13, 14] Therapy is the same as for infections with these agents at other sites. Kaposi's sarcoma involving the esophagus has been documented in up to 7% of AIDS patients with esophageal symptoms.[8, 10, 27]

REFERENCES

1. Rabeneck L, Popovic M, Gartner S, et al. Acute HIV infection presenting with painful swallowing and esophageal ulcers. JAMA. 1990;263:2318–2322.
2. Baehr PH, McDonald GB. Esophageal disorders caused by infection, systemic illness, medications, radiation, and trauma. In: Feldman M, Scharschmidt BF, Sleisenger MH, eds. *Gastrointestinal and Liver Disease*. 6th ed. Philadelphia: WB Saunders; 1998:519–539.
3. Kikendall JW. Pill-induced esophageal injury. Gastroenterol Clin North Am. 1991;20:835–846.
4. Monig SP, Schmidt R, Wolters U, Krug B. Esophageal tuberculosis: A differential diagnostic challenge. Am J Gastroenterol. 1995;90:153–154.
5. Mokoena T, Shama DM, Ngakane H, Bryer JV. Oesophageal tuberculosis: A review of eleven cases. Postgrad Med J. 1992;68:110–115.
6. Rosario MT, Raso CL, Comer GM. Esophageal tuberculosis. Dig Dis Sci. 1989;34:1281–1284.
7. Garcia Sepulcre MF, Casellas Valde JA, Alonso Maillo G, et al. Esophageal tuberculosis with fistula to mediastinum. Am J Gastroenterol. 1995;90:2074–2075.
8. Connolly GM, Hawkins D, Harcourt-Webster JN, et al. Oesophageal symptoms, their causes, treatment, and prognosis in patients with the acquired immunodeficiency syndrome. Gut. 1989;30:1033–1039.
9. El-Serag HB, Johnston DE. *Mycobacterium avium* complex esophagitis. Am J Gastroenterol. 1997;92:1561–1563.
10. Bonacini M, Young T, Laine L. The causes of esophageal symptoms in human immunodeficiency virus infection. A prospective study of 110 patients. Arch Intern Med. 1991;151:1567–1572.
11. Jacobs DH, Macher AM, Handler R, et al. Esophageal cryptococcosis in a patient with the hyperimmunoglobulin E–recurrent infection (Job's) syndrome. Gastroenterology. 1984;87:201–203.
12. Forsmark CE, Wilcox CM, Darragh TM, Cello JP. Disseminated histoplasmosis in AIDS: An unusual case of esophageal involvement and gastrointestinal bleeding. Gastrointest Endosc. 1990;36:604–605.
13. Poles MA, McMeeking AA, Scholes JV, Dieterich DT. *Actinomyces* infection of a cytomegalovirus esophageal ulcer in two patients with acquired immunodeficiency syndrome. Am J Gastroenterol. 1994;89:1569–1572.
14. Spencer GM, Roach D, Skucas J. Actinomycosis of the esophagus in a patient with AIDS: Findings on barium esophagograms. AJR Am J Roentgenol. 1993;161:795–796.
15. Kazlow PG, Shah K, Benkov KJ, et al. Esophageal cryptosporidiosis in a child with acquired immune deficiency syndrome. Gastroenterology. 1986;91:1301–1303.
16. Grimes MM, LaPook JD, Bar MH, et al. Disseminated *Pneumocystis carinii* infection in a patient with acquired immunodeficiency syndrome. Hum Pathol. 1987;18:307–308.
17. Sherman RA, Silva J Jr, Gandour-Edwards R. Fatal varicella in an adult: Case report and review of the gastrointestinal complications of chickenpox. Rev Infect Dis. 1991;13:424–427.
18. Gill RA, Gebhard RL, Dozeman RL, Sumner HW. Shingles esophagitis: Endoscopic diagnosis in two patients. Gastrointest Endosc. 1984;30:26–27.
19. Kitchen VS, Helbert M, Francis ND, et al. Epstein-Barr virus associated oesophageal ulcers in AIDS. Gut. 1990;31:1223–1225.
20. Edwards P, Turner J, Gold J, Cooper DA. Esophageal ulceration induced by zidovudine. Ann Intern Med. 1990;112:65–66.
21. Indorf AS, Pegram PS. Esophageal ulceration related to zalcitabine (ddC). Ann Intern Med. 1992;117:133–134.
22. Wilcox CM. Esophageal disease in the acquired immunodeficiency syndrome: Etiology, diagnosis, and management. Am J Med. 1992;92:412–421.
23. Baehr PH, McDonald GB. Esophageal infections: Risk factors, presentation, diagnosis, and treatment. Gastroenterology. 1994;106:509–532.
24. Tavitian A, Raufman JP, Rosenthal LE. Oral candidiasis as a marker for esophageal candidiasis in the acquired immunodeficiency syndrome. Ann Intern Med. 1986;104:54–55.
25. Bonacini M, Laine L, Gal AA, et al. Prospective evaluation of blind brushing of the esophagus for *Candida* esophagitis in patients with human immunodeficiency virus infection. Am J Gastroenterol. 1990;85:385–389.

26. Porro GB, Parente F, Cernuschi M. The diagnosis of esophageal candidiasis in patients with acquired immune deficiency syndrome: Is endoscopy always necessary? Am J Gastroenterol. 1989;84:143–146.
27. Smith PD, Eisner MS, Manischewitz JF, et al. Esophageal disease in AIDS is associated with pathologic processes rather than mucosal human immunodeficiency virus type 1. J Infect Dis. 1993;167:547–552.
28. Wingard JR, Merz WG, Rinaldi MG, et al. Increase in *Candida krusei* infection among patients with bone marrow transplantation and neutropenia treated prophylactically with fluconazole. N Engl J Med. 1991;325:1274–1277.
29. Andersen LI, Frederiksen HJ, Appleyard M. Prevalence of esophageal *Candida* colonization in a Danish population: Special reference to esophageal symptoms, benign esophageal disorders, and pulmonary disease. J Infect Dis. 1992;165:389–392.
30. Vermeersch B, Rysselaere M, Dekeyser K, et al. Fungal colonization of the esophagus. Am J Gastroenterol. 1989;84:1079–1083.
31. Decker CF, Tiernan R, Paparello SF. Esophageal candidiasis associated with acute infection due to human immunodeficiency virus. Clin Infect Dis. 1992;14:791.
32. Laine L, Bonacini M. Esophageal disease in human immunodeficiency virus infection. Arch Intern Med. 1994;154:1577–1582.
33. Frick T, Fryd DS, Goodale RL, et al. Incidence and treatment of candida esophagitis in patients undergoing renal transplantation. Data from the Minnesota prospective randomized trial of cyclosporine versus antilymphocyte globulin–azathioprine. Am J Surg. 1988;155:311–313.
34. Johnson R, Peitzman AB, Webster MW, et al. Upper gastrointestinal endoscopy after cardiac transplantation. Surgery. 1988;103:300–304.
35. McDonald GB, Sharma P, Hackman RC, et al. Esophageal infections in immunosuppressed patients after marrow transplantation. Gastroenterology. 1985;88:1111–1117.
36. Levine MS, Macones AJ Jr, Laufer I. *Candida* esophagitis: Accuracy of radiographic diagnosis. Radiology. 1985;154:581–587.
37. Altman C, Bedossa P, Dussaix E, Buffet C. Cytomegalovirus infection of esophagus in immunocompetent adult. Dig Dis Sci. 1995;40:606–608.
38. Wilcox CM, Diehl DL, Cello JP, et al. Cytomegalovirus esophagitis in patients with AIDS. A clinical, endoscopic, and pathologic correlation. Ann Intern Med. 1990;113:589–593.
39. McBane RD, Gross JB Jr. Herpes esophagitis: Clinical syndrome, endoscopic appearance, and diagnosis in 23 patients. Gastrointest Endosc. 1991;37:600–603.
40. Galbraith JC, Shafran SD. Herpes simplex esophagitis in the immunocompetent patient: Report of four cases and review. Clin Infect Dis. 1992;14:894–901.
41. Ramanathan J, Rammouni M, Baran J, Khatib R. Herpes simplex esophagitis in the immunocompetent host: Primary disease or reactivation? Abstract 279. Presented at the Thirty-sixth Annual Meeting of the Infectious Diseases Society of America, Denver, 1998.
42. Genereau T, Lortholary O, Bouchaud O, et al. Herpes simplex esophagitis in patients with AIDS: Report of 34 cases. The Cooperative Study Group on Herpetic Esophagitis in HIV Infection. Clin Infect Dis. 1996;22:926–931.
43. Wilcox CM, Schwartz DA, Clark WS. Esophageal ulceration in human immunodeficiency virus infection. Causes, response to therapy, and long-term outcome. Ann Intern Med. 1995;123:143–149.
44. Bach MC, Howell DA, Valenti AJ, et al. Aphthous ulceration of the gastrointestinal tract in patients with the acquired immunodeficiency syndrome (AIDS). Ann Intern Med. 1990;112:465–467.
45. Wilcox CM, Zaki SR, Coffield LM, et al. Evaluation of idiopathic esophageal ulceration for human immunodeficiency virus. Mod Pathol. 1995;8:568–572.
46. Wilcox CM, Schwartz DA. Comparison of two corticosteroid regimens for the treatment of HIV-associated idiopathic esophageal ulcer. Am J Gastroenterol. 1994;89:2163–2167.
47. Jacobson JM, Greenspan JS, Spritzler J, et al. Thalidomide for the treatment of oral aphthous ulcers in patients with human immunodeficiency virus infection. N Engl J Med. 1997;336:1487–1493.
48. Alexander JA, Brouillette DE, Chien MC, et al. Infectious esophagitis following liver and renal transplantation. Dig Dis Sci. 1988;33:1121–1126.
49. Wilcox CM, Straub RF, Schwartz DA. Cytomegalovirus esophagitis in AIDS: A prospective evaluation of clinical response to ganciclovir therapy, relapse rate, and long-term outcome. Am J Med. 1995;98:169–176.
50. Parente F, Bianchi Porro G. Treatment of cytomegalovirus esophagitis in patients with acquired immune deficiency syndrome: A randomized controlled study of foscarnet versus ganciclovir. Am J Gastroenterol. 1998;93:317–322.
51. Blanshard C, Benhamou Y, Dohin E, et al. Treatment of AIDS-associated gastrointestinal cytomegalovirus infection with foscarnet and ganciclovir: A randomized comparison. J Infect Dis. 1995;172:622–628.
52. Alexander LN, Wilcox CM. A prospective trial of thalidomide for the treatment of HIV-associated idiopathic esophageal ulcers. AIDS Res Hum Retroviruses. 1997;13:301–304.
53. Fichtenbaum CJ, Powderly WG. Refractory mucosal candidiasis in patients with human immunodeficiency virus infection. Clin Infect Dis. 1998;26:556–565.
54. Wilcox CM, Darouiche RO, Laine L, et al. A randomized, double-blind comparison of itraconazole oral solution and fluconazole tablets in the treatment of esophageal candidiasis. J Infect Dis. 1997:176:227–232.
55. Barbaro G, Barbarini G, Calderon W, et al. Fluconazole versus itraconazole for candida esophagitis in acquired immunodeficiency syndrome. Gastroenterology. 1996;111:1169–1177.

Chapter 83

Nausea, Vomiting, and Noninflammatory Diarrhea

RICHARD L. GUERRANT
DAVID A. BOBAK

The vast majority of acute gastrointestinal illnesses do not involve a recognizable inflammatory process.[1–4] Although there is considerable inflammatory enteritis during summer months in warm areas with poor sanitation, most cases of diarrhea in these areas are noninflammatory, which suggests an enterotoxic bacterial, viral, or noninvasive parasitic process.[2, 5–9]

EPIDEMIC DIARRHEA IN NEWBORN NURSERIES

Epidemic infantile diarrhea has long been recognized as a potentially serious problem that occurs in newborn nurseries. The mortality rate for this disease has been as high as 24 to 50%.[10, 11] Epidemic diarrhea among hospitalized newborns has been associated with certain "enteropathogenic" serotypes of *Escherichia coli* (EPEC). Enteropathogenic *E. coli* serotypes have been associated with diarrhea in hospitalized infants under 4 months of age.

The unusual susceptibility of newborns may be explained by their unique host status; they have not yet acquired a normal intestinal flora or specific immunity. In infants in special care nurseries, this situation is compounded by severe underlying diseases such as prematurity or congenital cardiac or pulmonary disease. The consequences of diarrhea in the newborn are unusually severe because of poorly developed homeostatic mechanisms and limited water and electrolyte reserves. Nosocomial transmission may occur because the newborn nurseries may be crowded with susceptible infants.[12] A nursery outbreak can go unrecognized because infants may develop diarrhea after being discharged.

The onset is insidious, with the development of listlessness, irritability, and poor feeding over a period of 3 to 6 days.[11, 13, 14] Vomiting and fever are infrequent, and the stools tend to be watery, yellow-green in color, and usually without mucus, pus, or blood. Early signs such as failure to gain weight or a slight weight loss and abdominal distention may be subtle. The disease may progress to more severe signs of dehydration and shock with depressed sensorium, drowsiness, coma, sunken eyes, circumoral cyanosis, and grayish discoloration of the skin. Shock without hyperpnea often occurs in this setting despite the development of severe acidosis. Poorly nourished infants with decreased protein and potassium reserves may have severe hypokalemia, hyponatremic dehydration, and paradoxical edema. The illness usually lasts 5 to 15 days but may persist or relapse over the course of several weeks. Complications may include intercurrent otitis media, pneumonia, bacteremia, peritonitis, and renal vein or cerebral sinus thrombosis. Dissemination of EPEC to the lungs has been demonstrated by immunofluorescence staining of tissue at autopsy.[15] Although the mortality may be quite high, as noted previously, South[16] and Kaslow and colleagues[17] have reported a milder illness with lower morbidity and mortality. However, in many areas such as South Africa and southern Brazil, EPEC organisms remain among the most common causes of diarrhea in infants and young children, especially during the summer months.[18–20] Endemic childhood diarrheal illness in areas like England and Canada also remain associated with EPEC in 6 to 18% of cases.[18, 19]

Several potentially life-threatening processes may mimic this infantile diarrhea syndrome. So-called parenteral diarrhea is the well-recognized but poorly understood tendency for systemic infections or localized infections elsewhere (such as otitis or meningitis) to be manifested clinically with diarrhea. Likewise, a strangulated hernia, intussusception, or torsion of an ovary or testis may be manifested by abdominal pain or diarrhea.

Appropriate antibiotic therapy must be tailored to the specific sensitivity pattern of the organism isolated.[16] If systemic infection is suspected, parenteral therapy should be started and should be tailored to the antibiotic sensitivity pattern of the organism isolated. Appropriate preventive measures include cohorting of nursery admissions, avoidance of overcrowding in nurseries, utilization of individual units and equipment, careful formula preparation, isolation of infants with diarrhea, and careful hand washing by hospital personnel.

The association of a certain strain of *E. coli* with infantile diarrhea was first demonstrated by slide agglutination by Bray and Beavan[21] in 1945 and reported in further detail in 1948. They identified serologically homogeneous *E. coli* organisms in most infants with summer diarrhea (87.5% versus 4% of the controls); half of the cases were hospital-acquired. Varela and associates[22] and Olarte and Varela[23] subsequently found this strain (called *E. coli*–"gomez" by Varela and associates) in cases of infantile diarrhea in Mexico. A second serotype, initially designated as *beta* to distinguish it from the earlier serotype called *alpha*, was described by Giles and Sangster[24] as the cause of an outbreak of infantile gastroenteritis in Aberdeen.

Escherichia coli strains are classified into a large number of serotypes on the basis of three major types of antigens: the "O" or heat-stable somatic antigen (lipopolysaccharide endotoxin), which forms the basis for 169 serogroups; an outer, heat-labile "capsular" antigen called "K," which may inhibit O agglutination; and, for motile organisms, the "H" or flagellar antigen, which is also heat-labile. Three different kinds of K antigens have been identified: L, A, and B, the latter being of importance in the identification of EPEC serotypes. The original α- and β-serotypes of *E. coli* were subsequently associated with several outbreaks of infantile epidemic gastroenteritis and were classified as serotypes O111:B4 and O55:B5, respectively, by Kaufmann and Dupont.[25] As shown in Table 83–1, exclusive of certain invasive serotypes (see Table 85–2 in Chapter 85), there are 14 classically recognized EPEC *E. coli* serotypes, beginning with O111:K58 (α), 055:K59 (β), O127:K63, O128:K67, O26:B6, O86:K61, O119:K69, O125:K70, O126:K71, O20:B7, and O44:K74. Additional serotypes recognized as causes of epidemic infantile diarrhea include O114,[10, 29, 30] O142,[12, 27] and O158.[28] *E. coli* O157:H7 and other enterohemorrhagic *E. coli* strains (EHEC) that make a Shiga-like toxin have caused hemorrhagic diarrhea with minimal inflammation and hemolytic-uremic syndrome (HUS) in several outbreaks as well as sporadic cases.[31–35]

TABLE 83–1 Enteropathogenic and Enterohemorrhagic *Escherichia coli* Serotypes Classically Recognized in Infantile Diarrhea Outbreaks*

Serotype	Difco Serogroup (with References)
Class I (EAF-positive) EPEC	
O55 : K59(B5) : H⁻/6/7	A (24–26)
O111ab : K58(B4) : H⁻/5/12	A (21–23, 25, 26)
O127a : K63(B8) : H6	A (26)
O119 : K69(B14)	B (26)
O125ac : K70(B15) : H21	B (26)
O126 : K71(B10) : H⁻/H2	B (26)
O128ab : K67(B12)	B (26)
O142	(12, 26, 27)
O158	(26, 28)
Class II (EAF-negative) EPEC	
O44 : K74	C (26)
O114	(10, 26, 29, 30)
O86a : K61(B7)	B (26)
O157 : H7	(31–33)
O26 : B6	A (26)

*See also Table 81–4.
Abbreviations: EAF, Enteroadherence factor probe for focal HEp-2 cell adherence plasmid pMAR2; EHEC, enterohemorrhagic *E. coli;* EPEC, enteropathogenic *E. coli.*

TABLE 83–2 Serotypes of *Escherichia coli* That Appear with Increased Frequency among Enterotoxigenic Isolates

LT *E. coli*	ST *E. coli*
O6 : K15 : H16	O78 : H11, O78 : H12
O8 : K40 : H9, O8 : K25 : H9	O115 : H40
LT + ST *E. coli*	O128 : H7
O11 : H27	O148 : H28
O15 : H22	O149 : H10
O20 : H⁻, O20 : H11	O153
O25 : K7 : H42,	O159 : H20
O25 : K98 : H⁻	O166, O167
O27 : H7	
O63 : H12	
O80, O85, O139	

Abbreviations: LT, Heat-labile; ST, heat-stable.

The mechanism by which most EPEC organisms cause disease involves a complex set of attachment and effacement traits, as detailed in Chapter 85. Although most are not invasive and do not produce conventionally recognized heat-labile or heat-stable enterotoxins, these organisms are capable of causing diarrheal disease in human volunteers, from whom the organism can be reisolated and in whom an antibody response can be documented.[13, 36] EPEC diarrhea continues to occur in some areas, especially urban hospitals in subtropical areas.[37, 38] Human volunteer studies in adults suggest that EPEC diarrhea may be more inflammatory than previously recognized.[39]

Epidemic infantile diarrhea may also be caused by enterotoxigenic organisms that are not limited to certain serotypes of *E. coli.* An outbreak has been described in which multiple serotypes of different organisms *(E. coli, Klebsiella,* and *Citrobacter)* that were demonstrated to be transiently enterotoxigenic were isolated,[40] which suggests the transmission of enterotoxigenicity among etiologic strains by plasmids[41] or by bacteriophages.[42] A subsequent outbreak of diarrhea on a cruise ship also documented the association of enterotoxigenic *Klebsiella* and *Citrobacter* as well as *E. coli* with watery diarrhea.[43] Another report of sporadic diarrhea among infants and children in Africa has shown that enteric organisms other than *E. coli* may produce an enterotoxin.[6] Enterotoxigenicity is not limited to specific serotypes, and most EPEC serotypes do not produce recognizable enterotoxins.[5–7, 44] However, a number of serotypes of *E. coli* are identified more often among enterotoxigenic isolates, as shown in Table 83–2.[26, 45] Whether these organisms are better recipients for enterotoxin plasmids or whether they are simply better adapted to maintaining these plasmids is not known.

A 9-month-long outbreak of diarrhea in the special care nurseries of a pediatric hospital has been reported in association with a multiple drug–resistant *E. coli* O78 that produced only the heat-stable type of enterotoxin.[46] Another outbreak of diarrhea lasting 3 months in a newborn nursery in Scotland was related to heat-stable enterotoxin–producing *E. coli* O159.[47]

Shigellosis[48] and epidemic salmonellosis[49, 50] may readily spread in the newborn nursery setting. Echoviruses,[51] coxsackieviruses,[52] adenoviruses,[53] and rotaviruses[54–56] are potential viral causes of epidemic infantile diarrhea. Echovirus 18 was isolated from 10 of 12 infants who had watery noninflammatory diarrhea in a 21-patient premature nursery. The virus was also isolated from two nurses, one of whom was implicated in the spread of the agent to five other babies in another ward.[51] Although there are conflicting interpretations of the significance of isolation of enteroviruses and adenoviruses among controls as well as patients, some authorities have postulated that these viruses may cause summer and winter gastroenteritis, respectively. Hospital acquisition of rotaviruses may be common among newborns; some investigators suggest that mild diarrhea develops relatively infrequently.[57] However, rotaviruses have been clearly implicated in epidemic neonatal diarrhea,[54–56] as well as in sporadic infantile diarrhea after the neonatal period.

WEANLING DIARRHEA

Weanling diarrhea usually occurs in the second year of life in areas where sanitation is poor. The greatest attack rate of diarrhea in the community occurs at the time of weaning, usually between 6 and 24 months of age.[9, 11, 12, 58] As noted in the previous chapter, weanling diarrhea is a major cause of mortality around the world. The increased susceptibility of a recently weaned infant relates to several factors.[59] In areas with poor sanitation, the infant ingests large numbers of many new organisms at the time of weaning. In developing countries, weaning foods prepared under conditions of poor hygiene are frequently found to be contaminated with large numbers of potential pathogens.[60, 61] A second contributing factor is the deteriorating nutritional status that may occur with weaning in many parts of the world.[62, 63] Finally, cellular and humoral factors passively transferred in human breast milk convey resistance to agents that commonly cause diarrhea in this age group.[64–68] Weanling diarrhea is manifested clinically as an acute, sporadic, watery diarrheal illness that occurs with increased frequency, especially in the summer months, in areas with poor sanitation. In the well-nourished infant, the disease is usually short-lived and resolves within 2 to 3 days with adequate hydration. A low-grade fever may be present, and vomiting is common.[5, 58] Diarrhea in the malnourished child tends to persist or to recur and is often much more severe.

Weanling diarrhea is usually an acute, noninflammatory process. Acute diarrhea in children 6 to 24 months of age has been commonly associated with rotaviruses[3–5] and with enterotoxigenic *E. coli*.[2, 6, 7] Shigellosis may also occur in this setting. From 16 to 83% of acute diarrheal illnesses among infants and young children have been associated with enterotoxigenic *E. coli*.[2, 6, 7, 69] Most of these reports involve studies of the summer peak of diarrhea in areas with poor sanitation. The presence of antibody to the heat-labile enterotoxin (LT) of *E. coli* in colostrum[64, 65] may provide some protection against LT-producing *E. coli* diarrhea among breast-fed infants exposed to unsanitary conditions. The demonstration of passive protection against experimental enterotoxigenic *E. coli* infections in human volunteers with immune bovine colostrum further documents the potential protective role of passive antibody in colostrum or milk.[70] The role of enterotoxigenic *E. coli* in causing infantile diarrhea in temperate climates is less clear. Enterotoxigenic *E. coli* serotypes were uncommon among children with diarrhea in studies from Massachusetts and Virginia.[71–73]

The ability of enteric organisms other than *E. coli* to produce enterotoxins has been suggested, but these organisms appear to be considerably less common than enterotoxigenic *E. coli*. Studies from Ethiopia suggested that young children with sporadic diarrhea may have *Klebsiella, Citrobacter, Aeromonas*, or *E. coli* that produce an LT-like toxin.[73a] However, in Brazil, enterotoxigenic *Klebsiella* organisms were found in only 2 of 40 patients, both of whom also had enterotoxigenic *E. coli*.[2] Diarrhea produced by LT shares the adenylate cyclase–activating mechanism with cholera toxin,[74–78] while the heat-stable toxin (STa) activates intestinal guanylate cyclase.[79–81]

The major nonbacterial causes of weanling diarrhea are rotaviruses. Although most adults have demonstrable antibody to rotaviruses that may protect against symptomatic disease, children less than 2 years of age throughout temperate and tropical climates appear to be highly susceptible to rotavirus diarrhea, which occurs most frequently in the winter or cooler, dry months[3, 5, 71, 82–88] and occasionally in the summer months.[89] Rotavirus diarrhea appears to be associated with low humidity and possibly indoor crowding to a greater extent than with low temperature or inadequate sanitation.[90–92] The illness is usually mild and without fever and is often associated with vomiting.[3, 5, 93] Rotaviruses have been associated with initial bouts of weanling diarrhea in aboriginal communities,[94] and antirotavirus antibody has been demonstrated in human colostrum among patients in Costa Rica and Brazil.[65, 67] There is a high frequency of rotavirus shedding or seroconversion among parents and other household contacts of cases of rotavirus-associated diarrhea.[5, 95, 96] Up to 40% of these infected adult contacts may develop mild abdominal cramps or diarrhea.[97]

The human rotaviruses demonstrate antigenic cross-reactivity with several animal strains, including the Nebraska calf diarrhea virus (NCDV), the agent of epizootic diarrhea of infant mice (EDIM), simian rotavirus (SA-11), and the "O" agent of monkeys.[5, 98] However, there are different antigenic types of rotaviruses,[99–102] so multiple attacks may occur.[103]

The laboratory diagnosis of rotavirus diarrhea may be made by examining the stool directly for viruses or the rotaviral RNA genome or by testing for an antibody titer increase in serum. Rotaviruses can be detected in fecal material by direct electron microscopy or by using immunologic techniques such as the enzyme-linked immunosorbent assay (ELISA),[104] radioimmunoassay,[105] counterimmunoelectrophoresis,[106] or fluorescence antibody staining of stool or biopsy specimens.[107, 108] Immunoassays for rotaviral antigen are available, with ELISA being the most sensitive. Simple rapid latex agglutination assays with 86% sensitivity and 95% specificity have been developed.[109] Detection of rotaviral genomic RNA in stools by means of "dot" hybridization using labeled RNA probes appears to be sensitive, specific, and convenient.[110] Methods for detecting serum antibody titers to rotaviruses use their cross-reactivity with NCDV, SA-11, or O agents of animals that can be cultivated in bovine embryonic kidney cells or in African green monkey kidney cells in tissue culture. Serum antibody has been measured by means of immunoelectron microscopy,[84, 111] complement fixation,[5, 84] and immunofluorescence[71] with one of the substitute antigens.

Much has been learned about the pathogenesis and the pathologic characteristics of intestinal rotavirus infections. Biopsy specimens from confirmed cases have shown transient, patchy, irregular inflammatory responses in the lamina propria and immature, cuboidal epithelium with 70- to 90-nm rotavirus particles in the distended cisternae of the endoplasmic reticulum.[82] Normal columnar epithelium at the villus tips was replaced by irregular cuboidal cryptlike cells. As would be expected from the destruction of villous-type epithelial cells, a transient brush border disaccharidase deficiency in the duodenal and upper jejunal mucosa and, despite the efficacy of oral therapy with glucose-electrolyte solutions, increased fecal-reducing substances have been noted in children with rotavirus diarrhea.[112–115] The degree of microvillus damage parallels the severity of diarrhea and dehydration.[116] As with transmissible gastroenteritis in piglets, studies of experimental rotaviral infections in animals confirm the shortened villi, reduced sucrase activity, increased thymidine kinase activity, no change in cyclic AMP concentrations, and blunted glucose-induced sodium absorption.[117, 118] As noted in Chapter 81, this loss of absorptive villus tip cells may be responsible for the fluid imbalance and nutritional impact of rotaviral infections.

Therapy should be directed first at the immediate restoration of fluid balance by intravenous or oral glucose-electrolyte therapy and then at restoration of the nutritional state to normal. Worldwide, rotavirus infection is the most serious cause of diarrhea in infants and young children, causing about 870,000 deaths per year and about 6% of all deaths in children younger than 5 years of age.[119–122] Few deaths due to rotavirus-associated diarrhea occur in the United States, but it is an important cause of morbidity in young children, accounting for about 30,000 hospitalizations per year.[123, 124] There is great interest, therefore, in the successful development of an effective rotavirus vaccine. Although several candidate live oral rotavirus vaccines (including bovine, rhesus monkey, and reassortant rotaviruses) show promise, earlier studies raised questions about their efficacy in infants (<1 year of age), especially in developing countries, and about the optimal means of delivery, age, and serotype to provide protection with minimal side effects.[125, 126] Recent studies in the United States, Finland, and Venezuela have shown that a live, orally administered tetravalent rotavirus vaccine has provided protection rates of 48 to 83% against any rotavirus-induced illness and rates of 70 to 95% against the most severe forms of such illness.[127–131] This vaccine has recently been approved for use in infants in the United States (see Chapters 139 and 312). Reasonable preventive measures include the provision of improved sanitation facilities and safe water supplies, as well as efforts to develop protective antibacterial, antitoxic, or antiviral immunity.[132]

ACUTE NAUSEA AND VOMITING (WINTER VOMITING DISEASE)

The syndrome of acute nausea and vomiting, "intestinal flu," or "viral gastroenteritis" commonly occurs in winter months in temperate climates. Although there is some overlap of this syndrome with rotavirus-associated infantile gastroenteritis, rotaviruses appear to be a relatively uncommon cause of winter vomiting disease in older children and adults. The Cleveland family studies of Dingle and coworkers[1] showed that enteritis was second only to upper respiratory infection as a cause of illness in homes. Gastrointestinal illnesses were most common between the ages of 1 and 10 years, when approximately two illnesses occurred per person per year. The peak season for these gastrointestinal illnesses was November through February, with June being the month of lowest frequency over this continuous study period. Most illnesses were of less than 1 to 3 days' duration; 20% occurred with respiratory symptoms, and 20% involved only diarrhea.

Illnesses tended to occur in one of two patterns: (1) mild afebrile illness with watery diarrhea or (2) a more severe febrile illness with vomiting, headache, and constitutional symptoms. Although etiologic agents were rarely identified, these two patterns of illness subsequently developed among volunteers who ingested filtrates prepared from the feces of ill patients.[133–135] Studies done in 1975–1977 in Charlottesville, Virginia, confirmed this pattern of winter illnesses, with clustering in families, highest attack rates in children, and the absence of identifiable etiologic agents in most cases despite the application of techniques for virologic and enterotoxin studies.[72, 73]

Although there has been little consistent documentation of enteroviruses in association with febrile winter vomiting disease, echovirus type 11 has been demonstrated in association with a small laboratory outbreak of febrile vomiting disease.[136] Abdominal pain and vomiting have been described with influenza B infections in children between the ages of 4 and 10 years.[137]

Careful evaluation of specimens from an outbreak of winter vomiting disease in an elementary school revealed a 27-nm parvovirus-like agent.[138–140] Typical winter vomiting disease, first described in 1929 by Zahorsky,[141] occurred over a 2-day period in late October 1968 in Norwalk, Ohio. Fifty percent of 232 students and teachers in an elementary school developed a mild illness characterized by nausea, vomiting, and abdominal cramps that usually lasted only 12 to 24 hours. Diarrhea occurred in fewer than half, and a low-grade fever occurred in approximately a third of affected persons. A remarkable 32% secondary attack rate in family contacts occurred approximately 48 hours later. A bacteria-free fecal suspension from a secondary case from the Norwalk outbreak caused an illness with low-grade fever and diarrhea in two of three volunteers. A second passage in volunteers produced either a febrile vomiting disease or an afebrile diarrheal disease, and illness was also produced in one of four volunteers who ingested an inoculum after three passages in human fetal intestinal organ culture.[139] From the stool of a second human passage in these volunteers, Kapikian and colleagues[140] used convalescent serum to identify a 27-nm agent by immunoelectron microscopy. Antibody in the convalescent serum of other volunteers and in three of five patients with naturally acquired illness was shown to coat and to aggregate these particles. Biopsy specimens revealed an intact small intestinal mucosa but blunted villi, shortened microvilli, and dilatation of the endoplasmic reticulum with intracellular multivesiculate bodies. Dilated mitochondria and intercellular spaces were observed.[142] There was a transient decrease in the activities of the brush border enzymes, alkaline phosphatase, sucrase, and trehalase. All laboratory values had returned to normal by 2 weeks after the illness. The colon is relatively spared, and fecal leukocytes are absent in this noninflammatory type of diarrhea.

The pathophysiologic features of winter vomiting disease caused by Norwalk-like agents may be parallel in some respects to those features mentioned in the previous section for rotaviruses. Both cause mucosal villus disruption and transient brush border enzyme deficiencies in the upper portion of the small bowel without any alteration in adenylate cyclase activity.[101, 143, 144] The roles of transient enzyme deficiency, malabsorption of xylose and lactose, and the slight increase in the number of bacteria present during the Norwalk illness remain unclear.[143, 145]

Similar outbreaks of vomiting disease have occurred elsewhere with either documented or suspected Norwalk-like agents. In March 1971, all four members of a household in Honolulu, Hawaii, developed a vomiting illness over a 4-day period with an apparent 44- to 48-hour incubation period, and in June 1971, another family of four in Montgomery County, Maryland, developed illnesses at 24- to 48-hour intervals that were characterized by vomiting, diarrhea, and occasional myalgias.[146] Fecal specimens from these patients revealed 27-nm Norwalk-like particles, and subsequent cross-challenge volunteer studies suggested that the Norwalk and Montgomery County agents were antigenically similar and conferred cross-immunity, whereas the Hawaii agent appeared to be antigenically different and failed to confer cross-immunity to the other agents.[146] Other Norwalk-like agents include the Snow Mountain and Taunton agents.[147] Clarke and associates[148] reported an outbreak from a boys' boarding school in Britain. The illness was transmitted to volunteers with filtered extracts of feces from one ill boy (W agent). Another outbreak in a primary school in Ditchling, England, in October 1975 revealed 26-nm particles that aggregated in convalescent serum and appeared to be antigenically similar to the W agent but different from the Hawaii and Norwalk agents.[149] Another 27-nm Norwalk-like agent, the Snow Mountain agent, was associated with an outbreak of gastroenteritis in a winter resort camp in Colorado.[150] From a convalescent hospital in Marin County, California, and a social gathering nearby, outbreaks of acute gastroenteritis have been associated with yet another viral agent capable of causing gastroenteritis, the Marin County agent.[151]

Several small (ranging from 20 to 35 nm in diameter), round (variably structured) viral agents of gastroenteritis have been grouped into four categories.[147, 152–154] The first three categories have a better-defined surface morphology: (1) Norwalk-like viruses (including Norwalk or Montgomery County agent and Hawaii, Snow Mountain, and Taunton agents); (2) caliciviruses, with characteristic "chalice-like" surface hollows (including agents described in the United Kingdom [UK1–4] and Japan); (3) astroviruses, with five- or six-pointed starlike surface structure (including Marin County, UK1–5, and Japan agents); and (4) other less well-defined, small round viruses (including Wollan, W or Ditchling, Cockle, Paramatta, and other agents). Except for certain astrovirus and calicivirus strains, these have not yet been cultivated in vitro, and the lack of a convenient animal model has restricted their study. The roles of other viral agents, including enteroviruses (especially echovirus types 11, 14, and 18), enteric adenoviruses (said to cause up to 9% of pediatric inpatient diarrhea[155]), human coronaviruses (isolated from infants with gastroenteritis[156, 157]), pestiviruses,[158] toroviruses,[159, 160] and picobirnaviruses,[161] are beyond the scope of this chapter. Over one third of outbreaks of nonbacterial gastroenteritis in the United States have been associated with the Norwalk virus.[162, 163] Astroviruses have been found to be among the most common causes of viral gastroenteritis in the pediatric age group.[164–167] Infection with astrovirus occasionally occurs in association with other enteric pathogens; in these cases the illness is more severe and protracted.[166] In a review of electron microscopy findings from 10 centers in the United States and Canada over 6 years, a viral agent was seen in 16% of cases, including rotavirus, adenovirus, small round virus (SRV), astroviruses, and caliciviruses, the latter three being associated with nosocomial diarrhea.[167]

Identification of Norwalk-like agents capable of causing winter vomiting disease requires immune electron microscopy[140] or radioimmunoassay for demonstration of a serologic response.[168] In vitro expression of the Norwalk virus capsid protein results in the production of capsid structures resembling clinical isolates of this agent.[169] These recombinant particles may facilitate generation of clinically useful diagnostic tests for Norwalk virus (see Chapter 163). It is clear that there are multiple antigenic types of these agents that are capable of causing similar disease and that resistance may relate to individual (genetic) differences rather than to lasting protective immunity after symptomatic infection.[169, 170] Methods for detection of other viral causes of gastroenteritis include monoclonal antibody-based enzyme immunoassay,[158, 171] tissue culture,[172] and gene probes.[173] Finally, additional viral agents are being recognized as potential causes of diarrhea in children in developing and developed areas.[159, 160]

ACUTE NONINFLAMMATORY DIARRHEA IN ADULTS

In temperate climates, acute noninflammatory diarrhea in adults may be caused by rotaviruses[174, 175] or by Norwalk-like viruses.[97, 101, 139, 174] The association of rotaviruses as well as adenoviruses, coxsackieviruses, and toxigenic *Clostridium difficile* with diarrhea, abdominal cramps, and a higher mortality among adult bone marrow transplant recipients has also been noted.[176] Additionally, several agents of food poisoning such as *Clostridium perfringens, Bacillus cereus*, or *Staphylococcus aureus* commonly cause noninflammatory diarrheal syndromes in adults (see Chapter 87).

In adults living in areas with poor sanitation, several other agents commonly cause sporadic noninflammatory diarrhea. In certain areas in South Asia, cholera is an endemic cause of severe watery diarrhea. With the increased infection-to-case ratio of El Tor cholera, the seventh pandemic has swept most of the continents of the Eastern Hemisphere, including Asia, Africa, and the Mediterranean portions of Europe.[177] Isolated cases have also occurred in the United States.[178, 179] Outbreaks have been related to contaminated mineral water[180] and to undercooked shellfish.[181, 182] Beginning in Madras, India, in late 1992 and rapidly spreading to Calcutta and Bangladesh in 1993, a new strain of non-O1 *Vibrio cholerae*—O139, called "Bengal"—is causing epidemic cholera gravis and may represent the beginning of an eighth pandemic.[183–187] Cholera should be suspected in any patient who has severe dehydration and watery diarrhea, especially if the patient has a history of recent travel to a cholera-endemic area. The disease can be so fulminant as to cause hypovolemic shock and death from the outpouring of fluid into the upper portion of the small bowel before the first diarrheal stool occurs.[188] As discussed in detail in Chapter 202, the entire dehydrating syndrome of cholera appears to be related to the activation of intestinal adenylate cyclase by the potent cholera enterotoxin.[74, 75] To make the diagnosis of cholera bacteriologically, stool specimens should be cultured onto thiosulfate citrate bile salts sucrose agar. Of prime importance in therapy is fluid replacement, accomplished either intravenously with isotonic fluids or orally with glucose-electrolyte solutions.

Patients from whom *V. cholerae* cannot be isolated may also have a cholera-like syndrome. In 1956, De and associates[189] demonstrated that *E. coli* isolated from adults and children with this syndrome caused fluid accumulation similar to that seen with *V. cholerae* in ligated rabbit ileal loops. In the early 1960s, Trabulsi,[190] working in São Paulo, reported similar findings with "toxigenic" *E. coli*. Subsequently, studies by Taylor and colleagues[191, 192] demonstrated that enterotoxigenicity correlated poorly with classic serotypes and that viable organisms were not required. Smith and Halls[193] identified several enterotoxigenic strains in association with animal diarrhea. Other workers showed that several adult cases of "acute undifferentiated diarrhea" in tropical Bengal were due to enterotoxigenic *E. coli* strains that were usually not of the classically recognized pathogenic serotypes.[194–197] These strains were transiently present during acute illness and elicited a net jejunal fluid secretion. The toxic material present in the culture filtrate of these *E. coli* strains was demonstrated to be heat-labile and nondialyzable and was precipitated in 40% ammonium sulfate. Subsequent studies have demonstrated that two types of enterotoxin are produced by *E. coli*: a heat-labile enterotoxin—that is, LT—and a heat-stable enterotoxin (ST).[198] Like cholera toxin, the *E. coli* LT activates mucosal adenylate cyclase.[63–65] LT is larger, inactivated by heating at 60°C for 30 minutes, and antigenically and mechanistically similar to cholera toxin, with a lag period before the activation of adenylate cyclase. LT is detected by several bioassay systems that use the adenylate cyclase–activating property of this toxin[199–201] or by immunoassay methods.[202] In contrast, STa activates guanylate cyclase,[79–81] has an earlier onset of action,[198] has greater tissue specificity,[81] and has a much lower molecular weight compared with LT.[203] It is assayed in suckling mice.[204] The role of yet a different type of enterotoxin, STb, that causes secretion in piglets without altering intestinal cyclic AMP or cyclic GMP remains unclear in humans at present.[205–207]

Methods for demonstrating enterotoxigenic *E. coli* are limited by the lack of a selective culture process (as routinely used, for example, to identify salmonellae or shigellae) and the necessity to pick a few random colonies of *E. coli* for enterotoxin testing. Data from a common-source outbreak of enterotoxigenic *E. coli* diarrhea in Crater Lake National Park in Oregon demonstrate the insensitivity of nonselective culture methods.[208] Fourteen patients in this outbreak had enterotoxigenic *E. coli* diarrhea by epidemiologic and clinical criteria, and each had multiple, random *E. coli* stool isolates tested for enterotoxin as well as paired sera examined for antitoxic immunity. Only 43% had enterotoxigenic *E. coli* identified, 36% had significant serum antitoxin antibody titer increases, and only 64% had either one or the other. Thirty-six percent of the cases could not be confirmed by current, nonselective methods. The lack of a serum antibody response in many patients with this intraluminal toxinosis is not surprising.

Other studies have shown that, in addition to the association with diarrhea in children, LT-only, ST-only, and LT-plus-ST–producing strains are associated with adult diarrhea.[4] Adults living in areas of poor sanitation may often carry LT-producing *E. coli* asymptomatically.[209, 210] In contrast, ST-producing *E. coli* strains are significantly associated with diarrheal disease and are less frequently present in asymptomatic control patients living in areas with poor sanitation. However, studies suggest that enterotoxigenic *E. coli* serotypes are uncommonly associated with diarrhea in the United States.[71, 72]

A cause of acute, noninflammatory, self-limited diarrhea among persons exposed to infected animals and patients is cryptosporidiosis.[211–213] The agent, a tiny coccidian protozoal parasite, causes more severe, watery, prolonged diarrhea in immunocompromised hosts.

Treatment of diarrhea in adults consists primarily of rehydration. If glucose or sucrose accompanies the isotonic fluid taken orally, the coupled absorption of sodium and water is often sufficient to replace fluid loss.[214] Bismuth subsalicylate (Pepto-Bismol) may reduce enterotoxin action,[215] and if there is no significant febrile or inflammatory process, low doses of antimotility agents may offer some relief with minimum risk if cramping is severe.

DIARRHEA IN PATIENTS WITH ACQUIRED IMMUNODEFICIENCY SYNDROME

Patients with the acquired immunodeficiency syndrome (AIDS) often develop or present with diarrhea. Among patients with AIDS in the United States, 30 to 60% present with diarrhea,[207, 208, 208a, 216–218] a number that reaches 95% in tropical developing areas such as Africa or Haiti.[217] In many of these patients, diarrhea becomes prolonged and life-threatening and may pose major difficulties in management. Although some investigators have reported an enteropathy without identifiable pathogens[219, 220] or with primary human immunodeficiency virus (HIV) infection of enterochromaffin cells in the bowel mucosal crypts and lamina propria,[211] others report one or more enteric pathogens in 55 to 85% of patients with AIDS and diarrhea.[218, 222, 223] Sexually promiscuous homosexual males often become infected with *Giardia lamblia, Entamoeba histolytica, Campylobacter jejuni, Shigella, Chlamydia trachomatis, C. difficile*, or (with proctitis) *Neisseria gonorrheae*, herpes simplex virus, or *Treponema pallidum*.[224] As shown in Table 83–3, the leading agents found in patients with AIDS and diarrhea are cytomegalovirus, *Cryptosporidium, Microsporidium, E. histolytica, G. lamblia, Salmonella, Campylobacter, Shigella, C. difficile, Vibrio parahaemolyticus*, and *Mycobacterium* spp.[222, 223, 225–227] *Cyclospora* and *Isospora belli* infections are also potentially treatable causes of persistent diarrhea in patients with AIDS, especially in tropical areas like Haiti.[218, 228–230] Even *Pneumocystis carinii* can occasionally involve the intestinal tract in this setting.[231] Although eradicative treatment may be difficult, most of these patients respond to specific antimicrobial or antiparasitic therapy, thus emphasizing the need to identify the etiologic agent in these infections whenever possible. The antiviral agent ganciclovir can transiently reverse intestinal cytomegalovirus infection,[232] and most bacterial and parasitic infections can be treated with the expectation of some improvement. *Cryptosporidium*, which infects 3 to 21% of patients with AIDS in the United States, can be found in as many as 50% of patients with AIDS and diarrhea in Africa and Haiti.[217] *Cryptosporidium* may also extend into the biliary tract as well in this setting. The same acid-fast stain that detects *Cryptosporidium* or *Mycobacterium* in fecal specimens may also reveal *I. belli* and *Cyclospora* in 2 to 15% of AIDS patients with diarrhea in the United States and Africa, respectively.[217, 218, 229, 230] *Cryptosporidium* and microsporidial infections are associated with villus atrophy, crypt hyperplasia, increased intraepithelial lymphocytes, and D-xylose malabsorption.[225] An increased yield for pathogens may be found when there is a 5- to 10-kg weight loss or an abnormal result on the Schilling test.[226] Nontyphoidal *Salmonella* infections occur with an estimated 20-fold increase in frequency, as well as with increased severity in patients with AIDS.[233–236] Enteric viruses have also emerged as significant potential pathogens seen with diarrhea in HIV-infected individuals. In one study, astrovirus, picobirnavirus, calicivirus, and adenovirus were found in 6 to 12% of HIV-positive patients with diarrhea.[237] Nevertheless, infections due to these pathogens, like those due to *C. jejuni* and other species, are treatable. Other common enteric infections include esophagitis or stomatitis with *Candida* or herpes simplex virus. A practical algorithmic approach to the diagnosis and management of diarrhea in the HIV-infected patient has been published. This approach involves the use of stool studies and potential empirical treatment trials before more invasive tests are implemented.[218]

TABLE 83–3 Possible Enteric Pathogens in Patients with Acquired Immunodeficiency Syndrome

Pathogen	Diarrhea (n = 181)	No Diarrhea (n = 28)
Cytomegalovirus	12–45%	15%
Cryptosporidium	14–30	0
Microsporidium	7.5–33	0
Entamoeba histolytica	0–15	0
Giardia lamblia	2–15	5
Salmonella spp.	0–15	0
Campylobacter spp.	2–11	8
Shigella spp.	5–10	0
Clostridium difficile toxin	6–7	0
Vibrio parahaemolyticus	4	0
Mycobacterium spp.	2–25	0
Isospora belli	2–6	0
Cyclospora	0–11	0
Blastocystis hominis	2–15	16
Candida albicans	6–53	24
Herpes simplex	5–18	40
Chlamydia trachomatis	11	13
Strongyloides	0–6	0
Intestinal spirochetes	11	11
One or more pathogens	55–86	39

Data from refs. 225, 226, 228, 229.

DIARRHEA IN INSTITUTIONS

Institutions provide special host and environmental settings for the acquisition of certain enteric pathogens. As with diarrhea in patients with AIDS and as with traveler's diarrhea, most cases of institution-acquired diarrhea are still noninflammatory; however, an increased frequency of certain causes of inflammatory diarrhea should prompt a careful search for fecal leukocytes in sporadic or clustered cases in hospitals, chronic care facilities, or daycare centers.[238]

Hospitals

Nosocomial diarrhea is among the most common of reported nosocomial outbreaks to the Centers for Disease Control and Prevention (CDC) and accounts for 21% of all 223 nosocomial outbreaks reported from 1956 to 1979.[239] However, its frequency is often overlooked, and it has been suggested to be the most common nosocomial infection in some areas.[240] Furthermore, nosocomial diarrhea appears to be a significant predisposing factor to other nosocomial infections such as urinary tract infection.[241] Overall rates range from 2.3 to 4.1 illnesses per 100 admissions on pediatric wards[240, 242] and from 7.7 per 100 admissions to 41% of adults hospitalized in intensive care units.[240, 243] From limited available data, *C. difficile* appears to be associated with most cases with a recognized etiology (45%), followed by *Salmonella* (12%).[244] In particular, *C. difficile*–associated diarrhea is an important emerging nosocomial infection worldwide, especially in elderly hospitalized patients.[245, 246] Most sporadic and outbreak cases of *C. difficile*–associated disease appear to be caused by exposure to contaminated environmental surfaces, rather than by direct contact with an index case.[247–249] There has also been a new appreciation of the significance of *C. difficile*–associated disease occurring on inpatient surgical wards.[250, 251] *Salmonella* is the most common cause among reported outbreaks of nosocomial gastroenteritis.[239] One study suggests that *Cryptosporidium* may be associated with cases of nosocomial diarrhea involving chronically ill, elderly patients in addition to HIV-positive patients.[252] In young children and in immunocompromised hosts, viral agents (rotaviruses, adenoviruses, coxsackieviruses, and others) are often found as well.[242, 253]

Chronic Care Facilities

Diarrheal illnesses also constitute a significant problem in extended care facilities for the elderly. A conservative estimate based on passively reported illness rates is that one third of patients in chronic care facilities experience diarrhea each year.[254–256] About one fourth of these patients have *C. difficile* cytotoxin, one third of whom are symptomatic with diarrhea.[257] Over 20% have fecal cytotoxin on admission, and a comparable number acquire cytotoxigenic *C. difficile* in the institution.[257] When patients with diarrhea are studied, 18 to 53% have cytotoxin or *C. difficile*, respectively.[258] The frequency of potentially transmissible enteric pathogens emphasizes the importance of careful hand washing in situations in which hygiene is often difficult. Similar problems have long been recognized in mental institutions, where hepatitis, *Strongyloides* infection, and amebiasis are readily acquired.

Daycare Centers

Another special institutional setting in which hygiene is difficult and enteric infections are increasingly appreciated is in daycare centers. Numerous outbreaks have been reported in association with viruses, bacteria, or parasites. Most common in infants and children younger than 2 years of age are rotaviruses, whereas older toddlers are more likely to acquire *G. lamblia*.[259] Newer diagnostic tests, based on immunoassays and reverse transcriptase polymerase chain reaction (RT-PCR), have been used to detect a greater number of etiologic agents, such as astrovirus, in many recent diarrhea outbreaks in daycare centers.[260, 261] A clinical syndrome of prolonged noninflammatory diarrhea may be associated with *Cryptosporidium* in daycare centers.[262–264] Outbreaks of inflammatory diarrhea in the daycare center setting include those due to *Shigella, C. jejuni*, and *C. difficile*.[265, 266]

TRAVELER'S DIARRHEA (TURISTA)

Whether it "arouses one from bed with a start at 4 A.M. for a record-breaking race to the bathroom to begin a staccato ballet"[267] or it produces the poetry of the Psalmist, "I am poured out like water . . . my heart like wax is melted in the midst of my bowels,"[268] traveler's diarrhea has a major impact each year on the 300 to 500 million international travelers and probably on the distribution of well over $100 billion in international tourism receipts.[269, 269a] Sixteen million people (8 million from the United States) travel from industrialized to developing countries. This type of diarrhea is by far the most common and among the most feared illnesses that threaten the traveler. Many studies have focused on North Americans and northern Europeans, who appear to be the groups at greatest risk when they travel to Latin America, southern Europe, Africa, or Asia.[270–273] Traveler's diarrhea, which may be severe and incapacitating (albeit rarely if ever fatal), is by far the most common health problem encountered with travel to developing countries.[274] The global nature of the problem and some suggested causal forces are illustrated by its more euphemistic names: "Delhi belly," "Gyppi tummy," "GIs," "Rome runs," "Greek gallop," "Turkey trots," "Montezuma's revenge," "Aztec two-step," "Aden gut," "San Franciscitis," "Basra belly," "la turista," "backdoor sprint," "summer complaint," "coeliac flux," "Canary disease," "passion," "Hong Kong dog," "Poona poohs," "Casablanca crud," "tourist trots," "Malta dog," and many more.

The onset in the vast majority of cases of traveler's diarrhea is usually between 5 and 15 days after arrival, with a range from 3 to 31 days in several reported series.[267, 275–281] The illness is typically manifested by malaise, anorexia, and abdominal cramps, followed by the sudden onset of watery diarrhea. Nausea and vomiting may accompany 10 to 25% of the illnesses. The diarrhea is usually noninflammatory, without blood or pus. A low-grade fever may be present in approximately a third of the cases. The duration is usually 1 to 5 days, but a significant number of people (19 to 50%) have an illness that continues beyond 5 to 10 days.

The attack rate ranges from 7% after 2 weeks in Aden[276] to 54% after 8 days in Mexico[270] and was 4 to 51% over a 14-day period among 17,280 Swiss tourists, depending on where they went.[273] One report of British tourists notes an attack rate ranging from 26% in Africa to 7.7% in North America. In descending order of risk after Africa in this study were the Middle East, southern Europe, central Europe, Asia (including India and Pakistan), South America, Australia, and North America.[281, 282] In general, it appears that the risk of acquiring turista during travel to a tropical country from a temperate climate for 2 weeks or more approaches 50%. The attack rate also appears to decrease with age after 25 years, an observation that may reflect different habits and exposures rather than inherent susceptibility.[267, 273] Expatriate residents appear to be at persistent risk for diarrhea of infectious causes; one study showed an attack rate of 49% per month during the first 2 years of residence in Nepal.[283]

For many years, the etiology of turista was an enigma; only infrequently have parasites or bacteria such as amebas, *Giardia, Salmonella*, or *Shigella* been identified. Likewise, viral studies have failed to elucidate significant viral causes of traveler's diarrhea. The first suggestion that an infectious bacterial process was likely came from the effective reduction in the attack rate by the use of prophylactic antimicrobial agents.[207, 213, 275, 281] Studies by Kean[267] suggested that *E. coli* of certain enteropathogenic serotypes might be involved in up to one third of the cases. The involvement of *E. coli* was further confirmed in an outbreak of traveler's diarrhea among the British troops in Aden, where *E. coli* O148 was identified among 54% of British troops with diarrhea.[276]

Subsequent studies have demonstrated ETEC in approximately 50% (range 20 to 75%) of cases of traveler's diarrhea in Latin America, Africa, and Asia (Table 83–4).[265, 266] The attack rate ranged from 20 to 100% (median 52 to 54%) in 26 studies reviewed (see Table 83–4).[282, 284] Enterotoxigenic *E. coli* organisms were almost never present before the travel; such organisms were acquired by only 14 of 111 (12.6%) fellow travelers who did not become ill.[278–280] The type of enterotoxin produced by *E. coli* associated with traveler's diarrhea may be the heat-labile type (LT), the heat-stable type (ST), or both LT and ST (Table 83–5). In contrast to adults who live in tropical areas and may often carry enterotoxigenic *E. coli* asymptomatically, the traveler appears to be susceptible to illness caused by enterotoxin-producing *E. coli*. Salmonellae, shigellae, or vibrios are present in only 1 to 16% of the patients with traveler's diarrhea. *Aeromonas* spp. have also been implicated in causing a small percentage of cases of traveler's diarrhea.[285, 286] Rotavirus infections have been described in 0 to 36% of cases of traveler's diarrhea, often in association with bacterial or parasitic pathogens.[287] In a study of Panamanian tourists to Mexico, rotavirus or Norwalk virus was found in 41%, *Campylobacter* in 11%, and ETEC in only one case of diarrhea.[288] *Cryptosporidium parvum* and *Cyclospora cayetanensis* may cause occasional cases of traveler's diarrhea.[289] *Blastocystis hominis* is commonly identified in the stools of persons traveling to developing countries. However, it has been difficult to ascertain whether this organism actually causes disease in this population or is merely a commensal.[290–292] Cholera is rarely a problem for U.S. travelers.[273, 293] A subset of patients will have persistent diarrhea for which no infectious agent can be implicated. Chronic idiopathic diarrhea, referred to as Brainerd diarrhea, has been reported

TABLE 83–4 Etiology of Traveler's Diarrhea

Characteristic	Latin America (15 Studies)	Africa (3 Studies)	Asia (8 Studies)
Duration of stay (d)	21 (2–42)*	28 (28–35)	(28–42)
Attack rate (%)	52 (21–100)	54 (36–62)	(39–57)
Percentage with			
Enterotoxigenic *Escherichia coli*	46 (28–72)	36 (31–75)	(20–34)
Shigella	0 (0–30)	0 (0–15)	(4–7)
Salmonella		0 (0–0)	(11–15)
Campylobacter jejuni	—	—	(2–15)
Vibrio parahaemolyticus	—	—	(1–13)
Rotavirus	23 (0–36)	0 (0–0)	—

*Median (range) from 26 studies.[285, 287]

TABLE 83–5 Frequency of Enterotoxigenic *Escherichia coli* in Association with Traveler's Diarrhea in Latin America, Africa, and Asia

	Reported Frequency				
Feature	***Gastroenterologists in Mexico*[159]**	***Peace Corps Volunteers in Kenya*[160]**	***Yale Glee Club in Latin America*[161]**	***Japanese Travelers Returning to Tokyo from India, Southeast Asia, Orient*[287]**	***Total***
Illness attack rate (%)	49% in 16 d	69% in 5 wk	74% in 1 mo	—	
Type of enterotoxin					
LT only (%)	16%	33%	25%	4.8%	21%
LT and ST (%)	16%	15%	12.5%	11.8%	38%
ST only (%)	9.8%	2%	19%	13.6%	41%
Total	21/51 cases	14/27 cases	9/16 cases	226/749 cases	270/843 cases
Percentage of illness with ETEC	41%	52%	56%	30.2%	32%

Abbreviations: ETEC, Enterotoxigenic *E. coli;* LT, heat-labile; ST, heat-stable.

to occur in outbreaks in the United States and, more recently, in a group of North American travelers to the Galapagos Islands.[294–297]

In contrast to the frequent identification of potential etiologic agents among travelers to tropical areas who develop diarrhea, careful studies of a group of marines who developed diarrhea upon arrival in temperate South Korea (21% in 3 weeks) failed to reveal any evidence of bacterial, parasitic, or rotaviral pathogens.[298] Travelers to certain areas such as Russia and national parks in the United States may be especially susceptible to development of the more insidious watery diarrhea seen with giardiasis or cryptosporidiosis.[299–302] Stronglyoidiasis may also be acquired in tropical areas and may cause noninflammatory diarrhea, abdominal pain, and eosinophilia.[303]

Several other potentially serious infections manifested initially by diarrhea or abdominal pain may be acquired by travelers. Malaria may be manifested initially as "gastroenteritis" with nausea, vomiting, diarrhea, or abdominal pain in 30 to 50% of the cases.[304] The physician caring for world travelers should also remember to consider typhoid fever and other infections that may be manifested with a "typhoidal pattern" including plague, melioidosis, typhus, and arboviral hemorrhagic fevers.[304, 305]

The desire to control the bothersome problem of diarrhea in travelers has led to extreme and sometimes irrational attempts at management.[267] Some travelers persist in using iodochlorhydroxquin (Entero-Vioform, clioquinol), which has been shown not only to be ineffective for traveler's diarrhea[270, 306] but also to carry a risk of severe subacute myelo-optic atrophy.[307] Other commonly used remedies such as diphenoxylate-atropine (Lomotil) and kaolin-pectin suspension were of no value in treating children with acute diarrhea in Guatemala.[308] The former and other antimotility agents may actually worsen the illness with inflammatory processes such as shigellosis.[309] Bismuth subsalicylate (Pepto-Bismol) has been shown to inhibit enterotoxin activity in experimental animal models[215] and has been recommended for symptomatic therapy and, in doses as low as 1.05 g/day (2 tablets bid), for prophylaxis.[309–311] The mainstay of therapy, as with any diarrheal illness, is adequate hydration with an oral glucose- or sucrose-electrolyte solution.

Prevention of traveler's diarrhea should be directed toward reducing the consumption of infectious agents in food and water. Salads, raw vegetables, and untreated water (or ice) are high-risk foods.[312] Bottled, noncarbonated water cannot be considered safe because outbreaks of cholera[180] and typhoid fever[313, 314] have been traced to bottled water and beverages, respectively. It has been suggested that even brief, 10-minute heating to 50 to 55°C (the temperature of some hot tap water, "too hot for the hand to tolerate") may kill many enteric bacterial and parasitic pathogens.[315] Care in eating and drinking may reduce one's risk even in highly endemic areas to less than 15%.[312, 316]

The efficacy of prophylactic antimicrobial agents has been documented in several studies.[275, 281, 317] However, multiple drug-resistant enterotoxigenic *E. coli* strains occur and have demonstrated cotransfer of enterotoxigenicity and drug resistance.[318, 319] The increased risk of acquiring a more severe infection such as salmonellosis,[370] the risk of drug side effects (such as photosensitivity in the tropics), and the emergence of drug-resistant organisms should preclude the widespread use of antibiotic prophylaxis at this time. Because treatment regimens combining loperamide with antibiotic are rapidly effective in controlling traveler's diarrhea (<10 hours), most experts consider prophylactic therapy only in travelers with special considerations (e.g., high risk of infection, importance to remain disease-free during the trip).[321, 322] Until more widespread resistance develops,[323, 324] treatment of traveler's diarrhea with a fluoroquinolone such as ciprofloxacin, norfloxacin, or ofloxacin for 1 to 3 days can significantly reduce the duration and severity of the disease.[286, 325–327]

Travelers to developing countries should be given a fluoroquinolone to use if needed.[322] Fluoroquinolone drugs are contraindicated in pregnant women (a nonabsorbable agent such as attapulgite can be tried[322, 326]) and children under the age of 16 years (combination therapy with trimethoprim-sulfamethoxazole and erythromycin has been suggested[322, 331]). The emergence of fluoroquinolone-resistant strains of *Campylobacter* spp. is of concern especially for travelers and military personnel deployed to Thailand.[332, 333]

DIFFERENTIAL DIAGNOSIS OF ACUTE NONINFLAMMATORY DIARRHEA

Acute noninflammatory diarrhea may also be the consequence of several noninfectious processes. As with agents that effect an osmotic diuresis, nonabsorbable agents such as sorbitol may cause diarrhea if consumed in excess. Ipecac fluid extract used by mistake instead of ipecac syrup may cause watery diarrhea instead of vomiting. Heavy metal poisoning (with As, Sn, Fe, Cd, Hg, Pb) is often associated with diarrhea, probably as a result of toxic effects on the rapidly growing mucosal epithelium. Endocrine causes of diarrhea that may share the adenylate cyclase–activating mechanism with enterotoxins include non–β-islet cell tumors, medullary carcinoma of the thyroid, carcinoid tumors, and others that are associated with increased serum prostaglandins or vasoactive intestinal polypeptide (VIP).[334] Patients with thyrotoxicosis and adrenal or parathyroid insufficiency may also have diarrhea. Congenital and acquired enzyme deficiencies include lactase deficiency and pancreatic or biliary insufficiency, in which inadequately degraded or absorbed nutrients may promote an osmotic diarrhea. A child with diarrhea as well as with edema, hypertension, or petechiae should be suspected of having HUS with or without enterohemorrhagic *E. coli* O157:H7. Patients with dermatitis herpetiformis may also have diarrhea that may respond to sulfone or sulfapyridine therapy or to a gluten-free diet.

CHRONIC NONINFLAMMATORY DIARRHEA

Syndromes of chronic noninflammatory diarrhea of infectious etiology include giardiasis, tropical spruelike syndromes, syndromes of bacterial "overgrowth," and *Cryptosporidium* or *I. belli* infection (especially in immunocompromised hosts).[211, 212, 217, 239, 335]

The patient with weight loss, malaise, and watery or fatty stools should be suspected of having giardiasis or some other cause of a malabsorption syndrome. This syndrome may also be associated with hypocalcemia, with iron or folate deficiency anemia, or with vitamin D, vitamin K, or protein deficiency.

Giardiasis may go undiagnosed for weeks. Although it is endemic throughout most of the United States and much of the world, giardiasis received attention when it was acquired in Rocky Mountain ski resorts and in Leningrad.[237, 238] Effective management requires a high index of suspicion followed by a careful search by a competent experienced person for the trophozoite or cyst of *G. lamblia* in multiple stool specimens or in a small bowel aspirate or "string" (Enterotest; Hedeco, Palo Alto, CA) sample. Recommended therapy is administration of metronidazole (Flagyl), 250 mg tid for 7 to 10 days, with a reported 70% cure rate.[335] Higher doses of metronidazole may be more effective. Furazolidone, which is available in liquid form for pediatric use, divided into three daily doses with meals (total, 8 mg/kg/day) for 10 days is often used in children.[336]

The diagnosis of *Cryptosporidium, Cyclospora*, or *I. belli* infection is best made by phase microscopic or modified Kinyoun acid-fast stain examination of fecal specimens with or without sugar flotation.[211, 217, 337] The diagnosis of *Cryptosporidium* and *Giardia* infections is also now facilitated by a fluorescence antibody test.

BACTERIAL OVERGROWTH SYNDROMES

Many syndromes have been described in which impaired absorption was attributed to abnormal bacterial colonization in the upper segment of the small bowel.[338] Whether these organisms are virulent pathogens or simply part of the normal colonic flora abnormally distributed is unclear at present.

Normally, the upper portion of the small bowel is relatively sparsely populated, with fewer than 10^5 organisms/ml; these are predominantly facultative gram-positive organisms (diphtheroids, streptococci, and lactobacilli).[339] The organisms most often incriminated in bacterial overgrowth syndromes in the small bowel are aerobic enteric coliforms (members of the family Enterobacteriaceae) and anaerobic gram-negative fecal flora (*Bacteroides* and other genera). Other organisms such as *Plesiomonas shigelloides* may occasionally be responsible.[340] Bacterial colonization in the upper part of the small bowel may be associated with malabsorption or chronic diarrhea in the absence of significant histopathologic changes. Small bowel overgrowth is usually associated with a predisposing bowel abnormality such as achlorhydria (from gastritis, pernicious anemia, or gastric surgery), blind-loop syndromes, cholangitis, impaired motility (scleroderma, diabetic neuropathy, vagotomy), surgery, strictures, diverticula, or radiation damage.[341, 342] Malnutrition, especially with protein, folate, or vitamin B_{12} deficiency, may also render the bowel more susceptible to microbial colonization and injury.[339, 343] An episode of acute infectious diarrhea may also provide the initiating event in the establishment of small bowel colonization and chronic diarrhea.[339, 344, 345] Lindenbaum and colleagues[346] described spruelike morphologic changes in the upper portion of the small bowel in association with increased numbers of bacteria and malabsorption among Peace Corps volunteers living in Pakistan.

The mechanism by which fecal flora in the small bowel cause malabsorption may involve bacterial binding or utilization of nutrients (such as vitamin B_{12} or carbohydrates, respectively), deconjugation of bile salts by bacteria such as enterococci and anaerobes,[347] or the toxic effects of bacterial products such as fatty acids or amines.[339] Indeed, *E. coli* organisms that lack other recognized virulence traits but that colonize the bowel have been shown to cause prolonged diarrhea in a rabbit model,[348] with an associated impairment in water and electrolyte absorption as well as disaccharidase activity.[349]

The approach to the patient suspected of having bacterial "overgrowth" as a cause of malabsorption or chronic diarrhea should include quantitative aerobic and anaerobic cultures of the upper small bowel contents obtained by intubation or "string" passage. Because the critical number of organisms appears to be approximately 10^5 organisms/ml, semiquantitative estimates from a Gram stain analogous to the urine Gram stain may also prove to be of value. Roberts and associates[344] have suggested that unexplained malnutrition in the elderly may be due to clinically inapparent bacterial overgrowth that can be detected by the ^{14}C-glycocholic acid breath test for bacterial deconjugation of bile salts. Tests for urinary indican (from bacterial conversion of tryptophan) have proved to be insensitive and nonspecific for bacterial overgrowth syndromes.[350]

Patients with diarrhea or malabsorption and bacterial overgrowth are potential candidates for antibiotic therapy, especially if predisposing conditions like achlorhydria, scleroderma, or diabetes are present. Depending on results of quantitative cultures of upper small bowel aspirates, therapy may need to be directed against anaerobes as well as aerobic coliform organisms.[339, 344] Although small amounts of antibiotics have been used to improve the nutritional status of animals and poultry and even of malnourished children,[351] the potential risks of widespread antibiotic use[352] must be weighed against potential benefits.

Noninfectious causes of chronic noninflammatory diarrhea should also be considered in the differential diagnosis. These include congenital deficiency syndromes and food allergies, certain neoplastic and endocrine processes, and less well-understood functional disorders. Causative disorders to be considered in the first two categories are milk allergies, disaccharidase deficiencies, gluten enteropathy, acrodermatitis enteropathica, β-lipoprotein deficiency, familial hyperchloremic alkalosis (congenital "chloridorrhea"), Leiner's disease, and Wiskott-Aldrich syndrome. Neoplastic and endocrine causes of diarrhea include carcinoid, Werner syndrome (multiple endocrine adenomatosis), Zollinger-Ellison syndrome (gastrinoma), "pancreatic cholera" syndromes, medullary carcinoma of the thyroid, and thyrotoxicosis. Patients with partial mechanical bowel obstruction or pellagra may also have chronic diarrhea. Finally, frequent small stools may suggest an irritable bowel syndrome of presumed functional etiology. However, a search for the infectious agents of treatable diarrheal illness reviewed in this chapter should always precede the latter diagnosis.

REFERENCES

1. Dingle JH, Badger GF, Jordan WS Jr. Illnesses in the Home: A Study of 25,000 Illnesses in a Group of Cleveland Families. Cleveland: Press of Western Reserve University; 1964.
2. Guerrant RL, Moore RA, Kirschenfeld PM, et al. Role of toxigenic and invasive bacteria in acute diarrhea of childhood. N Engl J Med. 1975;293:567.
3. Kapikian AZ, Kim H-W, Wyatt RG, et al. Human reovirus–like agent as the pathogen associated with "winter" gastroenteritis in hospitalized infants and young children. N Engl J Med. 1976;294:965.
4. Black RE, Merson MH, Huq I, et al. Incidence and severity of rotavirus and *E. coli* diarrhea in rural Bangladesh. Lancet. 1981;1:141.
5. Ryder TW, Sack DA, Kapikian AZ, et al. Enterotoxigenic *Escherichia coli* and reovirus-like agent in rural Bangladesh. Lancet. 1976;1:659.
6. Schorling JB, Wanke CA, Schorling SK, et al. A prospective study of persistent diarrhea among children in an urban Brazilian slum. Am J Epidemiol. 1990;132:144–156.
7. Sack RB, Hirschhorn N, Brownlee I, et al. Enterotoxigenic *Escherichia coli*–associated diarrheal disease in Apache children. N Engl J Med. 1975;292:1041.
8. Black RE, Brown KH, Becker S, et al. Longitudinal studies of infectious diseases and physical growth of children in rural Bangladesh. I. Patterns of morbidity. Am J Epidemiol. 1982;115:305.
9. Guerrant RL, Kirchoff LV, Shields DS, et al. Prospective study of diarrheal illnesses in northeastern Brazil: Patterns of disease, nutritional impact and risk factors. J Infect Dis. 1983;148:986.
10. Jacobs SI, Holzel A, Wolman B, et al. Outbreak of infantile gastroenteritis caused by *Escherichia coli* O114. Arch Dis Child. 1970;45:656.
11. Neter E. Enteritis due to enteropathogenic *Escherichia coli*: Present-day status and unsolved problems. J Pediatr. 1959;55:223.
12. Hone R, Fitzpatrick S, Keane C, et al. Infantile enteritis in Dublin caused by *Escherichia coli* O142. Med Microbiol. 1973;6:505.
13. Levine MM, Nalin DR, Hornick RB, et al. *Escherichia coli* strains that cause diarrhea but do not produce heat-labile or heat-stable enterotoxins and are noninvasive. Lancet. 1978;1:1119.
14. Nelson JD, Haltalin KC. Accuracy of diagnosis of bacterial diarrheal disease by clinical features. J Pediatr. 1971;78:519.

15. Drucker MM, Polliack A, Yeivin R, et al. Immunofluorescent demonstration of enteropathogenic *Escherichia coli* in tissues of infants dying with enteritis. Pediatrics. 1970;46:855.
16. South MA: Enteropathogenic *Escherichia coli* disease: New developments and perspectives. J Pediatr. 1971;79:1.
17. Kaslow RA, Taylor A, Dweck HS, et al. Enteropathogenic *Escherichia coli* infection in a newborn nursery. Am J Dis Child. 1974;128:797.
18. Levine MM, Edelman R. Enteropathogenic *Escherichia coli* of classic serotypes associated with infant diarrhea: Epidemiology and pathogenesis. Epidemiol Rev. 1984;6:31–51.
19. Gurwith M, Hinde D, Gross R, et al. A prospective study of enteropathogenic *E. coli* in endemic diarrheal disease. J Infect Dis. 1978;137:292.
20. Toledo MRF, Alvariza MCB, Murahovschi J, et al. Enteropathogenic *Escherichia coli* serotypes and endemic diarrhea in infants. Infect Immun. 1983;39:586–589.
21. Bray J, Beavan TED. Slide agglutination of *Bacterium coli* var. *Neopolitanum* in summer diarrhea. J Pathol Bacteriol. 1948;60:395.
22. Varela G, Aguirre A, Grillo J. *Escherichia coli*–gomez, nueva especie aislada de un caso mortal de diarrea. Bol Med Hosp Infantil Mexico. 1946;3:3.
23. Olarte J, Varela G. A complete somatic antigen common to *Salmonella adelaide, Escherichia coli*–gomez and *Escherichia coli* O111:B4. J Lab Clin Med. 1952;40:252.
24. Giles C, Sangster G. An outbreak of infantile gastro-enteritis in Aberdeen. J Hyg (Camb) 1948;46:1.
25. Kaufmann F, Dupont A. *Escherichia* strains from infantile epidemic gastroenteritis. Acta Pathol Microbiol Scand. 1950;27:552.
26. Ørskov I, Ørskov F, Jann B, et al. Serology, chemistry and genetics of O and K antigens of *Escherichia coli*. Bacteriol Rev. 1977;41:667.
27. Rowe B, Gion RJ. *Escherichia coli* O142 and infantile enteritis in Scotland. Lancet. 1971;1:649.
28. Rowe B, Gross J, Lindop R, et al. A new *E. coli* O group O158 associated with an outbreak of infantile enteritis. J Clin Pathol. 1974;27:832.
29. Rogers KB, Cracknell VM. Epidemic infantile gastro-enteritis due to *Escherichia coli* type O114. J Pathol Bacteriol. 1956;72:27.
30. Charter RE. *Escherichia coli* type O114 isolated from infantile diarrhea and calf scours. J Pathol Bacteriol. 1956;72:33.
31. Riley LW, Remis RS, Helgerson SD, et al. Outbreaks of hemorrhagic colitis associated with a rare *Escherichia coli* serotype. N Engl J Med. 1983;308:681.
32. Johnson WM, Lior H, Bezanson GS. Cytotoxic *Escherichia coli* O157:H7 associated with hemorrhagic colitis in Canada. Lancet. 1983;1:76.
33. Outbreak of hemorrhagic colitis—Ottawa, Canada. MMWR. 1983;32:133.
34. Slutsker LM, Ries AA, Greene KD, et al. *Escherichia coli* O157:H7 diarrhea in the United States: Clinical and epidemiologic features. Ann Intern Med. 1994;126:505–513.
35. Iida T, Naka A, Suthienkul O, et al. Measurement of fecal lactoferrin for rapid diagnosis of enterohemorrhagic *Escherichia coli* infection. Clin Infect Dis. 1997;25:167.
36. Neter E, Shumway CN: *E. coli* serotype D433: Occurrence in intestinal and respiratory tracts, cultural characteristics, pathogenicity, sensitivity to antibiotics. Proc Soc Exp Biol Med. 1950;74:504.
37. Thielman NM, Guerrant RL. Enteric *Escherichia coli* infections. In: Guerrant RL, Walker DA, Weller PF, eds. Tropical Infectious Diseases: Principles, Pathogens, and Practice. Philadelphia: WB Saunders; 1999.
38. Donnenberg MS. Enteropathogenic *Escherichia coli*. In: Blaser MJ, Smith PD, Ravdin JR, et al, eds. Infections of the Gastrointestinal Tract. New York: Raven; 1995:709–726.
39. Miller JR, Barrett LJ, Kotloff K, Guerrant RL. A rapid test for infectious and inflammatory enteritis. Arch Intern Med. 1994;154:2660–2664.
40. Guerrant RL, Dickens MD, Wenzel RP, et al. Toxigenic bacterial diarrhea: Nursery outbreak involving multiple bacterial strains. J Pediatr. 1976;89:885.
41. Skerman FJ, Formal SB, Falkow S. Plasmid-associated enterotoxin production in a strain of *Escherichia coli* isolated from humans. Infect Immun. 1972;5:622.
42. Takeda Y, Murphy J. Bacteriophage conversion of heat labile enterotoxin in *Escherichia coli*. J Bacteriol. 1978;133:172.
43. Wachsmith K, Wells J, Shipley P, et al. Heat-labile enterotoxin production in isolates from a shipboard outbreak of human diarrheal illness. Infect Immun. 1979;24:793–797.
44. Sack RB. Human diarrheal disease caused by enterotoxigenic *Escherichia coli*. Annu Rev Microbiol. 1975;29:333.
45. Merson MH, Black RE, Gross RJ, et al. Use of antisera for identification of enterotoxigenic *E. coli*. Lancet. 1980;2:222.
46. Ryder RW, Wachsmuth IK, Buxton AE, et al. Infantile diarrhea produced by heat-stable enterotoxigenic *Escherichia coli*. N Engl J Med. 1976;295:849.
47. Gross RJ, Rowe B, Henderson A, et al. A new *Escherichia coli* O-group, O159, associated with outbreaks of enteritis in infants. Scand J Infect Dis. 1976;8:195.
48. Haltalin KC. Neonatal shigellosis. Am J Dis Child. 1967;114:603.
49. Schroeder SA, Aserkoff B, Brachman PS. Epidemic salmonellosis in hospitals and institutions. N Engl J Med. 1968;279:674.
50. Rice PA, Craven PC, Wells JG: *Salmonella heidelberg* enteritis and bacteremia. An epidemic on two pediatric wards. Am J Med. 1976;60:509.
51. Eichenwald HF, Ababio A, Arky AM, et al. Epidemic diarrhea in premature and older infants caused by echo virus type 18. JAMA. 1958;166:1563.
52. Yow MD, Melnick JL, Blattner RJ, et al. The association of viruses and bacteria with infantile diarrhea. Am J Epidemiol. 1970;92:33.
53. Moffet HL, Shulenberger HK, Burkholder ER. Epidemiology and etiology of severe infantile diarrhea. J Pediatr. 1968;72:1.
54. Murphy AM, Albrey MB, Crew EB. Rotavirus infections of neonates. Lancet. 1977;2:1149.
55. Cameron DJS, Bishop RF, Davidson GP, et al. New virus associated with diarrhea in neonates. Med J Aust. 1976;1:85.
56. Bishop RF, Hewstone AS, Davidson GP, et al. An epidemic of diarrhea in human neonates involving a reoviruslike agent and "enteropathogenic" serotypes of *Escherichia coli*. J Clin Pathol. 1976;29:46.
57. Chrystie IL, Totterdell BM, Banatvala JE. Asymptomatic endemic rotavirus infections in the newborn. Lancet. 1978;1:1176.
58. Gordon JE, Chitkara ID, Wyon JB. Weanling diarrhea. Am J Med Sci. 1963;245:345.
59. Welsh JK, May JT. Anti-infective properties of breast milk. J Pediatr. 1979;94:1.
60. Motarjemi Y, Kaferstein F, Moy G, Quevedo F. Contaminated weaning food: A major risk factor for diarrhoea and associated malnutrition. Bull WHO. 1993;71:79–92.
61. King J, Ashworth A. Contemporary feeding practices in infancy and early childhood in developing countries. In: King J, Ashworth A, eds. Infant and Child Nutrition, Worldwide Issues and Perspectives. Boca Raton, Fla: CRC Press; 1991:141–174.
62. Gordon JE, Guzman MA, Ascoli W, et al. Acute diarrhoeal disease in less developed countries. Bull WHO. 1964;31:9.
63. Reddy V, Rashuramulu N, Bhaskaram C. Secretory IgA in protein-calorie malnutrition. Arch Dis Child. 1976;51:871.
64. Stollar OA, Kaniecki-Green E, Pelley RP, et al. Secretory IgA against enterotoxins in breast milk. Lancet. 1976;1:1258.
65. Brown SE III, Sauer KT, Nations MK, et al. Comparison of paired whole milk and dried filter paper samples for anti-enterotoxin and antirotavirus activities. J Clin Microbiol. 1982;16:103.
66. Bullen CL, Willis AT. Resistance of the breast-fed infant to gastroenteritis. BMJ. 1971;3:338.
67. Bullen JJ, Rogers HJ, Leigh L. Iron-binding proteins in milk and resistance of *Escherichia coli* infection in infants. BMJ. 1972;1:69.
68. Simhon A, Mata L. Anti-rotavirus antibody in human colostrum. Lancet. 1978;1:39.
69. Gorbach SL, Khurana CM. Toxigenic *Escherichia coli*: A cause of infantile diarrhea in Chicago. N Engl J Med. 1972;287:791.
70. Tacket CO, Losonsky G, Link H, et al. Protection by milk immunoglobulin concentrate against oral challenge with enterotoxigenic *Escherichia coli*. N Engl J Med. 1988;318:1240–1243.
71. Echeverria P, Blacklow NR, Smith DH. Role of heat-labile toxigenic *Escherichia coli* and reovirus-like agent in diarrhea in Boston children. Lancet. 1975;2:1113.
72. Hughes JM, Gwaltney JM, Hughes DH, et al. Acute gastrointestinal illness in Charlottesville: A prospective family study (Abstract). Clin Res. 1978;26:24.
73. Guerrant RL, Hughes JM, Lima NL, et al. Microbiology of diarrhea in developed and developing countries. Rev Inf Dis. 1990;12(Suppl):S41–S50.
73a. Wadstrom T, Aust-Kettis A, Habte D, et al. Enterotoxin-producing bacteria and parasites in stool of Ethiopian children with diarrheal disease. Arch Dis Child. 1976;51:865.
74. Chen LC, Rohde JE, Sharp GWG. Intestinal adenyl-cyclase activity in human cholera. Lancet. 1971;1:939.
75. Guerrant RL, Chen LC, Sharp GWG. Intestinal adenyl-cyclase activity in canine cholera: Correlation with fluid accumulation. J Infect Dis. 1972;125:377.
76. Evans DJ Jr, Chen LC, Curlin GT, et al. Stimulation of adenyl cyclase by *Escherichia coli* enterotoxin. Nature. 1972;236:137.
77. Guerrant RL, Ganguly U, Casper AGT, et al. Effect of *Escherichia coli* on fluid transport across canine small bowel: Mechanism and time course—with enterotoxin and whole bacterial cells. J Clin Invest. 1973;52:1707.
78. Kantor HS, Tao P, Gorbach SL. Stimulation of intestinal adenyl cyclase by *Escherichia coli* enterotoxin: Comparison of strains from an infant and an adult with diarrhea. J Infect Dis. 1974;129:1.
79. Hughes JM, Murad F, Chang B, et al. Role of cyclic GMP in the action of heat stable enterotoxin of *Escherichia coli*. Nature. 1978;271:755.
80. Field M, Graf LH Jr, Laird WJ, et al. Heat-stable enterotoxin of *Escherichia coli*: In vitro effects on guanylate cyclase activity, cyclic GMP concentration, and ion transport in small intestine. Proc Natl Acad Sci U S A. 1978;75:2800.
81. Guerrant RL, Hughes JM, Chang B, et al. Activation of intestinal guanylate cyclase by heat stable enterotoxin of *E. coli*: Studies of tissue specificity, potential receptors, and intermediates. J Infect Dis. 1980;142:220.
82. Bishop RF, Davidson GP, Holmes IH, et al. Virus particles in epithelial cells of duodenal mucosa from children with acute non-bacterial gastroenteritis. Lancet. 1973;2:1281.
83. Flewett TH, Bryden AS, Davies H. Virus particles in gastroenteritis. Lancet. 1973;2:1497.
84. Kapikian AZ, Kim HW, Wyatt RG, et al. Reoviruslike agent in stools: Association with infantile diarrhea and development of serologic tests. Science. 1974;185:1049.
85. Virus of infantile gastroenteritis (Editorial). BMJ. 1975;3:555.
86. Rotaviruses of man and animals (Editorial). Lancet. 1975;1:257.
87. Mata L, Simhon A, Padilla R, et al. Diarrhea associated with rotaviruses, enterotoxigenic *E. coli, Campylobacter*, and other agents in Costa Rican children, 1976–1981. Am J Trop Med Hyg. 1983;32:146.
88. Black RE, Merson MH, Rahman ASMM, et al. A two-year study of bacterial, viral, and parasitic agents associated with diarrhea in rural Bangladesh. J Infect Dis. 1980;142:660.
89. Echeverria P, Ho MT, Blacklow NR, et al. Relative importance of viruses and bacteria in the etiology of pediatric diarrhea in Taiwan. J Infect Dis. 1977;136:383.

90. Paul MO, Erinle EA. Influence of humidity on rotavirus prevalence among Nigerian infants and young children with gastroenteritis. J Clin Microbiol. 1982;15:212.
91. Brandt CD, Kim HW, Rodriguez WJ. Rotavirus gastroenteritis and weather. J Clin Microbiol. 1982;16:478.
92. Gurwith M, Wenman W, Gurwith D, et al. Diarrhea among infants and young children in Canada: A longitudinal study in three northern communities. J Infect Dis. 1983;147:685.
93. Shepherd RW, Truslow S, Walker-Smith JA. Infantile gastroenteritis: A clinical study of reovirus-like agent infection. Lancet. 1975;2:1082.
94. Sexton M, Davidson GP, Bishop RF, et al. Viruses in gastroenteritis. Lancet. 1974;2:355.
95. Tallett S, MacKenzie C, Middleton P, et al. Clinical, laboratory, and epidemiologic features of a viral gastroenteritis in infants and children. Pediatrics. 1977;60:217.
96. Kim HW, Brandt CD, Kapikian AZ, et al. Human reoviruslike agent infection. Occurrence in adult contacts of pediatric patients with gastroenteritis. JAMA. 1977;238:404.
97. Wenman WM, Hinde D, Feltham S, et al. Rotavirus infection in adults: Results of a prospective family study. N Engl J Med. 1979;301:303.
98. Kapikian AZ, Dienstag JL, Purcell RH. Immune electron microscopy as a method for the detection, identification, and characterization of agents not cultivable in an in vitro system. In: Rose NR, Friedman H, ed. Manual of Clinical Immunology. Washington, DC: American Society for Microbiology; 1976.
99. Zissis G, Lambert JP. Different serotypes of human rotaviruses. Lancet. 1978;1:38.
100. Beards GM, Pilford JN, Thouless ME, et al. Rotavirus serotypes by serum neutralization. J Med Virol. 1980;5:231.
101. Blacklow NR, Cukor G. Viral gastroenteritis. N Engl J Med. 1981;304:397.
102. Urasawa S, Urasawa T, Taniguchi K. Three human rotavirus serotypes demonstrated by plaque neutralization of isolated strains. Infect Immun. 1982;38:781.
103. Fonteyne J, Zissis G, Lambert JP. Recurrent rotavirus gastroenteritis. Lancet. 1978;1:983.
104. Yolken R, Kim HW, Clem T, et al. Enzyme immunoassay (ELISA) for the detection of human reovirus-like agent in human stools. Lancet. 1977;2:263.
105. Kalica AR, Purcell RH, Sereno NM, et al. Microtiter solid phase radioimmunoassay for detection of the human reovirus-like agent in stools. J Immunol. 1977;118:1275.
106. Middleton PJ, Petrie M, Hewitt CM, et al. Counter-immunoelectroosmophoresis for the detection of infantile gastroenteritis virus (orbi group) antigen and antibody. J Clin Pathol. 1976;29:191.
107. Middleton PJ, Szymanski MT, Abbott GD, et al. Orbivirus acute gastroenteritis of infancy. Lancet. 1974;1:1241.
108. Davidson GP, Goller I, Bishop RF, et al. Immunofluorescence in duodenal mucosa of children with acute enteritis due to a new virus. J Clin Pathol. 1975;28:263.
109. Thomas EE, Puterman ML, Kawano E, et al. Evaluation of seven immunoassays for detection of rotavirus in pediatric stool samples. J Clin Microbiol. 1988;26:1189–93.
110. Flores J, Purcell RH, Perez I, et al. A dot hybridization assay for detection of rotavirus. Lancet. 1983;1:555.
111. Flewett TH, Bryden AS, Davies H, et al. Relation between viruses from acute gastroenteritis of children and newborn calves. Lancet. 1974;2:61.
112. Guerrant RL. Pathophysiology of the enterotoxic and viral diarrhea. In: Chen LC, Scrimshaw NS, eds. Diarrhea and Malnutrition: Interactions, Mechanisms and Interventions. New York: Plenum; 1983;23–43.
113. Middleton PJ, Szymanski MT, Abbott GD, et al. Orbivirus acute gastroenteritis of infancy. Lancet. 1974;1:1241.
114. Davidson GP, Goller I, Bishop RF, et al. Immunofluorescence in duodenal mucosa of children with acute enteritis due to a new virus. J Clin Pathol. 1974;28:263.
115. Sack DA, Chowdhury AMAK, Eusof A, et al. Oral hydration in rotavirus diarrhea: A double blind comparison of sucrose with glucose electrolyte solution. Lancet. 1978;2:280.
116. Davidson GP, Barnes GL. Structural and functional abnormalities of the small intestine in infants and young children with rotavirus enteritis. Acta Paediatr Scand. 1979;68:181.
117. Shepherd RW, Butler DG, Cutz E, et al. The mucosal lesion in viral enteritis: Extent and dynamics of the epithelial response to virus invasion in transmissible gastroenteritis of piglets. Gastroenterology. 1979;76:770.
118. Davidson GP, Gall DG, Petric M, et al. Human rotavirus enteritis induced in conventional piglets: Intestinal structure and transport. J Clin Invest. 1977;60:1402.
119. Clark HF, Offit PA. Rotavirus vaccines. In: Plotkin SA, Offit PA, eds. Vaccines. 2nd ed. Philadelphia: WB Saunders; 1994.
120. Ardern S, Lennon D. Rotavirus gastroenteritis: Is vaccine prevention near at hand? N Z Med J. 1997;110:407–409.
121. Grimwood K, Carzino R, Barnes GL, Bishop RF. Patients with enteric adenovirus gastroenteritis admitted to an Australian pediatric teaching hospital from 1981 to 1992. J Clin Microbiol. 1995;33:131–136.
122. Bennet R, Hedlund KO, Ehrnst A, Eriksson M. Nosocomial gastroenteritis in two infant wards over 26 months. Acta Paediatr. 1995;84:667–671.
123. Parashar UD, Holman RC, Clarke MJ, et al. Hospitalizations associated with rotavirus diarrhea in the United States, 1993 through 1995—surveillance based on the new ICD-9-CM rotavirus-specific diagnostic code. J Infect Dis. 1998;177:13–17.
124. Laboratory-based surveillance for rotavirus—United States, July 1996–June 1997. MMWR Morb Mortal Wkly Rep. 1997;46:1092–1094.
125. Vesikari T, Isolauri E, D'Hondt E, et al. Protection of infants against rotavirus diarrhea: R1T 4237 attenuated bovine rotavirus vaccine. Lancet. 1984;1:977–980.
126. Edelman R. Perspective on the development and deployment of rotavirus vaccines. Pediatr Infect Dis. 1987;6:704.
127. Pereȥ-Schael I, Guntinas MJ, Perez M, et al. Efficacy of the rhesus rotavirus-based quadrivalent vaccine in infants and young children in Venezuela. N Engl J Med. 1997;337:1181–1187.
128. Glass RI, Gentsch J, Smith JC. Rotavirus vaccines: Success by reassortment? Science. 1994;265:1389–1391.
129. Bernstein DI, Glass RI, Rodgers G, et al. Evaluation of rhesus rotavirus monovalent and tetravalent reassortant vaccines in US children. US Rotavirus Vaccine Efficacy Group. JAMA. 1995;273:1191–1196.
130. Rennels MB, Glass RI, Dennehy PH, et al. Safety and efficacy of high-dose rhesus-human reassortant rotavirus vaccines—report of the National Multicenter Trial. United States Rotavirus Vaccine Efficacy Group. Pediatrics. 1996;97:7–13.
131. Vesikari T. Clinical experience with rotavirus vaccine in Finland. Presented at the Second Satellite Symposium of the Fourteenth Annual Meeting of the European Society for Paediatric Infectious Diseases, Elsinore, Denmark, June 18–21, 1996.
132. Glass RI, Kilgore PE, Holman RC, et al. The epidemiology of rotavirus diarrhea in the United States: Surveillance and estimates of disease burden. J Infect Dis. 1996;174(Suppl 1):S5–S11.
133. Gordon I, Ingraham HS, Korns RF. Transmission of epidemic gastroenteritis to human volunteers by oral administration of fecal filtrates. J Exp Med. 1947;86:409.
134. Jordan WS, Gordon I, Dorrance WR. A study of illness in a group of Cleveland families. VII. Transmission of acute nonbacterial gastroenteritis to volunteers: Evidence for two different etiologic agents. J Exp Med. 1953;98:461.
135. Kojima S, Fukumi H, Kusama H, et al. Studies on the causative agent of the infectious diarrhea; records of the experiments on human volunteers. Jpn Med J. 1948;1:467.
136. Klein JO, Lerner AM, Finland M. Acute gastroenteritis associated with echo virus, type II. Am J Med Sci. 1950;240:749.
137. Kerr AA, McQuillin J, Downham MAPS, et al. Gastric "flu" influenza B causing abdominal symptoms in children. Lancet. 1975;1:291.
138. Adler JL, Zickl R. Winter vomiting disease. J Infect Dis. 1969;119:668.
139. Dolin R, Blacklow NR, DuPont H, et al. Transmission of acute infectious nonbacterial gastroenteritis to volunteers by oral administration of stool filtrates. J Infect Dis. 1971;123:307.
140. Kapikian AZ, Wyatt RG, Dolin R, et al. Visualization by immune electron microscopy of a 27-nm particle associated with acute infectious nonbacterial gastroenteritis. J Virol. 1972;10:1075.
141. Zahorsky J. Hyperemesis heimis or the winter vomiting disease. Arch Pediatr. 1929;46:391.
142. Agus SG, Dolin R, Wyatt RG, et al. Acute infectious nonbacterial gastroenteritis. Intestinal histopathology. Ann Intern Med. 1973;79:18.
143. Schreiber DS, Trier JS, Blacklow NR. Recent advances in viral gastroenteritis. Gastroenterology. 1977;73:174.
144. Levy AG, Widerlite L, Schwartz CJ, et al. Jejunal adenylate cyclase activity in human subjects during viral gastroenteritis. Gastroenterology. 1976;70:321.
145. Blacklow NR, Dolin R, Fedson DS, et al. Acute infectious nonbacterial gastroenteritis: Etiology and pathogenesis. Ann Intern Med. 1972;76:993.
146. Wyatt RG, Dolin R, Blacklow NR, et al. Comparison of three agents of acute infectious nonbacterial gastroenteritis by cross-challenge in volunteers. J Infect Dis. 1974;129:709.
147. Dolin R, Treanor JJ, Madore HP. Novel agents of viral enteritis in humans. J Infect Dis. 1987;155:365–376.
148. Clarke SKR, Cook GT, Egglestone SI, et al. A virus from epidemic vomiting disease. BMJ. 1972;3:86.
149. Appleton H, Buckley M, Thom BT, et al. Virus-like particles in winter vomiting disease. Lancet. 1977;1:409.
150. Morens DM, Zweighaft RM, Vernon TM. A waterborne outbreak of gastroenteritis with secondary person-to-person spread. Lancet. 1979;1:964.
151. Oshiro LS, Haley CE, Roberto RR, et al. A 27-nm virus isolated during an outbreak of acute infectious nonbacterial gastroenteritis in a convalescent hospital: A possible new serotype. J Infect Dis. 1981;143:791.
152. Caul EO, Appleton H. The electron microscopical and physical characteristics of small round human fecal viruses: An interim scheme for classification. J Med Virol. 1982;9:257–265.
153. Caul EO. Viral gastroenteritis: Small round structured viruses, caliciviruses and astroviruses. Part I. The clinical and diagnostic perspective. J Clin Pathol. 1996;49:874–880.
154. Caul EO. Viral gastroenteritis: Small round structured viruses, caliciviruses and astroviruses. Part II. The epidemiological perspective. J Clin Pathol. 1996;49:959–964.
155. Brandt CD, Kim HW, Rodriguez WJ, et al. Adenoviruses and pediatric gastroenteritis. J Infect Dis. 1985;151:437–443.
156. Gerna G, Passarani N, Battaglia M, et al. Human enteric coronaviruses: Antigenic relatedness to human coronavirus OC43 and possible etiologic role in viral gastroenteritis. J Infect Dis. 1985;151:796–802.
157. Battaglia M, Passarani N, DiMatteo A, et al. Human enteric coronaviruses: Further characterization and immunoblotting of viral proteins. J Infect Dis. 1987;144:140–143.
158. Yolken R, Santosham M, Reid R, et al. Pestiviruses: Major etiological agents of gastroenteritis in human infants and children (Abstract). Clin Res. 1988;36:780.
159. Koopmans MG, Goosen ESM, Lima AAM, et al. Association of torovirus with acute and persistent diarrhea in children. Pediatr Infect Dis J. 1997;16:504–507.
160. Koopmans M, Petric M, Glass RI, Monroe SS. Enzyme-linked immunosorbent assay reactivity of torovirus-like particles in fecal specimens from humans with diarrhea. J Clin Microbiol. 1993;31:2738–2744.

161. Grohmann GS, Glass RI, Pereira HG, et al. Enteric viruses and diarrhea in HIV-infected patients. N Engl J Med. 1993;329:14–20.
162. Greenberg HB, Valdesuso J, Yolken RH, et al. Role of Norwalk virus in outbreaks of nonbacterial gastroenteritis. J Infect Dis. 1979;139:564.
163. Kaplan JE, Gary GW Jr, Baron RC, et al. Epidemiology of Norwalk gastroenteritis and the role of the Norwalk virus in outbreaks of nonbacterial gastroenteritis. Ann Intern Med. 1982;96:756.
164. Moe CL, Monroe SS, Gary HE Jr, et al. Detection of astrovirus in pediatric stool samples by immunoassay and RNA probe. J Clin Microbiol. 1991;29:2390–2396.
165. Lew JF, Moe CL, Monroe SS, et al. Astrovirus and adenovirus associated with diarrhea in children in day care settings. J Infect Dis. 1991;164:673–678.
166. Cruz JR, Bartlett AV, Herrmann JE, et al. Astrovirus-associated diarrhea among Guatemalan ambulatory, rural children. J Clin Microbiol. 1992;30:1140–1144.
167. Lew JF, Glass RI, Petric M, et al. Six-year retrospective surveillance of gastroenteritis virus identified at ten electron microscopy centers in the United States and Canada. Pediatr Infect Dis. 1990;9:709–714.
168. Greenberg HB, Wyatt RG, Valdesuso J, et al. Solid-phase microtiter radioimmunoassay for detection of the Norwalk strain of acute nonbacterial, epidemic gastroenteritis virus and its antibodies. J Med Virol. 1978;2:97.
169. Jiang X, Wang M, Graham DY, et al. Expression, self-assembly, and antigenicity of the Norwalk virus capsid protein. J Virol. 1992;66:6527–6232.
170. Parrino TA, Schreiber DS, Trier JS, et al. Clinical immunity in acute gastroenteritis caused by Norwalk agent. N Engl J Med. 1977;297:86–89.
171. Herrmann JE, Perron-Henry DM, Blacklow NR. Antigen detection with monoclonal antibodies for the diagnosis of adenovirus gastroenteritis. J Infect Dis. 1987;155:1167–1171.
172. Shinozaki T, Araki K, Ushijima H, et al. Use of Graham 293 cells in suspension for isolating enteric adenoviruses from the stools of patients with acute gastroenteritis. J Infect Dis. 1987;156:246.
173. Neil C, Gomes SA, Leite JPG, et al. Direct detection and differentiation of fastidious and nonfastidious adenoviruses in stools by using a specific nonradioactive probe. J Clin Microbiol. 1986;24:785–789.
174. von Bonsdorff CH, Hovi T, Makela P, et al. Rotavirus associated with acute gastroenteritis in adults. Lancet. 1976;2:423.
175. Wenman WM, Hinde D, Feltham S, et al. Rotavirus infection in adults. Results of a prospective study. N Engl J Med. 1979;301:306.
176. Yolken RH, Bishop CA, Townsend TR, et al. Infectious gastroenteritis in bone-marrow transplant recipients. N Engl J Med. 1982;306:1099.
177. Goodgame RW, Greenough WBIII. Cholera in Africa: A message for the west. Ann Intern Med. 1975;82:101.
178. Weissman JB, DeWitt WE, Thompson J, et al. A case of cholera in Texas, 1973. Am J Epidemiol. 1975;100:487.
179. Blake PA, Allegra DT, Snyder JD, et al. Cholera: A possible endemic focus in the United States. N Engl J Med. 1980;302:305.
180. Blake PA, Rosenberg ML, Florencia J, et al. Cholera in Portugal, 1974. II. Transmission by bottled mineral water. Am J Epidemiol. 1977;105:344.
181. Baine WB, Mazzotti M, Greco D, et al. Epidemiology of cholera in Italy in 1973. Lancet. 1974;2:1370.
182. Gitelson S. Gastrectomy, achlorhydria and cholera. Isr J Med Sci. 1971;7:663.
183. Ramamurthy T, Garg S, Sharma R, et al. Emergence of novel strain of *Vibrio cholerae* with epidemic potential in southern and eastern India (Letter). Lancet. 1993;341:703–704.
184. Albert MJ, Siddique AK, Islam MS, et al. Large outbreak of clinical cholera due to *Vibrio cholerae* non-O1 in Bangladesh (Letter). Lancet. 1993;341:704.
185. Bhattacharya MK, Bhattacharya SK, Garg S, et al. Outbreak of *Vibrio cholerae* non-O1 in India and Bangladesh (Letter). Lancet. 1993;341:1346–1347.
186. Shimada T, Nair GB, Deb BC, et al. Outbreak of *Vibrio cholerae* non-O1 in India and Bangladesh (Letter). Lancet. 1993;341:1347.
187. Centers for Disease Control and Prevention. Emerging infectious diseases: Imported cholera associated with a newly described toxigenic *Vibrio cholerae* O139 strain—California, 1993. MMWR Morb Mortal Wkly Rep. 1993;42:501–503.
188. Snow J. On the Mode of Communication of Cholera. 2nd ed. London: Churchill; 1855.
189. De SN, Bhattacharya K, Sarkar JK. A study of the pathogenicity of strains of *Bacterium coli* from acute and chronic enteritis. J Pathol Bacteriol. 1956;71:201.
190. Trabulsi LR. Revelaçáo de colibacilos associados as diarreias infantis pelo metodo da infecão experimental da alca ligade do intestino do coelho. Rev Inst Med Trop Sao Paulo. 1964;6:197.
191. Taylor J, Wilkins MP, Payne JM. Relation of rabbit gut reaction to enteropathogenic *Escherichia coli*. Br J Exp Pathol. 1961;42:43.
192. Taylor J, Bettleheim KA. The action of chloroform-killed suspensions of enteropathogenic *Escherichia coli* on ligated rabbit-gut segments. J Gen Microbiol. 1966;42:309.
193. Smith HW, Halls S. Studies on *Escherichia coli* enterotoxin. J Pathol Bacteriol. 1967;93:531.
194. Gorbach SL, Banwell JG, Chatterjee BD, et al. Acute undifferentiated human diarrhea in the tropics. I. Alterations in intestinal microflora. J Clin Invest. 1971;50:881.
195. Banwell JG, Gorbach SL, Pierce NF, et al. Acute undifferentiated human diarrhea in the tropics. II. Alterations in intestinal fluid and electrolyte movements. J Clin Invest. 1971;50:890.
196. Sack RB, Gorbach SL, Banwell JG, et al. Enterotoxigenic *Escherichia coli* isolated from patients with severe cholera-like disease. J Infect Dis. 1971;123:378.
197. DuPont HL, Formal SB, Hornick RB, et al. Pathogenesis of *Escherichia coli* diarrhea. N Engl J Med. 1971;285:1.
198. Evans DG, Evans DJ Jr, Pierce NF. Differences in the response of rabbit small intestine to heat-labile and heat-stable enterotoxins of *Escherichia coli*. Infect Immun. 1973;7:873.
199. Guerrant RL, Brunton LL, Schnaitman TC, et al. Cyclic adenosine monophosphate and alteration of Chinese hamster ovary cell morphology: A rapid, sensitive in vitro assay for the enterotoxins of *Vibrio cholerae* and *Escherichia coli*. Infect Immun. 1974;10:320.
200. Donta ST, Moon HW, Whipp SC. Detection of heat-labile *Escherichia coli* enterotoxin with the use of adrenal cells in tissue culture. Science. 1974;183:334.
201. Guerrant RL, Brunton LL. Characterization of the Chinese hamster ovary cell assay for the enterotoxins of *Vibrio cholerae* and *Escherichia coli* and for antitoxin: Differential inhibition by gangliosides, specific antisera, and toxoid. J Infect Dis. 1977;135:720.
202. Honda T, Arita M, Takeda Y, et al. Further evaluation of the Biken test (modified Elek test) for detection of enterotoxigenic *E. coli* producing heat-labile enterotoxin and application of the test to sampling of heat-stable enterotoxin. J Clin Microbiol. 1982;16:60.
203. Alderete JF, Robertson DC. Purification and chemical characterization of the heat-stable enterotoxin produced by porcine strains of enterotoxigenic *Escherichia coli*. Infect Immun. 1978;19:1021.
204. Dean AG, Ching YC, Williams RG, et al. Test for *Escherichia coli* enterotoxin using infant mice: Application in a study of diarrhea in children in Honolulu. J Infect Dis. 1972;125:407.
205. Gyles CL. Limitation of the infant mouse test for *E. coli* heat-stable enterotoxin. Can J Comp Med. 1979;43:371–379.
206. Kennedy DJ, Greenberg RN, Dunn JA, et al. Effects of *Escherichia coli* heat stable enterotoxin STb on intestines of mice, rats, rabbits and piglets. Infect Immun. 1984;46:639–643.
207. Weikel CS, Mellans HN, Guerrant RL. In vivo and in vitro effects of a novel enterotoxin, STb, produced by *Escherichia coli*. J Infect Dis. 1986;153:893–901.
208. Rosenberg ML, Koplan JP, Wachsmuth IK, et al. Epidemic diarrhea at Crater Lake from enterotoxigenic *Escherichia coli*. A large, waterborne outbreak. Ann Intern Med. 1977;86:714.
209. Korzeniowski OM, Dantas W, Trabulsi LR, et al. A controlled study of endemic sporadic diarrhea among adult residents of southern Brazil. Trans R Soc Trop Med Hyg. 1984;78:363–369.
210. Hughes JM, Rouse JD, Barada FA, et al. Etiology of summer diarrhea among the Navajo. Am J Trop Med Hyg. 1980;29:613.
211. Current WL, Reese NC, Ernst JV, et al. Human cryptosporidiosis in immunocompetent and immunodeficient persons. N Engl J Med. 1983;308:1252.
212. Tzipori S. Cryptosporidiosis in animals and humans. Microbiol Rev. 1983;47:84.
213. Wolfson JS, Richter JM, Waldron MA, et al. Cryptosporidiosis in immunocompetent patients. N Engl J Med. 1985;312:1278–1282.
214. Palmer DL, Koster FT, Islam AFMR, et al. A comparison of sucrose and glucose in oral electrolyte therapy of cholera and other severe diarrheas. N Engl J Med. 1977;297:1107.
215. Ericsson CD, Evans DG, DuPont HL, et al. Bismuth subsalicylate inhibits activity of crude toxins of *Escherichia coli* and *Vibrio cholerae*. J Infect Dis. 1977;136:693.
216. Gelb A, Miller S. AIDS and gastroenterology. Am J Gastroenterol. 1986;81:619–622.
217. Soave R, Johnson WD. *Cryptosporidium* and *Isospora belli* infections. J Infect Dis. 1988;157:225–229.
218. Guerrant RL, Thielman NM. Emerging enteric protozoa: *Cryptosporidium, Cyclospora* and microsporidia. In: Scheld WM, Armstrong D, Hughes JM, eds. Emerging Infections. Washington, DC: ASM Press; 1997:233–245.
219. Kotler DP, Goetz HP, Lange M, et al. Enteropathy associated with the acquired immunodeficiency syndrome. Ann Intern Med. 1984;101:421–428.
220. Gillin JS, Shike M, Alcock N, et al. Malabsorption and mucosal abnormalities of the small intestine in the acquired immunodeficiency syndrome. Ann Intern Med. 1985;102:619–622.
221. Nelson JA, Reynolds-Kohler G, Margaretten W, et al. Human immunodeficiency virus detected in bowel epithelium from patients with gastro-intestinal symptoms. Lancet. 1988;1:259–262.
222. Smith PD, Lance C, Gill VJ, et al. Intestinal infections in patients with the acquired immunodeficiency syndrome (AIDS). Ann Intern Med. 1988;108:328–333.
223. Laughon BE, Druckman DA, Vernon A, et al. Prevalence of enteric pathogens in homosexual men with and without acquired immunodeficiency syndrome. Gastroenterology. 1988;94:984.
224. Quinn TC, Stamm WE, Goodell SE, et al. The polymicrobial origin of intestinal infections in homosexual men. N Engl J Med. 1983;309:576–582.
225. Kotler DP, Francisco A, Clayton F, et al. Small intestinal injury and parasitic diseases in AIDS. Ann Intern Med. 1990;113:444–449.
226. Connolly GM, Forbes A, Gazzard BG. Investigation of seemingly pathogen-negative diarrhoea in patients infected with HIV1. Gut 1990;31:886–889.
227. Guerrant RL, Bobak DA. Bacterial and protozoal gastroenteritis. N Engl J Med 1991;325:327–340.
228. DeHovitz JA, Pape JW, Boncy M, Johnson WD Jr. Clinical manifestations and therapy of *Isospora belli* infection in patients with the acquired immunodeficiency syndrome. N Engl J Med. 1986;315:87–90.
229. Pape JW, Verdier RI, Boncy M, et al. *Cyclospora* infection in adults infected with HIV. Clinical manifestations, treatment, and prophylaxis. Ann Intern Med. 1994;121:654–657.
230. Guerrant RL, Thielman NM. Emerging enteric protozoa: *Cryptosporidium, Cyclospora*, and Microsporidia. In: Scheld WM, Armstrong D, Hughes JM, eds. Emerging Infections. Washington, DC: ASM Press; 1998:233–245.

231. Carter TR, Cooper PH, Petri WA Jr, et al. *Pneumocystis carinii* infection of the small intestine in a patient with acquired immune deficiency syndrome. Am J Clin Pathol. 1988;89:679–683.
232. Chachoua A, Dieterich D, Krasinski K, et al. 9-(1,3-Dihydroxy-2-propoxy-methyl)-guanine (ganciclovir) in the treatment of cytomegalovirus gastrointestinal disease with the acquired immunodeficiency syndrome. Ann Intern Med. 1987;107:133–137.
233. Celum CL, Chaisson RE, Rutherford GW, et al. Incidence of salmonellosis in patients with AIDS. J Infect Dis. 1987;156:998–1002.
234. Jacobs JL, Gold JWM, Murray HW, et al. *Salmonella* infections in patients with the acquired immunodeficiency syndrome. Ann Intern Med. 1985;102:186–188.
235. Glaser JB, Morton-Kute L, Berger SR, et al. Recurrent *Salmonella typhimurium* bacteremia associated with the acquired immunodeficiency syndrome. Ann Intern Med. 1985;102:189–193.
236. Sperber SJ, Schleupner CJ: Salmonellosis during infection with human immunodeficiency virus. Rev Infect Dis. 1987;9:925–934.
237. Grohman GS, Glass RI, Pereira HG, et al. Enteric viruses and diarrhea in HIV-infected patients. N Engl J Med. 1993;329:14–20.
238. Guerrant RL, Hughes JM, Lima NL, et al. Microbiology of diarrhea in developed and developing countries. Rev Infect Dis. 1990;12(Suppl):S41–S50.
239. Stamm WE, Weinstein RA, Dixon RE. Comparison of endemic and epidemic nosocomial infections. Am J Med. 1981;70:393–397.
240. Lima N, Searcy M, Guerrant R. Nosocomial diarrhea rates exceed those of other nosocomial infections on ICU and pediatric wards. Abstract 1050. Presented at the Twenty-sixth Interscience Conference on Antimicrobial Agents and Chemotherapy, New Orleans, La, 1986.
241. Lima NL, Guerrant RL, Kaiser DL, et al. Nosocomial diarrhea: A possible risk factor for nosocomial infections (Abstract). Clin Res. 1988;36:580.
242. Welliver RC, McLaughlin S. Unique epidemiology of nosocomial infection in a children's hospital. Am J Dis Child. 1984;138:131–135.
243. Kelly WJ, Patrick MR, Hilman KM. Study of diarrhea in critically ill patients. Crit Care Med. 1983;1:7–9.
244. Hughes JM, Jarvis WR. Nosocomial gastrointestinal infections. In: Wenzel RP, ed. Prevention and Control of Nosocomial Infections. Baltimore: Williams & Wilkins; 1987.
245. Karlstrom O, Fryklund B, Tullus K, Burman LG. A prospective nationwide study of *Clostridium difficile*–associated diarrhea in Sweden. The Swedish *C. difficile* Study Group. Clin Infect Dis. 1998;26:141–145.
246. Barbut F, Corthier G, Charpak Y, et al. Prevalence and pathogenicity of *Clostridium difficile* in hospitalized patients. A French multicenter study. Arch Intern Med. 1996;156:1449–1454.
247. Samore MH, Venkataraman L, DeGirolami PC, et al. Clinical and molecular epidemiology of sporadic and clustered cases of nosocomial *Clostridium difficile* diarrhea. Am J Med. 1996;100:32–40.
248. McFarland LV. Epidemiology, risk factors, and treatments for antibiotic-associated diarrhea. Dig Dis. 1998;16:292–307.
249. Samore MH, Bettin KM, DeGirolami PC, et al. Wide diversity of *Clostridium difficile* types at a tertiary referral hospital. J Infect Dis. 1994;170:615–621.
250. Kent KC, Rubin MS, Wroblewski L, et al. The impact of *Clostridium difficile* on a surgical service: A prospective study of 374 patients. Ann Surg. 1998;227:296–301.
251. Brown E, Talbot GH, Axelrod P, et al. Risk factors for *Clostridium difficile* toxin-associated diarrhea. Infect Control Hosp Epidemiol. 1990;11:283–290.
252. Neill MA, Rice SK, Ahmad NV, Flanigan TP. Cryptosporidiosis: An unrecognized cause of diarrhea in elderly hospitalized patients. Clin Infect Dis. 1996;22:168–170.
253. Yolken RJ, Bishop CA, Towsend R, et al. Infectious gastroenteritis in bone marrow transplant recipients. N Engl J Med. 1982;306:1009–1012.
254. Farber BF, Brennen JC, Puntereri AJ, et al. A prospective study of nosocomial infections in a chronic care facility. J Am Geriatr Soc. 1984;32:499.
255. Nicolle LE, McIntyre M, Zacharias H, et al. Twelve-month surveillance of infections in institutionalized eldery men. J Am Geriatr Soc. 1984;32:513.
256. Sims RV, Hauser RJ, Adewale AO, et al. Acute gastroenteritis in three community-based nursing homes. J Gerontol. 1994;M252–M256.
257. Bender BS, Laughon BE, Gaydos C, et al. Is *Clostridium difficile* endemic in chronic-care facilities? Lancet. 1986;2:1279.
258. Treolar AJ, Kalra L. Mortality and *Clostridium difficile* diarrhoea in the elderly. Lancet. 1987;2:1279.
259. Pickering LK, Evans DG, Dupont HL, et al. Diarrhea caused by *Shigella*, rotavirus and *Giardia* in day care centers: Prospective study. J Pediatr. 1981;99:51–56.
260. Mitchell DK, Monroe SS, Jiang X, et al. Virologic features of an astrovirus diarrhea outbreak in a day care center revealed by reverse transcriptase–polymerase chain reaction. J Infect Dis. 1995;172:1437–1444.
261. Mitchell DK, Van R, Morrow AL, et al. Outbreaks of astrovirus gastroenteritis in day care centers. J Pediatr. 1993;123:725–732.
262. Centers for Disease Control and Prevention. Cryptosporidiosis among children attending day-care centers: Georgia, Pennsylvania, Michigan, California, New Mexico. MMWR Morb Mortal Wkly Rep. 1984;33:599.
263. Alpert G, Bell LM, Kirkpatrick CE, et al. Crystosporidiosis in a day-care center. N Engl J Med. 1984;311:860–861.
264. Taylor JP, Perdue JN, Dingley D, et al. Cryptosporidiosis outbreak in a day-care center. Am J Dis Child. 1985;139:1023–1025.
265. Bartlett AV, Moore M, Gary GW, et al. Diarrheal illness among infants and toddlers in daycare centers. I. Epidemiology and pathogens. J Pediatr. 1985;107:495–502.
266. Guerrant RL, Lohr JA, Williams EK. Acute infectious diarrhea. I. Epidemiology, etiology, and pathogenesis. Pediatr Infect Dis. 1986;5:353–359.
267. Kean BH. The diarrhea of travelers to Mexico. Summary of five-year study. Ann Intern Med. 1963;59:605.
268. Psalms 22:14.
269. Consensus development conference statement on travelers' diarrhea. Rev Infect Dis. 1986;8(Suppl):227–233.
269a. Keystone JS, Kozarsky PE. Health Advice for International Travel. In: Guerrant RL, Walker DH, Weller PF, eds. Tropical Infectious Diseases: Principles, Pathogens and Practice. Philadelphia: WB Saunders; 1999.
270. Lowenstein MS, Balows A, Gangarosa EJ. Turista at an international congress in Mexico. Lancet. 1973;1:529.
271. The diarrhea of travelers: Turista (Editorial). JAMA. 1962;180:402.
272. Higgens AR. Observations on the health of United States personnel living in Cairo, Egypt. Am J Trop Med Hyg. 1955;4:970.
273. Steffen R. Epidemiologic studies of travelers' diarrhea, severe gastrointestinal infections, and cholera. Rev Infect Dis. 1986;8(Suppl 2):122–130.
274. Steffen R, Rickernbach M, Wilhelm U, et al. Health problems after travel to developing countries. J Infect Dis. 1987;156:84–91.
275. Kean BH, Schaffner W, Brennan RW. The diarrhea of travelers. V. Prophylaxis with phthalylsulfathiazole and neomycin sulphate. JAMA. 1962;180:367–71.
276. Rowe B, Taylor J, Bettelheim KA. An investigation of travelers' diarrhea. Lancet. 1970;1:1.
277. Gorbach SL, Kean BH, Evans DG, et al. Travelers' diarrhea and toxigenic *Escherichia coli*. N Engl J Med. 1975;292:933.
278. Merson MH, Morris GK, Sack DA, et al. Travelers' diarrhea in Mexico, a prospective study of physicians and family members attending a congress. N Engl J Med. 1976;294:1299.
279. Sack DA, Kaminsky DC, Sack RB, et al. Enterotoxigenic *Escherichia coli* diarrhea of travelers: A prospective study of American Peace Corps volunteers. Johns Hopkins Med J. 1977;141:63.
280. Guerrant RL, Rouse JD, Hughes JM. Turista among members of the Yale Glee Club in Latin America. Am J Trop Med Hyg. 1980;29:895.
281. Turner AC. Travelers' diarrhoea: A survey of symptoms, occurrence, and possible prophylaxis. BMJ. 1967;4:453–454.
282. Black RE. Pathogens that cause travelers' diarrhea in Latin America and Africa. Rev Infect Dis. 1986;8(Suppl 2):131–135.
283. Hoge CW, Shlim DR, Echeverria P, et al. Epidemiology of diarrhea among expatriate residents living in a highly endemic environment. JAMA. 1996;275:533–538.
284. Taylor DN, Echeverria P. Etiology and epidemiology of travelers' diarrhea in Asia. Rev Infect Dis. 1986;8(Suppl 2):136–141.
285. Castelli F, Carosi G. Epidemiology of traveler's diarrhea. Chemotherapy. 1995;41(Suppl)32.
286. Wolfe MS. Protection of travelers. Clin Infect Dis. 1997;25:177–184.
287. Bolivar R, Conklin RH, Vollet JJ, et al. Rotavirus in travelers' diarrhea: Study of an adult student population in Mexico. J Infect Dis. 1978;137:324.
288. Ryder RW, Oquist CA, Greenberg H, et al. Travelers' diarrhea in Panamanian tourists in Mexico. J Infect Dis. 1981;144:442.
289. Jelinek T, Lotze M, Eichenlaub S, et al. Prevalence of infection with *Cryptosporidium parvum* and *Cyclospora cayetanensis* among international travellers. Gut. 1997;41:801–804.
290. Shlim DR, Hoge CW, Rajah R, et al. Is *Blastocystis hominis* a cause of diarrhea in travelers? A prospective controlled study in Nepal. Clin Infect Dis. 1995;21:97–101.
291. Keystone JS. *Blastocystis hominis* and traveler's diarrhea (Editorial). Clin Infect Dis. 1995;21:102–103.
292. Jelinek T, Peyerl G, Loscher T, et al. The role of *Blastocystis hominis* as a possible intestinal pathogen in travellers. J Infect. 1997;35:63–66.
293. Snyder JD, Blake PA. Is cholera a problem for US travelers? JAMA. 1982;247:2268.
294. DuPont HL. Pathogenesis of traveler's diarrhea. Chemotherapy. 1995;41(Suppl)9.
295. Osterholm MT, MacDonald KL, White KE, et al. An outbreak of a newly recognized chronic diarrhea syndrome associated with raw milk consumption. JAMA. 1986;256:484–490.
296. Parsonnet J, Trock SC, Bopp CA, et al. Chronic diarrhea associated with drinking untreated water. Ann Intern Med. 1989;110:985–991.
297. Mintz ED, Weber JT, Guris D, et al. An outbreak of Brainerd diarrhea among travelers to the Galapagos Islands. J Infect Dis. 1998;177:1041–1045.
298. Echeverria P, Hodge FA, Blacklow NR, et al. Travelers' diarrhea among United States marines in South Korea. Am J Epidemiol. 1978;108:68.
299. Wolfe MS. Current concepts in parasitology. Giardiasis. N Engl J Med. 1978;298:319.
300. Brodsky RE, Spencer HC Jr, Schultz MG. Giardiasis in American travelers to the Soviet Union. J Infect Dis. 1974;130:319.
301. Soave R, Armstrong D. *Cryptosporidium* and cryptosporidiosis. Rev Infect Dis. 1986;8:1012–1023.
302. Jokipii L, Pohjola S, Jokipii AMM. *Cryptosporidium*: A frequent finding in patients with gastrointestinal symptoms. Lancet. 1983;2:358–360.
303. Kean BH, Reilly PC. Malaria—the mime. Recent lessons from a group of civilian travelers. Am J Med. 1976;61:159.
304. Pearson RD, Hewlett EL, Guerrant RL. Tropical diseases in North America. Dis Mon. 1984;30:1–68.
305. Hill DR, Pearson RD. Health advice for international travel. Ann Intern Med. 1988;108:839–852.
306. Kean BH, Waters SR. Diarrhea of travelers. III. Drug prophylaxis in Mexico. N Engl J Med. 1959;261:71.

307. Oakley GP. The neurotoxicity of the halogenated hydroxyquinolines. JAMA. 1973;225:395.
308. Portnoy BL, DuPont HL, Pruitt D, et al. Antidiarrheal agents in the treatment of acute diarrhea in children. JAMA. 1976;236:844.
309. DuPont HL, Hornick RB. Adverse effect of Lomotil therapy in shigellosis. JAMA. 1973;226:1525.
310. DuPont HL, Sullivan P, Pickering LK, et al. Symptomatic treatment of diarrhea with bismuth subsalicylate among students attending a Mexican university. Gastroenterology. 1977;73:715.
311. Steffen R, Heusser R, DuPont HL. Prevention of travelers' diarrhea by nonantibiotic drugs. Rev Infect Dis. 1986;8:(Suppl 2):151–159.
312. Blaser MJ. Environmental interventions for the prevention of travelers' diarrhea. Rev Infect Dis. 1986;8(Suppl 2):142–150.
313. Gonzales-Cortez A, Gangarosa EJ, Parrilla C, et al. Bottled beverages and typhoid fever: The Mexican epidemic of 1972–3. Am J Public Health. 1982;72:844.
314. Harris JR. Are bottled beverages safe for travelers? Am J Public Health. 1982;72:787.
315. Neumann HH. Travellers' diarrhea. Lancet. 1970;1:420.
316. Tjoa W, DuPont HL, Sullivan P, et al. Location of food consumption and travelers' diarrhea. Am J Epidemiol. 1977;106:61.
317. Sack DA, Kaminsky DC, Sack RB, et al. Prophylactic doxycycline for travelers' diarrhea, results of a prospective double-blind study of Peace Corps volunteers in Kenya. N Engl J Med. 1978;298:758.
318. Echeverria P, Verhaert L, Ulyangco CV, et al. Antimicrobial resistance and enterotoxin production among isolates of *Escherichia coli* in the Far East. Lancet. 1978;2:589.
319. Murray BE. Resistance of *Shigella, Salmonella* and other selected enteric pathogens. Rev Infect Dis. 1986;8(Suppl 2):172–181.
320. Mentzing LO, Ringertz O. *Salmonella* infection in tourists. 2. Prophylaxis against salmonellosis. Acta Pathol Microbiol Scand. 1968;74:405.
321. Ericsson CD, DuPont HL, Matthewson JJ et al. Treatment of travelers' diarrhea with sulfamethoxazole and trimethoprim and loperamide. JAMA. 1990;263:257–261.
322. DuPont HL, Ericsson CD. Prevention and treatment of travelers' diarrhea. N Engl J Med. 1993;328:1821–1826.
323. Murray BE, Rensimer ER, DuPont HL. Emergence of high level trimethoprim resistance in fecal *E. coli* during oral administration of trimethoprim or trimethoprim/sulfamethoxazole. N Engl J Med. 1982;306:130.
324. Tiemens KM, Shipley PL, Correia RA, et al. Sulfamethoxazole-trimethoprim resistant *Shigella flexneri* in northeastern Brazil. Antimicrob Agents Chemother. 1984;25:653–654.
325. DuPont HL, Reves RR, Galindo E, et al. Treatment of travelers' diarrhea with trimethoprim/sulfamethoxazole and with trimethoprim alone. N Engl J Med. 1983;307:841–844.
326. Statement on travellers' diarrhea. Committee to Advise on Tropical Medicine and Travel. CMAJ. 1995;152:205–212.
327. Petruccelli BP, Murphy GS, Sanchez JL, et al. Treatment of traveler's diarrhea with ciprofloxacin and loperamide. J Infect Dis. 1992;165:557–560.
328. Ericsson CD, DuPont HL, Sullivan P, et al. Bicozamycin, a poorly absorbable antibiotic, effectively treats travelers' diarrhea. Ann Intern Med. 1983;98:20.
329. Ericsson CD, Johnson PC, DuPont HL, et al. Ciprofloxacin or trimethoprim-sulfamethoxazole as initial therapy for travelers' diarrhea. Ann Intern Med. 1987;106:216–220.
330. Bandres JC, Mathewson JJ, Ericsson CD, et al. Trimethoprim/sulfamethoxazole remains active against enterotoxigenic *Escherichia coli* and *Shigella* species in Guadalajara, Mexico. Am J Med Sci. 1992;303:289–291.
331. Gough A, Barsoum NJ, Mitchell L, et al. Juvenile canine drug-induced arthropathy. Toxicol Appl Pharmacol. 1979;51:177–187.
332. Sack RB, Rahman M, Yunus M, Khan EH. Antimicrobial resistance in organisms causing diarrheal disease. Clin Infect Dis. 1997;24(Suppl):5.
333. Murphy GS Jr, Echeverria P, Jackson LR, et al. Ciprofloxacin- and azithromycin-resistant *Campylobacter* causing traveler's diarrhea in U.S. troops deployed to Thailand in 1994. Clin Infect Dis. 1996;22:868–869.
334. Said SI, Faloona GR. Elevated plasma and tissue levels of vasoactive intestinal polypeptide in the watery diarrhea syndrome due to pancreatic, bronchogenic, and other tumors. N Engl J Med. 1975;293:155.
335. Wolff MS. Giardiasis. JAMA. 1975;233:1362.
336. Murphy TV, Nelson JD. Five vs ten days' therapy with furazolidone for giardiasis. Am J Dis Child. 1983;137:267.
337. Ma P, Soave R. Three-step stool examination for cryptosporidiosis in 10 homosexual men with protracted watery diarrhea. J Infect Dis. 1983;147:824.
338. Donaldson RM Jr. Small bowel bacterial overgrowth. Adv Intern Med. 1970;16:191.
339. Gorbach SL. Intestinal microflora. Gastroenterology. 1971;60:1110.
340. Penn RG, Giger DK, Knoop FC, et al. *Plesiomonas shigelloides* overgrowth in the small intestine. J Clin Microbiol. 1982;15:869.
341. Scott AJ, Khan GA. Partial biliary obstruction with cholangitis producing a blind loop syndrome. Gut. 1968;9:187.
342. Vantrappen G, Janssens J, Hellemans J, et al. Interdigestive motor complex of normal subjects and patients with bacterial overgrowth of the small intestine. J Clin Invest. 1977;59:1158.
343. Heyworth B, Brown J. Jejunal microflora in malnourished Gambian children. Arch Dis Child. 1975;50:27.
344. Roberts SH, James O, Jarvis EH. Bacterial overgrowth syndrome without "blind loop": A cause for malnutrition in the elderly. Lancet. 1977;2:1193.
345. Ruiz-Palacios GM, DuPont HL. Bacterial overgrowth syndrome after acute nonspecific diarrhoea. Lancet. 1978;1:337.
346. Lindenbaum J, Kent TH, Sprinz H. Malabsorption and jejunitis in American Peace Corps volunteers in Pakistan. Ann Intern Med. 1955;65:1201.
347. Shimada K, Bricknell KS, Finegold SM. Deconjugation of bile acids by intestinal bacteria: Review of literature and additional studies. J Infect Dis. 1969;119:273.
348. Wanke CA, Guerrant RL. Small bowel colonization alone is a cause of diarrhea. Infect Immun. 1987;55:1924–1926.
349. Schlager TA, Wanke CA, Guerrant RL. Net fluid secretion and impaired villous function induced by small intestinal colonization by non-toxigenic, colonizing *E. coli*. Infect Immun. 1990;58:1337.
350. Hamilton JD, Dyer NH, Dawson AM, et al. Assessment and significance of bacterial overgrowth in the small bowel. Q J Med. 1970;39:265.
351. MacDougall LG. The effect of aureomycin on undernourished African children. J Trop Pediatr. 1957;3:74.
352. Levy SB, FitzGerald GB, Macone AB. Changes in intestinal flora of farm personnel after introduction of a tetracycline-supplemented feed on a farm. N Engl J Med. 1976;295:583.

Chapter 84

Antibiotic-Associated Colitis

NATHAN M. THIELMAN

Diarrhea is one of the most common complications associated with antibiotic therapy, and colitis is one of the most serious. Attack rates vary depending on the antimicrobial used, the epidemiologic setting, and the host. Overall, attack rates for antibiotic-associated diarrhea in hospitals range from 3.2 to 29%.[1, 2] Nearly 15% of hospitalized patients receiving β-lactam antibiotics develop diarrhea,[2] and rates for those receiving clindamycin range from 10 to 25%.[3] Predisposing host factors and circumstances affecting the frequency and severity of disease include advanced age, underlying illness, recent surgery, and recent administration of bowel motility–altering drugs.

Clostridium difficile is now recognized as a frequent cause of antibiotic-associated diarrhea and colitis.[4] It is implicated in 20 to 30% of patients with antibiotic-associated diarrhea,[5–7] in 50 to 75% of those with antibiotic-associated colitis,[4] and in more than 90% of those with antibiotic-associated pseudomembranous colitis.[5–7] In a recent Swedish study, *C. difficile*–associated diarrhea was almost twice as prevalent as all diagnosed domestic cases of reportable bacterial and protozoal diarrhea combined.[8]

The etiology of antibiotic-associated diarrhea and colitis *not* caused by *C. difficile* is poorly understood. *Staphylococcus aureus*, once implicated as the agent of antibiotic-associated colitis, is now rarely appreciated (see "Historical Overview"). Receiving more attention in the last decade has been a possible link with *Candida* spp., particularly among hospitalized elderly patients.[9–12] In most[12] but not all[10] patients, colitis is absent, and in nearly all reported cases, therapy with oral nystatin leads to improvement. Definitive data establishing the pathogenicity of *Candida* in diarrhea, however, are lacking, and dense colonization has been observed in the absence of diarrhea.[13] Enterotoxigenic *Clostridium perfringens* has also been cited as a possible cause of antibiotic-associated diarrhea,[14, 15] and recent antibiotic exposure has emerged as a distinct risk factor in both sporadic cases and outbreaks of salmonellosis.[16–19] Changes in carbohydrate and short-chain fatty acid metabolism may also play a role in antibiotic-associated diarrhea not caused by infectious agents.[20–22]

Although the morbidity and economic burden of broadly characterized antibiotic-associated diarrhea are difficult to quantify, relevant data for *C. difficile*–associated diarrhea have been reported. A prospective case-control analysis conducted in a geriatric population documented significantly higher death rates and increased hospital costs—in excess of $5000 per case—among patients with *C. difficile*–associated diarrhea hospitalized in Britain.[23] In the United States, charges incurred when the admitting diagnosis was *C. difficile*–associated diarrhea averaged $5000 per case in 1991 in a community hospital, and charges for cases acquired in the hospital were nearly $2000 per patient.[24] It is not surprising that several studies have reported substantial increases in length of hospital stay associated with this disease.[23, 25, 26]

HISTORICAL OVERVIEW

Paradoxically, the major pathologic feature of antibiotic-associated colitis—pseudomembrane formation—was first described in the preantibiotic era. Finney[27] reported the case of a 22-year-old woman who, 10 days after gastric surgery, developed hemorrhagic diarrhea and eventually died; the autopsy report described "diphtheritic colitis." This historic description, published more than 40 years prior to the introduction of antibiotics, illustrates the importance of abdominal surgery, hospitalization, and impaired intestinal motility (following administration of opiates) in the pathogenesis of this process. As early as 1948, staphylococci were implicated in a case of fatal enteritis in an infant following administration of oral streptomycin.[28] Thereafter, Bennett and colleagues at Johns Hopkins Hospital resectioned and reexamined the original pathologic specimens from Finney's case and found "myriads of gram-positive cocci."[29] In the 1950s and 1960s, several reports of staphylococcal enterocolitis were based on merely culturing staphylococci in diarrheal stools or pathology specimens[28, 30–33]; in other reports, the organism was actually demonstrated within pseudomembranes or intestinal tissue sections (Fig. 84–1).[34–37] Noting the absence of *S. aureus* in 11 of 18 patients with pseudomembranous enterocolitis, Dearing and associates[32] concluded that such findings "cast doubt on the concept that all cases of pseudomembranous enteritis are produced by *S. aureus* in the intestine." Since the late 1960s, and following the discovery of *C. difficile* as the major cause of antibiotic-associated colitis in 1977, antibiotic-associated staphylococcal diarrhea has virtually disappeared from the medical literature, with only a few purported cases in the United States and Japan.[38] There are least three potential explanations for this dramatic decline in the number of reported cases of staphylococcal enterocolitis: (1) Staphylococci were wrongly implicated and actually played no role in pseudomembranous enterocolitis[39]; (2) the actual incidence of the disease decreased dramatically following the introduction of β-lactamase–stable penicillins[40]; or (3) the entity still exists but is ignored because of the emphasis on *C. difficile* toxin testing and the use of empirical vancomycin for antibiotic-associated diarrhea.[38]

The literature from the mid-1970s emphasized the attack rates for diarrhea and pseudomembranous colitis associated with the use of individual antibiotics. Several studies reported clindamycin (and lincomycin)-associated diarrhea rates ranging from 7 to 21%[41–44] and those for ampicillin from 4 to 17%.[41, 45, 46] In a now classic prospective clinical investigation, Tedesco and associates found diarrhea in 21% of 200 patients receiving clindamycin and described "clindamycin colitis" in fully 10%.[46] Although proctoscopic examination confirmed the presence of pseudomembranous colitis in the latter group, the investigators found little to suggest an underlying bacterial cause, and results of cultures of plaque-like lesions, mucosal smears, and stool for staphylococci were negative.[47] Prompted by these data and additional reports, in 1979 the Committee on Safety of Medicines in the United Kingdom recommended that clindamycin and lincomycin "should in general be reserved for severe or life-threatening conditions where other antibiotic therapy is ineffective or undesirable"; similar warnings had already been issued in the United States.[40, 48, 49]

In the late 1970s, a series of investigations established toxigenic *C. difficile* as the cause of pseudomembranous colitis. First, Larson and colleagues,[50] in attempts to isolate viruses from the feces of a 12-year-old girl with a prior history of penicillin exposure, diarrhea, negative results on stool cultures, and endoscopically proven pseudomembranous colitis, suggested a role for bacterial toxins in this process. Fecal suspensions from the patient (and subsequently those from four of five others with pseudomembranous colitis) demonstrated cytopathic effects on HeLa cells, Rhesus monkey kidney cells, and human embryonic lung fibroblast cells (Fig. 84–2).[50] Within a short period of time, several other reports subsequently shed light on this observation. Bartlett and coworkers,[51] using a Syrian hamster model of clindamycin-associated enterocolitis, found that intracecal material transferred the disease from affected hamsters

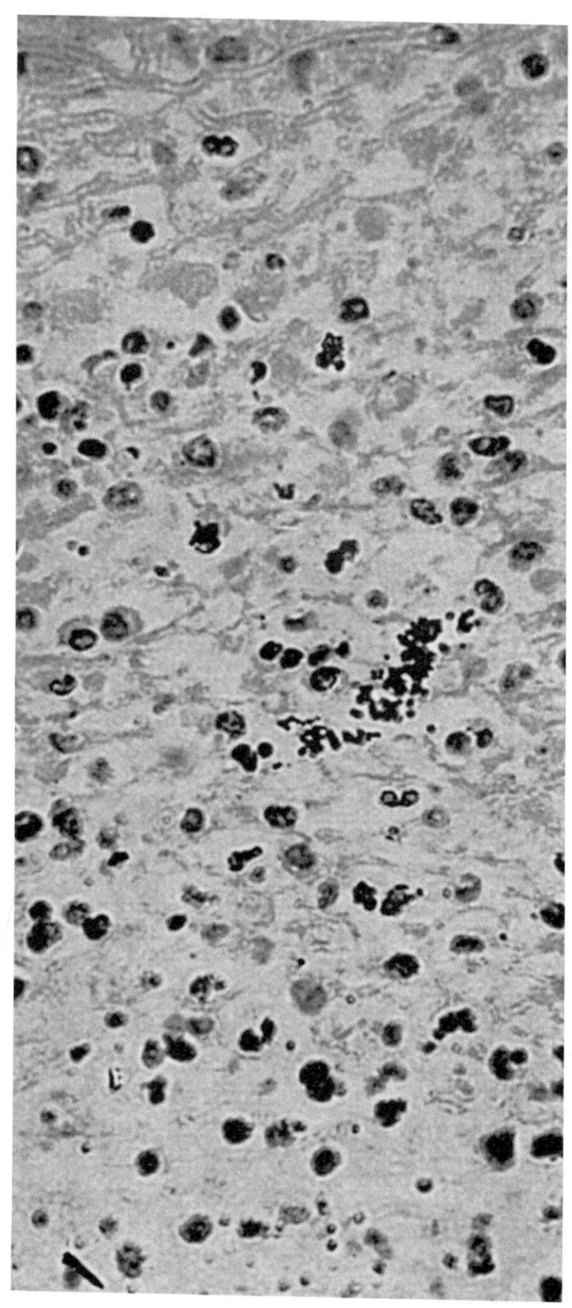

FIGURE 84–1. Section of pseudomembrane demonstrating inflammatory cells, fibrin, and gram-positive cocci from a 1956 report of a fatal case of staphylococcal pseudomembranous enteritis. (From Corridan M. Antibiotic-resistant staphylococcal pseudomembranous enteritis. J Clin Pathol. 1956;9:131–135.)

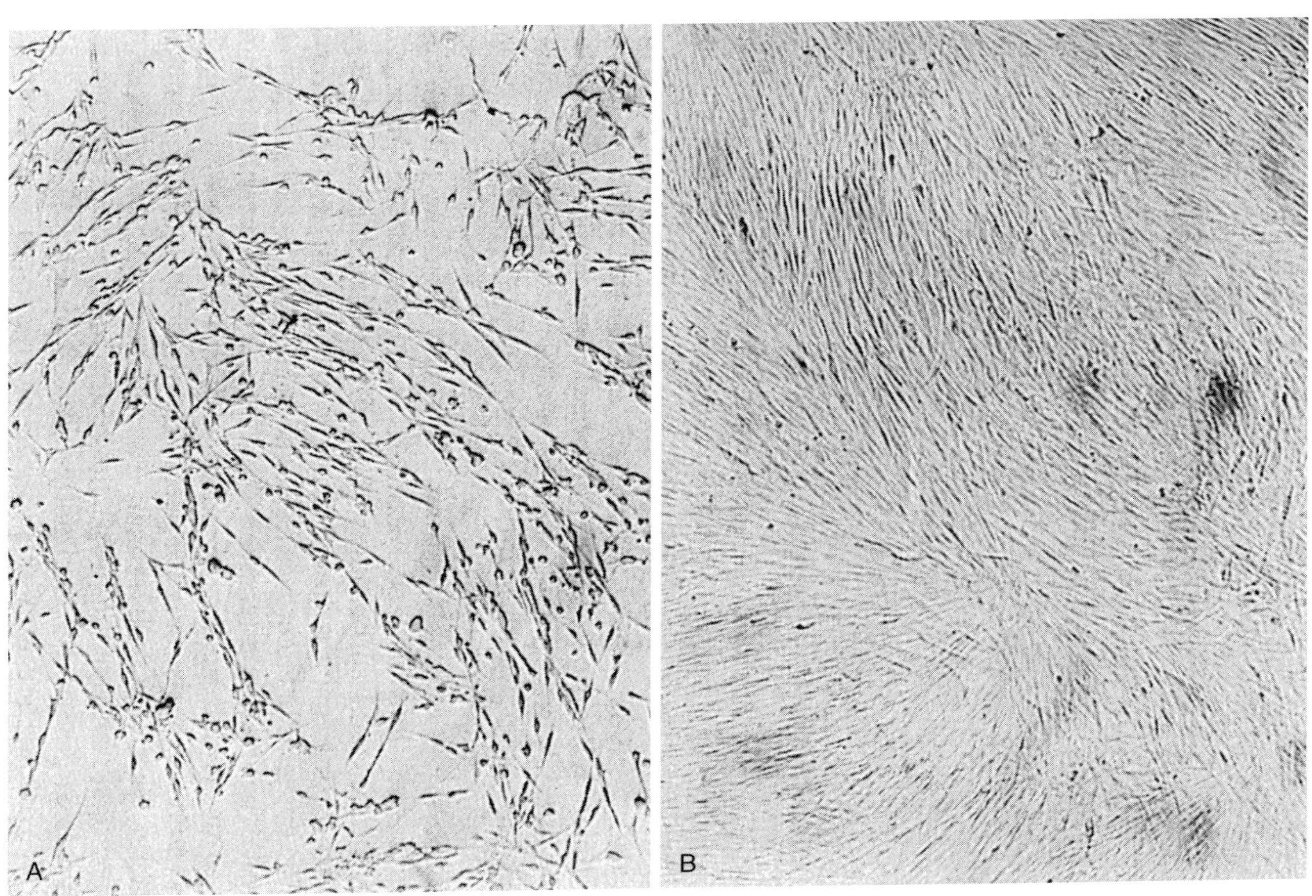

FIGURE 84–2. *A*, Toxic cytopathic effect of fecal suspension in human embryonic lung fibroblasts (MRC 5 cells) from 12-year-old girl with pseudomembranous colitis. *B*, Uninoculated tissue cultures. These figures accompanied one of the first reports to implicate a bacterial toxin in pseudomembranous colitis; 7 months later, the same investigators reported that this effect was neutralized by *Clostridium sordellii* antitoxin.[53] (From Larson HE, Perry JV, Price AB, et al. Undescribed toxin in pseudomembranous colitis. BMJ. 1977;1:1246–1248.)

to healthy ones, that broth cultures of clostridia and their cell-free supernatants produced this disease, and that this activity was neutralized by gas gangrene antiserum. Rifkin and associates[52] reported around the same time that stool filtrates from humans with pseudomembranous colitis were lethal for hamsters; caused edema, hemorrhage, and increased vascular permeability in rabbit skin; and possessed cytotoxic activity that was neutralized by *Clostridium sordellii* antitoxin. Larson and colleagues' original observation was followed by identification of a toxin in stool neutralized by *C. sordelli* antitoxin in nine of nine patients with pseudomembranous colitis and two of two others with antibiotic-associated nonspecific colitis.[53] Other investigators soon implicated the species *C. difficile*, demonstrating the presence of toxigenic strains from the stool of patients with pseudomembranous colitis.[54–56]

MICROBIOLOGY

Forty-three years before *C. difficile* was established as a pathogen, Hall and O'Toole[57] isolated this organism during a study of intestinal flora of newborn infants. They described an obligate anaerobic, spore-producing, gram-positive rod that was toxigenic, and "because of the unusual difficulty which was encountered in its isolation and study" it was first named *Bacillus difficilis*.[58] (Three years later it was renamed *Clostridium difficile*.) Unlike with most other toxigenic clostridia, the production of spores by this organism is not associated with toxin production. Some strains produce thin capsules, and some produce fimbria-like structures, but neither is clearly a virulence determinant.[59]

Cycloserine, cefoxitin, and fructose agar in an egg-yolk agar base are the constituents of CCFA medium, described by George and colleagues soon after *C. difficile* was discovered to be of medical importance.[60] The medium is both selective and differential for *C. difficile*, detecting as few as 2000 organisms in a total of 6×10^{10} bacteria per gram of wet feces.[61] This medium was recently reevaluated and demonstrated growth characteristics (in plates anaerobically reduced for 4 hours before use) that were superior to those for cycloserine-mannitol blood agar.[62] As with many clostridial species, *C. difficile* gives off a distinctive odor, characterized as a "horse dung" odor, particularly when grown on agar. Once growth is sustained on CCFA, if colonial morphology and Gram stain do not presumptively identify the organism, commercial identification kits are typically used.

EPIDEMIOLOGY

Prevalence of Symptomatic Disease in Hospitals and Extended-Care Facilities and among Outpatients

The incidence of antibiotic-associated diarrhea and colitis varies greatly, depending on the offending antibiotic and its spectrum of activity and pharmacokinetic properties, as well as the epidemiologic setting. Toxigenic *C. difficile* remains the most common cause of nosocomial diarrhea and is implicated in 10 to 30% of such cases. Local nosocomial diarrhea prevalence rates may vary considerably depending on antibiotic prescribing patterns, endemic strains, and criteria used to define antibiotic-associated diarrhea.[5, 6, 63, 64] The reported frequency of *C. difficile* colitis among acute care hospitalized patients ranges between 1 in 1000 and 10 in 1000 discharges.[65, 66] In a given hospital this may vary considerably over time, as evidenced in a 10-year prospective study at the Veterans Administration Hospital in Minneapolis, where the annual rate of *C. difficile*–associated diarrhea ranged from 3.2 to 9.9 cases per 1000 discharges.[67, 68]

Although colonization with toxigenic *C. difficile* is frequent among residents of some extended-care and rehabilitation facilities (see later on), only a minority of infected patients develop symptomatic disease.[69–72] Conversely, *C. difficile* infection was recently identified in 25% of patients undergoing diagnostic evaluation for diarrhea in two rehabilitation hospitals.[73] In contrast, among outpatients exposed to antibiotics, clinically recognized *C. difficile*–associated diarrhea is uncommon. A retrospective cohort study of a 265,000-member health maintenance organization revealed an overall risk of less than 1 case per 10,000 antibiotic prescriptions.[74] The rate of hospitalization in this study was 0.5 to 1 hospital admission per 100,000 person-years, a rate similar to that previously reported.[74, 75]

Inciting Agents

Although almost all antibiotic classes have been associated with the disease (Table 84–1), reports of large clinical series most commonly implicate clindamycin, penicillins, and cephalosporins.[45, 64, 76, 77] Whereas several noteworthy studies primarily implicated clindamycin and ampicillin in the 1970s,[41–43, 46, 47] more recent reports have emphasized an association with cephalosporins.[76–81] Third-generation cephalosporins have been implicated in particular and appear to predispose to *C. difficile*–associated disease more commonly than narrow-spectrum penicillins (i.e., penicillin V and penicillin G) and beta-lactamase–stable penicillins.[77, 78] Ticarcillin-clavulanate appears to be associated infrequently with the disease. In a 2-year retrospective study of 61,000 courses of ticarcillin-clavulanate therapy, no *C. difficile*–induced disease was identified.[78] Other studies, however, report an association.[66, 82] Several case reports and a case-control study have also implicated fluoroquinolones in *C. difficile* disease.[65, 83, 84] In the hamster model, the following drugs regularly produce lethal hemorrhagic cecitis due to *C. difficile*: ampicillin, carbenicillin, cefamandole, cefaclor, cefazolin, cefoxitin, cephalexin, cephaloridine, cephalothin, cephradine, clindamycin, oral gentamicin, imipenem, metronidazole, nafcillin, penicillin, and ticarcillin; only rarely do tetracyclines, chloramphenicol, sulfonamides, and trimethoprim-sulfamethoxazole produce disease.[3, 85]

Changes in antibiotic restriction policies have generally been associated with varying *C. difficile*–associated diarrhea attack rates,[66] and limiting the use of clindamycin[86, 87] and cefotaxime[88] in different hospital outbreaks has reduced the number of new cases. Because the reduction in new cases seen in some outbreaks is greater than that predicted by the number of patients for whom the antimicrobial was avoided, a "herd immunity" model of *C. difficile*–associated diarrhea has recently been proposed.[89] This paradigm takes into account the risk of the disease with use of certain antimicrobials for an entire population rather than solely for individuals.

A number of antineoplastic agents, particularly those with modest antibacterial activity, have been associated with *C. difficile* diarrheal disease, including doxorubicin, cisplatin, cyclophosphamide, 5-fluorouracil, chlorambucil, and methotrexate.[90–96]

Rarely, the disease occurs without exposure to agents known to alter the microecology of the gut.[97–101]

TABLE 84–1 Antimicrobial and Chemotherapeutic Agents Implicated in *Clostridium difficile*–Associated Diarrhea or Colitis

More Frequently Implicated	Less Frequently Implicated
Cephalosporins	Ticarcillin-clavulanate
Ampicillin and amoxicillin	Chloramphenicol
Clindamycin	Metronidazole
Other penicillins, including β-lactamase–stable penicillins	Amphotericin B
Erythromycin and other macrolides	Quinolones
Tetracyclines	Rifampin
Trimethoprim-sulfamethoxazole	5-Fluorouracil
	Methotrexate
	Doxorubicin
	Cyclophosphamide
	Aminoglycosides
	Sulfonamides

Data from Bartlett,[3] Kelly et al.,[7] and Thielman and Guerrant.[354]

Contributing Factors

In addition to the use of antimicrobials, certain host and environmental factors also predispose to *C. difficile*–associated disease. In a comprehensive prospective study of risk factors in hospitalized patients, McFarland and associates identified advanced age and severity of underlying illness as factors associated with increased risk of *C. difficile* carriage and diarrhea and found that agents that alter normal intestinal motility, specifically enemas and gastrointestinal stimulants, as well as stool softeners, also contributed to the risk of *C. difficile*–associated diarrhea.[76] Other investigators report that critically ill burned patients,[102] uremic patients,[103, 104] patients with hematologic malignancies,[105, 106] and those undergoing gastrointestinal surgery[107, 108] are at increased risk for *C. difficile* diarrhea and colitis.

Human immunodeficiency virus (HIV) infection per se does not appear to predispose to *C. difficile* colonization,[109] and specific risk factors for *C. difficile*–associated disease among HIV-infected patients appear to be similar to HIV-seronegative persons.[110] Patients with very low $CD4^+$ counts (<50/mm³) may be at increased risk by virtue of their increased exposure to antibiotics.[111, 112] Although some reports[112, 113] suggest that *C. difficile* disease is more severe in HIV-infected patients, others found that the disease behaves no differently in this group than in HIV-negative controls.[114, 115]

Reservoirs

The source of *C. difficile* may be either endogenous or environmental. Following Hall and O'Toole's original description of the organism in healthy neonates,[57] subsequent studies have documented the prevalence of *C. difficile* (or one of its toxins) in 15 to 70% of stools of healthy neonates.[63, 116–121] Despite the presence of toxin-producing organisms in this population, the prevalence of *C. difficile* colitis remains relatively low.[63, 118, 121] Enhanced chemotactic responses of granulocytes to toxin A in older persons[122] and the absence of high-affinity receptors for toxin A in neonates (in a rabbit model)[123] have been cited as possible reasons for this age-dependent susceptibility (see "Pathogenesis").

In healthy adults, intestinal carriage rates of toxigenic *C. difficile* are typically 3% or less and not greater than 8%.[77, 124, 125] Asymptomatic intestinal carriage rates are higher, around 20%, among hospitalized adults, particularly those who have received antibiotics.[3, 63] The prevalence of *C. difficile* colonization has been documented in particular patient populations, including 13% of patients (70% of whom were seropositive for HIV) on admission to an infectious diseases ward; 2 to 8% of elderly nursing home residents; and 7 to 14% of elderly hospitalized patients.[72, 109, 126] It is important to note that although *C. difficile* carriage rates may be quite high in asymptomatic adults, rarely do these persons harbor significant quantities of toxin A or toxin B in stool (the basis for the clinical diagnosis in most cases).

The frequency of extraintestinal carriage of this organism is not yet clearly defined. Whereas *C. difficile* was isolated from the vast majority of urethral and vaginal cultures in men and women attending a sexually transmitted diseases clinic,[127] other studies have reported vaginal carriage in fewer than 18% of pregnant women,[128] and still others were unable to detect urogenital colonization at all.[129]

Clearly, a preexisting endogenous reservoir of *C. difficile* is not a prerequisite for symptomatic infection, and the majority of disease-causing organisms appear to be acquired from exogenous sources. In a prospective cohort study of patients admitted to a Seattle teaching hospital, acquisition of the organism was documented in 21% of 399 patients who initially had negative culture results; of these patients, 37% developed diarrhea.[130] Arguing for the significance of environmental acquisition of *C. difficile* is the number of outbreaks that have been reported in hospitals,[80, 131–137] chronic-care facilities,[71, 136, 138] and daycare centers.[139] Even the classic "clindamycin colitis" study[47] is now retrospectively recognized as a report of the first confirmed hospital epidemic—owing to the unusually high rates of *C. difficile* toxin in subsequent stool analysis.[4] In such settings, *C. difficile* is readily cultured from multiple inanimate environmental sources and from the hands of hospital personnel.[130, 140] Among hospital personnel caring for patients shedding *C. difficile*, 59% had positive results on culture for *C. difficile* from their hands in one report.[130]

In addition, *C. difficile* is found in many sources outside the hospital and has been cultured from soil, swimming pools, and beaches, as well as sea, river, and tap water, and from several animals.[141] Carriage rates in household pets such as dogs and cats range from 20 to 40%, and some authorities propose that it may be zoonotically acquired.[141–143] Foodborne transmission has also been suggested, but neither this nor zoonotic transmission has been definitively documented.[144]

Epidemic Strains

Numerous outbreaks featuring a predominant strain or a closely related group of *C. difficile* strains have been reported,[86, 87, 110, 136, 137, 145, 146] possibly reflecting antimicrobial use patterns, increased virulence or resistance among particular strains, or breakdowns in infection control.[147] Molecular typing analysis—using restriction enzyme analysis, pulsed-field gel electrophoresis, and arbitrarily primed polymerase chain reaction (PCR)—implicated either a single strain or a set of genetically closely related strains among multiple isolates in five of six outbreaks in different regions in North America.[145] Similar methodology resolved a few distinct and genetically stable serogroup C strains associated with outbreaks in Belgium, France, and Benin spanning more than a decade.[146] Despite this evidence for several unique outbreak strains, a high incidence of *C. difficile* diarrhea in a given facility does not necessarily suggest a clonal outbreak. Significant clonal diversity was recently documented at a New England hospital, with 55 distinct types isolated from 106 patients including asymptomatic patients with culture-proven colonization and those with diarrhea,[148] and divergent strains predominated in a recent typing analysis of endemic *C. difficile* isolates from patients and the environment on an oncology ward[149] and among elderly residents in a long-term care facility.[72]

CLINICAL MANIFESTATIONS

Infection with toxigenic *C. difficile* causes a spectrum of disease ranging from asymptomatic carriage (particularly in neonates) to a fulminant, relapsing, and occasionally fatal colitis. When *C. difficile* produces clinical disease, the onset of signs and symptoms is typically after 5 to 10 days of antibacterial treatment, but diarrhea may develop as early as the first day of therapy or as late as 10 weeks after cessation of therapy.[150] *C. difficile*–associated diarrhea may be brief and self-limited or cholera-like, resulting in more than 20 stools per day.[3] Accompanying findings often include fever (30 to 50% of patients),[64, 151, 152] leukocytosis (50 to 60%),[64, 78, 152] and abdominal pain or cramping (20 to 33%).[151–154] Nausea, malaise, anorexia, hypoalbuminemia, occult colonic bleeding, and dehydration are also reported.[3, 7, 155] Infrequently, *C. difficile* colitis presents without diarrhea as an acute abdominal syndrome or toxic megacolon (Fig. 84–3).[156–160] In one report, 5 of 97 patients with *C. difficile* disease (only 1 of whom had profuse diarrhea) presented initially with marked leukocytosis (white blood cell count of ≥25,000/mm^3) and right lower quadrant peritoneal signs mimicking those of acute peritonitis.[160] Toxic megacolon is suggested by acute dilatation of the colon to a diameter greater than 6 cm, associated systemic toxicity, and the absence of mechanical obstruction[161] and carries a high mortality rate (64% in one series of 11 patients).[162]

Other intra-abdominal complications include colonic perforation,[163, 164] transverse volvulus,[165] protein-losing enteropathy,[166] and recurrent *C. difficile*–associated diarrhea, the last occurring in approximately 20% of patients.[167–171]

Extraintestinal manifestations occur more rarely and include bacteremia, often with concurrent isolation of other constituent organisms in the bowel flora,[82, 106, 172–176] splenic abscess,[172, 177, 178] and osteomyelitis.[179–182] In addition, multiple reports describe reactive arthritis or tenosynovitis or both,[183–194] some cases including features of Reiter's syndrome[188, 195] and others occurring in patients with preexisting Reiter's syndrome.[185, 195, 196] As with other reactive arthritides following enteric infections, in many of these cases, patients are HLA-B27 antigen–positive.[183, 187–189, 193, 194]

Considerations in the differential diagnosis of antibiotic-associated colitis include diarrhea caused by other enteric pathogens (especially *Salmonella*[18]), adverse reactions to other medications, ischemic colitis, inflammatory bowel disease, and intra-abdominal sepsis.[155]

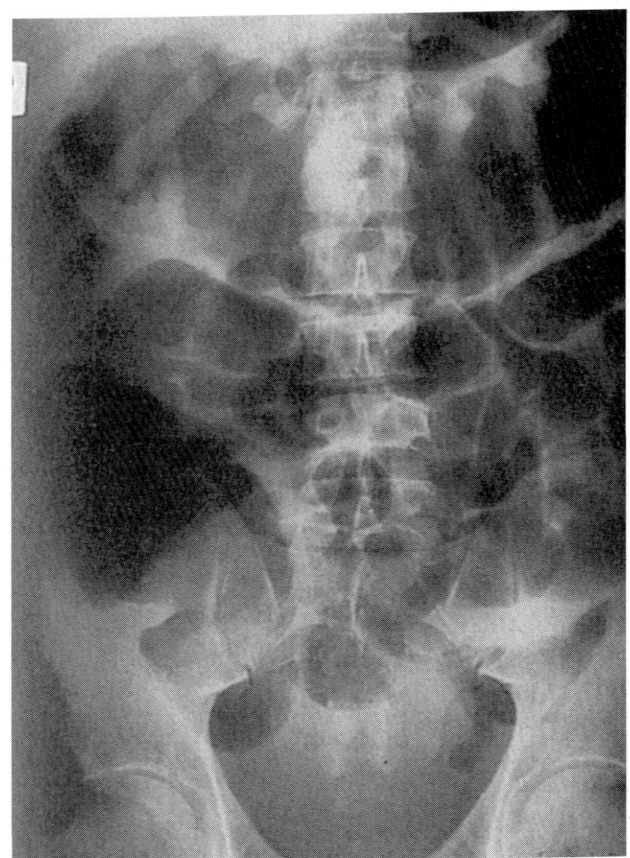

FIGURE 84–3. Abdominal radiograph demonstrating markedly dilated colon, wall edema, and loss of haustration in a patient with *Clostridium difficile*–associated pseudomembranous colitis complicated by toxic megacolon. (From Agnifili A, Gola P, Manno M, et al. The role and timing of surgery in the treatment of pseudomembranous colitis. A case complicated by toxic megacolon. Hepatogastroenterology. 1994;41:394–396.)

PATHOGENESIS

Key steps in the pathogenesis of *C. difficile*–mediated diarrhea and colitis include (1) disruption of normal colonic flora by antibiotics or antineoplastic agents with antibacterial activity, (2) colonization with *C. difficile*, (3) elaboration of toxin A and toxin B, both of which mediate cytoskeletal derangement in target cells, and (4) mucosal injury and inflammation.

The indigenous microflora of the gut constitutes a complex and poorly understood host defense system. This dense biomass, which may contain as many as 10^{12} bacteria per gram of stool, includes 400 to 500 species of bacteria, belonging to over 30 genera.[7, 197] Animal models demonstrate that these organisms en masse confer resistance to *C. difficile* colonization,[198] and that disruption of this microbial ecosystem with antibiotics is a prerequisite for establishing *C. difficile* disease.[4, 85, 199–201]

Once antibiotics have rendered the gut more susceptible to *C. difficile* infection, colonization occurs by fecal-oral transmission. Whereas most vegetative cells are killed in the acidic environment of the stomach, acid-resistant spores pass through relatively undamaged and convert to vegetative forms in the small bowel following exposure to primary bile acid.[197, 202] Colony counts of greater than 10^8 colony-forming units (CFUs) are typical in patients with *C. difficile* disease, and it appears more likely that the organism grows throughout the lumen of the colon, rather than attaching to specific colonocyte receptors.[203] Although some *C. difficile* strains possess fimbriae, the role of this morphologic feature in colonization and virulence remains unclear.[204]

As pathogenic *C. difficle* organisms reach the late logarithmic and early stationary stages of growth in the colon, they begin to release two potent toxins that ultimately mediate diarrhea and colitis. These large exotoxins—toxin A, a 308-kD enterotoxin, and toxin B, a 269-kD cytotoxin[205]—rank among some of the most lethal bacterial toxins studied[206] and have proved active against the more than 20 different cell lines from different mammalian species and tissues tested to date.[58, 207] These toxins, which exhibit an overall homology of greater than 45% at the amino acid level, contain a complex series of contiguous repeated units at the carboxyl terminus.[203] For toxin A, these repeating units appear to be responsible for carbohydrate receptor binding.[208] In humans and rodents, toxin A binds to specific carbohydrate receptors containing the carbohydrate moiety galactose-β-1,4-*N*-acetylglucosamine.[209] Three carbohydrate antigens bearing this structure—Lewis I, X, and Y, which exist on human intestinal epithelium—bind toxin A.[209, 210] The receptors for toxin B have not yet been identified.

Once the toxins gain access to the cytoplasm, both toxin A and toxin B inactivate Rho proteins, a family of small guanosine triphosphate (GTP)-binding proteins that regulate actin cytoskeleton and various signal transduction processes.[211–213] Specifically, using uridine diphosphate (UDP)-glucose as cosubstrate, the toxins catalyze monoglucosylation of Rho at the threonine 37 position.[213, 214] Ultimately, the toxin-induced dysregulation of Rho leads to cytoskeletal disruption, cell rounding and retraction, and apoptosis in cultured cell lines[215, 216] and probably explains the profound effect of toxin A on intercellular tight junctions of epithelial cell monolayers.[217, 218]

In intact animal models, *C. difficile* toxin A causes intestinal fluid secretion, mucosal injury, and inflammation. When instilled in equimolar amounts to ligated loops of rabbit small intestine, toxin A stimulates fluid secretion as efficiently as cholera toxin, although the mechanisms of action for the two are completely different.[219] A sequential study[220] of early histopathologic changes in rabbit small intestine exposed to toxin A revealed an initial diffuse lymphocytic infiltrate in the lamina propria, followed by edema and bulging of the lamina propria in the apical portions of villi and, eventually, cytolysis and separation of the basal portions of the apical epithelial cells. An acute inflammatory response also occurs, with polymorphonuclear leukocyte and mononuclear cell infiltration into the lamina propria.[221]

Key mediators implicated in the inflammatory and secretory responses of toxin A include arachidonic acid metabolites (prostaglandins, leukotrienes, and platelet-activating factor),[222–225] substance P,[226, 227] and, potentially, monocyte-derived interleukins IL-8 and IL-6, tumor necrosis factor (TNF), and IL-1.[216, 228–232]

Neutrophils, found within pseudomembranes and within the intestinal mucosal layer underneath pseudomembranes, play a pivotal role in the pathophysiology of this disease.[201, 233–235] Via a pertussis toxin–inhibitable G protein, toxin A directly activates human granulocytes in vitro, inducing a transient rise in unbound cytosolic calcium that is both rapid and dose-dependent, while promoting chemotaxis and chemokinesis.[236] Monoclonal antibodies directed against the neutrophil adhesion molecule CD11/18 markedly inhibit both neutrophil infiltration and intestinal secretory responses in a rabbit model of *C. difficile* disease.[237] Mast cells also participate in these responses in mouse and rat models in pathways that appear to involve substance P.[227, 238]

Although toxin B has no demonstrable effect on permeability, fluid secretion, neutrophil migration, or changes in intestinal morphology in the rabbit model,[221, 239] like toxin A it disrupts tight junctions in human epithelial cell monolayers,[240] and it is approximately 10 times more potent on a molar basis than toxin A in mediating damage to human colonic mucosa in the Ussing chamber model.[241] In a rat model of neutrophil migration, toxin B also stimulates intense neutrophil recruitment via macrophage-derived TNF-α and lipoxygenase.[242]

PATHOLOGY

A distinct macroscopic appearance characterizes pseudomembranous colitis at endoscopy (Fig. 84–4). The colonic mucosa is studded with adherent raised white and yellowish plaques. Initially, these lesions are small and discrete and are easily dislodged; the intervening mucosa may be inflamed and covered with mucus but often appears entirely normal.[243, 244] With progression of disease, pseudomembranous plaques may enlarge and coalesce. Pseudomembranes can exist

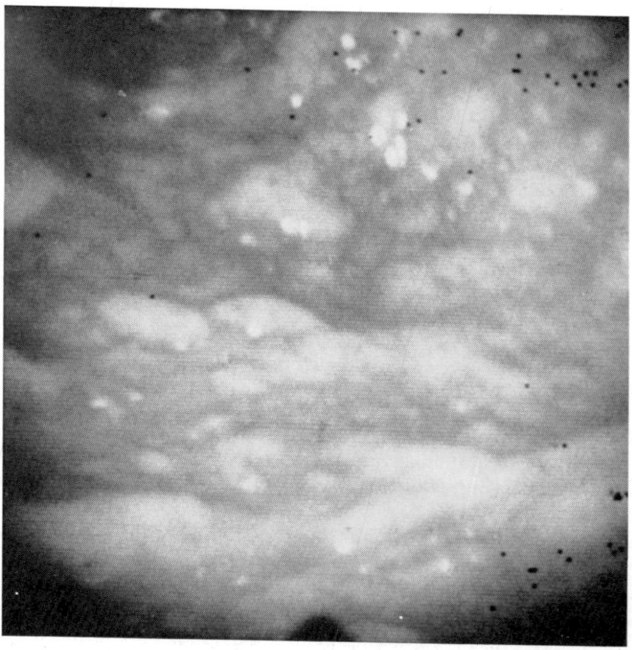

FIGURE 84–4. Proctoscopic view of pseudomembranous colitis in a patient who received clindamycin. Note the 4–8 mm raised white plaques overlying an erythematous mucosa. (From Tedesco FJ, Barton RW, Alpers DH. Clindamycin-associated colitis. Ann Intern Med. 1974;81:429–433.)

throughout the entire colon, but they are usually most pronounced in the rectosigmoid colon; rarely does the disease progress proximal to the ileocecal valve.[245]

Histologic criteria for pseudomembranous colitis and a method for grading lesions have been described.[246] The principal features are inflamed mucosa with a neutrophilic predominance and mucin-distended glands. Attached pseudomembranes are composed of a loose network of mucin, neutrophils, fibrin, and nuclear debris.[243, 246]

DIAGNOSIS

C. difficle–associated disease should be suspected in patients with diarrhea who have received antibiotics within the previous 2 months or whose diarrhea begins 72 hours after hospitalization.[155] In most instances, toxin testing or *C. difficile* culture of a single stool specimen effectively establishes the diagnosis; however, repeat testing or endoscopy, or both, may be necessary. Table 84–2 summarizes characteristics of the different tests used in the diagnosis of *C. difficile*–associated diarrhea.

Detection of *C. difficile* Toxins

The most widely utilized means of diagnosing *C. difficile*–associated diarrhea and colitis clinically is detection of *C. difficile* toxins in stool specimens. The cytotoxicity assay is considered the optimal diagnostic modality by most studies evaluating enzyme immunoassay (EIA) and other, newer techniques.[247] As in the original descriptions of *C. difficile* cytotoxin assays,[50, 52] stool filtrates are incubated with a mammalian tissue culture cell line with and without toxin-neutralizing antibody. If cytotoxic activity, usually manifested as rounding of cultured cells, is noted in the well with the stool filtrate but not in the well containing both stool filtrate and toxin-neutralizing antibody, the test result for the specimen is considered to be positive (see Fig. 84–2).[50] Used in the appropriate clinical setting, this test is both sensitive and specific. More than 90% of patients with pseudomembranous colitis have cytotoxic activity in their stools detected by this assay.[207] Sensitivity may vary, however, with the use of different cell lines, and because of potential inactivation of toxin B during storage and handling of samples.[248] Additional disadvantages of the cytotoxicity assay include its expense, lack of standardization, slow turnaround time (up to 2 days), and, in most cases, the need for a tissue culture facility (use of some commercial kits may not require this). Finally, although the cytotoxicity assay is widely considered the best single test for *C. difficile*–associated enteric disease, its sensitivity has been cited as low as 67% when a combination of clinical and laboratory criteria was used to confirm the diagnosis.[249]

At least eight commercial enzyme-linked immunosorbent assay (ELISA) kits that detect toxin A or B are available, and their performance characteristics have been studied extensively.[250–258] A recent review succinctly summarizes the published performance characteristics of these tests.[247] In general, they are rapid, relatively inexpensive, and specific but lack the sensitivity of the technically more cumbersome cytotoxin assays. Against the strictest diagnostic criteria that include clinical diarrhea, along with positive cytotoxin assay and positive culture results, sensitivity ranges from 63% to 94%, with a specificity of 75 to 100%.[259] As with many laboratory tests, those with greatest sensitivity often have poorer specificity, and some have a relatively broad indeterminate range,[258] necessitating either repeat testing or use of a different method on the same sample. Because rare *C. difficile* isolates (serogroup F) produce toxin B without producing toxin A, testing schemes that detect only toxin A may miss a small proportion of *C. difficile* isolates.[260]

Culture for *C. difficile*

Anaerobic culture for *C. difficile*, the most sensitive test in many laboratories, remains essential for epidemiologic studies of outbreaks. Cost and convenience issues, however, have driven many hospital laboratories to replace routine cultures with the more rapid and less expensive ELISA-based assays, sometimes in combination with cytotoxin assays. Most clinical microbiology laboratories are not equipped to distinguish between toxigenic and nonpathogenic, nontoxigenic strains, and testing schemes that rely solely on *C. difficile* cultures yield a significant number of false-positive results (in some hospitals, 20 to 25% of *C. difficile* isolates are nontoxigenic[149]). Testing for stool toxin simultaneously or the use of in vitro toxin production assays may help to resolve this problem,[259] but at considerable additional expense.

Additional Tests for *C. difficile*

The latex agglutination test is rapid and simple but relatively insensitive and nonspecific. Originally thought to detect toxin A, this inexpensive test actually detects glutamate dehydrogenase, a protein that has no definable role in enteric disease,[261, 262] and organisms other than *C. difficile* produce antigens that cross-react with the antibody used in this assay.[263] Because of its overall poor performance and the availability of other rapid tests that are more sensitive and specific, use of the latex agglutination test is not recommended.[259]

PCR amplification utilizing specific primers for toxin B[264, 265] and toxin A,[266] and a two-step procedure using both *C. difficile* 16S ribosomal RNA (rRNA) and toxin B sequences[267] have been designed. The clinical potential for these techniques will remain uncertain until PCR technology becomes more widely used in hospital diagnostic laboratories.

The Role of Endoscopy

Direct visualization of exudative plaques, or pseudomembranes, on colonic mucosa establishes the diagnosis of pseudomembranous colitis. The pathognomonic lesion is characteristically raised, yellowish, and usually 2 to 10 mm in diameter with "skip" areas of normal mucosa, but in severe disease, lesions may coalesce to form plaques.[155] Ninety percent or more of patients with pseudomembranous colitis demonstrate either *C. difficile* or its toxin in stool samples.[5, 6, 151, 268]

Flexible sigmoidoscopy alone will not detect up to 10% of cases without colonoscopy.[269] When *C. difficile* colitis is not accompanied

TABLE 84–2 Sensitivity and Specificity of Tests for Diagnosis of *Clostridium difficile*–Associated Disease

Test	Sensitivity* (%)	Specificity* (%)	Clinical Utility
Endoscopy	51	≈100	Diagnostic of PMC
Culture for *C. difficile*	89–100	84–99	Highly sensitive; confirmation of organism toxicity optimal
Cell culture cytotoxin test	67–100	85–100	With clinical data, diagnostic of CDAD
EIA toxin test	63–99	75–100	With clinical data, diagnostic of CDAD
Latex test for *C. difficile* antigen	58–92	80–96	Less sensitive and specific than other tests; rapid results
PCR toxin gene detection	Undetermined	Undetermined	Research test

*Using both clinical and test-based criteria.
Abbreviations: CDAD, *Clostridium difficile*–associated disease; EIA, enzyme immunoassay; PCR, polymerase chain reaction; PMC, pseudomembranous colitis.
Modified from Gerding DN, Johnson S, Peterson LR, et al. *Clostridium difficile*–associated diarrhea and colitis. Infect Control Hosp Epidemiol. 1995;16:459–477.

by pseudomembrane formation, endoscopic findings are relatively nonspecific, but biopsy may reveal changes typical of pseudomembranous colitis.[248]

Because of its cost, risk to the patient, and the availability of other diagnostic tests, endoscopy is usually reserved for special situations. The American College of Gastroenterology Guidelines[155] recommend endoscopy for situations such as the following: (1) when a rapid diagnosis is needed and either test results are delayed or insensitive tests are used, (2) when the patient has an ileus and stool is not available, or (3) when other colonic diseases that can be diagnosed with endoscopy are being considered.

Testing Strategies

The proper use of the aforementioned tests necessitates an understanding of which patients should be tested. According to a clinical prediction rule derived and validated in a relatively narrow patient population, hospitalized patients without both a history of antimicrobial use within the past 30 days *and* either significant diarrhea (defined as ≥3 stools of decreased consistency within 24 hours) or abdominal pain would be expected to have a negative result on cytotoxin assay for *C. difficile*.[153, 154] The clinical utility of this rule is its negative predictive value: 94 to 97% of such patients are cytotoxin-negative; therefore, in such circumstances, cytotoxin testing generally is not required. Katz and associates[153, 154] calculated that on the basis of this rule, 29 to 39% of cytotoxin tests ordered in such study populations could have been avoided or deferred. In addition, *C. difficile* testing is not recommended for patients with nondiarrheal stool specimens (unless ileus due to *C. difficile* is suspected); for infants less than 1 year of age (clinical illness does not correlate with presence of toxin in stools); or for "test of cure."[147, 249, 259]

No single best laboratory testing scheme for the diagnosis of *C. difficile*–associated diarrhea and colitis has been established. The Society for Healthcare Epidemiology Association (SHEA)[259] and other authorities[249, 270] recommend combining tissue culture cytotoxin testing with stool culture for optimal diagnostic sensitivity (culture) and specificity (cytotoxin assay). Many laboratories, however, no longer culture *C. difficile*,[247, 271] and stool cytotoxin testing is costly and time-consuming. Although toxin ELISAs sacrifice some sensitivity, because of their relatively good specificity, rapid turnaround time, convenience, and cost, they are considered reasonable alternatives to cytotoxin assays and are widely used.[7, 147, 155, 259, 272] A combination of EIA testing and cytotoxin testing is used sequentially in some laboratories.[152, 247, 273] Manabe and coworkers found that the addition of a tissue culture assay to EIA testing improved the diagnostic sensitivity of the first stool specimen from 72% to 81%.[152] If initial stool studies are negative, and the patient's diarrhea persists without any other obvious cause, repeating the studies may increase the rate of detection significantly[152, 274] and has been recommended,[155] although not all authorities support this practice.[275]

Because stool toxin testing may take up to 2 to 3 days to perform (depending on the assay used), in some instances, testing for the presence of fecal inflammatory markers may assist with clinical decision making. For *C. difficile*–associated disease, the sensitivity of the fecal lactoferrin assay ranges from 75 to 90%,[152, 276] but the test is not very specific (46% in one study).[276] In comparison, microscopy for fecal leukocytes is less sensitive (28 to 40%) but more specific (92%).[276, 277]

TREATMENT

General Considerations

Both the American College of Gastroenterology and the Society for Healthcare Epidemiology of America have prepared recent management recommendations for *C. difficile*–associated disease (Table 84–3).[155, 259] Initial therapy of patients with pseudomembranous colitis should include discontinuation of the offending antibiotic regimen, if possible, and replacement of fluid and electrolyte losses. In a prospective treatment trial, the diarrhea resolved prior to initiation of therapy in 23% of 149 patients,[278] but most patients require specific antibacterial therapy. If the offending antibiotic cannot be discontinued or cannot be safely replaced by another antibiotic less likely to predispose to *C. difficile*–associated disease (see Table 84–1), antibacterial therapy with either oral metronidazole or oral vancomycin should be considered.

TABLE 84–3 Recommendations for Treatment of *Clostridium difficile*–Associated Diarrhea and Colitis

1. If the clinical situation allows, discontinue the offending antibiotic and/or modify the regimen to include an agent less commonly associated with *C. difficile* disease (see Table 84–1).
2. Replace fluid and electrolyte losses.
3. Avoid antiperistaltic agents.
4. If the foregoing conservative measures are either not effective or not practical, institute specific therapy with oral metronidazole, 250 mg qid for 10 days.
5. Do treat asymptomatic patients colonized with *C. difficile*.
6. Retreat first-time recurrences with the same regimen used to treat the initial episode.
7. Avoid vancomycin use, if possible.*

*In general, vancomycin should be reserved for patients who (a) fail to respond to or cannot take metronidazole (because of, e.g., intolerance, coadministration of ethanol-containing solutions, pregnancy, age less than 10 years), (b) have *C. difficile* disease associated with metronidazole-resistant strains, or (c) are critically ill because of *C. difficile*–associated disease.
Adapted from the American College of Gastroenterology Practice Guidelines as reported by Fekety R. Am J Gasteroenterol. 1997;92:739–750; and from the Society for Healthcare Epidemiology Association position paper presented by Gerding DN, Johnson S, Peterson LR, et al. *Clostridium difficile*–associated diarrhea and colitis. Infect Control Hosp Epidemiol. 1995;16:459–477.

Oral Metronidazole

Although metronidazole and vancomycin are equally effective for treating *C. difficile*–associated disease,[278] metronidazole is now considered the drug of choice for most cases because of cost and concerns regarding the emergence of vancomycin-resistant enterococci.[7, 155, 259, 279] The vast majority of *C. difficile* isolates are highly susceptible to metronidazole, with the minimal inhibitory concentration for 90% of the organisms (MIC_{90}) ranging from 0.25 to 1.0 μg/ml in several studies from various geographic regions.[280–285] Equally important, in patients with *C. difficile*–associated diarrhea, bactericidal fecal levels are readily achievable; in one study, nine patients had bactericidal fecal concentrations of metronidazole (mean 9.3 ± 7.5 μg/g of wet stool) and of its hydroxymetabolite during therapy for *C. difficile*–associated diarrhea.[286] As the patients' diarrhea abated, metronidazole and hydroxymetronidazole levels fell, with neither detectable following recovery. In other settings, after administration of oral metronidazole, patients with severe Crohn's disease have higher intraluminal levels than in those with more quiescent disease,[287] and fecal levels are either undetectable or minimally detectable in healthy volunteers[288] and in asymptomatic *C. difficile* carriers.[70] The decline in fecal levels of metronidazole during therapy parallels expected decreases in mucosal inflammation and may be explained by decreased exudation of metronidazole through less inflamed mucosa. It is also possible that with clinical improvement, decreased intestinal motility increases metronidazole transit time, enabling more complete absorption.[286] This phenomenon has been invoked as a potential explanation for the relapses seen with metronidazole.

Despite these concerns, oral metronidazole is highly effective clinically, with cure rates of between 94 and 95% and relapse rates of 5 to 16% in two prospective randomized trials.[278, 289] The largest recorded experience with metronidazole comes from the Minneapolis Veterans Affairs Hospital, where from 1982 to 1991, oral metronidazole therapy was used in 632 patients with *C. difficile*–associated diarrhea. Metronidazole was judged to be highly effective in this observational report, with intolerance, failure, and relapse rates of 1%, 2%, and 7%, respectively.[68]

Oral Vancomycin

Multiple randomized comparative studies have documented the efficacy of oral vancomycin for *C. difficile*–associated diarrhea and colitis,[278, 289–292] and despite concerns for cost and the emergence of vancomycin-resistant enterococci, it remains the preferred drug for severe disease.[155, 272, 279] Most *C. difficile* isolates are susceptible to a MIC of 1 μg/ml, and virtually all are susceptible to 16 μg/ml, levels that are orders of magnitude lower than the intraluminal levels achieved with oral vancomycin.[293] Oral vancomycin is rarely absorbed to any appreciable degree, and multiple studies report levels in stool in excess of 1000 to 3000 μg/ml,[290, 294–296] which, unlike those of metronidazole, are maintained for the duration of antimicrobial therapy. Although higher doses may achieve greater fecal concentrations,[294, 295] it remains unclear if higher dosing regimens (which are considerably more expensive) offer any clinical benefit. Doses of 125 mg qid for 10 days effected no fewer cures than doses at 500 mg qid in one study, but the trial lacked sufficient statistical power to prove equivalence of the two regimens.[297] One case report documents enteral absorption of vancomycin leading to significant serum levels (up to 20 μg/ml) in a patient with pseudomembranous colitis and renal failure.[298]

Comparative prospective studies with various doses of vancomycin document clinical response rates of 86 to 100%, with relapses in 15 to 33%.[289–292, 297] A retrospective review[299] of clinical outcome in 189 patients receiving oral vancomycin (at dosages ranging from 0.5 to 2.0 g/day, usually for 7 to 14 days) identified treatment failures in only 3%. Overall treatment response was judged to be good (i.e., prompt improvement and recovery without a change in the specific therapy) in 87%, with relapses noted in 24%.[299]

Oral vancomycin therapy is a significant risk factor for colonization and infection with vancomycin-resistant enterococci,[300–302] and the Hospital Infection Control Practice Advisory Committee (HICPAC) recommends vancomycin for antibiotic-associated colitis only when metronidazole fails or when the disease is severe and potentially life-threatening.[279] It should be noted, however, that some of these same studies have also identified metronidazole use as a risk factor for vancomycin-resistant enterococci colonization or infection.[301, 302]

Second-Line Agents

A number of other antibacterials and toxin-binding preparations have been evaluated for the treatment of primary *C. difficile* disease. The results of prospective randomized studies[290, 291] using oral bacitracin are summarized in Table 84–4. Given the overall relatively poor efficacy of this agent compared with that of oral vancomycin and metronidazole, its higher cost (which is increased by the need for compounding by a pharmacist), and lack of palatability, oral bacitracin should be considered only in rare circumstances when oral metronidazole or vancomycin cannot be used. Oral teicoplanin and fusidic acid, neither of which is available in the United States, have demonstrated efficacy similar to that of oral vancomycin and metronidazole in two small but well-designed clinical studies. Experience with these glycopeptides for *C. difficile* disease, however, remains limited. The anion-exchange resins cholestyramine and colestipol, which bind *C. difficile* cytotoxin,[303] have been proposed for potential nonantibiotic treatment for milder cases or for consolidation therapy, after the use of first-line agents, for relapses.[293] The following findings argue against their routine use: Only 5 of 14 patients with either toxin- or culture-positive diarrhea responded to colestipol in a prospective evaluation[304]; unsatisfactory results were reported retrospectively in 37% of 19 patients receiving cholestyramine[299]; and systemic absorption of cholestyramine has been documented.[305]

Therapy for Patients Who Lack Oral Access

In patients unable to take or tolerate oral metronidazole or vancomycin because of paralytic ileus, nasogastric suctioning, intestinal obstruction, or diversion, no single regimen has demonstrated superiority. After intravenous administration of metronidazole, three patients with documented *C. difficile*–associated diarrhea responded clinically, and fecal concentrations of metronidazole and its hydroxymetabolite were documented at concentrations well in excess of the MIC for *C. difficile*.[286] Intravenous metronidazole was also used successfully in six patients with acute abdomen, antibiotic-associated colitis (pseudomembranous in five), and positive results on latex agglutination testing for *C. difficile* (three also received vancomycin via nasogastric tube).[158] Parenteral metronidazole failures have also been reported.[306–308]

Fewer clear-cut treatment successes with intravenous vancomycin are reported,[309] and failures have been clearly documented.[306, 310] In one such failure, fecal levels of vancomycin could not be detected despite five days of parenteral therapy.[310] Anecdotal reports of adjunctive therapy with rectal vancomycin (coadministered with intravenous or nasogastric vancomycin or metronidazole) pepper the literature,[311–316] and the drug has been administered both as an enema and through a long catheter placed during colonoscopy.[312, 317] The safety and efficacy of this practice, however, have not been established; systemic absorption after long-catheter colonic instillation of vancomycin has been reported.[313]

The absence of controlled prospective trials of treatment in patients who lack oral access precludes definitive treatment recommen-

TABLE 84–4 Efficacy and Cost of Oral Antibiotics for *Clostridium difficile*–Associated Diarrhea and Colitis

Drug and Range of Dosing Regimens Reported	Response Rate (%)	Relapse Rate (%)	No. of Days to Improvement or Resolution (mean)	Cost*
Metronidazole 250 mg qid to 500 mg tid × 10 d	94–95	5–16	2.4–3.2	$0.70†
Vancomycin 125 mg qid × 7 days to 500 mg qid × 10 d	86–100	15–33	2.6–4.2	$100‡
Bacitracin 20,000–25,000 U qid × 7–10 d	76–80	42	2.4–4.1	$76§
Teicoplanin 100–400 mg bid × 10 d	96–98	8	2.8–3.4	NA
Fusidic acid 500 mg tid × 10 d	93	28	3.8	NA

*University Health Consortium cost to pharmacy, Medical University of South Carolina, 1998.
†Cost for 250 mg PO qid for 10 days.
‡Cost for 125 mg PO qid for 10 days.
§Estimated cost for 25,000 U PO qid for 10 days, including pharmacist's compounding fee.
Abbreviation: NA, Not available in United States.
Data from prospective, randomized trials reported by Teasley,[278] Young,[290] Dudley,[291] de Lalla,[292] Fekety,[297] and Wenisch[355] and their respective coworkers.

dations; however, the use of intravenous metronidazole (500 mg every 6 to 8 hours), vancomycin via nasogastric tube (500 mg every 6 hours), or vancomycin retention enemas (500 mg every 4 to 8 hours) or vancomycin via colonic catheter should be considered.[309, 318] Rarely, extremely ill patients with ileus may benefit from surgical decompression and direct instillation of vancomycin or metronidazole via the stoma.[318]

Antimotility Agents

Antiperistaltic agents, such as loperamide and diphenoxylate hydrochloride with atropine, should be avoided. There is little evidence that such agents lead to symptomatic improvement, and in one study predating the discovery of *C. difficile* as a pathogen,[319] diarrhea was actually more common among patients receiving diphenoxylate-atropine plus lincomycin than among those receiving placebo plus lincomycin. Several anecdotes and case series have associated the use of diphenoxylate, and of loperamide and other antiperistaltic agents, with the development of toxic megacolon in patients with *C. difficile* disease[157, 159, 162] or pseudomembranous colitis.[320] Because these agents promote colonic stasis, there is a theoretical risk of further damage and inflammation with prolonged mucosal exposure to *C. difficile* toxins. In addition, colonic stasis may actually favor the growth of anaerobes, including *C. difficile*.[293]

Surgery

Although rarely necessary, surgical intervention may be lifesaving, particularly in cases complicated by toxic megacolon or colonic perforation. Reported rates of surgery necessitated by *C. difficile* disease range from 0.39% of 3300 toxin-positive assays in a 6-year survey at Johns Hopkins[321] to 3.6% of 138 such cases during a 6-month outbreak in Dublin.[322] Various surgical approaches for management of toxic megacolon have been described, including diversion of the fecal stream by ileostomy, cecostomy, or decompressive colostomy or by subtotal colectomy. The last-named has been advocated as the procedure of choice for serious disease, including fulminant toxic megacolon associated with pseudomembranous colitis.[164, 321, 323] Two patterns of perforation have been described: multiple perforations involving a large portion of the colon, associated with a higher mortality rate, and a single perforation, associated with relatively lower mortality.[164] With localized perforation, limited segmental resection may be successful. The overall mortality rate in cases requiring surgery is around 30 to 35%,[164, 321] although some series report mortality rates in excess of 50%.[162, 322]

RECURRENT DISEASE

Despite initial adequate antimicrobial treatment, recurrent *C. difficile*–associated diarrhea has been reported in 5 to 50% of patients in several small studies[170, 171, 278, 290, 291]; in 24% of 189 patients who had received vancomycin therapy, as determined by retrospective analysis[299]; and in 7% of 754 patients in whom either metronidazole or vancomycin treatment was initially successful in the Minneapolis experience.[68] A multiple relapse pattern characterized by five or more relapses following intervening treatments has been described and may be seen in 5 to 8% of patients who receive specific drug therapy.[4, 68, 324] Risk factors for recurrent disease identified in prospective studies include increased age, recent abdominal surgery, increased number of *C. difficile* diarrheal episodes, and, oddly, onset of initial disease in spring.[168, 170] Additional risk factors suggested by retrospective analysis include leukocytosis, chronic renal failure, initial presentation of community-acquired disease, infection with certain immunoblot types, and female gender.[167, 168]

The leading explanation for relapsing *C. difficile* disease has been persistence of *C. difficile* spores, which may survive even high intraluminal levels of vancomycin and remain cultivable from feces during and after therapy.[171, 294, 325, 326] In the case of metronidazole, the declining drug levels seen over the course of treatment may permit germination of residual *C. difficile* spores.[325] Alternatively, patients with recurrent disease may reacquire the original strain from exogenous environmental sources or may acquire a new strain altogether. Although one recent study found the same strain type in both first and second episodes in 7 of 8 cases,[167] in other studies using varied typing analyses, new strains were implicated in approximately 50% of recurrences.[311, 327, 328]

Patients who experience relapses usually respond to a repeated course of either metronidazole or vancomycin[3, 68]; the best course for such relapses, however, has yet to be established. The only critical comparative trial for treatment of relapsing *C. difficile* disease evaluated the effectiveness of the yeast *Saccharomyces boulardii*. This multicenter, placebo-controlled trial demonstrated that 4 weeks of *S. boulardii* administered orally, in addition to standard antimicrobial therapy, yielded significantly fewer treatment failures in recurrent but not initial *C. difficile* disease.[329] A variety of other approaches have been reported anecdotally, including usual therapy followed by an extended course of cholestyramine[330–332]; intravenous immune globulin (particularly when low levels of circulating antitoxin A immunoglobulin G [IgG] are documented)[333–335]; tapering doses of vancomycin followed by pulse therapy[336]; vancomycin combined with rifampin[337]; oral administration of *Lactobacillus* GG (gamma globulin)[338–340]; oral bacteriotherapy with a nontoxigenic *C. difficile* strain[341]; oral IgA[342]; whole-bowel irrigation with a polyethylene glycol solution[343]; bacterial enemas incorporating various facultatively aerobic and anaerobic bacteria[344]; and even rectal infusion of normal feces.[344, 345] In most of these reports, the interventions were used following multiple failed attempts with traditional therapy or as adjunctive therapy. Some are riskier than others, and insufficient scientific rigor precludes specific recommendations. Some authorities, however, favor vancomycin with rifampin[147]; vancomycin or metronidazole followed by cholestyramine, lactobacilli, or low-dose vancomycin[3]; or tapering doses of vancomycin.[272]

PREVENTION

The prevention and control of *C. difficile*–associated diarrhea and colitis have been thoroughly reviewed in the Society for Healthcare Epidemiology of America position paper.[259] Simple infection control measures such as scrupulous glove use during the handling of any body substance[346] and replacing electronic thermometers with single-use disposable ones[347] are of proven benefit for decreasing *C. difficile* transmission in health care settings. Good handwashing and environmental cleaning and disinfection are prudent for many reasons and may be effective in reducing the incidence of *C. difficile* disease.[130] Screening to identify asymptomatic carriers for specific drug therapy is neither practicable nor enduringly effective. In one study, although treatment with vancomycin was temporarily effective in eradicating asymptomatic *C. difficile* excretion in hospitalized patients, they began to excrete the organism again soon after cessation of therapy.[70]

Limiting the use of certain antimicrobials (particularly those associated with *C. difficile* disease in a given insitution) has proved an effective means of controlling some outbreaks.[86, 87, 348] In particular, restriction of clindamycin use in outbreaks due to clindamycin-resistant strains resulted in fewer *C. difficile* infections[86, 87] and was associated with a return of clindamycin susceptibility and overall cost savings.[87]

Introduction of competing, nonpathogenic organisms into the intestinal tract may be useful in preventing antibiotic-associated diarrhea.[349] In two double-blind placebo-controlled trials involving 393 patients, *S. boulardii* decreased the overall incidence of antibiotic-associated diarrhea by around 50% but did not significantly affect *C. difficile*–associated diarrhea rates.[2, 350] Preparations containing lactobacilli, *Bifidobacterium*, and lactic acid–producing *Enterococcus faecium* SF68 have also been evaluated in smaller trials.[351–353] Additional well-designed trials are needed to establish the role of such therapy, if any, in the prevention of antibiotic-associated diarrhea.

REFERENCES

1. McFarland LV. Diarrhea acquired in the hospital. Gastroenterol Clin North Am. 1993;22:563–577.
2. McFarland LV, Surawicz CM, Greenberg RN, et al. Prevention of beta-lactam–associated diarrhea by *Saccharomyces boulardii* compared with placebo. Am J Gastroenterol. 1995;90:439–448.
3. Bartlett JG. Antibiotic-associated diarrhea. Clin Infect Dis. 1992;15:573–581.
4. Bartlett JG. *Clostridium difficile*: Clinical considerations. Rev Infect Dis. 1990;12:S243–S251.
5. George WL, Rolfe RD, Finegold SM. *Clostridium difficile* and its cytotoxin in feces of patients with antimicrobial agent–associated diarrhea and miscellaneous conditions. J Clin Microbiol. 1982;15:1049–1053.
6. Bartlett JG, Taylor NS, Chang T, Dzink J. Clinical and laboratory observations in *Clostridium difficile* colitis. Am J Clin Nutr. 1980;33:2521–2526.
7. Kelly CP, Pothoulakis C, LaMont JT. *Clostridium difficile* colitis. N Engl J Med. 1994;330:257–262.
8. Karlstrom O, Fryklund B, Tullus K, Burman LG. A prospective nationwide study of *Clostridium difficile*–associated diarrhea in Sweden. The Swedish *C. difficile* Study Group. Clin Infect Dis. 1998;26:141–145.
9. Levine J, Dykoski RK, Janoff EN. *Candida*-associated diarrhea: A syndrome in search of credibility. Clin Infect Dis. 1995;21:881–886.
10. Margolis BD, Tsang TK, Kuo D. Persistent diarrhea secondary to *Candida* overgrowth. Am J Gastroenterol. 1990;85:329–330.
11. Danna PL, Urban C, Bellin E, Rahal JJ. Role of candida in pathogenesis of antibiotic-associated diarrhoea in elderly inpatients. Lancet. 1991;337:511–514.
12. Gupta TP, Ehrinpreis MN. *Candida*-associated diarrhea in hospitalized patients. Gastroenterology. 1990;98:780–785.
13. Cohen R, Roth FJ, Delgado E, et al. Fungal flora of the normal human small and large intestine. N Engl J Med. 1969;280:638–641.
14. Borriello SP, Larson HE, Welch AR, et al. Enterotoxigenic *Clostridium perfringens*: A possible cause of antibiotic-associated diarrhoea. Lancet. 1984;1:305–307.
15. Schwartz JN, Hamilton JP, Fekety R, et al. Ampicillin-induced enterocolitis: Implication of toxigenic *Clostridium perfringens* type C. J Pediatr. 1980;97:661–663.
16. Pavia AT, Shipman LD, Wells JG, et al. Epidemiologic evidence that prior antimicrobial exposure decreases resistance to infection by antimicrobial-sensitive *Salmonella*. J Infect Dis. 1990;161:255–260.
17. Neal KR, Briji SO, Slack RC, et al. Recent treatment with H_2 antagonists and antibiotics and gastric surgery as risk factors for *Salmonella* infection. BMJ. 1994;308:176.
18. Spika JS, Waterman SH, Hoo GW, et al. Chloramphenicol-resistant *Salmonella newport* traced through hamburger to dairy farms. A major persisting source of human salmonellosis in California. N Engl J Med. 1987;316:565–570.
19. Borgnolo G, Barbone F, Scornavacca G, et al. A case-control study of *Salmonella* gastrointestinal infection in Italian children. Acta Paediatr. 1996;85:804–808.
20. Clausen MR, Bonnen H, Tvede M, Mortensen PB. Colonic fermentation to short-chain fatty acids is decreased in antibiotic-associated diarrhea. Gastroenterology. 1991;101:1497–1504.
21. Rao SS, Edwards CA, Austen CJ, et al. Impaired colonic fermentation of carbohydrate after ampicillin. Gastroenterology. 1988;94:928–932.
22. Hove H, Tvede M, Mortensen PB. Antibiotic-associated diarrhoea, *Clostridium difficile*, and short-chain fatty acids. Scand J Gastroenterol. 1996;31:688–693.
23. Wilcox MH, Cunniffe JG, Trundle C, Redpath C. Financial burden of hospital-acquired *Clostridium difficile* infection. J Hosp Infect. 1996;34:23–30.
24. Kofsky P, Rosen L, Reed J, Tolmie M, Ufberg D. *Clostridium difficile*—a common and costly colitis. Dis Colon Rectum. 1991;34:244–248.
25. McCarter MD, Abularrage C, Velasco FT, et al. Diarrhea and *Clostridium difficile*–associated diarrhea on a surgical service. Arch Surg. 1996;131:1333–1337.
26. Macgowan AP, Brown I, Feeney R, et al. *Clostridium difficile*–associated diarrhoea and length of hospital stay. J Hosp Infect. 1995;31:241–244.
27. Finney J. Gastro-enterostomy for cicatrizing ulcer of the pylorus. Johns Hopkins Hospital Bulletin. 1893;4:53–55.
28. Kramer IRH. Fatal staphylococcal enteritis developing during streptomycin therapy by mouth. Lancet. 1948;1:646–647.
29. Bennett IL, Wood JS, Yardley HH. Staphylococcal pseudomembranous enterocolitis in chinchillas: A clinico-pathologic study. Trans Assoc Am Physician. 1956;69:116.
30. Altemeier WA, Hummel RP, Hill EO. Staphylococcal enterocolitis following antibiotic therapy. Ann Surg. 1963;157:847–858.
31. Cook J, Elliott C, Elliot-Smith A, et al. Staphylococcal diarrhoea with an account of two outbreaks in the same hospital. BMJ 1957;1:542–547.
32. Dearing WH, Baggenstoss AH, Weed LA. Studies on the relationship of *Staphylococcus aureus* to pseudomembranous enteritis and to postantibiotic enteritis. Gastroenterology. 1960;38:441–451.
33. Hummel RP, Altemeier WA, Hill EO. Iatrogenic staphylococcal enterocolitis. Ann Surg. 1964;160:551–560.
34. Brown WJ, Winston R, Sommers SC. Membranous staphylococcal enteritis after antibiotic therapy; report of two cases. Am J Dig Dis. 1953;20:73.
35. Corridan M. Antibiotic-resistant staphylococcal pseudomembranous enteritis. J Clin Pathol. 1956;9:131–135.
36. Wakefield RF, Sommers SC. Fatal membranous staphylococcal enteritis in surgical patients. Ann Surg. 1953;138:249.
37. Williams E. Staphylococcal pseudomembranous enterocolitis complicating treatment with aureomycin. Lancet. 1954;1:999.
38. Fekety R. Staphylococcal diarrhea and enterocolitis. In: Crossley KB, Archer GL, eds. The Staphylococci in Human Disease. New York: Churchill Livingstone; 1997:545–563.
39. Bartlett JG, Gorbach SL. Pseudomembranous enterocolitis (antibiotic-related colitis). Adv Intern Med. 1977;22:455–476.
40. Willis TA. Historical aspects. In: Rolfe RD, Finegold SM, eds. *Clostridium difficile*: Its Role in Intestinal Disease. San Diego: Academic Press; 1988:15–28.
41. Lusk RH, Fekety FR Jr, Silva J Jr, et al. Gastrointestinal side effects of clindamycin and ampicillin therapy. J Infect Dis. 1977;135(Suppl):S111–S119.
42. Gurwith MJ, Rabin HR, Love K. Diarrhea associated with clindamycin and ampicillin therapy: Preliminary results of a cooperative study. J Infect Dis. 1977;135(Suppl):S104–S110.
43. Swartzberg JE, Maresca RM, Remington JS. Clinical study of gastrointestinal complications associated with clindamycin therapy. J Infect Dis. 1977;135(Suppl):S99–S103.
44. Neu HC, Prince A, Neu CO, Garvey GJ. Incidence of diarrhea and colitis associated with clindamycin therapy. J Infect Dis. 1977;135(Suppl):S120–S125.
45. Robertson MB, Breen KJ, Desmond PV, et al. Incidence of antibiotic-related diarrhoea and pseudomembranous colitis: A prospective study of lincomycin, clindamycin and ampicillin. Med J Aust. 1977;1:243–246.
46. Tedesco FJ. Ampicillin-associated diarrhea—a prospective study. Am J Dig Dis. 1975;20:295–297.
47. Tedesco FJ, Barton RW, Alpers DH. Clindamycin-associated colitis. Ann Intern Med. 1974;81:429–433.
48. Colitis associated with clindamycin. Med Lett Drugs Ther. 1974;16:73–74.
49. Warning on antibiotic-induced colitis. Lancet. 1979;1:1306.
50. Larson HE, Parry JV, Price AB, et al. Undescribed toxin in pseudomembranous colitis. BMJ. 1977;1:1246–1248.
51. Bartlett JG, Onderdonk AB, Cisneros RL, Kasper DL. Clindamycin-associated colitis due to a toxin-producing species of *Clostridium* in hamsters. J Infect Dis. 1977;136:701–705.
52. Rifkin GD, Fekety FR, Silva J Jr. Antibiotic-induced colitis: Implication of a toxin neutralised by *Clostridium sordellii* antitoxin. Lancet. 1977;2:1103–1106.
53. Larson HE, Price AB. Pseudomembranous colitis: Presence of clostridial toxin. Lancet. 1977;2:1312–1314.
54. George RH, Symonds JM, Dimock F, et al. Identification of *Clostridium difficile* as a cause of pseudomembranous colitis. BMJ. 1978;1:695.
55. Bartlett JG, Chang TW, Gurwith M, et al. Antibiotic-associated pseudomembranous colitis due to toxin-producing clostridia. N Engl J Med. 1978;298:531–534.
56. Bartlett JG, Moon N, Chang TW, et al. Role of *Clostridium difficile* in antibiotic-associated pseudomembranous colitis. Gastroenterology. 1978;75:778–782.
57. Hall IC, O'Toole E. Intestinal flora in new-born infants. Am J Dis Child. 1935;49:390–402.
58. Thielman NM, Guerrant RL. *Clostridium difficile* and its toxins. In: Moss J, Iglewski B, Vaughn M, Tue AT, eds. Bacterial Toxins and Virulence Factors in Disease. New York: Marcel Dekker; 1995:327–366.
59. Borriello SP, Davies HA, Kamiya S, et al. Virulence factors of *Clostridium difficile*. Rev Infect Dis. 1990;12(Suppl 2):S185–S191.
60. George WL, Sutter VL, Citron D, Finegold SM. Selective and differential medium for isolation of *Clostridium difficile*. J Clin Microbiol. 1979;9:214–219.
61. Lyerly DM, Allen SD. The clostridia. In: Emmerson AM, Hawkey PM, Gillespie SH, eds. Principles and Practice of Clinical Bacteriology. Chichester: John Wiley & Sons; 1997:599–623.
62. Mundy LS, Shanholtzer CJ, Willard KE, et al. Laboratory detection of *Clostridium difficile*. A comparison of media and incubation systems. Am J Clin Pathol. 1995;103:52–56.
63. Viscidi R, Willey S, Bartlett JG. Isolation rates and toxigenic potential of *Clostridium difficile* isolates from various patient populations. Gastroenterology. 1981;81:5–9.
64. Gerding DN, Olson MM, Peterson LR, et al. *Clostridium difficile*–associated diarrhea and colitis in adults. A prospective case-controlled epidemiologic study. Arch Intern Med. 1986;146:95–100.
65. Lai KK, Melvin ZS, Menard MJ, et al. *Clostridium difficile*–associated diarrhea: Epidemiology, risk factors, and infection control. Infect Control Hosp Epidemiol. 1997;18:628–632.
66. Ho M, Yang D, Wyle FA, Mulligan ME. Increased incidence of *Clostridium difficile*–associated diarrhea following decreased restriction of antibiotic use. Clin Infect Dis. 1996;23(Suppl 1):S102–S106.
67. Manian FA, Meyer L. CDAD rates. Infect Control Hosp Epidemiol. 1995;16:63–65.
68. Olson MM, Shanholtzer CJ, Lee JT Jr, Gerding DN. Ten years of prospective *Clostridium difficile*–associated disease surveillance and treatment at the Minneapolis VA Medical Center, 1982–1991. Infect Control Hosp Epidemiol. 1994;15:371–381.
69. Thomas DR, Bennett RG, Laughon BE, et al. Postantibiotic colonization with *Clostridium difficile* in nursing home patients. J Am Geriatr Soc. 1990;38:415–420.
70. Johnson S, Homann SR, Bettin KM, et al. Treatment of asymptomatic *Clostridium difficile* carriers (fecal excretors) with vancomycin or metronidazole. A randomized, placebo-controlled trial. Ann Intern Med. 1992;117:297–302.
71. Bender BS, Bennett R, Laughon BE, et al. Is *Clostridium difficile* endemic in chronic-care facilities? Lancet. 1986;2:11–13.

72. Simor AE, Yake SL, Tsimidis K. Infection due to *Clostridium difficile* among elderly residents of a long-term care facility. Clin Infect Dis. 1993;17:672–678.
73. Yablon SA, Krotenberg R, Fruhmann K. *Clostridium difficile*–related disease: Evaluation and prevalence among inpatients with diarrhea in two freestanding rehabilitation hospitals. Arch Phys Med Rehabil. 1993;74:9–13.
74. Hirschhorn LR, Trnka Y, Onderdonk A, et al. Epidemiology of community-acquired *Clostridium difficile*–associated diarrhea. J Infect Dis. 1994;169:127–133.
75. Stergachis A, Perera DR, Schnell MM, Jick H. Antibiotic-associated colitis. West J Med. 1984;140:217–219.
76. McFarland LV, Surawicz CM, Stamm WE. Risk factors for *Clostridium difficile* carriage and *C. difficile*–associated diarrhea in a cohort of hospitalized patients. J Infect Dis. 1990;162:678–684.
77. Aronsson B, Möllby R, Nord CE. Antimicrobial agents and *Clostridium difficile* in acute enteric disease: Epidemiological data from Sweden, 1980–1982. J Infect Dis. 1985;151:476–481.
78. Anand A, Bashey B, Mir T, Glatt AE. Epidemiology, clinical manifestations, and outcome of *Clostridium difficile*–associated diarrhea. Am J Gastroenterol. 1994;89:519–523.
79. Starr JM, Impallomeni M. Risk of diarrhoea, *Clostridium difficile* and cefotaxime in the elderly. Biomed Pharmacother. 1997;51:63–67.
80. Cartmill TD, Panigrahi H, Worsley MA, et al. Management and control of a large outbreak of diarrhoea due to *Clostridium difficile*. J Hosp Infect. 1994;27:1–15.
81. Watanakunakorn PW, Watanakunakorn C, Hazy J. Risk factors associated with *Clostridium difficile* diarrhea in hospitalized adult patients: A case-control study—sucralfate ingestion is not a negative risk factor. Infect Control Hosp Epidemiol. 1996;17:232–235.
82. Feldman RJ, Kallich M, Weinstein MP. Bacteremia due to *Clostridium difficile*: Case report and review of extraintestinal *C. difficile* infections. Clin Infect Dis. 1995;20:1560–1562.
83. Bauwens JE, McFarland LV, Melcher SA. Recurrent *Clostridium difficile* disease following ciprofloxacin use. Ann Pharmacother. 1997;31:1090.
84. Dan M, Samra Z. *Clostridium difficile* colitis associated with ofloxacin therapy. Am J Med. 1989;87:479.
85. Small JD. Drugs used in hamsters with a review of antibiotic-associated colitis in the laboratory hamster. In: Van Hoosier GL, McPherson CW, eds. Laboratory Hamsters. Orlando: Academic Press; 1987:179–199.
86. Pear SM, Williamson TH, Bettin KM, et al. Decrease in nosocomial *Clostridium difficile*–associated diarrhea by restricting clindamycin use. Ann Intern Med. 1994;120:272–277.
87. Climo MW, Israel DS, Wong ES, et al. Hospital-wide restriction of clindamycin: Effect on the incidence of *Clostridium difficile*–associated diarrhea and cost. Ann Intern Med. 1998;128:989–995.
88. Impallomeni M, Galletly NP, Wort SJ, et al. Increased risk of diarrhoea caused by *Clostridium difficile* in elderly patients receiving cefotaxime. BMJ. 1995;311:1345–1346.
89. Starr JM, Rogers TR, Impallomeni M. Hospital-acquired *Clostridium difficile* diarrhoea and herd immunity. Lancet. 1997;349:426–428.
90. George WL. Antimicrobial Agent–Associated Diarrhea in Adult Humans. New York: Academic Press; 1988:31–44.
91. Cudmore MA, Silva J Jr, Fekety R, et al. *Clostridium difficile* colitis associated with cancer chemotherapy. Arch Intern Med. 1982;142:333–335.
92. Silva J, Fekety R, Werk C, et al. Inciting and etiologic agents of colitis. Rev Infect Dis. 1984;6:S214–S221.
93. Bartlett JG. Antimicrobial agents implicated in *Clostridium difficile* toxin–associated diarrhea or colitis. Johns Hopkins Med J. 1981;149:6–9.
94. Emoto M, Kawarabayashi T, Hachisuga MD, et al. *Clostridium difficile* colitis associated with cisplatin-based chemotherapy in ovarian cancer patients. Gynecol Oncol. 1996;61:369–372.
95. Anand A, Glatt AE. *Clostridium difficile* infection associated with antineoplastic chemotherapy: A review. Clin Infect Dis. 1993;17:109–113.
96. Ramos A, Martinez-Taboacla VM, Fito C, Rodriguez-Valverde V. *Clostridium difficile*–associated diarrhea in rheumatoid arthritis patients who are receiving therapy with low-dose chlorambucil. Arthritis Rheum. 1997;40:2090–2091.
97. Colarian J. *Clostridium difficile* colitis following antiviral therapy in the acquired immunodeficiency syndrome. Am J Med. 1988;84:1081.
98. Moskovitz M, Bartlett JG. Recurrent pseudomembranous colitis unassociated with prior antibiotic therapy. Arch Intern Med. 1981;141:663–664.
99. Peikin SR, Galdibini J, Bartlett JG. Role of *Clostridium difficile* in a case of nonantibiotic-associated pseudomembranous colitis. Gastroenterology. 1980;79:948–951.
100. Wald A, Mendelow H, Bartlett JB. Nonantibiotic associated pseudomembranous colitis due to toxin producing clostridia. Ann Intern Med. 1980;92:798–799.
101. Ellis ME, Watson BM, Milewski PJ, Jones G. *Clostridium difficile* colitis unassociated with antibiotic therapy. Br J Surg. 1983;70:242–243.
102. Grube BJ, Heimbach DM, Marvin JA. *Clostridium difficile* diarrhea in critically ill burned patients. Arch Surg. 1987;122:655–661.
103. Leung AC, Orange G, McLay A, Henderson IS. *Clostridium difficile*–associated colitis in uremic patients. Clin Nephrol. 1985;24:242–248.
104. Aronsson B, Barany P, Nord CE, et al. *Clostridium difficile*–associated diarrhoea in uremic patients. Eur J Clin Microbiol. 1987;6:352–356.
105. Heard SR, Wren B, Barnett MJ, et al. *Clostridium difficile* infection in patients with haematological malignant disease. Risk factors, faecal toxins and pathogenic strains. Epidemiol Infect. 1988;100:63–72.
106. Rampling A, Warren RE, Bevan PC, et al. *Clostridium difficile* in haematological malignancy. J Clin Pathol. 1985;38:445–451.
107. Keighley MR, Burdon DW, Alexander-Williams J, et al. Diarrhoea and pseudomembranous colitis after gastrointestinal operations. A prospective study. Lancet. 1978;2:1165–1167.
108. Pierce PF Jr, Wilson R, Silva J Jr, et al. Antibiotic-associated pseudomembranous colitis: An epidemiologic investigation of a cluster of cases. J Infect Dis. 1982;145:269–274.
109. Hutin Y, Casin I, Lesprit P, et al. Prevalence of and risk factors for *Clostridium difficile* colonization at admission to an infectious diseases ward. Clin Infect Dis. 1997;24:920–924.
110. Hutin Y, Molina JM, Casin I, et al. Risk factors for *Clostridium difficile*–associated diarrhoea in HIV-infected patients. AIDS. 1993;7:1441–1447.
111. Barbut F, Meynard JL, Guiguet M, et al. *Clostridium difficile*–associated diarrhea in HIV-infected patients: Epidemiology and risk factors. J Acquir Immune Defic Syndr Hum Retrovirol. 1997;16:176–181.
112. Tumbarello M, Tacconelli E, Leone F, et al. *Clostridium difficile*–associated diarrhoea in patients with human immunodeficiency virus infection: A case-control study. Eur J Gastroenterol Hepatol. 1995;7:259–263.
113. Cappell MS, Philogene C. *Clostridium difficile* infection is a treatable cause of diarrhea in patients with advanced human immunodeficiency virus infection: A study of seven consecutive patients admitted from 1986 to 1992 to a university teaching hospital. Am J Gastroenterol. 1993;88:891–897.
114. Cozart JC, Kalangi SS, Clench MH, et al. *Clostridium difficile* diarrhea in patients with AIDS versus non-AIDS controls. Methods of treatment and clinical response to treatment. J Clin Gastroenterol. 1993;16:192–194.
115. Lu SS, Schwartz JM, Simon DM, Brandt LJ. *Clostridium difficile*–associated diarrhea in patients with HIV positivity and AIDS: A prospective controlled study. Am J Gastroenterol. 1994;89:1226–1229.
116. Snyder ML. The normal fecal flora of infants between two weeks and one year of age. J Infect Dis. 1940;66:1–16.
117. Bolton RP, Tait SK, Dear PR, Losowsky MS. Asymptomatic neonatal colonisation by *Clostridium difficile*. Arch Dis Child. 1984;59:466–472.
118. Donta ST, Myers MG. *Clostridium difficile* toxin in asymptomatic neonates. J Pediatr. 1982;100:431–434.
119. Holst E, Helin I, Mårdh PA. Recovery of *Clostridium difficile* from children. Scand J Infect Dis. 1981;13:41–45.
120. Al-Jumaili IJ, Shibley M, Lishman AH, Record CO. Incidence and origin of *Clostridium difficile* in neonates. J Clin Microbiol. 1984;19:77–78.
121. el-Mohandes AE, Keiser JF, Refat M, Jackson BJ. Prevalence and toxigenicity of *Clostridium difficile* isolates in fecal microflora of preterm infants in the intensive care nursery. Biol Neonate. 1993;63:225–229.
122. Triadafilopoulos G, Shah MH, Pothoulakis C. The chemotactic response of human granulocytes to *Clostridium difficile* toxin A is age dependent. Am J Gastroenterol. 1991;86:1461–1465.
123. Eglow R, Pothoulakis C, Itzkowitz S, et al. Diminished *Clostridium difficile* toxin A sensitivity in newborn rabbit ileum is associated with decreased toxin A receptor. J Clin Invest. 1992;90:822–829.
124. Marrie TJ, Furlong M, Faulkner RS, et al. *Clostridium difficile*: Epidemiology and clinical features. Can J Surg. 1982;25:438–442.
125. Nakamura S, Mikawa M, Nakashio S, et al. Isolation of *Clostridium difficile* from the feces and the antibody in sera of young and elderly adults. Microbiol Immunol. 1981;25:345–351.
126. Rudensky B, Rosner S, Sonnenblick M, et al. The prevalence and nosocomial acquisition of *Clostridium difficile* in elderly hospitalized patients. Postgrad Med J. 1993;69:45–47.
127. Hafiz S, Morton R, McEntegart M, et al. *Clostridium difficile* in the urogenital tract of males and females. Lancet. 1975;1:420–421.
128. Tabaqchali S, O'Farrell S, Nash JQ, Wilks M. Vaginal carriage and neonatal acquisition of *Clostridium difficile*. J Med Microbiol. 1984;18:47–53.
129. Larson HE, Barclay FE, Honour P, Hill ID. Epidemiology of *Clostridium difficile* in infants. J Infect Dis. 1982;146:727–733.
130. McFarland LV, Mulligan ME, Kwok RY, Stamm WE. Nosocomial acquisition of *Clostridium difficile* infection. N Engl J Med. 1989;320:204–210.
131. Greenfield C, Burroughs A, Szawathowski M, et al. Is pseudomembranous colitis infectious? Lancet. 1981;1:371–372.
132. Testore GP, Pantosti A, Cerquetti M, et al. Evidence for cross-infection in an outbreak of *Clostridium difficile*–associated diarrhoea in a surgical unit. J Med Microbiol. 1988;26:125–128.
133. Delmee M, Bulliard G, Simon G. Application of a technique for serogrouping *Clostridium difficile* in an outbreak of antibiotic-associated diarrhoea. J Infect. 1986;13:5–9.
134. Poxton IR, Aronsson B, Möllby R, et al. Immunochemical fingerprinting of *Clostridium difficile* strains isolated from an outbreak of antibiotic-associated colitis and diarrhoea. J Med Microbiol. 1984;17:317–324.
135. Han VK, Sayed H, Chance GW, et al. An outbreak of *Clostridium difficile* necrotizing enterocolitis: A case for oral vancomycin therapy? Pediatrics. 1983;71:935–941.
136. Cartmill TD, Shrimpton SB, Panigrahi H, et al. Nosocomial diarrhoea due to a single strain of *Clostridium difficile*: A prolonged outbreak in elderly patients. Age Ageing. 1992;21:245–249.
137. Nath SK, Thornley JH, Kelly M, et al. A sustained outbreak of *Clostridium difficile* in a general hospital: Persistence of a toxigenic clone in four units. Infect Control Hosp Epidemiol. 1994;15:382–389.
138. Bennett RG, Laughon BE, Mundy LM, et al. Evaluation of a latex agglutination test for *Clostridium difficile* in two nursing home outbreaks. J Clin Microbiol. 1989;27:889–893.

139. Kim K, DuPont HL, Pickering LK. Outbreaks of diarrhea associated with *Clostridium difficile* and its toxin in day-care centers: Evidence of person-to-person spread. J Pediatr. 1983;102:376–382.
140. Fekety R, Kim KH, Brown D, et al. Epidemiology of antibiotic-associated colitis: Isolation of *Clostridium difficile* from the hospital environment. Am J Med. 1981;70:906–908.
141. al Saif N, Brazier JS. The distribution of *Clostridium difficile* in the environment of South Wales. J Med Microbiol. 1996;45:133–137.
142. Riley TV, Adams JE, O'Neill GL, Bowman RA. Gastrointestinal carriage of *Clostridium difficile* in cats and dogs attending veterinary clinics. Epidemiol Infect. 1991;107:659–665.
143. Borriello SP, Honour P, Turner T, Barclay F. Household pets as a potential reservoir for *Clostridium difficile* infection. J Clin Pathol. 1983;36:84–87.
144. Gurian L, Ward TT, Katon RM. Possible foodborne transmission in a case of pseudomembranous colitis due to *Clostridium difficile*: Influence of gastrointestinal secretions on *Clostridium difficile* infection. Gastroenterology. 1982;83:465–469.
145. Samore M, Killgore G, Johnson S, et al. Multicenter typing comparison of sporadic and outbreak *Clostridium difficile* isolates from geographically diverse hospitals. J Infect Dis. 1997;176:1233–1238.
146. van Dijck P, Avesani V, Delmee M. Genotyping of outbreak-related and sporadic isolates of *Clostridium difficile* belonging to serogroup C. J Clin Microbiol. 1996;34:3049–3055.
147. Johnson S, Gerding DN. *Clostridium difficile*–associated diarrhea. Clin Infect Dis. 1998;26:1027–1036.
148. Samore MH, Bettin KM, DeGirolami PC, et al. Wide diversity of *Clostridium difficile* types at a tertiary referral hospital. J Infect Dis. 1994;170:615–621.
149. Cohen SH, Tang YJ, Muenzer J, et al. Isolation of various genotypes of *Clostridium difficile* from patients and the environment in an oncology ward. Clin Infect Dis. 1997;24:889–893.
150. Tedesco FJ. Pseudomembranous colitis. Med Clin North Am. 1982;66:655–664.
151. Gebhard RL, Gerding DN, Olson MM, et al. Clinical and endoscopic findings in patients early in the course of *Clostridium difficile*–associated pseudomembranous colitis. Am J Med. 1985;78:45–48.
152. Manabe YC, Vinetz JM, Moore RD, et al. *Clostridium difficile* colitis: An efficient clinical approach to diagnosis. Ann Intern Med. 1995;123:835–840.
153. Katz DA, Lynch ME, Littenberg B. Clinical prediction rules to optimize cytotoxin testing for *Clostridium difficile* in hospitalized patients with diarrhea. Am J Med. 1996;100:487–495.
154. Katz DA, Bates DW, Rittenberg E, et al. Predicting *Clostridium difficile* stool cytotoxin results in hospitalized patients with diarrhea. J Gen Intern Med. 1997;12:57–62.
155. Fekety R. Guidelines for the diagnosis and management of *Clostridium difficile*–associated diarrhea and colitis. American College of Gastroenterology, Practice Parameters Committee. Am J Gastroenterol. 1997;92:739–750.
156. Edwards DP, Saleemi MA, Grundy C, Chisholm EM. *Clostridium difficile* toxic megacolon following splenectomy. J R Army Med Corps. 1997;143:167–168.
157. Walley T, Milson D. Loperamide-related toxic megacolon in *Clostridium difficile* colitis. Postgrad Med J. 1990;66:582.
158. Triadafilopoulos G, Hallstone AE. Acute abdomen as the first presentation of pseudomembranous colitis. Gastroenterology. 1991;101:685–691.
159. Burke GW, Wilson ME, Mehrez IO. Absence of diarrhea in toxic megacolon complicating *Clostridium difficile* pseudomembranous colitis. Am J Gastroenterol. 1988;83:304–307.
160. Drapkin MS, Worthington MG, Chang TW, Razvi SA. *Clostridium difficile* colitis mimicking acute peritonitis. Arch Surg. 1985;120:1321–1322.
161. Markowitz IP, Nichols RL. Surgical aspects of therapy. In: Rolfe RD, Finegold SM, eds. *Clostridium difficile*: Its Role in Intestinal Disease. San Diego: Academic Press; 1988:359–366.
162. Trudel JL, Deschenes M, Mayrand S, Barkun AN. Toxic megacolon complicating pseudomembranous enterocolitis. Dis Colon Rectum. 1995;38:1033–1038.
163. Snooks SJ, Hughes A, Horsburgh AG. Perforated colon complicating pseudomembranous colitis. Br J Surg. 1984;71:291–292.
164. Morris JB, Zollinger R Jr, Stellato TA. Role of surgery in antibiotic-induced pseudomembranous enterocolitis. Am J Surg. 1990;160:535–539.
165. Yaseen ZH, Watson RE, Dean HA, Wilson ME. Case report: Transverse colon volvulus in a patient with *Clostridium difficile* pseudomembranous colitis. Am J Med Sci. 1994;308:247–250.
166. Rybolt AH, Bennett RG, Laughon BE, et al. Protein-losing enteropathy associated with *Clostridium difficile* infection. Lancet. 1989;1:1353–1355.
167. Do AN, Fridkin SK, Yechouron A, et al. Risk factors for early recurrent *Clostridium difficile*–associated diarrhea. Clin Infect Dis. 1998;26:954–959.
168. Fekety R, McFarland LV, Surawicz CM, et al. Recurrent *Clostridium difficile* diarrhea: Characteristics of and risk factors for patients enrolled in a prospective, randomized, double-blinded trial. Clin Infect Dis. 1997;24:324–333.
169. Sutphen JL, Grand RJ, Flores A, et al. Chronic diarrhea associated with *Clostridium difficile* in children. Am J Dis Child. 1983;137:275–278.
170. Young GP, Bayley N, Ward P, et al. Antibiotic-associated colitis caused by *Clostridium difficile*: Relapse and risk factors. Med J Aust. 1986;144:303–306.
171. Walters BA, Roberts R, Stafford R, Seneviratne E. Relapse of antibiotic-associated colitis: Endogenous persistence of *Clostridium difficile* during vancomycin therapy. Gut. 1983;24:206–212.
172. Studemeister AE, Beilke MA, Kirmani N. Splenic abscess due to *Clostridium difficile* and *Pseudomonas paucimobilis.* Am J Gastroenterol. 1987;82:389–390.
173. Genta VM, Gilligan PH, McCarthy LR. *Clostridium difficile* peritonitis in a neonate. A case report. Arch Pathol Lab Med. 1984;108:82–83.
174. Gerard M, Defresne N, Van der Auwera P, Meunier F. Polymicrobial septicemia with *Clostridium difficile* in acute diverticulitis. Eur J Clin Microbiol Infect Dis. 1989;8:300–302.
175. Spencer RC, Courtney SP, Nicol CD. Polymicrobial septicaemia due to *Clostridium difficile* and *Bacteroides fragilis.* BMJ [Clin Res]. 1984;289:531–532.
176. Byl B, Jacobs F, Struelens MJ, Thys JP. Extraintestinal *Clostridium difficile* infections. Clin Infect Dis. 1996;22:712.
177. Stieglbauer KT, Gruber SA, Johnson S. Elevated serum antibody response to toxin A following splenic abscess due to *Clostridium difficile.* Clin Infect Dis. 1995;20:160–162.
178. Saginur R, Fogel R, Begin L, et al. Splenic abscess due to *Clostridium difficile.* J Infect Dis. 1983;147:1105.
179. Riley TV, Karthigasu KT. Chronic osteomyelitis due to *Clostridium difficile.* BMJ [Clin Res]. 1982;284:1217–1218.
180. Incavo SJ, Muller DL, Krag MH, Gump D. Vertebral osteomyelitis caused by *Clostridium difficile.* A case report and review of the literature. Spine. 1988;13:111–113.
181. Gaglani MJ, Murray JC, Morad AB, Edwards MS. Chronic osteomyelitis caused by *Clostridium difficile* in an adolescent with sickle cell disease. Pediatr Infect Dis J. 1996;15:1054–1056.
182. Pron B, Merckx J, Touzet P, et al. Chronic septic arthritis and osteomyelitis in a prosthetic knee joint due to *Clostridium difficile.* Eur J Clin Microbiol Infect Dis. 1995;14:599–601.
183. Atkinson MH, McLeod BD. Reactive arthritis associated with *Clostridium difficile* enteritis. J Rheumatol. 1988;15:520–522.
184. Boice JL. Reactive arthritis induced by *Clostridium difficile.* West J Med. 1994;160:171–172.
185. Cope A, Anderson J, Wilkins E. *Clostridium difficile* toxin-induced reactive arthritis in a patient with chronic Reiter's syndrome. Eur J Clin Microbiol Infect Dis. 1992;11:40–43.
186. Cron RQ, Gordon PV. Reactive arthritis to *Clostridium difficile* in a child. West J Med. 1997;166:419–421.
187. Hannonen P, Hakola M, Mottonen T, Oka M. Reactive oligoarthritis associated with *Clostridium difficile* colitis. Scand J Rheumatol. 1989;18:57–60.
188. Hayward RS, Wensel RH, Kibsey P. Relapsing *Clostridium difficile* colitis and Reiter's syndrome. Am J Gastroenterol. 1990;85:752–756.
189. Mermel LA, Osborn TG. *Clostridium difficile*–associated reactive arthritis in an HLA-B27 positive female: Report and literature review. J Rheumatol. 1989;16:133–135.
190. Putterman C, Rubinow A. Reactive arthritis associated with *Clostridium difficile* pseudomembranous colitis. Semin Arthritis Rheum. 1993;22:420–426.
191. Sensini A, Marroni M, Bassotti G, et al. *Clostridium difficile*–associated reactive arthritis in an HLA-B27 negative male. J Clin Gastroenterol. 1993;16:354–355.
192. Wright TW, Linscheid RL, O'Duffy JD. Acute flexor tenosynovitis in association with *Clostridium difficile* infection: A case report. J Hand Surg [Am]. 1996;21:304–306.
193. Lofgren RP, Tadlock LM, Soltis RD. Acute oligoarthritis associated with *Clostridium difficile* pseudomembranous colitis. Arch Intern Med. 1984;144:617–619.
194. Abbott WG, Caughey DE. Reactive arthritis due to *Clostridium difficile.* N Z Med J. 1982;95:287.
195. McCluskey J, Riley TV, Owen ET, Langlands DR. Reactive arthritis associated with *Clostridium difficile.* Aust N Z J Med. 1982;12:535–537.
196. Case records of the Massachusetts General Hospital. Weekly clinicopathological exercises. Case 19-1998. A 70-year-old man with diarrhea, polyarthritis, and a history of Reiter's syndrome. N Engl J Med. 1998;338:1830–1836.
197. Wilson KH. The microecology of *Clostridium difficile.* Clin Infect Dis. 1993;16(Suppl 4):S214–S218.
198. Wilson KH, Silva J, Fekety FR. Suppression of *Clostridium difficile* by normal hamster cecal flora and prevention of antibiotic-associated cecitis. Infect Immun. 1981;34:626–628.
199. Borriello SP. The influence of the normal flora on *Clostridium difficile* colonisation of the gut. Ann Med. 1990;22:61–67.
200. Corthier G, Muller MC, Wilkins TD, et al. Protection against experimental pseudomembranous colitis in gnotobiotic mice by use of monoclonal antibodies against *Clostridium difficile* toxin A. Infect Immun. 1991;59:1192–1195.
201. Czuprynski CJ, Johnson WJ, Balish E, Wilkins T. Pseudomembranous colitis in *Clostridium difficile*–monoassociated rats. Infect Immun. 1983;39:1368–1376.
202. Wilson KH, Sheagren JN, Freter R. Population dynamics of ingested *Clostridium difficile* in the gastrointestinal tract of the Syrian hamster. J Infect Dis. 1985;151:355–361.
203. Lyerly DM, Wilkins TD. *Clostridium difficile.* In: Blaser MJ, Smith PD, Ravdin JI, et al., eds. Infections of the Gastrointestinal Tract. New York: Raven; 1995:867–891.
204. Borriello SP, Davies HA, Barclay FE. Detection of fimbriae amongst strains of *Clostridium difficile.* FEMS Microbiol Lett. 1988;49:65–67.
205. von Eichel-Streiber C, Laufenberg-Feldmann R, Sartingen S, et al. Comparative sequence analysis of the *Clostridium difficile* toxins A and B. Mol Gen Genet. 1992;233:260–268.
206. Gill DM. Bacterial toxins: A table of lethal amounts. Microbiol Rev. 1982;46:86–94.
207. Lyerly DM, Krivan HC, Wilkins TD. *Clostridium difficile*: Its disease and toxins. Clin Microbiol Rev. 1988;1:1–18.
208. Price SB, Phelps CJ, Wilkins TD, Johnson JL. Cloning of the carbohydrate-binding portion of the toxin A gene of *Clostridium difficile.* Curr Microbiol. 1987;16:55–60.

209. Tucker KD, Wilkins TD. Toxin A of *Clostridium difficile* binds to the human carbohydrate antigens I, X, and Y. Infect Immun. 1991;59:73–78.
210. Smith JA, Cooke DL, Hyde S, et al. *Clostridium difficile* toxin A binding to human intestinal epithelial cells. J Med Microbiol. 1997;46:953–958.
211. Hippenstiel S, Kratz T, Krull M, et al. Rho protein inhibition blocks protein kinase C translocation and activation. Biochem Biophys Res Commun. 1998;245:830–834.
212. Just I, Fritz G, Aktories K, et al. *Clostridium difficile* toxin B acts on the GTP-binding protein Rho. J Biol Chem. 1994;269:10706–10712.
213. Just I, Wilm M, Selzer J, et al. The enterotoxin from *Clostridium difficile* (ToxA) monoglucosylates the Rho proteins. J Biol Chem. 1995;270:13932–13936.
214. Just I, Selzer J, Wilm M, et al. Glucosylation of Rho proteins by *Clostridium difficile* toxin B. Nature. 1995;375:500–503.
215. Fiorentini C, Fabbri A, Falzano L, et al. *Clostridium difficile* toxin B induces apoptosis in intestinal cultured cells. Infect Immun. 1998;66:2660–2665.
216. Mahida YR, Makh S, Hyde S, et al. Effect of *Clostridium difficile* toxin A on human intestinal epithelial cells: Induction of interleukin 8 production and apoptosis after cell detachment. Gut. 1996;38:337–347.
217. Moore R, Pothoulakis C, LaMont JT, et al. *C. difficile* toxin A increases intestinal permeability and induces Cl^- secretion. Am J Physiol. 1990;259:G165–G172.
218. Hecht G, Pothoulakis C, LaMont JT, Madara JL. *Clostridium difficile* toxin A perturbs cytoskeletal structure and tight junction permeability of cultured human intestinal epithelial monolayers. J Clin Invest. 1988;82:1516–1524.
219. Lima AA, Lyerly DM, Wilkins TD, et al. Effects of *Clostridium difficile* toxins A and B in rabbit small and large intestine in vivo and on cultured cells in vitro. Infect Immun 1988;56:582–588.
220. Lima AA, Innes D Jr, Chadee K, et al. *Clostridium difficile* toxin A. Interactions with mucus and early sequential histopathologic effects in rabbit small intestine. Lab Invest. 1989;61:419–425.
221. Triadafilopoulos G, Pothoulakis C, O'Brien MJ, LaMont JT. Differential effects of *Clostridium difficile* toxins A and B on rabbit ileum. Gastroenterology. 1987;93:273–279.
222. Fonteles M, Fang G, Thielman NM, et al. Role of platelet activating factor in the inflammatory and secretory effects of *Clostridium difficile* toxin A. J Lipid Mediat Cell Signal. 1995;11:133–143.
223. Beubler E, Schirgi-Degen A, Pabst MA, et al. Effects of purified *Clostridium difficile* toxin A in the small intestine of the rat in vivo. Nat Toxins. 1993;1:369–375.
224. Burakoff R, Zhao L, Celifarco AJ, et al. Effects of purified *Clostridium difficile* toxin A on rabbit distal colon. Gastroenterology. 1995;109:348–354.
225. Triadafilopoulos G, Pothoulakis C, Weiss R, et al. Comparative study of *Clostridium difficile* toxin A and cholera toxin in rabbit ileum. Gastroenterology. 1989;97:1186–1192.
226. Castagliuolo I, Keates AC, Qiu B, et al. Increased substance P responses in dorsal root ganglia and intestinal macrophages during *Clostridium difficile* toxin A enteritis in rats. Proc Natl Acad Sci U S A. 1997;94:4788–4793.
227. Pothoulakis C, Castagliuolo I, LaMont JT, et al. CP-96,345, a substance P antagonist, inhibits rat intestinal responses to *Clostridium difficile* toxin A but not cholera toxin. Proc Natl Acad Sci U S A. 1994;91:947–951.
228. Steiner TS, Flores CA, Pizarro TT, Guerrant RL. Fecal lactoferrin, interleukin-1beta, and interleukin-8 are elevated in patients with severe *Clostridium difficile* colitis. Clin Diagn Lab Immunol. 1997;4:719–722.
229. Rocha MF, Maia ME, Bezerra LR, et al. *Clostridium difficile* toxin A induces the release of neutrophil chemotactic factors from rat peritoneal macrophages: Role of interleukin-1beta, tumor necrosis factor alpha, and leukotrienes. Infect Immun. 1997;65:2740–2746.
230. Linevsky JK, Pothoulakis C, Keates S, et al. IL-8 release and neutrophil activation by *Clostridium difficile* toxin–exposed human monocytes. Am J Physiol. 1997;273(6 Pt 1):G1333–G1340.
231. Melo Filho AA, Souza MH, Lyerly DM, et al. Role of tumor necrosis factor and nitric oxide in the cytotoxic effects of *Clostridium difficile* toxin A and toxin B on macrophages. Toxicon. 1997;35:743–752.
232. Flegel WA, Muller F, Daubener W, et al. Cytokine response by human monocytes to *Clostridium difficile* toxin A and toxin B. Infect Immun. 1991;59:3659–3666.
233. Sumner HW, Tedesco FJ. Rectal biopsy in clindamycin-associated colitis. An analysis of 23 cases. Arch Pathol. 1975;99:237–241.
234. Onderdonk AB, Cisneros RL, Bartlett JG. *Clostridium difficile* in gnotobiotic mice. Infect Immun. 1980;28:277–282.
235. Dailey DC, Kaiser A, Schloemer RH. Factors influencing the phagocytosis of *Clostridium difficile* by human polymorphonuclear leukocytes. Infect Immun. 1987;55:1541–1546.
236. Pothoulakis C, Sullivan R, Melnick DA, et al. *Clostridium difficile* toxin A stimulates intracellular calcium release and chemotactic response in human granulocytes. J Clin Invest. 1988;81:1741–1745.
237. Kelly CP, Becker S, Linevsky JK, et al. Neutrophil recruitment in *Clostridium difficile* toxin A enteritis in the rabbit. J Clin Invest. 1994;93:1257–1265.
238. Wershil BK, Castagliuolo I, Pothoulakis C. Direct evidence of mast cell involvement in *Clostridium difficile* toxin A–induced enteritis in mice. Gastroenterology. 1998;114:956–964.
239. Mitchell TJ, Ketley JM, Haslam SC, et al. Effect of toxin A and B of *Clostridium difficile* on rabbit ileum and colon. Gut. 1986;27:78–85.
240. Hecht G, Koutsouris A, Pothoulakis C, et al. *Clostridium difficile* toxin B disrupts the barrier function of T84 monolayers. Gastroenterology. 1992;102:416–423.
241. Riegler M, Sedivy R, Pothoulakis C, et al. *Clostridium difficile* toxin B is more potent than toxin A in damaging human colonic epithelium in vitro. J Clin Invest. 1995;95:2004–2011.
242. Souza MH, Melo-Filho AA, Rocha MF, et al. The involvement of macrophage-derived tumour necrosis factor and lipoxygenase products on the neutrophil recruitment induced by *Clostridium difficile* toxin B. Immunology. 1997;91:281–288.
243. Gerding DN, Gebhard RL, Sumner HW, Peterson LR. Pathology and Diagnosis of *Clostridium difficile* Disease. New York: Academic Press; 1988:260–286.
244. Burdon DW. Spectrum of disease. In: Borriello SP, ed. Antibiotic Associated Diarrhea and Colitis. Boston: Martinus Nijhoff; 1984:9–23.
245. Fekety R. Antibiotic-associated colitis. In: Mandell GL, Bennett JE, Dolin R, eds. Mandell, Douglas, and Bennett's Principles and Practice of Infectious Diseases. 4th ed. New York: Churchill Livingstone; 1995:978–987.
246. Price AB, Davies DR. Pseudomembranous colitis. J Clin Pathol. 1977;30:1–12.
247. Groschel DH. *Clostridium difficile* infection. Crit Rev Clin Lab Sci. 1996;33:203–245.
248. Fekety R, Shah AB. Diagnosis and treatment of *Clostridium difficile* colitis. JAMA 1993;269:71–75.
249. Peterson LR, Kelly PJ. The role of the clinical microbiology laboratory in the management of *Clostridium difficile*–associated diarrhea. Infect Dis Clin North Am. 1993;7:277–293.
250. Arrow SA, Croese L, Bowman RA, Riley TV. Evaluation of three commercial enzyme immunoassay kits for detecting faecal *Clostridium difficile* toxins. J Clin Pathol. 1994;47:954–956.
251. Doern GV, Coughlin RT, Wu L. Laboratory diagnosis of *Clostridium difficile*–associated gastrointestinal disease: Comparison of a monoclonal antibody enzyme immunoassay for toxins A and B with a monoclonal antibody enzyme immunoassay for toxin A only and two cytotoxicity assays. J Clin Microbiol. 1992;30:2042–2046.
252. Delmee M, Mackey T, Hamitou A. Evaluation of a new commercial *Clostridium difficile* toxin A enzyme immunoassay using diarrhoeal stools. Eur J Clin Microbiol Infect Dis. 1992;11:246–249.
253. De Girolami PC, Hanff PA, Eichelberger K, et al. Multicenter evaluation of a new enzyme immunoassay for detection of *Clostridium difficile* enterotoxin A. J Clin Microbiol. 1992;30:1085–1088.
254. Borriello SP, Vale T, Brazier JS, et al. Evaluation of a commercial enzyme immunoassay kit for the detection of *Clostridium difficile* toxin A. Eur J Clin Microbiol Infect Dis. 1992;11:360–363.
255. Altaie SS, Meyer P, Dryja D. Comparison of two commercially available enzyme immunoassays for detection of *Clostridium difficile* in stool specimens. J Clin Microbiol. 1994;32:51–53.
256. DiPersio JR, Varga FJ, Conwell DL, et al. Development of a rapid enzyme immunoassay for *Clostridium difficile* toxin A and its use in the diagnosis of *C. difficile*–associated disease. J Clin Microbiol. 1991;29:2724–2730.
257. Merz CS, Kramer C, Forman M, et al. Comparison of four commercially available rapid enzyme immunoassays with cytotoxin assay for detection of *Clostridium difficile* toxin(s) from stool specimens. J Clin Microbiol. 1994;32:1142–1147.
258. Whittier S, Shapiro DS, Kelly WF, et al. Evaluation of four commercially available enzyme immunoassays for laboratory diagnosis of *Clostridium difficile*–associated diseases. J Clin Microbiol. 1993;31:2861–2865.
259. Gerding DN, Johnson S, Peterson LR, et al. *Clostridium difficile*–associated diarrhea and colitis. Infect Control Hosp Epidemiol. 1995;16:459–477.
260. Depitre C, Delmee M, Avesani V, et al. Serogroup F strains of *Clostridium difficile* produce toxin B but not toxin A. J Med Microbiol. 1993;3:434–441.
261. Lyerly DM, Wilkins TD. Commercial latex test for *Clostridium difficile* toxin A does not detect toxin A. J Clin Microbiol. 1986;23:622–623.
262. Lyerly DM, Ball DW, Toth J, Wilkins TD. Characterization of cross-reactive proteins detected by Culturette Brand Rapid Latex Test for *Clostridium difficile*. J Clin Microbiol. 1988;26:397–400.
263. Wongwanich S, Kusum M, Phan-Urai R. Reactivity of the CD D-1 latex test with *Clostridium difficile* and other bacteria. Southeast Asian J Trop Med Public Health. 1994;25:321–323.
264. Wolfhagen MJ, Fluit AC, Torensma R, et al. Rapid detection of toxigenic *Clostridium difficile* in fecal samples by magnetic immuno PCR assay. J Clin Microbiol. 1994;3:1629–1633.
265. Gumerlock PH, Tang YJ, Weiss JB, Silva J Jr. Specific detection of toxigenic strains of *Clostridium difficile* in stool specimens. J Clin Microbiol. 1993;31:507–511.
266. Tang YJ, Gumerlock PH, Weiss JB, Silva J Jr. Specific detection of *Clostridium difficile* toxin A gene sequences in clinical isolates. Mol Cell Probes. 1993;8:463–467.
267. Kuhl SJ, Tang YJ, Navarro L, et al. Diagnosis and monitoring of *Clostridium difficile* infections with the polymerase chain reaction. Clin Infect Dis. 1993;16(Suppl 4):S234–S238.
268. George WL, Rolfe RD, Harding GK, et al. *Clostridium difficile* and cytotoxin in feces of patients with antimicrobial agent–associated pseudomembranous colitis. Infection. 1982;10:205–208.
269. Tedesco FJ, Corless JK, Brownstein RE. Rectal sparing in antibiotic-associated pseudomembranous colitis: A prospective study. Gastroenterology. 1982;83:1259–1260.
270. Fang FC, Gerding DN, Peterson LR. Diagnosis of *Clostridium difficile* colitis. Ann Intern Med. 1996;125:515; discussion 516.
271. Vinetz J, Manabe Y, Bartlett J. Diagnosis of *Clostridium difficile* colitis. Ann Intern Med. 1996;125:516.
272. Kelly CP, LaMont JT. *Clostridium difficile* infection. Annu Rev Med. 1998;49:375–390.
273. Schleupner MA, Garner DC, Sosnowski KM, et al. Concurrence of *Clostridium difficile* toxin A enzyme-linked immunosorbent assay, fecal lactoferrin assay, and

clinical criteria with *C. difficile* cytotoxin titer in two patient cohorts. J Clin Microbiol. 1995;33:1755–1759.

274. Aronsson B, Mollby R, E. NC. Diagnosis and epidemiology of *Clostridium difficile* enterocolitis in Sweden. J Antimicrob Chemother. 1984;14(suppl D):85–95.
275. Renshaw AA, Stelling JM, Doolittle MH. The lack of value of repeated *Clostridium difficile* cytotoxicity assays. Arch Pathol Lab Med. 1996;120:49–52.
276. Yong WH, Mattia AR, Ferraro MJ. Comparison of fecal lactoferrin latex agglutination assay and methylene blue microscopy for detection of fecal leukocytes in *Clostridium difficile*–associated disease. J Clin Microbiol. 1994;32:1360–1361.
277. Marx CE, Morris A, Wilson ML, Reller LB. Fecal leukocytes in stool specimens submitted for *Clostridium difficile* toxin assay. Diagn Microbiol Infect Dis. 1993;16:313–315.
278. Teasley DG, Gerding DN, Olson MM, et al. Prospective randomised trial of metronidazole versus vancomycin for *Clostridium difficile*–associated diarrhoea and colitis. Lancet. 1983;2:1043–1046.
279. Recommendations for preventing the spread of vancomycin resistance. Recommendations of the Hospital Infection Control Practices Advisory Committee (HICPAC). MMWR Morb Mortal Wkly Rep. 1995;44(RR-12):1–13.
280. Chow AW, Cheng N, Bartlett KH. In vitro susceptibility of *Clostridium difficile* to new beta-lactam and quinolone antibiotics. Antimicrob Agents Chemother. 1985;28:842–844.
281. Nord CE, Hagelback A. Susceptibility of anaerobic bacteria to PD 131628. Eur J Clin Microbiol Infect Dis. 1992;11:68–71.
282. Rolfe RD, Finegold SM. Comparative in vitro activity of new beta-lactam antibiotics against anaerobic bacteria. Antimicrob Agents Chemother. 1981;20:600–609.
283. Dzink J, Bartlett JG. In vitro susceptibility of *Clostridium difficile* isolates from patients with antibiotic-associated diarrhea or colitis. Antimicrob Agents Chemother. 1980;17:695–698.
284. Bacon AE, McGrath S, Fekety R, Holloway WJ. In vitro synergy studies with *Clostridium difficile.* Antimicrob Agents Chemother. 1991;35:582–583.
285. Levett PN. Antimicrobial susceptibility of *Clostridium difficile* determined by disc diffusion and breakpoint methods. J Antimicrob Chemother. 1988;22:167–173.
286. Bolton RP, Culshaw MA. Faecal metronidazole concentrations during oral and intravenous therapy for antibiotic-associated colitis due to *Clostridium difficile.* Gut. 1986;27:1169–1172.
287. Krook A, Lindstrom B, Kjellander J, et al. Relation between concentrations of metronidazole and *Bacteroides* spp in faeces of patients with Crohn's disease and healthy individuals. J Clin Pathol. 1981;34:645–650.
288. Arabi Y, Dimock F, Burdon DW, et al. Influence of neomycin and metronidazole on colonic microflora of volunteers. J Antimicrob Chemother. 1979;5:531–537.
289. Wenisch C, Parschalk B, Hasenhundl M, et al. Comparison of vancomycin, teicoplanin, metronidazole, and fusidic acid for the treatment of *Clostridium difficile*–associated diarrhea. Clin Infect Dis. 1996;22:813–818.
290. Young GP, Ward PB, Bayley N, et al. Antibiotic-associated colitis due to *Clostridium difficile*: Double-blind comparison of vancomycin with bacitracin. Gastroenterology. 1985;89:1038–1045.
291. Dudley MN, McLaughlin JC, Carrington G, et al. Oral bacitracin vs vancomycin therapy for *Clostridium difficile*–induced diarrhea. A randomized double-blind trial. Arch Intern Med. 1986;146:1101–1104.
292. de Lalla F, Nicolin R, Rinaldi E, et al. Prospective study of oral teicoplanin versus oral vancomycin for therapy of pseudomembranous colitis and *Clostridium difficile*–associated diarrhea. Antimicrob Agents Chemother. 1992;36:2192–2196.
293. Finegold SM, George WL. Therapy directed against *Clostridium difficile* and its toxins: Complications of therapy. In: Rolfe RD, Finegold SM, eds. *Clostridium difficile*: Its Role in Intestinal Disease. San Diego: Academic Press; 1988:341–366.
294. Baird DR. Comparison of two oral formulations of vancomycin for treatment of diarrhoea associated with *Clostridium difficile.* J Antimicrob Chemother. 1989;23:167–169.
295. Keighley MR, Burdon DW, Arabi Y, et al. Randomised controlled trial of vancomycin for pseudomembranous colitis and postoperative diarrhoea. BMJ. 1978;2:1667–1669.
296. Mogg GA, Arabi Y, Youngs D, et al. Therapeutic trials of antibiotic associated colitis. Scand J Infect Dis Suppl. 1980;22(Suppl):41–45.
297. Fekety R, Silva J, Kauffman C, et al. Treatment of antibiotic-associated *Clostridium difficile* colitis with oral vancomycin: Comparison of two dosage regimens. Am J Med. 1989;86:15–19.
298. Spitzer PG, Eliopoulos GM. Systemic absorption of enteral vancomycin in a patient with pseudomembranous colitis. Ann Intern Med. 1984;100:533–534.
299. Bartlett JG. Treatment of antibiotic-associated pseudomembranous colitis. Rev Infect Dis. 1984;6(Suppl 1):S235–S241.
300. Handwerger S, Raucher B, Altarac D, et al. Nosocomial outbreak due to *Enterococcus faecium* highly resistant to vancomycin, penicillin, and gentamicin. Clin Infect Dis. 1993;16:750–755.
301. Shay DK, Maloney SA, Montecalvo M, et al. Epidemiology and mortality risk of vancomycin-resistant enterococcal bloodstream infections. J Infect Dis. 1995;172:993–1000.
302. Morris JG Jr, Shay DK, Hebden JN, et al. Enterococci resistant to multiple antimicrobial agents, including vancomycin. Establishment of endemicity in a university medical center. Ann Intern Med. 1995;123:250–259.
303. Taylor NS, Bartlett JG. Binding of *Clostridium difficile* cytotoxin and vancomycin by anion-exchange resins. J Infect Dis. 1980;141–92–97.
304. Keighley MRB. Antibiotic-associated pseudomembranous colitis: Pathogenesis and management. Drugs. 1980;20:49–56.
305. McDonald GB, Vracko R. Systemic absorption of oral cholestyramine. Gastroenterology. 1984;87:213–215.
306. Oliva SL, Guglielmo BJ, Jacobs R, Pons VG. Failure of intravenous vancomycin and intravenous metronidazole to prevent or treat antibiotic-associated pseudomembranous colitis. J Infect Dis. 1989;159:1154–1155.
307. Guzman R, Kirkpatrick J, Forward K, Lim F. Failure of parenteral metronidazole in the treatment of pseudomembranous colitis. J Infect Dis. 1988;158:1146–1147.
308. Brown JR. Metronidazole and antibiotic-associated colitis. BMJ [Clin Res]. 1981;283:1334.
309. Cohen H, Brocavich JM. Managing *Clostridium difficile* colitis in patients who lack oral access. Infect Med. 1996;13:101–109.
310. Tedesco F, Markham R, Gurwith M, et al. Oral vancomycin for antibiotic-associated pseudomembranous colitis. Lancet 1978;2:226–228.
311. Johnson S, Adelmann A, Clabots CR, et al. Recurrences of *Clostridium difficile* diarrhea not caused by the original infecting organism. J Infect Dis. 1989;159:340–343.
312. Pasic M, Jost R, Carrel T, et al. Intracolonic vancomycin for pseudomembranous colitis. N Engl J Med. 1993;329:583.
313. Pasic M, Carrel T, Opravil M, et al. Systemic absorption after local intracolonic vancomycin in pseudomembranous colitis. Lancet. 1993;342:443.
314. Goodpasture HC, Dolan PJ Jr, Jacobs ER, Meredith WT. Pseudomembranous colitis and antibiotics. Kans Med. 1986;87:133, 146.
315. Griebie M, Adams GL. *Clostridium difficile* colitis following head and neck surgery. Report of cases. Arch Otolaryngol. 1985;111:550–553.
316. Osler T, Lott D, Bordley JT, et al. Cefazolin-induced pseudomembranous colitis resulting in perforation of the sigmoid colon. Dis Colon Rectum. 1986;29:140–143.
317. Bublin JG, Barton TL. Rectal use of vancomycin. Ann Pharmacother. 1994;28:1357–1358.
318. Peterson LR, Gerding DN. Antimicrobial agents in *Clostridium difficile*–associated intestinal diseases. In: Rambaud J, Ducluzeau R, eds. *Clostridium difficile*–Associated Intestinal Diseases. Paris: Springer-Verlag; 1990:115–127.
319. Novak E, Lee JG, Seckman CE, et al. Unfavorable effect of atropine-diphenoxylate (Lomotil) therapy in lincomycin-caused diarrhea. JAMA. 1976;235:1451–1454.
320. Hoogland T, Cooperman AM, Farmer RG, Fazio VW. Toxic megacolon—unusual complication of pseudomembranous colitis. Cleve Clin Q. 1977;44:149–155.
321. Lipsett PA, Samantaray DK, Tam ML, et al. Pseudomembranous colitis: A surgical disease? Surgery. 1994;116:491–496.
322. Synnott K, Mealy K, Merry C, et al. Timing of surgery for fulminating pseudomembranous colitis. Br J Surg. 1998;85:229–231.
323. Agnifili A, Gola P, Marino M, et al. The role and timing of surgery in the treatment of pseudomembranous colitis. A case complicated by toxic megacolon. Hepatogastroenterology. 1994;41:394–396.
324. Bartlett JG. Treatment of *Clostridium difficile* colitis. Gastroenterology. 1985;89:1192–1195.
325. Levett PN. Time-dependent killing of *Clostridium difficile* by metronidazole and vancomycin. J Antimicrob Chemother. 1991;27:55–62.
326. Wilcox MH, Spencer RC. *Clostridium difficile* infection: Responses, relapses and re-infections. J Hosp Infect. 1992;22:85–92.
327. McKay I, Coia JE, Poxton IR. Typing of *Clostridium difficile* causing diarrhoea in an orthopaedic ward. J Clin Pathol. 1989;42:511–515.
328. O'Neill GL, Beaman MH, Riley TV. Relapse versus reinfection with *Clostridium difficile.* Epidemiol Infect. 1991;107:627–635.
329. McFarland LV, Surawicz CM, Greenberg RN, et al. A randomized placebo-controlled trial of *Saccharomyces boulardii* in combination with standard antibiotics for *Clostridium difficile* disease. JAMA. 1994;271:1913–1918.
330. Pruksananonda P, Powell KR. Multiple relapses of *Clostridium difficile*–associated diarrhea responding to an extended course of cholestyramine. Pediatr Infect Dis J. 1989;8:175–178.
331. Kunimoto D, Thomson AB. Recurrent *Clostridium difficile*–associated colitis responding to cholestyramine. Digestion. 1986;33:225–228.
332. Moncino MD, Falletta JM. Multiple relapses of *Clostridium difficile*–associated diarrhea in a cancer patient. Successful control with long-term cholestyramine therapy. Am J Pediatr Hematol Oncol. 1992;14:361–364.
333. Leung DY, Kelly CP, Boguniewicz M, et al. Treatment with intravenously administered gamma globulin of chronic relapsing colitis induced by *Clostridium difficile* toxin. J Pediatr. 1991;118:633–637.
334. Salcedo J, Keates S, Pothoulakis C, et al. Intravenous immunoglobulin therapy for severe *Clostridium difficile* colitis. Gut. 1997;41:366–370.
335. Warny M, Denie C, Delmee M, Lefebvre C. Gamma globulin administration in relapsing *Clostridium difficile*–induced pseudomembranous colitis with a defective antibody response to toxin A. Acta Clin Belg. 1995;50:36–39.
336. Tedesco FJ, Gordon D, Fortson WC. Approach to patients with multiple relapses of antibiotic-associated pseudomembranous colitis. Am J Gastroenterol. 1985;80:867–868.
337. Buggy BP, Fekety R, Silva J Jr. Therapy of relapsing *Clostridium difficile*–associated diarrhea and colitis with the combination of vancomycin and rifampin. J Clin Gastroenterol. 1987;9:155–159.
338. Gorbach SL. Lactic acid bacteria and human health. Ann Med. 1990;22:37–41.
339. Biller JA, Katz AJ, Flores AF, et al. Treatment of recurrent *Clostridium difficile* colitis with *Lactobacillus* GG. J Pediatr Gastroenterol Nutr. 1995;21:224–226.
340. Gorbach SL, Chang TW, Goldin B. Successful treatment of relapsing *Clostridium difficile* colitis with *Lactobacillus* GG. Lancet. 1987;2:1519.
341. Seal D, Borriello SP, Barclay F, et al. Treatment of relapsing *Clostridium difficile* diarrhoea by administration of a nontoxigenic strain. Eur J Clin Microbiol. 1987;6:51–53.
342. Tjellstrom B, Stenhammar L, Eriksson S, Magnusson KE. Oral immunoglobulin A

supplement in treatment of *Clostridium difficile* enteritis. Lancet. 1993;341:701–702.

343. Liacouras CA, Piccoli DA. Whole-bowel irrigation as an adjunct to the treatment of chronic, relapsing *Clostridium difficile* colitis. J Clin Gastroenterol. 1996;22:186–189.
344. Tvede M, Rask-Madsen J. Bacteriotherapy for chronic relapsing *Clostridium difficile* diarrhoea in six patients. Lancet. 1989;1:1156–1160.
345. Schwan A, Sjölin S, Trottestam U, Aronsson B. Relapsing *Clostridium difficile* enterocolitis cured by rectal infusion of normal faeces. Scand J Infect Dis. 1984;16:211–215.
346. Johnson S, Gerding DN, Olson MM, et al. Prospective, controlled study of vinyl glove use to interrupt *Clostridium difficile* nosocomical transmission. Am J Med. 1990;88:137–140.
347. Brooks SE, Veal RO, Kramer M, et al. Reduction in the incidence of *Clostridium difficile*–associated diarrhea in an acute care hospital and a skilled nursing facility following replacement of electronic thermometers with single-use disposables. Infect Control Hosp Epidemiol. 1992;13:98–103.
348. Brown E, Talbot GH, Axelrod P, et al. Risk factors for *Clostridium difficile* toxin–associated diarrhea. Infect Control Hosp Epidemiol. 1990;11:283–290.
349. Elmer GW, Surawicz CM, McFarland LV. Biotherapeutic agents. A neglected modality for the treatment and prevention of selected intestinal and vaginal infections. JAMA. 1996;275:870–876.
350. Surawicz CM, Elmer GW, Speelman P, et al. Prevention of antibiotic-associated diarrhea by *Saccharomyces boulardii*: A prospective study. Gastroenterology. 1989;96:981–988.
351. Colombel JF, Cortot A, Neut C, Romond C. Yoghurt with *Bifidobacterium longum* reduces erythromycin-induced gastrointestinal effects. Lancet. 1987;2:43.
352. Gotz V, Romankiewicz JA, Moss J, Murray HW. Prophylaxis against ampicillin-associated diarrhea with a lactobacillus preparation. Am J Hosp Pharm. 1979;36:754–757.
353. Wunderlich PF, Braun L, Fumagalli I, et al. Double-blind report on the efficacy of lactic acid–producing *Enterococcus* SF68 in the prevention of antibiotic-associated diarrhoea and in the treatment of acute diarrhoea. J Int Med Res. 1989;17:333–338.
354. Thielman NM, Guerrant RL. *Clostridium difficile*. In: Burg FD, Ingelfinger JR, Wald ER, Polin RA, eds. Gellis and Kagan's Current Pediatric Therapy. 15th ed. Philadelphia: WB Saunders; 1995:584–586.
355. Wenisch C, Etzersdorfer E, Breyer S, Graninger W. Intravenous teicoplanin does not prevent *Clostridium difficile*–associated diarrhea. Clin Invest. 1994;72:922–924.

Chapter 85

Inflammatory Enteritides

RICHARD L. GUERRANT
ALDO A. M. LIMA

The acute inflammatory enteritides include several specific distal small bowel and colonic infections such as campylobacteriosis, salmonellosis, shigellosis, and amebiasis, as well as the syndromes of necrotizing enteritis and antibiotic-associated pseudomembranous enterocolitis. Several other infectious agents cause chronic enteric inflammatory processes that may result in syndromes of abdominal pain, weight loss, diarrhea, or malabsorption. These include such processes as gastrointestinal mycoses, mycobacterioses, bacterial infections, and certain parasitic infections such as coccidiosis.

ACUTE DYSENTERY: HISTORY, EPIDEMIOLOGY, AND DIAGNOSIS

Syndromes of acute dysentery with fecal blood and pus have been well recognized since the days of Hippocrates. Dysentery is defined as frequent, small bowel movements accompanied by blood and mucus with tenesmus or pain on defecation. This syndrome implies an inflammatory invasion of the colonic mucosa resulting from bacterial, cytotoxic, or parasitic destruction.

The pathologic changes of inflammatory colitis range from a superficial intense exudative inflammatory process involving the colonic mucosa, as in infection by shigellae or invasive *Escherichia coli* organisms, to deeper, penetrating, "flask-shaped" ulcers with undermined edges, as seen in amebic dysentery. The pathogenesis of the inflammatory colitides may involve cytotoxic products of shigellae,[1] certain *E. coli* strains,[2] clostridia, or other organisms.

The epidemiologic patterns of acute dysenteric syndromes are influenced by the unusually low inoculum required by organisms such as shigellae or amebae for infection. As few as 100 shigellae or as few as 10 cysts of enteric parasites such as *Entamoeba coli* or *Giardia lamblia* have been found to result in infection in adult volunteers.[3, 4] Consequently, there is a substantial risk of person-to-person spread in daycare centers,[5] institutions, or other areas where nonhygienic conditions may allow direct fecal-oral spread. The cysts of parasites such as *Entamoeba histolytica* or *Balantidium coli* often resist chlorination and therefore may cause waterborne outbreaks of dysenteric illnesses. Saltwater or seafood exposure should lead to consideration of *Vibrio parahaemolyticus* as a cause of inflammatory colitis, and farm or domestic animal exposure might lead to consideration of nontyphoid *Salmonella* spp., *Campylobacter jejuni*, or *Yersina enterocolitica*. In addition, when typhoid fever is present with diarrhea in an endemic area, the diarrhea is often inflammatory, with many fecal polymorphonuclear leukocytes seen on microscopic examination.[6] A history of travel to areas of poor sanitation may implicate any of the aforementioned pathogens. Finally, venereal exposure, particularly among male homosexuals, may implicate *gonococci*, herpes simplex virus, *Chlamydia trachomatis*, or *Treponema pallidum* as a cause of proctitis or *Campylobacter, Shigella, C. trachomatis* (lymphogranuloma venereum serotypes), *E. histolytica*, or *Clostridium difficile* as a cause of colitis.[7]

Examination for fecal leukocytes often reveals sheets of polymorphonuclear leukocytes in clumps of mucus even in the absence of gross blood in the stool specimen (Fig. 85–1).[8, 9] Fewer pyknotic leukocytes are reported in amebic dysentery;[10–12] this may be attributable to the deeper, undermining ulcers characteristic of intestinal amebiasis or to a contact-dependent cytolytic effect of the ameba on leukocytes. The use of fresh specimens promptly plated onto appropriate enteric culture media is very important in the isolation of shigellae.[13] Specialized techniques are required to isolate *Vibrio* (thiosulfate citrate bile salts [TCBS] agar),[14] *Yersinia* (cold enrichment),[15] or *C. jejuni*.[16] The identification of toxigenic *C. difficile* is done by immunoassay or cell culture cytotoxicity assay for *C. difficile* toxin A or B, respectively.[17–19] Leukocytosis or even a leukemoid reaction has been described in colitis due to *C. difficile*. Sigmoidoscopic examination, especially with biopsy, may be useful in the diagnosis of a pseudomembranous enterocolitis or in the identification of parasites such as *E. histolytica* (with special periodic acid–Schiff [PAS] stain) or *Balantidium coli*. Amebic colitis is associated with discrete

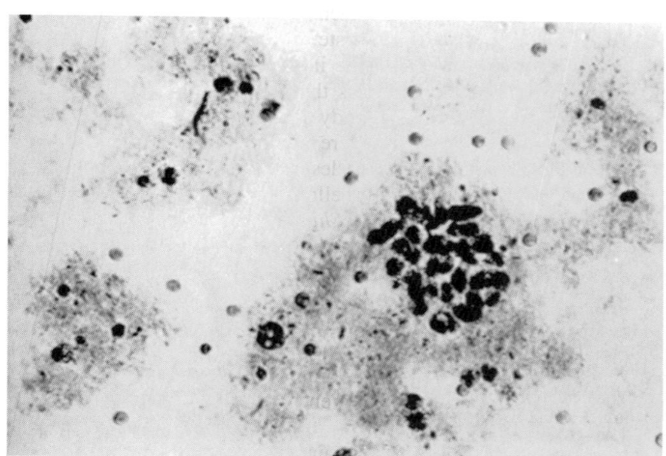

FIGURE 85–1. Methylene blue stain of fecal leukocytes found in colitis. This exudative response may be seen in shigellosis, salmonellosis, *Campylobacter* infection, and colitis due to invasive *Escherichia coli*.

TABLE 85–1 Differential Diagnosis of Acute Dysentery and Inflammatory Enterocolitis

Specific infectious processes
- Bacillary dysentery (*Shigella dysenteriae, Shigella flexneri, Shigella sonnei, Shigella boydii;* invasive *Escherichia coli*)
- Campylobacteriosis (*Campylobacter jejuni*)
- Amebic dysentery (*Entamoeba histolytica*)
- Ciliary dysentery (*Balantidium coli*)
- Bilharzial dysentery (*Schistosoma japonicum, Schistosoma mansoni*)
- Other parasitic infections (*Trichinella spiralis*)
- Vibriosis (*Vibrio parahaemolyticus*)
- Salmonellosis (*Salmonella typhimurium*)
- Typhoid fever (*Salmonella typhi*)
- Enteric fever (*Salmonella choleraesuis, Salmonella paratyphi*)
- Yersiniosis (*Yersinia enterocolitica*)
- Spirillar dysentery (*Spirillum* spp.)

Proctitis
- Gonococcal (*Neisseria gonorrhoeae*)
- Herpetic (herpes simplex virus)
- Chlamydial (*Chlamydia trachomatis*)
- Syphilitic (*Treponema pallidum*)

Other syndromes
- Necrotizing enterocolitis of the newborn
- Enteritis necroticans
- Pseudomembranous enterocolitis (*Clostridium difficile*)
- Diverticulitis
- Typhlitis

Syndromes without known infectious etiology
- Idiopathic ulcerative colitis
- Crohn's disease
- Radiation enteritis
- Ischemic colitis
- Allergic enteritis

small ulcerations with undermined edges amid relatively normal mucosa. Acute shigellosis causes more widespread, shallow, 3- to 7-mm ulcers with a more intense inflammatory exudate. Barium studies are unnecessary and are relatively contraindicated in toxic patients with acute colitis. Therapy consists of careful supportive fluid management with specific antimicrobial therapy directed at a specific pathogen if suspected on the basis of the epidemiologic setting or culture results.

The potential causes of acute dysentery are listed in Table 85–1.

Shigellosis and Enteroinvasive *Escherichia coli*

It is estimated that *Shigella* spp. infect over 200 million people and cause 650,000 deaths each year worldwide.[20] The four *Shigella* spp. are classified in subgroups A to D: *Shigella dysenteriae, Shigella flexneri, Shigella sonnei*, and *Shigella boydii*, respectively. Shigellae are facultative intracellular pathogens and may cause acute bloody dysentery with high fever and systemic manifestations of malaise, headache, and abdominal pain. The incubation period ranges from 6 hours to 9 days but is usually less than 72 hours. *Shigella* spp. are the most common cause of bloody diarrhea in children, and the syndrome may be particularly severe in poorly nourished children.[21]

Despite the intense superficial destructive process in the colonic epithelium that typifies acute shigellosis, bacteremia and disseminated infection are relatively rare.[22] *Shigella* infection (especially with *S. dysenteriae* type 1) is associated with enteric protein loss that ceases after appropriate antimicrobial therapy.[23] This protein loss may contribute to increased susceptibility to secondary infections or growth stunting.[24, 25] A complication of severe shigellosis in childhood is a hemolytic-uremic syndrome (HUS) that may be associated with a leukemoid reaction, pseudomembranous colitis, circulating immune complexes, and circulating endotoxin, usually in the absence of demonstrable bacteremia.[26]

Intestinal obstruction, which occurs in about 3% of patients, is a poor prognostic sign, not infrequently associated with death or the development of HUS.[27] Other, more common extraintestinal manifestations of shigellosis are headache, meningismus, and even seizures, especially in children.[28] These findings may be attributable to a neurotoxin that has been demonstrated with *S. dysenteriae* type 1.[1, 29] A serious arthritis similar to that seen in Reiter's syndrome has been described in up to 10% of cases 2 to 5 weeks after the dysenteric illness that characteristically occurs in patients with histocompatibility antigen HLA-B27.[30, 31] Culture-positive conjunctivitis during acute shigellosis has also been described and may represent autoinoculation of the conjunctiva analogous to that induced in guinea pigs in the Sereny test.[32] Arthritis syndromes have also been described after inflammatory colitis with *Y. enterocolitica, Salmonella enteritidis*, or *C. difficile*, again in association with HLA-B27.[33, 34]

Certain *E. coli* strains may produce an identical syndrome to that seen with acute shigellosis. The incubation period is usually 2 to 3 days after ingestion. Although invasive *E. coli* organisms appear to be limited to certain serotypes (Table 85–2),[32, 35–37] to confirm the presence of such organisms, their invasive potential should be demonstrated in the guinea pig conjunctivitis (Sereny) test[38] or in Hela cells,[39] or the 120- to 140-MD plasmid that is associated with invasiveness in *Shigella* and invasive *E. coli* should be identified.[40–42] Invasive *E. coli* organisms were responsible for a single widespread outbreak of dysentery associated with imported French Camembert cheese.[37, 43] Although they have been identified as occasional causes of diarrhea in Brazil,[32] invasive *E. coli* organisms do not appear to be frequent causes of sporadic diarrhea in the United States. Because they are often slow to ferment lactose in the laboratory, invasive *E. coli* organisms may be initially mistaken for shigellae,[32, 37, 44] to which they are closely related. Invasive *E. coli* organisms are also usually lysine-negative and often nonmotile[45] and are antigenically related to *Shigella*.[46]

Enterohemorrhagic *Escherichia coli* Diarrhea

Although the frequency with which it causes inflammatory diarrhea is not clear, a significant cause of bloody diarrhea and potentially fatal HUS is now recognized to be enterohemorrhagic *E. coli* organisms (EHEC) that produce relatively large amounts of Shiga-like toxin (Vero cytotoxin) of two forms, SLT I and SLT II.[2, 47] These organisms have attracted particular attention with widespread outbreaks in popular hamburger chain restaurants.[48–50] While they account for only 0.8 to 3.0% of all cases of diarrhea in the United States and Canada, EHEC (of serotype O157) are estimated to account for 15 to 36% of cases of bloody diarrhea.[2, 51] The majority of recognized EHEC strains are of serotype O157; others include O26:K60:H11; O103:H2; O91:H2; O145:H–; O111:K58:H–; O38:H21; O6:H–; O5:H–; O128; O139; O113:K75; O121; and O172.[2, 36, 51–54] EHEC were the most commonly recognized cause of diarrhea (3%) among 5415 patients studied in Calgary in Alberta, Canada, where such cases showed a summer seasonal peak.[51] In addition to causing 15 to 36% of all cases of bloody diarrhea, including outbreaks of hemorrhagic colitis, EHEC are associated with 75 to 90% of cases of HUS in North America, a complication that develops in 8% of EHEC infections.[2]

The pathogenesis of EHEC infections involves attachment to and effacement of the gut epithelium by the organism in delivery of Shiga-like toxin.[55, 56] This inhibits protein synthesis, destroys epithe-

TABLE 85–2 Enteroinvasive *Escherichia coli* Serotypes

Serotype	*Difco Serogroup*	Reference(s)
O28 ac	C	32, 35
O29		36
O112 a,c	C	35
O124	B	32, 35, 37
O136	C (Trabulsi's 193-T-64)	35, 37
O143		35
O144		35, 37
O152	(Trabulsi's 185-T-64)	35, 37

lial cells, and causes vascular necrosis and edema of the intestinal tract. Some patients develop full-blown HUS.[52, 53] The diagnosis is suggested by the clinical findings and confirmed by serotyping sorbitol-negative *E. coli* insolates or by using tissue culture or gene probes to detect the cytotoxin.

Campylobacter Enteritis

C. jejuni (formerly *Campylobacter fetus* or *"Vibrio fetus"*) systemic infections have been recognized for many years. Although the majority of *Campylobacter* blood stream infections in humans are with *C. fetus* (old subspecies, *intestinalis*),[57] *C. jejuni* commonly causes an enteric infection in all age groups. This organism was recognized many years ago as a cause of swine dysentery.[58] Commercially available techniques of fecal culture have enabled the culture of *C. jejuni* on highly selective media at 42°C from fecal specimens of patients with diarrhea.[16, 59] This organism causes a syndrome of severe abdominal pain, fever, and acute inflammatory enteritis that may range from watery diarrhea to severe dysentery with blood and pus in the stools.[59–61] This infection has also been associated with sequelae of reactive arthritis and Guillain-Barré syndrome.[62] Reports from Belgium, England, and central Africa reveal that in 5 to 14% of unselected cases of diarrhea, *C. jejuni* is present,[60, 61, 63] and outbreaks of *Campylobacter* enteritis have been associated with ingestion of contaminated water, raw milk, or uncooked meat or poultry. The roles of toxins, adhesins, and lipopolysaccharides in the pathogenesis of *Campylobacter* enteritis remain uncertain.[64]

Amebic Dysentery

There are two morphologically identical *Entamoeba* species named *E. histolytica* and *Entamoeba dispar.*[65] The former is a pathogen and is responsible for invasive amebiasis, whereas the latter is a gut commensal. *E. histolytica* cysts are ingested, pass through the gastric acidity, and undergo digestion of the capsule in the small bowel. Trophozoites then invade the colonic mucosa and produce shallow, flask-shaped undermining ulcers. The capacity of this parasite to invade tissue has been attributed to histolytic enzymes, but invasion probably also involves contact-dependent cytolysis of target cells, especially polymorphonuclear leukocytes, which then discharge their cytolytic contents.[66–72] After their invasion of the intestine, amebae may then seed the liver via the portal vein, from which extension may occur to the skin, diaphragm, lung, or pericardium. Although extraintestinal amebiasis occurs with less than one-tenth the frequency of symptomatic intestinal amebic dysentery, dissemination is reportedly more common in states of undernutrition, with cytotoxic or steroid medication, during late pregnancy, and with carcinoma or other overwhelming systemic diseases. Asymptomatic cyst carriage occurs in 1 to 5% of the population in the southern United States. The frequency of amebiasis is greater in rural and lower socioeconomic groups and in institutions where fecal-oral spread of this human parasite may occur.[73] Fulminant amebic colitis is a rare disease but may be associated with diabetes mellitus and chronic alcoholism.[74]

Ciliary Dysentery

B. coli is the only ciliate parasite that is pathogenic for humans. The most common reservoir is swine. Like *E. histolytica*, this parasite excysts in the small bowel, invades the terminal ileum and colon, and may cause appendicitis or a dysenteric syndrome with rectosigmoid ulceration (with heaped-up edges around 1.5- to 3-cm ulcers) and secondary bacteremia. However, there is no extraintestinal extension of *B. coli* infection, as may be seen with amebiasis. The diagnosis is made by scraping the margin of the ulcer and examining microscopically for the ciliate trophozoite. Mucosal invasion is usually limited to the rectal vault. Symptoms may last for 1 to 4 weeks and may recur several times a year if the infection goes untreated. Therapy with tetracycline is usually successful.

Bilharzial Dysentery

Schistosomiasis may cause acute bloody diarrhea, abdominal pain, and weight loss when the adult schistosomes (usually *Schistosoma japonicum* or *Schistosoma mansoni*) migrate to the intestinal tract, where they begin egg deposition. This occurs 3 to 8 weeks after initial skin exposure to the cercariae and may last for several weeks. Fecal examination reveals blood, pus, and numerous ova. Fever, leukocytosis, and increasing eosinophilia may be associated with this illness, and hepatosplenic disease may follow. *S. mansoni* may also cause chronic blood or protein loss via inflammatory "polyps."

Other Parasitic Infections

Another potential parasitic cause of inflammatory enteritis is acute trichinosis. Approximately 24 hours after the ingestion of infested pork, the larvae excyst and invade the intestinal mucosa, often resulting in nausea, vomiting, diarrhea, and abdominal pain. This precedes the systemic manifestation of periorbital edema, fever, myositis, and eosinophilia by 1 to 2 weeks.

Vibriosis

In addition to classic and El Tor *Vibrio cholerae* O1, non-O1 *V. cholerae* and several halophilic *Vibrio* species are now recognized to cause diarrhea and occasional wound or blood stream infection.[75, 76] The most common and best characterized is *V. parahaemolyticus. V. parahaemolyticus* has been recognized since 1950 in Japan and was identified as a vibrio in 1963. *V. parahaemolyticus* is a cause of seafood poisoning, with onset of signs and symptoms 9 to 25 hours after the ingestion of inadequately cooked fish or shellfish. This has been reported throughout the coastal areas of the United States and on cruise ships and is the most common form of food poisoning in Japan, where raw seafood is commonly eaten.[77] Diarrhea may be explosive and watery or may be characterized by full-blown dysentery with blood and pus and superficial ulceration on proctoscopic examination.[78, 79] The latter syndrome may be associated with cramps, nausea, vomiting, headache, and fever. The illness usually is self-limited, resolving within 3 to 4 days. The pathogenic Kanagawa-positive strains from patients produce β-hemolysis on special (Wagatsuma) medium—in contrast to environmental isolates—and are best isolated as blue-green colonies (alkaline) on TCBS agar.[14]

Other halophilic vibrios include *Vibrio alginolyticus, Vibrio fluvialis, Vibrio hollisae, Vibrio damsela*, and *Vibrio vulnificus*, which have been associated with enteric, wound, or systemic infections in humans.[75, 76] *V. vulnificus* has been associated with life-threatening septicemia occurring within 24 hours of ingesting raw oysters.[76, 80]

Salmonellosis

Salmonella enterocolitis is characterized by fever, cramping, abdominal pain, and diarrhea that begins 8 to 48 hours after ingestion of an infective dose, usually with food, and usually lasts 3 to 5 days. The diarrheal stools of patients with salmonellosis often contain a moderate number of polymorphonuclear leukocytes, usually fewer than is typical of shigellosis.

Although *Salmonella* enteritis predominantly involves the lamina propria in the small bowel, several reports have noted *Salmonella typhimurium* as a cause of colitis, with crypt abscesses and erosion and ulcerations of the colonic mucosa, resulting in blood and pus in the stool.[81–85] Certain other strains of salmonella (*Salmonella choleraesuis* and *Salmonella paratyphi*), like *Salmonella typhi*, tend to elicit a mononuclear response and cause a bacteremia characteristic of enteric fever.

Typhoid Fever

Typhoid fever may lead to an erosion of the blood vessels in Peyer's patches that without appropriate treatment may result in gross blood in the feces in 10 to 20% of the patients. Severe intestinal hemorrhage may complicate approximately 2% of the cases late in the course of untreated typhoid fever. Such intestinal bleeding may precede perforation, another complication of typhoid fever.[86]

Yersiniosis

Y. enterocolitica is another increasingly recognized enteric pathogen that may be responsible for an enteric fever-like illness, mesenteric adenitis (that may mimic acute appendicitis), or an inflammatory ileitis or ulcerative colitis syndrome with fecal neutrophils and mononuclear cells.[87–89] *Yersinia* infection may also be associated with migratory polyarthritis, Reiter's syndrome, or erythema nodosum. A syndrome of acute diarrhea and vomiting is especially common in young children.[90] The organism may cause disseminated abscesses in the liver and spleen[91] or an inflammatory colitis.[92] The causative agent, a gram-negative member of the family Enterobacteriaceae, is in the same genus as the plague bacillus *Yersinia pestis* and is sometimes mistaken for *Proteus* on initial culture plates. Cultivation may require cold enrichment techniques.[15]

Gonococcal Proctitis

Neisseria gonorrhoeae may be the cause of ulcerative proctitis, usually acquired by venereal exposure.[7] The resultant purulent proctitis is accompanied by an erythematous friable mucous membrane in the rectal vault and occasional abscess or fistula formation. Although copious purulent discharge, tenesmus, and burning rectal pain may be noted, two thirds of the culture-positive patients with anorectal gonococcal infection are asymptomatic.[93, 94] Additional diagnostic possibilities in cases of venereally acquired proctitis are syphilitic, herpetic, and chlamydial proctitis.[95]

Spirillar Dysentery

"Spirillar" or "spirochetal" dysentery has been reported to occur in southern France and has been attributed to *Spirillum* spp.[96] Although severe mucoid diarrhea or dysentery has been associated with intestinal spirochetes, their frequency and role in causing enteric disease is unclear.[97] A DNA probe for the 16S recombinant RNA (rRNA) of the agent of swine dysentery, *Treponema hyodysenteriae* has been developed and may open new approaches to the recognition of similar infections in humans.[98]

Other unusual or emerging causes of colitis include brucellosis[99] and adenovirus infections.[100, 101]

Approach to Diagnosis and Treatment of Acute Dysentery

Any of the aforementioned microorganisms may cause an acute dysentery syndrome with blood and pus in the stool; examination for leukocytes or for indirect evidence such as fecal lactoferrin[102] may suggest the specific disorder even if blood is not present in the stool on gross examination. Other considerations in the differential diagnosis of inflammatory colitis are pseudomembranous enterocolitis, which may be associated with antibiotic use, and the potentially rapidly progressive necrotizing enterocolitis syndromes, which are discussed elsewhere. These diagnoses are suggested by the clinical course, history, and findings on radiologic and proctoscopic examinations. Noninfectious syndromes that may be manifested as acute inflammatory enterocolitis include idiopathic ulcerative colitis and Crohn's disease.

Presumptive therapy for the inflammatory colitides varies greatly with the different organisms and is influenced by the increasing resistance of enteric pathogens to antimicrobial therapy[103] (see p. 1086 in Chapter 81). For example, an acute febrile dysenteric illness in a young child with daycare exposure or in an area where shigellosis is common should be treated with an antimicrobial agent such as one of the fluoroquinolones. If the *Shigella* organism is sensitive, prompt therapy can successfully stop the diarrhea, alleviate systemic symptoms, and reduce shedding of the organisms in the feces.[104–106] Because shigellae are increasingly multi-antibiotic-resistant,[107, 108] the practitioner must be familiar with the local resistance pattern of shigellae to appropriately treat acute shigellosis when it is first suspected. Although the fluoroquinolones are not approved at present for use in children in the United States, the available data suggest that a short course of therapy is safe.[109] The quinolone antibiotics offer a considerable advance in treating inflammatory diarrhea. Not only are they effective in treating otherwise resistant shigellosis, but they reduce fecal shedding and the duration of illness with *C. jejuni* infection and, although they do not necessarily eradicate the organism, may shorten the clinical course even with *Salmonella* infections.[110–112] Recent studies in adults with *Campylobacter* enteritis have shown that treatment with ciprofloxacin (when sensitive) or azithromycin may reduce the duration of symptoms.[113] Vitamin A has also been used to reduce both severity and mortality from shigellosis.[114]

Amebic dysentery is usually diagnosed by direct examination of wet mounts of fresh fecal or proctoscopic specimens, which reveal *E. histolytica* trophozoites or cysts in 60 to 80% of the cases. The cysts and trophozoites are characterized by four or fewer delicate nuclei with central karyosomes. Additional patients may be diagnosed by biopsy, where PAS-positive trophozoites or cysts may be found in the undermining ulcer in the lamina propria, or by a serum indirect hemagglutinating antibody (IHA) test, which is positive in approximately 90% of the patients with intestinal amebiasis.[115] Although the systemic amebicide metronidazole is effective in eradicating hepatic amebiasis and may eradicate intestinal disease, the iodoquinol may be required to eradicate intestinal infection. The therapy for balantidiasis is administration of tetracycline or iodoquinol. Praziquantel is used for significant schistosomal infections. The optimal therapies for *V. parahaemolyticus, Y. enterocolitica*, and *C. jejuni* infections are not well established and should be tailored to the specific sensitivity pattern of the organism isolated.

As with all diarrheas, the therapy for *Salmonella* gastroenteritis is supportive fluid management. With the apparent exception of ciprofloxacin,[110] oral antibiotics are of no benefit and may actually prolong shedding of the organism and even be associated with increased risk of relapse in children.[116, 117]

NECROTIZING ENTEROCOLITIS IN THE NEWBORN

The syndrome of diffuse fulminating necrotizing colitis has been increasingly recognized among infants since reports by Waldhausen and associates[118] in 1963 and Mizrahi and colleagues[119] in 1965. This syndrome probably represents the same entity described as "spontaneous" intestinal perforation and peritonitis as early as 1838.[120–122] Although milder forms of the syndrome doubtless exist, the syndrome of necrotizing enterocolitis (NEC) is defined by the presence of air in the wall of the intestine, portal venous system, or peritoneal cavity or by necrosis of the bowel wall with mucosal sloughing. This fulminant syndrome often leads to intestinal perforation, peritonitis, and bacteremia. It is a major cause of mortality in low-birth-weight infants ($<$1500 g) after the first week of life.[123] The diffuse necrotic changes that characterize this syndrome most often occur in the terminal ileum but may be seen in the colon or in the proximal portion of the gastrointestinal tract.

The pathogenesis of NEC appears to involve mucosal injury that is most often of ischemic origin from hypoxemic or hypotensive episodes that may occur in premature infants or in the presence of complicating factors such as an umbilical vein exchange transfusion. Ischemia may also result from the effects of endotoxemia followed by the effects of epinephrine, to which the vessels supplying the terminal ileum may be especially sensitive. Other factors predisposing to mucosal ischemia include asphyxia in association with hyaline membrane disease in premature infants or cyanotic heart disease. Increased intraluminal pressures may contribute to ischemia and pneumatosis, a process that may also play a role in previously normal infants who develop necrotizing colitis after protracted periods of diarrhea.[124] Some investigators have suggested a localized Shwartzman reaction to endotoxemia or gram-negative bacteria.[125] The absence of lysozyme (normally present in human breast milk) may allow overgrowth of gram-negative bacilli. McKay and Wahle[126] have reported the association of "enteropathogenic" *E. coli* serotype O111:B4 with NEC. Because of the association with use of umbilical vein polyvinylchloride catheters and feeding tubes, the toxic effect of plasticizers leached from the polyvinylchloride materials has been suggested.[127] Reports of outbreaks of NEC in newborn intensive care units[128–131] have led to a careful search for infectious agents including viral, fungal, or bacterial pathogens.[132–134] Among bacteria, *Pseudomonas, Klebsiella,*[132, 133] certain *E. coli* strains,[126, 135, 136] *Salmonella,*[137] and *Clostridium butyricum*[130] have been implicated. The roles of both ischemia and bacteria have been suggested by Barlow and colleagues[138] with work in an experimental rat model of NEC, in which breast milk was also shown to be protective. On the basis of acidic intraluminal pH (<5.0) and organic acids in human neonates with NEC,[139] increased numbers of lactose-fermenting *Klebsiella* organisms have been postulated to play a role in the pathogenesis.[140] Other investigators have suggested a role for platelet-activating factor (PAF),[141] and protection by superoxide dismutase or by endogenous nitric oxide.[141–143]

Clinical features of this serious condition in newborn infants include apneic spells, vomiting, abdominal distention, and occasionally bloody diarrhea. Most infants are less than 1 week of age, and there is an association with prematurity, maternal infections during delivery (such as amnionitis with prolonged post–ruptured membranes status), and exchange transfusion via the umbilical vein. There is no gender or seasonal predilection. The disease often progresses rapidly to intestinal perforation, shock, septicemia, and pneumatosis intestinalis. Air may also be evident in the portal venous system or biliary tract on plain roentgenograms. This syndrome is associated with a mortality rate that is often in excess of 70%.

The diagnosis of NEC should be considered in any premature infant with altered gastrointestinal function, abdominal distention, or apneic spells. Further investigation should include examination of the stool for occult blood and for the presence of reducing substances.[144] Plain abdominal roentgenograms may reveal air in the bowel wall, peritoneal cavity, or portal venous system, and there may be bloody diarrhea late in the course of the disease. Management must be initiated early and aggressively for any infant suspected of having NEC. Umbilical catheters should be removed, oral feeding should be stopped, and nasogastric aspiration should be initiated. Intravenous fluid therapy is of paramount importance. Laparotomy and excision of the necrotic bowel are often necessary and should be done aggressively if there is any evidence of peritonitis or obstruction.[145]

Prevention of NEC includes avoidance of risk factors and careful infection control measures in newborn intensive care units. Hypertonic elemental formulas have been implicated and should be avoided in high-risk patients.[146] NEC rarely occurs in breast-fed infants. Explanations of the advantage of human breast milk include the presence of lysozyme, antibodies, and cellular elements that may play a protective role against potential infectious agents. Although oral prophylactic nonabsorbable antibiotics have been suggested,[147] serious questions remain about the use of prophylactic antibiotics, even in high-risk newborn infants weighing less than 1500 g.[148]

DARMBRAND, PIG-BEL, NECROTIZING ENTERITIS IN ADULTS (ENTERITIS NECROTICANS)

First described as *Darmbrand* (meaning "fire bowels") in epidemics of enteritis necroticans in northern Germany in the immediate postwar period in the mid-1940s,[149] a severe necrotizing jejunitis has also been recognized in both epidemic and sporadic forms after pork feasting in the highlands of Papua New Guinea.[150] *Pig-bel* was the name given to the syndrome of abdominal discomfort that followed a large pork meal, commonly eaten after a large "pig kill," which takes place every 3 to 10 years among the highland Melanesians of Papua New Guinea. Sporadic cases have been reported from other parts of the world, including the United States.[151, 152]

The pathologic findings are those of acute patchy, necrotizing disease of the small bowel in previously healthy people that may proceed rapidly to segmental gangrene with small amounts of gas in the mucosa, mesentery, or nodes.

Several theories of pathogenesis have been suggested, most of which involve the toxic products of *Clostridium perfringens* type C, including α- and β-toxins. Sporadic cases of NEC have been noted in association with nutritional disorders, alcoholism, and malabsorption and after pancreatic or gastric resection.[153, 154] After gastric surgery, increased numbers of *C. perfringens* organisms and increased levels of α-toxin have been noted in the upper small bowel and stomach.[155] Whether α- or β-toxins are capable of causing the necrotizing enteritis alone or whether they initiate the invasion of the mucosa by other organisms such as gram-negative rods is currently unclear. An attractive hypothesis has been suggested by Lawrence and Walker[154] that could explain the association of necrotizing enteritis with poor nutrition and episodic dietetic overindulgence. The low-protein diet of Papua New Guinea highlanders is associated with low levels of digestive proteases in the intestinal lumen, which can be shown to inactivate the β-toxin. The proteases can be further blocked by the oral intake of trypsin inhibitors, which are found in such dietary staples as sweet potatoes in this population. Proteases return with improved diet,[156] as occurred in postwar Germany. This hypothesis has been confirmed in an animal model that required protease inhibitors for symptomatic infection.[157]

The clinical syndromes of necrotizing enteritis range from anorexia, vomiting, severe abdominal pain, and bloody diarrhea to fulminant toxemia and shock. Acute complications that necessitate emergency surgery include paralytic ileus, strangulation, and bowel perforation with peritonitis. These complications are common in the first 2 weeks of illness. Later complications that may also necessitate surgery include scarring leading to stenosis, obstruction, malabsorption, or fistulas. Necrotizing enteritis occurs with greater frequency and greater severity in children under 10 years of age. In contrast to European controls, 70% of the healthy adults in Papua New Guinea have demonstrable antibody to clostridial β-toxin.[150, 154]

The syndrome is defined by the pathologic findings but should be suspected in patients who develop severe abdominal pain, bloody diarrhea, ileus, and toxemia. The course is often too fulminant for radiographic detection of air in the bowel wall to be of any diagnostic value.

Etiologic agents held responsible for necrotizing enteritis include *C. perfringens* type C, once designated as type F in the older classification of *Clostridium welchii*. The majority of surgically resected bowel specimens from patients with necrotizing enteritis contain *C. perfringens*, over half of which are type C. Furthermore, 12 of 21 cases described had a significant change in serum β-antitoxin titer after illness with pig-bel in Papua New Guinea.[150] Although polyvalent gas gangrene antiserum was ineffective, administration of type C antiserum resulted in a 30% decrease in the need for surgery and a reduced mortality, from 43% to 19%.[150] Furthermore, active immunization against the β-toxin has also proved effective in preventing pig-bel.[158, 159]

Some authorities have suggested that type A *C. perfringens*, staphylococci, or even hepatitis virus may be responsible for necrotizing enteritis.[160] The syndrome of "enteritis gravis" has been described in association with infectious hepatitis, although no viral etiology has been documented.

Considerations in the differential diagnosis of necrotizing enteritis include acute shigellosis, acute food poisoning syndromes, antibiotic-associated pseudomembranous colitis, and acute ulcerative colitis. The absence of colonic involvement, the epidemiologic setting, especially in poorly nourished patients, and the rapid progression to toxemia and shock are strongly suggestive of necrotizing enteritis.

Therapy for NEC includes careful supportive care and bowel decompression. Fluid requirements may be substantially greater than what is indicated by fecal output. Resection of the involved bowel must be considered if there is a persistence of paralytic ileus, a rapid increase in signs of toxemia, localized or diffuse signs of peritonitis, persistent pain, or a palpable mass lesion. If subacute obstruction or malabsorption is suspected on the basis of weight loss, elective surgery may be required up to 6 months after the acute illness. Raw peanut or soybean diets should be avoided because they contain trypsin inhibitors. *C. perfringens* type C antiserum containing β-antitoxin or the active β-toxin vaccine should be available for use in areas where necrotizing enteritis may be expected to occur.

PSEUDOMEMBRANOUS ENTEROCOLITIS (*CLOSTRIDIUM DIFFICILE* COLITIS)

First reported by Coats[161] in 1883 and described by Finney[162] as postoperative diphtheritic enteritis in 1893, the syndrome of pseudomembranous enterocolitis has received increasing attention in recent years as different host and etiologic factors have been unraveled. Pettet and colleagues[163] characterized pseudomembranous enterocolitis as occurring typically 4 to 5 days after abdominal surgery, often for colonic obstruction due to a carcinoma. The association of pseudomembranous enterocolitis with antibiotics was first noted by Reiner and associates[164] in 1952. Although this disease occurred in the preantibiotic era in association with intestinal obstruction, surgery, uremia, pneumonia, myocardial infarction, and sepsis,[165, 166] most reports in the last 2 decades have identified an association with the administration of antimicrobial agents, especially those with a broad antianaerobic spectrum. Diarrhea constitutes a major side effect of many antibiotics. From 4 to 50% of the patients taking tetracycline, chloramphenicol, penicillin, ampicillin, lincomycin, or clindamycin will develop diarrhea. Furthermore, each of these antibiotics has also been associated with the potentially life-threatening pseudomembranous enterocolitis.

Pseudomembranous enterocolitis is defined by the proctoscopic appearance of small, 1- to 5-mm, raised, whitish-yellow plaques of "pseudomembrane" that may become confluent and that overlie an erythematous, minimally friable colonic mucosa (Fig. 85–2).[167] It is often necessary to remove a thick layer of mucus to identify the characteristic pseudomembrane. Ulcers and erosions as seen in amebic, bacillary, or ulcerative colitis are usually absent in pseudomembranous enterocolitis. The pseudomembrane is composed microscopically of epithelial debris, fibrin, and polymorphonuclear leukocytes and may be found on biopsy if the whole plaque is obtained.[168] The appearance of filling defects or "thumb-printing" on plain and barium roentgenograms is inconstant and not reliable for diagnosis.

The pathophysiology of *C. difficile* infections involves alterations of indigenous colonic flora by antimicrobial agents or anticancer chemotherapy and subsequent ingestion of spores and colonization by the organism, followed by release of the enterotoxin (toxin A is the major cause of intestinal effects of *C. difficile*). Recent studies indicate that toxin B, the cytotoxin, is also active in human colon, and both toxins stimulate a potent inflammatory response.[169, 170]

The cloning and sequencing of toxin A and B genes and the identification of the guanosine triphosphate (GTP)-binding protein Rho as their intracellular target represent major advances in our understanding of the mode of action of these toxins.[171] Important characteristics of *C. difficile* infection are the dramatic inflammatory and secretory effects seen in antibiotic-associated and pseudomembranous colitis. Several studies now support the concept that an interplay between lamina propria neuro-immune cells and intestinal epithelial cells may be crucial in the pathogenesis of this toxin-mediated inflammatory response.[172]

Although *Candida* often appears in the stools of patients taking broad-spectrum antibiotics and may be associated with diarrhea,[173] a double-blind, controlled trial of antifungal therapy failed to reduce

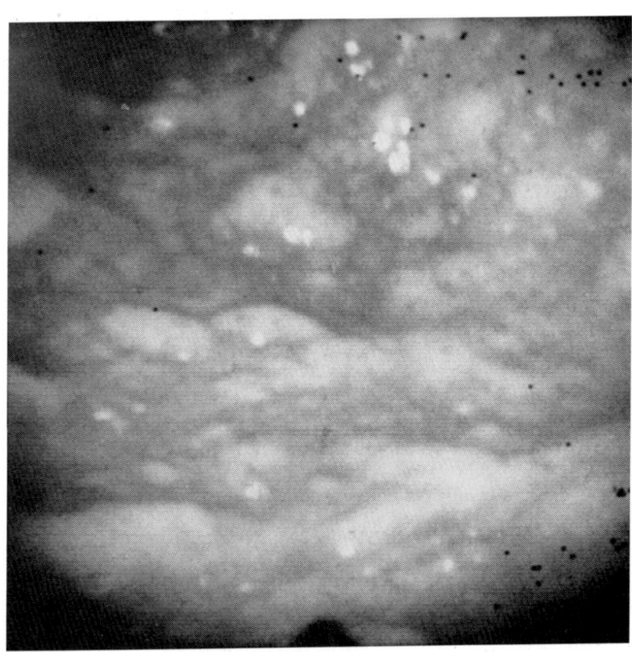

FIGURE 85–2. Proctoscopic view of pseudomembranous colitis in a patient who received clindamycin. Note the 4–8-mm raised, white plaques overlying an erythematous mucosa. (From Tedesco FJ, Barton RW, Alpers DH. Clindamycin-associated colitis. Ann Intern Med. 1974; 81:429.)

the high frequency of gastrointestinal symptoms with oral tetracycline.[174] Pseudomembranous colitis in humans and animals has been associated with overgrowth of staphylococci in the stool.[175, 176] Although there is debate about their role in causing colitis,[177] staphylococci are capable of producing a cytotoxic Δ-toxin that causes tissue destruction and cell damage and elicits a net secretory response in animal models.[178]

The onset of clinical illness is usually abrupt, often with fever and abdominal pain. Although most patients develop symptoms after receiving antibiotics for 4 to 9 days, several cases have been reported to begin 2 to 4 weeks after the discontinuation of clindamycin therapy. With early diagnosis discontinuation of treatment usually results in resolution of symptoms within 1 week. However, the continuation of the drug or the occurrence of colitis after a full course of antibiotic may lead to diarrhea of 6 to 10 weeks' duration that may cause severe electrolyte abnormalities and protein loss with significant mortality.

Therapy, after discontinuing treatment with the antibiotic, is mainly supportive. Most patients will improve within 1 week. The potential risk of *increased* diarrheal symptoms when antimotility drugs are used has been documented with lincomycin-associated colitis.[179] Metronidazole is usually used for treating pseudomembranous enterocolitis. Vancomycin should be used only when symptoms persist or worsen. The emergence of vancomycin-resistant enterococci also poses potential risks of excessive vancomycin use.[180] Antibiotic therapy is by far the most important risk factor for colonization and infection with *C. difficile*.[181] Thus, the three main elements of prevention are (1) restricing the overuse of antibiotics, (2) strict enteric precautions, and (3) meticulous cleaning of clinical areas.[182] (See Chapter 84 for a complete discussion of diagnosis and therapy.)

CHRONIC INFLAMMATORY PROCESSES

Chronic inflammatory enteritides are often indolent, slowly progressive infections. Often there is a history over weeks or months of fever, abdominal pain, weight loss, or other systemic manifestations. Recurring or relapsing symptoms may be seen with *C. jejuni* or *Salmonella* gastroenteritis. In addition, 16% of cases of shigellosis may become prolonged, lasting for 3 weeks or longer.[183] Any diarrheal illness that extends beyond 2 weeks is considered severe and is associated with a high risk of nutritional morbidity in children who live in tropical, developing areas.[184–186]

Enteropathogenic and Enteroaggregative *Escherichia coli*

Enteropathogenic *E. coli* organisms that cause acute diarrhea in infants by largely unknown mechanisms may rarely be associated with an insidious persistent or relapsing illness.[187] *E. coli* organisms in O groups 1, 2, 4, 7, and 75 that produce hemolysin and necrotoxin have been isolated from patients with ulcerative colitis. These toxic organisms were not present in healthy people or in patients with acute diarrheal syndromes.[188] In addition, enteroaggregative *E. coli* organisms are increasingly recognized as a cause of persistent diarrhea in India, Brazil, and Mexico.[189–191] Enteroaggregative *E. coli* (EAggEC) infections are an emerging problem, and enteropathogenic *E. coli* (EPEC) infections remain important in many parts of the world.[192] Enteroaggregative *E. coli* organisms have been associated with intestinal inflammation and malnutrition, even in the absence of diarrhea.[193] The effects of antibiotic treatment constitute a topic of current interest, and such therapy may be feasible.[194]

Syphilis

Syphilis can also involve the gastrointestinal tract, usually in the upper part of the small bowel or stomach. An acute erosive and infiltrative gastritis with motile spirochetes and a positive specific response on treponemal immunofluorescence testing has been reported in late secondary syphilis.[195] The initial complaints are upper abdominal pain, vomiting, and weight loss. More classic are the late gastrointestinal manifestations of lues: pyloric obstruction, "hourglass" constriction, and linitis plastica of the stomach. Less commonly, gumma may be seen in the small bowel or colon.

Gastrointestinal Tuberculosis

Intestinal tuberculosis, once considered common, had become a relatively rare disease but is now reemerging in association with acquired immunodeficiency syndrome (AIDS) and with multidrug-resistant tuberculosis.[196] Intestinal involvement with tuberculosis may be either *primary*, from ingestion of the organisms or from spread of miliary tuberculosis, or *secondary*, usually from a pulmonary source.

Primary intestinal tuberculosis without pulmonary disease often results in hypertrophic mucosal changes. Sixty-four percent of the cases of acute miliary tuberculosis may also have gastrointestinal involvement.[197] Patients with primary intestinal tuberculosis may present with abdominal pain, fever, and a tender, fixed palpable mass in the ileocecal area.[198] Primary hypertrophic intestinal tuberculosis continues to occur in the Near East[199] and in India,[200] where infection is most often due to the human strain *Mycobacterium tuberculosis*.[201]

Intestinal involvement secondary to pulmonary tuberculosis may result from swallowing infected sputum or from biliary excretion of the organism from an infected liver. The frequency of secondary intestinal tuberculosis increases to 25 to 80% with far-advanced pulmonary disease.[202] Hippocrates stated that "diarrhea attacking a person with phthisis is a mortal symptom."[203]

Tuberculosis may involve any part of the gastrointestinal tract, but most ulcerative and hypertrophic types occur in the ileocecal region, where there is a predominance of submucosal lymphatic tissue.[204] The most common features are fever and abdominal pain that is often relieved by defecation or vomiting. Weight loss is more common in secondary intestinal tuberculosis. Only one third of the patients with gastrointestinal tuberculosis have diarrhea. Diarrhea may be related to exacerbations of abdominal pain and occasionally occurs with extensive involvement of the small intestine, which may cause steatorrhea and a malabsorption syndrome. Although ulceration and mucous diarrhea are relatively common with secondary intestinal tuberculosis, hemorrhage and the presence of gross blood in the stool are distinctly uncommon, perhaps because of the associated obliterative endarteritis.

The diagnosis of gastrointestinal tuberculosis may be very difficult radiologically and even histologically. It must be distinguished from regional enteritis, sarcoidosis, actinomycosis, ameboma, carcinoma, and periappendiceal abscess. In contrast to Crohn's disease, gastrointestinal tuberculosis rarely causes anal lesions, fistulas, or perforation; it is often associated with miliary nodules on the serosa, rarely causes strictures longer than 3 cm, and may cause circumferential transverse ulcers. Tuberculosis may also cause fibrosis of the muscularis mucosa, pyloric metaplasia, and epithelial regeneration.[205] There may be minimal or no radiologic changes in the bowel mucosa. Small mucosal ulcerations may result in tiny calcified nodules in the mucosa in association with calcified mesenteric lymph nodes analogous to the pulmonary Ghon complex. The ileocecal region often reveals radiologic evidence of irritability and hypermotility, with hypersegmentation of the mucosal folds or poor filling of the ileocecal region detected by barium enema. Occasionally, frank ulcerations can be noted on contrast studies, and late in the course there is scarring. The diagnosis requires a careful examination of involved tissue for acid-fast bacilli by special stain and culture. Caseous necrosis is more frequently found in the mesenteric nodes than in intestinal tissue itself. Complications of intestinal tuberculosis include perforation, peritonitis, and obstruction from either hypertrophy, scarring, or tuberculoma.

Gastrointestinal Mycosis

Candida albicans can cause ulcerations in any part of the gastrointestinal tract.[206] Although shallow invasion of gastric or duodenal ulcers may have no obvious clinical consequence in the nonimmunosuppressed patient,[207] ulcerations anywhere from the distal third of the esophagus to the rectum may be deeply invaded and numerous in the neutropenic patient, constituting an important entry site for hematogenously disseminated candidiasis. Patients infected with human immunodeficiency virus type 1 (HIV-1) are prone to esophageal candidiasis, but dissemination from that site is rare.[208] Several reports have implicated *Candida* spp. as a cause of diarrhea.[209–211] Although *Candida* organisms may reach high concentrations in the stool of patients receiving antimicrobial agents, this agent has no established role in causing diarrhea.

Whereas gastrointestinal involvement with the North American blastomycosis is quite rare, South American blastomycosis (due to *Paracoccidioides brasiliensis*) is often manifested as lesions of the skin, oral mucosa, or intestinal tract, where it causes granulomatous or ulcerative disease.[212] The most common intestinal sites of involvement are the appendix, cecum, and anorectal areas. There is often abscess formation and lymphatic spread to regional nodes and to the spleen, the liver, or even the lungs. The major symptoms are abdominal pain and ulcerative, granulomatous lesions, especially in the oropharynx. Palpable, tender abdominal masses in the ileocecal region may be noted on physical examination. Peritoneal signs are often absent. Diagnosis is made by biopsy, stain, and culture of the ulcerative lesion.

Other fungi usually involve the intestinal tract as only one feature of disseminated granulomatous disease; some of these pathogens may be acquired through a gastrointestinal portal of entry. Phycomycetes (*Absidia, Rhizopus*, and *Mucor* spp.) may invade the predisposed host via the gastrointestinal tract,[213] or phycomycosis may involve the gastrointestinal tract by hematogenous spread and cause abdominal pain, diarrhea, gastrointestinal bleeding, and peritonitis.[214]

Histoplasmosis may also involve the intestinal tract as a part of disseminated infection. In the gastrointestinal tract, histoplasmosis is manifested as ulceration, bleeding, obstruction, or, rarely, protein-losing enteropathy.[215–217] Lesions tend to be single and may be considered initially to be neoplastic.

Parasitic Enteritis

Parasitic enteritides that should be considered among causes of chronic inflammatory bowel processes include coccidiosis, chronic or recurrent amebiasis, and the rare invasive, inflammatory form of giardiasis.

Human coccidiosis is an upper small bowel inflammatory process caused by *Isospora belli* that should be considered in patients with chronic diarrhea of obscure origin and eosinophilia,[218, 219] especially in AIDS patients.[209, 220] Weight loss, fever, headache, and colicky abdominal pain may also be present, with steatorrhea and malabsorption. This infection is common in Chile and has occurred in nontraveling U.S. residents. It probably often goes unrecognized. The causative unicellular sporazoan parasite undergoes asexual schizogony in the intestinal epithelial cells, from which merozoites are released. Like malarial plasmodia, merozoites may then invade other cells and repeat the asexual schizogony cycle or may mature into sexual gametocytes and form zygotes and then sporulated oocysts that rupture to yield sporozoites that restart the enterocyte cycle. Sporulated oocysts are the infective form and have caused laboratory-acquired infections. The diagnosis is made by careful examination of multiple serial sections of intestinal biopsy specimens for any stage of the parasite or by examining small bowel contents for oocysts. Stool oocysts may be seen after staining with a modified acid-fast stain as for *Cryptosporidium*[220] or may rarely be demonstrated with some difficulty by incubating a specimen at room temperature for 1 to 2 days to permit their maturation before examination using a concentration technique such as zinc sulfate flotation. Although many therapeutic agents have been used unsuccessfully (including quinacrine, nitrofurantoin, tetracycline, and metronidazole), sulfamethoxazole-trimethoprim or pyramethamine and sulfadiazine in combination have been effective even in AIDS patients, in whom multiple courses or suppressive therapy may be required.[219–221]

The related protozoan parasite *Cryptosporidium* is a cause of severe chronic diarrhea in immunosuppressed persons.[220, 222, 223] It may also cause diarrhea that is self-limited in normal people.[223] Unlike *Isospora* organisms, cryptosporidia usually infect only the surface of the mucosal epithelium, and the process is usually noninflammatory. The organism may be identified by sugar flotation or modified acid-fast stains of fecal specimens.[220, 224] A newly recognized sporozoan parasite, *Cyclospora* (these organisms are also called *cynobacterium-like bodies*) has also now been associated with persistent diarrhea in travelers, those living in tropical areas, health care workers, and AIDS patients.[225–227]

Invasive syndromes may occur over a long period of time or in a recurring pattern with intestinal amebiasis. This syndrome may even extend into an entity called *ulcerative postdysenteric colitis* that may no longer respond to antiamebic therapy.[228]

Inflammatory small bowel disease may occur with unusually severe *G. lamblia* infection. This may result in severe villus atrophy, with dense plasma cell infiltration and acute inflammation in the lamina propria.[229]

Considerations in the differential diagnosis of chronic inflammatory diarrhea include several syndromes of noninfectious or unknown causes. Idiopathic inflammatory bowel disease including regional enteritis, granulomatous colitis, and ulcerative colitis may be difficult to distinguish from infectious enteritides. Other conditions that often require biopsy and culture to exclude infectious processes include intestinal involvement with sarcoidosis, lymphoma, or carcinoma. Radiation enterocolitis, ischemic colitis, and diverticulitis may also be manifested as chronic inflammatory diarrhea.

REFERENCES

1. Keusch GT, Jacewicz M. The pathogenesis of *Shigella* diarrhea. V. Relationship of Shiga enterotoxin, neurotoxin and cytotoxin. J Infect Dis. 1975;131(Suppl):33.
2. Edelman R, Karmali MA, Fleming PA. Summary of the International Symposium and Workshop on Infections Due to Verocytotoxin (Shiga-like Toxin)-Producing *Escherichia coli*. J Infect Dis. 1988;157:1102–1104.
3. Blacklow NR, Dolin R, Fedson DS, et al. Acute infectious nonbacterial gastroenteritis: Etiology and pathogenesis. Ann Intern Med. 1972;76:993.
4. Rendtorff RC. The experimental transmission of human intestinal protozoan parasites. Am J Hyg. 1954;59:196.
5. Weissman JB, Schmerler A, Gangarosa EJ, et al. Shigellosis in day-care centres. Lancet. 1975;1:88.
6. Roy SK, Speelman P, Butler T, et al. Diarrhea associated with typhoid fever. J Infect Dis. 1985;151:1138–1143.
7. Quinn TC, Stamm WE, Goodell SE, et al. The polymicrobial origin of intestinal infections in homosexual men. N Engl J Med. 1983;309:576.
8. Korzeniowski OM, Barada FA, Rouse JD, et al. Value of examination for fecal leukocytes in the early diagnosis of shigellosis. Am J Trop Med Hyg. 1979;28:1031.
9. Pickering LK, DuPont HL, Olarte J, et al. Fecal leukocytes in enteric infections. Am J Clin Pathol. 1977;68:562–565.
10. Haugwout FG. The microscopic diagnosis of the dysenteries at their onset. JAMA. 1924;83:1156.
11. Guerrant RL, Brush JE, Ravdin JI, et al. Interaction between *Entamoeba histolytica* and human polymorphonuclear neutrophils. J Infect Dis. 1981;143:83–93.
12. Speelman P, McGlaughlin R, Kabir I, et al. Differential clinical features and stool findings in shigellosis and amebic dysentery. Trans R Soc Trop Med Hyg. 1987;81:549–551.
13. Rahaman MM, Khan MM, Azi KMS, et al. An outbreak of dysentery caused by *Shigella dysenteriae* type I on a coral island in the Bay of Bengal. J Infect Dis. 1975;132:15.
14. Feeley JC, Balows A. *Vibrio*. In: Lennette EH, Spaulding EH, Truant JP, eds. Manual of Clinical Microbiology. Washington, DC: American Society for Microbiology; 1974;238–245.
15. Morris GK, Feeley JC, Martin WT, et al. Isolation and identification of *Yersinia enterocolitica*. Public Health Lab. 1977;35:217.
16. Skirrow MB. *Campylobacter enteritis*: A "new" disease. BMJ. 1972;2:9.
17. Lyerly DM, Krivan HC, Wilkins TD. *Clostridium difficile*: Its disease and toxins. J Clin Microbiol. 1988;1:1–18.
18. Doern GV, Coughlin RT, Wu L. Laboratory diagnosis of *Clostridium difficile*–associated gastrointestinal disease: Comparison of a monoclonal antibody enzyme immunoassay for toxins A and B with a monoclonal antibody enzyme immunoassay for toxin A only and two cytotoxicity assays. J Clin Microbiol. 1992;30;2042–2046.
19. Lima AAM, Lyerly DM, Wilkins TD, et al. Effects of *Clostridium difficile* toxins A and B in rabbit small and large intestine *in vitro* and on cultured cells *in vitro*. Infect Immun. 1988;56:582–588.
20. Lindberg AA, Pal T. Strategies for development of potential candidate *Shigella* vaccines. Vaccine. 1993;11:168–179.
21. Townes JM, Quick R, Gonzales OY, et al. Etiology of bloody diarrhea in Bolivian children: Implications for empiric therapy. J Infect Dis. 1997;175:1527–1530.
22. Struelens MJ, Mondal G, Roberts M, et al. Role of bacterial and host factors in the pathogenesis of *Shigella* septicemia. Eur J Clin Microbiol Infect Dis. 1990;9:337–344.
23. Bennish ML, Salam MA, Wahed MA. Enteric protein loss during shigellosis. Am J Gastroenterol. 1993;88:53–57.
24. Black RE, Brown KH, Becker S. Effects of diarrhea associated with specific enteropathogens on the growth of children in rural Bangladesh. Pediatrics. 1984;73:799–805.
25. Henry FJ, Alam N, Aziz KMS, et al. Dysentery, not watery diarrhea, is associated with stunting in Bangladeshi children. Hum Nutr Clin Nutr. 1987;41C:243–249.
26. Koster F, Levin J, Walker L, et al. Hemolytic uremic syndrome after shigellosis. Relation to endotoxemia and circulating immune complexes. N Engl J Med 1978;298:927.
27. Bennish ML, Azad AK, Yousefzadeh D. Intestinal obstruction during shigellosis: Incidence, clinical features, risk factors, and outcome. Gastroenterology. 1991;101:626–634.
28. Barrett-Connor E, Connor JD. Extraintestinal manifestations of shigellosis. Am J Gastroenterol. 1970;53:234.
29. Keusch GT, Grady GF, Mata LJ, et al. The pathogenesis of *Shigella* diarrhea. I. Enterotoxin production by *Shigella dysenteriae* 1. J Clin Invest. 1972;51:1212.
30. Calin A, Fries JF. An "experimental" epidemic of Reiter's syndrome revisited. Follow-up evidence on genetic and environmental factors. Ann Intern Med. 1976;84:564.
31. Aho K, Ahvonen P, Alkio P, et al. HLA-27 in reactive arthritis following infection. Ann Rheum Dis. 1975;34(Suppl):29.
32. Trabulsi LR, Fernandes MFR, Zuliani ME. Noval bacterias pathogenicas para o intestino do homn. Rev Inst Med Trop Sao Paulo. 1967;9:31.
33. Hayward RS, Wensel RH, Kibsey P. Relapsing *Clostridium difficile*, colitis and Reiter's syndrome. Am J Gastroenterol. 1990;85:752–756.
34. Mermel LA, Osborn TG. *Clostridium difficile* associated reactive arthritis in an HLA-B27 positive female: Report and literature review. J Rheumatol. 1989;16:133–135.
35. Ørskov F. Virulence factors of the bacterial cell surface. J Infect Dis. 1978;137:630.
36. Levine MM. *Escherichia coli* that cause diarrhea: Enterotoxigenic, enteropathogenic, enteroinvasive, enterohemorrhagic, and enteroadherent. J Infect Dis. 1987;155:377–389.
37. Tulloch EF Jr, Ryan KJ, Formal SB, et al. Invasive enteropathic *Escherichia coli* dysentery. An outbreak in 28 adults. Ann Intern Med. 1973;79:13.

38. Sereny B. Experimental shigella keratoconjunctivitis: A preliminary report. Acta Microbiol Acad Sci Hung. 1955;2:293.
39. DuPont HL, Formal SB, Hornick R. Pathogenesis of *E. coli* diarrhea. N Engl J Med. 1971;285:1–9.
40. Harris JR, Wachsmuth IK, Davis BF, et al. High molecular weight plasmid correlates with *E. coli* enteroinvasiveness. Infect Immun. 1982;37:1295–1298.
41. Sansonetti PS, d'Hauteville H, Ecobiochon C. Molecular comparison of virulence in *Shigella* and enteroinvasive *E. coli* (Abstract). Ann Microbiol (Paris). 1983;134:295–318.
42. Silva RM, Toledo MRF, Trabulsi LR. Correlations of invasiveness with plasmids in enteroinvasive strains of *E. coli*. J Infect Dis. 1982;146:706.
43. Marier R, Wells JG, Swanson RC, et al. An outbreak of enteropathogenic *Escherichia coli* foodborne disease traced to imported French cheese. Lancet. 1973;2:1376.
44. DuPont HL, Formal SB, Hornick RB, et al. Pathogenesis of *Escherichia coli* diarrhea. N Engl J Med. 1971;285:1.
45. Silva RM, Toledo MRF, Trabulsi LF. Biochemical and cultural characteristics of invasive *Escherichia coli*. J Clin Microbiol. 1980;11:441.
46. Pal T, Pasca S, Emody L, et al. Antigenic relationship among virulent enteroinvasive *E. coli, Shigella flexneri* and *Shigella sonnei* detected by ELISA. Lancet. 1983;2:102.
47. O'Brien AD, Newland JW, Miller SF, et al. Shiga-like toxin–converting phages from *Escherichia coli* strains that cause hemorrhagic colitis or infantile diarrhea. Science. 1984;226:694–696.
48. Riley LW, Remis RS, Helgerson SD, et al. Outbreak of hemorrhagic colitis associated with a rare *E. coli* serotype. N Engl J Med. 1983;308:681–685.
49. Griffin PM, Tauxe RV. The epidemiology of infections caused by *Escherichia coli* O157:H7, other enterohemorrhagic *E. coli*, and the associated hemolytic uremic syndrome. Epidemiol Rev. 1991;13:60–98.
50. Centers for Disease Control and Prevention. Preliminary Report: Foodborne outbreak of *Escherichia coli* O157:H7 infections from hamburgers—western United States, 1993. MMWR. 1993;42:85–86.
51. Pai CH, Ahmed N, Lior H, et al. Epidemiology of sporadic diarrhea due to verocytotoxin-producing *Escherichia coli*: A two-year prospective study. J Infect Dis. 1988;157:1054–1057.
52. Moon HW. Comparative histopathology of intestinal infections. Adv Exp Med Biol. 1997;412:1–19.
53. Obrig TG. *Shiga* toxin mode of action in *E. coli* O157:H7 disease. Front Biosci. 1997;2:D635–D642.
54. Orskov I, Wachsmuth IK, Taylor DN, et al. Two new *Escherichia coli* O groups: O172 from "Shiga-like" toxin II–producing strains (EHEC) and O173 from enteroinvasive E. coli (EIEC). Acta Patho Microbiol Immunol Scand. 1991;99:30–32.
55. Obrig TG, Moran TP, Brown JE. The mode of action of shigatoxin on peptide elongation of eukaryotic protein synthesis. Biochem J. 1987;244:287–294.
56. Takeda Y, Yutsudo T, Igarashi K, et al. Mode of action of Vero toxins (VT1 and VT2) from *Escherichia coli* and of Shiga toxin. Williamsburg, Va: Twenty-third US–Japan Joint Conference on Cholera; 1987:104.
57. Guerrant RL, Lahita RG, Winn WC, et al. Campylobacteriosis in man: Pathogenic mechanisms and review of 91 bloodstream infections. Am J Med. 1978;65:584.
58. Doyle LP. A vibrio associated with swine dysentery. Am J Vet Res. 1944;5:3.
59. Dekeyser P, Gossuin-Detrain M, Butzler JP, et al. Acute enteritis due to related *Vibrio*: First positive stool cultures. J Infect Dis. 1972;125:390.
60. Butzler JP, Dekeyser P, Detrain M, et al. Related vibrio in stools. J Pediatr. 1973;82:493.
61. Blaser MJ, Reller LB. *Campylobacter* enteritis. N Engl J Med. 1981;305:1444.
62. Scott DA. Vaccines against *Campylobacter jejuni*. J Infect Dis 1997;2:S183–S188.
63. DeMol P, Bosmans E. *Campylobacter* enteritis in Central Africa. Lancet. 1978;1:604.
64. Perez-Perez GL, Cohn DL, Guerrant RL, et al. Clinical and immunologic significance of choleralike toxin and cytotoxin production by *Campylobacter* species in patients with acute inflammatory diarrhea in the USA. J Infect Dis. 1989;160:460–467.
65. Jackson TF. *Entamoeba histolytica* and *Entamoeba dispar* are distinct species; clinical, epidemiological and serological evidence. Int J Parasitol. 1998;1:181–186.
66. Ravdin JI, Croft BY, Guerrant RL. Cytopathologic mechanisms of *Entamoeba histolytica*. J Exp Med. 1980;152:377.
67. Lynch EC, Rosenberg IM, Gitler C. An ion-channel forming protein produced by *Entamoeba histolytica*. EMBO J. 1982;1:801.
68. Young JDE, Young TM, Lu LP, et al. Characterization of a membrane pore-forming protein from *Entamoeba histolytica*. J Exp Med. 1982;156:1677.
69. Ravdin JI, Guerrant RL. A review of the parasite cellular mechanisms involved in the pathogenesis of amebiasis. Rev Infect Dis. 1982;4:1185–1207.
70. Wittner M, Rosenbaum RM, Role of bacteria in modifying virulence of *Entamoeba histolytica*: Studies of amebae from axenic cultures. Am J Trop Med Hyg. 1970;19:755.
71. Bracha R, Mirelman D. Virulence of *Entamoeba histolytica* trophozoites. Effects of bacteria, microaerobic conditions and metronidazole. J Exp Med. 1984;160:353.
72. Petri WA Jr, Chapman MD, Snodgrass T, et al. Subunit structure of the galactose and *N*-acetyl-D-galactosamine–inhibitable adherence lectin of *Entamoeba histolytica*. J Biol Chem. 1989;264:3007–3012.
73. Krogstad DJ, Spencer HC Jr, Healy GR, et al. Amebiasis: Epidemiologic studies in the United States, 1971–1974. Ann Intern Med. 1978;88:89.
74. Takahashi T, Gamboa-Dominguez A, Gomez-Mendez TJ, et al. Fulminant amebic colitis: Analysis of 55 cases. Dis Colon Rectum. 1997;40:1362–1367.
75. Blake PA. Disease of humans (other than cholera) caused by vibrios. Annu Rev Microbiol. 1980;34:341.
76. Morris JG, Black RE. Cholera and other vibrioses in the United States. N Engl J Med. 1985;312:343.
77. Hughes JM, Boyce JM, Aleen ARMA, et al. *Vibrio parahemoliticus* enterocolitis in Bangladesh: Report of an outbreak. Am J Trop Med Hyg. 1978;27:106.
78. Bolen JL, Zamiska SA, Greenough WB III. Clinical features in enteritis due to *Vibrio parahemolyticus*. Am J Med. 1974;57:638.
79. Barker WH. *Vibrio parahemolyticus* outbreaks in the United States. Lancet. 1974;1:551.
80. Blake PA, Merson MH, Weaver RE, et al. Disease caused by a marine vibrio: Clinical characteristics and epidemiology. N Engl J Med. 1979;300:1.
81. Mandal BK, Mani V. Colonic involvement in salmonellosis. Lancet. 1976;1:887.
82. Thomas M, Tillett H. Colonic involvement in salmonellosis. Lancet. 1976;1:1129.
83. Boyd JF. Colonic involvement in salmonellosis. Lancet. 1976;1:1415.
84. Appelbaum PC, Scragg J, Schonland MM. Colonic involvement in salmonellosis. Lancet. 1976;2:102.
85. Radsel-Medvescek A, Zargi R, Acko M, et al. Colonic involvement in salmonellosis. Lancet. 1977;1:601.
86. Rowland HAK. The complications of typhoid fever. J Trop Med Hyg. 1961;64:143.
87. Sonnenwirth AC, Weaver RE. *Yersinia enterocolitica*. N Engl J Med. 1970;283:1468.
88. Black RE, Jackson RJ, Tsai T, et al. Epidemic *Yersinia enterocolitica* infection due to contaminated chocolate milk. N Engl J Med. 1978;298:76.
89. Leino R, Kalliomaki JL. Yersiniosis as an internal disease. Ann Intern Med. 1974;81:458.
90. Ahvonen P. Human yersiniosis in Finland. II. Clinical features. Ann Clin Res. 1972;4:39.
91. Rabson AR, Hallett AF, Koornhof HJ. Generalized *Yersinia enterocolitica* infection. J Infect Dis. 1975;131:447.
92. Bradford WD, Noce PS, Gutman LT. Pathologic features of enteric infection with *Yersinia enterocolitica*. Arch Pathol. 1974;98:7.
93. Kilpatrick AM. Medical intelligence—current concepts: Gonorrheal proctitis. N Engl J Med. 1972;287:967.
94. Klein EJ, Fisher LS, Chow AW. Anorectal gonococcal infection. Ann Intern Med. 1977;86:340.
95. Quinn TC, Stamm WE, Gardell SE. The polymicrobial etiology of intestinal infections in homosexual men. N Engl J Med. 1983;309:576–582.
96. Dantec LE. Dysenterie spirillaire. C R Soc Biol. 1903;55:617.
97. Lee FD, Kraszewski A, Gordon J, et al. Intestinal spirochaetosis. Gut. 1971;12:126.
98. Jensen NS, Casey TA, Stanton TB. Detection and identification of *Treponema hyodysenteriae* by using oligodeoxynucleotide probes complementary to 16S rRNA. J Clin Microbiol. 1990;28:2717–2721.
99. Stermer E, Levy N, Potasman I, et al. Brucellosis as a cause of severe colitis. Am J Gastroenterol. 1991;86:917–919.
100. Krajden M. Brown M, Petrasek A, et al. Clinical features of adenovirus enteritis: A review of 127 cases. Pediatr Infect Dis J. 1990;9:636–641.
101. Janoff EN, Orenstein JM, Manischewitz JF, et al. Adenovirus colitis in the acquired immunodeficiency syndrome. Gastroenterology. 1991;100:976–979.
102. Guerrant RL, Araujo V, Cooper WH, et al. Measurement of fecal lactoferrin as a marker of fecal leukocytes and inflammatory enteritis. J Clin Microbiol. 1992;30:1238–1242.
103. Nataro JP. Treatment of bacterial enteritis. Pediatr Infect Dis. 1998;17:420–421.
104. Haltalin KC, Nelson JD, Ring R III, et al. Double-blind treatment study of shigellosis comparing ampicillin, sulfadiazine, and placebo. J Pediatr. 1967;70:970.
105. Tong MJ, Martin DG, Cunningham JJ, et al. Clinical and bacteriological elevation of antibiotic treatment in shigellosis. JAMA. 1970;214:1841.
106. Barada FA, Guerrant RL. Sulfamethoxazole-trimethoprim versus ampicillin in treatment of acute invasive diarrhea in adults. Antimicrob Agents Chemother. 1980;17:961.
107. Farrar WE Jr, Eidson M: Antibiotic resistance to *Shigella* mediated by R factors. J Infect Dis. 1971;123:477.
108. Ross S, Controni G, Khan W. Resistance of shigellae to ampicillin and other antibiotics. Its clinical and epidemiological implications. JAMA. 1972;221:45.
109. Salam MA, Dhar U, Khan WA, Bennish ML. Randomised comparison of ciprofloxacin suspension and pivmecillinam for childhood shigellosis. Lancet. 1998;352:522–527.
110. Pichler HET, Diridl G, Stickler K, et al. Clinical efficacy of ciprofloxacin compared with placebo in bacterial diarrhea. Am J Med. 1987;82(Suppl 4A):329–332.
111. DuPont HL, Ericsson CD, Robinson A, et al. Current problems in antimicrobial therapy for bacterial enteric infection. Am J Med. 1987;82(Suppl 4A):324–328.
112. Neill MA, Opal SM, Heelan J, et al. Failure of ciprofloxacin to eradicate convalescent fecal excretion after acute salmonellosis: Experience during an outbreak in health care workers. Ann Intern Med. 1991;114:195–199.
113. Kuschner RA, Trofa AF, Thomas RJ, et al. Use of azithromycin for the treatment of *Campylobacter* enteritis in travelers to Thailand, an area where ciprofloxacin resistance is prevalent. Clin Infect Dis. 1995;21:536–541.
114. Hossain S, Biswas R, Kabir I, et al. Single dose vitamin A treatment in acute shigellosis in Bangladesh children: Randomised double blind controlled trial. BMJ. 1998;316:422–426.
115. Healy GR. Laboratory diagnosis of amebiasis. Bull NY Acad Med. 1971;47:478.
116. Aserkoff B, Bennett JV. Effect of antibiotic therapy in acute salmonellosis on the fecal excretion of salmonellae. N Engl J Med. 1969;281:636.
117. Nelson JD, Jusmiesz H, Jackson LH, et al. Treatment of *Salmonella* gastroenteritis with ampicillin, amoxicillin or placebo. Pediatrics. 1980;65:1125.

118. Waldhausen JA, Herendeen T, King H. Necrotizing colitis of the newborn: Common cause of perforation of the colon. Surgery. 1963;54:365.
119. Mizrahi A, Barlow O, Berdon W, et al. Necrotizing enterocolitis in premature infants. J Pediatr. 1965;66:697.
120. Simpson JY. Peritonitis in the fetus in uterus. Edinb Med Surg J. 1838;15:390.
121. Genersich A. Bauchfellentzondung beim Neugeboreneh in Folg von Perforation des Ileums. Arch Pathol Anat. 1891;126:485.
122. Thelander HE. Perforation of the gastrointestinal tract of the newborn infant. Am Dis J Child. 1939;58:371.
123. Wilson R, Kanto WP, McCarthy BJ, et al. Epidemiologic characteristics of necrotizing enterocolitis: A population-based study. Am J Epidemiol. 1981;114:880.
124. Fairborn RA. Etiology os necrotizing enterocolitis. Lancet. 1977;1:956.
125. Hermann RE. Perforation of the colon from necrotizing colitis in the newborn: Report of a survival and new etiologic concept. Surgery. 1965;58:436.
126. McKay DG, Wahle GH. Epidemic gastroenteritis due to *Escherichia coli* O111B4. Arch Pathol. 1955;60:679.
127. Rogers AF, Dunn PM. Intestinal perforation, exchange transfusion and P.V.C. Lancet. 1969;2:1246.
128. Virnig NL, Reynolds JW. Epidemiological aspects of neonatal necrotizing enterocolitis. Am J Dis Child. 1974;128:186.
129. Book LS, Overall JC, Herbst JJ, et al. Clustering of necrotizing enterocolitis. Interruption by infection-control measures. N Engl J Med. 1977;297:984.
130. Howard FM, Flynn DM, Bradley JM, et al. Outbreak of necrotizing enterocolitis caused by *Clostridium butyricum*. Lancet. 1977;2:1099.
131. Ryder RW, Buxton AE, Wachsmuth IK. Heat-stable enterotoxigenic *Escherichia coli* and necrotizing enterocolitis: Lack of an association. J Pediatr. 1977;91:302.
132. Olarte J, Ferguson WW, Henderson NI, et al. *Klebsiella* strains isolated from diarrheal infants. Am J Dis Child. 1961;101:763.
133. Frantz ID, L'Heureux P, Engel RR, et al. Necrotizing enterocolitis. J Pediatr. 1975;86:259.
134. Levin SE, Isaacson C. Spontaneous perforation of the colon in the newborn infant. Arch Dis Child. 1960;35:378.
135. Speer ME, Taber LH, Yow MD, et al. Fulminant neonatal sepsis and necrotizing enterocolitis associated with a "nonenteropathogenic" strain of *Escherichia coli*. J Pediatr. 1976;89:91.
136. Drucker MM, Polliack A, Yeivin R, et al. Immunofluorescent demonstration of enteropathogenic *Escherichia coli* in tissue of infants dying with enteritis. Pediatrics. 1970;46:855.
137. Stein H, Beck J, Solomon A, et al. Gastroenteritis with necrotizing enterocolitis in premature babies. BMJ. 1972;2:616.
138. Barlow B, Santulli TV, Heird WC, et al. An experimental study of acute neonatal enterocolitis—the importance of breast milk. J Pediatr Surg. 1974;9:587.
139. Clark DA, Thompson JE, Weiner LB, et al. Necrotizing enterocolitis: Intraluminal biochemistry in human neonates and a rabbit model. Pediatr Res. 1985;19:919–921.
140. Carbonaro CA, Clark DA, Elseviers D. A bacterial pathogenicity determinant associated with necrotizing enterocolitis. Microb Pathogen. 1988;5:427–436.
141. Miller MJ, McNeill H, Mullane KM. SOD prevents damage and attenuates eicosanoid release in a rabbit model of necrotizing enterocolitis. Am J Physiol. 1988;255:G556–G565.
142. Clark DA, Fornabaio DM, McNeill H, et al. Contribution of oxygen-derived free radicals to experimental necrotizing enterocolitis. Am J Pathol. 1988;130:537–542.
143. MacKendrick W, Caplan M, Hsueh W. Endogenous nitric oxide protects against platelet-activating factor–induced bowel injury in the rat. Pediatr Res. 1993;34:222–228.
144. Book LS, Herbst JJ, Jung AL: Carbohydrate malabsorption in necrotizing enterocolitis. Pediatrics. 1975;57:201.
145. Stevenson JK, Oliver TK, Graham CB, et al. Aggressive treatment of neonatal necrotizing enterocolitis: Thirty-eight patients with 25 survivors. J Pediatr Surg. 1971;6:28.
146. Book LS, Herbst JJ, Atherton SO, et al. Necrotizing enterocolitis in low-birth-weight infants fed on elemental formula. J Pediatr. 1975;87:602.
147. Egan EA, Mantilla G, Nelson RM, et al. A prospective controlled trial of oral kanamycin in the prevention of neonatal necrotizing enterocolitis. J Pediatr. 1976;89:467.
148. Nelson JD. Commentary. J Pediatr. 1976;89:471.
149. Hansen K, Jeckeln E, Jochims J, et al. Darmbrand-Enteritis Necroticans. Stuttgart: Georg Thieme Verlag; 1949.
150. Murrell TGC, Roth L, Egerton J, et al. Pig-bel: Enteritis necroticans. Lancet. 1966;1:217.
151. Patterson M, Rosenbaum HD. Enteritis necroticans. Gastroenterology. 1952;21:110.
152. Fick KA, Wolken AP. Necrotic jejunitis. Lancet. 1949;1:519.
153. Williams MR, Pullan JM. Necrotising enteritis following gastric surgery. Lancet. 1953;2:1013.
154. Lawrence G, Walker PD. Pathogenesis of enteritis necroticans in Papua New Guinea. Lancet. 1976;1:125.
155. Howie JW, Duncan IBR, Mackie LM. Growth of *Clostridium welchii* in the stomach after partial gastrectomy. Lancet. 1953;2:1018.
156. Kumar R, Banks PA, George PK, et al. Early recovery of exocrine pancreatic function in adult protein-calorie malnutrition. Gastroenterology. 1975;68:1593.
157. Lawrence G, Coake R. Experimental pigbel: The production and pathology of necrotizing enteritis due to *Clostridium welchii* type C in the guinea pig. Br J Exp Pathol. 1980;61:261–271.
158. Lawrence G, Shann F, Frestone DS, et al. Prevention of necrotising enteritis in Papua New Guinea by active immunization. Lancet. 1979;1:227–230.
159. Lawrence GW, Lehmann D, Anian G, et al. Impact of active immunization against enteritis necroticans in Papua New Guinea. Lancet. 1990;336:1165–1167.
160. Kravetz RE, Brazenas NV. Viral hepatitis associated with enteritis gravis. Arch Intern Med. 1963;112:179.
161. Coats J. A Manual of Pathology. Philadelphia: Henry C Lea's Sons; 1883:567.
162. Finney JMT. Gastroenterostomy for cicatrizing ulcer of the pylorus. Bull Johns Hopkins Hosp. 1893;4:53.
163. Pettet JD, Baggenstoss AH, Dearing WH, et al. Postoperative pseudomembranous enterocolitis. Surg Gynecol Obstet. 1954;98:546.
164. Reiner L, Schlesinger MJ, Miller GM. Pseudomembranous colitis following aureomycin and chloramphenicol. Arch Pathol. 1952;54:39.
165. Hardaway RM, McKay DG. Pseudomembranous enterocolitis. Are antibiotics wholly responsible? Arch Surg. 1959;78:446.
166. Goulston SJM, McGovern VJ. Pseudo-membranous colitis. Gut. 1965;6:207.
167. Tedesco FJ, Barton RW, Alpers DH. Clindamycin-associated colitis. Ann Intern Med. 1974;81:429.
168. Summer HW, Tedesco FJ. Rectal biopsy in clindamycin-associated colitis. Arch Pathol. 1975;99:237.
169. Rocha MF, Maia ME, Bezerra LR, et al. *Clostridium difficile* toxin A induces the release of neutrophil chemotactic factors from rat peritoneal macrophages: Role of interleukin-1 beta, tumor necrosis factor alpha, and leukotrienes. Infect Immun. 1997;65:2740–2746.
170. Souza MH, Melo-Filho AA, Rocha MF, et al. The involvement of macrophage-derived tumor necrosis factor and lipoxygenase products on the neutrophil recruitment induced by *Clostridium difficile* toxin B. Immunology. 1997;91:281–288.
171. Pothoulakis C. Pathogenesis of *Clostridium difficile*–associated diarrhea. Eur J Gastroenterol Hepatol. 1996;8:1041–1047.
172. Guerrant RL, Lima AAM, Thielman NM, et al. Diarrhea, demography and cell signaling: Lessons from microbial toxins. Am Clin Climat Assn. 1997;108:149–164.
173. Kane JG, Chretien JH, Garagusi VF. Diarrhoea caused by *Candida*. Lancet. 1976;1:335.
174. Comparisons of side-effects of tetracycline and tetracycline plus nystatin. Report of the Research Committee of the British Tuberculosis Association by the Clinical Trials Subcommittee. BMJ. 1968;4:411.
175. Dearing WH, Baggenstoss AH, Weed LA. Studies on the relationship of *Staphylococcus aureus* to pseudomembranous enteritis and to postantibiotic enteritis. Gastroenterology. 1960;38:441.
176. Bennett IL, Wood JS Jr, Yardley JH. Staphylococcal pseudomembraneous enterocolitis in chinchillas: A clinico-pathologic study. Trans Assoc Am Physicians. 1956;69:116.
177. Bartlett JG, Chang TW, Taylor NS, et al. Colitis induced by *Clostridium difficile*. Rev Infect Dis. 1979;1:370.
178. Kapral FA, O'Brien AD, Ruff PD, et al. Inhibition of water absorption in the intestine by *Staphylococcus aureus* delta toxin. Infect Immun. 1976;13:140.
179. Novak E, Lee JG, Seckman CE, et al. Unfavorable effect of atropine-diphenoxylate (Lomotil) therapy in lincomycin caused diarrhea. JAMA. 1976;235:1451.
180. Frieden TR, Munsiff SS, Low DE, et al. Emergence of vancomycin-resistant enterococci in New York City. Lancet. 1993;342:76–79.
181. Jumaa P, Wren B, Tabaqchali S. Epidemiology and typing of *Clostridium difficile*. Eur J Gastroenterol Hepatol. 1996;8:1035–1040.
182. Worsley MA. Infection control and prevention of *Clostridium difficile* infection. J Antimicrob Chemother. 1998;41(Suppl):C59–C66.
183. Black RE, Merson MH, Rahaman SMM, et al. Prospective study of bacterial, viral, and parasitic agents associated with diarrhea in rural Bangladesh. J Infect Dis. 1980;142:660.
184. McAuliffe JF, Shields DS, de Souza MA, et al. Prolonged and recurring diarrhea in the northeast of Brazil: Examination of cases from a community-based study. J Pediatr Gastroenterol Nutr. 1986;5:902–906.
185. Schorling JB, Wanke CA, Schorling SK, et al. A prospective study of persistent diarrhea among children in an urban Brazilian slum. Am J Epidemiol. 1990;132:144–156.
186. Guerrant RL, Schorling JB, McAuliffe JF, et al. Diarrhea as a cause and effect of malnutrition: Diarrhea prevents catch-up growth and malnutrition increases diarrhea frequency and duration. Am J Trop Med Hyg. 1992;47:28–35.
187. Nelson JD, Haltalin KC. Accuracy of diagnosis of bacterial diarrheal disease by clinical features. J Pediatr. 1971;78:519.
188. Cooke EM. Properties of strains of *Escherichia coli* isolated from the feces of patients with ulcerative colitis, patients with acute diarrhea and normal persons. J Pathol Bacteriol. 1968;95:101.
189. Bhan MK, Raj P, Levine MM, et al. Enteroaggregative *Escherichia coli* associated with persistent diarrhea in a cohort of rural children in India. J Infect Dis. 1989;159:1061–1064.
190. Wanke CA, Schorling JB, Barrett LJ, et al. Adherence traits of *Escherichia coli*, alone and in association with other stool pathogens: Potential role in pathogenesis of persistent diarrhea in an urban Brazilian slum. Pediatr J Infect Dis. 1991;10:746–751.
191. Carvioto A, Tello A, Navarro A, et al. Association of *Escherichia coli* Hep-2 adherence patterns with type and duration of diarrhoea. Lancet. 1991;337:262–264.
192. Nataro JP, Kaper JB. Diarrheagenic *Escherichia coli*. Clin Microbiol Rev. 1998;11:142–201.
193. Steiner TS, Lima AA, Nataro JP, Guerrant RL. Enteroaggregative *Escherichia coli* produce intestinal inflammation and growth impairment and cause interleukin-8 release from intestinal epithelial cells. J Infect Dis. 1998;177:88–96.
194. Wanke CA, Mayer H, Weber R, et al. Enteroaggregative *Escherichia coli* as a

potential cause of diarrheal disease in adults infected with human immunodeficiency virus. J Infect Dis. 1998;178:185–190.
195. Sachar DB, Klein RS, Swerdlow F. Erosive syphilitic gastritis: Dark-field and immunofluorescent diagnosis from biopsy specimen. Ann Intern Med. 1974;80:512.
196. Fischl MA, Daikos GL, Uttamchandani RB, et al. Clinical presentation and outcome of patients with HIV infection and tuberculosis caused by multiple-drug-resistant bacilli. Ann Intern Med. 1992;117:184–190.
197. Cullen JH. Intestinal tuberculosis—a clinicopathologic study. Q Bull Sea View Hosp. 1940;5:143.
198. Davis AA. Hypertrophic intestinal tuberculosis. Surg Gynecol Obstet. 1933;56:907.
199. Hamandi WJ, Thamer MA. Tuberculosis of the bowel in Iraq: A study of 86 cases. Dis Colon Rectum. 1965;8:158.
200. Anand SS. Hypertrophic ileo-cecal tuberculosis in India with a record of fifty hemicolectomies. Ann R Coll Surg Engl. 1956;19:205.
201. Blacklock JWS. Tuberculous diseases in children. Medical Research Council, Spec Rep Ser 1972. London: His Majesty's Stationery Office; 1932.
202. Blumberg A. Pathology of intestinal tuberculosis. J Lab Clin Med. 1928;13:405.
203. Walsh J. Diagnosis of intestinal tuberculosis. Trans Natl Assoc Prev Tuberc Lond. 1909;5:217.
204. Paustian FF, Monto GL. Tuberculosis of the intestines. In: Bockus HL, ed. Gastroenterology. v 2. Philadelphia: WB Saunders; 1976;750–777.
205. Tandon HD, Prakach A. Pathology of intestinal tuberculosis and its distinction from Crohn's disease. Gut. 1972;13:260.
206. Eras P, Goldstein MJ, Sherlock P. *Candida* infection of the gastrointestinal tract. Medicine (Baltimore). 1972;51:367.
207. Bensaude A, Breging E. Examen anorecto-sigmoidien au cours des colopathies a *Candida albicans*. Ann Gastroenterol Hepatol. 1972;8:199.
208. Smith PD, Lane C, Gill VJ, et al. Intestinal infections in patients with the acquired immunodeficiency syndrome (AIDS): Etiology and response to therapy. Ann Intern Med. 1988;108:328–333.
209. Gupta TP, Ehrinpreis MN. *Candida* associated diarrhea in hospitalized patients. Gastroenterology. 1990;98:780–785.
210. Margolis BD, Tsang TK, Kuo D. Persistent diarrhea secondary to *Candida* overgrowth (Letter). Am J Gastroenterol. 1990;85:329–330.
211. Zaidi M, Ponce de Leon S, Ortiz RM, et al. Hospital-acquired diarrhea in adults: A prospective case-controlled study in Mexico. Infection Control Hosp Epidemiol. 1991;12:349–355.
212. Restrepo A, Robledo M, Gutierrey F, et al. Paracoccidioidomycosis (South American blastomycosis). Am J Trop Med Hyg. 1970;19:68.
213. Satir AA, Alla MD, Mahgoub S, et al. Systemic phycomycosis. BMJ. 1971;1:440.
214. Smith JMB. Mycoses of the alimentary tract. Gut. 1969;10:1035.
215. Bank S, Trey C, Gans I, et al. Histoplasmosis of the small bowel with "giant" intestinal villi and secondary protein-losing enteropathy. Am J Med. 1965;39:492.
216. Shull HJ. Human histoplasmosis. Disease with protean manifestations, often with digestive system involvement. Gastroenterology. 1953;25:582.
217. Kirk ME, Lough J, Warner HA. *Histoplasma* colitis: An electron microscopic study. Gastroenterology. 1971;61:46.
218. Brandborg LL, Goldberg SB, Breidenbach WC. Human coccidiosis—a possible cause of malabsorption. The life cycle in small-bowel mucosal biopsies as a diagnostic feature. N Engl J Med. 1970;24:1306.
219. Trier JS, Moxey PC, Schimmel EM, et al. Chronic intestinal coccidiosis in man: Intestinal morphology and response to treatment. Gastroenterology. 1974;66:923.
220. Soave R, Johnson WD Jr. *Cryptosporidium* and *Isospora belli* infections. J Infect Dis. 1988;157:225.
221. Pape JW, Verdier R, Johnson WD. Treatment and prophylaxis of *Isospora belli* infection in patients with the acquired immunodeficiency syndrome. N Engl J Med. 1989;320:1044–1047.
222. Tzipori S. Cryptosporidiosis in animals and humans. Microbiol Rev. 1983;47:84.
223. Current WL, Reese NC, Ernst JV, et al. Human cryptosporidiosis in immunocompetent and immunodeficient persons. N Engl J Med. 1983;308:1252.
224. Ma P, Soave R. Three-step stool examination for cryptosporidiosis in homosexual men with protracted watery diarrhea. J Infect Dis. 1983;147:824.
225. Soave R, Dubey JP, Ramos LJ, et al. A new intestinal pathogen? Clin Res. 1986;34:533A.
226. Long EG, Ebrahimzadeh A, White EH, et al. Alga associated with diarrhea in patients with acquired immunodeficiency syndrome and in travelers. J Clin Microbiol. 1990;28:1101–1104.
227. Ortega YR, Sterling CR, Gilman RH, et al. *Cyclospora* sp—a new protozoan pathogen of humans. N Engl J Med. 1993;328:1308–1312.
228. Powell SJ, Wilmot AJ. Ulcerative post-dysenteric colitis. Gut. 1966;7:438.
229. Blenkinsopp WK, Gibson JA, Haffenden GP. Giardiasis and severe jejunal abnormality. Lancet. 1978;1:994.

Chapter 86

Enteric Fever and Other Causes of Abdominal Symptoms with Fever

RICHARD D. PEARSON
RICHARD L. GUERRANT

Typhoid fever and several other enteric infections are characterized by clinical syndromes of abdominal pain and fever distinct from acute gastroenteritis. The portal of entry of the responsible infectious agents is usually the gastrointestinal tract. After a systemic phase, these infections may subsequently involve intestinal tissue and are then manifest as one of three clinical syndromes. (1) Enteric fever, characterized by sustained fever, headache, abdominal pain, splenomegaly, bacteremia, and occasionally skin rash, is the most serious of these syndromes and may result from infection by several bacteria. A number of systemic bacterial, rickettsial, viral, fungal, and parasitic infections, such as malaria, may mimic enteric fever, and a delay in diagnosis can be life-threatening. They are discussed later in the chapter. (2) Mesenteric adenitis, a syndrome that may mimic acute appendicitis, can be caused by several bacteria. (3) Eosinophilia, associated with abdominal cramps or diarrhea often accompanied by fever, may be caused by a number of parasites, usually helminths, several diseases of unknown cause, and neoplasms.

We focus on the differential diagnosis of these syndromes. Important clinical and epidemiologic features, appropriate diagnostic approaches, and antimicrobial therapeutic considerations are discussed.

ENTERIC FEVER

The classic syndrome of enteric fever is an acute illness, the first typical manifestations of which are fever, headache, abdominal pain, relative bradycardia, splenomegaly, and leukopenia.[1] The prototype of the syndrome is typhoid fever caused by *Salmonella typhi* (see Chapter 210). Fever is present in 75 to 100% of cases[2,3] and is often initially of the remittent type, rising in a stepwise fashion during the first week of illness, after which it becomes sustained.[4,5] Typhoid fever is a major problem for people living in developing areas where there is poor sanitation and fecal contamination of food and water. In the United States, 2445 cases were reported to the Centers for Disease Control and Prevention between 1985 and 1994, 72% of which were imported, most frequently from Mexico or India.[6,7] In addition, outbreaks occur in the United States.[7,8]

Pathogenesis

Salmonella typhi and other bacteria that cause the enteric fever syndrome are ingested and survive exposure to gastric acid before gaining access to the small bowel, where they penetrate the intestinal epithelium possibly via microfold cells over Peyer's patches. They multiply in intestinal lymphoid tissue and then disseminate via the lymphatic or hematogenous route. *Salmonella* spp. grow intracellularly, primarily in reticuloendothelial cells in lymph nodes, spleen, liver, and bone marrow. Animal models for this syndrome in which mice are infected orally with *Salmonella enteritidis* or *Yersinia enterocolitica* have been developed.[9]

Clinical Features

The organism classically responsible for the enteric fever syndrome is *S. typhi.* Other salmonellae, especially *Salmonella paratyphi* A, *Salmonella schottmuelleri* (formerly *S. paratyphi* B), *Salmonella hirschfeldii* (formerly *S. paratyphi* C), and *S. choleraesuis,* may cause a similar clinical syndrome (Table 86–1). Other diseases that may mimic enteric fever and that must be included in the differential diagnosis of enteric fever are also summarized in Table 86–1; important clinical and epidemiologic clues to these specific diagnoses are indicated.

Symptoms

Classic "typhoidal" fever begins with a remittent fever pattern that becomes sustained over the first few days of illness. The frequencies of reported symptoms from several series of patients infected by *S. typhi* and *S. paratyphi* A and *S. schottmuelleri* are summarized in Table 86–2. Most patients report fever and headache. Although reports from the preantibiotic era suggest that constipation occurred more frequently than diarrhea (79 versus 43%),[5] more recent reports suggest that these symptoms occur with approximately equal frequency[2, 10] or that diarrhea may be more common.[11–13] Extraintestinal symptoms reported by patients include cough and conjunctivitis. Although enteric fever caused by salmonellae other than *S. typhi* is usually less severe and of shorter duration than typhoid fever,[14, 15] the syndromes are not sufficiently different to permit clinical separation of individual case.

Physical Findings

In evaluating patients with possible enteric fever syndrome, the physical examination should focus on characteristics of the fever curve and accompanying pulse, skin, eyes, oral cavity and oropharynx, chest, abdomen, and lymph nodes. The frequencies of commonly reported physical findings are summarized in Table 86–2. Fever is present in most series in over 90% of the cases. However, bacteriologic confirmation of typhoid fever has been obtained in patients who were afebrile when the culture was obtained.[11, 12] Classically, the fever is remittent during the first week, rising in a stepwise fashion in both naturally acquired infection[5] and volunteer studies[4, 16]; after the first week, the fever usually becomes sustained. Deviations from this classic pattern frequently occur, particularly in endemic areas. In two studies from India, fever was remittent in 30 and 60% of the cases, sustained in 22 to 25%, and intermittent in 15 to 46%.[3, 13] Relative bradycardia suggests the diagnosis of enteric fever. The presence of rose spots, although not pathognomonic, is extremely helpful in confirming the impression of enteric fever[17]; however, they are observed in less than half of the patients and are even less common in dark-skinned people.[5] Rose spots may be observed more frequently in infection caused by *S. typhi* than in other forms of enteric fever.[14, 18] Conjunctivitis has been reported in up to 44% of the patients with enteric fever,[10] but it is usually less common.[5] Pharyngitis is infrequent and usually not a prominent feature. Rales may be present on examination of the chest. Abdominal tenderness may be diffuse or localized, most often in the right lower quadrant. Splenomegaly is noted more frequently than hepatomegaly. Two physical findings, lymphadenopathy and herpes simplex labialis, are useful in suggesting alternative diagnoses because they rarely occur in patients with enteric fever.

Laboratory Findings

The definitive diagnosis of enteric fever is made by isolating *S. typhi* or another *Salmonella* spp. from blood, bone marrow, stool, or urine. Cultures of blood as well as stool and urine should be obtained before the initiation of antimicrobial therapy. If multiple blood cultures are obtained, 73 to 97% of the cases will be confirmed.[5, 10] Patients with severe disease are the most likely to have positive cultures. Culture of the blood clot after the serum is removed has been reported to yield more positive results.[2, 10, 19] Bone marrow cultures may be positive when blood cultures are negative, even after antibiotics have been administered.[14, 20, 21] Stool cultures are positive in less than half the patients,[5, 20] and urine cultures are even less frequently positive.[5, 20] If patients have received antimicrobial therapy, blood cultures are often negative. Cultures of biopsy specimens of rose spots have been reported to be positive in nearly two thirds of patients, including some who previously received antimicrobial therapy.[20]

The Widal test has been used to detect anti–*S. typhi* antibodies for more than 100 years, but its role in the diagnosis of typhoid fever is limited.[22] The minimal titers defined as positive for the O (surface polysaccharide) antigens and H (flagellar) antigens must be determined for individual geographic areas and are higher in developing regions than in the United States.[11] Cross-reactions occur with both non–*S. typhi* group D salmonellae[23] and salmonellae from other groups.[24] When paired acute and convalescent samples are studied, a fourfold or greater increase is considered positive.

The Widal test has been reported to be positive in 46 to 94% of patients with typhoid fever.[3, 11, 22–29] The test is most reliable in areas in which data on the titers in control groups without enteric fever are available; the sensitivity of the test can be improved when diseases such as rheumatoid arthritis, which are associated with false-positive reactions, are ruled out by other assays. Although the criteria vary, a single elevated titer for O equal to or greater than (1:320) or H equal to or greater than (1:640) is considered positive. A fourfold or greater titer rise demonstrated in paired serum specimens obtained 2 to 3 weeks apart is also diagnostic, but it is of no value in the acute setting. The potential for either false-positive or false-negative responses limits the value of the Widal test in the diagnosis of typhoid fever.[22, 27–29] Finally, the Widal test is not helpful in the diagnosis of enteric fever caused by organisms other than *S. typhi.*

A number of other assays have been used to detect antibodies against other *S. typhi* antigens or circulating antigens themselves. They include an enzyme-linked immunosorbent assay (ELISA) using a cell envelope antigen or lipopolysaccharide of *S. typhi*[29, 30] or purified Vi antigen.[5, 31] Countercurrent immunoelectrophoresis has been used to detect *S. typhi* antigens in blood or urine, but a lack of sensitivity and specificity has limited their use.[32–34] Finally, polymerase chain reaction assays appear promising as rapid diagnostic tests but are now available only in research settings.[35–37]

Additional laboratory tests that may be of value include the white blood cell count and differential, liver function tests, urinalysis, and chest radiograph. Leukopenia is reported in 16 to 46% of the cases.[11, 12] In two series, two thirds of patients had no eosinophils on peripheral smear,[3, 10] a finding that may be helpful in areas in which helminthic diseases are prevalent and eosinophilia is common. Liver function tests may reveal a mildly elevated bilirubin level[10] and a slight to threefold elevation in alkaline phosphatase and transaminase levels in from one to two thirds of the patients[10, 12]; on occasion, hepatic manifestations may be prominent.[38] Urinalysis frequently reveals proteinuria, pyuria, and casts[5, 10]; immune complex glomerulonephritis with red blood cell casts occasionally occurs.[39] Coagulation abnormalities compatible with mild disseminated intravascular coagulation are common, but the syndrome is rarely clinically apparent.[40] Chest radiographic films reveal infiltrates in 2 to 11% of the cases.[2, 5] In patients with diarrhea, a methylene blue stain of a fresh stool specimen for fecal leukocytes may reveal mononuclear cells.[41]

Epidemiology

Certain epidemiologic data may be of value in the diagnosis of enteric fever. Typhoid fever is more common in children and adolescents both in the United States[6] and abroad.[10, 11, 42] In the United States, cases occur throughout the year. Since humans are the only reservoir for *S. typhi,* a history of being abroad in settings where

TABLE 86–1 Clinical, Epidemiologic, and Laboratory Clues to the Causes of Enteric Fever and Conditions That May Mimic Enteric Fever

Etiologic Agent or Disease	Clinical Clues in Addition to Fever	Epidemiologic Clues	Laboratory Clues
Causes of Enteric Fever			
Salmonella typhi *Salmonella paratyphi* A *Salmonella schottmuelleri* *Salmonella choleraesuis*	Relative bradycardia, splenomegaly, rose spots, conjunctivitis	Young adults, travel, especially to India, Mexico, and other tropical areas,* exposure to known carrier	Cultures (B, BM, U, F), serology, leukopenia
Yersinia enterocolitica *Yersinia pseudotuberculosis*	Chronic liver or other underlying disease, arthritis, erythema nodosum	Older adults, ± pet exposure	Cultures (B, F, J), serology
Campylobacter fetus	Stigmata or chronic liver disease, phlebitis	Older adults, ± farm or small-animal contact	Cultures (B, F), serology
Brucellosis (*Brucella* spp.)	Paucity of physical findings	Occupation (abattoir employee, butcher), animal contact (goats, sheep, cattle), diet (unpasteurized cheese)	Cultures (B, BM), serology, leukopenia
Typhoidal tularemia (*Francisella tularensis*)	Severe prostration, splenomegaly	Animal contact (especially rabbits), vector exposure (ticks)	Serology
Conditions That May Mimic Enteric Fever			
Bacterial infections			
Septicemic plague (*Yersinia pestis*)	Severe prostration	Rodent contact, vector exposure (fleas), travel	Cultures (B), serology
Intestinal anthrax (*Bacillus anthracis*)	Severe prostration	Travel,* diet (undercooked meat)	Cultures (B, F)
Septicemia melioidosis (*Burkholderia pseudomallei*)	Severe prostration, pustular skin lesions	Travel,* especially Southeast Asia	Cultures (B), serology, chest radiograph
Acute bartonellosis (*Bartonella bacilliformis*)	Severe prostration, hemolysis, renal failure	Travel to Andean valleys in Peru, Ecuador, and Columbia,* vector exposure (sand fly)	Cultures (B), blood smear, acute hemolysis
Leptospirosis (*Leptospira* spp.)	Relative bradycardia, conjunctival suffusion	Occupation (farmers, abattoir and sewer workers, veterinarians), animal contact (especially cattle, dogs), swimming†	Cultures (B, CSF, U), serology, hepatorenal dysfunction
Relapsing fever (*Borrelia* spp.)	Fever pattern, conjunctival suffusion, splenomegaly, skin rash	Travel, especially to Southeast Asia, Far East, Ethiopia, and the western United States),* vector exposure (louse, tick)	Blood smear
Legionellosis (*Legionella* spp.)	Pneumonia, CNS symptoms	Normal or compromised host	Chest radiograph, purulent sputum, DFA of sputum, urine antigen
Intestinal tuberculosis (*Mycobacterium tuberculosis, Mycobacterium avium-intracellulare*)	Stigmata of tuberculosis or AIDs	Exposure to known case, ± travel* ± diet (unpasteurized milk and milk products), malnourished children, HIV infection	Cultures (S, G, BM, L), radiograph (UGI, SBFT)
Abdominal actinomycosis (*Actinomyces* spp.)	Abdominal mass, fistula	Men	Culture (FD, A), radiograph (UGI, SBFT), CT with oral contrast medium
Intra-abdominal abscess	Spiking daily fever, reduced diaphragmatic excursion, intraabdominal or diaphragmatic pain	Previous surgery, bowel or biliary tract disease	Leukocytosis, CT, gallium scan, sonography, fluoroscopy
Rat bite fever			
Streptobacillus moniliformis	Headache, nausea, vomiting, rash, myalgia, polyarthritis	Rat bite or foot-borne outbreak	Culture (B, J), serology
Spirillum minus	Headache, nausea, adenopathy, roseolar-urticarial rash	Rat bite	Serology
Mycoplasma pneumoniae	Cough, headache, bullous myringitis	Children and adolescents	Serology
Chlamydia psittaci	Headache, nausea, vomiting, arthralgias, cough	Exposure to parrots, parakeets, related birds	Serology
Bacterial pneumonia (*Streptococcus pneumoniae, Haemophilus influenzae* spp.)	Cough, sputum, rales, headache, delirium, pulmonary infiltrates	Older adults, smoking, underlying diseases	Sputum Gram stain, culture (S, B), chest radiograph
Viral infections			
Hepatitis	Jaundice, arthritis (with hepatitis B)	Exposure to known case, drug abuse, travel*	Liver dysfunction, antibody and/or antigen detection
Dengue	Relative bradycardia, myalgia, conjunctival suffusion, rash	Travel,* vector exposure (mosquito)	Culture (B), serology, leukopenia, thrombocytopenia
Infectious mononucleosis	Pharyngitis, lymphadenopathy, splenomegaly, rash	Young adults	Serology, lymphocyte morphology
Rickettsial infections			
Rocky Mountain spotted fever	Rash, headache, myalgias	Travel,* vector exposure (tick)	Serology, skin biopsy
Epidemic typhus	Conjunctival suffusion, rash, severe prostration	Travel,* vector exposure (louse)	Serology
Brill-Zinsser disease	Rash	Older adults, remote travel* history	Serology
Endemic typhus	Conjunctival suffusion, rash, splenomegaly	Rat contact, vector exposure (flea)	Serology
Scrub typhus	Conjunctival suffusion, rash, lymphadenopathy	Travel,* vector exposure (mites)	Serology
Q fever	Pneumonia, hepatitis	Animal contact (especially livestock), ± travel, ± diet (especially unpasteurized milk)	Serology, chest radiograph, liver dysfunction
Ehrlichiosis	Headache, myalgia, rash (occasional)	Travel,* vector exposure (tick)	Serology, leukopenia, thrombocytopenia
Mycotic infections			
Disseminated histoplasmosis	Mucocutaneous lesions, adrenal insufficiency	Travel,* animal contact (chicken, birds, bats), hobby (cave exploration)	Culture (B, BM, L, MM), biopsy (BM, L, MM), chest radiograph, urine antigen
Penicillium marneffei	Umbilicated skin lesions, lymphadenopathy, cough, hepatomegaly	Travel,* concurrent AIDS	Culture (B, BM, LN), chest radiograph

TABLE 86–1 Clinical, Epidemiologic, and Laboratory Clues to the Causes of Enteric Fever and Conditions That May Mimic Enteric Fever *Continued*

Etiologic Agent or Disease	Clinical Clues in Addition to Fever	Epidemiologic Clues	Laboratory Clues
Parasitic infections			
Malaria	Fever pattern, splenomegaly	Travel,* vector exposure (mosquito)	Blood smear
Amebiasis	Colitis, liver abscess	Travel*	Stool examination, serology, liver scan, sonography, CT, colon biopsy
Babesiosis	Paucity of physical findings	Travel,* splenectomy, vector exposure (tick)	Blood smear, serology
Toxoplasmosis	Lymphadenopathy	Animal contact (cat); diet (undercooked pork)	Serology, biopsy (lymph node)
Trichinosis	Periorbital edema, muscle tenderness	Diet (undercooked pork or bear meat)	Serology, eosinophilia, biopsy (muscle)
Katayama fever (acute schistosomiasis)	Urticaria, lymphadenopathy	Travel,* swimming or other freshwater exposure	Eosinophilia, serology, stool O&P
Visceral larva migrans	Hepatosplenomegaly, rash, bronchospasm, ocular lesions	Young children with history of pica, animal contact (dog, cat)	Serology, biopsy (L), eosinophilia
Noninfectious causes			
Malignancy	Adenopathy, anergy, weight loss	Family history or prior malignancy	Sonography, CT, gallium scan, biopsy
Collagen vascular or granulomatous disease (e.g., sarcoidosis, granulomatous hepatitis, ulcerative colitis, Crohn's disease, Still's disease, vasculitis, etc.)	Skin lesions, arthritis, serositis, multiple organ involvement	Family history	Biopsy of involved tissue, serology (ANA, C′), exclusion of other causes

*Travel to endemic areas, either domestic or foreign.
†Swimming in contaminated surface water.
Abbreviations: A, Abscess; AIDS, acquired human immunodeficiency syndrome; ANA, antinuclear antibody; B, blood; BM, bone marrow; C′, complement; CNS, central nervous system; CSF, cerebrospinal fluid; CT, computed tomography; DFA, direct fluorescent antibody test; F, feces; FD, fistula drainage; G, gastric aspirate; HIV, human immunodeficiency virus; J, joint fluid; L, liver; LN, lymph node; MM, mucous membrane; N, nasal; O&P, ova and parasite; S, sputum; T, throat; U, urine; UGI, SBFT, upper gastrointestinal tract with small bowel follow-through.

sanitation is poor or with a known typhoid case or carrier is useful, but a specific contact is identified in a minority of cases.[6, 7] The proportion of the cases in the United States that were acquired abroad has increased dramatically; during 1985–1994, 72% of the cases were acquired abroad.[7] Six countries accounted for 80% of the cases: Mexico (28%), India (25%), the Philippines (10%), Pakistan (8%), El Salvador (5%), and Haiti (4%). The percentage of cases associated with visiting Mexico decreased from 46% in 1985 to 23% in 1994, whereas the percentage of cases associated with visiting the Indian subcontinent increased from 25% in 1985 to 37% in 1994. The incidence among U.S. citizens traveling to the Indian subcontinent was at least 18 times higher than to any other geographic region.[7] Patients who acquire infection abroad are usually older than those who acquire disease in the United States.[6]

The importance of the microbiology laboratory as a source of domestic *S. typhi* infection has also been recognized.[43, 44] In most laboratory-acquired cases, *S. typhi* had been used for proficiency testing or research.[43] Most patients with enteric fever caused by *S. paratyphi* A or *S. schottmuelleri* acquire their infection abroad; *S. schottmuelleri* is only occasionally and *S. paratyphi* A rarely isolated in the United States.

TABLE 86–2 Frequency of Symptoms and Physical Findings in Patients with Enteric Fever

	Typhoid Fever* (%)	Paratyphoid A and B† (%)
Symptoms		
Fever	39–100	92–100
Headache	43–90	60–100
Nausea	23–36	33–58
Vomiting	24–35	22–45
Abdominal cramps	8–52	29–92
Diarrhea	30–57	17–68
Constipation	10–79	2–29
Cough	11–86	10–68
Physical findings		
Fever	98–100	100
Abdominal tenderness	33–84	6–29
Splenomegaly	23–65	0–74
Hepatomegaly	15–52	16–32
Relative bradycardia	17–50	11–100
Rose spots	2–46	0–3
Rales or rhonchi	4–84	2–87
Epistaxis	1–21	2–13
Meningismus	1–12	0–3

*Data from refs. 2, 3, 5, 10–13.
†Data from refs. 10, 14, 18.

Differential Diagnosis

Enteric Fever–like Syndromes Caused by Other Bacteria

Yersinia enterocolitica, Yersinia pseudotuberculosis, and *Campylobacter fetus* can each produce an illness characterized by fever, headache, and abdominal pain that may be clinically indistinguishable from enteric fever caused by *S. typhi* or other salmonellae (see Table 86–1). However, certain features of these infections may differentiate them from true enteric fever. Acute diarrhea is often a prominent feature of enteric fever–like illnesses caused by *Y. enterocolitica*[45, 46] and occasionally *Y. pseudotuberculosis.*[47, 48] Diarrhea is less frequent in enteric fever–like illness caused by *C. fetus;* the acute gastrointestinal symptoms of nausea, vomiting, abdominal cramps, and diarrhea were present in only 27% of bacteremic illnesses caused by *C. fetus.*[49] A clue to the diagnosis of *Campylobacter* infection is associated phlebitis.[49–51]

The enteric fever–like syndromes caused by *Y. enterocolitica, Y. pseudotuberculosis,* and *C. fetus* tend to occur in patients with significant underlying disease. Of 31 patients with *Y. enterocolitica* bacteremia for whom information was available, 12 had cirrhosis of the liver; 4 others had thalassemia and 1 had kwashiorkor.[46] Only 5 were known to be free of underlying disease. In another series, 5 of 7 patients with the acute septicemic or typhoidal form of *Y. enterocolitica* infection had evidence of liver disease; in addition all 6 patients with the subacute, localized form of the disease characterized by hepatic and splenic abscesses had cirrhosis of the liver.[45] Of 20 patients with the enteric fever–like syndrome caused by *Y. pseudotuberculosis,* 11 had evidence of significant underlying disease; the liver was involved in 10 of these patients.[47] In a series of patients with bacteremia *C. fetus* illness, 73% had a significant underlying disease, frequently involving the liver.[49]

Epidemiologic clues in differentiating true enteric fever from these enteric fever–like syndromes include the patient's age, residence, and recent travel history. Patients with *Salmonella*-induced enteric fever are most often younger than 30 years,[6] whereas the vast majority of patients with non-*Salmonella* enteric fever–like syndromes are older than 40.[45–52] As with typhoid fever, men are more frequently affected than women. Patients with *Salmonella*-induced enteric fever frequently have a history of recent foreign travel, most often to developing countries. Diseases caused by *Y. enterocolitica* and *Y. pseudotuberculosis* appear to be common in Europe, particularly in Scandinavia,[53, 54] and are not frequently reported from developing countries. Infections due to both *Y. enterocolitica* and *Y. pseudotuberculosis* may be acquired in the United States as well.[55–58] Although bacteremic *C. fetus* infection is relatively rarely documented, the majority of cases have been reported from the United States, and foreign travel has not appeared to be a significant predisposing factor.[49, 52]

A pulse-temperature deficit similar to that observed in typhoid fever has been reported in enteric fever–like illness caused by *Y. enterocolitica*[46, 57–59] and *Y. pseudotuberculosis*[47, 55] but not in that caused by *C. fetus*.[49] An additional clue may be provided by the fever pattern. In contrast to *Salmonella*-induced enteric fevers in which sustained fever is common, intermittent fever throughout the illness caused by *Y. enterocolitica* has been reported.[60] Because of the increased frequency of chronic liver disease in patients with these enteric fever–like syndromes, physical examination is more likely to reveal stigmata of chronic liver disease such as spider angiomas, gynecomastia, ascites, and testicular atrophy. In addition, hepatomegaly is frequent and may be more pronounced than in patients with typhoid fever.[46] Both erythema nodosum and polyarthritis may occur in patients with illnesses caused by *Y. enterocolitica* and *Y. pseudotuberculosis;* in one series, 55% of the patients with yersiniosis had arthritis, and 88% of those had multiple joint involvement.[53] Nonsuppurative arthritis is more common in infections caused by *Y. enterocolitica* (43%) than in those caused by *Y. pseudotuberculosis* (10%).[61] Patients with bacteremic infection caused by *Y. enterocolitica* and *C. fetus* may also have acute septic arthritis,[46, 52, 57, 59] a condition that is infrequently found in patients with classic enteric fever. Erythema nodosum has been reported in 15 to 24% of patients with *Yersinia* and may be slightly more common with *Y. pseudotuberculosis* infection than with *Y. enterocolitica* infection.[53, 61] Thrombophlebitis has been reported in patients with *C. fetus* bacteremia and may be an additional diagnostic clue.[49–51, 62]

As in the *Salmonella*-induced enteric fevers, blood cultures are the key to the diagnosis. Each of the three organisms is more frequently isolated from blood than from other specimens.[45–49, 52] The isolation rate from stool cultures is improved if cold-enrichment techniques are used for *Yersinia*[63] and if special selective media are used for *Campylobacter*.[64, 65] However, because of its sensitivity to cephalosporins, *C. fetus* cannot be cultured from stool on commonly used *Campylobacter jejuni* selective agars if they contain cephalosporins. In addition, serologic tests are available for documenting infection with *Y. enterocolitica* and *Y. pseudotuberculosis* and appear to be more sensitive and more specific than those for *Salmonella* infection.[54, 66] Polymerase chain reaction–based assays for *Y. enterocolitica, Y. pseudotuberculosis,* and *C. fetus* appear promising, but they are available only in research settings.

Leukopenia is infrequent in patients with enteric fever–like syndromes; its presence suggests that salmonellae are responsible. Findings on abdominal computed tomography (CT) or ultrasonography suggestive of hepatic or splenic abscesses favor the diagnosis of yersiniosis.[45, 67] Glomerulitis complicating both typhoid fever and *Y. enterocolitica* has been reported; therefore, the presence of protein, red blood cells, and red blood cell casts in the urine is compatible with either of these syndromes.[39, 68]

Patients with typhoidal tularemia may be clinically indistinguishable from those with enteric fever. The epidemiologic history may be of value. A history of rabbit or tick exposure within 7 days before the onset of illness supports the diagnosis of tularemia.[69] Although potentially dangerous, *Francisella tularensis* may be isolated from blood if the appropriate medium is used. More often, serologic tests are used to confirm the diagnosis.

Acute brucellosis may manifest with fever, myalgias, and splenomegaly.[70] As in typhoid fever, white blood cell counts are frequently normal or low. Skin lesions are uncommon in brucellosis. Blood and bone marrow cultures and serologic testing permit separation of these entities.

Systemic Infections That May Mimic Enteric Fever

A number of other serious infections may be initially confused with enteric fever. These are particularly important because several are potentially fatal if not promptly recognized and treated. Among the most common serious febrile illnesses associated with travel to tropical areas is malaria, which should be considered even in individuals who claim to have been compliant in avoiding mosquitoes and taking malarial prophylaxis. It is characterized by fever, headache, myalgias, and, in some patients, gastrointestinal complaints. Intestinal and extraintestinal amebiases may present as acute or subacute febrile illnesses. Dengue fever can begin up to 9 days after exposure in an endemic area. Other, less common infectious causes of fever and enteric symptoms are discussed later. Some are endemic in North America, whereas others are not. In addition, persons with pneumococcal, *Legionella,* or *Mycoplasma* pneumonia may have enteric symptoms along with respiratory complaints.

Septicemic plague can mimic enteric fever. The diagnosis of plague is suggested by a sudden onset and rapid progression of illness. The history may again provide a clue to the diagnosis; plague is present in wild rodents in the southwestern United States and in endemic areas abroad. A history of travel to those areas, particularly if there is exposure to rodents during the previous 2 weeks, supports the diagnosis of plague.[71] Blood cultures, methylene blue stains of peripheral blood,[72] and serologic testing aid in the diagnosis.

Intestinal anthrax may be characterized by fever and severe abdominal pain. It is typically acute in onset and rapid in progression. Patients usually die during the first few days of their illness. A history of ingesting raw or undercooked meat in an area where anthrax is endemic suggests the diagnosis.[73]

Acute septicemic melioidosis may be confused clinically with enteric fever; this disease is endemic in Southeast Asia. Physical findings that support the diagnosis of melioidosis include pustular skin lesions.[74] The chest radiograph may reveal nodular pulmonary densities. Blood cultures and serologic studies again permit differentiation from typhoid fever.

Acute bartonellosis (Oroya fever) may manifest with fever, headache, and abdominal pain. Because this disease occurs only in certain valleys in the Andes mountains of Peru, Ecuador, and Colombia, a lack of travel in the preceding month is helpful in excluding this possibility.[75] Evidence of acute hemolysis suggests the diagnosis. The causative organisms may be seen on a stained peripheral blood smear. Because Oroya fever predisposes to *Salmonella*-induced bacteremia, both infections may be encountered simultaneously.[76]

Rat-bite fever caused by *Streptobacillus moniliformis* may mimic enteric fever when the rat puncture site is not clinically evident or when the infection is foodborne.[77] This illness may also mimic enteric fever–like syndromes. History of a recent rat bite suggests the diagnosis.[77] Cultures of blood and joint fluid may confirm the diagnosis; serologic tests may also be helpful. The other cause of rat-bite fever, *Spirillum minus,* causes subacute fever, headache, nausea, and vomiting, often with an urticarial rash (sodoku), 1 to 4 weeks after a rat bite. There is usually regional adenopathy.[78, 79] Spirillary fever causes a false-positive serologic test for syphilis in the majority of cases. *Spirillum minus* requires mouse inoculation for its isolation or demonstration of the 2- to 5-μm twisted gram-negative rod in tissue or blood for diagnosis. Like syphilis and relapsing fever, spirillary fever is often associated with a Herxheimer's reaction when treatment with penicillin G is initiated.

Leptospirosis frequently manifests with fever and headache and is most prevalent in young adults. Abdominal pain occurs in approximately 30% of cases.[80] Diarrhea and constipation are less frequent. Muscle pain and tenderness occur in nearly 70% of the patients, more frequently than in enteric fever. Additional differentiating features are the fever curve and clinical course; leptospirosis is characteristically a biphasic illness.[81] Evidence of liver dysfunction is present in approximately 50% of the patients with leptospirosis.[80] Although conjunctival suffusion is characteristic of leptospirosis and is reported in one third of patients, conjunctivitis occurs in enteric fever as well. Two findings that would favor the diagnosis of leptospirosis are azotemia (26% of cases) and cerebrospinal fluid pleocytosis (47% of cases).[80] Serologic tests are of value in confirming the diagnosis of leptospirosis.

Relapsing fever due to *Borrelia hermsii* may be confused with enteric fever. The history of travel during the previous 3 weeks to an area where louse-borne relapsing fever is endemic (Ethiopia, South America, Far East) raises the possibility of this diagnosis. Tick-borne relapsing fever can also be acquired in the western United States.[82] Conjunctivitis, rash, and hepatosplenomegaly are common. However, in contrast to patients with enteric fever, patients with tick-borne relapsing fever have a fever that resolves in a crisis during the first week only to recur later.[83] Giemsa or Wright stain of peripheral blood during a febrile episode may confirm the presence of spirochetes.

Patients with intestinal tuberculosis may have fever and findings referable to the gastrointestinal tract. The areas most commonly affected are jejunoileum and ileocecum. Radiologic studies of the terminal ileum may show evidence of a terminal ileitis that can be confused with the terminal ileitis of typhoid fever or *Y. enterocolitica* infection. Imaging features that suggest tuberculosis include cecal amputation, ileocecal thickening and inflammation, mesenteric adenopathy, and evidence of associated peritonitis.[84] Intestinal tuberculosis, once a rare disease in the United States, has become more common as a consequence of the acquired immunodeficiency syndrome epidemic, and it remains an important problem in developing areas.[85] Evidence of active pulmonary tuberculosis, which is present in approximately 20% of cases, and a positive purified protein derivative test support the diagnosis.

Abdominal actinomycosis may also mimic enteric fever. Physical examination may reveal an abdominal mass; the presence of a draining sinus tract strongly favors this diagnosis.[86] The diagnosis is confirmed by culture.

Intra-abdominal pyogenic abscesses can pose difficult diagnostic challenges and remain high on the list of undiagnosed causes of fever.[87] They should be suspected when fever persists or recurs and may be detected by sonography, CT, or magnetic resonance imaging.

Patients with *Mycoplasma pneumoniae* infection rarely have a course suggestive of enteric fever. Fever and headache may be prominent. The presence of tracheobronchitis with severe, nonproductive cough or pneumonia identified by physical examination or on the chest radiograph suggests this diagnosis, although infiltrates may also occur in patients with enteric fever due to *S. typhi.* The presence of bullous myringitis suggests *M. pneumoniae* infection.[88] The appearance of upper or lower respiratory illness in friends or members of the patient's family also favors this diagnosis. Serologic studies can be used to confirm *M. pneumoniae* infection.

Patients with psittacosis frequently have an illness characterized by fever, headache, myalgia, abdominal pain, vomiting, and diarrhea. On physical examination a faint macular rash may be noted; splenomegaly occurs in some patients.[89] A history of exposure to birds suggests the diagnosis, and serologic testing is helpful in confirmation.

Several rickettsial infections, especially epidemic typhus, Brill-Zinsser disease, endemic typhus, Rocky Mountain spotted fever, and scrub typhus as well as Q fever are characterized by fever, headache, myalgia, and, except in Q fever, skin rash. Of these, Rocky Mountain spotted fever is the most likely to be encountered in the United States.[90, 91] The gastrointestinal manifestations of Rocky Mountain spotted fever include abdominal pain, diarrhea, vomiting, and upper gastrointestinal tract bleeding, and a diagnosis of appendicitis, cholecystitis, or gastroenteritis may initially be considered.[92–94] A history of recent tick exposure suggests the diagnosis. Although failure of the characteristic rash to develop may lead to a fatal delay in diagnosis and treatment,[95] once the characteristic rash associated with these illnesses appears, the diagnostic confusion is lessened. Serologic testing provides documentation of rickettsial infections. In addition, fluorescent antibody techniques can be used to demonstrate *Rickettsia rickettsii* in biopsy specimens of involved skin.[96] Sporadic cases of epidemic typhus associated with flying squirrels have been reported in the United States since 1976.[97, 98] The majority of these have occurred in southeastern states during the winter months. Q fever is associated with cattle and sheep exposure or the ingestion of unpasteurized milk.[99]

Monocytotropic and granulocytotropic ehrlichiosis, other tick-borne diseases, may also present with typhoid-like symptoms including fever, myalgias, vomiting, diarrhea, headache, and, in some cases, rash, with elevated liver enzyme levels, leukopenia, and anemia[100, 101] A history of tick exposure in an endemic area is helpful. The diagnosis can be confirmed by serologic tests.

Legionella infections in normal or immunocompromised hosts may present with gastrointestinal symptoms of abdominal pain, nausea, vomiting, or diarrhea that is usually watery and noninflammatory.[102–104] Patients with disseminated histoplasmosis may have fever, abdominal pain, nausea, vomiting, and diarrhea.[105] The diagnosis may be suggested by the presence of mucous membrane lesions or adrenal insufficiency. Biopsy specimens and cultures of liver, blood, urine, and bone marrow may be useful in confirming the diagnosis.

Several acute viral infections have gastrointestinal manifestations. Abdominal pain, nausea, and vomiting are frequent symptoms in patients with hepatitis. However, the severity of jaundice and the extent of elevation of transaminase levels are much greater than those observed in enteric fever. Influenza (particularly type B) may manifest with fever, headache, and abdominal pain. Serologic studies and, in the case of influenza, nasopharyngeal swabs are useful in distinguishing these illnesses. Infectious mononucleosis may mimic enteric fever, particularly when acute pharyngitis is not prominent. Examination of the peripheral blood smear and studies for heterophil or Epstein-Barr virus–specific antibodies are helpful in differentiating this illness from enteric fever.

In dengue fever, an important mosquito-borne viral disease in the tropics, headache, severe myalgias, and leukopenia are common. The maculopapular skin rash that characteristically appears on the trunk on the third to fifth day of illness and subsequently spreads peripherally, the biphasic clinical course, and a history of recent travel (within the previous 9 days) to areas in which dengue is endemic suggest the diagnosis.

A number of protozoal and helminthic infections can also mimic typhoid fever. Malaria is endemic in many areas of the world in which typhoid fever is also relatively common. Both diseases may present with fever, headache, abdominal pain, and other gastrointestinal symptoms. Two thirds of 25 cases of malaria in one series presented with prominent gastrointestinal symptoms (nausea, vomiting, abdominal pain, or diarrhea) that might have misled physicians from an early diagnosis of malaria.[106] When present, intermittent fever suggests the diagnosis of malaria, but it is not observed in the majority of nonimmune individuals with the disease. Peripheral blood smears confirm the diagnosis of malaria.

Fever, chills, and hemolytic anemia in a person with exposure to an area with *Ixodes scapularis* ticks and white-footed mice (*Peromyscus* spp.) or white-tailed deer (*Odocoileus virginianus*) may be due to infection with *Babesia microti,* especially in an asplenic patient.[107, 108]

Either intestinal or hepatic amebiasis may mimic acute enteric fever. In patients with hepatic abscesses, documentation of a single abscess cavity favors the diagnosis of amebiasis.[109] The diagnosis may be confirmed by means of a positive indirect hemagglutination test. Patients with visceral leishmaniasis frequently present with fever, malaise, hepatosplenomegaly, weight loss, anemia, thrombocytopenia and leukopenia. Massive splenomegaly suggests visceral leishmaniasis. The diagnosis is made by identifying leishmanial amastigotes within mononuclear phagocytes in aspirates of the spleen or bone marrow or by culturing leishmania from those specimens.

Several helminthic infections may cause an enteric fever–like syndrome, but they are usually associated with eosinophilia as discussed later. Patients with trichinosis typically present with fever, headache, myalgias, abdominal pain, diarrhea, periorbital edema, and rash. The presence of eosinophilia, rather than the eosinopenia frequently noted in enteric fever, helps in the differentiation. The history of recent ingestion of raw or undercooked pork suggests trichinosis. It can be confirmed by acute and convalescent serologic tests or biopsy, but the latter is seldom necessary.

Patients with visceral larva migrans may also have fever and hepatomegaly. In more severe infections, splenomegaly, rash, and pneumonitis may also occur. In contrast to enteric fever, visceral larva migrans is typically associated with pronounced eosinophilia. The diagnosis is suggested by a history of pica. Serologic tests may confirm the diagnosis of *Toxocara* spp. infection.

Patients with acute schistosomiasis (Katayama fever) may also present with an enteric fever syndrome. Again, eosinophilia is helpful in separating these possibilities. The history of swimming in fresh water during the previous month in areas where schistosomiasis is endemic further suggests schistosomiasis. The diagnosis is suggested by serologic tests and confirmed by the eventual identification of ova in the stool.

Noninfectious causes of fever and abdominal pain such as eosinophilic gastroenteritis; hematologic and other malignancies involving abdominal lymph nodes or the intestine; vasculitides; and granulomatous diseases must also be considered. Diagnosis in such cases often requires radiographic studies, biopsy of involved tissues, and the exclusion of other processes as discussed later. See Chapter 44 for a discussion of the differential diagnosis of fever of unknown origin.

Therapy of Enteric Fever

In patients with the enteric fever syndrome, it is advisable to consider empirical antimicrobial therapy for typhoid fever before the diagnosis is confirmed by culture. Multiple-drug–resistant isolates of *S. typhi* unresponsive to ampicillin, trimethoprim-sulfamethoxazole, and chloramphenicol are increasingly prevalent around the world.[110–113] Fluoroquinolones, such as ciprofloxacin or ofloxacin,[114–116] are now widely used, but resistance to them has been reported in a number of areas.[117–119] The fluoroquinolones achieve high concentration in phagocytic cells and in bile. They are usually well tolerated, and provided the infecting strain is sensitive, result in faster defervescence than cephalosporins. Fluoroquinolones are not approved for use in children in the United States because of their potential to damage cartilage and tendons. Third-generation cephalosporins, such as ceftriaxone,[120–122] and the monobactam aztreonam are also effective.[123] For sensitive *S. typhi,* ampicillin, trimethoprim-sulfamethoxazole, or chloramphenicol can be used. Strains may occasionally acquire resistance during therapy.[124] A patient's recent travel and exposure history should be considered in selecting additional empirical antimicrobial drugs to cover other possible causes of the enteric syndrome, pending the results of cultures and other diagnostic tests.

MESENTERIC ADENITIS

Patients with mesenteric adenitis typically have a history of fever and abdominal pain, frequently with localization to the right lower quadrant. The illness is similar to acute appendicitis. Few data are available on the incidence of this syndrome, and it may vary with the geographic location. In one series of hospitalized patients, 50 of 651 (7.7%) admitted with a diagnosis of appendicitis had a discharge diagnosis of mesenteric adenitis.[125]

Etiologic Agents and Pathogenesis

The most frequently reported causes of the syndrome of mesenteric adenitis are *Y. enterocolitica* and *Y. pseudotuberculosis.* These organisms seem to be more prevalent in Europe than in the United States. Among 2861 consecutive patients undergoing appendectomy for suspected appendicitis in a Belgian hospital, *Y. enterocolitica* was isolated from the appendix or stool in 3.6%. Of those with histologically confirmed mesenteric adenitis or terminal ileitis without appendicitis, or both, *Y. enterocolitica* was cultured in 75%.[126] In another report, five of eight patients (63%) who had mesenteric adenitis confirmed at surgery also had serologic evidence of recent *Y. enterocolitica* infection.[127] Of 20 patients with mesenteric adenitis reported by Mair and associates, 17 were adequately studied; 3 (18%) had evidence of infection with *Y. pseudotuberculosis.*[128] In a school-related outbreak of *Y. pseudotuberculosis* among 34 children in Finland, 3 children went to surgery for suspected appendicitis and were found to have mesenteric lymphadenitis.[129] In a mouse model, after intragastric administration of *Y. enterocolitica*, polymorphonuclear leukocytes appeared in Peyer's patches within 24 hours. The infection then spread to the mesenteric lymph nodes, where abscesses developed.[130]

Mesenteric adenitis can theoretically occur with any pathogen that affects lymph nodes. It has also been associated with nontyphoidal *Salmonella* spp. infections,[131, 132] *S. typhi* infections,[132] tuberculous mesenteric lymphadenitis, intestinal anthrax, and, in children with human immunodeficiency virus infections in Southeast Asia, *Penicillium marneffei* infection.[133]

In the preantibiotic era, hemolytic streptococci were frequently reported as etiologic agents. In one study, 19 of 36 patients (53%) with mesenteric adenitis in whom cultures were obtained grew hemolytic streptococci and 4 (11%) grew *Escherichia coli.* Of interest is the fact that 37 of 39 patients (97%) had throat cultures positive for hemolytic streptococci, and 35 of these had a history of a recent sore throat.[134] Although now uncommon, hemolytic streptococci have been isolated in a few cases of mesenteric adenitis in the antibiotic era as well.[128, 135–136] Asch and colleagues reported on one patient from whom β-hemolytic streptococci were isolated from an inflamed mesenteric node and in whom subsequent studies revealed an elevated anti–streptolysin O titer.[135] *Staphylococcus aureus* alone or with β-hemolytic streptococci has also been isolated from inflamed mesenteric nodes in the absence of appendicitis.[136] In a report of two patients with mesenteric abscesses secondary to suppurative mesenteric adenitis, one had enterococci and an unidentified hemolytic bacillus isolated from an abscess, whereas the other had *Bacteroides* and *Clostridium* spp.; in both cases the appendix was normal.[137] A viral cause has also been suspected for mesenteric adenitis but has not been well documented.

Clinical Features of Mesenteric Lymphadenitis Due to *Yersinia* Species

Symptoms

Yersinia enterocolitica produces a spectrum of disease, including acute enterocolitis, terminal ileitis, and mesenteric adenitis. *Yersinia pseudotuberculosis,* which commonly infects animals, is a less frequent cause of human disease. It typically produces mesenteric adenitis, especially in older children and adults.

Regardless of the cause, persons with mesenteric adenitis present with fever and right lower quadrant pain, making the syndrome indistinguishable from acute appendicitis.[138] The symptoms reported by persons in four common-source outbreaks of *Yersinia* infection are summarized in Table 86–3.[139–141] Fever, abdominal pain, vomiting, and diarrhea were frequent. In a series of 37 sporadic cases of *Yersinia*-induced enteritis reported from Belgium, 84% of the patients had abdominal pain, 78% had diarrhea, 43% had fever, and 22% reported anorexia; 13% had nausea, and 8% vomiting.[142] Patients with mesenteric adenitis caused by *Yersinia* may have a history of biphasic illness.[143] Consumption of raw pork in the 2 weeks before illness has been associated with *Y. enterocolitica* infection in the most highly endemic country, Belgium.[144]

TABLE 86-3 Symptoms in Four Outbreaks of Mesenteric Adenitis Caused by *Yersinia enterocolitica*

Location	Japan (139)	Japan (140)	Japan (140)	United States (141)
Serotype	03	03	03	08
Number ill	198	188	544	38
Percentage with				
Abdominal pain	76	86	64	97
Fever	61	76	50	100
Diarrhea	36	60	32	47
Vomiting	12	4	11	—
Percentage undergoing appendectomy	2	—	—	42

Physical Examination

The physical findings of mesenteric adenitis typically include fever, right lower quadrant tenderness, and often rebound tenderness. Rectal tenderness was present in nearly one third of people examined in one epidemic.[141] In contrast to the enteric fever syndromes, a pulse-temperature deficit is not found.

Laboratory Findings

Leukocytosis is usually present in patients with *Yersinia*-associated mesenteric adenitis[143–148]; white blood cell counts typically are between 10,000 and 15,000/mm^3. Examination of feces may reveal polymorphonuclear leukocytes.[149] Blood cultures are rarely positive, but *Y. enterocolitica* or *Y. pseudotuberculosis* may be isolated from stool cultures. The frequency of isolation is improved by the use of cold-enrichment techniques.[150] Stool cultures were positive in 56% of hospitalized patients with the syndrome in one common-source outbreak[141]; the isolation of *Y. pseudotuberculosis* from feces seems to occur less frequently, but has been reported.[151] Serologic testing may be helpful in the diagnosis, but agglutinins are rarely present during the first week of illness,[142] and cross-reactions can occur with *Brucella* spp., *Vibrio* spp., and some Enterobacteriaceae. Serologic confirmation was obtained in 84% of the hospitalized patients in one outbreak.[143] The isolation of *Y. enterocolitica* from a stool culture should be considered significant; the organism was isolated from only 1 out of 974 controls in one study and from none of 545 controls in another.[152, 153]

Sonographic, radiographic contrast studies or CT examination may provide clues that are helpful in differentiating mesenteric lymphadenitis from appendicitis. Of 170 patients presenting with a clinical syndrome suggesting acute appendicitis or mesenteric lymphadenitis who underwent sonography using graded compression, 14 had only enlarged mesenteric nodes with mural thickening of the terminal ileum (without visualization of the appendix); none of the 14 had appendicitis; and 8 (of 9 cultured) had *Y. enterocolitica* in the stool.[154] In another study of 609 patients with suspected appendicitis, graded ultrasonography suggested a spectrum of other diseases in addition to appendicitis, but in three cases there were incorrect sonographic diagnoses with serious sequelae.[155] In a series of 37 adult patients who had documented *Y. enterocolitica* infection, 40% had symptoms compatible with appendicitis, 21 of the 24 patients studied with radiographic contrast material had abnormalities of the terminal ileum consisting of coarse mucosal folds in 67%, nodularity in 45%, or ulceration in 45%.[142] Although radiologic studies of the colon were normal in these patients, sigmoidoscopic or colonoscopic examination in 13 revealed evidence of colitis in 6 and aphthoid ulceration in 2, indicating that colonic involvement may occur. In another series of 25 patients with *Yersinia* infection who were given the clinical diagnosis of acute appendicitis and underwent appendectomy, acute terminal ileitis was confirmed at surgery. When these patients were examined within 1 week of surgery by a barium contrast study of the small bowel, abnormalities were confined to the distal 20 cm of the ileum. The lesions evolved from an initial nodular pattern to an edematous pattern before resolution within 10 weeks in all cases.[155]

Helical appendiceal CT can also be used to diagnose appendicitis. An enlarged appendix with periappendiceal fat stranding occurs in 93% of cases of appendicitis. Less common, but specific changes are cecal apical changes and an appendolith or appendoliths.[156] In a series of 18 patients with a discharge diagnosis of mesenteric lymphadenitis, the CT scan showed three or more nodes measuring 5 mm in the shortest axis clustered in the right lower quadrant, with a normal appendix.[125] Eight patients had associated ileal or ileocecal wall thickening. As promising as sonography, radiography, and CT appear, they are still not sufficiently sensitive and specific to preclude surgery in most instances.

At surgery, patients with mesenteric adenitis may also have evidence of acute appendicitis, but the organ is rarely severely inflamed or ruptured. Patients may also have evidence of acute terminal ileitis.[127, 138, 145, 148, 155] Culture of the terminal ileum at surgery may yield the organism.[147] Histopathologic examination of resected mesenteric lymph nodes in cases of *Y. enterocolitica* infection frequently reveals histiocytic infiltration and the presence of large pyroninophilic cells; abscesses are typically absent.[157, 158] In contrast, although reticulum cell hyperplasia is frequently seen in nodes infected with *Y. pseudotuberculosis,* granulomas, polymorphonuclear leukocyte infiltration, and abscess formation are more frequent.[128, 147, 157, 159] In both infections, tissue Gram stain may reveal the bacteria. Two fatal cases occurred in a *Y. enterocolitica* outbreak among four families in North Carolina.[160] Postmortem examination revealed extensive ulceration and necrosis extending from the stomach or small bowel to the colon. Mesenteric lymph nodes were necrotic in one case, and the sinusoids were filled with leukocytes and mononuclear cells. In the second case, the lymph nodes were large, firm, and edematous. There was reticuloendothelial hyperplasia with abundant histiocytes and plasma cells within the sinusoids.[149]

Epidemiology

Mesenteric adenitis caused by *Y. enterocolitica* or *Y. pseudotuberculosis* is a syndrome of children and young adults, is most frequent in people between 5 and 14 years of age, is more common in boys, and is most often encountered during the winter and spring. This seasonal pattern is reported from both the preantibiotic[134] and antibiotic eras.[145, 161]

The mode of transmission of *Y. enterocolitica* and *Y. pseudotuberculosis* has not been well defined; outbreaks involving several members of several families[160] or people from the same school have been reported. In these and other episodes of *Yersinia* infection, simultaneous documentation of infection in family pets has been obtained[162]; whether these animals were the source of the human infection or merely acquired the infection simultaneously is unknown. Person-to-person spread to family members does occur.[153] Large common-source outbreaks of mesenteric adenitis have also been reported[139–141, 163, 164]; in one of these, chocolate milk was the vehicle of transmission.[141] *Yersinia enterocolitica* has been isolated from drinking water,[165, 166] but water-borne transmission of these organisms has not been well documented. Results of one study in Wisconsin suggested that *Y. enterocolitica* infection was more common in rural areas.[167]

Differential Diagnosis

The major consideration in the differential diagnosis of mesenteric adenitis is acute appendicitis. Other infectious diseases characteristically involving the terminal ileum or mesenteric lymph nodes, or both, such as tuberculosis, nontyphoidal *Salmonella* infections,[131, 132] *Salmonella typhi* infections,[132] actinomycosis, *Mycobacterium avium-intracellulare* infection in patients with acquired immunodeficiency syndrome,[168] or *P. marneffei* infections in children with human immunodeficiency virus infection in Southeast Asia[133] must be considered. Viruses have been occasionally implicated as causes of mesenteric lymphadenitis, including parvovirus B19 as a cause of pseudoappendicitis,[169] and Epstein-Barr virus as a cause of mesenteric lymphadenopathy.[170] Adenovirus infection has been associated with mesenteric lymph node hypertrophy and intussusception.[171] *Angiostrongylus costaricensis* may produce an appendicitis-like syndrome but usually is associated with eosinophilia as described later.[172]

Therapy

Mesenteric adenitis is a self-limited illness in the vast majority of cases. Specific antimicrobial therapy is often not required. In patients who are severely ill or who have evidence of systemic disease, the selection of an antimicrobial agent should be based, if possible, on the results of antimicrobial sensitivity tests. When these data are not available, therapeutic agents to be considered for *Y. enterocolitica* include trimethoprim-sulfamethoxazole, second- and third-generation cephalosporins, ciprofloxacin and other fluoroquinolones, piperacillin, imipenem, tetracycline, and chloramphenicol.[173–175] *Yersinia enterocolitica* is often resistant to amoxicillin, cefazolin, and macrolides.[173–175] Although *Y. enterocolitica* isolates may be sensitive in vitro to aminoglycosides,[176] these drugs should not be the initial choice for treatment because of the reported failure of these agents to eradicate systemic infection.[45] *Yersinia pseudotuberculosis* is usually sensitive to tetracycline, cephalosporins, aminoglycosides and chloramphenicol.

SYNDROME OF ABDOMINAL PAIN OR DIARRHEA WITH EOSINOPHILIA

The differential diagnosis and etiologic considerations for the syndrome of abdominal pain, diarrhea, and eosinophilia as well as useful diagnostic tests are summarized in Table 86–4. Most cases are caused by helminths. Additional diagnostic considerations include eosinophilic gastroenteritis, dermatitis herpetiformis, polyarteritis nodosa, regional enteritis, and ulcerative colitis. In addition, lymphomas and some solid tumors may manifest with abdominal pain and eosinophilia. Epidemiologic data, particularly dietary and travel histories, may provide important clues to the diagnosis. Valuable laboratory tests in these patients include examination of stool and small bowel contents for ova and parasites, specific serologic tests, and, in some cases, radiologic studies or biopsy.

Differential Diagnosis

Strongyloides stercoralis is unique among intestinal nematodes in its ability to persist for many years through autoinfection and to produce life-threatening hyperinfection in immunocompromised hosts.[177] It infects people in areas where sanitation is poor. Patients with strongyloidiasis frequently have abdominal pain, diarrhea, or a sense of bloating and eosinophilia. Pain is often epigastric, although some patients report pain in the right upper and right lower quadrants or in the periumbilical region. Ninety percent of those infected have eosinophilia. Cases of hyperinfection have occurred in persons who are immunosuppressed after organ transplantation and in association with malnutrition, lymphoma, cimetidine therapy, or human immunodeficiency virus infection, although hyperinfection has been observed less commonly than expected with human immunodeficiency virus infection.[177–180] Strongyloides hyperinfection can result in secondary bacteremia, meningitis, urinary tract infection, or pneumonia due to enteric bacteria on the surface of migrating larvae.

In the United States, strongyloidiasis is most often diagnosed in immigrants, residents of the Southeast, or veterans who served in endemic areas abroad. Prolonged infections have been demonstrated in troops and former prisoners of World War II who served in Southeast Asia.[181–184] A prospective study in rural Tennessee documented *S. stercoralis* in 6.1% of patients at a Veterans Affairs hospital and in 2.6% of their household contacts.[185] The diagnosis of strongyloidiasis can be confirmed by demonstration of larvae in fresh stool specimens, but the sensitivity is low. The sensitivity can be enhanced by studying multiple specimens or by using the Baermann funnel gauze test[186, 187] or the agar plate method, which is probably the diagnostic measure of choice.[188] Larvae can also be identified in some cases in duodenal contents[189] and in sputum in some patients with disseminated hyerinfection. Immunofluorescence assay or ELISA can be used to detect anti-*Strongyloides* antibodies,[190–192] but both false-positive and false-negative results can occur. Eosinophilia is often absent in immunocompromised patients, particularly those taking corticosteroids.[178, 179]

Most patients infected with *Ascaris lumbricoides* are asymptomatic. Although ascariasis is not usually associated with diarrhea, severe abdominal pain may occur when patients with heavy worm burdens develop intestinal obstruction or adult worms migrate into or occlude the biliary or pancreatic ducts.[193–195] These complications are most frequent in young children. It is estimated that acute intestinal obstruction due to *Ascaris* may occur in as many as 1 in 1000 persons in endemic areas. Ascariasis is most common in areas where sanitation is poor. Eggs are ingested in contaminated food or water or, by children, in dirt. In the United States, *Ascaris* infection was once common in the southeastern states, but symptomatic infections are now rare. Eosinophilia may or may not be present. The diagnosis is made by the demonstration of ova in stool specimens. Because a single worm produces large numbers of eggs, concentration of feces is not necessary. In patients with intestinal or biliary tract obstruction, sonographic, radiologic, or CT studies may reveal the presence of an adult worm, and there may be elevations of liver or pancreatic enzyme levels.[195]

Patients with toxocariasis (visceral larva migrans) caused by animal nematodes such as *Toxocara canis* may present with abdominal pain and eosinophilia. In temperate climates, *T. canis* is the most important etiologic agent.[196] The abdominal pain may be associated with the presence of tender hepatomegaly. Clinical clues to the diagnosis include the simultaneous occurrence of splenomegaly or pneumonitis with bronchospasm.[197–199] Patients may have pruritic rashes on the trunk or lower extremities. The presence of a granuloma in the ocular fundus or other evidence of ocular inflammation, high titers of isoagglutinins, and hypergammaglobulinemia provide additional diagnostic clues. The total white count is often elevated, and eosinophils may exceed 50%. Patients are usually young children; additional epidemiologic clues are a history of pica or close contact with dogs. As many as 10 to 30% of the soil samples in public playgrounds and parks in the United States have been found to be contaminated with *Toxocara* eggs.[196] Serologic tests are available; ELISA seems to be the most sensitive and specific.[197–199] On rare occasions, larvae are identified in biopsies of the liver or other organs.

The onset of infection with *Trichinella spiralis* may be characterized initially by diarrhea, which occurs in approximately 40% of the cases; abdominal pain, which occurs in approximately 20%; or constipation.[200, 201] The intestinal symptoms, which are attributed to the presence of adult worms or invading larvae in the intestinal tract, occur during the first week of illness and may precede the appearance of eosinophilia. Approximately 100 cases of trichinosis are reported annually in the United States.[202] Infection occurs by the ingestion of raw or undercooked pork or pork products such as sausage, bear meat, or horse meat, and occasionally by other vehicles such as

TABLE 86-4 Etiologic Agents and Useful Laboratory Studies in the Differential Diagnosis of Infectious Causes of the Syndrome of Abdominal Pain and/or Diarrhea with Eosinophilia

Etiologic Agents or Disease	Stool Examination	Small Bowel Fluid Examination or Biopsy	Tissue Biopsy	Serology	Radiologic and Other Studies
Nematodes					
Strongyloides stercoralis	+	+	−	+	−
Ascaris lumbricoides	+	±	−	−	± (small bowel)
Visceral larva migrans (*Toxocara canis, Toxocara cati,* and others)	−	−	+ (liver)	+	−
Trichinella spiralis	−	−	+ (muscle)	+	−
Anisakiasis (*Anisakis* spp. and other genera)	−	−	−	−	+ (endoscopy)
Capillaria philippinensis	+	+	−	−	−
Angiostrongylus costaricensis	−	−	+ (ileum, colon)	+	+ (UGI series; small bowel)
Trematodes					
Schistosoma spp.	+	−	+ (rectum)	+	−
Clonorchis sinensis (Chinese liver fluke)	+	−	−	−	± (biliary tract abnormalities)
Opisthorchis spp. (Southeast Asian liver fluke)	+	−	−	−	± (biliary tract abnormalities)
Metorchis conjunctus (North American liver fluke)	+	−	−	+	−
Fasciola hepatica (sheep liver fluke)	+	−	−	−	+ (ultrasound, liver CT scan)
Fasciolopsis buski (intestinal fluke)	+	−	−	−	−
Heterophyes heterophes (intestinal fluke)	+	−	−	−	−
Metagonimus yokogawi (intestinal fluke)	+	−	−	−	−
Nanophyetus salmincola (intestinal fluke)	+	−	−	−	−
Cestodes					
Echinococcosis	−	−	−	+	+ (chest radiograph, abdominal ultrasound or CT scan)
Protozoa					
Isospora belli	+	+	−	−	−
Dientamoeba fragilis	+	−	−	−	−
Diseases of unknown cause					
Eosinophilic gastroenteritis	−	+	−	−	+ (UGI series; small bowel CT scan)
Polyarteritis nodosa and other forms of vasculitis	−	−	+ (skin, muscle, kidney)	−	+ (angiography)
Inflammatory bowel disease	−	−	+ (colon)	−	+ (small bowel, colonoscopy)
Malignancies	−	−	+ (lymph nodes, liver, bone marrow)	−	+ (UGI Series, barium enema, CT scan, ultrasound)

Abbreviations: +, Feature present; −, feature absent; CT, computed tomography; UGI, upper gastrointestinal.

ground beef contaminated during processing with pork.[201–205] Myalgias, periorbital edema, muscle tenderness, splinter hemorrhages, and evidence of myocarditis or central nervous system involvement with eosinophilia further suggest the diagnosis. Prolonged diarrhea has been the dominant symptom among Inuit inhabitants of northern Canada who become reinfected with *Trichinella nativa* after eating contaminated, uncooked walrus meat. Myalgia and muscle weakness are less prominent complaints in that setting.[206–207] The diagnosis of trichinosis is usually made on clinical grounds and confirmed by serologic tests, but antibodies do not typically become positive until several weeks into infection.[208] A definitive diagnosis may be made by the demonstration of larvae in muscle, although biopsy is seldom necessary.

Patients with anisakiasis caused by nematodes of the family Anisakidae and related parasites of fish may have an acute illness characterized by epigastric pain, nausea, and vomiting or a chronic illness characterized by abdominal pain and fever. The disease is caused by larvae that migrate from the viscera to the muscle of fish after they are caught and penetrate the human gastrointestinal tract after fish is eaten raw or inadequately cooked. The stomach, small bowel, or colon may be involved. Necrotizing eosinophilic granulomatous inflammation with peripheral eosinophilia occur at the sites where larvae attempt to invade.[209–211] The pathologic and radiologic manifestations may resemble regional enteritis[212]; mass lesions resembling malignancies may also occur.[213] The disease is rarely reported in the United States; it is most common in the Netherlands and Japan. The infection is acquired by the ingestion of raw or undercooked marine fish such as cod, salmon, and herring. In Japan, raw or pickled marine fish are common vehicles; in the Netherlands, raw or slightly salted herring is the most common source of infection.[209, 210] Therefore, the travel or a dietary history may suggest the diagnosis. Confirmation is obtained by identification of the larvae by endoscopy or in tissue specimens. Eustrongylidiasis is another helminthic infection associated with abdominal pain, diarrhea, and eosinophilia after the ingestion of contaminated uncooked fish or minnows.[214]

Capillaria philippinensis is a rare, but important cause of intestinal disease in endemic regions of the Philippines. Sporadic cases have also been reported from Thailand, Egypt, and other areas of the world. Those infected typically give a history of vague abdominal pain and voluminous watery diarrhea.[215] The illness is characterized by a protein-losing enteropathy and malabsorption, which may be severe. Electrolyte abnormalities and hypoproteinemia are common. Weight loss, muscle wasting, weakness, hyporeflexia, and edema occur.[216, 217] Worms are found in the small bowel, especially in the jejunum, and the adults are partially embedded in the mucosa. The intestinal villi are flattened in focal areas.[218] The life cycle involves birds and freshwater fish, which appear to be the vehicle of transmission when eaten raw or poorly cooked.[219] The finding of eggs, adult worms, and larvae in small bowel contents suggests that autoinfection may occur. Travel and dietary histories may provide a clue to the diagnosis. The diagnosis is confirmed by identifying ova of *C. philippinensis* in fecal specimens.

Angiostrongylus costaricensis lives in the lumen of mesenteric arteries of the ileocecal region of rodents and occasionally involves the same site in humans.[220–222] Eggs form emboli to terminal branches of the mesenteric arteries. Disease, usually encountered in children, may present as an acute abdominal infection with fever, nausea, vomiting, pain, and sometimes a right lower quadrant mass. Leukocytosis and eosinophilia (11 to 82%) are common. In some cases it may be impossible to distinguish infection with *A. costaricensis* from acute appendicitis on clinical grounds.[221] Humans become infected by ingesting material contaminated by infected slugs or land snails, which are intermediate hosts. *Angiostrongylus costaricensis* is endemic in areas of Central and South America. Infection has also been acquired in the United States.[222] The diagnosis is suggested by the clinical syndrome and history of exposure. Antibodies can be detected by ELISA or latex agglutination tests.[221] The diagnosis is frequently made after surgical exploration and resection by identifying adult worms and eggs in tissue.

Patients with schistosomiasis and other trematode infections may present with gastrointestinal complaints and eosinophilia. Katayama fever, a serum sickness–like syndrome characterized by fever, headache, diarrhea, hepatosplenomegaly, generalized lymphadenopathy, urticaria, and eosinophilia, can occur within 4 to 8 weeks after primary exposure to schistosomes. The syndrome is seen in persons with heavy infections. It occurs most frequently with *Schistosoma japonicum*, less frequently with *Schistosoma mansoni*, and rarely with *Schistosoma haematobium* infections.[223] The acute manifestations of schistosomiasis are usually self-limited, although death may occur. The diagnosis of Katayama fever should be suspected in patients with a serum sickness–like illness accompanied by eosinophilia who have had exposure to schistosomes during the previous 4 to 8 weeks through swimming or bathing in fresh water in an endemic area.[224, 225] Serologic tests provide suggestive evidence of disease. The diagnosis is confirmed by the demonstration of ova in feces[223] or in a rectal biopsy specimen.

Acute infections with the Chinese fluke, *Clonorchis sinensis,* the Southeast Asian liver fluke, *Opisthorchis viverrini*, or the North American liver fluke, *Metorchis conjunctus*, are acquired through the ingestion of raw or inadequately cooked freshwater fish.[226–228] Persons infected may present with fever, abdominal pain, diarrhea, hepatomegaly, and eosinophilia. Those with established *C. sinensis* and *O. viverrini* infections are usually free of abdominal discomfort and eosinophilia, but they are at increased risk of ascending cholangitis and cholangiocarcinoma. Acute infection with *Fasciola hepatica,* the sheep liver fluke, is endemic in many cattle- and sheep-raising areas of the world. It is characterized by fever and pain in the right upper quadrant, hepatomegaly, and often marked eosinophilia.[229–231] Human infections are acquired by the ingestion of metacercariae that encyst on aquatic plants such as wild watercress. Infections have been reported from South America, Africa, Europe, China, and Australia. The diagnosis is confirmed by the identification of characteristic ova in the feces or bile. Concentration techniques increase the likelihood of finding ova.

Several trematodes that inhabit the gastrointestinal tract can produce abdominal pain, diarrhea and eosinophilia. Infection with *Heterophyes heterophyes, Metagonimus yokogawai,* and *Nanophyetus salmincola* are acquired through the ingestion of raw or undercooked freshwater fish,[232–235] *Fasciolopsis buski* is acquired through the ingestion of water chestnuts or the peeling of other freshwater plants with the teeth before ingestion.[232] Infection with these flukes may be asymptomatic, but patients with heavy infections often develop both abdominal pain and diarrhea. The diagnosis is suggested by a history of exposure in an endemic area and the dietary history. The diagnosis is made by the demonstration of ova in feces and may require concentration techniques. *Echinostoma* spp. may cause a similar syndrome after ingestion of raw, infected snails, amphibians, or fish.[236]

Adult tapeworm infestations with *Taenia solium*, the pork tapeworm, *Taenia saginata,* the beef tapeworm, *Diphyllobothrium latum*, the fish tapeworm, and *Hymenolepis nana,* the dwarf tapeworm, are usually asymptomatic, but they can on occasion be associated with abdominal discomfort, diarrhea, or eosinophilia.[237] In patients with echinococcosis, eosinophilia may occur in conjunction with abdominal pain or occasionally anaphylaxis when cysts leak.[238] The diagnosis of echinococcosis should be suspected in patients who have lived or traveled in endemic areas. The diagnosis is usually made on the basis of sonographic or CT findings and serologic studies.[239]

Patients with enteric protozoal infections (e.g., *Entamoeba histolytica*) usually do not have eosinophilia. *Isospora belli* is an exception.[240, 241] It can cause abdominal pain, watery diarrhea, and malabsorption in association with eosinophilia. Infection is usually encountered in the tropics where sanitation is poor. In healthy adults, *I. belli* produces a self-limited disease, but it is an important cause of severe, chronic diarrhea and weight loss in Haitians and others with acquired immunodeficiency syndrome.[242] The diagnosis is suggested by a history of potential exposure and confirmed by the demonstration of oocysts in feces; concentration techniques and acid-fast staining are helpful.[243, 244] Examination of duodenal contents or small-bowel biopsy specimens are more sensitive diagnostic techniques. *Dientamoeba fragilis* is another protozoan that can cause diarrhea and abdominal discomfort. It has been associated with pinworm infection and eosinophilia.[245, 246]

Eosinophilic gastroenteritis is a rare disease of uncertain cause characterized by eosinophilic infiltration of the gastrointestinal tract, peripheral eosinophilia in the majority of cases, and clinical manifestations that may include abdominal pain, diarrhea, protein-losing enteropathy, malabsorption, or gastric outlet obstruction in the absence of documented helminthic infestion.[247] The clinical manifestations depend both on the portion of bowel involved (stomach, duodenum, jejunum, or ileum) and on the layer involved (mucosa, muscular layer, or submucosa). The stomach and small intestine are the most common sites, but eosinophilic ileocolitis has also been reported.[248] Patients frequently have a history of allergic diathesis.[247–249] The sedimentation rate is usually normal or only mildly elevated, and Charcot-Leyden crystals may be seen in the stool.[249] Radiologic studies may reveal polypoid gastric or duodenal mucosal folds and rigid dilated loops of jejunum with a sawtooth mucosal pattern.[250] The diagnosis is usually made by endoscopic biopsy. Histologic examination of involved tissue reveals eosinophilia in the absence of both granulomas, vasculitis, and helminths.[249] Since the involvement may be patchy, multiple biopsies should be taken. Biopsies may be negative if the disease involves only the muscular or subserosal layers. In the latter case, the presence of eosinophils in ascitic fluid is suggestive of the diagnosis.[249] Eosinophilic gastroenteritis is chronic and occasionally fatal,[251] but most patients respond to corticosteroid therapy.[247, 249] As previously discussed, a number of intestinal helminths that infect humans, such as the dog hookworm *Ancylostoma caninum*, which can produce eosinophilic enteritis in humans, and nematodes of fish that cause anisakiasis can produce eosinophilic enteritis or gastroenteritis and must be excluded before a diagnosis of idiopathic eosinophilic gastroenteritis is made.

Gastrointestinal involvement with eosinophilia can also occur as manifestations of vasculitis.[252–254] Up to 25% of the patients with polyarteritis nodosa have involvement of the gastrointestinal tract. It is the initial manifestation of disease in 15% of patients.[253, 254] Abdominal pain is a prominent symptom, and eosinophilia is frequent. The clue to the diagnosis, which may be confirmed by biopsy or angiography, is provided by the systemic nature of the disease with frequent involvement of the kidneys, heart, and musculoskeletal and nervous systems. In allergic angiitis and granulomatosis of the Churg-Strauss syndrome type, lung involvement is pronounced, patients manifest prominent eosinophilia, and there is a strong allergic diathesis, often with asthma.[252] Some of the patients with this syndrome also have abdominal involvement and have been classified as having a polyangiitis overlap syndrome.[255, 256]

Abdominal pain and diarrhea accompanied by eosinophilia may occur in patients with regional enteritis, Whipple's disease, or ulcerative colitis.[257, 258] In one series, 32% of the patients with radiologically or surgically proven regional enteritis had eosinophilia on more than one occasion.[257] The average elevated eosinophil count was 6.2%; the range was from 4 to 22%.[257] On occasion the extraintestinal manifestations of inflammatory bowel diseases provide clues to their diagnosis.

Patients with solid tumors and lymphomas may also have abdominal pain, diarrhea, and eosinophilia.[259–261] Eosinophilia is most commonly associated with solid tumors after metastasis has occurred.[259, 260] Among solid tumors, frequently implicated malignancies are gastric, colonic, lung, pancreatic, and uterine carcinomas.[259, 261] A history of weight loss and the presence of melena or guaiac-positive stools and anemia suggest the diagnosis of cancer in the gastrointestinal tract, which may be confirmed by appropriate radiographic or endoscopic studies. Both Hodgkin's disease and non-Hodgkin's lymphomas may also be associated with eosinophilia, diarrhea, and abdominal pain when the bowel or abdominal or retroperitoneal nodes are involved.

REFERENCES

1. Christie AB. Typhoid and paratyphoid fevers. In: Infectious Diseases: Epidemiology and Clinical Practice. 2nd ed. New York: Churchill Livingstone; 1974:55–130.
2. Walker W, ed. The Aberdeen typhoid outbreak of 1964. Scott Med J. 1965;10:466–479.
3. Gulati PD, Saxena SN, Gupta PS, et al. Changing pattern of typhoid fever. Am J Med. 1968;45:544–548.
4. Hornick RB, Greisman SE, Woodward TE, et al. Typhoid fever: Pathogenesis and immunologic control. N Engl J Med. 1970;283:686–691.
5. Stuart BM, Pullen RL: Typhoid: Clinical analysis of three hundred and sixty cases. Arch Intern Med. 1946;78:629–661.
6. Ryan CA, Hargrett-Bean NT, Blake PA. *Salmonella typhi* infections in the United States, 1975–1984: Increasing role of foreign travel. Rev Infect Dis. 1989;11:1–8.
7. Mermin JH, Townes JM, Gerber M, et al. Typhoid fever in the United States, 1985–1994: Changing risks of international travel and increasing antibiotic resistance. Arch Intern Med. 1998;158:633–638.
8. Birkhead GS, Morse DL, Levine WC, et al. Typhoid fever at a resort hotel in New York: A large outbreak with an unusual vehicle. J Infect Dis. 1993;167:1228–1232.
9. Carter PB, Collins FM. The route of enteric infection in normal mice. J Exp Med. 1974;139:1189–1203.
10. Kamat SA, Herzog C. Typhoid: Clinical picture and response to chloramphenicol: Prospective study in Bombay (1972). Infection. 1977;5:85–91.
11. Wicks ACB, Holmes GS, Davidson L. Endemic typhoid fever: A diagnostic pitfall. Q J Med. 1971;40:341–354.
12. Hoffman TA, Ruiz CJ, Counts GW, et al. Waterborne typhoid fever in Dade County, Florida: Clinical and therapeutic evaluation of 105 bacteremic patients. Am J Med. 1975;59:481–487.
13. Samantray SK, Johnson SC, Chakrabarti AK. Enteric fever: An analysis of 500 cases. Practitioner. 1977;218:400–408.
14. Wahab MFA, Robertson RP, Raasch FO. Paratyphoid A fever, Cairo, Egypt. Ann Intern Med. 1969;70:913–917.
15. Black PH, Kunz LJ, Swartz MN. Salmonellosis: A review of some unusual aspects. N Engl J Med. 1960;262:811–817.
16. Sprinz H, Gangarosa EJ, Williams M, et al. Histopathology of the upper small intestines in typhoid fever: Biopsy study of experimental disease in man. Am J Dig Dis. 1966;11:615–624.
17. Litwack KD, Hoke AW, Borchardt KA. Rose spots in typhoid fever. Arch Dermatol. 1972;105:252–255.
18. Meals RA. Paratyphoid fever: A report of 62 cases with several unusual findings and a review of the literature. Arch Intern Med. 1976;136:1422–1428.
19. Watson KC. Laboratory and clinical investigation of recovery of *Salmonella typhi* from blood. J Clin Microbiol. 1978;7:122–126.
20. Gilman RH, Terminel M, Levine MM, et al. Relative efficacy of blood, urine, rectal swab, bone-marrow, and rose-spot cultures for recovery of *Salmonella typhi* in typhoid fever. Lancet. 1975;1:1211–1213.
21. Gasem MH, Dolmans WM, Isbandrio BB, et al. Culture of *Salmonella typhi* and *Salmonella paratyphi* from blood and bone marrow in suspected typhoid fever. Trop Geogr Med. 1995;47:164–167.
22. Shukla S, Patel B, Chitnis DS. 100 years of Widal test and its reappraisal in an endemic area. Indian J Med Res. 1997;105:53–57.
23. Schroeder SA. Interpretation of serologic tests for typhoid fever. JAMA. 1968;206:839–840.
24. Reynolds DW, Carpenter RL, Simon WH. Diagnostic specificity of Widal's reaction for typhoid fever. JAMA. 1970;214:2192–2193.
25. Senewiratne B, Chir B, Senewiratne K. Reassessment of the Widal test in the diagnosis of typhoid. Gastroenterology. 1977;73:233–236.
26. Brodie J: Antibodies and the Aberdeen typhoid outbreak of 1964. I. The Widal reaction. J Hyg. 1977;79:161–180.
27. Buck RL, Escamilla J, Sangalang RP, et al. Diagnostic value of a single, pretreatment Widal test in suspected enteric fever cases in the Philippines. Trans R Soc Trop Med Hyg. 1987;81:871–873.
28. Levine MM, Grados O, Gilman RH, et al. Diagnostic value of the Widal test in areas endemic for typhoid fever. Am J Trop Med Hyg. 1978;27:795–800.
29. Editorial: Typhoid and its serology. BMJ. 1978;1:389.
30. Beasley WJ, Joseph SW, Weiss E: Improved serodiagnosis of *Salmonella* enteric fevers by an enzyme-linked immunosorbent assay. J Clin Microbiol. 1981;13:106–114.
31. Barrett TJ, Blake PA, Brown SL, et al. Enzyme-linked immunosorbent assay for detection of human antibodies to *Salmonella typhi* Vi antigen. J Clin Microbiol. 1983;17:625–627.
32. Tsang RSW, Chau PY. Serological diagnosis of typhoid fever by counterimmunoelectrophoresis. BMJ. 1981;282:1505–1507.
33. Sundararaj T, Ilango B, Subramanian S. A study on the usefulness of counter immuno-electrophoresis for the detection of *Salmonella typhi* antigen in the sera of suspected cases of enteric fever. Trans R Soc Trop Med Hyg. 1983;77:194–197.
34. Taylor DN, Harris JR, Barrett TJ, et al. Detection of urinary Vi antigen as a diagnostic test for typhoid fever. J Clin Microbiol. 1983;18:872–876.
35. Song JH, Cho H, Park MY, et al. Detection of *Salmonella typhi* in the blood of patients with typhoid fever by polymerase chain reaction. J Clin Microbiol. 1993;31:1439–1443.
36. Hashimoto Y, Itho Y, Fujinaga Y, et al. Development of nested PCR based on the ViaB sequence to detect *Salmonella typhi*. J Clin Microbiol. 1995;33:775–777.
37. Chaudhry R, Laxmi BV, Nisar N, et al. Standardization of polymerase chain reaction for the detection of *Salmonella typhi* in typhoid fever. J Clin Pathol. 1997;50:437–439.
38. Ramachandran S, Godfrey JJ, Perera MVF. Typhoid hepatitis. JAMA. 1974;230:236–242.
39. Sitprija V, Pipatanagul V, Boonpucknavig V, et al. Glomerulitis in typhoid fever. Ann Intern Med. 1974;81:210–213.
40. Butler W, Bell WR, Levin J, et al. Typhoid fever: Studies of blood coagulation, bacteremia, and endotoxemia. Arch Intern Med. 1978;138:407–410.
41. Harris JC, DuPont HL, Hornick RB. Fecal leukocytes in diarrheal illness. Ann Intern Med. 1972;76:697–703.
42. Misra S, Diaz PS, Rowley AH. Characteristics of typhoid fever in children and adolescents in a major metropolitan area in the United States. Clin Infect Dis. 1997;24:998–1000.
43. Blaser MJ, Hickman FW, Farmer JJ III, et al. *Salmonella typhi:* The laboratory as a reservoir of infection. J Infect Dis. 1980;142:934–938.
44. Blaser MJ, Lofgren JP. Fatal salmonellosis originating in a clinical microbiology laboratory. J Clin Microbiol. 1981;13:855–858.
45. Rabson AR, Hallett AF, Koornhof JH. Generalized *Yersinia enterocolitica* infection. J Infect Dis. 1975;131:447–451.
46. Spira TJ, Kabins SA. *Yersinia enterocolitica* septicemia with septic arthritis. Arch Intern Med. 1976;136:1305–1308.
47. Marlon A, Gentry L, Merigan TC. Septicemia with *Pasteurella pseudotuberculosis* and liver disease. Arch Intern Med. 1971;127:947–949.
48. Ljungberg P, Valtonen M, Harjola VP, et al. Report of four cases of *Yersinia pseudotuberculosis* septicemia and a literature review. Eur J Clin Microbiol Infect Dis. 1995;14:804–810.
49. Guerrant RL, Lahita RG, Winn WC Jr, et al. Campylobacteriosis in man: Pathogenic mechanisms and review of 91 bloodstream infections. Am J Med. 1978;65:584–592.
50. Schmidt U, Chmel H, Kaminski Z, et al. The clinical spectrum of *Campylobacter fetus* infection: Report of 5 cases and review of the literature. Q J Med. 1980;49:431–442.
51. Carbone KM, Heinrich MC, Quinn TC. Thrombophlebitis and cellulitis due to *Campylobacter fetus* spp *fetus*. Medicine. 1984;64:244–250.
52. Bokkenheuser V. *Vibrio fetus* infection in man. I. Ten new cases and some epidemiologic observations. Am J Epidemiol. 1970;91:400–409.
53. Leino R, Kalliomäki JL. Yersiniosis as an internal disease. Ann Intern Med. 1974;81:458–461.
54. Ahvonen P. Human yersiniosis in Finland. I. Bacteriology and serology. Ann Clin Res. 1972;4:30–38.
55. Hubbert WT, Petenyi CW, Glasgow LA, et al. *Yersinia pseudotuberculosis* infection in the United States: Septicemia, appendicitis, and mesenteric lymphadenitis. Am J Trop Med Hyg. 1971;20:679–684.
56. Yamashiro KM, Goldman RH, Harris D, et al. *Pasteurella pseudotuberculosis:* Acute sepsis with survival. Arch Intern Med. 1971;128:605–608.
57. Keet EE. *Yersinia enterocolitica* septicemia: Source of infection and incubation period identified. N Y State J Med. 1974;74:2226–2230.
58. Sonnenwirth AC. Bacteremia with and without meningitis due to *Yersinia enterocolitica, Edwardsiella tarda, Comamonas terrigena,* and *Pseudomonas maltophilia.* Ann N Y Acad Sci. 1970;174:488–502.
59. Taykor BG, Zafarzai MZ, Humphreys DW, et al. Nodular pulmonary infiltrates and septic arthritis associated with *Yersinia enterocolitica* bacteremia. Am Rev Respir Dis. 1977;116:525–529.
60. Bliddal J, Kaliszan S. Prolonged monosymptomatic fever due to *Yersinia enterocolitica.* Acta Med Scand. 1977;201:387–389.
61. Ahvonen P. Human yersiniosis in Finland. II. Clinical features. Ann Clin Res. 1972;4:39–48.
62. Franklin B, Ulmer DD. Human infection with *Vibrio fetus.* West J Med. 1974;120:200–204.
63. Greenwood JR, Flanigan SW, Pickett MJ, et al. Clinical isolation of *Yersinia enterocolitica:* Cold temperature enrichment. J Clin Microbiol. 1975;2:559–560.
64. Skirrow MB. *Campylobacter* enteritis: A "new" disease. BMJ. 1977;2:9–11.
65. Lauwers S, DeBoeck M, Butzler JP. *Campylobacter* enteritis in Brussels. Lancet. 1978;1:604–605.
66. Bokkenheuser V. *Vibrio fetus* infection in man: A serological test. Infect Immun. 1972;5:222–226.
67. Reinicke V, Korner B. Case report: Fulminant septicemia caused by *Yersinia enterocolitica.* Scand J Infect Dis. 1977;9:249–251.
68. Forrsstrom J, Viander M, Lehtonen A, et al. Case report: *Yersinia enterocolitica* infection complicated by glomerulonephritis. Scand J Infect Dis. 1977;9:253–256.
69. Guerrant RL, Humphries MK Jr, Butler JE, et al. Tickborne oculoglandular tularemia. Arch Intern Med. 1976;136:811–813.
70. Buchanan TM, Faber LC, Feldman RA. Brucellosis in the United States, 1960–

1972: An abattoir-associated disease. I. Clinical features and therapy. Medicine. 1974;53:403–413.
71. Reed WP, Palmer DL, Williams RC Jr, et al. Bubonic plague in the southwestern United States: A review of recent experience. Medicine. 1970;49:465–486.
72. Cantey JR. Plague in Vietnam: Clinical observations and treatment with kanamycin. Arch Intern Med. 1974;133:280–283.
73. Nalin DR, Sultana B, Sahunja R, et al. Survival of a patient with intestinal anthrax. Am J Med. 1977;62:130–132.
74. Brundage WG, Thuss CJ Jr, Walden DG. Four fatal cases of melioidosis in US soldiers in Vietnam: Bacteriologic and pathologic characteristics. Am J Trop Med Hyg. 1968;17:183–191.
75. Schwartzman W. Bartonella (Rochalimaea) infections: Beyond cat scratch. Ann Rev Med. 1996;47:355–364.
76. Cuadra M. Salmonellosis complication in human bartonellosis. Tex Rep Biol Med. 1956;14:97–113.
77. Cunningham BB, Paller AS, Katz BZ. Rat bite fever in a pet lover. J Am Acad Dermatol. 1998;38:330–332.
78. Kowal J. Spirillum fever: Report of a case and review of the literature. N Engl J Med. 1961;264:123–128.
79. Anderson LC, Leary SL, Manning PJ. Rat bite fever in animal research laboratory personnel. Lab Anim Sci. 1983;33:292–294.
80. Heath CW Jr, Alexander AD, Galton MM. Leptospirosis in the United States: Analysis of 483 cases in man, 1949–1961. N Engl J Med. 1965;273:857–864.
81. Edwards GA, Domm BM. Human leptospirosis. Medicine. 1960;39:117–156.
82. Trevejo RT, Schriefer ME, Gage KL, et al. An interstate outbreak of tick-borne relapsing fever among vacationers at a Rocky Mountain cabin. Am J Trop Med Hyg. 1998;58:743–747.
83. Dworkin MS, Anderson DE Jr, Schwan TG, et al. Tick-borne relapsing fever in the northeastern United States and southeastern Canada. Clin Infect Dis. 1998;26:122–131.
84. Jadvar H, Mindelzun RE, Olcott EW, et al. Still the great mimicker: Abdominal tuberculosis. AJR Am J Roentgenol. 1997;168:1455–1460.
85. Horvath KD, Whelan RL. Intestinal tuberculosis: Return of an old disease. Am J Gastroenterol. 1998;93:692–696.
86. Smego RA Jr, Foglia G. Actinomycosis. Clin Infect Dis. 1998;26:1255–1261.
87. Larson EB, Featherstone HJ, Petersdorf RG. Fever of undetermined origin: Diagnosis and follow-up of 105 cases, 1970–1980. Medicine. 1982;61:269–292.
88. Murray HW, Masur H, Senterfit LB, et al. The protean manifestations of *Mycoplasma pneumoniae* infection in adults. Am J Med. 1975;58:229–242.
89. Gregory DW, Schaffner W. Psittacosis. Semin Respir Infect. 1997;12:7–11.
90. Walker DH. Rocky Mountain spotted fever: A seasonal alert. Clin Infect Dis. 1995;20:1111–1117.
91. Dalton MJ, Clarke MJ, Holman RC, et al. National surveillance for Rocky Mountain spotted fever, 1981–1992: Epidemiologic summary and evaluation of risk factors for fatal outcome. Am J Trop Med Hyg. 1995;52:405–413.
92. Walker DH. Gastroenterology of Rocky Mountain spotted fever. Practical Gastroenterol. 1986;10:25–39.
93. Jiminez J, Byrne WJ, Seibert JJ, et al. Gastrointestinal symptoms in Rocky Mountain spotted fever: Histopathologic finding of ulcerative enteritis with vasculitis. Clin Pediatr. 1982;21:581–584.
94. Middleton DB. Rocky Mountain spotted fever: Gastrointestinal and laboratory manifestations. South Med J. 1978;71:629–632.
95. Westerman EL. Rocky Mountain spotted fever: A dilemma for the clinician. Arch Intern Med. 1982;142:1106–1107.
96. Woodward TE, Pedersen CE Jr, Oster CN, et al. Prompt confirmation of Rocky Mountain spotted fever: Identification of rickettsiae in skin tissues. J Infect Dis. 1976;134:297–301.
97. Duma RJ, Sonenshine DE, Bozeman FM, et al. Epidemic typhus in the United States associated with flying squirrels. JAMA. 1981;245:2318–2323.
98. Centers for Disease Control and Prevention. Epidemic typhus associated with flying squirrels: United States. MMWR Morb Mortal Wkly Rep. 1982;31:555–561.
99. Marrie TJ, Schlech WF III, Williams JC, et al. Q fever pneumonia associated with exposure to wild rabbits. Lancet. 1986;1:427–429.
100. Bakken JS, Krueth J, Wilson-Nordskog C, et al. Clinical and laboratory characteristics of human granulocytic ehrlichiosis. JAMA. 1996;275:199–205.
101. Jacobs RF, Schultz GE. Ehrlichiosis in children. J. Pediatr. 1997;131:184–192.
102. Yu VL, Kroboth FJ, Shonnard J, et al. Legionnaires' disease: New clinical perspective from a prospective pneumonia study. Am J Med. 1982;73:357–361.
103. Kirby BD, Snyder KM, Meyer RD, et al. Legionnaires' disease: Report of 65 nosocomially acquired cases and a review of the literature. Medicine. 1980;59:188–205.
104. Chow JW, Lu VL. New perspectives on *Legionella* pneumonia: Diagnosis, management and prevention. J Crit Illness. 1988;3:17–27.
105. Sturim HS, Kouchonkos NT, Ahlvin RC. Gastrointestinal manifestations of disseminated histoplasmosis. Am J Surg. 1965;110:435–440.
106. Gordon S, Brennessel DJ, Goldstein JA, et al. Malaria: A city hospital experience. Arch Intern Med. 1988;148:1569–1571.
107. Gorenflot A, Moubri K, Precigout E, et al. Human babesiosis. Ann Trop Med Parasitol. 1998;92:489–501.
108. Boustani MR, Gelfand JA. Babesiosis. Clin Infect Dis. 1996;22:611–615.
109. Lee KC, Yamazaki O, Hamba H, et al. Analysis of 69 patients with amebic liver abscess. J Gastroenterol. 1996;31:40–45.
110. Butler T, Arnold K, Linh NN, et al. Chloramphenicol-resistant typhoid fever in Vietnam associated with R factor. Lancet. 1973;2:983–991.
111. Brown JD, Mo DH, Rhoades ER. Chloramphenicol-resistant *Salmonella typhi* in Saigon. JAMA. 1975;231:162–166.
112. Olarte J, Galindo E. *Salmonella typhi* resistant to chloramphenicol, ampicillin and other antimicrobial agents: Strains isolated during an extensive typhoid fever epidemic in Mexico. Antimicrob Agents Chemother. 1973;4:597–603.
113. Bhutta ZA, Naqvi SH, Razzaq RA, et al. Multidrug-resistant typhoid in children. Presentation and clinical features. Rev Infect Dis. 1991;13:832–836.
114. Chew SK, Monteiro EH, Lim YS, et al. A 7-day course of ciprofloxacin for enteric fever. J Infect. 1992;25:267–271.
115. Uwaydah AK, al Soub H, Matar I. Randomized prospective study comparing two dosage regimens of ciprofloxacin for the treatment of typhoid fever. J Antimicrob Chemother. 1992;30:707–711.
116. Dutta P, Rasaily R, Saha MR, et al. Ciprofloxacin for treatment of severe typhoid fever in children. Antimicrob Agents Chemother. 1993;37:1197–1199.
117. Murdock DA, Banatvala NA, Bone A, et al. Epidemic ciprofloxacin-resistant *Salmonella typhi* in Tajikistan. Lanet. 1998;351:339.
118. Wain J, Hoa NT, Chinh NT, et al. Quinolone-resistant *Salmonella typhi* in Viet Nam: Molecular basis of resistance and clinical response to treatment. Clin Infect Dis. 1997;25:1401–1410.
119. Rowe B, Ward LR, Threlfall EJ. Multidrug-resistant *Salmonella typhi*: A worldwide epidemic. Clin Infect Dis. 1997;24(Suppl):S106–S109.
120. Lasserre R, Sangalang RP, Santiago L. Three-day treatment of typhoid fever with two different doses of ceftriaxone, compared to 14-day therapy with chloramphenicol: A randomized trial. J Antimicrob Chemother 1991;28:765–772.
121. Soe GB, Overturf GD. Treatment of typhoid fever and other systemic salmonellosis with cefotaxime, ceftriaxone, cefoperazone and other newer cephalosporins. Rev Infect Dis. 1987;9:719–736.
122. Memon IA, Billoo AG, Memon HI. Cefixime: An oral option for the treatment of multidrug-resistant enteric fever in children. South Med J. 1997;90:1204–1207.
123. Girgis NI, Sultan Y, Hammad O, et al. Comparison of the efficacy, safety and cost of cefixime, ceftriaxone and aztreonam in the treatment of multi-drug resistant *Salmonella typhi* septicemia in children. Pediatr Infect Dis J. 1995;14:603–605.
124. Datta N, Richards H, Datta C. *Salmonella typhi* in vivo acquires resistance to both chloramphenicol and co-trimoxazole. Lancet. 1981;1:1181–1183.
125. Rao PM, Rhea JT, Novelline RA. CT diagnosis of mesenteric adenitis. Radiology. 1997;202:145–149.
126. Van Noyen R, Selderslaghs R, Bekaert J, et al. Causative role of *Yersinia* and other enteric pathogens in the appendicular syndrome. Eur J Clin Microbiol Infect Dis. 1991;10:735–741.
127. Winblad S, Nilehn B, Sternby NJ. *Yersinia enterocolitica* (Pasteurella X) in human enteric infections. BMJ. 1966;2:1363–1366.
128. Mair NS, Mair HJ, Stirk EM, et al. Three cases of acute mesenteric lymphadenitis due to *Pasteurella pseudotuberculosis*. J Clin Pathol. 1960;13:432–439.
129. Tertti R, Vuento R, Mikkola P, et al. Clinical manifestations of *Yersinia pseudotuberculosis* infection in children. Eur J Clin Microbiol Infect Dis. 1989;8:587–591.
130. Carter PB. Pathogenicity of *Yersinia enterocolitica* for mice. Infect Immun. 1975;11:164–170.
131. Garcia-Corbeira P, Ramos JM, Aguado JM, et al. Six cases in which mesenteric lymphadenitis due to non-typhi *Salmonella* caused an appendicitis-like syndrome. Clin Infect Dis. 1995;21:231–232.
132. Lee JH, Rhee PL, Lee JK, et al. The etiology and clinical characteristics of mesenteric adenitis in Korean adults. J Korean Med Sci. 1997;12:105–110.
133. Ukarapol N, Sirisanthana V, Wongsawasdi L. *Penicillium marneffei* mesenteric lymphadenitis in human immunodeficiency virus–infected children. J Med Assoc Thai. 1998;81:637–640.
134. Collins DC. Mesenteric lymphadenitis in adolescents simulating appendicitis. Can Med Assoc J. 1936;34:402–405.
135. Asch MJ, Amoury RA, Touloukian RJ, et al. Suppurative mesenteric lymphadenitis: A report of two cases and review of the literature. Am J Surg. 1968;115:570–573.
136. Constantinides CG, Davies MRQ, Cywes S. Suppurative mesenteric lymphadenitis in children: Case reports. S Afr Med J. 1981;60:629–631.
137. Dudley HAF, MacLaren IF. Primary mesenteric abscess. Lancet. 1956;2:1182–1184.
138. Jepsen OB, Korner B, Lauritsen KB, et al. *Yersinia enterocolitica* infection in patients with acute surgical abdominal disease: A prospective study. Scand J Infect Dis. 1976;8:189–194.
139. Zen-Yoji H, Maruyama T, Sakai S, et al. An outbreak of enteritis due to *Yersinia enterocolitica* occurring at a junior high school. Jpn J Microbiol. 1973;17:220.
140. Asakawa Y, Akahane S, Kagata N, et al. Two community outbreaks of human infection with *Yersinia enterocolitica*. J Hyg (Lond). 1973;71:715–23.
141. Black RE, Jackson RJ, Tsai T, et al. Epidemic *Yersinia enterocolitica* infection due to contaminated chocolate milk. N Engl J Med. 1978;298:76–79.
142. Vantrappen G, Agg HO, Ponette E, et al. *Yersinia* enteritis and enterocolitis: Gastroenterological aspects. Gastroenterology. 1977;72:220–227.
143. Jansson E, Wallgren GR, Ahvonen P. *Yersinia enterocolitica* as a cause of acute mesenteric lymphadenitis. Acta Paediatr Scand. 1968;57:448–450.
144. Tauxe RV, Vandepitte J, Wauters G, et al. *Yersinia enterocolitica* infections and pork: The missing link. Lancet. 1987;1:1129–1132.
145. Knapp W. Mesenteric adenitis due to *Pasteurella pseudotuberculosis* in young people. N Engl J Med. 1958;259:776–778.
146. Randall KJ, Mair NS. Family outbreak of *Pasteurella pseudotuberculosis* infection. Lancet. 162;1:1042–1043.
147. Weber J, Finlayson NB, Mark JBD. Mesenteric lymphadenitis and terminal ileitis due to *Yersinia pseudotuberculosis*. N Engl J Med. 1970;283:172–174.

148. Saari TN, Triplett DA. *Yersinia pseudotuberculosis* mesenteric adenitis. J Pediatr. 1974;85:656–659.
149. Bradford WD, Noce PS, Gutman LT. Pathologic features of enteric infection with *Yersinia enterocolitica.* Arch Pathol. 1974;98:17–22.
150. Weissfeld AS, Sonnenwirth AC. *Yersinia enterocolitica* in adults with gastrointestinal disturbances: Need for cold enrichment. J Clin Microbiol. 1980;11:196–197.
151. Daniëls JJHM. Enteral infection with *Pasteurella pseudotuberculosis:* Isolation of the organism from human feces. BMJ. 1961;2:997.
152. Niléhn B, Sjostrom B. Studies on *Yersinia enterocolitica* occurrence in various groups of acute abdominal disease. Acta Pathol Microbiol Scand. 1967;71:612–628.
153. Marks MI, Pai CH, Lafleur L, et al. *Yersinia enterocolitica* gastroenteritis: A prospective study of clinical, bacteriologic, and epidemiologic features. J Pediatr. 1980;96:26–31.
154. Puylaert JB. Mesenteric adenitis and acute terminal ileitis: Ultrasound evaluation using graded compression. Radiology. 1986;161:691–695.
155. Ekberg O, Sjöström B, Brahme F. Radiological findings in *Yersinia* ileitis. Radiology. 1977;123:15–19.
156. Rao PM, Rhea JT, Novelline RA. Sensitivity and specificity of the individual CT signs of appendicitis: Experience with 200 helical appendiceal CT examinations. J Comput Assist Tomogr. 1997;21:686–692.
157. Ahlqvist J, Ahvonen P, Räsänen JA, et al. Enteric infection with *Yersinia enterocolitica*: Large pyroninophilic cell reproduction in mesenteric lymph nodes associated with early production of specific antibodies. Acta Pathol Microbiol Scand A. 1971;79:109–122.
158. Braunstein H, Tucker EB, Gibson BC. Mesenteric lymphadenitis due to *Yersinia enterocolitica:* Report of a case. Am J Clin Pathol. 1971;55:506–510.
159. El-Maraghi NRH, Mair NS. The histopathology of enteric infection with *Yersinia pseudotuberculosis.* Am J Clin Pathol. 1979;71:631–639.
160. Gutman LT, Ottesen EA, Quan TJ, et al. An inter-familial outbreak of *Yersinia enterocolitica* enteritis. N Engl J Med. 1973;288:1372–1377.
161. Arvastson B, Damgaard K, Winblad S. Clinical symptoms of infection with *Yersinia enterocolitica.* Scand J Infect Dis. 1971;3:37–40.
162. Wilson HD, McCormick JB, Feeley JC. *Yersinia enterocolitica* infection in a 4-month-old infant associated with infection in household dogs. J Pediatr. 1976;89:767–768.
163. Tacket CO, Narain JP, Sattin R, et al. A multistate outbreak of infections caused by *Yersinia enterocolitica* transmitted by pasteurized milk. JAMA. 1984;251:483–486.
164. Nolan C, Harris N, Ballard J, et al. Outbreak of *Yersinia enterocolitica:* Washington State. MMWR Morb Mortal Wkly Rep. 1982;31:562.
165. Laasen J. *Yersinia enterocolitica* in drinking-water. Scand J Infect Dis. 1972;4:125–127.
166. Highsmith AK, Feeley JC, Skaliy P, et al. Isolation of *Yersinia enterocolitica* from well water and growth in distilled water. Appl Environ Microbiol. 1977;34:745–750.
167. Snyder JD, Christenson E, Feldman RA. Human *Yersinia enterocolitica* infections in Wisconsin. Am J Med. 1982;72:768–774.
168. Berkowitz FE, Nesheim S. Chylous ascites caused by *Mycobacterium avium* complex and mesenteric lymphadenitis in a child with the acquired immunodeficiency syndrome. Pediatr Infect Dis J. 1993;12:99–101.
169. Morinet F, Monsuez JJ, Roger P, et al. Parvovirus B19 associated with pseudoappendicitis (Letter). Lancet. 1987;2:1466.
170. Chen CM, Chao K, Su IJ. Acute primary Epstein-Barr virus infection presenting as acute abdomen. Peditr Infect Dis J. 1991;10:471–473.
171. Bhisitkul DM, Tod KM, Listernick R. Adenovirus infection and childhood intussusception. Am J Dis Child. 1992;146:1331–1341.
172. Loría-Cortés R, Lobo-Sanahuja JF. Clinical abdominal angiostrongylosis: A study of 116 children with intestinal eosinophilic granuloma caused by *Angiostrongylus costaricensis.* Am J Trop Med Hyg. 1980;29:538–544.
173. Gutman LT, Wilfert CM, Quan T. Susceptibility of *Yersinia enterocolitica* to trimethoprim-sulfamethoxazole. J Infect Dis. 1973;128(Suppl):S538.
174. Hornstein MJ, Jupeau AM, Scavizzi MR, et al. In vitro susceptibilities of 126 clinical isolates of *Yersinia enterocolitica* to 21 β-lactam antibiotics. Antimicrob Agents Chemother. 1985;27:806–811.
175. Stolk-Engelaar VM, Meis JF, Mulder JA, et al. In-vitro antimicrobial susceptibility of *Yersinia enterocolitica* isolates from stools in The Netherlands from 1982–1991. J Antimicrob Chemother. 1995;36:839–843.
176. Hammerberg S, Sorger S, Marks MI. Antimicrobial susceptibilities of *Yersinia enterocolitica* biotype 4, serotype O:3. Antimicrob Agents Chemother. 1977;11:566–568.
177. Mahmoud AAF. Strongyloidiasis. Clin Infect Dis. 1996;23:949–952.
178. Scowden EB, Schaffner W, Stone WJ. Overwhelming strongyloidiasis: An unappreciated opportunistic infection. Medicine. 1978;57:527–544.
179. Morgan JS, Schaffner W, Stone WJ. Opportunistic strongyloidiasis in renal transplant recipients. Transplantation. 1986;42:518–524.
180. Cadranel JF, Eugene C. Another example of *Strongyloides stercoralis* infection associated with cimetidine in an immunosuppressed patient. Gut. 1986;27:1229.
181. Pelletier LL Jr, Baker CB, Gam AA, et al. Diagnosis and evaluation of treatment of chronic strongyloidiasis in ex-prisoners of war. J Infect Dis. 1988;157:573–576.
182. Gill GV, Bell DR. *Strongyloides stercoralis* infection in former Far East prisoners of war. BMJ. 1979;2:572–574.
183. Grove DI. Strongyloidiasis in Allied ex-prisoners of war in south-east Asia. BMJ. 1980;280:598–601.
184. Pelletier LL Jr. Chronic strongyloidiasis in World War II Far East ex-prisoners of war. Am J Trop Med Hyg. 1984;33:55–61.
185. Berk SL, Verghese A, Alvarez S, et al. Clinical and epidemiologic features of strongyloidiasis: A prospective study in rural Tennessee. Arch Intern Med. 1987;147:1257–1261.
186. Lima JP, Delgado PG. Diagnosis of strongyloidiasis: Importance of Baermann's method. Am J Diagn Dis. 1961;6:899.
187. De Kaminsky RG. Evaluation of three methods for laboratory diagnosis of *Strongyloides stercoralis* infection. J Parasitol. 1993;79:277–280.
188. Salazar SA, Gutierrez C, Berk SL. Value of the agar plate method for the diagnosis of intestinal strongyloides. Diagn Microbiol Infect Dis. 1995;23:141–145.
189. Beal CB, Viens P, Grant RGL, et al. A new technique for sampling duodenal contents: Demonstration of upper small bowel pathogens. Am J Trop Med Hyg. 1970;19:399–352.
190. Grove DI, Blair AJ. Dignosis of human strongyloidiasis by immunofluorescence using *Strongyloides ratti* and *S. stercoralis* larvae. Am J Trop Med Hyg. 1981;30:344–349.
191. Kagen IG, Maddison SE. Parasitic immunodiagnosis. In Strickland GT, ed: Hunter's Tropical Medicine. 7th ed. Philadelphia: WB Saunders; 1991:1090–1095.
192. Gam AA, Neva FA, Krotoski WA. Comparative sensitivity and specificity of ELISA and IHA for serodiagnosis of strongyloidiasis with larval antigens. Am J Trop Med Hyg. 1987;37:157–161.
193. Blumenthal DS, Schultz MG. Incidence of intestinal obstruction in children infected with *Ascaris lumbricoides.* Am J Trop Med Hyg. 1975;24:801–805.
194. Akgun Y. Intestinal obstruction caused by *Ascaris lumbricoides.* Dis Colon Rectum. 1996;39:1159–1163.
195. Krige JEJ, Lewis G, Bornman PC. Recurrent pancreatitis caused by a calcified ascaris in the duct of Wirsung. Am J Gastroenterol. 1987;82:256–257.
196. Schantz PM, Glickman LT. Toxocaral visceral larva migrans. N Engl J Med. 1978;298:436–439.
197. Glickman LT, Magnaval JF. Zoonotic roundworm infections. Infect Dis Clin North Am. 1993;7:717.
198. Thompson DE, Bundy DAP, Cooper ES, et al. Epidemiological characteristics of *Toxocara canis* zoonotic infection of children in a Caribbean community. Bull World Health Organ. 1986;64:283–290.
199. Glickman LT, Magnaval J-F, Domanski LM, et al. Visceral larva migrans in French adults: A new disease syndrome. Am J Epidemiol. 1987;125:1019–1034.
200. Grove DI, Warren KS, Mahmoud AAF. Algorithms in the diagnosis and management of exotic diseases. VII. Trichinosis. J Infect Dis. 1975;132:485–488.
201. Campbell WC. Trichinella and Trichinosis. New York: Plenum; 1983.
202. Bailey TM, Schantz PM. Trends in the incidence and transmission patterns of trichinosis in the United States: Comparisons of the periods 1975–1981 and 1982–1986. Rev Infect Dis. 1990;12:5–11.
203. Singal M, Schantz PM, Werner SB. Trichinosis acquired at sea: Report of an outbreak. Am J Trop Med Hyg. 1976;25:675–681.
204. Petri WA Jr, Holsinger JR, Pearson RD. Common-source outbreak of trichinosis associated with eating raw home-butchered pork. South Med J. 1988;81:1056–1058.
205. Trichinosis outbreaks associated with horsemeat. Parasitol Today. 1986;2:295.
206. Viallet J, MacLean JD, Goresky CA, et al. Arctic trichinosis presenting as prolonged diarrhea. Gastroenterology. 1986;91:938–946.
207. MacLean JD, Poirier L, Gyorkos TW, et al. Epidemiologic and serologic definition of primary and secondary trichinosis in the Arctic. J Infect Dis. 1992;165:908–912.
208. Kagan IG. Serodiagnosis of trichinosis. In: Cohen S, Sadun EH, eds. Immunology of Parasitic Infections. Oxford: Blackwell Scientific; 1976:143–151.
209. Kwee HG, Sautter RL. Anisakiasis. Am Fam Physician. 1987;36:137–140.
210. Smith JW, Wooten R. Anisakis and anisakiasis. Adv Parasitol. 1978;16:93–163.
211. Pinkus GS, Coolidge C. Intestinal anisakiasis: First case report from North America. Am J Med. 1975;59:114–120.
212. Richman RH, Lewicki AM. Right ileocolitis secondary to anisakiasis. Am J Roentgen Rad Ther Nucl Med. 1973;119:329–331.
213. Yokogawa M, Yoshimura H. Clinicopathologic studies on larval anisakiasis in Japan. Am J Trop Med Hyg. 1967;16:723-734.
214. Whittner M, Turner JW, Jacquette G, et al. Eustrongylidiasis—a parasitic infection acquired by eating sushi. N Engl J Med. 1989;320:1124–1126.
215. Cross JH. Intestinal capillariasis. Clin Microbiol Rev. 1992;5:120.
216. Donda F, Chaves F, Sanz A, et al. Human intestinal capillariasis in an area of nonendemicity: Case report and review. Clin Infect Dis. 1993;17:909.
217. Watten RH, Beckner WM, Cross JH, et al. Clinical studies of capillariasis philippinensis. Trans R Soc Trop Med Hyg. 1972;66:828–834.
218. Fresh JW, Cross JH, Reyes V, et al. Necropsy findings in intestinal capillariasis. Am J Trop Med Hyg. 1972;21:169–173.
219. Cross JH, Banzon T, Clarke MD, et al. Studies on the experimental transmission of *Capillaria philippinensis* in monkeys. Trans R Soc Trop Med Hyg. 1972;66:819–827.
220. Morera P, Perez F, Mora F, et al. Visceral larva migrans–like syndrome caused by *Angiostrongylus costaricensis.* Am J Trop Med Hyg. 1982;31:67–70.
221. Morera P. Abdominal angiostrongyliasis. Clin Trop Med Commun Dis. 1987;2:747–754.
222. Hulbert TV, Larsen RA, Chandrasoma PT. Abdominal angiostrongyliasis mimicking acute appendicitis and Meckel's diverticulum: Report of a case in the United States and review. Clin Infect Dis. 1992;14:836–840.
223. Mahmoud AA. Schistosomiasis. N Engl J Med. 1977;297:1329–1331.
224. Elliot DE. Schistosomiasis. Pathophysiology, diagnosis, and treatment. Gastroenterol Clin North Am. 1996;25:599–625.
225. Farid Z, Trabolsi B, Hafez A. Acute schistosomiasis mansoni (Katayama syndrome). Ann Trop Med Parasitol. 1986;80:563–564.

226. Brockelman WY, Upatham ES, Viyanant V, et al. Measurement of incidence of the human liver fluke, *Opisthorchis viverrini*, in northeast Thailand. Trans R Soc Trop Med Hyg. 1987;81:327–335.
227. MacLean JD, Arthur JR, Ward BJ, et al. Common-source outbreak of acute infection due to the North American liver fluke *Metorchis conjunctus*. Lancet. 1996;347:154–158.
228. Liu LX, Harinasuta KT. Liver and intestinal flukes. Gastroenterol Clin North Am. 1996;25:627–636.
229. Arjona R, Riancho JA, Aguado JM, et al. Fasioliasis in developed countries: A review of class and aberrant forms of the disease. Medicine. 1995;74:13–23.
230. Han JK, Choi BI, Cho JM, et al. Radiographic findings of human fascioliasis. Abdom Imaging. 1993;18:261–264.
231. Jones EA, Kay JM, Milligan HP, et al. Massive infection with *Fasciola hepatica* in man. Am J Med. 1977;63:836–842.
232. Warren KS, Mahmoud AAF. Algorithms in the diagnosis and management of exotic diseases. XXI. Liver, intestinal and lung flukes. J Infect Dis. 1977;135:692–696.
233. Adams KO, Jungkind DL, Bergquist EJ, et al. Intestinal fluke infection as a result of eating sushi. Am J Clin Pathol. 1986;86:688–689.
234. Goldsmith RS. Chronic diarrhea in returning travelers: Intestinal parasite infection with the fluke *Metagonimus yokogawai*. South Med J. 1978;71:1513–1515.
235. Harrell LW, Deardorff TL. Human nanophyetiasis: Transmission by handling naturally infected coho salmon (*Oncorhynchus kisutch*). J Infect Dis. 1990;161:146–148.
236. Huffman JE, Fried B. *Echinostoma* and echinostomiasis. Adv Parasitol. 1990;29:215–269.
237. Schantz PM. Tapeworms (cestodiasis). Gastroenterol Clin North Am. 1996;25:637–653.
238. Ammann RW, Eckert J. Cestodes. *Echinococcus*. Gastroenterol Clin North Am. 1996;25:655–689.
239. Craig PS, Rogan MT, Allan JC. Detection, screening and community epidemiology of taeniid cestode zoonoses; cystic echinococcosis, alveolar echinococcosis and neurocysticercosis. Adv Parasitol. 1996;38:169–250.
240. Ackers JP. Gut coccidia—*Isospora, Cryptosporidium, Cyclospora* and *Sarcocystis*. Semin Gastrointest Dis. 1997;8:33–44.
241. Soave R. *Cyclospora*: An overview. Clin Infect Dis. 1996;23:429–435.
242. DeHovitz JA, Page JW, Boncy M, et al. Clinical manifestations and therapy of *Isospora belli* infection in patients with the acquired immunodeficiency syndrome. N Engl J Med. 1986;315:87–90.
243. Guerrant RL, Bobak DA. Bacterial and protozoal gastroenteritis. N Engl J Med. 1991;325:327–340.
244. Pape JW, Verdier R, Johnson WD. Treatment and prophylaxis of *Isospora belli* infection in patients with the acquired immunodeficiency syndrome. N Engl J Med. 1989;320:1044–1047.
245. Butler WP. *Dientamoeba fragilis*. An unusual intestinal pathogen. Dig Dis Sci. 1996;41:1811–1813.
246. Cuffari C, Oligny L, Seidman EG. *Dientamoeba fragilis* masquerading as allergic colitis. J Pediatr Gastroenterol Nutr. 1998;26:16–20.
247. Lee M, Hodges WG, Huggins TL, Lee EL. Eosinophilic gastroenteritis. South Med J. 1996;89:189–194.
248. Schoonbroodt D, Horsmans Y, Laka A, et al. Eosinophilic gastroenteritis presenting with colitis and cholangitis. Dig Dis Sci. 1995;40:308–314.
249. Klein NC, Hargrove L, Sleisenger MH, et al. Eosinophilic gastroenteritis. Medicine. 1970;49:299–319.
250. Goldberg HI, O'Kieffe D, Jenis EH, et al. Diffuse eosinophilic gastroenteritis. Am J Roentgenol Radium Ther Nucl Med. 1973;119:342–51.
251. Tytgat GN, Grijm R, Dekker W, et al. Fatal eosinophilic enteritis. Gastroenterology. 1976;71:479–483.
252. Cupps TR, Fauci AS. The Vasculitides. Philadelphia: WB Saunders; 1981.
253. Mowrey FH, Lundberg EA. The clinical manifestations of essential polyangiitis (periarteritis nodosa), with emphasis on the hepatic manifestations. Ann Intern Med. 1954;40:1145–1164.
254. Nightingale EJ. The gastroenterological aspects of periarteritis nodosa. Am J Gastroenterol. 1959;31:152–165.
255. Leavitt RY, Fauci AS. Polyangiitis overlap syndrome. Am J Med. 1986;81:79–85.
256. Lhote F, Cohen P, Guillevin L. Polyarteritis nodosa, microscopic polyangiitis and Churg-Strauss syndrome. Lupus. 1998;7:238–258.
257. Haeberle MG, Griffen WO Jr. Eosinophiia and regional enteritis: A possible diagnostic aid. Am J Dig Dis. 1972;17:200–204.
258. Benfield GF, Asquith P. Blood eosinophilia and ulcerative colitis—influence of ethnic origin. Postgrad Med J. 1986;62:1101–1105.
259. Isaacson NJ, Rapoport P. Eosinophilia in malignant tumors: Its significance. Ann Intern Med. 1946;25:893–902.
260. Banerjee RN, Narang RM. Haematological changes in malignancy. Br J Haematol. 1967;13:829–843.
261. Beeson P. Cancer and eosinophilia. N Engl J Med. 1983;309:792–793.

Chapter 87

Foodborne Disease

ROBERT V. TAUXE
DAVID L. SWERDLOW
JAMES M. HUGHES

Foodborne disease syndromes result from ingestion of a wide variety of foods contaminated with pathogenic microorganisms, microbial toxins, or chemicals. From 1973 to 1992, a mean of approximately 500 outbreaks of foodborne disease affecting 16,000 persons in the United States were reported annually to the Centers for Disease Control and Prevention (CDC).[1, 2] These figures certainly underestimate the magnitude of the problem. The actual incidence of foodborne disease is unknown, but estimates range from 6,500,000 to 81,000,000 illnesses annually.[3, 4] The annual economic burden has been estimated at 5 billion dollars.[4]

Although a wide variety of microorganisms and toxins can cause foodborne disease, this discussion focuses on foodborne disease syndromes that are acute (onset of symptoms usually within 72 hours of ingestion) and whose clinical features include gastrointestinal manifestations. The diseases to be discussed and the frequency with which outbreaks were reported to the CDC from 1973 to 1992 are indicated in Table 87–1.

The spectrum of foodborne diseases has expanded in recent years.[5] New foodborne agents causing severe disease have emerged (e.g., *Escherichia coli* O157:H7, *Cyclospora cayatenensis*)[6–8]; previously uncommon food vehicles such as fresh fruits and vegetables have become important sources of foodborne disease; and *Salmonella* and *Campylobacter* have become increasingly resistant to antimicrobial drugs. Important food sources have been defined for other established pathogens, such as *Vibrio cholerae* O1 and *Listeria monocytogenes*. Postinfectious syndromes have been recognized as important sequelae of foodborne infections, including hemolytic uremic syndrome after infections with *E. coli* O157:H7,[7] Reiter's syndrome after salmonellosis,[9] and Guillain-Barré syndrome after campylobacteriosis.[10] Centralization of the food supply increases the risk for nationwide outbreaks. Globalization of the food supply has facilitated exposure to foodborne pathogens from other parts of the world. The growing population of persons with immunosuppressive conditions or treatments and the increasing number of institutionalized elderly persons mean that more of the population is exquisitely susceptible to microbial contamination of food.

PATHOGENESIS AND CLINICAL FEATURES

Foodborne disease can appear as an isolated sporadic case or, less frequently, as an outbreak of illnesses affecting a group of people after a common food exposure. The diagnosis of foodborne disease should be considered when an acute illness with gastrointestinal or neurologic manifestations affects two or more persons who have shared a meal during the previous 72 hours. Important clues to the etiologic agent are provided by both the symptoms and the incubation period.

Foodborne Disease Caused by Microbial Agents or Their Toxins

The toxic mechanisms of foodborne bacterial disease are summarized in Table 87–2.

Nausea and Vomiting within 1 to 6 Hours. The major etiologic considerations are *Staphylococcus aureus* and *Bacillus cereus*. The

TABLE 87–1 Foodborne Disease Outbreaks and Outbreak-Associated Cases of Known Cause Reported to the Centers for Disease Control and Prevention, 1973–1992

Etiologic Agent	Outbreaks Number	Outbreaks %	Cases Number	Cases %
Bacterial				
Bacillus cereus	80	2	1559	1
Campylobacter	80	2	2279	1
Clostridium botulinum	288	7	619	0
Clostridium perfringens	231	6	16626	10
Escherichia coli	21	1	1431	1
Listeria monocytogenes	3	0	223	0
Salmonella	1343	35	77339	47
Shigella	128	3	20579	13
Staphylococcus aureus	418	11	18958	12
Streptococcus, group A	14	0	2052	1
Vibrio cholerae O1 or O139	10	0	950	1
Vibrio parahaemolyticus	27	1	556	0
Yersinia enterocolitica	5	0	767	0
Other bacterial	23	1	459	0
Chemical				
Ciguatoxin	276	7	1228	1
Heavy metals	50	1	782	0
Histamine fish poisoning	278	7	1730	1
Monosodium glutamate	18	0	58	0
Mushrooms	66	2	187	0
Paralytic shellfish poisoning (PSP)	26	1	225	0
Other chemical	127	3	1174	1
Parasitic				
	15	0	362	0
Trichinella spiralis	138	4	1038	1
Other parasitic	7	0	30	0
Viral				
Hepatitis A	154	4	5406	3
Norwalk virus	15	0	6474	4
Other viral	12	0	1315	1
Total	3853	100	164406	100

relatively short incubation period reflects the fact that these diseases are caused by a preformed enterotoxin. Staphylococcal food poisoning is characterized by vomiting (76% of cases) and diarrhea (77%); fever is relatively uncommon (23%).[11] Staphylococci responsible for episodes of food poisoning produce one or more enterotoxins; five immunologically distinct heat-stable proteins (A, B, C, D, and E) with molecular weights ranging from 28,000 to 35,000 Da have been identified.[12] Another staphylococcal protein, enterotoxin F, is produced by the majority of *S. aureus* strains causing toxic shock syndrome[13] but has not been reported to cause foodborne disease. Although the mechanism of action of these enterotoxins in humans has not been clarified, studies in monkeys and cats suggest that the enterotoxin produces its emetic action after interaction with abdominal viscera.[14, 15] The sensory stimulus is carried to the vomiting center in the brain by the vagus and sympathetic nerves.[14] Other studies suggest that diarrhea may result from inhibition of water and sodium absorption in the small intestine by enterotoxin.[16]

Enterotoxigenic staphylococci isolated from implicated foods in outbreaks are most often lysed by group III phages; less commonly, they are lysed by both group I and group III phages or by group I phages alone.[17] More than 99% of enterotoxigenic staphylococci associated with food poisoning are coagulase positive; occasionally, an outbreak caused by enterotoxigenic *Staphylococcus epidermidis* is reported.[18] In the past, strains producing type A enterotoxin alone accounted for 44 to 69% of the reported outbreaks of staphylococcal food poisoning in the United States and England.[19, 20] Strains producing type D enterotoxin, either alone or in combination with type A, were the next most frequently implicated. Strains producing enterotoxins B, C, or E alone accounted for fewer than 10% of the outbreaks. During 1979–1981, all reported staphylococcal foodborne outbreaks in the United States of known toxin type were caused by strains producing type A enterotoxin alone.[21]

B. cereus strains can cause two types of food poisoning syndromes, one characterized primarily by nausea and vomiting with an incubation period of 1 to 6 hours (short-incubation "emetic" syndrome) and a second manifested primarily by abdominal cramps and diarrhea with an incubation period of 8 to 16 hours (long-incubation "diarrhea" syndrome).[22, 23] The short-incubation syndrome, characterized by vomiting (100% of cases), abdominal cramps (100%), and, less frequently, diarrhea (33%),[24] is caused by a heat-stable toxin that is produced by some *B. cereus* strains and is capable of causing vomiting when fed to monkeys.[25] The mechanism and site of action of this toxin, which has a molecular weight of less than 5000 Da, are unknown.[26]

Another clue to the cause of both staphylococcal and short-incubation *B. cereus* outbreaks is provided by the fact that the illnesses are of short duration, usually lasting less than 12 hours.[11, 24]

Abdominal Cramps and Diarrhea within 8 to 16 Hours. The major etiologic considerations for this syndrome, which is also enterotoxin mediated, are *Clostridium perfringens* and *B. cereus*. In contrast to staphylococcal food poisoning and the short-incubation *B. cereus* disease, which are caused by ingestion of preformed enterotoxins in food, *C. perfringens* and long-incubation *B. cereus* food poisoning are caused by toxins produced in vivo, accounting for the longer incubation period. In *C. perfringens* food poisoning, the most common symptoms are diarrhea and abdominal cramps. Although nausea may occur, vomiting and fever are uncommon, occurring in less than 10% of the patients.[27, 28] Although five types of *C. perfringens* toxin have been described, type A is almost always the toxin causing this food poisoning syndrome.[28, 29] *C. perfringens* enterotoxin is a heat-labile protein with a molecular weight of approximately 35,000 Da[30] synthesized by the vegetative cells of *C. perfringens* in the gastrointestinal tract; the enterotoxin is produced during sporulation.[31] Studies in rabbits and rats indicate that the enterotoxin is active throughout the small intestine, with greatest activity in the ileum, in which net secretion of sodium and fluid and inhibition of chloride and glucose absorption occur.[32, 33] The enterotoxin damages brush borders of epithelial cells at villus tips.[33]

B. cereus strains, which cause a similar long-incubation syndrome that produces diarrhea (96%) and abdominal cramps (75%), sometimes vomiting (33%), and rarely fever,[24] elaborate a heat-labile enterotoxin with a molecular weight of approximately 50,000 Da[26] that activates intestinal adenylate cyclase and results in intestinal

TABLE 87–2 Pathogenic Mechanisms in Bacterial Foodborne Disease

Preformed Toxin	Toxin Production In Vivo	Tissue Invasion	Toxin Production and/or Tissue Invasion
Staphylococcus aureus *Bacillus cereus* (short incubation) *Clostridium botulinum*	*Clostridiuim perfringens* *B. cereus* (long incubation) *C. botulinum* (infant botulism) Enterotoxigenic *Escherichia coli* *Vibrio cholerae* O1 or O139 *V. cholerae* non-O1 Shiga toxin-producing *E. coli*	*Campylobacter jejuni* *Salmonella* *Shigella* Invasive *E. coli*	*Vibrio parahaemolyticus* *Yersinia enterocolitica*

fluid secretion.[34] This enterotoxin appears also to have cytotoxic properties in rabbit small intestine and guinea pig skin.[26, 34]

Although nausea occurs in many patients with *C. perfringens* and long-incubation *B. cereus* food poisoning, vomiting occurs infrequently. In fact, occurrence of vomiting in more than one third of affected people suggests that these organisms are not involved. Although these illnesses last longer than staphylococcal and short-incubation *B. cereus* food poisoning do, symptoms usually resolve within 24 hours.[24, 35] However, in some long-incubation *B. cereus* outbreaks, the mean duration of illness can be more than 2 days, and occasionally illness may last several weeks.[36–38]

Fever, Abdominal Cramps, and Diarrhea within 16 to 48 Hours. The major etiologic considerations for this syndrome are salmonellae, shigellae, *Campylobacter jejuni, Vibrio parahaemolyticus,* and invasive *E. coli.* These organisms cause this syndrome after tissue invasion.[39–42] Vomiting occurs in 35 to 80% of the patients.[43–46] These illnesses usually resolve within 2 to 7 days.

C. jejuni is the most common foodborne bacterial pathogen.[47, 48] The frequency of findings of fecal blood and polymorphonuclear leukocytes[49] and colitis[50] suggests that this organism also causes this syndrome after tissue invasion. In contrast to the illnesses caused by other organisms in this group, *C. jejuni* food poisoning is characterized by vomiting in only 15 to 25% of cases[49, 51, 52] and by a longer incubation period of 1 to 7 days.[47] The duration of illness is usually less than 1 week, but relapses may occur in untreated patients.[53] In one milk-associated outbreak, *L. monocytogenes* caused a febrile gastroenteritis in previously healthy persons, characterized by watery frequent diarrhea, abdominal cramps, headache, and myalgias, with a median incubation period of 20 hours.[54]

The diarrhea experienced by patients with *V. cholerae* non-O1 infection is sometimes bloody, and fever may be present.[54–56]

Abdominal Cramps and Watery Diarrhea within 16 to 72 Hours. The major etiologic considerations in this syndrome are enterotoxigenic strains of *E. coli, V. parahaemolyticus, V. cholerae* non-O1, and, in endemic areas, *V. cholerae* O1 and O139; *C. jejuni*, salmonellae, and shigellae may also cause this syndrome. Enterotoxins synthesized in vivo are responsible for the syndrome caused by *V. cholerae* O1,[57] *V. cholerae* non-O1,[58, 59] and enterotoxigenic strains of *E. coli*;[60] enterotoxigenic or cytotoxic substances, or both, may also play a role in the pathogenesis of this syndrome when it is caused by salmonellae,[61, 62] shigellae,[63–65] or *V. parahaemolyticus*.[66, 67]

Severe cholera manifests as a profuse, watery diarrhea accompanied by vomiting and muscular cramps. With the other infections, fever and vomiting occur in a minority of cases.[68–71] With the exception of cholera, which may last for 5 days, and disease caused by *V. cholerae* non-O1, which may last for 2 to 12 days, these illnesses usually resolve within 72 to 96 hours. However, in one documented enterotoxigenic *E. coli* outbreak, the median duration of illness was 7 days.[72]

Foodborne transmission of the Norwalk agent and related 27-nm viruses may be common.[73–76] In contrast to the illness produced by bacterial agents causing this syndrome, vomiting and headache are prominent features of Norwalk agent gastroenteritis and occur in the majority of cases.[73] The duration of illness is usually 24 to 48 hours. The occurrence of secondary cases in close contacts not exposed to the suspected food is an important clue to the possibility of infection by a Norwalk agent. A group of related viruses, called the small round structured viruses or human caliciviruses, cause similar illnesses[77] (see Chapter 163).

Fever and Abdominal Cramps within 16 to 48 Hours. *Yersinia enterocolitica* has been incriminated as a cause of foodborne outbreaks in the United States and is a more common cause of foodborne disease in Northern Europe and Canada.[78–82] Although some strains of this organism have been reported to produce a heat-stable enterotoxin,[83, 84] the frequent occurrence of fever and mesenteric adenitis suggests that this organism causes disease as a result of tissue invasion. In younger children, febrile diarrhea is the most common presentation.[78, 80, 86] In older children and adults, the clinical illness may be prolonged, and one syndrome may closely resemble acute appendicitis; nausea and vomiting are relatively uncommon, occurring in less than 25 to 40% of the cases.[79, 85] Duration of the illness may range from 24 hours to 4 weeks.[81, 85]

Bloody Diarrhea without Fever within 72 to 120 Hours. The distinctive syndrome of hemorrhagic colitis has been linked to Shiga toxin–producing strains of *E. coli*, most often serotype O157:H7.[6, 87, 88] These strains produce cytotoxins that affect Vero kidney cell cultures, are neutralized by antiserum to Shiga toxin, and have been called Shiga-like toxins or verotoxins.[89, 90] A new nomenclature calls them all Shiga toxins.[91] The bacteria are noninvasive. The toxins are absorbed from the gut and damage vascular endothelial cells in target organs such as the gut and kidney.[92] The illness is characterized by severe abdominal cramping and diarrhea, which is initially watery but later grossly bloody.[88] Patients with uncomplicated infection usually remain afebrile. The mean incubation period in outbreaks is 3 to 8 days. The duration of uncomplicated illness ranges from 1 to 12 days. The development of fever and leukocytosis may herald complications, which include hemolytic uremic syndrome, thrombotic thrombocytopenic purpura, and death.[88, 93–95] Hemolytic uremic syndrome can occur in 2 to 7% of infections, with onset 5 to 10 days after the beginning of the diarrheal illness.[93] The case-fatality rate in outbreaks has been 0 to 2%, with rates as high as 16 to 35% in nursing homes.[6, 93, 94] Other *E. coli* serotypes that produce Shiga toxins can also cause hemorrhagic colitis and hemolytic uremic syndrome, and two serotypes, O104:H21 and O111:NM, have caused outbreaks.[94, 95]

Nausea, Vomiting, Diarrhea, and Paralysis within 18 to 36 Hours. The occurrence of acute gastrointestinal symptoms simultaneously with or just before the onset of descending weakness or paralysis strongly suggests the diagnosis of foodborne botulism. Constipation is common once the neurologic syndrome is well established, but nausea and vomiting occur at onset in 50% of the patients, and diarrhea occurs in approximately 20 to 25%.[96–98] The pathogenesis of the acute gastrointestinal symptoms is not understood; the botulinal toxins, which inhibit acetylcholine release from nerve endings,[99, 100] do not appear to be responsible. The disease in humans is usually caused by one of three immunologically distinct heat-labile protein neurotoxins, designated A, B, and E,[101] which are produced after germination of *Clostridium botulinum* spores in inadequately processed foods. The disease in older children and adults results from ingestion of preformed toxin. The syndrome of infant botulism results from ingestion of spores with subsequent toxin production in vivo.[102–104] Both illnesses last from several weeks to several months. Clinical suspicion is critical if the disease is to be correctly diagnosed.[105]

Guillain-Barré syndrome has been associated with serologic evidence of recent infection with *C. jejuni*.[10] In a multicenter study of 118 patients in the United States with Guillain-Barré syndrome, 36% had serologic evidence of a preceding *C. jejuni* infection.[10] When preceding diarrheal illness is reported, it typically occurs 1 to 3 weeks before the onset of neurologic symptoms.[10] In contrast to botulism, this syndrome is usually manifested by an ascending paralysis accompanied by sensory findings and abnormal nerve conduction velocity.

Foodborne Disease Caused by Nonbacterial Toxins

Nausea, Vomiting, and Abdominal Cramps within 1 Hour. The major etiologic considerations for this syndrome are heavy metals; copper, zinc, tin, and cadmium have caused foodborne outbreaks.[106–110] Incubation periods most often range from 5 to 15 minutes. Nausea, vomiting, and abdominal cramps result from irritation of the gastric mucosa and usually resolve within 2 to 3 hours after removal of the offending agent during emesis.

TABLE 87–3 Fish and Shellfish Poisoning Syndromes

Syndrome	Incubation Period	Duration	Geographic Location*	Season
Histamine fish poisoning (scombroid)	5 min–1 h	Few hours	Primarily coastal areas (Hawaii, California)	Year round
Ciguatera	1–6 h	Few days–few months	35°N–35°S latitude (Hawaii, Florida)	Feb.–Sept.
Paralytic shellfish poisoning	5 min–4 h	Few hours–few days	Above 30°N and below 30°S latitude (New England, West Coast)	May–Nov.
Neurotoxic shellfish poisoning	5 min–4 h	Few hours–few days	Gulf and Atlantic coasts of Florida (Florida)	Spring, Fall
Amnesic shellfish poisoning	15 min–6 h	Few days–permanent	Coastal areas?	Uncertain

*Location of U.S. outbreaks in parentheses.

Paresthesias within 1 Hour. When patients have this symptom, fish poisoning, shellfish poisoning (Table 87–3), the so-called Chinese restaurant syndrome, and niacin poisoning are the major possibilities. Histamine fish poisoning (scombroid) is characterized by symptoms resembling those of a histamine reaction. Burning of the mouth and throat, flushing, headache, and dizziness are common; abdominal cramps, nausea, vomiting, and diarrhea also occur in most cases.[111] In severe cases, urticaria and bronchospasm may also occur. Symptoms are thought to result from histamine and inhibitors of histamine degradation produced in fish flesh by the enzymatic decarboxylation of histidine by certain marine bacteria.[112] In an outbreak traced to tuna sashimi, a strain of *Klebsiella pneumoniae* capable of producing large quantities of histamine was implicated.[113] Symptoms usually resolve in a few hours.

Three types of shellfish poisoning should be considered: paralytic (PSP), neurotoxic (NSP), and amnesic (ASP).[114, 115] PSP is characterized by paresthesias of the mouth, lips, face, and extremities.[116–119] In severe cases, dyspnea, dysphagia, muscle weakness or frank paralysis, ataxia, and respiratory insufficiency may occur.[118, 119] Respiratory failure may occur during the first 12 hours of the illness.[118] Some patients also have nausea, vomiting, and diarrhea.[114] The disease is caused by neurotoxic substances in dinoflagellates, one of which is known as *saxitoxin*. Bivalve mollusks feed on these dinoflagellates; the toxins are concentrated in their flesh but do not affect the mollusks.[116] Saxitoxin appears to be the only neurotoxin produced by *Gonyaulax catenella*, whereas *Gonyaulax tamarensis* produces saxitoxin and several additional neurotoxic substances.[120–122] The structure of saxitoxin has been determined;[123] it is heat stable and blocks the propagation of nerve and muscle action potentials by interfering with the increase in sodium permeability by acting at a metal cation-binding site in the sodium channels or nerve membranes.[124–126] The mechanisms of action of the other neurotoxins are unknown. Duration of the illness ranges from a few hours to a few days.[114]

Although many patients with PSP experience the onset of symptoms within 1 hour of ingestion, the incubation period is often inversely related to the amount of toxin ingested. A European outbreak involved 120 patients who ingested contaminated mussels; the median incubation period in this outbreak was 3.5 hours, with a range of 1 to 10 hours.[117]

The clinical features of NSP are similar to those of PSP, but paralysis does not occur.[114, 116] Several poorly characterized neurotoxins responsible for this illness are found in *Gymnodinium breve*, the responsible dinoflagellate.[127, 128] One of these neurotoxins stimulates postganglionic cholinergic nerve fibers.[129] Duration of the illness ranges from a few hours to a few days.[114]

The clinical features of ASP are initially nonspecific and include vomiting, abdominal cramping, and diarrhea. Confusion, amnesia, coma, and cardiovascular instability follow within hours in severe cases; these signs tend to occur in older persons and in persons with underlying renal disease. The hallmark of the disease is antegrade amnesia, which was reported in 25% of affected persons in a large Canadian outbreak.[115] The disease is caused by domoic acid, a toxin produced by the dinoflagellate *Nitzchia pungens* and concentrated in the flesh of mollusks. Amnesia can be permanent and is the result of bilateral destruction of the hippocampi by the toxin.[130]

The Chinese restaurant syndrome is characterized by a burning sensation in the neck, chest, abdomen, or arms and by a sensation of tightness over the face and chest.[131] Headache, flushing, diaphoresis, lacrimation, weakness, nausea, abdominal cramps, and thirst frequently occur.[131, 132] Symptoms appear to be caused by excessive amounts of monosodium L-glutamate in foods, although other undefined substances may also play a role.[131, 132] The illness usually resolves within several hours.

Niacin poisoning produces a burning facial erythema within 20 minutes of ingestion, which rapidly resolves.[133]

Paresthesias within 1 to 6 Hours. The major diagnostic considerations for this syndrome are PSP and ciguatera fish poisoning (see Table 87–3). Ciguatera is characterized by the onset of abdominal cramps, nausea, vomiting, and diarrhea preceded or followed by numbness and paresthesias of the lips, tongue, and throat.[134–136] Malaise, headache, pruritus, dry mouth, metallic taste, myalgias, arthralgias, blurred vision, photophobia, and transient blindness have also been reported.[137–139] Sharp shooting pains in the legs and a sensation of looseness and pain in the teeth are characteristic.[135] In severe cases, reversal of hot and cold temperature sensations, sinus bradycardia, hypotension, cranial nerve palsies, and respiratory paralysis may occur.[136, 137, 140]

The illness is caused by ciguatoxin, a poorly characterized lipid-soluble, relatively heat-stable compound[141] that is acquired by fish through the food chain.[142] The dinoflagellate *Gambierdiscus toxicus* and other algae that grow on reefs have been identified as the source of the toxin in the food chain.[143] Ciguatoxin inhibits red blood cell cholinesterase activity,[144] increases membrane sodium permeability,[145] and changes the electrical potential of cells through its action on sodium channels.[146, 147] Duration of the acute illness ranges from a few days to a few months; pain in the extremities has been reported to occur intermittently for years after an episode of ciguatera. Other natural marine toxins have been associated with similar syndromes, including searitoxin, maitotoxin, and palytoxin.[143]

Miscellaneous Mushroom Poisoning Syndromes with Onset within 2 Hours. At least five clinical syndromes may occur within 2 hours of ingestion of toxic mushrooms (Table 87–4).[148–151] Species containing ibotenic acid and muscimol cause an illness mimicking acute alcoholic intoxication that is characterized by confusion, restlessness, and visual disturbances followed by lethargy; symptoms resolve within 24 hours. Species containing muscarine cause an illness characterized by evidence of parasympathetic hyperactivity (e.g., salivation, lacrimation, diaphoresis, blurred vision, abdominal cramps, diarrhea). Some patients experience miosis, bradycardia, and bronchospasm. Symptoms usually resolve within 24 hours. Species containing the toxic substances psilocybin and psilocin cause an acute psychotic reaction manifested by hallucinations and inappropriate behavior, which usually resolves within 12 hours. The mushroom *Coprinus atramentarius* contains a disulfiram-like substance that can result in headache, flushing, paresthesias, nausea, vomiting, and tachycardia if alcohol is consumed during the 48-hour period after

TABLE 87–4 Mushroom Poisoning Syndromes

Syndrome	Mushroom Species	Toxins
Short incubation		
Delirium	*Amanita muscaria, Amanita pantherina*	Ibotenic acid, muscimol
Parasympathetic hyperactivity	*Inocybe* spp. *Clitocybe* spp.	Muscarine
Hallucinations	*Psilocybe* spp. *Panaeolus* spp.	Psilocybin, psilocin
Disulfiram reaction	*Coprinus atramentarius*	Disulfiram-like substance
Gastroenteritis	Many	?
Long incubation		
Gastroenteritis, hepatorenal failure	*Amanita phalloides* *Aminosa virosa* *Amanita verna* *Galerina autumnalis* *Galerina marginata* *Galerina venenata*	Amatoxins, phallotoxins
Gastroenteritis, hepatic failure, hemolysis, seizures, coma	*Gyromitra* spp.	Gyromitrin

ingestion. The fifth clinical syndrome is characterized by nausea, vomiting, abdominal cramps, and diarrhea after the ingestion of mushrooms containing gastrointestinal irritants that are not well characterized.

Abdominal Cramps and Diarrhea within 6 to 24 Hours, Followed by Hepatorenal Failure. Species of poisonous mushrooms containing amatoxins and phallotoxins are responsible for this syndrome (see Table 87–4).[148, 149, 151] The most common implicated species are *Amanita phalloides, Amanita virosa*, and *Amanita verna*.[152, 153] The illness is typically biphasic; the abdominal cramps and diarrhea, which may be severe, usually resolve within 24 hours. The patient then remains well for 1 to 2 days before evidence of hepatic and renal failure supervenes. A mortality rate of 30 to 50% has been reported.[154, 155]

A similar clinical syndrome occurs after ingestion of mushrooms of the *Gyromitra* genus, which contain the toxic substance gyromitrin. Hemolysis, seizures, and coma can occur, but this toxin does not cause acute renal failure.[156]

Persistent Diarrhea within 1 to 3 Weeks. Two distinctive persistent diarrheal syndromes can be foodborne: cyclosporiasis and Brainerd diarrhea. Cyclosporiasis emerged as a major foodborne infection in the United States in 1996, when it caused many outbreaks related to imported raspberries. The diarrhea is often intermittent and relapsing; is associated with anorexia, weight loss, nausea and profound fatigue; and begins after a median incubation period of 7 days.[8] A distinctive chronic watery diarrhea, known as Brainerd diarrhea, was first described in persons who had consumed raw milk.[157] After a mean incubation period of 15 days, affected persons developed acute, watery diarrhea with marked urgency and abdominal cramping. Diarrhea persisted for a mean of 2 years. No etiologic agent was identified. A restaurant-associated outbreak of a similar illness suggests that food vehicles other than raw milk may also be involved.[158]

Waterborne Disease. The evaluation of a suspected foodborne outbreak may reveal that water was the vehicle. Pathogens incriminated in waterborne outbreaks are different from those most often responsible for foodborne disease; the responsible etiologic agents for waterborne outbreaks reported to the CDC from 1972 through 1994 are shown in Table 87–5.[160–177] *Giardia lamblia* is the most frequently recognized pathogen in the United States and has been reponsible for several large outbreaks traced to municipal water supplies.[174–177] This illness is characterized by abdominal pain, bloating, flatulence, and occasionally malabsorption. The incubation period is typically 1 to 4 weeks, and the duration of illness may be several weeks. Large waterborne outbreaks caused by *Cryptosporidium parvum*,[178] *E. coli* O157:H7,[179] shigellae,[180] hepatitis A,[181] *Salmonella* Typhi,[182] nontyphoid salmonellae,[183] enterotoxigenic *E. coli*,[184] *C. jejuni*,[185, 186] Brainerd diarrhea,[187] the Norwalk agent,[188, 189] and the Snow Mountain agent, a Norwalk-like virus,[190] have been reported. The majority of waterborne outbreaks are of unknown cause.

Miscellaneous Foodborne Infections. This discussion has focused on diseases often transmitted by foods and manifested primarily by gastrointestinal or neurologic symptoms and signs. Some foodborne diseases manifest largely as invasive infections in immunocompromised patients. Listeriosis typically affects pregnant women, fetuses, and persons with compromised cellular immunity, who present with fever, myalgias, and primary bacteremia or meningitis. Identified sources are most often foods, including coleslaw, dairy products, and cold processed meats. The incubation period is prolonged, ranging from 2 to 6 weeks, and the case-fatality rate is 23%.[191] *Vibrio vulnificus* infections cause fulminant myonecrosis or primary bacteremia after ingestion of raw oysters. This severe syndrome is seen almost exclusively in patients with underlying liver disease, especially if associated with iron-overload states.[192]

Other infectious diseases with primary symptoms outside the gastrointestinal and neurologic systems that are occasionally or usually transmitted by foods include group A β-hemolytic streptococci (most commonly in potato and egg salads), typhoid fever (shellfish), brucellosis (goat's milk cheese), anthrax (meat), tularemia (water), tuberculosis (milk), Q fever (milk), hepatitis A (shellfish, fresh produce), trichinosis (pork), toxoplasmosis (beef), anisakiasis (fish), and tapeworms (beef, pork, and fish).

TABLE 87–5 Waterborne Disease Outbreaks of Known Cause, Associated With Drinking Water, Reported to the Centers for Disease Control and Prevention, 1972–1994

Etiologic Agent	Outbreaks	
	Number	%
Giardia lamblia	109	37.5
Shigella	34	11.7
Hepatitis A	21	7.2
Norwalk-like agents	16	5.5
Campylobacter jejuni	15	5.2
Nontyphoid salmonella	13	4.5
Cryptosporidium	10	3.4
Salmonella Typhi	5	1.7
Vibrio cholerae	2	0.7
Enterotoxigenic *Escherichia coli*	1	0.3
Escherichia coli O157 : H7	1	0.3
Yersinia enterocolitica	1	0.3
Rotavirus	1	0.3
Entamoeba histolytica	1	0.3
Miscellaneous chemicals	61	21.0
Total	291	100

EPIDEMIOLOGY

In addition to the clinical syndrome and incubation period, other clues to the cause of an outbreak of foodborne disease may be provided by the type of food responsible and the setting in which it is eaten (Table 87–6).

Foods

Outbreaks of staphylococcal food poisoning are associated with foods of high protein content, such as ham, poultry, potato and egg salads, and cream-filled pastries, which are thought to be contaminated during preparation by a food handler. In the classic staphylococcal foodborne outbreak a food handler has a purulent skin lesion on his or her hand, but this is true in only a minority of outbreaks. In contrast, outbreaks of *B. cereus* food poisoning of the short-incubation type are most often associated with fried rice that has been cooked and held warm for extended periods. The growth of *B. cereus* under similar experimental conditions in rice has been well documented.[193]

C. perfringens outbreaks usually occur after the ingestion of meat (especially beef and poultry) and gravies; organisms have been isolated from 16 to 85% of raw meat, poultry, and fish specimens.[195] Outbreaks are more likely to occur when these items are prepared in large quantities for banquets or in institutional settings, with food prepared well in advance without adequate final reheating.[196] Long-incubation *B. cereus* food poisoning is also frequently associated with meat or vegetable dishes. In addition to the frequent contamination of raw meats, vegetables, and milk products with *B. cereus*, the organism has been isolated from 25% of dried foods such as seasoning mixes, spices, and dried potatoes[197] and from more than 50% of dried beans and cereals.[198] A long-incubation *B. cereus* outbreak was traced to a "meals on wheels" operation in which food was held at and above room temperature for an extended period.[199]

E. coli O157:H7 outbreaks typically occur after consumption of undercooked ground beef or raw milk,[93] foods that are derived from cattle. However, more recent *E. coli* O157 outbreaks have been traced to a broad range of foods, including lettuce, apple cider, alfalfa sprouts, venison, and salami. Produce may become contaminated with *E. coli* O157:H7 through use of manure as fertilizer or use of contaminated water in processing. Outbreaks have also been caused by waterborne exposures and by person-to-person transmission in daycare centers.[7, 93, 200]

Salmonella foodborne outbreaks most frequently occur after ingestion of poultry, beef, egg, or dairy products. Internally contaminated shell eggs cause many outbreaks of infections with *Salmonella* Enteritidis.[201] Foods made with raw or undercooked shell eggs are now a dominant source of outbreaks and sporadic cases of salmonellosis in the United States.[202, 203] The role of raw milk in the transmission of *Salmonella* infections persists.[204] Outbreaks also have been traced to fresh produce, including melons, tomatoes, unpasteurized orange juice, and alfalfa sprouts.[205–208] Large international outbreaks have been caused by contaminated chocolate candy and peanut snacks.[209, 210] *Shigella* outbreaks are most often associated with cool, moist foods, such as potato and egg salads, that require much handling after cooking. Outbreaks have been caused by fresh produce, including raw vegetables at a salad bar, green scallions, and lettuce.[211–213] *C. jejuni* infection most often follows the ingestion of undercooked poultry.[47] *V. parahaemolyticus* outbreaks in the United States are associated with the ingestion of bivalve mollusks and crustaceans.[214, 215]

V. cholerae O1 and non-O1 outbreaks have been traced to contaminated shellfish eaten raw or inadequately cooked.[216] Crabs, shrimp, and raw oysters were implicated as the vehicles of transmission of a unique strain of *V. cholerae* O1 in Louisiana.[217] Crabs brought in travelers' luggage from Latin America have caused outbreaks of cholera in the United States.[218] Sporadic cases of diarrhea associated with *V. cholerae* non-O1 strains in the United States have also been linked to shellfish ingestion.[54, 55]

Foodborne infections with *Y. enterocolitica* have been caused by consumption of raw pork and contaminated milk and by cross-contamination from the preparation of pork chitterlings in the household.[78–82] A foodborne outbreak caused by invasive *E. coli* occurred after the ingestion of cheese.[46] Travelers' diarrhea caused by enterotoxigenic *E. coli* was associated with consumption of salads in Mexico,[219] and a foodborne outbreak of enterotoxigenic *E. coli* occurred after ingestion of imported cheese.[220] In recent years, out-

TABLE 87–6 Etiology of Foodborne Disease Outbreaks by Food, Season, and Geographic Predilection

Etiology	Foods	Season	Geographic Predilection
Bacterial			
Salmonella	Beef, poultry, eggs, dairy products, produce	Summer, fall	None
Staphylococcus aureus	Ham, poultry, egg salads, pastries	Summer	None
Campylobacter jejuni	Poultry, raw milk	Spring, summer	None
Clostridium botulinum	Vegetables, fruits, fish, honey (infants)	Summer, fall	None
Clostridium perfringens	Beef, poultry, gravy, Mexican food	Fall, winter, spring	None
Shigella	Egg salads, lettuce	Summer	None
Vibrio parahaemolyticus	Shellfish	Spring, summer, fall	Coastal states
Bacillus cereus	Fried rice, meats, vegetables	Year round	None
Yersinia enterocolitica	Milk, tofu, port chitterlings	Winter	Unknown
Vibrio cholerae O1	Shellfish	Variable	Tropical, Gulf Coast, Latin America
V. cholerae non-O1	Shellfish	Unknown	Tropical, Gulf Coast
Shiga toxin–producing *Escherichia coli*	Beef, raw milk, fresh produce	Summer, fall	Northern States
Viral			
Norwalk-like agents	Shellfish, salads	Year round	None
Chemical			
Ciguatera	Barracuda, snapper, amberjack, grouper	Spring, summer (in Florida)	Tropical reefs
Histamine fish poisoning (scombroid)	Tuna, mackerel, bonito, skipjack, mahi-mahi	Year round	Coastal
Mushroom poisoning	Mushrooms	Spring, fall	Temperate
Heavy metals	Acidic beverages	Year round	None
Monosodium-L-glutamate	Chinese food	Year round	None
Paralytic shellfish poisoning	Shellfish	Summer, fall	Temperate coastal zones
Neurotoxic shellfish poisoning	Shellfish	Spring, fall	Subtropical

breaks of "travelers' diarrhea at home" related to consumption of fresh produce have become more common.[221]

Botulism outbreaks are most often associated with the ingestion of low-acid (pH ≥4.4) home-canned vegetables, fruits, and fish. Outbreaks of botulism have occurred after ingestion of unusual vehicles, including baked potatoes, sauteed onions, and chopped garlic.[105, 222] Honey was the source of *C. botulinum* in some cases of infant botulism.[223] In Norwalk agent outbreaks, shellfish[74, 75, 224, 225] and salads[226] have been implicated. In one large multistate outbreak, steamed shellfish from the Gulf Coast were implicated. These were probably contaminated by ill oystermen themselves, who, lacking toilet facilities on their oysterboats, defecated and vomited directly into the shallow oyster beds.[227] Contamination of food by an ill food handler has been documented.[228] Foodborne transmission of the Snow Mountain agent has been associated with clams.[77] In 1996 and 1997, large outbreaks of *Cyclospora* infections followed consumption of raspberries imported from Central America.[8] Outbreaks have been associated with mesclun mix lettuce and a basil sauce.[229, 230]

Outbreaks of heavy metal poisoning are most often associated with acidic beverages such as lemonade, fruit punch, and carbonated drinks that have been stored in corroded metallic containers such as punch bowls[108] or that have been in contact with metallic tubing (e.g., in vending machines)[231] for periods sufficient to leach the metallic ions from the container.

Histamine fish poisoning outbreaks are associated with scombroid fish, the most common of which are tuna, mackerel, bonito, and skipjack. In addition, the nonscombroid fish mahi-mahi has caused outbreaks of scombroid-like fish poisoning. Ciguatera fish poisoning has been associated with more than 400 species of fish. Barracuda, red snapper, amberjack, and grouper are most commonly implicated. The disease is more often associated with large fish; in one study, 69% of red snapper weighing 2.8 kg or more were toxic, compared with only 18% of smaller fish.[232] PSP, NSP, and ASP occur after ingestion of bivalve mollusks, most often oysters, clams, and mussels. The most common food item associated with the Chinese restaurant syndrome is soup, which is frequently the first item ingested at a meal; the absorption of monosodium L-glutamate is most rapid when the stomach is empty.[131]

Although it is unlikely, the possibility that foodborne illness could be the result of an intentional contamination should also be considered. An outbreak of salmonellosis in Oregon in 1984 involved 751 persons who ate or worked at 10 area restaurants. Epidemiologic investigation determined that illness was associated with eating from salad bars, but no single item was implicated. A subsequent criminal investigation revealed that members of a religious commune had deliberately contaminated the salad bars.[233] In 1996, an outbreak of *Shigella dysenteriae* type 2 affecting 12 laboratory workers was caused by consumption of deliberately contaminated muffins.[234] The use of botulinum toxin by terrorists has also become a concern.[96]

Changes in the Population

The increasing average age in many countries means that more of the population has a heightened susceptibility to severe foodborne infections. In the United States, a growing segment of the population has immune impairment as a consequence of infection with the human immunodeficiency virus (HIV) or underlying chronic disease. People with compromised immunity due to infection with HIV have higher reported rates of salmonellosis, campylobacteriosis, and listeriosis than do persons not infected with HIV.[235, 236] *Salmonella* and possibly *Campylobacter* infections are more likely to be severe, recurrent, or persistent in such patients. Furthermore, extraintestinal disease caused by *Salmonella* and *L. monocytogenes* infection are more likely to be reported among HIV-infected persons than in the general population.[235, 236]

Seasonality

The time of year may also provide a clue to the cause of a foodborne outbreak. Outbreaks caused by the bacterial pathogens *S. aureus, Salmonella*, and *Shigella* are most common during the summer months. *C. jejuni* outbreaks are more common during the spring and fall. *C. perfringens* outbreaks occur throughout the year but least often during the summer months, and botulism outbreaks are more common during the summer and fall. Shellfish-associated *Vibrio* infections are largely limited to late summer and early fall and are closely related to the temperature of the water in the oyster beds.[237] *Y. enterocolitica* is typically a winter infection, often occurring after winter holidays at which pork chitterlings are served.[78]

In general, chemical food poisoning occurs throughout the year. Exceptions are PSP, which often occurs in association with a red tide[238] and is most common in the summer and fall; ciguatera, which is most common in the spring and summer in Florida;[239] and mushroom poisoning, which is most common in the spring, late summer, and fall.

Geographic Location

The geographic setting may also provide a clue to the cause of foodborne disease. *E. coli* O157:H7 infections are more common in the northern tier of states bordering on Canada, for unexplained reasons.[48] *Salmonella* Enteritidis infections have been most common in the Northeast but are increasing in frequency in the Southwest as well.[240] *V. parahaemolyticus* outbreaks are most frequently reported from coastal states.[214, 215] An outbreak of cholera and sporadic cases of *V. cholerae* O1 and non-O1 infection have been reported from the Gulf Coast of the United States.[217] Type A botulism outbreaks are most common west of the Mississippi River, whereas type B outbreaks are most common in the East and type E outbreaks are most common in Alaska.[101]

Ciguatera outbreaks occur in tropical and subtropical regions between 35°N and 35°S latitudes. More than 90% of outbreaks in the United States have been reported from Florida or Hawaii.[114] Ciguatera is common in the West Indies,[240] and travelers who return with the characteristic syndrome should be questioned regarding fish consumption. PSP and NSP outbreaks occur in coastal areas.

Epidemiologic Assessment

If an outbreak of foodborne disease is suspected, public health authorities should be contacted so that it can be investigated. Investigating the outbreak is important to identify and rapidly control the source and to prevent similar outbreaks from happening again. Once a common meal is identified through interviews with ill people, food-specific attack rates should be determined for all foods and beverages served at the meal (Table 87–7). People who were present at the same meal but did not become ill must also be interviewed to serve as controls. Food-specific attack rates may identify the responsible vehicle of transmission. To be adequately incriminated, a food must have a significantly higher attack rate for those who ate it than for those who did not, and most of those who became ill must have eaten the food. On occasion, more than one food item may be incriminated. On these occasions, simple cross-table analysis may indicate whether both items were contaminated by the etiologic agent or whether both were eaten by most people at the meal (e.g., meat and gravy) (see Table 87–7). For example, if meatloaf and gravy were both incriminated, subsequent analysis may indicate that attack rates were high for those who ate meatloaf regardless of whether they ate gravy, and were low for those who did not eat meatloaf regardless of whether they ate gravy, indicating that the meatloaf alone was responsible for the outbreak.

Once a food vehicle for the infections is identified, the investigation turns to the question of how contamination is likely to have occurred. Steps of food preparation are reviewed with the chef, and the safety of the various ingredients and the hygienic circumstances in the kitchen are assessed. In complex outbreaks, detailed epidemiologic investigation into the sources of food ingredients and replication of the cooking protocol may be needed to explain the event.

TABLE 87–7 Example of Use of Food-Specific Attack Rates and Cross-Table Analysis to Identify Food Vehicle in a Foodborne Outbreak

	Food-Specific Attack Rates					
	No. of People Eating Food			***No. of People Not Eating Food***		
Food	*Total*	*Ill*	*Percent Ill*	*Total*	*Ill*	*Percent Ill*
Meatloaf	100	88	88*	10	2	20*
Gravy	80	80	100†	30	10	33†
Potatoes	95	78	82	15	12	80
Salad	90	74	82	20	16	80
Water	70	58	82	40	32	80
	Cross-Table Analysis					
	No. of People Eating Meatloaf			***No. of People Not Eating Meatloaf***		
	Total	*Ill*	*Percent Ill*	*Total*	*Ill*	*Percent Ill*
No. eating gravy	75	67	89‡	5	1	20§
No. not eating gravy	25	21	84‡	5	1	20§

*$p < .05$ (Fisher's exact test).
†$p < .05$ (chi-square analysis).
‡$p > .05$ (chi-square analysis).
§$p > .05$ (Fisher's exact test).

LABORATORY DIAGNOSIS

Appropriate specimens for laboratory confirmation vary with the etiologic agents but include feces, vomitus, serum, and blood (Table 87–8). In addition, cultures of the leftover food, the food preparation environment, and food handlers may be indicated. The laboratory should be alerted to suspected causes so that special techniques can be used for identification of *C. perfringens*, vibrios, *C. jejuni, E. coli* O157:H7, *Cyclospora*, and *Y. enterocolitica* and so that organisms considered part of the normal flora (other *E. coli, B. cereus*) are not overlooked.

Careful specimen collection and transport is critical to successful diagnosis.[241] Rectal swabs for bacteriologic diagnosis should be collected from patients not already treated with antimicrobials and should be transported under refrigeration to the laboratory in Cary-Blair or another suitable medium. They should be frozen if they cannot be plated within 48 hours. For optimum viral diagnosis, liquid stools should be collected as early as possible in the illness and transported under refrigeration without freezing. Parasitic diagnosis depends on collection of a stool sample and its transport in specialized parasitic transport media.

Outbreaks of staphylococcal food poisoning may be confirmed by the isolation of *S. aureus* of the same phage type from vomitus or feces of ill people and from the incriminated food or a skin lesion on the hand of a food handler; by the isolation of more than 10^5 *S. aureus* organisms per gram of incriminated food; or by the demonstration of staphylococcal enterotoxin in the food by gel diffusion, radioimmunoassay (RIA), or the enzyme-linked immunosorbent assay (ELISA).[242]

B. cereus outbreaks may be documented by the isolation of organisms from the feces of ill people who shared the same meal or by the isolation of 10^5 or more *B. cereus* per gram of incriminated food. Serotyping, if available, may be of value in confirming that isolates were derived from a common source, since 14% of healthy adults have been reported to have transient gastrointestinal colonization with *B. cereus*.[243] Plasmid analysis may also be useful.[244] Commercial immunoassays are available for the diarrheagenic toxin of *B. cereus*.[245]

The laboratory confirmation of *C. perfringens* outbreaks is more difficult. Because both heat-sensitive and heat-resistant strains of *C. perfringens* type A have been implicated as causes of food poisoning, selective isolation procedures involving heat treatment of food and fecal specimens should not be used. Because *C. perfringens* organisms are part of the normal flora in most healthy people, organisms of the same serotype[246–248] or bacteriocin type[249] should be demonstrated in stools of ill people and in the incriminated food—or in stools of ill people and not in those of people who ate the same meal but did not become ill—or median counts of 10^6 or more *C. perfringens* spores per gram of feces obtained within 48 hours after onset of illness should be demonstrated.[246, 250] Alternatively, counts of 10^5 or more organisms per gram of food provide etiologic confirmation. Demonstration of *C. perfringens* enterotoxin in stools of ill people and not in those of control subjects is possible with ELISA or latex agglutination.[251–253] For serotyping, approximately 90 *C. perfringens* antisera, including the original 13 Hobbs serotypes, are available, but many isolates cannot be typed. In the United Kingdom, serotyping implicates a specific serotype in almost two thirds of

TABLE 87–8 Appropriate Laboratory Specimens for Documentation of the Cause of a Foodborne Outbreak

	Patient			**Food Handler**				
	Stools	*Vomitus*	*Blood*	*Stools*	*Nose*	*Hands*	**Food**	**Food-Preparation Environment**
Bacterial								
Salmonella	C		C	C			C	C
Staphylococcus aureus	C	C			C	C	C, T	
Campylobacter jejuni	C			C			C	C
Clostridium botulinum	C, T	C, T	T				C, T	
Clostridium perfringens	C, T						C	
Shigella	C			C			C	
Vibrio parahaemolyticus	C						C	C
Bacillus cereus	C	C					C	
Yersinia enterocolitica	C		S	C			C	C
Vibrio cholerae O1 and non-O1	C		S	C			C	C
Shiga toxin–producing *Escherichia coli*	C, T		S	C			C	
Viral								
Norwalk agent	I, P		S	I, P			P	
Chemical								
Ciguatera							T	
Histamine fish poisoning (scombroid)							T	
Mushroom	T	T	T				T	
Heavy metals							T	
Monosodium-L-glutamate							T	
Paralytic shellfish poisoning							T	
Neurotoxic shellfish poisoning							T	

Abbreviations: C, Culture; I, immune electron microscopy; P, polymerase chain reaction probe; S, serology; T, toxin testing.

outbreaks,[247] whereas in the United States serotyping is helpful in only approximately 20% of outbreaks.[254]

Salmonella, Shigella, C. jejuni, V. cholerae O1 and non-O1, *V. parahaemolyticus*, and *Y. enterocolitica* outbreaks may be confirmed by isolation and serotyping of the organisms from the feces of ill people. In *Salmonella* outbreaks in which it is uncertain whether a common vehicle is responsible, pulsed field gel electrophoresis (PFGE), plasmid profiling, or determination of phage type may be necessary.[210, 255–257] Strains of *V. parahaemolyticus* isolated from patients are hemolytic on special blood agar medium (Kanagawa-positive strains). Isolation and serotyping of salmonellae, shigellae, *C. jejuni*, vibrios, and *Y. enterocolitica* from the incriminated food may also be confirmatory. Molecular characterization of *V. cholerae* O1 may help to define the geographic origins of the infecting organism.[258] Because *V. parahaemolyticus* in low numbers are a frequent contaminant of shellfish, counts of 10^5 or more organisms per gram are required for confirmation; food isolates are usually Kanagawa negative. Serologic testing of acute and convalescent sera may be helpful in confirming the diagnosis in patients in *Y. enterocolitica*, cholera, and typhoid fever outbreaks but currently plays no important role in the investigation of nontyphoid *Salmonella, Shigella, C. jejuni*, and *V. parahaemolyticus* outbreaks.

Infection with *E. coli* O157:H7 can be diagnosed by isolating sorbitol-negative *E. coli* from stools of ill persons on sorbitol-MacConkey medium and confirming the serotype.[259] *E. coli* O157:H7 strains can be usefully subtyped by determination of PFGE pattern in a new network being implemented in public health laboratories around the country, called PulseNet. Information is available on the World Wide Web at http://www.cdc.gov/ncidod/dbmd/pulsenet/pulsenet.htm. Infection with other Shiga toxin–producing *E. coli* can be diagnosed by demonstration of free Shiga toxin in stools, or by isolation of other Shiga toxin–producing strains from stools from ill persons.[95] In the outbreak setting, enterotoxigenic *E. coli* can be identified by examining samples of *E. coli* from ill and well persons. Useful assays include gene probe for the toxin gene[260] and detection of the toxins themselves: heat-labile enterotoxin by tissue culture assays,[261] ELISA,[262] or the Biken test[263] and heat-stable enterotoxin by the suckling mouse assay.[264] Enteroinvasive *E. coli* strains may be identified by gene probe[265] or by the Sereny test.[266] Because *E. coli* serotypes have been shown to cause diarrhea in volunteers in the absence of detectable enterotoxin production or invasiveness, the *E. coli* adherence factor (EAF) gene probe for enteropathogenic *E. coli*[267] and serotyping of *E. coli* isolates from both patients and controls may also be useful in outbreak settings if affected persons are found to have a serotype absent from controls.

Botulism outbreaks may be confirmed by the demonstration of botulinal toxin in the serum or stool of ill people or in incriminated food by the mouse neutralization test, or by the isolation of *C. botulinum* from the feces of ill people or from the incriminated food.[268, 269] Laboratory confirmation by testing of clinical specimens can be obtained in approximately 70 to 75% of the cases of botulism.[268, 269] Outbreaks of Norwalk agent or other human caliciviruses may be confirmed by the detection of viral genes in stools of ill persons by a polymerase chain reaction–based gene probe[270] or by demonstration of a serologic response by a biotin-avidin immunoassay procedure.[271] Laboratory diagnosis of parasitic pathogens typically depends on visualization of characteristic forms in the feces. The enteric parasites *Cyclospora* and *Cryptosporidium* are identified after specialized concentration and staining methods.[272, 273] Further information is available on the World Wide Web at http://www.dpd.cdc.gov/dpdx/.

Outbreaks caused by heavy metals may be documented by demonstration of the metallic ion in the incriminated food. Histamine fish poisoning may be confirmed by demonstration of histamine in the fish; concentrations of 100 mg in 100 g of fish flesh correlate with toxicity. The diagnosis of ciguatera is based on the clinical picture. However, ciguatera outbreaks may be documented by demonstration of ciguatoxin in the incriminated fish using ELISA techniques.[274] Shellfish poisoning may be confirmed either by demonstration of the toxin in mollusks by the mouse bioassay technique or by finding elevated numbers of the responsible dinoflagellate in the water from which the mollusks were obtained. Outbreaks of Chinese restaurant syndrome may be confirmed by demonstration of elevated monosodium L-glutamate levels in the food. Mushroom poisoning may be confirmed either by the identification of the responsible toxin in gastric contents, blood, urine, or fecal specimens by thin-layer chromatography or RIA or by the identification of the mushroom by a mycologist.

More than 50% of the reported foodborne disease outbreaks in the United States are of unknown cause. In some cases, appropriate diagnostic procedures are not conducted. In others, diagnostic specimens are not collected or transported properly. In still others, no agent is identified despite testing, raising the possibility that other etiologic agents are responsible. Possibilities include enterotoxigenic *E. coli, Plesiomonas shigelloides*, rotaviruses, and Norwalk-like agents. Although enterococci and gram-negative rods (*Aeromonas hydrophila, Klebsiella, Enterobacter, Proteus, Citrobacter*, and *Pseudomonas* spp.) have been reported as causes of foodborne outbreaks on rare occasions, their role has not been well documented, and they may be present in foods without causing illness. Because these organisms may be part of the normal fecal flora, documentation of their presence in ill people and their absence from well people is required to confirm their role in foodborne outbreaks.

THERAPY

Supportive measures are the mainstay of therapy in most cases of food poisoning. Most diarrheal diseases can be managed with oral rehydration.[275] Antiemetics and antiperistaltic agents offer symptomatic relief, although the latter are contraindicated in patients with high fever, bloody diarrhea, or fecal leukocytes indicative of an invasive infection. Fatalities can still occur. The most lethal foodborne diseases are botulism, listeriosis (affecting neonates and immunocompromised persons), *V. vulnificus* infection (in those with impaired hepatic function), paralytic shellfish poisoning, and long-incubation mushroom poisoning (Table 87–9). With other pathogens, fatalities may occur because the patient is extremely young, is extremely old, or has compromised host defenses; because the dose is overwhelming; or because the pathogen is resistant to treatment.

In any diarrheal illness, gastrointestinal fluid losses should be replaced either orally or parenterally. Antimicrobial agents may be used in the treatment of shigellosis and cholera, and are lifesaving in invasive salmonellosis and typhoid fever, but should be avoided in uncomplicated gastrointestinal infection caused by nontyphoid salmonellae. Tetracycline shortens both the duration of clinical cholera and the excretion of *V. cholerae* O1. Erythromycin eradicates carriage of *C. jejuni* and can shorten the duration of illness if given early in the disease. *Cyclospora* infection can be treated with high-dose trimethoprim-sulfamethoxazole. The role of antimicrobial agents in the management of food poisoning caused by *V. parahaemolyticus*; by enterotoxigenic, Shiga toxin–producing, or invasive *E. coli*; or by *Y. enterocolitica* is unsettled but probably minimal. Patients with *E. coli* O157:H7 infection should be evaluated expectantly for the development of hemolytic uremic syndrome, which often requires transfusion, renal dialysis, and prolonged intensive care.[276] Antimicrobial agents are of no value in the management of staphylococcal, *C. perfringens*, or *B. cereus* food poisoning. Patients with botulism present several additional therapeutic problems, which are discussed in Chapter 235.

A multiple-drug–resistant strain of *Salmonella*, called *Salmonella* serotype Typhimurium definitive type 104 (DT104), has emerged in the United Kingdom and United States. By 1996, DT104 was the second most common cause of human salmonellosis in England and Wales, and accounted for 8% of all salmonellosis in the United States; 4006 isolates were reported from humans in that year alone.[277, 278] More than 90% of all DT104 isolates were resistant

TABLE 87–9 Number of Deaths and Death-to-Case Ratios in Foodborne Disease Outbreaks Reported to the Centers for Disease Control and Prevention, 1973–1992

Etiologic Agent	No. of Deaths	Death-to-Case Ratio*
Bacterial		
Bacillus cereus	0	0.0
Campylobacter	4	1.8
Clostridium botulinum	57	92.1
Clostridium perfringens	13	0.8
Escherichia coli	4	2.8
Listeria monocytogenes	71	318.4
Salmonella	132	1.7
Shigella	4	0.2
Staphylococcus aureus	4	0.2
Streptococcus, Group A	0	0.0
Vibrio parahemolyticus	0	0.0
Vibrio cholerae O1 or O139	13	13.7
Yersinia enterocolitica	0	0.0
Other bacterial	5	10.9
Chemical		
Ciguatoxin	3	2.4
Histamine fish poisoning	1	0.6
Mushrooms	8	42.8
Paralytic shellfish poisoning (PSP)	3	13.3
Other chemical	9	4.5
Parasitic		
Trichinella spiralis	5	4.8
Other parasitic	0	0.0
Viral		
Hepatitis A	10	1.8
Other viral	0	0.0
Unknown	30	0.2
Total	376	

*per 1000 cases.

to ampicillin, chloramphenicol, streptomycin, sulphonamides, and tetracycline (R-type ACSSuT), and 30% of strains also showed resistance to trimethoprim and ciprofloxacin.[277] Surveillance for DT104 infections in the United Kingdom indicates high hospitalization and fatality rates compared with infections caused by other *Salmonella* serotypes. In one study, 41% of patients with multiresistant DT104 infection required hospitalization, and 3% died.[279] The appearance of this highly resistant strain can complicate treatment for any infection, because an inapparent subclinical DT104 infection can be changed to severe salmonellosis by exposure to an antimicrobial agent to which DT104 is resistant.[280] The emergence of this resistant strain is probably related to agricultural uses of antimicrobials. This highlights the interconnected pool of pathogens between animal reservoirs and people and underlines the need for prudent use of antimicrobials in both sectors.

Patients with PSP and some patients with ciguatera may require ventilatory support, usually for only a few days. Reports suggest that intravenous mannitol may ameliorate the acute neurologic symptoms of severe ciguatera and that tocainide may improve persistent dysesthesias.[281, 282] Therapy is otherwise supportive; no antitoxins are available. If not contraindicated by the presence of ileus, enemas or cathartics may be administered in an effort to remove unabsorbed toxin from the intestinal tract. Because of the severe dysesthesias associated with ciguatera, analgesics may also be required. Symptoms of histamine fish poisoning may be relieved by antihistamines. In severe cases with bronchospasm, epinephrine or aminophylline may be required.

Therapy for short-incubation types of mushroom poisoning is primarily supportive.[283] Patients who have ingested species containing pharmacologically active amounts of muscarine and who manifest evidence of parasympathetic hyperactivity may be treated with atropine. Patients who are severely ill after ingestion of species containing ibotenic acid and muscimol may be treated with physostigmine. Therapy for the long-incubation illness includes cathartics and enemas to remove unabsorbed toxin and a number of specific and supportive measures.[283] Because hypoglycemia often occurs, intravenous glucose may be required. Liver failure may ultimately require transplantation. α-Lipoic acid (thioctic acid) is an experimental drug that appears to be an effective antidote in these patients[153]; the drug may be obtained from Burton M. Berkson, MD, PhD, in Las Cruces, New Mexico (505–524–3720 or 505–521–1609). Pyridoxine is indicated in the management of patients poisoned with *Gyromitra* spp.

Therapy for acute heavy metal poisoning is supportive. Emesis should be induced if it does not occur spontaneously. Antiemetics are contraindicated, because retention of the toxic ions in the gut and subsequent systemic absorption may result. In severe cases with systemic manifestations of heavy metal toxicity, use of specific antidotes may be considered, but it is rarely necessary in these outbreaks.

SURVEILLANCE

Public health authorities monitor trends in specific diseases through reports of diagnosed cases provided by clinicians and microbiologists. These reports are the starting point for public health activities that can prevent further cases from occurring, such as education, identification of potentially hazardous events, and epidemiologic investigation. Increasingly, public health notification occurs most rapidly through the clinical laboratory. For *Salmonella, Shigella*, and *E. coli* O157:H7, the bacterial isolate itself is often referred to a public health laboratory for serotyping or molecular subtyping. Although knowing the specific serotype is rarely of importance in the management of a single case, it is fundamental to the recognition of outbreaks and to monitoring of the success of control efforts. This means that ordering the diagnostic tests needed to determine the nature of the illness is of benefit not only to the patient but to society as a whole. A single case of illness reported from a daycare center or family gathering not infrequently leads to discovery of an entire outbreak. Outbreaks can be apparent even though the specific diagnosis is not in hand, and investigation can succeed in identifying and controlling a source even without knowing the cause. This means that the astute clinician or microbiologist who calls the public health department epidemiologist to discuss a potential outbreak plays an important role in the control of foodborne and other diseases.

In addition to routine collection of notifiable disease reports and laboratory subtype-based surveillance, more information about sporadic cases of foodborne illness has been gathered since 1996 through a new active surveillance program called FoodNet.[284] Further information is available on the World Wide Web at http://www.cdc.gov/ncidod/dbmd/foodnet/foodnet.htm. This program gathers data actively, through regular contact with clinical laboratories, so that all cases that are diagnosed are counted. This provides accurate information concerning the numbers of cases, regardless of whether they are reported through the notifiable disease system. In 1997, seven sentinel sites, comprising approximately 6% of the U.S. population, participated in FoodNet. This system provides the most accurate and timely information about the actual burden of specific bacterial pathogens that are often foodborne (Table 87–10).

PREVENTION

Prevention of foodborne disease depends on careful handling of raw products and finished foods all the way from the farm to the table and on technologies that reduce or eliminate contamination in food.[285] Raw animal products, including meat, milk, eggs, and shellfish, are common sources of contamination leading to foodborne diseases. Contamination of raw animal products can be reduced by better animal production and slaughter practices. Monitoring of the safety of industrial food processing is increasingly important as the nation's food supply becomes more centralized and preprocessed for the

TABLE 87-10 Annual Incidence of Diagnosed Infections Identified through Active Surveillance in FoodNet, 1996

Pathogen	Incidence per 100,000 Population
Campylobacter	23.5
Salmonella	14.5
Shigella	8.9
Escherichia coli O157 : H7	2.7
Yersinia enterocolitica	1
Listeria monocytogenes	0.5
Vibrio spp.	0.1

From Centers for Disease Control and Prevention. Results of active surveillance with FoodNet, 1997. MMWR Morb Mortal Wkly Rep. 1998; 47:782–785.

convenience of the consumer. One approach to risk reduction, called the Hazard Analysis Critical Control Point (HACCP) program, was originally developed to ensure the safety of foods used in the space program. This approach requires a food producer to identify points where the risk of contamination can be controlled and to use production systems that eliminate these hazards. HACCP programs focus on preventing food contamination rather than relying on a final inspection step to detect it after it has occurred. Milk pasteurization and commercial canning practices are early examples of technologies that make foods safe. Strategies being explored now include provision of microbiologically safe food and water to animals, acid rinses and steam scalding of carcasses, and gamma and electron-beam irradiation of meats and produce.[286]

Renewed efforts are also being focused on identification of sites and sources of contamination of fresh produce harvested in the United States, Mexico, and Central America. There are many points where produce can become contaminated during growth and harvesting, processing and washing, transport, and final processing.[287] The surface of plants and fruits may be contaminated by soil, manure, or feces of animals or agricultural workers. It is unknown whether contamination is more likely to occur when produce is grown outside the United States; however, water quality in the developing world is a particular concern. Unclean water supplies can lead to contamination because water is used to irrigate and wash produce and to make the ice that is used to keep produce cool during trucking. The extra handling required to prepare salads and salad bars, and the time delay between preparation and consumption associated with salad bars, may increase the potential for produce to cause illness.[288] Pasteurizing juice and implementing HACCP programs will help decrease the risk associated with consumption of produce.

Much foodborne disease can be prevented if food is selected, prepared, and stored properly. In large kitchens and in homes, careful cooking and storage are necessary to kill pathogens and to prevent their growth when food is recontaminated after cooking. Because they serve high-risk populations, the kitchens of hospitals and nursing homes must pay particular attention to food safety. For example, routine use of pasteurized eggs instead of shell eggs prevents many nosocomial outbreaks of foodborne salmonellosis. In outbreaks reported to the CDC, the most common error is storage of food at inappropriate temperatures; this error is most often identified in staphylococcal, short- and long-incubation *B. cereus, C. perfringens,* and *Salmonella* outbreaks. Bacterial pathogens grow in food at temperatures ranging from 40°F to 140°F; growth may be prevented if cold food is adequately refrigerated and hot food is held at temperatures higher than 140°F before serving.

The usual source of contamination for *Salmonella, Campylobacter, C. perfringens*, vibrios, *Y. enterocolitica*, and other zoonoses is raw foods of animal origin, not infected food handlers.[289] However, poor personal hygiene by food handlers frequently contributes to *Staphylococcus, Shigella*, hepatitis A, and Norwalk agent–like outbreaks. Although thorough cooking of food just before consumption eliminates the risk of many illnesses, protection against staphylococcal food poisoning is not provided, because the staphylococcal enterotoxins are heat stable. Inadequate heat processing of canned foods can lead to botulism, and the use of contaminated equipment such as knives and meat slicers can result in *E. coli* O157:H7 infections and nontyphoid salmonellosis.[290, 291] Particular care in handling and cooking of raw poultry, beef, pork, shellfish, and eggs is important to prevent many foodborne diseases. Avoiding consumption of raw milk is important to prevent *Salmonella, E. coli* O157:H7, and *C. jejuni* infections.[7, 204, 292]

Food-handling errors resulting in chemical intoxication are different from those leading to bacterial outbreaks. Heavy metal poisoning occurs when acidic beverages are stored in defective metallic containers or when valves in vending machines malfunction. Ciguatera and shellfish poisoning occur when fish or shellfish are obtained from unsafe sources. Items contaminated with these toxins appear and taste normal; in addition, cooking of these items does not provide protection, because the toxins are heat stable.

The role of the clinician goes beyond that of diagnosis and treatment to prevention. This means warning high-risk patients (e.g., those infected with HIV, infants and the elderly, those with chronic medical conditions) of the hazards of raw oysters, raw eggs, and unpasteurized milk.[236, 293] Clinicians and microbiologists are also important in the detection of outbreaks, in particular in obtaining appropriate diagnostic tests for foodborne pathogens and reporting them to public health authorities.[294] Public health surveillance of foodborne infections and outbreaks is important in understanding the magnitude and complexity of the problem and guiding targeted prevention efforts. Reporting is essential if investigations are to be conducted to identify the source of the outbreak so that it can be corrected. Prompt reporting may also lead to the prevention of additional cases; there are well-documented outbreaks of botulism,[105, 295] salmonellosis,[296] and *E. coli* O157:H7[297] in which recognition and reporting of the initial illness could have prevented many subsequent cases. Diagnosing and reporting of illnesses with the potential for intrafamilial spread, or for spread within institutions such as childcare centers (e.g., shigellosis, *E. coli* O157:H7 infection) can prevent secondary transmission.[298, 299] Reporting is critical to stimulate concerted action to control major new hazards, such as *Salmonella* Enteritidis in eggs, or *E. coli* O157:H7 in beef. As we approach the 21st century, clinicians, laboratory workers, public health authorities, food safety officials, and members of industry can all play critical roles in decreasing the burden of foodborne illnesses.

REFERENCES

1. Bean NH, Griffin PM. Foodborne disease outbreaks in the United States, 1973–1987: Pathogens, vehicles and trends. J Food Protection. 1990;53:804–817.
2. Bean NH, Goulding JS, Lao C, et al. Surveillance for foodborne-disease outbreaks—United States, 1988–1992. MMWR Morb Mortal Wkly Rep. 1996;45:1–66.
3. Bennett JV, Holmberg SD, Rogers MF, et al. Infectious and parasitic diseases. In: Amler RW, Dull HB, eds. Closing the Gap: The Burden of Unnecessary Illness. New York: Oxford University Press; 1987:102–114.
4. Archer DL, Kvenberg JE. Incidence and cost of foodborne diarrheal disease in the United States. J Food Protection. 1985;48:887–894.
5. Tauxe RV. Emerging foodborne diseases: An evolving public health challenge. Emerg Infect Dis. 1997;3:425–434.
6. Lederberg J, Shope RE, Oaks SC Jr, eds. Emerging infections: Microbial threats to health in the United States. Washington, DC: National Academy Press; 1992.
7. Griffin PM, Tauxe RV. The epidemiology of infections caused by *Escherichia coli* O157:H7, other enterohemorrhagic *E. coli,* and the associated hemolytic uremic syndrome. Epidemiol Rev. 1991;13:60–98.
8. Herwaldt BL, Ackers ML, and the *Cyclospora* Working Group. An outbreak in 1996 of cyclosporiasis associated with imported raspberries. N Engl J Med. 1997;336:1548–1556.
9. Swerdlow DL, Lee LA, Tauxe RV, et al. Reactive arthropathy following a multistate outbreak of *Salmonella typhimurium* infections (Abstract 916). 30th Interscience Conference on Antimicrobial Agents and Chemotherapy. Atlanta, October 21–24, 1990.
10. Mishu B, Ilyas AA, Kosli CL, et al. Serologic evidence of previous *Campylobacter jejuni* infections in patients with the Guillain-Barré syndrome. Ann Intern Med. 1993;118:947–953.
11. Feig M. Staphylococcal food poisoning. A report of two related outbreaks, and a discussion of the data presented. Am J Public Health. 1950;40:279.

12. Bergdoll MS. The enterotoxins. In: Cohen JO, ed. The Staphylococci. New York: Wiley; 1972:301.
13. Bergdoll MS, Crass BA, Reiser RF, et al. A new staphylococcal enterotoxin, enterotoxin F, associated with toxic-shock-syndrome *Staphylococcus aureus* isolates. Lancet. 1981;1:1017.
14. Sugiyama H, Hayama T. Abdominal viscera as site of emetic action for staphylococcal enterotoxin in the monkey. J Infect Dis. 1965;115:330.
15. Clark WG, Vanderhooft GF, Borison HL. Emetic effect of purified staphylococcal enterotoxin in cats. Proc Soc Exp Biol Med. 1962;111:205.
16. Elias J, Shields R. Influence of staphylococcal enterotoxin on water and electrolyte transport in the small intestine. Gut. 1976;17:527.
17. Gilbert RJ. Staphylococcal food poisoning and botulism. Postgrad Med J. 1974;50:603.
18. Breckinridge JC, Bergdoll MS. Outbreak of foodborne gastroenteritis due to a coagulase-negative enterotoxin-producing staphylococcus. N Engl J Med. 1971;284:541.
19. Merson MH. The epidemiology of staphylococcal foodborne disease. Proc Staph Foods Conf. University Park, PA: Pennsylvania State University; 1973:20.
20. Šimkovičova M, Gilbert RJ. Serological detection of enterotoxin from food-poisoning strains of *Staphylococcus aureus.* J Med Microbiol. 1971;4:19.
21. Holmberg SD, Blake PA. Staphylococcal food poisoning in the United States: New facts and old misconceptions. JAMA. 1984;251:487.
22. Mortimer PR, McCann G. Food-poisoning episodes associated with *Bacillus cereus* in fried rice. Lancet. 1974;1:1043.
23. Midura T, Gerber M, Wood R, et al. Outbreak of food poisoning caused by *Bacillus cereus.* Public Health Rep. 1970;85:45.
24. Terranova W, Blake PA. *Bacillus cereus* food poisoning. N Engl J Med. 1978;298:143.
25. Melling J, Capel BJ, Turnbull PCB, et al. Identification of a novel enterotoxigenic activity associated with *Bacillus cereus.* J Clin Pathol. 1976;29:938.
26. Turnbull PCB, Kramer JM, Jorgensen K. Properties and production characteristics of vomiting, diarrheal, and necrotizing toxins of *Bacillus cereus.* Am J Clin Nutr. 1979;32:219.
27. Hobbs BC, Smith ME, Oakley CL, et al. *Clostridium welchii* food poisoning. J Hyg. 1953;51:75.
28. Shandera WX, Tacket CO, Blake PA. Food poisoning due to *Clostridium perfringens* in the United States. J Infect Dis. 1983;147:167.
29. Smith LDS. *Clostridium perfringens.* The Pathogenic Anaerobic Bacteria. Springfield, IL: Charles C Thomas; 1975:115.
30. Stark RL, Duncan CL. Purification and biochemical properties of *Clostridium perfringens* type A enterotoxin. Infect Immun. 1972;6:662.
31. Rood JI, Cole ST. Molecular genetics and pathogenesis of *Clostridium perfringens.* Microbiol Rev. 1990;55:621–648.
32. McDonel JL, Duncan CL. Regional localization of activity of *Clostridium perfringens* type A enterotoxin in the rabbit ileum, jejunum, and duodenum. J Infect Dis. 1977;136:661.
33. McDonel JL. The molecular mode of action of *Clostridium perfringens* enterotoxin. Am J Clin Nutr. 1979;32:210.
34. Turnbull PCB. Studies on the production of enterotoxins by *Bacillus cereus.* J Clin Pathol. 1976;29:941.
35. Loewenstein MS. Epidemiology of *Clostridium perfringens* food poisoning. N Engl J Med. 1972;286:1026.
36. Giannella RA, Brasile L: A hospital food-borne outbreak of diarrhea caused by *Bacillus cereus.* Clinical, epidemiologic, and microbiologic studies. J Infect Dis. 1979;139:366.
37. Granum PE. *Bacillus cereus* and food hygiene. Norsk Vet Tidskr. 1994;106:911–914.
38. Granum PE, Næstvold A, Gundersby KN. *Bacillus cereus* food poisoning during Norwegian Ski Championship for juniors. Norsk Vet Tidskr. 1995;107:945–948.
39. Giannella RA, Formal SB, Dammin GJ, et al. Pathogenesis of salmonellosis: Studies of fluid secretion, mucosal invasion, and morphologic reaction in the rabbit ileum. J Clin Invest. 1973;52:441.
40. Rout WR, Formal SB, Giannella RA, et al. Pathophysiology of shigella diarrhea in the rhesus monkey: Intestinal transport, morphological, and bacteriological studies. Gastroenterology. 1975;68:270.
41. Boutin BK, Townsend SF, Scarpino PV, et al. Demonstration of invasiveness of *Vibrio parahaemolyticus* in adult rabbits by immunofluorescence. Appl Environ Microbiol. 1979;37:647.
42. Tulloch EF, Ryan KJ, Formal SB, et al. Invasive enteropathic *Escherichia coli* dysentery: An outbreak in 28 adults. Ann Intern Med. 1973;79:13.
43. Horwitz MA, Pollard RA, Merson MH, et al. A large outbreak of foodborne salmonellosis on the Navaho Nation Indian Reservation: Epidemiology and secondary transmission. Am J Public Health. 1977;67:1071.
44. Weissman JB, Williams SV, Hinman AR, et al. Foodborne shigellosis at a country fair. Am J Epidemiol. 1974;100:178.
45. Chatterjee BD, Neogy KN, Gorbach SL. Studies of *Vibrio parahaemolyticus* from cases of diarrhea in Calcutta. Indian J Med Res. 1970;58:234.
46. Marier R, Wells JG, Swanson RC, et al. An outbreak of enteropathogenic *Escherichia coli* foodborne disease traced to imported French cheese. Lancet. 1973;2:1376.
47. Tauxe RV. Epidemiology of *Campylobacter jejuni* infections in the United States and other industrialized nations. In: Nachamkin I, Blaser ML, Tompkins L, eds. *Campylobacter jejuni*: Current Status and Future Trends. Washington, DC: American Society of Microbiology; 1992;9–19.
48. Slutsker L, Ries AA, Greene KD, et al. *Escherichia coli* O157:H7 diarrhea in the United States: Clinical and epidemiologic features. Ann Intern Med. 1997;126:505.
49. Blaser MJ, Wells JG, Feldman RA. *Campylobacter* enteritis in the United States: A multicenter study. Ann Intern Med. 1983;98:360.
50. Lambert ME, Schofield PF, Ironside AG, et al. *Campylobacter* colitis. BMJ. 1979;1:857.
51. Taylor DN, Porter BW, Williams CA, et al. *Campylobacter* enteritis: A large outbreak traced to commercial raw milk. West J Med. 1982;137:365.
52. Blaser MJ, Checko P, Bopp C, et al. *Campylobacter* enteritis associated with foodborne transmission. Am J Epidemiol. 1982;116:886.
53. Blaser MJ, Berkowitz ID, LaForce FM, et al. *Campylobacter* enteritis: Clinical and epidemiologic features. Ann Intern Med. 1979;91:179.
54. Dalton CB, Austin CC, Sobel J, et al. An outbreak of gastroenteritis and fever due to *Listeria monocytogenes* in milk. N Engl J Med. 1997;336:100.
55. Morris JG Jr. Non-O1 group 1 *Vibrio cholerae* strains not associated with epidemic disease. In: Wachsmuth IK, Blake PA, Olsvik O, eds. *Vibrio cholerae* and Cholera: Molecular to Global Perspectives. Washington DC: American Society for Microbiology; 1994:103–116.
56. Wilson R, Lieb S, Roberts A, et al. Non-O group 1 *Vibrio cholerae* gastroenteritis associated with eating raw oysters. Am J Epidemiol. 1981;114:293.
57. Kaper JB, Fasano A, Trucksis M. Toxins of *Vibrio cholerae.* In: Wachsmuth IK, Blake PA, Olsvik O, eds. *Vibrio cholerae* and Cholera: Molecular to Global Perspectives. Washington, DC: American Society for Microbiology; 1994:145–176.
58. Zinnaka Y, Carpenter CCJ Jr. An enterotoxin produced by noncholera vibrios. Johns Hopkins Med J. 1972;131:403.
59. Craig JP, Yamamoto K, Takeda Y, et al. Production of cholera-like enterotoxin by a *Vibrio cholerae* non-O1 strain isolated from the environment. Infect Immun. 1981;34:90.
60. Sack RB. Human diarrheal disease caused by enterotoxigenic *Escherichia coli.* Annu Rev Microbiol. 1975;29:333.
61. Sandefur PD, Peterson JW. Neutralization of *Salmonella* toxin-induced elongation of Chinese hamster ovary cells by cholera antitoxin. Infect Immun. 1977;15:988.
62. Sedlock DM, Deibel RH. Detection of *Salmonella* enterotoxin using rabbit ileal loops. Can J Microbiol. 1978;24:268.
63. Keusch GT, Donta ST. Classification of enterotoxins on the basis of activity in cell culture. J Infect Dis. 1975;131:58.
64. Keusch GT, Jacewicz M. The pathogenesis of *Shigella* diarrhea. IV. Toxin and antitoxin in *Shigella flexneri* and *Shigella sonnei* infections in humans. J Infect Dis. 1977;135:552.
65. O'Brien AD, Gentry MK, Thompson MR, et al. Shigellosis and *Escherichia coli* diarrhea: Relative importance of invasive and toxigenic mechanisms. Am J Clin Nutr. 1979;32:229.
66. Honda T, Shimizu M, Takeda Y, et al. Isolation of a factor causing morphological changes of Chinese hamster ovary cells from the culture filtrate of *Vibrio parahaemolyticus.* Infect Immun. 1976;14:1028.
67. Carruthers MM. Cytotoxicity of *Vibrio parahaemolyticus* in HeLa cell culture. J Infect Dis. 1975;132:555.
68. Banwell JG, Gorbach SL, Pierce NF, et al. Acute undifferentiated human diarrhea in the tropics. II. Alterations in intestinal fluid and electrolyte movements. J Clin Invest. 1971;50:890.
69. Barker WH Jr, Mackowiak PA, Fishbein M, et al. *Vibrio parahaemolyticus* gastroenteritis outbreak in Covington, Louisiana, in August 1972. Am J Epidemiol. 1974;100:316.
70. Aldova E, Lázničková K, Stěpanková E, et al. Isolation of nonagglutinable vibrios from an enteritis outbreak in Czechoslovakia. J Infect Dis. 1968;118:25.
71. Carpenter CCJ Jr, Mitra PP, Sack RB. Clinical studies in Asiatic cholera. I. Preliminary observations, November 1962–March 1963. Bull Johns Hopkins Hosp. 1966;118:165.
72. Taylor WR, Schell WL, Wells JG, et al. A foodborne outbreak of enterotoxigenic *Escherichia coli* diarrhea. N Engl J Med. 1982;306:1093.
73. Kaplan JE, Gary GW, Baron RC, et al. Epidemiology of Norwalk gastroenteritis and the role of Norwalk virus in outbreaks of acute nonbacterial gastroenteritis. Ann Intern Med. 1982;96:756.
74. Murphy AM, Grohmann GS, Christopher PJ, et al. An Australia-wide outbreak of gastroenteritis from oysters caused by Norwalk virus. Med J Aust. 1979;2:329.
75. Morse DL, Guzewich JJ, Hanrahan JP, et al. Widespread outbreaks of clam- and oyster-associated gastroenteritis: Role of Norwalk virus. N Engl J Med. 1986;314:678–681.
76. Kaplan JE, Feldman R, Campbell DS, et al. The frequency of a Norwalk-like pattern of illness in outbreaks of acute gastroenteritis. Am J Public Health. 1982;72:1329–32.
77. Kapikian AZ, Estes MK, Chanock RM. Norwalk group of viruses. In: Fields BN, Knipe DM, Howley PM, eds. Virology. 3rd ed. Philadelphia: Lippincott-Raven; 1995:783.
78. Lee LA, Gerber AR, Lonsway DR, et al. *Yersinia enterocolitica* O:3 infections in infants and children, associated with household preparation of chitterlings. N Engl J Med. 1990;322:984–987.
79. Black RE, Jackson RJ, Tsai T, et al. Epidemic *Yersinia enterocolitica* infection due to contaminated chocolate milk. N Engl J Med. 1978;298:76.
80. Tacket CO, Narain JP, Sattin R, et al. A multistate outbreak of infections caused by *Yersinia enterocolitica* transmitted by pasteurized milk. JAMA. 1984;251:483.
81. Ostroff SM, Kapperud G, Lassen J, et al. Clinical features of sporadic *Yersinia enterocolitica* infections in Norway. J Infect Dis. 1992;166:812–817.
82. Tauxe RV, Vandepitte J, Wauters G, et al. *Yersinia enterocolitica* infections and pork: The missing link. Lancet. 1987;1:1129–32.

83. Pai CH, Mors V. Production of enterotoxin by *Yersinia enterocolitica.* Infect Immun. 1978;19:908.
84. Boyce JM, Doyle DJ Jr, Evans DG, et al. Production of heat-stable, methanol-soluble enterotoxin by *Yersinia enterocolitica.* Infect Immun. 1979;25:532.
85. Asakawa Y, Akahane S, Kagata N, et al. Two community outbreaks of human infection with *Yersinia enterocolitica.* J Hyg (Camb). 1973;71:715.
86. Arvastson B, Damgaard K, Winblad S. Clinical symptoms of infection with *Yersinia enterocolitica.* Scand J Infect Dis. 1971;3:37.
87. Riley LW, Remis RS, Helgerson SD, et al. Hemorrhagic colitis associated with a rare *Escherichia coli* serotype. N Engl J Med. 1983;308:681.
88. Griffin PM, Ostroff SM, Tauxe RV, et al. Illnesses associated with *Escherichia coli* O157:H7 infections: A broad clinical spectrum. Ann Intern Med. 1988;109:705–12.
89. Johnson WM, Lior H, Bezanson GS. Cytotoxic *Escherichia coli* O157:H7 associated with haemorrhagic colitis in Canada. Lancet. 1983;1:76.
90. O'Brien AD, Lively TA, Chen ME, et al. *Escherichia coli* O157:H7 strains associated with haemorrhagic colitis in the United States produce a *Shigella dysenteriae* 1 (shiga) like cytotoxin. Lancet. 1983;1:702.
91. Calderwood SB, Acheson DWK, Keusch GT, et al. Proposed new nomenclature for SLT (VT) family. ASM News. 1996;62:118–119.
92. Lingwood CA, Mylvaganam M, Arab S, et al. Shiga toxin (verotoxin) binding to its receptor glycolipid. In: Kaper JB, O'Brien AD, eds. *Escherichia coli* O157:H7 and Other Shiga Toxin–Producing *E. coli* Strains. Washington, DC: American Society for Microbiology; 1998:129–139.
93. Boyce TG, Swerdlow DL, Griffin PM. *Escherichia coli* O157:H7 and the hemolytic-uremic syndrome. N Engl J Med. 1995;333:364–367.
94. Centers for Disease Control and Prevention. Outbreak of acute gastroenteritis attributable to *Escherichia coli* serotype O104:H21—Montana. MMWR Morb Mortal Wkly Rep. 1995;44:501–504.
95. Banatvala N, Debeukelaer MM, Griffin PM, et al. Shiga-like toxin–producing *Escherichia coli* O111 and associated hemolytic uremic syndrome: A Family outbreak. Pediatr Infect Dis J. 1996;15:1008–1011.
96. Shapiro RL, Hatheway C, Swerdlow DL. Botulism in the United States: A clinical and epidemiologic review. Ann Intern Med. 1998;129:221–228.
97. Woodruff BA, Griffin PM, McCroskey LM, et al. Clinical and laboratory comparison of botulism from toxin types A, B, and E in the United States, 1975–1988. J Infect Dis. 1992;166:1281–1286.
98. Hughes JM, Blumenthal JR, Merson MH, et al. Clinical features of types A and B food-borne botulism. Ann Intern Med. 1981;95:442.
99. Kao I, Drachman DB, Price DL. Botulinum toxin: Mechanism of presynaptic blockade. Science. 1976;193:1256.
100. Simpson LL. The origin, structure, and pharmacological activity of botulinum toxin. Pharmacol Rev. 1981;33:155.
101. Horwitz MA, Hughes JM, Merson MH, et al. Food-borne botulism in the United States, 1970–1975. J Infect Dis. 1977;136:153.
102. Midura TF, Arnon SS. Infant botulism: Identification of *Clostridium botulinum* and its toxins in feces. Lancet. 1976;2:934.
103. Arnon SS. Infant botulism. In: Feigen RD, Cherry JD, eds. Textbook of Pediatric Infectious Diseases. 4th ed. Philadelphia: WB Saunders; 1998:1570–1577.
104. Sugiyama H, Mills DC. Intraintestinal toxin in infant mice challenged intragastrically with *Clostridium botulinum* spores. Infect Immun. 1978;21:59.
105. St Louis ME, Shaun HS, Peck MB, et al. Botulism from chopped garlic: Delayed recognition of a major outbreak. Ann Intern Med. 1988;108:363–368.
106. Semple AB, Parry WH, Phillips DE. Acute copper poisoning: An outbreak traced to contaminated water from a corroded geyser. Lancet. 1960;2:700.
107. Brown MA, Thom JV, Orth GL, et al. Food poisoning involving zinc contamination. Arch Environ Health. 1964;8:657.
108. Centers for Disease Control and Prevention. Illness associated with elevated levels of zinc in fruit punch: New Mexico. MMWR Morb Mortal Wkly Rep. 1983;32:257.
109. Barker WH Jr, Runte V. Tomato juice-associated gastroenteritis, Washington and Oregon, 1969. Am J Epidemiol. 1972;96:219.
110. Baker TD, Hafner WG. Cadmium poisoning from a refrigerator shelf used as an improvised barbecue grill. Public Health Rep. 1961;76:543.
111. Merson MH, Baine WB, Gangarosa EJ, et al. Scombroid fish poisoning: Outbreak traced to commercially canned tuna fish. JAMA. 1974;228:1268.
112. Taylor SL. Histamine food poisoning: Toxicology and clinical aspects. CRC Crit Rev Toxicol. 1986;17:91–128.
113. Taylor SL, Guthertz LS, Leatherwood M, et al. Histamine production by *Klebsiella pneumoniae* and an incident of scombroid fish poisoning. Appl Environ Microbiol. 1979;37:274.
114. Hughes JM, Merson MH. Fish and shellfish poisoning. N Engl J Med. 1976;295:1117.
115. Perl TM, Bedard L, Kosatsky T, et al. An outbreak of toxic encephalopathy caused by eating mussels contaminated with domoic acid. New Engl J Med. 1990;322:1775–80.
116. Halstead BW, Courville DA. Poisonous and Venomous Marine Animals of the World, v. 1. Invertebrates. Washington, DC: Government Printing Office; 1965:157.
117. Zwahlen A, Blanc MH, Robert M. Epidémie d'intoxication par les moules ("Paralytic Shellfish Poisoning"). Schweiz Med Wochenschr. 1977;107:226.
118. Acres J, Gray J. Paralytic shellfish poisoning. Can Med Assoc J. 1978;119:1195.
119. Rodriguez DC, Etzel RA, Hall S, et al. Lethal paralytic shellfish poisoning in Guatemala. Am J Trop Med Hyg. 1990;42:267–71.
120. Proctor NH, Chan SL, Trevor AJ: Production of saxitoxin by cultures of *Gonyaulax catenella.* Toxicon. 1975;13:1.
121. Ghazarossian VE, Schantz EJ, Schnoes HK, et al. Identification of a poison in toxic scallops from a *Gonyaulax tamarensis* red tide. Biochem Biophys Res Comm. 1974;59:1219.
122. Shimizu Y, Buckley LJ, Alam M, et al. Structures of gonyautoxin II and III from the East Coast toxic dinoflagellate *Gonyaulax tamarensis.* J Am Chem Soc. 1976;98:5414.
123. Schantz EJ, Ghazarossian VE, Schnoes HK, et al. The structure of saxitoxin. J Am Chem Soc. 1975;97:1238.
124. Henderson R, Ritchie JM, Strichartz GR. The binding of labelled saxitoxin to the sodium channels in nerve membranes. J Physiol. 1973;235:783.
125. Henderson R, Ritchie JM, Strichartz GR. Evidence that tetrodotoxin and saxitoxin act at a metal cation binding site in the sodium channels of nerve membrane. Proc Natl Acad Sci U S A. 1974;71:3936.
126. Catterall WA. Neurotoxins that act on voltage-sensitive sodium channels in excitable membranes. Annu Rev Pharmacol Toxicol. 1980;20:15.
127. Spiegelstein MY, Paster Z, Abbott BC. Purification and biological activity of *Gymnodinium breve* toxins. Toxicon. 1973;11:85.
128. Kim YS, Padilla GM. Purification of the ichthyotoxic component of *Gymnodinium breve* (red tide dinoflagellate) toxin by high pressure liquid chromatography. Toxicon. 1976;14:379.
129. Grunfeld Y, Spiegelstein MY. Effects of *Gymnodinium breve* toxin on the smooth muscle preparation of guinea-pig ileum. Br J Pharmacol. 1974;51:67.
130. Teitlebaum JS, Zatorre RJ, Carpenter S, et al. Neurologic sequelae of domoic acid intoxication due to the ingestion of contaminated mussels. N Engl J Med. 1990;322:1781–7.
131. Schaumburg HH, Byck R, Gerstl R, et al. Monosodium L-glutamate: Its pharmacology and role in the Chinese restaurant syndrome. Science. 1969;163:826.
132. Reif-Lehrer L. A questionnaire study of the prevalence of Chinese restaurant syndrome. Fed Proc. 1977;36:1617.
133. Hudson PJ, Vogt RL. A foodborne outbreak traced to niacin overenrichment. J Food Protection. 1985;48:249–251.
134. Barkin RM. Ciguatera poisoning: A common source outbreak. South Med J. 1974;67:13.
135. Halstead BW. Fish poisoning: The diagnosis, pharmacology and treatment. Clin Pharmacol Ther. 1964;5:615.
136. Russell FE. Ciguatera poisoning: A report of 35 cases. Toxicon. 1975;13:383.
137. Halstead BW, Courville DA. Poisonous and Venomous Marine Animals of the World, v. 1. Vertebrates. Washington, DC: Government Printing Office; 1967:63.
138. Engleberg NC, Morris JG Jr, Lewis J, et al. Ciguatera fish poisoning: A major common-source outbreak in the U.S. Virgin Islands. Ann Intern Med. 1983;98:336.
139. Bagnis R, Kuberski T, Laugier S. Clinical observations on 3,009 cases of ciguatera (fish poisoning) in the South Pacific. Am J Trop Med Hyg. 1979;28:1067.
140. Morris JG Jr, Lewin P, Hargrett NT, et al. Clinical features of ciguatera fish poisoning: A study of the disease in the U.S. Virgin Islands. Arch Intern Med. 1982;142:1090.
141. Scheuer PJ, Takahashi W, Tsutsumi J, et al. Ciguatoxin: Isolation and chemical nature. Science. 1967;155:1267.
142. Helfrich P, Banner AH. Experimental induction of ciguatera: Toxicity in fish through diet. Nature. 1963;197:1025.
143. Morris JG Jr. Natural toxins associated with fish and shellfish. In: Blaser MJ, Smith PD, Ravdin JI, eds. Infections of the Gastrointestinal Tract. New York: Raven Press; 1995:251–256.
144. Li K-M. Ciguatera fish poison: A cholinesterase inhibitor. Science. 1965;147:1580.
145. Halstead BW. Current status of marine biotoxicology: An overview. Clin Toxicol. 1981;18:1.
146. Le Grand AM, Galonnier M, Bagnis R. Studies on the mode of action of ciguateric toxins. Toxicon. 1982;20:311–315.
147. Bidard JN, Vijverberg HPM, Frelin C, et al. Ciguatoxin is a novel type of Na^+ channel toxin. J Biol Chem. 1984;259:8353–7.
148. Lampe KF. Current concepts of therapy in mushroom intoxication. Clin Toxicol. 1974;7:115.
149. Becker CE, Tong TG, Boerner U, et al. Diagnosis and treatment of *Amanita phalloides*–type mushroom poisoning: Use of thioctic acid. West J Med. 1976;125:100.
150. Hall AH, Spoerke DG, Rumack BH. Mushroom poisoning: identification, diagnosis, and treatment. Pediatr Rev. 1987;8:291–298.
151. Lampe KF. Toxic fungi. Annu Rev Pharmacol Toxicol. 1979;19:85.
152. Paaso B, Harrison DC. A new look at an old problem: Mushroom poisoning. Am J Med. 1975;58:505.
153. Hughes JM, Horwitz MA, Merson MH, et al. Foodborne disease outbreaks of chemical etiology in the United States, 1970–1974. Am J Epidemiol. 1977;105:233.
154. Editorial: Death-cap poisoning. Lancet. 1972;1:1320.
155. Centers for Disease Control and Prevention: Mushroom poisoning among Laotian refugees: 1981. MMWR Morb Mortal Wkly Rep. 1982;31:287.
156. Wieland T, Wieland O. The toxic peptides of *Amanita* species. In: Kadis S, Ciegler A, Aji SJ, eds. Microbiol Toxins, v. 8. Fungal Toxins. New York: Academic Press; 1972:249.
157. Osterholm MT, MacDonald KL, White KE, et al. An outbreak of a newly recognized chronic diarrhea syndrome associated with raw milk consumption. JAMA. 1986;256:484–90.
158. Martin DL, Hoberman LJ. A point source outbreak of chronic diarrhea in Texas: No known exposure to raw milk. JAMA. 1986;256:469.
159. Mintz ED, Weber JT, Guris D, et al. An outbreak of Brainerd diarrhea among travellers to the Galapagos Islands. J Infect Dis. 1998;177:1041.
160. Merson MH, Barker WH Jr, Craun GF, et al. Outbreaks of waterborne disease in the United States, 1971–1972. J Infect Dis. 1974;129:614.

161. Hughes JM, Merson MH, Craun GF, et al. Outbreaks of waterborne disease in the United States, 1973. J Infect Dis. 1975;132:336.
162. Horwitz MA, Hughes JM, Craun GF. Outbreaks of waterborne disease in the United States, 1974. J Infect Dis. 1976;133:588.
163. Black RE, Horwitz MA, Craun GF. Outbreaks of waterborne disease in the United States, 1975. J Infect Dis. 1978;137:370.
164. Centers for Disease Control and Prevention. Foodborne and Waterborne Disease Outbreaks Annual Summary 1976. October 1977.
165. Centers for Disease Control and Prevention. Foodborne and Waterborne Disease Surveillance Annual Summary 1977. August 1979.
166. Centers for Disease Control and Prevention. Water-Related Disease Outbreaks Surveillance Annual Summary 1978. May 1980.
167. Centers for Disease Control and Prevention. Water-Related Disease Outbreaks Surveillance Annual Summary 1979. September 1981.
168. Centers for Disease Control and Prevention. Water-Related Disease Outbreaks Surveillance Annual Summary 1980. February 1982.
169. Centers for Disease Control and Prevention. Water-Related Disease Outbreaks Surveillance Annual Summary 1981. September 1982.
170. Centers for Disease Control and Prevention. Water-Related Disease Outbreaks Surveillance Annual Summary 1982. Centers for Disease Control. 1983;1–15.
171. Centers for Disease Control and Prevention. Water-Related Disease Outbreaks Surveillance Annual Summary 1983. 1984;1–15.
172. Centers for Disease Control and Prevention. Water-Related Disease Outbreaks Surveillance Annual Summary 1984. 1985;1–15.
173. St Louis ME. Water-Related Disease Outbreaks, 1985. CDC surveillance summaries. MMWR Morb Mortal Wkly Rep. 1986;37(No. SS-2):15–24.
174. Levine WC, Stephenson WT, Craun GF. Waterborne disease outbreaks, 1986–1988. Centers for Disease Control Surveillance Summaries, March 1990. MMWR Morb Mortal Wkly Rep. 1990;39(No. SS-1):1–13.
175. Herwaldt BL, Craun GF, Stokes SL, et al. Waterborne disease outbreaks, 1989–1990. Centers for Disease Control Surveillance Summaries, December 1991. MMWR Morb Mortal Wkly Rep. 1991;40(No. SS-3):1–21.
176. Moore AC, Herwaldt BL, Craun GC, et al. Surveillance for waterborne disease outbreaks—United States, 1991–1992. MMWR Morb Mortal Wkly Rep. 1993;42(SS-5):1.
177. Kramer MH, Herwaldt BL, Craun GC, et al. Surveillance for waterborne disease outbreaks—United States, 1993–1994. MMWR Morb Mortal Wkly Rep. 1996;45(SS-1):1.
178. MacKenzie WR, Hoxie NJ, Proctor ME, et al. A massive outbreak in Milwaukee of *Cryptosporidium* infection transmitted through the public water supply. N Engl J Med. 1994;331:161.
179. Swerdlow DL, Woodruff BA, Brady RC, et al. A waterborne outbreak in Missouri of *Escherichia coli* O157:H7 associated with bloody diarrhea and death. Ann Intern Med. 1992;117:812–819.
180. Weissman JB, Craun GF, Lawrence DN, et al. An epidemic of gastroenteritis traced to a contaminated public water supply. Am J Epidemiol. 1976;103:391.
181. Mosley JW. Water-borne infectious hepatitis. N Engl J Med. 1959;261:703.
182. Feldman RE, Baine WB, Nitzkin JL, et al. Epidemiology of *Salmonella typhi* infection in a migrant labor camp in Dade County, Florida. J Infect Dis. 1974;130:334.
183. A collaborative report. A waterborne epidemic of salmonellosis in Riverside, California, 1965: Epidemiologic aspects. Am J Epidemiol. 1971;93:33.
184. Rosenberg ML, Koplan JP, Wachsmuth IK, et al. Epidemic diarrhea at Crater Lake from enterotoxigenic *Escherichia coli*: A large waterborne outbreak. Ann Intern Med. 1977;86:714.
185. Vogt RL, Sours HE, Barrett T, et al. *Campylobacter* enteritis associated with contaminated water. Ann Intern Med. 1982;96:292.
186. Palmer SR, Gully PR, White JM, et al. Water-borne outbreak of *Campylobacter* gastroenteritis. Lancet. 1983;1:287.
187. Parsonnet J, Trock SC, Bopp CA, et al. Chronic diarrhea associated with drinking untreated water. Ann Intern Med. 1989;110:985–91.
188. Wilson R, Anderson LJ, Holman RC, et al. Waterborne gastroenteritis due to the Norwalk agent: Clinical and epidemiologic investigation. Am J Public Health. 1982;72:72.
189. Kaplan JE, Goodman RA, Schonberger LB, et al. Gastroenteritis due to Norwalk virus: An outbreak associated with a municipal water system. J Infect Dis. 1982;146:190.
190. Morens DM, Zweighaft RM, Vernon TM, et al. A waterborne outbreak of gastroenteritis with secondary person-to-person spread. Lancet. 1979;1:964.
191. Jackson LA, Wenger JD. Listeriosis: A foodborne disease. Infections Med. 1993;10:61–66.
192. Blake PA, Merson MH, Weaver RE, et al. Disease caused by a marine *Vibrio*: Clinical characteristics and epidemiology. N Engl J Med. 1979;300:1–5.
193. Gilbert RJ, Stringer MF, Peace TC. The survival and growth of *Bacillus cereus* in boiled and fried rice in relation to outbreaks of food poisoning. J Hyg (Camb). 1974;73:433.
194. Granum PE. *Bacillus cereus*. In: Doyle MP, Beuchat LR, Montville TJ, eds. Food Microbiology: Fundamentals and Frontiers. Washington, DC: American Society for Microbiology; 1997:327–336.
195. McClane B. *Clostridium perfringens*. In: Doyle MP, Beuchat LR, Montville TJ, eds. Food Microbiology: Fundamentals and Frontiers. Washington, DC: American Society for Microbiology; 1997:305–326.
196. Petersen LR, Mshar R, Cooper GH Jr, et al. A large *Clostridium perfringens* foodborne outbreak with an unusual attack rate pattern. Am J Epidemiol. 1988;127:605–611.
197. Kim HU, Goepfert JM. Enumeration and identification of *Bacillus cereus* in foods. I. 24-hour presumptive test medium. Appl Microbiol. 1971;22:581.
198. Blakey LJ, Priest FG. The occurrence of *Bacillus cereus* in some dried foods including pulses and cereals. J Appl Bacteriol. 1980;48:297.
199. Jephcott AE, Barton BW, Gilbert RJ, et al. An unusual outbreak of food-poisoning associated with meals-on-wheels. Lancet. 1977;2:129.
200. Griffin PM. Epidemiology of Shiga toxin-producing *Escherichia coli* infections in humans in the United States. In: Kaper JB, O'Brien AD, eds. *Escherichia coli* O157:H7 and Other Shiga Toxin–Producing *E. coli* Strains. Washington, DC: American Society for Microbiology; 1998:15–22.
201. St Louis ME, Morse DL, Potter ME, et al. The emergence of grade A eggs as a major source of *Salmonella enteritidis* infections. JAMA. 1988;259:2103–2107.
202. Centers for Disease Control and Prevention: Outbreaks of *Salmonella* serotype Enteritidis infections associated with consumption of raw shell eggs—United States, 1994–1995. MMWR Morb Mortal Wkly Rep. 1996;45:737.
203. Hogue A, White P, Guard-Petter J, et al. Epidemiology and Control of Egg-Associated *Salmonella* Enteritidis in the United States of America. Washington, DC: Office International des Épizooties, Scientific and Technical Review; 1997;16:542–553.
204. Headrick ML, Korangy S, Bean NH, et al. The epidemiology of raw milk-associated foodborne disease outbreaks reported in the United States, 1973 through 1992. Am J Public Health. 1998;88:1219–1221.
205. Ries AA, Zaza S, Langkop C, et al. A multistate outbreak of *Salmonella chester* linked to imported canteloupe (Abstract). Proceedings of the 30th Interscience Conference on Antimicrobial Agents and Chemotherapy. Washington, DC: American Society for Microbiology; 1990:38.
206. Wood RC, Hedberg C, White K, et al. A multi-state outbreak of *Salmonella javiana* infections associated with raw tomatoes (Abstract). Proceedings of the 40th Annual Conference of the Epidemic Intelligence Service. Atlanta, GA: Centers for Disease Control and Prevention; 1991:69.
207. Cook KA, Swerdlow DL, Dobbs T, et al. Fresh squeezed *Salmonella*: An outbreak of *Salmonella hartford* associated with unpasteurized orange juice in Florida (Abstract). In: Program and Abstracts of the 36th Interscience Conference on Antimicrobial Agents and Chemotherapy. Washington, DC: American Society for Microbiology; 1996:258.
208. Mahon BE, Pönkä A, Hall WN, et al. An international outbreak of *Salmonella* infections caused by alfalfa sprouts grown from contaminated seeds. J Infect Dis. 1997;175:876–882.
209. Gill ON, Bartlett CLR, Sockett PN, et al. Outbreak of *Salmonella napoli* infection caused by contaminated chocolate bars. Lancet. 1983;1:574.
210. Killalea D, Ward LR, Roberts D, et al. An outbreak of *Salmonella agona* infection in England and the United States caused by contamination of a ready-to-eat savoury snack. BMJ. 1996;313:1105–1107.
211. Centers for Disease Control and Prevention. Hospital-associated outbreak of *Shigella dysenteriae* type 2: Maryland. MMWR Morb Mortal Wkly Rep. 1983;32:250.
212. Cook KA, Boyce T, Langkop C, et al. Scallions and shigellosis: A multistate outbreak traced to imported green onions (Abstract). Proceedings of the 44th Annual Conference of the Epidemic Intelligence Service. Atlanta, Ga: Centers for Disease Control and Prevention; 1995:36.
213. Frost JA, McEvoy MB, Bentley CA, et al. An outbreak of *Shigella sonnei* infection associated with consumption of iceberg lettuce. Emerg Infect Dis. 1995;1:6–9.
214. Barker WH Jr. *Vibrio parahaemolyticus* outbreaks in the United States. Lancet. 1974;1:551.
215. Centers for Disease Control and Prevention. Outbreak of *Vibrio parahaemolyticus* infections associated with eating raw oysters—Pacific Northwest, 1997. MMWR Morb Mortal Wkly Rep. 1998;47:457–462.
216. Mintz ED, Popovic T, Blake PA. Transmission of *Vibrio cholerae* O1. In: Wachsmuth IK, Blake PA, Olsvik O, eds. *Vibrio cholerae* and Cholera: Molecular to Global Perspectives. Washington, DC: American Society for Microbiology; 1994:345–356.
217. Blake PA. Endemic cholera in Australia and the United States. In: Wachsmuth IK, Blake PA, Olsvik O, eds. *Vibrio cholerae* and Cholera: Molecular to Global Perspectives. Washington, DC: American Society for Microbiology; 1994:309–320.
218. Finelli L, Swerdlow D, Mertz K, et al. Outbreak of cholera associated with crab brought from an area with epidemic disease. J Infect Dis. 1992;166:1433–1435.
219. Merson MH, Morris GH, Sack DA, et al. Travelers' diarrhea in Mexico. N Engl J Med. 1976;294:1299.
220. MacDonald KL, Eidson M, Strohmeyer C, et al. A multistate outbreak of gastrointestinal illness caused by enterotoxigenic *Escherichia coli* in imported semisoft cheese. J Infect Dis. 1985;151:716–20.
221. Dalton C, Mintz ED, Wells JG, et al. Outbreaks of enterotoxigenic *Escherichia coli* infection in American adults: A clinical and epidemiologic profile. Epidemiol Infect. 1999. In press.
222. MacDonald KL, Cohen ML, Blake PA. The changing epidemiology of adult botulism in the United States. Am J Epidemiol. 1986;124:794–799.
223. Spika JS, Shaffer N, Hargrett-Bean N. Risk factors for infant botulism in the United States. Am J Dis Child. 1989;143:828–832.
224. Linco SJ, Grohmann GS. The Darwin outbreak of oyster-associated viral gastroenteritis. Med J Aust. 1980;1:211.
225. Gunn RA, Janowski HT, Lieb S, et al. Norwalk virus gastroenteritis following raw oyster consumption. Am J Epidemiol. 1982;115:348.
226. Griffin MR, Surowiec JJ, McCloskey DI, et al. Foodborne Norwalk virus. Am J Epidemiol. 1982;115:178.
227. Kohn MA, Farley TA, Ando T, et al. An outbreak of Norwalk virus gastroenteritis associated with eating raw oysters. JAMA. 1995;273:466–471.

228. Reid JA, Caul EO, White OG, et al. Role of infected food handler in hotel outbreak of Norwalk-like viral gastroenteritis: Implications for control. Lancet. 1988;2:321–323.
229. Centers of Disease Control and Prevention. Update: Outbreaks of cyclosporiasis. MMWR Morb Mortal Wkly Rep. 1997;46:521–523.
230. Centers of Disease Control and Prevention. Outbreaks of cyclosporiasis—Northern Virginia/Washington, DC/Baltimore, Maryland Metropolitan Area, 1997. MMWR Morb Mortal Wkly Rep. 1997;46:689–691.
231. Hopper SH, Adams HS. Copper poisoning from vending machines. Public Health Rep. 1958;73:910.
232. Hesse IDW, Halstead BW, Peckham NH. Marine biotoxins. I. Ciguatera poison: Some biological and chemical aspects. Ann N Y Acad Sci. 1960;90:788–797.
233. Török TJ, Tauxe RV, Wise RP, et al. A large community outbreak of salmonellosis caused by intentional contamination of restaurant salad bars. JAMA. 1997;278:389–395.
234. Kolavic SA, Kimura A, Simons SL, et al. An outbreak of *Shigella dysenteriae* type 2 among laboratory workers due to intentional food contamination. JAMA. 1997;278:396–398.
235. Altekruse SF, Hyman FH, Klontz KC, et al. Foodborne bacterial infections in individuals with the human immunodeficiency virus. South Med J. 1994;87:169–173.
236. Angulo FJ, Swerdlow DL. Bacterial enteric infections in persons infected with human immunodeficiency virus. Clin Infect Dis. 1995;21(Suppl 1):S84–S93.
237. Shapiro RL, Altekruse S, Hutwagner L, et al. The role of Gulf Coast oysters harvested in warmer months in *Vibrio vulnificus* infections in the United States, 1988–1996. J Infect Dis. 1998;178:752–759.
238. Collins JC, Bicknell WJ. The red tide: A public-health emergency. N Engl J Med. 1974;288:1126.
239. Lawrence DN, Enriquez MB, Lumish RM, et al. Ciguatera fish poisoning in Miami. JAMA. 1980;244:254.
240. Morris JG Jr, Lewin P, Smith CW, et al. Ciguatera fish poisoning: Epidemiology of the disease on St. Thomas, U.S. Virgin Islands. Am J Trop Med Hyg. 1982;31:574.
241. Lew JF, LeBaron CW, Glass RI, et al. Recommendations for collection of laboratory specimens associated with outbreaks of gastroenteritis. MMWR Morb Mortal Wkly Rep. 1990;39(No.RR 14):1–13.
242. Jablonski LM, Bohach GA. *Staphylococcus aureus.* In: Doyle MP, Beuchat LR, Montville TJ, eds. Food Microbiology: Fundamentals and Frontiers. Washington, DC: ASM Press; 1997:353–375.
243. Ghosh AC. Prevalence of *Bacillus cereus* in the faeces of healthy adults. J Hyg (Lond). 1978;80:233.
244. De Buono BA, Brondum J, Kramer JM, et al. Plasmid, serotypic, and enterotoxin analysis of *Bacillus cereus* in an outbreak setting. J Clin Microbiol. 1988;26:1571–1574.
245. Notermans S, Beumer R, Rombouts F. Detecting foodborne pathogens and their toxins: Conventional versus rapid and automated methods. In: Doyle MP, Beuchat LR, Montville TJ, eds. Food Microbiology: Fundamentals and Frontiers. Washington, DC: ASM Press; 1997:697–710.
246. Hauschild AHW. Criteria and procedures for implicating *Clostridium perfringens* in food-borne outbreaks. Can J Public Health. 1975;66:388.
247. Stringer MF, Turnbull PCB, Gilbert RJ. Application of serological typing to the investigation of outbreaks of *Clostridium perfringens* food poisoning, 1970–1978. J Hyg (Lond). 1980;84:443.
248. Harmon SM, Kautter DA, Hatheway CL. Enumeration and characterization of *Clostridium perfringens* spores in the feces of food poisoning patients and normal controls. J Food Protection. 1986;49:23–28.
249. Watson GN, Stringer MF, Gilbert RJ, et al. The potential of bacteriocin typing in the study of *Clostridium perfringens* food poisoning. J Clin Pathol. 1982;35:1361.
250. Schiemann DA. Laboratory confirmation of an outbreak of *Clostridium perfringens* food poisoning. Health Lab Sci. 1977;14:35–38.
251. Harmon SM, Kautter DA. Evaluation of a reversed passive latex agglutination test kit for *Clostridium perfringens* enterotoxin. J Food Protection. 1986;49:523–525.
252. McClane BA, Strouse RJ. Rapid detection of *Clostridium perfringens* type A enterotoxin by enzyme-linked immunosorbent assay. J Clin Microbiol. 1984;19:112–115.
253. Birkhead G, Vogt RL, Heun EM, et al. Characterization of an outbreak of *Clostridium perfringens* food poisoning by quantitative fecal culture and fecal enterotoxin measurement. J Clin Microbiol. 1988;26:471–474.
254. Hatheway CL, Whaley DN, Dowell VR Jr. Epidemiological aspects of *Clostridium perfringens* foodborne illness. Food Technol. 1980;34:77.
255. Centers for Disease Control and Prevention. Multistate outbreak of *Salmonella* serotype Agona infections linked to toasted oats cereal—United States. MMWR Morb Mortal Wkly Rep. 1998;47:462–464.
256. Riley LW, Cohen ML. Plasmid profiles and *Salmonella* epidemiology. Lancet. 1982;1:573.
257. Rodriguez DC, Cameron DN, Puhr ND, et al. Comparison of plasmid profiles, phage types, and antimicrobial resistance patterns of *Salmonella enteritidis* isolates in the United States. J Clin Microbiol. 1992;30:854–857.
258. Wachsmuth IK, Evins GM, Fields PI, et al. The molecular epidemiology of cholera in Latin America. J Infect Dis. 1993;167:621–626.
259. March SB, Ratnam S. Latex agglutination test for detection of *Escherichia coli* serotype O157:H7. J Clin Microbiol. 1989;27:1675–1677.
260. Murray B, Mathewson J, Dupont H, et al. Utility of oligodeoxyribonucleotide probes for detecting enterotoxigenic *Escherichia coli.* J Infect Dis. 1987;155:809–811.
261. Guerrant RL, Brunton LL, Schnaitman TC, et al. Cyclic adenosine monophosphate and alteration of Chinese hamster ovary cell morphology: A rapid, sensitive in vitro assay for the enterotoxins of *Vibrio cholerae* and *Escherichia coli.* Infect Immun. 1974;10:320.
262. Svennerholm AM, Wiklund G. Rapid GM1-enzyme-linked immunosorbent assay with visual reading for identification of *Escherichia coli* heat-labile enterotoxin. J Clin Microbiol. 1983;17:596.
263. Honda T, Arita M, Takeda Y, et al. Further evaluation of the Biken test (modified Elek test) for detection of enterotoxigenic *Escherichia coli* producing heat-labile enterotoxin and application of the test to sampling of heat-stable enterotoxin. J Clin Microbiol. 1982;16:60.
264. Giannella RA. Suckling mouse model for detection of heat-stable *Escherichia coli* enterotoxin: Characteristics of the model. Infect Immun. 1976;14:95.
265. Venkatesen M, Buysse J, Vandendries E, et al. Development and testing of invasion-associated DNA probes for detection of *Shigella* spp and enteroinvasive *Escherichia coli.* J Clin Microbiol. 1988;26:261–266.
266. Sereny B. Experimental *Shigella* keratoconjunctivitis: A preliminary report. Acta Microbiol Hung. 1955;2:293.
267. Jerse A, Martin W, Galen J, et al. Oligonucleotide probe for the detection of enteropathogenic *Escherichia coli* (EPEC) adherence factor of localized adherent EPEC. J Clin Microbiol. 1990;28:2842–4.
268. Dowell VR Jr, McCroskey LM, Hatheway CL, et al. Coproexamination for botulinal toxin and *Clostridium botulinum.* JAMA. 1977;238:1829.
269. Mann JM, Hatheway CL, Gardiner TM. Laboratory diagnosis in a large outbreak of type A botulism. Am J Epidemiol. 1982;115:598.
270. Ando T, Monroe SS, Gentsch JR, et al. Detection and differentiation of antigenically distinct small round structured viruses (Norwalk-like viruses) by reverse transcription-PCR and Southern hybridization. J Clin Microbiol. 1995;33:64.
271. Gary GW Jr, Kaplan JE, Stine SE, et al. Detection of Norwalk virus antibodies and antigen with a biotin-avidin immunoassay. J Clin Microbiol. 1985;22:274–8.
272. Eberhard ML, Pieniazek NJ, Arrowood MJ. Laboratory diagnosis of *Cyclospora* infections. Arch Pathol Lab Med. 1997;121:792.
273. Garcia LS, Bruckner DA. Diagnostic medical parasitology. 3rd ed. Washington, DC: American Society for Microbiology; 1997:66–69.
274. Hokama Y, Abad MA, Kimura LH. A rapid enzyme-immunoassay for the detection of ciguatoxin in contaminated fish tissues. Toxicon. 1983;21:817–824.
275. Duggan C, Santosham M, Glass RI. The management of acute diarrhea in children: Oral rehydration maintenance and nutritional therapy. MMWR Morb Mortal Wkly Rep. 1992;41(RR-16):1.
276. Meyers KEC, Schulman SL, Kaplan BS. Principles of the treatment of Shiga toxin–associated hemolytic uremic syndrome: Pay meticulous attention to detail and do no harm. In: Kaper JB, O'Brien AD, eds. *Escherichia coli* O157:H7 and Other Shiga Toxin–Producing *E. coli* Strains. Washington, DC: American Society for Microbiology; 1998:364.
277. Wall PG, Ross D, Van Somern P, et al. Features of the epidemiology of multidrug resistant *Salmonella typhimurium* DT 104 in England and Wales. Proceedings of *Salmonella* and Salmonellosis '97. Ploufragan France, 1997:565–567.
278. Glynn MK, Bopp C, DeWitt W, et al. Emergence of multidrug-resistant *Salmonella enterica* serotype Typhimurium DT 104 infections in the United States. N Engl J Med. 1998;338:1333–1338.
279. Wall PG, Morgan D, Lamden K, et al. A case control study of infection with an epidemic strain of multiresistant *Salmonella typhimurium* DT 104 in England and Wales. Commun Dis Rep. 1994;4:R130–135.
280. Cohen ML, Tauxe RV. Drug-resistant *Salmonella* in the United States. An epidemiologic perspective. Science. 234:964–969, 1986;234:964–969.
281. Swift AEB, Swift TR. Ciguatera. Clin Toxicol. 1993;31:1–29.
282. Lange WR, Kreider SD, Hatwick M, et al. Potential benefit of tocainide in the treatment of ciguatera: Report of three cases. Am J Med. 1988;84:1087–1088.
283. Mitchel DH. *Amanita* mushroom poisoning. Ann Rev Med. 1980;31:51.
284. Centers for Disease Control and Prevention. Results of active surveillance with FoodNet, 1997. MMWR Morb Mortal Wkly Rep. 1998;47:782–785.
285. Osterholm MT, Potter ME. Irradiation pasteurization of solid foods: Taking food safety to the next level. Emerg Infect Dis. 1997;3:575–577.
286. Steele JH, Engel RE. Radiation processing of foods. J Am Vet Med Assoc. 1992;201:1522–1529.
287. Tauxe RV, Kruse H, Hedberg C, et al. Microbial hazards and emerging issues associated with produce; A preliminary report to the National Advisory Committee on Microbiologic Criteria for Foods. J Food Protect. 1997;60:1400–1408.
288. Hedberg CW, MacDonald KL, Osterholm MT. Changing epidemiology of foodborne disease: A Minnesota perspective. Clin Infect Dis. 1994;18:671–682.
289. Cruickshank JG, Humphrey TJ. The carrier food-handler and non-typhoid salmonellosis. Epidemiol Infect. 1987;98:223–230.
290. Jordan MC, Powell KE, Corothers TE, et al. Salmonellosis among restaurant patrons: The incisive role of a meat slicer. Am J Public Health. 1973;63:982.
291. Banatvala N, Magnano AR, Cartter ML, et al. Meat grinders and molecular epidemiology: Two supermarket outbreaks of *Escherichia coli* O157:H7 infections. J Infect Dis. 1996;173:480–483.
292. Potter ME, Kauffman AF, Blake PA, et al. Unpasteurized milk: The hazards of a health fetish. JAMA. 1984;252:2048–2052.
293. Tuttle J, Kellerman S, Tauxe RV. The risks of raw shellfish: What every transplant patient should know. J Transplant Coord. 1994;4:60–63.
294. Dupont HL. How safe is the food we eat? JAMA. 1992;268:3240.
295. Horwitz MA, Marr JS, Merson MH, et al. A continuing common-source outbreak of botulism in a family. Lancet. 1975;2:861.
296. Payne DJH, Scudamore JM. Outbreaks of salmonella food poisoning over a period of eight years from a common source. Lancet. 1977;1:1249.

297. Cieslak PR, Noble SJ, Maxson DJ, et al. Hamburger-associated *Escherichia coli* O157:H7 infection in Las Vegas: A hidden epidemic. Am J Public Health. 1997;87:176–180.
298. Mohle-Boetani JC, Stapleton M, Finger R, et al. Communitywide shigellosis: Control of an outbreak and risk factors in child day-care centers. Am J Public Health. 1995;85:812–816.
299. Swerdlow DL, Griffin PM. Duration of fecal shedding of *Escherichia coli* O157:H7 among children in day-care centres (Commentary). Lancet. 1997;349:745–746.

Chapter 88

Tropical Sprue/Enteropathy

CHRISTINE A. WANKE
RICHARD L. GUERRANT

Tropical sprue, also called *postinfectious tropical malabsorption,* is a syndrome of enigmatic origin that is characterized by a prolonged diarrheal illness and malabsorption of two or more substances in persons in the tropics who have no other obvious reason for malabsorption. Tropical sprue has been recognized since the second or third century AD, when Aretaeus of Cappadocchia reported on "The Coeliac Affection." The first mention of sprue in the modern medical literature was in 1747, when Dr. William Hillary emigrated from England to Barbados and published his observations on a prolonged tropical diarrheal disease in native islanders. The English term *sprue* is an adaptation from the Dutch *sprouw,* which was originally used to refer to persistent diarrheal disease in Holland (probably celiac disease). The term *sprue* was first used in 1880 by Manson for the persistent wasting diarrhea that occurred in tropical countries.[1] Knowledge about the cause or pathogenesis of sprue did not advance significantly until investigations were begun after recognized outbreaks during World War II. The distinction between celiac sprue and tropical sprue was not truly clear until the early 1970s.

EPIDEMIOLOGY

Although sprue is considered a disease of tropical locales, there are distinct geographic areas of risk within the tropics. Tropical sprue has been most readily identified in Asia and the Caribbean islands, and there are isolated areas of particular risk within both hemispheres. Sprue is relatively common among the indigenous populations of Puerto Rico, Haiti, the Dominican Republic, and Cuba, but it is not seen in the rest of the Caribbean islands and is no longer recognized in Barbados.[2, 3] It is seen in northern South America, in Venezuela and Colombia, but rarely in Central America or Mexico. It is common on the Indian subcontinent, from the Himalayas to the south and it has been recognized in Mayanmar and the Philippines.[4–6] Little tropical sprue was documented in Africa until the 1970s; cases have been recognized in Rhodesia and South Africa, and tropical sprue has developed among expatriates living in Nigeria.[7] There may be endemic foci of tropical sprue in the Middle East as well, with a spruelike illness recognized in Turkey.

Unlike other endemic diarrheal illnesses in the tropical world, tropical sprue is a disease mainly of adults. Children are thought to be relatively spared, although clearly disease has been documented in all age groups. Very young children have not been found to have tropical sprue; this may represent a beneficial effect of breast-feeding. In studies of family outbreaks of tropical sprue in South India, even older children developed disease at a significantly lower rate than adults.[8] The reason for this is not clear. Certainly persistent diarrhea develops in children more commonly in parts of the world where the environment is contaminated more heavily with potentially disease-causing microorganisms.[9] Tropical sprue may be one of the causes of prolonged diarrhea and wasting in this age group as well, but etiologic studies such as small bowel intubation and cultures or biopsy have shown conflicting results regarding the correlation of small bowel colonization with persistent diarrhea.[10, 11, 12]

Some patterns of disease expression are of particular interest in tropical sprue. There are clear epidemics of the disease, which have been best documented in families and villages in South India.[8] There have been descriptions of sprue houses, in which successive tenants have developed disease, and an outbreak was described in which more than half of the exposed persons in an isolated extended family developed tropical sprue within 3 months of onset of disease in the index case. Well-documented outbreaks of sprue affecting entire villages have also been reported, mostly from the Indian subcontinent. Such an epidemic pattern suggests an underlying infectious cause.

There has been a seasonal variation in outbreaks of tropical sprue as well. An increased rate of mild tropical sprue in the setting of an increased rate of diarrheal disease was seen more often from March to July than at other times of the year for at least 4 years at an American military base in the Philippines.[6] In these outbreaks, sprue occurred among American military personnel and their dependents, who were eating a well-balanced, Western-style diet. A seasonal variation has also been documented in the rate of occurrence of tropical sprue in the indigenous population of Puerto Rico.[3] Such a seasonal variation also lends credence to the possibility of an underlying infectious cause.

As suggested by the outbreaks among American military personnel, tropical sprue occurs among expatriates living in endemic areas.[13] Tropical sprue was originally recognized among expatriates and British colonists in India in the early 19th century and subsequently among the Dutch in Java, the French in Indochina, and Americans in the Philippines, Vietnam, and Puerto Rico. Tropical sprue or malabsorption with jejunitis ("tropical enteropathy") has been described among Peace Corps volunteers and has occurred sporadically among travelers.[14] Generally tropical sprue develops in an expatriate who has lived for a prolonged time, 6 months to 1 year, in an endemic area. Rare cases also have been described among short-term travelers.[15] Tropical sprue is also recognized among immigrants who leave endemic areas, although they may not complain of gastrointestinal symptoms until they have been out of the endemic area for a prolonged period.[16, 17] These exposure data also suggest an infectious origin for tropical sprue.

ETIOLOGY

There is a strong presumption that tropical sprue is caused by an enteric infection, perhaps with a component of nutritional deficiency. The facts lending support to this theory include the following: (1) often the prolonged episode of tropical sprue is initiated by an episode of acute diarrheal disease; (2) there is an epidemic and seasonal nature to the epidemiology of the disease, as discussed previously; and (3) the disease responds most often to treatment with antibiotics with or without nutritional supplements. The precise nature of the infection that leads to development of tropical sprue is less clear.

Multiple studies in Asia and the Caribbean have demonstrated small bowel bacterial overgrowth in patients with tropical sprue.[14, 18, 19] Although some bacteria normally live in the upper small bowel of healthy persons, the organisms isolated from this region of the gut in healthy asymptomatic individuals are most often gram-positive. Streptococci, staphylococci, and lactobacilli are among the common isolates, and these are present in small numbers. In the distal small bowel, the cecum, and the colon, anaerobes and facultative gram-negative organisms predominate in normal persons. Small bowel cultures from travelers with tropical sprue demonstrate increased numbers of gram-negative rods, including *Alcaligenes, Enterobacter aerogenes*, and *Hafnia* spp. In small bowel cultures from persons with tropical sprue who were native to India, Haiti, or Puerto Rico, *Klebsiella, Escherichia coli*, and *Enterobacter cloacae* were the most common organisms. However, carefully done studies in South Africa and India documented similar organisms in similar concentrations in the small bowel of asymptomatic control patients and in patients with tropical sprue, suggesting that environmental contamination may predispose to increased small bowel flora.[14, 18, 19] In another series of patients from India, the numbers of organisms found in the small bowel of tropical sprue patients was the same as that found in the small bowel of healthy controls, but the type of organisms isolated varied.[18] Other organisms, especially *Enterobacter* and *Veillonella*, were isolated more frequently from the small bowel of patients with tropical sprue than from healthy controls.[20]

Gram-negative organisms isolated from the small bowel of tropical sprue patients in Haiti were found to have a secretory effect, presumably by toxin production, in rabbit ileal loops and rat perfusion studies.[21, 22] These supposedly enterotoxigenic organisms have not been studied for the presence of any of the recognized secretory toxins by currently available methodology such as DNA probes or enzyme-linked immunosorbent assay; nor have these organisms been studied for the presence of colonizing factors, such as pili or the hydrophobic surface proteins that are found in many enteric pathogens. *E. coli* and *Klebsiella* isolated from Indian patients with tropical sprue were not found to produce heat-stable or heat-labile enterotoxins when they were tested.[23] Other in vivo data have suggested that small bowel overgrowth by colonizing nontoxigenic *E. coli* can produce a secretory diarrheal syndrome if the level of colonization reaches a high enough concentration within the small bowel.[24, 25]

More recent data further suggest that enteroaggregative *E. coli* are associated with malnutrition, with or without persistent diarrhea, and with intestinal inflammation and cytokine production.[26–30] In addition to its association with persistent diarrhea among children in tropical developing areas, enteroaggregative *E. coli* in patients with the acquired immunodeficiency syndrome (AIDS) is associated with persistent diarrhea that improves with antimicrobial therapy.[31, 32]

The presence of bacteria in the small bowel may potentiate the symptoms caused by the small bowel parasite *Giardia lamblia*, and the interaction of small bowel bacteria and parasites has been considered as a possible cause of tropical sprue.[33] Infection with hookworm or *Strongyloides stercoralis* has also been discussed as a possible cause for tropical sprue. Reports of tropical sprue occurring in the setting of the presence of orthomyxovirus or coronavirus particles in the stool have also appeared in the literature. Cases of tropical sprue have been reported after an intestinal infection with either fungus or the blue-green algae *Prototheca*,[34, 35] but the traditional definition of tropical sprue would exclude those patients with diarrhea on the basis of recognized pathogens.

That small bowel overgrowth, as it occurs spontaneously in a certain segment of the population in the less developed countries or after an acute enteric infection, may precipitate a series of intestinal insults that proceed to full-blown tropical sprue in susceptible persons is at present the most likely etiologic explanation for tropical sprue. The predisposition for progression from intestinal insult to tropical sprue is less easy to explain. Malnutrition may be a predisposing factor, but it is neither necessary nor sufficient, as demonstrated by the occurrence of tropical sprue among well-nourished military personnel and their dependents. Small bowel overgrowth may alter intestinal transit time and promote further overgrowth and intestinal stasis, but it cannot explain the initial colonization that induces the episode.

In vitro data suggest that small bowel colonization by *E. coli* may be increased by low levels of cytokines, as might be expected in chronic parasitic infections in the developing world.[36] As noted previously, certain organisms such as enteroaggregative *E. coli* can alter the intestinal environment by the induction of intestinal proinflammatory cytokines and intestinal inflammation.[26] Furthermore, some have suggested that human immunodeficiency virus (HIV) infection may be associated with increased colonization by gram-negative bacilli.[36a] There has been no genetic predisposition noted for tropical sprue as there has been for celiac sprue.

The processes that control the normal colonization of the small bowel are not well understood; therefore, the forces that may disrupt these normal processes to permit abnormal colonization are even less well understood. However, some of the factors that can affect the normal small bowel colonization process include gastric acidity, which controls the entry of viable organisms into the small bowel, and intestinal mucin glycoprotein, which contains receptors for and specifically binds a variety of bacteria within the small bowel lumen.[37] *Helicobacter pylori*, for example, may impair gastric acidity and thereby predispose to small bowel colonization or persistent diarrhea.[38, 39]

Bacterial binding to mucin is presumed to promote clearance of pathogenic organisms to protect the small bowel, but it may promote colonization by nonpathogenic organisms or promote small bowel colonization by pathogens when the mucin is damaged by malnutrition, an inflammatory process, or bacterial proteases or mucinases. Some loss of the protective mucin layer in tropical sprue is suggested by evidence that the bacteria visualized are often tightly associated within the mucosa rather than being free within the lumen of the gut.[1] Damage to the protective mucin layer may also permit epithelial cell damage by food or other small bowel antigens. The presence of free bile acids within the upper small bowel can alter intestinal bacterial growth rates and colonization, but bile acid concentrations have not been abnormal in patients with tropical sprue, and the bacterial organisms that have been cultured from patients with tropical sprue are not those that classically alter bile salt metabolism.[23]

Intestinal immunologic dysfunction has been suggested as a factor that might predispose to abnormal bacterial colonization in tropical sprue. Patients with deficiencies of secretory immunoglobulin A (IgA) are subject to more frequent and severe bouts of enteric infections. In addition to secretory IgA, lymphoid tissue is present throughout the small bowel focally in Peyer's patches and diffusely as mucosal lymphocytes. When small bowel lymphocytes were characterized in patients with tropical sprue and in control patients with irritable bowel syndrome in southern India, there was no difference in the number of IgA-, IgG-, or IgM-producing lymphocytes between the two groups.[40, 41] Patients with sprue had increased numbers of lymphocytes in the crypt epithelium, with a higher percentage of immunoblasts and a higher mitotic index.[42] These data can be interpreted as evidence that lymphoid activation does occur in tropical sprue but that it is probably secondary to whatever primary process institutes the disease rather than being an inciting process itself.

It has also been postulated that dietary fat might play a role in tropical sprue. Similar to the permissive effect of protein ingestion in the pathogenesis of pig bel, the intake of long-chain fatty acids has been studied as a potential etiologic factor for tropical sprue.[43] The seasonal epidemic occurrence of tropical sprue in Puerto Rico immediately follows a traditional holiday feast of pork, which is rich in long-chain fatty acids.[44] There are several mechanisms by which these long-chain fatty acids might contribute to the production of clinical tropical sprue. Long-chain fatty acids can alter intestinal motility and delay intestinal transit time. Plasma levels of enteroglucagon and motilin are significantly increased in patients with tropical sprue; motilin slows gastric emptying, and enteroglucagon slows intestinal transit.[45] Intubation studies have demonstrated that intestinal infusions of fat increase plasma enteroglucagon levels and decrease intestinal motor activity. Fat within the gut lumen also inhibits both the mucosal sodium-potassium fluxes and the magnesium adenosine triphosphatases, which can contribute to malabsorption of water and electrolytes in the intestine and raise the pH of the mucosal microenvironment.[43, 46] The elevated mucosal pH produced by intestinal fats has also been associated with increased growth of gram-negative bacteria in the lumen of the small bowel.[15, 47]

The elevation of mucosal pH and the presence of fatty acids within the lumen of the gut may also impair the ability of the intestine to absorb folate; folate deficiency may then potentiate the intestinal dysfunction that precedes it.[48] Folate deficiency leads to a decreased number of gut epithelial cells, as assessed by DNA concentrations, and to villus atrophy. Additional structural alterations are seen in the intestine with folate deficiency; these include crypt hypertrophy, villus blunting, and megaloblastic changes in the epithelial cells. These changes are somewhat nonspecific and are similar to those seen with vitamin B_{12} deficiency or with tropical sprue. Functionally, the folate-deficient gut is less efficient in absorbing water, electrolytes, and carbohydrates than the normal small bowel.[49] It is likely that whatever the initial insult to the gut may be in tropical sprue, the resulting folate malabsorption and deficiency contribute to the further pathogenesis of disease (Fig. 88–1).

CLINICAL MANIFESTATIONS

The classic clinical features of tropical sprue are nonspecific and simply reflect the symptoms of malabsorption. These symptoms include prolonged diarrhea, abdominal cramping, and anorexia, with or without nausea and secondary weight loss. Other associated but less common symptoms, also related to the malabsorption of nutrients and subsequent malnutrition, include peripheral edema, glossitis, stomatitis, and dermatitis.[15, 16] Fever may occur at the onset of diarrhea (especially in Asia); although the presence of fever has been suggested as a means to distinguish Caribbean from Asian sprue, this distinction has not consistently been observed. Fever rarely persists for the course of disease, which may span months to years. Signs and symptoms related to anemia may also occur; pallor and weakness are most common early in disease. Later in the course of tropical sprue, peripheral neuropathy, confusion, and, if the anemia is severe enough, congestive symptoms reflecting high-output failure may occur.

Many patients can pinpoint the onset of disease; tropical sprue rarely has an insidious onset and is far more often associated with an obvious acute episode of diarrhea that then becomes prolonged. Persons with tropical sprue may recall other people with similar acute illnesses or being exposed to someone with an acute illness just before getting sick themselves. Because the operative definition of tropical sprue implies that the function of the gut was normal before the development of the disease, ideally the alteration of bowel habits from a normal pattern by the inciting episode of acute diarrheal disease should be notable. In practice, especially in the developing world, the distinction between normal and abnormal bowel habits may not be so clear.

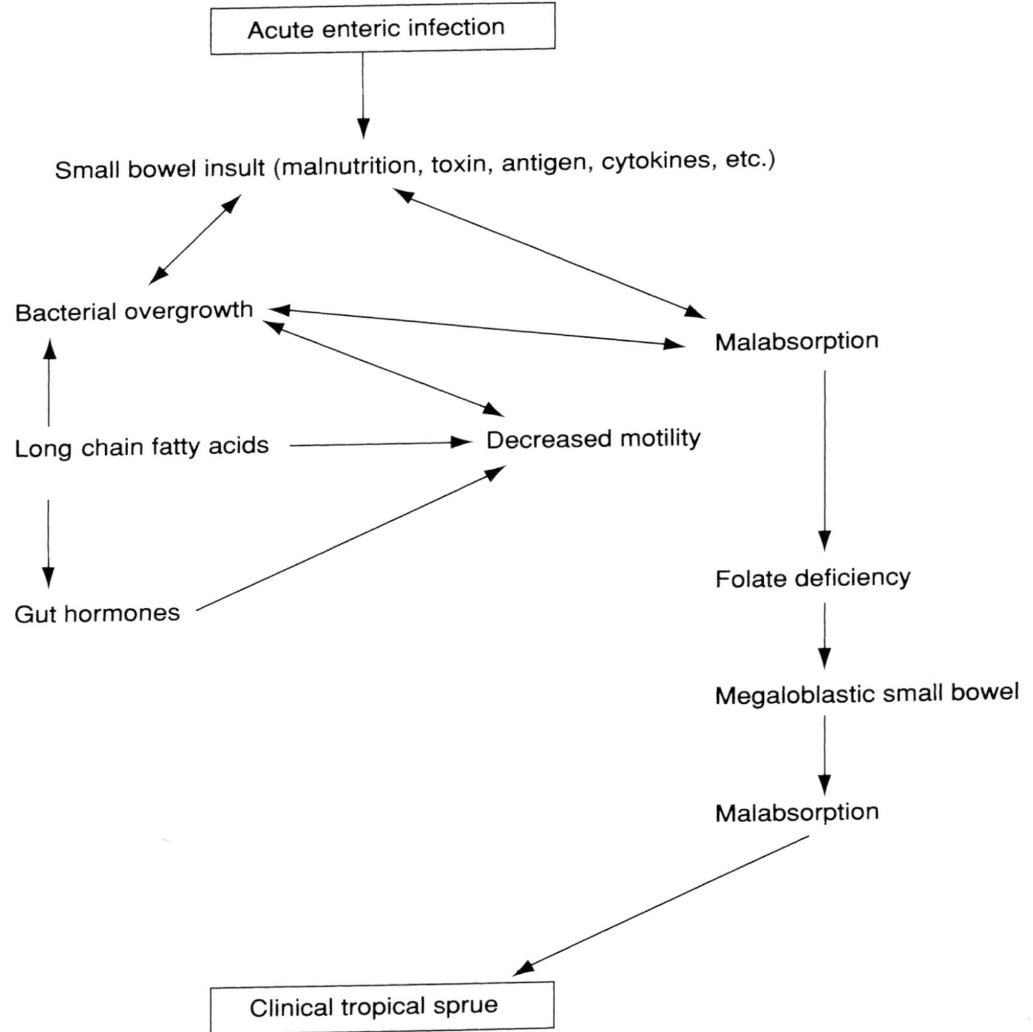

FIGURE 88–1. Proposed pathogenesis of tropical sprue. The complex vicious cycle of small bowel insult that results in bacterial overgrowth and malabsorption and further small bowel damage by luminal long-chain fatty acids and dysregulation of intestinal hormones may promote disease in susceptible persons after an acute enteric infection.

Patients describe crampy abdominal pain, multiple soft or loose stools daily often with mucus, and the exacerbation of symptoms with food consumption. Patients may also complain of nausea and bloating that lead to decreased appetite and decreased oral intake. The precise presentation of a patient with tropical sprue depends on the duration of illness and the extent of malabsorption.

Malabsorption of specific nutrients may lead to other symptoms and syndromes.[50] Lactose intolerance often develops early in the course of tropical sprue. The anemia of tropical sprue is most often macrocytic and related to vitamin B_{12} and folate malabsorption. Iron deficiency may also occur, again related to malabsorption, and may turn a macrocytic anemia into a normocytic anemia. Impaired absorption of calcium, vitamin D, and magnesium may occur, with resulting osteopenia.[51] Patients with tropical sprue also malabsorb fats and, depending on the severity of fat malabsorption, may complain of bulky, floating, or foul-smelling stools.

Spontaneous recovery may occur, but this is not inevitable. Spontaneous recovery is more common in travelers to areas endemic for tropical sprue who return to their native environments. Persons who have emigrated from endemic areas and those living in endemic areas often require medical therapy to alleviate symptoms. Because the clinical manifestations of tropical sprue are nonspecific, symptomatic response to specific therapy can be considered additional evidence that the patient had tropical sprue.

INTESTINAL ABNORMALITIES

Although the secretory and malabsorptive syndrome seen in tropical sprue suggests preferential damage to the small bowel, which has greater nutrient absorptive capabilities and a greater secretory capacity than the colon, functional abnormalities are seen in both the small and the large bowel in tropical sprue. Functional changes in the small bowel mirror the morphologic changes seen and are most prominent in the ileum and jejunum. In tropical sprue, the jejunum is in a net secretory state, with active secretion of water, sodium, and chloride[52]; however, glucose-linked absorption remains intact, as it does for many other secretory infectious diarrheal syndromes.[53] In tropical sprue, the ileum malabsorbs bile acids and vitamin B_{12}. Bile acid malabsorption leads to fat malabsorption and malabsorption of the fat-soluble vitamins D, A, K, and E. Brush-border enzymes are decreased functionally and are less efficient in digesting and absorbing disaccharides such as lactose.[54, 55] Xylose, glucose, and folate malabsorption occur, as does malabsorption of minerals such as calcium and magnesium. Amino acid malabsorption occurs; protein metabolism is further complicated by loss of albumin in the lumen of the damaged small bowel.[56]

Most of the functional changes in tropical sprue may be related to small bowel mucosal damage represented by the morphologic changes seen, but the hormonal regulation of the gut is dysfunctional in this disease as well.[57] Postprandial insulin and gastric inhibitory peptide are reduced in tropical sprue; enteroglucagon and motilin levels are increased. In chronic tropical sprue, gastric acid secretion and secretion of intrinsic factor may also be affected. Transit time through the small bowel is slowed, as measured by breath hydrogen testing.[58, 59]

The colon normally serves as a storage and absorptive organ, absorbing 4 to 7 liters of water and 100 to 160 mmol of carbohydrates per day. In the few studies of colonic function in tropical sprue that have been done, the ability of the colon to absorb water is decreased in patients compared with controls. There is speculation that the dysfunction of colonic cells may be related to damage by excess fatty acids in the gut lumen or bacterial toxins or infection. Although there is physiologic confirmation of the ability of fatty acids to disturb the absorptive function of colonocytes and small bowel enterocytes, data suggesting that colonic infections are of importance in the pathogenesis of tropical sprue are lacking.

MORPHOLOGY

Partial villus atrophy is the hallmark histologic change seen in the small bowel in tropical sprue, as opposed to the flattened mucosa that is characteristic of coeliac sprue.[60] The villi in tropical sprue progressively shorten and thicken, forming fused leaves after about 4 months of illness. These histologic changes are seen in the jejunum and the ileum, where the changes in absorption also are localized. These histologic changes are not specific for tropical sprue but may be present in severe folate deficiency or with bacterial overgrowth.

Microscopically, the mucosa is thin, with an infiltrate of chronic inflammatory cells consisting of plasma cells, histiocytes, lymphocytes, and eosinophils. As mentioned previously, these lymphocytes have been characterized, and IgA, IgG, and IgM lymphocytes are present in numbers equal to those of asymptomatic control patients.[40, 41] An increased mitotic index can be seen in the crypt cells; the nuclei of the crypt cells may also appear megaloblastic.[56, 61] An increased number of goblet cells may be present, and lipoid vacules have been seen within the basement membrane. To date, there is no convincing evidence that tropical sprue is an immunologically mediated disease.

DIAGNOSIS

Because the symptom complex of tropical sprue is nonspecific, the travel and exposure history of the patient is of prime importance in making the diagnosis. Tropical sprue should certainly be considered in a patient who presents with chronic diarrhea, weight loss, and evidence of malabsorption. Attempts should be made to elicit the onset of the diarrheal illness, its duration, the degree of weight loss, the frequency and character of the stool, and any other systemic complaints such as prolonged fever, jaundice, or itching that might suggest alternative explanations for the diarrheal illness. Information regarding travel to, residence in, or immigration from the tropics should be requested; although there are sporadic case reports of mild sprue-like illnesses occurring after diarrheal illnesses in temperate climates, this so-called temperate sprue is rare, and a history of exposure to an endemic area should be present to entertain the diagnosis of tropical sprue.[44]

Pertinent medical history should also be obtained, with particular emphasis on any surgical procedures that may have altered the anatomy of the bowel, predisposing to a blind loop syndrome, or any medications that may predispose to small bowel overgrowth. Social history, in addition to travel and exposures, should include questions relating to possible HIV exposures, because HIV infection is a major risk factor for the development of chronic diarrhea.[62] History pertaining to symptoms of specific nutrient deficiencies, such as night blindness secondary to malabsorption of vitamin A, would be expected only in very prolonged disease.

There are no diagnostic physical findings for tropical sprue. The physical examination should document presence or absence of fever, volume status by any orthostatic changes, body weight, evidence of weight loss such as temporal wasting, and presence or absence of significant lymphadenopathy or abdominal masses. Hyperactive bowel sounds may be the only pertinent abdominal finding. Signs of anemia, such as pallor, are notoriously nonspecific but can be looked for. Signs of specific nutrient deficiencies may also be present on physical examination: cheilosis, stomatitis, glossitis, rashes, dermatitis, koilonychia, muscle pain or weakness, peripheral neuropathy, or edema can suggest deficiencies of iron, zinc, vitamin B_{12}, folate, vitamins D and E, or protein. Deficiencies of any of these nutrients could be present in tropical sprue because of malabsorption by the damaged small bowel.

Laboratory evaluation of the patient with suspected tropical sprue can be minimal or extensive, depending on the degree of suspicion and the urgency for diagnosis. A simple complete blood count demonstrating a macrocytic anemia in a high-risk patient in the appropriate clinical setting could be sufficient to proceed with other, more confirmatory diagnostic tests such as a small bowel biopsy. A more complete laboratory evaluation would include serum vitamin B_{12} level and red blood cell folate levels, serum carotene concentration, or, preferably, a 72-hour fecal fat determination. Stool examination to exclude *Giardia* is very useful; stool culture looking for bacterial pathogens is less likely to be helpful in chronic diarrhea.

Ultimately, a small bowel series with small bowel follow-through showing flattened mucosal folds, luminal dilatation, or flocculation of the barium meal can be suggestive of tropical sprue.[62] An upper endoscopy with duodenal aspirate for parasites, biopsy, and quantitative small bowel culture, if available, can be diagnostic of tropical sprue in the appropriate clinical setting. Documentation of abnormal transit time by small bowel follow-through or breath hydrogen testing, which can also imply bacterial overgrowth, is suggestive but not diagnostic of tropical sprue. The differential diagnosis that must be considered in a patient with chronic diarrhea, weight loss, and malabsorption, even in a clinical setting consistent with tropical sprue, should include giardiasis, cryptosporidiosis, coccidiosis *(Isosospora belli)*, capillariasis, strongyloidiasis coeliac sprue (gluten enteropathy), lymphoma, intestinal tuberculosis, the blind loop syndrome, pancreatic tumors, Whipple's disease, and microsporidia associated HIV enteropathy.

TREATMENT

Treatment with folate alone improves the symptoms of tropical sprue but does not cure the diarrhea. Combination therapy with tetracycline and folate seems to be most effective in symptom resolution and cure of diarrhea with promotion of weight gain.[63, 64] Treatment with 250 mg of tetracycline four times daily and 5 mg of folate daily for 1 month has been effective for travelers with tropical sprue, but therapy must be prolonged for 6 months or longer for residents of the tropics who have had long-term disease. Even with prolonged therapy, relapses have been seen in this population, although these may have been caused by reexposure to an infecting organism and represent recurrent rather than relapsing disease.[65] Reports have suggested that tropical sprue in the Caribbean is more amenable to therapy than sprue in India, but these studies are difficult to compare.[62] Poorly absorbed sulfa drugs are an acceptable alternative to tetracycline in children or pregnant women.[66] A favorable symptomatic response to therapy with folate and antibiotics can provide additional evidence that tropical sprue was the cause of chronic diarrhea and malabsorption in a patient; however, even this is not specific, because bacterial overgrowth in a blind loop syndrome would also be expected to respond.

REFERENCES

1. Bartholomew C. William Hillary and sprue in the Caribbean: 230 years later. Gut Festschr. 1989;30:17–21.
2. Klipstein FA, Samloff IM, Smarth G, et al. Treatment of overt and subclinical malabsorption in Haiti. Gut. 1969;10:315–322.
3. Klipstein FA, Corcino JJ. Seasonal occurrence of overt and subclinical tropical malabsorption in Puerto Rico. Am J Trop Med Hyg. 1974;23:1189–1196.
4. Gorbach SL, Banwell JG, Jacobs B, et al. Tropical sprue and malnutrition in West Bengal. Am J Clin Nutr. 1970;23:1515–1558.
5. Mathan VI, Baker SJ. Epidemic tropical sprue and other epidemics of diarrhea in South Indian villages. Am J Clin Nutr. 1968;21:1077–1087.
6. Jones TC, Dean AG, Parker GW. Seasonal gastroenteritis and malabsorption at an American military base in the Philippines. Am J Epidemiol. 1973;95:128–139.
7. Thomas G, Clain DJ, Wicks CB. Tropical enteropathy in Rhodesia. Gut. 1976;17:888–894.
8. Mathan VI, Ignatius M, Baker SJ. A household epidemic of tropical sprue. Gut. 1966;7:490.
9. Schorling JB, Wanke CA, Schorling SK, et al. A prospective study of persistent diarrhea among children in an urban Brazilian slum. Am J Epidemiol. 1990;132:144–156.
10. Wanke CA, Guerrant RL. Pathogenesis of persistent diarrhea. In: Guerrant RL, de Souza MA, Nations MK, eds. At the Edge of Development: Health Crises in a Transitional Society, 1st ed. Durham, NC: Carolina Academic Press; 1996:177–201.
11. Lima AA, Fang G, Schorling JB, et al. Persistent diarrhea in northeast Brazil: Etiologies and interactions with malnutrition. Acta Paediatr Scand Suppl. 1992;381:39–44.
12. Penny ME, Scotland SM, Smith HR, et al. Virulence properties of Enterobacteriaceae isolated from the small intestine of children with diarrhea. Pediatr Infect Dis J. 1992;11:623–630.
13. Klipstein FA. Tropical sprue in travelers and expatriates living abroad. Gastroenterology. 1981;80:590.
14. Lindenbaum J, Kent TH, Sprine H. Malabsorption and jejunitis in American Peace Corps volunteers in Pakistan. Ann Intern Med. 1966;65:1201.
15. Davis JS, Klipstein FA. Tropical sprue in visitor to Mexico. Lancet. 1985;1:454.
16. Klipstein FA, Falaiye JM. Tropical sprue in expatriates from the tropics living in the continental United States. Medicine (Baltimore). 1969;48:475.
17. Montgomery RD, Beale DJ, Sammons HG, et al. Postinfective malabsorption: A sprue syndrome. BMJ. 1973;2:265–268.
18. Appelbaum PC, Moshal MG, Hift W, et al. Intestinal bacteria in patients with tropical sprue. S Afr Med J. 1980;57:1081.
19. Bhat P, Shantakumari S, Rajan D, et al. Bacterial flora of the gastrointestinal tract in southern Indian control subjects and patients with tropical sprue. Gastroenterology. 1972;62:11.
20. Tomkins AM, Drasbar BS, James WPT. Bacterial colonisation of jejunal mucosa in acute tropical sprue. Lancet. 1975;1:59.
21. Klipstein FA, Engert RF, Short HB. Enterotoxigenicity of colonising coliform bacteria in tropical sprue and blind-loop syndrome. Lancet. 1978;342.
22. Klipstein FA, Holdeman LV, Corcino JJ. Enterotoxigenic intestinal bacteria in tropical sprue. Ann Intern Med. 1973;79:632–641.
23. Ramakrishna BS, Mathan VI. Role of bacterial toxins, bile acids, and free fatty acids in colonic water malabsorption in tropical sprue. Dig Dis Sci. 1987;32:500–505.
24. Wanke CA, Guerrant RL. Small-bowel colonization alone is a cause of diarrhea. Infect Immun. 1987;55:1924–1926.
25. Schlager TA, Wanke CA, Guerrant RL. Net fluid secretion and impaired villous function induced by colonization of the small intestine by non-toxigenic, colonizing *E. coli*. Infect Immun. 1990;58:1337–1343.
26. Steiner TS, Lima AM, Nataro JP, et al. Enteroaggregative *Escherichia coli* produce intestinal inflammation and growth impairment and cause interleukin-8 release from intestinal epithelial cells. J Infect Dis. 1998;177:88–96.
27. Nataro JP, Steiner TS, Guerrant RL. Enteroaggregative *Escherichia coli* (EAEC): An emerging cause of diarrhea and malnutrition. Emerg Infect Dis. 1998;4:251–261.
28. Bhan MK, Raj P, Levine MM, et al. Enteroaggregative *Escherichia coli* associated with persistent diarrhea in a cohort of rural children in India. J Infect Dis. 1989;159:1061–1064.
29. Cravioto A, Tello A, Navarro A, et al. Association of *Escherichia coli* HEp-2 adherence patterns with type and duration of diarrhoea. Lancet. 1991;337:262–264.
30. Wanke CA, Schorling JB, Barrett LJ, et al. Potential role of adherence traits of *Escherichia coli* in persistent diarrhea in an urban Brazilian slum. Pediatr Infect Dis J. 1991;10:746–751.
31. Wanke CA, Mayer H, Weber R, et al. Enteroaggregative *Escherichia coli* as a potential cause of diarrheal disease in adults infected with human immunodeficiency virus. J Infect Dis. 1998;178:185–190.
32. Wanke CA, Gerrior J, Blais V, et al. Successful treatment of diarrheal disease associated with enteroaggregative *E. coli* in adults infected with human immunodeficiency virus. J Infect Dis. 1998;178:1369–1372.
33. Tomkins AM, Wright SG, Drasbar BS, et al. Bacterial colonization of jejunal mucosa in giardiasis. Trans R Soc Trop Med Hyg. 1978;72:33.
34. Klipstein FA, Schneider R. Prototheca and sprue. Gastroenterology. 1975;69:1372.
35. Swanson VL, Haley LD, Wheby MS. Mycological study of jejunal biopsy specimens from patients with tropical sprue. Am J Trop Med Hyg. 1965;14:1066.
36. Wanke CA, Cronan S, Bistrian B. Recombinant tumor necrosis factor and recombinant murine IL-1 alter binding of *Escherichia coli* to intestinal mucin and the HT29 intestinal cell line. Nutrition. 1997;13:959–964.
36a. Arrington RG, Thielman NM, Guerrant RL. Bacterial colonization susceptibility of buccal epithelial cells in HIV-seropositive patients [Abstract]. Student National Medical Association, 32nd Annual Medical Education Conference, New Orleans, LA, March 27–30, 1997.
37. Wanke CA, Cronan S, Goss C, et al. Characterization of binding of *Escherichia coli* strains which are enteropathogens to small-bowel mucin. Infect Immun. 1990;58:794–800.
38. Graham D, Alpert L, Smith J, et al. Iatrogenic *Campylobacter pylori* infection is a cause of epidemic achlorhydria. Am J Gastroenterol. 1988;83:974.
39. Nurko SS, García-Aranda JA, Consuelo A, et al. Is *Helicobacter pylori* a significant risk factor for persistent diarrhea in Mexican children? Gastroenterology. 1993;104:A160.
40. Malik AK, Mehta SK, Chandrashekhar Y, et al. Quantitation of immunoglobin-containing cells in the jejunal lamina propria in tropical sprue. J Clin Gasterol. 1992;14:163–166.
41. Marsh MN. Functional and structural aspects of the epithelial lymphocyte, with implications for coeliac disease and tropical sprue. Scand J Gastroenterol. 1985;115:55–75.
42. Marsh MN, Mathan M, Mathan VI. Studies of intestinal lymphoid tissue: VII. The secondary nature of lymphoid cell "activation" in the jejunal lesion of tropical sprue. Am J Pathol. 1983;112:302–312.
43. Tiruppathi C, Balasubramanian KA, Hill PG, et al. Faecal free fatty acids in tropical sprue and their possible role in the production of diarrhoea by inhibition of ATPases. Gut. 1983;24:300–305.
44. Glynn J. Tropical sprue: Its aetiology and pathogenesis. J R Soc Med. 1986;79:599.

45. Cook GC. Aetiology and pathogenesis of postinfective tropical malabsorption (tropical sprue). Lancet. 1984;1:721.
46. Ramakrishna BS, Mathan VI. Absorption of water and sodium and activity of adenosine triphosphatases in the rectal mucosa in tropical sprue. Gut. 1988;29:665–668.
47. Lucas ML, Mathan VI. Jejunal surface pH measurements in tropical sprue. Trans R Soc Trop Med Hyg. 1989;83:138–142.
48. Kesavan V, Noronha JM. An ATPase dependent, radio sensitive, acidic microclimate essential for folate absorption. J Physiol. 1978;280:1–7.
49. Davidson GP, Townley RRW. Structural and functional abnormalities of the small bowel due to nutritional folate deficiency in infancy. J Pediatr. 1977;90:590–594.
50. Chacko A, Begum A, Mathan VI. Absorption of nutrient energy in southern Indian control subjects and patients with tropical sprue. Am J Clin Nutr. 1984;40:771–775.
51. Haddock L, Vazquez MDC, Rivera R, et al. The kinetics of D3-3H metabolism in tropical sprue. P R Health Sci J. 1985;4:47.
52. Tompkins A. Tropical malabsorption: Recent concepts in pathogenesis and nutritional significance. Clin Sci. 1981;60:131–137.
53. Rolston DDK, Mathan VI. Jejunal and ileal glucose-stimulated water and sodium absorption in tropical enteropathy: Implications for oral rehydration therapy. Digestion. 1990;46:55–60.
54. Batt RM, Bush BM, Peters TJ. Subcellular biochemical studies of a naturally occurring enteropathy in the dog resembling chronic tropical sprue in human beings. Am J Vet Res. 1993;44:1492.
55. Cook GC, Menzies IS. Intestinal absorption and unmediated permeation of sugars in post-infective tropical malabsorption (tropical sprue). Digestion. 1986;33:109–116.
56. Westergaard H. Southwestern Internal Medicine Conference: The sprue syndromes. Am J Med Sci. 1985;290:249–262.
57. Besterman HS, Cook GC, Sarson DL, et al. Gut hormones in tropical malabsorption. BMJ. 1979;1252–1255.
58. Cook GC. Delayed small-intestinal transit in tropical malabsorption. BMJ. 1978;2:238–240.
59. Jayanthi V, Chacko A, Gani IK, et al. Intestinal transit in healthy southern Indian subjects and in patients with tropical sprue. Gut. 1989;30:35–38.
60. Tawil SC, Brandt LJ, Bernstein LH. Scalloping of the valvulae conniventes and mosaic mucosa in tropical sprue. Gastroenterology. 1991;37:365.
61. Mathan MM, Ponniah J, Mathan VI. Epithelial cell renewal and turnover and relationship to morphologic abnormalities in jejunal mucosa in tropical sprue. Dig Dis Sci. 1986;31:586–592.
62. Thielman NM, Guerrant RL. An algorithmic approach to the workup and management of HIV-related diarrhea. J Clin Outcomes Management. 1997;4:36–47.
62. Scully RE, Mark EJ, McNeely WF, et al. Weekly clinicopathologic exercises: Case 15–1990. N Engl J Med. 1990;322:1067–1075.
63. Guerra R, Wheby MS, Bayless TM. Long-term antibiotic therapy in tropical sprue. Ann Intern Med. 1965;63:619.
64. Rickles FR, Klipstein FA, Tomasini J, et al. Long-term follow-up of antibiotic-treated tropical sprue. Ann Intern Med. 1972;76:203–210.
65. Gerson CD, Kent TH, Saha JR, et al. Recovery of small-intestinal structure and function after residence in the tropics: II. Studies in Indians and Pakistanis living in New York City. Ann Intern Med. 1971;75:41–48.
66. Maldonado N, Horta E, Guerra R, Perez-Santiago H: Poorly absorbed sulfonamides in the treatment of tropical sprue. Gastroenterology. 1969;57:559.

Chapter 89

Whipple's Disease

THOMAS MARTH

Whipple's disease (WD), or intestinal lipodystrophy, first described in 1907 by George Hoyt Whipple,[1] is a rare infectious disorder. This chronic and systemic disease affects mostly middle-aged white men, who usually present with weight loss, arthralgia, diarrhea, and abdominal pain. Due to the systemic nature of the disease, a variety of other clinical symptoms including involvement of the heart, lung, and central nervous system (CNS) are frequent. The disease is often diagnosed by small bowel biopsy, which is characterized by periodic acid–Schiff (PAS)–positive inclusions representing the causative bacteria. These organisms have a distinct electron-microscopic structure and can be found in a high frequency free within the lamina propria and within macrophages of the gastrointestinal tract. Recently, the causative organisms have been phylogenetically classified as actinomycetes by amplification of bacterial 16-S ribosomal RNA[2, 3]; the proposed name is *Tropheryma whippelii*.[3] Newer studies have shown that in active and inactive WD patients there are subtle defects of cell-mediated immunity that may predispose individuals to infection with *T. whippelii*. Whereas most patients respond well to antibiotic treatment, some treated patients with relapsing disease may have a poor prognosis, and untreated patients have a uniformly downhill course.

ETIOLOGY AND PATHOGENESIS

In his original report, G. H. Whipple found rod-shaped structures in the silver stain but noted: "Whether this is the active agent in this peculiar pathological complex cannot be determined from the study of this single case but its distribution in the glands is very suggestive."[1] As noted in 1961 by two groups, a characteristic rod-shaped (0.25×1.5 to 2.5 μm) organism can be observed by electron microscopy within cells in various stages of degradation and in the extracellular space in florid disease (Fig. 89–1).[4, 5] The organism possesses a trilaminar plasma membrane, a surrounding homogeneous cell wall of 20-nm thickness, and an outer trilaminar membrane-like structure.[6] Although the latter feature can be seen in gram-negative bacteria, other characteristics including the central location of tubules and vesicles are rather typical of gram-positive organisms, and the light microscopic staining pattern is indeed gram-positive.[6, 7] The bacillus can be found typically in macrophages of the lamina propria of the small intestine and its lymphatic drainage but has also been observed in endothelial and epithelial cells, muscle cells, and various cells of the immune system including polymorphonuclear leukocytes, plasma cells, mast cells, and intraepithelial lymphocytes; in addition, it has been found in a number of other cell types.[6–8] The fact that the typical organisms disappear from the lamina propria on antibiotic-induced clinical improvement has long argued strongly for their etiologic significance.[9] Furthermore, in addition to its characteristic appearance in electron microscopy, the unique nature of the WD organism was suggested by its distinct cross-reactivity with streptococcal (groups A, B, and G) and *Shigella* (group B) antisera on fixed tissues as confirmed by a number of investigators.[10, 11] It has not yet been possible with standard techniques to isolate, culture, and define an organism in vitro from patients or to transfer the disease to laboratory animals in order to fulfill the classic Koch's postulates. However, two important steps toward this goal have been made.

First, specific segments of bacterial 16-S ribosomal RNA from lesions of diseased patients were amplified using the polymerase chain reaction (PCR).[2, 3] Thus, with the use of broad-range and specific primers as well as sequence analysis, it was possible to classify the causative organism phylogenetically as a new genus and species,[2, 3] and the name *Tropheryma whippelii* (*trophe*, for "nourishment"; *eryma*, for "barrier") was proposed.[3] *Tropheryma whippelii* has been placed phylogenetically within the subdivision of gram-positive bacteria with high guanine and cytosine content, the actinomycetes, and is in close relationship to several actinobacteria, nocardioforms, and cellulomonads including organisms such as *Dermatophilus congolensis, Arthrobacter globiformis, Terrabacter tumescens, Cellulomonas cellasea, Corynebacterium aquaticus* as well as to *Rhodococcus* species.[2, 3, 12] *Tropheryma whippelii* is more weakly related to *Streptomyces* and *Mycobacterium* species (including *Mycobacterium avium-intracellulare complex*).[2, 3, 12] *T. whippelii* occurs, like some of its phylogenetic relatives, in the environment.[13] Many studies since the first reports were capable of identifying *T. whippelii* with the use of the original PCR primers in a variety of tissues, and newer work has shown that alternative primer pairs may be useful in diagnostic procedures as well.[14, 15]

Second, in 1997, *T. whippelii* was reported to be propagated in a special cell culture system. In this system, human phagocytes were deactivated with cytokines (using interleukin-4 and interleukin-10) and then infected with the bacillus from heart valve tissue.[16] If confirmed in future studies and with bacteria from other tissue

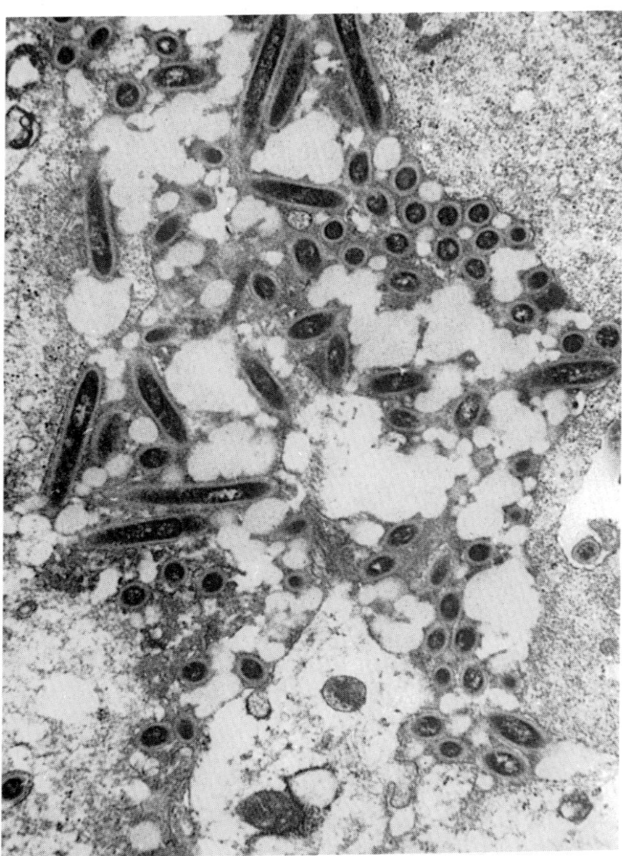

FIGURE 89–1. Electron microscopic view of the Whipple bacillus, designated as *Tropheryma whippelii*. The characteristic, rod-shaped (0.25 × 1.5–2.5 μm) organism can be observed in the extracellular space in florid disease, or within cells in various stages of degradation. The bacillus is found typically and in the highest frequency in macrophages of the lamina propria of the small intestine and its lymphatic drainage. *T. whippelii* is characterized by a trilaminar plasma membrane, a surrounding homogeneous cell wall of 20-nm thickness, and an outer trilaminar membrane-like structure usually seen in gram-negative bacteria. Other characteristics, including the central location of tubules and vesicles, however, are rather typical of gram-positive organisms. (×20,000.)

types, this technique could be helpful in further characterization of *T. whippelii*.

For reasons that are not yet apparent, this rare disease occurs primarily in elderly white persons (mean age at diagnosis approximately 55 years) and eight times more often in men than in women.[8, 17] A specific genetic susceptibility is also suggested by the fact that approximately 30% of the patients are HLA-B27–positive, although familial cases have only rarely been reported.[8, 18] Moreover, the disease may have a chronic-relapsing course, and the organism may persist in the affected tissues for a long period of time despite prolonged antibiotic therapy.[8, 17] Collectively, these observations suggest that a host factor, putatively of immunologic nature, plays a role in the occurrence of the disease.

The presumed immunologic defect in WD has been studied with increasing interest since the 1970s and is likely to be subtle and quite specific for the WD organism, since patients with the disease are usually not predisposed to infections with other organisms. This holds true for the majority of patients, although some newer case reports have pointed out that WD may also occur in a setting of immune deficiency or immune suppression (e.g., in one individual with acquired immunodeficiency disease).[19, 20]

The immunohistologic features of the lamina propria in WD are unique since the intestinal tissue contains reduced numbers of differentiated B cells (i.e., plasma cells) and shows a relative paucity of lymphocytic infiltration despite the massive influx of macrophages.[7, 21–23] Although the lack of lymphocytic infiltrate in WD could be partially attributed to a loss of lymphocytes secondary to an intestinal lymphangiectasia, many studies have found a more profound phenotypic and functional alteration of immunologic features in WD patients. A number of studies have shown that both lamina propria and circulating T-cell populations in active WD are characterized by a reduced CD4/CD8 T-cell ratio, a shift toward mature T-cell subpopulations (e.g., CD45RO expression increased, CD45RA expression decreased), and increased cell activation markers.[23–25] These changes are accompanied by disturbed function of peripheral T cells, that is, by reduced T-cell proliferative responses to a variety of stimuli (phytohemagglutinin, concanavalin A, and anti-CD2 antibodies), and in a number of instances yet-unidentified serum factors have been found that downregulate T-cell–mediated responses.[18, 24, 26, 27] In addition, impaired delayed-type hypersensitivity reaction to skin antigens (mostly recall antigens) can be detected in many patients.[24, 27] Although these alterations are present most clearly in acutely ill patients, they are found in many patients with long-standing remission. Studies have found reduced numbers of B cells positive for immunoglobulin A (IgA) but increased numbers of surface IgM–positive B cells in the lamina propria.[23, 28] Secretory IgA levels determined from intestinal aspirates have been found to be normal.[8] Humoral immune responses to infectious agents in the periphery as well as total serum IgG levels are usually normal, whereas IgM is often decreased and IgA increased in acute stages of the disease.[8, 29] One recent report showed decreased levels of IgG2 subclass, the IgG subclass that is produced in response to infection with encapsulated bacteria and is presumably regulated by cell-mediated immune responses and interferon-γ.[30] Peripheral macrophages from WD patients manifested decreased intracellular degradation of several organisms in one study,[31] and intestinal macrophages showed some decrease of phagocytosis in another.[32] It has been demonstrated that patients with active and inactive WD have reduced numbers of circulating cells expressing CD11b, the α-chain of complement receptor 3, which serves on macrophages as a facilitator of microbial phagocytosis, plays a role in antigen processing, and mediates interferon-γ–induced intracellular killing of ingested bacteria.[24] During active disease, intestinal macrophages do not express CD11b.[33] In addition, the impaired function of antigen-presenting cells in WD may also be related to reduced macrophage interleukin-12 production,[30] a cytokine that has important functions in regulating cell-mediated immune responses and interferon-γ. Underlining the pathogenetic relevance of impaired cellular immunity, a recent study reported that in one patient with WD refractory to antibiotic regimens and with reduced interferon-γ levels in vitro, treatment with antimicrobials and recombinant interferon-γ led to a clearance of the infection and to a correction of the immune deficits.[34] Thus, a reduction in monocyte CD11b expression or interleukin-12 production may herald a decrease in the ability to cope with intracellular infection and go along with the observation that *T. whippelii* can be grown in cytokine-deactivated macrophages.[16] Although many of the immunologic features argue for a primary defect in WD, an immune suppression secondary to the infection with *T. whippelii* has not been excluded.

PATHOLOGY OF WHIPPLE'S DISEASE

On gross inspection, the duodenum and jejunum, which are the sites most frequently affected, often appear thickened and edematous.[21] The infiltration of the bowel wall is associated with a widening and flattening of the villi and with dilated lacteals containing yellow lipid deposits that represent the result of a villous lymphatic blockade. Based on these and similar observations in the mesenteric lymph nodes, G. H. Whipple assumed a disorder of fat metabolism and suggested the name *intestinal lipodystrophy*.[1] Pathophysiologically, the disturbance of the villous architecture is presumably the cause of the steatorrhea and the subsequent malabsorption syndrome that accompany the disease. In addition, the intestinal lymphangiectasia and protein-losing enteropathy seem to be mainly secondary to lymphatic blockage within intestinal tissues.

Light-microscopic examination usually reveals infiltration of the lamina propria with large macrophages (also called *sickle-form particle-containing* cells) containing granular-foamy PAS-positive, diastase-resistant, silver-positive inclusions that represent more or less intact remnants of ingested bacteria.[7, 21, 35, 36] The PAS reaction represents a cross-reaction with bacterial glycoproteins located in the cell wall (first reported in 1949).[36] In florid disease, undigested extracellular bacteria are seen as well.[7, 9] Although it would be reasonable to assume that the route of infection is through the intestinal lumen, resulting in a secondary accumulation of *T. whippelii* in the lamina propria, the possibility that the bacterium could penetrate via other sites and access the lamina propria through the intestinal lymphatics must be considered because in one study the most viable organisms were seen at the base and not the apex of the epithelial cells.[7]

As WD is a systemic disease, PAS-positive macrophages and electron microscopically detectable bacilli have been demonstrated in many cell types, as noted previously, and in almost all organs, including the heart, lung, CNS, eye, liver, spleen, lymph nodes, endocrine glands, joints, and bone marrow.[4, 7, 8, 21] The involvement of heart valves deserves special mention because it leads to clinical symptoms and is present in more than one third of the autopsy cases. Other frequent pathologic features include peri- or myocarditis; pleuritis; hepatosplenomegaly; ascites or polyserositis; uveitis as well as ependymitis; cortical atrophy; and demyelination of the CNS.[8, 21] Involvement of the lamina propria and lymphatic tissues can be accompanied by noncaseating, epithelioid cells (sarcoid-like) granulomas.[37] Infection with *Rhodococcus equii* and *Mycobacterium avium-intracellulare* complex in patients with acquired immunodeficiency syndrome is histologically similar to WD, and the latter can be ruled out by a Ziehl-Neelsen stain, which does not stain *T. whippelii*.[38]

TABLE 89–1 Signs and Symptoms in Whipple's Disease

	Approximate Frequency (%)*
Major clinical features	
Weight loss	95 (85–100)
Arthropathy	85 (70–100)
Diarrhea	75 (70–85)
Abdominal pain	65 (50–90)
Frequent signs and symptoms	
Fever	50 (40–60)
Lymphadenopathy	50 (40–60)
Hyperpigmentation	45 (35–60)
Hypotension	40 (30–80)
Peripheral edema	35 (20–45)
Cardiac murmurs	35 (30–40)
Occult bleeding	25 (20–30)
Myalgia	25
Abdominal mass	20 (15–25)
Chronic cough	20
Splenomegaly	15 (5–20)
Hepatomegaly	15
Ascites	10
Other clinical features	
Pleuritis	
Pleural effusion	
Endocarditis	
Muscle wasting	
Glossitis	
Peripheral neuropathy	
Eye involvement (e.g., visual loss, uveitis, retinitis)	
CNS involvement (e.g., dementia, ophthalmoplegia, myoclonus, ataxia, nystagmus)	
Organ-specific symptoms	
Gastrointestinal tract	100 (95–100)
Cardiovascular system	55 (35–65)
Respiratory system	50 (35–60)
CNS	25 (20–30)
Eye	10 (5–15)

*In parentheses are the approximate frequencies reported in the literature.[8, 17, 21, 39, 49]
Abbreviation: CNS, Central nervous system.

CLINICAL FEATURES AND DIAGNOSIS

The leading symptoms of WD are weight loss, diarrhea, and arthropathies, and in 75% of cases, these symptoms are found together by the time of diagnosis.[8, 17, 39, 40] However, the clinical presentation of the patients may vary to a great extent because of the differential organ involvement and the stage of the disease. In most instances (63% in one large series),[17] the disease begins insidiously with arthropathy. This symptom (in 30% associated with positivity for HLA-B27) may precede the diagnosis by a very considerable length of time and consists usually of chronic migratory, nondestructive, and seronegative joint disease involving predominantly the peripheral joints; in addition, it is often accompanied by myalgias.[8, 17, 18, 39] Gastrointestinal symptoms, which usually begin later and ultimately often lead to diagnosis, consist of episodic and watery diarrhea or steatorrhea in many cases accompanied by colicky abdominal pain and, in 20 to 30% of patients, occult blood in the stool.[8, 17, 39, 40] These symptoms and concomitant anorexia may lead to the full picture of a malabsorption syndrome with severe weight loss, weakness, cachexia, and the associated secondary signs and symptoms (Table 89–1).

Systemic symptoms occur quite frequently in WD. These consist of intermittent, mostly low-grade fever, night sweats, and peripheral and abdominal lymphadenopathy. A frequent feature of WD is skin hyperpigmentation, particularly affecting light-exposed areas. No major organ is excluded from infection by *T. whippelii*, and chronic nonproductive cough indicative of lung involvement, cardiac murmurs, hypotension, edema, ascites, or polyserositis as well as hepatomegaly and splenomegaly are among other more frequently found signs and symptoms (see Table 89–1).[8, 39, 40]

A major and frequently overlooked area of involvement in WD is the CNS. This manifests as memory disorders, personality changes, dementia, ophthalmoplegia, disturbed sleep patterns, myoclonias, nystagmus, ataxia, seizures, symptoms of cerebral compression due to hydrocephalus, and a variety of cranial nerve symptoms such as hearing loss and blurred vision.[8] In some patients, an oculomasticatory myorhythmia has been described.[41] Such CNS symptoms can occur with minimal or even absent gastrointestinal involvement.[42]

The diagnosis of WD is usually made by upper endoscopy showing whitish or yellowish plaques distributed on a friable mucosa.[43] Small bowel biopsies should be taken from both the proximal and the distal duodenum or the jejunum, since involvement can be patchy. The diagnosis usually can be established if the characteristic PAS-positive material is present in the lesions. However, a specific diagnostic test is now recommended in every newly identified patient, and is mandatory in doubtful cases. Both electron microscopy and the PCR can be considered specific diagnostic tests for WD. Formerly, electron-microscopic examination of the biopsy material was often helpful to confirm the diagnosis. However, a considerable amount of experience has been gained with the diagnostic use of the PCR. Thus, a PCR should now be routinely performed on small bowel tissue and additionally (in patients with long-standing systemic involvement or with suspected CNS manifestation) on cerebrospinal fluid.[14, 15, 44] Biopsies from abdominal or peripheral lymph nodes or from other organs may yield diagnostic material as well. Biopsies taken from the colon or the rectum, sites that are only infrequently involved, can be misleading because of other conditions that are accompanied by PAS-positive cells (such as melanosis coli)[8] and only should be regarded diagnostic if Whipple bacilli are demonstrated by other techniques. The question whether the diagnosis of WD can be established with the highly sensitive PCR from the peripheral blood cannot be answered yet; whereas genetic material has been found in the whole blood or in blood cells in a few patients,[45] this diagnostic approach seems to have its limitations.[46]

Radiographic findings before the diagnosis of WD may reveal abdominal lymphomas, specific organ involvement, or the presence of a thickening of the mucosal folds (e.g., in conventional radiography, sonography, computed tomography, nuclear magnetic resonance tomography).[39] Laboratory testing often reveals evidence of malabsorption and protein-losing enteropathy: reduced serum levels of β-carotene, various vitamins (B_{12}, D, K, and folic acid), albumin, cholesterol, and electrolytes; and lymphocytopenia; additionally, stool fat excretion may be elevated, and D-xylose absorption may be reduced.[8, 39] For unexplained reasons, some WD patients have eosinophilia and abnormalities of serum immunoglobulin levels such as low IgM or high IgA levels.[8, 28] Finally, other and less specific laboratory abnormalities in WD include an elevated erythrocyte sedimentation rate, thrombocytosis, elevated acute-phase proteins such as C-reactive protein, and hypochromic anemia.

TREATMENT AND PROGNOSIS

WD was considered to be a uniformly fatal disorder until successful treatment with antibiotics (first with chloramphenicol) was reported in the 1950s.[47] The basis of this empirical regimen was later solidified by observations concerning the bacterial cause of the disease.

In most patients with WD, antibiotic therapy leads to a rapid improvement of the clinical status and to a lasting remission. Diarrhea and fever may disappear within 1 week of therapy, whereas arthropathy and other symptoms are often improved after 2 to 4 weeks. Laboratory findings often normalize over a period of several weeks. Clinical improvement is usually accompanied by a gradual reconstitution of the villous architecture of the small intestine and by a disappearance of the bacteria over a period of several months. Finally, immunologic parameters such as increased IgA or shifts in T-cell subpopulations return to normal within several months, and some immune parameters may be helpful to determine the duration of therapy in single cases.[24] In contrast, the subtle defect in cell-mediated immunity persists for years, if not indefinitely.[24, 27]

A variety of antibiotic regimens have been proved beneficial in WD patients including penicillin alone, penicillin plus streptomycin, tetracycline, chloramphenicol, ceftriaxone, and trimethoprim-sulfamethoxazole.[8] Most patients up to the 1980s were treated with a 2-week systemic course of penicillin plus streptomycin followed by oral tetracycline. Several retrospective studies have, however, shown that this treatment regimen may be associated with a higher frequency of relapses, particularly relapses involving the CNS.[17, 48, 49] The institution of trimethoprim-sulfamethoxazole seems to be clinically superior to tetracycline for patients both with and without CNS symptoms as the primary treatment as well as for the treatment of relapse.[17, 48] There are, however, no prospective studies available yet on the choice or the duration of antibiotic therapy.

Antibiotic treatment of proven efficacy is trimethoprim-sulfamethoxazole (160/800 mg orally twice daily), which should be given for at least 1 year. This should be preceded, especially in the severely ill patient, by a 2-week course of parenteral therapy with ceftriaxone, 2 g per day intravenously. In the case of intolerance to oral sulfonamides, second-line regimens including oral penicillin (e.g., penicillin V, 1 to 1.5 g daily), minocycline, tetracycline, or chloramphenicol (up to a 30-g cumulative dose) can be instituted. Rarely, a Jarisch-Herxheimer reaction has been described after the initiation of penicillin therapy in WD.[8, 9]

In the case of a good clinical response, it is sufficient to follow the patient with duodenal biopsies 6 months and 1 year after diagnosis. If no bacteria are detected by electron microscopy or by PCR and if no PAS-positive material is found after 1 year, antibiotic treatment can be stopped. Even in successfully treated patients in whom therapy has been discontinued, we recommend follow-up biopsies (at increasingly longer intervals) approximately up to 5 years after the establishment of the diagnosis. In the case that bacteria persist after 1 year of treatment (as determined, for example, by PCR), therapy must be continued. An alternative antibiotic regimen should be considered. In cases with long-standing persistence of PAS-positive material (>30 months) without detectable intact bacteria, a continuation of therapy seems to be justified, because we observed a higher percentage of relapses in such patients (Marth et al, unpublished); therapy can be stopped, however, if the histologic appearance has been stationary for over 2 years.[17]

In the severely ill patient, nutritional replacement therapy is indicated. This includes fat-soluble vitamins (A, D, E, K) and calcium supplementation in the case of steatorrhea; fluid and electrolyte replacement in the cachectic patient; iron in anemic patients; and a high calorie, high-protein, high-vitamin diet.

Cerebral manifestations of WD are not infrequent at the time of diagnosis, occur more frequently in a relapse, and may lead progressively to death.[8, 17, 39] When such manifestations have been documented, antimicrobials with good penetration into the CNS such as a course of ceftriaxone (2 g intravenously daily) or chloramphenicol (1 g daily) have been used, but optimal treatment still needs to be defined. The follow-up of these patients includes analysis of the cerebrospinal fluid in 6-month intervals until bacterial material is undetectable. Chronic CNS involvement may be associated with tissue gliosis and thus may be resistant to antibiotic treatment.

Relapses become evident mostly within a few years after diagnosis and are accompanied by the reappearance of extracellular organisms.[8, 9] They seem to occur less frequently after treatment with trimethoprim-sulfamethoxazole than with tetracycline therapy and are usually treated successfully with reinstitution of the primary antibiotic regimen.[8, 17] There are, however, patients with an antibiotic-refractory disease course and a combination of antibiotic treatment and immunotherapy (e.g., therapy with recombinant interferon-γ, which reconstitutes the cellular immune functions), as shown in one case report, could become a therapeutic option in these patients.[30, 34]

REFERENCES

1. Whipple GH. A hitherto undescribed disease characterized anatomically by deposits of fat and fatty acids in the intestinal and mesenteric lymphatic tissues. Johns Hopkins Hosp Bull. 1907;18:382–391.
2. Wilson KH, Blitchington R, Frothingham R, et al. Phylogeny of the Whipple's disease-associated bacterium. Lancet. 1991;338:474–475.
3. Relman DA, Schmidt TM, Macdermott RP, et al. Identification of the uncultured bacillus of Whipple's disease. New Engl J Med. 1992;327:293–301.
4. Yardley JH, Hendrix TR. Combined electron and light microscopy in Whipple's disease—Demonstration of "bacillary bodies" in the intestine. Johns Hopkins Hosp Bull. 1961;109:80–98.
5. Chears WC, Ashworth CT. Electron microscopy study of the intestinal mucosa in Whipple's disease—Demonstration of encapsulated bacilliform bodies in the lesion. Gastroenterology. 1961;41:129–138.
6. Silva MT, Macedo PM, Nunes JFM. Ultrastructure of bacilli and bacillary origin of the macrophagic inclusions in Whipple's disease. J Gen Microbiol. 1985;131:1001–1013.
7. Dobbins WO III, Ruffin JM. A light- and electron-microscopic study of bacterial invasion in Whipple's disease. Am J Pathol. 1967;51:225–242.
8. Dobbins WO III: Whipple's Disease. Springfield, Ill: Charles C Thomas; 1987.
9. Trier JS, Phelps PC, Eidelmann S, et al. Whipple's disease: Light and electron microscope correlation of jejunal mucosal histology with antibiotic treatment and clinical status. Gastroenterology. 1965;48:684–707.
10. Keren DF. Whipple's disease: A review emphasizing immunology and microbiology. Crit Rev Clin Lab Sci. 1981;14:75–108.
11. Kent SP, Kirkpatrick PM. Whipple's disease: Immunological and histochemical studies of eight cases. Arch Pathol Lab Med. 1980;104:544–547.
12. Maiwald M, Ditton HJ, von Herbay A, et al. Reassessment of the phylogenetic position of the bacterium associated with Whipple's disease and determination of the 16S–23S ribosomal intergenic spacer sequence. Int J Syst Bacteriol. 1996;46:1078–1082.
13. Maiwald M, Schuhmacher F, Ditton, HJ, et al. Environmental occurrence of the Whipple's disease bacterium (*Tropheryma whippelii*). Appl Environ Microbiol. 1998;64:760–762.
14. Von Herbay A, Ditton HJ, Maiwald M. Diagnostic application of a polymerase chain reaction assay for the Whipple's disease bacterium to intestinal biopsies. Gastroenterology. 1996;110:1735–1743.
15. Ramzan NN, Loftus E, Burgart LJ, et al. Diagnosis and monitoring of Whipple's disease by polymerase chain reaction. Ann Intern Med. 1997;126:520–527.

16. Schoedon G, Goldenberger D, Forrer R, et al. Deactivation of macrophages with interleukin-4 is the key to the isolation of *Tropheryma whippelii*. J Infect Dis. 1997;176:672–677.
17. Feurle GE, Marth T. An evaluation of antimicrobial treatment for Whipple's disease—Tetracycline versus trimethoprim-sulfamethoxazole. Dig Dis Sci. 1994;39:1642–1648.
18. Feurle GE, Dörken B, Schöpf E, et al. HLA-B27 and defects in the T-cell system in Whipple's disease. Eur J Clin Invest. 1979;9:385–389.
19. Maiwald M, Meier-Willersen HJ, Hartmann M, et al. Detection of *Tropheryma whippelii* DNA in a patient with AIDS. J Clin Microbiol. 1995;33:1354–1356.
20. Meier-Willersen HJ, Maiwald M, von Herbay A. Whipple's disease associated with opportunistic infections. Dtsch Med Wochenschr. 1993;118:854–860.
21. Enzinger FM, Helwig EB. Whipple's disease: A review of the literature and report of 15 patients. Virchows Arch. 1963;336:238–268.
22. Maxwell JD, Ferguson A, McCay AM, et al. Lymphocytes in Whipple's disease. Lancet. 1968;1:887–889.
23. Ectors N, Geboes K, De Vos R, et al. Whipple's disease: A histological, immunocytochemical and electronmicroscopic study of the immune response in the small intestinal mucosa. Histopathology. 1992;21:1–12.
24. Marth T, Roux M, von Herbay A, et al. Persistent reduction of complement receptor 3 alpha-chain expressing mononuclear blood cells and transient inhibitory serum factors in Whipple's disease. Clin Immunol Immunopathol. 1994;72:217–226.
25. Von Herbay A, Windler F, Heckmayr M, et al. Abdominaler Pseudotumor als klinische Manifestation eines Morbus Whipple. Dtsch Med Wochenschr. 1987;112:1621–1625.
26. Groll A, Valberg LS, Simon JB, et al. Immunological defect in Whipple's disease. Gastroenterology. 1972;63:943–950.
27. Martin FF, Vilseck J, Dobbins WO III, et al. Immunological alterations in patients with treated Whipple's disease. Gastroenterology. 1972;63:6–18.
28. Eck M, Kreipe H, Harmsen D, et al. Invasion and destruction of mucosal plasma cells by *Tropheryma whippelii*. Hum Pathol. 1997;28:1424–1428.
29. Dobbins WO III. Is there a immune deficit in Whipple's disease? Dig Dis Sci. 1981;26:247–252.
30. Marth T, Neurath M, Cuccherini BA, et al. Defects of monocyte interleukin-12 production and humoral immunity in Whipple's disease. Gastroenterology. 1997;113:442–448.
31. Bjerkness R, Odegaard S, Bjerkvig R, et al. Whipple's disease: Demonstration of a persisting monocyte and macrophage dysfunction. Scand J Gastroenterol. 1988;23:611–619.
32. Lukacs G, Dobi S, Szabo M. A case of Whipple's disease with repeated operations for ileus and complete cure. Acta Hepatogastroenterol. 1978;25:238–242.
33. Ectors N, Geboes K, Rutgeerts P, et al. RFD7-RFD9 coexpression by macrophages points to T cell–macrophage interaction deficiency in Whipple's disease. Gastroenterology. 1992;106:A676.
34. Schneider T, Stallmach A, von Herbay A, et al. Treatment of refractory Whipple's disease with interferon-gamma. Ann Intern Med. 1998;129:875–877.
35. Sieracki JC, Fine G. Whipple's disease—Observation on systemic involvement. II. Gross and histological observations. Arch Pathol. 1959;67:81–93.
36. Black-Schaffer B. Tinctorial demonstration of a glycoprotein in Whipple's disease. Proc Soc Exp Biol Med. 1949;72:225–227.
37. Rodarte JR, Garrison CO, Holley KE, et al. Whipple's disease simulating sarcoidosis. Arch Intern Med. 1972;129:479–482.
38. Strom RL, Gruninger RP. AIDS with *Mycobacterium avium–intracellulare* lesions resembling those of Whipple's disease. N Engl J Med. 1983;309:1323–1324.
39. Fleming JL, Wiesner RH, Shorter RG. Whipple's disease: Clinical, biochemical and histopathological features and assessment of treatment in 29 patients. Mayo Clin Proc. 1988;63:539–551.
40. Marth T, Strober W. Whipple's disease. Semin Gastrointest Dis. 1996;7:41–48.
41. Adler CH, Galetta SL. Oculo-facial-skeletal myorhythmia in Whipple's disease: Treatment with ceftriaxone. Ann Intern Med. 1990;112:467–469.
42. Feurle GE, Volk B, Waldherr R. Cerebral Whipple's disease with negative jejunal histology. N Engl J Med. 1979;300:907–908.
43. Geboes K, Ectors N, Heidbuchel H, et al. Whipple's disease: The value of upper gastrointestinal endoscopy for the diagnosis and follow-up. Acta Gastroenterol Belg. 1992;55:209–219.
44. Von Herbay A, Ditton HJ, Schuhmacher F, et al. Whipple's disease: Staging and monitoring by cytology and polymerase chain reaction of cerebrospinal fluid. Gastroenterology. 1997;113:434–441.
45. Lowsky R, Archer GL, Fyles G, et al. Diagnosis of Whipple's disease by molecular analysis of peripheral blood. N Engl J Med. 1994;331:1343–1346.
46. Marth T, Fredericks D, Strober W, et al. Limited role for PCR-based diagnosis of Whipple's disease from peripheral blood mononuclear cells. Lancet. 1996;348:66–67.
47. Paulley JW. A case of Whipple's disease (intestinal lipodystrophy). Gastroenterology. 1952;22:128–133.
48. Keinath RD, Merrell DE, Vlietstra R, et al. Antibiotic treatment and relapse in Whipple's disease. Gastroenterology. 1985;88:1867–1873.
49. Von Herbay A, Otto HF. Whipple's disease: A report of 22 patients. Klin Wochenschr. 1988;66:533–539.

SECTION K

BONE AND JOINT INFECTIONS

Chapter 90

Infectious Arthritis

JAMES W. SMITH
M. SHAHBAZ HASAN

An inflammatory reaction in the joint space (arthritis) follows infection with many different microorganisms. Bacterial invasion of the joint generally leads to a suppurative arthritis, principally of one joint (monarticular). Certain bacteria may produce symptoms in multiple joints during bacteremia, and some, such as *Neisseria gonorrhoeae*, may induce inflammation in the neighboring tendon sheaths. Viral infections frequently involve multiple joints and demonstrate inflammation without suppuration. A chronic granulomatous monarticular arthritis due to either mycobacteria or fungi must be differentiated from chronic monarticular arthritis with other causes. A sterile arthritis may occur early in the infection, as with hepatitis B, or later, as with a postinfectious arthritis. Infectious arthritis has a low case-fatality rate but can leave residual symptoms if not recognized and treated promptly. Any person with an inflamed joint must have infection included as a diagnostic possibility. Distinction between infectious and reactive arthritis can be difficult unless the joint is aspirated.

PATHOGENESIS AND PREDISPOSING FACTORS

Infectious arthritis usually follows hematogenous inoculation of pathogenic organisms.[1–3] In infants younger than 1 year, capillaries perforate the epiphyseal growth plate, providing a conduit from bone to joint space. After 1 year of age, the capillaries recede and infection is usually limited to the bone because the growth plate contains the infection.[4] Patients with preexisting arthritis are predisposed to infectious arthritis, especially those with more debilitating arthritis who require intra-articular injection (Table 90–1).[5, 6] Intra-articular injection or trauma may lead to infection because capillary integrity is interrupted so that microbial seeding takes place during bacteremia.[2] Other systemic conditions predisposing to infectious arthritis include immunosuppressive therapy and chronic debilitating illnesses such as diabetes mellitus or malignancies.[1, 6–8] Extra-articular infections such as skin infections, predispose to bacterial arthritis.[6, 7]

Synovial tissue is highly vascular and lacks a basement membrane and thus is susceptible to hematogenous seeding by bacteria.[8] The most common pathogen, *Staphylococcus aureus*, has been demonstrated in vitro to bind to bone sialoprotein, a glycoprotein found in joints.[9] In experimental arthritis produced by the intra-articular injection of *S. aureus*, this organism is destructive to cartilage because of the production of chondrocyte proteases.[10] In rabbits, early pathologic changes were noted on the surface and in the matrix of the superficial zone of the articular surface by electron microscopy within 24 hours.[11] At this time, the joint cavity showed polymorphonuclear leukocytes, and lysosomal bodies were present in the synovial cells. By 3 days, the destruction of articular cartilage was more extensive and was even visible with light microscopy. The matrix appeared loose in the superficial zones, and degeneration of chondrocytes was noted in deeper zones.

Endocrine factors appear to be important in the genesis of the disseminated gonococcal syndrome and viral arthritis.[12, 13] Gonococcal infections tend to occur in women during pregnancy and during menstruation.[12] Rubella arthritis principally occurs in postpubertal women, whereas mumps arthritis is seen exclusively in postpubertal men.[13]

Immunologic response accounts for the clinical expression of arthritis with hepatitis B, meningococci, and lymphocytic choriomeningitis virus.[14–16] Arthritis in patients with hepatitis B infection relates to the transient appearance of complement-fixing complexes in patients with arthritis.[14] Reiter's syndrome can develop in persons after sexually transmitted diseases or after enteric infections with *Shigella, Salmonella, Campylobacter*, and *Yersinia*.[17, 18] The presence of the specific histocompatibility antigen HLA-B27 increases the likelihood of postinfectious arthritis 50-fold and has been reported to predispose to more severe diseases.[18]

TABLE 90–1 Predisposing Factors in Bacterial Arthritis

Preexisting arthritis	Prior intravascular catheterization
Age	Other infections (skin, urinary tract)
Diabetes mellitus	Intra-articular injections
Immunosuppression	Areas endemic for Lyme disease and coccidioidomycosis
Intravenous drug abuse	Sexually transmitted diseases

Data from refs. 3, 6, and 7.

CLINICAL FEATURES

Septic Arthritis

The reported incidence of septic arthritis varies from 2 to 5 per 100,000 per year in the general population to 28 to 38 per 100,000 per year in patients with rheumatoid arthritis and 40 to 68 per 100,000 per year in patients with a joint prosthesis.[6] Children and adults with bacterial arthritis present with fever in 60 to 80% of cases, and with monarticular involvement in 90%.[1, 19, 20] Most have mild temperature elevation, with only 30 to 40% having a temperature exceeding 39°C.[1, 8, 19] Joint motion is limited, and swelling representing synovial effusion is visible in peripheral joints. Joint tenderness may vary from minimal to severe. The knee is the most commonly affected joint in both children and adults with bacterial arthritis, as well as infections with *Mycobacterium tuberculosis* (Table 90–2).[21] The hip is the next most commonly involved joint, but correct diagnosis of bacterial infection of the hip and shoulder joints is frequently delayed because effusions may be difficult to demonstrate.[1] Interphalangeal joints of the hand are infrequently involved with bacterial arthritis except for *N. gonorrhoeae* and *M. tuberculosis* and after human and animal bites. Infection of the sacroiliac joint may be difficult to distinguish from septic arthritis of the hip. Pyogenic sacroiliitis is usually due to *S. aureus* or *Streptococcus* groups A, B, C, and G and often occurs in infants, children, or young adults and presents with fever and pain on ambulation.[22, 23] Pain on flexion, abduction, external rotation, and extension of the ipsilateral hip (FABERE test) plus tenderness over the sacroiliac joint should prompt a bone scan or magnetic resonance imaging of the sacroiliac joint. The sacroiliac joint is a favored site for brucella arthritis, a more indolent infection.[24] The sternoclavicular joint is infrequently infected except when parenteral drug abuse is a predisposing factor.[8] Most patients with bacterial arthritis have an acute presentation, but

TABLE 90–2 Frequency (Percentages) of Joint Involvement in Infectious Arthritis*

Joint	Bacterial (Suppurative)		Mycobacterial	Viral
	Children	*Adults*		
Knee	41	54	24	60
Hip	23	16	20	4
Ankle	14	7	12	30
Elbow	12	3	8	20
Wrist	4	7	20	55
Shoulder	4	8	4	5
Interphalangeal and metacarpal	1.4	4	12	75
Sternoclavicular	0.4	<1	0	0
Sacroiliac	0.4	<1	0	0

*More than one joint may be involved, so the percentages exceed 100 percent.
Data from refs. 1, 4, 13, and 19–21.

a prolonged duration of symptoms has been reported with neisserial infections.[15] Infections with mycobacteria and certain fungi such as *Sporothrix schenckii* have such an insidious onset that a diagnosis of infection may not be considered.[25]

Infection of multiple joints is observed in 10 to 20% of patients, especially those with rheumatoid arthritis.[7] Infectious arthritis of viral cause (e.g., rubella virus) tends to involve multiple joints, with most patients having symptoms in the interphalangeal joints of the hands and wrist, as well as the knees, ankles, and elbows (see Table 90–2).[13, 26] Inflammation of multiple tendon sheaths (tenosynovitis) causes pain on joint motion and must be distinguished from arthritis. Acute tenosynovitis often accompanies the disseminated gonococcal syndrome (Fig. 90–1)[12] and also may be seen with infections due to *Moraxella* and rubella virus. Chronic tenosynovitis may occur in extracutaneous sporotrichosis and infections with nontuberculous mycobacteria. Carpal tunnel syndrome (paresthesias of the hands), with or without joint symptoms, occurs with rubella virus and nontuberculous mycobacteria.

Septic Bursitis

Acute septic olecranon bursitis is due to *S. aureus* in 95% of cases and can be distinguished from arthritis of the elbow by the location of inflammation proximal to the olecranon process and the absence of joint pain on motion.[27] Bursae over the patella or tibial tubercle may also be infected by *S. aureus*, often after minor trauma. Bursitis also may be the first manifestation of infectious arthritis in patients with rheumatoid arthritis. The olecranon and prepatellar bursae are the usual sites. Chronic infectious olecranon bursitis presents with firm swelling and little tenderness. Infection follows minor trauma, which inoculates organisms of low-grade virulence into the bursa, including *Prototheca*, nontuberculous mycobacteria, and agents of phaeohyphomycosis.

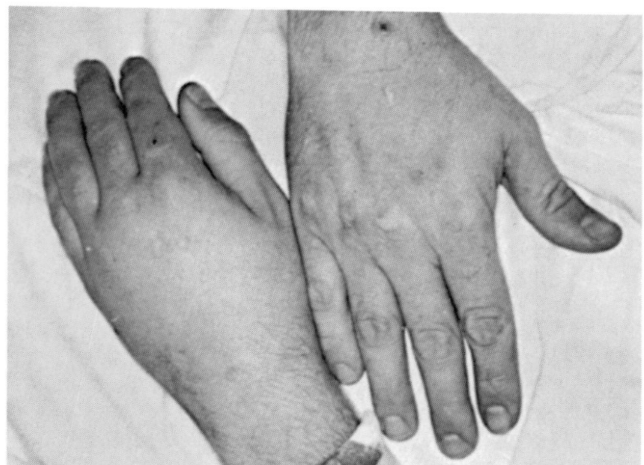

FIGURE 90–1. Patient with chronic gonococcemia with swollen hand and skin lesions over dorsal surface of wrist. (From Smith JW. Infectious arthritis. Curr Prescribing, April 1979.)

LABORATORY FINDINGS

Patients with infectious arthritis, whether bacterial, viral, or caused by *M. tuberculosis*, usually have an elevated erythrocyte sedimentation rate. The sedimentation rate is higher in those with bacterial infection and can be helpful in the assessment of patients with rheumatoid arthritis; however, it lacks sensitivity and specificity.[7] Children with bacterial arthritis tend to have elevated white blood cell counts with a predominance of polymorphonuclear leukocytes, whereas many adults have minimal or no elevation of the peripheral blood leukocyte count.[1, 7]

Examination of synovial fluid from inflamed joints is essential to distinguish infectious from noninfectious arthritis. Joint fluid from monarticular bacterial arthritis generally appears turbid or purulent, although 10 to 20% of patients have serosanguineous fluid. The synovial leukocyte count usually exceeds 50,000/mm^3, and most have a differential count of more than 75% polymorphonuclear leukocytes.[1, 28] However, this finding is not specific for bacterial arthritis, because synovial fluid in rheumatoid arthritis and crystalline joint disease also shows a preponderance of polymorphonuclear leukocytes; furthermore, bacterial infections in patients who have malignancy, are on corticosteroids, or are intravenous drug abusers do not elicit as high a synovial fluid leukocyte count (half below 28,000 cells/mm^3), although their percentage of segmented neutrophils exceeds 90%.[28] Protein levels are generally elevated, but this has little specificity for joint infection. A low synovial fluid glucose level is neither sensitive nor specific for bacterial arthritis.[19, 29] Viral arthritis may be associated with a modest elevation of the synovial fluid leukocyte count.[13] In most instances, the preponderant cell is mononuclear, although some cases with proven rubella arthritis have had a majority of polymorphonuclear leukocytes.[26] Leukocyte counts exceeding 1000/mm^3 are characteristic of staphylococcal bursitis.[27]

In persons with bacterial arthritis, smears of joint fluid stained for bacteria show the organisms in one third of the cases.[4] The Gram stain can give false-positive results (positive test results not confirmed by positive cultures). Both blood and joint fluid should be cultured for bacteria aerobically and anaerobically. Pharyngeal, rectal, and cervical or urethral cultures should be plated on gonococcal media if the disseminated gonococcal syndrome is considered.[18, 19] Blood cultures have been positive in 10 to 60% of adults and in 29% of children with bacterial arthritis.[1, 4, 19] Joint cultures are positive in up to 90% of those with nongonococcal bacterial arthritis, but in less than 50% of those with gonococcal arthritis.[7] For mycobacterial and fungal infection, cultures of synovial tissue produce higher yields than synovial fluid.[21, 25] Recent advances in diagnostic testing include the application of polymerase chain reaction technology for the detection of bacterial DNA within the synovial fluid and synovial tissue. This is particularly useful in infections due to fastidious organisms or in partially treated patients. Among the microorganisms detected by polymerase chain reaction are *Yersinia* spp., *Chlamydia* spp., *Mycoplasma* and *Ureaplasma* spp., *Borrelia burgdorferi* and *N. gonorrhoeae*.[7]

RADIOLOGIC AND IMAGING EVALUATION

Routine radiographic studies are much less useful than computed tomography or magnetic resonance imaging in the diagnosis of infectious arthritis. Computed tomography has the advantage of good definition of contiguous bone lesions and the ability to guide needle aspiration. Magnetic resonance imaging better defines the soft tissues, such as distended joint spaces and extension to periarticular structures. Effusions in axial joints such as the hip and sacroiliac joints are better defined radiologically with magnetic resonance imaging than with conventional radiographs.[30] Narrowing of the joint space is seen in adults, whereas in children, displacement of the ossific nucleus within cartilage or destruction of cartilage can be seen.[30] Rapid destruction of the joint is a hallmark of untreated pyogenic arthritis.[31] Radiographs of the joint in those with mycobacterial infection show minimal joint space narrowing with marginal erosions and extensive demineralization as common features (Phemister's triad).[31] Viral infections rarely produce radiographic changes unless significant quantities of fluid are present and result in distention of the joint capsule.

Radionuclide imaging with the three-phase bone scan is also helpful in evaluating joint infection in the setting of suspected osteomyelitis or in detecting bacterial sacroiliitis.[23, 30, 31] Although bone and gallium scans are frequently positive with asymmetric uptake in patients with septic arthritis, these scans are of little use in distinguishing inflamed from infected joints.[30]

HISTOPATHOLOGY

Synovial tissue removed by surgery or arthroscopy can be diagnostic on culture or special stains for bacteria, fungi, or mycobacteria. The inflammatory response in the synovium is not usually helpful in distinguishing infectious from noninfectious arthritis.

SYNDROMES OF INFECTIOUS ARTHRITIS

Acute Bacterial Arthritis

The frequencies of the etiologic agents that induce bacterial arthritis vary with age. *Haemophilus influenzae* type b was the preponderant causative organism in children younger than 2 years. It has virtually disappeared since the introduction of the conjugate vaccine. In infants younger than 1 month, group B streptococci, gram-negative bacilli, and *S. aureus* are causative organisms. *S. aureus* is the most frequent organism causing bacterial arthritis in children older than 2 years[4] and is the causative organism in the vast majority of cases of suppurative arthritis in adults.[1, 4, 19, 20] *N. gonorrhoeae* is the preponderant cause of bacterial arthritis in adults younger than 30 years.[19] The frequency of streptococcal infections as a cause of bacterial arthritis is relatively constant from childhood through the adult years (13 to 27%). Previously, the most frequently isolated type in both children and adults was group A β-hemolytic streptococci; however, the non–group A streptococci (groups B, C, and G) are also being recognized as significant pathogens.[7] *Streptococcus pneumoniae* is rarely encountered now as a cause of suppurative arthritis but has been noted to be the causative organism of septic arthritis in children with sickle cell disease.[32]

Infectious arthritis due to gram-negative bacilli is seen in 9 to 20% of cases of infectious arthritis.[1, 7, 19] The presence of comorbid conditions, such as intravenous drug abuse, chronic arthritis, and extra-articular infections (urinary tract infection, infected decubiti), predispose to joint infections due to these microorganisms.[7] Septic arthritis due to *Salmonella* spp. occurs preponderantly in children but bears no association with sickle cell disease, unlike *Salmonella* osteomyelitis.

Gonococcal arthritis, one of the more commonly recognized features of disseminated gonococcal infections, is caused by organisms with protein 1-A serotype, which are also resistant to serum.[12, 33] The syndrome exists in either of two forms. In one form, patients have systemic symptoms with fever, shaking chills, skin lesions, and a polyarticular syndrome. Blood cultures are frequently positive, particularly within 2 days of the onset of symptoms, whereas synovial fluid cultures are rarely positive. *N. gonorrhoeae* can be recovered from cultures of genital, rectal, and pharyngeal areas. The skin lesions begin as tiny erythematous papules, frequently petechiae, and may evolve to become vesicles or pustules (see Fig. 90–1). These lesions are fairly transient and last 3 to 4 days. An occasional patient who fails to come to medical attention may have recurrent episodes of skin lesions and polyarthralgias for periods up to 3 months (as in the case in Fig. 90–1). The organism is occasionally recovered from scrapings of the skin lesion, although more frequently organisms are recovered from blood. Other microorganisms to be considered in the differential diagnosis of patients with skin rash and arthritis include *H. influenzae, Moraxella osloenis, Streptobacillus moniliformis*, and *Neisseria meningitidis*.

In the other form of gonococcal infection, patients have a monarticular suppurative infection with recovery of the organism from joint fluid.[12] These patients may give a history of having had transient polyarthralgias before the monarticular arthritis developed and may even have a history of skin lesions; however, skin lesions are rarely present in those with a monarticular arthritis. Infection with *N. meningitidis* may mimic the disseminated gonococcemia syndrome; patients with more than 100 skin lesions have a high probability of meningococcal infection.[34] In addition, patients with meningococcemia may develop joint effusions 5 to 10 days after the onset of the infection. Sterile effusions are found in multiple joints and resolve rather rapidly. An uncommon variety of meningococcal infection is chronic meningococcemia in which symptoms are present for more than 1 week without meningeal involvement.[15] These patients have low-grade fever; a rash that may be macular, papular, or petechial; joint involvement; and headache. Two thirds of the patients have polyarthralgias, and one third have arthritis with joint effusions.

Septic arthritis of the metacarpophalangeal joint after human bites can be caused by oral microbes or after cat or dog bites, by *Pasteurella multocida* or *Capnocytophaga* spp. (Table 90–3).[35, 36] Infections with *S. moniliformis* occur 2 to 3 days after rat bites with the onset of chills, a macular rash of the palms and soles, and arthralgias in large joints.[37] The organism, a pleomorphic gram-negative bacillus, can be grown in blood cultures but not from joint fluid. The arthritis of Lyme disease is characterized by intermittent attacks of a migratory polyarticular arthritis lasting weeks to months, usually in large joints, that occur late in the course of the disease.[38] This spirochetal infection transmitted by tick bite (see Chapter 231) also rarely can result in a long-standing chronic arthritis of the knee joint.[38] Brucella arthritis manifests as either an acute or a chronic infection and most commonly affects the sacroiliac joint, followed by the knee and the hip joint.[24, 39] The diagnosis is most frequently made by a *Brucella* agglutination test on serum.

Obligate anaerobic bacteria, principally gram-positive cocci, are rarely the causative agents in bacterial arthritis, even when anaerobic

TABLE 90–3 Epidemiologic Associations in Infectious Arthritis

Organism	Epidemiologic Association
Neisseria gonorrhoeae	Female during menstrual cycle or pregnancy; multiple skin lesions[12]
Organisms from oral flora (*Eikenella corrodens, Fusobacterium nucleatum*)	Human bite[35]
Pasteurella multocida, Capnocytophaga spp.	Cat or dog bite[36]
Streptobacillus moniliformis	Rat bite[37]
Borrelia burgdorferi (Lyme disease)	Tick exposure[38]
Brucella spp.	Ingestion of unpasteurized dairy products[39]
Staphylococcus aureus and *Pseudomonas aeruginosa*	Intravenous drug abuse[7]
Mycoplasma hominis and *Ureaplasma urealyticum*	Postpartum women and hypogammaglobulinemia[40]
Sporothrix schenckii	Outdoor work, including farming[25]
Mycobacterium marinum	Trauma in aquatic environment[41]
Aerobic gram-negative bacilli	Immunocompromise[7]
	Urinary tract infection

cultures are performed routinely on joint fluid.[8] *Bacteroides* spp. are rarely encountered. The most frequent anaerobic pathogen in arthritis of children is *Clostridium* spp.[4]

An acute septic arthritis occurs with *Mycoplasma hominis* and *Ureaplasma urealyticum* in postpartum women and immunocompromised (hypogammaglobulinemic) individuals.[7, 40]

Chronic Monarticular Arthritis

Mycobacteria

Chronic monarticular arthritis with a granulomatous reaction on pathologic examination may be caused by a variety of organisms (Table 90–4). Mycobacterial infections of the joint are chronic, slowly progressive monarticular infections that may also involve the tendon sheaths, particularly the carpal tunnel area of the wrist.[21] A granulomatous reaction of the synovium is seen pathologically in young adults with tuberculosis, although only 60% of elderly patients had granulomas histologically.[21] Patients younger than 60 years with tuberculous infections principally presented with arthritis of a single weight-bearing joint such as the knee and few systemic symptoms, whereas those older than 60 years had systemic symptoms, other foci of tuberculosis, and arthritis of non–weight-bearing joints such as the shoulder.[21] Concomitant active pulmonary tuberculosis is usually not evident.

Nontuberculous mycobacteria also produce infections of the joints (see Table 90–4). Among these, *Mycobacterium kansasii, Mycobacterium marinum*, and *Mycobacterium avium-intracellulare* complex are the most common causes of monarticular synovitis.[41] These organisms have a propensity to involve the wrist and hands and to cause flexor tenosynovitis, carpal tunnel syndrome, and, rarely, olecranon bursitis.[41] The organisms can localize to a joint after trauma or spread from a pulmonary focus. Rarely, the patients have documented extra-articular infection. *M. marinum* would be suspected in a patient with arthritis who develops the infection after exposure to tropical fish aquariums or marine environments.

Synovial tissue from a patient with a chronic monarticular arthritis should be cultured for mycobacteria, inspected at a few days (to recognize *Mycobacterium fortuitum*, a rapid grower), and incubated at 30°C (*M. marinum* grows better at this temperature than at 37°C). Patients with lepromatous leprosy may have a symmetric polyarthritis of wrist, metacarpal, and small joints of the hands, especially patients with erythema nodosum leprosum.[42] Juxta-articular erosions are seen in the carpal bones.

Fungi

Fungal arthritis can be caused by a number of fungi with some variation based on geographic localization. *S. schenckii* causes infections of one or more peripheral joints in previously normal persons, particularly those with outdoor occupations.[43] The chest radiograph is usually normal. The most commonly affected joint is the knee, followed by the wrist and the elbow (Figs. 90–2 and 90–3). The joint is boggy, with a decreased range of motion, but not red or tender. On radiographs, progressive cartilage erosion and a loss of definition of trabecular bone in adjacent long bones and carpal bones become evident over months and years. The infection may be manifest in contiguous bursae or, in the knee, in a Baker's cyst. Diagnosis is by culture of fluid or tissue; fungal elements of *Sporothrix* are infrequent in tissue and difficult to find in pathologic specimens.

A chronic monarticular or oligoarticular arthritis is common with disseminated coccidioidomycosis, an infection acquired by inhalation of arthroconidia in endemic areas.[44] The knee is the most frequently involved joint. The joint fluid may show either a polymorphonuclear or a lymphocytic cellular response, but smears and cultures are often negative. Radiographs of bone may be normal initially but often show a contiguous osteolytic lesion many months later. Diagnosis is made by culture of synovial biopsy or, less often, of joint fluid. Patients' sera also have positive complement fixation responses with *Coccidioides* antigen. Joint infection in patients with blastomycosis primarily spreads from osteomyelitis.[23] The diagnosis can be made by examination of synovial tissue and by appropriate culture of surgical material. Paracoccidioidomycosis affects rural workers in endemic areas, usually involving the joints of the long bones, and may occur with or without pulmonary involvement.[45]

Infections of the joints with *Candida*, principally *Candida albicans*, generally have an acute onset after hematogenous spread of the organism; rarely, the fungus may be introduced during intra-

TABLE 90–4 Infectious Causes of Chronic Monarticular Arthritis

Bacterial	Fungi
Brucella spp.	*Sporothrix schenckii*
Tropherema whippelii	*Coccidioides immitis*
Mycobacteria and Nocardia	*Blastomyces dermatitidis*
Mycobacterium tuberculosis	*Paracoccidioides brasiliensis*
M. kansasii	*Candida albicans*
M. marinum	*Pseudallescheria boydii*
M. avium-intracellulare complex	
M. fortuitum	
M. haemophilum	
M. leprae	
Nocardia asteroides	

FIGURE 90–2. Wrist of patient who had sporotrichosis of wrist and olecranon bursa. (From Smith JW. Infectious arthritis. Curr Prescribing, April 1979.)

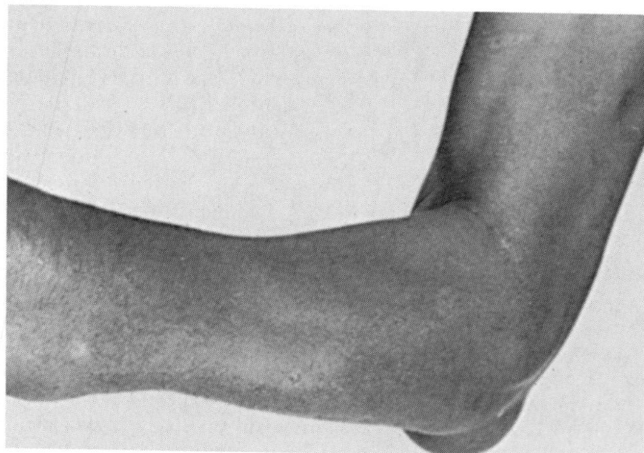

FIGURE 90–3. Elbow of patient who had sporotrichosis of wrist and olecranon bursa. (From Smith JW. Infectious arthritis. Curr Prescribing, April 1979.)

TABLE 90–5 Viral Agents Associated with Arthritis

Group	Virus
DNA viruses	
Poxvirus	Small pox
	Vaccinia*
Adenovirus	Adenovirus*
Herpesvirus	Varicella*
	Epstein-Barr (infectious mononucleosis)*
	Cytomegalovirus*
Parvovirus B19	Erythema infectiosum
Hepadnavirus	Hepatitis B
RNA viruses	
Paramyxovirus	Mumps
	Rubeola*
Orthomyxovirus	Influenza*
Picornavirus	Echovirus*
Togavirus	
Alphavirus	Chikungunya
	O'nyong-nyong
	Sindbis
	Mayaro virus
	Ross River virus
Rubivirus	Rubella
Arenavirus	Lymphocytic choriomeningitis virus
Lentivirus	
Retrovirus	Human T-lymphotropic virus type 1
	Human immunodeficiency virus type 1

*Unusual manifestation of infection.

articular corticosteroid injection.[25] In low-birth-weight neonates, catheter-acquired candidemia may lead to acute arthritis of the knee, with or without meningitis or brain abscess. Culture of synovial fluid typically has increased neutrophils, but only a few *Candida* colonies may grow. In adults, any peripheral joint can be involved, but multiple joint infection is observed in up to 37%.[25] Migratory polyarthritis, usually in association with skin lesions or erythema nodosum and erythema multiforme, has been seen with acute histoplasmosis.[25] Arthritis is rare in cryptococcosis or aspergillosis. Carpal tunnel syndrome has also been noted rarely in patients with disseminated histoplasmosis. *Pseudallescheria boydii, Scedosporium prolificans*, and dematiaceous fungi such as *Curvularia* and *Exophiala jeanselmei* have caused monarticular arthritis after penetrating trauma of the knee.[25]

Viral Arthritis

Viral agents associated with symptoms and signs of arthritis are listed in Table 90–5. Arthritis is a reasonably frequent event of infection with rubella virus and mumps virus, whereas it is an atypical manifestation of infection with varicella virus, adenovirus, echovirus, and rubeola virus.[13] A polyarthritis due to rubella virus occurs principally in adult women (Table 90–6).[46] The onset of joint symptoms occurs either with the rash or within 3 days after the eruption in 52% of females.[46] The small joints of the hand are most frequently involved, with knees, wrists, and ankles less commonly affected. Synovial fluid shows a predominance of mononuclear cells, and virus is rarely isolated from the joint fluid. The course is self-limited in most people, although some have recurrent episodes of joint symptoms up to 6 months after infection.[46] Rubella vaccine induces joint symptoms in 41% of susceptible postpubertal women.[46] In late winter and spring, outbreaks of epidemic erythema infectiosum, an infection caused by parvovirus B19, are associated with a symmetric arthritis in adults, particularly in women.[47] Arthritis occurs in association with mumps with a frequency of 0.44% and is seen more commonly in men.[48] The arthritis begins from 1 day before to 15 days after the onset of parotitis, with multiple large and small joints affected. Effusions are infrequent. Symptoms subside within 2 weeks, although arthritis may persist for up to 3 months.[48]

TABLE 90–6 Clinical or Epidemiologic Characteristics of Viral Agents Causing Arthritis

Virus	Characteristic
Rubella virus	Women with tenosynovitis
Parvovirus B19	Women with erythema infectiosum
Mumps virus	Men
Hepatitis B virus	Preicteric phase
Lymphocytic choriomeningitis virus	Adults with aseptic meningitis
Chikungunya virus	East Africa, India
O'nyong-nyong virus	East Africa
Mayaro virus	South America, Caribbean
Ross River virus	Australia
Barmah Forest virus	Australia

Up to 20% of patients with hepatitis B have been noted to develop arthritis, frequently in association with urticaria 2 days to 6 weeks before the onset of jaundice.[14] In the great majority, the symptoms disappear with the onset of the jaundice.[14] The arthritis is symmetric with a predilection for the hands followed by knees and ankles; joint effusions are scanty when present and reveal predominantly mononuclear cells. Hepatitis C is rarely associated with arthritis, except when the virus induces a cryoglobulinemic state.[49]

Lymphocytic choriomeningitis, caused by an arenavirus, was associated with arthritis in one outbreak among laboratory personnel.[16] The development of a severe influenza-like disease with headache and arthritis may be due to lymphocytic choriomeningitis virus rather than influenza, a disease in which arthritis is an uncommon complication.

A number of alphaviruses of the togavirus family, which are arthropod borne, have arthritis as a frequent manifestation of the illness they cause. Chikungunya derives its name from its characteristic clinical finding (that which bends up). This disease is characterized by an abrupt onset of fever, chills, and severe incapacitating pain in the large joints, although hot, swollen joints are infrequently seen.[13] Maculopapular eruption occurs over the trunk and extensor surfaces of the extremities in 80% of those with the disease. A similar illness in Uganda in 1959 was given the name *O'nyong-nyong fever* (weakening of the joints).[13] The onset of O'nyong-nyong fever was also abrupt, with symmetric involvement of most of the large joints with excruciating pain. All eventually made a full recovery. Sindbis virus and Sindbis-related diseases have been noted to have arthritis as a prominent manifestation of the illness.[50] In Australia, epidemics of polyarthritis with rash have been observed that are due to two different alphaviruses, the Ross River virus and the Barmah Forest virus.[51, 52]

Patients with human T-lymphotropic virus type 1 have a chronic persistent oligoarthritis. This is a proliferative synovitis involving large joints with atypical lymphocytes in synovial fluid and proviral DNA within tissue cells.[53] Human immunodeficiency virus type 1 infection has been associated with arthralgias of multiple joints, and, rarely, a monarticular reactive or septic arthritis.[54]

Parasites

Joint manifestations are not a feature of any of the commonly recognized parasitic infections. However, in the Sepik district of Papua New Guinea, arthritis in association with filarial infections was the most frequent cause of arthritis.[55] The knee was the most frequently involved joint and showed warmth, tenderness, and limitation of motion. Joint effusions were present in slightly less than one half of the cases, and the fluid aspirated was creamy yellow. Radiographs showed no articular destruction, only soft tissue swelling. Microfilariae were present in the blood. A reactive polyarthropathy is seen with schistosomiasis characterized by high immunoglobulin E levels, an inflammatory exudate, and low complement in synovial fluid.[56]

DIFFERENTIAL DIAGNOSIS

Bacterial infection should be suspected in any patient with acute monarticular arthritis, even in the absence of fever. However, a number of noninfectious conditions may involve single joints, including acute rheumatoid arthritis, gout, and chondrocalcinosis (pseudogout). As stated earlier, all these illnesses can cause an inflammatory arthritis with more than 75% polymorphonuclear leukocytes.[29] Hence, the ultimate diagnosis must be based on Gram stain and culture of joint fluid and blood. Synovial fluid from any adult with monarticular arthritis should be examined for negatively birefringent (uric acid) and positively birefringent (calcium pyrophosphate) crystals. Simultaneous bacterial infection and crystalline joint disease has been reported.[57] Serologic studies including rheumatoid factor tests, antinuclear antibody tests, and acute and convalescent studies for antistreptolysin O should be performed if more than one joint is affected. Any hot, tender joints with a fluid collection in a rheumatoid patient should be aspirated and the fluid submitted for smear and culture. Gonococcal arthritis, Reiter's syndrome, or acute rheumatic fever should be suspected in any adult having fever and multiple joint involvement; characteristic skin lesions and tenosynovitis suggest the disseminated gonococcal syndrome. The other features of the triad of Reiter's syndrome, conjunctivitis and urethritis, may not be apparent initially. Frequently, the only way to distinguish between gonococcal infection and Reiter's syndrome is to observe the response to treatment with antibiotics appropriate for *N. gonorrhoeae*: If a new joint becomes affected after the second day of therapy, then Reiter's syndrome is the more likely diagnosis. HLA-B27 testing is not helpful in individual cases of Reiter's syndrome.

When a monarticular arthritis has a chronic course, an infectious cause should also be considered uppermost in the differential diagnosis. The leading infectious cause has been infection with nontuberculous mycobacteria, followed closely by *S. schenckii*. Infection with *M. tuberculosis* predominates in some countries,[21] and the occurrence of tuberculosis in association with human immunodeficiency virus could presage a rise in extrapulmonary tuberculosis, including arthritis.[41, 54] Synovial fluid cultures for acid-fast bacteria and fungi should be performed in any patient who is immunocompromised, is on immunosuppressive therapy, or has a persistent effusion. A synovial biopsy culture should be done for fungus and acid-fast organisms in any person with a chronic monarticular involvement whose synovial fluid cultures are negative or with tenosynovitis as a prominent feature. In addition, Lyme arthritis should be considered if the patient is from an endemic area.[38] In Lyme arthritis, the infectious agent can be demonstrated by Dieterle's silver stain in up to 25% of cases, but serologic examination and polymerase chain reaction tests of joint fluid are more helpful.[7] A diagnosis of viral arthritis should be considered if a person presents with multiple joint involvement and systemic manifestations consistent with a viral infection. It is frequently not possible to isolate virus from the joint fluid, so serologic confirmation of the infection is necessary using acute and convalescent sera. In general, the course is the major determinant in distinguishing between viral arthritis and rheumatic disorders such as adult Still's disease, since the former has a self-limited course with no residual joint abnormalities.

ANTIMICROBIAL THERAPY

Empirical antimicrobial therapy for presumed bacterial arthritis should be given after obtaining blood for culture and withdrawing synovial fluid for culture, Gram stain, a leukocyte count, and chemistry tests. The choice of drug depends on the Gram stain result and the patient's age and sexual activity.

If *S. aureus* is suspected clinically or by Gram stain, appropriate initial therapy is an intravenous penicillinase-resistant penicillin such as nafcillin, 9 g/day intravenously in every-4-hour doses in adults and 150 mg/kg/day divided into every-4-hour to every-6-hour doses in children. Vancomycin, 1 g every 12 hours intravenously for adults, with modifications for renal function, would be preferred if the patient is penicillin allergic or comes from a population in which methicillin-resistant *S. aureus* is commonly encountered. If the Gram stain suggests streptococci, intravenous penicillin 12 to 18 million units/day for an adult, given every 4 hours, would be the drug of choice, with alternatives including cefazolin or vancomycin. If gram-negative cocci are seen, ceftriaxone 1 to 2 g intravenously daily for adults or 50 mg/kg daily for children would be indicated. Cefotaxime 6 to 8 g/day for an adult, divided into 8-hourly doses, would be an alternative. If the Gram stain is negative in community-acquired acute septic arthritis, then ceftriaxone or cefotaxime are reasonable for initial coverage of gonococci, streptococci and *S. aureus*, pending culture and susceptibility results. Ampicillin-sulbactam intravenously, 6 to 9 g of ampicillin per day for adults divided into every-4-hour doses, would be useful for empirical therapy of septic arthritis after a dog or cat bite because ampicillin, like penicillin, has excellent activity against *Pasteurella* and *Capnocytophaga* spp. The range of possibilities is broad in arthritis after surgery or in a prosthetic joint, beyond the scope of this chapter. Recommendations for the treatment of infections in prosthetic joints are given in Chapter 92.

The usual course of therapy for suppurative arthritis is 2 weeks for *H. influenzae*, streptococci, or gram-negative cocci and 3 weeks for staphylococci or gram-negative bacilli.[58] The gonococcal arthritis-dermatitis syndrome is treated with parenteral antibiotics for 2 days after clinical improvement. This can then be changed to oral therapy to complete 7 to 10 days of treatment. Gonococcal septic arthritis requires 3 weeks of parenteral antibiotics.[7] Intra-articular injections of drugs used to treat suppurative bacterial arthritis are unnecessary. Most agents used to treat suppurative arthritis reach sufficient levels in the joint when given intravenously.[59, 60] The inclusion of antibiotics in solutions used to irrigate the joint is not indicated. The reader is referred to the relevant chapters of this text for the treatment of other specific organisms such as *Brucella*, fungi, mycobacteria, and Lyme borreliosis.

OTHER THERAPEUTIC MODALITIES

Most people with suppurative arthritis respond adequately to appropriate antimicrobial agents after an initial joint aspiration for diagnosis. Early treatment in experimental infectious arthritis reduces the loss of collagen and erosion of articular surface and therefore should minimize the need for ancillary treatment.[61] Repeated needle aspiration for recurrent joint effusions has been used with success during the first 5 to 7 days of treatment.[8, 62] If the volume of synovial fluid, the cell count, and the percentage of polymorphonuclear leukocytes decrease with each aspiration, then the combination of antimicrobial therapy and aspiration as needed is probably adequate. Surgical drainage may be necessary when the response to therapy is poor or needle aspiration is unsuccessful because of thick exudate or loculation. Surgical drainage is generally thought to be required for the hip joint, with the exception of gonococcal arthritis.[7] The shoulder requires either computed tomography–guided aspiration or surgical drainage. If open surgical drainage is performed, continued irrigation of the joint after drainage is of little value. The duration of treatment with systemic antimicrobial agents depends on the pathogen but is generally given for 2 weeks for nongonococcal arthritis. Parenteral therapy should be continued for at least 1 week after open drainage.

Arthroscopy has emerged as an alternative to open surgical drainage. It allows the visualization of joint tissue and the ability to lyse adhesions, drain pus pockets, and débride necrotic material with considerably less morbidity. The wounds heal faster and rehabilitation time is reduced.[63]

In the usual case of septic arthritis, immobilization of the infected joint is not necessary, although weight bearing should be avoided until signs of inflammation and pain have disappeared. The joint should be maintained in the functional position, and passive motion may be instituted early, once the symptoms of pain have subsided. As the inflammation diminishes, active exercises may be instituted,

TABLE 90–7 Predictors of Poor Outcome with Bacterial Arthritis

Age >60 yr
Infection in hip and shoulder
Duration of symptoms before treatment >1 wk
>4 joints
Preexisting rheumatoid arthritis
Persistently positive culture after 7 d of appropriate therapy

Data from refs. 1, 7, and 20.

and weight bearing may be permitted when all signs of inflammation have disappeared and no evidence of effusion is present.[8]

Staphylococcal bursitis also responds to antibiotics and one or more aspirations. Surgical drainage is not recommended, although bursae that are repeatedly or chronically infected may need to be excised when infection has resolved.

PROGNOSIS

Although some persons with bacterial arthritis recover without long-term residual abnormalities, certain persons have a poor long-term response (Table 90–7). Elderly patients do poorly, especially with infections of the hip and with underlying joint disease.[64, 65] The frequency of sequelae in children was shown to be 27%,[66] including a slight limitation of movement, impairment of ambulation, and shortening of the extremity. These residua were more common with hip and ankle infection. In adults, up to 50% had limitation of motion or persistence of pain.[19] Most with septic arthritis immediately after arthroscopy did well with few sequelae.[67] Infectious causes of chronic monarticular arthritis are occasionally associated with substantial residua even after maximal therapy.[25, 41] Synovectomy has been combined with chemotherapy to improve the therapeutic outcome.[44]

REFERENCES

1. Cooper C, Cawley MID. Bacterial arthritis in an English health district: A 10 year review. Ann Rheum Dis. 1986;45:458–463.
2. McCarty DJ. Joint sepsis: A chance for cure. JAMA. 1982;247:835.
3. Smith JW, Piercy EA. Infectious arthritis. Clin Infec Dis. 1995;20:225–231.
4. Jackson MA, Nelson JD. Etiology and medical management of acute suppurative bone and joint infections in pediatric patients. J Pediatr Orthop. 1982;2:313–323.
5. Ostensson A, Geborek P. Septic arthritis as a non-surgical complication in rheumatoid arthritis: Relation to disease severity and therapy. Br J Rheum. 1991;30:35–38.
6. Kaandorp CJE, van Schaardenburg D, Krijnen P, et al. Risk factors for septic arthritis in patients with joint disease. Arthritis Rheum. 1995;38:1819–1825.
7. Pioro MH, Mandell BF. Septic arthritis. Rheum Dis Clin North Am. 1997;23:239–258.
8. Goldenberg DL, Reed JI. Bacterial arthritis. N Engl J Med. 1985;312:764–771.
9. Bremell T, Lange S, Yacoub A, et al. Experimental *Staphylococcus aureus* arthritis in mice. Infect Immun. 1991;59:2615–2623.
10. Williams RJ III, Smith RL, Schurman DJ. Septic arthritis: Staphylococcal induction of chondrocyte proteolytic activity. Arthritis Rheum. 1990;33:533–541.
11. Roy S, Bhawan J. Ultrastructure of articular cartilage in pyogenic arthritis. Arch Pathol. 1975;99:44–47.
12. O'Brien JPP, Goldenberg DL, Rice PA. Disseminated gonococcal infection: A prospective analysis of 49 patients and a review of pathophysiology and immune mechanisms. Medicine. 1983;62:395–406.
13. Smith JW, Sanford JP. Viral arthritis. Ann Intern Med. 1967;67:651–659.
14. Inman RD. Rheumatic manifestations of hepatitis B virus infection. Semin Arthritis Rheum. 1982;11:406–420.
15. Kidd BL, Hart HH, Grigor RR. Clinical features of meningococcal arthritis: A report of four cases. Ann Rheum Dis. 1985;44:790–792.
16. Baum SG, Lewis AM Jr, Rowe WP, et al. Epidemic nonmeningitis lymphocytic-choriomeningitis-virus infection. N Engl J Med. 1966;274:934–936.
17. Fryden A, Bengtsson A, Foberg U, et al. Early antibiotic treatment of reactive arthritis associated with enteric infections: Clinical and serological study. Br Med J. 1990;301:1299–1302.
18. Keat A. Sexually transmitted arthritis syndromes. Med Clin North Am. 1990;74:1617–1631.
19. Sharp JT, Lidsky MD, Duffy J, et al. Infectious arthritis. Arch Intern Med. 1979;139:1125–1130.
20. Ho G Jr, Su EY. Therapy for septic arthritis. JAMA. 1982;247:797–800.
21. Garrido G, Gomez-Reino J, Fernandez-Dapica P, et al. A review of peripheral tuberculous arthritis. Semin Arthritis Rheum. 1988;18:142–149.
22. Bohay DR, Gray JM. Sacroiliac pyarthrosis. Orthop Rev. 1993;22:817–823.
23. Vyskocil JJ, McIlroy MA, Brennan TA, et al. Pyogenic infection of the sacroiliac joint. Case reports and review of the literature. Medicine. 1991;70:188–197.
24. Ariza J, Pujol M, Nolla JM, et al. Brucellar sacroiliitis: Findings in 63 episodes and current relevance. Clin Infect Dis. 1993;16:761–765.
25. Cuellar ML, Silveira LH, Espinoza LR. Fungal arthritis. Ann Rheum Dis. 1992;51:690–697.
26. Medical Staff Conference: Arthritis caused by viruses. Calif Med. 1973;119:38–44.
27. Zimmerman B, Mikolich DJ, Ho G. Septic bursitis. Semin Arthritis Rheum. 1995;24:391–410.
28. McCutchan HJ, Fisher RC. Synovial leukocytosis in infectious arthritis. Clin Orthop. 1990;257:226–230.
29. Shemerling RH, Delbanco TL, Tosetson ANA, et al. Synovial fluid tests. JAMA. 1990;264:1009–1014.
30. Brower AC. Septic arthritis. Radiol Clin North Am. 1996;34:293–309.
31. Forrester DM, Feske WI. Imaging of infectious arthritis. Semin Roentgenol. 1996;31:239–249.
32. Syrogiannopoulos GA, McCracken GH Jr, Nelson JD. Osteoarticular infections in children with sickle cell disease. Pediatrics. 1986;78:1090–1096.
33. Hook EW. Septic arthritis: Gonococcal arthritis is much more common in the USA than in the UK. Br J Rheumatol. 1990;29:283.
34. Rompalo AM, Hook EW, Roberts PL, et al. The acute arthritis-dermatitis syndrome. The changing importance of *Neisseria gonorrhoeae* and *Neisseria meningitidis*. Arch Intern Med. 1987;147:281–283.
35. Resnick D, Pineda CJ, Weisman MH, et al. Osteomyelitis and septic arthritis of the hand following human bites. Skeletal Radiol. 1985;14:263–266.
36. Ewing R, Fainstein V, Musher DM, et al. Articular and skeletal infections caused by *Pasteurella multocida*. South Med J. 1980;73:1349–1352.
37. Holroyd KJ, Reiner AP, Dick JD. *Streptobacillus moniliformis* polyarthritis mimicking rheumatoid arthritis: An urban case of rat bite fever. Am J Med. 1988;85:711–714.
38. Goldings EA, Jericho J. Lyme disease. Clin Rheum Dis. 1986;12:343–367.
39. Khateeb MI, Araj GF, Majeed SA, Lulu AR. Brucella arthritis: A study of 96 cases in Kuwait. Ann Rheum Dis. 1990;49:994–998.
40. Luttrell LM, Kanj SS, Corey GR, et al. *Mycoplasma hominis* septic arthritis: Two case reports and review. Clin Infect Dis. 1994;19:1067–1070.
41. Meier JL. Mycobacterial and fungal infections of bone and joints. Curr Opin Rheumatol. 1994;6:408–414.
42. Atkin SL, El-Ghobarey A, Kamel M, et al. Clinical and laboratory studies of arthritis in leprosy. Br Med J. 1989;298:1423–1425.
43. Bayer AS, Scott VJ, Guze LB. Fungal arthritis. III. Sporotrichal arthritis. Semin Arthritis Rheum. 1979;9:66–74.
44. Bayer AS, Guze LB. Fungal arthritis. II. Coccidioidal synovitis: Clinical, diagnostic, therapeutic, and prognostic considerations. Semin Arthritis Rheum. 1979;8:200–211.
45. Amstalden EM, Xavier R. Paracoccidioidomycosis of bones and joints. A clinical, radiological and pathological study of 9 cases. Medicine. 1996;75:213–225.
46. Tingle AJ, Allen M, Petty RE, et al. Rubella-associated arthritis. I. Comparative study of joint manifestations associated with natural rubella infection and RA 27/3 rubella immunization. Ann Rheum Dis. 1986;45:110–114.
47. Garcia-Tapia AM, Fernandez-Gutierrez C, Giron JA, et al. Spectrum of parvovirus B19 infection: Analysis of an outbreak of 43 cases in Cadiz, Spain. Clin Infect Dis. 1995;21:1424–1430.
48. Gordon SC, Lauter CB. Mumps arthritis: A review of the literature. Rev Infect Dis. 1984;6:388–444.
49. Naides SJ. Viral arthritis including HIV. Curr Opin Rheumatol. 1995;7:337–342.
50. Niklasson B, Espmark A, Lundstrom J. Occurrence of arthralgia and specific IgM antibodies three to four years after Ockelbo disease. J Infect Dis. 1988;157:832–835.
51. Fraser JRE. Epidemic polyarthritis and Ross River virus disease. Clin Rheum Dis. 1986;12:369–388.
52. Phillips DA, Murray JR, Aaskov JG, et al. Clinical and subclinical Barmah Forest virus infection in Queensland. Med J Aust. 1990;152:463–466.
53. Sato K, Maruyama I, Maruyama Y, et al. Arthritis in patients infected with human T lymphotropic virus type I. Clinical and immunopathologic features. Arthritis Rheum. 1991;34:714–721.
54. Monteagudo I, Rivera J, Lopez-Longo J, et al. AIDS and rheumatic manifestations in patients addicted to drugs. An analysis of 106 cases. J Rheumatol. 1991;18:1038–1041.
55. Salfield S. Filarial arthritis in the Sepik District of Papua New Guinea. Med J Aust. 1975;1:264–267.
56. Kamal M, Safwat E, Eltayeb S. Bilharzial arthropathy. Scand J Rheumatol. 1989;18:315–319.
57. Baer PA, Tenenbaum J, Fam AG, et al. Coexistent septic and crystal arthritis. Report of four cases and literature review. J Rheumatol. 1986;13:604–607.
58. Syrogiannopoulos GA, Nelson JD. Duration of antimicrobial therapy for acute suppurative osteoarticular infections. Lancet. 1988;1:37–40.
59. Nelson JD. Antibiotic concentration in septic joint effusions. N Engl J Med. 1971;284:349–353.
60. Sattar MA, Barrett SP, Cawley MID. Concentrations of some antibiotics in synovial fluid after oral administration, with special reference to antistaphylococcal activity. Ann Rheum Dis. 1983;42:67–74.
61. Smith RL, Schurman DJ, Kajiyama G, et al. The effect of antibiotics on the destruction of cartilage in experimental infectious arthritis. J Bone Joint Surg. 1987;69A:1063–1068.

62. Rosenthal J, Giles GB, Robinson WD. Acute nongonococcal infectious arthritis. Evaluation of risk factors, therapy, and outcome. Arthritis Rheum. 1980;23:889–897.
63. Parisien JS, Shafer B. Arthroscopic management of pyoarthrosis. Clin Orthop. 1992;275:243–247.
64. Cooper C, Cawley MID. Bacterial arthritis in the elderly. Gerontology. 1986;32:222–227.
65. McGuire NM, Kauffman CA. Septic arthritis in the elderly. J Am Geriatr Soc. 1985;33:170–174.
66. Howard JG, Highgenboten CL, Nelson JD. Residual effects of septic arthritis in infancy and childhood. JAMA. 1976;236:932–935.
67. Armstrong RW, Bolding F, Joseph R. Septic arthritis following arthroscopy: Clinical syndrome and analysis of risk factors. J Arthrosc. 1992;8:213–223.

Chapter 91

Osteomyelitis

JON T. MADER
JASON CALHOUN

GENERAL CONCEPT OF OSTEOMYELITIS

Bone infections are classified by the system of Waldvogel and colleagues[1–3] as either hematogenous osteomyelitis or osteomyelitis secondary to a contiguous focus of infection. Contiguous-focus osteomyelitis has been further subdivided into osteomyelitis with or without vascular insufficiency. Hematogenous and contiguous-focus osteomyelitis have been further divided into acute or chronic disease. Acute disease presents as a suppurative infection accompanied by edema, vascular congestion, and small vessel thrombosis. In early acute disease, the vascular supply to the bone is compromised by infection extending into the surrounding soft tissue. When both the medullary and periosteal blood supplies are compromised, large areas of dead bone (sequestra) may be formed. Within this necrotic and ischemic tissue, the bacteria may be difficult to eradicate even after an intense host response, surgery, or antibiotic therapy, or all of these. Clinically, acute osteomyelitis evolves into chronic disease. The hallmarks of chronic disease are a nidus of infected dead bone or scar tissue, an ischemic soft tissue envelope, and a refractory clinical course.[4]

The term *cure* is not used in osteomyelitis, since the bone infection may recur years after apparently successful treatment of the disease. If the patient suffers trauma in the involved area or the host response to the infection is suppressed, or both, the organism or organisms may again proliferate and lead to an exacerbation of the infection. Therefore, in osteomyelitis treatment the infection is said to be *arrested* rather than *cured.*

An alternative classification system has been developed by Cierny and Mader.[5, 6] This classification takes into consideration the quality of the host, the anatomic nature of the disease, treatment factors, and prognostic factors (Table 91–1). This staging system combines four anatomic disease types (Fig. 91–1) and three physiologic host categories to define 12 discrete clinical stages of osteomyelitis.

Stage 1, or medullary, osteomyelitis, equates with early hematogenous osteomyelitis in which the primary lesion is endosteal. Pediatric stage 1 usually can be treated with antibiotics alone. Adult stage 1 osteomyelitis is usually treated with cortical unroofing and intramedullary reaming. An infected intramedullary rod in a stable bone is another example of stage 1 osteomyelitis. In this case the infected intramedullary rod must be removed, followed by intramedullary reaming.

We thank Mike Cripps, Mark Shirtliff, and Donna Milner Mader for manuscript research and preparation and Dr. Leonard Swischuk for radiologic interpretation and review.

In stage 2, or superficial, osteomyelitis, the bone infection results from an adjacent soft tissue infection and represents a true contiguous-focus lesion. An exposed, infected necrotic outer surface of the bone lies at the base of a soft tissue wound. Stage 2 osteomyelitis requires superficial débridement and coverage with a local or microvascular flap.

Stage 3, or localized, osteomyelitis is characterized by full-thickness cortical sequestration that can be surgically removed without compromising stability of the infected bone. Stage 3 osteomyelitis requires débridement, saucerization, and possibly a bone graft to improve stability.

Stage 4, or diffuse, osteomyelitis, represents a through and through section of the bone and usually requires segmental resection of the bone. The stage 4 patient may also have bone infection on both sides of a nonunion or a major joint. Diffuse osteomyelitis includes those infections with a loss of bony stability either before or after débridement surgery. Stage 4 osteomyelitis require débridement, dead space management, and stabilization.

In this system, patients are classified as A, B, or C hosts. A hosts are those patients with normal physiologic, metabolic, and immunologic capabilities. B hosts (see Table 91–1) are patients who are locally compromised, systematically compromised, or both. It is important to improve the factors and diseases that made the patient a B host. The goal of host modification is to make a B host as much like an A host as possible. The final category, or C host, represents the patient for whom the treatment of the bone infection is worse than the osteomyelitis itself.

This staging system has been used to determine optimal treatment protocols and prognoses and to compare therapy results between institutions. The stages are dynamic and may be altered by the outcome of therapy or a change in the host's status. The traditional Waldvogel classification system is used throughout this chapter, but references to the Cierny-Mader classification are made when appropriate.

HEMATOGENOUS OSTEOMYELITIS

Primary hematogenous osteomyelitis occurs mainly in infants and children. The metaphyses of the long bones (tibia, femur) are most

TABLE 91–1 Cierny and Mader Classification System

Anatomic type
Stage 1, medullary osteomyelitis
Stage 2, superficial osteomyelitis
Stage 3, localized osteomyelitis
Stage 4, diffuse osteomyelitis
Physiologic class
A host: normal host
B host:
Systemic compromise (Bs)
Local compromise (Bl)
C host: treatment worse than disease
Systemic or local factors that affect immune surveillance, metabolism, and local vascularity
Systemic (Bs)
Malnutrition
Renal, liver failure
Diabetes mellitus
Chronic hypoxia
Immune disease
Malignancy
Extremes of age
Immunosuppression or immune deficiency
Tobacco abuse
Local (Bl)
Chronic lymphedema
Venous stasis
Major vessel compromise
Arteritis
Extensive scarring
Radiation fibrosis
Small vessel disease
Complete loss of local sensation

FIGURE 91–1. Anatomic classification of adult long bone osteomyelitis, etiology, and treatment. *Abbreviation:* ORIF, Orthopedic rod internal fixation.

Stage I (Medullary Osteomyelitis)

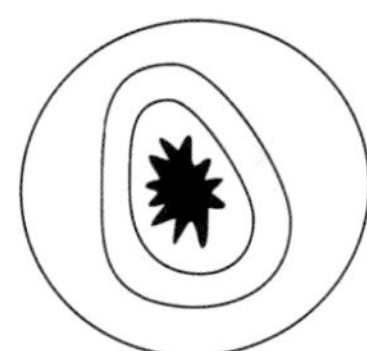

Necrosis limited to medullary contents and endosteal surfaces.
Etiology: Hematogenous
Treatment:
Early: Antibiotics/ Host alteration
Late: Unroofing, intramedullary reaming

Stage II (Superficial Osteomyelitis)

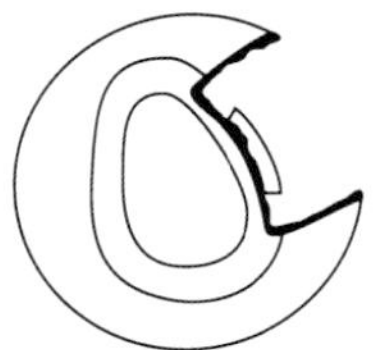

Necrosis limited to exposed surfaces.
Etiology: Contiguous soft tissue infection
Treatment:
Early: Antibiotics/ Host alteration
Late: Superficial debridement/ Coverage
Possible ablation

Stage III (Localized Osteomyelitis)

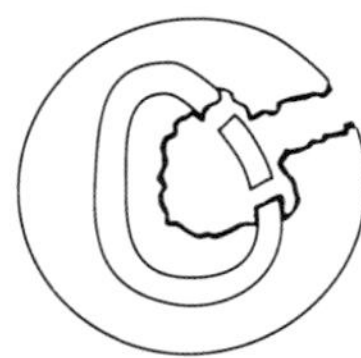

Well marginated and stable before and after debridement.
Etiology: Trauma, evolving stages I and II, Iatrogenic
Treatment:
Antibiotics/ Host alteration
Debridement, Dead space management
Temporary stabilization, Bone graft optional

Stage IV (Diffuse Osteomyelitis)

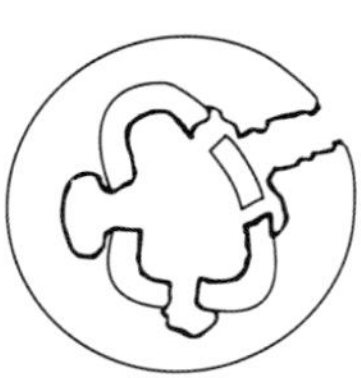

Circumferential and/or permeative.
Unstable prior to or after debridement
Etiology: Trauma, evolving stages I and II and III, Iatrogenic
Treatment:
Antibiotics/ Host alteration
Stabilization - ORIF, External fixation (Ilizarov)
Debridement, Dead space management
Possible ablation

frequently involved (Fig. 91–2). The anatomy of the metaphyseal region seems to explain this clinical localization.[7] Nonanastamosing capillary ends of the nutrient artery make sharp loops under the growth plate and enter a system of large venous sinusoids where the blood flow becomes slow and turbulent. These capillary loops are essentially "end-artery" branches of the nutrient artery. Any end-capillary obstruction can lead to an area of avascular necrosis. The metaphyseal capillaries lack phagocytic lining cells, and sinusoidal veins contain functionally inactive phagocytic cells.[8] The infant or child is predisposed to infection by minor trauma that produces a small hematoma, vascular obstruction, and subsequent bone necrosis. The area is then susceptible to inoculation from a transient bacteremia.[9] The acute infection initially produces a local cellulitis that results in an infiltration with leukocytes, increased bone pressure, decreased pH, and decreased oxygen tension. The cumulative effects of these physiologic factors further compromise the medullary circulation and enhance the spread of infection. The infection may proceed laterally through the haversian and Volkmann canal systems, perforate the bony cortex, and lift the periosteum from the surface of the bone. When this occurs in the presence of medullary extension, both the periosteal and endosteal circulations are lost, and large segments of dead cortical and cancellous bone are formed. In the infant, medullary infection may spread to the epiphysis and joint surfaces through capillaries that cross the growth plate. In the child older than 1 year, since the growth plate is avascular, the infection is confined to the metaphysis and diaphysis. The joint is spared unless the metaphysis is intracapsular. Thus, cortical perforation at the proximal radius, humerus, or femur infects the elbow, shoulder, or hip joint, respectively, regardless of the age of the patient.

Primary hematogenous osteomyelitis is also found in the adult population. The infection usually begins in the diaphysis but may spread to involve the entire medullary canal (Fig. 91–3). Extension into the joint may occur since the growth plate has matured and once again shares vessels with the metaphysis. As the periosteum is firmly adherent to the bone, cortical penetration usually leads to a soft tissue abscess. In time, sinus tracts connecting the sequestered nidus of infection to the skin via soft tissue extension may form.

Secondary hematogenous infections in adults are more common and represent reactivation of a quiescent focus of hematogenous osteomyelitis initially developed in infancy or childhood. Secondary hematogenous osteomyelitis in adults generally has a metaphyseal localization.

A single pathogenic organism is almost always recovered from the bone. In infants, *Staphylococcus aureus*, *Streptococcus agalac-*

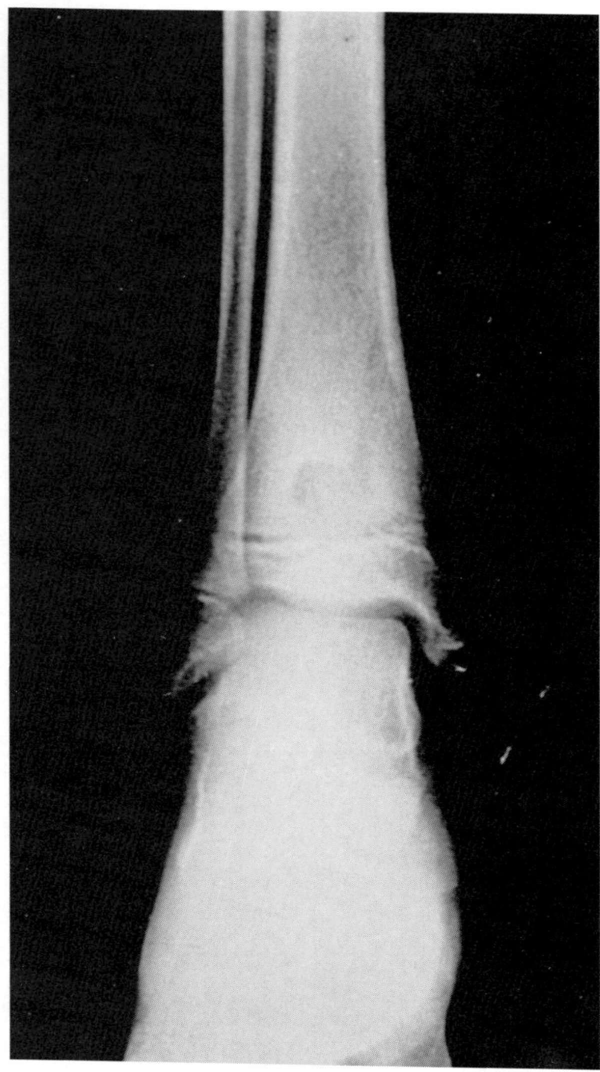

FIGURE 91–2. Hematogenous osteomyelitis in a child. There is bony involvement with lytic changes in the metaphysis of the distal tibia.

tiae, and *Escherichia coli* are most frequently isolated from blood or bones, whereas in children older than 1 year, *Staph. aureus, Streptococcus pyogenes*, and *Haemophilus influenzae* are most commonly isolated. The incidence of *H. influenzae* infection decreases after the age of 4 years. However, the overall incidence of *H. influenzae* as a cause of osteomyelitis is decreasing because of the new *H. influenzae* vaccine now given to children.[10] In adults, *S. aureus* is the most common organism isolated.

Neonatal osteomyelitis is characterized by a paucity of systemic and local findings.[11] Local findings include edema and decreased motion of a limb. A joint effusion adjacent to the bone infection is present in approximately 60% of the patients.

Children with hematogenous osteomyelitis may present with abrupt fever, irritability, lethargy, and local signs of inflammation 3 weeks or less in duration.[12] However, 50% of children present with vague complaints, including pain of the involved limb 1–3 months in duration and minimal if any temperature elevation.

Infants and children with hematogenous osteomyelitis usually have normal soft tissue enveloping the infected bone and are capable of a very efficient metabolic response to infection. Therefore, children have the potential to resorb large sequestra and generate a significant periosteal response to the infection. This latter feature leads to substantial formation of bone formed at the margin of the infection (involucrum). The involucrum affords skeletal continuity and the maintenance of function during the healing phase. If antimicrobial therapy directed at the responsible pathogen is begun before extensive bone necrosis, the patient has an excellent probability of disease arrest.

Adults usually present with vague complaints consisting of nonspecific pain and few constitutional symptoms 1–3 months in duration. However, acute clinical presentations with fever, chills, swelling, and erythema over the involved bone or bones are occasionally seen.

VERTEBRAL OSTEOMYELITIS

Pyogenic vertebral osteomyelitis is usually hematogenous in origin. An arterial route rather than Batson's venous plexus is believed to be the most likely route of infection.[13] The segmental arteries supplying the vertebrae usually bifurcate to supply two adjacent bony segments.[14, 15] Therefore, the disease usually involves two adjacent vertebrae and the intervertebral disk. In the normal host, *S. aureus* remains the most commonly isolated organism.[16] However, in intravenous drug users, *Pseudomonas aeruginosa* is the most commonly isolated organism.[17, 18] Other sources of infection include the genitourinary tract, skin and soft tissue, respiratory tract, infected intravenous sites, endocarditis, dental infection, or unknown sources.[19–21]

Localized pain and tenderness of the involved bone segments are present in at least 90% of the patients. The pain is usually insidious and slowly progresses over 3 weeks to 3 months.

Fever and peripheral leukocytosis are absent in approximately 50% of the patients. The erythrocyte sedimentation rate is usually elevated and may be used as a prognostic guide during treatment. Posterior extension of the infection may lead to epidural and subdural abscesses or even to meningitis. Extension anteriorly or laterally may lead to paravertebral, retropharyngeal, mediastinal, subphrenic, or retroperitoneal abscesses. Motor and sensory neurologic defects can be detected in 6 to 15% of the patients.[16] The lumbar region is affected in at least 45% of the patients with hematogenous vertebral osteomyelitis, followed by the thoracic spine (35%) and the cervical spine (20%).[13]

CONTIGUOUS-FOCUS OSTEOMYELITIS WITHOUT GENERALIZED VASCULAR INSUFFICIENCY

In contiguous-focus osteomyelitis, the organisms may be directly inoculated into the bone at the time of trauma, spread by nosocomial contamination during perioperative or intraoperative procedures, or extend from an adjacent soft tissue infection (Fig. 91–4). Common predisposing factors include surgical reduction and internal fixation of fractures, prosthetic devices, open fractures, and chronic soft tissue infections. In contrast to hematogenous osteomyelitis, multiple organisms are usually isolated from the infected bone. *S. aureus* remains the most commonly isolated pathogen. However, gram-negative bacilli and anaerobic organisms are frequently isolated.

The infection usually occurs within 1 month after inoculation of the organism from trauma, surgery, or a soft tissue infection. The patient presents with low-grade fever, pain, and drainage. Loss of bone stability, bone necrosis, and soft tissue damage frequently occur, making this form of osteomyelitis difficult to treat.

CONTIGUOUS-FOCUS OSTEOMYELITIS WITH GENERALIZED VASCULAR INSUFFICIENCY

The majority of the patients in this category of osteomyelitis have diabetes mellitus. The small bones of the feet are commonly involved in this type of infection (Figs. 91–5, 91–6*A–C*). Blunting of the local tissue response because of inadequate tissue perfusion predisposes the patient to infection. Commonly, the infection is initiated by minor

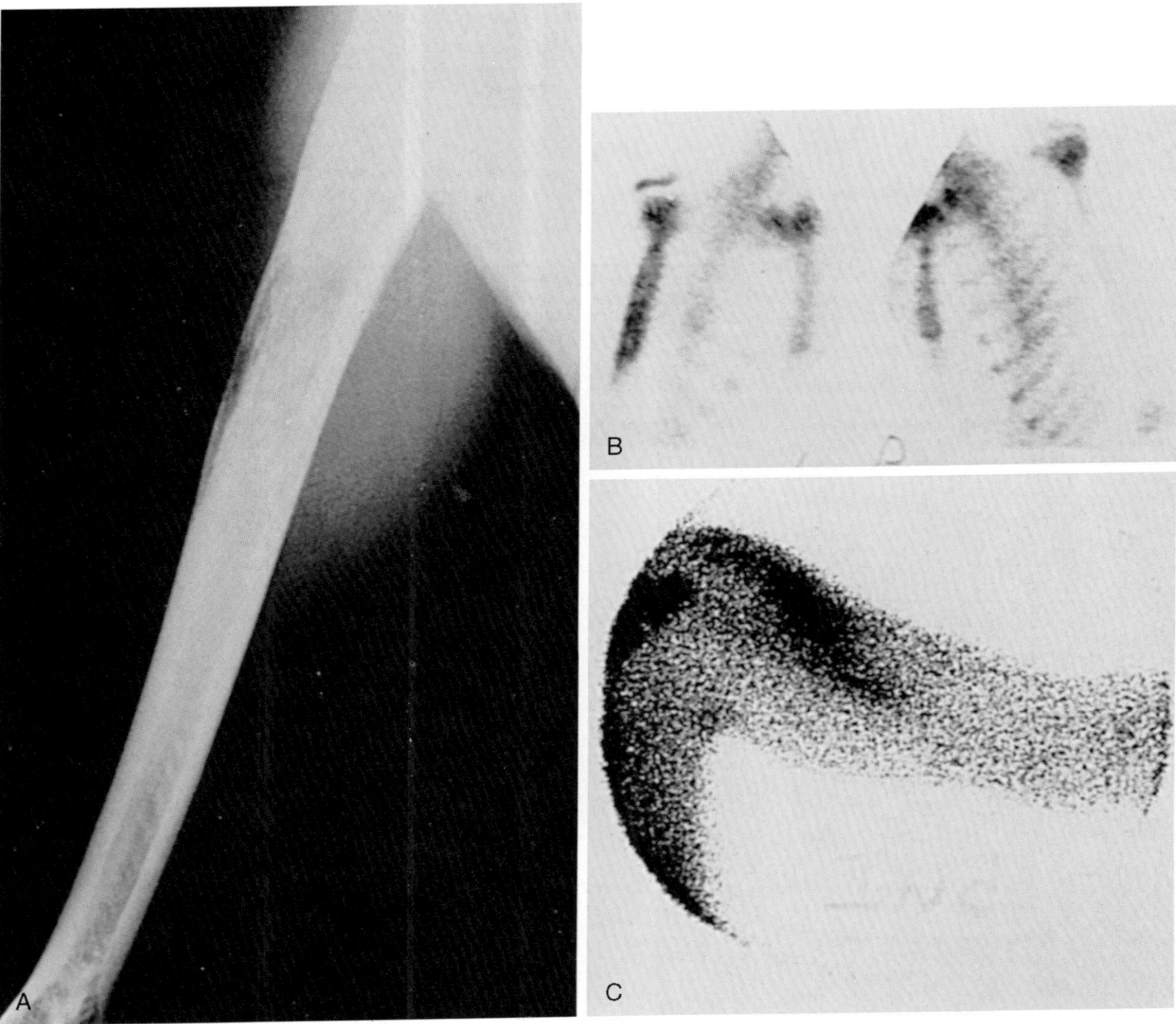

FIGURE 91–3. *A*, Hematogenous osteomyelitis in the diaphysis of the humerus of a 28-year-old man. There is involvement of the intramedullary canal with cortical extension to the periosteum and soft tissue. *B*, ^{99m}Technetium polyphosphate scan showing involvement of the humerus. In our experience the technetium scan tends to show more bony involvement than is surgically present. Minor trauma may also cause a positive technetium scan result. *C*, Indium chloride scan showing involvement of the intramedullary canal of the humerus with extension to the adjacent soft tissue.

trauma of the feet. Multiple organisms are usually isolated from the infected bone. The most common organisms are coagulase-positive and -negative staphylococci, *Streptococcus* spp., *Enterococcus* spp., gram-negative bacilli, and anaerobes. Aerobic gram-negative bacilli are usually a part of a mixed infection.

Osteomyelitis in vascularly compromised patients can be difficult to diagnose. The patient may present with an ingrown toenail, a perforating foot ulcer, cellulitis, or a deep space infection. Concurrent peripheral neuropathy mutes the patient's perception of pain. Fever and systemic toxicity are often absent. Examination shows decreased dorsalis pedis and posterior tibial pulses, poor capillary refill, and decreased sensation. Osteomyelitis should be considered to be present when bone is exposed in the ulcer bed either before or after débridement or if probing the ulcer encounters bone. Radiologic evidence of osteomyelitis is a late finding.

Although arrest of the infection is desirable, a more attainable treatment goal is to suppress the infection and maintain the functional integrity of the involved limb. Recurrent or new bone infections occur in the majority of the patients even after appropriate treatment. Resection of the infected area is almost always necessary.

CHRONIC OSTEOMYELITIS

Both hematogenous and contiguous-focus osteomyelitis can progress to a chronic condition. Local bone loss, persistent drainage, sinus tracts, or all of these, are common.[22] The nidus of the persistent contamination must be removed before the infection will start to regress. Antibiotic therapy alone is usually unsuccessful in the treatment of chronic osteomyelitis. Prospects of arresting the infection are reduced when the integrity of surrounding soft tissue is poor, the bone is unstable secondary to an infected nonunion, or there is an adjacent septic joint.

The patient usually presents with chronic pain and drainage. If present, fever is low grade. The sedimentation rate is usually elevated, reflecting chronic inflammation, but the leukocyte count is usually normal. The chronic disease is usually nonprogressive or

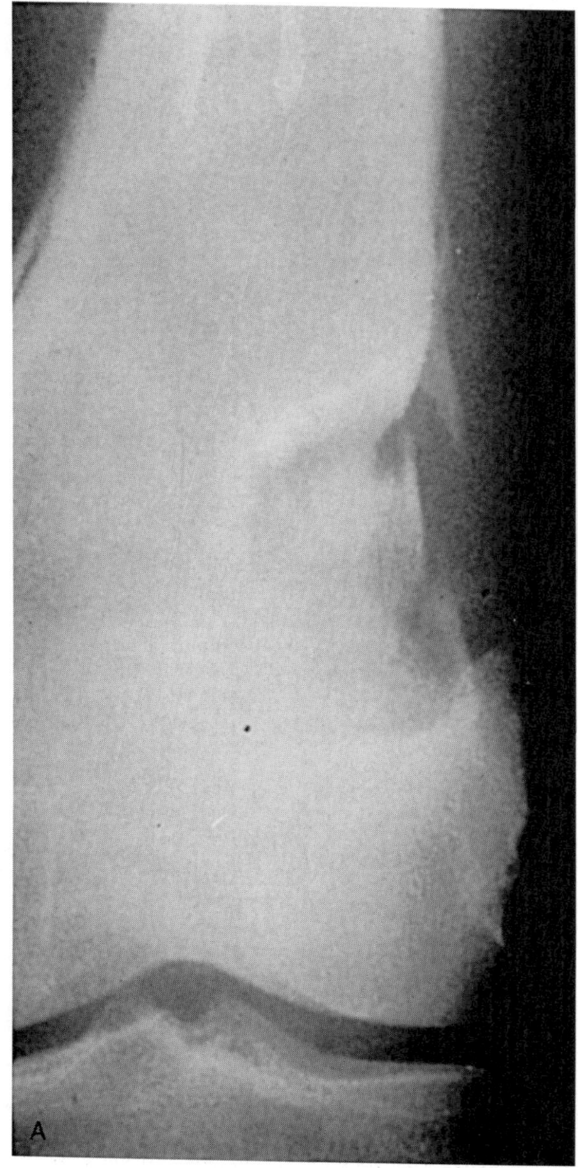

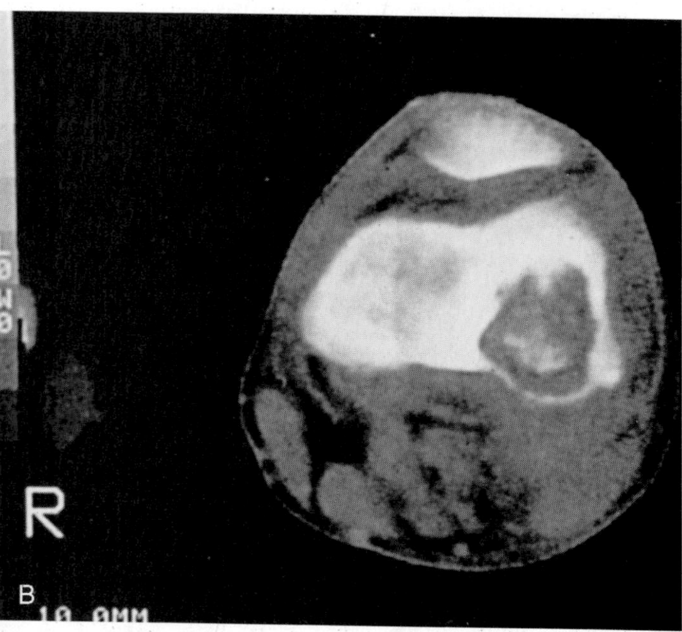

FIGURE 91–4. *A*, Contiguous focus osteomyelitis in a 20-year-old man. The radiograph shows a large sequestrum in the distal femur. *B*, A computed tomography scan showing the large sequestrum in the distal femur. The femur was saucerized, and the resulting defect was bone grafted.

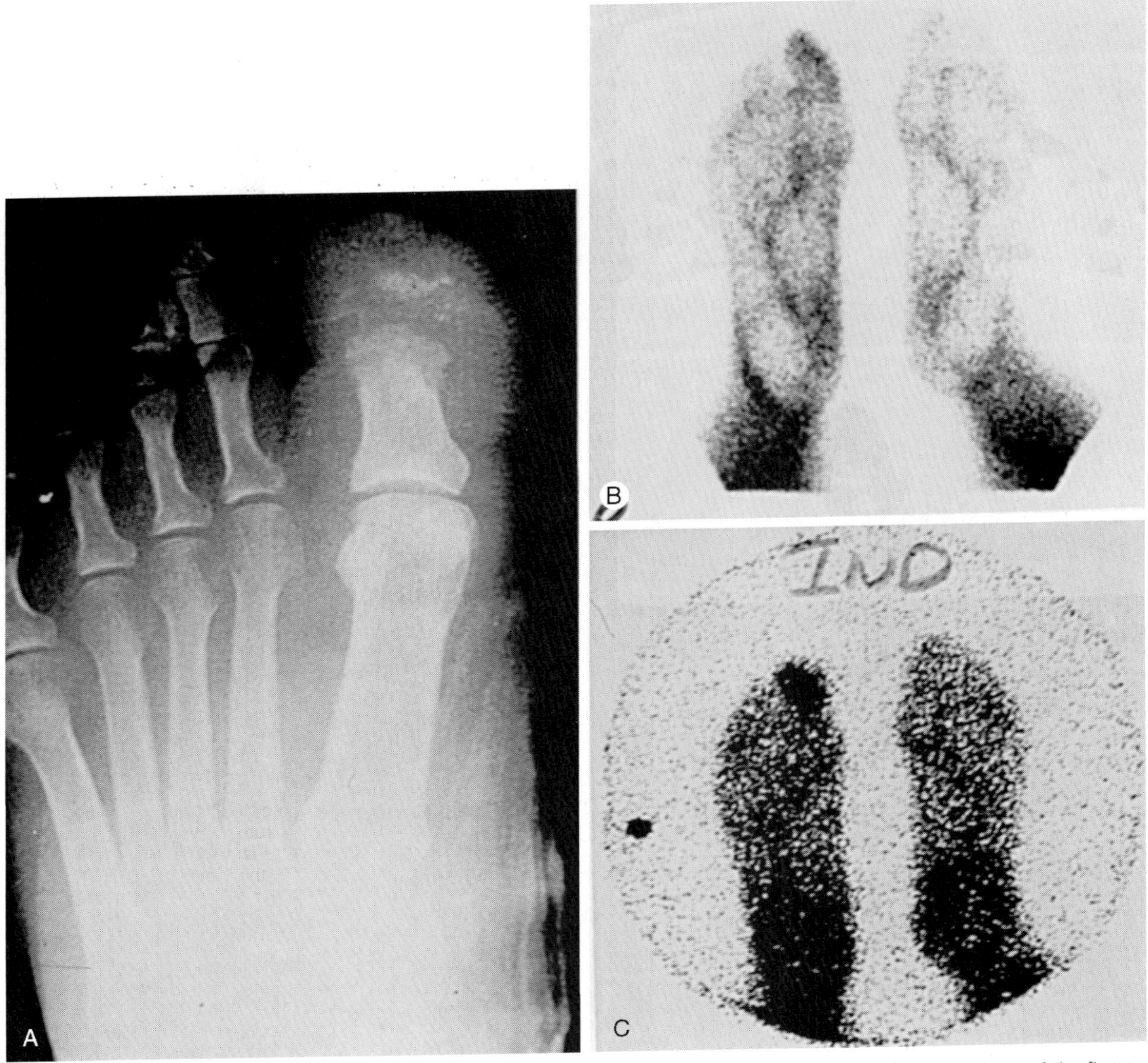

FIGURE 91–5. *A*, Contiguous focus osteomyelitis in a 40-year-old man with diabetes mellitus. The proximal and distal phalanges of the first toe around the proximal interphalangeal joint show bony destruction. *B*, A 3-minute ^{99m}technetium polyphosphate scan (venous pool) of the first toe showing increased uptake consistent with osteomyelitis. *C*, Indium chloride scan showing increased uptake in the bones of the first toe. The indium scan is consistent with (inflammation) osteomyelitis of the first toe. Comparison of the technetium and indium scans supports osteomyelitis of the first toe. A more diffuse pattern on both scans would suggest a soft tissue process.

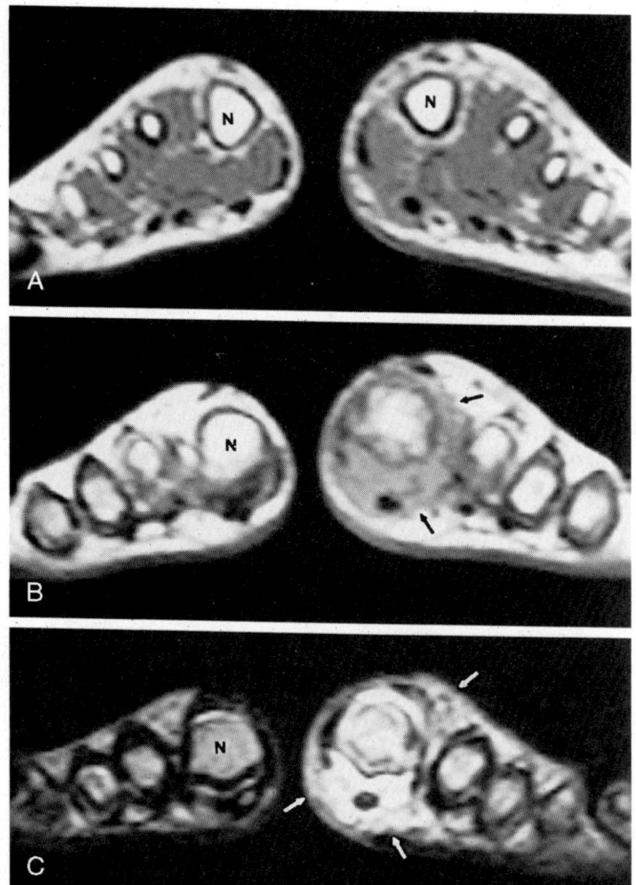

FIGURE 91–6. *A*, Bilateral first metatarsals demonstrate normal high signal (N) of fatty marrow on this T_1-weighted image. *B*, T_1-weighted image. On the normal side (N) high signal remains but the signal through the bone marrow on the abnormal side is altered and expanded. Furthermore, the surrounding low signal cortex is irregular. The metatarsal is also surrounded by a wide rim of low signal edema (*arrows*). The black oval inferiorly is the tendon. *C*, T_2-weighted image demonstrates that the normal fatty marrow (N) now loses its signal, but on the abnormal side high signal is present in the marrow signifying that it has been replaced by purulent exudate. In addition, the surrounding edema and inflammatory process (*arrows*) now produce high signal.

slowly progressive. If a sinus tract becomes obstructed, the patient may present with a localized abscess or a soft tissue infection or both. Squamous cell carcinoma at the site of tissue drainage and amyloidosis are rare complications of chronic osteomyelitis.

DIAGNOSIS OF OSTEOMYELITIS

The diagnosis of long bone osteomyelitis rests on the obligatory isolation of the pathogen from the bone lesion or blood culture. In hematogenous osteomyelitis, positive blood cultures can often obviate the need for a bone biopsy when there is radiographic evidence of osteomyeiitis.

Sinus tract cultures are reliable for *S. aureus* but not for predicting gram-negative organisms causing osteomyelitis.[23, 24] In most cases, antibiotic treatment of osteomyelitis should be based on meticulous cultures taken at débridement surgery or from deep bone biopsies and antibiotic susceptibility tests.[4]

Sedimentation rates and leukocyte counts are frequently elevated before therapy in acute disease, but the leukocyte count rarely exceeds 15,000/mm³, and it is usually normal in patients with chronic osteomyelitis. Elevated sedimentation rates and leukocyte counts may fall with appropriate therapy. However, both values may elevate acutely around each débridement surgery. A sedimentation rate that returns to normal during the course of therapy is a favorable prognostic sign. However, in the compromised host, this laboratory determination is not reliable since these patients are constantly challenged by minor illnesses and peripheral lesions that may elevate this index.

Diagnosis of Long Bone Osteomyelitis

Radiograph Studies

In acute hematogenous osteomyelitis, radiographic changes accurately reflect the destructive process but lag at least 2 weeks behind the evolution of infection. The earliest changes are swelling of the soft tissue, periosteal thickening or elevation, or both, and focal osteopenia (see Figs. 91–2 and 91–3*A*). At least 50 to 75% of the bone matrix must be destroyed before radiographs show lytic changes (Fig. 91–7*A*). The more diagnostic lytic changes are delayed and often associated with an indolent infection of several months' duration. Radiographic improvement may lag behind clinical recovery, even when the patient is receiving appropriate antimicrobial therapy.[25] In contiguous-focus and chronic osteomyelitis, the radiographic changes are subtle, often found in association with other nonspecific radiographic findings, and require a careful clinical correlation to achieve diagnostic significance (see Figs. 91–4*A* and 91–5*A*).

Radionuclide Studies

Radionuclide scans may be obtained when the diagnosis of osteomyelitis is ambiguous or to help gauge the extent of bone and soft tissue inflammation. In general, it is not usually necessary to obtain these scans for the diagnosis of long bone osteomyelitis. The actual mechanism of bone labeling with radiopharmaceuticals is still unclear. The technetium Tc 99 m polyphosphate scan demonstrates increased isotope accumulation in areas of increased blood flow and reactive new bone formation (see Figs. 91–3*B* and 91–5*B*).[26] In biopsy-confirmed cases of hematogenous osteomyelitis, it is usually positive as early as 48 hours after the initiation of the bone infection.[27] Negative ^{99m}Tc scans in documented cases of osteomyelitis may reflect impaired blood supply to the infected area.[28]

A second class of radiopharmaceuticals used for the evaluation of osteomyelitis includes gallium citrate. Gallium attaches to transferrin, which leaks from the blood stream into areas of inflammation. The gallium scan also shows increased isotope uptake in areas concentrating polymorphonuclear leukocytes, macrophages, and malignant tumors.[29] Since the gallium citrate scan does not show bone detail well, it is often difficult to distinguish between bone and soft tissue inflammation; a comparison with a ^{99m}Tc scan helps to resolve this problem (see Figs. 91–3*B* and 91–5*B*).[30] Gallium citrate is found to accumulate in areas of reactive bone.[29]

Indium-labeled leukocyte scans are less useful in the evaluation of osteomyelitis. Indium leukocyte scans are positive in approximately 40% of patients with acute osteomyelitis and 60% of patients with septic arthritis.[31] Patients who have chronic osteomyelitis, bony metastases, and degenerative arthritis often have negative scans.

Computed Tomography

Computed axial tomography (CT) may play a role in the diagnosis of osteomyelitis. Increased marrow density occurs early in the infection,[32] and intramedullary gas has been reported in patients with hematogenous osteomyelitis.[33] The CT scan can also help to identify areas of necrotic bone and to assess the involvement of the surrounding soft tissues (see Fig. 91–4*B*). In a recalcitrant infection, the CT scan may assist in identifying the surgical approach and augment débridement.[32, 34] One disadvantage of this study is the scatter phe-

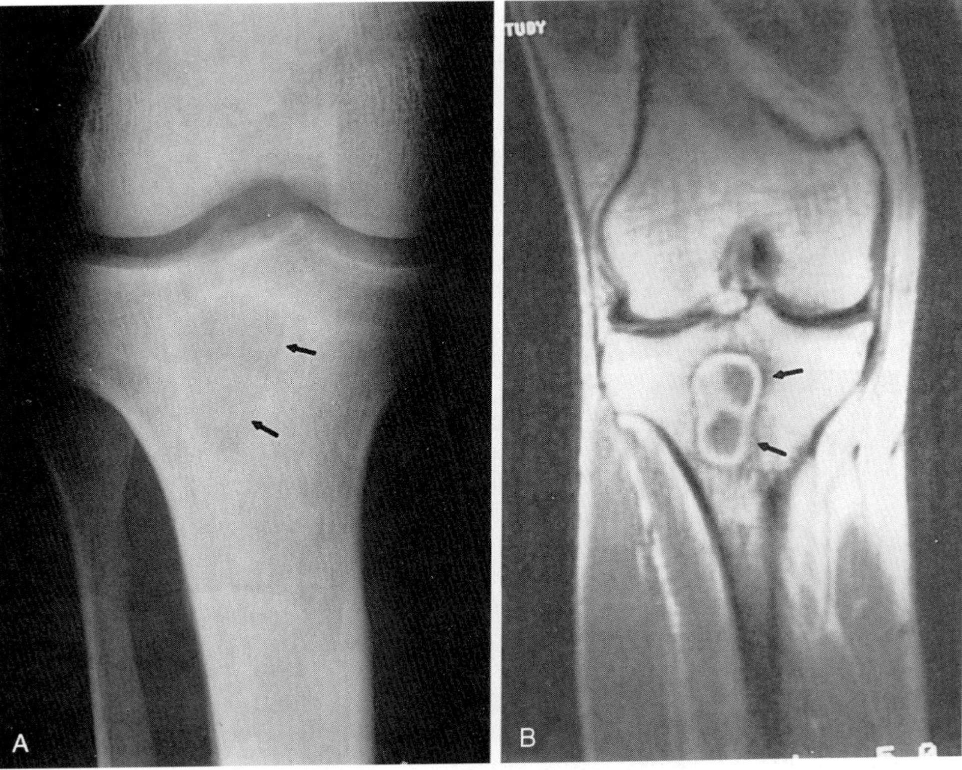

FIGURE 91–7. *A*, Note the typical lytic lesion (*arrows*) in the upper tibia. *B*, A magnetic resonance T_1-weighted image with contrast demonstrates the area of osteomyelitis (*arrows*). The central two lobules show abnormal low signal, but the normal fatty marrow in the surrounding upper tibia shows high signal. A high signal enhancing rim is seen around the lesion.

nomenon, which occurs when metal is present in or near the area of bone infection. This scatter results in a significant loss of image resolution.

Magnetic Resonance Imaging

Magnetic resonance imaging (MRI) has been recognized as a useful modality for diagnosing the presence and scope of musculoskeletal sepsis.[35–37] The spatial resolution of MRI makes it useful in differentiating between bone and soft tissue infection, often a problem with radionuclide studies.[38] Unlike the radionuclide studies, MRI is not useful for whole-body examinations. Metallic implants in the region of interest may produce focal artifacts, thereby decreasing the utility of the image.[39] Initial MRI screening usually consists of a T_1-weighted and a T_2-weighted spin-echo pulse sequence. In a T_1-weighted study, edema is dark and fat is bright. In a T_2-weighted study, the reverse is true. The typical appearance of osteomyelitis is a localized area of abnormal marrow with decreased signal intensity on T_1-weighted images and increased signal intensity on T_2-weighted images (see Figs 91–6*A*, *B*, and 6*C* and 91–7*B*). On occasion, there may be decreased signal intensity on T_2-weighted images.[39] Post-traumatic or surgical scarring of the marrow is seen as a region of decreased signal intensity on T_1-weighted images with no change of the T_2-weighted image. Sinus tracts are seen as areas of high signal intensity on the T_2-weighted image extending from the marrow and bone through the soft tissues and out of the skin. Cellulitis is seen as diffuse areas of intermediate signal in the T_1-weighted images of the soft tissues, with increased signal on the T_2-weighted images of the same area. Since differentiation of infection from neoplasm on the basis of the MRI may be difficult, clinical and radiographic confirmation is necessary.[39]

Vertebral Osteomyelitis

Anteroposterior and lateral radiographic views of the spine reveal intervertebral disk space narrowing, with destruction and new bone formation at the anterior edge of the vertebral disk (Fig. 91–8*A*). A CT or MRI scan can demonstrate evidence of osteomyelitis before radiographic changes occur, showing early evidence of paravertebral soft tissue swelling and bone destruction (see Fig. 91–8*B* and 8*C*).[40–42]

The technetium Tc 99m polyphosphate scan also can detect spinal abnormalities in the early stages of infection, even before radiographic changes are seen.[43] The gallium scan is difficult to interpret due to the high concentration of hematopoietic tissue in vertebral bodies. However, a positive gallium scan is suggestive of vertebral osteomyelitis.[44]

A definitive diagnosis of vertebral osteomyelitis rests on the isolation of the organism from bone. A bone biopsy is generally required, since blood cultures are usually sterile. The biopsy should be performed under fluoroscopy or CT scan for guidance into the infected areas. In addition to aerobic and anaerobic bacterial cultures, the specimens should be sent for fungal and mycobacterial stains and cultures, as well as histologic examination. If the original cultures are negative, an open surgical biopsy should be performed before empirical antibiotic therapy is started.

TREATMENT

The components of osteomyelitis treatment include evaluation of the patient, staging assessment, the identification and sensitivity of the microorganism or microorganisms, the administration of antibiotics, débridement surgery, dead space management, and, if necessary, stabilization.[4, 45, 46] Reconstruction is considered at the first surgery.

Acute Hematogenous Osteomyelitis

In children, acute hematogenous osteomyelitis is primarily a medical disease. In the adult, débridement surgery, bone unroofing, intramedullary reaming, incision and drainage of soft tissue abscesses, or all of these, are often required. Identification of the causative pathogen

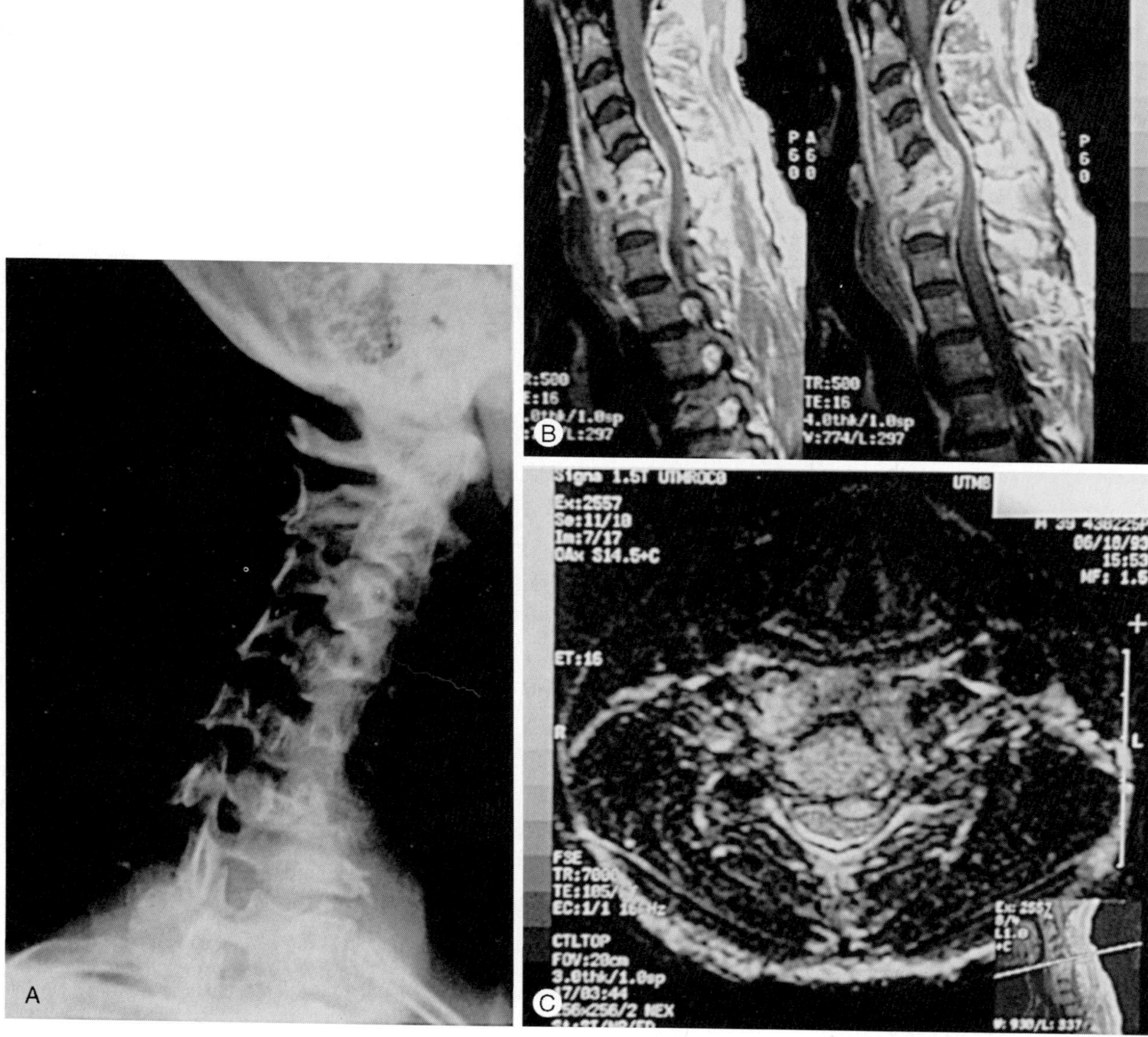

FIGURE 91–8. *A*, Cervical spine film showing involvement of the C5–6, C6–7 cervical vertebral disk spaces. There is destructive involvement of the body of C6. *B*, Magnetic resonance imaging (MRI) showing involvement of C5–6 and C6–7 disk spaces. There is destruction of the body of C6. There is an associated extension of the infection into the prevertebral and epidural areas. *C*, MRI cross-section at C6. There is osteomyelitis of the body of C6 and epidural extension of the infection.

is essential. The infection is usually susceptible to specific antimicrobial therapy. Mismanagement with inappropriate antibiotics encourages extension of disease, necrosis, and sequestra formation. Surgical intervention is indicated if the patient has not responded to specific antimicrobial therapy within 48 hours, has evidence of a persistent soft tissue abscess, or has diagnosed or suspected joint sepsis. A bone biopsy for culture is necessary unless the patient has positive blood cultures along with radiographic findings consistent with osteomyelitis. After samples for culture are obtained, a parenteral antimicrobial regimen is begun to cover the clinically suspected pathogens. Once the organism is identified, the antibiotic regimen may be continued or changed on the basis of sensitivity results.[47] The patient is treated for 4 to 6 weeks with appropriate parenteral antimicrobial therapy, dated from the initiation of therapy or after the last major débridement surgery. If the initial medical management fails and the patient is clinically compromised by a recurrent infection, medullary or soft tissue débridement, or both, will be necessary in conjunction with another 4- to 6-week course of antibiotics.

Oral antibiotic therapy can be utilized for the treatment of childhood osteomyelitis. However, it is recommended that the patient initially receive 2 weeks of parenteral antibiotic therapy before changing to an oral regimen.[48, 49] In addition, the patient must be compliant and have close outpatient follow-up. Absorption and activity of the orally administered antibiotic should be monitored. Pediatric patients should not be given oral antimicrobial therapy with quinolones.[50, 51]

Vertebral Osteomyelitis

Biopsy and débridement cultures dictate the choice of antibiotic or antibiotics. The antibiotics are given for 4 to 6 weeks and are dated from the initiation of therapy or from the last major débridement surgery. Open surgical therapy is usually not necessary, except in cases in which the patient develops an extension of the infection, such as paravertebral or epidural abscesses, when medical management fails, or when instability is pending. Percutaneous transpedicular débridement and diskectomy by removing infected necrotic bone accelerates healing and prevents the progression of bone destruction and deformity in the early stages of vertebral osteomyelitis and spondylodiscitis.[52] The procedure is ineffective in the presence of excessive bone destruction with spinal deformity. The percutaneous transpedicular approach, performed under fluoroscopic guidance, is through a pedicle that is caudal to the affected disk. The approach avoids the exiting nerve roots. Following a Steinmann pin guide, a biopsy tool is passed into the affected disk. The larger lumen allows the passage of various instruments through the biopsy tool.

The neurologic status of the patient must be closely monitored. Surgical fusion of the involved vertebrae is usually not required, as spontaneous bony fusion occurs in 1 to 12 months after appropriate antibiotic therapy. The success of patients treated with bed rest alone is not substantially different from that of those who are ambulatory and stabilized with a cast, a corset, or a brace.

Osteomyelitis Secondary to Contiguous-Focus Infection or Chronic Osteomyelitis

In contiguous-focus and chronic osteomyelitis, the primary problem is infected necrotic bone having a poorly perfused surrounding soft tissue envelope. The infection cannot be arrested until the nidus for the persistent contamination is removed. Adequate drainage, thorough débridement, obliteration of dead space, hardware removal, wound protection, and specific antimicrobial therapy are the mainstays of treatment.[53]

If possible, antibiotic therapy should not be initiated until the results of the bone bacterial culture and sensitivity tests are known. However, if immediate débridement surgery is required, empirical broad-spectrum antibiotic therapy can be started. The antibiotics may be modified, if necessary, when results of the débridement cultures and sensitivity tests are available. Surgical exposure is direct, atraumatic, and designed to avoid unnecessary devitalization of bone and soft tissue. The wound is débrided until all nonviable tissue and superfluous hardware have been removed. To ensure antibiotic perfusion and avoid continued sequestration, the cancellous and cortical bone remaining in the wound after débridement must bleed uniformly.

Since it takes 3 to 4 weeks for bone to revascularize after débridement surgery, antibiotics are used to treat live infected bone and to protect bone undergoing revascularization. The patient is treated with 4 to 6 weeks of antimicrobial therapy dated from the last major débridement surgery.[45, 46] Outpatient intravenous therapy with long-term intravenous access catheters such as the Hickman or Groshong catheters makes outpatient intravenous antibiotic treatment possible.[54–56] Outpatient intramuscular antibiotic administration is also feasible. Oral therapy using quinolones for gram-negative organisms is currently being utilized in adult patients with osteomyelitis.[57–59] The older quinolones (ciprofloxacin, ofloxacin) have poor activity against *Streptococcus* spp., Enterococcus spp., and anaerobic bacteria.[60] Later quinolones (levofloxacin, sparfloxacin) have excellent *Streptococcus* spp. activity but minimal anaerobic coverage.[61] The newest quinolones (trovafloxacin, grepafloxacin) have excellent *Streptococcus* spp. and anaerobic organism coverage.[61, 62] None of the currently available quinolones have reliable *Enterococcus* spp. coverage. The current quinolones have variable *S. aureus* and *Staphylococcus epidermidis* coverage, and resistance to the second-generation quinolones is increasing.[63] For methicillin-sensitive *S. aureus*, oral clindamycin is an alternative. Before changing to an oral regimen, it is recommended that the patient initially receive 2 weeks of parenteral antibiotic therapy and that the organism or organisms be sensitive to the oral regimen. The patient must be compliant and have close outpatient follow-up.

A combination of parenteral and oral antibiotics has been used in some situations. Methicillin-sensitive and methicillin-resistant *S. aureus* osteomyelitis have been successfully treated with a semisynthetic penicillin–rifampin and vancomycin–rifampin, respectively.[64]

In general, it is not necessary to follow antibiotic levels,[65] because most treatment failures are due to a lack of adequate surgical débridement rather than antibiotic efficacy.[45] It may be necessary to follow antibiotic serum levels in cases of relatively resistant organisms.

Appropriate management of any dead space created by débridement surgery is mandatory to arrest the disease and to maintain the integrity of the bone part (Fig. 91–9). The goal of dead space management is to replace dead bone and scar tissue with durable vascularized tissue.[45, 46] Secondary intention healing is discouraged, since the scar tissue that fills the defect may later become avascular. Suction irrigation systems are not recommended because of the high incidence of associated nosocomial infections and the unreliability of these setups.[66, 67] Complete wound closure should be attained whenever possible. Local tissue flaps or free flaps may be used to fill dead space.[68–70] An alternative technique is to place cancellous bone grafts beneath local or transferred tissues where structural augmentation is necessary. Careful preoperative planning is critical to the conservation of the patient's limited cancellous bone reserves. Open cancellous grafts without soft tissue coverage are useful when a free tissue transfer is not a treatment option and local tissue flaps are inadequate.[71] Antibiotic-impregnated acrylic beads may be used to sterilize and temporarily maintain dead space (Fig. 91–10). The beads are usually removed within 2 to 4 weeks and replaced with a cancellous bone graft.[45, 46, 72–77] Antibiotics (clindamycin, amikacin) have also been delivered directly into dead space with an implantable pump.[78]

If movement is present at the site of infection, measures must be taken to achieve permanent stability of the bone. Stability may be achieved with plates, screws, rods, or an external fixator. The Ilizarov external fixator allows bone reconstruction of segmental defects and difficult infected nonunions.[79] The Ilizarov external fixation method uses distraction or compression histogenesis, a process of bone regeneration to fill bone defects or to compress nonunions and correct malunion. In one clinical series,[80] 92% of patients with chronic osteomyelitis with segmental defects, ranging from simple nonunions to 8-cm gaps, were successfully reconstructed. The technique is labor intensive and requires an extended period of treatment averaging 8.5 months in the device. The Ilizarov pins usually become infected, and the device is painful.

Osteomyelitis Secondary to Contiguous-Focus Infection with Vascular Diseases

Because of the relative inability of the host to participate in the eradication of the infectious process, this type of osteomyelitis is difficult to treat. These infections are insidious and are often beyond simple salvage by the time the patient seeks medical therapy.

Determination of the vascular status of the tissue at the infection site is crucial in the evaluation of these patients. Measurement of pulse pressures is one common method. Hyperbaric oxygen therapy may facilitate healing in areas where borderline or low oxygen tensions are present (see Chapter 38).

The patient may be managed with suppressive antibiotic therapy, local débridement surgery, or ablative surgery. The decision regarding treatment options used is based on tissue oxygen perfusion at the infection site, the extent of the osteomyelitis, and the patient's preference.[81–83]

The patient can be offered long-term suppressive antibiotic therapy when a definitive surgical procedure would lead to unacceptable

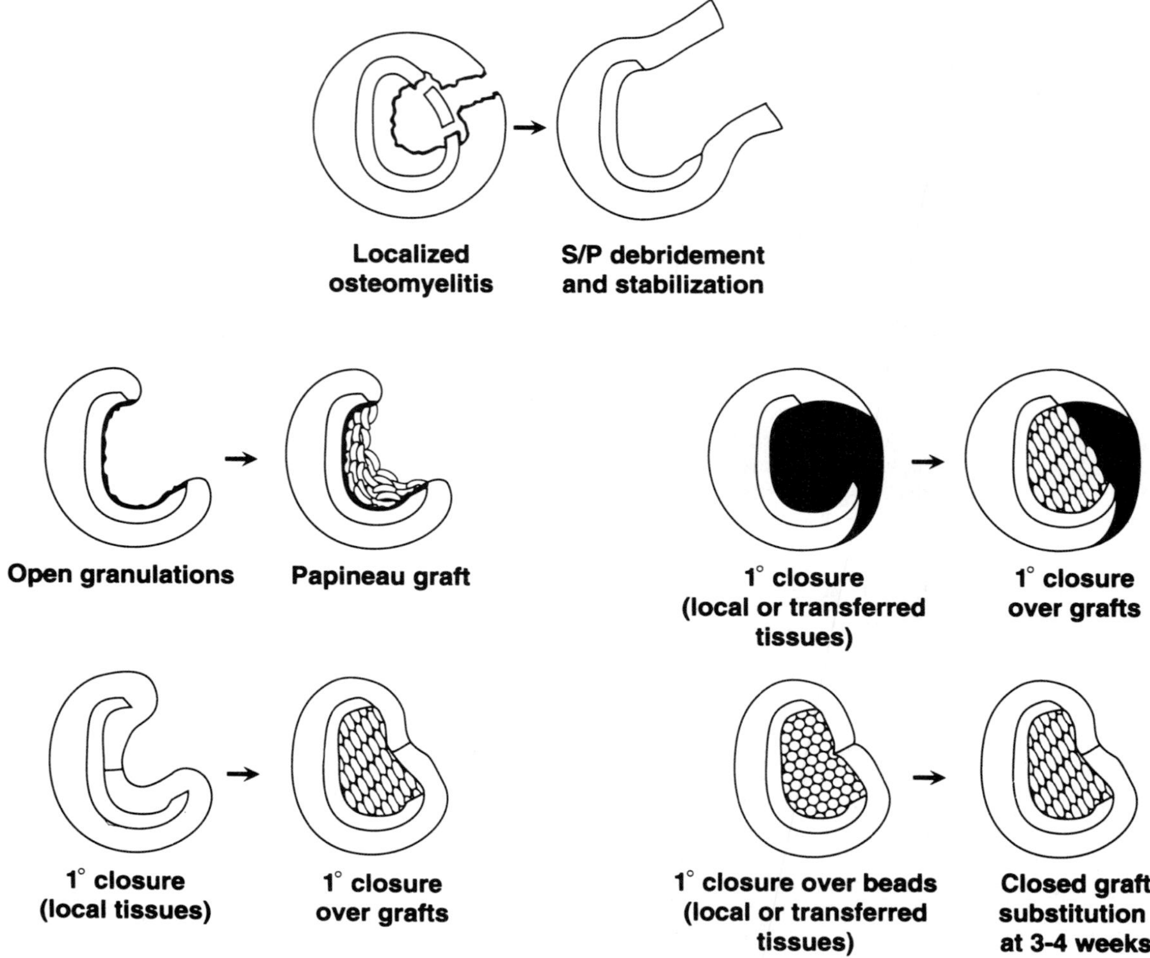

FIGURE 91–9. Dead space management of long bone osteomyelitis.

morbidity or disability or in cases in which the patient refuses local débridement or ablative surgery. Even with suppressive antibiotic therapy, in time, most of these patients require an amputation of the involved bone.

Local débridement surgery and a 4-week course of antibiotics may be employed in the patient who has localized osteomyelitis in the larger bones of the foot and ankle such as the talus, calcaneus, and distal tibia and fibula. Unless good oxygen tensions are present in the area of débridement surgery, the wound will fail to heal and ultimately result in an ablative procedure.

The patient with extensive osteomyelitis and poor tissue oxygen perfusion usually requires some type of ablative surgery. Digital and ray resections (toe and corresponding metatarsal), transmetatarsal amputations, midfoot disarticulations, and Syme's amputations (amputation of the foot with retention of the heel pad) permit the patient to ambulate without a prosthesis. The amputation level is determined by the vascularity of the tissues proximal to the site of infection and the requirements of a thorough débridement. The patient is given 4 weeks of antibiotics when infected bone is surgically transected. Two weeks of antibiotics are given when the infected bone is completely excised, but some residual soft tissue infection remains. When the amputation is performed proximal to the bone and soft tissue infection, the patient is given 1 to 3 days of antibiotic therapy.

Bone Concentrations

Because of the need for prolonged therapy, antibiotics employed in the treatment of bone and joint infection must be nontoxic, convenient to administer, and cost-effective. Bone concentration of the treatment antibiotic may be an important factor in eradicating the organism from the bone. There are still no standardized methods for measuring bone concentrations, but most investigators use an elution technique to recover antibiotic from bone. Using a rabbit model for *S. aureus* osteomyelitis, we found clindamycin to have the greatest bone serum ratio followed by vancomycin, nafcillin, tobramycin, cefazolin, and cephalothin (Table 91–2).[84] The significance of bone antibiotic concentrations is unclear, but clindamycin gave the best treatment results in experimental *S. aureus* osteomyelitis.[85]

Hyperbaric Oxygen Therapy

The results of several open clinical trials have shown that adjunctive hyperbaric oxygen (HBO) therapy (see Chapter 38) may be useful in the treatment of chronic osteomyelitis.[86] Morrey and associates[87] reported on 40 patients with chronic osteomyelitis who met all of the following criteria: the infection had persisted longer than 1 month; at least one surgical débridement had been performed; at least 2 weeks of parenteral antibiotics had been administered; and the patients had been followed for at least 1 year after treatment. All patients had chronic refractory osteomyelitis with a recurrence of this infection despite previous aggressive antibiotic therapy and surgical treatment. After HBO therapy, appropriate surgery, and treatment with antibiotics, 34 patients (85%) remained clinically free of disease, and six experienced recurrences of their osteomyelitis. Using the same criteria, Davis and coworkers[88] evaluated 38 patients who

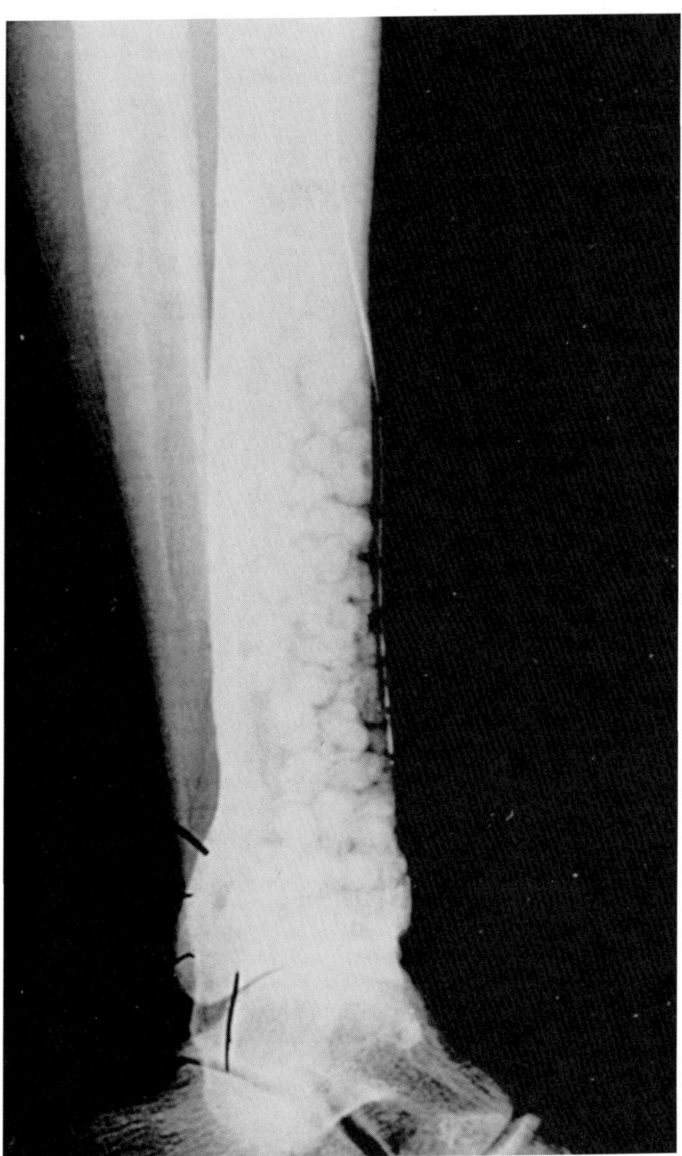

FIGURE 91–10. Osteomyelitis of the distal tibia. Following débridement surgery, antibiotic-impregnated (vancomycin and tobramycin) polymethylmethacrylate (PMMA) beads were placed. The antibiotic-impregnated beads were removed at 3 weeks and the dead space replaced with cancellous bone graft.

were treated with adjunctive HBO. Of these 38 patients, 34 remained free of clinical signs of osteomyelitis. Although the results of these clinical trials are encouraging, the adjunctive role of HBO in the treatment of osteomyelitis is difficult to assess because of the multiple patient, surgical, organism, bone, and antibiotic variables.

Animal studies performed in an experimental *S. aureus* osteomyelitis model have shown that HBO administered under standard treatment conditions was as effective as cephalothin in eradicating *S. aureus* from infected bone.[89] Osteomyelitic bone in this experimental model has decreased blood flow and greatly decreased the partial pressure of oxygen. Hyperoxia did not directly affect this strain of *S. aureus*. HBO was found to restore intramedullary oxygen tensions to physiologic or supraphysiologic tensions but did not acutely increase blood flow in osteomyelitic bone. HBO was effective in *S. aureus* osteomyelitis because it increased intramedullary oxygen to tensions at which phagocytic killing may proceed more efficiently.[90] In a *P. aeruginosa* osteomyelitis model, HBO potentiated the aminoglycoside tobramycin.[91–93]

Wound healing is a dynamic process that requires an adequate oxygen tension to proceed.[94, 95] In the ischemic or infected wound, HBO provides oxygen to promote collagen production, angiogenesis, and ultimately wound healing.

OTHER CLINICAL SITUATIONS

Osteomyelitis in Hemodialysis Patients

Osteomyelitis sometimes occurs as a complication of hemodialysis. Since *S. aureus* and *S. epidermidis* are common blood isolates in hemodialysis patients in whom indwelling cannulae allow portals for bacterial entry, bone infections are probably hematogenous in origin. The ribs and the thoracic vertebral column are the most common sites of involvement. The diagnosis of osteomyelitis is usually made 12 to 72 months after the initiation of hemodialysis. Surgical intervention and antibiotic treatment can result in an arrest of the infection. The infection may not be recognized, as the clinical signs and radiographs may mimic those of renal osteodystrophy.

Osteomyelitis in Patients with Sickle Cell Disease

One large series reviewing sickle cell disease and osteomyelitis reported that 20 of 70 patients with complete hemoglobin defects had at least one hospitalization for the treatment of osteomyelitis during a 10-year period.[96] In essentially all cases, the infecting organisms were gram-negative rods. *Salmonella* spp. accounted for approximately 80% of the gram-negative organisms. In the same hospital series, 1 of 117 patients with normal hemoglobin levels who had osteomyelitis exhibited a *Salmonella* spp. infection of the bone. In a second series of osteomyelitis patients with sickle cell disease, *S. aureus* was the most common pathogen followed by *Salmonella* spp. and *Proteus mirabilis*.[97]

It is often difficult to differentiate thrombotic marrow crisis from osteomyelitis in patients with sickle cell disease. Often a history of bone pain and fever followed in 1 to 2 weeks by the onset of spiking fever, chills, and leukocytosis is suggestive of osteomyelitis after a crisis. Patients with sickle cell disease may present with multiple sites of bone infection. Since the presenting symptoms are often insidious and mimic those of marrow crisis, early cultures of blood and stool offer clues to the correct diagnosis. Presumptive antibiotic therapy in patients suspected of having osteomyelitis should include antibiotics effective against *Salmonella* spp.

TABLE 91–2 Infected Bone Concentrations of Drug after Antibiotic Administration in Experimental *Staphylococcus aureus* Osteomyelitis in Rabbits

Antibiotic (conc. in mg/kg)	Serum (μg/ml)	Infected Bone (μg/g)	Serum (%)
Clindamycin (70)	12.1 ± 0.6	11.9 ± 1.9	98.3
Vancomycin (30)	36.4 ± 4.6	5.3 ± 0.8	14.5
Nafcillin (40)	21.8 ± 4.6	2.1 ± 0.3	9.6
Tobramycin (5)	14.3 ± 1.3	1.3 ± 0.1	9.1
Cefazolin (15)	67.2 ± 2.6	4.1 ± 0.7	6.1
Cefazolin (5)	45.6 ± 3.2	2.6 ± 0.2	5.7

Osteomyelitis in Heroin-Addicted Patients

Osteomyelitis is a complication of intravenous drug addiction.[98–100] Clinical symptoms and signs of infection may be subtle and include localized pain. Fever is often absent. The infection is commonly found in the vertebrae, pubis, and clavicles but may occur in any bone. *S. aureus*, *S. epidermidis*, gram-negative rods, and *Candida* spp. are the most commonly isolated pathogens. Since the initial films are often normal, serial radiographs of the involved area may be necessary. Unless blood cultures are positive along with radiographic evidence of osteomyelitis, bone cultures are mandatory to make a correct bacteriologic diagnosis.

Brodie's Abscess

Brodie's abscess is the name given to a chronic localized bone abscess. Subacute cases may present with fever, pain, and periosteal elevation, whereas chronic cases are often afebrile and present with long-standing dull pain. The most common site of involvement is the distal part of the tibia. The lesion is typically single and located near the metaphysis. About 75% of the patients are less than 25 years of age. Surgical débridement and culture-directed antibiotics are often curative.[101–102]

Diskitis

The question whether the intervertebral disk is the primary seat of a disease or whether its involvement is always secondary to involvement of the bone continues to be debated. [103] It is now known that the intervertebral disk is not an avascular structure.[104] Thus, the disk can be infected by the hematogenous route and also by direct inoculation of organisms. Clinical presentations of diskitis include childhood "diskitis," adult disk space infection, postsurgical disk space infection, and direct infection (trauma) of the intervertebral disk. The management of postsurgical disk space infection and direct infection of the intervertebral disk is comparable to that of vertebral osteomyelitis.

The term *diskitis* is used to describe a usually benign disorder in children that causes intervertebral disk inflammation.[105] It is characterized clinically by severe back pain and radiographically by disk space narrowing and involvement of the adjacent vertebral end plates. A single vertebral space is usually involved. The disease is usually self-limited with a clinical recovery within 72 hours.[106] Complete or partial restoration of the height of the involved disk space is seen in most children within 6 weeks to 1 year.[107] *S. aureus* is the predominant clinical isolate, although many patients have negative cultures. An antecedent viral illness has been noted by some investigators. Primary diskitis occurs in adults. However, adults are not assured of the benign outcome that is associated with childhood disease.[108] Treatment is controversial since most children and many adults improve without antibiotics. Some physicians have advocated withholding antibiotics unless the patient appears systemically ill or a specific organism is recovered or both. If an organism is isolated at biopsy, the patient is treated with 4 to 6 weeks of culture-directed antibiotic therapy.

Skeletal Tuberculosis

Skeletal tuberculosis is the result of hematogenous spread of *Mycobacterium tuberculosis* early in the course of a primary infection. Rarely, skeletal tuberculosis may be a contiguous infection from an adjacent caseating lymph node. If the primary bone infection is not initially arrested, or a quiescent primary bone infection is reactivated, an inflammatory reaction is produced, followed by the development of granulation tissue. The granulation tissue erodes and destroys the cartilage and cancellous bone. Eventually, the infection causes bone demineralization and necrosis. Proteolytic enzymes that can destroy cartilage are not produced in skeletal tuberculosis. Cartilage is destroyed slowly by granulation tissue, preserving the joint or disk space for considerable periods of time. Healing of the infection involves deposition of fibrous tissue. Pain is the most frequent clinical complaint.

Any bone may be involved in skeletal tuberculosis, but the infection usually involves one site. In children or adolescents, the metaphysis of the long bones is most frequently infected. In the adult, the axial skeleton followed by the proximal femur, knee, and small bones of the hands and feet are most often involved. In the axial skeleton, the thoracic vertebral bodies are most frequently infected, followed by the lumbar and cervical vertebral bodies. Vertebral infection usually begins in the anterior portion of a vertebral body and is adjacent to an intervertebral disk. The infection produces destruction of the nearby bone and the intervertebral disk. Adjacent vertebral bodies may become involved, and a paravertebral abscess may develop. Generally, pyogenic osteomyelitis involves the disk early on and produces rapid sclerosis by 3 to 4 months. Tubercular spondylitis progresses slowly, over a period of years. Sixty percent of the patients with skeletal tuberculosis have evidence of extraosseous tuberculosis.[109]

Tissue for culture and histologic examination is almost always required for the diagnosis of skeletal tuberculosis. Cultures for *M. tuberculosis* are positive in approximately 60% of the patients. But since weeks may be required for the growth and identification of the organism,[110, 111] histologic studies showing granulomatous tissue compatible with tuberculosis and a positive tuberculosis skin test are sufficient to begin therapy. However, a negative skin test does not rule out skeletal tuberculosis.[112] Therapy for skeletal tuberculosis involves prolonged chemotherapy and in some cases surgical débridement.

Nontuberculous Mycobacterial Infections

Osteoarticular infections with nontuberculous mycobacteria fall into three distinct types: tenosynovitis, synovitis, and osteomyelitis. Diverse species, including *Mycobacterium tuberculosis*, *M. marinum*, *M. avium-intracellulare*, *M. fortuitum*, *M. chelonae*, *M. ulcerans*, *M. kansasii*, and *M. xenopi* have been associated with infection. Many of these infections seem to respond well to surgery alone. The role of antituberculous therapy, particularly with organisms like *M. avium-intracellulare*, is not clear.[113]

Fungal Osteomyelitis

Bone infections may be caused by a variety of mycoses, including coccidioidomycosis, blastomycosis, cryptococcosis, candidiasis, and sporotrichosis. The most common presentation is a cold abscess overlying osteolytic lesion. Joint space extension may occur in coccidioidomycosis and blastomycosis. Therapy for fungal osteomyelitis involves surgical débridement and antifungal chemotherapy.[114]

REFERENCES

1. Waldvogel FA, Medoff G, Swartz MN. Osteomyelitis: A review of clinical features, therapeutic considerations, and unusual aspect. N Engl J Med. 1970;282:198–206,260–266,316–322.
2. Waldvogel FA, Vasey H. Osteomyelitis: The past decade. N Engl J Med. 1980;303:360–370.
3. Lew DP, Waldvogel FA. Current concepts of osteomyelitis. N Engl J Med. 1997;336:999–1007.
4. Cierny G, Mader JT. Adult chronic osteomyelitis. Orthopedics. 1984;7:1557–1564.
5. Cierny G, Mader JT, Pennick H. A clinical staging system of adult osteomyelitis. Contemp Orthop. 1985;10:17–37.
6. Mader JT, Shirtliff M, Calhoun JH. Staging and staging application osteomyelitis. Clin Infect Dis. 1997;25:1303–1309.
7. Trueta J, Morgan JD. The vascular contribution to osteogenesis. I. Studies by the injection method. J Bone Joint Surg Br. 1960;42:97–109.
8. Hobo T, Zur Pathogenese de akuten haematogenen Osteomyelitis, mit Berucksichtigung der Vitalfarbungslehre. Acta Sch Med Univ Imp Kioto. 1922;4:1–29.

9. Morrissy RT, Haynes DW. Acute hematogenous osteomyelitis: A model with trauma as an etiologic agent (Abstract). Kappa Delta Paper 2. Presented at American Academy of Orthopaedic Surgeons 51st Annual Meeting, Atlanta, Ga, 1984.
10. De Jonghe M, Glaesener G: Type B *Haemophilus influenzae* infection. Experience at the pediatric hospital of Luxembourg. Bull Soc Sci Med Grand Duche Luxemb. 1995;132:17–20.
11. Ish-Horowicz MR, McIntyre P, Nade S. Bone and joint infections caused by multiply resistant *Staphylococcus aureus* in a neonatal intensive care unit. Pediatr Infect Dis J. 1992;11:82–87.
12. Morrey BF, Peterson HA. Hematogenous pyogenic osteomyelitis in children. Orthop Clin North Am. 1975;6:935–951.
13. Batson OV. The function of the vertebral veins and their role in the spread of metastases. Ann Surg. 1940;112:138–140.
14. Wiley AM, Trueta J. The vascular anatomy of the spine and its relationship to pyogenic vertebral osteomyelitis. J Bone Joint Surg. Br. 1959;41:796–804.
15. Croke HV, Goldwasser M. Anatomic studies of the circulation in the region of the vertebral end-plate in adult greyhound dogs. Spine. 1984;9:702–706.
16. Sapico FL, Montgomerie JZ. Pyogenic vertebral osteomyelitis: Report of nine cases and review of the literature. Rev Infect Dis. 1979;1:754–776.
17. Holzman RS, Bishko F. Osteomyelitis in heroin addicts. Ann Intern Med. 1971;75:693–696.
18. Sapico FL, Montgomerie JZ. Vertebral osteomyelitis in intravenous drug abusers: Report of three cases and review of the literature. Rev Infect Dis. 1980;2:196–206.
19. Lee YH, Kerstein MD. Osteomyelitis and septic arthritis: A complication of subclavian venous catheterization. N Engl J Med. 1971;285:1179–1180.
20. Leonard A, Comty CM, Shapiro FL, et al. Osteomyelitis in hemodialysis patients. Ann Intern Med. 1973;78:651–658.
21. Watanakunakorn C. Vertebral osteomyelitis as a complication of *P. aeruginosa* pneumonia. South Med J. 1975;68:173–176.
22. Gruber HE. Bone and the immune system. Proc Soc Exp Biol Med. 1991;197: 219–225.
23. Mackowiak PA, Jones SR, Smith JW. Diagnostic value of sinus tract cultures in chronic osteomyelitis. JAMA. 1978;239:2772–2775.
24. Perry CR, Pearson RL, Miller GA. Accuracy of cultures of material from swabbing of the superficial aspect of the wound and needle biopsy in the preoperative assessment of osteomyelitis. J Bone Joint Surg Am. 1991;73:745–749.
25. Butt WP. The radiology of infection. Clin Orthop. 1973;96:20–30.
26. Jones AG, Francis MD, Davis MA. Bone scanning: Radionuclide reaction mechanisms. Semin Nucl Med. 1976;6:3–18.
27. Treves S, Khettry J, Broker FH, et al. Osteomyelitis: Early scintigraphic detection in children. Pediatrics. 1976;57:173–186.
28. Russin LD, Staab EV. Unusual bone-scan findings in acute osteomyelitis: Case report. J Nucl Med. 1976;17:617–619.
29. Deysine M, Rafkin H, Teicher I, et al. Diagnosis of chronic and postoperative osteomyelitis with gallium 67 citrate scans. Am J Surg. 1975;129:632–635.
30. Lisbona R, Rosenthall L. Observations of the sequential use of ^{99m}Tc phosphate complex and ^{67}Ga imaging in osteomyelitis, cellulitis, and septic arthritis. Radiology. 1977;123:123–129.
31. Propst-Proctor SL, Dillingham MF, McDougall IR, et al. The white blood cell scan in orthopedics. Clin Orthop. 1982;168:157–165.
32. Kuhn JP, Berger PE. Computed tomographic diagnosis of osteomyelitis: Radiology. 1979;130:503–506.
33. Ram PC, Martinez S, Korobkin M, et al. CT detection of intraosseous gas: A new sign of osteomyelitis. Am J Roentgenol. 1981;137:721–723.
34. Seltzer SE. Value of computed tomography in planning medical and surgical treatment of chronic osteomyelitis. J Comput Assist Tomogr. 1984;8:482–487.
35. Ma LD, Frassica FJ, Bluemke DA, et al. CT and MRI evaluation of musculoskeletal infection. Crit Rev Diagn Imaging 1997;38:535–568.
36. Erdman WA, Tamburro F, Jayson HT, et al. Osteomyelitis: Characteristics and pitfalls of diagnosis with MR imaging. Radiology. 1991;180:533–539.
37. Tehranzadeh J, Wang F, Mesgarzadeh M. Magnetic resonance imaging of osteomyelitis. Crit Rev Diagn Imaging. 1992;33:495–534.
38. Unger E, Moldofsky P, Gatenby R, et al. Diagnosis of osteomyelitis by MR imaging. Am J Roentgenol. 1988;150:605–610.
39. Modic MT, Pflanze W, Feiglin DHI, et al. Magnetic resonance imaging of musculoskeletal infections. Radiol Clin North Am. 1986;24:247–258.
40. Golimbu C, Firooznia H, Rafii M. CT of osteomyelitis of the spine. Am J Roentgenol. 1984;142:159–163.
41. Post MJ, Quencer RM, Montalvo BM, et al. Spinal infection: Evaluation with MR imaging and intraoperative US. Radiology. 1988;169:765–771.
42. Post MJ, Sze G, Quencer RM, et al. Gadolinium-enhanced MR in spinal infection. J Comput Assist Tomogr. 1990;14:721–729.
43. Adatepe MH, Powell OM, Isaacs GH, et al. Hematogenous pyogenic vertebral osteomyelitis: Diagnostic value of radionuclide bone imaging. J Nucl Med. 1986;27:1680–1685.
44. Hadjipavlou AG, Cesani-Vazquez F, Villaneuva-Meyer J, et al. The effectiveness of gallium citrate Ga 67 radionuclide imaging in vertebral osteomyelitis revisited. Am J Orthop. 1998;27:179–183.
45. Cierny G, Mader JT. The surgical treatment of adult osteomyelitis. In: Evarts CMC, ed. Surgery of the Musculoskeletal System, v.11. New York: Churchill Livingstone; 1983:15–35.
46. Mader JT, Ortiz M, Calhoun JH. Update on the diagnosis and management of osteomyelitis. Clin Podiatr Med Surg. 1996;13:53–61.
47. Ericoson HM, Sherris JC. Antibiotic sensitivity testing: Report of an international collaborative study. Acta Pathol Microbiol Scand. 1971;227(Suppl B):1–90.
48. Tetzloff TR, McCracken GH, Nelson FD. Oral antibiotic therapy for skeletal infections in children. II. Therapy of osteomyelitis and suppurative arthritis. J Pediatr. 1978;92:485–490.
49. Nelson JD. A critical review of the role of oral antibiotics in the management of hematogenous osteomyelitis. In: Remington RS, Swartz MN, eds. Current Clinical Topics in Infectious Diseases, v. 4. New York: McGraw-Hill; 1983:64–74.
50. Christ W, Lehnert T, Ulbrich B. Specific toxicologic aspects of the quinolones. Rev Infect Dis. 1988;10(Suppl 1):141–146.
51. Mayer DG. Overview of toxicological studies. Drugs 1987;34(Suppl 1):150–153.
52. Hadjipavlou AG, Crow WN, Borowski A, et al. Percutaneous transpedicular discectomy and drainage in pyogenic spondylodiscitis. Am J Orthopaed, 1988;27: 188–197.
53. Anthony JP, Mathes SJ. Update on chronic osteomyelitis. Clin Plast Surg. 1991;18:515–523.
54. Hickman RO, Buckner CD, Clift RA, et al. A modified right atrial catheter for access to the venous system in marrow transplant recipients. Surg Gynecol Obstet. 1979;148:871–875.
55. Couch L, Cierny G, Mader JT. Inpatient and outpatient use of the Hickman catheter for adults with osteomyelitis. Clin Orthop. 1987;219:226–235.
56. Graham DR, Keldermans MM, Klemm LW, et al. Infectious complications among patients receiving home intravenous therapy with peripheral, central, or peripherally placed central venous catheters. Am J Med. 1991;91:95S–100S.
57. Mader JT. Fluoroquinolones in bone and joint infections. In: Sanders WE Jr, Sanders CC, eds. Fluoroquinolones in the Treatment of Infectious Diseases. Glenview, Ill: Physicians & Scientists; 1990:71–86.
58. Lew DP, Waldvogel FA. Quinolones and osteomyelitis: State-of-the-art. Drugs 1995;49(Suppl 2):100–111.
59. Mader JT, Cantrell JS, Calhoun JH. Oral ciprofloxacin compared with standard parenteral antibiotic therapy for chronic osteomyelitis in adults. J Bone Joint Surg. Am. 1990;72:104–110.
60. Schamberg DR, Dillon WI, Terpenning MS, et al. Increasing resistance of enterococci to ciprofloxacin. Antimicrob Agents Chemother. 1992;36:2533–2535.
61. Ernst ME, Ernst EJ, Klepser ME: Levofloxacin and trovafloxacin: The next generation of fluoroquinolones Am J Health Syst Pharm 1997;54:2569–2584.
62. Wagstaff AJ, Balfour JA. Grepafloxacin. Drugs. 1997;825–827.
63. Blumberg HM, Rimland D, Carroll DJ, et al. Rapid development of ciprofloxacin resistance in methicillin-susceptible and -resistant *Staphylococcus aureus*. J Infect Dis. 1991;163:1279–1285.
64. Norden CW, Bryant R, Palmer D, et al. Chronic osteomyelitis caused by *Staphylococcus aureus*: Controlled clinical trial of nafcillin therapy and nafcillin-rifampin therapy. South Med J. 1986;79:947–951.
65. Reller LB, Stratton CW. Serum dilution test for bactericidal activity. II. Standardization and correlation with antimicrobial assays and susceptibility tests. J Infect Dis. 1977;136:196–204.
66. Clawson DK, Davis FJ, Hansen ST. Treatment of chronic osteomyelitis with emphasis on closed suction–irrigation technique. Clin Orthop. 1973;96:88–97.
67. Letts RM, Wong E. Treatment of acute osteomyelitis in children by closed-tube irrigation: A reassessment. Can J Surg. 1975;18:60–63.
68. Ruttle PE, Kelley PJ, Arnold PG, et al. Chronic osteomyelitis treated with a muscle flap. Orthop Clin North Am. 1984;451–459.
69. May JW Jr, Jupiter JB, Gallico GG 3d, et al. Treatment of chronic traumatic bone wounds. Microvascular free tissue transfer: A 13-year experience in 96 patients. Ann Surg. 1991;214:241–250.
70. Anthony JP, Mathes SJ, Alpert BS. The muscle flap in the treatment of chronic lower extremity osteomyelitis: Results in patients over 5 years after treatment. Plast Reconstr Surg. 1991;88:311–318.
71. Papineau LJ, Alfageme A, Dalcourt JP, et al. Chronic osteomyelitis: Open excision and grafting after saucerization. Int Orthop. 1979;3:165–176.
72. Scott DM, Rotschafer JC, Behrens F. Use of vancomycin and tobramycin polymethylmethacrylate impregnated beads in the management of chronic osteomyelitis. Drug Intell Clin Pharmacol. 1988;22:480–483.
73. Wilson KJ, Cierny G, Adams KR, et al. Comparative evaluation of the diffusion of tobramycin and cefotaxime out of antibiotic-impregnated polymethylmethacrylate beads. J Orthop Res. 1988;6:279–286.
74. Adams K, Couch MSL, Cierny G, et al. In vitro and in vivo evaluation of antibiotic diffusion from antibiotic-impregnated polymethylmethacrylate (PMMA) beads. Clin Orthop. 1992;276:244–252.
75. Calhoun JH, Mader JT. Antibiotic beads in the management of surgical infection. Am J Surg. 1989;157:443–449.
76. Henry SL, Seligson D, Mangino P, et al. Antibiotic-impregnated beads. Part I. Bead implantation versus systemic therapy. Orthop Rev. 1991;20:242–247.
77. Popham GJ, Mangino P, Seligson D, et al. Antibiotic-impregnated beads. Part II. Factors in antibiotic selection. Orthop Rev. 1991;20:331–337.
78. Perry CR, Davenport K, Vossen MK. Local delivery of antibiotics via an implantable pump in the treatment of osteomyelitis. Clin Orthop. 1988;226:222–230.
79. Green SA. Osteomyelitis. The Ilizarov perspective. Orthop Clin North Am. 1991;22:515–521.
80. Calhoun JH, Anger DM, Mader JT. The Ilizarov technique in the treatment of osteomyelitis. Tex Med. 1991;87:56–59.
81. Matsen FA, Wyss CR, Pedegana LR, et al. Transcutaneous oxygen tension measurement in peripheral vascular disease. Surg Gynecol Obstet. 1980;150:525–528.
82. Calhoun JH, Cantrell J, Lacy J, et al. Treatment of diabetic foot infection. Wagner classification, and outcome. Foot Ankle. 1988;9:101–106.
83. Calhoun JH, Mader JT. Osteomyelitis of the diabetic foot. In: Frykberg SRG, ed.

The High Risk Foot in Diabetes Mellitus. New York: Churchill Livingstone; 1991:213–239.
84. Mader JT, Adams KR. Experimental osteomyelitis. In: Schlossberg D, ed. Orthopedic Infection. New York: Springer-Verlag; 1988:39–48.
85. Mader JT, Adams KR, Morrison L. Comparative evaluation of cefazolin and clindamycin in the treatment of experimental *Staphylococcus aureus* osteomyelitis in rabbits. Antimicrob Agent Chemother. 1989;33:1760–1764.
86. Mader JT, Adams KR, Sutton TE. Infectious diseases: Pathophysiology and mechanisms of hyperbaric oxygen. J Hyperbaric Med. 1987;2:133–140.
87. Morrey BF, Dunn JM, Heimbach RD, et al. Hyperbaric oxygen and chronic osteomyelitis. Clin Orthop. 1979;144:121–127.
88. Davis JC, Heckman JD, DeLee JC, et al. Chronic non-hematogenous osteomyelitis treated with adjuvant hyperbaric oxygen. J Bone Joint Surg Am. 1986;68:1210–1217.
89. Mader JT, Guckian JC, Glass DL, et al. Therapy with hyperbaric oxygen for experimental osteomyelitis due to *Staphylococcus aureus* in rabbits. J Infect Dis. 1978;138:312–318.
90. Mader JT, Brown GL, Guckian JC, et al. A mechanism for the amelioration by hyperbaric oxygen of experimental staphylococcal osteomyelitis in rabbits. J Infect Dis. 1980;142:915–922.
91. Verklin RM, Mandell GL. Alteration of effectiveness of antibiotics by anaerobiosis. J Lab Clin Med. 1977;89:65–71.
92. Reynolds. AV, Hamilton-Miller JMT, Brumfittt W. Diminished effect of gentamicin under anaerobic and hypercapnic conditions. Lancet. 1976;1:447–449.
93. Mader JT, Adams KR, Couch LA, et al. Potentiation of tobramycin by hyperbaric oxygen in experimental *Pseudomonas aeruginosa* osteomyelitis. Abstract 1331. In: Abstracts of the 27th Interscience Conference on Antimicrobial Agents and Chemotherapy. Washington, DC: American Society for Microbiology; 1987.
94. Hunt TK, Pai MP. The effect of varying ambient oxygen tensions on wound metabolism and collagen synthesis. Surg Gynecol Obstet. 1972;135:756–758.
95. Hunt TK, Zederfeldt B, Goldstick TK. Oxygen and healing. Am J Surg. 1969;118:521–525.
96. Engh C, Hughes J, Abrams R, et al. Osteomyelitis in the patient with sickle cell disease. J Bone Joint Surg Am. 1971;53:1–15.
97. Epps CH Jr, Bryant DD 3d, Coles MJ, et al. Osteomyelitis in patients who have sickle-cell disease: Diagnosis and management. J Bone Joint Surg Am. 1991;73:1281–1294.
98. Gifford DB, Patzakis M, Ivler D, et al. Septic arthritis due to *Pseudomonas* in heroin addicts. J Bone Joint Surg Am. 1975;57:631–635.
99. Roca RPP, Yoshikawa TT. Primary skeletal infections in heroin users: A clinical characterization, diagnosis, and therapy. Clin Orthop. 1979;144:238–248.
100. Chandrasekar PH, Narula AP. Bone and joint infections in intravenous drug abusers. Rev Infect Dis. 1986;8:904–911.
101. Miller W, Murphy W, Gilula L. Brodie abscess: Reappraisal. Radiology. 1979;132:15–23.
102. Dunn EC, Singer L. Operative treatment of Brodie's abscess. J Foot Surg. 1991;30:443–445.
103. Freedman E. The behavior of the intervertebral disc in certain spine lesions. Radiology. 1935;22:219–235.
104. Ratcliffe JFA. Anatomic basis for the pathogenesis and radiologic features of vertebral osteomyelitis and its differentiation from childhood discitis: A microarteriographic investigation. Acta Radiol Diagn. 1985;26:137–143.
105. Menelaus MB. Discitis: An inflammation affecting the intervertebral discs in children. J Bone Joint Surg Br. 1964;46:16–23.
106. Hensey OJ, Coad N, Carty HM. Juvenile discitis. Arch Dis Child 1983;58:983–987.
107. Bonfiglio N, Lange TA, Kim YM. Pyogenic vertebral osteomyelitis: Disk space infections. Clin Orthop. 1973;96:234–247.
108. Kemp HBS, Jackson JW, Jeremiah, JD, et al. Pyogenic infections occurring primarily in intervertebral discs. J Bone Joint Surg Br. 1973;55:698–714.
109. Falk A. Results of long-term chemotherapy in spinal tuberculosis. XVII. A follow-up study of 235 patients. Am Rev Respir Dis. 1967;95:1–5.
110. Wallace R, Cohen AS. Tuberculosis arthritis: A report of two cases with review of biopsy and synovial fluid findings. Am J Med. 1976;61:277–282.
111. Gorse GJ, Pais MJ, Kusske JA, et al. Tuberculosis spondylitis: A report of six cases and a review of the literature. Medicine. 1983;62:178–193.
112. Davidson PT, Horowitz I. Skeletal tuberculosis: A review with patient presentations and discussion. Am J Med. 1970;48:77–84.
113. Marchevsky A, Damsker B, Green S, et al. The clinicopathological spectrum of non-tuberculous mycobacterial osteoarticular infection. J Bone Joint Surg Am. 1985;67A:925–929.
114. Gathe J Jr, Harris R, Garland B, et al. *Candida* osteomyelitis: Report of 5 cases and review of the literature. Am J Med. 1987;82:927–937.

Chapter 92

Infections with Prostheses in Bones and Joints

BARRY D. BRAUSE

Prosthetic replacement surgery for hip, knee, shoulder, and elbow joints has become commonplace because of the magnificent success of these procedures in restoring function to persons disabled by arthritis. Patients receiving total joint replacements number in the hundreds of thousands each year worldwide, and millions of people have indwelling prosthetic articulations. One to 5% of indwelling prostheses become infected; this is a calamity for the patient and is associated with significant morbidity and occasionally death. Prosthesis removal, which usually is necessary to treat these infections, produces large skeletal defects, shortening of the extremity, and severe functional impairment. The health care cost of treating a single septic prosthetic joint has been estimated conservatively at $50,000, with an extrapolated expenditure of more than $100 million per year in the United States alone.[1] The patient faces protracted hospitalization, sizable financial expense, and potentially renewed disability.

PATHOGENESIS

Certain patient populations have been identified as being predisposed toward infection of their prosthetic joints, including patients with prior surgery at the site of the prosthesis, rheumatoid arthritis, immunocompromised states, diabetes mellitus, poor nutritional status, obesity, psoriasis, or extremely advanced age.[2–4] Infection usually occurs in osseous tissue adjacent to the foreign body. Because most prostheses are cemented in place with polymethylmethacrylate, infection develops at the bone-cement interface. Sepsis involving cementless prostheses develops in the bone contiguous with the metallic alloy.

Prosthetic joints become infected by two different pathogenetic routes: locally introduced and hematogenous types of osteomyelitis. The locally introduced form of infection is the result of wound sepsis contiguous to the prosthesis or operative contamination. Any factor or event that delays wound healing increases the risk of infection. Ischemic necrosis, infected wound hematomas, wound infection (with or without identifiable cellulitis), and suture abscesses are common preceding events for joint replacement sepsis. During the early postimplantation period, when these superficial infections develop, the fascial layers have not yet healed and the deep, periprosthesis tissue is not protected by the usual physical barriers. Generally these infections are caused by a single pathogen, but polymicrobial sepsis with as many as five different organisms is also observed. Coagulase-negative staphylococci are the most common etiologic agents in this clinical setting. Infrequently, latent foci of chronic, quiescent osteomyelitis are reactivated by the disruption of tissue associated with implantation surgery. Although bone cultures at the time of the joint replacement operation may be sterile, old *Staphylococcus aureus* and *Mycobacterium tuberculosis* infections can recrudesce postoperatively.[3]

Any bacteremia can induce infection of a total joint replacement by the hematogenous route.[5–7] Dentogingival infections and manipulations are known causes of viridans streptococcal and anaerobic *(Peptococcus, Peptostreptococcus)* infections in prostheses. Pyogenic skin processes can cause staphylococcal *(S. aureus, Staphylococcus epidermidis)* and streptococcal (groups A, B, C, and G streptococci) infections of joint replacements. Genitourinary and gastrointestinal tract procedures or infections are associated with gram-negative bacillary, enterococcal, and anaerobic infections of prostheses.

Twenty to 40% of prosthetic joint infections arise by the hematogenous route, the remainder being of the locally introduced type.

The frequency of specific etiologic microorganisms in prosthetic joint sepsis varies among the published studies, but a general view of the spectrum of this bacteriology and the prominence of certain microbial groups, is given in Table 92–1. Staphylococci (coagulase-negative staphylococci and *S. aureus*) are the principal causative agents; aerobic streptococci and gram-negative bacilli are each responsible for 20 to 25%; and anaerobes represent 10% of these infections. The spectrum of microbial agents capable of causing prosthetic joint infection is unlimited and includes organisms ordinarily considered "contaminants" of cultures, such as corynebacteria, propionibacteria, and *Bacillus* spp. Rarely have infections with fungi (particularly *Candida*) or mycobacteria been described.[3]

As foreign bodies, the indwelling metallic prosthesis and the polymethylmethacrylate cement, which binds the metal alloy to adjacent bone, predispose both joint space and osseous tissue to septic processes. Foreign substances contribute to local sepsis experimentally by decreasing the quantity of bacteria necessary to establish infection and by permitting pathogens to persist on their avascular surface, sequestered from circulating immunologic defenses (leukocytes, antibodies, and complement) and from systemic antibiotics.[3, 8] Polymethylmethacrylate cement appears to predispose toward infection to an extent beyond that of other inert foreign substances. The cement in unpolymerized form has been shown to inhibit phagocytic, lymphocytic, and complement function in vitro.[9, 10] The polymerization process itself appears to enhance the risk of infection, possibly because of the substantial heat generated by this in vivo reaction.[9] In an effort to provide total joint replacement without polymethylmethacrylate, cementless prostheses have been designed. These devices have textured surfaces to provide fixation by the growth of adjacent bone into the "porous" interface of the prosthesis. The performance and durability of this form of arthroplasty is uncertain.

Host responses to methylmethacrylate also may play a role in the pathogenesis of infection. Fibronectin, a connective tissue and plasma glycoprotein, appears to enhance *S. aureus* adherence to polymethylmethacrylate in vivo and thus may contribute to the occurrence of sepsis.[11] Microbial products may assist the development and persistence of infection in association with foreign substances. In the presence of prosthetic devices, many bacteria elaborate a fibrous exopolysaccharide material called *glycocalyx*. Organisms can grow within this matrix and form thick biofilms that are protected at least in part from host defense mechanisms.[2, 12] Bacteria adherent to biomaterials demonstrate decreased quantitative susceptibility to antibiotics both in vitro and in vivo.[13, 14]

CLINICAL PRESENTATION

Prosthetic joint sepsis produces the cardinal symptoms of inflammation with a wide spectrum of severity. Most patients present with a long, indolent course characterized by a progressive increase in joint pain and occasionally by the formation of cutaneous draining sinuses, but not by fever, soft tissue swelling, or systemic toxicity. Others present with an acute, fulminant illness with high fever, severe joint pain, local swelling, and erythema. The frequencies of these presenting symptoms are listed in Table 92–2.[15]

TABLE 92–1 Bacteriology of Prosthetic Joint Infection

Pathogens	Frequency (%)
Coagulase-negative staphylococci	22
Staphylococcus aureus	22
Viridans streptococci	9
β-Hemolytic streptococci groups A, B, G	5
Enterococci	7
Gram-negative aerobic bacilli	25
Anaerobes	10

TABLE 92–2 Presenting Symptoms of Prosthetic Joint Infection

Symptom	Frequency (%)
Joint pain	95
Fever	43
Periarticular swelling	38
Wound or cutaneous sinus drainage	32

The pattern of clinical presentation is determined largely by three factors: the virulence of the infecting pathogen, the nature of the host tissue in which the microorganism grows, and the route of infection. *S. aureus* is a particularly virulent pathogen in this setting and usually produces a fulminant infection (occasionally with septic shock). β-Hemolytic streptococci and aerobic gram-negative bacilli are also capable of causing this clinical picture. Alternatively, the relatively avirulent but tenacious coagulase-negative staphylococci are consistently associated with an indolent course.

Characteristics of the involved tissue can influence the type of presentation on the basis of their support of microbial growth. Wound hematomas (as well as seromas and hemarthroses), fresh operative wounds, ischemic wounds, and tissues in diabetic and steroid-treated patients all enhance the ability of bacteria to multiply rapidly in expansive tissue planes. These factors promote the development of a more fulminant infection when a large inoculum of bacteria is allowed access to deep tissue compartments during surgery or in a slowly healing wound postoperatively.

The hematogenous route of infection theoretically seeds the bone-cement interface with a relatively small number of organisms. When a bloodborne infection arises in a prosthetic joint several months or years after implantation surgery, the fully healed connective tissue often is capable of restricting the septic process to a relatively small but critical focus at the bone-cement interface. Joint pain is the principal symptom of deep tissue infection irrespective of the mode of presentation and suggests either acute inflammation of periarticular tissue or loosening of the prosthesis as a result of subacute erosion of bone at the bone-cement interface.

DIAGNOSIS

The clinical manifestations previously described (i.e., joint pain, swelling, erythema, and warmth) all reflect an underlying inflammatory process in the surrounding tissues but are not specific for infection. When a painful prosthesis is accompanied by a fever or purulent drainage from overlying cutaneous sinuses, infection may be presumed, pending further confirmatory tests. However, in most cases, infection must be differentiated from aseptic and mechanical problems (e.g., hemarthrosis, gout, bland loosening, dislocation, metallic debris–induced synovitis or osteolysis), which are more common causes of pain and inflammatory symptoms in these patients.

Constant joint pain is suggestive of infection, whereas mechanical loosening commonly causes pain only with motion and weight bearing.[2] Plain radiographs can reveal (1) abnormal lucencies greater than 2 mm in width at the bone-cement interface, (2) changes in the position of prosthetic components, (3) cement fractures, (4) periosteal reaction, or (5) motion of components on stress views. In addition, the intra-articular injection of dye (arthrography) may reveal abnormal communications between the joint space and multiple defects in the bone-cement interface. These radiologic abnormalities (Fig. 92–1) are found in 50% of septic prostheses. They are generally related to the duration of infection, because it may require 3 to 6 months to manifest such changes. When both distal and proximal components of a prosthetic joint demonstrate radiographic pathology, sepsis is more likely than is simple mechanical loosening. However, these changes seen on radiographs are not specific for infection because they are also seen frequently with aseptic processes.

Radioisotopic scans with technetium diphosphonate demonstrate

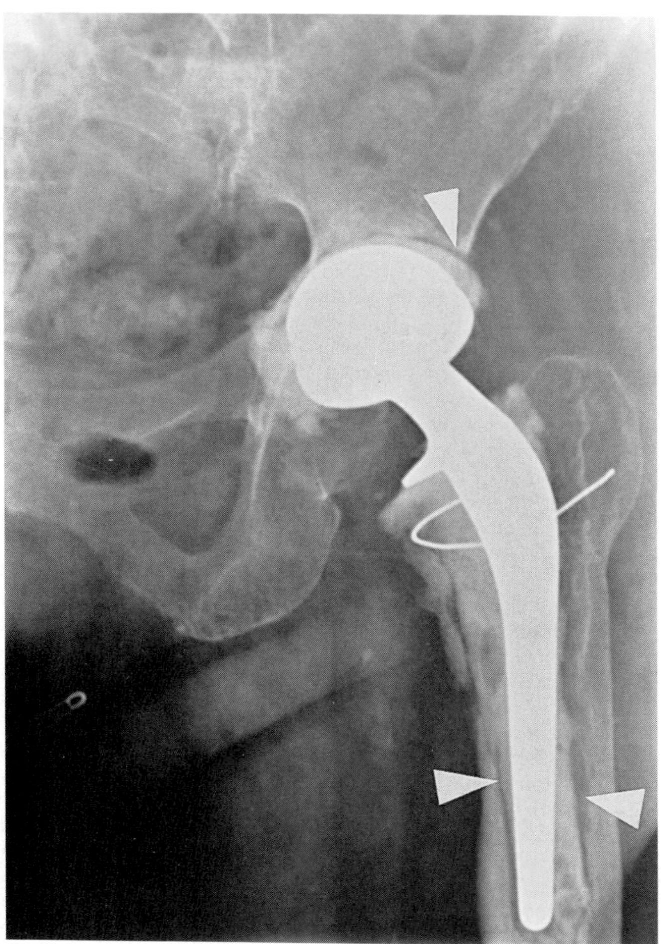

FIGURE 92–1. A plain radiograph of an infected total hip prosthesis demonstrates lucencies at the bone-cement interface of both femoral and acetabular components *(arrowheads)*.

increased uptake in areas of bone with enhanced blood supply or increased metabolic activity. Increased technetium uptake is seen routinely around normal prostheses for 6 months after arthroplasty. Positive scan findings after this period are abnormal and reflect inflammation and possible loosening but not specifically infection of the implant. Sequential technetium-gallium bone scanning is also nondiagnostic because of unacceptable sensitivity (66%) and specificity (81%).[16] Indium-labeled leukocyte scanning, although very sensitive, also provides only nonspecific results.[17] Therefore, normal or negative technetium or indium leukocyte scan findings can be considered strong evidence against the presence of infection, but they are not definitive in establishing the diagnosis. Elevated peripheral leukocyte counts, erythrocyte sedimentation rates, and C-reactive protein levels, although suggestive, also are inadequate to diagnose sepsis in this clinical setting.[18]

The specific diagnosis of joint replacement infection depends, in large part, on isolation of the pathogen by aspiration of joint fluid or by culture of tissue obtained at arthrotomy.[19] Analysis of joint fluid often reveals a high leukocyte count (mainly polymorphonuclear cells), a high protein content, and a low glucose concentration. However, these changes are only variably present and are neither prerequisites for making the diagnosis of joint replacement infection nor specific for this entity. Histopathologic examination of periprosthetic tissue frequently reveals an infiltration of polymorphonuclear leukocytes, indicative of an acute inflammatory reaction, but this parameter is only variably present (probably because of the sampling limitations of frozen-section histopathology) and also may not be sufficiently specific. Therefore, the single observation that delineates the presence of implant infection is isolation of the pathogen by arthrocentesis or surgical débridement.

Because fastidious microorganisms, including anaerobes, may be etiologic agents in prosthetic arthroplasty infections, multiple specimens should be obtained and rapidly cultured in appropriate media. Arthrocentesis demonstrates the pathogen in 85 to 98% of cases.[19, 20] Gram staining is positive in 32% of cases. Fluoroscopic guidance and arthrography are useful to document accurate needle placement. If difficulty is encountered in obtaining intra-articular fluid, irrigation with sterile normal saline solution (without antiseptic preservative additives) can be used to provide the necessary fluid for culture. If initial cultures reveal a relatively avirulent organism (*S. epidermidis*, corynebacteria, propionibacteria, or *Bacillus* spp.), a second aspirate should be considered to reconfirm the bacteriologic diagnosis and to eliminate the possibility that the isolate is artifactual. Multiple positive operative cultures are definitively diagnostic of infection; therefore, the patient should not receive antimicrobial therapy for several weeks before the procedure. Several (five to seven) specimens of tissue and fluid should be submitted for culture. The results of these microbiologic techniques should confirm the presence and nature of the infection and allow for optimal treatment. In the uncommon circumstance in which the clinical suggestion of sepsis is strong but the cultures are sterile, fastidious organisms (particularly anaerobes) should be suspected. To design the most efficacious and least toxic antimicrobial therapy, the patient's infecting strain of bacteria must first be available for in vitro evaluation (described later).

THERAPY

Successful treatment of a total joint arthroplasty infection depends on extensive and meticulous surgical débridement and effective antimicrobial therapy. Simple surgical drainage (with retention of the prosthesis in situ) followed by antibiotic therapy has been successful in only 20% of cases.[21] More recent attempts at treating early postoperative infections (<1 month after implantation) without prosthesis removal have had variable results. Success rates of approximately 70% have been reported in small numbers of patients receiving a single débridement followed by 4 to 6 weeks of antibiotic therapy.[22, 23] Success with longer courses (3 to 6 months) of antibiotic therapy using rifampin in combination with other antimicrobial agents has been reported in selected patients with retained orthopedic implants.[24] However, most of these infected implants were fracture fixation devices and not septic total joint prostheses, for which infections appear more difficult to cure. In addition, antibiotic therapy with prosthesis retention eradicated only 36% of *S. aureus* infections in a separate study.[25] For more predictably effective treatment of prosthetic joint infection, complete removal of all foreign materials (metallic prosthesis, cement, and any accompanying biofilm) is essential. Prosthesis extraction and reimplantation can be accomplished in a single-stage (exchange) procedure or in a more efficacious two-stage approach.

The most successful protocol incorporates standardized antimicrobial therapy with a two-stage surgical procedure. Removal of the prosthesis and cement is followed by a 6-week course of bactericidal antibiotic therapy chosen on the basis of quantitative in vitro susceptibility studies. Reimplantation is performed at the conclusion of the 6-week antibiotic course. Use of methylmethacrylate cement impregnated with an antimicrobial agent (usually tobramycin or gentamicin) has not been subjected to controlled trials and is not approved by the U.S. Food and Drug Administration but is commonly practiced. The antimicrobial agent leaches out from the hardened plastic (cement) to produce variable but high initial release, and protracted diffusion, of antibiotic into surrounding tissues at the bone-cement interface.[26] Antibiotic-loaded polymethylmethacrylate is also commonly used in cement spacers inserted after prosthesis removal to facilitate delayed reimplantation. With this protocol a 90 to 96% success rate has been achieved in total hip replacement infections, and a 97% success rate has been obtained in total knee replacement infections.[4, 27–31] The success of this regimen relies on thorough débridement techniques and effective antimicrobial therapy. In this manner, both gram-positive bacteria (including multidrug-resistant staphylococci and enterococci) and gram-negative bacteria (including *Pseudomonas aeruginosa*) can be eliminated if the specific sensitivity of each isolate allows eradication. The empiric selection of a 6-week duration of antibiotic therapy may be critical for efficacy. Others have employed a similar approach to therapy but with only a 2-week course of antibiotic treatment before reinsertion of the prosthesis.[32] With this protocol, the pathogen was eradicated in only 79% of the cases, and only 35% of the patients obtained good function in the new prosthesis.

The alternative method of treatment involves extraction of the metallic joint and cement with immediate reimplantation of a new prosthesis in a one-stage surgical procedure (exchange operation) accompanied by antimicrobial therapy. Antibiotic-loaded methylmethacrylate cement is used during reimplantation. The protocol is effective in 70 to 80% of cases.[4, 33–35] When the exchange operation is repeated (in those for whom the first replacement failed) and antibiotic-laden cement is used, the success rate is increased to 90%.[34] It has been suggested that this mode of therapy is applicable only to infections with the less virulent microorganisms, because high failure rates are observed when the pathogen is *S. aureus* or a gram-negative bacillus.[36] Systemic antibiotics are administered rarely and without standardization in this regimen. Moreover, the selection of an aminoglycoside as a component in the recementing phase of these operations may not reflect the susceptibility of the pathogen being treated. Although the two-stage removal-reimplantation approach is more effective, the one-stage procedure is often employed in elderly or infirm patients who might not tolerate protracted bed rest and a second major operation.[37]

Present therapeutic interventions include the most efficacious parts of these two protocols, combining a 6-week antibiotic regimen and two-stage prosthesis removal-reimplantation surgery with the incorporation of antibiotic-impregnated cement during arthroplasty reinsertion.[30, 31] In those clinical situations in which adequate antimicrobial potency cannot be achieved, arthrodesis or resection arthroplasty is recommended rather than an attempt at prosthesis reimplantation. However, with the advent of antibiotic-impregnated cement incorporating new antimicrobial agents, even patients in these difficult cases may be candidates for another total joint arthroplasty.

SUPPRESSIVE ANTIBIOTIC THERAPY

Although removal of the implanted prosthesis is necessary to confidently eradicate deep infection associated with these devices, this therapeutic approach is not always available. Occasionally surgical excision is contraindicated as a result of medical and surgical conditions or patient refusal. Because it is likely that the pathogen will be able to persist at the undébrided bone-cement interface despite high-dose, finite systemic antimicrobial therapy, lifelong oral antibiotic treatment can be considered to suppress the infection and retain the usefulness of the total joint replacement. In selected cases in which (1) prosthesis removal is not possible, (2) the pathogen is relatively avirulent, (3) the pathogen is exquisitely sensitive to an orally absorbed antibiotic, (4) the patient can tolerate an appropriate oral antibiotic, and (5) the prosthesis is not loose, suppressive oral antimicrobial therapy may be of value. Successful retention of a functioning hip arthroplasty has been seen in 63% of patients when all these five criteria are fulfilled.[38] However, when similar therapy is employed in total knee replacements infected with a variety of microorganisms (both virulent and relatively avirulent), successful joint function is maintained in only 26%.[39] The suppressive approach is not without risk. Serial radiographs are needed over the course of treatment to monitor for progressive bone resorption at the bone-cement interface, which could reduce the success of any future revision surgery. Secondary resistance can emerge, and despite continual antibiotic therapy, the localized septic process can extend into adjacent tissue compartments or become a systemic infection.[24] Moreover, the patient is subjected to the potential side effects of chronic antibiotic administration.

PREVENTION OF JOINT PROSTHESIS INFECTION

In view of the catastrophic effects of prosthetic arthroplasty infection, prevention of these septic processes is of prime importance. In anticipation of elective total joint replacement surgery, the patient should be evaluated for the presence of pyogenic dentogingival pathology, obstructive uropathy, and dermatologic conditions that might predispose to infection and bacteremia. Strong consideration should be given to reducing the risks represented by these factors (i.e., dental extraction, prostatic resection, control of dermatitis) before insertion of the prosthesis. Perioperative antibiotic prophylaxis has been shown to reduce deep wound infection effectively in total joint replacement surgery.[40] Oxacillin or cefazolin is commonly administered as an antistaphylococcal agent immediately before the operation and for 1 to 2 days thereafter. The use of aminoglycoside-impregnated cement during implantation may additionally decrease the incidence of infection.[41] Filtered laminar airflow systems in the operating room further reduce infection rates, especially when whole-body, exhaust-ventilated suits are worn by the operating team.[42, 43]

For patients with indwelling joint prostheses, early recognition and prompt therapy for infection in any location is critical to reduce the risk of seeding the joint implant hematogenously. Situations likely to cause bacteremia should be avoided. The use of prophylactic antibiotics in anticipation of bacteremic events (i.e., dental surgery, cystoscopy, colonoscopic biopsy, surgical procedures on infected or contaminated tissues) has been suggested on the same empiric basis on which endocarditis prophylaxis is recommended.[3, 6] This approach to prevention is controversial, and no data are available with which to determine the adequacy or the cost-effectiveness of such measures. The American Dental Association and the American Academy of Orthopedic Surgeons have jointly advised that a single dose of prophylactic antibiotic be given to selected patients undergoing dental procedures associated with significant bleeding (including periodontal scaling).[44] The selected patient populations include patients with inflammatory arthropathies, immunosuppression, diabetes mellitus, malnutrition, hemophilia, or previous prosthetic joint infection and all others undergoing these procedures within 2 years after joint replacement. Clinical decisions regarding prophylactic antibiotics for expected bacteremias in patients with prosthetic joints should be made on an individual basis.

REFERENCES

1. Sculco TP. The economic impact of infected total joint arthroplasty. Instructional Course Lectures, v. 42. Rosemont, Ill: American Academy of Orthopaedic Surgeons: 1993:349–351.
2. Gristina AG, Kolkin J. Total joint replacement and sepsis. J Bone Joint Surg Am. 1983;65:128–134.
3. Brause BD. Prosthetic joint infections. Curr Opin Rheumatol. 1989;1:194–198.
4. Hanssen AD, Rand JA. Evaluation and treatment of infection at the site of a total hip or knee arthroplasty. J Bone Joint Surg Am. 1998;80:910–922.
5. Ahlberg A, Carlsson AS, Lindberg L. Hematogenous infection in total joint replacement. Clin Orthop. 1978;137:69–75.
6. Maderazo EG, Judson S, Pasternak H. Late infections of total joint prostheses: A review and recommendations for prevention. Clin Orthop. 1988;229:131–142.
7. Lindqvist C, Slatis P. Dental bacteremia: A neglected cause of arthroplasty infections? Acta Orthop Scand. 1985;56:506–508.
8. Petty W, Spanier S, Shuster JJ, et al. The influence of skeletal implants on incidence of infection. J Bone Joint Surg Am. 1985;67:1236–1244.
9. Petty W. The effect of methylmethacrylate on bacterial inhibiting properties of normal human serum. Clin Orthop. 1978;132:266–277.
10. Petty W. The effect of methylmethacrylate on bacterial phagocytosis and killing by human polymorphonuclear leukocytes. J Bone Joint Surg Am. 1978;60:752–757.
11. Vaudaux P, Suzuki R, Waldvogel FA, et al. Foreign-body infection: Role of fibronec-

tin as a ligand for the adherence of *Staphylococcus aureus*. J Infect Dis. 1984;150:546–553.
12. Costerton JW, Irvin RT, Cheng K-J. The bacterial glycocalyx in nature and disease. Annu Rev Microbiol. 1981;35:299–324.
13. Gristina AG, Jennings RA, Naylor PT, et al. Comparative in vitro antibiotic resistance of surface-colonizing coagulase-negative staphylococci. Antimicrob Agents Chemother. 1989;33:813–816.
14. Widmer AF, Frei R, Rajacic Z, et al. Correlation between in vivo and in vitro efficacy of antimicrobial agents against foreign body infections. J Infect Dis. 1990;162:96–102.
15. Inman JN, Gallegos KV, Brause BD, et al. Clinical and microbial features of prosthetic joint infection. Am J Med. 1984;77:47–53.
16. Merkel KD, Brown ML, Fitzgerald RH. Sequential technetium-99m HMDP-gallium-67 citrate imaging for the evaluation of infection in the painful prosthesis. J Nucl Med. 1986;27:1413–1417.
17. Pring DJ, Henderson RG, Rivett AG, et al. Autologous granulocyte scanning of painful prosthetic joints. J Bone Joint Surg Br. 1986;68:647–652.
18. Spangehl MJ, Younger ASE, Masri BA, et al. Diagnosis of infection following total hip arthroplasty. J Bone Joint Surg Am. 1997;79:1578–1588.
19. O'Neill DA, Harris WH. Failed total hip replacement: Assessment by plain radiographs, arthrograms and aspiration of the hip joint. J Bone Joint Surg Am. 1984;66:540–546.
20. Eftehar NS. Wound infection complicating total hip joint arthroplasty. Orthop Rev. 1979;8:49–64.
21. Fitzgerald RH, Nolan DR, Ilstrup DM, et al. Deep wound sepsis following total hip arthroplasty. J Bone Joint Surg Am. 1977;59:847–855.
22. Tsukayama DT, Estrada R, Gustilo RB. Infection after total hip arthroplasty. J Bone Joint Surg Am. 1996;78:512–523.
23. Mont MA, Waldman B, Banerjee C, et al. Multiple irrigation, debridement, and retention of components in infected total knee arthroplasty. J Arthroplasty. 1997;12:426–433.
24. Zimmerli W, Widmer AF, Blatter M, et al. Role of rifampin for treatment of orthopedic implant-related staphylococcal infections. JAMA. 1998;279:1537–1541.
25. Brandt CM, Sistrunk WW, Duffy MC, et al. *Staphylococcus aureus* prosthetic joint infection treated with debridement and prosthesis retention. Clin Infect Dis. 1997;24:914–919.
26. Wininger DA, Fass RJ. Antibiotic impregnated cement and beads for orthopedic infections. Antimicrob Agents Chemother. 1996;40:2675–2679.
27. Callaghan JJ, Salvati EA, Brause BD, et al. Reimplantation for salvage of the infected hip. The Hip: Proceedings of the 14th Open Scientific Meeting of The Hip Society. St Louis: CV Mosby; 1986:65–94.
28. Windsor RE, Insall JN, Urs WK, et al. Two-stage reimplantation for the salvage of total knee arthroplasty complicated by infection. J Bone Joint Surg Am. 1990;72:272–278.
29. Salvati EA, Chekofsky KM, Brause BD, et al. Reimplantation in infection. Clin Orthop. 1982;170:62–75.
30. Lieberman JR, Callaway GH, Salvati EA, et al. Treatment of the infected total hip arthroplasty with a two-stage reimplantation protocol. Clin Orthop. 1994;301:205–212.
31. Garvin KL, Salvati EA, Brause BD. Role of gentamicin-impregnated cement in total joint arthroplasty. Orthop Clin North Am. 1988;19:605–610.
32. Rand JA, Bryan RS. Reimplantation for the salvage of an infected total knee arthroplasty. J Bone Joint Surg Am. 1983;65:1081–1086.
33. Buchholz HW, Elson RA, Lodenkamper H. The infected joint implant. In: McKibbin B, ed. Recent Advances in Orthopedics. Edinburgh: Churchill Livingstone; 1979:139–161.
34. Buchholz HW, Elson R, Engelbrecht E. Management of deep infection of total hip replacement. J Bone Joint Surg Br. 1981;63:342–353.
35. Carlsson AS, Josefsson G, Lindberg L. Revision with gentamicin-impregnated cement for deep infection in total hip arthroplasties. J Bone Joint Surg Am. 1978;60:1059–1064.
36. Fitzgerald RH, Jones DR. Hip implant infection. Am J Med. 1986;78(Suppl 6B):225–228.
37. Garvin KL, Hanssen AD. Infection after total hip arthroplasty. J Bone Joint Surg Am. 1995;77:1576–1588.
38. Goulet JA, Pellicci PM, Brause BD, et al. Prolonged suppression of infection in total hip arthroplasty. J Arthroplasty. 1988;3:109–116.
39. Ayers DC, Dennis DA, Johanson NA, et al. Common complications of total knee arthroplasty. J Bone Joint Surg Am. 1997;79:278–311.
40. Norden C. A critical review of antibiotic prophylaxis in orthopedic surgery. Rev Infect Dis. 1983;5:928–932.
41. Espehaug B, Engesaeter LB, Vollset SE, et al. Antibiotic prophylaxis in total hip arthroplasty. J Bone Joint Surg Br. 1997;79:590–595.
42. Lidwell O, Lowbury E, Whyte E. Effect of ultraclean air in operating rooms on deep sepsis in the joint after total hip or total knee replacement. BMJ. 1982;285:10–14.
43. Salvati EA, Robinson RP, Zeno SM, et al. Infection rates after 3175 total hip and total knee replacements performed with and without a horizontal unidirectional filtered air-flow system. J Bone Joint Surg Am. 1982;64:525–535.
44. American Dental Association; American Academy of Orthopaedic Surgeons, Advisory Statement. Antibiotic prophylaxis for dental patients with total joint replacements. J Am Dental Assoc. 1997;128:1004–1007.

SECTION L

DISEASES OF THE REPRODUCTIVE ORGANS AND SEXUALLY TRANSMITTED DISEASES

Chapter 93

Genital Skin and Mucous Membrane Lesions

MICHAEL F. REIN

The skin of the genital area is subject to many of the same diseases that affect other anatomic sites. Nonvenereal and noninfectious conditions can involve the genital epithelium alone or as part of a more generalized disease process.[1–5] Among adults, sexually transmitted diseases (STDs) are a frequent cause of genital lesions, and a thorough history including sexual history and diligent search for confirmatory manifestations of STD should be a part of the initial workup.

HISTORY

Pediatric Age Group

Candida albicans or herpes simplex virus (HSV) can infect the neonatal genitalia, and herpetic vulvitis occurs occasionally in young children as the initial manifestation of exposure to the virus. Molluscum contagiosum is a common pediatric infection that only occasionally involves the genitalia, probably by autoinfection. The presence of sexually transmitted lesions such as herpes genitalis in an older child[6, 7] or condylomata acuminata[8] or exclusively genital molluscum contagiosum[9] in a child should prompt an evaluation for, but does not prove, sexual abuse.[10, 11]

Sexual History

Exposure to multiple partners increases the risk of sexually acquired infection. Orogenital contact can inoculate sexually transmitted pathogens into the oral or pharyngeal mucosa.[12–15] Receptive anal intercourse predisposes to perianal, anal, and rectal infection.[13–17] A history of genital symptoms in, or recent treatment of, a sexual partner may be helpful diagnostically. Specific sexual practices such as particularly vigorous coitus or masturbation[18] or a history of being bitten by a sexual partner should be sought.

Incubation Period

The clinician can sometimes estimate the incubation period of a sexually transmitted infection by obtaining the history of a single sexual contact or exposure to a new partner. Genital lesions developing within hours of sexual exposure suggest trauma, chemical irritation, or hypersensitivity.[1, 18–20] Localized penile edema occurring within hours of vigorous coitus has been reported.[18] The swelling decreased spontaneously, and no specific therapy was required. Incubation periods of less than 24 hours are occasionally observed in chancroid.[21, 22] Some patients experience reactivation of herpes genitalis within 12 hours after coitus.[13, 14, 23]

Somewhat longer incubation periods of 2 to 5 days are usually seen with chancroid[21, 22] or herpes genitalis,[13, 14, 23] although the mean incubation period for primary genital herpes is actually about 6 days.[13, 14, 23] Clinical manifestations may follow infection by as long as 2 to 3 weeks later for either of these diseases. An incubation period of 1 to 3 weeks is usually seen with syphilis,[15] although this may rarely extend up to 12 weeks. An incubation period of 4 to 12 weeks usually precedes the development of genital warts,[17] and the symptoms of pubic lice[24] and scabies generally follow infection by about 4 weeks (see Chapters 283 and 284). The incubation period for molluscum contagiosum is not well documented and apparently ranges from 2 to 26 weeks.[25, 26] The incubation period for donovanosis is also poorly defined but appears to average around 1 to 4 weeks.[27, 28]

Residence and Travel

The most common causes of genital ulcers in the United States are, in decreasing order, genital herpes, primary syphilis, and chancroid.[29] Lymphogranuloma venereum is considerably more common in Africa and the Far East than in the United States. Chancroid has been diagnosed in 12 to 90% of patients with genital ulcerations in various parts of the developing world.[21, 22, 29, 30] Donovanosis is endemic in India, Papua New Guinea, the West Indies, and some parts of Africa and South America.[27, 28] Dual or multiple infections, in which some combination of *Treponema pallidum, Haemophilus ducreyi, Calymmatobacterium granulomatis,* and HSV is isolated from a single lesion, are frequently reported in the developing world and may result in partial responses to therapy aimed at only a single organism. Whereas lymphogranuloma venereum and donovanosis are distinctly rare in the United States, chancroid became far more common in major metropolitan areas[21, 22] during the 1980s, often occurring in localized epidemics, especially in association with prostitute contact.[31] The incidence of chancroid has recently decreased in the United States.[22]

Use of Antimicrobials

Antimicrobials and other drugs have been reported to cause fixed drug eruptions (FDEs) that occasionally involve the genitalia.[1, 32–36] The tetracyclines, commonly used in the treatment of STDs, are incriminated with particular frequency as a cause of genital FDE.[33] Such lesions may take several forms but are frequently manifested as yellow ulcerations. Antimicrobials may predispose to the development of candidiasis and may alter or completely eliminate the lesions of syphilis,[37] chancroid, or lymphogranuloma venereum.

Underlying Diseases

Immunodeficiency states predispose to a variety of genital lesions. Balanitis—inflammation of the glans penis—due to *Candida*[38] or gram-negative bacteria[39] has been reported in neutropenic patients wearing condom catheters.

The acquired immunodeficiency syndrome (AIDS) is associated with chronic necrotizing and recurrent genital[40] and perianal[41] HSV infections and recalcitrant genital candidiasis as well.[42] In the setting of AIDS, the genital and disseminated lesions of syphilis may become progressive, nodular, and necrotizing,[43, 44] resulting in a condition known as *lues maligna.* Molluscum contagiosum proliferates, often involving the face.[25] In patients with AIDS, fungal infection, particularly cryptococcosis, can produce lesions morphologically indistinguishable from those of molluscum contagiosum.[45] Genital herpes can produce hypertrophic lesions,[46] and donovanosis[27] and chancroid[22] take longer to heal. It is now well established that the presence of genital ulcer disease increases the risk of transmission of human immunodeficiency virus (HIV)[47–49]

Mode of Onset and Course

Because lesions often change over time, a history of the initial manifestation may be helpful in making the diagnosis. Thus, the patient with genital ulcerations who can state with surety that the lesions began as vesicles has helped to confirm a diagnosis of herpes genitalis. Vesicles often rupture quickly, so that this stage of the lesions can go unnoticed by women.[23] A prodrome of local paresthesia preceding the appearance of lesions is reported by 50 to 90% of patients with recurrent genital herpes.[13, 14, 50, 51] The papuloulcerative primary lesion of lymphogranuloma venereum heals quickly and is usually overlooked by the patient.[52] Venereal warts and molluscum contagiosum may remain relatively static for long periods of time after their initial appearance. The lesions of syphilis often last for many weeks and then heal without antibiotic intervention.[15] Pearly penile papules, appearing in single or multiple rows around the penile corona at puberty, are a completely benign condition.[53]

Stereotypical recurrences of the lesions at intervals strongly suggest genital herpes. The rate of recurrence varies strikingly among affected persons, but the average rate of recurrence among patients genitally infected with HSV type 2 is 0.33 per month, whereas genital infections with HSV type 1 recur at an average rate of only 0.02 per month.[54] Indeed, whereas 90% of patients with symptomatic initial type 2 genital infections report a recurrence within 1 year, recurrences are experienced by only 25% of the symptomatic patients genitally infected with HSV type 1.

Pain

Although the syphilitic chancre is usually described as nontender, up to 30% of the patients with primary syphilis experience either pain or tenderness of the lesions.[37] The relative indolence of the lesions of donovanosis[27, 28] sometimes results in long delays before the patient seeks medical attention. Pain usually accompanies the lesions of chancroid,[21, 22] herpes genitalis,[13, 14, 23] tularemia,[55, 56] and amebiasis.[57–59]

Pruritus

Itching is associated with herpes genitalis and is described by 50 to 90% of patients with recurrent disease,[13, 14, 23, 51] particularly in the prodromal period. Pruritus accompanies 90% of infestations with pubic lice,[24] and severe itching, increased by warming the skin either in bed or when taking a bath, suggests scabies. Although *severe* pruritus is uncommon in secondary syphilis,[15] 42% of patients describe at least mild itching.[60] Pruritus also characterizes candidal balanitis, which is observed occasionally in male sexual partners of women with vulvovaginal candidiasis in men who have taken antibiotics.[36, 61, 62]

Vaginal Discharge

Several infectious vaginitides are associated with vulvar lesions. The vulvovaginitis syndrome is discussed in Chapter 95.

Fever

Fever occurs in 5 to 8% of the patients with secondary syphilis[15, 60] and in many patients with disseminated gonococcal infection.[63] Fever accompanies primary herpes genitalis in 70% of women and 40% of men but is uncommon in recurrent disease.[13, 14, 23, 50]

Other Features

Sacral root neurologic symptoms suggest herpes,[13, 14, 23] and a urethral discharge suggests gonorrhea or, less commonly, Reiter's syndrome (see Chapter 94). Inguinal adenopathy may accompany syphilis, chancroid, herpes genitalis, and lymphogranuloma venereum, in which lesions involve the vulva, distal two thirds of the vagina, shaft of the penis, or scrotum. The cervix and proximal third of the vagina and the glans penis drain to the iliac rather than the inguinal nodes, and lesions in these regions are not associated with palpable adenopathy. The adenopathy of herpes genitalis or chancroid is usually tender, whereas the adenopathy of syphilis is characteristically indolent.

MORPHOLOGIC CHARACTERISTICS OF GENITAL LESIONS

Careful examination of the entire genital area is essential and is facilitated by a good light source and use of a hand lens. A definitive diagnosis can often be made on the basis of the morphologic characteristics of genital lesions, but variations from the typical appearance and clinical overlap among the various diseases are unfortunately common.[29, 37, 64–67] A differential diagnosis for genital ulcers based on clinical appearance presents perhaps the greatest challenge,[29, 39, 64–69] with the most common error involving the overdiagnosis of herpes as chancroid.[29, 68] Nonetheless, the morphologic characteristics of genital lesions often supply the first clue to their cause. Table 93–1 provides a classification of genital lesions but can serve only as a rough guide.

The absence of lesions does not rule out active disease. From 1 to 8% of asymptomatic persons attending STD clinics are shedding herpes simplex virus.[70] About 60% of infected persons give no prior history of genital lesions,[71, 72] although with instruction some 50% can recognize subsequent symptomatic outbreaks.[73] In one study, only 22% of blood donors with antibody to HSV type 2 had a history of genital herpes.[74] Subclinical carriage of human papillomavirus (HPV) is common, and the rate of occurrence greatly exceeds that indicated by the presence of visible warts.[75, 76] Subclinical HPV lesions stain white when 5% acetic acid is applied for several minutes. The cause of such "acetowhite" lesions must be confirmed by biopsy, because several other inflammatory conditions produce the same reaction.[77, 78] Although long challenged, the asymptomatic carriage of *H. ducreyi* appears to have been demonstrated by polymerase chain reaction.[79]

Vesicles or Bullae

The classic initial lesions of genital herpes are grouped vesicles on an erythematous base.[13, 14] Umbilications are sometimes observed.[13, 14] The vesicles have often ruptured by the time the patient seeks medical attention, and only ulcers are observed. The initial manifestations of infection with varicella-zoster virus may be lesions in the

TABLE 93–1 Morphologic Classification of Genital Lesions

Ulcers	Vesicles and bullae
Herpes genitalis	Scabies
Syphilis	Herpes genitalis
Trauma	Diffuse erythema
Chancroid	Candidiasis
Fixed drug eruption	Trauma
Lymphogranuloma venereum	Contact dermatitis
Tularemia	Fixed drug eruption
Behçet's syndrome	Crusts
Malignancy	Herpes genitalis
Donovanosis (granuloma inguinale)	Scabies
Candidiasis	Miscellaneous findings
Histoplasmosis	Linear tracks: scabies
Mycobacterioses	Reddish flecks: crab louse excreta
Amebiasis	Maculae ceruleae (sky-blue spots): crab lice
Gonorrhea	Nits: crab lice
Trichomoniasis	Hypertrophic: donovanosis
Papules	
Venereal warts	
Scabies	
Molluscum contagiosum	
Candidiasis	
Syphilis	

genital area.[80] Scabies occasionally is manifested as vesicular or bullous lesions.[81]

Genital Ulcers

As noted earlier, the causes of genital ulcers vary markedly in different parts of the world. Chancroid has become far more common in major metropolitan areas of the United States,[21, 22, 29, 31] and the practitioner can no longer reject a clinical diagnosis of chancroid.[64] Tuberculosis,[82–84] histoplasmosis,[85] and amebiasis[57–59] are rare causes of destructive penile ulcerations. Genital ulcers have assumed particularly ominous importance, for it appears that they can serve as a portal of entry for HIV.[47–49]

The diagnostic information in the following sections should be applied with caution, as no single clinical features are specific for any etiologic diagnosis. DiCarlo and Martin have shown that the classic descriptive clinical patterns have relatively high specificity for syphilis (marked induration, limited tenderness, clean base: 98%), chancroid (undermined edges, tenderness, purulent base: 94%), and herpes (three or more shallow, tender lesions: 94%), but these patterns are seen in only about one third of the cases of each infection.[29, 30]

Number

The classic chancre of primary syphilis is a single lesion (Figs. 93–1 and 93–2)[15, 86]; however, in some series, almost half of all the patients with proven primary syphilis had more than one penile ulcer.[37, 86] Chancroid is usually said to present as multiple ulcerations, yet in some series, 40 to 70% of affected men had but a single lesion.[21, 22, 87] The genital lesion of tick-borne tularemia is solitary.[55] Herpes genitalis characteristically produces multiple ulcerations in groups surrounded by an erythematous border (Fig. 93–3).[13, 14, 23, 50] The vagina per se is involved in only 4% of cases.[13, 14, 23] A rare cause of recurrent, multiple genital ulcerations in the United States is Behçet's syndrome,[88, 89] an inflammatory disease of unknown etiology that usually also involves the oral, conjunctival, and synovial membranes. Behçet's ulcers occur on the scrotum and vulva more frequently than on the penis, anus, or vagina, and scars from previous episodes may be present.[88] Ulcers are occasionally observed in vulvovaginal or penile candidiasis. Intravaginal ulcers may follow tampon use,[90] but infectious and neoplastic causes must be ruled out in these cases.

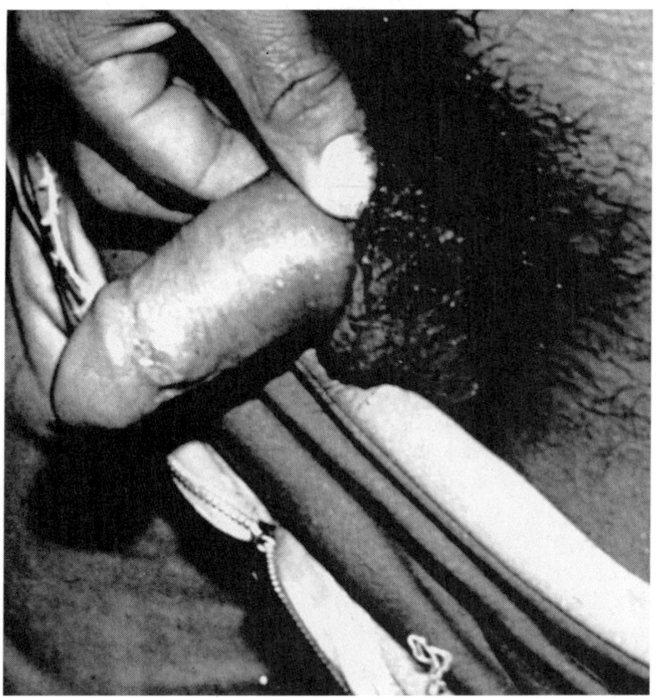

FIGURE 93–1. Primary syphilitic chancre of the penis.

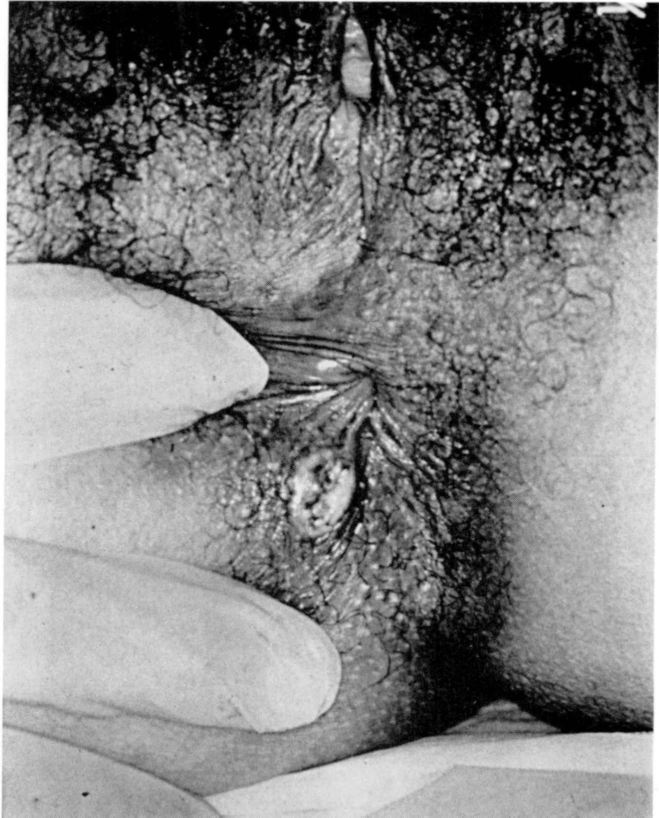

FIGURE 93–2. Primary syphilitic chancre of the perineum.

Size

The multiple ulcers of HSV tend to be of the same size, although individual ulcers may coalesce to form what appear to be larger lesions. The lesions of chancroid, however, are more variable on presentation, with ulcers ranging in size from 3 to 20 mm across.[21, 22, 52] Chancroidal lesions, too, may coalesce to form so-called "giant chancroid."[52]

Tenderness

Tenderness to palpation may be extreme with herpes genitalis,[13, 14, 23] and chancroid,[21, 22] is present in 30% of syphilitic chancres,[37] and characterizes tularemia.[55] Even massive, ulcerated lesions of donovanosis are nontender, however.[27, 28]

Ulcer Base

The lesions of chancroid are usually ragged and have a necrotic base.[21, 22, 29] Conversely, syphilitic and herpetic ulcers are relatively clean (see Figs. 93–1 to 93–3). The ulcers of Behçet's syndrome often have a yellow, necrotic base.[89] Donovanosis results in ulcers with granulation tissue at the base, yielding beefy red lesions that often become exuberantly hypertrophic and produce large, friable, ulcerated masses projecting above the skin.[27, 28]

Ulcer Edge

The ulcers of chancroid are characteristically undermined,[21, 22] a helpful finding,[29] but the edge is not indurated,[21, 22, 29] giving rise to the informal name "soft chancre." A markedly indurated lesion

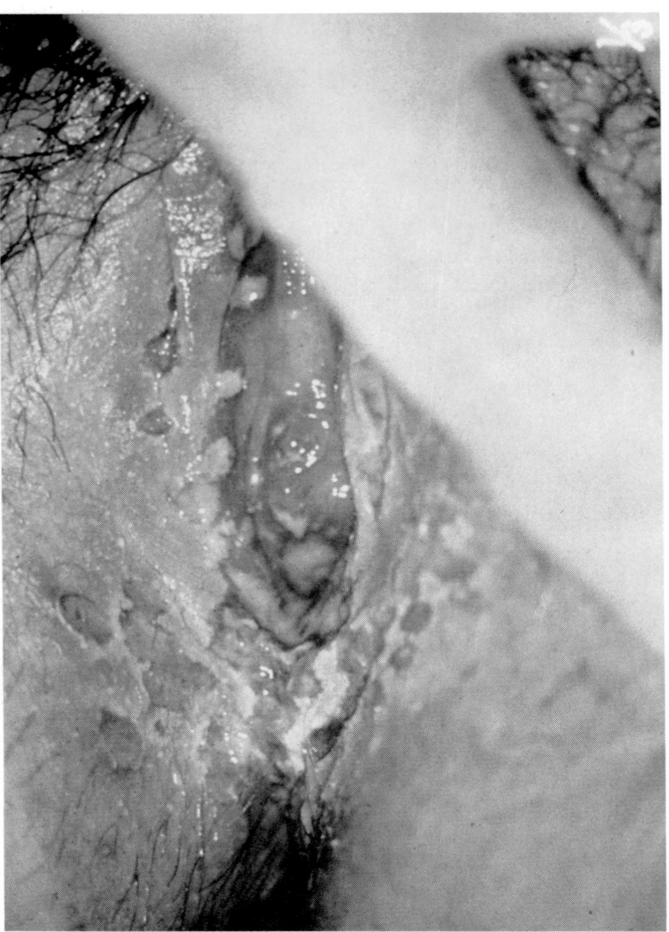

FIGURE 93–3. Herpes (HSV2) infection of the vulva.

suggests syphilis[15, 29] and occurs in 47 to 92% of infected patients.[29, 37] An erythematous border is seen both with herpes[13, 14, 23] and with chancroid.[21, 22] The border of the lesion in donovanosis may be stark white, which is characteristic of no other genital infection.[27, 28] Lesions of donovanosis also often manifest a thickening of the edge that yields a rolled appearance.[27, 28] Serpiginous lesions, progressing in one area as they heal in another, are characteristic of donovanosis[27, 28] and less so of chancroid.

Genital Papules

Careful examination of the papules with the aid of a hand lens often suggests a specific etiologic diagnosis. Papules may be the transient, initial manifestation of a variety of genital infections, including syphilis,[37] scabies,[91] lymphogranuloma venereum,[92] chancroid,[21, 22] and herpes.[13, 14, 23] Early condylomata acuminata usually appear as simple papules that can be identified when the hand lens reveals the beginning of a verrucous cap or tiny blood vessels at the base. Papular or papulosquamous lesions are seen on the external genitalia in most patients with secondary syphilis.[15, 50, 65, 66]

Pearly penile papules are a normal finding, occurring in 8 to 25% of men, and usually appear at puberty.[53] They are found more commonly in uncircumcised men and manifest as one or more rows of grayish-white or pink papules along the corona or in the coronal sulcus. Patients concerned about venereal disease occasionally notice the lesions and seek medical attention. Although their histologic appearance is characteristic, biopsy is rarely warranted because the diagnosis can be made clinically.

Umbilication

The hand lens will reveal tiny umbilications at the vertex of the lesions of molluscum contagiosum (see Chapter 123).[25, 26] The umbilications often appear to contain keratin plugs (Fig. 93–4). These 1- to 5-mm papules occur singly or in small clusters on the penile shaft, glans, labia majora, thighs, and buttocks. The lesions may be particularly abundant and disseminated in patients with AIDS,[93] but almost identical lesions are also seen in disseminated cryptococcosis in the same population.[45, 94] The lesions of molluscum contagiosum are nonpruritic and may coalesce to form larger masses.[25, 26] Squeezing a lesion expresses caseous material from the umbilication. If the diagnosis is in doubt, a papule can be removed and crushed between two microscope slides. Wright or Giemsa stain reveals cells distended by intracytoplasmic inclusions (see Chapter 123).

Verrucous Lesions

Verrucous papules suggest a diagnosis of condylomata acuminata (venereal warts). The lesions are usually multiple and may show a satellite phenomenon, wherein a larger wart is surrounded by smaller lesions. Stalked or sessile, the warts can be found anywhere on the external genitalia and in the vagina or on the cervix. Perianal warts in women may occur as a result of the spread from a genital focus. Perianal condylomata in men, however, are associated with receptive anal intercourse,[16, 17, 95] and men with these lesions should be evaluated for intra-anal warts and other anorectal infections. Perianal warts in men should prompt the clinician to recommend immediate serologic testing for HIV. Inside the vagina, warts may become relatively elongated.

Condylomata acuminata must be differentiated from the moist lesions of secondary syphilis, condylomata lata. The syphilitic lesions tend to be flatter and more grayish than viral warts.[15] Definitive diagnosis is best made by carefully abrading the lesions and performing a darkfield examination; condylomata lata are teeming with spirochetes. Unfortunately, anaerobic spirochetes occasionally superinfect condylomata acuminata, giving an initial appearance of darkfield positivity.

Venereal warts, particularly flat warts of the cervix, are strongly associated with cervical intraepithelial neoplasia and cancer (see Chapter 133),[96] and culposcopy or biopsy may be indicated for suspicious lesions.

Although acetic acid applications have long been used to identify subclinical HPV infections of the cervix and vagina, the technique is now also employed to detect otherwise invisible lesions in men.[77, 78, 97–101] Acetic acid, 3 to 5%, is applied to the penis for 3 to 5

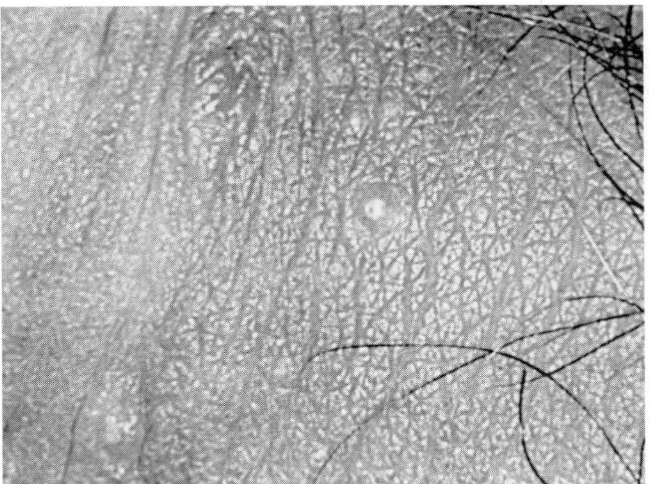

FIGURE 93–4. Molluscum contagiosum: Penile lesions displaying characteristic keratin-plugged umbilications.

minutes, and the skin is examined with the colposcope. Flat white lesions are revealed in 40 to 80% of the male partners of women with warts, and HPV is identified in 60 to 80% of such lesions by biopsy.[78, 97–101] Thus, the mere presence of acetowhite lesions does not confirm the diagnosis of HPV infection; other inflammatory conditions also yield a similar reaction with acetic acid.

Crusted Lesions

Herpetic ulcers heal by crusting over. Crusts are also characteristic of scabies (see Chapter 284) and may be accompanied by moist papules and burrows. These threadlike lesions, often stippled, are 1 to 10 mm long and are specific for scabies. They may be dramatically demonstrated by covering a papule with ink (as from a fountain pen) and then wiping it off with an alcohol swab. In about two thirds of cases, the burrow, now filled with ink, is readily visualized.[102]

Diffuse Erythematous Lesions

Superficial infection with the dermatophytes responsible for tinea or with *Candida* causes diffusely erythematous, intensely pruritic lesions of the groin. Candidal lesions are often more intensely erythematous and moist, whereas the lesions of tinea are usually somewhat brown, are frequently lichenified, and may show central clearing. Involvement of the scrotum and the appearance of small papules or pustules beyond the main border of the erythema (satellite lesions) suggest candidal infection.

Candidal balanitis occurs in some men who are the sexual partners of women with candidal vulvovaginitis[36, 61, 62] and is sometimes manifested as pruritic plaques of the glans, foreskin, or shaft of the penis. Other causes of balanitis or balanoposthitis (involvement of the internal surface of the prepuce) include group A[36, 103, 104] and group B[61, 104, 105] streptococci, anaerobic bacteria,[36, 106] gram-negative rods,[106] *Gardnerella vaginalis,*[36, 107] *Trichomonas vaginalis,*[36, 108, 109] mycobacteria,[36] amebae,[36, 57–59] and even mycoplasmas.[109] Staphylococcal balanitis has been associated with toxic shock syndrome.[110] HPV should be considered as a cause of recurrent or intractable patchy balanitis[111]; the diagnosis is confirmed histologically. Atopic dermatitis and reaction to soaps have also been implicated.[104]

Pubic Hair Findings

Crab lice are usually present in very small numbers, an average infestation consisting of fewer than 10.[112] Some lice are, however, observed in 97% of infested patients who have not treated the infection before seeking medical attention.[24] Examination of the pubic hair with a hand lens reveals the lice as gray-brown creatures climbing along the shafts or partially buried at the bases. They are found in perianal hair in about 50% of patients and in abdominal hair in about 17%.[24] If the organisms themselves are not observed, the diagnosis can still be made in 80% of patients by recognizing the eggs (nits) as 0.5-mm ovoids adherent to the hair shafts. A careful examination will reveal tiny reddish spots of louse excreta at the base of the hair or in the underwear of about 15% of patients.[24] Louse bites sometimes result in round to oval, 0.5- to 1.5-mm, bluish-red macules called *maculae ceruleae,* or sky-blue spots.[24, 113]

EXTRAGENITAL DERMATOLOGIC MANIFESTATIONS OF SEXUALLY TRANSMITTED DISEASES

Patients should be questioned about orogenital and receptive anal sexual practices, because these may result in direct inoculation of sexually transmitted pathogens into extragenital sites. Additionally, sexually transmitted infections sometimes disseminate, producing secondary extragenital manifestations.

Mouth

Direct inoculation of sexually transmitted viruses can cause oral lesions. Intraoral condylomata acuminata[23] and molluscum contagiosum[114] are reported, and lesions resemble those of the genital area. HSV has been transmitted from the genital tract to the mouth and vice versa.[13, 14, 23, 54] Genital lesions produced by HSV type 1 are indistinguishable from those produced by HSV type 2. Likewise, oral inoculation can result in fever blisters, a primary gingivostomatitis, or a herpangina-like picture, with clusters of vesicles and ulcers on the hard palate.[13, 14, 23, 115]

Although the oral mucosa is generally resistant to gonococcal infection, occasional cases of gonococcal stomatitis, presumably resulting from direct inoculation, have been reported.[116] Syphilitic chancres of the lip, buccal mucous membranes, gingiva, and tonsils are becoming relatively more common. They are usually painless and may be difficult to diagnose, because the normal presence of oral spirochetes confounds the darkfield examination.[15, 86]

Disseminated infections may also affect the mouth. Mucous patches occur in about 20% of patients with secondary syphilis and appear on the oral mucous membranes and the tongue as painless, relatively clean, shallow ulcerations, often with a yellow or gray base and a small amount of surrounding erythema.[15, 60, 86] Atypical presentations are described in patients with AIDS.[117] Palatal petechiae may accompany gonococcal bacteremia. Recurrent oral and genital ulcers suggest Behçet's syndrome.[88]

Anorectum

Perianal warts[16, 17, 95] and herpetic lesions[41, 118] are seen in homosexual men and also women who practice receptive anal intercourse. In women, however, the lesions may also have extended to the anus from a primary genital focus. Among patients with AIDS, herpetic proctitis may be chronic and relentlessly destructive.[41] Necrotizing perianal lesions occasionally result from amebiasis in endemic areas.[57, 59]

Other Skin

The generalized rash of secondary syphilis frequently involves the genitalia. In fact, a generalized eruption sparing the genital area and the oral mucous membranes is unlikely to be syphilis.[15] The rash is highly variable, and the differential diagnosis is challenging.[15, 65, 86] Secondary syphilis should be a consideration in the differential diagnosis for any generalized, relatively indolent eruption, particularly if the palms and soles are involved, if there is accompanying generalized lymphadenopathy (70 to 86%), or if there is patchy hair loss.[15, 50] The lesions are usually macular, maculopapular (70%), or papulosquamous and are symmetrically distributed.[15, 50] Vesicular or markedly pruritic lesions in an adult are unlikely to represent syphilis.

About 33 to 50% of patients with disseminated gonococcal infection will have a small number of skin lesions, which are usually found on the distal portions of the extremities and occasionally on the palms and the soles. Some patients with very large numbers of lesions have also been reported, but in these cases, meningococcemia must also be considered.[119] Lesions are relatively pleomorphic and may be macular, maculopapular, petechial, vesicular, pustular, or necrotic.[63] The typical lesion is an erythematous or hemorrhagic spot, 2 to 5 mm in diameter, that is surmounted by a gray pustule, sometimes displaying a small eschar in its center.[63] The lesions of subacute meningococcemia may be similar—an important consideration in the differential diagnosis.[119]

The interdigital webs, wrists, and ankles are often involved in scabies.[120] Secondary papular lesions, thought to represent a hypersensitivity phenomenon, may occur on the abdomen or in the pelvic girdle area. Burrows, described previously, are pathognomonic for scabies.[102] Maculae ceruleae (see earlier) are occasionally observed on the anterior and lateral portions of the abdomen and thorax of patients with crab lice.[113]

Herpes genitalis involves the thigh or buttock in some 15% of infected women.[121–123] Many of these women simultaneously shed virus from genital sites.[123] Patients with AIDS demonstrate a variety of skin lesions, including Kaposi's sarcoma, at some distance from sexual orifices (see Chapter 108).

LABORATORY EXAMINATION

Sufficiently accurate etiologic diagnoses can often be made on the basis of clinical examination when genital lesions are classic in presentation. In many situations, particularly in the etiologic diagnosis of genital ulcers, laboratory examination is required.[29, 52]

Direct Microscopic Examination

Any ulcerated genital lesion or hypertrophic lesion in a moist area may be examined by darkfield microscopy (see Chapter 227), which in experienced hands has a sensitivity for syphilis of 70 to 95%.[29, 124] The diagnosis of chancroid can sometimes be confirmed by cleaning the lesion with gauze and swabbing material from the undermined edge. Gram staining of this material may reveal chains of streptobacilli suggestive of *H. ducreyi*,[21, 22] but the smear technique has a low sensitivity and specificity and is not useful in a clinical setting.[33, 34–88, 124]

A smear of material from the base of a freshly ruptured vesicle may be stained with Wright or Giemsa stain and examined for the multinucleated giant cells that are diagnostic of herpetic infection—the Tzanck test.[13, 14, 23] This test is not generally helpful, however, because the presence of vesicles is essentially diagnostic of herpetic infection, and the test is insensitive on genital ulcers, with positive results in fewer than 40% of culture-proven cases.[125]

Bits of tissue from a hypertrophic lesion may be crushed between microscope slides, treated with Wright or Giemsa stain, and examined for the characteristic intracytoplasmic bacterial inclusions of donovanosis.[27, 28] Papular lesions may be scraped, crushed, stained with a variety of agents, and examined for the balloon-like cells of molluscum contagiosum.[25, 26] Heating skin scrapings with 10% potassium hydroxide will destroy the squamous elements and may reveal the dermatophytes responsible for tinea, *Candida,* or the mites or larvae of scabies.[91] Mixing scrapings with mineral oil rather than potassium hydroxide may give an advantage in the diagnosis of scabies, because unlike potassium hydroxide, mineral oil preserves mite fecal pellets and motility.[126] Scrapings or aspirates of the peripheral lesions of disseminated gonococcal infection reveal the organisms only infrequently by Gram stain but may be subjected to immunofluorescence microscopy, which will be diagnostic in about half the cases.[63, 127]

REFERENCES

1. Wilson JF. The nonvenereal diseases of the genitals: Their differentiation from venereal lesions. Med Clin North Am. 1964;48:787.
2. Hillman RJ, Wladron S, Walker MM, et al. Granuloma annulare of the penis. Genitourin Med. 1992;68:47–49.
3. Hillman RJ, Walker MM, Harris JRW, et al. Penile dermatoses: A clinical and histopathological study. Genitourin Med. 1992;68:166–169.
4. Shen RN, Cybulska RA, Thin RN, et al. Vulval Crohn's disease mimicking genital herpes. Int J STD AIDS. 1993;4:54–55.
5. Steinbach F, Essbach U, Florschutz A, et al. Ulcerative balanoposthitis as the initial manifestation of acute promyelocytic leukemia. J Urol. 1998;160:1430–1431.
6. Hibbard RA. Herpetic vulvovaginitis and child abuse. Am J Dis Child. 1985;139:542–545.
7. Dyson C, Hosein IK. The role of the microbiology laboratory in the investigation of child sexual abuse. J Med Microbiol. 1996;45:313–318.
8. Moscicki AB. Genital HPV infections in children and adolescents. Obstet Gynecol Clin North Am. 1996;23:675–697.
9. Bargman H, Schachner L, Hankim D. Is genital molluscum contagiosum a cutaneous manifestation of sexual abuse in children? J Am Acad Dermatol. 1986;14:847–849.
10. Ross JD, Scott GR, Busuttil A. Condylomata acuminata in prepubertal children. Med Sci Law. 1993;33:78–82.
11. Cohen BA, Honig P, Androphy E. Anogenital warts in children. Clinical and virological evidence for sexual abuse. Arch Dermatol. 1990;126:1575–1580.
12. Choukass NC, Toto PD. Condyloma acuminatum of the oral cavity. Oral Surg. 1982;54:480.
13. Corey L, Adams HG, Brown ZA, et al. Genital herpes simplex infection: Clinical manifestations, course, and complications. Ann Intern Med. 1983;98:958.
14. Mertz GJ. Genital herpes simplex virus infections. Med Clin North Am. 1990;74:1433–1454.
15. Stokes HJ, Beerman H, Ingraham NR. Modern Clinical Syphilology. 3rd ed. Philadelphia: WB Saunders; 1944.
16. Carr G, William DC. Anal warts in a population of gay men in New York City. Sex Transm Dis. 1977;4:56.
17. Oriel JD. Genital warts. Sex Transm Dis. 1981;8:326.
18. Wilde H, Canby JP. Penile venereal edema. Arch Dermatol. 1973;108:263.
19. Fried FA. Glans penis dermatitis after treatment of wife's vaginitis. JAMA. 1981;245:2532.
20. Gochfeld M, Burger J. Sexual transmission of nickel and poison oak contact dermatitis. Lancet. 1983;1:589.
21. Trees Dl, Morse SA. Chancroid and *Haemophilus ducreyi:* An update. Clin Microbiol Rev. 1995;8:357–375.
22. Marrazzo JM, Handsfield HH. Chancroid: New developments in an old disease. Curr Clin Top Infect Dis. 1995;15:129–152.
23. Pazin GJ. Management of oral and genital herpes simplex virus infections: Diagnosis and treatment. Dis Mon. 1986;32:725–824.
24. Chapel TA, Katta T, Kuszmar T, et al. Pediculosis pubis in a clinic for sexually transmitted diseases. Sex Transm Dis. 1979;6:257.
25. Lewis EJ, Lam M, Crutchfield CE. An update on molluscum contagiosum. Cutis. 1997;60:29–34.
26. Brown ST, Nalley JF, Kraus SJ. Molluscum contagiosum. Sex Transm Dis. 1981;8:227.
27. Jamkhedkar PP, Hira SK, Shroff HJ, Lanjewar DN. Clinico-epidemiologic features of granuloma inguinale in the era of acquired immunodeficiency syndrome. Sex Transm Dis. 1998;25:196–200.
28. Hart G. Donovanosis. Clin Infect Dis. 1997;25:24–30.
29. DiCarlo RP, Martin DH. The clinical diagnosis of genital ulcer disease in men. Clin Infect Dis. 1997;25:292–298.
30. Ronald A. Genital ulceration and clinical acumen. Clin Infect Dis. 1997;25:299–300.
31. DiCarlo RP, Armentor BS, Martin DH. Chancroid epidemiology in New Orleans men. J Infect Dis. 1995;172:446–452.
32. Talbot MD. Fixed genital drug eruption. Practitioner. 1980;224:823.
33. Dodds PR, Chi TN. Balanitis as a fixed drug eruption to tetracycline. J Urol. 1981;133:1044–1045.
34. Cohen HA, Ashkenazi A, Nussinovitch M, et al. Fixed drug eruption of the scrotum due to methylphenidate. Ann Pharmacother. 1992;26:1378.
35. Lacey HB, Ness A, Mandal BK. Vulval ulceration associated with foscarnet. Genitourin Med. 1992;68:182.
36. Edwards S. Balanitis and balanoposthitis: a review. Genitourin Med. 1996;72:155–159.
37. Chapel TA. The variability of syphilitic chancres. Sex Transm Dis. 1978;5:68.
38. Morrissey R, Xavier A, Nguyen N, et al. Invasive candidal balanitis due to a condom catheter in a neutropenic patient. South Med J. 1985;78:1247–1249.
39. Manian FA, Alford RH. Nosocomial infectious balanoposthitis in neutropenic patients. South Med J. 1987;80:909–911.
40. Maier JA, Bergman A, Ross MG. Acquired immunodeficiency syndrome manifested by chronic primary genital herpes. Am J Obstet Gynecol. 1986;155:756–758.
41. Siegal FP, Lopez C, Hammer GS, et al. Severe acquired immunodeficiency in male homosexuals manifested by chronic perianal herpes simplex lesions. N Engl J Med. 1981;305:1439–1444.
42. Imam N, Carpenter CCJ, Mayer KH, et al. Hierarchical pattern of mucosal *Candida* infections with HIV seropositive women. Am J Med. 1990;89:142.
43. Don PC, Rubenstein R, Christie S. Malignant syphilis (lues maligna) and concurrent infection with HIV. Int J Dermatol. 1995;34:403–407.
44. Sands M, Markus A. Lues maligna, or ulceronodular syphilis, in a man with human immunodeficiency virus: Case report and review. Clin Infect Dis. 1995;20:387–390.
45. Munoz-Perez MA, Colmenero MA, Rodriguez-Pichardo A, et al. Disseminated cryptococcosis presenting as molluscum-like lesions as the first manifestation of AIDS. Int J Dermatol. 1996;35:646–648.
46. Tong P, Mutasim DF. Herpes simplex virus infection masquerading as condyloma acuminatum in a patient with HIV disease. Br J Dermatol. 1996;134:797–800.
47. O'Farrell N. Global eradication of donovanosis: An opportunity for limiting the spread of HIV-1 infection. Genitourin Med. 1995;71:27–31.
48. Hayes RJ, Schulz KF, Plummer FA. The cofactor effect of genital ulcers on the per-exposure risk of HIV transmission in sub-saharan Africa. J Trop Med Hyg. 1995;98:1–8.
49. Wasserheit JN. Epidemiological synergy: Interrelationship between HIV infection and other STDs. Sex Transm Dis. 1992;19:61–77.
50. Guinan ME, MacCalman J, Kern ER, et al. The course of untreated recurrent genital herpes simplex infection in 27 women. N Engl J Med. 1981;304:759.
51. Brookes JL, Haywood S, Green J. Prodromal symptoms in genital herpes simplex infection. Genitourin Med. 1992;68:347–348.
52. Rosen T, Brown TJ. Cutaneous manifestations of sexually transmitted diseases. Med Clin North Am. 1998;82:1081–1104.
53. Rehbein HM. Pearly penile papules: Incidence. Cutis. 1977;19:54.
54. Lafferty WE, Coombs RW, Benedetti J, et al. Recurrences after oral and genital

herpes simplex virus infection. Influence of site of infection and viral type. N Engl J Med. 1987;316:1444–1449.
55. Dienst FT. Tularemia: A perusal of 339 cases. J La State Med Soc. 1963;115:114.
56. Evans ME, Gregory DW, Schaffner W, et al. Tularemia: A 30 year experience with 88 cases. Medicine. 1985;64:251–269.
57. Parkash S, Ramakrishnan K, Ananthakrishnan N, et al. Amoebic ulcer of the penis. Postgrad Med J. 1982;58:375.
58. Veliath AJ, Bansal R, Sankaran V, et al. Genital amebiasis. Int J Gynaecol Obstet. 1987;25:249–256.
59. O'Leary RK, Posen J. Amoebiasis of the penis. S Afr Med J. 1984;65:113–116.
60. Chapel TA. The signs and symptoms of secondary syphilis. Sex Transm Dis. 1980;7:161.
61. Abdullah AN, Drake SM, Wade AA, Walzman M. Balanitis (balanoposthitis) in patients attending a department of genitourinary medicine. Int J STD AIDS. 1992;3:128–129.
62. Dockerty WG, Sonnex C. Candidal balano-posthitis: A study of diagnostic methods. Genitourin Med 1995;71:407–409.
63. Cucurull E, Espinoza LR. Gonococcal arthritis. Rheum Dis Clin North Am. 1998;24:305–322.
64. Chapel TA, Brown WJ, Jeffries C, et al. How reliable is the morphologic diagnosis of penile ulcerations? Sex Transm Dis. 1977;4:150.
65. Chapel TA. Physician recognition of the signs and symptoms of secondary syphilis. JAMA. 1981;246:250.
66. Dangor Y, Ballard RC, Exposto FDL, et al. Accuracy of clinical diagnosis of genital ulcer disease. Sex Transm Dis. 1990;17:184–189.
67. O'Farrell N, Hoosen AA, Coetzee KD, et al. Genital ulcer disease: Accuracy of clinical diagnosis and strategies to improve control in Durban, South Africa. Genitourin Med. 1994;70:7–11.
68. Ndinya-Achola JO, Kihara AN, Fisher LD, et al. Presumptive specific clinical diagnosis of genital ulcer disease (GUD) in a primary health care setting in Nairobi. Int J STD AIDS 1996;7:201–205.
69. Verdich J. *Haemophilus ducreyi* infection resembling granuloma inguinale. Acta Dermatol Venereol. 1984;64:452–455.
70. Guinan ME, Wolinsky SM, Reichman RC. Epidemiology of genital herpes simplex virus infection. Epidemiol Rev. 1985;7:127–146.
71. Koutsky LA, Stevens CE, Holmes KK, et al. Underdiagnosis of genital herpes by current clinical and viralisolation procedures. N Engl J Med. 1992;326:1533–1539.
72. Koutsky LA, Ashley RL, Holmes KK, et al. The frequency of unrecognized type 2 herpes simplex virus infection among women. Implications for the control of genital herpes. Sex Transm Dis. 1990;17:90–94.
73. Langenberg A, Benedetti J, Jenkins J, et al. Development of clinically recognizable genital lesions among women previously identified as having "asymptomatic" herpes simplex virus type 2 infection. Ann Intern Med. 1989;110:882–887.
74. Cowan FM, Johnson AM, Ashley R, et al. Relationship between antibodies to herpes simiplex virus (HSV) and symptoms of HSV infection. J Infect Dis. 1996;174:470–475.
75. Horn JE, McQuillan GM, Shah KV, et al. Genital human papillomavirus infection in patients attending an inner-city STD clinic. Sex Transm Dis. 1991;18:183–187.
76. Kiviat NB, Koutsky LA, Paavonen JA, et al. Prevalence of genital papillomavirus infection among women attending a college student health clinic or a sexually transmitted disease clinic. J Infect Dis. 1989;159:293–302.
77. Wikstrom A, Hedblad MA, Johansson B, et al. The acetic acid test in evaluation of subclinical genital papillomavirus infection: A comparative study on penoscopy, histopathology, virology and scanning electron microscopy findings. Genitourin Med. 1992;68:90–99.
78. Hippeläinen MI, Syrjänen, Hippeläinen MJ, et al. Diagnosis of genital human papillomavirus (HPV) lesions in the male: Correlation of penoscopy, histology, and in situ hybridisation. Genitourin Med. 1993;69:346–351.
79. Hawkes S, West B, Wilson S, et al. Asymptomatic carriage of *Haemophilus ducreyi* confirmed by the polymerase chain reaction. Genitourin Med. 1995;71:224–227.
80. Simon HK, Steele DW. Varicella: Pediatric genital/rectal vesicular lesions of unclear origin. Ann Emerg Med. 1995;25:111–114.
81. Veraldi S, Scarabelli G, Zerboni R, et al. Bullous scabies. Acta Derm Venereol. 1996;76:167–168.
82. Vekataramaiah NR, van Raate JA, Dutta SN. Tuberculous ulcer of the penis. Postgrad Med J. 1982;58:59.
83. Nishigori C, Taniguchi S, Hayakawa M, et al. Penis tuberculosis: Papulonecrotic tuberculosis on the glans penis. Dermatologica. 1986;172:93–97.
84. Kumar B, Skarma VK. Papulonecrotic tuberculids on glans penis. Dermatologica. 1987;174:151–153.
85. Carroll PR, Cattokica EV, Turzan CW, et al. Necrotizing soft-tissue infections of the perineum and genitalia. Etiology and early reconstruction. West J Med. 1986;144:174–178.
86. Hutchinson CVM, Hook EW 3d. Syphilis in adults. Med Clin North Am. 1990;74:1389–1416.
87. D'Costa LJ, Bowmer I, Nsanze H, et al. Advances in the diagnosis and management of chancroid. Sex Transm Dis. 1986;13:189–191.
88. Shmmizu T, Ehrlich GE, Inaba G, et al. Behçet disease (Behçet syndrome). Semin Arthritis Rheum. 1979;8:223.
89. Lee S. Diagnostic criteria of Behçet's disease: Problems and suggestions. Yonsei Med J. 1997;38:365–369.
90. Weissberg SM, Dodson MG. Recurrent vaginal and cervical ulcers associated with tampon use. JAMA. 1983;250:1430.
91. Shelley WB, Wood MG. Larval papule as a sign of scabies. JAMA. 1976;236:1144.
92. Schachter J, Dawson CR. Human Chlamydial Infection. Littleton, Mass: PSG Publishing; 1978:45.
93. Schwartz JJ, Myskowski PI. Molluscum contagiosum in patients with human immunodeficiency virus infection. A review of twenty-seven patients. J Am Acad Dermatol. 1992;27:583–588.
94. Ghigliotti G, Carrega G, Farris A, et al. Cutaneous cryptococcosis resembling molluscum contagiosum in a homosexual man with AIDS. Report of a case and review of the literature. Acta Derm Venereol. 1992;72:182–184.
95. Oriel JD. Genital warts. Sex Transm Dis. 1977;4:153.
96. Koutsky LA, Holmes KK, Critchlow CW, et al. A cohort study of the risk of cervical intraepithelial neoplasia grade 2 or 3 in relation to papillomavirus infection. N Engl J Med. 1992;327:1272–1278.
97. Rosenberg SK. Subclinical papilloma viral infection of male genitalia. Urology. 1985;26:554–557.
98. Sand PK, Baven LW, Blischke PA, et al. Evaluation of male consorts of women with genital human papilloma virus infections. Obstet Gynecol. 1986;68:679–681.
99. Schultz RE, Skelton HG. Value of acetic acid screening for flat genital condylomata in men. J Urol. 1988;139:777–975.
100. Krebs HB, Schneider V. Human papillomavirus–associated lesions of the penis: Colposcopy, cytology, and histology. Obstet Gynecol. 1987;70:299–304.
101. Sedlack TV, Cunnane M, Carpiniello V. Colposcopy in the diagnosis of penile condyloma. Am J Obstet Gynecol. 1986;154:494–496.
102. Woodley D, Saurat JH. The burrow ink test and the scabies mite. J Am Acad Dermatol. 1981;4:715.
103. Kyriazi NC, Costenbader CL. Group A beta-hemolytic streptococcal balanitis: It may be more common than you think. Pediatrics. 1991;88:154–156.
104. Birley HDL, Walker MM, Luzzi GA, et al. Clinical features and management of recurrent balanitis: Association with atopy and genital washing. Genitourin Med. 1993;69:400–403.
105. Lucks DA, Venezio FR, Lakin CM. Balanitis caused by group B streptococcus. J Urol. 1986;135:1015.
106. Sonnex C, Croucher PE, Dockerty WG. Balanposthitis associated with the presence of subpreputial "smegma stones." Genitourin Med. 1997;73:567.
107. Burdge DR, Bowie WR, Chow A. *Gardnerella vaginalis*–associated balanoposthitis. Sex Transm Dis. 1986;13:159–162.
108. Krieger JN. Epidemiology and clinical manifestations of urogenital trichomoniasis in men. In: Honigberg BM, ed. Trichomonads Parasitic in Humans. New York: Springer Verlag; 1990:235–245.
109. Vohra S, Badlani G. Balanitis and balanoposthitis. Urol Clin North Am. 1992;19:143–147.
110. Daher A, Fortenberry JD. *Staphylococcus*–induced toxic shock following balanitis. Clin Pediatr. 1995;34:172–174.
111. Arumainayagam JT, Sumathipala AH, Smallman LA, et al. Flat condylomata of the penis presenting as patchy balanoposthitis. Genitourin Med. 1990;66:251–253.
112. Ackerman A. Crabs: The resurgence of *Phthirus pubis*. N Engl J Med. 1968;278:950.
113. Miller RA. Maculae ceruleae. Int J Dermatol. 1986;25:383–384.
114. Whitaker SB, Wiegand SE, Budnick SD. Intraoral molluscum contagiosum. Oral Surg Oral Med Oral Pathol. 1991;72:334–336.
115. Chang TW. Herpetic angina following orogenital exposure. J Am Vener Dis. 1975;1:163.
116. Jamsky RJ, Christen AG. Oral gonococcal infections. Oral Surg. 1982;53:358.
117. Ficarra G, Zaragoza AM, Stendardi L, et al. Early oral presentation of lues maligna in a patient with HIV infection. Oral Surg Oral Med Oral Pathol. 1993;75:728–732.
118. Goodell SE, Quinn TC, Mkrtichian PAC, et al. Herpes simplex virus proctitis in homosexual men. Clinical, sigmoidoscopic and histopathological features. N Engl J Med. 1983;308:868.
119. Rompalo AM, Hook EW 3rd, Roberts PL, et al. The acute arthritis dermatitis syndrome. The changing importance of *Neisseria gonorrhoeae* and *Neisseria meningitidis*. Arch Intern Med. 1987;147:281–283.
120. Burkhart CG. Scabies: An epidemiologic reassessment. Ann Intern Med. 1983;98:498.
121. Weisman K, Secher L, Hjorth N. Recurrent genital herpes on the buttocks: "Herpes disciformis." Cutis. 1987;40:166–168.
122. Wickett WH, Miller RD. Sites of multiple lesions in recurrent genital herpes. Am Fam Physician. 1985;32:145–152.
123. Mead PB, Amstey MS, Gail SA, et al. Report on asymptomatic genital excretion of herpes simplex virus (HSV) in 21.9% of 41 women with clinical buttock herpes. J Reprod Med. 1991;36:831–834.
124. Cummings MC, Lukehart SA, Marra C, et al. Comparison of methods for the detection of *Treponema pallidum* in lesions of early syphilis. Sex Transm Dis. 1996;23:366–369.
125. Brown ST, Jaffe HW, Zaidi A, et al. Sensitivity and specificity of diagnostic tests for genital infection with *Herpesvirus hominis*. Sex Transm Dis. 1979;6:10.
126. Austin VH, Topham EB. Mineral oil versus KOH for *Sarcoptes*. J Am Acad Dermatol. 1982;7:555.
127. Tronca E, Handsfield HH, Wiesner PJ, et al. Demonstration of *Neisseria gonorrhoeae* with fluorescent antibody in patients with disseminated gonococcal infection. J Infect Dis. 1974;129:583.

Chapter 94

Urethritis

WILLIAM M. McCORMACK
MICHAEL F. REIN

Urethritis is a very common condition that was described in the earliest recorded histories of humankind. Two recent reviews present a historical overview of urethritis.[1, 2]

The symptoms of urethritis range from the trivial and often overlooked to the disabling. Urethral discharge may be apparent at all times during the day and may be present in sufficient quantity to stain undergarments, or it may be so scanty that it is noted by the patient only on arising as a small bead of moisture or crust at the meatus. It may be completely clear, mucopurulent, or frankly purulent, and it may be white, yellow, green, or brown. Some patients complain only of a deviation of the first morning urine stream. Occasionally, urethral discharge comes to the attention of the patient through the observation of mucus strands in the urine specimen.

The urine stream transiently eliminates most inflammatory discharges; thus, scanty discharges are best observed on arising before the passage of any urine. Micturition immediately preceding urethral examination may completely eliminate signs of infection.

The discomfort of urethritis can take several forms. Dysuria is common, and men variously localize it to the meatus, the distal portion of the penis, or anywhere along the shaft. Discomfort is sometimes increased by the acidity or solute content of the urine and therefore may be most marked during the passage of a concentrated first morning urine. Dysuria may be increased in the presence of irritants such as alcohol, which is an observation that sometimes leads the patient to attribute his disease to the ingestion of specific foods or fluids. Discomfort may persist between micturitions and is perceived as pain, itching, frequency, urgency, or a feeling of heaviness in the genitals.

Discomfort experienced only during ejaculation, deep pelvic pain, or pain radiating to the back is infrequent in uncomplicated urethritis and suggests prostatitis or inflammation involving other portions of the urogenital tract such as the epididymis. Hematuria, particularly if painless, or blood in the ejaculate is uncommon in urethritis. The persistence of hematuria after cure of urethritis demands a thorough urologic evaluation.

EXAMINATION OF THE URETHRA

Men should stand before the seated examiner so that the external genitalia are at approximately eye level. Alternatively, the genitalia can be examined while the patient is supine. A good light source is essential. The patient should remove his trousers and underwear so that the entire genital area can be observed. The underwear may reveal stains of dried discharge, suggesting that it is being produced in large amounts. This observation is particularly useful if the patient has recently urinated.

The patient is preferably examined at least 2 hours after his last micturition. If advised to restrict his fluids during the day preceding the examination, he may be able to present for evaluation before passing the first urine of the day, which sometimes permits the recovery of very small amounts of discharge.[3]

The entire genital area should be carefully examined because other sexually transmitted infections are relatively common in patients with urethritis. Inguinal adenopathy should be sought, and tenderness should be noted. The skin of the entire pubic area, scrotum, groin, and penis should be examined for lesions, and the hair should be examined for nits. The testes, epididymides, and spermatic cords should be palpated for masses or tenderness. The foreskin should be completely retracted and the glans examined. The urethral meatus should be inspected for dried crusts, redness, and spontaneous discharge. If no discharge is present, the urethra should be gently stripped as follows: The examiner places the gloved thumb along the ventral surface of the base of the penis and the forefinger on the dorsum and then applies gentle pressure; the hand is moved slowly toward the meatus. This maneuver will frequently expel a discharge that may be collected on a swab for examination as described later on.

If no discharge is delivered by this maneuver, the third and fourth fingers should be used to grip the penis lightly from above, just behind the glans. The thumb and forefinger can then spread open the meatus to examine for urethral redness or the presence of small amounts of discharge. Unless the patient has recently urinated or has been in a state of sexual arousal, virtually no fluid should be expressible from the urethra or observed by spreading the meatus.

If expressed material cannot be collected at the meatus, a specimen must be recovered from inside the urethra. This is best accomplished with a calcium alginate urethral or nasopharyngeal swab.[4] The swab should be inserted gently at least 2 cm into the urethra with care taken not to attempt to force the tip past an obstruction. The patient should be warned that the examination is uncomfortable; also, the insertion and removal of the swab should be accomplished as quickly as possible. Patients may tolerate the examination better if they are supine. If additional specimens are required for multiple examinations or cultures, separate swabs should be used, and each one should be inserted at least 1 cm deeper than the one preceding it.

Regular cotton swabs should not be used for urethral examination, because their larger diameter makes insertion extremely uncomfortable and because of the possibility that the cotton or the wooden shaft may be toxic to some fastidious pathogens. A small platinum loop is effective, but it must be sterilized in a flame and carefully cooled between uses.

A woman's urethra is best examined when she is in the lithotomy position. The entire genital area should be examined for lesions, and the vagina should be examined as described in Chapter 95. The urethral meatus may be directly visualized, and the urethra may be stripped by placing the gloved finger inside the vagina and gently moving it along the urethra. A calcium alginate swab may be inserted a short distance into the meatus to obtain a urethral specimen.

EXAMINATION OF THE URETHRAL SPECIMEN

A swab that contains material from the urethra should be rolled across a clean microscope slide. Rolling rather than streaking the swab brings all its surfaces into contact with the slide and better preserves cellular morphologic characteristics. The material may be air-dried and fixed by gentle heating or by rinsing with methanol. Gram staining of urethral material is particularly useful in the workup of urethritis, and the specimen should be examined by using the oil-immersion objective. Specimens obtained from within the urethra generally reveal urethral epithelial cells. When recovered from near the meatus, these are typical squamous cells with a very large cytoplasmic-nuclear ratio, or when obtained from further within the urethra they are cuboidal epithelial cells, which are smaller and have relatively larger, less dense nuclei.

Urethral material from patients with acute urethritis will contain polymorphonuclear neutrophils (PMNs). The area of the smear that contains the most PMNs should be sought. More than four PMNs per oil-immersion microscopic field is always abnormal and is seen in 60 to 90% of all patients with acute symptomatic urethritis.[4–6] However, 16 to 50% of all men with documented urethral infection will not show four PMNs in maximally dense oil-immersion fields.[7–12] The number of PMNs in the smear is reduced by recent micturition[13]; also, there often is considerable observer variation in the number of PMNs detected in a single specimen.[14] Thus, although purulent discharges may reveal sheets of PMNs, the minimal number of these cells that indicates disease is not known. In general, the presence of even rare PMNs suggests infection, particularly in the patient who has urethral symptoms or who is found to have a small amount of discharge on examination.

The distal centimeter of the urethra is colonized by normal skin or introital flora. The smear will usually contain a variety of gram-positive and gram-negative organisms that have no particular significance. Of great diagnostic value, however, is the presence of typical gram-negative, "intracellular" diplococci (Fig. 94–1). These organisms are not randomly distributed among the cells but are seen in large numbers in a few PMNs. They will be observed in more than 95% of all symptomatic patients with gonococcal urethritis and in fewer than 2% of all symptomatic men who cannot be shown to have gonorrhea by culture.[15–17] Some strains of *Neisseria gonorrhoeae* are inhibited by the concentrations of vancomycin that usually are employed in selective isolation media; these organisms will not be recovered by standard culture techniques.[18] Extracellular diplococci indicate gonorrhea in only 10 to 29% of all cases, and this predictive value is reduced even further in populations with a low prevalence of gonorrhea.[17] A shortcoming of the Gram-stained smear is that it cannot diagnose coincidental nongonococcal urethritis (NGU) in the presence of gonorrhea. Although a smear containing PMNs that does not reveal gram-negative intracellular diplococci strongly suggests NGU, a smear revealing these organisms does not rule out NGU.

Candida organisms may be recognized as gram-positive or beaded, oval bodies about 3 by 6 μm. Observing small numbers of yeast cells does not prove a candidal origin for the urethritis, because *Candida* may be recovered from normal patients, particularly if they are uncircumcised.

Trichomonads are very difficult to identify on Gram-stained smears. Urethral material may be mixed with a small amount of saline and observed as a wet mount with the substage condenser racked down or the substage diaphragm partially closed. Motile trichomonads occasionally are observed but are rarely seen unless the urethral material for examination is obtained before the first voiding. Positive findings on a wet mount are diagnostic of trichomoniasis, but findings on the wet mount are often negative in infected men. Endourethral cultures or cultures of first-void urine sediment in media such as modified Diamond's medium constitute the preferred method for diagnosis of trichomoniasis in men.[19, 20]

After the patient's urethra has been carefully examined, he may be asked to provide a divided urine specimen. The patient delivers the first 10 ml of urine into one container and a midstream urine specimen into a second. The presence of mucus strands in the first fraction that clear in the second portion suggests urethritis. Equal aliquots of the fractions may be centrifuged and the sediments examined as wet mounts. Observing more white blood cells in the initial than in the second fraction suggests urethritis, while observing equal numbers of white cells in both fractions suggests cystitis or infection higher in the urinary tract.[3] A total of more than 15 white blood cells in five 400× microscopic fields of the sediment from the initial fraction strongly suggests urethritis,[4, 7, 10] but the minimum significant number of white blood cells is unknown. A PMN count of more than 10 per high-power field is found in 90% of all men with chlamydial urethritis.[7]

The presence of white blood cells in the initial urine fraction provides no clue to the cause of the urethritis. Such a finding, however, may allow an objective diagnosis of urethritis to be made in a man whose Gram-stained smear does not contain PMNs.

Many men who are infected with *N. gonorrhoeae* or *Chlamydia trachomatis* have no symptoms. Such men often have pyuria that can be detected by examination of the first 10-ml urine sample by either microscopy or leukocyte-esterase "dipstick" testing. This approach provides a noninvasive, inexpensive method for screening men for urethral infection. Men found to have pyuria are candidates for further examination, including examination of endourethral specimens for gonococci and chlamydia.[21]

If the urine specimen is a first morning micturition, motile trichomonads may be observed in the sediment. In one study, *Trichomonas vaginalis* organisms were recovered by culture of urethral swabs in 80% and first-void urine in 68% of infected patients. When combined, these two cultures detected 49 (98%) of 50 infected men.[19] Trichomonads are recovered less frequently from patients who have already voided during the day.

Material recovered from the urethra can be cultured with appropriate media for *N. gonorrhoeae*. Culture systems for *C. trachomatis* are not widely available. Nonculture tests such as enzyme-linked immunosorbent assay (ELISA) and gene amplification techniques such as polymerase chain reaction for identifying *C. trachomatis* in genital specimens have been developed (see Chapter 168) and are changing our approach to these infections. Although ELISA, DNA probes, and direct immunofluorescence tests are less sensitive than cultures, gene amplification tests appear to be more sensitive than chlamydial cultures while retaining high specificity.[22–25] Gene amplification techniques will probably replace cell culture as the standard modality for identification of *C. trachomatis* organisms.

Cultures for *Ureaplasma urealyticum* should not be performed. Their interpretation is complicated by the high prevalence of colonization in asymptomatic, sexually active people. Although present in the distal urethra, normal skin organisms (such as *Staphylococcus epidermidis*, α-hemolytic streptococci, and propionibacteria) and vag-

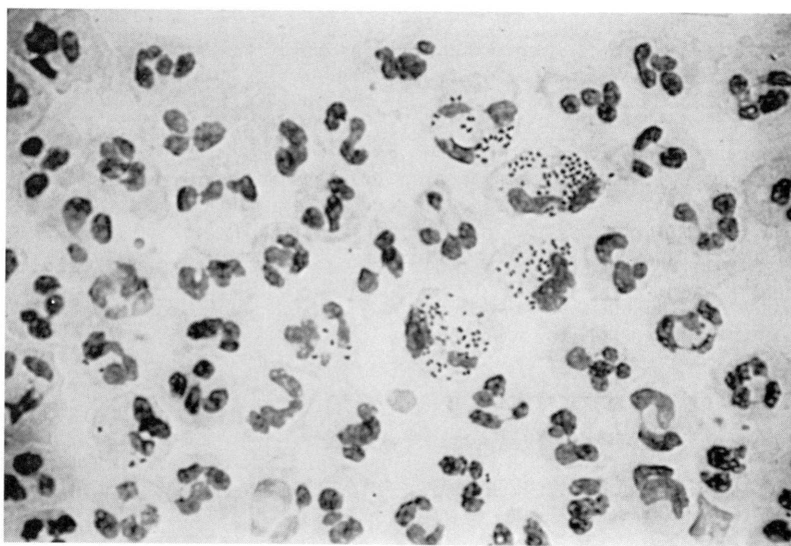

FIGURE 94–1. Gram stain of urethral exudate from a man with gonorrhea. Several neutrophils contain many gram-negative cell-associated diplococci.

inal organisms (such as *Candida albicans,* lactobacilli, *Escherichia coli,* and *Gardnerella vaginalis*) are of no diagnostic significance.[26, 27]

NONINFECTIOUS URETHRITIS

So psychologically important is the genital tract that trivial symptoms often receive patients' frightened attention. The "worried well" make up a significant fraction of men who are seen in venereal disease clinics and in private practices. Sympathetic questioning as to why the patient thinks he has contracted a genital infection may reveal guilt over an act such as masturbation, which does not put the patient at significant risk of infection. The urethral specimen in these cases usually reveals normal epithelial cells and no white blood cells. Some patients confuse dried remnants of semen with inflammatory discharge. Microscopic examination again fails to reveal inflammatory cells, but spermatozoa may be recognized on the Gram stain as gram-positive ovoids whose coloration fades gradually toward the acrosomal cap or may be recognized on the wet mount. However, the physician must remember that symptoms and signs of true urethritis can be trivial and that microscopic examination may miss minimal inflammation, particularly if the patient has recently voided. Symptomatic patients with negative examination results should have urethral specimens examined for gonococci and chlamydiae and be asked to return in several days, by which time the symptoms may have resolved or examination may provide a diagnosis. Antimicrobial treatment of symptomatic men who have neither objective evidence of urethritis nor positive cultures for urethral pathogens is inadvisable and may serve to reinforce psychosomatic contributions to their symptoms.[28] An occasional patient who complains of a discharge is really suffering from urinary incontinence.

Chronic irritation of the urethra can elicit a clear, mucoid discharge. Occasional patients, concerned that they may have contracted a venereal disease, vigorously strip the urethra looking for a discharge. After several days of this, a clear discharge obligingly appears that may contain a few white blood cells. A history of vigorous urethral stripping is helpful diagnostically. Patients who are receiving treatment for other forms of urethritis should be cautioned not to examine themselves too vigorously for fear that such a traumatic discharge may confuse the clinical picture. Very rarely, patients will insert foreign bodies into the urethra and produce a mechanical urethritis.[29] This sort of self-instrumentation should be considered in retarded or psychotic persons.

A heavy precipitation of crystals in the urine can suggest a discharge, and the presence of large amounts of crystalline material or calculous gravel may produce urinary discomfort. The intermittent nature of pain associated with the passage of gravel or the obvious presence of crystals on microscopic examination of the urine sediment usually confirms this diagnosis. White blood cells may be present.

Urethritis may accompany noninfectious systemic disease such as Stevens-Johnson syndrome or Wegener's granulomatosis.

Chemicals may irritate the urethra, and alcohol has long been known to produce mild dysuria. The ingestion of alcohol during the treatment for gonorrhea was at one time thought to be responsible for the syndrome of postgonococcal urethritis, discussed later, although it is now known to have an infectious etiology. An occasional patient may develop urethral symptoms on contact with vaginal chemicals such as spermicides used by a sexual partner. The history of discomfort immediately after sexual contact may be suggestive. This condition should be diagnosed only after other possible causes have been excluded.

INFECTIOUS URETHRITIS

Gonococcal and Nongonococcal Urethritis

The classic specific etiologic agent of acute urethritis is *N. gonorrhoeae.* Urethral inflammation of all other causes is referred to collectively as NGU. As with gonorrhea, most cases of NGU are sexually acquired. NGU is more common than gonorrhea in the United States and in much of the developed world as well. In some underdeveloped areas, however, gonorrhea accounts for 80% of the cases of acute urethritis. As with many other sexually transmitted diseases (STDs), gonococcal urethritis and NGU have an increased incidence during the summer months, presumably because of a seasonal increase in sexual activity. The ratio of cases of NGU to gonococcal urethritis is greater among groups of higher socioeconomic status in the United States. Thus, most of the urethritis cases seen among college students are nongonococcal in origin, whereas gonorrhea is the most common cause of urethritis in most urban STD clinics.[30–32]

Compared with gonococci, the organisms that cause NGU are relatively less prevalent among homosexual than among heterosexual men with urethritis. Examining consecutive men attending an STD clinic, Stamm and colleagues[9] recovered gonococci from 12% of heterosexual and 25% of homosexual men, whereas they recovered chlamydiae from 14% of heterosexual but only 5% of homosexual men. Recent studies have associated fellatio with the acquisition of gonococcal urethritis and NGU in homosexual but not in heterosexual men.[33, 34]

Historically, there has been considerable interest in the possible contribution of circumcision to the epidemiology of STD. Such studies are difficult to interpret, because certain behavioral factors are associated with circumcision.[35] The presence of a foreskin may mask a urethral discharge and delay patients from presenting for evaluation, but other roles remain speculative.[35]

The clinical spectrum of gonorrhea differs from that of NGU, but there is sufficient overlap that an accurate diagnosis must be based on examination of the urethral specimen. Seventy-five percent of men who acquire urethral gonorrhea develop symptoms within 4 days,[3] and 80 to 90% within 2 weeks.[30, 36, 37] The incubation period for NGU is much more variable and is often longer, usually between 7 and 14 days, but incubation periods ranging from 2 to 35 days have been described,[30, 32, 36] and almost 50% of men with NGU developed urethral symptoms within 4 days.[3, 30, 36] Thus, an incubation period of less than 1 week is not a reliable factor in the differential diagnosis.[3, 30, 36] The incubation period of either infection can be prolonged by the ingestion of subcurative doses of antibiotics.[38]

The urethral discharge is described as frankly purulent in three fourths of the patients with gonorrhea but in only 11 to 33% of the patients with NGU.[15, 32, 39] A purulent discharge issuing from the meatus obtained without stripping the urethra correlates strongly with the diagnosis of gonorrhea but is also seen in 4% of patients with NGU.[15, 39] Mucopurulent discharge, consisting of thin cloudy fluid or mucoid fluid with purulent flecks, is seen in about 50% of the patients with NGU but in only 25% of the patients with symptomatic gonorrhea.[15, 39] The discharge is completely clear and moderately viscid in 10 to 50% of the patients with NGU, principally those who are minimally symptomatic, but in only 4% of symptomatic patients with gonorrhea.[15, 39, 40] A diagnosis based on the clinical characteristics of the urethral discharge is unreliable and correctly identifies the causative disorder in only 73% of all cases, even under optimal circumstances.[39] Microscopic examination always should be part of the initial evaluation.

Dysuria has been described in 53 to 75% of the patients with NGU and in 73 to 88% of the patients with symptomatic gonorrhea.[15, 41] Only about 10% of the patients complaining of dysuria without discharge have gonorrhea; the remainder suffer from NGU.[15] A combination of dysuria and discharge is seen in 71% of the patients with gonococcal urethritis but in only 38% of the patients with NGU. Thus, the combination of discharge and dysuria is associated with gonorrhea, while the appearance of one without the other is more frequently seen with NGU. The association is insufficiently specific for differentiating these two entities. Urethral discomfort may mimic cystitis in men and women and result in urinary frequency and urgency.

Symptoms of gonorrhea often begin abruptly, and the patient may remember the specific time of day when they were first noted. NGU usually has a less acute onset, with symptoms increasing over several days. A urethral discharge may appear days in advance of dysuria; the symptoms may wax and wane, even to the point of transiently disappearing before the patient seeks therapy. The mildness and variability of the symptoms may erroneously convince the patient with NGU that he or she does not have a significant disease; such patients often delay seeking medical attention.[15, 41]

The symptoms of infectious urethritis will, in most cases, resolve even if the causative disorder remains untreated. Ninety-five percent of patients with acute gonococcal urethritis who do not receive treatment will be free of symptoms 6 months after contracting the disease,[37] and the symptoms of NGU gradually subside over a period of 1 to 3 months in 30 to 70% of the patients.[42] How many of these asymptomatic patients remain infected and potentially infectious is unknown. Untreated gonococcal urethritis may subside to a chronic state characterized by little or no urethral discomfort and a small amount of mucoid discharge called *gleet.* This discharge contains small numbers of gonococci and PMNs.

So great is the clinical overlap between NGU and gonococcal urethritis that a diagnosis should not be made on clinical grounds alone. Gram staining of urethral discharge material will reveal typical, gram-negative, "intracellular" diplococci in about 95% of the cases of gonococcal urethritis and will be negative in about 97% of the patients with NGU.[15–17] Thus, in a population in which about 50% of the cases of acute urethritis are gonococcal, a positive result on Gram staining suggests gonorrhea, and a negative result on Gram staining suggests NGU with 98% accuracy.[15, 17] The finding of typically shaped extracellular diplococci diagnoses gonorrhea with an accuracy of 10 to 30%.[17] Such results on Gram staining are known or *equivocal* and are found in about 15% of patients with symptomatic urethritis.[15]

The sensitivity of the culture for *N. gonorrhoeae* is less than 100%, partly because some gonococci are inhibited by the vancomycin concentrations used in selective media. The chances of isolating the organism are further reduced if the patient has recently taken antibiotics or if there is a delay in processing the culture. Thus, it seems likely that most of the few patients with positive findings on Gram staining and negative cultures actually have gonorrhea. In most cases of acute symptomatic urethritis, culture is unnecessary to confirm Gram stain findings diagnostic of gonorrhea. It must be remembered that results on Gram staining will be negative in as many as 5% of such patients who have gonorrhea, so Gram stain findings suggestive of NGU should be confirmed with a culture for gonococci, although therapy need not be delayed until the results are known. Results on Gram staining cannot be used to make a diagnosis of simultaneous NGU in the presence of gonorrhea. Because of the frequency with which trichomonads may be missed with direct microscopic techniques, patients in whom trichomonal urethritis is suspected should be evaluated by culture of urethral or first-void urine specimens, or both, as well as by wet mount.[19]

There is no doubt that urethritis is sexually transmitted. It occurs most frequently during the ages of peak sexual activity and in groups with a high prevalence of other STDs. It is found with increased frequency in persons with a history of other sexually transmitted genital infections.[30, 32] It frequently follows sexual exposure to a new partner and is almost never seen in virgins except as a part of some systemic conditions. As the etiologic agents of urethritis have been defined, they have been isolated with high frequency from the female and homosexual male sexual partners of infected men by whom, however, they usually are carried asymptomatically.

Recognizing urethritis as an STD is important for several practical reasons. It allows definition of a population at very high risk for carrying the causative agents, namely, the sexual partners of infected patients. The prevalence of infection with these agents is sufficiently high among sexual partners to justify their treatment on epidemiologic grounds, even if they are asymptomatic. Many episodes of recurrent NGU are terminated only by the treatment of an asymptomatic sexual partner of the infected patient. Because persons with one STD are at increased risk for others, it is important to screen patients with urethritis for other STDs.

Etiology of Nongonococcal Urethritis

The organism most clearly associated with NGU, *C. trachomatis,* is discussed in detail in Chapter 168. This obligate intracellular parasite causes as many as 50% of cases of NGU.[7, 26, 31, 43] Effective *Chlamydia* control programs may reduce the proportion of men with NGU who are infected with *C. trachomatis.*[44] *C. trachomatis* is susceptible to several antimicrobial agents, including the tetracyclines, sulfonamides, and erythromycin. Significantly, it is not reliably eradicated by penicillins, cephalosporins, fluoroquinolones, or spectinomycin in the single doses used to treat uncomplicated gonorrhea.

Chlamydiae are not recovered from at least 50% of men with NGU. Although the clinical features of *Chlamydia*-negative NGU are very similar to those of *Chlamydia*-positive NGU,[30, 45] some workers have suggested that less discharge is produced in patients who are positive for *Chlamydia* than in those who are not, and the mean incubation period may be slightly shorter.[30, 45]

The agents responsible for *Chlamydia*-negative NGU remain, to some extent, unidentified. *U. urealyticum,* formerly known as the *T-strain mycoplasma,* has been recovered from 81% of men with *Chlamydia*-negative NGU, which is significantly higher than the 60% isolation rate from asymptomatic controls.[26, 46, 47] Furthermore, *U. urealyticum* can be recovered in larger numbers from men with *Chlamydia*-negative NGU than from control subjects.[46, 48] Supporting the hypothesis that these agents (see Chapter 172) cause some cases of NGU is the observation that sulfonamides and rifampin, to which the organisms are insensitive, fail to cure most patients with *Chlamydia*-negative NGU.[49, 50] Conversely, spectinomycin, which is active against ureaplasmas but inactive against *Chlamydia,* cures patients with NGU from whom only *U. urealyticum* has been isolated.[49] Additional support comes from experiments in which two investigators inoculated themselves with ureaplasmas; both developed NGU.[51] Furthermore, some patients with NGU show rises in IgM and IgG antibody titers against *U. urealyticum.*[52] Thus, the weight of evidence favors an etiologic role for *U. urealyticum* organisms in NGU. Accurate assessment of the relative contribution of ureaplasmas is hindered by the ubiquity of the organisms that can be recovered from urethral cultures from many sexually experienced men who have no evidence of urethritis.[53, 54] *Mycoplasma hominis* is not a cause of NGU,[53, 54] whereas *Mycoplasma genitalium* has been recovered from patients with NGU.[55] Recent studies in which this fastidious organism was identified with use of polymerase chain reaction assays have associated *M. genitalium* with NGU.[56, 57] Determination of the proportion of cases of NGU that are caused by *M. genitalium* requires further research.

As is *Chlamydia,* the ureaplasmas are susceptible to erythromycin and, usually, tetracyclines—the agents that have been most successful in treating NGU. Some patients, however, are infected with tetracycline-resistant *U. urealyticum*[5, 58–61]; such patients may not be cured by tetracycline therapy. A significant minority of men with NGU do not carry either *C. trachomatis* or *U. urealyticum,*[49, 50, 62, 63] and it would not be surprising if other agents were in the future identified as causes of NGU. Patients with nonchlamydial, nonureaplasmal NGU have a higher recurrence rate after therapy than do men with chlamydial urethritis.[50, 62, 63]

Uncommon Causes of Nongonococcal Urethritis

Dysuria is described by 83% of women and 44% of men with primary herpes simplex genital infection. Some men notice a clear, mucoid discharge that seems disproportionately mild relative to the degree of dysuria that they experience. Herpes simplex virus (HSV) is recovered from the urethras of about 80% of women and 30% of men with primary infection, and HSV must be regarded as a cause of some cases of NGU. In most such instances, however, the diagnosis of HSV is obvious because of genital lesions. Urethral involvement is less common in recurrent disease, and dysuria is described by only 27% of women and 9% of men.[64]

Trichomonas vaginalis has been isolated from patients with NGU,[19, 20, 27] and it causes a small percentage of the cases. The syndrome is not clinically distinguishable from NGU of other causes, although the discharge often is so scant that it may be noticed by the patient only as a small bead at the meatus on arising in the morning.

Preexisting urethral stricture, particularly in the presence of other infectious agents, may (it is said) produce a urethritis-like syndrome. Urethral infection with gram-negative bacilli can be seen in men with diabetes or who practice insertive anal intercourse and may occur in patients with phimosis or with urethral trauma after instrumentation or indwelling catheterization.[65] Periurethral abscesses may occur in this setting. Somewhat fewer than 3% of the cases of urethritis are due to infection higher up in the urinary tract. Syphilis, with an endourethral chancre, and intraurethral condylomata acuminata occasionally cause a urethral discharge. *N. meningitidis* organisms have been isolated from some patients who had urethritis.[66]

A few investigators have attributed some cases of NGU to *Clostridium difficile, Branhamella catarrhalis, Haemophilus influenzae,* corynebacteria, *G. vaginalis, Bacteroides ureolyticus,*[67] adenoviruses,[68] and schistosomes. Most of these observations, however, are uncontrolled for the presence of such important pathogens as *C. trachomatis* and *U. urealyticum,* and the role of these organisms must be considered unproven. Indeed, other studies have reported the recovery of corynebacteria, *G. vaginalis,* and anaerobes less frequently from patients with NGU than from asymptomatic controls.[26, 46, 69]

POSTGONOCOCCAL URETHRITIS

Some patients who receive single-dose treatment for acute gonococcal urethritis experience prompt resolution followed in a few days by a recurrence of symptoms—usually a mucoid or mucopurulent discharge and sometimes mild dysuria. Other patients may note that their symptoms have never entirely disappeared and, after initial rapid improvement, stabilized at a low level. This syndrome is referred to as *postgonococcal urethritis* (PGU) and should be suspected if signs, symptoms, or laboratory evidence of urethritis is found 4 to 7 days after single-dose treatment for gonorrhea.[70, 71] It is a manifestation of dual urethral infection. Gonococci and the agents of NGU are extremely prevalent in sexually active populations, and they are carried simultaneously and asymptomatically by many women. Male sexual partners of these women may acquire both agents during the same sexual exposure. In the presence of gonorrhea, coincident NGU cannot be diagnosed with Gram staining. Single-dose treatment of gonorrhea with cephalosporins, quinolones, or spectinomycin eradicates the gonococci (eliminating the symptoms of gonorrhea), but it usually spares the agents of NGU. When the incubation period of NGU is exceeded, the patient experiences a recurrence or persistence of milder symptoms that is consistent with the latter infection.

Although PGU was originally thought to result from the consumption of alcohol or other irritants during therapy for gonorrhea, dual infection is now well established as the explanation for PGU. *C. trachomatis* has been recovered from 11 to 50% of men with gonorrhea[43]; 75 to 100% of patients with gonorrhea who are also culture-positive for *Chlamydia* will develop PGU if their gonorrhea is treated with an agent that does not eradicate *Chlamydia.*[70–74] *C. trachomatis* can be recovered from almost 50% of the patients with PGU, which is similar to the recovery rate in NGU. PGU, however, also develops in 20 to 50% of the patients with gonorrhea from whom chlamydiae are not recovered[70, 71, 73]; some of these cases appear to be associated with ureaplasmal infection.[71] As might be expected, if gonorrhea is treated with a regimen active against the agents of NGU, the incidence of PGU is lower.[74–76] Accordingly, current treatment schedules for gonorrhea include a second agent such as doxycycline or azithromycin.

Patients suffering persistence or recurrence of urethral symptoms after therapy for acute gonococcal urethritis may indeed have PGU, but the physician also should remember the possibilities of gonococcal reinfection or frank treatment failure. The patient who is experiencing recurrent urethritis must be evaluated as a new patient to differentiate gonococcal from nongonococcal infection.

ASYMPTOMATIC URETHRAL INFECTION

Many patients without specific complaints that are referable to the urethra will be found to have signs of urethritis on physical examination; sexually transmitted pathogens can be recovered from some patients who have neither symptoms nor signs of urethritis. Infected adolescents are less likely to complain of urethral symptoms than are adults.[77]

The importance of asymptomatic urethral gonococcal infection in men is well recognized.[78] Prolonged asymptomatic urethral carriage of gonococci occurs in about 2 to 3% of newly infected men[78]; however, because these men do not seek treatment, the prevalence of asymptomatic urethral gonococcal infections is distinctly higher than 3% and may have considerable epidemiologic significance. Random screening of asymptomatic populations is unrewarding[78] except in high-risk populations.[79] Most cases of asymptomatic urethral infection are detected when gonorrhea is diagnosed in female sexual partners or if complications subsequently develop in the infected man. Asymptomatic urethral infection is therefore particularly prevalent among the male sexual partners of women who develop symptomatic complications of gonorrhea or when gonorrhea is detected by screening.[78] Up to 40% of the asymptomatic sexual partners of women with disseminated gonococcal infection or pelvic inflammatory disease are found to be infected[78]; 60% of the infected men may be asymptomatic. Asymptomatic urethral infection also is prevalent among men with gonococcal dermatitis-arthritis syndrome.[78] Asymptomatic gonorrhea may be diagnosed by examination of Gram-stained urethral material collected on a swab with a sensitivity of about 70%.[78]

Part of the controversy over the etiologic role of *U. urealyticum* is its recovery from 59% of sexually active, asymptomatic men attending venereal disease clinics.[26, 46] *C. trachomatis* is recovered from about 3% of such men.[26, 46] Many men harboring trichomonads are asymptomatic,[20] and represent an important vector of infection.

Asymptomatic urethritis in many cases can be rapidly detected by observing PMNs in material recovered from the urethra with a swab or loop. About 25% of asymptomatic men with four or more PMNs per oil-immersion microscopic field were found to carry *C. trachomatis* in their urethras.[80] Endourethral sampling, however, is uncomfortable and is poorly accepted by asymptomatic men. Examination of first-void urine for leukocytes or leukocyte esterase[24] or for evidence of gonococcal or chlamydial infection with nucleic acid amplification techniques[25] may provide an acceptable means of examining men for asymptomatic urethral infection.

Because of the frequency of asymptomatic, sexually transmitted urethral infections in men, asymptomatic sexual partners of infected women or homosexual men should always be evaluated. Because immediate diagnostic techniques are of relatively low sensitivity, such men should receive treatment at the time of their initial presentation (epidemiologic treatment).

URETHRAL SYNDROME AND RELATED DISEASES OF WOMEN

Dysuria, frequency, urgency, and nocturia are frequent symptoms of bacterial cystitis in women. A similar syndrome occurs in women who do not have classic bacterial infection of the lower urinary tract. Such women are said to have the acute urethral syndrome.[81] The usual workup for bacterial urinary tract infection is unrewarding because fewer than 10^5 organisms are recovered from each milliliter of urine. If the urine sediment contains PMNs, the symptoms frequently respond to antimicrobial therapy. Some of these patients appear to suffer from bacterial cystitis, although bacteria are recovered from the urine in smaller than usual numbers.[81, 82] Other patients' symptoms, however, appear to be related to urethritis rather than to cystitis. *Escherichia coli* sometimes apparently causes urethritis in the absence of cystitis.[83] When ordinary bacterial pathogens associated with urinary tract infections are not isolated (even in small numbers), the condition is often due to sexually transmitted agents.[81, 82] If pyuria is absent, cultures for enteric bacteria and agents of STD are less likely to be positive, and antimicrobial treatment is less likely to be effective; a noninfectious explanation for urethral symptoms should be sought in such patients.

N. gonorrhoeae can affect the urethra in women as it does in men, and it occasionally causes the urethral syndrome.[84] Gently stripping the urethra may deliver a purulent discharge that on Gram staining will reveal typical gram-negative, cell-associated diplococci. The Gram-stained smear from the female urethra has a sensitivity of about 50% for gonorrhea.[85] In about three fourths of affected women, gonococci are recovered from the endocervix as well.[84] The syndrome responds to standard therapy for uncomplicated anogenital gonorrhea (see Chapter 200).

C. trachomatis may be recovered from the urethra in women with dysuria, frequency, and pyuria.[81, 82] Indeed, urinary tract symptoms are described by 53% of women in whom *C. trachomatis* is isolated from the urethra.[86, 87] This association suggests that in some cases the urethral syndrome is the clinical counterpart in women of NGU. In such patients, if initial drug therapy includes antimicrobial agents that are active against chlamydiae (e.g., tetracyclines, amoxicillin, fluoroquinolones, sulfonamides, sulfamethoxazole-trimethoprim [SMX-TMP]), clinical improvement with resolution of symptoms is likely. Relapses, however, are frequent and may reflect reinfection from an asymptomatic male sexual partner. In most studies, *U. urealyticum* has not been statistically associated with the urethral syndrome,[81, 82, 86–88] although one group found an association with more than 10^3 organisms per milliliter and pyuria.[89] The acute urethral syndrome, which is associated with pyuria, must be differentiated from the chronic urethral syndrome. The latter is not associated with pyuria and responds poorly to antimicrobial therapy.[90–93]

Dysuria is a common complaint of women with trichomoniasis. The parasite is recovered from the urethra and periurethral glands in over 90% of women with the infection (see Chapter 270) and is associated with pyuria.[94] Dysuria also may result from vulvar irritation such as that accompanying vaginal candidiasis. It is far less common in patients with bacterial vaginosis.

The urethral syndrome has been treated with steroids[82] or with urethral dilatation and other types of instrumentation. Among sexually active women, however, gonococcal, chlamydial, and trichomonal infection should be ruled out before other therapies are tried.

TREATMENT OF SEXUAL PARTNERS OF MEN WITH NONGONOCOCCAL URETHRITIS

C. trachomatis can be recovered from the endocervix of 45 to 90% of the sexual partners of infected men[31, 42, 95–97] and from the urethra alone in about 15 to 25% of these women.[86, 94, 98, 99] Although infected women usually are asymptomatic, the organism is far from benign (see Chapter 167). Chlamydial infection can be documented in as many as 50% of women with mucopurulent cervicitis who are attending an STD clinic. Indeed, cervical abnormalities, often mild, may be seen in many women from whom *C. trachomatis* is recovered. *C. trachomatis* is a cause of acute salpingitis. In addition, babies born to infected women may develop chlamydial conjunctivitis or pneumonia, and asymptomatic women undoubtedly are a reservoir for recurrent NGU. The carriage of ureaplasmas has been linked to infertility,[100] although the causal nature of the relationship is controversial.[53, 54] These considerations support the routine treatment of female sexual partners of men with NGU.

COMPLICATIONS OF URETHRITIS

Both *N. gonorrhoeae* and *C. trachomatis* have been identified as causes of acute epididymitis among sexually active men.[101] Epididymitis could conceivably lead to infertility, although an association between infectious epididymitis and infertility in men has not been convincingly demonstrated.[102] In 20 to 30% of men with NGU, prostatic involvement is documented; however, it is usually asymptomatic[5, 103] and responds to standard treatments. The role of chlamydia in the development of chronic nonbacterial prostatitis remains unproved. The organism has been recovered from some men with chronic nonbacterial prostatitis,[104–106] and in some patients the condition appeared to respond to treatment with tetracyclines. The role of *U. urealyticum* is even more controversial. The organism has been associated with prostatitis in some series but not in others.[53, 54] An association with infertility and abnormal semen specimens has been described,[100, 107] but this also is regarded as controversial.[54] Stricture may follow gonococcal urethritis or NGU. *C. trachomatis* can infect the conjunctiva. Also, an oculogenital syndrome consisting of NGU and conjunctivitis may be seen in about 4% of patients with NGU[108, 109]; it responds to standard therapy with tetracyclines and must be differentiated from Reiter's syndrome (see later discussion).

THERAPY

Specific forms of urethritis including chlamydial and ureaplasmal infections, gonorrhea, trichomoniasis, and syphilis should be treated as discussed in the appropriate chapters in Part III. As a syndrome, NGU has been treated with a variety of regimens, but doxycycline and azithromycin are the current drugs of choice.

Tetracyclines are usually prescribed for 7 days; there is little convincing evidence that full-dose regimens exceeding 7 days have any additional benefits.[110–113] Tetracycline hydrochloride is given in doses of 500 mg four times a day.[110–113] The patient should be instructed to take the drug on an empty stomach and not accompanied by milk or antacids. Alternatively, doxycycline can be administered in a dose of 100 mg orally twice daily for 7 days. This drug is highly effective, well tolerated by patients, and can be taken with food. Twice-daily administration and fewer side effects are probably associated with better compliance.[114] Because inexpensive generic preparations are now available, doxycycline is the tetracycline of choice for treatment of NGU. Administration of doxycycline may be associated with photosensitivity reactions. Minocycline has no apparent advantages over doxycycline, and it produces dizziness in many patients.[63]

Azithromycin is an azalide antimicrobial agent with a prolonged half-life that is active against *C. trachomatis* and *U. urealyticum.* A single 1.0-g oral dose is effective against chlamydial infections[115] and in syndromic NGU.[116]

Both doxycycline and azithromycin are highly effective and well tolerated. Generic doxycycline is inexpensive, but compliance with the 7-day regimen will not be complete in all instances.[117] Azithromycin is more expensive, but compliance can be assured if the drug is given under direct observation.

Erythromycin is as effective as tetracycline in chlamydial infections[8] and is active against tetracycline-resistant ureaplasmas.[5, 61] Erythromycin has the additional theoretic advantage of producing higher prostatic levels than those obtainable with tetracycline hydrochloride, and it may be of use in the retreatment of patients whose symptoms are relieved by tetracycline but return after therapy is completed. Such patients may have a prostatic focus of infection that is not cured by tetracycline.[8, 118] Gastrointestinal discomfort is an unfortunately common adverse effect of erythromycin therapy. Patients who cannot tolerate a dose of 500 mg four times daily for 7 days can be given 250 mg four times daily for 14 days, a regimen that is almost as effective in NGU.[8]

Fluoroquinolone antimicrobial agents have been evaluated in chlamydial urethritis and in syndromic NGU. Ciprofloxacin was ineffective,[119] whereas ofloxacin (300 mg twice daily for 7 days) was effective.[120] Sulfonamides including sulfisoxazole and SMX-TMP can be used to treat chlamydial NGU but are less effective in *Chlamydia*-negative NGU.[49]

Even if the condition is untreated, the symptoms of NGU will resolve within 2 weeks in 14 to 30% of patients[110]; up to 70% of patients will have a complete resolution of symptoms within 6 months.[42] Resolution of symptoms does not, of course, mean that the infection is cured; asymptomatic patients may remain infected and infectious. Conversely, the inflammatory response accompanying NGU may take some time to resolve, even after the pathogens have been eliminated.[51]

During treatment, the symptoms of NGU frequently resolve before the patient has completed the therapy. Patients should be cautioned to complete the entire course of antibiotics, because relapse is considerably more common if therapy is aborted. To differentiate reliably a relapse from reinfection and to protect sexual partners, patients undergoing treatment for urethritis should refrain from coitus or should use condoms until both partners have completed their medication regimens and their symptoms have resolved.

Because coincident chlamydial infection is very common in men with gonorrhea, the Centers for Disease Control and Prevention has suggested that uncomplicated gonococcal urethritis should be treated with a combined regimen consisting of a single dose of a suitable cephalosporin or fluoroquinolone antibiotic followed by 7 days of doxycycline (100 mg orally twice daily) or by azithromycin (in a single 1.0-g oral dose). These regimens have the advantage of providing effective single-dose therapy for gonorrhea and effective therapy for coincident, undiagnosed NGU.[121] Disadvantages include increased cost and the potential for adverse reactions. It is also prudent to use one of these combined regimens to treat urethritis of undetermined etiology. Fluoroquinolone-resistant strains of *Neisseria gonorrhoeae* are widespread in many countries in Asia and have been reported in the United States.[122] Increased prevalance of gonococci with decreased susceptibility to fluoroquinolones may necessitate revision of current treatment guidelines.

Patients who are receiving treatment for urethritis should be examined for other STDs and should be tested serologically for syphilis at the initial visit. An initial workup for trichomoniasis probably is not indicated in most settings because the infection accounts for a small proportion of cases.[20] Additionally, direct microscopic examination of a urethral specimen for trichomonads usually is unrewarding unless the patient can be seen before the first morning micturition. If the patient's urethritis has not been cured by previous antibacterial therapy or if symptoms or signs in the sexual partner suggest trichomonal infection, the patient's first-void urine sediment can be examined as a wet mount or can be cultured on suitable media.[19] Empirical treatment for trichomoniasis with oral metronidazole may be warranted in some patients.

In men whose symptoms and signs do not resolve or in whom clinical manifestations recur following appropriate treatment for urethritis, urethral Gram-stained specimens or first-void urine sediments should be examined to establish the existence of persistent urethritis. Symptoms and signs may persist in the absence of objective evidence of urethritis. Antimicrobial treatment in symptomatic men who do not have objective evidence of urethritis is of questionable value.[28]

Patients who initially receive treatment for NGU but in whom urethritis is not eliminated by doxycycline should be suspected of having infection with *Trichomonas* or doxycycline-resistant *Ureaplasma*.[5, 58, 59, 61] Because these infections may be impossible to differentiate clinically, such patients may be given empirical treatment with a single 2-g dose of metronidazole followed by erythromycin, 500 mg orally four times daily for 7 days.[122] It is, of course, important that their sexual partners receive the same regimen.

Some men report that their urethral symptoms disappeared while they were taking a tetracycline but reappeared days to weeks after completing therapy. Such recurrences with objective evidence of urethritis are seen in about 20% of patients with chlamydial NGU and in about 40% of patients with nonchlamydial infection. Among NGU patients from whom neither chlamydiae nor ureaplasmas are isolated, the recurrence rate is greater than 50%.[50, 62, 63] Eighty percent of cases of recurrent NGU occur in patients in whom neither organism is initially recovered,[63] and 70 to 80% of men with recurrent NGU are culture-negative for both organisms at the time of recurrence.[85]

Men with recurrent urethritis should be questioned closely about the possibility of reexposure, and attention should be given to ensuring simultaneous treatment of all sexual partners. If reexposure is likely, retreatment with the initial doxycycline or azithromycin regimen may be given. If the patient has not been reexposed, a recurrence of urethritis suggests the possibility that some pathogens remained in a relatively antibiotic-protected site. Prostatic involvement is common in NGU. It is possible that some men may have a prostatic focus of infection. In men with repeated relapses, occasionally treatment with a 3-week course of erythromycin in successful.[123] Patients whose relapses are not eliminated by these maneuvers should be referred for urologic evaluation to rule out anatomic abnormalities.[118] Such men probably are not infected with *Chlamydia* or *Ureaplasma*. About one fourth will be found to have a partial obstruction to urine flow, and about half of these will have urethral strictures.[118] They and their sexual partners do not appear to be at significant risk for infectious complications.[124] Long-term antimicrobial suppression is useful in this setting.[124]

Sexual partners of patients with sexually transmitted urethritis should receive treatment simultaneously. A woman who has been the sexual partner of a man with urethritis of undetermined etiology should be given a regimen that is effective against gonococci, chlamydiae, and ureaplasmas. A regimen combining a cephalosporin or a fluoroquinolone with doxycycline as described previously is suitable in nonpregnant women. Erythromycin, amoxicillin,[125] or clindamycin[126] may be substituted for doxycycline in pregnancy. Asymptomatic male sexual partners of women known to have gonorrhea, chlamydial infection, or trichomoniasis should receive treatment even in the absence of abnormalities on direct microscopic examination.

REITER'S SYNDROME

Some cases of NGU appear as one element of Reiter's syndrome, which also includes arthritis, uveitis, and often, lesions of the skin and mucous membranes. The syndrome complicates 1 to 2% of the cases of NGU[127] and is thought to be the most common peripheral inflammatory arthritis in young men.[128] Its pathogenesis is unclear, but it probably represents an abnormal host response to any of a number of infectious agents.[129] The idiosyncratic nature of the host's response is supported by a strong correlation between the development of Reiter's syndrome and the presence of the HLA-B27 histocompatibility antigen. This antigen has been found in 90 to 96% of patients with Reiter's syndrome,[127, 128, 130, 131] and it also has been related to uveitis and sacroiliitis.[127] Although possibly providing a clue to pathogenesis, the presence of this antigen is not diagnostic.[132]

The inciting infection is of two types. Reiter's syndrome may follow sexually transmitted urethritis, and most cases in North America and Europe seem to occur in sexually active young people.[133, 134] Many cases occur after contact with a new partner, and some cases have been epidemiologically linked.[127, 135] In one series, 9% of cases followed gonococcal urethritis, although 50% of affected patients subsequently developed PGU.[136] *C. trachomatis* is strongly implicated in the pathogenesis of Reiter's syndrome.[137] It has been recovered from the urethras of 16 to 44% of patients with Reiter's syndrome and from 69% of those men who had signs of urogenital inflammation at the time of examination.[134, 138, 139] Antibodies to *C. trachomatis* have been detected in 46 to 67% and *Chlamydia*-specific cell-mediated immunity in 72% of patients with Reiter's syndrome.[129, 139, 140] *Chlamydiae* have been isolated from synovial biopsies in 15 of 29 patients from a number of small series and from a smaller proportion of synovial fluid specimens.[141] Chlamydial nucleic acids have been identified in the synovial membranes,[142, 143] and chlamydial elementary bodies have been observed in joint fluid[144] in a few patients. Mycoplasmas have ostensibly been isolated from synovial fluid in even rarer reports.[145] The significance of these observations is not yet defined, and other attempts to isolate or identify organisms in affected joints have not been successful.[141]

Reiter's syndrome also follows bacterial gastroenteritis and has been repeatedly described following infection with *Salmonella, Shigella, Yersinia,* and *Campylobacter.*[127, 128, 130, 136, 146–150] A few cases suggest that Reiter's syndrome may follow antibiotic-associated colitis[151] or cryptosporidiosis.[152] Postdysenteric Reiter's syndrome has been reported in 0.24 to 1.50% of patients after epidemics of gastrointestinal infection[147, 149]; it is considerably more common among patients who are HLA-B27–positive. Short peptides shared by HLA-B27 and enteric pathogens have raised the question of a contribution of molecular mimicry to pathogenesis.[153, 154] Antibodies reacting with *Yersinia* proteins appear in the sera of many patients with Reiter's syndrome,[155] synovial fluid lymphocytes react with antigens from enteric pathogens,[156] and bacterial antigens have been identified in affected joints.[145]

Clinically, Reiter's syndrome after genital infection is indistinguishable from that following bacterial gastroenteritis; indeed, 12 to 80% of patients with postdysenteric Reiter's syndrome have genital symptoms.[127, 157] The age- and gender-specific attack rates, however, are different; 94 to 99% of the cases of Reiter's syndrome following sexually transmitted infections occur in men. However, up to 10% of the cases of postdysenteric Reiter's syndrome occur in women.[133, 149] It has also been reported in sexually inexperienced children.[133, 148, 158]

Reiter's syndrome is encountered with some frequency in HIV-infected persons.[159–161] It is said to be the most common rheumatologic complication of acquired immunodeficiency syndrome (AIDS). The spectrum of clinical manifestations is similar to that in other patients, but the arthritis and mucocutaneous lesions are more severe and may require more intense therapy.

The syndrome has been observed as a complication of bladder instillation of Calmette-Guérin bacillus.[162] Small numbers of cases suggest the possibility of Reiter's syndrome following respiratory infection with *Chlamydia psittaci* or *Chlamydia pneumoniae.*[163, 164]

Clinical Features

NGU is the initial manifestation of Reiter's syndrome in 80% of the patients.[127, 128] As with other forms of NGU, it usually occurs 7 to 14 days after sexual exposure.[127] The urethritis may be mild and may go unnoticed by the patient, being detectable only by physical examination performed before the first morning micturition. Gonococcal urethritis sometimes precedes Reiter's syndrome,[136] but coinfection with an agent of NGU is difficult to rule out. The urethral discharge may be purulent or mucopurulent, and patients may or may not complain of dysuria. Accompanying prostatitis, usually asymptomatic, has been described by some authors.[128, 157, 165] Cystitis without urethritis has also been reported and may be a manifestation, particularly in women.[157] Cervicitis may represent female genital infection with the inciting microorganism.

The other features of Reiter's syndrome develop 1 to 5 weeks after the onset of urethritis.[157] Arthritis begins within 4 weeks of the onset of urethritis in four fifths of patients,[127] but it precedes urethritis in about 15%.[133] The knees are most frequently involved, followed by the ankles and small joints of the feet. Sacroiliitis, either symmetric[157] or, more frequently, asymmetric,[133, 148, 165] develops in up to two thirds of patients.[157] It is more frequent in patients with the HLA-B27 antigen.[148] Ankylosing spondylitis, which occurs in only about 1% of the general population, complicates a significant minority of cases of Reiter's syndrome,[127, 131, 148, 166] and back pain is reported by 60% of all patients.[128] Many patients with Reiter's syndrome and the HLA-B27 antigen developed ankylosing spondylitis,[166, 167] which is rare in patients without the antigen. Calcaneal spurring may be seen in up to one fourth of the patients with Reiter's syndrome[133, 165] and may produce heel pain. A dactylitis resulting in sausage-shaped swelling of the digits is also characteristic.[133] Arthritis is the most persistent feature of the syndrome and may last for months to years after other manifestations have disappeared.[133, 157]

Mild bilateral conjunctivitis, iritis, keratitis, or uveitis is sometimes present but often lasts for only a few days.[157, 165, 168, 169] Unlike the conjunctivae in direct infection with *C. trachomatis,* the inflamed conjunctivae in Reiter's syndrome do not manifest follicular hypertrophy. The uveitis is usually anterior, acute, and unilateral.[169]

Dermatologic manifestations occur in up to 50% of the patients.[127, 128] The initial lesions are waxy papules, which often display a central yellow spot and occur most frequently on the soles and palms[157] and with decreasing frequency on the nails, scrotum, scalp, and trunk. The papules epithelialize and thicken to produce keratoderma blenorrhagicum in about 10 to 25% of the patients.[128] Circinate balanitis is usually painless and occurs in about 25 to 40% of all patients.[127, 128, 157] Circinate and ulcerative vulvitis also are described.[170] Painless erosions on the dorsum of the tongue and fauces occur most commonly with the initial episode and less frequently with recurrence.[153] Incomplete Reiter's syndrome, consisting of urethritis and arthritis or arthritis alone, has been reported.[128, 146, 171]

The initial episode of Reiter's syndrome usually lasts for 2 to 6 months, but episodes lasting for 1 year have been described.[128, 157, 165] Most patients feel completely well after the attack subsides, but the disease recurs in many cases at a rate of about 15% in each 5-year period after the initial attack.[127, 128, 133, 144, 166, 172] During recurrence, the genital symptoms are usually less marked and may be entirely absent.[172–174] Over half of the patients will have active disease 15 to 20 years after the initial episode,[128, 131, 166, 172] the risk of residua being somewhat higher among patients with the HLA-B27 antigen.[175] Almost 50% of affected persons develop some degree of permanent disability.[131, 166]

Rare complications of Reiter's syndrome include pericarditis, myocarditis, first-degree antrioventricular block, and aortic insufficiency.[131, 157, 165, 176] Thrombophlebitis, radiculitis, myelopathy, and seizures are occasionally described.[177, 178]

Laboratory Features

Anemia is common,[128] and the erythrocyte sedimentation rate is elevated in about 50% of patients.[133] Findings in fluid recovered at the same time from different joints may be dissimilar.[157] Synovial fluid usually contains 1000 to 200,000 white blood cells per ml, more than two thirds of which are PMNs.[157] The glucose level in joint fluid is low in about 50% of affected joints.[157] Synovial biopsy specimens reveal nonspecific inflammatory changes.

Therapy

Treatment of Reiter's syndrome remains controversial. Because of the possibility that the inciting infection may be sexually transmitted NGU, standard antichlamydial treatment is recommended[179] and has been claimed by some authorities to reduce or eliminate urethritis.[180] Others, however, have seen no effect on the arthritis or on the overall course of the disease.[173, 179] The relative safety of antichlamydial therapy and the frequency with which chlamydiae are isolated from patients with Reiter's syndrome make such treatment reasonable. Among a population in Greenland with a high prevalence of HLA-B27, treatment of patients who had urethritis or cervicitis with a tetracycline or erythromycin was associated with a lower incidence of subsequent arthritis than was treatment with penicillin or no treatment at all.[181]

Long-term antichlamydial treatment (e.g., with a tetracycline for 3 months) has been suggested, and its use is supported by a double-blind, placebo-controlled trial that demonstrated an ameliorating effect on *Chlamydia*- but not enteropathogen-associated disease.[182] The effectiveness of long-term tetracycline therapy in other arthritides[183] raises the question of whether the drug is working through an antibacterial effect on persistent, viable microorganisms or through an anti-inflammatory action. That the tetracyclines are more effective in *Chlamydia*–associated than in other reactive arthritides suggests the former.

Administration of nonsteroidal anti-inflammatory drugs (NSAIDs) is the most effective treatment.[128] Indomethacin or tolmetin is favored by some workers,[184] and all of these agents are superior to salicylates or corticosteroids. Sulfasalazine may be beneficial for patients whose symptoms do not respond to an NSAID. Cytotoxic agents such as methotrexate[184] or immunosuppressive agents such as cyclosporine[185] may be of value in recalcitrant cases.

REFERENCES

1. Oriel JD. The history of non-gonococcal urethritis. Genitourin Med. 1996;72:374–379.
2. Taylor-Robinson D. The history of nongonococcal urethritis. Thomas Parran Award Lecture Sex Transm Dis. 1996;23:86–91.
3. Swartz SL. Diagnosis of nongonococcal urethritis. In: Hobson D, Holmes KK, eds. Nongonococcal Urethritis and Related Infections. Washington, DC: American Society for Microbiology; 1977:15–18.
4. Bowie WR. Comparison of Gram stain and first-voided urine sediment in the diagnosis of urethritis. Sex Transm Dis. 1978;5:39–42.
5. Root TE, Edwards LD, Spengler PJ. Nongonococcal urethritis: A survey of clinical and laboratory features. Sex Transm Dis. 1980;7:59–65.
6. Swartz SL, Kraus SJ, Herrmann KL, et al. Diagnosis and etiology of nongonococcal urethritis. J Infect Dis. 1978;138:445–454.
7. Desai K, Robson HG. Comparison of the Gram-stained urethral smear and first-voided urine sediment in the diagnosis of nongonococcal urethritis. Sex Transm Dis. 1982;9:21–25.
8. Scheibel JH, Kristensen JK, Hentzer B, et al. Treatment of chlamydial urethritis in men and *Chlamydia trachomatis*–positive female partners: Comparison of erythromycin and tetracycline in treatment courses of one week. Sex Transm Dis. 1982;9:128–131.
9. Stamm WE, Koutsky LA, Benedetti JK, et al. *Chlamydia trachomatis* urethral infections in men. Prevalence, risk factors, and clinical manifestations. Ann Intern Med. 1984;100:47–51.
10. Perera SAB. Use of Kova-Slide II with grid and uncentrifuged segmented urine specimens in the diagnosis of nongonococcal urethritis: A quantitative technique. Sex Transm Dis. 1985;12:14–18.
11. Veeravahu M, Smyth RW, Clay JC. Detection of leukocyte esterase in urine: A new screening test for nongonococcal urethritis compared with two microscopic methods. Sex Transm Dis. 1987;14:180–184.
12. Perera SAB, Jones C, Srikantha V, et al. Leukocyte esterase test as rapid screen for non-gonococcal urethritis. Genitourin Med. 1987;63:380–383.
13. Simmons PD. Evaluation of the early morning smear investigation. Br J Vener Dis. 1978;54:128–129.
14. Willcox JR, Adler MW, Belsey EM. Observer variation in the interpretation of Gram-stained urethral smears. Br J Vener Dis. 1981;57:134–136.
15. Jacobs NF Jr, Kraus SJ. Gonococcal and nongonococcal urethritis in men. Clinical and laboratory differentiation. Ann Intern Med. 1975;82:7–12.
16. Kraus SJ. Semiquantitation of urethral polymorphonuclear leukocytes as objective evidence of nongonococcal urethritis. Sex Transm Dis. 1982;9:52–55.
17. Goodhart ME, Ogden J, Zaidi AA, Kraus SJ. Factors affecting the performance of smear and culture tests for the detection of *Neisseria gonorrhoeae*. Sex Transm Dis. 1982;9:63–69.
18. Haberberger RL Jr, Mikhail IA, Fox E, et al. Predominance of vancomycin-sensitive strains of *Neisseria gonorrhoeae* in Djibouti. Lancet 1989;2:683.
19. Krieger JN, Verdon M, Siegel N, et al. Risk assessment and laboratory diagnosis of trichomoniasis in men. J Infect Dis. 1992;166:1362–1366.
20. Krieger JN, Jenny C, Verdon M, et al. Clinical manifestations of trichomoniasis in men. Ann Intern Med. 1993;118:844–849.
21. Shafer M-A, Schachter J, Moscicki AB, et al. Urinary leukocyte esterase screening test for asymptomatic chlamydial and gonococcal infections in males. JAMA. 1989;262:2562–2566.
22. Lee HH, Chernesky MA, Schachter J, et al. Diagnosis of *Chlamydia trachomatis* genitourinary infection in women by ligase chain reaction assay of urine. Lancet. 1995;345:213–216.
23. Howell MR, Quinn TC, Brathwaite W, Gaydos CA. Screening women for *Chlamydia trachomatis* in family planning clinics: The cost-effectiveness of DNA amplification assays. Sex Transm Dis. 1998;25:108–117.
24. Puolakkainen M, Hiltunen-Back E, Reunala T, et al. Comparison of performances of two commercially available tests, a PCR assay and a ligase chain reaction test, in detection of urogenital *Chlamydia trachomatis* infection. J Clin Microbiol. 1998;36:1489–1493.
25. Jaschek G, Gaydos CA, Welsh LE, et al. Direct detection of *Chlamydia trachomatis* in urine specimens from symptomatic and asymptomatic men by using a rapid polymerase chain reaction assay. J Clin Microbiol. 1993;31:1209–1212.
26. Bowie WR, Pollock HM, Forsyth PS, et al. Bacteriology of the urethra in normal men and men with nongonococcal urethritis. J Clin Microbiol. 1977;6:482–488.
27. Wong JL, Hines PA, Brasher MD, et al. The etiology of nongonococcal urethritis in men attending a venereal disease clinic. Sex Transm Dis. 1977;4:4–8.
28. Augenbraun MH, Cummings M, McCormack WM. Management of chronic urethral symptoms in men. Clin Infect Dis. 1992;15:714–715.
29. Pec J, Straka S, Novomesky F, et al. Mechanical urethritis and ascendent genitourinary infections due to sexual stimulation of the urethra by inserted foreign bodies. Genitourin Med. 1992;68:399–400.
30. McCutchan JA. Epidemiology of venereal urethritis: Comparison of gonorrhea and nongonococcal urethritis. Rev Infect Dis. 1984;6:669–688.
31. Judson FN. Epidemiology and control of nongonococcal urethritis and genital chlamydial infections: A review. Sex Transm Dis. 1981;8:117–126.
32. McChesney JA, Zedd A, King H, et al. Acute urethritis in male college students. JAMA. 1973;226:37–39.
33. Lafferty WE, Hughes JP, Handsfield HH. Sexually transmitted diseases in men who have sex with men. Acquisition of gonorrhea and nongonococcal urethritis by fellatio and implications for STD/HIV prevention. Sex Transm Dis. 1997;24:272–278.
34. Schwartz MA, Lafferty WE, Hughes JP, Handsfield HH. Risk factors for urethritis in heterosexual men. The role of fellatio and other sexual practices. Sex Transm Dis. 1997;24:449–455.
35. Smith GL, Greenup R, Takafuji ET. Circumcision as a risk factor for urethritis in racial groups. Am J Public Health. 1987;77:452–454.
36. Boyd JT, Csonka GW, Oates JK. Epidemiology of non-specific urethritis. Br J Vener Dis. 1958;34:40–43.
37. Holmes KK. Gonococcal infection. Clinical, epidemiologic and laboratory perspectives. Adv Intern Med. 1974;19:259–285.
38. Harrison WO, Hooper RR, Wiesner PJ, et al. A trial of minocycline given after exposure to prevent gonorrhea. N Engl J Med. 1979;300:1074–1080.
39. Rothenberg R, Judson FN. The clinical diagnosis of urethral discharge. Sex Transm Dis. 1983;10:24–28.
40. Lee Y-H, Rosner B, Alpert S, et al. Clinical and microbiological investigation of men with urethritis. J Infect Dis. 1978;138:798–803.
41. Volk J, Kraus SJ. Nongonococcal urethritis. A venereal disease as prevalent as epidemic gonorrhea. Arch Intern Med. 1974;134:511–514.
42. Oriel JD. Treatment of nongonococcal urethritis. In: Hobson D, Holmes KK, eds. Nongonococcal Urethritis and Related Infections. Washington, DC: American Society for Microbiology; 1977:38–42.
43. Johannisson G, Lowhagen G-B, Nilsson S. *Chlamydia trachomatis* and urethritis in men. Scand J Infect Dis. 1982;32(Suppl):87–92.
44. van Duynhoven YT, Van de Laar MJ, Fennema JS, et al. Development and evaluation of screening strategies for *Chlamydia trachomatis* infections in an STD clinic. Genitourin Med. 1995;71:375–381.
45. Jacobs NF Jr, Arum ES, Kraus SJ. Nongonococcal urethritis: The role of *Chlamydia trachomatis*. Ann Intern Med. 1977;86:313–314.
46. Bowie WR, Wang S-P, Alexander ER, et al. Etiology of nongonococcal urethritis. Evidence for *Chlamydia trachomatis* and *Ureaplasma urealyticum*. J Clin Invest. 1977;59:735–742.
47. Viarengo J, Hebrant F, Piot P. *Ureaplasma urealyticum* in the urethra of healthy men. Br J Vener Dis. 1980;56:169–172.
48. Hunter JM, Smith IW, Peutherer JF, et al. *Chlamydia trachomatis* and *Ureaplasma urealyticum* in men attending a sexually transmitted diseases clinic. Br J Vener Dis. 1981;57:130–133.
49. Bowie WR, Floyd JF, Miller Y, et al. Differential response of chlamydial and ureaplasma-associated urethritis to sulphafurazole (sulfisoxazole) and aminocyclitols. Lancet. 1976;2:1276–1278.
50. Coufalik ED, Taylor-Robinson D, Csonka GW. Treatment of nongonococcal urethritis with rifampicin as a means of defining the role of *Ureaplasma urealyticum*. Br J Vener Dis. 1979;55:36–43.
51. Taylor-Robinson D, Csonka GW, Prentice MJ. Human intraurethral inoculation of ureaplasmas. Q J Med. 1977;46:309–326.
52. Brown MB, Cassell GH, Taylor-Robinson D, et al. Measurement of antibody to *Ureaplasma urealyticum* by an enzyme-linked immunosorbent assay and detection of antibody responses in patients with nongonococcal urethritis. J Clin Microbiol. 1983;17:288–295.
53. Cassell GH, Cole BC. Mycoplasmas as agents of human disease. N Engl J Med. 1981;304:80–89.
54. Taylor-Robinson D, McCormack WM. The genital mycoplasmas. N Engl J Med. 1980;302:1003–1010, 1063–1067.
55. Tully JG, Cole RM, Taylor-Robinson D, et al. A newly discovered mycoplasma in the human urogenital tract. Lancet. 1981;1:1288–1291.
56. Taylor-Robinson D, Furr PM. Genital mycoplasma infections. Wien Klin Wochenschr. 1997;109:578–583.
57. Busolo F, Camposampiero D, Bordignon G, Bertollo G. Detection of *Mycoplasma*

genitalium and *Chlamydia trachomatis* DNAs in male patients with urethritis using the polymerase chain reaction. New Microbiol. 1997;20:325–332.
58. Magalhaes M. Persistent nongonococcal urethritis associated with a minocycline-resistant strain of *Ureaplasma urealyticum:* A case report. Sex Transm Dis. 1983;10:151–152.
59. Arya OP, Pratt BC. Persistent urethritis due to *Ureaplasma urealyticum* in conjugal or stable partnerships. Genitourin Med. 1986;62:329–332.
60. Magalhaes M, Veras A. Minocycline resistance among clinical isolates of *Ureaplasma urealyticum.* J Infect Dis. 1984;149:117.
61. Stimson JB, Hale J, Bowie WR, Holmes KK. Tetracycline-resistant *Ureaplasma urealyticum:* A cause of persistent nongonococcal urethritis. Ann Intern Med. 1981;94:192–194.
62. Bowie WR. Urethritis and infections of the lower urogenital tract. Urol Clin North Am. 1980;7:17–28.
63. Bowie WR, Alexander ER, Stimson JB, et al. Therapy for nongonococcal urethritis. Double-blind, randomized comparison of two doses and two durations of minocycline. Ann Intern Med. 1981;95:306–311.
64. Corey L, Adams HG, Brown ZA, et al. Genital herpes simplex virus infection: Clinical manifestations, course, and complications. Ann Intern Med. 1983;98:958–972.
65. Nacey JN, Tulloch AGS, Ferguson AF. Catheter-induced urethritis: A comparison between latex and silicone catheters in a prospective clinical trial. Br J Urol. 1985;57:325–328.
66. Conde-Glez CJ, Calderon E. Urogenital infection due to meningococcus in men and women. Sex Transm Dis. 1991;18:72–75.
67. Fontaine EAR, Bryant TN, Taylor-Robinson D, et al. A numerical taxonomic study of anaerobic gram-negative bacilli classified as *Bacteroides ureolyticus* isolated from patients with non-gonococcal urethritis. J Gen Microbiol. 1986;132:3137–3146.
68. Swenson PD, Lowens MS, Celum CL, Hierholzer JC. Adenovirus types 2, 8, and 37 associated with genital infections in patients attending a sexually transmitted disease clinic. J Clin Microbiol. 1995;33:2728–2731.
69. Woolley PD, Kinghorn GR, Talbot MD, Duerden BI. Microbiological flora in men with non-gonococcal urethritis with particular reference to anaerobic bacteria. Int J STD AIDS. 1990;1:122–125.
70. Arya OP, Mallinson H, Pareek SS, et al. Post-gonococcal cervicitis and postgonococcal urethritis. A study of their epidemiological correlation and the role of *Chlamydia trachomatis* in their aetiology. Br J Vener Dis. 1981;57:395–399.
71. Bowie WR, Alexander ER, Holmes KK. Etiologies of postgonococcal urethritis in homosexual and heterosexual men: Roles of *Chlamydia trachomatis* and *Ureaplasma urealyticum.* Sex Transm Dis. 1978;5:151–154.
72. Terho P. *Chlamydia trachomatis* in gonococcal and postgonococcal urethritis. Br J Vener Dis. 1978;54:326–329.
73. Oriel JD, Ridgway GL, Reeve P, et al. The lack of effect of ampicillin plus probenecid given for genital infections with *Neisseria gonorrhoeae* on associated infections with *Chlamydia trachomatis.* J Infect Dis. 1976;133:568–571.
74. Stamm WE, Guinan ME, Johnson C, et al. Effect of treatment regimens for *Neisseria gonorrhoeae* on simultaneous infection with *Chlamydia trachomatis.* N Engl J Med. 1984;310:545–549.
75. Patrone P, Negosanti M, Ghetti P, et al. A combined treatment in prevention of postgonococcal urethritis. Dermatologica. 1984;168:300–302.
76. Holmes KK, Johnson DW, Floyd TM, et al. Studies of venereal disease. II. Observations on the incidence, etiology, and treatment of the postgonococcal urethritis syndrome. JAMA. 1967;202:467–473.
77. Chambers CV, Shafer M-A, Adger H, et al. Microflora of the urethra in adolescent boys: Relationships to sexual activity and nongonococcal urethritis. J Pediatr. 1987;110:314–321.
78. Handsfield HH, Lipman TO, Harnisch JP, et al. Asymptomatic gonorrhea in men. Diagnosis, natural course, prevalence and significance. N Engl J Med. 1974;290:117–123.
79. Smith JA, Linder CW, Jay MS, et al. Isolation of *Neisseria gonorhoeae* from the urethra of asymptomatic adolescent males. Clin Pediatr (Phila). 1986;25:566–568.
80. Swartz SL, Kraus SJ. Persistent urethral leukocytosis and asymptomatic chlamydial urethritis. J Infect Dis. 1979;140:614–617.
81. Stamm WE. Etiology and management of the acute urethral syndrome. Sex Transm Dis. 1981;8:235–238.
82. Stamm WE, Wagner KF, Amsel R, et al. Causes of the acute urethral syndrome in women. N Engl J Med. 1980;303:409–414.
83. Fihn SD, Johnson C, Stamm WE. *Escherichia coli* urethritis in women with symptoms of acute urinary tract infection. J Infect Dis. 1988;157:196–199.
84. Curran JW. Gonorrhea and the urethral syndrome. Sex Transm Dis. 1977;4:119–121.
85. Goh BT, Varia KB, Ayliffe PF, et al. Diagnosis of gonorrhea by Gram-stained smears and cultures in men and women: Role of the urethral smear. Sex Transm Dis. 1985;12:135–139.
86. Paavonen J. *Chlamydia trachomatis*–induced urethritis in female partners of men with nongonococcal urethritis. Sex Transm Dis. 1979;6:69–71.
87. Paavonen J, Vesterinen E. *Chlamydia trachomatis* in cervicitis and urethritis in women. Scand J Infect Dis. 1982;32(Suppl):45–54.
88. Hunter JM, Young H, Harris AB. Genitourinary infection with *Ureaplasma urealyticum* in women attending a sexually transmitted disease clinic. Br J Vener Dis. 1981;57:338–342.
89. Stamm WE, Running K, Hale J, et al. Etiologic role of *Mycoplasma hominis* and *Ureaplasma urealyticum* in women with the acute urethral syndrome. Sex Transm Dis. 1983;10:318–322.
90. Fihn SD, Stamm WE. The urethral syndrome. Semin Urol. 1983;1:121–129.
91. Latham RH, Stamm WE. Urethral syndrome in women. Urol Clin North Am. 1984;11:95–101.
92. Scotti RJ, Ostergard DR. The urethral syndrome. Clin Obstet Gynecol. 1984;27:515–529.
93. Bump RC, Copeland WE Jr. Urethral isolation of the genital mycoplasmas and *Chlamydia trachomatis* in women with chronic urologic complaints. Am J Obstet Gynecol. 1985;152:38–41.
94. Feldman RG, Johnson AL, Schober PC, et al. Aetiology of urinary symptoms in sexually active women. Genitourin Med. 1986;62:333–341.
95. Ghadirian FD, Robson HG. *Chlamydia trachomatis* genital infections. Br J Vener Dis. 1979;55:415–418.
96. Paavonen J, Kousa M, Saikku P, et al. Examination of men with nongonococcal urethritis and their sexual partners for *Chlamydia trachomatis* and *Ureaplasma urealyticum.* Sex Transm Dis. 1978;5:93–96.
97. Thelin I, Mardh P-A. Contact tracing in genital chlamydial infection. Scand J Infect Dis. 1982;32(Suppl):163–166.
98. Johannison G, Lowhagen G-B, Lycke E. Genital *Chlamydia trachomatis* infection in women. Obstet Gynecol. 1980;56:671–675.
99. Wallin JE, Thompson SE, Zaidi A, et al. Urethritis in women attending an STD clinic. Br J Vener Dis. 1981;57:50–54.
100. Toth A, Lesser ML, Brooks C, et al. Subsequent pregnancies among 161 couples treated for T-mycoplasma genital-tract infection. N Engl J Med. 1983;308:505–507.
101. Berger RE. Acute epididymitis. Sex Transm Dis. 1981;8:286–289.
102. Ness RB, Markovic N, Carlson CL, Coughlin MT. Do men become infertile after having sexually transmitted urethritis? An epidemiologic examination. Fertil Steril. 1997;68:205–213.
103. Holmes KK, Hansfield HH, Wang SP, et al. Etiology of nongonococcal urethritis. N Engl Med. 1975;292:1199–1205.
104. Bruce AW, Chadwick P, Willett WS, O'Shaughnessy M. The role of chlamydiae in genitourinary disease. J Urol. 1981;126:625–629.
105. Mardh P-A, Ripa KT, Colleen S, et al. Role of *Chlamydia trachomatis* in non-acute prostatitis. Br J Vener Dis. 1978;54:330–334.
106. Nilsson S, Johannisson G, Lycke E. Isolation of *Chlamydia trachomatis* from the urethra and from prostatic fluid in men with signs and symptoms of acute urethritis. Acta Dermatol Venereol (Stockh). 1981;61:456–459.
107. Cassell GH, Younger JB, Brown MB, et al. Microbiologic study of infertile women at the time of diagnostic laparoscopy. Association of *Ureaplasma urealyticum* with a defined subpopulation. N Engl J Med. 1983;308:502–505.
108. Mordhorst CH. Clinical epidemiology of oculogenital *Chlamydia* infection. In: Hobson D, Holmes KK, eds. Nongonococcal Urethritis and Related Infections. Washington, DC: American Society for Microbiology; 1977:126–134.
109. Ronnerstam R, Persson K. Chlamydial eye infection in adults. Scand J Infect Dis. 1982;32(Suppl):111–115.
110. Holmes KK, Johnson DW, Floyd TM. Studies of venereal disease. III. Double-blind comparison of tetracycline hydrochloride and placebo in treatment of nongonococcal urethritis. JAMA. 1967;202:474–476.
111. Arya OP, Alergant CD, Annels EH, et al. Management of non-specific urethritis in men. Evaluation of six treatment regimens and effect of other factors including alcohol and sexual intercourse. Br J Vener Dis. 1978;54:414–421.
112. Thambar IV, Simmons PD, Thin RN, et al. Double-blind comparison of two regimens in the treatment of nongonococcal urethritis. Seven-day vs 21-day courses of triple tetracycline (Deteclo). Br J Vener Dis. 1979;55:284–288.
113. Bowie WR, Yu JS, Fawcett A, et al. Tetracycline in nongonococcal urethritis. Comparison of 2 g and 1 g daily for seven days. Br J Vener Dis. 1980;56:332–336.
114. Jordan WC. Doxycycline vs. tetracycline in the treatment of men with gonorrhea: The compliance factor. Sex Transm Dis. 1981;8:105–109.
115. Martin DH, Mroczkowski TF, Dalu ZA, et al. A controlled trial of a single dose of azithromycin for the treatment of chlamydial urethritis and cervicitis. N Engl J Med. 1992;327:921–925.
116. Stamm WE, Hicks CB, Martin DH, et al. Azithromycin for empirical treatment of the nongonococcal urethritis syndrome in men. A randomized, double-blind study. JAMA. 1995;274:545–549.
117. Augenbraun M, Bachmann L, Wallace T, et al. Compliance with doxycycline therapy in sexually transmitted disease clinics. Sex Transm Dis. 1998;25:1–4.
118. Krieger JN, Hooton TM, Brust PJ, et al. Evaluation of chronic urethritis. Defining the role for endoscopic procedures. Arch Intern Med. 1988;148:703–707.
119. Hooton TM, Rogers ME, Medina TG, et al. Ciprofloxacin compared with doxycycline for nongonococcal urethritis. Ineffectiveness against *Chlamydia trachomatis* due to relapsing infection. JAMA. 1990;264:1418–1421.
120. Mogabgab WJ, Holmes B, Murray M, et al. Randomized comparison of ofloxacin and doxycycline for chlamydia and ureaplasma urethritis and cervicitis. Chemotherapy. 1990;36:70–76.
121. Centers for Disease Control and Prevention. 1998 guidelines for treatment of sexually transmitted diseases. MMWR Morb Mortal Wkly Rep. 1998;47(No RR-1):1–116.
122. Gordon SM, Carlyn CJ, Doyle LT, et al. The emergence of *Neisseria gonorrhoeae* with decreased susceptibility to ciprofloxacin in Cleveland, Ohio: Epidemiology and risk factors. Ann Intern Med. 1996;125:465–470.
123. Hooton TM, Wong ES, Barnes RC, et al. Erythromycin for persistent or recurrent nongonococcal urethritis. A randomized placebo-controlled trial. Ann Intern Med. 1990;113:21–26.
124. Berger RE. Recurrent nongonococcal urethritis. JAMA. 1983;249:409.
125. Crombleholme WR, Schachter J, Grossman M, et al. Amoxicillin therapy for *Chlamydia trachomatis* in pregnancy. Obstet Gynecol. 1990;75:752–756.

126. Campbell WR, Dodson MG. Clindamycin therapy for *Chlamydia trachomatis* in women. Am J Obstet Gynecol. 1990;162:343–347.
127. Keat A. Reiter's syndrome and reactive arthritis in perspective. N Engl J Med. 1983;309:1606–1615.
128. Arnett FC Jr. Reiter's syndrome. Johns Hopkins Med J. 1982;150:39–44.
129. Ford DK, deRoza DM, Schulzer M. The specificity of synovial mononuclear cell responses to microbiological antigens in Reiter's syndrome. J Rheumatol. 1982;9:561–567.
130. Lehman DH. Postdysenteric Reiter's syndrome. West J Med. 1977;126:405–407.
131. Sairanen E, Paronen I, Mahonen H. Reiter's syndrome: A follow-up study. Acta Med Scand. 1969;185:57–63.
132. Kahn MA, Kahn MK. Diagnostic value of HLA-B27 testing in ankylosing spondylitis and Reiter's syndrome. Ann Intern Med. 1982;96:70–76.
133. Hawkes JG. Clinical and diagnostic features of Reiter's disease: A follow-up study of 39 patients. N Z Med J. 1973;78:347–353.
134. Kousa M, Saikku P, Richmond S, et al. Frequent association of chlamydial infection with Reiter's syndrome. Sex Transm Dis. 1978;5:57–61.
135. Rustin MHA, Wedzicha JA, Keat AC, et al. Sexually transmitted arthritis? Two informative cases. J Rheumatol. 1982;9:646.
136. Leirisalo M, Skylv G, Kousa M, et al. Followup study on patients with Reiter's disease and reactive arthritis, with special reference to HLA-B27. Arthritis Rheum. 1982;25:249–259.
137. Is Reiter's syndrome caused by chlamydia? (Editorial). Lancet. 1985;1:317–319.
138. Keat AC, Thomas BJ, Taylor-Robinson D, et al. Evidence of *Chlamydia trachomatis* infection in sexually acquired reactive arthritis. Ann Rheum Dis. 1980;39:431–437.
139. Kousa M. Evidence of chlamydial involvement in the development of arthritis. Scand J Infect Dis. 1982;32(Suppl):116–121.
140. Inman RD, Johnston MEA, Chiu B, et al. Immunochemical analysis of immune response to *Chlamydia trachomatis* in Reiter's syndrome and nonspecific urethritis. Clin Exp Immunol. 1987;69:246–254.
141. Hughes RA, Keat AC. Reiter's syndrome and reactive arthritis: A current view. Semin Arthritis Rheum. 1994;24:190–210.
142. Taylor-Robinson D, Gilroy CB, Thomas BJ, Keat ACS. Detection of *Chlamydia trachomatis* DNA in joints of reactive arthritis patients by polymerase chain reaction. Lancet. 1992;340:81–82.
143. Beutler AM, Schumacher HR Jr, Whittum-Hudson JA, et al. Case report: *In situ* hybridization for detection of inapparent infection with *Chlamydia trachomatis* in synovial tissue of a patient with Reiter's syndrome. Am J Med Sci. 1996;310:206–213.
144. Keat A, Dixey J, Sonnex C, et al. *Chlamydia trachomatis* and reactive arthritis: The missing link. Lancet. 1987;1:72–75.
145. Bartholomew LE. Isolation and characterization of mycoplasmas (PPLO) from patients with rheumatoid arthritis, systemic lupus erythematosus and Reiter's syndrome. Arthritis Rheum. 1965;8:376–387.
146. Jones RAK. Reiter's disease after *Salmonella typhimurium* enteritis. BMJ 1977;1:1391.
147. Noer HR. An "experimental" epidemic of Reiter's syndrome. JAMA. 1966;198:693–698.
148. Calin A. Reiter's syndrome. Med Clin North Am. 1977;61:365–376.
149. Paronon I. Reiter's disease. A study of 344 cases observed in Finland. Acta Med Scand. 1948;131(Suppl 212):1–112.
150. Urman JD, Zurier RB, Rothfield NF. Reiter's syndrome associated with *Campylobacter fetus* infection. Ann Intern Med. 1977;86:444–445.
151. Hayward RS, Wensel RH, Kibsey P. Relapsing *Clostridium difficile* colitis and Reiter's syndrome. Am J Gastroenterol. 1990;85:752–756.
152. Cron RQ, Sherry DD. Reiter's syndrome associated with cryptosporidial gastroenteritis. J Rheumatol. 1995;22:1962–1963.
153. Scofield RH, Kurien B, Gross T, et al. HLA-B27 binding of peptide from its own sequence and similar peptides from bacteria: Implications for spondyloarthropathies. Lancet. 1995;345:1542–1544.
154. Scofield RH, Warren WL, Koelsch G, Harley JB. A hypothesis for the HLA-B27 immune dysregulation in spondyloarthropathy: Contributions from enteric organisms, B27 structure, peptides bound by B27, and convergent evolution. Proc Natl Acad Sci USA. 1993;90:9330–9334.
155. Kobayashi S, Ogasawara M, Maeda K, et al. Antibodies against *Yersinia enterocolitica* in patients with Reiter's syndrome. J Lab Clin Med. 1985;105:380–389.
156. Ford DK. Lymphocytes from the site of disease in reactive arthritis indicate antigen-specific immunopathology. J Infect Dis. 1991;164:1032–1033.
157. Weinberger HW, Ropes MW, Kulka JP, et al. Reiter's syndrome, clinical and pathologic observations. A long term study of 16 cases. Medicine (Baltimore). 1962;41:35–91.
158. Zivony D, Nocton J, Wortmann D, Esterly N. Juvenile Reiter syndrome: A report of four cases. J Am Acad Dermatol. 1998;38:32–37.
159. Weitzul S, Duvic M. HIV-related psoriasis and Reiter's syndrome. Semin Cutan Med Surg. 1997;16:213–218.
160. Stein CM, Davis P. Arthritis associated with HIV infection in Zimbabwe. J Rheumatol. 1996;23:506–511.
161. Kaye BR. Rheumatologic manifestations of HIV infections. Clin Rev Allergy Immunol. 1996–7;14:385–416.
162. Saporta L, Gumus E, Karadag H, et al. Reiter syndrome following intracavity BCG administration. Scand J Urol Nephrol 1997;31:211–212.
163. Lanham JG, Doyle DV. Case report: Reactive arthritis following psittacosis. Br J Rheumatol. 1984;23:225–226.
164. Braun J, Laitko S, Treharne J, et al. *Chlamydia pneumoniae*—a new causative agent of reactive arthritis and undifferentiated oligoarthritis. Ann Rheum Dis. 1994;53:100–105.
165. Good AE. Reiter's disease. Postgrad Med. 1977;61:153–158.
166. Marks JS, Holt PJL. The natural history of Reiter's disease—21 years of observations. Q J Med. 1986;60:685–697.
167. Morris R, Metzger AL, Bluestone R, et al. HL-A W27-A clue to the diagnosis and pathogenesis of Reiter's syndrome. N Engl J Med. 1974;290:554–556.
168. Mark DB, McCulley JB. Reiter's keratitis. Arch Ophthalmol. 1982;100:781–784.
169. Lyons JL, Rosenbaum JT. Uveitis associated with inflammatory bowel disease compared with uveitis associated with spondyloarthropathy. Arch Ophthalmol. 1997;115:61–64.
170. Daunt SON, Kotowski KE, O'Reilly AP, et al. Ulcerative vulvitis in Reiter's syndrome. A case report. Br J Vener Dis. 1982;58:405–407.
171. Arnett FC, McClusky OE, Schacter BZ, et al. Incomplete Reiter's syndrome: Discriminating features and HL-A W27 in diagnosis. Ann Intern Med. 1976;84:8–12.
172. Csonka GW. Recurrent attacks in Reiter's disease. Arthritis Rheum. 1960;3:164–169.
173. Catterall RD. The role of microbial infection in Reiter's syndrome. In: Dumont DC, ed. Infection and Immunology in the Rheumatic Diseases. Oxford: Blackwell Scientific Publications; 1976:147–150.
174. Butler MJ, Russell AS, Percy JS, et al. A follow-up study of 48 patients with Reiter's syndrome. Am J Med. 1979;67:808–810.
175. Calin A, Fried JF. An "experimental" epidemic of Reiter's syndrome revisited. Ann Intern Med. 1976;84:564–566.
176. Ruppert GB, Lindsay J, Barth WF. Cardiac conduction abnormalities in Reiter's syndrome. Am J Med. 1982;73:335–340.
177. Montanaro A, Bennett RM. Myelopathy in Reiter's disease. J Rheumatol. 1984;11:540–541.
178. Wollschlaeger B. Epileptic seizures as a neurological complication of Reiter disease. J Am Board Fam Pract. 1995;8:233–236.
179. Bardin T, Schumacher HR. Should we treat postvenereal Reiter's syndrome by antibiotics? (Editorial). J Rheumatol. 1991;18:1780–1781.
180. Ford DK. Reiter's syndrome: Current concepts of etiology and pathogenesis. In: Hobson D, Holmes KK, eds. Nongonococcal Urethritis and Related Infections. Washington, DC: American Society for Microbiology; 1977:64–66.
181. Bardin T, Enel C, Cornelis F, et al. Antibiotic treatment of venereal disease and Reiter's syndrome in a Greenland population. Arthritis Rheum. 1992;35:190–194.
182. Lauhio A, Leirisalo-Repo M, Lähdevirta J, et al. Double-blind, placebo-controlled study of three-month treatment with lymecycline in reactive arthritis, with special reference to *Chlamydia* arthritis. Arthritis Rheum. 1991;34:6–14.
183. Toussirot E, Despaux J, Wending D. Do minocycline and other tetracyclines have a place in rheumatology? Rev Rhum Engl Ed. 1997;64:474–480.
184. Treating Reiter's syndrome (Editorial). Lancet. 1987;2:1125–1126.
185. Kiyohara A, Takamori K, Niizuma N, Ogawa H. Successful treatment of severe recurrent Reiter's syndrome with cyclosporine. J Am Acad Dermatol. 1997;36:482–483.

Chapter 95

Vulvovaginitis and Cervicitis

MICHAEL F. REIN

NORMAL VAGINA

Under the influence of estrogens, the vaginal epithelium becomes cornified and supports a prodigious microbial flora. This adult microenvironment may develop transiently in neonates because of transplacentally acquired maternal estrogens[1] but resolves within several weeks as they are metabolized. The prepubescent vagina supports a flora rich in anaerobic bacteria, in particular, more *Bacteroides* spp. than are commonly found in the adult.[2] *Staphylococcus epidermidis* is frequently recovered,[2] and yeasts and *Gardnerella vaginalis* are isolated from 10% of girls.[2, 3] The vagina again matures in the immediate premenarchal period.

In its mature state, the vagina is colonized by a variety of bacteria,[4–8] primarily obligate and facultative anaerobes. More than 10^5 lactobacilli per milliliter of vaginal material are recovered from three fourths of women. These are primarily *Lactobacillus crispatus* and *Lactobacillus jensonii*.[9] Viridans streptococci and *S. epidermidis* are isolated from almost one half of asymptomatic women of childbearing age. Large numbers (10^5) of *Bacteroides* and *Prevotella* spp. were recovered from only one sixth of these women,[4, 5, 7, 8] and *G. vaginalis* from 30 to 90%.[10, 11] *Staphylococcus aureus* is recovered from the vaginas of only about 5% of healthy women.[12] Pregnancy has little effect on the distribution of most of the bacteria,[6, 7, 13] although the flora varies slightly during the menstrual cycle.[4] Yeasts are carried by about 15 to 20% of healthy women.[14] With the onset of sexual activity, statistically significant increases are observed in the prevalence of *G. vaginalis,* lactobacilli, mycoplasmas, and ureaplasmas, but the prevalences of group B streptococci, *S. aureus,* and yeasts are not significantly altered.[15] It is of interest that ureaplasmas and *G. vaginalis* are recovered from 20 to 25% of young women who have not commenced sexual activity.[15]

Although our descriptive knowledge of vaginal microbiology has increased, our understanding of the factors controlling the flora remains primitive.[13, 16] Changes in the level of gestational hormones influence the relative numbers of organisms of various species.[13, 17] Specific and nonspecific vaginal host defenses have been cataloged, but again, their precise significance is unclear.[18, 19] The metabolic products of some bacteria, for example, the hydrogen peroxide produced by some lactobacilli, may suppress the growth of other organisms such as anaerobes[19–22] but not yeasts.[22, 23] The vaginal microflora remains remarkably stable even through repeated douching,[13] and exposure to nonoxinol 9.[24]

Mucoid endocervical secretions combine with sloughed vaginal epithelial cells and normal bacteria to form a physiologic vaginal discharge. This material is usually unnoticed but may produce symptomatic "leukorrhea." It is often increased during pregnancy or with the use of oral contraceptives.

VULVOVAGINITIS

Vulvovaginitis is a common clinical syndrome and is diagnosed in more than one fourth of women attending sexually transmitted disease clinics.[25] Its incidence appears to be increasing.[26, 27] Treatment should be based on a specific etiologic diagnosis that can usually be made at the time of the initial evaluation (Table 95–1).[28] Symptoms alone are inadequate for differential diagnosis,[29] and the use of over-the-counter antifungal therapy is therefore slightly treacherous.[30] Multiple infections are not rare.[31]

TABLE 95–2 Organisms Associated with Vulvovaginal Yeast Infections in a Vaginitis Clinic Population

Species	Percentage of All Vaginal Fungal Infections
Candida albicans	91
Candida glabrata	7
Candida parapsilosis	1
Candida tropicalis	1
Candida krusei	Rare
Candida pseudotropicalis	Rare
Candida kefir	Rare
Candida lusitaniae	Rare
Candida rugosa	Rare
Saccharomyces cerevisiae	Rare

From Spinillo A, Capuzzo E, Gulminetti R, et al. Prevalence of and risk factors for fungal vaginitis caused by non-*albicans* species. Am J Obstet Gynecol. 1997;176:138–141.

Candidiasis

The archaic term *moniliasis* should be discarded.[32] *Candida albicans* is isolated from about 80 to 90% of patients with vulvovaginal candidiasis, and other yeasts account for up to 15% of cases (Table 95–2).[26, 33–39] *Candida tropicalis* is isolated from about 1 to 5% and may be associated with a higher rate of recurrence after standard treatments.[39, 40] *Candida* (formerly *Torulopsis*) *glabrata* accounts for about 10% of vaginal yeast isolates.[10, 26, 33, 34, 36, 38, 39, 41] Symptomatic vaginitis caused by this organism is associated with less intense itching and dyspareunia[36] than that caused by other *Candida* spp., but the organism may be harder to eradicate with standard therapies.[39, 41] The relative incidence of vaginitis caused by fungi other than *C. albicans* appears to be increasing, accounting for up to 18% of infections in some populations.[27, 39] Non-*albicans* infections are associated with recurrent disease (21 versus 12% of initial infections) and with human immunodeficiency virus infections (22 versus 12% of infections in human immunodeficiency virus–negative women), especially in those human immunodeficiency virus–infected women who receive prophylaxis with imidazoles or triazoles.[39] It is thought that the widespread use of topical antifungals, especially in short courses, may contribute to selection for non-*albicans* yeasts, which are less susceptible to these agents than is *C. albicans.* Cases of vaginitis caused by *Saccharomyces cerevisiae* have been reported

TABLE 95–1 Typical Features of the Common Infectious Vaginitides

Symptoms	Physiologic	Trichomonal	Candidal	Bacterial Vaginosis
Vulvar irritation	–	+ +	+ +	– to +
Dysuria	–	20%	+	–
Odor	–	– to +	–	+ +
Signs				
Labial erythema	–	– to +	– to +	–
Satellite lesions	–	–	+	–
Discharge				
Consistency	Floccular	Frothy 25%	± Curdy	Homogeneous, ± frothy
Color	White	Yellow-green 25%	White	Gray, white
Adherence to vaginal walls	–	–	+	+
pH	≤4.5	± (4.7	≤4.5	≥4.7
Microscopy				
Epithelial cells	Normal	Normal	Normal	Clue cells
PMNs per epithelial cell	≤1	≥1	Variable	≤1
Bacteria	Gram + rods	Gram + rods	Gram + rods	Gram-variable coccobacilli
Pathogens	–	Trichomonads 70%	Yeasts and pseudohyphae 50%	Coccobacilli and motile rods
Bimanual examination				
Vaginal tenderness	–	+	+	–
Rugal hypertrophy	–	+	– to +	–
Adnexal tenderness	–	Occasionally	–	–

Abbreviation: PMN, Polymorphonuclear neutrophil.

and may be associated with baking.[37, 42, 43] Vulvovaginal candidiasis (VC) accounts for about one third of the vaginitis cases seen in private practice and is increasing in clinics specializing in vaginitis.[39] Some workers have estimated that 75% of adult women suffer at least one episode of VC during their lifetimes.[14] Yeast carried vaginally in small numbers and producing no symptoms may be considered part of the normal vaginal flora. VC may result if conditions in the vagina change so as to give the yeast an advantage over competing normal vaginal bacteria and induce an inflammatory response. Inhibition of normal bacterial flora by broad-spectrum antibiotics favors the growth of yeasts,[44] although cases are seen after the use of antimicrobials that do not suppress lactobacilli.[45] Thus, yeasts were isolated from about 10% of women before but from 30% of women after 2- to 3-week courses of various tetracyclines.[10] VC sometimes follows courses of vaginal antimicrobials used to treat trichomoniasis and bacterial vaginosis.

Overgrowth of yeasts is apparently favored by high estrogen levels, although such levels also promote the growth of lactobacilli.[13, 17, 46] VC is more common in pregnancy; it occurs in 10% of first-trimester women and 36 to 55% of women in their third trimesters.[10] Symptomatic disease has eventually developed in 60 to 90% of pregnant carriers, and old inoculation studies confirm the increased susceptibility of pregnant women.[10] Some nonpregnant women note recurrent or increasing symptoms preceding each menstrual period. The prevalence of vaginal carriage of *Candida* is higher among users of oral contraceptives than among women using other methods of birth control, but regimens based on lower estrogen doses are associated with a lower incidence of disease.[26, 44, 46] Small series and anecdotal reports suggest that some patients with recurrent VC can be cured only when oral contraceptives are discontinued.[10, 44] The mechanism of estrogenic predisposition is unclear, although some investigators have suggested that increased vaginal glycogen stores may play a role[10] or that estrogens influence vaginal pH in a way that makes the milieu more hospitable to the fungi.[14] Estrogens induce changes in vaginal epithelial cells that increase the adherence of yeasts[26] and may directly affect the organism. An estrogen receptor is found in the cytosol of *C. albicans,*[47] and estrogens induce the formation of filamentous forms.[17] The mechanism of increased glycogen stores has also been adduced to explain the association of VC with poorly controlled diabetes mellitus, and tight glycemic control decreases the frequency of symptomatic infection,[48] but testing for diabetes in women with recurrent VC is not cost-effective.[44]

It has been suggested that tight, insulating clothing predisposes to VC by increasing vulvar warmth and moisture. In prospective studies, a higher prevalence of candidal carriage and higher concentrations of organisms were found among women who wore tight rather than loose clothing.[49–51] Impairment of phagocytic cells or cell-mediated immunity (e.g., transplantation, chemotherapy) also predisposes to VC, and severe, refractory disease plagues some women with the acquired immunodeficiency syndrome,[52, 53] although some studies have failed to show an overall increase in the prevalence of VC in this population.[54]

The contribution of sexual transmission is probably small. VC increases in incidence with the onset of sexual activity,[54–56] but the incidence is also increased by the use of oral contraceptives,[26, 44, 46] the contraceptive sponge,[54] and the intrauterine device,[54] the use of any of which might coincide. The incidence of infection is not associated with having multiple sexual partners, but recurrences have been associated with the practices of receptive oral or anal intercourse.[57]

The mechanism by which *Candida* produces disease is not well defined. Although it is postulated that differences in virulence must exist,[44] in the laboratory, strains isolated from symptomatic women are not demonstrably different from isolates from asymptomatic carriers.[58] Filamentous forms (hyphae and pseudohyphae) are associated with active disease.[32] Pseudohyphae have been observed to penetrate the vaginal epithelial cells[59] and are more adherent to cells than are blastospores.[60] Adherence appears to be an important pathogenic feature of *Candida* spp.,[61] and sublethal concentrations of antifungals may ameliorate disease by reducing adherence.[62]

The severity of symptoms in VC is not directly related to the number of yeasts present.[10] Indeed, very small numbers of yeasts may be present in vaginal material recovered from highly symptomatic women.[10, 44] An immunologic reaction has been suggested as the mechanism for symptomatic disease in such women,[26, 63] and a small series suggests that desensitization may decrease the frequency of symptomatic episodes.[64]

Clinical Features

Patients with candidal vulvovaginitis generally complain of perivaginal pruritus, often with little or no discharge. Dysuria is occasionally noted and is likely to be perceived as vulvar rather than urethral. The labia may be pale or erythematous, and excoriation is often present. Shallow, radial, linear ulcerations, especially on the posterior portion of the introitus, are common. Tiny papules or papulopustules, called *satellite lesions*, just beyond the main area of erythema are helpful diagnostically. The vaginal walls may be erythematous. Candidal discharge is classically thick and adherent and contains curds. It may, however, be thin and loose and thus resemble the discharge of other vaginitides.

Diagnosis

The vaginal pH is generally normal (approximately 4.5) for women of childbearing age in women with VC[65–67] in contrast to the pH in trichomoniasis or bacterial vaginosis, in which it is characteristically elevated. Thus, demonstrating a normal pH (see Table 95–1) in a woman with signs and symptoms of vaginitis suggests that she has candidiasis rather than one of the other infections. The addition of 10% potassium hydroxide (KOH) to vaginal discharge on a slide or in the speculum (see Table 95–1) fails to elicit a fishy odor in most women with VC. Such an odor (a positive "whiff" test) suggests trichomoniasis or bacterial vaginosis.

An attempt should be made to demonstrate the organism on a wet mount of vaginal discharge. Adding 10 to 20% KOH to the specimen destroys the cellular elements and facilitates recognition of the fungi. Although classic descriptions and most textbook pictures suggest that one sees extensive tangles of filamentous forms, many patients in fact carry only small numbers of yeasts. Indeed, direct microscopic examination fails to reveal fungi in 30 to 50% of infected women,[14, 68, 69] and a presumptive diagnosis must be made on the basis of the clinical features, a normal pH, a negative whiff test, and microscopic examination negative for other pathogens. A commercially available latex agglutination test has a limited sensitivity of about 60%.[70–72] The discharge usually contains relatively few polymorphonuclear neutrophils.

Treatment

Currently available regimens are listed in Table 95–3.

Topical Therapy. VC may be treated with the topical application of an antifungal agent. The striking variety of available drugs and regimens attests to the size of the market and the lack of a clear superiority of one product over another.

Commercially available preparations are characterized by safety in pregnancy and high acceptability by patients. Most of the commercially available drugs are imidazoles (e.g., clotrimazole, miconazole, butoconazole, tioconazole, and econazole) or triazoles (terconazole). They are available in a variety of forms, including creams, tablets, and coated tampons.[67] Nystatin is the only polyene antifungal currently available for vaginal use in the United States. It is difficult to compare therapies directly, because of the variety of protocols used in various studies. Early studies suggest that imidazoles cure about 90% of infections and are superior to polyenes, which cure about

TABLE 95-3 Regimens for the Treatment of Vulvovaginal Candidiasis

Duration	Drug	Regimen
Single dose	Miconazole	1200-mg suppository
	Clotrimazole	500-mg suppository
		10% cream, 5 g
	Tioconazole	6.5% ointment, 4.6 g
3 days	Miconazole	200-mg suppository qhs
	Clotrimazole	200-mg suppository qhs
	Butoconazole	2% cream, 5 g qhs
	Econazole	150-mg suppository qhs
	Terconazole	0.8% cream, 5 g qhs
		80-mg suppository qhs
7 days	Miconazole	2% cream, 5 g qhs
		100-mg suppository qhs
	Clotrimazole	100-mg suppository qhs
		1% cream, 5 g qhs
	Terconazole	0.4% cream, 5 g qhs
	Fenticonazole	2% cream, 5 g qhs*
14 days	Nystatin	100,000 U suppository qhs
Oral—varied times	Ketoconazole	200 mg PO bid for 3–5 d†
		200 mg PO for 3 d†,‡
	Fluconazole	150 mg PO for 1 d
	Itraconazole	200 mg PO bid for 1 d†,‡
		200 mg PO qd for 3 d†,‡

*Not currently available in the United States.
†Not approved by the Food and Drug Administration for this use.
‡Clinical data are limited.

80%.[73] There are no significant differences among currently available topical preparations or between delivery systems consisting of creams or vaginal tablets.[74]

Current interest centers on shorter courses of therapy. Seven-day regimens with an imidazole yield cure rates ranging from 80 to 94%.[10] Newer, 3-day regimens produce approximately equivalent cure rates,[75–77] although some reviews suggest marginally better results with 7 days of therapy.[78] Because patients' compliance is likely to be better with a 3-day course, it seems reasonable to recommend that regimen.[79]

Single-dose treatments with larger amounts of imidazoles, such as 500 mg of clotrimazole,[80–84] may be preferred for the sake of convenience in the treatment of mild infections. Cure rates obtained with these regimens have not quite matched those obtained with longer courses. Treatment in pregnancy is more often unsuccessful, and the longer regimens may be preferred in this setting.

Nystatin is a polyene that has been used in the United States for many years in a regimen consisting of one 100,000-unit tablet inserted intravaginally daily for 14 days, and that yields cure rates approximately equivalent to those obtained with the imidazoles.[10] It must be remembered, however, that treatment with nystatin requires 2 weeks compared with shorter regimens now recommended for the imidazoles.

Oral Therapy. Several orally administered and well-absorbed imidazoles and triazoles are effective in the treatment of VC.[10, 85–100] A number of studies strongly support the efficacy of the Food and Drug Administration (FDA)–approved single oral dose of 150 mg of fluconazole for VC.[88–94] Results are not substantially superior to those obtained with topical regimens, and the clinician must carefully consider the need for systemic therapy for VC in view of the potential toxicities and possible teratogenicity of the drugs (see Chapter 35). Oral therapy may be particularly useful when a possible response to therapy may be mimicked by the nonspecific soothing effect of the topical carrier or when VC complicates herpetic infection. Fourteen percent of women with primary genital herpes develop VC during the second week of infection.[101, 102] Treatment of these secondary infections, however, must be done carefully, because the topical antifungal miconazole cream appears to be associated with delayed healing of genital herpetic lesions.[103] Indeed, the application of any occlusive preparation to herpetic lesions should probably be avoided,[101, 102] and therapy of accompanying VC with an oral imidazole or triazole would be preferred in this setting.

Other Therapies. Gentian violet, a classic treatment, has suffered from low patient acceptability because it stains clothing. Newer delivery systems, such as impregnated tampons, may be easier to use.[104] Povidone-iodine cures about 65% of infections.[105] It should probably be avoided in pregnancy because absorption of iodine might suppress fetal thyroid development.[106] Treatment with 600 mg of boric acid powder in gelatin capsules intravaginally each evening or as vaginal suppositories used twice daily for 14 days cured 85 to 92% of women.[104, 107] This regimen may have a role in the treatment of infection with species of yeast, other than *C. albicans*, which are relatively resistant to the topical imidazoles[34, 41, 104] but should be used with caution because experience is limited, and toxicity may well result from chronic use. Treatment of VC with various topical and oral *Lactobacillus* preparations has long been recommended in published anecdotes and in the lay press.[108, 109] Theoretically acting by restoring a normal bacterial flora that can successfully compete with yeasts, these regimens have not been evaluated in well-controlled trials. Indeed, the lactobacillary flora remains intact in most patients with vulvovaginal candidiasis,[22, 23] and so the therapeutic value of repopulating the vagina with orally administered lactobacilli[109] has little theoretical support.

Recurrent Infection. When samples from patients treated for VC are recultured 3 to 6 weeks after the completion of therapy, a sizable proportion are found once again to harbor the yeasts. Results from many studies suggest a late recolonization rate of 21 ± 12% (mean ± SD),[10, 83, 95, 110] which is largely independent of the regimen used and often precedes symptomatic recurrence by 1 to 2 months.[44, 85] Recurrent symptomatic infection is a major problem. The mechanisms of recurrence remain obscure, but what is known has been analyzed by Sobel and others.[14, 44, 111] Specific candidal anergy is postulated to play a role.[44] Recurrence does not appear to result from the development of resistance to antifungals.[14, 26, 33, 44, 112]

Some studies have suggested that about 40% of women with recurrent disease are infected with new strains of *Candida*[14, 44]; however, more recent work supports the contention that most recurrences involve the same strain,[112–114] sometimes displaying minor genetic differences [114] or increased resistance to antifungals.[113] Obviously, women whose recurrence is associated with reappearance of the same strain might have suffered either recurrence or reinfection. The source of putative reinfection is poorly defined. Sexual transmission may be implicated in some cases, but its overall contribution to recurrent disease is unclear and probably low.[26, 44] Only about 15% of women associate recurrences with sexual contact.[14, 44] Yeasts are carried by 5 to 26% of male partners,[14, 33] and 80% of the female partners of infected men are vaginally colonized.[14, 44] Conjugal partners usually carry the same strain.[14, 114, 115] Simultaneous treatment of male partners, however, does not delay symptomatic recurrence,[116] and the effect on vaginal recolonization is minimal.[85, 95] Reinfection from contaminated douche equipment has also been proposed.[14] Contaminated underwear appears to play no role.[111]

Vaginal reinfection from a persistent rectal focus has been alleged, but support for this contention is weak. Admittedly, 40 to 70% of women with VC have positive rectal cultures, and 80% of doubly colonized women carry the same strain in rectal and vaginal sites,[14, 33, 44, 117] but simultaneous treatment of a rectal focus with oral nystatin or systemic ketoconazole[85–87] does not significantly lower recolonization or recurrence rates over vaginal therapy alone. One large study does suggest a benefit of adding oral nystatin to topical therapy, showing decreased colonization and symptomatic relapse rates. The study suffers from a relatively short (3- to 7-week) follow-up period and a poorly defined subject population.[118] Care must therefore be taken in interpreting these results. Whether selected women might benefit from simultaneous gastrointestinal therapy is unclear.

Endogenous vaginal relapse from small numbers of yeasts that survive chemotherapy has also been suggested.[12, 44] This contention is supported by the rapidity with which vaginal cultures return to positive after treatment and the frequency with which recurring strains are the same as those causing the previous infection.[44] Intracellular residence may protect some fungal cells from antimycotic agents.[14, 33, 44] Small numbers of yeasts would certainly be invisible on wet mount and even by culture,[14] so early post-treatment evaluation might erroneously suggest a cure. As Lossick has remarked,[119] the frequency with which *Candida* is carried asymptomatically suggests that the mere reintroduction of yeasts into the vagina is not an adequate cause of symptomatic recurrence; host susceptibility or responsiveness must also play a role.[44] In addition to the risk factors described previously, some women with recurrent VC appear to be mildly zinc deficient[120] or have defective cell-mediated immunity to yeasts[121–123] or lack vaginal secretion of anticandidal antibody. The significance of these findings is unclear. Tolerance may be induced by chronic infection rather than serving as its cause.[14, 44]

If our lack of understanding of recurrence is dispiriting, our lack of effective therapy is intensely frustrating to patients and clinicians. One should attempt to reduce or eliminate the aforementioned risk factors. Short courses of topical antifungal therapy administered on days 5 to 11 of the menstrual cycle or immediately preceding[85, 86] or following[124–126] menses reduce but by no means eliminate symptomatic recurrences. Likewise, 200 mg of itraconazole orally on days 5 and 6 of the menstrual cycle suppresses symptoms for the duration of therapy.[127] Such treatment is apparently not curative and rapidly becomes oppressively expensive. Simultaneous treatment of a rectal focus with oral nystatin or systemic treatment with ketoconazole does not significantly reduce the relapse rate.[87, 128, 129] In some cases of frequently recurrent VC, a switch to lower-dose oral contraceptives or even a discontinuance of oral contraceptives may be indicated. Oral glucose tolerance tests in such women have very low yield and are not routinely recommended.[14, 44] Rarely, examination of sexual partners may reveal candidal balanitis, which could conceivably be a source of exogenous reinfection.

A prospective, much publicized study reported that the daily ingestion of yogurt containing live *Lactobacillus acidophilus* decreased the rate of vaginal recolonization and symptomatic relapse in women with frequently recurrent disease.[130] The study is flawed by a small sample size, a lack of suitable design (i.e., double blinding) and controls (i.e., yogurt lacking live organisms), and possible biases.[131] Although the oral administration of lactobacilli does increase the lactobacillary content of the intestine,[109] its value in preventing VC remains highly speculative. In addition, most yogurt in the United States is pasteurized and contains no live organisms.

Continuous daily treatment with ketoconazole[86] or fluconazole[44] prevents recurrences for the duration of treatment, and almost half of the women so treated have prolonged freedom from symptoms. Some workers have postulated that prolonged clearance of candida from the vagina reduces local hypersensitivity and restores a more protective form of local immunity.[44]

Disease in Men

The sexual transmission of vaginal candidiasis is apparently considerably less than that of other forms of vaginitis. Balanitis, however, has been reported in 3 to 10% of the male sexual partners of women with candidal vulvovaginitis, and this condition is clearly sexually transmitted.[14, 47, 132, 133] It responds to antifungal creams or ointments and treatment of the involved women. Some men develop pruritus within minutes of sexual contact. Symptoms usually resolve by the following day, and this syndrome may result from hypersensitivity to a partner's vaginal yeast.[14]

Trichomoniasis

The incidence of trichomoniasis in the United States appears to be decreasing. The disease is almost always sexually acquired and usually produces a combination of vaginal discharge and vulvovaginal irritation. About 25% of the women carrying trichomonads are asymptomatic. The infection is discussed in detail in Chapter 270.

Bacterial Vaginosis

Most women presenting to their physicians with vaginal symptoms have a specific condition first described by Gardner and Dukes in 1955.[134] This condition is now usually referred to, perhaps unfortunately from a linguistic standpoint,[135] as *bacterial vaginosis* (BV).[136, 137] Inflammation and perivaginal irritation are considerably milder than in trichomoniasis or candidiasis. Dysuria and dyspareunia are correspondingly rare. Affected women are usually sexually active and often complain predominantly of vaginal odor. This odor is described as "fishy" in the textbooks more frequently than by the patients. About 90% of patients also notice a mild to moderate discharge. Abdominal discomfort is occasionally present, but it is usually mild and should prompt evaluation for coincident infections, including salpingitis.

Discharge is often present at the introitus and visible on the labia minora. The labia and vulva are generally not erythematous or edematous. On speculum examination, the vaginal walls usually appear uninflamed. The vagina often contains a grayish, thin, homogeneous discharge manifesting small bubbles. This discharge differs from normal, physiologic discharge in that the latter has a floccular appearance, and bubbles are absent. Although the discharge may be heavy enough to pool in the posterior fornix, it is usually present in smaller amounts. In some patients, the discharge may be so slight that it does not conspicuously pool. Because it is relatively thin but adherent to the vaginal walls, it is often apparent only as an increased light reflex, giving rise to the impression that the vaginal walls are too wet. A distinct, pungent odor may be noted by the examiner.

The endocervix is unaffected by the process, and the cervical discharge should be physiologic and therefore mucoid. The presence of a purulent cervical discharge or frank cervicitis is not rare but results from coincident gonococcal, chlamydial, or herpetic infection.[138] Abnormalities on bimanual examination are unusual in uncomplicated BV and should prompt a search for other pathologic processes, because there is an increased risk of endometritis and salpingitis among women with BV.[139–142]

Other vaginal infections may closely resemble BV; an accurate differential diagnosis depends on laboratory examination of the genital specimen. The pH of vaginal discharge is elevated above the normal of 4.5 in about 90% of women with BV.[134, 143, 144] Although the pH may also be elevated in trichomoniasis, it is usually normal in VC. A vaginal pH of 5 or higher strongly suggests infection.[145] If 10 to 20% KOH is added to vaginal discharge samples either in the speculum blade or on a microscope slide, a distinctively pungent, fishy odor is generated.[10, 143, 146, 147] This positive whiff test has been used as part of the case definition of BV by some workers and has been found to be positive in about 70% of cases in other series.[143, 146] The accuracy of this test appears to improve with experience,[147] but the test is also positive in some patients with trichomoniasis, and its predictive value is therefore limited in populations with a high prevalence of the protozoal infection.

BV is perhaps most easily differentiated from trichomoniasis on the basis of direct microscopic examination of vaginal discharge. A wet mount of the discharge from patients with BV reveals clue cells, which are vaginal epithelial cells studded with tiny coccobacilli. These organisms are best appreciated at the edges of the cell (Fig. 95–1) but may be dense enough to obscure the nucleus partially. Not all cells in the specimen are clue cells, but some clue cells are seen in over 90% of patients with BV.[147, 148] Predominant bacterial flora can also be assessed on a wet mount slide. In healthy women, the predominant morphotype is a large rod (presumably *Lactobacillus* spp.). In the discharge from a patient with BV, these rods have been completely supplanted by clumps of coccobacilli. Similar discrimination can be made on the basis of a Gram stain of the vaginal

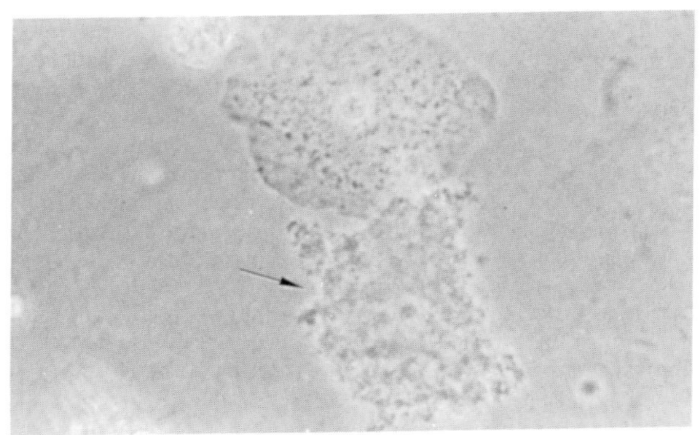

FIGURE 95–1. A wet mount of vaginal discharge from a patient with bacterial vaginosis shows epithelial cells, neutrophils, and trichomonads *(arrows)*. (Phase microscopy, ×400.)

discharge[10, 137, 149–152] or on cervical cytologic examination.[153–155] Discharge in BV contains few polymorphonuclear neutrophils (PMNs). This may in part explain the absence of the green or yellow color that frequently characterizes the discharge in trichomoniasis. Up to about one PMN per epithelial cell is considered normal in a vaginal wet mount. Finding increased numbers of PMNs in a patient with BV sometimes suggests the presence of a second inflammatory process, possibly coincidental cervicitis.[138]

Culture for *G. vaginalis* is easily accomplished on a variety of media (see Chapter 214). The organism is isolated from 92 to 98% of women with BV,[10, 137, 147, 156] but it is also recovered in smaller numbers from up to 70% of some populations of asymptomatic women,[2, 3, 10, 15, 137, 156–158] and its presence does not therefore prove that the patient has BV or suggest a need for treatment. Thin-layer chromatography, gas-liquid chromatography, and enzyme assays can be used to diagnose BV by identifying specific bacterial products.[137, 144, 159–161] These techniques are not routinely performed, but they provide insight into the pathophysiology of BV.

Amsel and associates have suggested that the clinician look for a pH greater than 4.5; a homogeneous, white, adherent vaginal discharge; a positive whiff test; and clue cells.[147] Finding any three of these four signs strongly supports the diagnosis of BV, although an abnormal discharge, an elevated pH, and a positive whiff test often accompany trichomoniasis as well. These criteria have become somewhat standardized in the literature, but several reasonable modifications have been suggested, and studies confirm that the finding of clue cells is the most specific of the criteria.[137, 162] Rather than rigidly adhering to statistical criteria, however, the clinician should base the final diagnosis and decision to treat on a complete evaluation of the patient.

Epidemiology

Bacterial vaginosis was initially described in sexually active women and is common in populations with a high prevalence of sexually transmitted diseases. Its prevalence is increased in women using intrauterine devices.[163] The precise contribution of sexual transmission to the overall epidemiology of the condition remains controversial. Support for a significant role for sexual transmission includes the following observations: (1) BV is more prevalent among women with greater numbers of recent and lifetime sexual partners.[164–167] (2) Its presence is associated with a higher prevalence of other sexually transmitted diseases, including nongonococcal urethritis[168] and infection with *Chlamydia trachomatis,*[167, 169] *Neisseria gonorrhoeae,*[169] and human papillomavirus.[170] (3) Symptoms first develop in many women shortly after they become sexually active.[134] (4) Vaginal recolonization with *G. vaginalis* is far more common in women reexposed to untreated male partners than to those who are not.[143] (5) *Gardnerella vaginalis* is recovered from the urethras of more than 80% of the male sexual partners of infected women,[134, 143] and the isolates are almost always of the same biotype.[137] Surprisingly, the prevalence is apparently high in lesbians,[171, 172] among whom other sexually transmitted diseases are relatively uncommon.

Several observations argue against exclusively sexual transmission: (1) *Gardnerella vaginalis* can be isolated from prepubescent girls[2, 3] and sexually inactive women.[10, 11] (2) The syndrome of bacterial vaginosis has been recognized in virgins.[173] (3) Recurrences are observed in the absence of sexual reexposure. (4) Initial, simultaneous treatment of sexual partners cannot be shown to reduce recurrence rates.[174–183] (5) The age and racial distribution of BV differ from those of gonorrhea, being relatively more likely to occur in older, white women.[27] (6) The organisms associated with BV can be cultured from the rectum, from which site, it is speculated, they might colonize the vagina.[184] (7) Nonvenereal risk factors include douching [22] and the use of an intrauterine device.[163]

The association of bacterial vaginosis with sexual transmission is, however, sufficiently well established that clinicians diagnosing bacterial vaginosis should screen affected women for other sexually transmitted diseases, such as gonococcal or chlamydial infections,[167, 169] or human immunodeficiency virus,[21, 185] which may be clinically silent but of greater eventual medical significance.

Although it is not demonstrably necessary to treat male sexual partners of women with an initial diagnosis of BV,[180–182] some women suffering from frequently recurring BV can be cured only if sexual partners are treated as well. Still, the factors leading to recurrence are not completely understood, and recurrence should not be considered diagnostic of reinfection. The possible contribution of sexual contact to recurrent disease in an individual case may be difficult to determine, but the need for treating sexual partners might be supported by a history of symptoms recurring only after contact with a particular partner.

Pathophysiology

Microscopic examination of vaginal discharge in BV characteristically reveals a predominant flora of coccobacilli. On the basis of its morphology, this organism was originally called *Haemophilus vaginalis.*[134] It has now been given its own genus and is called *Gardnerella vaginalis* in honor of Dr. Gardner's initial observations (see Chapter 214).[186] Several observations suggest a less than straightforward relationship between *G. vaginalis* and BV. Although Gardner and Dukes regularly produced BV by inoculating fresh vaginal discharge from BV patients into the vaginas of healthy volunteers, inoculation of a pure culture of *G. vaginalis* was far less likely to produce disease.[134] In addition, *G. vaginalis* is isolated from 30 to 40% of asymptomatic women,[2, 3, 10, 11, 15, 147, 156–158] and only 50% of women with heavy vaginal colonization by *G. vaginalis* actually have BV.[158] Finally, the in vitro sensitivity of *G. vaginalis* to antimicrobial agents does not match the effectiveness of these agents in clinical disease. Metronidazole is highly effective therapy for BV[143, 179, 187–191] despite the fact that *G. vaginalis* is relatively resistant to the drug in vitro.[143, 188, 192]

An explanation for all these observations is that *G. vaginalis* is not the single cause of BV. There is considerable experimental support for the hypothesis that BV is actually a synergistic infection involving not only *G. vaginalis* but certain anaerobic bacteria as well.[8, 10, 19, 137, 143, 144, 146, 161, 191, 193] The total number of such organisms is dramatically increased in the vaginas of women with BV. Various *Bacteroides* and *Prevotella* species other than *B. fragilis* and various peptococci are principally involved. Asymptomatic carriers of *G. vaginalis* might lack the anaerobic synergants. Pure cultures of *G. vaginalis* would not be able to produce clinical disease in patients lacking the other necessary bacteria, but the vaginal discharge from symptomatic women would be expected to contain all the necessary bacterial components. Drugs relatively inactive against *G. vaginalis* might still cure the disease if they acted against the other bacteria, and metronidazole is highly active against most strict anaerobes. The characteristic odor of BV is due to various aromatic amines such as triethylamine, putrescine, and cadaverine, which are produced by anaerobes but not by *G. vaginalis*.[144] These aromatic diamines are volatilized at basic pH, which explains the positive whiff test associated with the infection.

Most cases of BV are also associated with motile, curved anaerobic rods that are gram-negative or gram-variable.[137, 184, 194–201] These organisms, classified into the new genus *Mobiluncus*,[202] are sensitive to ampicillin, but some species are relatively resistant to metronidazole.[197, 200] The precise pathogenic role of these organisms remains to be elucidated, but antibody to them can be demonstrated in many patients with BV.[203]

Mycoplasma hominis[20, 156, 204–206] and *Ureaplasma urealyticum*[21] are isolated from the vaginas of many women with BV. Their role in the production of BV has not been established, but sialidases elaborated by *Ureaplasma*[21] and *Prevotella*[207] species may destroy mucin and immunoglobulin A (IgA) and enhance bacterial adherence.[208]

Hydrogen peroxide–producing lactobacilli appear to play a major role in limiting *Gardnerella* and the anaerobic flora of the vagina.[20, 22, 139, 156] These lactobacilli are present in the vaginas of 60% of normal women but in only 5% of women with BV.[156, 209, 210] This relationship is not absolute, and some women with BV carry hydrogen peroxide–producing lactobacilli[211] and some women lacking these organisms remain asymptomatic.[21] Many workers now believe that an undefined change in the vaginal milieu permits the replacement of protective lactobacilli with *G. vaginalis*, and the resulting failure of suppression allows a variety of pathogens to achieve large numbers, possibly sequentially.[212] Recent work suggests the presence of a sexually transmissible bacteriophage that can kill lactobacilli and set the stage for BV.[212a] The process is at times reversible, and some women with BV spontaneously recover.[213, 214]

Treatment

Applicable regimens are summarized in Table 95–4. Many studies have shown that BV is successfully treated with metronidazole,[143, 174, 187–191, 215, 216] 500 mg orally twice daily, 250 mg orally three times daily, or 750 mg in an extended-release tablet once daily[217] for 7 days. Cure rates of 80 to 90% are reported, although very limited data suggest that the effectiveness of the single daily tablet may be somewhat lower.[217] Several good studies suggest that single doses of metronidazole are inadequate.[10, 160, 174, 178, 188–190, 215, 216] Clindamycin is active against anaerobes and *G. vaginalis* in vitro, and 300 mg orally twice daily for 7 days is effective therapy for BV.[218] Although ampicillin is highly active in vitro against *G. vaginalis*, experience reveals inadequate efficacy in treating the disease.[143, 187, 190, 191] The inferiority of ampicillin to metronidazole probably derives in part from its inactivation by penicillinase elaborated by *Bacteroides* or *Prevotella* spp. in the vagina[91, 143]; however, the combination of amoxicillin with clavulanic acid is still inferior to metronidazole.[190]

TABLE 95–4 Regimens for the Treatment of Bacterial Vaginosis

Oral regimens
- Metronidazole, 500 mg PO bid for 7 d
- Metronidazole, 250 mg PO tid for 7 d
- Metronidazole, 750 mg extended-release tablet PO qd for 7 d*
- Metronidazole, 2 g PO as single dose†
- Clindamycin, 300 mg PO bid for 7 d*
- Cephalexin, 250 mg PO qid for 7 d‡
- Cefadroxil, 500 mg PO bid for 7 d*

Vaginal regimens
- Clindamycin 2% vaginal cream, 5 g vaginally qhs for 7 d
- Metronidazole 0.75% vaginal gel, 5 g vaginally bid or qhs for 5 d

*Limited clinical data.
†Not as effective as the 7-day regimens.
‡Principally anecdotal data.

Ampicillin, amoxicillin, and, transiently, clindamycin[45] block recolonization of the vagina by normal lactobacilli, whereas metronidazole does not.[45, 191] Recolonization with lactobacilli is part of the process of recovery from BV.

The value of oral cephalosporins for BV remains somewhat controversial. Gardner and Dukes praised them anecdotally,[134, 219] as do other workers. Indeed, cephalexin, 500 mg taken four times daily for 1 week, has cured some women whose disease relapsed after repeated treatments with metronidazole. Limited data also suggest a role for cefadroxil, 500 mg twice daily for 7 days.[220] Oral therapy with tetracyclines, erythromycin, or the fluoroquinolones has been disappointing.[10, 221]

Topical therapies have proved effective and are of use in women who prefer not to take oral medications. Clindamycin 2% cream used in an intravaginal regimen of 5 g nightly for seven doses yields cure rates of about 75 to 95%, results that are not significantly different from those obtained with oral metronidazole in the same studies.[180, 222–229] Metronidazole 0.75% vaginal gel is applied as 5 g once or twice daily for 5 days, yielding cure rates of about 80 to 90%, again comparable to the results obtained with oral metronidazole.[228, 230–232] VC occurred in some women receiving topical treatments, more frequently with metronidazole than with clindamycin.[228] Absorption of metronidazole from the vagina produces serum levels approximately 4% of those following a single 500-mg oral dose, and steady-state levels after multiple doses are about 275 ng/ml.[233] Clindamycin is also absorbed from the vagina, yielding peak serum levels of about 16 ng/ml on the last day of treatment.[234] *Clostridium difficile* colitis has followed topical clindamycin therapy for BV.[235, 236] The cost of the topicals is currently considerably higher than that of oral metronidazole.

Povidone-iodine has an unacceptably low cure rate.[10] Triple sulfa preparations have been used topically for some decades, but small series suggest that the compounds are ineffective.[143, 237] Topical therapy with acetic acid has no value.[238, 239] On the other hand, a small experience supports the value of a topical lactate gel.[240, 241]

Topical treatment with yogurt, in an effort to reinstitute a lactobacillary flora, has yielded inconsistent results in very small studies.[239, 242] Further study is required before such treatment can be recommended, and it should be noted that the lactobacillary species in commercial yogurt are not those found in the vagina.[9] Various commercially available topical *Lactobacillus* preparations have yielded variable success,[243, 244] and several other commercially available topical *Lactobacillus*-containing products have not been subject to clinical trial, may be microbiologically unsuitable because they are likely to contain *Lactobacillus* spp. that do not produce hydrogen peroxide, and are frequently contaminated with other bacteria.[245] Very limited data support the use of a 3% hydrogen peroxide douche.[246]

There are no data supporting the need to treat asymptomatic male sexual partners initially.[10, 179–183] Some women, however, suffer from frequently relapsing disease that can be controlled only by the simultaneous treatment of male sexual partners. The drug of choice for the treatment of such partners has not been defined; each of the drugs metronidazole, clindamycin, or even amoxicillin has advocates. Vaginal carriage of *G. vaginalis* in the absence of signs or symptoms of BV is common and need not be treated. The treatment of asymptomatic women with BV diagnosed on examination has been controversial,[247] but current data on complications favor such treatment, which should be undertaken in women about to undergo instrumentation of the upper genital tract[160, 247] or in pregnancy.

Treatment in pregnancy is the same as in nonpregnant women.[248] Clindamycin cream should not, however, be used, because of an apparently increased risk of preterm birth.[248–250]

Complications of Bacterial Vaginosis

The reader is referred to Chapter 214 for a description of other infections caused by *G. vaginalis*. The organism is recovered from the urethras of asymptomatic men; it does not cause urethritis.

Bacterial vaginosis cannot be considered a benign condition.

Among women with BV there is a significantly increased risk of endometritis[142, 251]; of salpingitis,[139–141] particularly following abortion[252, 253]; and of vaginal cuff and wound infection after hysterectomy.[139, 254, 255] BV is associated with postpartum fever, endometritis, and salpingitis.[222, 252, 256–260] Amnionitis [250, 261] and premature labor and delivery[250, 258, 262–272] occur more frequently in women with BV than in other women. A true pathogenic role for BV in these settings is supported by the recovery of microorganisms associated with BV from amniotic fluid, wound infections, and blood.[270, 272] BV has also been associated with late-term miscarriage.[273] These observations give added impetus to the treatment of BV in pregnancy.

Other Vaginal Infections

Staphylococci

S. aureus is recovered from the vaginas of only about 5% of healthy women.[11] The organism is isolated, however, from most women with catamenial toxic shock syndrome (see Chapter 183).[274, 275] A history of vaginitis is associated with an increased incidence of toxic shock syndrome.[276] The disease is usually characterized by vulvar edema and vulvar and vaginal erythema.[275] A vaginal discharge, purulent but often scanty, is observed in about one fourth to one third of these patients,[274, 275] and vaginal ulceration was noted in about 7%.[274] The pathogenesis of the vaginitis is not entirely understood. Toxic shock syndrome is manifested as a polymucositis, and vaginitis is also reported in about one third of women who have nonmenstrual toxic shock syndrome, sometimes with the staphylococcal source at sites other than the vagina. Thus, the vaginitis may reflect direct infection or may be a secondary effect of staphylococcal toxin. The ulcerations sometimes observed may result from tampon use, with which toxic shock syndrome is associated.

Foreign Body Vaginitis

Secondary anaerobic infections may be associated with foreign bodies in the vagina. In adults, the most common of these are the forgotten vaginal tampon and various contraceptive devices such as a diaphragm, a cervical cap, or a condom that has slipped off during coitus. Objects apparently used in masturbation are occasionally implicated.[277] In children and the mentally incompetent, a variety of objects may be found.[1] These infections often produce an intensely foul odor, and the discharge is usually scanty and contains small amounts of blood. Therapy often requires only the removal of the offending object, but oral metronidazole may speed recovery.

Tampon use affects the vaginal mucosa.[278–281] Extended tampon use, particularly of superabsorbent tampons, may produce local drying and peeling of the vaginal mucosa and result in frank ulceration of the vaginal wall and endocervix. Tampon fibers have been observed within ulcerations.[280] Microscopic ulcers have been noted in up to one fifth of women using tampons,[278] and larger lesions are occasionally observed.[279, 281] Ulceration may be associated with vaginal bleeding and pain on insertion of the tampons. Because of possible confusion with other ulcerating vaginal diseases, including malignancy, a thorough workup is essential.[281]

Herpes Simplex Virus

The adult vaginal epithelium is relatively resistant to herpetic infection. Vaginal lesions have been observed in only about 4% of infected women.[101, 102]

Human Papillomavirus

Genital warts inside the vagina often assume a more filiform shape than do those on the vulva. Micropapillomatosis manifests as sheets of tiny warts (see Chapter 133). Human papillomavirus infection may be associated with vestibular adenitis (see later).

Less Common Infections

True vaginal infections with other specific agents such as *Mycobacterium tuberculosis,* salmonellae, and Enterobacteriaceae, are rare and usually occur in patients with underlying diseases or who are systemically ill. Group A streptococcal vaginitis has been described in children aged 3 to 5 years. It presents with a blood-tinged discharge, "fiery red" vaginal mucosae, and dysuria. A Gram stain is usually negative, and the disease responds promptly to penicillin G.[282–285] Group B streptococci occasionally cause frank vaginitis,[283, 286, 287] especially in children, but are usually carried asymptomatically. *Haemophilus influenzae* has been rarely reported to cause pediatric vaginitis.[283, 285]

Preexisting lesions due to other diseases may become secondarily infected with a mixed anaerobic flora of fusobacteria and spirochetes. Such "fusospirochetal" infections can progress rapidly. Metronidazole, 250 mg orally three times daily, is recommended therapy.

Pinworms are an occasional cause of perivaginal itching, especially in children.[1, 285] Perianal pruritus that becomes worse at night may suggest this diagnosis. True vaginal infestation has been described.[288]

Neisseria gonorrhoeae or *C. trachomatis* can cause frank vaginitis in prepubescent girls.[289]

"Döderlein's cytolysis" or "cytolytic vaginosis," a condition characterized by irritative symptoms exacerbated in the premenstrual interval and theoretically caused by microbially induced hyperacidity, is poorly substantiated. It is said to result from an overgrowth of lactobacilli and to be diagnosed by finding abnormally large numbers of rods, "bare or naked intermediate [cell] nuclei," and relatively few PMNs on a vaginal wet mount. The vaginal pH is reportedly below 4.5. The condition is said to respond to alkalinizing douches.[290]

Noninfectious Vulvovaginitis

Genital neoplasm may result in an abnormal vaginal discharge. Such conditions are more common in older women and are usually manifested by the gradual onset of a thin, often foul-smelling discharge that may be blood tinged. In postmenopausal women, the absence of estrogen stimulation results in atrophy of the vaginal epithelium, which may lead to an atrophic vaginitis. The vaginal walls become secondarily infected with a number of different organisms, but treatment of the primary disease often requires estrogenic supplementation.[54]

Occasional cases of vulvovaginal inflammation from chemicals,[291] including deodorant sprays,[292] and allergic reactions to semen,[293] nickel,[294] and even dust mites[295] have been reported. Fixed drug eruptions frequently involve the genitalia, particularly in association with oral tetracyclines or sulfonamides. Lesions usually consist of dusky red to purple plaques that may be surmounted by ulcers. Patients with episodic genital lesions should be carefully questioned about recent oral medications. Acquired immunodeficiency syndrome patients may develop aphthous ulcerations of the vagina[296] in addition to the gastrointestinal tract.

Desquamative or purulent vaginitis is characterized by a vaginal discharge containing large numbers of PMNs. The cause and therapy of the condition are unknown, but lichen planus should be considered in the differential diagnosis.[297–299] Treatment is not well defined, but anecdotal experience supports the use of topical steroids.[299] A subset of women with this condition have a streptococcal vaginal flora and respond to topical clindamycin. [300]

Related Considerations and Conditions

Physiologic or normal vaginal discharge is sometimes referred to as *leukorrhea* and generally consists of cervical mucus combined with desquamated vaginal epithelial cells. This material passes through the vaginal introitus, where it is perceived by the patient as a vaginal discharge. Neonates may have a transient physiologic discharge until transplacentally acquired maternal estrogens are metabolized. In the adult, the output of the endocervical glands is highly responsive to hormonal levels and sometimes increases at the time of ovulation or in the immediate premenstrual period. Oral contraceptives may increase the cervical component, and women sometimes note a new discharge when they start to use these agents. This leukorrhea may cause considerable concern since it often begins coincidentally with first sexual exposures, thus raising the specter of venereal disease. It may be heavy enough to stain underwear and may dry to a brown residue, which patients sometimes associate with infectious vaginitis. Unlike most infections, it is usually not associated with perineal burning or pruritus, dyspareunia, or dysuria, but an odor is sometimes described.[301] Abdominal pain does not occur unless another process is present. Microscopic examination reveals normal vaginal flora and few PMNs. More than one PMN per epithelial cell is unusual in physiologic vaginal discharge.

Infectious cervicitis due to any of several different organisms may result in an inflammatory cervical discharge that passes through the vagina. This condition is discussed in a later section of this chapter. A variety of inflammatory diseases confined to the perineum may produce symptoms suggesting vaginitis to the patient. The lesions of herpes genitalis or chancroid produce considerable perineal discomfort. Intertrigo may result in burning, an unpleasant odor, and staining of underwear. Infections of Bartholin's glands and Skene's glands sometimes produce perineal discomfort and a discharge and are discussed in a later section of this chapter. Inflammatory diseases of the rectum occasionally result in a discharge that suggests vaginitis to the patient. Internal dysuria may be a symptom of urinary tract infection.

Of interest is a condition referred to as *vulvar vestibulitis, focal vulvitis,* or *vestibular adenitis,* which may be more common than previously suspected.[302–304] Affected women suffer vulvar pain and significant dyspareunia. They are sometimes unable to sit comfortably or wear tight clothing. These women frequently undergo repeated treatments for vulvovaginal candidiasis, and they are often thought to be neurotic. Physical examination reveals rather subtle but exquisitely tender, erythematous patches, usually along the posterior portion of the introital ring. Biopsy demonstrates nonspecific lymphocytic inflammation of vestibular glands[302, 305, 306] and the presence of mast cells. The condition may be associated with interstitial cystitis.[307, 308] Current therapy is surgical excision[309–311] or laser ablation[310] of the affected areas, with relief of discomfort obtained in about two thirds of cases. Failure may result from inadequately aggressive ablation.[312, 313] An infectious cause has not been convincingly demonstrated for all cases and remains controversial,[314] but the presence of human papillomavirus can be demonstrated in about 50% of cases.[315–319] Very limited data suggest that when associated with human papillomavirus infection, vulvar vestibulitis appears to respond to intralesional[317, 320] or even to systemic interferon therapy.[321] Biopsy and DNA probes may be required to differentiate between the conditions. Psychosexual findings are recognized in some affected women.[322–324]

Vaginitis emphysematosa is an uncommon condition in which the vaginal walls contain submucosal gas-filled cysts.[325–328] The endocervix too may be involved.[329] This benign but dramatic condition is frequently associated with trichomoniasis or with bacterial vaginosis and resolves after treatment of the accompanying infection.

Obstruction of the pelvic nodes is a rare cause of lymphatic weeping of the vagina. Massive lymphedema of the lower extremities usually accompanies this finding, and the diagnosis is not difficult to make.

There are small numbers of women who complain of vaginal discharge, discomfort, or odor without any objective findings.[330] Such women may be motivated by a neurotic fear of uncleanliness, guilt concerning sexual activities (or a desire to avoid them), or anxiety about venereal disease, whether or not sexual exposure has actually taken place. Such patients often seek advice from numerous physicians, and their symptoms fail to respond to a variety of standard therapies. They require careful and complete medical evaluation. The diagnosis of "worried well" must not be made without a thorough examination for physical disease. Women with psychosomatic complaints may respond to a careful and sympathetic explanation of the results of the examination and to psychotherapy.[330]

Scabies, pediculosis, or enterobiasis may produce intense perivaginal itching and soreness.

APPROACH TO THE PATIENT WITH VAGINAL COMPLAINTS

History

The etiologic diagnosis of vaginitis depends on a careful evaluation of the history, physical examination, and immediate laboratory tests. Historical features are relatively nonspecific,[10, 29] but they may direct clinical suspicion toward certain causes.

Age

Neonates can acquire trichomonal or candidal vulvovaginitis during passage through an infected birth canal, an argument for treating these infections in pregnant women before term. Neonatal vaginal thrush responds promptly to topical antifungal medications.[1] Neonatal trichomoniasis can be treated with metronidazole.[331] After the neonatal period, any vaginal discharge is abnormal and should prompt a vigorous search for disease. Sexual abuse may also be a consideration. Prepubescent vaginal epithelium is not cornified, and the entire vagina is susceptible to infection with *N. gonorrhoeae* or *C. trachomatis.* Gonococcal vulvovaginitis often causes profuse vaginal discharge, and the rectum is almost always involved. Vaginal candidiasis is extremely rare in prepubescent girls.[332] Immediately before menarche, physiologic discharge reappears. A diagnosis of sexually transmitted disease in a young girl should raise the suspicion of child abuse, although some agents have been transmitted to children in the absence of frank sexual contact.

Patients in the sexually active years are more likely to have a sexually transmitted disease. Genital neoplasia is more common among older women, and postmenopausal women are more likely to have atrophic vaginitis.

Mode of Onset

An abrupt and identifiable time of onset of symptoms suggests infection. Vaginal discharge associated with neoplasia, estrogen depletion, or a foreign body often has a subacute onset, with symptoms progressing over a period of weeks. Symptoms beginning during or immediately after the menstrual period are somewhat suggestive of trichomoniasis, and a premenstrual onset more frequently accompanies candidiasis.

Quantity of Discharge

The amount of discharge is highly variable in all conditions. Patients with candidiasis often have scanty discharge or note no discharge at all. Atrophic or neoplastic discharges are commonly scanty unless infection has supervened.

Perineal Irritation

Physiologic discharge is rarely associated with perineal discomfort. Pruritus with a scanty or absent discharge is frequently seen in candidiasis and less commonly with trichomoniasis. Perineal discomfort is an infrequent complaint in BV. Severe episodic perineal pain sometimes preventing urination is strongly suggestive of herpes genitalis, which affects the labia but usually spares the vagina per se.[49, 50] Chronic discomfort, often interfering with sexual activity, should prompt consideration of vulvar vestibulitis.

Odor

An unpleasant odor accompanies many vaginal infections and sometimes physiologic discharge as well.[301] Vaginal odor in the absence of other symptoms is the initial complaint in many cases of BV. A feculent odor may accompany anaerobic superinfection of genital lesions or may be noted in the presence of a foreign body.

Abdominal Pain

Abdominal discomfort is rare in uncomplicated vulvovaginitis except for occasional cases of trichomoniasis. Women complaining of abdominal pain should be examined carefully for evidence of coincidental infections, including cystitis and pelvic inflammatory disease.

Sexual History

Exposure to a new sexual partner increases the likelihood of sexually transmitted disease. A history of genital symptoms in a sexual partner is helpful diagnostically. The commencement of oral contraceptive use may be associated with increased physiologic discharge. The use of tampons, particularly the prolonged use of superabsorbent tampons, may be associated with ulcerative vaginitis.[278–281]

Other Diseases

Diabetes mellitus, acquired immunodeficiency syndrome, malignancy and the treatment thereof, and possibly hypoparathyroidism increase the risk of candidal vaginitis. Diseases known to impair host defenses may predispose to otherwise rare infections. Other diseases may be treated with drugs that predispose to vaginal infection.

Medication

Systemic or local medication influences the spectrum of vaginal infection. Antibiotics, particularly tetracyclines and ampicillin, are active against much of the normal bacterial flora of the vagina, and their use predisposes to candidal vaginitis. Metronidazole is active against vaginal anaerobes and also predisposes to candidal infection, but less frequently than many other antimicrobials. Low doses of many antibiotics can interfere with the isolation of *N. gonorrhoeae* and possibly *C. trachomatis*. Low-dose antibiotics may result in the development of atypical syphilitic chancres or may entirely eliminate the primary stage of syphilis. Patients taking corticosteroids or oral contraceptives are at increased risk for developing vulvovaginal candidiasis. Oral contraceptive use may also be associated with the development of a physiologic vaginal discharge. Local medication including vaginal douches rarely produce a chemical vaginitis, but douching immediately before examination makes etiologic diagnosis difficult.

Examination of the Female Genitalia

With the patient supine on the examining table, the pubic hair should be examined for the presence of crab lice or nits. The inguinofemoral areas are palpated for adenopathy. Suprapubic and lower abdominal tenderness or masses are sought by palpation. With the patient in the lithotomy position, the labia and the perineum should be examined for erythema, lichenification, excoriation, or discrete lesions. Diffuse perineal erythema may accompany trichomoniasis or candidiasis. Diffuse reddening with small satellite lesions, usually papular or papulopustular, suggests candidiasis. The degree of perineal irritation is quite variable with all infections, but severe perivaginal irritation is uncommon with BV. Labial edema may accompany severe irritation.

Careful examination of all the extravaginal surfaces may reveal lesions of herpes genitalis, syphilis, condyloma acuminata, molluscum contagiosum, scabies (which are discussed in Chapter 93), or vulvar vestibulitis. Even though the patient's chief complaint may strongly suggest a true vaginitis, examination of the external genitalia for coincident infections is very important because multiple, coexistent sexually transmitted diseases are common.

Applying a 3 to 5% solution of acetic acid to the vulva may reveal white areas where no lesions were grossly visible. Such acetowhite staining suggests the possibility of human papillomavirus infection. Several other conditions, such as lichen planus, psoriasis, acute inflammation, or healing tissue, may also stain acetowhite. Diagnosis must be based on the histologic appearance of a biopsy specimen.[333] Acetic acid staining is not indicated as part of the routine gynecologic examination but may be a useful adjunct in evaluating the patient with vulvar symptoms or known human papillomavirus infection.

By spreading the labia with the gloved hand, one may examine the urethral meatus. The urethra may be gently stripped with the finger placed inside the introitus. Urethral discharge is not a common finding, but if delivered, such material should be examined microscopically and cultured. The introitus and the internal surfaces of the labia minora should be examined for lesions. Vaginal discharge is sometimes observed on the labia or actually running out onto the perineum. Such copious discharge is usually associated with trichomoniasis but may accompany other infections.

If the patient has had a hysterectomy, a calcium alginate urethral swab should be inserted gently into the urethra and the recovered material inoculated for gonococcal culture. Urethral culture is unnecessary if the cervix is present since gonococci are more often recovered from the cervix than from the urethra. The urethra is in 25% of cases the only site from which *C. trachomatis* can be recovered.

A vaginal speculum moistened with warm water is gently inserted. In the presence of severe herpes genitalis or, occasionally, trichomoniasis or candidiasis, insertion of the speculum may be impossible because of the patient's discomfort. In such a case, a primary diagnosis is sometimes made from material recovered on a cotton swab gently inserted into the vagina. After the speculum has been inserted, the vaginal walls are examined. Candidal or trichomonal vaginitis is often accompanied by erythema of the vaginal walls. The degree of erythema, however, is often very difficult to assess in an individual patient. Punctate hemorrhages of the vaginal walls strongly suggest trichomoniasis. A diffuse sheen, manifested by an increased light reflex, may be caused by thin discharge adhering to the walls. This is seen most frequently with BV but may accompany other infections. Finger-like projections within the vagina may be condylomata acuminata, but these must be differentiated from hymeneal tags. The latter are normal but are usually found only near the introitus.

The surface of the cervix may be inflamed. Punctate hemorrhages are only rarely observed with the naked eye in patients with severe trichomoniasis (colpitis macularis, strawberry cervix), although they are revealed by colposcopy in almost 50% of cases.[334] Cervical ulcerations may be present in herpes genitalis. Mucoid material is normally observed at the cervical os and is present in increased amounts in women taking oral contraceptives. A normal cervical discharge may be clear or white, but purulent or mucopurulent discharge is associated with infectious cervicitis, primarily chlamydial, gonococcal, or herpetic.

Acetic acid staining of the vagina and cervix is useful as an adjunct to colposcopy but is not indicated during the routine genital examination.

Bimanual examination for adnexal tenderness and masses should be a part of the evaluation. Adnexal tenderness is sufficiently uncommon with local vaginal infections that its presence suggests salpingitis.

Other Bedside Evaluation

After the speculum is withdrawn, the pH of vaginal secretions can be determined by inserting a strip of indicator paper into the material collected in the lower lip of the speculum. I have found Nitrazine paper with a pH range of 4.5 to 7 to be useful. A normal pH of 4.5 is seen in most patients with vulvovaginal candidiasis, whereas a pH elevated to 5.0 or above is associated with BV and trichomoniasis. Several drops of 10% KOH are then added to the material on the speculum. A resultant pungent, fishy, amine-like odor constitutes a positive whiff test. The whiff test is positive in more than 90% of patients with BV and in many patients with trichomoniasis. It is negative in women with vulvovaginal candidiasis. The whiff test may also be evaluated on a slide that has been prepared for KOH microscopic examination.

Laboratory Examination

A wet mount is of greatest value in the differential diagnosis of a vaginal discharge, and the specimen may be prepared in several ways. A swab of vaginal discharge may be agitated in a tube containing about 0.5 ml of normal saline. One drop of the resulting suspension is put on a microscope slide, and a coverslip is applied. Alternatively, the examiner may place a drop of saline on the slide and mix in a loop full of vaginal material, after which a coverslip is applied. The slide is examined initially under low power (×100) and then under high power (×400) on a bright-field microscope with the substage condenser racked down and the substage diaphragm closed down to increase the contrast. Phase-contrast microscopy is becoming more widely available in clinical settings and provides an excellent means of evaluating vaginal wet mounts. The relative numbers of epithelial cells and PMNs should be noted. PMNs are present in physiologic endocervical discharge that collects in the vagina,[335] so small numbers of PMNs may be observed in the vaginal material recovered from healthy women. Finding many more than one PMN per epithelial cell should raise the examiner's suspicion of cervical or vaginal inflammation, although this is not a specific finding.[336] Observing relatively few PMNs does not rule out vaginal infection. Vaginal candidiasis often produces a discharge containing only small numbers of PMNs.[66] The relative absence of PMNs is characteristic of the discharge of BV.[10, 337] In fact, finding many PMNs in the vaginal discharge of a patient with BV should prompt the examiner to search for simultaneous infection such as trichomoniasis, gonorrhea, or chlamydial cervicitis. Large clumps of pseudohyphae suggest vaginal candidiasis, but the examiner often sees only moderate or even very small numbers of yeasts in this condition. Indeed, some patients with VC have organisms identified only by culture. The wet preparation should be scanned for motile trichomonads.

Normal squamous epithelial cells have transparent cytoplasm and small nuclei. Epithelial cells covered with tiny coccobacillary forms (see Fig. 95–1) are called *clue cells* and are associated with BV. Clue cells are best recognized by observing the edges of epithelial cells, which may be obscured by the adherent coccobacilli. Some cells are so heavily encrusted that the nuclei are obscured. Trichomonads (Fig. 95–2) are best be recognized by their characteristic twitching motility. The flagella and undulating membrane may be observed by carefully focusing the microscope and adjusting the light source. Trichomonad motility is improved by gently warming the preparation. Unfortunately, the wet mount is negative in about 30% of the women with trichomoniasis (see Chapter 270), and a negative wet mount does not rule out this infection, particularly in relatively asymptomatic women. A negative wet mount should be confirmed with a culture. Small numbers of yeasts are frequently observed and do not necessarily indicate that the patient's vaginitis has a fungal cause.

The bacterial flora can be assessed on the wet mount. Normal vaginal flora consists primarily of rods. In BV, the predominant flora is tiny coccobacilli. Spermatozoa may be observed as long as 10 days after the last coitus, but motile sperm suggest sexual contact within the preceding 24 hours.[338]

Combining a drop of 10 or 20% KOH with the vaginal material

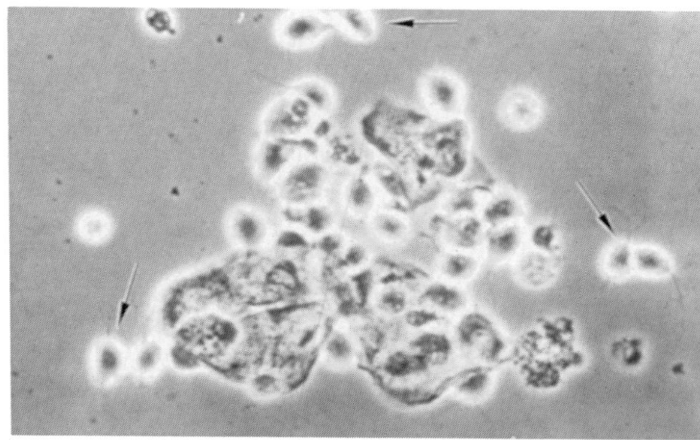

FIGURE 95–2. A wet mount of vaginal discharge from a patient with trichomonal vaginitis shows epithelial cells, neutrophils, and trichomonads *(arrows)*. (Phase microscopy, ×400.)

on a microscope slide, applying a coverslip, and gently heating destroys cellular elements but leaves the bacteria and fungi unscathed. The KOH preparation cannot be used for a microscopic diagnosis of trichomoniasis or BV, but elaboration of a fishy odor from the slide suggests either of these infections.

A Gram stain of vaginal material is somewhat less useful for differential diagnosis than is the wet mount, because although *G. vaginalis* and *Candida* spp. are readily recognized on the Gram-stained smear, trichomonads are very difficult to identify. Normal vaginal flora consists primarily of gram-positive rods, which are presumably lactobacilli. In BV the normal flora is replaced by sheets of gram-variable coccobacilli, which often overly the surface of epithelial cells. Small numbers of yeasts are occasionally observed as dense, gram-positive or beaded ovoids, and women with active vaginal candidiasis sometimes have large numbers of budding yeasts and pseudohyphae recognizable as thick gram-positive or beaded tubes. Unfortunately, the Gram stain is positive in less than one third of the women from whom *Candida* can be cultured.[68]

Material recovered from the endocervix can be Gram stained. Cervical discharge always contains moderate numbers of PMNs, and their presence is not necessarily an indication of specific inflammation.[335] Large numbers of PMNs indicate cervicitis. Gram-negative, intracellular diplococci accurately diagnose gonorrhea (see Chapter 200), but extracellular diplococci are of no significance, since nonpathogenic *Neisseria* is part of the normal flora of the female genital tract. Unfortunately, the cervical Gram stain is positive in only about one half of the women with cervical gonorrhea, and a negative Gram stain does not rule out the infection.[68] Trichomonads are only infrequently found in the endocervix, and cervical material should not be used to examine for trichomoniasis. Cervical material recovered from women at risk should be cultured for *N. gonorrhoeae* and evaluated for *C. trachomatis.* The Papanicolaou smear may reveal *Trichomonas vaginalis* or clue cells, but neither of these findings is sufficiently sensitive for a negative result to rule out infection. Direct staining of cervical specimens using the Giemsa or Papanicolaou methods is insufficiently sensitive for the diagnosis of chlamydial cervicitis (see Chapter 168).

CERVICITIS

Under the influence of estrogens, the normal vaginal epithelium cornifies and becomes relatively resistant to infection with a number of pathogens. The endocervix, however, is lined with columnar epithelium, which remains susceptible to many of these infections. Therefore, the examiner frequently finds infectious cervicitis in the absence of vaginitis and vice versa. Studies of the cause of cervicitis have been hampered by the lack of a reliable definition of the syndrome.[136, 339, 340] Erythema around the cervical os may indicate infection or may merely represent cervical ectropion (previously called *erosion* or *eversion*), a term indicating migration of endocervical epithelium over the surface of the cervix. This lesion is usually symmetric about the os and is not particularly friable. It is accompanied by a mucoid cervical discharge. Ectropion is more common in women taking oral contraceptives, and the increased amount of exposed columnar epithelium may contribute to the greater risk of chlamydial infection among women taking oral contraceptives. It is often impossible on clinical grounds alone to differentiate ectropion from true infection. *Hypertrophic cervicitis,* on the other hand, is manifested as an intensely erythematous, raised, irregular lesion that bleeds easily.[138, 339–341] This lesion is often associated with chlamydial infection.[138, 339–341]

Normal cervical discharge is clear and mucoid. Purulent or mucopurulent discharge is associated with gonococcal or chlamydial infection.[138, 342–344] The nature of the cervical discharge can be assessed by obtaining endocervical material on a swab and comparing its consistency and color against a well-illuminated sheet of white paper or cloth.

PMNs are normally present in the endocervix,[335] but abnormally increased numbers can be detected crudely on a Gram stain of endocervical material. After the endocervix has been cleaned off, a swab is inserted into the cervix and gently rotated, and the recovered material is applied to a microscope slide by rolling the swab over an area about 1 × 2 cm. The specimen is then Gram stained. Observation of 10 to 30 PMNs per oil-immersion field in the densest portion of the slide correlates statistically with the presence of gonococci or chlamydiae,[138, 343, 345–349] but the sensitivity and positive predictive value of the observation (both 25 to 45% in a high-risk population) are far too low for a definitive diagnosis. The presence of inflammation on cervical cytologic examination suggests a need for further investigation, but only about 25 to 50% of high-risk women with inflammation on cervical cytologic examination have infection with *N. gonorrhoeae, C. trachomatis,* or human papillomavirus.[350–355] Increased numbers of PMNs in the vaginal wet mount are a poor predictor of cervical abnormality.[336]

Specific Causes of Acute Cervicitis

The clinical features of specific cervical infections overlap too much to permit an accurate etiologic diagnosis without laboratory assistance.[138, 339, 356] Multiple infections are common[356] and may be missed if the diagnosis is attempted on clinical grounds alone.

Acute gonococcal cervicitis has been known for hundreds of years. The endocervix is the site from which gonococci are most frequently isolated in women with uncomplicated gonococcal infections. In typical cases, the cervical os is reddened and produces a purulent discharge.[357] A Gram stain of this material reveals typical gram-negative cell-associated diplococci in only about 50 to 75% of the infected women (Fig. 95–3),[68, 347] and a negative Gram stain must never be used as an argument against treating women for uncomplicated gonorrhea. Examination for gonococcal cervicitis must include an appropriate culture. The sensitivity of the endocervical culture is disputed but is generally held to be on the order of 90%. Most women with uncomplicated gonococcal cervicitis are asymptomatic, but about one third note vaginal discharge.[357] *Chlamydia trachomatis* can be recovered from the endocervix of 60 to 90% of the sexual partners of men with chlamydial urethritis.[339–341, 358, 359] Cervical abnormalities, often subtle, have been observed in 80 to 90% of chlamydia-positive women,[339–341, 358, 359] but about one third note a discharge from the vagina that actually originates in the inflamed cervix. Chlamydiae have been isolated from 50 to 90% of sexually active patients with hypertrophic cervicitis. Only 19 to 32% of women with chlamydial cervical infection manifest hypertrophic cervicitis, and only about 30% have a mucopurulent or purulent cervical discharge.[339, 340, 342, 360] On examination, 20 to 70% of infected women are found to have a completely normal cervix.[342, 260] Therefore, physical examination never adequately excludes chlamydial infection, similar to the situation with gonococcal cervicitis. Female partners of men with nongonococcal urethritis should be epidemiologically treated even before the diagnosis of chlamydial infection is confirmed by laboratory techniques.

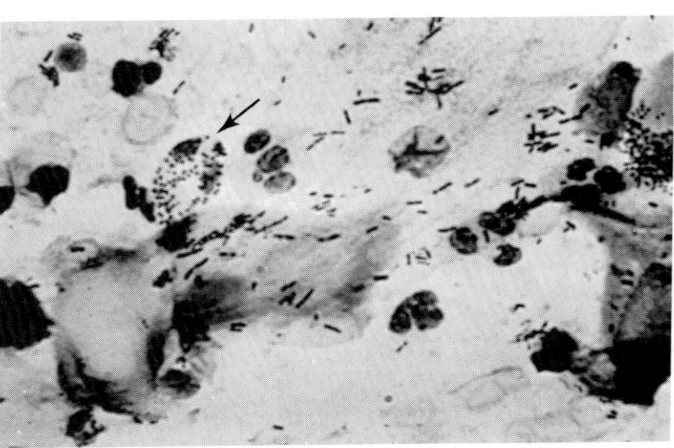

FIGURE 95–3. Gram stain of cervical exudate from a woman with gonorrhea. A neutrophil contains many gram-negative diplococci. Other bacteria are normal vaginal flora. (×1000.)

Chlamydiae can be identified in cervical specimens from 75 to 95% of infected women by using immunofluorescence microscopy, enzyme immunoassays, DNA probes, polymerase chain reaction, and the ligase chain reaction (see Chapter 167).

Herpes simplex virus is isolated from the cervix of 88% of women with primary infection but only from 12% of women with recurrent herpetic infection.[101, 102] Herpetic cervicitis may be present without external lesions. Cervicitis is seen on physical examination in about 90% of women whose cervical cultures are positive for herpes simplex virus.[101, 102] The cervix usually displays diffuse friability and, less frequently, frank ulcers or necrosis.[101] Cervical discharge is usually mucoid, but it is occasionally mucopurulent, and in one series herpetic cervical infection caused 8% of cases of mucopurulent cervicitis.[138] Affected patients may have lower abdominal pain, but inguinal adenopathy is rare unless the disease is accompanied by lesions of the external genitalia[361] because lymphatic drainage of the cervix involves the external iliac rather than the inguinofemoral nodes. The diagnosis of herpetic cervicitis may be made cytologically by observing multinucleated giant cells, often with intranuclear inclusions.[362] In the presence of severe necrosis, however, cellular architecture is so distorted that cytologic examination becomes insensitive, and other methods such as culture, DNA probe, or polymerase chain reaction are more useful (see Chapter 124).

Human papillomavirus, particularly certain subtypes, frequently infects the cervix.[363] It has been observed since 1837 that cancer of the cervix behaves epidemiologically as if it were a sexually transmitted disease.[364] The strongest infectious association with cancer of the cervix has been established for some types of human papillomavirus (see Chapter 133).[365]

Other organisms occasionally considered causes of cervicitis include adenovirus,[366] measles virus,[367] cytomegalovirus,[368] *Enterobius vermicularis,*[369] amoebae,[370] *M. tuberculosis,*[371] group B streptococci,[372] *N. meningitidis,*[373] and actinomycetes,[374] the last usually in association with the use of intrauterine contraceptive devices. The chancre of syphilis sometimes manifests as a cervical lesion.[375]

Therapeutic Approach to Cervicitis

Specifically diagnosed gonococcal cervicitis should be treated as recommended in Chapter 200. Because 30 to 60% of women with gonococcal cervicitis also have chlamydial infection, simultaneous treatment for both infections is advised when gonorrhea is diagnosed.[248] Cervicitis in patients who are the sexual partners of men with nongonococcal urethritis should be treated with the same regimen as their partners (see Chapter 168). Cervicitis of unknown cause should be treated with a regimen that is adequate for gonorrhea and chlamydial infection. Management of cervicitis due to herpes simplex is discussed in Chapter 125.

INFECTIONS OF BARTHOLIN'S AND SKENE'S GLANDS

Bartholinitis

In the adult, Bartholin's gland is a 1-cm structure on each side of the vagina near the base of the labia minora. The healthy gland is not palpable and nontender. A 2-cm-long duct lined with columnar epithelium opens on the inner surface of the labia minora at the junction of the posterior and middle thirds. Inflammation of the duct can produce blockage resulting in the development of a sterile cyst, and infection of the duct is said to be more common than infection of the gland itself.[376] Infection of the gland behind a blocked duct can result in the development of a Bartholin's gland abscess.

The frequency with which specific organisms infect Bartholin's glands is incompletely defined. Anaerobic and polymicrobic infections are common.[377] Rees recovered gonococci from the glands of 28% of women with gonorrhea, most of whom were asymptomatic,[376] but later workers recovered gonococci from only 5 to 12% of a series of patients with Bartholin's gland abscess.[378, 379] Gonococcal bartholinitis is usually asymptomatic, but about 1 in 5 women has a palpable enlargement or tenderness of the glands, and 1 in 20 has edema.[376] The examiner should attempt to palpate the glands during the pelvic examination. If material can be expressed from the duct opening, it should be examined with the Gram stain, and it should be cultured.

Chlamydia trachomatis causes occasional cases of bartholinitis,[380] although its incidence is apparently low. Infection with normal genital flora is also significant. Single or mixed species of anaerobes have been recovered from up to 90% of the infected glands.[377, 378, 381, 382] *Escherichia coli* and *Proteus mirabilis* are also frequently recovered.[378, 382–384] *Staphylococcus aureus* is apparently a rare cause of abscess, but streptococci are frequently isolated.[378, 384, 385] *Haemophilus influenzae* has been recovered.[386]

Lee and colleagues recovered *U. urealyticum* from two thirds of Bartholin's gland abscesses.[378] Occasionally, herpes genitalis involves the duct and produces a transient but recurrent swelling of the gland.

Bartholinitis accompanying gonococcal infection can be treated like acute gonorrhea,[376] although longer treatment or surgical drainage may be required if there is obstruction of the duct. The optimal initial therapy for bartholinitis of uncertain cause is not known. A combination of ofloxacin, in doses adequate for chlamydial infection, with clindamycin might be considered. Doxycycline alone has been used traditionally with good anecdotal results. A failure of bartholinitis to respond to antibiotic therapy suggests the need for surgical drainage of the abscess.[387, 388] Complications of bartholinitis include toxic shock,[385] septic shock,[389] and necrotizing fasciitis.[390]

Skenitis

Skene's glands are small structures that empty into the urethra. Dysuria is the usual complaint of patients with infection of these glands, and sometimes a bead of pus can be expressed. The gonococcus is felt to produce some cases of skenitis, but the role of other potential pathogens has not been determined. Empirical therapy should probably resemble that for bartholinitis.

REFERENCES

1. Lang WR. Pediatric vaginitis. N Engl J Med. 1955;253:1153.
2. Hammerschlag MR, Alpert S, Onderdonk AB, et al. Anaerobic microflora of the vagina in children. Am J Obstet Gynecol. 1978;131:853–860.
3. Hammerschlag MR, Alpert S, Rosner I, et al. Microbiology of the vagina in children: Normal and potentially pathogenic organisms. Pediatrics. 1978;62:57–62.
4. Levison ME, Corman LC, Carrington ER, et al. Quantitative microflora of the vagina. Am J Obstet Gynecol. 1977;127:80.
5. Tashijan JH, Coulam CB, Washington JA. Vaginal flora in asymptomatic women. Mayo Clin Proc. 1976;51:557.
6. Brown WJ. Variations in the bacterial flora: A preliminary report. Ann Intern Med. 1982;96:131.
7. Larsen B, Galask RP. Vaginal microbial flora: Composition and influences of host physiology. Ann Intern Med. 1982;96(Suppl 6):926.
8. Spiegel CA, Amsel R, Eschenbach D, et al. Anaerobic bacteria in nonspecific vaginitis. N Engl J Med. 1980;303:601.
9. Giorgi A, Torriani S, Dellaglio F, et al. Identification of vaginal lactobacilli from asymptomatic women. Microbiologia. 1987;10:377–384.
10. Rein MF, Holmes KK. "Nonspecific vaginitis," vulvovaginal candidiasis, and trichomoniasis. In: Remington JS, Swartz MN, eds. Current Clinical Topics in Infectious Diseases, v. 4. New York: McGraw-Hill; 1983:281.
11. Easmon CSF, Ison CA. *Gardnerella vaginalis.* Lancet. 1983;2:343.
12. Guinan ME, Dan BB, Guidotti RJ, et al. Vaginal colonization with *Staphylococcus aureus* in healthy women: A review of four studies. Ann Intern Med. 1982;94:944.
13. Larsen B. Vaginal flora in health and disease. Clin Obstet Gynecol. 1993;36:107–121.
14. Sobel JD. Epidemiology and pathogenesis of recurrent vulvovaginal candidiasis. Am J Obstet Gynecol. 1985;1523:924–935.
15. Shafer MA, Sweet FL, Ohm-Smith MJ, et al. Microbiology of the lower genital tract in postmenarchal adolescents girls: Differences in sexual activity, contraception, and presence of nonspecific vaginitis. J Pediatr. 1985;107:974–981.
16. Hill GB, Eschenbach DA, Holmes KK. Bacteriology of the vagina. Scand J Urol Nephrol. 1984;18:(Suppl 86):23–30.
17. Sonnex C. Influence of ovarian hormones on urogenital infection. Sex Transm Infect. 1998;74:11–19.
18. Cohen MS, Black JR, Proctor RA, et al. Host defenses and the vaginal mucosa: A reevaluation. Scand J Urol Nephrol. 1984(Suppl 86):13–22.
19. Eschenbach DA, Davick PR, Williams BL, et al. Prevalence of hydrogen peroxide–producing *Lactobacillus* species in normal women and women with bacterial vaginosis. J Clin Microbiol. 1989;27:251.
20. Thorsen P, Jensen IP, Jeune B, et al. Few microorganisms associated with bacterial vaginosis may constitute the pathologic core: A population-based microbiologic study among 3596 pregnant women. Am J Obstet Gynecol. 1998;178:580–587.
21. Hillier SL. The vaginal microbial ecosystem and resistance to HIV. AIDS Res Human Retroviruses. 1998;14(Suppl 1):S17–S21.
22. Hawes SE, Hillier SL, Benedetti J, et al. Hydrogen peroxide–producing lactobacilli and acquisition of vaginal infections. J Infect Dis. 1996;174:1058–1063.
23. Sobel JD, Chaim W. Vaginal microbiology of women with acute recurrent vulvovaginal candidiasis. J Clin Microbiol. 1996;34:2497–2499.
24. Richardson BA, Marin HL Jr, Stevens CE, et al. The use of nonoxynol-9 and changes in vaginal lactobacilli. J Infect Dis. 1998;178:441–445.
25. Centers for Disease Control and Prevention. Nonreported sexually transmitted diseases. MMWR Morb Mortal Wkly Rep. 1979;28:61.
26. Sobel JD. Candidal vulvovaginitis. Clin Obstet Gynecol. 1993;36:153–165.
27. Kent HL. Epidemiology of vaginitis. Am J Obstet Gynecol. 1991;165:1168–1176.
28. Sweet RL. Importance of differential diagnosis in acute vaginitis. Am J Obstet Gynecol. 1985;152:921–923.
29. Schaaf VM, Perez-Stable EJ, Borchardt K. The limited value of symptoms and signs in the diagnosis of vaginal infections. Arch Intern Med. 1990;150:1929–1933.
30. Taylor CA, Lipsky MS. Physicians' perceptions of the impact of the reclassification of vaginal antifungal agents. J Fam Pract. 1994;38:157–160.
31. Redondo-Lopez V, Meriwether C, Schmitt C, et al. Vulvovaginal candidiasis complicating recurrent bacterial vaginosis. Sex Transm Dis. 1990;17:51–53.
32. Odds FC. *Candida* and Candidosis. Baltimore: University Park; 1979:4.
33. O'Connor MI, Sobel JD. Epidemiology of recurrent vulvovaginal candidiasis: Identification and strain differentiation of *Candida albicans.* J Infect Dis. 1986;154:358–363.
34. Sobel JD, Chaim W. Treatment of *Torulopsis glabrata* vaginitis: A retrospective review of boric acid therapy. Clin Infect Dis. 1997;24:649–652.
35. Nyirjesy P, Seeney SM, Terry Grody MH, et al. Chronic fungal vaginitis: The value of cultures. Am J Obstet Gynecol. 1995;173:820–823.
36. Geiger AM, Foxman B, Sobel JD. Chronic vulvovaginal candidiasis: Characteristics of women with *Candida albicans, C. glabrata* and no candida. Genitourin Med. 1995;75:304–307.
37. Nyirjesy P, Vazquez JA, Ufberg DD, et al. *Saccharomyces cerevisiae* vaginitis: Transmission from yeast used in baking. Obstet Gynecol. 1995;86:326–329.
38. Spinillo A, Capuzzo E, Egbe TO, et al. *Torulopsis glabrata* vaginitis. Obstet Gynecol. 1995;85:993–998.
39. Spinillo A, Capuzzo E, Gulminetti R, et al. Prevalence of and risk factors for fungal vaginitis caused by non-albicans species. Am J Obstet Gynecol. 1997;176:138–141.
40. Horowitz BJ, Edelstein SW, Lippman L. *Candida tropicalis* vulvovaginitis. Obstet Gynecol. 1985;66:229–232.
41. Redondo-Lopez V, Lynch M, Schmitt CA, et al. *Torulopsis glabrata* vaginitis: Clinical aspects and susceptibility to antifungal agents. Obstet Gynecol. 1990;76:651.
42. Sobel JD, Vazquez J, Lynch M, et al. Vaginitis due to *Saccharomyces cerevisiae:* Epidemiology, clinical aspects, and therapy. Clin Infect Dis. 1993;16:93–99.
43. McCullough MJ, Clemons KV, Farina C, et al. Epidemiological investigation of vaginal *Saccharomyces cerevisiae* isolates by a genotypic method. J Clin Microbiol. 1998;36:557–562.
44. Sobel JD. Pathogenesis and treatment of recurrent vulvovaginal candidiasis. Clin Infect Dis. 1992;14(Suppl 1):S148–S153.

45. Agnew KJ, Hillier SL. The effect of treatment regimens for vaginitis and cervicitis on vaginal colonization with lactobacilli. Sex Transm Dis. 1995;22:269–273.
46. Spinillo A, Capuzzo E, Nicola S, et al. The impact of oral contraception on vulvovaginal candidiasis. Contraception. 1995;51:293–297.
47. Powell BL, Frey CL, Drutz DJ. Estrogen receptor in *Candida albicans*. A possible explanation for hormonal influences in vaginal candidiasis. Abstract 751. In: Proceedings of the 23rd Interscience Conference on Antimicrobial Agents and Chemotherapy. Las Vegas, September, 1983.
48. Anonymous. Adverse events and their association with treatment regimens in the diabetes control and complications trial. Diabetes Care. 1995;18:1415–1427.
49. Elgebe IA, Botu M. A preliminary study on dressing patterns and incidence of candidiasis. Am J Public Health. 1982;72:176.
50. Elgebe IA, Elgebe I. Quantitative relationships of *Candida albicans* infections and dressing patterns in Nigerian women. Am J Public Health. 1983;73:450–452.
51. Heidrich FE, Berg AO, Bergman JJ. Clothing factors and vaginitis. J Family Pract. 1984;19:491–494.
52. Rhoads JL, Wright DC, Redfield RR, et al. Chronic vaginal candidiasis in women with human immunodeficiency virus infection. JAMA. 1987;257:3105–3109.
53. Imam N, Carpenter CCJ, Mayer KH, et al. Hierarchical pattern of mucosal *Candida* infections with HIV seropositive women. Am J Med. 1990;89:142.
54. Sobel JD. Vaginitis. N Engl J Med. 1997;337:1896–1903.
55. Gieger AM, Foxman B, Gillespie BW. The epidemiology of vulvovaginal candidiasis among university students. Am J Public Health. 1995;85:1146–1148.
56. Gieger AM, Foxman B. Risk factors in vulvovaginal candidiasis: A case controlled study among university students. Epidemiology. 1996;7:182–187.
57. Hellberg D, Zdolsek B, Milsson S, Mårdh P-A. Sexual behavior of women with repeated episodes of vulvovaginal candidiasis. Eur J Epidemiol. 1995;11:575–579.
58. Odds FC. Genital candidosis. Clin Exp Dermatol. 1982;7:345–354.
59. Garcia-Tamayo J, Castillo G, Martinez AJ. Human genital candidiasis: Histochemistry, scanning and transmission electron microscopy. Acta Cytol. 1982;26:7.
60. Kimura LH, Pearsal NH. Relationship between germination of *Candida albicans* and increased adherence to human buccal epithelial cells. Infect Immun. 1980;28:464.
61. King RD, Lee JC, Morris AL. Adherence of *Candida albicans* and other *Candida* species to mucosal epithelial cells. Infect Immun. 1980;27:667.
62. Sobel JD, Muller G. Ketoconazole in the prevention of experimental candidal vaginitis. Antimicrob Agents Chemother. 1984;25:281–282.
63. Fidel PJ Jr, Sobel JD. Immunopathogenesis of recurrent vulvovaginal candidiasis. Clin Microbiol Rev. 1996;9:335–348.
64. Rigg D, Miller MM, Motzger WJ. Recurrent allergic vulvovaginitis treatment with *Candida albicans* allergen immunotherapy. Am J Obstet Gynecol. 1990;162:232.
65. Drake SM, Evans BA, Gerken A. Vaginal pH and microflora related to yeast infections and treatment. Br J Vener Dis. 1980;56:107.
66. Peeters F, Snauwaert R, Segers J, et al. Observations on candidal vaginitis: Vaginal pH, microbiology. Am J Obstet Gynecol. 1972;112:80.
67. Baldson MJ. Comparison of miconazole-coated tampons with clotrimazole vaginal tablets in the treatment of vaginal candidosis. Br J Vener Dis. 1981;57:275.
68. Rothenberg RB, Simm R, Chipperfield E, et al. Efficacy of selected diagnostic tests for sexually transmitted diseases. JAMA. 1976;235:49.
69. Pattman RS. Evaluation of a culture in the diagnosis of vaginal candidosis. Br J Vener Dis. 1981;57:67.
70. Rajakumar R, Lacey CJN, Evans EGV, et al. Use of a slide latex agglutination test for rapid diagnosis of vaginal candidosis. Genitourin Med. 1987;63:192–195.
71. Sobel JD, Schmitt C, Meriwether C. A new slide agglutination test for the diagnosis of acute *Candida* vaginitis. Am J Clin Pathol. 1990;94:323–325.
72. Reed BD, Pierson CL. Evaluation of a latex agglutination test for identification of *Candida* species in vaginal discharge. J Am Board Fam Pract. 1992;5:375–380.
73. Odds FC. Cure and relapse with antifungal therapy. Proc R Soc Med. 1977;70(Suppl 4):24.
74. Doering PL, Santiago TM. Drugs for treatment of vulvovaginal candidiasis: Comparative efficacy of agents and regimens. DICP. 1990;24:1078–1083.
75. Anonymous. Butoconazole for vulvovaginal candidiasis. Med Lett Drugs Ther. 1986;28:68.
76. Bradbeer CS, Mayhew SR, Barlow D. Butoconazole and miconazole in treating vaginal candidiasis. Genitourin Med. 1985;61:270–272.
77. Droegemuller W, Adamson DG, Brown D, et al. Three-day treatment with butoconazole nitrate for vulvovaginal candidiasis. Obstet Gynecol. 1984;64:530–534.
78. Weisberg M. Treatment of vaginal candidiasis in pregnant women. Clin Ther. 1986;8:563–567.
79. Nixon SA. Vulvovaginitis: The role of patient compliance in treatment success. Am J Obstet Gynecol. 1991;165:1207–1209.
80. Lebherz T, Guess E, Wolfson N. Efficacy of single-versus multiple-dose clotrimazole therapy in the management of vulvovaginal candidiasis. Am J Obstet Gynecol. 1985;152:965–967.
81. Heary F, Hughes D, Floyd R. Therapeutic results obtained in vaginal mycoses after single-dose treatment with 500 mg clotrimazole vaginal tablets. Am J Obstet Gynecol. 1985;152:968–970.
82. Loendersloot EW, Goormans E, Wieshann E, et al. Efficacy and tolerability of single-dose versus six-day treatment of candidal vulvovaginitis with vaginal tablets of clotrimazole. Am J Obstet Gynecol. 1985;152:953–955.
83. Cohen L. Single dose treatment of vaginal candidosis: Comparison of clotrimazole and isoconazole. Br J Vener Dis. 1984;60:40–42.
84. Milson I, Forssman L. Treatment of vaginal candidosis with a single 500 mg clotrimazole pessary. Br J Vener Dis. 1982;58:124.
85. Sobel JD. Management of recurrent vulvovaginal candidiasis with intermittent ketoconazole prophylaxis. Obstet Gynecol. 1985;65:435–440.
86. Sobel JD. Recurrent vulvovaginal candidiasis. A prospective study of the efficacy of maintenance ketoconazole therapy. N Engl J Med. 1986;315:1455–1458.
87. Eschenbach DA, Hummel D, Gravett MG. Recurrent and persistent vulvovaginal candidiasis: Treatment with ketoconazole. Obstet Gynecol. 1985;66:248–254.
88. Houang ET, Chappatte O, Byrne D, et al. Fluconazole levels in plasma and vaginal secretions of patients after a 150-milligram single oral dose and rate of eradication of infection in vaginal candidiasis. Antimicrob Agents Chemother. 1990;34:909–910.
89. Van Heusden AM, Merkus HMWM, Corbeij RSACM, et al. Single-dose oral fluconazole versus single-dose topical miconazole for the treatment of acute vulvovaginal candidosis. Acta Obstet Gynecol Scand. 1990;69:417–422.
90. Boag FC, Houang ET, Westrom R, et al. Comparison of vaginal flora after treatment with a clotrimazole 500 mg pessary or a fluconazole 150 mg capsule for vaginal candidosis. Genitourin Med. 1991;67:232–234.
91. Salem HT, Salah M, Farid A, et al. Oral versus local treatment of vaginal candidosis. Int J Gynaecol Obstet. 1989;30:57–62.
92. Osser S, Haglund A, Westrom L. Treatment of candidal vaginitis: A prospective randomized investigator-blind multicenter study comparing topically applied econazole with oral fluconazole. Acta Obstet Gynecol Scand. 1991;70:73–78.
93. Brammer KW. Single-dose oral fluconazole in the treatment of vaginal candidosis. Ann N Y Acad Sci. 1988;544:561–563.
94. Phillips RJ, Watson SA, McKay FF. An open multicentre study of the efficacy and safety of a single dose of fluconazole 150 mg in the treatment of vaginal candidiasis in a general practice. Br J Clin Pract. 1990;44:219–222.
95. Calderon-Marquez JJ. Itraconazole in the treatment of vaginal candidosis and the effect of treatment of the sexual partner. Rev Infect Dis. 1987;9(Suppl 1):143–145.
96. Tobin JM, Loo P, Granger SE. Treatment of vaginal candidosis: A comparative study of the efficacy and acceptability of itraconazole and clotrimazole. Genitourin Med. 1992;68:36–38.
97. Stein GE, Mummaw N. Placebo-controlled trial of itraconazole for treatment of acute vaginal candidiasis. Antimicrob Agents Chemother. 1992;37:89–92.
98. Silva-Cruz A, Andrade L, Sobral L, et al. Itraconazole versus placebo in the management of vaginal candidiasis. Int J Gynecol Obstet. 1991;36:229–232.
99. Roongpisuthipong A, Sentrakul P, Bhiraleus P, et al. Itraconazole in the treatment of acute vaginal candidosis. J Med Assoc Thai. 1992;75:30–34.
100. Wesel S. Itraconazole: A single-day oral treatment for acute vulvovaginal candidosis. Br J Clin Pract Symp Suppl. 1990;71:S77–S80.
101. Corey L, Adams HG, Brown AZ, et al. Genital herpes simplex virus infections. Clinical manifestations, course, and complications. Ann Intern Med. 1983;98:958.
102. Pazin GH. Management of oral and genital herpes simplex viral infections: Diagnosis and treatment. Disease a Month. 1986;32:725–784.
103. Corey L, Holmes KK. The use of 2-deoxy-D-glucose for genital herpes. JAMA. 1980;243:29.
104. Jovanovic R, Congema E, Nguyen HT. Antifungal agents vs. boric acid for treating chronic mycotic vulvovaginitis. J Reprod Med. 1991;36:593–597.
105. Clayton YM. Antifungal drugs in current use. A review. Proc R Soc Med. 1977;70(Suppl 4):15.
106. Vorherr H, Vorherr UF, Mehta P, et al. Vaginal absorption of povidone-iodine. JAMA. 1980;244:2628.
107. Van Slyke KK, Michel VP, Rein MF. Treatment of vulvovaginal candidiasis with boric acid powder. Am J Obstet Gynecol. 1981;141:145–148.
108. Podolsky S, Tauber AI. Yogurt for candidal vaginitis. Ann Intern Med. 1992;117:345–346.
109. Shalev E, Battino S, Weiner E, et al. Ingestion of yogurt containing *Lactobacillus acidophilus* compared with pasteurized yogurt as prophylaxis for recurrent candidal vaginitis and bacterial vaginosis. Arch Fam Med. 1996;5:593–596.
110. Cohen L. Is more than one application of an antifungal necessary in the treatment of acute vaginal candidiasis. Am J Obstet Gynecol. 1985;152:961–964.
111. Rashid S, Collins M, Kennedy RJ. A study of candidosis: The role of fomites. Genitourin Med. 1991;67:137–142.
112. Vazquez JA, Sobel JD, Demitriou R, et al. Karyotyping of *Candida albicans* isolates obtained longitudinally in women with recurrent vulvovaginal candidiasis. J Infect Dis. 1994;170:1566–1569.
113. Maffei CM, Paula CR, Mazzocato TS, Franceschini S. Phenotype and genotype of *Candida albicans* strains isolated from pregnant women with recurrent vaginitis. Mycopathologia. 1997;137:87–94.
114. Lockhart SR, Reed BD, Pierson CL, Soll DR. Most frequent scenario for recurrent *Candida* vaginitis is strain maintenance with "substrain shuffling": Demonstration by sequential DNA fingerprinting with probes Ca3, C1, and CARE2. J Clin Microbiol. 1996;34:767–777.
115. Schmidt J, Rotman M, Reed B, et al. Genetic similarity of *Candida albicans* strains from vaginitis patients and their partners. J Clin Microbiol. 1993;31:39–46.
116. Fong IW. The value of treating the sexual partners of women with recurrent vaginal candidiasis with ketoconazole. Genitourin Med. 1992;68:147–146.
117. Hill LVH, Embil JA. Vaginitis. Current microbiological and clinical concepts. Can Med Assoc J. 1986;134:3221–3231.
118. Nystatin Multicenter Study Group. Therapy of candidal vaginitis: The effect of eliminating intestinal *Candida*. Am J Obstet Gynecol. 1986;155:651–655.
119. Lossick JG. Sexually transmitted vaginitis. Semin Adolesc Med. 1985;2:131–142.
120. Edman J, Sobel JD, Taylor ML. Zinc status in women with recurrent vulvovaginal candidiasis. Am J Obstet Gynecol. 1986;155:1082–1085.
121. Witkin SS, Yu IR, Ledger WJ. Inhibition of *Candida albicans*–induced lymphocyte proliferation by lymphocytes and sera from women with recurrent vaginitis. Am J Obstet Gynecol. 1983;147:809–811.
122. Witkin SS, Hirsch J, Ledger WJ. A macrophage defect in women with recurrent *Candida* vaginitis and its reversal by prostaglandin inhibitors. Am J Obstet Gynecol. 1986;155:790–795.

123. Hilton E, Chandrasekaran V, Rindos P, Isenberg HD. Association of recurrent candidal vaginitis with inheritance of Lewis blood group antigens. J Infect Dis. 1995;172:1616–1619.
124. Davidson F, Mould RF. Recurrent genital candidosis in women and the effect of intermittent prophylactic treatment. Br J Vener Dis. 1978;54:176.
125. Roth AC, Milson I, Forssman L, et al. Intermittent prophylactic treatment of recurrent vaginal candidiasis by postmenstrual application of a 500 mg clotrimazole tablet. Genitourin Med. 1990;66:357–360.
126. Sobel JD, Schmitt C, Meriwether C. Clotrimazole treatment of recurrent and chronic *Candida* vulvovaginitis. Obstet Gynecol. 1989;73:330–334.
127. Van Heusden AM, Merkus JM. Chronic recurrent vaginal candidiasis: Easy to treat, difficult to cure. Results of treatment with a new oral antifungant. Eur J Obstet Gynecol Reprod Biol. 1990;35:75–83.
128. Milne JD, Warnock DW. Effect of simultaneous oral and vaginal treatment on the rate of cure and relapse in vaginal candidosis. Br J Vener Dis. 1979;55:362.
129. Velupillai S, Thin RN. Treatment of vulvovaginal yeast infection with nystatin. Practitioner. 1977;219:897.
130. Hilton E, Isenberg HD, Alperstein P, et al. Ingestion of yogurt containing *Lactobacillus acidophilus* as prophylaxis for candidal vaginitis. Ann Intern Med. 1992;116:353–357.
131. Drutz DJ. *Lactobacillus* prophylaxis for *Candida* vaginitis. Ann Intern Med. 1992;116:419–420.
132. Waugh MA. Clinical presentation of candidal balanitis—its differential diagnosis and treatment. Chemotherapy. 1982;28(Suppl 1):56–60.
133. Oriel JD, Partridge BM, Denny MJ, et al. Genital yeast infections. BMJ. 1972;4:761.
134. Gardner HL, Dukes CD. *Haemophilus vaginalis* vaginitis: A newly defined specific infection previously classified "non-specific" vaginitis. Am J Obstet Gynecol. 1955;69:962.
135. Huth EJ. Style note. Bacterial vaginosis or vaginal bacteriosis. Ann Intern Med. 1989;111:553–554.
136. Mardh PA, Taylor-Robinson D, eds. Bacterial vaginosis. Scand J Urol Nephrol. 1984;18(Suppl 86):1–270.
137. Speigel CA. Bacterial vaginosis. Clin Microbiol Rev. 1991;4:485–502.
138. Brunham RC, Pavonen J, Stevens CE, et al. Mucopurulent cervicitis—the ignored counterpart in women of urethritis in men. N Engl J Med. 1984;311:1–6.
139. Eschenbach DA. Bacterial vaginosis and anaerobes in obstetric-gynecologic infections. Clin Infect Dis. 1993;16(Suppl 4):S282–S287.
140. Peipert JF, Mantagno AB, Cooper AS, Sung CJ. Bacterial vaginosis as a risk factor for upper genital tract infection. Am J Obstet Gynecol. 1997;177:1184–1187.
141. Sweet RL. Role of bacterial vaginosis in pelvic inflammatory disease. Clin Infect Dis. 1995;20(Suppl 2):S271–S275
142. Korn AP, Bolan G, Padian N, Ohm-Smith M, et al. Plasma cell endometritis in women with symptomatic bacterial vaginosis. Obstet Gynecol. 1995;85:387–390.
143. Pheifer TA, Forsyth PS, Durfee MA, et al. Nonspecific vaginitis: Role of *Haemophilus vaginalis* and treatment with metronidazole. N Engl J Med. 1978;298:1429.
144. Chen KCS, Forsyth PS, Buchman TM, et al. Amine content of vaginal fluid from untreated and treated patients with nonspecific vaginitis. J Clin Invest. 1979;63:828.
145. Hanna NF, Taylor-Robinson D, Kalodiki-Karammanoki M, et al. The relation between vaginal pH and the microbiological status in vaginitis. Br J Obstet Gynaecol. 1985;92:1267–1271.
146. Vontver LA, Eschenbach DA. The role of *Gardnerella vaginalis* in nonspecific vaginitis. Clin Obstet Gynecol. 1981;24:439.
147. Amsel R, Totten PA, Spiegel CA, et al. Nonspecific vaginitis: Diagnostic criteria and microbial and epidemiological associations. Am J Med. 1983;74:14.
148. Bhattycharyya MN, Jones BM. *Haemophilus vaginalis* infection: Diagnosis and treatment. J Reprod Med. 1980;24:71.
149. Spiegel CA, Amsel R, Holmes KK. Diagnosis of bacterial vaginosis by direct Gram stain of vaginal fluid. J Clin Microbiol. 1983;18:170–177.
150. Thomasen JL, Andersen RJ, Gelbart SM, et al. Simplified Gram stain interpretative methods for diagnosis of bacterial vaginosis. Am J Obstet Gynecol. 1992;167:16–19.
151. Nugent RP, Krohn MA, Hillier SI. Reliability of diagnosing bacterial vaginosis is improved by a standardized method of Gram stain interpretation. J Clin Microbiol. 1991;29:297–301.
152. Schwebke JR, Hillier SL, Sobel JD, et al. Validity of the vaginal Gram stain for the diagnosis of bacterial vaginosis. Obstet Gynecol. 1996;88:573–576.
153. Platz-Christensen JJ, Larsson PG, Sundstrom E, et al. Detection of bacterial vaginosis in Papanicolaou smears. Am J Obstet Gynecol. 1995;158:953–959.
154. Giacomini G, Calcinai A, Moretti D, Cristofani R. Accuracy of cervical/vaginal cytology in the diagnosis of bacterial vaginosis. Sex Transm Dis. 1998;25:24–27.
155. Davis JD, Connor EE, Clerk P, et al. Correlation between cervical cytological results and Gram stain as diagnostic tests for bacterial vaginosis. Am J Obstet Gynecol. 1997;177:532–535.
156. Hillier SL, Krohn MA, Rabe LK, et al. The normal vaginal flora, H_2O_2-producing lactobacilli to bacterial vaginosis in pregnant women. Clin Infect Dis. 1993;16(Suppl 4)S273–S281.
157. Ratnam S, Fitzgerald BL. Semiquantitative culture of *Gardnerella vaginalis* in laboratory determination of nonspecific vaginitis. J Clin Microbiol. 1983;18:344.
158. Totten PA, Amsel R, Hale J, et al. Selective differential human blood bilayer media for isolation of *Gardnerella* (*Haemophilus*) *vaginalis*. J Clin Microbiol. 1982;15:141–147.
159. Schoonmaker JN, Lunt BD, Lawellin DW, et al. A new proline aminopeptidase assay for the diagnosis of bacterial vaginosis. Am J Obstet Gynecol. 1991;165:737–742.
160. Biswas MK. Bacterial vaginosis. Clin Obstet Gynecol. 1993;36:166–176.
161. Chen KCS, Amsel R, Eschenbach DA, et al. Biochemical diagnosis of vaginitis: Determination of diamines in vaginal fluid. J Infect Dis. 1982;145:337.
162. Thomason JL, Gelbart SM, Andersen RJ, et al. Statistical evaluation of diagnostic criteria for bacterial vaginosis. Am J Obstet Gynecol. 1990;102:155–160.
163. Haukkamaa M, Stranden P, Jouosimses-Somer H, et al. Bacterial flora of the cervix in women using different methods of contraception. Am J Obstet Gynecol. 1986;154:520–524.
164. Larsson PG, Platz-Christensen JJ, Sundstrom E. Is bacterial vaginosis a sexually transmitted disease? Int J STD AIDS. 1991;2:362–364.
165. Barbone F, Austin H, Louv WC, et al. A follow-up study of methods of contraception, sexual activity, and rates of trichomoniasis, candidiasis, and bacterial vaginosis. Am J Obstet Gynecol. 1990;163:510–514.
166. Avonts D, Sercu M, Heyetick P, et al. Incidence of uncomplicated genital infections in women using oral contraception or an intrauterine device: A prospective study. Sex Transm Dis. 1990;17:23–29.
167. Nilsson U, Hellberg D, Shoubnikova M, et al. Sexual risk factors associated with bacterial vaginosis and *Chlamydia trachomatis* infection. Sex Transm Dis. 1997;24:241–246.
168. Keane FE, Thomas BJ, Whitaker L, et al. An association between non-gonococcal urethritis and bacterial vaginosis and the implications for patients and their sexual partners. Genitourin Med. 1997;73:373–377.
169. Joesoef MR, Wiknjosastro G, Norojono W, et al. Coinfection with chlamydia and gonorrhoeae among pregnant women with bacterial vaginosis. Int J STD AIDS. 1996;7:61–64.
170. Sikstrom B, Hellberg D, Nilsson S, et al. Gynecological symptoms and vaginal wet smear findings in women with cervical human papillomavirus infection. Gynecol Obstet Invest. 1997;43:49–52.
171. Skinner CJ, Stokes J, Kirlew Y, et al. A case controlled study of the sexual health needs of lesbians. Genitourin Med. 1996;72:277–280.
172. Berger BJ, Kolton S, Zenilman JM, et al. Bacterial vaginosis in lesbians: A sexually transmitted disease. Clin Infect Dis. 1995;21:1402–1405.
173. Bump RC, Buesching WJ III. Bacterial vaginosis in virginal and sexually active adolescent females: Evidence against exclusive sexual transmission. Am J Obstet Gynecol. 1988;158:935–939.
174. Swedberg J, Steiner JF, Deiss F, et al. Comparison of single-dose vs one-week course of metronidazole for symptomatic bacterial vaginosis. JAMA. 1985;254: 1046–1049.
175. Mengel MB, Berg AD, Weaver CH, et al. The effectiveness of single-dose metronidazole therapy for patients and their partners with bacterial vaginoses. J Fam Pract. 1989;28:163–171.
176. Vutyavanich T, Pongsuthirak P, Vannareumol P, et al. A randomized double-blind trial of tinidazole treatment of the sexual partners of females with bacterial vaginosis. Obstet Gynecol. 1993;82:550–554.
177. Holst E, Wathne B, Hovelins B, Mårdh PA. Bacterial vaginosis: Microbiology and clinical findings. Eur J Clin Microbiol. 1987;6:536–541.
178. Jones BM, Geary I, Alawattegama AB, et al. *In vitro* and *in vivo* activity of metronidazole against *Gardnerella vaginalis, Bacteroides* spp and *Mobiluncus* spp in bacterial vaginosis. J Antimicrob Chemother. 1985;16:189–197.
179. Lugo-Miro VI, Green M, Mazur L. Comparison of different metronidazole regimens for bacterial vaginosis. JAMA. 1992;268:92–95.
180. Colli E, Landoni M, Parazzini F. Treatment of male partners and recurrence of bacterial vaginosis: A randomized trial. Genitourin Med. 1997;73:267–270.
181. Moi H, Erkkola R, Jerve F, et al. Should male consorts of women with bacterial vaginosis be treated? Genitourin Med. 1989;65:263–268.
182. Vejtorp M, Bollerup AC, Vejtorp L, et al. Bacterial vaginosis: A double-blind randomized trial of the effect of treatment of the sexual partner. Br J Obstet Gynecol. 1988;95:920–926.
183. Joesoef MR, Schmidt GP. Bacterial vaginosis: Review of treatment options and potential clinical indications for therapy. Clin Infect Dis. 1995;20(Suppl 1):S72–S79.
184. Holst E. Reservoir of four organisms associated with bacterial vaginosis suggests lack of sexual transmission. J Clin Microbiol. 1990;28:2035–2039.
185. Sewankambo N, Gray RH, Wawer MJ, et al. HIV-1 infection associated with abnormal vaginal flora morphology and bacterial vaginosis. Lancet. 1997;350:546–550.
186. Greenwood JR, Picket MJ. Transfer of *Haemophilus vaginalis* to a new genus, *Gardnerella: G. vaginalis* (Gardner and Dukes) com nov. Int J Syst Bacteriol. 1980;30:170.
187. Malouf M, Fortier M, Morin G, et al. Treatment of *Hemophilus vaginalis* vaginitis. Obstet Gynecol. 1980;57:711.
188. Monhanty KC, Deighton R. Comparison of 2 g single dose of metronidazole, nimorazole and tinidazole in the treatment of vaginitis associated with *Gardnerella vaginalis*. J Antimicrob Chemother. 1987;19:393–399.
189. Monhanty KC, Deighton R. Comparison of two different metronidazole regimens in the treatment of *Gardnerella vaginalis* infection with or without trichomoniasis. J Antimicrob Chemother. 1985;16:799–803.
190. Van der Meijden WI, Piot P, Loriaux SM, et al. Amoxycillin, amoxycillin-clavulanic acid and metronidazole in the treatment of clue cell positive discharge. A comparative clinical and laboratory study. J Antimicrob Chemother. 1987;20:735–742.
191. Amsel R, Critchlow CW, Spiegel CA, et al. Comparison of metronidazole, ampicillin, and amoxicillin for treatment of bacterial vaginosis (nonspecific vaginitis): Possible explanation for the greater efficacy of metronidazole. In: Finegold S, ed. United States Metronidazole Conference. Proceedings from a Symposium, Tarpon Springs, Florida, February 18–20, 1982. New York: Biomedical Information; 1982;225.
192. Shander S, Munro R. Sensitivity of *Gardnerella vaginalis* to metabolites of metronidazole and tinidazole. Lancet. 1982;1:167.
193. Taylor E, Blackwell AL, Barlow D, et al. *Gardnerella vaginalis,* anaerobes, and vaginal discharge. Lancet. 1982;1:1376.
194. Hillier SL, Critchlow CW, Stevens CE, et al. Microbiological, epidemiological and clinical correlates of vaginal colonization by *Mobiluncus* species. Genitourin Med. 1991;67:26–31.

195. Darieux R, Dublanchet A. Les "vibrions" anaerobics des leucorrhees. I. Technique d'isolement et sensibilité aux antibiotiques. Med Mal Infect. 1980;10:109.
196. Sprott MS, Pattman RS, Ingham HR, et al. Anaerobic curved rods in vaginitis. Lancet. 1982;1:54.
197. Hjelm E, Hallen A, Forsum U, et al. Motile anaerobic curved rods in nonspecific vaginitis. Lancet. 1982;1:9.
198. Spiegel CA, Eschenbach DA, Amsel R, et al. Curved anaerobic bacteria in bacterial vaginosis and their response to antimicrobial therapy. J Infect Dis. 1983;148:817.
199. Thomason JL, Schreckenberger PC, Spellacy WN, et al. Clinical and microbiological characterization of patients with nonspecific vaginosis associated with motile, curved anaerobic rods. J Infect Dis. 1984;149:801–809.
200. Spiegel CA. New developments in the etiology and pathogenesis of bacterial vaginosis. Adv Exp Med Biol. 1987;224:127–134.
201. Thomason JL and the Working Group. Diagnosis of infection with anaerobic cervical rods. Scand J Urol Nephrol. 1984;18(Suppl 86):261–262.
202. Spiegel CA, Roberts M. *Mobiluncus* gen nov, *Mobiluncus curtisii* subspecies *curtisii* sp nov, *Mobiluncus curtisii* subspecies *holmesii* subsp nov, and *Mobiluncus mulieris* sp nov, curved rods from the human vagina. Int J Syst Bacteriol. 1984;34:177–184.
203. Schwebke JR, Morgan SC, Hillier SL. Humoral antibody to *Mobiluncus curtisii,* a potential marker for bacterial vaginosis. Clin Diagn Lab Immunol. 1996;3:567–569.
204. Eschenbach DA, Gravett MG, Chen KCS, et al. Bacterial vaginosis during pregnancy: An association with prematurity and postpartum complications. Scand J Urol Nephrol. 1984;18(Suppl 86):213–222.
205. Paavonen J, Miettinen A, Stevens CE, et al. *Mycoplasma hominis* in nonspecific vaginitis. Sex Transm Dis. 1983;10:271–275.
206. Mårdh P-A, Alshibly S, Kallings I, Hellberg D. Vaginal flora changes associated with *Mycoplasma hominis.* Am J Obstet Gynecol. 1997;176:173–178.
207. Cauci S, Dirussi S, Monte R, et al. Immunoglobulin A response against *Gardnerella vaginalis* hemolysin and sialidase activity in bacterial vaginosis. Am J Obstet Gynecol. 1998;178:511–515.
208. Cauci S, Scrimin F, Driussi S, et al. Specific immune response against *Gardnerella vaginalis* hemolysin in patients with bacterial vaginosis. Am J Obstet Gynecol. 1996;175:1601–1605.
209. Eschenbach DA, Davick PR, Williams BL, et al. Prevalence of hydrogen peroxide–producing *Lactobacillus* species in normal women and women with bacterial vaginosis. J Clin Microbiol. 1989;27:251–256.
210. Hillier SL, Krohn MA, Klebanoff SJ, et al. The relationship of hydrogen-peroxide–producing lactobacilli to bacterial vaginosis and genital microflora in pregnant women. Obstet Gynecol. 1992;79:369–373.
211. Rosenstein IJ, Fontaine EA, Morgan DJ, et al. Relationship between hydrogen–peroxide producing of lactobacilli and vaginosis-associated bacterial species in pregnant women. Eur J Clin Microbiol Infect Dis. 1997;16:517–522.
212. Rosenstein IJ, Morgan DJ, Sheehan M, et al. Bacterial vaginosis in pregnancy. Distribution of bacterial species in different gram-stain categories of the vaginal flora. J Med Microbiol. 1996;45:120–126.
212a. Pavlova SI, Kilic AO, Clarridge JE, Tao L. Phage infection and transmission in vaginal lactobacilli: Initial evidence. Abstract D/B-20. Session 32, 99th annual meeting of the American Society for Microbiology, Chicago, May 30–June 3, 1999, p 213.
213. Gratacos E, Fihuras F, Barranco M, et al. Spontaneous recovery from bacterial vaginosis in pregnancy is not associated with an improved perinatal outcome. Acta Obstet Gynecol Scand. 1998;77:37–40.
214. Hay PE, Ugwumadu A, Chowns J. Sex, thrush and bacterial vaginosis. Int J STD AIDS. 1997;8:603–608.
215. Alawattengama AB, Jones BM, Kinghorn GR, et al. Single-dose versus seven-day metronidazole in *Gardnerella vaginalis* associated with nonspecific vaginitis. Lancet. 1984;1355–1357.
216. Eschenbach DA, Critchlow CW, Watkins H, et al. A dose-duration study of metronidazole for the treatment of nonspecific vaginosis. Scand J Infect Dis. 1983;40(Suppl):73–80.
217. Baker DA, McGregor JA, Monif GRG. Once daily modified-release oral metronidazole is more effective than clindamycin vaginal cream in the treatment of bacterial vaginosis. Abstract. 2nd Annual Meeting, Infectious Disease Society for Obstetrics and Gynecology, April 25–27, 1997, Las Vegas, Nevada.
218. Greaves WL, Chungfung J, Morris B, et al. Clindamycin versus metronidazole in the treatment of bacterial vaginosis. Obstet Gynecol. 1988;72:799–802.
219. Gardner H. *Hemophilus vaginalis* vaginitis after twenty-five years. Am J Obstet Gynecol. 1980;137:385–392.
220. Wathne B, Hovelius B, Holst E. Cefadroxil as an alternative to metronidazole in the treatment of bacterial vaginosis. Scand J Infect Dis. 1989;21:585–586.
221. Nayagam AT, Smith MD, Ridgeway GL, et al. Comparison of ofloxacin and metronidazole for the treatment of bacterial vaginosis. Int J STD AIDS. 1992;3:204–207.
222. Hillier S, Krohn MA, Watts P, et al. Microbiological efficacy of intravaginal clindamycin cream for the treatment of bacterial vaginosis. Obstet Gynecol. 1990;76:407–413.
223. Livengood CH, Thomason JL, Hill GB. Bacterial vaginosis: Treatment with topical intravaginal clindamycin phosphate. Obstet Gynecol. 1990;76:118–123.
224. Schmitt C, Sobel JD, Meriwether C. Bacterial vaginosis: Treatment with clindamycin cream versus oral metronidazole. Obstet Gynecol. 1992;79:1020–1023.
225. Livengood CH III, Thomason JL, Hill GB. Bacterial vaginosis: Diagnostic and pathologic findings during topical clindamycin therapy. Am J Obstet Gynecol. 1990;163:515–520.
226. Andres FJ, Parker R, Hosein I, et al. Clindamycin cream versus oral metronidazole in the treatment of bacterial vaginosis: A prospective, double-blind clinical trial. South Med J. 1992;85:1077–1080.
227. Mikamo H, Kawazoe K, Izumi K, et al. Comparative study on vaginal or oral treatment of bacterial vaginosis. Chemotherapy. 1997;43:60–68.
228. Ferris DG, Litaker MS, Woodward L, et al. Treatment of bacterial vaginosis: A comparison of oral metronidazole, metronidazole vaginal gel, and clindamycin vaginal cream. J Fam Pract. 1995;41:443–449.
229. Mikamo H, Kawazoe K, Izumi K, et al. Bacteriological epidemiology and treatment of bacterial vaginosis. Chemotherapy. 1996;42:78–84.
230. Galask RP, Bowdler N. Open label evaluation of 0.75% metronidazole gel in the treatment of bacterial vaginosis. Presented at annual meeting of the Infectious Disease Society for Obstetrics and Gynecology, August 6–8, 1992, San Diego.
231. McGregor JA, Livengood C III, French JI, et al. Intravaginal metronidazole gel (0.75%) for bacterial vaginosis: Results of a double-blinded, randomized, placebo-controlled trial. Presented at annual meeting of the Infectious Disease Society for Obstetrics and Gynecology, August 6–8, 1992, San Diego.
232. Hillier SL, Lipinski C, Briselden AM, et al. Efficacy of intravaginal 0.75% metronidazole gel for the treatment of bacterial vaginosis. Obstet Gynecol. 1993;81:963–967.
233. Curatek Pharmaceuticals. MetroGel-Vaginal Clinical Monograph. Elk Grove Village, Ill. Curatek; 1992;13–14.
234. Borin MT, Powley GW, Tackwell KR, Batts DH. Absorption of clindamycin after intravaginal application of clindamycin phosphate 2% cream. J Antimicrob Chemother. 1995;35:833–841.
235. Meadowcroft AM, Diaz PR, Latham GS. *Clostridium difficile* toxin–induced colitis after use of clindamycin phosphate vaginal cream. Ann Pharmacother. 1998;32:309–311.
236. Trexler MF, Fraser TG, Jones MP. Fulminant pseudomembranous colitis caused by clindamycin phosphate vaginal cream. Am J Gastroenterol. 1997;92:2112–2113.
237. Piot P, Van Dyck E, Godts P, et al. A placebo-controlled, double-blind comparison of tinidazole and triple sulfonamide cream for the treatment of nonspecific vaginitis. Am J Obstet Gynecol. 1983;147:85–89.
238. Fredricsson B, Englund K, Weintraub L, et al. Bacterial vaginosis is not a simple ecological disorder. Gynecol Obstet Invest. 1989;28:156–160.
239. Neri A, Sabah G, Samra Z. Bacterial vaginosis in pregnancy treated with yoghurt. Acta Obstet Gynecol Scand. 1993;72:17–19.
240. Holst E, Brandberg A. Treatment of bacterial vaginosis in pregnancy with a lactate gel. Scand J Infect Dis. 1990;22:625–626.
241. Andersch B, Lindell D, Dahlen I, et al. Bacterial vaginosis and the effect of intermittent treatment with an acid lactate gel. Gynecol Obstet Invest. 1990;30:114–119.
242. Fredricsson B, Englund K, Weintraub L, et al. Ecological treatment of bacterial vaginosis. Lancet. 1987;1:276.
243. Hallen A, Jarstrand C, Pahlson C. Treatment of bacterial vaginosis with lactobacilli. Sex Transm Dis. 1992;19:146–148.
244. Parent D, Bossens M, Bayot D, et al. Therapy of bacterial vaginosis using exogenously applied *Lactobacilli acidophili* and a low dose of estriol: A placebo-controlled multicentric clinical trial. Arzneimittelforschung. 1996;46:68–73.
245. Hughes VL, Hillier SL. Microbiologic characteristics of *Lactobacillus* products used for colonization of the vagina. Obstet Gynecol. 1990;75:244–248.
246. Ahmed-Jushuf IH, Shahmanesh M, Arya OP. The treatment of bacterial vaginosis with a 3 day course of 2% clindamycin cream: Results of a multicenter, double blind, placebo controlled trial. Genitourin Med. 1995;71:254–256.
247. Thomason JL, Gelbart SM, Scaglione NJ. Bacterial vaginosis: Current review with indications for asymptomatic therapy. Am J Obstet Gynecol. 1991;165:1210–1217.
248. Centers for Disease Control and Prevention. 1998 Guidelines for the treatment of sexually transmitted diseases. MMWR Morb Mortal Wkly Rep. 1998;47 (No. RR-1):1–116.
249. McGregor JA, French JL, Jones W, et al. Bacterial vaginosis is associated with prematurity and vaginal fluid mucinase and sialidase: Results of a controlled trial of topical clindamycin cream. Am J Obstet Gynecol. 1994;171:1048–1060.
250. Joesoef MR, Hillier SL, Wiknjosastro G, et al. Intravaginal clindamycin treatment for bacterial vaginosis: Effects on preterm delivery and low birth weight. Am J Obstet Gynecol. 1995;173:1527–1531.
251. Hillier SL, Kiviat NB, Hawes SE, et al. The role of bacterial vaginosis–associated microorganisms in endometritis. Am J Obstet Gynecol. 1996;175:435–441.
252. Larsson P-G, Platz Christensen J-J, Thejls H, et al. Incidence of pelvic inflammatory disease after first-trimester legal abortion in women with bacterial vaginosis after treatment with metronidazole: A double-blind, randomized study. Am J Obstet Gynecol. 1992;166:100–103.
253. Larsson P-G, Bergman B, Forsum U, et al. *Mobiluncus* and clue cells as predictors of PID after first trimester abortion. Acta Obstet Gynecol Scand. 1989;68:217–220.
254. Soper DE, Bump RC, Hurt WG. Bacterial vaginosis and trichomoniasis vaginitis are risk factors for cuff cellulitis after abdominal hysterectomy. Am J Obstet Gynecol. 1990;163:1016–1023.
255. Larsson P-G, Platz-Christensen J-J, Forsum U, et al. Clue cells in predicting infections after abdominal hysterectomy. Obstet Gynecol. 1991;77:450.
256. Rosene K, Eschenbach DA, Tompkins LS, et al. Polymicrobial early postpartum endometritis with facultative and anaerobic bacteria, genital mycoplasma, and *Chlamydia trachomatis:* Treatment with piperacillin or cefoxitin. J Infect Dis. 1986;153:1028–1037.
257. Lamey JR, Eschenbach DA, Mitchell SH, et al. Isolation of mycoplasmas and bacteria from the blood of postpartum women. Am J Obstet Gynecol. 1982;143:104–112.
258. Gravett MG, Hummel DH, Eschenbach DA, et al. Preterm labor associated with subclinical amniotic fluid infection and with bacterial vaginosis. Obstet Gynecol. 1986;67:229–237.
259. Reimer LG, Reller LB. *Gardnerella vaginalis* bacteremia: A review of 30 cases. Obstet Gynecol. 1984;65:180–182.

260. Watts DH, Krohn MA, Hillier SL, et al. Bacterial vaginosis as a risk factor for postcesarian endometritis. Obstet Gynecol. 1990;75:52–58.
261. Newton AA, Piper J, Peairs W. Bacterial vaginosis and intraamniotic infection. Am J Obstet Gynecol. 1997;176:672–677.
262. McGregor JA, French JI, Richter R, et al. Antenatal microbiologic and maternal risk factors associated with prematurity. Am J Obstet Gynecol. 1990;163:1465–1473.
263. Krohn MA, Hillier SL, Lee ML, et al. Vaginal *Bacteroides* species are associated with an increased risk of preterm delivery among women in preterm labor. J Infect Dis. 1991;164:88–93.
264. Kurki T, Sivonen A, Renkonen OV, et al. Bacterial vaginosis in early pregnancy and pregnancy outcome. Obstet Gynecol. 1992;80:173–177.
265. Goldenberg RL, Iams JD, Mercer BM, et al. The preterm prediction study. The value of new vs standard risk factors in predicting early and all spontaneous preterm births. NICHD MFMU Network. Am J Public Health. 1998;88:233–238.
266. McDonald HM, O'Loughlin JA, Vigneswaran R, et al. Impact of metronidazole therapy on preterm birth in women with bacterial vaginosis flora (*Gardnerella vaginalis*): A randomized, placebo controlled trial. Br J Obstet Gynecol. 1997;104:1391–1397.
267. Goldenberg RL, Andrews WW, Yuan AC, et al. Sexually transmitted diseases and adverse outcomes of pregnancy. Clin Perinatol. 1997;24:23–41.
268. Chaim W, Mazor M, Leiberman FF. The relationship between bacterial vaginosis and preterm birth. Arch Gynecol Obstet. 1997;259:51–58.
269. Hillier SL, Nugent RP, Eschenbach DA, et al. Association between bacterial vaginosis and preterm delivery of a low-birthweight infant. N Engl J Med. 1995;333:1737–1742.
270. Morales WJ, Schorr S, Albritton J. Effect of metronidazole in patients with preterm birth in preceding pregnancy and bacterial vaginosis: A placebo-controlled, double-blind study. Am J Obstet Gynecol. 1994;171:345–347.
271. Meis PJ, Goldenberg RL, Mercer B, et al. The preterm prediction study: Significance of vaginal infections. National Institute of Child Health and Human Development Maternal-Fetal Medicine Units network. Am J Obstet Gynecol. 1995;173:1231–1235.
272. Hauth JC, Goldenberg RL, Andrews WW, et al. Reduced incidence of preterm delivery with metronidazole and erythromycin in women with bacterial vaginosis. N Engl J Med. 1995;333:1732–1736.
273. Llahi-Camp JM, Rai R, Ison C, et al. Association of bacterial vaginosis with a history of second trimester abortion. Hum Reprod. 1996;11:1575–1578.
274. Shands KN, Schmid GP, Dan BB, et al. Toxic shock syndrome in menstruating women. Association with tampon use and *Staphylococcus aureus* and clinical features in 52 cases. N Engl J Med. 1980;303:1436.
275. Tofte RW, Williams DN. Clinical and laboratory manifestations of toxic shock syndrome. Ann Intern Med. 1982;96:843.
276. Lanes SF, Poole C, Dreyer NA. Toxic shock syndrome, contraceptive methods, and vaginitis. Am J Obstet Gynecol. 1986;154:989–991.
277. Zaaijman JD, deBeer J. An unusual vaginal foreign body. S Afr Med J. 1982;61:33.
278. Friedrich EG, Siegesmund KA. Tampon associated vaginal ulcerations. Obstet Gynecol. 1980;55:149.
279. Friedrich EG. Tampon effects on vaginal health. Clin Obstet Gynecol. 1981;24:295.
280. Jimerson SD, Becker JD. Vaginal ulcers associated with tampon usage. Obstet Gynecol. 1980;56:97.
281. Weissberg SM, Dodson MG. Recurrent vaginal and cervical ulcers associated with tampon use. JAMA. 1983;250:1430.
282. Ginsburg CM. Group A streptococcal vaginitis in children. Pediatr Infect Dis. 1982;1:36.
283. Cox RA. *Haemophilus influenzae:* An underrated cause of vulvovaginitis in young girls. J Clin Pathol. 1997;50:765–768.
284. Jones R. Childhood vulvovaginitis and vaginal discharge in general practice. Fam Pract. 1996;13:369–372.
285. O'Brien TJ. Paediatric vulvovaginitis. Australas J Dermatol. 1995;36:216–218.
286. Koumantakis EE, Hassan EA, Deligeoroglou EK, Creatsas GK. Vulvovaginitis during childhood and adolescence. J Pediatr Adolesc Gynecol. 1997;10:39–43.
287. Maniatis AN, Palermos J, Kantzanou M, et al. *Streptococcus agalactiae:* A vaginal pathogen? J Med Microbiol. 1996;44:199–202.
288. Symmers W. Pathology of oxyuriasis. Arch Pathol. 1950;50:475.
289. Dump RC. *Chlamydia trachomatis* as a cause of prepubertal vaginitis. Obstet Gynecol. 1985;65:384–388.
290. Cibley LJ, Cibley LJ. Cytolytic vaginosis. Am J Obstet Gynecol. 1991;165:1245–1249.
291. Sharp HC. Vulvovaginal conditions mimicking vaginitis. Clin Obstet Gynecol. 1993;36:129–136.
292. Fisher AA. Allergic reactions to feminine hygiene sprays. Arch Dermatol. 1973;108:801.
293. Chang T. Familial allergic seminal vulvovaginitis. Am J Obstet Gynecol. 1976;126:442.
294. Gochfeld M, Burger J. Sexual transmission of nickel and poison oak contact dermatitis. Lancet. 1983;1:589.
295. Moraes PS. Allergic vulvovaginitis induced by house dust mites: A case report. J Allergy Clin Immunol. 1998;101:557–558.
296. Schuman P, Christensen C, Sobel JD. Aphthous vaginal ulceration in two women with acquired immunodeficiency syndrome. Am J Obstet Gynecol. 1996;174:1660–1663.
297. Gardner HL. Desquamative inflammatory vaginitis: A newly defined entity. Am J Obstet Gynecol. 1968;102:1102–1105.
298. Edwards L, Friedrich EG. Desquamative vaginitis: Lichen planus in disguise. Obstet Gynecol. 1988;71:832–836.
299. Oates JK, Rowen D. Desquamative inflammatory vaginitis. A review. Genitourin Med. 1990;66:274–279.
300. Sobel JD. Desquamative inflammatory vaginitis: A new subgroup of purulent vaginitis responsive to topical 2% clindamycin therapy. Am J Obstet Gynecol. 1994;171:1215–1220.
301. Huggins GR, Preti G. Vaginal odors and secretions. Clin Obstet Gynecol. 1981;24:355.
302. Peckham BM, Maki DG, Patterson JJ, et al. Focal vulvitis: A characteristic syndrome and cause of dyspareunia. Features, natural history, and management. Am J Obstet Gynecol. 1986;154:855–864.
303. Goetsch MF. Vulvar vestibulitis: Prevalence and historic features in a general gynecologic practice population. Am J Obstet Gynecol. 1991;164:1609–1614.
304. Marinoff SC, Turner ML. Vulvar vestibulitis syndrome. Dermatol Clin. 1992;10:435–444.
305. Pyka RE, Wilkinson EJ, Friedrich EG, et al. The histopathology of vulvar vestibulitis syndrome. Int J Gynecol Pathol. 1988;7:249.
306. Prayson RA, Stoler MH, Hart WR. Vulvar vestibulitis. A histopathological study of 36 cases, including human papillomavirus *in situ* hybridization analysis. Am J Surg Pathol. 1995;19:154–160.
307. Chaim W, Meriwether C, Gonik D, et al. Vulvar vestibulitis subjects undergoing surgical intervention: A descriptive analysis and histopathological correlates. Eur J Obstet Gynecol Reprod Biol. 1996;68:165–168.
308. McCormack WM. Two urogenital sinus syndromes: Interstitial cystitis and focal vulvitis. J Reprod Med. 1990;35:873–876.
309. Mann MS, Kaufman RH, Brown DJ, et al. Vulvar vestibulitis: Significant clinical variables and treatment outcome. Obstet Gynecol. 1992;79:122–125.
310. Micklewitz H, Kennison RD, Turksoy RN, et al. Vulvar vestibulitis: Subgroup with Bartholin gland duct inflammation. Obstet Gynecol. 1989;73:410–413.
311. Bergeron S, Bouchard C, Fortier M, et al. The surgical treatment of vulvar vestibulitis syndrome: A follow-up study. J Sex Marital Ther. 1997;23:317–325
312. Bornstein J, Goldik Z, Alter Z, et al. Persistent vulvar vestibulitis: The continuing challenge. Obstet Gynecol Surv. 1998;53:39–44.
313. Bornstein J, Zarfati D, Goldik Z, Abramovici H. Perineoplasty compared with vestibuloplasty for severe vulvar vestibulitis. Br J Obstet Gynecol. 1995;102:652–655.
314. Dennerstein GJ, Scurry JP, Garland SM, et al. Human papillomavirus vulvitis: A new disease or an unfortunate mistake? Br J Obstet Gynecol. 1994;101:992–998.
315. Reid R, Greenberg MD, Daoud MA. Colposcopic findings in women with vulvar pain syndromes: A preliminary report. J Reprod Med. 1988;33:523.
316. Potkul RK, Lancaster WD, Kurman RJ, et al. Vulvar condylomas and squamous vestibular micropapilloma: Differences in appearance and response to treatment. J Reprod Med. 1990;35:1019–1022.
317. Umpierre SA, Kaufman RH, Adam E, et al. Human papillomavirus DNA in tissue biopsy specimens of vulvar vestibulitis patients treated with interferon. Obstet Gynecol. 1991;78:693–695.
318. Bornstein J, Shapiro S, Goldshmid N, et al. Severe vulvar vestibulitis. Relation to HPV infection. J Reprod Med. 1997;42:514–518.
319. Bornstein J, Shapiro S, Rahat M, et al. Polymerase chain reaction search for viral etiology of vulvar vestibulitis syndrome. Am J Obstet Gynecol. 1996;175:139–144.
320. Horowitz BJ. Interferon therapy for condylomatous vulvitis. Obstet Gynecol. 1989;73:446–448.
321. Bornstein J, Pascal B, Abramovici H. Intramuscular β-interferon treatment for severe vulvar vestibulitis. J Reprod Med. 1993;38:117–120.
322. Nunns D, Mandal D. Psychological and psychosexual aspects of vulvar vestibulitis. Gentourin Med. 1997;73:541–544.
323. Jantos M, White G. The vestibulitis syndromes. Medical and psychosexual assessment of a cohort of patients. J Reprod Med. 1997;42:145–152.
324. Van Lankveld JJ, Weijenborg PT, ter Kuile MM. Psychologic profiles of and sexual function in women with vulvar vestibulitis and their partners. Obstet Gynecol. 1996;88:65–70.
325. Gardner HL, Fernet P. Etiology of vaginitis emphysematosa: Report of ten cases and review of the literature. Am J Obstet Gynecol. 1946;88:680–694.
326. Kramer K, Jobon H. Vaginitis emphysematosa. Arch Pathol Lab Med. 1987;111:746–711.
327. Josey WE, Campbell WG. Vaginitis emphysematosa: Report of four cases. J Reprod Med. 1990;35:974–977.
328. Riethdorf L, Nehmzow M, Straube W, Lorenze G. Vaginitis emphysematosa during immunosuppressive therapy. Arch Gynecol Obstet. 1995;256:39–41.
329. McCallion JS, Parkin DE. Emphysematous vaginitis masquerading as carcinoma of the cervix. Case report. Br J Obstet Gynaecol. 1988;95:309–311.
330. Dodson MG, Friedrich EG. Psychosomatic vulvovaginitis. Obstet Gynecol. 1978;51(Suppl):23.
331. Danesh IS, Stephen JM, Gorbach J. Neonatal *Trichomonas vaginalis* infection. J Emerg Med. 1995;13:51–54.
332. Paradise JE, Campos JM, Friedman HM, et al. Vulvovaginitis in premenarchal girls. Clinical features and diagnostic evaluation. Pediatrics. 1982;70:193.
333. Nuovo GJ. Human papillomavirus DNA in genital tract lesions histologically negative for condylomata: Analysis by in situ, Southern blot hybridization and polymerase chain reaction. Am J Surg Pathol. 1990;14:643–651.
334. Wolner-Hanssen P, Krieger JN, Stevens CE, et al. Clinical manifestations of vaginal trichomoniasis: Implications for strategies for diagnosis and control of the infection. JAMA. 1989;261:571–576.
335. Stern JE, Givan AL, Gonzalez JL, et al. Leukocytes in the cervix: A quantitative evaluation of cervicitis. Obstet Gynecol. 1998;91:987–992.
336. Majeroni BA, Schank JN, Horwitz M, Valenti J. Use of the wet mount to predict *Chlamydia trachomatis* and *Neisseria gonorrhoeae* cervicitis in primary care. Fam Med. 1996;28:580–583.

337. Rein MF, Shih LM, Miller JR, Guerrant RL. Utility of a lactoferrin assay in the differential diagnosis of female genital tract infections and implications for the pathophysiology of bacterial vaginosis. Sex Transm Dis. 1996; 23:517–521.
338. Silverman EM, Silverman AG. Persistence of spermatozoa in the lower genital tracts of women. JAMA. 1978;240:1875.
339. Tait IA, Rees E, Hobson D, et al. Chlamydial infection of the cervix in contacts of men with nongonococcal urethritis. Br J Vener Dis. 1980;56:37.
340. Mardh PA, Moller BR, Paavonen J. Chlamydial infection of the female genital tract with emphasis on pelvic inflammatory disease. A review of Scandinavian studies. Sex Transm Dis. 1981;8:140.
341. Paavonen J, Vesterinen E. *Chlamydia trachomatis* in cervicitis and urethritis in women. Scand J Infect Dis. 1982;32(Suppl):45.
342. Spence MR, Barbacci M, Kappus E, et al. A correlative study of Papanicolaou smear, fluorescent antibody, and culture for the diagnosis of *Chlamydia trachomatis*. Obstet Gynecol. 1986;68:691–695.
343. Paavonen J, Critchlow CW, DeRouen T, et al. Etiology of cervical inflammation. Am J Obstet Gynecol. 1986;154:556–564.
344. Harrison HR, Costin M, Meder JB, et al. Cervical *Chlamydia trachomatis* infection in university women: Relationship to history, contraceptives, ectopy, and cervicitis. Am J Obstet Gynecol. 1985;153:224–251.
345. Moscicki B, Shafer MA, Millstein SG, et al. The use and limitations of endocervical Gram stain and mucopurulent cervicitis as predictors for *Chlamydia trachomatis* in female adolescents. Am J Obstet Gynecol. 1987;157:65–71.
346. Nugent RP, Hillier SL. Mucopurulent cervicitis as a predictor of chlamydial infection and adverse pregnancy outcome. Sex Transm Dis. 1992;19:198–202.
347. Knud-Hansen CR, Dallabetta GA, Reichart C, et al. Surrogate methods to diagnose gonococcal and chlamydial cervicitis: Comparison of leukocyte esterase dipstick, endocervical Gram stain, and culture. Sex Transm Dis. 1991;18:211–216.
348. Katz BP, Caine VA, Jones RB. Diagnosis of mucopurulent cervicitis among women at risk for *Chlamydia trachomatis* infection. Sex Transm Dis. 1989;16:103–106.
349. Sellors J, Howard M, Pickard L, et al. Chlamydial cervicitis: Testing the practice guidelines for presumptive diagnosis. CMAJ. 1998;158:41–46.
350. Dimian C, Nayagam M, Bradbeer C. The association between sexually transmitted diseases and inflammatory cervical cytology. Genitourin Med. 1992;68:305–306.
351. Bertolino JG, Rangel JE, Blake RL Jr, et al. Inflammation on the cervical Papanicolaou smear: The predictive value for infection in asymptomatic women. Fam Med. 1992;241:447–452.
352. Lowley TB, Lee RB, Kapela R. The significance of moderate and severe inflammation on class I Papanicolaou smear. Obstet Gynecol. 1990;76:997–999.
353. Singh V, Gupta MM, Satyanarayana L, et al. Association between reproductive tract infections and cervical inflammatory epithelial changes. Sex Transm Dis. 1995;22:25–30.
354. Rantala I, Kivinen S. Demonstration of *Chlamydia trachomatis* in Papanicolaou-stained gynecological smears. Eur J Clin Microbiol Infect Dis. 1998;17:46–48.
355. Eckert LO, Koutsky LA, Kiviat NB, et al. The inflammatory Papanicolaou smear: What does it mean? Obstet Gynecol. 1995;86:360–366.
356. Wentworth BB, Bonin P, Holmes KK, et al. Isolation of viruses, bacteria and other organisms from venereal disease clinic patients: Methodology and problems associated with multiple isolations. Health Lab Sci. 1973;10:75.
357. Curran JW, Rendtorff RC, Chandler RW, et al. Female gonorrhea: Its relationship to abnormal uterine bleeding, urinary tract symptoms and cervicitis. Obstet Gynecol. 1975;45:195.
358. Hilton AL, Richmond SJ, Milne JD, et al. Chlamydia A in the female genital tract. Br J Vener Dis. 1974;50:1.
359. Oriel JD, Powis PA, Reeve P, et al. Chlamydial infection of the cervix. Br J Vener Dis. 1974;50:11.
360. Quinn TC, Gupta PK, Burkman RT. Detection of *Chlamydia trachomatis* cervical infections: A comparison of Papanicolaou and immunofluorescent staining with cell cultures. Am J Obstet Gynecol. 1987;157:394–399.
361. Willcox RR. Necrotic cervicitis due to primary infection with the virus of herpes simplex. BMJ. 1968;1:610.
362. Morse AR, Coleman DV, Gardner SD. An evaluation of cytology in the diagnosis of herpes simplex virus infection and cytomegalovirus infection of the cervix uteri. J Obstet Gynecol Br Common. 1974;81:393.
363. Reid R, Greenberg M, Jensen AB, et al. Sexually transmitted papillomavirus infections. I. The anatomic distribution and pathologic grade of neoplastic lesions associated with different viral types. Am J Obstet Gynecol. 1987;156:212–222.
364. Waugh MA. History of clinical developments in sexually transmitted diseases. In: Holmes KK, Mardh P-A, Sparling PF, et al, eds. Sexually Transmitted Diseases. 2nd ed. New York: McGraw-Hill; 1990:3–16.
365. Koutsky LA, Holmes KK, Critchlow CW, et al. A cohort study of the risk of cervical intraepithelial neoplasia grade 2 or 3 in relation to papillomavirus infection. N Engl J Med. 1992;327:1272–1278.
366. Laverty CR, Russell P, Black J, et al. Adenovirus infection of the cervix. Acta Cytol. 1977;21:114.
367. Heimann A, Scanlon R, Gentile J, et al. Measles cervicitis. Report of a case with cytologic and molecular biologic analysis. Acta Cytol. 1992;36:727–730.
368. Deppisch LM. Cytomegalovirus inclusion body endocervicitis. Significance of CMV inclusions in endocervical biopsies. Mt Sinai J Med. 1981;48:418.
369. Wong JV, Becker SN. *Enterobius vermicularis* ova in routine cervicovaginal smears. Light scanning electron microscopic observations. Acta Cytol. 1982;26:484.
370. Arroyo G, Elgueta R. Squamous cell carcinoma associated with amoebic cervicitis. Acta Cytol. 1989;33:301–304.
371. Chakraborty P, Roy A, Battacharya S, et al. Tuberculous cervicitis: A clinicopathological and bacteriological study. J Indian Med Assoc. 1995;93:167–168.
372. Buttigieg G. Cervicitis and urethritis caused by group B streptococcus: Case report. Genitourin Med. 1985;61:343–344.
373. Conde-Glez CJ, Calderon E. Urogenital infection due to meningococcus in men and women. Sex Transm Dis. 1991;18:72–75.
374. Mao K, Guillebaud J. Influence of removal of intrauterine contraceptive devices on colonization of the cervix by *Actinomyces*-like organisms. Contraception. 1984;30:535–544.
375. Gutmann EJ. Syphilitic cervicitis simulating stage II cervical cancer. Report of two cases with cytological findings. Am J Clin Pathol. 1995;104:643–647.
376. Rees E. Gonococcal bartholinitis. Br J Vener Dis. 1967;43:150.
377. Brook I. Aerobic and anaerobic microbiology of Bartholin's abscess. Surg Gynecol Obstet. 1989;169:32–34.
378. Lee Y-H, Rankin JS, Alpert S, et al. Microbiological investigation of Bartholin's gland abscesses and cysts. Am J Obstet Gynecol. 1977;129–150.
379. Blecker OP, Smalbraak DJ, Schutte MF. Bartholin's abscess: The role of *Chlamydia trachomatis*. Genitourin Med. 1990;66:24–25.
380. Davies JA, Rees E, Hobson D, et al. Isolation of *Chlamydia trachomatis* from Bartholin's duct. Br J Vener Dis. 1978;54:409.
381. Swenson RM, Michaelson TC, Dayl MJ, et al. Anaerobic bacterial infections of the female genital tract. Obstet Gynecol. 1973;42:538.
382. Kubitz R, Hoffman K. Bartholin's gland abscess in an infant. A case report. J Reprod Med. 1986;31:67–69.
383. Carson GD, Smith LP. *Escherichia coli* endotoxic shock complicating Bartholin's gland abscess. Can Med Assoc J. 1980;122:1397.
384. Morton BD, McCarthy LR. Bartholinitis: An unusual etiologic agent. Obstet Gynecol. 1980;55:(Suppl):97.
385. Shearin RS, Boehlke J, Karanth S. Toxic shock-like syndrome associated with Bartholin's gland abscess: Case report. Am J Obstet Gynecol. 1989;160:1073–1044.
386. Van Bosterhaut B, Buts R, Veys A, et al. *Haemophilus influenzae* bartholinitis. Eur J Clin Microbiol Infect Dis. 1990;9:442.
387. Azzan BB. Bartholin's cyst and abscess: A review of treatment of 53 cases. Br J Clin Pract. 1978;32:101.
388. Anderson PG, Christensen S, Detlefsen GU, et al. Treatment of Bartholin's abscess. Marsupializtion versus incision, curettage and suture under antibiotic cover. A randomized study with six months' follow up. Acta Obstet Gynecol Scand. 1992;71:59–62.
389. Lopez-Zeno JA, Ross E, O'Grady JP. Septic shock complicating drainage of a Bartholin gland abscess. Obstet Gynecol. 1990;76:915–916.
390. Frolich EP, Schein M. Necrotizing fasciitis arising from Bartholin's abscess. Case report and review of the literature. Isr J Med Sci. 1989;25:644–64 7.

Chapter 96

Infections of the Female Pelvis

PHILIP B. MEAD

Infections of the female pelvis constitute a diverse group of both community- and hospital-acquired infections. They are conveniently considered in three categories: infections related to pregnancy; infections occurring after gynecologic surgery; and sexually transmitted pelvic inflammatory disease.

INTRAPARTUM, POSTPARTUM, AND POSTABORTAL INFECTIONS

Intra-amniotic Infection Syndrome

Intra-amniotic infection syndrome (IAIS), known also as *chorioamnionitis*, is a clinically detectable infection of the uterus and its contents during pregnancy.[1] IAIS occurs in 1 to 2% of patients with full-term pregnancies and in up to 25% of women with preterm labor. Most cases of IAIS are ascending in origin, occurring after prolonged rupture of the membranes or labor in patients with multiple vaginal examinations. A few cases, most notably those caused by *Listeria monocytogenes*, result from transplacental hematogenous spread in mothers with bacteremia.[2] Rare cases have been reported after diagnostic amniocentesis, intrauterine transfusion, or percutaneous umbilical blood sampling. Intrauterine infection also occurs after cervical cerclage in 1 to 2% of patients, and this risk may be as high as 25%

if the cerclage is carried out after prolapse of the membranes into the vagina. Risk factors for IAIS include prolonged duration of labor or rupture of membranes, multiple vaginal examinations, young age, low socioeconomic class, nulliparity, and preexisting bacterial vaginosis.[3]

The organisms most commonly isolated from amniotic fluid in cases of IAIS are anaerobes, genital mycoplasmas, group B streptococci, and *Escherichia coli*. The latter two are found most commonly when maternal or neonatal bacteremia complicates intra-amniotic infection. Two constellations of organisms have been noted. In one, presumed to be from a vaginal source, *Gardnerella vaginalis, Mycoplasma hominis*, and anaerobes are associated. In the other, enterococci, *E. coli*, and other aerobic gram-negative bacilli are associated, suggesting an intestinal source.

Maternal manifestations of IAIS are fever, tachycardia, and uterine tenderness. Foul-smelling or grossly purulent amniotic fluid is an uncommon finding. Fetal heart rate abnormalities, primarily tachycardia and decreased variability, are important markers of intrauterine infection. Approximately 5 to 10% of women with preterm labor and intact membranes have symptomatic chorioamnionitis, and another 10% have subclinical infection. In patients with preterm premature rupture of the membranes, the frequency of subclinical infection at the time of admission may be as high as 25%. In full-term pregnancies, chorioamnionitis typically causes dysfunctional labor. About 75% of infected women require augmentation of labor with oxytocin, and about 40% require cesarean delivery, usually because of arrest of progress in labor.

Although diagnosis is based largely on clinical findings, amniotic fluid Gram staining, leukocyte esterase activity, and glucose concentration have been shown to be useful in supporting the clinical impression.[4] Microbial invasion of the amniotic cavity is frequently accompanied by the presence of high amniotic fluid concentrations of proinflammatory cytokines such as interleukin-1, tumor necrosis factor, interleukin-6, and interleukin-8.[5] In the future, the measurement of these substances may help to identify intra-amniotic infections in women with preterm labor.

Management of IAIS is based on the principles that antibiotic therapy should be started as soon as the diagnosis is made and that delivery is essential to cure. Antibiotic administration seeks to reduce the frequency of neonatal pneumonia and bacteremia and to cure the maternal infection. Because group B streptococci and *E. coli* are the most common isolates from infected newborns, a combination of ampicillin plus gentamicin is a reasonable initial regimen for IAIS. In patients who deliver vaginally, this regimen is usually sufficient to treat the mother as well. If cesarean delivery is required, however, 20 to 30% of operative patients given only ampicillin and gentamicin experience treatment failure. These patients probably require better anaerobic coverage, and accordingly a drug such as clindamycin should be added to the treatment regimen. Other broad-spectrum regimens may be equally effective. Gibbs and colleagues[6] documented improved neonatal and maternal outcome when antibiotic therapy is begun as soon as the diagnosis of IAIS is made, rather than immediately postpartum. This is currently the standard of care.

Although delivery is essential to cure, no critical diagnosis-to-delivery interval beyond which the frequency of neonatal complications escalates dramatically has been identified. Accordingly, labor must be managed actively, but cesarean delivery should be performed only for accepted obstetric indications.

Postpartum Endometritis

Postpartum infection of the uterus, the most common cause of puerperal fever, is designated *endometritis, endomyometritis*, or *endoparametritis* depending on the extent of disease. Cesarean delivery, particularly after labor or rupture of the membranes of any duration, is the dominant predictor of postpartum endometritis (PPE).[7] After vaginal delivery, the reported incidence of PPE ranges from 0.9 to 3.9%, and the incidence after cesarean section ranges from 10% or less in most private services to 50% or more in large teaching services caring for indigent patients. Postulated secondary predictors of postcesarean endometritis include duration of labor or rupture of membranes, presence of bacterial vaginosis, number of vaginal examinations, and use of internal fetal monitoring.[8–10]

Although prolonged membrane rupture, midforceps delivery, anemia, and maternal soft tissue trauma are commonly mentioned as factors predisposing to endometritis after vaginal delivery, these events are not identified in most patients with such infections and are probably relative risk factors. Indigent patients are at substantially higher risk for PPE after either vaginal or abdominal delivery, for reasons that have not been fully delineated.

PPE is a polymicrobial infection caused by a wide variety of bacteria. Group B streptococci, enterococci, other aerobic streptococci, *G. vaginalis, E. coli, Prevotella bivia, Bacteroides* spp., and peptostreptococci are the most common endometrial isolates, with group B streptococci and *G. vaginalis* the most common isolates from blood.[11–13]

The isolation of *Ureaplasma urealyticum* and *M. hominis* from endometrium and blood suggests that these organisms can cause PPE, although good clinical responses have been obtained in patients with mycoplasmas cultured from blood who were treated with antibiotics not active against these organisms.

Chlamydia trachomatis has been associated with a late form of PPE occurring more than 2 days to 6 weeks postpartum among women who deliver vaginally.[14] Group A β-hemolytic streptococcal endometritis is rare; it is epidemiologically unique because its source is exogenous infection (usually in a caregiver), and it is characterized by early onset and rapid progression with poor localization.

The diagnosis of PPE is suggested by the development of fever, usually on the first or second postpartum day. Significant fever is defined as an oral temperature of 38.5°C or higher in the first 24 hours after delivery or 38°C or higher for at least 4 consecutive hours 24 or more hours after delivery. Other consistently associated findings are lower abdominal pain, uterine tenderness, and leukocytosis.

Patients with suspected PPE should undergo a bimanual pelvic examination to determine uterine size, consistency, and tenderness. The presence of an adnexal mass can also be ascertained at this time.

The value of transvaginally obtained uterine cultures and the optimal method of obtaining such cultures are currently matters of controversy. Although cultures obtained transvaginally are often difficult to interpret because of contaminants, they may be useful in those patients in whom initial therapy fails.[15] It is important to obtain blood cultures because 10 to 20% of patients have a documentable bacteremia. Bacteremia does not predict the severity of clinical illness or a prolonged recovery, however. Cultures or rapid antigen detection tests for *Chlamydia* should be obtained from patients with late-onset PPE and from those with PPE who are at high risk for chlamydial infection (e.g., teenage pregnancy). *Mycoplasma* cultures are presently a research tool only.

Based on findings of general systemic toxicity, patterns of pulse and fever, and clinical course, some patients are classified as having severe PPE. Clindamycin plus gentamicin has proved to be an effective regimen for these patients, especially if they developed PPE after cesarean section. PPE of mild to moderate severity is typically treated with one of the extended-spectrum penicillins or second-generation cephalosporins (e.g., cefotetan, cefoxitin, ampicillin/sulbactam, ticarcillin/clavulanic acid). Parenteral therapy should be continued until the patient's temperature has remained lower than 37.5°C for 24 hours, the patient is pain free, and the leukocyte count is normal. The use of oral antibiotics after discharge has been shown to be unnecessary. Women with positive cultures for *Chlamydia* should receive a course of azithromycin or doxycycline therapy even if they have had an initial clinical response to one of the previously mentioned regimens.

Failure of antimicrobial therapy usually results from either enterococcal superinfection or inadequate coverage of a multidrug-resistant anaerobe. Enterococcal superinfection is suggested when patients fail to respond or relapse after treatment with regimens that are not effective against enterococci (e.g., cephalosporins; clindamycin plus gentamicin), particularly when this organism is isolated in pure culture or heavy growth from an endometrial specimen. If enterococcal superinfection is suspected, one of the following regimens should be employed: clindamycin or metronidazole plus ampicillin plus gentamicin; ampicillin/sulbactam; cefoxitin or cefotetan plus ampicillin; ticarcillin/clavulanic acid; piperacillin; or mezlocillin. Antimicrobial failure due to lack of coverage of a multidrug-resistant anaerobe can often be corrected by a regimen containing either metronidazole or clindamycin.

If fever persists despite apparently appropriate antimicrobial therapy, the differential diagnosis includes a wound or pelvic abscess, puerperal ovarian vein thrombosis, and noninfectious fever (e.g., drug fever, breast engorgement).

Prophylactic antimicrobial agents can be expected to decrease the postcesarean endometritis rate in a given institution by 50%[16, 17] and are currently the standard of care for any patient who requires a cesarean section after labor or rupture of the membranes of any duration.[10] PPE develops in about 15% of women undergoing nonelective cesarean section despite antimicrobial prophylaxis,[9] possibly because of unrecognized subclinical infection at the time of cesarean delivery.[18]

PPE caused by group A β-hemolytic streptococci has special epidemiologic significance.[19–20] The Centers for Disease Control and Prevention recommends that health care worker screening should be undertaken when an episode of postpartum group A streptococcus (GAS) infection is identified. All health care workers present at the delivery and those who performed vaginal examinations before delivery should be screened with cultures of the nares, throat, vagina, rectum, and skin. Any health care worker who is culture-positive for GAS should refrain from patient care for the first 24 hours of antimicrobial therapy. If surveillance identifies additional patients or health care workers with positive cultures for GAS, the isolates should be typed by sequencing the variable portion of M-protein gene, serologic, or other molecular methods to identify the strain.[21]

Puerperal Ovarian Vein Thrombophlebitis

Puerperal ovarian vein thrombophlebitis is a syndrome resulting from acute thrombosis of one or both ovarian veins in the postpartum period. It can occur after either cesarean or vaginal delivery and is rare, with a reported incidence of 1 case per 2000 deliveries, or 1 to 2 cases per 100 patients with postpartum infection. Puerperal ovarian vein thrombophlebitis is usually associated with postcesarean endometritis but may occur in the absence of infection. Onset is variable but most often occurs 2 to 4 days after delivery.

Clinical symptoms have an acute onset, and patients appear ill. Most have a moderate temperature elevation and complain of lower abdominal pain, usually on the right side. Many patients have previously been diagnosed with PPE that failed to respond to appropriate antibiotics.

The pulse rate usually is elevated, often disproportionately compared with the temperature. Temperature elevations persist and often are accompanied by shaking chills. On physical examination a tender, sausage-shaped or ropelike abdominal mass can be palpated in one half to two thirds of patients. The mass usually originates centrally near the right uterine cornua and extends laterally and cephalad toward the upper abdomen. An ileus is frequently present. Tachypnea, stridor, and other signs of respiratory distress may be present if pulmonary embolization has occurred.[22]

In the absence of a thrombosed vessel palpable abdominally, the diagnosis is one of exclusion based on the clinical history. Computed tomography, duplex Doppler ultrasonography, and magnetic resonance imaging have all been used to confirm the presence of puerperal ovarian vein thrombophlebitis.[23, 24]

Therapy consists of broad-spectrum antibiotics, effective against the common pelvic pathogens, and continuous intravenous heparin anticoagulation. The optimal duration of anticoagulation is unknown, but, in the absence of pulmonary embolization, most clinicians have used a course of 7 to 10 days, concurrent with antibiotic administration. Even though blood cultures are usually sterile in these women, evidence for an infection-related cause is convincing, because resected thrombi usually contain microorganisms, a hectic fever course is common, and treatment with heparin alone is not successful in all cases.[23]

Episiotomy Infections

Infection of the episiotomy site is an uncommon occurrence. Overall only 0.1% of episiotomies become infected, although this rate increases to 1 to 2% for episiotomies complicated by third- or fourth-degree extensions.

Shy and Eschenbach[25] have classified episiotomy infections into four categories, depending on the depth of infection (Fig. 96–1). The *simple episiotomy infection* is a local infection that is limited to the skin and superficial fascia along the episiotomy incision. In contrast to deeper infection, the associated skin changes of edema and erythema occur only adjacent to the episiotomy. The simple episiotomy infection should be opened, explored, and débrided under adequate anesthesia to exclude a hematoma or previously unrecognized rectovaginal communication. If the superficial fascial layer is extensively infected, antibiotic administration is appropriate to inhibit streptococci, staphylococci, Enterobacteriaceae, and anaerobes, including *Bacteroides fragilis.* Ramin and colleagues showed that, with proper preoperative care, simple episiotomy infection is not a contraindication to early repair of dehiscence.[26]

Two infections of the two layers of the superficial fascia may occur. The more common is *superficial fascia infection without necrosis*, the clinical presentation of which is neither striking nor distinctive. The skin may be erythematous and edematous, but severe systemic manifestations do not occur. If response to broad-spectrum antibiotic therapy does not occur in 24 to 48 hours, or if the clinical condition worsens during antibiotic therapy, then the episiotomy should be surgically explored.

Infection of the superficial fascia with necrosis, most commonly referred to as *necrotizing fasciitis*, is an infection of the subcutaneous tissues (i.e., the superficial fascia) that spreads in the fascial clefts overlying the deep fascia. The deep fascia usually, but not always, is spared; skin involvement results only secondarily after the nutrient vessels to the skin thrombose. Because the skin is not primarily involved, the episiotomy wound may appear normal, making early recognition difficult and causing fatal delay in treatment. Despite the minimal local findings, patients may appear severely ill, with marked local pain, high fever, and prominent systemic manifestations. Most patients are diabetic. Definitive diagnosis is made at surgery when the operator discovers extensive undermining of surrounding tissues and lack of resistance in the superficial fascial plane to probing with a blunt instrument. Treatment includes broad-spectrum antibiotics (e.g., clindamycin plus ampicillin plus gentamicin) and radical débridement to include removal of all necrotic and pale tissue.

In the extremely rare event of infection beneath the deep fascia, muscle may be involved, resulting in the fourth type of episiotomy infection, *myonecrosis*. Myonecrosis is most commonly caused by *Clostridium perfringens*, although it can occur from a neglected necrotizing fasciitis infection that invades deep fascia. Myonecrosis of the subgluteal muscles surrounding the hip joint or the psoas muscles can also occur from bacteria introduced into this deep space by a paracervical or pudendal needle. These patients experience severe hip pain associated with marked limitation of motion.

Both myonecrosis and clostridial infection should be treated with surgical resection and antibiotic therapy. For clostridial infection, high-dose penicillin is the therapy of choice. Radical wide excision may be necessary. Hyperbaric oxygen therapy is at best an adjunctive

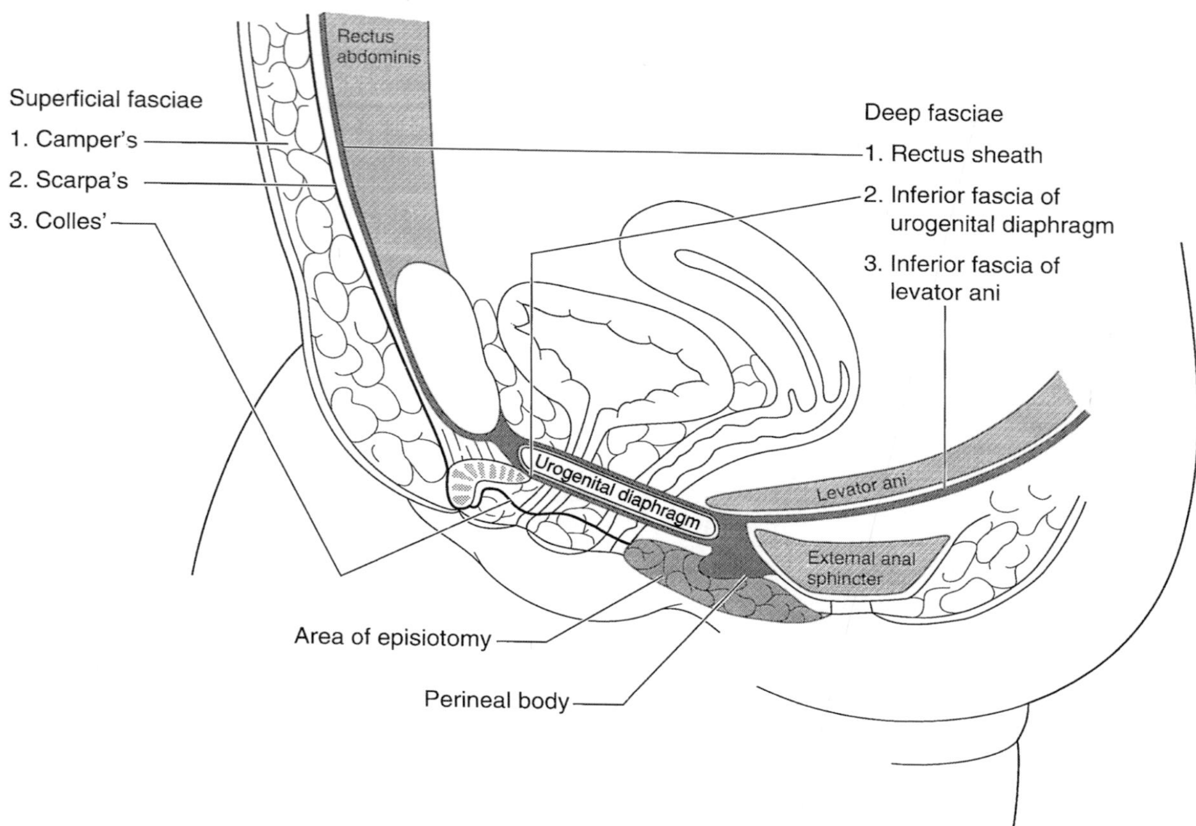

FIGURE 96–1. Diagrammatic representation of the fascial layers of the lower abdomen and perineum in paramedian sagittal section. (From Shy KK, Eschenbach DA. Fatal perineal cellulitis from an episiotomy site. Obstet Gynecol. 1979;54:292–298.)

measure to surgical débridement. Polyvalent gas gangrene antitoxin is probably ineffective (see Chapter 236).

Soper[27] reported an unusually severe form of clostridial myonecrosis arising from an episiotomy caused by *Clostridium sordelli*. The patient had a distinctive course characterized by sudden onset of severe and unrelenting hypotension associated with marked, generalized tissue edema and third spacing, with increased hematocrit, marked leukemoid reaction, absence of rash or fever, and a rapid fatal course. This syndrome was subsequently reported in association with retention of a vaginal pack, degeneration of a cervical myoma, and postpartum endometritis.[28, 29]

Postabortal Infection

Infection after abortion is an ascending process and occurs more commonly in the presence of retained products of conception or operative trauma. Risk factors include greater duration of pregnancy, technical difficulties, and the unsuspected presence of sexually transmitted pathogens.

Symptoms include fever, chills, abdominal pain, and vaginal bleeding, often with the passage of placental tissue. Postabortal infection typically has its onset within 4 days of the procedure.

Physical findings include an elevated temperature, tachycardia, tachypnea, and abdominal tenderness. In the presence of bacteremia, hypotension or frank shock may occur, and the patient may be agitated or disoriented. Pelvic examination reveals a sanguinopurulent discharge and uterine tenderness, with or without adnexal and parametrial tenderness. It is important to look for cervical or vaginal lacerations, especially with a suspected illegal abortion.

Septic abortion caused by *C. perfringens* infection has a characteristic clinical presentation. In severe cases, massive intravascular hemolysis produces jaundice, mahogany-colored urine, and severe anemia.

Laboratory evaluation for patients with more than early uncomplicated postabortal endometritis should include complete blood count, urinalysis, culture, and Gram staining of cervical material; blood cultures; anteroposterior radiographs of the abdomen and pelvis; and upright chest roentgenograms.

Simple endometritis, defined as low-grade fever associated with mild uterine tenderness after uncomplicated elective abortion, can be treated with oral doxycycline. Patients with established infection, as indicated by fever greater than 38°C, pelvic peritonitis, or tachycardia, should be hospitalized for parenteral antibiotic therapy and prompt uterine evacuation. Stubblefield and Grimes[30] have reviewed the management of these cases.

Surgical removal of infected tissue is essential in all but the mildest of postabortal infections. Pelvic ultrasound can be employed to confirm the presence of retained tissue. In most cases, prompt curettage controls the infection. When the uterus is too large to allow suction curettage, oxytocin administration is often successful. Prostaglandin E_2 suppositories are contraindicated in the presence of acute pelvic infection. Concurrent laparoscopy may be needed for curettage of a uterus perforated at the time of abortion.

Indications for laparotomy and hysterectomy include failure to respond to uterine evacuation and appropriate medical therapy, perforation and infection with suspected bowel injury, pelvic and adnexal abscess, and clostridial necrotizing myometritis (gas gangrene). Isolation of *C. perfringens* does not mandate hysterectomy. Initial treatment should be with high-dose penicillin, curettage, supportive therapy, and intensive cardiovascular monitoring. Laparotomy is indicated if there is deterioration or no response.

Avoidance of unwanted pregnancies by making contraceptives

available is the most important preventive measure. Screening for sexually transmitted diseases before performance of elective abortion is optimal but often impractical. A meta-analysis revealed a substantial protective effect of antibiotics in all subgroups of women undergoing induced abortion, even women in low-risk groups. Routine use of periabortal antibiotics in the United States may prevent up to half of all cases of postabortal infection.[31]

INFECTION AFTER GYNECOLOGIC SURGERY

Pathogens

The normal vaginal flora consists of lactobacilli, various species of streptococci, *G. vaginalis*, strains of Enterobacteriaceae, and anaerobes. Anaerobes predominate numerically, with a ratio of 10:1.[32] The normal flora mirrors the major pathogens in nonvenereal infections of the female pelvis (Table 96–1), supporting an endogenous route of infection as postulated by Schottmueller[33] more than 80 years ago. Unexplained exceptions to this association are *Fusobacteria* and *B. fragilis*, both infrequent members of the normal vaginal flora.

Many factors alter the vaginal flora and may indirectly predispose to postoperative infection. Ohm and Galask[34, 35] showed that, after abdominal or vaginal hysterectomy, *E. coli, Klebsiella, Proteus, Enterobacter, B. fragilis*, and enterococci are more common in 5-day postoperative vaginal cultures than in preoperative cultures from the same patients. Although several studies have documented increased enterococcal colonization after perioperative cephalosporin prophylaxis, other factors must be involved, because placebo groups show increased enterococcal colonization as well. Hospitalization appears to exert a profound effect on the vaginal flora, regardless of surgery or antibiotic prophylaxis, and this change tends to be in the direction of more virulent organisms, including enterococci, *B. fragilis*, and resistant Enterobacteriaceae.

Other factors that affect the vaginal flora include use of nonoxynol-9–containing vaginal contraceptive preparations,[36, 37] douching,[38] use of the female condom,[39] and the phase of the menstrual cycle. The significance of these factors in relation to infection after gynecologic surgery is unknown.

The animal model of intra-abdominal infection devised by Weinstein and colleagues[40, 41] clarified the distinctive roles played by different bacteria in the natural history of pelvic infection. These investigators documented a biphasic response to infection consisting of an early-onset phase with high rates of sepsis and death, in which gram-negative aerobic bacteria predominate (peritonitis stage), and a late-onset phase with abscess formation, in which anaerobes predominate (abscess stage).

TABLE 96–1 Endogenous Pathogens Commonly Isolated from Postoperative Pelvic Infections

Aerobic gram-positive cocci
Viridans and nongroup A, B, and D streptococci
Group B streptococci
Enterococcus faecalis
Staphylococcus aureus
Staphylococcus epidermidis
Aerobic gram-negative bacilli
Escherichia coli
Klebsiella species
Proteus mirabilis
Gardnerella vaginalis
Anaerobic organisms
Peptostreptococcus species
Bacteroides fragilis group
Prevotella bivia
Prevotella disiens
Fusobacterium species
Mycoplasmas
Mycoplasma hominis
Ureaplasma urealyticum

Risk Factors

Several factors, many beyond the surgeon's control, influence the likelihood of development of a postoperative infection. Febrile morbidity is more common after abdominal than after vaginal hysterectomy.[42] The incidence of postoperative infection is higher in patients of lower socioeconomic status, regardless of the surgical approach. Age has inconsistently been shown to be a risk factor after hysterectomy, with premenopausal women shown to be at increased risk in some studies, especially after vaginal hysterectomy. It is not known whether this increased risk in younger women is caused by estrogen-mediated influences on vaginal flora and host response[43] or by greater difficulty in obtaining hemostasis. Duration of surgery is directly correlated with postoperative infection rates. For infections of the operative site (i.e., "deep" as opposed to incisional infections), duration of surgery probably reflects the degree of technical difficulty of a procedure, the skill of the surgeon, or both.

Bacterial vaginosis has been associated with an increased risk of infection after abdominal hysterectomy.[44, 45] Patients scheduled for elective hysterectomy should be screened for bacterial vaginosis 1 month before the planned procedure. Those found to have bacterial vaginosis should be treated and allowed several weeks to reestablish a normal lactobacillus-dominant flora before surgery.

Pelvic Cellulitis

The most common infection after hysterectomy is pelvic cellulitis. Patients complain of increasing lower abdominal and pelvic pain that is usually more severe on one side. Symptoms typically develop on the second or third postoperative day, and the temperature is greater than 38.5°C. Direct tenderness over the parametrial area is elicited by abdominal and confirmed by bimanual examinations.

The value of obtaining a culture from the vaginal cuff is controversial. Some believe that cultures can identify the responsible pathogens, especially when an infection has not responded to the initial antimicrobial regimen. Others argue that the inevitable contamination with vaginal flora renders such cultures uninterpretable.

Pelvic cellulitis usually responds promptly to single-agent parenteral antibiotic therapy. Successful regimens include cefotetan, cefoxitin, ampicillin/sulbactam, and ticarcillin/clavulanic acid. Patients with true allergy to β-lactam antibiotics and those for whom initial therapy has failed can be treated with a regimen of clindamycin plus gentamicin. Parenteral therapy is continued until the patient has been afebrile for 24 to 36 hours. Hager and associates[46] showed that oral outpatient antibiotic therapy after successful parenteral therapy is unnecessary.

Not all patients who are febrile after hysterectomy are infected. Hemsell[47] observed that 17% of women undergoing vaginal hysterectomy and 35% of those undergoing abdominal hysterectomy have recurrent temperature elevations on the second or third postoperative day but have normal abdominal and pelvic examinations and no pain. These patients become afebrile without therapy.[47]

Cuff Cellulitis

An inflammatory response at the margins of the vaginal cuff incision is a normal part of the healing process in the early postoperative period. Host defense mechanisms quickly resolve this cellulitis in most patients without need for antibiotic administration. In a small number of cases, however, cuff cellulitis after hysterectomy requires antibiotic therapy. These cases usually occur in the 10-day period after discharge from the hospital. Patients complain of increasing central lower abdominal or pelvic pain, increased vaginal discharge, and low-grade temperature elevation. Abdominal examination is normal or elicits only slight suprapubic tenderness to deep palpation. On bimanual examination only the vaginal surgical margin is tender, and no masses are palpable. Women with cuff cellulitis have been treated successfully as outpatients with oral antibiotics such as amoxicillin/clavulanic acid. Patients should monitor their temperatures at home, and clinical reevaluation must be carried out at 72 hours.

Cuff Abscess

A few patients develop a well-localized collection just above the vaginal cuff. They usually become febrile on the second or third postoperative day and may complain of a sense of fullness in the lower abdomen. Drainage facilitates cure and may be accomplished in a treatment room. Any purulent material recovered should be cultured for aerobic and anaerobic pathogens. Parenteral antibiotics should be given until the patient has been afebrile for 24 to 36 hours.[48]

Pelvic Abscess

The most serious late postoperative complication is an adnexal abscess. These infections are rare, occur almost exclusively in premenopausal women, occur despite the use of prophylactic antibiotics, and often have a latent period of many weeks between surgery and onset of symptoms.[49, 50]

Patients may have had no apparent infection during their initial hospitalization, or, alternatively, they may have appeared to respond rapidly to the initial selection of antibiotics for presumed pelvic cellulitis, only to relapse after discharge. Typically the fever curve is characterized by a high spike late in the afternoon or early evening. The leukocyte count is often in the range of 20,000/mm^3, and the erythrocyte sedimentation rate is markedly elevated. Patients with postoperative adnexal abscesses often have a palpable mass high in the pelvis. Ultrasonography and computed tomography scans both confirm the presence of the mass and help to determine whether it is loculated, related to an intraperitoneal structure, or drainable percutaneously.

Identification of a postoperative pelvic abscess does not mandate immediate drainage if it is inaccessible, because antibiotic therapy alone is often successful in the treatment of this complication. The frequent isolation of *B. fragilis* from these abscesses warrants the use of clindamycin, metronidazole, or other agents effective against gram-negative anaerobes. A regimen of clindamycin plus gentamicin is frequently employed. In patients whose infection fails to respond to appropriate antibiotic therapy, drainage is necessary. Ledger and colleagues[51] showed that most such antibiotic failures are caused not by antimicrobial resistance but by the unique environment of the abscess, which inhibits antibiotic effectiveness.

If the abscess is located in the posterior cul-de-sac, colpotomy drainage can be attempted under ultrasound guidance.[52] The abscess cavity should be completely evacuated and a drain placed to prevent reaccumulation of fluid. Abscesses not located in the cul-de-sac may be drained percutaneously if they are located adjacent to the abdominal wall or are determined to be accessible by computed tomographic scanning. A pigtail or equivalent catheter should remain in place until drainage ceases, usually 4 to 8 days.[53–57] Patients with suspected postoperative pelvic abscess that fails to respond to antibiotic therapy and cannot be drained by one of the previously mentioned techniques require laparotomy. The least extensive operation compatible with cure should be used. If the abscess is amenable to extraperitoneal drainage, this alone should suffice. If not, as in a postoperative adnexal abscess, extirpation may be necessary.

Purulent material obtained at drainage procedures should be submitted for culture in an anaerobic transport vial. Fluid should be inoculated through the rubber diaphragm, and tissue, such as a specimen of abscess wall, may be placed into the vial after the cap has been briefly removed. Introduction of oxygen into the vial is not a problem if tissue or pus is being cultured. Material placed in an anaerobic transport vial is adequate for every type of culture, including aerobes, anaerobes, fungi, and mycobacteria. For most purposes several milliliters of pus or a 0.5-cm cube of tissue is adequate.

Parenteral antibiotics should be administered until the patient has remained afebrile for 48 to 72 hours, the leukocyte count is normal, and the signs and symptoms have resolved. Controversy exists as to the need for postdischarge oral antibiotics for patients with pelvic abscesses that have responded to parenteral therapy and when the abscess was neither excised nor drained. Some clinicians choose to treat these patients for 7 days after discharge with oral agents such as amoxicillin/clavulanic acid or metronidazole. Regardless of whether they receive such therapy, all patients should be reexamined 2 weeks after discharge to ensure that recurrence or reaccumulation of the abscess has not occurred. Sauer and Paulson[58] reported the unusual case of a pelvic abscess complicating transcervical embryo transfer.

Septic Pelvic Thrombophlebitis

Pelvic vein thrombophlebitis may manifest as the so-called enigmatic fever syndrome, a rare cause of obscure postoperative fever.[22, 59] This condition is almost always associated with a diagnosed operative site infection and typically has a gradual onset 4 to 8 days after surgery. Antibiotic therapy is started, and the patient, unlike those with puerperal ovarian vein thrombophlebitis (discussed previously), usually experiences definite improvement in all clinical parameters except temperature. They do not appear to be acutely ill, and positive physical findings are usually limited to recurrent temperature elevations, often as high as 39.4°C to 40.0°C, and tachycardia proportional to the fever. Pain, tenderness, palpable mass, and adynamic ileus usually are not present. Because there is no obvious source for the recurrent temperature elevations, this syndrome is aptly described as "enigmatic fever." The diagnosis of septic pelvic thrombophlebitis should be suspected in any patient with a recent soft tissue pelvic infection and recurrent temperature elevations that persist despite appropriate broad-spectrum antibiotic therapy. Differential diagnoses include drug fever, viral illness, collagen-vascular disease, and pelvic or incisional abscess. The diagnosis of septic pelvic thrombophlebitis is almost invariably one of exclusion and is verified by observing defervesence after therapeutic anticoagulation with heparin.[60]

Osteomyelitis Pubis

Osteomyelitis of the pubis is a rare infection that results from either bacteremic seeding or extension of a contiguous focus of infection. Most cases in women occur after urethral suspension, radical vulvectomy, or pelvic exenteration. In the study conducted by Hoyme and colleagues,[61] symptoms, consisting of pubic bone pain and tenderness, avoidance of ambulation, and pain on abduction, did not appear until more than 8 weeks after the initial operation. Wound drainage, low-grade fever, moderate leukocytosis, and an elevated erythrocyte sedimentation rate or alkaline phosphatase level may be present. Blood and bone biopsy specimens or aspirated material should be cultured.

The radiograph or computed tomogram of the pubic bone often shows rarefaction, erosion, osteolytic lesions, or irregularities of the bone margins with separation of the symphysis. Later in the course of disease there is evidence of bone repair, with new bone formation or sclerosis of the symphysis. Radioactive scanning techniques may show increased activity.

Antimicrobial therapy must be prolonged and capable of covering both *Staphylococcus aureus* and aerobic gram-negative bacteria, the usual pathogens, unless a specific organism is isolated. Surgical débridement may be necessary as well.[61]

Sacral osteomyelitis as a complication of abdominal sacral colpopexy has been reported.[62]

PELVIC INFLAMMATORY DISEASE

The term *acute pelvic inflammatory disease* (PID) refers to the clinical syndrome, unrelated to pregnancy or surgery, that results when cervical microorganisms ascend to the endometrium, fallopian tubes, and contiguous pelvic structures producing one or more of the following inflammatory conditions: endometritis, salpingitis, pelvic peritonitis, or tuboovarian abscess. Each year approximately 1 million women in the United States experience an episode of symptomatic PID. Many women with PID have minimal or no symptoms.

PID results from direct canalicular spread of organisms from the endocervix to the endometrial and fallopian tube mucosa. Both *Neisseria gonorrhoeae* and *C. trachomatis* commonly cause endocervicitis, and 10 to 40% of women with these infections who do not receive adequate treatment develop clinical symptoms of acute PID. In addition to *N. gonorrhoeae* and *C. trachomatis*, a wide variety of bacteria have been isolated from the upper genital tracts of women with acute PID, including anaerobes, gram-negative rods, streptococci, and mycoplasmas. Barham and associates[63] reported a rare case of acute salpingitis caused by group A β-hemolytic streptococci infection after endometrial biopsy.

Risk Factors

Age is inversely related to the rate of PID, with sexually experienced teenagers three times more likely to be diagnosed with PID than are 25- to 29-year-old women. A history of multiple sexual partners, an increased rate of acquisition of new partners within the previous 30 days,[64] and frequent intercourse with a single partner[65] are all associated with an increased risk of PID. Contraceptive choice modifies PID risk in a complex manner: mechanical and chemical barriers decrease risk; oral contraceptives have a variable effect; and intrauterine devices confer a slightly increased risk of nonsexually transmitted PID in the first months after insertion. Other suggested associations with PID include bacterial vaginosis,[66] douching,[67] menses, cigarette smoking,[68] and substance abuse.

Although an association between the use of an intrauterine contraceptive device (IUD) and increased risk of PID has been documented for many years, newer studies suggest that the magnitude of this association has been overestimated.[69, 70] Contamination of the endometrial cavity at insertion apparently results in a slightly increased risk of acute PID that is limited to the first 4 months of IUD use. Infections occurring after 4 months are believed to be the result of acquired sexually transmitted pathogens, not of the IUD itself.

A unique role for *Actinomyces* organisms in IUD-associated PID has been suggested, but this relationship remains unclear. Although as many as 4 to 8% of IUD users have *Actinomyces*-like organisms identified on a Papanicolaou (Pap) smear, their presence has not been equated with pelvic actinomycosis, nor has the risk of subsequent pelvic infection been quantified.[71]

Diagnosis

Minimum clinical criteria for acute PID include direct lower quadrant tenderness, cervical motion tenderness, and adnexal tenderness. Additional criteria that support a diagnosis of PID include mucopurulent cervicitis, laboratory documentation of cervical infection with *N. gonorrhoeae* or *C. trachomatis*, oral temperature greater than 38.3°C, and elevated erythrocyte sedimentation rate or C-reactive protein level.[72] Definitive criteria for PID include histopathologic evidence of endometritis on endometrial biopsy,[73] transvaginal sonography or other imaging techniques showing thickened fluid-filled tubes with or without free pelvic fluid or tubo-ovarian complex,[74] and laparoscopic abnormalities consistent with PID.

Asymptomatic PID may be a common occurrence. Gump and coworkers[75] found that two thirds of patients with evidence of old PID on laparoscopy or hysterosalpingography could not recall a history of PID and yet had sufficient residual disease to impair fertility. Walters and colleagues[76] found that only 18% of women with ectopic pregnancies and detectable antichlamydial antibody or inflammatory tubal damage reported a history of PID.

Clinical diagnosis and grading of PID has poor specificity.[77] Patients with atypical clinical presentations, those with other suspected diagnoses, and those for whom empiric therapy has failed should undergo laparoscopy for definitive diagnosis.

Although rare, acute salpingitis can occur in the proximal stump of patients who have undergone surgical sterilization.[78–80]

Management of Acute Pelvic Inflammatory Disease

There is no consensus on the need to carry out treatment of PID in the hospital. The Centers for Disease Control and Prevention (CDC) recommends hospitalization of patients with acute PID in the following situations: surgical emergencies such as appendicitis cannot be excluded; the patient is pregnant; the patient does not respond clinically to oral antimicrobial therapy; the patient is unable to follow or tolerate an outpatient oral regimen; the patient has severe illness, nausea and vomiting, or high fever; the patient has a tubo-ovarian abscess; or the patient is immunodeficient.

Treatment consists of bed rest, pelvic rest, and antibiotics. The antimicrobial regimen of choice has not been established by randomized clinical trials. No single agent is active against the entire spectrum of potential pathogens. A variety of combination antimicrobial regimens are highly effective in producing clinical and microbiologic cures. Uncertainties regarding the effectiveness of antimicrobial therapy in preventing late sequelae and the appropriateness of ambulatory treatment further complicate therapeutic decisions. The CDC has published antibiotic treatment guidelines for acute PID (Tables 96–2 and 96–3).[64, 72, 81, 82]

All patients treated as outpatients should be clinically reevaluated within 72 hours. Those not responding favorably should be hospitalized. All male sex partners of women with acute PID should be evaluated for sexually transmitted diseases and empirically treated with regimens effective against *C. trachomatis* and *N. gonorrhoeae* if they had sexual contact with the patient during the 60 days preceding onset of symptoms in the patient.

TABLE 96–2 Oral Treatment Regimens for Acute Pelvic Inflammatory Disease

Regimen A		
Ofloxacin, 400 mg orally twice daily for 14 d	PLUS	Metronidazole, 500 mg orally twice daily for 14 d
Regimen B		
Ceftriaxone, 250 mg IM OR Cefoxitin, 2 g IM, PLUS Probenecid, 1 g orally in a single dose concurrently once OR Other parenteral third-generation cephalosporin (e.g., ceftizoxime, cefotaxine)	PLUS	Doxycycline, 100 mg orally twice daily for 14 d

From Centers for Disease Control and Prevention. 1998 Guidelines for treatment of sexually transmitted diseases. MMWR Morb Mortal Wkly Rep. 1998;47(No. RR-1):79–86.

TABLE 96-3 Parenteral Treatment Regimens for Acute Pelvic Inflammatory Disease

Regimen A		
Cefotetan, 2 g IV every 12 h OR Cefoxitin, 2 g IV every 6 h	PLUS	Doxycycline, 100 mg IV or orally every 12 h
Regimen B		
Clindamycin, 900 mg IV every 8 h	PLUS	Gentamicin loading dose IV or IM (2 mg/kg) followed by maintenance dose (1.5 mg/kg) every 8 h (single daily dosing may be substituted)
Parenteral therapy may be discontinued 24 h after clinical improvement. Continuing oral therapy should consist of doxycycline 100 mg orally twice a day or clindamycin 450 mg orally four times a day to complete a total of 14 d of therapy.		
Alternative Regimens		
Ofloxacin, 400 mg IV every 12 h OR	PLUS	Metronidazole, 500 mg IV every 8 h
		Doxycycline, 100 mg orally or IV every 12 h
Ampicillin/Sulbactam, 3 g IV every 6 h OR	PLUS	Doxycycline, 100 mg orally or IV every 12 h
Ciprofloxacin, 200 mg IV every 12 h	PLUS	Metronidazole, 500 mg IV every 8 h plus doxycycline, 100 mg orally or IV every 12 h

From Centers for Disease Control and Prevention. 1998 Guidelines for treatment of sexually transmitted diseases. MMWR Morb Mortal Wkly Rep. 1998;47(No. RR-1):79–86.

Management of Suspected Tubo-ovarian Abscess

Patients suspected of having a tubo-ovarian abscess should be hospitalized and given broad-spectrum antimicrobial drugs that include adequate coverage for gram-negative anaerobes.[83] Failure of response to medical therapy is suggested by lack of defervescence within 72 hours or increase in the size of the mass. Eighty-five percent of abscesses with a diameter of 4 to 6 cm respond to antibiotics alone, but only 40% of those 10 cm or larger respond.[84]

Surgical intervention for a tubo-ovarian abscesses that does not respond to antimicrobial therapy can be carried out laparoscopically,[85, 86] percutaneously,[53–55, 57, 87] transvaginally,[52, 56, 88] or by laparotomy. Patients with a suspected leaking or ruptured abscess should undergo immediate laparotomy after rapid stabilization and institution of broad-spectrum antibiotics.

Prognosis

After one episode of PID a woman's risk of ectopic pregnancy increases sevenfold. Approximately 13% of women are infertile after a single episode of PID, 25 to 35% after two episodes, and 50 to 75% after three or more episodes.[64, 89] If a true tubo-ovarian abscess is present, only 7 to 14% of patients are able to conceive after treatment. After treatment for a tubo-ovarian complex, a less restrictive diagnostic category than tubo-ovarian abscess, approximately two thirds of women attempting pregnancy are unable to conceive.[90] Other sequelae associated with PID include dyspareunia, pelvic adhesions, and chronic pelvic pain.[91]

REFERENCES

1. Gibbs RS, Duff P. Progress in pathogenesis and management of clinical intra-amniotic infection. Am J Obstet Gynecol. 1991;164:1317–1326.
2. Liner RI. Intrauterine *Listeria* infection: Prenatal diagnosis by biophysical assessment and amniocentesis. Am J Obstet Gynecol. 1990;163:1596–1597.
3. Newton ER, Piper J, Peairs W. Bacterial vaginosis and intraamniotic infection. Am J Obstet Gynecol. 1997;176:672–677.
4. Gauthier DW, Meyer WJ. Comparison of Gram stain, leukocyte esterase activity, and amniotic fluid glucose concentration in predicting amniotic fluid culture results in preterm premature rupture of membranes. Am J Obstet Gynecol. 1992;167:1092–1095.
5. Greig PC, Murtha AP, Jimmerson CJ, et al. Maternal serum interleukin-6 during pregnancy and during term and preterm labor. Obstet Gynecol. 1997;90:465–469.
6. Gibbs RS, Dinsmoor MJ, Newton ER, Ramamurthy RS. A randomized trial of intrapartum versus immediate postpartum treatment of women with intraamniotic infection. Obstet Gynecol. 1988;72:823–828.
7. Seaward PG, Hannah ME, Myhr TL, et al. International multicentre term prelabor rupture of membranes study: Evaluation of predictors of clinical chorioamnionitis and postpartum fever in patients with prelabor rupture of membranes at term. Am J Obstet Gynecol. 1997;177:1024–1029.
8. Watts DH, Krohn MA, Hillier SL, et al. Bacterial vaginosis as a risk factor for post-cesarean endometritis. Obstet Gynecol. 1990;75:52–58.
9. Chang PL, Newton ER. Predictors of antibiotic prophylactic failure in post-cesarean endometritis. Obstet Gynecol. 1992;80:117–122.
10. Hemsell DL. Prophylactic antibiotics in gynecologic and obstetric surgery. Rev Infect Dis. 1991;13(10):S821–S41.
11. Watts DH, Eschenbach DA, Kenny GE. Early postpartum endometritis: The role of bacteria, genital mycoplasmas, and *Chlamydia trachomatis*. Obstet Gynecol. 1989;73:52–60.
12. Eschenbach DA, Rosene K, Tompkins LS, et al. Endometrial cultures obtained by a triple-lumen method from afebrile and febrile postpartum women. J Infect Dis. 1986;153:1038–1045.
13. Watts DH, Hillier SL, Eschenbach DA. Upper genital tract isolates at delivery as predictors of post-cesarean infection among women receiving antibiotic prophylaxis. Obstet Gynecol. 1991;77:287–292.
14. Hoyme UB, Kiviat N, Eschenbach DA. The microbiology and treatment of late postpartum endometritis. Obstet Gynecol. 1986;68:226–232.
15. Martens MG, Faro S, Hammil HA, et al. Transcervical uterine cultures with a new endometrial suction curette: A comparison of three sampling methods in postpartum endometritis. Obstet Gynecol. 1989;74:273–276.
16. Faro S, Martens MG, Hammill HA, et al. Antibiotic prophylaxis: Is there a difference? Am J Obstet Gynecol. 1990;162:900–909.
17. Polk BF. Antimicrobial prophylaxis to prevent mixed bacterial infection. J Antimicrob Chemother. 1981;8(D):115–129.
18. Gonik B, Shannon RL, Shawar R, et al. Why patients fail antibiotic prophylaxis at cesarean delivery: Histologic evidence for incipient infection. Obstet Gynecol. 1992;79:179–184.
19. Noronha S, Yue C, Sekosan M. Puerperal group A-beta hemolytic streptococcal toxic shock-like syndrome. Obstet Gynecol. 1996;88:728.
20. Meis JF, Muytjens HC, van den Berg PP, et al. Analysis of an outbreak of puerperal fever due to group A streptococci by random amplified polymorphic DNA fingerprinting. Infect Dis Obstet Gynecol. 1997;5:232–236.
21. Centers for Disease Control and Prevention. Nosocomial group A streptococcal infections associated with asymptomatic health care workers—Maryland and California, 1997. MMWR Morb Mortal Wkly Rep. 1999;48:163–166.
22. Duff P, Gibbs RS. Pelvic vein thrombophlebitis: Diagnostic dilemma and therapeutic challenge. Obstet Gynecol Surv. 1983;38:365–373.
23. Brown CEL, Lowe TW, Cunningham FG, Weinreb JC. Puerperal pelvic thrombophlebitis: Impact on diagnosis and treatment using x-ray computed tomography and magnetic resonance imaging. Obstet Gynecol. 1986;68:789–794.
24. Witlin AG, Sibai BM. Postpartum ovarian vein thrombosis after vaginal delivery: A report of 11 cases. Obstet Gynecol. 1995;85:775–780.
25. Shy KK, Eschenbach DA. Fatal perineal cellulitis from an episiotomy site. Obstet Gynecol. 1979;54:292–298.
26. Ramin SM, Ramus RM, Little BB, et al. Early repair of episiotomy dehiscence associated with infection. Am J Obstet Gynecol. 1992;167:1104–1107.
27. Soper DE. Clostridial myonecrosis arising from an episiotomy. Obstet Gynecol. 1986;68:26S–28S.
28. McGregor JA, Soper DE, Lovell G, Todd JK. Maternal deaths associated with *Clostridium sordelli* infection. Am J Obstet Gynecol. 1989;161:987–995.
29. Spera RV, Kaplan MH, Allen SL. *Clostridium sordelli* bacteremia: Case report and review. Clinical Infect Dis. 1992;15:950–954.
30. Stubblefield PG, Grimes DA. Septic abortion. N Engl J Med. 1994;331:310–314.
31. Sawaya GF, Grady D, Kerlikowske K, et al. Antibiotics at the time of induced abortion: The case for universal prophylaxis based on a meta-analysis. Obstet Gynecol. 1996;87:884–890.

32. Bartlett JG, Moon NE, Goldstein PR, et al. Cervical and vaginal bacterial flora: Ecologic niches in the female lower genital tract. Am J Obstet Gynecol. 1978;130:658–661.
33. Schottmueller H. Significance of several anaerobes in pathology, especially in puerperal illnesses. Mitt Grenzt Med Chir. 1910;21:450.
34. Ohm MJ, Galask RP. The effect of antibiotic prophylaxis on patients undergoing vaginal operations. Am J Obstet Gynecol. 1975;123:597–604.
35. Ohm MJ, Galask RP. The effect of antibiotic prophylaxis on patients undergoing total abdominal hysterectomy. Am J Obstet Gynecol. 1976;125:448–454.
36. McGroarty JA, Tomeczek L, Pond DG, et al. Hydrogen peroxide production by *Lactobacillus* species: Correlation with susceptibility to the spermicidal compound nonoxynol-9. J Infect Dis. 1992;165:1142–1144.
37. Klebanoff SJ. Effects of the spermicidal agent nonoxynol-9 on vaginal microbial flora. J Infect Dis. 1992;165:19–25.
38. Onderdonk AB, Delaney ML, Hinkson PL, DuBois AM. Quantitative and qualitative effects of douche preparations on vaginal microflora. Obstet Gynecol. 1992;80:333–338.
39. Soper DE, Brockwell NJ, Dalton HP. Evaluation of the effects of a female condom on the female lower genital tract. Contraception. 1991;44:21–29.
40. Weinstein WM, Onderdonk AB, Bartlett JG, Gorbach SI. Experimental intraabdominal abscesses in rats: Development of an experimental model. Infect Immun. 1974;10:1250–1255.
41. Bartlett JG, Onderdonk AB, Louie T, et al. Lessons from an animal model of intraabdominal sepsis. Arch Surg. 1978;113:853–857.
42. Dicker RC, Greenspan JR, Strauss LT, et al. Complications of abdominal and vaginal hysterectomy among women of reproductive age in the United States. Am J Obstet Gynecol. 1982;144:841–848.
43. Styrt B, Sugarman B. Estrogens and infection. Rev Infect Dis. 1991;13:1139–1150.
44. Soper DE, Bump RC, Hurt WG. Bacterial vaginosis and trichomoniasis are risk factors for cuff cellulitis after abdominal hysterectomy. Am J Obstet Gynecol. 1990;163:1016–1023.
45. Larsson P-G, Platz-Christensen J-J, Forsum U, Pahlson C. Clue cells in predicting infections after abdominal hysterectomy. Obstet Gynecol. 1991;77:450–452.
46. Hager WD, Pascuzzi M, Vernon M. Efficacy of oral antibiotics following parenteral antibiotics for serious infections in obstetrics and gynecology. Obstet Gynecol. 1989;73:326–329.
47. Hemsell DL. Posthysterectomy cuff and pelvic cellulitis. In: Mead PB, Hager WD, eds. Infection Protocols for Obstetrics and Gynecology. Montvale, NJ: Medical Economics Publishing; 1992:283–287.
48. Hemsell DL, Nobles B, Heard MC. Recognition and treatment of post-hysterectomy pelvic infections. Infect Surg. 1988;7:47–68.
49. Livengood CH, Addison WA. Adnexal abscess as a delayed complication of vaginal hysterectomy. Am J Obstet Gynecol. 1982;143:596–597.
50. Ledger WJ, Campbell C, Wilson JR. Postoperative adnexal infection. Obstet Gynecol. 1968;31:83–89.
51. Ledger WJ, Moore DE, Lowensohn RI, Gee CL. A fever index evaluation of chloramphenicol or clindamycin in patients with serious pelvic infections. Obstet Gynecol. 1977;50:523–530.
52. Rubenstein PR, Mishell DR, Ledger WJ. Colpotomy drainage of pelvic abscess. Obstet Gynecol. 1976;48:142–145.
53. Tyrrel RT, Murphy FB, Bernardino ME. Tubo-ovarian abscesses: CT-guided percutaneous drainage. Radiology. 1990;175:87–89.
54. Mueller PR, Van Sonnenberg E. Interventional radiology in the chest and abdomen. N Engl J Med. 1990;322:1364–1374.
55. Martin EC, Karlson KB, Fankuchen EI, et al. Percutaneous drainage of postoperative intra-abdominal abscesses. AJR Am J Roentgenol. 1982;138:13–15.
56. Loy RA, Gallup DG, Hill JA, et al. Pelvic abscesses. Examination and transvaginal drainage guided by real-time ultrasonography. South Med J. 1989;82:788–790.
57. Casola G, Van Sonnenberg E, D'Agostino HB, et al. Percutaneous drainage of tuboovarian abscesses. Radiology. 1992;182:399–402.
58. Sauer MV, Paulson RJ. Pelvic abscess complicating transcervical embryo transfer. Am J Obstet Gynecol. 1992;166:148–149.
59. Dunn LJ, Van Voorhis LW. Enigmatic fever and pelvic thrombophlebitis. N Engl J Med. 1967;276:265–268.
60. Josey WE, Staggers SR. Heparin therapy in septic pelvic vein thrombophlebitis: A study of 46 cases. Am J Obstet Gynecol. 1974;120:228–233.
61. Hoyme UB, Tamimi HK, Eschenbach DA, et al. Osteomyelitis pubis after radical gynecologic operations. Obstet Gynecol. 1984;63:47S–53S.
62. Weidner AC, Cundiff GW, Harris RL, et al. Sacral osteomyelitis: An unusual complication of abdominal sacral colpopexy. Obstet Gynecol. 1997;90:689–691.
63. Barham WB, Haberberger RL, Decker CF. Group A streptoccal sepsis secondary to acute salpingitis. Clin Infect Dis. 1993;16:444–445.
64. Centers for Disease Control and Prevention. Pelvic inflammatory disease: Guidelines for prevention and management. MMWR Morb Mortal Wkly Rep. 1991;40:1–25.
65. Lee NC, Rubin GL, Grimes DA. Measures of sexual behavior and the risk of pelvic inflammatory disease. Obstet Gynecol. 1991;77:425–430.
66. Eschenbach DA, Hillier S, Critchlow C, et al. Diagnosis and clinical manifestations of bacterial vaginosis. Am J Obstet Gynecol. 1988;158:819–828.
67. Wolner-Hanssen P, Eschenbach DA, Paavonen J, et al. Association between vaginal douching and acute pelvic inflammatory disease. JAMA. 1990;263:1936–1941.
68. Scholes D, Daling JR, Stergachis AS. Cigarette smoking and risk of pelvic inflammatory disease. Am J Epidemiol. 1990;132:759.
69. Centers for Disease Control and Prevention. IUD Safety: Report of a nationwide physician survey. MMWR Morb Mortal Wkly Rep. 1997;46:969–974.
70. Lee NC, Rubin GL, Borucki R. The intrauterine device and pelvic inflammatory disease revisited: New results from the Women's Health Study. Obstet Gynecol. 1988;72:1–6.
71. Fiorino AS. Intrauterine contraceptive device–associated actinomycotic abscesses and *Actinomyces* detection on cervical smear. Obstet Gynecol. 1996;87:142–149.
72. Centers for Disease Control and Prevention. 1998 Guidelines for treatment of sexually transmitted diseases. MMWR Morb Mortal Wkly Rep. 1998;47(No. RR-1):79–86.
73. Paavonen J, Aine T, Teisala K, et al. Comparison of endometrial biopsy and peritoneal fluid cytologic testing with laparoscopy in the diagnosis of acute pelvic inflammatory disease. Am J Obstet Gynecol. 1985;151:645–650.
74. Cacciatore B, Leminen A, Ingman-Friberg S, et al. Transvaginal sonographic findings in ambulatory patients with suspected pelvic inflammatory disease. Obstet Gynecol. 1992;80:912–916.
75. Gump DW, Gibson M, Ashikaga T. Evidence of prior pelvic inflammatory disease and its relationship to *Chlamydia trachomatis* antibody and intrauterine contraceptive device use in infertile women. Am J Obstet Gynecol. 1983;146:153–159.
76. Walters MD, Eddy CA, Gibbs RS, et al. Antibodies to *Chlamydia trachomatis* and risk for tubal pregnancy. Am J Obstet Gynecol. 1988;159:942–946.
77. Livengood CH, Hill GB, Addison WA. Pelvic inflammatory disease: Findings during inpatient treatment of clinically severe, laparoscopy-documented disease. Am J Obstet Gynecol. 1992;166:519–524.
78. Fletcher V. Proximal stump salpingitis. Am J Obstet Gynecol. 1986;155:496–500.
79. Vermesh M, Confino E, Boler LR, et al. Acute salpingitis in sterilized women. Obstet Gynecol. 1987;69:265–267.
80. Green MM, Vicario SJ, Sanfilippo JS, Lochhead SA. Acute pelvic inflammatory disease after surgical sterilization. Ann Emerg Med. 1991;20:344–347.
81. Peterson HB, Walker CK, Kahn JG, et al. Pelvic inflammatory disease. JAMA. 1991;266:2605–2611.
82. Landers DV, Wolner-Hanssen P, Paavonen J, et al. Combination antimicrobial therapy in the treatment of acute pelvic inflammatory disease. Am J Obstet Gynecol. 1991;164:849–858.
83. Reed SD, Landers DV, Sweet RL. Antibiotic treatment of tuboovarian abscess. Am J Obstet Gynecol. 1991;164:1556–1561.
84. Amstey MS, Sweet RL. Definition of pelvic abscess (Letter). Am J Obstet Gynecol. 1993;168:740–741.
85. Henry-Suchet J, Soler A, Loffredo V. Laparoscopic treatment of tuboovarian abscesses. J Reprod Med. 1984;29:579–582.
86. Reich H. Role of laparoscopy in treating TOA and pelvic abscess. Contemp OB/GYN. 1989;34(June):91–102.
87. Shulman A, Maymon R, Shapiro A, Bahary C. Percutaneous catheter drainage of tubo-ovarian abscesses. Obstet Gynecol. 1992;80:555–557.
88. Teisala K, Heinonen PK, Punnonen R. Transvaginal ultrasound in the diagnosis and treatment of tubo-ovarian abscess. Br J Obstet Gynaecol. 1990;97:178–180.
89. Westrom L. Effect of acute pelvic inflammatory disease on fertility. Am J Obstet Gynecol. 1975;121:707–713.
90. Brumsted JR, Clifford PM, Nakajima ST, Gibson M. Reproductive outcome after medical management of complicated pelvic inflammatory disease. Fertil Steril. 1988;50:667–669.
91. Safrin S, Schachter J, Dahrouge D, et al. Long-term sequelae of acute pelvic inflammatory disease. Am J Obstet Gynecol. 1992;166:1300–1305.

Chapter 97

Prostatitis, Epididymitis, and Orchitis

JOHN N. KRIEGER

ANATOMY AND PHYSIOLOGY OF THE TESTES AND MALE ACCESSORY SEX ORGANS

The testicle has two functional components, seminiferous tubules and interstitial cells. Sperm production is the primary function of the seminiferous tubules. Interstitial cells, located between the seminiferous tubules, are primarily responsible for hormone production. After spermatogenesis, spermatozoa are transported from the testis into the epididymis (Fig. 97–1). Sperm then move into the vas deferens, a muscular tube approximately 12 inches long that is easily palpable in the scrotum. Fructose from the seminal vesicles is the major energy source for ejaculated sperm. In addition, the seminal vesicles provide proteins that cause coagulation of the ejaculate. Liquefaction

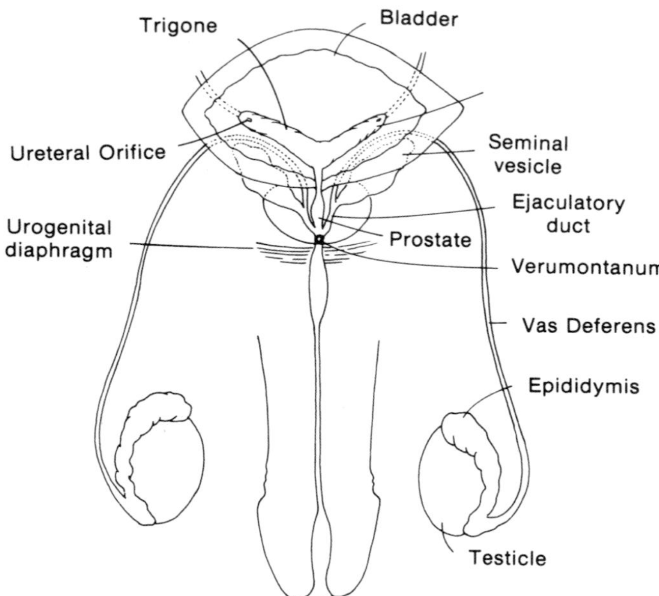

FIGURE 97–1. Anatomy of the male sex organs and lower urinary tract.

of the semen occurs within 5 to 30 minutes after ejaculation as a result of proteolytic enzymes from the prostate.

HOST DEFENSES OF THE MALE LOWER UROGENITAL TRACT

Organisms that ascend through the urethra cause most infections of the urogenital ducts and accessory sex organs.[1] Thus, mechanical factors such as the flushing action of micturition and ejaculation should provide some protection against infection, although the relative significance of such defenses is unclear.

A zinc-containing polypeptide known as the *prostatic antibacterial factor* is the most important antimicrobial substance secreted by the prostate.[1,2] Men with well-documented chronic bacterial prostatitis have significantly lower levels of zinc in their prostatic fluid than those in healthy men, but their serum zinc levels are within normal limits.[2] Other findings suggesting that bacterial prostatitis is associated with generalized secretory dysfunction include increased pH of prostatic fluid; reduced calcium, citric acid, and spermine concentrations; and changes in prostatic fluid enzymes.[3] It is unclear whether reduced zinc concentrations precede the development of prostatic infection or represent a secretory dysfunction resulting from such infections. Prostatic secretions of patients with bacterial prostatitis contain high concentrations of immunoglobulins.[4] Several studies have demonstrated antigen-specific antibody coating of bacteria isolated from the lower urinary tracts of patients with prostatitis syndromes. The antigen-specific antibody response in prostatic secretions (predominantly secretory IgA) is significantly greater in magnitude than is the serologic response.

The presence of leukocytes is characteristic of many conditions of the male lower urinary tract, including prostatitis.[5] Phagocytosis of abnormal sperm by leukocytes has been observed in infertile men with pyosemina.

PROSTATITIS

Classification of Prostatitis

The term *prostatitis* is employed clinically to describe a condition in a large group of adult men with a variety of complaints referable to the lower urogenital tract and perineum.[1,6] It has been estimated that 50% of men will experience symptoms of prostatitis at some time in their lives.[2] Among otherwise healthy young men, prostatitis may be the most common urologic diagnosis.[7] A national survey of physician visits found that there were almost 2 million visits annually for prostatitis, accounting for 8% of visits to urologists and 1% of visits to primary care physicians in the United States.[8]

The crucial clinical issue is to distinguish patients with lower urinary tract complaints associated with bacteriuria—that is, patients who may have bacterial prostatitis—from the larger number of patients without bacteriuria. Further classification of patients with prostatitis depends on careful bacteriologic assessment of the lower urinary tract, which is based on sequential cultures obtained during micturition (Table 97–1).[8,9] Prostatitis syndromes may be classified into four major groups: acute bacterial prostatitis, chronic bacterial prostatitis, chronic prostatitis/chronic pelvic pain syndrome, and asymptomatic inflammatory prostatitis (Table 97–2).[9] In addition, rare patients develop granulomatous prostatitis.

Bacterial prostatitis is a frequent diagnosis in clinical practice, but well-documented bacterial infections of the prostate, whether acute or chronic, are uncommon.[1] The great majority of patients with a diagnosis of prostatitis are adult men with perineal, lower back, or lower abdominal pain or ejaculatory complaints.[9] Most have no history of bacteriuria, and there is little objective evidence of bacterial infection of the prostate. Thus, most patients with prostatitis may be classified as having chronic prostatitis/chronic pelvic pain syndrome, concerning which there are few firm data on which to base therapeutic decisions.

Acute Bacterial Prostatitis

Acute bacterial prostatitis is seldom a subtle or difficult diagnosis. Patients complain of symptoms associated with lower urinary tract infection such as urinary frequency and dysuria. Patients may also experience lower urinary tract obstruction owing to acute edema of the prostate. Signs of systemic toxicity are common. On physical examination, patients may have a high temperature and lower abdominal or suprapubic discomfort due to bladder infection. Findings on rectal examination are frequently impressive, with an exquisitely tender, tense prostate on palpation. Results of urinalysis are abnormal, with pyuria, and cultures are positive. Bacteremia may be present spontaneously or may result from excessively vigorous rectal examinations.

Results of antimicrobial therapy for acute bacterial prostatitis are often dramatic. Many drugs that do not penetrate into the prostate under normal conditions are effective in acute bacterial prostatitis.[1] Thus, drugs that would be appropriate in patients with bacteremia caused by members of the family Enterobacteriaceae, pseudomonads, and enterococci should be administered once specimens have been obtained for urine and blood cultures. Urinary retention is best managed with a suprapubic cystostomy, rather than a transurethral

TABLE 97–1 Lower Urinary Tract Localization Using Sequential Urine Cultures*

Specimen	Symbol	Description
Voided bladder 1	VB_1	Initial 5–10 ml of urinary stream
Voided bladder 2	VB_2	Midstream specimen
Expressed prostatic secretions	EPS	Secretions expressed from prostate by digital massage after midstream specimen
Voided bladder 3	VB_3	First 5–10 ml of urinary stream immediately after prostatic massage

*Unequivocal diagnosis of bacterial prostatitis requires that the colony count in the VB_3 specimen greatly exceed the count in the VB_1 specimen, preferably by at least 10-fold. Many patients who have chronic bacterial prostatitis, however, harbor only small numbers of bacteria in the prostate. In such patients, direct culture of prostatic secretions is particularly useful. Microscopic examination of the EPS is useful for identifying white blood cells and "oval fat bodies," large lipid-laden macrophages characteristic of the prostatic inflammatory response.[1]

TABLE 97–2 Classification of Prostatitis Syndromes on the Basis of Lower Urinary Tract Localization Studies

Condition	Bacteriuria*	Infection Localized to Prostate†	Inflammatory Response‡	Abnormal Rectal Examination of Prostate§	Systemic Illness‖
Acute bacterial prostatitis	+	+	+	+	+
Chronic bacterial prostatitis	+	+	+	–	–
Chronic prostatitis/chronic pelvic pain syndrome					
Inflammatory subtype¶	–	–	+	–	–
Noninflammatory subtype**	–	–	–	–	–
Asymptomatic inflammatory prostatitis	–	–	+	±	–

*Documented with an identical organism that is shown to localize to a prostatic focus when the midstream urine culture is negative.
†Refer to the text for diagnostic criteria.
‡In expressed prostatic secretions, semen, post-massage urine, or prostate tissue.
§Abnormal findings include exquisite tenderness and swelling that may be associated with signs of lower urinary tract obstruction.
‖Systemic findings frequently include fever and rigors and may include signs of bacteremia.
¶Formerly termed "nonbacterial prostatitis."
**Formerly termed "prostatodynia."

catheter, to avoid obstructing drainage of infected prostatic secretions into the urethra. General measures including hydration, analgesics, and bed rest are also indicated. The most important complications of acute bacterial prostatitis are prostatic abscess, prostatic infarction, chronic bacterial prostatitis, and granulomatous prostatitis.

Chronic Bacterial Prostatitis

Chronic bacterial prostatitis is an important cause of bacterial persistence in the male lower urinary tract. Characteristically, patients experience recurrent bacterial urinary tract infections caused by the same organism.[1] Patients are generally asymptomatic between episodes of bladder bacteriuria. The prostate gland is usually normal on either rectal or endoscopic evaluation. Thus, careful lower urinary tract localization studies constitute the cornerstone on which to base a diagnosis of chronic bacterial prostatitis (see Tables 97–1 and 97–2).[1] Diagnosis of chronic bacterial prostatitis based solely on symptoms, the number of leukocytes in expressed prostatic secretions, or the use of prostate biopsy specimens is inadequate.

Gram-negative rods (members of Enterobacteriaceae or pseudomonads) are by far the most important pathogens in chronic bacterial prostatitis. Gram-positive cocci such as *Enterococcus faecalis* or, perhaps, *Staphylococcus saprophyticus* may be the etiologic organisms in a few cases. Reports implicating many other organisms are generally difficult to evaluate owing to methodologic problems with case definition or a lack of documentation of bacteriuria by the alleged pathogen.

Medical management is effective in curing or suppressing bacterial infections of the prostate. Trimethoprim has two useful characteristics: it achieves good levels in the prostatic parenchyma, and it is effective against most of the common bacterial pathogens.[1] Available studies have most commonly employed the combination of trimethoprim and sulfamethoxazole for treating well-documented chronic bacterial prostatitis. Long treatment courses result in symptomatic and bacteriologic cure in approximately one third of patients, symptomatic improvement while receiving therapy in roughly another third of patients who relapse after therapy is stopped, and no improvement in the remaining patients.[10] The newer quinolones are promising alternative agents for treatment of bacterial prostatitis.[11, 12]

Bacteria isolated from patients with chronic bacterial prostatitis, even after multiple episodes of symptomatic bacteriuria and prolonged courses of antibiotics, are generally antibiotic-sensitive strains.[1, 10] However, *Escherichia coli* strains that cause prostatitis tend to possess urovirulence profiles similar to strains isolated from women with acute pyelonephritis, especially hemolysin and cytotoxic necrotizing factor,[13] with many strains exhibiting multiple virulence factors.[14] Several findings may explain the disappointing results with antibiotic therapy, including poor diffusion of many drugs into the prostatic parenchyma, changes in prostatic fluid pH level associated with infection, and infected calculi, which may serve as persistent foci for bacteria.[10]

Patients with chronic bacterial prostatitis who are not cured may be rendered asymptomatic by long-term, suppressive treatment. Because patients are usually asymptomatic between episodes of bacteriuria, the goal of suppressive therapy is to prevent symptomatic episodes despite the persistence of bacteria in the prostate. Very low doses of agents such as penicillin, tetracycline, nitrofurantoin, nalidixic acid, trimethoprim-sulfamethoxazole, or newer quinolones are remarkably effective in preventing episodes of symptomatic bladder infection in patients with chronic bacterial prostatitis.[1, 11]

Chronic Prostatitis/Chronic Pelvic Pain Syndrome

Patients with chronic prostatitis/chronic pelvic pain syndrome are the largest population of patients with prostatitis, representing more than 90% of patients evaluated in our clinic.[15] These patients have no history of bacteriuria and lack objective evidence of bacterial infection of their prostatic secretions on careful lower urinary tract localization studies (see Table 97–2).[16] Such patients may complain of a variety of perineal and pelvic symptoms, especially pain.[9, 17, 18] Pain or vague discomfort may be perineal, suprapubic, infrapubic, scrotal, or inguinal in location and may be exacerbated by ejaculation. Other complaints include voiding difficulty and erectile dysfunction. The discomfort may be described as either continuous or spasmodic and is commonly described as a "dull ache." Occasional patients complain of increased urinary frequency or dysuria, and ejaculatory complaints are common. Systemic symptoms or signs are absent. Physical examination is generally unremarkable. Some patients with chronic prostatitis/chronic pelvic pain syndrome have leukocytes in their expressed prostatic secretions, post–prostate massage urine (VB-3), or semen (in the inflammatory subtype, formerly termed "nonbacterial prostatitis"[1]) whereas others have no objective evidence of inflammation (in the noninflammatory subtype, formerly termed "prostatodynia"; see Table 97–2[9]).

The causes of chronic prostatitis/chronic pelvic pain syndrome remain uncertain. Mardh and Colleen[19] and Mardh and associates[20] found no evidence for an etiologic role for *Neisseria gonorrhoeae, Trichomonas vaginalis, Ureaplasma urealyticum, Mycoplasma hominis, Candida albicans,* anaerobic bacteria, *Chlamydia trachomatis,* or viruses in these syndromes. However, other researchers have reported that many patients with "subacute or chronic prostatitis" are infected with *C. trachomatis*[21–23] or *U. urealyticum.*[24] The techniques, control groups, and findings in these later studies have been questioned by other workers.[1, 25, 26] Some authorities have proposed that nonbacterial prostatitis is not an infectious disease.[17, 27] In poorly controlled studies, prostaglandins, autoimmunity, psychological abnormalities, neuromuscular dysfunction of the bladder neck or urogenital diaphragm, and allergy to environmental agents all have been suggested as etiologic factors.[28–31] Recent culture and molecular biology data suggest that patients with inflammatory chronic prostatitis are significantly more likely to have evidence of bacteria in their prostatic parenchyma than are patients with noninflammatory chronic prostatitis/chronic pelvic pain syndrome.[32, 33]

Current therapy for symptomatic patients with chronic prostatitis/chronic pelvic pain syndrome is unsatisfactory. There is little objective evidence that patients benefit from empirical antimicrobial therapy.

Asymptomatic Inflammatory Prostatitis

The new National Institutes of Health consensus classification of prostatitis includes a category for patients who have diagnosable prostatitis but who have no genitourinary tract symptoms. These patients have prostate inflammation but have none of the usual symptoms associated with other prostatitis syndromes. For example, it is common for patients with elevated prostate-specific antigen levels to undergo prostate biopsy for evaluation of possible prostate cancer.[34, 35] The most common benign pathologic diagnosis is "prostatitis," based on the histologic finding of inflammatory infiltrates in the prostatic parenchyma.[35] Some clinicians recommend a course of antimicrobial or anti-inflammatory therapy in this situation. These recommendations are based on the observations that acute bacterial prostatitis and exacerbations of chronic bacterial prostatitis are associated with elevations of both serum prostate-specific antigen and acid phosphatase. Whether antimicrobial therapy is beneficial for asymptomatic patients with histologic evidence of prostatitis remains uncertain.

Histologic evidence of prostatic inflammation may also be noted in patients with no clinical history of prostatitis who have benign prostate tissue removed during surgical procedures for treatment of bladder outflow obstruction. Animal studies suggest that chronic inflammation may promote prostatic hyperplasia.[36] Asymptomatic inflammatory prostatitis may be diagnosed among men undergoing evaluation for infertility (reviewed in ref. 37). Many of these men have no genitourinary tract symptoms. On semen analysis, increased numbers of "round cells" may prompt a diagnosis of prostatitis. Other terms used in the infertility literature include "asymptomatic male genital tract infection," "male accessory gland infection," "prostatoseminal vesiculitis," "leukocytospermia," and "pyosemia." Some specialists recommend antimicrobial therapy, but the proportion of these patients who have active genital tract infections is poorly defined.[37, 38] Thus, it would appear prudent to diagnose a specific genitourinary tract pathogen before recommending antimicrobial therapy for asymptomatic men who present for infertility evaluation.

Granulomatous Prostatitis

Granulomatous prostatitis is a characteristic histologic reaction of the prostate to a variety of insults, with granulomas containing lipid-laden histiocytes, plasma cells, and scattered giant cells. In most cases, granulomatous prostatitis follows an episode of acute bacterial prostatitis.[6, 39] There are also a number of specific infectious causes of granulomatous reaction by the prostate. Tuberculous prostatitis is usually secondary to tuberculosis elsewhere in the genital tract.[40, 41] Most patients have no symptoms referable to prostatic infection. At biopsy, the granulomas may contain typical Langhans giant cells and exhibit caseous necrosis. Such infections are caused most often by *Mycobacterium tuberculosis* but have also been reported with nontuberculous mycobacteria.[42] Iatrogenic mycobacterial prostatitis may develop in patients who receive with intravesicular Calmette-Guérin bacillus for treatment of transitional cell carcinoma of the bladder.[43, 44] Prostatitis may be secondary to systemic involvement with many of the deep mycoses.[45] Most cases of mycotic prostatitis reported have been associated with blastomycosis,[45] coccidioidomycosis,[46] and cryptococcosis.[47] The prostate may be a focus of persistent cryptococcosis in patients with acquired immunodeficiency syndrome (AIDS).[48] Rarely, prostatic histoplasmosis occurs in this population.[49]

Granulomatous prostatitis is most important in the differential diagnosis for an indurated, firm, or nodular prostate. Findings on rectal examination in such patients raise the suspicion of prostatic carcinoma. Biopsy is usually necessary for diagnosis, and it is important that appropriate stains be used for the detection of specific etiologic agents.

Prostatic Abscess

Prostatic abscess is a rare complication in patients who receive appropriate treatment for acute bacterial prostatitis.[50] Most prostatic abscesses occur in patients with diabetes, in immunocompromised patients, and in patients who have not received appropriate therapy for acute prostatitis.[51] Foreign bodies and urinary tract obstruction are other predisposing factors. In the past, *N. gonorrhoeae* was a common pathogen, but most cases are now caused by the common uropathogens. Infection generally occurs by the ascending route.[51] On occasion, *Staphylococcus aureus* is the pathogen, which suggests the possibility of hematogenous infection. Patients are usually febrile with irritative voiding symptoms, and they may have signs of urosepsis. Thus, the clinical presentation closely resembles that of acute bacterial prostatitis. Classically, the abscess presents as a fluctuant area in the prostate palpated during rectal examination. However, the presentation may be more subtle. The use of ultrasonography,[52] computed tomography,[53] or magnetic resonance imaging of the pelvis is helpful for confirming the diagnosis or in patients with equivocal clinical findings. Treatment includes draining the abscess, through either a perineal or a transurethral route, besides appropriate antimicrobial therapy.

EPIDIDYMITIS

Epididymitis is an inflammatory reaction of the epididymis to a variety of infectious agents or to local trauma. Epididymitis is common, accounting for over 600,000 visits to physicians per year in the United States. Acute epididymitis is responsible for more days lost from military service than any other disease and is responsible for 20% of urologic hospital admissions in military populations.[54]

Patients with epididymitis usually complain of painful swelling of the scrotum. The onset may be acute over 1 or 2 days or more gradual and is often accompanied by dysuria or irritative lower urinary tract symptoms. Many patients have a urethral discharge.[55] Specific attention should be directed to eliciting a past history of genitourinary tract disease or sexual exposure. Some patients may have only a nonspecific finding of fever or other signs of infection. This is particularly frequent in hospitalized patients who have undergone recent urinary tract manipulation and who may be obtunded by medication.

Tender swelling, frequently accompanied by erythema, generally unilateral, may be noted primarily in the posterior aspect of the scrotum. If the patient is examined early in the course of the disease, the swelling may be localized to one portion of the epididymis. Later, involvement of the ipsilateral testis is frequent, producing an epididymo-orchitis, and it may be difficult to distinguish the testicle from the epididymis within the inflammatory mass. Scrotal examination commonly reveals the presence of a hydrocele, caused by the secretion of inflammatory fluid between the layers of the tunica vaginalis. Urethral discharge may be apparent on inspection or "stripping" of the urethra.

There are two common types of epididymitis: nonspecific bacterial epididymitis and sexually transmitted epididymitis. In addition, epididymitis may occur rarely after genital trauma or with disseminated infections.

Nonspecific Bacterial Epididymitis

The most common cause of epididymitis in men over 35 years old is infection with coliform or *Pseudomonas* species.[55, 56] In most series, gram-negative aerobic rods caused over two thirds of the cases of bacterial epididymitis.[55–57] However, gram-positive cocci are also important pathogens and were the most common organisms in some reports.[58]

Many patients who develop bacterial epididymitis have underlying urologic pathology or have a history of recent genitourinary tract manipulation.[54, 55] The development of epididymitis after surgery or urethral catheterization may occur weeks or rarely months after the manipulation. Epididymitis is particularly likely in patients who undergo urinary tract surgery or instrumentation while they are bacteriuric. Acute and chronic bacterial prostatitis are other important predisposing conditions for the development of bacterial epididymitis.

Bacterial epididymitis may be an important focus of organisms causing bacteremia and local morbidity in patients with indwelling transurethral catheters. Genitourinary tract complications of acute bacterial epididymitis include testicular infarction, scrotal abscess, pyocele, a chronic draining scrotal sinus, chronic epididymitis, and infertility.[59, 60]

Tuberculous epididymitis is the most common manifestation of male genital tuberculosis, with orchitis and prostatitis less commonly seen. The usual symptom is a sensation of heaviness or swelling. There is characteristic scrotal swelling with "beadlike" enlargement of the vas deferens. Chronic draining scrotal sinuses may be a feature. The systemic mycoses may rarely cause epididymitis; blastomycetes are the most common pathogen and may also cause a draining sinus through the scrotal wall.

Medical management is appropriate for most patients with bacterial epididymitis. Initial empirical treatment with agents appropriate for both gram-negative rods and gram-positive cocci should be initiated pending urine culture and sensitivity results.[61] Nonspecific measures such as bed rest, scrotal elevation, analgesics, and local ice packs are helpful. Surgery may be necessary for management of complications of acute epididymal infections but has no role in treating tuberculous or fungal epididymitis.

Sexually Transmitted Epididymitis

Sexually transmitted epididymitis is the most common type of epididymitis in young men. *C. trachomatis* and *N. gonorrhoeae* are the major pathogens in this population.[61] Chlamydiae have been identified as the most common cause of epididymitis in younger, sexually active populations.[62] Such patients were formerly considered to have "idiopathic," nonspecific epididymitis. Berger and coworkers[55] documented infections with *C. trachomatis* in 17 of 34 cases of epididymitis in patients less than 35 years old and only 1 of 16 cases of epididymitis in patients older than 35. Patients with chlamydial epididymitis frequently do not complain of urethral discharge. However, 11 of 17 patients with epididymitis caused by chlamydiae had demonstrable discharge, usually the scant, watery discharge characteristic of nonspecific urethritis. The median interval from the last sexual exposure was 10 days, with a range of 1 to 45 days. Thus, patients may carry chlamydiae for long periods before the development of overt epididymitis.

Before the availability of penicillin, it was estimated that epididymitis occurred in 10 to 30% of men with gonococcal urethritis. In more recent studies, *N. gonorrhoeae* was identified as the cause of acute epididymitis in 16% of cases in military populations[63] and in 21% of cases of epididymitis in civilians less than 35 years old.[55] Many patients with gonococcal epididymitis do not have a history of urethral discharge, and a discharge may be demonstrable in only 50% of such patients.

Underlying genitourinary tract abnormalities are uncommon in patients with sexually transmitted epididymitis. Diagnosis depends on a high index of clinical suspicion, evaluation for presence of urethritis (which may be asymptomatic), and appropriate cultures. Specific antibiotic therapy, generally employing drugs appropriate for both chlamydial and gonococcal infections (i.e., tetracycline, 500 mg PO four times daily for at least 10 days), is the most important aspect of treatment.[60, 61, 64] Patients should be evaluated for other sexually transmitted diseases (STDs), and treatment of sexual partners is important. In general, a complete urologic workup is not indicated for patients with uncomplicated sexually transmitted epididymitis. Complications of sexually transmitted epididymitis include abscess formation, testicular infarction, chronic epididymitis, and infertility. Ultrasonography, particularly color-flow Doppler ultrasonography, is useful for the differential diagnosis of complicated cases of epididymitis.[65, 66]

Follow-up. Failure of the signs and symptoms of epididymitis to subside within 3 days requires reevaluation of both the diagnosis and the therapy.[61] Persistent swelling and tenderness after completion of therapy suggest the need for comprehensive evaluation. Considerations in the differential diagnosis include abscess, infarction, testicular cancer, and tuberculous or fungal epididymitis.

ORCHITIS

Orchitis is significantly less common than either prostatitis or epididymitis. Orchitis differs from infections of the male accessory sex glands in two important respects: blood-borne dissemination is the major route of infection, and viruses are clearly implicated as important pathogens.

Viral Orchitis

Viral infections, particularly mumps, are associated with most cases of orchitis. Although mumps rarely causes orchitis in prepubertal boys, orchitis occurs in approximately 20% of postpubertal patients with mumps.[67] Testicular pain and swelling usually begin 4 to 6 days after the onset of parotitis but may occur without parotid involvement. Orchitis is unilateral in approximately 70% of cases. Contralateral testicular swelling may occur 1 to 9 days after involvement of the first side. The clinical course is variable and ranges from mild testicular discomfort and swelling to severe testicular pain and marked swelling accompanied by nausea, vomiting, prostration, high fever, and constitutional symptoms. Epididymitis and inflammation of the spermatic cord may be noted on physical examination. Resolution of mild cases may occur in 4 to 5 days. More severe cases usually resolve in 3 to 4 weeks. In approximately half of the cases, the involved testes undergo some degree of atrophy. In older series, sterility was reported in 25% of patients with bilateral disease. However, more recent studies have found that mumps orchitis seldom results in infertility.[67] Coxsackie B virus produces a disease that clinically and histologically resembles mumps orchitis.

Bacterial Orchitis

With the exception of viral diseases, acute genitourinary tract infections involving only the testis are distinctly unusual. Pyogenic bacterial orchitis usually occurs because of the contiguous spread from an inflammatory process in the epididymis to cause an epididymo-orchitis. Thus, most cases of pyogenic orchitis are caused by *Escherichia coli, Klebsiella pneumoniae, Pseudomonas aeruginosa,* staphylococci, or streptococci. Occasionally, acute orchitis may be caused by other organisms as a result of metastatic seeding.

The patient with pyogenic orchitis appears acutely ill, with a high fever and marked discomfort and swelling of the involved testicle. Generally the pain is described as radiating to the inguinal canal, and it is frequently accompanied by nausea and vomiting. On examination, there is usually an acute hydrocele, and the testis is swollen and exquisitely tender. The overlying scrotal skin is generally erythematous and edematous. Complications of pyogenic bacterial orchitis include testicular infarction, abscess formation, and pyocele of the scrotum.[60] Surgery is usually required for treatment of these conditions. Orchitis can be caused by tuberculosis and blastomycosis, but by extension from the epididymis. Involvement of the testicle without palpable abnormality in the adjacent epididymis has rarely been observed with these agents.

PROSTATITIS, EPIDIDYMITIS, AND ORCHITIS IN MEN WITH HUMAN IMMUNODEFICIENCY VIRUS TYPE 1 INFECTION

One study of 80 autopsied AIDS patients found that 2 of 11 cases with systemic toxoplasmosis involved the testes; 4 of 48 cases of systemic cytomegalovirus infection involved the prostate, and 1 involved the testes; and 1 of 27 cases of systemic candidiasis involved the prostate.[68] Other opportunistic infections involving the male genital tract include those due to *Mycobacterium avium* complex,[69] cryptococcosis,[70] toxoplasmosis,[71] *Haemophilus parainfluenzae* infections,[72] candidiasis,[73] and *Aspergillus fumigatus* infections.[74] The testes characteristically exhibit azospermia, marked spermatogenic arrest, germ cell degeneration, peritubular fibrosis, and Leydig cell depletion. These nonspecific findings probably reflect the severe systemic disease in these patients. Focal accumulations of leukocytes in the connective tissue stroma of the testes and epididymides may represent a portal of entry for human immunodeficiency virus type 1 (HIV-1) into the semen.[75]

Urologic Manifestations

Other urologic manifestations in patients with AIDS and HIV-1 infections reflect involvement of related organ systems. For example, bladder dysfunction may occur in patients with HIV-1–associated neurologic disorders. Such bladder dysfunction increases the risk of urinary tract infection. Urinary tract infections were diagnosed in 14 to 20% of HIV-1–seropositive patients.[76, 77] In another study, bacterial prostatitis was diagnosed in 17 (8%) of 209 men hospitalized for treatment of HIV-1–related infections.[78] The most common presentation of prostatitis was fever plus irritative lower tract symptoms associated with bacteriuria.

Semen

The relative contributions of behavioral and clinical risk factors to transmission of HIV-1 are incompletely understood, but clearly, sexual activity alone provides a limited explanation for transmission of HIV. Expressing risk as a function of frequency and types of sexual contacts has not yielded straightforward patterns.[79–82] This probably reflects biologic factors that determine infectiousness as well as the vulnerable partner's susceptibility.[83] Stage of disease and viral load,[84] viral characteristics such as syncytia-inducing capability, and antiviral treatment have been linked to greater and lesser degrees of infectivity.[85, 86]

A number of studies document that treating other STDs reduces sexual transmission of HIV.[82, 87–89] Such infections are believed to increase susceptibility to HIV infection by recruiting target cells and disrupting epithelial barriers. In addition, genital ulcer diseases and urethritis (both gonococcal and nongonococcal) increase the HIV viral load in semen. In contrast, STD treatment reduces HIV shedding.

Epidemiologic studies suggest that direct contact with semen is the most important route for sexual transmission of HIV-1.[69, 75] HIV-1 was first isolated by cocultivation of seminal cells and donor lymphocytes.[90, 91] Shedding of HIV-1 in semen was associated with no significant changes in semen parameters that assess fertility in one study of 50 semen specimens from asymptomatic or minimally symptomatic HIV-1–seropositive men.[92] In contrast, three men with AIDS all had pyosemia and grossly abnormal sperm. Thus, abnormalities in HIV-1–seropositive men's semen reflect severity of disease and therapies that are toxic to the seminiferous epithelium but do not correlate with seminal shedding of HIV-1.

Semen is composed of cell-free seminal plasma and seminal cells (mature spermatozoa, immature sperm forms, leukocytes, and epithelial cells). Two types of approach have been used to determine the likely sources of HIV within the semen. The first approach is to fractionate and analyze ejaculated semen specimens.[93–96] These studies suggest that most viable (i.e., culturable) HIV in semen is cell-associated, particularly with T lymphocytes and macrophages but not with motile spermatozoa. The second approach is anatomic, based on the observations that vasectomy causes dramatic reductions in seminal cells and also eliminates secretions from proximal sites in the male reproductive tract.[97] HIV RNA was assayed in seminal plasma and HIV DNA in seminal cells from 46 asymptomatic, seropositive men before and after vasectomy. Vasectomy produced no significant change in HIV RNA or HIV DNA levels, supporting the conclusion that most seminal HIV is not associated with germinal cells but arises from distal sites in the male reproductive tract.

Several lines of evidence support the idea that the male genital tract may be distinct from the systemic immune compartment.[98–101] Qualitative and quantitative virologic measurements between blood and genital compartments suggest lack of association between culturability of virus in semen and viral RNA level in blood, discordant distribution of phenotypes, discordant viral RNA levels, a weak correlation between viral RNA level in semen and $CD4^+$ cell count in blood, differences in the biologic variability of viral RNA levels, and differences in the viral load response to antiretroviral therapy.[98] Some but not all studies suggest a weak correlation between HIV-1 RNA levels in the blood plasma and HIV RNA levels in the seminal plasma. However, neither HIV-1 RNA blood level nor the $CD4^+$ count reliably predicts either shedding of culturable virus or detection of viral RNA in the semen.[98, 99, 101–103] Factors that may influence the HIV viral load in seminal fluid include systemic illness, antiretroviral therapy, male genital tract inflammation, reactivation of genital herpes virus infection, and seminal shedding of cytomegalovirus or other viruses.[88, 89, 101, 102, 104] If the male reproductive tract is indeed a distinct immunologic compartment, then factors determining infectiousness of semen may differ substantially from the factors determining HIV levels in blood, lymphatic tissue, or central nervous system.[98, 100, 101]

REFERENCES

1. Stamey TA. Pathogenesis and Treatment of Urinary Tract Infections. Baltimore: Williams & Wilkins; 1980:1, 342.
2. Fair WR, Couch J, Wehner N. Prostatic antibacterial factor: Identity and significance. Urology. 1976;7:169.
3. Meares EM Jr. Prostatitis syndromes: New perspectives about old woes. J Urol. 1980;123:141.
4. Shortliffe LMD, Wehner N, Stamey TA. Use of solid-phase radioimmunoassay and formalin-fixed whole bacterial antigen in the detection of antigen-specific immunoglobulin in prostatic fluid. J Clin Invest. 1981;67:780.
5. Schaeffer AJ, Wendel EF, Dunn JK, et al. Prevalence and significance of prostatic inflammation. J Urol. 1981;125:215.
6. Krieger JN. Prostatitis syndromes: Pathophysiology, differential diagnosis and treatment. Sex Transm Dis. 1984;11:100.
7. Drabick JJ, Gambel JM, Mackey JF. Prostatodynia in the United Nations peacekeeping forces in Haiti. Mil Med. 1997;162:380–383.
8. McNaughton-Collins M, Stafford RS, O'Leary MP, Barry MJ. How common is prostatitis? A national survey of physician visits. J Urol. 1998;159:1224–1228.
9. Krieger JN, Egan KJ, Ross SO, et al. Chronic pelvic pains represent the most

prominent urogenital symptoms of "chronic prostatitis." Urology. 1996;48:715–721.
10. Fair WR, Crane DB, Schiller N, et al. Re-appraisal of treatment in chronic bacterial prostatitis. J Urol. 1979;121:437.
11. Naber KG: Use of quinolones in urinary tract infections and prostatitis. Rev Infect Dis. 1989:11(Suppl 5):S1321.
12. Weidner W, Schiefer HG, Brahler E: Refractory chronic bacterial prostatitis: A re-evaluation of ciprofloxacin treatment after a median followup of 30 months. J Urol. 146:350.
13. Andreu A, Fernandez F, Stamm WE. Urovirulence determinants in *Escherichia coli* strains causing prostatitis. J Infect Dis. 1997;176:464–469.
14. Terai A, Yamamoto S, Mitsumori K, et al. *Escherichia coli* virulence factors and serotypes in acute bacterial prostatitis. Int J Urol. 1997;4:289–294.
15. Krieger JN, Egan KJ. Comprehensive evaluation and treatment of 75 men referred to chronic prostatitis clinic. Urology. 1991;38:11–19.
16. Drach GW, Meares EM, Fair WR, et al. Classification of benign diseases associated with prostatic pain: Prostatitis or prostatodynia? J Urol. 1978;120:266.
17. Egan KJ, Krieger JN. Chronic abacterial prostatitis—a urological chronic pain syndrome. Pain. 1997;69:213–218.
18. Moon TD. Questionnaire survey of urologists and primary care physicians' diagnostic and treatment practices for prostatitis. Urology. 1997;50:543–547.
19. Mardh PA, Colleen S. Search for uro-genital tract infections in patients with symptoms of prostatitis. Scand J Urol Nephrol. 1975;9:8.
20. Mardh PA, Ripa KT, Colleen S, et al. Role of *Chlamydia trachomatis* in nonacute prostatitis. Br J Vener Dis. 1978;54:330.
21. Weidner W, Arens M, Krauss H, et al. *Chlamydia trachomatis* in "abacterial" prostatitis: Microbiological, cytological, and serological studies. Urol Int. 1983;38:146.
22. Poletti F, Medici MC, Alinovi A, et al. Isolation of *Chlamydia trachomatis* from the prostatic cells in patients affected by nonacute abacterial prostatitis. J Urol. 1985;134:691.
23. Bruce AW, Chadwick P, Willet WS, O'Shaughnesey M. The role of chlamydiae in genitourinary disease. J Urol. 1981;126:625.
24. Weidner W, Brunner H, Krause W. Quantitative culture of *Ureaplasma urealyticum* in patients with chronic prostatitis or prostatosis. J Urol. 1980;124:622.
25. Schacter J. Is *Chlamydia trachomatis* a cause of prostatitis? J Urol. 1985;134:711.
26. Doble A, Walker TMM, Harris JRW, et al. The role of *Chlamydia trachomatis* in chronic abacterial prostatitis: A study using ultrasound guided biopsy. J Urol. 1989;141:332.
27. Segura JW, Opitz JL, Green L. Prostatosis prostatitis or pelvic floor tension myalgia? J Urol. 1979;122:168.
28. Nickel JC. Prostatitis: Myths and realities. Urology. 1998;51:362–366.
29. Mayo ME, Ross SO, Krieger JN. Few patients with "chronic prostatitis" have significant bladder outlet obstruction. Urology. 1998;52(3):417–421.
30. Orsilles MA, Depiante-Depaoli M. Oxidative stress–related parameters in prostate of rats with experimental autoimmune prostatitis. Prostate. 1998;34:270–274.
31. Barbalais GA, Nikiforidis G, Liatsikos EN. Alpha-blockers for the treatment of chronic prostatitis in combination with antibiotics. J Urol. 1998;159:883–887.
32. Krieger JN, Riley DE, Roberts MC, Berger RE. Prokaryotic DNA sequences in patients with chronic idiopathic prostatitis. J Clin Microbiol. 1996;34:3120–3128.
33. Berger RE, Krieger JN, Rathman I, Muller CH. Bacteria in the prostate tissue of men with idiopathic prostatic inflammation. J Urol. 1997;157:863–865.
34. Tchetgen MB, Oesterling JE. The effect of prostatitis, urinary retention, ejaculation, and ambulation on the serum prostate-specific antigen concentration. Urol Clin North Am. 1997;24:283–291.
35. Ornstein DK, Smith DS, Humphrey PA, Catalona WJ. The effect of prostate volume, age, total prostate specific antigen level and acute inflammation on the percentage of free serum prostate specific antigen levels in men without clinically detectable prostate cancer. J Urol. 1998;159:1234–1237.
36. Kessler OJ, Keiseri Y, Servadio C, Abramovici A. Role of chronic inflammation in the promotion of prostatic hyperplasia in rats. J Urol. 1998;159:1049–1053.
37. Krieger JN, Berger RE, Ross SO, et al. Seminal fluid findings in men with nonbacterial prostatitis and prostatodynia. J Androl. 1996;17:310–318.
38. Branigan EF, Muller CH. Efficacy of treatment and recurrence rate of leukocytospermia in infertile men with prostatitis. Fertil Steril. 1994;62:P580–P584.
39. Stillwell TJ, Engen DE, Farrow GM. The clinical spectrum of granulomatous prostatitis: A report of 200 cases. J Urol. 1987;138:320.
40. Venema RJ, Lattimer, JK. Genital tuberculosis in the male. J Urol. 1957;78:65.
41. Simon HB. Genitourinary tuberculosis: Clinical features in a general hospital population. Am J Med. 1977;63:410.
42. Brooker WJ, Aufderheide AC. Genitourinary tract infections due to atypical mycobacteria. J Urol. 1980;124:242.
43. Oates RD, Stilmant MM, Freedlund MC, Siroky MB. Granulomatous prostatitis following bacillus Calmette-Guérin immunotherapy for bladder cancer. J Urol. 1988;140:751.
44. Miyashita H, Troncoso P, Babaian RJ. BCG-induced granulomatous prostatitis: A comparative ultrasound and pathologic study. Urology. 1992;39:364.
45. Inoshita T, Youngberg GA, Boelen LJ, Langston J. Blastomycosis presenting with prostatic involvement: Report of 2 cases and review of the literature. J Urol. 1983;130:160–216.
46. Price MJ, Lewis EL, Carmalt JE. Coccidioidomycosis of prostate gland. Urology. 1982;19:653.
47. Hinchley WW, Someren A. Cryptococcal prostatitis. Am J Clin Pathol. 1981;75:257.
48. Bozzette SA, Larsen RA, Chiu J, et al. Fluconazole treatment of persistent *Cryptococcus neoformans* prostatic infection in AIDS. Ann Intern Med. 1991;115:285–286.
49. Zighelboim J, Goldfarb RA, Mody D, et al. Prostatic abscess due to *Histoplasma capsulatum* in a patient with the acquired immunodeficiency syndrome. J Urol. 1992;147:166.
50. Meares EM Jr. Prostatic abscess. J Urol. 1986;136:1281.
51. Weinberger M, Cytron S, Servadio C, et al. Prostatic abscess in the antibiotic era. Rev Infect Dis. 1988;10:239.
52. Suago H, Takiuchi H, Sakurai T. Transrectal longitudinal ultrasonography of prostatic abscess. J Urol. 1986;136:1316.
53. Vaccaro JA, Belville WD, Kiesling VJ Jr, et al. Prostatic abscesses: Computerized tomography scanning as an aid to diagnosis and treatment. J Urol. 1986;136:1318.
54. Bormel P. Current concepts on the etiology and treatment of epididymitis. Med Bull US Army Europe. 1963;20:332.
55. Berger RE, Alexander ER, Harnisch JP, et al. Etiology, manifestations and therapy of acute epididymitis: Prospective study of 50 cases. J Urol. 1979;121:750.
56. Berger RE, Alexander ER, Monda GD, et al. *Chlamydia trachomatis* as a cause of acute "idiopathic" epididymitis. N Engl J Med. 1978;298:301.
57. Mittemeyer BT, Lennox KW, Borski AA. Epididymitis—a review of 610 cases. J Urol. 1966;95:390.
58. Nilsson S, Obrant KD, Persson PS. Changes in the testes parenchyma caused by acute nonspecific epididymitis. Fertil Steril. 1968;19:748.
59. Witherington R, Harper WM IV. The surgical management of acute bacterial epididymitis with emphasis on epididymotomy. J Urol. 1982;128:722.
60. Krieger JN. Epididymitis, orchitis, and related conditions. Sex Transm Dis. 1984;11:173.
61. Centers for Disease Control and Prevention. 1998 guidelines for treatment of sexually transmitted diseases. MMWR Morbid Mortal Wkly Rep. 1998;47(RR-1):1–111.
62. Harnisch JP, Berger RE, Alexander ER, et al. Aetiology of acute epididymitis. Lancet. 1977;1:819.
63. Watson RA. Gonorrhea and acute epididymitis. Milit Med. 1979;144:785.
64. Drotman PD. Epidemiology and treatment of epididymitis. Rev Infect Dis. 1982;4(Suppl):788.
65. Krieger JN, Wang K, Mack L. Preliminary evaluation of color Doppler imaging for investigation of intrascrotal pathology. J Urol. 1990;140:904.
66. Erden MI, Ozbeck SS, et al. Color-Doppler imaging in acute scrotal disorders. Urol Int. 1993;50:39.
67. Beard CM, Benson RC, Kelalis PP, et al. The incidence and outcome of mumps orchitis in Rochester, Minn. Mayo, 1935–1974. Mayo Clin Proc. 1977;52:3.
68. Shevchuk M, de Silza M, Armenakas N, et al. The male genital tract in AIDS. J Urol. 141:354, 1989.
69. Mikolich DJ, Mates SM. Granulomatous prostatitis due to *Mycobacterium avium* complex. Clin Infect Dis. 1992;14:589.
70. Adams JRJ, Mata JA, Culkin DJ, et al. Acquired immunodeficiency syndrome manifesting as prostate nodule secondary to cryptococcal infection. Urology. 1992;39:289.
71. Haskell L, Fusco MJ, Ares L. Disseminated toxoplasmosis presenting as symptomatic orchitis and nephrotic syndrome. Am J Med Sci. 1989;298:185.
72. Clairmont GJ, Zon LI, Groopman JE. *Hemophilus parainfluenzae* prostatitis in a homosexual man with chronic lymphadenopathy syndrome and HTLV-III infection. Am J Med. 1987;82:175.
73. Swartz DA, Harrington P, Wilcox R. Candidal epididymitis treated with ketoconazole. N Engl J Med. 1988;319:1485.
74. Hood SV, Bell D, McVey R, et al. Prostatitis and epididymo-orchitis due to *Aspergillus fumigatus* in a patient with AIDS. Clin Infect Dis. 1998;26:229–231.
75. Pudney J, Anderson D. Orchitis and human immunodeficiency virus type 1–infected cells in reproductive tissues from men with the acquired immune deficiency syndrome. Am J Pathol. 1991;139:149.
76. Miles BJ, Melser M, Farah R, et al. The urological manifestations of the acquired immunodeficiency syndrome. J Urol. 1989;142:771.
77. Kaplan MS, Wechsler M, Benson MC. Urologic manifestations of AIDS. Urology. 30:1987.
78. Leport C, Rousseau F, Perronne C, et al. Bacterial prostatitis in patients infected with the human immunodeficiency virus. J Urol. 1989;141:334.
79. Skurnick JH, Kennedy CA, Perez G, et al. Behavioral and demographic risk factors for transmission of human immunodeficiency virus type 1 in heterosexual couples: Report from the heterosexual HIV transmission study. Clin Infect Dis. 1998;26:855–864.
80. Padian NS, Shiboski SC, Jewell NP. The effect of number of exposures on the risk of heterosexual HIV transmission. J Infect Dis. 1990;161:883–887.
81. Downs AM, DeVincenzi I, for the European Study Group on Heterosexual Transmission of HIV. Probability of heterosexual transmission of HIV: Relationship to the number of unprotected sexual contacts. J Acquir Immune Defic Syndr Hum Retrovirol. 1996;11:388–396.
82. Deschamps M-M, Pape JW, Hafner A, Johnson WD Jr. Heterosexual transmission of HIV in Haiti. Ann Intern Med. 1996;125:324–330.
83. Holmberg SD, Horsburgh CR, Jr, Ward JW, Jaffe HW. Biologic factors in the sexual transmission of human immunodeficiency virus. J Infect Dis. 1989;160:116–125.
84. Saracco A, Musicco M, Nicolosi A, et al. Man-to-woman sexual transmission of HIV: Longitudinal study of 343 steady partners of infected men. J Acquir Immune Defic Syndr. 1993;6:497–502.
85. Conlon CP, Klenerman P, Edwards A, et al. Heterosexual transmission of human

immunodeficiency virus type 1 variants associated with ziduvidine resistance. J Infect Dis. 1994;169:411–415.
86. Musicco M, Lazzarin A, Nicolosi A, et al. Antiretroviral treatment of men infected with human immunodeficiency virus type 1 reduces the incidence of heterosexual transmission. Italian Study Group on HIV Heterosexual Transmission. Arch Intern Med. 1994;154:1971–1976.
87. Figuerosa JP, Brathwaite A, Morris J, et al. Rising HIV-1 prevalence among sexually transmitted disease clinic attenders in Jamaica: Traumatic sex and genital ulcers as risk factors. J Acquir Immune Defic Syndr. 1994;7:310–316.
88. Cohen MS, Hoffman IF, Royce RA, et al. Reduction of concentration of HIV-1 in semen after treatment of urethritis: Implications for prevention of sexual transmission of HIV-1. Lancet. 1997;349:1868–1873.
89. Moss GB, Overbaugh J, Welch M, et al. Human immunodeficiency virus DNA in urethral secretions in men: Association with gonococcal urethritis and CD4+ cell depletion. J Infect Dis. 1995;172:1469–1474.
90. Ho DD, Schooley R, Rota T, et al. HTLV-III in the semen and blood of a healthy homosexual man. Science. 1984;226:451.
91. Zagury D, et al. Evidence for HTLV-III in T-cells from semen of AIDS patients. Cancer Res. 1985;45(S):4595.
92. Krieger JN, Coombs RW, Collier AC, et al. Fertility parameters in men infected with human immunodeficiency virus. J Infect Dis. 1991;164:464.
93. Delwart EL, Mullins JI, Gupta P, et al. Human immunodeficiency virus type 1 populations in blood and semen. J Virol. 1998;72:617–623.
94. Quayle AJ, Xu C, Mayer KH, Anderson DJ. T lymphocytes and macrophages, but not motile spermatozoa, are a significant source of human immunodeficiency virus in semen. J Infect Dis. 1997;176:960–968.
95. Hamed KA, Winters MA, Holodiy MA, et al. Detection of human immunodeficiency virus type 1 in semen: Effects of disease stage and nucleoside therapy. J Infect Dis. 1993;167:798–802.
96. Krieger JN, Coombs RW, Collier AC, et al. Recovery of human immunodeficiency virus type 1 from semen: Minimal impact of stage of infection and current antiviral chemotherapy. J Infect Dis. 1991;163:386.
97. van Voorhis BJ, Martinez A, Mayer K, Anderson DJ. Detection of human immunodeficiency virus type 1 in semen from seropositive men using culture and polymerase chain reaction deoxyribonucleic acid amplification techniques. Fertil Steril. 1991;55:588–594.
98. Coombs RW, Speck CE, Hughes JP, et al. Association between culturable human immunodeficiency virus type 1 (HIV-1) in semen and HIV-1 RNA levels in semen and blood: Evidence for compartmentalization of HIV-1 between semen and blood. J Infect Dis. 1998;177:320–330.
99. Liuzzi G, Chirianni A, Clementi M, et al. Analysis of HIV-1 load in blood, semen and saliva: Evidence for different viral compartments in a cross-sectional and longitudinal study. AIDS. 1996;10:F51–F56.
100. Zhu T, Wang N, Carr A, et al. Genetic characterization of human immunodeficiency virus type 1 in blood and genital secretions: Evidence for viral compartmentalization and selection during sexual transmission. J Virol. 1996;70:3098–3107.
101. Krieger JN, Coombs RW, Collier AC, et al. Seminal shedding of human immunodeficiency virus type 1 and human cytomegalovirus: Evidence for different immunological controls. J Infect Dis. 1995;171:1018–1022.
102. Anderson DJ, O'Brien TR, Politch JA, et al. Effects of disease stage and zidovudine therapy on the detection of human immunodeficiency virus type 1 in semen. JAMA. 1992;267:2769.
103. Gupta P, Mellors J, Kingsley L, et al. High viral load in semen of human immunodeficiency virus type 1–infected men at all stages of disease and its reduction by therapy with protease and nonnucleoside reverse transcriptase inhibitors. J Virol. 1997;71:6271–6275.
104. Dyer JR, Eron JJ, Hoffman IF, et al. Association of CD4+ cell depletion and elevated blood and seminal plasma human immunodeficiency virus type 1 (HIV-1) RNA concentrations with genital ulcer disease in HIV-1–infected men in Malawi. J Infect Dis. 1998;177:224–227.

SECTION M

EYE INFECTIONS

Chapter 98

Conjunctivitis

TERRENCE P. O'BRIEN

The conjunctiva is a nonkeratinized, goblet cell–containing, stratified squamous epithelium with an underlying substantia propria. Conjunctivitis is the most common ocular inflammation; it involves all ages and occurs worldwide. The principal causes of acute conjunctivitis are infections, allergens, and irritative substances. Acute conjunctivitis is defined by onset within 3 weeks of presentation. Chronic conjunctivitis is defined by persistence for at least 3 weeks. Accurate diagnosis and management of conjunctivitis requires differentiation between an acute or chronic pace of inflammation, identification of any precipitating events, consideration of the role of any antecedent medications, and use of the principal ocular signs with identification of the key distinctive conjunctival signs. The principal clinical signs in patients with conjunctivitis include skin and mucous membrane involvement, orbital involvement, regional lymphadenopathy, type and amount of conjunctival discharge, morphologic pattern of conjunctival inflammation, and type of corneal epithelial or stromal abnormality. Infectious conjunctivitis may cause significant morbidity, depending in part on the type of invading organism and local ocular defense mechanisms. The many organisms that can cause conjunctivitis are listed in Table 98–1.

CLINICAL MANIFESTATIONS

The clinical findings and the course of infection are influenced by the pathogenic features of the exogenous microorganisms. The most obvious clinical manifestation of conjunctivitis is hyperemia of the conjunctiva. The dilatation and congestion of the vessels are greater near the periphery of the bulbar conjunctiva and become less marked as the corneal margin (limbus) is approached.

The presence of secretion is almost always a feature of conjunctivitis. It is caused by an exudation of inflammatory cells and a fibrin-rich, edematous fluid from the blood. The exudate is combined with denuded epithelial cells and mucus. The secretion may be purulent, mucopurulent, fibrinous, or serosanguineous, depending on the cause and severity of the disease. When the exudate dries, the eyelids may stick together. Conjunctival edema (chemosis) may be present in parts of the conjunctiva that are freely movable over the globe and lids. The normal transparency of the conjunctiva may be lost, and it may appear thickened because of the infiltration of the tissues with leukocytes. If there is diffuse leukocytic infiltration of the conjunctival stroma with hyperplasia of the overlying epithelium, papillae may form. A papilla contains a central blood vessel in its core. This vessel branches on the surface of the papilla. Papillae usually occur in the tarsal conjunctiva. The conjunctiva may have a velvety appearance from numerous small papillae. When large, the papillae have the appearance of cobblestone excrescences. This is unusual in acute infectious conjunctivitis but more common in allergic and chronic conjunctivitis. Papillae are nonspecific conjunctival signs but are most commonly observed with bacterial infection and allergy.

The conjunctiva contains lymphatic tissue that may be stimulated by various microbial antigens to form a follicle. A normal conjunctiva has an occasional follicle in its substantia propria, especially in the fornices. In certain forms of conjunctivitis, especially viral, chlamydial, or toxic, a follicular reaction may predominate. Follicles and papillae are differentiated clinically by appearance, with follicles resembling smooth, glistening bumps and papillae being smaller (<1 mm) and red with a central vascular core.

Membrane formation is also seen in some cases of conjunctivitis, especially with viral and some bacterial causes. This membrane consists of a superficial fibrinous layer connected to subconjunctival granulation tissue. When this membrane is excised, a raw, bleeding surface is exposed.

Corneal involvement may occur in conjunctivitis, especially viral conjunctivitis, owing to the close proximity of the corneal epithelium to the inflamed tarsal and limbal conjunctivae. Symptoms of corneal involvement include a gritty foreign-body sensation, photophobia, diminished vision, and pain. The various forms of conjunctivitis have many of the aforementioned signs and symptoms in common. Awareness of the principal ocular signs with selection of the most

TABLE 98–1 Etiologic Agents of Conjunctivitis

Bacteria
- *Streptococcus pneumoniae*
- *Streptococcus pyogenes*
- Streptococci of the viridans group
- *Staphylococcus aureus*
- *Haemophilus influenzae* (includes *Haemophilus aegyptius*)
- *Neisseria gonorrhoeae*
- *Haemophilus ducreyi*
- *Neisseria meningitidis*
- *Proteus vulgaris*
- *Moraxella lacunata*
- *Corynebacterium diphtheriae*
- *Mycobacterium tuberculosis*
- *Francisella tularensis*
- *Treponema pallidum*
- *Moraxella catarrhalis*
- *Shigella flexneri*
- *Yersinia enterocolitica*
- *Staphylococcus epidermidis*
- *Acinetobacter* spp.
- *Aeromonas hydrophila*
- *Peptostreptococcus*
- *Bartonella (Rochalimaea) henselae* (cat-scratch bacillus)

Viruses
- Adenoviruses
- Poxviruses (variola, vaccinia, molluscum contagiosum)
- Herpesviruses (herpes simplex, varicella-zoster, Epstein-Barr virus)
- Papillomaviruses
- Influenza A and B viruses
- Paramyxoviruses (measles, mumps, Newcastle disease virus)
- Picornaviruses (echovirus, enterovirus, coxsackievirus, and poliovirus)

Chlamydia trachomatis

Fungi
- *Candida* spp.
- *Sporothrix schenckii*
- *Rhinosporidium seeberi*

Parasites
- *Onchocerca volvulus*
- *Loa loa*
- *Wuchereria bancrofti*
- *Oestrus ovis* (myiasis)
- Microsporidiosis
  - *Nosema* spp.
  - *Encephalitozoon* spp.
- *Toxocara canis*

distinctive conjunctival sign can narrow the differential diagnosis and guide more specific therapy.

Bacterial Conjunctivitis

Bacterial conjunctivitis is a common type of ocular infection. Typically, pathogenesis involves exogenous routes of infection via airborne fomites, contact with upper respiratory tract infections, hand-to-eye contact, and contact with genital secretions. Less frequently, contiguous infection may spread to the conjunctiva from the face, eyelids, lacrimal drainage apparatus, or paranasal sinuses. Hematogenous routes of infection in acute bacterial conjunctivitis are rare.

The principal causes of acute bacterial conjunctivitis in the normal host include *Staphylococcus aureus, Streptococcus pneumoniae, Neisseria gonorrhoeae,* and *Haemophilus influenzae.* Age-related factors are important determinants of causative organisms. In neonates, clinical signs are altered by the immature immune system. In the newborn, *Chlamydia trachomatis* and *N. gonorrhoeae* are the most common causes.[1, 2] *Neisseria cinerea* can cause conjunctivitis in neonates or very young children and may be misidentified as *N. gonorrhoeae.*[3] In young children, *H. influenzae* can cause severe conjunctivitis.[4, 5] Successful immunization with conjugated vaccine may be protective against *H. influenzae* type B conjunctivitis. *Streptococcus pneumoniae, Pseudomonas aeruginosa,* and *S. aureus* may also cause acute conjunctivitis in neonates or children.[6, 7] In sexually active teenagers and adults, *C. trachomatis* and *N. gonorrhoeae* are encountered.

In adults, the most common bacterial isolates from an acute conjunctivitis are *S. pneumoniae, S. aureus,* and perhaps *Staphylococcus epidermidis.*[8] Although leptospirosis commonly causes conjunctival suffusion, this infection is a rare cause of actual conjunctivitis. Staphylococcal toxic shock is also accompanied by conjunctival suffusion without exudate. Although *C. trachomatis* clearly causes chronic conjunctivitis, whether other organisms play a role is unclear.[9]

Investigations into the cause of institutional outbreaks of bacterial conjunctivitis have encountered *Serratia marcescens,*[10] *S. pneumoniae, P. aeruginosa,*[11] and *Moraxella* spp.[12] *H. influenzae* biogroup *aegyptius* has caused community outbreaks of purulent conjunctivitis in children, followed by sepsis. Because the disease was encountered in rural Brazil and was accompanied by petechiae, the illness was originally called Brazilian purpuric fever (see Chapter 212).

In acute bacterial conjunctivitis, it is helpful to assess the severity of inflammation based on the rate of evolution of certain distinctive signs, including corneal involvement. In less severe bacterial conjunctivitis, there is minimal to no lid edema, scant purulent discharge with mild to moderate conjunctival hyperemia, and a normal cornea. In contrast, severe conjunctivitis is characterized often by marked lid edema with copious purulent discharge, marked conjunctival hyperemia, chemosis, membrane formation, and suppurative or nonsuppurative keratitis.

The principal causes of less severe bacterial conjunctivitis are *S. aureus, S. pneumoniae, Haemophilus* spp. in older children, and *Moraxella* spp. Severe bacterial conjunctivitis is most often caused by *Neisseria* spp., *H. influenzae* in young children, *Streptococcus pyogenes,* and *S. aureus.*

Severe conjunctivitis caused by *N. gonorrhoeae*[13] or *Neisseria meningitidis*[14] deserves special recognition. Infection with *Neisseria* may result in markedly swollen eyelids, extreme hyperemia and chemosis, and a profuse purulent discharge.[13] The massively swollen conjunctiva, infiltrated with polymorphonuclear neutrophils, may become draped over the peripheral cornea at the limbus. The action of lytic enzymes from the neutrophils can cause serious complications in untreated gonococcal conjunctivitis, including corneal ulceration with subsequent perforation. Occasionally, gonococcal conjunctivitis has a prolonged, asymptomatic course, in a manner similar to some of the genital infections. Coinfection with *C. trachomatis* may occur. Gonococcal conjunctivitis can rarely occur without sexual transmission, although a healthy suspicion for possible sexual abuse should be maintained in prepubertal children.[15]

N. meningitidis is an uncommon cause of acute bacterial conjunctivitis. In 84 cases of primary meningococcal conjunctivitis, the male-female ratio was 1.76:1, with 9 neonates, 55 children, and 20 adults.[14] Systemic meningococcal disease developed in 17.8% of the patients, and the overall mortality rate was 13.3%. Other *Neisseria* spp., including *N. cinerea,* may cause acute purulent conjunctivitis.[3, 16]

Membrane formation may be seen in any severe infection of the conjunctiva, but it is typically present in infections with streptococci, *Corynebacterium diphtheriae,* and adenovirus. These membranes may lead to a spectrum of changes from fine corneal scarring to obliteration of the fornices and permanent dry-eye states. In contrast to most other types of conjunctivitis, pain is a common symptom with *C. diphtheriae* infection. Diphtheritic conjunctivitis does not occur as the sole manifestation of diphtheria, and so other manifestations of the disease should be sought. Widespread immunization programs have made diphtheritic conjunctivitis extremely rare.[17]

Moraxella lacunata produces a localized, "angular" conjunctivitis associated with fissuring and dermatitis of the external canthi and a scanty conjunctival discharge. *Moraxella* conjunctival infection may be incorrectly diagnosed as chlamydial, epidemic keratoconjunctivitis, or herpes simplex infection. Although *Moraxella* conjunctivitis is associated with adolescent girls, 13 of 27 female patients with culture-proven *Moraxella* infection (48%) were 20 years of age or older.[18] *Moraxella* conjunctivitis can occur in epidemics as a result of sharing of contaminated eye makeup.[12] *Serratia, Pseudomonas,* and other gram-negative organisms can also be transmitted in makeup.

Certain nonpyogenic organisms (*Mycobacterium tuberculosis, Francisella tularensis, Treponema pallidum*) produce an atypical clinical picture characterized by unilateral conjunctival nodules that tend to ulcerate. Moderate localized conjunctival injection, minimal discharge, and a palpable preauricular lymph node on the affected side are present. Infection with *Borrelia burgdorferi* has reportedly caused conjunctivitis in association with Lyme disease.[19, 20]

The cat-scratch disease bacillus, *Bartonella (Rochalimeae) henselae,* produces a unilateral follicular conjunctivitis associated with prominent enlargement of the ipsilateral preauricular lymph node (see Chapter 224). Reiter's syndrome, which can follow *Yersinia* infection, may be accompanied by self-limited conjunctivitis.[21] *Yersinia enterocolitica* has also been associated with an isolated conjunctivitis.[22]

Haemophilus ducreyi,[23] *Pasteurella multocida,*[24] *F. tularensis,*[25] *Acinetobacter* spp.,[26] and *Aeromonas hydrophila*[27] have caused isolated cases of acute conjunctivitis.

Fungal Conjunctivitis

Primary fungal conjunctivitis is infrequently encountered clinically (see Table 98–1). *Candida* conjunctivitis is most often seen in patients receiving long-term corticosteroid eyedrops. Blastomycosis involving the eyelid may cause a granulomatous conjunctivitis.[28] Lid or conjunctival nodules are the usual form of ocular involvement with *Sporothrix schenckii. Rhinosporidium seeberi* may cause a characteristic granulomatous inflammatory mass in the conjunctiva, which may become pedunculated (see Chapter 259).

Viral Conjunctivitis

Viral conjunctivitis is common, causing 20% of nonepidemic cases of conjunctivitis in one study in children[29] and 14% of adult cases in another study.[30] The morphology of associated corneal changes, time course, systemic involvement, and epidemic characteristics usually permit presumptive clinical diagnosis of viral conjunctivitis. The actual causative virus usually cannot be determined by ocular morphologic characteristics alone, and definitive diagnosis requires culture. Polymerase chain reaction is being used in research laboratories.[31, 32] Most cases of viral conjunctivitis are self-limited but highly contagious, with potential for causing considerable morbidity. The discharge is usually serous rather than mucoid or purulent. A generalized conjunctival hyperemia, moderate tearing, and mild itching are present. Follicle formation may be prominent. Regional lymphadenopathy with preauricular and submandibular node enlargement is common, and occasionally the conjunctivitis is associated with an upper respiratory tract infection. The preauricular node is usually exquisitely tender to palpation.

Adenoviruses are most frequently responsible for epidemics of viral conjunctivitis in the United States and are a major occupational hazard for eye care professionals. The serotypes of adenoviruses most often associated with pharyngoconjunctival fever are 3 and 7, with occasional involvement by types 1, 2, 4, 5, 6, 8, and 14. The clinical complex of pharyngitis, fever, and conjunctivitis, inferior forniceal follicles, and, rarely, keratitis may help to identify this conjunctivitis. Spontaneous resolution within 1 to 2 weeks is the rule (see Chapter 132). Outbreaks among children may occur after swimming pool inoculation or hand-to-eye contact.[33]

Epidemic keratoconjunctivitis has most commonly resulted from infection with adenovirus serotype 8, but types 2, 3, 4, 7, 9, 10, 11, 14, 16, 19, 29, and 37 have been reported.[34] The clinical picture frequently includes regional (preauricular and submandibular) lymphadenopathy and follicular conjunctivitis, and there is a 7- to 10-day incubation period with a 5- to 12-day interval before characteristic (but inconsistent) corneal subepithelial infiltrates develop. These epidemics are sometimes propagated by eye health care personnel. Despite a wide spectrum of symptoms ranging from severe photophobia to mild irritation only, this disease is usually self-limited and is rarely associated with visual loss from corneal changes. Occasional reports have described raised intraocular pressure,[35] chronic keratitis, and Stevens-Johnson syndrome[36] as a result of epidemic keratoconjunctivitis. Chronic adenovirus conjunctivitis has also been reported.[37]

Enterovirus 70 is an important cause of epidemic hemorrhagic conjunctivitis.[38] Coxsackievirus A24[39] and adenovirus 11 have resulted in a similar clinical picture (Fig. 98–1). This consists of bilateral follicular conjunctivitis of sudden onset, with (rarely) corneal changes and systemic symptoms, a short symptomatic course (4 to 5 days), and bulbar conjunctival hemorrhages. Spontaneous resolution with low morbidity is the usual course, although occasional reports have described Bell's palsy, radiculomyelitis, cranial nerve palsies, and other types of central nervous system involvement.[40]

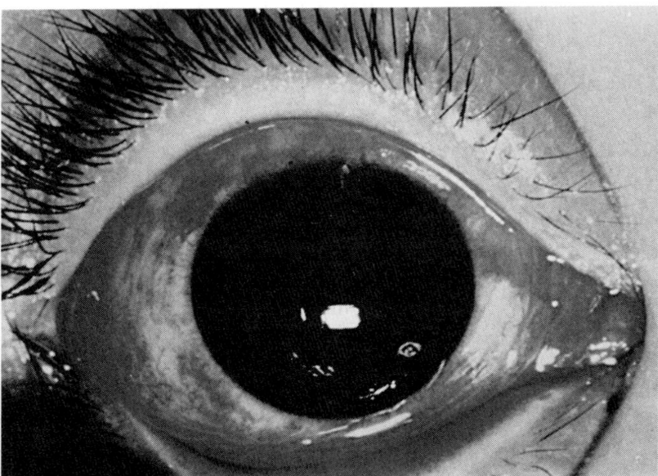

FIGURE 98–1. Acute hemorrhagic conjunctivitis due to enterovirus 70. (From Kono R, Miyamura K, Yamazaki S, et al. Seroepidemic studies of acute hemorrhagic conjunctivitis virus [enterovirus type 70] in West Africa. II. Studies with human sera collected in West African countries other than Ghana. Am J Epidemiol. 1981;114:274–283.)

Ocular infection with vaccinia virus occurs when the virus is accidentally transferred from the site of medical inoculation to the eye. Vesicles appear on the lid margin, and a conjunctivitis may follow. Conjunctivitis without lid lesions can also occur.

Molluscum contagiosum virus produces small, waxy, elevated nodules on the lid margin with umbilicated centers that are associated with a chronic follicular conjunctivitis.[41]

Herpes simplex virus types 1 and 2, varicella-zoster virus, and Epstein-Barr virus can cause conjunctivitis. Primary herpes simplex is responsible for the majority of cases of nonepidemic follicular conjunctivitis in young children. Vesicular lid lesions, preauricular lymphadenopathy, and transient keratitis may be noted. The conjunctivitis is self-limited and is rarely associated with significant morbidity.

In patients with chickenpox, papules may develop on the lids and conjunctiva and at the corneal limbus during the infection. These papules may become pustules and ulcerate. Vesicles may be found on the conjunctiva, particularly on the semilunar fold. Four percent of patients with chickenpox have conjunctival and corneal manifestations.[42] In herpes zoster ophthalmicus, a follicular conjunctivitis with regional adenopathy occurs but is rare. In less than 5% of patients with infectious mononucleosis, a mild conjunctivitis is present.[43]

Human papillomavirus may produce lesions on the tarsal and bulbar conjunctivae and on the lid margin. A catarrhal conjunctivitis may result, and the cornea may show multiple punctate erosions. The presence of viral antigen and DNA sequences in some dysplastic epithelial lesions of the conjunctiva has raised concern that the virus may have a role in the development of conjunctival epithelial malignancies, similar to its role in the female genital tract[44] (see Chapter 133).

Congenital rubella is associated with numerous ocular abnormalities. Rubella in young children has produced a follicular conjunctivitis associated with occasional corneal epithelial changes.

Influenza viruses often cause catarrhal conjunctivitis and occasionally an acute follicular conjunctivitis. This ocular manifestation of influenza has been reported in 48 to 60% of patients.

Infections caused by measles (rubeola) virus may be associated with mild paralimbal conjunctival epithelial erosion; the epithelia contain measles antigens that develop during the prodrome before the skin rash. An epithelial keratitis with photophobia may occur after the skin rash occurs. Koplik spots may be found on the semilunar fold.

Conjunctivitis occurs rarely with mumps. Newcastle disease virus (which causes a fatal pneumoencephalitis in fowl) may produce a self-limited, unilateral follicular conjunctivitis in humans. Echovirus 11 and poliovirus have occasionally been described as a cause of follicular conjunctivitis. Echovirus more commonly causes keratoconjunctivitis.[45]

Parinaud's oculoglandular syndrome is a clinical complex of conjunctivitis, prominent preauricular lymphadenopathy, and a febrile illness with various possible causes, including infectious mononucleosis, cat-scratch disease, syphilis, tuberculosis, and sarcoidosis. Sporotrichosis causes similar findings but without fever.

Chlamydial Conjunctivitis

Trachoma, one of the leading causes of blindness in the world, is caused by *C. trachomatis.*[46] In the United States, the disease is confined largely to certain Native American populations that are characterized by poverty and poor communal hygiene. Repeated or chronic infections appear necessary to establish clinical trachoma.[47] Trachoma conjunctivitis is characterized by a follicular reaction in the superior tarsal conjunctiva that is often associated with a concurrent papillary response. As follicles resolve, they appear to be replaced with fine subconjunctival scars. The degree of scarring seems to be related to the intensity of the follicular response and also to the presence of secondary bacterial infection. The subconjunctival scarring may in time lead to distortion of the tarsal plate and result in trichiasis. *C. trachomatis* serotypes A, B, Ba, and C have been most commonly found in hyperendemic areas of trachoma. Also associated with trachoma is the development of a superior limbic pannus with opacification of the corneal stroma and neovascularization. Follicles may occur in the limbus, and when these resolve a clear depression persists (Herbert's pit).

Inclusion conjunctivitis is a disease of adults caused by *C. trachomatis* (serovars D through H). Infection is most often transmitted by conjunctival contact with genital secretions from a sexual partner who has urethritis or cervicitis. In an infant who has acquired *C. trachomatis* by passage through an infected birth canal, the conjunctivitis is grouped together with gonococcal conjunctivitis and called *ophthalmia neonatorum.* Because the conjunctiva in the newborn does not form follicles, the injected appearance of this conjunctivitis in newborns is nonspecific. In adults, numerous papillae and follicles form on the tarsal conjunctiva and are more pronounced on the lower lid. Bulbar conjunctival follicles may appear, and their presence is highly suggestive of chlamydial infection. *Chlamydia psittaci* and *Chlamydia pneumoniae* also appear to be causes of chronic follicular conjunctivitis, although little is known about the incidence or epidemiology.[46] The disease is usually bilateral, acute, and accompanied by a profuse mucopurulent discharge. Inclusion conjunctivitis is differentiated from trachoma by two important features: (1) corneal scarring rarely occurs; and (2) in trachoma the upper tarsal conjunctiva is more involved than the lower, although occasionally inclusion conjunctivitis may take on the characteristics of trachoma and various corneal changes have been described in inclusion conjunctivitis. Conjunctivitis is a rare manifestation of systemic lymphogranuloma venereum caused by certain immunotypes (L-1, L-2, L-3) of *C. trachomatis.* Moderate unilateral conjunctival injection, slight conjunctival discharge, and extreme edema of the upper and lower lids are present. In addition, ipsilateral preauricular, parotid, and submaxillary lymphadenopathy is present.

Lymphogranuloma venereum conjunctivitis has caused marginal keratitis with corneal perforation in a patient with human immunodeficiency virus (HIV) infection.[48]

Parasitic Conjunctivitis

A number of ocular parasites can cause conjunctivitis. Blepharoconjunctivitis may be caused by *Leishmania donovani* in association with nodules of post–kala azar dermal leishmaniasis, with infection of the conjunctiva by spread from contaminated fingers.[49] Parasites are being recovered in increasing frequency from the conjunctiva of persons with the acquired immunodeficiency syndrome (AIDS). Microsporidia are small, ubiquitous, obligate intracellular parasites that usually cause infections in animals and rarely in humans. *Encephalitozoon* species may cause a mild conjunctivitis with punctate keratopathy in patients with AIDS.[50] The symptoms may mimic those of blepharitis or dry eye and may be accompanied by chronic sinusitis or clinically silent disseminated infection (see Chapter 274). Cryptosporidial conjunctivitis has been reported.[51] Conjunctival involvement with fly larvae,[52] nematodes, and trematodes has been described.

Ophthalmia Neonatorum

The incidence of acute conjunctivitis of the newborn (ophthalmia neonatorum) is reported to be as high as 12% of all newborns.[53] It previously was most commonly the result of mild chemical irritation after ocular silver nitrate prophylaxis. This self-limited chemical conjunctivitis appears within the first 24 hours, and it lasts 1 to 2 days. However, chlamydial conjunctivitis has become much more common, with an incidence of approximately 2.8% of all births at one clinic, and occurring in more than 35% of infants born to mothers with proven chlamydial cervicitis.[54] The onset generally occurs within 5 to 19 days after delivery, with no pathologic features except for an association with other systemic chlamydial infections such as pneumonia and otitis media. It has been suggested that the organism in these cases gains entry to the neonate through the conjunctival mucosa. There have been reports of chlamydial conjunctivitis in infants delivered by cesarean section.

Bacterial conjunctivitis of the newborn is most often the result of *S. aureus* infection, with *S. pneumoniae* and *H. influenzae* also seen.[6] There are no pathognomonic features of these infections, and they may occur as early as 24 hours after birth. Streptococcal infections may be associated with acute dacryocystitis of the newborn. *Pseudomonas* spp. have been reported as an occasional cause and may cause a subsequent pseudomonal sepsis. Cases of staphylococcal scalded skin syndrome have been attributed to primary staphylococcal conjunctivitis. *Shigella flexneri* has caused ethmoiditis and conjunctivitis. *Moraxella catarrhalis* and *N. cinerea* conjunctivitis are being more frequently diagnosed and have been confused with true gonococcal ophthalmia neonatorum.[3]

The current incidence of gonococcal ophthalmia neonatorum is not known, but it is usually seen 1 to 2 days after birth and is characterized by a florid course and the threat of corneal ulceration and perforation. Infants born to mothers with herpes simplex virus cervicitis may develop a conjunctivitis within a few days of birth. The conjunctivitis is usually self-limited but may be associated with corneal epithelial changes and, rarely, stromal keratitis.

Noninfectious Conjunctivitis

Conjunctival inflammation (chemosis, injection, and discharge) is seen as a result of many noninfectious conditions, but particularly as an allergic mucosal response. The agents responsible include drugs and devices such as hard and soft contact lenses, contact lens sterilizing solutions (usually the preservative thimerosal), and prostheses, which can cause giant papillary conjunctivitis. Other agents implicated include topical timolol, atropine, antiviral agents, cosmetics, and external allergens that cause vernal keratoconjunctivitis. Conjunctivitis may occur as a response to irritating agents such as gentian violet, latex, and ultraviolet irradiation. Phlyctenular keratoconjunctivitis has occurred in rare patients with acute coccidioidomycosis.

The precise mechanisms eliciting conjunctivitis in numerous other conditions with fairly specific clinical features have not been conclusively identified. These include keratoconjunctivitis sicca, superior limbic keratoconjunctivitis, ligneous conjunctivitis, mucocutaneous lymph node syndrome, and Reiter's syndrome. Immune-mediated conjunctivitis has been implicated in mucous membrane pemphigoid (ocular cicatricial pemphigoid) and in the conjunctivitis associated with graft-versus-host disease in bone marrow transplant recipients.

DIFFERENTIAL DIAGNOSIS

Other serious, sight-threatening conditions that present as "red eye" may superficially resemble a conjunctivitis. The points of difference are highlighted in Table 98–2. Chronic, unilateral conjunctivitis in which a specific diagnosis is not made should alert the physician to the possibility of a meibomian gland carcinoma.

LABORATORY INVESTIGATIONS

Mild conjunctivitis is not routinely investigated and is often treated empirically without benefit of microbial culture. Reports differ on the value of culturing in suspected bacterial conjunctivitis. In mild conjunctivitis, a calcium alginate swab dipped in trypticase soy broth or a culturette device may be used to obtain material from the conjunctival sacs. Cultures should be obtained from both eyes, moistened with transport medium, and transported as soon as possible to the microbiology laboratory for plating on selected bacteriologic media. In severe conjunctivitis, scrapings of the superior and inferior

TABLE 98–2 Comparison of Conjunctivitis and Other Conditions

Characteristics	Conjunctivitis	Uveitis	Acute Angle-Closure Glaucoma
Prominent symptoms	Discharge, irritation	Photophobia, visual loss	Pain, visual loss
Vision	Usually normal	Normal and occasionally decreased	Markedly reduced
Ocular injection	Conjunctival injection generalized	Paralimbal injection	Paralimbal injection
Cornea	Usually clear	Usually clear	Edematous and cloudy
Pupil	Normal	May be normal or small	Usually mid-dilated, irregular, and immobile
Intraocular pressure	Normal	Normal or elevated	Markedly elevated

tarsal conjunctiva should be taken after the administration of topical proparacaine HCl, 0.5% to obtain material for smears as well as microbial culture. Cultures are occasionally taken separately from both lids in suspected conjunctivitis, although the value of this practice is uncertain. Chlamydial cultures are usually taken with a dry calcium alginate swab, which is then placed in special *Chlamydia* transport medium before it is processed for cell culture. Rapid culture methods are available for adenovirus (see Chapter 14).

In all cases of suspected ophthalmia neonatorum, cultures and smears should be performed for bacteria, *Chlamydia,* and herpes simplex virus. Acute and convalescent serologic tests for adenovirus and some enteroviruses may help in diagnosing epidemic conjunctivitis, but these are generally not required because of the self-limited nature of the infection, the nonspecific treatment available, and the diagnostic characteristics of the epidemic features. Serodiagnostic testing of tears and serum by microimmunofluorescence has been described for patients with *C. trachomatis* inclusion conjunctivitis.

In a conjunctival scraping from a normal, healthy eye, epithelial cells and occasional goblet cells are present. In acute bacterial infection, the scraping shows large numbers of neutrophils. Bacteria may be present within or outside leukocytes. In chronic bacterial infections, there is a decrease in neutrophils and an increase in lymphocytes and large mononuclear cells. In viral conjunctivitis, lymphocytes and monocytes are predominant. In herpes simplex infections, multinucleated epithelial cells may be seen. In chlamydial infections, a mixed inflammatory cell population (polymorphonuclear leukocytes and lymphocytes) is present, and basophilic intracytoplasmic inclusion bodies may be seen in epithelial cells; the latter finding is common in children and less common in adults. Immunofluorescent techniques provide more sensitivity in identification. Topically applied fluorescein does not appear to have an effect on fluorescent monoclonal antibodies in the diagnosis of chlamydial conjunctivitis. In allergic conjunctivitis, scrapings characteristically reveal eosinophils. They are found in greatest abundance in vernal conjunctivitis. Between attacks of vernal conjunctivitis, mast cells and no eosinophils are seen.

Scrapings from patients with keratoconjunctivitis sicca or superior limbic keratoconjunctivitis reveal keratinized epithelial cells or condensed chromatin patterns with the Papanicolaou staining technique. Impression cytology may offer an alternative to the conjunctival scraping method.

TREATMENT

Most types of mild bacterial conjunctivitis and most types of viral conjunctivitis are self-limited, benign conditions that perhaps require no treatment. Topical gentamicin or tobramycin for gram-negative rod infections and erythromycin, bacitracin, polymyxin B/trimethoprim, or neomycin/polymyxin for gram-positive infections, given every 2 to 4 hours for 7 to 10 days, are usually effective. Topical fluoroquinolone solutions are also effective alternatives for severe conjunctivitis and keratitis. Often an organism reported to be resistant to a specific antibiotic in the laboratory based on achievable serum levels nevertheless responds to that antibiotic clinically because of the high concentrations that are achieved in the tear film by topical application.

Therapy for suspected bacterial conjunctivitis occurring in children should include coverage against *H. influenzae, S. pneumoniae,* and *S. aureus.* Polymyxin B–bacitracin combination therapy provides a suitable broad spectrum but is available only as a fixed-combination ointment preparation. Polymyxin B–trimethoprim, applied 4 times daily for 1 week, can be effective broad-spectrum therapy for nonsevere conjunctivitis, although the coverage against gram-positive organisms provided by trimethoprim is for some species less than optimal. Aminoglycoside drops (gentamicin 0.3% and tobramycin 0.3%) are inherently less active against gram-positive organisms and have a low therapeutic-toxic ratio as topical agents. Neomycin–polymyxin B–gramicidin drops or neomycin–polymyxin B–bacitracin ointment provides broad-spectrum coverage, but neomycin poses a 10% risk of hypersensitivity reaction with contact dermatitis. Fluoroquinolones, although active against a variety of gram-positive and gram-negative organisms, also may be ineffective against some isolates of *Streptococcus, Enterococcus,* and *Staphylococcus.* Fluoroquinolones have not proved to be more effective than aminoglycosides in treating bacterial conjunctivitis. Erythromycin is ineffective against *H. influenzae* and should not be used as initial therapy.

Therapy for suspected bacterial conjunctivitis in adults is primarily directed against staphylococcal species but should include activity against *S. pneumoniae* and *H. influenzae.* Fluoroquinolone solutions (ciprofloxacin, levofloxacin, norfloxacin, and ofloxacin) have been investigated and found effective, yet no more effective than aminoglycosides, in treating bacterial conjunctivitis. If there is associated blepharitis, bacitracin ointment applied to the eyelids and conjunctiva twice daily for 1 week provides excellent coverage against *Staphylococcus* species. Erythromycin is a less desirable alternative, because some *S. aureus* isolates are only moderately susceptible.

Gonococcal conjunctivitis requires urgent parenteral therapy with a broad-spectrum cephalosporin such as cefotaxime or ceftriaxone. Frequent instillations of normal saline solution for ocular lavage can dilute the effects of released toxins on ocular tissues. A single intramuscular dose of 125 mg of ceftriaxone has resulted in a 100% cure rate for gonococcal ophthalmia neonatorum without the need for concomitant topical therapy.

Herpes simplex virus conjunctivitis may be treated with topical trifluridine every 2 hours for 7 days, although this condition is usually benign and self-limited. Vidaribine ointment (Vira-A) applied 5 times daily for 7 days may be used as an alternative. Systemic acyclovir, famciclovir, or valacyclovir may also be effective in patients with allergy or sensitivity to topically applied antiviral agents.

Adult inclusion conjunctivitis is treated systematically and requires a 1-week course of doxycycline, 100 mg twice daily; in pregnant or lactating women, erythromycin or azithromycin may be substituted orally.[55] Adjunctive topical tetracycline or erythromycin ointment may also be prescribed. A similar therapy is effective in treating trachoma, but prevention of reinfection and bacterial superinfection are equally important. Macrolide antibiotics with long serum half-lives and favorable tissue penetration (e.g., azithromycin,[56, 57] clarithromycin, roxithromycin) may also be used.

Allergic and immune-mediated conjunctivitis respond best to topical corticosteroids. The long-term use of topical steroids may be associated with glaucoma and cataracts, whereas short-term use may aggravate herpes simplex epithelial keratitis. Nonsteroidal anti-inflammatory agents such as aspirin and cromolyn sodium, diclofenac, ketorolac tromethamine, and others are useful adjunctive measures.

Topical combination products containing histamine receptor antagonists and mast cell stabilizing agents have been useful in twice-daily dosing for allergic conjunctivitis.

PROPHYLAXIS OF OPHTHALMIA NEONATORUM

There is considerable debate over the relative efficacy of 1% silver nitrate versus topical antibiotics such as 0.5% erythromycin or 1% tetracyclines. Silver nitrate is still extremely effective, particularly against gonococcal infection, but it has little impact on the increasing incidence of chlamydial infections. It also has a 5-fold greater incidence of toxicity than erythromycin. Topical erythromycin seems to be the most effective agent in preventing this infection.[58] In infants born to mothers with known genital chlamydial infection, the routine use of erythromycin ointment eliminates chlamydial conjunctivitis, but systemic erythromycin estolate is preferred to prevent nasopharyngeal colonization.[59, 60] Neonatal *Chlamydia* infections require treatment with oral erythromycin, 50 mg/kg/day in 4 divided doses for 10 to 14 days. Topical povidone-iodine 2.5% may also be an effective agent for prophylaxis including activity against *Chlamydia.*

REFERENCES

1. deToledo AR, Chandler JW. Conjunctivitis of the newborn. Infect Dis Clin North Am. 1992;6:807–813.
2. Ratelle S, Keno D, Hardwood M, Etkind PH. Neonatal chlamydial infections in Massachusetts, 1992–1993. Am J Prev Med. 1997;13:221–224.
3. Dolter J, Wong J, Janda JM. Association of *Neisseria cinerea* with ocular infections in paediatric patients. J Infect. 1998;36:49–52.
4. Trottier S, Stenberg K, VonRosen IA, et al. *Haemophilus influenzae* causing conjunctivitis in day-care children. Pediatr Infect Dis J. 1991;10:578–584.
5. Weiss A, Brinser JH, Nazar-Stewart V. Acute conjunctivitis in childhood. J Pediatr. 1993;122:10–14.
6. Iroha EO, Kesah CN, Egri-Okwaji MT, Odugbemi TO. Bacterial eye infection in neonates: A prospective study in a neonatal unit. West Afr J Med. 1998;17:168–172.
7. Shah SS, Gallagher PG. Complications of conjunctivitis caused by *Pseudomonas aeruginosa* in a newborn intensive care unit. Pediatr Infect Dis J. 1998;17:97–102.
8. Seal DV, Barrett SP, McGill JI. Aetiology and treatment of acute bacterial infection of the external eye. Br J Ophthalmol. 1982;66:357.
9. Syed MA, Hyndiuk RA. Infectious conjunctivitis. Infect Dis Clin North Am. 1992;6:789–805.
10. Van Ogtrop ML, Van Zoeren-Groggen D, Verbakel-Salomons EM, Van Boven CP. *Serratia marcescens* infections in neonatal departments: Description of an outbreak and review of the literature. J Hosp Infect. 1997;36:95–103.
11. King S, Devi SP, Mindroff C, et al. Nosocomial *Pseudomonas aeruginosa* conjunctivitis in a pediatric hospital. Infect Control Hosp Epidemiol. 1988;9:77–80.
12. Schwartz B, Harrison LH, Motter JS, et al. Investigation of an outbreak of *Moraxella* conjunctivitis at a Navajo boarding school. Am J Ophthalmol. 1988;107:341–347.
13. Valenton MJ, Abendanio R. Gonorrhea conjunctivitis. Can J Ophthalmol. 1973;8:421.
14. Barquet N, Gasser I, Domingo P, et al. Primary meningococcal conjunctivitis: Report of 21 patients and review. Rev Infect Dis. 1990;12:838–847.
15. Lewis LS, Glauser TA, Joffe E. Gonococcal conjunctivitis in pre-pubertal children. Am J Dis Child. 1990;144:546–548.
16. Au YK, Reynolds MD, Rambin ED, et al. *Neisseria cinerea* acute purulent conjunctivitis. Am J Ophthalmol. 1990;109:96–97.
17. Boralkar AN. Diphtheritic conjunctivitis: A rare case report in Indian literature. Indian J Ophthalmol. 1989;37:49–50.
18. Kowalski RP, Hardwick JC. Incidence of *Moraxella* conjunctivial infection. Am J Ophthalmol. 1986;101:437–440.
19. Flach AJ, Lavoie PE. Episcleritis, conjunctivitis and keratitis as ocular manifestations of Lyme disease. Ophthalmology. 1990;97:973–975.
20. Mombaerts IM, Maudgal P, Knockaert DC. Bilateral follicular conjunctivitis as a manifestation of Lyme disease. Am J Ophthalmol. 1991;112:96–97.
21. Saari KM, Laitinen O, Leirisalo M, et al. Ocular inflammation associated with *Yersinia* infection. Am J Ophthalmol. 1980;89:84.
22. Crichton EP. Suppurative conjunctivitis caused by *Yersinia enterocolitica.* Can Med J. 1978;118:22.
23. Gregory JE, Henderson RW, Smith R. Conjunctivitis due to *Haemophilus ducreyi* infection. Br J Vener Dis. 1980;56:414.
24. Eschete ML, Rambin ED, West BC. *Clostridium pseudotetanicum* bacteremia in a patient with *Pasteurella multocida* conjunctivitis. J Clin Microbiol. 1978;8:509.
25. Guerrant RL, Humphries MK, Butler JE, et al. Tickborne oculoglandular tularemia: Case report and review of seasonal and vectorial associations in 106 cases. Arch Intern Med. 1976;136:811.
26. Abel R, Shulman J, Boyle GL, et al. *Herellea vaginicola* and ocular infections. Ann Ophthalmol. 1975;7:1485.
27. Smith JA. Ocular *Aeromonas hydrophila.* Am J Ophthalmol. 1980;89:449.
28. Slack JW, Hyndiuk RA, Harris GJ, et al. Blastomycosis of the eyelid and conjunctiva. Ophthal Plast Reconstr Surg. 1992;8:143–149.
29. Gigliotti F, Williams WT, Hayden FG, et al. Etiology of acute conjunctivitis in children. J Pediatr. 1981;98:531.
30. Leibowitz HM, Pratt MV, Flagstad IJ, et al. Human conjunctivitis: A diagnostic evaluation. Arch Ophthalmol. 1976;94:1747.
31. Cooper RJ, Yeo AC, Bailey AS, Tullo AB. Adenovirus polymerase chain reaction assay for rapid diagnosis of conjunctivitis. Invest Ophthalmol Vis Sci. 1999;40:90–95.
32. Hidalgo R, Melon S, de Ona M, et al. Diagnosis of herpetic keratoconjunctivitis by nested polymerase chain reaction in human tear film. Eur J Clin Microbiol Infect Dis. 1998;17:120–123.
33. Outbreak of pharyngoconjunctival fever at a summer camp, North Carolina, 1991. Infect Control Hosp Epidemiol. 1992;13:499–500.
34. Curtis S, Wilkinson GW, Westmoreland D. An outbreak of epidemic keratoconjunctivitis caused by adenovirus type 37. J Med Microbiol. 1998;47:91–94.
35. Hara J, Ishibashi T, Fujimoto F, et al. Adenovirus type 10 keratoconjunctivitis with increased intraocular pressure. Am J Ophthalmol. 1980;90:481.
36. Kiernan JP, Schanzlin DJ, Leveille AS. Stevens-Johnson syndrome associated with adenovirus conjunctivitis. Am J Ophthalmol. 1981;92:543.
37. Pettit TH, Holland GN. Chronic keratoconjunctivitis associated with ocular adenovirus infection. Am J Ophthalmol. 1979;88:748.
38. Shulman LM, Manor Y, Azar R, et al. Identification of a new strain of fastidious enterovirus 70 as the causative agent of an outbreak of hemorrhagic conjunctivitis. J Clin Microbiol 1997;35:2145–2149.
39. Christopher S, Theogaraj S, Godbole S, et al. An epidemic of acute hemorrhagic conjunctivitis due to coxsackievirus A24. J Infect Dis. 1982;146:16.
40. John TJ, Christopher S, Abraham J. Neurological manifestation of acute haemorrhagic conjunctivitis due to enterovirus 70. Lancet. 1981;2:1283.
41. Denis J, Chauvaud D, Savoldelli M, et al. Fine structure of palpebral molluscum contagiosum and its secondary conjunctival lesions. Graefes Arch Clin Exp Ophthalmol. 1978;208:207.
42. Stucchi CA, Bianchi G. Complications oculaires graves postvaricelleuses chez l'adulte. Ophthalmologica. 1970;161:108.
43. Wilhelmus KR. Ocular involvement in infectious mononucleosis. Am J Ophthalmol. 1981;91:117.
44. McDonnell JM, McDonnell PK, Green WR, et al. Demonstration of papillomavirus capsid antigen in human conjunctival neoplasia. Arch Ophthalmol. 1986;104:1801.
45. Kaye SB, Morton DE, Tong CY, O'Donnell NP. Echovirus keratoconjunctivitis. Am J Ophthalmol. 1998;125:187–190.
46. Lietman T, Brooks D, Moncada J, et al. Chronic follicular conjunctivitis associated with *Chlamydia psittaci* or *Chlamydia pneumoniae.* Clin Infect Dis. 1998;26:1335–1340.
47. Bobo LD, Novak N, Munoz B, et al. Severe disease in children with trachoma is associated with persistent *Chlamydia trachomatis* infection. J Infect Dis. 1997;176:1524–1530.
48. Buus DR, Pflugfelder SC, Schachter J, et al. Lymphogranuloma venereum conjunctivitis with a marginal corneal perforation. Ophthalmology. 1988;95:799–802.
49. Nandy A, Addy M, Chowdhury AB. Leishmanial blepharoconjunctivitis. Trop Geogr Med. 1991;43:303–306.
50. Friedberg TN, Stenson SM, Orenstein JM, et al. Microsporidian keratoconjunctivitis in acquired immunodeficiency syndrome. Arch Ophthalmol. 1990;108:504–508.
51. Green ST, Scott V, McMenamin J, et al. Cryptosporidial enteritis complicated by conjunctivitis. Ann Rheum Dis. 1991;50:526.
52. Wong D. External ophthalmomyiasis caused by the sheep bot *Oestrus ovis.* Br J Ophthalmol. 1982;66:786.
53. Pierce JM, Ward ME, Seal DV. Ophthalmia neonatorum in the 1980's: Incidence, aetiology and treatment. Br J Ophthalmol. 1982;66:728.
54. Schachter J, Holt J, Goodner E, et al. Prospective study of chlamydial infection in neonates. Lancet. 1979;2:377.
55. Nakagawa H. Treatment of chlamydial conjunctivitis. Ophthalmologica. 1997;211 (Suppl 1):25–28.
56. Hammerschlag MR, Gelling M, Roblin PM, et al. Treatment of neonatal chlamydial conjunctivitis with azithromycin. Pediatr Infect Dis J. 1998;17:1049–1050.
57. Bailey RL, Arullendran P, Whittle HC, Mabey DC. Randomised controlled trial of single-dose azithromycin in treatment of trachoma. Lancet. 1993;342:453–456.
58. Hammerschlag MR, Chandler JW, Alexander ER, et al. Erythromycin ointment for ocular prophylaxis of neonatal chlamydial infection. JAMA. 1980;244:2291.
59. Patamasucon P, Rettig PJ, Faust KL, et al. Oral versus topical erythromycin therapies for chlamydial conjunctivitis. Am J Dis Child. 1982;136:817.
60. Rees E, Tait A, Hobson D, et al. Persistence of chlamydial infection after treatment for neonatal conjunctivitis. Arch Dis Child. 1981;56:193.

Chapter 99

Keratitis

TERRENCE P. O'BRIEN

Keratitis, or inflammation of the cornea, may be produced by infectious organisms and by noninfectious causes. Microbial keratitis is a common, potentially sight-threatening ocular infection that may be caused by bacteria, fungi, viruses, or parasites. In one survey of 5845 eyes with suspected infectious keratitis, a microbial agent was identified in 49%, with 82% being bacteria, 16% fungi, and 2% parasites.[1] The challenge for the clinician is to distinguish microbial keratitis from other noninfectious inflammatory conditions of the cornea resulting from trauma, hypersensitivity, and other immune-mediated reactions. There are no absolutely specific clinical signs that confirm infection, yet the clinician should assess and define distinctive corneal signs based on the status of the epithelium (intact or ulcerated), type of stromal inflammation (nonsuppurative or suppurative), and site of stromal inflammation (focal, diffuse, multifocal, or marginal). With advanced corneal infection or severe host-inflammatory response, permanent structural alterations such as thinning, perforation, or scleral extension may be present and may require surgical intervention.

Because the corneal and conjunctival epithelia are continuous, forming the ocular surface, agents causing conjunctival disease may also affect the cornea. Before most infectious agents and some mediators of the immune reaction can invade the corneal stroma, a defect in the ocular surface must usually be present. This defect can be caused by various kinds of external trauma, including trauma from contact lenses, trichiasis, entropion, or abnormal lid margins. Radial keratotomy, a procedure now infrequently performed, has been reported to be followed by infection in 0.25 to 0.7% of cases, but that estimate may be low because prolonged follow-up is necessary.[2] About half the infections in radial keratotomy sites occur during the first 2 weeks postoperatively[2] and are frequently bilateral following simultaneous bilateral keratotomy.[3, 4] Later infections, mostly from bacteria[5] but occasionally from fungi,[6] herpes simplex virus,[7] or *Acanthamoeba,*[8, 9] occur from months to 10 years later.[10] Predisposing factors are postoperative contact lens use, reoperation, and micropenetration during surgery.[2] Epithelial fragility in the incision site or altered tear distribution has been postulated to account for the late infections.[11, 12] Late complications of the more current methods of refractive surgery are less clear, although early infections are rare with photoreactive keratectomy using the excimer laser. In a series of 1019 eyes undergoing laser in situ keratomileusis for myopia, infectious keratitis was reported in only one case.[13] Nocardia keratitis has been reported as a complication of laser in situ keratomileusis.[14] Corneal surface defects may also result from chronic problems in severely dry eyes, bullous keratopathy,[15] exposure, or neurogenic corneal anesthesia. Comatose patients receiving ventilatory support,[16] particularly those with chemosis that prevents lid occlusion, and leprosy patients with lagophthalmos or trichiasis (see Chapter 241) are prone to bacterial keratitis. Systemic disease such as diabetes mellitus or immunodeficiency states decrease the corneal host resistance when the ocular surface has been broached by one of the preceding mechanisms.

Any corneal inflammation should be considered potentially sight-threatening and in need of prompt management. Corneal perforation and loss of the eye can occur rapidly after a severe inflammatory episode or infection with virulent organisms. Even minor corneal ulcerations occurring in the central visual axis can disrupt visual acuity.

ETIOLOGIC AGENTS

The various agents known to cause keratitis are listed in Table 99–1. The organisms most commonly identified in microbial keratitis vary geographically depending on the climate, soil, and individual patient factors. Under the appropriate opportunistic conditions, any organism can cause keratitis.

CLINICAL MANIFESTATIONS

Because of the rich innervation of the cornea, the most common symptom of ulcerative inflammatory lesions of the cornea is pain. The movement of the eyelids over the ulcerated corneal epithelium increases the pain. Examination of patients with microbial keratitis is greatly facilitated by first instilling a drop of topical anesthetic.

Unlike conjunctival infections, keratitis is usually accompanied by a variable decrease in vision. Discharge, which is a distinctive feature of conjunctivitis, is generally absent in patients with keratitis unless a purulent bacterial keratitis is present. Reflex tearing, photophobia, and blepharospasm are common.

Because the cornea is normally a clear, avascular tissue, the clinical appearance of an inflammatory reaction is different from that observed in other tissues. After a noxious agent enters the cornea, inflammatory cells migrate into the cornea from dilatated limbal vessels and from the preocular tear film. An early sign of keratitis is therefore a subtle loss of corneal transparency, localized or generalized, and frequently a focal epithelial defect that is best observed with a cobalt blue light after instillation of fluorescein using a sterile strip. Signs distinctive for microbial keratitis include an ulceration of the epithelium with suppurative stromal inflammation that is either focal or diffuse. Multifocal suppurative keratitis is suggestive of mixed infection (polymicrobial keratitis). Occasionally, manifestations of microbial keratitis are an intact epithelium and nonsuppurative multifocal stromal inflammation. Perhaps the most important result of the inflammatory reaction with invasion by microbial pathogens is loss of corneal substance (keratolysis), which may rapidly lead to perforation if untreated or sometimes to a corneal scar (leukoma) even if successful therapy is promptly initiated.

In severe keratitis, there is frequently an invasion of the cornea by blood vessels (neovascularization). After the inflammation subsides, residual microscopic empty blood channels (ghost vessels) may be the only evidence of a previous inflammatory condition.

Some degree of corneal edema accompanies almost all inflammatory conditions of the cornea, leading to a loss of corneal transparency and a resultant decrease in vision. Edema fluid may also accumulate under the corneal epithelium and form bullae that cause severe "foreign body" pain. Rupture of the bullae disrupts the epithelium and provides a portal of microbial entry.

An associated intraocular inflammation is common. Early inflammatory changes may be discernible only by careful slit-lamp biomicroscopic examination (flare and cells). Severe inflammation may lead to layering of fibrin and white blood cells in the inferior portion of the anterior chamber (hypopyon) by gravity (Fig. 99–1). There may also be hyphema, extensive synechiae, and glaucoma. The aqueous and vitreous humors remain sterile in most microbial keratitis until a late stage when infective endophthalmitis may occur.

BACTERIAL KERATITIS

Bacterial keratitis accounts for 65 to 90% of all microbial corneal infections.[17–21] Four principal groups of bacterial pathogens responsible for the majority of infective keratitis include the Micrococcaceae *(Staphylococcus, Micrococcus),* the *Streptococcus* spp., the *Pseudomonas* spp., and the Enterobacteriaceae *(Citrobacter, Klebsiella, Enterobacter, Serratia, Proteus).* Eighty-seven percent of cases of bacterial keratitis are caused by organisms in these four groups.[17] The prevalence of organisms incriminated in bacterial keratitis has shifted somewhat over the past several decades. *Streptococcus pneumoniae*

TABLE 99–1 Some Infectious Agents That Cause Keratitis

Bacteria
- Gram-positive cocci
  - *Staphylococcus aureus*
  - *Staphylococcus epidermidis*
  - *Streptococcus pneumoniae*
  - Streptococci of the viridans group
  - *Streptococcus pyogenes* (group A)
  - *Enterococcus faecalis*
  - *Peptostreptococcus* spp.
- Gram-negative bacilli
  - *Pseudomonas, Burholderia,* and *Stenotrophomonas* spp.
  - *Comamonas acidovorans*
  - *Proteus mirabilis*
  - *Morganella morganii*
  - *Klebsiella pneumoniae*
  - *Serratia marcescens*
  - *Escherichia coli*
  - *Aeromonas hydrophila*
  - *Bartonella henselae*
- Gram-negative coccobacilli
  - *Moraxella catarrhalis*
  - *Moraxella lacunata*
  - *Moraxella nonliquefaciens*
  - *Acinetobacter* spp.
  - *Pasteurella multocida*
  - *Neisseria gonorrhoeae*
- Gram-positive bacilli
  - *Bacillus cereus*
  - *Bacillus coagulans*
  - *Bacillus laterosporus*
  - *Bacillus licheniformis*
  - *Bacillus brevis*
  - *Corynebacterium diphtheriae*
  - *Clostridium perfringens*
  - *Clostridium tetani*
- Spirochetes
  - *Treponema pallidum*
  - *Borrelia burgdorferi*
- Mycobacteria
  - *Mycobacterium tuberculosis*
  - *Mycobacterium fortuitum*
  - *Mycobacterium chelonae*
  - *Mycobacterium gordonae*
  - *Mycobacterium avium-intracellulare*
- Actinomycetes
  - *Nocardia* spp.

Chlamydia
- *Chlamydia trachomatis*
- Viruses
- Herpes simplex virus
- Adenovirus
- Varicella-zoster virus
- Epstein-Barr virus
- Poxviruses (vaccinia, molluscum contagiosum)
- Rubeola (measles)

Fungi
- *Acremonium* spp.
- *Fusarium* spp.
- *Bipolaris* spp.
- *Candida* spp.
- *Aspergillus* spp.
- *Pseudallescheria boydii*
- *Penicillium* spp.
- *Alternaria* spp.
- *Neurospora* spp.
- *Phialophora* spp.
- *Curvularia* spp.

Parasites
- *Onchocerca volvulus*
- *Acanthamoeba polyphaga*
- *Acanthamoeba castellani*
- *Leishmania brasiliensis*
- *Trypanosoma* spp.
- *Nosema* spp.
- *Encephalitozoon* spp.

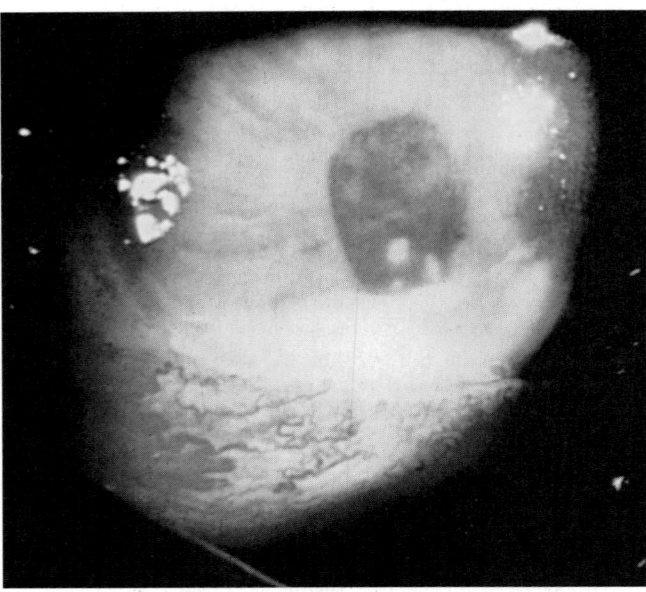

FIGURE 99–1. Hypopyon, corneal clouding, and conjunctival hyperemia due to *Capnocytophaga canimorsus* keratitis.

was the predominant cause of microbial keratitis in the past, often in association with chronic dacryocystitis. In most large series, gram-positive organisms continue to be the predominant cause of microbial keratitis. *Staphylococcus aureus* is now the most commonly isolated agent in microbial keratitis, especially in the northern and northeastern United States and Canada. In a reported series from New York City,[18] *S. aureus* was the most common organism, followed by *Moraxella, Pseudomonas aeruginosa,* and *S. pneumoniae.* In London,[22] the most common organisms were *S. aureus, S. pneumoniae, Pseudomonas,* and *Moraxella.* Streptococcal species are still commonly isolated causative organisms in eastern and western United States.

Opportunistic commensals are now frequently isolated. In addition to bacteria, fungi and mycobacteria other than *Mycobacterium tuberculosis* have been reported with increasing frequency. *P. aeruginosa* is an increasingly frequent organism encountered in infectious keratitis, especially among contact lens wearers. *P. aeruginosa* is more common in the South than *S. aureus.*[19, 23] *Pseudomonas* and *Streptococcus* are the main pathogens in previously healthy eyes in the southern United States. In a series from South Florida, there were 238 bacterial corneal infections among 663 patients with suspected microbial keratitis.[19] *P. aeruginosa* was the single most common organism (31%) and was observed frequently in association with hard or soft contact lens wear. *S. aureus* and *S. pneumoniae* combined caused 22% of the total bacterial keratitis cases.

Any apparent changes that have occurred result from improved isolation techniques from the cornea, an increase in the population of patients who are systemically immunosuppressed, an increase in topical steroid administration, and an increase in the use of soft contact lenses,[20, 24, 25] especially for extended wear.[26, 27] There have been occasional cases of bacterial keratitis as a result of organ-cultured and MK medium–stored corneal buttons used for corneal transplantation.[28]

The pathogenesis of bacterial keratitis involves several routes of inoculation. Direct penetration of intact corneal epithelium occurs only by organisms releasing special toxins, enzymes, and other virulent factors (*Neisseria gonorrhoeae, Neisseria meningitidis, Corynebacterium diphtheriae, Listeria,* and *Shigella* spp.). An enormous variety of organisms may cause keratitis when introduced through a corneal epithelial defect or a gap in epithelial bridges occurring by mechanical, thermal, or chemical injury or epithelial erosion secondary to ocular conditions, including eyelid abnormalities, tear dysfunction states, corneal anesthesia, or decreased adherence of the corneal epithelium as in bullous keratopathy, damage to the epithelial basement membrane and Bowman's membrane, and some dystrophies. The inoculation of organisms into the corneal stroma may occur via obvious trauma, such as scratches,[29] or more often via inapparent inoculation of minor corneal epithelial abrasions such as by contaminated mascara.[30, 31]

S. aureus and *Staphylococcus epidermidis* may reach the cornea from body sites in which they are resident colonizers.[21, 32] *S. epidermidis* and streptococci can cause corneal ulceration, usually in immunocompromised hosts and occasionally in association with chronic dacryocystitis.[33, 34] *P. aeruginosa* is recognized for its particular swift suppurative course to perforation because of its proteolytic enzyme production (see Chapter 207), which degrades the corneal stroma. *Pseudomonas* may produce characteristic inflammatory rings consisting of polymorphonuclear leukocytes within the corneal stroma.[35] Similar stromal ring infiltrates may be observed in fungal, viral, and *Acanthamoeba* keratitis. Host-derived enzymes also contribute in the pathogenesis of *Pseudomonas* corneal infection.[36] Enzymes from neutrophils may contribute to destruction of the corneal collagen matrix in ground substance. The extent of visual impairment is directly related to severity of inflammatory cell infiltration, phagocytic activity, cell death, release of proteolytic enzymes, and damage to corneal endothelium.

In comatose patients with corneal exposure and tracheostomies colonized by *P. aeruginosa,* the danger of corneal infection is greatly increased.[37] Extension of the keratitis into the sclera may occur.[38, 39] Other related species such as *Comamonas (Pseudomonas) acidovorans* and *Pseudomonas stutzeri* have caused bacterial keratitis with a less malignant course.[40] Infectious keratitis due to *Morganella morganii* may be clinically indistinguishable from *Pseudomonas* ulcerative keratitis. *Serratia marcescens* corneal ulcerations have been associated with contact lens wear[41] and contaminated eyedrops.[42] *Moraxella* keratitis has been described in debilitated alcoholic patients in whom the organism is also frequently a nasopharyngeal commensual[43] and in otherwise well patients when chronic ocular surface disease is present.[44] The infrequency of isolation of this bacteria may perhaps be explained by its fastidious nature and culture and the inhibitory topical anesthetic agent instilled before obtaining corneal scrapings for microbial cultures.

N. gonorrhoeae may cause a keratitis during an episode of untreated or inadequately treated conjunctivitis. It is one of the few organisms that can penetrate an intact corneal epithelium. *Neisseria* spp. can produce marked conjunctival chemosis and infiltration of the conjunctiva with polymorphonuclear neutrophils. The edematous, infiltrated conjunctiva may drape over the peripheral cornea with resultant exposure to lytic enzymes capable of producing epithelial ulceration. It is essential that the presence of the gonococcus be verified by culture because *Acinetobacter,* which is morphologically identical to the gonococcus, can also cause corneal perforation.

Gram-positive aerobic bacilli are widespread in nature and are of low virulence. They produce infections of the cornea when host resistance is lowered.[45] *Bacillus cereus* is an aerobic, gram-positive rod that may produce an extremely virulent course following introduction after foreign body injury (see Chapter 196). *C. diphtheriae* may also penetrate intact corneal epithelium to produce keratitis.[46]

Primary tuberculous keratitis is now extremely rare. Mycobacteria other than *M. tuberculosis*, particularly *Mycobacterium fortuitum* and *Mycobacterium chelonae,* are increasingly recognized as agents of keratitis, especially after injury with a foreign body or following office surgical procedures.[47–51] These mycobacteria cause chronic indolent corneal ulcerations. *Mycobacterium gordonae* and *Mycobacterium avium-intracellulare* are rare causes of ulcerative keratitis.

The incidence of ocular lesions of leprosy varies from about 15% of patients with tuberculoid leprosy to about 100% of the patients with long-standing lepromatous leprosy. Lagophthalmos, or the inability of the lids to occlude the cornea, and trichiasis, which is distortion of the lids so that lashes scratch the cornea, are complications of leprosy that predispose to keratitis (Chapter 241).

Organisms less frequently causing bacterial keratitis include *Moraxella catarrhalis,*[52] *Aeromonas hydrophila,*[53] *Pasteurella multocida,*[54] *Clostridium perfringens,*[55] *Bacillus licheniformis,*[56] *Bacillus thuringiensis,*[57] *Peptostreptococcus*, *Peptococcus,*[58] and *Propionibacterium acnes*. Polymicrobial keratitis was seen in about 78% of cases in one series of bacterial and fungal keratitis and is associated with the use of therapeutic soft "bandage" contact lenses in diseased corneas.

FUNGAL KERATITIS

More than 70 genera of filamentous fungi and yeast forms have been identified in fungal keratitis.[19, 59] The septate filamentous fungi are the most common causes of fungal keratitis, with a variable geographic distribution generally occurring in the southern and southwestern United States.[60, 61] *Fusarium solanae* is the most common causative organism and has been isolated in up to 62% of cases.[60, 62] The most common predisposing factor to keratitis from filamentous fungi is corneal injury, usually by tree branches or vegetative material. In a series of 125 cases, trauma, including wearing contact lenses, preceded fungal keratitis in 44%.[62] In a series of 211 cases of fungal keratitis in children younger than 16 years of age living in India, trauma was the predisposing factor in 55%, systemic illness in 11%, and ocular surgery in 10%.[61] *Aspergillus* spp. were the most common (40%), followed by *Fusarium* (11%), *Alternaria* (10%), *Curvularia* (7%), and *Penicillium* (7%). Filamentous fungi can infect the cornea of patients with soft contact lenses, especially when the lens is used therapeutically as a "bandage" for a diseased cornea.

Distinctive signs of fungal keratitis in early nonsevere infection include either an intact or an ulcerated epithelium with nonsuppurative stromal inflammation, often with fine feathery infiltrates. Inflammation early in the course may be minimal and either focal or multifocal "satellite" stromal infiltrates. In advanced severe fungal keratitis, the epithelium may be ulcerated with diffuse suppurative stromal inflammation. Deep stromal invasion is common enough that lamellar keratoplasty is often inadequate excision. Invasion of the anterior chamber with endophthalmitis is a late complication. Descemet's membrane is a partial barrier to posterior extension from the cornea.

Candida and other yeasts are more commonly isolated in cooler climates from patients with previous existent disease. Risk factors for *Candida* keratitis include protracted epithelial ulceration, topical corticosteroid therapy, keratoplasty treated with topical corticosteroids, and therapeutic soft contact lens wear. In patients with local ocular surface abnormalities such as dry eyes, exposure keratitis, and previous herpes simplex keratitis or with systemic immunosuppression, infection with *Candida* is more common. In contrast to filamentous keratitis, *Candida* keratitis typically causes a small oval ulceration of the corneal epithelium with an expanding, discrete, sharply demarcated, dense yellow-white stromal suppuration lacking the delicate features observed with filamentous organisms. Indeed, *Candida* keratitis may closely mimic a gram-positive bacterial keratitis, such as that caused by *S. aureus* or *S. pneumoniae.* The inflammatory reaction in *Candida* keratitis is somewhat less marked than in bacterial keratitis, often sparing the periphery of the cornea and less often associated with hypopyon.

Nocardia[63] and *Corynebacterium matruchotii*[64] are rare causes of bacterial keratitis but are mentioned here because the lesions are indistinguishable from those of a fungal origin. Rare causes of fungal keratitis, not listed in Table 99–1, include include *Absidia corymbifera,*[62] *Fonsecaea pedrosoi,*[66] *Paecilomyces lilacinus,*[67] *Scedosporium,*[68] *Phialophora bubakii,*[69] and *Tritirachium* spp.[70] Because these agents can also be isolated from the environment, it is often difficult to be sure of their role when isolated from an infected cornea.

PARASITIC KERATITIS

Parasitic keratitis is a major cause of blindness in some tropical areas. Sclerosing keratitis and stromal opacification occur from invasion of the corneal stroma by microfilariae of *Onchocerca volvulus*.[71–73] Black fly vectors are found in Africa and in scattered areas of Central and South America. The gravid female fly deposits her eggs on rocks and vegetation in rivers and streams, hence the common term *river blindness*. Onchocerciasis is one of the leading causes of blindness worldwide.[74] The ocular lesions in onchocerciasis are the direct result of microfilarial invasion of the anterior segment of the eye. Excessive tearing, conjunctival hyperemia, and photophobia are early symptoms of infection. Living microfilaria are well tolerated by the host and are often seen floating in the anterior chamber or traversing slowly through the cornea near Bowman's membrane.[75] Once the intracorneal microfilariae dies, a severe inflammatory reaction ensues.[76] Sclerosing keratitis is the blinding complication that usually occurs following a high-intensity infection of several years' duration.

Leishmania may produce a keratitis similar to that observed in onchocerciasis.[77] *Leishmania* are obligate intracellular parasites transmitted by the bites of infected sand flies. Depending on the parasite species, human infection can result in cutaneous, mucocutaneous, or visceral disease. Infection of the eyelids and conjunctiva may result in edema, ulceration, and scarring. Corneal involvement begins with superficial phlyctenules that may progress to abscess formation and ultimately result in corneal perforation.

Acanthamoeba is now a worldwide infectious agent being recognized more frequently as the cause of painful, recalcitrant keratitis, frequently leading to loss of vision or even loss of the eye.[78] These free-living amoebae may be isolated from fresh water, well water, brackish water, soil, and even air. There are many different species, of which at least seven have been associated with human keratitis. *Acanthamoeba* exist in nature and tissue in two forms. The trophozoite form is a uninucleated, motile stage that reproduces by conventional mitosis. The cystic form is double-walled with a wrinkled outer wall (ectocyst) and a stellate, polygonal inner wall (endocyst). The ability of the trophozoite to encyst under adverse conditions renders *Acanthamoeba* highly resistant to freezing, desiccation, standard chlorination of water supplies, and a variety of antimicrobial agents.

A risk factor for *Acanthamoeba* keratitis is contact lens wear, especially extended or daily wear soft contact lenses.[79, 80] Contaminated homemade saline solutions, failure of cold contact lens sterilization, and a predilection for substrate of gram-negative organisms are additional risk factors. *Acanthamoeba* keratitis may follow corneal trauma, especially with contaminated water.

The clinical features of *Acanthamoeba* keratitis early in the course may be nonspecific with patchy corneal epithelial irregularity or focal or multifocal, pleomorphic epithelial ulceration. Early in the course of infection, the epithelial abnormality may mimic dendritic ulceration, as seen with herpes simplex keratitis. Established infection typically develops a ring-shaped corneal stromal infiltrate that may be partial or complete. The patient typically complains of severe pain, and there may be an associated nodular, diffuse, or posterior scleritis. Presence of risk factors and intense pain should suggest the diagnosis. Although a stromal ring infiltrate is diagnostically helpful, it may not be seen early in the course. *Acanthamoeba* can be seen in smear and cultured by appropriate techniques.

Microsporidia are ubiquitous small obligate intracellular parasites. The two main genera causing keratitis are *Nosema* and *Encephalitozoon*. Corneal nosematosis has been observed in a 26-year-old woman in Africa,[81] in an 11-year-old boy with ulceration in India,[82] and in a 9-year-old boy in Japan with granulomatous meningoencephalitis, chorioretinitis, and meningitis.[83] Patients with acquired immunodeficiency syndrome may experience mild conjunctivitis with punctate keratitis due to *Encephalitozoon* spp.[84] Symptoms may be subtle and mimic dry eye syndromes or blepharitis. A high index of suspicion in any patient with acquired immunodeficiency syndrome is necessary to make the clinical diagnosis of microsporidial corneal infection.

African trypanosomiasis, or African sleeping sickness, is caused by hemoflagellates that are transmitted to humans via the bite of tsetse flies of the genus *Glossina*. Unilateral conjunctivitis, periorbital edema, and preauricular lymphadenopathy may be observed. Interstitial keratitis similar to that observed in syphilitic keratitis with iritis and conjunctival hyperemia has been observed.[85]

OTHER CAUSES OF KERATITIS

Corneal changes secondary to trachoma conjunctivitis are major causes of blindness worldwide.[86] Trachoma affects approximately 500 million persons in the world and represents a major health problem in both developing and highly industrialized countries. The major clinical eye diseases caused by *Chlamydia trachomatis* include trachoma, adult inclusion conjunctivitis, and neonatal inclusion conjunctivitis. In developed countries, sexually transmitted *C. trachomatis* infection rarely mimics the morphologic characteristics of true trachoma, which requires chronicity. Trachoma begins as an acute follicular conjunctivitis, which may progress to a chronic phase. The cicatricial phase of the disease causes conjunctival and lid reformation (entropion and trichiasis), which ultimately leads to corneal ulceration and opacification, often long after active infection has subsided. The disease is often characterized by repeated reinfection. Bacterial superinfection may prolong and exacerbate inflammation.

Perhaps the most common cause of keratitis is a hypersensitivity reaction to the exotoxin of *Staphylococcus*. Typically, inferior punctate corneal epithelial defects, marginal corneal stromal infiltrates, and ulcers are clinical manifestations of this allergy. Histologically, lymphocytes and plasma cells are present in the peripheral cornea, but the cornea is free of infectious organisms. Marginal keratitis associated with inflammation of the lid margin from staphylococcal blepharitis has two principal forms: (1) marginal infiltrative or ulcerative keratitis, or both, is presumably caused by a hypersensitivity reaction (type III, immune complex–mediated) to staphylococcal exotoxins or other antigens and (2) phlyctenular keratitis is presumably caused by a hypersensitivity reaction (type IV, cell-mediated) to staphylococci and other organisms.

Ring ulcerations of the cornea may give the appearance of coalesced marginal ulcerative keratitis. These ulcers may progress to total corneal destruction. The precise cause is uncertain, but these ulcerations are sometimes associated with acute systemic diseases such as influenza, bacillary dysentery, brucellosis, gonococcal arthritis, dengue, herpes zoster ophthalmicus, diabetes mellitus, and hookworm. The ring ulcerations may also be associated with a number of autoimmune connective tissue diseases such as periarteritis nodosa, rheumatoid arthritis,[87] Wegener's granulomatosis,[88] systemic lupus erythematosus, and giant cell arteritis.[89]

The two major types of interstitial keratitis encountered clinically are due to syphilis and tuberculosis. About 90% of all cases of interstitial keratitis are caused by congenital syphilis. Mycobacteria other than *M. tuberculosis* rarely cause a similar keratitis. The best explanation for the occurrence of interstitial keratitis in these two main conditions is as a host immune response rather than an active microbial infection.

Ocular involvement with syphilis may be acquired or congenital. The chancre of acquired primary syphilis has been reported to have occurred in the conjunctiva.[90] Among patients with acquired secondary syphilis, the incidence of ocular complications is 4.5%.[91] These complications include papulosquamous lesions of the skin of the lids, temporary loss of the eyebrows, diffuse papillary conjunctivitis, scleroconjunctivitis, interstitial keratitis, iritis, chorioretinitis,[92, 93] and optic[94] and retrobulbar[95] neuritis. The most common eye lesion in secondary syphilis is iridocyclitis, which accounts for about 75% of all eye lesions of the early acquired disease.[96] In almost all cases of iridocyclitis, there are other manifestations of early syphilis. Iridocyclitis can also be a late manifestation of acquired syphilis.[97]

Interstitial keratitis is a rare complication of acquired primary or secondary syphilis. Less than 3% of all cases of interstitial keratitis are due to acquired syphilis. Interstitial keratitis is also rare in early congenital syphilis. However, it is the most common lesion of late congenital syphilis and occurs in about 52% of untreated patients. It typically occurs in the early teens, with most of the cases occurring in patients between the ages of 5 and 20 years. In the acute stage, patients have decreased visual acuity, photophobia, pain, blepharospasm, and lacrimation. The corneal stroma becomes hazy within a few days and has a ground-glass appearance with marked reduction in vision. A severe iridocyclitis is present in the early stages. Over a period of months, new vessels grow into the corneal stroma from the limbus at all levels. When the vessels meet in the center of the cornea, there is a dramatic regression of the disease; the corneal infiltrates are resorbed, and the vessels are partially obliterated. The final visual prognosis in some of these patients is surprisingly good. Seventy percent have 20/20 to 20/100 acuity, and only 10% have poorer than 20/200 acuity. Nonsyphilitic spirochetal infection of the cornea may occur in Lyme disease. An interstitial keratitis similar to that observed in syphilis may be caused by the spirochete *Borrelia burgdorferi*.[98]

Cogan's syndrome is a systemic vasculitis with acute interstitial keratitis and vestibuloauditory dysfunction, usually affecting young adults. Besides interstitial keratitis, other infrequent eye findings include episcleritis, scleritis, uveitis, and optic disk edema. Ocular involvement in Cogan's syndrome[99] must be differentiated from that occurring in congenital and acquired syphilis, chlamydial infection, mumps, herpes zoster, herpes simplex, and rubeola.

A deep, nonsuppurative stromal keratitis of uncertain pathogenesis may simulate herpes simplex stromal keratitis and may follow penetrating keratoplasty and is caused by gram-negative bacilli including *Methylobacterium mesophilicum, Capnocytophaga* spp., and *Alcaligenes xylosooxidans* subspecies *denitrificans*.

A severe liquefactive keratitis may develop secondary to decreased tear production, which may be idiopathic[100, 101] or due to decreased corneal sensation after local corneal disease (e.g., herpes zoster infection), to neurologic lesions of the ophthalmic division of the trigeminal nerve, or to medullary infarction. This problem is greatly compounded when associated with inadequate lid closure.

Infectious crystalline keratopathy is a distinct clinical entity caused by a variety of bacteria. In one series of 18 patients with positive cultures, 5 were caused by gram-negative bacilli, 10 were caused primarily by gram-positive cocci, and 3 were caused primarily by yeasts.[102] There were no distinguishing features among the different organisms.

VIRAL KERATITIS

About 20% of infants born with herpes simplex virus type 1 or type 2 infection have ocular changes.[103] Seven percent have keratitis with punctate keratopathy, dendritic ulcers, or disciform keratitis. Of these, 30% are infected by herpes simplex type 1. Occasionally, keratouveitis is present at the time of birth. Prophylactic silver nitrate use is not uniformly successful in preventing ocular disease in neonates born to mothers with genital herpes simplex. Atypically, the primary keratitis may present as subepithelial dendritic opacities.[104] Morphologically, the lesions of herpes simplex types 1 and 2 are identical.

Ocular herpes simplex acquired during childhood usually manifests as a follicular conjunctivitis and is frequently undiagnosed. Transient epithelial lesions are common. However, changes similar to those described further on in adults may also be encountered.[105]

In adults with documented previous corneal herpetic infection, the recurrence rates are approximately 25% within 12 months of the last attack and 33% within 24 months.[106] Another study suggested a 40% recurrence rate for all cases of corneal epithelial herpes and a 25% recurrence rate in the form of stromal disease or keratouveitis.[107] Six percent experience visual loss secondary to stromal scarring. The clinical forms of herpes simplex epithelial keratitis include a punctate (nondendritiform) that may occur with or without conjunctivitis. The more classic form of herpes simplex virus epithelial keratitis is the linear, dendritic figure. There also may be geographic macroulceration of the epithelium. In the nonlinear and dendritic forms, active viral replication in the ulcer margin has been documented in the epithelium. The geographic type is notable for a prolonged course. Dendritic and geographic epithelial keratitis is known to heal spontaneously within 10 to 14 days in 80% of cases. Stromal involvement is usually seen in recurrent attacks, and the cornea has not been shown conclusively to harbor active viral particles. Herpes simplex virus stromal involvement (disciform keratitis) is an immune-mediated reaction. The process frequently results in some stromal scarring, commonly with thinning and occasionally with perforation. An associated uveitis is common. Recurrent ocular herpes simplex is thought to result from reactivation of latent herpes in the trigeminal ganglion and centripetal spread to the eye.[108] Herpes simplex viral DNA has been detected using the polymerase chain reaction. Corneal hypesthesia,[109] which worsens with repeated attacks, is common.

The pattern of disease is different in immunosuppressed patients.[110, 111] They may have bilateral corneal involvement, which is seen in only 5% of other patients, and may also have extensive and multiple lesions on the cornea and conjunctiva. These lesions tend to persist or recur with topical antiviral therapy until immunosuppressive therapy is reduced.

The precise mechanisms for viral reactivation are incompletely understood, yet some of the factors that may precipitate recurrent episodes are exposure to sunlight, menstruation, psychiatric disturbances, fever, and other acute stresses.[112] Acute illnesses may temporarily suppress the immune mechanisms, and the most common cause of a unilateral red eye in a hospitalized patient is herpes simplex keratitis. Topical and systemic steroids and immunosuppressive agents may provoke recurrences in corneal epithelium, and they enhance replication in established lesions.[113]

The subepithelial corneal opacities occurring in epidemic keratoconjunctivitis caused by adenovirus probably represent an immune phenomenon. These opacities tend to appear approximately 10 to 14 days after the symptoms commence. The natural course of the corneal lesions is resolution over 2 to 3 weeks, although patients may be very photophobic during this period. The lesions tend to clear dramatically with the use of topical corticosteroids, with occasional reappearance when the steroid therapy is discontinued.

In about 10% of the patients with herpes zoster infections, the ophthalmic division of the trigeminal nerve is involved. The various ocular manifestations include vesicles on the lid and conjunctiva, iridocyclitis, secondary glaucoma, ophthalmoplegia, neuroretinitis, optic neuritis, and retinal vascular occlusion.[114, 115] Corneal findings include decreased corneal sensation, epithelial and subepithelial punctate keratitis, dendritic figures, disciform keratitis, segmental keratitis, and corneal vascularization. The corneal disease may occur after the skin eruption has healed, and it can be prolonged.[116] Visual loss may result from peripheral and central stromal involvement.[117]

In varicella infections (chickenpox), ocular involvement is usually limited to the appearance of vesicles on the lids, conjunctiva, and limbus. Superficial punctate keratitis, interstitial and disciform keratitis, and uveitis have also been reported.[118] Epithelial dendritic figures that are identical to those seen in herpes zoster keratitis may occur immediately or up to several months after the skin eruption.[119] A scleritis may also accompany varicella disciform keratitis.[120] Vaccinia infections of the eye occur from accidental autoinoculation.[121] Corneal complications occur in one third of the patients with ocular vaccinia and may consist of superficial punctate keratitis, epithelial ulcers, and rarely disciform keratitis. The epithelial ulcers may superficially resemble herpetic keratitis.[122, 123]

The keratitis that is occasionally associated with measles (rubeola) infection causes punctate or dendritic epithelial defects in the cornea.[124] In one adult population study, all rubeola patients had epithelial keratitis that followed a benign course.[125] The changing immune status of the population after vaccination programs is changing the pattern of clinical disease—from a childhood illness to an adult disease and perhaps a different ocular expression of measles infection. In developing countries, vitamin A deficiency and malnutrition sometimes make measles keratitis a blinding disease with secondary bacterial infection and perforation of the globe.

Epstein-Barr virus infections may cause a spectrum of ocular involvement, including dacryoadenitis, oculoglandular syndrome, follicular conjunctivitis, punctate and dendritic epithelial keratitis, and stromal keratitis. Cranial nerve palsies, papilledema, and optic neuritis may also be observed. The stromal keratitis may affect the subepithelial region,[126] the anterior and midstroma, or the deep stroma.[127]

There have been occasional reported cases of Jakob-Creutzfeldt disease[128] and rabies transmission[129] from the use of infected donor tissue in corneal transplantation. Human immunodeficiency virus has been demonstrated within the corneal epithelium.[130] All potential donors of corneas considered for transplantation are screened for possible human immunodeficiency virus infection and the hepatitis viruses.

LABORATORY INVESTIGATIONS FOR DIAGNOSIS

Because the morphologic features of infectious and noninfectious keratitis are sometimes indistinguishable, diagnostic laboratory evaluation of corneal scrapings is imperative if there is suspicion of microbial keratitis. One of the basic principles of laboratory investigation is to follow a standard set plan for all suspected cases of microbial keratitis. The ophthalmologist and clinical microbiology laboratory should establish a routine method for obtaining diagnostic material and maintaining standard materials for collection, transport, and culture.[131] Other basic principles include maintaining complete patient control to ensure adequate sampling of the area of corneal suppuration. This can be achieved through administration of local anesthesia to achieve akinesia in uncooperative adults or general anesthesia in children if necessary. Multiple samples from areas of suppuration should be obtained for *each* stain and media. The smears of corneal scrapings on glass slides should be fixed promptly in methyl alcohol. Material from corneal scrapings should also be directly inoculated to fresh culture media, which has been warmed to room temperature. Special stains and media should be used if directed by clinical signs or results of prior studies. Methods for obtaining material and techniques for culture vary considerably. Proparacaine hydrochloride (0.5%) is less antiseptic than are other topical anesthetics and is the preferred topical anesthetic for performing corneal scrapings. Corneal scraping can be achieved using a blunt platinum (Kimura) spatula, sterile surgical blade (Bard-Parker), or calcium alginate swab dipped in trypticase soy broth. The calcium alginate swab dipped in trypticase soy broth may cause corneal pathogens to adhere better than the platinum spatula, thereby increasing the yield of diagnostic corneal scrapings. Superficial keratectomy may be helpful in dry nonsuppurative infections and is aided by the use of a sharp sterile blade or scissors and forceps. Corneal biopsy[132] may assist in diagnosis in dry, nonsuppurative infections if the surface of the cornea is spared. A corneal shave biopsy can be completed with a sterile surgical blade, or adequate corneal biopsy may be performed with a 1.5- or 2.0-mm trephine and unguarded diamond blade. Corneal biopsy can usually be performed at the slit-lamp biomicroscope, although some patients may require the operating room and adjunctive anesthesia for controlled biopsy. Lamellar keratoplasty is typically unnecessary for diagnostic purposes. A penetrating therapeutic keratoplasty may be required for diagnosis and therapy of progressive, destructive keratitis if the cause is not determined by other methods.

Corneal scrapings are transferred to clean glass slides for Gram, Giemsa, acid-fast and calcofluor white, or methenamine silver stains. Multiple inoculations of the corneal scraping with the spatula or calcium alginate swab are completed on blood agar, chocolate agar, thioglycolate or Schaedler broth, brain-heart infusion or Sabouraud's agar, and blood agar incubated anaerobically. Special methods are required to recover *Chlamydia* or *Acanthamoeba.* For mycobacteria, Lowenstein-Jensen agar at 35°C, Middlebrook 7H10 or 7H11, or commercial radiometric broth (Bactec) medium is appropriate (see Chapter 14). In many cases, concomitant cultures of the conjunctiva and lid on the affected and unaffected eye are obtained to ascertain the person's flora and to assist in assessing the significance of positive corneal cultures taken from the area of ulceration. The type and number of positive cultures needed to support a microbial diagnosis are still unsettled.[133, 134] Negative cultures obtained from corneal scrapings in the face of a suspicious ulcerative keratitis should lead to a superficial keratectomy or corneal biopsy. These investigations may prove positive when superficial scrapings were previously negative because fungi and *Acanthamoeba* are characteristically deep in corneal parenchyma and conspicuously absent on the surface.[131, 132] Viral keratitis may not require culture because diagnosis can be made by appearance of the lesions. Careful débridement of the corneal epithelium and transfer to viral transport media usually suffices to grow herpes simplex virus types 1 and 2 and adenovirus. Herpes zoster virus is rarely isolated from corneal lesions. In doubtful cases, transmission electron microscopy may occasionally be helpful in establishing the viral cause.[132, 135]

The majority of aerobic bacteria causing keratitis grow on the standard media within 48 hours, and sometimes a pathogen may be recognized in 12 to 15 hours. Some criteria suggested for confirming an infectious corneal process include growth of an organism in two or more media, confluent growth of a known ocular pathogen in one solid medium, or growth in one medium of an organism identified on routine stain.

Once a corneal pathogen has been identified from the appropriate media, antimicrobial susceptibility testing should proceed according to the usual laboratory techniques. Laboratory antifungal sensitivity testing currently lacks optimal standardization and reproducibility.

TREATMENT

Because of the rapid evolution to perforation in keratitis due to virulent pathogens and visual loss secondary to central scarring, many patients with bacterial keratitis and significant ulceration need to be hospitalized. The high frequency and intense dosage scheduling of antimicrobial therapy often requires the assistance of trained nursing personnel.

In infectious keratitis, aggressive antibiotic therapy is the mainstay, and there are several routes of administration, including topical antibiotic drops and ointments, continuous lavage, antibiotic-soaked collagen corneal shields or therapeutic soft contact lenses, iontophoresis, subconjunctival injection, and parenteral administration. The objective of therapy in bacterial keratitis is to eliminate the infective organism or organisms in a rapid fashion, reduce the inflammatory response, prevent structural damage to the tissue, and promote healing. Selection of the appropriate antibiotic agent requires a thorough understanding of the inherent antimicrobial properties, spectrum of microbiologic efficacy, tissue pharmacokinetics, and clinical effectiveness.

With suspected infectious keratitis, the clinician has the option of initiating specific directed or broad-spectrum antimicrobial therapy, deferring treatment pending the results of laboratory investigation, or monitoring the clinical signs. In general, because of the potential rapid destruction of corneal tissue that may accompany bacterial keratitis, if there is a clinical suspicion suggestive of a bacterial pathogen, the patient should be treated appropriately for bacterial keratitis until a definitive diagnosis is substantiated.

A basic plan for therapy of severe suppurative keratitis depends on the results of Gram stains on smears from diagnostic corneal scrapings. If a single type of bacterium is observed with microscopic analysis of smears and the patient has not been on antecedent therapy, a single specific antibacterial agent is selected. If two or more types of bacteria are present on Gram stain, combined specific antibacterial therapy is recommended. If a single bacterium is observed on Gram stain, however, and the patient has received prior therapy, a broad-spectrum antibacterial therapeutic regimen is recommended.

The decision to base initial antibiotic therapy on the results of Gram stain requires a high technical proficiency on the part of the microbiology laboratory. With optimal conditions, the microbiology laboratory can identify the pathogen on Gram stain in 75% of monobacterial keratitis cases and 37% of polybacterial keratitis cases. If the Gram stain is equivocal or there is uncertainty in interpretation of diagnostic smears, broad-spectrum antibiotic coverage should be initiated in the initial treatment of all cases of severe suppurative microbial keratitis because the consequences of inappropriate or inadequate therapy can be devastating.[136]

A solution of topical antibiotic is administered frequently and in high concentration. Solutions are preferred over ointments because solutions can penetrate into ocular tissues to achieve higher concentration in ocular tissues than can be achieved with ointment preparations. Hospital pharmacies can readily prepare highly concentrated (fortified) solutions by using commercially available ocular lubricants and parenteral antibiotic formulations.[137]

Subconjunctival administration of antibiotics, although painful, provides a transient peak concentration of drug within the corneal stroma, yet equivalent drug levels may be attained with highly concentrated antibiotic solutions administered topically at great frequency.[138]

Continuous lavage of the cornea with antibiotics has been described.[139] The advantages of this method include potentially increased drug levels obtained within the aqueous humor,[140] as well as a lack of dependence on nursing personnel for frequent drop instillations.

Soft hydrophilic contact lenses have been used as drug delivery systems to achieve higher intraocular drug concentrations than can be obtained with frequent topical administration.[141, 142] Collagen corneal shields soaked in antibiotic solutions have also been shown to increase antibiotic penetration compared with therapeutic soft contact lenses.[143, 144] Use of collagen corneal shields as adjuncts in the therapy of bacterial keratitis has been experimentally documented.[145] No controlled clinical trials documenting efficacy and safety have been completed. Polymer inserts have also been designed to prolong the presence of drug in the tear film. Liposomal systems have been designed to improve the interaction of drugs with the corneal surface.[146, 147] Transcorneal iontophoresis of antibiotics has also been employed to increase attainable drug concentrations and increase efficacy of antibacterial therapy.[148] Other strategies to improve drug delivery to the cornea include placement of temporary punctal occlusion plugs to maintain more antibiotic in the preocular tear film.

Parenteral (intramuscular or intravenous) administration of antibiotics is reserved for severe suppurative keratitis with impending perforation. Intravenous antibiotic administration is also recommended for contiguous spread of infection to involve the sclera (sclerokeratitis).

Factors that frequently guide the choice of appropriate antibiotic for systemic infection are not necessarily applicable to the topical therapy of ocular infections. The minimal inhibitory concentration determinations in antimicrobial susceptibility testing are based on achievable serum levels and do not directly apply to topical therapy of infective keratitis. Other factors important in the therapy of systemic infections such as distribution space, mode of excretion, influence of renal or hepatic failure, and absorption characteristics are also not directly applicable to ocular infections. The antimicrobial agent selected for initial therapy should have bactericidal activity against common corneal pathogens, low rates of acquired resistance, favorable solubility characteristics to enhance penetration, and minimal toxicity to ocular tissues. Initial broad-spectrum therapy for suspected bacterial keratitis has traditionally been with a topical first-generation cephalosporin (e.g., cefazolin) and an aminoglycoside (gentamicin, tobramycin, or amikacin).

Many classes of antibiotics have been used for the directed specific therapy of bacterial keratitis. Gram-positive keratitis, especially from staphylococcal species, is most often treated with topical cephalosporin antibiotics. If there is suspected resistance of the staphylococcal species to cephalosporins or semisynthetic penicillins, topical vancomycin should be considered. Penicillin G is the therapy of choice for pneumococcal keratitis.

Gentamicin has been the therapy of choice for gram-negative keratitis and can be administered by topical, subconjunctival, and parenteral routes. Ophthalmic solutions (eyedrops) of 0.3% are commercially available and can be fortified to 1.3 to 1.5%. Tobramycin is similar. The aminoglycosides may be synergistic with ticarcillin or piperacillin against *Pseudomonas* and *Proteus* spp., but they may be inactivated if mixed in the same solution.

Three fluoroquinolones are commercially available as 0.3% ophthalmic solutions: ciprofloxacin, norfloxacin, and ofloxacin. The have similar antimicrobial spectra that includes most aerobic gram-negative and some gram-positive bacteria.[149] Fluoroquinolones are highly active against most Enterobacteriaceae. In particular, fluoroquinolones are highly active against *P. aeruginosa*, including strains that are resistant to other bacterial agents. Ciprofloxacin has the most potent in vitro activity of the ophthalmic fluoroquinolones currently commercially available against *P. aeruginosa*.

Although fluoroquinolones are active against *P. aeruginosa*, they are less active against other *Pseudomonas* spp. and the related species, *Stenotrophomonas maltophilia* and *Burkholderia (Pseudomonas) cepacia*. Most strains of *Acinetobacter* are susceptible to ciprofloxacin or ofloxacin. Norfloxacin is considerably less active. Ciprofloxacin and ofloxacin are the most active of the commercially available ophthalmic agents against several gram-positive species. Streptococci, including *Streptococcus pyogenes* (group A), *Streptococcus agalactiae* (group B), *S. pneumoniae* and viridans streptococci, and *Enterococcus faecalis* (enterococci) are only moderately susceptible to ciprofloxacin and ofloxacin, even considering topical concentrations. Norfloxacin is even less active. *Haemophilus influenzae*, *Haemophilus ducreyi*, *N. gonorrhoeae*, *N. meningitidis*, and *M. catarrhalis* are all highly susceptible to the fluoroquinolones, including β-lactamase–producing strains of these organisms. Ciprofloxacin and ofloxacin have clinically useful activity against some nontuberculous mycobacteria, such as *Mycobacterium fortuitum* and, to a lesser extent, *M. chelonae*.[150] Ciprofloxacin and ofloxacin also have activity in vitro against *C. trachomatis*. Newer fluoroquinolones, such as trovafloxacin, have substantial activity against anaerobic bacteria. Ciprofloxacin and ofloxacin demonstrate no useful activity against these species.

There is considerable clinical experience with treatment of bacterial keratitis with fluoroquinolones. A randomized, double-blind comparison of ciprofloxacin solution 0.3% versus cefazolin 5.0% with tobramycin 1.3% in 324 patients at 28 centers found equal efficacy and less ocular discomfort with ciprofloxacin.[151] A similarly designed trial compared ofloxacin 0.3% versus gentamicin 1.5% with cefuroxime 5.0% in 122 patients and found no difference in efficacy.[152] Ofloxacin 0.3% also compared favorably with a combination of tobramycin 1.5% with cefazolin 10% in a large, multicenter, double-blind, randomized trial.[153] The ofloxacin-treated patients complained less of ocular burning and stinging. It is useful to note the frequency with which the solutions were instilled, starting with every 15 minutes then slowly progressing to every 6 hours by the sixth day. Crystalline, white ciprofloxacin precipitates were observed in the area of epithelial ulceration in 16% of patients. Such crystalline drug precipitation occurs with higher frequency in eyes treated with ciprofloxacin than in those treated with norfloxacin[154] or ofloxacin, consistent with differences in fluoroquinolone compound pH solubility profiles. The crystalline deposition has the potential disadvantage of decreasing visualization of the stromal infiltrate immediately deep to the precipitate for clinical monitoring of therapeutic progress. The crystalline corneal precipitates of ciprofloxacin usually spontaneously resolve with cessation of therapy. Both the solution and ointment are commercially available as 0.3% ciprofloxacin.

Norfloxacin is also available as a 0.3% topical ophthalmic solution. Norfloxacin is generally less active in vitro and in vivo against gram-positive organisms and most gram-negative organisms as compared with ciprofloxacin and ofloxacin. Topical norfloxacin ophthalmic solution has U.S. Food and Drug Administration approval for the treatment of bacterial conjunctivitis, but not for keratitis. Topical norfloxacin exhibits greater corneal epithelial toxicity than does topical ciprofloxacin or ofloxacin, similar to the toxicity profile observed with the combination of a cephalosporin and aminoglycoside.

The spectrum and safety of ciprofloxacin and ofloxacin ocular solutions make them attractive alternatives for empirical use in keratitis that is not vision-threatening. Fluoroquinolone monotherapy is not recommended for empirical therapy of sight-threatening bacterial keratitis. Therapy directed toward the pathogen, which can be more than one organism, is essential in such patients. Forster has put all these ideas together and offered the following recommendations for the management of keratitis:

1. Perform corneal scrapings in selected patients with suspected infectious keratitis when risk factors are present, when there is a large central infiltrate, or when empirical therapy has failed.
2. Continue to culture all cases of suspected infectious keratitis in community- and hospital-based practices.
3. Use fortified antibiotics for more severe keratitis.
4. Use monotherapy with a fluoroquinolone or other commercially available antibiotics, or both, for mild keratitis.
5. As an alternative, combine fortified cefazolin with a fluoroquinolone.[1]

Supportive therapy in the treatment of infectious keratitis consists of topical cycloplegics to reduce photophobia, enzyme inhibitors, metalloproteinase inhibitors, therapeutic soft contact lenses, collagen corneal shields, and topical corticosteroids. Because severe anterior chamber inflammatory reaction may occur with bacterial keratitis, cycloplegics should be administered to prevent the formation of synechiae and to relieve the discomfort of ciliary spasm.

If corneal ulceration is marked, the temporary use of a therapeutic soft contact lens or "bandage" lens may facilitate stromal repair and promote reepithelialization by protecting the corneal surface from mechanical trauma of lid movement. Topical medication may be continued after the contact lens insertion, and drug delivery to the cornea may also be enhanced.

The use of topical corticosteroids in the management of bacterial keratitis is somewhat controversial. It has been suggested that steroids in conjunction with specific antibacterial therapy minimize the inflammatory sequelae of bacterial keratitis. A number of experimental studies have concluded that corticosteroid therapy does not adversely affect results of antibiotic therapy in bacterial keratitis.[155, 156] *Pseudomonas* keratitis requires long-term high-dose antibiotic therapy prior to cautious introduction of corticosteroid therapy.

Signs of clinical improvement are based on frequent slit-lamp examination. Clinical changes may be difficult to appreciate in the early course of therapy because of the effects of diagnostic corneal scraping and frequent topical antibiotic therapy. After the first 48 hours, the frequency of antibiotic administration can usually be decreased gradually. Highly concentrated antibiotic solutions may be converted to commercial-strength drops after several days. The therapeutic end point in ulcerative keratitis is epithelial healing, yet concentrated antibiotics may retard reepithelialization.

The research and development of effective antifungal compounds for ocular mycotic infections has lagged behind that for antibacterial agents. Therapy for fungal keratitis generally requires prolonged use of topical antifungal agents and occasionally adjunctive parenteral therapy. An ophthalmic preparation of natamycin (pimaricin) is no longer available in the United States. Amphotericin B desoxycholate (Fungizone) can be prepared in the pharmacy in sterile water as 1.5 mg/ml. Amphotericin B has also been compounded as 5 mg/g in white vasoline for ophthalmic ointment.[157] Amphotericin B is active against fungi, particularly *Candida,* although the desoxycholate formulation is toxic to the corneal epithelium. Itraconazole has been used orally for fungal keratitis, but experience is meager. Fluconazole is available as a sterile solution for intravenous use and has been used topically for a few cases of *Candida* keratitis. Chlorhexidine gluconate 0.2% compared favorably with natamycin 2.5% in a randomized comparison carried out in 71 patients in Bangladesh.[158] The most common fungi encountered in those patients were *Aspergillus* and *Fusarium.* Caution must be exercised when adding topical corticosteroid to therapy when a response to the antifungal agent has been observed to help reduce corneal destruction caused by host response. In severe cases of fungal keratitis, corneal transplantation, keratoplasty, or conjunctival flaps may be needed to stabilize the eye. Penetrating keratoplasty and conjunctival flaps were the main defense against fungal keratitis prior to antifungal chemotherapy.

Medical therapy for *Acanthamoeba* keratitis remains unsatisfactory (see Chapter 263). *Acanthamoeba* keratitis has most often been treated with multiple agents. Polyhexamethylene biguanide, a polymeric biguanide and environmental biocide, has been shown to have clinical efficacy in the therapy of keratitis.[159] Cationic antiseptics, such as chlorhexidine gluconate, in combination with aromatic diamidines, such as propamidine (Brolene) or hexamidine (Desomedine) have been used. Many cases of *Acanthamoeba* keratitis require both medical therapy and therapeutic keratoplasty to eradicate the cyst effectively from the corneal tissue.

Diethylcarbamazine is no longer recommended for therapy of onchocerciasis. Ivermectin is highly effective and less toxic with fewer ocular complications than seen with diethylcarbamazine[160] (see Chapter 278). Because syphilitic interstitial keratitis is a manifestation of an immune phenomenon, specific antitreponemal therapy does not greatly affect the course of the acute inflammation. However, therapy reduces the chances of recurrence from 27% in untreated cases to 3.6% in treated cases. Treatment also reduces the likelihood of bilateral ocular involvement. Topical steroids are used during the acute stages of the keratitis to avoid severe postinflammatory sequelae. Because Lyme keratitis is a manifestation of a systemic infection having potentially protean manifestations, including neurologic, cardiologic, rheumatologic, and dermatologic complications, a course of systemic parenteral therapy with intravenous ceftriaxone is indicated. Topical corticosteroids to reduce interstitial inflammation should be applied and may require a prolonged taper.

The treatment of epithelial keratitis in herpes simplex viral infections consists of minimal wiping débridement of the epithelium[161] and use of a topical antiviral agent; this is effective in most cases of corneal dendritic ulcerations. Extensive involvement, central lesions, geographic macroulcerations, or resistant lesions are usually treated with a 10-day course of topical antiviral agents. Trifluridine ophthalmic solution (commercially available) and acyclovir are the agents used topically because of their lower corneal toxicity. The use of corticosteroids is contraindicated in isolated herpes simplex epithelial keratitis. Active epithelial keratitis generally resolves within 5 to 10 days, and judgment of activity is aided clinically by the use of rose bengal solution, which also has antiviral activity. Concurrent prophylactic antibacterial antibiotics are generally not indicated, as they may enhance ocular toxicity. Corticosteroids are the only effective therapeutic measure for herpes simplex virus stromal keratitis. Use and dosage is determined by the severity of the stromal inflammation, presence of prior epithelial keratitis, interval since any prior epithelial keratitis, and antecedent corticosteroid use. Use of a concurrent topical antiviral agent as prophylaxis against recurrent epithelial keratitis is recommended when corticosteroid therapy is administered more often than once daily. The role of oral acyclovir in combination with topical steroids has not been shown to be beneficial in control of stromal keratitis. Oral acyclovir, 400 mg twice daily taken for 1 year, reduced the incidence of recurrent herpes simplex virus stromal keratitis from 28% in placebo recipients to 14%.[162] Because recurrences are common and may impair vision, long-term oral acyclovir prophylaxis appears useful. Uncontrolled herpetic stromal keratitis and secondary stromal scarring may require corneal transplantation.[163, 164]

Stromal keratitis caused by herpes zoster frequently requires corticosteroids to reduce the inflammatory response and resultant corneal destruction, including neovascularization and lipid deposition along with permanent endothelial dysfunction.

Oral acyclovir or topical antiviral agents are not indicated for therapy of herpes zoster stromal keratitis even with concomitant corticosteroid administration. Oral corticosteroids may be required for concurrent scleritis.

Epidemic keratoconjunctivitis from adenovirus rarely requires therapy beyond supportive measures such as artificial tears and mild cycloplegics. Severe photophobia, incapacitating irritation, and decreased vision during acute episodes may be relieved with topical corticosteroids. It is unclear whether their use prolongs the course of the disease. Ocular involvement in infectious mononucleosis also typically requires only the use of ocular lubricants or mild corticosteroids to control the stromal keratitis.

REFERENCES

1. Forster RK. Conrad Berens lecture. The management of infectious keratitis as we approach the 21st century. CLAO J. 1998;24:175–180.
2. Jain S, Azar DT. Eye infections after refractive keratotomy. J Refract Surg. 1996;12:148–155.
3. Duffey RJ. Bilateral *Serratia marcescens* keratitis after simultaneous bilateral radial keratotomy. Am J Ophthalmol. 1995;119:233–236.
4. Szerenyi K, McDonnell JM, Smith RE, et al. Keratitis as a complication of bilateral, simultaneous radial keratotomy. Am J Ophthalmol. 1994;117:462–467.
5. Procope JA. Delayed-onset *Pseudomonas* keratitis after radial keratotomy. J Cataract Refract Surg. 1997;23:1271–1272.
6. Heidemann DG, Dunn SP, Watts JC. Aspergillus keratitis after radial keratotomy. Am J Ophthalmol. 1995;120:254–256.
7. Santos CR. Herpetic corneal ulcer following radial keratotomy. Ann Ophthalmol. 1983;15:82–85.
8. Friedman RF, Wolf TC, Chodosh J. *Acanthamoeba* infection after radial keratotomy. Am J Ophthalmol. 1997;123:409–410.
9. Gussler JR, Miller D, Jaffe M, et al. Infection after radial keratotomy. Am J Ophthalmol. 1995;119:798–799.
10. Lu Y, Snibson GR. Delayed microbial keratitis following radial keratotomy. Aust NZ J Ophthalmol. 1997;25:231–232.
11. Mandelbaum S, Waring GO 3d, Forster RK, et al. Late development of ulcerative keratitis in radial keratotomy scars. Arch Ophthalmol. 1986;104:1156–1160.
12. McClellan KA, Bernard PJ, Gregory-Roberts JC, et al. Suppurative keratitis: A late complication of radial keratotomy. J Cataract Refract Surg. 1988;14:317–320.
13. Lin RT, Maloney RK. Flap complications associated with lamellar refractive surgery. Am J Ophthalmol. 1999;127:129–136.
14. Perez-Santonja JJ, Sakla HF, Abad JL, et al. Nocardial keratitis after laser in situ keratomileusis. J Refract Surg. 1997;13:314–317.
15. Luchs JI, Cohen EJ, Rapuano CJ, et al. Ulcerative keratitis in bullous keratopathy. Ophthalmology. 1997;104:816–822.
16. Parkin B, Turner A, Moore E, et al. Bacterial keratitis in the critically ill. Br J Ophthalmol. 1997;81:1060–1063.
17. Jones DB. Polymicrobial keratitis. Trans Am Ophthalmol Soc. 1981;79:153.
18. Asbell P, Stenson S. Ulcerative keratitis. Survey of 30 years laboratory experience. Arch Ophthalmol. 1982;100:77.
19. Liesegang TJ, Forster RK. Spectrum of microbial keratitis in South Florida. Am J Ophthalmol. 1980;90:38.
20. Eichenbaum JW, Feldstein M, Podos SM. Extended-wear aphakic soft contact lenses in corneal ulcers. Br J Ophthalmol. 1982;66:663.
21. Wang AG, Wu CC, Liu JH. Bacterial corneal ulcer: A multivariate study. Ophthalmologica. 1998;212:126–132.
22. Coster DJ, Wilhelmus KR, Peacock J, et al. Suppurative keratitis in London. In: Trevor-Roper T, ed. European Society of Ophthalmology. The Cornea, Health, and Disease. London: Academic Press; 1981:395.
23. Ostler HB, Okumoto M, Wilkey C. The changing pattern of the etiology of central bacterial corneal (hypopyon) ulcer. Trans Pacific Coast Oto-Ophthalmol Soc. 1976;57:235.
24. Wilson LA, Schlitzer RL, Ahearn DG. *Pseudomonas* corneal ulcers associated with soft contact lens wear. Am J Ophthalmol. 1981;92:546.
25. Krachmer JH, Purcell JJ. Bacterial corneal ulcers in cosmetic soft contact lens wearers. Arch Ophthalmol. 1978;96:57.
26. Schein OD, Poggio EC, Seddon JM, et al. The incidence of ulcerative keratitis among extended contact lens wearers. N Engl J Med. 1989;321:773.
27. Glynn RJ, Schein OD, Seddon JM, et al. The incidence of ulcerative keratitis among aphakic contact lens wearers in New England. Arch Ophthalmol. 1991;109:104–107.
28. Escapini H Jr, Olson RJ, Kaufman HE. Donor cornea contamination with McCarey-Kaufman medium preservation. Am J Ophthalmol. 1979;88:59.
29. Udell IJ, Kelly CG, Woolf TC, et al. Cat scratch keratitis. Ophthalmology. 1987;94(Suppl):124.
30. Wilson LA, Ahearn DG. *Pseudomonas* induced corneal ulcers associated with contaminated eye mascaras. Am J Ophthalmol. 1977;84:112.
31. Reid PR, Wood TO. *Pseudomonas* corneal ulcer. The causative role of contaminated eye cosmetics. Arch Ophthalmol. 1979;97:1640.
32. Locatcher-Khorazo D, Gutierrez E. Bacteria typing of *Staphylococcus aureus*. A study of normal, infected eyes in environment. Arch Ophthalmol. 1960;63:774.
33. Kim HB, Ostler HB. Marginal corneal ulcer due to beta-*Streptococcus*. Arch Ophthalmol. 1977;95:454.
34. Cohn H, Mondino BJ, Brown SI, et al. Marginal corneal ulcers with acute beta-streptococcal conjunctivitis in chronic dacryocystitis. Am J Ophthalmol. 1979;87:541.
35. Belmont JB, Ostler HB, Chandler RD, et al. Non-infectious ring-shaped keratitis associated with *Pseudomonas aeruginosa*. Am J Ophthalmol. 1982;93:338.
36. Kessler E, Mondino BJ, Brown SI. The corneal response to *Pseudomonas aeruginosa:* Histopathological and enzymatic characterization. Invest Ophthalmol Vis Sci. 1977;16:116.
37. Hutton WL, Sexton RR. Atypical *Pseudomonas* corneal ulcers in semi-comatose patients. Am J Ophthalmol. 1972;73:37.
38. Codere F, Brownstein S, Jackson WB. *Pseudomonas aeruginosa* scleritis. Am J Ophthalmol. 1981;91:706.
39. Raber IM, Laibson PR, Kurz GH, et al. *Pseudomonas* corneoscleral ulcers. Am J Ophthalmol. 1981;92:353.
40. Brinser JH, Torczynski E. Unusual *Pseudomonas* corneal ulcers. Am J Ophthalmol. 1977;84:462.
41. Lass JH, Haaf J, Foster CS, et al. Visual outcome in eight cases of *Serratia marcescens* keratitis. Am J Ophthalmol. 1981;92:384.
42. Templeton WC, Eiferman RA, Snyder JW, et al. *Serratia* keratitis transmitted by contaminated eyedroppers. Am J Ophthalmol. 1982;93:723.
43. Baum J, Fedukowicz HB, Jordan A. A survey of *Moraxella* corneal ulcers in a derelict population. Am J Ophthalmol. 1980;90:476.
44. Cobo LM, Coster DJ, Peacock J. *Moraxella* keratitis in a nonalcoholic population. Br J Ophthalmol. 1981;65:683.
45. vanBusterveld OP, Richards RD. Bacillus infection of the cornea. Arch Ophthalmol. 1965;74:91.
46. Chandler JW, Milam DF. Diphtheria corneal ulcers. Arch Ophthalmol. 1978;96:53.
47. Turner L, Stinson I. *Mycobacterium fortuitum* as a cause of corneal ulcer. Am J Ophthalmol. 1965;60:329.
48. Meisler DM, Friedlaender MH, Okumoto M. *Mycobacterium chelonei* keratitis. Am J Ophthalmol. 1982;94:398.
49. Gangadharam PRJ, Lanier JD, Jones DB. Keratitis due to *Mycobacterium chelonei*. Tubercle. 1978;59:55.
50. Lazar M, Nemet P, Bracha R, et al. *Mycobacterium fortuitum* keratitis. Am J Ophthalmol. 1974;78:530.
51. Newman PE, Goodman RA, Waring GA, et al. A cluster of cases of *Mycobacterium chelonei* keratitis associated with outpatient office procedures. Am J Ophthalmol. 1984;97:344.
52. Wilhelmus KR, Peacock J, Coster BJ. *Branhamella* keratitis. Br J Ophthalmol. 1980;64:892.
53. Feaster FT, Nisbet RN, Barber JC. *Aeromonas hydrophilia* corneal ulcer. Am J Ophthalmol. 1978;85:114.
54. Purcell JJ, Krachmer JH. Corneal ulcer caused by *Pasteurella multocida*. Am J Ophthalmol. 1977;83:540.
55. Stern GA, Hodes BL, Stock EL. *Clostridium perfringens* corneal ulcer. Arch Ophthalmol. 1979;97:661.
56. Tabbara KF, Taraba VN. *Bacillus licheniformis* corneal ulcer. Am J Ophthalmol. 1979;87:717.
57. Samples JR, Buettner H. Corneal ulcer caused by a biologic insecticide (*B. thuringiensis*). Am J Ophthalmol. 1983;95:258.
58. Ostler HB, Okumoto M. Anaerobic streptococcal corneal ulcer. Am J Ophthalmol. 1976;81:518.
59. Jones DB. Opportunistic fungal infections in ophthalmology. Fungal keratitis. In: Chic ED, Balows A, Furcolow ML, eds. Opportunistic Fungal Infections. Springfield, Ill: Charles C Thomas; 1975:103.
60. Jones DB, Forster RK, Rebell G. *Fusarium solani* keratitis treated with natamycin (pimaricin): 18 consecutive cases. Arch Ophthalmol. 1972;88:147.
61. Panda A, Sharma N, Das G, et al. Mycotic keratitis in children: Epidemiologic and microbiologic evaluation. Cornea. 1997;16:295–299.
62. Rosa RH Jr, Miller D, Alfonso EC. The changing spectrum of fungal keratitis in south Florida. Ophthalmology. 1994;101:1005–1013.
63. Hirst LW, Harrison GK, Merz EG, et al. *Nocardia asteroides* keratitis. Br J Ophthalmol. 1979;63:449.
64. Wilhelmus KR, Robinson NN, Jones DB. *Bacterionema matruchotii* ocular infections. Am J Ophthalmol. 1979;87:143.
65. Marshall DH, Brownstein S, Jackson WB, et al. Post-traumatic corneal mucormycosis caused by *Absidia corymbifera*. Ophthalmology. 1997;104:1107–1111.
66. Barton K, Miller D, Pflugfelder SC. Corneal chromoblastomycosis. Cornea. 1997;16:235–239.
67. Okhravi N, Dart JK, Tower, HM, et al. *Paecilomyces lilacinus* endophthalmitis with

secondary keratitis: A case report and review of the literature. Arch Ophthalmol. 197;115:11320–11324.

68. Kumar B, Crawford GJ, Morlet GC. *Scedosporium prolificans* corneoscleritis: A successful outcome. Aust N Z J Ophthalmol. 1997;25:169–171.
69. Eiferman RA, Snyder JW, Barbee JV Jr. Corneal chromomycosis. Am J Ophthalmol. 1982;95:255.
70. Rodrigues MM, Laibson P, Kaplan W. Exogenous corneal ulcer caused by *Tritirachium roseum.* Am J Ophthalmol. 1979;80:804.
71. Taylor HR. Treatment of onchocerciasis in the 1980's. Onchocerciasis is one of the leading causes of blindness worldwide. Postgrad Doctor AFR. 1983;5:74.
72. Buck AA, ed. Onchocerciasis: Symptomatology, Pathology, Diagnosis. Geneva: World Health Organization; 1974.
73. Gibson DW, Heggie C, Connor DA. Clinical and pathologic aspects of onchocerciasis. Pathol Ann. 1980;15:195.
74. Thylefors B. Ocular onchocerciasis. Bull World Health Organ. 1978;56:63.
75. Fuglsang JA. Living microfilariae of *Onchocerca volvulus* in the cornea. Br J Ophthalmol. 1983;57:712.
76. Rodger FC, Chir M. The pathogenesis and pathology of ocular onchocerciasis. Am J Ophthalmol. 1960;49:104.
77. Roizenblatt J. Interstitial keratitis caused by American (mucocutaneous) leishmaniasis. Am J Ophthalmol. 1979;87:175.
78. Jones DB, Visvesvara GS, Robinson NM. *Acanthamoeba polyphaga* keratitis and *Acanthamoeba* uveitis associated with fatal meningoencephalitis. Trans Ophthalmol Soc UK. 1975;95:221.
79. Ma P, Willaert E, Juechter KB, et al. A case of keratitis due to *Acanthamoeba* in New York, and features of ten cases. J Infect Dis. 1981;143:662.
80. Mannis NJ, Tamaro R, Roth AM, et al. *Acanthamoeba* scleral keratitis. Determining diagnostic criteria. Arch Ophthalmol. 1986;104:1313–1317.
81. Pinnolis M, Egbert PR, Font RL, et al. Nosematosis of the cornea. Arch Ophthalmol. 1981;99:1044.
82. Ashton N, Wirasinha P. Encephalitozoonosis (nosematosis) of the cornea. Br J Ophthalmol. 1973;57:669.
83. Matsubayashi H, Koike T, Mikata I, et al. A case of encephalitozoon-like body infection in man. Arch Pathol. 1959;67:181.
84. Friedberg DN, Stenson SM, Orenstein JM, et al. Microsporidial keratoconjunctivitis in acquired immunodeficiency syndrome. Arch Ophthalmol. 1990;108:504–508.
85. Neame H. Parenchymatous keratitis in trypanosomiasis in cattle and in dogs and in man. Br J Ophthalmol. 1927;11:209.
86. Dawson CR, Jones BR, Tarizzo ML. Guide to Trachoma Control in Programs for the Prevention of Blindness. Geneva: World Health Organization; 1981.
87. Eiferman RA, Carothers DJ, Yangeelow JA. Peripheral rheumatoid ulceration and evidence for conjunctival collagenase production. Am J Ophthalmol. 1979;87:703.
88. Austin P, Green WR, Sallyer DC, et al. Peripheral corneal degeneration and occlusive vasculitis in Wegener's granulomatosis. Am J Ophthalmol. 1978;85:311.
89. Gerstle CC, Friedman AH. Marginal corneal ulceration (limbal guttering) as a presenting sign of temporal arteritis. Ophthalmology. 1980;87:1173.
90. Duke-Elder S. System of Ophthalmology, v. 8. Diseases of the Outer Eye. St. Louis: CV Mosby; 1965:237, 259, 539, 828, 829, 1032.
91. Woods AC. Syphilis of the eye. Am J Syph Gonor Vener Dis. 1943;27:133.
92. Ballantyne AJ, Michaelson IC. Textbook of the Fundus of the Eye. Baltimore: Williams & Wilkins; 1962:564.
93. Knapp A. Bilateral circumpapillary chorioretinitis with detachment of the retina in syphilis. Trans Am Acad Ophthalmol Otolaryngol. 1920;25:132.
94. Stokes JH, Beerman H, Ingraham NR. Modern Clinical Syphilology. Philadelphia: WB Saunders; 1949:59.
95. Carrol FD. Retrobulbar neuritis. Arch Ophthalmol. 1940;24:44.
96. Hogan MJ, Zimmerman LE, et al. In: Spencer WH, ed. Ophthalmic Pathology, 3rd ed. Philadelphia: WB Saunders; 1968:397.
97. Moore JE. Syphilitic iritis. Am J Ophthalmol. 1931;14:110.
98. Baum J, Bavza M, Weinstein P, et al. Bilateral keratitis as a manifestation of Lyme disease. Am J Ophthalmol. 1988;105:75.
99. Vollerstein RS, McDonald TJ, Younge BR, et al. Cogan's syndrome: 18 cases and a review of the literature. Mayo Clin Proc. 1986;61:344–361.
100. Krachmer JH, Laibson PR. Corneal Thinning and Perforation in Sjögren's syndrome. Am J Ophthalmol. 1974;78:917.
101. Pfister RR, Murphy GE. Corneal ulceration and perforation associated with Sjögren's syndrome. Arch Ophthalmol. 1980;98:89.
102. Khater TT, Jones DB, Wilhelmus KR. Infectious crystalline keratopathy caused by gram-negative bacteria. Am J Ophthalmol. 1997;124:19–23.
103. Nahmias AJ, Visintine AM, Caldwell DR, et al. Eye infections with herpes simplex viruses in neonates. Surv Ophthalmol. 1976;21:100.
104. Stern DA, Zam ZS, Gutgesell VJ. Primary herpes simplex subepithelial dendritic keratitis. Am J Ophthalmol. 1981;91:496.
105. Poirier RH. Herpetic ocular infections of childhood. Arch Ophthalmol. 1980;98:704.
106. Shuster JJ, Kaufman HE, Nesburn AB. Statistical analysis of the rate of recurrence of herpes virus ocular epithelial disease. Am J Ophthalmol. 1981;91:328.
107. Wilhelmus KR, Coster DJ, Donovan HC, et al. Prognostic indicators of herpetic keratitis. Analysis of a five year observation after corneal ulceration. Arch Ophthalmol. 1981;99:1578.
108. Baringer J, Swoveland P. Recovery of herpes simplex virus from human trigeminal ganglions. N Engl J Med. 1973;288:648.
109. Norn MS. Dendritic (herpetic keratitis), IV. Follow-up examination of corneal sensitivity. Acta Ophthalmol. 1970;48:383.
110. Bloomfield SE, Lopez C. Herpes infections in the immunosuppressed host. Ophthalmology. 1980;87:1226.
111. Howcroft MJ, Breslin CW. Herpes simplex keratitis in renal transplant recipients. Can Med Assoc J. 1981;124:292.
112. Cleobury JF, Skinner GRB, Thouless ME, et al. Association between psychopathic disorder in serum antibody to herpes simplex virus (type I). BMJ. 1971;261:438.
113. Patterson A, Jones BR. Management of ocular herpes. Trans Ophthalmol Soc UK. 1967;87:59.
114. Womack LW, Liesegang TJ. Complications of herpes zoster ophthalmicus. Arch Ophthalmol. 1983;101:42.
115. Hedges TR III, Elbert DM. The progression of ocular abnormalities of herpes zoster. Histopathologic observations of nine cases. Ophthalmology. 1982;89:165.
116. Edgerton AE. Herpes zoster ophthalmicus: Report of cases and review of literature. Arch Ophthalmol. 1945;34:40.
117. Mondino BJ, Brown SI, Mondzelewski JP. Peripheral corneal ulcers with herpes zoster ophthalmicus. Am J Ophthalmol. 1978;86:611.
118. Strachman J. Uveitis associated with chicken pox. J Pediatr. 1955;46:327.
119. Uchida Y, Kaneko M, Hyashi K. Varicella dendritic keratitis. Am J Ophthalmol. 1980;89:259.
120. Threlkeld AB, Elliot D, O'Brien TP. Scleritis in varicella-zoster disciform keratitis. Am J Ophthalmol. 1992;113:721.
121. Frampton G, Smith C. Primary vaccinia of the eyelid. Br J Ophthalmol. 1952;36:214.
122. Bedell AJ. Multiple vaccination of the eyelids. Trans Am Ophthalmol Soc. 1919;17:273.
123. Darrell RW, Vrabec F. Vaccinia virus infection of the rabbit cornea. Arch Ophthalmol. 1971;86:568.
124. Sachs U, Marcus M. Bilateral herpetic keratitis during measles. Am J Ophthalmol. 1981;91:796.
125. Deckard PS, Bergstrom TJ. Rubeola keratitis. Ophthalmology. 1981;88:810.
126. Pinnolis M, McCulley JP, Urman JD. Nummular keratitis associated with infectious mononucleosis. Am J Ophthalmol. 1980;89:791.
127. Matoba AY, Wilhelmus KR, Jones DB. Epstein-Barr viral stromal keratitis. Ophthalmology. 1986;93:746–751.
128. Manuelidis EE, Angelo JN, Gorgacz EJ, et al. Experimental Creutzfeldt-Jacob disease transmitted via the eye with infected cornea. N Engl J Med. 1977;296:1334.
129. Houff SA, Burton RC, Wilson RW, et al. Human to human transmission of rabies virus by corneal transplant. N Engl J Med. 1979;300:603.
130. Salahuddin SZ, Palestine AG, Heck E, et al. Isolation of the human T-cell leukemia/lymphotropic virus type III from the cornea. Am J Ophthalmol. 1986;101:149–152.
131. Jones DB, Liesegang TJ, Robinson NM. Cumitech 13, laboratory diagnosis of ocular infections. In: Washington JA II, Brewer NS, eds. Laboratory Procedures in Clinical Microbiology. Washington, DC: American Society for Microbiology; 1981:1–27.
132. Lee P, Green WR. Corneal biopsy: Indications, techniques and a report of 87 cases. Ophthalmology. 1990;97:718–721.
133. Forster RK, Rebell G. The diagnosis and management of keratomycoses, II. Medical and surgical management. Arch Ophthalmol. 1975;93:1134.
134. Jones DB. Decision making in the management of microbial keratitis. Ophthalmology. 1981;88:814.
135. Boerner CF, Lee FK, Wichliffe CL, et al. Electron microscopy for the diagnosis of ocular viral infections. Ophthalmology. 1981;88:1377.
136. Baum JL. Initial therapy of suspected microbial corneal ulcers, I. Broad antibiotic therapy based on prevalence of organisms. Surv Ophthalmol. 1979;24:97.
137. Chaudhuri PR, Godfrey B. Treatment of bacterial corneal ulcers with concentrated antibiotic eyedrops. Trans Ophthalmol Soc UK. 1982;102:11.
138. Baum JL, Barza M. Topical versus subconjunctival treatment of bacterial corneal ulcers. Ophthalmology. 1983;90:162.
139. Hessburg PC. Treatment of *Pseudomonas* keratitis in humans. Am J Ophthalmol. 1966;61:896.
140. Golden B, Fingerman LH, Allen HF. *Pseudomonas* corneal ulcers in contact lens wearers. Arch Ophthalmol. 1971;85:543.
141. Waltman SR, Kaufman HE. Use of hydrophilic contact lenses to increase ocular penetration of topical drugs. Invest Ophthalmol. 1970;9:250–255.
142. Matoba AI, McCulley JP. The effect of therapeutic soft contact lenses on antibiotic delivery to the cornea. Ophthalmology. 1985;92:97–99.
143. O'Brien TP, Sawusch MR, Dick JD, et al. Use of collagen corneal shields versus soft contact lenses to enhance penetration of topical tobramycin. J Cataract Refract Surg. 1988;14:505–507.
144. Unterman SR, Rootman DS, Hill JM, et al. Collagen shield drug delivery: Therapeutic concentrations of tobramycin in the rabbit cornea and aqeuous humor. J Cataract Refract Surg. 1988;14:500–503.
145. Sawusch MR, O'Brien TP, Dick JD, et al. Use of collagen corneal shields in the treatment of bacterial keratitis. Am J Ophthalmol. 1988;106:279–281.
146. Smolin G, Okumoto M, Feiler S, et al. Idoxuridine-liposome therapy for herpes simplex keratitis. Am J Ophthalmol. 1981;91:220–225.
147. Schaeffer HE, Krohn DL. Liposomes in topical drug delivery. Invest Ophthalmol Vis Sci. 1982;22:220–227.
148. Rootman DS, Hobden JA, Jantzen JA, et al. Iontophoresis of tobramycin for the treatment of experimental *Pseudomonas* keratitis in the rabbit. Arch Ophthalmol. 1988;106:262–265.
149. Bower KS, Kowalski RP, Gordon YJ. Fluoroquinolones in the treatment of bacterial keratitis. Am J Ophthalmol. 1996;121:712–715.
150. Hu FR, Luh KT. Topical ciprofloxacin for treating nontuberculous mycobacterial keratitis. Ophthalmology. 1998;105:269–272.

151. Hyndiuk RA, Eiferman RA, Caldwell DR, et al. Comparison of ciprofloxacin ophthalmic solution 0.3% to fortified tobramycin-cefazolin in treating bacterial corneal ulcers. Ciprofloxacin Bacterial Keratitis Study Group. Ophthalmology. 1996;103:1854–1862; see discussion on pages 1862–1863.
152. Ofloxacin Study Group. Ofloxacin monotherapy for the primary treatment of microbial keratitis: A double-masked, randomized, controlled trial with conventional dual therapy. Ophthalmology. 1997;104:1902–1909.
153. O'Brien TP, Maguire MG, Fink NE, et al. Efficacy of ofloxacin vs cefazolin and tobramycin in the therapy for bacterial keratitis. Report from the Bacterial Keratitis Study Research Group. Arch Ophthalmol. 1995;113:1257–1265.
154. Castillo A, Benitez del Castillo JM, Toledano N, et al. Deposits of topical norfloxacin in the treatment of bacterial keratitis. Cornea. 1997;16:420–423.
155. Leibowitz HM, Kupferman A. Topically administered corticosteroids: Effect on antibiotic-treated bacterial keratitis. Arch Ophthalmol. 1980;98:1287–1290.
156. Badenoch PR, Hay GJ, McDonald PJ, et al. A rat model of bacterial keratitis: Effect of antibiotics and corticosteroids. Arch Ophthalmol. 1985;103:718–722.
157. Hirose H, Terasaki H, Awaya S, et al. Treatment of fungal corneal ulcers with amphotericin B ointment. Am J Ophthalmol. 1997;124:836–838.
158. Rahman MR, Johnson GJ, Husain R, et al. Randomised trial of 0.2% chlorhexidine gluconate and 2.5% natamycin for fungal keratitis. Br J Ophthalmol. 1998;82:919–925.
159. Larkin DFP, Kilingman S, Dart JKG. Treatment of *Acanthamoeba* keratitis with polyhexamethylene biguanide. Ophthalmology. 1992;99:185–191.
160. White AT, Newland HS, Taylor HR, et al. Controlled trial and dose-finding study of ivermectin for treatment of onchocerciasis. J Infect Dis. 1987;156:463–470.
161. LaLau C, Oosterhuis A, Versteeg J, et al. Acyclovir and trifluorothymidine in herpetic keratitis; A multicentre trial. Br J Ophthalmol. 1982;66:506.
162. Herpetic Eye Disease Study Group. Acyclovir for the prevention of recurrent herpes simplex virus eye disease. N Engl J Med. 1998;339:300–306.
163. Foster CS, Duncan J. Penetrating keratoplasty for herpes simplex keratitis. Am J Ophthalmol. 1981;92:336.
164. Liesegang TJ. Corneal complications from herpes zoster ophthalmicus. Ophthalmology. 1985;92:316.

Chapter 100

Endophthalmitis

TERRENCE P. O'BRIEN

Endophthalmitis is an inflammatory process involving the ocular cavity and adjacent structures. Based on the clinical setting in which the disease occurs, endophthalmitis can be classified according to the type of etiologic agent, the mode of entry, and the location within the eye. Infectious etiologic agents include bacteria, fungi, viruses, protozoa, and parasites (Table 100–1). Infectious microorganisms may be introduced directly into the eye, as in cases of surgical and nonsurgical trauma, or may reach the eye via hematogenous spread from a distant site of infection. Noninfectious stimuli causing endophthalmitis include retained lens material after cataract surgery, foreign materials introduced at the time of surgery, intraocular blood, and neoplasms. The inflammatory process may be localized to specific tissues within the eye or may involve the intraocular contents in a generalized fashion. Inflammation involving all ocular tissue layers, including the episclera, is termed *panophthalmitis.* Pain with movement of the eye is a prominent feature of panophthalmitis.

BACTERIAL ENDOPHTHALMITIS

Bacteria are the most common causative infectious agents of endophthalmitis. The typical clinical course of bacterial endophthalmitis develops suddenly with rapid progression.[1] Symptoms and signs of ocular inflammation are most commonly manifested in the first 24 to 48 hours after surgical or nonsurgical trauma. Patients undergoing extracapsular cataract extraction may have onset of symptoms up to the fifth postoperative day.[1] Routine scheduling of visits on postoperative days 1 and 4 has been advised to detect the earliest ocular finding of endophthalmitis.[1] Development of increasing pain with progressive blurred vision, accompanied by exaggerated conjunctival hyperemia, chemosis, lid edema, and corneal edema with anterior chamber and vitreous inflammatory cell reaction, is highly suggestive of bacterial endophthalmitis. Careful slit-lamp biomicroscopic examination and direct or indirect ophthalmoscopy are necessary to detect the earliest signs of endophthalmitis.

Most cases of bacterial endophthalmitis develop after intraocular surgery. In one large series, the overall incidence of postoperative endophthalmitis was 0.093%.[2] The incidences in that series were

TABLE 100–1 Infectious Agents That Cause Endophthalmitis

Bacteria
Aerobic
Gram-positive cocci
Staphylococcus aureus, Staphylococcus epidermidis
Streptococcus pneumoniae, other *Streptococcus* and *Enterococcus* spp.
Gram-positive bacilli
Bacillus cereus, Bacillus subtilis, and other *Bacillus* spp.
Corynebacterium pseudodiphtheriticum (Corynebacterium hofmannii)
Corynebacterium spp.
Listeria monocytogenes
Gram-negative cocci
Neisseria meningitidis
Gram-negative bacilli
Acinetobacter spp.
Alcaligenes faecalis
Enterobacter spp.
Escherichia coli
Flavobacterium meningosepticum
Haemophilus influenzae
Klebsiella spp.
Moraxella spp.
Proteus spp.
Pseudomonas aeruginosa
Salmonella typhimurium
Serratia marcescens
Anaerobic
Clostridium spp.
Propionibacterium acnes
Never grown in vitro
Whipple's disease bacillus ("*Tropheryma whippelii*")
Spirochetes
Treponema pallidum
Higher bacteria
Actinomyces israelii
Mycobacterium tuberculosis, Mycobacterium leprae, other nontuberculous mycobacteria
Fungi
Acremonium (Cephalosporium) spp.
Aspergillus spp.
Blastomyces dermatitidis
Candida spp., including *Candida (Torulopsis) glabrata*
Cladosporium spp.
Coccidioides immitis
Cryptococcus neoformans
Exophiala jeanselmei
Fusarium spp.
Graphium spp.
Histoplasma capsulatum
Mucor spp.
Neurospora sitophila
Rhizopus spp.
Paecilomyces spp.
Penicillium spp.
Pneumocystis carinii
Pseudallescheria (Petriellidium) boydii (Scedosporium apiospermum)
Sporothrix schenckii
Trichosporon spp.
Volutella spp.
Virus
Herpes simplex virus
Herpes zoster virus
Cytomegalovirus
Rubella
Rubeola
Parasites
Onchocerca volvulus
Taenia solium (cysticercosis)
Toxocara canis and *Toxocara cati*
Toxoplasma gondii

as follows: cataract extraction, with or without implantation of an intraocular lens, (IOL) 0.082% (54/58123); pars plana vitrectomy, 0.046% (3/6557); penetrating keratoplasty, 0.178% (5/2805); secondary implantation of an IOL, 0.366% (5/1367); and glaucoma surgery, 0.124% (4/3233).[2] As these numbers show, the frequency of cataract surgery makes this procedure the most common cause of postoperative endophthalmitis. The usefulness of prophylactic antiseptics and antibiotics applied topically or subconjunctivally before, during, or after surgery remains unproved, although preoperative topical antibiotics are widely used. The ocular surface microflora are responsible for the majority of infections and probably gain access to the eye during surgery. The techniques of molecular epidemiology implicate the patient's external ocular tissue as the source of the infecting organism in a majority of cases of acute postoperative endophthalmitis.[3] Conjunctival preparation with povidone-iodine appears to reduce the incidence of postoperative endophthalmitis.[4]

Virtually any bacterial microorganism, including those previously considered saprophytic, can cause endophthalmitis (see Table 100–1). In postoperative infections, gram-positive organisms predominate, particularly *Staphylococcus epidermidis.*[1, 5] *Staphylococcus aureus* infections are less common but more severe. Visual acuity after recovery from postoperative endophthalmitis tends to be poor, with the median being 20/200,[2] but the outcome is better when the infecting organism is *S. epidermidis* or *Propionibacterium acnes* rather than *S. aureus,* streptococci, or gram-negative bacilli.[5]

The incidence of endophthalmitis after cataract extraction is about the same with extracapsular extraction or phacoemulsification (0.22% versus 0.30%).[5] Secondary implantation of an IOL has a higher risk than cataract extraction.[1] Delayed-onset endophthalmitis after cataract extraction in patients with an IOL can have a chronic course, with recurrent low-grade inflammation.[6, 7] The spectrum of organisms include most notably *P. acnes, S. epidermidis,* nontuberculous mycobacteria, and *Corynebacterium* spp. Contamination of intraocular lenses or viscoelastic material used in cataract surgery has produced endophthalmitis.[8]

Surgical creation of filtering blebs is used to treat glaucoma and, rarely, is an unintended surgical complication. Both early and late postoperative infections can result from bacteria entering the eye through this portal. The term "blebitis" or "conjunctival blebitis" has been introduced to refer to inflammation limited to the bleb and the immediate surrounding area, which may include the anterior chamber. Bleb-related endophthalmitis manifests with rapidly worsening visual acuity, ocular pain, diffuse conjunctival injection, intense inflammation in the anterior chamber with or without hypopyon, florid vitritis, and an opalescent bleb.[9, 10] Visual outcome after treatment is usually poor.[9] The organism in blebitis usually is not recovered, and about half of the vitreous cultures are negative in patients with endophthalmitis.[9] In one series of patients with bleb-related endophthalmitis occurring before postoperative week 6, four of six patients with positive vitreous cultures had *S. epidermidis* infection. In the 27 late cases, *Streptococcus* species and gram-negative organisms comprised 48% of isolates. In another series of cases of bleb-related endophthalmitis, all occurring 1 month or later after operation, streptococcal species were cultured from 15 of 32 eyes (47%).[10] Postoperative use of contact lenses may increase the incidence of bleb-related endophthalmitis in patients with unintended filtering blebs.

Extensive use of radial keratotomy for correction of visual refractive errors has made evident the low but significant incidence of infectious complications. Keratitis is discussed in Chapter 99. Endophthalmitis is rare but can be either an early or late complication.[11]

Bacterial endophthalmitis can result from penetrating nonsurgical trauma. In one series of 403 penetrating injuries, endophthalmitis developed in 4.2% of cases and was more common with posterior pole injury (7%) than with corneal injury (2.1%).[12] Infection was more common in the presence of a foreign body (15%). *S. epidermidis* was the most common organism (23.4%). The outcome was evisceration or absent light perception in 82.3%. *Bacillus* species are common pathogens in some series.[13]

Sudden onset of endophthalmitis in an unoperated, nontraumatized eye suggests hematogenous spread from a distant focus of infection. The clinical picture of endogenous endophthalmitis is similar to that seen in postoperative bacterial endophthalmitis, except that the posterior segment of the eye is usually involved and the patients are usually extremely ill and often immunologically compromised. Common clinical features of endogenous endophthalmitis include decreased visual acuity, pain, hypopyon, severe anterior uveitis, and conjunctival hyperemia. Often a focal chorioretinitis may develop within hours of metastatic seeding. Vitreous infection and finally an acute panophthalmitis may follow. Patients with meningitis caused by *Haemophilus influenzae, Streptococcus pneumoniae,* or *Neisseria meningitidis* may present with hematogenous endophthalmitis.[14] Abdominal infection, endocarditis, pneumonia, otitis media, breast abscess, paronychia, pharyngitis, or lymphangitis may be the source of bacteremia. Occasionally the patient was previously healthy and a focus cannot be found.[15] Dental procedures occasionally precede the development of bacterial endophthalmitis. Neonates and women in the puerperal period may also occasionally develop endogenous endophthalmitis. Whenever the source of the bacteremia cannot be found, a careful search for subacute bacterial endocarditis should be considered, including echocardiography.

Because the etiologic agents are usually of low virulence in subacute bacterial endocarditis, ocular findings may be minimal. Conjunctival and retinal hemorrhage are the most frequent findings. Retinal hemorrhages with white centers, called *Roth spots,* may represent septic retinitis. These lesions are characteristic but not pathognomonic of subacute bacterial endocarditis, because most hemorrhages with white centers are caused by the accumulation of platelets and fibrin. Rapidly progressive bacterial endophthalmitis caused by *Bacillus cereus* may occur after trauma, after transfusion with contaminated blood, or after intravenous heroin injection (see Chapter 197). In miliary tuberculosis, small, elevated yellow-white choroidal nodules with indistinct borders may be observed.

In congenital syphilis, a severe chorioretinitis leads to extensive chorioretinal scarring with a variety of patterns. In secondary and late acquired syphilis, iridocyclitis is the most frequent ocular finding. Other inflammatory features include retinal vasculitis, phlebitis, periarteritis, panuveitis, "posterior uveitis," multifocal choroiditis ("salt-and-pepper fundus"), chorioretinitis, papillitis, and neuroretinitis (see Chapter 227).

In immunocompromised patients, the possibility of *Nocardia* endophthalmitis should be kept in mind,[16] although the list of possible organisms is broad. The patients complain of blurred vision and pain. Ophthalmoscopic examination discloses central or paracentral foci of necrotizing chorioretinitis. Discrete detachments of the retinal pigment epithelium may occur in early cases. A vitreous abscess may ensue.

Endogenous bacterial endophthalmitis may occur in Whipple's disease, and macrophages with phagocytosed bacilli in varying stages of breakdown have been observed in the vitreous cavity and retina (see Chapter 89).

FUNGAL ENDOPHTHALMITIS

The incidence of systemic fungal infections has increased over the past several decades, perhaps in part because of the widespread use of antibiotics, corticosteroids, chemotherapy, and immunosuppressive therapy; increased intravenous narcotic abuse; and hyperalimentation. Fungi generally considered to be saprophytes can cause endophthalmitis. More than 20 different fungal organisms have been isolated from cases of intraocular mycoses.

Fungal endophthalmitis may occur as a result of exogenous or endogenous routes of organism entry. Exogenous sources include extension of a fungal keratitis with or without perforation and surgical or nonsurgical trauma; there have been outbreaks of fungal endophthalmitis caused by contaminated ophthalmic irrigation solution.[17] The principal clinical difference between bacterial and fungal endophthalmitis after trauma or surgery is the time of onset of symptoms and signs. Typically, in a fungal endophthalmitis the onset of symptoms and signs is delayed, compared with bacterial endophthalmitis. After intraocular surgery, there may be a lapse of several weeks before the development of ocular pain, ciliary injection, and signs of a nonspecific uveitis. On slit-lamp examination, a localized gray-white area may be seen in the anterior vitreous adjacent to the pupillary border. A transient hypopyon may occur, and additional satellite lesions occur in the anterior vitreous. In rare instances, the site of infection and abscess formation may be in the anterior chamber, usually near the chamber angle.

The incidence of fungal endophthalmitis after cataract surgery is very low. In one series of 36,000 cataract extractions, only 2 cases of fungal infection were reported.[18] An outbreak of fungal endophthalmitis has occurred after implantation of intraocular lenses contaminated with *Paecilomyces lilacinus.*[19] Fungal infections are rare complications of many other ocular surgical procedures and include fungal species that otherwise have not been identified as a cause of disease in humans (see Table 100–1).

After penetrating nonsurgical trauma, signs of fungal endophthalmitis may develop in an indolent fashion many weeks later. Presence of a foreign body, implanted at the time of the trauma, predisposes to infection. Trauma may also cause fungal keratitis, which can lead to endophthalmitis.

Hematogenous endophthalmitis is caused by a much more restricted range of pathogens than mycoses arising from surgery or trauma. *Candida* species are the most common, accounting for 17 of 20 eyes in 18 patients.[20] In that series, *Aspergillus* accounted for the remaining cases. *Candida* was also the most common mycosis in an autopsy series of 14 patients who died with a deep mycosis and were found to have endophthalmitis: 11 had *Candida,* 2 *Aspergillus,* and 2 *Cryptococcus* infection.[21] In hematogenous fungal endophthalmitis, ocular involvement may be the first or only manifestation of disseminated mycosis.

Candida endophthalmitis may occur in otherwise healthy persons after intravenous injection of a contaminated anesthetic,[22] although most cases originate with catheter-acquired candidemia. The ocular symptoms generally become manifest after a latent period of many days after *Candida* is recovered from the blood, although retinal lesions usually are visible much earlier. Symptoms include blurred vision, pain, and redness of the eyes. Frequently, the patient does not report early symptoms because of concomitant grave illness, endotracheal intubation, or depressed mentation. Fluffy yellow-white retinal, chorioretinal, or vitreoretinal lesions are seen. Although the border of the lesions eventually may become cloudy because of vitreous extension, early lesions resemble the cotton-wool spots of diabetes mellitus, retinal lesions of human immunodeficiency virus 1 (HIV-1) angiopathy, a Roth spot of subacute bacterial endocarditis, or the cytoid body of systemic lupus erythematosus. Gradual enlargement over a few days aids in distinguishing *Candida* endophthalmitis, although *Candida* lesions may regress spontaneously. Ocular lesions are unilateral in one half of the cases. Spread of retinal infection into the vitreous leads to a vitreous abscess, which is later obscured by diffuse inflammation and clouding of the vitreous. Occasionally patients present with an abscess of the iris or ciliary body. More commonly, extension of *Candida* endophthalmitis into the anterior chamber is a late finding. Prognosis for the return of normal visual acuity in an eye with a *Candida* vitreous abscess is guarded despite appropriate therapy. Recognition of an early ophthalmoscopic lesion not only may preserve vision but may provide useful evidence of disseminated candidiasis or *Candida* endocarditis.[23] Periodic ophthalmoscopic examinations are indicated in patients with known or suspected candidemia.

Aspergillus endophthalmitis occurs in patients who are seriously immunosuppressed, such as patients with solid organ transplants,[24] high-dose corticosteroid therapy, or late-stage HIV-1 infection. Intravenous injection of illicit drugs is another cause of *Aspergillus* endophthalmitis.[25] The most common sign is an iridocyclitis or a vitritis with associated yellow-white retinal lesions. Retinal hemorrhages, hypopyon, scleritis, and panophthalmitis also are seen.

Patients with endophthalmitis caused by *Cryptococcus neoformans, Blastomyces dermatitidis, Histoplasma capsulatum,* or *Coccidioides immitis* usually have other evidence of disseminated infection. Occasionally, endophthalmitis is the only evidence of the infection.[26] In mucormycosis, the orbit is involved by direct extension from infection of the sinuses.

In a report of 17 cases of ophthalmic infections caused by *Pseudallescheria boydii,* 7 were endophthalmitis.[27] Predisposing factors included were trauma (3 cases) and immunosuppression (3 cases), but in 1 patient there were no predisposing factors.

Pneumocystis carinii has caused choroidopathy in a small number of patients, most of whom have a history of *Pneumocystis* pneumonia. The lesions are one-third to two disk diameters in size, creamy white or yellow, round or oval, and usually multifocal and bilateral. The vitreous is clear.[28–30] Ocular lesions respond to the same drugs used to treat pulmonary pneumocystosis (see Chapter 260).

VIRAL INFECTIONS

Necrotizing Herpetic Retinopathies

Herpes simplex virus, varicella-zoster virus, and cytomegalovirus can cause a spectrum of diseases extending from acute retinal necrosis (ARN), occurring predominantly in previously healthy persons, to progressive outer retinal necrosis (PORN), occurring mostly in severely immunocompromised patients. In a review of 216 reported cases of ARN, only 16% clearly had impaired immunity.[31] Although cultures from vitrectomy specimens have rarely been positive, polymerase chain reaction (PCR) has been used to identify the virus.[32] Varicella-zoster virus appears to account for the majority of ARN and PORN cases. Acute retinal necrosis typically begins peripherally and extends centrally; it is characterized by a marked anterior chamber reaction, marked vitritis, retinal and choroidal vasculitis, and full-thickness retinal necrosis. Retinal detachment occurs in 70 to 80%. PORN is characterized by multifocal retinal necrosis that extends rapidly with little or no inflammation. The vitreous remains clear. Bilateral disease develops in approximately two thirds of patients; retinal detachment occurs in about 70%.

Herpes Simplex

In herpes simplex keratitis, usually from herpes simplex virus type 1, intraocular inflammation in the form of a persistent, nongranulomatous iridocyclitis may be present. Occasionally, an iridocyclitis is seen in the absence of keratitis. In a few cases, herpes simplex virus has been isolated from the aqueous humor.

The intraocular inflammation from herpes simplex is usually located in the anterior segment of the eye. However, posterior involvement has been documented, especially in the newborn, usually as a result of herpes simplex virus type 2 infection. Large patches of yellow-white retinal exudates accompanying perivascular and vitreous inflammatory infiltrates are present. The posterior pole of the fundus usually is more extensively involved than is the periphery. When the lesions heal, sharply circumscribed, punched-out chorioretinal scars that may be confused with toxoplasmic scars are seen.

Varicella-Zoster Virus

Herpes-zoster keratitis is commonly followed by iridocyclitis. A diffuse choroiditis may occur. The characteristic histopathologic feature of ocular herpes zoster infection is a chronic, nongranulomatous infiltration around posterior ciliary nerves and vessels. Occlusive vasculitis may lead to iris and ciliary body necrosis and to anterior chamber hemorrhage. A perivasculitis and vasculitis of retinal vessels may lead to hemorrhagic retinopathy. In varicella infections, uveitis may develop either during the acute infection stage or during convalescence.

Cytomegalovirus

Congenital cytomegalovirus (CMV) infection is a well-recognized cause of chorioretinitis and occurs in 23 to 29% of neonates with the disease. Iritis, cataracts, and optic atrophy may also accompany congenital infections.

CMV retinitis in adults was uncommon before the acquired immunodeficiency syndrome (AIDS) epidemic. It occurs in patients receiving chemotherapy for acute leukemia and malignant lymphomas.[33] However, it most frequently occurs in patients who have advanced HIV-1 infection and $CD4^+$ T-lymphocyte counts lower than 100 cells/mm^3. Patients whose CD4 count has risen from this level during protease inhibitor therapy may still be at risk.[34] CMV retinitis occasionally occurs in solid organ and bone marrow transplant recipients. Patients usually complain of blurred vision, floaters, and scotomas. Initially, this visual impairment is mild, but, with progression of the disease, severe and permanent visual loss occurs. Ocular pain usually is not present. Ophthalmoscopic examination discloses retinal edema, scattered intraretinal hemorrhages, yellow-white exudates, vessel attenuation, and sheathing. The picture of a branch retinal vein occlusion or a necrotizing vasculitis may be simulated. As the initial lesions heal, retinal and pigment epithelial atrophy occurs. Adjacent areas of active infection may be seen to progress through the same exudative, hemorrhagic, and atrophic stages. The appearance of the fundus and the maintenance of a clear vitreous humor is quite distinctive and usually is the only clinical sign of CMV infection other than fever. Urine and often blood contain CMV, indicating that dissemination is usual. Regular ophthalmoscopic examinations should be performed in all patients with advanced HIV-1 infection or organ transplantation. A typical recommendation is examination by an ophthalmologist every 3 to 4 months once the CD4 count has fallen below 50/mm^3. There is currently no agreement about the impact of highly active antiretroviral therapy (HAART) on the incidence of initial CMV retinitis, though the median time to relapse with maintenance therapy clearly seems prolonged.[35] Patients with CMV retinitis who respond to HAART may have spontaneous improvement in their retinitis.[36] Other patients with inactive CMV retinitis who respond to HAART may have a decrease in vision due to a newly described entity, called *immune recovery vitritis*. In a series of 30 HAART responders with CMV retinitis and CD4 counts rising higher than 60/mm^3, symptomatic vitritis in the absence of active retinitis developed in 19 patients (63%) who were observed for a median of 13.5 months while receiving HAART.[37] Inflammation is in the eye with prior CMV retinitis.[38] The syndrome must be distinguished from anterior iritis arising from intravenous cidofovir therapy, which is bilateral.[39]

Rubeola and Rubella

Measles (rubeola) retinopathy occurs 6 to 12 days after the skin rash; it is clinically manifested by acute blindness caused by macular involvement. It may or may not accompany measles encephalitis. In the early stages, retinal edema, attenuated vessels, and a stellate macular figure are seen in the fundus. In the later stages of the disease, there is frequently a return of useful vision and the occurrence of a secondary pigmentary retinopathy that may have a "salt-and-pepper" appearance.

Subacute sclerosing panencephalitis is a progressive, invariably fatal disease of childhood caused by measles virus, and it appears years after the attack of clinical measles. Chorioretinitis is a common ocular complication occurring in about 30% of the patients. Optic atrophy, papilledema, and cortical blindness may also occur.

The ocular complications of congenital rubella virus infection include cataracts, glaucoma, and a pigmentary retinopathy.

PARASITIC ENDOPHTHALMITIS

Toxoplasma gondii is a protozoan that causes retinochoroiditis. Because *Toxoplasma* organisms are found primarily in an area of coagulative necrosis of the retina, with a secondary granulomatous choroiditis, the term *retinochoroiditis* is applied to the ocular lesion. Ocular involvement is present in both congenital and acquired forms of the disease. A retinochoroiditis usually affecting the macula is present in 80% of the patients with congenital toxoplasmosis. The eye is rarely affected in the acquired form of the disease, and it has been suggested that almost all cases of ocular toxoplasmosis are congenital.

In the active stage, the fundus lesion is yellow-white, with indistinct borders and an overlying hazy vitreous. In recurrent disease, an active focus of inflammation is present at the border of an area of an inactive healed scar of retinochoroiditis. An iridocyclitis is usually present, and posterior vitreous detachment with vitreous precipitates on its detached surface is common. As the activity of the retinochoroiditis subsides, its color changes from yellow-white to gray and the vitreous haze recedes. Glaucoma, cataract, vitreous hemorrhage, and retinal detachment are possible complications.

Toxoplasma retinochoroiditis in the immunodeficient patient results in more extensive tissue destruction, may be more difficult to diagnose and treat, may produce single or multifocal lesions in one or both eyes, and may cause diffuse retinal necrosis. The disease responds to conventional antiparasitic therapy, but continued treatment is probably necessary to prevent reactivation.[40, 41]

The nematode *Toxocara* is the most common parasitic cause of endophthalmitis. The second-stage larva of this nematode is responsible for endophthalmitis with or without visceral larva migrans. The average age of the patients is 7.5 years, with a range of 2 to 31 years. Children become infected by the ingestion of ova present in soil contaminated with the excrement of dogs or cats. Nematode endophthalmitis was diagnosed in 2% of 1000 eyes enucleated in children younger than 15 years of age and is thought to be responsible for 10% of the cases of uveitis in children.

Infection may manifest as a diffuse chronic endophthalmitis, as a posterior-pole granuloma, or as a peripheral granuloma in a quiet eye. A cloudy vitreous, cyclitic membrane, and posterior synechiae may be present. A *Toxocara* granuloma is typically white with a diameter roughly equal to or larger than the optic disk (1.5 mm). It is primarily located in the retina. It may be present at the macula or at the periphery of the fundus. Other ocular manifestations of *Toxocara* infestation include a localized vitreous abscess, papillitis, pars planitis, and iridocyclitis. Nematode granulomas in the eye may be confused with retinoblastoma, and the differential diagnosis is critical.

Diffuse unilateral neuroretinitis is a syndrome characterized by a loss of vision, vitritis, papillitis, and recurrent crops of gray-white retinal lesions; the syndrome progresses to optic atrophy, retinal vessel narrowing, and diffuse pigmentary changes. Diffuse unilateral neuroretinitis may be caused by at least two different nematodes.

Ocular infestation with *Cysticercus cellulosae* may occur in 13% of patients with cysticercosis (see Chapter 280). The parasite may be found in the vitreous cavity, anterior chamber, or subretinal space. Ocular inflammation and characteristic retinal tracks may be seen with fly larvae (myiasis). Onchocerciasis (river blindness) is usually manifested in the eye as keratitis, but iridocyclitis, glaucoma, and choroiditis also may occur (see Chapter 278).

LABORATORY FINDINGS

Early recognition of distinctive clinical signs and prompt and accurate microbiologic investigation to assist with rapid diagnosis of the etiologic agent are essential if functional vision is to be salvaged in acute bacterial endophthalmitis. Although initial selection of antimicrobial therapy is not dependent on microbiologic results, subsequent modification and specification of treatment require proper identification of the microbial pathogen and antimicrobial susceptibility pattern. The vitreous humor is the intraocular site from which microbial isolation has the highest yield. Conjunctival cultures are inadequate and often misleading in bacterial endophthalmitis. The anterior chamber, vitreous cavity, wound abscesses, and wound dehiscences are all potential sites from which material should be obtained for culture on appropriate media.

In cases of suspected infectious endophthalmitis occurring after trauma or after surgical intervention, both aqueous and vitreous aspiration for microbial culture and smear should be performed. In a study of 140 cases of endophthalmitis, a microbial agent was isolated by vitreous and aqueous paracentesis in 78 cases. In 27 of these, the organism was isolated from the vitreous alone, with a negative aqueous culture. The vitreous specimen should be specially prepared for cytology, and centrifugal cytology may be helpful.

Smears of material from each site should be separately stained with Gram, Giemsa, and periodic acid–Schiff (PAS) stains and cultured for aerobic and anaerobic bacteria, mycobacteria, and fungi. Vitreous irrigation material from vitrectomy fluid can be centrifuged and smeared or passed through a millipore filter that can then be stained and cultured. Care must be taken to exclude contamination by airborne fungi, because they could be suspected of causing endophthalmitis. For the same reason, slides should be cleaned with alcohol to remove organisms before smears are made. Calcofluor white staining for fungi and fluorochrome staining for mycobacteria aid in detecting small numbers of those organisms. In patients with leukocoria and suspected nematode endophthalmitis, microscopic cytologic examination of aqueous humor disclosing eosinophils and normal lactate dehydrogenase levels may prevent enucleation as a result of a misdiagnosis of retinoblastoma. Enzyme-linked immunosorbent assay or PCR testing of aqueous humor material may also aid in the diagnosis.

TREATMENT

Successful outcome of management of endophthalmitis requires a low threshold of clinical suspicion for diagnosing infectious endophthalmitis. Acute bacterial endophthalmitis represents a true ophthalmologic emergency, and effective therapy requires early diagnostic aspirates, immediate initial broad-spectrum antimicrobial coverage, appropriate therapy to reduce the host immune and anti-inflammatory response, and, finally, modification of the antibiotic therapy based on results of identification of organisms in microbial culture, susceptibility testing, and clinical response to therapy. Surgical removal (pars plana vitrectomy) of vitreous infected by certain organisms may facilitate diagnosis and cure.

Animal and human studies demonstrate that the visual outcome is greatly influenced by the virulence of the infectious etiologic agent. *S. epidermidis* endophthalmitis, which appears to be increasing in frequency, responds well to relatively conservative therapy with vancomycin, with or without corticosteroids.

Reliable and rapid diagnosis of the etiologic organism can sometimes be challenging. Destruction of the eye by virulent pathogens such as *Pseudomonas aeruginosa, B. cereus,* and *S. aureus* may occur within 24 hours, so aggressive therapy is warranted if these organisms are suspected. Improvements in understanding of the role of the vitreous humor and pathogenesis of acute bacterial endophthalmitis have resulted in an evolving preference toward early mechanical vitrectomy with intravitreal administration of broad-spectrum antibiotics. There is currently no consensus, however, on what constitutes appropriately aggressive therapy. It may include early mechanical vitrectomy; intravitreal antibiotics; early systemic, topical, and perhaps intravitreal corticosteroids; and intravenous broad-spectrum antibiotics, most commonly including a third-generation cephalosporin. Selection of the optimal agent for intravitreal administration includes consideration of maximum efficacy against the suspected pathogens and potential toxicity of the intravitreal antibiotic preparation. Because of the potential extreme toxicity of aminoglycoside antibiotics to the retina, there has been a trend toward use of third-generation cephalosporins having activity against gram-negative pathogens. In cases of oxacillin-resistant *S. aureus,* intravitreal vancomycin may be the agent of choice. In cases of post-traumatic endophthalmitis, intravitreal and systemic clindamycin therapy should be considered because of the risk of *B. cereus* endophthalmitis.

The Endophthalmitis Vitrectomy Study (EVS) was designed to answer two questions related to the treatment of endophthalmitis: (1) Combined with injection of antibiotics, is immediate vitrectomy a better approach than vitreous tap or biopsy (tap-biopsy)? and (2) Are systemic antibiotics beneficial?[42] Patients were eligible for the EVS if they had signs and symptoms of endophthalmitis occurring within 6 weeks of cataract surgery or secondary intraocular lens implantation (early postoperative endophthalmitis) and visual acuity ranging from 20/50 to light perception (LP). A total of 420 patients entered the study and underwent two-way randomization into four treatment groups; 392 patients completed nine months of follow-up.

Overall, the visual acuity outcome was quite good in the EVS. More than 50% of patients achieved 20/40 or better vision, and about 75% had 20/100 or better vision, whereas only 12% ended up with severe vision loss, defined as 5/200 or worse. Patients that received systemic antibiotics did not have a better visual outcome, and there was no difference between the immediate vitrectomy and the tap-biopsy groups for achieving 20/100 or better vision; however, patients who had immediate vitrectomy were less likely to have severe vision loss. Subgroup analysis showed that this result for the entire patient population was caused by a beneficial effect of vitrectomy in patients who presented with LP vision, whereas there was no difference in outcome for the two treatment approaches in patients who presented with hand motions or better vision. The two major conclusions of the EVS were as follows. If vision was better than LP, the best regimen was vitreous tap or biopsy plus intravitreous injection of antibiotics. Patients who presented with LP vision benefited by immediate vitrectomy. Also, the systemic antibiotics used, ceftazidime and amikacin, did not improve visual outcome.

Effective management of *P. acnes* infection may require adjunctive surgical removal of all residual lens material and capsule when the organism is sequestered in the lens capsule. Intravitreal as well as systemic antibiotic therapy may be necessary. The organism is susceptible to a wide variety of agents, including penicillins and cephalosporins.

The rationale for the use of early corticosteroids as an addition to antimicrobial therapy is based on the recognition of the visually destructive secondary processes that can occur from host inflammatory and immune response to the causative organism. Unlike various extraocular infections, effective elimination of the organism is not the only criterion for successful treatment of endophthalmitis. If vision is to be retained, control of the inflammatory and immune response, in addition to elimination of the organism, is crucial.

Therapy for suspected fungal endophthalmitis remains challenging because of delays in diagnosis and less information available on pharmacokinetics and sensitivity testing of preferred antifungal agents. Intravenous amphotericin B and intravitreous injections of 5 to 10 μg of amphotericin B have been the therapy most broadly used. This should be combined with mechanical vitrectomy if any intravitreal abscess is present.

Candida endophthalmitis appears to be best treated with intravenous amphotericin B. Systemic fluconazole also has been efficacious in hematogenous *Candida* endophthalmitis, particularly for patients without vitritis.[43] Once vitreous invasion is present, significant intraocular morbidity occurs despite appropriate antifungal therapy. Vitreous organization and traction leading to retinal detachment may occur. *Candida* infection in the retina not involving the vitreous may sometimes resolve spontaneously without antifungal treatment. Presumably, these patients have relatively intact immunologic systems. Once extension to the vitreous or anterior chamber occurs, progression to blindness is anticipated in the absence of appropriate therapy. Pars plana vitrectomy is both a diagnostic and a therapeutic modality that may be used in the management of *Candida* endophthalmitis. It facilitates diagnosis by making tissue available for culture and microscopic evaluation. It plays a therapeutic role by removing replicating fungi in the vitreous body, by improving the diffusion of systematically administered antifungal agents into the vitreous cavity, and by preventing future vitreoretinal traction.

High-dose intravenous amphotericin B is the treatment of choice for *Aspergillus* endophthalmitis, although the prognosis remains grave. Successful treatment of endogenous *Aspergillus* endophthalmitis usually requires surgical removal of infected vitreous combined with aggressive administration of intravenous amphotericin B. High-dose oral itraconazole may have some role late in the course of treatment, after the infection has become more indolent.

Intravenous amphotericin B is the drug of choice for endophthalmitis caused by *C. neoformans, C. immitis,* and *Histoplasma capsulatum.*

Topical corticosteroids and cycloplegics are used to reduce the inflammation and accompanying photophobia in herpetic keratouveitis and herpes zoster iridocyclitis.

In the treatment of CMV infection in immunosuppressed adults, early reduction or discontinuation of immunosuppressive therapy, if possible, should help in limiting the progression of the ocular and systemic infection. Therapy for AIDS patients with CMV retinitis is discussed in Chapters 116 and 127. Therapy for ARN has been with intravenous acyclovir, 500 mg/m^2 every 8 hours for 10 to 14 days. Results with treatment of PORN have been dismal, leading to use of a variety of regimens.[44]

In the treatment of ocular toxoplasmosis, mydriatics, topical corticosteroids, systemic and/or periocular depot administration of corticosteroids, and pyrimethamine with sulfonamides have been recommended. Some authorities recommend treatment of only those cases with extensive involvement and those in which the macula is threatened with involvement. Clindamycin has been combined with pyrimethamine to treat intracerebral toxoplasmosis and might be considered for treatment of ocular toxoplasmosis in patients who are allergic to sulfonamides (see Chapter 268).

Intraocular inflammation develops when the *Toxocara* larvae die within the eye. Therefore, systemic or periocular injection of corticosteroids is the usual therapy of choice. Removal of the encysted larvae, lysis of traction bands, and removal of epiretinal membranes can be helpful. Ivermectin is the drug of choice for onchocerciasis, although repeated courses must be given.

REFERENCES

1. Lam SR, Tuli R, Menezes et al. Bacterial endophthalmitis following extracapsular cataract extraction: Recommendations for early detection. Can J Ophthalmol. 1997;32:311–314.
2. Aaberg TM Jr, Flynn HW Jr, Schiffman J, Newton J. Nosocomial acute-onset postoperative endophthalmitis survey: A 10-year review of incidence and outcomes. Ophthalmology. 1998;105:1004–1010.
3. Speaker MG, Milch FA, Shah MK, et al. Role of external bacterial flora in the pathogenesis of acute postoperative endophthalmitis. Ophthalmology. 1991;98:639–650.
4. Speaker MG, Menikoff JA. Prophylaxis of endophthalmitis with topical povidone-iodine. Ophthalmology. 1991;98:1769–1775.
5. Somani S, Grinbaum A, Slomovic AR. Postoperative endophthalmitis: Incidence, predisposing surgery, clinical course and outcome. Can J Ophthalmol. 1997;32:303–310.
6. Fox GM, Joondeph BC, Flynn HW Jr, et al. Delayed-onset pseudophakic endophthalmitis. Am J Ophthalmol. 1991;111:163–173.
7. Sawusch MR, Michels RG, Stark WJ, et al. Endophthalmitis due to *Propionibacterium acnes* sequestered between IOL optic and posterior capsule. Ophthalmic Surg. 1989;20:90–92.
8. Roy M, Chen JC, Miller M, et al. Epidemic *Bacillus* endophthalmitis after cataract surgery I: Acute presentation and outcome. Ophthalmology. 1997;104:1768–1772.
9. Ciulla TA, Beck AD, Topping TM, Baker AS. Blebitis, early endophthalmitis, and late endophthalmitis after glaucoma-filtering surgery. Ophthalmology. 1997;104:986–995.
10. Kangas TA, Greenfield DS, Flynn HW Jr, et al. Delayed-onset endophthalmitis associated with conjunctival filtering blebs. Ophthalmology. 1997;104:746–752.
11. Heidemann DG, Dunn SP, Haimann M. Endophthalmitis after radial keratotomy enhancement. J Cataract Refract Surg. 1997;23:951–953.
12. Duch-Samper AM, Menezo JL, Hurtado-Sarrio M. Endophthalmitis following penetrating eye injuries. Acta Ophthalmol Scand. 1997;75:104–106.
13. Affeldt JC, Flynn HW, Forster RK, et al. Microbial endophthalmitis resulting from ocular trauma. Ophthalmology. 1987;94:407.
14. Barnard T, Das A, Hickey S. Bilateral endophthalmitis as an initial presentation in meningococcal meningitis. Arch Ophthalmol. 1997;115:1472–1473.
15. Piczenik Y, Kjer B, Fledelius HC. Metastatic bacterial endophthalmitis: A report of four cases all leading to blindness. Acta Ophthalmol Scand. 1997;75:466–469.
16. Davitt B, Gehrs K, Bowers T. Endogenous *Nocardia* endophthalmitis. Retina 1998;18:71–73.
17. McCray E, Rampell N, Solomon SL, et al. Outbreak of *Candida parapsilosis* endophthalmitis after cataract extraction and intraocular lens implantation. J Clin Microbiol. 1986;24:625.
18. Allen HF. Amphotericin-B and exogenous mycotic endophthalmitis after cataract extraction. Arch Ophthalmol. 1972;88:640.
19. Pettit TH, Olsen RJ, Foos RY, et al. Fungal endophthalmitis following intraocular lens implantation. Arch Ophthalmol. 1980;98:1025.
20. Essman TF, Flynn HW, Smiddy WE, et al. Treatment outcomes in a 10-year study of endogenous fungal endophthalmitis. Ophthalmic Surg Lasers. 1997;28:184–194.
21. McDonnell PJ, McDonnell JM, Brown RH, et al. Ocular involvement in patients with fungal infections. Ophthalmology. 1985;92:706.
22. Daily MJ, Dickey JB, Packo KH. Endogenous *Candida* endophthalmitis after intravenous anesthesia with propofol. Arch Ophthalmol. 1991;109:1081–1084.
23. Shmuely H, Kremer I, Sagie A, Pitlik S. *Candida tropicalis* multifocal endophthalmitis as the only initial manifestation of pacemaker endocarditis. Am J Ophthalmol. 1997;123:559–560.
24. Anteby I, Kramer M, Rahav G, Benezra D. Necrotizing choroiditis-retinitis as presenting symptom of disseminated aspergillosis after lung transplantation. Eur J Ophthalmol. 1997;7:294–296.
25. Doft BH, Clarkson JG, Febell G, et al. Endogenous *Aspergillus* endophthalmitis in drug abusers. Arch Ophthalmol. 1980;98:859.
26. Li S, Perlman JI, Edward DP, Weiss R. Unilateral *Blastomyces dermatitidis* endophthalmitis and orbital cellulitis: A case report and literature review. Ophthalmology. 1998;105:1466–1470.
27. McGuire TW, Bullock JD, Bullock JD Jr, et al. Fungal endophthalmitis: An experimental study with a review of 17 human ocular cases. Arch Ophthalmol. 1991;109:1289–1296.
28. Dugel PU, Rao NA, Forster DJ, et al. *Pneumocystis carinii* choroiditis after long-term aerosolized pentamidine therapy. Am J Ophthalmol. 1990;110:113–117.
29. Freeman WR, Gross JG, Labelle J, et al. *Pneumocystis carinii* choroidopathy: A new clinical entity. Arch Ophthalmol. 1989;107:863–867.
30. Macher AM, Bardenstein DS, Zimmerman LE, et al. *Pneumocystis carinii* choroiditis in a male homosexual with AIDS and disseminated pulmonary and extrapulmonary *P. carinii* infection. N Engl J Med. 1987;316:1092.
31. Guex-Crosier Y, Rochat C, Herbort CP. Necrotizing herpetic retinopathies: A spectrum of herpes virus-induced diseases determined by the immune state of the host. Ocul Immunol Inflamm. 1997;5:259–265.
32. Knox CM, Chandler D, Short GA, Margolis TP. Polymerase chain reaction–based assays of vitreous samples for the diagnosis of viral retinitis: Use in diagnostic dilemmas. Ophthalmology. 1998;105:37–44.
33. Papanicolaou GA, Meyers BR, Fuchs WS, et al. Infectious ocular complications in orthotopic liver transplant patients. Clin Infect Dis. 1997;24:1172–1177.
34. Jacobson MA, Zegans M, Pavan PR, et al. Cytomegalovirus retinitis after initiation of highly active antiretroviral therapy. Lancet. 1997;349:1443–1445.
35. Casado JL, Perez-Elias MJ, Marti-Belda P, et al. Improved outcome of cytomegalovirus retinitis in AIDS patients after introduction of protease inhibitors. J Acquir Immune Defic Syndr Hum Retrovirol. 1998;19:130–134.
36. Whitcup SM, Cunningham ET Jr, Polis MA, Fortin E. Spontaneous and sustained resolution of CMV retinitis in patients receiving highly active antiretroviral therapy. Br J Ophthalmol. 1998;82:845–846.
37. Karavellas MP, Plaummer DJ, Macdonald JC, et al. Incidence of immune recovery vitritis in cytomegalovirus retinitis patients following institution of successful highly active antiretroviral therapy. J Infect Dis. 1999;179:697–700.
38. Zegans ME, Walton RC, Holland GN, et al. Transient vitreous inflammatory reactions associated with combination antiretroviral therapy in patients with AIDS and cytomegalovirus retinitis. Am J Ophthalmol. 1998;125:292–300.
39. Akler ME, Johnson DW, Burman WJ, Johnson SC. Anterior uveitis and hypotony after intravenous cidofovir for the treatment of cytomegalovirus retinitis. Ophthalmology. 1998;105:651–657.
40. Holland GN, Engstrom RE, Glasgow BJ. Ocular toxoplasmosis in patients with the acquired immunodeficiency syndrome. Am J Ophthalmol. 1988;106:653–657.
41. Heineman MH, Gold JMW, Maisel JM. Bilateral *Toxoplasma* retinochoroiditis in a patient with the acquired immunodeficiency syndrome. Retina. 1986;6:224–226.
42. Endophthalmitis Vitrectomy Study Group. Results of the endophthalmitis vitrectomy study: A randomized trial of immediate vitrectomy and of intravenous antibiotics for the treatment of postoperative bacterial endophthalmitis. Arch Ophthalmol. 1995;13:1479–1496.
43. Akler ME, Vellend H, McNeely DM, et al. Use of fluconazole in the treatment of candidal endophthalmitis. Clin Infect Dis. 1995;20:657–664.
44. Perez-Blazquez E, Traspas R, Mendez Marin I, et al. Intravitreal ganciclovir treatment in progressive outer retinal necrosis. Am J Opthalmol. 1997;124:418–421.

Chapter 101

Periocular Infections

TERRENCE P. O'BRIEN

Serious ocular and systemic complications may result from microbial infections of the orbit and ocular adnexa. Prevention of complications requires early recognition of distinctive clinical features, prompt microbiologic investigation, aggressive antimicrobial therapy, and proper adjunctive surgery.

The principal periocular structures susceptible to microbial infection include the eyelids, the components of the lacrimal apparatus, the orbit, and the paranasal and cavernous sinuses.

EYELIDS

The eyelids display signs of inflammation quite readily because of the overlying thin skin and a subcutaneous layer composed of loose strands of connective tissue without fat. Bacteria are the principal pathogens responsible for most infections of the eyelids, with *Staphylococcus* spp. being the most common cause.[1] The term *blepharitis* connotes inflammation of the lid margins, which is typically chronic and bilateral.[2] There are two main types: anterior (staphylococcal) and posterior (meibomian gland dysfunction). Both forms have similar symptoms, including chronic irritation, a burning sensation, mild redness, and occasional itching of the lid margins.

Staphylococcal blepharitis may be acute and ulcerative caused by infection of the skin of the eyelids, ciliofollicles, or accessory glandular structures by *Staphylococcus aureus.* Chronic blepharitis and blepharoconjunctivitis involving the anterior lid margin is most commonly caused by infection with *S. aureus* and *Staphylococcus epidermidis.* Chronic infection is often manifested by hyperemia with small ulcerations along the lid margins, crusted exudate in the form of dry scales around the base of the lashes, and even loss of the lashes (madarosis).

Other bacteria less frequently implicated in anterior blepharitis include *Pseudomonas* spp.,[3] *Proteus mirabilis,*[4] and *Capnocytophaga ochracea.*[5] *Pseudomonas* blepharitis in the neutropenic patient may progress rapidly, with extensive necrosis.[3] Anterior blepharitis may be secondary to contact allergies caused by agents such as cosmetics.[6] Mascara use has been implicated in some cases of blepharitis.

Molluscum contagiosum may cause unilateral red, irritated eyes with an associated waxy, dome-shaped nodule that becomes umbilicated. These nodules may be hidden between the eyelashes and contribute to a toxic conjunctivitis often with diffuse fine punctate epithelial keratitis. Hair follicle mites *Demodex folliculorum* and *Demodex brevis* have been associated with blepharitis, although their precise role in pathogenesis is unclear.[7–9]

Infestation of the anterior lid margins (phthiriasis palpebrarum) by the pubic or "crab" louse *(Phthirus pubis)* causes itching and red swollen lid margins. Nits (0.5 to 1 mm) and adult lice (3 mm) may be observed on and between the lashes with red or rust-colored flecks on the lid margin (lice excreta). An irritating bloody blepharitis is sometimes experienced. Phthiriasis palpebrarum is often transmitted sexually.[10]

Posterior lid margin disease (meibomian gland dysfunction) is caused by a complex abnormality of meibomian secretion with alterations of meibomian ductal epithelium and surrounding tissues. The posterior inflammation is probably not due to direct infection, although bacterial flora lipases may play a role in breaking down meibum into irritating free fatty acids.

A chalazion is a nontender, sterile, chronic lipogranulomatous inflammation of the meibomian gland that has a tendency to recur. It presents as a lid nodule and may begin with inflammation and tenderness. Once fully developed, the chalazion is characterized by an absence of acute inflammatory signs. If a chalazion becomes secondarily infected, signs of acute inflammation are evident. The majority of these lesions point toward the conjunctival surface of the lid, and they may be large enough to press on the globe and distort vision. Because sebaceous gland carcinoma of the lid may be confused clinically with a chalazion, any recurrent chalazion should be examined histopathologically. The main histopathologic feature of a chalazion is a chronic granulomatous inflammatory reaction centered around clear spaces. These spaces represent areas of lipid material that are dissolved out during tissue processing.

If a chalazion ruptures through the tarsal conjunctiva, there may be an outgrowth of granulation tissue that results in a rapidly enlarging, painless polypoid mass called a *granuloma pyogenicum.* Histopathologically, it is composed of capillaries in a radiating pattern and is separated by loose connective tissue with an acute and chronic inflammatory cell infiltrate.

The skin around the eyelids is thin and may become inflamed (dermatoblepharitis). This condition may be due to infection, allergy, connective tissue disease, or other dermatologic disease. Rosacea, also called acne rosacea, is a common disease of the facial skin of adults that often extends to the lids and conjunctiva. The facial lesions primarily affect the malar and nasal areas and are characterized by flushing, erythema, papules, pustules, and telangiectasia. Rhinophyma is a late complication.[11] The lid margins are often involved, and mild conjunctivitis, with grittiness, a burning sensation, and edema of the periocular skin may also be seen.[12, 13]

Infectious dermatoblepharitis may be caused by primary or secondary infection with herpes simplex virus (type 1 or 2).[14] Herpes simplex virus dermatoblepharitis is more commonly seen in children younger than 6 years of age but may occur in adolescents or adults. Primary infection may be associated with symptoms of upper respiratory tract infection. Ocular signs include ipsilateral preauricular lymphadenopathy, follicular conjunctivitis, and pleomorphic epithelial keratitis. Herpes simplex virus can cause acute, subacute, or recurrent blepharoconjunctivitis in adults.[15, 16] Occasionally, the infection is bilateral.[15] Subacute inflammation can lead to fusion of portions or all of the lid (ankyloblepharon).[17]

Varicella-zoster virus may cause dermatoblepharitis in a characteristic dermatomal distribution involving the ophthalmic division of the trigeminal nerve. Usually all three branches (frontal, lacrimal, nasociliary) are involved, but isolated branch involvement may occur. Nasociliary involvement does not necessarily predict ocular involvement. Laboratory diagnosis is often not necessary unless there is a question of immune compromise of the host, dissemination, or atypical features. Human immunodeficiency virus testing is recommended in young patients with any potential risk factors.

Dermatoblepharitis of bacterial etiology (impetigo) results from skin infection caused by *S. aureus* or occasionally *Streptococcus pyogenes.* Impetigo is most common in children younger than 6 years of age and may complicate preexisting skin lesions in varicella, herpes simplex virus infection, or eczema.

Erysipelas is acute cellulitis caused by *S. pyogenes,* less commonly other streptococci, and *S. aureus.* Erysipelas presumably occurs by invasion of the organism into the subcutaneous tissue through an abrasion or inflammatory ulceration and is often accompanied by marked lymphatic involvement. Clinical features include an elevated, erythematous skin plaque with a brawny indurated appearance that progresses to sharply demarcated, bright-red, or crimson erythema with marked edema of the eyelids. A high temperature (39.44°C to 40°C [103°F to 104°F]), leukocytosis, chills, and malaise may occur. Extensive necrosis and therapeutic failure can be seen.[18]

A hordeolum is a common acute purulent infection of the glands of the eyelids that is usually caused by *S. aureus.* Depending on the glands affected, a hordeolum can be classified into two types—internal and external.

A internal hordeolum is an infection of the meibomian glands. Hordeola may be associated with diffuse lid swelling, erythema, and tenderness. They may point toward the skin or the conjunctival surface of the lid.

An external hordeolum (or stye) is an infection of the glands of Zeis, which are small sebaceous glands connected with the follicles of the eyelashes and the glands of Moll, which are apocrine sweat glands near the lid margin. External hordeola are smaller and more superficial than internal hordeola. They are discrete, elevated, erythematous, tender pustules and point toward the skin surface of the lid, usually near the margin. Warm compresses may provide localized hyperthermia to promote drainage, and systemic or topical antibiotics are rarely indicated.

LACRIMAL APPARATUS

The lacrimal apparatus has two major functions. The main lacrimal gland (located anteriorly in the superotemporal quadrant of the orbit) and the accessory lacrimal glands of Krause and Wolfring (located in the conjunctiva) produce the aqueous component of the tear film. The lacrimal puncta, the superior and inferior canaliculi, the common canaliculus, the lacrimal sac, and the nasolacrimal duct are concerned with the drainage of tears from the conjunctival sac and tear lake to the nasal cavity. Pathologic processes affecting the main and accessory lacrimal glands result in diminished tear production, whereas those affecting the lacrimal drainage apparatus cause obstruction resulting in excessive tearing (epiphora).

Canaliculitis is a low-grade chronic inflammation in the canaliculi that is usually due to infection from the anaerobic, gram-positive filamentous organisms *Propionibacterium propionicus* and species of *Actinomyces.* Characteristically, these organisms form gritty casts composed of organisms that lie within and obstruct the lacrimal duct.[19] Other organisms that infect the lacrimal tract include *Malassezia (Pityrosporum) pachydermatis,*[20] herpes simplex virus,[20, 21] and herpes zoster virus.[21] Inflammation leads to obstruction of the lumen of the canaliculus,[22] which results in epiphora, chronic conjunctivitis, and a tender swollen nasal lid margin. This condition may go undiagnosed for years. Typically, the punctum has a slightly distended appearance. Trachoma and medications (antiviral agents, silver nitrate, miotics, and systemic fluorouracil,[23] or thiotepa) may contribute to canalicular scarring that can predispose to infection.

Dacryocystitis is inflammation of the lacrimal sac. It is clinically useful to divide dacryocystitis into chronic and acute forms. Chronic dacryocystitis is usually caused by a single site of partial or complete obstruction within the lacrimal sac or within the nasolacrimal duct. The infection is usually the result and not the cause of the obstruction.

There are many causes of obstruction. Small silicone plugs implanted in the lacrimal puncta to relieve symptoms of dry eyes can migrate down into and obstruct the canaliculus. [24] In about 5% of all newborns, the distal end of the nasolacrimal duct is not patent at birth, but in most cases there is spontaneous opening of the duct during the first few days or weeks of life.[25, 26]

Trauma causing fractures in the nasoethmoid region may obstruct the drainage system at the junction of the lacrimal sac and the nasolacrimal duct. Infection of the lacrimal sac by *Aspergillus, Candida albicans,* or *Actinomyces* may occur. Benign and malignant tumors of the lacrimal sac may cause obstruction of the outflow system. Obstruction in the area of the sac-duct junction from a silicone implant used for an orbital floor fracture repair has been reported; a chronic dacryocystitis developed.[27]

Streptococcus pneumoniae is most commonly isolated from cases of chronic dacryocystitis. However, a mixed infection with *Staphylococcus, Streptococcus,* and *Pseudomonas aeruginosa* can occur. Sarcoidosis[28] and *Chlamydia trachomatis*[29] may cause a chronic recurrent dacryocystitis.

Epiphora may be the only clinical finding in patients with chronic dacryocystitis. On palpation of the tear sac area, a mucoid discharge may be expressed through the lacrimal puncta.

Acute dacryocystitis occurs when both the proximal and distal ends of the drainage system become partially or totally obstructed. The obstruction may be due to trauma, dacryoliths acting as ball valves, or flare-up of a chronic dacryocystitis or lacrimal sac sarcoidosis. The major symptom in patients with acute dacryocystitis is pain in the tear sac area. On palpation, tenderness in the lacrimal sac area is present, and purulent material can be expressed in a retrograde fashion through the lacrimal puncta. Localized cellulitis may progress to dacryocystopyocele and orbital abscess. A serious complication of acute dacryocystitis is orbital cellulitis (see farther on).[30, 31] This occurs if the inflammation process involving the lacrimal sac spreads posteriorly through the orbital septum; this is more likely in older patients with attenuated septa.[32]

The common pathogens in acute dacryocystitis are *S. aureus, Streptococcus* spp. and, in unvaccinated children, *Haemophilus influenzae.*[30]

Histopathologic study of bone from the area adjacent to the lacrimal sac showed normal bone in approximately one half of patients undergoing dacryocystorhinostomy for acute or chronic dacryocystitis. The other half of the bone samples revealed evidence of bone remodeling or woven bone, but no inflammation. The periosteum of the lacrimal fossa may help prevent bony changes in dacryocystitis.[32]

Dacryoadenitis refers to inflammation of the main lacrimal gland. Acute dacryoadenitis is characterized by localized tenderness and swelling of the outer half of the upper eyelid, producing S-curved deformity of the lid margin. There may be associated conjunctivitis and periorbital edema. Acute bacterial infections of the gland are uncommon. Infections may occur from an exogenous site on the skin, or the gland may be seeded during a bacteremia. Local trauma is a predisposing factor. The palpebral extension of the gland is more frequently involved than is the orbital portion. Pyogenic bacteria such as *S. aureus* and streptococci are the bacteria most often implicated as causes. Rarely, gonococcal bacteremia may result in an acute dacryoadenitis. Dacryocystitis due to *Cysticercus cellulosae* has been reported.[33] Viral infections of the lacrimal gland cause acute inflammation and usually occur in children. The two viral diseases that most often involve the gland are mumps[34] and infectious mononucleosis. Clinically inapparent infection of the lacrimal gland may occur with cytomegalovirus, coxsackievirus A, echoviruses, or varicella-zoster virus infections.[35] Patients with acute dacryoadenitis complain of severe pain in the lacrimal gland region, and signs of inflammation including erythema of overlying skin, swelling, and tenderness on palpation of the region are noted. Ocular motility defects such as combined abduction and elevation deficiency or isolated abduction deficiency may be seen. In some cases (particularly in children), fever and leukocytosis occur.[35]

Chronic infections of the lacrimal gland may be bilateral with minimal eyelid edema. Infectious causes include tuberculosis,[36] syphilis, leprosy, cysticercosis, and schistosomiasis.[37] Clinically, painless enlargement of one or both lacrimal glands may occur, and signs of acute inflammation are not present. Similar clinical features may be present in noninfectious causes, including sarcoidosis.[38] Fungal infections involving the lacrimal gland are rare but include blastomycosis, histoplasmosis, nocardiosis, and sporotrichosis.

Chronic dacryoadenitis of unknown cause is a nonspecific inflammatory condition, occurring mainly in men older than 40 years of age, that is characterized by mild tenderness, bulbar conjunctival stasis, and chemosis.[39, 40] There is slight exophthalmos and good visual acuity. The cause, although presumed to be an immune disorder, remains unknown.

ORBIT AND CAVERNOUS SINUS

Preseptal cellulitis is infection confined anterior to the orbital septum. Distinctive features include hyperemia of the skin of the eyelids, distention of the soft tissue, and absence of signs of orbital congestion. The source may be the ethmoid sinus but is often occult. *H. influenzae* type B preseptal cellulitis, once common in children and often accompanied by positive blood cultures, has all but disappeared in the United States as a result of immunization.[41] In 59 children with preseptal cellulitis seen at Vanderbilt Hospital, blood cultures were positive in only 6 (10%); 5 had streptococci and one, an unimmunized child, had *H. influenzae*.[41] When an organism can be obtained from the tissue or blood, *S. aureus* and streptococci now predominate. In 14 patients from India, aged 2 to 55 years, in whom cultures were obtained, *S. aureus* was found in 7, *S. pyogenes* in 2, and *Pseudomonas* in 1.[42] Preseptal cellulitis from *Moraxella catarrhalis* has been described.[43] The prognosis is good when appropriate intravenous antibiotics are given, although complications include streptococcal toxic shock syndrome,[44, 45] lid abscess, ectropion, and lagophthalmos.[42]

Postseptal (orbital) cellulitis is an acute infection of the orbital contents. It is a serious infection because of the risk of visual loss and the possibility of posterior spread to involve the cavernous sinus, which may lead to thrombosis and death. There are many causes of orbital cellulitis.[46] Most cases occur by spread from contiguous structures such as the paranasal sinuses.[47, 48] The potentially serious nature of this condition is frequently underestimated. Any of the sinuses may be involved. The lamina papyracea separating the ethmoid air cells from the orbit is thin and may permit the spread of infection. Congenital or traumatic breaks may further compromise this barrier. In addition, the anterior and posterior ethmoid foramina allow communication between the sinus and orbit. In children, because the ethmoid sinuses are the first to pneumatize, ethmoiditis is the most common source.[49] In one large series, 84% of the children with orbital cellulitis had roentgenographic evidence of sinusitis. This sinusitis was bilateral in almost half the cases.[50] In adults, extensions from the frontal sinusitis also occur.

Direct inoculation of organisms may occur after puncture wounds to the orbit when they perforate the orbital septum. Retained orbital foreign bodies are another source of infection. Orbital cellulitis may occur as a complication of orbital fractures, even in the absence of adjacent sinusitis.[51] Certain surgical procedures can rarely cause orbital infections. These include exploration for orbital tumors, retinal reattachment procedures, and strabismus operations.[52] Foreign materials such as sutures, encircling ocular bands, and sponges may serve as the nidus in postoperative orbital infections, and such materials must be removed to eliminate the infection.[53] Acute dacryocystitis[54] or posterior perforation of the lacrimal sac during therapeutic probing may result in orbital cellulitis. Rare cases from bites by house pets and rats have been reported.[55] Dental and intracranial infections may extend into the orbit and produce an orbital cellulitis.

In adults, infection of the orbit by blood-borne bacterial metastases from a distant site is extremely rare.[56] *Enterococcus faecalis* causing a bacteremia with the subsequent development of orbital cellulitis has also been reported.[57] Anaerobes are frequently present in cases of chronic sinusitis and should be suspected in orbital cellulitis associated with long-standing sinus disease. Multiple anaerobic strains may be found.[58] Trauma with resultant inoculation of earthen material is a cause of orbital cellulitis due to *Clostridium perfringens*.[59]

The bacteria most commonly causing orbital cellulitis are *S. aureus, S. pyogenes,* and *S. pneumoniae*.[49] Of these, *S. aureus* is the most common causative agent in adults. In eight children with positive cultures at Vanderbilt Hospital, four had streptococccal species and none had *S. aureus*.[41] If crepitation is present, the possibility of cellulitis secondary to clostridial organisms should be considered. In patients receiving immunosuppressive drugs, nontuberculous mycobacteria may rarely cause orbital cellulitis.

Regardless of the source of the infection, many of the symptoms and signs of orbital cellulitis are distinctive. However, in some cases it may be difficult to establish an early diagnosis. For example, after severe injuries, hemorrhage and edema in the lids and orbit may prevent early recognition of the signs of infection. Likewise, nonseptic inflammation after intraorbital surgical procedures often mimics bacterial cellulitis with the presence of lid edema, chemosis, orbital edema, and restricted ocular motion. These factors may contribute to a delay in diagnosis. Therefore, it is imperative that the clinician maintain a high index of suspicion of the possibility of infection in such cases and perform magnetic resonance imaging (MRI) or thin-section computed tomography (CT) of the orbit.[46, 47] After trauma, symptoms and signs of orbital cellulitis usually begin within 48 to 72 hours. However, occasionally a retained intraorbital foreign body may reveal signs of infection only several months later.

Fever, lid edema, and rhinorrhea are the most frequent early signs. They are followed by orbital pain, tenderness on palpation of the lids, and headache. Vision is usually normal during the early stages. As the infection progresses, the lids acquire a dark red discoloration and increased warmth. Conjunctival hyperemia, chemosis, and proptosis follow. The direction of proptosis may help to indicate the primary site of involvement in the orbit. There is limitation of ocular motility, with pain on attempted motion and increased resistance to retropulsion of the globe. Increased orbital pressure, reduced corneal sensation, congestion of retinal veins, and chorioretinal striae may be present later in the course of the infection. In severe cases of orbital cellulitis, gangrene and sloughing of the lids have been reported. Acute infarction of the choroid and retina from involvement of the posterior ciliary vessels and ophthalmic artery may rarely occur. A leukocytosis with a white blood cell count greater than 15,000/mm^3 is usually present.

A different clinical course is seen in "posterior" orbital cellulitis. Patients with this condition manifest an orbital apex syndrome in which profound visual loss and ophthalmoplegia develop with minimal external inflammatory signs. This condition occurs as a result of contiguous spread into the orbit from an adjacent sphenoidal or ethmoidal sinusitis. The cause of visual loss in posterior orbital cellulitis is probably due to vascular compromise, for example, to the ophthalmic artery or the rete of vessels within the optic sheath. In addition to CT and MRI, color Doppler (orbital ultrasonography with Doppler) can help define the anatomy of such cases.[60] In the few cases reported, the visual loss has been almost uniformly irreversible. Posterior orbital cellulitis is less common than is orbital cellulitis.[61]

Preseptal and postseptal (orbital) cellulitis secondary to paranasal sinusitis may be classified into five clinical stages.[62] In the first stage (preseptal cellulitis), bacteria are not present within the orbit, but inflammatory orbital edema produced by the proximity of a suppurative sinusitis is present. During the second stage, there is a direct extension through bone, with infiltration of the orbital contents by bacteria and inflammatory cells. The third stage occurs after the infection has extended beneath bone, thereby leading to formation of a subperiosteal abscess. The fourth stage is reached when the infection within the orbit consolidates as an abscess. This may be verifiable clinically by the subcutaneous induration of the lids, as mentioned earlier, and by fluctuance in the orbit that is detectable on retropulsion of the globe. This is unlike the usual loss of resiliency and the difficulty in retropulsion that accompanies orbital cellulitis without abscess formation. Occasionally, the abscess may rupture through the orbital septum and appear beneath the skin of the lid. The fifth stage is the uncommon late complication of cavernous sinus thrombosis.

Before antibiotics became available, about 19% of the patients with orbital cellulitis died of intracranial complications. About 20% of the patients were blinded in the involved eye, and an additional 13% suffered some visual loss from the infection.[63] Additional complications include osteomyelitis, strabismus, an afferent pupillary defect, a chronic draining sinus, and a scarred upper eyelid. With antibiotic therapy, the prognosis in cases of orbital cellulitis has markedly improved.

Tuberculous involvement of the orbit is very rare, occurs by a hematogenous route, and is unassociated with miliary tuberculosis. The patients are apparently healthy, without pulmonary disease or other signs of systemic tuberculosis.

Syphilitic gummas in the orbit are rare. They may occur in the extraocular muscles, the orbital nerves, and the optic nerve.

The most common fungal infections causing orbital infection are mucormycosis (see Chapter 249), aspergillosis (see Chapter 248), and phaeohyphomycosis (see Chapter 259). Orbital infection results from infection in the ethmoid sinus, although other sinuses may be involved. Allergic fungal sinusitis may be due to *Aspergillus* but is more commonly caused by dark-walled fungi, that is, the agents of phaeohyphomycosis. Patients with chronic allergic rhinitis, particularly those with nasal polyps, are predisposed. A history of years of seasonal or intermittent nasal obstruction and sinus discomfort, sometimes with episodes of bacterial sinusitis, is typical. Orbital involvement is signaled by painless proptosis, as the lamina papyracea protrudes into the orbit. CT shows the ethmoid sinus to be packed full of soft tissue with bulging lateral walls and eroded septa. Other ipsilateral sinuses are usually opacified as well. The syndrome and its management is described in Chapter 259. Patients with late-stage human immunodeficiency virus infection are prone to indolent invasive fungal sinusitis, usually due to *Aspergillus*.[64] Patients with persistent and profound neutropenia are prone to rapidly invasive fungal sinusitis, which may spread to the orbit, hard palate, facial skin, nose, and brain. The usual cause is *Aspergillus fumigatus* or *Aspergillus flavus*. Agents of mucormycosis can cause the same syndrome in profoundly immunosuppressed patients but also in patients receiving deferoxamine or with poorly controlled diabetes mellitus. The diagnosis of mucormycosis is usually not considered until orbital extension occurs but is preceded by fever and dull sinus pain. Proptosis and chemosis are rapidly followed by external ophthalmoplegia and decreasing visual acuity. Indolent cases of craniofacial mucormycosis have been described.[65]

The nematode *Trichinella spiralis* may invade the extraocular muscles and result in periorbital edema and pain on movement of the eyes.

Cavernous sinus thrombosis may be difficult to distinguish from mucormycosis and orbital cellulitis. Most often, cavernous sinus thrombosis results from blood-borne infection from the face, nasal cavity, paranasal sinuses, and ear. It may also occur as a rare complication of orbital cellulitis. The symptoms and signs of cavernous sinus thrombosis are graver than those of orbital cellulitis. The early onset of internal and external ophthalmoplegia is a suggestive feature. Decreased sensation around the eye, indicating involvement of the trigeminal nerve, and signs of bilaterality with paretic muscles in the contralateral eye are strong evidence of cavernous sinus thrombosis. Altered consciousness and other signs of meningitis indicate the seriousness of this clinical entity. Diagnosis and management of suppurative intracranial phlebitis is discussed in Chapter 77.

LABORATORY FEATURES

Patients with blepharitis may often be more symptomatic than the clinical findings seem to warrant. In such cases, bacteriologic culture of the lid margins may reveal a dense population of *Staphylococcus*.

Microscopic examination of concretions from the lacrimal canaliculus discloses tangled masses of *P. propionicus* or *Actinomyces* hyphae. These branching filamentous organisms are gram- and periodic acid–Schiff–positive. Anaerobic cultures should be obtained for confirmation, but the organisms may be difficult to isolate (see Chapter 14).

When obstruction of the lacrimal drainage system is suspected, several procedures are available to evaluate its patency. When the drainage apparatus is fully patent, 2% fluorescein dye instilled in the conjunctival sac may usually be collected on a nasal applicator passed beneath the inferior turbinate (Jones I test). If no dye is recovered, the fornices are irrigated to remove residual fluorescein. The nasolacrimal sac is then cannulated and irrigated with saline (Jones II test). If dye is recovered with the Jones II test when none could be recovered with the Jones I test, a partial nasolacrimal duct obstruction is probably present. Probing of the lacrimal passages may provide information regarding the site of the obstruction.

Several other techniques have been devised to assess the patency and status of the lacrimal drainage system. Thermography, a process by which body surface temperatures are recorded in the form of thermal images, has been used to study lacrimal system obstructions and inflammations. Inflammation induces hyperthermia, and canaliculitis and acute dacryocystitis may be demonstrated by comparisons to a normal contralateral side. Radiographic studies that have been used to evaluate the patency of the drainage system include plain film dacryocystography with contrast injection (distention dacryocystography), macrodacryocystography, scintillography, and tomography (including CT).[66–68] CT of the outflow system after topical instillation of a contrast agent is useful as a physiologic test with good anatomic resolution.

In cases of orbital cellulitis, the isolation of the causative agent is often difficult because external drainage is often absent and aspiration of fluid from the orbit is contraindicated (unless an abscess is present). Blood cultures should always be obtained, but results are variable. Most patients require ethmoidectomy and, although this may be performed later, the organism may be recovered from pus and necrotic tissue removed at surgery, despite intervening antibiotic therapy. CT and MRI are the preferred techniques for imaging patients with suspected orbital cellulitis.[46, 47, 69] CT sections spaced 5 mm apart with and without intravenous contrast are helpful. A correlation of computed tomographic findings with the clinical stages of orbital cellulitis mentioned previously has been proposed.[69] In stage II disease (orbital cellulitis without abscess), a low-density fluid collection is present between the periosteum and the adjacent rectus muscle. In stage III (subperiosteal abscess), the periosteum is elevated and the rectus muscle displaced by an abscess defined by an enhancing periosteal border. An orbital abscess (stage IV) is manifested by a homogeneous, heterogeneous, or ringlike mass within the orbital space.[70] Computed tomography will also delineate sinus and bony abnormalities and most orbital foreign bodies. MRI is excellent for visualizing orbital and sinus inflammation but provides less resolution of bony structures.

In cases of suspected cavernous sinus thrombosis, MRI is the imaging modality of choice. Carotid arteriography is of diagnostic usefulness but is potentially dangerous. Orbital venography is effective in the region of the cavernous sinus, and modification of this technique by digital subtraction has also been used to diagnose thrombosis. Contrast-enhanced CT has been beneficial in some cases of cavernous sinus thrombosis but is inferior to MRI.[71] The cerebrospinal fluid often shows pleocytosis with an abundance of polymorphonuclear cells and an increased protein level, although this is of little diagnostic utility. Cultures of the cerebrospinal fluid are almost always negative in cases of cavernous sinus thrombosis.

Paranasal sinus aspergillosis with orbital extension is best diagnosed by tissue removed from the paranasal sinus. Fungal cultures of sinus tissue alone are not diagnostic because the molds also can be airborne contaminants. Septated hyphae can be readily visualized in resected tissue if Gomori methenamine silver or periodic acid–Schiff staining is performed. In cases of mucormycosis, positive cultures are often difficult to obtain, and the diagnosis is usually made by histologic examination of excised tissue. Otolaryngologic consultation is necessary, and a biopsy and scraping samples from any necrotic area of the nasal mucosa or palate are essential. On tissue sections, nonseptate branching hyphae that are large (6 to 20 μm wide) with an irregular diameter are found in mucormycosis.

TREATMENT

In staphylococcal blepharitis, the use of a topical antibiotic (bacitracin, erythromycin, or sulfacetamide) or antibiotic-steroid combination ointment and lid scrubs with or without diluted shampoo applied to the lid margins may decrease lid inflammation. Topical corticosteroid drops are occasionally used briefly to decrease ocular surface inflammation. Caution must be exercised to avoid complications from long-term steroid use, including cataract formation and possible glaucoma. Rosacea on the lid margins is improved by lid hygiene and topical metronidazole gel applied to the lid margin.[72] Accompanying conjunctivitis responds less well but may respond in adults treated with long-term oral tetracycline.[73]

Any internal or external hordeolum should be treated with warm compresses until the inflammation subsides. The use of topical and systemic antibiotics is rarely indicated, and surgical drainage is seldom required.

Because most chalazia infrequently subside spontaneously, typically having chronic or subacute inflammation, surgical curettage and excision may be performed. However, simple observation is reasonable because chalazia tend to decrease in size with time. The use of intralesional long-acting corticosteroids (e.g., triamcinolone acetate) has been suggested. One should be concerned about the possibility of a sebaceous gland carcinoma in older individuals with recurrent chalazia. *P. pubis* infestation usually affects body hair in addition to the lashes and should be treated with a pediculocide, such as gamma benzene hexachloride (Lindane) shampoo, applied to the body hair of the patient and that of other family members and sexual contacts (see Chapter 283). Care should be taken to keep the pediculocide out of the eyes. Application of a thick layer of petrolatum jelly to the eyelid margins twice daily for 8 days will asphyxiate the lice. Alternatively, 1% yellow oxide of mercury can be applied to the lid margins for 2 weeks.

The value of topical antiviral ointment to treat ulcerative herpes simplex blepharitis is unclear, although a short course of topical trifluridine is reasonable in an effort to prevent inoculation of the ocular surface with herpes simplex virus.

Antibiotic irrigation of the canaliculi combined with topical antibiotic eyedrops is useful in the treatment of canaliculitis. Penicillin G (160,000 units/ml as an irrigant, 60,000 units/ml as drops) is used for *P. propionicus* and *Actinomyces* spp. When concretions are present, they should be removed by canaliculotomy and curettage. The canaliculus should then be reconstructed; silicone intubation may be needed.[74] Cases of canicular obstruction associated with herpes simplex virus infection may require surgical intervention more frequently than do cases caused by bacteria. A possible explanation is that with herpes, the epithelial lining of the canaliculus is damaged, with resultant adherence of the subepithelial layers with scar formation. In the cases of bacterial infection, however, the epithelium remains intact, and the obstruction is due to edema, which is more reversible.

Parents of infants with nasolacrimal duct obstruction should be taught to massage the lacrimal sac area firmly several times daily. Topical antibiotic eyedrops may be used for crusted exudate on the lids. If symptoms persist for 6 to 8 months, the lacrimal drainage apparatus should be irrigated and possibly probed. Probing is more successful in cases of lacrimal duct obstruction due to membranous obstruction than in cases due to narrowing of the duct. If probing is unsuccessful, repeat probing is performed a few months later. Silicone intubation of the drainage apparatus is performed if the repeat probing also fails to succeed.[19]

In adults with acute dacryocystitis, treatment with warm compresses and systemic antibiotics should be given. If *S. pyogenes* is isolated or suspected, oral penicillin or amoxicillin is used. Staphylococci are best treated with an oral penicillinase-resistant penicillin such as cloxacillin or dicloxacillin. After the acute infection is controlled, the patient should be taught to perform digital massage of the lacrimal sac, and topical antibiotic drops should be used. If epiphora persists, a dacryocystorhinostomy is performed in most cases to obtain adequate tear drainage.

Bacterial dacryoadenitis is treated with systemic antibiotics. If an orbital abscess forms, surgical drainage is necessary.

Management of preseptal cellulitis includes clinical assessment of the degree and evolution of conjunctival injection and chemosis, presence or absence of proptosis, limitation of or pain on extraocular movement, visual acuity, and pupillary reaction. A CT or an MRI scan of the orbit should be performed if there is any question of orbital involvement. In post-traumatic preseptal cellulitis, wound sites should be cultured on appropriate media and Gram staining performed. If gram-positive cocci are observed on diagnostic smears, intravenous nafcillin or oxacillin or, in milder cases, oral cloxacillin or dicloxacillin are recommended. Intravenous cefazolin or oral cephalexin may be administered to nonanaphylactic penicillin-allergic patients. If there is a history of anaphylactic penicillin allergy, intravenous vancomycin is recommended. If gram-negative rods are observed on diagnostic smears or if empirical therapy is necessary, intravenous ceftriaxone, cefotaxime, or cefepime can be started. Once clinical improvement is seen and the patient is afebrile for 24 hours, oral therapy with amoxicillin-clavulanate or levofloxacin can be considered.

In treating orbital cellulitis, appropriate intravenous antibiotics are urgently required, as well as CT or MRI. An otolaryngology and ophthalmology consultation should be sought. Paranasal sinus surgery may be necessary. The bacterial agents most commonly responsible for this infection were mentioned earlier. In adults, an initial regimen might include ceftriaxone 1 g every 12 hours with or without vancomycin 1 g every 12 hours, depending on the incidence of ceftriaxone-resistant pneumococci in the community. If the infection progresses and the clinical situation deteriorates despite adequate intravenous antibiotic therapy, it is probably due to the development of a subperiosteal or orbital abscess. Repeat CT is indicated. Surgical drainage may be imperative. Material obtained from such drainage should have the complete microbiologic evaluation mentioned previously. In cases of radiographically suspected subperiosteal abscess that seem to be responding to conservative measures, surgery may be deferred, but inflammatory signs may persist much longer than in patients treated by drainage.[69, 75, 76]

If the management of patients with orbital mucormycosis is to be successful, the combined efforts of internists, mycologists, otolaryngologists, and ophthalmologists are essential. The underlying disease, for example, diabetic ketoacidosis, should be treated. Intravenous amphotericin B 1.0 to 1.5 mg/kg daily is of value. For diabetics with preexisting renal disease, amphotericin B lipid complex, 5 mg/kg intravenously daily may be substituted. Surgical débridement of devitalized tissue is extremely important. Frequently, the affected eye may need to be sacrificed to obtain adequate orbital débridement.

In the treatment of chronic orbital aspergillosis or phaeohyphomycosis, surgical excision appears to be the best method. Amphotericin B is only of ancillary help.

REFERENCES

1. Smolin G, Okumoto M. Staphylococcal blepharitis. Arch Ophthalmol. 1977;95:812.
2. Smith RE, Flowers CW Jr. Chronic blepharitis: A review. CLAO J. 1995;21:200–207.
3. Giagounidis AA, Meckenstock G, Flacke S, et al. *Pseudomonas aeruginosa* blepharoconjunctivitis during cytoreductive chemotherapy in a woman with acute lymphocytic leukemia. Ann Hematol. 1997;75:121–123.
4. Parunovic A. *Proteus mirabilis* causing necrotic inflammation of the eyelid. Am J Ophthalmol. 1973;76:543.
5. Wasserman D, Asbell PA, Friedman AJ, et al. *Capnocytophaga ochracea* chronic blepharoconjunctivitis. Cornea. 1995;14:533–535.
6. Van Ketel WG, Liem DH. Eyelid dermatitis from nickel contaminated cosmetics. Contact Dermatitis. 1981;4:217.
7. Junk AK, Lukacs A, Kampik A. Topical administration of metronidazole gel as an effective therapy alternative in chronic *Demodex* blepharitis—a case report. Klin Monatsbl Augenheilkd. 1998;213:48–50.
8. Rufli T, Mumcuoglu Y. The hair follicle mites *Demodex folliculorum* and *Demodex brevis:* Biology and medical importance. A review. Dermatologica. 1981;162:1.
9. Roth AM. *Demodex folliculorum* in hair follicles of eyelid skin. Ann Ophthalmol. 1979;11:37.
10. Couch JM, Green WR, Hirst LW, et al. Diagnosing and treating *Phthirus pubis* palpebrarum. Surv Ophthalmol. 1982;26:219.
11. Chalmers DA. Rosacea: Recognition and management for the primary care provider. Nurse Pract. 1997;22:18, 23–28, 30.
12. Chen DM, Crosby DL. Periorbital edema as an initial presentation of rosacea. J Am Acad Dermatol. 1997;37(2 Pt 2):346–348.

13. Bourrat E, Rybojad M, Deplus S, et al. Rosacea with ocular involvement in a child. Ann Dermatol Venereol. 1996;123:664–665.
14. Egerer I, Stary A. Erosive-ulcerative herpes simplex blepharitis. Arch Ophthalmol. 1980;98:1760.
15. Parisi ML. A case of recurrent, isolated, simultaneous, bilateral herpes simplex lid infection. J Am Optom Assoc. 1998;69:49–56.
16. Robinson J. Photo quiz. Blepharitis due to herpes simplex virus type 1. Clin Infect Dis. 1997;24:17.
17. Campanella PC, Rosenwasser GO, Sassani JW, et al. Herpes simplex blepharoconjunctivitis presenting as complete acquired ankyloblepharon. Cornea. 1997;16:360–361.
18. Kranish JW, McLeish WM. Eyelid necrosis and perioribital necrotizing fasciitis. Report of a case and review of the literature. Ophthalmology. 1991;95:92–98.
19. McKellar MJ, Aburn NS. Cast-forming *Actinomyces israelii* canaliculitis. Aust N Z J Ophthalmol. 1997;25:301–303.
20. Romano A, Segal E, Blumenthal M. Canaliculitis with isolation of *Pityrosporum pachydermatis*. Br J Ophthalmol. 1978;62:732.
21. Bouzas AG. Canalicular inflammation in ophthalmic cases of herpes zoster and herpes simplex. Am J Ophthalmol. 1965;60:713–716.
22. Harris GJ, Hyndiuk RA, Fox MJ, et al. Herpetic canicular obstruction. Arch Ophthalmol. 1981;99:282–283.
23. Lee V, Bentley CR, Olver JM. Sclerosing canaliculitis after 5-fluorouracil breast cancer chemotherapy. Eye. 1998;12(Pt 3a):343–349.
24. Rumelt S, Remulla H, Rubin PA. Silicone punctal plug migration resulting in dacryocystitis and canaliculitis. Cornea. 1997;16:377–379.
25. Kushner BJ. Congenital nasolacrimal system obstruction. Arch Ophthalmol. 1982;100:597.
26. Berlin AJ, Ruth R, Rich L. Lacrimal system dacryoliths. Ophthalmic Surg. 1980;11:435.
27. Mauriello JA, Fiore PM, Kotch M. Dacryocystitis—late complications of orbital floor fracture repaired with implant. Ophthalmology. 1987;94:248–250.
28. Harris GJ, Williams GA, Clarke GP. Sarcoidosis of the lacrimal sac. Arch Ophthalmol. 1981;99:1198.
29. Bahnasawi SA, Abdalla MI, Ghaly AF, et al. Trachoma of the lacrimal sac. Bull Ophthalmol Soc Egypt. 1976;69:619.
30. Hurwitz JJ, Rodgers KJA. Management of acquired dacryocystitis. Can J Ophthalmol. 1983;18:213–216.
31. Ahrens-Palumbo MJ, Ballen PH. Primary dacryocystitis causing orbital cellulitis. Ann Ophthalmol. 1982;14:600.
32. Hinton P, Hurwitz JJ, Cruickshank B. Nasolacrimal bone changes and diseases of the lacrimal drainage sytsem. Ophthalmic Surg. 1984;15:516–521.
33. Sen DK. Acute suppurative dacryocystitis caused by a *Cysticercus cellulosae*. J Pediatr Ophthalmol Strabismus. 1982;19:100.
34. Riffenburgh RS. Ocular manifestations of mumps. Arch Ophthalmol. 1961;56:739.
35. Jakobiec FA, Jones IS. Orbital inflammations. In: Duan CD, ed. Clinical Ophthalmology, v. 2. Philadelphia: Harper & Row; 1987;65.
36. Baghdassarian SA, Zakharia H, Asdourian KK. Report of a case of bilateral caseous tuberculous dacryocystitis. Am J Ophthalmol. 1972;74:744.
37. Jakobiec FA, Gess L, Zimmerman LE. Granulomatous dacryoadenitis caused by *Schistosoma haematobium*. Arch Ophthalmol. 1977;95:278.
38. Obernauf CD, Shaw HE, Sydnor CJ, et al. Sarcoidosis and its ophthalmic manifestations. Am J Ophthalmol. 1978;86:8648.
39. Amemiya T, Mori H, Koizumi K. Clinical and histocytopathological study of chronic dacryoadenitis. Graefes Arch Clin Exp Ophthalmol. 1983;220:229–232.
40. Mcnally L, Jakobiec FA, Knowles DM. Clinical, morphologic, immunophenotypic, and molecular genetic analysis of bilateral ocular adnexal lymphoid neoplasms in 17 patients. Am J Ophthalmol. 1987;103:555.
41. Donahue SP, Khoury JM, Kowalski RP. Common ocular infections. A prescriber's guide. Drugs. 1996;52:526–540.
42. Rao VA, Hans R, Mehra AK. Pre-septal cellulitis—varied clinical presentations. Indian J Ophthalmol. 1996;44:225–227.
43. Rotta AT, Asmar BI. *Moraxella catarrhalis* bacteremia and preseptal cellulitis. South Med J. 1994;87:541–542.
44. Ingraham HJ, Ryan ME, Burns JT, et al. Streptococcal preseptal cellulitis complicated by the toxic *Streptococcus* syndrome. Ophthalmology. 1995;102:1223–1226.
45. Meyer MA. Streptococcal toxic shock syndrome complicating preseptal cellulitis. Am J Ophthalmol. 1997;123:841–843.
46. Hershey BL, Roth TC. Orbital infections. Semin Ultrasound CT MR. 1997;18:448–459.
47. Curtin HD, Rabinov JD. Extension to the orbit from paraorbital disease. The sinuses. Radiol Clin North Am. 1998;36:1201–1213.
48. Diaz I, Bamberger DM. Acute sinusitis. Semin Respir Infect. 1995;10:14–20.
49. Noel LP, Clark WN, Peacocke TA. Periorbital and orbital cellulitis in children. Can J Ophthalmol. 1981;16:178.
50. Weiss A, Friendly D, Eglin K, et al. Bacterial periorbital and orbital cellulitis in children. Ophthalmology. 1983;90:195.
51. Goldfarb MS, Hoffman DS, Rosenberg S. Orbital cellulitis and orbital fractures. Ann Ophthalmol. 1987;19:97–99.
52. Wilson ME, Paul TO. Orbital cellulitis following strabismus surgery. Ophthalmic Surg. 1987;18:92–94.
53. Penland RL, Wilhelmus KR. *Stenotrophomonas maltophilia* ocular infections. Arch Ophthalmol. 1996;114:433–436.
54. Ntountas I, Morschbacher R, Pratt D, et al. An orbital abscess secondary to acute dacryocystitis. Ophthalmic Surg Lasers. 1997;28:758–761.
55. Diwan R, Sen DK, Sood GC. Rat bite orbital cellulitis. Br J Ophthalmol. 1970;54:211.
56. Biedner BZ, Marmur U, Yassur Y. *Streptococcus faecalis* orbital cellulitis. Ann Ophthalmol. 1986;18:194–195.
57. Hornblass A, Herschorn BJ, Stern RK, et al. Orbital abscess. Surv Ophthalmol. 1984;29:169–178.
58. Partamian LG, Jay WM, Fritz KL. Anaerobic orbital cellulitis. Ann Ophthalmol. 1983;15:123–126.
59. Crock GW, Heriot WJ, Janakiraman P, et al. Gas gangrene infection of the eyes and orbits. Br J Ophthalmol. 1985;69:143–148.
60. Sanchez TG, Cahali MB, Murakami MS. Septic thrombosis of orbital vessels due to cutaneous nasal infection. Am J Rhinol. 1997;11:429–433.
61. Slavin ML, Glaser JS. Acute severe irreversible visual loss with sphenoethmoiditis—"posterior" orbital cellulitis. Arch Ophthalmol. 1987;105:345–348.
62. Chandler JR, Langenbrunner DJ, Stevens ER. The pathogenesis of orbital complications in acute sinusitis. Laryngoscope. 1970;80:1414–1428.
63. Birch-Hirshfield, cited by Duke-Elder S. The ocular abscess. In: Duke-Elder S, ed. Textbook of Ophthalmology, v. 5. St. Louis: CV Mosby; 1952:5420–5444.
64. Johnson TE, Casiano RR, Kronish JW, et al. Sino-orbital aspergillosis in acquired immunodeficiency syndrome. Arch Ophthalmol. 1999;117:57–64.
65. Harril WC, Stewart MG, Lee AG, et al. Chronic rhinocerebral mucormycosis. Laryngoscope. 1996;106:1292–1297.
66. Galloway JE, Kavic TA, Raflo GT. Digital subtraction macrodacryocystography: A new method of lacrimal system imaging. Ophthalmology. 1984;91:956.
67. Rossomondo RM, Carlton WH, Trueblood JH, et al. A new method of evaluating lacrimal drainage. Arch Ophthalmol. 1972;88:523.
68. Freeman LN, Zinreich SJ, Iliff NT. Radiography of the lacrimal system using topical CT dacryocystography (Abstract). Ophthalmology. 1987;94:142.
69. Eustis HS, Amstrong DC, Buncie JR, et al. Staging of orbital cellulitis in children: Computed tomography characteristics and treatment guidelines. J Pediatr Ophthalmol Strabismus. 1986;23:246–251.
70. Harr DL, Quencer RM, Abrams GW. Computed tomography and ultrasound in the evaluation of orbital infection and pseudotumor. Radiology. 1982;152:395.
71. Savino PJ, Grossman RI, Schatz NJ, et al. High-field magnetic resonance imaging in the diagnosis of cavernous sinus thrombosis. Arch Neurol. 1986;43:1081–1082.
72. Barnhorst DA Jr, Foster JA, Chern KC, et al. The efficacy of topical metronidazole in the treatment of ocular rosacea. Ophthalmology. 1996;103:1880–1883.
73. Seal DV, Wright P, Ficker L, et al. Placebo controlled trial of fusidic acid gel and oxytetracycline for recurrent blepharitis and rosacea. Br J Ophthalmol. 1995;79:42–45.
74. Campbell CB, Flanagan JC, Schaefer AJ. Acquired lacrimal disorders. In: Smith BC, Della Rocca RC, Nesi FA, eds. Ophthalmic Plastic and Reconstructive Surgery. St. Louis: CV Mosby; 1987:956.
75. Gold SC, Arrigg PG, Hedges TR. Computed tomography in the management of acute orbital cellulitis. Ophthalmic Surg. 1987;18:753–756.
76. Harris GJ. Subperiosteal inflammation of the orbit: A bacteriological analysis of 17 cases. Arch Ophthalmol. 1988;106:947–952.

SECTION N

HEPATITIS

Chapter 102

Acute Viral Hepatitis

HIROSHI KAWAI
STEPHEN M. FEINSTONE

BACKGROUND

Major Causative Agents of Acute Viral Hepatitis

Acute viral hepatitis is a self-limiting disease characterized by necro-inflammatory responses in the affected liver. This disease was traditionally separated into two types based on clinical and epidemiologic characteristics: type A or "infectious" hepatitis, caused by the hepatitis A virus (HAV), and type B or "serum" hepatitis, caused by the hepatitis B virus (HBV).[1–4] Over the past 30 years, at least five hepatitis viruses have been identified: the hepatitis A virus (HAV)[5]; the hepatitis B virus (HBV)[6, 7]; the hepatitis delta or hepatitis D virus (HDV)[8–11]; the hepatitis C virus (HCV), which is the cause of parenterally transmitted, classic non-A, non-B hepatitis as well as community-acquired non-A, non-B hepatitis[12–14]; and an enterically transmitted, epidemic non-A, non-B hepatitis agent called hepatitis E virus (HEV).[15–17] Further vigorous efforts to identify novel hepatitis viruses have led to the identification of other candidate viruses: hepatitis F virus, hepatitis GB virus C (HGBV-C),[18, 19] and hepatitis G virus (HGV).[20] Hepatitis F virus was discovered from the feces of a patient with hepatitis and was transmitted to primates.[21] However, this finding has not been confirmed, and the role of this virus is still unclear. Also of importance are the novel candidate blood-borne hepatitis viruses provisionally called GBV-C or HGV, which were discovered by two groups independently and are regarded as different isolates of the same virus. Virologic and epidemiologic studies of GBV-C and HGV have not yet reached consensus regarding their significance as hepatitis viruses[22–24] (see Chapter 144). Another novel candidate virus for hepatitis, called TTV, has also been identified.[25] TTV is a DNA virus identified from the serum of patients with non–A–G post-transfusion hepatitis. As with GBV-C/HGV, there is uncertainty about its pathogenicity[26] (see Chapter 144). Despite the variety of causative viruses, clinical symptoms of acute viral hepatitis are almost identical, with several exceptions. Therefore, etiologic diagnosis now depends on serologic assays specific for each of the different viruses.

Minor Causative Agents of Acute Viral Hepatitis

The five recognized hepatitis viruses infect primarily the liver, resulting in hepatic inflammation and hepatocellular necrosis without major pathologic involvement of other organs. Many other known viral agents can also infect the liver and induce a viral hepatitis-like syndrome, but they do so in the context of a more widespread pathologic picture. For instance, yellow fever virus (YFV) frequently causes severe hepatic necrosis, but it is a systemic viral infection with widespread pathology affecting multiple organs. Other common hepatitis-inducing agents in the United States are the Epstein-Barr virus (EBV) and cytomegalovirus (CMV), and liver disease also can result from infections with herpes simplex viruses, varicella-zoster virus, measles, rubella, rubeola, coxsackie B viruses, and adenoviruses. Although these agents can cause diagnostic confusion by producing some degree of liver inflammation and dysfunction, they are not primary causes of acute or chronic viral hepatitis.

A minority of patients have a viral hepatitis-like syndrome without serologic evidence of infection by any of the recognized agents. These patients may have disease caused by one of the five known viral agents but have levels of antigen or antibody that are undetectable by any of the specific serologic tests, or they may be infected by other, unidentified viruses; alternatively, there may be a noninfectious cause accounting for their clinical condition.

Trends of Acute Viral Hepatitis

Acute viral hepatitis is a common disease. In the United States during the 1984–1994 period, the Centers for Disease Control and Prevention estimated that the total number of annual acute infections for HAV was 125,000 to 200,000; HBV, 140,000 to 320,000; HCV, 35,000 to 180,000; and HDV, 6,000 to 13,000. Among these, 84,000 to 134,000 of HAV, 70,000 to 160,000 of HBV, and 25 to 30% of acute HCV infections were estimated to result in symptomatic infections. The relative contributions of major hepatitis viruses to acute hepatitis in the United States during 1982–1993 period were hepatitis A, 47%; hepatitis B, 34%; hepatitis C, 16%; and hepatitis non–A–C, 3%. Although hepatitis B cases have been declining since a peak in 1985, hepatitis A cases have been increasing, especially in the western United States. Acute hepatitis C is a very underreported disease, and because specific tests have been available only since 1990, the trends in incidence are difficult to determine. Hepatitis C has been virtually eliminated as a cause of transfusion-associated hepatitis since the institution of donor screening in 1990, and the overall rate of acute disease may be declining. The rates of reported cases of hepatitis A, hepatitis B, and non-A non-B hepatitis are presented in Figure 102–1. The risk factors associated with acute viral hepatitis A, B, and C are listed in Table 102–1. The similarity in risk factors for hepatitis B and C reflects their similar modes of transmission, which are largely parenteral and sexual and which differ from the fecal-oral transmission associated with HAV.

Fulminant Hepatitis

Acute viral hepatitis can be a serious disease. Although it is a rare complication, the overall mortality rate for icteric viral hepatitis is approximately 1%. The mortality rate is higher in older persons, and some of the reported variation relates to the age of the affected patients. The frequency of fulminant hepatitis also depends on the cause of the hepatitis. Fulminant disease occurs more commonly in hepatitis B and D than in the other forms of acute viral hepatitis. In various outbreaks of delta hepatitis, the mortality rate has been reported to be between 2 and 20%.[9, 27] A striking characteristic of type E hepatitis is an increased incidence of fulminant disease and a high mortality rate (about 10%) in pregnant women, especially during the third trimester.[17]

In addition to morbidity and mortality from the acute disease, the progression of viral hepatitis B, C, and D from an acute to a chronic state can also lead to serious sequelae, including chronic liver disease, cirrhosis, and hepatocellular carcinoma; in addition, polyarteritis nodosa, cryoglobulinemia, glomerulonephritis, and aplastic anemia have been associated with either acute or chronic

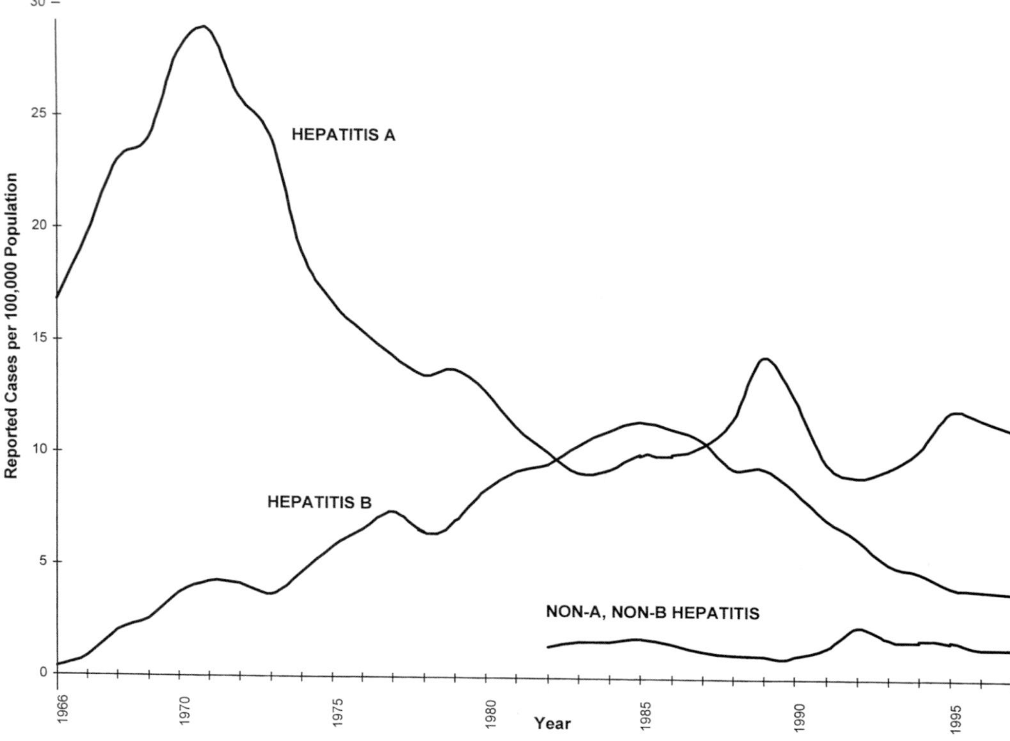

FIGURE 102–1. Reported cases of viral hepatitis A, B and non-A, non-B (mostly hepatitis C) by year in the United States. 1966–1997. The first hepatitis B vaccine was approved in 1982. The first test for antibody to hepatitis C virus was introduced in 1990 for screening blood donors. Although this test has limited utility for the diagnosis of acute hepatitis C, it has made specific diagnosis possible when properly applied. However, acute hepatitis C remains the most underreported type of acute viral hepatitis. (From Centers for Disease Control surveillance data.)

infection[28–30] (see Chapter 135). In the United States and Western Europe, chronic viral hepatitis is probably the second most frequent cause of cirrhosis, second only to alcohol abuse. The chronic forms of hepatitis B, delta hepatitis, and hepatitis C are common causes of terminal liver disease for which hepatic transplantation is performed. On a worldwide scale, chronic HBV infection is the most important cause of cirrhosis and is a major cause of cancer mortality. It is estimated that 5% of the world's population has chronic HBV infection (the chronic carrier state), and hepatocellular carcinoma resulting from such chronic infections is among the most common malignancies worldwide.[31] Chronic infection by HCV is also associated with a greatly increased risk of liver cancer.[32–35]

Major advances during the past 25 years have been made in defining the agents that are capable of causing hepatitis; this has translated into means of accurately detecting and preventing these infections. Less progress has been made in the realm of specific treatment to prevent complications such as chronicity. Serologic markers have now been developed for all five forms of viral hepatitis and have had a major impact in preventing post-transfusion hepatitis and in defining the epidemiology, natural history, and means of control of community-acquired viral hepatitis. A safe, highly effective hepatitis B vaccine made from hepatitis B surface antigen (HBsAg) purified from the plasma of chronic carriers has been available since 1982, and safe and highly effective vaccines prepared from bioengineered recombinant yeast expressing HBsAg have been available since 1986.[36] Both killed and live attenuated vaccines against hepatitis A have been developed. A formalin-inactivated hepatitis A vaccine has been demonstrated to be highly effective in protecting against clinically apparent infection.[37–41] Now, two hepatitis A vaccines are available in the United States for high-risk individuals older than 2 years of age. For persons who have been exposed to HAV and have not previously been given HAV vaccine, a single intramuscular dose of immune globulin should be used no longer than 2 weeks after exposure (see Chapters 161 and 312).

CLINICAL MANIFESTATIONS

Symptoms

The clinical presentation of acute viral hepatitis ranges from asymptomatic disease to fulminant hepatic failure with its attendant high

TABLE 102–1 Risk Factors Associated with Acute Viral Hepatitis A, B, and C

Hepatitis A	% of Total	Hepatitis B	% of Total	Hepatitis C	% of Total
Personal contact	24	Heterosexual contact	41	Injection drug use	43
Day care–associated	15.1	Injection drug use	15	Sexual contact	15
Foreign travel	5.5	Homosexual contact	9	Other	14
Outbreak-associated	4.7	Household	2	Past drug use (>6 mo)	11
Male homosexual	3.8	Health care workers	1	Cocaine snorting	5
Injection drug use	2.4	Other	1	Occupation	4
Unknown	44.5	Unknown	31	Transfusion	4*
				Household	3

*Since 1995, transfusion-associated hepatitis C has virtually disappeared.
From Centers for Disease Control and Prevention. Hepatitis surveillance data.

mortality rate. There are no clinical features that unequivocally distinguish the individual types of hepatitis from each other, although certain epidemiologic patterns of transmission may suggest a particular etiology. Acute viral hepatitis is conveniently separated into four clinical stages: incubation period, preicteric phase, icteric phase, and convalescence. The timing and major symptoms of each of these stages are shown diagrammatically in Figure 102–2.

The incubation period of acute viral hepatitis varies from as short as a few weeks to as long as 6 months, depending on the particular infecting virus. The incubation period of hepatitis A averages about 21 days (range, 15 to 45 days); type B hepatitis, about 70 days (range, 30 to 180 days); type C hepatitis (classic non-A, non-B hepatitis), 50 days (range, 15 to 150 days); and type E hepatitis (epidemic non-A, non-B hepatitis), about 40 days (range, 15 to 60 days). The incubation period of delta hepatitis has not been well documented. Because delta hepatitis invariably occurs in conjunction with hepatitis B, its incubation period probably is similar. Because there is considerable overlap in the incubation periods of each of the viruses, one cannot reliably ascertain the etiologic agent based on such information. During the incubation period, the patient is asymptomatic and feels well.

The initial symptoms of acute hepatitis are nonspecific; typically, the patient develops malaise and weakness, followed shortly by anorexia, nausea, vomiting, and a vague, dull, right upper quadrant pain. These symptoms of the preicteric phase usually last 3 to 10 days. The onset of jaundice or dark urine, or both, then ushers in the icteric phase. It is these symptoms that usually bring the patient to the doctor. The patient may begin to feel better even while jaundice persists.

Although this sequence represents the "typical" case, there is considerable variation in the clinical presentation. Clinically evident icterus accounts for only 20 to 50% of hepatitis virus infections. The remainder pass unnoticed, without symptoms or with such mild symptoms that they are dismissed as inconsequential ("indigestion" or "the flu"). The spectrum of clinical disease ranges from inapparent, to anicteric (but symptomatic), to icteric, to fulminant.

The onset of viral hepatitis can be sudden (most typical of hepatitis A) or insidious (more typical of type B or C). At least 25% of the patients with viral hepatitis describe the onset of their disease as an "influenza-like" illness with weakness, headaches, myalgias, chills, and fever. This onset is most common with hepatitis A. Symptoms of an upper respiratory infection, such as a sore throat and cough, may be present. These symptoms are short-lived (1 to 3 days) and are replaced by the more typical symptoms of anorexia, nausea, and then jaundice. Fever, in particular, rarely persists into the icteric phase. Jaundice with high fever is *not* characteristic of viral hepatitis.

Malaise is the earliest and most common (approximately 95%) symptom of this disease. It usually is the first symptom to appear and the last to leave. *Anorexia* is frequently present in symptomatic viral hepatitis, but it typically is one of the first symptoms to abate. There may be a change in taste and smell with a concomitant aversion to food and often to cigarettes. This dysgeusia is not specific for viral hepatitis and may be seen with any form of acute hepatitis. *Nausea* and vomiting occur in about 80% of patients with symptomatic viral hepatitis. The nausea is typically intermittent and rarely intractable. Nausea, like malaise, may be absent early in the day and then appear and worsen as the day progresses. Mild weight loss is common during viral hepatitis. Abdominal *pain* can accompany acute viral hepatitis (about 60%), and it usually consists of a mild, dull, right upper quadrant, aching discomfort that is unaffected by meals, antacids, stool patterns, or position.

A minority of patients with acute hepatitis (5 to 15%) experience a "serum sickness–like syndrome" at the onset of their illness.[42, 43] This consists of a triad of symptoms: fever, rash, and arthritis. It is a manifestation of immune complex (virus-antibody) deposition. This syndrome occurs during the preicteric phase and almost invariably resolves dramatically with the onset of jaundice. *Fever* is usual but

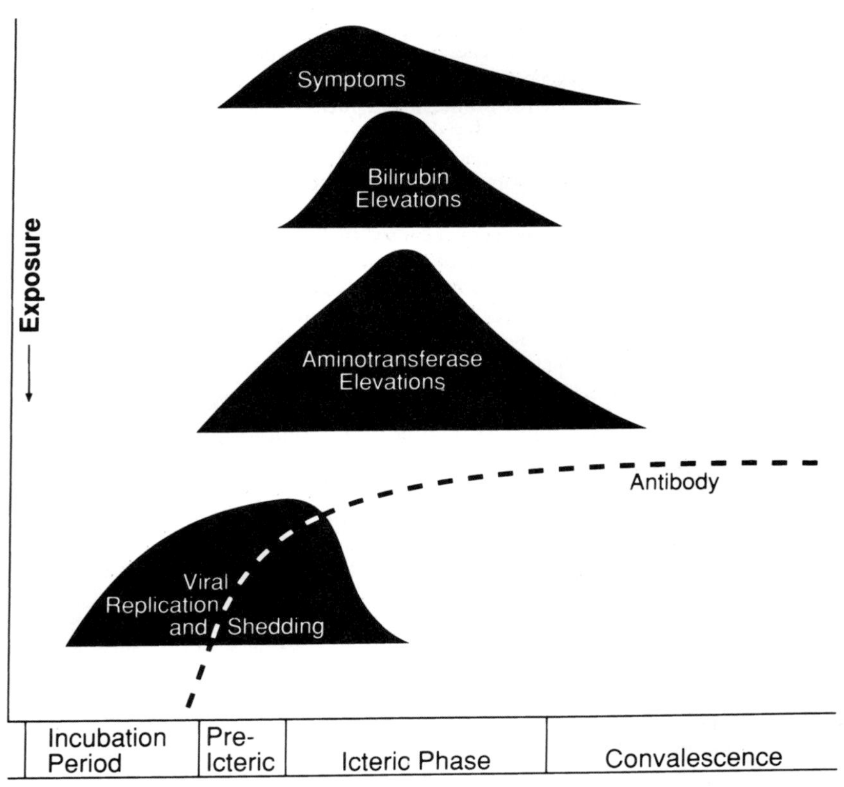

FIGURE 102–2. The course of acute viral hepatitis. The timing of the clinical symptoms related to laboratory findings, virologic events, and development of serum antibodies is shown.

not invariable. The *rash* is typically urticarial, with pruritic hives appearing and disappearing in a largely peripheral distribution. More exanthem-like macular-papular lesions can also occur, as can fleeting, irregular patches of erythema. The *arthritis* is mild to moderate, nondeforming, polyarticular, and migratory. Major joints involved are the elbows, wrists, knees, and small joints of the hands. Arthralgias probably are more common than frank arthritis. This syndrome is most common with hepatitis B, but it also has been reported in hepatitis A. In children with hepatitis B, a condition perhaps related to this syndrome—papular acrodermatitis (Gianotti's disease)—has been described. It is characterized by skin eruptions, lymphadenopathy and lymphadenitis, and mild, usually anicteric, acute viral hepatitis.[44]

Jaundice and dark urine are the most distinctive symptoms of acute hepatitis, but they can be unreliable. Scleral icterus may go unnoticed, even with a serum bilirubin level as high as 10 mg/dl. *Dark urine* often is more noticeable than scleral icterus. The presence of dark urine is also helpful in indicating that the jaundice is accompanied by conjugated (direct) hyperbilirubinemia, which is not found with jaundice caused by hemolysis or Gilbert's syndrome. Although jaundice and dark urine usually occur after a 4- to 10-day preicteric phase, some patients have jaundice only and deny any prodrome of malaise, anorexia, or nausea. Light-colored stools also can occur with the jaundice of viral hepatitis, reflecting the lack of bile pigments being added to the intestinal contents. The lightening of stool color in viral hepatitis usually is not as great as in obstructive jaundice, and white or chalky stools are uncommon. Persons with prominent jaundice also often complain of *pruritus.* Approximately 40% of jaundiced patients complain of itching at the peak of icterus or some time into convalescence.

In addition to a serum sickness–like syndrome, there are other immune complex–mediated diseases that have been described in association with acute (and chronic) viral hepatitis. Polyarteritis nodosa, associated with HBV infection, leads to a small-, medium-, and large-vessel arteritis that affects multiple organs. Symptoms include fever, abdominal pain, arthralgias, mononeuritis, renal disease, hypertension, central nervous system abnormalities, and skin rashes. Studies show that up to 69% of patients with established polyarteritis nodosa are HBsAg-positive.[45] Both hepatitis B and hepatitis C have been associated with glomerulonephritis, which is thought to be caused by immune complex deposition of viral antigen or antibody (or both) within the glomerular basement membrane, leading to membranous and membranoproliferative glomerulonephritis.[46–48] Not infrequently, the severity of the renal disease overshadows the hepatitis. Mixed cryoglobulinemia, caused by the production of antibodies with altered physical characteristics such that they form a precipitate when subjected to lower temperatures, has been associated with HBV and, more recently, with HCV infection.[49, 50] The rare occurrence of other manifestations, such as Raynaud's phenomenon, bullous formation, and erythema nodosa, also has been described in acute hepatitis.

Fulminant viral hepatitis is the most ominous manifestation of viral hepatitis. It is defined as severe acute liver failure with hepatic encephalopathy occurring within 8 weeks after the onset of symptoms with jaundice.[51, 52] Late-onset hepatic failure is defined as severe acute liver failure occurring from 8 to 12 weeks after the onset of symptoms with jaundice. Approximately 75% of cases of fulminant hepatic failure are caused by viral hepatitis, with HBV being responsible for 30 to 60% of all cases. Up to 30 to 40% of patients with fulminant hepatic failure caused by HBV also test positive for the delta virus and presumably are co-infected. HAV infection is an uncommon cause, with less than 0.1% of cases progressing to hepatic failure. HCV has not by itself been implicated as a cause of acute fulminant hepatic failure, although it may act as a cofactor in patients who are co-infected with another virus, such as HBV. Although the role of GBV-C/HGV in viral hepatitis is still being investigated and many researchers now regard it as a nonhepatitis virus,[53, 54] there is evidence that links HGV to fulminant hepatitis.[55–57] Fulminant hepatic failure can occur at any time—early or late—during the course of the disease. The first symptoms usually are lethargy, somnolence, and a change in personality. Patients may be excited, euphoric, and unruly. These symptoms are followed in more severe cases by stupor and then coma.

Physical Findings

The physical findings in acute viral hepatitis are few. Vital signs are normal, although bradycardia can occur when significant hyperbilirubinemia is present. Icterus can be detected if the bilirubin level exceeds 2.5 to 3.0 mg/dl. It is seen most easily in the sclera or under the tongue. In light-skinned people, the skin may have a yellowish hue. Palpation of the abdomen often demonstrates a slightly enlarged and tender liver. A spleen tip is felt in 5 to 25% of the patients. Signs of portal hypertension are not seen in acute hepatitis except in late, severe disease (as with subacute hepatic necrosis). Adenopathy, if present, is not prominent.

There are several skin findings in acute viral hepatitis. Vascular spiders often are found in light-skinned persons, but they are few and small. Severe pruritus may lead to excoriations. One should search for forearm venipuncture marks suggesting drug addiction, a common source of hepatitis virus infection. Patients with the serum sickness–like syndrome have urticaria or a mild, fleeting erythematous rash and (occasionally) red, warm, and tender joints. Finally, acne-prone persons may exhibit an exacerbation of this condition with acute hepatitis.

When fulminant hepatitis supervenes, signs of hepatic encephalopathy appear. These consist of lethargy, somnolence, untidiness, confusion, forgetfulness, and then stupor and full coma. Typical of hepatic encephalopathy is asterixis—the asynchronous, irregular flapping of the forcibly dorsiflexed, outstretched hands. In stage I coma, mild mental changes are present, but asterixis is minimal or absent. Stage II coma is marked by worsening of mental changes and definite asterixis. In stage III coma, the patient develops stupor and semicoma but can still be roused. With stage IV coma, the patient no longer is arousable, and there may or may not be a response to deep pain stimuli. Patients with hepatic failure may demonstrate other neurologic signs: flapping of the tongue, involuntary movements, long-tract signs, and decerebrate posturing. They also may demonstrate the distinctive sweetish smell of fetor hepaticus.

Laboratory Findings

Although the symptoms and signs of acute viral hepatitis are frequently nonspecific or vague, laboratory findings are characteristic (Fig. 102–3). Most distinctive of viral hepatitis are the dramatic elevations in the aminotransferases—aspartate aminotransferase (AST) and alanine aminotransferase (ALT). In acute viral hepatitis, concentrations of both of the aminotransferases are elevated, usually to more than eight times normal at the time of the appearance of jaundice. The AST-ALT ratio is usually less than 1 in viral hepatitis, whereas it usually exceeds 1.5 in alcoholic liver disease.[58–60] The alkaline phosphatase and other serum enzyme levels that denote biliary obstruction or cholestasis (gamma glutamyl transferase, 5′-nucleotidase) are only mildly increased (1 to 3 times normal). The lactic dehydrogenase (LDH) concentration usually is mildly elevated in acute viral hepatitis (1 to 3 times normal). The dramatic increase in both AST and ALT, with only mild elevation in alkaline phosphatase and LDH, is virtually diagnostic of "acute hepatitis" or "acute necroinflammatory disease of the liver." Given this enzyme pattern, the only question to resolve is whether this acute hepatitis is caused by a hepatitis virus, a hepatotoxic drug, a toxin, or a nonspecific liver injury (e.g., anoxia, shock, severe heart failure).

The AST and ALT become abnormal during the late incubation period of this disease. They are invariably abnormal once symptoms

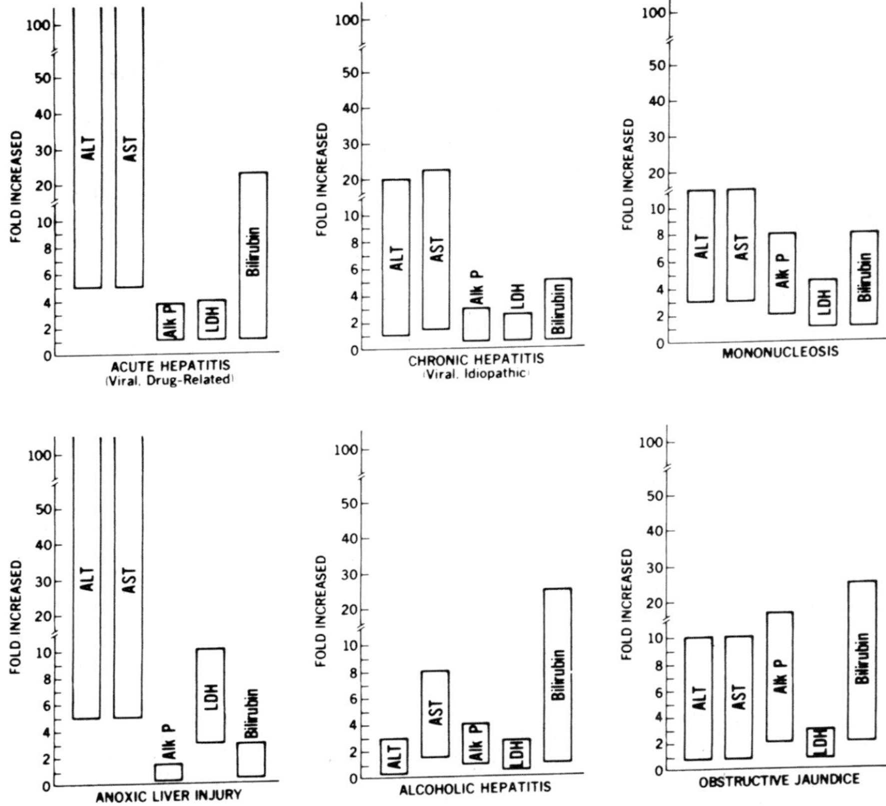

FIGURE 102–3. The range of elevation of key serum enzyme levels in acute viral hepatitis and other common liver diseases. *Abbreviations:* Alk P, Alkaline phosphate; ALT, alanine aminotransferase; AST, aspartate aminotransferase; LDH, lactic dehydrogenase.

occur, usually rise during the preicteric phase, and peak early in the icteric phase. With recovery, the aminotransferase levels quickly fall but almost always remain slightly abnormal for several weeks after the jaundice and symptoms have abated.

The bilirubin level is variably elevated in icteric viral hepatitis. This elevation involves both the direct and indirect fractions, with the ratio being approximately equal. Disproportionate elevations in direct bilirubin concentration suggest cholestasis, whereas the preponderance of indirect bilirubin (>80%) suggests hemolysis. Persons with underlying hemolytic states (glucose-6-phosphate dehydrogenase deficiency or sickle cell disease) may have accelerated hemolysis with many viral infections and especially with viral hepatitis.[61] These persons may become markedly jaundiced and yet have relatively mild symptoms and increased aminotransferase levels.

The prothrombin time typically is normal in acute viral hepatitis, and when it is prolonged, suspicion should be raised of more severe liver necrosis that may progress to fulminant hepatic failure. Any elevation should be regarded as a serious sign. When the prothrombin time is longer than 100 seconds, or longer than 50 seconds in association with a bilirubin level higher than 17.6 mg/dl in a patient who is younger than 11 or older than 40 years of age, the probability that spontaneous recovery will occur is low and the patient should promptly be considered for liver transplantation.[62] The partial thromboplastin time is not as sensitive or as reliable a measure as the prothrombin time.

Other laboratory test results rarely are abnormal. The serum albumin and globulin levels usually are normal in acute viral hepatitis, as are hemoglobin values. The leukocyte count is either normal or slightly low. A mild lymphocytosis can occur. The platelet count remains normal except with fulminant hepatitis, in which case disseminated intravascular coagulation can supervene. Patients with acute viral hepatitis often develop low levels of anti-DNA and smooth muscle antibodies (SMA). Biologic false-positive Venereal Disease Research Laboratory (VDRL) test reactions are rare. The sedimentation rate is normal or minimally increased. Serum immunoglobulin levels usually are normal except in hepatitis A, in which case the serum level of immunoglobulin M (IgM) may double during the course of the disease.

Pathologic Findings

The clinical history, pattern of serum enzyme levels, and serologic findings in acute viral hepatitis are sufficiently characteristic that a percutaneous liver biopsy specimen is rarely indicated for diagnosis. However, when several possible causes of acute liver disease are present or when therapy is a consideration, a liver biopsy can be helpful. The typical liver biopsy findings of acute viral hepatitis are lobular disarray, ballooning and eosinophilic degeneration, liver cell necrosis, mononuclear cell infiltration of the parenchyma and portal tracts, and variable degrees of cholestasis.[63] These changes are diffuse and generalized; therefore, sampling error from needle biopsy usually is not a problem. Lobular disarray refers to a loss of the orderly pattern of hepatic sinusoidal cords, the result of widespread anisocytosis, liver cell degeneration, regeneration, or death (Fig. 102–4). Liver cells demonstrate two forms of degeneration: ballooning degeneration (in which there is swelling of the liver cell and rarefaction of the cytoplasm) and eosinophilic degeneration (in which the cell shrinks and becomes a deeper red and more angular). The end result of eosinophilic degeneration is the free hyaline body (Fig. 102–5). There also may be "smudging" of hepatocytes with indistinctness of cell outline as well as cell "dropout," with or without associated inflammatory cell reaction. Kupffer's cells appear to be more numerous and enlarged. Areas of lymphocytic infiltration are common both in the parenchyma and in portal tracts. Polymorphonuclear leukocytes are not numerous. A few plasma cells and eosinophils may be found, but a prominence of portal tract plasma cells suggests chronic hepatitis; also, unusual numbers of eosinophils suggest drug addiction or a drug-related hepatitis. Cholestasis (bile

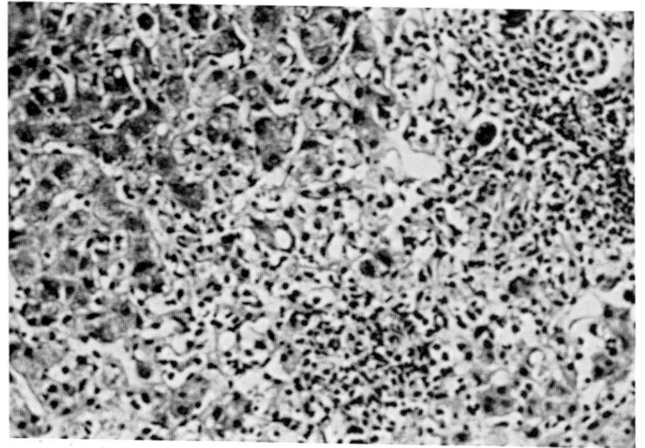

FIGURE 102–4. Liver biopsy specimen from a patient with acute viral hepatitis. Note the lobular disarray; the occurrence of eosinophilic degeneration, free hyaline bodies, and spotty hepatocellular necrosis; and the prominent mononuclear cell infiltrates in the portal zone and areas of parenchyma (H&E, × 240). (Photomicrograph courtesy of Dr. Kamal Ishak, Washington, DC.)

staining of liver cells and bile "plugs") may be seen on liver biopsy specimens and generally correspond in degree to the height of the serum bilirubin level. The portal bile ducts, however, usually appear to be normal.

In typical viral hepatitis, cell necrosis is spotty and focal. More severe hepatitis may be accompanied by coalescent or bridging necrosis (between portal zones or from portal zones to central veins), multilobular necrosis, or massive necrosis.[63–66] Bridging necrosis found during acute viral hepatitis indicates a serious lesion that can progress to postnecrotic cirrhosis. Multilobular or massive necrosis is seen in severe and fulminant disease.

DIFFERENTIAL DIAGNOSIS

The specific etiologic diagnosis of acute viral hepatitis depends primarily on serologic testing once it has been demonstrated that acute necroinflammatory disease (acute hepatitis) is present. This is based largely on the pattern of serum enzyme concentrations—dramatic increases in aminotransferase levels with mild increases in

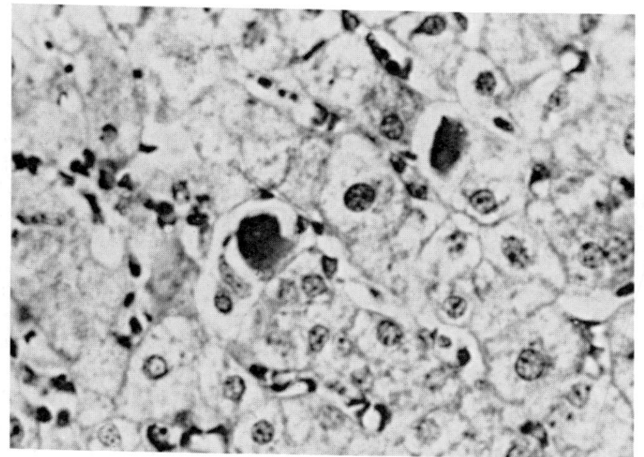

FIGURE 102–5. The free hyaline body and eosinophilic degeneration typical of acute viral hepatitis (H&E, × 660). (Photomicrograph courtesy of Dr. Kamal Ishak, Washington, DC.)

the alkaline phosphatase level. The differential diagnosis of acute hepatitis includes other infectious diseases as well as noninfectious forms of liver disease. These include bacterial infections (pneumococcal pneumonia, leptospirosis), various drugs (acetaminophen, isoniazid), toxins (alcohol, carbon tetrachloride), and nonspecific injury (shock, ischemia). These types of acute hepatitis usually can be excluded by a careful history with some support from laboratory data. In addition to the identification of the responsible viral agent using serologies, identification of the source of infection should also be attempted. Most cases of acute viral hepatitis are caused by one of five agents: HAV, HBV, HCV, HDV, or HEV. Although these agents are virologically distinct, the diseases that they cause are quite similar. They overlap so much in symptoms and severity that they cannot be reliably distinguished on clinical grounds, by biochemical tests, or even by liver biopsy findings. Specific serologic assays can usually separate and identify these five types of viral hepatitis, but in some circumstances diagnostic uncertainties remain. The use of specific serologic tests is summarized in Figure 102–6. Among the cases of diagnostic uncertainty without positive specific antibody tests are patients in the window period, when antibodies have not yet developed, patients infected with viruses that escape antibody assay because of mutation, and the cases in which specific antibody assays are not yet available.

Hepatitis A

Hepatitis A is an acute, self-limited disease that only rarely causes death (see Chapter 161). Hepatitis A characteristically has an acute, sudden, influenza-like onset with a prominence of myalgia, headache, fever, and malaise.[1, 67–69] The ratio of anicteric to icteric hepatitis is high, particularly in children. Hepatitis A usually is not as severe nor as long-lasting as hepatitis B. However, a transient relapsing course has been reported,[70] and a prolonged cholestasis appearing late in the acute phase and lasting for several months may be seen.[71, 72] Both of these unusual forms of hepatitis A are usually benign; the mortality rate of hepatitis A is low (about 2 per 1000 icteric cases),[68, 73] and the disease ultimately resolves. Hepatitis A never leads to a chronic hepatitis or a carrier state.[74]

Epidemiologic features can be helpful in distinguishing hepatitis A from other forms of viral hepatitis.[75, 76] Hepatitis A is spread predominantly by the fecal-oral route. It is highly contagious and spreads rapidly to close contacts. Hepatitis A can occur in outbreaks that may have an identifiable point source (often a person in the incubation period of acute disease). Hepatitis A has been shown to be spread by contaminated water, milk, or food[77]; after breakdown in usual sanitary conditions or after floods or natural disasters[78] by ingestion of raw or undercooked shellfish (oysters, clams, and mussels) from contaminated waters[78] during travel to areas of the world with poor hygienic conditions where hepatitis A is endemic[79]; among institutionalized children and adults[1]; and after exposure to recently imported chimpanzees or apes.[80]

Three other epidemiologic sources have been shown to be important in spread of hepatitis A: exposure to children in day care centers,[76, 81] male homosexuality,[82] and intravenous drug addiction.[75, 76] Day care centers can serve as sources of outbreaks of hepatitis A, especially when there are children who are not toilet trained in the centers. Male homosexuals may have a high incidence of hepatitis A that probably is related to sexual practices. Some cases occur without any known point source of infection. Blood transfusion is a very rare mode of transmission of hepatitis A.[75]

The clinical, virologic, and serologic course of a typical case of hepatitis A is shown in Figure 102–7. Fecal shedding of HAV is found during both the incubation period and the early symptomatic phase of illness but may no longer may be detectable at the time of onset of jaundice. Antibody to HAV (anti-HAV) is detectable in serum by the time of onset of disease. Initially, the anti-HAV consists of both IgG and IgM antibodies. After 3 to 12 months, IgM anti-HAV disappears, whereas IgG anti-HAV persists in high titer, confer-

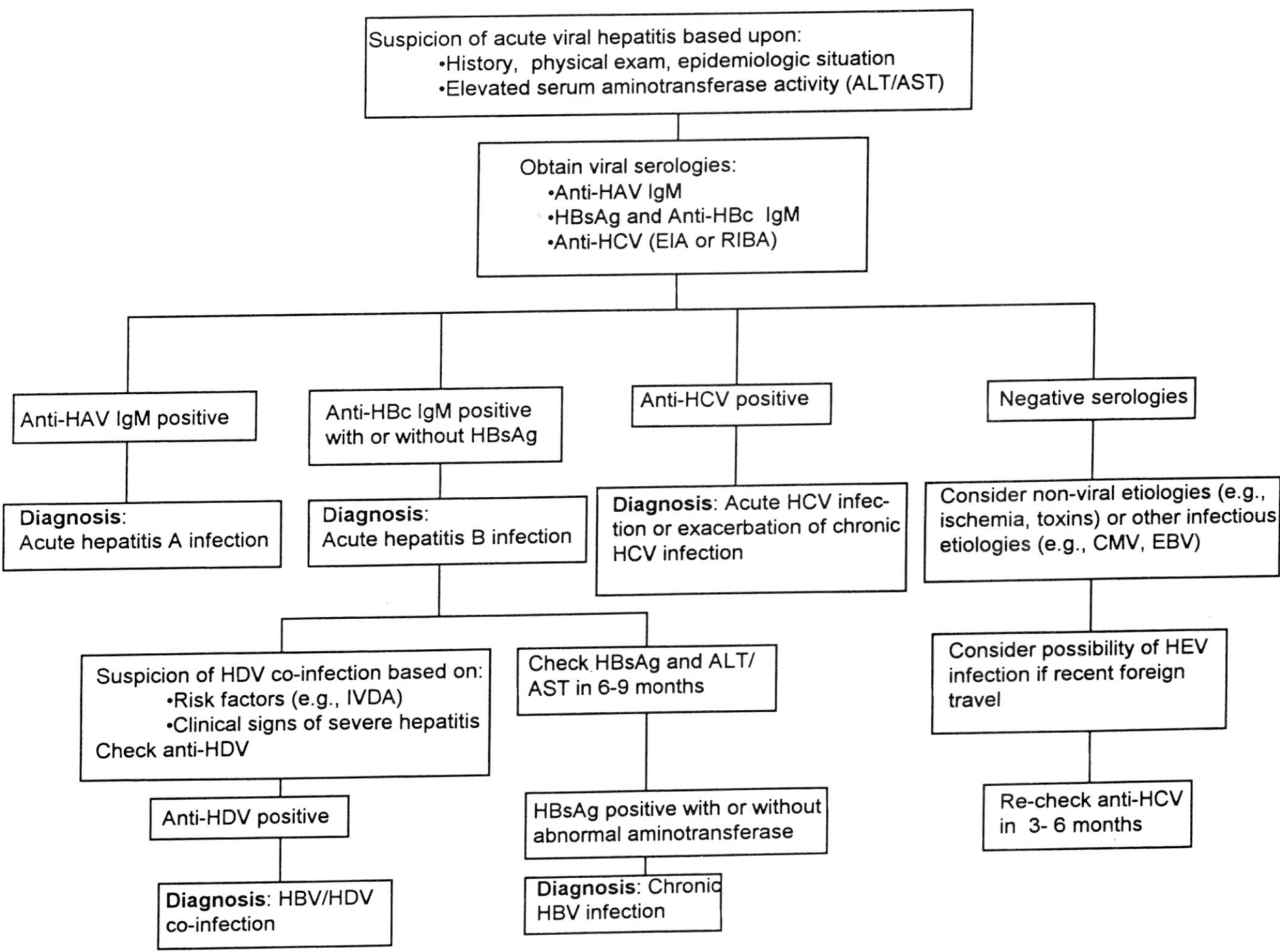

FIGURE 102–6. A flow diagram showing the use of specific serologic tests for the diagnosis of acute viral hepatitis in relation to the clinical and epidemiologic setting. Coinfections and superinfections of chronic hepatitis B or C patients should always be considered in cases that do not fit well with the clinical or serologic picture.

ring lifelong immunity. Therefore, the diagnosis of acute hepatitis A is made by the finding of IgM anti-HAV in a patient with either clinical symptoms or biochemical evidence of acute hepatitis (see Fig. 102–6).[83] Immunoassays are now available for IgM anti-HAV and for total anti-HAV. These assays allow for both diagnosis (IgM anti-HAV) of hepatitis A and assessment of immunity (total anti-HAV) to hepatitis A. For purposes of diagnosis of acute hepatitis A, only the IgM anti-HAV measurement is necessary.

Hepatitis B

Hepatitis B appears to be a more serious disease than hepatitis A, and it has a definite propensity for chronicity. It usually has a more insidious onset and a more prolonged course than hepatitis A (see Chapter 135). In the individual case, however, hepatitis B cannot be distinguished from hepatitis A or from hepatitis C on clinical grounds alone. The occurrence of the serum sickness–like syndrome of fever, rash, and polyarthritis during the preicteric phase favors the diagnosis of hepatitis B.

Epidemiologic features can suggest HBV infection. This disease has a long incubation period (40 to 180 days) and is more likely to occur as sporadic rather than epidemic hepatitis.[1] Whether apparent or not, HBV is spread predominantly by the parenteral route. On a worldwide basis, the most common forms of spread are from mother to child during or soon after birth and by sexual contact. In the United States, hepatitis B often occurs in persons with exposure to blood or blood products (multiply transfused patients, hemophiliacs, renal dialysis and oncology ward patients), with exposure to contaminated needles and syringes (medical personnel with accidental needlesticks, drug addicts), with multiple sexual contacts (homosexuals, prostitutes, the sexually active),[84] or with exposure to saliva or other potentially infectious excreta (children in institutions for the mentally retarded).[1] Risk factors for acute hepatitis B are summarized in Table 102–1. Heterosexual activity (41%) and injection drug use (15%) were the leading factors in the United States. However, these same epidemiologic features also can be found in cases of non-A, non-B hepatitis (hepatitis C) and occasionally also in hepatitis A. In at least 50% of acute hepatitis B cases, no history of parenteral exposure is uncovered. Whether these cases were acquired by "nonparenteral" routes or by inapparent parenteral routes is not known. At the present time, with screening of all blood donors for high-risk behavior and the testing of all donated blood and source plasma for HBsAg and antibody to the core antigen (anti-HBc) as well as specific viral inactivation of most plasma-derived products, the transmission of HBV by these biologicals is now rare.

The diagnosis of hepatitis B should rest on specific serologic testing, with the finding of HBsAg in the serum during the acute disease (Fig. 102–6). The clinical, virologic, and serologic course of

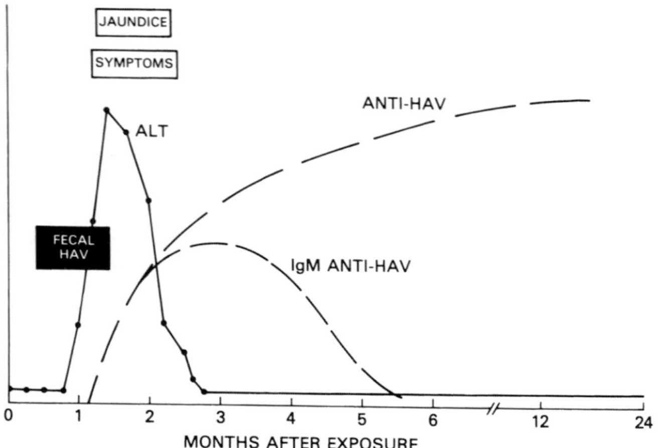

FIGURE 102–7. The clinical, virologic, and serologic courses of a typical case of hepatitis A. *Abbreviations:* ALT, Alanine aminotransferase; ANTI-HAV, antibody to hepatitis A virus; HAV, hepatitis A virus.

a cause of acute hepatitis B is presented in Figure 102–8. HBsAg appears in the serum during the incubation period, 2 to 7 weeks before the onset of symptoms. It usually persists in the blood throughout the illness and disappears with convalescence.[85, 86] The majority of patients (95%) are HBsAg positive at the onset of symptoms and jaundice. In some patients, however, HBsAg is cleared rapidly and may be absent by the time the patient is tested. In this situation, tests for antibody must be used to make the diagnosis. Antibody to HBsAg (anti-HBs) usually arises during convalescence from hepatitis B and, indeed, may not be detectable for some time into the recovery phase. Antibody to hepatitis B core antigen (anti-HBc) is a more reliable marker of HBV infection and usually appears at or about the time of onset of symptoms. Sensitive and specific immunoassays are now available for assaying both anti-HBs and anti-HBc. However, neither of these assays is definitive in the serodiagnosis of acute hepatitis B, because both anti-HBs and anti-HBc are long-lived. The finding of either of these antibodies in the serum of a patient with acute hepatitis does not prove that the disease is caused by HBV infection, because infection with another virus might have occurred in a patient previously infected with HBV. However, immunoassays for IgM anti-HBc have been developed that are very useful in the diagnosis of hepatitis B. IgM anti-HBc arises early in the illness of patients with acute HBV infection but rapidly decreases in titer and no longer may be detectable 6 to 24 months after the illness.[87] Both false-positive and false-negative results can occur with the IgM anti-HBc test, but they are rare.

Patients with acute hepatitis B also develop hepatitis B "early" antigen (HBeAg) as well as direct markers for the presence of HBV in serum, such as HBV-DNA (as detected by molecular hybridization or polymerase chain reaction [PCR]) and DNA polymerase (the endogenous polymerase of this virus). These markers of active viral replication are detected early in the course of acute hepatitis. By the peak of clinical illness and jaundice, levels of HBV in serum usually are decreasing or absent. Indeed, the seroconversion from HBeAg to antibody to HBeAg (anti-HBe) may be a favorable serologic sign indicating that the height of the viral replication has passed and the infection is on the wane.

From 5 to 10% of patients with HBV infection do not clear HBsAg but become HBsAg carriers.[1, 86, 88] These people typically have mild, often anicteric and asymptomatic disease, which may explain why most chronic HBsAg carriers do not give a history of acute hepatitis. As many as 0.2 to 1.0% of adults in the United States are chronic HBsAg carriers. The prevalence of the carrier state is even higher in "high-risk" populations such as male homosexuals (6%), intravenous drug abusers (7%), hemophiliacs (7%), and renal dialysis patients (2 to 15%).[86] Most chronic HBsAg carriers are asymptomatic and have minimal or no accompanying liver injury.

The development of the chronic HBsAg carrier state as a result of symptomatic acute viral hepatitis occurs less commonly than with asymptomatic disease. Progression to a chronic carrier state should be suspected if the patient remains HBeAg positive or if HBsAg persists beyond 6 months after acute infection.[85]

The presence of the chronic HBsAg carrier state also can create diagnostic confusion in the serodiagnosis of acute viral hepatitis. A

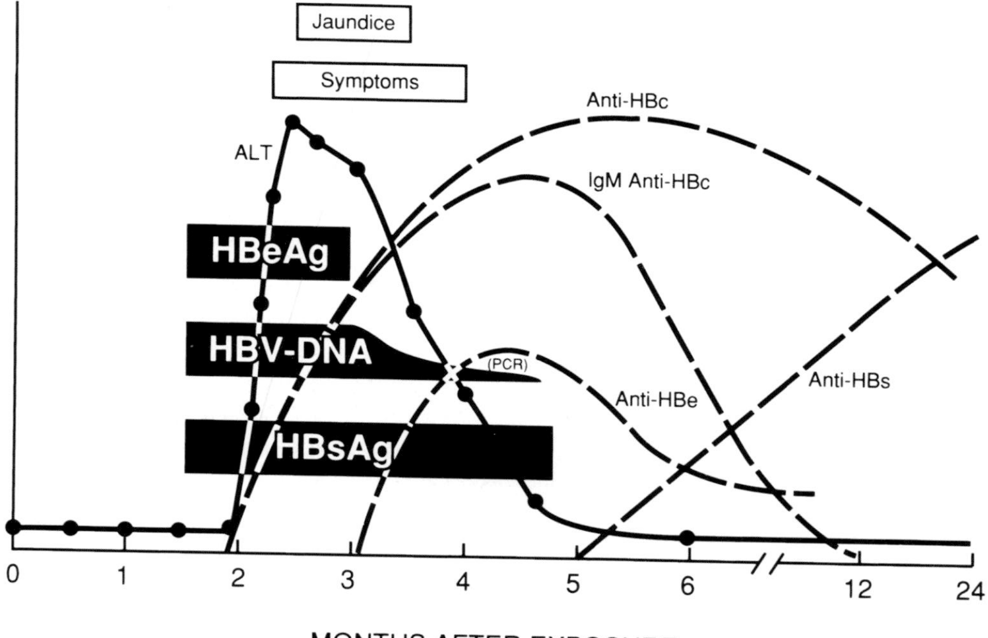

FIGURE 102–8. The clinical, virologic, and serologic courses of a typical case of acute hepatitis B. *Abbreviations:* anti-HBc, Antibody to hepatitis B core antigen; anti-HBe, antibody to hepatitis B e antigen; anti-HBs, antibody to hepatitis B surface antigen; DNA-pl, hepatitis B DNA polymerase activity; HBeAg, hepatitis B e antigen; HBsAg, hepatitis B surface antigen; HBV-DNA, hepatitis B DNA.

patient with acute viral hepatitis who is HBsAg positive does not necessarily have acute hepatitis B; the patient may be a chronic HBsAg carrier and have a superimposed and unrelated form of acute liver injury. This possibility is not as unlikely as it may seem. People who are at high risk for development of hepatitis B and the chronic HBsAg carriers state often are at high risk for other forms of acute viral hepatitis; delta hepatitis represents just this phenomenon of an acute viral hepatitis being superimposed on the chronic HBsAg carrier state.[9] In this situation, testing for IgM anti-HBc can be helpful. This marker of acute type B hepatitis should be absent if the patient is a chronic HBsAg carrier with another form of acute hepatocellular injury.[87]

Hepatitis D (Delta Hepatitis)

Delta hepatitis is unusual in that it absolutely requires co-infection with HBV. It is a defective RNA virus that uses HBsAg for its structural protein shell[9, 89] (see Chapter 135). HDV infection occurs only in patients who have HBsAg in serum and therefore have either acute or chronic HBV infection. In the United States and Western Europe, delta hepatitis occurs most commonly in persons who have multiple parenteral exposures, such as intravenous drug addicts, hemophiliacs, and persons who have had multiple transfusions.[89] HDV infection is uncommon in medical care workers and male homosexuals. There are several areas of the world with a high prevalence of HDV infection among HBV carriers, including the Amazon basin in South America, central Africa, southern Italy, and Middle Eastern countries. Why HDV infection became established among HBsAg carriers in those particular areas of the world and not in others such as China and Southeast Asia (where hepatitis B is very common) is not known. Acute HDV infection occurs in two forms depending on the state of the underlying HBV infection: (1) as co-infection in which acute delta hepatitis occurs simultaneously with acute hepatitis B and (2) as superinfection in which acute delta hepatitis is superimposed on a chronic hepatitis B[90] (Fig. 102–9). Delta antigen can sometimes be detected in the serum during the early phase of acute delta hepatitis; with disappearance of the antigen, anti-HDV arises.[91] However, the appearance of anti-HDV may be delayed, short-lived, and low in titer. For this reason, many

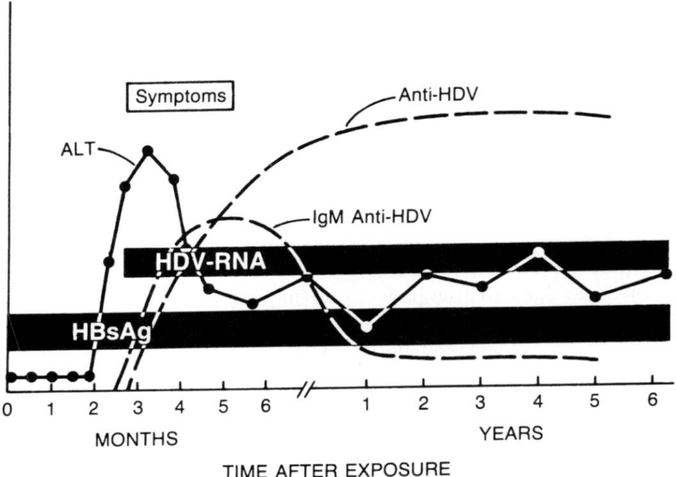

FIGURE 102–9. The clinical, virologic, and serologic courses of a typical case of acute hepatitis D (delta hepatitis) superinfection in a patient with a chronic hepatitis B infection leading to chronic HDV infection. *Abbreviations:* ALT, Alanine aminotransferase; anti-HDV, antibody to HDV; HBsAg, hepatitis B surface antigen; HDV, hepatitis D virus.

patients with acute delta hepatitis test negative for anti-HDV during the acute illness and become positive only in convalescence and then only in low titer. A radioimmunoassay for anti-HDV is commercially available,[92] but anti-HDV tests are not always reliable for diagnosis of acute HDV infection.

Most patients with acute delta co-infection recover. As the hepatitis B resolves and HBsAg is cleared from the serum, the HDV infection also resolves. Less than 5% of cases of acute HDV coinfection result in chronic delta hepatitis. In contrast, most patients with delta superinfection are left with chronic delta hepatitis; because HBsAg persists, the HDV infection can persist. More than 70% of cases of delta superinfection result in chronic hepatitis (see Fig. 102–9).[91] The diagnosis of chronic HDV infection is easier than that of acute type D hepatitis; high titers of anti-HDV (>1:100 by commercial radioimmunoassay) indicate ongoing delta infection. Furthermore, patients with chronic delta hepatitis have HDV antigen detectable by immunohistochemical techniques in the liver and persistence of IgM anti-HDV in serum.[91]

Two research assays have provided information regarding the natural history and biology of HDV infection: tests of HDV antigen in serum and liver using immunoblotting[93] and tests for HDV RNA in serum and liver using molecular hybridization technology with probes made from cloned cDNA or RNA.[94] The finding of HDV antigen or RNA in serum is a direct demonstration of the presence of virus and indicates active viral replication. HDV antigen and RNA are typically present transiently during the early phases of acute delta hepatitis and for prolonged periods in chronic delta hepatitis. The sensitivity of these assays is still not well documented; only 50 to 80% of patients with chronic delta hepatitis (as shown by the presence of delta antigen in liver by immunoperoxidase) have detectable HDV antigen or RNA in serum. The use of the PCR for the detection of HDV RNA has improved the sensitivity over that achieved with molecular hybridization.

Clinically, delta hepatitis tends to be a severe illness. Acute delta hepatitis has a mortality rate of 2 to 20%.[89] The illness also often has a biphasic and protracted course. Chronic delta hepatitis is also a severe illness and is more likely to result in serious morbidity or mortality than chronic hepatitis B alone or chronic hepatitis C. In large series, 60 to 70% of patients with chronic delta hepatitis eventually developed cirrhosis, and the majority of these patients died of liver disease.[95] The progression to cirrhosis usually takes 10 to 15 years, but it can occur as quickly as 2 years after the onset of infection.[89]

The epidemiology of delta hepatitis indicates that it is usually spread by parenteral exposures, which explains why this disease is common among drug addicts and hemophiliacs. Other modes of spread are less well defined. In some areas of the world intrafamilial spread has been documented in addition to spread between sexual partners.[96] Delta hepatitis often occurs in indolent, prolonged severe epidemics that strike susceptible populations (i.e., populations with a high HBsAg carrier rate).[27] Epidemics of delta hepatitis have been described in the Amazon basin, in central Africa, and among communities of drug addicts and institutionalized, mentally handicapped children.[89]

The diagnosis of delta hepatitis should be suspected in any HBsAg-positive patient with acute or chronic hepatitis, especially if the disease is severe or the patient is a drug addict or has had multiple parenteral exposures. The diagnosis can be made by the finding of HBsAg and anti-HDV in serum, rising titers of antibody indicating acute and sustained high titers indicating chronic infection. Confirmation of the diagnosis rests on finding HDV antigen or RNA in serum or liver.

Hepatitis C

Hepatitis C is the designation for what had been referred to as parenterally transmitted or classic non-A, non-B hepatitis until the causative agent of this disease was identified and named HCV (see Chapter 143). Although acute hepatitis caused by HCV obviously occurs clinically, it manifests much more frequently as a chronic hepatitis diagnosed on the basis of blood chemistry testing. The singular feature that distinguishes disease caused by HCV from the other hepatotropic viral infections is the propensity toward development of chronic infection. The original description of the existence of a non-A, non-B form of viral hepatitis was made in 1974 and 1975 when Prince and colleagues studied a group of patients who had non-B post-transfusion hepatitis for which the incubation periods clearly exceeded the range accepted for hepatitis A infections.[96a] Feinstone and colleagues showed that non-B transfusion-associated hepatitis was serologically unrelated to infection by HAV, and the term non-A, non-B hepatitis was introduced.[12] Attempts to identify the non-A, non-B hepatitis agent were undertaken by many investigators during the following 15 years without convincing success until 1989, when Choo and coworkers, using advanced molecular biology techniques, identified the etiologic agent of non-A, non-B hepatitis and named it HCV.[13] Molecular cloning, sequencing, and analysis of the HCV genome have enabled characterization and classification of the virus.[97, 98] The expression and synthesis of specific viral proteins by recombinant technology have led to the development of clinically useful diagnostic tests based on the detection of serum antibody to these viral antigens in infected persons.[14]

HCV is the most common cause of post-transfusion hepatitis, accounting for 70 to 95% of cases. With the implementation of universal donor testing by the new assays for antibody to HCV, HCV infection, like HBV, is rapidly becoming a rare event after blood transfusion. However, the majority of HCV infections occur in people without previous transfusions, and it appears that parenteral exposure from illicit drug use and needle sharing constitutes the major means of transmission in the United States. A large proportion of such sporadically acquired infections also are unassociated with obvious risk factors such as parenteral exposure, and there may be means of transmission that have not been fully defined. Risk factors for acute hepatitis C are summarized in Table 102–1. Sexual activity is less frequent (15%) as a risk factor for acute hepatitis C than for acute hepatitis B (50%). In American surveys, HCV was considered to be the cause of 65 to 90% of cases of sporadic acute viral hepatitis.[76, 98–100] Surveys of the seroprevalence of antibodies to HCV indicate that between 0.2 and 0.6% of volunteer blood donors in the United States are infected. However, much higher prevalence rates have been found among high-risk populations; for example, 18% of all patients seen in a major inner city emergency room in Baltimore were seropositive.[101] In part because hepatitis C is associated with a high rate of chronicity, there is a very large reservoir of infected and infectious persons among the general population.

Approximately 25% of cases of acute hepatitis C are icteric, and the mortality rate during acute infection is less than 1%.[97] There is a high rate of subclinical acute infection, because most persons with sporadically acquired chronic infection do not recall any previous history suggestive of acute hepatitis. On average, hepatitis C has a more indolent and prolonged course than hepatitis B. Serum aminotransferases often fluctuate widely and peak at levels (10 to 20 times normal) somewhat lower than those seen in hepatitis B (20 to 50 times normal) (Fig. 102–10). The onset also tends to be more insidious than in hepatitis B.

In prospective studies, 50 to 70% of persons with acute hepatitis C have persistent abnormalities in liver enzymes indicative of progression to chronic hepatitis.[97, 102] Liver biopsy shows evidence of chronic hepatitis that may progress to chronic active disease, fibrosis, and cirrhosis. The chronicity rate tends to be just as high after sporadic as after transfusion-related infections.[100] Chronic hepatitis C is frequently indolent and often silent. However, long-term follow-up studies of patients with this disease have shown that 20 to 25% ultimately develop cirrhosis of the liver.[102] It is often with the development of end-stage liver disease that symptoms first appear in patients infected by HCV. Chronic hepatitis C is one of the major causes of cirrhosis in the United States and is one of the most common indications for liver transplantation in adults. Chronic HCV infection may also be a major cause of hepatocellular carcinoma worldwide.

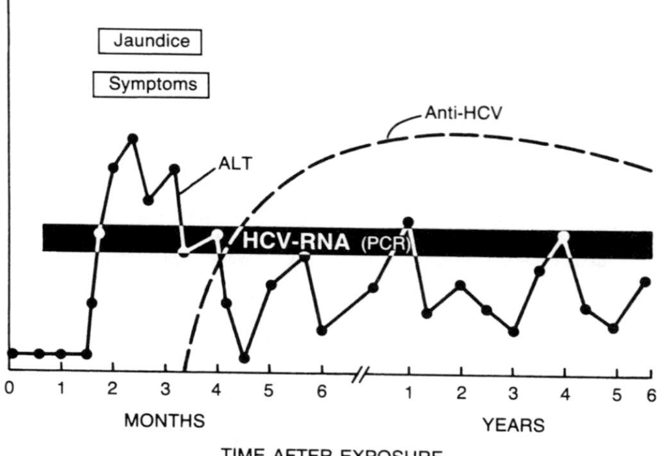

FIGURE 102–10. The clinical, virologic, and serologic courses of a typical case of acute hepatitis C. *Abbreviations:* ALT, Alanine aminotransferase; anti-HCV, antibody to HCV; HCV-RNA, hepatitis C virus RNA as determined by polymerase chain reaction.

Antibodies to HCV (anti-HCV) can be detected by immunoassays that use recombinant or synthesized antigens based on the deduced genomic sequence of the virus. The commercially available diagnostic tests for HCV detect antibodies to recombinant viral antigens and are most useful for screening blood donors who are chronic HCV carriers diagnosing chronic infection. Because seroconversion may not occur early in acute infection, the antibody tests cannot be relied on for diagnosis of acute HCV infection. However, anti-HCV almost invariably appears later in the course of the disease, and a patient with an initially seronegative sample during acute disease should be retested in 3 to 6 months. In addition, a positive antibody test does not distinguish between an acute and a chronic infection, and antibody may persist in a minority of patients who have cleared the infection.

Hepatitis E

In certain developing countries of the world, both large outbreaks and sporadic cases of non-B hepatitis have occurred in persons already immune to HAV.[103] These outbreaks did not fit the epidemiologic picture of what we now call hepatitis C and were therefore thought to represent a second form of non-A, non-B hepatitis, termed *enterically transmitted* non-A, non-B hepatitis. The causative agent was originally identified in much the same way as HAV, by the use of immune electron microscopy on stool samples of an infected patient. In this case, the patient was the investigator, who ingested a stool filtrate that he had collected during his investigations of an outbreak.[15] The genome of this virus has now been molecularly cloned; the virus has been characterized as calicivirus-like and has been named HEV[16] (see Chapter 165).

Epidemiologically, hepatitis E resembles hepatitis A; both are transmitted by the fecal-oral route, and disease tends to occur both in epidemics and as sporadic cases. Outbreaks of hepatitis E have been described from India, Pakistan, Russia, China, central and northern Africa, Peru, and Mexico.[17] Most outbreaks have been linked to fecal contamination of the water supply. The outbreaks were distinctive in that they largely affected young adults and produced an unusually high mortality rate in pregnant women.[104, 105] Secondary cases in families were uncommon, and the outbreaks were generally self-limited. No outbreaks of this disease have been described in the United States or Western Europe but cases have occurred among travelers returning from endemic areas.

Clinically, hepatitis E is characterized as an acute, self-limited disease that is often cholestatic. Serum aminotransferase levels tend to be lower in this disease than in other forms of acute viral hepatitis, but serum alkaline phosphatase tends to be somewhat higher.[104] Prolonged jaundice can occur. Like hepatitis A, hepatitis E does not lead to chronic hepatitis or a carrier state.

The HEV is a small RNA virus that is found in the stools of patients during the incubation period and in the early acute phase of illness.[15, 105] The amount of HEV shedding in stool is generally not as great as in hepatitis A. HEV may also be more labile in the environment than HAV. These features may explain the low rate of secondary spread of HEV infection.

Antibody to HEV (anti-HEV) can be detected by immune electron microscopy, by inhibition of immunofluorescence detection of HEV antigen in hepatocyte cytoplasm,[105, 106] and, more recently, by enzyme immunoassays (EIA) using antigen expressed in recombinant DNA systems. These techniques have shown that antibody develops early during the course of illness. Cases of hepatitis associated with large-scale epidemics of enterically transmitted, non-A, non-B hepatitis have invariably demonstrated the development of anti-HEV. In contrast, none of a large number of cases of sporadic non-A, non-B hepatitis from the United States demonstrated anti-HEV reactivity. These preliminary results suggest that HEV, which may be a common cause of jaundice and acute hepatitis in the developing world, is still a very rare cause of hepatitis in the United States.

GBV-C/HGV and TTV

GBV-C/HGV (now called HGV) was independently identified as a candidate hepatitis virus by two groups.[19, 20] HGV is a positive and single-stranded RNA virus that has one open leading frame and is classified as a member of the Flaviviridae, like HCV.[18, 20] However, HGV is distinct from HCV in that it has neither a core protein nor a hypervariable region in its envelope glycoproteins.[107, 108] HGV RNA has been detected by reverse transcriptase–PCR in various population groups; 1 to 2% in the general population, 3.1% in maintenance hemodialysis patients, 19.8% in hemophiliacs, and 24.5% in intravenous drug users.[20, 109–111] These observations imply that this virus can spread by parenteral routes. The high prevalence of HGV RNA among prostitutes implies that it can also be transmitted by sexual intercourse.[112] There is also evidence that this virus can be transmitted from mother to infant.[113] Although several studies indicated a possible connection between HGV and fulminant hepatitis,[55–57] this issue remains controversial. It is possible that the detection of HGV in fulminant hepatitis is the result of contamination from the use of blood products to treat the patients.[114–117] Furthermore, epidemiologic studies conducted in the United States failed to show a significant correlation between infection with HGV and post-transfusion hepatitis[22] or sporadic hepatitis.[24] HGV shares risk factors with HCV and is prevalent in patients infected with HCV. However, co-infection with HGV does influence the clinical features, liver histology, response to interferon therapy, or risk for development of hepatocellular carcinoma in patients infected with HCV.[118–122] Based on these observations, HGV is now generally regarded as a nonhepatitis virus that shares pathways of parenteral spread with other hepatitis viruses.[53, 54] However, the issue of its pathogenicity is not fully settled (see Chapter 144).[123]

TTV is another candidate hepatitis virus. TTV, a non-enveloped, single-stranded DNA virus, was isolated from serum of a patient (TT) with post-transfusion hepatitis.[25] In the initial report from Japan, TTV DNA was detected in sera from three of the five patients with post-transfusion non–A–G hepatitis, implying that this agent may be a novel, transfusion-transmissible hepatitis pathogen.[25] Fecal excretion of TTV has been reported.[124] Although TTV is a DNA virus, it has a wide range of sequence divergence (up to 30%), which has led to its classification into two genotypes.[125] Reports from Japan detected DNA of TTV in 47 and 46% of patients with acute and chronic non–A–G hepatitis, respectively, and in 12% of Japanese blood donors.[124] In England, TTV DNA was present in 10% of a normal population[126] and was detected in samples from patients with fulminant hepatitis.[127] It has been postulated that TTV replicates in the liver, but definitive data are lacking.[125] The role, if any, of TTV as a cause of hepatitis remains to be defined (see Chapter 144).[26, 116]

Serodiagnosis of Acute Viral Hepatitis

A guide to the serodiagnosis of acute viral hepatitis is presented in Figure 102–6. Patients in whom acute hepatitis is suspected based on history, physical examination, and elevated serum aminotransferase activity should be tested for IgM anti-HAV, HBsAg and IgM anti-HBc, and anti-HCV. The presence of IgM anti-HAV establishes the diagnosis of acute hepatitis A. The presence of HBsAg suggests the diagnosis of hepatitis B but does not differentiate between acute and chronic disease. The presence of IgM anti-HBc confirms the diagnosis of *acute* hepatitis B; its absence suggests that the patient is actually a chronic carrier of HBsAg and that the acute hepatitis is caused by either an exacerbation of the underlying chronic hepatitis B or superinfection with another hepatitis agent. Patients with chronic hepatitis B may have low levels of IgM anti-HBc as long as viral replication persists; however, the commercial assays for IgM anti-HBc detect this antibody only when it is present in high titer.[88]

Anti-HDV should be sought only when evidence of HBV infection is found, since delta hepatitis can occur only in the presence of hepatitis B. The presence of anti-HDV suggests the diagnosis of delta hepatitis co-infection, although it is not conclusive and does not indicate whether the delta infection is resolved, ongoing, acute, or chronic. The titer of anti-HDV can help to separate acute hepatitis D (low or rising titers) from chronic delta hepatitis (sustained high titers $> 1{:}100$).

Hepatitis C can be diagnosed on the basis of finding anti-HCV antibodies in serum, although the presence of such antibodies does not distinguish between acute and chronic HCV infections. Because of the fluctuating nature of the transaminase elevations seen in association with chronic hepatitis C, it may be difficult to determine whether the patient is acutely infected or is having a flare of chronic disease unless a source of infection (e.g., contaminated blood) is found or previous chemistries indicate ongoing liver inflammation. Antibody is not always detectable early in the course of the acute infection, and assays to detect IgM anti-HCV are not clinically available. The first-generation HCV immunodetection assays were insensitive in diagnosing acute infection and frequently did not detect antibodies until as long as 6 to 12 months after injection; the current, second-generation assays have shortened the window period to about 8 to 12 weeks. There remain patients who are antibody negative during early acute infection; they should be retested 3 to 6 months later if there is a suspicion of HCV infection. Because of the high incidence of chronicity associated with hepatitis C, acutely infected patients should always be observed for 6 to 12 months to determine whether chronic hepatitis C has developed. Mixed infections of hepatitis C with any of the other viruses are always a possibility and should be considered. Many research centers use the PCR to obtain direct evidence for the presence of HCV. At present this is the only technology available with the sensitivity required to detect HCV (as opposed to antibodies to HCV) in clinical samples. However, it has been difficult to bring PCR technology to the clinical diagnostic laboratory, and it remains a research tool.

Anti-HEV testing is rarely necessary in the United States or Western Europe, because the only cases of HEV infections in these areas to date have been among travelers returning from endemic areas. Immunoassays to detect anti-HEV antibody are not commercially available in the United States. This situation may change, and diagnostic tests could be made available based on present technology.

Chronic Hepatitis

Chronic hepatitis with an acute exacerbation can mimic acute viral hepatitis and can represent a significant problem in the differential diagnosis. This is best demonstrated for HBsAg-positive chronic hepatitis. These patients are sometimes asymptomatic except for recurrent bouts of jaundice and symptoms of hepatitis that can occur with almost seasonal regularity. Several features should suggest the presence of chronic hepatitis. These include previous bouts of hepatitis or jaundice, a prolonged and indolent preicteric phase of disease, protracted and only mild-to-moderate increases in aminotransferase and serum bilirubin levels (Fig. 102–3), and increased globulin and decreased serum albumin levels. In most instances the presence of HBsAg with the absence of IgM anti-HBc confirms the diagnosis of chronic infection. In the final analysis, however, differentiation requires the test of time. The persistence of symptoms or abnormal serum enzyme levels for more than 6 months indicates chronic hepatitis. A liver biopsy specimen usually is helpful if it demonstrates chronic hepatitis with fibrosis, piecemeal necrosis, or ground-glass cells; it can also be helpful in determining the severity and aggressiveness of the hepatic inflammatory process. However, it may not clearly differentiate acute from chronic hepatitis at the height of an acute exacerbation. Chronic hepatitis is more extensively discussed in Chapter 103.

Acute Hepatitis Caused by Other Viruses

Several other common viral infections can secondarily affect the liver and cause an acute, hepatitis-like picture. The liver disease associated with these infections usually is mild, self-limited, subclinical, and overshadowed by the other symptoms in these diseases.

Of prime importance as a secondary cause of viral hepatitis is the Epstein-Barr virus (EBV), the agent of heterophile-positive infectious mononucleosis. Mild increases in serum aminotransferase levels (2 to 5 times normal) in the absence of symptoms suggestive of liver disease are very common in acute mononucleosis. This syndrome generally presents no diagnostic confusion with acute viral hepatitis; the liver disease is mild and subclinical. However, on rare occasions, EBV infection can manifest as acute icteric hepatitis without the usual symptoms of mononucleosis.[58] Physical examination may reveal little or no evidence of pharyngitis or lymphadenopathy. Several features of the hepatitis should suggest that it is caused by EBV infection. First, fever that is prominent and persistent into the icteric phase suggests mononucleosis; fever is low grade in acute viral hepatitis. Second, the serum enzyme levels in mononucleosis are not entirely typical of those in acute viral hepatitis. The alkaline phosphatase and LDH levels usually are higher than expected from the degree of jaundice and aminotransferase elevation (see Fig. 102–3). Most suggestive, however, is the presence of a significant lymphocytosis (>50%) with atypical lymphocytes (>20%). Without this finding, hepatitis cannot readily be ascribed to EBV infection. Finally, the mononucleosis slide test or heterophile antibody is usually but not invariably reactive. Absolute confirmation of EBV infection rests on the appearance (see Chapter 128) of specific anti-EBV antibody responses, such as a 4-fold rise in titer when acute and convalescent sera are tested. Liver biopsy findings in acute mononucleosis hepatitis are quite characteristic but are not usually required for diagnosis. A diagnosis of EBV-induced acute hepatitis requires only a typical pattern of serum enzyme levels, atypical lymphocytosis, a positive heterophile test, and serologic exclusion of other causes of viral hepatitis.

The role of CMV infection in causing a hepatitis in adults still is subject to debate, especially as it relates to post-transfusion hepatitis.[102, 128–130] The problem centers on relating changes in anti-CMV titers or excretion of the virus to an episode of hepatitis. Such changes can occur in totally asymptomatic patients and are common after blood transfusions regardless of the occurrence of hepatitis.[128] There is no doubt that primary CMV infection can cause a heterophile-negative mononucleosis syndrome that frequently is accompanied by hepatosplenomegaly and minor elevations of serum aminotransferases.[128–130] Whether CMV can induce a purely hepatitis-like syndrome is unclear. If it can, it probably is rare in adults. The diagnosis rests either on the finding of atypical lymphocytosis with acute liver injury, absence of heterophile antibody, and a significant titer rise of anti-CMV antibodies (without anti-EBV rise) or on the excretion of the virus in urine or oropharyngeal secretions (see Chapter 127).

Several other common human viruses (including rubella, rubeola, mumps viruses, and coxsackie B viruses) can induce mild abnormalities in liver enzymes.[131] These changes are not common and rarely are accompanied by jaundice. In the immunosuppressed host, however, several usually benign viruses can cause a disseminated infection, part of which may include hepatic involvement. Chief among these are herpes simplex virus, CMV, and varicella-zoster virus.[128–132] These are all herpesviruses that are very common and usually result in relatively benign infections in humans. In the patient with poor host defenses, however, dissemination with these viruses can occur. Hepatic necrosis, marked elevations in serum aminotransferases, icterus, and even death from hepatic failure have been described. In the immunosuppressed host with fulminant hepatic failure, a search for these viruses should be made. Liver biopsy specimens may demonstrate inclusion bodies or intranuclear herpesvirus particles. These viruses, however, are not common causes of sporadic acute hepatitis in the otherwise healthy host.

Although yellow fever has not been reported in the United States for more than 40 years, it is still enzootic in Central America, South America, and central Africa, and the mosquito vector exists in the United States. Yellow fever is marked by a short incubation period (3 to 7 days), severe hepatitis with high aminotransferase levels, and a high mortality rate (approximately 20%).[133] It need be considered only in the recent traveler to enzootic areas who has not received adequate immunization. The diagnosis is made by isolating the virus from the blood, by finding a significant rise in antibody titers on paired sera, or by characteristic pathologic findings in the liver (see Chapter 142).

Hepatitis Caused by Nonviral Infectious Diseases

Increased serum enzyme levels and liver dysfunction can occur with many nonviral infectious diseases caused by bacteria, mycobacteria, rickettsia, and fungi. Jaundice with mild elevations in the aminotransferases and in alkaline phosphatase (2 to 5 times normal) can be seen with sepsis and with pneumococcal pneumonia.[58, 134] Furthermore, minor elevations of liver enzymes without jaundice often are seen with many severe infections that usually do not primarily involve the liver, including pulmonary and miliary tuberculosis,[135–139] brucellosis, tularemia, plague, gram-negative sepsis, and legionnaires' disease. Liver biopsy specimens usually show nonspecific changes and focal areas of necrosis. However, at times (e.g., in miliary tuberculosis), a liver biopsy specimen can be very helpful in establishing the primary diagnosis.

Three nonviral infectious agents that can produce an acute hepatitis-like syndrome deserve special note: syphilis, leptospirosis, and Q fever. Early syphilis, either primary or early secondary, can be accompanied by significant increases in serum aminotransferase concentrations (3 to 8 times normal).[140] Jaundice is rare, and the chancre of primary syphilis or the rash of secondary syphilis should be present. Liver enzyme tests, as in mononucleosis hepatitis, show atypically high elevations of alkaline phosphatase (4 to 8 times normal) when compared with the extent of aminotransferase abnormalities. Diagnosis is established by the finding of a reactive VDRL and fluorescent treponemal antibody and by the typical clinical setting and response to treatment (see Chapter 228).

Leptospirosis is an unusual cause of jaundice and hepatitis in the United States. The disease is caused by at least 15 serotypes of *Leptospira interrogans*.[141] The serotypes that are responsible for most of the infections in this country are *icterohemorrhagiae* (30 to 40%), which is enzootic in rats; *canicola* (30%), enzootic in dogs; and *pomona* (10 to 20%), enzootic in cattle and swine. The history usually points to exposure to these animals or their urine (e.g., lake water, swimming holes). The clinical manifestations include malaise, fever, chills, severe myalgias, and headache.[141] Later symptoms of cough, sputum production, prostration, and hepatic and renal involvement appear. Hepatic involvement is most common with the serotype *icterohemorrhagiae*. Evaluation may demonstrate fever, prostration, severe muscle tenderness, hepatosplenomegaly, and pneumonitis. Laboratory abnormalities include leukocytosis and a left shift in the differential count. The urinalysis may show albuminuria, casts, and white and red blood cells. In severe cases, the urine output falls and the blood urea nitrogen level rises; central nervous system manifestations and pneumonitis also may appear. Liver function tests reveal jaundice that is often out of proportion to the degree of serum enzyme elevations. As with the jaundice of pneumococcal pneumonia,[134] the jaundice in leptospirosis appears to result from a defect in bilirubin excretion rather than hepatic necrosis.[141] The diagnosis is made by finding a high titer or a significant rise in leptospiral agglutinins. Because of the variable course of this disease, the value of antibiotic therapy has been difficult to demonstrate. Nevertheless, a 1-week course of intravenous penicillin or ampicillin in moderate or severe cases or oral doxycycline, ampicillin, or amoxicillin in milder cases is recommended and should commence as early in the disease as possible (see Chapter 229).

Q fever is a third nonviral infectious disease that may be mistaken for acute viral hepatitis. This disease is caused by the rickettsial agent, *Coxiella burnetii,* and is uncommon in the United States. In this disease, as in leptospirosis, constitutional symptoms are prominent, with fever, chills, and pneumonitis. Overt jaundice occurs in only about 5% of the cases, although subclinical hepatic involvement is common. In rare cases, hepatitis without pneumonitis occurs, and a differentiation from acute viral hepatitis may be difficult.[142] Epidemiologic features should reveal exposure to farm or wild animals (cows, goats, sheep). Clinically, persistent fever, pneumonitis, and prostration are more prominent than in viral hepatitis. Liver function tests reveal jaundice with only mild elevations in aminotransferases (2 to 5 times normal) and sometimes marked elevations in the alkaline phosphatase concentration. The diagnosis is made by demonstration of a rise in agglutination titers against *C. burnetii* in paired sera. Early treatment with tetracycline for 2 weeks is usually recommended (see Chapter 177).

It has been reported that some bacterial toxins can cause fulminant hepatic failure in previously healthy adults.[143] An emetic toxin of *B. cereus* was shown to cause fulminant hepatic failure with microvesicular steatosis and midzonal necrosis by inhibiting hepatic mitochondrial fatty-acid oxidation.

Drug-Related Acute Hepatitis

The major differential diagnosis in acute hepatitis is often between viral and drug-related hepatitis. Every patient with hepatitis should be questioned carefully about all medications used and should specifically be asked about over-the-counter products. Drug-related acute liver injury is not nearly as common as acute viral hepatitis, but it often is much more serious and is a prominent cause of fulminant hepatic failure.[144] Drug-related acute liver injury may act synergistically with acute viral hepatitis to increase the severity of liver necrosis. Many drugs and toxins have been shown to induce hepatic injury, but few have been repeatedly implicated as causing an acute hepatitis-like syndrome. The major common medications available in the United States that are associated with significant hepatotoxicity are listed in Table 102–2 by the type of injury usually seen and with an approximate incidence. This is not an exhaustive list. Any patient who develops hepatitis while taking a drug that is a known or potential hepatotoxin should have the medication stopped until the full clinical picture can be evaluated. The most serious mistake that can be made in caring for patients with acute hepatic injury is to underestimate the role of drugs and to continue administering them in the face of acute hepatitis. Suspicion of drug-induced liver injury should be greatest when the epidemiologic features are not absolutely typical of acute viral hepatitis, as in the elderly, in patients with underlying diseases, and in patients who develop fulminant hepatitis. However, even when epidemiologic features are appropriate for acute viral hepatitis, the role of drugs should not be dismissed: the renal dialysis patient taking methyldopa or the drug addict receiving isoniazid who develops acute hepatitis should have treatment with these medications stopped until adequate evaluation of the cause and course of the disease.

Some of the most commonly encountered causes of drug-related acute hepatitis are acetylsalicylic acid (aspirin), acetaminophen, isoniazid, rifampin, phenytoin, and the anesthetic halothane. Aspirin can cause moderate elevations in serum enzymes (2 to 5 times normal), but it rarely causes jaundice. Aspirin hepatotoxicity seems to occur only with a high maintenance dosage, usually with serum salicylate levels of 20 mg/dl or greater. Characteristically, the biochemical abnormalities subside rapidly on withdrawal of the drug. Acetaminophen overdose, both purposeful and accidental, has become a major cause of fulminant hepatic failure.[145–147] The liver disease appears 2 to 5 days after the overdose. Every patient with evidence of severe hepatic injury should be carefully questioned regarding acetaminophen use, since the liver injury can be averted if the patient is treated within 10 hours of the overdose with large doses of *N*-acetylcysteine (Mucomyst). Liver injury from chronic use of acetaminophen in high doses also has been described.[145] Both isoniazid and rifampin have been implicated in causing an acute hepatitis-like syndrome; both have been associated with fulminant hepatic failure. Rifampin hepatic injury usually has its onset within the first weeks of therapy, whereas isoniazid hepatotoxicity is most common after 1 to 2 months of therapy. The incidence of isoniazid hepatotoxicity is approximately 1%, but it is definitely higher in older age groups and approaches 10% in patients older than 40 years of age. Treatment with these drugs should be discontinued if symptoms of hepatitis or jaundice appear or if aminotransferase concentrations are persistently elevated more than 5 times normal. Phenytoin can cause an acute hepatitis, usually within 1 to 6 weeks of starting the medication and associated with other manifestations of hypersensitivity such as fever, rash, lymphadenopathy, and eosinophilia. It has a mortality rate of approximately 10%. A cooperative study on halothane-induced hepatitis suggested that approximately 1 in 10,000 patients given this anesthetic for the first time and 1 in 1000 given it more than once develop fulminant hepatic necrosis.[148–151] Clinically, halothane-related jaundice appears within 3 to 14 days after its use and resembles an acute, severe viral hepatitis. Fever is characteristic early in the course, and many patients have an accompanying leukocytosis and eosinophilia. Halothane-induced hepatitis usually is not confused with post-transfusion hepatitis because of its early onset after surgery and anesthesia.

Anoxic Liver Injury

A syndrome resembling acute viral hepatitis can occur after anoxic injury to the liver caused by a period of hypotension, severe left- or right-sided heart failure, or cardiopulmonary arrest.[152] An inciting event is frequently obvious, but in some cases no clear history of an anoxic episode is obtained, or the patient is brought to the hospital comatose and unable to give an adequate history. In these situations, a diagnosis usually can be made on the basis of serum enzymes. Within hours of an anoxic episode, there are marked elevations of aminotransferase concentrations into the range seen with acute viral hepatitis (Fig. 102–3). The LDH level is dramatically elevated (as is the creatine phosphatase), and may be most helpful in suggesting this diagnosis. Most typical of anoxic liver injury, however, is the rapid resolution of these enzyme abnormalities. The aminotransferase levels can fall from 50 to 100 times higher than normal to normal

TABLE 102–2 Common Causes of Drug-Related Liver Injury

Agent Class	Agent	Frequency of Occurrence*	Type of Injury
Analgesic	Acetaminophen	Dose-related	Hepatitis
	Aspirin	Dose-related	Hepatitis
Anesthetic	Halothane	Rare (0.01–0.1%)	Hepatitis
	Methoxyflurane	Rare	Hepatitis
Antiarthritic	Allopurinol	Rare	Granuloma/hepatitis
	Indomethacin	Very rare	Hepatitis
	Phenylbutazone	Rare	Granuloma/mixed
Antibacterial	Carbenicillin	Low†	Hepatitis
	Erythromycin estolate	Low	Cholestasis
	Nitrofurantoin	Rare	Mixed
	Oxacillin	Rare	Hepatitis
	Sulfonamides/sulfones	Rare	Hepatitis
	Tetracycline	Dose-related	Steatosis/necrosis
Antifungal	Ketoconazole	Rare	Hepatitis
Antineoplastic	Azathioprine	Rare†	Cholestasis
	6-Mercaptopurine	Common† (10–35%)	Hepatitis
	Methotrexate	Dose-related	Fibrosis
	Mithromycin	Rare†	Necrosis
Antituberculosis	Isoniazid	Low (1%)	Hepatitis
	Para-aminosalicyclic acid	Low (0.1–1%)	Hepatitis
	Rifampin	Low	Hepatitis
Cardiovascular	Methyldopa	Low	Hepatitis
	Quinidine	Rare	Granuloma/hepatitis
	Thiazides	Very rare	Mixed
	Amiodarone	Low (1–3%)	Steatosis/necrosis
Endocrinologic	17-Alkylated androgens	Dose-related	Cholestasis
	Chlorpropamide	Rare	Cholestasis
	Oral contraceptives	Rare	Cholestasis
	Propylthiouracil	Rare	Cholestasis
	Tolbutamine	Very rare	Hepatitis
	Dantrolene	Low (1–2%)	Cholestasis
			Hepatitis
Neuropharmacologic and psychopharmacologic	Monoamine oxidase inhibitors	Low	Hepatitis
	Phenothiazines	Low (1–2%)	Cholestasis
	Phenytoin	Rare	Hepatitis
	Valproic acid	Low (1–2%)	Steatosis/necrosis

*The frequency of occurrence is an estimate from the literature[144]: common, >2%; low, 0.1–2%; rare, <0.1%; very rare, isolated case reports only.
†Dose-related to some degree.

within 1 week. Jaundice is uncommon and mild. In some cases, aminotransferases remain elevated (2 to 5 times normal) for 5 to 14 days after the injury, in which case differentiation from acute viral hepatitis may be difficult and may require liver biopsy (which will show a bland centrozonal necrosis). Although a liver biopsy specimen is diagnostic, it generally is not needed for the diagnosis when the clinical history and pattern of enzyme levels are typical.

Alcoholic Liver Disease

Alcohol abuse is the most common cause of serious liver disease in the United States. Acute alcoholic hepatitis may be confused with viral hepatitis. Alcoholic patients have gradual and imprecisely dated onset of malaise, anorexia, weight loss, nausea and vomiting, fever and chills, abdominal swelling, and jaundice or dark urine. The history of alcohol intake should suggest the diagnosis, but many patients conceal or underestimate the amount of alcohol they consume. The lower limit of alcohol intake said to lead to alcoholic liver disease is 80 g/day—equivalent to a half pint of 86-proof whiskey, four conventional cocktails, five to six cans beer, or 1 quart of wine each day.[149, 153] Alcoholic liver disease is rarely manifested until after 10 or more years of excessive drinking.

Clinically, the patient usually appears chronically ill. Fever and tachycardia are common. Examination may reveal evidence of chronic liver disease and alcohol abuse that is not seen with acute viral hepatitis: wasting, parotid enlargement, palmar erythema, vascular spiders, gynecomastia, testicular atrophy, significant hepatomegaly, and signs of portal hypertension. The laboratory data may be helpful.[58] The leukocyte count usually is increased with a left shift. The hematocrit may be slightly decreased, and the red blood cell indices reveal macrocytosis (with or without folate deficiency). Liver function tests reveal hyperbilirubinemia and, typically, a low albumin level and a prolonged prothrombin time. The aminotransferase values are most characteristic (see Fig. 102–3) in that the AST is elevated out of proportion to the ALT (which can be slightly elevated, normal, or even low); in viral hepatitis, the ALT and AST are comparably elevated.

Cholestatic Liver Disease

The term *cholestatic liver disease* refers to a host of diseases marked by bile retention. Cholestasis can result from extrahepatic biliary obstruction (gallstones, stricture, pancreatitis, or tumor) or from intrahepatic causes (primary biliary cirrhosis, several childhood cholestatic syndromes, and drug-induced cholestasis from phenothiazines or methyltestosterone). These patients have the nonspecific symptoms of acute liver disease with jaundice, but the signs and symptoms of cholestasis are prominent: the degree of jaundice, lightening of stools, and itching overshadow the amount of anorexia or malaise. Laboratory data are confirmatory and show modest abnormalities in aminotransferase concentrations but marked elevations in alkaline phosphatase (Fig. 102–3).

Other Liver Diseases

Few other causes of jaundice pose a problem in the differential diagnosis of acute hepatitis. Rare causes of an acute hepatitis-like syndrome include Wilson's disease,[154] sickle cell crisis,[155] acute Budd-Chiari syndrome or veno-occlusive disease,[156] and massive replacement of the liver by tumor.[157] These causes usually are associated with a fulminant or severe hepatitis. Patients with hemolytic anemia may have vague, nonspecific symptoms and jaundice, but the urine contains no bilirubin, and the aminotransferase levels are normal. Patients with congenital disorders of bilirubin metabolism (Gilbert's and Dubin-Johnson syndromes) may become notably jaundiced, especially during intercurrent viral illnesses, but serum enzyme levels should be normal.

MANAGEMENT

Supportive Care

There is limited specific therapy for acute viral hepatitis. Good management consists of supportive measures, relief of symptoms, and avoidance of further injury. An important role of the physician is to identify and carefully follow the rare patient who develops fulminant hepatic failure; early consultation and referral to a liver transplant center is essential in such cases.

Hospitalization. Most patients with acute viral hepatitis do not require hospitalization. Usually, little can be done in the hospital that is not available at home. Hospitalization is advisable for any patient who is in danger from dehydration due to poor oral intake, whose prothrombin time shows any prolongation, who has a rising bilirubin level (>15 to 20 mg/dl), or who has any clinical evidence of hepatic failure. The duration of hospitalization varies with the severity of illness. Once symptoms have abated, the patient usually can be discharged to continue convalescence at home. There is no need to continue hospitalization until laboratory values return to normal.

Rest. Bed rest should be prescribed for patients with acute viral hepatitis during the period of symptoms. However, the bed rest should not be absolute; use of the bathroom and periods of being up each day should be encouraged. Traditionally, it has been recommended that bed rest be continued until recovery is complete and liver function values have returned to normal. Although most patients are willing to remain at bed rest for the duration of the symptoms, many—and especially the young—are anxious to return to normal activity once symptoms abate. Controlled studies have shown that, after the symptoms have cleared, normal activity and even strenuous exercise does not slow recovery, induce relapses, or predispose to chronic liver disease.[158] It is unnecessarily restrictive to insist on bed rest until the aminotransferase levels return to normal or until HBsAg is negative. A gradual return to activity with monitoring of liver function test values is warranted once symptoms have abated. Relapses of symptoms should be treated with a return to bed rest.

Alcohol Avoidance. Alcohol should be avoided during the acute illness. However, there are no data to suggest that moderate alcohol intake after recovery leads to a worsening of acute hepatitis or predisposes to chronic hepatitis. Although it is prudent to advise abstinence during the acute symptomatic phase of viral hepatitis, the recommendation of total abstinence for 6 to 12 months after viral hepatitis is unnecessarily strict.

Diet Management. There is little evidence that any dietary regimen affects the course of acute hepatitis. A generally nutritious diet should be encouraged. During the symptomatic phase, patients frequently are anorexic and may have distinct likes and dislikes. The patient with anorexia cannot be forced to eat; however, some encouragement can come from the use of frequent, small feedings and a diet low in fat but high in carbohydrates. Forced or nasogastric tube feedings should be avoided.

Drugs. Most medications are best avoided during acute hepatitis. In particular, sedatives should not be given, because their elimination is altered in patients with hepatic disease. Antibiotics are not indicated. Immune serum globulin has no effect. Symptomatic therapy for nausea, pain, or sleeplessness may be needed at times. Antiemetics can be helpful, but chlorpromazine (because of its potential to cause intrahepatic cholestasis) should be avoided. Among analgesics, acetaminophen is preferable to aspirin (because of its reduced effects on platelet function and the gastric mucosa) and to codeine or morphine derivatives (because of their sedative effects). Previous data suggested that estrogens might worsen the course of typical acute viral hepatitis; however, prospective studies of women with acute viral hepatitis who were taking oral contraceptives have failed to support this finding.[159] Nevertheless, it is advisable that treatment with all but the most necessary medications be discontinued during the acute phase of viral hepatitis. Vitamins often are given but have not been shown to be beneficial in patients with acute hepatitis. If the prothrombin time is prolonged, a trial of vitamin K (1 to 5 mg intramuscularly) can be given. However, the administration of vitamin K has little or no effect on the prothrombin time in typical viral hepatitis unless there has been prolonged cholestasis.

Treatment

There are no well-accepted, specific therapies for acute viral hepatitis. Corticosteroids have not been shown to shorten the course or to aid in healing of acute viral hepatitis.[160, 161] Some studies have indicated that corticosteroids may predispose to more prolonged illness, more relapses, and more chronic liver disease.[161] Therefore, corticosteroids definitely are not indicated for the typical uncomplicated case of acute viral hepatitis.

Corticosteroids have sometimes been recommended for two situations in acute viral hepatitis: cholestatic hepatitis and fulminant hepatic failure. In prolonged cholestasis after acute viral hepatitis, corticosteroids can decrease serum bilirubin levels and ameliorate symptoms of fatigue and itching. Use of corticosteroids in this situation, however, should be limited to cases of hepatitis A, in which there is no possibility of transition to chronic hepatitis. In fulminant hepatitis, corticosteroids are often used, frequently because no other options are available. However, controlled clinical trials have failed to demonstrate any benefit of corticosteroids in acute viral hepatitis, and some studies indicated that the adverse side effects of high doses of corticosteroids outweigh their potential benefit.[161]

Interferon-α has been demonstrated to be efficacious as therapy in chronic viral hepatitis B and C[162–165]; it may also hold promise for treatment of acute disease. However, the only studies of antiviral treatment in severe acute viral hepatitis have involved small numbers of patients. In a study from Israel,[166] five patients with fulminant hepatitis were treated with interferon-α and three survived, which led the authors to suggest that antiviral therapy might be helpful in a subset of patients with severe or fulminant hepatitis. However, in a later study from Spain, only 2 of 12 patients with fulminant hepatitis B or hepatitis B plus delta hepatitis who were treated with high doses of parenteral interferon-α survived, indicating that this medication is unlikely to be of benefit in reversing fulminant viral hepatitis.[167] The absence of a beneficial effect of therapy in fulminant hepatitis does not necessarily indicate that the therapy will have no effect in patients with less advanced or less severe hepatic injury. There is some evidence in a limited number of patients with acute hepatitis C that treatment with natural interferon-β may reduce the likelihood of chronic hepatitis C.[158] It has not been determined whether treatment with recombinant interferon-α may be associated with similarly positive results.

Monitoring

Monitoring during acute viral hepatitis should be regular and specific. If the patient is so ill that hospitalization is necessary, a once- or twice-daily check on major symptoms is important. The patient should be examined for the degree of icterus, liver size, and the presence of asterixis or other evidence of hepatic encephalopathy. The ALT, AST alkaline phosphatase, and bilirubin levels and the prothrombin time should be monitored once or twice a week during hospitalization and every 1 to 2 weeks thereafter until they return to normal. Initially, the patient should be tested for HBsAg. If positive, the test is best repeated every 1 to 2 months until HBsAg disappears. The continued presence of HBsAg 4 to 6 months after acute viral hepatitis indicates establishment of the chronic HBsAg carrier state. If all initial serology results are negative, antibodies to hepatitis C should be rechecked in 6 months; if that test result is positive, the patient should be further monitored for the probable development of chronic hepatitis C.

A percutaneous liver biopsy specimen in acute viral hepatitis may establish the diagnosis, but usually it is not necessary. However, liver biopsy is indicated in several situations: when the diagnosis is in doubt and diagnostic confusion remains despite clinical, biochemical, and serologic data; if more than one explanation of acute liver injury exists; if drug-related acute hepatitis is a possibility; and when specific therapy is being considered.

Management of Fulminant Viral Hepatitis

The management of fulminant viral hepatitis should begin with its early recognition. The initial signs and symptoms of hepatic encephalopathy may be subtle (nightmares, slight changes in personality, restlessness) or dramatic (unexpected aggressive physical or sexual activity). It is important to recognize these signs for what they are and not respond to them by using sedative or physical restraints.

At the first sign of encephalopathy, vigorous management should be started.[51, 52, 169–171] This should include bed rest, a low-protein diet (20 to 30 g/day), the administration of enemas to cleanse the bowel, and the use of oral neomycin (0.5 to 1.0 g every 6 hours) or lactulose (30 to 60 ml in sorbitol every 2 to 6 hours until loose stools are achieved). Treatment with all sedatives is contraindicated. With deepening coma, the patient should be monitored in an intensive care unit and may require intravenous fluids, a central venous pressure line, a nasogastric tube, and a urinary bladder catheter. Coagulation defects may require correction with the use of fresh-frozen plasma (the coagulation-factor concentrates such as fibrinogen and prothrombin complex should not be used). The patient should be monitored carefully for gastrointestinal bleeding. Cimetidine (300 to 500 mg intravenously every 6 hours) or vigorous antacid therapy may be begun to help prevent upper gastrointestinal bleeding. Most important is careful attention to all the details of "routine" medical management (fluid and electrolyte balance, acid-base balance, pulmonary toilet, intravenous and bladder catheter care, skin care, and monitoring for signs of blood loss or superinfection). More aggressive experimental approaches such as exchange transfusions, "total body washout," charcoal hemoperfusion, cross-circulation with a human or baboon liver, and immunotherapy with antibody to HBsAg each have had their advocates, but none has been shown repeatedly to be more effective than "conventional" medical management.

The most promising new therapy for fulminant hepatic failure is emergency liver transplantation.[169–172] Since the introduction of cyclosporin A as an immunosuppressive agent in the early 1980s, liver transplantation has become a successful and well accepted approach to severe liver disease. At present more than 2500 liver transplants are done yearly in the United States in 40 to 50 different medical centers. Approximately 7% of patients undergo liver transplantation for fulminant or subacute hepatic failure. The 1- to 2-year survival rates have ranged between 60 and 90%.[171]

The major reason to avoid liver transplantation in fulminant hepatic failure is the possibility of spontaneous recovery. The survival rate of patients with fulminant hepatitis in stage III to IV coma averages 20 to 30%. Features that predict a poor outcome include age (<10 or >40 years), medications as a cause of the liver injury, and a prothrombin time longer than 100 seconds or longer than 50 seconds in association with a bilirubin level higher than 17.6 mg/dl.[173] The decision for transplantation needs to be made before severe complications supervene—in particular, severe intracranial hypertension with decerebration, after which recovery is unlikely even with transplantation. Fulminant hepatitis does not recur in the transplanted liver, although reinfection by the virus may occur.[174, 175] Therefore, at the first sign of hepatic failure, the physician should refer the patient with acute viral hepatitis to a liver transplantation center. The criteria for transplantation in fulminant hepatitis are evolving, and the decision for transplantation should be made by a team of physicians with experience in treating fulminant hepatic failure.

Prevention

Prevention of viral hepatitis is discussed in the chapters dealing with the individual viral agents and in Chapter 312. Needlestick injuries in hospital employees are discussed in Chapter 295. Certain nonspecific measures regarding the patient with acute hepatitis should be stressed here.

A patient who is hospitalized should be placed in enteric isolation to prevent the spread of type A hepatitis. Even with lax precautions, such spread is very rare; most patients with hepatitis A are no longer excreting virus once they have become symptomatic. Nevertheless, there are exceptions, and isolation is prudent. Health care personnel should use universal blood and secretion precautions when handling specimens. Labeling of blood specimens, as from a patient with hepatitis, is a common practice. However, all blood from any patient should be handled as if potentially infectious.

If at home, the patient should be advised about care in personal hygiene—use of a private bathroom, if possible, and careful hand washing. Attention also should be paid to blood and blood products and to the handling of cuts and lacerations.

Recommendations regarding prevention of acute hepatitis are governed by the type of viral hepatitis that is being considered. In the case of acute hepatitis A, all family members and close personal contacts should receive immune serum globulin at a dose of 0.02 to 0.06 ml/kg intramuscularly as soon as possible after exposure. Office, factory, and school contacts do not need to be treated. Immune serum globulin can be given for up to 4 weeks after exposure, but it probably is effective only if given within 7 to 14 days. For prevention of hepatitis A in travelers, vaccination is an attractive option if the first dose can be given at least 4 weeks before travel. In the case of acute hepatitis B, prophylaxis needs to be provided only for "regular" sexual contacts. Combined passive-active immunization is the preferable method of prophylaxis. Hepatitis B immune globulin (HBIG) at a dosage of 0.06 ml/kg intramuscularly as soon as possible and again 1 month later has been the conventional recommendation in this situation. However, the efficacy of HBIG in preventing the sexual spread of acute hepatitis B has not been well proved.[176, 177] In addition, there is now evidence that postexposure immunization with HBV vaccine can attenuate or prevent acute hepatitis B.[178–181] In view of this, the combined approach dictates that vaccine should be given at the recommended dose as soon as possible and then 1 month and 6 months later. In the case of acute delta hepatitis, no specific immunoprophylaxis is available, and efforts should be directed toward prevention of hepatitis B. In the case of non-A, non-B hepatitis (hepatitis C), there is little or no information concerning the efficacy of any mode of prevention. Immune globulin (0.06 ml/kg) can be administered as soon as possible after percutaneous exposure, but there are no data demonstrating that this approach is efficacious. Similarly, there are no data on the efficacy of immune globulin prophylaxis for sexual or household contacts of patients with hepatitis C; however, in view of epidemiologic studies showing that there is a very low rate of transmission of hepatitis C to household or even regular sexual contacts of chronically infected patients, it is unlikely that passive prophylaxis will greatly affect the already low rate of transmission.

There is often a delay between diagnosis of acute viral hepatitis and determination of whether the disease is caused by HAV, HBV, HCV, or HDV. The recommendations already described require that prophylaxis of family members and intimate contacts of patients be postponed until the results of serologic testing are known. A simplified approach to prophylaxis is to administer immune serum globulin immediately to all family, household, and intimate contacts and to begin HBV vaccination of sexual contacts if the disease is subsequently shown to be type B (or delta) hepatitis. This schema could be modified if the hepatitis is obviously not caused by HAV (e.g., post-transfusion hepatitis). This approach is appealing because of its simplicity and also because the titers of anti-HBs (the protective antibody in hepatitis B) in standard preparations of immune serum globulin have been increasing over the past 10 to 15 years.[176, 179] Therefore, the immune serum globulin that is currently being produced may be partially effective in preventing hepatitis B.

Finally, it should be stressed that viral hepatitis is a reportable disease. Once the diagnosis is verified and serologic testing data are available, patients should be reported to the local or state department of health.

REFERENCES

1. Krugman S, Giles JP. Viral hepatitis. New light on an old disease. JAMA. 1970;212:1019.
2. Carey WD, Patel G. Viral hepatitis in the 1990s: Part I. Current principles of management. Cleve Clin J Med. 1992;59:317–325.
3. Carey WD, Patel G. Viral hepatitis in the 1990s: Part II. Hepatitis B and delta virus. Cleve Clin J Med. 1992;59:393–401.
4. Carey WD, Patel G. Viral hepatitis in the 1990s: Part III. Hepatitis C, hepatitis E, and other viruses. Cleve Clin J Med. 1992;59:595–601.
5. Feinstone SM, Kapikian AZ, Purcell RH. Hepatitis A: Detection by immune electron microscopy of a virus-like antigen associated with acute illness. Science. 1973;182:1026.
6. Blumberg BS, Alter HJ, Visnich S. A "new" antigen in leukemia sera. JAMA. 1965;191:541.
7. Tiollais P, Pourcel C, Dejean A. The hepatitis B virus. Nature. 1985;317:489.
8. Rizzetto M, Canese MG, Arico S, et al. Immunofluorescence detection of a new antigen-antibody system (delta/anti-delta) associated with hepatitis B virus in liver and serum of HBsAg carriers. Gut. 1977;18:997.
9. Rizzetto M. The delta agent. Hepatology. 1983;3:729.
10. Thomas HC, Karayiannis P, Monjardino J, McNair A. Hepatitis delta virus and the host response: current status and future perspectives. Prog Clin Biol Res. 1993;382:431–435.
11. Karayiannis P, Saldanha J, Monjardino J, et al. Prevention and treatment of hepatitis delta virus infection. Prog Clin Biol Res. 1991;364:377–383.
12. Feinstone SM, Kapikian AZ, Purcell RH, et al. Transfusion-associated hepatitis not due to viral hepatitis type A or B. N Engl J Med. 1975;292:767.
13. Choo Q-L, Kuo G, Weiner AJ, et al. Isolation of a cDNA clone from a blood-borne non-A non-B viral hepatitis genome. Science. 1989;244:329–362.
14. Kuo G, Choo Q-L, Alter HJ, et al. An assay for circulating antibodies to a major etiologic virus of human non-A, non-B hepatitis. Science. 1989;244:262–264.
15. Balayan MS, Andjaparidze AG, Savinskaya SS, et al. Evidence for a virus in non-A/non-B hepatitis transmitted via the fecal oral route. Intervirology. 1983;20:23.
16. Reyes GR, Purdy MA, Kim JP. Isolation of cDNA from the virus responsible for enterically transmitted non-A, non-B hepatitis. Science. 1990;247:1335–1339.
17. Gust ED, Purcell RH. Waterborne non-A, non-B hepatitis. J Infect Dis. 1987;156:630.
18. Leary TP, Muerhoff AS, Simons JN, et al. Sequence and genomic organization of GBV-C: A novel member of the Flaviviridae associated with human non–A–E hepatitis. J Med Virol. 1996;48:60–67.
19. Simons JN, Leary TP, Dawson GJ, et al. Isolation of novel virus-like sequences associated with human hepatitis. Nat Med. 1995;1:564–569.
20. Linnen J, Wages J Jr, Zhang-Keck ZY, et al. Molecular cloning and disease association of hepatitis G virus: A transfusion-transmissible agent. Science. 1996;271:505–508.
21. Deka N, Sharma MD, Mukerjee R. Isolation of the novel agent from human stool samples that is associated with sporadic non-A, non-B hepatitis. J Virol. 1994;68:7810–7815.
22. Alter HJ, Nakatsuji Y, Melpolder J, et al. The incidence of transfusion-associated hepatitis G virus infection and its relation to liver disease [see comments]. N Engl J Med. 1997;336:747–754.
23. Miyakawa Y, Mayumi M. Hepatitis G virus: A true hepatitis virus or an accidental tourist? [editorial; comment] [see comments]. N Engl J Med. 1997;336:795–796.
24. Alter MJ, Gallagher M, Morris TT, et al. Acute non-A-E hepatitis in the United States and the role of hepatitis G virus infection. Sentinel Counties Viral Hepatitis Study Team [see comments]. N Engl J Med. 1997;336:741–746.
25. Nishizawa T, Okamoto H, Konishi K, et al. A novel DNA virus (TTV) associated with elevated transaminase levels in posttransfusion hepatitis of unknown etiology. Biochem Biophys Res Commun. 1997;241:92–97.
26. Cossart Y. TTV: A common virus, but pathogenic? Lancet. 1998;352:164.
27. Hadler SC, de Monzon M, Ponzetto A, et al. An epidemic of severe hepatitis due to delta virus infection in Yucpa Indians of Venezuela. Ann Intern Med. 1984;100:339.
28. Hoofnagle JH, Shafritz DA, Popper H. Chronic hepatitis B and the "healthy" HBsAg carrier state. Hepatology. 1987;7:758.
29. Zeldis JB, Dienstag JL, Gale RP. Aplastic anemia and non-A, non-B hepatitis. Am J Med. 1983;74:64.
30. Beasley RP, Hwang LY, Lin CC, et al. Hepatocellular carcinoma and hepatitis B virus: A prospective study of 22,707 men in Taiwan. Lancet. 1981;2:1129.
31. Beasley RP. Hepatitis B virus as the etiologic agent in hepatocellular carcinoma: Epidemiologic considerations. Hepatology. 1982;2(Suppl):21.
32. Saito I, Miyamura T, Ohbayashi A, et al. Hepatitis C virus infection is associated with the development of hepatocellular carcinoma. Proc Natl Acad Sci U S A. 1990;87:6547–6549.
33. Nishioka K, Watanabe J, Furuta S. A high prevalence of antibody to hepatitis C virus in patients with hepatocellular carcinoma in Japan. Cancer. 1991;67:429–433.
34. Kaklamani E, Trichopoulos D, Tzonou A. Hepatitis B and C viruses and their interaction in the origin of hepatocellular carcinoma. JAMA. 1991;265:1974–1976.
35. Simonetti RG, Camma C, Fiorello F. Hepatitis C virus infection as a risk factor for hepatocellular carcinoma in patients with cirrhosis: A case-controlled study. Ann Intern Med. 1992;115:97–102.
36. Stevens CE, Taylor PE. Hepatitis B vaccine: Issues, recommendations, and new developments. Semin Liver Dis. 1986;6:23.
37. Werzberg A, Mensch B, Kuter B, et al. A controlled trial of a formalin-inactivated hepatitis A vaccine in healthy children. N Engl J Med. 1992;327:453–457.
38. Kane MA. Perspectives on the control of hepatitis A by vaccination. Vaccine. 1992;10(Suppl 1):S93–S96.
39. Margolis HS. Prevention of acute and chronic liver disease through immunization: Hepatitis B and beyond. J Infect Dis. 1993;168:9–14.
40. Steffen R. Hepatitis A and hepatitis B: Risks compared with other vaccine preventable diseases and immunization recommendations. Vaccine. 1993;11:518–520.
41. Gardner P, Schaffner W. Immunization of adults. N Engl J Med. 1993;328:1252–1258.
42. Alpert E, Isselbacher KJ, Schur PH. The pathogenesis of arthritis associated with viral hepatitis. N Engl J Med. 1971;285:185.
43. Heermann KH, Gerlich WH. Immunology of hepatitis B virus infections. Rheumatol Int. 1989;9:167–173.
44. Gianotti F. Hepatitis B antigen in papular acrodermatitis of children. BMJ. 1974;3:169.
45. Michalak T. Immune complexes of hepatitis B surface antigen in the pathogenesis of periarteritis nodosa. Am J Pathol. 1978;90:619.
46. Eknoyan G, Gyorkey F, Dicheso C, et al. Renal morphological and immunological changes associated with acute viral hepatitis. Kidney Int. 1972;1:413.
47. Kneiser MR, JHenis EH, Lowenthal DT, et al. Pathogenesis of renal disease associated with viral hepatitis. Arch Pathol. 1974;97:193.
48. Johnson RJ, Gretch DR, Yamabe H, et al. Membranoproliferative glomerulonephritis associated with hepatitis C virus infection. N Engl J Med. 1993;328:7.465–470.
49. Levo Y, Gorevic PD, Kassab HJ, et al. Liver involvement in the syndrome of mixed cryoglobulinemia. N Engl J Med. 1977;296:1501.
50. Agnello V, Chung RT, Kaplan LM. A role for hepatitis C virus infection in type II cryoglobulinemia. N Engl J Med. 1992;327:1490–1495.
51. Bernuau J, Rueff B, Benhamou JP. Fulminant and subfulminant liver failure: Definition and causes. Semin Liver Dis. 1985;6:97–106.
52. Katelaris PH, Jones DB. Fulminant hepatic failure. Med Clin North Am. 1989;73:955–970.
53. Nagata I, Tzampouras N, Chokshi S, et al. Hepatitis GB virus-C/hepatitis G virus infection in liver disease. Arch Dis Child. 1997;77:223–226.
54. Theodore D, Lemon SM. GB virus C, hepatitis G virus, or human orphan flavivirus? Hepatology. 1997;25:1285–1286.
55. Yoshiba M, Okamoto H, Mishiro S. Detection of the GBV-C hepatitis virus genome in serum from patients with fulminant hepatitis of unknown aetiology. Lancet. 1995;346:1131–1132.
56. Heringlake S, Osterkamp S, Trautwein C, et al. Association between fulminant hepatic failure and a strain of GBV virus C. Lancet. 1996;348:1626–1629.
57. Tameda Y, Kosaka Y, Tagawa S, et al. Infection with GB virus C (GBV-C) in patients with fulminant hepatitis. J Hepatol. 1996;25:842–847.
58. Zimmerman HG. The differential diagnosis of jaundice. Med Clin North Am. 1968;52:1417.
59. Frank BB. Clinical evaluation of jaundice: A guideline of the Patient Care Committee of the American Gastroenterological Association. JAMA. 1989;262:3031–3034.
60. Elias E. Clinical and biochemical diagnosis of jaundice. Baillieres Clin Gastroenterol. 1989;3:357–385.
61. Salen G, Goldstein F, Haurani F, et al. Acute hemolytic anemia complicating viral hepatitis in patients with glucose-6-phosphate dehydrogenase deficiency. Ann Intern Med. 1966;65:1210.
62. O'Grady JG, Alexander GJ, Hayllar KM, Williams R. Early indicators of prognosis in fulminant hepatic failure. Gastroenterology. 1989;97:439–445.
63. Ishak KG. Light microscopic morphology of viral hepatitis. Am J Clin Pathol. 1976;65:787.
64. Boyer JL, Klatskin G. Pattern of necrosis in acute viral hepatitis: Prognostic value of bridging (subacute hepatic necrosis). N Engl J Med. 1970;283:1063.
65. Lefkowitch JH, Schiff ER, Davis GL, et al. Pathological diagnosis of chronic hepatitis C: A multicenter comparative study with chronic hepatitis B. The Hepatitis Interventional Therapy Group. Gastroenterology. 1993;104:595–603.
66. Mathiesen LR, Fauerholt L, Moller Am, et al. Immunofluorescence studies for

hepatitis A virus and hepatitis B surface and core antigen in liver biopsies from patients with acute viral hepatitis. Gastroenterology. 1979;77:623.
67. Boggs JD, Melnick JL, Conrad ME, et al. Viral hepatitis, clinical and tissue culture studies. JAMA. 1970;214:1041.
68. Lemon S. Type A viral hepatitis: New developments in an old disease. N Engl J Med. 1985;313:1059.
69. Koff RS. Clinical manifestations and diagnosis of hepatitis A virus infection. Vaccine. 1992;10(Suppl 1):S15–S17.
70. Sjogren MH, Tanno H, Fay O, et al. Hepatitis A virus in stool during clinical relapse. Ann Intern Med. 1987;106:221.
71. Gordon SC, Reddy KR, Schiff L, et al. Prolonged intrahepatic cholestasis secondary to acute hepatitis A. Ann Intern Med. 1984;101:635–637.
72. Schiff ER. Atypical clinical manifestations of hepatitis A. Vaccine. 1992;10(Suppl 1):S18–S20.
73. O'Grady J. Management of acute and fulminant hepatitis A. Vaccine. 1992;10(Suppl 1):S21–S23.
74. Rakela A, Redeker AF, Edwards VM, et al. Hepatitis A virus infection in fulminant hepatitis and chronic active hepatitis. Gastroenterology. 1978;74:879.
75. Centers for Disease Control. Hepatitis surveillance report no. 51. Atlanta: CDC; 1987:13.
76. Francis DP, Hadler SC, Prendergast TJ, et al. Occurrence of hepatitis A, B, and non-A, non-B hepatitis in the United States: CDC Sentinel County hepatitis study I. Am J Med. 1984;76:69.
77. Dienstag JL, Routenberg JA, Purcell Rh, et al. Foodhandler-associated out-break of hepatitis type A: An immune electron microscopic study. Ann Intern Med. 1975;83:647.
78. Mackowiak PA, Caraway CT, Portnoy EL. Oyster-associated hepatitis: Lessons from the Louisiana experience. Am J Epidemiol. 1976;103:181.
79. Woodson RD, Clinton JJ. Hepatitis prophylaxis abroad: Effectiveness of immune serum globulin in protecting Peace Corps volunteers. JAMA. 1968;109:1053.
80. Pattison CP, Maynard JE, Bryan JS. Subhuman primate-associated hepatitis. J Infect Dis. 1975;132:478.
81. Hadler SC, Erben JJ, Francis DP, et al. Risk factors for hepatitis A in daycare centers. J Infect Dis. 1982;145:255.
82. Corey L, Holmes KK. Sexual transmission of hepatitis A in homosexual men: Incidence and mechanism. N Engl J Med. 1980;302:435.
83. Decker RH, Kosakowski SM, Vanderbilt AS, et al. Diagnosis of acute hepatitis A by Havab-M, a direct radioimmunoassay for IgM anti-HAV. Am J Clin Pathol. 1981;76:140.
84. Szmuness W, Much MI, Prince AM, et al. On the role of sexual behavior in the spread of hepatitis B infection. Ann Intern Med. 1975;83:489.
85. Krugman S, Overby LR, Mushahwar IK, et al. Viral hepatitis type B: Studies on the natural history and prevention reexamined. N Engl J Med. 1979;300:101.
86. Hoofnagle JH, Seeff LB, Bales ZB, et al. Serologic responses in hepatitis B. In: Vyas GN, Cohen SN, Schmid R, eds. Viral Hepatitis. Philadelphia: Franklin Institute Press; 1978:219–244.
87. Chau KH, Hargie MP, Decker RH, et al. Serodiagnosis of recent hepatitis B infection by IgM class anti-HBc. Hepatology. 1983;3:142.
88. Hoofnagle JH, Di Bisceglie AM. Serologic diagnosis of acute and chronic viral hepatitis. Semin Liver Dis. 1991;11:73–83.
89. Rizzetto M, Gerin JL, Purcell RH, eds. Hepatitis Delta Virus and Its Infection. New York: Alan R Liss; 1987.
90. Hoofnagle JH. Type D hepatitis. JAMA. 1989;261:1321.
91. Farci P, Gerin JL, Aragona M, et al. Diagnostic and prognostic significance of the IgM antibody to the hepatitis delta virus. JAMA. 1986;255:1443.
92. Mushawar IK, Decker RH. Prevalence of delta antigen and anti-delta detected by immunoassays in various HBsAg positive populations. In: Vyas GN, Dienstag JL, Hoofnagle JH, eds. Viral Hepatitis and Liver Disease. Orlando, Fla: Grune & Stratton; 1984:617.
93. Bergmann KF, Gerin JL. Antigens of hepatitis delta virus in the liver and serum of humans and animals. J Infect Dis. 1986;514:702.
94. Smedile A, Baroudy BM, Bergmann KF, et al. Clinical significance of HDV RNA in HDV disease. In: Rizzetto M. Gerin JL, Purcell RH, eds. Hepatitis Delta Virus and Its Infection. New York: Alan R Liss; 1987:31–34.
95. Rizzetto M, Verme G, Recchia S, et al. Chronic HBsAg hepatitis with intrahepatic expression of delta antigen: An active and progressive disease unresponsive to immunosuppressive treatment. Ann Intern Med. 1983;98:437.
96. Rocca G, Poli G, Gerardo P, et al. Familial clustering of delta infection. In: Verme G, Bonino F, Rizzetto M, eds. Viral Hepatitis and Delta Infection. New York: Alan R Liss; 1984:133–137.
96a. Prince AM, Brotman B, Grady GF, et al. Long-incubation post-transfusion hepatitis without serological evidence of exposure to hepatitis-B virus. Lancet. 1974;2:241–246.
97. Esteban JI, Genesca J, Alter HJ. Hepatitis C: Molecular biology, pathogenesis, epidemiology, clinical features, and prevention. Prog Liver Dis. 1992;10:253–282.
98. Houghton M, Weiner A, Han J, et al. Molecular biology of the hepatitis C viruses: Implications for diagnosis, development and control of viral disease. Hepatology. 1991;14:381–388.
99. Alter MJ, Hadler SC, Judson FN, et al. Risk factors for acute non-A, non-B hepatitis in the United States and association with hepatitis C virus infection. JAMA. 1990;264:2231–2235.
100. Alter MJ, Gerety RJ, Smallwood LA, et al. Sporadic non-A, non-B hepatitis: Frequency and epidemiology in an urban U.S. population. J Infect Dis. 1982;145:886.
101. Kelen GD, Green GB, Purcell RH. Hepatitis B and hepatitis C in emergency department patients. N Engl J Med. 1992;326:1399–1404.
102. Alter HJ, Hoofnagle JH. Non-A, non-B: Observations on the first decade. In: Vyas GN, Dienstag JL, Hoofnagle JH, eds. Viral Hepatitis and Liver Disease. Orlando, Fla: Grune & Stratton; 1984:345–355.
103. Wong DC, Purcell RH, Sreenivasan MA, et al. Epidemic and endemic hepatitis in India: Evidence for non-A/non-B hepatitis virus etiology. Lancet. 1980;2:876.
104. Khuroo SM. Study of an epidemic of non-A, non-B hepatitis: Possibility of another human hepatitis virus distinct from post-transfusion non-A, non-B type. Am J Med. 1980;68:818.
105. Kane MA, Bradley DW, Shrestha SM, et al. Epidemic non-A, non-B hepatitis in Nepal: Recovery of a possible etiologic agent and transmission studies in marmoset. JAMA. 1984;252:3140.
106. Kraczynski K, Bradley DW, Kane MA. Virus associated antigen of epidemic non-A, non-B hepatitis and specific antibodies in outbreaks and in sporadic cases of NANB hepatitis. Hepatology. 1988;8:1223.
107. Simons JN, Desai SM, Schultz DE, et al. Translation initiation in GB viruses A and C: Evidence for internal ribosome entry and implications for genome organization. J Virol. 1996;70:6126–6135.
108. Erker JC, Simons JN, Muerhoff AS, et al. Molecular cloning and characterization of a GB virus C isolate from a patient with non-A-E hepatitis. J Gen Virol. 1996;77:2713–2720.
109. Aikawa T, Sugai Y, Okamoto H. Hepatitis G infection in drug abusers with chronic hepatitis C. N Engl J Med. 1996;334:195–196.
110. Kinoshita T, Miyake K, Nakao H, et al. Molecular investigation of GB virus C infection in hemophiliacs in Japan. J Infect Dis. 1997;175:454–457.
111. Masuko K, Mitsui T, Iwano K, et al. Infection with hepatitis GB virus C in patients on maintenance hemodialysis. N Engl J Med. 1996;334:1485–1490.
112. Wu JC, Sheng WY, Huang YH, et al. Prevalence and risk factor analysis of GBV-C/HGV infection in prostitutes. J Med Virol. 1997;52:83–85.
113. Zanetti AR, Tanzi E, Romano L, et al. Multicenter trial on mother-to-infant transmission of GBV-C virus. The Lombardy Study Group on Vertical/Perinatal Hepatitis Viruses Transmission [published erratum appears in J Med Virol 1998;54:328]. J Med Virol. 1998;54:107–112.
114. Moaven LD, Locarnini SA, Bowden DS, et al. Hepatitis G virus and fulminant hepatic failure: Evidence for transfusion-related infection. J Hepatol. 1997;27:613–619.
115. Kanda T, Yokosuka O, Ehata T, et al. Detection of GBV-C RNA in patients with non-A-E fulminant hepatitis by reverse-transcription polymerase chain reaction. Hepatology. 1997;25:1261–1265.
116. Kuroki T, Nishiguchi S, Tanaka M, et al. Does GBV-C cause fulminant hepatitis in Japan? Lancet. 1996;347:908.
117. Sallie R, Shaw J, Mutimer D. GBV-C virus and fulminant hepatic failure. Lancet. 1996;347:1552.
118. Martinot M, Marcellin P, Boyer N, et al. Influence of hepatitis G virus infection on the severity of liver disease and response to interferon-alpha in patients with chronic hepatitis C. Ann Intern Med. 1997;126:874–881.
119. Saiz JC, Ampurdanes S, Olmedo E, et al. Hepatitis G virus infection in chronic hepatitis C: Frequency, features and response to interferon therapy. J Hepatol. 1997;26:787–793.
120. Bralet MP, Roudot-Thoraval F, Pawlotsky JM, et al. Histopathologic impact of GB virus C infection on chronic hepatitis C. Gastroenterology. 1997;112:188–192.
121. Kubo S, Nishiguchi S, Kuroki T, et al. Poor association of GBV-C viremia with hepatocellular carcinoma. J Hepatol. 1997;27:91–95.
122. Lightfoot K, Skelton M, Kew MC, et al. Does hepatitis GB virus-C infection cause hepatocellular carcinoma in black Africans? Hepatology. 1997;26:740–742.
123. Tanaka T, Takeuchi T, Inoue K, et al. Acute hepatitis caused by sexual or household transmission of GBV-C. J Hepatol. 1997;27:1110–1112.
124. Okamoto H, Akahane Y, Ukita M, et al. Fecal excretion of a nonenveloped DNA virus (TTV) associated with posttransfusion non-A-G hepatitis. J Med Virol. 1998;56:128–132.
125. Okamoto H, Nishizawa T, Kato N, et al. Molecular cloning and characterization of a novel DNA virus (TTV) associated with posttransfusion hepatitis of unknown etiology. Hepatol Res. 1998;10:1–6.
126. Naoumov NV, Petrova EP, Thomas MG, Williams R. Presence of a newly described human DNA virus (TTV) in patients with liver disease. Lancet. 1998;352:195–197.
127. Simmonds P, Davidson F, Lycett C, et al. Detection of a novel DNA virus (TTV) in blood donors and blood products [see comments]. Lancet. 1998;352:191–195.
128. Purcell RH, Walsh IH, Holland PV, et al. Seroepidemiological studies of transfusion-associated hepatitis. J Infect Dis. 1981;123:406.
129. Lamb SG, Stern H. Cytomegalovirus hepatitis. Lancet. 1966;2:1003.
130. Laskus T, Lupa E, Cianciara J, Slusarczyk J. Cytomegalovirus infection presenting as hepatitis. Digestion. 1990;47:167–171.
131. Gavish D, Kleinman Y, Morag A, et al. Hepatitis and jaundice associated with measles in young adults. Arch Intern Med. 1983;143:674.
132. Shalev-Zimels H, Weizman Z, Lotan C, et al. Extent of measles hepatitis in various ages. Hepatology. 1988;8:1138.
133. Francis TI, Moore DL, Edington GM, et al. A clinicopathological study of human yellow fever. Bull World Health Organ. 1972;46:659.
134. Zimmerman HG, Fang M, Utili R, et al. Jaundice due to bacterial infection. Gastroenterology. 1979;77:362.
135. Bowry S, Chan CH, Weiss H, et al. Hepatic involvement in pulmonary tuberculosis. Histologic and functional characteristics. Am Rev Respir Dis. 1970;101:941.
136. Godwin JE, Coleman AA, Sahn SA. Miliary tuberculosis presenting as hepatic and renal failure. Chest. 1991;99:752–754.
137. Kielhofner MA, Hamill RJ. Focal hepatic tuberculosis in a patient with acquired immunodeficiency syndrome. South Med J. 1991;84:401–404.

138. Asada Y, Hayashi T, Sumiyoshi A, et al. Miliary tuberculosis presenting as fever and jaundice with hepatic failure. Hum Pathol. 1991;22:92–94.
139. Oliva A, Duarte B, Jonasson O, Nadimpalli V. The nodular form of local hepatic tuberculosis: A review. J Clin Gastroenterol. 1990;12:166–173.
140. Lee RV, Thornton GF, Conn HO. Liver disease associated with secondary syphilis. N Engl J Med. 1971;284:1423.
141. Heath CW Jr, Alexander AD, Galton MM. Leptospirosis in the United States: Analysis of 483 cases in man, 1949–1961. N Engl J Med. 1965;273:857.
142. Bernstein M, Edmondson HA, Barhour BH. The liver lesion in Q fever: Clinical and pathologic features. Arch Intern Med. 1965;116:491.
143. Mahler H, Pasi A, Kramer JM, et al. Fulminant liver failure in association with the emetic toxin of *Bacillus cereus.* N Engl J Med. 1997;336:1142–1148.
144. Zimmerman HJ. Hepatotoxicity: The Adverse Effects of Drugs and Other Chemicals on the Liver. New York: Appleton-Century-Crofts; 1978.
145. Johnson GK, Tolman KG. Chronic liver disease and acetaminophen. Ann Intern Med. 1977;87:302.
146. Janes J, Routledge PA. Recent developments in the management of paracetamol (acetaminophen) poisoning. Drug Saf. 1992;7:170–177.
147. Nelson SD. Molecular mechanisms of the hepatotoxicity caused by acetaminophen. Semin Liver Dis. 1990;10:267–278.
148. Subcommittee on the National Halothane Study of the Committee on Anesthesia. Possible association between halothane anesthesia and postoperative hepatic necrosis. JAMA. 1966;197:775.
149. Ray DC, Drummond GB. Halothane hepatitis. Br J Anaesth. 1991;67:84–99.
150. Kenna JG. The molecular basis of halothane-induced hepatitis. Biochem Soc Trans. 1991;19:191–195.
151. Neuberger JM. Halothane and hepatitis: Incidence, predisposing factors and exposure guidelines. Drug Saf. 1990;5:28–38.
152. Bynum TE, Boinoit JK, Maddrey WC. Ischemic hepatitis. Am J Dig Dis. 1979;24:129.
153. Lieber CS. Biochemical and molecular basis of alcohol-induced injury to the liver and other tissues. N Engl J Med. 1988;319:1639.
154. Roche-Sicot J, Benhamou JP. Acute intravascular hemolysis and acute liver failure associated as a first manifestation of Wilson's disease. Ann Intern Med. 1977;86:301.
155. Rosenblate HJ, Eisenstein R, Halmes AW. The liver in sickle cell anemia. Arch Pathol Lab Med. 1970;90:235.
156. Parker RGF. Occlusion of the hepatic veins in man. Medicine (Baltimore). 1959;38:369.
157. Harrison HB, Middleton HM, Crosby JH, et al. Fulminant hepatic failure: An unusual presentation of metastatic liver disease. Gastroenterology. 1981;80:820.
158. Repsher LH, Freebern RK. Effects of early and vigorous exercise on recovery from infectious hepatitis. N Engl J Med. 1969;281:1393.
159. Schweitzer IL, Weiner JM, McPeak CM, et al. Oral contraceptives in acute viral hepatitis. JAMA. 1975;233:979.
160. Blum AL, Stutz R, Haemmerli UP, et al. A fortuitously controlled study of steroid therapy in acute viral hepatitis: I. Acute disease. Am J Med. 1969;47:82.
161. Gregory PB, Knauer CM, Miller R, et al. Steroid therapy in severe viral hepatitis. N Engl J Med. 1976;294:681.
162. Perrillo RP, Schiff ER, Davis GL, et al. A randomized, controlled trial of interferon alfa-2b alone and after prednisone withdrawal for the treatment of chronic hepatitis B. The Hepatitis Interventional Therapy Group. N Engl J Med. 1990;323:295–301.
163. Davis GL, Balart LA, Schiff ER, et al. Treatment of chronic hepatitis C with recombinant interferon alfa: A multicenter randomized, controlled trial. Hepatitis Interventional Therapy Group. N Engl J Med. 1989;321:1501–1506.
164. Davis GL. Recombinant alpha-interferon treatment of non-A, and non-B (type C) hepatitis: Review of studies and recommendations for treatment. J Hepatol. 1990;11(Suppl 1):S72–S77.
165. Hoofnagle JH, Di Bisceglie AM. Treatment of chronic type C hepatitis with alpha interferon. Semin Liver Dis. 1989;9:259–263.
166. Levin S, Hahn T. Interferon system in acute viral hepatitis. Lancet. 1982;1:592.
167. Sanchez-Tapias JM, Mas A, Costal J, et al. Recombinant alpha 2c interferon therapy in fulminant viral hepatitis. J Hepatol. 1987;5:205.
168. Omata M, Yokosuka O, Takano S, et al. Resolution of acute hepatitis C after therapy with natural beta interferon. Lancet. 1991;338:914–915.
169. Peleman RR, Gavaler JS, Van Thiel DH, et al. Liver transplantation for acute and subacute hepatic failure. Hepatology. 1985;5:1045.
170. Mutimer DJ, Elias E. Liver transplantation for fulminant hepatic failure. Prog Liver Dis. 1992;10:349–367.
171. Lidofsky SD. Liver transplantation for fulminant hepatic failure. Gastroenterol Clin North Am. 1993;22:257–269.
172. Vickers C, Neuberger J, Buckels J, et al. Transplantation of the liver in adults and children with fulminant hepatic failure. J Hepatol. 1988;7:143.
173. Bernuau J, Gordeau A, Poynard T, et al. Multivariate analysis of prognostic factors in fulminant hepatitis. Hepatology. 1986;6:648.
174. Auslander MO, Gitnick GL. Vigorous medical management of acute fulminant hepatitis. Arch Intern Med. 1977;137:599.
175. Katelaris PH, Jones DB. Fulminant hepatic failure. Med Clin North Am. 1989;73:955–970.
176. Seeff LB, Hoofnagle JH. Immunoprophylaxis of viral hepatitis. Gastroenterology. 1979;77:161.
177. Margolis HS. Prevention of acute and chronic liver disease through immunization: Hepatitis B and beyond. J Infect Dis. 1993;168:9–14.
178. Centers for Disease Control. Post-exposure prophylaxis of hepatitis B. Ann Intern Med. 1984;101:351.
179. Catterall AP, Murray-Lyon IM. Strategies for hepatitis B immunisation. Gut. 1992;33:576–579.
180. Hadler SC, Margolis HS. Hepatitis B immunization: Vaccine types, efficacy, and indications for immunization. Curr Clin Top Infect Dis. 1992;12:282–308.
181. Beasley RP, Hwang LY, Lee GC, et al. Prevention of perinatally transmitted hepatitis B virus infections with hepatitis B immune globulin and hepatitis B vaccine. Lancet. 1983;2:1099.

Chapter 103

Chronic Hepatitis

THOMAS A. SHAW-STIFFEL

Chronic hepatitis is a descriptive term used to denote ongoing inflammation of the hepatic parenchyma. Of the various etiologies of chronic hepatitis (Table 103–1), the leading cause worldwide remains viral. Approximately 5% of the world's population (or 350 million people) are infected with the hepatitis B virus (HBV) and 1% (or 60 million people) with the hepatitis C virus (HCV). In the United States alone, it is estimated that more than 1.5 million people have chronic hepatitis B and more than 4 million chronic hepatitis C. The social and economic consequences of chronic viral hepatitis are indeed staggering. Because both diseases lead to cirrhosis, portal hypertension, and hepatocellular carcinoma in a sizable proportion of those infected, chronic viral hepatitis ranks as the fifth most common cause of death worldwide. In the United States alone, the economic burden of HBV and HCV together has been estimated to be well over $1 billion. The problems with chronic HCV are only bound to worsen over the coming years. According to the Centers for Disease Control and Prevention (CDC), about 10,000 people now die annually in the United States from HCV-related disease and the mortality rate is expected to triple in the next two decades. The term "killer" epidemic has been applied to the evolving situation with chronic HCV infection and with some justification.[1–3]

Apart from HBV and HCV, other hepatotropic viruses have been identified as potential causes of chronic hepatitis. One of these, the hepatitis G virus (HGV), has not yet been linked to any significant liver damage[4] (see Chapter 144). The clinical implications of another novel transfusion-transmissible virus (TTV) also remain to be determined[5] (see Chapter 144). Hepatitis D virus (HDV) requires the presence of hepatitis B surface antigen (HBsAg) in order to survive, and it may cause fulminant hepatitis and acute liver failure when it coinfects or superinfects patients with acute or chronic HBV infection.[2, 3] Although cytomegalovirus, Epstein-Barr virus, hepatitis A virus (HAV), and hepatitis E virus (HEV) are important causes of

TABLE 103–1 Major Etiologies of Chronic Hepatitis

Etiology
Chronic viral hepatitis
Hepatitis B
Hepatitis C
Hepatitis D
Autoimmune hepatitis and variant syndromes
Hereditary hemochromatosis
Wilson's disease
α-Antitrypsin deficiency
Fatty liver and nonalcoholic steatohepatitis
Alcoholic liver disease
Drug-induced liver disease
Hepatic granulomas
Infectious
Drug induced
Neoplastic
Idiopathic

acute hepatitis, they have not been shown to result in chronic disease.[3] Sometimes, however, HAV can lead to a syndrome of prolonged cholestasis with elevated serum levels of alkaline phosphatase and total bilirubin that persist for several months and, even more rarely, to a chronic relapsing course that is thought to result from incomplete clearance of HAV. This usually resolves within a year.[6, 7] A variant form of autoimmune hepatitis may also be triggered by HAV and lead to what is mistakenly considered a case of "chronic" hepatitis A.[8] One study suggests that the mortality rate with HAV may be higher in patients chronically infected with HCV (but not HBV), and immunization against HAV is recommended for these patients.[9]

In general, the diagnosis of chronic hepatitis has serious implications, because chronic hepatitis may lead to cirrhosis and other adverse outcomes if left unchecked. As a result, a new classification system for chronic hepatitis has been adopted in order to include features that are now thought to predict more accurately the long-term risk of developing cirrhosis. It should also help in assessing the benefits of any new therapies.[10] Previously, chronic hepatitis had simply been defined as a condition in which serum levels of hepatic enzymes, namely aspartate aminotransferase (AST; formerly known as serum glutamic-oxaloacetic transaminase), alanine aminotransferase (ALT, previously serum glutamic-pyruvic transaminase), or both, were found to be elevated for more than 6 months. By this definition, patients with normal aminotransferase levels were not considered to have chronic hepatitis or to be at any risk for long-term complications. Furthermore, in patients with chronic hepatitis, the long-term prognosis was thought to be determined for the most part by specific features on liver biopsy that corresponded to the histopathologic entities *chronic persistent*, *chronic lobular*, and *chronic active hepatitis*, with chronic active hepatitis as the most predictive of an adverse outcome such as cirrhosis.[10, 11]

However, in prospective studies of patients chronically infected with HCV, many of those who initially had only chronic persistent hepatitis on biopsy (presumed to be a favorable prognostic indicator) were later found to have developed cirrhosis during the ensuing years. In addition, the previous emphasis placed on *piecemeal necrosis* (now better termed *interface hepatitis*, because the most likely cause is hepatocyte apoptosis or programmed cell death rather than necrosis or cellular destruction) was also misguided, because other forms of cell damage such as *bridging necrosis* are equally, if not more, important in prognosis.[11] Furthermore, it has now become evident that certain hepatotropic viruses such as HBV and HCV are rarely, if ever, cleared completely from the liver, even though serum ALT levels have returned to normal and circulating viral particles (HCV RNA) are no longer detectable with ultrasensitive techniques such as the reverse transcriptase–polymerase chain reaction (RT-PCR) or the signal amplification branched-chain DNA (bDNA) assay.[12, 13]

Consequently, the term chronic hepatitis should be applied not solely on the basis of disease duration or the presence or absence of *interface hepatitis* on liver biopsy but rather on what has been identified as the most likely cause (e.g., viral, autoimmune, drug). In most instances, this revised classification of chronic hepatitis (now based on etiology alone) should help to indicate the prognosis and dictate appropriate therapeutic interventions. Moreover, on liver biopsy, the grade of necroinflammatory activity (portal or periportal versus lobular) and the stage of fibrosis should be graded using specific scoring systems. This has been shown to help in prediction of long-term outcome in the absence of specific therapy or removal of any inciting factors and to help monitor improvements at future time intervals with these interventions.[14]

CHRONIC HEPATITIS B

It was estimated that by the year 2000 there would be more than 400 million people (or 5% of the world's population) with some form of chronic HBV infection.[2, 3, 15] Currently, in the United States, close to 1.25 million people are chronic carriers and health-related costs are estimated to be more than $650 billion annually.[2, 15] Thus, HBV has become one of the major causes of chronic hepatitis, cirrhosis, and hepatocellular carcinoma worldwide, with more than 1 million deaths caused by HBV each year.[16] Unfortunately, treatment of chronic HBV infection with interferon-α (IFN-α) has been of limited benefit and, despite safe and effective HBV vaccines, immunization has not yet been widely applied.[17] However, a report from Taiwan suggested that the incidence of hepatocellular carcinoma can be reduced significantly through a universal HBV vaccination program.[18] In the United States, immunization of neonates and adolescents is now the standard of care.[19]

Virology

A detailed discussion of the virology of HBV is presented in Chapter 135. In brief, HBV is a member of the Hepadnaviridae family of DNA viruses that infect humans as well as certain animals such as the woodchuck, ground squirrel, and duck.[2, 20] All these viruses have similar replication cycles that primarily involve the liver and lead to chronic hepatitis, cirrhosis, and hepatocellular carcinoma. The main genes of HBV are as follows: *S*, which stands for the surface or envelope gene that produces HBsAg; *C*, for the core gene that produces hepatitis B core antigen (HB_cAg) and hepatitis B e antigen (HB_eAg), a circulating viral peptide derived from HB_cAg; *P*, for the DNA polymerase gene (P protein) involved in viral replication (reverse transcriptase activity) and subsequent viral assembly; and *X*, for the *X* gene, which appears to encode two transcription transactivators crucial for viral replication and which may be involved in promoting hepatocellular carcinoma.[2, 20, 21] The Dane particle circulates as a 42-nm sphere that consists of HBsAg surrounding the nucleocapsid or core (HB_cAg) and viral DNA.

Effective clearance of HBV by the host's immune system appears to depend mostly on expression of the HB_cAg-derived peptides that are located on the hepatocyte surface membrane and that trigger potent cytotoxic T-cell ($CD8^+$) responses. HB_eAg is a viral peptide (closely related to HB_cAg) that is found in the circulation of almost every individual with active HBV replication. Precore mutants lack the ability to produce complete HB_eAg peptides because of a defective *pre-C* gene. As a result, in patients with precore mutants, circulating HB_eAg is absent although viral replication persists and thus HBV DNA remains detectable. It has been shown that precore mutants lead to more aggressive hepatic inflammation and in some cases acute liver failure, as well as resistance to IFN-α therapy and a higher likelihood of graft loss after liver transplantation.[22] Therefore, apart from the occasional precore mutant, HB_eAg is an inexpensive marker of the presence of immune tolerance because of the close relationship of HB_eAg to HB_cAg, the putative target of the host's immune response. Long-term immunity is conferred by antibody that is specifically directed at HBsAg (anti-HB_s) via either natural exposure to the intact virus or vaccination with recombinant HBsAg.[2]

HBV also has several viral antigenic subdeterminants, one of which is known as *a*, found in all individuals with HBsAg, and others termed *d*, *y*, *w*, and *r*, which combine with *a* to produce four main HBV subtypes (adw, ayw, adr, and ayr). In general, these subtypes have no clinical significance apart from the mutants that emerge with changes at the *a* subdeterminant during hepatitis B immune globulin (HBIG) prophylaxis and cause HBV recurrence after transplantation. These subtypes may also help epidemiologists to track common-source outbreaks and other related issues. On occasion, two or more viral subtypes may coinfect a single individual, which may partly explain the rare phenomenon in which HBsAg and anti-HBs are detected simultaneously.[2, 20, 21]

Epidemiology

The prevalence rate of chronic HBV infection is highest in the Far East (Southeast Asia, China, the Philippines, Indonesia), the Middle

East, Africa, and parts of South America. In some of these areas, more than 50% of the general population have serologic markers of previous HBV infection and up to 15% are chronic carriers. In the United States, the highest rate of chronic HBV infection is found in Pacific Islanders and Alaskan natives, who have a prevalence rate of 6.4%. In other areas of the world where HBV is common, transmission usually occurs via vertical (mother-to-neonate) routes but also by horizontal routes (from one child to another), although less frequently. This may also apply to children of certain ethnic or immigrant groups who now live in the United States. However, the most common mode of HBV transmission in the United States is the sexual route, especially in adolescents and young adults.[2, 23–25]

High-risk groups for chronic HBV infection in the United States include injection drug users, men who have sex with other men, other individuals with multiple sexual partners, household contacts and sexual partners of HBV carriers, health care workers, patients receiving chronic hemodialysis, and organ transplant recipients.[24–26] Transmission from a surgeon to his patients has been reported.[27] However, about 20 to 30% of individuals infected with HBV have no apparent risk factors.[2, 15, 16, 19] The epidemiology of HBV is discussed in more detail in Chapter 135.

Pathophysiology and Natural History

In most instances, HBV is not directly cytopathic. Instead, the host's immune system is thought to play a major role in the acute hepatic injury and long-term sequelae of HBV, namely, chronic hepatitis and cirrhosis. Active hepatic inflammation occurs as part of the "innocent bystander" phenomenon with cell injury and apoptosis, related to the immune response's attempt to clear the virus. The duration of ongoing HBV replication also depends primarily on the maturity of the host's immune system.[2, 18–21, 24] After exposure to HBV, more than 95% of neonates born to mothers who are HBsAg positive become asymptomatic chronic carriers, whereas only about 5% of adults become carriers.[28] Horizontal spread in children may also be an important source of infection.[29, 30] Children infected after the neonatal period but before age 6 become carriers about 30% of the time.[31] Although chronic HBV in childhood is usually subclinical and mild, the long-term consequences are significant, with cirrhosis, liver failure, and hepatocellular carcinoma seen in substantial numbers.[2, 21, 24, 31]

The life cycle of HBV can be divided into four stages as shown in Table 103–2.[2, 21, 24] The first two stages are part of the *replicative* phase, with active viral replication, whereas stages 3 and 4 form the *integrative* phase, with viral integration into the host's genome. The duration of each stage depends on the individual's genetic predisposition, gender, age at HBV acquisition, status of the immune system, viral coinfections, appearance of HBV mutants, and other important contributors. During stage 1, immune tolerance of HBV by the host permits continued viral replication without any obvious clinical manifestations. Serum aminotransferases remain normal. In healthy adults, this stage (also known as the incubation period) usually lasts for 2 to 4 weeks before viral clearance begins (stage 2), whereas in neonates it may continue for decades. Fortunately, hepatic inflammation is minimal and the progression to cirrhosis is rare. In stage 2, the host's immune response is probably triggered by the stimulation of cytotoxic T lymphocytes ($CD8^+$) directed against HBV proteins, HB_cAg in particular, that are present on the hepatocyte cell membrane. The main concern is that in stage 2, ongoing hepatic inflammation, specifically when prolonged in duration and severe in intensity, places the individual at high risk for cirrhosis and hepatocellular carcinoma. In most adults who go on to clear HBV, this stage lasts for 3 to 4 weeks, whereas in chronic carriers it may persist for 10 years or more.[21, 22, 31–37] Ongoing hepatic inflammation can lead to cirrhosis in about 50% of individuals within 5 years, although 71% remain alive at 5 years unless major liver decompensation occurs.[36]

Stage 3 begins when viral replication has begun to fall significantly in response to the host's vigorous immune response. In the serum, HB_eAg is cleared, antibody to HB_eAg (anti-HB_e) becomes detectable, and levels of HBV DNA fall precipitously. Active HBV infection has now ended. However, small amounts of viral DNA may still be detected in the serum with sensitive RT-PCR techniques. With abatement of the immune response and associated improvement in hepatic inflammation, serum aminotransferases become normal. For extented periods of time, however, serum HBsAg may remain detectable because the *S* gene is probably integrated into the hepatocyte genome. In stage 4, full host immunity to HBV has occurred with clearance of serum HBsAg and the development of anti-HB_s. HBV DNA is no longer detectable in the circulation even by RT-PCR, although it may be found in the liver. Rarely, such as after systemic chemotherapy, organ transplantation, or human immunodeficiency virus (HIV) infection, HBV may be reactivated in these individuals and lead to recurrence of hepatic inflammation and the risk of further damage.[2, 24]

TABLE 103–2 Stages of Hepatitis B Virus Infection

	Replicative Phase		Integrative Phase	
Stage	*1*	*2*	*3*	*4*
HBsAg	Positive	Positive	Positive	Negative
Antibody to HBsAg	Negative	Negative	Negative	Positive
Antibody to HB_cAg	Positive	Positive	Positive	Positive
HB_eAg	Positive	Positive	Negative	Negative
Antibody to HB_eAg	Negative	Negative	Positive	Positive
HBV DNA	Strongly +	Positive	Negative (+ by PCR)	Negative
AST and ALT	Normal	Elevated	Normal	Normal

Abbreviations: ALT, Alanine aminotransferase; AST, aspartate aminotransferase; HB_cAg, hepatitis B core antigen; HB_eAg, hepatitis B e antigen; HBsAg, hepatitis B surface antigen; HBV, hepatitis B virus; PCR, polymerase chain reaction.

Adapted with permission from Lee WM. Hepatitis B virus infection. N Engl J Med. 1997;337:1733–1745. Copyright © 1997 Massachusetts Medical Society. All rights reserved.

TABLE 103–3 Extrahepatic Manifestations of Hepatitis B Virus Infection

Polyarteritis nodosa
Membranous or membranoproliferative glomerulonephritis
Leukocytoclastic vasculitis
Erythema nodosum
Arthritis and serum sickness (usually acute HBV infection)
Raynaud's phenomenon
Polyneuropathy (mononeuritis multiplex, usually with PAN)
Guillain-Barré syndrome (rare)
Pericarditis (rare)
Pancreatitis (rare)

Abbreviations: HBV, Hepatitis B virus; PAN, polyarteritis nodosa.

Clinical Features

There are no specific clinical findings to indicate that a given individual has chronic HBV infection, because most patients remain asymptomatic until the ravages of end-stage liver disease and its sequelae become evident. However, a variety of clinical syndromes have been associated with chronic HBV (Table 103–3). These may be the initial reason for presentation, and the diagnosis of HBV may not be suspected unless there is a high index of suspicion. Nonspecific symptoms of fatigue and right upper quadrant discomfort are not uncommon with chronic HBV, especially in those with active hepatic inflammation as seen in stage 2 (discussed earlier). However, any symptoms such as jaundice, weight loss, ascites, or worsening abdominal pain should prompt a workup for a complication such as hepatocellular carcinoma, which may appear acutely or in a more indolent manner associated with various paraneoplastic syndromes. An algorithm for the management of patients with chronic HBV is presented in Figure 103–1. Because the field is changing so rapidly,

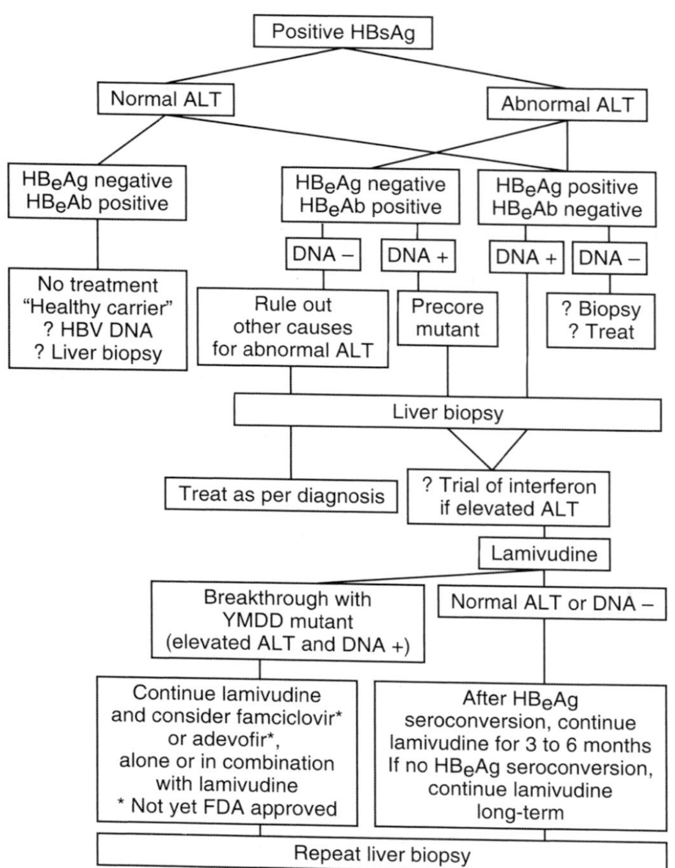

FIGURE 103–1. Algorithm for the management of patients with chronic hepatitis B virus infection.

local or national experts in addition to the most recent publications on HBV should be consulted for up-to-date recommendations on the workup and management of these patients.[24, 38, 39]

Treatment of Chronic Hepatitis B Virus Infection with Interferons

Effective treatment of chronic HBV infection is based on a knowledge of the natural history of HBV disease if left untreated, balanced by the benefits and side effects of antiviral therapy. The main complications of long-term HBV infection are cirrhosis, liver failure, and hepatocellular carcinoma.[31–37, 40] Individuals from high-endemicity regions of the world in which vertical transmission of HBV has occurred early in life have a much higher risk of developing cirrhosis (relative risk up to 80 in HBV carriers versus control subjects) and hepatocellular carcinoma (relative risk as high as 148 in Alaska or 98 in the Far East).[23, 25] Early treatment of these patients should be a priority whenever active viral replication is confirmed, because clearance of HBsAg rarely occurs spontaneously (0.4 to 2% per year in western countries, where HBV infection is transmitted mostly in adults, versus only 0.1 to 0.8% per year in Alaska or in Asian countries such as Taiwan, where infection occurs at birth or during the first 5 years of life). Spontaneous clearance of HB_eAg is reported to occur at a rate of 8 to 12% per year.[31–37, 40]

Several factors play a role in determining the need for treatment and the likelihood of response, including the patient's current age, age at HBV acquisition, geographic and genetic predisposition, and stage of viral infection.[2, 24] As already noted, individuals in stage 2 of HBV infection, especially those with long-standing or aggressive hepatic inflamation, have the highest risk of a poor outcome and should receive early and more intensive therapy. However, many individuals with chronic HBV infection (particularly those who acquired HBV infection by vertical transmission, early in life, or both) may still be in stage 1 (the immune tolerant phase), a stage in which immunostimulants such as IFN-α are usually not effective.[40] Antiviral agents that inhibit viral replication, such as lamivudine, might be more appropriate. On the other hand, some chronic carriers may have already made the transition from stage 2 to stage 3, in which case viral replication has waned and the use of IFN-α or antivirals would be of limited benefit. Patients in stage 4 are immune to HBV and do not require any form of therapy.[2, 38, 39]

Until recently, IFN-α has been the only therapy for chronic hepatitis B approved by the Food and Drug Administration (FDA) (see Table 103–4). (For more details of the IFN-α products currently available in the United States to treat chronic HCV infection, see "Treatment of Chronic Hepatitis C Virus Infection with Interferons" and Chapter 36.) IFN-α was first noted in the 1970s to be beneficial in the treatment of chronic HBV infection, even though only minute amounts were available for study.[41] Later, with sufficient quantities of the drug produced via recombinant engineering, IFN-α was shown in preliminary trials to clear HB_eAg and even HBsAg from the serum of chronic HBV carriers in a significant proportion of cases. Improvement in liver histology was also noted.[42–45] Subsequently, several large randomized controlled trials in Europe, Asia, and the United States demonstrated the efficacy of IFN-α in chronic HBV carriers, primarily those in stage 2 of the replicative phase.[46–48] In general, HB_eAg seroconversion occurred in only 10 to 20% of control subjects versus 25 to 40% of unselected patients treated for a minimum of 4 months with IFN-α.[2, 24, 38, 39, 41–50] Features that were found to predict a favorable response included elevated serum aminotransferase levels and low levels of circulating HBV DNA at baseline.[51–57] In fact, most patients do not respond to IFN-α if they have normal or minimally elevated serum ALT levels, which is often the case for patients infected at birth or in childhood, such as those from Asia and other regions of high endemicity.[40, 52]

TABLE 103–4 Alpha Interferons for Chronic Hepatitis B and C

Product	Hepatitis B	Hepatitis C
Interferon-alfa2a (Roferon A, Hoffmann-LaRoche)	5 MU daily or 10 MU tiw SC	3 MU tiw SC for 12–18 months if tolerated well SVR of 10–20% in treatment-naive patients; ? more after >18 mo SVR much less in relapsers Nonresponders rarely if ever respond to higher or daily doses for longer time
Interferon-alfa2b (Intron A, Schering-Plough)	5 MU daily or 10 MU tiw SC Approved by the FDA for use in children older than 1 year with chronic HBV infection	Same as above Fewer antibodies to IFN-α reported (? clinical impact)
Interferon alfacon (Infergen, Amgen)	Not indicated	9 μg tiw SC for 6 mo in treatment-naive patients with SVR of 10–15% 15 μg tiw SC for 6–12 mo in relapsers; SVR 28–58% Nonresponders need higher or daily doses
Interferon-alfa2b + ribavirin (Intron A 3 MU tiw SC + Rebetol 1000–2000 mg/d) (Rebetron, Schering-Plough)	Not indicated	Treatment-naive need 6–12 mo with SVR 30–38% Patients with relapses need 6 mo; SVR 49% versus 5% with interferon monotherapy Nonresponders?

Abbreviations: FDA, Food and Drug Administration; MU, million units; SC, subcutaneously; SVR, sustained virologic response (hepatitis C virus DNA negative at end of treatment and at 6 mo); tiw, three times a week.

The therapeutic benefit of IFN-α was also confirmed in a meta-analysis[50] that considered more than 800 chronic HBV carriers (derived from 15 randomized controlled trials) treated with IFN-α in varying doses from 5 million units (MU) daily to 10 MU three times a week (tiw) for at least 3 months and with at least 6 months of follow-up after the completion of therapy. IFN-α for a minimum of 4 months led to a loss of circulating HBV DNA in 37% of those treated versus only 17% of control subjects, loss of HB_eAg in 33% of those treated versus 21% of control subjects, and loss of HBsAg in 8% of those treated versus 2% of control subjects. Normalization of ALT also occurred more often in those who received IFN-α. Similarly to what occurs during spontaneous HB_eAg seroconversion, a favorable response to IFN-α leads to resolution of hepatic inflammation, and the risks of developing cirrhosis and hepatocellular carcinoma diminish significantly.[2] Once HBV seroconversion has been achieved, active viral replication rarely recurs unless the patient becomes immunosuppressed (e.g., with systemic chemotherapy, HIV disease, or organ transplantation).[56]

Cost-effectiveness analyses have also confirmed the benefits of IFN-α therapy for chronic HBV infection. One study[57] addressed the hypothetic situation of treating a 35-year-old HBV carrier with chronic hepatitis but without cirrhosis using IFN-α at 10 MU TIW versus no treatment. In this model, IFN-α therapy was shown to decrease health care costs and improve quality-adjusted life expectancy. In addition, IFN-α decreased the cumulative lifetime risk of developing cirrhosis, liver decompensation or hepatocellular carcinoma by 13, 9, and 4%, respectively. Furthermore, 7 patients would have to be treated to prevent each case of cirrhosis, 11 to prevent each case of decompensation, and 26 to prevent each case of hepatocellular carcinoma. Similar results were found in another cost-effectiveness analysis using cohorts of HBV DNA–positive chronic carriers 25 to 35 years of age.[58]

As expected from what is seen during spontaneous HB_eAg seroconversion, a favorable response to IFN-α is associated with a "flare" in serum aminotransferases to levels two to five times above baseline. This may last for up to 3 months. Patients are usually asymptomatic during this period, although in some instances they may develop jaundice and even frank liver failure. As a result, IFN-α is contraindicated for patients with advanced end-stage liver disease because urgent liver transplantation may be required for salvage if these patients deteriorate. These patients are also more likely to develop infectious or bleeding complications.[2, 24, 38, 39] However, there may be some benefit and fewer risks in using low-dose, titratable IFN-α for patients with advanced HBV disease.[59]

A number of strategies have been proposed to enhance the response rates seen with IFN-α therapy. One approach is to select patients using specific pretreatment criteria. Favorable prognostic indicators include a short duration of disease, low serum levels of HBV DNA, histology compatible with active hepatitis, and high serum levels of aminotransferases, all of which suggest an already primed immune system.[40, 41, 51] Initially, chronic HBV carriers from Asian countries did not appear to respond as well as those from the West, probably because they acquired HBV at an early age and thus remained in stage 1 of the replicative phase.[33] However, when Asian HBV carriers with elevated serum ALT levels were treated with IFN-α, the response rates were similar to those seen in other non-Asian groups.[60, 61] Coinfection with HIV appears to have a minimal impact on the severity of liver disease related to HBV, although HIV infection may reduce the likelihood of a favorable response to IFN-α therapy.[62–64]

Another approach that has been used in an attempt to improve response rates is a short course of corticosteroids that are withdrawn just before initiating standard IFN-α therapy (steroid priming). However, study results have been conflicting and at present this strategy remains controversial.[46, 65, 66] In fact, steroid therapy was shown in clinical trials in the 1970s to decrease survival in patients with chronic HBV, probably by increasing viral replication via a steroid-responsive receptor. Prolonged use of steroids may also delay the seroconversion from HB_eAg to anti-HB_e.[67, 68] Nevertheless, steroid priming may have a role specifically for individuals with a normal or minimally elevated serum ALT level (i.e., less than 100 IU/liter) before IFN-α therapy, because these chronic HBV carriers are most likely to be in stage 1 of the viral replication phase and thus require a certain degree of "immune priming." Because HB_eAg is detectable in these patients, they can be readily differentiated from those in stage 3 (i.e., with no detectable HB_eAg), who do not require therapy. Other immunomodulators, including thymosin-α_1, IFN-β, IFN-γ, or interleukin-2 plus prostaglandin E, have not been shown to be of benefit in controlled and uncontrolled clinical trials, nor have other antiviral agents such as ribavirin, acyclovir, or ara-AMP conjugated with lactosominated human serum albumin.[2, 24, 38, 39, 69–72] The benefits of lamivudine and other antivirals in chronic HBV are discussed in the section "Other Drug Therapies for Chronic Hepatitis B."

In children, the use of IFN-α for chronic HBV has remained controversial.[73] Initial trials with this drug in Asian children yielded poor response rates,[33, 40, 49, 52] probably because the subjects had high levels of circulating HBV DNA and low levels of serum ALT (as noted earlier). However, subsequent series indicated that children with elevated serum ALT levels responded as well to IFN-α as did adults.[49, 73–77] Steroid priming does not provide additional benefit.[78, 79] A multinational randomized controlled trial[77] demonstrated significant benefits with interferon-alfa-2b (IFN-α2b) for 24 weeks at a dose of 6 MU/m^2 three times a week in children between the ages of 1 and 17 years. On the basis of this and other similar studies, the FDA has approved the use of IFN-α-2b for children with chronic HBV.

Knowledge regarding the clinical pharmacology of IFN-α is limited, but it appears to be distributed and cleared via relatively simple kinetics (see Chapter 36).[80] IFN-α must be given parenterally and is associated with significant side effects (see Table 103–5).[24, 80–83] Most side effects are dose dependent and diminish significantly with continued therapy. During the first 2 to 4 weeks of IFN-α treatment, flulike symptoms (fever, chills, myalgias, fatigue, and arthralgias) predominate. They usually occur 4 to 6 hours after drug administration and can be avoided by taking IFN-α before bedtime along with acetaminophen or a nonsteroidal anti-inflammatory drug such as ibuprofen. These symptoms usually resolve after a few weeks of continued therapy. Missing a dose or several doses can cause them to recur. In fact, daily dosing seems to be better tolerated and may have an ameliorative effect on viral clearance. Many of these side effects may be avoided in the future with pegylated IFN-α, a new formulation of the drug with a long half-life (see "Treatment of Chronic Hepatitis C Virus Infection with Interferons").

Of the other side effects seen with IFN-α, the most common are cytopenias, alopecia, thyroid dysfunction, and depression.[24, 80–83] Most of these are reversible. Careful monitoring of platelet and neutrophil counts is important, especially at the start of therapy. Periodic monitoring of thyroid-stimulating hormone levels during IFN-α therapy is helpful in detecting problems early on. Thyroid replacement therapy

TABLE 103–5 Alpha Interferons: Major Side Effects

- Flulike symptoms (malaise, myalgias, fever, chills)
- Gastrointestinal upset (nausea, weight loss)
- Cytopenias
  - Low white blood count (neutropenia)
  - Low platelet count
- Thyroid dysfunction
  - Hypothyroidism
  - Hyperthyroidism
- Hyperlipidemia (hypertriglyceridemia)
- Depression (suicidal ideation)
- Alopecia
- Miscellaneous
  - Skin rash
  - Neuro-ophthalmic changes
  - Dyspnea
  - Allograft rejection (mostly renal)

TABLE 103–6 Contraindications to the Use of Interferon-α

History of severe depression, especially suicide attempt
Uncontrolled thyroid disorders
Decompensated chronic hepatitis B virus infection
Low platelet count (less than 100,000/mm^3 for HBV or 70,000/mm^3 for HCV)
Low white cell count (absolute neutrophil count less than 1500/mm^3)
Organ transplant recipient (primarily renal)
Coronary artery disease
Terminal HIV infection
Recent history of malignancy

Abbreviations: HBV, Hepatitis B virus; HCV, hepatitis C virus; HIV, human immunodeficiency virus.

should be prescribed whenever necessary, but cases of hyperthyroidism may also occur. Depression is one of the more common side effects with IFN-α therapy and suicides have been reported. The onset of depressive symptoms usually occurs during the third or fourth month of IFN-α therapy. Monthly or more frequent visits are advisable for all patients receiving IFN-α and particularly for those who have a significant prior psychiatric history. For selected patients, psychiatric consultation is advisable before the initiation of IFN-α therapy, with close monitoring during the drug treatment. One should maintain a high index of suspicion for atypical symptoms and antidepressants should be prescribed as needed. Dose reduction or temporary discontinuation is required for any serious or ongoing adverse effects. Patients often have a recurrence of flulike symptoms upon resuming IFN-α and should be warned of this ahead of time. Specific contraindications to the use of interferon-α are listed in Table 103–6.

Other Drug Therapies for Chronic Hepatitis B

Several antiviral drugs that inhibit the replication of HBV have been evaluated as therapies for chronic hepatitis B. They include ganciclovir, lamivudine, famciclovir, adefovir, lobucavir, and BMS-200475.[84–93] Many of the new antivirals act as reverse transcriptase inhibitors and inhibit the replication of both HIV and HBV (Table 103–7). More specifically, during reverse transcription, lamivudine works as an RNA chain terminator by substituting for deoxycytidine, whereas adefovir, lobucavir, and other purine-based analogues serve primarily as blockers of protein priming at the 5′ end of genomic RNA.[90–93]

In contrast to HIV and other retroviruses, HBV does not integrate into the host's genome as part of its replication cycle. As a result, genomic and subgenomic transcripts of HBV are synthesized solely from "episomal" or nonintegrated covalently closed circular DNA (cccDNA). Because lamivudine acts primarily as a reverse transcriptase inhibitor, the cccDNA template remains intact and serves as a reservoir for new HBV virions when lamivudine is stopped.[90–94] Evidence for this comes from studies in humans in which in situ hybridization showed that HBV DNA persists unchanged in the liver as cccDNA even after 1 year of lamivudine therapy.[94] Perhaps with a longer duration of antiviral therapy using lamivudine alone or in combination with other agents, cccDNA might be reduced significantly or eliminated entirely through turnover of infected hepatocytes, thus preventing new replication cycles and recurrent infection with HBV.[89]

A potentially serious problem with the long-term administration of lamivudine is the emergence of viral escape mutants (about 15 to 30% per year of lamivudine therapy). Also, because chronic HBV infection lasts for decades, integration of cccDNA (or more often its fragments) into the hepatocyte genome occurs and may play an important role in carcinogenesis.[95] Whether lamivudine or any of the other nucleoside analogues can alter viral integration is unknown, although most of the evidence suggests that this is not the case.[89] With this background in mind, the therapeutic potential of individual antiviral agents in treating chronic HBV is discussed next.

Lamivudine

Lamivudine is the (−) enantiomer of β-L-2′,3′dideoxy-3′-thiacytidine, a nucleoside analogue that has potent activity as a reverse transcriptase inhibitor of both HIV and HBV.[91–94, 96–99] Lamivudine has been approved by the FDA for treating HIV[98] and for chronic hepatitis B (Epivir-HBV, Glaxo Wellcome, Research Triangle Park, N.C.). Lamivudine is rapidly absorbed, has excellent bioavailability, and is excreted almost entirely unchanged in the urine. Thus, dose adjustments are necessary for patients with renal failure. The active metabolite, lamivudine triphosphate, appears to act as an RNA chain terminator in HBV reverse transcription.[90–93] Lamivudine is a poor substrate for hepatocyte nuclear and mitochondrial DNA polymerases, and thus it does not share the toxicity of nucleoside analogues such as fialuridine that caused deaths from lactic acidosis, coagulopa-

TABLE 103–7 Antivirals for Chronic Hepatitis B Virus Infection

Drug Name	Mechanism of Action	Clinical Efficacy Reported to Date	Food and Drug Administration Status (United States)
Lamivudine (Epivir HBV, Glaxo Wellcome)	LAM triphosphate acts mostly as an RNA chain terminator in HBV DNA reverse transcription.	Rapid fall in serum HBV DNA levels with HB_eAg seroconversion in 16% at 1 year vs 4% in control subjects Concerns with YMDD mutants after long-term use before and after transplantation	Approved for chronic HBV infection Also approved for HIV infection, alone or in combination with zidovudine
Famciclovir (Famvir, SmithKline Beecham)	Primarily affects priming of RNA template with minor effects on RNA chain termination.	Converted intracellularly to active drug penciclovir Less effective than LAM for HBV but may be helpful in combination with LAM or other antivirals, especially after transplantation	Approved for herpesviruses (varicella and herpes simplex)
Adefovir dipivoxil (Gilead Sciences)	Inhibits protein priming of RNA template during HBV reverse transcription. May have important immunomodulatory effects.	Trials to date show potent effects on HBV replication May have synergistic effects when used in combination with LAM by reducing the risk of selecting out YMDD escape mutants	Phase III trials in progress
Lobucavir (Bristol-Myers Squibb)	Inhibits protein priming of RNA template.	Trials to date show potent effects on HBV replication May have synergistic effects when used in combination with LAM	Phase III trials stopped in May 1999 owing to higher rate of hepatoma
BMS-200475	Inhibits RNA priming and elongation.	Limited trials to date show considerable promise	Phase I/II trials in progress

Abbreviations: HBV, Hepatitis B virus; HIV, human immunodeficiency virus; LAM, lamivudine.

thy, and liver and renal failure as a result of mitochondrial poisoning.[100] Lamivudine is well tolerated with minimal if any side effects that are not dose limiting. The only clinical important drug interaction is with trimethoprim-sulfamethoxazole.[91–94, 98, 101–109]

In short-term phase II trials, lamivudine led to a rapid fall in serum levels of HBV DNA by over 90% (as measured by sensitive RT-PCR assays), even in patients who had not responded previously to therapy with IFN-α.[101–106] The suppression of HBV replication was almost complete within 2 to 3 weeks. Histologic evidence of piecemeal necrosis also improved after 6 months of lamivudine.[107] On the basis of these and subsequent trials, the minimum effective dose was found to be 100 mg/day. The degree of viral suppression was similar in Asian and non-Asian patients.[107–109] However, viral replication resumed rapidly after short-term therapy was stopped, and a sustained loss of HBV DNA and HB_eAg occurred in only 5 to 12% of patients receiving lamivudine.[103, 105, 107] Drug cessation was accompanied by a rebound in serum HBV DNA levels in some patients. During lamivudine therapy, serum ALT levels also rose significantly in about 40% of patients, possibly because of triggering of the immune system during viral clearance, as occurs with IFN-α.[107–111] Otherwise, only minimal elevations in creatinine kinase, amylase, and lipase have been noted, without any associated symptoms or other serious adverse side effects.[94, 102–109] In some patients, the flare in serum ALT levels may also occur after lamivudine has been stopped. This may be related to the emergence of viral escape mutants during lamivudine therapy that have a higher replicative potential and more efficient antigen production when antiviral treatment is withheld, although recurrence of wild-type virus may also lead to more aggressive liver damage.[110]

In several phase III trials, lamivudine has been used for a longer duration (12 months or more) with further evidence that it consistently suppresses HBV DNA replication, improves liver histology, and increases the rate of HB_eAg seroconversion.[94, 107–109] In a multicenter, randomized, placebo-controlled trial in China[94] in patients with active viral replication (defined as detectable HBsAg, HB_eAg, and HBV DNA for at least 6 months before enrollment), 358 Chinese patients were randomized to receive lamivudine (25 or 100 mg/day) or placebo. There were significant improvements in liver histology during 12 months of lamivudine therapy at both doses as compared with placebo, especially in patients with a more severe hepatitis score (Knodell's histologic activity index). Lamivudine at 100 mg/day also reduced the rate of progression to fibrosis, led to a sustained normalization of ALT, and, most important, resulted in HB_eAg seroconversion (defined as the loss of HB_eAg, development of anti-HB_e antibody, and undetectable HBV DNA) in 16% of patients receiving therapy compared with only 4% receiving placebo. When the study was extended for another 12 months as an open-label trial in 334 patients,[108] the HBV DNA clearance rate at the end of treatment was 52% in the patients who continued to take lamivudine (100 mg/day) for a full 2 years, compared with only 5% in those who were switched over to placebo after only 1 year of lamivudine. The end-of-treatment HB_eAg seroconversion rate was 27% after 2 years of lamivudine versus only 17% after 1 year of therapy. There were few study dropouts (more than 90% of patients completed the trials), and lamivudine was well tolerated with a side effect profile similar to that of placebo.

Essentially identical results were obtained in a U.S. multicenter trial[109] involving 137 patients with active HBV replication who were randomized to receive lamivudine at 100 mg/day or placebo for 52 weeks and followed up for 16 weeks after treatment. Even though serum HBV DNA levels were higher at baseline in the treated group than in control subjects, lamivudine led to end-of-treatment HB_eAg seroconversion (defined as undetectable HB_eAg, development of anti-HB_e antibody, and undetectable HBV DNA) in 17% compared with 6% for placebo. The end-of-treatment clearance rate of HB_eAg alone from the serum (without regard to the other defined components of HB_eAg seroconversion) was 32% for patients receiving lamivudine versus 11% for those given placebo. Of the patients in whom HB_eAg cleared by the end of treatment, more than 80% remained HB_eAg negative after 16 weeks of follow-up. Elevations of serum ALT levels (up to 10 times baseline) were seen in a minority of patients during therapy as well as after its completion.[110, 111] Otherwise, lamivudine was well tolerated. In general, the seroconversion of HB_eAg to HB_eAb with lamivudine appears to be durable.[112] Preliminary reports suggest that lamivudine may also be useful for patients with HBV precore mutants (detectable serum HBV DNA but no detectable serum HB_eAg), which are thought to cause more aggressive disease.[113, 114] The encouraging results of studies using lamivudine therapy before and after liver transplantation are discussed in "Hepatitis B Virus Infection and Liver Transplantation."

The optimal duration of lamivudine therapy for patients with HBV remains uncertain. Preliminary data suggest that immunohistochemical staining for HB_cAg on liver biopsy may be of help in deciding when to discontinue lamivudine.[115] However, the main problem with long-term lamivudine therapy is the emergence of genotypic resistance because of base pair substitution at specific sites within the YMDD locus of the DNA polymerase gene.[116–118] Most, if not all, of these mutations involve amino acid residue 552 or 558 and interfere with binding of lamivudine to viral reverse transcriptase.[119] Even though these mutations do not involve the *S* gene or envelope protein synthesis, HBV replication and viremia rapidly recur. In one preliminary report, escape mutants were found in 36% of the patients who had received lamivudine for over 26 weeks.[118] However, in trials involving more patients, YMDD mutants were detected in only 15% of those treated with lamivudine for up to 52 weeks. The mutants tended to emerge later in therapy (after 36 weeks) and were associated with a rise in serum ALT and HBV DNA levels but not back to baseline values.[94, 108, 120] Of concern is the fact that when lamivudine was used to treat recurrent HBV after liver transplantation, YMDD mutants were noted in 30% of patients after only 1 year of therapy.[121]

In patients who have developed escape mutants, continuing lamivudine therapy may still be helpful because HB_eAg seroconversion has been reported in some cases.[122] However, lamivudine escape mutants may also cause significant liver disease. In one report, three patients with recurrent HBV after transplantation went on to develop fibrosing cholestatic hepatitis and liver failure after the emergence of lamivudine-induced mutants. Famciclovir was of no benefit, although ganciclovir helped to save two of the three patients.[123] On the other hand, as noted earlier, stopping lamivudine therapy may actually cause a rebound in HBV replication and an acute exacerbation of liver disease with possible decompensation.[110] In most instances, therefore, lamivudine should not be stopped unless HB_eAg seroconversion has been confirmed, as this approach avoids HBV reactivation upon lamivudine withdrawal.[84–88] Nevertheless, in one report, discontinuing lamivudine temporarily was found to permit the restoration of wild-type virus as the predominant species, after which lamivudine could be re-introduced to control HBV replication successfully before new mutants recurred.[124]

Another therapeutic strategy being actively explored is to combine lamivudine with IFN-α in an attempt to enhance the clearance of virally infected hepatocytes and also to reduce the risk of developing viral escape mutants. In a preliminary report of a multicenter trial from Canada, Europe, and Australia,[125] 226 treatment-naive patients with chronic hepatitis B were randomized to receive lamivudine at 100 mg/day for 52 weeks, IFN-α2b at 10 MU three times a week for 16 weeks, or lamivudine at 100 mg/day initially for 8 weeks followed by lamivudine plus IFN-α2b at 10 MU three times a week for another 16 weeks (combination therapy). The rate of HB_eAg seroconversion (i.e, undetectable HB_eAg and HBV DNA, detectable anti-HB_e antibody) was similar in the three groups at weeks 52 and 64. Even though a somewhat higher seroconversion rate was seen with combination therapy, it did not reach statistical significance. There were also no major differences in the degree of histologic improvement among the three groups.[125]

In terms of patients with chronic hepatitis B who have not

responded to a standard course of IFN-α, one study[126] assessed nine such patients who were given IFN-α at 10 MU three times a week plus lamivudine at 100 mg/day for 16 weeks but found no benefit in sustained virologic response or immune function or T helper responses in particular. In a large trial involving IFN-α nonresponders,[127] 238 patients with chronic HBV were randomized to receive placebo for 68 weeks, lamivudine at 100 mg/day initially for 8 weeks followed by the same dose of lamivudine plus IFN-α2b at 10 MU three time a week for the next 16 weeks, or lamivudine at 100 mg/day for the first 52 weeks followed by randomization at week 52 to lamivudine at 100 mg/day or placebo until week 68. Liver biopsies were performed before treatment and again at week 52 to assess histologic response. At week 52, histologic response, sustained ALT normalization, and HB_eAg loss were best in the lamivudine monotherapy group. There was also a trend for HB_eAg seroconversion to HB_e antibody to occur more frequently in this group, but it did not reach statistical significance. Primary treatment comparisons were made at week 52, and this may have led to a bias in favor of the lamivudine monotherapy group because the combination therapy group had completed treatment much earlier at week 24. Combination therapy also resulted in substantially more adverse events.

In summary, lamivudine monotherapy is well tolerated and offers considerable benefit in terms of HB_eAg seroconversion for both IFN-α naive patients and those who have not responded to previous IFN-α therapy. Asian and non-Asian individuals appear to respond equally well. Trials are in progress to compare IFN-α monotherapy directly with lamivudine, because combination therapy does not appear to offer any particular advantage. However, long-term selection of escape mutants is a concern.

Famciclovir

Another antiviral agent effective against herpesviruses as well as HBV is famciclovir, the oral prodrug of penciclovir, an acyclic deoxyguanosine analogue[84–88, 90–92, 128] (see Chapter 36). Hepatocyte cellular enzymes catalyze the phosphorylation of penciclovir to its active form, penciclovir triphosphate.[129–132] The mechanism of action of this agent is uncertain, although it may inhibit reverse transcription by preventing priming of nascent strands or short-circuit HBV replication as a secondary chain terminator.[128] In all of the studies to date, famciclovir has been shown to have minimal, if any, side effects.[128, 129] Famciclovir (Famvir, SmithKline Beecham, Philadelphia, Pa.) has been approved by the FDA for the treatment of varicella-zoster and herpes simplex virus infections. However, famciclovir appears to be less potent than lamivudine for HBV.[84–88, 128–132]

Famciclovir has been shown to be reasonably effective against HBV. In a small trial[133] in nontransplant patients, famciclovir led to a dose-dependent inhibition of HBV replication with a fall in serum HBV DNA levels by more than 90% in 6 of the 11 patients studied. Data on HB_eAg and HBsAg were not reported. In a larger multicenter placebo-controlled trial with 333 HBV-positive patients,[128, 134] a 16-week course of famciclovir caused a significant fall in serum HBV DNA levels and a rapid normalization of serum ALT levels. The rate of HB_eAg seroconversion was 14% in treated patients compared with only 3% in those receiving placebo. As with IFN-α therapy for chronic HBV, high pretreatment serum ALT levels predicted a favorable response to famciclovir. However, compared with IFN-α therapy, famciclovir led to better response rates in Asian patients, in patients who acquired HBV by vertical transmission, and in nonresponders to IFN-α. Furthermore, there was no flare in serum ALT levels when the drug was stopped, although HBV replication recurred rapidly. In this study, the minimal effective dose of famciclovir was found to be 500 mg orally three times a day. For the most part, famciclovir was well tolerated.

Combining famciclovir (or penciclovir) with lamivudine may overcome some of the problems that may arise with escape mutants, because the drugs appear to work by different mechanisms. Lamivudine triphosphate has been shown to cause chain termination of nascent DNA strands by substituting for deoxycytidine, thereby inhibiting the RNA- and DNA-dependent HBV polymerases.[84, 90, 94] On the other hand, penciclovir triphosphate not only leads to chain termination and destabilization or defunctioning of viral genomes but also competes with guanosine triphosphate for the priming of reverse transcription and the synthesis of the DNA strand.[84, 86, 128–132] In a study using primary duck hepatocyte cultures from ducklings congenitally infected with duck HBV, penciclovir but not lamivudine inhibited the production of cccDNA and also prevented the expression of pre-S antigen (which is thought to be important in HBV binding and entry into uninfected hepatocytes). However, there were significant synergistic effects on HBV replication when both drugs were used in combination.[135] One note of caution: sequential rather than concurrent use of nucleoside analogues should be avoided, as it may predispose to the emergence of multidrug-resistant mutants, as occurs with HIV.[136]

Another potentially effective approach is to use an immunomodulatory drug in combination with famciclovir. In one report, thymosin-α_1 at 1.6 mg subcutaneously twice weekly plus famciclovir at 500 mg three times a day for 26 weeks led to a greater reduction in serum HBV DNA levels and to more frequent HB_eAg seroconversion than famciclovir used alone.[137]

Adefovir Dipivoxil

Adefovir dipivoxil (ADV, Gilead Sciences, Foster City, Calif.), the oral prodrug of phosphonyl-methoxyladenine, an acyclic nucleotide analogue of deoxyadenosine monophosphate, has been shown to be active against retroviruses, hepadnaviruses, and herpesviruses.[91, 92] In a phase I-II trial,[138] 20 HB_eAg-positive patients (13 coinfected with HIV) were randomized to receive ADV at 125 mg/day or placebo by mouth for 28 days, followed by 12 weeks of observation. The 15 patients receiving ADV had a significant reduction in their serum HBV DNA levels during therapy compared with the 5 patients given placebo. However, HB_eAg seroconversion was not observed in either group. A rise in serum ALT levels occurred in three patients while taking ADV and in four after the completion of therapy, mostly in HIV-negative individuals. Otherwise, the drug was tolerated well. In an extension of this trial,[139] 15 HB_eAg-positive patients from the original study (10 coinfected with HIV and 5 previous placebo recipients) were randomized to receive ADV at 60 or 120 mg/day for 24 weeks. A marked rise in serum ALT levels occurred in one patient given ADV, but the drug was held for 2 weeks and resumed with alternate-day dosing without any further problems. At the end of treatment, 4 of the 15 patients had undetectable serum HBV DNA; 3 had cleared HB_eAg, and 2 of these were anti-HB_e positive.

In a phase II dose-ranging study,[140] HB_eAg-positive patients with elevated serum ALT levels were randomized to receive placebo or 5, 30, or 60 mg of ADV daily for 12 weeks. All doses of ADV significantly reduced serum HBV DNA levels compared with placebo ($p<.001$), with the greatest reduction (a 4 $\log_{10}$ fall from baseline) observed with 30 and 60 mg/day. At 36 weeks of follow-up, HB_eAg seroconversion had occurred in 20% of patients receiving ADV at 30 or 60 mg/day versus none with placebo. A lower pretreatment serum HBV DNA level correlated with a higher likelihood of seroconversion. Four of the six HB_eAg seroconversions occurred during ADV therapy and were preceded by an elevation in serum ALT levels in all but one patient. In this report, 14 additional patients, all with normal serum ALT levels at baseline, were given ADV at 30 mg/day or placebo. However, no patient had HB_eAg seroconversion. Another study[141] has shown that the rise in ALT levels noted during therapy with ADV, especially in patients who go on to HB_eAg seroconversion, correlates with activation of the immune response, and this seems to occur more often in patients who have significant virus-specific T-cell reactivity before treatment with ADV. Nevertheless, other studies indicated that the rapid viral clearance seen with ADV may result from the nearly complete inhibition of HBV replication rather than the induction of accelerated viral clearance.[142]

In terms of viral cross-resistance, in preliminary studies the escape mutants that develop with lamivudine or famciclovir appeared to remain sensitive to ADV.[143–145] This is probably related to the different mechanisms by which these drugs affect viral reverse transcription. ADV blocks HBV protein priming, whereas lamivudine causes chain termination of nascent DNA strands by substituting for deoxycytidine, and famciclovir works by both mechanisms.[91, 92, 143–145] Thus, combining ADV with other nucleoside analogues may provide additional benefit.

Lobucavir

Lobucavir (Bristol-Myers Squibb, Princeton, N.J.) is another guanosine analogue with a broad spectrum of antiviral activity against HBV and all herpesviruses. This drug alters HBV replication primarily by blocking protein priming of the RNA template during reverse transcription.[86, 91, 92] In a double-blind, placebo-controlled trial in the United States and Canada,[146] 22 patients with chronic HBV infection were randomized to receive lobucavir at 200 mg by mouth, twice a day or four times a day, or placebo for 28 days. Both doses of lobucavir led to a significant 2 to 4 log reduction in serum HBV DNA levels, although the levels returned to baseline in all but one patient after the drug was stopped. Two of the patients treated with the higher dose of lobucavir had post-treatment elevations in serum ALT levels that subsequently returned to baseline. Overall, lobucavir was well tolerated.

In another phase II trial,[147] 95 patients (92% HB_eAg positive, 42% Asian, and 28% treated previously with IFN-α) were randomized to receive placebo or lobucavir at 200, 400, or 800 mg/day for 12 weeks, followed by 24 weeks of observation. All doses of lobucavir significantly reduced serum HBV DNA levels compared with placebo ($p<.001$), with a median 3 $\log_{10}$ fall from baseline. At 12 weeks, 68% of patients receiving lobucavir had undetectable serum HBV DNA versus only 9% on those given placebo. Data on HB_eAg seroconversion were not reported. Mild to moderate side effects were observed with lobucavir, but they were not any more severe or frequent than those with placebo. Lobucavir caused a rise in serum ALT levels but to a similar extent as placebo. After therapy, serum HBV DNA levels returned to baseline but without the rebound effect that has been seen with other antivirals. Similar results were observed in another study with lobucavir given at 200 mg/day for up to 6 months.[148] Unfortunately, the trials with lobucavir were discontinued when a higher rate of hepatoma was noted.

Miscellaneous Strategies

A novel carbocyclic nucleoside related to lobucavir, BMS-200475, has potent anti-HBV activity and is currently undergoing phase II clinical trials.[149] Other compounds of the L-nucleoside family such as the 5-fluoro congener of lamivudine, *cis*-5-fluoro-1-[2-(hydroxymethyl)-1,3-oxathiolan-5-yl]-cytosine, β-L-5-fluoro-2′,3′-dideoxycytidine, and 1-(2-fluoro-5-methyl-β-L-arabinofuranosyl)-uracil are being studied in patients with chronic HBV.[150–153] The safety and efficacy of combination therapies such as famciclovir plus IFN-α have not yet been assessed. Therapeutic vaccines against small "major" HBsAg (S) and pre-S2 or against the HB_cAg epitope attached to a T helper peptide such as tetanus toxoid are being studied, as are specific cytokines such as interleukin-2, interleukin-12, tumor necrosis factor-α, and IFN-γ.[154–158] Because proinflammatory cytokines alter the expression of viral transcripts in hepatocytes, combining them with nucleoside analogues may also prove useful for enhancing viral clearance. Adoptive transfer to boost the immune response has not been practical to date. Antisense oligonucleotides directed against conserved regions of HBV RNA may modulate HBV replication effectively, although the delivery of large concentrations of these molecules has been difficult in vivo, a problem similar to that encountered with the use of ribozymes or dominant negative mutants to deactivate RNA and DNA during viral replication.[159, 160]

Hepatitis B Virus Infection and Liver Transplantation

One of most challenging areas involves HBV-infected patients with end-stage liver disease who undergo liver transplantation.[24, 161–166] Currently in the United States, about 25% of liver transplantations are performed for viral hepatitis, and close to 25% of these involve HBV-positive patients.[161, 162] The number of such patients is sizable and the costs of allograft failure enormous, because HBV recurrence is almost universal without prophylaxis. The sources for reinfection of the allograft are thought to be preexisting virions in the circulation or those derived from extrahepatic reservoirs such as bone marrow and peripheral blood mononuclear cells.[167] Immunosuppression, especially with corticosteroids, appears to enhance HBV replication after transplantation. In most patients, HBV recurrence is tolerated reasonably well,[166] but in some, cirrhosis may occur as soon as 8 months after transplantation.[168] A particularly aggressive form, fibrosing cholestatic hepatitis, may develop in nearly 25%.[169] Retransplantation leads to dismal results, and allograft failure and death almost invariably occur.[170] Precore mutants may also be associated with a more serious outcome.[171]

The risk of HBV recurrence in the liver allograft correlates closely with pretransplantation levels of circulating HBV DNA in the recipient. In patients with active replication who are HB_eAg and HBV DNA positive, nearly 100% of allografts become infected within days or weeks after transplantation versus only 30% in nonreplicators.[172–175] Patients who undergo liver transplantation for fulminant hepatic failure related to acute HBV infection and those with HBV who are coinfected with HDV usually have a low recurrence rate, probably because minimal levels of circulating HBV DNA are present at the time of the transplantation.[176] Recipients who are positive for antibody to HB_cAg (anti-HB_c) before liver transplantation appear to be at low risk for HBV recurrence after transplantation, because the major source of any residual cccDNA is removed during the transplantation operation itself. However, a significant risk of HBV transmission has been documented in recipients who receive organs from anti-HB_c–positive donors.[177, 178]

In a study from four major U.S. liver transplantation centers,[177] among 932 HBsAg-negative donors, 36 (3.7%) were found to be anti-HB_c positive. Of the 23 evaluable liver recipients, 19 (83%) became HBsAg positive after 3.2 years of follow-up. All 19 developed chronic infection and 18 became HB_eAg positive. Although the numbers were small, positive anti-HB_s in the recipient de novo or after HBV vaccination did not confer any protection. On liver biopsy, 12 of 14 patients had minimal changes after 1 year, but at later time intervals more than 60% had active inflammation. Donors with anti-HB_c as their only marker of HBV replication probably have latent hepatic HBV infection as well as levels of systemic viremia that are too low to be detected by currently available methods. Consequently, most experts recommend prophylaxis with lamivudine or high-dose polyclonal anti-HB_s immunoglobulin (HBIG) or both, similarly to recipients who are HBsAg positive before transplantation (see later). However, the duration of therapy remains uncertain. Fortunately, HBV acquired de novo via the allograft appears to be less severe than recurrent HBV infection after transplantation.[177, 178]

In patients who are HBsAg positive before transplantation, the risk of recurrent HBV infection after transplantation has been reduced from about 75% to less than 35% with long-term administration of HBIG. Serum levels of anti-HB_s should be maintained above 100 IU/liter and preferably above 250 IU/liter. However, large intravenous doses of HBIG are required at the time of transplantation, daily during the first postoperative week, and then on a monthly basis. Fever, chills, and myalgias are common with HBIG administration but can be minimized with appropriate preliminary medications. Another problem is the expense of HBIG, estimated at more than $20,000 a year.[161, 162, 167, 172–175] For convenience and lower cost, some centers now use intramuscular HBIG, although it has not yet been approved by the FDA for that purpose.[162] Despite the widespread use of high-dose HBIG, nearly 20% of patients have a recurrence of detectable HBsAg after transplantation and a significant proportion develop hepatic inflammation without any detectable HBsAg.[172, 173] This breakthrough phenomenon may occur as a result of inadequate anti-HB_s titers and unusually high viral loads. However, the primary reason appears to be mutations in the *a* determinant region of the *S* gene induced or selected for by immune pressure related to HBIG.[179–181] In addition, as noted earlier, de novo acquisition caused by reactivation of HBV in recipients of livers from anti-HB_c–positive donors has been found to be another important source of HBV infection after transplantation.[177, 178]

Several therapeutic modalities other than HBIG have been used to prevent or treat HBV recurrence after transplantation, but most have not yet had a major impact. IFN-α can rarely be given before transplantation because of the risk of inducing a rapid deterioration in liver function associated with immunologic flare in patients with end-stage HBV disease.[182] One strategy has been to use IFN-α instead after liver transplantation. In one study,[183] 14 patients with recurrent HBV after transplantation were treated with IFN-α2b at 3 MU three times a week. Four patients cleared HBV DNA (by bDNA assay), but only one lost HB_eAg and another lost both HB_eAg and HBsAg. One patient had evidence of graft rejection while receiving IFN-α. Concerns have been raised that IFN-α may trigger graft rejection because of its ability to enhance human leukocyte antigen presentation on hepatocytes.[184] In another report,[185] two patients (one with HDV) responded favorably to high-dose IFN-α therapy.

A promising strategy for preventing as well as treating recurrent HBV infection after transplantation is the use of antivirals, either alone or in combination with HBIG. Of these, lamivudine has shown the most promise to date.[186–192] Lamivudine may also forestall the need for liver transplantation in selected cases.[190, 191] More details regarding the use of this drug in nontransplantation patients with chronic hepatitis B can be found in "Other Drug Therapies for Chronic Hepatitis B." In a preliminary study in the United Kingdom using a "preemptive" strategy with lamivudine, 10 patients began this drug before receiving a liver transplant and continued to take lamivudine for at least 24 weeks after transplantation. Despite the fact that HBIG prophylaxis was not used in the study protocol, HBV recurrence was documented in only 1 of the 10 patients after transplantation.[186]

In a larger preemptive trial in the United States and Canada,[190] 78 patients awaiting a liver transplant for end-state HBV cirrhosis who had detectable serum HBsAg (detectable HB_eAg in 49% and HBV DNA in 29%) began lamivudine at 100 mg/day at variable time points before transplantation and continued it for 52 weeks after transplantation. In 19 cases, the patient's liver disease stabilized to such a degree with lamivudine that transplantation could be postponed indefinitely. Of the 78 patients enrolled, 42 went on to transplantation. Lamivudine was continued after transplantation but HBIG prophylaxis was not given, according to the study protocol. The preliminary analysis included 38 patients treated with lamivudine for a median of 32 days before transplantation and for at least 6 months after transplantation. Of the 34 patients evaluated at week 24 after transplantation, all (100%) had cleared serum HBV DNA. However, 2 of the 12 patients tested at week 52 (18%) had elevated serum HBV DNA levels, probably related to the emergence of escape mutants. Ten of the 12 (83%) evaluable patients remained clear of both HB_eAg and HBsAg by week 52. Of the original 38 patients, only 5 went on to develop YMDD escape mutants while taking lamivudine (three before and two after transplantation). Overall, lamivudine therapy was well tolerated and of the 14 study withdrawals, none was related to the drug.

For the treatment of HBV recurrence after transplantation, the most extensive trial reported to date used lamivudine at 100 mg/day in 67 liver recipients who were found to be HBsAg positive after transplantation.[191] After 6 weeks of lamivudine, all 52 evaluable patients (100%) had cleared serum HBV DNA. After 52 weeks of therapy, 75% of the 51 evaluable patients remained clear of HBV DNA; 35% had cleared HB_eAg and 7% had cleared HBsAg. Serum ALT levels and histology also improved significantly with lamivudine. However, by the end of therapy, 14 patients (30%) had developed breakthrough HBV replication, and 7 of them had an increase in serum ALT levels, although none deteriorated clinically. All 14 of these patients were found to have YMDD escape mutants. Nevertheless, lamivudine was well tolerated and only 1 of the 11 study withdrawals was directly linked to the drug.

In a small trial involving 12 liver recipients,[192] lamivudine at 100 mg/day was started within 8 weeks of HBsAg reappearance after transplantation and the patients were observed for a mean of 68 weeks. Lamivudine led to a sustained inhibition of viral replication and normalization of serum ALT levels in the majority. Almost 75% cleared HBV DNA by bDNA and 45% became HBsAg negative. However, breakthrough replication occurred in three of the five HBsAg-negative patients as a result of viral resistance. Although these studies are not directly comparable, it appears that lamivudine is best started before transplantation, because half as many patients developed escape mutants with this approach as when lamivudine was begun after transplantation and HBV recurred in the allograft.[193–195]

The reason for the higher mutation rate after transplantation remains unknown, although a higher viral load resulting from concurrent immunosuppression probably plays a major role. Another possibility is that surgical removal of the recipient's liver, which is predominantly infected with cccDNA, may permit other HBV virions (presumably escape mutants) derived from extrahepatic sources to infect the donor liver at the time of transplantation, when cccDNA has not yet had sufficient time to regain a foothold.[162, 167] Whatever the case, a dilemma arises: starting lamivudine too early before transplantation may lead to a higher rate of viral mutation, which in the long run could make the management of HBV both before and after transplantation even more challenging because of escape mutants. On the other hand, waiting too long to begin lamivudine therapy may permit further deterioration of liver function, prompting urgent transplantation for survival. Ongoing studies should help clarify the best timing for lamivudine in patients with chronic HBV infection.[167, 196, 197]

In terms of other antiviral agents, ganciclovir was promising in a small study of HBV recurrence after transplantation, but this drug has significant myelosuppressant effects.[198] Famciclovir has been used with some success as prophylaxis,[167, 199, 200] as well as to treat recurrent HBV after transplantation.[167, 201–204] In a pilot study[201] of 11 transplant recipients who were reinfected with HBV despite HBIG prophylaxis, famciclovir at 500 mg by mouth three times a day for a minimum of 12 weeks led to a 90% fall in serum HBV DNA levels by 6 months of therapy, clearance of HBV DNA in 50% of patients by conventional bDNA, and normalization of serum ALT levels in 33%. A subsequent trial[202] involving 107 patients with recurrent HBV after transplantation showed similar results when famciclovir was used for up to 4 years. By the end of the first year, HBV DNA levels had fallen by a median of 95%, and after 2 years, they had fallen by close to 99%, with significant improvements in serum ALT levels and liver histology. Several smaller studies confirmed the safety and efficacy of famciclovir for recurrent HBV.[203–206]

As with lamivudine, escape mutants have been reported during the long-term use of famciclovir but they involve mostly the B domain of the HBV polymerase gene rather than the C domain (YMDD motif), more characteristic of lamivudine.[207–210] In a study of eight patients with recurrent HBV after transplantation treated with lamivudine after nonresponse, low response, or breakthrough to famciclovir, all patients responded initially to lamivudine with no evidence of cross-resistance. As well, there were no uniform mutations in the B or C domains of the polymerase gene, which correlated with the type of initial response to famciclovir. However, of three patients who later developed breakthrough YMDD mutants resistant to lamivudine, two initially had mutation L528M, which has been associated with famciclovir resistance.[211] Combination therapy with various antiviral agents has also shown some promise in preliminary reports. Lamivudine given before and continued after transplantation in conjunction with HBIG prophylaxis after transplantation may be more effective than lamivudine used alone. In one study,[212] 14 patients who underwent liver transplantation for HBV-related disease (4 of them HBV DNA positive initially and 1 at transplantation) were started with lamivudine at 150 mg/day before or at the time of transplantation and maintained with it indefinitely after transplantation. HBIG was given in the standard manner at the time of transplantation and thereafter. At a median follow-up of 1.1 years after transplantation, none of the 13 surviving patients had detectable circulating HBV DNA. One patient died from unrelated causes. All five HBV DNA–positive patients became negative by a median of 28 days after starting lamivudine.

However, despite the potential of HBIG passive immunity to inhibit viral replication and prevent the emergence of lamivudine-resistant mutants, the overlapping reading frames of the polymerase and envelope HBV genes may actually lead to further problems. Mutations in the polymerase gene induced by lamivudine may change the antigenicity of HBsAg with reduced efficacy of HBIG prophylaxis, whereas HBIG-induced mutations in the envelope gene may induce HBV polymerase resistance to lamivudine.[90, 165, 167]

CHRONIC HEPATITIS C

Around the world, chronic infection with HCV has reached epidemic proportions.[213] In the United States alone, nearly 4 million Americans are seropositive for HCV. This represents about 1.8% of the general population.[214–216] Among those acutely infected with HCV, more than 85% remain viremic in the long term. Of concern is a study that showed that, even in the 10 to 20% of individuals who have cleared the virus from the blood stream (determined by ultrasensitive RT-PCR), HCV persists indefinitely in the liver in 90% of cases.[12, 13] Another important problem with chronic hepatitis C is its seemingly indolent course with minimal if any symptoms. However, given sufficient time, chronic infection with HCV in the United States has been shown to cause almost 60% of the cases of chronic liver disease and result in 8000 to 10,000 deaths each year from end-stage liver disease and its complications, including hepatocellular carcinoma.[1, 214, 217, 218] Furthermore, the CDC estimated that the number of deaths caused by HCV-related disease will triple in the next 10 to 20 years.[219]

In terms of the burden to society, the annual costs for patients with HCV in the United States were estimated to be more than $600 million in 1992, almost the same as that for patients with HBV, $660 million (CDC, unpublished data). Furthermore, more than 30% of liver transplantations now performed in the United States are for patients with end-stage liver disease related to chronic HCV. When patients with alcoholic liver disease coinfected with HCV are included, the figure is perhaps as high as 45%.[220] Despite FDA approval of three interferons as well as ribavirin (in combination with IFN-α), current antiviral therapy remains of limited benefit and is associated with significant side effects. However, the crystalline structure of the HCV serine protease has been described,[221–224] and therapeutic agents specifically targeted at viral replication are under development.

Virology

Details of the virology of HCV are discussed in Chapter 143. Briefly, HCV is a member of the Flaviviridae family and is a spherical, enveloped, single-stranded RNA virus that is 9.4 kb in length. The HCV genome has a single open reading frame that codes for a precursor polypeptide of nearly 3010 amino acids. This is split into at least three structural proteins (core and two envelope) at the 5′ end and several nonstructural proteins (including helicase, RNA polymerase, and serine protease) at the 3′ end.[225] Because of the critical role of the serine protease in splitting off other proteins needed for HCV replication, this enzyme is an attractive target for future anti-HCV therapy, an approach similar to that used with many of the newer anti-HIV agents.[221–224] There are at least six main HCV genotypes and more than 40 subtypes within these types. Genotype 1b tends to cause more aggressive liver disease, is more resistant to therapy with interferons, and may lead to a worse outcome after liver transplantation. The viral genotypes tend to follow a discrete geographic distribution, with type 1 being the most common in the United States (about 75% of all genotypes) and 1a almost equal in frequency to 1b, whereas in Japan and Europe genotypes other than 1 predominate. These local variation in HCV genotype must be taken into consideration when analyzing the results of therapeutic trials or assessing the potential risks for complications such as cirrhosis and hepatocellular carcinoma.[226–228]

HCV replication results in frequent errors in RNA transcription. HCV may mutate readily in response to host immunologic pressure, and as a result the virus often exists in a heterogeneous population of closely related, although slightly different, genetic sequences called *quasispecies*. This may be one of the reasons why so many patients remain chronically infected. Quasispecies can change rapidly in response to the host's immunologic pressure, which permits viral escape. This phenomenon may also explain the reported variation in long-term outcome exclusive of other factors such as viral genotype and viral load. The number of HCV quasispecies has been found to be low in immunocompromised individuals, which suggests that the immunologic pressure on HCV to mutate is minimal in these patients.[229]

Epidemiology

Over the past few years, various population-based and sentinel surveillance studies have helped define the epidemiology of acute and chronic HCV infection and disease. An estimated 4 million Americans (or 1.8% of the general population) have a positive test for HCV antibody in the serum, according to the Third National Health and Nutrition Examination Survey conducted in the United States from 1988 to 1994 with a sample of noninstitutionalized civilians.[217, 218, 230, 231] Studies have also shown serologic evidence that HCV infection is present in as many as one of every five individuals evaluated in inner-city emergency departments[232, 233] and in one of every three prisoners.[234, 235] Furthermore, 85 to 100% of intravenous drug users in some areas of the United States may be infected with HCV.[1, 219] For acute HCV, the highest incidence rate at present is in young adults between the ages of 20 and 39 years, with a slight male preponderance, and in more Hispanics than in representatives of other ethnic or racial groups. In contrast, chronic HCV has the highest prevalence rates in African American males between the ages of 30 and 49 years.[214, 215, 217–219]

The dramatic 80% fall in the incidence of acute HCV infection correlates well with the introduction of surrogate testing of blood products in 1986 and HCV antibody testing in 1989, as well as the decline in acute cases associated with injection drug use, although the reason for the latter remains unknown.[236] The use of blood products remained the most common cause of acute and chronic HCV, or "non-A, non-B" hepatitis as it was called,[237] until 1989, when innovative molecular biology techniques were developed to identify specific antibodies to the structural and nonstructural proteins produced by HCV.[238, 239] Screening for hepatitis A and B had begun in the early 1970s and screening for HIV in 1985. An elevated serum ALT level in a blood donation was first used as a surrogate marker for non-A, non-B hepatitis in the United States starting in 1986. This reduced the incidence of new cases of post-transfusion hepatitis to a significant extent. However, in Canada, where surrogate testing was not adopted, nearly 80,000 people became infected with HCV between 1986 and 1990.[240, 241]

With the availability of screening HCV serologic tests after 1989, acute HCV infection was found to be the cause of more than 80% of cases of post-transfusion hepatitis.[214–217, 236] After widespread screening for HCV in all blood products in the United States, the incidence of acute HCV, which had reached a peak in the 1980s at about 180,000 cases per year, fell by more than 80% to less than 30,000 cases per year by 1995.[242] Although the relative risk of acquiring HCV was only 0.45% per unit transfused, most individuals received two or more blood transfusions. As a result, 10 to 20% of individuals who had received multiple blood transfusions or plasma products before serologic testing for HCV were later found to be HCV antibody positive.[214] In the United States, with current screening techniques, the risk has now fallen significantly to about 1 in 100,000 units transfused, or a 0.001% chance.[217, 242] A small residual risk of acquiring HCV from blood products remains at present, because even the most sensitive immunoassay tests for HCV antibody take 3 to 4 months to become positive after an individual is exposed to HCV. The use of more sensitive tests such as RT-PCR to screen blood donations for HCV would probably reduce the risk even further but at considerable expense.[243]

The worldwide prevalence of HCV determined by serologic tests of blood donors using second- or third-generation immunoassays is thought to be close to 1%. However, the prevalence in blood donors varies widely from less than 1% in the United States, Canada, and northern Europe, to intermediate higher rates (1.4 to 2.1%) in Thailand, Malaysia, and India, to the highest rates in Ukraine (9.2%) and in northern and sub-Saharan Africa and Arabic countries, including Egypt (14.5%). Immigrants to the United States from countries with high endemicity (such as Africa, the Middle East, and countries of the former Soviet Union) should be screened for chronic HCV because reusable syringes or needles and various other local practices may have put them at higher than usual risk.[214, 228]

In a CDC study of the sentinel countries, important risk factors for HCV other than blood products have been identified (Table 103–8). Intravenous drug use is now one of the most common causes in the United States, but intranasal cocaine use ("snorting"), a previously unidentified factor, may prove to be the most frequent source of HCV infection because of its widespread popularity. Cocaine snorting appears to result in nasal ulceration and bleeding, which serves as a source for HCV transmission, and could explain the high number of cases in the previously "unknown" risk category of patients with chronic hepatitis C.[216–219]

Sexual transmission of HCV has been reported but at a considerably lower rate than for HBV. This is probably related to the fact that HCV RNA has not been detected in semen, vaginal fluid, urine, or stool,[244, 245] although low levels of HCV RNA are found in saliva.[246, 247] Other important contributors to HCV transmission between couples may include the shared use of razor blades or toothbrushes[219] or other risk factors such as injection drug use in one of the partners.[248] For heterosexual couples living in a monogamous relationship for 10 to 20 years, studies from the United States and Europe have demonstrated that the risk of HCV transmission is about 5%,[217, 219, 248–256] although higher rates (7 to 28%) have been reported from Asia.[228, 253, 257] Nevertheless, a study from Japan showed that the risk of HCV transmission remains insignificant for heterosexual couples even after living together for 30 years, and the risk rose only slightly thereafter.[258] In a study from Italy that used sensitive viral typing techniques to assess couples in which both partners were infected with HCV, each partner was actually found to have a different viral subtype.[259] Therefore, each person probably acquired the infection from a source other than his or her partner.[260]

Although the risk associated with a single sexual encounter appears to be small, a history of multiple sexual partners before the age of 25 was found to be a risk factor in the sentinel countries study.[214–219] Another study confirmed that the relative risk of HCV infection increases with the number of sexual partners, especially when there is no history of parenteral exposure.[261] Prostitutes are more likely to be HCV seropositive, particularly if they have additional risk factors such as a high number of sexual partners, traumatic sexual activity, failure to use a condom, injection drug use, and a positive test for syphilis.[262–265] Therefore, safe sex practices should be strongly advised for these people and those in other age categories at risk for a similar reason. Gay men are not at more risk for HCV acquisition even when they have a higher number of sexual partners.[266] Furthermore, the prevalence of HCV seropositivity is similar in heterosexual and homosexual partners.[249] In terms of coinfection with HIV, one study showed an increased risk of HCV transmission from 4 to 9%.[251]

There have been no reports of any direct transmission through nonsexual household contact. In health care workers, the risk of acquiring HCV from a random needlestick injury is about 0.1% and rises to 5 to 10% if the index case has confirmed HCV viremia.[217–219] Overall, about 2% become viremic or develop anti-HCV antibodies. HCV transmission appears to be more likely with hollow cannula devices than with solid needles.[267] Simultaneous transmission of HIV and HCV has been documented after a needlestick injury, with rapid progression to liver failure and death.[268] Colonoscopes and barbershop razors have been reported as unusual modes of transmission, probably related to inadequate sterilization of the equipment.[269, 270]

The risk of HCV transmission from mother to infant appears to be low, reported at about 5%, whereas with active HBV infection transmission rates may reach 90%.[217–219, 271] As with HBV, transmission of HCV probably occurs during labor and delivery rather than in utero, because HCV RNA has been detected in puerperal fluid.[271] The risk of HCV transmission also appears to correlate with the level of circulating HCV RNA in the mother.[272, 273] Thus, with HIV-positive mothers, whose circulating HCV RNA levels tend to be higher than those of HIV-negative mothers, the rate of mother-to-infant transmission of HCV may be as high as 22%.[272, 273] However, if HCV RNA is absent in maternal blood, the risk of HCV transmission to the infant is extremely low.[274–279] It is important to note that anti-HCV antibody should not be used to screen infants because there may be passive transplacental transfer of this antibody. Instead, qualitative testing for HCV RNA by the sensitive RT-PCR technique provides the best approach to confirming HCV transmission in neonates and infants. In one study, HCV RNA was found in the cord blood of 40% of neonates born to mothers with anti-HCV antibody.[280] To date, HCV RNA has not been detected in breast milk and there are no reports of HCV transmission via breast-feeding.[217, 281]

TABLE 103–8 Major Risk Factors for Acquiring Hepatitis C

Injection drug use
Blood transfusions before 1992
Clotting factor concentrates before 1985 (factor VIII) or 1987 (factor IX)
Intranasal cocaine use (snorting)
Multiple sexual partners (not with long-term monogamous relationship)
Lower socioeconomic status
Perinatal (especially if mother is HIV positive)
Miscellaneous (e.g., tattoos, occupational, multiple STDs)

Abbreviations: HIV, Human immunodeficiency virus; STD, sexually transmitted disease.

Pathogenesis

For the most part, liver injury caused by HCV appears to be mediated via direct viral cytopathic effects rather than immunologic events, in contrast to the case of HBV, where the reverse applies. However, evidence suggests a significant correlation between host cytotoxic T-lymphocyte responses and the degree of hepatocellular injury.[282] Immunoregulatory cytokines also appear to play an important role in facilitating the immune response and clearing the virus through T helper ($CD4^+$) cell activation. Most individuals with acute HCV infection who clear the virus and do not progress to chronic viremia demonstrate a strong Th1 (cell-mediated) response with little or no Th2 (humoral) response, whereas those with chronic hepatitis C viremia show the reverse.[283–286] This suggests that an enhanced humoral immune response may prevent immune clearance of HCV. The degree of liver injury has also been linked to enhanced expression of the Th1 cytokines interleukin-2 and IFN-γ, because patients with advanced disease or cirrhosis have higher levels of these cytokines than control subjects or those with milder disease.[286]

In terms of immunomodulatory therapy, IFN-α tends to decrease Th2 cytokines such as interleukin-10.[287] As a result, IFN-α may downregulate the immune-inhibiting effects of the Th2 immune response and thereby restore the Th1 immune response to normal, which leads to HCV clearance. Nevertheless, despite Th2 downregulation, an enhanced Th1 cytokine profile is not seen uniformly in all interferon responders. This could explain the high relapse rate after IFN-α is stopped. Mechanisms other than immune modulation may therefore be operative. Clearly, iron and iron-binding proteins alter the degree to which chronic HCV infection leads to hepatocellular damage as well as the response to antiviral therapy, although the exact role of iron remains unclear.[288] Multicenter trials are in progress to answer this important question. A major problem in studying HCV has been the absence of an in vitro cell culture system, which has limited studies of pathogenesis as well as inhibited the development of antiviral drugs.[289–291]

Natural History

In a study by Seeff and colleagues[292] of veterans infected with HCV via blood transfusions, the risk of dying because of liver complications was only slightly increased, even though 20% already had cirrhosis on liver biopsy. Subsequent studies suggest a more aggressive and serious problem with chronic HCV.[293] It is now estimated that 10 to 30% of patients infected with HCV progress to cirrhosis over the course of 20 to 30 years, and 1 to 5% develop hepatocellular carcinoma.[294–296] However, the degree and rapidity of progression are difficult to predict for any individual.[297] Various factors appear to play a role, including gender, viral load, duration of infection, mode of infection, hepatic iron content, and alcohol consumption. Cirrhosis appears to be more common in patients who acquired HCV from blood transfusions than in injection drug users, even accounting for disease duration.[298, 299] Patients infected when very young or very old appear to fare less well. Although genotype 1b has been thought to be an important factor in the development of cirrhosis,[300] studies suggest that this genotype was the most common one found in the 1960s. Therefore, genotype 1b may not in itself cause more severe liver disease, apart from being associated with a longer disease duration than that of other genotypes.[301, 302]

Excess alcohol ingestion also worsens the outcome of patients with chronic HCV. In general, up to 25% of alcoholics are infected with HCV when tested via antibody screening.[303] The severity of liver disease in these patients and the long-term risk of progression of diseased correlate well with the presence of HCV antibody.[304] Although not conclusive, several studies have shown that active alcohol intake may increase serum HCV RNA levels even when alcohol is consumed in "social" amounts and worsen the severity of histologic damage and fibrosis.[305–307] Habitual drinkers with chronic HCV are more likely to develop fibrosis than nonhabitual drinkers.[307] In a large study in Italy,[308] the frequency of cirrhosis was increased 10-fold and that of hepatocellular carcinoma 5-fold in chronic alcoholics infected with HCV compared with those who were not. Similar results were found in another large study, this time in France.[298]

A U.S. retrospective study[303] confirmed that patients infected with HCV who had previously consumed significant amounts of alcohol (>40 g/day in women or >60 g/day in men for more than 5 years) had a two- to three-fold greater risk of cirrhosis and decompensation, independent of viral load, mode of transmission or gender, than those who did not consume such a high amount. By the second decade of follow-up, cirrhosis had developed in 58% of the group who drank heavily versus only 10% of the nonalcohol group. An Australian study[309] also showed that cirrhosis correlated best with the estimated total consumption of alcohol both during the patient's lifetime and throughout the duration of HCV infection. Average daily alcohol consumption appeared to be less helpful in predicting an adverse outcome. Differences in hepatic iron content associated with excess alcohol consumption may also explain some of these results (see later).

The main dilemma with treatment of chronic HCV remains that patients who might benefit from antiviral therapy are usually asymptomatic and in the earlier stages of the disease. When the disease progresses to more advanced stages, antiviral therapy may be contraindicated or less effective. In most cases, the progression to cirrhosis takes approximately 20 years, although the duration ranges from as little as 13 years in men who acquire HCV after age 40 to as much as 42 years in women who acquire HCV before age 40 and who do not consume alcohol. Without treatment, 33% of HCV patients had an expected median time to cirrhosis of less than 20 years, whereas 31% never progress to cirrhosis over a 50-year period. Certain characteristics, such as age, alcohol consumption, and male sex, are more strongly associated with the development of cirrhosis than are virologic factors.[24, 217–219, 310]

Another major concern is the risk of hepatocellular carcinoma, which may develop in 5% or more of patients with HCV after 30 years.[296, 301, 310–314] However, studies suggest that the risk of developing hepatoma may be attenuated to some degree with IFN-α therapy.[311–314] In two studies[311, 312] involving hundreds of patients with chronic hepatitis C, only 5% of those who were IFN-α complete or partial responders developed hepatoma at 5 years versus 20% of nonresponders, whether or not they had cirrhosis to begin with. Another study from France has also shown that patients with HCV who have developed cirrhosis may still benefit from IFN-α therapy to prevent hepatoma.[314]

Clinical Features and Diagnostic Studies

As with HBV, most individuals with chronic HCV remain asymptomatic until the ravages of end-stage liver disease and its sequelae supervene. Patients may occasionally recall a remote episode of jaundice and malaise, which was diagnosed as some other type of hepatitis. Risk factors for HCV acquisition should be addressed (see Table 103–8) and appropriate serologic studies ordered, depending on the individual's risk category. The serologic diagnosis of chronic HCV is discussed in Chapter 143. With post-transfusion hepatitis now so uncommon, a direct link to this risk factor is rare indeed. A variety of clinical syndromes have been associated with chronic HCV, as noted in Table 103–9. These may be the initial reason for presentation, and the diagnosis of HCV may not be suspected unless there is a high index of suspicion. Nonspecific symptoms of fatigue, malaise, or right upper quadrant discomfort are common with chronic HCV. However, any unusual symptoms such as fever, jaundice, weight loss, worsening abdominal pain, or ascites should prompt a workup for a complication such as hepatocellular carcinoma.

Management of patients with chronic HCV is dictated by the likelihood of disease progression and the need for antiviral treatment (for a management algorithm see Fig. 103–2). An essential part of the workup for those with confirmed viremia remains a liver biopsy in order to determine the severity of disease at baseline. If therapy is not warranted by these findings, most experts recommend a repeated liver biopsy in 4 or 5 years to evaluate for any progression.

TABLE 103–9 Syndromes Associated with Chronic Hepatitis C Infection
Persistently normal serum alanine aminotransferase
Essential mixed cryoglobulinemia (vasculitis)
Monoclonal gammopathies
Renal involvement (membranoproliferative glomerulonephritis)
Porphyria cutanea tarda
Sjögren's syndrome

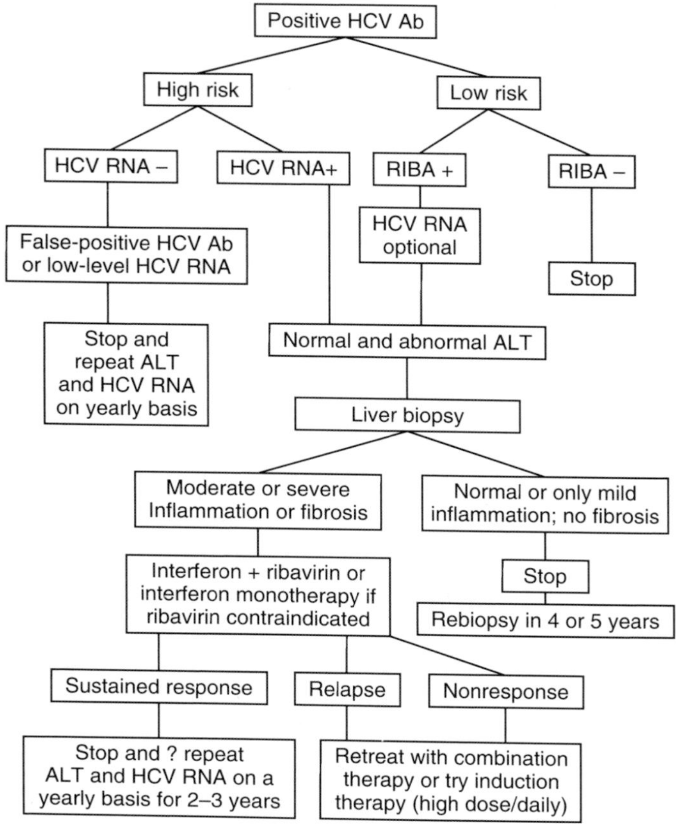

FIGURE 103–2. Algorithm for the management of patients with chronic hepatitis C virus infection.

One study[315] showed that empirical IFN-α monotherapy *without* a liver biopsy had marginal cost-effectiveness within the bounds of other commonly accepted therapies and missed none of the potentially sustained responders. However, this model used only a 6-month course with a standard dose of IFN-α, and thus the results may not apply to a longer duration of IFN-α monotherapy or combination therapy (IFN-α plus ribavirin). Because the field is changing so rapidly, local or national experts in addition to the most recent publications on HCV should be consulted for up-to-date recommendations on the workup and management of these patients.[1, 24, 219, 316–323]

Treatment of Chronic Hepatitis C Virus Infection with Interferons

For the foreseeable future and until specific inhibitors of HCV replication are introduced, IFN-α will remain the primary treatment modality for chronic HCV, either alone (as monotherapy) or together with the antiviral ribavirin (as combination therapy). After 12 to 18 months of standard-dose IFN-α therapy, about 15 to 20% of patients with chronic HCV achieve a long-term or sustained virologic response, as defined in the following.[316–323] Evidence suggests that patients who respond can expect prolonged clearance of HCV RNA from the serum[324] as well as a lowered risk of developing cirrhosis and hepatocellular carcinoma.[311–314] Nevertheless, IFN-α has important drawbacks in terms of cost (in the United States more than $700 a month) and side effects (see Table 103–5). Furthermore, more than two thirds of the patients treated with IFN-α do not achieve a sustained response, and most have relapses after IFN-α is stopped. About 15% may never respond despite repeated courses of IFN-α. However, studies have confirmed the safety and improved efficacy of combination therapy (IFN-α plus ribavirin) over IFN-α monotherapy in patients who have had relapses.[325] The new "consensus" interferon may be superior to combination therapy in efficacy for specific subgroups such as those with cirrhosis or genotype 1b or both.[326–331] Clinical trials are in progress to compare the two forms of therapy. It remains to be seen whether daily doses of IFN-α for the first month or two (so-called induction therapy) with or without ribavirin will provide additional benefit as initial therapy or for treating relapsers or nonresponders or both.[332–334]

Although the mechanisms of action of IFN-α in viral hepatitis remain uncertain, there is evidence that, in patients with chronic HCV, IFN-α clears virus by preventing de novo infection of susceptible hepatocytes rather than by inhibiting intracellular viral replication.[335–340] In patients who respond favorably to IFN-α, the balance between the Th1 (proinflammatory) and the Th2 (anti-inflammatory) immune response may be tipped in favor of Th1. Furthermore, patients who manifest primarily a Th2 response to HCV may be more likely to develop chronic viremia and respond less favorably to IFN-α.[282, 287] IFN-α may also work in chronic HCV infection by reducing viral heterogeneity so that there are fewer circulating quasispecies and less opportunity for HCV to escape the host immune response.[335]

Standard and Novel Types of Interferons Used for Treating Hepatitis C Virus Infection

In the United States, three α-interferons have been approved by the FDA for treating chronic HCV infection: IFN-α2b (IntronA, Schering-Plough, Kenilworth, NJ), IFN-α2a (Roferon-A, Hoffman-LaRoche, Nutley, NJ), and interferon alfacon-1, also known as consensus interferon (CIFN, Infergen, Amgen, Thousand Oaks, Calif.). IFN-α2b and IFN-α2a are human recombinant interferons produced by using a strain of *Escherichia coli* bearing genetically engineered plasmids that contain an IFN-α2b or IFN-α2a gene derived from human leukocytes.[316] In contrast, CIFN is a synthetic interferon developed by selecting the most common amino acid at each position from 11 naturally occurring IFN-α subtypes with the most activity against HCV.[326] CIFN has been reported to have 10-fold greater in vitro activity against HCV than IFN-α2b or IFN-α2a.[341] It is also important to note that the dose of CIFN is measured in micrograms rather than million units (MU). In general, a 9-μg dose of CIFN is equivalent to 3 MU of IFN-α2b or IFN-α2a, whereas 15 μg corresponds to 5 MU.[326–332] These α interferons are administered subcutaneously three times a week and each has its own FDA-approved indications (see Table 103–4).

Another new IFN-α is interferon alfa-n1 (IFN-αn1), which is derived from a human B lymphoid cell line after induction by the Sendai virus (Wellferon, Glaxo Wellcome, Research Triangle Park, NC). This unique IFN-α consists of over 22 components, 18 of which are similar to other IFN-α subtypes, and at least two additional proteins that are glycosylated, in contrast to IFN-α2b and IFN-α2a, which are single unglycosylated proteins.[342, 343] The optimal dosing schedule appears to be 3 MU subcutaneously three times a week for 12 months,[343] which may actually be more effective than standard-dose IFN-α2b or IFN-α2a.[344–346] Higher doses of IFN-αn1 may lead to more adverse effects.[343, 346, 347]

A long-acting formulation of IFN-α termed pegylated interferon (PEG-IFN) has been developed by covalently binding hairlike strands of an inert polymer, polyethylene glycol (PEG), to standard IFN-α by a process called pegylation. This modification delays the recognition of PEG-IFN as a foreign substance by the immune system, thus prolonging its half-life in the circulation. As a result, PEG-IFN can be administered only once a week, which may reduce many of the initial side effects as well as minimize the surges in serum HCV RNA levels seen with thrice-weekly dosing.[348–351] One type of PEG-IFN, pegylated-40k IFN-α2a (PEGASYS, developed by Hoffman-LaRoche and Shearwater Polymers) has shown promise in a phase II trial in which 155 noncirrhotic HCV-positive patients were randomized to receive PEGASYS in doses of 45, 90, 180, or 270 μg, or standard-dose IFN-α2a. More than 75% had genotype 1a or 1b, the HCV genotypes that are the most difficult to treat. The overall sustained virologic response (undetectable HCV RNA after 48 weeks of therapy and a 24-week observation period) with PEGASYS was 36% versus only 3% with standard-dose IFN-α2a. PEGASYS was tolerated to the same degree as standard-dose IFN-α2a, although neutrophil and platelet counts were lower with PEGASYS.[351] Currently, PEGASYS and other types of PEG-IFN are being evaluated in clinical trials in the United States and Europe.

Antiviral Treatment Response Scenarios

The terms therapeutic "response," "relapse," and "nonresponse" after a course of IFN-α need to be carefully defined. A response to therapy can be measured in one of three ways: biochemical (normalization of an elevated serum ALT level), virologic (clearance of circulating HCV RNA), or both. Early studies of chronic HCV therapy used only a biochemical end point of treatment (see later). However, about 10% of patients whose ALT levels become normal during IFN-α therapy continue to have detectable serum HCV RNA, and about 10% of patients who lose HCV RNA still have an abnormal ALT level, perhaps because of fatty liver, medications, or alcohol consumption, as noted earlier.[352] Thus, at present, the "gold standard" indicator of a treatment response is clearance of serum HCV RNA assessed by RT-PCR (qualitative or quantitative) rather than normalization of ALT levels alone, as was the case in earlier studies.[316–320]

The time point at which these indicators of a therapeutic response are assessed also has a direct bearing on the likelihood of a favorable long-term outcome. For instance, the response rate at the end of treatment is considerably higher than the sustained response rate measured at a future point in time, often taken to be at 6 or 12 months after therapy. This is the case because viral relapse tends to resume shortly after IFN-α is stopped, usually during the first few weeks after therapy. With time, the incidence of viral relapse appears to reach a plateau by the end of the first 6 to 12 months after drug cessation. Therefore, a sustained virologic response is defined as the absence of detectable circulating HCV RNA at the end of treatment, as well as on at least two occasions subsequently, during an observation period of 6 months or more.[316–320]

With IFN-α therapy, a number of clinical scenarios can be anticipated. Some patients respond within 2 to 4 weeks with normalization of ALT and rapid clearance of serum HCV RNA, although these may not always occur simultaneously. Of these two indicators, the more predictive of a sustained response is thought to be the clearance of HCV RNA.[353] Even though ALT may remain elevated, HCV recurrence is infrequent when HCV RNA remains consistently negative. In these cases, other causes of a persistently elevated ALT despite a negative HCV RNA should be explored, such as fatty liver; alcoholic liver disease; nonalcoholic steatohepatitis; and autoimmune, viral, metabolic, or other etiologies. Occasionally, a liver biopsy may be needed.

A sustained virologic response has now been identified as the best predictor of a favorable long-term outcome.[354, 355] In a retrospective study in France,[324] of 80 patients who had a sustained virologic response after a course of IFN-α (3 MU three times a week for 6 months in the majority), more than 95% remained clear of HCV infection (defined as no detectable circulating HCV RNA by bDNA) for a mean of 4 years and some for as long as 7 years. None of the 27 sustained virologic responders who had a follow-up liver biopsy were found to have any HCV RNA detectable in liver tissue. Evidence is also mounting that a sustained response to therapy, whatever the weekly dose or type of IFN-α used, has significant benefit in terms of reducing the risk of hepatocellular carcinoma.[311–314, 356, 357] In most instances, therefore, a sustained virologic response remains the gold standard of therapy at present.

Another possible scenario during IFN-α therapy is viral "breakthrough," in which a patient, after having had an initially favorable response to IFN-α therapy with complete clearance of circulating HCV RNA, has a recurrence despite continuing to take IFN-α. Patients with this pattern of response deserve more study. In a true viral relapse, circulating HCV RNA is no longer detectable at the end of IFN-α therapy but reappears later after treatment has been stopped. In contrast, nonresponse is defined as persistence of circulating HCV RNA despite a 12-week course of standard-dose IFN-α. With these definitions in mind, we can now assess key studies relevant to IFN-α therapy for patients with chronic HCV who have never been treated before (treatment naive), those who have had relapses after previously successful therapy (relapsers), and those who have not responded to any previous therapy (nonresponders).

Interferon Monotherapy Strategies for Treatment-Naive Patients

IFN-α was first shown to be of benefit for treatment-naive patients even before HCV was identified as the virus that causes post-transfusion (non-a, non-B) hepatitis.[358] Subsequent trials have confirmed the efficacy of IFN-α therapy in normalizing serum ALT levels and improving histologic changes on liver biopsy.[359–361] A few studies have also suggested additional long-term benefits such as reducing the risk of progression to cirrhosis or development of hepatocellular carcinoma.[311–314, 356, 357] These early studies looked almost exclusively at patients with chronic HCV infection who had abnormal ALT levels (usually more than 1.5 times normal) and those who fulfilled other entry criteria such as the presence on liver biopsy of severe necroinflammatory activity and advancing fibrosis assessed by a variety of scoring systems. However, accurate methods for detecting circulating HCV RNA levels with RT-PCR had not yet been developed and thus were not used in these trials.[316]

These early studies found that IFN-α2b or IFN-α2a at a dose of 3 MU three times a week usually for 6 months (so-called standard IFN-α therapy) led to a biochemical response (i.e., normalization of ALT levels) in well over 50% of treatment-naive patients. Unfortunately, after IFN-α therapy was stopped, more than half of these patients had relapses during the subsequent 6 months with a return of serum ALT levels to baseline.[316–320] Thus, the overall biochemical response rate with standard IFN-α therapy in these trials was at best 20 to 25%. However, these studies overestimated the actual response rates that were seen in clinical practice, because they included many patients who were more likely to respond to IFN-α to begin with, namely, those with HCV genotypes other than 1.[1, 24, 316–320]

Subsequent studies have shown that the sustained virologic response rate after standard IFN-α therapy with IFN-α2b or IFN-α2a (3 MU three times a week for 6 months) is only 10 to 15% in treatment-naive patients selected to be more representative of those living in the United States.[316–320, 362] CIFN has been shown to lead to similar response rates when given for 6 months.[326–332] In a multicenter, double-blind, controlled study,[328] 704 patients with chronic HCV were randomized to receive two different doses of CIFN (3 or 9 μg three times a week) or IFN-α2b at 3 MU three times a week for 6 months, followed by another 6 months of observation. Even though there were more patients with cirrhosis in the CIFN-treated groups, the sustained virologic response rate with CIFN at 9 μg (12%) was equivalent to that with IFN-α2b at 3 MU (11%) and better than that with CIFN at 3 μg. However, in patients with genotype 1 and a high viral load (HCV RNA by RT-PCR greater than 4.75×10^6 copies/ml), CIFN appeared more effective than IFN-α2b. CIFN also induced a significantly greater fall in serum HCV RNA than IFN-α2b ($p < .01$). Other studies have indicated favorable results with CIFN.[326, 327, 330–332]

Prolonging IFN-α therapy to a total of 12 to 18 months (or longer) has been shown to improve sustained biochemical and virologic response rates further, perhaps to as high as 20 to 25%, but at incremental cost and possibly with more side effects.[362–364] On the basis of these findings, for treatment-naive patients, the duration of therapy with either IFN-α2a or IFN-α2b was approved by the FDA for 12 to 18 months. Higher initial doses of IFN-α given three times a week have not been shown to provide additional benefit over standard doses.[24, 316–320] However, daily induction therapy with IFN-α for the first month, perhaps followed by combination therapy with ribavirin, may enhance sustained virologic response rates by preventing rapid mutation of HCV and subsequent quasispecies escape. Clinical trials are planned to address this issue. The role of combination therapy with IFN-α2b plus ribavirin in treatment-naive patients is reviewed in "Ribavirin and Combination Therapy for Hepatitis C Virus Infection." Even for nonresponders, preliminary data suggest that there may be significant benefits associated with IFN-α therapy such as lowering serum HCV RNA levels and improving histologic activity scores.[352, 353] Continuous treatment with IFN-α (perhaps at low doses) may ultimately prove effective in preventing or delaying histologic progression or other long-term complications even in those who do not respond according to the usual criteria.[364]

Because only a limited proportion (30% at best) of treatment-naive patients respond to standard IFN-α therapy for 12 months or longer, this leaves 70% or more who are nonresponders, relapsers, or breakthroughs. As a result, several pretreatment criteria have been studied in order to identify the patients who are most likely to respond to IFN-α and perhaps to target therapy to these patients in the future.[323, 352–355] HCV RNA levels (greater than 1×10^5 genome equivalents/ml by bDNA or 1×10^6 copies/ml by RT-PCR) and genotype (other than 1) have been found to be the most important predictors of a sustained virologic response.[316–320, 352–355] In fact, nearly 40% of patients with HCV genotype 2 or 3 have a sustained response after standard-dose IFN-α, whereas less than 10% of patients with genotype 1 respond to such therapy.[316–320]

Altered iron metabolism is another important factor affecting response rates to IFN-α.[365, 366] In one study of patients with chronic viral hepatitis, around 40% had abnormal serum iron parameters but, for the most part, these patients had normal hepatic iron concentrations.[367] In subsequent studies, however, patients with chronic viral hepatitis who failed to respond to IFN-α therapy were found to have higher hepatic iron concentrations than those who responded favorably.[368–370] Nonresponders also had more iron deposited in their Kupffer cells than responders, even though overall hepatic iron concentrations did not differ.[371] One syndrome associated with both chronic HCV infection and iron overload is *porphyria cutanea tarda*, which responds well to IFN-α as well as to phlebotomy, to deplete the excess iron stores that frequently exacerbate the condition (for further details, see "Chronic Hepatitis C: Other Issues").[372]

These observations led to several preliminary studies that also considered phlebotomy as an adjunctive therapy for other HCV-seropositive patients, specifically those who had failed to respond initially to IFN-α. Iron reduction with phlebotomy consistently improved serum ALT levels but had no effect on circulating HCV RNA levels.[373–376] Because the hepatic iron concentration correlates well with the degree of hepatic inflammation, IFN-α itself may reduce hepatic iron indirectly by reducing inflammation.[377] Nevertheless, other potentially beneficial effects of IFN-α may play a role, such as the downregulation of transferrin receptor expression on hepatic macrophages or the upregulation of major histocompatibility complex class I proteins that result in a net decrease in iron absorption from the gut or uptake via the *HFE* gene.[378] Several large-scale prospective trials are in progress to address this issue.

Apart from these generalizations, however, one cannot predict whether any given patient will or will not respond to IFN-α. As a result, unless there are specific contraindications to the use of IFN-α (see Table 103–6), all treatment-naive patients should be considered for a course of therapy as long as they are confirmed to have active viremia (detectable HCV RNA) as well as appropriate liver biopsy findings to suggest aggressive disease, including moderate to severe necroinflammatory activity, early fibrosis, or both. Previous studies have shown that patients meeting these criteria have a high risk of progression to cirrhosis without any therapy.[310] The 1997 National Institutes of Health Consensus Development Conference on the Management of Hepatitis C (National Institutes of Health Consensus Conference) advocated performing liver biopsies only for patients with elevated serum ALT levels and treating these patients with IFN-α only if they had the abnormal liver biopsy findings just mentioned. However, subsequent studies suggest that this may be too conservative an approach (as discussed later in "Persistently Normal Serum Alanine Aminotransferase Levels").

Of additional concern is a study that questions the validity of using viral clearance as an important measure of the outcome of therapy.[12, 13] In this study, of patients whose HCV RNA had cleared from the circulation without any IFN-α therapy (and whose chronic HCV infection was thus presumed to have resolved spontaneously), 90% were found to have residual HCV RNA on liver biopsy using ultrasensitive RT-PCR techniques. Thus, it may not be possible to achieve complete eradication of systemic HCV, at least for the foreseeable future.[379, 380] However, these patients have an excellent prognosis because most have minimal changes on liver biopsy. Studies have shown that the majority of patients who achieve a sustained virologic response have done so after 3 months of IFN-α therapy.[316–320, 381–383] After that, few if any are expected to respond. Some studies even report that a virologic response to IFN-α can be seen in as little as 4 weeks.[329, 355, 382] For now, however, the standard procedure is to recheck HCV RNA after 3 months of therapy. With this cutoff point, patients who have a minimal chance of responding to further IFN-α therapy can be saved the additional expense, or side effects, or both.

Interferon Monotherapy Strategies for Relapsers and Nonresponders

Unfortunately, relapse and nonresponse to standard IFN-α therapy are all too frequent problems and more than two thirds of treatment-naive patients do not achieve a sustained response after an initial course of standard IFN-α therapy, even when it is administered for 12 months or longer. As noted earlier, patients who do not respond after at least 12 weeks of IFN-α therapy are termed nonresponders, although in certain cases (when the patient has several predictors of a favorable response such as a low pretreatment HCV RNA titer, a steady fall in viral titer during therapy, female gender, or recent acquisition of disease), continued therapy for another 2 to 3 months may be advisable before considering the patient a true nonresponder. Nonresponders infrequently respond to further courses of IFN-α, although CIFN at 15 μg three times a week for 48 weeks has been shown to result in a 13% sustained virologic response at 48 weeks (see later)[326] and higher dose IFN-α2b monotherapy may achieve a 10 to 15% sustained virologic response after 6 to 12 months of therapy (10 MU three times a week followed by 6 MU three times a week, 6 MU three times a week, or 5 MU daily for 2 weeks and then tapering doses for a total of 12 months).[384, 385]

Because the strict definitions of response, relapse, and nonresponse have just been adopted, interpreting the response profile of earlier studies and comparing them with more recent ones is problematic. For example, when ALT normalization was used alone as a measure of response in early studies, a substantial number of patients thought to have relapses were in fact virologic nonresponders. Because nonresponders have been shown to respond rarely, if ever, to further courses of standard-dose IFN-α, inadvertently including nonresponders in these early studies led to very low response rates for patients who were presumed to have relapsed (0 to 5%). In studies since then that have used HCV RNA clearance rather than ALT normalization to differentiate true relapsers from nonresponders, somewhat higher response rates (5 to 10%) were seen in true relapsers with standard IFN-α therapy of 3 MU three times a week for 6 months.[325]

Although re-treatment of relapsers with a standard IFN-α regimen for 6 months offers no real benefit, a longer duration of IFN-α therapy for 12 to 24 months at standard or even higher doses may increase sustained response rates significantly. In some reports, the overall virologic sustained response rate was only 7% after 6 months of IFN-α2b at 3 MU three times a week but increased to 20% after 12 months and 59% after 24 months of therapy. In other studies, more intensive regimens improved the outcome for relapsers such that in one study, higher doses of IFN-α2b (6 or 12 MU three times a week) led to sustained ALT response rates of nearly 40%, compared with only 9 to 18% with the same therapy given initially.[386–390] In an important study in France,[391] a sustained response was not observed in patients who had relapses after an initial course of IFN-α at 3 MU three times a week when they were treated again with the same dose. However, when they were retreated with a higher dose of 5 MU three times a week for 6 to 12 months, the sustained response rate rose to about 30%. Re-treatment of nonresponders with either dose of IFN-α led to a 50% fall in serum HCV RNA levels, although no long-term sustained responses were observed.

The FDA has approved CIFN at 15 μg three times a week for 24 to 48 weeks for relapsers and nonresponders, and this therapy has shown some promise for these individuals. In the multicenter, open-label U.S. trial that led to FDA approval,[326, 327] patients who had not responded to or had had relapses after previous therapy with IFN-α2b at 3 MU three times a week or CIFN at 9 μg three times a week for 24 weeks were randomized to receive CIFN at 15 μg three times a week for 24 weeks versus 48 weeks, followed by a 24-week observation period. For relapsers, the virologic sustained response rate was 58% after 48 weeks of CIFN compared with 28% at 24 weeks of CIFN, whereas for previous nonresponders, the virologic sustained response rates were 13 and 5%, respectively. This dose of CIFN was safe and well tolerated.[326, 327]

By comparison, combination therapy (IFN-α2b at 3 MU three times a week plus ribavirin) for 24 weeks in relapsers led to a sustained response of around 45% versus 5% in nontreated control subjects.[325] Extrapolation of other data from a European meta-analysis suggested a 60% sustained response in relapsers after 48 weeks of IFN-α2b at 3 MU three times a week.[392] However, because 15 μg of CIFN is probably equivalent to 5 MU rather than 3 MU of IFN-α2b and the subjects may have differed in their baseline characteristics, these results cannot be directly compared with the data from other studies of relapsers and nonresponders. Clinical trials to compare CIFN with combination therapy are in progress.

Other approaches for treating chronic HCV have been tried but without much success. In an uncontrolled study,[393] amantadine led to improvements in serum ALT and HCV RNA levels, but subsequent studies have not shown any benefit with amantadine with or without IFN-α.[394–396] Although more active and better tolerated than amantadine, rimantadine had no effect on serum ALT and HCV RNA levels in patients with recurrent HCV after liver transplantation.[397] Interleukin-2 and interleukin-12 have shown encouraging results in pilot studies.[398, 399] Because of the poor sustained response rates seen with available therapies, many patients with chronic HCV have looked to alternative medicines for help. The most commonly used agent is silymarin, derived from milk thistle, or *Silybum marianum*.[400] Although silymarin is nontoxic and improves serum ALT levels, it has no effects on HCV RNA. Oral thymic extract was shown in a controlled trial to be of no benefit for patients with chronic HCV.[401]

Ribavirin and Combination Therapy for Chronic Hepatitis C Virus Infection

Ribavirin is a guanosine nucleoside analogue that is active against many RNA and DNA viruses[402, 403] (see Chapter 36). Several clinical trials have shown that ribavirin when used together with IFN-α2b improves both biochemical and virologic sustained response rates.[403–409] Combination therapy appears to work by reducing the rate of viral relapse after the completion of therapy rather than by enhancing end-of treatment response rates, as may be the case with a longer duration of IFN-α therapy. The FDA approved combination therapy (Rebetron with its two components: oral ribavirin, Rebetol, and injectable IFN-α2b, Intron A, Schering Corporation, Kenilworth, NJ) for treatment-naive patients and those who have had relapses after previous therapy with IFN-α. It remains to be seen whether combination therapy will be safe and effective for others such as nonresponders, patients with HIV or chronic renal failure, or organ transplant recipients.

The precise mechanism of action of ribavirin in chronic hepatitis C is not well understood. Ribavirin appears to enhance host clearance of HCV primarily via intracellular virustatic effects and immunomodulation rather than by any direct virucidal effect.[410–415] In most clinical trials to date, ribavirin has been shown to clear circulating HCV RNA only when the drug is used in combination with IFN-α.[403–409] High concentrations of ribavirin monophosphate are found in erythrocytes, because they are less able than other cells to hydrolyze this compound to its inactive form.[416–418] This is probably why hemolysis is seen with such frequency in patients taking ribavirin. Ribavirin and its metabolites are eliminated by the kidneys and the liver, and dose reductions should be made in patients with significant renal or hepatic impairment.[416] No major interactions have been reported apart from possible interactions with azathioprine, zidovudine, stavudine, and zalcitobine.[419, 420]

Ribavirin was initially studied as monotherapy for chronic HCV.[421–427] At doses of 600 to 1200 mg/day for 12 to 48 weeks, ribavirin lowered serum ALT levels significantly compared with placebo, and ALT levels returned to normal in almost 40% of treated patients. This was associated with significantly less necroinflammatory activity on sequential liver biopsies. However, in a further study comparing ribavirin monotherapy and IFN-α monotherapy, ribavirin was found to be less effective than IFN-α in normalizing serum ALT levels.[427] Furthermore, in most trials to date, ribavirin has not had any significant effect on serum HCV RNA titers and patients did not clear HCV RNA during treatment or thereafter.[423–426] Moreover, in one study, although serum HCV RNA levels decreased slightly during ribavirin therapy, after the completion of therapy a rebound effect in HCV RNA was noted to levels above those at baseline.[428]

In contrast, when ribavirin is given together with IFN-α as combination therapy, there appears to be a synergistic effect with sustained response rates significantly better than those seen with IFN-α alone.[403–409, 429–433] As noted earlier, IFN-α monotherapy for 6 to 12 months at standard doses results in a sustained virologic response (no detectable HCV RNA for 6 months after treatment cessation) in only 10 to 20% of treatment-naive patients, although by extending therapy for 18 to 24 months the sustained virologic response rate can be increased to about 30%.[316, 322] When ribavirin is combined with IFN-α for treatment-naive patients, the sustained virologic responses are markedly improved, as seen in two open-label trials. After only 6 months of combination therapy, a sustained response (defined as a normal serum ALT or no detectable serum HCV RNA 12 to 24 months after therapy) was noted in over 40% of treatment-naive patients compared with less than 10% of similar patients treated with IFN-α alone.[429, 430] As with IFN-α monotherapy, the sustained response rates with combination therapy depend on the patient's viral genotype: a 20% response was seen in patients with genotype 1b, 40% in genotype 2a, and 75% in genotype 3.[405, 429, 430]

Besides viral genotype, other factors such as pretreatment viral load and liver histology may alter the response rates with combination therapy in treatment-naive patients. In a double-blind, placebo-controlled trial in Sweden,[431] 100 treatment-naive patients were randomized to receive 6 months of either IFN-α2b at 3 MU three times a week plus ribavirin at 1000 or 1200 mg/day based on body weight or the same IFN-α2b regimen plus placebo, with follow-up at 6 and 12 months after treatment. By intention-to-treat analysis, at 6 months after treatment, the difference in sustained virologic response rates barely reached statistical significance in favor of combination therapy, 36% versus 18% ($p<.047$). However, at 12 months after treatment, significantly fewer patients who had received combination therapy ended up with a viral relapse, and the sustained virologic response rate was 42% for combination therapy versus 20% for IFN-α2b alone ($p=.03$).

This study included a retrospective analysis that showed that the main predictor of a sustained virologic response was the pretreatment viral load.[431] Consequently, for serum HCV RNA levels greater than 4 million copies/ml (measured by RT-PCR with the Superquant assay, National Genetics Institute, Culver City, Calif.), the sustained virologic response rate was significantly better with combination therapy than with IFN-α2b alone (44% versus 8%, respectively, $p = .008$), whereas with a viral load less than 4 million copies/ml, the response rate did not differ (28% for each group). Overall, there were no significant differences in sustained virologic response rates for the various genotypes, apart from those seen in patients with genotype 3a, who fared best with combination therapy. Pretreatment liver histology did not help predict the sustained virologic response rate, although none of the cirrhotic patients responded to IFN-α2b alone.

Two multicenter, randomized, placebo-controlled studies[432, 433] involving treatment-naive patients have confirmed that combination therapy leads to a significant improvement in virologic sustained response rates over those seen with IFN alone, especially in patients with HCV genotypes other than 1. The U.S. study[432] had four treatment arms: combination therapy (IFN-α2b at 3 MU three times a week plus ribavirin at 1000 to 1200 mg/day based on body weight) for either 24 or 48 weeks and IFN-α2b at 3 MU three times a week plus ribavirin matched placebo for either 24 or 48 weeks. With combination therapy for 24 or 48 weeks, the sustained virologic responses were 31 and 38%, respectively, versus 6 and 13% with IFN-α2b alone. In the patients with genotypes other than 1, the sustained response at 24 weeks was as high as 69% versus only 16% for IFN-α2b monotherapy. Prolonging combination therapy to 48 weeks led to no additional benefit.[432] Similar results were seen in another large international study,[433] although it did not have a 24-week IFN-α2b monotherapy arm. Again, 48 weeks of combination therapy appeared best for patients with genotype 1 and a viral load greater than 2 million copies/ml, whereas 24 weeks was sufficient for those with genotypes other than 1 and a viral load less than 2 million copies/ml. Both studies included well over 1700 enrolled patients, who were mostly men (66%) with genotype 1 (66% or more) and a viral load over 2 million copies/ml (66% or more). Few patients had cirrhosis.[432, 433]

The low overall sustained response rates seen with IFN-α monotherapy may be related to both a poor initial response to therapy and a higher risk of relapse after treatment.[403, 405] In a meta-analysis of 186 patients from four different European trials,[434] a sustained response (defined in this study as having both a normal serum ALT level and undetectable serum HCV RNA) was found by odds-ratio analysis to occur 3.3 times more often at the end of therapy in patients receiving combination therapy than those given IFN-α monotherapy and 7.3 times more often at 6 months after drug cessation. This meta-analysis included a mix of 45 treatment-naive patients and 141 relapsers and nonresponders. When these groups were analyzed separately, the estimated probabilities of achieving a sustained response (as just defined) after 6 months of combination therapy were as follows: 52% for treatment-naive patients, 52% for relapsers, and 19% for nonresponders. Overall, patients with genotype 1 were predicted to fare worst. When the data were extrapolated to 12 months, the estimated probabilities of a sustained response for relapsers and nonresponders were 60 and 20%, respectively, with combination therapy, compared with 30 and 0%, respectively with IFN-α monotherapy.[393, 434, 435] However, caution is advised because the results presented in the study are only estimates based on extrapolations derived from the original meta-analysis.

In terms of patients with chronic HCV who have had relapses after previous IFN-α monotherapy, the FDA approved combination therapy for these patients on the basis of results of two large multicenter, randomized, placebo-controlled trials, one conducted in the United States and the other in Canada, Europe, Israel, and Australia.[325, 416] The studies were combined to give a total of 345 patients who had relapses after one or two previous courses of recombinant (IFN-α2b or IFN-α2a) or lymphoblastoid (IFN-αn1) IFN-α monotherapy at 3 to 6 MU three times a week for at least 20 weeks and for no more than 18 months. The patients also had to meet strict entry criteria, including elevated serum ALT levels, chronic hepatitis on liver biopsy, and minimal hemoglobin levels. Thus, only 345 of 495 screened patients were included. Eligible patients were randomly assigned to receive 6 months of either combination therapy (IFN-α2b at 3 MU three times a week plus ribavirin at 1000 or 1200 mg/day on the basis of body weight) or IFN-α monotherapy (IFN-α2b at 3 MU three times a week plus placebo). Both groups were well matched in terms of age, sex, pretreatment HCV RNA levels, and degree of fibrosis and cirrhosis, but both groups had fewer patients with genotype 1 than usual (55 or 57%).

Re-treatment with combination therapy led to a sustained virologic response rate of 49% versus only 5% in those retreated with IFN-α2b alone ($p < .001$). The low response rates seen with IFN-α2b monotherapy in this study were not unexpected and have been seen in other studies using IFN-α alone to treat relapsers.[24, 316–320] However, the lower number of genotype 1 patients may have led to more favorable results in this trial.[355] On the other hand, the number of true relapsers is unknown because HCV RNA levels were not available for recruited patients after their previous courses of therapy, and a significant proportion of patients may in fact have been nonresponders. Patients with lower viral loads (HCV RNA less than 2 million copies/ml) had higher response rates in both groups, although those with viral genotypes other than 1 had sustained responses only with combination therapy. Overall, combination therapy was well tolerated, although a predictable fall in hemoglobin levels occurred (mean fall of 2.0 g/dl).

To date, no study has compared the sustained response rates with combination therapy with those with CIFN or PEG-IFN. As noted in "Treatment of Chronic Hepatitis C Virus Infection with Interferons," a study with CIFN showed considerable promise for relapsers, although the number of patients treated was small and there was no control group for comparison. CIFN at 15 μg three times a week led to a 28% sustained virologic response rate after 6 months of therapy and 58% after 12 months.[326, 327] Head-to-head trials are currently in progress to determine any differences in efficacy, safety, and cost between combination therapy and CIFN or PEG-IFN.

Other promising roles for combination therapy include the prevention or treatment of HCV recurrence after liver transplantation (see "Hepatitis C Virus Infection and Liver Transplantation"). However, studies have yet to assess the efficacy and safety of combination therapy in HCV patients coinfected with other viruses, including HBV and HIV,[419] and those awaiting liver or kidney transplantation. Future studies should also help to clarify whether induction therapy with daily doses of IFN-α for the first 2 to 4 weeks during combination therapy will enhance the sustained virologic response rate. Although combination therapy appears to work best when ribavirin is begun together with IFN-α at the start of therapy rather than later on, conclusive data in this respect are lacking at present.[436] The potential benefit of maintenance therapy with ribavirin alone after an initial course of combination therapy also needs further study.[403–409]

On the whole, ribavirin has minimal side effects apart from hemolysis, which occurs to some degree in nearly all patients receiving this drug.[325, 393, 403–409, 416, 431–435] In most studies, ribavirin has caused a mean fall in serum hemoglobin of 2 to 3 g/dl, although in about 10% of patients the reduction may be to levels less than 10 g/dl. As a result, ribavirin is usually contraindicated for patients with underlying hemolytic disorders such as hemoglobinopathies (thalassemia and sickle cell anemia). Patients with renal impairment may also have more severe hemolysis because of higher serum concentrations of ribavirin, as this drug is renally cleared. The main brunt of hemolysis seems to occur within the first 2 to 4 weeks of therapy, after which the patient's bone marrow tends to adapt. For a few patients, adjustments in dose or temporary discontinuation of ribavirin may be required, and in rare instances, severe anemia may exacerbate angina pectoris or lead to myocardial ischemia or infarction. Consequently, patients with known cardiac risk factors should have a cardiology opinion before they start to take ribavirin and require more careful monitoring while they continue to have therapy with the drug.[416] A sudden fall in hemoglobin may precipitate hepatic encephalopathy in some patients with cirrhosis.[405]

Leukopenia does not appear to be any worse with combination therapy than with IFN-α alone, and platelet counts may actually rise.[416] Other reported side effects include dyspnea, pulmonary infiltrates, pneumonitis and pneumonia, irritability, insomnia, depression, and vertigo.[405, 409, 416] Mild elevations in serum bilirubin and uric acid are common (secondary to hemolysis). Psychiatric adverse events are common and may occur even in patients without a previous psychiatric history. Serious neuro-ophthalmologic disorders have also been reported and diabetic or hypertensive patients require a vision examination before ribavirin is started. Most important of all, ribavirin has been shown to be teratogenic and embryocidal in animal models, and it can impair spermatogenesis. Therefore, strict contraceptive techniques are mandatory in women of childbearing potential while they are receiving ribavirin and for at least 6 months after drug cessation. The same constraints apply to men taking ribavirin and for 6 months after treatment if they have sexual partners who are women of childbearing potential.[416]

Hepatitis C Virus Infection and Liver Transplantation

End-stage liver disease secondary to chronic HCV infection has become the leading indication for liver transplantation in the United States, and if patients with alcoholic liver disease infected with HCV are included, nearly 45% of all liver transplantations are performed for this reason.[220] HCV has been shown to recur in over 90% of patients by the end of the first year after transplantation and usually within a few weeks, if sensitive RT-PCR techniques are used to detect HCV RNA.[437–442] Because of immunosuppression, high levels of viremia may lead in some cases to a direct cytopathic effect of HCV on the transplanted liver, and severe cholestasis and fibrosis develop in about 5% of patients, similar to the fibrosing cholestatic hepatitis seen in HBV recurrence after transplantation.[443–453] Retransplantation for severe recurrent HCV has a poor outcome, especially in patients with renal failure.[454]

Nevertheless, controversy persists about the overall impact of HCV recurrence on long-term outcome. If only patients with abnormal serum aminotransferases after transplantation are suspected to have recurrent HCV, poor outcomes may be overestimated.[438] To date, most short-term studies have not shown any major adverse effects on graft loss or patients' survival, probably because these studies did not include enough patients to provide statistical power, nor was follow-up long enough to detect any significant differences in outcome.[437–442] Other factors that may affect outcome include the age of the patient; the type, degree, and duration of immunosuppression; the pretransplantation level of viremia; the level of hepatic HCV RNA; and the severity of liver disease at the time of transplantation.[437–442, 450] In a study from the National Institute of Diabetes and Digestive and Kidney Diseases Database,[443] high pretransplantation serum HCV RNA levels were strongly associated with poorer survival rates among HCV-positive recipients, although long-term survival rates of patients and grafts did not differ on the whole from those of patients who had transplants for other indications. Similar results were seen in a study from Germany in which patients were observed for over 10 years.[444] However, some long-term studies have shown that 50% of HCV-positive liver transplant recipients may develop chronic hepatitis within 2 years and 35% may have chronic active hepatitis or cirrhosis within 5 years.[447] In one study that used strict protocol biopsies for a mean of 32 months after transplantation, cirrhosis developed in 15% after 1 year and 28% after 4 to 5 years, and the risk of developing cirrhosis was linked to the number of graft rejection episodes. Findings on liver biopsy at 1 year after transplantation were predictive of a more rapid progression to cirrhosis.[449]

In terms of antiviral therapy, IFN-α can rarely be given to patients before transplantation because of the advanced nature of their liver disease, which has prompted the need for transplantation in the first place. As a result, these patients often have relative or absolute contraindications to IFN-α such as a low platelet count or a low white cell count. In addition, the response rate to IFN-α in patients with cirrhosis is stated to be less than 10% (compared with a 20 to 30% rate in patients without cirrhosis) and these patients appear to be at higher risk for infections when treated with IFN-α. However, one of the primary goals of the treatment of HCV before transplantation would be to lower HCV RNA levels to a minimum, because this may lead to a better outcome after transplantation, as noted earlier. Therefore, low-dose, titratable IFN-α therapy may be an appropriate option before transplantation for selected individuals.[392, 437–442]

After transplantation, when HCV has recurred, IFN-α monotherapy appears to offer no major benefit and ductopenic rejection has been documented in some studies.[455–461] However, a U.S. randomized trial assessed the role of prophylactic IFN-α2b in preventing recurrent HCV after transplantation.[462] Starting at 2 weeks after transplantation, 86 patients were randomized to receive IFN-α2b at 3 MU three times a week for 1 year versus no treatment. Data for 71 patients who survived longer than 3 months were analyzed. Recurrence was based solely on liver biopsy findings when performed at 1 year or to evaluate abnormal liver enzymes. After a mean follow-up of almost 2 years, fewer patients treated with IFN-α2b than control subjects had recurrent HCV noted on liver biopsy ($p = .017$) and the risk of recurrence was reduced with IFN-α2b by a factor of 0.4 ($p = .04$) At 1 year, piecemeal necrosis was also a less common finding on liver biopsy in patients who received IFN-α2b. Patients' survival at the 1- and 2-year intervals was no different between the groups. Of note, the number and severity of rejection episodes were similar in both groups. However, in patients with two or more rejection episodes, the risk of recurrence was increased by a factor of 2.17 ($p = .05$). However, interpretation of this study is limited because it was not placebo controlled or "blinded," and the less sensitive bDNA assay was used to measure circulating HCV RNA levels, which may have resulted in underestimating the number of patients with a virologic recurrence despite normal liver biopsy findings. Furthermore, only 56% of the patients treated with IFN-α2b completed a full year of therapy because of low platelet counts and other adverse effects.

Ribavirin monotherapy has been shown to normalize serum ALT levels but it has no apparent effect on HCV RNA levels in transplant recipients with recurrent HCV.[463–466] In a preliminary study in Canada,[463, 464] ribavirin monotherapy (800 to 1200 mg/day) was begun at a median of 6 months after transplantation and continued for almost 2 years in 18 patients with biochemical and liver biopsy evidence of recurrent HCV hepatitis. The long-term response rate was compared to that in 33 untreated historical control subjects. Initially, ribavirin led to a favorable biochemical response (improvement in serum ALT levels), but after a median of 15 months, most patients had significant worsening of liver fibrosis and 22% actually developed cirrhosis. Ribavirin had no discernible effects on serum HCV RNA levels.

In a study of recurrent HCV after transplantation from the United Kingdom,[467] ribavirin alone was compared with IFN-α alone. Ribavirin (up to 1200 mg/day) or IFN-α (3 MU three times a week) was begun at least 6 months after liver transplantation. Some ameliorative effects were noted: ribavirin improved serum ALT levels and reduced lobular inflammation, whereas IFN-α reduced serum HCV RNA levels. However, compared with IFN-α monotherapy, ribavirin monotherapy caused a significant decline in both total leukocyte and total lymphocyte counts, as well as some degree of hemolysis in all patients, with a fall in serum hemoglobin to less than 10 g/dl in 50%.

To date, combination therapy with IFN-α plus ribavirin has shown the most promise for patients with recurrent HCV after transplantation. In a pilot study from France,[468] 21 liver recipients with recurrent HCV (defined as persistently elevated serum ALT levels, a positive HCV RNA by RT-PCR, and confirmed active hepatitis without rejection on liver biopsy) were given IFN-α2b (3 MU three times a week) plus ribavirin (1200 mg/day), but therapy was begun only after a mean of 9 months after transplantation (range 3 to 24 months) to permit initial adjustments in immunosuppressive therapy and reduce the potential risk of rejection noted previously with IFN-α monotherapy. Combination therapy was administered for 6 months, followed by another 6 months of ribavirin alone (1200 mg/day).

By the end of combination therapy, all 21 patients had a normal serum ALT level and in 10 of 21 (48%) HCV RNA had been cleared from the serum, although the remaining patients had a significant fall in HCV RNA. Liver histologic scores improved in all patients after combination therapy. However, during the subsequent 6 months with ribavirin alone, 5 of the 10 initial responders had a viral relapse, although HCV RNA levels were lower than those at baseline. In all but 1 of the 18 patients who tolerated a complete course of ribavirin through 12 months, serum ALT levels remained normal and liver histology improved further. The main side effect was hemolytic anemia, and in three patients significant hemolysis led to discontinuation of ribavirin. However, the drug was reintroduced successfully in two patients by using concomitant erythropoietin. No episodes of rejection were documented.

In a preliminary follow-up report of this study,[469] a total of 30 patients with recurrent HCV after transplantation (genotype 1b in 27) were treated with combination therapy for 6 months followed by ribavirin alone for a mean of 28 months. At the completion of combination therapy, 28 had responded biochemically and 16 had cleared HCV RNA. After a mean of 28 months with ribavirin alone, 11 of the 16 remained negative for HCV RNA. Ribavirin was discontinued, and all but one of the 10 patients continued to be HCV RNA negative after a mean of 9 months without ribavirin. Liver histology in 6 of the 10 showed no evidence of relapse, and histologic scores were improved over those before treatment. There were no episodes of acute or chronic rejection, although ribavirin had to be discontinued for 6 of the 30 patients because of significant hemolysis.

There may be some merit to starting combination therapy as early as possible after transplantation in a so-called preemptive strategy to prevent HCV reinfection of the allograft and improve outcome. This has some merit because extrahepatic sites of HCV replication probably contribute little to the phenomenon of recurrence and the half-life of HCV appears to be only 4 hours in the perioperative setting.[470] In a pilot study from Italy,[471] 21 HCV-positive liver recipients (genotype 1b in 19) who had undergone transplantation for small hepatomas were given IFN-α2b (3 MU three times a week) plus ribavirin (10 mg/kg/day) starting as early as week 3 after transplantation, whether or not they had evidence of HCV-related liver damage. Patients were observed every 2 weeks and liver biopsies performed at 6 months and 1 year after transplantation or when liver enzymes rose to levels two to three times normal.

Survival of patients and graft survival were both 95% after a median of 12 months (1 of the 21 patients died of recurrent hepatocellular carcinoma). After 1 year of combination therapy, 9 of 21 patients (41%) became seronegative for HCV RNA both in serum and in liver tissue, after a median of only 37 days of treatment. Eight of the nine patients were infected with genotype 1b. On treatment, 17 of 21 (81%) remained free of any liver biopsy evidence of hepatitis. Of the four (19%) who developed some form of hepatitis, only one (5%) had chronic active hepatitis and none had cirrhosis. Overall, combination therapy was deemed a success in 95% of patients (9 of 21 remained HCV RNA negative and 11 of 21 had a completely normal graft although they were HCV RNA positive). However, some degree of toxicity occurred in 62% of patients and dosage reductions were required in 43% (mostly because of hemolytic anemia). Of interest, four of the nine patients with moderate to severe toxicity ended up clearing HCV. There were no reported episodes of rejection.[471]

Therefore, combination therapy might be used in one or more of the following strategies: (1) before transplantation to prevent complications such as hepatoma, (2) just before liver transplantation to prevent recurrence after transplantation, (3) early after transplantation in a preemptive manner (within 4 weeks after transplantation), or (4) when HCV recurs after transplantation. Ongoing clinical trials are addressing which of these strategies (alone or in combination) is ideal. For now, patients should be treated only in the context of a clinical trial.

Chronic Hepatitis C: Other Issues

Persistently Normal Serum Alanine Aminotransferase Levels

The National Institutes of Health Consensus Conference did not recommend liver biopsies or treatment with IFN-α for individuals with persistently normal ALT levels (PNAL).[472, 473] In part this was due to a report suggesting that IFN-α therapy in these patients could lead to elevations in serum ALT levels.[474] However, to date, HCV-seropositive patients with PNAL have not received sufficient scrutiny, because by the nature of the histologic definition used in most clinical trials (moderate to severe inflammation, or advancing fibrosis, or both), patients with PNAL were excluded.[472, 473] Although selection bias may also be a problem in any histopathologic study, a sizable proportion of HCV-seropositive patients with PNAL do have some degree of chronic hepatitis on initial liver biopsy and a few patients may even have cirrhosis. As a result, there is a growing consensus that, whenever feasible, a liver biopsy should be performed at baseline for most, if not all, patients with PNAL. Some of these patients may also benefit from IFN-α with or without ribavirin.

The extent of this problem may be more serious than was first suspected. Although one of the hallmarks of chronic infection with HCV is the periodic fluctuation in serum ALT levels, studies have shown that 25 to 40% (or more) of HCV-seropositive individuals have PNAL.[475–479] By general consensus, PNAL has been defined as normal ALT levels on three to six occasions during a 6-month period in individuals who have a positive serum antibody to HCV as well as detectable circulating HCV RNA.[472] Two logistic issues make this definition less than ideal: the upper limit of normal for ALT varies from one laboratory to the next, and even though a certain ALT value may be within the "normal" range, it may actually be elevated for an individual whose ALT was considerably lower before the acquisition of HCV.

Most individuals with PNAL are asymptomatic. Several studies report a preponderance of nondrinking women, attributed perhaps to higher alcohol consumption by men or perhaps hormonal differences in the immunologic response to chronic HCV infection.[473–480] Otherwise, individuals with PNAL do not differ from those with abnormal ALT levels in terms of symptoms, source of infection, age at diagnosis or acquisition, circulating HCV RNA levels, viral genotype, or quasispecies heterogeneity.[472, 475–483] However, studies in Italy have suggested a link between genotype 2a or 2c and PNAL.[484, 485] Markedly elevated HCV RNA titers have also been noted in some cases of PNAL.[482] Most often, these individuals are diagnosed at the time of a blood donation, because up to 60% of potential blood donors with chronic HCV infection fit the criteria for PNAL. Approximately 65% of these individuals are viremic.[472, 480]

The long-term prognosis for individuals with PNAL is unknown but seems favorable, judging from the limited data available to date.[472, 476, 480, 486–488] A review of 11 studies[480] with a total of 290 cases with PNAL showed minimal or no changes on liver biopsy in 27%, chronic hepatitis with mild inflammation and minimal or no necrosis in 54%, and chronic hepatitis with moderately active necroinflammatory activity in 19%. Cirrhosis was seen in only one case and fibrosis was absent or minimal in the vast majority. In another study,[486] sequential liver biopsies were performed for HCV-seropositive individuals, one group with PNAL and the other with abnormal ALT levels. The two groups were well matched for age, sex, duration of and age at infection, ethnic origin, mode of acquisition, and alcohol consumption. This was the first such study to match the groups in this manner to avoid bias. Although only 66% of the PNAL group had detectable HCV RNA by RT-PCR versus 97% of the abnormal-ALT group, other factors such as viral titer and genotype did not differ between the two groups. The important finding was that histologic activity on liver biopsy was considerably less severe in the PNAL group ($p<.0001$). Likewise, the median progression rate of fibrosis was much lower in the patients with PNAL, even after the patients who had no detectable circulating HCV RNA were excluded from the analysis ($p<.001$). Severe fibrosis was found to be associated only with high alcohol consumption.

Other studies have been less favorable regarding the risk of progression.[487] One study of 10 HCV-seropositive patients with PNAL and detectable circulating HCV RNA showed that 9 had chronic hepatitis and 1 had established cirrhosis on biopsy.[488] In another report,[489] close to 20% of HCV-infected individuals with PNAL were found to have cirrhosis on liver biopsy, but no data were provided with respect to alcohol consumption, frequency of serum ALT levels, or mean ALT levels. In a subsequent study,[479] 46 HCV RNA–positive patients with PNAL (most of whom were women, asymptomatic, and with few risk factors) had significant liver damage on biopsy with a grade of inflammation and stage of fibrosis similar to those of a group of 52 HCV RNA–positive patients with abnormal ALT levels. There were also no differences between the two groups in terms of symptoms or circulating HCV RNA levels, although genotype 2a was more common in the patients with PNAL.

In a study from the United States[476] of 303 patients screened for chronic HCV infection, 50 (or 16.5%) were found to have PNAL and a positive recombinant immunoblot assay II or HCV RNA by RT-PCR. Most of the patients (68%) had known risk factors for HCV and relatively few were initially diagnosed at the time of a blood donation. The mean circulating HCV RNA level was 380,000 copies/ml. On liver biopsy, seven patients (14%) had established cirrhosis and only three (6%) had normal findings. Most of the others had some degree of chronic hepatitis ("persistent" in 50% and "active" in 30%). Close to half (19 of 50) had inflammation of grade 3 and 20% (10 of 50) had fibrosis of stage 3 or 4. Most were female nondrinkers and none were HIV positive or receiving any immunosuppressants.

A connection with female gender has also been seen in pregnancy; HCV-infected women have been shown to have a significant fall in elevated serum ALT levels during the third trimester with ALT levels returning to baseline after delivery.[490] Altered T-cell–mediated cytotoxicity may play a role because a correlation has been found between serum ALT levels and the number of $CD8^+$ cytotoxic T cells in the hepatic lobules on liver biopsy.[491] Furthermore, markedly elevated HCV RNA titers are frequently seen in individuals with PNAL. One reason for this may be that these individuals have a limited if not absent Th1 (proinflammatory) immune response directed at the HCV-infected hepatocytes.[472, 491]

In terms of the potential benefit of IFN-α therapy for HCV-seropositive patients with PNAL, controversy rages. The response rates (no detectable HCV RNA) in these individuals have been variable in most uncontrolled studies to date, ranging from 0 to 38%.[492–494] However, the sustained response rate may be similar to that seen in patients with elevated ALT levels: 19% at 6 to 12 months after drug cessation.[316, 472] Higher doses of IFN-α2b (5 MU daily for 6 to 12 months) have also resulted in some benefit but may be risky.[495, 496] A pilot randomized controlled study from Italy showed no benefit with IFN-α2a at 3 MU three times a week for 6 months in patients with PNAL.[497] At the end of therapy, 94% of the treated group had detectable HCV RNA versus 93% of those not treated. Serum ALT levels flared in 10 of the treated patients but in only one of the control subjects. However, half of the episodes occurred during therapy, the other half after drug cessation. This has been a common phenomenon during other trials and may be related to enhanced recognition of HCV-related cell surface antigens by $CD8^+$ cytotoxic T cells.[480, 497]

Until there is more evidence in favor of IFN-α therapy and the concerns regarding a flare in serum ALT levels with IFN-α are adequately addressed, individuals with PNAL should usually be treated only in the context of a clinical trial. However, they should be offered a liver biopsy. If the liver biopsy is normal, no treatment is warranted, although close follow-up is recommended, perhaps with a biopsy in another 3 to 5 years to assess any progression in disease. IFN-α with or without ribavirin may be worth considering for individuals with significant histologic findings or symptomatic cryoglobulinemia or women planning a pregnancy.[416, 472, 498, 499]

Hepatitis C Virus–Associated Cryoglobulinemia

Of the various extrahepatic manifestations associated with chronic HCV infection such as arthritis, keratoconjunctivitis sicca (Sjögren's syndrome), lichen planus, and glomerulonephritis, by far the most serious is *essential mixed cryoglobulinemia* (EMC). A systemic vasculitis marked by fatigue, myalgias, arthralgias, palpable purpura, peripheral neuropathy, glomerulonephritis, and hepatosplenomegaly, EMC can be incapacitating and even fatal through progressive renal failure. Most patients have hypocomplementemia. The long-term prognosis is determined by the degree of end-organ damage, primarily that involving the kidneys.[498–517]

Although cryoglobulins are found in nearly one third of HCV-seropositive patients, only about 1 to 2% of these patients develop EMC. There may be genetic differences in the host that predispose to EMC. However, the exact cause remains uncertain.[500–507] One hypothesis is that infection of B-cell lymphocytes by HCV leads to monoclonal B-cell expansion,[508] and an association between chronic HCV infection and non-Hodgkin's lymphoma has been reported.[509] Circulating HCV–host lipoprotein complexes may also serve as a chronic stimulant for production of monoclonal rheumatoid factors. However, nonantigenic B-cell stimulation by HCV may occur.[510] HCV-encoded nucleocapsid protein has been reported to stimulate cell proliferation by inhibiting apoptotic cell death.[511] This might explain the rare case of transformation to malignancy. Early treatment of EMC with IFN-α may reverse end-organ damage.[500] In one study,[512] monoclonal gammopathies were reported in 11% of HCV-positive patients versus only 1% of HCV-negative patients ($p=.004$), with genotype 2a/c predominating in 50% of those with monoclonal gammopathies compared with only 18% without ($p=.009$).

Nephrotic syndrome is the most common presentation for renal involvement in EMC. In a study of eight patients with glomerulonephritis and chronic HCV infection, all had membranoproliferative glomerulonephritis on renal biopsy and five had cryoglobulinemia. In three of these five patients, the cryoprecipitates contained HCV RNA and anti-HCV antibodies, indicating a disorder related to immune complex deposition. Four of the patients were treated with IFN-α. Renal disease improved and circulating HCV RNA disappeared in all four.[513, 514] IFN-α was first used in the 1980s for its antiproliferative effect, because EMC was thought to be a low-grade malignancy. After IFN-α2b at 3 MU daily for 3 months followed by 3 MU three times a week, 77% of patients responded favorably and for a prolonged duration.[515]

Subsequently, in a prospective randomized trial of HCV-seropositive patients with EMC, 75% of whom had renal disease, 27 received IFN-α for 24 weeks and 26 control subjects were treated with low-dose prednisone and other supportive measures. Of the 27 who received IFN-α, 15 cleared circulating HCV RNA by the end of treatment and this was associated with significant improvements in their skin lesions, with the purpuric lesions resolving completely in 6. Serum levels of creatinine, cryoglobulin, and rheumatoid factor also improved significantly. However, none of the controls had clearance of circulating HCV RNA or manifested any clinical improvement. When IFN-α therapy was stopped, the syndrome recurred in the 15 virologic responders within 6 to 13 months, and most had severe symptomatic cryoglobulinemia. Four of these patients were re-treated for another 6 months with another excellent response.[516] The addition of 6-methylprednisolone at 16 mg/day for a year to IFN-α therapy does not seem to provide further benefit and should be avoided because HCV RNA levels rise with steroids.[517, 518] However, plasmapharesis may help to resolve the nephrotic syndrome in more severe cases.[500]

Chronic Renal Disease

Infection with HCV is a common and potentially serious problem in patients with chronic renal disease, particularly after renal transplantation.[519–525] Besides causing more significant liver damage in these patients for unknown reasons, HCV also leads to a variety of kidney disorders such as membranoproliferative glomerulonephritis and cryoglobulinemia-related disease (as discussed earlier). With second-generation HCV antibody tests, up to 38% of patients with end-stage renal disease in general and nearly 55% of those receiving chronic hemodialysis are seropositive, whereas patients receiving peritoneal dialysis are at much less risk.[526, 527] The gold standard method for confirming HCV infection in these patients is determination of serum HCV RNA by RT-PCR (qualitative or quantitative), because the level of anti-HCV antibody is often too low to be detected, even with later-generation assays.[528, 529]

Serum ALT levels are normal in more than two thirds of these patients, as with other immunosuppressed patients.[530–533] This may occur even more frequently in patients receiving hemodialysis because serum ALT is cleared efficiently, leading to falsely normal serum levels. Previously, when the decision to treat with IFN-α was based primarily on abnormal ALT levels, many patients went without appropriate therapy, a major concern because liver histology is abnormal in most hemodialysis patients with chronic HCV.[524, 525] Although less than 10% of these patients have cirrhosis, up to 100% have some degree of chronic hepatitis.[530, 534, 535] As noted earlier, there is a poor correlation between serum ALT levels and the grade of inflammation seen on liver biopsy.[530, 535] In one study, only one in three patients with chronic hepatitis confirmed by liver biopsy had abnormal serum ALT levels,[528] and in another study, only 43% had sustained elevations in ALT.[535] Therefore, all HCV-positive patients with significant renal disease should be evaluated with a liver biopsy, whether or not the serum ALT level is elevated, because of the rapid progression of hepatic disease in most patients and the important prognostic information determined only by histologic assessment.

Treatment for HCV in these patients should be initiated after a baseline liver biopsy, preferably before renal transplantation, because IFN-α may cause allograft rejection even several years after transplantation.[536, 537] Unfortunately, IFN-α therapy may be less effective in patients receiving hemodialysis.[521, 538] It may also be associated with more side effects, including fatigue, dyspnea, and anorexia, so that discontinuation rates are higher.[538] Combination therapy with IFN-α plus ribavirin has not been adequately assessed in renal patients to permit any recommendations at present. However, utmost care is necessary because ribavirin is cleared via the kidneys, leading to a prolonged half-life in patients with significant renal impairment.[416–418] In addition, many of these patients have concomitant disorders such as diabetes mellitus, cardiac disease, hypertension, and anemia, which may preclude combination therapy in general.[416] In addition, ribavirin has not yet been approved by the FDA for use in patients with chronic renal failure. The best monitors of therapeutic response are HCV RNA titers rather than serum ALT levels.[530]

HCV-related liver disease can be particularly serious in patients who undergo renal transplantation, because liver-related deaths have been reported in up to 28% of long-term survivors.[539, 540] This is similar to the situation with transplant recipients in general because of the enhanced HCV replication associated with immunosuppression in these patients. Unfortunately, no studies to date have compared the outcome for HCV-seropositive patients after long-term hemodialysis with that after renal transplantation.[521–524] Nevertheless, all patients with confirmed hepatitis C viremia who are being considered for renal transplantation should be evaluated in detail by a gastroenterologist or hepatologist. A liver biopsy is mandatory to assess the extent of liver damage and ongoing inflammation.[541] Advanced fibrosis or cirrhosis usually precludes renal transplantation because HCV-related liver disease progresses more rapidly after transplantation, leading to liver failure.[542] Patients with milder degrees of liver damage should be considered for IFN-α monotherapy (or possibly combination therapy), as long as there are no specific contraindications.[542–553] The use of organs from HCV-positive donors remains controversial. With the worsening organ shortage, there may be no choice but to use these organs in the future. However, superinfection with the dominant genotype (usually type 1) may lead to more serious liver disease in the recipient, and treatment options are limited.[524, 538]

In patients with chronic HCV who proceed to renal transplantation, significant liver disease is a major problem.[538, 554–556] In one study, more than 40% of renal transplant recipients had features of chronic active hepatitis on liver biopsy.[555] The 5-year survival for grafts and patients has not been shown to differ between HCV-seropositive and -seronegative patients,[524, 538] although a case-control study showed that at 10 years after transplantation survival rates for grafts and patients were significantly worse in HCV-seropositive patients and independently associated with biopsy-proven cirrhosis, either before or after transplantation.[539, 540] To date, there have been no controlled trials to assess the efficacy of IFN-α therapy after renal transplantation, and the risk of graft rejection has been reported to range between 40 and 100%.[521, 538, 542] Some experts feel that IFN-α may precipitate an episode of rejection by upregulating the cell surface expression of major histocompatibility complex class II antigens.[524, 556] Therefore, therapy with IFN-α should not be used after transplantation unless absolutely necessary, such as in patients with confirmed viremia and moderate to severe chronic hepatitis, advanced fibrosis, or both on liver biopsy.[524, 538]

Although strict universal precautions (now referred to as standard precautions) should be applied to all patients receiving hemodialysis, the CDC does not currently recommend using segregated areas or dedicated machines for HCV-seropositive patients. Participation in dialyzer reuse programs is also permissible.[521, 524, 538] However, nosocomial spread of HCV infection has been reported,[532, 533] and patients receiving chronic hemodialysis may benefit from monthly checks of serum ALT levels to detect exposure to HCV. Because ALT levels are frequently normal even in cases of confirmed HCV infection in these patients, periodic screening with HCV RNA tests may be advisable, although it is expensive. Routine screening of dialysis personnel is not recommended.[219, 524, 538, 542]

Porphyria Cutanea Tarda

The most common type of porphyria, porphyria cutanea tarda (PCT), is often associated with chronic HCV infection. Most patients present with a vesiculobullous eruption on the face and hands caused by deposits in the skin of uroporphyrins and heptacarboxyporphyrins that are light sensitive. Excess production of these porphyrins by the liver may result from decreased activity of hepatic uroporphyrinogen decarboxylase (Uro-D) or altered provision of porphyrin substrates for pathways involving and not involving uroporphyrinogen decarboxylase. In most instances, however, additional factors are required for PCT to develop, notably excess hepatic iron or chronic liver disease secondary to alcohol or HCV.[557–559] The prevalence of HCV in patients with PCT varies from a high of 71 to 91% in southern Europe to a low of 0 to 18% in northern or central Europe, Australia, and New Zealand.[557–560] In a study[560] of 70 unselected patients from the United States with typical PCT, 56% had evidence of HCV infection. On the other hand, 15% of HCV patients without PCT were found to have elevated urinary porphyrins, but these were not the porphyrins usually seen in PCT, which suggests that preclinical PCT is rare in patients with chronic HCV in the United States.

However, altered iron metabolism may also play an important role in PCT. Most patients with PCT have some degree of excess hepatic iron, and iron reduction therapy improves the clinical features of PCT. The HFE gene mutations (C282T and H63D) that cause hereditary hemochromatosis have been noted in about 45% of European and 73% of U.S. individuals with PCT.[560–562] Alcohol and estrogen have been identified as additional risk factors. As discussed earlier in "Treatment of Chronic Hepatitis C Virus Infection with Interferons," excess hepatic iron may worsen the liver disease resulting from HCV and blunt the response to IFN-α therapy. In PCT, iron may increase the production of uroporphyrinogen decarboxylase substrates as well as inhibit uroporphyrinogen decarboxylase activity. The management of PCT includes the removal of inciting factors such as iron supplements, alcohol, and estrogens as well as iron reduction therapy with phlebotomy. Additional potential benefits of phlebotomy include an improved response to IFN-α therapy.[557–560, 563, 564]

Coinfection with Hepatitis B Virus or Human Immunodeficiency Virus

Because of similar modes of transmission, coinfection with other viruses is a common problem in patients with chronic HCV.[565] In terms of HBV and HCV coinfection, these patients have more aggressive liver disease and may be at higher risk for developing hepatocellular carcinoma, even though HCV appears to inhibit HBV replication.[566–569] Because coinfected patients tend to have a lower level of hepatitis B viremia, more sensitive assays such as PCR for HBV DNA are required to exclude HBV. One report suggests that when this method is used, hepatitis B viremia can be readily detected in coinfected patients from areas in which HBV is highly endemic, even in those who are HB_sAg negative.[570] On the other hand, HCV replication appears to be enhanced by HBV and the chance of responding to IFN-α may be reduced.[571, 572] Nevertheless, patients coinfected with HBV and HCV should always be considered for treatment. Most experts advise treating HBV first with IFN-α monotherapy (i.e., 5 MU daily) for 6 months. This may also clear HCV infection, but if not, combination therapy with IFN-α plus ribavirin for 6 months or longer is warranted.[565, 567]

With the advent of highly active antiretroviral therapy, most patients with HIV can now expect a more favorable outcome. However, HIV coinfection appears to worsen HCV-related liver disease and has a less adverse impact on HBV.[573–575] The reverse effect of these viruses on the progression of HIV remains unclear.[565, 576, 577] A rapidly progressive form of cholestasis has been reported in HIV-positive patients coinfected with HCV who have severely compromised immune function, and a rising alkaline phosphatase may predict imminent death.[565, 578] Drug-induced hepatotoxicity must always be suspected in these patients, because it can be seen with the protease inhibitors (e.g., indinavir and ritonavir) and with the non-nucleoside reverse transcriptase inhibitor nevirapine.[565, 576]

In terms of antiviral therapy, patients with HIV should be treated for the HIV before starting additional therapy for HCV or HBV, perhaps 2 to 3 months later. Most patients with HBV tend to be receiving lamivudine already as part of their highly active antiretroviral therapy.[98, 565] If lamivudine needs to be discontinued, it should always be tapered to avoid a flare in HBV infection. IFN can also be used effectively for HBV, as long as baseline serum ALT levels are elevated significantly (see "Treatment of Chronic Hepatitis B Virus Infection with Interferons"). Although $CD4^+$ cell counts above 500/μl and the absence of opportunistic infections may be important in determining the outcome of HCV treatment, they appear to be less helpful than first thought.[565, 576, 577] Nevertheless, standard-dose IFN-α monotherapy led to lower sustained virologic response rates (0 to 44% after 6 to 12 months) in HIV-HCV–coinfected patients than in HIV-negative patients, although therapy was tolerated well with no increase in the risk of opportunistic infections.[576–579] The variable rates of response with IFN-α are probably related to differences in the degree of immunosuppression and in the type of therapy. Longer duration and higher doses lead to more favorable response rates,[576, 577] although a sudden and dramatic fall in the $CD4^+$ cell count may occur in up to 5% of patients when IFN-α is initiated.[580, 581]

Because liver damage tends to be rapidly progressive in HIV-HCV–coinfected patients, more aggressive approaches such as combination therapy (IFN-α plus ribavirin) or daily induction IFN-α monotherapy may be warranted, although studies are still in progress. Of note, ribavirin has been shown to inhibit HIV replication as well as HIV-1 reverse transcriptase in vitro,[582, 583] but clinical benefit has not been observed.[419, 577, 584, 585] Drug interactions between ribavirin and zidovudine or stavudine have been reported in vitro, but they are not likely to be a problem in clinical practice.[416, 565, 577, 586, 587] Interferon and zidovudine may have additive adverse effects on bone marrow function.[565] In some studies, highly active antiretroviral therapy may actually reduce HCV RNA levels and potentially reduce the risk of progression to cirrhosis, but more long-term studies are required.[577, 588]

CHRONIC HEPATITIS D

First identified in 1977 as the delta agent,[589] HDV is a defective, 37-nm single-stranded, 1700-nucleotide RNA virus that requires the presence of HB_sAg in order to replicate efficiently[590] (see Chapter 135). HDV affects almost 15 million people worldwide. High-prevalence areas include Italy, eastern Europe, the Amazon basin, western Asia, and some Pacific islands. Transmission of HDV occurs in a manner similar to transmission of HBV, primarily via parenteral routes. In low-frequency areas such as the United States, intravenous drug use is the most common risk factor, whereas in areas of high endemicity, such as Italy, vertical transmission predominates. Sexual transmission of HDV appears to be less efficient than that of HBV.[591] The geographic distribution of HDV tends to parallel that of chronic HBV infection, although not completely, which suggests that other factors such as age at acquisition may be important. In fact, individuals infected with HBV in infancy (e.g., in Italy) seem at less risk of acquiring HDV than older individuals (e.g., in the United States).[591, 592] This may be related, however, to different modes of transmission and associated risks of acquiring other viral infections. Three genotypes of HDV have been proposed; type 1 is the most common one identified worldwide. Type 2 is found in Taiwan and type 3 in South America. The incidence of HDV infection is falling in the United States, where it previously caused more than 7500 infections a year. Although HDV is a less frequent cause of chronic hepatitis than the other viruses, HDV is more likely to lead to fulminant hepatitis or chronic progressive liver disease and cirrhosis.[589–594]

Acute HDV infection may occur in one of three ways: concurrently in a patient with acute HBV infection (coinfection), in a patient already infected with HBV (superinfection), and after liver transplantation when latent HDV infection in the allograft occurs before overt HBV reinfection of the graft.[593, 595] Coinfection usually results in clinical features similar to those seen in acute infection with HBV alone, although for unknown reasons fulminant hepatitis is more common. In one study, 34% of patients with fulminant HBV had evidence of HDV, compared with only 4% of those with nonfulminant acute HBV infection. Coinfection with HDV does not appear to increase the risk of developing chronic HBV infection. On the other hand, superinfection of chronic HBV carriers leads to progressive liver disease in as many as 90% of cases and fulminant liver failure is also common.[589–596]

HDV infection should always be suspected in patients with HBV who have seroconverted and become anti-HB_e antibody positive but continue to manifest chronic hepatitis, because liver inflammation usually resolves rapidly after HBV seroconversion.[594] HDV should also be considered in stable HB_sAg-positive patients with a significant flare in serum ALT or aspartate aminotransferase levels but no change in HB_eAg status or in those with rapidly progressive disease and early onset of cirrhosis. However, the diagnosis of acute HDV is problematic because anti-HDV immunoglobulin G (IgG) may take several weeks to become positive. Anti-HDV IgM levels are usually detected before the appearance of anti-HDV IgG. In chronic cases, anti-HDV IgG levels remain elevated and anti-HDV IgM persists indefinitely, as in the case of chronic HBV replication. On liver biopsy, HDV antigen can be detected by immunohistochemistry or in situ hybridization.[589–596]

HDV antigen may also be found in the serum in 20% of acute cases, but in most patients with chronic disease HDV antigen disappears because it binds to anti-HDV. However, low levels of circulating HDV antigen may remain detectable in low titer in patients who are immunodeficient or immunosuppressed. Coinfection cannot be differentiated from superinfection by using anti-HDV IgM levels, and anti-HB_c IgM levels are the most helpful in this respect. Patients with acute coinfection have detectable HDV viral markers accompanied by anti-HB_c IgM, whereas in cases with superinfection, HDV markers are present but circulating anti-HB_c IgM is absent, probably because of the suppression of HBV replication by HDV. High titers of anti-HDV IgG ($>$ 1:1000) usually indicate ongoing viral replication. Although still a research tool, HDV RNA may also be helpful in determining the presence or absence of active HDV infection.[589–596]

In terms of treatment, IFN-α has been the agent used most often to date but with only limited success.[589, 597–606] No specific factors predict a response to IFN-α, although a shorter duration of disease, as is the case with intravenous drug users, may be a more favorable predictor.[593, 598] Pilot studies using standard doses of IFN-α for 3 to 4 months led initially to biochemical and histologic improvement in most patients accompanied by a fall in or disappearance of markers of HDV replication. However, these effects were only transitory. In contrast, higher doses of IFN-α given for prolonged periods may improve sustained response rates significantly.[597–606] In a multicenter trial in Italy,[605] IFN-α at 9 MU three times a week for 12 months led to a remission (normalization of serum ALT levels and clearance of serum HDV RNA) in 36% of treated patients, whereas a lower dose of 3 MU three times a week was not effective. Both treated groups, however, had a higher rate of response than control subjects, among whom there were no responders. Viral relapse occurred in all upon drug cessation.

Slow tapering of IFN-α after completion of a 12-month course of therapy does not appear to prevent relapse, because breakthrough was noted in serum ALT levels when the IFN-α dose was lowered from 5 to 3 MU three times a week.[597, 599] Furthermore, unlike the situation with HBV or HCV, in which a sustained virologic response can usually be predicted within the first 2 to 4 months of therapy, it may take 10 months or more for patients with HDV to respond adequately. Therefore, a minimum of 12 months of IFN-α therapy at 9 MU three times a week or 5 MU daily is recommended for most patients with HDV. With this, up to 15 to 25% have sustained improvements, usually accompanied by disappearance of HB_sAg from the serum.[597]

Because of similar modes of transmission, patients with HDV and HBV are often coinfected with HIV.[589, 591] The long-term prognosis may be worse for these patients.[607–610] IFN-α therapy may also be less effective,[597, 599] although in one study[606] selection of patients for prolonged IFN-α therapy using specific criteria led to a favorable response in a sizable number. In terms of other therapies for HDV patients in general, although suramin and ribavirin are active against HDV in a primary woodchuck hepatocyte model, suramin has been found to be toxic and ribavirin has shown no benefit in preliminary trials.[597] Whether the enhanced clearance rate of HB_sAg with lamivudine or other nucleoside analogues will have a favorable impact on the management of HDV remains to be determined.

As with patients with HBV-related cirrhosis, IFN-α is contraindicated in advanced cases of end-stage HDV-related liver disease, because of the risks of precipitating further decompensation related to a flare in necroinflammatory activity during viral clearance. Instead, these patients should be listed for liver transplantation. As mentioned earlier, after transplantation, latent HDV infection of the allograft may occur before overt reinfection of the graft with HBV.[593] However, unlike patients with HBV infection alone, those with HDV have a better outcome after liver transplantation, because HDV tends to inhibit HBV replication and lower the rate of reinfection after transplantation by half (from 67 to 32%), which is associated with a significantly better 3-year survival rate (88 versus 44% in favor of HDV-coinfected patients).[597, 606] Transplantation for acute HDV fulminant hepatitis also carries a more favorable prognosis, with a 3-year survival rate of about 65%.[594, 597] For patients with chronic HDV who undergo liver transplantation, prophylactic HBIG remains an effective means of preventing recurrence of HBV as well as HDV in the allograft. In a study of HDV patients given HBIG prophylactically, the recurrence rate of HBV was only 10%, considerably less than that seen in patients who had HBV alone. Survival was also improved.[611]

HEPATIC GRANULOMAS

Granulomatous hepatitis is a misnomer because the classic inflammatory responses involved in granuloma formation are rarely identified in this condition and significant hepatocellular dysfunction ("hepatitis") is uncommon.[612] A better term is hepatic granulomas. They are found in a variety of conditions, which can be grouped into four main categories (Table 103–10): infectious, drug induced, neoplastic, and miscellaneous.[613, 614] Despite extensive investigations, the exact cause cannot be identified in a sizable proportion of cases, ranging from 5 to 50%, the higher figure coming from a study at a tertiary care center.[615, 616] On the other hand, in a classic paper published more than 20 years ago, 74% of hepatic granulomas were related to a systemic process, 21% were primarily related to neither a systemic nor a hepatic process, and 4% were not associated with any other disease.[617]

Granulomas form in the liver as a cell-mediated response to a variety of antigens, many of which are unknown. Macrophages are recruited to the site of acute inflammation and attempt to clear antigens and other inflammatory by-products. In the case of tuberculosis, these consist of mycobacterial lipids. Schistosome eggs can elicit the same responses. In contrast, nonmicrobial compounds (silica or metal salts) act via nonimmunologic mechanisms. If macrophages are unsuccessful in clearing residual antigen, additional monocytes are attracted from the blood stream and bone marrow to form tissue epithelioid histiocytes, which then fuse to become multinucleated giant cells.[614, 618] These unusual cells lose their phagocytic properties and instead take on secretory functions. In the case of sarcoidosis, they are thought to be the origin of the angiotensin-converting enzyme activity characteristic of this condition.[619] Cytokines of the Th1 immune response then attract $CD4^+$ and $CD8^+$ T lymphocytes, which ultimately constitute the periphery of the granulomas. Systemic recognition and sensitization of the antigen result in activation of the Th2 immune response with subsequent necrosis or caseation.[620] The Kveim test elicits many of these responses but it is no longer commercially available.[621]

Unfortunately, with hepatic granulomas, there are no pathognomonic symptoms, signs, or physical findings to suggest that a patient might have the condition. Fever is a major manifestation of hepatic granulomas, and in many cases hepatic granulomas are detected as part of a diagnostic workup for fever of unknown origin.[622] On liver biopsy, the granulomas consist of discrete nodular infiltrates of epithelioid cells within the liver lobules (not the portal triads) with varying numbers of mononuclear cells. The epithelioid cells may often coalesce to form typical multinucleated giant cells, although the latter need not be present to make the diagnosis. These histopathologic features are clearly distinct from those seen in the much

TABLE 103–10 Hepatic Granulomas: Major Causes

Infectious	Drug Induced	Neoplastic	Miscellaneous
Bacteria	Allopurinol	Hodgkin's disease	Sarcoidosis
Tuberculosis	Carbamazepine	Non-Hodgkin's lymphoma	Primary biliary cirrhosis
Mycobacterium avium-intracellulare	Diltiazem	Renal cell cancer	Talc
Brucellosis	Gold		Berylliosis
Listeriosis	Hydralazine		Whipple's disease
Tularemia	Methyldopa		Inflammatory bowel disease
Leprosy	Nitrofurantoin		Idiopathic
Rickettsiae	Phenytoin		
Coxiella burnetii (Q fever)	Procainamide		
Secondary syphilis	Quinidine		
Fungi	Sulfonamides		
Histoplasmosis			
Cryptococcosis			
Parasites			
Toxoplasmosis			
Schistosomiasis			

more common chronic hepatitis, in which mononuclear cells (and polymorphonuclear cells) infiltrate the portal triads. When hepatic granulomas are identified, however, the exact cause must be looked for diligently in order to direct appropriate therapy and improve outcome. Corticosteroids quickly resolve noninfectious causes of hepatic granulomas but would be contraindicated for most infectious causes, for which antimicrobials are instead the primary treatment modality.[612–614]

Worldwide, the most common cause of hepatic granulomas is tuberculosis. With the HIV epidemic, tuberculosis and atypical mycobacteria are now top contenders in the United States.[622] Miliary tuberculosis is associated with hepatic granulomas in almost all cases, and the granulomas in this condition may grow to more than 2 mm in diameter and spread throughout the liver parenchyma. In contrast, hepatic granulomas are rarely found in patients with predominantly lung involvement by tuberculosis and are seen in only 75% of those with extrapulmonary disease.[613, 622] The hepatic granulomas encountered in tuberculosis are confined to the periportal areas much as in sarcoidosis, making the distinction between the two sometimes difficult. Acid-fast stains are insensitive in hepatic tuberculosis, and cultures give a higher yield.[623] In suspicious cases, antituberculous therapy should be instituted promptly because cultures may take several weeks to become positive.

In HIV-positive patients, hepatic granulomas are most often associated with typical and atypical mycobacteria. They are usually noncaseating and consist of large foamy macrophages with few lymphocytes. The presence of granulomas may indicate a more active immune system in these HIV-positive patients and a better prognosis.[623] Cultures are more likely to be positive despite a negative stain.[624] Fungi, cytomegalovirus, talc, and lymphoma should be considered as other causes for hepatic granulomas in these patients.[613] Leprosy and schistosomiasis are endemic in some areas of the world and may cause granulomas in the liver in a high percentage of cases.[615]

Although rare, other infectious causes of hepatic granulomas include brucellosis, Q fever, boutonneuse fever, and syphilis. Brucellosis classically presents with undulating fevers, arthralgias, myalgias, and hepatosplenomegaly, although the kidneys, heart valves, and joints may also be involved. The granulomas in brucellosis tend to be scattered throughout the liver lobule rather than confined to the periportal areas.[622] They are usually few in number except in some cases in which exuberant Kupffer cell hyperplasia and nonepithelioid granulomas may occur.[625] Specific serologic tests for brucellosis are required. In Q fever, there is a striking degree of lymphoid hyperplasia in the portal triads with destruction of the limiting plate. The granulomas in Q fever also have a classic "doughnut" or "fibrin ring" appearance because of a halo that results from an area of fibrin enclosing a clear space of necrosis.[626] However, these ring granulomas may also be found with boutonneuse fever, visceral leishmaniasis, Hodgkin's lymphoma, drug hypersensitivity (e.g., allopurinol), or with cytomegalovirus disease.[613]

Sarcoidosis is a systemic granulomatous disease that frequently involves the liver. Serum alkaline phosphatase and aminotransferases are elevated to a mild to moderate degree. Severe cholestasis rarely occurs. Most of the time, the hepatic granulomas in sarcoidosis are found in the portal areas and are nondescript. Rarely they may be associated with significant fibrosis and portal hypertension and its complications. Marked hepatomegaly has been reported, especially in African Americans between the ages of 20 and 50, in which biliary fibrosis or cirrhosis is more common.[622, 627] Involvement of small bile ducts is infrequent, but this may make differentiation from primary biliary cirrhosis and primary sclerosing cholangitis difficult.[628, 629] On occasion, sarcoidosis may overlap with these conditions and antimitochondrial antibody may actually be positive in some cases. Angiotensin-converting enzyme may point toward sarcoidosis if it is elevated significantly.[630]

Of the other unusual causes of hepatic granulomas (see Table 103–10), drugs should always be considered in the differential diagnosis. These include allopurinol, sulfonamides, hydralazine, quinidine, and any other drug, for that matter.

When the etiology of the disease process remains obscure, a systematic approach to establishing the diagnosis directed at the possible causes outlined in Table 203–10 should be undertaken. The liver biopsy specimen should be cultured for bacterial fungal, mycobacterial, and viral agents. Stains for microbial agents, including silver-impregnated stains, should be used. Skin tests for *Mycobacterium tuberculosis* (purified protein derivative) should be applied. Serologic tests for syphilis, Q fever, brucellosis, schistosomiasis, Epstein-Barr virus, and cytomegalovirus should be conducted. A similar systematic approach should be used to exclude the noninfectious causes listed in Table 103–10.

Treatment of hepatic granulomas should be directed at the specific etiology, if identified. The resolution of the granulomas correlates with the therapeutic response to the underlying disease. In cases in which infectious and other causes have been excluded as far as possible, the use of corticosteroids should be considered. Because of the risk of administering corticosteroids in the presence of untreated tuberculosis, an empirical course of treatment for tuberculosis before the use of corticosteroids has been suggested. If a clinical response is observed, treatment is continued to complete the course. If no clinical response is seen after 2 months, antituberculous treatment should be stopped and steroids begun. If the patient is positive with purified protein derivative, isoniazid is continued with the corticosteroids. In cases in which symptoms are mild, treatment may be deferred and the patient observed carefully.[612–614, 622, 623]

REFERENCES

1. Gross JB Jr. Clinician's guide to hepatitis C. Mayo Clin Proc. 1998;73:355–361.
2. Lee MW. Hepatitis B virus infection. N Engl J Med. 1997;337:1733–1745.

3. Maddrey WC, Schiff ER. The diagnosis and management of chronic viral hepatitis: Update 1998. Clin Cour. 16(49):September 1998.
4. Karayiannis P, Thomas HC. Hepatitis G virus: Identification, prevalence and unanswered questions. Gut. 1997;40:294–296.
5. Simmonds P, Davidson F, Lycett C, et al. Detection of a novel DNA virus (TTV) in blood donors and blood products. Lancet. 1998;352:191–195.
6. Schiff E. Atypical clinical manifestations of hepatitis A. Vaccine. 1992;10(Suppl 1):S18–S23.
7. Glikson M, Galun E, Oren, R et al. Relapsing hepatitis A: Review of 14 cases and literature survey. Medicine (Baltimore). 1992;71:14–22.
8. Vento S, Garofano T, DiPerri G, et al. Identification of hepatitis A virus as a trigger for autoimmune chronic hepatitis type 1 in susceptible individuals. Lancet. 1991;2:1183–1185.
9. Vento S, Garofano T, Renzini C, et al. Fulminant hepatitis associated with hepatitis A virus superinfection in patients with chronic hepatitis C. N Engl J Med. 1998;338:286–290.
10. Hübscher SG. Histological grading and staging in chronic hepatitis: Clinical applications and problems. J Hepatol. 1998;29:105–1022.
11. Scheuer PJ, Davies SE, Dhillon AP. Histopathological aspects of viral hepatitis. J Viral Hepatol. 1996;3:277–283.
12. Hayden GH, Jarvis LM, Blair CS, et al. Clinical significance of intrahepatic hepatitis C virus levels in patients with chronic HCV infection. Gut. 1998;42:570–575.
13. Berenguer M, Wright TL. Is the hepatocyte a Trojan horse for hepatitis C virus? Gut. 1998;42:456–458.
14. Desmet VJ, Gerber M, Hoofnagle JH, et al. Classification of chronic hepatitis: Diagnosis, grading and staging. Hepatology. 1994;19:1513–1520.
15. Alter MJ, Gallagher M, Morris TT, et al. Acute non-A–E hepatitis in the United States and the role of hepatitis G virus infection. N Engl J Med. 1997;336:741–746.
16. Margolis H, Alter M, Hadler S. Hepatitis B: Evolving epidemiology and implications for control. Semin Liver Dis. 1991;11:84–95.
17. Francis DP. The public's health unprotected: Reversing a decade of underutilization of hepatitis B vaccine. JAMA. 1995;274:1242–1243.
18. Chang M-H, Chen C-J, Lai M-S, et al. Universal hepatitis B vaccination in Taiwan and the incidence of hepatocellular carcinoma in children. N Engl J Med. 1997;336:1855–1859.
19. Update: Recommendations to prevent hepatitis B virus transmission—United States. JAMA. 1995;274:603–604.
20. Lau JYN, Wright TL. Molecular virology and pathogenesis of hepatitis B. Lancet. 1993;342:1335–1340.
21. Moradpour D, Wands JR. Understanding hepatitis B virus infection. N Engl J Med. 1995;332:1092–1093.
22. Angus PW, Locarnini SA, McCaughan GW, et al. Hepatitis B virus precore mutant infection is associated with severe recurrent disease after liver transplantation. Hepatology. 1995;21:14–18.
23. McMahon B, Bulkow L, et al. Early detection of hepatocellular carcinoma in HBsAg-positive carriers: A 15-year prospective population-based study in Alaska. Hepatology. 1998;28(Suppl 1):388A.
24. Terrault NA, Wright TL. Viral hepatitis A through G. In: Feldman M, Scharschmidt BF, Sleisinger MH, eds. Gastrointestinal and Liver Disease. 6th ed. Philadelphia: WB Saunders; 1998;1123–1170.
25. Alter M, Mast E. The epidemiology of hepatitis in the United States. Gastroenterol Clin North Am. 1994;23:437–445.
26. Alter M, Hadler S, Margolis H, et al. The changing epidemiology of hepatitis B in the United States: Need for alternative vaccination strategies. JAMA. 1990;263:1218–1221.
27. Harpaz R, Von Seidlin L, Averhoff FM, et al. Transmission of hepatitis B virus to multiple patients from a surgeon without evidence of inadequate infection control. N Engl J Med. 1996;334:549–554.
28. Chen HL, Chang MH, Ni YH, et al. Seroepidemiology of hepatitis B virus infection in children. JAMA. 1996;276:906–908.
29. Davis LG, Weber DJ, Lemon SM. Horizontal transmission of hepatitis B virus. Lancet. 1993;1:889–893.
30. Leichtner A, Leclair J, Goldmann DA, et al. Horizontal nonparenteral spread of hepatitis B among children. Ann Intern Med. 1993;94:346–349.
31. Bortolotti F, Cadrobbi P, Crivellaro C, et al. Long-term outcome of chronic type B hepatitis in patients who acquire hepatitis B virus infection in childhood. Gastroenterology. 1990;99:805–810.
32. Fattovich G, Giustina G, Schalm SW, et al. Occurrence of hepatocellular carcinoma and decompensation in western European patients with cirrhosis type B. Hepatology. 1995;21:77–82.
33. Lok ASF, Lai C-L. A longitudinal follow-up of asymptomatic hepatitis B surface–positive Chinese children. Hepatology. 1988;8:1130–1133.
34. Fattovich G, Brollo L, Alberti A, et al. Long-term follow-up of anti-HBe–positive chronic active hepatitis B. Hepatology. 1988;8:1651–1654.
35. DeJongh FE, Janssen HLA, deMan RA, et al. Survival and prognostic indicators in hepatitis B surface antigen–positive cirrhosis of the liver. Gastroenterology. 1992;103:1630–1635.
36. Fattovich G, Giustina G, Sanchez-Tapias J, et al. Delayed clearance of serum HBsAg in compensated cirrhosis B: Relation to interferon alpha therapy and disease prognosis. Am J Gastroenterol. 1998;93:896–900.
37. Villeneuve J-P, Desrochers M, Infante-Rivard C, et al. A long-term follow-up study of asymptomatic hepatitis B surface antigen–positive carriers in Montreal. Gastroenterology. 1994;106:1000–1005.
38. Hoofnagle JH, DiBisceglie AM. The treatment of chronic viral hepatitis. N Engl J Med. 1997;336:347–356.
39. DiBisceglie AM, Hoofnagle JH. Chronic viral hepatitis. In: Zakim D, Boyer TD, eds. Hepatology—A Textbook of Liver Disease. Philadelphia: WB Saunders; 1996;1299–1329.
40. Lok ASF, Lai C-L, Wu P-C, Leung EKY. Long-term follow-up in a randomised controlled trial of recombinant α2-interferon in Chinese patients with chronic hepatitis B infection. Lancet. 1988;2:298–302.
41. Greenberg HB, Pollard RB, Lutwick LI, et al. Effect of human leukocyte interferon on hepatitis B virus infection in patients with chronic active hepatitis. N Engl J Med. 1976;295:517–522.
42. Dusheiko G, DiBisceglie A, Bowyer S, et al. Recombinant leukocyte interferon treatment of chronic hepatitis B. Hepatology. 1985;5:556–561.
43. Dooley JS, Davis GL, Peters M, et al. Pilot study of recombinant human alpha-interferon for chronic type B hepatitis. Gastroenterology. 1986;90:150–155.
44. Hoofnagle JH, Peters M, Mullen KD, et al. Randomized, controlled trial of recombinant human alpha-interferon in patients with chronic hepatitis B. Gastroenterology. 1988;95:1318–1322.
45. Alexander GJ, Brahm J, Fagan FA, et al. Loss of HBsAg with interferon therapy in chronic hepatitis B virus infection. Lancet. 1987;2:66–68.
46. Perrillo RP, Schiff ER, Davis GL, et al. A randomized, controlled trial of interferon alfa-2b alone and after prednisone withdrawal for the treatment of chronic hepatitis B. N Engl J Med. 1990;323:295–301.
47. DiBisceglie AM, Fong T, Fried MW, et al. A randomized, controlled trial of recombinant alpha-interferon therapy for chronic hepatitis B. Am J Gastroenterol. 1993;88:1887–1892.
48. Krogsgaard K. The long-term effect of treatment with interferon-α2a in chronic hepatitis B. The Long-term Follow-up Investigator Group. The European Study Group on Viral Hepatitis (EUROHEP). Executive Team on Anti-Viral Treatment. J Viral Hepat. 1998;5:389–397.
49. Lok ASF, Chung H-T, Liu VWS, et al. Long-term follow-up of chronic hepatitis B patients treated with interferon alfa. Gastroenterology. 1993;105:1833–1838.
50. Wong DKH, Cheung AM, O'Rourke K, et al. Effect of alpha-interferon treatment in patients with hepatitis B e antigen–positive chronic hepatitis B: A meta-analysis. Ann Intern Med. 1993;119:312–323.
51. Brook MG, Karayiannis P, Thomas HC. Which patients will respond to α interferon therapy? A statistical analysis of predictive factors. Hepatology. 1989;10:761–763.
52. Lai CL, Lok AS, Lin HJ, et al. Placebo-controlled trial of recombinant alpha 2 interferon in Chinese HBsAg carrier children. Lancet. 1987;2:877–880.
53. Perrillo R, Brunt E. Hepatic histologic and immunohistochemical changes in chronic hepatitis B after prolonged clearance of hepatitis B e antigen and hepatitis B surface antibody. Ann Intern Med. 1991;115:113–118.
54. Carreño V, Castillo I, Molina J, et al. Long-term follow-up of hepatitis B chronic carriers who responded to interferon therapy. J Hepatol. 1992;15:102–106.
55. Korenman J, Baker B, Waggoner J, et al. Long-term remission of chronic hepatitis B after alpha-interferon therapy. Ann Intern Med. 1991;114:629–634.
56. Niederau C, Heintges T, Lange S, et al. Long-term follow-up of HBeAg-positive patients treated with interferon alfa for chronic hepatitis B. N Engl J Med. 1996;334:1422–1427.
57. Wong JB, Koff RS, Tine F, Pauker SG. Cost-effectiveness of interferon-α2b treatment for hepatitis B e antigen–positive chronic hepatitis B. Ann Intern Med. 1995;122:644–675.
58. Dusheiko G, Roberts J. Treatment of chronic type B and C hepatitis with interferon alfa: An economic appraisal. Hepatology. 1995;22:1863–1866.
59. Perrillo R, Tamburro C, Regenstein F, et al. Low dose, titratable interferon alfa in decompensated liver disease caused by chronic infection with hepatitis B virus. Gastroenterology. 1995;109:908–916.
60. Martin P, Hann HW, Westerberg S, et al. Interferon alpha-2b therapy is efficacious in Asian-Americans with chronic hepatitis B infection: A prospective controlled trial. Dig Dis Sci. 1998;43:875–882.
61. Carrithers RL Jr. Effect of interferon on hepatitis B. Lancet. 1998;351:157–159.
62. Lutwick LI. Clinical interactions between human immunodeficiency virus and the human hepatitis viruses. Infect Dis Clin Pract. 1999;8:9–20.
63. Gilson RJ, Hawkins AE, Beecham MR, et al. Interactions between HIV and hepatitis B virus in homosexual men: Effects on the natural history of infection. AIDS. 1997;11:597–606.
64. Sinicco A, Raiteri R, Sciandra M, et al. Coinfection and superinfection of hepatitis B in patients with human immunodeficiency virus: No evidence of faster progression to AIDS. Scand J Infect Dis. 1997;29:111–115.
65. Perez V, Tanno H, Vallamil F, Fay O. Recombinant interferon alfa-2b following prednisone withdrawal in the treatment of chronic type B hepatitis. J Hepatol. 1990;11:S113–S115.
66. Krogsgaard K, Marcellin P, Trepo C, et al. Prednisolone withdrawal therapy enhances the effect of human lymphoblastoid interferon in chronic hepatitis B. J Hepatol. 1996;25:803–813.
67. Steroids in chronic B-hepatitis. A randomized, double-blind, multinational trial on the effect of low-dose, long-term treatment on survival. A trial group of the European Association for the Study of the Liver. Liver. 1986;6:227–230.
68. Nair PV, Tong MJ, Stevenson D, et al. Effects of short-term, high-dose prednisone treatment of patients with HBsAg-positive chronic active hepatitis. Liver. 1985;5:8–11.
69. Mutchnick M, Appelman HD, Chung H, et al. Thymosin treatment of chronic hepatitis B: A placebo-controlled pilot trial. Hepatology. 1991;14:409–415.
70. Mutchnick M, Lindsay K, Schiff E, et al. Thymosin alpha 1 treatment of chronic

hepatitis B: A multicenter, randomized, placebo-controlled double-blind study. Gastroenterology. 1995;108:A1127.
71. Chien R-N, Liaw Y-F, Chen T-C, et al. Efficacy of thymosin α_1 in patients with chronic hepatitis B: A randomized, controlled trial. Hepatology. 1998;27:1383–1387.
72. Fried MW, Fong T, Swain MG, et al. Therapy of chronic hepatitis B with a 6-month course of ribavirin. J Hepatol. 1994;21:145–149.
73. Conjeevaram HS, DiBesceglie AM. Management of chronic viral hepatitis in children. J Pediatr Gastroenterol Nutr. 1995;20:365–375.
74. Moreno MR, Rua MJ, Molina J, et al. Prospective, randomized trial of interferon in children with chronic hepatitis B. Hepatology. 1991;13:1035–1039.
75. Sokal EM, Wirth S, Goyens P, et al. Interferon alfa 2b therapy in children with chronic hepatitis B. Gut. 1993;34(Suppl):S87–S90.
76. Barbera C, Bortolotti F, Crivellaro C, et al. Recombinant interferon alpha 2a hastens the rate of HBeAg clearance in children with chronic hepatitis B. Hepatology. 1994;20:287–290.
77. Sokal EM, Conjeevaram HS, Roberts EA, et al. Interferon alfa therapy for chronic hepatitis B in children: A multinational randomized controlled trial. Gastroenterology. 1998;114:988–995.
78. Utili R, Sagnelli E, Gaeta GB, et al. Treatment of chronic hepatitis B in children with prednisone followed by alfa interferon: A controlled randomized study. J Hepatol. 1994;20:163–167.
79. Gregorio GV, Jara P, Hierro L, et al. Lymphoblastoid interferon alfa with and without steroid pretreatment in children with chronic hepatitis B: A multicenter controlled trial. Hepatology. 1996;23:700–707.
80. Marcellin P, Loriot M, Boyer N, et al. Recombinant human interferon in patients with chronic active hepatitis B: Pharmacokinetics, tolerance and biological effects. Hepatology. 1990;12:155–161.
81. Okanoue T, Sakamoto S, Itoh Y, et al. Side effects of high-dose interferon therapy for chronic hepatitis C. J Hepatol. 1996;25:283–291.
82. Fattovich G, Giustina G, Favarato S, et al. A survey of adverse events in 11,241 patients with chronic viral hepatitis treated with alfa interferon. J Hepatol. 1996;24:38–47.
83. Mohr DC, Goodkin DE, Likosky W, et al. Treatment of depression improves adherence to interferon beta-1b therapy for multiple sclerosis. Arch Neurol. 1997;54:531–533.
84. Nicoll A, Locarnini S. Review: Present and future directions in the treatment of chronic hepatitis B infection. J Gastroenterol Hepatol. 1997;12:843–854.
85. Terrault NA. Treatment of chronic hepatitis B and chronic hepatitis C. Rev Med Virol. 1996;6:215–222.
86. Zoulim F, Trepo C. Drug therapy for chronic hepatitis B: Antiviral efficacy and influence of hepatitis B virus polymerase mutations on the outcome of therapy. J Hepatol. 1998;29:151–168.
87. Schalm SW, de Man RA, Heijtink RA, Niesters HG. New nucleoside analogues for chronic hepatitis B. J Hepatol. 1995;1:52–56.
88. Hoofnagle JH, Lau D. New therapies for chronic hepatitis B. J Viral Hepat. 1997;4(Suppl 1):41–50.
89. Omata M. Treatment of chronic hepatitis B infection (Editorial). N Engl J Med. 1998;339:114–115.
90. Shaw T, Locarnini S. Hepatic purine and pyrimidine metabolism: Implications for antiviral chemotherapy of viral hepatitis. Liver. 1995;15:169–184.
91. Lee J-Y, Colledge D, Locarnini S. Pathogenic effects of antiviral therapy in chronic hepatitis B virus infection. In: Schinazi RF, Sommadossi J-P, Thomas HC, eds. Therapies for Viral Hepatitis. Atlanta: International Medical Press; 1998:285–302.
92. Furman PA, Schinazi RF. The mechanism of action and cellular pharmacology of anti–hepatitis B virus agents. In: Schinazi RF, Sommadossi J-P, Thomas HC, eds. Therapies for Viral Hepatitis. Atlanta: International Medical Press; 1998:273–283.
93. Wong WWS, Tyrrell DLJ. Treatment of hepatitis B virus with lamivudine. In: Schinazi RF, Sommadossi J-P, Thomas HC, eds. Therapies for Viral Hepatitis. Atlanta: International Medical Press; 1998:353–363.
94. Lai C-L, Chien R-N, Leung NWY, et al. A one-year trial of lamivudine for chronic hepatitis B. N Engl J Med. 1998;339:61–68.
95. Shafritz DA, Shouval D, Sherman HI, et al. Integration of hepatitis B virus DNA into the genome of liver cells in chronic liver disease and hepatocellular carcinoma: Studies in percutaneous liver biopsies and post-mortem tissue specimens. N Engl J Med. 1981;305:1067–1073.
96. Doong S-L, Tsai C-H, Schinazi RF, et al. Inhibition of the replication of hepatitis B virus in vitro by 2′,3′-dideoxy-3′thiacytidine and related analogues. Proc Natl Acad Sci U S A. 1991;88:8495–8499.
97. Tyrrell DLJ, Fischer K, Savani K, et al. Treatment of chimpanzees and ducks with lamivudine, 2′,3′-dideoxy-3′-thiacytidine, results in a rapid suppression of hepadnaviral DNA in sera. Clin Invest Med. 1993;16(Suppl 4):B77.
98. Moyle GJ, Gazzard BG, Lamivudine in the management of adults with human immunodeficiency virus type 1 infection. Antiviral Ther. 1998;3:7–18.
99. Severini A, Liu X-Y, Wilson J, Tyrrell D. Mechanism of inhibition of duck hepatitis B virus polymerase by (−)-β-L-2′,3′-dideoxy-3′-thiacytidine. Antimicrob Agents Chemother. 1995;39:1430–1435.
100. McKenzie R, Fried MW, Sallie R, et al. Hepatic failure and lactic acidosis due to fialuridine (FIAU), an investigational nucleoside analogue for chronic hepatitis B. N Engl J Med. 1995;333:1099–1105.
101. Van Leeuwen R, Katlama C, Kitchen V, et al. Evaluation of safety and efficacy of 3TC (lamivudine) in patients with advanced human immunodeficiency virus infection. J Infect Dis. 1995;171:1438–1447.
102. Tyrrell D, Mitchell M, De Man R, et al. Phase II trial of lamivudine for chronic hepatitis B. Hepatology. 1993;18(Suppl):112A.
103. Benhamou Y, Katlama C, Lunel F, et al. Effects of lamivudine on replication of hepatitis B virus in HIV-infected men. Ann Intern Med. 1996;125:705–712.
104. Dienstag JL, Perrillo RP, Schiff ER, et al. A preliminary trial of lamivudine for chronic hepatitis B infection. N Engl J Med. 1995;333:1657–1661.
105. Honkoop P, de Man RA, Zondervan PE, Schalm SW. Histological improvement in patients with chronic hepatitis B virus infection treated with lamivudine. Liver. 1997;2:103–106.
106. Lai C-L, Ching C-K, Tung AK-M, et al. Lamivudine is effective in suppressing hepatitis B virus DNA in Chinese hepatitis B surface antigen carriers: A placebo-controlled trial. Hepatology. 1997;25:241–244.
107. Nevens F, Main J, Honkoop P, et al. Lamivudine therapy for chronic hepatitis B: A six month randomized dose-ranging study. Gastroenterology. 1997;113:1258–1263.
108. Liaw YF, Lai CL, Leung NWY, et al. Two-year lamivudine therapy in chronic hepatitis B infection: Results of a placebo controlled multicenter study in Asia. Gastroenterology. 1998;114:A1289.
109. Dienstag J, Schiff E, Wright T, et al. Lamivudine treatment for one year in previously untreated US hepatitis B patients: Histologic improvement and hepatitis Be-antigen (HBeAg) seroconversion. Gastroenterology. 1998;114:A1235.
110. Honkoop P, de Man RA, Heijtink RA, et al. Hepatitis B reactivation after lamivudine. Lancet. 1995;346:1156–1157.
111. Naoumov NV, Perrillo RP, Chokshi S, et al. Reduction in hepatitis B virus quasispecies during lamivudine treatment is associated with enhanced viral replication and hepatocytolysis. Hepatology. 1995;22(Suppl 1):328A.
112. Schiff E, Cianciara J, Kowdley K, et al. Durability of HBeAg seroconversion after lamivudine monotherapy in controlled phase II and III trials. Hepatology. 1998;28(Suppl 1):163A.
113. Lau DT-Y, Doo E, Ghany MG, et al. Lamivudine for chronic hepatitis B with typical and atypical serology. Hepatology. 1997;26(Suppl 1):429A.
114. Tassopoulos NC, Volpes R, Pastore G, et al. Lamivudine therapy in patients with anti-HBe positive chronic hepatitis B: End of treatment analysis. J Hepatol. 1998;28(Suppl 1):43.
115. Watanabe H, Izumi N, Simizu M, et al. Disappearance of HBcAg in the liver is a clinically useful marker for discontinuation of lamivudine therapy in patients with chronic hepatitis B. Gastroenterology. 1998;114:A1363.
116. Tipples GA, Ma MM, Fischer KP, et al. Mutation in HBV RNA-dependent DNA polymerase confers resistance to lamivudine *in vivo*. Hepatology. 1996;24:714–717.
117. Naoumov NV, Chokshi S, Smith HM, Williams R. Emergence and characterization of lamivudine-resistant hepatitis B virus variant. Hepatology. 1996;24(Suppl):282A.
118. Honkoop P, Niesters HGM, de Man RAM, et al. Lamivudine resistance in immunocompetent chronic hepatitis B: Incidence and patterns. J Hepatol. 1997;26:1393–1395.
119. Allen MI, Deslauriers M, Andrews CW, et al. Identification and characterization of mutations in hepatitis B virus resistant to lamivudine. Hepatology. 1998;27:1670–1677.
120. Lai CL, Liaw YF, Leung NWY, et al. Genotypic resistance to lamivudine in a prospective, placebo-controlled multicenter study in Asia of lamivudine therapy for chronic hepatitis B infection: Incidence, kinetics of emergence, and correlation with disease parameters. Hepatology. 1997;26(Suppl 1):259A.
121. Perrillo R, Rakela J, Martin P, et al. Long term lamivudine therapy of patients with recurrent hepatitis B post liver transplantation. Hepatology. 1997;26(Suppl 1):177A.
122. Garrett L, Dienstag JL, Gauthier J, et al. Hepatitis e-antigen (HBeAg) seroconversion in two patients with evidence of genotypic resistance following extended lamivudine treatment. Hepatology. 1997;26(Suppl 1):431A.
123. Shields PL, Ling R, Harrison T, et al. Management and outcome of lamivudine resistant hepatitis B virus infection after liver transplantation. Hepatology. 1997;26(Suppl 1):260A.
124. Chayama K, Suzuki Y, Kobayashi M, et al. Emergence and takeover of YMDD motif mutant hepatitis B virus during long-term lamivudine therapy and re-takeover by wild type after cessation of therapy. Hepatology. 1998;27:1711–1716.
125. Heathcote J, Schalm SW, Ciancara J, et al. Lamivudine and Intron A combination treatment in patients with chronic hepatitis B infection. J Hepatol. 1998;28(Suppl 1):43.
126. Marinos G, Naoumov N, Williams R. Impact of complete inhibition of viral replication on the cellular immune response in chronic hepatitis B virus infection. Hepatology. 1996;24:991–995.
127. Schiff E, Karayalçin S, Grimm I, et al. A placebo controlled study of lamivudine and interferon alpha-2b in patients with chronic hepatitis B who previously failed interferon therapy. Hepatology. 1998;28(Suppl):388A.
128. Trepo C, Zoulim F. Treatment of chronic hepatitis B with famciclovir. In: Schinazi RF, Sommadossi J-P, Thomas HC, eds. Therapies for Viral Hepatitis. Atlanta: International Medical Press; 1998:365–370.
129. Cirelli R, Herne SD, McCrary M, et al. Famciclovir: Review of clinical efficacy and safety. Antiviral Res. 1996;29:141–151.
130. Korba BE, Boyd MR. Penciclovir is a selective inhibitor of hepatitis B virus replication in cultured human hepatoblastoma cells. Antimicrob Agents Chemother. 1996;40:1282–1284.
131. Shaw T, Mok S, Locarnini S. Inhibition of hepatitis B virus DNA polymerase by enantiomers of penciclovir triphosphate and metabolic basis for selective inhibition of HBV replication by penciclovir. Hepatology. 1996;24:996–1002.
132. Fontana RJ, Lok ASF. Combination therapy for chronic hepatitis B (Editorial). Hepatology. 1997;26:234–237.
133. Main J, Brown JL, Karayiannis P, et al. A double-blind, placebo-controlled study to assess the effect of famiciclovir on virus infection in patients with chronic hepatitis B virus infection. J Viral Hepat. 1996;3:211–215.

134. Trepo C, Jezek P, Atkinson GF, Boon RJ. Long term efficacy of famiciclovir (FCV) in chronic hepatitis B: Results of a phase IIB study. J Hepatol. 1997;26(Suppl 1):74.
135. Colledge D, Locarnini S, Shaw T. Synergistic inhibition of hepadnaviral replication by lamivudine in combination with penciclovir in vitro. Hepatology. 1997;26:216–225.
136. Richman DD. Drug resistance and its implications in the management of HIV infection. Antiviral Ther. 1997;2(Suppl 4):41–58.
137. Lau GKK, Kwok A, Karlberg J, et al. A twenty-six weeks trial of thymosin-α1 plus famciclovir in the treatment of Chinese immune tolerant adult patients with chronic hepatitis B. Hepatology. 1998;28(Suppl 1):216A.
138. Gilson RJC, Chopra K, Murray-Lyon I, et al. A placebo-controlled phase I/II study of adefovir dipivoxil (bis-POM PMEA) in patients with chronic hepatitis B infection. Hepatology. 1996;24(Suppl 1):281A.
139. Gilson RJC, Murray-Lyon IM, Nelson MR, et al. Extended treatment with adefovir dipivoxil in patients with chronic hepatitis B virus infection. Hepatology. 1998;28(Suppl 1):491A.
140. Heathcote EJ, Jeffers L, Wright T, et al. Loss of serum HBV DNA and HBeAg and seroconversion following short-term (12 weeks) adefovir dipivoxil therapy in chronic hepatitis B: Two placebo-controlled phase II studies. Hepatology. 1998;28(Suppl 1):317A.
141. Chokshi S, Papakonstantinou A, Gilson RJC, et al. Hepatitis flares in patients treated with adefovir dipivoxil correlate with activation of hepatitis B core-specific T cell reactivity. Hepatology. 1998;28(Suppl 1):589A.
142. Tsiang M, Dale B, Rooney J, et al. Dynamics of hepatitis B virus clearance from the serum of patients treated with adefovir dipivoxil for 12 weeks. Hepatology. 1998;28(Suppl 1):492A.
143. Xiong X, Flores C, Yang H, et al. Mutations in hepatitis B DNA polymerase associated with resistance to lamivudine do not confer resistance to adefovir *in vitro*. Hepatology. 1998;28:1669–1673.
144. Ono-Nita SK, Kato N, Shiratori Y, et al. Susceptibility of lamivudine resistant hepatitis B virus to other antivirals: Adefovir and lobucavir. Hepatology. 1998;28(Suppl 1):165A.
145. Xiong X, Yang H, Westland CE, et al. Human hepatitis B virus DNA polymerases which contain mutations arising during famciclovir treatment remain sensitive to adefovir. Hepatology. 1998;28(Suppl 1):491A.
146. Bloomer J, Chan R, Sherman M, et al. A preliminary study of lobucavir for chronic hepatitis B. Hepatology. 1997;26(Suppl 1):428A.
147. Heathcote J, Chan R, McHutchison J, et al. A phase 2 multi-center study of oral lobucavir for treatment of chronic hepatitis B. Hepatology. 1998;28(Suppl 1):318A.
148. Bloomer J, Brennan-Rowe N, Denisky G, et al. Extended treatment of chronic hepatitis B with oral lobucavir: Safety and efficacy. Hepatology. 1998;28(Suppl 1):486A.
149. Innaimo SF, Seifer M, Bisacchi GS, et al. Identification of BMS-200475 as a potent and selective inhibitor of hepatitis B virus. Antimicrob Agent Chemother. 1997;41:1444–1448.
150. Condreay L, Condreay J, Jansen R, et al. (−)-*cis*-5-Fluoro-1-(2-hydroxymethyl)-1,3-oxathiolan-5-yl) cytosine (524W91) inhibits hepatitis B virus replication in primary human hepatocytes. Antimicrob Agents Chemother. 1996;40:520–523.
151. Zoulim F, Dannaoui E, Borel C, et al. 2′,3′-dideoxy-β-L-5-fluorocytidine inhibits duck hepatitis B virus reverse transcription and suppresses viral DNA synthesis in hepatocytes, both *in vitro* and *in vivo*. Antimicrob Agents Chemother. 1996;40:448–453.
152. Aguesse-Germon S, Liu SH, Chevallier M, et al. Inhibitory effect of 2′-fluoro-5-methyl-β-L-arabinofuranosyl-uracyl on duck hepatitis B virus replication. Antimicrob Agents Chemother. 1998;42:369–376.
153. Chu CK, Boudinot FD, Peek SF, et al. Preclinical investigation of L-FMAU as an anti–hepatitis B virus agent. In: Schinazi RF, Sommadossi J-P, Thomas HC, eds. Therapies for Viral Hepatitis. Atlanta: International Medical Press; 1998:303–312.
154. Vitiello A, Ishioka G, Grey HM, et al. Development of a lipopeptide-based therapeutic vaccine to treat chronic HBV infection. I. Induction of a primary cytotoxic T lymphocyte response in humans. J Clin Invest. 1995;95:341–349.
155. Koziel MJ. The immunopathogenesis of hepatitis B virus infection. In: Schinazi RF, Sommadossi J-P, Thomas HC, eds. Therapies for Viral Hepatitis. Atlanta: International Medical Press; 1998:53–64.
156. Donnelly JJ, Ulmer JB, Shiver JW, Liu MA. DNA vaccines. Annu Rev Immunol. 1997;15:617–648.
157. Guilhot S, Guidotti L, Chisari F. Interleukin-2 downregulates hepatitis B virus gene expression in transgenic mice by a posttranscriptional mechanism. J Virol. 1993;67:7444–7449.
158. Cavanaugh VJ, Guidotti L, Chisari FV. Interleukin-12 inhibits hepatitis B virus replication in transgenic mice. J Virol. 1997;71:3236–3243.
159. Zern MA, Kresina T. Hepatic drug delivery and gene therapy. Hepatology. 1997;25:484–491.
160. von Weizsacker F, Wieland S, Kock J, et al. Gene therapy for chronic viral hepatitis: Ribozymes, antisense oligonucleotides, and dominant negative mutants. Hepatology. 1997;26:251–255.
161. Terrault NA, Wright TL. Hepatitis B virus infection and liver transplantation. Gut. 1997;40:568–571.
162. Poterucha JJ, Wiesner RH. Liver transplantation and hepatitis B. Ann Intern Med. 1997;126:805–807.
163. Ben-Ari Z, Tur-Kaspa R. New trends in liver transplantation for viral hepatitis. Am J Gastroenterol. 1997;92:2155–2159.
164. Grellier L, Dusheiko GM. Hepatitis B virus and liver transplantation: Concepts in antiviral prophylaxis. J Viral Hepat. 1997;4(Suppl 1):111–116.
165. Angus PW. Hepatitis B and liver transplantation. J Gastroenterol Hepatol. 1997;12:217–223.
166. O'Grady JG, Smith HM, Davies SE, et al. Hepatitis B virus reinfection after orthotopic liver transplantation: Serological and clinical implications. J Hepatol. 1992;14:104–111.
167. Kruger M, Manns MP. Liver transplantation and hepatitis B: Prophylaxis and treatment of reinfection with new antiviral agents. In: Schinazi RF, Sommadossi J-P, Thomas HC, eds. Therapies for Viral Hepatitis. Atlanta: International Medical Press; 1998:403–412.
168. Lautz HV, Muller R, Wittekind C, et al. Unusually rapid development of HBsAg-positive liver cirrhosis after transplantation. Klin Wochenschr. 1989;67:1061–1065.
169. Davies SE, Portman BC, O'Grady JG, et al. Hepatic histological findings after transplantation for chronic hepatitis B virus infection, including a unique pattern of fibrosing cholestatic hepatitis. Hepatology. 1991;13:150–157.
170. Crippin J, Foster B, Carlen S, et al. Retransplantation in hepatitis B: A multicenter experience. Transplantation. 1994;57:823–826.
171. Angus PW, Locarnini SA, McCaughan GW, et al. Hepatitis B virus precore mutant infection is associated with severe recurrent disease after liver transplantation. Hepatology. 1995;21:14–18.
172. Samuel D, Muller R, Alexander G, et al. Liver transplantation in European patients with the hepatitis B surface antigen. N Engl J Med. 1993;329:1842–1847.
173. Konig V, Hopf U, Neuhaus P, et al. Long-term follow-up of hepatitis B virus–infected recipients after orthotopic liver transplantation. Transplantation. 1994;58:553–559.
174. Samuel D, Bismuth A, Mathieu D, et al. Passive immunoprophylaxis after liver transplantation in HBsAg-positive patients. Lancet. 1991;337:813–815.
175. McGory R, Ishitani M, Oliveira W, et al. Improved outcome of orthotopic liver transplantation for chronic hepatitis B cirrhosis with aggressive passive immunization. Transplantation. 1996;61:1358–1364.
176. Sheil AGR, McCaughan GW, Isai H, et al. Acute and subacute fulminant hepatic failure: The role of liver transplantation. Med J Aust. 1991;154:724–728.
177. Dickson RC, Everhart JE, Lake JR, et al. Transmission of hepatitis B by transplantation of livers from donors positive for antibody to hepatitis B core antigen. The National Institute of Diabetes and Digestive and Kidney Diseases Liver Transplantation Database. Gastroenterology. 1997;113:1668–1674.
178. Uemoto S, Inomata Y, Sannomiya A, et al. Posttransplant hepatitis B infection in liver transplantation with hepatitis B core antibody–positive donors. Transplant Proc. 1998;30:134–135.
179. Terrault NA, Zhou S, McCory RW, et al. Incidence and clinical consequences of surface and polymerase gene mutations in liver transplant recipients on hepatitis B immunoglobulin. Hepatology. 1998;28:555–561.
180. Ghany MG, Ayola B, Villamil FG, et al. Hepatitis B virus S mutants in liver transplant recipients who were reinfected despite hepatitis B immune globulin prophylaxis. Hepatology. 1998;27:213–222.
181. Locarnini SA. Hepatitis B virus surface antigen and polymerase gene variants: Potential virological and clinical significance. Hepatology. 1998;27:294–297.
182. Marcellin P, Samuel D, Areias J, et al. Pretransplantation interferon treatment and recurrence of hepatitis B virus infection after liver transplantation for hepatitis B–related end-stage liver disease. Hepatology. 1994;19:6–12.
183. Terrault NA, Holland CC, Ferrell L, et al. Interferon-alfa for recurrent hepatitis B infection after liver transplantation. Liver Transplant Surg. 1997;2:132–138.
184. Pignatelli M, Waters J, Brown D, et al. HLA class I antigens on the membrane during recovery from acute hepatitis B virus infection and during interferon therapy in chronic hepatitis B virus infection. Hepatology. 1986;6:349–353.
185. Ben-Ari Z, Shmueli D, Shapiro Z, et al. Loss of serum HBsAg following interferon-alfa therapy in liver transplant patients with recurrent hepatitis-B infection. Liver Transplant Surg. 1997;3:394–397.
186. Grellier L, Mutimer D, Ahmed M, et al. Lamivudine prophylaxis against reinfection in liver transplantation for hepatitis B cirrhosis. Lancet. 1996;348:1212–1215.
187. Ben-Ari Z, Shmueli D, Mor E, et al. Beneficial effect of lamivudine in recurrent hepatitis B after liver transplantation. Transplantation. 1997;3:393–396.
188. Bain VG, Kneteman NM, Ma MM, et al. Efficacy of lamivudine in chronic hepatitis B patients with active viral replication and decompensated cirrhosis undergoing liver transplantation. Transplantation. 1996;62:1456–1462.
189. Villeneuve J-P, Bilodeau M, Fenyves D, et al. Suppression of hepatitis B virus replication by lamivudine results in improvement of liver function in patients with severe cirrhosis. Hepatology. 1997;26(Suppl 1):430A.
190. Perrillo R, Rakela J, Martin P, et al. Lamivudine for suppression and/or prevention of hepatitis B when given pre/post liver transplantation. Hepatology. 1997;26(Suppl 1):260A.
191. Perrillo R, Rakela J, Martin P, et al. Long term lamivudine therapy of patients with recurrent hepatitis B post liver transplantation. Hepatology. 1997;26(Suppl 1):177A.
192. Andreone P, Caraceni P, Grazi GL, et al. Lamivudine treatment for acute hepatitis B after liver transplantation. J Hepatol. 1998;29:985–989.
193. Ling R, Mutimer D, Ahmed M, et al. Selection of mutations in the hepatitis B virus polymerase during therapy of transplant recipients with lamivudine. Hepatology. 1996;24:711–713.
194. Bartholomew MM, Jansen RW, Jeffers LJ, et al. Hepatitis B virus resistance to lamivudine given for recurrent infection after orthotopic liver transplantation. Lancet. 1997;340:20–22.
195. Schalm SW. Clinical implications of lamivudine resistance by HBV. Lancet. 1997;349:3–4.
196. Aye TT, Bartholomeusz A, Shaw T, et al. Hepatitis B virus polymerase mutations

during antiviral therapy in a patient following liver transplantation. J Hepatol. 1997;26:1148–1153.
197. Petit MA, Buffello D, Roche B, et al. Residual hepatitis B virus (HBV) infection in liver transplant patients under treatment with lamivudine (3TC): Assessment by quantitation of HBV DNA by PCR and assay of pres antigens. Hepatology. 1997;26:315A.
198. Gish RG, Lau JYN, Brooks L, et al. Ganciclovir treatment of hepatitis B virus infection in liver transplant recipients. Hepatology. 1996;23:1–7.
199. Manns M, Neuhaus P, Schoenborn H, et al. Famciclovir treatment of hepatitis B infection in patients with end-stage liver disease. J Hepatol. 1998;28(Suppl 1):114.
200. Singh N, Grayowski T, Wannstedt CF, et al. Pretransplant famciclovir as prophylaxis for hepatitis B recurrence after liver transplantation. Transplantation. 1997;63:1415–1419.
201. Kruger M, Tillmann HL, Trautwein C, et al. Famciclovir treatment of hepatitis B virus recurrence after liver transplantation: A pilot study. Liver Transplant Surg. 1996;2:253–262.
202. Neuhaus P, Manns M, Atkinson G. Safety and efficacy of famciclovir for the treatment of recurrent hepatitis B in liver transplant recipients. Hepatology. 1997;26(Suppl 1):260A.
203. Rabinovitz M, Dodson F, Rakela J. Famciclovir for recurrent hepatitis B (HBV) infection after liver transplantation. Hepatology. 1996;24(Suppl 1):282A.
204. Prieto M, Cordoba J, Berenguer M, et al. Famciclovir treatment of hepatitis B virus (HBV) infection after liver transplantation: A pilot study. Hepatology. 1996;24(Suppl 1):419A.
205. Klein M, Geoghehan J, Schmidt K, et al. Conversion of recurrent delta-positive hepatitis B infection to seronegativity with famciclovir after liver transplantation. Transplantation. 1997;64:162–163.
206. McCaughan G, Angus P, Bowden S, et al. Retransplantation for precore mutant–related chronic hepatitis B infection: Prolonged survival in a patient receiving sequential ganciclovir/famciclovir therapy. Liver Transplant Surg. 1996;2:472–474.
207. Aye TT, Bartholomeusz AI, Shaw T, et al. Hepatitis B virus polymerase mutations during famciclovir therapy in patients following liver transplantation. Hepatology. 1996;24(Suppl 1):285A.
208. Tillmann HL, Trautwein C, Bock T, et al. Response and mutations in patients sequentially treated with lamivudine and famciclovir for recurrent hepatitis B after liver transplantation. Hepatology. 1997;26(Suppl 1):429A.
209. Locarnini SA, Aye TT, Shaw T, et al. The emergence of famciclovir resistant mutations in the hepatitis B virus polymerase during therapy in patients following liver transplantation. Hepatology. 1997;26:368A.
210. Zoulim F, Pichoud C, Wang Z, et al. Hepatitis B virus genome variability during famciclovir therapy. Hepatology. 1997;26:428A.
211. Jochum C, Holtmann G, Hoffmann P, et al. Ganciclovir and lamivudine combination therapy after orthotopic liver transplantation. Gastroenterology. 1998;114:A1266.
212. Markowitz JS, Martin P, Conrad AJ, et al. Prophylaxis against hepatitis B recurrence following liver transplantation using combination lamivudine and hepatitis B immune globulin. Hepatology. 1998;28:585–589.
213. National Institutes of Health Consensus Development Conference Panel statement: Management of hepatitis C. Hepatology. 1997;26(Suppl 1):2S–10S.
214. World Health Organization. Hepatitis C: Global prevalence. Wkly Epidemiol Rec 1997;72:341–344.
215. Alter MJ. The epidemiology of acute and chronic hepatitis C. Clin Liver Dis. 1997;1:559–568.
216. McQuillan G, Alter M, Moyer L, et al. A population based serologic study of hepatitis C virus infection in the United States. In: Rizzetto M, Purcell RH, Gerin JL, Verme G, eds. Viral Hepatitis and Liver Disease. Turin: Edizioni Minerva Medica; 1997:267–270.
217. Alter MJ. Epidemiology of hepatitis C in the West. Semin Liver Dis. 1995;15:5–14.
218. Alter MJ. Epidemiology of hepatitis C. Hepatology. 1997;26(Suppl 1):62S–65S.
219. Centers for Disease Control and Prevention. Recommendations for prevention and control of hepatitis C virus (HCV) infection and HCV-related chronic disease. MMWR Morb Mortal Wkly Rep. 1998;47(RR-19):1–39.
220. Detre KM, Belle SH, Lombardero M. Liver transplantation for chronic viral hepatitis. Viral Hepat Rev. 1997;2:219–228.
221. Love RA, Parge HE, Wiekersham JA, et al. The crystal structure of hepatitis C virus NS3 proteinase reveals a trypsin-like fold and structural zinc binding site. Cell. 1996;87:331–342.
222. Yao N, Hesson T, Cable M, et al. Structure of hepatitis C virus RNA helicase domain. Nat Struct Biol 1997;4:463–467.
223. Blight KJ, Kolykhalov AA, Reed KE, et al. Molecular virology of hepatitis C virus: An update with respect to potential antiviral targets. In: Schinazi RF, Sommadossi J-P, Thomas HC, eds. Therapies for Viral Hepatitis. Atlanta: International Medical Press; 1998:207–217.
224. Littlejohn M, Locarnini S, Bartholomeusz A. Targets for inhibition of hepatitis C virus replication. In: Schinazi RF, Sommadossi J-P, Thomas HC, eds. Therapies for Viral Hepatitis. Atlanta: International Medical Press; 1998:219–227.
225. Sharara AI, Hunt CM, Hamilton JD. Hepatitis C. Ann Intern Med. 1996;125:658–668.
226. Simmonds P, Alberti A, Alter HJ, et al. A proposed system for the nomenclature of hepatitis C viral genotypes. Hepatology. 1994;19:1321–1324.
227. Simmonds P, Mellor J, Craxi A, et al. Epidemiological, clinical and therapeutic association of hepatitis C types in western European patients. J Hepatol. 1996;24:517–524.
228. Heintges T, Wands JR. Hepatitis C: Epidemiology and transmission. Hepatology. 1997;26:521–526.
229. Bukh J, Miller RH, Purcell RH. Genetic heterogeneity of hepatitis C virus: Quasispecies and genotypes. Semin Liver Dis. 1995;15:41–63.
230. Alter MJ, Hadler SC, Judson FN, et al. Risk factors for acute non-A, non-B hepatitis in the United States and association with hepatitis C virus infection. JAMA. 1990;264:2231–2235.
231. Williams AE, Thomson RA, Schreiber GB, et al. Estimates of infectious disease risk factors in US blood donors. JAMA. 1997;277:967–972.
232. Kelen GD, Green GB, Purcell RH, et al. Hepatitis B and hepatitis C in emergency department patients. N Engl J Med. 1992;1399–1402.
233. Weiss S, Afridi S, Maisel J, et al. Prevalence of hepatitis B and C and HIV at a community hospital. Gastroenterology. 1994;106:A2007.
234. Vlahov D, Nelson KE, Quinn TC, Kendig N. Prevalence and incidence of hepatitis C virus infection among male prison inmates in Maryland. Eur J Epidemiol. 1993;9:566–569.
235. Reindollar RW. Hepatitis C in the correctional population. In: Maddrey WC, Schiff ER, eds. The Clinician's Companion II: Part 2: Assessment of Special Patient Populations. Secaucus, NJ: Monograph. Projects in Knowledge; 1998:10–13.
236. Donahue JG, Munoz A, Ness PM, et al. The declining risk of post-transfusion hepatitis C virus infection. N Engl J Med. 1992;327:369–373.
237. Feinstone SM, Kapikian AZ, Purcell RH, et al. Transfusion-associated hepatitis not due to viral hepatitis A or B. N Engl J Med. 1975;292:767–770.
238. Choo QL, Kuo G, Weiner AJ, et al. Isolation of a cDNA clone derived from a blood-borne non-A, non-B viral hepatitis genome. Science. 1989;244:359–362.
239. Kuo G, Choo QL, Alter HJ, et al. An assay for circulating antibodies to a major etiologic virus of non-A, non-B viral hepatitis genome. Science. 1989;244:362–364.
240. McGregor M. The hepatitis C disaster. Can Med Assoc J. 1998;158:1461–1462.
241. Hoey J. Hepatitis C as medical misadventure. Can Med Assoc J. 1998;158:1463–1464.
242. Schreiber GB, Busch MP, Kleinmann SH, Korelitz JJ. The risk of transfusion-transmitted viral infections. N Engl J Med. 1996;334:1685–1690.
243. Conry-Cantilena C, VanRaden M, Gibble J, et al. Routes of infection, viremia, and liver disease in blood donors found to have hepatitis C virus infection. N Engl J Med. 1996;334:1691–1696.
244. Dienstag JL. Sexual and perinatal transmission of hepatitis C. Hepatology. 1997;26(Suppl 1):66S–70S.
245. Lissen E, Alter HJ, Abad MA, et al. Hepatitis C virus infection among sexually promiscuous groups and the heterosexual partners of hepatitis C virus infected index cases. Eur J Clin Microbiol Infect Dis. 1993;12:827–831.
246. Fried MW, Shindo M, Fong T-S, et al. Absence of hepatitis C viral RNA from saliva and semen in patients with chronic hepatitis C. Gastroenterology. 1992;102:28–31.
247. Wang JT, Wang TH, Sheu JC, et al. Hepatitis C virus RNA in saliva of patients with posttransfusion hepatitis and low efficiency of transmission amongst spouses. J Med Virol. 1992;36:28–31.
248. Gordon SC, Patel AH, Kulesza GW, et al. Lack of evidence for the heterosexual transmission of hepatitis C. Am J Gastroenterol. 1992;87:1849–1851.
249. Tong MJ, Lai PPC, Hwang S-J, et al. Evaluation of sexual transmission in patients with hepatitis C infection. Clin Diagn Virol. 1995;3:39–47.
250. Everhart JE, DiBisceglie AM, Murray LM, et al. Risk for non-A, non-B (type C) hepatitis through sexual or household contact with chronic carriers. Ann Intern Med. 1990;112:544–545.
251. Eyster ME, Alter HJ. Aledort LM, et al. Heterosexual cotransmission of hepatitis C virus (HCV) and human immunodeficiency virus (HIV). Ann Intern Med. 1991;115:764–768.
252. Brettler DB, Mannucci PM, Gringeri A, et al. The low risk of hepatitis C virus transmission among sexual partners of hepatitis C–infected males: An international, multicenter study. Blood. 1992;80:540–543.
253. Chayama K, Kobayashi M, Tsubota A, et al. Molecular analysis of intraspousal transmission of hepatitis C virus. J Hepatol. 1995;22:431–439.
254. Soto B, Rodrigo L, Garcia-Bengoechea M, et al. Heterosexual transmission of hepatitis C virus and the possible role of coexistent human immunodeficiency virus infection in the index case. A multicenter study of 423 pairings. J Intern Med. 1994;236:515–519.
255. Meisel H, Relp A, Faltus B, et al. Transmission of hepatitis C virus to children and husbands by women infected with contaminated anti-D immunoglobulin. Lancet. 1995;345:1209–1211.
256. Nakashima S, Ikematsu H, Hayashi J. et al. Intrafamilial transmission of hepatitis C virus among the population of an endemic area in Japan. JAMA. 1995;274:1459–1461.
257. Akahane Y, Kojima M, Sugai Y, et al. Hepatitis C virus infection in spouses of patients with type C chronic liver disease. Ann Intern Med. 1994;120:748–752.
258. Kiyosawa K, Tanaka E, Sodeyama T, et al. Transmission of hepatitis C in an isolated area in Japan: Community-acquired infection. Gastroenterology. 1994;106:1596–1602.
259. Chiaramonte M, Stroffolino T, Lorenzoni U, et al. Risk factors in community-acquired chronic hepatitis C virus infection: A case-control study in Italy. J Hepatol. 1996;24:129–134.
260. Power JP, Davidson F, O'Riordan J, et al. Hepatitis C infection from anti-D immunoglobulin (Letter). Lancet. 1995;346:372–373.
261. Thomas DL, Zenilman JM, Alter HJ, et al. Sexual transmission of hepatitis C virus among patients attending sexually transmitted diseases clinics in Baltimore—An analysis of 309 sex partnerships. J Infect Dis. 1995;171:768–775.
262. Alter MJ, Gerety RJ, Smallwood L, et al. Sporadic non-A, non-B hepatitis: Frequency and epidemiology in an urban United States population. J Infect Dis. 1982;145:886–893.

263. Alter MJ, Coleman PJ, Alexander WJ, et al. Importance of heterosexual activity in the transmission of hepatitis B and non-A, non-B hepatitis. JAMA. 1989;262:1201–1205.
264. Salleras L, Buguera M, Vidal J, et al. Importance of sexual transmission of hepatitis C virus in seropositive pregnant women: A case-control study. J Med Virol. 1997;52:164–167.
265. Wu JC, Lin HC, Jeng FS, et al. Prevalence, infectivity, and risk factor analysis of hepatitis C infection in prostitutes. J Med Virol. 1993;39:312–317.
266. Melbye M. Biggar RJ, Wantzin P, et al. Sexual transmission of hepatitis C: A cohort study (1981–9) among European homosexual men. Br Med J. 1990;301:210–212.
267. Puro V, Petrosillo N, Ippolito G. Risk of hepatitis C seroconversion after occupational exposures in health care workers. Am J Infect Control. 1995;23:273–277.
268. Ridzon R, Gallagher K, Ciesielski C, et al. Simultaneous transmission of human immunodeficiency virus and hepatitis C virus from a needle-stick injury. N Engl J Med. 1997;336:919–922.
269. Bronowicki JP, Venard V, Botte C, et al. Patient-to-patient transmission of hepatitis C virus during colonoscopy. N Engl J Med. 1997;337:237–240.
270. Gitlin N, Nolte FS, Weiss M. Hepatitis C: Risk of a haircut. Ann Intern Med. 1997;126:410–411.
271. Kurauchi O, Furui T, Itakura A, et al. Studies on transmission of hepatitis C virus from mother-to-child in the perinatal period. Arch Gynecol Obstet. 1993;253:121–126.
272. Reinus JF, Leikin EL, Later HJ, et al. Failure to detect vertical transmission of hepatitis C virus. Ann Intern Med. 1992;117:881–886.
273. Ohto H, Terazawa S, Sasaki N, et al. Transmission of hepatitis C from mothers to infants. N Engl J Med. 1994;330:744–750.
274. Lin HH, Kao JH, Hsu HY, et al. Absence of infection in breast-fed infants born to hepatitis C virus infected mothers. J Pediatr. 1995;126:589–591.
275. Zanetti AR, Tanzi E, Paccagnini S, et al. Mother-to-infant transmission of hepatitis C virus. Lombardy Study Group on Vertical HCV Transmission. Lancet. 1995;345:289–291.
276. Paccagnini S, Principi N, Massironi E, et al. Perinatal transmission and manifestation of hepatitis C virus infection in a high risk population. Pediatr Infect Dis J. 1995;14:195–199.
277. Thomas DL, Villano SA, Riester KA, et al. Perinatal transmission of hepatitis C virus from human immunodeficiency virus type-1 mothers. Womens and Infants Transmission Study. J Infect Dis. 1998;177:1480–1488.
278. Granovsky MO, Minkoff HL, Tess BH, et al. Hepatitis C virus infection in the mothers and infants cohort study. Pediatrics. 1998;102:355–359.
279. Roudot-Thoraval F, Pawlotsky JM, Thiers V, et al. Lack of mother-to-infant transmission of hepatitis C virus in HIV-negative women: A prospective study with hepatitis C virus RNA testing. Hepatology. 1993;17:772–777.
280. Silverman NS, Snyder M, Hodinka RL, et al. Detection of hepatitis C virus ribonucleic acid sequences in cord bloods from a heterogeneous prenatal population. Am J Obstet Gynecol. 1995;173:1396–1400.
281. Lin HH, Kao JH, Hsu HY, et al. Absence of infection in breast-fed infants born to hepatitis C virus-infected mothers. J Pediatr. 1995;126:589–591.
282. Nelson DR, Marousis CG, Davis GL, et al. The role of hepatitis C virus–specific cytotoxic T lymphocytes in chronic hepatitis C. J Immunol. 1997;158:1473–1481.
283. Tsai SL, Liaw YF, Chen MH, et al. Detection of type 2-like T-helper cells in hepatitis C virus infection: Implications for hepatitis C virus chronicity. Hepatology. 1997;25:449–457.
284. Reiser M, Marousis CG, Nelson D, et al. Serum interleukin-4 and interleukin-10 levels in patients with chronic hepatitis C virus infection. J Hepatol. 1997;26:471–478.
285. Napoli J, Bishop GA, McGuinness PH, et al. Progressive liver injury in chronic hepatitis C infection correlates with increased intrahepatic expression of Th_1-associated cytokines. Hepatology. 1996;24:759–765.
286. Cacciarelli TV, Martinez OM, Gish RG, et al. Immunoregulatory cytokines in chronic hepatitis C virus infection: Pre- and post-treatment with interferon alfa. Hepatology. 1996;24:6–8.
287. Silva M. The role of cytokines in hepatitis C. In: Maddrey WC, Schiff ER, eds. The Clinician's Companion: Expert Perspectives on Contemporary Clinical Issues in Hepatitis C. Secaucus, NJ: Projects in Knowledge; 1997:46–47.
288. Bonkovsky HL, Banner BF, Rothman AL. Iron and chronic viral hepatitis. Hepatology. 1997;25:759–768.
289. Kolykhalov AA, Agapov EV, Blight KJ, et al. Transmission of hepatitis C by intrahepatic inoculation with transcribed RNA. Science. 1997;277:570–574.
290. Major ME, Feinstone SM. The molecular virology of hepatitis C. Hepatology. 1997;25:1527–1538.
291. Shehab TM, Moseley RH. Viral hepatitis. Curr Opin Gastroenterol. 1998;14:228–233.
292. Seeff LB, Buskell-Bales Z, Wright EC, et al. Long term mortality after transfusion-associated nonA, nonB hepatitis. N Engl J Med. 1992;27:1906–1911.
293. Tassopoulos NC. Patterns of progression: Unpredictability and risk of decompensated cirrhosis. Dig Dis Sci. 1996;41:41S–48S.
294. Tong MJ, El-Farra NS, Reikes AR, Co RL. Clinical outcomes after transfusion-associated hepatitis C. N Engl J Med. 1995;332:1463–1466.
295. DiBisceglie AM, Goodman ZD, Ishak KG, et al. Long-term clinical and histopathological follow-up of chronic posttransfusion hepatitis. Hepatology. 1991;14:969–974.
296. Takahashi M, Yamada G, Miyamoto R, et al. Natural course of chronic hepatitis C. Am J Gastroenterol. 1993;88:240–243.
297. Dienstag JL. The natural history of chronic hepatitis C and what we should do about it. Gastroenterology. 1997;112:651–655.
298. Roudot-Thoraval F, Bastie A, Pawlotsky JM, Dhumeaux D. Epidemiological factors affecting the severity of hepatitis C virus–related liver disease: A French survey of 6,664 patients. Hepatology. 1997;26:485–490.
299. Gordon SC, Ellaway RS, Long JC, Dmuchowski CF. Pathology of hepatitis C as function of mode of transmission: Blood transfusions vs intravenous drugs. Hepatology. 1993;18:1338–1343.
300. Silini E, Bono F, Cividini A, et al. Differential distribution of hepatitis C virus genotypes in patients with and without liver function abnormalities. Hepatology. 1995;21:285–290.
301. Yamada M, Kakumu S, Yoshida K, et al. Hepatitis C virus genotypes are not responsible for development of serious liver disease. Dig Dis Sci. 1994;39:234–239.
302. Befrits R, Hedman M, Blomquist L, et al. Chronic hepatitis C in alcoholic patients: Prevalence, genotypes and correlation to liver disease. Scand J Gastroenterol. 1995;30:1113–1118.
303. Wiley TE, McCarthy M, Breidi L, et al. Impact of alcohol on the histological and clinical progression of hepatitis C infection. Hepatology. 1998;28:805–809.
304. Mendenhall CL, Seeff L, Diehl AM, et al. Antibodies to hepatitis B virus and hepatitis C virus in alcoholic hepatitis and cirrhosis: Their prevalence and clinical relevance. Hepatology. 1991;14:581–589.
305. Anand BS, Valez M. Does alcohol abuse influence hepatitis C virus replication. Gastroenterology. 1997;112:A1211.
306. Oshita M, Hayashi N, Kasahara A, et al. Increased serum hepatitis C virus RNA among alcoholic patients with chronic hepatitis C. Hepatology. 1994;20:1115–1120.
307. Pessione F, Degos F, Marcellin P, et al. Effect of alcohol consumption on serum hepatitis C virus RNA and histological lesions in chronic hepatitis C. Hepatology. 1998;27:1717–1722.
308. Bellentani S, Tiribelli C, Sarroccio G, et al. Prevalence of chronic liver disease in the general population of northern Italy. The Dionysos Study. Hepatology. 1994;20:1442–1449.
309. Ostapowicz G, Watson KJR, Locarnini SA, Desmond PV. Role of alcohol in the progression of liver disease caused by hepatitis C virus infection. Hepatology. 1998;27:1730–1735.
310. Poynard T, Benossa P, Opolon P. Natural history of liver fibrosis progression in patients with chronic hepatitis C. The OBSVIRC, METAVIR and DOSVIRC groups. Lancet. 1997;349:825–832.
311. Kasahare A, Hayashi N, Chazovillères O, et al. Risk factors for hepatocellular carcinoma and its incidence after interferon treatment in patients with chronic hepatitis C. Hepatology. 1998;27:1394–1402.
312. International Interferon-α Hepatocellular Carcinoma Study Group. Effect of interferon-α on progression of cirrhosis to hepatocellular carcinoma: A retrospective cohort study. Lancet. 1998;351:1535–1539.
313. Imai Y, Kawata S, Tamura S, et al. Relation of interferon therapy and hepatocellular carcinoma in patients with chronic hepatitis C. Ann Intern Med. 1998;129:94–99.
314. Serfaty L, Aumaitre H, et al. Determinants of outcome of compensated hepatitis C virus–related cirrhosis. Hepatology. 1998;27:1435–1440.
315. Wong JB, Bennett WG, Koff RS, Pauker SG. Pretreatment evaluation of chronic hepatitis C: Risks, benefits and costs. JAMA. 1998;280:2088–2093.
316. Lindsay KL. Therapy of hepatitis C: Overview. Hepatology. 1997;26(Suppl 1):71S–77S.
317. Levine RA. Treating histologically mild chronic hepatitis C: Monotherapy, combination therapy, or tincture of time? Ann Intern Med. 1998;129:323–326.
318. National Institutes of Health Consensus Development Conference Panel statement: management of hepatitis C. Hepatology. 1997;26(Suppl 1):2S–10S.
319. Davis GL. Interferon treatment for chronic hepatitis C. Am J Med. 1994;96:41S–46S.
320. Fried MW, Hoofnagle JH. Therapy of hepatitis C. Semin Liver Dis. 1995;15:82–91.
321. Esteban JI, Genesca J, Alter HJ. Hepatitis C: Molecular biology, pathogenesis, epidemiology, clinical features, and prevention. Prog Liver Dis. 1992;10:253–282.
322. Poynard T, Bedossa P, Chevalier M, et al. A comparison of three α-2b interferon regimens for long-term treatment of chronic non-A, non-B hepatitis. N Engl J Med. 1995;332:1457–1462.
323. Maddrey WC, Schiff ER: The Clinician's Companion: Expert Perspectives on Contemporary Clinical Issues in Hepatitis C—Monograph. Secaucus, NJ: Projects in Knowledge; 1997.
324. Marcellin P, Boyer N, Gervais A, et al. Long-term histologic improvement and loss of detectable intrahepatic HCV RNA in patients with chronic hepatitis C and sustained response to interferon-α therapy. Ann Intern Med. 1997;127:875–881.
325. Davis GL, Esteban-Mur R, Rustgi V, et al. Interferon alfa-2b alone or in combination with ribavirin for the treatment of chronic hepatitis C. N Engl J Med. 1998;339:1493–1499.
326. Heathcote EJL, Keeffe EB, Lee SS, et al. Re-treatment of chronic hepatitis C with consensus interferon. Hepatology. 1998;27:1136–1143. [Erratum. Hepatology. 1998;28:599.]
327. Heathcote J. Consensus interferon: A novel interferon for the treatment of hepatitis C. J Viral Hepatitis. 1998;5(Suppl 1):13–18.
328. Keeffe EB, Hollinger FB, Consensus Interferon Study Group. Therapy of hepatitis C: Consensus interferon trials. Hepatology. 1997;26(Suppl 1):101S–107S.
329. Tong MJ, Reddy KR, Lee WM, et al. Treatment of chronic hepatitis C with consensus interferon: A multicenter, randomized, controlled trial. Hepatology. 1997;26:747–754.
330. Tong MJ, Blatt LM, Resser K, et al. Treatment of patients with chronic HCV infection with a novel type-1 interferon, consensus interferon. Hepatology. 1993;18:150A.
331. Craig JR, Bain VG, Black M, et al. Liver histology improvement is associated

with ALT and HCV RNA response following treatment with consensus interferon (CIFN). Gastroenterology. 1996;110:A1175.
332. Jones C, Agrawal R, Tibaldi N, et al. A preliminary study of high dose consensus interferon in the treatment of chronic hepatitis C. Am J Gastroenterol. 1998;93:A1677.
333. Shiffman ML. Use of high-dose interferon in the treatment of chronic hepatitis C. Semin Liver Dis. 1999;19(Suppl 1):25–33.
334. Lam NP, Neumann AU, Gretch DR, et al. Dose-dependent clearance of hepatitis C genotype 1 virus with interferon alpha. Hepatology. 1997;26:226–231.
335. Yun ZB, Odeberg J, Lundeberg J, et al. Restriction of hepatitis C virus heterogeneity during prolonged interferon-alpha therapy in relation to changes in virus load. J Infect Dis. 1996;173:992–998.
336. Isaacs A, Lindenmann J. Virus interference. I. The interferon. Proc R Soc 1957;147:258–261.
337. Sen GC, Ransohoff RM. Interferon-induced anti-viral actions and their regulation. Adv Virus Res. 1993;42:57–60.
338. Ransohoff RM. Cellular responses to interferons and other cytokines: The JAK-STAT paradigm. N Engl J Med. 1998;338:616–618.
339. Cavanaugh VJ, Guidotti LG, Chisari FV. Interleukin-12 inhibits hepatitis B virus replication in transgenic mice. J Virol. 1997;71:3236–3243.
340. Guidotti LG, Borrow P, Hobbs MV, et al. Viral cross talk: Intracellular inactivation of the hepatitis B virus during an unrelated viral infection of the liver. Proc Natl Acad Sci U S A. 1996;93:4589–4594.
341. Blatt LM, Davis JM, Klein SB, Taylor MW. The biologic activity and molecular characterization of a novel synthetic interferon-alpha species, consensus interferon. J Interferon Cytokine Res. 1996;16:489–499.
342. Zoon KC, Miller D, Bekicz J, et al. Purification and characterization of multiple components of human lymphoblastoid interferon-α. J Biol Chem. 1002;1267:15210–15216.
343. Farrell GC. Therapy of hepatitis C: Interferon alfa-n1 trials. Hepatology. 1997;26(Suppl 1):96S–100S.
344. Bardelli F, Messori A, Rampazzo R, et al. Effect of recombinant or lymphoblastoid interferon-α on alanine aminotransferase in patients with chronic hepatitis C or chronic non-A non-B hepatitis. A meta-analysis. Clin Drug Invest. 1995;9:239–254.
345. Rumi M, Del Ninno E, Parravicini ML, et al. A prospective randomized trial comparing lymphoblastoid to recombinant interferon alfa 2a as therapy for chronic hepatitis C. Hepatology. 1996;24:1366–1370.
346. Farrell G, Bacon B, Goldin R. Lymphoblastoid interferon alfa-n1b improves the long-term response to a 6-month course of treatment in chronic hepatitis C compared with recombinant interferon-α 2b: Results of an international randomized controlled trial. Hepatology. 1998;27:1121–1127.
347. Benhamou JP, Hopf U, Rizzetto M, et al. A randomized, double-blind, controlled, multicentre trial of human lymphoblastoid interferon alpha in the treatment of adults with chronic hepatitis non-A, non-B (C). J Hepatol. 1994;21:173A.
348. Xu R. Pharmacokinetic/pharmacodynamic modeling of PEG-IFN. Faculty 2000 Exchange Forum, Naples, Fla, September 7, 1997.
349. Zeuzem S, Schmid JM, Lee JH, et al. Dynamics of hepatitis C virus turnover in vivo. Hepatology. 1995;22:287A.
350. Hoffman J. Pegylated interferon α-2a: Preliminary phase II safety and efficacy results. Faculty 2000 Exchange Forum, Naples, Fla, September 7, 1997.
351. Reddy R. Pegyated interferon. International Symposium on Hepatitis, Palm Beach, Fla, November 2, 1998.
352. Gross J Jr, Hassanein T, Herrera J, et al. Management of Interferon Treatment Failures in Chronic Hepatitis C. Littleton, Colo: Postgraduate Institute for Medicine; April 1998:6.
353. Schiffman ML, Hoffmann CM, Thompson EB, et al. Relationship between biochemical, virological, and histological response during interferon treatment of chronic hepatitis C. Hepatology. 1997;26:780–785.
354. Tsubota A, Chayama K, Arase Y, et al. Factors useful in predicting the response to interferon therapy in chronic hepatitis C. J Gastroenterol Hepatol. 1993;8:535–539.
355. Tong MJ, Blatt LM, McHutchinson J, et al. Prediction of response during interferon alfa 2b therapy in chronic hepatitis C patients using viral and biochemical characteristics: A comparison. Hepatology. 1997;26:1640–1645.
356. Nishiguchi S, Kuroki T, Nakatami S, et al. Randomized controlled trial of effects of interferon-alfa in the incidence of hepatocellular carcinoma. Lancet. 1995;346:1051–1053.
357. DiBisceglie AM. Hepatitis C and hepatocellular carcinoma. Hepatology. 1997;26(Suppl 1):34S–38S.
358. Hoofnagle JH, Mullen KD, Jones DB, et al. Treatment of chronic non-A, non-B hepatitis with recombinant human alpha interferon: A preliminary report. N Engl J Med. 1986;315:1575–1580.
359. DiBisceglie A, Marin P, Kassianides C, et al. Recombinant interferon alfa therapy for chronic hepatitis C: A randomized, double-blind, placebo-controlled trial. N Engl J Med. 1989;321:1506–1511.
360. Davis G, Balart L, Schiff E, et al. Treatment of chronic hepatitis C with recombinant interferon alfa. N Engl J Med. 1989;321:1501–1505.
361. Tine F, Magrin S, Craxi S, et al. Interferon for non-A, non-B chronic hepatitis: A meta-analysis of randomized clinical trials. J Hepatol. 1991;12:192–198.
362. Poynard T, Leroy V, Cohard M, et al. Meta-analysis of interferon randomized trials in the treatment of viral hepatitis C: Effects of dose and duration. Hepatology. 1996;24:778–789.
363. Lindsay KL, Davis GL, Schiff ER, et al. Response to higher doses of interferon alfa-2b in patients with chronic hepatitis C: A randomized multicenter trial. Hepatology. 1996;24:1034–1040.
364. Kasahara A, Hayashi N, Hiramatsu N, et al. Ability of prolonged interferon treatment to suppress relapse after cessation of therapy in patients with chronic hepatitis C: A multicenter randomized controlled trial. Hepatology. 1995;21:291–296.
365. Bacon BR. Iron and hepatitis C (Editorial). Gut. 1997;41:127–128.
366. Bonkovsky HL. Therapy of hepatitis C: Other options. Hepatology. 1997;26(Suppl 1):143S–151S.
367. DiBisceglie AM, Axiotis CA, Hoofnagle JH, Bacon BR. Measurement of iron status in patients with chronic hepatitis. Gastroenterology. 1992;102:2108–2113.
368. Van Thiel DH, Friedlander L, Fagiuoli S, et al. Response to interferon-α therapy is influenced by the iron content of the liver. J Hepatol. 1994;20:410–415.
369. Olynyk JK, Reddy KR, DiBisceglie AM, et al. Hepatic iron concentration as a predictor of response to interferon alfa therapy in chronic hepatitis C. Gastroenterology. 1995;108:1104–1109.
370. Piperno A, Sampietro M, D'Alba R, et al. Iron stores, response to interferon therapy and effect of iron depletion in chronic hepatitis C. Liver. 1996;16:248–254.
371. Barton AL, Banner BF, Cable EE, Bonkovsky HL. Distribution of iron in the liver predicts the response of chronic hepatitis C infection to interferon therapy. Am J Clin Pathol. 1995;103:419–424.
372. DeCastro M, Sanchez J, Herrera JF, et al. Hepatitis C virus antibodies and liver disease in patients with porphyria cutanea tarda. Hepatology. 1993;17:551–557.
373. Hayashi H, Takikawa T, Nishumara N, et al. Improvement of serum aminotransferase levels after phlebotomy in patients with chronic active hepatitis C and excess hepatic iron. Am J Gastroenterol. 1994;89:986–988.
374. Bacon BR, Rebholz AE, Fried M, DiBisceglie AM. Beneficial effect of iron reduction therapy in patients with chronic hepatitis C who failed to respond to interferon-α. Hepatology. 1993;18:150A.
375. Van Thiel DH, Friedlander L, Malloy P, et al. Retreatment of hepatitis C interferon nonresponders with larger doses of interferon with and without phlebotomy. Gastroenterology. 1994;106:A1002.
376. Hayashi H, Takikawa T, Nishimura N, Yano M. Serum aminotransferase levels as an indicator of the effectiveness of venesection for chronic hepatitis C. J Hepatol. 1995;22:268–271.
377. Caraceni P, Fagiuoli S, Van Thiel DH. Iron reduction therapy: Simply camouflage, or a real weapon? Am J Gastroenterol. 1994;89:970–973.
378. Boucher E, Bourienne A, Adams P, et al. Liver iron concentration and distribution in chronic hepatitis C before and after interferon treatment. Gut. 1997;41:115–120.
379. Shindo M, Arai K, Sokawa Y, et al. Hepatic hepatitis C virus RNA as a predictor of a long-term response to interferon alfa therapy. Ann Intern Med. 1995;122:586–592.
380. Balart L, Perrillo R, Roddenberry J, et al. Hepatitis C RNA in liver of chronic hepatitis C patients before and after interferon alfa treatment. Gastroenterology. 1993;104:1472–1478.
381. Colloredo G, Beliati A, Ricci A, et al. HCV-RNA as a predictor of relapse after interferon therapy for chronic hepatitis C. Hepatology. 1996;24:156A.
382. Karino Y, Toyota J, Sugawara M, et al. Early loss of serum hepatitis C virus RNA can predict a sustained response to interferon therapy in patients with chronic hepatitis C. Am J Gastroenterol. 1997;92:61–65.
383. Chemello L, Cavalletto L, Casarin C, et al. Persistent hepatitis C viremia predicts late relapse after sustained response to interferon-alfa in chronic hepatitis C. Ann Intern Med. 1996;124:1058–1060.
384. Payen JL, Izopet, J, Galindo V, et al. A comparison of three interferon alfa-2b regimens for retreatment (RTT) of patients with chronic hepatitis C with prior complete response followed by a relapse: A controlled, randomized trial. Hepatology. 1996;24:273A.
385. Rolachon A, Kezachian G, Causse X, et al. Interest of a higher dose of interferon alpha in non-responder patients with chronic hepatitis C: A prospective randomized study. Hepatology. 1996;24(Suppl):569A.
386. Kawanishi H. A therapeutic trial of alpha (α) interferon (IFN) monitored by serum HCV–RNA levels for patients with chronic hepatitis (CH), C who failed the treatment with 3 MU standard dose of αIFN. Hepatology. 1995;22:437A.
387. Marcellin P, Boyer N, Pouteau M, et al. Retreatment with interferon-α of chronic hepatitis C infection. Lancet. 1994;344:690–691.
388. Tong M, Blatt LM, Tong L, et al. Retreatment of chronic HCV patients who previously failed 24 weeks of interferon alfa 2b with longer duration therapy. Hepatology. 1997;26(Suppl 1):418A.
389. Picciotto A, Brizzolara R, Campo N, et al. Two year interferon retreatment may induce a sustained response in relapsing patients with chronic hepatitis C. Hepatology. 1996;24:273A.
390. Toyoda H, Nakano S, Takeda I, et al. Retreatment of chronic hepatitis C with interferon. Am J Gastroenterol. 1994;89:1453–1457.
391. Chow W-C, Boyer N, Marcellin P, et al. Re-treatment with interferon alfa of patients with chronic hepatitis C. Hepatology. 1998;27:1144–1148.
392. Schalm SW, Fattovich G, Brouwer JT. Therapy of hepatitis C: Patients with cirrhosis. Hepatology. 1997;26:128S–132S.
393. Smith JP. Treatment of chronic hepatitis C with amantadine. Dig Dis Sci. 1997;42:1681–1687.
394. Olmeda M, Khalili M, Perrillo RP. Amantadine monotherapy in patients with chronic hepatitis C. Gastroenterology. 1998;114:A1316.
395. Wiley TE, Mihalov M, O'Riordan K, et al. Amantadine is not effective in clearing HCV from the serum in patients who are not candidates for interferon therapy. Gastroenterology. 1998;114:A1365.
396. Khalili M, Olmeda M, Yantsos VA, Perrillo RP. Pilot study of Intron-A and ribavirin vs Intron-A and amantadine in interferon non-responders with chronic hepatitis C. Gastroenterology. 1998;114:A1271.
397. Sherman KE, Sickler J, Aranda-Michel J, et al. Rimantadine for treatment of

hepatitis C infection in liver transplant recipients. Liver Transplant Surg. 1999;5:25–28.
398. Teuber G, Berg T, Rodig S, et al. Interleukin-12 (IL-12) therapy in patients with chronic hepatitis C. Gastroenterology. 1998;114:A1354.
399. Schlaak JF, Radecke K, Meyer zum Buschenfelde K-H, Gerken G. Low-dose, non-toxic IL-2 therapy is effective in the treatment of HIV/HBV and HIV/HCV coinfection. Gastroenterology. 1998;114:A1336.
400. Flora K, Hahn M, Rosen H, Benner K. Milk thistle *(Silybum marianum)* for the therapy of liver disease. Am J Gastroenterol. 1998;93:139–143.
401. Raymond RS, Fallon MB, Abrams GA. Oral thymic extract for chronic hepatitis C in patients previously treated with interferon: A randomized, double-blind, placebo-controlled trial. Ann Intern Med. 1998;129:797–800.
402. Sidwell RW, Hoffmann JH, Khare GP, et al. Broad-spectrum anti-viral activity of Virazole: 1-β-D-ribofuranosyl-1,2,4-triazole-3-carboxamide. Science. 1972; 177:705–709.
403. Moussalli P, Opolon P, Poynard T. Management of hepatitis C. J Viral Hepat. 1998;5:73–82.
404. Gish RG: Liver Disease Digest, v. 2. Parsippany, NJ: Applied Clinical Communications; 1998.
405. Interferon Alfa-2b/Ribavirin Combination Therapy: A Promising Step Toward the Treatment of Chronic Hepatitis C—Monograph. New York: Long Island Jewish Medical Center, Albert Einstein College of Medicine; 1998.
406. Maddrey WC, Schiff ER. The Clinician's Companion: Expert Perspectives on Contemporary Clinical Issues in Hepatitis C—Monograph. Secaucus, NJ: Projects in Knowledge; 1997.
407. Maddrey WC, Schiff ER. Beyond Monotherapy: Next Generation Therapies for Chronic Hepatitis C—Monograph. Secaucus, NJ: Projects in Knowledge; 1998.
408. Treating Chronic Hepatitis C: New Strategies for Nonresponders and Relapsers—AASLD Meeting Highlights. Secaucus, NJ: Projects in Knowledge; 1998.
409. Reichard O. Combination therapy. In: Maddrey WC, Schiff ER, eds. The Clinician's Companion: Expert Perspectives on Contemporary Clinical Issues in Hepatitis C. Secaucus, NJ: Projects in Knowledge; 1997:23.
410. Browne MJ. Mechanism and specificity of action of ribavirin. Antimicrob Agents Chemother. 1978;15:747–753.
411. Patterson JL, Fernandez-Larsson R. Molecular action of ribavirin. Rev Infect Dis. 1990;12:1139–1146.
412. Goswami BB, Borek E, Sharma OK. The broad spectrum antiviral agent ribavirin inhibits capping of mRNA. Biochem Biophys Res Commun. 1979;89:830–836.
413. Powers CN, Peavy DL, Knight V. Selective inhibition of functional lymphocyte subpopulations by ribavirin. Antimicrob Agents Chemother. 1982;22:108–112.
414. Heagy W, Crumpacker C, Lopez PA, et al. Inhibition of immune functions by antiviral drugs. J Clin Invest. 1991;87:1916–1919.
415. Ning Q, Brown D, Parodo J, et al. Ribavirin inhibits viral-induced macrophage production of tumor necrosis factor, interleukin-1, and procoagulant fg12 prothrombinase and preserves Th1 cytokine production but inhibits Th2 cytokine response. J Immunol. 1998;160:3487–3493.
416. Package insert. Rebetron. Schering-Plough, Kenilworth, NJ.
417. Stoffa R, Burgess SJ, Peters M. Clinical pharmacology of anti-viral agents. In: Zakim D, Boyer TD, eds. Hepatology—A Textbook of Liver Disease 3rd ed. Philadelphia: WB Saunders; 1996:1293–1299.
418. Connor J. Ribavirin pharmacokinetics. Pediatr Infect Dis J. 1990;9:S91–S93.
419. Zylberberg H, Landau A, Chaix M-L, et al. Ribavirin does not modify HIV replication in HCV-HIV coinfected subjects under antiretroviral regimen. Hepatology. 1998;28(Suppl 1):479A.
420. Thevenot T, Mathurin P, Moussalli J, et al. Effects of cirrhosis, interferon and azathioprine on adverse events in patients with chronic hepatitis C treated with ribavirin. J Viral Hepat. 1997;4:243–253.
421. Poynard T, Moussali J, Thevenot T, et al. Treatment of chronic hepatitis C with interferon: 1998 update. In: Schinazi RF, Sommadossi J-P, Thomas HC, eds. Therapies for Viral Hepatitis. Atlanta: International Medical Press; 1998:371–378.
422. Reichard O, Andersson J, Schvarcz R, Weiland O. Ribavirin treatment for chronic hepatitis. C. Lancet. 1991;337:1058–1061.
423. DiBisceglie A, Shindo M, Fong TL, et al. A pilot study of ribavirin therapy for chronic hepatitis C. Hepatology. 1992;16:649–654.
424. Bodenheimer HC, Lindsay KL, Davis GL, et al. Tolerance and efficacy of oral ribavirin treatment of chronic hepatitis C: A multicenter trial. Hepatology. 1997;26:473–477.
425. DiBisceglie AM, Conjeevaram HS, Fried MW, et al. Ribavirin as therapy for chronic hepatitis C. A randomized, double-blind, placebo-controlled trial. Ann Intern Med. 1995;123:897–903.
426. Brouwer JT, Nevens F, Michielsen P, et al. What options are left when hepatitis C does not respond to interferon? Placebo-controlled Benelux multicenter retreatment trial on ribavirin monotherapy versus combination with interferon. J Hepatol. 1994;21:S17.
427. Dusheiko G, Main J, Thomas H, et al. Ribavirin treatment for patients with chronic hepatitis C: Results of a placebo-controlled study. J Hepatol. 1996;25:591–598.
428. Kakuma S, Yoshioka K, Wakita T, et al. A pilot study of ribavirin and interferon beta for treatment of chronic hepatitis C. Gastroenterology. 1993;105:507–512.
429. Chemello L, Cavaletto L, Bernardinello E, et al. The effect of interferon alfa and ribavirin combination therapy in naïve patients with chronic hepatitis C. J Hepatol. 1995;23(Suppl 2):8–12.
430. Lai M-Y, Kao J-H, Yang P-M, et al. Long-term efficacy of ribavirin plus interferon alfa in the treatment of chronic hepatitis C. Gastroenterology. 1996;111:1307–1312.
431. Reichard O, Norkrans G, Fryden A, et al. Randomized double-blind placebo-controlled trial of interferon-α2b with and without ribavirin for chronic hepatitis C. Lancet. 1998;351:83–87.
432. McHutchison JG, Gordon SC, Schiff E, et al. Interferon alfa-2b alone or in combination with ribavirin as initial treatment for chronic hepatitis C. N Engl J Med. 1998;339:1485–1492.
433. Poynard T, Marcellin P, Lee SS, et al. Randomised trial of interferon α2b plus ribavirin for 48 weeks or for 24 weeks versus interferon α2b plus placebo for 48 weeks for treatment of chronic infection with hepatitis C. Lancet. 1998;352:1426–1432.
434. Schalm SW, Brouwer JT. Anti-viral therapy of hepatitis C. Scand J Gastroenterol Suppl 1991;223:46–49.
435. Schalm SW, Brouwer JT, Chemello L, et al. Interferon-ribavirin combination therapy for chronic hepatitis C. Dig Dis Sci. 1996;41:131S–134S.
436. Sostegni R, Ghisetti V, Pittaluga F, et al. Sequential versus concomitant administration of ribavirin and interferon alfa-n3 in patients with chronic hepatitis C not responding to interferon alone. Results of a randomized controlled trial. Gastroenterology. 1998;114:A1344.
437. Berenguer M, Wright TL. Hepatitis C virus in the transplant setting. In: Schinazi RF, Sommadossi J-P, Thomas HC, eds. Therapies for Viral Hepatitis. Atlanta: International Medical Press; 1998:389–402.
438. Davern TJ, Lake JR. Recurrent disease after liver transplantation. Semin Gastrointest Dis. 1998;9:86–109.
439. Brumage LK, Wright TL. Treatment for recurrent viral hepatitis after liver transplantation. J Hepatol. 1997;26:440–445.
440. Araya V, Rakela J, Wright T. Hepatitis C after orthotopic liver transplantation. Gastroenterology. 1997;112:575–582.
441. Imperial JC, Keeffe EB. Liver transplantation for chronic viral hepatitis: Prevention and management of recurrent disease. Pract Gastroenterol. 1997;21:12–29.
442. Wright TL, Donegan E, Hsu HH, et al. Recurrent and acquired hepatitis C viral infection in liver transplant recipients. Gastroenterology. 1992;103:317–322.
443. Charlton M, Seaberg E, Wiesner R, et al. Predictors of patient and graft survival following liver transplantation for hepatitis C. Hepatology. 1998;28:823–830.
444. Boker KH, Dalley G, Bahr MJ, et al. Long-term outcome of hepatitis C virus infection after liver transplantation. Hepatology. 1997;25:203–210.
445. Gane EJ, Portmann BC, Naoumov NV, et al. Long-term outcome of hepatitis C infection after liver transplantation. N Engl J Med. 1996;334:815–820.
446. Vierling JM, Villamil FG, Rojter SE, et al. Morbidity and mortality of recurrent hepatitis C infection after orthotopic liver transplantation. J Viral Hepat. 1997;4(Suppl 1):117–124.
447. Greenson JK, Svoboda-Newman SM, Merion RM, et al. Histologic progression of recurrent hepatitis C in liver transplant allografts. Am J Surg Pathol. 1996;20:731–738.
448. Gordon FD, Poterucha JJ, Germer J, et al. Relationship between hepatitis C genotype and severity of recurrent hepatitis C after liver transplantation. Transplantation. 1997;63:1419–1423.
449. Prieto M, Berenguer M, Rayon JM, et al. High incidence of allograft cirrhosis in hepatitis C virus genotype 1b infection following transplantation: Relationship with rejection episodes. Hepatology. 1999;29:250–256.
450. DiMartino V, Feray C, Saurini F, et al. The level of liver HCV RNA is a predictor of chronic active hepatitis (CAH) after liver transplantation (Abstract). Hepatology 1996;24:296A.
451. Schluger LK, Sheiner PA, Thung SN, et al. Severe recurrent cholestatic hepatitis C following orthotopic liver transplantation. Hepatology. 1996;23:971–976.
452. Dickson RC, Caldwell SH, Ishitani MB, et al. Clinical and histologic patterns of early graft failure due to recurrent hepatitis C in four patients after liver transplantation. Transplantation. 1996;61:701–705.
453. Lim HL, Lau GKK, Davis GL, et al. Cholestatic hepatitis leading to hepatic failure in a patient with organ-transmitted hepatitis C infection. Gastroenterology. 1994;106:248–251.
454. Sheiner PA, Schluger LK, Emre S, et al. Retransplantation for recurrent hepatitis C. Liver Transplant Surg. 1997;3:130–136.
455. Wright HI, Gavaler JS, Van Thiel DH, et al. Preliminary experience with α2b-interferon therapy of viral hepatitis in liver allograft recipients. Transplantation. 1992;53:121–124.
456. Wright TL, Combs C, Kim M, et al. Interferon-therapy for hepatitis C virus infection after liver transplantation. Hepatology. 1994;20:773–779.
457. Feray C, Samuel D, Gigou M, et al. An open trial of interferon alfa recombinant for hepatitis C after liver transplantation: Antiviral effects and risk of rejection. Hepatology. 1995;22:1084–1089.
458. Terrault NA, Holland CC, Ferrell L, et al. Interferon alfa for recurrent hepatitis B after liver transplantation. Liver Transplant Surg. 1996;2:132–138.
459. Singh N, Gayowski T, Wannstedt CF, et al. Interferon-alpha therapy for hepatitis C recurrence after liver transplantation: Long-term response with maintenance therapy. Clin Transplant. 1996;10:348–351.
460. Wright TL. Liver transplantation for chronic hepatitis C viral infection. Gastroenterol Clin North Am. 1993;22:231–242.
461. Vargas V, Charco R, Castells L, et al. Alpha-interferon for acute hepatitis C in liver transplant patients. Transplant Proc. 1995;27:1222–1223.
462. Sheiner PA, Boros P, Klion FM, et al. The efficacy of prophylactic interferon alfa-2b in preventing recurrent hepatitis C after liver transplantation. Hepatology. 1998;28:831–838.
463. Cattral MS, Krajden M, Wanless IR, et al. A pilot study of ribavirin therapy for recurrent hepatitis C virus infection after liver transplantation. Transplantation. 1996;61:1483–1488.
464. Cattral MS, Hemming AW, Wanless IR, et al. Outcome of long-term ribavirin

therapy for recurrent hepatitis C after liver transplantation. Transplantation. 1999;67:1277–1280.

465. Gane EJ, Tibbs CJ, Ramage JK, et al. Ribavirin therapy for hepatitis C recurrence following liver transplantation. Transpl Int. 1995;8:61–64.
466. Bizollon T, Adahm M, Ducerf C, et al. New approaches to treatment of recurrent hepatitis C virus following liver transplantation using ribavirin. Transplant Proc. 1996;28:2842–2843.
467. Gane EJ, Lo S-K, Riordan S, et al. A randomized study comparing ribavirin and interferon alfa monotherapy for hepatitis C recurrence after liver transplantation. Hepatology. 1998;27:1403–1407.
468. Bizollon T, Palazzo U, Ducerf C, et al. Pilot study of the combination of interferon alfa and ribavirin as therapy of recurrent hepatitis C after liver transplantation. Hepatology. 1997;26:500–504.
469. Bizollon T, Ducerf C, Chevallier M, et al. Maintenance ribavirin monotherapy after interferon combination therapy in HCV recurrence after OLT: Follow-up after two years of ribavirin and natural evolution of HCV RNA negative patients after cessation of treatment. Abstract 111. Presented at the Transplantation Society XVII World Congress, Montreal, July 13, 1998.
470. Fukumoto T, Berg T, Ku Y, et al. Kinetics of hepatitis C viremia after orthotopic liver transplantation. Transplant Proc. 1997;29:511–513.
471. Mazzaferro V, Regalia E, Pulvirenti A, et al. Prophylaxis against HCV recurrence after liver transplantation: Effect of interferon and ribavirin combination. Transplant Proc. 1997;29:519–521.
472. Marcellin P, Levy S, Erlinger S. Therapy of hepatitis C: Patients with normal aminotransferase levels. Hepatology. 1997;26(Suppl 1):133S–136S.
473. Pawlotsky J-M. Chronic hepatitis C virus infection with repeatedly normal aminotransferase levels: Disease or not disease? (Editorial). Am J Gastroenterol. 1997;92:1775–1777.
474. Sangiovanni A, Spinzi G, Ceriani R, et al. Randomized controlled trial of HCV healthy carriers with interferon (Abstract). Hepatology 1995;22:290A.
475. Shakil AO, Conry-Cantilena C, Alter HJ, et al. Volunteer blood donors with antibody to hepatitis C virus: Clinical, biochemical, virologic and histologic features. Ann Intern Med. 1995;123:330–337.
476. Gholson CF, Morgan K, Catinis G, et al. Chronic hepatitis C with normal aminotransferase levels: A clinical histologic study. Am J Gastroenterol. 1997;92:1788–1792.
477. Morales TG, Sampliner RE, Bhattacaryya A, et al. Liver histology in anti-HCV positive persons with normal or minimally elevated aminotransferases. J Clin Gastroenterol. 1995;21:301–305.
478. Naito M, Hayashi N, Hagiwara H, et al. Serum hepatitis C virus RNA quantity and histological features of hepatitis C virus carriers with persistently normal ALT levels. Hepatology. 1994;19:871–875.
479. Puoti C, Magrini A, Stati T, et al. Clinical, histological and virological features of hepatitis C virus carriers with persistently normal or abnormal alanine transaminase levels. Hepatology. 1997;26:1393–1398.
480. Marcellin P, Levy S, Benhamou JP, et al. Management of the asymptomatic HCV carrier with normal ALT levels. Rev Viral Hepatitis. 1996;2:277–283.
481. Prieto M, Olaso C, Verdù C, et al. Does the healthy hepatitis C virus carrier state really exist? An analysis using polymerase chain reaction. Hepatology. 1995;22:413–417.
482. Martinot-Peignoux M, Marcellin PO, Gournay J, et al. Detection and quantitation of serum HCV-RNA by branched DNA amplification in anti-HCV positive blood donors. J Hepatol. 1994;20:676–678.
483. Shindo M, Arai K, Sokawa Y, Okuno T. The virological and histological states of anti-hepatitis C virus positive subjects with normal liver biochemical values. Hepatology. 1995;22:418–425.
484. Silini E, Bono F, Cividini A, et al. Differential distribution of hepatitis C virus genotypes in patients with and without liver function abnormalities. Hepatology. 1995;21:285–290.
485. Prati D, Capelli C, Zanella A, et al. Influence of different hepatitis C virus genotypes on the course of asymptomatic hepatitis C virus infection. Gastroenterology. 1996;110:178–183.
486. Mathurin P, Moussali J, Cadranel J-F, et al. Slow progression rate of fibrosis in hepatitis C virus patients with persistently normal alanine transaminase activity. Hepatology. 1998;27:868–872.
487. Healey CJ, Chapmann RWG, Fleming KA. Liver histology in hepatitis C infection: A comparison between patients with persistently normal or abnormal transaminases. Gut. 1995;37:274–278.
488. Alberti A, Morsica G, Chemello L, et al. Hepatitis C viraemia and liver disease in symptom-free individuals with anti-HCV. Lancet. 1992;340:697–698.
489. Stanley AJ, Haydon GH, Piris J, et al. Assessment of liver histology in patients with normal transaminase levels. Eur J Gastroenterol Hepatol. 1996;8:869–872.
490. Grangé JD, Abergel A, Amiot X, et al. Interactions between chronic viral hepatitis C and pregnancy. Gastroenterol Clin Biol. 1995;19:520–524.
491. Ballardini G, Groff P, Pontisso P, et al. Hepatitis C virus (HCV) genotype, tissue HCV antigens, hepatocellular adhesion-1 molecules: Clues to pathogenesis of hepatocellular damage and response to interferon treatment in patients with chronic hepatitis C. J Clin Invest. 1995;95:2067–2075.
492. Serfaty L, Chazouilleres O, Pawlotsky J-M, et al. Interferon alfa therapy in patients with chronic hepatitis C and persistently normal aminotransferase activity. Gastroenterology. 1996;110:291–295.
493. Silverman AL, Piquette DL, Filipiak CL, et al. Alfa interferon treatment of hepatitis C virus RNA–positive patients with normal or near-normal alanine aminotransferase levels. Am J Gastroenterol. 1997;92:1793–1795.
494. Montalto G, Zignego AL, Ruggeri MI, et al. Serum HCV-RNA and liver histologic findings in patients with long-term normal transaminases. Dig Dis. 1997;42:1703–1707.
495. Orito E, Mizokami M, Suzuki K, et al. Interferon alpha therapy for individuals with normal serum alanine aminotransferase levels before treatment. J Gastroenterol Hepatol. 1996;12:58–61.
496. Van Thiel DH, Caraceni P, Molloy PJ, et al. Chronic hepatitis C in patients with normal or near normal alanine aminotransferase levels. The role of interferon α2b therapy. J Hepatol. 1995;23:503–508.
497. Sangiovanni A, Morales R, Spinzi G, et al. Interferon alfa treatment of HCV RNA carriers with persistently normal transaminase levels: A pilot randomized controlled study. Hepatology. 1998;27:853–856.
498. Schiff ER, Tagle FM. Treatment of HCV: Approach to difficult cases. Clin Liver Dis. 1997;3:647–662.
499. Hoofnagle JH. Hepatitis C: The clinical spectrum of disease. Hepatology. 1997;26(Suppl 1):15S–20S.
500. Agnello V, Romain PL. Mixed cryoglobulinemia secondary to hepatitis C virus infection. Rheumatol Dis Clin North Am. 1996;22:1–21.
501. Booth JCL. Chronic hepatitis C: The virus, its discovery and the natural history of the disease. J Viral Hepat. 1998;5:213–222.
502. Ábel G, Zhang Q-X, Agnello V. Hepatitis C virus infection in type II mixed cryoglobulinemia. Arthritis Rheum. 1993;36:1341–1345.
503. Lunel F, Musset L. Hepatitis C virus infection and cryoglobulinemia. Viral Hepat Rev. 1996;2:111–124.
504. Disdier P, Harle J-R, Weiller P-J. Cryoglobulinemia and hepatitis C infection. Lancet. 1991;338:1151–1152.
505. Misiani R, Bellavita P, Fenili D. Hepatitis C virus infection in patients with essential mixed cryoglobulinemia. Ann Intern Med. 1992;117:573–576.
506. Agnello V, Chung RT, Kaplan LM. A role of hepatitis C virus infection in type II cryoglobulinemia. N Engl J Med. 1992;327:1490–1495.
507. Marcellin P, Descamps V, Marinot-Peignoux M, et al. Cryoglobulinemia with vasculitis associated with hepatitis C virus infection. Gastroenterology. 1993;104:272–277.
508. Ferri C, Monti M, LaCivita L, et al. Infection of peripheral blood mononuclear cells by hepatitis C virus in mixed cryoglobulinemia. Blood. 1993;82:3701–3704.
509. Mazzaro C, Zagonel V, Monfardini S, et al. Hepatitis C virus and non-Hodgkin's lymphomas. Br J Haemotol. 1996;94:544–550.
510. Schott P, Pott C, Ramadori G, Hartmann H. Hepatitis C virus infection–associated non-cryoglobulinaemic monoclonal IgMκ gammopathy responsive to interferon-α treatment. J Hepatol. 1998;29:310–315.
511. Ray RB, Meyer K, Ray R. Suppression of apoptotic cell death by hepatitis C virus core protein. Virology. 1996;226:176–182.
512. Andreone P, Zignego AL, Cursaro C, et al. Prevalence of monoclonal gammopathies in patients with hepatitis C virus infection. Ann Intern Med. 1998;129:294–298.
513. Johnson RJ, Gretch DR, Yamabe H, et al. Membranoproliferative glomerulonephritis associated with hepatitis C virus infection. N Engl J Med. 1993;328:465–470.
514. Bichard P, Ounanian A, Girard M, et al. High prevalence of hepatitis C virus RNA in the supernatant and the cryoprecipitate of patients with essential and secondary type II mixed cryoglobulinemia. J Hepatol. 1994;21:58–63.
515. Bonomo L, Casato M, Afeltra A, et al. Treatment of idiopathic mixed cryoglobulinemia with alpha interferon. Am J Med. 1987;83:726–730.
516. Casato M, Lagana B, Antonelli G, et al. Long-term results of therapy with interferon-α for type II essential mixed cryoglobulinemia. Blood. 1991;78:3142–3144.
517. Misiani R, Bellavita P, Fenili D, et al. Interferon alfa-2a therapy in cryoglobulinemia associated with hepatitis C virus. N Engl J Med. 1994;330–334.
518. Dammacco F, Sansonno D, Han JH. Natural interferon versus its combination with 6-methyl-prednisolone in the therapy of type II mixed cryoglobulinemia: A long-term, randomized, controlled study. Blood. 1994;84:3336–3339.
519. Pereira BJG, Levey AS. Hepatitis C virus infection in dialysis and renal transplantation. Kidney Int. 1997;51:981–999.
520. Puoti M, Sandrini S, Zaltron S. Impact of hepatitis C virus infection on patients with chronic renal failure. J Nephrol. 1995;8:291–299.
521. Roth D. Hepatitis C virus: The nephrologist's view. Am J Kidney Dis. 1995;25:3–16.
522. Roth D. The significance of hepatitis C virus infection in the care of patients with renal disease. In: Epstein M, ed. The Kidney in Liver Disease. 4th ed. Philadelphia: Hanley & Belfus; 1996:151–166.
523. Davis CL, Gretch DR, Carrithers RL. Hepatitis C virus in renal disease. Curr Opin Nephrol Hypertens. 1994;3:164–173.
524. Pessoa MG, Wright TL. Hepatitis C infection in transplantation. Clin Liver Dis. 1998;3:663–690.
525. Umlauft F, Gruenewald KM, Weiss G, et al. Patterns of hepatitis C viremia in patients receiving hemodialysis. Am J Gastroenterol. 1997;92:73–77.
526. Cantu P, Mangano S, Masini M, et al. Prevalence of antibodies against hepatitis C virus in a dialysis unit. Nephron. 1992;61:337–338.
527. Chan TM, Lok AS, Cheng IKP. Prevalence of hepatitis C virus infection in hemodialysis patients: A longitudinal study comparing the results of RNA and antibody assays. Hepatology. 1993;17:5–8.
528. Lau J, Davis G, Brunson M, et al. Hepatitis C virus infection in kidney transplant recipients. Hepatology. 1993;18:1027–1031.
529. Lau J, Qian K, Mizokami M, et al. Significance of serum hepatitis C virus RNA levels in chronic hepatitis C. Lancet. 1993;341:1501–1504.
530. Pol S, Romeo R, Zins B, et al. Hepatitis C virus RNA in anti-HCV positive

hemodialyzed patients: Significance and therapeutic implications. Kidney Int. 1993;44:1097–1100.
531. Garcia G, Terrault NA, Wright TL. Hepatitis C virus infection in the immunocompromised patient. Semin Gastrointest Dis. 1995;6:35–45.
532. Jadoul M, Cornu C, van Ypersele de Strihou C, et al. Incidence and risk factors for hepatitis C seroconversion in hemodialysis: A prospective study. Kidney Int. 1993;44:1322–1326.
533. Munro J, Briggs J, McCruden E. Detection of a cluster of hepatitis C infections in a renal transplant unit by analysis of sequence variation of the *NS5a* gene. J Infect Dis. 1996;174:177–180.
534. Alfurayh O, Sobh M, Buali A, et al. Hepatitis C virus infection in chronic hemodialysis patients, a clinicopathologic study. Nephrol Dial Transplant. 1992;7:327–332.
535. Caramelo C, Ortiz A, Aguilera B, et al. Liver disease patterns in hemodialysis patients with antibodies to hepatitis C virus. Am J Kidney Dis. 1993;22:822–828.
536. Ichikawa Y, Kyo M, Hanafusa T, et al. A 20-year case study of a kidney transplant recipient with chronic active hepatitis C: Clinical course and successful treatment for late acute rejection induced by interferon therapy. Transplantation. 1998;65:134–138.
537. Rostaing L, Modesto A, Baron E, et al. Acute renal failure in kidney transplant patients treated with interferon alpha 2b for chronic hepatitis C. Nephron. 1996;74:512–516.
538. Carithers RL Jr. Hepatitis C in patients with renal failure. In: Maddrey WC, Schiff ER, eds. The Clinician's Companion II: Part 2: Assessment of Special Patient Populations—Monograph. Secaucus, NJ: Projects in Knowledge; 1998:14–16.
539. Mathurin P, Mouquet C, Poynard T, et al. Impact of hepatitis B and C virus on kidney transplantation outcome. Hepatology. 1999;29:257–263.
540. Kellerman S, Alter MJ. Preventing hepatitis B and hepatitis C virus infections in end-stage renal disease patients: Back to basics (Editorial). Hepatology. 1999;29:291–293.
541. Rao K, Anderson W, Kasiske B, et al. Value of liver biopsy in the evaluation and management of chronic liver disease in renal transplant recipients. Am J Med. 1993;94:241–250.
542. Terrault NA, Wright TL, Pereira BJ. Hepatitis C in the transplant recipient. Infect Dis Clin North Am. 1995;9:943–964.
543. Koenig P, Vogel W, Umlauft F, et al. Interferon treatment for chronic hepatitis C virus infection in uremic patients. Kidney Int. 1994;45:1507–1509.
544. Pol S, Thiers V, Camot F, et al. Efficacy and tolerance of alpha-2b interferon therapy on hepatitis C virus infection of hemodialyzed patients. Kidney Int. 1995;47:1412–1418.
545. Duarte R, Huraib S, Said R, et al. Interferon-alpha facilitates renal transplantation in hemodialysis patients with chronic viral hepatitis. Am J Kidney Dis. 1995;25:40–45.
546. Raptopoulou-Gigi M, Spaia S, Garifallos S, et al. Interferon-alpha 2b treatment of chronic hepatitis C in haemodialysis patients. Nephrol Dial Transplant. 1995;10:1834–1837.
547. Casanovas TT, Baliellas C, Sese E, et al. Interferon may be useful in hemodialysis patients with hepatitis C virus chronic infection who are candidates for kidney transplant. Transplant Proc. 1995;27:2229–2230.
548. Chan TM, Lok AS, Cheng IK, Ng IO. Chronic hepatitis C after renal transplantation. Treatment with alpha-interferon. Transplantation. 1993;56:1095–1098.
549. Rostaing L, Izopet J, Baron E, et al. Preliminary results of treatment of chronic hepatitis C with recombinant interferon alpha in renal transplant patients. Nephrol Dial Transplant. 1995;10:93–96.
550. Rostaing L, Izopet J, Baron E, et al. Treatment of chronic hepatitis C with recombinant interferon alpha in kidney transplant recipients. Transplantation. 1995;59:1426–1431.
551. Ghalib R, Qian P, Ritter J, et al. Treatment of HCV after solid organ transplant with alfa 2b interferon. Hepatology. 1995;22:132A.
552. Rostaing L, Izopet J, Baron E, et al. Treatment of chronic hepatitis C with recombinant interferon alpha 2b in kidney transplant patients: Preliminary results and side effects. Transplant Proc. 1995;27:948–950.
553. Ozgur O, Boyacioglu S, Telatar H, Haberal M. Recombinant alpha-interferon in renal allograft recipients with chronic hepatitis C. Nephrol Dial Transplant. 1995;10:2104–2106.
554. Mahony J. Long term results and complications of transplantation: The kidney. Transplant Proc. 1989;21:1433–1434.
555. Haem J, Berthoux P, Cecillon S, et al. HCV renal disease in renal transplantation: A clinical and histological study. Nephrol Dial Transplant. 1996;11:48–51.
556. Rao K, Ma J. Chronic viral hepatitis enhances the risk of infection but not acute rejection in renal transplant recipients. Transplantation. 1996;62:1765–1769.
557. Elder GH. Porphyria cutanea tarda. Semin Liver Dis. 1998;18:67–75.
558. Bonkovsky HL, Banner BF, Lambrecht RW, Rubin RB. Iron in liver diseases other than hemochromatosis. Semin Liver Dis. 1996;16:65–82.
559. Bonkovsky HL, Banner BF, Rothman AL. Iron and chronic viral hepatitis. Hepatology. 1997;25:759–768.
560. Han S-H, Fong T-L, Valinchuk B, et al. Randomized controlled trial of the effect of iron depletion on aminotransferase levels, HCV RNA and response to interferon therapy in patients with chronic hepatitis C virus. Hepatology. 1995;22:180A.
561. Roberts AG, Whatley SD, Morgan RR, et al. Increased frequency of the haemochromatosis Oys282Tyr mutation in sporadic porphyria cutanea tarda. Lancet. 1997;349:321–323.
562. Santos M, Clevers HC, Marx JM. Mutations of the hereditary hemochromatosis candidate gene *HLA-H* in porphyria cutanea tarda. N Engl J Med. 1997;336:1327–1328.
563. DeCastro M, Sanchez J, Herrera JF, et al. Hepatitis C virus antibodies and liver disease in patients with porphyria cutanea tarda. Hepatology. 1993;17:551–557.
564. Murphy A, Dooley S, Hillary IB, Murphy GM. HCV infection in porphyria cutanea tarda. Lancet. 1993;341:1534–1535.
565. Dietrich DT. Coinfections: Hepatitis C, hepatitis B, and HIV. In: Maddrey WC, Schiff ER, eds. The Clinician's Companion II: Part 2: Assessment of Special Patient Populations—Monograph. Secaucus, NJ: Projects in Knowledge; 1998:1–5.
566. Weltmann MD, Brotodihardjo A, Crewe EB, et al. Coinfection with hepatitis B and C or B, C and delta viruses results in severe chronic liver disease and responds poorly to interferon-alpha treatment. J Viral Hepat. 1995;2:39–45.
567. Bonino F, Olivieri F, Colombatto P, Brunetto MR. Impact of interferon-alpha therapy on the development of hepatocellular carcinoma in patients with liver cirrhosis: Results of an international survey. J Viral Hepat. 1997;4(Suppl 2):70–82.
568. Sato S, Fujiyama S, Tanaka M, et al. Coinfection of hepatitis C virus in patients with chronic hepatitis B infection. J Hepatol. 1994;21:159–166.
569. Mimms LT, Mosley J, Hollinger FB, et al. Effect of concurrent infection with hepatitis C virus on acute hepatitis B virus infection. Br Med J. 1993;307:1095–1097.
570. Lee DS, Huh K, Lee EH, et al. HCV and HBV coexist in HBsAg-negative patients with HCV viraemia: Possibility of coinfection in these patients must be considered in HBV-high endemic area. J Gastroenterol Hepatol. 1997;12:855–861.
571. Uchida T, Kaneita Y, Gotoh K, et al. Hepatitis C virus is frequently coinfected with serum marker–negative hepatitis B virus: Probable replication promotion of the former by the latter demonstrated by in vitro cotransfection. J Med Virol. 1997;52:399–405.
572. Zignego AL, Fontana R, Puliti S, et al. Impaired response to alpha interferon in patients with an inapparent hepatitis B and hepatitis C virus coinfection. Arch Virol. 1997;142:535–544.
573. Scharschmidt BF, Held MJ, Hollander HH, et al. Hepatitis B in patients with HIV infection: Relationship to AIDS and patient survival. Ann Intern Med. 1992;117:837–838.
574. Zylberberg H, Pol S. Reciprocal interactions between human immunodeficiency virus and hepatitis C virus infections. Clin Infect Dis. 1996;23:1117–1125.
575. Eyster ME, Diamondstone LS, Lien JM, et al. Natural history of hepatitis C virus infection in multitransfused hemophiliacs: Effect of coinfection with human immunodeficiency virus. The Multicenter Hemophilia Cohort Study. J Acquir Immune Defic Syndr. 1993;6:602–610.
576. Collier J, Heathcote J. Hepatitis C viral infection in the immunosuppressed patient. Hepatology. 1998;27:2–6.
577. Spengler U, Rockstron JK. Hepatitis C in the patient with human immunodeficiency virus. J Hepatol. 1998;29:1023–1030.
578. Rockstroh JK, Spengler U, Sudhop T, et al. Immunosuppression may lead to progression of hepatitis C virus associated liver disease in hemophiliacs coinfected with HIV. Am J Gastroenterol. 1996;91:2563–2568.
579. Ramos Paesa C, Arazo Garces P, Pascular Catalan A, et al. Interferon treatment of chronic hepatitis C in human immunodeficiency virus infected patients. Rev Clin Esp. 1998;198:221–225.
580. Soriano V, Garcia-Samaniego J, Bravo R, et al. Efficacy and safety of alpha-interferon treatment of chronic hepatitis C in HIV-infected patients. J Infect. 1995;31:9–13.
581. Vento S, DiPerri G, Cruciano M, et al. Rapid decline of $CD4^+$ cells after IFN alpha treatment in HIV-1 infection (Letter). Lancet. 1993;341:958–959.
582. McCormick JB, Getchell JP, Mitchell SW, Hicks DR. Ribavirin suppresses replication of lymphadenopathy-associated virus in cultures of human adult T-lymphocytes. Lancet. 1984;15:1367–1369.
583. Fernandes-Larsson R, Patterson JL. Ribavirin is an inhibitor of human immunodeficiency virus reverse transcriptase. Mol Pharmacol. 1990;38:766–770.
584. Roberts RB, Dickinson GM, Haseltine PN, et al. Multicenter clinical trial of oral ribavirin in HIV-infected patients with lymphadenopathy. J Acquir Immun Defic Syndr. 1990;3:884–892.
585. Bernier R, Tremblay M, Tsoukas C, Bergeron MG. Drug sensitivity of human immunodeficiency virus type 1 isolates after ribavirin. J Infect Dis. 1997;175:176–178.
586. Vogt MW, Hartshorn KL, Furman PA, et al. Ribavirin antagonizes the effect of azidothymidine on HIV replication. Science. 1987;235:1376–1379.
587. Japour AJ, Lertora JJ, Meehan PM, et al. A phase-I study of the safety, pharmacokinetics, and antiviral activity of combination didanosine and ribavirin in patients with HIV-1 disease. J Acquir Immune Defic Syndr. 1996;13:235–246.
588. Rutschmann OT, Negro F, Hirschel B, et al. Impact of treatment with human immunodeficiency virus (HIV) protease inhibitors on hepatitis C viremia in patients coinfected with HIV. J Infect Dis. 1998;177:783–785.
589. Rizzetto M, Verme G, Recchia S, et al. Immunofluorescence detection of a new antigen-antibody system (delta-antidelta) associated to the hepatitis virus in the liver and the serum of HBsAg carriers. Gut. 1977;18:996–999.
590. Purcell RH, Rizzetto M, Gerin JL. Hepatitis delta virus infection of the liver. Semin Liver Dis. 1984;4:340–346.
591. Alter M, Mast E. The epidemiology of viral hepatitis in the United States. Gastroenterol Clin North Am. 1994;23:437–448.
592. Hoofnagle JH. Type D (delta) hepatitis. JAMA. 1989;261:1321–1325 [Erratum. JAMA. 1989;261:3552.]
593. Ottobrelli A, Marzano A, Smedile A, et al. Patterns of hepatitis delta virus reinfection and disease after liver transplantation. Gastroenterology. 1991;101:1649–1655.
594. Govindarajan S, Chin K, Redecker A, et al. Fulminant B viral hepatitis: Role of delta agent. Gastroenterology. 1984;86:1417–1421.

595. Negro F, Rizzetto M. Diagnosis of hepatitis delta virus infection. J Hepatol. 1995;22(Suppl 1):136–139.
596. Smedile A, Rizzetto M, Denniston K, et al. The clinical significance of hepatitis D RNA in serum as detected by a hybridization-based assay. Hepatology. 1986;6:1297–1301.
597. Hoofnagle JH. Therapy of acute and chronic viral hepatitis. Adv Intern Med. 1994;39:241–275.
598. Rosina F, Pintus C, Meschievitz C, Rizzetto M. A randomized controlled trial of a 12-month course of recombinant human interferon-α in chronic delta (type D) hepatitis: A multicentric Italian study. Hepatology. 1991;13:1052–1056.
599. Rosino F, Cozzolongo R. Interferon for HDV infection. Antiviral Res. 1994;24:165–173.
600. Farci P, Mandas A, Coiana A, et al. Treatment of chronic hepatitis D with interferon alpha-2a. N Engl J Med. 1994;330:88–94.
601. Porres JC, Carreno V, Bartolomé J, et al. Treatment of chronic delta infection with recombinant human interferon alpha 2c at high doses. J Hepatol. 1989;9:338–344.
602. DiBisceglie AM, Martin P, Lisker-Melman M, et al. Therapy of chronic delta hepatitis with interferon alpha-2b. J Hepatol. 1990;11(Suppl 1):151–154.
603. Buti M, Esteban R, Roget M, et al. Long-term treatment with interferon alpha-2b in patients with chronic delta hepatitis and HIV antibodies. J Hepatol. 1990;11(Suppl 1):174.
604. Hadziyannis SJ. Use of α-interferon in the treatment of chronic delta hepatitis. J Hepatol. 1991;13(Suppl 1):21–26.
605. Madejon A, Cotonat T, Bartolomé J, et al. Treatment of chronic hepatitis D virus infection with low and high doses of IFN-α2a: Utility of polymerase chain reaction in monitoring antiviral response. Hepatology. 1994;19:1331–1336.
606. Puoti M, Rossi S, Forleo MA, et al. Treatment of chronic hepatitis D with interferon alpha-2b in patients with human immunodeficiency virus infection. J Hepatol. 1998;29:45–52.
607. Novick DM, Farci P, Croxson TS, et al. Hepatitis D virus and human immunodeficiency virus antibodies in parenteral drug abusers who are hepatitis B surface antigen positive. J Infect Dis. 1988;158:795–803.
608. Housset C, Pol S, Carbot F, et al. Interactions between human immunodeficiency virus-1, hepatitis delta virus and hepatitis B virus infections in 260 chronic carriers of hepatitis B virus. Hepatology. 1992;15:578–583.
609. Buti M, Jardi R, Allende H, et al. Chronic delta hepatitis: Is the prognosis worse when associated with hepatitis C virus and human immunodeficiency virus? J Med Virol. 1996;49:66–69.
610. Eyster ME, Sanders JC, Battegay M, DiBisceglie AM. Suppression of hepatitis C virus (HCV) replication by hepatitis D virus (HDV) in HIV-infected hemophiliacs with chronic hepatitis B and C. Dig Dis Sci. 1995;40:1583–1588.
611. Samuel D, Zignego AL, Reynes M, et al. Long term clinical and virological outcome after liver transplantation for cirrhosis caused by chronic delta hepatitis. Hepatology. 1995;21:333–339.
612. Chung RT, Friedman LS. Liver abscess and bacterial, parasitic, fungal, and granulomatous liver disease. In: Feldman M, Scharschmidt BF, Sleisinger MH, eds. Gastrointestinal and Liver Disease. 6th ed. Philadelphia: WB Saunders; 1998:1170–1188.
613. Weiss SA, Davis GL, Shaw-Stiffel TA. Hepatic sarcoidosis presenting as acute abdominal pain. Gastroenterologist. 1994;2:247–253.
614. Fauci AS, Hoffman GS. Granulomatous hepatitis. In: Mandell, Bennett JE, Dolin R, eds. Principles and Practice of Infectious Diseases. 4th ed. New York: Churchill Livingstone; 1995;1159–1164.
615. Neville A, Pyasena KHG, James PG. Granulomas of the liver. Postgrad Med J. 1975;51:361–365.
616. Sartin JS, Walker RD. Granulomatous hepatitis: A retrospective reivew of 88 cases at the Mayo Clinic. Mayo Clin Proc. 1991;66:914–918.
617. Klatskin G. Hepatic granulomata: Problems in interpretation. Ann N Y Acad Sci. 1976;278:427–433.
618. Williams GGT, Williams WJ. Granulomatous inflammation—A review. J Clin Pathol. 1983;36:723–730.
619. Gronhagen-Riska C, Fyhrquist F, von Willebrand E. Angiotensin I converting enzyme: A marker of highly differentiated monocytic cells. Ann N Y Acad Sci. 1986;465:242–249.
620. Berman JS, Beer DJ, Bernardo J, et al. A proposed model for the accumulation of helper/inducer lymphocytes in sarcoidosis: The role of lymphocyte subset–specific chemoattractant lymphokines. Ann N Y Acad Sci. 1986;465:98–109.
621. Tierstein AS. The Kveim test after Siltzbach. Ann N Y Acad Sci. 1986;465:744–747.
622. Reynolds TF, Campra JL, Peters RL. Granulomatous liver disease. In: Zakim D, Boyer TD, eds. Hepatology—A Textbook of Liver Disease. 3rd ed. Philadelphia: WB Saunders; 1996;1472–1489.
623. Maddrey WC. Granulomatous liver disease: Clinical aspects. In: Seeff LB, Lewis JH, eds. Current Perspectives in Hepatology. New York: Plenum; 1989:309–326.
624. Bach N, Thiese ND, Schaffner F. Hepatic histopathology in the acquired immunodeficiency syndrome. Semin Liver Dis. 1992;12:205–212.
625. Cervantes F, Burguera M, Carbonell J, et al. Liver disease in brucellosis. A clincial and pathological study of 40 cases. Postgrad Med J. 1982;58:346–351.
626. Hoffman CF, Heaton JW. Q fever hepatitis. Clinical manifestations and pathological findings. Gastroenterology. 1982;83:474–480.
627. Rudzki G, Ishak KG, Zimmerman HJ. Chronic intrahepatic cholestasis of sarcoidosis. Am J Med. 1975;59:373–379.
628. Leff JA, Ready JB, Repetto C, et al. Coexistence of primary biliary cirrhosis and sarcoidosis. West J Med. 1990;153:439–441.
629. Ilan Y, Rappaport I, Feigin R, et al. Primary sclerosing cholangitis in sarcoidosis. J Clin Gastroenterol. 1993;16:326–328.
630. Johnson DA, Diehl AM, Sjogren MH, et al. Serum angiotensin converting enzyme activity in evaluation of patients with liver disease. Am J Med. 1987;83:256–260.

SECTION O

ACQUIRED IMMUNODEFICIENCY SYNDROME

Chapter 104

Global Perspectives on Human Immunodeficiency Virus Infection and Acquired Immunodeficiency Syndrome

PETER PIOT
MICHAEL H. MERSON

Almost 2 decades after the recognition of acquired immunodeficiency syndrome (AIDS) in the United States, the global epidemiologic pattern of human immunodeficiency virus (HIV) infection has changed dramatically. Whereas the disease was originally confined primarily to North America, Western Europe, and parts of sub-Saharan Africa, HIV has now spread throughout the world, with major epidemic foci in all continents. In addition, on a worldwide scale, the epidemic is now evolving into a mainly heterosexually transmitted disease of the developing world, and, increasingly, of underprivileged populations in the industrialized world. In this aspect, HIV infection now resembles the "classic" infectious diseases, disproportionately affecting those most socially and economically vulnerable.

This chapter focuses on specific features of the epidemiology and impact of HIV infection and AIDS in the developing world, as well as the response to the epidemic. Although two serotypes of HIV are currently recognized, namely HIV-1 and HIV-2, the term *HIV* is used in this chapter to designate HIV-1, which is the major virus.

SIZE OF THE PROBLEM

As of the end of 1998, the Joint United Nations Programme on HIV/AIDS (UNAIDS) estimated that more than 33 million adults and children were living with HIV/AIDS, from a cumulative total of well over 47 million persons infected since the beginning of the epidemic. Figure 104–1 shows global estimates of the HIV/AIDS epidemic.[1]

More than 90% of infected persons live in the developing world, and 70% of cases have occurred in Africa. These figures keep increasing at a staggering rate, with approximately 16,000 new infections per day. In 1998 alone, it is estimated that almost 6 million people became infected, with a majority of these new infections occurring in sub-Saharan Africa and Asia. Half of all new infections occur in young people between 10 and 24 years of age.[1, 2]

EUROPE

The epidemiology of HIV/AIDS in North America is extensively discussed in Chapter 105; except for this section, this chapter deals mainly with the situation in the developing world. In 1997, a total of 14,874 AIDS cases had been reported in the 12 countries of the European Community—a 38% drop from 1995 (Fig. 104–2).[3] In general, in the industrialized countries of Europe, Australia, and New Zealand, there has been a marked fall in AIDS incidence, and in some cases of HIV incidence, among homosexual and bisexual men. Heterosexual transmission is slowly rising, however, in part because of rising infection rates among drug users, who often have sex with noninjectors. In some Scottish cities, up to one third of new infections now occur through heterosexual intercourse, and among women attending antenatal clinics in some neighborhoods of London, HIV prevalence ranged between 1 and 5 per 1000.

In 1997, most new cases of AIDS in Europe were identified in injecting drug users. This population contributes particularly to the epidemic in Spain, Italy, and France, which together contain more than two thirds of all cases reported in the European Community.[3] However, homosexual and bisexual men still represent a large proportion of AIDS cases in Europe, reflecting the high incidence of infection in these populations a decade ago.

In the previous edition of this textbook, HIV incidence in Eastern Europe was reported as being low, but with a potential for an "uncontrolled epidemic." Until the mid-1990s, mass screening of various populations indicated extremely low levels of HIV infection. However, between 1994 and 1997, HIV infections increased sixfold in the former socialist economies of Eastern Europe and Central Asia, totaling approximately 200,000 adults by the end of 1997. Particularly the Russian Federation, Ukraine, Belarus, and Moldavia have experienced enormous growth in HIV infection rates, most related to injection drug use (Fig. 104–3). For example, in Ukraine in 1994 approximately 1500 people were infected, but by 1998 well over 100,000 were estimated to be HIV positive.[2]

This rapid spread of HIV infection in Eastern Europe parallels epidemics of sexually transmitted diseases and of injection drug use. Syphilis rates in four countries of the region have skyrocketed in the 1990s. However, the bulk of spread has been among injection drug users, who account for about 80% of newly diagnosed cases, as illustrated in Figure 104–3 for the Russian Federation.

AFRICA

Sub-Saharan Africa remains by far the worst affected region, with 8% of all adults younger than 45 years of age being HIV positive,

- **People living with HIV/AIDS** .... **33.4 million**
- **New HIV infections in 1998** .... **5.8 million**
- **Deaths due to HIV/AIDS in 1998** .... **2.5 million**
- **Cumulative number of deaths due to HIV/AIDS** .... **13.9 million**

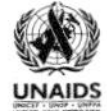

WAD-EN 1998
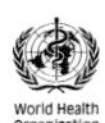

FIGURE 104–1. Global summary of HIV/AIDS epidemic in December 1998. (Data from ref. 1.)

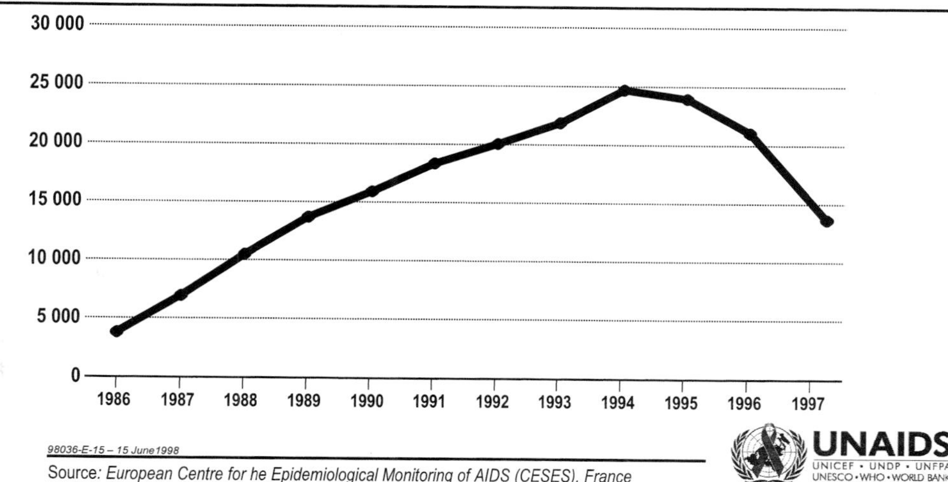

FIGURE 104–2. Number of new AIDS cases, Western Europe, 1986–1997. (Data from ref. 3.)

and in four countries (Botswana, Zimbabwe, Namibia, and Swaziland) more than one in four adults are infected. In cities such as Harare, Zimbabwe, and Gaborone, Botswana, as many as 40% of all sexually active adults are infected, and this is even the case now in some rural areas as well. However, the HIV prevalence rate is still well below 1 to 2% in countries such as Madagascar and Senegal.[1, 2, 4]

In most parts of Africa, the epidemic is still expanding. Figure 104–4 shows the evolution of HIV prevalence among pregnant women in various African cities. In general, prevalence of HIV infection is highest in eastern and southern Africa, although in Côte d'Ivoire and surrounding countries in West Africa it is now rapidly increasing. Infection rates are rising very rapidly in girls and young women, who often are infected by older men and are biologically more vulnerable to sexual acquisition of HIV. For example, in Lusaka, Zambia, as many as one in four 18-year-old women are infected with HIV, compared with 5% of 18-year-old men.[5] Prevalence rates are generally highest among the sexually most active parts of the population, as illustrated by the age distribution of HIV infections, which peak between the ages of 20 and 40 years; by very high infection rates among men with a sexually transmitted disease (STD); and by high rates among prostitutes. Even in areas where HIV infection is still relatively uncommon in the population as a whole, prevalence rates well over 10% can be found in these higher-risk populations. It is now increasingly common in Africa to find HIV prevalence rates exceeding 80% among prostitutes and 50% among STD patients, particularly when the latter have genital ulcers. However, studies in antenatal clinics in Rwanda, Kenya, and Malawi demonstrate that the HIV epidemic is not limited any longer to people with high-risk sexual behavior.[6–8] They also show that sexual behavior of the partner is an equally important risk factor in HIV infection.

This fact is further illustrated by annual HIV incidence rates of 0.3% to as high as 5% in cohorts thought to be representative of the general population.[9] Among highly exposed female prostitutes, such incidence rates may be as high as 12 to 50% per year.[10, 11]

Amidst this gloomy picture, there are also the first signs of the impact of prevention efforts. This is well documented in urban Uganda, where HIV prevalence rates among antenatal clinic attendees declined from 25 to 30% in 1991 to 15% in 1996 (Fig. 104–5).[12, 13] A similar reduction in HIV prevalence has been found in northern Tanzania,[14] where, in the town of Bukoba, the prevalence among young women (15 to 24 years old) fell from 28% in 1987 to 11% in 1993. The prevalence of HIV stabilized at 5 to 10% between 1990 and 1997 in some Congolese populations.[9] However, it should be kept in mind that "stable" prevalence still implies active spread of HIV, but at a rate more or less equaling the rate of death from AIDS in that population.[15] Overall, about equal numbers of men and women are infected, although, as mentioned previously, women become infected at a much earlier age than men.

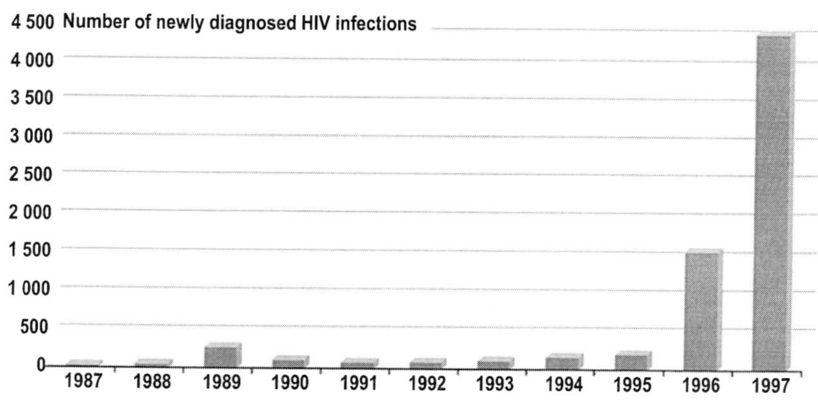

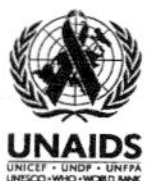

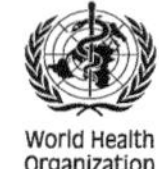

FIGURE 104–3. Number of newly diagnosed HIV infections, Russian Federation, 1987–1997. (Data from Russian AIDS Centre, Moscow.)

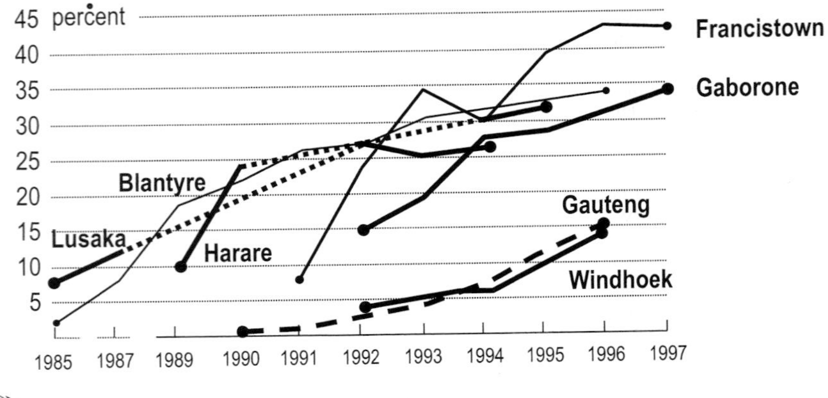

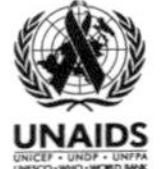

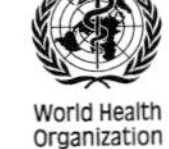

FIGURE 104–4. HIV prevalence among pregnant women in selected southern African cities, 1985–1997. (Data from ref. 1.)

The disease burden of HIV infection in sub-Saharan Africa is high and will grow considerably higher. In 1998 alone, 2 million Africans died from AIDS, constituting 80% of the global total.[2] In addition, more than half a million children were born with HIV. The enormous impact of AIDS on health services, individuals, and communities is discussed in later sections of this chapter.

A second human immunodeficiency virus, HIV-2, is found in West Africa and, to a much lesser extent, in Angola and Mozambique.[16] The highest HIV-2 prevalence rates are found in Guinea-Bissau, where almost 10% of the sexually active population are infected.[17] In the other countries where HIV-2 infection is found, prevalence rates are usually lower than 2% among pregnant women.[16]

HIV-2 seems to spread more slowly and the average age of infection appears to be higher than with HIV-1 infection in the same population.[18, 19] On the other hand, STD patients and prostitutes have the highest risk of HIV-2 infection, indicating that transmission of this virus also is mainly sexual. However, mother-to-child transmission and HIV-2 infection of infants and children are unusual.[20] Overall, the risk of transmission of HIV-2 appears to be significantly less than that of HIV-1. Similarly, the rate of disease development is reduced after HIV-2 infection, compared with HIV-1.[21]

Dually-reactive sera for both HIV-1 and HIV-2 antibodies occur frequently in HIV-2–prevalent populations. One third to one half of such cases are caused by concomitant infection with both viruses.[22, 23]

Although information about HIV infection in North Africa and the Middle East is very limited, HIV spread appears to have been limited.

ASIA

In recent years HIV has spread considerably in South and Southeast Asia, where more than 6.7 million people were living with HIV by 1998[1]; at the same time, less than 900,000 cases of AIDS were reported from Asia. India was the country with the largest number of infected persons in 1998, 3 to 5 million. The countries of Southeast Asia, with the exception of Indonesia, the Philippines, and Laos, are comparatively hard hit.

The extent of the spread of HIV in Asia is critical for the future of the pandemic, because more than half of the world's population lives on this continent. In addition, the full consequences of HIV infection in Asia will begin to be seen only after the year 2000, when many of the persons currently infected with HIV will have progressed to AIDS.

HIV-1 spread was first detected in Asia among injection drug users. The virus has spread fulminantly among drug users in selected areas of Thailand, Myanmar, northeast India, and Malaysia, where HIV seroprevalence levels of 50% are not uncommon in such populations. The situation is similar in some parts of southern China, Malaysia, and Vietnam.[24–27]

In a simultaneously occurring epidemic, the virus has also been

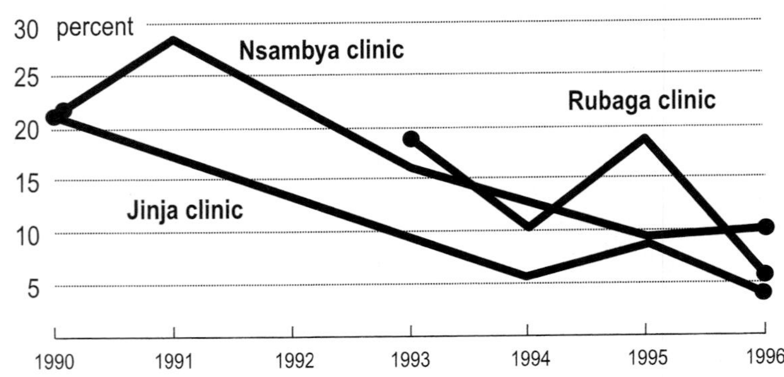

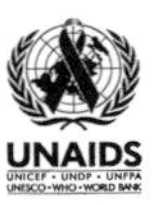

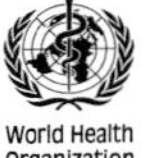

FIGURE 104–5. Declining HIV prevalence among urban pregnant women aged 15–19 years, Uganda, 1990–1996. (From Asiinwe-Okiroz G, Oppio AA, Musinguzi J, et al. Change in sexual behaviour and decline in HIV infection among young pregnant women in urban Uganda. AIDS. 1997; 11:1757–1764.)

spreading heterosexually, and this is now the main mode of transmission of HIV in Asia. As in Africa, it was initially among female prostitutes that HIV infection rates increased most dramatically. In Bombay, India, HIV seroprevalence rates among prostitutes appear to have increased from zero in 1987 to more than 40% in 1995. Molecular and serologic techniques support the separate introduction of a different HIV virus subtype among prostitutes and injection drug users in Thailand.[28] In contrast, as of 1997, HIV had not yet spread or had spread to only a very limited extent among prostitutes in cities such as Calcutta, India, or in countries such as Korea, the Philippines, and Taiwan.

In Thailand, HIV has now spread well beyond the most vulnerable groups, as illustrated by an HIV antibody prevalence rate of almost 6% among military recruits in the Thai Army in mid-1992, up from 0.5% in 1989,[27] and an overall prevalence rate of 2.3% in the adult population in 1997. Similarly, in Tamil Nadu state in India, in 1998, 1% of the rural adult population was HIV positive, as compared with 0.7% of urban adults. These figures illustrate the depth of HIV spread into the general adult population of Thailand and India.

China is still relatively little affected by HIV, with approximately 400,000 infected individuals. HIV is spreading mainly in two ways in China: among injection drug users in the southwest and heterosexually, especially along the prosperous eastern seaboard, where STDs such as gonorrhoea and syphilis are on the rise.

Prevention efforts have resulted in a well documented decline of HIV incidence among young Thai men, associated with a decrease in commercial sex and increased condom use[20–32] (Fig. 104–6).

LATIN AMERICA AND THE CARIBBEAN

Spread of HIV in the Caribbean and Latin America probably started at about the same time as in the United States. By 1997, approximately 630,000 cases of AIDS had occurred in this region, and 1.7 million adults were infected with HIV.[1] Certain islands in the Caribbean have some of the highest cumulative incidence rates of AIDS in the world. Eight percent of pregnant women were infected with the virus in 1993 in Haiti and in one site in 1996 in the Dominican Republic.

Epidemiologic patterns in the region have been diverse and are changing over time. In general, homosexual and bisexual activity has been the main mode of spread since the beginning of the epidemic, but heterosexual intercourse and injection drug use have become increasingly important routes of transmission since the late 1980s in many countries.[33–35] For instance, in Brazil the proportion of AIDS cases attributable to homosexual or bisexual transmission decreased from approximately 79% in 1980–1986 to less than 35% in 1992,[34] and whereas in 1986 1 AIDS patient in 17 was a woman, the figure became 1 in 4 by 1997. Bisexual behavior of their male partners is an important source of HIV infection for women in several Latin American countries.[36] Also, there is clear evidence of increasing infection among poorer and less educated members of the population.[2, 35]

HIV infection in the Caribbean is a true mosaic of different epidemiologic patterns determined by the local interaction of various risk determinants of HIV transmission.[33] Male homosexual transmission predominates in Trinidad, Tobago, Barbados, and Guyana. Injection drug use and sex for drugs (mainly cocaine/crack) are major risk factors in the Bahamas, Bermuda, Puerto Rico, and Trinidad. Finally, heterosexual transmission is predominant in Haiti and in the neighboring Dominican Republic. Haiti was one of the first countries in which a sustained AIDS epidemic in a heterosexual population was documented.[37] Other nearby countries, such as Honduras, may rapidly catch up.

DYNAMICS OF THE SPREAD OF THE HUMAN IMMUNODEFICIENCY VIRUS

There is no difference between modes of transmission of HIV in the developing world and the industrialized countries. Selected aspects of HIV transmission in the developing world, and other determinants of HIV spread are reviewed briefly here.

Modes of Transmission

Worldwide, HIV infection is basically a sexually transmitted infection. Unprotected heterosexual intercourse accounts for the large majority of cases of HIV infection in the developing world, but the situation is different in North America and western Europe.

The low efficiency of penile-vaginal intercourse for transmission of HIV has now been well documented, especially for transmission from women to men. A sustained and fulminant heterosexual epidemic can be explained only by a common occurrence of factors amplifying heterosexual transmission, possibly in addition to high-risk sexual behavior patterns.

Factors that may enhance the efficiency of heterosexual transmission of HIV include higher viremia or more advanced immunodeficiency in the infecting partner, receptive anal intercourse, sex during menses, and the presence of other STDs. Other factors that may increase the risk of heterosexual transmission but are less well

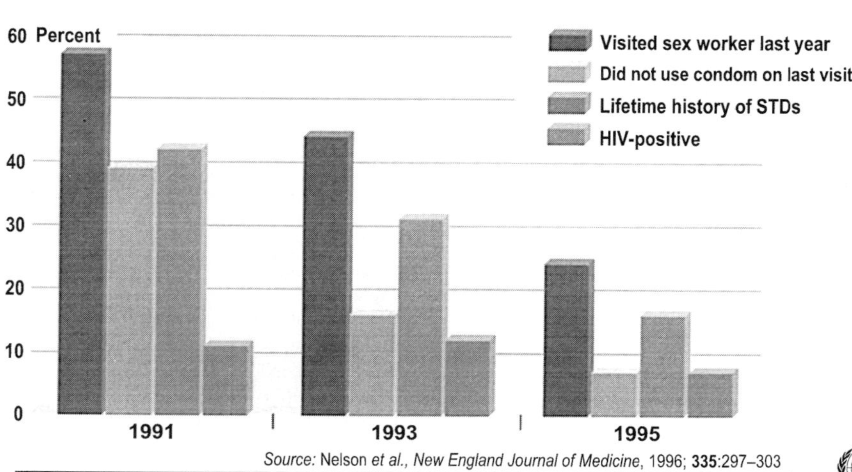

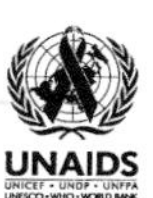

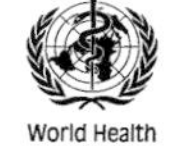

FIGURE 104–6. Sexual behavior, sexually transmitted diseases, and HIV infection in 21-year-old men, Northern Thailand, 1991–1995. (From Nelson K, Gelentano D, Eiumtrakol S, et al. Changes in sexual behaviour and a decline in HIV infection among young men in Thailand. N Engl J Med. 1996;335:297–303.)

documented include lack of circumcision in men, the use of various desiccating vaginal agents, traumatic sexual intercourse, and cervical ectopy.[38–40]

Conventional STDs have attracted the most attention as a risk factor, because many are curable with relatively inexpensive antibiotics, leading to public health interventions for HIV prevention.[40, 41] There is now convincing evidence from prospective studies that particularly genital ulcers (e.g., chancroid, syphilis, genital herpes) but also the more common nonulcerative STDs (e.g., gonorrhea, chlamydial infection) enhance the sexual transmission of HIV. This has been extensively documented in Africa, mainly in Kenya and the Democratic Republic of Congo.[10, 42] Finally, a conclusive randomized trial in northern Tanzania demonstrated that community-based treatment of bacterial STDs reduced the spread of HIV.[43]

Cohort studies in Nairobi, Kenya, found that the adjusted relative risks of genital ulcers (mainly chancroid) for HIV transmission were 3 to 8, but it is plausible that these lesions increase the risk of HIV transmission during a single sexual act by a factor between 10 and 100.[42] In addition, people with HIV infection with declining immunity have more genital ulcers; this probably increases their infectiousness during sexual intercourse, because HIV can often be detected in ulcer material obtained from such persons.

The relative risks of gonorrhea and chlamydial infection for HIV acquisition in women are smaller than those of genital ulcers.[10] However, because these STDs are far more common in most populations than genital ulcers, their contribution to the heterosexual spread of HIV may also be greater.[41] Several studies have found that genital shedding of HIV is greatly enhanced in the presence of urethral, cervical, or vaginal inflammation.[44, 45]

Globally, mother-to-child transmission during pregnancy, delivery, or breast-feeding is a second major mode of spread of HIV. Studies on mother-to-child transmission of HIV have consistently found higher rates of transmission in Africa than in North America or Europe (approximately 30 to 40% versus 15 to 20%, respectively).[46, 47]

Breast-feeding probably explains most of this higher risk of transmission in Africa.[48] Several studies have shown that the risk of transmission through breast-feeding is approximately 15% but can be as high as 29% for women who acquire HIV infection after delivery.[48–50]

Maternal vitamin A deficiency, high plasma HIV viral load, low $CD4^+$ T-lymphocyte count, chorioamnionitis, prolonged rupture of membranes, biologic phenotype of the virus, and vaginal delivery, rather than cesarean section, have also been associated with increased risk for mother-to-child transmission.[51–55] In contrast to the richer countries, pregnant women in most developing countries rarely have access to interventions to prevent mother-to-child transmission of HIV.

As mentioned, HIV has spread considerably among injection drug users in parts of Asia, Latin America, and the Caribbean; this has sometimes occurred where injecting has replaced smoking and inhaling as a way of administering drugs.[19] Sharing of injection equipment and imprisonment were the strongest predictors of HIV infection in Thailand.[56]

Transfusion with HIV-contaminated blood continues to be a source of HIV infection in some parts of the developing world, particularly in sub-Saharan Africa.[57–59] This illustrates tragically that mere availability of technology (i.e., serologic tests for HIV antibody) is not sufficient to solve a public health problem. It was estimated that in 1995, in Africa, one quarter of all blood donations were not tested for HIV antibody.[58]

Nosocomial transmission of HIV via injection with nonsterile syringes and needles occurs, but its contribution to the spread of HIV in the developing world is not well documented, although it is probably low.[60, 61] However, outbreaks of injection-associated nosocomial HIV infection in the former Soviet Union and in Romania show that injections for medical purposes may be a source of HIV infection in the community.[62, 63]

Factors Influencing the Spread of the Human Immunodeficiency Virus

The HIV/AIDS epidemic is still in a dynamic phase in most parts of the world, with continuing geographic spread and changing epidemiologic patterns. Moreover, there is substantial heterogeneity in the epidemiology of HIV throughout the world.[35]

A multitude of variables influence the spread of HIV. It is the complex mix and interaction of these direct (behavioral) and indirect (demographic) risk and vulnerability factors that determine how and when HIV spreads in the population.[64]

Sexual Behavior

Sexual behavior is undoubtedly the most important determinant of HIV spread. Such behavior is very heterogeneous among and within populations. Sexual behavior surveys in Africa and Asia have documented this heterogeneity in terms of number of partners, age of sexual debut, and rates of casual and commercial sex.[64–66] In addition, these studies found that men have generally more partners than women and that in some societies higher socioeconomic status is associated with a higher number of partners. However, according to mathematical models, sexual mixing patterns are equally important in determining the spread of HIV, particularly in early stages of the epidemic.[67] The "core group" concept postulates that a relatively small proportion of the population is contributing to maintenance of the epidemic; this pattern was first described in the 1970s with respect to the epidemiology of gonorrhoea in the United States.[68] However, for a chronic viral infection such as HIV, this concept is probably more relevant during the emerging phase of the epidemic than for "mature" epidemics with high levels of HIV infection already occurring among persons at a very young age and with relatively low-risk behavior.

The behavior of one's partner is as relevant for the risk of HIV infection as one's own behavior. This seems particularly true for women, who often become infected by their stable male partner. Data suggest that an increasing proportion of women with HIV infection in Africa, Thailand, and India have their husbands as their only sexual contact.[6–8]

Sexual practices, in particular the frequency of anal intercourse, which is the most efficient mode of sexual transmission of HIV, may also vary among populations. Heterosexual anal intercourse and male bisexual behavior appear to be more frequent in some Latin American countries.[36]

Last, but not least, the rate of condom use plays a major role in the extent of HIV spread. Despite much early scepticism, condoms have become increasingly popular in many parts of the developing world, particularly where social marketing programs are active.[69] The use of condoms has played a role in the significant reduction of HIV incidence among intensively counseled discordant couples in the Democratic Republic of Congo; in large populations of men and women in Thailand, Uganda, and Senegal; and among sex workers in Kenya, the Democratic Republic of Congo, and Bolivia[13, 32, 70–74] (Fig. 104–7). These "success stories" demonstrate that effective HIV prevention is possible, even under the difficult conditions of poor resource settings.

There is increasing awareness that personal behavior is critically influenced and conditioned by the social, economic, and cultural context.[35, 75]

Demography and Social Context

One of the most striking differences between the industrialized and the developing world is the age structure of the population; a much higher proportion of people in developing countries belong to the sexually most active age group. This by itself often results in higher incidence rates of sexually transmitted infections such as HIV infection.

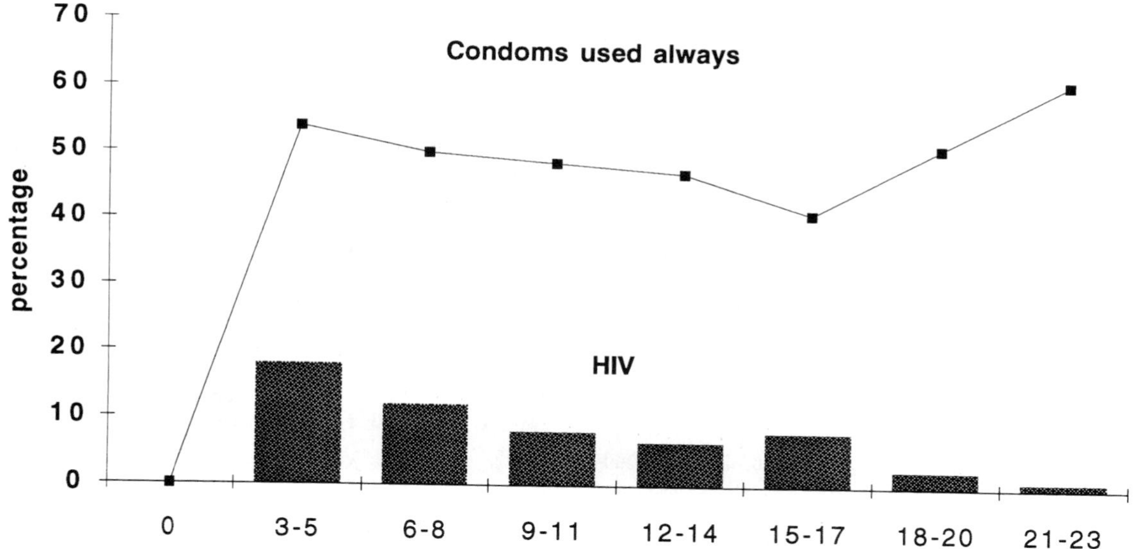

FIGURE 104–7. Increase in condom use and decrease in new infections among female prostitutes in Kinshasa. (Adapted from Laga M, Alary M, Nzila N, et al. Condom promotion and STD treatment, and declining incidence of HIV-1 infection in female Zairian Sex Workers. Lancet. 1994;344:2446–2448. © by The Lancet Ltd, 1994.)

Traditionally, migration and rapid urbanization have been associated with higher rates of STD. Both rural-to-urban and international migrations occur all over the developing world and have played a major role in the spread of HIV in southern Africa.[76]

An imbalance in numbers between the sexes may be an important determinant of HIV epidemiology, because cities with such an imbalance appear to experience a more rapid spread of HIV.[66, 77] Migration of male labor into the cities of the developing world may create such situation, but also social constraints on sexual behavior, such as disapproval of premarital and extramarital sex among women and late marriage by men for economic reasons, may be contributing factors. These demographic and social patterns may be associated with a higher rate of prostitute contacts by men.

Biologic Variables

As mentioned previously, several studies have documented a higher efficiency of heterosexual transmission of HIV in the presence of more advanced immunodeficiency in the index case, owing to higher levels of viremia and virus excretion. In populations that have experienced an HIV epidemic for a longer time, this may imply an increased overall efficiency of heterosexual and perinatal transmission of HIV. Such higher rates of transmission have been observed in Africa.

African HIV isolates exhibit a higher degree of genetic variability than American or European isolates.[78, 79] It is not known whether such viral variation has implications for the epidemiology of HIV, through strain differences in infectivity and cell tropism or in capacity to reach higher levels of viremia. However, it has been shown that differences in these features play a role in the different epidemiologic patterns seen with HIV-1 and HIV-2 infection.

Just as STDs enhance the efficiency of sexual transmission of HIV, their prevalence in a population also partly determines its vulnerability for the spread of HIV. Prevalence rates for various STDs vary widely among populations but are generally higher in the developing world, particularly in urban Africa. They may be particularly high in the populations most vulnerable to STD and HIV infection, such as sex workers and their clients, truck drivers, fishermen, and the military. Most important, high levels of STDs are a result not only of unsafe sexual behavior but also of inadequate care for patients with STDs.[80] Lack of circumcision in men, if confirmed as a risk factor for HIV transmission, may also play a role in the differential spread of HIV, because male circumcision is practiced to varying degrees throughout the world.

Impact of Prevention Programs

The effectiveness of national responses to the AIDS pandemic will ultimately determine how extensively HIV will spread. This requires, in the first place, political commitment to HIV/AIDS prevention, which is often insufficient. In addition, many countries need about 5 to 10 times more financial resources than they presently available to control the AIDS epidemic.

In many developing countries, public health care systems have deteriorated during the past three decades, and the introduction of user fees has resulted in declining access to health services and poorer management of people with STDs. In Nairobi, Kenya, after introduction of user fees at the main STD clinic, the attendance of men decreased significantly, to 40% of what it was before fees were levied.[81]

Lastly, poverty is not only a consequence of epidemics but also one of the major driving forces. It is associated with prostitution, homeless adults and street children, low rate of literacy, migration and separated families, and low status of women, all of which provide fertile ground for an HIV epidemic and make it more difficult for individuals and communities to cope with the consequences of HIV infection. Therefore programs that concentrate solely on reducing epidemiologic risk factors without addressing simultaneously what makes people vulnerable to HIV are likely to be insufficiently effective.[66, 82, 83]

CLINICAL EXPRESSION

The clinical manifestations and opportunistic diseases associated with HIV infection differ from one geographic area to another. First, there are indications that the progression to disease among persons with HIV infection may be more rapid in Africa.[84, 85] In a rural cohort in Uganda, the rate of disease progression was as high as 12.4% per year,[86] and the median time to AIDS after infection has been between 5 and 7.5 years in African studies.[84–86] This may be explained by a lack of medical care and prophylaxis for opportunistic infections (particularly tuberculosis) and by a higher occurrence of other endemic diseases such as parasitoses and tuberculosis, which depress the immune response. A study in Haiti found that chemoprophylaxis with isoniazid in patients infected with both HIV and *Mycobacterium tuberculosis* considerably extended life expectancy, supporting both hypotheses.[87]

However, the most striking difference in the natural history of HIV infection in adults is the short survival time of AIDS patients in Africa—in general as short as 1 year—compared with patients in the industrialized world.[88] This is obviously a consequence of inadequate medical care for most patients in Africa.

Although all opportunistic diseases may occur in AIDS patients throughout the world, the relative importance of specific diseases may be different in different locations. For instance, major opportunistic diseases in North America, such as *Pneumocystis carinii* pneumonia and Kaposi's sarcoma, are less common in African AIDS patients.[84, 89] In contrast, tuberculosis, chronic diarrhoea, and bacteremia due to pathogens such as *Salmonella typhimurium* and *Streptococcus pneumoniae* are very common.[90] In southeast Asia, systemic infection with *Penicillium marneffei* is a common opportunistic mycosis in patients with HIV infection. In Chiang Mai, northern Thailand, penicillinosis was diagnosed in 140 (35%) of 400 consecutive AIDS patients and specific prophylaxis with itraconazole was able to prevent development of penicillinosis marneffei.[91] An almost pathognomonic generalized papular pruritic skin eruption, mainly on the extremities, is observed in about 20% of African patients with HIV infection but rarely in patients from other continents.[92] Its cause is unknown.

Tuberculosis is not only the leading opportunistic infection among adult AIDS patients in Africa, but it itself is greatly affected by the HIV epidemic, with rising incidence rates wherever HIV has become endemic.[93, 94] This rise in incidence is probably entirely attributable to the spread of HIV infection in populations in which 50 to 80% of all adults are infected with *M. tuberculosis.* A new tuberculosis epidemic is now accompanying the AIDS epidemic in many countries and is one of the major public health consequences of HIV infection in the developing world.

In Africa and Haiti, between 30 and 75% of tuberculosis patients are now infected with HIV. In other developing countries, the HIV prevalence is still low among tuberculosis patients, but usually higher than in the general population. However, because pulmonary tuberculosis may develop across a broad spectrum of HIV-associated immunodeficiency in tuberculosis-endemic populations, it is of limited use as an AIDS-defining illness.[95]

Additional consequences of dual HIV–*M. tuberculosis* infection include a high mortality rate among tuberculosis patients with HIV infection (mostly from HIV-related illness), a growing rate of multidrug resistance of *M. tuberculosis,* and an increase of up to 10-fold in severe skin reactions, including Stevens-Johnson syndrome, during thiacetazone therapy in HIV-positive patients.[93, 94]

The cause of death in patients with HIV infection in the developing world is not well studied.[89] In a large study of a representative sample of patients who died during hospitalization in Abidjan, Côte d'Ivoire, tuberculosis, bacteremia with gram-negative rods, and cerebral toxoplasmosis caused 53% of the deaths.[96] Tuberculosis was found in half of the cadavers with an AIDS-defining pathology, compared with only 4% for *P. carinii* pneumonia. In this population, where both HIV-1 and HIV-2 occur, patients with HIV-2 infection more often had severe cytomegalovirus infection and HIV-associated encephalitis than did patients with HIV-1 infection; this finding is compatible with the more prolonged course of disease associated with HIV-2 infection.

IMPACT OF THE HIV/AIDS EPIDEMIC

The impact of the AIDS epidemic on many parts of the developing world is already severe, but it will undoubtedly become worse as the number of people with AIDS and HIV-related illness continues to increase over the next decades. AIDS not only affects individual patients and their relatives but also communities at large, with a long-term impact on households, on the health sector, on demography, and on the economic and social systems.[35, 97]

Perhaps the most visible aspect of the burden of AIDS is the large number of men and women with AIDS in the hospitals of many African countries, where they now make up at least 50% of all patients. AIDS has also become the major cause of death among hospitalized patients.[98, 99] By the early 21st century, several Asian and Latin American cities will probably face the same problem as Africa today.

With a growing number of persons with HIV infection developing AIDS, the demand for health services will expand rapidly. In Thailand, it is estimated that by the year 2000, 12% of all hospital bed days will be required to care for patients with AIDS.[100] Absorbing this growing burden of patients is a major challenge for health care systems in the developing world.

The long-term demographic impact of AIDS is becoming clearer. As a result of AIDS, life expectancy at birth is declining by 10 to 15 years in the most affected countries, and overall population growth will slow[2] (Fig. 104–8).

AIDS is now the leading cause of death among adults in many African cities,[98] and in Thailand it is estimated that by the year 2000 almost 30% of all deaths will be caused by AIDS.[101] AIDS is also doubling to quadrupling the mortality rate in children younger than

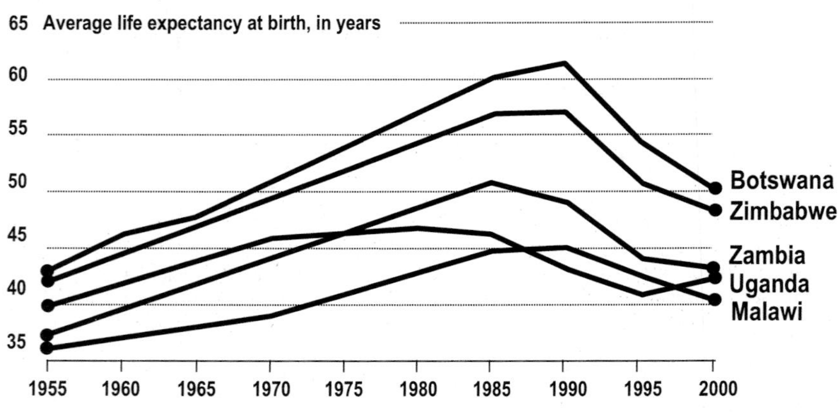

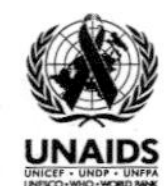

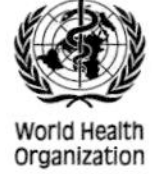

FIGURE 104–8. Changes in life expectancy in selected African countries with high HIV prevalence, 1995–2000. (Data from United Nations Population Division, 1996.)

5 years of age, leading to a reversal of the benefits of child survival initiatives in many high-prevalence areas. In addition, the number of orphans of parents who died from AIDS is growing at a staggering rate in the worst affected countries, with cumulatively 1.7 million AIDS orphans in 1998 in Uganda alone, and almost 9 million worldwide.

In economic terms, AIDS is now among the top five causes of healthy life lost in urban sub-Saharan Africa. Because HIV infection occurs mostly in adults in their most productive years, it profoundly affects the economic and social sectors.[102, 103] The gross domestic product of severely affected countries will decline because of loss of productivity in agriculture, industry, and services. In Tanzania it is estimated that the real rate of growth of the gross domestic product will decline by 15 to 28% as a result of AIDS between 1995 and 2010.[104]

To paraphrase the World Bank's World Development Report 1993, "Historians will look back on the latter half of this century as having had one great medical triumph, the eradication of smallpox, and one great medical tragedy, AIDS."[97]

REFERENCES

1. UNAIDS and WHO. AIDS Epidemic Update: December 1998, Geneva, UNAIDS, 1998.
2. UNAIDS and WHO. Report on the Global HIV/AIDS Epidemic. Geneva, UNAIDS, June 1998.
3. European Centre for the Epidemiological Monitoring of AIDS. AIDS Surveillance in the European Community and COST countries. Paris: March 1998.
4. Laga M, ed. AIDS in Africa, 2nd ed. London: Rapid Science Publishers; 1997.
5. Fylkesnes K, Kasumba K, Ndhlovu Z, Musonda RM. Comparing sentinel surveillance and population-based HIV prevalence rates in Zambia. In: Laga M, ed. AIDS in Africa. London: Rapid Science Publishers; 1997:12.
6. Allen S, Lindan C, Serufila A, et al. Human immunodeficiency virus infection in urban Rwanda: Demographic and behavioural correlates in a representative sample of child bearing women. JAMA. 1991;226:1657–1663.
7. Temmerman M, Mohammed Ali F, Ndinya-Achola JO, et al. Rapid increase of both HIV-1 infection and syphilis among pregnant women in Nairobi, Kenya. AIDS. 1992;6:1181–1185.
8. Dallabetta GA, Miotti PG, Chiphangui JD, et al. High socio-economic status is a risk factor for human immunodeficiency virus type 1 (HIV-1) infection but not for sexually transmitted diseases in women in Malawi: Implications for HIV-1 control. J Infect Dis. 1993;167:36–42.
9. Tarantola D, Schwartländer B. HIV/AIDS epidemics in sub-Saharan Africa: Dynamism, diversity and discrete declines. Laga M, ed. AIDS in Africa, 2nd ed. London: Rapid Science Publishers; 1997:5–22.
10. Laga M, Manoka A, Kivuvu M, et al. Non-ulcerative sexually transmitted diseases as risk factors for HIV-1 transmission in women: Results from a cohort study. AIDS. 1993;7:95–102.
11. Ngugi EN, Plummer FA, Simonsen JN, et al. Prevention of HIV transmission in Africa: The effectiveness of condom promotion and health education among high-risk prostitutes. Lancet. 1988;2:887–890.
12. Asiinwe-Okiroz G, Oppio AA, Musinguzi J, et al. Change in sexual behaviour and decline in HIV infection among young pregnant women in urban Uganda. AIDS. 1997;11:1757–1764.
13. UNAIDS. A measure of success in Uganda: The value of monitoring both HIV prevalence and sexual behaviour. Geneva: UNAIDS Best Practice Collection, UNAIDS; 1998.
14. Kwesigabo G, Killewo J, Godoy C, et al. Decline in the prevalence of HIV-1 infection in young women in the Kagera region of Tanzania. J Acquir Immun Defic Syndr Hum Retrovirol. 1998;17:262–268.
15. Anderson RM, May RM, Boily MC, et al. The spread of HIV-1 in Africa: Sexual contact patterns and the predicted demographic impact of AIDS. Nature. 1991;352:581–589.
16. De Cock KM, Brun-Vézinet F, Soro B. HIV-1 and HIV-2 infections and AIDS in West Africa. AIDS. 1991;5(Suppl 1):S21–S28.
17. Poulsen AG, Krinesdal B, Aaby P, et al. Prevalence of and mortality from human immunodeficiency virus type 2 in Bissau, West Africa. Lancet. 1989;1:827–831.
18. Kanki PJ, Travers K, Mboup S, et al. Slower heterosexual spread of HIV-2 than HIV-1. Lancet. 1994;343:943–946.
19. De Cock KM, Adjorlolo G, Ekpini E, et al. Epidemiology and transmission of HIV-2: Why there is no HIV-2 pandemic. JAMA. 1993;270:2083–2086.
20. Andreasson PA, Dias F, Nauclér A, et al. A prospective study of vertical transmission of HIV-2 in Bissau, Guinea-Bissau. AIDS. 1993;7:989–994.
21. Marlink R, Kanki P, Thior I, et al. Reduced rate of disease development after HIV-2 infection as compared to HIV-1. Science. 1994;265:1587–1590.
22. George R, Ou C-Y, Parekh B, et al. Prevalence of HIV-1 and HIV-2 mixed infections in Côte d'Ivoire. Lancet. 1992;1:338–339.
23. Peeters M, Gershy-Damet GM, Fransen K, et al. Virological and polymerase chain reaction studies of HIV-1/HIV-2 dual infection in Côte d'Ivoire. Lancet. 1992;1:339–340.
24. Kaldor JM, ed. AIDS in Asia and the Pacific. 2nd ed. London: Rapid Science Publishers; 1998.
25. Brown T, Chan R, Mugrditchian D, et al, eds. Sexually transmitted diseases in Asia and the Pacific. Armidale, Australia, Venereology Publishing Inc.; 1998.
26. Des Jarlais DC, Friedman SR, Choopanyq K, et al. International epidemiology of HIV and AIDS among injecting drug users. AIDS. 1992;6:1053–1068.
27. Weinger BG, Limpakarnjanarat K, Ungchusok K, et al. The epidemiology of HIV infection and AIDS in Thailand. AIDS. 1991;5(Suppl 2):S71–S85.
28. Ou C-Y, Auwanet W, Pan C-P, et al. Wide distribution of two subtypes of HIV-1 in Thailand. AIDS Res Hum Retroviruses. 1992;8:1471–1472.
29. Anupong C, Werasit S, Brown T, Mugrditchian D. Thailand. In: Brown T, Chan R, Mugrditchian D, et al, eds. Sexually Transmitted Diseases in Asia and the Pacific. Armidale, Venereology Publishing Inc., 1998.
30. Nelson K, Celentano D, Eiumtrakol S, et al. Changes in sexual behaviour and a decline in HIV infection among young men in Thailand. N Engl J Med. 1996;335:297–303.
31. Wiput R, Hanenberg R. The 100% condom programme in Thailand. AIDS. 1996;10:1–7.
32. UNAIDS. Connecting lower HIV infection rates with changes in sexual behaviour in Thailand: Data collection and comparison. Geneva: UNAIDS Best Practice Collection, UNAIDS; 1998.
33. Hospedales J, White F, Gayle C, et al. Epidemiology of HIV/AIDS in the Caribbean. In: Lamptey P, White F, Figueroa JP, et al. eds. The Handbook for AIDS Prevention in the Caribbean. Research Triangle Park, NC: Family Health International; 1992:1–23.
34. Boletim Epidemiológico AIDS 1992. Brasilia: Programo Nacional de Doencas Sexualmente Transmissiveis/AIDS; 1992.
35. Mann J, Tarantola D, eds. AIDS in the World II. New York: Oxford University Press; 1996.
36. Parker RG, Tawil O. Bisexual behaviour and HIV transmission in Latin America. In: Tielman R, Carballo M, Hendriks A, eds. Bisexuality and HIV/AIDS. New York: Prometheus Press; 1991;59–63.
37. Pape J, Liautand B, Thomas F, et al. Characteristics of the acquired immunodeficiency syndrome (AIDS) in Haiti. N Engl J Med. 1983;309:945–950.
38. Bongaarts J, Reining P, Way P, et al. The relationship between male circumcision and HIV infection in African populations. AIDS. 1989;3:373–377.
39. Clemetson DBA, Moss GB, Willerford DM, et al. Detection of HIV DNA in cervical and vaginal secretions: Prevalence and correlates among women in Nairobi, Kenya. JAMA. 1993;269:2860–2864.
40. Wasserheit JN. Epidemiological synergy: Interrelationships between HIV infection and other STDs. Sex Transm Dis. 1992;19:61–77.
41. Laga M, Nzila N, Goeman J. The interrelationship of sexually transmitted diseases and HIV infection: Implications for the control of both epidemics in Africa. AIDS. 1991;5(Suppl 1):S55–S64.
42. Cameron DW, Simonsen JN, D'Costa LJ, et al. Female to male transmission of human immunodeficiency virus type 1: Risk factors for seroconversion in man. Lancet. 1989;2:401–407.
43. Grosskurth H, Mosha F, Todd J, et al. Impact of improved treatment of sexually transmitted diseases on HIV infection in rural Tanzania: Randomised controlled trial. Lancet. 1995;346:530–536.
44. Ghys P, Fransen K, Diallo MO, et al. The association between cervicovaginal HIV shedding, sexually transmitted diseases and immunosuppression in female sex workers in Abidjan, Côte d'Ivoire. AIDS. 1997;11:F85–F93.
45. Cohen MS, Hoffman IF, Royce R, et al. Reduction of concentration of HIV-1 in semen after treatment of urethritis: Implications for prevention of sexual transmission of HIV-1. Lancet. 1997;349:1863–1873.
46. The Working Group on Mother-to-Child Transmission of HIV. Rates of mother-to-child transmission of HIV-1 in Africa, America and Europe: Results from 13 perinatal studies. J Acquir Immune Defic Syndr 1995;8:506–510.
47. Wiktor SZ, Ekpini E, Nduati RW. Prevention of mother-to-child transmission of HIV-1 in Africa. In: Laga M, ed. AIDS in Africa, 2nd edition. London: Rapid Science Publishers; 1997:79–87.
48. Dunn DT, Newell ML, Ades AE, et al. Risk of human immunodeficiency virus type 1 transmission through breast feeding. Lancet. 1992;1:585–588.
49. Ekpini E, Wiktor SZ, Satten GA, et al. Late postnatal transmission of HIV-1 in Abidjan, Côte d'Ivoire. Lancet. 1997;349:1054–1059.
50. Van de Perre P, Simonon A, Msellati P, et al. Postnatal transmission of human immunodeficiency virus in infants born to seropositive mothers. N Engl J Med. 1991;325:593–599.
51. St Louis ME, Kamenga M, Brown C, et al. Risk for perinatal HIV-1 transmission according to maternal immunologic, virologic and placental factors. JAMA. 1993;269:2853–2859.
52. Ryder RW, Nsa W, Hassig SE, et al. Perinatal transmission of the human immunodeficiency virus type 1 to infants of seropositive women in The Democratic Republic of Congo. N Engl J Med. 1989;302:1637–1642.
53. Nduati RW, John GC, Richardson BA, et al. Human immunodeficiency virus type 1-infected cells in breast milk from HIV-1 infected women: Association with immunosuppression and vitamin A deficiency. J Infect Dis. 1995;172:1461–1468.
54. John GC, Nduati RW, Mbori ND, et al. Genital shedding of human immunodeficiency virus type 1 DNA during pregnancy: Association with immunosuppression, abnormal cervical or vaginal discharge, and severe vitamin A deficiency. J Infect Dis. 1997;175:57–62.
55. Semba RD, Miotti PG, Chiphangui JD, et al. Infant mortality and maternal vitamin

A deficiency during human immunodeficiency virus infection. Clin Infect Dis. 1995;21:966–972.
56. Choopanya K, Vanichseni S, Des Jarlais DC, et al. Risk factors and HIV seropositivity among injecting drug users in Bangkok. AIDS. 1991;5:1509–1513.
57. Colebunders R, Ryder R, Francis H, et al. Seroconversion rate, mortality and clinical manifestations associated with the receipt of a human immunodeficiency virus infected blood transfusion. J Infect Dis. 1991;164:450–456.
58. Gershy-Damet GM, Tarantola D. HIV screening of blood donations in sub-Saharan Africa, 1995. In: Laga M, ed. AIDS in Africa, 2nd ed. London: Rapid Science Publishers; 1997:94–95.
59. Jäger H, N'galy B, Perriëns J, et al. Prevention of transfusion-associated HIV transmission in Kinshasa, The Democratic Republic of Congo: HIV screening is not enough. AIDS. 1990;4:571–574.
60. Berkeley S. Parenteral transmission of HIV in Africa. AIDS. 1991;5(Suppl 1):S163–S168.
61. Lepage P, Van de Perre P. Nosocomial transmission of HIV in Africa: What tribute is paid to contaminated blood transfusions and medical injections? Infect Control Hosp Epidemiol. 1989;9:200–203.
62. Pokrovsky VV, Eramone EV. Nosocomial outbreak of HIV infection in Elista, USSR. Abstract WA 05. Fifth International Conference on AIDS, Montreal, June 1989.
63. Hersh BS, Popovici F, Apetrei RC, et al. Acquired immunodeficiency syndrome in Romania. Lancet. 1991;1:645–649.
64. Caraël M, Cleland J, Adeokun L. Overview and selected findings of sexual behaviour surveys. AIDS. 1991;5(Suppl 1):S65–S74.
65. Anderson RM, May RM. Transmission dynamics of HIV infection. Nature. 1987;26:137–142.
66. Caraël M, Buvé A, Awusabo-Asare K. The making of HIV epidemics: What are the driving forces? In: Laga M, ed. AIDS in Africa, 2nd ed. London: Rapid Science Publishers; 1997:23–32.
67. Boily MC, Anderson RM. Sexual contact patterns between men and women and the spread of HIV-1 in urban centres in Africa. IMA J Math Appl Med Biol. 1991;8:221–247.
68. Yorke JA, Heathcote HW, Nold A. Dynamics and control of the transmission of gonorrhoea. Sex Transm Dis. 1978;5:31–37.
69. Lamptey PR, Kamenga MC, Weir SS. Prevention of sexual transmission of HIV in sub-Saharan Africa: Lessons learned. In: Laga M, ed. AIDS in Africa, 2nd ed. London: Rapid Science Publishers; 1997:63–77.
70. Kamenga M, Ryder RW, Jingu M, et al. Evidence of marked sexual behaviour change associated with low HIV-1 seroconversion in 149 married couples with discordant HIV-1 status: Experiences at an HIV counselling centre in The Democratic Republic of Congo. AIDS 1991;5:61–67.
71. Trends in HIV incidence and prevalence: Natural course of the epidemic or results of behavioral change? Geneva: UNAIDS, 1999.
72. Moses S, Plummer FA, Ngugi E, et al. Controlling HIV in Africa: Effectiveness and cost of an intervention in a high-frequency STD transmitter core group. AIDS. 1991;5:407–411.
73. Laga M, Alary M, Nzila N, et al. Condom promotion and STD treatment, and declining incidence of HIV-1 infection in female Zairian sex workers. Lancet. 1994;344:2446–2448.
74. Levine WC, Revallo R, Kaune V, et al. Decline in sexually transmitted disease prevalence in female Bolivian sex workers: Impact of an HIV prevention project. AIDS. 1998;12:1899–1906.
75. UNAIDS. Expanding the global response to HIV/AIDS through focused action: Reducing risk and vulnerability. Definitions, rationale and pathways. Geneva: UNAIDS Best Practice Collection, UNAIDS; 1998.
76. Hunt CW. Migrant labor and sexually transmitted diseases: AIDS in Africa. J Health Soc Behav. 1989;30:353–373.
77. Larson A. Social context of HIV transmission in Africa: Historical and cultural bases of East and Central African sexual relations. Rev Infect Dis. 1989;11:71–73.
78. Louwagie J, McCutchan FE, Peeters M, et al. Comparison of *gag* genes from sixty one international HIV-1 isolates provides evidence for multiple genetic subgroups. AIDS. 1993;7:769–780.
79. Janssens W, Buvé A, Nbengason JN. The puzzle of subtypes in Africa. AIDS. 1997;11:705–712.
80. Dallabetta G, Laga M, Lamptey P, ed. Control of sexually transmitted diseases: A handbook for the design and management of programs. Arlington, Va: Family Health International; 1996.
81. Moses S, Manji F, Bradley JE, et al. Impact of user fees on attendance at a referral centre for sexually transmitted diseases in Kenya. Lancet. 1992;340:463–466.
82. Tawil O, Verster A, O'Reilly KR. Enabling approaches for HIV/AIDS prevention: Can we modify the environment and minimize the risk? AIDS. 1995;9:1299–1306.
83. World Bank. Confronting AIDS: Public priorities in a global epidemic. New York: Oxford University Press; 1997.
84. Grant AD, Djomand G, De Cock KM. Natural history and spectrum of disease in adults with HIV/AIDS in Africa. In: Laga M, ed. AIDS in Africa, 2nd ed. London: Rapid Science Publishers; 1997:43–54.
85. Anzala OA, Nagelkerke NJ, Bwayo JL, et al. Rapid progression to disease in African sex workers with human immunodeficiency virus type 1 infection. J Infect Dis. 1995;171:686–689.
86. Mulder DW, Nunn AJ, Wagner HU, et al. HIV-1 incidence and HIV-1 associated mortality in a rural Ugandan population cohort. AIDS. 1994;8:87–92.
87. Pape JW, Simone S, Ho J, et al. Effect of isoniazid prophylaxis on incidence of active tuberculosis and progression of HIV infection. Lancet. 1993;342:268–272.
88. Colebunders RL, Latif AS. Natural history and clinical presentation of HIV-1 infection in adults. AIDS. 1991;5(Suppl 1):S103–S112.
89. Lucas SB, Odida M, Wabinga H. The pathology of severe morbidity and mortality due to HIV infection in Africa. AIDS. 1991;5(Suppl 1):S143–S148.
90. Gilks CF, Brindle RJ, Otieno LS, et al. Life-threatening bacteremia in HIV-1 seropositive adults admitted to hospital in Nairobi, Kenya. Lancet. 1990;336:545–549.
91. Supparatpinyo K, Periens J, Nelson KE, Sirisanthana T. A controlled trial of itraconazole to prevent relapse of *Penicillium marneffei* infection in patients infected with the human immunodeficiency virus. N Engl J Med. 1998;339:1739–1743.
92. Colebunders R, Mann JM, Francis H, et al. Generalized pustular pruritic eruption in African patients with human immunodeficiency virus infection. AIDS. 1987;1:117–121.
93. Raviglione MC, Snider DE Jr, Kochi A. Global epidemiology of tuberculosis: Morbidity and mortality of a worldwide epidemic. JAMA. 1995;275:220–226.
94. De Cock KM, Soro B, Koulibaly IM, et al. Tuberculosis and HIV infection in sub-Saharan Africa. JAMA. 1992;268:1581–1587.
95. Mukadi Y, Perriëns JH, St Louis ME, et al. Spectrum of immunodeficiency in HIV-1 infected patients with pulmonary tuberculosis in The Democratic Republic of Congo. Lancet. 1993;342:143–146.
96. Lucas SB, Hounnou A, Peacock C, et al. The mortality and pathology of HIV infection in a West African city. AIDS. 1993;7:1569–1579.
97. The World Bank. World Development Report 1993: Investing in Health. New York: Oxford University Press; 1993.
98. De Cock KM, Barrere B, Diaby L, et al. AIDS: The leading cause of adult death in the West African city of Abidjan, Ivory Coast. Science. 1990;249:793–796.
99. Hassig SE, Perriens J, Baende E, et al. An analysis of the economic impact of HIV infection among patients at Mama Yemo Hospital, Kinshasa, The Democratic Republic of Congo. AIDS. 1990;4:883–887.
100. Viravoidy M, Obremsky S, Myers C. The Economic Impact of AIDS on Thailand. Working Paper No. 4. Cambridge, MA: Harvard School of Public Health, Department of Population and International Health; 1992.
101. Werasit S, Brown T, Obremskey S, et al. Projection of HIV/AIDS in Thailand and Social and Demographic Impacts. Paper presented at the Workshop on Population Programme Policies: New Directions, National Economic and Social Development Board, Chiang Mai, Thailand, September 11, 1992.
102. Whiteside A, Stover J. The demographic and economic impact of AIDS in Africa. In: Laga M, ed. AIDS in Africa, 2nd ed. London: Rapid Science Publishers; 1997:55–61.
103. Barnett T, Blaikie P. AIDS in Africa: Its Present and Future Impact. London: Bellhaven Press; 1992.
104. The World Bank. Tanzania: AIDS Assessment and Planning Study. Washington, DC: The World Bank; 1992.

Chapter 105

Epidemiology and Prevention of Acquired Immunodeficiency Syndrome and Human Immunodeficiency Virus Infection

CARLOS DEL RIO
JAMES W. CURRAN

Acquired immunodeficiency syndrome (AIDS) is the most severe manifestation of a clinical spectrum of illness caused by infection with human immunodeficiency virus (HIV). The syndrome is defined by the development of serious opportunistic infections, neoplasms, or other life-threatening manifestations resulting from progressive HIV-induced immunosuppression. AIDS was first recognized in mid-1981, when unusual clusters of *Pneumocystis carinii* pneumonia and Kaposi's sarcoma were reported in young, previously healthy homosexual men in New York City, Los Angeles, and San Francisco.[1, 2] The subsequent documentation of cases among persons with hemophilia, blood transfusion recipients, and heterosexual injecting drug users and their sex partners suggested that a transmissible agent was the primary cause of the immunologic defects characteristic of AIDS. In 1983, 2 years after the first reports of AIDS, a cytopathic retrovirus was isolated from persons with AIDS and associated conditions such as chronic lymphadenopathy. By 1985, serologic tests to detect evidence of infection with HIV had been developed and licensed.

Recent data suggest that HIV originated in Africa. Blood obtained in 1959 from an adult Bantu man in the Democratic Republic of Congo represents the oldest known case of HIV-1 infection in the world.[3] HIV infection has become a pandemic affecting every region of the world and is a major cause of morbidity and mortality, particularly among young adults. HIV is spread primarily through heterosexual contact, with women accounting for approximately half of new HIV infections in adults.[4] Even in many developed countries, where transmission through male homosexual contact predominated for the first decade, the number of persons infected through heterosexual contact and injecting drug use is increasing. In contrast, transmission through transfusion of blood and blood products has been virtually eliminated in countries that have systematically instituted HIV antibody screening of donated blood and plasma and heat treatment of clotting factors. The epidemiology of AIDS has been affected by the increasing use of antiretroviral therapies, particularly combination therapy with protease inhibitors, and other treatment strategies that have delayed the development of certain opportunistic conditions, such as *P. carinii* pneumonia, in infected persons. In comparison, the HIV epidemic has contributed to a marked and alarming increase in tuberculosis infection in the United States and other countries, which has been further complicated by the development of multidrug-resistant strains of *Mycobacterium tuberculosis*.

Now more than ever, control and prevention of HIV infection, whether on a global or an individual scale, must be grounded in an understanding of the changing epidemiology of HIV.

HIV AND AIDS SURVEILLANCE IN THE UNITED STATES

All 50 states, the District of Columbia, and all U.S. territories require reporting of AIDS cases to local health authorities, which in turn use a uniform surveillance case definition and case report form to report cases to the Centers for Disease Control and Prevention (CDC). Health department staff members actively survey case reports submitted from physicians, hospitals, and other medical care facilities and from record systems such as death certificates and tumor registries. Along with HIV serologic surveys and HIV infection reporting, the AIDS surveillance system serves as a major resource to monitor and anticipate trends in HIV morbidity.

The initial AIDS surveillance case definition, which was established soon after the first reports of unexplained illnesses associated with cellular immunodeficiency in homosexual or bisexual men, formally listed the opportunistic infections and neoplasms indicative of underlying immunosuppression.[5] In the absence of previously described causes of immunosuppression, a diagnosis of one of these conditions was defined as AIDS. The definition did not include the less severe manifestations of HIV infection and was designed to be highly specific and to provide a standard means to monitor trends of severe immunodeficiency caused by what was then an unknown agent.

One of the initial uses of AIDS surveillance was to search medical records and death certificates retrospectively for previously unrecognized or unreported cases of similar immunodeficiency. This review identified only 125 cases of AIDS diagnosed between 1977 and 1981 and provided evidence that the condition was a new disease in the United States. Although a few isolated cases compatible with AIDS have been retrospectively diagnosed from the 1950s and 1960s, the AIDS epidemic in the United States essentially began in the late 1970s.[6, 7]

The AIDS surveillance case definition was modified in 1985, in 1987, and again in 1993.[8–10] These revisions were made to reflect the development of serologic tests to detect HIV in 1985, the recognition of additional clinical illnesses associated with or directly caused by HIV infection, and changes in the clinical management of HIV-infected persons. Each revision to the AIDS surveillance case definition has subsequently resulted in a higher proportion of HIV-infected persons being defined as having AIDS.

The 1985 and 1987 revisions added several new diseases to the AIDS surveillance definition for persons with diagnosed HIV infection. The 1985 revision included disseminated histoplasmosis, chronic isosporiasis, and certain non-Hodgkin's lymphomas. After this revision, the number of AIDS cases reported increased by an estimated 3 to 4%.[11] The 1987 revision incorporated HIV encephalopathy, wasting syndrome, and other AIDS-indicator diseases that are diagnosed presumptively (i.e., without definitive laboratory evidence). As a result of this revision, an estimated additional 10 to 15% of HIV-infected persons became reportable as having AIDS, and AIDS cases increased by as much as 28% in some areas.[12, 13] The increase in AIDS case reporting resulting from these revisions was greatest for women, blacks, Hispanics, and injecting drug users.[12, 13]

In 1993, the AIDS surveillance definition was expanded to include HIV-infected adolescents and adults with severe immunosuppression ($<$200 CD4$^+$ T lymphocytes/μl or a CD4$^+$ T-lymphocyte percentage of total lymphocytes of less than 14), pulmonary tuberculosis, recurrent (i.e., two or more episodes in a 12-month period) bacterial pneumonia, and invasive cervical cancer (Table 105–1). The inclusion of measurements of CD4$^+$ T lymphocytes in the 1993 revised case definition was necessary because the results of this test had by then become an integral part of the clinical and therapeutic management of HIV-infected persons. Initiation of antiretroviral therapy was recommended for persons with CD4 T-lymphocyte counts of less than 500 cells/μl, and prophylaxis against *P. carinii* pneumonia was recommended for all persons with CD4 T-lymphocyte counts of less than 200 cells/μl.[14–17] These clinical interventions have delayed or prevented the development of previous AIDS-defining opportunistic illnesses in many HIV-infected patients, which in turn has directly affected the timeliness and representativeness of AIDS case reporting.[18] Inclusion of these immunologic criteria allows for

TABLE 105–1 Conditions Included in the 1993 AIDS Surveillance Case Definition

Condition
Bacterial infections, multiple or recurrent*
Candidiasis of bronchi, trachea, or lungs
Candidiasis, esophageal
Cervical cancer, invasive†
Coccidioidomycosis, disseminated or extrapulmonary
Cryptococcosis, extrapulmonary
Cryptosporidiosis, chronic intestinal (>1-mo duration)
Cytomegalovirus disease (other than liver, spleen, or nodes)
Cytomegalovirus retinitis (with loss of vision)
Encephalopathy, HIV related
Herpes simplex, chronic ulcer(s) (>1-mo duration); or bronchitis, pneumonitis, or esophagitis
Histoplasmosis, disseminated or extrapulmonary
Isoporiasis, chronic intestinal (>1-mo duration)
Kaposi's sarcoma
Lymphoid interstitial pneumonia and/or pulmonary lymphoid hyperplasia*
Lymphoma, Burkitt's (or equivalent term)
Lymphoma, immunoblastic (or equivalent term)
Lymphoma, primary, of brain
Mycobacterium avium-intracellulare complex or *Myobacterium kansasii*, disseminated or extrapulmonary
Mycobacterium tuberculosis, any site (pulmonary† or extrapulmonary)
Mycobacterium, other species or unidentified species, disseminated or extrapulmonary
Pneumocystis carinii pneumonia
Pneumonia, recurrent†
Progressive multifocal leukoencephalopathy
Salmonella septicemia, recurrent
Toxoplasmosis of brain
Wasting syndrome of HIV infection

*Children younger than 13 years.
†Added in the 1993 expansion of the AIDS surveillance case definition for adolescents and adults.

more accurate representation of the number of persons with severe HIV-related immunosuppression. The clinical conditions added to the 1993 surveillance case definition have been shown to be important health problems for HIV-infected persons. Persons coinfected with HIV and *M. tuberculosis* have a much greater likelihood of progression to clinical tuberculosis, and diagnosis and treatment may be more difficult in such patients than in non–HIV-infected persons.[19, 20] Other than the conditions in the 1987 surveillance definition, pneumonia is the leading cause of serious illness, hospitalization, and death in HIV-infected persons.[21–23] Cervical dysplasia, a precursor lesion that may progress to cervical cancer, is common among HIV-infected women and increases in severity as immunosuppression worsens.[24–26] The addition of invasive cervical cancer to the definition emphasizes the importance of gynecologic care for HIV-infected women and will allow for assessment of trends in the diagnosis of this condition as the number of HIV-infected women increases (see Chapter 113).

Evaluation studies have shown that AIDS surveillance has provided complete and timely information on diagnosed cases of AIDS. A national multicenter study published in 1992 used computerized medical records in six areas to determine that 92% of persons with AIDS-defining conditions were reported to local health departments.[27] Of these previously reported cases, 67% were reported to local health departments within 2 months of the date of diagnosis. Studies of state and local death certificate information and national vital statistics found that completeness of reporting of persons with AIDS ranged from 80 to 96% and that 70 to 90% of HIV-related deaths were reported to AIDS surveillance groups.[21, 22, 28] Completeness of reporting for AIDS has been comparable with or higher than that in other disease surveillance systems.[29, 30] In recent years, as a result of more effective treatments, diagnosis and treatment of HIV infection are more often confined to outpatient settings, which has traditionally been associated with less complete reporting.

Twenty-seven states require confidential reporting by name of persons with confirmed HIV infection, in addition to AIDS reporting.[31] HIV infection reporting in conjunction with HIV serosurveys is a useful adjunct to AIDS case surveillance and can assist efforts to plan, implement, and evaluate HIV prevention and medical intervention programs.[31–33] HIV infection reporting provides a minimum estimate of the number of persons known to be infected in a given area and also provides information regarding more recently infected persons than those reported with AIDS.[32] In states where HIV infection is a reportable condition, the number of persons reported with HIV infection is on average twice that of persons reported with AIDS. In addition, in line with more recent trends in HIV transmission, persons reported with HIV infection are more likely than those reported with AIDS to be women, adolescents, and racial and ethnic minorities.[32]

With the increasing effectiveness of antiretroviral therapy to modify the natural history of HIV infection and decrease mortality from AIDS,[34] case surveillance data will become less useful and it will be more appropriate to have a surveillance system that emphasizes HIV infection rather than AIDS case reporting.[35]

Concurrent with revision of the AIDS surveillance case definition in 1993, the CDC implemented a revised classification system for HIV-infected adolescents and adults.[10] The system reflected the evolving knowledge about the spectrum and progression of HIV infection and standards of medical care at the time for infected persons. The system is based on a combination of three ranges of CD4 T-lymphocyte counts and three clinical categories (Table 5–2). Dividing the continuum of HIV infection into mutually exclusive and descriptive categories serves many useful purposes, including increased awareness of the spectrum of clinical manifestations of HIV infection; facilitation of surveillance and reporting for AIDS and HIV infection; provision of information for designing, standardizing, and evaluating drug and vaccine trials and epidemiologic and natural history studies and for formulating health policy and strategy; and facilitation of scientific communication.[36–38] The public health orientation of the CDC's classification system is complemented by other proposed systems for classifying the natural history of HIV infection, including prognostic staging systems,[38–40] prognostic scoring indices,[41] and systems that can be adapted to settings throughout the world that lack testing for sophisticated laboratory markers.[37]

HIV INFECTION AND AIDS IN ADULTS

Incidence and Prevalence of AIDS in the United States

As of December 31, 1997, 534,532 adolescents and adults have been reported with AIDS in the United States.[42] Since 1981, when the first cases were reported,[1, 2] the number of persons with AIDS has increased rapidly. As a result of this rapid growth, the first 100,000 AIDS cases were reported during an 8-year period (1981–1989), whereas the second 100,000 cases were reported in just over 2 years (1989–1991).[43]

In the early 1990s, the number of persons reported with AIDS in the United States increased substantially, in part because of expansion of the surveillance definition for AIDS,[10] primarily the inclusion of markers of severe HIV-related immunosuppression. As a result of this expansion, the number of reported AIDS cases increased by more than 100% in 1993 versus 1992.[44] Because of improved survival of AIDS patients as a consequence of more effective therapies,[34, 45] the number of persons living with AIDS in the United States has also increased in recent years. In 1997 it was estimated that 260,000 persons in the United States were living with AIDS.

Serologic Monitoring of the HIV Epidemic

Because AIDS is the most advanced manifestation of HIV infection and the period between infection with HIV and the development of AIDS is long, surveillance systems for HIV infection are needed to supplement the information available through AIDS case surveillance. Various methods have been periodically used to estimate the prevalence and incidence of HIV infection over the course of the epidemic. The U.S. Public Health Service has estimated that approximately 650,000 to 900,000 U.S. residents are infected with HIV (0.3% of the U.S. population), with at least 41,000 new infections occurring annually.[46, 47]

HIV seroprevalence surveys describe patterns of current HIV infection. These surveys have been conducted on (1) specimens not linked to personal identifiers and collected for other purposes, (2) name-identified specimens, and (3) specimens collected from populations subject to routine or mandatory HIV screening, such as blood donors or military personnel. In general, the patterns of HIV transmission observed in these studies in the United States are similar to those observed through AIDS case surveillance—higher rates of HIV infection are found among men than women, among blacks and Hispanics than whites, and among persons 20 to 45 years old than persons in other age groups. The highest incidence remains among men who have sex with men; however, the absolute number of new infections is greater among heterosexuals. In addition, it is estimated that approximately 0.6% of men and 0.1% of women are infected in the United States. However, the prevalence is much higher for African Americans, in whom 2% of men and 0.6% of women are estimated to be infected.[47]

Homosexual and bisexual men remain a major population with an increased prevalence of HIV infection. Of surveys conducted primarily in sexually transmitted disease clinics in the early to mid-1980s, HIV seroprevalence rates in homosexual and bisexual men ranged from 10 to 70%, with most rates falling between 20 and 50%.[48] Although the highest rates were found in New York City and San Francisco, areas of high to moderate HIV seroprevalence are dispersed throughout the country.[48, 49] In 1997, a study of unlinked serologic specimens collected from homosexual/bisexual men attending sexually transmitted disease clinics in 17 cities had a median seroprevalence rate of 19.3%, with rates among black men approxi-

TABLE 105–2 1993 Revised Classification System for HIV Infection and Expanded AIDS Surveillance Case Definition for Adolescents and Adults*

	Clinical Categories		
	A	*B*	*C*†
CD4+ T-Cell Categories	*Asymptomatic, Acute (Primary) HIV, or PGL*	*Symptomatic, Not A or C Conditions*	*AIDS-Indicator Conditions*
1. ≥500/μl	A1	B1	C1
2. 200–499/μl	A2	B2	C2
3. <200/μl AIDS-indicator T-cell count*	A3	B3	C3

*Shading indicates conditions included in the 1993 AIDS surveillance case definitions for adolescents and adults.
†Clinical conditions in category C are listed in Table 105–1.
Abbreviation: PGL, Persistent generalized lymphadenopathy.
From Centers for Disease Control and Prevention. 1993 Revised classification system for HIV infection and expanded surveillance case definition for AIDS among adolescents and adults. MMWR Morb Mortal Wkly Rep. 1992;41(RR-17):1–19.

mately twice those of white men who had sex with men[50] (Fig. 105–1). Among homosexual and bisexual men attending sexually transmitted diseases clinics in the United States from 1988 to 1992, the overall HIV seroprevalence was 33% (range, 5 to 52%).[51] The HIV seroprevalence rate in this population decreased over time, especially among white homosexual and bisexual men, from 32% in 1989 to 22% in 1992, thus suggesting a decrease in HIV infection incidence.[52] The incidence of HIV infection among homosexual/bisexual men in some cohort studies dropped in the mid to late 1980s.[48, 53, 54] However, the prevalence of HIV infection remains high, and new infections continue to occur because not all men in this population have adopted or sustained safer sexual practices.[55, 56] Adolescent and young adult homosexual/bisexual men appear to be at particular risk for acquiring HIV.[56]

In contrast to the epidemic among homosexual/bisexual men, the epidemic among injecting drug users has been more concentrated geographically within the United States. Among injecting drug users, the initial HIV seroprevalence studies demonstrated very high rates of HIV infection in the Northeast and along the Atlantic coast of the United States and low rates on the western coast and in cities in other areas.[48, 57, 58] Although the highest rates of HIV infection continue to be observed in northeast cities, the rate of HIV infection among drug users in other cities has increased. Studies conducted in the late 1980s in Atlanta, Chicago, and Baltimore have shown HIV seroprevalence rates greater than 12%.[59–61] Surveys conducted in drug treatment centers in 1997 showed a median HIV seroprevalence rate of 14.8% (range 0 to 37.7%) among injecting drug users entering drug treatment programs[50] (Fig. 105–2). Similar findings have been noted in subsequent studies: HIV seroprevalence among injecting drug users admitted to drug treatment canters in Baltimore (25%) and Newark (24%) was high whereas it was low in San Francisco (7%), Seattle (5%), Denver (2%), and Detroit (1%).[62–64]

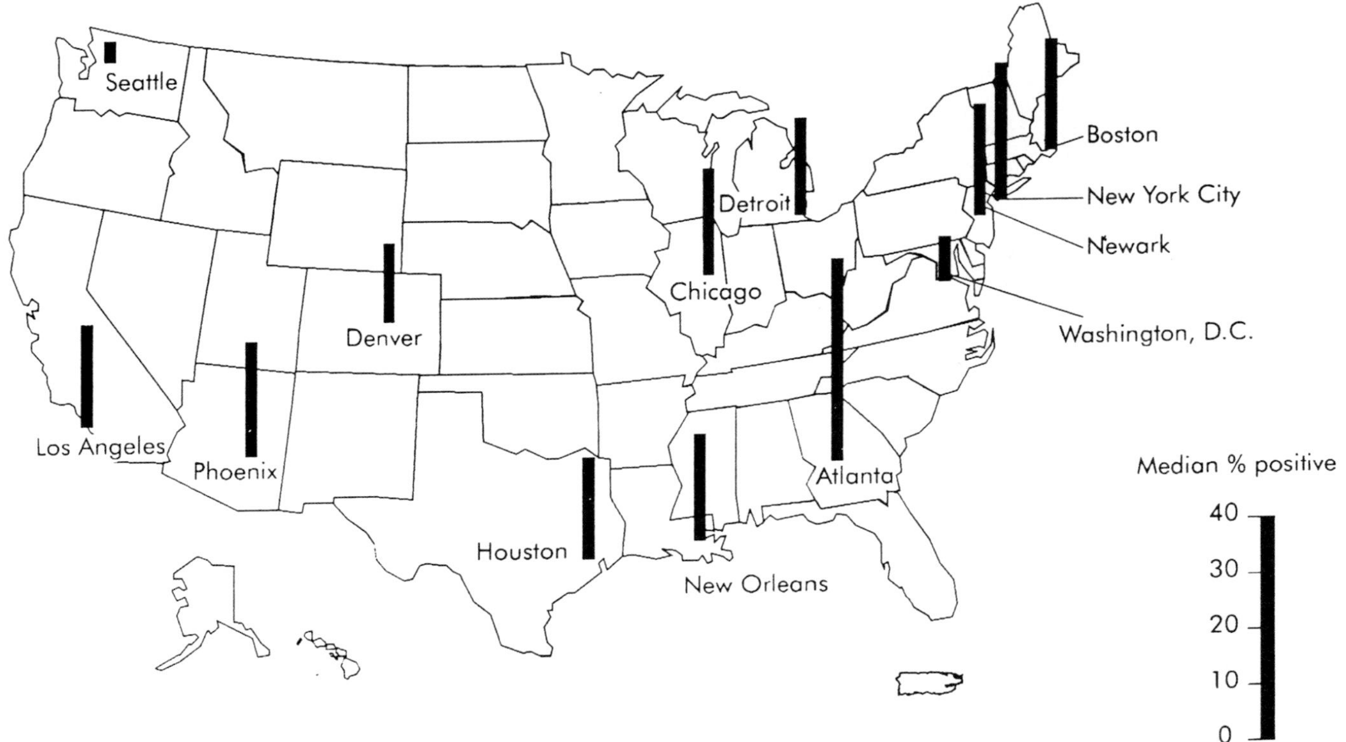

FIGURE 105–1. HIV seroprevalence in men having sex with men, sexually transmitted disease clinic surveys, 1997. (From Centers for Disease Control and Prevention [CDC]. National HIV Prevalence Surveys, 1997 Summary. Atlanta: Centers for Disease Control and Prevention; 1998:1–25.)

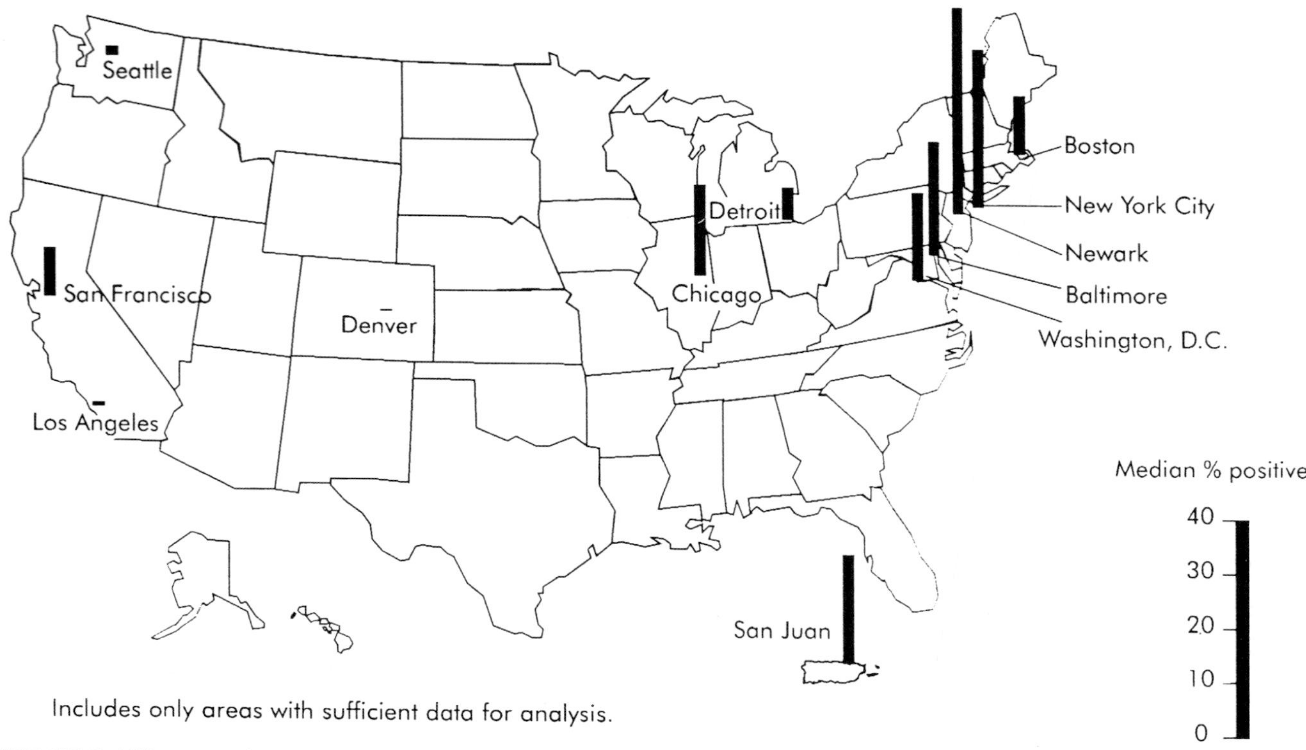

FIGURE 105–2. HIV seroprevalence in injecting drug users, drug treatment center surveys, 1997. (From Centers for Disease Control and Prevention [CDC]. National HIV Prevalence Surveys, 1997 Summary. Atlanta: Centers for Disease Control and Prevention; 1998:1–25.)

The reasons for the geographic differences in HIV seroprevalence among injecting drug users in the United States remain poorly understood inasmuch as cities with low prevalence rates have many injecting drug users who practice high-risk behaviors.[64] Studies in sexually transmitted disease clinics have also shown elevated rates of HIV infection among heterosexual injecting drug users in comparison to other heterosexual men and women.[51, 52] Although heroin injection is typically associated with parenteral transmission of HIV, injectors of cocaine and other drugs also have increased rates of HIV infection.[61–66] Cocaine injection, especially the use of "speedballs" (cocaine or amphetamines with heroin), injection in a "shooting gallery," and sexual risk behavior are associated with HIV infection among injecting drug users.[66, 67] Preliminary evidence suggests that HIV seroprevalence among injecting drug users in some cities such as New York may be decreasing.[68]

Some populations of heterosexual men and women who do not inject drugs also have appreciable rates of HIV infection. In 1988–1989, studies conducted in sexually transmitted disease clinics with heterosexual persons who do not inject drugs but have other sexually transmitted diseases found a median seroprevalence of 2.3% with a range of 0 to 14%.[52] Although men in these clinics typically had higher rates than women did, in some areas adolescent women had higher rates of HIV infection than adolescent men did. Nearly one third of persons infected heterosexually are estimated to have been infected as adolescents.[69]

HIV infection acquired through heterosexual contact is the source of an increasing number of AIDS cases. Of persons infected heterosexually, sexual contact with an injecting drug user is the most frequently reported risk. Accordingly, the geographic distribution of HIV rates among persons who acquired their infection through heterosexual contact and among injecting drug users is similar.[70] In addition, persons who use smokable forms of cocaine ("crack cocaine") and other noninjected illicit drugs have elevated risks for HIV infection as a result of exchanging sex for drugs or money and the presence of other sexually transmitted diseases.[67, 71–74] Some persons infected through heterosexual contact may not report a risk of HIV infection because they are unaware of the serostatus of their heterosexual partners.[42, 52, 71]

Female commercial sex workers (prostitutes) are at increased risk for HIV infection because of injecting drug use and multiple sex partners. In a 1987 multicenter study of prostitutes in various settings in selected cities, 65 (10%) of 670 women tested positive for HIV antibody.[75] Seroprevalence rates for HIV infection ranged from 0% for prescreened prostitutes in Nevada to 69% for prostitutes being treated for drug addiction in New Jersey. Among prostitutes who were studied, the major risk factor was injecting drug use. In a study in south Florida in 1987, 37 (41%) of 90 inner-city sex workers were HIV antibody positive, including 29 (46%) of 63 women who reported drug use and 8 (30%) of 27 women who denied using drugs.[76] From 1987 to 1991, the prevalence of HIV infection among female sex workers in south Florida remained relatively stable at approximately 24%. However, the incidence of HIV infection among female sex workers in this area who received multiple HIV tests increased from 0.3% per 100 person-years in 1987 to 15% in 1991.[77]

Surveys conducted in some clinical settings indicate that the HIV infection rate is higher than in a more representative sample of the general population.[78–80] In a 1989–1991 survey of persons admitted to 20 hospitals, an HIV seroprevalence of 4.7% (range, 0.2 to 14.2%) was observed; in one hospital, 24% of men 15 to 54 years old were infected with HIV.[78] Data from this survey were used to estimate that 225,000 HIV-infected persons were hospitalized in 1990; 72% of these persons were admitted for conditions other than HIV infection or AIDS. A 1990–1992 survey of patients seen in primary care practices revealed an HIV seroprevalence rate of 0.45%, with the seroprevalence among men (0.96%) being higher than the rate among women (0.22%).[79]

In many areas, persons with tuberculosis have high rates of HIV infection. Among 27 tuberculosis treatment clinics in 15 metropolitan areas surveyed between 1988 and 1995, HIV seroprevalence ranged from 0.6 to 42.9%, with a median rate of 8.9%.[80] The highest rates were found in the Northeast and in Atlantic coast areas and among U.S.-born persons 30 to 39 years old, who had a median seroprevalence of 30.1%. High rates were also noted among persons with extrapulmonary disease.

Studies of HIV seroprevalence in entrants to correctional facilities have indicated a wide range of rates, with the highest in areas with a moderate to high incidence of AIDS.[81] From 1991 to 1992, the median HIV seroprevalence was 2.9% (range, 0 to 15%) in 35 correctional facilities in 17 metropolitan areas.[60] Rates ranged from 1 to 12.5% for men and 0 to 24% for women, which is a reflection of the high rates of drug use in these persons. Among New York state prison entrants between 1987 and 1997, 12% of men and 18% of women were infected with HIV.[82]

HIV seroprevalence data are more available for large groups of persons who are tested for HIV infection on a routine basis. These groups include blood donors, applicants for military service, military personnel, and applicants to U.S. Department of Labor Job Corps training programs.[60, 83–90] These surveys are valuable but are limited in generalizability in that many persons at risk for HIV infection are excluded from some populations (e.g., potential blood donors and military applicants). Among U.S. blood donors, the level of HIV infection was 1.4 per 10,000 up to 1992.[83]

The overall prevalence of HIV infection among 2.3 million applicants for military service was 1.31 per 1000 between October 1985 and September 1989.[84] HIV infection rates in this population were higher for men (1.42/1000) than women (0.66/1000), for black non-Hispanic men (3.7/1000) than white men (0.61/1000), and for persons from large metropolitan areas, particularly those with higher rates of AIDS case reporting. The seroprevalence rate among teenage military applicants (0.34/1000) was lower than the median rate for all applicants; the male-to-female ratio was nearly 1 to 1 and the rate of infection among 17- and 18-year-old females exceeded that of same-age males.[85] Overall, the prevalence of HIV infection in applicants has decreased from approximately 0.15% in 1985 to 0.045% (1 positive for every 2200 applicants tested) in 1997.[50] Rates are particularly high for black male military applicants (0.15%). Because HIV-positive applicants and drug users are not accepted into the military, a self-selection bias among persons in high-risk categories may occur, and thus certain populations may be underrepresented among military applicants.[50]

Among U.S. Army active-duty personnel, approximately 220 new HIV infections are diagnosed each year,[86] with an HIV seroconversion rate of 0.39 per 1000 person-years.[89] The rate of seroconversion decreased from 0.49 per 1000 person-years in 1985–1987 to 0.29 per 1000 person-years in 1988–1989. However, a reduction in the seroconversion rate was not observed for black soldiers, thus suggesting a higher rate of continued transmission in this population.

Students who enter Job Corps training programs tend to be economically disadvantaged school-aged youths drawn from racial and ethnic minority communities in both rural and urban areas. For students aged 16 to 21 years who entered training from January 1990 through December 1996, 2.3 per 1000 were infected with HIV, a rate almost 10 times that seen among applicants for military service, with statewide prevalence rates ranging from 0.0 to 0.8% in 1997.[50, 90] Among Job Corps applicants, the infection rate increased with age. HIV prevalence was higher for women than for men (2.8 per 1000 versus 2.0 per 1000). HIV seroprevalence rates were highest for African American women (4.9 per 1000). From 1990 through 1996, HIV prevalence rates for women and men declined from 2.8 per 1000 in 1990 to 1.4 per 1000 in 1996. The highest rates were observed in students from large northeast urban centers and also among students from rural and smaller urban centers in the South.

Another type of broad population survey was the survey of childbearing women, which provided unbiased population-based estimates of HIV infection in women giving birth in the United States. HIV antibody prevalence for childbearing women was ascertained by blinded surveys conducted on residual blood samples collected on filter paper from newborns for routine metabolic screening such as that for phenylketonuria.[91] HIV seroprevalence among childbearing women remained stable nationwide from 1987 through 1994 at values ranging from 1.5 to 1.7 per 1000 women.[92] Seroprevalence decreased over this time in the Northeast and increased in the South. In 1994, HIV seroprevalence rates among African American childbearing women were 2 to 20 times higher than those among white women. The findings of seroprevalence studies of women seeking reproductive care services have also shown the highest HIV rates to be in clinics located along the Atlantic coast area and in Puerto Rico.[50, 93] If HIV seroprevalence rates among childbearing women were similar for all women of reproductive age in the United States, in 1994 approximately 84,000 women in this age group would have been infected with HIV.[91] The survey of childbearing women was halted in 1995 in light of Congressional concerns about blinded surveys in this population.

Exposure Categories

Since the first cases of AIDS were reported in 1981, cases in men who have sex with men and heterosexual injecting drug users have consistently represented the largest number of AIDS cases reported. The rate of growth in the total number of AIDS cases and in these two exposure categories was most rapid through 1986.[94, 95] In 1987, the rate of increase in AIDS reporting began to slow for homosexual/bisexual men, particularly in cities where AIDS was first recognized. This slowing in case reporting was related to several events, including the increasing use of therapies such as zidovudine and prophylaxis against *P. carinii* pneumonia, which delayed the development of AIDS-defining conditions; a decrease in the number of new HIV infections, which in part reflects the impact of prevention programs; and a decline in the completeness of reporting.[46, 53, 96, 97] As a result of this slowing in case reporting, the proportion of AIDS cases among homosexual/bisexual men decreased from 65 to 35% of the total cases reported from 1987 to 1997. In contrast, the proportion of cases reported among heterosexual drug users increased from 17% of all cases to 25% during the same time period.

Cases of AIDS among recipients of blood or blood components and among persons with hemophilia increased dramatically during the mid-1980s, but since 1987 the numbers have declined and these persons represented less than 1% of the AIDS cases reported in 1997. After implementation of HIV antibody testing in March 1985, no more than 5 cases of transfusion-associated HIV infection per year were reported to the CDC during the subsequent years as compared with 714 cases in 1984.[95] Since the initiation of HIV antibody screening of donated blood and plasma and heat treatment of clotting factors, transmission of HIV through blood and blood products has been reported only rarely.[98] Almost all cases of transfusion-associated AIDS diagnosed in 1991 with known transfusion dates were the result of transfusions received before 1986.[95]

Heterosexual contact cases consist of persons who report heterosexual exposure to a person with or at increased risk for HIV infection (e.g., an injecting drug user) or persons born in countries where heterosexual transmission is the major route of HIV infection (e.g., areas of sub-Saharan Africa and some Caribbean countries). AIDS cases associated with heterosexual contact have been increasing steadily and in 1997 represented 13% of all cases reported among adults. Since 1986, the annual percent increase in this group has been higher than that of any other exposure category and has been most striking for women. In 1992, the number of cases diagnosed among women infected through heterosexual contact exceeded the number infected through injecting drug use for the first time and represented 38% of cases among women reported in 1997.[22, 99] African Americans and Hispanics accounted for 75% of all persons reported with AIDS attributed to heterosexual contact.[100]

For AIDS cases reported in 1997, most of the source partners for persons with heterosexually acquired AIDS were injecting drug users (27%). However, this number could be larger because the risk of the partner was not specified for 65%. Persons with sex partners of unknown HIV infection or risk status are classified in the undetermined category (see later). Selected follow-up and investigation of heterosexual contact cases has identified other sources of exposure to HIV infection for some persons, especially men.[101] Nonetheless, it is unlikely that such misclassification bias has significantly influenced national trends.[94]

Of the 60,161 adults and adolescents with AIDS reported in 1997, 15% had two or more reported risk factors for infection. The largest overlaps occurred in men who reported both having sex with men and injecting drugs (7% of all cases). Except for this group, persons with more than one reported mode of exposure to HIV are counted only once in a hierarchy of exposure categories.[42]

In 1997, 22% of AIDS cases were reported with no history of exposure to HIV through any of the modes listed in the hierarchy of exposure categories. Most of these cases represent persons whose risk status is currently under investigation by local health department officials. Investigation of 90,837 cases of AIDS reported in adolescents and adults through December 1997 has thus far resulted in the reclassification of 41,391 (45.6%). Data from previous years indicate that when follow-up information is obtained, an established exposure mode can be identified for over 90% of these persons, and they are subsequently reclassified into the appropriate exposure category.[102] Although surveillance and investigation of cases with an undetermined risk can assist in detecting unusual modes of transmission (e.g., transplantation), such instances remain rare.[103]

AIDS Trends

The 1993 change in the AIDS case definition[10] dramatically changed AIDS incidence trends as a result of a large increase in reported AIDS cases. In 1993, the first year that the new case definition was used, 103,500 AIDS cases were reported to the CDC among persons 13 years or older as compared with 49,016 cases in 1992.[44] In 1994, 1995, and 1996, the number of AIDS cases reported annually decreased in contrast to the artificial peak in the number of cases reported in 1993. Since implementation of the revised case definition more than half of all cases are reported on the basis of a CD4 T-lymphocyte count less than 200 cells/μl. However, from 1995 to 1996, for the first time in the epidemic, the occurrence of AIDS-defining opportunistic illnesses and death among persons with AIDS decreased 7 and 25%, respectively.[44, 104] Reported AIDS incidence and deaths decreased again from 1996 to 1997 (Fig. 105–3). This decrease was largely due to the increasing use of combination antiretroviral therapy.[34]

Demographic Characteristics

Men accounted for 78% of AIDS cases reported in 1997, and AIDS case rates were much higher for men (44 per 100,000) than women (11.5 per 100,000) because of the large number of persons with AIDS among men who have had sex with other men (Table 105–3). However, the number of women reported with AIDS is increasing more rapidly than the number of men, and the proportion of total AIDS cases who are women has increased from 8% in 1988 to 22% in 1997.[31] Most of the increase in AIDS cases among women is due to heterosexual transmission of HIV.

Through December 1997, 63% of reported AIDS cases occurred in persons 20 to 39 years old. Persons who acquired their infections through transfusion of blood or blood products had the highest average age (53 years), similar to that of all transfusion recipients in the United States. Information from HIV infection reporting suggests that adolescents and young adults, particularly young black women, have a high rate of recently acquired infection.[32] Since 1991, 11% of AIDS cases have been reported among persons 50 years or older.[105]

In 1997, 53% of persons reported with AIDS were white, 47% were black non-Hispanic (40% of reported cases among men and 60% among women), and 21% were Hispanic (see Table 105–3). The rate of AIDS among blacks and Hispanics has increased disproportionately in comparison to whites[106]: the rate was approximately eight times greater for blacks and three times greater for Hispanics. Black women were 15 times and Hispanic women 10 times more likely to have AIDS than were white women. Cases reported among

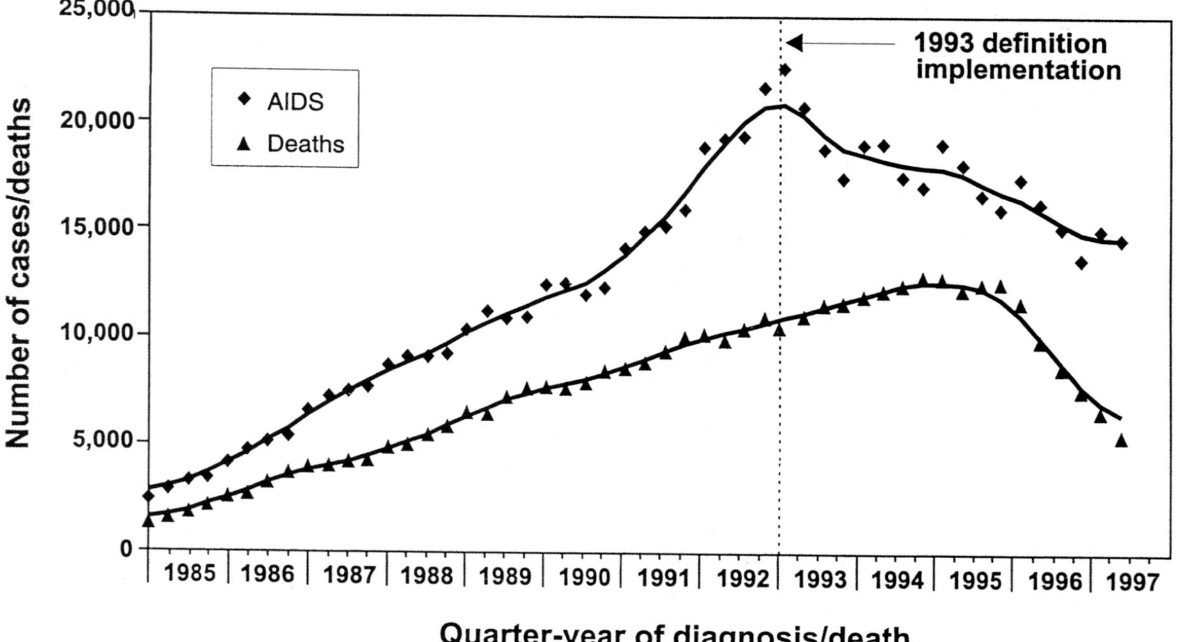

FIGURE 105–3. Estimated incidence of AIDS and deaths of persons with AIDS, adjusted for delays in reporting, by quarter-year of diagnosis/death, United States, January 1985 through June 1997. (From Centers for Disease Control and Prevention. HIV/AIDS Surveillance Report. 1997;9:39.)

TABLE 105–3 Characteristics of Persons Reported with AIDS and Rates by Year of Report, United States, 1995 and 1997

	1996		1997	
	Number (n = 69,151)	*Rate**	*Number (n = 60,634)*	*Rate**
Sex†				
Male	54,997 (79.5%)	51.9	47,312 (78%)	44.0
Female	14,154 (20.5%)	12.3	13,322 (22%)	11.5
Race/ethnicity				
White	26,327	13.5	20,197	10.4
Black	28,775	89.7	27,075	83.7
Hispanic	13,111	41.3	12,466	37.7
Asian/Pacific Islander	562	5.9	448	4.5
American Indian/Alaska Native	210	10.7	206	10.4

*Per 100,000 population extrapolating from the official 1980 and 1990 census counts (1996 census estimates published in U.S. Bureau of Census Publication PE-101PL-57 and 1997 census estimates published in U.S. Bureau of Census Publication PPL-91).
†Rates by sex are only for adult/adolescent cases of AIDS.
From Centers for Disease Control and Prevention. HIV/AIDS Surveillance Report. 1996;8:(2):1–39; and Centers for Disease Control and Prevention. HIV/AIDS Surveillance Report. 1997;9(2):1–43.

American Indians and Alaskan Natives have significant increased; however, only 206 cases (0.3% of the total) were reported in 1997 in these populations.

Hispanics with AIDS represent different countries of origin and cultures.[107] Among Hispanic AIDS cases reported in 1997, Puerto Rican–born Hispanics represented 27%. Puerto Ricans have been disportionately affected by the epidemic, and the rate of AIDS is highest for Hispanics in the Northeast and in Puerto Rico. Injecting drug use is the predominant exposure mode in Puerto Rican–born men and women with AIDS residing in either Puerto Rico or the U.S. mainland. The AIDS rate among Hispanics is lowest in the West. Hispanics with AIDS in this area are primarily from Mexico or Central and South America and are less likely to report a history of injecting drug use.

Geographic Distribution of AIDS Cases

The first cases of AIDS reported in the United States were clustered among homosexual/bisexual men and injecting drug users in the major metropolitan areas of the East and West coasts.[1, 2] Since then, AIDS cases have been reported from all 50 states, the District of Columbia, Puerto Rico, the Virgin Islands, and Guam. However, these cases are distributed unevenly across the United States.[31, 42] The populous northeastern states and metropolitan areas with greater than 1 million persons have the highest rates of AIDS. In 1997, AIDS incidence rates by state varied from 1.5 per 100,000 population in Wyoming to 233.3 per 100,000 population in the District of Columbia (Figs. 105–4 and 105–5).

The geographic distribution of AIDS is changing over time. Five states—New York, California, Florida, Texas, and New Jersey—have reported 57% of all AIDS cases. However, the proportion of cases from these states had decreased from 54% of the 50,316 cases reported before 1988 to 43% of the 60,634 cases reported in 1997 alone.[31] This change reflects a slowing in case reporting from these areas and a greater increase in the number of persons with AIDS reported from other areas of the United States. The southern region of the United States accounted for 34% of the cases reported through December 1997 and 37% of the cases reported that year alone.[108] In 1997, the rate of AIDS cases reported in metropolitan areas with a population of 500,000 or more was 29.3 per 100,000. In metropolitan areas with a population of 50,000 to 500,000, the rate was 13.2 per 100,000, whereas in nonmetropolitan areas it was 8.0 per 100,000 population. The cities with the highest AIDS rates per 100,000 population were New York (114.9), Jersey City (92.5), Miami (81.8), San Francisco (78), Newark (69.8), and Fort Lauderdale (69). Regional variations in AIDS case reporting reflect temporal differences in the introduction of HIV, the rate of new HIV infections over time, migration of HIV-infected persons, and local reporting practices.[96, 109]

The geographic trends observed in population-based HIV seroprevalence studies are similar to those for AIDS case reporting.[84, 86, 88–92]

The geographic distribution of persons with AIDS also varies by the reported mode of HIV transmission and reflects multiple epidemics among different populations in different regions of the country. Men who have sex with men represent a large percentage of AIDS cases in some states, although they are distributed throughout all regions of the United States.[110] Injecting drug use is the second most frequently reported risk behavior for HIV infection in states along the Atlantic coast of the United States. In 1995, 25,860 (35%) of the AIDS cases reported that year were associated with injecting drug use,[111] but this mode of transmission accounted for greater than 50% of the cases reported from Delaware, Connecticut, Maryland, Rhode Island, and Puerto Rico. Although the highest rates of AIDS associated with injecting drug use continue to occur in the Northeast, the rate there has slowed down and the number of cases in the South and West has increased at a faster rate.

All areas of the country have had an increase in the number of men and women with AIDS reportedly infected through heterosexual contact, but the largest increase in recent years has occurred in the South.

AIDS cases reported among persons infected with HIV through the receipt of blood or blood products correlates with the rate of all other AIDS cases.[112]

Clinical Manifestations of HIV Infection

Spectrum and Progression of HIV Infection

The spectrum of HIV infection ranges from an asymptomatic state to severe immunodeficiency and associated serious secondary infections, neoplasms, and other conditions.[23, 113] Initial or primary infection with HIV can be followed by an acute mononucleosis-like illness. Features of this acute illness associated with seroconversion include fever, lymphadenopathy, sweats, myalgia, arthralgia, rash, malaise, lethargy, sore throat, anorexia, nausea, vomiting, diarrhea, headache, photophobia, and mucocutaneous ulcers.[114, 115] Less common manifestations have also been reported, including a variety of neurologic conditions (e.g., aseptic meningitis, myelopathy, radiculopathy, peripheral neuropathy, and Guillain-Barré syndrome),[116] *Candida* esophagitis,[117] and mucocutaneous ulcerations (see Chapter 108).

Estimates of the frequency of symptoms among those with primary HIV infection range from 40 to 90%. The signs and symptoms of acute HIV infection are usually manifested days to weeks after exposure.[115, 118, 119] In a comprehensive review of primary HIV infection, the interval between exposure and symptomatic illness was reported to range on average between 2 and 4 weeks, with the duration of illness lasting from 1 to 2 weeks.[117] However, the diagno-

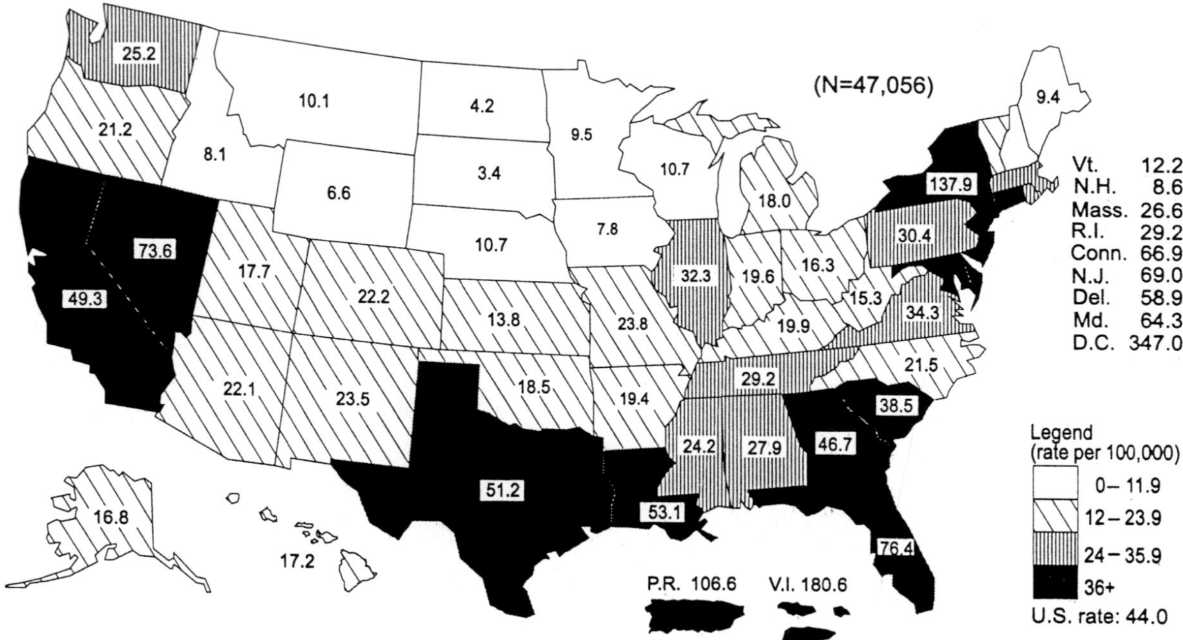

FIGURE 105–4. Male adolescent/adult AIDS annual rates per 100,000 population, for cases reported in 1997, United States. (From Centers for Disease Control and Prevention. HIV/AIDS Surveillance Report. 1997;9:39.)

sis of acute HIV infection is frequently missed. In a group of 23 persons at risk of HIV infection, 87% were symptomatic and 95% of them sought medical care, yet few had the correct diagnosis made at the first clinic visit.[114] Acute HIV infection should therefore be included in the correct setting in the differential diagnosis of any unexplained febrile illness.[115]

The diagnosis of acute HIV infection cannot be made with the standard serologic tests used to diagnose HIV infection because these tests detect antibodies and become positive approximately 3 weeks after the initial infection.[120] Studies of homosexual men,[121, 122] persons with hemophilia,[121, 123] and intravenous drug users[124] have consistently demonstrated the development of detectable HIV antibodies within 3 to 12 weeks after infection. Epidemiologic studies and case reports, as well as modeling techniques,[121] suggest that seroconversion beyond 6 months is very uncommon. Currently, the only test licensed for the detection of HIV infection before the presence of detectable antibodies is the p24 antigen test, now used routinely in the screening of blood donors.[125, 126] Detection of HIV genomic sequences by

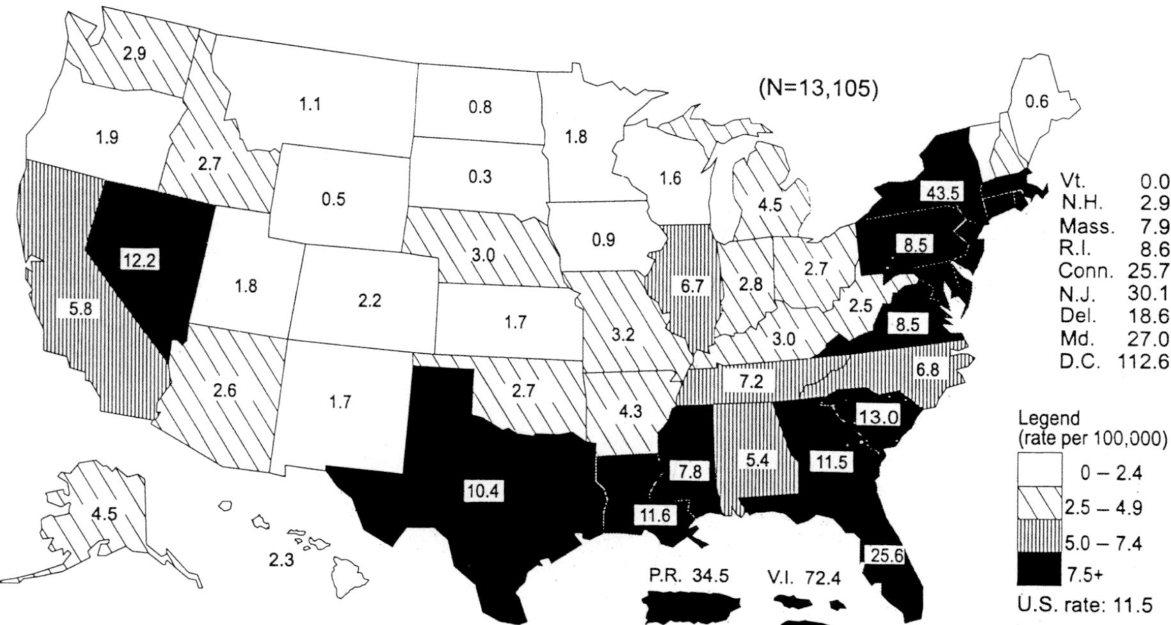

FIGURE 105–5. Female adult/adolescent AIDS annual rates per 100,000 population, for cases reported in 1997, United States. (From Centers for Disease Control and Prevention. HIV/AIDS Surveillance Report. 1997;9:39.)

polymerase chain reaction (PCR) has also been used for the diagnosis of acute HIV infection, but the test is not currently licensed for this diagnostic use.[115] However, the presence of viral p24 antigen or high-titer HIV RNA in a patient with a negative test for HIV-1 antibodies establishes the diagnosis of acute HIV infection (see Chapter 106).

Since 1989, cases of severe cellular immunodeficiency and associated opportunistic conditions in the absence of detectable HIV infection have been reported.[127] A provisional surveillance case definition was subsequently developed and based on the common feature of CD4+ T-lymphocyte depletion; this condition was termed *idiopathic CD4+ T lymphocytopenia.*[128] Extensive laboratory and epidemiologic investigations have determined that these cases do not represent occult HIV infection and do not appear to be etiologically linked, nor is there evidence to support a new transmissible agent.[129]

After primary infection with HIV, the risk for disease progression increases with the duration of infection. Most cohort studies that have evaluated the natural history of HIV infection have been conducted in the United States and Europe and show that AIDS develops in less than 5% of HIV-infected adults within 2 years of infection; without therapy, AIDS develops in approximately 20 to 25% within 6 years of infection and in 50% within 10 years.[130–133] Approximately 5 to 8% of HIV-infected individuals remain clinically asymptomatic with normal CD4 T-lymphocyte counts for more than 8 years after infection. These individuals are called "long-term nonprogressors."[134–136]

Differences in the rate of progression may be due to the route of infection, the size of the viral inoculum, the pathogenicity of the infecting viral strain, or the immunologic status of the host. For example, in one analysis of nearly 700 HIV-infected transfusion recipients, the estimated risk for the development of AIDS was 33% for persons within 5 years of infection and 49% within 7 years of infection.[137] Among recipients infected for similar periods, AIDS developed more rapidly in those who received blood from donors who progressed to AIDS soon after donation (50%) than in those who received blood from other HIV-infected donors (26%). In the same study, recipients in whom AIDS developed had received significantly more units of blood at the time of infection than did HIV-infected recipients without AIDS, which raises the possibility that the underlying clinical status leading to multiple transfusions, particularly the degree of immunosuppression, or exposure to other viral cofactors may also have affected disease progression.

The role of exogenous biologic and behavioral cofactors in the progression to AIDS remains uncertain. Coinfection with other viruses, use of tobacco, and injecting or recreational drug use have not been consistently associated with acceleration of HIV disease.[138–141] Several studies have suggested that the risk of development of AIDS increases significantly with age.[131, 141, 142] Pregnancy has not been shown to affect the progression of HIV infection.[143]

Because the natural history of HIV infection can vary considerably from person to person, clinical and laboratory predictors of progression are helpful. Oral candidiasis,[144] oral hairy leukoplakia,[145] and severe, recurrent herpes zoster[146] have been associated with an increased likelihood of development of AIDS. Measures of CD4+ T lymphocytes are the most specific laboratory markers of HIV-related immunosuppression and are strongly predictive of disease progression.[147] Recently, the quantity of HIV RNA present in serum or plasma (the "viral load") has been found to be the single best predictor of progression to AIDS and death among HIV-infected individuals.[148, 149] When both the viral load and CD4 T-cell count are combined, the prognosis is more accurately defined, and thus both parameters are important in the evaluation of HIV-infected persons.[150]

AIDS-Indicator Diseases

The relative frequency of individual AIDS-indicator diseases is most representative for those diseases diagnosed at the time of the initial case report to national AIDS surveillance because subsequent diagnoses are much less completely reported (Table 105–4).

Three clinical conditions accounted for more than three fourths of all initial AIDS-indicator conditions reported in 1992: *P. carinii* pneumonia (42%), HIV wasting syndrome (20%), and candidiasis of the esophagus (15%). The prevalence of several AIDS-indicator diseases was higher in men who have sex with men than in either heterosexual men or women. In general, the reported frequency of AIDS-indicator diseases is similar for men and women with similar modes of exposure to HIV. However, among injecting drug users, esophageal candidiasis, cytomegalovirus disease and retinitis, and herpes simplex virus disease have been reported more frequently for women than men.[151]

Because most AIDS-indicator infections result from the endogenous reactivation of previously acquired pathogens, the frequency of reported opportunistic infections probably reflects in part the geographic-specific prevalence of endemic infections. For example, toxoplasmosis and cryptococcosis are more likely to develop in African and Haitian patients.[152] Similarly, the risk of extrapulmonary tuberculosis among foreign-born persons with AIDS in the United States is highest in persons from Haiti, the Philippines, Central America, and Africa.[153] Among U.S.-born persons, those at increased risk for extrapulmonary tuberculosis include residents of the South and Northeast, blacks and Hispanics, and injecting drug users.[154]

Expansion of the surveillance case definition for AIDS in the United States in 1993 to include immunologic criteria (CD4 T-lymphocyte cell count less than 200/μl) caused a substantial distortion in the trend in the incidence of AIDS-defining diseases. Therefore, the CDC developed a procedure for estimating the incidence of AIDS-defining opportunistic infections among persons reported solely on the basis of immunologic criteria; this procedure allowed trends in the incidence of opportunistic infections in persons with AIDS to be estimated as though the case definition had not changed.[154] Changes in incidence and prevalence trends of AIDS-defining diseases between 1991 and 1996 demonstrated that for homosexual/bisexual men, significant decreasing trends occurred for 11 opportunistic infections, including *Mycobacterium avium-intracellulare* disease, *P. carinii* pneumonia, cytomegalovirus retinitis, Kaposi's sarcoma, esophageal candidiasis, cytomegalovirus disease, extrapulmonary cryptococcosis, toxoplasmic encephalitis, tuberculosis, herpes simplex, and disseminated histoplasmosis. In contrast, for injecting drug users, decreasing trends were seen for only five opportunistic infections (*P. carinii* pneumonia, esophageal candidiasis, tuberculosis, chronic herpes simplex, and chronic cryptosporidiosis), and an increase occurred for recurrent pneumonia.[155] The decreasing trend for some AIDS-defining opportunistic infections such as *P. carinii* pneumonia is probably related to the increasing use of antiretroviral therapy and prophylaxis against *P. carinii* pneumonia. For example, among adults and adolescents with a single AIDS-defining disease reported through 1996, the proportion with *P. carinii* pneumonia decreased from 50% in 1988 to 39% in 1996. Although declines were seen in all persons with AIDS during this period, it was most striking for homosexual/bisexual men and persons with hemophilia or a coagulation disorder. Differences in trends for homosexual/bisexual men and injecting drug users may reflect differences in socioeconomic status, access to medical care, or adherence to preventive medications. Increasing use of effective antiretroviral therapy, which began in 1995–1996, had caused, by the end of 1996, a dramatic decrease in the incidence of AIDS-defining opportunistic illnesses,[34, 156] and the incidence of AIDS could no longer be reliably estimated. The decline in AIDS-defining opportunistic illnesses that began in 1996 continued in 1997. Despite this trend, 23,527 AIDS-defining opportunistic illnesses were reported in 1997 among adolescents and adults, and *P. carinii* pneumonia continues to be the most common AIDS-defining infection.[31] With the increasing use of effective antiretroviral therapy, AIDS-defining illnesses are occurring mainly among persons with newly diagnosed HIV infection at the time of AIDS, among those known to be infected but who do not seek or receive care, and among those for whom treatment has failed.[157–160]

In 1993, three new AIDS-defining illnesses were added to the

TABLE 105–4 AIDS-Indicator Diseases in Adults/Adolescents and Children Reported in 1997, United States*

AIDS-Indicator Diseases	No. Adults/Adolescents (%) (n = 60,161)	No. Children (%) (n = 473)
Pneumocystis carinii pneumonia		
Definitive diagnosis	5763 (10)	77 (16)
Presumptive diagnosis	3382 (6)	44 (9)
Wasting syndrome	4212 (7)	73 (15)
Kaposi's sarcoma		
Definitive diagnosis	1088 (2)	—
Presumptive diagnosis	412 (1)	
Candidiasis, esophageal		
Definitive diagnosis	2057 (3)	30 (6)
Presumptive diagnosis	1255 (2)	20 (4)
Mycobacterium avium-intracellulare complex, extrapulmonary		
Definitive diagnosis	941 (2)	22 (5)
Presumptive diagnosis	183 (<1)	10 (2)
Cytomegalovirus disease	827 (1)	30 (6)
Cytomegalovirus, retinitis		
Definitive diagnosis	551 (1)	4 (1)
Presumptive diagnosis	260 (<1)	5 (1)
HIV encephalopathy	1196 (2)	108 (23)
Herpes simplex disease	1250 (2)	15 (3)
Cryptococcosis, extrapulmonary	1168 (2)	5 (1)
Toxoplasmosis of brain		
Definitive diagnosis	576 (1)	1 (<1)
Presumptive diagnosis	497 (1)	2 (<1)
Cryptosporidiosis, chronic	314 (1)	10 (2)
Lymphoma, immunoblastic	518 (1)	3 (1)
Candidiasis, pulmonary	534 (1)	11 (2)
Mycobacterium tuberculosis		
Extrapulmonary	491 (1)	2 (<1)
Pulmonary	1621 (3)	NA†
Mycobacterial disease, other, extrapulmonary	301 (1)	2 (<1)
Histoplasmosis, extrapulmonary	208 (<1)	1 (<1)
Lymphoma, Burkitt's	162 (<1)	2 (<1)
Progressive multifocal leukoencephalopathy	213 (<1)	1 (<1)
Lymphoma, brain, primary	170 (<1)	1 (<1)
Isosporiasis, chronic	100 (<1)	22 (5)
Coccidioidomycosis, extrapulmonary	74 (<1)	1 (<1)
Salmonella, septicemia	68 (<1)	NA†
Bacterial infections, multiple or recurrent	NA‡	84 (18)
Carcinoma, invasive cervical	144 (<1)	
	NA†	
Histoplasmosis, disseminated or extrapulmonary	208 (<1)	1 (<1)
Lymphoid interstitial pneumonia and/or pulmonary lymphoid hyperplasia	NA‡	80 (17)
Pneumonia, recurrent	1347 (2)	NA†
Immunosuppression, severe, HIV related§	36,634 (61)	NA†

*Percentages exceed 100% because some persons were reported with more than one AIDS-indicator disease.
‡Not applicable as indicator of AIDS in adults/adolescents.
†Not applicable as indicator of AIDS in children.
§Defined as a CD4 T-lymphocyte count of less than 200 cells/µl or a CD4 percentage less than 14 in adults/adolescents.
From Centers for Disease Control and Prevention. HIV/AIDS Surveillance Report. 1997;9(2):1–43.

surveillance case definition: recurrent bacterial pneumonia, invasive cervical carcinoma, and pulmonary tuberculosis.[10] Several studies have shown that persons with HIV-related immunosuppression are at increased risk of bacterial pneumonia,[23, 161] which can result in significant morbidity and mortality.[21, 22] One study among injecting drug users found that the annual incidence rate of bacterial pneumonia was five times higher in those who were infected with HIV than in those who were seronegative injecting drug users.[161] *Streptococcus pneumoniae* is the most commonly isolated bacterial pathogen and has been reported to precede the onset of other AIDS-defining conditions in 57 to 81% of persons with HIV infection.[162] In a population-based survey in San Francisco, the rate of pneumococcal bacteremia (89% of HIV-infected patients with bacteremia had pneumonia as a major clinical syndrome) among persons with AIDS was nearly 100 times higher than rates reported before the HIV epidemic.[163] The risk of pneumonia in HIV-infected patients is inversely related to their CD4 T-lymphocyte count[23] (see Chapter 109).

Precursor lesions to invasive cervical cancer such as cervical dysplasia, neoplasia, and genital papillomavirus infection are more commonly diagnosed in HIV-infected women than in other women.[24, 164] In a prospective clinic-based study of more than 500 women, HIV-infected women were nearly three times more likely to have colposcopy or biopsy-confirmed cervical intraepithelial neoplasia than were HIV-seronegative women.[165] This risk was independent of other potentially confounding factors such as sexual behavior. In this same study, although HIV-infected women had an increased prevalence (52%) of human papillomavirus when compared with uninfected women (22%), human papillomavirus infection was strongly associated with cervical intraepithelial neoplasia in both groups of women.[165, 166] The increased risk for human papillomavirus and the development of cervical intraepithelial neoplasia in HIV-infected women was related to the degree of HIV-related immunosuppression.[24, 166] Whether the increased frequency of these precursor conditions will translate into a significantly increased frequency of invasive cervical cancer is the subject of current study.

HIV Infection and Tuberculosis

After several decades of declining incidence, the number of new cases of tuberculosis in the United States began to increase in 1986.[167] Many factors contributed to the resurgence of tuberculosis, but the HIV/AIDS epidemic is, in large part, a major cause of these excess cases of tuberculosis.[168] It is estimated that 6000 to 9000 new cases of tuberculosis occur annually in the United States among

HIV-infected persons[169]; however, the full spectrum of the overlap between HIV and tuberculosis is not known, and more than 100,000 persons in the United States are thought to be coinfected with HIV and *M. tuberculosis.*[167, 168] Comparisons of AIDS and tuberculosis registries conducted by the 50 states and Puerto Rico revealed that 14% of persons with tuberculosis in 1993–1994 (27% among those 25 to 44 years old) also appeared in the AIDS registry.[170] The overlap in demographic and geographic characteristics of the two diseases is evident by surveys of HIV seroprevalence in tuberculosis clinics, as well as by the fact that 80% of persons with tuberculosis and AIDS were found in New York, California, Florida, Georgia, New Jersey, Illinois, and Texas. Both tuberculosis and HIV infection disproportionately affect racial/ethnic minorities and the urban poor.[167] In one analysis, black and Hispanic adults who died with AIDS were nearly three times more likely than whites to also have tuberculosis.[171]

HIV infection is a strong risk factor for the development of active tuberculosis in persons with latent *M. tuberculosis* infection. In a prospective study of injecting drug users with documented positive tuberculin skin tests, the observed incidence of active tuberculosis was 7.9 per 100 person-years for 49 HIV-infected persons versus no cases among 62 HIV-seronegative persons.[19] The risk of active tuberculosis in HIV-seropositive persons in this study—14% over 2 years[19]—contrasts strikingly with the estimated 10% lifetime risk in HIV-negative persons with latent tuberculosis infection.[172] In addition, HIV-infected persons are at increase risk for the development of active, symptomatic tuberculosis after their initial exposure and subsequent infection with *M. tuberculosis.*[173] Outbreaks of tuberculosis among HIV-infected individuals in correctional facilities, AIDS clinics, and hospital wards suggest that the development of active tuberculosis after exposure is greatly increased among HIV-infected persons. Finally, molecular epidemiology studies conducted in San Francisco and New York suggest that one third of cases in San Francisco and 40% in New York are due to recent transmission rather than reactivation.[174, 175]

Drug-resistant tuberculosis is more common in persons with HIV infection than in those with tuberculosis but without HIV infection.[170] In a multivariate analysis conducted by the CDC between 1993 and 1996, being infected with HIV was a risk factor for isoniazid and rifampin monoresitance, as well as multidrug-resistant tuberculosis.[176] In a study conducted in New York City, the proportion of isolates resistant to one or more antituberculosis drugs increased from 10% in 1982–1984 to 23% in 1991.[177] Among isolates of *M. tuberculosis* with primary resistance to isoniazid or rifampin, 75% came from patients known to be infected with HIV.[177] The increased risk of drug-resistant tuberculosis among HIV-infected persons may reflect a higher proportion of disease resulting from recently acquired drug-resistant strains,[174, 175] as well as other factors such as decreased absorption of oral antimycobacterial drugs among HIV-infected persons.[178] Outbreaks of multidrug-resistant tuberculosis (e.g., resistant to both isoniazid and rifampin and/or other drugs) have been characterized by (1) a high prevalence of HIV infection among the outbreak cases (range, 20 to 100%), (2) a high mortality rate among persons infected with resistant strains (range, 72 to 89%), (3) a short median interval between diagnosis and death (range, 4 to 16 weeks), and (4) nosocomial transmission to health care workers.[170, 179–181]

Mortality of Persons with HIV Infections and AIDS

Through December 31, 1997, 61% of the 633,000 adolescents and adults in whom AIDS had been diagnosed in the United States were reported to have died.[31] The estimated number of deaths among persons with AIDS increased steadily through 1995, when approximately 50,000 persons were estimated to have died of AIDS in the United States. In 1996, the estimated number of deaths from AIDS decreased to 37,525 and again dropped to 21,909 in 1997[31] (see Fig. 105–3). These declines in AIDS mortality have been more rapid among whites and among homosexual/bisexual men but have occurred in all populations.

In 1993, HIV infection became the most common cause of death among persons aged 25 to 44 years.[182] In 1994, 72% of HIV-related deaths occurred in persons aged 25 to 44 years, in whom it was the leading cause of death and accounted for 19% of the deaths in this age group. After 1996, when AIDS mortality began to decline, AIDS was no longer the leading cause of death in this age group.

To put in perspective the impact of AIDS-related mortality, the years of potential life lost before the age of 65 because of AIDS have been calculated.[183] From 1989 to 1990, the years of potential life lost before the age of 65 years that could be attributed to AIDS and HIV infection increased by 13%. In 1993, AIDS had become the fifth leading cause of years of potential life lost before age 65, and in 1994 it became the fourth. That year it was estimated that approximately 49,500 persons died of AIDS.[182]

AIDS IN CHILDREN

Through December 31, 1997, a total of 8086 cases of AIDS in children younger than 13 years had been reported in the United States.[31] Pediatric cases of AIDS include children who have one of a broad range of "indicator" diseases[10] (see Table 105–1). Although the spectrum of AIDS-defining opportunistic infections and malignancies in children overlaps considerably with those that are included in the surveillance case definition for adults and adolescents, some differences can be noted[184] (see Chapter 114). Three important exceptions for children younger than 13 years are the inclusion of lymphoid interstitial pneumonia and/or pulmonary lymphoid hyperplasia and recurrent bacterial infections and the exclusion of a threshold CD4 T-lymphocyte count (e.g., <200 $CD4^+$ T lymphocytes/μl). Longitudinal evaluations of lymphocyte subsets in both HIV-infected and HIV-uninfected children suggest some measure of prognostic value.[185, 186] However, because normal newborns and young infants have a prominent lymphocytosis,[187] moderate declines in $CD4^+$ T lymphocytes by adult standards can represent significant impairment in young children.[185, 188]

Pediatric cases are ordered into a hierarchy of mutually exclusive exposure categories,[31] and most children reported with AIDS acquired HIV infection perinatally from their mothers.[189] Of the 473 children reported in 1997, only 1 had hemophilia or another coagulation disorder; 91% were born to mothers either with or at risk for HIV infection; 2 received a transfusion of blood, blood components, or tissue; and 8% had an undetermined risk. Similar to adults, when follow-up information is available, most children who are initially reported with an undetermined risk are reclassified. In one study, half of the children who were reclassified had mothers who used injecting drugs or were partners of men who used injecting drugs.[190] Of the 432 children reported with AIDS in 1997 who were born to mothers with or at risk for HIV infection, 39% had mothers who reported injecting drugs or having sex with an injecting drug user. The remaining mothers acquired their infection through heterosexual contact with infected men other than injecting drug users (26%), received a transfusion of blood or blood components (2%), or had an undetermined risk for HIV infection (34%). Because most children acquire HIV infection from their mothers, the racial/ethnic and geographic distribution of children with AIDS parallels that of women with AIDS. Sixty-two percent of pediatric AIDS cases diagnosed in 1997 were African American and 23% were Hispanic. In addition to cases of AIDS, 258 cases of pediatric HIV infection have been reported from states with confidential HIV reporting. The exposure category and race/ethnicity of these cases parallel that of pediatric AIDS cases.

From 1984 through 1992, the estimated number of children with perinatally acquired AIDS diagnosed each year increased and peaked at 905 in 1992.[189] In 1994, as a result of a clinical trial that demonstrated the efficacy of zidovudine in reducing perinatal HIV transmission by two thirds,[191] the Public Health Service issued recommendations for the use of zidovudine and for counseling and HIV testing of pregnant women in the United States.[192, 193] With the implementation of these recommendations, the number of children with perinatally acquired HIV infection has decreased dramatically in the United States, with 432 cases diagnosed in 1997 (Fig. 105–6). The Northeast (44%) and the South (36%) account for most of the cases of perinatally acquired HIV infection.[194] For children in whom perinatally acquired AIDS is diagnosed when younger than 1 year the incidence has declined 39% from 8.4 to 5.1 per 100,000 live births.[194]

Among children reported with AIDS in 1996–1997, the most prevalent AIDS-indicator diseases reported were *P. carinii* pneumonia (24%), HIV encephalopathy (19%), lymphoid interstitial pneumonitis (19%), recurrent bacterial infections (19%), HIV wasting syndrome (15%), and *Candida* esophagitis (12%).

The relative frequency of certain AIDS-indicator diseases appears to vary with age. For example, lymphoid interstitial pneumonitis is more common in older children. Of children reported with AIDS in 1991–1992 in whom the syndrome was diagnosed before or at 12 months of age, 7% had lymphoid interstitial pneumonitis as compared with 36% of children in whom AIDS was diagnosed at 1 to 4 years of age. In contrast, in children in whom AIDS was diagnosed before or at 12 months of age, 58% had *P. carinii* pneumonia versus 14% of those aged 1 to 4 years. This early age at onset, as well as the high mortality rate associated with *P. carinii* pneumonia in infants and children, reinforces recommendations that HIV infection in infants should be diagnosed as soon as possible after birth so that prophylaxis can be promptly initiated when indicated.[195]

Overall, 58% of children with AIDS detected through national surveillance are reported to have died. Survival in HIV-infected children is closely related to age at the initial diagnosis of AIDS and to the specific AIDS-defining condition. The shortest duration of survival, ranging from 1 to 9 months, has been reported for children with an initial AIDS diagnosis of *P. carinii* pneumonia.[196–198] In contrast, longer median survival times ranging from 65 to 72 months have been reported for lymphoid interstitial pneumonitis.[196, 197] In a longitudinal evaluation of 789 children enrolled in the New York State Medicaid Programs, the proportion of children younger than 6 months at diagnosis who survived 1 year after AIDS was diagnosed (40 to 54%) was substantially less than that for children older than 6 months (70 to 85%), irrespective of the AIDS-indicator disease.[197] Similar to adults, effective antiretroviral treatment for children, *P. carinii* prophylaxis, and intravenous immunoglobulin have had a positive impact on survival by delaying disease progression. Implementation of recent recommendations by the Public Health Service for the treatment of HIV-infected women during pregnancy with combination antiretroviral therapy has undoubtedly had a positive impact in reducing perinatal HIV transmission and may further decrease the number of HIV-infected children born in this country every year.[198]

MODES OF TRANSMISSION

More than a decade after the initial studies were conducted to determine the ways in which HIV is transmitted, surveillance and epidemiologic data throughout the world continue to support strongly three primary modes of transmission: sexual contact; exposure to blood, largely through injecting drug use and transfusion; and perinatal transmission from infected mothers to their infants.

Sexual Transmission

Sexual contact is the predominant mode of HIV transmission throughout the world. However, the geographic distribution of cases attributable to homosexual and heterosexual transmission varies markedly.[199] Whereas heterosexual transmission is the major mode of spread of HIV infection in Africa, most of South America, and the Caribbean, it accounts for a smaller, albeit growing proportion of AIDS cases in North America and Europe, where male-to-male sexual transmission continues to account for a major proportion of reported cases of AIDS.[200]

The likelihood of acquiring or transmitting HIV infection through a single sexual contact is directly related to certain correlates of exposure, such as the number of partners and the prevalence of HIV

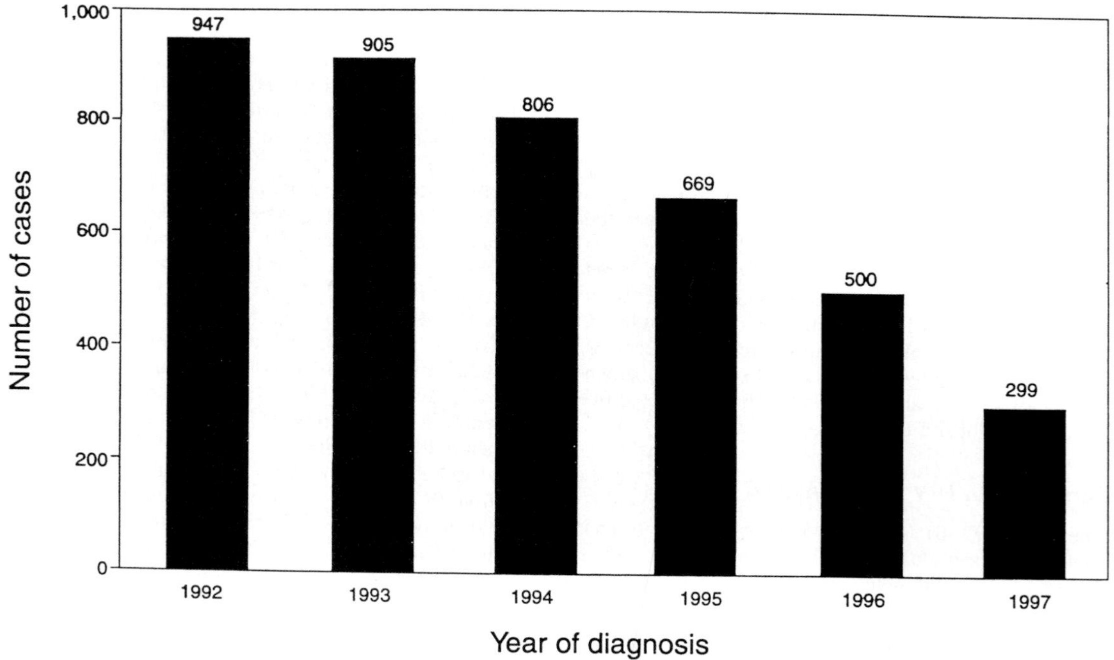

FIGURE 105–6. Estimated pediatric AIDS incidence by year of diagnosis, 1992 through 1997, United States. These numbers do not represent actual cases of children diagnosed with AIDS. Rather, these numbers are point estimates based on cases diagnosed using the 1987 definition, adjusted for reporting delays. The 1993 AIDS surveillance case definition affected only the adult/adolescent cases, not pediatric cases. (From Centers for Disease Control and Prevention. HIV/AIDS Surveillance Report 1998;10:1–40.)

infection in the population. Sexual transmission of HIV is relatively inefficient, but behavioral and biologic factors influence the likelihood of HIV transmission in a given sexual encounter. For example, anal sex has been consistently found to be more risky that vaginal sex, which in turn is higher risk than oral sex,[201] and the coexistence of a sexually transmitted infection (most notably the presence of genital ulcerative disease) greatly increase the infectiousness as well as the susceptibility of the individual.[202, 203]

Infectiousness of the Source Partner

Variability in the infectiousness of the source partner has been suggested by observations that some persons appear to be highly efficient transmitters of HIV through sexual contact. Such efficiency is manifested by the infection of a high proportion of an individual's sexual partners,[204] often after only a single contact.[205, 206]

Multiple lines of evidence indicate that HIV transmission appears to be more efficient late in the course of HIV infection.[207–211] This association was first suggested in a prospective study of infected hemophilic men and their female sex partners.[208] Subsequent epidemiologic studies have supported the correlation of advanced disease stage, as measured by diseases indicative of AIDS or decreased numbers of peripheral CD4+ T lymphocytes, with an increased likelihood of transmission to sexual partners.[209–212] Furthermore, this association has been observed for male-to-male, male-to-female, and female-to-male transmission. These observations correlate well with laboratory studies demonstrating that both the ability to isolate HIV from semen and the concentration of virus in plasma are inversely proportional to the number of CD4+ T-lymphocyte.[213–215] In another study, HIV was isolated more frequently from the cervicovaginal secretions of women with AIDS than from those of women in earlier stages of disease.[216] In addition, primary HIV infection may also be a period associated with increased infectiousness.[217] From a public health point of view, this association could be extremely important because increased infectivity would precede recognition of infection by the individual. With the availability of assays that allow measurement of the quantity of HIV present in plasma, blood, or genital secretions, it is now possible to attempt to correlate infectiousness with the quantity of HIV RNA present in genital secretions. In general, HIV is more readily detected and also present at higher concentrations in individuals with more advanced disease[218]; however, this correlation is not found in all studies.[216, 219] These findings notwithstanding, all infected persons must be presumed to be capable of sexually transmitting HIV, regardless of their stage of infection.

Antiretroviral therapy may influence infectivity and the subsequent risk of transmission through sexual contact. Treatment with zidovudine alone has been associated with decreased detection of HIV in semen,[214] and an epidemiologic study has demonstrated that antiretroviral therapy was associated with a 50% reduction in sexual transmission of HIV among discordant heterosexual couples.[220] However, even with the use of combination antiretroviral therapy and in the presence of suppression of HIV RNA in plasma, proviral DNA has been detected in the seminal cells of infected men[221] and genital secretions of women.[222] Thus, any protective effect of antiretrovirals on sexual transmission of HIV is likely to be partial and not render an individual completely noninfectious.[223, 224]

Because HIV is present in both blood cells and cervicovaginal secretions, sexual contact with an HIV-infected woman during menstruation somewhat increases the risk of female-to-male HIV transmission,[209] as well as the woman's risk of acquiring HIV infection.[210] Nonmenstrual vaginal and penile bleeding have also been reported to be associated with HIV transmission.[225, 226]

The probability of saliva from HIV-infected persons transmitting HIV through oral-oral or oral-genital sexual contact is probably low but real.[227] HIV is found in very low concentrations in the saliva of infected persons,[228, 229] and since 1987, 21 case reports of 42 potential instances of oral transmission of HIV have appeared.[227] Such transmissions are difficult to prove or rule out because most persons with HIV and a history of oral sexual contact report genital contact as well.

Epidemiologic and laboratory data indicate that genital ulcer disease in the source partner is an important factor facilitating HIV transmission. The higher rates of heterosexual transmission in Africa may be explained in part by the higher prevalence of genital ulcer disease and other sexually transmitted infections in many developing countries, including Africa, than in countries in North America and Europe.[230] Genital ulcers probably increase the infectiousness of both male and female source partners.[231, 232] In a prospective study of over 400 men who acquired a sexually transmitted disease (including HIV infection) from a group of prostitutes in Nairobi, Kenya, seroconversion to HIV was independently associated with the concurrent acquisition of genital ulcer disease.[233] Genital ulcer disease may have augmented the women's infectiousness by increasing viral shedding in the female genital tract through a local inflammatory response mediated by the recruitment and activation of HIV-infected macrophages and lymphocytes to the disrupted mucosal surface.[233, 234] The recovery of HIV from genital ulcers in HIV-infected women supports this hypothesis.[235]

Nonulcerative sexually transmitted diseases may also enhance sexual transmission of HIV. Among men, urethritis and gonorrhea are associated with increased detection of HIV in semen,[236, 237] and appropriate antibiotic treatment diminishes the amount of HIV present in genital secretions.

Susceptibility of the Recipient Partner

As previously mentioned, the presence of genital and anorectal ulceration or mucosal disruption secondary to infection has emerged as one of the most consistent and biologically plausible factors affecting the transmission and acquisition of HIV infection through sexual contact. Although ulcerations that disrupt the genital epithelium can serve simply as a portal of entry for HIV, ulcerations may have a more complex role in HIV transmission. Genital ulcerations cause an inflammatory response that in turn may increase the number of stimulated T lymphocytes at the surface of the ulceration and thus increase the number of susceptible cells.[234]

A number of epidemiologic studies have demonstrated that a history of genital ulcer disease in the recipient partner is a risk factor for acquiring HIV in both heterosexual and homosexual men[234, 238] and women.[232, 238] Although this association may not be surprising, two seroepidemiologic studies of homosexual men have convincingly demonstrated that genital ulcer disease is not simply a marker for increased sexual activity.[234, 239] Rather, infection with HIV was independently associated with serologic evidence of prior syphilis or infection with herpes simplex virus type 2, the two most common causes of genital ulcers among homosexual men in the United States. In another study among female prostitutes in Nairobi, 60% of seroconverting women experienced one or more episodes of genital ulcers before seroconverting.[232]

Nonulcerative sexually transmitted diseases such as gonorrhea and chlamydial infection also facilitate the acquisition of HIV infection by causing mucosal disruption of the genital tract.[232] Other nonulcerative sexually transmitted diseases (e.g., urethritis, cervicitis, balanitis, bacterial vaginosis, and genital warts) also increase the risk of acquiring HIV infection.[240–242] The higher frequency of balanitis in uncircumcised men has been postulated as a partial explanation for the increased risk of HIV observed among uncircumcised men in developing countries.[233, 243, 244]

Noninfectious causes of ulcerations of the genital tract may also pose a risk for sexual transmission of HIV. For example, frequent use of the nonoxynol 9 contraceptive sponge by female prostitutes in Nairobi was associated with increased rates of genital ulcers, vulvitis, and HIV seroconversion in one study.[245] The increased risk for HIV acquisition may be attributable to chemical irritation from the spermicide or to mechanical trauma, both of which can result in inflammation and ulceration.[246] The importance of the treatment of sexually transmitted infections in the HIV epidemic was made evident by a study in Tanzania that showed that prompt management of sexually transmitted infections decreased the incidence of HIV infection by 42%.[247] Certain traumatic sexual practices that result in rectal mucosal disruption and lesions have been associated with HIV infection. Early epidemiologic studies of homosexual men found that receptive anal intercourse, "fisting," and douching increased the risk of HIV transmission.[248–250] Subsequent studies have both supported these findings and extended the association of receptive anal intercourse to heterosexual transmission of HIV.[209, 218, 226]

Although cases of AIDS have been reported among lesbian and bisexual women, most were infected through injecting drug use practices.[251] Female-to-female transmission of HIV appears to be very rare.[252] However, at least four such instances have been reported.[253–255]

No consistent association between oral contraceptive use by women and acquisition of HIV infection has been found. In one study, women who reported taking oral contraceptives had a reduced risk of HIV infection.[210] However, in a longitudinal cohort study of Nairobi prostitutes and a cross-sectional study of sex partners at a sexually transmitted disease clinic in Nairobi, oral contraceptive use was an independent risk factor for HIV seroconversion and for prevalent infection, respectively.[232, 256] In contrast, a study of prostitutes in Zaire[238] and a study of pregnant women in a rural U.S. community with a high prevalence of HIV infection[72] found no association between HIV infection and the use of oral contraceptives. The presence of cervical ectopy has been associated with an increased risk of HIV seropositivity among long-term female partners of HIV-positive men in Nairobi.[256] Because oral contraceptives are associated with higher rates of ectopy, the relationship, if any, between oral contraceptives and HIV requires further study.

Although anal and vaginal intercourse are the two sex practices associated with the greatest risk of transmission, other sexual activities involving exposure to semen or blood also carry a potential risk of transmission. For example, seroconversion for HIV antibody has been documented after receptive oral intercourse with ejaculation.[227]

Finally, a mutation in the chemokine receptor gene has recently been identified that may render the rare homozygous host relatively resistant to HIV infection (see Chapter 157). When this mutation is present in the heterozygous state, it does not prevent infection.[257] The presence of this mutation varies according to race, with 11% and 1.7% homozygosity among whites and African Americans, respectively.[217]

Transmission through Injecting Drug Use

Among injecting drug users, HIV is transmitted by parenteral exposure to HIV-infected blood through the use of contaminated needles and other injection equipment. Specific factors that have been associated with HIV infection among injecting drug users include the duration of injecting drug use since 1977, frequency of needle sharing, number of needle-sharing partners, number of injections, median number of injections in "shooting galleries," and prevalence of HIV infection in the area of residence.[48, 58, 258, 259] The rate of HIV infection among injecting drug users varies widely among different geographic areas. In the United States, the rate of HIV infection has been highest in the Northeast.[61, 63]

Most studies have found higher rates of HIV infection associated with cocaine and heroin injection than with heroin injection alone, probably because of the greater frequency of cocaine injections.[65, 260, 261] Among injecting drug users, poor socioeconomic conditions, homelessness, and minority race/ethnicity are associated with an increased frequency of risk behavior and higher rates of HIV infection.[50, 67, 262, 263] Among injecting drug users enrolled in a study in Baltimore from 1988 to 1989, the 703 HIV-infected users were more likely to have a history of syphilis (16.8%) than were the 2218 uninfected injecting drug users (11.3%).[264] The higher rates of sexually transmitted disease among HIV-infected injecting drug users than among uninfected users suggests that some infections are transmitted through unsafe sexual practices.[264, 265]

Many injecting drug users have changed their drug use behavior to reduce their risk of HIV infection.[266, 267] Drug abuse treatment, street outreach programs, needle and syringe exchange programs, AIDS educational efforts, and HIV counseling and testing programs have all been shown to be effective in reducing, but not eliminating the risk of HIV transmission in these population.[268]

Transmission by Blood and Other Tissues

Recipients of unscreened blood or blood products from HIV-infected donors are at high risk for HIV infection. HIV has been transmitted through receipt of whole blood, blood cellular components, plasma, and clotting factors.[269, 270] The likelihood of a person becoming infected with HIV after receiving a single-donor blood product documented to be HIV positive approaches 100%.[271, 272] Other blood or plasma products, such as hepatitis B immune globulin, immune serum globulin, Rh(D) immune globulin, and hepatitis B vaccine, are prepared by using one of several fractionation processes that inactivate HIV; use of these products has not been associated with transmission.[273, 274]

Before serologic testing for HIV was begun in 1985, 0.04% of 1,200,000 donations in the United States were estimated to be HIV positive.[275] During this time an estimated 29,000 blood or blood product recipients were exposed to HIV; because many died of underlying conditions, 12,000 of these persons were estimated to survive long enough for AIDS to develop.[276] Confidential unit exclusion and direct donor deferral, as well as the institution of HIV antibody screening in 1985, followed by additional tests for antibodies to HIV-2 and p24 antigen in 1996, have markedly decreased the risk of HIV infection through blood or blood products. Currently, the risk of HIV transmission through transfusion of screened blood has been estimated to be 1 in 200,000 to 1 in 2,000,000 per unit transfused in the United States.[277, 278] The risk of HIV infection for patients with hemophilia who received concentrated clotting factors composed of blood components from potentially thousands of donors was substantial before 1984–1985,[279, 280] but now it is quite low. HIV transmission by transplantation of liver, heart, kidney, pancreas, bone, and possibly skin has been reported.[103, 281, 282] Relatively avascular tissues such as corneas and processed tissues have not been associated with transmission.[103, 283, 284] AIDS developed in several transplant recipients after receiving a variety of organs from a single HIV-negative cadaver donor. The donor was subsequently found to be HIV infected by culture and PCR.[103]

Perinatal Transmission

Vertical transmission of HIV from an infected woman to her infant can occur during gestation (in utero), at the time of delivery (intrapartum), or postpartum through breast-feeding. Significant progress has been made in elucidating risk factors that influence transmission during these three periods, in detecting infection in the newborn earlier and more reliably, and in the prevention of perinatal transmission with the use of antiretroviral drugs (see Chapter 113).

The occurrence of intrauterine infection is supported by the detection of HIV both in fetal tissue as early as 8 weeks' gestation[285] and in placental tissue infected in vivo and in vitro.[286] In addition, the 30 to 50% of infected infants who test positive by PCR or HIV culture at birth[287–289] also suggests intrauterine transmission of HIV. The proportion of infants who become infected in each trimester of pregnancy is unknown, but transmission to the infant early in pregnancy would presumably allow for viral replication to reach a level sufficient for detection by culture or PCR.[290] HIV-infected infants who test negative by PCR or HIV culture at birth may have become infected late in pregnancy or during the intrapartum period. Accumulating information suggests that a sizable proportion of vertical transmission may occur during the intrapartum period.[291, 292] Both vaginal and cesarean delivery present frequent and varied opportunities for the infant to be exposed to infected maternal blood and cervicovaginal fluids. Although many studies have found statistically similar rates of transmission for vaginal and cesarean section delivery,[293–296] a recent meta-analysis found that elective cesarean section reduces the risk of perinatal HIV transmission even when accounting for the use of antiretrovirals.[297] The isolation of HIV from breast milk,[298] as well as reports of breast-feeding mothers who infected their infants after they had acquired HIV infection through postpartum blood transfusions, provided initial evidence for postnatal HIV transmission.[299] Subsequent evaluation has focused on estimating the added, or attributable, risk of perinatal transmission conveyed by breast-feeding. Several prospective cohort studies that compared breast-fed and bottle-fed infants have detected higher rates of HIV infection in breast-fed children.[292–294, 300, 301] The attributable risk of transmission through breast-feeding ranges from 14 to 29% and was determined on the basis of data from developing countries where antiretroviral therapy has not been used.[302] Mothers who themselves acquired HIV infection in the postpartum period were more efficient transmitters, presumably because of the increased viral burden associated with primary HIV infection.[303, 304] For these reasons, it has been recommended since 1985 in the United States that HIV-infected women abstain from breast-feeding their infants. Epidemiologic studies[301] and mathematic models[305] have evaluated the competing risks of acquiring HIV infection by breast-feeding and the increased morbidity and mortality associated with alternatives to breast-feeding in developing countries. Both approaches have found that for children in many developing countries, the benefits from breast-feeding outweigh the risk of HIV transmission through breast-feeding. However, the risk of "not breast-feeding" varies greatly between and within developing countries, and thus the situation needs to be considered on an individual basis.

Prospective studies of infants born to women with HIV infection before the use of antiretrovirals have found rates of transmission ranging from 13 to 40%,[293–295, 306] with the highest rates of perinatally acquired HIV infection, which approach 40%, reported from Africa.[306] The disparity in these rates most likely reflects differences in the severity of maternal disease stage, nutritional status, rates of breast-feeding, study design, completeness and length of follow-up, and use of different diagnostic criteria.[188] The risk of perinatal transmission appears to vary by the disease stage of the mother. Mothers at both extremes of the clinical spectrum of HIV infection with either acute, primary infection[291] or advanced, symptomatic disease[303, 306] have been reported to be more likely to transmit HIV to their infants than have asymptomatic seropositive women. Data regarding the correlation of maternal HIV viral load with the risk of perinatal transmission have been conflicting. A higher viral load has been observed among women who transmitted HIV to their infants.[307] However, transmission has been observed across the entire range of HIV RNA levels, and an HIV RNA threshold below which transmission does not occur has not been found.[308]

In addition to maternal risk factors, placental factors that disrupt the maternal-fetal barrier can increase perinatal transmission. In one study conducted among Zairean women, the presence of histologic chorioamnionitis and funisitis was associated with an overall twofold increase in transmission risk.[309] Preterm delivery and prolonged rupture of membranes (greater than 4 hours) are also associated with increased risk for perinatal HIV transmission.[310]

Infants born to HIV-infected mothers have passively acquired maternal antibody to HIV that persists for 12 to 18 months. For infants 0 to 6 months of age, PCR and virus culture offer the greatest sensitivity and specificity for detecting HIV infection[311] (see Chapters 106 and 114). Nonetheless, these tests can detect only one half or fewer of perinatally infected infants, which is a reflection of very low viral burden, sequestration of the virus in other tissues, or recent transmission to the infant either late in the third trimester or at the time of delivery.[312] Other options for diagnosing HIV infection in infants include HIV-specific IgA assays and an in vitro antibody production assay such as the ELISPOT (a method for quantifying specific and total antibody-secreting cells[312a]).[290] However, the overall sensitivity and specificity of these tests are less than those of PCR and viral culture, especially for infants younger than 3 months.

Transmission of HIV in Health Care Settings

Percutaneous, mucous membrane, and cutaneous exposure to blood-contaminated body fluids can occur frequently in the health care setting.[313–315] Such exposure has resulted in occupationally acquired HIV infection in health care workers[316–320] (see Chapter 296). Data from several prospective surveillance projects among health care workers indicate that the average risk of seroconversion after a needlestick injury with HIV-infected blood is approximately 0.3%.[316–318] Transmission of HIV has been reported after mucous membrane and cutaneous exposure to blood, although too few seroconversions have occurred in prospective studies to quantify the risk precisely. As of June 1998, a total of 54 health care workers have been reported to the CDC with documented HIV seroconversion after occupational exposure.[31] Of these 54 cases, 46 had a percutaneous exposure, 5 had a mucocutaneous exposure, and 2 had both percutaneous and mucocutaneous exposure. In addition, 133 cases of possible occupational transmission of HIV have been reported to the CDC; in these cases, HIV seroconversion temporally associated with an occupational exposure was not documented.

Because health care workers are more likely than patients to have contact with blood in the health care setting, the risk of HIV transmission from patient to health care worker clearly exceeds that of health care worker to patient.[321, 322] Transmission of HIV from a health care worker to patients has been documented in two instances, in a dental practice in Florida[323, 324] and in a recent case from an orthopedic surgeon in France.[325] In the cluster of cases in Florida, the precise events that resulted in the dentist transmitting HIV to 6 of approximately 1100 patients tested for HIV in this practice remain unknown. However, the six patients had no other confirmed exposure to HIV other than receiving treatment from the dentist, and each was infected with a viral strain that was very similar to that of the dentist but dissimilar to those from other HIV-infected persons in the local area.[323, 324] The very small risk of a health care worker transmitting HIV to a patient probably depends on several factors, including the type of procedure; the technique, skill, and medical condition of the health care worker; and the titer of circulating virus.[321, 326, 327] Aside from these two instances, investigation of 22,759 patients of 53 other HIV-infected health care workers has not identified other episodes of health care worker–to–patient transmission of HIV.[328]

Two patients undergoing nuclear medicine procedures have been reported to have been infected through inadvertent intravenous injections of blood or other material from HIV-infected patients.[329] Also, transmission of HIV through percutaneous or mucocutaneous exposure to blood or other body substances has occurred in homes in which health care has been provided.[330, 331] Transmission of HIV from patient to patient through improper sterilization or reuse of contaminated needles and syringes has been reported in Romania and the former Soviet Union.[332, 333] Similarly, a report from Australia suggested that a breach in infection-control precautions caused HIV to be transmitted from one patient to four other patients during minor surgical procedures performed on the same day by an HIV-negative surgeon.[334] A more detailed review of transmission in the health care setting can be found in Chapter 296.

Other Modes of Transmission

Although HIV has been isolated from a variety of body fluids,[218, 229, 298, 335–337] only contact with blood, semen, other genital secretions, and breast milk has been implicated as sources of infection. HIV infection is acquired through exposure to blood, principally through injecting drug use and receipt of contaminated blood, blood products, organs, and tissues. Exposure of nonintact skin to blood after a motor vehicle accident and a sports injury has been reported to result in HIV infection, but these occurrences are rare.[338, 339]

Vaginal and anal intercourse is the predominant way in which persons are exposed to HIV-infected semen and cervicovaginal fluids. However, transmission of HIV through intravaginal insemination with unprocessed donor semen[340, 341] and through intrauterine insemination with processed semen[342] has been reported. Although data regarding the magnitude of the risk are conflicting,[340–342] there is no evidence that any procedure can reliably eliminate HIV from semen.[342]

Laboratory and epidemiologic studies indicate that the infectivity of saliva from HIV-infected persons through human bites or occupational contact is extremely low. Furthermore, definitive attribution of HIV transmission to contact with saliva is difficult because saliva is often commingled with blood in these settings. The low risk of saliva-mediated HIV transmission is probably attributable to the very low concentrations of HIV in the saliva of infected persons,[228, 229] as well as the presence of HIV inhibitory activity in saliva.[343] One case report of two siblings infected with HIV suggested a bite as the route of transmission for the previously uninfected child.[344] However, because the bite did not break the skin or result in bleeding, the precise mode of transmission remains uncertain. Multiple epidemiologic studies, including occupational and household contact studies, have found no evidence of transmission via a human bite.[345] Similarly, studies of health care workers monitored prospectively after percutaneous, mucous membrane (e.g., during the administration of cardiopulmonary resuscitation), or nonintact skin exposure to saliva from HIV-infected patients have not detected any instances of HIV antibody seroconversion.[317, 346]

To examine the risk of HIV transmission through casual contact, studies have evaluated more than 1000 nonsexual household contacts of both adults and children with HIV infection.[345, 347–349] In these households, transmission of HIV was found only among sex partners, children born to infected mothers, and persons who themselves had risk factors for HIV infection. However, eight case reports have described household transmission of HIV unassociated with sexual contact, injecting drug use, or breast-feeding. Five of the eight reports were associated with documented or probable blood contact.[331, 350–352] Two reports involved nursing care of terminally ill persons with AIDS in which blood exposure might have occurred but was not documented; in both reports, skin contact with other secretions and excretions occurred.[331, 353] In the last report, a bite was suggested but not documented to have resulted in transmission.[344]

Laboratory and epidemiologic studies have produced no evidence of replication of HIV within insects, in vitro mechanical transmission of HIV, or transmission through biting or bloodsucking insects.[354–356] The potential role of insect-mediated HIV infection was evaluated in a study of residents in a southern Florida community with a high rate of HIV infection.[357] HIV seropositivity was not associated with either epidemiologic or laboratory evidence of exposure to mosquitoes, as measured by the presence of antibodies to five arboviruses. Additional studies in Africa failed to establish an association between the presence of malaria antibodies and HIV.[358]

HIV INFECTION AND AIDS OUTSIDE THE UNITED STATES

HIV infection is a pandemic affecting almost all countries. Through November 1997, the World Health Organization (WHO) had received reports of more than 1.7 million cases of AIDS from 197 countries.[359] However, the WHO estimates that the number of reported AIDS cases worldwide is less than 15% of the total estimated number of AIDS cases that have occurred throughout the epidemic. The United Nations Global Programme on AIDS (UNAIDS) estimated that by December 1998, the number of people living with HIV or AIDS worldwide totaled approximately 33.4 million, with more than 95% of all HIV-infected people living in the developing world[360] (see Chapter 104). Modes of transmission of HIV are similar throughout the world, but the relative frequency varies considerably between countries and regions. In Western Europe, North America, and Australia, as well as some parts of South America and the Caribbean, homosexual/bisexual men and injecting drug users remain the predominantly affected groups.[361] In northern Europe, most AIDS cases have occurred among homosexual and bisexual men, whereas in southern Europe, more than 60% of persons with AIDS are injecting drug users.[362] The sex partners of injecting drug users have been particularly affected by heterosexual transmission of HIV. The proportion of infections attributed to heterosexual transmission has increased over time, particularly in Brazil and other countries in South America, where infection rates among injecting drug users are relatively high.[362–364]

In sub-Saharan Africa and some areas of the Caribbean, heterosexual contact is the most common mode of transmission.[361, 365–371] High rates of HIV infection among pregnant women have resulted in a substantial number of children with perinatally acquired HIV.[359, 371] The highest rates of HIV infection in Africa and some Caribbean countries are found among female prostitutes and persons treated for other sexually transmitted diseases.[236, 370, 372–376] Injecting drug use is less common in developing countries than in some areas of the United States.[361] In contrast, receipt of contaminated blood products remains a major source of HIV transmission in many developing countries, and medical injections with contaminated medical devices continue to result in some HIV infections.[358, 361, 377]

HIV was introduced later (middle to late 1980s) in Asia, the Middle East, North Africa, and Eastern Europe than in other regions. Progression of the HIV epidemic in South and Southeast Asia has been quite rapid, with an explosive increase in HIV infection among injecting drug users, prostitutes, and other populations of young adults in Thailand, Myanmar, India, Malaysia, Cambodia, and Vietnam.[378–386] India is now the country believed to have the highest number of HIV-infected persons, with an estimated 2 to 5 million people currently infected. Korea and Japan continue to have low rates of HIV infection among their populations at risk.[387, 388]

In Eastern Europe and the newly independent states of the former Soviet Union, HIV infections are rapidly increasing, primarily in association with injecting drug use, and the prevalence of HIV among persons who inject drugs is growing. In the Czech Republic, Estonia, and Bulgaria, HIV infections are typically caused by sexual transmission. In the former Soviet Union and Romania, outbreaks of HIV had been related to contaminated blood products and medical equipment; however, rising trends for syphilis and other sexually transmitted infections have given origin to an explosive HIV epidemic in Russia and many of the newly independent states.[389] In 1990, several thousand Romanian children were infected after receiving multiple injections with improperly cleaned needles and syringes and transfusions of unscreened blood.[332] In Russia, a nosocomial outbreak of HIV infection among 152 hospitalized children was associated with the multiple use of unsterilized syringes.[333]

The HIV epidemic is expected to continue to grow in the coming years, with an increasing proportion of infected persons residing in developing countries. The UNAIDS/WHO estimates that 5.8 million cases of HIV infection and 2.5 million deaths from AIDS occurred during 1998.[360] A more extensive discussion of AIDS in the developing world is presented in Chapter 104.

HIV-2

A second retrovirus, HIV-2, can result in severe immunosuppression and the development of serious opportunistic diseases that are clinically indistinguishable from those caused by HIV-1. Infection with HIV-2 was first reported in West Africa in 1986.[390] Although cases of HIV-2 infection have since been reported in other parts of Africa, several European countries, Canada, the United States, Brazil, and India,[391] the virus continues to be found mostly among heterosexual persons in West Africa.[392] Differences in the geographic distribution of HIV-1 and HIV-2 may reflect differences in viral load, which in turn can affect transmissibility and the duration of infectiousness.[392] Data from surveillance and serologic surveys indicate that the prevalence of HIV-2 infection in the United States is extremely low.[369, 370] In 1992, the U.S. Food and Drug Administration recommended that all blood donations be screened with serologic assays for HIV-1 and HIV-2. Serologic testing of more than 24 million blood donations found no HIV-2–infected persons.[370] Similarly, surveys conducted among persons presumably at increased risk of infection with retroviruses through sexual contact and injecting drug use have found very low rates of HIV-2 infection.[391, 393] In a survey performed during 1988 to 1990, of 31,533 persons at high risk for HIV infection in the United States, 10% were found to be infected with HIV-1, but only 2 persons (0.006%) were seropositive for HIV-2.[394]

Accumulating information suggests that the modes of transmission for HIV-1 and HIV-2 are similar. Worldwide, HIV-2 infections have been diagnosed predominantly in men and women infected through heterosexual contact and, to a lesser extent, in homosexual men, injecting drug users, transfusion recipients, and persons with hemophilia.[391, 395] In general, the patterns of HIV-1 and HIV-2 transmission within a country are similar. Although perinatal transmission of HIV-2 has been reported, numerous studies suggest that HIV-2 is transmitted less efficiently than HIV-1 from mother to child.[395–398] The natural histories of HIV-1 and HIV-2 infection appear similar in that both are characterized by a broad spectrum of disease. However, the incubation period from the time of initial infection to the eventual development of AIDS may be longer for HIV-2.[395, 399–401]

HIV-1 and HIV-2 are genetically and immunologically distinct. However, nucleotide sequence analysis indicates that HIV-1 and HIV-2 share a similar genomic organization, thus suggesting a common evolutionary origin.[402] Overall, the nucleotide sequence homology for HIV-1 and HIV-2 is approximately 40%; the *gag* and *pol* genes for the two viruses are approximately 60% homologous.[402] These genetic similarities can result in frequent serologic cross-reactions between HIV-1 and HIV-2. HIV-1 antibody tests using whole virus lysate enzyme immunoassay will detect 41 to 91% of HIV-2–infected persons.[403] Similarly, because the *gag* and *pol* proteins of HIV-1 and HIV-2 are antigenically cross-reactive, HIV-2–infected persons may have an indeterminate HIV-1 Western blot.[404] The available HIV-2 enzyme immunoassay tests have a reported sensitivity of greater than 99%,[391] and criteria for the diagnosis of HIV-2 infection by Western blot have been established.[405] Although dual infection with both HIV-1 and HIV-2 has been reported, in one study among persons in Côte d'Ivoire with antibodies to both retroviruses, PCR and viral isolation results suggested that more than half were probably infected with HIV-1 alone.[406] Preliminary data suggest that HIV-2 infection might protect against subsequent infection with HIV-1.[407]

Currently, blood donations in the United States are tested for evidence of both HIV-1 and HIV-2 antibodies. The very low prevalence of HIV-2 infection in the United States does not warrant routine testing for HIV-2 in settings other than blood centers. The CDC has recommended that tests for both HIV-1 and HIV-2 be performed in two HIV-testing situations: (1) if demographic or behavioral information suggests that HIV-2 infection might be present, for example, sexual or blood contact with a person from a country where HIV-2 is endemic or with a person known to be infected with HIV-2, or (2) when clinical evidence suggests HIV disease in the absence of a positive test for antibodies to HIV-1 or in the presence of an HIV-1 Western blot with only *gag* and *pol* bands.[391] Detailed HIV-2 testing and counseling algorithms have been developed.[391] In general, preventive counseling and medical management for persons infected with HIV-2 are similar to those for persons in whom HIV-1 infection is diagnosed.

PREVENTION OF HIV INFECTION IN THE COMMUNITY

Prevention of HIV infection must be based on strategies that interrupt sexual, blood-borne, and perinatal transmission of the virus. Such strategies must be grounded in an understanding of the epidemiology of HIV infection and knowledge of the science of human behavior. These science-based strategies are the foundation for the design, implementation, and evaluation of prevention efforts.

Prevention of Sexual Transmission

Strategies for the prevention of sexual transmission of HIV have focused on reducing unsafe sexual behavior (by promoting sexual abstinence or decreasing the number of partners), encouraging condom use, and treating sexually transmitted infections.[408] Consistent use of latex condoms has been shown to be effective for the prevention of HIV transmission at both an individual and population level.[409, 410] Multiple epidemiologic studies of heterosexual couples in which one partner is HIV positive and the other is HIV negative indicate that the correct and consistent use of condoms can significantly reduce transmission of HIV and other sexually transmitted diseases.[411–414]

In one prospective study of 342 HIV-seronegative women who had no exposure to HIV other than participation in a stable, monogamous relationship with an infected man, 19 seroconversions were detected for an incidence rate of 3.6 per 100 person-years.[413] The risk of acquiring HIV infection was sixfold greater for women whose partners were inconsistent (i.e., never or not always) condom users than for women who reported that their partners always used condoms. A second longitudinal study of heterosexual HIV-serodiscordant couples reported similar findings: no seroconversions occured among 124 partners who always used condoms, whereas 12 of 121 partners who were irregular condom users seroconverted for an incidence rate of 4.8 per 100 person-years.[414] Deriving precise and consistent estimates of condom efficacy is often hindered by the inability to control for potentially important confounders that may significantly affect transmission, including the presence of other concurrent sexually transmitted diseases, the frequency of sex, the duration of the partnership, anal intercourse, and the source partner's degree of immunosuppression.[412] Two large prospective studies of serodiscordant couples have demonstrated that among partners who do not use condoms regularly, the risk of transmission increases with advanced stages of HIV infection in the index partner and with the presence of a genital tract infection in the HIV-negative partner.[413, 414] Such information reinforces the need for ongoing counseling of persons involved in long-term partnerships with infected partners whose clinical condition may change over time.

In Thailand, a program of "100% condom use" in commercial sex establishments led to an enormous increase in condom use and substantial changes in sexual behavior with parallel declines in HIV seroprevalence and sexually transmitted infections.[415, 416]

The effectiveness of condoms in reducing the risk of HIV transmission can be affected by condom breakage, leakage, and slippage. Although condom breakage can occur, it appears to be uncommon, particularly in developed countries, where studies have found breakage rates of 2% or less for vaginal or anal intercourse.[410, 411] Similarly, low rates of slippage (i.e., less than 1%) have been reported.[417] In vitro testing of intact latex condoms to detect leakage of HIV-sized particles suggests that condoms, when properly used, can act as an effective physical barrier and substantially reduce contact with fluid containing HIV-sized particles, even if leakage were to occur.[418]

Intravaginal pouches ("female condoms"), advocated as a "female-controlled" barrier prevention method, also require correct and consistent use.[419, 420] The female condom has been shown to be as effective as the male condom for the prevention of sexually transmitted infections,[420, 421] and its contraceptive failure rate has ranged from 11 to 26% depending on the consistency and correctness of usage.[421] However, a condom's contraceptive failure rate may not accurately reflect its effectiveness in reducing heterosexual HIV transmission.[410, 411]

Whether data on the protective effect of spermicides against a variety of sexually transmitted diseases apply to HIV as well has not been determined.[422] The irritative effects of spermicides on the vaginal epithelium may in fact facilitate, rather than reduce HIV transmission.[246, 422] In a randomized trial among prostitutes in Kenya, the use of a vaginal sponge containing a high dose of nonoxynol 9 was associated with an increased risk of HIV transmission.[245] Topical microbicides and other female-controlled methods to prevent HIV and sexually transmitted diseases that can be safely and effectively used by women must be developed.

Despite the demonstrated benefits of condom use, multiple studies have found relatively low rates of consistent condom use among sexually active homosexual men and heterosexual men and women. Factors that influence condom use are complex.[423] Concern about decreased sexual pleasure or a partner's noncooperation, inadequate communication skills, the temporal effects of drugs or alcohol, use of other methods for contraception, and cultural influences have been correlated with low rates of condom use.[423–426]

Among homosexual and bisexual men, significant reductions in certain high-risk behavior such as sex with nonsteady partners and insertive anal intercourse have been achieved, and reductions in incident HIV infections have been observed.[53, 427] However, coincident with these observation is accumulating evidence that such risk reduction behavior has not been universally adopted and is difficult to maintain over extended periods.[428] In cross-sectional studies of homosexual and bisexual men, younger men aged 18 to 25 years,[429] blacks,[425] and men from cities with a low AIDS prevalence[430] reported the highest rates of unprotected anal intercourse. Two longitudinal studies of men who adopted safer sexual practices found that 12% of participants in San Francisco[431] and 47% in Chicago[432] acknowledged relapsing to unprotected receptive anal intercourse. One study of men who engaged in receptive anal intercourse found that heavy alcohol ingestion, moderate to heavy drug use, and younger age were associated with subsequent seroconversion.[433] Collectively, these studies highlight the diversity among men who have sex with men, the challenges in preventing new HIV infection, and the need for continued commitment to the development, implementation, and targeting of intervention and education programs suitable for different age, racial/ethnic, socioeconomic, and geographic populations.[434]

The data available suggest that changes in sexual behavior by heterosexual men and women at risk for HIV infection have been limited. In the United States, the HIV epidemic among heterosexual men and women has its roots in injecting drug use, crack cocaine use, and the exchange of sex for drugs.[100, 435] Prevention of heterosexually acquired HIV will require efforts to prevent HIV transmission associated with drug use, especially injecting drug use, as well as the prevention and treatment of other sexually transmitted diseases that facilitate HIV transmission.[264, 435, 436]

Partner notification is another mechanism to assist in the prevention of sexual transmission of HIV. Even though many HIV-infected individuals will cooperate in notifying at least some of their sex partners, others do not.[437, 438] Although the effectiveness of contact tracing and partner notification has been hotly debated,[439] it is probably an effective prevention strategy,[440] particularly when targeted to primary HIV infection. The efficacy of contact tracing for preventing incident HIV infection or reducing high-risk behavior by both infected persons and their partners has not been evaluated extensively,[440] but it must be carefully weighed against other activities and be conducted with special attention to confidentiality concerns.

The control of sexually transmitted infections is also an important intervention to reduce the sexual transmission of HIV. Data from a study in Tanzania in which a syndromic approach was used in the treatment of symptomatic sexually transmitted infections led to a 42% decrease in HIV incidence.[247] In contrast, in the Rakai district of Uganda, a recently completed community-based trial of mass treatment for sexually transmitted infections failed to show a difference between the treated and the control arms.[441] The reasons for the lack of consistency in the results of these two trials are multiple and not yet fully explained.

More recently and based on the rationale that zidovudine treatment decreases the risk of infection after occupational exposure to HIV,[442] the use of antiretrovirals has been proposed as a way to reduce the risk of HIV transmission after sexual exposure.[443] The probability of HIV infection per episode of receptive anal intercourse is estimated at 0.1 to 3%, whereas the risk after receptive vaginal intercourse is estimated at 0.1 to 0.2%,[444] which is similar to the estimated risk of HIV transmission after a contaminated needlestick injury.[317] The most frequently administered treatment, which is based on that used for occupational exposure, is zidovudine (200 mg orally three times per day) and lamivudine (150 mg orally twice a day) for 4 weeks, with consideration of the addition of a protease inhibitor in selected cases.[444] Most experts do not recommend initiating treatment more than 72 hours after exposure. However, no data exist regarding the efficacy of this preventive therapy, and costs and side effects must be considered. Until further evidence of its effectiveness is obtained, preventive therapy should be considered an unproven clinical intervention.

Prevention of Transmission by Injecting Drug Use

Prevention and treatment of injecting drug use are critical for reducing HIV transmission among injecting drug users,[445] and several studies have documented that significantly lower rates of drug use and related risk behavior are practiced by injecting drug users who are in treatment.[446] However, an estimated 80% of active drug users in the United States are not in treatment because of either choice or the unavailability of treatment.[447] This situation has necessitated the development of a creative blend of educational and alternative therapeutic approaches, including the removal of restrictions on the purchase of needles and syringes,[448] needle and syringe exchange programs,[449] proper use of bleach for disinfection of drug injection equipment,[450] and interim methadone maintenance programs.[451] Improvement in selected drug use behavior has been reported, including a decrease in sharing of drug-injecting equipment and an increase in the use of bleach for cleaning equipment,[262, 452] although the duration of such behavior has not been studied extensively. Evidence is increasing that social change processes, particularly peer influence, are important in HIV risk reduction among injecting drug users.[455, 456] Recent reviews of needle exchange programs have found that these programs do not result in increased drug use among participants or in the recruitment of first-time users and that they reduce the transmission of HIV among injecting drug users.[455, 456] Use of bleach was not found to be effective in studies in New York City and Baltimore.[457, 458] As previously mentioned for sexual exposure to HIV, it has been proposed that antiretroviral therapy be considered for persons exposed to HIV through injection drug use,[443, 444] but no data are available on the effectiveness of this approach for the prevention of HIV infection among injecting drug users.

Prevention of Transmission through Blood and Other Tissues

The first report of transfusion-associated AIDS was in 1982. In 1983, blood banks initiated the voluntary self-exclusion of donors with risks for HIV infection. In 1985, the first serologic assays for HIV antibody became available, and the use of these HIV serologic tests to screen blood donations dramatically decreased the risk of transfusion-associated HIV transmission.[276, 277] Serologic identification of repeat donors with HIV infection (including the detection of p24 antigen), screening of blood for hepatitis C and human T-lymphotropic virus types I and II, and reductions in the number of transfusions performed have also lowered transmission risks.[277, 278] In addition to HIV antibody testing of plasma donors and deferral procedures for donors with risks for HIV infection, the implementation of viral inactivation procedures such as heat and solvent/detergent treatments and purification with monoclonal antibody has virtually eliminated the risk of HIV transmission through pooled plasma products for persons with hemophilia. In 1993, a recombinant factor VIII product obtained from hamster cells containing the gene for human factor VIII became available as an alternative therapy to pooled human plasma products. Organ and tissue donors should be evaluated and serologically screened in a manner similar to blood donors.[459, 460] In addition, donations of semen and bone from a living donor may be quarantined until subsequent testing has definitively ruled out the possibility of delayed seroconversion in the donor.

Prevention of Transmission in the Health Care Setting

Effective prevention of HIV transmission in the health care setting requires a multifaceted approach to reduce the frequency of occupational blood exposure among health care workers. Such a strategy includes engineering controls that do not rely on worker compliance (e.g., self-sheathing needles), safe work practices and techniques, personal protective equipment, and training.[461] In particular, a reduction in percutaneous injuries will require the development of puncture-resistant gloves, the redesign of needles and other sharp instruments, or both. In 1987, the CDC recommended that the principles of "universal precautions" be incorporated in programs for infection control.[462] Under universal precautions, blood and certain other body fluids from *all* patients are considered to be potentially infective. Universal precautions include the appropriate use of hand washing and protective barriers, care in the use and disposal of needles and other sharp instruments, and appropriate disinfection and sterilization of reusable equipment. For occupational exposure to HIV among health care workers, the CDC recommended in 1990 the use of zidovudine for postexposure prophylaxis.[463] This recommendation was further supported by a case-control study involving health care workers from the United States, France, Italy, and the United Kingdom that showed that the risk of HIV seroconversion after occupational exposure was decreased by approximately 81% with the use of zidovudine.[442] Subsequent recommendations have incorporated the newer antiretroviral drugs, as well as risk stratification for the type of exposure, in the management of occupational exposure to HIV.[464] A detailed discussion of the prevention of transmission of HIV in the health care setting is presented in Chapter 296.

Prevention of Perinatal Infection

Primary prevention of perinatally acquired HIV infection must center on routine, voluntary counseling and HIV antibody testing and on the availability of reproductive health services for women of reproductive age[465, 466] (see Chapter 113). Because a substantial proportion of women may not initially acknowledge high-risk behavior or know the infection status of their partners, routine HIV testing and counseling must be considered a standard of care, especially in areas of high prevalence,[467] and not be reserved only for women with self-reported risk histories. In 1994, results of a randomized, double-blind clinical trial (Pediatric AIDS Clinical Trials Group Protocol 076) found that zidovudine therapy administered to HIV-infected pregnant women during pregnancy, at the time of labor, and postpartum to their infants was associated with a 67.5% reduction in the risk of perinatal HIV transmission.[191] Based on these results, a Public Health Service task force issued recommendations for the use of zidovudine for the reduction of perinatal HIV-1 transmission.[192] Several subsequent studies have confirmed the benefits of zidovudine for the prevention of perinatal HIV-1 transmission even when the drug is given for a much shorter period than in the original Protocol 076 trial.[468, 469] These encouraging results include a study conducted in Thailand in which no intravenous zidovudine was administered during labor, which makes the intervention more applicable in developing countries.[469] The exact mechanism of action of zidovudine in preventing perinatal transmission is not full understood. Implementation of these recommendations has resulted in significant public health benefits; for example, the number of cases of perinatal HIV infection decreased 43% in the United States between 1992 and 1996.[194] These regimens, however, are not applicable in the vast majority of the developing world where most perinatal HIV transmission occurs, and simpler, shorter, and less costly regimens are urgently needed.[470] Advances in understanding the pathogenesis of HIV infection and the availability of laboratory tests to monitor the disease (such as HIV RNA) and better antiretroviral drugs have led to a recent update in the recommendations for the use of antiretroviral drugs in pregnant women.[198]

Prevention of postnatal transmission of HIV infection through breast-feeding must take into account the likelihood of competing risks for morbidity and mortality associated with feeding alternatives in developing countries. In 1985, after the first case report implicating HIV transmission from breast milk and the isolation of HIV from breast milk, the CDC recommended that HIV-seropositive women not breast-feed their infants.[471] This recommendation was intended for mothers in the United States, where alternative, safe, and nutritious substitute feeding methods are readily available.[299] In 1992, the WHO and the United Nations International Children's Emergency Fund developed a consensus statement on HIV transmission related to breast-feeding and stated that "In settings where the primary causes of infant deaths are infectious diseases and malnutrition, breastfeeding should remain the standard advice to pregnant women, including those who are HIV-infected."[472] By 1996, UNAIDS published a revised statement that supported breast-feeding in all populations, irrespective of HIV infection rates, but recommended counseling for women about the risks of HIV transmission through breast-feeding[473]:

> *When children born to women living with HIV can be ensured uninterrupted access to nutritionally adequate breast-milk substitutes that are safely prepared and fed to them, they are at less risk of illness and death if they are not breast-fed. However, when these conditions are not fulfilled, in particular in an environment where infectious diseases and malnutrition are the primary causes of death during infancy, artificial feeding substantially increases children's risk of illness and death.*

Preliminary results of a UNAIDS-sponsored trial of zidovudine plus lamivudine for the prevention of perinatal HIV transmission suggest that this drug combination is effective in a breast-feeding population in Africa.[474]

COUNSELING AND HIV ANTIBODY TESTING

Early recognition of HIV infection through HIV antibody testing has been one of the primary objectives of HIV prevention efforts. However, with the availability of more effective therapies, HIV testing has become an even more important preventive intervention. The major benefits of HIV testing programs are (1) referral of HIV-seropositive persons for medical evaluation, treatment, and other social services and (2) counseling to promote the behavior change necessary to reduce HIV transmission.

Physicians have an essential role in this public health effort. As the principal providers of primary health care, they are most frequently named by the general public as the desired source for HIV testing.[475] The number of people who have been tested for HIV antibodies is quite large, and it has been estimated that in the United States, 65% of homosexual/bisexual men, 50% of injecting drug users, and 30% of heterosexuals with multiple partners know their HIV antibody status.[476]

Indications for HIV Testing

Knowledge of the behavior that places persons at risk for HIV infection, the clinical conditions associated with HIV infection, and the estimated rate of HIV infection in the community served by the health care facility or practitioner is necessary to target effectively HIV counseling and testing. Specific populations or clinical settings in which testing is recommended include the following[465, 477, 478]:

1. *Persons with behavioral risks for HIV infection.* Persons at risk for HIV infection include men who have had sex with other men, persons who have injected drugs, male and female prostitutes, sex partners of persons with or at increased risk for HIV infection, and other persons who consider themselves at risk. To identify risks associated with HIV transmission, physicians should interview patients regarding their sexual and drug use practices. Injecting drug users are at increased risk of HIV infection through contact with contaminated needles or syringes. HIV counseling can provide these persons with information on safer sexual and needle-sharing practices that can further reduce HIV transmission, as well as with referrals for substance abuse treatment and preventive services.
2. *Persons with clinical conditions associated with HIV infection.* The HIV antibody test is a useful diagnostic tool for evaluating persons with generalized lymphadenopathy; unexplained weight loss, fever, diarrhea, or dementia; diseases such as tuberculosis, generalized herpes simplex, and chronic candidiasis; and other conditions suggestive of HIV infection.[10]
3. *Persons who received blood or blood products between 1978 and 1985.* Persons who received transfusions of blood or blood components from 1978 to 1985 are at increased risk of transfusion-associated HIV transmission. The risk of transfusion-associated transmission is greatest for persons who received relatively large numbers of units in geographic areas with high rates of AIDS and HIV infection.[479] Because clotting factor concentrates are derived from many donors nationwide, all persons with hemophilia who received clotting factor concentrate during this time are considered to be at risk for HIV infection.
4. *Persons with other sexually transmitted diseases.* HIV testing should be considered for persons with other sexually transmitted diseases because many of these persons have probably practiced behaviors that place them at risk for HIV infection.
5. *Women of reproductive age.* Women at risk for HIV infection include those with the behavioral risks outlined earlier and all women living in communities or born in countries where the prevalence of HIV infection among women is known or suspected to be high. Offering HIV testing to all women, especially pregnant women, is particularly important in view of the availability of effective interventions to prevent perinatal transmission.[192, 198]
6. *Children born to mothers with HIV infection or at increased risk.* Children born to infected mothers should be evaluated as early as possible after delivery for laboratory and clinical evidence of HIV infection so that appropriate prophylactic and therapeutic interventions can begin. Infected infants often have life-threatening complications of HIV infection in the first few months of life.
7. *Patients 15 to 54 years old in acute health care settings with high rates of unsuspected HIV infection.* High rates of unrecognized HIV infection have been found among patients at some U.S. hospitals and associated clinics.[78, 314] In anonymous unlinked serologic surveys, 0.2 to 8.9% of persons receiving care in emergency departments and 0.1 to 7.8% of persons admitted to hospitals were HIV antibody positive. In two studies that collected data on previous HIV testing, many persons were unaware of their HIV infection before hospital admission.[78] Thus, testing of persons on the basis of acknowledged risk behavior or clinical signs and symptoms will recognize only a minority of HIV-infected persons. To address this shortcoming, routine, voluntary HIV counseling and testing programs are recommended for hospitals and associated clinics with a high rate of HIV infection. A high rate of HIV infection is defined as an estimated HIV seroprevalence rate of at least 1% or an AIDS diagnosis rate of 1.0 or higher per 1000 discharges. The AIDS diagnosis rate is the annual number of patients in whom AIDS is diagnosed and reported to the health department divided by the annual number of discharges times 1000. Acute care facilities and other health care institutions such as mental health facilities or private medical practitioners' offices with high rates of HIV infection should strongly consider routinely offering HIV counseling and testing to all patients 15 to 54 years old.
8. *Persons who sustain occupational exposures that may place them at risk of HIV infection.* Occupational exposures that may place a worker at risk of HIV infection include percutaneous injuries and contact of mucous membranes or skin (especially when the skin is chapped, abraded, or afflicted with dermatitis or the contact is prolonged or involves an extensive area) with blood and other body fluids to which universal precautions apply.[464]
9. *Health care workers who perform exposure-prone procedures.* Health care workers who perform invasive procedures that are considered exposure prone (e.g., procedures that include digital palpation of a needle tip in a body cavity or the simultaneous presence of the health care worker's fingers and a needle or other sharp object in a poorly visualized or highly confined anatomic site) should know their HIV antibody status. Mandatory testing of health care workers for HIV antibody is not recommended.[480]

Guidelines for HIV Counseling and Testing

Testing for HIV infection should be voluntary, with informed consent obtained in accordance with local laws.[478] Confidentiality and the avoidance of discrimination toward persons who test positive must be ensured. Mandatory testing is not recommended except in the limited setting of tissue and organ donation. HIV testing for purposes other than immediate medical care should be deferred until a later time for persons who are too severely ill to give informed consent. Testing patients to reduce the risk of HIV transmission within health care settings has not been shown to be effective and is not a substitute for universal precautions.[313, 481]

Although study results have differed, voluntary HIV counseling and testing have been found to reduce the prevalence of high-risk behavior such as unprotected intercourse and is thus an effective intervention that can help reduce HIV transmission.[482–486] Counseling should be performed in accordance with existing CDC recommendations by health care providers knowledgeable about HIV infection.[465, 478, 487] HIV testing should be preceded by information about the testing policies of the physician or institution, the medical implications of the test, an assessment of risk, and the opportunity to receive additional information. After testing, HIV-seronegative persons should be informed that continued high-risk sexual or drug use behavior could result in HIV infection. Seronegative persons concerned about a recent exposure should be advised to seek repeated testing at least 6 months after the exposure.

Counseling of HIV-seropositive persons should be tailored for each individual and include an interpretation of the test results and a discussion of the medical, social, and psychological implications of a positive test result. HIV-infected persons should also be instructed to notify sex or needle-sharing partners and to refer them for HIV counseling and testing. If HIV-infected persons are reluctant to inform their partners directly, physicians may offer to inform partners or seek local health department assistance. Confidentiality is very important to protect individuals and not discourage persons from seeking HIV testing.

Persons found to be HIV seropositive should be referred for medical evaluation, including immunologic (CD4 T-lymphocyte cell counts) and virologic (quantitation of HIV RNA) monitoring, screening for other sexually transmitted diseases, prophylaxis against certain opportunistic illnesses, vaccinations, antiretroviral therapy, and other preventive and therapeutic services.[488] Physicians who offer HIV testing should be able to provide these services or have an effective referral mechanism.

REFERENCES

1. Centers for Disease Control and Prevention. *Pneumocystis* pneumonia—Los Angeles. MMWR Morb Mortal Wkly Rep. 1981;30:250–252.
2. Centers for Disease Control and Prevention. Kaposi's sarcoma and *Pneumocystis* pneumonia among homosexual men—New York City and California. MMWR Morb Mortal Wkly Rep. 1981;30:305–308.
3. Zhu T, Korber BT, Nahmias AJ, et al. An African HIV-1 sequence from 1959 and implications for the origin of the epidemic. Nature. 1998;391:594–597.
4. UNAIDS. Report on the Global HIV/AIDS Epidemic. December 1997.
5. Centers for Disease Control and Prevention: Update on acquired immune deficiency syndrome (AIDS)—United States. MMWR Morb Mortal Wkly Rep. 1982;31:507–508, 513–514.
6. Garry RF, Witte MH, Gottlieb AA, et al. Documentation of an AIDS virus infection in the United States in 1968. JAMA. 1988;260:2085–2087.
7. Huminer D, Rosenfeld JB, Pitlik SD. AIDS in the pre-AIDS era. Rev Infect Dis. 1987;9:1102–1108.
8. Centers for Disease Control and Prevention. Revision of the case definition of acquired immunodeficiency syndrome for national reporting—United States. MMWR Morb Mortal Wkly Rep. 1985;34:373–375.
9. Centers for Disease Control and Prevention. Revision of the CDC surveillance case definition for acquired immunodeficiency syndrome. MMWR Morb Mortal Wkly Rep. 1987;36(Suppl):S1–S15.
10. Centers for Disease Control and Prevention. 1993 Revised classification system for HIV infection and expanded surveillance case definition for AIDS among adolescents and adults. MMWR Morb Mortal Wkly Rep. 1992;41(RR-17):1–19.
11. Centers for Disease Control and Prevention. Update: Acquired immunodeficiency syndrome—United States, 1981–1988. MMWR Morb Mortal Wkly Rep. 1989;38:229–236.
12. Selik RM, Buehler JW, Karon JM, et al. Impact of the 1987 revision of the case definition of the acquired immunodeficiency syndrome in the United States. J Acquir Immune Defic Syndr. 1990;3:73–82.
13. Payne SF, Rutherford GW, Lemp GF, et al. Effect of the revised AIDS case definition on AIDS reporting in San Francisco: Evidence of increased reporting in intravenous drug users. AIDS. 1990;4:335–339.
14. National Institutes of Health. State-of-the-art conference on azidothymidine therapy for early HIV infection. Am J Med. 1990;89:335–344.
15. Volberding PA, Lagakos SW, Koch MA, et al. Zidovudine in asymptomatic human immunodeficiency virus infection: A controlled trial in persons with fewer than 500 CD4-positive cells per cubic millimeter. The AIDS Clinical Trials Group of the National Institute of Allergy and Infectious Diseases. N Engl J Med. 1990;322:941.
16. Centers for Disease Control and Prevention. Recommendations for prophylaxis against *Pneumocystis carinii* pneumonia for adults and adolescents infected with human immunodeficiency virus. MMWR Morb Mortal Wkly Rep. 1992;41(RR-4):1–11.
17. El Sadr W, Oleshe JM, Agins BD, et al. Evaluation and Management of Early HIV Infection. Clinical Practice Guideline No. 7, Publication No. 940572. Rockville, Md: Agency for Health Care Policy and Research, Public Health Service, U.S. Department of Health and Human Services; 1994:28.
18. Brookmeyer R. Reconstruction and future trends of the AIDS epidemic in the United States. Science. 1991;253:37–42.
19. Selwyn PA, Hartel D, Lewis VA, et al. A prospective study of the risk of tuberculosis among intravenous drug users with human immunodeficiency virus infection. N Engl J Med. 1989;320:545–550.
20. Selwyn PA, Sckell BM, Alcabes P, et al. High risk of active tuberculosis in HIV infected drug users with cutaneous anergy. JAMA. 1992;268:504–509.
21. Buehler JW, Devine OJ, Berkelman RL, et al. Impact of the human immunodeficiency virus epidemic on mortality trends in young men, United States. Am J Public Health. 1990;80:1080–1086.
22. Chu SY, Buehler JW, Berkelman RL. Impact of the human immunodeficiency virus epidemic on mortality in women of reproductive age, United States. JAMA. 1990;264:225–229.
23. Farizo KM, Buehler JW, Chamberland ME, et al. Spectrum of disease in persons with human immunodeficiency virus infection in the United States. JAMA. 1992;267:1798–1805.
24. Schafer A, Friedmann W, Mielke M, et al. The increased frequency of cervical dysplasia-neoplasia in women infected with the human immunodeficiency virus is related to the degree of immunosuppression. Am J Obstet Gynecol. 1991;164:593–599.
25. Feingold AR, Vermund SH, Burk RD, et al. Cervical cytologic abnormalities and papillomavirus in women infected with human immunodeficiency virus. J Acquir Immune Defic Syndr. 1990;3:896–903.
26. Maiman M, Fruchter RG, Serur E, et al. Human immunodeficiency virus infection and cervical neoplasia. Gynecol Oncol. 1990;38:377–382.
27. Rosenblum LS, Buehler JW, Morgan MW, et al. The completeness of AIDS case reporting, 1988: A multisite collaborative surveillance project. Am J Public Health. 1992;82:1495–1499.
28. Buehler JW, Berkelman RL, Stehr-Green JK. The completeness of AIDS surveillance. J Acquir Immune Defic Syndr. 1992;5:257–264.
29. Thacker SB, Choi K, Brachman PS. The surveillance of infectious disease. JAMA. 1983;249:1181–1185.
30. Vogt RL, Clark SW, Kappel S. Evaluation of the state surveillance system using hospital discharge diagnoses, 1982–83. Am J Epidemiol. 1986;123:197–198.
31. Centers for Disease Control and Prevention. HIV/AIDS Surveillance Report. 1997;9:39.
32. Fleming PL, Ward JW, Morgan MW, et al. Mandatory HIV reporting: Characteristics of adults reported with HIV compared to AIDS in the United States (Abstract WSC172). In: Abstracts of the IXth International Conference on AIDS/IVth STD World Congress, v. 1. Berlin: 1993:98.
33. Centers for Disease Control and Prevention. Public health uses of HIV-infection reports—South Carolina, 1986–1991. MMWR Morb Mortal Wkly Rep. 1992;41:245–249.
34. Palella FJ, Delaney KM, Moorman AC, et al. Declining morbidity and mortality among patients with advanced human immunodeficiency virus infection. N Engl J Med. 1998;338:853–860.
35. Gastin LO, Ward JW, Baker AC. National HIV case reporting in the United States. A defining moment in the history of the epidemic. N Engl J Med. 1997;337:1162–1167.
36. Solomon SL, Curran JW. Public health applications of a classification system for human immunodeficiency virus infection (Editorial). Ann Intern Med. 1987;106:319–321.
37. World Health Organization. Interim proposal for a WHO staging system for HIV infection and diseases. Wkly Epidemiol Rec. 1990;65:221–224.
38. Royce RA, Luckmann RS, Fusaro RE, Winkelstein W Jr. The natural history of HIV-1 infection: Staging classifications of disease. AIDS. 1991;5:355–364.
39. Redfield RR, Wright DC, Tramont EC. The Walter Reed staging classification for HTLV-III/LAV infection. N Engl J Med. 1986;314:131–132.
40. Zolla-Pazner S, DesJarlais DC, Friedman SR, et al. Nonrandom development of immunologic abnormalities after infection with human immunodeficiency virus: Implications for immunologic classification of the disease. Proc Natl Acad Sci U S A. 1987;84:5404–5408.
41. Justice AC, Feinstein AR, Wells CK. A new prognostic staging system for the acquired immunodeficiency syndrome. N Engl J Med. 1989;320:1388–1393.
42. Centers for Disease Control and Prevention. HIV/AIDS Surveillance Report. 1998;10:1–40.
43. Centers for Disease Control and Prevention. The second 100,000 cases of acquired immunodeficiency syndrome—United States, June 1981–December 1991. MMWR Morb Mortal Wkly Rep. 1992;41:28–29.
44. Centers for Disease Control and Prevention. Update: Impact of the expanded AIDS surveillance case distribution for adolescents and adults on case reporting—United States, 1993. MMWR Morb Mortal Wkly Rep. 1994;43:160–161, 167–170.
45. Carpenter CC, Fischl MA, Hammer SM, et al. Antiretroviral therapy for HIV infection in 1998: Updated recommendations of the International AIDS Society—USA Panel. JAMA. 1998;280:78–86.
46. Karon JM, Rosenberg PS, McQuillan G, et al. Prevalence of HIV infection in the United States, 1984 to 1992. JAMA. 1996;276:126–131.
47. Holmberg SD. The estimated prevalence and incidence of HIV in 96 large US metropolitan areas. Am J Public Health. 1996;86:627–628.
48. Centers for Disease Control and Prevention. Human immunodeficiency virus infection in the United States: A review of current knowledge. MMWR Morb Mortal Wkly Rep. 1987;36(Suppl 6):S1–S48.
49. Selik RM, Chu SY, Buehler JW. Human immunodeficiency virus (HIV) infection as a leading cause of death among young adults in U.S. cities and states. JAMA. 1993;269:2991–2994.
50. Centers for Disease Control and Prevention (CDC). National HIV Prevalence Surveys, 1997 Summary. Atlanta: Centers for Disease Control and Prevention; 1998:1–25.
51. Weinstock HS, Sidhu J, Gwinn M, et al. Trends in HIV seroprevalence among persons attending sexually transmitted diseases clinics in the United States. J Acquir Immune Defic Syndr. 1995;9:514–522.
52. McCray E, Onorato IM, the Field Services Branch. Sentinel surveillance of human immunodeficiency virus infection in sexually transmitted disease clinics in the United States. Sex Transm Dis. 1992;19:235–241.
53. Winkelstein W Jr, Wiley JA, Padian NS, et al. The San Francisco Men's Health Study: Continued decline in HIV seroconversion rates among homosexual/bisexual men. Am J Public Health. 1988;78:1472–1474.
54. Kingsley LA, Bacellar H, Zhou S, et al. Temporal trends in HIV seroconversion: A report from the multicenter AIDS cohort study (MACS) (Abstract F.C.550). In: Final Program and Abstracts of the VIth International Conference on AIDS, v. 2. San Francisco: 1990:218.
55. Katz MH, McFarland W, Guillin V, et al. Continuing high prevalence of HIV and risk behaviors among young men who have sex with men: The young men's survey in the San Francisco Bay Area in 1992 to 1993 and in 1994 to 1995. J Acquir Immune Defic Syndr Hum Retroviral. 1998;19:178–181.
56. Hernandez SR, Kellogg TA, Wilson MJ, et al. Prevalance of HIV-1 among homosexual and bisexual men in the San Francisco Bay area: Evidence of infection among young gay men (Abstract W.C.3010). In: Abstracts of the VIIth International Conference on AIDS, v. 2. Florence, Italy: 1991:298.
57. Hahn RA, Onorato IM, Jones TS, et al. Prevalence of HIV infection among intravenous drug users in the United States. JAMA. 1989;261:2677–2684.
58. Des Jarlais DC, Friedman SR, Novick DM, et al. HIV-1 infection among intravenous drug users in Manhattan, New York City, from 1977 through 1987. JAMA. 1989;261:1008–1012.
59. Weibel W, Lampinen T, Chene D, et al. HIV-1 seroconversion in a cohort of street intravenous drug users in Chicago (Abstract F.C.556). In: Final Program and Abstracts of the VIth International Conference on AIDS, v. 2. San Francisco: 1990:220.
60. Centers for Disease Control and Prevention (CDC): National HIV Serosurveillance

Summary—Results through 1992. Publication No. HIV/NCID/1193/036. Atlanta: U.S. Department of Health and Human Services, Public Health Service; 1993.
61. Allen DM, Onorato IM, Green TA, et al. HIV infection in intravenous drug users entering drug treatment, United States, 1988 to 1989. Am J Public Health. 1992;82:541–546.
62. Murill C, Weeks HR, Lambert S, et al. Age-specific trends in seroprevalence of HIV and hepatitis B and C virus among injecting drug users admitted to drug treatment in six US cities Abstract 13224. Presented at the Twelfth International Conference on AIDS. Geneva, 1998.
63. Prevosts DR, Allen DM, Lehman JS, et al. Trends in human immunodeficiency virus seroprevalence among injection drug users entering drug treatment centers, United States 1988–1993. Am J Epidemiol. 1996;143:733–742.
64. Battjes RJ, Pickens RW, Brown LS Jr. HIV infection and AIDS risk behaviors among injecting drug users entering methadone treatment: An update J Acquir Immune Defic Syndr. 1995;10:90–96.
65. Chaisson RE, Bacchetti P, Osmond D, et al. Cocaine use and HIV infection in intravenous drug users in San Francisco. JAMA. 1989;261:561–565.
66. Battjes RJ, Pickens RW, Haverkos HW, Slobada Z. HIV risk factors among injection drug users in five US cities. AIDS. 1994;8:6817.
67. Kral AH, Bluthenthal RN, Booth RE, Watters JK. HIV seroprevalence among street-recruited injection drug and crack cocaine users in 16 US municipalities. Am J Public Health. 1998;88:108–113.
68. DesJarlais DC, Perlis T, Friedman SR, et al. Declining seroprevalence in a very large HIV epidemic: Injection drug users in New York City, 1991 to 1996. Am J Public Health. 1998;88:1801.
69. Byers RH, Lindegren ML, Hanson IC, et al. AIDS patients infected during adolescence, United States Abstract 284. Presented at the Thirty-Second Interscience Conference on Antimicrobial Agents and Chemotherapy, Anaheim, Calif, October 11–14, 1992.
70. Dondero TJ, Allen DM, McCray D, et al. Injected drug use: The driving force for much of the U.S. epidemic (Abstract WC 3356). In: Abstracts of the VIIth International Conference on AIDS, v. 2. Florence, Italy: 1991:385.
71. Chaisson MA, Stoneburner RL, Hildebrandt DS, et al. Heterosexual transmission of HIV-1 associated with the use of smokable freebase cocaine (crack). AIDS. 1991;5:1121–1126.
72. Ellerbrock TV, Lieb S, Harrington PE, et al. Heterosexually transmitted human immunodeficiency virus infection among pregnant women in a rural Florida community. N Engl J Med. 1992;327:1704–1709.
73. Jones D, Irwin KL, Inciardi J, et al. The high-risk sexual practices of crack-smoking sex workers recruited from the streets of three American cities. The Multicenter Crack Cocaine and HIV Infection Study Team. Sex Transm Dis. 1998;25:184–193.
74. Stoneburner RL, Chaisson MA, Weisfuse IB, et al. The epidemic of AIDS and HIV-1 infection among heterosexuals in New York City. AIDS. 1990;4:99–106.
75. Darrow WW, Cohen JB, French J, et al. Multicenter study of HIV antibody in U.S. prostitutes. Abstract W.2.1. Presented at the Third International Conference on AIDS. Washington, DC, June 1–5, 1987.
76. Fischl MA, Dickinson GM, Flanagan S, et al. Human immunodeficiency virus (HIV) among female prostitutes in south Florida. Abstract W.2.2. Presented at the Third International Conference on AIDS. Washington, DC, June 1–5, 1987.
77. Onorato IM, Klaskala W, Morgan M. High and rising HIV incidence in female sex workers in Miami, Florida, despite stable HIV prevalence over time. Abstract 285. Presented at the Thirty-Second Interscience Conference on Antimicrobial Agents and Chemotherapy, Anaheim, Calif, October 11–14, 1992.
78. Janssen RS, St. Louis ME, Satten GA, et al. HIV infection among patients in U.S. acute care hospitals: Strategies for the counseling and testing of hospital patients. N Engl J Med. 1992;327:445–452.
79. Miller RS, Green LA, Nutting PA, et al. Human immunodeficiency virus seroprevalence in community-based primary care practices, 1990–1992. A report from the Ambulatory Sentinel Practice Network. Arch Fam Med. 1995;4:1042–1047.
80. Schneider E, McCray E, Onorato IM. HIV seroprevalence among TB clinic patients in the US, 1988–1995. Abstract 145. Presented at the Thirty-sixth Interscience Conference on Antinicrobial Agents and Chemotherapy, New Orleans, La, 1996.
81. Withum DG, Guerena-Burgueno F, Gwinn M, et al. High HIV prevalence among female and male prisoners in the United States, 1989–1992: Implications for prevention and treatment strategies (Abstract POC213115). In: Abstracts of the IX International Conference on AIDS/STD World Congress, v. II. Berlin: 1993:736.
82. Mikl J, Dzierbicki A, Smith PF, et al. Trends in HIV infection rates among New York State prison entrants, 1987–97. Abstract 2356. Presented at the Twelfth International Conference on AIDS, Geneva, 1998.
83. Kennedy M, Petersen L, Doll L, et al: Five year trends in HIV seroprevalence and risk behaviors among U.S. blood donors: A multicenter study (Abstract POC213118). In: Abstracts of the IXth International Conference on AIDS/STD World Congress, v. II. Berlin: 1993:737.
84. Brundage JF, Burke DS, Gardner LI, et al. Tracking the spread of the HIV infection epidemic among young adults in the United States: Results of the first four years of screening among civilian applicants for U.S. military service. J Acquir Immune Defic Syndr. 1990;3:1168–1180.
85. Burke DS, Brundage JF, Goldenbaum M, et al. Human immunodeficiency virus infections in teenagers. JAMA. 1990;263:2074–2074.
86. Withers BG, Kelley PW, McNeil JG. A brief review of the epidemiology of HIV in the U.S. Army. Mil Med. 1992;157:80–84.
87. Cowan DN, Pomerantz RS, Wann ZF, et al. Human immunodeficiency virus infection among members of the reserve components of the U.S. Army: Prevalence, incidence, and demographic characteristics. J Infect Dis. 1990;162:827–836.
88. Kelley PW, Miller RN, Pomerantz R, et al. Human immunodeficiency virus seropositivity among members of the active duty U.S. Army 1985–89. Am J Public Health. 1990;80:405–410.
89. McNeil JG, Brundage JF, Gardner LI, et al. Trends of HIV seroconversion among young adults in the U.S. Army, 1985 to 1989. JAMA. 1991;265:1709–1714.
90. Valleroy LA, MacKellar DA, Karon JM, et al. HIV infection in disadvantaged out-of-school youth: Prevalence for US Job Corps entrants, 1990 through 1996. J Acquir Immune Defic Syndr Hum Retrovirol. 1998;19:67–73.
91. Pappaioanou M, George RJ, Hannon WH, et al. HIV seroprevalence surveys of childbearing women: Objectives, methods, and uses of the data. Public Health Rep. 1990;105:147–152.
92. Fisher-Davis S, Rosen DH, Steinberg S, et al. Trends in HIV prevalence among childbearing women in the United States, 1989–1994. J Acquir Immun Defic Syndr Hum Retrovirol. 1998;19:158–164.
93. Sweeney PA, Onorato IM, Allen DM, et al. Sentinel surveillance of human immunodeficiency virus infection in women seeking reproductive health services in the United States, 1988–1989. Obstet Gynecol. 1992;79:503–510.
94. Green TA, Karon JM, Nwanyanwu OC. Changes in AIDS incidence trends in the United States. J Acquir Immune Defic Syndr. 1992;5:547–555.
95. Selik RM, Ward JW, Buehler JW. Trends in transfusion-associated acquired immune deficiency syndrome in the United States, 1982 through 1991. Transfusion. 1993;33:890–893.
96. Berkelman R, Karon J, Thomas P, et al. Are AIDS cases among homosexual men leveling. Abstract W.A.O.13. Presented at the Fifth International Conference on AIDS. Montreal: June 4–9, 1989.
97. Gail MH, Rosenberg PS, Goedert JJ. Therapy may explain recent deficits in AIDS incidence. J Acquir Immune Defic Syndr. 1990;3:296–306.
98. Conley LJ, Holmberg SD. Transmission of AIDS from blood screened negative for antibody to the human immunodeficiency virus (Letter). N Engl J Med. 1992;326:1499–1500.
99. Centers for Disease Control and Prevention: Update: Acquired immunodeficiency syndrome—United States, 1992. MMWR Morb Mortal Wkly Rep. 1993;42:547–551, 557.
100. Neal JJ, Fleming PL, Green TA, Ward JW. Trends in heterosexually acquired AIDS in the United States, 1988 through 1995. J Acquir Immune Defic Syndr. Hum Retrovirol. 1997;14:465–474.
101. Nwanyanwu OC, Conti LA, Ciesielski CA, et al. Increasing frequency of heterosexually transmitted AIDS in southern Florida: Artifact or reality? Am J Public Health. 1993;83:571–573.
102. Castro KG, Lifson AR, White CR, et al. Investigations of AIDS patients with no previously identified risk factors. JAMA. 1988;259:1338–1342.
103. Simonds RJ, Holmberg SD, Hurwitz RL, et al. Transmission of human immunodeficiency virus type 1 from a seronegative organ and tissue donor. N Engl J Med. 1992;326:726.
104. Centers for Disease Control and Prevention. Update: Trends in AIDS incidence, deaths and prevalence—United States, 1996. MMWR Morb Mortal Wkly Rep. 1997;46:165–173.
105. Centers for Disease Control and Prevention. AIDS among persons aged greater than or equal to 50 years—United States, 1991–1996. MMWR Morb Mortal Wkly Rep. 1998;47:21–27.
106. Centers for Disease Control and Prevention. AIDS among racial/ethnic minorities—United States, 1993. MMWR Morb Mortal Wkly Rep. 1994;43:644–655.
107. Diaz T, Buehler JW, Castro KG, et al. AIDS trends among Hispanics in the United States. Am J Public Health. 1993;83:504–509.
108. Centers for Disease Control and Prevention: Risks for HIV infection among persons residing in rural areas and small cities—selected sites, Southern United states, 1995–1996. MMWR Morb Mortal Wkly Rep. 1998;47:974–978.
109. Thomas PA, Hindin R, Greenberg A, et al. Decreased incidence of reported AIDS cases, New York City (Abstract Th.C.707). In: Abstracts of the VIth International Conference on AIDS, v. 1. San Francisco: 1990:301.
110. Karon J, Berkelman RL. The geographic and ethnic diversity of AIDS incidence trends in homosexual/bisexual men in the United States. J Acquir Immune Defic Syndr. 1991;4:1179–1189.
111. Centers for Disease Control and Prevention. AIDS associated with injecting drug use—United States, 1995. MMWR Morb Mortal Wkly Rep. 1996;45:392–396.
112. Selik RM, Ward JW, Buehler JW. Demographic differences in cumulative incidence rates of transfusion-associated acquired immunodeficiency syndrome. Am J Epidemiol. 1994;140:105–112.
113. Greenberg AE, Thomas PA, Landesman SH, et al. The spectrum of HIV-1–related disease among outpatients in New York City. AIDS. 1992;6:849–859.
114. Schacker T, Collier AC, Hughes J, et al. Clinical and epidemiological features of primary HIV infection. Ann Intern Med. 1996;125:257–264.
115. Kahn JO, Walker BD. Current concepts: Acute human immunodeficiency virus type 1 infection. N Engl J Med. 1998;339:33–39.
116. Hardy WD, Daar ES, Sokolov RT Jr, et al. Acute neurologic deterioration in a young man. Rev Infect Dis. 1991;13:745–750.
117. Tindall B, Cooper DA. Primary HIV infection: Host responses and intervention strategies. AIDS. 1991;5:1–14.
118. Fox R, Eldred LJ, Fuchs EJ, et al. Clinical manifestations of acute infection with human immunodeficiency virus in a cohort of gay men. AIDS. 1987;1:35–38.
119. Pedersen C, Lindhardt BO, Jensen BL, et al. Clinical course of primary HIV infection: Consequences for subsequent course of infection. BMJ. 1989;299:154–157.
120. Busch MP, Lee LL, Shatten GA, et al. Time course of detection of viral and

serologic markers preceding human immunodeficiency virus type 1 seroconversion: Implications for screening of blood and tissue donors. Transfusion. 1995;35:91–97.
121. Horsburgh CR Jr, Ou CY, Jason J, et al. Duration of human immunodeficiency virus infection before detection of antibody. Lancet. 1989;2:637–640.
122. Pan LZ, Sheppard HW, Winkelstein W, et al. Lack of detection of human immunodeficiency virus in persistently seronegative homosexual men with high or medium risks for infection. J Infect Dis. 1991;164:962–964.
123. Simmonds P, Lainson FAL, Cuthbert R, et al. HIV antigen and antibody detection: Variable responses to infection in the Edinburgh haemophiliac cohort. BMJ. 1988;296:593–598.
124. Yerly S, Chamot E, Deglon JJ, et al. Absence of chronic human immunodeficiency virus infection without seroconversion in intravenous drug users: A prospective and retrospective study. J Infect Dis. 1991;164:965–968.
125. Daar ES, Moudgil T, Meyer RD, et al. Transient high levels of viremia in patients with primary immunodeficiency virus type 1 infection. N Engl J Med. 1991;324:961–964.
126. Alter HJ, Epstein JS, Swenson SG, et al. Prevalence of human immunodeficiency virus type 1 p24 antigen in the US blood donors—an assessment of the efficacy of testing in donor screening. The HIV-Antigen Study Group. N Engl J Med. 1990;323:1312–1317.
127. Laurence J, Siegal FP, Schattner E, et al. Acquired immunodeficiency syndrome without evidence of infection with human immunodeficiency virus types 1 and 2. Lancet. 1992;340:273–274.
128. Centers for Disease Control and Prevention: Unexplained CD4+ T-lymphocyte depletion in persons without evident HIV infection—United States. MMWR Morb Mortal Wkly Rep. 1992;41:541–545.
129. Smith DK, Neal JJ, Holmberg SD, et al. Unexplained opportunistic infections and CD4+ T-lymphocytopenia without HIV infection. An investigation of cases in the United States. N Engl J Med. 1993;328:373–379.
130. Centers for Disease Control and Prevention: Projections of the number of persons diagnosed with AIDS and the number of immunosuppressed HIV-infected persons—United States, 1992–1994. MMWR Morb Mortal Wkly Rep. 1992;41(RR-18):1–29.
131. Ragni MV, Kingsley LA. Cumulative risk for AIDS and other HIV outcomes in a cohort of hemophiliacs in western Pennsylvania. J Acquir Immune Defic Syndr. 1990;3:708–713.
132. Kuo JM, Taylor JMG, Detels R. Estimating the AIDS incubation period from a prevalent cohort. Am J Epidemiol. 1991;133:1050–1057.
133. Rutherford GW, Lifson AR, Hessol NA, et al. Course of HIV-1 infection in a cohort of homosexual and bisexual men: An 11 year follow up study. BMJ. 1990;301:1183–1188.
134. Lifson AR, Buchbinder SP, Sheppard HW, et al. Long-term human immunodeficiency virus infection in asymptomatic homosexual and bisexual men with normal CD4+ lymphocyte counts: Immunologic and virologic characteristics. J Infect Dis. 1991;163:959–965.
135. Learmont J, Tindall B, Evans L, et al. Long-term symptomless HIV-1 infection in recipients of blood products from a single donor. Lancet. 1992;340:863–867.
136. Ashton JJ, Carr A, Cunningham PM, et al. Predictors of progression in long-term non-progressors. Australian Long-term Nonprogressor Study Group. AIDS Res Hum Retrovirus. 1998;14:117–121.
137. Ward JW, Bush TJ, Perkins HA, et al. The natural history of transfusion-associated infection with human immunodeficiency virus. N Engl J Med. 1989;321:947–952.
138. Selwyn PA, Alcabes P, Hartel D, et al. Clinical manifestations and predictors of disease progression in drug users with human immunodeficiency virus infection. N Engl J Med. 1992;327:1697–1703.
139. Coates RA, Farwell VT, Raboud J, et al. Cofactors of progression to acquired immunodeficiency syndrome in a cohort of male sexual contacts of men with human immunodeficiency virus disease. Am J Epidemiol. 1990;132:717–722.
140. Kaslow RA, Blackwelder WC, Ostrow DG, et al. No evidence for a role of alcohol or other psychoactive drugs in accelerating immunodeficiency in HIV-1 positive individuals. A report from the Multicenter AIDS Cohort Study. JAMA. 1989;261:3424–3429.
141. Goedert JJ, Kessler CM, Aledort LM, et al. A prospective study of human immunodeficiency virus type 1 infection and the development of AIDS in subjects with hemophilia. N Engl J Med. 1989;321:1141–1148.
142. Mariotto AB, Mariotti S, Pezzotti P, et al. Estimation of the acquired immunodeficiency syndrome incubation period in intravenous drug users: A comparison with male homosexuals. Am J Epidemiol. 1992;135:428–437.
143. Vermund SH, Galbraith MA, Ebner SC, et al. Human immunodeficiency virus/acquired immunodeficiency syndrome in pregnant women. Ann Epidemiol. 1992;2:773–803.
144. Klein RS, Harris CA, Small CB, et al. Oral candidiasis in high-risk patients as the initial manifestation of the acquired immunodeficiency syndrome. N Engl J Med. 1984;311:354–358.
145. Greenspan D, Greenspan JS, Hearst NG, et al. Relation of oral hairy leukoplakia to infection with the human immunodeficiency virus and the risk of developing AIDS. J Infect Dis. 1987;155:475–481.
146. Melbye M, Grossman RJ, Goedert JJ, et al. Risk of AIDS after herpes zoster. Lancet. 1987;1:728–731.
147. Stein DS, Korvick JA, Vermund SH. CD4+ lymphocyte cell enumeration for prediction of clinical course of human immunodeficiency virus disease: A review. J Infect Dis. 1992;165:352–363.
148. Mellors JW, Rinaldo CR, Gupta P, et al. Prognosis in HIV-1 infection predicted by the quantity of virus in plasma. Science. 1996;272:1167–1170.
149. Saag MS, Holodniy M, Kuritzkes DR, et al. HIV viral load markers in clinical practice. Nat Med. 1996;2:625–629.
150. Mellors JW, Muñoz A, Giorgi JV, et al. Plasma viral load and CD4+ lymphocytes as prognostic markers of HIV-infection. Ann Intern Med. 1997;126:946–954.
151. Fleming PL, Ciesielski CA, Byers RH, et al. Gender differences in reported AIDS-indicative diagnoses. J Infect Dis. 1993;168:61–67.
152. Kreiss JK, Castro KG. Special considerations for managing suspected human immunodeficiency virus infection and AIDS in patients from developing countries. J Infect Dis. 1990;162:955–960.
153. Slutsker L, Castro KG, Ward JW, et al. Epidemiology of extrapulmonary tuberculosis among persons with AIDS in the United States. Clin Infect Dis. 1993;16:513–518.
154. Karon JM, Green TA, Hanson DL, Ward JW. Estimating the number of AIDS-defining opportunistic illness diagnoses from data collected under the 1993 AIDS surveillance definition. J Acquir Immune Defic Syndr Hum Retroviral. 1997;16:116–121.
155. Jones JL, Hanson DL, Dworkin MS, et al. Trends in AIDS-related opportunistic infections among men who have sex with men and among injecting drug users, 1991–96. J Infect Dis. 1998;178:114–120.
156. Cohn DL, Davidson AJ, Coca VJ, et al. Decreases in HIV-related morbidity, mortality and healthcare utilization related to highly active antiretroviral therapy (HAART). Abstract 13239. Presented at the Twelfth International Conference on AIDS, Geneva, 1998.
157. Holtzer CD, Jacobson MA, Hadley WK, et al. Decline in the rate of specific opportunistic infections at the San Francisco General Hospital, 1994–1997. AIDS. 1998;12:1931–1933.
158. Maniar J, Saple DG, Kurimura T. Changing pattern of opportunistic infections. Abstract 13245. Presented at the Twelfth International Conference on AIDS, Geneva, 1998.
159. Jacobson MA, Franch M. Altered natural history of AIDS-related opportunistic infections in the era of potent combination antiretroviral therapy. AIDS. 1998;12(Suppl A):S157–S163.
160. Mouron Y, Alfandari S, Valette M, et al. Impact of protease inhibitors on AIDS-defining events and hospitalizations in 10 French AIDS reference centers. AIDS. 1997;11:F101–F105.
161. Selwyn PA, Feingold AR, Hartel D, et al. Increased risk of bacterial pneumonia in HIV-infected intravenous drug users without AIDS. AIDS. 1988;2:167–172.
162. Janoff EN, Breiman RF, Daley CL, et al. Pneumococcal disease during HIV infection. Epidemiologic, clinical, and immunologic perspectives. Ann Intern Med. 1992;117:314–324.
163. Redd SC, Rutherford GW III, Sande MA, et al. The role of human immunodeficiency virus infection in pneumococcal bacteremia in San Francisco residents. J Infect Dis. 1990;162:1012–1017.
164. Laga M, Icenogle JP, Marsella R, et al. Genital papillomavirus infection and cervical dysplasia—opportunistic complications of HIV infection. Int J Cancer. 1992;50:45–48.
165. Ellerbrock T, Wright TC, Chiasson MA, et al. Strong independent association between HIV infection and cervical intraepithelial neoplasia (CIN) (Abstract WSB075). In: Abstracts of the IX International Conference on AIDS/IVth STD World Congress, v. 1. Berlin: 1993:50.
166. Wright T, Sun X, Ellerbrock T, et al. Human papillomavirus infections in HIV+ and HIV− women: Prevalence, association with cervical intraepithelial neoplasia, and impact of CD4+ count (Abstract WSB172). In: Abstracts of the IX International Conference on AIDS/IVth STD World Congress, v. 1. Berlin: 1993:60.
167. Barnes PF, Bloch AB, Davidson PT, et al. Tuberculosis in patients with human immunodeficiency virus infection. N Engl J Med. 1991;324:1644–1650.
168. Raviglione MC, Narain JP, Kochi A. HIV-associated tuberculosis in developing countries: Clinical features, diagnosis, and treatment. Bull World Health Organ. 1992;70:515–526.
169. Markowitz N, Harnsen NI, Hopewell PC, et al. Incidence of tuberculosis in the United States among HIV-infected persons. Ann Intern Med. 1997;126:123–132.
170. Centers for Disease Control and Prevention: Prevention of tuberculosis among patients infected with human immunodeficiency virus: Principles of therapy and revised recommendations. MMWR Morb Mortal Wkly Rep. 1998;47(RR = 20):1–58.
171. Braun MM, Cote TR, Rabkin CS. Trends in death with tuberculosis during the AIDS era. JAMA. 1993;269:2865–2868.
172. Rieder HL, Snider DE Jr. Tuberculosis and the acquired immunodeficiency syndrome (Editorial). Chest. 1986;90:469–470.
173. Havlir DV, Barnes PF. Tuberculosis in patients with human immunodeficiency virus infection. N Engl J Med. 1998;340:367–373.
174. Small PM, Hopewell PC, Singh SP, et al. The epidemiology of tuberculosis in San Francisco: A population based study using conventional and molecular methods. N Engl J Med. 1994;330:1703.
175. Alland D, Kalbut GE, Moss AR, et al. Transmission of tuberculosis in New York City: An analysis of DNA fingerprinting and conventional epidemiologic methods. N Engl J Med. 1994;330:1710.
176. Moore M, Onorato IM, McCoy E, Castro KG. Trends in drug-resistant tuberculosis in the United States, 1993–1996. JAMA. 1997;278:833–837.
177. Frieden TR, Sterling T, Pablos-Mendez A, et al. The emergence of drug-resistant tuberculosis in New York City. N Engl J Med. 1993;328:521–526.
178. Peloquin C, MacPhee AA, Berning SE. Malabsorption of antimycobacterial medications (Letter). N Engl J Med. 1993;329:1122.
179. Edlin BR, Tokars JI, Grieco MH, et al. An outbreak of multidrug-resistant tuberculosis among hospitalized patients with the acquired immunodeficiency syndrome. N Engl J Med. 1992;326:1514–1521.

180. Pearson ML, Jereb JA, Frieden TR, et al. Nosocomial transmission of multidrug-resistant *Mycobacterium tuberculosis*. A risk to patients and health care workers. Ann Intern Med. 1992;117:191–196.
181. BeckSague C, Dooley SW, Hutton MD, et al. Hospital outbreak of multidrug-resistant *Mycobacterium tuberculosis* infections. Factors in transmission to staff and HIV-infected patients. JAMA. 1992;268:1280–1286.
182. Centers for Disease Control and Prevention: Update: Mortality attributable to HIV-infection among persons aged 25–44 years—United States—1994. MMWR Morb Mortal Wkly Rep. 1996;45:121–125.
183. Centers for Disease Control and Prevention: Years of potential life lost before age 65—United States, 1990 and 1991. MMWR Morb Mortal Wkly Rep. 1993;42:251–252.
184. Turner BJ, Eppes S, McKee LJ, et al. A population-based comparison of the clinical course of children and adults with AIDS. AIDS. 1995;9:65–72.
185. Duliege AM, Messiah A, Blanche S, et al. Natural history of human immunodeficiency virus type 1 infection in children: Prognostic value of laboratory tests on the biomodal progression of the disease. Pediatr Infect Dis J. 1992;11:630–635.
186. McKinney RE Jr, Wilfert CM. Lymphocyte subsets in children younger than 2 years old: Normal values in a population at risk for human immunodeficiency virus infection and diagnostic and prognostic application to infected children. Pediatr Infect Dis J. 1992;11:639–644.
187. Waecker NJ Jr, Ascher DP, Robb ML, et al. Age-adjusted CD4+ lymphocyte parameters in healthy children at risk for infection with human immunodeficiency virus. Clin Infect Dis. 1993;17:123–125.
188. Quinn TC, Ruff A, Modlin J. HIV infection and AIDS in children. Annu Rev Public Health. 1992;13:1–30.
189. Centers for Disease Control and Prevention: AIDS among children—United States, 1996. MMWR Morb Mortal Wkly Rep. 1996;45:1005–1010.
190. Lifson AR, Rogers MF, White C, et al. Unrecognized modes of transmission of HIV: Acquired immunodeficiency syndrome in children reported without risk factors. Pediatr Infect Dis. 1987;6:292–293.
191. Connor EM, Sperling RS, Gelber R, et al. Reduction of maternal-infant transmission of human immunodeficiency virus type 1 with zidovudine treatment. N Engl J Med. 1994;331:1173–1180.
192. Centers for Disease Control and Prevention: Recommendations of the US Public Health Service Task Force on the use of zidovudine to reduce perinatal transmission of human immunodeficiency virus. MMWR Morb Mortal Wkly Rep. 1994;43(RR-11):1–20.
193. Centers for Disease Control and Prevention: US Public Health Service Recommendations for human immunodeficiency virus counseling and testing for pregnant women. MMWR Morb Mortal Wkly Rep. 1995;44(RR-7):1–15.
194. Centers for Disease Control and Prevention: Update: Perinatally acquired HIV/AIDS—United States, 1997. MMWR Morb Mortal Wkly Rep. 1997;46:1086–1092.
195. Centers for Disease Control and Prevention: Guidelines for prophylaxis against *Pneumocystis carinii* pneumonia for children infected with human immunodeficiency virus. MMWR Morb Mortal Wkly Rep. 1991;40(RR-2):1–13.
196. Scott GB, Hutto C, Makuch RW, et al. Survival in children with perinatally acquired human immunodeficiency virus type 1 infection. N Engl J Med. 1989;321:1791–1796.
197. Turner BJ, Denison M, Eppes SC, et al. Survival experience of 789 children with the acquired immunodeficiency syndrome. Pediatr Infect Dis J. 1993;12:310–320.
198. Centers for Disease Control and Prevention: Public Health Service recommendations for the use of antiretroviral drugs in pregnant women infected with HIV-1 for maternal health and for reducing perinatal HIV-1 transmission in the United States. MMWR Morb Mortal Wkly Rep. 1998;47(RR-2):1–30.
199. Padian NS. Heterosexual transmission of acquired immunodeficiency syndrome: International perspectives and national projections. Rev Infect Dis. 1987;9:947–960.
200. Chin J, Sato PA, Mann JM. Projections of HIV infections and AIDS cases to the year 2000. Bull World Health Organ. 1990;68:1–11.
201. Samuel MC, Hessol N, Shiboski S, et al. Factors associated with human immunodeficiency virus seroconversion in homosexual men in three San Francisco cohorts. J Acquir Immun Defic Syndr. 1993;6:303.
202. Cohen MS. Sexually transmitted diseases enhance HIV transmission: No longer a hypothesis. Lancet. 1998;351:(Suppl 3):S5–S7.
203. Quinn TC. Association of sexually transmitted diseases and infection with the human immunodeficiency virus: Biological cofactors and markers of behavioral interventions. Int J STD AIDS. 1996;7(Suppl 2):S17–S24.
204. Clumeck N, Taelman H, Hermans P, et al. A cluster of HIV infection among heterosexual people without apparent risk factors. N Engl J Med. 1989;321:1460–1462.
205. Peterman TA, Stoneburner RL, Allen JR, et al. Risk of human immunodeficiency virus transmission from heterosexual adults with transfusion-associated infections. JAMA. 1988;59:55–58.
206. Johnson AM, Petherick A, Davidson SJ, et al. Transmission of HIV to heterosexual partners of infected men and women. AIDS. 1989;3:367–372.
207. Seidlin M, Vogler M, Lee E, et al. Heterosexual transmission of HIV in a cohort of couples in New York City. AIDS. 1993;7:1247.
208. Goedert JJ, Eyster ME, Bigger RJ, et al. Heterosexual transmission of human immunodeficiency virus: Association with severe depletion of T-helper lymphocytes in men with hemophilia. AIDS Res Hum Retroviruses. 1987;3:355–361.
209. European Study Group on Heterosexual Transmission of HIV. Comparison of female to male and male to female transmission of HIV in 563 stable couples. BMJ. 1992;304:809–813.
210. Lazzarin A, Saracco A, Musicco M, et al. Man-to-woman sexual transmission of the human immunodeficiency virus. Risk factors related to sexual behavior, man's infectiousness, and woman's susceptibility. Arch Intern Med. 1991;151:2411–2416.
211. Laga M, Taelman H, Van der Stuyft P, et al. Advanced immunodeficiency as a risk factor for heterosexual transmission of HIV. AIDS. 1989;3:361–366.
212. Seage GR III, Mayer KH, Horsburgh CR Jr. Risk of human immunodeficiency virus infection from unprotected receptive anal intercourse increases with decline in immunologic status of infected partners. Am J Epidemiol. 1993;137:899–908.
213. Anderson DJ, Hill JA. CD4 (T4+) lymphocytes in semen of healthy heterosexual men: Implications for the transmission of AIDS (Letter). Fertil Steril. 1987;48:703–704.
214. Anderson DJ, O'Brien TR, Politch JA, et al. Effects of disease stage and zidovudine therapy on the detection of human immunodeficiency virus type 1 in semen. JAMA. 1992;267:2769–2774.
215. Ho DD, Moudgil T, Alam M. Quantitation of human immunodeficiency virus type 1 in the blood of infected persons. N Engl J Med. 1989;321:1621–1625.
216. Hénin Y, Mandelbrot L, Henrion R, et al. Virus excretion in the cervical secretions of pregnant and nonpregnant HIV-infected women. J Acquir Immune Defic Syndr. 1993;6:72–75.
217. Boyce RA, Seña A, Cates W, Cohen MS. Sexual transmission of HIV. N Engl J Med. 1997;336:1072–1078.
218. Vernezza PL, Eron JJ, Cohen MS, et al. Detection and biologic characterization of infectious HIV-1 in semen of seropositive men. AIDS. 1994;8:1325–1329.
219. Krieger JM, Coombs RW, Collier AC, et al. Recovery of human immunodeficiency virus type 1 from semen: Minimal impact of stage of infection and current antiviral chemotherapy. J Infect Dis. 1991;163:386–388.
220. Musicco M, Lazzarin A, Nicolasi A, et al. Antiretroviral treatment of men infected with human immunodeficiency virus type 1 reduces the incidence of heterosexual transmission: Italian Study Group on HIV Heterosexual Transmission. Arch Intern Med. 1994;154:1971–1976.
221. Zhang H, Dornadula G, Beumont M, et al. Human immunodeficiency virus type 1 in the semen of men receiving highly active antiretroviral therapy. N Engl J Med. 1998;339:1803–1809.
222. Rasheed S, Li Z, Xu D, Kovacs A. Presence of cell-free human immunodeficiency virus in cervicovaginal secretions is independent of viral load in the blood in human immunodeficiency virus–infected women. Am J Obstet Gynecol. 1996;175:122–129.
223. Eron JJ, Vernazza PL, Johnston DM, et al. Resistance of HIV-1 to antiretroviral agents in blood and seminal plasma: Implications for transmission. AIDS. 1998;12:F181–F189.
224. Haase AT, Schacker TW. Potential for transmission of HIV-1 despite highly active antiretroviral therapy. N Engl J Med. 1998;339:1846–1848.
225. Padian NS, Shiboski SC, Jewell NP. Female-to-male transmission of human immunodeficiency virus. JAMA. 1991;266:1664–1667.
226. Padian NS, Shiboski SC, Jewell NP. The effect of number of exposures on the risk of heterosexual HIV transmission. J Infect Dis. 1990;161:883–887.
227. Rothenberg RB, Scarlett M, del Rio C, et al. Oral transmission of HIV. AIDS. 1998;12:2095–2105.
228. Goto Y, Yeh CK, Notkins AL, et al. Detection of proviral sequences in saliva of patients infected with human immunodeficiency virus type 1. AIDS Res Hum Retroviruses. 1991;7:343–347.
229. Levy JA, Greenspan D. HIV in saliva (Letter). Lancet. 1988;2:1248.
230. Piot P, Plummer PA. Genital ulcer adenopathy syndrome. In: Holmes KK, Mardh PA, Sparling PF, eds. Sexually Transmitted Diseases. 2nd ed. New York: McGraw-Hill; 1990:711–716.
231. Piot P, Laga M. Genital ulcers, other sexually transmitted diseases, and the sexual transmission of HIV. The first two may be important risk factors for the third. BMJ. 1989;298:623–624.
232. Plummer FA, Simonsen JN, Cameron DW, et al. Cofactors in male-female sexual transmission of human immunodeficiency virus type 1. J Infect Dis. 1991;163:233–239.
233. Cameron DW, Simonsen JN, D'Costa LJ, et al. Female to male transmission of human immunodeficiency virus type 1: Risk factors for seroconversion in men. Lancet. 1989;2:403–407.
234. Stamm WE, Handsfield HH, Rompalo AM, et al. The association between genital ulcer disease and acquisition of HIV infection in homosexual men. JAMA. 1988;260:1429–1433.
235. Kreiss KJ, Coombs R, Plummer F, et al. Isolation of human immunodeficiency virus from genital ulcers in Nairobi prostitutes. J Infect Dis. 1989;160:380–384.
236. Moss GB, Overbaugh J, Welch M, et al. Human immunodeficiency virus DNA in urethral secretions in men: Association with gonococcal urethritis and CD4 depletion. J Infect Dis. 1995;172:1469–1474.
237. Atkins MC, Carlin EM, Emery VC, et al. Fluctuations of HIV load in semen of HIV positive patients with newly acquired sexually transmitted diseases. BMJ. 1996;313:341–342.
238. Greenblatt RM, Lukehart SA, Plummer FA, et al. Genital ulceration as a risk factor for human immunodeficiency virus infection. AIDS. 1988;2:47–50.
239. Holmberg SD, Stewart JA, Gerber AR, et al. Prior herpes simplex virus type 2 infection as a risk factor for HIV infection. JAMA. 1988;259:1048–1050.
240. Laga M, Manoka A, Kivuvu M, et al. Non-ulcerative sexually transmitted diseases as risk factor for HIV-1 transmission in women: Results from a cohort study. AIDS. 1993;7:95–102.
241. Kapiga SH, Shao JF, Lwihula GK, et al. Risk factors for HIV infection among women in Dar-es-Salaam, Tanzania. J Acquir Immune Defic Syndr. 1994;7:301–309.
242. Cohen CR, Duerr A, Pruithithada N, et al. Bacterial vaginosis and HIV seropreva-

lence among female commercial sex workers in Chaing Mai, Thailand. AIDS. 1995;9:1093–1097.
243. Hira SK, Kamanga J, Macuacua R, et al. Genital ulcers and male circumcision as risk factors for acquiring HIV-1 in Zambia (Letter). J Infect Dis. 1990;161:584–585.
244. Jessamine PG, Plummer FA, Achola JON, et al. Human immunodeficiency virus, genital ulcers and the male foreskin: Synergism in HIV-1 transmission. Scand J Infect Dis. 1990;69(Suppl):S181–S186.
245. Kreiss J, Ngugi E, Holmes K, et al. Efficacy of nonoxynol 9 contraceptive sponge use in preventing heterosexual acquisition of HIV in Nairobi prostitutes. JAMA. 1992;268:477–482.
246. Stone KM, Peterson HB. Spermicides, HIV, and the vaginal sponge (Editorial). JAMA. 1992;268:521–523.
247. Grosskurth H, Mosha F, Todd J, et al. Impact of improved treatment of sexually transmitted diseases on HIV infection in rural Tanzania: Randomized controlled trial. Lancet. 1995;346:530–536.
248. Darrow WW, Echenberg DF, Jaffe HW, et al. Risk factors for human immunodeficiency virus (HIV) infections in homosexual men. Am J Public Health. 1987;77:479–483.
249. Winkelstein W, Lyman DM, Padian N, et al. Sexual practices and risk of infection by the human immunodeficiency virus. The San Francisco Men's Health Study. JAMA. 1987;257:321–325.
250. Kingsley LA, Detels R, Kaslow R, et al. Risk factors for seroconversion to human immunodeficiency virus among male homosexuals. Results from the Multicenter AIDS Cohort Study. Lancet. 1987;1:345–349.
251. Chu SY, Hammett TA, Buehler JW. Update: Epidemiology of reported cases of AIDS in women who report sex only with other women, United States, 1980–1991. AIDS. 1992;6:518.
252. Petersen LR, Doll L, White C, et al. No evidence for female-to-female HIV transmission among 960,000 female blood donors. J Acquir Immune Defic Syndr. 1992;5:853–855.
253. Marmor M, Weiss LR, Lyden M, et al. Possible female-to-female transmission of human immunodeficiency virus (Letter). Ann Intern Med. 1986;105:969.
254. Monzon OT, Capellan JMB. Female-to-female transmission of HIV (Letter). Lancet. 1987;2:40–41.
255. Rich JD, Buck A, Tuomala RE, et al. Transmission of human immunodeficiency virus infection presumed to have occurred via female-homosexual contact. Clin Infect Dis. 1993;17:1003.
256. Moss GB, Clemetson D, D'Costa L, et al. Association of cervical ectopy with heterosexual transmission of human immunodeficiency virus: Results of a study of couples in Nairobi, Kenya. J Infect Dis. 1991;164:588–591.
257. Dean M, Carrington M, Winkler C, et al. Genetic restriction of HIV-1 infection and progression to AIDS by a deletion allele of the CKR5 structural gene. Science. 1996;273:1856–1862.
258. Schoenbaum EE, Hartel D, Selwyn PA, et al. Risk factors for human immunodeficiency virus infection in intravenous drug users. N Engl J Med. 1989;321:874–879.
259. Lange WR, Synder FR, Lozovsky D, et al. The geographic distribution of human immunodeficiency virus markers in parenteral drug abusers. Am J Public Health. 1988;78:443–446.
260. Anthony JC, Vlahov D, Nelson KE, et al. New evidence on intravenous cocaine use and the risk of infection with human immunodeficiency virus type 1. Am J Epidemiol. 1991;134:1175–1189.
261. Koblin BA, McCusker J, Lewis BF, et al. Racial/ethnic differences in HIV-1 seroprevalence and risky behaviors among intravenous drug users in a multisite study. Am J Epidemiol. 1990;132:837–846.
262. Selik RM, Castro KG, Pappaioanou M, et al. Birthplace and the risk of AIDS among Hispanics in the United States. Am J Public Health. 1989;79:836–839.
263. McCusker J, Koblin B, Lewis BF, et al. Demographic characteristics, risk behaviors, and HIV seroprevalence among intravenous drug users by site of contact: Results from a communitywide HIV surveillance project. Am J Public Health. 1990;80:1062–1067.
264. Nelson KE, Vlahov D, Cohn S, et al. Sexually transmitted diseases in a population of intravenous drug users: Association with seropositivity to the human immunodeficiency virus (HIV). J Infect Dis. 1991;164:457–463.
265. Rolfs RT, Goldberg M, Sharrar RG. Risk factors for syphilis: Cocaine use and prostitution. Am J Public Health. 1990;80:853–857.
266. Magura S, Grossman JI, Lipton DS, et al. Determinants of needle sharing among intravenous drug users. Am J Public Health. 1989;79:459–462.
267. Guydish JR, Abramowitz A, Woods W, et al. Changes in needle sharing behavior among intravenous drug users: San Francisco, 1986–88. Am J Public Health. 1990;80:995–997.
268. Neaigus A, Sufian M, Friedman SR, et al. Effects of outreach intervention on risk reduction among intravenous drug users. AIDS Educ Prev. 1990;2:253–271.
269. Curran JW, Lawrence DN, Jaffe H, et al. Acquired immunodeficiency syndrome (AIDS) associated with transfusions. N Engl J Med. 1984;310:69–75.
270. Evatt BL, Ramsey RB, Lawrence DN, et al. The acquired immunodeficiency syndrome in patients with hemophilia. Ann Intern Med. 1984;100:499–504.
271. Donegan E, Stuart M, Niland JC, et al. Infection with human immunodeficiency virus type 1 (HIV1) among recipients of antibody-positive blood donations. Ann Intern Med. 1990;113:733–739.
272. Ward JW, Deppe DA, Samson S, et al. Risk of human immunodeficiency virus infection from blood donors who later developed the acquired immunodeficiency syndrome. Ann Intern Med. 1987;106:61–62.
273. Centers for Disease Control and Prevention: Safety of therapeutic immune globulin preparations with respect to transmission of human T-lymphocytropic virus type III/lymphadenopathy-associated virus infection. MMWR Morb Mortal Wkly Rep. 1986;35:231–233.
274. Wells MA, Wittek AE, Epstein JS, et al. Inactivation and partition of human T-cell lymphotrophic virus, type III, during ethanol fractionation of plasma. Transfusion. 1986;26:210–213.
275. Ward JW, Grindon AJ, Feorino PM, et al. Laboratory and epidemiologic evaluation of an enzyme immunoassay for antibodies to HTL V-III. JAMA. 1986;256:357–361.
276. Peterman TA, Lui KJ, Lawrence DN, et al. Estimating the risks of transfusion-associated acquired immune deficiency syndrome and human immunodeficiency virus infection. Transfusion. 1987;27:371–374.
277. Lackritz EM, Satten GA, Aberle-Grasse J, et al. Estimated risk of transmission of the human immunodeficiency virus by screened blood in the United States. N Engl J Med. 1995;333:1721–1725.
278. Schreiber GB, Bush MP, Kleinman SH, Korelitz JJ. The risk of transfusion-transmitted viral infections. N Engl J Med. 1996;334:1635–1690.
279. StehrGreen JK, Jason JM, Evatt BL, et al. Geographic variability of hemophilia-associated AIDS in the United States: Effect of population characteristics. Am J Hematol. 1989;32:178–183.
280. Eyster ME, Gail MH, Ballard ID, et al. Natural history of human immunodeficiency virus infection in hemophiliacs: Effects of T-cell subsets, platelet counts and age. Ann Intern Med. 1987;107:1–6.
281. Erice A, Rhame FS, Heussner RC, et al. Human immunodeficiency virus infection in patients with solid-organ transplants: Report of five cases and review. Rev Infect Dis. 1991;13:537–547.
282. Clarke JA. HIV transmission and skin grafts. Lancet. 1987;1:983.
283. Pepose JS, McRae S, Quinn TC, et al. Serologic markers after the transplantation of corneas from donors infected with human immunodeficiency virus. Am J Ophthalmol. 1987;103:798–801.
284. Glasser DB. Serologic testing of cornea donors. Cornea. 1998;17:123–128.
285. Lewis SH, Reynolds-Kohler C, Fox HE, et al. HIV-1 in trophoblastic and villous Hofbauer cells, and haematological precursors in eight-week fetuses. Lancet. 1990;335:565–568.
286. Douglas GC, King BF. Maternal-fetal transmission of human immunodeficiency virus: A review of possible routes and cellular mechanisms of infection. Clin Infect Dis. 1992;15:678–691.
287. Krivine A, Firtion G, Cao L, et al. HIV replication during the first weeks of life. Lancet. 1992;339:1187–1189.
288. Rogers MF, Ou CY, Rayfield M, et al. Use of the polymerase chain reaction for early detection of the proviral sequences of human immunodeficiency virus in infants born to seropositive mothers. N Engl J Med. 1989;320:1649–1654.
289. Burgard M, Mayaux MJ, Blanche S, et al. The use of viral culture and p24 antigen testing to diagnose human immunodeficiency virus infection in neonates. N Engl J Med. 1992;327:1192–1197.
290. Rogers MF, Schochetman G, Hoff R. Advances in diagnosis of HIV infection in infants. In: Pizzo PA, Wilfert CM, eds. Pediatric AIDS: The Challenge of HIV Infection in Infants, Children and Adolescents. 2nd ed. Baltimore: Williams & Wilkins; 1994:219–238.
291. Ehrnst A, Lindgren S, Dictor M, et al. HIV in pregnant women and their offspring: Evidence for late transmission. Lancet. 1991;338:203–207.
292. European Collaborative Study. Risk factors for mother-to-child transmission of HIV-1. Lancet. 1992;339:1007–1012.
293. Gabiano C, Tovo PA, de Martino M, et al. Mother-to-child transmission of human immunodeficiency virus type 1: Risk of infection and correlates of transmission. Pediatrics. 1992;90:369–374.
294. Blanche S, Rouzioux C, Moscato MLG, et al. A prospective study of infants born to women seropositive for human immunodeficiency virus type 1. N Engl J Med. 1989;320:1643–1648.
295. Hutto C, Parks WP, Lai S, et al. A hospital-based prospective study of perinatal infection with human immunodeficiency virus type 1. J Pediatr. 1991;118:347–353.
296. Goedert JJ, Duliege AM, Amos CI, et al. High risk of HIV-1 infection for firstborn twins. Lancet. 1991;338:1471–1475.
297. The International Perinatal HIV Group. The mode of delivery and the risk of vertical transmission of human immunodeficiency virus type 1—a meta-analysis of 15 prospective cohort studies. N Engl J Med. 1999;340:977–987.
298. Thiry L, Sprecher-Goldberger S, Jonchkheer T, et al. Isolation of AIDS virus from cell-free breast milk of three healthy virus carriers (Letter). Lancet. 1985;2:891–892.
299. Oxtoby MJ. Human immunodeficiency virus and other viruses in human milk: Placing the issues in broader perspective. Pediatr Infect Dis J. 1988;7:825–835.
300. Phuapradit W. Timing and mechanism of perinatal human immunodeficiency virus-1 infection. Aust N Z J Ostet Gynaecol. 1998;38:293–297.
301. Ryder RW, Manzila T, Baende E, et al. Evidence from Zaire that breastfeeding by HIV-1 seropositive mothers is not a major route for perinatal HIV-1 transmission but does decrease morbidity. AIDS. 1991;5:709–714.
302. Dunn DT, Newell ML, Ades AE, et al. Risk of human immunodeficiency virus type 1 transmission through breastfeeding. Lancet. 1992;340:585–588.
303. Van de Perre P, Simonon A, Msellati P, et al. Postnatal transmission of human immunodeficiency virus type 1 from mother to infant. A prospective cohort study in Kigali, Rwanda. N Engl J Med. 1991;325:593–598.
304. Palasithran P, Ziegler JB, Stewart GJ, et al. Breastfeeding during primary human immunodeficiency virus infection and risk of transmission from mother to infant. J Infect Dis. 1993;167:441.
305. Hu DJ, Heyward WL, Byers RH Jr, et al. HIV infection and breastfeeding: Policy implications through a decision analysis model. AIDS. 1992;6:1505–1513.

306. Ryder RW, Nsa W, Hassig SE, et al. Perinatal transmission of the human immunodeficiency virus type 1 to infants of seropositive women in Zaire. N Engl J Med. 1989;320:1637–1642.
307. Dickover RE, Garratty EM, Horman SA, et al. Identification of levels of maternal HIV-1 RNA associated with risk of perinatal transmission: Effect of maternal zidovudine treatment on viral load. JAMA. 1996;275:599–605.
308. Sandberg RS, Shapiro DE, Coombs RW, et al. Maternal viral load, zidovudine treatment and the risk of transmission of human immunodeficiency virus type 1 from mother to infants. N Engl J Med. 1996;335:1621–1629.
309. St. Louis ME, Kamenga M, Brown C, et al. Risk for perinatal HIV-1 transmission according to maternal immunologic, virologic, and placental factors. JAMA. 1993;269:2853–2859.
310. Kuhn L, Steketee RW, Weedon J, et al. Distinct risk factors for intrauterine and intrapartum human immunodeficiency virus transmission and consequences for disease progression in infected children. J Infect Dis. 1999;179:52–58.
311. Borkowsky W, Krasinski K, Pollack H, et al. Early diagnosis of human immunodeficiency virus infection in children <6 months of age: Comparison of polymerase chain reaction, culture, and plasma antigen capture techniques. J Infect Dis. 1992;166:616–619.
312. Report of a Consensus Workshop, Siena, Italy, January 17–18, 1992. Early diagnosis of HIV infection in infants. J Acquir Immune Defic Syndr. 1992;5:1169–1178.
312a. Nesheim S, Lee F, Sawyer M, et al. Diagnosis of human immunodeficiency virus infection by enzyme-linked immunospot assays in a prospectively followed cohort of infants of human immunodeficiency virus-seropositive women. Pediatr Infect Dis J. 1992;11:635–639.
313. Tokars JI, Bell DM, Culver DH, et al. Percutaneous injuries during surgical procedures. JAMA. 1992;267:2899–2904.
314. Marcus R, Culver DH, Bell DM, et al. Risk of human immunodeficiency virus infection among emergency department workers. Am J Med. 1993;94:363–370.
315. Wong ES, Stotka JL, Chinchilli VM, et al. Are universal precautions effective in reducing the number of occupational exposures among health care workers? A prospective study of physicians on a medical service. JAMA. 1991;265:1123–1128.
316. Tokars JI, Marcus R, Culver DH, et al. Surveillance of HIV infection and zidovudine use among health care workers after occupational exposure to HIV-infected blood. Ann Intern Med. 1993;118:913–919.
317. Henderson DK, Fahey BJ, Willy M, et al. Risk for occupational transmission of human immunodeficiency virus type 1 (HIV 1) associated with clinical exposures. A prospective evaluation. Ann Intern Med. 1990;113:740–746.
318. Gerberding JL. Incidence and prevalence of human immunodeficiency virus, hepatitis B virus, hepatitis C virus and cytomegalovirus among health care personnel at risk for blood exposure: Final report from a longitudinal study. J Infect Dis. 1994;170:1410–1417.
319. Ippolito G, Puro V, De Carli G. The risk of occupational human immunodeficiency virus infection in health care workers. Italian multicenter study. Arch Intern Med. 1993;153:1451–1458.
320. Chamberland ME, Conley LJ, Bush TJ, et al. Health care workers with AIDS. National surveillance update. JAMA. 1991;266:3459–3462.
321. Chamberland ME, Bell DM. HIV transmission from health care worker to patient: What is the risk (Editorial). Ann Intern Med. 1992;116:871–873.
322. Gerberding J. Provider-to-patient HIV transmission: How to keep it exceedingly rare. Ann Intern Med. 1999;130:1–6.
323. Ciesielski C, Marianos D, Ou CY, et al. Transmission of human immunodeficiency virus in a dental practice. Ann Intern Med. 1992;116:798–805.
324. Centers for Disease Control and Prevention: Update: Investigations of patients who have been treated by HIV-infected healthcare workers—United States. MMWR Morb Mortal Wkly Rep. 1993;42:329–337.
325. Lot F, Séguier JC, Fégueux S, et al. Probable transmission of HIV from an orthopedic surgeon to a patient in France. Ann Intern Med. 1999;130:1–6.
326. Ou CY, Ciesielski CA, Myers G, et al. Molecular epidemiology of HIV transmission in a dental practice. Science. 1992;256:1165–1171.
327. Bell DM, Shapiro CN, Gooch BF. Preventing HIV transmission to patients during invasive procedures. J Public Health Dent. 1993;53:170–173.
328. Robert LM, Chamberland ME, Cleveland JL, et al. Investigations of patients of health care workers infected with HIV: the Centers for Disease Control and Prevention database. Ann Intern Med. 1995;122:653.
329. Centers for Disease Control and Prevention. Patient exposures to HIV during nuclear medicine procedures. MMWR Morb Mortal Wkly Rep. 1992;41:575–578.
330. Centers for Disease Control and Prevention. HIV infection in two brothers receiving intravenous therapy for hemophilia. MMWR Morb Mortal Wkly Rep. 1992;41:228–231.
331. Centers for Disease Control and Prevention. Human immunodeficiency virus transmission in household settings—United States. MMWR Morb Mortal Wkly Rep. 1994;43:347, 353–356.
332. Hersh BS, Popovici F, Apetrei RC, et al. Acquired immunodeficiency syndrome in Romania. Lancet. 1991;338:645–649.
333. Pokrovsky VV, Eramova EU. Nosocomial outbreak of HIV infection in Elista, USSR. Abstract W.A.O.5. Presented at the Fifth International Conference on AIDS. Montreal, June 4–9, 1989.
334. Chant K, Lowe D, Rubin G, et al. Patient-to-patient transmission of HIV in private surgical consulting rooms (Letter). Lancet. 1993;342:1548–1549.
335. Fujikawa LS, Salahuddin SZ, Palestine AG, et al. Isolation of human T-lymphotropic virus type III from the tears of a patient with the acquired immunodeficiency syndrome. Lancet. 1985;2:529–530.
336. Ho DD, Rota TR, Schooley RT, et al. Isolation of HTL V-III from cerebrospinal fluid and neural tissues of patients with neurologic syndromes related to the acquired immunodeficiency syndrome. N Engl J Med. 1985;313:1493–1497.
337. Mundy DC, Schinazi RF, Gerber AR, et al. Human immunodeficiency virus isolated from amniotic fluid (Letter). Lancet. 1987;2:459–460.
338. Hill DR. HIV infection following motor vehicle trauma in central Africa. JAMA. 1989;261:3282–3283.
339. Torre D, Sampietro C, Ferraro G, et al. Transmission of HIV-1 infection via sports injury (Letter). Lancet. 1990;335:1105.
340. Stewart GJ, Tyler JPP, Cunningham AL, et al. Transmission of human T-cell lymphotropic virus type III (HTL V-III) by artificial insemination by donor. Lancet. 1985;2:581–585.
341. Chiasson MA, Stoneburner RL, Joseph SC. Human immunodeficiency virus transmission through artificial insemination. J Acquir Immune Defic Syndr. 1990;3:69–72.
342. Centers for Disease Control and Prevention: HIV-1 infection and artificial insemination with processed semen. MMWR Morb Mortal Wkly Rep. 1990;39:249, 255–256.
343. Yeh CK, Handelman B, Fox PC, et al. Further studies of salivary inhibition of HIV-1 infectivity. J Acquir Immun Defic Syndr. 1992;5:898–903.
344. Wahn V, Kramer HH, Voit T, et al. Horizontal transmission of HIV infection between two siblings (Letter). Lancet. 1986;2:694.
345. Rogers MF, White CR, Sanders R, et al. Lack of transmission of human immunodeficiency virus from infected children to their household contacts. Pediatrics. 1990;85:210–214.
346. Saviteer SM, White GC, Cohen MS, et al. HTLV-III exposure during cardiopulmonary resuscitation (Letter). N Engl J Med. 1985;313:1606–1607.
347. Lifson AR. Do alternate modes for transmission of human immunodeficiency virus exist? A review. JAMA. 1988;259:1353–1356.
348. Gershon RRM, Vlahov D, Nelson KE. The risk of transmission of HIV-1 through nonpercutaneous, nonsexual modes—A review. AIDS. 1990;4:645–650.
349. Lusher JM, Operskalski EA, Aledort LM, et al. Risk of human immunodeficiency virus type 1 infection among sexual and nonsexual household contacts of persons with congenital clotting disorders. Pediatrics. 1991;88:242–249.
350. Centers for Disease Control and Prevention: Apparent transmission of human T-lymphotrophic virus type III/lymphadenopathy-associated virus from a child to a mother providing health care. MMWR Morb Mortal Wkly Rep. 1986;35:76–79.
351. Centers for Disease Control and Prevention: HIV transmission between two adolescent brothers with hemophilia. MMWR Morb Mortal Wkly Rep. 1993;42:948–951.
352. Fitzgibbon JE, Gaur S, Frenkel LD, et al. Transmission from one child to another of human immunodeficiency virus type 1 with a zidovudine-resistance mutation. N Engl J Med. 1993;329:1835–1846.
353. Grint P, McEvoy M. Two associated cases of the acquired immunodeficiency syndrome (AIDS). Commun Dis Rep. 1985;42:4.
354. Srinivasan A, York D, Bohan C. Lack of HIV replication in arthropod cells (Letter). Lancet. 1987;1:1094–1095.
355. Miike L. Do Insects Transmit AIDS? Washington, DC: Health Program, Office of Technology Assessment, U.S. Congress; 1987:1–43.
356. Webb PA, Happ CM, Maupin GO, et al. Potential for insect transmission of HIV: Experimental exposure of *Cimex hemipterus* and *Toxorhynchites amboinensis* to human immunodeficiency virus. J Infect Dis. 1989;160:970–977.
357. Castro KG, Lieb S, Jaffe HW, et al. Transmission of HIV in Belle Glade, Florida: Lessons for other communities in the United States. Science. 1988;239:193–197.
358. Greenberg AE, Nguyen-Dinh P, Mann JM, et al. The association between malaria, blood transfusions, and HIV seropositivity in a pediatric population in Kinshasa, Zaire. JAMA. 1988;259:545–549.
359. World Health Organization. Global AIDS Surveillance. Wkly Epidemiol Rec. 1997;72:357–364.
360. UNAIDS and WHO. AIDS Epidemic Update: December 1998. Geneva, Switzerland.
361. World Health Organization. Global AIDS surveillance. Part II. Wkly Epidemiol Rec. 1997;72:356–372.
362. Mertens TE, Belsey E, Stoneburner RL, et al. Global estimates of HIV infections and AIDS: Further heterogeneity in spread and impact. AIDS. 1995;9(Suppl 1):S251.
363. Mann JM, Tarantola DJM, eds. AIDS in the World: II. Cambridge: Oxford University Press; 1996:61.
364. Cortes E, Detels R, Aboulafia D, et al. HIV-1, HIV-2, and HTLV-I infection in high risk groups in Brazil. N Engl J Med. 1989;320:953–958.
365. Torrey BB, Way PO. Seroprevalence of HIV in Africa: Winter 1990. CIR staff paper No. 55. Washington, DC: Center for International Research, U.S. Bureau of the Census; 1990.
366. Rwandan HIV Seroprevalence Study Group. Nationwide community based serological survey of HIV-1 and other human retrovirus infections in a central African country. Lancet. 1989;1:941–943.
367. Serwadda D, Wawer MJ, Musgrave SD, et al. HIV risk factors in three geographic strata of rural Rakai District, Uganda. AIDS. 1992;6:983–989.
368. Miotti PG, Dallabetta GA, Ndovi E, et al. HIV-1 and pregnant women: Associated factors, prevalence, estimate of incidence and role in fetal wastage in Central Africa. AIDS. 1990;4:733–736.
369. Allen S, Lindan C, Serufilira A, et al. Human immunodeficiency virus infection in urban Rwanda: Demographic and behavioral correlates in a representative sample of childbearing women. JAMA. 1991;226:1657–1663.
370. N'Galy B, Ryder RW. Epidemiology of HIV infection in Africa. J Acquir Immune Defic Syndr. 1988;1:551–558.
371. Dallabetta GA, Miotti PG, Chiphangwi JD, et al. High socioeconomic status is a

risk factor for human immunodeficiency virus type 1 (HIV-1) infection but not for sexually transmitted diseases in women in Malawi: Implications for HIV-1 control. J Infect Dis. 1993;167:36–42.
372. Piot P, Plummer FA, Rey MA, et al. Retrospective seroepidemiology of AIDS virus infections in Nairobi populations. J Infect Dis. 1987;155:1108–1112.
373. Simonsen JN, Plummer FA, Ngugi EN, et al. HIV infection among lower socioeconomic strata prostitutes in Nairobi. AIDS. 1990;4:139–144.
374. Simonsen JN, Cameron W, Gakinya MN, et al. Human immunodeficiency virus infection among men with sexually transmitted diseases. N Engl J Med. 1988;319:274–278.
375. Pape JW, Stanback ME, Pamphile M, et al. Prevalence of HIV infection and high-risk activities in Haiti. J Acquir Immune Defic Syndr. 1990;3:995–1001.
376. Diallo MO, Ackah AN, Lafontaine MF, et al. HIV-1 and HIV-2 infections in men attending sexually transmitted disease clinics in Abidjan, Cote D'Ivoire. AIDS. 1992;6:581–585.
377. Lackritz EM. Prevention of HIV transmission by blood transfusion in the developing world: Achievements and continuing challenges. AIDS. 1998;12(Suppl A):S81.
378. Weniger BG, Limpakarnjanarat K, Ungchusak K, et al. The epidemiology of HIV infection and AIDS in Thailand. AIDS. 1991;5(Suppl 2):S71–S85.
379. Ou CY, Takebe Y, Weniger BG, et al. Independent introduction of two major HIV-1 genotypes into distinct high-risk populations in Thailand. Lancet. 1993;341:1171–1174.
380. Sirisopana N, Torugsa K, Carr J, et al. Prevalence of HIV-1 infection in young men entering the Royal Thai Army (Abstract POCO82778). In: Abstracts of the IXth International Conference on AIDS/IVth STD World Congress, v. 2. Berlin: 1993:680.
381. Jain MK, John JT, Keusch GT. Epidemiology of HIV and AIDS in India. AIDS. 1994;8(Suppl 2):S61–S75.
382. Ryan CA, Vathiny OV, Gorbach PM, et al. Explosive spread of HIV-1 and sexually transmitted diseases in Cambodia. Lancet. 1998;351:1175.
383. Singh YN, Malaviya AN, Tripathy SP, et al. HIV serosurveillance among prostitutes and patients from a sexually transmitted diseases clinic in Delhi, India. J Acquir Immune Defic Syndr. 1990;3:287–289.
384. Singh S, Crofts N, Gertig D. HIV infection among IDU's in northeast Malaysia (Abstract POCO82777). In: Abstracts of the IXth International Conference on AIDS/IVth STD World Congress, v. 2. Berlin: 1993:680.
385. Zheng X, Thian C, Zhang J, et al. Rapid spread of HIV among drug users and their wives in southwest China (Abstract POCO82766). In: Abstracts of the IXth International Conference on AIDS/IVth STD World Congress, v. 2 Berlin: 1993:678.
386. Lindan CP, Lieu TX, Giang LT, et al. Rising HIV infection rates in Ho Chi Minh City herald emerging AIDS epidemic in Vietnam. AIDS. 1997;11(Suppl 1):S513.
387. Oh Md, Choe K, Shin Y, et al. Current status of HIV/AIDS epidemic in South Korea (Abstract POCO82769). In: Abstracts of the IXth International Conference on AIDS/IVth STD World Congress, v. 2. Berlin: 1993:678.
388. Soda K, Fukutomi K, Hashimoto S, et al. Temporal trend and projections of HIV/AIDS epidemic in Japan (Abstract POCO82779). In: Abstracts of the IXth International Conference on AIDS/IVth STD World Congress, v. 2. Berlin: 1993:680.
389. Gromyko A. Challenge of HIV/AIDS and STD rising trends in Eastern Europe. Abstract 60107. Presented at the Twelfth International Conference on AIDS, Geneva, 1998.
390. Clavel F, Guetard D, Brun-Vezinet F, et al. Isolation of a new human retrovirus from West African patients with AIDS. Science. 1986;233:343–346.
391. Centers for Disease Control and Prevention: Testing for antibodies to human immunodeficiency virus type 2 in the United States. MMWR Morb Mortal Wkly Rep. 1992;41(RR-12):1–9.
392. DeCock KM, Adjorlolo G, Ekpini E, et al. Epidemiology and transmission of HIV-2: Why there is no HIV-2 pandemic. JAMA. 1993;270:2083–2086.
393. O'Brien TR, George JR, Holmberg SD. Human immunodeficiency virus type 2 infection in the United States: Epidemiology, diagnosis, and public health implications. JAMA. 1992;267:2775–2779.
394. Onorato IM, O'Brien TR, Schable CA, et al. Sentinel surveillance for HIV-2 infection in high-risk US populations. Am J Public Health. 1993;83:515–519.
395. Markovitz DM. Infection with the human immunodeficiency virus type 2. Ann Intern Med. 1993;118:211–218.
396. Poulsen AG, Kvinesdal BB, Aaby P, et al. Lack of evidence of vertical transmission of human immunodeficiency virus type 2 in a sample of the general population in Bissau. J Acquir Immune Defic Syndr. 1992;5:25–30.
397. Del Mistro A, Chotard J, Hall AJ, et al. HIV-1 and HIV-2 seroprevalence rates in mother-child pairs living in The Gambia (West Africa). J Acquir Immune Defic Syndr. 1992;5:19–24.
398. Adjorlolo-Johnson G, DeCock KM, Ekpini E, et al. Prospective comparison of mother-to-child transmission of HIV-1 and HIV-2 in Abidjan, Ivory Coast. JAMA. 1994;272:462.
399. Dufoort G, Courouce AM, Ancelle-Park R, et al. No clinical signs 14 years after HIV-2 transmission via blood transfusion (Letter). Lancet. 1988;2:510.
400. Pepin J, Morgan G, Dunn D, et al. HIV-2–induced immunosuppression among asymptomatic. West African prostitutes: Evidence that HIV-2 is pathogenic, but less so than HIV-1. AIDS. 1991;5:1165–1172.
401. Marlink R, Thior I, Travers K, et al. Reduced virulence of HIV-2 compared to HIV-1. Science. 1994;265:1587.
402. Guyader M, Emerman M, Sonigo P, et al. Genome organization and transactivation of the human immunodeficiency virus type 2. Nature. 1987;326:662–669.
403. George JR, Rayfield MA, Phillips S, et al. Efficacies of US Food and Drug Administration–licensed HIV-1–screening enzyme immunoassays for detecting antibodies to HIV-2. AIDS. 1990;4:321–326.
404. Myers RA, Patel JD, Joseph JM. Identifying HIV-2 seropositive individuals by reevaluating HIV-1 indeterminate sera. J Acquir Immune Defic Syndr. 1992;5:417–423.
405. World Health Organization: Recommendations for interpretation of HIV-2 Western blot results. Wkly Epidemiol Rec. 1990;10:74.
406. Peeters M, Gershy-Damet GM, Fransen K, et al. Virological and polymerase chain reaction studies of HIV-1/HIV-2 dual infection in Cote d'Ivoire. Lancet. 1992;340:339–340.
407. Travers K, Mboup S, Marlink R, et al. Natural protection against HIV-1 infection provided by HIV-2. Science. 1995;268:1612.
408. Chen MS, Dellabeta G, Laga M, Holmes KK. A new deal in HIV prevention: Lessons from the global approach. Ann Intern Med. 1994;120:340–341.
409. Johnson AM. Condoms and HIV transmission. N Engl J Med. 1994;331:391–392.
410. Centers for Disease Control and Prevention: Update: Barrier protection against HIV infection and other sexually transmitted diseases. MMWR Morb Mortal Wkly Rep. 1993;42:589–591.
411. Thompson JL, Yager TJ, Martin JL. Estimated condom failure and frequency of condom use among gay men. Am J Public Health. 1993;83:1409–1413.
412. Weller SC. A metaanalysis of condom effectiveness in reducing sexually transmitted HIV. Soc Sci Med. 1993;36:1635–1644.
413. Saracco A, Musicco M, Nicolosi A, et al. Man-to-women sexual transmission of HIV: Longitudinal study of 343 steady partners of infected men. J Acquir Immune Defic Syndr. 1993;6:497–502.
414. De Vincenzi I. A longitudinal study of human immunodeficiency virus transmission by heterosexual partners. European Study Group on Heterosexual Transmission of HIV. N Engl J Med. 1994;331:341–346.
415. Nelson KE, Celentano DD, Eiumtrakol S, et al. Changes in sexual behavior and a decline in HIV infection among young men in Thailand. N Engl J Med. 1996;335:297–303.
416. Hanenberg RS, Rojanapithayakoron W, Kunasol P, Sokal DC. Impact of Thailand's HIV-control programme as indicated by the decline of sexually transmitted diseases. Lancet. 1994;344:243–245.
417. Trussell J, Warner DL, Hatcher R. Condom performance during vaginal intercourse: Comparison of TrojanEnz and Tactylon condoms. Contraception. 1992;45:11–19.
418. Carey RF, Herman WA, Retta SM, et al. Effectiveness of latex condoms as a barrier to human immunodeficiency virus–sized particles under conditions of simulated use. Sex Transm Dis. 1992;19:230–234.
419. Rosenberg MJ, Gollub EL. Commentary: Methods women can use that may prevent sexually transmitted disease, including HIV. Am J Public Health. 1992;82:1473–1478.
420. French P, Latka M, Gollub EL, et al. Female condoms as effective as male condoms in preventing sexually transmitted diseases. Abstract 60730. Presented at the Twelfth International Conference on AIDS, Geneva, 1998.
421. Fontanet AL, Saba J, Chandelying V, et al. Protection against sexually transmitted diseases by granting sex workers in Thailand the choice of using the male or female condom: Results from a randomized controlled trial. AIDS. 1998;12:1851–1859.
422. Cates W Jr, Stewart FH, Trussell J. Commentary: The quest for women's prophylactic methods—hopes vs science. Am J Public Health. 1992;82:1479–1482.
423. Roper WL, Peterson HB, Curran JW. Commentary: Condoms and HIV/STD prevention—clarifying the message. Am J Public Health. 1993;83:501–503.
424. Centers for Disease Control and Prevention: Heterosexual behaviors and factors that influence condom use among patients attending a sexually transmitted disease clinic—San Francisco. MMWR Morb Mortal Wkly Rep. 1990;39:685–689.
425. Peterson JL, Coates TJ, Catania JA, et al. High-risk sexual behavior and condom use among gay and bisexual African-American men. Am J Public Health. 1992;82:1490–1494.
426. Catania JA, Coates TJ, Kegeles S, et al. Condom use in multiethnic neighborhoods of San Francisco: The population-based AMEN (AIDS in multiethnic neighborhoods) study. Am J Public Health. 1991;81:284–287.
427. Osmond DH, Page K, Wiley J, et al. HIV infection in homosexual and bisexual men 18 to 29 years of age: The San Francisco Young Men's Health Study. Am J Public Health. 1994;84:1933–1937.
428. Stall R, Ekstrand M, Polleck L, et al. Relapse from safer sex: The next challenge for AIDS prevention efforts. J Acquir Immune Defic Syndr. 1990;3:1181–1187.
429. Hays RB, Kegeles SM, Coates TJ. High HIV risk-taking among young gay men. AIDS. 1990;4:901–907.
430. St. Lawrence JS, Hood HV, Brasfield T, et al. Differences in gay men's AIDS risk knowledge and behavior patterns in high and low AIDS prevalence cities. Public Health Rep. 1989;104:391–395.
431. Ekstrand ML, Coates TJ. Maintenance of safer sexual behaviors and predictors of risky sex: The San Francisco Men's Health Study. Am J Public Health. 1990;80:973–977.
432. Adib SM, Joseph JG, Ostrow DG, et al. Relapse in sexual behavior among homosexual men: A 2-year follow-up from the Chicago MACS/CCS. AIDS. 1991;5:757–760.
433. Penkower L, Dew MA, Kingsley L, et al. Behavioral, health and psychosocial factors and risk for HIV infection among sexually active homosexual men: The Multicenter AIDS Cohort Study. Am J Public Health. 1991;81:194–196.
434. Lifson AR. Men who have sex with men: Continued challenges for preventing HIV infection and AIDS (Editorial). Am J Public Health. 1992;82:166–167.
435. Chirgwin K, DeHovitz JA, Dillon S, et al. HIV infection, genital ulcer disease,

and crack cocaine uses among patients attending a clinic for sexually transmitted diseases. Am J Public Health. 1992;81:1576–1579.
436. Centers for Disease Control and Prevention: Condom use among male injecting-drug users—New York City, 1987–1990. MMWR Morb Mortal Wkly Rep. 1992;41:617–620.
437. Marks G, Richardson JL, Maldonado N. Self-disclosure of HIV infection to sexual partners. Am J Public Health. 1991;81:1321–1323.
438. Landis SE, Schoenbach VJ, Weber DJ, et al. Results of a randomized trial of partner notification in cases of HIV infection in North Carolina. N Engl J Med. 1992;326:101–106.
439. Bayer R, Toomey KE. HIV prevention and the two faces of partner notification. Am J Public Health. 1992;82:1158–1164.
440. Pavia AT, Benyo M, Niler L, et al. Partner notification for control of HIV: Results after 2 years of a statewide program in Utah. Am J Public Health. 1993;83:1418–1424.
441. Wawer MJ, Sewankambo NK, Serwadda D, et al. Control of sexually transmitted diseases and AIDS prevention in Uganda: A randomized community trial. Lancet. 1999;353:525–535.
442. Cardo DM, Colver DH, Ciesielski CA, et al. A case-control study of HIV seroconversion in health-care workers after percutaneous exposure. N Engl J Med. 1997;337:1485–1490.
443. Centers for Disease Control and Prevention: Management of possible sexual, injecting-drug-use, or other nonoccupational exposure to HIV, including considerations related to antiretroviral therapy. Public Health Service Statement. MMWR Morb Mortal Wkly Rep. 1998;47(RR-17):1–14.
444. Katz MH, Gerberding JL. Posexposure treatment of people exposed to the human immunodeficiency virus through sexual contact or injection-drug use. N Engl J Med. 1997;336:1097–1100.
445. The Twin Epidemics of Substance Use and HIV. Washington, DC: National Commission on AIDS; 1991.
446. Metzger DS, Navaline H, Woody GE. Drug-abuse treatment as AIDS Prevention. Public Health Rep. 1998;113(Suppl 1):S97–S106.
447. Centers for Disease Control and Prevention: Update: Reducing HIV transmission in intravenous-drug users not in drug treatment—United States. MMWR Morb Mortal Wkly Rep. 1990;39:97–101.
448. Groseclose SL, Weinstein B, Jones S, et al. Legal purchase of clean needles and syringes in Connecticut: Do they make a difference? (Abstract POD274185). In: Abstracts of the IX International Conference on AIDS/IVth STD World Congress, v. 2. Berlin: 1993:915.
449. U.S. General Accounting Office. Needle Exchange Programs: Research Suggests Promise as an AIDS Prevention Strategy. Washington, DC: USGAO, Human Resources Division; 1993. Report to the Chairman, Select Committee on Narcotics Abuse and Control, House of Representatives.
450. Centers for Disease Control and Prevention: Use of bleach for disinfection of drug injection equipment. MMWR Morb Mortal Wkly Rep. 1993;42:418–419.
451. Yancovitz SR, Des Jarlais DC, Peyser NP, et al. A randomized trial of an interim methadone maintenance clinic. Am J Public Health. 1991;81:1185–1191.
452. Stephens RC, Feucht TE, Roman SW. Effects of an intervention program on AIDS-related drug and needle behavior among intravenous drug users. Am J Public Health. 1991;81:568–571.
453. Negigus A, Friedman SR, Curtis R, et al. Relevance of drug injectors' social networks and risk networks for understanding and preventing HIV infection. Soc Sci Med. 1994;38:67.
454. Des Jarlais DC, Friedman SR, Friedman P, et al. HIV/AIDS related behavior change among injecting drug users in different national settings. AIDS. 1995;9:611.
455. The Public Health Impact of Needle Exchange Programs in the United States and Abroad. Summary, Conclusions, and Recommendations. Report prepared for the Centers for Disease Control and Prevention, September 1993.
456. Vlahov D, Junge B. The role of needle exchange programs in HIV prevention. Public Health Rep. 1998;113(Suppl 1):S75–S80.
457. Titus S, Marmor M, Des Jarlais DC, et al. Bleach use and HIV seroconversion among New York City injection drug users. J Acquir Immune Defic Syndr. 1994;7:700.
458. Vlahov D, Astemborski J, Soloman L, Nelson KE. Field effectiveness of needle disinfection among injecting drug users. J Acquir Immune Defic Syndr. 1994;7:760.
459. Centers for Disease Control and Prevention: Semen banking, organ and tissue transplantation, and HIV antibody testing. MMWR Morb Mortal Wkly Rep. 1988;37:57–58, 63.
460. Centers for Disease Control and Prevention: Transmission of HIV through bone transplantation: Case report and public health recommendations. MMWR Morb Mortal Wkly Rep. 1988;37:597–599.
461. Bell DM. Human immunodeficiency virus transmission in health care settings: Risk and risk reduction. Am J Med. 1991;91(Suppl 3B):S294–S300.
462. Centers for Disease Control and Prevention: Recommendations for prevention of HIV transmission in healthcare settings. MMWR Morb Mortal Wkly Rep. 1987;36(Suppl 2S):S1–S18.
463. Centers for Disease Control and Prevention: Public Health Service statement on management of occupational exposure to human immunodeficiency virus, including considerations regarding zidovudine postexposure use. MMWR Morb Mortal Wkly Rep. 1990;39(RR-1):1–14.
464. Centers for Disease Control and Prevention: Public Health Service guidelines for the management of health-care worker exposures to HIV and recommendations for postexposure prophylaxis. MMWR Morb Mortal Wkly Rep. 1998;47(RR-7):1–33.
465. Centers for Disease Control and Prevention: Public Health Service guidelines for counseling and antibody testing to prevent HIV infection and AIDS. MMWR Morb Mortal Wkly Rep. 1987;36:509–515.
466. Working Group on HIV Testing of Pregnant Women and Newborns. HIV infection, pregnant women, and newborns. JAMA. 1990;264:2416–2420.
467. Lindsay MK, Peterson HB, Feng TI, et al. Routine antepartum human immunodeficiency virus infection screening in an inner-city population. Obstet Gynecol. 1989;74:289–294.
468. Wade NA, Birkhead GS, Warren BL, et al. Abbreviated regimens of zidovudine prophylaxis and perinatal transmission of the human immunodeficiency virus. N Engl J Med. 1998;339:1409–1414.
469. Centers for Disease Control and Prevention: Administration of zidovudine during late pregnancy and delivery to prevent perinatal HIV transmission—Thailand, 1996–1998. MMWR Morb Mortal Wkly Rep. 1998;47:1551–1554.
470. Mofenson LM. Mother-child HIV-1 transmission: Timing and determinants. Obstet Gynecol Clin North Am. 1997;24:759–784.
471. Centers for Disease Control and Prevention: Recommendations for assisting in the prevention of perinatal transmission of human T-lymphotrophic type III/lymphadenopathy-associated virus. MMWR Morb Mortal Wkly Rep. 1985;34:721–726, 731–732.
472. World Health Organization. Consensus statement from the WHO/UNICEF consultation on HIV transmission and breast-feeding. Wkly Epidemiol Rec. 1992;67:177–179.
473. UNAIDS. HIV and infant feeding: An interim statement. Wkly Epidemiol Rec. 1996;71:289–291.
474. Saba J (on behalf of the PETRA trial study team). Interim analysis of the efficacy of three short ZVD/3TC combination regimens to prevent mother-to-child transmission of HIV-1: The PETRA trial. Abstract S7. Presented at the Sixth Conference on Retroviruses and Opportunistic Infections, Chicago, 1999.
475. Valdiserri RO, Holtgrave DR, Brackbill RM. American adults' knowledge of HIV testing availability. Am J Public Health. 1993;83:525–528.
476. Berrios DC, Hearst N, Cotes TJ, et al. HIV antibody testing among those at risk for infection: The National AIDS Behavioral Surveys. JAMA. 1993;270:1576–1580.
477. Ward J. Testing for retroviral infections: Medical indications and ethical considerations. In: Schochetman G, George JR, eds. AIDS testing. Methodology and Management Issues. New York: Springer-Verlag; 1992:6–17.
478. Centers for Disease Control and Prevention: Recommendations for HIV testing services for inpatients and outpatients in acute-care hospital settings. MMWR Morb Mortal Wkly Rep. 1993;42(RR-2):1–17.
479. Centers for Disease Control and Prevention: Human immunodeficiency virus infection in transfusion recipients and their family members. MMWR Morb Mortal Wkly Rep. 1987;36:137–140.
480. Centers for Disease Control and Prevention: Recommendations for preventing transmission of human immunodeficiency virus and hepatitis B virus to patients during exposure-prone invasive procedures. MMWR Morb Mortal Wkly Rep. 1991;40(RR-8):1–9.
481. Gerberding JL, Littell C, Tarkington A, et al. Risk of exposure of surgical personnel to patients' blood during surgery at San Francisco General Hospital. N Engl J Med. 1990;322:1788–1793.
482. Higgins DL, Galavotti C, O'Reilly KR, et al. Evidence for the effects of HIV antibody counseling and testing on risk behaviors. JAMA. 1991;266:2419–2429.
483. Sangiwa G, Balmer D, Furlonge C, et al. Voluntary HIV counseling and testing reduces risk behavior in developing countries: Results from the voluntary counseling and testing study. Abstract 133/33269. Presented at the Twelfth International Conference on AIDS, Geneva, 1998.
484. Otten MW, Zaidi AA, Wroten JE, et al. Changes in sexually transmitted disease rates after HIV testing and posttest counseling, Miami 1988 to 1989. Am J Public Health. 1993;83:529–533.
485. Zenilman JM, Erickson B, Fox R, et al. Effect of HIV posttest counseling on STD incidence. JAMA. 1992;267:843–845.
486. Holtgrave DR, Valdiserri RO, Gerber AR, et al. Human immunodeficiency virus counseling, testing, referral, and partner notification services: A cost-benefit analysis. Arch Intern Med. 1993;153:1225–1230.
487. Centers for Disease Control and Prevention: Technical guidance on HIV counseling. MMWR Morb Mortal Wkly Rep. 1993;42(RR-2):11–17.
488. Jewett JF, Hecht FM. Preventive health care for adults with HIV infection. JAMA. 1993;269:1144–1153.

Chapter 106

Detection of Human Immunodeficiency Virus Infection

LISA M. DEMETER
RICHARD C. REICHMAN

Infections with human immunodeficiency virus types 1 and 2 (HIV-1 and HIV-2) affect more than 30 million people.[1] HIV-1 is the major cause of the acquired immunodeficiency syndrome (AIDS) in the United States. HIV-2 also causes AIDS and has been found principally in West African countries as well as in other parts of Africa, South America, and West India. It is becoming increasingly important to establish the diagnosis of HIV infection before the development of AIDS, because of advances in the therapy for HIV infection and prevention of perinatal transmission. In addition, early and sensitive detection of HIV infection is essential to the maintenance of a safe blood supply. This chapter summarizes the methods currently available for detecting HIV infection and discusses approaches to the diagnosis of these retroviral infections in different clinical settings.

HUMAN IMMUNODEFICIENCY VIRUS STRUCTURE AND REPLICATION CYCLE

A brief overview of HIV structure and replication is necessary to put into perspective the different methods for detecting HIV in clinical specimens (a detailed discussion of these topics can be found in Chapter 157). HIV-1 and HIV-2 are retroviruses, which are enveloped viruses containing positive-sense, single-stranded RNA that is reverse transcribed to DNA and integrated into the host cell genome. HIV virions contain two copies of genomic RNA and a number of viral proteins, as shown in Figure 106–1. The most common viral protein that is directly assayed is the core (p24) antigen. Antibody responses to a number of viral proteins can be detected, including products of the viral genes *env* (glycoprotein [gp] 160, gp120, and gp41), *gag* (p24, p17, p7, p9), and *pol* (p32, p66, p51, and p11).[2] HIV-1 and HIV-2 share approximately 40 to 60% homology at the amino acid level.[2] Strains of HIV-1 can be divided into two groups, M (which stands for major) and O (for outlier). Group M is further subdivided into 10 different subtypes or clades (A to J). Group O, which is endemic in West and central Africa, includes strains that share amino acid homology of 55 to 70% with other subtypes of HIV-1.[2]

The major target of HIV infection is the $CD4^+$ T cell, although HIV can also infect other cell types such as macrophages. After fusion of the virion with the cell membrane, uncoating and reverse transcription of the viral RNA genome occur. The reverse-transcribed double-stranded DNA genome is then transported to the nucleus, where it is integrated into the host cell genome. Productive infection of lymphocytes (both in peripheral blood and in other tissue compartments) results in the extracellular release of virions. Direct detection of viral nucleic acids is performed using the polymerase chain reaction (PCR) to amplify virion RNA from the plasma or extracellular space and proviral DNA from lymphoid cells.

EARLY EVENTS IN HUMAN IMMUNODEFICIENCY VIRUS INFECTION

The utility and performance characteristics of the different methods for detecting HIV infection are best understood in the context of early events in HIV infection (Fig. 106–2). Approximately 50 to 70% of patients with primary HIV infection present with an acute mononucleosis-like syndrome approximately 2 to 6 weeks after initial infection.[3–5] High levels of plasma viremia, which can be detected by both culture and reverse transcriptase–PCR (RT-PCR) assays, characterize this period of time.[4, 5] During acute infection, p24 antigen is also detectable in plasma. Antibodies to core and envelope proteins can be demonstrated within 2 to 6 weeks after the onset of symptoms and generally persist throughout the course of infection.[6–8] Plasma viremia and p24 antigen levels decrease dramatically in temporal association with the emergence of host immune responses, although viral RNA remains detectable by RT-PCR in the majority of patients. During the asymptomatic period of HIV infection, p24 antigen is generally undetectable and plasma cultures are usually negative. In some patients, p24 antigen and plasma viremia again rise to detectable levels with the onset of clinical AIDS.

TESTS FOR THE DETECTION OF HUMAN IMMUNODEFICIENCY VIRUS INFECTION

Serologic Assays

Antibodies to HIV do not develop until after the initial decline in HIV viremia and can first be detected within 2 to 8 weeks after infection. Thus, serologic assays are generally not useful in the diagnosis of acute or primary HIV infection. Persistently undetectable antibodies more than 3 months after infection are rare, and initial reports of prolonged serologically negative HIV-infected patients have not been confirmed.

Seroconversion usually begins with an immunoglobulin M (IgM) response to Gag proteins, with a switch from IgM to IgG antibodies occurring over 1 to 41 weeks.[9] The IgM response overlaps the viremic period and is followed within 5 to 7 days by an IgG response.[9] Most studies reported that IgG responses to p24 and gp120 proteins develop first, followed by antibodies to gp41 and to viral proteins with molecular masses between 50 and 65 kD. The rise in antibody to p24 coincides with a decline in detectable p24 antigen. IgG antibody titers generally increase over the first few months after infection and then stabilize. Late in infection, p24 antibody titers can decline in association with rising p24 antigen; antibodies against other viral proteins generally persist for life.

In adults, testing for HIV antibodies is considered positive when a repeatedly reactive enzyme-linked immunosorbent assay (ELISA) is confirmed by a more specific assay, such as a Western blot.[10] This finding should generally be considered to indicate current infection with HIV. An exception to this rule is a volunteer who has received an experimental HIV vaccine; a discussion of the approach to diagnosing HIV infections in these individuals is outlined in more detail in a later section. In addition, because of passive transfer of maternal antibodies, serologic testing is not useful in diagnosing HIV infection in a neonate or infant born to an HIV-infected mother.

Enzyme-Linked Immunosorbent Assay

The primary approach to screening for established HIV infection in adults involves the use of ELISAs for the detection of antibodies. Most approved procedures utilize immobilized HIV antigens to bind IgG antibodies in the patient's sample. Bound HIV antibodies are then complexed with enzyme-labeled anti-human IgG and are detected in a colorimetric reaction. The resulting color change is quantitated spectrophotometrically and is proportional to the concentration of antibodies in the original sample. An absorbance cutoff is determined for each assay on the basis of standardized positive and negative control samples. These assays originally utilized whole-virus lysate as the antigen. Subsequent use of recombinant viral proteins and peptides has resulted in increased sensitivity and improved specificity.[2, 9] Infections with non–subtype B strains may be missed because of the decreased affinity of antibodies for the anti-

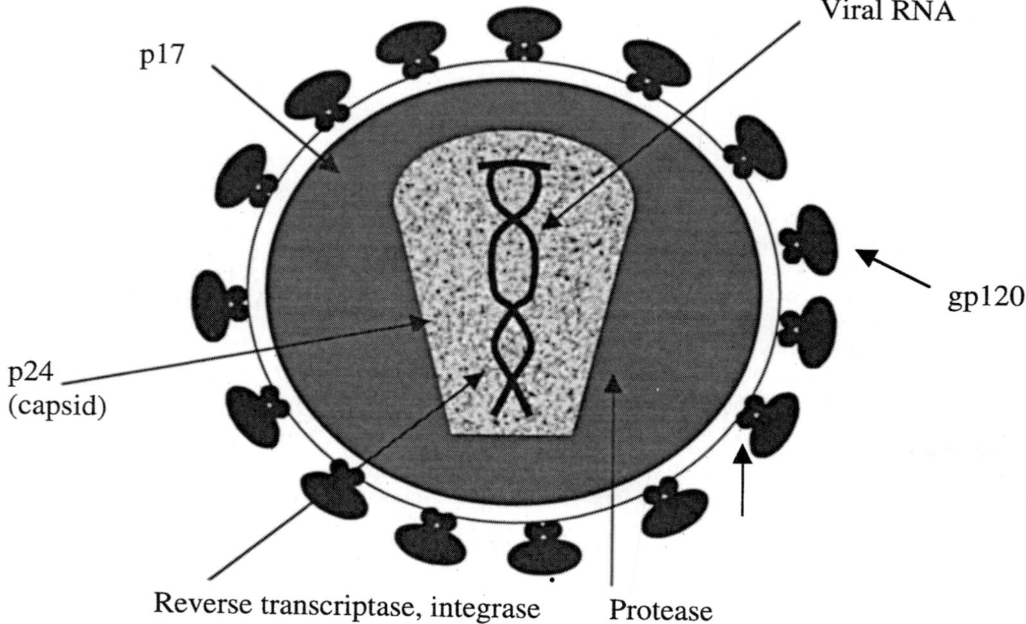

FIGURE 106–1. Locations of viral proteins and nucleic acids in the HIV-1 virion.

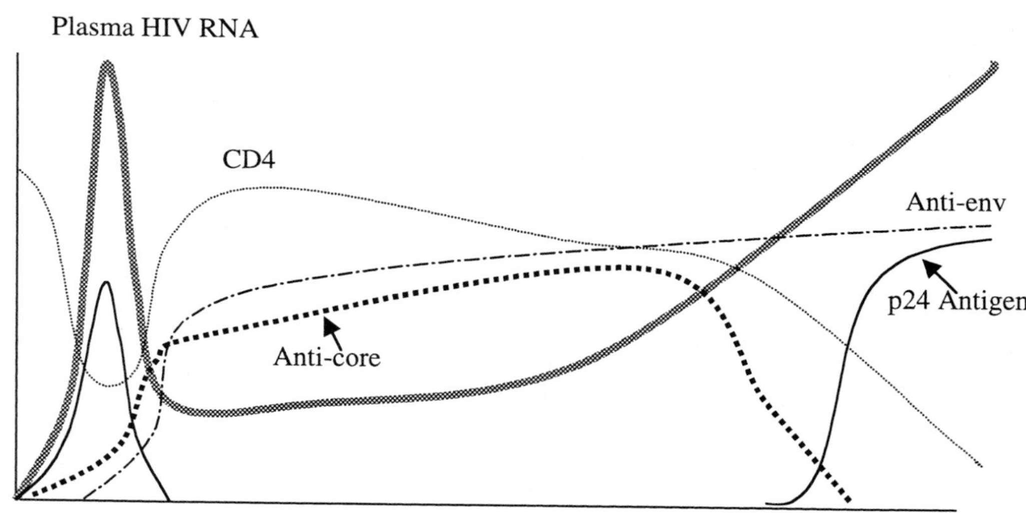

FIGURE 106–2. Course of human immunodeficiency virus infection.

gens usually included in these assays.[11] Inclusion of group O antigens in ELISAs since 1994 has increased the sensitivity for detecting infection with variant strains,[12] although the marked heterogeneity among group O strains still results in some false-negative reactions.[13, 14] ELISAs utilizing peptide antigens appear to be less sensitive for detecting group O strains than ELISAs utilizing viral proteins.[14, 15]

In general, the sensitivity of ELISAs ranges from 93 to 100%; the reported sensitivity for licensed tests under optimal experimental conditions is greater than 99%.[9] Falsely negative ELISA results can occur during primary HIV infection,[16] in immunosuppressed patients (including occasional patients with late-stage AIDS),[17] and with errors in specimen labeling or handling.[9] In addition, HIV-1 ELISAs are relatively insensitive to HIV-2 infection; the rate of reactivity with sera from patients known to be HIV-2 infected ranges from 60 to 90%.[18, 19] Addition of recombinant HIV-2 antigens has resulted in ELISAs that are sensitive to the detection of both retroviruses.[18, 20]

The specificity of a repeatedly reactive ELISA is approximately 99%.[9, 18] Causes of false-positive ELISAs include human error, hemodialysis, a reactive rapid plasmin reagin test, and concomitant medical problems such as autoimmune disorders, multiple myeloma, hemophilia, and alcoholic hepatitis.[9] Because of the clinical implications of a false-positive ELISA result, current recommendations for the serologic diagnosis of HIV infection include a repeatedly reactive ELISA that is confirmed by a second assay.[10] The second assay is most commonly a Western blot (see later), although the World Health Organization has stated that equivalent sensitivity and specificity may be obtained if the diagnosis is made using two ELISAs that contain different antigens and rely on different testing principles.[21] This latter approach may be more cost-effective for developing countries.

A rapid ELISA to detect HIV antibodies is also commercially available in the United States (Single Use Diagnostic System or SUDS, Murex Diagnostics). The patient's serum or plasma is added to a mixture of latex beads coated with HIV-1 antigens. Positive results must be confirmed with another test, such as a Western blot, but negative results are available in 10 to 15 minutes. This rapid ELISA appears highly sensitive and specific, although false positives can occur with inadequate centrifugation or with problems in specimen processing.[22]

Modifications of the standard ELISA and Western blot assay have resulted in tests that can accurately detect HIV antibodies in saliva, obviating the need for phlebotomy.[23–25] These saliva tests appear to have sensitivities and specificities similar to those of tests performed on serum or plasma.

Western Blot

The assay most commonly used to confirm ELISA reactivity is the Western blot. This test involves incubation of the patient's serum with a nitrocellulose strip on which have been blotted viral proteins that have been electrophoretically separated. Human antibodies directed against specific HIV proteins can be identified by binding to enzyme-linked anti-human IgG, as in the ELISA method. A positive Western blot is defined by the Centers for Disease Control and Prevention and the Association of State and Territorial Public Health Laboratory Directors as the presence of any two of the p24, gp41, and gp120/160 bands.[10] The absence of any reactive bands is considered to be a negative result. A Western blot with reactive bands that do not meet the criteria for a positive test is termed indeterminate.

The Western blot can reliably detect antibodies against subtype B strains of HIV-1, although it is less sensitive than ELISA during the early stages of seroconversion. Commercial assays do not include group O proteins and may miss infections with non–subtype B strains of HIV-1.[26, 27] Approximately 20% of HIV-2–positive sera may give negative results with Western blot, and approximately 10% of HIV-1 group O sera are negative by Western blot.[2]

False-positive Western blot results have been reported in patients with hyperbilirubinemia, connective tissue disorders, and polyclonal gammopathies.[9] Studies of blood donors with persistent indeterminate Western blots who were at low risk for HIV infection have found no evidence for HIV-1 or HIV-2 infection.[28–30] Patients with a repeatedly reactive ELISA and indeterminate Western blot require serologic and clinical follow-up to determine whether HIV infection is present. There are no clear patterns of antigen reactivity that predict a higher likelihood of seroconversion in patients with indeterminate Western blots.[31] Additional testing for HIV infection using PCR or culture methods or both may be indicated, depending on the clinical picture and risk factors for HIV infection.

Assays for Direct Detection of Human Immunodeficiency Virus Infection

There are currently no assays approved by the Food and Drug Administration (FDA) for the direct detection of HIV in a clinical setting. However, there are situations in which serologic assays for HIV infection are neither sensitive nor specific enough to diagnose HIV infection reliably. In these cases, many clinicians utilize one or more assays for direct detection of viral proteins or nucleic acids. It is important for the clinician to become familiar with the methods used by the testing laboratory and to interpret the results of the assays in the context of the patient's clinical condition and risk of infection, because these tests are not FDA approved for HIV diagnosis and because not all assays are standardized. Ideally, HIV infection should be confirmed using more than one assay type.

p24 Antigen Detection

Detection of p24 capsid antigen is performed using ELISA. p24 antigen ELISAs are based on the principle of solid-phase antigen capture, in which immobilized monoclonal or polyclonal anti-p24 antibodies bind antigen present in the test sample. The presence of p24 antigen is detected through binding of enzyme-linked anti-HIV IgG, followed by a colorimetric assay. Absorbance, measured spectrophotometrically, is directly proportional to antigen concentration. Available assays can reliably detect more than 10 pg/ml p24 antigen. Modifications of the p24 antigen assay are available that can detect immune-complexed p24 antigen; these assays are approximately twofold more sensitive for detection of HIV than standard p24 antigen assays.[32]

p24 antigen can be detected in serum or plasma during the acute phase of primary HIV infection and during late symptomatic stages of infection. Only 4% of asymptomatic HIV-infected adults have detectable p24 antigen. This proportion rises to 70% in patients with advanced AIDS.[9] p24 antigen detection can also be used to diagnose HIV infection in infants born to HIV-positive mothers. The overall sensitivity of p24 antigen testing for the detection of HIV infection in infants is 50 to 75% and the specificity is greater than 95%.[33, 34] The sensitivity of the assay decreases in asymptomatic children and in children younger than 6 months of age and ranges from 0 to 20% in the first month of life.[33–35] Children who are p24 antigen positive are more likely to progress clinically.[35]

Quantitation of p24 antigen was used in the past to demonstrate responses to antiretroviral agents; however, this assay has been supplanted by quantitative RT-PCR assays for plasma HIV RNA. Although p24 antigen assays are very specific for HIV infection, they are relatively insensitive compared with PCR assays for viral nucleic acids, and a negative p24 antigen result does not rule out the presence of HIV infection. p24 antigen detection is also commonly used to detect viral replication in culture supernatants; this method of HIV detection is discussed in more detail later.

Nucleic Acid Detection and Quantification

Detection of Proviral DNA

Highly sensitive detection of proviral DNA can be accomplished using the PCR, which involves the enzymatic amplification of a segment of DNA using specific oligonucleotide primers. A kit to amplify a short segment of the *gag* region of HIV-1 is commercially available (Amplicor assay, Roche Molecular Systems), although it is not currently FDA-approved for this purpose. This assay is normally performed on peripheral blood mononuclear cells (PBMCs) isolated from whole blood using a lysis technique. Of particular relevance to developing countries, this assay also appears to be highly effective when performed on dried blood spot specimens.[36]

The sensitivity of the Amplicor assay for detecting established HIV-1 infection is greater than 95% and the specificity is greater than 98%.[37, 38] The sensitivity of this assay for detection of HIV-1 infection in infants younger than 2 years of age ranges from 75 to 97% in different studies.[37, 39] The sensitivity of PCR in infants from 1 to 6 months of age is lower than in older children.[39] Causes of false-negative results that should be considered include errors in specimen labeling, handling, or processing; sequence variation in the primer binding sites; and low proviral DNA copy number.[37, 40] Testing laboratories may use their own internal PCR assays for the detection of HIV-1; such assays may differ in sensitivity and specificity of HIV-1 detection from the Amplicor assay. In addition, studies using standardized "blinded" panels have demonstrated interlaboratory variability and the need for quality assurance programs.[41, 42] PCR assays that are optimized to amplify group M strains of HIV-1 may not efficiently amplify group O strains. Specific group O primers have been developed for this purpose.[43, 44]

Detection and Quantification of Plasma Human Immunodeficiency Virus Type 1 RNA

A number of different assays are commercially available for the detection and quantification of plasma HIV RNA. Three assays are widely used at present: two are based on use of enzymatic amplification of target nucleic acids (Amplicor Monitor assay, Roche Molecular Systems; and NASBA, Organon Technika) and the third utilizes branched-chain DNA hybridization signal amplification (branched-chain DNA, Chiron). The Amplicor Monitor assay is the only assay that is currently FDA-approved for the purpose of determining the prognosis for HIV-1 infection.

Because of its availability, detection of plasma HIV RNA has been used by some clinicians to detect the presence of HIV infection in patients with acute HIV infection or in those who have reactive ELISAs and indeterminate Western blots, although the test is not FDA-approved for this indication. This method appears to be quite sensitive for the detection of HIV infection in these circumstances, although false positive results, usually with low copy numbers, have been reported.[45] There have been reports that RT-PCR assays give lower plasma RNA copy numbers than the branched-chain DNA assay in patients infected with non–subtype B HIV infections[46]; the impact of this reduced sensitivity on the ability to detect acute infection with these subtypes has not been studied systematically. Modification of the amplification primers in the RT-PCR assay has improved the sensitivity of this assay for the quantification of non–subtype B infections.

Human Immunodeficiency Virus Culture

HIV culture can be performed using either the patient's plasma or PBMCs. Plasma HIV cultures are rarely positive in asymptomatic disease, and PBMC cultures are most commonly utilized to diagnose HIV infection. A number of different cell culture systems and methods for detecting HIV replication have been used. The assays most commonly used to detect HIV in clinical samples are based on a consensus methodology standardized within the National Institutes of Health–sponsored AIDS Clinical Trials Group. The patient's PBMCs are isolated using density gradient centrifugation and incubated with phytohemagglutinin- and interleukin-2–stimulated PBMCs from an HIV-negative donor. Cocultivation of patient's and donor's PBMCs in the presence of interleukin-2 results in the production of progeny virions from infected cells. Culture supernatants are sampled on a weekly or twice-weekly basis to assay for p24 antigen production, using an ELISA assay. HIV-negative donor PBMCs are replenished on a weekly basis.

A positive culture is defined as one in which there is a sustained rise in p24 antigen production. The majority of cultures from HIV-positive untreated patients become positive within the first 3 weeks of incubation.[47] Factors that can increase the time to a positive culture or reduce the frequency of positive cultures include a low HIV viral load (either in patients who are long-term nonprogressors or as a result of suppression of viral load by antiretroviral therapy), low numbers of input PBMCs, and problems with reagent quality or incubation conditions.[48] In addition, factors that influence the reactivity of p24 antigen ELISAs can also cause falsely negative cultures. Viral replication in cell cultures can also be detected by assaying reverse transcriptase activity. In one report, there was a suggestion that reverse transcriptase assays may be more sensitive than p24 antigen assays in detecting replication of non–subtype B HIV isolates.[49]

HIV PBMC culture is a highly sensitive but labor-intensive method for detecting HIV infection in infants. In one study, DNA PCR was equivalent to and perhaps more sensitive than culture in detecting HIV infection in infants born to HIV-infected mothers.[39] HIV PBMC cultures are positive in only half of HIV-infected neonates during the first month of life.[35] Infants with negative HIV PBMC cultures are usually also PCR negative and are thought to have been infected late in pregnancy or during delivery rather than earlier in pregnancy.

CLINICAL USES OF HUMAN IMMUNODEFICIENCY VIRUS TESTING

Primary Human Immunodeficiency Virus Infection

The most important factor in diagnosing primary HIV infection is maintaining a high index of clinical suspicion.[50] Testing for HIV infection should be strongly considered for sexually active persons or illicit drug users with a compatible clinical syndrome. In addition, the diagnosis of primary HIV infection should be considered in asymptomatic patients with indeterminate serologic testing for HIV antibodies.

Because patients with primary HIV infection may not yet have mounted an antibody response, ELISA and Western blot assays may be negative or indeterminate. The most sensitive assay for the detection of acute HIV infection is plasma HIV RNA testing, although the test is currently not licensed for diagnostic indications. Patients with primary HIV infection have high levels of viremia (usually 10^5 to 10^6 copies per milliliter of plasma).[4, 5] It is important to note that false-positive RNA PCR test results can be obtained in the absence of HIV infection, as noted earlier. The diagnosis of acute HIV infection should be questioned if the plasma HIV RNA concentration is less than 2000 copies/ml. PCR to detect HIV proviral DNA is also positive in a high percentage of people with acute HIV infection. p24 antigen can be positive[51] but is significantly less sensitive than RNA or DNA PCR assays; therefore, a negative p24 antigen assay does not rule out primary HIV infection. Although direct detection of HIV proteins or nucleic acids is essential to make a prompt diagnosis of acute HIV infection, it should be borne in mind that these assays are not approved for this indication. All patients with suspected primary HIV infection should have follow-up studies to confirm seroconversion; this occurs in the majority of patients within 3 to 6 months of presentation.

Pediatric Human Immunodeficiency Virus Infection

The diagnosis of HIV infection in neonates and infants younger than 2 years born to HIV-infected mothers is complicated by the persistence of maternal antibodies. Thus, using serologic assays, one can establish perinatal transmission of HIV infection only retrospectively. DNA PCR and PBMC culture assays are the most sensitive methods for establishing the diagnosis of HIV infection in infants. These assays have a similar sensitivity, which is approximately 50% during the first month of life and nearly 100% in infants older than 6 months. One analysis suggested that the sensitivity of DNA PCR is higher than suggested by other studies, with approximately 38% of infected neonates positive within the first 2 days of birth and 90% positive within the first month.[52] A positive direct assay for HIV should be confirmed with a second assay, preferably of a second type performed on a sample obtained on a separate day. RT-PCR to detect plasma RNA also appears to have a sensitivity similar to that of PBMC culture and DNA PCR.[53]

Established Human Immunodeficiency Virus Infection in Adults

In general, the diagnosis of established HIV infection in adults is relatively straightforward and can be made serologically. A reactive ELISA that is confirmed with a Western blot is generally diagnostic for HIV infection, and direct detection of viral antigens or nucleic acids is not necessary to establish the diagnosis. A negative ELISA should be repeated in 3 to 6 months for someone at risk for acquiring HIV infection, as false-negative ELISAs can occur during the sero-negative window of primary HIV infection. In someone with a clinical picture strongly suggestive of AIDS and a negative ELISA, consideration should be given to pursuing the diagnosis of infection with unusual subtypes of HIV-1 or HIV-2, which may not be detected in the serologic assays used. Patients who are sexually active or users of illicit drugs who present with symptoms compatible with primary HIV infection should be evaluated with serologic assays and a method for directly detecting viral antigens or nucleic acids (such as plasma HIV RNA concentration, HIV DNA PCR, p24 antigen, or HIV culture). Any tests suggestive of HIV infection should be confirmed, and the ultimate diagnosis of HIV infection requires the demonstration of serologic conversion. Healthy volunteers who have received experimental vaccines may have reactive ELISAs or Western blots or both. These patients' serologic responses reflect immune responses to the vaccine antigens and do not necessarily reflect HIV infection. If there are concerns about HIV infection in such patients, direct testing for HIV, using PCR, antigen detection, or culture methods, should be performed.

REFERENCES

1. World Health Organization. The Current Global Situation of the HIV/AIDS Pandemic. Geneva: World Health Organization; 1996.
2. Gurtler L. Difficulties and strategies of HIV diagnosis. Lancet. 1996;348:176–179.
3. Schacker T. Primary HIV infection. Early diagnosis and treatment are critical to outcome. Postgrad Med. 1997;102(4):143–146, 149–151.
4. Clark SJ, Saag MS, Decker WD, et al. High titers of cytopathic virus in plasma of patients with symptomatic primary HIV-1 infection. N Engl J Med. 1991;324:954–960.
5. Daar ES, Moudgil T, Meyer RD, Ho DD. Transient high levels of viremia in patients with primary human immunodeficiency virus type 1 infection. N Engl J Med. 1991;324:961–964.
6. Horsburgh CR Jr, Ou CY, Jason J, et al. Duration of human immunodeficiency virus infection before detection of antibody. Lancet. 1989;2:637–640.
7. Gaines H, Non Sydow M, Sonnerborg A, et al. Antibody response in primary human immunodeficiency virus infection. Lancet. 1987;2:1249–1253.
8. Allain JP, Laurian Y, Paul DA, Senn D. Serological markers in early stages of human immunodeficiency virus infection in haemophiliacs. Lancet. 1986;2:1233–1236.
9. Bylund DJ, Ziegner UH, Hooper DG. Review of testing for human immunodeficiency virus. Clin Lab Med. 1992;12:305–333.
10. Centers for Disease Control. Interpretation and use of the Western blot assay for serodiagnosis of human immunodeficiency virus type 1 infections. MMWR Morb Mortal Wkly Rip. 1989;38(S-7):1–7.
11. Engelbrecht S, de Jager GJ, van Rensburg EJ. Evaluation of commercially available assays for antibodies to HIV-1 in serum obtained from South African patients infected with HIV-1 subtypes B, C, and D. J Med Virol. 1994;44:223–228.
12. Bachmann P, Beyer J, Brust S, et al. Multicentre study for diagnostic evaluation of an assay for simultaneous detection of antibodies to HIV-1, HIV-2 and HIV-1 subtype O (HIV-0). Infection. 1995;23:322–333.
13. Gurtler LG, Zekeng L, Simon F, et al. Reactivity of five anti-HIV-1 subtype O specimens with six different anti-HIV screening ELISAs and three immunoblots. J Virol Methods. 1995;51:177–183.
14. Loussert-Ajaka I, Ly TD, Chaix ML, et al. HIV-1/HIV-2 seronegativity in HIV-1 subtype O infected patients. Lancet. 1994;343:1393–1394.
15. Brennan CA, Lund JK, Golden A, et al. Serologic and phylogenetic characterization of HIV-1 subtypes in Uganda. AIDS. 1997;11:1823–1832.
16. Farzadegan H, Taylor E, Hardy W, et al. Performance of serological assays for early detection of human immunodeficiency virus type 1 seroconversion. J Clin Microbiol. 1989;27:1882–1884.
17. Farzadegan H, Polis MA, Wolinsky SM, et al. Loss of human immunodeficiency virus type 1 (HIV-1) antibodies with evidence of viral infection in asymptomatic homosexual men. A report from the Multicenter AIDS Cohort Study. Ann Intern Med. 1988;108:785–790.
18. Ayres L, Avillez F, Garcia-Benito A, et al. Multicenter evaluation of a new recombinant enzyme immunoassay for the combined detection of antibody to HIV-1 and HIV-2. AIDS. 1990;4:131–138.
19. George JR, Rayfield MA, Phillips S, et al. Efficacies of US Food and Drug Administration–licensed HIV-1–screening enzyme immunoassays for detecting antibodies to HIV-2. AIDS. 1990;4:321–326.
20. McAlpine L, Gandhi J, Parry JV, Mortina PP. Thirteen current anti–HIV-1/HIV-2 enzyme immunoassays: How accurate are they? J Med Virol. 1994;42(2):115–118.
21. Carvalho MB, Hamerschlak N, Vaz RS, Ferreira OC Jr. Risk factor analysis and serological diagnosis of HIV-1/HIV-2 infection in a Brazilian blood donor population: Validation of the World Health Organization strategy for HIV testing. AIDS. 1996;10:1135–1140.
22. Kassler WJ, Haley C, Jones WK, et al. Performance of a rapid, on-site human immunodeficiency virus antibody assay in a public health setting. J Clin Microbiol. 1995;33:2899–2902.
23. Emmons WW, Paparello SF, Dreker CF, et al. A modified ELISA and Western blot accurately determine anti–human immunodeficiency virus type 1 antibodies in oral fluids obtained with a special collecting device. J Infect Dis. 1995;171:1406–1410.
24. Emmons W. Accuracy of oral specimen testing for human immunodeficiency virus. Am J Med. 1997;102(4A):15–20.
25. Gallo D, George JR, Fitchen JH, et al. Evaluation of a system using oral mucosal transudate for HIV-1 antibody screening and confirmatory testing. OraSure HIV Clinical Trials Group. JAMA. 1997;277:254–258.
26. Gurtler LG, Zekeng L, Tsaque JM, et al. HIV-1 subtype O: Epidemiology, pathogenesis, diagnosis, and perspectives of the evolution of HIV. Arch Virol Suppl. 1996;11:195–202.
27. Jaffe HW, Schochetman G. Group O human immunodeficiency virus-1 infections. Infect Dis Clin North Am. 1998;12:39–46.
28. Jackson JB, MacDonald KL, Cadwell J, et al. Absence of HIV infection in blood donors with indeterminate Western blot tests for antibody to HIV-1. N Engl J Med. 1990;322:217–222.
29. Busch MP, Kleinman SH, Williams AE, et al. Frequency of human immunodeficiency virus (HIV) infection among contemporary anti–HIV-1 and anti–HIV-1/2 supplemental test–indeterminate blood donors. The Retrovirus Epidemiology Donor Study. Transfusion. 1996;36(1):37–44.
30. Sherman MP, Dock NL, Ehrlich GD, et al. Evaluation of HIV type 1 Western blot–indeterminate blood donors for the presence of human or bovine retroviruses. AIDS Res Hum Retroviruses. 1995;11:409–414.
31. Davey RT Jr, Deyton LR, Metcalf JA, et al. Indeterminate Western blot patterns in a cohort of individuals at high risk for human immunodeficiency virus (HIV-1) exposure. J Clin Immunol. 1992;12(3):185–192.
32. Bollinger RC Jr, Kline RL, Francis HL, et al. Acid dissociation increases the sensitivity of p24 antigen detection for the evaluation of antiviral therapy and disease progression in asymptomatic human immunodeficiency virus–infected persons. J Infect Dis. 1992;165:913–916.
33. Borkowsky W, Krasinski K, Paul D, et al. Human immunodeficiency virus type 1 antigenemia in children. J Pediatr. 1989;114:940–945.
34. Andiman WA, Silva TJ, Shapiro TD, et al. Predictive value of the human immunodeficiency virus 1 antigen test in children born to infected mothers. Pediatr Infect Dis J. 1992;11:436–440.
35. Burgard M, Mayaux MJ, Blarche S, et al. The use of viral culture and p24 antigen testing to diagnose human immunodeficiency virus infection in neonates. The HIV Infection in Newborns French Collaborative Study Group. N Engl J Med. 1992;327:1192–1197.
36. Cassol S, Butcha A, Kinard S, et al. Rapid screening for early detection of mother-to-child transmission of human immunodeficiency virus type 1. J Clin Microbiol. 1994;32:2641–2645.
37. Barlow KL, Tosswill JH, Parry JV, Clewley JP. Performance of the Amplicor human immunodeficiency virus type 1 PCR and analysis of specimens with false-negative results. J Clin Microbiol. 1997;35:2846–2853.
38. Khadir A, Coutlee F, Saint-Antoine P, et al. Clinical evaluation of Amplicor HIV-1 test for detection of human immunodeficiency virus type 1 proviral DNA in peripheral blood mononuclear cells. J Acquir Immune Defic Syndr Hum Retrovirol. 1995;9(3):257–263.
39. Bremer JW, Lew JF, Cooper E, et al. Diagnosis of infection with human immunodeficiency virus type 1 by a DNA polymerase chain reaction assay among infants enrolled in the Women and Infants' Transmission Study. J Pediatr. 1996;129(2):198–207.

40. Barlow KL, Tosswill JH, Clewley JP. Analysis and genotyping of PCR products of the Amplicor HIV-1 kit. J Virol Methods. 1995;52(1–2):65–74.
41. Defer C, Agut H, Gabarg-Chenon A, et al. Multicentre quality control of polymerase chain reaction for detection of HIV DNA. AIDS. 1992;6:659–663.
42. Jackson JB, Drew J, Lin HJ, et al. Establishment of a quality assurance program for human immunodeficiency virus type 1 DNA polymerase chain reaction assays by the AIDS Clinical Trials Group. ACTG PCR Working Group, and the ACTG PCR Virology Laboratories. J Clin Microbiol. 1993;31:3123–3128.
43. Janssens W, Fransen K, Loussert-Ajaka I, et al. Diagnosis of HIV-1 group O infection by polymerase chain reaction (Letter). Lancet. 1995;346:451–452.
44. Respess RA, Butcher A, Wang H. Detection of genetically diverse human immunodeficiency virus type 1 group M and O isolates by PCR. J Clin Microbiol. 1997;35:1284.
45. Brown AE, Jackson B, Fuller SA, et al. Viral RNA in the resolution of human immunodeficiency virus type 1 diagnostic serology. Transfusion. 1997;37:926–929.
46. Debyser Z, Van Wijngaerden E, Van Laethem K, et al. Failure to quantify viral load with two of the three commercial methods in a pregnant woman harboring an HIV type 1 subtype G strain. AIDS Res Hum Retroviruses. 1998;14:453–459.
47. Fiscus SA, Welles SL, Spector SA, Lathey JL. Length of incubation time for human immunodeficiency virus cultures. J Clin Microbiol. 1995;33:246–247.
48. Burke DS, Fowler AK, Redfield RR, et al. Isolation of HIV-1 from the blood of seropositive adults: Patient stage of illness and sample inoculum size are major determinants of a positive culture. The Walter Reed Retroviral Research Group. J Acquir Immune Defic Syndr. 1990;3:1159–1167.
49. Corrigan GE, Al-Khalili L, Malmsten A, et al. Differences in reverse transcriptase activity versus p24 antigen detection in cell culture, when comparing a homogeneous group of HIV type 1 subtype B viruses with a heterogeneous group of divergent strains. AIDS Res Hum Retroviruses. 1998;14:347–352.
50. Kahn JO, Walker BD. Acute human immunodeficiency virus type 1 infection. N Engl J Med. 1998;339:33–39.
51. Clark SJ, Kelen GD, Henrard DR, et al. Unsuspected primary human immunodeficiency virus type 1 infection in seronegative emergency department patients. J Infect Dis. 1994;170:194–197.
52. Dunn DT, Brandt CD, Krivine A, et al. The sensitivity of HIV-1 DNA polymerase chain reaction in the neonatal period and the relative contributions of intra-uterine and intra-partum transmission. AIDS. 1995;9(9):F7–F11.
53. Delamare C, Burgard M, Mayaux MJ, et al. HIV-1 RNA detection in plasma for the diagnosis of infection in neonates. The French Pediatric HIV Infection Study Group. J Acquir Immune Defic Syndr Hum Retrovirol. 1997;15(2):121–125.

Chapter 107

The Immunology of Human Immunodeficiency Virus Infection

OREN COHEN
CLAUDIA CICALA
MAURO VACCAREZZA
ANTHONY S. FAUCI

The interactions between the human immunodeficiency virus (HIV) and the human immune system are extraordinarily complex, as evidenced by the highly variable rates of disease progression observed in HIV-infected individuals. Indeed, even individuals who were infected from a common source may experience widely divergent clinical outcomes.[1] HIV subverts the immune system by infecting CD4$^+$ T cells that normally orchestrate immune responses and by activating the immune system and inducing a cytokine milieu that the virus uses to its own replicative advantage. The discovery that certain chemokine receptors function as HIV coreceptors for HIV entry into target cells has expanded the scope of host factors that play a role in the pathogenesis of HIV-induced disease. Understanding the immunoregulation of expression of chemokine receptors and their cognate ligands provides insight into disease pathogenesis and offers the potential for new avenues of therapeutic intervention.[2]

The lack of correlates of protective immunity in HIV infection continues to hamper vaccine development and immunotherapeutic approaches. Robust HIV-specific immune responses, both humoral and cell mediated, are mounted by most infected individuals. It remains unclear why the vast majority of HIV-infected individuals experience inexorable immunodeficiency and disease progression despite the presence of these robust antiviral immune responses. In this regard, qualitative as well as quantitative aspects of virus-specific immune responses may be important in the containment of viral replication.

The rate of progress that has been made to date in understanding the pathogenesis of HIV infection is unparalleled; however, fundamental questions regarding the cause of immunodeficiency in HIV infection remain unanswered. It is clear that HIV induces dysfunction of nearly all elements of the immune system and that the pathogenesis of HIV disease is multifactorial.[3] Although mechanisms of CD4$^+$ T-cell depletion and dysfunction in vitro have been elucidated, it remains uncertain which of these mechanisms are responsible for clinically relevant immune deficiency in vivo. Similarly, a great deal is known about HIV-induced dysregulation of the cytokine network; however, to manipulate this enormously complex and pleiotropic cytokine network to inhibit HIV replication without untoward effects is a daunting task.

MOLECULES OF THE IMMUNE SYSTEM NECESSARY FOR ENTRY OF HUMAN IMMUNODEFICIENCY VIRUS

HIV gains entry into cells through interactions with the CD4 molecule and one of a number of seven-transmembrane G-protein–coupled chemokine coreceptors. CD4 was identified as the major receptor for HIV fusion and entry in 1984.[4–6] Transfection of CD4 into CD4-negative human cells renders them infectable with HIV[7]; however, expression of human CD4 in murine cells does not render these cells susceptible to HIV infection, even though the HIV envelope glycoprotein gp120 binds to CD4 in this setting. This result suggested that other factors were necessary for HIV fusion and entry[8, 9]; however, these additional factors remained elusive for several years.

In late 1995 and early 1996, several lines of investigation into diverse areas of HIV pathogenesis converged to yield critical insight into the process of HIV entry. Investigators studying HIV suppressor factors secreted by CD8$^+$ T cells[10] reported in 1995 that the CC-chemokines (i.e., chemoattractant cytokines involved in regulating inflammation), macrophage inflammatory protein-1α (MIP-1α), MIP-1β, and RANTES (regulated on activation, normal T cell expressed and secreted) were major components of CD8$^+$ T-cell–derived HIV suppressor activity[11] (see the next section). These chemokines in combination inhibited the infection of activated CD4$^+$ T cells by certain strains of HIV-1, HIV-2, and simian immunodeficiency virus. Of note, these CC-chemokines potently inhibited infection of cells by macrophage-tropic (M-tropic) strains of HIV but did not block infection with T-cell line–tropic (T-tropic) strains. In a somewhat unrelated line of investigation, a gene was identified that allowed HIV envelope–mediated cell fusion in the presence of CD4.[12, 13] The protein, called fusin (later renamed CXC chemokine receptor 4, or CXCR4), is a seven-transmembrane G-protein–coupled chemokine receptor. This receptor, together with CD4, was required for cell fusion with envelope protein from T-tropic strains of HIV but was not used by envelope from M-tropic strains. The natural ligand for CXCR4 was later determined to be stromal cell–derived factor type 1 (SDF-1).[14, 15]

In a separate line of research, Paxton and coworkers were studying a population of individuals who had been multiply exposed to HIV-infected partners but remained uninfected (i.e., "exposed-uninfected").[16] They identified two subjects whose CD4$^+$ T cells were refractory to infection with M-tropic strains of HIV but were easily infectable with T-tropic strains. In addition, cells from these individuals produced high levels of MIP-1α, MIP-1β, and RANTES, the same chemokines previously identified as suppressors of infection with M-tropic strains of HIV. Subsequently, a new CC-chemokine receptor, CC-chemokine receptor type 5 (CCR5), was identified; interestingly, the natural ligands that bind to this receptor were identified as MIP-1α, MIP-1β, and RANTES.[17–19] In light of the previous work showing that the CCR5 ligands inhibit cellular entry of M-tropic strains of HIV, the obvious question that arose was whether CCR5 might function as a coreceptor for such strains. A series of five papers simultaneously showed such to be the case[20–24] (Fig. 107–1). Other chemokine receptors, including CCR1, CCR2b, and CCR3, were also identified in these reports as potential coreceptors for certain HIV strains. Recently, still other chemokine receptors have been shown to be potential HIV coreceptors.[25–30]

The interactions between the HIV envelope, CD4, and the relevant coreceptor molecule that is necessary for HIV entry are complex. M-tropic HIV envelope molecules bind first to CD4; this interaction creates a high-affinity binding site for CCR5, presumably as a consequence of a conformational change.[31–36] Although the chemokine ligands of CCR5 appear to interact only with the receptor's second extracellular loop, HIV envelope can interact with multiple CCR5 domains; in fact, the HIV coreceptor activity of CCR5 maps to all of the receptor's extracellular domains, including the N-terminal domain and all three extracellular loops.[37–46] Multiple points of contact may be made between the coreceptor and HIV envelope molecules; however, clearly, the V3 loop of the HIV envelope is critical in mediating this interaction.[31, 32, 34–36, 47–49] Importantly, HIV coreceptor activity and chemokine-mediated signal transduction are distinct properties of CCR5.[38, 41, 47, 50, 51] Many of the characteristics of the interactions between HIV envelope, CD4, and CCR5 appear to be operative in the case of CXCR4 as well. T-tropic HIV envelope molecules appear to interact with CD4 and CXCR4,[52] with multiple domains of CXCR4 playing a role in binding.[53] Of note, T-tropic HIV envelope molecules have a higher affinity for CD4 than do M-tropic envelope molecules.[54]

Transmission of HIV is almost always associated with replication of M-tropic strains of HIV in a newly infected individual.[55, 56] The reasons for this "bottleneck" in transmission are unclear but may be due to the expression of CCR5 and lack of expression of CXCR4 on cells that may serve as initial targets of HIV infection (i.e., Langerhans cells in genital mucosa).[57] Progression of HIV disease is sometimes associated with a switch in tropism of viral isolates from predominantly M-tropic or "non–syncytium inducing" to "syncytium inducing"; this latter terminology is based on the ability of a viral isolate to induce multinucleated giant cell, or syncytium, formation in certain cell lines in vitro. A non–syncytium-inducing to syncytium-inducing switch is a strong predictor of a decline in CD4 T-cell counts and clinical disease progression.[58–61] In addition, a non–syncytium-inducing to syncytium-inducing switch correlates with an expanded spectrum of coreceptor utilization by viral isolates, from exclusively CCR5 to CCR2b, CCR3, and/or CXCR4 in addition to CCR5.[62]

The critical role of CCR5 in the ability of HIV to be transmitted hinted at a possible explanation for individuals who were exposed to HIV but remained uninfected (see earlier). Indeed, two exposed, uninfected individuals were shown to be homozygous for identical 32–base pair deletions in the *CCR5* gene (*CCR5-Δ32*); this deletion resulted in a truncated version of the receptor that was not expressed at the cell surface and therefore does not serve as a functional coreceptor for HIV infection.[63] Molecular epidemiologic studies in HIV-uninfected populations have found that approximately 20% of white individuals of northern and western European background are heterozygous for this mutation and 1% are homozygous; the frequency of the *CCR5-Δ32* allele appears to be exceedingly low in Asian and African populations.[64–67] Among HIV-infected white individuals, no subjects homozygous for *CCR5-Δ32* were initially identified, thus suggesting complete protection from infection[64–67]; however, rare cases of infection of homozygous individuals have subsequently been reported, probably a reflection of rare transmission of T-tropic strains of HIV.[68–71] Although *CCR5-Δ32* heterozygotes are not protected against HIV infection, they are afforded a modest degree of protection against disease progression and are overrepresented among cohorts of HIV-infected long-term nonprogressors.[65–67, 72–74] The mechanism of delayed disease progression in *CCR5-Δ32* heterozygotes may involve a lower viral load "setpoint" after acute HIV infection and a slower rate of $CD4^+$ T-cell depletion.[66] These effects may be due to a decrease in expression of CCR5 on $CD4^+$ cells from *CCR5-Δ32* heterozygotes[75, 76] that allows less efficient spreading of HIV infection to new target cells[77]; however, it is clear that *CCR5-Δ32* is not the sole determinant of delayed progression of HIV disease.[73]

Mutations in chemokine receptor and chemokine genes other than *CCR5-Δ32* can confer protection against HIV infection or partial protection against disease progression. A rare point mutation in the *CCR5* gene (m303) results in a premature stop codon that prevents expression of a functional coreceptor; the *CCR5-Δ32/m303* genotype confers a high degree of resistance to HIV infection, similar to that afforded by homozygosity for *CCR5-Δ32*.[78] A mutation in the *CCR2* gene involving a conservative amino acid change in a transmembrane domain of the receptor results in a significant delay in disease

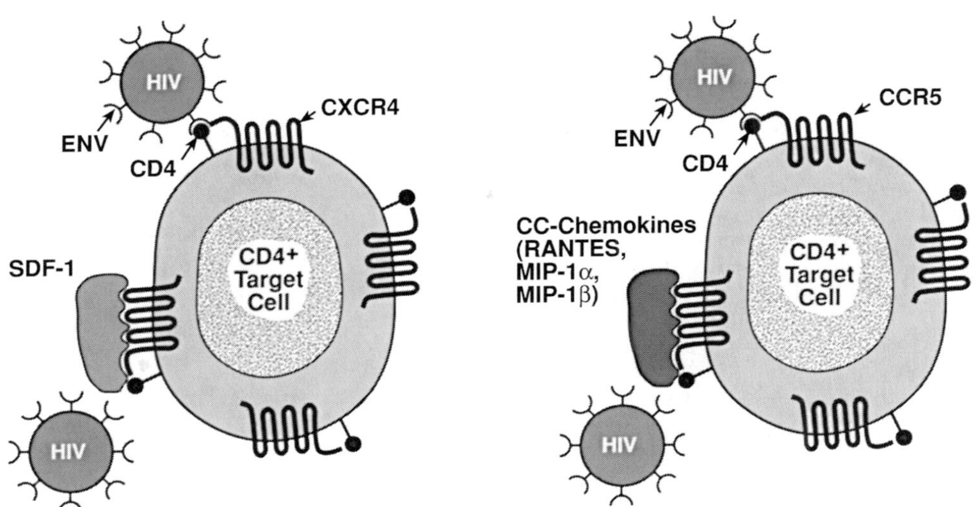

FIGURE 107–1. Model of CCR5 and CXCR4 usage and strain-specific inhibition of human immunodeficiency virus (HIV) binding by coreceptor ligands. Entry of M-tropic strains of HIV is blocked by the CCR5 ligands MIP-1α, MIP-1β, and RANTES. Entry of T-tropic strains of HIV is blocked by the CXCR4 ligand SDF-1. (Adapted with permission from Fauci AS. Host factors and the pathogenesis of HIV-induced disease. Nature. 1996;384:529–534. Copyright 1996, Macmillan Magazines Ltd.)

progression among HIV-infected individuals.[79–81] This result was surprising given the apparently trivial nature of the mutation and the fact that it occurred in a coreceptor gene considered to be of marginal pathogenic significance. However, the recent discovery that this mutation is always associated with a mutation in the promoter region of the nearby *CCR5* gene[80, 82] suggests that the *CCR2b* mutation is a marker for what is perhaps a more significant mutation in the *CCR5* gene. A mutation in the 3′ untranslated region of the *SDF1* gene, *SDF1-3′A,* also plays a role in protecting against disease progression in HIV-infected individuals.[83] Homozygosity for the *SDF1-3′A* allele may be associated with high levels of expression of SDF-1, which may occupy CXCR4 and thereby inhibit replication of T-tropic strains of HIV. Consistent with this hypothesis, the protective effect of the *SDF1* mutation is observed late in the course of HIV disease, when T-tropic strains may predominate.

Genetic polymorphisms in the chemokine-chemokine receptor axis genes represent only one of a number of possible mechanisms responsible for resistance to HIV infection or delayed disease progression. In this regard, downregulation of coreceptor expression and/or upregulation of chemokines may recapitulate phenotypes similar to those created by the genetic polymorphisms just described. Levels of CCR5 expression exhibit considerable interindividual variability, and these levels correlate with infectability of cells with M-tropic strains of HIV in vitro.[76] CCR5 expression occurs predominantly in previously activated, memory T cells[75]; treatment of cells with interleukin-2 (IL-2) slowly upregulates CCR5 expression,[75] whereas stimulation of cells through CD3 and CD28 abrogates CCR5 expression.[84] In contrast to CCR5, CXCR4 is expressed on naive, resting T cells,[75] and its regulation is reciprocal to that of CCR5 in many respects.[75, 84] Whether constitutive low-level expression of these coreceptors is associated with a favorable prognosis in HIV infection remains to be determined; in this regard, the more favorable prognosis of *CCR5-Δ32* heterozygotes should be relevant. Conflicting data exist regarding a possible role for high expression of chemokines in protecting against HIV disease progression. Measurement of serum and plasma concentrations of chemokines has not generally shown any association with progression of HIV disease.[85–87] Although two studies showed no correlation between levels of chemokines secreted by various cellular subsets in response to activating stimuli in vitro and clinical disease status,[88, 89] other data suggest a protective role for overproduction of chemokines. High levels of CC-chemokines were secreted by mitogen-stimulated peripheral blood mononuclear cells (PBMCs)[90] and $CD4^+$ T cells[16] from some exposed-uninfected individuals. Interestingly, $CD4^+$ T-cell clones from some exposed-uninfected individuals secrete high levels of CC-chemokines in response to a peptide derived from a conserved region of the HIV envelope.[91] Additional data support a role for overproduction of CC-chemokines by cellular subsets in protecting against HIV disease progression in HIV-infected individuals.[92–94]

Delineation of the role of chemokine receptors as HIV entry cofactors and the role of the chemokine ligands of these receptors as potential inhibitors of HIV cellular entry has led to the development of new therapeutic strategies.[2] Chemokine analogues that bind to HIV coreceptors and prevent entry of virus without transducing an intracellular signal represent an attractive class of compounds in that they are unlikely to elicit inappropriate inflammatory signals. Such a strategy is highlighted by two RANTES analogues that bind to CCR5 and block infection of cells with M-tropic strains of HIV without delivering intracellular signals.[95, 96] Several small molecules (AMD3100, a bicyclam; T22, a peptide derivative of polyphemusin II; and ALX40-4C, a highly cationic oligopeptide) that compete with SDF-1 for binding to CXCR4 have also been developed. These compounds bind specifically to CXCR4 and inhibit cellular entry of T-tropic strains of HIV; they also inhibit SDF-1–mediated intracellular calcium mobilization.[97–99] Finally, a molecular genetic approach has been taken to prevent cell surface expression of HIV coreceptors, thus recapitulating the *CCR5-Δ32* phenotype. In this approach, chemokine genes are modified to contain a KDEL endoplasmic reticulum retention signal sequence. Expression of these modified chemokine genes, or intrakines, results in accumulation of the chemokine in the endoplasmic reticulum, where it can bind to its receptor and thus prevent cell surface expression of that receptor. This strategy has been developed for MIP-1α/CCR5,[100] RANTES/CCR5,[100] and SDF-1/CXCR4.[101]

Many caveats must be heeded in the development of new therapeutic strategies that target HIV entry through the chemokine-chemokine receptor axis. The efficacy of any of these approaches depends on the spectrum of coreceptor utilization of the predominant viral population replicating in vivo. In this regard, exogenous and endogenous CC-chemokines suppress HIV replication in vitro in PBMCs from asymptomatic HIV-infected individuals harboring predominantly M-tropic strains of HIV,[102] but not in PBMCs from individuals with more advanced disease harboring predominantly T-tropic strains of HIV.[102, 103] Similarly, HIV isolates obtained longitudinally from individuals with rapid disease progression exhibit reduced sensitivity to inhibition by CC-chemokines in vitro over time.[62, 103] In addition, the effects of ligation of chemokine receptors in different cell types must be considered inasmuch as CC-chemokines may actually enhance the replication of M-tropic strains of HIV in monocyte/macrophages.[104] Unanticipated effects of manipulating the chemokine-chemokine receptor axis have also been observed, including CC-chemokine–mediated upregulation of CXCR4 expression and enhancement of replication of T-tropic strains of HIV in vitro.[105, 106] Finally, CXCR4 plays an essential role in normal hematopoiesis, cerebellar development, and gastrointestinal tract vascularization,[107–109] further highlighting potential caveats associated with manipulating chemokine receptors to inhibit HIV infection.

IMMUNE RESPONSES AGAINST HUMAN IMMUNODEFICIENCY VIRUS

Development of effective immunotherapies and vaccines for HIV infection has been hampered by the absence of known correlates of protective immunity (Fig. 107–2). Some immune responses to HIV may actually be harmful to the host. Certain anti-envelope gp41 antibodies present in the sera of HIV-infected individuals actually enhance HIV replication in vitro[110, 111]; the presence of these HIV-enhancing antibodies correlates with progression to acquired immunodeficiency syndrome (AIDS).[112] In addition, antibody responses to a specific epitope within the carboxy terminus of gp120 are associated with disease progression.[113] Anti-HIV cytotoxic T-lymphocyte (CTL) responses may be pathogenic in HIV-related inflammatory syndromes such as lymphocytic alveolitis.[114, 115] It has also been suggested that HIV-specific CTLs may play a central role in HIV pathogenesis by killing HIV-infected antigen-presenting cells in lymph nodes, bone marrow, and thymus, thus impairing the generation of immune responses.[116]

Most data, however, support a salutary role for most HIV-specific immune responses. The profound decrease in plasma viremia after acute HIV infection is associated with the appearance of HIV-specific cellular[117–119] and humoral[120–123] immune responses (Fig. 107–3*A* and *B*). The correlation of slow progression with vigorous HIV-specific immune responses also argues strongly in favor of a salutary role for these responses.[124]

Humoral Immune Responses

Antibodies against the viral core protein p24 develop within weeks of acute HIV infection and may play a role in the decline of plasma viremia associated with primary infection.[120, 122, 125, 126] Loss of anti-p24 antibodies is associated with progression of HIV disease.[120, 122, 125–128]

Antibodies that neutralize HIV infectivity in vitro may be responsible for partial control of viral replication in vivo.[122, 128–132] Neutralizing antibodies may be type specific (i.e., specific for one viral isolate)

Neutralizing Antibody

Cytotoxic CD8+ T Lymphocyte

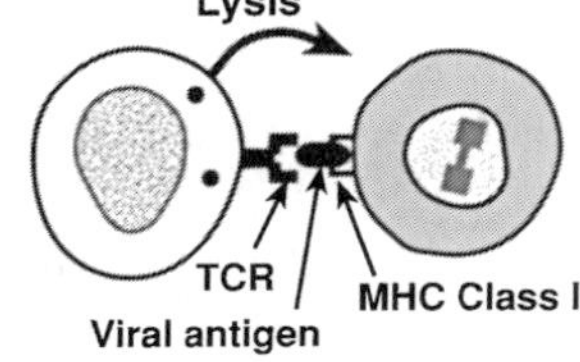

Bystander Killing

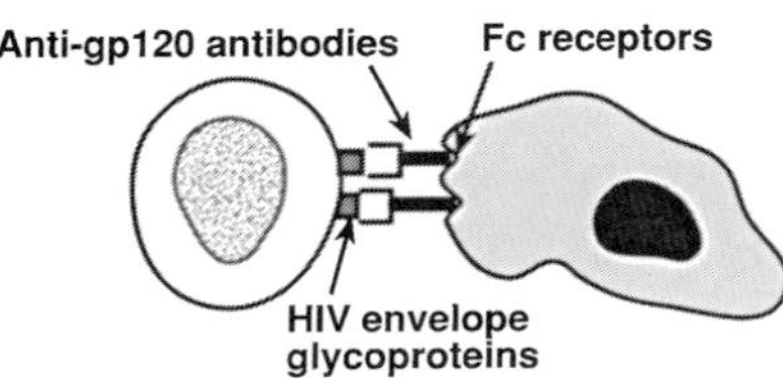

Helper CD4+ T Lymphocyte

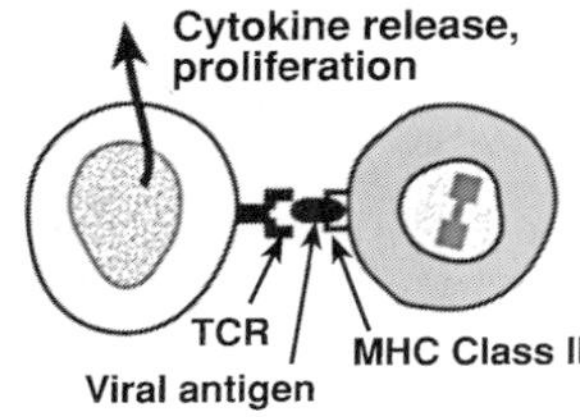

Natural Killer Cell Lysis

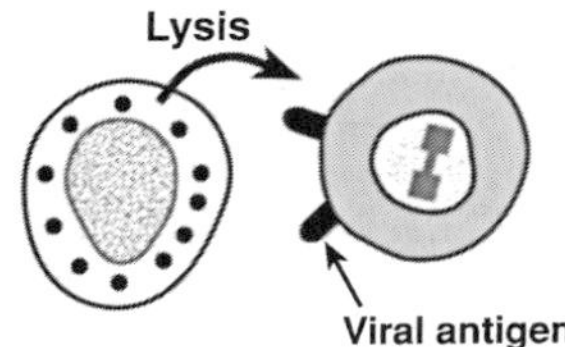

FIGURE 107–2. Immune responses against the human immunodeficiency virus (HIV). Neutralizing antibodies bind to virion components and prevent attachment to target cells. CD8+ cytotoxic T lymphocytes recognize viral antigens on the surface of infected cells in the context of MHC class I presentation and are able to directly lyse these cells. ADCC results in Fc receptor–mediated elimination of infected cells as well as uninfected cells that are coated HIV antigen-antibody complexes. CD4+ T cells may recognize viral antigens in the context of major histocompatibility complex (MHC) class II presentation, resulting in the release of cytokines and cellular proliferation. Natural killer cells may also directly lyse HIV-infected cells. *Abbreviation*: TCR, T-cell receptor. (Adapted from Fauci AS, Lane HC. Human immunodeficiency virus [HIV] disease: AIDS and related disorders. In: Fauci AS, Braunwald E, Isselbacher KJ, et al, eds. Harrison's Principles of Internal Medicine. 14th ed. New York: McGraw-Hill; 1998:1791–1856.)

or group specific (i.e., specific for a broad range of viral isolates). Most type-specific neutralizing antibodies recognize the V3 region of the HIV envelope gp120 protein.[133–138] These neutralizing anti–V3 loop antibodies may prevent the cleavage and conformational changes within gp120 necessary for HIV entry or for cell-cell fusion.[136, 139–142] Group-specific neutralizing antibodies recognize epitopes within the HIV envelope gp41 protein,[143–145] discontinuous conformational epitopes around the CD4 binding site of gp120,[146–149] or carbohydrate determinants.[150] Both type- and group-specific neutralizing antibodies are more efficient in neutralizing laboratory strains of HIV grown in T-cell lines as opposed to primary isolates grown in PBMCs, probably because of differential exposure of the V3 loop and CD4 binding domain epitopes.[151–154] Some neutralizing antibodies interfere with the interaction between the HIV envelope and CCR5, thereby inhibiting cellular entry of M-tropic strains of HIV.[31, 32]

The type of neutralizing antibody most relevant to the course of HIV infection is antibody that neutralizes autologous viral isolates.[155–157] The regularity with which viral variants emerge that resist neutralization suggests that such autologous neutralizing antibodies are potent impediments to viral replication.[155, 158–160] This cycle of neutralization followed by escape may be continuous over the course of infection in that serum from a given time point may neutralize contemporaneously isolated virus but not virus isolated at a later point.[158, 159, 161]

Disagreement surrounds the potential correlation between the presence of HIV neutralizing antibodies and the clinical course of disease, which is not surprising given the many different types of neutralizing antibodies that can be detected and the wide variety of assays for neutralization. Several studies do, however, suggest that the presence of neutralizing antibodies with broad specificity is correlated with a more favorable prognosis.[121, 132, 162–165]

Some anti-HIV antibodies bind to IgG Fc receptor–positive cells and sensitize them to mediate antibody-dependent cell-mediated cytotoxicity (ADCC) against HIV-infected or HIV-coated cells.[166–169] Most of these antibodies are directed against HIV envelope gp120 or gp41 proteins.[166, 168–172] CD16+ natural killer (NK) cells are important mediators of ADCC,[169, 173] although monocytes may also mediate this activity.[174] Anti-HIV ADCC antibodies develop soon after primary infection and are detectable throughout the course of HIV disease, with some decrease in titers with the onset of AIDS.[175–177]

ADCC may also represent an immunopathogenic immune response that may be responsible for CD4+ T-cell depletion during the course of HIV infection. In this regard, a combination of high levels of plasma viremia with high HIV envelope–specific ADCC activity is correlated with rapid CD4+ T-cell depletion; this correlation may reflect ADCC-mediated "innocent bystander" killing of gp120-coated, but uninfected CD4+ T cells.[178]

Cellular Immune Responses

Cytotoxic T Lymphocytes

In HIV-infected individuals, classic major histocompatibility complex (MHC) class I–restricted, HIV-specific CD8+ CTL responses have been demonstrated[179–181] against a variety of HIV target proteins,[182] including core proteins,[183, 184] reverse transcriptase,[185–187] envelope proteins,[187–190] and regulatory proteins.[191] An extraordinarily high frequency of HIV-specific CTLs and CTL precursors (up to 1% of peripheral blood T cells) has been observed in asymptomatic HIV-infected patients.[192–195]

A critical role for CTLs in the suppression of viral replication in HIV-infected individuals is suggested by the close correlation between emergence of an HIV-specific CTL response and downregulation of viremia after acute infection,[117–119] the inverse correlation between HIV-specific CTL activity and levels of plasma viremia,[195] the decline in HIV-specific CTL activity with disease progression,[179, 192] and the association of vigorous HIV-specific CTL responses with slow progression of HIV disease.[119, 162, 196–200] A beneficial role for HIV-specific CTLs is also suggested by their presence in the peripheral blood of individuals who are frequently exposed to HIV yet remain uninfected[201] and by the depletion of HIV-specific CTLs from lymph nodes of patients with advanced HIV disease.[202] These data argue against an immunopathogenic role for CTLs in HIV disease,[116] although as previously noted, CTL responses may be involved in the pathogenesis of some of the HIV-related inflammatory syndromes.[114, 115]

Although data support a salutary role for CTLs in HIV disease, the paradox of why disease progression occurs despite a vigorous CTL response remains unexplained. In this regard, qualitative aspects of the HIV-specific CTL response may also be important determinants of the efficacy of these responses in controlling viral replica-

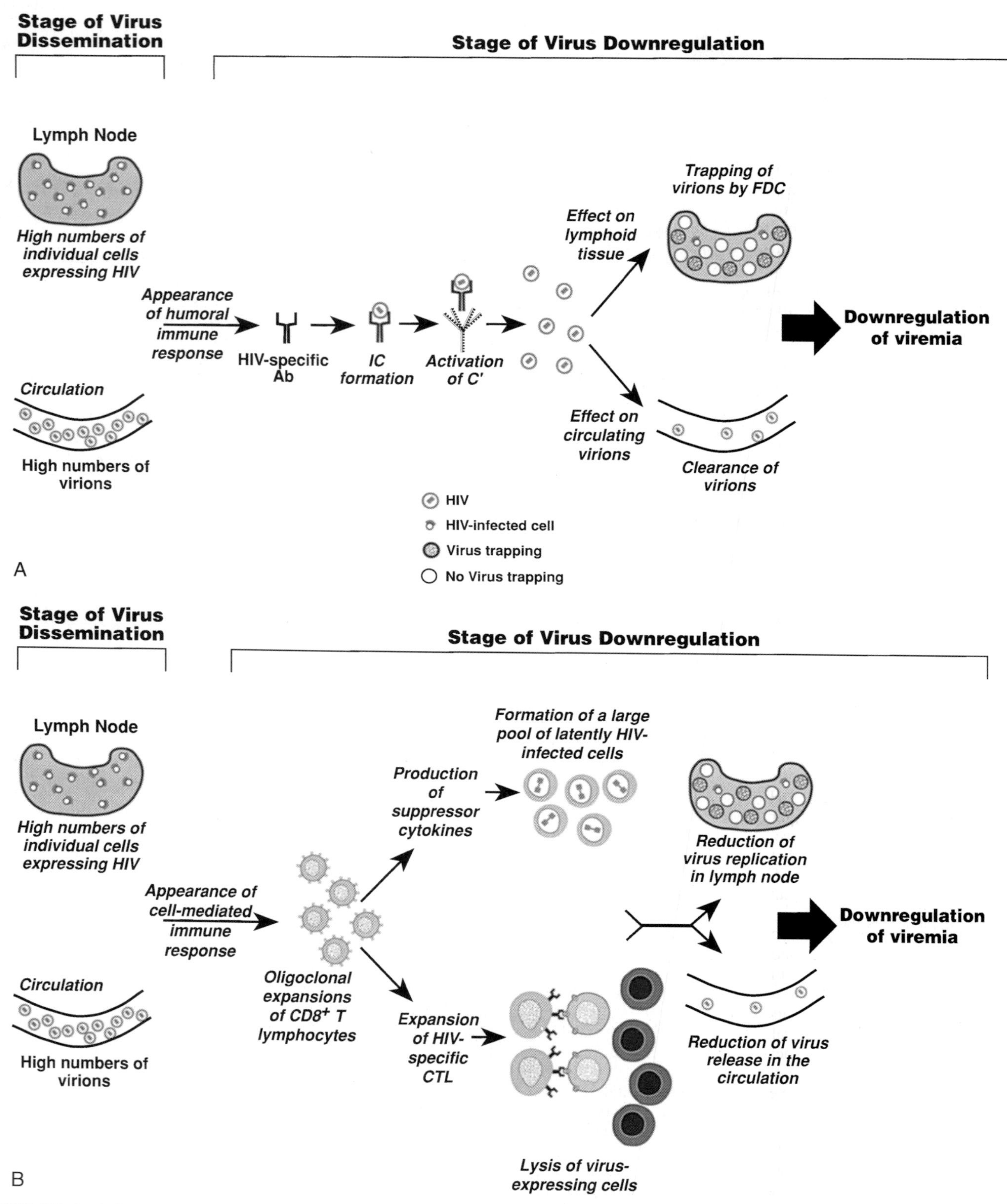

FIGURE 107–3. *A,* Downregulation of plasma viremia and adherence of virus-containing immune complexes to follicular dendritic cells in lymphoid tissue. Human immunodeficiency virus (HIV)–specific antibodies (Ab) combine with virions to form immune complexes (IC). Complement (C′) binds to the immune complexes, which are then trapped in the follicular dendritic cell (FDC) network by complement receptors. *B,* Downregulation of plasma viremia and establishment of a viral reservoir in lymphoid tissue after primary HIV infection. Emergence of cell-mediated immune responses against HIV leads to elimination of a large number of productively infected cells, causing a decrease in the source of plasma viremia. *Abbreviation.* CTL, Cytotoxic T lymphocyte. (Adapted with permission from Pantaleo G, Graziosi C, Demarest JF, et al. Role of lymphoid organs in the pathogenesis of human immunodeficiency virus [HIV] infection. Immunol Rev. 1994;140:105–130. © 1994, Munksgaard International Publishers Ltd. Copenhagen, Denmark.)

tion. Maintenance of CTL responses specific for viral core proteins is associated with a decreased risk of disease progression[199, 200, 203]; similar associations have been observed less often for CTL responses against other viral proteins.[119] CTL recognition of immunodominant HIV epitopes presented by certain MHC class I alleles may result in potent anti-HIV activity[204] and may in part explain the association of certain MHC class I alleles with slower progression of HIV disease.[205–207]

Molecular analysis has demonstrated that clones of HIV-specific $CD8^+$ CTLs initially expand during primary HIV infection and then decrease after their initial expansion. $CD8^+$ T-cell subsets can be categorized according to the expression of different variable (V) regions of the T-cell receptor V_β chain (V_β). Twenty-four V_β families in the T-cell receptor repertoire have been differentiated. Three patterns of $CD8^+$ CTL expansions may occur during the acute stages of HIV infection, and these patterns correlate with rates of disease progression. In the first pattern of CTL expansion, major expansion of one or two V_β families occurs; this pattern of expansion is associated with rapid disease progression, with AIDS often developing within 1 to 2 years. The second pattern of CTL expansion includes smaller expansions of three or four V_β families and is associated with a more moderate rate of disease progression. The third pattern, with minor, diffuse, or no significant expansions of V_β families, is associated with the most favorable prognosis.[208] Thus, the ability to recruit an HIV-specific CTL response composed of a diverse group of V_β families during primary infection is associated with better control of viral replication and an improved prognosis when compared with restricted CTL expansion from only one or two V_β families.

The loss of HIV-specific CTL activity in patients with progressive disease is probably a result of several factors. The viral accessory proteins Tat, Nef, and Vpu can downregulate cellular expression of the MHC class I molecules that are necessary for CTL recognition of infected cells.[209–212] Another mechanism responsible for the loss of CTL activity is the selective accumulation of $CD8^+$, DR^+ HIV-specific CTLs that lack the IL-2 receptor and are defective in clonogenic potential.[184, 213, 214] The ability of HIV to escape CTL responses by viral mutation or by exhaustion of CTL clones as a result of a high concentration of antigen also helps explain the loss of CTL-mediated control over viral replication (see later).

The host CTL response against HIV is constrained by the ability of MHC class I alleles to bind to various viral epitopes, whereas the virus is constrained by the degree to which an escape mutation impairs viral fitness. These host-virus dynamics are extraordinarily complex given the large number of permutations of viral epitopes and MHC class I alleles. Viral mutations within CTL recognition epitopes (i.e., "escape mutants") are associated with increased levels of viral replication and progression of HIV disease.[215–219] These viral escape mutants appear to emerge under the selective pressure exerted by the host CTL response[217–219]; they may thrive because of the release of CTL control over their replication and may also inhibit CTL responses against the pre-escape viral epitope.[220, 221] Some viral escape mutations are costly to viral fitness. In this regard, diffuse infiltrative CD8 lymphocytosis associated with HIV infection is associated with certain HLA types that apparently constrain evolution of viral sequence diversity in the envelope V3 loop.[222] Other studies have highlighted the constraints on the host CTL response imposed by MHC class I alleles. Kalams and coworkers demonstrated in an HIV-infected individual that CTL clones specific for an HLA-B14–restricted epitope of gp41 displayed very limited diversity of T-cell receptor utilization.[223] These investigators further demonstrated the limited plasticity of certain CTL responses in individuals with viral escape mutants, in whom the dominant CTL response may remain largely directed at the pre-escape viral epitope[224, 225]; these data are consistent with the "original antigenic sin" model.[226] Other studies demonstrated that increased plasticity of the CTL response (i.e., generation of vigorous escape mutant–specific CTLs) may allow the host to maintain more continuous and effective control over viral replication.[227, 228] A mathematic model of CTL-virus dynamics was provided by Nowak and coworkers, who described disease progression as a result of viral sequence variation that escapes an immunodominant CTL response and shifts the host response toward a weaker epitope.[229] In this scenario, disease progression may be the result of fitness of viral escape mutants outpacing the plasticity of the host CTL response, with slow progression resulting from CTL plasticity overpowering viral escape mutants with limited fitness.

A further mechanism for loss of CTL control over viral replication may be clonal exhaustion. This mechanism appears to be a strategy for viral persistence used by other viruses, such as certain strains of lymphocytic choriomeningitis virus that rapidly and completely mobilize the host CTL response and thereby result in CTL exhaustion (i.e., high zone tolerance).[230] CTL exhaustion may also occur to some degree in HIV infection: the disappearance of some CTL clonotypes can be demonstrated in the absence of viral escape mutations that might otherwise explain the phenomenon.[231]

Soluble Human Immunodeficiency Virus Suppressor Factors Secreted by $CD8^+$ T Cells

$CD8^+$ T cells may suppress HIV replication by both cytolytic and noncytolytic mechanisms.[232] A variety of soluble antiviral factors are elaborated by $CD8^+$ T cells. CD8 antiviral factor[10, 233, 234] is noncytolytic, acts in a non–MHC-restricted manner, inhibits viral replication at the level of HIV long terminal repeat transcription,[235–237] and lacks identity to known cytokines.[238] CD8 antiviral factor activity decreases with disease progression but remains potent in long-term nonprogressors.[92, 164, 239] RANTES, MIP-1α, and MIP-1β (the natural ligands for CCR5, a major coreceptor for M-tropic strains of HIV) are also important soluble antiviral factors secreted by $CD8^+$ T cells and other cell types.[11, 102] These CC-chemokines inhibit viral replication primarily at the level of cell entry. Conflicting data have been obtained regarding a relationship between levels of these chemokines and progression of HIV disease[85, 86, 88, 89, 92, 240–242]; recent reports, however, support a role for CC-chemokines in protecting against HIV infection and disease progression[90, 91, 93, 94] (see the previous section). Macrophage-derived chemokine is a recently discovered CC-chemokine that can potently suppress the replication of M- and T-tropic strains of HIV in vitro[243]; the role of macrophage-derived chemokine in controlling HIV replication in vivo is uncertain. Finally, IL-16 has been reported to be a soluble antiviral factor[244]; however, a relationship between IL-16 production and disease progression remains to be established.[88, 92]

$CD4^+$ T-Cell Responses

HIV proteins contain helper T-cell epitopes that may be presented by MHC class II alleles.[245–247] Recognition of these epitopes by $CD4^+$ T cells results in IL-2 secretion and cellular proliferation. These responses decrease with HIV disease progression.[248] The IL-2 that is produced during these responses may augment HIV-specific CTL responses; however, IL-2 may also indirectly enhance HIV replication by inducing the secretion of proinflammatory cytokines.[249] Whether $CD4^+$ T-cell proliferative responses to HIV play any protective or deleterious role in HIV-specific immunity remains uncertain; however, a recent study found vigorous HIV-specific $CD4^+$ T-cell responses in patients who were able to maintain low levels of plasma viremia in the absence of treatment.[250] A broader survey of patients in the chronic stage of HIV infection revealed an inverse correlation between the magnitude of the HIV-specific $CD4^+$ T-cell response and levels of plasma viremia; furthermore, strong $CD4^+$ T-cell responses may be preserved by potent antiretroviral therapy given during acute HIV infection.[250]

IMMUNE DYSFUNCTION DURING HUMAN IMMUNODEFICIENCY VIRUS INFECTION

A wide array of immune system deficits is associated with HIV infection. Abnormalities in the function of all limbs of the immune system, including T and B lymphocytes, antigen-presenting cells, NK cells, and neutrophils, have been described (see later). Immunodeficiency may become sufficiently profound in the late stages of disease that the HIV-specific antibody and cytolytic T-lymphocyte responses diminish in the face of high levels of ongoing viral replication.

The immunodeficiency induced by HIV can be best appreciated in the context of the microenvironment in which immune responses are generated. Advanced stages of HIV infection are marked by striking disruption of lymphoid tissue architecture.[251–258] Follicular involution, hypervascularity, and fibrosis are some of the pathologic changes evident in lymph nodes from patients with advanced HIV disease. The loss of follicular dendritic cells, which results in follicular involution, has important implications with regard to the pathogenesis of HIV-related immunodeficiency. The ability to mount immune responses against new antigens and the ability to maintain memory responses are severely impaired in the absence of an intact follicular dendritic cell network.[259] This loss of functional substrate for the generation and maintenance of immune responses results in loss of containment of HIV replication and enhanced susceptibility to opportunistic infections.

CD4⁺ T Cells

CD4⁺ T-cell dysfunction, both quantitative and qualitative, is the hallmark of HIV disease. The opportunistic infections observed with advancing disease are primarily due to defects in T-cell number and function that result directly or indirectly from HIV infection. Direct effects of HIV on CD4⁺ T-cell function include infection and resultant cytotoxicity with loss of absolute cell numbers. Indirect effects of HIV infection result in decreased CD4⁺ T-cell proliferation and differentiation, dysregulation and decreased production of IL-2 and other cytokines, decreased IL-2 receptor expression, and defective T-cell colony formation and other precursor defects (reviewed in ref. 260). The loss of immune competence during the course of HIV disease progression can be gauged by the sequential loss of in vitro proliferative responses of peripheral blood lymphocytes to recall antigens, alloantigens, and finally, mitogens.[261]

T cells from HIV-infected individuals manifest a variety of phenotypic abnormalities. In addition to the decrease in IL-2 production and IL-2 receptor expression, the percentage of CD4⁺ T cells expressing CD28 (i.e., the major costimulatory receptor that is necessary for normal activation of T cells) is reduced during HIV infection in comparison to cells from uninfected individuals.[262] CD28⁻ cells do not respond to activation signals, including anti-CD3 monoclonal antibodies or mitogens, and express markers of terminal activation, including HLA-DR, CD38, and CD45RO.[263] CD4⁺ T cells from HIV-infected individuals express abnormally low levels of CD40 ligand,[264] which may in part explain the dysregulation of B-cell function that is observed during the course of disease.

A variety of mechanisms, both directly and indirectly related to HIV infection of CD4⁺ T cells, are probably responsible for the observed defects in T-cell colony formation, autologous mixed lymphocyte reactions, expression of IL-2 receptors, and IL-2 production (reviewed in ref. 260). Interference with CD4 expression by HIV gp120,[265] Nef,[266] and Vpu[267, 268] may impair the ability of an infected CD4⁺ T cell to interact with appropriate MHC class II molecules. Preferential infection by HIV of CD4⁺CD45RO⁺ memory cells, the preferential susceptibility of these cells to the cytopathic effects of HIV infection, or both may in part explain the loss of memory responses to soluble antigens and the consequent increase in the risk of infection with opportunistic organisms.[269–271]

The relatively small fraction of T cells that are infected with HIV in seropositive subjects argues against direct infection as the sole mediator of the immunopathogenesis of HIV infection.[272] In addition, CD4⁺ T-cell dysfunction is evident even in the early stages of HIV infection, before quantitative depletion of this key cellular subset.[273] A role for HIV envelope in the immunopathogenesis of HIV disease has been suggested by a number of studies (reviewed in ref. 274). The presence of measurable levels of circulating soluble gp120 in HIV-infected subjects[275, 276] and accumulation of high concentrations of virions (both infectious and defective) in lymphoid tissue[258, 277, 278] underscore the potential for envelope to contribute to T-cell dysfunction in a process distinct from infection of CD4⁺ T cells.

HIV envelope glycoproteins bind with high affinity to the CD4 molecule and to a number of coreceptors (see earlier). Evidence of aberrant intracellular signaling induced by HIV has been available for a number of years.[279, 280] Intracellular signals transduced by HIV-1 envelope have been implicated in several immunopathogenic processes, including anergy,[281–284] syncytium formation,[285] apoptosis,[286, 287] and inappropriate cell trafficking.[288] The molecular mechanisms responsible for these abnormalities include dysregulation of the T-cell receptor phosphoinositide pathway,[289] p561ck activation,[281, 290–292] downregulation of the costimulatory molecules CD40 ligand and CD80,[293] and activation of the ras signaling pathway.[282] Most of these aberrant signals were presumed to result from interactions between HIV envelope glycoproteins and CD4; however, more recently it has become clear that HIV envelope may also transduce intracellular signals through coreceptor molecules such as CCR5.[288, 294, 294a]

Another incisive view of the qualitative nature of the immunodeficiency that occurs during the course of HIV infection is provided by study of the CD4⁺ T-cell receptor V_β repertoire. Disruptions in the V_β repertoire are seen with increased frequency in CD4⁺ T cells from patients with advanced-stage HIV disease, particularly with CD4⁺ T-cell counts of less than 200 cells/μl[295, 296]; these disruptions are caused by severe depletion of cells with various specificities, thus creating "holes" in the immunologic repertoire (Fig. 107–4). The degree to which the V_β repertoire can be reconstituted with antiretroviral therapy remains an important and controversial issue[295, 297] that has important implications regarding whether prophylaxis against opportunistic infections can be discontinued in individuals whose CD4⁺ T-cell counts rise to greater than 200 cells/μl during therapy.[298, 299]

A. Normal Vβx profile

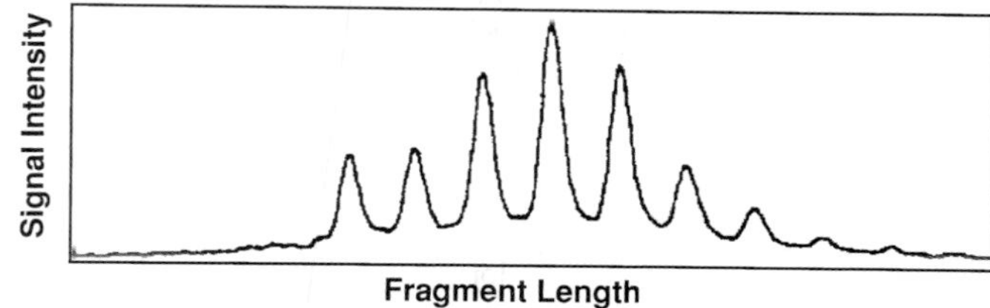

B. Skewed Vβx profile

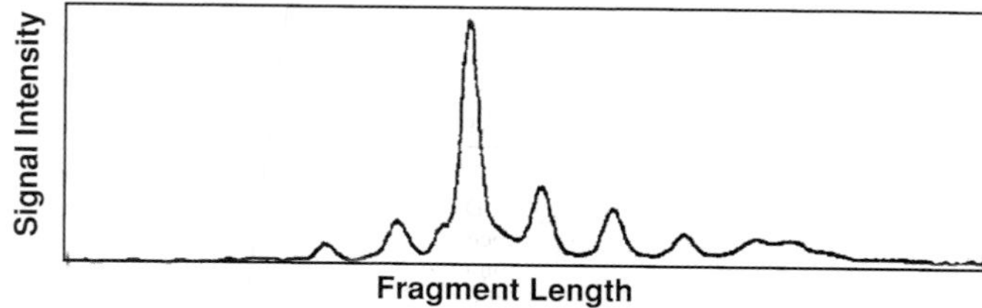

FIGURE 107–4. Polymerase chain reaction (PCR) amplication across the CDR3 region of T-cell receptor Vβ cDNA yields products of about eight different lengths; this is due to recombination, which alters the VDJ junction length by six to eight amino acids. A normal T-cell receptor profile *(A)* reveals a normal distribution of VDJ fragment lengths due to the random nature of recombination. Deletion of T cells with certain clonotypes (and therefore particular VDJ fragment lengths) yields a skewed Vβ profile, as shown in *B*.

Mechanisms of CD4+ T-Cell Depletion

Direct Infection

The observations that CD4+ T cells are the principal targets of HIV infection in vivo and that HIV infection of CD4+ T cells in vitro causes cytopathicity[300–307] led to a reasonable assumption that direct infection of CD4+ T cells in vivo results in their depletion. However, quantitative studies of the frequency of HIV-infected cells in vivo suggest that single-cell killing by direct infection with HIV may not be the predominant mechanism of CD4+ T-cell depletion. In this regard, the proportion of HIV-infected peripheral blood CD4+ T cells in individuals in the early asymptomatic stage of HIV infection is typically in the range of 1 in 1000 to 1 in 100,000.[272, 308] Although this frequency increases with disease progression, the proportion of HIV-infected peripheral blood CD4+ T cells rarely exceeds 1 in 100 even in patients with AIDS.[308–312] Viral burden and levels of virus expression are far greater in lymphoid tissue than in peripheral blood[258, 272, 313]; however, these levels, even in lymphoid tissue, do not appear to be sufficiently high to account for CD4+ T-cell depletion solely by direct mechanisms.

Multiple mechanisms of cell death appear to be operative after infection of a CD4+ T cell with HIV (Table 107–1). Early events in the viral life cycle, such as accumulation of reverse-transcribed viral DNA in the cytoplasm, may contribute to cell killing in HIV infection[302]; however, this mechanism is clearly not the only one responsible for single-cell killing by HIV.[314] High levels of viral RNA and aberrant RNA molecules are also present in the cytoplasm of infected cells and possibly interfere with normal cellular RNA processing.[315, 316]

The intracellular concentration of envelope gp120 molecules is high during the process of virion assembly in an HIV-infected cell. Several studies have suggested that intracellular gp120 may interact with intracellular CD4 molecules and that this interaction may induce cell death.[305, 317] The mechanism of cell death as a consequence of this intracellular gp120-CD4 interaction may be autofusion events that disrupt the integrity of the cell membrane.[318] Cell membrane integrity may also be compromised by the budding of virions from an infected cell[319, 320] and by HIV-induced increases in the concentration of intracellular monovalent cations.[321]

HIV-infected cells may also die as a consequence of viral-specific immune responses that occur before the cell succumbs directly to viral infection. Multiple effector mechanisms may be involved in the killing of HIV-infected cells, including CTL responses, ADCC, and NK cell responses.

Indirect Mechanisms

Syncytium Formation. HIV envelope glycoprotein molecules are inserted into the host cell membrane during virion assembly and are also shed by infected cells into the surrounding milieu. Interaction of these HIV envelope glycoprotein molecules with uninfected cells may be an important immunopathogenic mechanism of HIV infection.

The molecular events associated with viral entry that lead to fusion between the viral coat and cell membrane involve the interaction of HIV envelope glycoprotein, CD4, and a coreceptor molecule (see previous discussion). Similar events may occur when an infected cell bearing HIV envelope glycoprotein molecules on its surface encounters an uninfected CD4+ cell with an appropriate coreceptor. Fusion between infected and uninfected cells with the formation of multinucleated giant cells, or syncytia, has long been observed in vitro.[304, 306, 307, 322] Other molecules implicated in syncytium formation include LFA-1,[323, 324] CD7,[325] and HLA class I molecules.[326] Syncytia have been observed only rarely in tissues obtained from HIV-infected individuals[255, 327–332]; thus, it is unlikely that syncytium formation is a major pathogenic mechanism of CD4+ T-cell depletion.

Autoimmunity. Autoimmunity may occur during the course of HIV infection as a result of molecular mimicry by viral components. Highly homologous regions exist in the carboxy terminus of the HIV-1 envelope glycoprotein and the amino-terminal domains of different HLA-DR and DQ alleles.[333] Sera from a substantial number of HIV-infected individuals react with the shared determinant of gp41 and MHC class II; these sera can inhibit normal antigen-specific proliferative responses and also eliminate class II–bearing cells by ADCC.[334] Similar instances of molecular mimicry between HIV-1 envelope constituents and host proteins that may result in pathogenic autoimmune responses include the collagen-like region of complement component C1q-A,[335] MHC class I heavy chains,[336] HLA-DR4 and DR2 alleles,[337] variable regions of the T-cell receptor α-, β-, and γ-chains,[337] Fas,[337] functional domains of IgG and IgA,[337] denatured collagen,[338] and a number of nuclear antigens.[339, 340]

Superantigens. Superantigens are able to bind to the T-cell receptor V_β chain and an MHC class II molecule and are therefore able to stimulate virtually any T cell from a particular V_β family. The consequences of superantigenic stimulation involve perturbations (expansions, deletions, functional impairment) of cells from particular T-cell receptor V_β families. The discovery that the pathogenesis of murine leukemia virus–induced immunodeficiency syndrome in mice was linked to the presence of a virally encoded superantigen[341] led to the investigation of a similar scenario in HIV infection. Depletion of various sets of T-cell receptor V_β families in peripheral blood from HIV-infected patients further suggested that HIV may encode superantigens.[342] Anergy of $V_\beta8^+$ T cells in HIV-infected individuals and the preferential infectability of CD4+, $V_\beta12^+$ T cells with HIV also supported a possible role for a superantigen.[343–346] However, these latter observations were shown to be due to a putative cytomegalovirus-encoded superantigen rather than one encoded by HIV itself.[347] The superantigen-mediated pathogenesis hypothesis in HIV infection is tenuous given the number of studies that have found no evidence of superantigen-like effects in HIV-infected patients. Several studies have found no selective loss of particular V_β families of T cells during HIV infection.[348, 349] Other studies have found variable perturbations of the T-cell receptor V_β repertoire that are inconsistent with superantigen-mediated effects.[208, 295, 350, 351]

Innocent Bystander Phenomena. Immune responses that target HIV determinants on infected cells may also contribute to the elimination of uninfected cells bearing HIV proteins (e.g., gp120) on their surface. Targeting of such "innocent bystander" cells by antibody and cellular immune responses has been described.[352–354]

Apoptosis. Apoptosis is the morphologic description of a form of programmed cell death critical to physiologic homeostasis in virtually every organ system (reviewed in refs. 355 and 356). Apoptotic cell death is characterized by plasma membrane blebbing, nuclear condensation, DNA fragmentation, and release of cellular contents in the form of small, dense apoptotic bodies. Ingestion of apoptotic bodies by phagocytes completes the apoptotic death process without

TABLE 107–1 Mechanisms of CD4+ T-Cell Dysfunction and Depletion

Mechanisms
Direct mechanisms
Accumulation of unintegrated viral DNA
Interference with cellular RNA processing
Intracellular gp 120-CD4 autofusion events
Loss of plasma membrane integrity because of viral budding
Elimination of HIV-infected cells by virus-specific immune responses
Indirect mechanisms
Aberrant intracellular signaling events
Syncytium formation
Autoimmunity
Superantigenic stimulation
Innocent bystander killing of viral antigen–coated cells
Apoptosis
Inhibition of lymphopoiesis

the inflammation associated with spillage of cellular contents that occurs in nonphysiologic necrotic cell death. A wide array of physiologic stimuli serve as positive and negative regulators of apoptosis. Important inhibitors of apoptosis include growth factors, extracellular matrix, and CD40 ligand, whereas important activators of apoptosis include CD95 (Fas) ligand, tumor necrosis factor (TNF), transforming growth factor-β (TGF-β), neurotransmitters, and withdrawal of growth factor. The discoveries that the *bcl*-2 gene plays an important pathogenic role in lymphomagenesis through its ability to prevent cells from undergoing apoptosis[357–359] and that the *p53* gene is necessary for initiation of apoptosis[360–362] established the paradigm that diseases associated with increased cell survival or increased cell death may result from dysregulation of the normal pathways of apoptosis.

Several investigators suggested that aberrant intracellular signals transduced by HIV might prime CD4+ T cells for apoptosis and thereby result in depletion of these cells during the course of HIV infection.[363, 364] Acute infection of T cells with HIV in vitro was shown to induce apoptosis,[365, 366] and T cells from HIV-infected patients were demonstrated to undergo enhanced rates of apoptosis in vitro when compared with normal T cells, particularly after activation.[367, 368] Cross-linking of CD4 followed by ligation of the T-cell receptor is sufficient to induce apoptosis, which suggests that uninfected CD4+ T cells could be depleted inappropriately upon encountering antigen if CD4 had been cross linked by gp120.[286, 369] The viral Tat protein can also lead to apoptotic cell death, possibly by upregulating CD95 ligand, by enhancing activation of cyclin-dependent kinases, or both.[287, 370]

It remains uncertain whether HIV-induced apoptosis plays an important role in vivo in CD4+ T-cell depletion. The frequency of apoptotic CD4+ and CD8+ T cells, as well as B cells, is significantly higher in lymphoid tissue from HIV-infected individuals than uninfected controls.[371] The intensity of apoptosis is related to the degree of immune activation and is observed predominantly in uninfected "bystander" cells.[371, 372] Although some data support a positive correlation between the stage of HIV disease and susceptibility of peripheral blood T cells to apoptosis,[373] another study found no such correlation[374]; Muro-Cacho and colleagues found that the intensity of apoptosis in lymphoid tissue was independent of the peripheral CD4+ T-cell count and level of plasma viremia.[371] Perhaps the most compelling evidence that apoptosis may play a role in HIV pathogenesis is that an increased frequency of apoptosis in CD4+ T cells is seen in HIV-infected humans and in primates infected with pathogenic strains of simian immunodeficiency virus, but not in primates infected with nonpathogenic strains.[375]

Human Immunodeficiency Virus–Mediated Inhibition of Hematopoiesis. Failure of normal hematopoiesis is an obvious candidate mechanism to account for depletion of CD4+ T cells during HIV infection. A subset of CD34+ progenitor cells express CD4 and are infectable in vitro with HIV-1.[376–378] It is controversial whether CD34+ progenitor cells represent a substantial in vivo reservoir for HIV. A number of studies have failed to detect HIV-infected CD34+ progenitor cells in most HIV-infected individuals[379–382]; however, a large study by Stanley and associates showed that a substantial minority of HIV-infected patients with severe CD4+ T-cell depletion have a reservoir of HIV-infected CD34+ progenitor cells.[383] Recent reports demonstrating expression of HIV coreceptors on CD34+ progenitor cells[384, 385] suggest that the CD4+ subset of these cells may be infectable with HIV, further substantiating the earlier findings of Stanley and coworkers.

Although the role of direct infection of CD34+ progenitor cells in HIV pathogenesis remains controversial, a large body of evidence suggests that viral proteins and HIV-induced cytokines can impair the survival and clonogenic potential of these cells.[382, 386–393]

Disruption of the thymic microenvironment[394] and HIV-induced thymocyte depletion may also contribute to the failure of CD4+ T-cell replenishment. Thymic epithelial cells normally secrete IL-6, which can in turn increase HIV replication in infected cells.[395] Subpopulations of thymic CD3−, CD4−, CD8− cells (i.e., "triple-negative" cells) are susceptible to infection with HIV in vitro,[396] and thymic CD3−, CD4+, CD8− progenitor cells from HIV-infected patients are infected in vivo. Finally, uninfected thymocytes from HIV-infected individuals are primed for apoptotic death, thus suggesting that indirect mechanisms of defective thymopoiesis are operative as well.[397]

CD8+ T Cells

Dysregulation of CD8+ T-cell numbers and function is evident throughout the course of HIV disease. After acute primary infection, CD8+ T-cell counts usually rebound to supranormal levels and may remain elevated for prolonged periods. Increases in CD8+ T cells during all but the late stages of disease may in part reflect the expansion of HIV-specific CD8+ CTLs.

During HIV disease progression, CD8+ T cells acquire an abnormal phenotype characterized by the expression of certain activation markers and the absence of expression of the CD25 IL-2 receptor. Alterations in the phenotype of CD8+ T cells in HIV-infected individuals may have prognostic significance. In this regard, individuals whose CD8+ T cells express HLA-DR but not CD38 after seroconversion experience stabilization of their CD4+ T-cell counts and a less fulminant disease course, whereas individuals whose CD8+ T cells express both HLA-DR and CD38 experience a more aggressive course with rapid CD4+ T-cell depletion and have a poorer prognosis.[398–400] CD8+ T cells lacking CD28 expression are also increased in HIV disease,[401] possibly reflecting expansion of the CD8−, CD28−, CD57+ T-cell subset containing in vivo activated CTLs.[402] The loss of CTL activity with disease progression is not restricted to HIV-specific CTLs; a loss of cytotoxic activity to other common antigens, including Epstein-Barr virus and *Mycobacterium tuberculosis,* has also been observed.[403, 404] In addition to CTL activity, other CD8+ T-cell functions are impaired during HIV disease progression, including loss of noncytolytic non–MHC-restricted CD8+ T-cell–derived suppressor activity against HIV.[239]

Oligoclonal expansions of CD8+ T cells are characteristic of HIV infection (see earlier). These expansions are largely composed of HIV-specific CTLs.[351, 405] The disappearance of CTLs with particular specificity can be due to a number of factors, including mutation of the virus within the CTL recognition epitope. Another cause of the disappearance of some CTLs, however, is clonal exhaustion. This phenomenon, wherein high concentrations of antigen completely mobilize a CTL response, occurs in lymphocyte choriomeningitis virus infection[230]; deletion of the CTLs results with persistence of antigen. CTL exhaustion may occur to some extent during HIV infection, where disappearance of some CTLs is observed in the absence of viral escape mutations that would otherwise explain the phenomenon.[231]

Monocytes-Macrophages

Cells of the monocyte-macrophage lineage play key roles in the immunopathogenesis of HIV disease. These cells serve as reservoirs of viral infection and are responsible for a variety of tissue-specific pathologic processes. Dysfunction of these cells contributes to CD4+ T-cell dysfunction and also to impaired host defense against intracellular pathogens.[3, 406]

Monocytic cells express CD4 and numerous HIV coreceptors on their surface, including CCR5, CXCR4, and CCR3,[407–410] and serve as targets of HIV infection. Unlike infection of CD4+ T cells, HIV is relatively noncytopathic for cells of the monocyte-macrophage lineage, and HIV can replicate extensively in these cells.[411, 412] Chronically infected macrophages may be long lived, and current antiretroviral agents are not capable of targeting chronically infected cells; these cells therefore represent a formidable challenge to eradication of HIV.[413] Circulating monocytes are rarely found to be infected in vivo and are difficult to infect in vitro[412, 414, 415]; however, infection can readily be demonstrated in tissue macrophages, including resident microglial cells in the brain, pulmonary alveolar macrophages, and mature macrophages derived from blood monocytes in vitro.[180, 416–418] Infection of monocytic precursors in bone marrow may be directly or indirectly responsible for certain of the hematologic abnormalities observed in HIV-infected individuals. Lymphoid tissue macrophages can be prolific producers of HIV in the setting of opportunistic infections, during which the cytokine milieu in the tissue favors a highly productive state of HIV infection.[419]

Cells of the monocyte-macrophage lineage are central to the pathogenesis of HIV-induced central nervous system disease. HIV infection of brain microglial cells, derived from the monocytic lineage, may lead to encephalopathy and neuropathy,[420] astrocytosis,[421] and cerebral vasculitis.[422, 423] Levels of monocyte chemotactic protein type 1 (MCP-1) are markedly elevated in the cerebrospinal fluid of AIDS patients with HIV or cytomegalovirus encephalitis.[424, 425] A major source of these high levels of MCP-1 is likely HIV-infected macrophages.[425] MCP-1 in turn recruits and activates monocytes, which elaborate proinflammatory cytokines and thereby enhance HIV replication and induce neuropathologic disease.[426]

Infection of monocyte-macrophages with HIV or exposure of these cells to viral proteins, including envelope glycoproteins and Tat, leads to a number of functional abnormalities. Impaired accessory cell function[427, 428] may result from decreased MHC class II expression, decreased IL-12 secretion, and increased IL-10 secretion[428, 429]; this HIV-induced dysregulation of antigen presentation may in turn be a significant cause of hyporesponsiveness of $CD4^+$ T cells.[430] Defects in the ADCC function of monocyte-macrophages, possibly related to low levels of expression of Fc and complement receptors, have also been observed in HIV infection.[431–433] Finally, HIV-associated abnormalities in antigen uptake, oxidative burst, and chemotaxis have been described in monocyte-macrophages.[429, 434–437] As a consequence of these HIV-induced functional abnormalities, monocyte-macrophages exhibit poor intracellular killing of *Candida* species yeast forms,[432, 438] *Toxoplasma gondii,*[439] and *Histoplasma capsulatum.*[440]

Dendritic Cells

Dendritic cells are among the first cells to encounter HIV after mucosal exposure and are probably responsible for transporting the virus to lymphoid organs, thus facilitating infection of $CD4^+$ T cells and viral dissemination. Dendritic cells express several different chemokine receptors that can be used as HIV coreceptors for entry.[57, 441, 442] Studies of dendritic cells from HIV-infected individuals have yielded conflicting results: some authors have found high levels of infection in dendritic cells isolated ex vivo from peripheral blood,[443] whereas others have not.[444, 445] A number of studies have demonstrated that productive infection of tissue dendritic cells with HIV is rare. It is generally agreed that Langerhans cells (dendritic cells resident in the epidermis) from the skin of HIV-infected individuals are occasionally infected; however, such infection occurs at a very low frequency, rarely approaching the level of infection found in peripheral blood $CD4^+$ T cells and often 10 to 100 times less.[446–450] Dendritic cells in lymphoid organs also appear to be infrequently infected with HIV in vivo.[451, 452]

It has been reported that infectability of Langerhans cells may be dependent on viral subtype.[453] Clade B viruses, which are predominant in the United States and Europe, replicate poorly in Langerhans cells in vitro, whereas clade E viruses, which are predominant in Southeast Asia, replicate well in these cells.[453] It has been hypothesized that this finding may in part explain the differences in the epidemiology of HIV infection in the United States and Europe versus sub-Saharan Africa, Asia, and India. In the United States and Europe, the majority of HIV infections occur in homosexuals and injection drug users, whereas in sub-Saharan Africa, Asia, and India, more than 90% of infections are spread via heterosexual contact.[454] Thus, an HIV subtype that can replicate well in Langerhans cells, probably a major cell type involved in the initiation of viral infection through mucosal contact,[455] may be more efficiently transmitted heterosexually. It should be pointed out that these these findings are controversial[456, 457] and further studies are required to establish whether preferential cellular tropism of different clades of HIV plays a role in the global epidemiology of HIV spread.

It is controversial whether dysfunction of dendritic cells occurs during HIV infection.[443, 458, 459] A number of studies have suggested that HIV infection can impair the ability of dendritic cells to activate T cells[443, 460–462]; however, other studies have found no or minimal HIV-induced dendritic cell dysfunction.[450, 459] Interpretation of these studies is complicated by the use of different dendritic cell purification techniques, the existence of multiple dendritic cell subsets, and differential culture conditions used by investigators. Therefore, further studies are needed to clarify the possible role of dendritic cell depletion and dysfunction in the pathogenesis of HIV disease.

B Lymphocytes

HIV infection is almost invariably associated with hypergammaglobulinemia and B lymphocyte hyperactivation. A large component of the immunoglobulin specificity, at least in early-stage disease, is directed against HIV antigens. It has been suggested that a majority of activated B cells produce antibodies directed against HIV during this stage of infection (reviewed in ref. 463). In spite of the observed B-cell hyperactivation, the ability of B cells to respond to antigens is reduced. B cells from HIV-infected individuals express abnormally low levels of HLA-DR on their surface[464] and also fail to normally upregulate CD70 after stimulation with activated T cells[264]; this latter defect is associated with impaired CD70-dependent immunoglobulin synthesis.[264] Dysregulation of B-cell activation and the decreased ability of these cells to respond to antigen are probably responsible in part for the increase in certain bacterial infections seen in advanced HIV disease in adults, as well as for the morbidity and mortality associated with bacterial infections in HIV-infected children who cannot mount an adequate humoral response to common bacterial pathogens.

B cells from HIV-infected individuals secrete increased amounts of TNF-α and IL-6, cytokines known to enhance HIV replication,[465–467] and express surface-bound TNF-α, which can induce the production of HIV from infected $CD4^+$ T cells.[468] The secretion of proinflammatory cytokines and the expression of surface-bound TNF-α by B cells in the lymphoid microenvironment may contribute to T-cell activation and HIV replication in these tissues.

HIV gp120 has been observed to directly bind to an immunoglobulin variable chain (V_H3) and activate these B cells in much the same manner as a superantigen.[469, 470] This antigen-independent polyclonal activation leads in part to the hypergammaglobulinemia and B-lymphocyte hyperactivation of HIV infection. Other portions of HIV, including gp41, directly activate B cells in a non–superantigen-mediated manner.[471] Correlates of B-cell dysfunction observed in HIV-infected individuals include an increase in susceptibility to Epstein-Barr virus transformation in vitro and may contribute to the observed increased frequency of Epstein-Barr virus–induced lymphomas.[472–474]

Several studies have found an overall increase in IgE levels among HIV-infected individuals, probably reflecting a spectrum of IgE regulatory dysfunction.[475, 476] An association between elevated levels of IgE and emergence of syncytium-inducing strains of viruses has been noted.[477] In HIV-infected children, an expanded minor population of B lymphocytes has been identified that does not express CD23 (IgE receptor) and CD62L (L-selectin) and that may be involved in the pathogenesis of IgE dysregulation.[478]

Neutrophils

Dysregulation of neutrophil function occurs at all stages of HIV infection. Neutrophils isolated from asymptomatic HIV-infected individuals have an increase in nitroblue tetrazolium reduction, which suggests a state of increased cellular activation.[479] Activation of neutrophils from healthy, uninfected individuals by plasma from such individuals indicates the presence of a plasma neutrophil activating factor. In addition, plasma from the same individuals was found to be low in *N*-acetylcysteine, indicating that depletion of antioxidants may occur as a result of increased oxygen radical production.[480] The oxidative capacity of neutrophils after priming with granulocyte-macrophage colony-stimulating factor is also increased in HIV-infected individuals.[481] Further evidence of neutrophil hyperactivation in HIV infection includes increased expression of adhesion molecules, decreased expression of CD62L, and increased actin polymerization and H_2O_2 production.[479] The opsonizing activity of neutrophils is significantly impaired in HIV infection, and the degree of impairment correlates with disease progression.[482] Neutrophils from AIDS patients undergo apoptosis at an increased rate in comparison to those from normal controls.[483] Neutrophils from HIV-infected individuals also produce more TNF-α and IL-6 in response to lipopolysaccharide or *Candida* antigen than do neutrophils from normal donors.[484]

Dysfunction of neutrophils in HIV-infected individuals has several clinical implications. HIV infection, especially in women, is characterized by an increase in the incidence and severity of *Candida* infections. In a study comparing the ability of neutrophils from HIV-infected patients and normal controls to phagocytize and kill *Candida albicans,* neutrophils from AIDS patients showed an increased ability to phagocytose the organism, a similar ability to generate reactive oxygen, but a decreased ability to kill *Candida,* which suggests a defect in nonoxidative killing.[485] A potential mechanism for the decreased ability of neutrophils to kill *Candida* organisms has been suggested by the finding that IL-10, shown in some studies to be increased in HIV disease, inhibits neutrophil killing of *Candida.*[486]

Natural Killer Cells

Abnormalities of NK cells are observed throughout the course of HIV disease, and these abnormalities increase with disease progression. Most studies report that NK cells are normal in number and phenotype in HIV-infected individuals; however, decreases in numbers of the $CD16^+/CD56^+$ subpopulation of NK cells with an associated increase in activation markers have been reported.[487, 488] NK cells from HIV-infected individuals are defective in their ability to kill typical NK target cells, as well as gp160-expressing cells. The abnormality in NK cell lysis is thought to occur after binding of the NK cell to its target.[489] Otherwise, the NK lytic machinery appears to be capable of functioning normally because NK cells from HIV-infected individuals are able to mediate ADCC.[490] A possible mechanism for defective NK activity includes a lack of cytokines necessary for optimal function. Addition of either IL-2, IL-12, or IFN-α to cultures enhances the defective in vitro NK cell function of HIV-infected individuals.[491]

NK cells are an important source of HIV inhibitory CC-chemokines in HIV-infected individuals.[492] NK cells isolated from HIV-infected individuals produce high constitutive levels of MIP-1α, MIP-1β, and RANTES; high levels of chemokine production are also seen when these cells are stimulated by IL-2, IL-15, or CD16 cross-linking or during lytic killing.[492] Thus, NK cells, like $CD8^+$ T cells, may inhibit HIV replication by cell-mediated killing, as well as by secretion of soluble HIV inhibitory factors.

ROLE OF CELLULAR ACTIVATION IN THE PATHOGENESIS OF HUMAN IMMUNODEFICIENCY VIRUS

The end result of HIV infection is profound immunodeficiency; however, paradoxically, HIV infection is associated with hyperactivation of the immune system through most of the course of disease (Table 107–2). HIV subverts the immune system by inducing immune activation and using this milieu toward its own replicative advantage.[124, 363, 493, 494]

TABLE 107–2 Manifestations of an Activated Immune System in Human Immunodeficiency Virus Disease

Hyperactivation of B cells
Hypergammaglobulinemia
Spontaneous lymphocyte proliferation
Activation of monocytes with secretion of proinflammatory cytokines
Increased expression of activation markers on T cells
Follicular hyperplasia of lymphoid tissue
Elevated circulating levels of neopterin, β_2-microglobulin, acid-labile interferon, and soluble IL-2 receptors
Autoimmune phenomena

The replicative cycle of HIV infection is most efficiently achieved in activated cells.[495, 496] Cytokines that induce T-cell activation can further contribute to viral replication by inducing a state of productive infection in latently infected resting T cells.[497] Several lines of evidence suggest that HIV replication in vivo is dependent on antigen-driven activation of $CD4^+$ T cells. HIV-infected individuals with intercurrent infections experience transient increases in plasma viremia that correlate with the degree of immune activation that was induced; similar observations have been made in simian immunodeficiency virus–infected macaques and in HIV-infected individuals who received immunizations against various pathogens.[498–504] The amount of viral replication observed after vaccination with influenza vaccine or tetanus toxoid or during active infection with *M. tuberculosis* correlated inversely with the stage of HIV disease.[501–504] Individuals with late-stage HIV disease had a moderate increase in viral replication, whereas individuals with early-stage disease had a much greater increase in plasma viremia over baseline, which suggests a correlation between the ability of the immune system to respond to antigen and the magnitude of viral induction.[501–503] Furthermore, when PBMCs from tetanus toxoid–immunized, HIV-infected individuals were stimulated in vitro with tetanus antigen or when PBMCs from purified protein derivative–positive, HIV-infected individuals were stimulated in vitro with purified protein derivative or live *M. tuberculosis,* subjects with early-stage disease manifested a much stronger proliferative response to the respective antigens and had a larger increase in viral replication in vitro than did individuals with advanced-stage disease.[502–505] These studies suggest that the level of viral replication correlates with the level of immune system activation in response to an antigen.

Analysis of viral quasispecies and immune responses within lymphoid tissue from HIV-infected individuals suggests that HIV replication in vivo may not be driven by sustained high levels of immune activation. Within individual splenic white pulps a restricted number of individual antigen-specific immune responses occurred (defined by analysis of T-cell receptor V_β gene usage), and each of the immune responses contained a single or limited number of HIV quasispecies.[506] These data support the theory that within the context of individual antigen-specific immune responses, a single quasispecies of HIV that was present at the initiation of the reaction spread among the newly activated T cells. Thus, it is likely that continuous daily production of HIV occurs in newly activated $CD4^+$ T cells that are being driven by antigen-specific activation.[506, 507]

CYTOKINES AND HUMAN IMMUNODEFICIENCY VIRUS DISEASE: DYSREGULATION OF CYTOKINE PRODUCTION

Chronic immune activation induced by HIV infection and associated opportunistic infections results in dysregulation of the host cytokine network. Many of the observed alterations in cytokine production contribute to HIV pathogenesis by further stimulating viral replication, suppressing the ability of the immune system to mount an efficient antiviral response, and inducing cytokine-mediated cytopathic effects.[124, 493, 508–510]

HIV infection is associated with increased expression of proinflammatory cytokines, especially during the later stages of disease.[124, 509] High levels of TNF-α, IL-1β, and IL-6 are secreted by PBMCs and macrophages from HIV-infected subjects and are found at elevated levels in serum, cerebrospinal fluid, and tissues.[124, 509] High levels of expression of these cytokines, as well as interferon-γ (IFN-γ)[511–514] and IL-10,[513, 514] are particularly evident in lymphoid tissue, a major site of HIV replication throughout the course of disease.[258, 272, 277, 313] Chronically activated CD8$^+$ T cells[513, 515] and macrophages[510, 516] are thought to be major contributors to the elevated cytokine levels observed in HIV-infected subjects.

In addition to alterations in cytokine production caused by chronic immune activation, HIV-specific upregulation of certain cytokines may occur. In this regard, production of proinflammatory cytokines can be upregulated in PBMCs, lymph node mononuclear cells, and macrophages after acute HIV infection in vitro or after treatment with HIV proteins such as envelope gp120 and tat.[124, 509]

Another major disruption in the cytokine pattern observed in HIV disease is a progressive loss of the ability to produce immunoregulatory cytokines such as IL-2 and IL-12.[273, 430, 517, 518] IL-2 and IL-12 are critical for effective cell-mediated immune responses because they stimulate proliferation and lytic activity of CTLs and NK cells. These cell-mediated immune effectors represent the primary mechanism whereby most viral infections are cleared. In addition, IL-12 is essential for stimulating the production of type 1 T-helper (Th1) cytokines, including IL-2 and IFN-γ cytokines that favor the development of cell-mediated immune responses.[519–521] Although it is clear that the Th1 limb of cellular immune responses is impaired during the course of HIV infection,[518, 522–525] controversy surrounds the proposed dominance of Th2-like responses (i.e., secretion of IL-4, IL-5, and IL-10) during progression of HIV disease. Clerici and associates showed that stimulated PBMCs from HIV-infected patients exhibit a preferential Th2 pattern of cytokine secretion with disease progression,[518, 522, 523, 526] and other investigators have found that CD4$^+$ T cells from HIV-infected patients shift their cytokine secretion profile from a Th1-like to a Th2-like pattern during the course of disease progression.[527] However, still other investigators have found a skewing of the cytokine secretion pattern of T cells from HIV-infected patients toward a Th0 state (i.e., secretion of cytokines characteristic of both Th1 and Th2 patterns) rather than toward a Th2 state.[513, 524, 525] In either case, the finding that HIV replication is more efficient in Th0 than in Th1 clones[524, 528] suggests that depletion of Th1-like cells and a predominance of Th0-like cells may provide more suitable targets for HIV infection and replication during the course of disease progression.[529]

EFFECT OF CYTOKINES ON HUMAN IMMUNODEFICIENCY VIRUS REPLICATION

The effects of cytokines on HIV replication were recognized in early studies wherein activated PBMCs,[530] macrophages,[531, 532] and B cells[467] were shown to produce soluble factors that could dramatically upregulate HIV expression in acutely and chronically infected cells of the lymphocytic and macrophage lineages. These observations led to the identification of numerous cytokines that can directly influence HIV replication in infected cells[509, 510] (Fig. 107–5). Cytokines that have been reported to upregulate HIV replication in vitro include IL-1β, IL-2, IL-3, IL-6, IL-7, IL-12, IL-15, TNF-α, TNF-β, and macrophage and granulocyte-macrophage colony-stimulating factors (reviewed in refs. 509 and 533–536). IFN-α, IFN-β, and IL-16[537, 538] are primarily suppressors of HIV production, whereas other cytokines such as IL-4,[539, 540] IL-10,[541, 542] IL-13,[539] IFN-γ, and TGF-β reduce or enhance viral replication, depending on the infected cell type and the culture conditions.[509, 510] Many cytokines can influence HIV replication in both T cells and macrophages, such as the interferons and TNF-α, whereas others are cell lineage specific, such as macrophage colony-stimulating factor. The effects of a particular cytokine are often greatly influenced by the activity of other cytokines present in the microenvironment. In this regard, certain cytokines have been demonstrated to act in a synergistic[541, 543, 544] or in

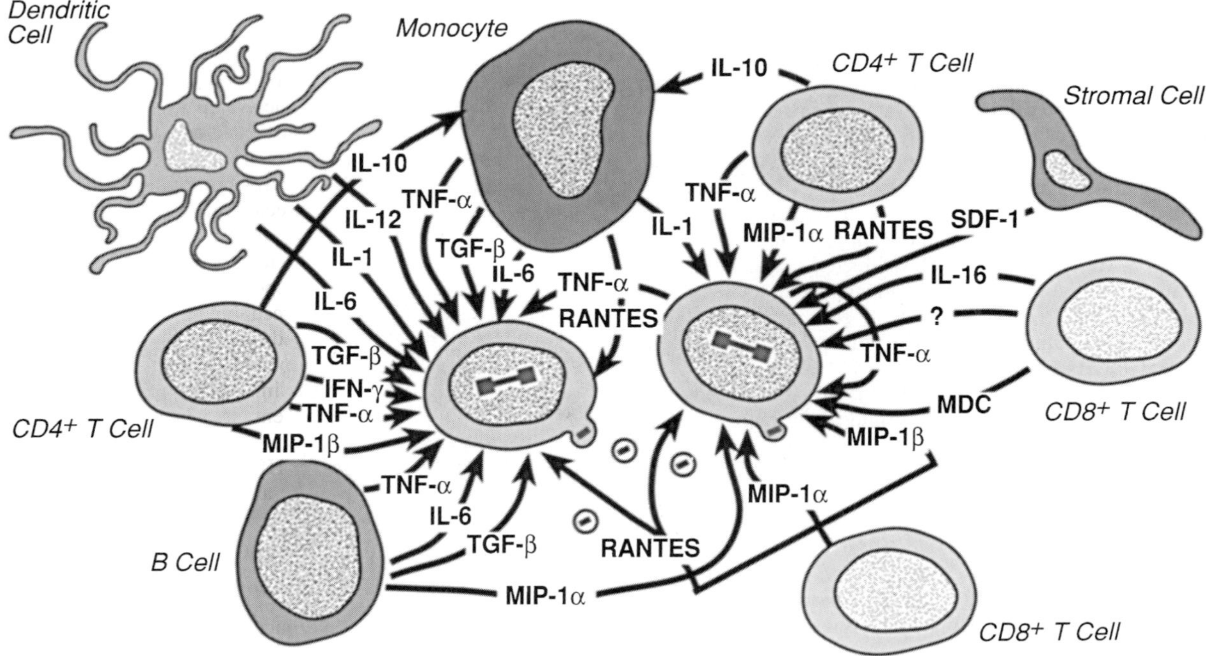

FIGURE 107–5. Cytokine networks that regulate human immunodeficiency virus (HIV) replication. The proinflammatory cytokines tumor necrosis factor (TNF)-α, interleukin (IL)-1β, and IL-6 strongly enhance viral replication. Transforming growth factor (TGF)-β and IL-10 downregulate viral replication; in the case of IL-10 this occurs at least in part owing to downregulation of the proinflammatory cytokines. The CC-chemokines inhibit M-tropic strains of HIV, SDF-1 inhibits T-tropic strains, and MDC-1 inhibits both M- and T-tropic strains. (Adapted with permission from Fauci AS. Host factors and the pathogenesis of HIV-induced disease. Nature. 1996;384:529–534. Copyright 1996, Macmillan Magazines Ltd.)

an antagonistic[411, 545] manner with other cytokines in regulating HIV replication. Finally, cytokines are pleiotropic, and the overall effects of a particular cytokine on HIV replication often reflect the balance of both HIV-inducing and HIV-inhibiting activities.

Proinflammatory cytokines, particularly TNF-α, are considered the most potent HIV-inducing cytokines, and their mechanism of action is relatively well understood. Both TNF-α and IL-1β activate the cellular nuclear transcription factor NFκB,[546, 547] a strong inducer of HIV long terminal repeat–mediated transcription. IL-6 increases HIV expression primarily by a post-transcriptional mechanism; however, IL-6 can synergize with NFκB-inducing cytokines to enhance HIV transcription.[543] The role of endogenous proinflammatory cytokines in the regulation of HIV replication has been demonstrated in several cellular systems in vitro. The production of HIV by macrophages or PBMCs stimulated by physiologic inducers of proinflammatory cytokine production such as bacterial endotoxin or IL-2 can be partially or nearly completely abrogated by the addition of anti-proinflammatory cytokines,[548, 549] neutralizing antibodies to the cytokines, or receptor antagonists such as IL-1ra.[535] In cultures of HIV-infected macrophages, the viral suppressive activity of several cytokines such as IL-10 and TGF-β is largely attributable to their ability to inhibit the secretion or activity of HIV-inducing proinflammatory cytokines.[411, 545, 548, 550] HIV production by infected T cells is sensitive to both the anti-proinflammatory and the antiproliferative activity of such cytokines.[551]

Although the role of proinflammatory and anti-proinflammatory cytokines in the regulation of HIV replication in vivo has not been demonstrated conclusively, several lines of evidence suggest that these cytokines may be involved in regulating viral production. Administration of pentoxifylline, an inhibitor of the secretion and activity of TNF, to HIV-infected individuals was found to reduce HIV viremia in concert with a reduction in plasma levels of TNF-α.[552, 553] The kinetics of HIV suppression in vivo correlated with a dramatic reduction in the ability of cells from these subjects to secrete TNF-α and IL-1β in vitro. Furthermore, IL-10 has been found to inhibit acute HIV infection in severe combined immunodeficiency mice engrafted with human fetal thymus and liver.[554] The ability of IL-10 to suppress T-cell activation and proliferation probably also plays a prominent role in its ability to suppress HIV replication in vivo.[555–557]

In addition to the use of immunosuppressive cytokines, which may depress HIV-inducing immune responses, cytokines that stimulate T cells or antigen-presenting cells have been administered to HIV-infected subjects for a number of years. The use of cytokine-based therapies aimed at immune reconstitution in HIV disease has expanded over the past several years, particularly with the development of potent antiretroviral therapies that limit the potential for cytokine-mediated increases in viral replication. In this regard, administration of IL-2 to asymptomatic HIV-infected subjects receiving concomitant antiretroviral therapy results in significant and sustained increases in CD4$^+$ T-cell numbers with no concomitant sustained increases in viremia.[558] Similar immune reconstitution therapies are being developed for IL-12, IL-13, and IL-15.[536, 559–565] New studies are continuing to expand the list of cytokines for use as potential immunotherapeutic agents. A particularly interesting cytokine-based immunotherapeutic approach has been suggested by a recent report demonstrating that transfection of a CD4$^+$ T-cell line with DNA encoding the 130–amino acid form of IL-16 renders cells virtually resistant to HIV infection.[537] IL-16–mediated inhibition of HIV in this system appears to be due to interference with viral transcription.[537, 538] This effect may be due to the ability of IL-16 to suppress T-cell activation.[566, 567] The combination of IL-2 and IL-16 is a particularly attractive option that may synergistically enhance the expansion of CD4$^+$ T cells.[568]

Numerous cell types produce a variety of chemokines,[569, 570] and modulation of the production of these factors may influence HIV replication in a strain-specific manner. Therefore, the overall effect of immune activation and the secretion of proinflammatory or immunoregulatory cytokines on HIV replication must now be considered in the context of potential influences on chemokine production, chemokine coreceptor expression, and the predominant viral quasispecies that is replicating in vivo (Fig. 107–6). Chemokine production, induced during inflammation, is enhanced by several cytokines, including TNF-α, IL-1β, and immunoregulatory cytokines such as IL-2 and IL-15.[569, 571–573] Thus, in HIV-infected subjects in the early stages of disease, the ability of TNF-α to stimulate CC-chemokine production and thereby suppress M-tropic viral entry may override its HIV-inducing effects; however, in individuals harboring predominantly T-tropic viral quasispecies in the later stages of HIV disease, only the HIV-inducing activity of TNF-α would be influential. In fact, TNF-α–mediated induction of CC-chemokine secretion may actually enhance the entry and replication of T-tropic strains of HIV.[105, 106]

Immunoregulatory aspects of chemokine receptor expression may also exert variable strain-dependent effects on HIV replication and spread. In this regard, IL-2 has been shown to upregulate expression of the M-tropic coreceptor CCR5.[75] In contrast, stimulation of CD4$^+$ T cells through CD3 and CD28 protects cells from HIV infection and potently downregulates HIV replication in infected cells[574–576]; this effect appears to be due in part to downregulation of CCR5.[84] The puzzling bottleneck in HIV transmission that so heavily favors the emergence of M-tropic, non–syncytium-inducing strains of virus in the new host[55, 56] may in part be due to the differential regulatory patterns of the relevant HIV coreceptors.[75, 577] In this regard, CCR5 expression is predominantly seen in previously activated, memory T cells (i.e., CD26^{high}, CD45RA^{low}, CD45RO$^+$), whereas CXCR4 expression is seen in naive, unactivated cells (i.e., CD26^{low}, CD45RA$^+$, CD45RO$^-$). It is therefore plausible that the profound degree of immune activation that occurs during acute HIV infection may result in high expression of CCR5 and low expression of CXCR4.[578] Similarly, coinfection with various other pathogens may differentially modulate the expression of HIV coreceptors and thereby exert selective pressure on HIV strains that use the coreceptors in question.[579]

Although in vitro culture systems and cell line models have allowed investigators to identify numerous host factors that influence HIV replication and to delineate the mechanisms whereby these factors suppress or enhance viral replication, it is difficult to anticipate how manipulation of these factors will ultimately influence HIV replication in vivo. It is clear that host factors function within the context of an interactive, immunoregulatory cytokine network and can have pleiotropic effects on HIV replication, some of which are viral strain specific. Nevertheless, numerous host factors provide real or potential immunotherapeutic benefit that should be further explored and pursued clinically for the treatment of HIV disease.

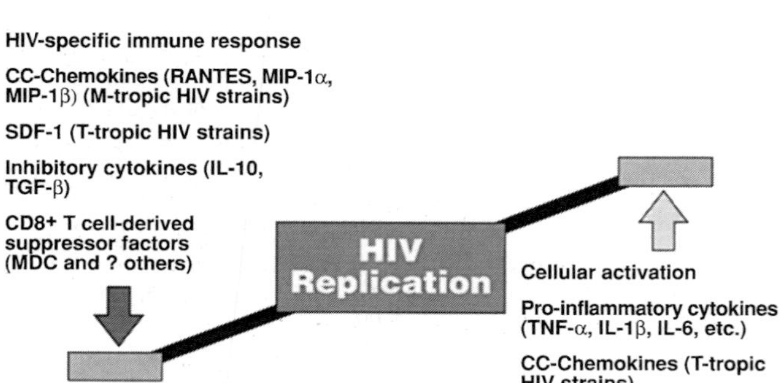

FIGURE 107–6. A delicate balance of host factors influences the net rate of viral replication. *Abbreviations:* HIV, Human immunodeficiency virus; MDC, monocyte-depleted cell; MIP, macrophage inflammatory protein; RANTES, regulated on activation, normal T-cell expressed and secreted; SDF, stromal-derived factor; TGF, transforming growth factor; TNF, tumor necrosis factor. (Adapted with permission from Fauci AS. Host factors and the pathogenesis of HIV-induced disease. Nature. 1996;384:529–534. Copyright 1996, Macmillan Magazines Ltd.)

LONG-TERM NONPROGRESSORS AND "EXPOSED-UNINFECTED" INDIVIDUALS

In recent years it has become clear that in a small percentage of HIV-infected individuals, no evidence of disease progression can be detected over a prolonged period (reviewed in ref. 124). Definitions of long-term nonprogression are somewhat arbitrary; however, a reasonable consensus definition includes documentation of HIV infection for more than 7 years, a CD4 T-cell count greater than 600 cells/μl without significant decline over time, no symptoms of HIV-induced disease, and no history of antiretroviral therapy. Although a minority of cases of long-term nonprogressive HIV infection may be associated with attenuated strains of HIV,[580–584] most data suggest that viral attenuation is rare among long-term nonprogressors and that host factors play a dominant role in determining the state of nonprogression.[162, 164, 585–587]

Host genetic factors influence the rate of disease progression in HIV infection. A number of different mechanisms may be responsible for the associations observed between certain HLA haplotypes and different rates of HIV disease progression.[205–207, 588] The ability of certain HLA molecules to efficiently present immunodominant viral epitopes in order to generate cell-mediated immune responses may explain an association with slow disease progression. Conversely, other HLA molecules may promote immunopathogenic responses associated with more rapid disease progression. In a recent study, HLA-B27, B57, and B51 were most strongly associated with slow progression of HIV disease, whereas HLA-A23, B37, and B49 were associated with rapid progression.[207] An HLA profile was developed that distinguished a sixfold difference between rates of disease progression in rapid versus slow progressors. Genetic polymorphisms in the recently described HIV coreceptors and their ligands may also have a significant impact on the course of HIV disease progression. As mentioned (see earlier), individuals who are homozygous for a 32–base pair inactivating mutation within the *CCR5* gene (*CCR5-Δ32*) are afforded a high degree of protection against HIV infection, whereas HIV-infected heterozygotes are partially protected against disease progression. Other mutations that limit the availability of functional coreceptors are also associated with protection against HIV infection and/or partial protection against disease progression (see previous discussion).

Recognition of immunodominant CTL epitopes presented by particular MHC class I alleles may result in potent anti-HIV activity[204] and may in part explain the association of certain MHC class I alleles with slower progression of HIV disease.[205–207] The presence of HIV-specific CTLs in exposed-uninfected individuals[201, 589] and the persistence of vigorous CTL responses in long-term nonprogressors[119, 162, 196–200] argue strongly for a salutary role of CTL in HIV infection; this conclusion is further bolstered by the demonstration of an inverse correlation between CTL activity and plasma viremia.[195]

Studies of long-term nonprogressors have demonstrated more potent $CD8^+$ T-cell–derived soluble antiviral responses than found in progressors.[92, 164] Hypersecretion of CC-chemokines, downregulation of HIV coreceptors, or both may play a role in protecting some exposed-uninfected individuals against HIV infection[90, 91, 590] and in protecting against disease progression in HIV-infected individuals.[93, 94]

Certain humoral immune responses may also protect against HIV infection, disease progression, or both. HIV-specific mucosal IgA has been detected in women who have been exposed to HIV yet remain uninfected.[591] The presence of circulating neutralizing antibodies to primary HIV isolates and to autologous virus is associated with nonprogression.[132, 163]

The morphologic abnormalities of lymphoid tissue associated with HIV disease progression are important determinants of immunodeficiency.[251–258] Despite the long period of HIV infection in long-term nonprogressors, histopathologic examination of lymph node biopsy tissue from these individuals revealed only mild HIV-related abnormalities such as follicular hyperplasia.[258] Follicular involution, fibrosis, and lymphocyte depletion, associated with progressive HIV disease, were found to be lacking in lymph nodes from nonprogressors. The degree of follicular hyperplasia, and thus lymphoid tissue activation, seen in nonprogressors is significantly lower than that seen in progressors and qualitatively distinct as well, without evidence of large geographic germinal centers extending into the nodal medulla.[258] It is likely that preservation of lymphoid architecture in nonprogressors is a reflection of the lower levels of viral replication over time in these individuals. Regardless of the mechanisms responsible for lower levels of viral replication in nonprogressors, preservation of lymphoid tissue architecture is a critical component of the immunocompetence observed. This observation further highlights the need to understand the mechanisms responsible for the destruction of lymphoid tissue architecture during progression of HIV disease. If immunorestorative strategies in advanced HIV infection are to be successful, substrate for the generation of immune responses (i.e., intact lymphoid tissue) must be present, thus necessitating prevention or reversal of the histopathologic abnormalities of lymphoid tissue associated with HIV disease progression.

CONCLUSIONS

The pathogenesis of HIV infection is a multifactorial process consisting of aberrant cellular activation and dysregulation of certain cytokines. Disease progression is intimately related to virus replication, and the net amount of virus replication reflects a balance among factors that either induce or downregulate virus expression and thereby lead by to quantitative and qualitative abnormalities of the immune system by direct and/or indirect mechanisms.

The discovery that certain chemokine receptors function as necessary cofactors for HIV entry into target cells has expanded the scope of host factors critical in the pathogenesis of HIV infection. CCR5 and CXCR4 appear to be the major coreceptors for M- and T-tropic strains of HIV. Other receptors can function as HIV coreceptors in vitro; however, it remains uncertain to what extent these other receptors are used in vivo. HIV coreceptors represent new potential targets of therapeutic intervention. Agents that might be expected to be of therapeutic value would downregulate coreceptor expression, sterically hinder access of HIV to the coreceptor, or upregulate expression of the natural ligands of the coreceptors. However, many caveats must be considered when manipulating the chemokine-chemokine receptor axis. In this regard, chemokine receptor antagonists may perturb the normal regulation of inflammation by preventing signal transduction by chemokines through the chemokine receptor. Chemokine receptor agonists might also dysregulate inflammation by transmitting aberrant intracellular signals; these signals might also actually *enhance* the replication of certain strains of HIV.

Progression of HIV disease in the setting of vigorous anti-HIV immune responses remains a central paradox in the pathogenesis of HIV infection. Elements of both the humoral and cell-mediated immune responses against HIV have been implicated in the partial control of virus replication. However, the lack of correlates of protective immunity in HIV infection continues to be a major obstacle to the rational development of immunotherapeutic approaches and vaccine development. In this regard, studies of the immune responses to HIV mounted by individuals who are exposed to HIV and yet remain uninfected and studies of HIV-infected long-term nonprogressors should provide valuable insight into mechanisms of immune containment of HIV replication.

HIV is the quintessential opportunist, as illustrated by its ability to subvert activation of the immune system to its own replicative advantage. The virus is able to disarm multiple components of the host immune attack by both direct and indirect mechanisms. Understanding more about interactions between the virus and host that lead to dysfunction and depletion of the immune system should aid in the development of preventive and therapeutic strategies.

REFERENCES

1. Liu S-L, Schacker T, Musey L, et al. Divergent patterns of progression to AIDS after infection from the same source: Human immunodeficiency virus type 1 evolution and antiviral responses. J Virol. 1997;71:4284–4295.
2. Baggiolini M, Moser B. Blocking chemokine receptors. J Exp Med. 1997;186:1189–1191.
3. Fauci A. Multifactorial nature of human immunodeficiency virus diseases: Implications for therapy. Science. 1993;262:1011–1018.
4. Dalgleish AG, Beverly PC, Clapham PR, et al. The CD4(T4) antigen is an essential component of the receptor for the AIDS retrovirus. Nature. 1984;312:763–767.
5. Klatzmann D, Barre-Sinoussi F, Nugeyre MT, et al. Selective tropism of lymphadenopathy-associated virus (LAV) for helper-inducer T-lymphocytes. Science. 1984;225:59–63.
6. Klatzmann D, Champagne E, Chamaret S, et al. T-lymphocyte T4 molecule behaves as receptor for human retrovirus LAV. Nature. 1984;312:767–768.
7. Maddon PJ, Dalgleish AG, McDougal JS, et al. The T4 gene encodes the AIDS virus receptor and is expressed in the immune system and the brain. Cell. 1986;47:333–348.
8. Broder CC, Berger EA. Fusogenic selectivity of the envelope glycoprotein is a major determinant of human immunodeficiency virus type 1 tropism for CD4+ T-cell lines vs. primary macrophages. Proc Natl Acad Sci U S A. 1995;92:9004–9008.
9. Alkhatib G, Broder CC, Berger EA. Cell type–specific fusion cofactors determine human immunodeficiency virus type 1 tropism for T-cell lines versus primary macrophages. J Virol. 1996;70:5487–5494.
10. Walker CM, Moody DJ, Stites DP, et al. CD8+ lymphocytes can control HIV infection in vitro by suppressing virus replication. Science. 1986;234:1563–1566.
11. Cocchi F, DeVico A, Garzino-Demo A, et al. Identification of RANTES, MIP-1α, and MIP-1β as the major HIV suppressive factors produced by CD8+ T cells. Science. 1995;270:1811–1815.
12. Feng Y, Broder C, Kennedy P, et al. HIV-1 entry cofactor: Functional cDNA cloning of a seven-transmembrane domain, G-protein coupled receptor. Science. 1996;272:872–877.
13. Berson J, Long D, Doranz B, et al. A seven-transmembrane domain receptor involved in fusion and entry of T-cell–tropic human immunodeficiency virus type 1 strains. J Virol. 1996;70:6288–6295.
14. Bleul CC, Farzan M, Choe H, et al. The lymphocyte chemoattractant SDF-1 is a ligand for LESTR/fusin and blocks HIV-1 entry. Nature. 1996;382:829–833.
15. Oberlin E, Amara A, Bachelerie F, et al. The CXC chemokine SDF-1 is the ligand for LESTR/fusin and prevents infection by T-cell-line–adapted HIV-1. Nature. 1996;382:833–835.
16. Paxton WA, Martin SR, Tse D, et al. Relative resistance to HIV-1 infection of CD4 lymphocytes from persons who remain uninfected despite multiple high-risk sexual exposures. Nat Med. 1996;2:412–417.
17. Samson M, Labbe O, Mollereau C, et al. Molecular cloning and functional expression of a new human CC-chemokine receptor gene. Biochemistry. 1996;35:3362–3367.
18. Combadiere C, Ahuja SK, Tiffany HL, et al. Cloning and functional expression of CC CKR5, a human monocyte CC chemokine receptor selective for MIP-1(alpha), MIP-1(beta), and RANTES. J Leukoc Biol. 1996;60:147–152.
19. Raport C, Gosling J, Schweickart V, et al. Molecular cloning and functional characterization of a novel human CC chemokine receptor (CCR5) for RANTES, MIP-1beta, and MIP-1alpha. J Biol Chem. 1996;271:17161–17166.
20. Deng H, Liu R, Ellmeier W, et al. Identification of a major co-receptor for primary isolates of HIV-1. Nature. 1996;381:661–666.
21. Dragic T, Litwin V, Allaway G, et al. HIV-1 entry into CD4+ cells is mediated by the chemokine receptor CC-CKR-5. Nature. 1996;381:667–673.
22. Alkhatib G, Combadiere C, Broder C, et al. CC CKR5: A RANTES, MIP-1α, MIP-1β receptor as a fusion cofactor for macrophage-tropic HIV-1. Science. 1996;272:1955–1958.
23. Choe H, Farzan M, Sun Y, et al. The β-chemokine receptors CCR3 and CCR5 facilitate infection by primary HIV-1 isolates. Cell. 1996;85:1135–1138.
24. Doranz B, Rucker J, Yi Y, et al. A dual-tropic primary HIV-1 isolate that uses fusin and the β-chemokine receptors CKR-5, CKR-3, and CKR-2b as fusion cofactors. Cell. 1996;85:1149–1158.
25. Alkhatib G, Liao F, Berger EA, et al. A new SIV co-receptor, STRL33. Nature. 1997;388:238.
26. Liao F, Alkhatib G, Peden KW, et al. STRL33, a novel chemokine receptor–like protein, functions as a fusion cofactor for both macrophage-tropic and T cell line–tropic HIV-1. J Exp Med. 1997;185:2015–2023.
27. Deng HK, Unutmaz D, KewalRamani VN, et al. Expression cloning of new receptors used by simian and human immunodeficiency viruses. Nature. 1997;388:296–300.
28. Choe H, Farzan M, Konkel M, et al. The orphan seven-transmembrane receptor apj supports the entry of primary T-cell-line–tropic and dualtropic human immunodeficiency virus type 1. J Virol. 1998;72:6113–6118.
29. Rucker J, Edinger AL, Sharron M, et al. Utilization of chemokine receptors, orphan receptors, and herpesvirus-encoded receptors by diverse human and simian immunodeficiency viruses. J Virol. 1997;71:8999–9007.
30. Horuk R, Hesselgesser J, Zhou Y, et al. The CC chemokine I-309 inhibits CCR8-dependent infection by diverse HIV-1 strains. J Biol Chem. 1998;273:386–391.
31. Trkola A, Dragic T, Arthos J, et al. CD4-dependent, antibody-sensitive interactions between HIV-1 and its co-receptor CCR-5. Nature. 1996;384:184–187.
32. Wu L, Gerard N, Wyatt R, et al. CD4-induced interaction of primary HIV-1 gp120 glycoproteins with the chemokine receptor CCR-5. Nature. 1996;384:179–183.
33. Hill CM, Deng H, Unutmaz D, et al. Envelope glycoproteins from human immunodeficiency virus types 1 and 2 and simian immunodeficiency virus can use human CCR5 as a coreceptor for viral entry and make direct CD4-dependent interactions with this chemokine receptor. J Virol. 1997;71:6296–6304.
34. Wyatt R, Kwong PD, Desjardins E, et al. The antigenic structure of the HIV gp120 envelope glycoprotein. Nature. 1998;393:705–711.
35. Kwong PD, Wyatt R, Robinson J, et al. Structure of an HIV gp120 envelope glycoprotein in complex with the CD4 receptor and a neutralizing human antibody. Nature. 1998;393:648–659.
36. Rizzuto CD, Wyatt R, Hernandez-Ramos N, et al. A conserved HIV gp120 glycoprotein structure involved in chemokine receptor binding. Science. 1998;280:1949–1953.
37. Wu L, LaRosa G, Kassam N, et al. Interaction of chemokine receptor CCR5 with its ligands: Multiple domains for HIV-1 gp120 binding and a single domain for chemokine binding. J Exp Med. 1997;186:1373–1381.
38. Atchison RE, Gosling J, Monteclaro FS, et al. Multiple extracellular elements of CCR5 and HIV-1 entry: Dissociation from response to chemokines. Science. 1996;274:1924–1926.
39. Kuhmann SE, Platt EJ, Kozak SL, et al. Polymorphisms in the CCR5 genes of African green monkeys and mice implicate specific amino acids in infections by simian and human immunodeficiency viruses. J Virol. 1997;71:8642–8656.
40. Rucker J, Samson M, Doranz BJ, et al. Regions in β-chemokine receptors CCR5 and CCR2b that determine HIV-1 cofactor specificity. Cell. 1996;87:437–446.
41. Alkhatib G, Ahuja SS, Light D, et al. CC chemokine receptor 5–mediated signaling and HIV-1 co-receptor activity share common structural determinants. Critical residues in the third extracellular loop support HIV-1 fusion. J Biol Chem. 1997;272:19771–19776.
42. Edinger AL, Amedee A, Miller K, et al. Differential utilization of CCR5 by macrophage and T cell tropic simian immunodeficiency virus strains. Proc Natl Acad Sci U S A. 1997;94:4005–4010.
43. Dragic T, Trkola A, Lin SW, et al. Amino-terminal substitutions in the CCR5 coreceptor impair gp120 binding and human immunodeficiency virus type 1 entry. J Virol. 1998;72:279–285.
44. Farzan M, Choe H, Vaca L, et al. A tyrosine-rich region in the N terminus of CCR5 is important for human immunodeficiency virus type 1 entry and mediates an association between gp120 and CCR5. J Virol. 1998;72:1160–1164.
45. Doranz BJ, Lu ZH, Rucker J, et al. Two distinct CCR5 domains can mediate coreceptor usage by human immunodeficiency virus type 1. J Virol. 1997;71:6305–6314.
46. Picard L, Simmons G, Power CA, et al. Multiple extracellular domains of CCR-5 contribute to human immunodeficiency virus type 1 entry and fusion. J Virol. 1997;71:5003–5011.
47. Oravecz T, Pall M, Norcross M. Beta-chemokine inhibition of monocytotropic HIV-1 infection. Interference with a postbinding fusion step. J Immunol. 1996;157:1329–1332.
48. Cocchi F, DeVico AL, Garzino-Demo A, et al. The V3 domain of the HIV-1 gp120 envelope glycoprotein is critical for chemokine-mediated blockade of infection. Nat Med. 1996;2:1244–1247.
49. Speck RF, Wehrly K, Platt EJ, et al. Selective employment of chemokine receptors as human immunodeficiency virus type 1 coreceptors determined by individual amino acids within the envelope V3 loop. J Virol. 1997;71:7136–7139.
50. Gosling J, Monteclaro FS, Atchison RE, et al. Molecular uncoupling of C-C chemokine receptor 5–induced chemotaxis and signal transduction from HIV-1 coreceptor activity. Proc Natl Acad Sci U S A. 1997;94:5061–5066.
51. Farzan M, Choe H, Martin KA, et al. HIV-1 entry and macrophage inflammatory protein-1beta–mediated signaling are independent functions of the chemokine receptor CCR5. J Biol Chem. 1997;272:6854–6857.
52. Lapham C, Ouyang J, Chadrasekhar B, et al. Evidence for cell-surface association between fusin and CD4-gp120 complex in human cell lines. Science. 1996;274:602–605.
53. Brelot A, Heveker N, Pleskoff O, et al. Role of the first and third extracellular domains of CXCR-4 in human immunodeficiency virus coreceptor activity. J Virol. 1997;71:4744–4751.
54. Kozak SL, Platt EJ, Madani N, et al. CD4, CXCR-4, and CCR-5 dependencies for infections by primary patient and laboratory-adapted isolates of human immunodeficiency virus type 1. J Virol. 1997;71:873–882.
55. Zhu T, Mo H, Wang N, et al. Genotypic and phenotypic characterization of HIV-1 in patients with primary infection. Science. 1993;261:1179–1181.
56. Zhang LQ, Mackenzie P, Cleland A, et al. Selection for specific sequences in the external envelope protein of human immunodeficiency virus type 1 upon primary infection. J Virol. 1993;67:3345–3356.
57. Zaitseva M, Blauvelt A, Lee S, et al. Expression and function of CCR5 and CXCR4 on human Langerhans cells and macrophages: Implications for HIV primary infection. Nat Med. 1997;3:1369–1375.
58. Tersmette M, Lange JMA, DeGoede REY, et al. Association between biological properties of human immunodeficiency virus variants and risk for AIDS and AIDS mortality. Lancet. 1989;1:983–985.
59. Tersmette M, Gruters RA, DeWolf F, et al. Evidence for a role of virulent human immunodeficiency virus (HIV) variants in the pathogenesis of acquired immunodeficiency syndrome: Studies on sequential HIV isolates. J Virol. 1989;63:2118–2125.
60. Cheng-Mayer C, Seto D, Tateno M, et al. Biologic features of HIV-1 that correlate with virulence in the host. Science. 1988;240:80–82.
61. Koot M, Keet IPM, Vos AHV, et al. Prognostic value of HIV-1 syncytium-inducing

phenotype for rate of CD4+ cell depletion and progression to AIDS. Ann Intern Med. 1993;118:681–688.
62. Connor RI, Sheridan KE, Ceradini D, et al. Change in coreceptor use correlates with disease progression in HIV-1–infected individuals. J Exp Med. 1997;185: 621–628.
63. Liu R, Paxton W, Choe S, et al. Homozygous defect in HIV-1 coreceptor accounts for resistance of some multiply-exposed individuals to HIV-1 infection. Cell. 1996;86:367–377.
64. Samson M, Libert F, Doranz B, et al. Resistance to HIV-1 infection in Caucasian individuals bearing mutant alleles of the CCR-5 chemokine receptor gene. Nature. 1996;382:722–725.
65. Dean M, Carrington M, Winkler C, et al. Genetic restriction of HIV-1 infection and progression to AIDS by a deletion allele of the CKR5 structural gene. Science. 1996;273:1856–1862.
66. Huang Y, Paxton W, Wolinsky S, et al. The role of a mutant CCR5 allele in HIV-1 transmission and disease progression. Nat Med. 1996;2:1240–1243.
67. Zimmerman P, Buckler-White A, Alkhatib G, et al. Inherited resistance to HIV-1 conferred by an inactivating mutation in CC chemokine receptor 5: Studies in populations with contrasting clinical phenotypes, defined racial backgrounds and quantified risks. Mol Med. 1997;3:23–36.
68. Biti R, French R, Young J, et al. HIV-1 infection in an individual homozygous for the CCR5 deletion allele. Nat Med. 1997;3:252–253.
69. Theodorou I, Meyer L, Magierowska M, et al. HIV-1 infection in an individual homozygous for CCR5Δ32. Lancet. 1997;349:1219–1220.
70. O'Brien T, Winkler C, Dean M, et al. HIV-1 infection in a man homozygous for CCR5Δ32. Lancet. 1997;349:1219.
71. Michael NL, Nelson JA, KewalRamani VN, et al. Exclusive and persistent use of the entry coreceptor CXCR4 by human immunodeficiency virus type 1 from a subject homozygous for CCR5 delta32. J Virol. 1998;72:6040–6047.
72. Michael N, Chang G, Louie L, et al. The role of viral phenotype and CCR-5 gene defects in HIV-1 transmission and disease progression. Nat Med. 1997;3:338–340.
73. Cohen O, Vaccarezza M, Lam G, et al. Heterozygosity for a defective gene for CC chemokine receptor 5 is not the sole determinant for the immunologic and virologic phenotype of HIV-infected long term non-progressors. J Clin Invest. 1997;100:1581–1589.
74. Eugen-Olsen J, Iversen AKN, Garred P, et al. Heterozygosity for a deletion in the CKR-5 gene leads to prolonged AIDS free survival and slower CD4 T cell fall in a cohort of HIV seropositive individuals. AIDS. 1997;11:305–310.
75. Bleul C, Wu L, Hoxie J, et al. The HIV coreceptors CXCR4 and CCR5 are differentially expressed and regulated on human T lymphocytes. Proc Natl Acad Sci U S A. 1997;94:1925–1930.
76. Wu L, Paxton WA, Kassam N, et al. CCR5 levels and expression pattern correlate with infectability by macrophage-tropic HIV-1, in vitro. J Exp Med. 1997;185:1681–1692.
77. Picchio G, Gulizia R, Mosier D. Chemokine receptor CCR5 genotype influences the kinetics of human immunodeficiency virus type 1 infection in human PBL-SCID mice. J Virol. 1997;71:7124–7127.
78. Quillent C, Oberlin E, Braun J, et al. HIV-1–resistance phenotype conferred by combination of two separate inherited mutations of CCR5 gene. Lancet. 1998;351:14–18.
79. Smith MW, Dean M, Carrington M, et al. Contrasting genetic influence of CCR2 and CCR5 variants on HIV-1 infection and disease progression. Science. 1997;277:959–965.
80. Kostrikis LG, Huang Y, Moore JP, et al. A chemokine receptor CCR2 allele delays HIV-1 disease progression and is associated with a CCR5 promoter mutation. Nat Med. 1998;4:350–353.
81. Rizzardi GP, Morawetz RA, Vicenzi E, et al. CCR2 polymorphism and HIV disease. Swiss HIV Cohort. Nat Med. 1998;4:252–253.
82. Mummidi S, Ahuja SS, McDaniel BL, et al. The human CC chemokine receptor 5 (CCR5) gene. Multiple transcripts with 5′-end heterogeneity, dual promoter usage, and evidence for polymorphisms within the regulatory regions and noncoding exons. J Biol Chem. 1997;272:30662–30671.
83. Winkler C, Modi W, Smith MW, et al. Genetic restriction of AIDS pathogenesis by an SDF-1 chemokine gene variant. Science. 1998;279:389–393.
84. Carroll RG, Riley JL, Levine BL, et al. Differential regulation of HIV-1 fusion cofactor expression by CD28 costimulation of CD4+ T cells. Science. 1997;276:273–276.
85. McKenzie S, Dallalio G, North M, et al. Serum chemokine levels in patients with non-progressing HIV infection. AIDS. 1996;10:29–33.
86. Zanussi S, D'Andrea M, Simonelli C, et al. Serum levels of RANTES and MIP-1α in HIV-positive long-term survivors and progressor patients. AIDS. 1996;10:1431–1432.
87. Krowka JF, Gesner ML, Ascher MS, et al. Lack of associations of chemotactic cytokines with viral burden, disease progression, or lymphocyte subsets in HIV-infected individuals. Clin Immunol Immunopathol. 1997;85:21–27.
88. Blazevic V, Heino M, Ranki A, et al. RANTES, MIP, and interleukin-16 in HIV infection. AIDS. 1996;10:1435–1436.
89. Clerici M, Balotta C, Trabattoni D, et al. Chemokine production in HIV-seropositive long-term asymptomatic individuals. AIDS. 1996;10:1432–1433.
90. Zagury D, Lachgar A, Chams V, et al. C-C chemokines, pivotal in protection against HIV type 1 infection. Proc Natl Acad Sci U S A. 1998;95:3857–3861.
91. Furci L, Scarlatti G, Burastero S, et al. Antigen-driven C-C chemokine–mediated HIV-1 suppression by CD4(+) T cells from exposed uninfected individuals expressing the wild-type CCR-5 allele. J Exp Med. 1997;186:455–460.
92. Scala E, D'Offizi G, Rosso R, et al. C-C chemokines, IL-16, and soluble antiviral factor activity are increased in cloned T cells from subjects with long-term nonprogressive HIV infection. J Immunol. 1997;158:4485–4492.
93. Ullum H, Lepri A, Victor J, et al. Production of beta-chemokines in human immunodeficiency virus (HIV) infection: Evidence that high levels of macrophage in inflammatory protein-1 beta are associated with a decreased risk of HIV disease progression. J Infect Dis. 1998;177:331–336.
94. Saha K, Bentsman G, Chess L, et al. Endogenous production of beta-chemokines by CD4+, but not CD8+, T-cell clones correlates with the clinical state of human immunodeficiency virus type 1 (HIV-1)-infected individuals and may be responsible for blocking infection with non-syncytium–inducing HIV-1 in vitro. J Virol. 1998;72:876–881.
95. Arenzana-Seisdedos F, Virelizier J-L, Rousset D, et al. HIV blocked by chemokine antagonist. Nature. 1996;383:400.
96. Simmons G, Clapham PR, Picard L, et al. Potent inhibition of HIV-1 infectivity in macrophages and lymphocytes by a novel CCR5 antagonist. Science. 1997;276:276–279.
97. Schols D, Struyf S, Van Damme J, et al. Inhibition of T-tropic HIV strains by selective antagonization of the chemokine receptor CXCR4. J Exp Med. 1997;186:1383–1388.
98. Murakami T, Nakajima T, Koyanagi Y, et al. A small molecule CXCR4 inhibitor that blocks T cell line–tropic HIV-1 infection. J Exp Med. 1997;186:1389–1393.
99. Doranz BJ, Grovit-Ferbas K, Sharron MP, et al. A small-molecule inhibitor directed against the chemokine receptor CXCR4 prevents its use as an HIV-1 coreceptor. J Exp Med. 1997;186:1395–1400.
100. Yang AG, Bai X, Huang XF, et al. Phenotypic knockout of HIV type 1 chemokine coreceptor CCR-5 by intrakines as potential therapeutic approach for HIV-1 infection. Proc Natl Acad Sci U S A. 1997;94:11567–11572.
101. Chen JD, Bai X, Yang AG, et al. Inactivation of HIV-1 chemokine co-receptor CXCR-4 by a novel intrakine strategy. Nat Med. 1997;3:1110–1116.
102. Kinter AL, Ostrowski M, Goletti D, et al. HIV replication in CD4+ T cells of HIV-infected individuals is regulated by a balance between the viral suppressive effects of endogenous beta-chemokines and the viral inductive effects of other endogenous cytokines. Proc Natl Acad Sci U S A. 1996;93:14076–14081.
103. Jansson M, Popovic M, Karlsson A, et al. Sensitivity to inhibition by β-chemokines correlates with biological phenotypes of primary HIV-1 isolates. Proc Natl Acad Sci U S A. 1996;93:15382–15387.
104. Schmidtmayerova H, Sherry B, Bukrinsky M. Chemokines and HIV replication. Nature. 1996;382:767.
105. Dolei A, Biolchini A, Serra C, et al. Increased replication of T-cell–tropic HIV strains and CXC-chemokine receptor-4 induction in T cells treated with macrophage inflammatory protein (MIP)-1alpha, MIP-1beta and RANTES beta-chemokines. AIDS. 1998;12:183–190.
106. Kinter A, Catanzaro A, Monaco J, et al. CC-chemokines enhance the replication of T-tropic strains of HIV-1 in CD4+ T cells: Role of signal transduction. Proc Natl Acad Sci U S A. 1998;95:11880–11885.
107. Tachibana K, Hirota S, Iizasa H, et al. The chemokine receptor CXCR4 is essential for vascularization of the gastrointestinal tract. Nature. 1998;393:591–594.
108. Zou YR, Kottmann AH, Kuroda M, et al. Function of the chemokine receptor CXCR4 in haematopoiesis and in cerebellar development. Nature. 1998;393: 595–599.
109. Ma Q, Jones D, Borghesani PR, et al. Impaired B-lymphopoiesis, myelopoiesis, and derailed cerebellar neuron migration in CXCR4- and SDF-1–deficient mice. Proc Natl Acad Sci U S A. 1998;95:9448–9453.
110. Robinson WE, Montefiori DC, Mitchell WM. Antibody-dependent enhancement of human immunodeficiency virus type 1 infection. Lancet. 1988;1:790–794.
111. Robinson WE, Kawamura T, Gorny MK, et al. Human monoclonal antibodies to the human immunodeficiency virus type 1 (HIV-1) transmembrane glycoprotein gp41 enhance HIV-1 infection in vitro. Proc Natl Acad Sci U S A. 1990;87:3185–3189.
112. Homsy J, Meyer M, Levy JA. Serum enhancement of human immunodeficiency virus (HIV) infection correlates with disease in HIV-infected individuals. J Virol. 1990;64:1437–1440.
113. Wong MT, Warren RQ, Anderson SA, et al. Longitudinal analysis of the humoral immune response to human immunodeficiency virus type 1 (HIV-1) gp160 epitopes in rapidly progressing and nonprogressing HIV-1–uninfected subjects. J Infect Dis. 1993;168:1523–1527.
114. Autran B, Mayaud CM, Raphael M, et al. Evidence for a cytotoxic T-lymphocyte alveolitis in human immunodeficiency virus–infected patients. AIDS. 1988;2: 179–183.
115. Guillon JM, Autran B, Denis M, et al. Human immunodeficiency virus–related lymphocytic alveolitis. Chest. 1988;94:1264–1270.
116. Zinkernagel RM, Hengartner H. T-cell–mediated immunopathology versus direct cytolysis by virus: Implications for HIV and AIDS. Immunol Today. 1994;15: 262–268.
117. Borrow P, Lewicki H, Hahn BH, et al. Virus-specific CD8+ cytotoxic T-lymphocyte activity associated with control of viremia in primary human immunodeficiency virus type 1 infection. J Virol. 1994;68:6103–6110.
118. Koup RA, Safrit JT, Cao Y, et al. Temporal association of cellular immune responses with the initial control of viremia in primary human immunodeficiency virus type 1 syndrome. J Virol. 1994;68:4650–4655.
119. Musey L, Hughes J, Schacker T, et al. Cytotoxic-T-cell responses, viral load, and disease progression in early human immunodeficiency virus type 1 infection. N Engl J Med. 1997;337:1267–1274.
120. Clark SJ, Saag MS, Decker WD, et al. High titers of cytopathic virus in plasma of

patients with symptomatic primary HIV-1 infection. N Engl J Med. 1991;324: 954–960.
121. Sei Y, Tsang PH, Roboz JP, et al. Neutralizing antibodies as a prognostic indicator in the progression of acquired immune deficiency syndrome (AIDS)-related disorders: A double-blind study. J Clin Immunol. 1988;8:464–472.
122. Sei Y, Tsang PH, Chu FN, et al. Inverse relationship between HIV-1 p24 antigenemia, anti-p24 antibody and neutralizing antibody response in all stages of HIV-1 infection. Immunol Lett. 1989;20:223–230.
123. Lathey JL, Pratt RD, Spector SA. Appearance of autologous neutralizing antibody correlates with reduction in virus load and phenotype switch during primary infection with human immunodeficiency virus type I. J Infect Dis. 1997;175: 231–232.
124. Cohen O, Kinter A, Fauci A. Host factors in the pathogenesis of HIV infection. Immunol Rev. 1997;159:31–48.
125. Allain JP, Laurian Y, Paul DA, et al. Serological markers in early stages of human immunodeficiency virus infection in haemophiliacs. Lancet. 1986;2:1233–1236.
126. Paul DA, Falk LA, Kessler HA, et al. Correlation of serum HIV antigen and antibody with clinical status in HIV-infected patients. J Med Virol. 1987;22: 357–363.
127. Hogervorst E, Jurriaans S, deWolf F, et al. Predictors for non- and slow progression in human immunodeficiency virus (HIV) type 1 infection: Low viral RNA copy numbers in serum and maintenance of high HIV-1 p24-specific but not V3-specific antibody levels. J Infect Dis 1995;171:811–821.
128. Weber JN, Clapham PR, Weiss RA, et al. Human immunodeficiency virus infection in two cohorts of homosexual men: Neutralizing sera and association of anti-gag antibody with prognosis. Lancet. 1987;1:119–122.
129. Weiss RA, Clapham PR, Cheingsong-Popov R, et al. Neutralization of human T-lymphotropic virus type III by sera of AIDS and AIDS-risk patients. Nature. 1985;316:69–72.
130. Robert-Guroff M, Brown M, Gallo RC. HTLV-III–neutralizing antibodies in patients with AIDS and AIDS-related complex. Nature. 1985;316:72–74.
131. Alesi DR, Ajello F, Lupo G, et al. Neutralizing antibody and clinical status of human immunodeficiency virus (HIV)-infected individuals. J Med Virol. 1989;27:7–12.
132. Fenyo EM, Putkonen P. Broad cross-neutralizing activity in serum is associated with slow progression and low risk of transmission in primate lentivirus infections. Immunol Lett. 1996;51:95–99.
133. Matthews TJ, Langlois AJ, Robey WG, et al. Restricted neutralization of divergent human T-lymphotropic virus type III isolates by antibodies to the major envelope glycoprotein. Proc Natl Acad Sci U S A. 1986;83:9709–9713.
134. Putney SD, Matthews TJ, Robey WG, et al. HTLV-III/LAV–neutralizing antibodies to an *E. coli*–produced fragment of the virus envelope. Science. 1986;234:1392–1395.
135. Palker TJ, Clark ME, Langlois AJ, et al. Type-specific neutralization of the human immunodeficiency virus with antibodies to env-encoded synthetic peptides. Proc Natl Acad Sci U S A. 1988;85:1932–1936.
136. Rusche JR, Javaherian K, McDanal C, et al. Antibodies that inhibit fusion of human immunodeficiency virus–infected cells bind a 24–amino acid sequence of the viral envelope, gp120. Proc Natl Acad Sci U S A. 1988;85:3198–3202.
137. Goudsmit J, Debouck C, Meloen RH, et al. Human immunodeficiency virus type 1 neutralization epitope with conserved architecture elicits early type-specific antibodies in experimentally infected chimpanzees. Proc Natl Acad Sci U S A. 1988;85:4478–4482.
138. Javaherian K, Langlois AJ, McDanal C, et al. Principal neutralizing domain of the human immunodeficiency virus type 1 envelope protein. Proc Natl Acad Sci U S A. 1989;86:6768–6772.
139. Kido H, Fukutomi A, Katunuma N. A novel membrane-bound serine esterase in human T4+ lymphocytes immunologically reactive with antibody inhibiting syncytia induced by HIV-1. Purification and characterization. J Biol Chem. 1990;265:21979–21985.
140. Clements GJ, Price-Jones MJ, Stephens PE, et al. The V3 loops of the HIV-1 and HIV-2 surface glycoproteins contain proteolytic cleavage sites: A possible function in viral fusion? AIDS Res Hum Retroviruses. 1991;7:3–16.
141. Freed EO, Myers DJ, Risser R. Identification of the principal neutralizing determinant of human immunodeficiency virus type 1 as a fusion domain. J Virol. 1991;65:190–194.
142. Niwa Y, Yano M, Futaki S, et al. T-cell membrane–associated serine protease, tryptase TL2, binds human immunodeficiency virus type 1 gp120 and cleaves the third-variable-domain loop of gp120. Neutralizing antibodies of human immunodeficiency virus type 1 inhibit cleavage of gp120. Eur J Biochem. 1996;237:64–70.
143. Muster T, Steindl F, Purtscher M, et al. A conserved neutralizing epitope on gp41 of human immunodeficiency virus type 1. J Virol. 1993;67:6642–6647.
144. Conley AJ, Kessler JA, Boots LJ, et al. Neutralization of divergent human immunodeficiency virus type 1 variants and primary isolates by IAM-41-2F5, an anti-gp41 human monoclonal antibody. Proc Natl Acad Sci U S A. 1994;91:3348–3352.
145. Reitz MS, Wilson C, Naugle C, et al. Generation of a neutralization-resistant variant of HIV-1 is due to selection for a point mutation in the envelope gene. Cell. 1988;54:57–63.
146. Back NK, Thiriart C, Delers A, et al. Association of antibodies blocking HIV1 gp160-sCD4 attachment with virus neutralizing activity in human sera. J Med Virol. 1990;31:200–208.
147. Steimer KS, Scandella C, Skiles PV, et al. Neutralization of divergent HIV-1 isolates by conformation-dependent human antibodies to Gp120. Science. 1991;254:105–108.
148. Ho DD, Fung MS, Cao YZ, et al. Another discontinuous epitope on glycoprotein gp120 that is important in human immunodeficiency virus type 1 neutralization is identified by a monoclonal antibody. Proc Natl Acad Sci U S A. 1991;88:8949–8952.
149. Thali M, Olshevsky U, Furman C, et al. Characterization of a discontinuous human immunodeficiency virus type 1 gp120 epitope recognized by a broadly reactive neutralizing human monoclonal antibody. J Virol. 1991;65:6188–6193.
150. Hansen JE, Clausen H, Nielsen C, et al. Inhibition of human immunodeficiency virus (HIV) infection in vitro by anticarbohydrate monoclonal antibodies: Peripheral glycosylation of HIV envelope glycoprotein gp120 may be a target for virus neutralization. J Virol. 1990;64:2833–2340.
151. Mascola JR, Snyder SW, Weislow OS, et al. Immunization with envelope subunit vaccine products elicits neutralizing antibodies against laboratory-adapted but not primary isolates of human immunodeficiency virus type 1. The National Institute of Allergy and Infectious Diseases AIDS Vaccine Evaluation Group. J Infect Dis. 1996;173:340–348.
152. Arendrup M, Akerblom L, Heegaard PM, et al. The HIV-1 V3 domain on field isolates: Participation in generation of escape virus in vivo and accessibility to neutralizing antibodies. Arch Virol. 1995;140:655–670.
153. Sullivan N, Sun Y, Li J, Hofmann W, et al. Replicative function and neutralization sensitivity of envelope glycoproteins from primary and T-cell line–passaged human immunodeficiency virus type 1 isolates. J Virol. 1995;69:4413–4422.
154. Bou-Habib DC, Roderiquez G, Oravecz T, et al. Cryptic nature of envelope V3 region epitopes protects primary monocytotropic human immunodeficiency virus type 1 from antibody neutralization. J Virol. 1994;68:6006–6013.
155. Albert J, Abrahamsson B, Nagy K, et al. Rapid development of isolate-specific neutralizing antibodies after primary HIV-1 infection and consequent emergence of virus variants which resist neutralization by autologous sera. AIDS. 1990;4: 107–112.
156. VonGegerfelt A, Albert J, Morfeldt-Manson L, et al. Isolate-specific neutralizing antibodies in patients with progressive HIV-1–related disease. Virology. 1991;185:162–168.
157. Lu W, Shih JW, Tourani JM, et al. Lack of isolate-specific neutralizing activity is correlated with an increased viral burden in rapidly progressing HIV-1–infected patients. AIDS. 1993;7(Suppl):S91–S99.
158. Arendrup M, Nielsen C, Hansen J-ES, et al. Autologous HIV-1 neutralizing antibodies: Emergence of neutralization-resistant escape virus and subsequent development of escape virus neutralizing antibodies. J Acquir Immune Defic Syndr. 1992;5:303–307.
159. Tremblay M, Wainberg MA. Neutralization of multiple HIV-1 isolates from a single subject by autologous sequential sera. J Infect Dis. 1990;162:735–737.
160. Tsang ML, Evans LA, McQueen P, et al. Neutralizing antibodies against sequential autologous human immunodeficiency virus type 1 isolates after seroconversion. J Infect Dis. 1994;170:1141–1147.
161. Wrin T, Crawford L, Sawyer L, et al. Neutralizing antibody responses to autologous and heterologous isolates of human immunodeficiency virus. J Acquir Immune Defic Syndr. 1994;7:211–219.
162. Pantaleo G, Menzo S, Vaccarezza M, et al. Studies in subject with long-term nonprogressive human immunodeficiency virus infection. N Engl J Med. 1995;332:209–216.
163. Montefiori DC, Pantaleo G, Fink LM, et al. Neutralizing and infection-enhancing antibody responses to human immunodeficiency virus type 1 in long-term nonprogressors. J Infect Dis. 1996;173:60–67.
164. Cao Y, Qin L, Zhang L, et al. Virologic and immunologic characterization of long-term survivors of human immunodeficiency virus type 1 infection. N Engl J Med. 1995;332:201–208.
165. Scarlatti G, Leitner T, Hodara V, et al. Interplay of HIV-1 phenotype and neutralizing antibody response in pathogenesis of AIDS. Immunol Lett. 1996;51:23–28.
166. Lyerly HK, Matthews TJ, Langlois AJ, et al. Human T-cell lymphotropic virus IIIB glycoprotein (gp120) bound to CD4 determinants on normal lymphocytes and expressed by infected cells serves as target for immune attack. Proc Natl Acad Sci U S A. 1987;84:4601–4605.
167. Ojo-Amaize EA, Nishanian P, Keith DE, et al. Antibodies to human immunodeficiency virus in human sera induce cell-mediated lysis of human immunodeficiency virus–infected cells. J Immunol. 1987;139:2458–2463.
168. Weinhold KJ, Lyerly HK, Matthews TJ, et al. Cellular anti-GP120 cytolytic reactivities in HIV-1 seropositive individuals. Lancet. 1988;1:902–905.
169. Tyler DS, Nastala CL, Stanley SD, et al. GP120 specific cellular cytotoxicity in HIV-1 seropositive individuals. Evidence for circulating CD16+ effector cells armed in vivo and cytophilic antibody. J Immunol. 1989;142:1177–1182.
170. Tyler DS, Stanley SD, Zolla-Pazner S, et al. Identification of sites within gp41 that serve as targets for antibody-dependent cellular cytotoxicity by using human monoclonal antibodies. J Immunol. 1990;145:3276–3282.
171. Koup RA, Sullivan JL, Levine PH, et al. Antigenic specificity of antibody-dependent cell-mediated cytotoxicity directed against human immunodeficiency virus in antibody-positive sera. J Virol. 1989;63:584–590.
172. Tanneau F, McChesney M, Lopez O, et al. Primary cytotoxicity against the envelope glycoprotein of human immunodeficiency virus-1: Evidence for antibody-dependent cellular cytotoxicity in vivo. J Infect Dis. 1990;162:837–843.
173. Murayama T, Cai Q, Rinaldo CR. Antibody-dependent cellular cytotoxicity mediated by CD16+ lymphocytes from HIV-seropositive homosexual men. Clin Immunol Immunopathol. 1990;55:297–304.
174. Jewett A, Giorgi JV, Bonavida B. Antibody-dependent cellular cytoxicity against HIV-coated target cells by peripheral blood monocytes from HIV seropositive asymptomatic patients. J Immunol. 1990;145:4065–4071.
175. Tyler DS, Stanley SD, Nastala CA, et al. Alterations in antibody-dependent cellular

cytotoxicity during the course of HIV-1 infection. Humoral and cellular defects. J Immunol. 1990;144:3375–3384.
176. Ljunggren K, Karlson A, Fenyo EM, et al. Natural and antibody-dependent cytotoxicity in different clinical stage of human immunodeficiency virus type 1 infection. Clin Exp Immunol. 1989;75:184–189.
177. Ojo-Amaize E, Nishanian PG, Heitjan DF, et al. Serum and effector-cell antibody-dependent cellular cytotoxicity (ADCC) activity remains high during human immunodeficiency virus (HIV) disease progression. J Clin Immunol. 1989;9:454–461.
178. Skowron G, Cole B, Zheng D, et al. gp120-directed antibody-dependent cellular cytotoxicity as a major determinant of the rate of decline in CD4 percentage in HIV-1 disease. AIDS. 1997;11:1807–1814.
179. Walker BD, Chakrabarti S, Moss B, et al. HIV-specific cytotoxic T lymphocytes in seropositive individuals. Nature. 1987;328:345–348.
180. Plata F, Autran B, Martins LP, et al. AIDS virus–specific cytotoxic T lymphocytes in lung disorders. Nature. 1987;328:348–351.
181. Koup RA, Sullivan JL, Levine PH, et al. Detection of major histocompatibility complex class I–restricted, HIV-specific cytotoxic T lymphocytes in the blood of infected hemophiliacs. Blood. 1989;73:1909–1914.
182. Riviere Y, Tanneau-Salvadori F, Regnault A, et al. Human immunodeficiency virus–specific cytotoxic responses of seropositive individuals: Distinct types of effector cells mediate killing of targets expressing gag and env proteins. J Virol. 1989;63:2270–2277.
183. Nixon DF, Townsend AR, Elvin JG, et al. HIV-1 gag-specific cytotoxic T lymphocytes defined with recombinant vaccinia virus and synthetic peptides. Nature. 1988;336:484–487.
184. Gotch FM, Nixon DF, Alp N, et al. High frequency of memory and effector gag specific cytotoxic T lymphocytes in HIV seropositive individuals. Int Immunol. 1990;2:707–712.
185. Walker BD, Flexner C, Paradis TJ, et al. HIV-1 reverse transcriptase is a target for cytotoxic T lymphocytes in infected individuals. Science. 1988;240:64–66.
186. Hosmalin A, Clerici M, Houghten R, et al. An epitope in human immunodeficiency virus 1 reverse transcriptase recognized by both mouse and human cytotoxic T lymphocytes. Proc Natl Acad Sci U S A. 1990;87:2344–2348.
187. Lieberman J, Fabry JA, Kuo MC, et al. Cytotoxic T lymphocytes from HIV-1 seropositive individuals recognize immunodominant epitopes in Gp160 and reverse transcriptase. J Immunol. 1992;148:2738–2747.
188. Koenig S, Earl P, Powell D, et al. Group-specific, major histocompatibility complex class I–restricted cytotoxic responses to human immunodeficiency virus 1 (HIV-1) envelope proteins by cloned peripheral blood T cells from an HIV-1–infected individual. Proc Natl Acad Sci U S A. 1988;85:8638–8642.
189. Hammond SA, Obah E, Stanhope P, et al. Characterization of a conserved T cell epitope in HIV-1 gp41 recognized by vaccine-induced human cytolytic T cells. J Immunol. 1991;146:1470–1477.
190. Clerici M, Lucey DR, Zajac RA, et al. Detection of cytotoxic T lymphocytes specific for synthetic peptides of gp160 in HIV-seropositive individuals. J Immunol. 1991;146:2214–2219.
191. Koenig S, Fuerst TR, Wood LV, et al. Mapping the fine specificity of a cytolytic T cell response to HIV-1 nef protein. J Immunol. 1990;145:127–135.
192. Hoffenbach A, Langlade-Demoyen P, Dadaglio G, et al. Unusually high frequencies of HIV-specific cytotoxic T lymphocytes in humans. J Immunol. 1989;142: 452–462.
193. Moss PA, Rowland-Jones SL, Frodsham PM, et al. Persistent high frequency of human immunodeficiency virus–specific cytotoxic T cells in peripheral blood of infected donors. Proc Natl Acad Sci U S A. 1995;92:5773–5777.
194. Altman JD, Moss PAH, Goulder PJR, et al. Phenotypic analysis of antigen-specific T lymphocytes. Science. 1996;274:94–96.
195. Ogg G, Jin X, Bonhoeffer S, et al. Quantitation of HIV-1 specific cytotoxic T lymphocytes and plasma load of viral RNA. Science. 1998;279:2103–2106.
196. Harrer T, Harrer E, Kalams SA, et al. Cytotoxic T lymphocytes in asymptomatic long-term nonprogressing HIV-1 infection. Breadth and specificity of the response and relation to in vivo viral quasispecies in a person with prolonged infection and low viral load. J Immunol. 1996;156:2616–2623.
197. Harrer T, Harrer E, Kalams SA, et al. Strong cytotoxic T cell and weak neutralizing antibody responses in a subset of persons with stable nonprogressing HIV type 1 infection. AIDS Res Hum Retroviruses. 1996;12:585–592.
198. Rinaldo C, Huang X-L, Fan Z, et al. High levels of anti–human immunodeficiency virus type 1 (HIV-1) memory cytotoxic T-lymphocyte activity and low viral load are associated with lack of disease in HIV-1–infected long-term nonprogressors. J Virol. 1995;69:5838–5842.
199. Klein MR, vanBaalen CA, Holwerda AM, et al. Kinetics of gag-specific cytotoxic T lymphocyte responses during the clinical course of HIV-1 infection: A longitudinal analysis of rapid progressors and long-term asymptomatics. J Exp Med. 1995;181:1365–1372.
200. Greenough TC, Brettler DB, Somasundaran M, et al. Human immunodeficiency virus type 1–specific cytotoxic T lymphocytes (CTL), virus load, and CD4 T cell loss: Evidence supporting a protective role for CTL in vivo. J Infect Dis. 1997;176:118–125.
201. Rowland-Jones S, Sutton J, Ariyoshi K, et al. HIV-specific cytotoxic T-cells in HIV-exposed but uninfected Gambian women. Nat Med. 1995;1:59–64.
202. Tenner-Racz K, Racz P, Thome C, et al. Cytotoxic effector cell granules recognized by the monoclonal antibody TIA-1 are present in CD8+ lymphocytes in lymph nodes of human immunodeficiency virus-1–infected patients. Am J Pathol. 1993;142:1750–1758.
203. Riviere Y, McChesney MB, Porrot F, et al. Gag-specific cytotoxic responses to HIV type 1 are associated with a decreased risk of progression to AIDS-related complex or AIDS. AIDS Res Hum Retroviruses. 1995;11:903–907.
204. Goulder PJ, Bunce M, Krausa P, et al. Novel, cross-restricted, conserved, and immunodominant cytotoxic T lymphocyte epitopes in slow progressors in HIV type 1 infection. AIDS Res Hum Retroviruses. 1996;12:1691–1698.
205. Klein MR, Keet IPM, D'Amaro J, et al. Associations between HLA frequencies and pathogenic features of human immunodeficiency virus type 1 infection in seroconverters from the Amsterdam Cohort of Homosexual Men. J Infect Dis. 1994;169:1244–1249.
206. Keet IP, Klein MR, Just JJ, et al. The role of host genetics in the natural history of HIV-1 infection: The needles in the haystack. AIDS. 1996;10(Suppl A): S59–S67.
207. Kaslow RA, Carrington M, Apple R, et al. Influence of combinations of human major histocompatibility complex genes on the course of HIV-1 infection. Nat Med. 1996;2:405–411.
208. Pantaleo G, Demarest JF, Schacker T, et al. The qualitative nature of the primary immune response to HIV infection is a prognosticator of disease progression independent of the initial level of plasma viremia. Proc Natl Acad Sci U S A. 1997;94:254–258.
209. Howcroft T, Strebel K, Martin M, et al. Repression of MHC class I gene promoter activity by two-exon tat of HIV. Science. 1993;260:1320–1322.
210. Schwartz O, Marechal V, Gall SL, et al. Endocytosis of major histocompatibility complex class I molecules is induced by the HIV-1 Nef protein. Nat Med. 1996;2:338–342.
211. Collins KL, Chen BK, Kalams SA, et al. HIV-1 Nef protein protects infected primary cells against killing by cytotoxic T lymphocytes. Nature. 1998;391: 397–401.
212. Kerkau T, Bacik I, Bennink JR, et al. The human immunodeficiency virus type 1 (HIV-1) vpu protein interferes with an early step in the biosynthesis of major histocompatibility complex (MHC) class I molecules. J Exp Med. 1997;185:1295–1305.
213. Pantaleo G, DeMaria A, Koenig S, et al. CD8+ T lymphocytes of patients with AIDS maintain normal broad cytolytic function despite the loss of human immunodeficiency virus–specific cytotoxicity. Proc Natl Acad Sci U S A. 1990;87:4818–4822.
214. Pantaleo G, Koenig S, Baseler M, et al. Defective clonogenic potential of CD8+ T lymphocytes in patients with AIDS. J Immunol. 1990;144:1696–1704.
215. Phillips RE, Rowland-Jones S, Nixon DF, et al. Human immunodeficiency virus genetic variation that can escape cytotoxic T cell recognition. Nature. 1991;354:433–434.
216. Koenig S, Conley AJ, Brewah YA, et al. Transfer of HIV-1–specific cytotoxic T lymphocytes to an AIDS patient leads to selection for mutant HIV variants and subsequent disease progression. Nat Med. 1995;1:330–336.
217. Borrow P, Lewicki H, Wei X, et al. Antiviral pressure exerted by HIV-1–specific cytotoxic T lymphocytes (CTLs) during primary infection demonstrated by rapid selection of CTL escape virus. Nat Med. 1997;3:205–211.
218. Goulder PJR, Phillips RE, Colbert RA, et al. Late escape from an immunodominant cytotoxic T-lymphocyte response associated with progression to AIDS. Nat Med. 1997;3:212–217.
219. Price DA, Goulder PJ, Klenerman P, et al. Positive selection of HIV-1 cytotoxic T lymphocyte escape variants during primary infection. Proc Natl Acad Sci U S A. 1997;94:1890–1895.
220. Klenerman P, Rowland-Jones S, McAdam S, et al. Cytotoxic T-cell activity antagonized by naturally occurring HIV-1 Gag variants. Nature. 1994;369:403–407.
221. Meier U-C, Klenerman P, Griffin P, et al. Cytotoxic T lymphocyte lysis inhibited by viable HIV mutants. Science. 1995;270:1360–1362.
222. Itescu S, Rose S, Dwyer E, et al. Certain HLA-DR5 and -DR6 major histocompatibility complex class II alleles are associated with a CD8 lymphocytic host response to human immunodeficiency virus type 1 characterized by low lymphocyte viral strain heterogeneity and slow disease progression. Proc Natl Acad Sci U S A. 1994;91:11472–11476.
223. Kalams SA, Johnson RP, Trocha AK, et al. Longitudinal analysis of T cell receptor (TCR) gene usage by human immunodeficiency virus 1 envelope–specific cytotoxic T lymphocyte clone reveals a limited TCR repertoire. J Exp Med. 1994;179:1261–1271.
224. Kalams SA, Johnson RP, Dynan MJ, et al. T cell receptor usage and fine specificity of human immunodeficiency virus 1–specific cytotoxic T lymphocyte clones: Analysis of quasispecies recognition reveals a dominant response directed against a minor in vivo variant. J Exp Med. 1996;183:1669–1679.
225. Wilson CC, Kalams SA, Wilkes BM, et al. Overlapping epitopes in human immunodeficiency virus type 1 gp120 presented by HLA A, B, and C molecules: Effects of viral variation on cytotoxic T-lymphocyte recognition. J Virol. 1997;71:1256–1264.
226. Klenerman P, Zinkernagel RM. Original antigenic sin impairs cytotoxic T lymphocyte responses to viruses bearing variant epitopes. Nature. 1998;394:482–485.
227. Wolinsky SM, Korber BTM, Neumann AU, et al. Adaptive evolution of human immunodeficiency virus-type 1 during the natural course of infection. Science. 1996;272:537–542.
228. Haas G, Plikat U, Debre P, et al. Dynamics of viral variants in HIV-1 Nef and specific cytotoxic T lymphocytes in vivo. J Immunol. 1996;157:4212–4221.
229. Nowak MA, May RM, Phillips RE, et al. Antigenic oscillations and shifting immunodominance in HIV-1 infections. Nature. 1995;375:606–611.
230. Moskophidis D, Lechner F, Pircher H, et al. Virus persistence in acutely infected immunocompetent mice by exhaustion of antiviral cytotoxic effector T cells. Nature. 1993;362:758–761.

231. Pantaleo G, Soudeyns H, Demarest J, et al. Evidence for rapid disappearance of initially expanded HIV-specific CD8+ T cell clones during primary HIV infection. Proc Natl Acad Sci U S A. 1997;94:9848–9853.
232. Yang OO, Kalams SA, Trocha A, et al. Suppression of human immunodeficiency virus type 1 replication by CD8+ cells: Evidence for HLA class I–restricted triggering of cytolytic and noncytolytic mechanisms. J Virol. 1997;71:3120–3128.
233. Walker CM, Levy JA. A diffusible lymphokine produced by CD8+ T lymphocytes suppresses HIV replication. Immunology. 1989;66:628–630.
234. Walker CM, Erickson AL, Hsueh FC, et al. Inhibition of human immunodeficiency virus replication in acutely infected CD4+ cells by CD8+ cells involves a noncytotoxic mechanism. J Virol. 1991;65:5921–5927.
235. Chen CH, Weinhold KJ, Bartlett JA, et al. CD8+ T lymphocyte–mediated inhibition of HIV-1 long terminal repeat transcription: A novel antiviral mechanism. AIDS Res Hum Retroviruses. 1993;9:1079–1086.
236. Copeland KF, McKay PJ, Rosenthal KL. Suppression of activation of the human immunodeficiency virus long terminal repeat by CD8+ T cells is not lentivirus specific. AIDS Res Hum Retroviruses. 1995;11:1321–1326.
237. Mackewicz C, Balckbourn DJ, Levy JA. CD8+ T cells suppress human immunodeficiency virus replication by inhibiting viral transcription. Proc Natl Acad Sci U S A. 1995;92:2308–2312.
238. Mackewicz CE, Oretega H, Levy JA. Effect of cytokines on HIV replication in CD4+ lymphocytes: Lack of identity with the CD8+ cell antiviral factor. Cell Immunol. 1994;153:329–343.
239. Mackewicz CE, Ortega HW, Levy JA. CD8+ cell anti-HIV activity correlates with the clinical state of the infected individual. J Clin Invest. 1991;87:1462–1466.
240. Chen Y, Gupta P. CD8+ T-cell–mediated suppression of HIV-1 infection may not be due to chemokines RANTES, MIP-1α, and MIP-1β. AIDS. 1996;10:1434–1435.
241. Vicenzi E, Bagnarelli P, Santagostino E, et al. Hemophilia and nonprogressing human immunodeficiency virus type 1 infection. Blood. 1997;89:191–200.
242. Rubbert A, Weissman D, Combadiere C, et al. Multifactorial nature of noncytolytic CD8+ T cell–mediated suppression of HIV replication: Beta-chemokine–dependent and –independent effects. AIDS Res Hum Retroviruses. 1997;13:63–69.
243. Pal R, Garzino-Demo A, Markham PD, et al. Inhibition of HIV-1 infection by the beta-chemokine MDC. Science. 1997;278:695–698.
244. Baier M, Werner A, Bannert N, et al. HIV suppression by interleukin-16. Nature. 1995;378:563.
245. Clerici M, Stocks NI, Zajac RA, et al. Interleukin-2 production used to detect antigenic peptide recognition by T-helper lymphocytes from asymptomatic HIV-seropositive individuals. Nature. 1989;339:383–385.
246. Schrier RD, Gnann JW, Landes R, et al. T cell recognition of HIV synthetic peptides in a natural infection. J Immunol. 1989;142:1166–1176.
247. Cease KB, Margalit H, Cornette JL, et al. Helper T-cell antigenic site identification in the acquired immunodeficiency syndrome virus gp120 envelope protein and induction of immunity in mice to the native protein using a 16-residue synthetic peptide. Proc Natl Acad Sci U S A. 1987;84:4249–4253.
248. Torseth JW, Berman PW, Merigan TC. Recombinant HIV structural proteins detect specific cellular immunity in vitro in infected individuals. AIDS Res Hum Retroviruses. 1988;4:23–30.
249. Kinter A, Fauci AS. Interleukin-2 and human immunodeficiency virus infection: Pathogenic mechanisms and potential for immunologic enhancement. Immunol Res. 1996;15:1–15.
250. Rosenberg ES, Billingsley JM, Caliendo AM, et al. Vigorous HIV-1–specific CD4+ T cell responses associated with control of viremia. Science. 1997;278:1447–1450.
251. Ioachim HL, Lerner CW, Tapper ML. The lymphoid lesions associated with the acquired immunodeficiency syndrome. Am J Surg Pathol. 1983;7:543–553.
252. Fernandez R, Mouradian J, Metroka C, et al. The prognostic value of histopathology in persistent generalized lymphadenopathy in homosexual men. N Engl J Med. 1983;309:185–186.
253. Janossy G, Pinching AJ, Bofill M, et al. An immunohistological approach to persistent lymphadenopathy and its relevance to AIDS. Clin Exp Immunol. 1985;59:257–266.
254. Biberfeld P, Chayt K, Marselle L, et al. HTLV-III expression in infected lymph nodes and relevance to pathogenesis of lymphadenopathy. Am J Pathol. 1986;125:436–442.
255. Racz P, Tenner-Racz K, Kahl C, et al. Spectrum of morphologic changes of lymph nodes from patients with AIDS or AIDS-related complexes. Prog Allergy. 1986;37:81–181.
256. Pallesen G, Gerstoft J, Mathiesen L. Stages in LAV/HTLV-III lymphadenitis: I. Histological and immunohistological classification. Scand J Immunol. 1987;25:83–91.
257. Turner R, Levine A, Gill P, et al. Progressive histopathologic abnormalities in the persistent generalized lymphadenopathy syndrome. Am J Surg Pathol. 1987;11:625–632.
258. Pantaleo G, Graziosi C, Demarest JF, et al. HIV infection is active and progressive in lymphoid tissue during the clinically latent stage of disease. Nature. 1993;362:355–358.
259. Tew JG, Burton GF, Kupp LI, et al. Follicular dendritic cells in germinal center reactions. Adv Exp Med Biol. 1993;329:461–465.
260. Pantaleo G, Fauci AS. Immunopathogenesis of HIV infection. Annu Rev Microbiol. 1996;50:825–854.
261. Clerici M, Stocks NI, Zajac RA, et al. Detection of three distinct patterns of T helper cell dysfunction in asymptomatic, human immunodeficiency virus–seropositive patients independent of CD4+ cell numbers and clinical settings. J Clin Invest. 1989;84:1892–1899.
262. Choremi-Papadopoulou H, Viglis V, Gargalianos P, et al. Downregulation of CD28 surface antigen on CD4+ and CD8+ T lymphocytes during HIV-1 infection. J Acquir Immune Defic Syndr. 1994;7:245–253.
263. Borthwick NJ, Bofill M, Gombert WM, et al. Lymphocyte activation in HIV-1 infection. II. Functional defects of CD28− T cells. AIDS. 1994;8:431–441.
264. Wolthers KC, Otto SA, Lens SM, et al. Functional B cell abnormalities in HIV type 1 infection: Role of CD40L and CD70. AIDS Res Hum Retroviruses. 1997;13:1023–1029.
265. Stevenson M, Meier C, Mann AM, et al. Envelope glycoprotein of HIV induces interference and cytolysis resistance in CD4+ cells: Mechanisms for persistence in AIDS. Cell. 1988;53:483–496.
266. Garcia JV, Miller AD. Serine phosphorylation–independent downregulation of cell-surface CD4 by nef. Nature. 1991;350:508–511.
267. Willey RL, Maldarelli F, Martin MA, et al. Human immunodeficiency virus type 1 Vpu protein induces rapid degradation of CD4. J Virol. 1992;66:7193–7200.
268. Yao XJ, Friborg J, Checroune F, et al. Degradation of CD4 induced by human immunodeficiency virus type 1 Vpu protein: A predicted alpha-helix structure in the proximal cytoplasmic region of CD4 contributes to Vpu sensitivity. Virology. 1995;209:615–623.
269. Schnittman SM, Lane HC, Greenhouse J, et al. Preferential infection of CD4+ memory T cells by human immunodeficiency virus type 1: Evidence for a role in the selective T-cell functional defects observed in infected individuals. Proc Natl Acad Sci U S A. 1990;87:6058–6062.
270. Chun T-W, Chadwick K, Margolick J, et al. Differential susceptibility of naive and memory CD4+ T cells to the cytopathic effects of infection with human immunodeficiency virus type 1 strain LAI. J Virol. 1997;71:4436–4444.
271. Spina CA, Prince HE, Richman DD. Preferential replication of HIV-1 in the CD45RO memory cell subset of primary CD4 lymphocytes in vitro. J Clin Invest. 1997;99:1774–1785.
272. Pantaleo G, Graziosi C, Butini L, et al. Lymphoid organs function as major reservoirs for human immunodeficiency virus. Proc Natl Acad Sci U S A. 1991;88:9838–9842.
273. Lane HC, Depper JM, Greene WC, et al. Qualitative analysis of immune function in patients with the acquired immunodeficiency syndrome. Evidence for a selective defect in soluble antigen recognition. N Engl J Med. 1985;313:79–84.
274. Chirmule N, Pahwa S. Envelope glycoproteins of human immunodeficiency virus type 1: Profound influences on immune functions. Microbiol Rev. 1996;60:386–406.
275. Oh SK, Cruickshank WW, Raina J, et al. Identification of HIV-1 envelope glycoprotein in the serum of AIDS and ARC patients. J Acquir Immune Defic Syndr. 1992;5:251–256.
276. Amadori A, De Silvestro G, Zamarchi R, et al. CD4 epitope masking by gp120/anti-gp120 antibody complexes. A potential mechanism for CD4+ cell function down-regulation in AIDS patients. J Immunol. 1992;148:2709–2716.
277. Fox C, Tenner-Rácz K, Rácz P, et al. Lymphoid germinal centers are reservoirs of human immunodeficiency virus type 1 RNA. J Infect Dis. 1991;164:1051–1057.
278. Sunila I, Vaccarezza M, Pantaleo G, et al. gp120 is present on the plasma membrane of apoptotic CD4 cells prepared from lymph nodes of HIV-1–infected individuals: An immunoelectron microscopic study. AIDS. 1997;11:27–32.
279. Gupta S, Vayuvegula B. Human immunodeficiency virus–associated changes in signal transduction. J Clin Immunol. 1987;7:486–489.
280. Linette GP, Hartzman RJ, Ledbetter JA, et al. HIV-1–infected T cells show a selective signaling defect after perturbation of CD3/antigen receptor. Science. 1988;241:573–576.
281. Hivroz C, Mazerolles F, Soula M, et al. Human immunodeficiency virus gp120 and derived peptides activate protein tyrosine kinase p561ck in human CD4 T lymphocytes. Eur J Immunol. 1993;23:600–607.
282. Tamma SML, Chirmule N, Yagura H, et al. CD4 cross-linking (CD4XL) induces RAS activation and tumor necrosis factor-alpha secretion in CD4+ T cells. Blood. 1997;90:1588–1593.
283. Oyaizu N, Chirmule N, Kalyanaraman VS, et al. Human immunodeficiency virus type 1 envelope glycoprotein gp120 produces immune defects in CD4+ T lymphocytes by inhibiting interleukin 2 mRNA. Proc Natl Acad Sci U S A. 1990;87:2379–2383.
284. Liegler TJ, Stites DP. HIV-1 gp120 and anti-gp120 induce reversible unresponsiveness in peripheral CD4 T lymphocytes. J Acquir Immune Defic Syndr. 1994;7:340–348.
285. Cohen DI, Tani Y, Tian H, et al. Participation of tyrosine phosphorylation in the cytopathic effect of human immunodeficiency virus-1. Science. 1992;256:542–545.
286. Banda NK, Bernier J, Kurahara DK, et al. Crosslinking CD4 by human immunodeficiency virus gp120 primes T cells for activation-induced apoptosis. J Exp Med. 1992;176:1099–1106.
287. Westendorp MO, Frank R, Ochsenbauer C, et al. Sensitization of T cells to CD95-mediated apoptosis by HIV-1 tat and gp120. Nature. 1995;375:497–500.
288. Weissman D, Rabin RL, Arthos J, et al. Macrophage-tropic HIV and SIV envelope proteins induce a signal through the CCR5 chemokine receptor. Nature. 1997;389:981–985.
289. Cefai D, Debre P, Kaczorek M, et al. Human immunodeficiency virus-1 glycoproteins gp120 and gp160 specifically inhibit the CD3/T cell–antigen receptor phosphoinositide transduction pathway. J Clin Invest. 1990;86:2117–2124.
290. Cefai D, Ferrer M, Serpente N, et al. Internalization of HIV glycoprotein gp120 is associated with down-modulation of membrane CD4 and p561ck together with impairment of T cell activation. J Immunol. 1992;149:285–294.
291. Goldman F, Jensen W, Johnson G, et al. gp120 ligation of CD4 induces p561ck

activation and TCR desensitization independent of TCR tyrosine phosphorylation. J Immunol. 1994;153:2905–2917.
292. Guntermann C, Dye J, Nye KE. Human immunodeficiency virus infection abolishes CD4-dependent activation of ZAP-70 by inhibition of p56lck. J Acquir Immune Defic Syndr Hum Retrovirol. 1997;14:204–212.
293. Chirmule N, McCloskey TW, Hu R, et al. HIV gp120 inhibits T cell activation by interfering with expression of costimulatory molecules CD40 ligand and CD80 (B7-1). J Immunol. 1995;155:917–924.
294. Davis CB, Dikic I, Unutmaz D, et al. Signal transduction due to HIV-1 envelope interactions with chemokine receptors CXCR4 or CCR5. J Exp Med. 1997;186:1793–1798.
294a. Cicala C, Arthos J, Ruiz M, et al. Induction of phosphorylation and intracellular association of CC chemokine receptor 5 and focal adhesion kinase in primary human CD4+ T cells by macrophage-tropic HIV envelope. J Immunol. 1999;163:420–426.
295. Connors M, Kovacs JA, Krevat S, et al. HIV infection induces changes in CD4+ T-cell phenotype and depletions within the CD4+ T-cell repertoire that are not immediately restored by antiviral or immune-based therapies. Nat Med. 1997;3:533–540.
296. Gea-Banacloche JC, Weiskopf EE, Hallahan C, et al. Progression of human immunodeficiency virus disease is associated with increasing disruptions within the CD4+ T cell receptor repertoire. J Infect Dis. 1998;177:579–585.
297. Gorochov G, Neumann AU, Kereveur A, et al. Perturbation of CD4+ and CD8+ T-cell repertoires during progression to AIDS and regulation of the CD4+ repertoire during antiviral therapy. Nat Med. 1998;4:215–221.
298. Macdonald JC, Torriani FJ, Morse LS, et al. Lack of reactivation of cytomegalovirus (CMV) retinitis after stopping CMV maintenance therapy in AIDS patients with sustained elevations in CD4 T cells in response to highly active antiretroviral therapy. J Infect Dis. 1998;177:1182–1187.
299. Vrabec TR, Baldassano VF, Whitcup SM. Discontinuation of maintenance therapy in patients with quiescent cytomegalovirus retinitis and elevated CD4+ counts. Ophthalmology. 1998;105:1259–1264.
300. Gallo R, Salahuddin S, Popovic M, et al. Frequent detection and isolation of cytopathic retroviruses (HTLV-III) from patients with AIDS and at risk for AIDS. Science. 1984;224:500–503.
301. Levy J, Hoffman A, Kramer S, et al. Isolation of lymphocytopathic retroviruses from San Francisco patients with AIDS. Science. 1984;225:840–842.
302. Shaw GM, Hahn BH, Arya SK, et al. Molecular characterization of human T-cell leukemia (lymphotropic) virus type III in the acquired immune deficiency syndrome. Science. 1984;226:1165–1171.
303. Popovic M, Sarngadharan M, Read E, et al. Detection, isolation, and continuous production of cytopathic retroviruses (HTLV-III) from patients with AIDS and pre-AIDS. Science. 1984;224:497–500.
304. Sodroski J, Goh WC, Rosen K, et al. Role of the HTLV-III/LAV envelope in syncytium formation and cytopathicity. Nature. 1986;322:470–474.
305. DeRossi A, Franchini G, Aldovini A, et al. Differential response to the cytopathic effects of human T-cell lymphotropic virus type III (HTLV-III) superinfection in T4+ (helper) and T8+ (suppressor) T-cell clones transformed by HTLV-1. Proc Natl Acad Sci U S A. 1986;83:4297–4301.
306. Lifson JD, Reyes GR, McGrath MS, et al. AIDS retrovirus induced cytopathology: Giant cell formation and involvement of CD4 antigen. Science. 1986;232:1123–1127.
307. Lifson JD, Feinberg MB, Reyes GR, et al. Induction of CD4-dependent cell fusion by the HTLV-III/LAV envelope glycoprotein. Nature. 1986;323:725–728.
308. Schnittman SM, Greenhouse JJ, Psallidopoulos MC, et al. Increasing viral burden in CD4+ T cells from patients with human immunodeficiency virus (HIV) infection reflects rapidly progressive immunosuppression and clinical disease. Ann Intern Med. 1990;113:438–443.
309. Bagnarelli P, Menzo S, Valenza A, et al. Molecular profile of human immunodeficiency virus type 1 infection in symptomless patients and in patients with AIDS. J Virol. 1992;66:7328–7335.
310. Connor RI, Mohri H, Cao Y, et al. Increased viral burden and cytopathicity correlate temporally with CD4+ T-lymphocyte decline and clinical progression in human immunodeficiency virus type 1–infected individuals. J Virol. 1993;67:1772–1777.
311. Michael NL, Vahey M, Burke RS, et al. Viral DNA and mRNA expression correlate with the stage of human immunodeficiency virus (HIV) type 1 infection in humans: Evidence for viral replication in all stages of HIV disease. J Virol. 1992;66:310–316.
312. Poznansky MC, Walker B, Haseltine WA, et al. A rapid method for quantitating the frequency of peripheral blood cells containing HIV-1 DNA. J Acquir Immune Defic Syndr. 1991;4:368–373.
313. Embretson J, Zupancic M, Ribas J, et al. Massive covert infection of helper T lymphocytes and macrophages by HIV during the incubation period of AIDS. Nature. 1993;362:359–362.
314. Bergeron L, Sodroski J. Dissociation of unintegrated viral DNA accumulation from single-cell lysis induced by human immunodeficiency virus type 1. J Virol. 1992;66:5777–5787.
315. Somasundaran M, Robinson HL. Unexpectedly high levels of HIV-1 RNA and protein synthesis in a cytocidal infection. Science. 1988;242:1554–1557.
316. Koga Y, Lindstrom E, Fenyo EM, et al. High levels of heterodisperse RNAs accumulate in T cells infected with human immunodeficiency virus and in normal thymocytes. Proc Natl Acad Sci U S A. 1988;85:4521–4525.
317. Koga Y, Sasaki M, Yoshida H, et al. Cytopathic effect determined by the amount of CD4 molecules in human cell lines expressing envelope glycoprotein of HIV. J Immunol. 1990;144:94–102.
318. Cao J, Park IW, Cooper A, et al. Molecular determinants of acute single-cell lysis by human immunodeficiency virus type 1. J Virol. 1996;70:1340–1354.
319. Leonard R, Zagury D, Desportes I, et al. Cytopathic effect of human immunodeficiency virus in T4 cells is linked to the last stage of virus infection. Proc Natl Acad Sci U S A. 1988;85:33570–3574.
320. Lynn WS, Tweedale A, Cloyd MW. Human immunodeficiency virus (HIV-1) cytotoxicity: Perturbation of the cell membrane and depression of phospholipid synthesis. Virology. 1988;163:43–51.
321. Voss TG, Fermin CD, Levy JA, et al. Alteration of intracellular potassium and sodium concentrations correlates with induction of cytopathic effects by human immunodeficiency virus. J Virol. 1996;70:5447–5454.
322. Yoffe B, Lewis DE, Petrie BL, et al. Fusion as a mediator of cytolysis in mixtures of uninfected CD4+ lymphocytes and cells infected by human immunodeficiency virus. Proc Natl Acad Sci U S A. 1987;84:1429–1433.
323. Hildreth JE, Orentas RJ. Involvement of a leukocyte adhesion receptor (LFA-1) in HIV-induced syncytium formation. Sciene. 1989;244:1075–1078.
324. Pantaleo G, Butini L, Graziosi C, et al. Human immunodeficiency virus (HIV) infection in CD4+ T lymphocytes genetically deficient in LFA-1: LFA-1 is required for HIV-mediated cell fusion but not for viral transmission. J Exp Med. 1991;173:511–514.
325. Sato AI, Balamuth FB, Ugen KE, et al. Identification of CD7 glycoprotein as an accessory molecule in HIV-1–mediated syncytium formation and cell free infection. J Immunol. 1994;152:5142–5152.
326. deSantis C, Robbioni P, Longhi R, et al. Role of HLA class I in HIV type 1–induced syncytium formation. AIDS Res Hum Retroviruses. 1996;12:1031–1040.
327. Sharer LR, Cho ES, Epstein LG. Multinucleated giant cells and HTLV-III in AIDS encephalopathy. Hum Pathol. 1985;16:760.
328. Maier H, Budka H, Lassmann H, et al. Vacuolar myelopathy with multinucleated giant cells in the acquired immune deficiency syndrome (AIDS). Light and electron microscopic distribution of human immunodeficiency virus (HIV) antigens. Acta Neuropathol. 1989;78:497–503.
329. Burke AP, Benson W, Ribas JL, et al. Postmortem localization of HIV-1 RNA by in situ hybridization in lymphoid tissues of intravenous drug addicts who died unexpectedly. Am J Pathol. 1993;142:1701–1713.
330. Burke AP, Anderson D, Mannan P, et al. Systemic lymphadenopathic histology in human immunodeficiency virus-1–seropositive drug addicts without apparent acquired immunodeficiency syndrome. Hum Pathol. 1994;25:248–256.
331. Frankel SS, Wenig BM, Burke AP, et al. Replication of HIV-1 in dendritic cell–derived syncytia at the mucosal surface of the adenoid. Science. 1996;272:115–117.
332. Teo I, Veryard C, Barnes H, et al. Circular forms of unintegrated human immunodeficiency virus type 1 DNA and high levels of viral protein expression: Association with dementia and multinucleated giant cells in the brains of patients with AIDS. J Virol. 1997;71:2928–2933.
333. Golding H, Robey FA, Gates FT, et al. Identification of homologous regions in human immunodeficiency virus I gp41 and human MHC class II beta 1 domain. I. Monoclonal antibodies against the gp41-derived peptide and patient's sera react with native HLA class II antigens, suggesting a role for autoimmunity in the pathogenesis of acquired immune deficiency syndrome. J Exp Med. 1988;167: 914–923.
334. Golding H, Shearer G, Hillman K, et al. Common epitope in human immunodeficiency virus (HIV)1 gp41 and HLA class II elicits immunosuppressive autoantibodies capable of contributing to immune dysfunction in HIV 1–infected individuals. J Clin Invest. 1989;83:1430–1435.
335. Metlas R, Skerl V, Veljkovic V, et al. Immunoglobulin-like domain of HIV-1 envelope glycoprotein gp120 encodes putative internal image of some common human proteins. Viral Immunol. 1994;7:215–219.
336. Grassi F, Meneveri R, Gullberg M, et al. Human immunodeficiency virus type 1 gp120 mimics a hidden monomorphic epitope borne by class I major histocompatibility complex heavy chains. J Exp Med. 1991;174:53–62.
337. Silvestris F, Williams RC, Dammacco F. Autoreactivity in HIV-1 infections: The role of molecular mimicry. Clin Immunol Immunopathol. 1995;75:197–205.
338. Grant MD, Weaver MS, Tsoukas C, et al. Distribution of antibodies against denatured collagen in AIDS risk groups and homosexual AIDS patients suggests a link between autoimmunity and the immunopathogenesis of AIDS. J Immunol. 1990;144:1241–1250.
339. Muller S, Richalet P, Laurent-Crawford A, et al. Autoantibodies typical of non–organ-specific autoimmune diseases in HIV-seropositive patients. AIDS. 1992;6:933–942.
340. Cassani F, Baffoni L, Raise E, et al. Serum non–organ specific autoantibodies in human immunodeficiency virus 1 infection. J Clin Pathol. 1991;44:64–68.
341. Hugin AW, Vacchio MS, Morse HC. A virus-encoded "superantigen" in a retrovirus-induced immunodeficiency syndrome of mice. Science. 1991;252:424–427.
342. Imberti L, Sottini A, Bettinardi A, et al. Selective depletion in HIV infection of T cells that bear specific T cell receptor V beta sequences. Science. 1991;254: 860–862.
343. Garcia S, Dadaglio G, Cilote V, et al. Evidence for an in vivo superantigenic activity in human immunodeficiency virus–infected individuals. Blood. 1996;88:2151–2161.
344. Laurence J, Hodtsev AS, Posnett DN. Superantigen implicated in dependence of HIV-1 replication in T cells on TCR V beta expression. Nature. 1992;358:255–259.
345. Posnett DN, Kabak S, Dobrescu D, et al. The HIV-1 reservoir in distinct V beta subsets of CD4 T cells: Evidence for a putative superantigen. J Clin Immunol. 1995;15(Suppl):18S–21S.

346. Dobrescu D, Kabak S, Mehta K, et al. Human immunodeficiency virus 1 reservoir in CD4+ T cells is restricted to certain V beta subsets. Proc Natl Acad Sci U S A. 1995;92:5563–5567.
347. Dobrescu D, Ursea B, Pope M, et al. Enhanced HIV-1 replication in V beta 12 T cells due to human cytomegalovirus in monocytes: Evidence for a putative herpesvirus superantigen. Cell. 1995;82:753–763.
348. Boyer V, Smith LR, Ferre F, et al. T cell receptor V beta repertoire in HIV-infected individuals: Lack of evidence for selective V beta deletion. Clin Exp Immunol. 1993;92:437–441.
349. Posnett DN, Kabak S, Hodtsev A, et al. T-cell antigen receptor V beta subsets are not perferentially deleted in AIDS. AIDS. 1993;7:625–631.
350. Boldt-Houle DM, Rinaldo CR, Ehrlich GD. Random depletion of T cells that bear specific T cell receptor V beta sequences in AIDS patients. J Leukoc Biol. 1993;54:486–491.
351. Pantaleo G, Demarest JF, Soudeyns H, et al. Major expansion of CD8+ T cells with a predominant V beta usage during the primary immune response to HIV. Nature. 1994;370:463–467.
352. Weinhold KJ, Lyerly HK, Stanley SD, et al. HIV-1 GP120-mediated immune suppression and lymphocyte destruction in the absence of viral infection. J Immunol. 1989;142:3091–3097.
353. Zarling JM, Ledbetter JA, Sias J, et al. HIV-infected humans, but not chimpanzees, have circulating cytotoxic T lymphocytes that lyse uninfected CD4+ cells. J Immunol. 1990;144:2992–2998.
354. Manca F, Habeshaw JA, Dalgleish AG. HIV envelope glycoprotein, antigen specific T-cell responses, and soluble CD4. Lancet. 1990;335:811–815.
355. Cohen JJ. Apoptosis. Immunol Today. 1993;14:126–130.
356. Thompson CB. Apoptosis in the pathogenesis and treatment of disease. Science. 1995;267:1456–1462.
357. Vaux DL, Cory S, Adams JM. Bcl-2 gene promotes haemopoietic cell survival and cooperates with c-myc to immortalize pre-B cells. Nature. 1988;335:440–442.
358. Nunez G, London L, Hockenbery D, et al. Deregulated Bcl-2 gene expression selectively prolongs survival of growth factor–deprived hemopoietic cell lines. J Immunol. 1990;144:3602–3610.
359. Hockenbery D, Nunez G, Milliman C, et al. Bcl-2 is an inner mitochondrial membrane protein that blocks programmed cell death. Nature. 1990;348:334–336.
360. Lowe SW, Schmitt EM, Smith SW, et al. p53 is required for radiation-induced apoptosis in mouse thymocytes. Nature. 1993;362:847–849.
361. Clarke AR, Purdie CA, Harrison DJ, et al. Thymocyte apoptosis induced by p53-dependent and independent pathways. Nature. 1993;362:849–852.
362. Lee JM, Bernstein A. p53 mutations increase resistance to ionizing radiation. Proc Natl Acad Sci U S A. 1993;90:5742–5746.
363. Ascher MS, Sheppard HW. AIDS as immune system activation. II. The panergic imnesia hypothesis. J Acquir Immune Defic Syndr. 1990;3:177–191.
364. Ameisen JC, Capron A. Cell dysfunction and depletion in AIDS: The programmed cell death hypothesis. Immunol Today. 1991;12:102–105.
365. Laurent-Crawford AG, Krust B, Muller S, et al. The cytopathic effect of HIV is associated with apoptosis. Virology. 1991;185:829–839.
366. Terai C, Kornbluth RS, Pauza CD, et al. Apoptosis as a mechanism of cell death in cultured T lymphoblasts acutely infected with HIV-1. J Clin Invest. 1991;87:1710–1715.
367. Groux H, Torpier G, Monte D, et al. Activation-induced death by apoptosis in CD4+ T cells from human immunodeficiency virus–infected asymptomatic individuals. J Exp Med. 1992;175:331–340.
368. Meyaard L, Otto SA, Jonker RR, et al. Programmed death of T cells in HIV-1 infection. Science. 1992;257:217–219.
369. Oyaizu N, McCloskey TW, Coronesi M, et al. Accelerated apoptosis in peripheral blood mononuclear cells (PBMCs) from human immunodeficiency virus type-1 infected patients and in CD4 cross-linked PBMCs from normal individuals. Blood. 1993;82:3392–3400.
370. Li CJ, Friedman DJ, Wang C, et al. Induction of apoptosis in uninfected lymphocytes by HIV-1 tat protein. Science. 1995;268:429–431.
371. Muro-Cacho CA, Pantaleo G, Fauci AS. Analysis of apoptosis in lymph nodes of HIV-infected persons. J Immunol. 1995;154:5555–5566.
372. Finkel TH, Tudor-Williams G, Banda NK, et al. Apoptosis occurs predominantly in bystander cells and not in productively infected cells of HIV- and SIV-infected lymph nodes. Nat Med. 1995;1:129–134.
373. Gougeon M-L, Lecoeur H, Dulioust A, et al. Programmed cell death in peripheral lymphocytes from HIV-infected persons. J Immunol. 1996;156:3509–3520.
374. Meyaard L, Otto SA, Keet IP, et al. Programmed death of T cells in human immunodeficiency virus infection. No correlation with progression to disease. J Clin Invest. 1994;93:982–988.
375. Estaquier J, Idziorek T, DeBels F, et al. Programmed cell death and AIDS: Significance of T-cell apoptosis in pathogenic and nonpathogenic primate lentiviral infections. Proc Natl Acad Sci U S A. 1994;91:9431–9435.
376. Folks TM, Kessler SW, Orenstein JM, et al. Infection and replication of HIV-1 in purified progenitor cells of normal human bone marrow. Science. 1988;242: 919–922.
377. Steinberg HN, Crumpacker CS, Chatis PA. In vitro suppression of normal human bone marrow progenitor cells by human immunodeficiency virus. J Virol. 1991;65:1765–1769.
378. Chelucci C, Hassan JH, Locardi C, et al. In vitro human immunodeficiency virus-1 infection of purified hematopoietic progenitors in single-cell culture. Blood. 1995;85:1181–1187.
379. vonLaer D, Hufert FT, Fenner TE, et al. CD34+ hematopoietic progenitor cells are not a major reservoir of the human immunodeficiency virus. Blood. 1990;76:1281–1286.
380. Davis BR, Schwartz DH, Marx JC, et al. Absent or rare human immunodeficiency virus infection of bone marrow stem/progenitor cells in vivo. J Virol. 1991;65:1985–1990.
381. Neal TF, Holland HK, Baum CM, et al. CD34+ progenitor cells from asymptomatic patients are not a major reservoir for human immunodeficiency virus-1. Blood. 1995;86:1749–1756.
382. Marandin A, Katz A, Oksenhendler E, et al. Loss of primitive hematopoietic progenitors in patients with human immunodeficiency virus infection. Blood. 1996;88:4568–4578.
383. Stanley SK, Kessler SW, Justement JS, et al. CD34+ bone marrow cells are infected with HIV in a subset of seropositive individuals. J Immunol. 1992;149:689–697.
384. Deichmann M, Kronenwett R, Haas R. Expression of the human immunodeficiency virus type-1 coreceptors CXCR-4 (fusin, LESTR) and CKR-5 in CD34+ hematopoietic progenitor cells. Blood. 1997;89:3522–3528.
385. Ruiz M, Cicala C, Arthos J, et al. Peripheral blood derived CD34+ progenitor cells: CXCR4 and CCR5 chemokine receptor expression and infection by HIV. J Immunol. 1998;161:4169–4176.
386. Zauli G, Re MC, Furlini G, et al. Evidence for an HIV-1 mediated suppression of in vitro growth of enriched (CD34+) hematopoietic progenitors. J Acquir Immune Defic Syndr. 1991;4:1251–1253.
387. Louache F, Henri A, Bettaieb A, et al. Role of human immunodeficiency virus replication in defective in vitro growth of hematopoietic progenitors. Blood. 1992;80:2991–2999.
388. DeLuca A, Teofili L, Antinori A, et al. Haemopoietic CD34+ progenitor cells are not infected by HIV-1 in vivo but show impaired clonogenesis. Br J Haematol. 1993;85:20–24.
389. Re MC, Zauli G, Gibellini D, et al. Uninfected haematopoietic progenitor (CD34+) cells purified from the bone marrow of AIDS patients are committed to apoptotic cell death in culture. AIDS. 1993;7:1049–1055.
390. Zauli G, Re MC, Furlini G, et al. Human immunodeficiency virus type 1 envelope glycoprotein gp120-mediated killing of human haematopoietic progenitors (CD34+ cells). J Gen Virol. 1992;73:417–421.
391. Zauli G, Davis BR, Re MC, et al. Tat protein stimulates production of transforming growth factor-β_1 by marrow macrophages: A potential mechanism for human immunodeficiency virus-1–induced hematopoietic suppression. Blood. 1992;80:3036–3043.
392. Zauli G, Vitale M, Gibellini D, et al. Inhibition of purified CD34+ hematopoietic progenitor cells by human immunodeficiency virus 1 or gp120 mediated by endogenous transforming growth factor beta 1. J Exp Med. 1996;183:99–108.
393. Maciejewski JP, Weichold FF, Young NS. HIV-1 suppression of hematopoiesis in vitro mediated by envelope glycoprotein and TNF-α. J Immunol 1994;153:4303–4310.
394. Stanley S, McCune J, Kaneshima H, et al. Human immunodeficiency virus infection of the human thymus and disruption of the thymic microenvironment in the SCID-hu mouse. J Exp Med. 1993;178:1151–1163.
395. Schnittman SM, Singer KH, Greenhouse JJ, et al. Thymic microenvironment induces HIV expression. Physiologic secretion of IL-6 by thymic epithelial cells up-regulates virus expression in chronically infected cells. J Immunol. 1991;147:2553–2558.
396. Valentin H, Nugeyre MT, Vuillier F, et al. Two subpopulations of human triple-negative thymic cells are susceptible to infection by human immunodeficiency virus type 1 in vitro. J Virol. 1994;68:3041–3050.
397. Su L, Kaneshima H, Bonyhadi M, et al. HIV-1–induced thymocyte depletion is associated with indirect cytopathogenicity and infection of progenitor cells in vivo. Immunity. 1995;2:25–36.
398. Giorgi JV, Ho H-N, Hirji K, et al. CD8+ lymphocyte activation at human immunodeficiency virus type 1 seroconversion: Development of HLA-DR+ CD38− CD8+ cells is associated with subsequent stable CD4+ cell levels. J Infect Dis. 1994;170:775–781.
399. Mocroft A, Bofill M, Lipman M, et al. CD8+, CD38+ lymphocyte percent: A useful immunological marker for monitoring HIV-1–infected patients. J Acquir Immune Defic Syndr Hum Retrovirol. 1997;14:158–162.
400. Liu Z, Hultin LE, Cumberland WG, et al. Elevated relative fluorescence intensity of CD38 antigen expression on CD8+ T cells is a marker of poor prognosis in HIV infection: Results of 6 years of follow-up. Cytometry. 1996;26:1–7.
401. Kammerer R, Iten A, Frei PC, et al. Expansion of T cells negative for CD28 expression in HIV infection. Relation to activation markers and cell adhesion molecules, and correlation with prognostic markers. Med Microbiol Immunol (Berl). 1996;185:19–25.
402. Vingerhoets JH, Vanham GL, Kestens LL, et al. Increased cytolytic T lymphocyte activity and decreased B7 responsiveness are associated with CD28 down-regulation on CD8+ T cells from HIV-infected subjects. Clin Exp Immunol. 1995;100:425–433.
403. Carmichael A, Jin X, Sissons P, et al. Quantitative analysis of the human immunodeficiency virus type 1 (HIV-1)-specific cytotoxic T lymphocyte (CTL) response at different stages of HIV-1 infection: Differential CTL responses to HIV-1 and Epstein-Barr virus in late disease. J Exp Med. 1993;177:249–256.
404. Forte M, Maartens G, Rahelu M, et al. Cytolytic T-cell activity against mycobacterial antigens in HIV. AIDS. 1992;6:407–411.
405. Wilson J, Ogg G, Allen R, et al. Oligoclonal expansions of CD8+ T cells in chronic HIV infection are antigen specific. J Exp Med. 1998;188:785–790.

406. Fauci A. The human immunodeficiency virus: Infectivity and mechanisms of pathogenesis. Science. 1988;239:617–622.
407. Cheng-Mayer C, Liu R, Landau NR, et al. Macrophage tropism of human immunodeficiency virus type 1 and utilization of the CC-CKR5 coreceptor. J Virol. 1997;71:1657–1661.
408. Rana S, Besson G, Cook DG, et al. Role of CCR5 in infection of primary macrophages and lymphocytes by macrophage-tropic strains of human immunodeficiency virus: Resistance to patient-derived and prototype isolates resulting from the delta ccr5 mutation. J Virol. 1997;71:3219–3227.
409. Di Marzio P, Tse J, Landau NR. Chemokine receptor regulation and HIV type 1 tropism in monocyte-macrophages. AIDS Res Hum Retroviruses. 1998;14: 129–138.
410. He J, Chen Y, Farzan M, et al. CCR3 and CCR5 are co-receptors for HIV-1 infection of microglia. Nature. 1997;385:645–649.
411. Schuitemaker H, Kootstra NA, Koppelman MHGM, et al. Proliferation-dependent HIV-1 infection of monocytes occurs during differentiation into macrophages. J Clin Invest. 1992;89:1154–1160.
412. Weinberg JB, Mathhews TJ, Cullen BR, et al. Productive human immunodeficiency virus type 1 (HIV-1) infection of nonproliferating human monocytes. J Exp Med. 1991;174:1477–1482.
413. Perelson AS, Essunger P, Cao Y, et al. Decay characteristics of HIV-1 infected compartments during combination therapy. Nature. 1997;387:188–191.
414. Schnittman SM, Psallidopoulos MC, Lane HC, et al. The reservoir for HIV-1 in human peripheral blood is a T cell that maintains expression of CD4. Science. 1989;245:305–308.
415. Valentin A, Gegerfelt AV, Matsuda S, et al. In vitro maturation of mononuclear phagocytes and susceptibility to HIV-1 infection. J Acquir Immune Defic Syndr Hum Retrovirol. 1991;4:751–759.
416. Collman R, Hassan NF, Walker R, et al. Infection of monocyte-derived macrophages with human immunodeficiency virus type 1 (HIV-1). Monocyte-tropic and lymphocyte-tropic strains of HIV-1 show distinctive patterns of replication in a panel of cell types. J Exp Med. 1989;170:1149–1163.
417. Koenig S, Gendelman HE, Orenstein JM, et al. Detection of AIDS virus in macrophages in brain tissue from AIDS patients with encephalopathy. Science. 1986;233:1089–1093.
418. Armstrong J, Horne R. Follicular dendritic cells and virus-like particles in AIDS-related lymphadenopathy. Lancet 1984;2:370–372.
419. Orenstein J, Fox C, Wahl S. Macrophages as a source of HIV during opportunistic infections. Science. 1997;276:1857–1861.
420. Britton CB, Miller JR. Neurological complications in acquired immunodeficiency syndrome (AIDS). Neurol Clin. 1984;2:315–339.
421. Neilson SL, Petito CK, Urmacher CD, et al. Subacute encephalitis in acquired immune deficiency syndrome: A postmortem study. Am J Clin Pathol. 1984;82:678–682.
422. Faulstich M. Acquired immune deficiency syndrome: An overview of central nervous system complications and neuropsychological sequelae. Int J Neurosci. 1986;30:249–254.
423. Gabuza DH, Ho DD, de la Monte SM, et al. Immunohistochemical identification of HTLV-III antigen in brains of patients with AIDS. Ann Neurol. 1986;20:289–295.
424. Bernasconi S, Cinque P, Peri G, et al. Selective elevation of monocyte chemotactic protein-1 in the cerebrospinal fluid of AIDS patients with cytomegalovirus encephalitis. J Infect Dis. 1996;174:1098–1101.
425. Cinque P, Vago L, Mengozzi M, et al. Elevated cerebrospinal fluid levels of monocyte chemotactic protein-1 correlate with HIV-1 encephalitis and local viral replication. AIDS. 1998;12:1327–1332.
426. Giulian D, Vaca K, Noonan CA. Secretion of neurotoxins by mononuclear phagocytes infected with HIV-1. Science. 1990;250:1593–1596.
427. Ennen J, Seipp I, Norley SG, et al. Decreased accessory cell function of macrophages after infection with human immunodeficiency virus type 1 in vitro. Eur J Immunol. 1990;20:2451–2456.
428. Yoo J, Chen H, Kraus T, et al. Altered cytokine production and accessory cell function after HIV-1 infection. J Immunol. 1996;157:1313–1320.
429. Polyak S, Chen H, Hirsch D, et al. Impaired class II expression and antigen uptake in monocytic cells after HIV-1 infection. J Immunol. 1997;159:2177–2188.
430. Meyaard L, Schuitemaker H, Miedema F. T-cell dysfunction in HIV infection: Anergy due to defective antigen-presenting cell function? Immunol Today. 1993;14:161–164.
431. Bender BS, Augor FA, Quinn TC, et al. Impaired antibody-dependent cell-mediated cytotoxic activity in patients with the acquired immunodeficiency syndrome. Clin Exp Immunol. 1986;64:166–172.
432. Baldwin GC, Fleischmann J, Chung Y, et al. Human immunodeficiency virus causes mononuclear phagocyte dysfunction. Proc Natl Acad Sci U S A. 1990;87:3933–3937.
433. Kent SJ, Stent G, Sonza S, et al. HIV-1 infection of monocyte-derived macrophages reduces Fc and complement receptor expression. Clin Exp Immunol. 1994;95: 450–454.
434. Poli G, Botazzi B, Acero R, et al. Monocyte function in intravenous drug abusers with lymphadenopathy syndrome and in patients with acquired immunodeficiency syndrome: Selective impairment of chemotaxis. Clin Exp Immunol. 1985;62: 136–142.
435. Muller F, Rollag H, Froland SS. Reduced oxidative burst responses in monocytes and monocyte-derived macrophages from HIV-infected individuals. Clin Immunol Immunopathol. 1990;82:10–15.
436. Spear GT, Kessler HA, Rothberg L, et al. Decreased oxidative burst activity of monocytes from asymptomatic HIV-infected individuals. Clin Immunol Immunopathol. 1990;54:184–191.
437. Lafrenie RM, Wahl LM, Epstein JS, et al. HIV-1–Tat protein promotes chemotaxis and invasive behavior by monocytes. J Immunol. 1996;157:974–977.
438. Crowe SM, Vardaxis NJ, Kent SJ, et al. HIV infection of monocyte-derived macrophages in vitro reduces phagocytosis of *Candida albicans.* J Leukoc Biol. 1994;56:318–327.
439. Biggs BA, Hewish M, Kent S, et al. HIV-1 infection of human macrophages impairs phagocytosis and killing of *Toxoplasma gondii.* J Immunol. 1995;154:6132–6139.
440. Chaturvedi S, Newman SL. Modulation of the effector function of human macrophages for *Histoplasma capsulatum* by HIV-1. Role of the envelope glycoprotein gp120. J Clin Invest. 1997;100:1465–1474.
441. Granelli-Piperno A, Moser B, Pope M, et al. Efficient interaction of HIV-1 with purified dendritic cells via multiple chemokine coreceptors. J Exp Med. 1996; 184:2433–2438.
442. Rubbert A, Combadiere C, Ostrowski M, et al. Dendritic cells express multiple chemokine receptors used as coreceptors for HIV entry. J Immunol. 1998;160:3933–3941.
443. Macatonia SE, Lau R, Patterson S, et al. Dendritic cell infection, depletion and dysfunction in HIV-infected individuals. Immunology. 1990;71:38–45.
444. Karhumaki E, Viljanen ME, Cottler-Fox M, et al. An improved enrichment method for functionally competent, highly purified peripheral blood dendritic cells and its application to HIV-infected blood samples. Clin Exp Immunol. 1993;91:482–488.
445. Hsia K, Tsai V, Zvaifler NJ, et al. Low prevalence of HIV-1 proviral DNA in peripheral blood monocytes and dendritic cells from HIV-1–infected individuals. AIDS. 1995;9:398–399.
446. Dezutter-Dambuyant C, Schmitt D. Epidermal Langerhans cells and HIV-1 infection. Immunol Lett. 1993;39:33–37.
447. Giannetti A, Zambruno G, Cimarelli A, et al. Direct detection of HIV-1 RNA in epidermal Langerhans cells of HIV-infected patients. J Acquir Immune Defic Syndr. 1993;6:329–333.
448. Muller H, Weier S, Kojouharoff G, et al. Distribution and infection of Langerhans cells in the skin of HIV-infected healthy subjects and AIDS patients. Res Virol. 1993;144:59–67.
449. Zambruno G, Giannetti A, Bertazzoni U, et al. Langerhans cells and HIV infection. Immunol Today. 1995;16:520–524.
450. Blauvelt A, Katz SI. The skin as target, vector, and effector organ in human immunodeficiency virus disease. J Invest Dermatol. 1995;105(Suppl):122S–126S.
451. McIlroy D, Autran B, Cheynier R, et al. Infection frequency of dendritic cells and CD4(+) T lymphocytes in spleens of human immunodeficiency virus–positive patients. J Virol. 1995;69:4737–4745.
452. Weissman D, Fauci AS. Role of dendritic cells in immunopathogenesis of human immunodeficiency virus infection. Clin Microbiol Rev. 1997;10:358–367.
453. Soto-Ramirez LE, Renjifo B, McLane MF, et al. HIV-1 Langerhans' cell tropism associated with heterosexual transmission of HIV. Science. 1996;271:1291–1293.
454. Quinn TC. Global burden of the HIV pandemic. The epidemiology of the acquired immunodeficiency syndrome in the 1990s. Lancet. 1996;348:99–106.
455. Spira AI, Marx PA, Patterson BK, et al. Cellular targets of infection and route of viral dissemination after an intravaginal inoculation of simian immunodeficiency virus into rhesus macaques. J Exp Med. 1996;183:215–225.
456. Pope M, Frankel SS, Mascola JR, et al. Human immunodeficiency virus type 1 strains of subtypes B and E replicate in cutaneous dendritic cell–T-cell mixtures without displaying subtype-specific tropism. J Virol. 1997;71:8001–8007.
457. Dittmar MT, Simmons G, Hibbitts S, et al. Langerhans cell tropism of human immunodeficiency virus type 1 subtype A through F isolates derived from different transmission groups. J Virol. 1997;71:8008–8013.
458. Ree HJ, Liau S, Yancovitz SR, et al. The number of CD1a+ large low-density cells with dendritic cell features is increased in the peripheral blood of HIV+ patients. Clin Immunol Immunopathol. 1994;70:190–197.
459. Cameron PU, Forsum U, Teppler H, et al. During HIV-1 infection most blood dendritic cells are not productively infected and can induce allogeneic CD4+ T cells clonal expansion. Clin Exp Immunol. 1992;88:226–236.
460. Chehimi J, Prakash K, Shanmugam V, et al. In-vitro infection of peripheral blood dendritic cells with human immunodeficiency virus-1 causes impairment of accessory functions. Adv Exp Med Biol. 1993;329:521–526.
461. Roberts M, Gompels M, Pinching AJ, et al. Dendritic cells from HIV-1 infected individuals show reduced capacity to stimulate autologous T-cell proliferation. Immunol Lett. 1994;43:39–43.
462. Macatonia SE, Gompels M, Pinching AJ, et al. Antigen-presentation by macrophages but not by dendritic cells in human immunodeficiency virus (HIV) infection. Immunology. 1992;75:576–581.
463. Amadori A, Chieco-Bianchi L. B-cell activation and HIV-1 infection: Deeds and misdeeds. Immunol Today. 1990;11:374–379.
464. Ginaldi L, De Martinis M, D'Ostilio A, et al. Changes in antigen expression on B lymphocytes during HIV infection. Pathobiology. 1998;66:17–23.
465. Kehrl JH, Rieckmann P, Kozlow E, et al. Lymphokine production by B cells from normal and HIV-infected individuals. Ann N Y Acad Sci. 1992;651:220–227.
466. Rieckmann P, Poli G, Fox CH, et al. Recombinant gp120 specifically enhances tumor necrosis factor-alpha production and Ig secretion in B lymphocytes from HIV-infected individuals but not from seronegative donors. J Immunol. 1991;147:2922–2927.
467. Rieckmann P, Poli G, Kehrl JH, et al. Activated B lymphocytes from human immunodeficiency virus–infected individuals induce virus expression in infected T cells and a promonocytic cell line, U1. J Exp Med. 1991;173:1–5.

468. Macchia D, Almerigogna F, Parronchi P, et al. Membrane tumour necrosis factor-alpha is involved in the polyclonal B-cell activation induced by HIV-infected human T cells. Nature. 1993;363:464–466.
469. Berberian L, Goodglick L, Kipps TJ, et al. Immunoglobulin V_H3 gene products: Natural ligands for HIV gp120. Science. 1993;261:1588–1591.
470. Goodglick L, Zevit N, Neshat MS, et al. Mapping the Ig superantigen–binding site of HIV-1 gp120. J Immunol. 1995;155:5151–5159.
471. Chirmule N, Kalyanaraman VS, Saxinger C, et al. Localization of B-cell stimulatory activity of HIV-1 to the carboxyl terminus of gp41. AIDS Res Hum Retroviruses. 1990;6:299–305.
472. Dolcetti R, Gloghini A, De Vita S, et al. Characteristics of EBV-infected cells in HIV-related lymphadenopathy: Implications for the pathogenesis of EBV-associated and EBV-unrelated lymphomas of HIV-seropositive individuals. Int J Cancer. 1995;63:652–659.
473. Monroe JG, Silberstein LE. HIV-mediated B-lymphocyte activation and lymphomagenesis. J Clin Immunol. 1995;15:61–68.
474. Yao QY, Tierney RJ, Croom-Carter D, et al. Frequency of multiple Epstein-Barr virus infections in T-cell–immunocompromised individuals. J Virol. 1996;70:4884–4894.
475. Wright DN, Nelson RP Jr, Ledford DK, et al. Serum IgE and human immunodeficiency virus (HIV) infection. J Allergy Clin Immunol. 1990;85:445–452.
476. Mazza DS, Grieco MH, Reddy MM, et al. Serum IgE in patients with human immunodeficiency virus infection. Ann Allergy Asthma Immunol. 1995;74: 411–414.
477. Vigano A, Balotta C, Trabattoni D, et al. Virologic and immunologic markers of disease progression in pediatric HIV infection. AIDS Res Hum Retroviruses. 1996;12:1255–1262.
478. Rodriguez C, Thomas JK, O'Rourke S, et al. HIV disease in children is associated with a selective decrease in CD23+ and CD62L+ B cells. Clin Immunol Immunopathol. 1996;81:191–199.
479. Elbim C, Prevot MH, Bouscarat F, et al. Impairment of polymorphonuclear neutrophil function in HIV-infected patients. J Cardiovasc Pharmacol. 1995;25(Suppl 2):S66–S70.
480. Jarstrand C, Akerlund B. Oxygen radical release by neutrophils of HIV-infected patients. Chem Biol Interact. 1994;91:141–146.
481. Meyer CN, Nielsen H. Priming of neutrophil and monocyte activation in human immunodeficiency virus infection. Comparison of granulocyte colony-stimulating factor, granulocyte-macrophage colony-stimulating factor and interferon-gamma. APMIS 1996;104:640–646.
482. Tachavanich K, Pattanapanyasat K, Sarasombath S, et al. Opsonophagocytosis and intracellular killing activity of neutrophils in patients with human immunodeficiency virus infection. Asian Pac J Allergy Immunol. 1996;14:49–56.
483. Pitrak DL, Tsai HC, Mullane KM, et al. Accelerated neutrophil apoptosis in the acquired immunodeficiency syndrome. J Clin Invest. 1996;98:2714–2719.
484. Torosantucci A, Chiani P, Quinti I, et al. Responsiveness of human polymorphonuclear cells (PMNL) to stimulation by a mannoprotein fraction (MP-F2) of *Candida albicans* enhanced production of IL-6 and tumour necrosis factor-alpha (TNF-alpha) by MP-F2–stimulated PMNL from HIV-infected subjects. Clin Exp Immunol. 1997;107:451–457.
485. Wenisch C, Parschalk B, Zedwitz-Liebenstein K, et al. Dysregulation of the polymorphonuclear leukocyte–*Candida* spp. interaction in HIV-positive patients. AIDS. 1996;10:983–987.
486. Tascini C, Baldelli F, Monari C, et al. Inhibition of fungicidal activity of polymorphonuclear leukocytes from HIV-infected patients by interleukin (IL)-4 and IL-10. AIDS. 1996;10:477–483.
487. Hu PF, Hultin LE, Hultin P, et al. Natural killer cell immunodeficiency in HIV disease is manifest by profoundly decreased numbers of CD16+CD56+ cells and expansion of a population of CD16dimCD56− cells with low lytic activity. J Acquir Immune Defic Syndr Hum Retrovirol. 1995;10:331–340.
488. Lucia B, Jennings C, Cauda R, et al. Evidence of a selective depletion of a CD16+ CD56+ CD8+ natural killer cell subset during HIV infection. Cytometry. 1995;22:10–15.
489. Ahmad A, Menezes J. Defective killing activity against gp120/41-expressing human erythroleukaemic K562 cell line by monocytes and natural killer cells from HIV-infected individuals. AIDS. 1996;10:143–149.
490. Ahmad A, Menezes J. Antibody-dependent cellular cytotoxicity in HIV infections. FASEB J. 1996;10:258–266.
491. Ullum H, Gotzsche PC, Victor J, et al. Defective natural immunity: An early manifestation of human immunodeficiency virus infection. J Exp Med. 1995;182:789–799.
492. Oliva A, Kinter AL, Vaccarezza M, et al. Natural killer cells from human immunodeficiency virus (HIV)-infected individuals are an important source of CC-chemokines and suppress HIV-1 entry and replication in vitro. J Clin Invest. 1998;102:223–231.
493. Fauci A. Host factors and the pathogenesis of HIV-induced disease. Nature. 1996;384:529–534.
494. Ascher M, Sheppard H. AIDS as immune system activation: A model for pathogenesis. Clin Exp Immunol. 1988;73:165–167.
495. Zack JA, Arrigo SJ, Weitsman SR, et al. HIV-1 entry into quiescent primary lymphocytes: Molecular analysis reveals a labile, latent viral structure. Cell. 1990;61:213–222.
496. Bukrinsky M, Stanwick T, Dempsey M, et al. Quiescent T lymphocytes as an inducible virus reservoir in HIV-1 infection. Science. 1991;254:423–427.
497. Chun T-W, Engel D, Ehler L, et al. Induction of HIV-1 replication in latently infected CD4(+) T cells using a combination of cytokines. J Exp Med. 1998;188:83–91.
498. Claydon EJ, Bennett J, Gor D, et al. Transient elevation of serum HIV antigen levels associated with intercurrent infection (Letter). AIDS. 1991;5:113–114.
499. Fultz PN, Gluckman JC, Muchmore E, et al. Transient increases in numbers of infectious cells in an HIV-infected chimpanzee following immune stimulation. AIDS Res Hum Retroviruses. 1992;8:313–317.
500. Ho DD. HIV-1 viraemia and influenza. Lancet. 1992;339:1549.
501. O'Brien WA, Grovit-Ferbas K, Namazi A, et al. Human immunodeficiency virus-type 1 replication can be increased in peripheral blood of seropositive patients after influenza vaccination. Blood. 1995;86:1082–1089.
502. Staprans S, Hamilton B, Follansbee S, et al. Activation of virus replication after vaccination of HIV-1–infected individuals. J Exp Med. 1995;182:1727–1737.
503. Stanley S, Ostrowski MA, Justement JS, et al. Effect of immunization with a common recall antigen on viral expression in patients infected with human immunodeficiency virus type 1. N Engl J Med. 1996;334:1222–1230.
504. Goletti D, Weissman D, Jackson RW, et al. Effect of *Mycobacterium tuberculosis* on HIV replication. Role of immune activation. J Immunol. 1996;157:1271–1278.
505. Ostrowski MA, Stanley SK, Justement JS, et al. Increased in vitro tetanus-induced production of HIV type 1 following in vivo immunization of HIV type 1–infected individuals with tetanus toxoid. AIDS Res Hum Retroviruses. 1997;13:473–480.
506. Cheynier R, Henrichwark S, Hadida F, et al. HIV and T cell expansion in splenic white pulps is accompanied by infiltration of HIV-specific cytotoxic T lymphocytes. Cell. 1994;78:373–387.
507. Grossman Z, Feinberg MB, Paul WE. Multiple modes of cellular activation and virus transmission in HIV infection: A role for chronically and latently infected cells in sustaining viral replication. Proc Natl Acad Sci U S A. 1998;95:6314–6319.
508. Miedema F. Immunological abnormalities in the natural history of HIV infection: Mechanisms and clinical relevance. Immunodefic Rev. 1992;3:173–193.
509. Poli G, Fauci A. Role of cytokines in the pathogenesis of human immunodeficiency virus infection. In: Aggarwal B, Puri R, eds. Human Cytokines: Their Role in Disease and Therapy. Cambridge, Mass: Blackwell Science; 1995:421–449.
510. Alonso K, Pontiggia P, Medenica R, et al. Cytokine patterns in adults with AIDS. Immunol Invest. 1997;26:341–350.
511. Emilie D, Peuchmaur M, Maillot MC, et al. Production of interleukins in human immunodeficiency virus-1–replicating lymph nodes. J Clin Invest. 1990;86: 148–159.
512. Boyle MJ, Berger MF, Tschuchnigg M, et al. Increased expression of interferon-gamma in hyperplastic lymph nodes from HIV-infected patients. Clin Exp Immunol. 1993;92:100–105.
513. Graziosi C, Pantaleo G, Gantt KR, et al. Lack of evidence for the dichotomy of TH1 and TH2 predominance in HIV-infected individuals. Science. 1994;265: 248–252.
514. Graziosi C, Gantt K, Vaccarezza M, et al. Kinetics of cytokine expression during primary human immunodeficiency virus type 1 infection. Proc Natl Acad Sci U S A. 1996;93:4386–4391.
515. Jassoy C, Harrer T, Rosenthal T, et al. Human immunodeficiency virus type 1–specific cytotoxic T lymphocytes release gamma interferon, tumor necrosis factor alpha (TNF-alpha), and TNF-beta when they encounter their target antigens. J Virol. 1993;67:2844–2852.
516. Esser R, vonBriesen H, Brugger M, et al. Secretory repertoire of HIV-infected human monocytes/macrophages. Pathobiology. 1991;59:219–222.
517. Schulick RD, Clerici M, Dolan MJ, et al. Limiting dilution analysis of interleukin-2–producing T cells responsive to recall and alloantigens in human immunodeficiency virus–infected and uninfected individuals. Eur J Immunol. 1993;23: 412–417.
518. Clerici M, Lucey D, Berzofsky J, et al. Restoration of HIV-specific cell-mediated immune responses by interleukin-12 in vitro. Science. 1993;262:1721–1724.
519. Romagnani S. Human TH1 and TH2 subsets: Regulation of differentiation and role in protection and immunopathology. Int Arch Allergy Immunol. 1992;98:279–285.
520. Hsieh CS, Macatonia SE, Tripp CS, et al. Development of TH1 CD4+ T cells through IL-12 produced by *Listeria*-induced macrophages. Science. 1993;260:547–549.
521. Trinchieri G. Interleukin-12 and its role in the generation of TH1 cells. Immunol Today. 1993;14:335–338.
522. Clerici M, Hakim F, Venzon D, et al. Changes in interleukin-2 and interleukin-4 production in asymptomatic, human immunodeficiency virus–seropositive individuals. J Clin Invest. 1993;91:759–765.
523. Clerici M, Wynn T, Berzofsky J, et al. Role of interleukin-10 in T helper cell dysfunction in asymptomatic individuals infected with the human immunodeficiency virus. J Clin Invest. 1994;93:768–775.
524. Maggi E, Mazzetti M, Ravina A, et al. Ability of HIV to promote a TH1 to TH0 shift and to replicate preferentially in TH2 and TH0 cells. Science. 1994;265: 244–248.
525. Meyaard L, Otto S, Keet I, vanLier R, et al. Changes in cytokine secretion patterns of CD4+ T-cell clones in human immunodeficiency virus infection. Blood. 1994;84:4262–4268.
526. Clerici M, Shearer G. A TH1-TH2 switch is a critical step in the etiology of HIV infection. Immunol Today. 1993;14:107–111.
527. Klein SA, Dobmeyer JM, Dobmeyer TS, et al. Demonstration of the Th1 to Th2 cytokine shift during the course of HIV-1 infection using cytoplasmic cytokine detection on single cell level by flow cytometry. AIDS. 1997;11:1111–1118.
528. Vyakarnam A, Matear P, Martin S, et al. Th1 cells specific for HIV-1 gag p24 are less efficient than Th0 cells in supporting HIV replication, and inhibit virus replication in Th0 cells. Immunology. 1995;86:85–96.
529. Clerici M, Balotta C, Meroni L, et al. Type 1 cytokine production and low prevalence of viral isolation correlate with long term non-progression in HIV infection. AIDS Res Hum Retroviruses. 1996;12:1053–1061.

530. Folks TM, Justement J, Kinter A, et al. Cytokine-induced expression of HIV-1 in a chronically infected promonocyte cell line. Science. 1987;238:800–802.
531. Clouse KA, Powell D, Washington I, et al. Monokine regulation of human immunodeficiency virus-1 expression in a chronically infected human T cell clone. J Immunol. 1989;142:431–438.
532. Clouse KA, Robbins PB, Fernie B, et al. Viral antigen stimulation of the production of human monokines capable of regulating HIV-1 expression. J Immunol. 1989;143:470–475.
533. Smithgall M, Wong J, Critchett K, et al. IL-7 up-regulates HIV-1 replication in naturally infected peripheral blood mononuclear cells. J Immunol. 1996;156:2324–2330.
534. Bayard-McNeeley M, Doo H, He S, et al. Differential effects of interleukin-12, interleukin-15, and interleukin-2 on human immunodeficiency virus type 1 replication in vitro. Clin Diagn Lab Immunol. 1996;3:547–553.
535. Kinter AL, Poli G, Fox L, et al. HIV replication in IL-2–stimulated peripheral blood mononuclear cells is driven in an autocrine/paracrine manner by endogenous cytokines. J Immunol. 1995;154:2448–2459.
536. Lucey DR, Pinto LA, Bethke FR, et al. In vitro immunologic and virologic effects of interleukin 15 on peripheral blood mononuclear cells from normal donors and human immunodeficiency virus type 1–infected patients. Clin Diagn Lab Immunol. 1997;4:43–48.
537. Zhou P, Goldstein S, Devadas K, et al. Human CD4+ cells transfected with IL-16 cDNA are resistant to HIV infection: Inhibition of mRNA expression. Nat Med. 1997;3:659–664.
538. Maciaszek J, Parada N, Cruikshank W, et al. IL-16 represses HIV-1 promoter activity. J Immunol. 1997;158:5–8.
539. Naif HM, Li S, Ho-Shon M, et al. The state of maturation of monocytes into macrophages determines the effects of IL-4 and IL-13 on HIV replication. J Immunol. 1997;158:501–511.
540. Valentin A, Lu W, Rosati M, et al. Dual effect of interleukin 4 on HIV-1 expression: Implications for viral phenotypic switch and disease progression. Proc Natl Acad Sci U S A. 1998;95:8886–8891.
541. Weissman D, Poli G, Fauci AS. IL-10 synergizes with multiple cytokines in enhancing HIV production in cells of monocytic lineage. J Acquir Immune Defic Syndr Hum Retrovirol. 1995;9:442–449.
542. Finnegan A, Roebuck KA, Nakai BE, et al. IL-10 cooperates with TNF-alpha to activate HIV-1 from latently and acutely infected cells of monocyte/macrophage lineage. J Immunol. 1996;156:841–851.
543. Poli G, Bressler P, Kinter A, et al. Interleukin 6 induces human immunodeficiency virus expression in infected monocytic cells alone and in synergy with tumor necrosis factor alpha by transcriptional and post-transcriptional mechanisms. J Exp Med. 1990;172:151–158.
544. Poli G, Kinter AL, Fauci AS. Interleukin 1 induces expression of the human immunodeficiency virus alone and in synergy with interleukin 6 in chronically infected U1 cells: Inhibition of inductive effects by the interleukin 1 receptor antagonist. Proc Natl Acad Sci U S A. 1994;91:108–112.
545. Poli G, Kinter AL, Justement JS, et al. Transforming growth factor beta suppresses human immunodeficiency virus expression and replication in infected cells of the monocyte/macrophage lineage. J Exp Med. 1991;173:589–597.
546. Osborn L, Kunkel S, Nabel GJ. Tumor necrosis factor alpha and interleukin 1 stimulate the human immunodeficiency virus enhancer by activation of the nuclear factor kappa B. Proc Natl Acad Sci U S A. 1989;86:2336–2340.
547. Duh EJ, Maury WJ, Folks TM, et al. Tumor necrosis factor alpha activates human immunodeficiency virus type 1 through induction of nuclear factor binding to the NF-kappa B sites in the long terminal repeat. Proc Natl Acad Sci U S A. 1989;86:5974–5978.
548. Goletti D, Kinter AL, Hardy EC, et al. Modulation of endogenous IL-1 beta and IL-1 receptor antagonist results in opposing effects on HIV expression in chronically infected monocytic cells. J Immunol. 1996;156:3501–3508.
549. Weissman D, Poli G, Fauci AS. Interleukin 10 blocks HIV replication in macrophages by inhibiting the autocrine loop of tumor necrosis factor alpha and interleukin 6 induction of virus. AIDS Res Hum Retroviruses. 1994;10:1199–1206.
550. Schuitemaker H. IL4 and IL10 as potent inhibitors of HIV1 replication in macrophages in vitro: A role for cytokines in the in vivo virus host range? Res Immunol. 1994;145:588–592.
551. Goletti D, Weissman D, Jackson RW, et al. The in vitro induction of human immunodeficiency virus (HIV) replication in purified protein derivative–positive HIV-infected persons by recall antigen response to *Mycobacterium tuberculosis* is the result of a balance of the effects of endogenous interleukin-2 and proinflammatory and antiinflammatory cytokines. J Infect Dis. 1998;177:1332–1338.
552. Wallis RS, Nsubuga P, Whalen C, et al. Pentoxifylline therapy in human immunodeficiency virus–seropositive persons with tuberculosis: A randomized controlled trial. J Infect Dis. 1996;174:727–733.
553. Clerici M, Piconi S, Balotta C, et al. Pentoxifylline improves cell-mediated immunity and reduces human immunodeficiency virus (HIV) plasma viremia in asymptomatic HIV-seropositive persons. J Infect Dis. 1997;175:1210–1215.
554. Kollmann TR, Pettoello-Mantovani M, Katopodis NF, et al. Inhibition of acute in vivo human immunodeficiency virus infection by human interleukin 10 treatment of SCID mice implanted with human fetal thymus and liver. Proc Natl Acad Sci U S A. 1996;93:3126–3131.
555. Masood R, Lunardi-Iskandar Y, Moudgil T, et al. IL-10 inhibits HIV-1 replication and is induced by tat. Biochem Biophys Res Commun. 1994;202:374–383.
556. Moore K, O'Garra A, de Waal Malefyt R, et al. Interleukin-10. Annu Rev Immunol. 1993;11:165–190.
557. Ho A, Moore K. Interleukin-10 and its receptor. Ther Immunol. 1994;1:173–185.
558. Kovacs JA, Vogel S, Albert JM, et al. Controlled trial of interleukin-2 infusions in patients infected with the human immunodeficiency virus. N Engl J Med. 1996;335:1350–1356.
559. Seder R, Grabstein K, Berzofsky J, et al. Cytokine interactions in human immunodeficiency virus–infected individuals: Roles of interleukin (IL)-2, IL-12, and IL-15. J Exp Med. 1995;182:1067–1077.
560. Kanai T, Thomas E, Yasutomi Y, et al. IL-15 stimulates the expansion of AIDS virus–specific CTL. J Immunol. 1996;157:3681–3687.
561. Lin S, Roberts R, Ank B, et al. Human immunodeficiency virus (HIV) type-1 GP120-specific cell-mediated cytotoxicity (CMC) and natural killer (NK) activity in HIV-infected (HIV+) subjects: Enhancement with interleukin-2 (IL-2), IL-12, and IL-15. Clin Immunol Immunopathol. 1997;82:163–173.
562. Chehimi J, Marshall J, Salvucci O, et al. IL-15 enhances immune functions during HIV infection. J Immunol. 1997;158:5978–5987.
563. McKenzie A, Zurawski G. Interleukin-13: Characterization and biologic properties. Cancer Treat Res. 1995;80:367–378.
564. Montaner L, Gordon S. Th2-mediated HIV1 virostatic state: Macrophage-specific regulation in vitro. Res Immunol. 1994;145:583–587.
565. Trinchieri G, Scott P. The role of interleukin 12 in the immune response, disease and therapy. Immunol Today. 1994;15:460–463.
566. Cruikshank W, Lim K, Theodore A, et al. IL-16 inhibition of CD3-dependent lymphocyte activation and proliferation. J Immunol. 1996;157:5240–5248.
567. Theodore A, Center D, Nicoll J, et al. CD4 ligand IL-16 inhibits the mixed lymphocyte reaction. J Immunol. 1996;157:1958–1964.
568. Parada NA, Center DM, Kornfeld H, et al. Synergistic activation of CD4+ T cells by IL-16 and IL-2. J Immunol. 1998;160:2115–2120.
569. Schall T. Biology of the RANTES/sis cytokine family. Cytokine. 1991;3:165–183.
570. Baggiolini M, Dewald B, Moser B. Human chemokines: An update. Annu Rev Immunol. 1997;15:675–705.
571. Nelson P, Kim H, Manning W, et al. Genomic organization and transcriptional regulation of the RANTES chemokine gene. J Immunol. 1993;151:2601–2612.
572. Rathanaswami P, Hachicha M, Sadick M, et al. Expression of the cytokine RANTES in human rheumatoid synovial fibroblasts. Differential regulation of RANTES and interleukin-8 genes by inflammatory cytokines. J Biol Chem. 1993;268:5834–5839.
573. Schall T, Bacon K. Chemokines, leukocyte trafficking, and inflammation. Curr Opin Immunol. 1994;6:865–873.
574. Levine BL, Mosca JD, Riley JL, et al. Antiviral effect and ex vivo CD4+ T cell proliferation in HIV-positive patients as a result of CD28 costimulation. Science. 1996;272:1939–1943.
575. Riley JL, Carroll RG, Levine BL, et al. Intrinsic resistance to T cell infection with HIV type 1 induced by CD28 costimulation. J Immunol. 1997;158:5545–5553.
576. Roederer M, Raju PA, Mitra DK, et al. HIV does not replicate in naive CD4 T cells stimulated with CD3/CD28. J Clin Invest. 1997;99:1555–1564.
577. Unutmaz D, Littman D. Expression pattern of HIV-1 coreceptors on T cells: Implications for viral transmission and lymphocyte homing. Proc Natl Acad Sci U S A. 1997;94:1615–1618.
578. Ostrowski M, Justement S, Catanzaro A, et al. Expression of chemokine receptors CXCR4 and CCR5 in HIV-1–infected and uninfected individuals. J Immunol. 1998;161:3195–3201.
579. Moriuchi H, Moriuchi M, Fauci AS. Factors secreted by human T lymphotropic virus type I (HTLV-I)-infected cells can enhance or inhibit replication of HIV-1 in HTLV-I–uninfected cells: Implications for in vivo coinfection with HTLV-I and HIV-1. J Exp Med. 1998;187:1689–1697.
580. Learmont J, Tindall B, Evans L, et al. Long-term symptomless HIV-1 infection in recipients of blood products from a single donor. Lancet. 1992;340:863–867.
581. Deacon NJ, Tsykin A, Solomon A, et al. Genomic structure of an attenuated quasi species of HIV-1 from a blood transfusion donor and recipients. Science. 1995;270:988–991.
582. Kirchhoff F, Greenough TC, Brettler DB, et al. Brief report: Absence of intact nef sequences in a long-term survivor with nonprogressive HIV-1 infection. N Engl J Med. 1995;332:228–232.
583. Iversen AKN, Shpaer EG, Rodrigo AG, et al. Persistence of attenuated rev genes in a human immunodeficiency virus type 1–infected asymptomatic individual. J Virol. 1995;69:5743–5753.
584. Michael NL, Chang G, D'arcy LA, et al. Defective accessory genes in a human immunodeficiency virus type 1–infected long-term survivor lacking recoverable virus. J Virol. 1995;69:4228–4236.
585. Michael NL, Chang G, D'arcy LA, et al. Functional characterization of human immunodeficiency virus type 1 nef genes in patients with divergent rates of disease progression. J Virol. 1995;69:6758–6769.
586. Huang Y, Zhang L, Ho DD. Characterization of nef sequences in long-term survivors of human immunodeficiency virus type 1 infection. J Virol. 1995;69:93–100.
587. Huang Y, Zhang L, Ho D. Biological characterization of nef in long term survivors of human immunodeficiency virus type 1 infection. J Virol. 1995;69:8142–8146.
588. Kaslow RA, Duquesnoy R, VanRaden M, et al. A1, Cw7, B8, DR3 HLA antigen combination associated with rapid decline of T-helper lymphocytes in HIV-1 infection. Lancet. 1990;335:927–930.
589. Pinto LA, Sullivan J, Berzofsky JA, et al. ENV-specific cytotoxic T lymphocyte responses in HIV seronegative health care workers occupationally exposed to HIV-contaminated body fluids. J Clin Invest. 1995;96:867–876.
590. Paxton WA, Liu R, Kang S, et al. Reduced HIV-1 infectability of CD4+ lymphocytes from exposed-uninfected individuals: Association with low expression of CCR5 and high production of beta-chemokines. Virology. 1998;244:66–73.
591. Mazzoli S, Trabattoni D, Lo Caputo S, et al. HIV-specific mucosal and cellular immunity in HIV-seronegative partners of HIV-seropositive individuals. Nat Med. 1997;3:1250–1257.

Chapter 108

General Clinical Manifestations of Human Immunodeficiency Virus Infection (Including Oral, Cutaneous, Renal, Ocular, and Cardiac Diseases)

RICHARD E. CHAISSON
TIMOTHY R. STERLING
JOEL E. GALLANT

Human immunodeficiency virus (HIV) infection results in a wide range of clinical consequences from asymptomatic carriage to life-threatening opportunistic disease. In persons infected with HIV, ongoing viral replication produces a sequential decline in and ablation of cell-mediated immunity, giving rise to diverse manifestations of opportunistic disease. The acquired immunodeficiency syndrome (AIDS) is the most advanced stage of this illness, in which the infected host can no longer control opportunistic organisms or malignancies that rarely cause illness in immunocompetent individuals. The clinical features of HIV may vary according to the individual's age, sex, race, geographic location, treatment status, and behavioral history. This chapter reviews selected clinical aspects of HIV infection from the acquisition of the virus to death with AIDS and discusses the classification and staging of this important viral pathogen.

HISTORY

Disease caused by HIV-induced immunosuppression was first described in late 1980 and early 1981, when physicians in Los Angeles, New York, and San Francisco observed opportunistic infections in homosexual men.[1–4] Simultaneously, an outbreak of Kaposi's sarcoma (KS), a previously rare malignancy, was reported in young homosexual men from the same three cities.[5, 6] These patients had a selective defect in cell-mediated immunity that was manifested by low numbers of CD4+ T lymphocytes and the development of opportunistic infections.

That opportunistic disease occurred in homosexual men who had previously been healthy suggested that immunodeficiency developed because of an acquired rather than a congenital trait. In 1982, the Centers for Disease Control (CDC) developed a case definition, based on the clinical, immunologic, and epidemiologic features of the first clusters of cases, for what was called the acquired immunodeficiency syndrome (see Chapter 105).[7] AIDS was defined as the occurrence of a reliably diagnosed disease at least moderately indicative of underlying cellular immunodeficiency in a person without a condition known to be associated with an increased incidence of diseases related to cellular immunodeficiency.[6, 8] AIDS became a reportable condition in the United States in 1983. Soon after the initial case reports of AIDS, additional cases were observed in persons other than homosexual men. In 1981 and 1982, heterosexual intravenous drug users and immigrants from Haiti were reported to have AIDS.[2, 9–12] AIDS cases in hemophiliacs, recipients of blood transfusions, and Africans were soon reported.[13, 14]

As the groups of persons at risk for AIDS expanded, clinicians noted an increasing spectrum of clinical manifestations of AIDS-associated immunodeficiency. Unexplained generalized lymphadenopathy, idiopathic thrombocytopenia, oral candidasis, herpes zoster, and a constitutional wasting syndrome were observed in persons from AIDS risk groups who had deficits in cellular immunity.[15–19] The term *AIDS-related complex* was coined to describe the signs and symptoms of immunodeficiency recognized with increasing frequency in persons at risk for AIDS.[20] In 1982 to 1983, several investigators postulated an asymptomatic carrier state of the AIDS agent in healthy homosexual men, heterosexual partners of intravenous drug users, and Haitians who were noted to have laboratory evidence of impaired cellular immunity.[21] After HIV was first described in 1983 to 1984,[22–24] serologic tests to identify persons infected with HIV were developed that allowed large serologic surveys of at-risk populations to estimate the number of individuals infected with the virus and to delineate the spectrum of HIV-associated diseases.

Retrospective studies of serum and tissue indicate that the virus was present in Africa as early as 1959 and that disease associated with HIV occurred in the United States in 1968.[25, 26] The CDC expanded its case definition of AIDS in 1985 and again in 1987 (see Chapter 105) to accommodate the increased number of manifestations of impaired cellular immunity that had become associated with HIV infection.[27, 28] The World Health Organization also promulgated a case definition for AIDS for use in developing countries that lacked sophisticated diagnostic resource.[29] The AIDS case definition and HIV staging system were revised again in 1993 to include individuals with advanced immunodeficiency and with several other clinical manifestations of HIV disease (see Chapter 105).[30] New insights into the pathogenesis of HIV disease have emphasized the critical role of viral dynamics in the natural history of HIV infection,[31–33] leading to clinical management schemata based largely on viral load and CD4+ cell levels, as discussed in the following.

CLASSIFICATION OF HIV DISEASE

HIV infection represents an underlying active viral process in a majority of untreated individuals associated with progressive immunodeficiency that is likely to result in serious clinical consequences. Although there may be a prolonged state of clinical latency, during which many patients are unaware of their infection, HIV infection is usually not virologically latent, and infection with the virus should be considered a disease state. Individuals who are infected but asymptomatic may not be ill, but do have a chronic and potentially progressive condition that without treatment may ultimately result in a significant impairment and death. Although distinguishing between HIV infection and AIDS has been historically useful for epidemiologic purposes, the distinction is somewhat arbitrary and is less meaningful from a clinical perspective in an era of potent antiretroviral drug therapy. As already noted, current clinical staging approaches favor use of the CD4+ lymphocyte counts and plasma viral load assays.

Several systems for classifying HIV infection and disease have been developed. The 1986 CDC classification system placed HIV-infected persons into four categories: group I, acute infection; group II, asymptomatic infection; group III, persistent generalized lymphadenopathy (PGL); and group IV, symptomatic HIV disease.[34] This system had limited prognostic utility and was supplanted by the 1993 classification system and revised case definition (see Chapter 105).[35] The 1993 CDC classification system for HIV categorizes HIV-infected individuals according to clinical and CD4+ cell count groupings. The clinical categories are group A, asymptomatic, acute HIV infection, or PGL; group B, symptomatic HIV disease; and group C, AIDS indicator conditions, encompassing the 1987 case definition with the addition of recurrent bacterial pneumonia, pulmonary tuberculosis, and invasive cervical cancer. The CD4+ cell levels are (1) 500/mm^3 or greater, (2) 200 to 499/mm^3, and (3) less than 200/mm^3. CD4+ cell percentages may be used in place of CD4+ cell number. As noted before, patients in all three clinical categories whose CD4+ cell count is less than 200/mm^3 or 14% (stages A3, B3, and C3) are now classified as having AIDS by the CDC surveillance definition, along with patients who have AIDS indicator conditions (stages C1, C2, and C3).

The 1993 CDC classification system for HIV infection recognized the prognostic significance of the CD4$^+$ cell count in individuals with HIV infection but was developed before the importance of viral load in the pathogenesis of HIV disease was known. Even so, it is important to recognize that there is considerable variation in risk of opportunistic complications and prognosis among individuals with CD4$^+$ cell counts below 200/mm^3. Those with CD4$^+$ counts below 50/mm^3, for example, are generally considered to have advanced HIV disease, and are at much higher risk for death and for development of opportunistic infections such as cytomegalovirus (CMV) disease or disseminated *Mycobacterium avium* complex infection. The CDC classification system was developed at a time when the inevitable course of HIV infection was progression toward advanced immunodeficiency and death and when drug therapy was of limited and transient efficacy in stemming the course of the disease. According to the CDC classification system, HIV-infected individuals are classified on the basis of the most advanced stage they have reached. In the present era, patients treated with combination antiretroviral therapy often experience marked improvement in cellular immune function and have a dramatically lower risk of developing opportunistic disease than they had before receiving treatment. There is no current mechanism for reclassifying patients on the basis of immunologic and clinical improvement resulting from antiretroviral therapy, a situation that understandably curtails use of the CDC and similar staging systems (e.g., the Walter Reed and World Health Organization systems). In areas where combination antiretroviral therapy is not available or in use, these classification schemes more reliably reflect the maturity and status of the HIV epidemic within populations.

NATURAL HISTORY OF HIV INFECTION

The clinical spectrum of HIV infection includes primary infection (the acute retroviral syndrome), asymptomatic infection, early symptomatic infection, and advanced immunodeficiency with opportunistic complications. Figure 108–1 shows a schematic diagram of the key immunologic, viral, and clinical features of HIV infection in untreated individuals. Viral load or viremia is monitored by measurement of HIV RNA in plasma, and immunologic status is reflected in the absolute number of CD4$^+$ lymphocytes or in the proportion of lymphocytes that express CD4. Primary HIV infection is characterized by a high concentration of HIV RNA in plasma and suppression of the CD4$^+$ cell count. Plasma viremia declines precipitously with antibody seroconversion and the development of an anti-HIV immune response, usually reaching a steady-state level within 6 to 12 months.[36, 37] In most untreated asymptomatic patients, the CD4$^+$ cell count declines gradually over several years. The slope of decline is a function of the plasma viral load. Plasma viremia increases, accompanied by a more rapid decline in CD4$^+$ count, before the onset of symptomatic disease. As the viral load rises and CD4$^+$ cell count falls, the risk of opportunistic infections, malignancies, wasting, neurologic complications, and death increases substantially.

There is considerable variation in the progression of HIV disease, with some individuals progressing from infection to AIDS in less than 5 years[38] and so-called long-term nonprogressors remaining asymptomatic without treatment or evidence of immunologic decline for many years.[39, 40]

Before the availability of effective antiretroviral therapy, the rate of progression from primary HIV infection to AIDS and from AIDS to death was estimated in a number of studies. Among homosexual men in San Francisco, the median time from seroconversion to AIDS by the 1987 CDC case definition was 9.8 years.[41] Other studies estimated the period from infection to AIDS (1987 definition) to be 7 years for transfusion recipients, 10 years for hemophiliacs, 10 years for injection drug users, and 8 to 12 years for homosexual men.[42] An important study of the natural history of HIV infection was the study of a cohort of homosexual and bisexual men by the San Francisco Department of Public Health and the CDC beginning early in the AIDS epidemic.[43] These subjects were originally enrolled in a study of hepatitis B vaccine in 1978 and had serologic studies and clinical evaluations that dated from that time. Of the 489 men for whom the time of HIV seroconversion could be reliably estimated, 13% developed AIDS within 5 years, 51% within 10 years, and 54% at 11 years. In addition, of those who had not developed AIDS within 11 years of seroconversion, 19% had symptomatic disease and another 29% had CD4$^+$ cell counts less than 200/mm^3. Thus, after 11 years of follow-up, more than three quarters of HIV-infected homosexual men had severe immunodeficiency, had AIDS, or had died. A number of laboratory tests have been correlated with progressive immunodeficiency, the development of AIDS, and mortality. Taken together, however, the CD4$^+$ lymphocyte count and plasma viral load are the best prognostic markers for subsequent disease course in an HIV-infected individual. The CD4$^+$ lymphocyte count, a specific test for cellular immunocompetence, is a sensitive

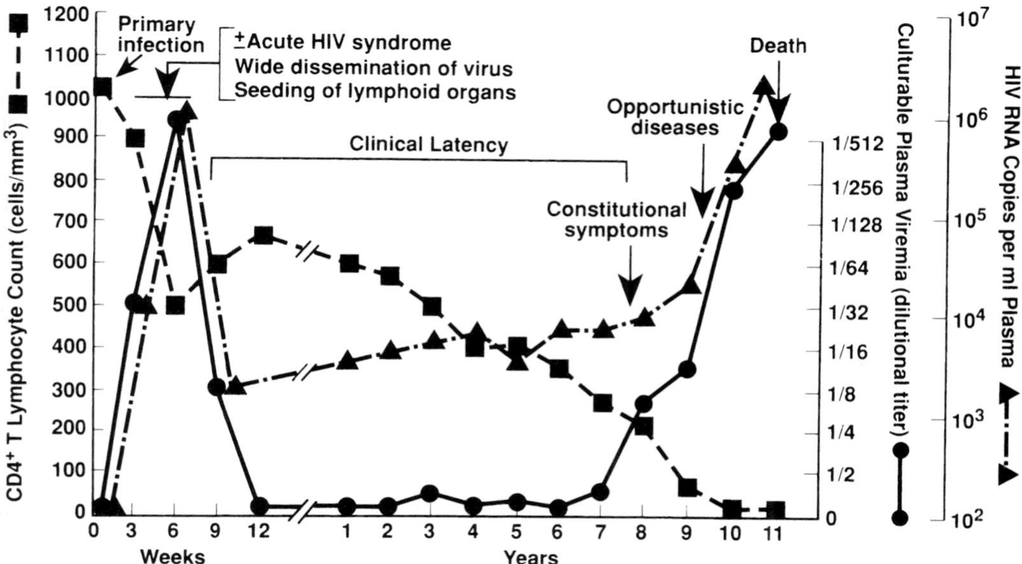

FIGURE 108–1. Natural history of human immunodeficiency virus (HIV) infection in the absence of therapy in a hypothetical patient. (From Fauci AS, Pantaleo G, Stanley S, Weissman D. Immunopathogenic mechanisms of HIV infection. Ann Intern Med. 1996;124:654–663.)

predictor of the development of symptomatic HIV infection and AIDS in the near term, as it reflects current immunologic capacity.[44–48] Conversely, the plasma viral load (HIV-1 RNA) is an extremely useful predictor of disease course over a more extended period of time and is strongly associated with the rate of subsequent CD4+ cell count decline.[49–57] A more rapid decline in CD4+ count, faster clinical progression, and decreased survival are all associated with a higher baseline viral load. In a study of HIV-infected gay or bisexual men enrolled in the Multicenter AIDS Cohort Study, the risk of progression to AIDS and death was highly correlated with plasma viral load at study entry, independent of CD4+ cell count.[49, 51] Baseline plasma viral load was a stronger predictor of progression and mortality than CD4+ count. Figure 108–2 shows the average annual decline in the CD4+ count of HIV-infected men according to their initial viral load, determined 10 years earlier. Using the viral load and CD4+ count together, however, gives the best prognostic estimate of subsequent clinical course (Table 108–1). Put in the context of HIV pathogenesis, the viral load measures the replicative rate of the infection and its destructive potential for the cellular immune system, and the CD4+ count gauges the extent of immune compromise and the present risk of opportunistic disease. A popular analogy of this situation proposed by John Coffin likens AIDS to an impending train wreck, with the viral load depicting the speed of the train and the CD4+ count reflecting the distance to the disaster.

In the absence of treatment, survival is short after the diagnosis of clinically defined AIDS. A study of survival of the first 505 patients with AIDS in San Francisco found a median survival of 9 months, with most patients dead within 2 years.[58] Patients diagnosed with an opportunistic infection had the most rapid mortality, whereas survival was significantly longer in patients initially diagnosed with KS. Similar results were noted in AIDS patients in New York City, although overall survival was slightly longer (median survival 12 months).[59] Subsequent studies revealed that survival after diagnosis of AIDS was directly related to the CD4+ cell level at diagnosis. In most studies before the availability of combination antiretroviral therapy, median survival after the diagnosis of AIDS was estimated to be between 12 and 18 months.[60] The mean survival time after a CD4+ count of 200/mm^3 was 38 to 40 months.[61, 62]

The rate of progression of HIV infection in population-based studies varied depending on age, with older individuals generally having a more rapidly progressive course.[63–67] Whether age differences in the pace of progression of HIV infection are the result of differences in viral setpoints, host immune responses, or both is unclear. Although studies have demonstrated differences in natural history or survival or both on the basis of sex, race, and risk category, these differences generally disappear when adjustment is made for age and quality of care.[64, 68–74] Patients who experience more severe or long-lasting symptoms during the acute retroviral syndrome tend to have higher viral loads after seroconversion and progress more rapidly than those who seroconvert without symptoms.[75] A sex difference in initial viral loads of HIV-infected individuals was reported, with women having lower viral loads than men, although they pro-

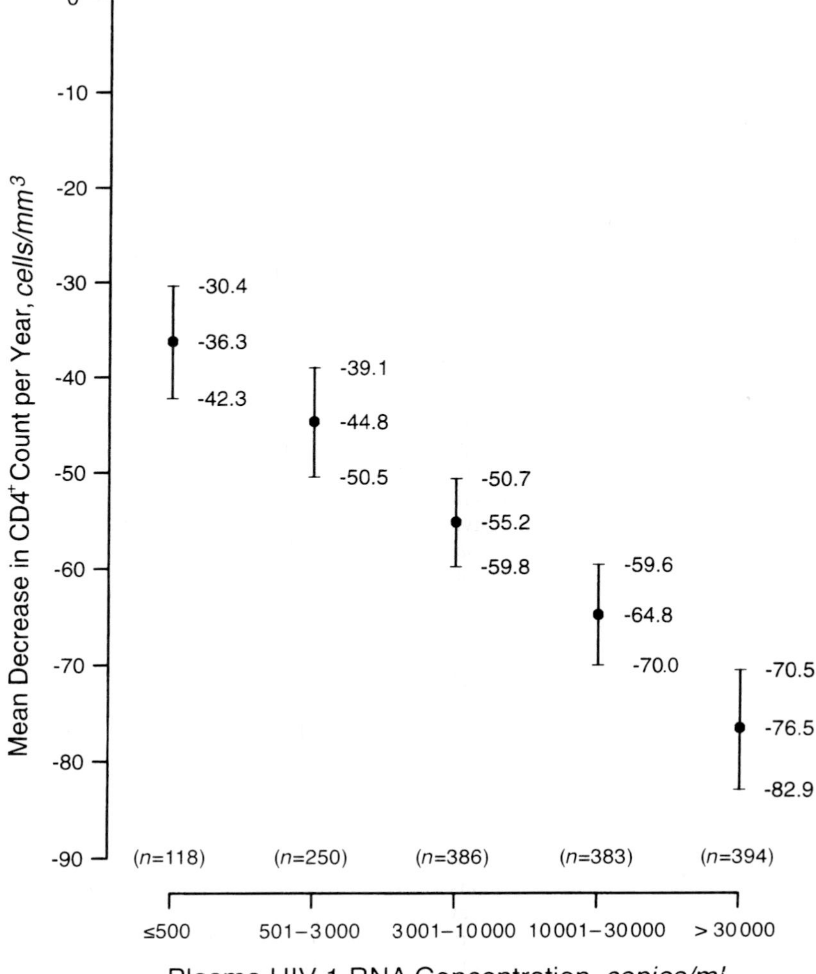

FIGURE 108–2. Annual rate of decline in CD4 cell count by baseline viral load in the Multicenter AIDS Cohort Study. Bars show 95% confidence intervals. (From Mellors JW, Munoz A, Giorgi JV, et al. Plasma viral load and CD4+ lymphocytes as prognostic markers of HIV-1 infection. Ann Intern Med. 1997;126:946–954.)

TABLE 108–1 Probability of Developing Acquired Immunodeficiency Syndrome (1987 Centers for Disease Control Case Definition) in 1604 Men in the Multicenter AIDS Cohort Study*

Baseline Viral Load†	Baseline CD4 Count‡	Number Studied	Number with AIDS	% AIDS at 3 Years	% AIDS at 6 Years	% AIDS at 9 Years
<500	>750	66	3	0	1.7	3.6
	<750	56	13	3.7	9.6	22.3
501–3000	Any	257	90	2.0	16.6	35.4
3001–10,000	>750	93	39	3.2	14.2	59.7
	<750	300	179	8.1	37.7	62.4
10,001–30,000	>750	64	42	9.5	36.7	62.4
	351–750	259	194	16.1	54.9	76.3
	≤350	73	63	40.1	72.9	86.2
>30,000	>500	141	105	32.6	66.8	76.3
	351–500	121	111	47.9	77.7	94.4
	201–350	104	92	64.4	89.3	92.9
	<200	70	67	85.5	97.9	100

*Based on baseline HIV branched-chain DNA viral load and CD4+ cell count.
†HIV RNA copies per milliliter of plasma by branched-chain DNA. Viral load determined by reverse transcriptase–polymerase chain reaction approximately twofold greater.
‡CD4+ cells per cubic millimeter.
Abbreviations: AIDS, Acquired immunodeficiency syndrome; HIV, human immunodeficiency virus.
From Mellors JW, Munoz A, Giorgi JV, et al. Plasma viral load and CD4+ lymphocytes as prognostic markers of HIV-1 infection. Ann Intern Med. 1997;126:946–954.

gressed to AIDS at the same rate.[76] Others have shown that at first presentation for clinical care, however, there is no sex difference in viral loads.[77]

Other laboratory studies that predict the development of AIDS in a seropositive individual include a total lymphocyte count less than 1000/mm³, a total white blood cell count less than 4000/mm³, a hematocrit less than 40 ml/dl, and a low percentage of CD4+ lymphocytes. Because the CD4+ percentage has a narrower range of variation in most clinical laboratories than the absolute CD4+ cell count, many clinicians favor using this measure for staging and monitoring of patients.[78] Other markers of HIV disease progression that have been validated in clinical studies include the HIV p24 antigen, serum β_2-microglobulin, neopterin, acid-labile interferon-α, anti-p24 antibody, and soluble CD8. These so-called surrogate markers are measures of either viral markers or host immune responses to HIV. However, these measures do not provide prognostic information independently of the viral load and have essentially been supplanted by quantitative plasma HIV-1 RNA monitoring.

The probability of an HIV-infected individual developing opportunistic disease is influenced by several factors. First, immunocompetence is a critical determinant of whether an infected individual can contain a potential pathogen. As discussed later, the CD4+ cell count appears to be the most clinically useful measure of host cellular immunocompetence and plays a central role in the staging of HIV disease. Second, exposure to potential pathogens is required before disease can result. Although some opportunistic pathogens are ubiquitous, resulting in latent infection in a large proportion of HIV-infected persons (e.g., *Pneumocystis carinii,* CMV), others are prevalent in a smaller proportion of individuals and cause disease less often (e.g., *Toxoplasma gondii, Mycobacterium tuberculosis*). Other opportunistic pathogens do not appear to be associated with latent reactivation but rather cause disease when a sufficiently immunocompromised host acquires new infection (e.g., *Cryptococcus neoformans, M. avium* complex). Third, the relative virulence of a potential pathogen is a factor that may determine which disease is likely to occur. For example, more virulent organisms such as *M. tuberculosis* or *Streptococcus pneumoniae* cause clinical illness in patients with less severe immunodeficiency, whereas less virulent organisms such as *P. carinii* or CMV cause illness in those with more severe immunodeficiency[79–81] Finally, whether a patient is taking chemoprophylactic agents with activity against specific pathogens influences the risk of disease. Figure 108–3 shows CD4+ cell counts at the time of diagnosis of opportunistic diseases in patients with CD4+ cell counts of 300/mm³ or less evaluated at the Johns Hopkins Hospital before 1996.[82] Although the range of CD4+ cell counts for some conditions is broad, most patients with truly opportunistic infections had CD4+ counts less than 100/mm³.

The incidence of specific opportunistic diseases has been determined for several large cohorts of HIV-infected individuals. In the Johns Hopkins study of more than 1200 patients with CD4+ cell counts less than 300/mm³, the 3-year probability of new opportunistic diseases (without highly active antiretroviral therapy [HAART]) was determined (Fig. 108-4*A* and *B*). In contrast to findings before the widespread use of prophylaxis, in which the most common opportunistic infection was *P. carinii* pneumonia,[83, 84] the most common opportunistic infection in this later cohort was *Candida* esophagitis (13.3 cases per 100 person-years). *P. carinii* pneumonia, disseminated *M. avium* complex, CMV disease, and the AIDS dementia complex occurred at rates of 5 to 9 cases per 100 person-years. Less common were toxoplasmosis, cryptococcal meningitis, herpes zoster, the wasting syndrome, and KS (2 to 4 cases per 100 person-years). The least common complications were non-Hodgkin's lymphoma, tuberculosis, progressive multifocal leukoencephalopathy, and cryptosporidiosis (1 to 2 per 100 cases person-years). In contrast, other investigators have found a decrease in the incidence of opportunistic conditions but no difference in the spectrum of diagnoses. In a retrospective analysis of 344 AIDS patients enrolled in the British Columbia Drug Treatment Program, declines in the incidence of HIV-related complications were seen between 1994 and 1996, but *P. carinii* pneumonia and KS remained the most common AIDS index diagnoses.[85]

The varying incidences of specific opportunistic infections have implications for prophylactic strategies (see Chapter 116). Chemoprophylaxis against *P. carinii* and *M. avium* complex is now recommended for all HIV-infected patients with severe enough immunodeficiency to elevate the risk of disease.[86] Conversely, prophylaxis against the less common pathogens *M. tuberculosis* and *T. gondii* is targeted at individuals known to be latently infected with these organisms (e.g., *T. gondii* immunoglobulin–seropositive persons or those with a positive tuberculin skin test).

Even before the era of HAART, it was clear that antiretroviral therapy and prophylaxis against *P. carinii* pneumonia had substantially altered the natural history of AIDS, prolonging the median survival of treated AIDS patients to 2 to 3 years.[87–91] Antiretroviral therapy and prophylaxis against *P. carinii* pneumonia and *M. avium* complex also prolonged the time from HIV infection to AIDS, decreased the incidence of opportunistic complications, and improved overall survival.[92–99] Changes in plasma viral and CD4+ cell counts resulting from antiretroviral drug treatment have been shown to be strong predictors of clinical progression (or regression) of HIV disease.[100, 101]

The use of combination antiretroviral therapy and the introduction of protease inhibitors in 1995 and 1996 led to a dramatic change in the natural history of treated HIV disease.[102–105] In the HIV Outpatient

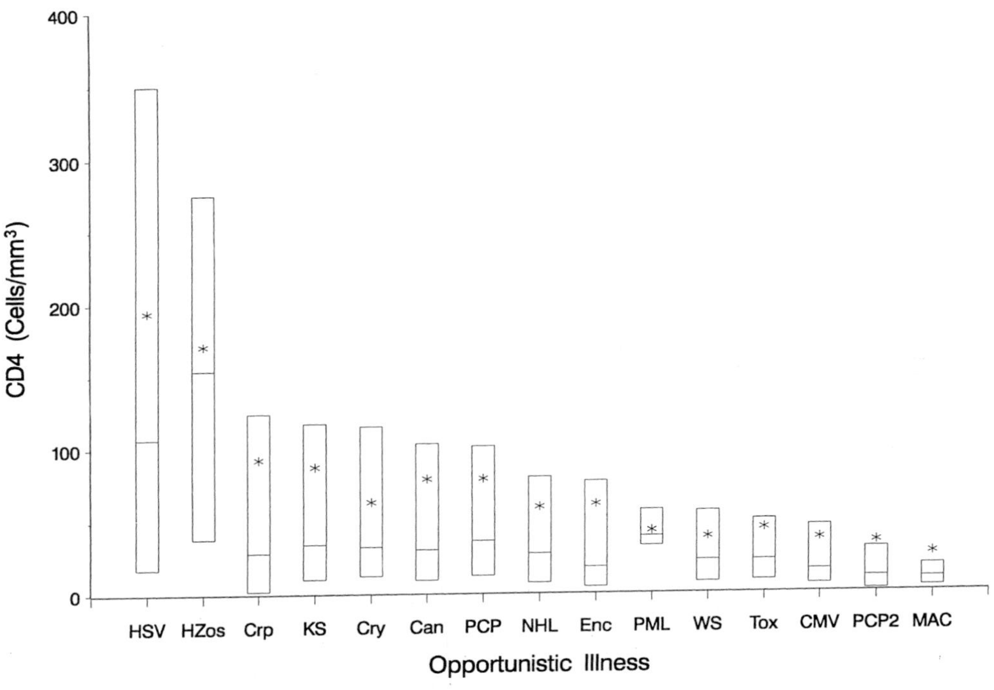

FIGURE 108–3. Range of CD4 lymphocyte counts at the time of diagnosis of opportunistic diseases in patients with human immunodeficiency virus (HIV) infection. Boxes represent the 25th to 75th percentiles, bars represent medians, and asterisks represent means. *Abbreviations*: Can, *Candida* esophagitis; CMV, cytomegalovirus; Crp, cryptosporidiosis; Cry, cryptococcosis; Enc, HIV encephalopathy; HSV, herpes simplex virus; Hzos, herpes zoster; KS, Kaposi's sarcoma; MAC, *Mycobacterium avium* complex; NHL, non-Hodgkin's lymphoma; PCP, first episodes of *Pneumocystis carinii* pneumonia; PCP2, recurrent *P. carinii* pneumonia; PML, progressive multifocal leukoencephalopathy; Tox, toxoplasmosis; WS, wasting syndrome. (From Moore RD, Chaisson RE. Natural history of opportunistic disease in an HIV-infected urban cohort. Ann Intern Med. 1996;124:633–642.)

Study, mortality declined from 29.4 deaths per 100 person-years in 1995 to 8.8 per 100 person-years in the second quarter of 1997 (Fig. 108–5).[106] This decline in mortality was accompanied by marked decreases in the incidence of *P. carinii* pneumonia, *M. avium* complex disease, and CMV retinitis: the incidence of any one of those three infections declined from 21.9 per 100 person-years in 1994 to 3.7 per 100 person-years by mid-1997 (Fig. 108–6). The degree of benefit was associated with the intensity of antiretroviral therapy: combination therapy resulted in an improved prognosis compared with monotherapy, and the use of a protease inhibitor in a combination regimen was associated with the greatest benefit. In the United States as a whole, deaths attributed to AIDS decreased by 23% in 1996 and by 44% in 1997.[107, 108]

Clinical findings may also predict disease progression in seropositive subjects. Oral candidiasis and oral hairy leukoplakia are early clinical markers of immunosuppression and herald the development of AIDS in many patients.[109–111] Generalized lymphadenopathy is also a clinical marker of HIV infection but does not predict progression to AIDS. In one study, the average $CD4^+$ cell count was higher in those with lymphadenopathy than in seropositive individuals without enlarged lymph nodes.[112] Most opportunistic diseases increase the risk of death independently of the $CD4^+$ cell count.[113, 114] This may be due not only to morbidity related to the complication itself but also to an increase in immune activation leading to upregulation of HIV replication with acceleration of HIV disease progression. A number of studies have demonstrated increases in HIV viral load in patients with acute opportunistic infections.[115–118]

As already noted, the availability of HAART has drastically altered the natural history of HIV disease in the industrialized world. Effective therapy has not only decreased the incidence of new opportunistic infections but also led to the resolution of preexisting conditions.[119] In some cases, the immune restoration resulting from HAART can alter the clinical presentation of specific opportunistic infections, as in the case of focal mycobacterial lymphadenitis or CMV vitritis.[120] It is becoming increasingly clear that the immunologic changes resulting from HAART represent at least a partial immune reconstitution, although the recovery of antigen-specific immunity appears to lag behind $CD4^+$ cell count increases.[121–124] The incidence of new opportunistic infections in patients who have had satisfactory virologic and immunologic responses to HAART is extremely low, even when primary prophylaxis has been discontinued.[125, 126] Moreover, reactivation of previously diagnosed opportunistic infections, such as *M. avium* complex infections and CMV retinitis, appears to be uncommon in patients with immune recovery who discontinue maintenance therapy.[127, 128]

Thus, over the past two decades the natural history of HIV infection has undergone considerable change, as has our understanding of it. The clinical course of HIV disease in individuals receiving combination antiretroviral therapy is likely to evolve further in the coming years, with additional manifestations and disease trajectories becoming apparent as larger numbers of patients are treated for longer periods of time.

DIAGNOSIS OF HIV INFECTION

As discussed in Chapter 106, the diagnosis of HIV infection is usually based on the serologic detection of specific anti-HIV antibodies. Serologic diagnosis of HIV infection using the combination of enzyme immunoassays and Western blotting is highly sensitive and specific (>99%). HIV serologic testing is indicated in numerous clinical settings, including screening of individuals at risk for infection, evaluating patients with symptoms or clinical findings suggestive of HIV infection (e.g., thrush, unexplained fever, thrombocytopenia, lymphadenopathy), and determining the status of patients with conditions seen with increased frequency in individuals with HIV infections (e.g., community-acquired pneumonia, tuberculosis, cervical dysplasia).

In the past, most patients with HIV infection were diagnosed after developing specific illnesses indicative of cellular immunodeficiency, such as *P. carinii* pneumonia. Although this situation remains the case in many developing countries, in industrialized countries HIV infection is increasingly diagnosed serologically among people without signs or symptoms of opportunistic disease who are tested on epidemiologic grounds. Because therapy for HIV infection is based on virologic and immunologic parameters more than clinical manifestations (and is more effective and durable when given before immunodeficiency is far advanced), early diagnosis of HIV infection is strongly encouraged. Individuals who should be tested for HIV

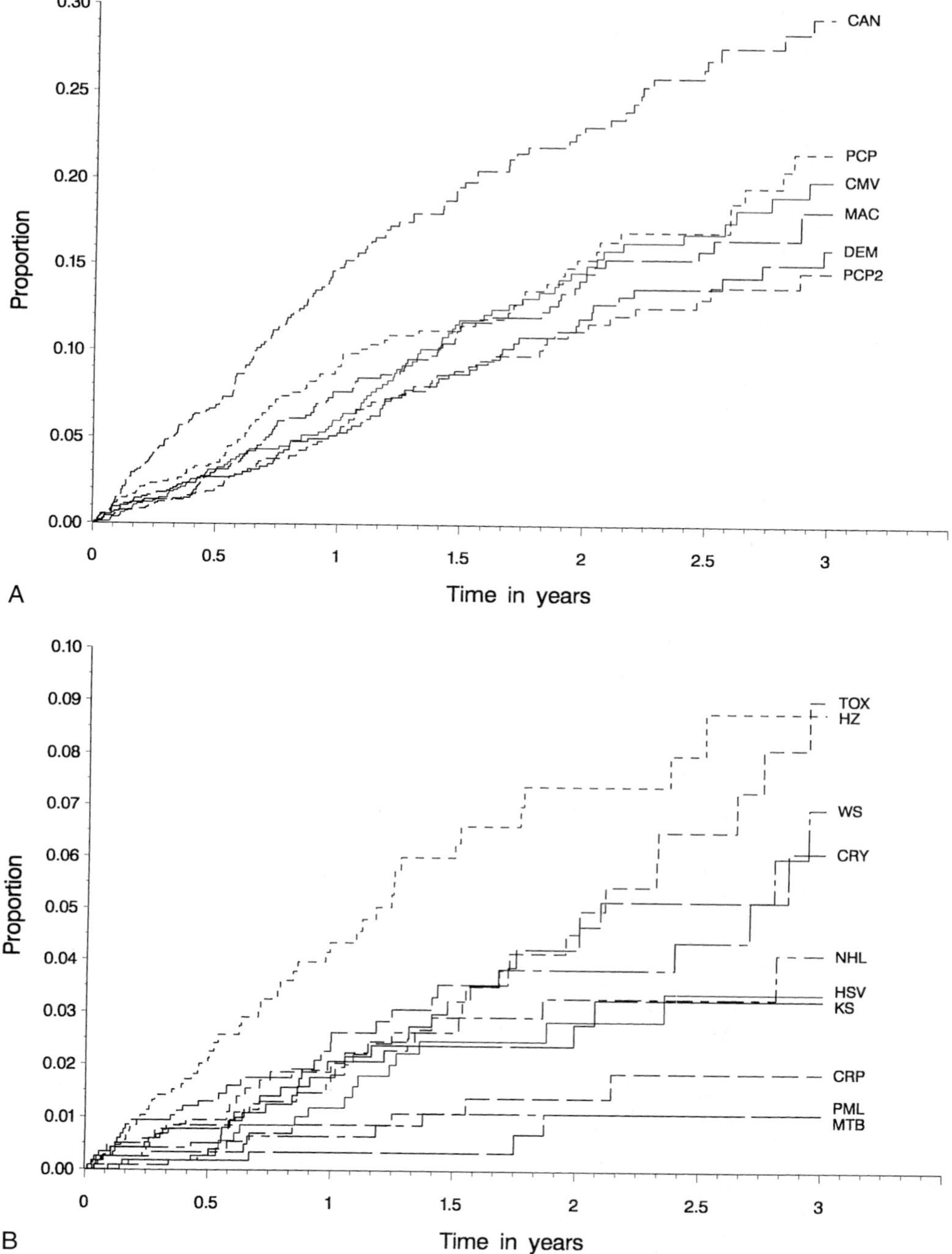

FIGURE 108–4. Incidence of opportunistic diseases in a cohort of 1246 patients with human immunodeficiency virus (HIV) infection and CD4 counts lower than 300/mm³ before the availability of combination antiretroviral therapy. *Abbreviations: A,* Can, *Candida* esophagitis; CMV, cytomegalovirus; DEM, HIV encephalopathy; MAC, *Mycobacterium avium* complex; PCP, first episodes of *Pneumocystis carinii* pneumonia; PCP2, recurrent *P. carinii* pneumonia. *B,* Crp, Cryptococcosis; HSV, herpes simplex virus; Hzos, herpes zoster; KS, Kaposi's sarcoma; MTB, tuberculosis; NHL, non-Hodgkin's lymphoma; PML, progressive multifocal leukoencephalopathy; Tox, toxoplasmosis; WS, wasting syndrome. (From Moore RD, Chaisson RE. Natural history of opportunistic disease in an HIV-infected urban cohort. Ann Intern Med. 1996;124:633–642.)

infection include those with known sexual or parenteral exposure to an HIV-infected individual, injection drug users, individuals treated with blood or blood products between 1977 and 1985, men who have or have had sex with men, and sexually active heterosexuals with multiple partners, particularly in areas with prevalent HIV infection. In addition, HIV serologic testing is recommended for all pregnant women in countries where the infection is prevalent and therapy to prevent maternal-infant transmission is available, for organ or tissue donors and recipients, for victims of sexual assault, and for health care workers who suffer needlestick or other exposures that may transmit HIV.

In certain situations, antibody testing for HIV infection is not diagnostic because of reduced sensitivity or specificity of the assays. In the acute retroviral syndrome that occurs in some patients with recent HIV infection, for example, clinical signs and symptoms occur before antibody seroconversion and enzyme immunoassays are negative. When acute HIV is suspected, detection of HIV p24 antigen with an antigen capture assay is a very sensitive test. In addition, during the acute retroviral syndrome, plasma HIV RNA measurement by polymerase chain reaction or branched-chain DNA testing usually reveals a viral load of more than 100,000 copies/ml. HIV RNA testing is not recommended for routine screening for HIV infection because both false-positive and false-negative result may be obtained. False-positive HIV RNA tests, however, usually show levels of less than 10,000 copies/ml; when viral loads greater than 100,000 copies/ml are detected in the clinical setting of acute viral illness, the test is diagnostic and extremely useful. HIV DNA polymerase chain reaction testing may be used to diagnose pediatric HIV infection in

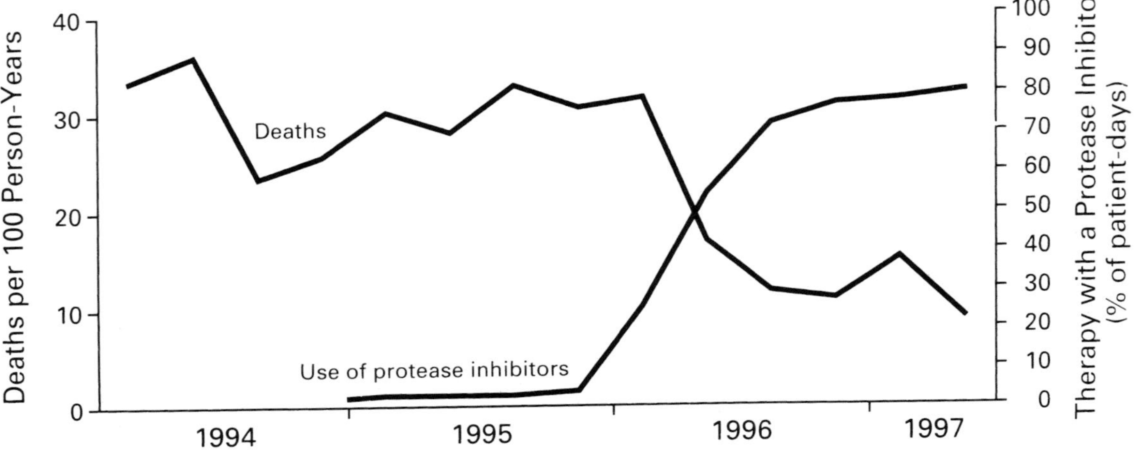

FIGURE 108–5. Incidence of death and use of protease inhibitors in patients with human immunodeficiency virus (HIV) infection and a CD4 count lower than 100/mm³ in the HIV Outpatient Study. (From Palella FJ, Delaney KM, Moorman AC, et al. Declining morbidity and mortality among patients with advanced human immunodeficiency virus infection. N Engl J Med. 1998;338:853–860. Copyright © 1998 Massachusetts Medical Society. All rights reserved.)

infants with maternal antibodies against HIV and is also sometimes useful in evaluating patients with indeterminate serologic results. HIV enzyme immunoassays are rarely falsely negative in patients with advanced HIV infection. In this setting, however, Western blots usually reveal specific anti-HIV bands and the HIV RNA test is almost always positive.

CLINICAL PRESENTATIONS OF HIV INFECTION

HIV infection causes disease manifestations of three principal types: an acute viral illness seen in the initial weeks of infection and associated with a high viral load and an intense host immune response, immunologically mediated processes related to host responses to chronic viral infection (e.g., lymphadenopathy, thrombocytopenia, HIV-related dementia), and opportunistic diseases resulting from impaired host responses as the cellular immune system is damaged or ablated. The major clinical syndromes most frequently seen in HIV-infected individuals fall into the last category, that is, opportunistic diseases that arise as a consequence of impaired cellular immunity in late-stage HIV infection. Potent antiretroviral therapy has added two new categories of clinical manifestations that may be commonly encountered in patients with HIV infection: immune reconstitution syndromes with exacerbations of previously silent or adequately treated infections, especially mycobacterial infections,[129] and a syndrome of lipodystrophy with fat loss and redistribution, elevated serum triglycerides and cholesterol, and insulin resistance seen in patients receiving HAART, especially with protease inhibitors.[130] The clinical features of these HIV-related disease processes are discussed in this and other chapters in this section.

CLINICAL FINDINGS

Acute Retroviral Syndrome

The initial manifestation of HIV infection in one half to two thirds of recently infected individuals is a mononucleosis-like illness referred to as the acute retroviral syndrome. The syndrome was first described in 1985 by Cooper and colleagues[131] as an acute mononucleosis-like syndrome in 11 of 12 homosexual men who seroconverted for HIV antibodies. In a follow-up study, 36 of 39 (92%) homosexual men with recent HIV infection recalled an illness consistent with the acute retroviral syndrome during the time when their tests showed seroconversion.[132] Forty percent of a seronegative control group also reported a mononucleosis-like illness, however. Similar descriptions of a characteristic syndrome have been reported in people infected with HIV through parenteral exposures, including health care workers exposed to accidental parenteral inoculation of HIV.[133]

The incidence of the acute retroviral syndrome is not precisely known. Retrospective studies of homosexual men infected with HIV

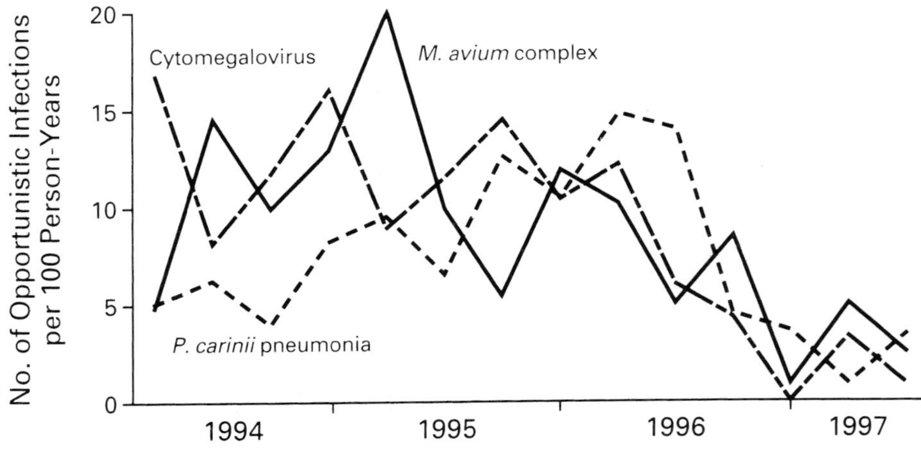

FIGURE 108–6. Incidence of selected opportunistic infections in patients with human immunodeficiency virus (HIV) infection and a CD4 count lower than 100/mm³ in the HIV Outpatient Study in the era before and after the introduction of protease inhibitors. (From Palella FJ, Delaney KM, Moorman AC, et al. Declining morbidity and mortality among patients with advanced human immunodeficiency virus infection. N Engl J Med. 1998;338:853–860. Copyright © 1998 Massachusetts Medical Society. All rights reserved.)

found a low frequency of seroconversion illness.[134, 135] A prospective study of homosexual men showed a 55% incidence of a mononucleosis-like illness in 22 subjects who became antibody positive, compared with 21% in 44 nonconverting control subjects.[136] Most health care workers with occupational acquisition of HIV had the acute retroviral syndrome after exposure.[133, 137] Overall, this syndrome is probably underreported and underdiagnosed, as noted in two series of patients, the majority of whom were not initially thought to have acute HIV infection.[138, 139]

The clinical features of the acute retroviral syndrome are nonspecific and variable.[140, 141] The onset of the illness ranges from 1 to 6 weeks after exposure to the virus but peaks at 3 weeks. Table 108–2 shows the signs and symptoms of the acute retroviral syndrome reported in 209 cases, reviewed by Niu and coworkers.[142] Fever, sweats, malaise, myalgias, anorexia, nausea, diarrhea, and a nonexudative pharyngitis are prominent symptoms.[142–149] Many patients report headaches, photophobia, and meningismus. Two thirds of patients may have a truncal exanthem that may be maculopapular, roseaola-like, or urticarial. Skin biopsies are nonspecific, with perivascular lymphocytic infiltrates and dermal mononuclear cell infiltrates.[150] In addition to aseptic meningitis, neurologic symptoms occur in a minority of patients and may include encephalitis, peripheral neuropathy, and an acute, ascending polyneuropathy (Guillian-Barré syndrome). Physical examination frequently reveals cervical, occipital, or axillary lymphadenopathy; rash; and, less commonly, hepatosplenomegaly. Oral aphthous ulcerations have been reported in several cases; these may involve the esophagus. Oral and esophageal candidiasis during the seroconversion illness has been reported. The remainder of the physical examination is usually unremarkable. Symptoms generally resolve in 10 to 15 days. A wide range of acute opportunistic infections have been reported in patients with the acute retroviral syndrome, including *P. carinii* pneumonia, cryptococcal meningitis, and *Candida* esophagitis. Their occurrence is probably due to the depression of the $CD4^+$ cell count that generally accompanies acute HIV infection.

Laboratory evaluation of patients with the syndrome reveals a reduced total lymphocyte count, elevated sedimentation rate, negative heterophile antibody test, and elevated transaminase and alkaline phosphatase levels.[142, 143] When lymphocyte phenotyping is performed, a characteristic pattern is observed.[151] Initially, the total lymphocyte count, including both $CD4^+$ and $CD8^+$ T lymphocytes, decreases with a normal ratio of $CD4^+$ to $CD8^+$ cells. Within several weeks, both the $CD4^+$ and $CD8^+$ cell populations begin to increase. The rise in $CD8^+$ cell numbers is relatively greater than that in $CD4^+$ cells, and the CD4/CD8 ratio is inverted. In the weeks that follow, the $CD8^+$ cell population increases rather markedly because of HIV-specific $CD8^+$ T lymphocytes. The ratio of $CD4^+$ to $CD8^+$ cells usually remains inverted as the acute illness resolves (primarily because of excess numbers of $CD8^+$ cells). In patients with neurologic symptoms, cerebrospinal fluid may show a lymphocytic pleocytosis with normal levels of protein and glucose.[152]

TABLE 108–2 Symptoms and Signs of the Acute Retroviral Syndrome in 209 Patients

Symptom or Sign	Number with Finding	Frequency (%)
Fever	200	96
Adenopathy	154	74
Pharyngitis	146	70
Rash	146	70
Myalgia or arthralgia	112	54
Thrombocytopenia	94	45
Leukopenia	80	38
Diarrhea	67	32
Headache	66	32
Nausea, vomiting	56	27
Elevated transaminases*	38	21
Hepatosplenomegaly	30	14
Thrush	24	12
Neuropathy	13	6
Encephalopathy	12	6

*Based on 178 subjects.

Adapted from Niu MT, Stein DS, Schnittman SM. Primary human immunodeficiency virus type 1 infection: Review of pathogenesis and early treatment intervention in human and animal retrovirus infections. J Infect Dis. 1993;168:1490–1501.

HIV core (p24) antigen may be detected in the serum and cerebrospinal fluid in about 75% of patients with primary HIV infection within 2 weeks of exposure, often coincidentally with the onset of symptoms.[152, 153] Antigenemia can persist for several weeks or months and generally resolves when antibodies to p24 are produced in sufficient quantity to form complexes with free antigen. The most sensitive marker for acute HIV infection, however, is plasma HIV RNA, which is markedly elevated in most patients.[154] Typical RNA levels range from 10^5 to more than 10^6 copies/ml of plasma, and the titers decline as the $CD8^+$ cytotoxic T-cell and antibody responses increase subsequently. As noted earlier, low-level ($<10^4$) false-positive HIV RNA tests may occur, but high-level viremia is virtually diagnostic of acute infection in the absence of anti-HIV antibodies. The enzyme immunoassay for HIV antibodies remains negative for an average of 2 to 6 weeks after the onset of symptoms despite the appearance of specific antibodies on a Western blot of the patient's serum. Anti-p24 appears on the Western blot shortly before seroconversion is detected by enzyme-linked immunosorblent assay and by the appearance of antibodies to other antigens.

The differential diagnosis of the acute retroviral syndrome includes a number of other illnesses: infectious mononucleosis; other viral infections such as influenza, viral hepatitis, measles, rubella, and primary herpes simplex infection; and secondary syphilis. Evaluation of patients presenting with an illness consistent with acute retroviral infection should include a careful history to elicit risks for HIV infection, laboratory tests to rule out mononucleosis and syphilis, HIV antibody and plasma RNA tests, and complete blood counts and differential. There is increasing interest in treating acute HIV with combination antiretroviral therapy, as there is evidence that this may both lower the viral setpoint and lead to enhanced $CD4^+$ and $CD8^+$ HIV-specific responses.[155] However, early treatment does not appear to prevent establishment of reservoirs of latently infected, resting $CD4^+$ cells.[156]

Persistent Generalized Lymphadenopathy

Infection with HIV is associated with a high prevalence of generalized lymphadenopathy, often beginning with the acute retroviral syndrome. In the early 1980s, PGL was recognized as a prodromal state to the development of AIDS in homosexual men who were otherwise healthy.[15, 16] The pathogenesis of generalized lymphadenopathy is related to the rapid infection of $CD4^+$ cells in lymph nodes by HIV after initial infection. The syndrome of PGL is defined as the presence of two or more extrainguinal sites of lymphadenopathy for a minimum of 3 to 6 months for which no other explanation could be found. Biopsy specimens of lymph nodes from such patients usually reveal a follicular hyperplasia without specific pathogens.

Approximately 50 to 70% of HIV-infected individuals develop PGL. The most frequently involved node groups are the posterior and anterior cervical, submandibular, occipital, and axillary chains; epitrochlear and femoral nodes may also be enlarged. Physical examination usually reveals symmetric, mobile, rubbery lymph nodes ranging from 0.5 to 2 cm. Pain and tenderness are uncommon. Localized (i.e., asymmetric) adenopathy and rapid nodal enlargement are not characteristic and suggest an infectious or malignant process. The remainder of the physical examination is often unremarkable, although other complications of HIV infection may be found such as thrush or hairy leukoplakia. Mediastinal and hilar adenopathy is not characteristic of the syndrome; however, abdominal computed tomography often reveals enlarged mesenteric and retroperitoneal adenopathy in HIV-infected persons. The natural history of HIV infection in individuals with PGL does not differ significantly from that of HIV infection without PGL.[157, 158] Involution of enlarged lymph nodes, with degeneration of follicular germinal centers and loss of hyperplasia, often accompanies progression of HIV infection to advanced disease.

In patients treated with highly active antiretroviral therapy, previously involuted lymph nodes may again enlarge as HIV-specific and other T cells are replenished. In addition, focal lymphadenitis with constitutional symptoms may occur in patients with previously silent mycobacterial infections 1 to 2 months after starting HAART. These "reversal" reactions or immune reconstitution syndromes are reminiscent of reversal reactions seen in multibacillary forms of leprosy, heralding a return of pathogen-specific T-cell responses.

The differential diagnosis of PGL includes HIV infection and a wide variety of other processes that are associated with generalized lymphadenopathy: sarcoid, secondary syphilis, and Hodgkin's disease, for example. In patients with HIV infection, lymphadenopathy may also be caused by mycobacterial infections, KS, and lymphoma.[159] An unusual cause of lymphadenopathy in patients with HIV infection is Castleman's disease.[160] Castleman's disease is an angioproliferative, hyperplastic process of lymph nodes and other lymphoid tissues showing characteristic histologic findings, with either hyaline vascular or plasma cell variants. In patients with HIV in particular, multicenter Castleman's disease is the most common presentation, with involvement of lymph nodes, liver, spleen, and other organs. Although the etiology of Castleman's disease is not fully understood, infection with human herpesvirus type 8 is thought to underlie a large proportion of cases.[161] Unlike PGL, Castleman's disease is associated with constitutional symptoms and multiorgan involvement in most HIV-infected patients. The diagnosis is established histopathologically.

In patients with clinical findings suggesting opportunistic disease, needle aspiration of lymph nodes may help establish a specific diagnosis.[162] Examination of aspirates with cytologic, acid-fast, and Gram stains is valuable in identifying infection or malignancy. If a specific diagnosis is not determined after staining and culture of node aspirates, then lymph node biopsy is indicated. Aspiration of lymph nodes in patients with PGL usually reveals benign cells. Biopsy specimens show follicular hyperplasia, with the normal architecture distorted by greatly expanded germinal centers composed of B lymphocytes. It is now known that active viral replication is occurring in these follicular cells and virus is trapped in dendritic cells, although the patient may appear well clinically.[163]

Most patients with PGL require no invasive evaluation and can be managed according to standard guidelines for HIV infection.

Constitutional Disease and Wasting

HIV infection is often completely asymptomatic; however, some patients complain of nonspecific constitutional symptoms in the months or years after primary infection but before opportunistic disease is diagnosed. Patients commonly complain of being easily fatigued and report the need to reduce their normal activities somewhat. Debilitating fatigue is uncommon in the early years of infection. Low-grade fevers (temperature $< 38°C$), occasional night sweats, and intermittent diarrhea are also reported. Severe wasting with loss of more than 10% of body weight is generally a finding of advanced HIV disease. The exact incidence of constitutional symptoms, fatigue, and weight loss is not known, and the etiology is varied and often multifactorial. The differential diagnosis of these findings includes intercurrent minor illnesses, endocrinologic abnormalities, anemia, and psychological or psychiatric disorders.

Anxiety and depression are common responses to the diagnosis of HIV infection,[164, 165] and studies suggest an increased prevalence of affective disorders among HIV-infected individuals. Injection drug users, in particular, have a high prevalence of affective disorders that may result in somatic complaints. Moreover, the physical effects of opiates and withdrawal from stimulants such as cocaine and amphetamines cause fatigue and other constitutional symptoms.

A number of metabolic and endocrinologic disturbances have been identified in patients with HIV.[166, 167] Hypogonadism, particularly depression of testosterone or dihydrotestosterone levels, is reported in both men and women with HIV infection and weight loss or wasting.[168] Elevated levels of myostatin-immunoreactive protein, a muscle catabolic agent, have been found in men with HIV and wasting.[169] In most clinical studies, however, wasting has been found in association with decreased caloric intake, elevated catabolism caused by opportunistic infections, or chronic diarrhea.[170–172] In advanced HIV, severe wasting, whatever the cause, is strongly associated with the risk of dying.[173]

In patients with more advanced HIV disease with high viral loads and severe depletion of $CD4^+$ cells, constitutional disease (fatigue, weight loss, malaise, fever) usually heralds the onset of opportunistic infections or malignancies. In one study of HIV-infected outpatients with fever, a specific etiology could be identified for 83%.[174] Common causes of fever in these patients included *P. carinii* pneumonia, *M. avium* complex bacteremia, catheter-related bacteremia, bacterial pneumonia, sinusitis, lymphoma, and drug reactions. Fever of greater than 2 weeks' duration was more often associated with AIDS-defining illnesses.

In African patients with HIV infection, a wasting illness, termed "slim" disease, has been described.[175] These patients have debilitating fatigue, fevers, sweats, protracted diarrhea, and severe weight loss. Opportunistic or conventional pathogens are not found, but the patients waste away and die of severe malnutrition and terminal secondary infections. This illness has been encountered in developed countries as well but far less commonly than in Africa—a pattern that suggests underdiagnosis of opportunistic diseases in Africa. Several studies of African patients with enteropathic slim disease found that most had enteric pathogens or microsporidia when a thorough evaluation was performed.[176, 177] In Abidjan, Côte d'Ivoire, 37% of patients who died with a diagnosis of slim disease were found at autopsy to have disseminated tuberculosis,[178] and the presence of tuberculosis at autopsy was strongly associated with the degree of wasting.[179] The definition of wasting syndrome in the United States is the presence of unexplained constitutional disease for more than 1 month with a temperature greater than 38.3°C, diarrhea, and loss of more than 10% of baseline body weight. A thorough evaluation to identify specific pathogens that would explain the symptoms and that might be amenable to treatment is essential before wasting syndrome is diagnosed, and usually a specific cause can be implicated.

Oral Disease

Abnormalities of the oral cavity occur throughout the course of HIV infection. Primary HIV infection has been associated with severe aphthous stomatitis and with oropharyngeal and esophageal candidiasis. As the infection progresses and immunologic impairment proceeds, numerous oral complications arise. In the late stages of disease, oral manifestations are highly prevalent and frequently severe.[180, 181] A number of studies have demonstrated that the occurrence of oral lesions such as candidiasis and hairy leukoplakia is associated with an increased risk of progression to AIDS.[182–184]

Oral Candidiasis

Candida infections of the hard and soft palates, buccal mucosa, tongue, pharynx, and hypophyarynx are observed frequently. *Candida albicans* is the species most commonly identified, but *Candida tropicalis, Candida glabrata,* and *Candida krusei* infections also occur. Contrary to systemic *Candida* infections, which appear to result from defects in phagocyte function and number, mucosal *Candida* infections result from impaired cellular immunity. The incidence of candidiasis increases with progressive cellular immunodeficiency, particularly as CD4$^+$ lymphocyte counts fall below 200 to 300/mm^3.[185] Because oral candidiasis itself is an opportunistic infection, it is predictive of the disease progression and development of other AIDS-related infections.

Several clinical manifestations of candidiasis have been described in HIV-infected patients. The most common form is thrush (pseudomembranous candidiasis). Characteristic "cottage cheese" plaques that can be removed with a tongue blade are seen on the soft palate, tonsils, and buccal mucosa. Less often, thrush involves the lateral and posterior aspects of the tongue, the hard palate, and the hypopharynx. *Candida* infection can produce flat, erythematous plaques distributed in the same way as the pseudomembranous form of the disease but without the characteristic white exudate. This atrophic form of candidiasis is underdiagnosed because many clinicians are unfamiliar with its appearance. Atrophic candidiasis of the tongue also occurs. Less frequently, *Candida* can cause a nonscrapable white plaque similar to that in hairy leukoplakia (see next section). Unlike the corrugated lesions and hairlike projections seen in oral hairy leukoplakia (OHL), candidal lesions are smooth. This hypertrophic form of disease may involve the lateral border of the tongue, the palate, and the buccal mucosa. *Candida* infection of the lateral lip (angular cheilitis) is another common complication. Angular cheilitis can cause pain, fissures, erythema, and difficulty opening the mouth. Physical examination, KOH preparation, and the response to antifungal therapy establish the diagnosis.

The diagnosis of candidiasis is frequently made on the basis of physical examination alone. A KOH preparation of scraped material from a plaque is diagnostic and can be performed easily in most clinical settings. Cultures for *Candida* are rarely necessary. A biopsy specimen of oral lesions can be used to distinguish various forms of leukoplakia. A therapeutic trial of antifungal agents can also help to establish a diagnosis. The widespread use of oral triazole antifungal agents has been accompanied by the emergence of disease caused by drug-resistant fungi.[186] Risk factors for fluconazole-resistant candidiasis include an extended duration of prior antifungal therapy and low CD4$^+$ count.[187] In addition, some species of *Candida,* such as *C. krusei* and *C. glabrata,* are frequently less sensitive to fluconazole.

Oral Hairy Leukoplakia

Originally described in 1984 by Greenspan and colleagues,[188] OHL is a raised, white lesion of the oral mucosa that is usually seen on the lateral margin of the tongue. The frequency of occurrence of OHL increases as the CD4$^+$ count decreases.[185] OHL appears to be caused by the replication of Epstein-Barr Virus in the epithelium of keratinized cells on the surface of the tongue and buccal mucosa.[189] Other herpesviruses have also been isolated from cultures of biopsy specimens of lesions; however, their role in the pathogenesis of OHL is unclear. HIV is not routinely cultured from specimens and is not found with DNA probes. The diagnosis of OHL is established by visual inspection, failure to scrape off the lesion with a tongue blade, failure of the lesion to respond to antifungal therapy, and biopsy material or scrapings in which Epstein-Barr Virus can be identified. Hairy leukoplakia is usually asymptomatic, although large lesions may impair taste, hinder eating, and cause discomfort. Lesions respond to high-dose acyclovir or ganciclovir, podophyllin, and isotretinoin, but only temporarily.

Gingivitis and Periodontitis

Severe gingivitis (linear gingival erythema) and periodontitis (necrotizing ulcerative periodontitis) have been observed in patients with HIV disease.[190] The onset of symptoms is often insidious but may be abrupt. Pain is often severe; patients may note foul breath, bleeding gums, and loosening of teeth. Physical examination may reveal a bright red marginal line on the gingiva, necrosis and ulceration of interdental papillae, gingival erosion, exfoliation of enamel, and loose teeth. The etiology of gingivitis and periodontitis is unclear. Cigarette smoking may be an important cofactor in the pathogenesis of periodontitis. Mixed cultures of aerobic and anaerobic flora have been obtained from gingival biopsy samples. More severe, ulcerating gingivitis can be caused by infections with gram-negative bacilli, particularly *Klebsiella pneumoniae* and *Enterobacter cloacae*. Infections tend to be chronic, but débridement, irrigation, and topical antiseptic agents or metronidazole therapy may control some cases.

Oral Ulcers

A number of ulcerative lesions may occur in the oral cavity of patients with HIV infection. Herpes simplex virus types 1 and 2 may cause primary or recurrent oral ulcers. These lesions generally appear as small, smooth ulcers on an erythematous base on the lips, buccal mucosa, hard palate, or gums. The ulcers may be single or multiple and are often painful. Episodes may last for several weeks; acyclovir may be beneficial. CMV may rarely cause solitary large ulcers in persons with disseminated CMV infection. Aphthous stomatitis is manifested by single or multiple painful ulcers, often with exudate or necrosis, that may appear on the buccal and labial mucosa and the lateral margin of the tongue. These ulcers do not occur more commonly than among HIV-seronegative persons, but episodes are more severe and prolonged.[191] They may be treated with topical steroids or thalidomide if persistent.[192, 193] The etiology of oral ulcers is best determined by biopsy and viral culture, although minor lesions may be observed without specific therapy in many cases. Several drugs have been reported to cause oral and gastrointestinal ulcers, including zalcitabine, zidovudine, and dapsone.

Other Oral Lesions

The purple-red lesions of KS may occur at any site in the mouth, but the palate is most common. Lesions may become large and nodular. Non-Hodgkin's lymphoma may present in the mouth as either a swelling or ulcers; biopsy is required for diagnosis. Oral warts caused by human papillomavirus infection may be seen; they are not malignant precursors. Ketoconazole and zidovudine can cause brown oral pigmentation. Salivary glands such as the parotid gland may be enlarged by infiltration with CD8$^+$ lymphocytes or benign lymphoepithelial cysts. These cysts often respond to antiretroviral therapy.[194]

Musculoskeletal Complications

Polymyositis complicates HIV infection in a small number of patients.[195] Clinical features include myalgias, weakness of the proximal muscles, muscle tenderness, wasting, and fatigue.[196] Creatinine kinase and other muscle enzyme concentrations are usually elevated, and electrophysiologic studies are consistent with a myopathy.[197] The pathogenesis is unknown; most patients respond clinically to a course of corticosteroids. The nucleoside analogue antiretroviral agent zidovudine is associated with a polymyositis-like clinical picture in a small proportion of patients who take this drug. The mechanism of this myopathy is inhibition of mitochondrial DNA, which is distinguished on electron microscopy by "ragged red" fibers.[198]

Pyomyositis has been reported in patients with advanced HIV. Skin flora, particularly *Staphylococcus aureus,* are usually recovered from wound cultures, and preexisting skin diseases such as prurigo nodularis are a risk factor.[199, 200]

Although rheumatologic findings in patients with HIV disease are not unusual, the extent to which HIV infection is associated with these disorders is not always clear. Defining a specific arthropathy caused by HIV is difficult because many patients with HIV infection are already at increased risk for inflammatory joint disease. Injection drug users, for example, may develop septic arthritis caused by pyogenic bacteria, particularly *S. aureus*. Homosexual men may have an increased risk for gonococcal arthritis or postinfectious reactive arthritis associated with genital or gastrointestinal tract infections (Reiter's syndrome). Immune complex deposition related to hepatitis B or C infection may also be associated with arthritis in patients with HIV infection. Thus, although some animal retroviruses are clearly associated with arthropathies, the situation with HIV remains somewhat clouded.

Data from three large cohort studies demonstrate that Reiter's syndrome does not occur with increased frequency among HIV-infected persons.[201, 202] The clinical course of Reiter's syndrome in HIV-infected persons may be prolonged and severe, however.[203] Patients with this syndrome are usually human leukocyte antigen HLA-B27 positive and present with an asymmetric oligoarticular arthritis, primarily of the large joints of the lower extremities, and sacroiliitis. Urethritis, conjunctivitis, keratoderma blennorrhagicum, and circinate balanitis may also be present. An enthesopathy of the Achilles tendon and plantar fascia can result in a characteristic gait in which weight is distributed to the lateral portion of the feet.[204] Aspirated synovial fluid is generally unremarkable, and synovial biopsy specimens show mononuclear cell infiltrates. Management is difficult, as the response to nonsteroidal anti-inflammatory drugs is limited and the use of the high doses of steroids often required further increases the risk of opportunistic infections. Methotrexate and azathioprine should also be avoided because of the resultant exacerbation of immune suppression.

Cutaneous Manifestations

Dermatologic consequences of HIV infection include primary cutaneous opportunistic infections and malignancies (which may also disseminate to the viscera) and systemic opportunistic diseases with skin involvement.[205]

Viral Infections of the Skin and Mucous Membranes

A wide range of viruses involve the skin in HIV-immunosuppressed patients. The exanthem of acute HIV infection is an erythematous morbilliform eruption of the trunk and upper arms that occurs 2 to 4 weeks after infection and is usually associated with fever, headache, arthralgias, night sweats, pharyngitis, or thrush.[206, 207] The rash resolves within 5 to 7 days. Herpes simplex viruses (HSVs) (see Chapter 125) frequently cause morbidity in patients with advanced HIV disease.[208] Serology shows previous infection with HSV-2 in more than 90% of homosexual men with HIV infection; it is less prevalent in other groups. Although HSV-2 recurs frequently even in nonimmunosuppressed hosts, it recurs more frequently and for prolonged periods in patients with HIV infection. HSV-2, a common pathogen of the sacral root dermatomes, often causes outbreaks in the buttocks, perineum, scrotum or vulva, and the shaft and glans of the penis. Characteristic lesions of herpes simplex appear first as painful erythematous papules; later they vesiculate and ulcerate, and pustules may form. Chronic ulcers may become granulated, verrucous, or bloody. Herpes simplex proctitis is associated with severe rectal pain, fever, tenesmus, and obstipation. External lesions may be absent, and the diagnosis is established by anoscopic or sigmoidoscopic examination and cultures. Giant perirectal ulcers and lesions at other sites that yield thymidine kinase–resistant strains of HSV-2 have occured in patients who were previously treated with acyclovir. HSV infections are diagnosed by the typical appearance and distribution of the lesions and culture. Tzanck preparations may show giant cells, which suggest HSV infection. Some physicians base their diagnosis on how patients respond to an empirical trial of acyclovir. Orolabial HSV infections in HIV-infected persons may be caused by either HSV-1 or HSV-2. Although primary infections may occur after patients acquire HIV, recurrences are the more common manifestation of HSV infection. Often, a prodrome of tingling and pain precedes the appearance of painful vesicles and ulcers. Lesions may be found on the lips, buccal mucosa, gingiva, soft palate, uvula, and tongue. HSV disease may recur chronically in patients with advanced immunosuppression.

In persons with HIV infection varicella-zoster virus (shingles) is often reactivated,[209] (see Chapter 126), typically when the $CD4^+$ level is 200 to 500 cells/mm^3. There have been reports of herpes zoster after initiation of highly active antiretroviral therapy,[210] suggesting a role of the host immune response in this clinical manifestation. Herpes zoster may occur early in the course of HIV infection, but the incidence in late HIV disease is 5 to 10% annually.[211–215] Dermatomal outbreaks are most common, and a substantial proportion of patients may have several dermatomes involved. Recurrent episodes at the same or different sites, chronic (nonremitting) zoster, and dissemination are often seen.[216] Shingles is often characterized by radicular pain and itching several days before erythematous papules appear, and vesiculation occurs within several days. Lesions are often extremely pruritic, and excoriation with secondary bacterial infection commonly occurs. Over a period of 4 to 7 days, lesions form bullae and crusts and begin to heal, although some patients have zoster chronically. Cranial and thoracic dermatomes, followed by lumbar and sacral roots, are most often involved. Outbreaks along the ophthalmic branch of the trigeminal nerve may result in corneal involvement and lead to scarring and opacification that impair vision. A substantial proportion of patients may experience postherpetic scarring and pain. In patients with HIV infection who acquire primary varicella (chickenpox), the acute infection may progress to a chronic form in a period of weeks to months.

Despite the frequency of disseminated CMV disease in late-stage AIDS, cutaneous manifestations are unusual. Vesicles, bullae, and hyperpigmented indurated plaques have all been described, however. Infections with human papillomavirus, the causative agent of condylomata acuminata, are more prevalent in HIV-infected persons than in the general population. In addition to genital lesions (Chapter 133), warts are often seen in periungual locations, on the feet (plantar warts), and in bearded areas of the face.

Molluscum contagiosum, a cutaneous poxvirus infection, is seen more often in HIV-infected persons than in other populations (see Chapter 123). Most patients have $CD4^+$ cell counts less than 200/mm^3. The agent is transmitted by sexual or other close contact; reactivation of remote infection may cause outbreaks in immunosuppressed hosts. Molluscum lesions are small, firm papules with a pearly white umbilicated surface distributed on the face, trunk, or genital areas. The lesions are usually painless and can be differentiated from herpetic lesions by the absence of erythema, smaller size, and resolution of lesions without ulcerating or crusting. Biopsy may be necessary to exclude more serious causes of cutaneous lesions such as cryptococcosis, pyogenic granuloma, and basal cell carcinoma. Liquid nitrogen is used effectively to treat this condition. Lesions may also resolve after initiation of HAART with a resultant increase in $CD4^+$ level.[217]

Bacillary Angiomatosis

Bacillary angiomatosis is associated with cutaneous and visceral involvement that produces lesions characterized by vascular proliferation, hemorrhage, and necrosis.[218–221] The disease was first described in 1983 in an AIDS patient with subcutaneous nodules with vascular proliferation and evidence of bacterial involvement by electron microscopy.[222] Subsequently, the etiology of bacillary angiomatosis was attributed to the organisms *Bartonella henselae* and *Bartonella quintana* (see Chapter 224). *B. henselae* infection has been associated with cat and flea exposure and *B. quintana* infection with low socioeconomic status, homelessness, and exposure to lice.[223] *Bartonella* organisms have been cultured from skin lesions, blood, liver, bone, and other sites.[218–221]

Patients with bacillary angiomatosis usually present with one or several cutaneous lesions, although disseminated disease is common.

The typical skin lesions are purple-red nodules or plaques that can ulcerate and crust. Lesions may be mistaken for cutaneous KS, skin tags, or basal cell carcinoma. Visceral disease may include hepatitis (bacillary peliosis), splenic or osseous lesions, bacillemia, pneumonitis, or, less often, involvement of other organs.[224] Bacillary peliosis is a characteristic illness in which patients present with fever, right upper quadrant pain, hepatomegaly, and elevation of liver enzymes, particularly alkaline phosphatase.[225, 226] Imaging studies of the liver may reveal echogenic defects; histologically, lesions have a cystic appearance, with vascular proliferation, hemorrhage, and necrosis.

The diagnosis of bacillary angiomatosis is best made by biopsy of involved sites. Hematoxylin and eosin stains of biopsy specimens from skin lesions show proliferation of small blood vessels in the dermis or cutis, enlarged endothelial cells with abundant cytoplasm, and necrotic and granulomatous changes. Warthin-Starry stains show perivascular accumulations of bacilli; these findings may be confirmed by electron microscopy, although this is not usually necessary. The diagnosis can also be established by culture of the organism in several special media or by detection of *Bartonella* DNA by polymerase chain reaction. Serologic assays for anti-*Bartonella* antibodies are available through the Special Pathogens Branch of the CDC. The natural history of the infection in patients with HIV is for relapses to occur in the absence of prolonged therapy with erythromycin or doxycycline. Fluoroquinolones, other macrolides, and trimethoprim-sulfamethoxazole also have activity against *Bartonella*.

Kaposi's Sarcoma

KS is a vascular neoplastic disorder that in the United States is seen predominantly in HIV-infected homosexual men. Human herpesvirus type 8, which is transmitted sexually, has been implicated in the pathogenesis of KS[227, 228] (see Chapters 112 and 130). Although KS also affects visceral organs, the characteristic findings are cutaneous red-purple nodules or plaques. Sites commonly involved include the legs, feet, mucous membranes, hard palate, nose, trunk, and scalp.[229] Lesions of KS are often difficult to distinguish from those of bacillary angiomatosis; biopsy is required for diagnosis.

Other Cutaneous Manifestations

A variety of other skin disorders have been described in HIV-infected patients. Seborrheic dermatitis, an inflammatory condition of sebaceous glands that may be associated with dermatophytic superinfection, is an early complication. Erythema and scaling of midline areas of the forehead, face, and groin are typical findings. Psoriasis occurs in 5% of HIV-infected persons, with scaly reddish plaques, onycholysis, nail pitting, and subungual hyperkeratosis. Associated psoriatic arthritis occurs more frequently than among HIV-seronegative persons with psoriasis. Tinea infections of the scalp, trunk, inguinal and perineal areas, extremities, and feet are also quite common. Onychomycoses, or fungal infections of the fingernails and toenails, are common although usually asymptomatic, causing only cosmetic changes. Bacterial folliculitis may be localized or disseminated in patients with HIV infection, and relapses frequently occur. *S. aureus* is the most common causative pathogen. Eosinophilic folliculitis is an inflammatory condition associated with raised, pruritic nodules with a pustular head on an erythematous base and is similar to bacterial folliculitis. Biopsy specimens of these lesions reveal intense infiltration of eosinophils and absence of polymorphonuclear cells and organisms. Xerosis and ichthyosis are also common in patients with more advanced HIV disease and may be refractory to therapy with emollients and anti-inflammatory agents. Prurigo nodularis appears as nodules and papules caused by chronic rubbing and scratching. This is precipitated by one of the many causes of pruritus in HIV-infected persons, such as xerosis, eosinophilic folliculitis, and atopic dermatitis.

Disseminated cryptococcosis and histoplasmosis may cause mucocutaneous papules, nodules, pustules, or ulcers. Biopsy and culture establish the diagnosis. In Thailand and Southern China, *Penicillium marneffei* is a common opportunistic fungal infectious agent in AIDS patients.[230] Patients can present with umbilicated papules, subcutaneous nodules, or morbilliform eruptions. Diagnosis is established by identifying the elliptic organism with central septation and characteristic red pigment production when grown in culture. Nontuberculous mycobacteria such as *M. avium* complex and *Mycobacterium haemophilum* may cause cutaneous papules, pustules, abscesses, lymphadenitis, or ulcerations. Culture is required for diagnosis.

Scabies

Sarcoptes scabiei var. *humanus* is the mite responsible for this common ectoparasitic infestation in HIV-infected persons. Scaly pruritic papules or hyperkeratotic plaques may occur on the palms, soles, trunk, or extremities. Characteristic burrows between the fingers and on the wrists are not always seen. Norwegian (crusted) scabies is a severe and highly contagious manifestation of this disease, seen particularly with advanced immunosuppression.[231] Permethrin 5% cream and ivermectin are effective therapies.[232]

Renal Disease

A number of renal abnormalities have been described in patients with HIV infection, including a specific HIV-related nephropathy.[233, 234] Ascribing renal dysfunction to HIV infection is problematic, however, because some patients with HIV have a high risk for renal disease of other causes. Intravenous drug use, hepatitis B and C infection, hypertension, fluid and electrolyte disorders, and concomitant opportunistic infections and malignancies are all associated with renal dysfunction. In addition, many drugs used to treat HIV infection and its associated opportunistic infections are nephrotoxic. Pentamidine, foscarnet, and the aminoglycosides can cause acute tubular necrosis, and indinavir, sulfadiazine, and intravenous acyclovir can cause intratubular obstruction by crystal formation. Thrombotic thrombocytopenic purpura/hemolytic uremic syndrome has been reported in HIV-infected persons. Hypertension may be a prominent feature, and the prognosis is poor.[235] Immune complex–mediated glomerular diseases, such as those associated with immunoglobulin A nephropathy[236] and hepatitis C virus infection,[237] have also been reported.

HIV-associated nephropathy was first reported in 1984 and occurs in 2 to 10% of HIV-infected persons.[233] Manifestations include proteinuria, mildly elevated serum creatinine levels, and focal and segmental glomerulosclerosis on histopathology. Although this entity is similar to heroin-associated nephropathy, only half of the patients studied had a history of intravenous drug use. In a review of 75 consecutive AIDS patients in Miami, 43% of the patients had proteinuria with more than 0.5 g of proteins per 24 hours; 9% had greater than 3 g per 24 hours.[238] In 36 autopsies, 17 (47%) had renal pathology, 5 had focal glomerulosclerosis, and 12 had mesangial proliferation. A subsequent review of the same population of patients found that patients with a history of intravenous drug use had the highest incidence of renal disease; however, other non–drug-using patients, including children, can develop HIV-related nephropathy. In another series of patients, renal disease was observed in 13 of 32 and included focal glomerulosclerosis, mesangial proliferation, and glomerulonephritis.[239] The pathogenesis of HIV-associated nephropathy is incompletely understood. Human and animal models have demonstrated proliferation of renal epithelial cells and apoptosis[240]; direct HIV-induced damage of glomerular and tubular epithelial cells may be involved. HIV-associated nephropathy is more commonly reported in blacks than in other racial groups, suggesting a biologic susceptibility to this disorder.

Renal dysfunction in patients with HIV disease is usually diagnosed incidentally when patients present with opportunistic infections and have CD4+ cell counts less than 200/mm^3.[241] Asymptomatic proteinuria, up to 5 g/day, is often the initial finding, and the serum creatinine level is often normal or only mildly elevated. The albumin concentration is almost always low (as is true for most AIDS patients with opportunistic infections), and the blood pressure is usually normal. Renal biopsy most often shows focal and segmental glomerulosclerosis ("collapsing" glomerulosclerosis) with severe tubulointerstitial disease and proliferative microcyst formation. Immunofluorescence studies often reveal deposits of immunoglobulin M and C3, and electron microscopy shows tubuloreticular inclusion bodies.

The clinical course of HIV-related nephropathy progresses quickly, usually because many other opportunistic processes occur simultaneously. Rao and coworkers[233] originally reported death with renal failure in 8 of 11 patients with HIV-related nephropathy in less than 4 months. Because nephropathy is usually diagnosed late in the course of HIV disease, it is difficult to determine the effect of renal dysfunction on survival. Some centers have reported that patients with AIDS respond poorly to maintenance by hemodialysis.[242] There is no proven effective therapy for HIV-associated nephropathy, although reports have suggested a benefit from corticosteroids,[243] angiotensin-converting enzyme inhibitors,[244] and cyclosporine.[245]

Ocular Complications

Ocular diseases are extremely common manifestations of HIV disease, with a wide variety of causes, ranging from a benign HIV retinopathy to sight-threatening viral opportunistic infections.[246, 246a] As HIV disease progresses, the risk of ocular complications rises appreciably.

HIV retinopathy occurs in one half to three fourths of all patients with HIV, with the prevalence higher in those with low CD4 counts. The most frequent finding is a cotton-wool spot, a small pale lesion that is thought to represent transient focal retinal ischemia. HIV retinopathy may also produce microaneurysms and retinal hemorrhages. The condition is generally benign, although some patients have developed visual defects attributed to this condition.

The most common and serious ocular complication of HIV disease is retinitis, most often caused by CMV. CMV is ubiquitous in patients with HIV infection and causes serious morbidity in AIDS. CMV is transmitted by the same routes as HIV, and almost all patients with sexually acquired HIV infection are also infected with CMV. Like other herpesviruses, CMV may infect cells latently and be reactivated when host defenses are impaired. Asymptomatic CMV viruria and viremia may be found in one third to one half of patients with advanced HIV disease. The risk of CMV retinitis is determined largely by the CD4+ cell count and CMV DNA level in the peripheral blood. For patients with CD4+ cell counts less than 200/mm^3, the annual risk is 4 to 12%. Further risk stratification is aided by CMV DNA measurements, with aviremic patients having less than 1% risk per year, even at low CD4+ cell counts.[247]

CMV has a unique predilection for the retina, with 90% of end-organ disease in patients with HIV infection being retinitis.[248] Other involved sites include the colon, esophagus, stomach, adrenals, pancreas, brain, and lungs. The onset of CMV retinitis may be insidious or rapid. Patients complain of painless, progressive visual loss, blurring, and "floaters." CMV retinitis usually presents unilaterally, although it may subsequently progress to the contralateral retina. Funduscopic examination of the involved eye typically reveals coalescing white exudates in a vascular pattern with surrounding hemorrhage and edema. Often, lesions are peripheral initially, involve the fovea later, and result in visual loss. Retinal detachment may occur as a late complication.

Fortunately, the advent of combination antiretroviral therapy has resulted in astonishing declines in the incidence of CMV retinitis. Several population-based studies have reported 60 to 90% reductions in the incidence of this disease. Improvement in cell-mediated immunity with antiretroviral therapy results in suppression of CMV DNA in plasma, with a subsequent fall in the risk of disease. Indeed, it appears that patients with treated CMV retinitis who receive HAART may safely discontinue anti-CMV therapy if their CD4+ counts rise to greater than 100 cells/mm^3.[249]

For patients with CD4+ counts less than 50 cells/mm^3, education regarding retinitis symptoms and regular ophthalmologic examinations are recommended. Patients complaining of ocular symptoms should undergo a thorough ophthalmologic examination. Retinal findings may include cotton-wool spots or lesions of infectious retinitis. Less common retinal infections include toxoplasmosis, pneumocystosis, varicella-zoster virus, and ocular syphilis, which is usually a diffuse intraocular process. Cotton-wool spots are prevalent in patients with AIDS but do not appear to predict the development of other retinal disease. The cotton-wool spots are distributed in a vascular pattern similar to that of CMV but do not have the irregular pattern of full retinal exudates and hemorrhages that is characteristic of CMV retinitis. An ophthalmologist or other highly trained observer should examine any patient with signs or symptoms of retinitis promptly, as delay in therapy can result in irreversible visual loss. Cultures of the blood and urine yield CMV in 60 and 80% of cases, respectively, although the diagnosis rarely rests on these results.

Patients who have had CMV retinitis frequently experience acute retinal detachments. Erosion of the retinal border at the site of a necrotic lesion allows the retina to be lifted off underlying tissues. Patients complain of sudden loss of vision, "like a curtain falling" in front of the affected eye. Surgical reattachment is often partially successful in restoring vision, although progressive visual loss may ensue.

Varicella-zoster retinitis is a severe necrotizing retinitis that may occur in patients with advanced HIV disease and low CD4+ cell counts, although some cases occur at earlier stages of HIV disease.[250] Patients most often note rapid visual loss. Funduscopic findings include peripheral necrosis, occlusive vasculopathy, optic neuritis, and vitreal and scleral inflammation, and the syndrome is termed acute retinal necrosis. Varicella-zoster retinitis usually occurs in the absence of zoster at other sites, but a history of varicella-zoster virus disease is common and the virus may be isolated from tissue samples in some patients.[251] Blindness ensues despite therapy in a majority of patients, although responses to acyclovir and foscarnet have been reported.

Ocular toxoplasmosis occurs in patients with advanced immunodeficiency, and many but not all have cerebral toxoplasmosis. *Toxoplasma* retinitis is characterized by discrete, rounded, pale exudates. Lesions are usually discrete foci of retinal inflammation without hemorrhage or vasculopathy. Vitreal inflammation is common. The diagnosis is made by observation by an experienced ophthalmologist.

P. carinii may cause a choroiditis that mimics CMV retinitis.[252] The lesions are typically posterior, yellow-orange in appearance, and do not cause vitreal inflammation. Choroidal pneumocystosis occurs most often in patients with previous *P. carinii* pneumonia, particularly in those taking aerosolized pentamidine for prophylaxis.

Cardiac Manifestations

Although early clinical observations suggested that HIV infection spared the heart, subsequent experience has shown that cardiac involvement in HIV and AIDS is not unusual.[253,254] Cardiac abnormalities in patients with HIV infection may include opportunistic infections or diseases of the myocardium (e.g., *T. gondii, Trypanosoma cruzi*) or pericardium (e.g., mycobacteria, KS), left ventricular dysfunction and dilated cardiomyopathy, cardiac autonomic abnormalities, and vascular heart disease such as pulmonary hypertension. Infectious endocarditis may also occur in patients with HIV infection, especially injection drug users, but there is little evidence to suggest that the risk is increased after accounting for behaviors. Marantic endocarditis is a manifestation of late-stage HIV disease and is sometimes noted at autopsy. Accelerated atherosclerosis with myocardial infarction has been reported in patients with HIV infection being treated with protease inhibitors and with elevated serum cholesterol and triglyceride levels.[255]

Myocardial disease in HIV-infected individuals is surprisingly common, particularly in late-stage disease. Infectious myocarditis has been reported with a number of opportunistic infections, notably *T. gondii*. In an autopsy-based study in France, for example, 12% of AIDS patients who died were found to have cardiac toxoplasmosis.[256] Most patients with cardiac toxoplasmosis also had cerebral involvement, although several patients had isolated toxoplasmic myocarditis. Myocarditis may be seen in acute *T. gondii* infection, and coincident toxoplasmic pneumonitis may present a clinical picture of diffuse pulmonary infiltrates and cardiac insufficiency. Other opportunistic agents causing myocardial involvement include mycobacteria and fungi.

A more common and underdiagnosed disorder in HIV-infected individuals is cardiomyopathy with left ventricular dysfunction, which may result in congestive heart failure.[257] Several large cohort studies have found that 8 to 12% of patients with HIV infection have echocardiographic evidence of left ventricular dysfunction, and the incidence of dilated cardiomyopathy with severe congestive heart failure (New York Heart Association class III or IV) is 15 to 18% per year.[258,259] Clinical evaluation of patients may reveal only complaints of fatigue and exertional dyspnea and physical examination may show tachycardia without rales or overt signs of congestive heart failure. Echocardiography shows global hypokinesis and enlargement of all four chambers with a modestly to severely reduced left ventricular ejection fraction and increased end-diastolic volume index. Chest radiography is frequently unhelpful. The etiology of HIV-related cardiomyopathies is multifactorial, with conflicting data on the role of cardiotropic viruses, vitamin deficiencies, and cardiotoxic drugs in causing disease. There is compelling evidence, however, that HIV itself is involved in the pathogenesis of cardiomyopathy in a large proportion of patients.[258,259] HIV has been identified in myocardial tissue by in situ hybridization in several studies and found to be positive in one third to two thirds of patients with myocarditis. In addition, an inflammatory cellular infiltrate composed of major histocompatibility complex class I–expressing $CD8^+$ cells is found in a large proportion of patients, suggesting an autoimmune mechanism in this process. Other viruses also implicated in dilated cardiomyopathy in patients with HIV infection include Epstein-Barr virus, coxsackieviruses, and CMV. Supportive treatment with digoxin, diuretics, and afterload reduction is usually of symptomatic benefit, and some patients with inflammatory myocarditis respond to corticosteroid therapy. Nonetheless, the prognosis for patients with this finding is poor,[260] although combination antiretroviral therapy might change this.

Pericardial effusions have been reported in varying proportions of patients in a number of studies, many of which suffer from selection bias. Among patients with more advanced illness in hospital-based settings, pericardial effusions can be quite common. A Portuguese study found, for example, that 41% of 181 HIV-infected patients had pericardial effusions.[261] Most effusions in this setting are asymptomatic or present with signs and symptoms of opportunistic disease at other sites. The etiology of pericardial disease in patients with HIV infection is diverse, but opportunistic infections and malignancies are the agents most commonly implicated. Mycobacterial infections, especially tuberculosis, are frequently associated with pericardial involvement in areas where coinfection with HIV and *M. tuberculosis* is common, and nontuberculous mycobacteria may also invade the pericardial space. Other infections seen in the pericardium include bacterial infections, fungal infections (e.g., *Cryptococcus*), and viral cardiopulmonary infections. KS and non-Hodgkin's lymphoma may cause pericardial effusion as well. Cardiac tamponade or cardiac dysfunction resulting from effusions is unusual in most series, and in most cases pericardiocentesis is not necessary as a therapeutic maneuver. One study, however, reported that 40% of patients with an HIV-related pericardial effusion had signs of tamponade.[262]

REFERENCES

1. Gottlieb MS, Schroff R, Schanker HM, et al. *Pneumocystis carinii* pneumonia and mucosal candidiasis in previously healthy homosexual men: Evidence of a new acquired cellular immunodeficiency. N Engl J Med. 1981;305:1425–1431.
2. Masur H, Michelis MA, Greene JB, et al. An outbreak of community-acquired *Pneumocystis carinii* pneumonia: Initial manifestation of cellular immune dysfunction. N Engl J Med. 1981;305:1431–1438.
3. Siegal FP, Lopez C, Hammer GS, et al. Severe acquired immunodeficiency in male homosexuals manifested by chronic perianal ulcerative herpes simplex lesions. N Engl J Med. 1981;305:1439–1444.
4. Follansbee SE, Busch DF, Wofsy CB, et al. An outbreak of *Pneumocystis carinii* pneumonia in homosexual men. Ann Intern Med. 1982;96:705–713.
5. Centers for Disease Control. Kaposi's sarcoma and *Pneumocystis* pneumonia among homosexual men—New York City and California. MMWR Morb Mortal Wkly Rep. 1982;30:305–308.
6. Centers for Disease Control. Opportunistic infections and Kaposi's sarcoma among Haitians in the United States. MMWR Morb Mortal Wkly Rep. 1982;31:353–361.
7. Centers for Disease Control. Update on acquired immunodeficiency syndrome (AIDS)—United States. MMWR Morb Mortal Wkly Rep. 1982;31:507–514.
8. Centers for Disease Control. Update on acquired immunodeficiency syndrome (AIDS)—United States. MMWR Morb Mortal Wkly Rep. 1985;34:245–248.
9. Centers far Disease Control. *Pneumocystis carinii* pneumonia among persons with hemophilia A. MMWR Morb Mortal Wkly Rep. 1982;31:365–367.
10. Centers far Disease Control. Update on acquired immune deficiency syndrome (AIDS) among patients with hemophilia A. MMWR Morb Mortal Wkly Rep. 1982;31:644–646, 652.
11. Pape JW, Liautaud B, Thomas F, et al. Characteristics of the acquired immunodeficiency syndrome (AIDS) in Haiti. N Engl J Med. 1983;309:945–950.
12. Pape JW, Liautaud B, Thomas F, et al. The acquired immunodeficiency syndrome in Haiti. Ann Intern Med. 1985;103:674–678.
13. Malebranche R, Annoux E, Guerin JM, et al. AIDS with severe gastrointestinal manifestations in Haiti. Lancet. 1983;2:873–878.
14. Centers for Disease Control. Possible transfusion-associated acquired immune deficiency syndrome AIDS—California. MMWR Morb Mortal Wkly Rep. 1982;31:652–654.
15. Abrams DI, Lewis BJ, Beckstead JP, et al. Persistent diffuse lymphadenopathy in homosexual men: Endpoint or prodrome? Ann Intern Med. 1984;100:801–808.
16. Metroka CE, Cunningham-Rundles S, Pollack MS, et al. Persistent generalized lymphadenopathy in homosexual men. Ann Intern Med. 1983;99:585.
17. Morris L, Distenfeld A, Amorosi E, et al. Autoimmune thrombocytopenic purpura in homosexual men. Ann Intern Med. 1982;96:714–717.
18. Walsh CM, Nardi MA, Karpatkin S. On the mechanism of thrombocytopenic purpura in sexually active homosexual men. N Engl J Med. 1984;311:635–639.
19. Abrams DI, Volberding PA, Linker CA, et al. Immune thrombocytopenic purpura in homosexual men: Clinical manifestations and treatment results (Abstract). Blood. 1983;62:1082.
20. Abrams DI. AIDS-related conditions. Clin Immunol Allergy. 1986;6:581.
21. Harris C, Small CB, Klein RS, et al. Immunodeficiency in female sexual partners of men with the acquired immunodeficiency syndrome. N Engl J Med. 1984;308:1181–1184.
22. Barre-Sinoussi F, Chermann JC, Rey F, et al. Isolation of a T-lymphotropic retrovirus from a patient at risk for acquired immunodeficiency syndrome (AIDS). Science. 1983;220:868–871.
23. Gallo RC, Salahudin SZ, Popovic M, et al. Frequent detection and isolation of cytopathic retroviruses (HTLV-III) from patients with AIDS and at risk for AIDS. Science. 1984;224:500–503.
24. Levy JA, Hoffman AD, Kramer SD, et al. Isolation of lymphocytopathic retrovirus from San Francisco patients with AIDS. Science. 1984;225:840–842.
25. Nzilambi N, DeCock KM, Forthal DN, et al. The prevalence of infection with human immunodeficiency virus over a 10-year period in rural Zaire. N Engl J Med. 1988;318:276.
26. Garry RF, Witte MH, Gottlieb AA, et al. Documentation of AIDS virus infection in the United States in 1968. JAMA. 1988;260:2085.
27. Centers for Disease Control. Revision of the CDC surveillance case definition for acquired immunodeficiency syndrome. MMWR Morb Mortal Wkly Rep. 1987;36:1S–15S.
28. Selik RM, Buehler JW, Karon JM, et al. Impact of the 1987 revision of the case definition of acquired immunodeficiency syndrome in the United States. J Acquir Immune Defic Syndr. 1990;3:73–82.
29. World Health Organization. Interim proposal for a WHO staging system for HIV infection and diseases. Wkly Epidemiol Rec. 1990;65:221–224.
30. Centers for Disease Control and Prevention. 1993 revised classification system for HIV infection and expanded surveillance case definition for AIDS among adolescents and adults. MMWR Morb Mortal Wkly Rep. 1992; 41:1–19.
31. Ho DD, Neumann AV, Perelson AS, et al. Rapid turnover of plasma virions and CD4 lymphocytes in HIV-1 infection. Nature. 1995;373:123–126.
32. Wei X, Ghosh SK, Taylor ME, et al. Viral dynamics in human immunodeficiency virus type 1 infection. Nature. 1995;373:117–122.
33. Perelson AS, Neumann AV, Markowitz M, et al. HIV-1 dynamics in vivo: Virion clearance rate, infected cell life-span, and viral generation time. Science. 1996;271:1582–1586.
34. Centers for Disease Control. Current trends: Classification system for human T lymphotropic virus type III/lymphadenopathy associated virus infections. MMWRM Morb Mortal Wkly Rep. 1986;35:334–339.

35. Centers for Disease Control and Prevention. 1993 revised classification system for HIV infection and expanded surveillance case definition for AIDS among adolescents and adults. MMWR Morb Mortal Wkly Rep. 1992;41:1–19.
36. Havlir DV, Richman DD. Viral dynamics of HIV: Implications for drug development and therapeutic strategies. Ann Intern Med. 1996;124:984–989.
37. Henrard DR, Phillips JF, Muenz LR, et al. Natural history of HIV-1 cell-free viremia. JAMA. 1995;274:554–558.
38. Phair J, Jacobson L, Detels R, et al. Acquired immune deficiency syndrome occurring within 5 years of infection with human immunodeficiency virus type 1: The Multicenter AIDS Cohort Study. J Acquir Immune Defic Syndr. 1992;5:490–496.
39. Sheppard HW, Lang W, Ascher MS, et al. The characteristics of non-progressors: Long term HIV-1 infection with stable CD4+ T-cell levels. AIDS. 1993;7:1159–1166.
40. Cao Y, Qin L, Zhang L, et al. Virologic and immunologic characterization of long-term survivors of human immunodeficiency virus type 1 infection. N Engl J Med. 1995;332:201–208.
41. Bacchetti P, Moss AR. Incubation period of AIDS in San Francisco. Nature. 1989;338:251–253.
42. Alcabes P, Munoz A, Vlahov D, Friedland GH. Incubation period of human immunodeficiency virus. AIDS. 1993;15:303–318.
43. Rutherford GW, Lifson AR, Hessol NA, et al. Course of HIV-1 infection in a cohort of homosexual and bisexual men: An 11 year follow-up study. BMJ. 1990; 301:1183–1188.
44. Goeddert JJ, Biggar RJ, Melbye M, et al. Effect of T4 count and cofactors on the incidence of AIDS in homosexual men infected with human immunodeficiency virus. JAMA. 1987;257:331–334.
45. Fahey JL, Taylor JM, Detels R, et al. The prognostic value of cellular and serologic markers in infection with human immunodeficiency virus type 1. N Engl J Med. 1990;322:166–172.
46. Muñoz A, Schrager L, Bacellar H, et al. Trends in the incidence of outcomes defining acquired immunodeficiency syndrome (AIDS) in the Multicenter AIDS Cohort Study: 1985–1991. Am J Epidemiol. 1993;137:423–438.
47. Polk BF, Fox R, Brookmeyer R, et al. Predictors of the acquired immunodeficiency syndrome developing in a cohort of seropositive homosexual men. N Engl J Med. 1987;316:61–66.
48. Moss AR, Bacchetti P, Osmond D, et al. Seropositivity for HIV and the development of AIDS or AIDS-related condition: Three year follow up of the San Francisco General Hospital Cohort. BMJ. 1988;296:745–750.
49. Mellors JW, Rinaldo CR, Phalguni G, et al. Prognosis in HIV-1 infection predicted by quantity of virus in plasma. Science. 1996;272:1167–1170.
50. Staszewski S, DeMasi R, Hill AM, Dawson D. HIV-1 RNA, CD4 cell count and the risk of progression to AIDS and death during treatment with HIV-1 reverse transcriptase inhibitors. AIDS. 1998;12:1991–1997.
51. Mellors JW, Muñoz A, Giorgi JV, et al. Plasma viral load and CD4+ lymphocytes as prognostic markers of HIV-1 infection. Ann Intern Med. 1997;126:946–954.
52. Mellors JW, Kingsley LA, Rinaldo CR, et al. Quantitation of HIV-1 RNA in plasma predicts outcome after seroconversion. Ann Intern Med. 1995;122:573–579.
53. Welles SL, Jackson JB, Yen-Lieberman B, et al. Prognostic value of plasma human immunodeficiency virus type 1 (HIV-1) disease and with little or no prior zidovudine therapy. J Infect Dis. 1996;174:696–703.
54. Yerly S, Perneger TV, Hirschel B, et al. A critical assessment of the prognostic value of HIV-1 RNA levels and CD4+ cell counts in HIV-infected patients. The Swiss HIV Cohort Study. Arch Intern Med. 1998;158:247–252.
55. O'Brien TR, Blattner WA, Waters D, et al. Serum HIV-1 RNA levels and time to development of AIDS in the multicenter hemophilia cohort study. JAMA. 1996;276:105–110.
56. Coombs RW, Welles SL, Hooper C, et al. Association of plasma human immunodeficiency virus type 1 RNA level with risk of clinical progression in patients with advanced HIV infection. J Infect Dis. 1996;174:705–712.
57. Lefrere J-J, Roudot-Thoraval F, Mariotti M. The risk of disease progression is determined during the first year of human immunodeficiency virus type 1 infection. J Infect Dis. 1998;177:1541–1548.
58. Bachetti P, Osmond D, Chaisson RE, et al. Patterns of survival in the acquired immunodeficiency syndrome. J Infect Dis. 1988;157:1044–1047.
59. Rothenberg R, Woelfel M, Stoneburner R, et al. Survival with the acquired immunodeficiency syndrome: Experience with 5833 cases in New York City. N Engl J Med. 1987;317:1297–1302.
60 Mocroft A, Johnson MA, Phillips AN. Factors affecting survival in patients with the acquired immunodeficiency syndrome. AIDS. 1996;10:1057–1065.
61. Osmond D, Harlebois E, Lang W, et al. Changes in AIDS survival time in two San Francisco cohorts of homosexual men, 1983 to 1993. JAMA. 1994;271:1083–1087.
62. Saravolatz L, Neaton J, Sacks L, et al. CD4+ lymphocyte counts and patterns of mortality among patients infected with human immunodeficiency virus who were enrolled in Community Programs for Clinical Research on AIDS. Clin Infect Dis. 1996;11:513–520.
63. Ehmann WC, Eyter ME, Wilson SE, et al. Relationship of CD4 lymphocyte counts to survival in a cohort of hemophiliacs infected with HIV. J Acquir Immune Defic Syndr. 1994;7:1095–1098.
64. Operskalski EA, Stram DO, Lee H, et al. Human immunodeficiency virus type 1 infection: Relationship of risk group and age to rate of progression to AIDS. J Infect Dis. 1995;172:648–655.
65. Eyster ME, Gail MH, Ballard JO, et al. Natural history of human immunodeficiency virus infections in hemophiliacs: Effects of T-cell subsets, platelet counts, and age. Ann Intern Med. 1987;107:1–6.
66. Mariotto AB, Mariotti S, Pezzotti P, et al. Estimation of the acquired immunodeficiency syndrome incubation period in intravenous drug users: A comparison with male homosexuals. Am J Epidemiol. 1992;135:428–437.
67. Moore RD, Keruly J, Richmann DD, et al. Natural history of advanced HIV disease in patients treated with zidovudine. AIDS. 1992;6:671–677.
68. Galai N, Vlahov D, Margolick JB, et al. Changes in markers of disease progression in HIV-1 seroconverters: A comparison between cohorts of injecting drug users and homosexual men. J Acquir Immun Defic Syndr Hum Retrovirol. 1995;8:66–74.
69. Melnick SM, Sherer R, Louis TA, et al. Survival and disease progression according to gender of patients with HIV infection. JAMA. 1994;272:1915–1921.
70. Vella S, Giuliano M, Floridia M, et al. Effect of sex, age and transmission category on the progression to AIDS and survival of zidovudine-treated symptomatic patients. AIDS. 1995;9;51–56.
71. Easterbrook PJ, Keruly JC, Creagh-Kirk T, et al. Racial and ethnic differences in outcome in zidovudine-treated patients with advanced HIV disease. JAMA. 1991;266:2713–2718.
72. Chaisson RE, Keruly JC, Moore RD. Race, sex, drug use, and progression of human immunodeficiency virus disease. N Engl J Med. 1995;333:751–751.
73. Poole WK, Fulkerson W, Lou Y, et al. Overall and cause-specific mortality in a cohort of homo-/bisexual men, injecting drug users, and female partners of HIV-infected men. AIDS. 1996;10:1257–1264.
74. Prins M, Veugelers, P. Comparison of progression and non-progression in injecting drug users and homosexual men with documented dates of HIV-1 seroconversion. AIDS. 1997;11:521–531.
75. Pedersen C, Katzenstein T, Nielsen C, et al. Prognostic value of serum HIV-RNA levels at virologic steady state after seroconversion: Relation to CD4 cell count and clinical course of primary infection. J Acquir Immun Defic Syndr Hum Retrovirol. 1997;16:93–99.
76. Farzadegan H, Hoover DR, Astemborski J, et al. Sex differences in HIV-1 viral load and progression to AIDS. Lancet. 1998;352:1510–1514.
77. Moore RD, Cheever L, Keruly JC, Chaisson RE. Lack of sex difference in CD4 to HIV-1 RNA viral load ratio (Letter). Lancet. 1999;353:463–464.
78. Taylor JM, Fahey JL, Detels R, et al. CD4 percentage, CD4 number, and CD4:CD8 ratio in HIV infection: Which to choose and how to use. J Acquir Immun Defic Syndr. 1989;2:114–124.
79. Masur H, Ognibene FP, Yarchoan R, et al. CD4 counts as predictors of opportunistic pneumonias in human immunodeficiency virus (HIV) infection. Ann Intern Med. 1992;111:223–231.
80. Janoff EN, Breiman RF, Daley CL, et al. Pneumococcal disease during HIV infection. Ann Intern Med. 1992;117:314–324.
81. Theuer CP, Hopewell PC, Elias D, et al. Human immunodeficiency virus infection in tuberculosis patients. J Infect Dis. 1990;162:8–12.
82. Moore RD, Chaisson RE. Natural history of opportunistic disease in an HIV-infected urban clinical cohort. Ann Intern Med. 1996;124:633–642.
83. Gallant JE, Moore RD, Chaisson RE. Prophylaxis for opportunistic infections in patients with HIV infection. Ann Intern Med. 1994;120:932–943.
84. Moore RD, Keruly J, Richmann DD, et al. Natural history of advanced HIV disease in patients treated with zidovudine. AIDS. 1992;6:671–677.
85. Forrest DM, Seminari E, Hogg RS, et al. The incidence and spectrum of AIDS-defining illnesses in persons treated with antiretroviral drugs. Clin Infect Dis. 1998;27:1379–1385.
86. USPHS/IDSA Prevention of Opportunistic Infections Working Group. 1997 USPHS/IDSA guidelines for the prevention of opportunistic infections in persons infected with human immunodeficiency virus. MMWR Morb Mortal Wkly Rep. 1997;46(RR-12):1–46.
87. Fischl MA, Richman DD, Grieco MH, et al. The efficacy of azidothymidine (AZT) in the treatment of patients with AIDS and AIDS-related complex: A double-blind, placebo-controlled trial. N Engl J Med. 1987;317:185–191.
88. Lemp GF, Payne SF, Temelso DN, et al. Survival trends for patients with AIDS. JAMA. 1990;264:402–405.
89. Harris JE. Improved short-term survival of AIDS patients initially diagnosed with *Pneumocystis carinii* pneumonia, 1984 through 1987. JAMA. 1990;263:397–405.
90. Moore RD, Hidalgo J, Sugland B, et al. Zidovudine and the natural history of the acquired immunodeficiency syndrome. N Engl J Med. 1991;324:1412–1416.
91. Chaisson RE, Keruly J, Richman DD, et al. *Pneumocystis* prophylaxis and survival in patients with advanced human immunodeficiency virus infection treated with zidovudine. Arch Intern Med. 1992;152:2009–2013.
92. Volberding PA, Lagakos SW, Koch MA, et al. Zidovudine in asymptomatic human immunodeficiency virus infection: A controlled trial in persons with fewer than 500 CD4-positive cells per cubic millimeter. N Engl J Med. 1990;322:941–949.
93. Graham NM, Zeger SL, Park LP, et al. Effect of zidovudine and *Pneumocystis carinii* pneumonia prophylaxis on progression of HIV-1 infection to AIDS. Lancet. 1991;338:265–269.
94. Graham NM, Zeger SL, Park LP, et al. The effects on survival of early treatment of human immunodeficiency virus infection. N Engl J Med. 1992;326:1037–1042.
95. Hammer S, Katzenstein DA, Hughes MD, et al. A trial comparing nucleoside monotherapy with combination therapy in HIV-infected adults with CD4 cell counts from 200 to 500 per cubic millimeter. N Engl J Med. 1996;335:1081–1090.
96. Delta Coordinating Committee. Delta: A randomized double-blind controlled trial comparing combinations of zidovudine plus didanosine or zalcitabine with zidovudine alone in HIV-infected individuals. Lancet. 1996;348:283–291.
97. Enger C, Graham N, Peng Y, et al. Survival from early, intermediate, and late stages of HIV infection. JAMA. 1996;275:1329–1334.
98. Fischl MA, Dickinson GM, La Voie L. Safety and efficacy of sulfamethoxazole

and trimethoprim chemoprophylaxis for *Pneumocystis carinii* pneumonia in AIDS. JAMA. 1988;259:1185–1189.
99. Pierce M, Crampton S, Henry D, et al. A randomized trial of clarithromycin as prophylaxis against disseminated *Mycobacterium avium* complex infection in patients with advanced acquired immunodeficiency syndrome. N Engl J Med. 1996;335:384–391.
100. Delta Coordinating Committee and Delta Virology Committee. HIV-1 RNA response to antiretroviral treatment in 1280 participants in the Delta Trial: An extended virology study. AIDS. 1999;13:57–65.
101. O'Brien WA, Hartigan PM, Martin D, et al. Changes in plasma HIV-1 RNA and CD4+ lymphocyte counts and the risk of progression to AIDS. N Engl J Med. 1996;334:426–431.
102. Brodt HR, Kamps BS, Gute P, et al. Changing incidence of AIDS-defining illnesses in the era of antiretroviral combination therapy. AIDS. 1997;11:1731–1738.
103. Torres RA, Barr M. Impact of combination therapy for HIV infection on inpatient census. N Engl J Med. 1997;336:1531–1532.
104. Centers for Disease Control and Prevention. Update: Trends in AIDS incidence, death, and prevalence—United States, 1996. MMWR Morb Mortal Wkly Rep. 1997;46:165–173.
105. Hogg RS, O'Shaughnessy MV, Gataric N, et al. Decline in deaths from AIDS due to new antiretrovirals. Lancet. 1997;349:1294.
106. Palella FJ, Delaney KM, Moorman AC, et al. Declining morbidity and mortality among patients with advanced human immunodeficiency virus infection. N Engl J Med. 1998;338:853–860.
107. Centers for Disease Control and Prevention. Update: Trends in AIDS incidence—United States, 1996. MMWR Morb Mort Wkly Rep. 1997;46:861–867.
108. Hogg RS, O'Shaughnessy MV, Gataric N, et al. Decline in deaths from AIDS due to new antiretrovirals (Letter). Lancet. 1997;349:1294.
109. Carne CA, Weller IVD, Loveday C, et al. From persistent generalized lymphadenopathy to AIDS: Who will progress? BMJ. 1987;294:868–869.
110. Polk BF, Fox R, Brookmeyer R, et al. Predictors of the acquired immunodeficiency syndrome developing in a cohort of seropositive homosexual men. N Engl J Med. 1987;316:61–66.
111. Greenspan D, Greenspan JS, Hearst NG, et al. Relation of oral hairy leukoplakia to infection with the human immunodeficiency virus and risk of developing AIDS. J Infect Dis. 1987;155:475–481.
112. Murray HW, Godbold JH, Jurica KB, Roberts RB. Progression to AIDS in patients with lymphadenopathy or AIDS-related complex: Reappraisal of risk and predictive factors. Am J Med. 1989;86:533–538.
113. Petruckevitch A, Del Amo J, Phillips AN, et al. Disease progression and survival following specific AIDS-defining conditions: A retrospective cohort study of 2048 HIV-infected persons in London. AIDS. 1998;12:107–113.
114. Chaisson RE, Gallant JE, Keruly JC, Moore RD. Impact of opportunistic disease on survival in patients with HIV infection. AIDS. 1998;12:29–33.
115. Donovan RM, Bush CE, Markowitz NP, et al. Changes in virus load markers during AIDS-associated opportunistic diseases in human immunodeficiency virus–infected persons. J Infect Dis. 1996;174:401–403.
116. Golletti D, Weissman D, Jackson RW, et al. Effect of *Mycobacterium tuberculosis* on HIV replication. Role of immune activation. J Immunol. 1996; 157:1271–1278.
117. Sulkowski M, Chaisson RE, Karp CL, et al. The effect of acute infectious illnesses on plasma human immunodeficiency virus (HIV) type 1 load and the expression of serologic markers of immune activation among HIV-infected adults. J Infect Dis. 1998;178:1642–1648.
118. Bush CE, Donovan RM, Markowitz NP, et al. A study of HIV RNA viral load in AIDS patients with bacterial pneumonia. J Acquir Immun Defic Syndr Hum Retrovirol. 1996;13:23–26.
119. Sepkowitz KA. Effect of HAART on natural history of AIDS-related opportunistic disorders. Lancet. 1998 351:228–229.
120. Race EM, Adelson-Mitty J, Kriegel GR, et al. Focal mycobacterial lymphadenitis following initiation of protease-inhibitor therapy in patients with advanced HIV-1 disease. Lancet. 1998;351:252–255.
121. Bisset LR, Cone RW, Huber W, et al. Highly active antiretroviral therapy during early HIV infection reverses T-cell activation and maturation abnormalities. AIDS. 1998;12:2115–2123.
122. Pakker NG, Kroon EDMB, Roos MTL, et al. Immune restoration does not invariably occur following long-term HIV-1 suppression during antiretroviral therapy. AIDS. 1999;13:203–212.
123. Powderly WG, Landay A, Lederman MM. Recovery of the immune system with antiretroviral therapy: The end of opportunism? JAMA. 1998;280:72–77.
124. Autran B, Carcelain G, Li TS, et al. Positive effects of combined antiretroviral therapy on CD4+ T cell homeostasis and function in advanced disease. Science. 1997;277:112–116.
125. Rodriguez-Guardado A, Maradona JA, Carton JA, et al. *Pneumocystis carinii* prophylaxis can be discontinued after CD4+ cell recovery over 200 × 106/l (Letter). AIDS. 1998;12:2355–2356.
126. Schneider M, Borleffs JC, Stolk RP, et al. Discontinuation of prophylaxis for *Pneumocystis carinii* pneumonia in HIV-1 infected patients treated with highly active antiretroviral therapy. Lancet. 1999;353:201–203.
127. Tural C, Romeu J, Sirera G, et al. Long-lasting remission of cytomegalovirus retinitis without maintenance therapy in human immunodeficiency virus–infected patients. J Infect Dis. 1998;177:1080–1083.
128. Martinez E, Miro JM, Gonzalez J, et al. Withdrawal of *Mycobacterium avium* complex suppressive therapy in HIV-1 infected patients on highly active antiretroviral therapy. AIDS. 1999;13:147–148.
129. Narita M, Ashkin D, Hollender ES, et al. Paradoxical worsening of tuberculosis following antiretroviral therapy in patients with AIDS. Am J Respir Crit Care Med. 1998;158:157–161.
130. Carr A, Samaras SK, Burton S, et al. Peripheral lipodystrophy, hyperlipidaemia and insulin resistance in patients receiving HIV protease inhibitors. AIDS. 1998;12:F51–F58.
131. Cooper DA, Gold J, Maclean P, et al. Acute AIDS retrovirus infeciton: Definition of a clinical illness associated with seroconversion. Lancet. 1985;1:537–540.
132. Tindall B, Barker S, Donovan B, et al. Characteristics of the acute clinical illness associated with human immunodeficiency virus infection. Arch Intern Med. 1988;148:945–949.
133. Tokars JI, Marcus R, Culver DH, et al. Surveillance of HIV infection and zidovudine use among health care workers after occupational exposure to HIV-infected blood. Ann Intern Med. 1993;118:913–919.
134. Moss AR, Osmond D, Bacchetti P, et al. Risk factors for AIDS and HIV seropositivity in homosexual men. Am J Epidemiol. 1987;125:1035–1047.
135. Jaffe HW, Hardy AM, Morgan WM, et al. The acquired immunodeficiency syndrome in gay men. Ann Intern Med. 1985;103:662–664.
136. Fox R, Eldred LJ, Fuchs EJ, et al. Clinical manifestations of acute infection with human immunodeficiency virus in a cohort of gay men. AIDS. 1987;1:35–38.
137. Anonymous: Needlestick transmission of HTLV-III from a patient infected in Africa. Lancet. 1984;2:1376–1377.
138. Schacker T, Collier AC, Hughes J, et al. Clinical and epidemiologic features of primary HIV infection. Ann Intern Med. 1996;125:257–264.
139. Clark SJ, Kelen GD, Henrard DR, et al. Unsuspected primary human immunodeficiency virus type 1 infection in seronegative emergency department patients. J Infect Dis 1994; 170:194–197.
140. Quinn TC. Acute primary HIV infection. JAMA. 1997;278:58–62.
141. Kahn JO, Walker BD. Acute human immunodeficiency virus type 1 infection. N Engl J Med 1998;339:33–39.
142. Niu MT, Stein DS, Schnittman SM. Primary human immunodeficiency virus type I infection: Review of pathogenesis and early treatment intervention in human and animal retrovirus infections. J Infect Dis. 1993;168:1490–1501.
143. Clark SJ, Saag MS, Decker WD, et al. High titers of cytopathic virus in plasma of patients with symptomatic primary HIV-1 infection. N Engl J Med. 1991;324:954–960.
144. Rustin MHA, Ridely CM, Smith MD, et al. The acute exanthem associated with seroconversion to human T-cell lymphotropic virus III in a homosexual man. J Infect Dis. 1986;12:161–163.
145. Carne CA, Tedder RS, Smith A, et al. Acute encephalopathy coincident with seroconversion for anti-HTLV-III. Lancet. 1985;2:1206–1208.
146. Denning DW, Anderson J, Rudge P, et al. Acute myelopathy associated with primary infection with human immunodeficiency virus. BMJ. 1987;294:143–144.
147. Elder G, Dalakas M, Pezeshkpour G, et al. Ataxic neuropathy due to ganglioneuritis after probable acute human immunodeficiency virus infection. Lancet. 1986;2:1275–1276.
148. Ho DD, Sarngadharan MG, Resnick L, et al. Primary human T-lymphotropic virus type II infection. Ann Intern Med. 1985;103:880–883.
149. Cooper DA, Imrie AA, Penny R. Antibody response to human immunodeficiency virus after primary infection. J Infect Dis. 1987;155:1113–1118.
150. Balslev E, Thomsen HK, Weismann K. Histopathology of acute human immunodeficiency virus exanthem. J Clin Pathol. 1990;43:201–202.
151. Cooper DA, Tindall B, Wilson E, et al. Characterization of T lymphocyte responses during primary HIV infection. J Infect Dis. 1987;157:889–896.
152. Goudsmit J, De Wolf F, Paul DA, et al. Expression of human immunodeficiency virus antigen (HIV-Ag) in serum and cerebrospinal fluid during acute and chronic infection. Lancet. 1986;2:177–180.
153. Kessler HA, Blaauw B, Spear J, et al. Diagnosis of human immunodeficiency virus infection in seronegative homosexuals presenting with an acute viral syndrome. JAMA. 1987;258:1196–1199.
154. Henrard DR, Phillips J, Windsor I, et al. Detection of human immunodeficiency virus type 1 p24 antigen and plasma RNA: Relevance to indeterminant serologic tests. Transfusion 1994 34:376–380.
155. Rosenberg ES, Billingsley JM, Caliendo AM, et al. Vigorous HIV-1-specific CD4+ T cell responses associated with control of viremia. Science. 1997;278:1447–1450.
156. Finzi D, Hermankova M, Pierson T, et al. Identification of a reservoir for HIV-1 in patients on highly active antiretroviral therapy. Science. 1997;278:1295–1300.
157. Murray HW, Godbold JH, Jurica KB, Roberts RB. Progression to AIDS in patients with lymphadenopathy or AIDS-related complex: Reappraisal of risk and predictive factors. Am J Med. 1989;86:533–538.
158. Osmond D, Chaisson RE, Moss A, et al. Lymphadenopathy in asymptomatic patients seropositive for HIV. N Engl J Med. 1987;317:246.
159. Bottles K, McPhaul LW, Volberding P. Fine-needle aspiration biopsy of patients with the acquired immunodeficiency syndrome (AIDS): Experience in an outpatient clinic. Ann Intern Med. 1988;108:42–45.
160. Oksenhendler E, Duarte M, Soulier J, et al. Multicenter Castleman's disease in HIV infection: A clinical and pathological study of 20 patients. AIDS. 1996;10:61–67.
161. Grandadaar M, Dupin N, Calvez V, et al. Exacerbations of clinical symptoms in human immunodeficiency virus type 1–infected patients with multicentric Castleman's disease are associated with a high increase in Kaposi's sarcoma herpesvirus DNA load in peripheral blood mononuclear cells. J Infect Dis. 1997;175:198–201.
162. Abrams DI. AIDS-related lymphadenopathy: The role of biopsy. J Clin Onccol. 1986;4:126–127.
163. Pantaleo G, Graziosi C, Demarest JF, et al. HIV infection is active and progressive in lymphoid tissue during the clinically latent stage of disease. Nature. 1993;362:355–358.

164. Miller EN, Selnes OA, McArthur JC, et al. Neuropsychological performance in HIV-1–infected homosexual men. Neurology. 1990;40;197–203.
165. Chuang HT, Devins GM, Hunsley J, et al. Psychosocial distress and well-being among gay and bisexual men with human immunodeficiency virus infection. Am J Psychiatry. 1989;146:876–880.
166. Grunfeld C, Feingold KR. Metabolic disturbances and wasting in the acquired immunodeficiency syndrome. N Engl J Med. 1992 327:329–337.
167. Dobs AS, Dempsey MA, Ladenson PW, et al. Endocrine disorders in men infected with human immunodeficiency virus. Am J Med. 1988;84:611–616.
168. Sattler F, Briggs W, Antonipillai I, et al. Low dihydrotestosterone and weight loss in the AIDS wasting syndrome. J Acquir Immune Defic Syndr Hum Retrovirol. 1998;18:246–251.
169. Gonzalez-Cadavid NF, Taylor WE, Yarasheski K, et al. Organization of the human myostatin gene and expression in healthy men and HIV-infected men with muscle wasting. Proc Natl Acad Sci USA. 1998;95:14938–14943.
170. Macallan DC, Noble C, Baldwin C, et al. Energy expenditure and wasting in human immunodeficiency virus infection. N Engl J Med. 1995;333:83–88.
171. Beaugerie L, Carbonnel F, Carrat F, et al. Factors of weight loss in patients with HIV and chronic diarrhea. J Acquir Immune Defic Syndr Hum Retrovirol. 1998;19:34–39.
172. Strawford A, Hellerstein M. The etiology of wasting in the human immunodeficiency virus and acquired immunodeficiency syndrome. Semin Oncol. 1998;25(2 Suppl 5):76–81.
173. Kotler DP. Wasting syndrome: Nutritional support in HIV infection. J Acquir Immune Defic Syndr Hum Retrovirol. 1994;10:931–934.
174. Sepkowitz KA, Telzak EE, Carrow M, et al. Fever among outpatients with advanced human immunodeficiency virus infection. Arch Intern Med. 1993;153:1909–1912.
175. Serwadda D, Mugerwa RD, Sewankambo NK, et al. Slim disease: A new disease in Uganda and its association with HTLV-III infection. Lancet. 1985;2:1849.
176. Sewankambo N, Mugerwa R, Goodgame R, et al. Enteropathic AIDS in Uganda: An endoscopic, histologic and microbiologic study. AIDS. 1987;1:9–14.
177. Chintu C, Dupont HL, Kaile T, et al. Human immunodeficiency virus–associated diarrhea and wasting in Zambia: Selected risk factors and clinical associations. Am J Trop Med Hyg. 1998;59:38–41.
178. DeCock KM, Soro B, Coulibably IM, et al. Tuberculosis and HIV infection in sub-Saharan Africa. JAMA. 1992;268:1581–1587.
179. Lucas SB, DeCock KM, Hounnou A, et al. Contribution of tuberculosis to slim disease in Africa. BMJ. 1994;308:1531–1533.
180. Greenspan D, Greenspan JS. HIV-related oral disease. Lancet. 1996;348:729–733.
181. Weinert M, Grimes RM, Lynch DP. Oral manifestations of HIV infection. Ann Intern Med. 1996;125:485–496.
182. Royce RA, Luckmann RS, Fusaro RE, et al. The natural history of HIV-1 infection: Staging classifications of disease. AIDS. 1991;5:355–364.
183. Klein RS, Harris CA, Small CB, et al. Oral candidiasis in high-risk patients as the initial manifestation of the acquired immunodeficiency syndrome. N Engl J Med. 1984;311:354–358.
184. Feigal DW, Katz MH, Greenspan D, et al. The prevalence of oral lesions in HIV-infected homosexual and bisexual men: Three San Francisco epidemiological cohorts. AIDS. 1991;5:519–525.
185. Lifson AR, Hilton JF, Westerhouse JL, et al. Time from HIV seroconversion to oral candidiasis or hairy leukoplakia among homosexual and bisexual men enrolled in three prospective cohorts. AIDS 1994;8:73–79.
186. Sanguineti A, Carmichael JK, Campbell K. Fluconazole-resistant *Candida albicans* after long-term suppressive therapy. Arch Intern Med. 1993;153:1122–1124.
187. Maenza JR, Keruly JC, Moore RD, et al. Risk factors for fluconazole-resistant candidiasis in human immunodeficiency virus–infected patients. J Infect Dis 1996;173:219–225.
188. Greenspan D, Greenspan JS, Conant M, et al. Oral "hairy" leukoplakia in male homosexuals: Evidence of association with both papillomavirus and a herpes-group virus. Lancet. 1984;2:831–834.
189. Greenspan JS, Greenspan D, Lennette ET, et al. Replication of Epstein-Barr virus within the epithelial cells of oral "hairy" leukoplakia and AIDS-associated lesion. N Engl J Med. 1985;313:1564–1571.
190. Rowland RW, Escobar MR, Friedman RB, et al. Painful gingivitus may be an early sign of infection with the human immunodeficiency virus. Clin Infect Dis. 1993;16:233–236.
191. MacPhail LA, Greenspan D, Greenspan JS. Recurrent aphthous ulcers in association with HIV infection: Diagnosis and treatment. Oral Surg Oral Med Oral Pathol. 1992;73:283–288.
192. Paterson DL, Georghiou PR, Allworth AM, et al. Thalidomide as treatment of refractory aphthous ulceration related to human immunodeficiency virus infection. Clin Infect Dis. 1995;20;250–254.
193. Jacobson JM, Greenspan JS, Spritzler J, et al. Thalidomide for the treatment of oral aphthous ulcers in patients with human immunodeficiency virus infection. N Engl J Med. 1997;336:1487–1493.
194. Craven DE, Duncan RA, Stram JR, et al. Response of lymphoepithelial parotid cysts to antiretroviral treatment in HIV-infected adults. Ann Intern Med. 1998;128:455–459.
195. Dalakas MC, Pezeshkpour GH, Gnavall M, et al. Polymyositis associated with AIDS retrovirus. JAMA. 1986;256:2381–2383.
196. Kaye BR. Rheumatologic manifestations of infection with human immunodeficiency virus (HIV). Ann Intern Med. 1989;111:158–167.
197. Dalakas MC, Pezeshkpour GH. Neuromuscular diseases associated with human immunodeficiency virus infection. Ann Neurol. 1988;23:S38–S48.
198. Dalakas MC, Illa I, Pezeshkpour GH, et al. Mitochondrial myopathy caused by long-term zidovudine therapy. N Engl J Med. 1990;322:1098–1105.
199. Schwartzman WA, Lambertus MW, Kennedy CA, et al. Staphylococcal pyomyositis in patients infected by the human immunodeficiency virus. Am J Med. 1991;90:595–600.
200. Widrow CA, Kellie SM, Saltzman BR. Pyomyositis in patients with the human immunodeficiency virus: An unusual form of disseminated bacterial infection. Am J Med. 1991;91:129–136.
201. Hochberg MC, Fox R, Nelson KE, et al. HIV infection is not associated with Reiter's syndrome: Data from the Johns Hopkins Multicenter AIDS Cohort Study. AIDS. 1990;4:1149–1151.
202. Clark MR, Solinger AM, Hochberg MC. Human immunodeficiency virus infection is not associated with Reiter's syndrome. Data from the three large cohort studies. Rheum Dis Clin North Am 1992;18:267–276.
203. Winchester R, Bernstein DH, Fischer HD, et al. The co-occurrence of Reiter's syndrome and acquired immunodeficiency syndrome. Ann Intern Med. 1987;106:19–26.
204. Kaye BR. Rheumatologic manifestations of HIV infections. Clin Rev Allergy Immunol. 1996;14:385–416.
205. Porras B, Costner M, Friedman-Kien AE, et al. Update on cutaneous manifestations of HIV infection. Med Clin North Am. 1998;82:1033–1080.
206. Tindall B, Barker S, Donovan B, et al. Characterization of the acute clinical illness associated with human immunodeficiency virus infection. Arch Intern Med. 1988;148:945–949.
207. Bollinger RC, Brookmeyer RS, Mehendale SM, et al. Risk factors and clinical presentation of acute primary HIV infection in India. JAMA. 1997;278:2085–2089.
208. Quinnan GV, Masur H, Rook AH, et al. Herpesvirus infections in the acquired immunodeficiency syndrome. JAMA. 1984;252:72–77.
209. Friedman-Kien AE, Lafleur FL, Gendler E, et al. Herpes zoster: A possible early clinical sign for development of acquired immunodeficiency syndrome in high-risk individuals. J Am Acad Dermatol. 1986;14:1023–1028.
210. Aldeen T, Hay P, Davison F, et al. Herpes zoster infection in HIV-seropositive patients associated with highly active antiretroviral therapy. AIDS. 1998;12:1719–1720.
211. Buchbinder SP, Katz MH, Hessol NA, et al. Herpes zoster and human immunodeficiency virus infection. J Infect Dis. 1992;166:1153–1156.
212. Glesby MJ, Moore RD, Chaisson RE. Herpes zoster in patients with advanced human immunodeficiency virus infection treated with zidovudine. J Infect Dis. 1993;168:1264–1268.
213. Melbye M, Grossman RJ, Goedert JJ, et al. Risk of AIDS after herpes zoster. Lancet. 1987:728–731.
214. Cohen PR, Beltrani VP, Grossman ME. Disseminated herpes zoster in patients with human immunodeficiency virus infection. Am J Med. 1988;84:1076–1080.
215. Grossman MC, Grossman ME. Chronic hyperkeratotic herpes zoster and human immunodeficiency virus infection. J Am Acad Dermatol. 1993;28:306–308.
216. Gilson IH, Barnett JH, Conant MA, et al. Disseminated ecthymatous varicella-zoster virus infection in patients with acquired immunodeficiency syndrome. J Am Acad Dermatol. 1989;20:637–642.
217. Horn CK, Scott GR, Benton EC. Resolution of severe molluscum contagiosum on effective antiretroviral therapy. Br J Dermatol. 1998;138:715–717.
218. Tappero JW, Mohle-Boetani J, Koehler JE, et al. The epidemiology of bacillary angiomatosis and bacillary peliosis. JAMA. 1993;269;770–775.
219. Relman DA, Loutit JS, Schmidt TM, et al. The agent of bacillary angiomatosis: An approach to the identification of uncultured pathogens. N Engl J Med. 1990;323:1576–1580.
220. Slater LN, Welch DF, Min KW. *Rochalimaea hensalae* causes bacillary angiomatosis and peliosis hepatitis. Arch Intern Med. 1992;152:602–606.
221. Koehler JE, Quinn FD, Berger TG, et al. Isolation of *Rochalimaea* species from cutaneous and osseous lesions of bacillary angiomatosis. N Engl J Med. 1992;327:1625–1631.
222. Stoler MH, Bonfiglio TA, Steigbigel RT, et al. An atypical subcutaneous infection associated with acquired immune deficiency syndrome. Am J Clin Pathol. 1983;80:714–718.
223. Koehler JE, Sanchez MA, Garrido CS, et al. Molecular epidemiology of *Bartonella* infections in patients with bacillary angiomatosis-peliosis. N Engl J Med. 1997;337:1876–1883.
224. Koehler JE, LeBoit PE, Egbert BM, et al. Cutaneous vascular lesions and disseminated cat-scratch disease in patients with the acquired immunodeficiency syndrome (AIDS) and AIDS-related complex. Ann Intern Med. 1988;109:449–455.
225. Koehler JE, Tappero JW. Bacillary angiomatosis and bacillary peliosis in patients infected with human immunodeficiency virus. Clin Infect Dis. 1993;17:612–624.
226. Mohle-Boetani JC, Koehler JE, Berger TG, et al. Bacillary angiomatosis and bacillary peliosis in patients infected with human immunodeficiency virus: Clinical characteristics in a case-control study. Clini Infect Dis. 1996;22:794–800.
227. Chang Y, Cesarman E, Pessin MS, et al. Identification of herpesvirus-like DNA sequences in AIDS-associated Kaposi's sarcoma. Science. 1994;266:1865–1869.
228. Martin JN, Ganem DE, Osmond DH, et al. Sexual transmission and the natural history of human herpesvirus 8 infection. N Engl J Med. 1998;338:948–954.
229. Beral V, Peterman TA, Berkelman RL, et al. Kaposi's sarcoma among persons with AIDS: A sexually transmitted infection. Lancet. 1990;335:123–128.
230. Supparatpinyo K, Khamwan C, Baosoung V, et al. Disseminated *Penicillium marneffei* infection in Southeast Asia. Lancet. 1994;344:110–113.
231. Schlesinger I, Oelrich DM, Tyring SK. Crusted (Norwegian) scabies in patients with AIDS: The range of clinical presentations. South Med J. 1994;87:352–356.

232. Meinking TL, Taplin D, Hermida JL, et al. The treatment of scabies with ivermectin. N Engl J Med. 1995;333:26–30.
233. Rao TKS, Filippone EJ, Nicastri AD, et al. Associated focal and segmental glomerulosclerosis in the acquired immunodeficiency syndrome. N Engl J Med. 1984;310:669–673.
234. Rao TK. Acute renal failure syndromes in human immunodeficiency virus infection. Semin Nephrol. 1998;18:378–395.
235. Kelleher P, Severn A, Tomson C, et al. The haemolytic uraemic syndrome in patients with AIDS. Genitourin Med. 1996;72:172–175.
236. Kimmel PL, Phillips TM, Ferreira-Centeno A, et al. HIV-associated immune-mediated renal disease. Kidney Int. 1993;44:1327.
237. Stokes MB, Chawla H, Brody RI, et al. Immune complex glomerulonephritis in patients coinfected with human immunodeficiency virus and hepatitis C virus. Am J Kidney Dis. 1997;29:514–525.
238. Pardo V, Aldana M, Colton RM, et al. Glomerular lesions in the acquired immunodeficiency syndrome. Ann Intern Med. 1984;101:429–434.
239. Rao TKS, Friedman EA, Nicastri AD. The types of renal disease in the acquired immunodeficiency syndrome. N Engl J Med. 1987;316:1062–1069.
240. Schwartz EJ, Klotman PE. Pathogenesis of human immunodeficiency virus (HIV)–associated nephropathy. Semin Nephrol. 1998;18:436–445.
241. Carbone L, D'Agati V, Cheng JT, et al. Course and prognosis of human immunodeficiency virus–associated nephropathy. Am J Med. 1989;87:389–395.
242. Ortiz C, Meneses R, Jaffe D, et al. Outcome of patients with human immunodeficiency virus on maintenance hemodialysis. Kidney Int. 1988;34:248–253.
243. Smith MC, Austen JL, Carey JT, et al. Prednisone improves renal function and proteinuria in human immunodeficiency virus–associated nephropathy. Am J Med. 1996;101:41–48.
244. Burns GC, Paul SK, Toth IR, et al. Effect of angiotensin-converting enzyme inhibition in HIV-associated nephropathy. J Am Soc Neprol 1997;8:1140–1146.
245. Inguilli E, Tejani AS, Fikrig S, et al. Nephrotic syndrome associated with acquired immune deficiency syndrome in children. J Pediatr. 1991;119:710.
246. Cunningham ET, Margolis TP. Current concepts: Ocular manifestation of HIV infection. N Engl J Med. 1998;339:236–244.
246a. Jabs DA. Ocular manifestations of HIV infection. Trans Am Ophthalmol Soc. 1995;93:623–683.
247. Spector SA, Wong R, Hsia K, et al. Plasma cytomegalovirus (CMV) DNA load predicts CMV disease and survival in AIDS patients. J Clin Invest. 1998;101:497–502.
248. Gallant JE, Moore RD, Richman DD, et al. Incidence and natural history of cytomegalovirus disease treated with zidovudine. J Infect Dis. 1992;166:1223–1227.
249. Whitcup SM, Fortin E, Nussenblatt RB, et al. Therapeutic effect of combination antiretroviral therapy on cytomegalovirus retinitis. JAMA. 1997;277:1519–1520.
250. Margolis TP, Lowder CY, Holland GN, et al. Varicella-zoster virus retinitis in patients with the acquired immunodeficiency syndrome. Am J Ophthalmol. 1991;112:119–131.
251. Bafisse D, Eliaszewicz M, Zazoun L, et al. Acute retinal necrosis in the course of AIDS: Study of 26 cases. AIDS. 1996;10:55–60.
252. Wasserman L, Haghighi P. Otic and ophthalmic pneumocystosis in acquired immunodeficiency syndrome. Arch Pathol Lab Med. 1992;116:500–503.
253. Lipschultz SE, ed. Cardiology in AIDS. New York; Chapman & Hall;1998.
254. Yunis NA, Stone VE. Cardiac manifestations of HIV/AIDS. J Acquir Immuno Defic Syndr Hum Retrovirol. 1998;18:145–154.
255. Henry K, Melroe H, Huebsch J, et al. Severe premature coronary artery disease with protease inhibitors. Lancet. 1998;351:1328.
256. Hofman P, Drici MD, Gibelin P, et al. Prevalence of *Toxoplasmas* myocarditis in patients with the acquired immunodeficiency syndrome. Br Heart J. 1993;70:376–381.
257. Herskowitz A, Wu T-C, Willoughby SB, et al. Myocarditis and cardiotropic viral infection associated with severe left ventricular dysfunction in late-stage infection with human immunodeficiency virus. J Am Coll Cardiol. 1994;24:1025–1032
258. Herskowitz A, Vlahov D, Willoughby S, et al. Prevalence and incidence of left ventricular dysfunction in patients with human immunodeficiency virus infection. Am J Cardiol. 1993;71:955–958.
259. Barbaro G, Di Lorenzo G, Grisoria B, et al. Incidence of dilated cardiomyopathy and detection of HIV in myocardial cells of HIV-positive patients. N Engl J Med. 1998;339:1093–1099.
260. Currie PF, Jacob AJ, Foreman AR, et al. Heart muscle disease related to HIV infection: Prognostic implications. BMJ. 1994;309:1605–1607.
261. Silva-Cardoso J, Moura B, Martins L, et al. Pericardial involvement in human immunodeficiency virus infection. Chest. 1999;115:418–422.
262. Chen Y, Brennessel D, Walters J, et al. Human immunodeficiency virus–associated pericardial effusion: Report of 40 cases and review of the literature. Am Heart J. 1999;137:516–521.

Chapter 109

Pulmonary Manifestations of Human Immunodeficiency Virus Infection

JUDITH FALLOON

EPIDEMIOLOGY AND IMPORTANCE

Pulmonary disease is the leading cause of morbidity and mortality in patients infected with the human immunodeficiency virus (HIV)[1–3] (Table 109–1). The incidence and spectrum of HIV-associated pulmonary disease is changing as a result of the use of both effective prophylaxis strategies against opportunistic infection and newer combination antiviral therapies, particularly protease inhibitor–containing regimens.[3–6] Even before the protease inhibitor era, deaths from *Pneumocystis carinii* pneumonia were declining, whereas deaths from bacterial pneumonia were rising. Pneumonia caused by unspecified organisms was the leading secondary cause of death among persons dying of HIV infection by 1992, surpassing *Pneumocystis* pneumonia.[3] Although less common in the United States, *Mycobacterium tuberculosis* infection is the most important HIV-associated

TABLE 109–1 Causes of Pulmonary Disease Associated with Human Immunodeficiency Virus Infection

Category	Pathogen or Entity
Mycobacterial	*M. tuberculosis*
	M. kansasii
	M. avium complex
	Other nontuberculous mycobacteria
Other bacterial	*Streptococcus pneumoniae*
	Staphylococcus aureus
	Haemophilus influenzae
	Enterobacteriaceae
	Pseudomonas aeruginosa
	Moraxella catarrhalis
	Group A *Streptococcus*
	Nocardia species
	Legionella species
	Rhodococcus equi
	Chlamydia pneumoniae
Fungal	*Pneumocystis carinii*
	Cryptococcus neoformans
	Histoplasma capsulatum
	Coccidioides immitis
	Aspergillus species
	Blastomyces dermatitidis
	Penicillium marneffei
Viral	Cytomegalovirus
	Herpes simplex virus
	Adenovirus
	Respiratory syncytial virus
	Influenza viruses
	Parainfluenza virus
Other	*Toxoplasma gondii*
	Strongyloides stercoralis
	Kaposi's sarcoma
	Lymphoma
	Lung cancer
	Lymphocytic interstitial pneumonitis
	Nonspecific interstitial pneumonitis
	Bronchiolitis obliterans with organizing pneumonia
	Pulmonary hypertension
	Emphysema-like or bullous disease
	Pneumothorax
	Congestive heart failure
	Diffuse alveolar damage
	Pulmonary embolus

pulmonary disease in the developing world.[7] Protease inhibitor–containing regimens may also alter the manifestations of opportunistic infections, with both improved prognoses and unusual manifestations having been reported.[7, 8]

ASSESSMENT AND DIAGNOSIS

In a new patient, the first task may be establishing a diagnosis of HIV infection. A high index of suspicion must be maintained because lack of awareness of HIV status and lack of regular care are important reasons for failure to prevent *Pneumocystis* pneumonia.[9, 10] The history and physical examination should attempt to delineate the patient's degree of immunosuppression, as well as the extent and severity of pulmonary disease, including assessment for extrapulmonary manifestations. Appropriate questions address symptoms and duration; HIV risk in a patient of unknown infection status (injection drug use, male homosexual sex, exposure to sex workers, multiple sex partners, incarceration, known infected sex partner); HIV disease status (opportunistic infections, CD4 cell count, viral burden); prior pulmonary disease; exposure to tuberculosis and purified protein derivative status; use of and compliance with medications, especially anti-*Pneumocystis* prophylaxis; smoking history; and travel history. A social history also provides clues; for instance, homelessness, incarceration, injection drug use, or origin from an area of endemicity suggests an increased risk of tuberculosis, whereas Kaposi's sarcoma is more common in men who have sex with men. Places of residence and travel are important; for example, within the United States the incidence of pulmonary mycoses such as coccidioidomycosis and histoplasmosis varies according to region, and *Penicillium marneffei* would be expected only in a patient with appropriate geographic exposure.

The extent of a patient's immunosuppression is an important clue to potential causes of pulmonary disease.[5, 11] Details about prior acquired immunodeficiency syndrome (AIDS)–associated conditions, CD4 cell counts and viral burden, and the presence or absence of signs such as thrush or wasting help delineate the degree of immunosuppression. In a patient without a known diagnosis of HIV infection or one who has not had recent immunologic monitoring, a depressed total lymphocyte count calculated from the complete blood count and differential may be a clue to immunosuppression.

A patient's CD4 cell count is very useful in the establishment of a differential diagnosis. Pulmonary disease at higher CD4 cell counts is more likely to be bacterial or tuberculous. *Pneumocystis* pneumonia is rare in patients with CD4 cell counts above 200 cells/μl. Patients with aspergillosis, *Mycobacterium avium* complex (MAC), or cytomegalovirus (CMV) disease have very low CD4 cell counts—usually below 50 cells/μl. Thus, the intensity of evaluation of a patient with cough and fever is often very different in a generally healthy patient with a CD4 cell count of 500 than in a patient with more advanced disease. Nonetheless, a CD4 cell count above 200 cells/μl does not exclude *Pneumocystis* pneumonia, especially in a patient with thrush or persistent fever or in a patient with a high viral burden, in whom CD4 cell counts may decline rapidly.[5, 11] *Pneumocystis* pneumonia is less common in patients receiving prophylaxis; breakthroughs are more common in patients treated by regimens other than trimethoprim-sulfamethoxazole and in patients with very low CD4 cell counts.

Although upper respiratory infections and acute bronchitis are very common in patients with HIV, so are life-threatening pulmonary infections.[1, 2] Physical examination is useful in directing the evaluation, but a normal result on lung examination is common in *Pneumocystis* pneumonia and should not be the deciding factor in whether to obtain a chest radiograph. A chest radiograph will not provide a specific diagnosis, and atypical manifestations are so common that the radiographic pattern is of limited use in diagnosis, but films help focus the diagnostic investigation.[12] The list of possible diagnostic tests is large, and the history, physical examination, and chest radiography should suggest which are appropriate and which can be deferred (Table 109–2). Chest computed tomography (CT) scans, especially high-resolution CT, can provide additional information by showing the extent of infiltration, lymphadenopathy, miliary nodules, occult cavitation, or ground-glass abnormalities.

TABLE 109–2 Diagnostic Studies to Be Considered in the Evaluation of Patients with Human Immunodeficiency Virus Infection and Pulmonary Disease

Category	Specific Tests to Consider
To Assess Severity and Extent of Disease	
Respiration	Respiratory rate and comfort
	Pulse oximetry and/or arterial blood gases at rest or with exercise
Imaging	Chest radiograph, chest CT scan
To Determine Etiology	
Nasopharyngeal wash	Rapid antigen tests; cultures for influenza, respiratory syncytial virus, adenoviruses, parainfluenza viruses
Respiratory specimens (sputum, induced sputum, bronchoalveolar lavage, pleural fluid)	Gram stain
	Pneumocystis carinii stain: immunofluorescence, toluidine blue, Giemsa, methenamine silver. PCR is investigational
	Fungal stain (wet mount) for *Histoplasma, Cryptococcus, Aspergillus, Coccidioides*
	Histoplasma polysaccharide antigen in lavage fluid
	Viral cultures (CMV, respiratory viruses)
	Mycobacterial stain
	Rapid nucleic acid test for *Mycobacterium tuberculosis*
	Modified acid-fast stain for *Nocardia*
	Cytopathology for tumor, cytomegalic cells, organisms
	Wet mount for *Strongyloides* larvae
	Giemsa stain or indirect immunofluorescence for *Toxoplasma*
	Culture for fungi, mycobacteria, aerobic bacteria, *Legionella*
Bronchoscopy for inspection of the bronchial tree	Endobronchial Kaposi's lesions
	Obstructive aspergillosis
	Herpetic tracheitis, endobronchial *Mycobacterium avium*
Biopsies for microscopy, culture	Transbronchial
	Transthoracic or transbronchial fine needle
	Open lung or video-assisted thoracoscopic
Urine	*Histoplasma* antigen
	Legionella pneumophila serogroup I antigen
	Fungal *(Cryptococcus)* and *Mycobacterium* culture
	Histoplasma polysaccharide antigen
	Mycobacterium
Blood	Culture (aerobic and anaerobic bacteria, mycobacteria, fungi)
	Peripheral blood or buffy coat smear for *Histoplasma* or *Toxoplasma*
	Cryptococcal antigen
	Histoplasma polysaccharide antigen
	Coccidioides serology
Stool	Examination for *Strongyloides*
Skin test	PPD

Abbreviations: CMV, Cytomegalovirus; CT, computed tomography; PCR, polymerase chain reaction; PPD, purified protein derivative.

An important part of the management of a patient with HIV infection and pulmonary disease is considering the diagnosis of tuberculosis and instituting appropriate precautions to prevent possible spread to both staff members and patients.[13] Medical personnel who are performing procedures such as induced sputum and bronchoscopy should follow recommended isolation procedures, but it is always appropriate to inform them when tuberculosis is suspected.

Empirical Therapy

The role of empirical therapy based on a presumptive diagnosis in the absence of immediate plans for diagnostic evaluation remains controversial.[14] Many clinicians would treat an acute focal pneumonia associated with the production of purulent sputum in a noncritically ill patient by using antibiotics directed against common bacterial pathogens such as *Streptococcus pneumoniae, Haemophilus influenzae, Mycoplasma pneumoniae, Chlamydia pneumoniae,* and *Legionella* species, particularly in a patient who does not have advanced AIDS. In a patient with advanced immunosuppression or with diffuse infiltrates, empirical management is difficult because the range of pathogens is too broad for empirical coverage and the risks of inappropriate therapy are great. Nonetheless, because *Pneumocystis* pneumonia has characteristic features and a slow progression, some clinicians have empirically treated reliable patients who appeared likely on clinical grounds to have *Pneumocystis* pneumonia.[14, 15] However, even experienced physicians will have made the wrong diagnosis in about 20% of patients clinically suspected of having *Pneumocystis* pneumonia.[16] In one decision analysis comparing the outcome of empirical treatment with early bronchoscopy, empirical therapy was found warranted when the probability of *Pneumocystis* pneumonia was at least 72%, although predicted survival differences were small even at low probabilities of *Pneumocystis* infection.[17] In another study, patients with care paid for by Medicaid were less likely than those with private insurance to have had bronchoscopy or a confirmed diagnosis of *Pneumocystis* pneumonia. After adjustment for severity of illness, these Medicaid-covered patients were almost 75% more likely to die during that admission, but with adjustment for confirmed diagnosis, their likelihood of death was no longer significantly greater.[18] Although payment issues may alter the aggressiveness of the approach to AIDS-associated pneumonia, such issues should not alter the fact that empirical therapy may be suboptimal in many cases. The limited data that exist are difficult to apply to the current era, where the incidence of *Pneumocystis* pneumonia is declining and prophylaxis is widespread. Thus, because clinical diagnosis can be difficult and errors in diagnosis contribute to morbidity and mortality, empirical management for suspected *Pneumocystis* pneumonia is becoming less appealing.

Because most empirical therapy is targeted against either common bacterial pathogens or *P. carinii,* it should not alter the ability to detect a fungal pathogen, and the limited data available suggest that a diagnosis of *P. carinii* infection is probably not significantly inhibited.[19, 20] Given the antituberculous activity of agents such as quinolones that might be used as empirical therapy, it is not clear how a diagnosis of tuberculosis would be affected.

A reasonable approach to a patient with suspected acute pulmonary infection includes using chest radiography, the CD4 cell count, and the severity of pulmonary disease to guide the need for a specific diagnosis. Patients with higher CD4 cell counts and those with clinical and radiographic features suggestive of acute bacterial pneumonia are better candidates for empirical treatment.

Diagnostic Procedures

Screening Tests to Detect Pulmonary Disease

Some centers use measures of pulmonary function to screen patients for the presence of pulmonary disease before bronchoscopy or induced sputum procedures. Pulmonary function measures are most likely to be useful in patients with mild symptoms and a normal, equivocal, or stably abnormal chest radiograph. Most algorithms that include screening tests have focused on early recognition and diagnosis of *Pneumocystis* pneumonia, an alveolar disease that alters respiratory function. Screening tests used include pulse oximetry, pulmonary function testing, carbon monoxide diffusing capacity, arterial blood gas, and arterial desaturation during exercise testing.[21] The cost-effectiveness of screening before the use of diagnostic procedures depends on the selection of patients for testing and the sensitivity, specificity, and cost of the test performed in comparison with that for induced sputum or bronchoalveolar lavage. Some physicians have found a highly sensitive screening test such as arterial oxygen desaturation during treadmill exercise testing to be an appealing strategy for the diagnosis of *Pneumocystis* pneumonia when both the prevalence of *Pneumocystis* pneumonia and the sensitivity of induced sputum are low in the screened population.[21] In one study, classic clinical symptoms consisting of dyspnea, cough, fever, a chest radiograph with obvious diffuse or perihilar interstitial infiltrates, and desaturation measured by pulse oximetry during exercise were strongly predictive of *Pneumocystis* pneumonia in patients without a prior episode; however, these findings lost their utility in patients who had prior *Pneumocystis* pneumonia.[15] The receipt of anti-*Pneumocystis* prophylaxis decreased the likelihood that the pulmonary disease was due to *Pneumocystis.* Tests such as spirometry and single-breath carbon monoxide diffusing capacity lack specificity. An abnormal diffusing capacity is common even without clinically significant pulmonary disease.[22, 23] Although an increase in the alveolar-to-arterial oxygen tension gradient or a lower percentage of saturation of hemoglobin is common in diffuse diseases such as *Pneumocystis* pneumonia, hypoxemia is not specific and not required for serious pulmonary disease.[15] Nonetheless, arterial blood gas testing is very important in the assessment of a patient with probable *Pneumocystis* pneumonia because it guides the practitioner in the use of concomitant corticosteroids in those with more than mild disease.

Gallium scanning, although sensitive for pulmonary disease, is expensive and nonspecific, and its pursuit delays more definitive testing. High-resolution CT scanning is being evaluated in some centers as an initial screening test. Patients with normal findings are unlikely to have *Pneumocystis* pneumonia.[24] CT scanning has the advantage of offering specific information that can help target the evaluation when an abnormality is found. Although lactate dehydrogenase is elevated in the blood in most patients with *Pneumocystis* pneumonia, elevated lactate dehydrogenase levels are nonspecific and not helpful.[25] Antibody testing is not useful in the diagnosis of most pulmonary diseases in AIDS because of ubiquitous exposure (as with *P. carinii*), poor sensitivity, and delayed return of results.

Induced Sputum

An appropriately processed induced sputum specimen obtained by an experienced respiratory therapist after the patient has inhaled a mist of hypertonic saline is a highly sensitive and specific means of making the diagnosis of *Pneumocystis* pneumonia in some institutions, especially if immunofluorescent staining is used.[26] Unfortunately, the techniques and yields from induced sputum vary widely among institutions. Although the sensitivity is over 90% at some institutions, others have far lower sensitivity, so the clinician needs to know the institution's procedures and success rates.[26] Negative induced sputum results do not exclude the diagnosis of *Pneumocystis* pneumonia. In a retrospective study of early bronchoscopy after negative induced sputum findings, half of the procedures resulted in a diagnosis, including *Pneumocystis* pneumonia in 32%.[27] A demonstration of *Pneumocystis* in the induced sputum also does not exclude the presence of a copathogen, which occurred in 18% of patients in one retrospective study.[12] Induced sputum has not been systematically assessed for most diagnoses other than *P. carinii* infection. Unless clinical suspicion is low (in which case the test should probably not have been performed) or another diagnosis has already been made, negative induced sputum results warrant further investigation by bronchoscopy.

Fiber-optic Bronchoscopy

Fiber-optic bronchoscopy with bronchoalveolar lavage is an important tool for the diagnosis of HIV-associated pulmonary disease.[12, 28] Numerous studies have demonstrated its high yield and safety. Most patients will have a fever after the procedure, and some will have a new infiltrate at the lavage site that resolves within 24 hours.[28] These should not be confused with disease progression. Bronchial brushing has a low yield for AIDS-associated infectious diagnoses and is rarely used. Because transbronchial biopsy not only prolongs the procedure but also increases the risk of pneumothorax and hemorrhage, the decision to perform a transbronchial biopsy with the initial bronchoscopy and lavage depends on the patient's clinical diagnosis and status (respiratory failure, coagulopathy) and on the preference of the bronchoscopist. Transbronchial lung biopsy will occasionally lead to a diagnosis of *Pneumocystis* pneumonia in a patient with negative bronchoalveolar lavage findings,[12, 28] but lavage without biopsy is highly sensitive and is the modality of choice in many institutions for the diagnosis of *Pneumocystis* pneumonia. A repeat procedure with biopsy is then performed only if the lavage has not provided a diagnosis. Although aerosolized pentamidine prophylaxis has been reported by some to decrease the sensitivity of bronchoalveolar lavage for the diagnosis of *Pneumocystis* pneumonia, others have found that it remains sensitive when upper lobe lavage is included.[29]

When diagnoses other than *Pneumocystis* pneumonia are considered probable, it may be appropriate to perform transbronchial biopsy with the initial procedure. Combining bronchoalveolar lavage with transbronchial biopsy leads to a very high yield for all pathogens (98% in one study).[29] Transbronchial biopsy can improve sensitivity or be required for a diagnosis of tuberculosis, CMV pneumonia, fungal pneumonia, lymphocytic or nonspecific interstitial pneumonitis, or malignancy other than Kaposi's sarcoma. The likelihood of different diagnostic possibilities and plans for samples and tests should be discussed with the bronchoscopist.

Biopsies

Percutaneous transthoracic needle aspiration or biopsy is useful in establishing a diagnosis in patients who have radiographic demonstration of nodules, masses, cavities, or adenopathy.[30] Open lung biopsy is now an uncommon procedure in patients with HIV infection, and the likelihood that it will result in a treatable diagnosis and thus its value have been points of controversy. It is rarely performed before bronchoscopy or needle biopsy. Indications are usually lack of diagnosis after bronchoscopy or needle biopsy or failure to respond to therapy for a diagnosis made at bronchoscopy. One study suggests that additional treatable diagnoses that affect outcome are not generally found in a patient who is deteriorating despite therapy for a diagnosis established by bronchoscopy.[31] However, in a selected group of patients, open biopsy can safely provide diagnoses of therapeutic importance.[32] The effect of lower-morbidity video-assisted thoracoscopic techniques on diagnostic strategies or success has not been systematically assessed.

DIFFERENTIAL DIAGNOSIS BY CHEST RADIOGRAPHIC MANIFESTATION

Focal Infiltrates

Patients who are mildly ill and who have sputum production and a focal infiltrate suggestive of a community-acquired bacterial pneumonia are commonly treated with empirical antibiotics with close assessment of response; however, a high index of suspicion has to be maintained for other diagnoses. Lack of symptomatic response with subsequent resolution on chest radiographs or progression despite therapy suggests the need for further evaluation. In a retrospective review of 53 HIV-infected patients hospitalized for community-acquired pneumonia with lobar or segmental consolidation, 35 had a specific diagnosis made.[33] Of these patients, 54% had typical bacterial pathogens (almost half were *Pneumococcus*), 34% had *Pneumocystis* pneumonia, and 11% had mycobacterial disease. Thus, *P. carinii* accounted for 23% of the focal infiltrates in this group of patients with predominantly low CD4 cell counts (median, 40 cells/μl). Kaposi's sarcoma, lymphoma, fungal infection, *Rhodococcus equi, Nocardia,* and *Aspergillus* infections can produce focal infiltrates. Upper lobe disease should bring to mind *Pneumocystis* pneumonia, tuberculosis, and *R. equi* pneumonia.

Diffuse Interstitial and Reticulonodular Infiltrates

Although diffuse interstitial infiltrates are associated with the diagnosis of *Pneumocystis* pneumonia, this pattern is nonspecific.[25, 34] Other important causes of a diffuse interstitial or reticulonodular pattern include tuberculosis or fungal disease, bacterial pneumonia (particularly *H. influenzae*), viral pneumonia, toxoplasmosis, and nonspecific interstitial pneumonitis. In one study of 351 patients presumed to have *Pneumocystis* pneumonia for the purpose of clinical trial enrollment, 81% had a confirmed diagnosis of *Pneumocystis* pneumonia made at bronchoscopy.[16] The second most common diagnosis was nonspecific interstitial pneumonitis, which occurred in about a quarter of those who did not have *Pneumocystis* infection.

Cavities and Abscesses

Many different diseases can produce pulmonary cavities in patients with HIV infection: tuberculosis and other mycobacterial infections, particularly infection with *Mycobacterium kansasii* (but only very rarely MAC); aspergillosis; pneumonia caused by *Pseudomonas, Staphylococcus, Rhodococcus,* or *Nocardia;* cryptococcosis; histoplasmosis; coccidioidomycosis; blastomycosis; and malignancies.[35] *Pneumocystis* causes thin-walled cysts, blebs, pneumatoceles, and rarely cavitary disease.[34] Intravascular infections should be considered, especially in injection drug users; such infections may be manifested as cavitated septic emboli.

In a review of 31 cases of HIV-associated lung abscess, all patients had advanced HIV disease with CD4 cell counts below 50 cells/μl, and most had a history of pulmonary infection.[36] Although bacteria were etiologic or contributory in 81%, *P. carinii,* fungal, and mixed infections also occurred. The most common bacterial pathogens were *Pseudomonas aeruginosa, S. pneumoniae, Klebsiella pneumoniae,* and *Staphylococcus aureus,* in that order. Anaerobic lung abscess should also be considered.

Pulmonary Nodules and Masses

Patients with HIV infection can have calcified, inactive pulmonary granulomas or hamartomas, but many nodules represent treatment-requiring illness. A rounded lesion could be a cryptococcoma, lymphoma, or a primary lung cancer.[37, 38] Primary lung cancer is greater than sixfold more likely in patients infected with HIV.[38] In a retrospective analysis of 10 Spanish patients with HIV infection and solitary pulmonary nodules, no single etiology predominated, but 70% were of infectious etiology.[39] Sputum samples were not diagnostic. For evaluation, chest CT is useful, and percutaneous transthoracic needle biopsy may be diagnostic.[23] Diagnoses other than malignancy include mycobacterial or fungal infections, Kaposi's sarcoma, septic emboli, and granulomatous *P. carinii* infection.

Pleural Effusion and Pneumothorax

Pleural effusion is common in hospitalized patients with HIV infection. In a retrospective analysis, 27% of 222 hospitalized patients with HIV infection had pleural effusion.[40] Most (66%) of these effusions were of infectious etiology, including bacterial infections caused by pneumococci, *Legionella, Mycoplasma,* gram-negative bacteria, *M. tuberculosis,* and *P. carinii.* Less common causes included septic emboli and *Nocardia, Cryptococcus,* and MAC infections. Noninfectious causes included hypoalbuminemia, cardiac failure, Kaposi's sarcoma, atelectasis, uremia, and adult respiratory distress syndrome. Large effusions were most commonly associated with tuberculosis.[40] Although not seen in this series, other considerations in an HIV-infected patient with effusion include histoplasmosis, toxoplasmosis, and lymphoma. Bloody effusion suggests Kaposi's sarcoma. Extrapulmonary pneumocystosis is a cause of pleural effusion; the organisms can be found on special stains of the fluid, and concentration can improve yield.[41]

Pneumothorax most often complicates acute or recent *Pneumocystis* infection. Aerosolized pentamidine prophylaxis and prior *Pneumocystis* pneumonia are risk factors for the development of pneumothorax.[42, 43] Active *Pneumocystis* infection is usually present.

Chest Radiograph without Infiltrates

In patients with a normal or subtly abnormal chest radiograph, attention is focused on the lung either because of pulmonary symptoms such as dyspnea or cough or because of fever without a known source. Patients with normal chest radiographs can present diagnostic difficulties, but a normal chest radiograph does not exclude diseases more commonly accompanied by radiographic abnormalities such as *Pneumocystis* pneumonia, tuberculosis, fungal disease, or nonspecific interstitial pneumonitis.[23, 25, 43, 44] A normal chest radiograph is seen in early *Pneumocystis* pneumonia, which is an optimal time for diagnosis and therapy. High-resolution CT scanning may be a useful technique in the case of normal, equivocal, or nonspecific chest radiographs. *Pneumocystis* pneumonia produces patchy or, less commonly, nodular ground-glass opacities.[24] High-resolution CT scanning has been sensitive but not specific because other pulmonary diseases also cause these types of opacities. CT scan also contributes to other diagnoses such as Kaposi's sarcoma, pulmonary edema, and pulmonary hypertension.[24]

A patient with dyspnea in the absence of infiltrates may have bullous disease that can be seen on CT scan. Although many of these patients will have had prior pulmonary infections, especially prior *Pneumocystis* pneumonia, these abnormalities plus abnormalities on pulmonary function testing have been reported in patients without prior known lung disease.[45] Dyspnea has also been the initial symptom in patients with pulmonary hypertension, which can be rapidly progressive.[46]

Adenopathy

Intrathoracic adenopathy is not usually a part of HIV-associated persistent generalized lymphadenopathy, and its presence warrants investigation. Tissue is generally required for diagnosis. The differential diagnosis includes tuberculosis and other mycobacterial infections, fungal infection, lymphoma, carcinoma, and Kaposi's sarcoma; rare causes include *P. carinii* and sarcoidosis.[34, 43, 47] A finding of low-density intrathoracic adenopathy, sometimes with a sharp rim of enhancement, on contrast-enhanced CT scan has been the most common pattern in tuberculosis.[48] The adenopathy is often massive.

SPECIFIC PATHOGENS AND ENTITIES

Bacterial Infections

Bacterial lower respiratory tract infection is the most frequent serious pulmonary disorder in HIV infection. It occurs more frequently in HIV-infected patients than in those without HIV infection, and it is most common among HIV-infected patients who are injection drug users.[1, 2, 49] Although the rate of bacterial pneumonia increases as the CD4 cell count decreases, bacteria are still the most likely cause of pneumonia in a patient with HIV infection and a high CD4 cell count.[49] In particular, pneumococcal pneumonia often occurs in a patient who has no history of opportunistic infection.

Although many pathogens are responsible for bacterial pneumonia, common ones include *S. pneumoniae, S. aureus, H. influenzae,* and gram-negative organisms, predominantly *Klebsiella* and *Pseudomonas.*[49] Pneumococcal pneumonia is typically manifested acutely in a manner similar to that in healthy hosts: fever, cough, chills, dyspnea and pleuritic chest pain with localized segmental, lobar, or multilobar consolidation. Pneumococcal bacteremia is more common in patients with HIV infection, and the diagnosis can be made by blood culture in about 60% of patients.[50] Although pneumococcal pneumonia can be characterized by interstitial infiltrates, *H. influenzae* pneumonia is more likely than pneumococcal pneumonia to resemble *Pneumocystis* pneumonia.[50] *P. aeruginosa* infection is an important and often community-acquired pathogen that is associated with advanced HIV disease; because it requires an antibiotic approach that differs from that for conventional community-acquired pathogens, it has an important place in the differential diagnosis of pneumonia in patients with AIDS. Pneumonia, both cavitary and noncavitary, has occurred in about one third to one half of HIV-associated *Pseudomonas* infections.[51–53] Both fulminant disease with sepsis syndrome and chronic or subacute disease have been described.[51] About half of the patients will be bacteremic, and relapse is common.[51–53] *Legionella* infection is an uncommon cause of HIV-associated pneumonia, but it should be considered, especially in cases of nosocomial pneumonia.[54]

Pulmonary nocardiosis is an uncommon diagnosis in patients with HIV infection; however, the lung is a primary target organ for nocardiosis in HIV.[55] Pulmonary nocardiosis is an acute, subacute, or chronic febrile illness with weight loss, cough, dyspnea, pleuritic chest pain, and sometimes hemoptysis. In a series of 21 patients, 82% had unilateral disease and two thirds had upper lobe disease. Although most had alveolar infiltrates, other patterns, including cavitation, were also seen. Empyema has occurred. The diagnosis is made by cultures of respiratory specimens from bronchoscopy or expectorated sputum, but growth of the organism is slow, and the observation of filamentous, beaded, branching, gram-positive, and modified acid-fast rods in respiratory specimens will speed the diagnosis.

R. equi is an important pulmonary pathogen in HIV-infected patients. Although an insidious onset of fever, cough, and chest pain plus cavitating pneumonia is typical, radiographic patterns are nonspecific and include infiltrate, pleural effusion, mass, and a normal chest radiograph.[56] Sputum, blood, bronchoalveolar lavage fluid, and tissue are useful specimens for culturing the organism. The diagnosis can be missed without a high index of suspicion because the organisms can be erroneously dismissed as insignificant normal flora or a contaminant. A pleomorphic, gram-positive coccobacillus on smear or aerobic culture should raise the question of a diagnosis of *R. equi* infection.

As with bacterial pneumonias in non-HIV–infected patients, Gram stain of expectorated sputum can provide a useful clue to the diagnosis (see Chapter 57). Culture of organisms in sputum or bronchoalveolar lavage specimens may be difficult to interpret. No specific criteria are known for the diagnosis of pneumonia from bronchoalveolar lavage fluid in patients with HIV infection, but semiquantitative cultures of lavage fluid have been used.[12]

Pneumocystis carinii Pneumonia

Pneumocystis pneumonia may have a more insidious onset in an HIV-infected patient than in others. Because the prognosis of *P. carinii* pneumonia worsens with more severe disease, early diagnosis and treatment have contributed to declines in mortality. Constitutional symptoms with fever, sweats, weight loss, fatigue, and nonproductive cough may have been present for weeks; dyspnea is at first exertional and then progresses as gas exchange is progressively impaired. Purulent sputum is not a feature of *Pneumocystis* pneumonia. A typical retrosternal discomfort on inspiration often occurs, and such discomfort can be the first symptom that a patient with prior *Pneumocystis* pneumonia recognizes as indicative of recurrence. Severe or pleuritic chest pain is uncommon. The chest examination is most often normal, although full inspiration may be inhibited. Although a bilateral diffuse interstitial infiltrate is the most frequent chest radiographic abnormality (occurring in about 80% of patients), abnormalities of all kinds have been described, including alveolar infiltrates, focal infiltrates, pleural effusions, nodules, atelectasis, cystic lesions, cavities, honeycombing, pneumatoceles, blebs, bullae, and in a significant number of patients with early disease, a normal chest radiograph[16, 25, 43] (Fig. 109–1). Upper lobe disease is more common in patients receiving aerosolized pentamidine prophylaxis, presumably because of the pattern of pulmonary disposition of the aerosol.[43] There is no assurance that any radiographic abnormality in a patient with HIV disease is not caused by this pathogen. In addition, *P. carinii* is commonly present with other pathogens, which further confuses its potential clinical manifestations.

The diagnosis of *Pneumocystis* pneumonia is made by examination of a respiratory specimen for cyst or trophozoite forms. Techniques vary according to the preference and expertise of the institution, but they include silver, Diff-Quik, toluidine blue O, and direct immunofluorescent antibody stains. A finding of *P. carinii* in a sputum or bronchoalveolar lavage specimen can be considered diagnostic of *Pneumocystis* pneumonia because true colonization with *P. carinii* has not been documented; however, the organism has been shown to persist for weeks after completion of successful treatment in some patients.[20] Polymerase chain reaction (PCR)-based tests are not yet widely available, although work on a PCR-based test of induced sputum and other specimens is ongoing.[57] PCR may offer no advantage in lavage specimens. No culture method is useful for detecting the organism.

Other Fungal Diseases

Although aspergillosis was removed from the list of AIDS-defining illnesses by the Centers for Disease Control and Prevention (CDC) after very few cases were reported, aspergillosis is now recognized as a significant problem in patients with advanced AIDS. It is generally seen in patients with very low CD4 cell counts and often, but not always, in the setting of neutropenia or high-dose corticosteroid therapy. The spectrum includes colonization, aspergilloma, invasive pulmonary aspergillosis, and tracheobronchial disease consisting of obstructing bronchial aspergillosis or pseudomembranous, ulcerative, and/or plaque-like bronchial aspergillosis.[58–60] Invasive pulmonary disease is characterized by fever and cough, usually nonproductive, by dyspnea, and by chest pain that is usually pleuritic. Hemoptysis is uncommon. In tracheobronchial disease, patients present with cough, at times with dyspnea, chest pain, or wheezing. In some cases of tracheobronchial disease, fungal casts are coughed up. In others, the diagnosis is established by the finding of fungal casts, mucoid impaction, pseudomembranes, mucosal inflammation with plaques, or ulceration at bronchoscopy.[58, 59] Endobronchial biopsies may show inflammation and invasive hyphal elements. About half of patients with tracheobronchial disease will have parenchymal lung involvement, and about 25% of cases of tracheobronchial disease are associated with disseminated disease.[58]

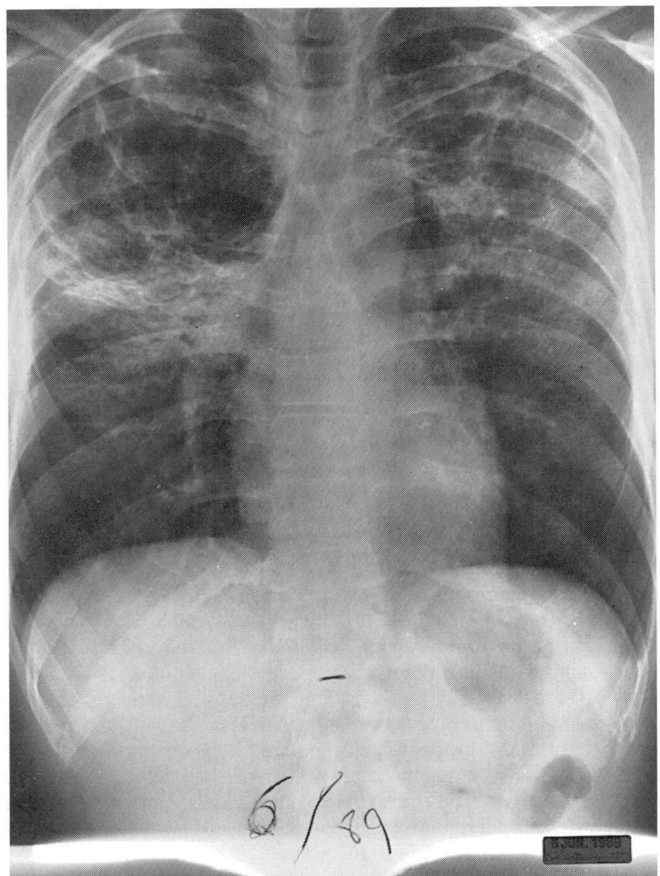

FIGURE 109–1. Chest radiograph in a patient with acute *Pneumocystis* pneumonia and multiple pulmonary cysts.

Chest radiographs in AIDS-associated pulmonary aspergillosis can show upper lobe thick- or thin-walled cavities, nodules, pleural-based lesions, and localized or diffuse infiltrates, particularly of the lower lobes, but radiographs are sometimes normal in patients with tracheobronchial disease. In invasive disease, transbronchial biopsy may be negative, but *Aspergillus* (most commonly *Aspergillus fumigatus*) is usually grown from bronchoalveolar lavage fluid. Because the recovery of *Aspergillus* species from respiratory specimens in the absence of aspergillosis represents disease in a minority of cases (11% in one series),[61] histopathologic evidence for tissue invasion with isolation is the gold standard for diagnosis. The organism is almost never grown from blood specimens.

Histoplasmosis most commonly occurs in endemic areas but can occur in patients who have moved from endemic to nonendemic areas. Most HIV-infected patients with histoplasmosis present with disseminated disease, and most patients with disseminated disease have advanced HIV disease.[62–64] Patients present with fever, weight loss, cough, and dyspnea. Pulmonary involvement is usually present in disseminated disease. Although the lungs may be involved despite normal chest radiographs, diffuse interstitial or reticulonodular infiltrates are commonly present.

Visualization of the organism on smear or detection by culture is diagnostic. Occasionally, *Histoplasma* is confused with *Pneumocystis* in tissue or on smears. In one study of 27 patients with AIDS and histoplasmosis, the organism was demonstrated by fungal stain of bronchoalveolar lavage fluid in 70% of patients and it was cultured from lavage fluid in 89% of patients, but weeks can elapse before a diagnosis is made by culture.[64] A test for *Histoplasma capsulatum* polysaccharide antigen provides a rapid diagnosis. Antigen has been detected in 93% of urine specimens, 89% of serum specimens, and 70% of unconcentrated bronchoalveolar fluid specimens from infected patients.[64] Although specificity is high, cross-reactions have occurred in patients with other mycoses. *Histoplasma* can also be cultured from blood, particularly if the lysis centrifugation system is used. Ninety-one percent of patients were culture positive by lysis centrifugation in one institution.[63] In fewer than one third of patients the organism can be seen on a carefully examined peripheral or buffy coat smear, which is a very rapid and noninvasive means of diagnosis.[62, 64] Extrapulmonary disease may be very prominent, and sepsis syndrome occurs.[63] Serologic analysis has limited diagnostic value.[63]

Pulmonary cryptococcosis is manifested primarily by cough and fever, and most but not all patients have diffuse interstitial abnormalities on chest radiographs[65] (Fig. 109–2). Demonstration of the organism by smear or culture in sputum or, more commonly, in bronchoalveolar lavage fluid generally provides the diagnosis. Culture is more sensitive than smear.[66] Extrapulmonary disease is common; thus, blood, urine, and cerebrospinal fluid examinations have also provided

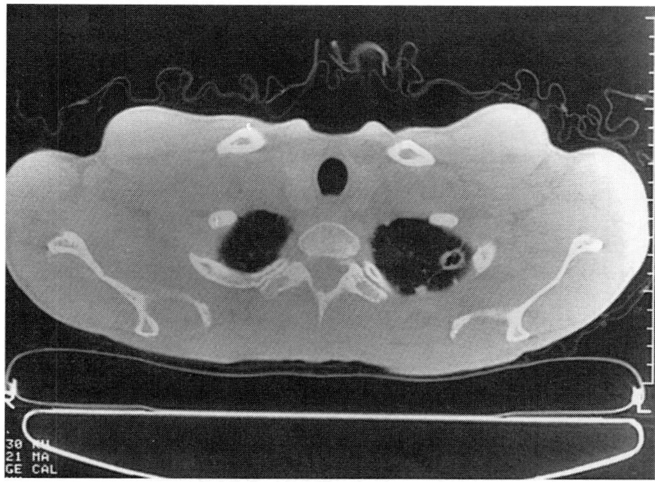

FIGURE 109–2. Chest computed tomography scan in a patient with an apical cavitary lesion caused by *Cryptococcus*. The diagnosis was made by observing yeast forms on bronchoalveolar lavage with confirmation by culture. (Courtesy Dr. Kirk Miller, National Institute of Allergy and Infectious Diseases, Bethesda MD 20892. From Miller KD, Mican JM, Davey RT. Asymptomatic solitary pulmonary nodules due to *Cryptococcus neoformans* in patients infected with human immunodeficiency virus. Clin Infect Dis. 1996;23:810–812.)

diagnoses, and these specimens should be obtained. Cryptococcal antigen in blood can be negative in patients with pulmonary disease, especially in the absence of meningitis.[37, 65, 66] Cryptococcal antigen testing of bronchoalveolar lavage and pleural fluid has been reported to be useful with high sensitivity, but the method is not standardized.[66]

Coccidioides immitis is a rare cause of HIV-associated pulmonary disease except in endemic areas.[67] The lung is the most frequent site of involvement, and fever, weight loss, and cough are the most common initial symptoms. Diffuse reticulonodular pulmonary infiltrates are present in one half to two thirds of patients with advanced HIV disease, but focal disease and a normal chest radiograph also occur.[67] The organism is seen on cytologic specimens in most sputum, bronchoalveolar lavage, and transbronchial biopsy samples, and cultures of respiratory specimens are also usually diagnostic. Blood cultures are infrequently (12%) positive.[68] Coccidioidal serologic studies were negative in 23% of patients in one report.[67] Evidence of prior infection as detected by reaction to spherulin skin testing was not predictive of the development of disease in one study, but the median follow-up was less than 1 year.[69] The diagnostic laboratory culturing specimens should be warned if coccidioidomycosis is suspected because the organism is a laboratory hazard.

Blastomycosis is an uncommon infection in patients with AIDS. In one series of 15 cases identified in 10 institutions, all patients had lived in an area endemic for *Blastomyces dermatitidis,* but one third of the infections were diagnosed in regions where blastomycosis is uncommon.[70] Eighty percent of the patients had pulmonary disease at the initial evaluation. Symptoms in these patients with pulmonary disease included fever, weight loss, and cough; almost all had CD4 cell counts below 200 cells/μl. In seven of the patients, the disease was limited to the lungs and pleura. Chest radiographs were abnormal but nonspecific; focal lobar, diffuse interstitial, bilateral nodular, cavitary, and pleural disease was seen.[70] Smear and culture of bronchoscopic specimens represent a common means of diagnosis. Serologic analysis is not useful, and no antigen testing is available, although limited data suggest cross-reactivity with *Histoplasma* antigen on testing.

Candida pneumonitis is rare, and the diagnosis should not be made in the absence of tissue invasion seen on a biopsy specimen. Because oral thrush is common, identification of *Candida* species on smear or culture of respiratory specimens is nonspecific and not useful for diagnosis. The diagnosis is difficult to establish. In an autopsy series, *Candida* pneumonitis was not diagnosed in four of four patients antemortem.[71]

P. marneffei is an important opportunistic infection in certain parts of Southeast Asia and China.[72] Disseminated disease with skin lesions is common, but about half of affected patients have cough. Chest radiographs show densities, abscesses, and cavities. The diagnosis is made by observing or culturing the organism from a number of specimens, most commonly skin and blood, but respiratory specimens are also used. Care must be taken to differentiate *P. marneffei* from *H. capsulatum,* another intracellular pathogen.

Mycobacterial Diseases

HIV infection is an important risk factor for the development of tuberculosis. Both an increased risk of reactivation of latent infection and an increased risk of clinical disease soon after infection occur.[7] Tuberculosis usually occurs without preexisting opportunistic infection.[73] Fever, weight loss, other constitutional symptoms, and cough, although nonspecific, should raise the question of tuberculosis. The diagnosis can be obscured by the frequency of atypical clinical and radiographic findings and overlap with other AIDS-associated infections, the likelihood of anergy on tuberculin testing, and the increased likelihood of a negative acid-fast smear of sputum. Because the diagnosis can be elusive and delayed diagnosis contributes to morbidity, mortality, and spread of disease, rapid evaluation for the purpose of substantiation or exclusion of the diagnosis should be undertaken in most patients with HIV-associated pulmonary disease. Empirical therapy may be needed while awaiting confirmation of the diagnosis.

Knowledge of the CD4 cell count of the patient is useful in considering tuberculosis: upper lobe disease and cavitation are associated with a higher CD4 cell count, and lower lobe infiltrates, miliary patterns, and mediastinal or hilar adenopathy are associated with a lower CD4 cell count.[44] Adenopathy, pleural effusion, or cavitation is an important clue to the diagnosis because they are rare in *Pneumocystis* pneumonia. Alveolar infiltrates suggestive of bacterial pneumonia, diffuse infiltrates mimicking *Pneumocystis* pneumonia, and normal chest radiographs occur. Acid-fast organisms are found on sputum smear in 40 to 67% of patients with HIV-associated tuberculosis, and sputum culture is positive in 74 to 95%.[7] The likelihood that a sputum sample will be smear positive for acid-fast bacilli decreases with decreasing CD4 cell counts, and a negative smear is more common with a normal chest radiograph.[7, 44] The presence of acid-fast organisms on a smear has a high positive predictive value for the diagnosis of tuberculosis even in areas where tuberculosis is less common, but patients with other mycobacterial infections, including MAC infection, can also have positive smears.[74] In general, smear-positive sputa should be considered more likely to be *M. tuberculosis* than MAC, a policy that would result in rapid treatment and infection-control measures for those who ultimately prove to have tuberculosis. Although HIV-infected patients have a significant (>25%) incidence of mycobacteremia, especially if the disease is disseminated, fewer are mycobacteremic in the setting of pulmonary but not disseminated disease.[7] Patients with more advanced HIV disease are more likely to have disseminated tuberculosis and mycobacteremia. In patients with smear-negative sputa, half or more of cases can be diagnosed by bronchoscopy. In this situation, transbronchial biopsy significantly contributes to the yield of the procedure. Pleural fluid smears are low yield, but pleural biopsy is diagnostic half the time.[7] Endobronchial needle aspiration of enlarged intrathoracic lymph nodes during bronchoscopy also produces specimens for diagnosis.

The newest tests used in the diagnosis of tuberculosis are those involving direct amplification of the nucleic acids of *M. tuberculosis*.[75, 76] The licensed tests are approved for use only in smear-positive specimens, where they provide a rapid clue to the likelihood that the organism is or is not *M. tuberculosis.* Although not approved, they are sometimes used in smear-negative specimens because of added sensitivity; however, a negative test does not exclude tuberculosis. Their interpretation in specimens from patients with HIV disease is still being assessed, but an understanding of the limitations of the tests, including the possibility of both false positives and false negatives, makes them very useful. Cultures are still needed for confirmation and susceptibility testing and because of the potential for mixed mycobacterial infections. Recent developments in culture systems and the use of nucleic acid hybridization assays for the identification of mycobacteria in culture have significantly decreased the time to grow and identify mycobacteria.[7]

Although sputum isolation of MAC is common, MAC-associated pulmonary disease in AIDS is rare.[77, 78] MAC isolated from sputum indicates an increased and substantial risk for the development of MAC bacteremia in a patient with a CD4 cell count below 50 cells/μl, but it is not diagnostic of pulmonary disease and does not in itself warrant treatment.[79] Criteria for the diagnosis of pulmonary disease caused by MAC in HIV infection are not well established, but for the diagnosis to be considered, patients should have MAC grown repeatedly from respiratory tract specimens, an infiltrate on chest radiograph, absence of other lung pathogens, and preferably biopsy specimens showing acid-fast organisms in abnormal lung tissue. Not all patients with MAC pneumonia will have disseminated MAC or MAC bacteremia. Endobronchial mass lesions caused by MAC have also been described.[80]

Of the nontuberculous mycobacteria, *M. kansasii* is the most important pulmonary pathogen in HIV disease. Patients have low CD4 cell counts (medians have been less than 50 cells/μl) and present with cough that is usually productive and constitutional symptoms of fever and weight loss.[81, 82] Dyspnea, chest pain, and hemoptysis occur. Radiographic abnormalities include interstitial or lobar infiltrates, cavities, hilar adenopathy, and nodules, but the chest radiograph is nonspecific. Because it is rarely attributable to colonization or contaminants, recovery of *M. kansasii* from respiratory specimens is usually diagnostic of pulmonary disease. Many patients will have no extrapulmonary involvement, so the diagnosis usually is made from respiratory tract specimens.[81]

Mycobacterium xenopi, Mycobacterium simiae, Mycobacterium scrofulaceum, and *Mycobacterium haemophilum* are unusual causes of HIV-associated pulmonary disease (see Chapter 243).

Viral Diseases

Upper respiratory tract illness and acute bronchitis are more common in HIV-infected patients, but influenza syndrome is not.[1, 2] Potential viral pathogens are sometimes isolated from respiratory specimens, and their significance can be difficult to determine. Although serious respiratory viral infections have been reported in patients with HIV infection, they appear to be uncommon. Because determining the significance of a cultured virus can be difficult, both isolation and confirmatory histopathology are used for diagnosis. The detection of influenza in a respiratory specimen indicates that it is the cause of respiratory disease, but such is not true for CMV or herpes simplex, where most isolates are not the causative agents of pulmonary disease. Other viruses reported to have been isolated from bronchoalveolar lavage specimens from patients with HIV infection include parainfluenza viruses, rhinoviruses, adenoviruses, and respiratory syncytial virus.[83]

Despite the fact that most isolates of CMV do not represent significant pulmonary disease, CMV is the most important AIDS-associated viral pulmonary pathogen. CMV pulmonary disease is a very late event in the course of HIV disease. Unfortunately, it is difficult to diagnose and the diagnosis can be missed. In one autopsy series, CMV was the most prevalent pulmonary pathogen, and 16 of 21 patients with significant CMV disease at autopsy did not have CMV disease diagnosed in life despite extensive evaluations for the disease in some.[71] In another 23 patients in this study, however, CMV inclusions were present but rare, and little inflammation was associated with the inclusions. These lesions were believed to be clinically insignificant. Thus, the clinician is left with a diagnostic dilemma. CMV pneumonitis cannot be distinguished from other entities on clinical grounds alone, but isolation of CMV from bronchoalveolar lavage specimens is common (>50%) and not diagnostic. Although the prognostic significance of CMV cultured from or detected in lavage fluid has been debated, it is not associated with an early diagnosis of CMV pneumonia.[84] Thus, pneumonia has to be defined by cytologic or histopathologic criteria.

Studies vary in their definition of CMV pneumonia. The most convincing diagnoses occur in the setting of clinical and radiographic evidence of pneumonia. Criteria include detection of CMV, absence of other pathogens, and confirmatory histopathology, preferably with both multiple CMV inclusions and associated inflammation. Criteria as rigid as these are likely to result in underdiagnosis because the disease can be patchy and it can occur in the presence of other pathogens. Neither CMV blood cultures nor serologic analysis adds to the diagnosis of CMV pneumonia. Isolation of CMV from lavage fluid should prompt a continued search for an etiology rather than the automatic use of anti-CMV agents.

Given the limitations in defining CMV pneumonia, case series also have their limitations. In one series, CMV pneumonia was diagnosed in 17 patients (8% of those who had undergone bronchoscopy) on the basis of infiltrates, CMV cultured from a bronchoscopy specimen, and CMV inclusions in tissue, with accompanying inflammation in all but 2 patients.[85] Symptoms included fever, shortness of breath, cough, and hypoxemia developing over days to weeks. Chest radiographs showed interstitial and alveolar infiltrates, generally bilateral, but eight of the patients had another concurrent pulmonary diagnosis. Most of them also had extrapulmonary CMV disease. In another retrospective study, CMV pneumonia was defined as inclusions in biopsy specimens in the absence of other pathogens.[86] Two percent of biopsy specimens met this definition. One third of the biopsies did not have accompanying inflammation. Patients had cough and dyspnea present for less than a month. Chest radiographs were normal in one third of patients; the others had an assortment of abnormalities, most of which were bilateral. Small pleural effusions were common. Half of the patients had extrapulmonary CMV disease.

The decision to treat for CMV pneumonia should be based on the aforementioned clinical and laboratory information in an individual patient and should take into account the limitations of data that are available from published reports (see Chapter 127).

Protozoan Diseases

Pulmonary toxoplasmosis has been more commonly reported in France than in the United States. In a review of 64 French cases, 39 patients had isolated pulmonary toxoplasmosis.[87] CD4 cell counts were below 50 cells/μl in 70%. Patients presented with fever, cough, dyspnea, and sometimes septic shock. Chest radiographs most frequently showed bilateral interstitial infiltrates, but nodules, pleural effusion, and a normal chest radiograph were also seen. Because it resembles *Pneumocystis* pneumonia, the diagnosis will be missed unless appropriate diagnostic techniques are performed. The diagnosis can be made by observation of tachyzoites on Giemsa stain or by indirect immunofluorescence assay performed on a bronchoalveolar lavage specimen, but in 11% of the patients, these tests were negative and the diagnosis was made by tissue culture or mouse inoculation, techniques that are not widely available.[87] An investigational PCR assay was also used. In 16 of 17 patients in whom peripheral blood buffy coat cells were examined, *Toxoplasma gondii* was observed. Almost all patients were seropositive for *T. gondii,* but seropositivity is not specific for the presence of disease associated with *T. gondii.*

Malignant and Noninfectious Causes of Pulmonary Disease

Pulmonary Kaposi's sarcoma, which can involve the tracheobronchial tree, lung parenchyma, and pleura, can be a difficult diagnosis to make. Although most patients have mucocutaneous disease that brings the diagnosis to mind, 16% of patients in a series of 168 cases had no mucocutaneous involvement.[88] Symptoms are nonspecific, mostly cough, dyspnea, and fever, but patients can be asymptomatic. Most patients have CD4 cell counts below 50 cells/μl. The major clue comes in its radiographic findings, where nodules and bronchial wall thickening often with extensive perihilar coalescence, air bronchograms, or both are seen. These findings can be accompanied by Kerley B lines and pleural effusions. Middle and lower lung zone abnormalities predominate.[88] Diffuse or upper lung zone involvement suggests a concomitant diagnosis, for example, *Pneumocystis* pneumonia. A typical CT scan shows bilateral perihilar infiltrates with soft tissue densities extending along perivascular and peribronchial pathways, sometimes with confluence[89] (Fig. 109–3). An experienced radiologist may suggest the diagnosis from characteristic radiographic findings; however, radiographic features can be variable.

Characteristic architecture rather than a specific cell type is needed for the diagnosis, and small pieces of tissue can result in both false-negative and false-positive interpretations. Crush artifact, hemorrhage, and other diagnoses can be misread as Kaposi's sarcoma. Thus, unequivocal tissue diagnosis requires a large tissue specimen that has not been crushed by biopsy forceps, and transbronchial biopsy is not usually sufficient.[90] Because of a desire to avoid highly invasive procedures such as an open lung biopsy, the diagnosis is generally considered confirmed when the bronchoscopist observes characteristic endobronchial erythematous or violaceous macules or papules consistent with Kaposi's sarcoma. These lesions are not usually biopsied because of low yield, risk of hemorrhage, and the difficulty of interpretation in the presence of crush artifact. Bronchoalveolar lavage is indicated to exclude concomitant pathogens. If an effusion is present, thoracenteses generally produce hemorrhagic fluid, but cytologic analysis is not diagnostic.[90]

HIV-associated pulmonary lymphoma can be manifested as infiltrates, masses, or nodules (Fig. 109–4). Bronchoalveolar lavage with cytology is not adequate for diagnosis. Transbronchial biopsy or open lung biopsy is generally needed unless the pleural fluid is diagnostic, although the diagnosis can sometimes be made by fine-needle aspiration.[91] In one series of 38 patients with non-Hodgkin's lymphoma and HIV infection, bronchoalveolar lavage and brushings did not provide a single diagnosis, and fine-needle aspiration was diagnostic in only 2 of 9 patients, whereas transbronchial biopsy, pleural cytology, and open lung biopsy were each diagnostic in over 50% of cases.[91]

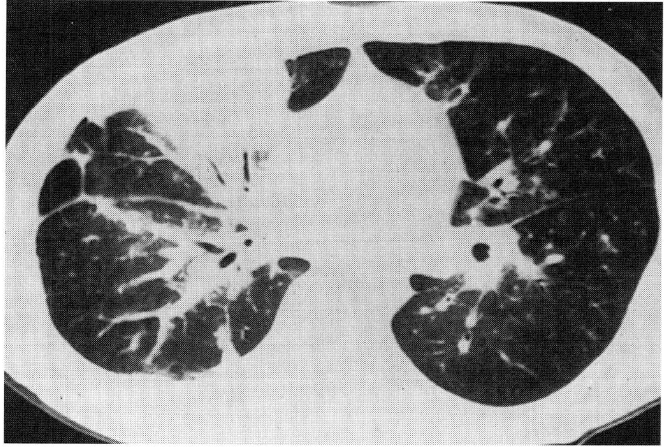

FIGURE 109–3. Computed tomography scan of the chest in a patient with pulmonary Kaposi's sarcoma. The peribronchovascular distribution of the infiltrate suggests the diagnosis. This patient also had dense consolidation of the right middle lobe caused by Kaposi's sarcoma. (Courtesy of Drs. Kirk Miller and Irwin Feuerstein. From Miller KD, Walker RE. A practical approach for diagnosing AIDS-associated pulmonary disease. The AIDS Reader. 1996. March/April; 58–65.)

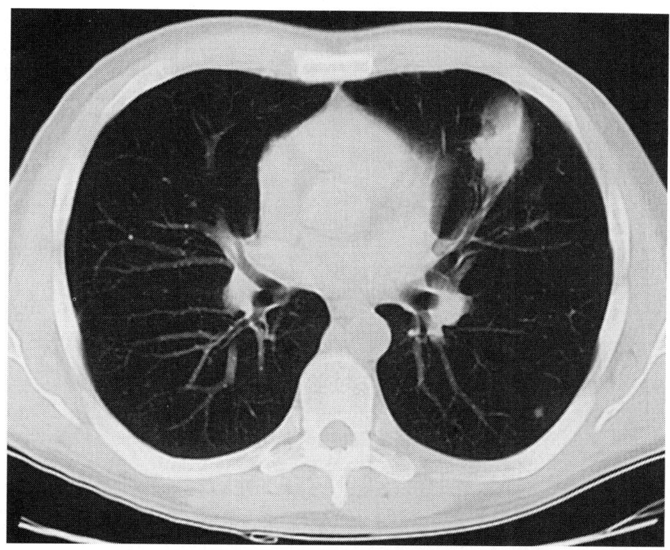

FIGURE 109–4. Chest computed tomography scan in a patient with diffuse large B-cell lymphoma of the lung that was diagnosed by open lung biopsy after the diagnosis was not obtained by transthoracic needle aspiration and bronchoscopy.

Nonspecific interstitial pneumonitis is a poorly understood entity diagnosed on either transbronchial or open lung biopsy specimens by histopathologic criteria.[92] The characteristic lesion is a mild to moderate interstitial mononuclear cell infiltrate that can be associated with interstitial edema, type II pneumocyte hyperplasia, increased alveolar macrophages, and nodular lymphoid aggregates.[92, 93] It occurred in 5% of patients given a presumptive diagnosis of *Pneumocystis* pneumonia on clinical grounds who subsequently underwent biopsy.[16] These patients had fever, cough, and dyspnea similar to the patients proved to have *Pneumocystis* pneumonia, but they had higher mean CD4 cell counts (492 versus 57 cells/μl) and less extensive pulmonary infiltrates. Patients with nonspecific interstitial pneumonitis improved spontaneously without treatment within about 1 week. The natural history has not been determined, but others have also noted spontaneous improvement without treatment. Nonspecific interstitial pneumonitis also occurs in asymptomatic patients. In one study in which 23 asymptomatic patients underwent transbronchial biopsy for research, almost half had nonspecific interstitial pneumonitis on biopsy.[23] Further research is needed to clarify the etiology, pathogenesis, and natural history of this lesion.

Other AIDS-associated pulmonary diseases are uncommon. Lymphocytic interstitial pneumonitis is a very rare diagnosis in HIV-infected adults, although it is more common in HIV-infected children.[93] It is a histopathologic diagnosis; thus, a tissue specimen is required, but a transbronchial biopsy is usually too small. Bronchiolitis obliterans with organizing pneumonia is also a histopathologic diagnosis.[94] It represents lung tissue response to a variety of insults and is typically manifested as multifocal alveolar opacities or nodular infiltrates. Other entities that affect the lung in AIDS include emphysema-like disease, pulmonary hypertension, pulmonary edema, and strongyloidiasis.[45, 46, 95] Pulmonary embolism is an important consideration in the differential diagnosis because of the potential for serious consequences if the diagnosis is missed. Pulmonary hemorrhage can complicate a variety of pulmonary lesions, and a search for an etiology should be made. In a review of almost 3000 hospitalized patients with HIV infection, hemoptysis occurred in less than 2%, and it had an infectious etiology in 80% of these patients.[96] Most episodes were caused by bacterial pneumonia. Kaposi's sarcoma was a rare cause.

PREVENTION

Patients must be aware of their HIV infection and receiving medical care to access preventive measures; thus, all health care workers must take advantage of opportunities for counseling and testing. Once identified, patients should be counseled about settings that might increase their risk of exposure to pulmonary pathogens such as *M. tuberculosis, Cryptococcus, Coccidioides,* or *Histoplasma,* and appropriate infection-control measures to diminish the spread of pathogens such as *M. tuberculosis* should be implemented.[5, 11, 13] Although the person-to-person transmissibility of *P. carinii* is not clear, isolating patients with HIV infection from others with acute *Pneumocystis* infection is not standard practice,[5] although advocated by some. Patients should not smoke cigarettes, and smoking cessation support should be offered as needed.[49] Annual influenza vaccine should be administered.[5] Patients latently infected with *M. tuberculosis* have an extraordinary risk of reactivation, but this risk can be reduced by preventive therapy. Thus, purified protein derivative–tuberculin skin testing should be conducted and prophylaxis administered according to CDC recommendations.[97] Yearly repeat testing should be considered for those who were initially negative and who belong to populations at risk for exposure to *M. tuberculosis.*[5] Pneumococcal vaccine should be administered as early in the course of HIV disease as possible to maximize antibody response.[5, 11, 98] The 23 vaccine serotypes account for almost 90% of strains isolated from HIV-infected patients.[50] *H. influenzae* type b vaccine is not routinely recommended for adults. Although the risk of invasive *H. influenzae* infection is increased in patients infected with HIV, it is still uncommon, and most of these infections are caused by non–type b strains, for which the vaccine would be ineffective.[98]

Although HIV can be grown from pulmonary specimens, no evidence of direct pathogenic consequences has emerged. Nonetheless, appropriate antiretroviral therapy and control of viral replication are key methods of prevention of pulmonary disease through their role in improving or maintaining immunologic function. Whether patients whose CD4 cell counts have risen from low to high values experience substantial reconstitution of their immune repertoire in response to antiretroviral therapy remains to be seen. Thus, although rates of hospitalization and opportunistic infection are declining and some data suggest immune reconstitution, experts recommend that prophylaxis be initiated and continued according to the patient's nadir CD4 cell count.[5, 11] Clinical trials are ongoing, and this recommendation may change.[8] For now, anti-*Pneumocystis* prophylaxis should be administered to all patients with a history of *Pneumocystis* pneumonia or with CD4 cell counts below 200/μl. In addition, patients with symptoms such as recurrent thrush or prior opportunistic infection are at increased risk and should receive prophylaxis despite higher CD4 counts.[5] Prophylaxis is most often omitted because of lack of knowledge of risk, and nonwhites and the uninsured are less likely to receive needed prophylaxis.[9, 10] Trimethoprim-sulfamethoxazole is the drug of choice for anti-*Pneumocystis* prophylaxis, and it provides an added benefit in reducing cases of bacterial pneumonia and toxoplasmosis.[5, 49] Because breakthrough disease is more common in patients treated by regimens other than trimethoprim-sulfamethoxazole, patients should not be labeled trimethoprim-sulfamethoxazole intolerant without considerable supporting data.

Patients with a CD4 lymphocyte count that has been below 50 cells/μl should receive chemoprophylaxis against MAC disease with either clarithromycin or azithromycin.[5] These drugs have added benefit in preventing bacterial respiratory infections. Although antifungal prophylaxis can reduce the frequency of cryptococcosis and histoplasmosis among patients with advanced HIV disease, it is not generally recommended because these diseases are uncommon and it has not been proved that antifungal prophylaxis improves survival. Widespread use of antifungal agents is also likely to contribute to the increasing problem of antifungal drug resistance. These drugs are costly, can result in drug-drug interactions, and have potential toxicity.[5]

Although neutropenia probably increases the risk of pulmonary infection, the role of colony-stimulating factors in preventing infections in HIV-infected patients is not defined, although they are widely used.[11, 99]

REFERENCES

1. Wallace JM, Rao AV, Glassroth J, et al. Respiratory illness in persons with human immunodeficiency virus infection. Am Rev Respir Dis. 1993;148:1523–1529.
2. Wallace JM, Hansen NI, Lavange L, et al. Respiratory disease trends in the pulmonary complications of HIV infection study cohort. Am J Respir Crit Care Med. 1997;155:72–80.
3. Selik RM, Chu SY, Ward JW. Trends in infectious diseases and cancers among persons dying of HIV infection in the United States from 1987 to 1992. Ann Intern Med. 1995;123:933–936.
4. Centers for Disease Control and Prevention. Update: Trends in AIDS incidence, deaths, and prevalence—United States, 1996. MMWR Morb Mortal Wkly Rep. 1997;46:165–172.
5. USPHS/IDSA Prevention of Opportunistic Infections Working Group. 1997 USPHS/IDSA guidelines for the prevention of opportunistic infections in persons infected with human immunodeficiency virus: Disease-specific recommendations. Clin Infect Dis. 1997;25(Suppl):S313–S334. This is also published in MMWR Morb Mortal Wkly Rep. 1997;46(RR-12):1–46.
6. Moore RD, Chaisson RE. Natural history of opportunistic disease in an HIV-infected urban clinical cohort. Ann Intern Med. 1996;124:633–642.
7. Shafer RW, Edlin BR. Tuberculosis in patients infected with human immunodeficiency virus: Perspective on the past decade. Clin Infect Dis. 1996;22:683–704.
8. Sepkowitz KA. Effect of HAART on natural history of AIDS-related opportunistic disorder. Lancet. 1998;351:228–230.
9. Gallant JE, McAvinue SM, Moore RD, et al. The impact of prophylaxis on outcome and resource utilization in *Pneumocystis carinii* pneumonia. Chest. 1995;107:1018–1023.
10. Schwarcz SK, Katz MH, Hirozawa A, et al. Prevention of *Pneumocystis carinii* pneumonia: Who are we missing? AIDS. 1997;11:1263–1268.
11. USPHS/IDSA Prevention of Opportunistic Infections Working Group. Preface to the 1997 USPHS/IDSA guidelines for the prevention of opportunistic infections in persons infected with human immunodeficiency virus. Clin Infect Dis. 1997; 25(Suppl):S299–S312.
12. Baughman RP, Dohn MN, Frame PT. The continuing utility of bronchoalveolar lavage to diagnose opportunistic infection in AIDS patients. Am J Med. 1994;97:515–522.
13. Centers for Disease Control. Guidelines for preventing the transmission of tuberculosis in health-care settings, with special focus on HIV-related issues. MMWR Morb Mortal Wkly Rep. 1990;39(RR-17):1–29.
14. Masur H, Shelhamer J. Empiric outpatient management of HIV-related pneumonia: Economical or unwise? Ann Intern Med. 1996;124:451–453.
15. Smith DE, Forbes A, Davies S, et al. Diagnosis of *Pneumocystis carinii* pneumonia in HIV antibody positive patients by simple outpatient assessments. Thorax. 1992;47:1005–1009.
16. Sattler F, Nichols L, Hirano L, et al. Nonspecific interstitial pneumonitis mimicking *Pneumocystis carinii* pneumonia. Am J Respir Crit Care Med. 1997;156:912–917.
17. Tu JV, Biem HJ, Detsky AS. Bronchoscopy versus empirical therapy in HIV-infected patients with presumptive *Pneumocystis carinii* pneumonia: A decision analysis. Am Rev Respir Dis. 1993;148:370–377.
18. Horner RD, Bennett CL, Rodriguez D, et al. Relationship between procedures and health insurance for critically ill patients with *Pneumocystis carinii* pneumonia. Am J Respir Crit Care Med. 1995;152:1435–1442.
19. De Gracia J, Miravitlles M, Mayordomo C, et al. Empiric treatments impair the diagnostic yield of BAL in HIV-positive patients. Chest. 1997;111:1180–1186.
20. Roger PM, Vandenbos F, Pugliese P, et al. Persistence of *Pneumocystis carinii* after effective treatment of *P. carinii* pneumonia is not related to relapse or survival among patients infected with human immunodeficiency virus. Clin Infect Dis. 1998;26:509–510.
21. Chouaid C, Housset B, Lebeau B. Cost-analysis of four diagnostic strategies for *Pneumocystis carinii* pneumonia in HIV-infected subjects. Eur Respir J. 1995;8:1554–1558.
22. Kvale PA, Rosen MJ, Hopewell PC, et al. A decline in the pulmonary diffusing capacity does not indicate opportunistic lung disease in asymptomatic persons infected with the human immunodeficiency virus. Am Rev Respir Dis. 1993;148:390–395.
23. Ognibene FP, Masur H, Rogers P, et al. Nonspecific interstitial pneumonitis without evidence of *Pneumocystis carinii* in asymptomatic patients infected with human immunodeficiency virus (HIV). Ann Intern Med. 1988;109:874–879.
24. Gruden JF, Huang L, Turner J, et al. High-resolution CT in the evaluation of clinically suspected *Pneumocystis carinii* pneumonia in AIDS patient with normal,

equivocal, or nonspecific radiographic findings. AJR Am J Roentgenol. 1997;169:967–975.

25. Opravil M, Marincek B, Fuchs WA, et al. Shortcomings of chest radiography in detecting *Pneumocystis carinii* pneumonia. J Acquir Immun Defic Syndr. 1993;7:39–45.
26. Kovacs JA, Ng VL, Masur H, et al. Diagnosis of *Pneumocystis carinii* pneumonia: Improved detection in sputum with use of monoclonal antibodies. N Engl J Med. 1988;318:589–593.
27. Huang L, Hecht FM, Stansell JD, et al. Suspected *Pneumocystis carinii* pneumonia with a negative induced sputum examination: Is early bronchoscopy useful? Am J Respir Crit Care Med. 1995;151:1866–1871.
28. Broaddus C, Dake MD, Stulbarg MS, et al. Bronchoalveolar lavage and transbronchial biopsy for the diagnosis of pulmonary infections in the acquired immunodeficiency syndrome. Ann Intern Med. 1985;102:747–752.
29. Yung RC, Weinacker AB, Steiger DJ, et al. Upper and middle lobe bronchoalveolar lavage to diagnose *Pneumocystis carinii* pneumonia. Am Rev Respir Dis. 1993;148:1563–1566.
30. Gruden JF, Klein JS, Webb WR. Percutaneous transthoracic needle biopsy in AIDS: Analysis in 32 patients. Radiology. 1993;189:567–571.
31. Bonfils-Roberts EA, Nickodem A, Nealon TF Jr. Retrospective analysis of the efficacy of open lung biopsy in acquired immunodeficiency syndrome. Ann Thorac Surg. 1990;49:115–117.
32. Miller RF, Pugsley WB, Griffiths MH. Open lung biopsy for investigation of acute respiratory episodes in patients with HIV infection and AIDS. Genitourin Med. 1995;71:280–285.
33. Amin Z, Miller RF, Shaw PJ. Lobar or segmental consolidation on chest radiographs of patients with HIV infection. Clin Radiol. 1997;52:541–545.
34. DeLorenzo LJ, Huang CT, Maguire GP, et al. Roentgenographic patterns of *Pneumocystis carinii* pneumonia in 104 patients with AIDS. Chest. 1987;91:323–327.
35. Gallant JE, Ko AH. Cavitary pulmonary lesions in patients infected with human immunodeficiency virus. Clin Infect Dis. 1996;22:671–682.
36. Furman AC, Jacobs J, Sepkowitz KA. Lung abscess in patients with AIDS. Clin Infect Dis. 1996;22:81–85.
37. Miller KD, Mican JM, Davey RT. Asymptomatic solitary pulmonary nodules due to *Cryptococcus neoformans* in patients infected with human immunodeficiency virus. Clin Infect Dis. 1996;23:810–812.
38. Parker MS, Leveno DM, Campbell TJ, et al. AIDS-related bronchogenic carcinoma: Fact or fiction? Chest. 1998;113:154–161.
39. Martinez-Marcos FJ, Viciana P, Canas E, et al. Etiology of solitary pulmonary nodules in patients with human immunodeficiency virus infection. Clin Infect Dis. 1997;24:908–913.
40. Joseph J, Strange C, Sahn SA. Pleural effusions in hospitalized patients with AIDS. Ann Intern Med. 1993;118:856–859.
41. Ingram RJH, Call S, Andrade A, et al. Management and outcome of pneumothoraces in patients infected with human immunodeficiency virus. Clin Infect Dis. 1996;23:624–627.
42. Sepkowitz KA, Telzak EE, Gold JWM, et al. Pneumothorax in AIDS. Ann Intern Med. 1991;114:455–459.
43. Kennedy CA, Goetz MB. Atypical roentgenographic manifestations of *Pneumocystis carinii* pneumonia. Arch Intern Med. 1992;152:1390–1398.
44. Perlman DC, El-Sadr WM, Nelson ET, et al. Variation of chest radiographic patterns in pulmonary tuberculosis by degree of human immunodeficiency virus–related immunosuppression. Clin Infect Dis. 1997;25:242–246.
45. Diaz PT, Clanton TL, Pacht ER. Emphysema-like pulmonary disease associated with human immunodeficiency virus infection. Ann Intern Med. 1992;116:124–128.
46. Mesa RA, Edell ES, Dunn WF, et al. Human immunodeficiency virus infection and pulmonary hypertension: Two new cases and a review of 86 reported cases. Mayo Clin Proc. 1998;73:37–45.
47. Lowery WS, Whitlock WL, Dietrich RA, et al. Sarcoidosis complicated by HIV infection: Three case reports and a review of the literature. Am Rev Respir Dis. 1990;142:887–889.
48. Pastores SM, Naidich DP, Aranda CP, et al. Intrathoracic adenopathy associated with pulmonary tuberculosis in patients with human immunodeficiency virus infection. Chest. 1993;103:1433–1437.
49. Hirschtick RE, Glassroth J, Jordan MC, et al. Bacterial pneumonia in persons infected with the human immunodeficiency virus. N Engl J Med. 1995;333:845–851.
50. Janoff NE, Breiman RF, Daley CL, et al. Pneumococcal disease during HIV infection. Epidemiologic, clinical, and immunologic perspectives. Ann Intern Med. 1992;117:314–324.
51. Baron AD, Hollander H. *Pseudomonas aeruginosa* bronchopulmonary infection in late human immunodeficiency virus disease. Am Rev Respir Dis. 1993;148:992–996.
52. Fichtenbaum CJ, Woeltje KF, Powderly WG. Serious *Pseudomonas aeruginosa* infections in patients infected with human immunodeficiency virus: A case-control study. Clin Infect Dis. 1994;19:417–422.
53. Dropulic LK, Leslie JM, Eldred LJ, et al. Clinical manifestations and risk factors of *Pseudomonas aeruginosa* infection in patients with AIDS. J Infect Dis. 1995;171:930–937.
54. Blatt SP, Dolan MJ, Hendrix CW, et al. Legionnaires' disease in human immunodeficiency virus–infected patients: Eight cases and review. Clin Infect Dis. 1994;18:227–232.
55. Uttamchandani RB, Daikos GL, Reyes RR, et al. Nocardiosis in 30 patients with advanced human immunodeficiency virus infection: Clinical features and outcome. Clin Infect Dis. 1994;18:348–353.
56. Harvey RL, Sunstrum JC. *Rhodococcus equi* infection in patients with and without human immunodeficiency virus infection. Rev Infect Dis. 1991;13:139–145.
57. Caliendo AM, Hewitt PL, Allega JM, et al. Performance of a PCR assay for detection of *Pneumocystis carinii* from respiratory specimens. J Clin Microbiol. 1998;36:979–982.
58. Denning DW, Follansbee SE, Scolaro M, et al. Pulmonary aspergillosis in the acquired immunodeficiency syndrome. N Engl J Med. 1991;324:654–662.
59. Kemper CA, Hostetler JS, Follansbee SE, et al. Ulcerative and plaque-like tracheobronchitis due to infection with *Aspergillus* in patients with AIDS. Clin Infect Dis. 1993;17:344–352.
60. Khoo SH, Denning DW. Invasive aspergillosis in patients with AIDS. Clin Infect Dis. 1994;19(Suppl 1):S41–S48.
61. Pursell KJ, Telzak EE, Armstrong D. *Aspergillus* species colonization and invasive disease in patients with AIDS. Clin Infect Dis. 1992;14:141–148.
62. Sarosi GA, Johnson PC. Disseminated histoplasmosis in patients infected with human immunodeficiency virus. Clin Infect Dis. 1992;14(Suppl 1):S60–S67.
63. Wheat LJ, Connolly-Stringfield PA, Baker RL, et al. Disseminated histoplasmosis in the acquired immune deficiency syndrome: Clinical findings, diagnosis and treatment, and review of the literature. Medicine (Baltimore). 1990;69:361–374.
64. Wheat JL, Connolly-Stringfield P, Williams B, et al. Diagnosis of histoplasmosis in patients with the acquired immunodeficiency syndrome by detection of *Histoplasma capsulatum* polysaccharide antigen in bronchoalveolar lavage fluid. Am Rev Respir Dis. 1992;145:1421–1424.
65. Meyohas M-C, Roux P, Bollens D, et al. Pulmonary cryptococcosis: Localized and disseminated infections in 27 patients with AIDS. Clin Infect Dis. 1995;21:628–633.
66. Baughman RP, Rhodes JC, Dohn MN, et al. Detection of cryptococcal antigen in bronchoalveolar lavage fluid: A prospective study of diagnostic utility. Am Rev Respir Dis. 1992;145:1226–1229.
67. Singh VR, Smith DK, Lawerence J, et al. Coccidioidomycosis in patients infected with human immunodeficiency virus: Review of 91 cases at a single institution. Clin Infect Dis. 1996;23:563–568.
68. Galgiani JN, Ampel NM. Coccidioidomycosis in human immunodeficiency virus–infected patients. J Infect Dis. 1990;162:1165–1169.
69. Ampel NM, Dols CL, Galgiani JN. Coccidioidomycosis during human immunodeficiency virus infection: Results of a prospective study in a coccidioidal endemic area. Am J Med. 1993;94:235–240.
70. Pappas PG, Pottage JC, Powderly WG, et al. Blastomycosis in patients with the acquired immunodeficiency syndrome. Ann Intern Med. 1992;116:847–853.
71. McKenzie R, Travis WD, Dolan SD, et al. The causes of death in patients with human immunodeficiency virus infection: A clinical and pathologic study with emphasis on the role of pulmonary diseases. Medicine (Baltimore). 1991;70:326–343.
72. Duong TA. Infection due to *Penicillium marneffei,* an emerging pathogen: Review of 155 reported cases. Clin Infect Dis. 1996;23:125–130.
73. Barnes PF, Bloch AB, Davidson PT, et al. Tuberculosis in patients with human immunodeficiency virus infection. N Engl J Med. 1991;324:1644–1650.
74. Yajko DM, Nassos PS, Sanders CA, et al. High predictive value of the acid-fast smear for *Mycobacterium tuberculosis* despite the high prevalence of *Mycobacterium avium* complex in respiratory specimens. Clin Infect Dis. 1994;19:334–336.
75. Catanzaro AB, Davidsonn L, Fujiwara PI, et al. Proceedings of the American Thoracic Society Workshop, "Rapid diagnostic tests for tuberculosis. What is the appropriate use?" Am J Respir Crit Care Med. 1997;155:1804–1814.
76. Barnes PF. Rapid diagnostic tests for tuberculosis: Progress but no gold standard. Am J Respir Crit Care Med. 1997;155:1497–1498.
77. Kalayjian RC, Toossi Z, Tomashefski JF Jr, et al. Pulmonary disease due to infection by *Mycobacterium avium* complex in patients with AIDS. Clin Infect Dis. 1995;20:1186–1194.
78. Hocqueloux L, Lesprit P, Herrmann J-L, et al. Pulmonary *Mycobacterium avium* complex disease without dissemination in HIV-infected patients. Chest. 1998;113:542–548.
79. Chin DP, Hopewell PC, Yajko DM, et al. *Mycobacterium avium* complex in the respiratory or gastrointestinal tract and the risk of *M. avium* complex bacteremia in patients with human immunodeficiency virus infection. J Infect Dis. 1994;169:289–295.
80. Packer SJ, Cesario T, Williams JH Jr. *Mycobacterium avium* complex infection presenting as endobronchial lesions in immunosuppressed patients. Ann Intern Med. 1988;109:389–393.
81. Levine B, Chaisson RE. *Mycobacterium kansasii:* A cause of treatable pulmonary disease associated with advanced human immunodeficiency virus (HIV) infection. Ann Intern Med. 1991;114:861–868.
82. Campo RE, Campo CE. *Mycobacterium kansasii* disease in patients infected with human immunodeficiency virus. Clin Infect Dis. 1997;24:1233–1238.
83. Connolly MG Jr, Baughman RP, Dohn MN, et al. Recovery of viruses other than cytomegalovirus from bronchoalveolar lavage. Chest. 1994;105:1775–1781.
84. Baughman RP. Cytomegalovirus: The monster in the closet? Am J Respir Crit Care Med. 1997;156:1–2.
85. Rodriguez-Barradas M, Stool E, Musher DM, et al. Diagnosing and treating cytomegalovirus pneumonia in patients with AIDS. Clin Infect Dis. 1996;23:76–81.
86. Salomon N, Gomez T, Perlman DC, et al. Clinical features and outcome of HIV-related cytomegalovirus pneumonia. AIDS. 1997;11:319–324.
87. Rabaud C, May T, Lucet JC, et al. Pulmonary toxoplasmosis in patients infected with human immunodeficiency virus: A French national survey. Clin Infect Dis. 1996;23:1249–1254.
88. Huang L, Schnapp LM, Gruden JF, et al. Presentation of AIDS-related pulmonary Kaposi's sarcoma diagnosed by bronchoscopy. Am J Respir Crit Care Med. 1996;153:1385–1390.

89. Naidich DP, Tarras M, Garay SM, et al. Kaposi's sarcoma: CT-radiographic correlation. Chest. 1989;96:723–728.
90. Ognibene FP, Steis RG, Macher AM, et al. Kaposi's sarcoma causing pulmonary infiltrates and respiratory failure in the acquired immunodeficiency syndrome. Ann Intern Med. 1985;102:471–475.
91. Eisner MD, Kaplan LD, Herndier B, et al. The pulmonary manifestations of AIDS-related non-Hodgkin's lymphoma. Chest. 1996;110:729–736.
92. Suffredini AF, Ognibene FP, Lack EE, et al. Nonspecific interstitial pneumonitis: A common cause of pulmonary disease in the acquired immunodeficiency syndrome. Ann Intern Med 1987;107:7–13.
93. Travis WD, Fox CH, Devaney KO, et al. Lymphoid pneumonitis in 50 adult patients infected with the human immunodeficiency virus: Lymphocytic interstitial pneumonitis versus nonspecific interstitial pneumonitis. Hum Pathol. 1992;23:529–541.
94. Leo Y-S, Pitchon HE, Messler G, et al. Bronchiolitis obliterans organizing pneumonia in a patient with AIDS. Clin Infect Dis. 1994;18:921–924.
95. Celedon JC, Mathur-Wagh U, Fox J, et al. Systemic strongyloidiasis in patients infected with the human immunodeficiency virus: A report of 3 cases and review of the literature. Medicine (Baltimore). 1994;73:256–263.
96. Nelson JE, Forman M. Hemoptysis in HIV-infected patients. Chest. 1996;110:737–743.
97. Centers for Disease Control and Prevention. Anergy skin testing and preventive therapy for HIV-infected persons: Revised recommendations. MMWR Morb Mortal Wkly Rep. 1997;46(RR-15):1–10.
98. Keller DW, Breiman RF. Preventing bacterial respiratory tract infections among persons infected with human immunodeficiency virus. Clin Infect Dis. 1995;21(Suppl 1):S77–S83.
99. Meynard J-L, Guiguet M, Arsac S, et al. Frequency and risk factors of infectious complications in neutropenic patients infected with HIV. AIDS. 1997;11:995–998.

Chapter 110

Gastrointestinal and Hepatobiliary Manifestations of Human Immunodeficiency Virus Infection

MARK S. SULKOWSKI
RICHARD E. CHAISSON

Diseases of the gastrointestinal system frequently complicate human immunodeficiency virus (HIV) infection and mark its progression to the acquired immunodeficiency syndrome (AIDS). Many HIV-related gastrointestinal diseases, such as *Candida* esophagitis, biliary cryptosporidiosis, and cytomegalovirus (CMV) colitis, represent opportunistic infections that are the result of advanced immunosuppression. Other gastrointestinal processes, such as chronic viral hepatitis and HIV-related medication toxicity, may occur at any stage of HIV disease. The likelihood and nature of gastrointestinal manifestations of HIV depend on both host and environmental factors, as infectious complications in particular are a product of both exposure to potential pathogens and immunocompetence. Over the course of their disease, however, most HIV-infected patients experience symptomatic gastrointestinal tract disease, and the broad range of diagnostic considerations mandates the systematic evaluation of gastrointestinal complaints among such patients.

DISORDERS OF THE ESOPHAGUS

Esophageal disease occurs commonly among HIV-infected persons, affecting up to one third of persons with AIDS[1] (also see Chapter 82). Esophageal abnormalities typically produce symptoms of dysphagia and odynophagia, which may be due to esophageal inflammation or ulceration caused by infectious pathogens or noninfectious processes. Esophagitis is most often due to infection with *Candida albicans* but may also be caused by viruses, such as herpes simplex virus, CMV, and varicella-zoster virus, and less commonly by other infectious agents, such as *Mycobacterium tuberculosis*, nontuberculous mycobacteria, *Histoplasma capsulatum*, *Pneumocystis carinii*, and primary HIV infection.[2, 3] Noninfectious processes, such as reflux esophagitis, pill esophagitis (zidovudine, zalcitabine, and doxycycline), and malignancy (carcinoma, lymphoma, and Kaposi's sarcoma), may be characterized by symptoms clinically indistinguishable from those of infections of the esophagus. Esophageal ulcerations are often caused by CMV (45%), idiopathic ulcers (40%), and herpes simplex virus (5%) and may involve symptoms of localized pain.[4]

In the era of effective antiretroviral therapy, the clinical spectrum of esophageal disease may be expected to change. The occurrence of CMV-related esophageal disease has decreased significantly, while the incidence of esophageal candidiasis has remained stable.[5] The frequency of idiopathic esophageal ulceration may also decrease with the effective treatment of HIV disease, although this is currently uncertain. Conversely, noninfectious esophageal disease, such as reflux and pill esophagitis, may account for an increasing proportion of esophageal symptoms.

Regardless of etiology, most esophageal processes are associated with dysphagia or odynophagia, and there may be persistent or intermittent retrosternal pain, nausea, anorexia, and weight loss. The onset of symptoms may be relatively acute but more typically follows an indolent course. Nonesophageal manifestations of disease may be found in patients with odynophagia; for example, oral candidiasis frequently accompanies *Candida* esophagitis, and active CMV infection may be found in other anatomic sites, such as the retina or colon.[6] However, the broad range of disease processes and the possibility of multiple etiologies mandate a methodical approach to the evaluation and management of esophageal symptoms in patients with HIV disease.

During the initial evaluation, medical history may suggest drug-induced esophagitis or gastroesophageal reflux disease, and physical examination may reveal oral candidiasis or CMV retinitis. The presence of oral candidiasis strongly suggests esophageal involvement and should prompt empirical antifungal therapy (fluconazole at 100 to 200 mg/day).[7] Presumptive oral antifungal therapy is highly effective for esophageal candidiasis and is usually preferable to diagnostic upper endoscopy or "blind" brushing of the esophagus via nasogastric tube.[8] If the esophageal symptoms resolve, the diagnosis of candidiasis can be established empirically. However, failure of symptoms to respond to empirical antifungal therapy within 7 to 10 days indicates a need for further evaluation.[9] Most patients (77%) who do not respond to antifungal therapy have esophageal ulceration rather than evidence of persistent esophageal candidiasis.[10] Upper endoscopy with biopsy is a highly sensitive procedure for establishing a specific diagnosis and is the preferred approach to the evaluation of patients with odynophagia or dysphagia who do not respond to empirical antifungal therapy. Upper gastrointestinal contrast radiography may reveal characteristic abnormalities, but these findings are relatively insensitive and nonspecific, whereas the symptom-specific use of upper endoscopy may yield a treatable pathologic diagnosis in as many as 78% of patients.[11]

The endoscopic appearance of esophageal candidiasis resembles cheesy friable plaques that may involve the entire esophagus, whereas viral esophagitis is usually associated with diffuse, erythematous ulceration of the mucosa. CMV esophagitis frequently causes numerous, large, shallow ulcerations, whereas herpes simplex virus esophagitis is typically seen as superficial, confluent ulcers in the distal esophagus and may be associated with concurrent nonesophageal lesions in 38% of patients.[12, 13] Idiopathic or apthous ulcers may have an endoscopic appearance similar to that of CMV ulcers and represent a diagnosis of exclusion. Less commonly, other infectious processes may be observed including those associated with *Mycobacterium avium* complex and *M. tuberculosis* and bacillary angiomatosis. Noninfectious processes, such as drug-induced ulcers and malignancies, may affect the esophagus, with the most common tumors being Kaposi's sarcoma, primary lymphoma, and adenocarcinoma. Persons with HIV infection may also have conventional esophageal pathology, such as reflux esophagitis, achalasia, esophageal strictures, and esophagotracheal fistulas.

For lesions visualized by endoscopy, a biopsy should be performed and tissue sections prepared for histopathologic stains to identify viral inclusion bodies (CMV), multinucleated giant cells (herpes simplex virus), or invasive fungi. Cultures for fungi and viruses may be helpful, although false-positive results may be seen with CMV and *C. albicans*. Antifungal drug sensitivity testing may be useful if azole-resistant candidiasis is suspected.[14] The yield of endoscopy with biopsy and culture is extremely high and more than one pathologic process may be found; nonetheless, multiple biopsies (more than three) may be needed to exclude the diagnosis of viral esophagitis.[15] Lesions that do not respond to appropriate therapy should be reevaluated by endoscopy with biopsy and culture to confirm the diagnosis and, if indicated, to perform drug sensitivity testing. Additional diagnostic procedures are usually not required but may be useful in special circumstances, such as when there is a clinical suspicion of esophageal dysmotility.

DISORDERS OF THE STOMACH

Gastric disorders in HIV-infected patients may be due to opportunistic infections but are often unrelated to HIV-induced immunodeficiency. Patients with gastric disease may present with protean complaints such as nausea, vomiting, early satiety, and anorexia; abdominal pain and hematemasis may also be present. Some disease processes such as CMV gastritis and gastrointestinal Kaposi's sarcoma may be associated with extragastric involvement.

Gastritis and gastroduodenal ulcers may be found in HIV-infected persons with upper gastrointestinal symptoms and may be due to *Helicobacter pylori* infection. However, several studies indicate that the prevalence of *H. pylori*–related disease is lower among persons with HIV disease than among the general population, possibly because of frequent antimicrobial therapy.[16–18] Varsky and coworkers[17] reported that only 5% of 497 HIV-infected patients with upper gastrointestinal complaints had endoscopic evidence of gastroduodenal ulcers, and *H. pylori* infection was found in only one third of these patients. *H. pylori* infection may be detected by serology, but the sensitivity (57%) is lower than that of histologic evaluation in patients with advanced immunodeficiency.[18] HIV-infected patients may also have altered gastric function, including decreased secretion of gastric acid and intrinsic factor.[19] Hypochlorhydria may impair the absorption of some medications, such as ketoconazole and itraconazole, and may also permit gastric bacterial overgrowth.[20, 21]

CMV may cause gastric inflammation or ulceration alone or in association with esophageal ulceration. The appearance of gastric CMV may be diverse and includes thickened, edematous gastric folds, erosive gastritis, and superficial or deep ulcerations. The radiographic features may be nonspecific and may even be masslike, suggestive of malignancy.[22] Other gastric infections have been reported, including infection with *Cryptosporidium*, *M. avium* complex infection, histoplasmosis, cryptococcosis, leishmaniasis, and syphilis. Malignant lesions involving the stomach may also be associated with upper gastrointestinal symptoms. Gastrointestinal Kaposi's sarcoma, associated with human herpesvirus type 8 infection, complicates cutaneous disease in as many as 50% of patients and most commonly involves the stomach.[23] Gastric Kaposi's sarcoma lesions may be asymptomatic but can also cause nausea, abdominal pain, and, rarely, severe hemorrhage.[24] AIDS-related lymphomas may also involve the gastrointestinal tract; these lesions tend to be multifocal but may rarely be gastric mucosa-associated lymphoid tissue lymphomas associated with *H. pylori*.[25, 26] In light of these diverse diagnostic considerations, patients with persistent upper gastrointestinal symptoms should be evaluated for opportunistic infection and malignancy, particularly those with CD4+ cell counts less than 200/mm^3.

The definitive diagnosis of upper gastrointestinal pathology often requires endoscopic evaluation with biopsy and cultures. Kaposi's sarcoma lesions typically appear as a violet-blue submucosal mass without ulceration or bleeding but may appear as linitis plastica. Biopsies of these lesions may fail to confirm Kaposi's sarcoma in up to two thirds of cases. However, when cutaneous Kaposi's sarcoma has been histologically confirmed, the endoscopic appearance of the lesion may be sufficient to establish the diagnosis.[23] Biopsy and immunohistochemical staining are needed for the diagnosis of gastric lymphoma. Biopsies of gastroduodenal ulcerations should be performed and specimens sent for viral culture and histologic staining for evidence of viral inclusions, fungi, and *H. pylori* infection. Multiple biopsies may be needed to exclude viral pathogens, and additional stains and cultures may be helpful in diagnosing specific infections, such as acid-fast stains and culture for *M. avium* complex.

DISORDERS OF THE BILIARY TREE AND GALLBLADDER

Diseases of the gallbladder and biliary tree affecting HIV-infected persons include non–HIV-associated conditions, such as cholelithiasis, and AIDS-associated conditions, such as acalculous cholecystitis and cholangiopathy. Patients typically present with postprandial pain, fever, right upper quadrant pain and tenderness, and an elevated serum alkaline phosphatase level. Ultrasonographic or computed tomographic imaging studies may reveal evidence of acute cholecystitis or cholangitis related to cholelithiasis, and in patients with advanced immunodeficiency, these studies may suggest acalculous cholecystitis or AIDS-associated cholangitis.[27] During acute or chronic acalculous cholecystitis, the gallbladder generally appears thickened and edematous with obliteration of the gallbladder lumen without evidence of gallstones. Nonvisualization of the gallbladder by randionuclide hepatobiliary scintigraphy is also suggestive of cholecystitis. If a cholecystectomy is performed, operative specimens should be sent for microbiologic and histopathologic evaluation, as opportunistic pathogens may be identified in more than 50% of cases.[28] CMV, *Cryptosporidium*, and microsporidians are the pathogens most commonly associated with acalculous cholecystitis; however, multiple organisms or other pathogens, such as *Isospora belli*, may be recovered. However, often no etiologic agent is identified after extensive microbiologic evaluation.[29–31] Although the exclusion of opportunistic infection is critical in the evaluation of HIV-infected patients with acute cholecystitis, cholelithiasis may account for a significant proportion of patients who undergo cholecystectomy.

If noninvasive, radiographic imaging indicates intra- or extrahepatic biliary ductal dilatation, endoscopic retrograde cholangiopancreatography may be necessary for the diagnosis and management of AIDS-associated cholangiopathy.[32] Cello[33] has described four common patterns of cholangiographic abnormalities revealed by endoscopic retrograde cholangiopancreatography: stenosis of the papilla of Vater with dilated extrahepatic biliary tract, sclerosing cholangitis, combination of sclerosing cholangitis and papillary stenosis, and choledochal long stenosis or strictures. Endoscopic retrograde cholangiopancreatography with collection of bile from the common bile duct and duodenal or papillary biopsy may identify an opportunistic pathogen or malignancy. Like acalculous cholecystitis, cholangitis is associated with opportunistic infections by CMV, *Cryptosporidium* or microsporidians in more than one half of cases.[30, 34, 35] Among 82 HIV-infected patients in whom cryptosporidiosis developed during a waterborne outbreak, 24 (29%) had evidence of biliary involvement. Biliary cryptosporidiosis was associated with CD4+ cell counts less than 50/mm^3, and patients were more likely to develop nausea, vomiting, and an elevated alkaline phosphatase level.[35] Other infectious pathogens, such as *Cryptococcus neoformans*, *I. belli*, and *P. carinii*, and biliary tree malignancies, including lymphoma and Kaposi's sarcoma, have been reported. In addition, bacterial superinfection may complicate any of these disease processes.

If papillary stenosis is present, endoscopic sphincterotomy may produce relief of symptoms and biochemical resolution of cholestasis, although in some case series the clinical effectiveness of this procedure has been disappointing.[36, 37]

DISORDERS OF THE LIVER

Hepatic abnormalities are quite common among HIV-infected persons and are often associated with elevated serum hepatic transaminase and alkaline phosphatase levels. Liver disease may be due to acute or chronic viral hepatitis, HIV-related opportunistic infections, or noninfectious processes, such as medication toxicity, alcohol, or malignancy (Table 110–1). Because of shared routes of transmission, chronic hepatitis B virus (HBV) and hepatitis C virus (HCV) infections frequently complicate HIV disease[38] (also see Chapter 103). Approximately 20% of HIV-infected persons who acquire acute HBV infection develop chronic HBV infection, characterized by hepatitis B surface antigenemia and active viral replication, compared with only 5% of HIV-negative persons. Spontaneous reactivation of HBV replication has been reported in anti–hepatitis B surface antibody–positive patients who develop severe immunosuppression.[39, 40] However, some reports indicate that HBV-related liver disease may be less severe among immunosuppressed patients as a result of attenuated immune-mediated hepatic injury, and chronic HBV infection does not appear to influence HIV disease progression.[41, 42]

Among HIV-infected persons with parenteral exposures, such as injection drug users and recipients of blood products, the prevalence of chronic HCV infection is high, ranging from 60 to 95% worldwide.[43] The majority of patients coinfected with HCV and HIV have asymptomatic elevations in serum hepatic transaminases; however, HCV infection may lead to the development of significant hepatic fibrosis or cirrhosis, which may be followed by hepatic decompensation or hepatocellular carcinoma or both.[44] HCV-infected patients with end-stage liver disease are profoundly symptomatic with manifestations of portal hypertension, including ascites, esophageal varices, and splenomegaly; decreased hepatic synthetic function, including hypoalbuminemia, thrombocytopenia, and coagulopathy; and hepatic encephalopathy. In addition, extrahepatic manifestations of hepatitis C infection, such as membranous glomerulonephritis, porphyria cutanea tarda, and mixed, type II cryoglobulinemia with or without vasculitis, may occur at any stage of disease.[45]

Studies of the natural history of HCV disease in HIV-infected persons demonstrate enhanced HCV replication and accelerated progression of liver disease, presumably because of HIV-related immunosuppression.[46] Darby and colleagues[47] reported a 6-fold higher risk of liver-related mortality among HIV-infected patients with hemophilia who received HCV-positive blood products than in those without HIV infection and a 94-fold higher risk than in the general population. Among HCV-infected injection drug users, HIV infection has been shown to be independently associated with the development of cirrhosis.[48] Conversely, chronic HCV infection does not appear to accelerate the clinical or immunologic progression of HIV disease, although the effect of HCV on HIV pathogenesis has not been fully characterized.[49] Nonetheless, the morbidity and mortality related to hepatitis C among HIV-infected persons are substantial, and the clinical importance of HCV may increase as effective antiretroviral therapies improve patients' longevity.

Hepatitis C infection is generally diagnosed by the detection of anti-HCV antibodies, but immunocompromised patients may have false-negative HCV antibody assays.[50] Most HIV-infected patients have evidence of active HCV replication, as indicated by plasma HCV RNA detection with molecular assays. Noninvasive radiographic imaging may reveal hepatic parenchymal abnormalities, mass lesions, or evidence of ascites, splenomegaly, or varices; however, imaging studies cannot reliably exclude the presence of significant histologic liver disease, such as piecemeal necrosis, advanced hepatic fibrosis, or cirrhosis. Liver biopsy is often required to determine the severity of HCV-related liver disease and may be useful to exclude other causes of hepatic disease, such as drug toxicity or opportunistic pathogens.[51]

Other infectious processes may involve the liver, leading to hepatocellular necrosis or granulomatous inflammation. Viral pathogens, such as CMV, Epstein-Barr virus, herpes simplex virus, and adenovirus, can cause hepatocellular damage, usually in the setting of disseminated disease. Other infectious pathogens, such as mycobacterial and fungal agents, may lead to granulomatous inflammation, characterized by elevated alkaline phosphatase levels and nonspecific hepatic granuloma. *M. avium* complex is the most common opportunistic pathogen affecting the liver and is associated with manifestations of systemic disease, including fever, abdominal pain, and wasting.[51] Extrapulmonary *M. tuberculosis* infection may be associated with hepatic involvement in 5 to 10% of HIV-related cases and, less commonly a tuberculosis abscess has been identified.[52] Disseminated fungal infections with organisms including *C. neoformans*, *H. capsulatum*, *Coccidioides immitis*, *Penicillium marneffei*, and *C. albicans* may produce a granulomatous response in liver. *C. neoformans* and *H. capsulatum* may be rapidly detected by evidence of polysaccharide capsular antigenemia; other causes of fungal hepatitis may be diagnosed by histologic and microbiologic evaluation of liver tissue.

P. carinii hepatic infection may occur, particularly during aerosolized pentamidine prophylactic therapy. *Bartonella henselae* can cause peliosis hepatis, a vascular proliferative liver infection, in the absence of cutaneous lesions. Peliosis hepatis occurs in patients with advanced immunodeficiency, who may present with fever, weight loss, and hepatosplenomegaly with an elevated serum alkaline phosphatase level. The diagnosis of bartonellosis is made by Warthin-Starry staining of biopsy specimens or culture of the blood or tissue plated on heart infusion agar with 5% rabbit blood[53] (see Chapter 224). Blood culture for acid-fast bacilli is usually sufficient to establish the diagnosis of disseminated mycobacterial infection. The evaluation of other potential causes of liver disease may require liver biopsy, which may rapidly yield a treatable diagnosis in more than 60% of HIV-infected patients with unexplained fever and liver abnormalities. Hepatic tissue should be sent for microbiologic evaluation and culture, as well as routine and specific histologic staining for acid-fast bacilli and fungal pathogens.[54]

Hepatic mass lesions are commonly due to malignancy, although radiographically, infectious processes may resemble mass lesions. The most common hepatic malignancy is Kaposi's sarcoma; hepatic involvement typically occurs in the setting of cutaneous disease and is often associated with hepatomegaly and abdominal pain. Abdominal imaging with contrast-enhanced computed tomography may reveal enhanced lesions located in the capsular, hilar, and portal areas with invasion into the liver parenchyma. The definitive diagnosis of

TABLE 110–1 Selected Causes of Hepatic Disease in Human Immunodeficiency Virus-Infected Persons

Viruses	Protozoa
Hepatitis A	*Toxoplasma gondii*
Hepatitis B	*Cryptosporidium parvum*
Hepatitis C	Microsporida spp.
Hepatitis D (with HBV)	*Schistosoma*
Epstein-Barr virus	Bacteria
Cytomegalovirus	*Bartonella henselae* (peliosis hepatis)
Herpes simplex virus	Malignancy
Adenovirus	Kaposi's sarcoma (HHV-8)
Varicella-zoster virus	Non-Hodgkin's lymphoma
Mycobacteria	Hepatocellular carcinoma
Mycobacterium avium complex	Medications
Mycobacterium tuberculosis	Zidovudine
Fungi	Didanosine
Histoplasma capsulatum	Ritonavir
Cryptococcus neoformans	Other HIV-1 protease inhibitors
Coccidioides immitis	Fluconazole
Candida albicans	Macrolide antibiotics
Pneumocystis carinii	Isoniazid
Penicillium marneffei	Rifampin
	Trimethoprim-sulfamethoxazole

Abbreviations: HBV, Hepatitis B virus; HHV-8, human herpesvirus type 8; HIV-1, human immunodeficiency virus type 1.

hepatic Kaposi's sarcoma requires biopsy with histologic examination; however, the risk of hemorrhage after a biopsy may be increased because of the vascular nature of the Kaposi's sarcoma lesion.

Non-Hodgkin's lymphomas may involve the liver, usually in association with lymph node or visceral involvement, or both, although primary hepatic lymphoma has been reported. Patients may present with "B" symptoms, including weight loss, fever, and night sweats, and abdominal pain; jaundice may occur with intra- or extrahepatic bile duct obstruction.[55] Radiographic imaging typically reveals solitary or multiple hepatic mass lesions and involvement of abdominal lymph nodes. Biopsy of the hepatic lesion or involved lymph nodes is needed to confirm the diagnosis of lymphoma. Hepatocellular carcinoma has been increasingly recognized in patients with cirrhosis related to chronic viral hepatitis; such patients may have evidence of advanced liver disease, elevated serum α-fetoprotein, and radiographic evidence of a mass lesion.

Hepatotoxicity associated with HIV-related medications is a common cause of liver abnormalities, and infection with HIV, HCV, or both may enhance the toxicity of some medications, such as antituberculosis drugs.[56] Patients typically present with elevated serum hepatic transaminases, although some drugs, such as macrolide antibiotics and trimethoprim-sulfamethoxazole, induce a cholestatic or mixed liver injury pattern. Drug-induced hepatotoxicity is often asymptomatic and detected through monitoring of serum liver enzymes. However, nucleoside analogues, such as zidovudine, have been associated with fatal hepatomegaly with severe steatosis and lactic acidosis.[57] HIV-1 protease inhibitors, particularly ritonavir, have been associated with severe hepatotoxicity after the initiation of therapy, which may be facilitated by concurrent chronic HBV or HCV infection.[58] HIV-infected patients should be monitored after initiating treatment with potentially hepatotoxic medications and treatment should be modified if drug-induced hepatotoxicity is suspected.

DISORDERS OF THE PANCREAS

Diseases involving the pancreas may be caused by processes unrelated to HIV infection, such as alcohol abuse, cholelithiasis, and hyperlipidemia, or may be due to HIV-related opportunistic infections or medication toxicity.[59] AIDS cholangiopathy caused by CMV, *Cryptosporidium*, or microsporidians may involve the juxta-ampullary portion of the pancreatic duct.[60] Mycobacterial infections of the pancreas have been described, including pancreatic abscess related to *M. tuberculosis* and disseminated *M. avium* complex.[61] Fungal pathogens, such as *C. neoformans* and *Candida* spp., *Toxoplama gondii*, *P. carinii*, and protozoal pathogens may involve the pancreas, typically in the setting of disseminated disease. Pancreatic CMV inclusions are frequently observed in autopsy specimens from patients with disseminated CMV disease, although clinical pancreatitis is infrequently recognized before death.[62]

Drug-induced pancreatic inflammation and dysfunction may occur in patients with HIV disease. Didanosine may cause asymptomatic hyperamylasemia; however, clinical pancreatitis has been observed in 1.2 to 6.7% of didanosine recipients, and fulminant pancreatic toxicity has been reported.[63] Patients with a prior history of pancreatitis are at higher risk for developing didanosine-related pancreatitis, and the drug should be avoided in this setting. Zalcitabine has also been associated with pancreatitis. Systemic pentamidine therapy for *P. carinii* pneumonia is toxic to pancreatic B islet cells and can cause pancreatitis and symptomatic hyperglycemia or hypoglycemia; in contrast, prophylaxis with aerosolized pentamidine rarely leads to pancreatic dysfunction.[64] The risk of pancreatitis in patients receiving intravenous pentamidine is dose related, with most cases occurring after 2 weeks of therapy. Other HIV-related medications, including megesterol acetate and HIV-1 protease inhibitors, have been associated with derangements of glucose homeostasis.[65, 66]

DISORDERS OF THE SMALL AND LARGE INTESTINE

Symptomatic disease of the small intestine and colon are common among HIV-infected individuals and may be caused by a diverse range of infectious agents. Small bowel diseases generally produce bloating, nausea, cramping, and profuse diarrhea and may be associated with malabsorption and weight loss. In contrast, colitis may produce lower abdominal discomfort and cramping, urgency, and tenesmus and typically causes frequent, small volume diarrhea. However, the clinical manifestations of small and large bowel infections may be indistinguishable, and some processes may cause panenteritis.[67]

The differential diagnosis for enterocolitis in an immunocompromised person is extensive and includes bacterial, protozoal, and viral pathogens (Table 110–2). Bacteria that are more common in HIV-infected patients include *Salmonella* spp, *Shigella*, *Campylobacter jejuni*, *Escherichia coli* (enterotoxigenic, enteroadherent, and enteroaggregative), and *Listeria monocytogenes*.[68] Salmonellosis is associated with bacteremia in one half of infections and may be recurrent in HIV-infected persons.[69] Less commonly, bacteremia may occur with *Shigella* and *Campylobacter* infection.[70] *C. difficile* toxin–associated diarrhea may also be more common among individuals with HIV disease, particularly among hospitalized patients and those who have recently received antibiotic therapy.[71] Small bowel overgrowth can occur and has been associated with hypochlorhydria and wasting. Other, less common bacterial causes of enterocolitis include *Aeromonas*, *Plesiomonas*, *Yersinia*, and *Vibrio* spp. Mycobacterial infections of the small bowel are usually associated with late-stage HIV disease and disseminated *M. avium* complex, although enteritis caused by *M. tuberculosis* has been reported.[72]

Parasites infecting the small and large bowel include spore-forming protozoa, *Cryptosporidium*, Microsporida spp. (such as *Enterocytozoon bieneusi* and *Septata intestinalis*), *Isospora*, and *Cyclospora*, as well as *Entamoeba histolytica* and *Giardia lamblia*. Amebic infection and giardiasis may occur at any stage of HIV disease and are commonly associated with conventional risk factors, such as sexual practices and travel-related exposures. Disease caused by *Crypto-*

TABLE 110–2 Causes of Lower Gastrointestinal Tract Disease in Patients with Human Immunodeficiency Virus

Causes of enterocolitis	Causes of proctitis
Bacteria	Bacteria
Campylobacter jejuni and other spp.	*Chlamydia trachomatis*
Salmonella spp.	*Neisseria gonorrhoeae*
Shigella flexneri	*Treponema pallidum*
Aeromonas hydrophila	Viruses
Plesiomonas shigelloides	Herpes simplex
Yersinia enterocolitica	Cytomegalovirus
Vibrio spp.	
Mycobacterium avium complex	
Mycobacterium tuberculosis	
Escherichia coli (enterotoxigenic, enteroadherent)	
Bacterial overgrowth	
Clostridium difficile (toxin)	
Parasites	
Cryptosporidium parvum	
Microsporida (*Enterocytozoon bieneusi, Septata intestinalis*)	
Isospora belli	
Entamoeba histolytica	
Giardia lamblia	
Cyclospora cayetanensis	
Viruses	
Cytomegalovirus	
Adenovirus	
Calicivirus	
Astrovirus	
Picobirnavirus	
Human immunodeficiency virus	
Fungi	
Histoplasma capsulatum	

sporidium is more common and severe in HIV-infected persons with advanced immunosuppression, leading to persistent infection (60%), biliary disease (29%) and even fulminant disease (8%).[35, 73] Similarly, microsporidiosis causes diarrhea in patients with advanced HIV disease (CD4$^+$ cell count <50/mm^3) and may be associated with cholangiopathy.[74] Less commonly, diarrhea caused by *Isospora* and *Cyclospora* has been reported in persons with advanced immunosuppression.[75, 76]

CMV is the most significant viral cause of enterocolitis, leading to fever, abdominal pain and tenderness, bloody diarrhea, and, rarely, intestinal perforation or toxic megacolon. As with its appearance in the esophagus, CMV enterocolitis occurs with severe immunodeficiency and produces mucosal inflammation with superficial ulceration.[77, 78] Other viral pathogens implicated as causes of diarrhea include adenovirus, which may cause a condition that mimics CMV colitis, as well as astrovirus, calicivirus, and picobirnavirus[79] (see Chapters 163 and 164).

Proctitis in patients with HIV disease typically reflects sexually transmitted infections, such as herpes simplex virus infection, *Chlamydia trachomatis* infection, syphilis, and gonorrhea, particularly among homosexual men.[80] However, advanced immunosuppression may be associated with more severe disease manifestations and recurrent infection. CMV proctitis is less common but may occur in the setting of extensive CMV colitis.

HIV-infected patients with diarrhea or other symptoms of enterocolitis should be carefully evaluated to identify treatable conditions. Historical assessments should focus on the nature and duration of the symptoms, concomitant medications, travel, and other exposures, such as through food, water, or sexual contact. The standard diagnostic evaluation should include stool leukocyte examination to identify inflammatory causes of diarrhea, such as bacterial pathogens and CMV, and guide empirical therapy; other infectious agents, such as protozoa and *M. avium* complex, are typically not associated with the finding of fecal leukocytes. Stool should be cultured for enteric bacterial pathogens, assayed for *C. difficile* toxin, and examined for ova and parasites. Stool specimens should be examined on at least three occasions with modified acid-fast stain to identify *Cryptosporidium*, *Cyclospora*, and *Isospora*. Special trichrome staining may be useful for the identification of microsporidians.[81]

If noninvasive stool studies are not diagnostic and symptoms persist, endoscopic evolution with biopsy may prove helpful, particularly in patients with chronic diarrhea and severe immunodeficiency (CD4$^+$ cells <100/mm^3).[82] Patients with signs and symptoms suggestive of large bowel involvement should undergo colonoscopy and biopsy. The sensitivity of endoscopic biopsy for the diagnosis for CMV disease is high, and colonoscopy may identify disease limited to the right side of the colon, which may be missed during flexible sigmoidoscopy.[83] Upper endoscopy with duodenal biopsy is useful for patients with symptoms of small bowel disease or those with persistent symptoms and negative evaluation of the lower gastrointestinal tract.[84] In addition to hematoxylin and eosin staining, duodenal histologic specimens should be stained with fungal stains and modified acid-fast stain for *Cryptosporidium* as well as undergo electron microscopy for microsporidians. Polymerase chain reaction assay of biopsy specimens may also prove valuable in the diagnosis of some pathogens, such as microsporidians.[85] Small bowel aspirates are generally not useful in the evaluation of unexplained diarrhea.

Approximately 20 to 50% of patients with chronic diarrhea have a negative gastrointestinal tract evaluation.[86] Patients without an identifiable cause of diarrhea may have HIV-associated enteropathy, the pathology of which is not fully understood. Histologic evaluation of small bowel biopsy specimens may reveal a decrease in villous surface area and crypt cell proliferation in the absence of inflammation.[87] No specific therapy is available, but highly active antiretroviral therapy may effectively control diarrhea in patients with HIV enteropathy, as well as those with microsporidiosis and cryptosporidiosis.[88] Furthermore, as diagnostic methods improve and additional pathogens are identified, the proportion of patients with unexplained diarrhea may decline.

REFERENCES

1. Connolly GM, Hawkins D, Harcourt-Webster JN, et al. Oesophageal symptoms, their causes, treatment, and prognosis in patients with the acquired immunodeficiency syndrome. Gut. 1989;30:1033–1039.
2. Bonacini M, Young T, Laine L. The causes of esophageal symptoms in human immunodeficiency virus infection. A prospective study of 110 patients. Arch Intern Med. 1991;151:1567–1572.
3. Rabeneck L, Popovic M, Gartner S, et al. Acute HIV infection presenting with painful swallowing and esophageal ulcers. JAMA. 1990;263:2318–2322.
4. Wilcox CM, Schwartz DA, Clark WS. Esophageal ulceration in human immunodeficiency virus infection. Causes, response to therapy, and long-term outcome. Ann Intern Med. 1995;123:143–149.
5. Pallela FJ, Delaney KM, Moorman AC, et al. Declining morbidity and mortality among patients with advanced human immunodeficiency virus infection. N Engl J Med. 1998;338:853–860.
6. Tavitian A, Raufman JP, Rosenthal LE. Oral candidiasis as a marker of esophageal candidiasis in the acquired immunodeficiency syndrome. Ann Intern Med. 1986;104:54–55.
7. Laine L, Dretler RH, Conteas CN, et al. Fluconazole compared with ketoconazole for the treatment of *Candida* esophagitis in AIDS. A randomized trial. Ann Intern Med. 1992;117:655–660.
8. Wilcox CM, Alexander LN, Clark WS, Thompson SE. Fluconazole compared with endoscopy for human immunodeficiency virus–infected patients with esophageal symptoms. Gastroenterology. 1996;110:1803–1809.
9. Wilcox CM. Short report: Time course of clinical response with fluconazole for *Candida* oesophagitis in patients with AIDS. Aliment Pharmacol Ther. 1994;8:347–350.
10. Wilcox CM, Straub RF, Alexander LN, Clark WS. Etiology of esophageal disease in human immunodeficiency virus–infected patients who fail antifungal therapy. Am J Med. 1996;101:599–604.
11. Bashir RM, Wilcox CM. Symptom-specific use of upper gastrointestinal endoscopy in human immunodeficiency virus infected patients yields high dividends. J Clin Gastroenterol. 1996;23:292–298.
12. Wilcox CM, Diehl DL, Cello JP, et al. Cytomegalovirus esophagitis in patients with AIDS. A clinical, endoscopic, and pathologic correlation. Ann Intern Med. 1990;113:589–593.
13. Genereau T, Lortholary O, Bouchaud O, et al. Herpes simples esophagitis in patients with AIDS: Report of 34 cases. The Cooperative Study Group on Herpetic Esophagitis in HIV Infection. Clin Infect Dis. 1996;22:926–931.
14. Maenza JR, Keruly JC, Moore RD, et al. Risk factors for fluconazole-resistant candidiasis in human immunodeficiency virus–infected patients. J Infect Dis. 1996;173:219–225.
15. Wilcox CM, Straub RF, Schwartz DA. Prospective evaluation of biopsy number for the diagnosis of viral esophagitis in patients with HIV infection and esophageal ulcer. Gastrointest Endosc. 1996;44:587–593.
16. Edwards PD, Carrick J, Turner J, et al. *Helicobacter pylori*–associated gastritis is rare in AIDS: Antibiotic effect or a consequence of immunodeficiency. Am J Gastroenterol. 1991;86:1761–1764.
17. Varsky CG, Correa MC, Sarmiento N, et al. Prevalence and etiology of gastroduodenal ulcer in HIV-positive patients: A comparative study of 497 symptomatic subjects evaluated by endoscopy. Am J Gastroenterol. 1998;93:935–940.
18. Fabris P, Bozzola L, Benedetti P, et al. *H. pylori* infection in HIV-positive patients. A serohistological study. Dig Dis Sci. 1997;42:289–292.
19. Lake-Bakaar G, Elsakr M, Hagag N, et al. Changes in parietal cell structure and function in HIV disease. Dig Dis Sci. 1996;41:1398–1408.
20. Lake-Bakaar G, Tom W, Lake-Bakaar D, et al. Gastropathy and ketoconazole malabsorption in the acquired immunodeficiency syndrome (AIDS). Ann Intern Med. 1988;15:471–473.
21. Belitsos PC, Greenson JK, Yardley JH, et al. Association of gastric hypoacidity with opportunistic infection in patients with AIDS. J Infect Dis. 1992;166:277–284.
22. Teixidor HS, Honig CL, Norsoph E, et al. Cytomegalovirus infection of the alimentary canal: Radiologic findings with pathologic correlation. Radiology. 1987;163:317–323.
23. Friedman SL, Wright TL, Altman DF. Gastrointestinal Kaposi's sarcoma in patients with acquired immunodeficiency syndrome. Endoscopic and autopsy findings. Gastroenterology. 1985;89:102–108.
24. Lew EA, Dieterich DT. Severe hemorrhage caused by gastrointestinal Kaposi's syndrome in patients with the acquired immunodeficiency syndrome: Treatment with endoscopic injection sclerotherapy. Am J Gastroenterol. 1992;87:1471–1474.
25. Cappell MS, Botros N. Predominantly gastrointestinal symptoms and signs in 11 consecutive AIDS patients with gastrointestinal lymphoma: A multicenter, multiyear study including 763 HIV-seropositive patients. Am J Gastroenterol. 1994;89:545–549.
26. Wotherspoon AC, Diss TC, Pan L, et al. Low grade gastric B-cell lymphoma of mucosa associated lymphoid tissue in immunocompromised patients. Histopathology. 1996;28:129–134.
27. Bonacini M. Hepatobiliary complications in patients with human immunodeficiency virus infection. Am J Med. 1992;92:404–411.

28. French AL, Beaudet LM, Benator DA, et al. Cholecystectomy in patents with AIDS: Clinicopathologic correlation in 107 cases. Clin Infect Dis. 1995;21:852–858.
29. Kavin H, Jonas RB, Chowdhury L, Kabins S. Acalculous cholecystitis and cytomegalovirus infection in the acquired immunodeficiency syndrome. Ann Intern Med. 1986;104:53–54.
30. Pol S, Romana CA, Richard S, et al. Microsporidia infection in patients with the human immunodeficiency virus and unexplained cholangitis. N Engl J Med. 1993;328:95–99.
31. Benator DA, French AL, Beaudet LM, et al. *Isospora belli* infection associated with acalculous cholecystitis in a patient with AIDS. Ann Intern Med. 1994;121:663–664.
32. Schneiderman DJ, Cello JP, Laing FC. Papillary stenosis and sclerosing cholangitis in the acquired immunodeficiency syndrome. Ann Intern Med. 1987;106:546–549.
33. Cello JP. Acquired immunodeficiency syndrome cholangiopathy: Spectrum of disease. Am J Med. 1989;86:539–546.
34. Benhamou Y, Caumes E, Gerosa Y, et al. AIDS-related cholangiopathy. Critical analysis of a prospective series of 26 patients. Dig Dis Sci. 1993;38:1113–1118.
35. Vakil NB, Schwartz SM, Buggy BP, et al. Biliary cryptosporidiosis in HIV-infected people after the waterborne outbreak of cryptosporidiosis in Milwaukee. N Engl J Med. 1996;334:19–23.
36. Cello JP, Chan MF. Long-term follow-up of endoscopic retrograde cholangiopancreatography sphincterotomy for patients with acquired immune deficiency syndrome papillary stenosis. Am J Med. 1995;99:600–603.
37. Ducreux M, Buffet C, Lamy P, et al. Diagnosis and prognosis of AIDS-related cholangitis. AIDS. 1995;9:875–880.
38. Kelen GD, Green GB, Purcell RH, et al. Hepatitis B and hepatitis C in emergency department patients. N Engl J Med. 1992;326:1399–1404.
39. Hadler SC, Judson FN, O'Malley PM, et al. Outcome of hepatitis B virus infection in homosexual men and its relation to prior human immunodeficiency virus infection. J Infect Dis. 1991;163:454–459.
40. Vento S, di Perri G, Luzzati R, et al. Clinical reactivation of hepatitis B in anti-HBs–positive patients with AIDS. Lancet. 1989;1:323.
41. Bodsworth N, Donovan B, Nightingale BN. The effect of concurrent human immunodeficiency virus infection on chronic hepatitis B: A study of 150 homosexual men. J Infect Dis. 1989;160:577–582.
42. Gilson RJ, Hawkins AE, Beecham MR, et al. Interaction between HIV and hepatitis B in homosexual men: Effects on the natural history of infection. AIDS. 1997;11:597–606.
43. Zylberberg H, Pol S. Reciprocal interactions between human immunodeficiency virus and hepatitis C virus infection. Clin Infect Dis. 1996;23:1117–1125.
44. Tong MJ, el-Farra NS, Reikes AR, Co RL. Clinical outcomes after transfusion associated hepatitis C. N Engl J Med. 1995;332:1436.
45. Gumber SC, Chopra S. Hepatitis C: A multifaceted disease. Review of extrahepatic manifestations. Ann Intern Med. 1995;123:615–620.
46. Thomas DL, Shih JW, Alter HJ, et al. Effect of human immunodeficiency virus on hepatitis C virus infection among injection drug users. J Infect Dis. 1996;174:690–695.
47. Darby SC, Ewart DW, Giangrande PL, et al. Mortality from liver cancer and liver disease in haemophilic men and boys in UK given blood products contaminated with hepatitis C. UK Haemophila Centre Directors' Organization. Lancet. 1997;350:1425–1431.
48. Pol S, Lamorthe B, Thi NT, et al. Retrospective analysis of the impact of HIV infection and alcohol use on chronic hepatitis C in a large cohort of drug users. J Hepatol. 1998;28:945–950.
49. Dorrucci M, Pezzotti P, Phillips AN, et al. Coinfection of hepatitis C virus with human immunodeficiency virus and progression to AIDS. Italian Seroconversion Study. J Infect Dis. 1995;172:1503–1508.
50. Marcellin P, Martinot-Peignoux M, Elias A, et al. Hepatitis C virus (HCV) viremia in human immunodeficiency virus–seronegative and –seropositive patients with indeterminate HCV recombinant immunoblot assay. J Infect Dis. 1994;170:433–435.
51. Poles MA, Dieterich DT, Schwarz ED, et al. Liver biopsy findings in 501 patients infected with human immunodeficiency virus (HIV). J Acquir Immune Defic Syndr Hum Retrovirol. 1996;11:170–177.
52. Chaisson RE, Schecter GF, Theuer CP, et al. Tuberculosis in patients with the acquired immunodeficiency syndrome. Clinical feature, response to therapy, and survival. Am Rev Respir Dis. 1987;136:470–474.
53. Koehler JE, Sanchez MA, Garrido CS, et al. Molecular epidemiology of *Bartonella* infection in patients with bacillary angiomatosis-peliosis. N Engl J Med. 1997;1337:1876–1883.
54. Cavicchi M, Pialoux G, Carnot F, et al. Value of liver biopsy for the rapid diagnosis of infection in human immunodeficiency virus–infected patients who have unexplained fever and elevated serum levels of alkaline phosphatase or gamma-glutamyl transferase. Clin Infect Dis. 1995;20:606–610.
55. Zeigler JL, Beckstead JA, Volberding PA, et al. Non-Hodgkin's lymphoma in 90 homosexual men. Relation to generalized lymphadenopathy and the acquired immunodeficiency syndrome. N Engl J Med. 1984;311:565–570.
56. Ungo JR, Jones D, Ashkin D, et al. Antituberculosis drug–induced hepatoxicity. The role of hepatitis C virus and the human immunodeficiency virus. Am J Respir Crit Care Med. 1998;157:1871–1876.
57. Freiman JP, Helfert KE, Hamrell MR, Stein DS. Hepatomegaly with severe steatosis in HIV-seropositive patients. AIDS. 1993;7:379–385.
58. Rodriguez-Rosado R, Garcia-Samaniego J, Soriano V. Hepatotoxicity after the introduction of highly active antiretroviral therapy. AIDS. 1998;12:1256.
59. Dutta SK, Ting CD, Lai LL. Study of the prevalence, severity, and etiological factors associated with acute pancreatitis in patients infected with human immunodeficiency syndrome. Am J Gastroenterol. 1997;92:2044–2048.
60. Farman J, Brunetti J, Baer JW, et al. AIDS-related cholangiopancreatographic changes. Abdom Imaging. 1994;19:417–422.
61. Jaber B, Gleckman R. Tuberculosis pancreatic abscess as an initial AIDS-defining disorder in a patient infected with the human immunodeficiency virus: Case report and review. Clin Infect Dis. 1995;20:890–894.
62. Wilcox CM, Forsmark CE, Grendell JH, et al. Cytomegalovirus-associated acute pancreatic disease with acquired immunodeficiency syndrome. Report of two patients. Gastroenterology. 1990;99:263–267.
63. Schindzielorz A, Pike I, Daniels M, et al. Rates and risk factors for adverse events associated with didanosine in the expanded access program. Clin Infect Dis. 1994;19:1076–1083.
64. Assan R, Perronne C, Assan D, et al. Pentamidine-induced derangements of glucose homeostasis. Determinant roles of renal failure and drug accumulation. A study of 128 patients. Diabetes Care. 1995;18:47–55.
65. Henry K, Rathgaber S, Sullivan C, McCabe K. Diabetes mellitus induced by megesterol acetate in a patients with AIDS and cachexia. Ann Intern Med. 1992;116:53–54.
66. Eastone JA, Decker CF. New onset diabetes mellitus associated with the use of protease inhibitor. Ann Intern Med. 1997;127:948.
67. Sharpstone D, Gazzard B. Gastrointestinal manifestation of HIV infection. Lancet. 1996;348:379–383.
68. Angulo FJ, Swerdlow DL. Bacterial enteric infections in persons with human immunodeficiency virus. Clin Infect Dis. 1996;21:S84–S93.
69. Glaser JB, Morton-Kute L, Berger SR, et al. Recurrent *Salmonella typhimurium* bacteremia associated with the acquired immunodeficiency syndrome. Ann Intern Med. 1985;102:189–193.
70. Tee W, Mijch A. *Campylobter jejuni* bacteremia in human immunodeficiency (HIV)–infected and non–HIV-infected patients: Comparison of clinical features and review. Clin Infect Dis. 1998;26:91–96.
71. Barbut F, Meynard JL, Guiguet M, et al. *Clostridium difficile*–associated diarrhea in HIV-infected patients: Epidemiology and risk factors. J Acquir Immune Defic Syndr Hum Retrovirol. 1997;16:176–181.
72. Damsker B, Bottone EJ. *Mycobacterium avium–Mycobacterium intracellulare* from the intestinal tracts of patients with the acquired immunodeficiency syndrome: Concepts regarding acquisition and pathogenesis. J Infect Dis. 1985;151:179–181.
73. Soave R, Danner RL, Honig CL, et al. Cryptosporidiosis in homosexual men. Ann Intern Med. 1984;200:504–511.
74. Rabeneck L, Gyorkey F, Genta RM, et al. The role of microsporidia in the pathogenesis of HIV-related chronic diarrhea. Ann Intern Med. 1993;119:895–899.
75. DeHovitz JA, Pape JW, Boncy M, Johnson WD Jr. Clinical manifestations and therapy of *Isospora belli* infection in patients with the acquired immunodeficiency syndrome. N Engl J Med. 1986;315:87–90.
76. Pape JW, Verdier RI, Boncy M, et al. *Cyclospora* infection in adults infected with HIV. Clinical manifestations, treatment, and prophylaxis. Ann Intern Med. 1994;121:654–657.
77. Dieterich DT, Rahmin M. Cytomegalovirus colitis in AIDS: Presentation in 44 patients and a review of the literature. J Acquir Immune Defic Syndr. 1991;4:S29–S35.
78. Mentec H, Leport C, Leport J, et al. Cytomegalovirus colitis in HIV-infected patients: A prospective research in 55 patients. AIDS. 1994;8:461–467.
79. Grohmann GS, Glass RI, Pereira HG, et al. Enteric viruses and diarrhea in HIV-infected patients. N Engl J Med. 1993;329:14–20.
80. Quinn TC, Stamm We, Goodell SE, et al. The polymicrobial origin of intestinal infections in homosexual men. N Engl J Med. 1983;309:576–582.
81. Goodgame RW. Understanding intestinal spore-forming protozoa: Cryptosporidia, microsporidia, isospora, and cyclospora. Ann Intern Med. 1996:124:429–441.
82. Wilcox CM, Schwartz DA, Cotsonis G, Thompson SE 3rd. Chronic unexplained diarrhea in human immunodeficiency virus infection: Determination of the best diagnostic approach. Gastroenterology. 1996;110:30–37.
83. Bini EJ, Weinshel EH. Endoscopic evaluation of chronic human immunodeficiency virus–related diarrhea: Is colonoscopy superior to flexible sigmoidoscopy? Am J Gastroenterol. 1998;93:56–60.
84. Bown JW, Savides TJ, Mathews C, et al. Diagnostic yield of duodenal biopsy and aspirate in AIDS-associated diarrhea. Am J Gastroenterol. 1996;91:2289–2292.
85. David F, Schuitema AR, Sarfati C, et al. Detection and species identification of intestinal microsporidia by polymerase chain reaction in duodenal biopsies from human immunodeficiency virus–infected patients. J Infect Dis. 1996;174:874–877.
86. Banshard C, Francis N, Gazzard BG. Investigation of chronic diarrhea in acquired immunodeficiency syndrome. A prospective study of 155 patients. Gut. 1996;39:824–832.
87. Greenson JK, Belitsos PC, Yardley JH, Bartlett JG. AIDS enteropathy: Occult enteric infections and duodenal mucosal alterations in chronic diarrhea. Ann Intern Med. 1991;114:366–372.
88. Carr A, Marriott D, Field A, et al. Treatment of HIV-1–associated microsporidiosis and cryptosporidiosis with combination antiretroviral therapy. Lancet. 1998;351:256–261.

Chapter 111

Neurologic Manifestations of Human Immunodeficiency Virus Infection

ROBERT G. HOLLOWAY, JR.
KARL D. KIEBURTZ

Neurologic complications occur frequently in persons infected with human immunodeficiency virus type 1 (HIV-1).[1, 2] There are many causes of neurologic disease in HIV-1–infected persons, including primary HIV infection–related syndromes, opportunistic processes, inflammatory conditions, and drug toxicity. Diagnosis and treatment of neurologic illness in the HIV-1–infected person are complicated. The risk of neurologic complications changes as the disease progresses, and multiple complications may coexist at the same time. Accurate diagnosis of neurologic complications in the HIV-infected person is crucial, as many complications are treatable and effective intervention can lead to increased survival or improved quality of life. This chapter reviews the most common neurologic complications in the HIV-infected person, with an emphasis on differential diagnosis and management.

EPIDEMIOLOGY

Neurologic complications occur in 39 to 70% of patients with acquired immunodeficiency syndrome (AIDS) and significantly affect functional capacity, quality of life, and survival.[2–4] Neuropathologic examination identifies abnormal neurologic conditions in over 90% of autopsies of AIDs patients.[5] The primary HIV-related syndromes occur in nearly 30% of those infected[6] and occur almost three times as often as the central nervous system (CNS) opportunistic processes.[7] The primary HIV-related syndromes—dementia, neuropathy, and myelopathy—have become common causes of neurologic disease in young people.[8]

Recent research suggests that a treatment regimen of HIV reverse transcriptase inhibitors and protease inhibitors reduces mortality and delays progression of disease.[9] The frequency and distribution of the neurologic complications seen in the HIV-infected population will probably change dramatically for those who have access to this treatment combination. Dramatic regression and stabilization of certain opportunistic infections (e.g., progressive multifocal leukoencephalopathy) have been reported with combination antiretroviral therapy.[10] The impact on the epidemiology of the primary HIV infection–related neurologic syndromes is not yet known.

NEUROINVASION AND ASYMPTOMATIC HIV-1 INFECTION OF THE CENTRAL NERVOUS SYSTEM

HIV-1 enters the CNS soon after primary infection. CNS penetration may occur either via infected monocytes or lymphocytes or via cell-free mechanisms.[11, 12] Macrophages and microglial cells are the predominant cells infected within the CNS and are largely responsible for virus replication within the brain. Neurons, astrocytes, and oligodendrocytes are only rarely infected, and HIV-1 can be detected in the latter cells only by highly sensitive methods.[13]

HIV-1 has been isolated from the cerebrospinal fluid (CSF) of HIV-infected persons prior to immunosuppression and from the CSF and brain of patients with AIDS, with and without neurologic symptoms.[14–20] In addition, many HIV-infected persons possess CSF abnormalities including increased lymphocytes, protein, immunoglobulins, and oligoclonal bands.[21, 22] These abnormalities are present not only in patients with symptomatic neurologic disease but in many asymptomatic persons during the early phases of infection. The crucial question remains of what triggers the conversion from this relatively asymptomatic state to progressive cognitive impairment as seen in HIV-associated dementia.

NEUROLOGIC COMPLICATIONS BASED ON THE STAGE OF INFECTION

The spectrum of neurologic disease seen in HIV-infected persons is tightly linked to the stage of infection and the competence of the immune system (Fig. 111–1). Monophasic inflammatory or autoimmune-related conditions predominate at the time of HIV-1 seroconversion, whereas the primary HIV-related syndromes and opportunistic conditions predominate in the later immunodeficient stages. During the often long asymptomatic stage of infection, the pattern of neurologic disease conforms more to that seen within a general population.

The Early and Asymptomatic Stage of Infection

A variety of neurologic complications have been described that occur several days to several months after the primary infection with HIV-1 (Table 111–1). Proposed mechanisms include the primary viremia and an autoimmune or inflammatory response seen after onset of the infection. Most of these disorders are monophasic and self-limited. Examples of reported complications include aseptic meningitis,[23, 24] meningoencephalitis,[25] ataxic neuropathy,[26] acute rhabdomyolysis,[27] Guillain-Barré syndrome,[28] acute myelopathy,[29] a multiple sclerosis–like illness,[30] acute brachial neuritis,[31] Bell's palsy,[32] and acute meningoradiculitis.[33] Their occurrence in high-risk persons should prompt a test for HIV-1 infection, with retesting in 3 to 6 months if the result of the original test is negative.[34]

During the minimally symptomatic stage of infection, the common conditions are those that affect other populations with chronic illnesses including headache, depression, drug abuse, pain syndromes, and anxiety. It is also in this stage that other neurologic conditions completely unrelated to HIV-1 infection, such as epilepsy, diabetic neuropathy, and herniated discs, may occur. Conditions with an incompletely defined association with this stage include headache,[35] neuromuscular syndromes,[36] multiple sclerosis,[30] vitamin B_{12} deficiency,[37] and neurosyphilis.[38]

Peripheral Neuropathy

Various neuromuscular complications of HIV infection have been described including demyelinating neuropathies, vasculitic neuropathies, polyradiculopathy, and myopathy.[39] The most common neuromuscular complication is a distal sensory polyneuropathy (DSP).[7] DSP is characterized by a predominance of sensory symptoms including pain, dysesthesias, and diminished sensation. Symptoms usually start in the feet and are typically confined to the distal limbs. Painful or dysesthetic sensations may be brought on by standing or walking or even by contact with bed sheets. Symptoms may be present throughout the day but often worsen in the evening. There may be associated mild weakness, but this is usually confined to the intrinsic muscles of the feet. The symptoms usually begin insidiously, initially being mild dysesthesias. The severity and frequency of the symptoms gradually progress over months. The clinical syndrome is typical for a toxic distal sensory neuropathy such as is observed with diabetes mellitus or alcohol abuse.

DSP is usually a complication of advanced HIV infection and is most commonly observed in patients with $CD4^+$ cell counts less than 100/mm^3.[7] In the Multicenter AIDS Cohort Study (MACS), the average incidence over 5 years was 1.6 cases per 100 person years, with a clear trend for a higher incidence in persons with lower $CD4^+$ cell counts. In addition, there appeared to be a temporal trend, with

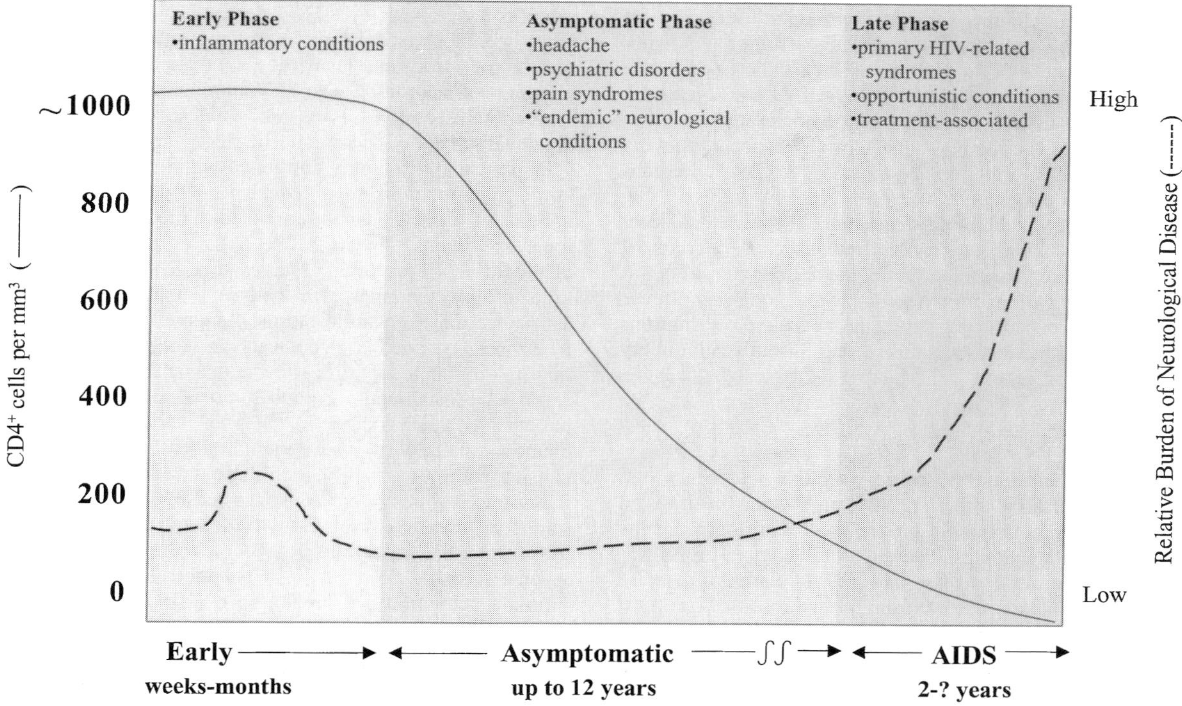

FIGURE 111–1. Major neurologic complications at different stages of HIV-1 infection.

an increasing incidence of neuropathy observed between 1989 and 1993. One possible cause of this increasing incidence was the introduction of antiretroviral agents that have been associated with the development of neuropathy. Both zalcitabine and didanosine can cause a painful neuropathy.[40–43] More recently developed antiretrovirals including lamivudine and stavudine may also be associated with a toxic neuropathy.[44] There has been no reported association between the protease inhibitors and DSP.

Pathologic specimens from patients with DSP demonstrate a range of findings from normal histologic features to infiltrates of mononuclear cells, predominantly macrophages, and nodules of Nageotte. HIV RNA sequences can be detected in the mononuclear cells and occasional neurons from the dorsal root ganglia of such patients.[45] The mechanism by which HIV infection causes DSP is unknown. However, active infection of neurons does not seem to be the most likely cause. A toxic effect of viral proteins or altered cytokine production may be responsible for nerve injury.[46, 47]

TABLE 111–1 Neurologic Complications of Early and Asymptomatic Human Immunodeficiency Virus Type 1 Infection

Early Infection (After Seroconversion)
Aseptic meningitis
Meningoencephalitis
Ataxic neuropathy
Acute rhabdomyolysis
Guillain-Barré syndrome
Acute myelopathy
Multiple sclerosis–like illness
Acute brachial neuritis
Bell's palsy
Acute meningoradiculitis
Asymptomatic Infection
Headache
Depression
Drug abuse
Pain syndromes
Anxiety
"Endemic" neurologic disease

A systematic diagnostic approach is useful in evaluating patients with pain and other sensory symptoms in the lower extremities, as such complaints are very common. The tempo of the illness, the distribution of the symptoms, and the antiviral drug regimen are all important to establishing the correct diagnosis. DSP related to HIV infection itself typically has a gradual, insidious onset; in contrast, antiretroviral toxic neuropathy typically develops more rapidly. The sensory findings in DSP are usually mild and consist of distal diminished response to light touch and vibration. Painful or dysesthetic sensation can sometimes be elicited by stimulation of the soles of the feet. Ankle reflexes are usually diminished or absent, and muscle weakness is usually not evident. The same findings are noted in antiretroviral neuropathy. The presence of prominent weakness or asymmetric sensory symptoms suggests an alternate diagnosis such as mononeuritis multiplex or demyelinating neuropathy. Early in the disease course, a non–HIV-related disorder is a more likely cause of DSP, such as lumbar disc disease or diabetic, nutritional (thiamine deficiency), or alcohol-related neuropathy. Routine screening laboratory tests should include determination of the serum vitamin B_{12} level, thyroid function tests, measurement of hemoglobin A_{1c}, and syphilis serologic studies. If there is concern regarding lumbar disc disease, lumbar imaging with computed tomography (CT) or magnetic resonance imaging (MRI) may be appropriate. Clear-cut asymmetric motor and sensory findings should prompt a neurologic referral for possible further evaluation including electrodiagnostic studies.

In patients in whom the history and physical findings suggest an antiretroviral cause of DSP, these agents should be temporarily suspended if possible. Symptoms may continue or even worsen for 2 to 3 weeks following cessation of the agent. After this, symptoms should gradually resolve, and some patients may be able to tolerate the reintroduction of the offending agent, sometimes at a lower dose. In patients who appear to have an HIV infection–related DSP, no specific intervention is required unless pain and other symptoms are problematic or functionally limiting. The pain and other symptoms associated with vasculitic neuropathy may be relieved by prednisone,[48] but prednisone does not appear to be effective in DSP. Standard therapeutic approaches for other painful neuropathies such as low-dose tricyclic antidepressants are commonly used. Typical starting doses of these agents are 10 to 25 mg at night, gradually increasing to doses of up to 50 to 100 mg nightly. Other therapeutic agents used are anticonvulsants and oral antiarrhythmic agents. A recent double-blind, placebo-controlled trial demonstrated that neither amitriptyline nor mexiletine was superior to placebo in relieving painful symptoms of HIV infection–related DSP.[49] Thus, clinicians must balance the anecdotal reports of some efficacy with tricyclic antidepressants with the results of this randomized trial. A randomized trial of peptide T also demonstrated no efficacy.[50] Trials of human recombinant nerve growth factor and the anticonvulsant lamotrigine for the treatment of painful neuropathy are ongoing. Better therapies are needed, because patients cite neurologic symptoms as a major cause of functional disability and diminished quality of life.[51, 52]

Cognitive Impairment

Clinicians and researchers have observed cognitive and behavioral decline in patients with HIV infection. Although it has been noted in all stages of HIV infection, this progressive neurologic decline usually happens in the later stages. The cognitive changes are different from those of Alzheimer's disease and are more similar to those observed with Parkinson's disease or Huntington's disease. The most common initial symptoms are decreased attention and concentration, as well as difficulty shifting cognitive tasks. Patients may compensate for these changes by writing down appointments and commitments and allowing more time to perform cognitive tasks. They may also focus attention on one task and complete it prior to moving to another task. Eventually, patients note difficulty following the content of reading material or media presentations. Associated behavioral changes include increased irritability, apathy, and a diminished desire for social contact. There may be concomitant neurologic difficulties including gait imbalance and upper extremity incoordination.[53, 54] The first major clinical and pathologic reports of this syndrome referred to it as the *AIDS dementia complex*.[55, 56] A revised nomenclature was proposed in 1991[57] and suggested the term *HIV-1–associated cognitive motor complex* to encompass both the cognitive and motor changes. *HIV-associated minor cognitive motor disorder* was proposed for milder forms of cognitive and motor impairment in which functional disability had not yet occurred. These terms have not become widely used. The more common terms in the literature are *HIV dementia* and, for the milder forms of the disorder, *HIV-associated cognitive impairment.*

Cognitive impairment is one of the more common and feared complications of HIV infection. Between 10% and 20% of HIV-infected people will develop some form of cognitive impairment prior to their death. The impact of therapy with protease inhibitors on the frequency of this complication is unknown. Follow-up of the patients in MACS revealed that cognitive performance, in general, was stable prior to AIDS, but after an AIDS-defining illness or $CD4^+$ count drop below 200/mm^3, there was a mild change in fine motor skills. In patients with more advanced HIV infection who went on to become clinically demented, there was a significant decline in all cognitive measures.[58] Although overt dementia is uncommon in early HIV infection, milder cognitive impairment in relatively early stages of HIV infection may be associated with increased work disability.[59] Development of cognitive impairment is a significant event, as multiple studies have found that it is an independent risk factor for death.[60, 61]

Brain specimens from patients who died with HIV dementia demonstrate mild to severe atrophy on gross examination. Microscopic abnormalities are seen chiefly in the white matter and subcortical gray matter, with relative sparing of the cortex. Perivascular lymphocytic and macrophagic infiltrates can be seen in the deep gray structures. Microglial nodules and multinucleated giant cells are also found in a similar distribution. Although there is no clear dropout of large numbers of cortical neurons, significant pruning of the dendritic arbor is associated with HIV dementia.[62] HIV proteins and RNA have been localized primarily to microglial cells and, to a lesser extent, to astrocytes. There does not appear to be any productive infection of neurons.[63] The HIV burden in the brain (measured by viral proteins or RNA titers) does not appear to be associated with the development of dementia. The frequency and presence of infected cells may be more highly correlated with multinucleated cell encephalitis,[64] the relationship of which to HIV dementia is unclear. The number of macrophages or activated microglial cells found in pathologic specimens appears to be a better predictor of a dementing disorder.[65, 66] These findings taken together suggest that the interactions of infected microglial cells and macrophages with activated astrocytes may constitute the mechanism of neurologic dysfunction. In support of such a hypothesis are the findings of elevated β_2-microglobulin, a measure of immune activation, and of increased levels of prostaglandin E_2 and tumor necrosis factor-α (TNF-α) in patients with HIV dementia.[67–69] There is also evidence that protein elements in the virus itself, including gp120 and tat, are capable of causing neurotoxicity, although these data are derived primarily from in vitro experiments.[70, 71] As suggested by preliminary findings, CSF viral load may be correlated with dementia severity in patients with advanced HIV infection.[72, 73] Studies are in progress to identify whether rising CSF viral load and increasing levels of markers of immune activation are predictors of HIV dementia or are epiphenomena.

The evaluation of the HIV-infected patient presenting with cognitive difficulties will differ according to whether the disease is in an early or advanced stage. In patients with early HIV infection, HIV-related cognitive impairment is very unusual. Depression and other psychiatric disorders, including alcohol and substance abuse, are more likely to be causes of cognitive impairment. In patients with $CD4^+$ cell counts below 200/mm^3 or, more frequently, below 100/mm^3, an opportunistic infectious or neoplastic process should also be suspected, particularly if the onset of the syndrome is acute or subacute. The presence of focal or asymmetric neurologic deficits always signals that HIV dementia is not the leading consideration in the differential diagnosis. The main diagnostic categories to consider aside from opportunistic infectious and neoplastic processes are metabolic derangements, drug-induced disorders, psychiatric disorders, vascular disease (especially in the protease inhibitor era), and HIV dementia (Table 111–2). Thrombotic thromborytopenic purpura (TTP) may also be a cause of confusion, disturbed consciousness, and seizures.

A routine evaluation of patients with advanced HIV infection and cognitive complaints should include a careful review of all drugs taken including nonprescription, prescription, and illicit. Withdrawal from narcotics, alcohol, and illicit drugs should also be considered as a potential cause of cognitive impairment. Taking a careful history to look for psychiatric disorders or for a family history of such

TABLE 111–2 Differential Diagnosis of Cognitive Impairment

Early to Mid-Stage HIV Disease
Depression
Alcohol and substance abuse
Medication-induced cognitive impairment
Metabolic encephalopathies
HIV-related cognitive impairment
Advanced HIV Disease ($CD4^+$ <100/mm^3)
Opportunistic infection of CNS
Neurosyphilis
CNS lymphoma
Progressive multifocal leukoencephalopathy
Depression
Metabolic encephalopathies
Medication-induced cognitive impairment
Stroke
HIV dementia

Abbreviations: CNS, Central nervous system; HIV, human immunodeficiency virus.

disorders is essential. Routine laboratory evaluations should include measurement of electrolyte concentrations and vitamin B_{12} level, thyroid and liver function tests, a serologic test for syphilis, and determination of cryptococcal serum antigen and *Toxoplasma* serum antibody titers. Screening neurologic examinations should be targeted to identify focal weakness or coordination difficulties. Such an examination should include assessment of finger tapping with both hands, hopping on each foot independently, finger-to-nose maneuvers, and the ability to stand with the feet together and the eyes closed. Difficulties with any of these tasks warrants a formal neurologic evaluation. Brain imaging is recommended in patients with a $CD4^+$ count below 200/mm^3, or in any patient with atypical or rapid progression of symptoms. MRI is the technique of choice for evaluation in HIV-infected patients. If the MRI scan reveals no mass lesions, CSF examination is important to exclude chronic meningitis and neurosyphilis.

Treatment options for HIV dementia are limited. The only reported placebo-controlled trial of an antiviral agent demonstrated that zidovudine in doses of 1000 to 2000 mg/day can improve cognitive performance.[74] More recent clinical trials have been targeted at assessment of agents that interrupt or interfere with the potential cascade of problems leading to neuronal injury.[75] A randomized trial of peptide T demonstrated no benefit in patients with HIV-associated cognitive impairment.[76] A pilot trial of an antioxidant medication, OPC-14117, in HIV dementia demonstrated no clear-cut benefit.[77] A small pilot trial of 38 patients found that the monoamine oxidase (MAO) B inhibitor selegiline at a dosage of 2.5 mg three times a week produced a modest improvement in attention and in the performance of timed cognitive tasks.[78] The same trial also assessed another antioxidant medication, α-lipoic acid, which showed no benefit. A trial of the calcium channel antagonist nimodipine showed no clear benefit, although some trends for improvement were noted.[79] Clinical trials are in progress to assess a platelet-aggregating factor antagonist, a TNF antagonist, and the weak glutamate receptor antagonist memantine. The impact of protease inhibitors on HIV dementia is unknown, although initial reports suggest that treatment initiation is associated with an improvement of cognitive function. Long-term impact has yet to be identified.

NEUROLOGIC SIDE EFFECTS OF DRUGS USED IN HUMAN IMMUNODEFICIENCY VIRUS TYPE 1 INFECTION

In addition to the neurologic complications caused by HIV-1 infection itself, antiviral treatments may induce neurologic complications (Table 111–3).

TABLE 111–3 Neurologic Side Effects from Drugs Used in Human Immunodeficiency Virus Infection

Drug	Neurologic Side Effects
Nucleoside Reverse Transcriptase Inhibitors	
Zidovudine	Myopathy, headache
Didanosine	Neuropathy
Zalcitabine	Neuropathy (high risk for this effect)
Stavudine	Neuropathy
Lamivudine	Headache, neuropathy rare
Non-nucleoside Reverse Transcriptase Inhibitors	
Nevirapine, delavirdine	Serious neurologic toxicity rare
Protease Inhibitors	Serious neurologic toxicity rare Lipid abnormalities and premature atherosclerosis
Others	
Trimethoprim-sulfamethoxazole	Headache
Foscarnet, ganciclovir	Lowered seizure threshold
Ethambutol	Retrobulbar neuritis

Nucleoside Reverse Transcriptase Inhibitors

Zidovudine

Zidovudine use has been associated with the development of myopathy. Zidovudine has been reported to interfere with mitochondrial function—potentially affecting mitochondrial DNA polymerase—and has been associated with muscle carnitine deficiency.[80–82] The clinical symptoms of zidovudine-induced myopathy are generally indistinguishable from the myopathy associated with HIV-1 infection, including symmetric primarily proximal weakness, myalgias, elevated serum creatine kinase (CK) levels, and normal sensory function. Electromyography may reveal fibrillation potentials, positive sharp waves, and complex repetitive discharges. Muscle biopsies have been reported to demonstrate the presence of ragged red fibers more frequently in zidovudine-associated myopathy.[83] Zidovudine-related myopathy can occur at any stage of the infection.

The standard therapeutic approach to zidovudine-induced myopathy has been to stop the potentially offending agent. Although there is some evidence that patients who receive this agent experience improvement in terms of improved strength, decreased myalgias, and lower serum CK levels,[84] some patients also spontaneously improve.[85] There is, therefore, controversy about the most appropriate approach to the management of patients with myopathy who are receiving zidovudine therapy. A clinical trial of prednisone versus withdrawal of zidovudine is in progress. At present the most prudent clinical management seems to be to stop zidovudine, with subsequent monitoring of the clinical course. If no other antiviral options are available, zidovudine can be reintroduced cautiously at lower levels. Clinical symptoms indicating a recurrence of myopathy include increased myalgias and an elevated serum CK level.

Zidovudine has also been associated with headache. In a double-blind, placebo-controlled study, headache was not significantly more common in the zidovudine treatment group, but the severity tended to be worse.[86] Zidovudine is not associated with the development of peripheral neuropathy, in contrast with the other reverse transcriptase inhibitors.

Didanosine

In early testing of didanosine, neuropathy was recognized as a dose-limiting complication, but this is uncommon at currently recommended doses.[42] The neuropathy is clinically very similar to the DSP associated with HIV-1 infection, as described previously. The symptoms are primarily sensory in nature and confined primarily to the lower extremities. There is minimal if any intrinsic foot muscle weakness. In comparison with that in HIV-1–related neuropathy, symptom onset may be more rapid. Other laboratory and electrodiagnostic tests are not generally useful in distinguishing antiviral-related toxic neuropathy from HIV-1–related neuropathy. Patients with a prior history of neuropathy may be more sensitive to the neurotoxic effects of antiretroviral drugs. Residual painful symptoms may respond to standard symptomatic treatment for neuropathy such as with tricyclic antidepressants.

Zalcitabine

Zalcitabine also causes a dose-dependent, primarily sensory neuropathy.[40, 87] In a large clinical trial comparing zalcitabine and didanosine, however, peripheral neuropathy was about twice as common in the zalcitabine group, suggesting that this agent at standard dosages may be more likely to produce neuropathy.[43] Vitamin B_{12} deficiency and prior alcohol use may be risk factors for developing this toxic neuropathy.[88] Other manifestations of neurologic toxicity are rarer with zalcitabine and include headache.[89]

Stavudine

Stavudine administered at high doses has also been associated with peripheral neuropathy, but this is rarely encountered as a clinical problem at currently recommended doses.[90]

Lamivudine

The development of peripheral neuropathy is extremely rare with lamivudine, although it has been shown to exacerbate preexisting peripheral neuropathy.[44] This drug is generally very well tolerated but can be associated with headache.

Non-nucleoside Reverse Transcriptase Inhibitors

The non-nucleoside reverse transcriptase–inhibiting agents, nevirapine and delavirdine, are relatively nontoxic, and available data on neurologic effects of these drugs are scarce. Peripheral neuropathy does not appear to be a complication of these drugs, and either agent may be a suitable alternative for combination therapy in persons who either have or are at increased risk for (e.g., owing to diabetes or alcohol use) peripheral neuropathy.

Protease Inhibitors

Little information is available on neurologic side effects of the protease inhibitors: saquinavir, ritonavir, indinavir, and nelfinavir. Although these agents do not appear to cause either a peripheral neuropathy or myopathy, ritonavir is commonly associated with circumoral paresthesias and occasionally headaches.[91] An emerging concern with the protease inhibitors is the potential for lipid abnormalities and accelerated atherosclerosis.[92] Drug interactions remain an important factor in their clinical use. Anxiolytic agents (e.g., triazolam, midazolam) should be used concomitantly with extreme caution, as the protease inhibitors may increase their bioavailability and cause excessive sedation.[89]

Other Commonly Used Drugs

Other therapeutic agents used in the treatment of HIV-related infections have also been reported to cause neuropathy: dapsone, isoniazid, vincristine, cisplatin, metronidazole, and nitrofurantoin. Other commonly used medications in the HIV population that are associated with headache include trimethoprim-sulfamethoxazole, fluconazole, itraconazole, azithromycin, and rifabutin. Finally, ethambutol is associated with optic neuropathy, and cycloserine, foscarnet, ganciclovir, and ethionamide may lower the seizure threshold.

OTHER MAJOR CATEGORIES OF NEUROLOGIC DISEASE

Headaches

Headaches are common in the HIV-1–infected person and increase in frequency as the disease progresses.[35, 93, 94] HIV infection–related headaches can occur at any time during the infection: at seroconversion, during the asymptomatic phase, in patients with symptomatic infection, or after an AIDS-defining illness. Causes of HIV infection–related headaches include HIV-1 infection itself, opportunistic infections, and HIV-specific medications. Recognized headache syndromes associated with HIV-1 infection include an acute aseptic meningitis, a chronic headache associated with a persistent pleocytosis, and a late-stage headache without a pleocytosis.[24, 95]

Opportunistic infections can be manifested as an isolated headache, although the absence of headache should never be used to rule out a diagnosis of a possible opportunistic CNS infection. For example, more than 10% of patients with cryptococcal meningitis and neurosyphilis, more than 40% of those with *Toxoplasma* encephalitis and tuberculous meningitis, and 70% of those with cytomegalovirus encephalitis do not have complaints of headache.[96–100]

Despite the underlying susceptibility to opportunistic conditions, the most common causes of headache in the HIV-1 population remain the primary headache syndromes: migraine headaches and tension-type headaches. Increased risk factors for developing headaches include anxiety, depression, psychiatric disease, and drug abuse.[101] Recognizing and referring or treating patients with concurrent mood and anxiety disorders may be the most important aspect of management in many of these patients.

In attempting pharmacologic therapy to control troubling headaches, the governing principle of choosing a medication (tricyclic antidepressant versus selective serotonergic reuptake inhibitor [SSRI]) should be based primarily on potential side effects, because the efficacy profiles of the prophylactic medications are similar. For example, antidepressants, such as amitriptyline, with sedative properties may not be appropriate for those patients with excessive fatigue and low energy levels. In contrast, patients with gastrointestinal complaints either from medications (e.g., protease inhibitors) or from chronic diarrhea would be less well served with the SSRIs.

Cerebrovascular Disease

HIV-infected persons are at an increased risk for developing strokes, and 8 to 34% of the cases in pediatric and adult autopsy series have cerebrovascular pathologic features.[102–104] The etiology of these strokes can be vascular occlusive disease or cardioembolism, both of which can be due to infectious conditions. Numerous opportunistic pathogens have been implicated in vasculopathy of infectious origin leading to stroke; *Treponema pallidum*,[105] *Myobacterium tuberculosis*,[106] cytomegalovirus (CMV),[107] varicella-zoster virus,[108] *Candida albicans*,[107] *Aspergillus fumigatus*, the agents of mucormycosis,[109] and HIV-1 itself;[102] lymphoma has also been reported as a cause of stroke in this population. Cardiac pathology is common in AIDS patients,[110] and cardiac emboli may arise with infective endocarditis, nonbacterial thrombotic endocarditis, congestive cardiomyopathy, or a patent foramen ovale.[104] AIDS patients also have a variety of hematologic abnormalities that can predispose to a hypercoagulable state including the presence of antiphospholipid antibodies[111] and deficient protein S and protein C levels.[112] For patients receiving protease inhibitor therapy, the possibility of raised lipid concentrations and accelerated atherosclerosis must be considered.[92] Intracerebral and subarachnoid hemorrhages are relatively infrequent but can be seen with illicit drug abuse, thrombocytopenia, and ruptured mycotic aneurysms.

Seizures

Seizures occur frequently in HIV-infected persons, although large-scale epidemiologic studies do not exist regarding the frequency of seizures in the various stages of HIV infection. Seizures were the presenting manifestation of HIV disease in 18 of 100 patients who had new-onset seizures, and generalized motor convulsions were more common than partial seizures.[113, 114] An identifiable cause is not found in 23 to 46% of patients, and the disorder is presumed to be secondary to HIV-1 infection itself. Other potential causes include *Toxoplasma* encephalitis, cryptococcal meningitis, primary CNS lymphoma, metabolic derangements, and cerebral infarctions. Anticonvulsant therapy should be strongly considered after the first seizure because recurrence is so frequent. Because of the high incidence of side effects and the potential for drug interactions with phenytoin,[113] phenobarbital may be an attractive first-line agent in new-onset seizures in the HIV-infected patient.

Opportunistic Infections

In opportunistic infections of the nervous system associated with HIV-1 infection, the presenting manifestations may be any of a variety of neurologic signs and symptoms. These most often involve the CNS and include headache, seizures, disturbance of cognitive function, and focal neurologic deficits.[115–117] The extent of immunosuppression in the patient is an important determinant of the likelihood that such an infection may be present. For example, toxoplasmosis, cryptococcosis, and progressive multifocal leukoencephalopathy (PML) occur largely in patients with CD4+ counts of less than 100/mm³, and often in patients with counts of less than 50/mm³.[115] Another important etiologic factor is intravenous substance abuse, which can lead to endocarditis, intravascular infections, and embolic phenomena involving the CNS.

A useful approach to the diagnosis of opportunistic infections of the CNS is to determine whether a focal or a diffuse (nonfocal) process is present. The use of neuroimaging techniques, particularly MRI, has enabled CNS lesions to be detected, localized, and characterized with great accuracy. With CD4+ counts of less than 50/mm³, more than 90% of focal lesions in the CNS will be shown to be either toxoplasmosis, PML, or primary CNS lymphoma[115] (see Chapter 112). Tuberculosis,[118] nocardiosis,[119] and aspergillosis can also present as focal CNS processes.

Opportunistic infections that usually present nonfocally include cryptococcal meningitis[120] and CMV encephalitis,[99] both of which usually occur in the setting of advanced immunosuppression. Unusual focal presentations of both cryptococcal and CMV infections[121] of the CNS have been reported as well. Meningitis caused by bacterial agents such as *M. tuberculosis* and, less commonly, *Streptococcus pneumoniae* and *Listeria monocytogenes* can also occur. Infection of the CNS with *T. pallidum*—that is, neurosyphilis—may be present in asymptomatic or symptomatic forms. The most common clinical presentation of neurosyphilis in this patient population is that of an acute syphilitic meningitis, or meningovascular syphilis. Other manifestations, including uveitis, sensorineural hearing loss, and tabes dorsalis, can also occur (see Chapter 227). A diffuse form of CNS toxoplasmosis ("toxoplasma encephalitis") can also occur and has a particularly fulminant course.[122] Viral encephalitis caused by herpes simplex virus or varicella-zoster virus may also have diffuse clinical presentations in AIDS patients. It should be noted that a low-grade mononuclear pleocytosis is a frequent CSF finding in both symptomatic and asymptomatic HIV-1–infected patients.[123] This has been attributed to direct CNS involvement with HIV-1 and can be a confounding variable in interpretation of CNS findings in HIV-1–infected patients.

A more detailed discussion of the diagnosis and management of opportunistic infections in patients with AIDS can be found in Chapter 116, as well as in chapters dealing with the individual microbial pathogens.

REFERENCES

1. Gabuzda DH, Hirsch MS. Neurologic manifestations of infection with human immunodeficiency virus: Clinical features and pathogenesis. Ann Intern Med. 1987;107:383–391.
2. Levy RM, Bredesen DE, Rosenblum ML. Neurological manifestations of the acquired immunodeficiency syndrome (AIDS): Experience at UCSF and review of the literature. J Neurosurg. 1985;62:475–495.
3. Snider WD, Simpson DM, Nielsen S, et al. Neurological complications of acquired immune deficiency syndrome: Analysis of 50 patients. Ann Neurol. 1983;14:403–418.
4. Wachtel T, Piette J, Mor V. Quality of life in persons with human immunodeficiency virus infection: Measurement by the medical outcomes study instrument. Ann Intern Med. 1992;116:129–137.
5. Budka H. Neuropathology of human immunodeficiency virus infection. Brain Pathol. 1991;1:163–175.
6. Nakagawa M, Maruyama Y, Sugita H, Osame M. Nationwide survey of neurologic manifestations of acquired immunodeficiency syndrome in Japan. Intern Med. 1997;36:175–178.
7. Bacellar H, Munoz A, Miller EN, et al. Temporal trends in the incidence of HIV-1–related neurologic diseases: Multicenter AIDS Cohort Study, 1985–1992. Neurology. 1994;44:1892–1900.
8. Janssen RS, Nwanyanwu OC, Selik RM, Stehr-Green JK. Epidemiology of human immunodeficiency virus encephalopathy in the United States. Neurology. 1992;42:1472–1476.
9. Carpenter CC, Fischl MA, Hammer SM. Antiretroviral therapy for HIV infection in 1997: Update recommendations of the international AIDS society—USA panel. JAMA. 1997;277:1962–1969.
10. Elliot B, Aromin I, Gold R, et al. 2.5 year remission of AIDS-associated progressive multifocal leukoencephalopathy with combined antiretroviral therapy. Lancet. 1997;349:850.
11. Resnick L, Berger JR, Shapshak P, Tourtellotte WW. Early penetration of the blood-brain barrier by HIV. Neurology. 1988;38:9–14.
12. Davis LE, Hjelle BL, Miller VE. Early viral brain invasion in iatrogenic human immunodeficiency virus infection. Neurology. 1992;42:1736–1739.
13. Gonzalez-Scarano F, Kolson DL, Albright AV. Viral receptors and cellular mechanisms of HIV-2 entry into the central nervous system. In: Gendelman HE, Lipton SA, Epstein L, Swindells S, eds. Neurology of AIDS. New York: Chapman & Hall; 1998:36–48.
14. Levy JA, Shimabukuro J, Hollander H, et al. Isolation of AIDS-associated retroviruses from cerebrospinal fluid and brain of patients with neurological symptoms. Lancet. 1985;2:586–588.
15. Ho DD, Rota TR, Schooley RT. Isolation of HTLV-III from cerebrospinal fluid and neural tissues of patients with neurological syndromes related to the acquired immunodeficiency syndrome. N Engl J Med. 1985;313:1493–1497.
16. Ghiodi F, Asjo B, Fanyo EM, et al. Isolation of HIV from cerebrospinal fluid of antibody-positive virus carrier without neurological symptoms. Lancet. 1986;2:1276–1277.
17. Goudsmit J, de Wolf F, Paul DA. Expression of human immunodeficiency virus antigen (HIV-ag) in serum and cerebrospinal fluid during acute and chronic infection. Lancet. 1986;2:177–180.
18. Resnick L, Dimarzo-Veronese F, Schupbach J. Intra-blood-brain-barrier synthesis of HTLV-III–specific IgG in patients with neurologic symptoms associated with AIDS or AIDS-related complex. N Engl J Med. 1985;313:1498–1504.
19. Chiodi F, Albert J, Olausson E. Isolation frequency of human immunodeficiency virus from cerebrospinal fluid and blood of patients with varying severity of HIV infection. AIDS Res Hum Retroviruses. 1988;4:351–358.
20. Hollander H, Levy JA. Neurologic abnormalities and recovery of human immunodeficiency virus from cerebrospinal fluid. Ann Intern Med. 1987;106:692–695.
21. Marshall DW, Brey RL, Cahill WT, et al. Spectrum of cerebrospinal fluid findings in various stages of human immunodeficiency virus infection. Arch Neurol. 1988;45:954–958.
22. McArthur JC, Cohen BA, Farzadegan H. Cerebrospinal fluid abnormalities in homosexual men with and without neuropsychiatric findings. Ann Neurol. 1988;23:S34–S37.
23. Ho DD, Sarngadharan MG, Resnick L, et al. Primary human T-lymphotropic virus type III infection. Ann Intern Med. 1985;103:880–883.
24. Hollander H, Stringari S. Human immunodeficiency virus–associated meningitis: Clinical course and correlations. Am J Med. 1987;83:813–816.
25. Carne CA, Tedder RS, Smith A. Acute encephalopathy coincident with seroconversion for anti-HTLV-III. Lancet. 1985;2:1206–1208.
26. Castellanos F, Mallada J, Ricart C, Zabala JA. Ataxic neuropathy associated with human immunodeficiency virus seroconversion. Arch Neurol. 1994;51:236.
27. Chariot P, Ruet E, Authier FJ, et al. Acute rhabdomyolysis in patients infected by human immunodeficiency virus. Neurology. 1994;44:1692–1696.
28. Hagberg L, Maimvail B, Svennerholm B, et al. Guillain-Barré syndrome as an early manifestation of HIV central nervous system infection. Scand J Infect Dis. 1986;18:591–592.
29. Denning DW, Anderson J, Rudge P, Smith H. Acute myelopathy associated with primary infection with human immunodeficiency virus. BMJ. 1987;294:143–144.
30. Berger AR, Sheremata W, Resnick L, et al. Multiple sclerosis–like illness occurring with human immunodeficiency virus infection. Neurology. 1987;39:324–329.
31. Calabresse LH, Proffitt MR, Levin KH, et al. Acute infection with the human immunodeficiency virus (HIV) associated with acute brachial neuritis and exanthematous rash. Ann Intern Med. 1987;107:849–851.
32. Wiselka MJ, Nicholson KG, Ward SC, Flower AJE. Acute infection with human immunodeficiency virus associated with facial nerve palsy and neuralgia. J Infect. 1987;15:189–194.
33. Paton P, Poly H, Gonnaud P. Acute meningoradiculitis concomitant with seroconversion to human immunodeficiency virus type 1. Res Virol. 1990;141:427–433.
34. Horsburgh CR, Ou CY, Jason J. Duration of human immunodeficiency virus infection before detection of antibody. Lancet. 1989;2:637–640.
35. Holloway RG, Kieburtz KD. Headache and the human immunodeficiency virus type 1 infection. Headache. 1996;35:245–255.
36. Lange DJ. Neuromuscular disease associated with HIV-1 infection. Muscle Nerve. 1994;17:16–30.
37. Robertson KR, Stern RA, Hall CD, et al. Vitamin B_{12} deficiency and nervous system disease in HIV infection. Arch Neurol. 1993;50:807–811.
38. Simon RP. Neurosyphilis. Neurology. 1994;44:2228–2230.
39. Fuller GN, Jacobs JM, Guiloff RJ. Nature and incidence of peripheral nerve syndrome in HIV infection. J Neurol Neurosurg Psychiatry. 1993;56:372–381.
40. Berger AR, Arezzo JC, Schaumburg HH, et al. 2′,3′-Dideoxycytidine (ddC) toxic neuropathy: A study of 52 patients. Neurology. 1993;43:358–362.
41. Blum AS, Dal Pan GJ, Feinberg J, et al. Low-dose zalcitabine–related toxic neuropathy: Frequency, natural history, and risk factors. Neurology. 1996;46:999–1003.
42. Kieburtz KD, Seidlin M, Lambert JS, et al. Extended follow-up of peripheral neuropathy in patients with AIDS and AIDS-related complex treated with dideoxyinosine. J Acquir Immune Defic Syndr. 1992;5:60–64.
43. Abrams DI, Goldman AI, Launer C, et al. A comparative trial of didanosine or zalcitabine after treatment with zidovudine in patients with human immunodeficiency virus infection. N Engl J Med. 1994;330:657–662.
44. Cupler EJ, Dalakas MC. Exacerbation of peripheral neuropathy by lamivudine. Lancet. 1995;345:460–461.
45. Brannagan TH, Nuovo GJ, Hays AP, Latov N. Human immunodeficiency virus

infection of dorsal root ganglion neurons detected by polymerase chain reaction in situ hybridization. Ann Neurol. 1997;42:368–372.
46. Yoshioka M, Shapshak P, Srivastava AK, et al. Expression of HIV-1 and interleukin-6 in lumbosacral dorsal root ganglia of patients with AIDS. Neurology. 1994;44:1120–1130.
47. Apostolski S, McAlarney T, Quattrini A, et al. The gp120 glycoprotein of human immunodeficiency virus type 1 binds to sensory ganglion neurons. Ann Neurol. 1993;34:855–863.
48. Bradley WG, Verma A. Painful vasculitic neuropathy in HIV-1 infection: Relief of pain with prednisone therapy. Neurology. 1996;47:1446–1451.
49. Kieburtz K, Yiannoutsos CP, Simpson D, AIDS Clinical Trials Group. A double-blind, randomized clinical trial of amitriptyline and mexiletine for painful neuropathy in human immunodeficiency virus infection (Abstract). Ann Neurol. 1997;42:429.
50. Simpson DM, Dorfman D, Olney RK, et al. Peptide T in the treatment of painful distal neuropathy associated with AIDS: Results of a placebo-controlled trial. Neurology. 1997;47:1254–1259.
51. Cleary PD, Fowler FJ, Weissman J, et al. Health-related quality of life in persons with acquired immune deficiency syndrome. Med Care. 1993;31:569–580.
52. Wilson IB, Cleary PD. Clinical predictors of functioning in persons with acquired immunodeficiency syndrome. Med Care. 1996;34:610–623.
53. Stern Y, Liu X, Marder K, et al. Neuropsychological changes in a prospectively followed cohort of homosexual and bisexual men with and without HIV infection. Neurology. 1995;45:467–472.
54. Marder K, Liu X, Stern Y, et al. Neurologic signs and symptoms in a cohort of homosexual men followed for 4.5 years. Neurology. 1995;45:261–267.
55. Navia BA, Jordan BD, Price RW. The AIDS dementia complex: I. Clinical features. Ann Neurol. 1986;19:517–524.
56. Navia BA, Cho E-S, Petito CK, Price RW. The AIDS dementia complex: II. Neuropathology. Ann Neurol. 1986;19:525–535.
57. American Academy of Neurology AIDS Task Force. Nomenclature and research case definitions for neurologic manifestations of human immunodeficiency virus type 1 (HIV-1) infection. Neurology. 1991;41:778–785.
58. Selnes OA, Galai N, Bacellar H, et al. Cognitive performance after progression to AIDS: A longitudinal study from the Multicenter AIDS Cohort Study. Neurology. 1995;45:267–275.
59. Albert SM, Marder K, Dooneief G, et al. Neuropsychologic impairment in early HIV infection. Arch Neurol. 1995;52:525–530.
60. Mayeux R, Tang M, Tocad G, et al. Mortality risks in gay men with human immunodeficiency virus infection and cognitive impairment. Neurology. 1993;43:176–182.
61. Ellis RJ, Deutsch R, Heaton RK, et al. Neurocognitive impairment is an independent risk factor for death in HIV infection. Arch Neurol. 1997;54:416–424.
62. Masliah E, Heaton RK, Marcotte TD, et al. Dendritic injury is a pathological substrate for human immunodeficiency virus–related cognitive disorders. Ann Neurol. 1997;42:963–972.
63. Takahashi K, Wesselingh SL, Griffin DE, et al. Localization of HIV-1 in human brain using polymerase chain reaction/in situ hybridization and immunonocytochemisty. Ann Neurol. 1996;39:705–711.
64. Brew BJ, Rosenblum M, Cronin K, Price RW. AIDS dementia complex and HIV-1 brain infection: Clinical-virological correlations. Ann Neurol. 1995;38:563–570.
65. Johnson RT, Glass JD, McArthur JC, Chesebro BW. Quantitation of human immunodeficiency virus in brains of demented and non-demented patients with acquired immunodeficiency syndrome. Ann Neurol. 1996;39:392–395.
66. Glass JD, Fedor H, Wesselingh SL, McArthur JC. Immunocytochemical quantitation of human immunodeficiency virus in the brain: Correlations with dementia. Ann Neurol. 1995;38:755–762.
67. McArthur JC, Nance-Sproson TE, Griffin DE, et al. The diagnostic utility of elevation in cerebrospinal fluid β_2-microglobulin in HIV-1 dementia. Neurology. 1992;42:1707–1712.
68. Griffin DE, Wesselingh SL, McArthur JC. Elevated central nervous system prostaglandins in human immunodeficiency virus–associated dementia. Ann Neurol. 1994;35:593–597.
69. Wilt SG, Milward E, Zhou JM, et al. In vitro evidence for a dual role of tumor necrosis factor-α in human immunodeficiency virus type 1 encephalopathy. Ann Neurol. 1995;37:381–394.
70. Lannuzel A, Barnier JV, Hery C, et al. Human immunodeficiency virus type 1 and its coat protein gp120 induce apoptosis and activate JNK and ERK mitogen-activated protein kinases in human neurons. Ann Neurol. 1997;42:847–856.
71. Magnuson DSK, Knudson BE, Geiger JD, et al. Human immunodeficiency virus type 1 tat activates non-*N*-methyl-D-aspartate excitatory amino acid receptors and causes neurotoxicity. Ann Neurol. 1995;37:373–380.
72. Ellis RJ, Hsia K, Spector SA, et al. Cerebrospinal fluid human immunodeficiency virus type 1 RNA levels are elevated in neurocognitively impaired individuals with acquired immunodeficiency syndrome. Ann Neurol. 1997;42:679–688.
73. McArthur JC, McClernon DR, Cronin MF, et al. Relationship between human immunodeficiency virus–associated dementia and viral load in cerebrospinal fluid and brain. Ann Neurol. 1997;42:689–698.
74. Sidtis JJ, Gatsonis C, Price RW, et al. Zidovudine treatment of the AIDS dementia complex: Results of a placebo-controlled trial. Ann Neurol. 1993;33:343–349.
75. Lipton SA, Gendelman HE. Dementia associated with the acquired immunodeficiency syndrome. N Engl J Med. 1995;332:934–940.
76. Heseltine PNR, Goodkin K, Atkinson JH, et al. Randomized double-blind placebo-controlled trial of peptide T for HIV-associated cognitive impairment. Arch Neurol. 1998;55:41–51.
77. The Dana Consortium. Safety and tolerability of the antioxidant OPC-14117 in HIV-associated cognitive impairment. Neurology. 1997;49:142–146.
78. The Dana Consortium. A randomized, double-blind, placebo-controlled trial of deprenyl and thioctic acid in human immunodeficiency virus–associated cognitive impairment. Neurology. 1998;50:645–651.
79. Navia BA, Dafni U, Simpson D, et al. A Phase I/II trial of nimodipine for HIV-related neurologic complications. Neurology. 1998;51:221–228.
80. Dalakas MC, Leon-Monzon ME, Bernardini I, et al. Zidovudine-induced mitochondrial myopathy is associated with muscle carnitine deficiency and lipid storage. Ann Neurol. 1994;35:482–487.
81. Mhiri C, Baudrimont M, Bonne G, et al. Zidovudine myopathy: A distinctive disorder associated with mitochondrial dysfunction. Ann Neurol. 1991;29:606–614.
82. Dalakas MC, Illa I, Pezeshkpour GH, et al. Mitochondrial myopathy caused by long-term zidovudine therapy. N Engl J Med. 1990;322:1098–1105.
83. Grau JM, Masanes F, Pedrol E, et al. Human immunodeficiency virus type 1 infection and myopathy: Clinical relevance of zidovudine therapy. Ann Neurol. 1993;34:206–211.
84. Simpson DM, Citak KA, Godfrey E, et al. Myopathies associated with human immunodeficiency virus and zidovudine: Can their effects be distinguished? Neurology. 1993;43:971–976.
85. Cupler EJ, Hench K, Jay CA, et al. The natural history of zidovudine (AZT)-induced mitochondrial myopathy (ZIMM). Neurology. 1994;44:132.
86. Richman DD, Fischl MA, Grieco MH. The toxicity of azidothymidine (AZT) in the treatment of patients with AIDS and AIDS-related complex. N Engl J Med. 1987;317:192–197.
87. Dubinsky RM, Yarchoan R, Dalakas M, Broder S. Reversible axonal neuropathy from the treatment of AIDS and related disorders with 2′,3′-dideoxycytidine (ddC). Muscle Nerve. 1989;12:856–860.
88. Fichtenbaum CJ, Clifford DB, Powederly WG. Risk factors for dideoxy-nucleoside-induced toxic neuropathy in patients with human immunodeficiency virus infection. J Acquir Immune Defic Syndr Hum Retrovirol. 1995;10:169–174.
89. Clifford DB. Antiretroviral therapies for HIV infection, implications for treatment for neurologic manifestations: An overview. In: Gendelman HE, Lipton SA, Epstein L, Swindells S, eds. Neurology of AIDS. New York: Chapman & Hall; 1998:353–363.
90. Browne MJ, Mayer KH, Chafee SB. 2′,3′-Didehydro-3′-deoxythymidine (d4t) in patients with AIDS or AIDS-related complex: A phase I trial. J Infect Dis. 1993;167:21–29.
91. Deeks SG, Smith M, Hologniy M, Kahn JO. HIV-1 protease inhibitors—a review for clinicians. JAMA. 1997;277:145–153.
92. Henry K, Melrose H, Huebsch J, et al. Severe premature coronary artery disease with protease inhibitors. Lancet. 1998;351:1328.
93. Goldstein J. Headache and acquired immunodeficiency syndrome. Neurol Clin. 1990;8:947–960.
94. Lipton RB, Feraru ER, Weiss G. Headache in HIV-1 related disorders. Headache. 1991;31:518–522.
95. Brew BJ, Miller J. Human immunodeficiency virus–related headache. Neurology. 1993;43:1098–1100.
96. Pons VG, Jacobs RA, Hollander H. Nonviral infections of the central nervous systems in patients with acquired immunodeficiency syndrome. In: Rosenblum ML, Levy RM, Bredesen DE, eds. AIDS and the Central Nervous System. New York: Raven Press; 1988:263–283.
97. Berenguer J, Moreno S, Laguna F. Tuberculous meningitis in patients infected with the human immunodeficiency virus. N Engl J Med. 1992;326:668–672.
98. Porter SB, Sande MA. Toxoplasmosis of the central nervous system in the acquired immunodeficiency syndrome. N Engl J Med. 1992;327:1643–1648.
99. Holland NR, Power C, Mathews VP, et al. Cytomegalovirus encephalitis in acquired immunodeficiency syndrome (AIDS). Neurology. 1994;44:507–514.
100. Katz DA, Berger JR, Duncan RC. Neurosyphilis: A comparative study of the effects of infection with human immunodeficiency virus. Arch Neurol. 1993;50:243–249.
101. Singer EJ, Kim J, Fahy-Chandon B, et al. Headache in ambulatory HIV-1 infected men enrolled in a longitudinal study. Neurology. 1996;47:487–494.
102. Mizusawa H, Hirano A, Llena JF, Shintaku M. Cerebrovascular lesions in acquired immune deficiency syndrome (AIDS). Acta Neuropathol. 1988;76:451–457.
103. Park YD, Belman AL, Kim TS. Stroke in pediatric acquired immunodeficiency syndrome. Adv Neurol. 1990;28:303–311.
104. Pinto AN. AIDS and cerebrovascular disease. Stroke. 1996;27:538–543.
105. Tyler KL, Sandberg E, Baum KF. Medial medullary syndrome and meningovascular syphilis: A case report in an HIV-infected man and a review of the literature. Neurology. 1994;44:2231–2235.
106. Dube MP, Holtom PD, Larsen RA. Tuberculous meningitis in patients with and without human immunodeficiency virus infection. Am J Med. 1992;93:520–524.
107. Kieburtz KD, Eskin TA, Ketonen L, Tuite MJ. Opportunistic cerebral vasculopathy and stroke in patients with the acquired immunodeficiency syndrome. Arch Neurol. 1993;50:430–432.
108. Morgello S, Block GA, Price RW, Petito CK. Varicella-zoster virus leukoencephalitis and cerebral vasculopathy. Arch Pathol Lab Med. 1988;112:173–177.
109. Cuadrado LM, Guerrero A, Asenjo LG, et al. Cerebral mucormycosis in two cases of the acquired immunodeficiency syndrome. Arch Neurol. 1988;45:109–111.
110. Roldan EO, Moskowitz L, Hensley GT. Pathology of the heart in AIDS. Arch Pathol Lab Med. 1987;111:943–946.

111. Naimi N, Plancherel C, Bosser C, et al. Anticardiolipin antibodies in HIV-negative and HIV-positive hemophiliacs. Blood Coagul Fibrinolysis. 1990;1:5–8.
112. Bissuel F, Berruyer M, Causee X, et al. Acquired protein S deficiency: Correlation with advanced disease in HIV-1–infected patients. J Acquir Immune Defic Syndr. 1987;294:143–144.
113. Holtzman DM, Kaku DA, So YT. New-onset seizures associated with human immunodeficiency virus infection: Causation and clinical features in 100 cases. Am J Med. 1989;87:173–177.
114. Wong MC, Suite NDA, Labar DR. Seizures in human immunodeficiency virus infection. Arch Neurol. 1990;47:640–642.
115. Price RW. Neurologic Diseases. In: Dolin R, Masur H, Saag MS (eds). AIDS Therapy. New York: Churchill-Livingstone; 1999:620–638.
116. Berger JR, Levy RM. AIDS and the Nervous System. 2nd ed. Philadelphia: Lippincott-Raven; 1997.
117. Gendelman HE, Lipton SA, Epstein L, et al. The Neurology of AIDS. New York: Chapman & Hall; 1998.
118. Dube MP, Holtman PD, Larsen RA. Tuberculous meningitis in patients with and without human immunodeficiency virus infection. Am J Med. 1992;93:520–524.
119. Kim J, Minamoto GY, Grieco MH. Nocardial infection as a complication of AIDS: Report of six cases and review. Rev Infect Dis. 1991;13:624–629.
120. Powderly NG. Cryptococcal meningitis and AIDS. Clin Infect Dis. 1993;17:837.
121. Masdeu JC, Small CB, Weiss L, et al: Multifocal cytomegalovirus encephalitis in AIDS. Ann Neurol. 1988;23:97.
122. Gary F, Gherardi R, Wingate E, et al. Diffuse "encephalitic" cerebral toxoplasmosis in AIDS: Report of four cases. J Neurol. 1989;236:273.
123. Appleman M, Marshall D, Brey R, et al. Cerebrospinal fluid abnormalities in patients without AIDS who are seropositive for the human immunodeficiency virus. J Infect Dis. 1988;158:193.

Chapter 112

Malignancies in Human Immunodeficiency Virus Infection

PHOEBE R. TRUBOWITZ
PAUL A. VOLBERDING

Malignancies in the setting of immunodeficiency were well described in the literature long before the advent of the human immunodeficiency virus (HIV) epidemic.[1–3] The incidence of malignancy is significantly increased in the setting of abnormal cell-mediated immunity.[1, 3, 4] This increase in incidence, however, does not apply to the cancers most commonly seen in the general population. Rather, in these immunosuppressed individuals a narrow spectrum of more unusual tumors are observed, such as Kaposi's sarcoma (KS) and non-Hodgkin's lymphoma (NHL).[3, 4] HIV infection also produces profound defects in cell-mediated immunity.[5] It is therefore not surprising that patients with HIV infection have a markedly increased risk of developing such neoplasms.

KS was the first cancer to be recognized as related to the acquired immunodeficiency syndrome (AIDS)[6, 7] and was designated as such by the Centers for Disease Control (CDC).[8] The CDC subsequently added primary central nervous system lymphoma (PCNSL), intermediate- and high-grade NHL, and invasive cervical cancer to the list of AIDS-defining conditions. The designation of invasive cervical cancer remains controversial as its high frequency may reflect individuals' lifestyles, and consequently high rates of human papillomavirus (HPV) infection, rather than impaired immunity.[9] Several other cancers have not been officially deemed AIDS defining by the CDC but their incidence appears to be increased in the HIV population.[10] These include anal cancer, Hodgkin's disease, leiomyosarcoma in children, testicular cancer, skin cancer, oral mucosa and head and neck cancer, and possibly lung cancer.[11–13] Regardless of the causal relationship between various malignancies and the underlying immunodeficiency state, the natural history of cancer may be altered in the setting of HIV infection.[14, 15] Patients tend to present with more advanced disease that is more rapidly progressive and responds less well to therapy than in the non–HIV-infected population. Lung cancer, particularly difficult to treat in the general population, is associated with an even worse clinical outcome in HIV-infected individuals. However, for neoplastic disease that is generally highly responsive to therapeutic intervention, such as testicular germ cell tumors, treatment can be highly successful in the setting of HIV infection.

Management of the HIV-infected individual with a malignancy imposes unique obstacles. The oncologist treating such an individual often has to risk further immunocompromise in order to administer adequate therapy for the treatment of an aggressive neoplasm. Poor bone marrow reserve and the risk of intercurrent opportunistic infections, problems frequently observed in this population of patients, can compromise the delivery of adequate dose intensity. Toxicities of chemotherapeutic agents, antibiotics, and radiation therapy are often severe, further impairing the physician's effectiveness.

This chapter focuses on the malignancies most commonly associated with AIDS from primarily a clinical perspective. KS, peripheral NHL, PCNSL, and anogenital neoplasia are discussed in relative detail. The natural history of and various therapeutic options for these malignancies are presented. Brief mention is made of other cancers in the setting of HIV infection.

KAPOSI'S SARCOMA

Epidemiology

Moritz Kaposi first described the entity Kaposi's sarcoma in 1872.[16] Before the advent of organ transplantation in the 1950s, KS was a rarely recognized disease, which, in the classic form, was confined largely to persons of Eastern European or Mediterranean descent. This variant, usually seen in elderly men, generally has an indolent course and primarily involves the skin over the lower extremities and feet.[17, 18] It can also be seen occasionally in gay men who remain HIV negative.[19] In central Africa, KS is much more prevalent; some of its variants are more aggressive and infiltrating, particularly in children, in whom the lymphadenopathic variant is rapidly fatal.

In the early 1970s, KS was occasionally seen in immunosuppressed allograft recipients.[2] In the early 1980s, cases of KS in young gay men helped alert the medical community to the AIDS epidemic. Several aspects of these cases were distinctly unusual. First, they affected a much younger population than prior (classic) KS in the United States. Second, the tumor was much more aggressive, with early and wide dissemination the rule. Finally, the patients often had the spectrum of unusual infections being diagnosed simultaneously in other gay men but had no known reason for immune deficiency. The combination of these striking findings in similar "risk" populations soon led to the recognition of the common underlying disease, AIDS.

KS is the most common neoplasm affecting HIV-infected individuals. It disproportionately affects HIV-infected gay men. In the first several years of the epidemic, 47% of gay and bisexual men with newly diagnosed AIDS had KS as compared with 3.9% of intravenous drug users.[20] KS is rarely reported in intravenous drug users or other HIV risk groups.[21, 22] The proportion of patients with KS as their AIDS-defining illness has changed with the epidemic.[23, 24] In New York City, KS was the initial AIDS diagnosis in 50% of gay men who were not intravenous drug users diagnosed between 1981 and 1983. Between 1984 and 1987, however, this proportion fell to 30%, well before the introduction of effective antiretroviral therapies. Similar trends have been reported in San Francisco.[25] Subsequent data from the Multicenter AIDS Cohort Study indicated a steady decline in the incidence of KS through January 1995 followed by a more precipitous fall from January 1995 to January 1997. This corresponds to the more widespread use of highly active antiretroviral therapy (HAART).[26] The number of new KS cases in the cohort fell from 25.6 per 1000 patient-years in the early 1990s to an average incidence of 7.5 per 1000 patient-years in 1996 to 1997.[26] Additional evidence suggesting a decline in the occurrence of KS in conjunction with widespread use of HAART has been reported from the San Francisco City Clinic Cohort Study[27] and the Adult Spectrum of HIV Disease Project.[28] Tumor registry data from San Francisco General Hospital demonstrate a decline in the number of newly diagnosed cases of KS from 103 in 1995 to 62 in 1996 to 36 in 1997.

Pathogenesis

The pathogenesis of KS in HIV-infected patients is complex and involves both viral processes and dysregulation of cytokine pathways. A sexually transmitted coinfection has long been suspected from the epidemiology of AIDS-related KS.[24, 29] In 1994, Chang and coworkers[30] discovered a new herpesvirus, human herpesvirus type 8 (HHV-8) or KS herpesvirus, in KS lesions (see Chapter 130). The virus is found predominantly in a latent form within the endothelial spindle cells of the lesions. It has been identified in all types of KS including classic KS, African or endemic KS, transplant-associated KS, and AIDS-related KS.[31] The virus can also be found in peripheral blood mononuclear cells in many patients with KS, and this not infrequently precedes the development of KS in AIDS patients.[32, 33]

HHV-8 is also associated with rare lymphoproliferative diseases most often seen in HIV-infected individuals, including Castleman's disease and a newly recognized form of NHL known as primary effusion or body cavity lymphoma.[34]

The transmissibility of this virus remains unclear. It has been detected in semen and prostate tissue.[35] Results of serologic studies remain controversial, as HHV-8 antibody testing remains to be refined, but seropositive rates are as expected given the epidemiology of KS[36]; that is, gay men with HIV or other active sexually transmitted diseases have the highest seropositivity rates.

The pathogenesis of KS is complex, with multiple putative pathways involving HHV-8, HIV, cytokines, integrins, and altered apoptosis and cell cycle controls.[37, 38] Cytokines released from spindle cells and inflammatory cells stimulate the growth of the tumors in complex autocrine and paracrine pathways, as does the HIV *tat* gene product. Finally, the HHV-8 genome encodes cyclin-D1– and interleukin-6–like proteins, which may play a role in the pathogenesis of the tumors.

The histopathology of KS is characterized by a proliferation of abnormal vascular structures. Three histologic variants have been reported: a spindle cell variant, an anaplastic form, and a mixed-cell form.[39–41] The mixed-cell variant is by far the most common of the three seen in AIDS patients. It is characterized by three features: proliferation within the tumor of vascular structures and slits, often lined by abnormally large, malignant-appearing endothelial cells; proliferation of surrounding spindle-shaped cells; and extravasation of erythrocytes. The spindle cell appears to originate from lymphatic endothelium.[42]

Clinical Manifestations

The natural history of AIDS-related KS is variable and thus difficult to predict. The disease can be present in patients with a wide range of $CD4^+$ cell counts but becomes increasingly common as immune function declines. Although an occasional individual has a spontaneous remission or long interval without disease progression, others have a rapidly progressive course.[43] Patients with limited disease and no symptoms suggestive of underlying infectious processes do reasonably well. More often, however, in the setting of uncontrolled HIV viral replication, KS progresses rapidly.

The skin is the most common first site of presentation. The lesions are generally painless and nonpruritic and appear as firm, slightly raised or nodular tumors. Cutaneous nodules ranging from 0.5 to 2.0 cm in diameter are frequently observed. In some patients, they may be barely visible or nonpalpable initially; in others, they may have the appearance of small ecchymoses. In more advanced disease, cutaneous lesions can coalesce to form large, plaquelike tumor masses involving extensive cutaneous surfaces, especially over the medial aspect of the upper thigh. In light-skinned individuals, the lesions are typically violaceous in color. In dark-skinned individuals, the lesions appear more brownish or even black. Lesions typically appear on the face and in the oral cavity or on the feet and lower extremities, although they may affect almost any site. KS frequently involves the plantar surfaces of the foot but rarely the palms. Other notable sites of disease include the tip of the nose, periorbital area, hard and soft palates, gingival areas of the mouth, external ear, conjunctiva, and penis. At autopsy, almost every organ system can demonstrate involvement. However, bone marrow disease and parenchymal brain disease are distinctly uncommon. KS is a multicentric tumor, and numerous lesions can appear simultaneously in widely scattered areas of the body. KS lesions tend to be circular, but those on the back or around the neck can be linear, following cutaneous lymphatic drainage patterns known as Langer's lines.

The disease may remain quiescent for many months, but this may be followed by a sudden rapid increase in disease activity with the appearance of numerous new lesions and enlargement of existing ones. Visceral involvement is extremely common, especially as the disease progresses, and may involve almost any site, most commonly the gastrointestinal tract. The head and neck are also sites of typical involvement, and careful inspection of the oral cavity frequently demonstrates evidence of KS lesions in up to 30% at the time of initial diagnosis. Oral involvement has been shown to correlelate with KS in the gastrointestinal tract.

KS does not commonly cause death of patients with HIV infection, except for those who develop diffuse pulmonary parenchymal involvement. Despite the relative lack of mortality associated with KS, morbidity associated with more advanced disease can be considerable. Bulky cutaneous lesions may become painful. Large, plaquelike lesions may coalesce and restrict movement. Lymphatic obstruction is common and may result in severe edema, usually involving the lower extremities or the face. Visceral spread of KS involving the gastrointestinal tract is rarely symptomatic. However, rare cases of obstruction, perforation, or gastrointestinal bleeding have been reported.[44] Finally, the social problems associated with this disfiguring neoplasm in the setting of an already socially stigmatizing disease cannot be overemphasized.

Pulmonary involvement is becoming an increasingly common complication of KS and thus deserves special attention. In contrast to KS at other visceral sites, pulmonary KS is generally symptomatic. Common symptoms include a barking cough, bronchospasm, and dyspnea. This complication tends to occur in the setting of advanced AIDS, with most individuals having $CD4^+$ cell counts of less than $100/mm^3$.[45] Pulmonary involvement tends to occur in individuals with more extensive cutaneous disease, such as those with more than 50 lesions. It can occur, however, in individuals with minimal and even absent cutaneous KS.[46] The disease is often rapidly progressive when it involves the lungs. Survival is relatively short in these patients; median survival times between 2 and 6 months have been reported.[45, 47] The radiographic appearance is variable with the characteristic reticulonodular pattern seen in approximately one third of patients.[47] Diffuse interstitial infiltrates are more commonly seen and may be difficult to distinguish from those in *Pneumocystis carinii* pneumonia.[45, 47, 48] Pleural effusions, usually cytologically benign, are frequently seen,[45, 47, 48] and hilar adenopathy is observed in approximately 50% of cases.[45] Respiratory failure resulting in death is not uncommon in patients with pulmonary KS.

Careful examination of the skin and oral cavity at each clinic visit is the key to early diagnosis. When lesions are identified, histologic confirmation should be obtained. This is particularly important because other cutaneous diseases, some of which can mimic

KS, are common in HIV-infected individuals. For cutaneous lesions, a small punch biopsy (2 to 4 mm) is usually adequate.

In the initial evaluation of a patient with KS, tumor extent should be determined by a complete skin examination. The oral cavity should also be carefully examined. Clinically important visceral KS, however, can occur in the absence of cutaneous or oral manifestations in approximately 15% of cases. If unexplained gastrointestinal or pulmonary symptoms are present, endoscopy should be performed. The classic appearance of small submucosal vascular nodules establishes the diagnosis of visceral KS. Biopsies are diagnostic in only a minority of cases of gastrointestinal KS because the tumors are generally submucosal, but biopsy specimens may exclude other diagnoses. In patients with suspected pulmonary KS, violaceous endobronchial lesions are typically observed on bronchoscopic examination. Endobronchial biopsy is discouraged because of the risk of hemorrhage. Bronchoscopic visualization of typical lesions is generally accepted for the purpose of diagnosis of pulmonary disease in patients who have had KS at other sites.[47] In patients for whom treatment with chemotherapy is anticipated for KS at other sites and who have respiratory symptoms or abnormal chest radiographs, gallium scanning can be sufficient to rule out a pulmonary opportunistic infection, making chemotherapy more acceptable. KS is not gallium avid.[47]

Although historically the most common cause of death in individuals with HIV and KS is opportunistic infection, there is evidence that, as survival is prolonged in individuals with HIV infection in the HAART era, pulmonary involvement with KS is becoming an increasingly common cause of death.

Treatment

With the exception of patients who develop pulmonary involvement, few patients' deaths are due directly to KS. It seems unlikely, therefore, that therapy directed toward this neoplasm would have a significant impact on survival. A retrospective review of 194 cases of KS by Volberding and colleagues[49] validated this point by demonstrating that there was no significant difference in survival time between a group of patients treated with chemotherapy (or interferon-alfa [IFN-alfa]) and those not treated.

The primary goals of treatment for patients with KS are palliation of symptoms and cosmesis. When to initiate treatment must be decided on a patient-by-patient basis, because even disease that appears to be medically uncomplicated may evoke powerful emotions for patients because of the social stigma associated with the disease. Treatment may range from potent HAART to systemic chemotherapy. KS must be considered a systemic disease, so systemic treatment is often the most appropriate choice of therapeutic modalities.

Treatment Modalities

Therapeutic options for AIDS-related KS can be divided into local and systemic approaches. Attempts to control HIV viral load should be made with or without the addition of local or systemic therapies.

Local Therapy

Radiotherapy has been the mainstay of local therapy for KS. A single dose of 800 cGy or an equivalent fractionated dose can be highly effective in achieving local palliation in selected patients.[50, 51] Maximal response to radiotherapy is generally seen over the course of several weeks to months after treatment.[50] Radiotherapy is best suited for patients with a single or a few locally symptomatic areas. Electron beam radiation applied to the entire face is highly effective in relieving facial edema. Radiotherapy can also be quite useful for treating dysphagia caused by pharyngeal lesions and tumor masses of the eye or the extremities.[51] Complications such as severe mucositis, radiotherapy fibrosis, loss of skin compliance, and chronic lymphedema are common and may result in significant discomfort after 6 to 12 months. In addition, complete disappearance of lesions is unusual at any site. As a result of the significant oral toxicity that has been observed with x-irradiation, laser surgery has been increasingly employed at San Francisco General Hospital for the treatment of intraoral lesions, with a lower incidence of morbidity.

Small cutaneous lesions can be treated with intralesional chemotherapy for cosmetic purposes.[52] This is generally accomplished by intralesional injection of 0.01 mg of vinblastine in 0.1 ml of sterile water using a tuberculin syringe. Repeated treatments may be necessary. A hyperpigmented area frequently remains after treatment.

Cryotherapy using liquid nitrogen has been used successfully for the treatment of isolated small KS lesions. For the treatment of cosmetically unsightly lesions, this modality has been particularly useful.

Lastly, photodynamic therapy utilizing intravenously administered porfimer sodium (Photofrin) has shown promise in phase I trials.[53] This approach is investigational at present but may be useful for small, cosmetically unsightly lesions in the future.

Systemic Therapy

The pathogenesis of KS indicates that it is a systemic disease. Systemic therapy consisting of antiretroviral therapy alone or in combination with KS-directed therapies is thus appropriate for the majority of patients. Several antineoplastic agents used alone or in combination are active against KS.

Advances in KS chemotherapy have come in the form of liposomal agents: liposomal doxorubicin (Doxil) and liposomal daunorubicin (DaunoXome). They are encapsulated anthracyclines and should be considered first-line treatment for relatively advanced KS as a result of their efficacy and low incidence of toxicity.

In a large randomized trial, Doxil produced a response rate nearly twice that of doxorubicin (Adriamycin), bleomycin, and vincristine (ABV), the once standard first-line therapy for advanced KS.[54] Liposome-encapsulated doxorubicin was also associated with a lower incidence of toxic effects such as nausea, fatigue, and alopecia. Neutropenia occurred as frequently with the liposomal agent as with the standard combination regimen.[55] In a similar study, liposomal daunorubicin was compared with Adriamycin, bleomycin, and vinblastine.[56] A lower incidence of alopecia, nausea, and neuropathy was noted with the liposomal agent. Response rates were similar in the two arms.

Paclitaxel (Taxol) has significant antitumor activity in patients with both previously untreated[57] and refractory KS.[57, 58] Response rates are greater than 50% regardless of prior therapy. Outstanding clinical responses have been seen in patients with advanced refractory symptomatic disease. The drug is well tolerated overall, with generally only mild toxicities reported. Paclitaxel is significantly myelosuppressive. Most patients in these trials have required adjunctive therapy with colony-stimulating factors (CSFs). This agent should be considered the treatment of choice for refractory KS.

Etoposide (VP-16), doxorubicin, vincristine, and bleomycin all have significant antitumor activity. Combinations such as Adriamycin, bleomycin, and vincristine have resulted in overall response rates up to 60% in patients with pulmonary KS. With the arrival of the newer agents, the earlier chemotherapeutics are now less often utilized because of their more severe toxicity.

The availability of the myeloid growth factors, granulocyte colony-stimulating factor (G-CSF), and granulocyte-macrophage colony-stimulating factor (GM-CSF) has made it possible to administer myelosuppressive chemotherapy to individuals for whom it might not have been possible in the past. Because many individuals with advanced KS have poor myeloid reserve, these agents can be valuable adjuncts to chemotherapy. For most individuals with KS, however, the use of a CSF is unnecessary. At San Francisco General Hospital, we reserve the use of CSFs for patients who require an anthracycline or paclitaxel as a part of their chemotherapeutic regimen and who have a neutrophil count less than 1500/mm^3 before any chemotherapy cycle is initiated. Although no specific guidelines exist, we generally begin administration of CSFs 1 to 4 days after chemotherapy administration. In our experience, a dose of 300 μg (5 μg/kg) administered on alternate days for a total of five doses is often adequate. Therapy should be individualized, however, and frequent neutrophil counts should be obtained during the first cycle of therapy to establish the optimal dosing regimen.

IFN-alfa is an active agent for the treatment of AIDS-related KS because it has both antiproliferative[59] and apparent anti-HIV activity.[60, 61] A large number of clinical trials of IFN-alfa as a single agent have demonstrated significant antitumor activity in AIDS-related KS.[59, 62–66] High doses (>20 million units/m^2) of IFN-alfa are more effective than lower doses in inducing antitumor responses.[63, 64, 66, 67] Several studies have shown that individuals with better immune function (higher CD4$^+$ cell counts) and without a prior history of opportunistic infection or systemic symptoms are more likely to respond to IFN-alfa than those with a more compromised immune status, history of a prior opportunistic infection, or clinical symptoms.[68, 69]

Despite objective responses and reports of long disease-free remissions, the use of IFN-alfa in high doses as a single agent has been significantly hampered by its toxicity profile. With chronic administration, many patients experience a flulike syndrome, with low-grade fever, anorexia, malaise, myalgias, and weight loss. Although many develop tachyphylaxis to these symptoms within the first several weeks, they can persist and become quite disabling. Treatment must then be reduced or discontinued altogether.

The combination of IFN-alfa and nucleoside analogues is being investigated in several phase I and phase II trials, and large clinical trials are continuing. The combination of IFN-alfa with a nucleoside analogue is attractive from the standpoint of antiretroviral therapy, as these agents appear to inhibit HIV-1 replication at different stages of the viral life cycle. The combination appears synergistic in inhibiting HIV-1 replication in vitro.[70] Several studies have looked at zidovudine and IFN-alfa and found response rates greater than 40%. Neutropenia has been a common dose-limiting toxicity. The use of another, less myelosuppressive antiretroviral agent, didanosine, in combination with IFN-alfa is being studied (AIDS Clinical Trial Group 206).

As tumor regression may take up to 8 weeks, appropriate candidates for therapy with IFN-alfa and antiretrovirals include patients with relatively intact immune function whose KS is minimally symptomatic. Clinical trials of INF-alfa with HAART are in progress.

The advent of HAART has had a significant impact on the management of patients with KS. These agents are probably the reason for the decline in the incidence of KS and appear to be altering the natural history of the neoplastic process itself. There have been several anecdotal reports[71–75] of anti-KS responses to antiretroviral therapy alone. Most clinicians caring for large numbers of patients with HIV disease recognize that in some patients, KS responds to the introduction of HAART in the absence of any specific KS-directed therapy. This phenomenon is generally associated with an effective antiviral response.[72] This is akin to the situation seen in the allograft population, wherein discontinuation of immunosuppressive therapy for iatrogenically immunosuppressed individuals often results in regression of KS. Thus, for patients with asymptomatic KS, a trial of HAART seems warranted and might prove effective enough to eliminate KS-specific therapy altogether.

After discontinuation of chemotherapy for patients whose KS has responded to therapy, no progression of KS was observed at a median follow-up of 10 weeks in patients receiving HAART.[76] These observations are significantly different from those in the pre-HAART era, when progression of KS after discontinuation of chemotherapy was the rule. Thus, it is now possible to discontinue KS-specific therapies in individuals who demonstrate a good virologic response to HAART, thereby eliminating the need for prolonged administration of chemotherapy for some patients.

Therapeutic Recommendations

Care of patients with KS should be individually tailored. KS should be thought of as a systemic disease, so in most cases, treatment should be systemic in nature. This may be defined as combination antiretroviral therapy, immunologic therapy, or systemic chemotherapy. Local therapeutic modalities such as intralesional vinblastine, radiotherapy, or laser surgery should be reserved for patients with minimal or locally symptomatic disease. These patients should be concurrently receiving some form of systemic therapy, including antiviral therapy. Patients with asymptomatic disease should be given combination antiretroviral therapy. If they are already receiving such a regimen, steps should be taken to maximize viral control as determined by viral load measurements. Such intervention alone may be effective therapy for KS in some patients.

For the relatively asymptomatic patient whose KS is not responding to antiretroviral therapy alone and for whom the KS is predominantly as issue of cosmesis, IFN-alfa is a good choice.

Chemotherapy is best utilized for patients with symptomatic disease when a more rapid response to therapy is needed. Treatment with antiretrovirals and IFN-alfa, although often effective, can be quite slow to produce a response. The liposomal anthracyclines (Doxil and DaunoXome) are considered first-line agents, and paclitaxel (Taxol) should be used for individuals with refractory disease.

NON-HODGKIN'S LYMPHOMA

The first cases of NHL in gay men were reported in 1982,[77] and increasing numbers have been reported since that time. NHL is the initial AIDS diagnosis in 2.5 to 5% of HIV-infected individuals[78] and has been estimated to occur eventually in approximately 8% of all HIV-infected individuals. The NHLs are a heterogeneous group of malignancies. Their biologic behavior ranges from indolent, requiring no therapy, to aggressive, with few long-term survivors.

The most commonly used classification for NHL[79] divides these malignancies into three major categories, low, intermediate, and high grade, according to pathologic characteristics of involved lymph nodes and morphologic criteria for the lymphoma cells. Approximately 70% of NHLs originate in B cells; another 20% derive from T cells.

The finding of an intermediate- or high-grade B-cell NHL in an HIV-infected individual constitutes an AIDS diagnosis as defined by the CDC.[80] Low-grade lymphomas occur infrequently in individuals with HIV infection and are not AIDS defining according to the CDC criteria. Advanced extranodal disease, poor response rates, high relapse rates, and short survival characterize the disease in the HIV-infected population.

Epidemiology

Individuals with impairment of cell-mediated immunity demonstrate a marked increase in the incidence of NHL.[1, 3] The best described of these groups are immunosuppressed allograft recipients, whose incidence of NHL is 30 to 50 times that of the general population.[3, 4, 81] Similar trends occur in populations at risk for HIV infection. Harnly and colleagues[82] demonstrated a statistically significant increase in the incidence of NHL among never-married men aged 25 to 44 years in San Francisco from 1980 to 1985. The increase in census tracts with a high incidence of AIDS was greater than the increase seen in other San Francisco census tracts. In 1985, the incidence of NHL was five times greater than the rate in 1980. Incidence rates for other neoplasms did not demonstrate such increases. The incidence of NHL in New York City follows similar trends.[68]

The Multicenter AIDS Cohort Study continues to demonstrate a 21% per year increase in cases of NHL since 1985.[26] From 1994 to 1997, the adult spectrum of the HIV Disease Project, which includes more than 40,000 individuals, documented no significant change in the incidence of systemic NHL. However, a significant decline in the incidence of PCNSL was seen.[28]

Pathogenesis

The molecular characteristics of AIDS-related NHL exhibit a great deal of heterogeneity, suggesting that lymphomagenesis may occur by a variety of different mechanisms. The large cell lymphomas, including intermediate-grade large cell lymphoma and high-grade immunoblastic lymphomas, account for about 60% of all lymphomas observed in HIV-infected individuals.[83] Within this histologic subtype, both monoclonal and polyclonal malignant lymphoproliferative processes have been demonstrated.[84–87] Autopsy data show these polyclonal processes to be as aggressive as typical monoclonal lymphomas.[68]

In immunosupressed allograft recipients, Epstein-Barr virus (EBV), seen in virtually all polyclonal NHLs, has been implicated as a causative agent in the development of this neoplasm.[46, 81, 88] In contrast to non-HIV NHL, in which EBV is ubiquitous, EBV DNA sequences are present in only 40% of systemic AIDS-related NHLs.[78, 89–91] However, the PCNSLs in HIV-infected individuals represent a subset of the large cell lymphomas and are a more homogeneous group. To date, virtually all PCNSLs studied have been monoclonal EBV-positive tumors.[87, 92] Another virus has been implicated in a rare type of HIV NHL. This subtype, referred to as a primary effusion lymphoma or body cavity lymphoma, is often seen with ascites or a pleural or pericardial effusion. It is quite aggressive and often refractory to chemotherapy. HHV-8 has been universally found in malignant cells, often in conjunction with EBV.

The question of a direct role for HIV in the lymphogenesis of HIV-associatcd T-cell lymphomas has been raised by the observation of a clonally integrated HIV genome in either the malignant T cells themselves or tumor-associated macrophages.[93, 94] HIV may act in a nonspecific way to enhance cytokine expression by infecting macrophages. Cytokine overexpression may then drive polyclonal B-cell proliferation. Cytokine dysregulation has been well documented, and there is evidence for expression of high levels of the lymphostimulatory cytokines interleukin-6 and interleukin-10 in AIDS-related large cell and immunoblastic lymphomas.[95–97]

The heterogeneity of molecular characteristics, including clonality and the presence or absence of EBV, suggests that lymphomagenesis may occur through several different mechanisms. Although EBV may be involved in the pathogenesis of some HIV NHLs, other viruses, cytokines, and even the underlying immune dysregulation itself may give rise to NHL.

Clinical Characteristics

As in other immunocompromised individuals, the vast majority of the NHLs observed in HIV-infected individuals are classified as B-cell neoplasms.[98–100] A small number of NHLs of other histologic and immunologic subtypes have been observed, including T-cell lymphoma[78, 101, 102] and others of uncertain lineage.[103] In 327 cases reported from five centers, 73% of the lymphomas were high grade, 24% were intermediate grade, and 3% were low grade.[78, 92, 104–106] Most B-cell lymphomas in these individuals are classified as diffuse large cell tumors of either intermediate-grade type or the high-grade immunoblastic type. In addition, one third of patients have tumors of the high-grade, small, noncleaved cell variety.

Systemic NHL occurs in individuals with widely ranging levels of immune function.[78, 107, 108] A median CD4+ cell count between approximately 100 and 180/mm³ has been reported.[78, 109] Seventy-five percent of cases occur in persons with a CD4+ count greater than 50/mm³ and 30% occur in persons with a CD4+ count greater than 200/mm³.[108] In a multicenter study of 192 patients with HIV NHL, the mean CD4+ cell count was 100/mm³ before treatment.[110] In contrast, persons who develop PCNSL almost universally have severe immunosuppression with CD4+ cell counts less than 50/mm³.

The hallmark of AIDS-related systemic NHL is widespread disease involving extranodal sites. Ziegler and coworkers[111] reported that 95% of patients from several institutions had evidence of extranodal disease, including 42% with CNS involvement and 33% with bone marrow involvement.

Similarly, Knowles and colleagues[92] reported extranodal disease in 87% of a series of 89 patients diagnosed at New York University. The most common sites of extranodal disease were the gastrointestinal tract, CNS, bone marrow, and liver. At San Francisco General Hospital, Kaplan and associates[78] reported that 31% of patients had extranodal disease alone, with no identifiable site of nodal disease. Several reports describe extensive extranodal involvement, stage IV disease, in 60 to 70% of HIV-infected persons at presentation.[78, 92, 107, 111]

Gastrointestinal NHL is among the most common forms in persons with HIV disease, occurring in up to 27% of patients. The majority of these cases involve the stomach,[112] but virtually any site in the gastrointestinal tract or hepatobiliary tree can be implicated. Other unusual sites include the subcutaneous and soft tissue, epidural space, gingiva, paranasal sinus,[92, 105, 107, 110, 111] heart, and pericardium.[111, 113]

Prognostic Features

Data for 192 prospectively enrolled patients in the AIDS Clinical Trial Group study,[114] a study of low-dose versus standard-dose chemotherapy, resemble those in the International Prognostic Index for aggressive NHL in nonimmunodeficient individuals. The factors gleaned from this study that were associated with poor prognosis included age older than 35 years, CD4+ cell count less than 100/mm³, history of intravenous drug use, and, for the first time, tumor bulk as deemed by stage of disease.[114] Advanced stage III or IV disease was associated with a poor outcome.

Treatment

Multiagent chemotherapeutic regimens have resulted in a dramatic improvement in the prognosis for non–HIV-infected individuals with NHL, intermediate- and high-grade types.[115] Such success has not been equaled with similar chemotherapeutic regimens in HIV-infected individuals. Complete response rates of 33 to 56% are significantly lower than the corresponding rates in the non–HIV-infected population, and survival times of 4 to 7 months have been observed (Table 112–1).

Ziegler and colleagues[111] reported the first large retrospective group of patients with AIDS-related NHL treated at multiple institutions. Of 66 evaluable patients, 53% achieved a complete response to combination chemotherapy. Of these complete responders, however, 54% subsequently had relapses. In a series of 65 patients treated with a variety of combination chemotherapeutic regimens at San Francisco General Hospital, 54% of 59 evaluable patients had complete responses to therapy.[78] Twenty-three percent of this group subsequently had relapses. Median survival for all patients receiving chemotherapy ($n = 65$) was only 5.5 months. However, subgroups of patients were identified within this population in whom survival was prolonged. Features identified as being predictive of a shorter survival time included the following: absolute CD4+ cell count less than 100/mm³, a prior AIDS diagnosis, Karnofsky's performance status less than 70% and the presence of an extranodal site of disease.

Morphologic subtype predicted response to chemotherapy and survival time in one series reported from New York University.[92] The best complete response rates and longest survival times were

TABLE 112-1 Response to Chemotherapy and Survival in Human Immunodeficiency Virus–Associated Non-Hodgkin's Lymphoma

Insitution*	No.	Treatment Regimen†	Complete Response (%)	Median Survival (mo)
USC	22	m-BACOD and others	45	NA
NYU	83	Various	33	5.0
UCSF	65	Various	54	5.5
MSKCC	30	Various	56	6.0
Pacific Medical Center	31	CHOP MACOP-B	39	7.0
Multicenter	66	Various	53	NA
AIDS Clinical Trials Group	36	m-BACOD‡	42	NA
Italian Cooperative Group	72	Various	35	4.0

*USC, University of Southern California; NYU, New York University; UCSF, University of California, San Francisco; MSKCC, Memorial Sloan-Kettering Cancer Center; Multicenter, UCSF, New York Hospital/Cornell, University of Texas/M.D. Anderson, NYU/Kaplan Cancer Center, MSKCC; A???for Clinical Trials Group, National Institutes of Health.

†Cyclophosphamide, doxorubicin, vincristine, and prednisone; m-BACOD, methotrexate, bleomycin, doxorubicin (Adriamycin), cyclophosphamide; vincristine, and dexamethasone.

‡Given at reduced doses.

From Ziegler J, Beckstead J, Volberding P, et al. Non-Hodgkin's lymphoma in 90 homosexual men: Relation to generalized lymphadenopathy and the acquired immunodeficiency syndrome. N Engl J Med. 1984;311:565–570.

reported for individuals classified as having large, noncleaved cell lymphoma (complete response, 52%; median survival, 7.5 months). Those having small, noncleaved cell and immunoblastic lymphomas had response rates of 26 and 21%, respectively, and median survivals of 5.5 and 2.0 months, respectively.

Contrary to the belief that more intensive chemotherapy provides an improved clinical outcome in non–HIV-infected individuals, retrospective data from two centers have suggested that survival may, in fact, be improved in HIV-infected individuals treated with less aggressive regimens.[78, 116] Kaplan and colleagues[78] reported that patients treated with chemotherapy regimens containing cyclophosphamide at 1 g/m^2 had a median survival time of only 4.6 months, whereas those treated with regimens containing cyclophosphamide at less than 1 g/m^2 had a median survival time of 12.2 months ($p = .02$). Similarly, in a study of nine patients treated with a novel, more aggressive chemotherapeutic regimen consisting of high-dose cytosine arabinoside, L-asparaginase, vincristine, prednisone, cyclophosphamide (high dose), methotrexate, and leucovorin, only three patients achieved complete remission.[117] This intensive regimen was associated with a high risk of mortality caused by opportunistic infection.

Dose intensity of chemotherapy in most studies has been significantly decreased by dose reduction and delay in administration. Cytopenias, related to poor bone marrow reserve, and intercurrent infections are the most commonly stated reasons for the decreased dose intensity. This may account for the high relapse rate and frequent deaths associated with poor control of the neoplastic process that have been reported in most series. As a result, two different approaches to the treatment of NHL in HIV-infected individuals have been pursued.

The first approach utilizes a lower dose, less aggressive chemotherapeutic regimen. A multicenter clinical trial evaluating the efficacy of a low-dose regimen enrolled 35 patients with AIDS-related NHL (mean CD4$^+$ cell count of 150/mm^3). They were treated with a modification of the standard methotrexate, bleomycin, doxorubicin (Adriamycin), cyclophosphamide, vincristine, and dexamethasone (m-BACOD) regimen. Cyclophosphamide and doxorubicin were administered at 300 and 25 mg/m^2, respectively, rather than 600 and 45 mg/m^2. Complete responses were observed in 42% of patients and the median survival of evaluable patients was 6.5 months. These results are similar to those reported from other institutions using a variety of more standard treatment regimens.[47]

The second approach to therapy has been to employ a colony-stimulating factor (GM-CSF or G-CSF) with higher or standard-dose chemotherapy regimens. Results from such a clinical trial in which standard doses of cyclophosphamide, doxorubicin, vincristine, and prednisone chemotherapy were used with or without GM-CSF demonstrated that individuals receiving GM-CSF had a significantly higher mean nadir neutrophil count and a significantly shorter duration of life-threatening neutropenia than those in the control arm. This corresponded to a significantly shorter period of hospitalization for fever and neutropenia in the group receiving GM-CSF, 5.9 days versus 18.6 days in the control group.[47]

Each of the aforementioned treatment approaches is effective in reducing myeloid toxicity and the complications of neutropenia. Which of the two will result in improved clinical outcome remains to be seen and speaks to the issue of dose intensity in the treatment of AIDS-related NHL.

In an effort to evaluate dose intensity, the AIDS Clinical Trials Group conducted a large, multicenter, clinical trial in which 198 individuals with HIV NHL were randomized to receive either standard-dose m-BACOD with adjunctive GM-CSF or the same low-dose m-BACOD regimen described earlier with GM-CSF administered as needed.[118] The results of this trial demonstrated no significant differences in complete response rate, response duration, or overall survival time. However, toxicity was more severe in the patients randomized to the standard-dose arm, particularly with respect to the occurrence of grade IV neutropenia (absolute neutrophil count <500). Results were similar for patients with CD4$^+$ cell counts above or below 100/mm^3, although overall survival times of those with CD4$^+$ counts greater than 100/mm^3 were longer in both treatment arms. These data suggest that immune function is of greater significance in predicting clinical outcome than choice of chemotherapy regimen and that most patients do not benefit from more toxic higher dose chemotherapy.

Another approach to therapy in HIV NHL is to use continuous infusion chemotherapy. Sparano and colleagues[119] treated 25 patients with a 96-hour continuous infusion of cyclophosphamide, doxorubicin, and etoposide. Antiretroviral therapy consisting of didanosine was given to every patient. A complete response of 58% and median survival of 18.4 months were described. These results raise the question of whether improved survival is the result of more effective chemotherapy or improved management of HIV disease. With the implementation of HAART, this question becomes increasingly important. Clinical trials are ongoing to help elucidate this point.

Intercurrent opportunistic infection during chemotherapy represents a significant problem in terms of both morbidity and mortality. Kaplan and colleagues[78] reported that 28% of 65 patients receiving combination chemotherapy developed *P. carinii* pneumonia. Current clinical trials include prophylactic antibiotic therapy in an effort to reduce the incidence of this complication and improve survival.

Variations in standard cytotoxic regimens will probably not have a major impact on survival. In the presence of the underlying immunodeficiency state, novel approaches are needed. Clinical trials are currently evaluating the use of monoclonal antibodies and immunotoxins directed toward cell surface determinants that are unique to AIDS-related NHL.

Treatment Recommendations

In selecting therapy for patients with AIDS-related NHL, the emphasis should be on individualizing therapy. Whereas standard-dose therapy may be appropriate for the patient with intact immune function (CD4$^+$ count 200/mm^3) and without prior history of an opportunistic infection, a lower dose regimen might be selected for a patient with more compromised immune function, marginal performance status, and prior opportunistic infection. For some patients who are severely ill, a decision to withhold therapy altogether may be appropriate. These decisions must take into account the individual's history and present condition as well as the individual's own desires concerning therapy.

Prophylactic, intrathecal chemotherapy is implemented for high-risk patients to decrease the likelihood of meningeal lymphoma.

Individuals at risk for meningeal disease, as identified in the nonimmunodeficient population, may have any of the following: small, noncleaved cell histology or other histology with bone marrow, epidural, perinasal sinus, or testicular involvement.

With the improvements in the overall status of HIV-infected individuals receiving HAART and *P. carinii* pneumonia prophylaxis, it is recommended that patients continue with their regimens or be given antiretroviral and prophylactic antibiotic therapy at the outset of chemotherapy. Utilizing fewer myelosuppressive antiretroviral agents is recommended. Ongoing studies are evaluating pharmacodynamics and pharmacokinetics in patients receiving HAART and combination chemotherapy. The impact of HAART on therapeutic outcome and tolerance of chemotherapy awaits elucidation.

PRIMARY CENTRAL NERVOUS SYSTEM LYMPHOMA

The incidence of PCNSL in HIV-infected individuals is 1000-fold higher than that in the general population.[83, 116, 120, 121] EBV is identified in virtually all PCNSLs. In one study, 100% of PCNSLs showed evidence of latent EBV infection, as reflected by detection of early antigen (EBER-1) by in situ hybridization.[122] Lymphomas that are seen as primary parenchymal lesions account for approximately 20% of all AIDS-related lymphomas.[105, 111, 123, 124] It is exceedingly rare for individuals who present with parenchymal brain lesions to have lymphoma outside the CNS.[83] As is true for many opportunistic infections, PCNSL occurs most often in the advanced stages of AIDS. In all reported series, the median CD4^{+} cell count of HIV-infected individuals diagnosed with PCNSL was less than 50/mm^3.[107, 120] Since the advent of HAART, a significant decline in the number of cases of PCNSL has occurred. Tumor registry data from San Francisco General Hospital demonstrate a decline from 18 cases in 1996 to 4 cases in 1997.

The most common presenting symptoms are confusion, lethargy, personality changes, and memory loss.[83, 116, 120, 125] Other symptoms include hemiparesis, aphasia, seizures, cranial nerve palsies, and headache. Single or multiple discrete contrast-enhanced lesions are the most common findings on computed tomographic or magnetic resonance imaging scans of the brain. The radiographic appearance of PCNSL is often quite difficult to distinguish from that of toxoplasmosis. Solitary lesions are observed in approximately 21% of magnetic resonance imaging scans of individuals with toxoplasmosis; therefore, solitary lesions are somewhat more likely to represent lymphoma. However, multiple lesions are present in 50% of cases of PCNSL, which creates a diagnostic dilemma.[126] Classic radiographic findings for PCNSL are lesions that are frequently hypo- or isodense and contrast enhanced. They may reveal central necrosis and their location is most often periventricular. Lesions can cross the midline, and subependymal involvement is almost pathognomonic.

Patients with neurologic symptoms should be evaluated promptly with computed tomographic or magnetic resonance imaging scans of the brain. If not contraindicated by the imaging studies, a lumbar puncture should be performed. Meningeal involvement with abnormal findings in the cerebrospinal fluid, including positive cytology for malignancy, is observed in roughly 20% of patients.[116] Serum should be tested for evidence of the cryptococcal antigen and *Toxoplasma* antibody. Toxoplasmosis is quite rare in patients with negative serologic tests.[127, 128] It is therefore prudent for clinicians to perform a brain biopsy in a timely fashion for patients who are seronegative for *Toxoplasma* antibody. For patients with focal intracerebellar lesions and positive toxoplasmosis serologic studies, anti-*Toxoplasma* therapy is initiated and the patients are observed closely for signs of improvement or deterioration.

Two less invasive techniques have been added to the clinician's armamentarium for diagnosing PCNSL: thallium-201 single photon emission computed tomographic scanning and polymerase chain reaction (PCR) to detect EBV DNA in the cerebrospinal fluid. In one series, thallium scans were negative for all 24 patients with toxoplasmosis and positive for all 12 patients with PCNSL.[25] In another series, nine individuals with PCNSL had positive thallium scans. Worrisome, however, was the fact that positive scans were also obtained for 3 of 10 patients with toxoplasmosis.[50] Clearly, data from larger studies are needed to identify the potential utility of this modality in diagnosing PCNSL. Observations made using PCR to detect EBV DNA in the cerebrospinal fluid are of even greater interest. De Luca and coworkers[129] showed that seven of eight individuals with documented PCNSL had positive PCR for EBV in cerebrospinal fluid. Of 11 individuals with brain lesions and no lymphoma, all had negative PCRs. Twenty-one individuals with AIDS but no CNS lesions were also all negative. In a second series, 17 individuals with PCNSL were all found to be positive for EBV by PCR, and 67 of 68 individuals with HIV and no lymphoma were negative.[130] Data from larger studies are confirmatory.[131] Together, these data demonstrate the strength of this minimally invasive technique as a diagnostic tool for PCNSL. In conjunction with thallium scanning and *Toxoplasma* serologic studies, EBV detection by PCR may be of particular value.

At present, the standard for diagnosing PCNSL is brain biopsy. Because treatment outcome hinges on early diagnosis and initiation of treatment, individuals with negative *Toxoplasma* titers, who are therefore quite unlikely to have toxoplasmosis, and negative cerebrospinal fluid cytology are urged to undergo an early brain biopsy. When the diagnosis of PCNSL is made, a slit-lamp examination is performed to evaluate for the presence of ocular lymphoma before initiation of therapy.

Treatment

PCNSL has been a particular therapeutic challenge. Many cases of PCNSL have been diagnosed at autopsy.[111] Cases observed before death were frequently in individuals with advanced AIDS who had suffered multiple previous bouts of opportunistic infections.[83]

In the largest published series to date, Baumgartner and coworkers[83] demonstrated significant clinical improvement in 78% of 29 individuals treated with whole-brain irradiation at 4000 cGY; 69% had a complete or partial radiographic response. Other institutions have had similar results with smaller series of patients. Despite good initial response rates, survival times remain short, with median survival times for treated patients between 2 and 5 months.[83, 120] The most common cause of death in these patients was opportunistic infection.[83, 120] In the series of Formenti and associates,[120] 50% of the deaths were due to opportunistic infections with only two deaths resulting from recurrent lymphoma.

Combined-modality therapy (chemo- and radiotherapy) has been investigated.[85, 132] In one series, 10 individuals had a complete response rate of 88%. None of these patients' deaths resulted from their lymphoma.[132] The median survival of 3.5 months, however, was no better than that in studies with radiotherapy alone. These results indicate that progress in the management of PCNSL will depend on advances in the management of both the neoplastic disease and the underlying HIV infection. With the addition of HAART, patients' overall survival has greatly improved, which makes the management of PCNSL of greater importance.

ANOGENITAL NEOPLASIA

Anogenital neoplasia, which includes both cervical and anal carcinomas and their likely precursor lesions, cervical and anal squamous intraepithelial lesions (SILs), is an increasingly common problem in HIV-infected individuals. Infection with the human papillomavirus is one of the most important risk factors associated with anogenital neoplasia. Both HIV and HPV are sexually transmitted with similar risk factors for acquisition. The pathogenesis of anogenital neoplasia in HIV-infected individuals may be related not only to the impairment of cell-mediated immunity caused by HIV but also to a direct interaction between these two viruses.

Considerable evidence links the development of anogenital carcinoma to HPV infection (see Chapter 133). At least 30 types of HPV have been noted to have a high predilection for the anogenital tract.[133] Specific types, such as HPV-6 and HPV-11, have been associated with benign disease including condyloma acuminatum and have been classified as low-risk types. High-risk or oncogenic genotypes (HPV-16, HPV-18, and HPV-31) are associated with high-grade cervical or anal SILs and cervical and anal carcinomas. HPV DNA has been demonstrated in more than 90% of cases of cervical squamous cell carcinoma.[134] Tumor tissues from the anal region also demonstrate the presence of HPV DNA, suggesting a similar causative role for this infection in anal carcinoma.[135] A recognized association exists between anogenital neoplasia and chronic immunodeficiency states. A high prevalence of HPV infection exists in immunosuppressed transplant recipients and probably accounts for their high incidence of anogenital carcinoma. The prevalence of HPV infection is 5 to 17 times greater in immunosuppressed transplant recipients than in the general population.[136]

Histopathology

Currently, most cervical and anal cytologic abnormalities are classified according to the Bethesda system.[137] At the benign end of the spectrum, histopathologic abnormalities secondary to HPV infection include condyloma and HPV-related cellular changes. Condyloma, koilocytosis, mild dysplasia, cervical intraepithelial neoplasia (CIN I), and anal intraepithelial neoplasia (AIN I) are all referred to as low-grade SIL (LSIL). At the other end of the spectrum, high-grade SIL (HSIL) encompasses moderate and severe dysplasia, CIN or AIN II, CIN or AIN III, and carcinoma in situ. Almost all of the invasive cancers arise from HSIL, not LSIL. The risk of developing invasive cancer increases with the severity of the dysplasia.

Although it is not clear that an actual increase in cervical or anal cancer exists among HIV-infected individuals, an increase in the prevalence of HPV infection and cervical SIL in HIV-infected women and anal SIL in HIV-infected men and women has been clearly demonstrated.

It is likely that cervical SIL and anal SIL are precursors of cervical and anal carcinoma, respectively, and these cancers are both theoretically preventable. Therefore, the development of adequate screening programs and treatment for precursor lesions are needed.

Cervical Neoplasia

Over the past 10 years, HIV infection has been identified as an important risk factor for HPV infection and the development of HPV-associated neoplasia of the female genital tract. This suggests that the immunodeficient status that results from HIV infection increases a woman's susceptibility to HPV infection and that HIV infection alters the natural history of HPV infection, making the development of anogenital neoplasia more likely.

In a large prospective cohort study,[138] the natural history of HIV infection was compared in HIV-infected and non–HIV-infected woman. In the New York City area, 220 HIV-infected and 221 non–HIV-infected woman were evaluated at two or more semiannual gynecologic examinations. Each examination included a test of cervicovaginal lavage specimens for HIV DNA. The investigators found that among women without neoplastic lesions identified at their first visit, HPV infection was more common and persistent among HIV-infected women. In addition, the high-risk, oncogenic HIV genotypes were more likely in the HIV-infected women.

In another study comparing HIV-infected and non–HIV-infected women, anal and cervical HPV infection and cytologic abnormalities were described.[139] In this cross-sectional study of 114 women, anal and cervical Papanicolaou smears, dot blot and PCR analysis for HPV, and CD4$^+$ cell counts were performed. Anal HPV infection was twice as common as cervical HPV infection and was more strongly associated with HIV infection. Cytologic abnormalities, both cervical and anal, were also strongly associated with HIV infection and with poor immune status as indicated by a lower CD4$^+$ cell count. The authors concluded that HPV-associated epithelial abnormalities were associated with immunodeficiency among HIV-infected women and that anal HPV infection was at least as common as cervical infection and disease among HIV-infected women.[139]

The importance of a cell-mediated response to HPV is clear. Persistence of HPV infection is thought to be requisite for the development of SILs. In an update concerning the New York cohort, the natural history of cervical HPV infection in HIV-infected women was described.[138] Persistent HPV infection with high-risk types was found in 20% of the seropositive women and 3% of the seronegative women. The likelihood of persistent infection was related to the level of immunosuppression, women with CD4$^+$ counts less than 200/mm^3 being more than twice as likely to have persistence of HPV infection as women with CD4$^+$ counts greater than 500/mm^3.

Maiman and coworkers[140] described a cohort of HIV-infected women in New York with invasive and preinvasive cervical neoplasia. In these women, compared with a group of non–HIV-infected women at the same institution, cervical neoplasia was more advanced at presentation, was more likely to recur, more frequently demonstrated perianal involvement, and was more often shown to have cytologic or histologic evidence of HPV infection. The authors also showed that with standard treatment approaches for advanced cervical cancer in HIV-infected women, there were significantly shorter intervals before disease recurrence and death than for the uninfected women. Maiman and coworkers[141] confirmed the elevated risk of cervical cancer recurrence in HIV-infected women in New York by examining the New York City cancer and AIDS registries from 1987 to 1995. The registry data indicate that 95% of the HIV-infected women who developed cervical cancer died from their disease.

Despite the high prevalence of cervical neoplasia in HIV-infected women, only a few cases of invasive cervical cancer have been reported.[140, 142–145] Experience with immunosuppressed transplant recipients suggests that a prolonged period of immunosuppression (approximately 3 months) may be necessary for the development of anogenital carcinoma.[99] In the pre-HAART era, a shorter period of immunodeficiency was common, and survival time may not have been long enough for cervical cancer to develop. With the advent of HAART and other medical therapies that can result in a longer duration of immunodeficiency, the frequency of cervical cancer may increase in women coinfected with HIV and HPV.

Anal Neoplasia

A relationship among HIV infection, HPV infection, and anal neoplasia also exists. The anal and cervical epithelia have similar embryologic origins and histology ranging from columnar epithelium to a transition zone, an area with increased metaplastic activity, and to a more differentiated squamous epithelium. Papanicolaou smears appear almost identical and are graded using the same criteria. The same HPV genotypes infect both the anal and cervical epithelia, producing similar manifestations ranging from condyloma to SIL to squamous carcinoma. Although anal cancer and its precursor lesion, anal SIL, have not been as well studied as cervical cancer and cervical SIL, similar evidence links HPV to anal cancer.

Palefsky and colleagues[87] assessed the prevalence of anal HPV infection and precancerous abnormalities of the anal epithelium in 97 severely immunodeficient, HIV-infected men. Abnormal anal cytology was found in 39% of the men, and 54% had HPV DNA in their anal cytologic specimens. Abnormalities on anal cytologic smears were significantly associated with the presence of HPV DNA (risk ratio, 4.6), and median CD4$^+$ cell counts in men with abnormal cytologic findings were significantly lower than those in men with normal cytologic findings ($p = .05$). Similar results have been obtained in a host of studies of this nature.

The natural history of anal HPV infection in gay or bisexual men is being characterized by an ongoing prospective study by Palefsky and colleagues in San Francisco in which 346 HIV-infected and 262 non–HIV-infected men have been enrolled. At baseline, 93% of the HIV-infected men and 61% of the non–HIV-infected men had anal HPV infection detected by PCR, with HPV-16 being the most common genotype in both groups. Infection with multiple genotypes of HPV was more common in the HIV-infected group, 73% versus 23%. The level of HPV infection and CD4+ cell count were inversely related in the HIV-infected individuals. Non–HIV-infected men who engaged in receptive anal intercourse were more likely to have anal HPV.[87]

Because cervical cancer is thought to develop from HSIL as opposed to LSIL, determining which individuals are at high risk for developing anal HSIL is particularly important. In a San Francisco cohort, new cases of HSIL developed in 38% of the HIV-infected men and 15% of the non–HIV-infected men over a 4-year period. HIV-infected men with LSIL or atypical cells at baseline were more likely to progress to HSIL than men with normal cytology and no visible lesion at baseline (57% versus 38%, $p = .001$). This association also held true for non–HIV-infected men (33% versus 14%, $p = .001$). Among both HIV-infected and noninfected men, risk factors for progression to HSIL were similar: infection with multiple HPV genotypes, persistent anal HPV infection, and a high level of infection with high-risk HPV genotypes.

Anal Cancer

Anal cancer is a rare malignancy. The incidence in the United States is about 0.8 per 100,000 persons, with almost twice as many women as men being affected. The relative risk in gay men is estimated to be 80-fold higher. This increase was noted before the AIDS epidemic.[9] The incidence in men with a history of receptive anal intercourse was estimated to be 35 in 100,000 before the AIDS epidemic. This rate is similar to the incidence of cervical cancer in women before the introduction of Papanicolaou smear screening and several times higher than current rates of cervical cancer in either HIV-infected or non–HIV-infected women (approximately 8 per 100,000 in the United States). It is not clear whether the incidence of anal cancer is higher in HIV-infected than non–HIV-infected gay men. At the 1998 AIDS Malignancy Conference, however, Biggar[146] reported that the risk of anal cancer in HIV-infected men doubled from 15- to 30-fold as immunosuppression worsened and an AIDS diagnosis was neared.

As with cervical cancer in HIV-infected women, Lorenz and colleagues, upon reviewing the surgical experience with anal carcinoma in HIV-infected men at the University of California, San Francisco, noted poor treatment outcomes and short survival times of HIV-infected men.[146a]

Holland and Swift[147] reported on a retrospective review of the anal cancer treatment outcomes of 7 HIV-infected individuals and 55 individuals with negative or unknown serostatus. The individuals were treated with standard radiotherapy with or without adjunctive chemotherapy. Treatment delays and hospitalizations for treatment-related toxicities occurred with much greater frequency in the HIV-infected population. This group also had a shorter mean time to treatment failure and higher incidence of relapse. The treatment regimen for anal carcinoma is quite toxic, and both HIV-infected and non–HIV-infected patients have difficulty and require medical assistance through the process. Both populations can benefit from standard treatment, and when HIV-related immunodeficiency is not advanced, standard treatment practices should be employed.

Clinical Implications of Human Immunodeficiency Virus–Related Anogenital Neoplasia

Because anogenital HPV infection and neoplasia are common in HIV-infected individuals, guidelines are needed for the management of cervical and anal neoplasia in this population. Information on the natural history of these conditions is limited, but it appears that these lesions are precancerous and likely to evolve into invasive cancer over time. As has been demonstrated with the successful use of the Papanicolaou smear in screening programs in the general population, early detection of preinvasive and minimally invasive cancers of the cervical region can provide the opportunity to cure these diseases. It therefore seems reasonable that some individuals with HIV infection, particularly those with relatively better prognoses, would benefit from early detection and treatment of anogenital neoplasia. Palefsky[86] has proposed guidelines (Table 112–2) for the management of cervical and anal neoplasia in HIV-infected individuals.

Palefsky is evaluating a large population of HIV-infected men with anal Papanicolaou smears and biopsies to validate the use of the Papanicolaou smear as a screening tool (J. Palefsky, personal communication). Recommendations about the widespread use of the anal Pap smear for screening purposes await the results of such trials.

As the AIDS epidemic progresses, anogenital carcinoma is likely to become more common. Extrapolating from observations of individuals with other immunosuppressed states, it seems plausible that as the duration of immunodeficiency is prolonged in HIV-infected individuals as a result of advanced antiretroviral and antibiotic treatments, the frequency of cervical and anal carcinoma may also increase.

Recommendations for Clinical Management

Cervical Squamous Intraepithelial Neoplasia

Abnormal cytology should be followed by colposcopy with biopsy of suspicious areas to determine the grade of lesions. Commonly, women with LSIL are evaluated every 3 to 6 months; lesions may regress spontaneously. Standard treatment should be utilized for women with HSIL. This consists of excision or ablation of the lesion with laser ablation, cryotherapy, a loop electrosurgical excision procedure, or cone biopsy. Routine, careful follow-up is necessary after therapy as an increased rate of recurrence among HIV-infected women is seen with all of these techniques.

TABLE 112–2 Papanicolaou Smears in Human Immunodeficiency Virus–Infected Individuals

Cervical Pap smears in HIV-infected women
- When HIV infection is first diagnosed, women *should* have a thorough gynecologic examination, including a Pap smear.
  - If the initial Pap smear is normal, a second Pap smear should be obtained at approximately 6 mos.
  - If both Pap smears are normal, annual Pap smears should follow.*
  - If any Pap smear reveals ASCUS or SIL, refer the individual for colposcopy with biopsy of abnormal area.

Anal Pap smears in HIV-infected women and gay or bisexual men
- When HIV infection is first diagnosed, an anal Pap smear *could* be part of the initial evaluation.
  - If the initial Pap smear is normal, a second Pap smear could be repeated at approximately 6 months.
  - If both Pap smears are normal, annual Pap smears could follow.*
  - If any Pap smear reveals ASCUS or SIL, refer the individual for colposcopy with biopsy of abnormal area.

Anal Pap smears in non–HIV-infected women and gay or bisexual men
- Men who have had anal warts or have receptive anal intercourse may benefit from an anal Pap smear. Women who have had anal warts, have a history of either cervical or vulvar HSIL or cancer, or have ever had receptive anal intercourse may benefit from an anal Pap smear.
  - If the initial Pap smear is normal, a second Pap smear could be repeated at approximately 6 months.
  - If both Pap smears are normal, individuals could have a Pap smear every 3 to 5 years.
  - If any Pap smear reveals ASCUS or SIL, refer the individual for colposcopy with biopsy of abnormal area.

*Some clinicians feel that individuals with a CD4+ cell count < 500/mm^3 should be monitored more frequently.

Abbreviations: ASCUS, Atypical squamous cells of unknown significance; HSIL, high-grade SIL; Pap, Papanicolaou; SIL, squamous intraepithelial lesion.

Cervical Cancer

Women with invasive cervical cancers should be managed according to the stage of their disease, regardless of their HIV status. Various modalities exist, including cone biopsy, radical hysterectomy, radiation therapy, and combined chemotherapy and radiation.

Anal Squamous Intraepithelial Neoplasia

At this time, there is no universally accepted standard of care for the treatment of anal SIL. As with cervical lesions, only individuals with high-grade disease, particularly those with severe dysplasia or AIN III, are referred for treatment. For both non–HIV-infected and HIV-infected individuals with a good functional status and a reasonable life expectancy, surgical excision or ablation should be considered. Individuals should be referred to an anal surgeon with experience in this setting.

As with cervical lesions, a high rate of recurrence or persistence of high-grade lesions is seen. At present, there are no medical therapies for HSIL that have proved efficacious. A number of protocols designed to investigate new therapies are under way.

OTHER NEOPLASMS ASSOCIATED WITH HUMAN IMMUNODEFICIENCY VIRUS DISEASE

Focusing on cancer incidence in single young men in San Franciso, Rabkin and associates[148] analyzed data from the Surveillance, Epidemiology, and End Results program. Except for KS and NHL, the incidence of all other cancers remained constant over the first decade of the HIV epidemic. (This program did not directly address the incidence of squamous cell skin cancer.)

Leiomyosarcoma

The occurrence of leiomyosarcomas and leiomyomas in children with HIV infection has been described in several case reports and small case series. Using molecular techniques, one group of investigators who studied these tumors found EBV genomes in all specimens evaluated.[149] In individuals with similar tumors but without HIV infection, the viral genome was not found. The authors speculated that in the setting of HIV-induced immunodeficiency, EBV may contribute to the pathogenesis of these smooth muscle tumors in children. It is possible that these tumors may some day be considered AIDS related.

Germ Cell Malignancy

Germ cell cancer is the most common malignancy in men younger than 40 years of age, the age range in which HIV infection most commonly occurs in men in the United States. No association between germ cell malignancies and immunodeficiency has been recognized. However, one epidemiologic cohort study suggested an increased incidence of seminoma in HIV-infected compared with non–HIV-infected men.[11]

Timmerman and coworkers[150] presented data on 15 men with HIV infection who were treated for germ cell tumors. The clinical presentations of these men were compared with those of 279 men with testicular cancer who were not at risk for HIV infection. These two populations were found to be quite similar with respect to stage of disease. Whereas most malignancies in this population tend to be seen at more advanced stages, behave more aggressively, and respond less well to standard chemotherapy regimens, these workers found the two populations to be quite similar with respect to stage of disease and response to chemotherapy. The HIV-infected men did not die as a result of the malignancy; if death occurred, it was found to be due to progression of their HIV disease.

Hodgkin's Disease

Hodgkin's disease is not an AIDS-defining illness. Controversy exists concerning the precise relationship between Hodgkin's disease and HIV infection. Initial epidemiologic data suggested that no relationship existed. Biggar and colleagues compared the rates of Hodgkin's disease in San Francisco[151] and New York[152] in the pre-AIDS period (1973 to 1978) with those early in the AIDS epidemic. No statistically significant increase in the odds ratio for Hodgkin's disease in single young men was observed.

Subsequent epidemiologic studies did suggest an increase in the risk of Hodgkin's disease among HIV-infected individuals. Hessol and associates[153] reviewed medical records of 6704 gay men who participated in the San Francisco City Clinic Cohort Study between 1978 and 1989. The study identified an excess risk attributable to HIV infection of 19.3 cases of Hodgkin's disease per 100,000 person-years. Reynolds and associates[154] also found a significantly increased incidence of Hodgkin's disease among people with AIDS.

Recent data from the Multicenter AIDS Cohort Study demonstrated an approximately fourfold increase in the risk of Hodgkin's disease in HIV-infected individuals.[155] The National Cancer Institute's AIDS Cancer Match Registry, which includes more than 300,000 cases in the United States, demonstrated an approximately 10-fold increase in the risk of Hodgkin's disease in HIV-infected individuals.[156] In the setting of HIV disease, in which the relative risk of Hodgkin's disease is markedly lower than the relative risk of NHL, it is not surprising that large numbers of individuals observed over extended periods of time would be required to demonstrate a significant increase in the risk of Hodgkin's disease.

Clinical observations suggest that Hodgkin's disease in HIV-infected individuals has a different natural history and therapeutic outcome than Hodgkin's disease in the general population. In large clinical series of Hodgkin's disease in nonimmunodeficient individuals diagnosed in the United States, nodular sclerosis was the most commonly encountered histologic subtype, occurring in 52 to 62% of all cases, with mixed cellularity accounting for approximately 24% and lymphocyte depleted in 3 to 6% of all individuals.[157] In individuals with HIV disease, these proportions are significantly shifted, with nearly all reported series indicating a high prevalence of mixed-cellularity disease and a significantly higher frequency of lymphocyte depletion.[158–162]

Advanced Hodgkin's disease (stage III or IV) also seems to occur with greater frequency in the HIV-infected population. Various series have demonstrated stage III or IV disease in 75 to 95% of HIV-infected individuals.[162, 163] In comparison, about 33% of non–HIV-infected individuals present with stage III or IV disease.[121]

The bone marrow appears to be one of the most common extranodal sites of involvement in HIV-associated Hodgkin's disease. Serrano and colleagues[161] identified bone marrow involvement in 10% of non–HIV-infected patients in Spain, compared with 50% of HIV-infected individuals.

Considering the multiplicity of unfavorable prognostic factors, such as advanced stage of disease, poor histologic subtype, greater extranodal involvement (particularly bone marrow and liver), and presence of B symptoms (unexplained fever >38°C, night sweats, weight loss >10% of body weight within the preceding 6 months), it is not surprising that HIV-infected individuals with Hodgkin's disease are less likely to have durable and complete responses. The outcome of therapy has been quite disappointing. Among 12 evaluable patients at San Francisco General Hospital, there were 7 complete responders to either nitrogen mustard, vincristine (Oncovorin), procarbazine, and prednisone (MOPP) or MOPP alternating with doxorubicin (Adriamycin), bleomycin, vinblastine, and dacarbazine (MOPP-ABVD).[163] Six of the complete responders subsequently had relapses. Eight patients (62%) developed *P. carinii* pneumonia during the course of treatment. There were no long-term survivors. None of these patients is alive. One half of the patients died with advanced Hodgkin's disease and the remaining patients died as a result of opportunistic infections. Median survival time was less than 1 year in this population, compared with 12 years in the control population. This dramatic difference in survival between the HIV-infected and the non–HIV-infected groups illustrates that the presence of HIV infection alters the natural history of the neoplasm.

The mean dose intensity of chemotherapy delivered to the patients was only 41% of the planned therapeutic dose. Poor bone marrow reserve and intercurrent opportunistic infections resulted in frequent dose reductions and delays in chemotherapy administration. This may account for the high relapse rate observed in complete responders.

Similar trends were reported by the Italian cooperative group for AIDS-related tumors.[159] Seventeen patients were treated with either MOPP, ABVD, ABV, or MOPP-ABVD. Only eight patients (30%) achieved complete remission. Of 13 patients who died, 7 (54%) died of opportunistic infections, 3 died of progression of Hodgkin's disease, and 2 died of disseminated intravascular coagulopathy. The median survival of the 17 patients who were treated was 15 months.

The poor therapeutic outcome and frequent toxicity associated with standard chemotherapy regimens in this population suggest that survival will not be improved with more aggressive chemotherapeutic regimens. Rather, less aggressive chemotherapeutic regimens or standard regimens with hematopoietic growth factors may be needed. Preliminary results of a clinical trial using a relatively nonmyelosuppressive combination chemotherapeutic regimen consisting of bleomycin, vincristine, streptozocin, and etoposide are encouraging.[164] Of the first five patients treated with this regimen, four had complete responses to chemotherapy alone and a fifth had a complete response after completion of chemotherapy and radiation therapy. Myelosuppression was not observed.

Levine and coworkers[165] studied the use of standard ABVD chemotherapy combined with G-CSF with the hope of reducing myelosuppression. Complete remission was seen in 60% of 21 patients treated, with a median survival of 19 months. Overall this regimen was tolerated well, although considerable hematologic toxicity occurred.

At present, sufficient data are not available to allow us to determine which chemotherapeutic regimen may be more efficacious. It is recommended that standard chemotherapy, usually ABVD, be employed with a CSF. For patients with poor hematologic reserve or severe immunosuppression ($CD4^+$ cell count <100/mm^3) or both, a dose-modified standard regimen or a less myelosuppressive chemotherapeutic combination as described earlier might be considered. In addition, prophylaxis against *P. carinii* pneumonia should be employed during treatment.

CONCLUSIONS

To date, all AIDS-defining malignancies have been associated in some way with a virus other than HIV. Although a direct link has not been identified, and thus the term virally induced malignancies is inappropriate, evidence is mounting in favor of a strong relationship between immune dysfunction; the presence of latent viruses, including EBV, HHV-8, and HPV; and the development of neoplasms in persons with HIV.

As oncogenesis continues to be investigated, discoveries about these various viruses and the host and immune status and responses should help us to understand and treat both those infected with HIV and those not infected. At present, it is important for the patients and the physicians caring for the patients to understand that all malignancies, AIDS defining or otherwise, tend to occur at a more advanced stage; behave more aggressively; and, although often responsive to medical intervention, recur more frequently. In addition to the behavior of the neoplasms, the individual's immune status presents a difficult baseline from which to initiate and maintain an intensive chemotherapeutic regimen. Poor bone marrow reserve, intercurrent opportunistic infections, and medication interactions are all factors that should be borne in mind while implementing often individualized treatment strategies.

REFERENCES

1. Frizzera G, Rosai J, Dehner L, et al. Lymphoreticular disorders in primary immunodeficiencies: New findings based on an up-to-date histologic classification of 35 cases. Cancer. 1980;46:692–699.
2. Harwood A, Osoba D, Hofstader S, et al. Kaposi's sarcoma in recipients of renal transplants. Am J Med. 1979;67:759–765.
3. Hoover R, Fraumeni J. Risk of cancer in renal transplant recipients. Lancet. 1973;2:55–57.
4. Penn I. The incidence of malignancies in transplant recipients. Transplant Proc. 1975;7:323–326.
5. Pinching A. The immunology of AIDS and HIV infection. Clin Immunol Allergy. 1986;6:645.
6. Ziegler J, Templeton AC, Vogel CL. Kaposi's sarcoma: A comparison of classical, endemic, and epidemic forms. Semin Oncol. 1984;11:47–52.
7. Friedman-Kien A, Laubenstein LJ, Rubinstein P, et al. Disseminated Kaposi's sarcoma in homosexual men. Ann Intern Med. 1982;96:693–700.
8. Centers for Disease Control. Revision of the Case Definition of AIDS Used by CDC for National Reporting (CDC Reportable AIDS), 1985. Atlanta: Department of Health and Human Services; 1985.
9. Biggar RJ, Rabkin CS. The epidemiology of AIDS-related neoplasms. Hematol Oncol Clin North Am. 1996;10:997–1010.
10. Melbye M, Rabkin C, Frisch M, Biggar RJ. Changing patterns of anal cancer incidence in the United States, 1940–1989. Am J Epidemiol. 1994;139:772–780.
11. Lyter DW, Bryant J, Thackeray R, et al. Incidence of human immunodeficiency virus–related and nonrelated malignancies in a large cohort of homosexual men. J Clin Oncol. 1995;13:2540–2546.
12. Remick S. Non–AIDS-defining cancers. Hematol Oncol Clin North Am. 1996;10:1203–1213.
13. Volm M, Von Roenn J. Non–AIDS-defining malignancies in patients with HIV infection. Curr Opin Oncol. 1996;8:386–391.
14. Ravalli S, Chabon A, Khan A. Gastrointestinal neoplasia in young HIV-positive patients. Am J Clin Pathol. 1989;91:458–461.
15. Tirelli U, Vaccher E, Sinicco A, et al. Forty-nine unusual HIV-related malignant tumors. Program of the 5th International Conference on AIDS, Montreal, 1989.
16. Braun M. Classics in oncology. Idiopathic multiple pigmented sarcoma of the skin by Kaposi. CA Cancer J Clin. 1982;32:340–347.
17. Kaposi M. Zur Nomenclatur des idiopathischen Pigmentsarkom Kaposi. Arch Dermatol Syph (Berl) 1894;29:164.
18. Koebner H. Kranken Vorstellung (idiopathisches multiples sarcoma Hemorrhagicum der Extremitaten). Arch Dermatol Syph (Berl) 1909;94:121.
19. Moore PS, Chang Y. Detection of herpes-like DNA sequences in Kaposi's sarcoma in patients with and without HIV infection. N Engl J Med. 1995;332:1181–1185.
20. DeJarlais D, Marmor M, Thomas P, et al. Kaposi's sarcoma among four different AIDS risk groups. Lancet. 1988;1:1119.
21. Mitsuyasu R, Groopman J. Biology and therapy of Kaposi's sarcoma. Semin Oncol. 1984;11:53–59.
22. Safai B. Pathophysiology and epidemiology of epidemic Kaposi's sarcoma. Semin Oncol. 1987;2(Suppl 3):7–12.
23. Des Jarlais D, Stoneburner R, Thomas P. Declines in proportion of Kaposi's sarcoma among cases of AIDS in multiple risk groups in New York City. Lancet. 1987;2:1024–1025.
24. Beral V, Peterman T, Berkelman R, Jaffe H. Kaposi's sarcoma among persons with AIDS: A sexually transmitted infection? Lancet. 1990;335:123–128.
25. Ruiz A, Ganz WI, Post MJ, et al. Use of thallium-201 brain SPECT to differentiate cerebral lymphoma from toxoplasma encephalitis in AIDS patients. AJNR. 1994;15:1885–1894.
26. Jacobson L. Impact of highly effective antiretroviral therapy on recent trends in cancer among HIV-infected individuals. Abstract S5. Presented at the Second National AIDS Malignancy Conference, Bethesda, Md, April 6–8, 1998.
27. Buchbinder S, Vittinghoff E, Colfax G, Holmberg S. Declines in AIDS incidence associated with highly active antiretroviral therapy (HAART) are not reflected in KS and lymphoma incidence. Abstract S7. Presented at the Second National AIDS Malignancy Conference, Bethesda, Md, April 6–8, 1998.
28. Jones J, Hanson D, Ward J. Effect of antiretroviral therapy on recent trends in cancer among HIV-infected persons. Abstract S3. Presented at the Second National AIDS Malignancy Conference, Bethesda, Md, April 6–8, 1998.
29. Jacobson L, Armenian H. An integrated approach to the epidemiology of Kaposi's sarcoma. Curr Opin Oncol. 1995;7:450–455.
30. Chang Y, Cesarman E, Pessin MS, et al. Identification of herpesvirus-like DNA sequences in AIDS-associated Kaposi's sarcoma. Science. 1994;266:1865–1869.
31. Schalling M, Ekman M, Kaaya EE, et al. A role for a new herpes virus (KSHV) in different forms of Kaposi's sarcoma. Nat Med. 1995;1:707–708.
32. Whitby D, Howard MR, Tenant-Flowers M, et al. Detection of Kaposi sarcoma associated herpesvirus in peripheral blood of HIV-infected individuals and progression to Kaposi's sarcoma. Lancet. 1995;346:799–802.
33. Humphrey RW, O'Brien TR, Newcomb FM, et al. Kaposi's sarcoma (KS)–associated herpesvirus-like KNA sequences in peripheral blood mononuclear cells: Association with KS and pesistence in patients receiving anti-herpesvirus drugs. Blood. 1996;88:297–301.
34. Soulier J, Grothet L, Oksenhendler E, et al. Kaposi's sarcoma–associated herpesvirus-like DNA sequences in multicentric Castleman's disease. Blood. 1995;86:1276–1280.
35. Monini P, de Lellis L, Fabris M, et al. Kaposi's sarcoma–associated herpesvirus

DNA sequences in prostate tissue and human semen. N Engl J Med. 1996;334:1168–1172.
36. Kedes DH, Operskalski E, Busch M, et al. The epidemiology of human herpesvirus 8 (Kaposi's sarcoma–associated herpesvirus): Distribution of infection in KS risk groups and evidence for sexual transmission. Nat Med. 1996;2:918–924.
37. Miles SA. Pathogenesis of AIDS-related Kaposi's sarcoma. Evidence of a viral etiology. Hematol Oncol Clin North Am. 1996;10:1011–1021.
38. Nickoloff B, Foreman K. Charting a new course through the chaos of KS (Kaposi's sarcoma). Am J Pathol. 1996;148:1323–1329.
39. Green TL, Beckstead JH, Lozada-Nur F, et al. Histopathologic spectrum of oral Kaposi's sarcoma. Oral Surg Oral Med Oral Pathol. 1984;58:306–314.
40. Dorfman R. Kaposi's sarcoma revisited. Hum Pathol. 1984;15:1013–1017.
41. McNeil C. HIV infection with Hodgkin's disease: The virus makes a difference (News). J Natl Cancer Inst. 1997;89:754–755.
42. Beckstead JH, Wood GS, Fletcher V. Evidence for the origin of Kaposi's sarcoma from lymphatic endothelium. Am J Pathol. 1985;119:294–300.
43. Conant MA, Opp KM, Poretz D, Mills RG. Reduction of Kaposi's sarcoma lesions following treatment of AIDS with ritonavir. AIDS. 1997;11:1300–1301.
44. Friedman SL. Gastrointestinal hepatobiliary neoplasms in AIDS. Gastroenterol Clin North Am. 1988;17:465–486.
45. Gill P, Akil B, Colletti P, et al. Pulmonary Kaposi's sarcoma: Clinical findings and results of therapy. Am J Med. 1989;87:57–61.
46. Hanto D, Gajl-Peczalkska K, Frizzera G, et al. Clinical spectrum of lymphoproliferative disorders in renal transplant recipients and evidence for the role of Epstein-Barr virus. Cancer Res. 1981;41:4253–4261.
47. Kaplan L, Hopewell P, Jaffe H. Kaposi's sarcoma involving the lung in patients with the acquired immunodeficiency syndrome. J Acquir Immune Defic Syndr. 1988;1:23–30.
48. Davis S, Henschke C, Chamides B, Westcott J. Intrathoracic Kaposi sarcoma in AIDS patients: Radiographic-pathologic correlation. Radiology. 1987;163:495–500.
49. Volberding P, Kusick P, Feigal D. Effects of chemotherapy for HIV-associated Kaposi's sarcoma on long-term survival (Abstract 11). Proc Am Soc Clin Oncol. 1989;8:3.
50. Chak L, Gill P, Levine A, et al. Radiation therapy for AIDS-related Kaposi's sarcoma. J Clin Oncol. 1988;6:863–867.
51. Hill D. The role of radiotherapy for epidemic Kaposi's sarcoma. Semin Oncol. 1987;14(Suppl 3):1207.
52. Newcomer VD. Human immunodeficiency virus infection and acquired immunodeficiency syndrome in the elderly (Letter). Arch Dermatol. 1997;133:1311–1312.
53. Bernstein Z, Wilson D, Summers K, et al. Pilot/phase I study—Photodynamic therapy (PDT) for treatment of AIDS-associated Kaposi's sarcoma (AIDS/KS). Proc Am Soc Clin Oncol. 1995;14:289.
54. Northfelt DW, Dezube BJ, Thommes JA, et al. Pegylated-liposomal doxorubicin versus doxorubicin, bleomycin, and vincristine in the treatment of AIDS-related Kaposi's sarcoma: Results of a randomized phase III clinical trial. J Clin Oncol. 1998;16:2445–2451.
55. Northfelt DW, Dezube BJ, Thommes JA, et al. Efficacy of pegylated-liposomal doxorubicin in the treatment of AIDS-related Kaposi's sarcoma after failure of standard chemotherapy. J Clin Oncol. 1997;15:653–659.
56. Gill P, Wernz J, Scadden D, et al. Randomized phase III trial of liposomal daunorubicin versus doxorubicin, bleomycin, and vincristine in AIDS-related Kaposi's sarcoma. J Clin Oncol. 1996;14:2353–2364.
57. Gill P, Hadienberg J, Espina B, et al. Low dose paclitaxel (Taxol) every two weeks over 3 hours is safe and effective in the treatment of advanced AIDS-related Kaposi's sarcoma. Abstract 1516. Presented at the American Society of Hematology (ASH), Thirty-ninth Annual Meeting, Seattle, December 2–5, 1995.
58. Saville M, Lietzau J, Pluda J, et al. Activity of placlitaxel (Taxol) as therapy for HIV-associated Kaposi's sarcoma. Lancet. 1995;346:26–28.
59. Krown S. The role of interferon in the therapy of epidemic Kaposi's sarcoma. Semin Oncol. 1987;14(Suppl 3):27–33.
60. Kovacs J, Lance H, Masur H, et al. A phase III, placebo-controlled trial of recombinant alpha-interferon in asymptomatic individuals seropositive for the acquired immunodeficiency syndrome. Clin Res. 1987;35:479A.
61. Lane H, Feinberg J, Davery V, et al. Anti-retroviral effects of interferon-alpha in AIDS-associated Kaposi's sarcoma. Lancet. 1988;2:1218–1222.
62. deWit R, Schatenkerk J, Boucher C, et al. Clinical and virological effects of high-dose recombinant interferon-alpha in disseminated AIDS-related Kaposi's sarcoma. Lancet. 1988;2:1214–1217.
63. Groopman J, Gottlieb M, Goodman J, et al. Recombinant alpha-2 interferon therapy for Kaposi's sarcoma associated with the acquired immunodeficiency syndrome. Ann Intern Med. 1984;100:671–676.
64. Real F, Oettgen H, Krown S. Kaposi's sarcoma and the acquired immunodeficiency syndrome: Treatment with high and low doses of leukocyte A interferon. J Clin Oncol. 1986;4:544–551.
65. Volberding P, Mitsuyasu R. Recombinant interferon alpha in the treatment of acquired immune deficiency syndrome–related Kaposi's sarcoma. Semin Oncol. 1985;2(Suppl 5):2–6.
66. Volberding P, Mitsuyasu R, Golando J, et al. Treatment of Kaposi's sarcoma with interferon alfa-2 (Intron A). Cancer. 1987;59:620–625.
67. Rios A, Mansell P, Newell G, et al. Treatment of acquired immunodeficiency syndrome–related Kaposi's sarcoma with lymphoblastoid interferon. J Clin Oncol. 1985;3:506–512.
68. Kristal A, Nasca P, Burnett W, Mikl J. Changes in the epidemiology of non-Hodgkin's lymphoma associated with epidemic human immunodeficiency virus (HIV) infection. Am J Epidemiol. 1988;128:711–718.
69. Vaccher E, Tirelli U, Spina M, et al. Age and serum lactate dehydrogenase level are independent prognostic factors in human immunodeficiency virus–related non-Hodgkin's lymphomas: A single-institute study of 96 patients. J Clin Oncol. 1996;14:2217–2223.
70. Hartshorn K, Vogt M, Chou T, et al. Synergistic inhibition of human immunodeficiency virus in vitro by azidothymidine and recombinant alpha A interferon. Antimicrob Agent Chemother. 1987;31:168–172.
71. Aboulafin D. Regression of acquired immunodeficiency syndrome–related pulmonary Kaposi's sarcoma after highly active antiretroviral therapy. Mayo Clin Proc. 1998;73:439–443.
72. Henry K, Worley J, Sullivan C, et al. Documented improvement in late stage manifestations of AIDS after starting ritonavir in combination with two reverse transcriptase inhibitors. Abstract 356. Presented at the Fourth Conference of Retroviruses and Opportunistic Infections, Chicago, January 22–26, 1997.
73. Parra R, Leal M, Delgrado J, et al. Regression of invasive AIDS-related Kaposi's sarcoma following antiretroviral therapy. Clin Infect Dis. 1998;26:218–219.
74. Wit FW, Sol CJ, Renwick N, et al. Regression of AIDS-related Kaposi's sarcoma associated with clearance of human herpesvirus-8 from peripheral blood mononuclear cells following initiation of antiretroviral therapy (Letter). AIDS. 1998;12:218–219.
75. Workman C, Lewis C, Smith D. Resolution of Kaposi's sarcoma associated with saquinavir therapy—case report. Abstract Tu.B.2217. Presented at the International Conference on AIDS, Vancouver, British Columbia, Canada, July 7–12, 1996.
76. Volm M, Wernz J. Patients with advanced AIDS-related Kaposi's sarcoma (KS) no longer require systemic therapy after introduction of effective antiretroviral therapy. Abstract 162. Presented at the Thirty-third Annual ASCO Meeting, Denver, May 17–20, 1997.
77. Ziegler J, Drew W, Miner R, et al. Outbreak of Burkitt's-like lymphoma in homosexual men. Lancet. 1982;2:631.
78. Kaplan LD, Abrams DI, Feigal E, et al. AIDS-associated non-Hodgkin's lymphoma in San Francisco. JAMA. 1989;261:719–724.
79. National Cancer Institute. NCI-sponsored study of classifications of non-Hodgkin's lymphoma: Summary and description of a working formulation for clinical usage. The Non-Hodgkin's Lymphoma Pathologic Classification Project. Cancer. 1982;49:2112–2135.
80. Centers for Disease Control. Revision of the case definition of acquired immunodeficiency syndrome for national reporting—United States. MMWR Morb Mortal Wkly Rep. 1985;4:373–374.
81. Penn I. Lymphomas complicating organ transplantation. Transplant Proc. 1983;15(Suppl 1):2790–2797.
82. Harnly M, Swan S, Holly E, et al. Temporal trends in the incidence of non-Hodgkin's lymphoma and selected malignancies in a population with a high incidence of acquired immunodeficiency syndrome (AIDS). Am J Epidemiol. 1988;128:261–267.
83. Baumgartner J, Rachlin J, Beckstead J, et al. Primary central nervous system lymphomas: Natural history and response to radiation therapy in 55 patients with acquired immunodeficiency syndrome. J Neurosurg. 1990;73:206–211.
84. Bais C, Santomasso B, Coso O, et al. G-protein–coupled receptor of Kaposi's sarcoma–associated herpesvirus is a vital oncogene and angiogenesis activator. Nature. 1998;391:86–89.
85. Chamberlain MC. Long survival in patients with acquired immune deficiency syndrome–related primary central nervous system lymphoma. Cancer. 1994; 73:1728–1730.
86. Palefsky J. Human papillomavirus infection among HIV-infected individuals. Hematol Oncol Clin North Am. 1991;5:357–370.
87. Palefsky J, Gonzales J, Greenblatt R, et al. Anal intraepithelial neoplasia and anal papillomavirus infection among homosexual males with group IV HIV disease. JAMA. 1990;263:2911–2916.
88. Shearer W, Ritz J, Finego M, et al. Epstein-Barr virus–associated B-cell proliferations of diverse clonal origins after bone marrow transplantation in a 12-year-old patient with severe combined immunodeficiency. N Engl J Med. 1985;312:1151–1159.
89. Meeker T, Shiramizu B, Kaplan L, et al. Evidence for molecular subtypes of HIV-associated lymphoma: Division into peripheral monoclonal, polyclonal and central nervous system lymphoma. AIDS. 1991;5:669–674.
90. Shiramizu B, Herndier B, Meeker T, et al. Molecular and immunophenotypic characterization of AIDS-associated EBV-negative polyclonal lymphoma. J Clin Oncol. 1992;10:383–389.
91. Subar M, Neri A, Inghirami G, et al. Frequent c-*myc* oncogene activation and infrequent presence of Epstein-Barr virus genome in AIDS-associated lymphoma. Blood. 1988;72:667–671.
92. Knowles D, Chamulak G, Subar M, et al. Lymphoid neoplasia associated with the acquired immunodeficiency syndrome (AIDS). Ann Intern Med. 1988;108:744–753.
93. Herndier B, Shiramizu B, Jewett N, et al. Acquired immunodeficiency syndrome–associated T-cell lymphoma: Evidence for human immunodeficiency virus type 1–associated T-cell transformation. Blood. 1992;79:1768–1774.
94. Shiramizu B, Herndier BG, McGrath MS. Identification of a common clonal human immunodeficiency virus integration site in human immunodeficiency virus–associated lymphomas. Cancer Res. 1994;54:2069–2072.
95. Emilie D, Coumbaras J, Raphael M, et al. Interleukin-6 production in high-grade B lymphomas: Correlation with the presence of malignant immunoblasts in acquired immunodeficiency syndrome and in human immunodeficiency virus–seronegative patients. Blood. 1992;80:498–504.
96. Emilie D, Touitou R, Raphael M, et al. In vivo production of interleukin-10 by malignant cells in AIDS lymphomas. Eur J Immunol. 1992;22:2937–2942.
97. McGrath M, Marsh J, Nolan T, Herndier B. Lymphokine gene expression and

effects on cell proliferation in AIDS-associated NHL (Abstract). J Cell Biochem Suppl. 1993;17E:270.
98. Kaplan L, Kahn J, Jacobson M, et al. Primary bile duct lymphoma in the acquired immmunodeficiency syndrome (AIDS). Ann Intern Med. 1989;110:162.
99. Penn I. Cancers of the anogenital region in renal transplant recipients: Analysis of 65 cases. Cancer. 1986;58:611–616.
100. Rogo K, Kavoo-Linge. Human immunodeficiency virus seroprevalence among cervical cancer patients. Gynecol Oncol. 1990;37:87–92.
101. Nasr S, Brynes R, Garrison C, Chan W. Peripheral T-cell lymphoma in a patient with acquired immunodeficiency syndrome. Cancer. 1988;61:947–951.
102. Presant C, Gala K, Wiseman C, et al, Human immunodeficiency virus–associated T-cell lymphoblastic lymphoma in AIDS. Cancer. 1987;60:1459–1461.
103. Knowles D, Inghirami G, Ubraico A, Dall-Favera R. Molecular genetic analysis of three AIDS-associated neoplasms of uncertain lineage demonstrates their B-cell derivation and the possible pathogenic role of Epstein-Barr virus. Blood. 1989;73:792–799.
104. Gill P, Levine A, Krail M, et al. AIDS-related malignant lymphoma: Results of prospective treatment trials. J Clin Oncol. 1987;5:1322–1328.
105. Lowenthal D, Straus D, Campbell S, et al. AIDS-related lymphoid neoplasia: The Memorial Hospital experience. Cancer. 1988;61:2325–2337.
106. Bermudez M, Grant K, Rodvien R, et al. Non-Hodgkin's lymphoma in a population with or at risk for acquired immunodeficiency syndrome: Indications for intensive chemotherapy. Am J Med. 1989;86:71–76.
107. Levine A, Sullivan-Halley J, Pike M, et al. Human immunodeficiency virus–related lymphoma: Prognostic factors predictive of survival. Cancer. 1991;68:2466–2472.
108. Northfelt D, Volberding P, Kaplan L. Degree of immunodeficiency at diagnosis of AIDS-associated non-Hodgkin's lymphoma. Proceedings of American Society of Clinical Oncology. San Diego, May 17–19, 1992.
109. Levin RJ, Henick DH, Cohen AF. Human immunodeficiency virus–associated non-Hodgkin's lymphoma presenting as an auricular perichondritis. Otolaryngol Head Neck Surg. 1995;112:493–495.
110. Kaplan L, Straus D, Testa M, et al. Randomized trial of standard-dose vs. low-dose mBACOD chemotherapy for HIV-associated non-Hodgkin's lymphoma. N Engl J Med. 1997;336:1641–1648.
111. Ziegler J, Beckstead J, Volberding P, et al. Non-Hodgkin's lymphoma in 90 homosexual men: Relation to generalized lymphadenopathy and the acquired immunodeficiency syndrome. N Engl J Med. 1984;311:565–570.
112. Burkes R, Meyer P, Gill P, et al. Rectal lymphoma in homosexual men. Arch Intern Med. 1986;146:913–915.
113. Tirelli U, Vaccher E, Rezza G, et al. Hodgkin's disease and infection with the human immunodeficiency virus in Italy. Ann Intern Med. 1988;108:309.
114. Straus DJ, Huang J, Testa MA, et al. Prognostic factors in the treatment of human immunodeficiency virus–associated non-Hodgkin's lymphoma: Analysis of AIDS Clinical Trials Group protocol 142—Low-dose versus standard-dose m-BACOD plus granulocyte-macrophage colony-stimulating factor. National Institute of Allergy and Infectious Diseases. J Clin Oncol. 1998;16:3601–3606.
115. De Vita V, Hubbard S, Young R, Longo D. The role of chemotherapy in diffuse aggressive lymphomas. Semin Hematol. 1988;25(Suppl 2):2–10.
116. Gill P, Levine A, Meyer R, et al. Primary central nervous system lymphoma in homosexual men: Clinical, immunologic and pathologic factors. Am J Med. 1985;78:742–748.
117. Gill P, Levine A, Krailo M, et al. AIDS-related malignant lymphoma: Results of prospective treatment trials. J Clin Oncol. 1987;5:1322.
118. Gill P, Naidu Y, Nakamur S, et al. IL-6 regulation by steroid hormones and autocrine activity in Kaposi's sarcoma. AIDS Res Hum Retroviruses. 1991;7:220.
119. Sparano JA, Wiernik PH, Hu X, et al. Pilot trial of infusional cyclophosphamide, doxorubicin, and etoposide plus didanosine and filgrastim in patients with human immunodeficiency virus–associated non-Hodgkin's lymphoma. J Clin Oncol. 1996;14:3026–3035.
120. Formenti S, Gill P, Rarick M, et al. Primary central nervous system lymphoma in AIDS: Results of radiation therapy. Cancer. 1989;63:1101–1107.
121. So Y, Beckstead J, Davis R. Primary central nervous system lymphoma in acquired immunodeficiency syndrome: A clinical and pathological study. Ann Neurol. 1986;20:566–572.
122. MacMahon E, Glass J, Hayward S, et al. Epstein-Barr virus in AIDS-related primary central nervous system lymphoma. Lancet. 1991;338:969.
123. Beral V, Peterman T, Berkelman R, Jaffe H. AIDS-associated non-Hodgkin's lymphoma. Lancet. 1991;337:805.
124. Levine A. Acquired immunodeficiency syndrome–related lymphoma. Blood. 1992;80:8.
125. Goldstein J, Dickson D, Moser F, et al. Primary central nervous system lymphoma in acquired immunodeficiency syndrome: A clinical and pathologic study with results of treatment with radiation. Cancer. 1991;67:2756.
126. Ciricillo S, Rosenblum M. Use of CT and MRI imaging to distinguish intracranial lesions and to define the need for biopsy in AIDS patients. J Neurosurg. 1990;73:720–724.
127. Grant I, Gold J, Armstron D. Risk of CNS toxoplasmosis in patients with acquired immune deficiency syndrome. Abstract 441. Program of the Interscience Conference on Antimicrobial Agents and Chemotherapy, New Orleans, September 28–October 1, 1986.
128. Porter S, Sande M. Toxoplasmosis of the central nervous system in the acquired immunodeficiency syndrome. N Engl J Med. 1992;327:1643–1648.
129. De Luca A, Antinori A, Cingolani A, et al. Evaluation of cerebrospinal fluid EBV-DNA and IL-10 as markers for in vivo diagnosis of AIDS-related primary central nervous system lymphoma. Br J Haematol. 1995;90:844–849. [Erratum. Br J Haematol. 1995;91:1035.]
130. Cinque P, Brytting M, Vago L, et al. Epstein-Barr virus DNA in cerebrospinal fluid from patients with AIDS-related primary lymphoma of the central nervous system. Lancet. 1993;342:398–410.
131. Cingolani A, De Luca A, Larocca LM, et al. Minimally invasive diagnosis of acquired immunodeficiency syndrome–related primary central nervous system lymphoma. J Natl Cancer Inst. 1998;90:364–369.
132. Forsyth PA, Yahalom J, DeAngelis LM. Combined-modality therapy in the treatment of primary central nervous system lymphoma in AIDS. Neurology. 1994;44:1473–1479.
133. Vernon S, Holmes K, Reeves W. Human papillomavirus infection and associated disease in persons infected with human immunodeficiency virus. Clin Infect Dis. 1995; (Suppl 1):S121–S124.
134. Pfister H. The role of human papillomavirus in anogential cancer. Obstet Gynecol Clin North Am. 1996;23:579–595.
135. Gal A, Saul S, Stoer M. In situ hybridization analysis of human papillomavirus in anal squamous cell carcinoma. Mod Pathol. 1989;2:439–443.
136. Sillman F, Sedlis A. Anogenital papillomavirus infection and neoplasia in immunodeficient women. Obstet Gynecol Clin North Am. 1987;14:537–538.
137. Committee TBSE. The Bethesda system for reporting cervical/vaginal cytologic diagnoses: Report of the 1991 Bethesda workshop. Hum Pathol. 1992;23:719–721.
138. Sun X, Kuhn L, Ellerbrock T, et al. Human papillomavirus infection in women infected with the human immunodeficiency virus. N Engl J Med. 1997;337:1343–1349.
139. Wright A, Darragh T, Vranizan, K, et al. Anal and cervical papillomavirus infection and risk of anal and cervical epithelial abnormalities in human immunodeficiency virus–infected women. Obstet Gynecol. 1997;89:76–80.
140. Maiman M, Fructer R, Serur E, et al. Human immunodeficiency virus infection and cervical neoplasia. Gynecol Oncol. 1990;38:377–382.
141. Maiman M, Fructer R, Clark M, et al. Cervical cancer as an AIDS-defining illness. Obstet Gynecol. 1997;89:76–80.
142. Maiman M, Fructer R, Guy L, et al. Human immunodeficiency virus infection and invasive cervical cancer. Cancer. 1993;71:402–406.
143. Monfardini S, Vaccher E, Pizzocaro G, et al. Unusual malignant tumors in 49 patients with HIV infection. AIDS. 1989;3:499–452.
144. Rellihan M, Dooley D, Burke T, et al. Rapidly progressing cervical cancer in a patient with human immunodeficiency virus infection. Gynecol Oncol. 1990;36:435–438.
145. Saccucci P, Mastrone M, Are P, et al. Rapidly progressive squamous cell carcinoma of the cervix in a patient with acquired immunodeficiency syndrome: Case report. Eur J Gyneaecol Oncol. 1996;17:306–308.
146. Biggar R. Cancers in AIDS: What types and what clues to etiology? Presented at the 1998 National AIDS Malignancy Conference, sponsored by the National Cancer Institute, Bethesda, Md, April 6–8, 1998.
146a. Lorenz HP, Wilson W, Leigh B, et al. Squamous cell carcinoma of the anus and HIV infection. Dis Colon Rectum. 1991;34:336–338.
147. Holland J, Swift P. Tolerance of patients with human immunodeficiency virus and carcinoma to treatment with combined chemotherapy and radiation therapy. Radiology. 1994;193:251–254.
148. Rabkin C, Biggar R, Horm J. Increased incidence of cancers associated with the human immunodeficiency virus epidemic. Int J Cancer. 1991;47:692–696.
149. McClain L, Leach C, Jenson H, et al. Association of Epstein-Barr virus with leiomyosarcomas in children with AIDS. N Engl J Med. 1995;332:12–18.
150. Timmerman J, Northfelt D, Small E. Malignant germ cell tumors in men infected with human immunodeficiency virus: Natural history and results of therapy. J Clin Oncol. 1996;13:1391–1397.
151. Biggar R, Horm J, Goedert J, et al. Cancer in a group at risk of acquired immunodeficiency syndrome (AIDS) through 1984. Am J Epidemiol. 1987;126:578.
152. Biggar R, Burnett W, Mikl J, et al. Cancer among New York men at risk of acquired immunodeficiency syndrome. Int J Cancer. 1989;43:979.
153. Hessol N, Katz M, Liu J, et al. Increased incidence of Hodgkin's disease in homosexual men with HIV infection. Ann Intern Med. 1992;117:309.
154. Reynolds P, Saunders L, Layefsky M, Lemp F. The spectrum of acquired immunodeficiency syndrome (AIDS)–associated malignancies in San Francisco, 1980–1987. Am J Epidemiol 1993;37:19.
155. Lyter D, Kingsley L, Rinaldo C, et al. Malignancies in the Multicenter AIDS Cohort Study (MACS), 1984–1994. Presented at the American Society of Clinical Oncology, Thirty-second Annual Meeting, Philadelphia, May 18–21, 1996.
156. Biggar R, Rabkin C. The epidemiology of AIDS-related neoplasms. In: Krown S, von Roenn, JH., eds. Hematologic and Oncologic Aspects of HIV Infection. Philadelphia: WB Saunders; 1996:997–1010.
157. Davis S, Dahlberg S, Nyers M, et al. Hodgkin's disease in the United States: A comparison of patient characteristics and survival in the centralized cancer patient data system and the surveillance, epidemiology, and end results program. J Natl Cancer Inst. 1987;78:471.
158. Monfardini S, Tirelli U, Vaccher E, et al. Hodgkin's disease in 63 intravenous drug users infected with human immunodeficiency virus. Ann Oncol. 1991;2(Suppl 2):201.
159. Ree H, Strauchen J, Hkan A, et al. Human immunodeficiency virus–associated Hodgkin's disease: Clinicopathologic studies of 24 cases and preponderance of mixed cellularity typed characterized by the occurrence of fibrohistiocytoid stromal cells. Cancer. 1991;67:1614.
160. Rubio R. Hodgkin's disease associated with human immunodeficiency virus infection. A clinical study of 46 cases. Cooperative Study Group of Malignancies Associated with HIV Infection of Madrid. Cancer. 1994;73:2400–2407.
161. Serrano M, Bellas C, Campo E, et al. Hodgkin's disease in patients with antibodies to human immunodeficiency virus. A study of 22 patients. Cancer. 1990;65:2248.

162. Tirelli U, Errante D, Vaccher E, et al. High frequency of Epstein-Barr virus genome detection in Hodgkin's disease of HIV positive patients. Int J Cancer. 1990;46:581.
163. Gold J, Altarac D, Ree H, et al. HIV associated Hodgkin's disease: A clinical study of 18 cases and review of the literature. Am J Hematol. 1991;36:93.
164. Kaplan L, Kahn J, Northfelt D, et al. Novel combination chemotherapy for Hodgkin's disease (HD) in HIV-infected individuals. Abstract 7 Proceedings of the American Society of Clinical Oncology, Houston, May 19–21, 1991.
165. Levine A, Cheung T, Tulpule A, et al. Preliminary results of AIDS Clinical Trials Group (ACTG) study # 149: Phase II trial of ABVD chemotherapy with G-CSF in HIV infected patients with Hodgkin's disease (HD) Abstract S7, National AIDS Malignancy Conference, Bethesda, Md, April 28–30, 1997.

Chapter **113**

Human Immunodeficiency Virus Infection in Women

SUSAN E. COHN
REBECCA A. CLARK

Human immunodeficiency virus (HIV) infection has had a profound impact on the health of women worldwide, and by the end of 1999, 41% of the more than 33 million people living with HIV infection, or 13.8 million, were women.[1] Women constitute the fastest-growing segment of the population with HIV infection in the United States, representing 7% of all cases of acquired immunodeficiency syndrome (AIDS) reported as of 1985; this proportion rose to 20% of all AIDS cases newly diagnosed in 1996.[2] This chapter addresses the epidemiology of HIV infection in women, transmission of HIV to women, pregnancy and risk of perinatal transmission, clinical manifestations of HIV infection in women, and management issues for women with HIV infection.

EPIDEMIOLOGY OF HUMAN IMMUNODEFICIENCY VIRUS INFECTION AND ACQUIRED IMMUNODEFICIENCY SYNDROME IN WOMEN

United States

When AIDS first was recognized in 1981, it was considered a disease of men who have sex with men and of persons who used injection drugs. Now, with the rapid increase in the number of women infected with HIV has come an increased understanding of the potential for heterosexual transmission of HIV infection in the United States. Between 1990 and 1994, the incidence of AIDS reported in women increased by 89%, three times the reported 29% increase in men.[3] In 1996, 14,154 cases of AIDS in women were reported, representing 20% of the 69,151 AIDS cases reported that year and 15% of the 581,429 cumulative cases reported as of the end of 1996.[2] A third of all women diagnosed with AIDS in the United States were diagnosed in 1995 and 1996.[2]

Increasingly, women are acquiring HIV infection through heterosexual contact, with a slowing of injection drug use (IDU)-associated cases since 1992. Since 1995, heterosexual contact has become the predominant mode of exposure for women in the United States.[4] Most cases due to heterosexual transmission were attributed to sex with an injection drug user (38%) or sex with an HIV-infected partner of risk not specified (53%).[4] Bisexually active men may also be contributing to the spread of HIV infection to women, because, at least in a Boston cohort, they were more likely to have unprotected sex with their female partners than with their male partners.[5, 6]

The AIDS epidemic has had a major impact on morbidity and mortality among young adult women. By 1992, AIDS was the fourth leading cause of death among women 25 to 44 years of age in the United States and was the leading cause of death among those in the same age group in 15 primarily East Coast cities.[7] By 1995, HIV infection was the third leading cause of death in women in this age group and the leading cause of death among African American women.[8] Deaths from AIDS peaked in 1994 and 1995 and then began decreasing in 1996.[9] In the first half of 1997, 12,040 Americans died of AIDS, compared with 21,460 in the first half of 1996.[9] Decreased mortality has been attributed to improved combination antiretroviral regimens, including protease inhibitors, rather than to advances in prevention of HIV transmission. These potent antiretroviral medication regimens have also been associated with decreased progression to AIDS, fewer opportunistic infections, fewer hospitalizations, and prolonged survival.[10, 11] Unfortunately, women have not benefited to the same degree as noted for men who acquired HIV infection through male-to-male sexual contact, presumably because women as a group have had less access to medical care and potent antiretroviral agents (see section entitled Human Immunodeficiency Virus Disease Progression).

HIV disproportionately affects women of color, with black and Hispanic women accounting for 78% of reported AIDS cases in 1996.[2] AIDS is predominantly a disease of childbearing women; 87% of affected women were diagnosed between 20 and 50 years of age. Women older than 50 have accounted for only 8% of all reported cases; however, underrecognition may be common, with older women typically presenting for medical attention with advanced disease and unaware of their risk for HIV infection.[2, 12, 13] A study of women older than 50 with AIDS found that they were more likely than younger women to live alone (24% versus 11%), to have not completed high school (63% versus 37%), to be tested for HIV infection while hospitalized (51% versus 32%), and to have never used a condom before diagnosis of HIV infection (86% versus 67%).[14]

The epidemiology of drug use affects the epidemiology of HIV infection among American women. In 1996, after exclusion of the 24% of women whose initial mode of transmission was not reported, two thirds of HIV-infected women reported injection drug use (45%) or heterosexual contact with an injection drug user (18%).[2] Over the past decade, heroin became less popular while cocaine and other drugs became increasingly used. When used intravenously, these newer drugs are typically injected more frequently and are associated with increased needle sharing.[7, 15] The use of smokable free-base ("crack") became widespread because of its low cost and high addictive potential, after its first appearance in New York City in 1985. Although smoking crack cocaine itself does not transmit HIV, the tendency of persons who use crack to engage in unsafe behaviors, including increased sexual activity with multiple partners and exchanging sex for drugs, has resulted in the increased spread of HIV infection and other sexually transmitted diseases including syphilis.[16, 17]

Five incidences of female-to-female sexual transmission of HIV have been documented in the literature.[7] In a review of 164 women with AIDS who reported having sexual contact only with women, 93% injected drugs and 7% had received a blood transfusion; no cases were attributable to female-to-female sexual transmission.[7, 18] In a study of 498 lesbian and bisexual women frequenting public venues in San Francisco and Berkeley, California, 6 (1.2%) were HIV-infected.[19] This population demonstrated high rates of high-risk behaviors (10% reported injecting drugs and 40% reported unprotected sex with men, some of whom were bisexual men and male injection drug users), and no evidence for sexual transmission between women was found. These data suggest that the frequency of female-to-female HIV transmission remains very low.

HIV transmission through intravaginal insemination of donor semen has been reported.[20–22] Because HIV has not been able to be removed effectively from semen, insemination with semen from HIV-infected men is currently not recommended.

Worldwide

New estimates from the World Health Organization (WHO) indicate that HIV infection is far more prevalent worldwide than previously thought.[1] As of December 1998, there were an estimated 33.4 million people living with HIV/AIDS, more than 40% of whom were women.[1] In 1998, there were on average 16,000 new HIV infections a day, 5600 (40%) of which were in adult women and 1600 were in children.[1] Worldwide, HIV infection is spread primarily through heterosexual contact, although IDU and its contribution to exposure to HIV varies geographically. Because female drug users have sexual partners who are themselves at high risk of HIV infection, and because drug use can lead to exchange of sex for drugs or money, there may be underrecognition and underreporting of cases spread through heterosexual contact.

The geographic region with the highest number of HIV-infected women is sub-Saharan Africa, where 7.4% of all women aged 15 to 49 are infected with HIV.[1a] Heterosexual transmission continues to be the predominant mode of HIV transmission in Africa. Concomitant with poor access to information and services for prevention of mother-to-child transmission in sub-Saharan Africa, 530,000 HIV-infected children were born there in 1997, representing about 90% of the new pediatric HIV infections in the world.[1a] By the year 2000, there are projected to be 6 million pregnant HIV-infected women in developing countries, especially in Asia and in sub-Saharan Africa.[23] In Botswana, the proportion of the adult population living with HIV has doubled over the last 5 years, and in 1997, 43% of pregnant women tested in the urban center of Francistown were HIV-infected.[1a] As in the United States, AIDS was initially concentrated in urban areas, but it is now spreading outward to smaller towns and rural areas, primarily along highways and truck routes.[24, 25]

The area with the largest growth in the HIV epidemic will probably be in Asia, where the epidemic is newer than in Africa.[1] Seroprevalence rates vary greatly, often with concurrent epidemics within a country; genetic analyses in China suggest little overlap between HIV epidemics among injection drug users and commercial sex workers.[1] Few countries in Asia have sophisticated systems for adequately monitoring the epidemic, and small differences in rates can alter estimates of numbers of infected persons greatly, given the enormous size of the combined population of China, India, and Southeast Asia.[1] Increasing rates of HIV seropositivity among female sex workers are still being reported in Vietnam, Malaysia, and India.[25] After an initial explosion in seroprevalence rates among female commercial sex workers in Thailand, recent government-sponsored prevention efforts have resulted in dramatically decreasing incidences.[1]

In Latin America and the Caribbean, the HIV epidemic has been concentrated in neglected populations living on the social and economic margins of society.[1] In Brazil, HIV seroprevalence is increasing among women and heterosexuals as the rates among drug users and their partners increase. The male-to-female ratio of AIDS cases has decreased from 16:1 in 1986 to 3:1 in 1996.[1a] Overall, seroprevalence rates ranging from 2% to 8% are reported in pregnant women in Latin America and the Caribbean.[25]

The high mortality rate for HIV/AIDS has had a major impact on families. Since the beginning of the epidemic, an estimated 8 million HIV-negative children and adolescents worldwide have been orphaned to AIDS, having lost their mother or both parents to AIDS.[1a] By the year 2000, these estimates are expected to double, with more than 80,000 youths left motherless in the United States.[26] Clearly, more effective strategies to prevent HIV transmission are needed.

TRANSMISSION OF HUMAN IMMUNODEFICIENCY VIRUS TO WOMEN

Heterosexual Transmission

Efficiency of Heterosexual Transmission of Human Immunodeficiency Virus

Globally, heterosexual transmission accounts for the spread of HIV infection in approximately 90% of persons living with AIDS and is the fastest-growing mode of HIV transmission in the United States.[27] However, mechanisms of heterosexual transmission remain poorly understood.[7] HIV has been isolated both from semen of HIV-infected men and from cervicovaginal secretions of HIV-infected women. Although heterosexual transmission appears more efficient from men to women than from women to men, HIV-infected women can spread HIV to their uninfected sexual partners.[28–30] The most likely explanation for this difference in ease of HIV spread from men to their partners relates to the larger volume of semen compared to cervicovaginal secretions, and to the higher concentration of HIV on average in seminal fluid.

HIV is not transmitted consistently by sexual contact. Whereas some persons become infected after a single sexual exposure or artificial insemination with HIV-infected semen,[21] others remain uninfected despite hundreds of exposures.[31–33] This lack of transmission may be due to the amount of virus, the host immune response, the relative virulence of HIV isolates, or some combination thereof.[34]

The efficiency of heterosexual transmission of HIV between women and men has not been fully characterized. The efficiency of transmission of gonorrhea, a well-studied sexually transmitted disease (STD), is approximately 25% after a single male contact with an infected female and close to 90% for transmission by infected males to uninfected female partners.[35, 36] HIV is much less efficiently transmitted; however, the extremely long incubation period of HIV disease has hindered specific inferences about the relative rates and efficiency of sexual transmission, because many persons do not learn of their infection until years after the relevant exposure. Estimates of infectivity for each sexual contact have ranged from 3 per 100 for the most efficient transmitters in a male homosexual cohort study[37] to less than 1 per 1000 contacts in studies of heterosexual couples discordant for HIV serostatus.[28, 31] In a California study of heterosexual HIV serostatus–discordant couples, the risk of male-to-female transmission was 17 times higher than the risk of female-to-male transmission.[29] An Italian study of 730 discordant heterosexual couples found the transmission of HIV from males to females to be twice as efficient as from females to males.[38]

Factors Associated with Heterosexual Transmission

Factors that have been associated with greater likelihood of transmitting HIV between heterosexual partners include viremia of greater magnitude or more advanced immunodeficiency in the infecting partner, the presence of any STD including both ulcerative and nonulcerative disease, sexual activity during menses, receptive anal sex, unprotected vaginal sex, traumatic sex, increased number of sexual contacts, and the infectivity of the HIV-infected partner.[39, 40] Other less well-documented factors that are thought to increase the risk of heterosexual transmission include lack of circumcision in men, cervical ectopy, certain contraceptive practices, and higher viral load in genital secretions (Table 113–1). The recently identified mutation in the chemokine receptor gene (32-base-pair deletion in *CCR5*) appears to confer resistance to HIV in persons who are homozygous for this trait.[39] Although persons with more advanced disease are more likely to transmit HIV, consistent with their increased viral burden, the data are incomplete. In some men receiving potent antiretroviral therapy, HIV was successfully cleared from the blood to below the level of detection of some laboratories (e.g., <400 copies per ml), but the men still were able to transmit HIV, suggesting a compartmentalization of HIV between semen and plasma.[41] Some investigators have found that treatment-induced changes in HIV viral load are generally associated with a corresponding change in the amounts of seminal and cervicovaginal HIV RNA, supporting the hypothesis that potent antiretroviral therapy may reduce the spread of HIV.[42–46]

STDs, particularly those associated with genital ulcers, increase both the efficiency of HIV transmission and susceptibility to HIV infection.[45] Genital ulcerative diseases, which include syphilis, chancroid, and genital herpes, are thought to enhance the access of HIV to mucosal tissues, lymphatic drainage, and systemic lymphocytes.[46, 47] HIV may also be transmitted through intact mucosal membranes, presumably by infecting dendritic cells within the

TABLE 113-1 Risk Factors Associated with Sexual Transmission of Human Immunodeficiency Virus

- Sexually transmitted infections
  - Ulcerative/nonulcerative diseases
- Genital tract inflammation
- HIV disease
  - Higher viral loads
  - Lower CD4+ levels
  - Acute HIV infection
  - Lack of effective antiretroviral therapy
  - Lack of heterozygosity or homozygosity for the inactivating 32-base-pair deletion in the chemokine receptor gene (*CCR5*)
- Anatomic factors
  - Lack of circumcision
  - Cervical ectopy
  - Leukocytospermia
  - ?Hormonal contraception
- Sexual practices
  - Sexual activity during menses
  - Receptive anal intercourse
  - Bleeding during intercourse (disruption of vaginal mucosa through trauma)
  - Lack of barrier protection
- HIV viral features
  - Syncytium formation
  - Certain viral clades

Abbreviation: HIV, Human immunodeficiency virus.

mucous membranes of the genital tract.[48] Epidemiologic studies suggest that both ulcerative and nonulcerative STDs increase the susceptibility to HIV infection; female sex workers in Zaire had an increased risk of HIV seroconversion if they had nonulcerative STDs,[49] and among HIV serostatus–discordant sex partners, seroconversion was more likely if the previously HIV-negative sex partner had both ulcerative and nonulcerative STDs.[50] Nonulcerative STDs such as gonorrhea, chlamydial infection, and trichomoniasis appear to increase the number of lymphocytes, monocytes, and Langerhans cells in the endocervix in susceptible seronegative women, thus providing more potential targets for HIV infection.[45] Similarly, nonulcerative STDs may increase the number of HIV-infected cells in the genital tracts of HIV-positive transmitters. Cohen and associates found that HIV-infected men with urethritis had seminal plasma of HIV type 1 (HIV-1) RNA 8 times those in seropositive men without urethritis.[51] Treatment of urethritis was associated with significant decreases in HIV-1 concentration in semen, suggesting a decrease in infectivity with successful STD treatment.

Human Immunodeficiency Virus Infection of the Genital Tract

Much research has been dedicated to isolation, identification, and quantification of the amount of HIV present within cervicovaginal secretions. The presence of HIV in the female genital tract is crucial for heterosexual transmission of HIV, as well as for perinatal transmission of HIV during labor and delivery. HIV-1 has been isolated from cervical and cervicovaginal secretions obtained using cervicovaginal lavage (CVL) and vaginal or cervical swabs.

It remains controversial whether plasma HIV viral load correlates with genital tract HIV levels. Some recent studies have suggested that elevated plasma HIV-1 viral levels and lower CD4+ cell counts are strong predictors of genital HIV-1 levels,[43, 52–54] whereas others have failed to document a clear association between the two compartments.[55, 56] A recent study of four HIV-infected women, using amino acid sequence analysis of cell-free HIV RNA in plasma and CVL virus, found CVL virus to be genotypically distinct from plasma HIV.[57] However, other studies have found strong similarities between virus genotypes from blood and cervical swab samples.[58] Cervicovaginal and seminal HIV viral loads are more likely to be high during acute HIV seroconversion and late in the course of HIV infection. Although viral loads in genital secretions tend to be lower following initiation of effective antiretroviral medications, detectable HIV in genital secretions has been reported in both men and women with undetectable plasma HIV levels.[53] Thus, patients with a low plasma virus burden may still potentially transmit HIV to a sexual partner or perinatally to an infant, although the risk is low.

HIV has been detected in menstrual blood, and having intercourse during menses increases the risk of infecting the male partner.[7] Menstruation introduces about 80 ml of blood into the genital tract over a 3- to 5-day period.[59] This menstrual blood is likely to contain HIV-infected cells as well as free virus, reflecting the HIV viral load of peripheral blood. Menstrual blood raises the pH in the vagina to the neutral range, improving the viability of HIV shed in menses and HIV in semen deposited in the vagina during intercourse.[60] Higher levels of HIV in the genital tract may be seen with conditions that raise the vaginal pH, such as blood in the vagina, bacterial vaginosis, menopause, intercourse, and possibly the use of some forms of birth control.[61]

Research is currently under way to develop intravaginal microbial agents capable of reducing the heterosexual and perinatal transmission of HIV-1.[62] Although nonoxynol-9, a commonly used spermicidal agent, has anti-HIV activity in vitro, there have been safety concerns following reports of vaginal ulceration and inflammation during clinical studies.[63, 64] Preliminary results from a placebo-controlled study of 400 women in Cameroon found similar rates of HIV seropositivity among women who inserted nonoxynol-9 or placebo in advance of and during sexual relations.[65] Cleansing the birth canal with chlorhexidine has been studied in Malawi and did not reduce perinatal HIV transmission[66] but did reduce early neonatal and maternal postpartum infectious problems.[67]

One early study showed that cervical shedding of HIV was associated with oral contraceptive pill use, cervical ectopy, and pregnancy.[68] Women with genital infection or cervicovaginal dysplasia have higher levels of proinflammatory cytokines in CVL fluid, which may affect local HIV replication and may influence their risk of acquisition or transmission of HIV.[69] More research is needed to identify risk factors associated with genital shedding of HIV including the role of hormonal contraceptive use and of potent antiretrovirals in decreasing HIV viral loads within the genital tract.

Risk of female-to-male transmission is also likely to be associated with the presence of HIV in cervicovaginal secretions of HIV-infected women.[70] In a study of 1201 female sex workers, cervicovaginal shedding of HIV-1 was more frequent in immunosuppressed women, in women with *Neisseria gonorrhoeae* or *Chlamydia trachomatis* infection, and in women with a cervical or vaginal ulcer.[71] HIV-1 shedding decreased from 42% to 21% in women whose STDs were cured, theoretically decreasing the infectivity of their secretions.[71] As our understanding of the relation between peripheral HIV viral load and HIV viral load within genital secretions broadens, so will our ability to more fully assess the infectivity of genital secretions.

Strategies to Prevent Heterosexual Transmission

Treatment of STDs is likely to decrease both transmission of HIV and susceptibility to HIV infection. In a Tanzanian clinical trial conducted among persons in rural communities, universal STD screening and treatment of symptomatic cases of STD resulted in a 40% reduction in HIV incidence from that in a village in which no STD screening or treatment was available.[72]

The role of hormonal contraception in the risk of HIV transmission remains uncertain.[30] Barrier contraceptives constitute an effective means of preventing HIV transmission. De Vincenzi found no heterosexual transmission among 124 HIV serostatus–discordant couples who used condoms consistently but a seroconversion rate of 4.8 per 100 person-years for the 121 discordant couples who used condoms inconsistently.[50] Thus, the use of barrier contraceptives such as condoms should be promoted both as a means of contraception and as partial protection against HIV and other STDs.

Perinatal Transmission

Our understanding of factors associated with increased perinatal transmission has increased greatly, and advances have led to earlier and more reliable detection of HIV infection in the newborn. Although antiretroviral medications used during pregnancy and delivery have resulted in dramatic decreases in perinatal transmission, much is still poorly understood about mechanisms and pathogenesis of mother-to-child transmission.

Prior to the use of antiretroviral medications, estimates of the frequency of perinatal transmission ranged from a low of 13% in Europe to a high of more than 60% in Africa, with frequencies of 14 to 33% reported in the United States.[73, 74] As the number of women who become HIV-infected during their childbearing years increases, so will the number of children who contract HIV perinatally without effective intervention. Practical, cost-effective strategies to reduce perinatal transmission are urgently needed.

Timing of Transmission

HIV can be transmitted from an HIV-infected woman to her infant during intrauterine gestation, at delivery, or in the postpartum period through breast feeding. HIV-1 has been isolated from fetal blood samples taken prior to elective terminations[75] and from fetal tissues at as early as 8 weeks of gestation.[76–79] In addition, in fetuses lost early in pregnancy, one study found that half had thymic tissue heavily infected with HIV, resulting in lymphoid depletion, epithelial injury, and precocious involution.[80] In half of the infants who eventually are proved to be HIV-infected, HIV-1 can be identified by either culture, polymerase chain reaction (PCR) assay, or p24 antigen detection at or shortly after birth, suggesting that they were infected in utero prior to delivery.[81] HIV-infected infants who test negative for HIV by PCR assay or culture at birth may have been infected late in pregnancy or during the birthing process. The differences in onset and progression of HIV infection in infants may reflect timing of infection, with infants infected earlier in pregnancy typically presenting with more rapid progression to AIDS than is noted in infants infected at birth, who present with asymptomatic HIV infection and have prolonged survival.[82, 83]

Perinatal transmission is thought to occur near or during delivery in the majority of cases.[73, 74, 84, 85] The French Collaborative Study, using virologic and serologic data, applied mathematical modeling to estimate the timing of perinatal transmission in non–breast-feeding women.[74, 86] The investigators estimated that 92% of all instances of transmission occurred during the last 2 months of pregnancy, with 65% (95% confidence interval of 22 to 92%) occurring during the intrapartum period.[86]

Twin studies have been used to further our understanding of the timing of perinatal HIV transmission. Goedert and coworkers studied 22 pairs of HIV seropositivity–discordant twins, and in 18 of the 22 pairs, the presenting twin was the infected sibling.[87] Data from the International Registry of HIV-Exposed Twins suggest that the risk of infection in the twin who is born first is twice that in the second (26% and 13%, respectively).[74, 87, 88] The greater infection rates of firstborn twins may be linked to increased contact with maternal secretions during birth.

Risk Factors for Increased Perinatal Transmission

Perinatal transmission is a multifactorial process, influenced by viral, immune, and clinical factors in both the mother and the infant (Table 113–2). Maternal plasma virus load seems to be the strongest predictor of the risk of transmitting HIV perinatally.[84, 89] Coll and colleagues studied 67 HIV-1–infected mothers during pregnancy and labor and their 69 newborns (including two sets of twins) and found a strong relationship between plasma viral RNA concentrations of greater than 10^5/ml (odds ratio OR 22, 95% confidence interval of 4.4–119.2, $p < .00001$) and $CD4^+$ cell counts of fewer than 400/mm^3, (odds ratio 4.1, 95% confidence interval 1.1–15.4, $p = .01$) and transmission of HIV.[90] Women with more advanced HIV disease and lower $CD4^+$ and higher $CD8^+$ T cell counts are at increased risk of transmitting HIV perinatally.[73, 91–93] In a nested case-control study within a prospectively followed cohort of HIV-infected women, Thea and colleagues found that high maternal viral load increased the likelihood of perinatal transmission in women without AIDS.[94] No threshold has been observed beyond which no transmission occurs; women with undetectable plasma HIV RNA have transmitted HIV perinatally.[89, 95] Maternal seroconversion associated with acute high-titer HIV viremia just prior to pregnancy or during breast feeding also appears to be associated with increased rates of transmission.

TABLE 113–2 Potential Factors Influencing Mother-to-Child Transmission of Human Immunodeficiency Virus

Maternal factors
Advanced HIV disease, as measured by
Clinical staging
Low $CD4^+$ lymphocyte count
Higher viral loads
p24 antigenemia
Primary HIV infection
Viral phenotype: syncytium-inducing
Viral genotype: virulent mutant strain of HIV
Coinfection with other sexually transmitted diseases
Firstborn twins
Obstetric events
Vaginal delivery
Invasive procedures or fetal monitoring during labor
Prolonged premature rupture of membranes (>4 hr)
Older maternal age
Cigarette smoking and illicit drug use during pregnancy
Breast-feeding
Unprotected sexual intercourse with multiple partners
Fetal or placental factors
Chorioamnionitis
Prematurity
Low birth weight
Labor or birth canal factors
Cervicovaginal viral load
Local HIV-specific immune response
Maternal-fetal transfusion of blood
Immune factors
Humoral
Neutralizing antibody
Antibody-dependent cellular cytotoxicity
gp120 V3 loop antibody
MHC concordance
Other
Cell-mediated
Cytotoxic T lymphocytes
CD8 suppression
Mucosal immunity

Abbreviations: HIV, Human immunodeficiency virus; MHC, major histocompatibility complex.
Adapted from Sprecher S, Soumenkoff G, Puissant F, et al. Vertical transmission in a 15 week fetus. Lancet. 1986;2:228, © by The Lancet Ltd, 1986; and Bryson YJ. Perinatal HIV-1 transmission: Recent advances and therapeutic interventions. AIDS. 1996;3:533–542.

Many reports have correlated perinatal transmission to virologic factors including p24 antigenemia,[73, 92] syncytium-inducing (SI) versus non-SI phenotype,[73] and persistently positive HIV-1 cultures.[91] Although production of autologous neutralizing antibody seems to be protective, with low levels associated with increased transmission, recent studies have reported conflicting results.[74] Recently, MacDonald and associates found that maternal-child major histocompatibility complex (MHC) discordance was associated with decreased perinatal transmission of HIV.[96]

Vitamin A deficiency in pregnant HIV-infected women has been associated with increased vaginal HIV-1 shedding[97] and increased perinatal transmission in nonindustrialized countries.[98] In a cohort of HIV-infected women in Malawi, low maternal levels of vitamin A during pregnancy were common; in a multivariate logistic regression analysis, vitamin A deficiency was an independent predictor of perinatal transmission.[98] Vitamin A helps promote epithelial cell regeneration, and low vitamin A levels may be associated with mucosal breaks and increased HIV shedding into genital secretions.[74, 99] Vitamin A deficiency is also associated with impaired immunity and increased susceptibility to infection. Given the possibility of teratogenicity of vitamin A when administered early in gestation,[100] and the finding that few pregnant women in the United States have vitamin A deficiency, vitamin A supplementation beyond that present in prenatal vitamins is not recommended at present. Many of the world's pregnant women may be at risk for vitamin A deficiency, however, and may benefit from supplementation.

Viral biologic phenotypes may influence transmission. Monocyte-macrophage–tropic (M-tropic) or non-SI viral isolates may be more likely to be transmitted than maternal T-cell–tropic or SI isolates.[74] Isolates obtained from infected infants tend to be of non–SI phenotype,[101] and neonatal macrophages are preferentially infected by non-SI M-tropic viral isolates.[74, 102]

HIV-1 can be classified into at least nine different genotypes (clades) based on differences in the envelope region of the viral genome.[74] The distribution of subtypes differs around the world: subtype B predominates in the United States and Europe; subtypes A, C, and D predominate in Africa; and subtypes B and E in Thailand.[74] The role of subtypes in perinatal transmission is as yet undefined, but some epidemiologic studies have suggested that subtype E may be more efficiently transmitted sexually than subtype B, perhaps accounting for at least some of the differences in transmission rates seen between countries.[74, 103]

Sociodemographic and lifestyle factors also appear to influence the risk of perinatal transmission. Maternal drug use, especially after the first trimester, may modify the risk of perinatal HIV-1 transmission.[100, 104] Several studies have suggested that the rate of perinatal transmission is increased with a higher frequency of unprotected vaginal intercourse after the first trimester of pregnancy even after controlling for maternal $CD4^+$ counts, zidovudine use, and higher frequency of STDs diagnosed during pregnancy.[100, 104, 105]

Obstetric factors are also thought to be associated with increased perinatal HIV-1 transmission. These include chorioamnionitis, placenta previa, and invasive interventions such as scalp monitoring, chorionic villus sampling, amniocentesis, cord blood sampling, and placental biopsy.[106, 107]

Elective cesarean section appears to reduce the risk of perinatal transmission of HIV-1. The protective benefit of elective cesarean section was demonstrated in two recent studies: (1) a large meta-analysis of 15 prospective North American and European cohort studies consisting of 8533 mother-child pairs[108] and (2) a prospective randomized clinical trial of elective cesarean section versus vaginal delivery among 370 mother-child pairs.[109] In the meta-analysis, after adjustment for receipt of antiretroviral therapy, maternal stage of disease, and infant birth weight, an elective cesarean section decreased the risk of perinatal transmission of HIV-1 by 50% (adjusted odds ratio, 0.43; 95% confidence interval of 0.33 to 0.56).[108] The transmission rate in the randomized prospective clinical trial within the cesarean section arm was only 1.8% (3 of 170 infants) compared with 10.5% (21 of 200 infants) in the vaginal delivery arm.[109] Although the data clearly demonstrate a protective benefit of elective cesarean section, it is important to note that these studies were performed in populations not receiving highly active antiretroviral therapy (HAART) with protease inhibitors or non-nucleoside reverse transcriptase inhibitors. The degree of protective efficacy that cesarean section offers to patients on HAART or with undetectable plasma viral loads is unknown. For HIV-positive women, cesarean section may be associated with increased risk of infection and other postoperative morbidity, especially in women with advanced HIV disease.[110] The morbidity from cesarean section was low in the prospective randomized trial, but postpartum fever was significantly more frequent in the women who delivered by elective cesarean section versus vaginal delivery (6.7% versus 1.1%, $p = 0.002$).[109] National guidelines regarding cesarean sectioning are pending, but HIV-infected women should be informed about these study results and the decision about mode of delivery should be individualized.

HIV transmission through breast milk is supported by known transmission of other viruses by milk, detection of HIV-1 in the cellular and acellular compartments of breast milk, and reports of transmission from mothers infected with HIV-1 during the postnatal period.[74, 111–114] A study in Rwanda found that 36 to 60% of breast-fed infants born to postnatally infected women became infected with HIV, and that seroconversion in infant and mother occurred during the same 3-month period.[112] These infants were presumably exposed to high viral titers, and no maternal HIV-1–specific humoral or cellular immune response was detected. A meta-analysis of studies published before 1992 suggested an attributable risk of transmission through breast milk by women who were infected prior to pregnancy of 14% and by postnatally infected women of 26%.[112, 115]

In summary, a variety of factors may increase the risk of perinatal transmission of HIV. Some of these factors may be amenable to modification, such as lowering viral load with antiretroviral agents or limiting the amount of time the infant is exposed to the genital secretions of the infected mother by delivery by cesarean section, shortening the labor process, decreasing the exposure to ruptured membranes, or limiting invasive procedures such as scalp monitoring.[107] Promotion of safer sexual practices, including condom use and limiting sexual partners, and abstaining from drug, tobacco, and alcohol use may also reduce the risk of perinatal transmission.

Impact of Pregnancy on Human Immunodeficiency Virus Infection

Although pregnancy and HIV infection are immunosuppressive conditions, large studies in the United States and Europe have failed to show that pregnancy accelerates HIV replication or disease progression.[116–119] Data from developing countries suggest that there may be a progression of HIV disease.[120] Differences in the impact of pregnancy on HIV infection across geographic areas may reflect differences in potential confounding issues such as poverty and nutrition, greater likelihood of advanced HIV disease at the time of pregnancy, and the impact of additional infectious disease.[80] Pregnancy does not appear to result in acceleration of HIV disease in most HIV-infected women; however, women with more advanced disease tend to experience progression of their disease over a shorter period than that typical of women with less advanced disease, suggesting that the pregnancy may enhance progression of HIV disease in such cases.[121]

Conflicting data exist regarding the effects of both HIV infection and pregnancy on T-cell function and phenotype.[121] Cellular immunity and $CD4^+$ lymphocyte levels are expected to decline during pregnancy but eventually return to baseline.[80, 121] In pregnancy complicated by HIV infection, the number of $CD4^+$ cells decreases, reaching their lowest levels in the third trimester. It is unclear whether these declines are due to the HIV infection, to pregnancy, or to hemodilution. Unlike in non–HIV-infected women, the $CD4^+$ cell counts rarely return to pre-pregnancy levels in HIV-infected women unless antiretroviral agents are taken. Determination of whether immunologic changes in HIV-positive women result in progression of HIV disease during pregnancy requires additional prospective, longitudinal studies.

Impact of Human Immunodeficiency Virus Infection on Pregnancy Outcome

Maternal HIV infection has not been associated with fetal anomalies, premature delivery, low birth weight, or specific pregnancy-related abnormalities in studies from industrialized countries.[80, 121] A dysmorphic syndrome associated with HIV infection was first reported in 1986. The clinical features included growth retardation, microcephaly, flattened nasal bridge, prominent forehead, obliquely placed eyes, and patulous lips.[122, 123] Subsequent reports, however, have not found an association between congenital anomalies and HIV serostatus.[124, 125] The original observations are now thought to be due to confounding variables such as drug and alcohol use. Because infection with HIV very early in pregnancy appears uncommon, embryopathy does not appear to be a major problem in pregnancies in women with HIV infection. Reports from various developing areas have noted an increased incidence of preterm deliveries and low-birth-weight infants.[80, 126] HIV infection does not seem to be a cause of spontaneous abortion; however, most published reports suggest a trend in that direction. In a large study from Malawi that tested 6605 consecutive women for HIV, HIV-seropositive women were more likely than HIV-seronegative women to have reported a history of spontaneous abortion (15% versus 7%).[127] Additional studies with adequate numbers of women are needed to elucidate more fully the impact of HIV infection on pregnancy outcome.

Use of Antiretroviral Drugs in Pregnancy to Reduce Perinatal Transmission

Zidovudine

Numerous studies are currently under way, in the United States and globally, to evaluate the use of antiretroviral agents to reduce perinatal transmission. Zidovudine (ZDV) was the first such agent studied, and in February 1994, the landmark study AIDS Clinical Trials Group Protocol 076 (ACTG 076) demonstrated that ZDV given to pregnant women after the first trimester and during labor and to newborns during their first 6 weeks could reduce perinatal transmission by 67.5%.[95, 128] Women with CD4+ cell counts higher than 200/mm³ were randomly assigned to a ZDV treatment group or to a control group in which placebo was given. The women in the treatment group received 100 mg of ZDV five times a day starting between 14 and 34 weeks of gestation and continued throughout pregnancy, followed by intrapartum ZDV (given as an intravenous loading dose of 2 mg/kg over 1 hour during labor and then a continuous intravenous infusion of 1 mg/kg/hour until delivery), with oral administration of ZDV to the infant (syrup 2 mg/kg every 6 hours) for 6 weeks. The rate of perinatal transmission was reduced to 8.3% in the 205 women who received ZDV, from a rate of 25.5% in the 204 women who received no antiretroviral therapy (p = .00006).[128] In August 1994, the U.S. Public Health Service Task Force issued recommendations for the use of ZDV for reduction of perinatal HIV-1 transmission,[129] followed in July 1995 by recommendations for universal prenatal HIV-1 counseling and HIV-1 testing with informed consent for all pregnant women in the United States.[130] Subsequent epidemiologic studies in the United States and France have demonstrated successful use of the ACTG 076 ZDV regimen in the "real" world to achieve dramatic reductions in perinatal transmission rates.[131–133]

The ZDV regimen chosen for ACTG 076 was well tolerated, and there were no significant differences in adverse events between the women receiving ZDV and those receiving placebo. The only evidence of toxicity observed more frequently in the treatment group was a lower hemoglobin concentration in neonates, which was not clinically significant; hemoglobin levels returned to those measured in infants born to mothers in the placebo group by week 12 postpartum. Prolonged exposure of adult rodents to high doses of ZDV has been associated with the development of noninvasive squamous epithelial vaginal tumors in 3 to 12% of females.[84] In humans, ZDV is extensively metabolized, and most of the drug excreted in urine is in the glucuronide form. In mice, however, ZDV excreted in the urine is mostly unmetabolized. The vaginal tumors are thought to form as a result of chronic exposure of the vaginal epithelium of rodents to unmetabolized ZDV, resulting from reflux of urine containing high concentrations of ZDV into the vaginal vault. This hypothesis was tested by administering 5 mg or 20 mg of ZDV per ml of saline into the vaginas of female mice; vaginal squamous cell carcinomas were documented at the higher concentration.[84] A National Institutes of Health (NIH) panel reviewed the data on ZDV toxicity in 1997 and concluded that the proven benefit of ZDV in reducing the risk for perinatal transmission outweighs the hypothetical concerns of carcinogenesis raised in the rodent studies.[134] No ZDV-associated tumors have been reported to date in studies of nearly 1000 children exposed to ZDV over an average follow-up period of 3 years.[134] Because the long-term effects of antiretroviral medication are unknown, all exposed children, regardless of HIV serostatus, should receive careful long-term follow-up evaluation.[135]

The mechanism by which ZDV reduces perinatal transmission remains undefined. The effect of ZDV on maternal HIV viral load is insufficient to explain fully its efficacy, especially when it is given to pregnant women with extensive prior ZDV experience.[95, 136] Preexposure prophylaxis of the fetus or infant may be important, and ZDV may be unique because, unlike didanosine (ddI) or zalcitabine (ddC), it is metabolized to the active triphosphate form within the placenta. The efficacy of ZDV chemoprophylaxis was evaluated in pregnant women with more advanced HIV disease than that affecting the women in ACTG 076 (i.e., ACTG 185), 23% of whom had received ZDV previously. All women received the same three-part ZDV regimen as outlined previously, combined with either infusions of hyperimmune HIV-1 immunoglobulin containing high levels of HIV-1 antibodies or standard intravenous immune globulin (IVIG). The study was stopped prematurely when women in both the treatment and the placebo groups were found to have similar low rates of perinatal transmission of 4.8%.[84]

The use of ZDV in accordance with the ACTG 076 regimen by HIV-infected pregnant women in the United States and Europe has resulted in marked declines in perinatal transmission rates, typically to as low as 3 to 4%. Unfortunately, because of the complexity of the regimen and the cost of the drug, ZDV has not been used in most developing countries where the majority of perinatal HIV-1 infection is occurring. Preliminary results from a study in Thailand indicate that a short-term antenatal regimen of ZDV can reduce the risk for perinatal HIV transmission by approximately 50%.[137] HIV-infected women were randomly assigned to receive either 300 mg of ZDV twice a day from 36 weeks of gestation until onset of labor, plus 300 mg every 3 hours from onset of labor until delivery, or a placebo. All women were given a supply of infant formula and counseled against breast-feeding, consistent with national guidelines for HIV-infected women in Thailand. Of 391 children born, 52 tested HIV-positive on PCR assay (17 in the ZDV group and 35 in the placebo group), all by the second-month visit. The estimated HIV transmission risk for the ZDV and placebo groups was 9.2% (95% confidence interval of 5.0 to 13.5%) and 18.6% (95% confidence interval of 13.0 to 24.0%), respectively, representing a 51% decrease in transmission risk.[137] Data from New York State indicated that the rate of perinatal HIV transmission among 939 HIV-exposed infants varied depending on when zidovudine prophylaxis was begun. When treatment was begun prenatally, the rate of HIV transmission was 6.1% (95% confidence interval, 4.1 to 8.9%); when begun intrapartum, the rate was 10.0% (95% confidence interval, 3.3 to 21.8%); when begun within 48 hours of life, the rate was 9.3% (95% confidence interval, 4.1 to 17.5%); and when begun on Day 3 of life or later, the rate was 18.4% (95% confidence interval, 7.7 to 34.3%).[138] Without zidovudine prophylaxis, the rate of HIV transmission was 26.6% (95% confidence interval, 21.1 to 32.7%).[138] Because it is not known precisely when ZDV confers efficacy, and because of theoretical benefits of ZDV administration during any of the three time periods, administration of partial ZDV regimens is preferred over no administration.

Concerns have been raised that ZDV use during pregnancy and delivery may be ineffective if the mothers have developed ZDV resistance. Although none of the women participating in ACTG 076 had high-level genotypic resistance to ZDV, low-level resistance was not associated with an increase in perinatal transmission, after adjusting for HIV RNA levels.[139] Frenkel and colleagues studied the HIV-1 viral isolates from 16 pregnant women who received ZDV and found 2 of 16 to be highly resistant to ZDV, with mutations at codons 41 and 215.[140] Two additional isolates had mutations at codon 70 (one susceptible and one moderately resistant to ZDV). One of the women with a highly resistant strain transmitted HIV to her infant, and the infant's isolate was also highly resistant to ZDV.[140]

Recent development of alternative antiretroviral strategies may somewhat mitigate these concerns.

Zidovudine monotherapy in pregnant women has been the standard of care since the release of results from ACTG 076 in 1994, and to date, no other antiretroviral medications have been demonstrated to safely reduce perinatal transmission. However, combination antiretroviral regimens are far superior to ZDV monotherapy in reducing HIV viral load and in prolonging survival.[10, 11] In mid-1997, two different panels convened by the U.S. Department of Health and Human Services, the NIH, and the International AIDS Society issued draft principles and guidelines on the use of antiretroviral agents in HIV-infected adults.[141, 142] Although there are no controlled clinical trials demonstrating safety or efficacy of most antiretrovirals during pregnancy, both panels recommended that antiretroviral therapy in pregnant women should generally be the same as for nonpregnant adults, unless clear fetal or maternal contraindications exist. In January 1998, the Centers for Disease Control and Prevention (CDC) revised its recommendations for the use of antiretroviral drugs in pregnant women infected with HIV-1.[84] This agency concluded that pregnancy is not a reason to defer standard therapy but outlined unique considerations for combination therapy use including the potential need to alter dosing as a result of physiologic changes associated with pregnancy, the potential for adverse short- or long-term effects on the fetus and newborn, and efficacy in reducing the risk of perinatal transmission. Therefore, women who are offered antitroviral medication during pregnancy should be informed about the known and unknown short- and long-term benefits and risks of such therapy for infected women and their infants. The current pharmacokinetic and safety data for the different antiretroviral agents are listed in Table 113–3. Further research is needed before combination antiretroviral therapy is determined to have enhanced ability to reduce perinatal transmission to rates below those achieved with ZDV monotherapy.

Nucleoside Reverse Transcriptase Inhibitors

Of the five currently approved nucleoside reverse transcriptase inhibitors (NRTIs), only ZDV, lamivudine (3TC), and ddI have been evaluated in clinical trials in pregnant women, to elucidate their pharmacokinetics.[84, 143] ZDV is well tolerated and does not require dose modification for use in pregnant women. The pharmacokinetics of 3TC do not appear to be altered by pregnancy, and no dose modification is indicated except in the young child, in whom the dose is decreased because of the reduced clearance of 3TC in infants 1 week of age. Although a study of 12 pregnant women found the clearance of IV and oral ddI given ante partum was greater than that observed at 6 weeks post partum, no dose modifications have yet been made.[143] All of these nucleoside analogue antiretroviral drugs are classified by the U.S. Food and Drug Administration (FDA) as FDA Pregnancy Category C agents, except for ddI, which is classified as a Category B drug.[84] Although all of the nucleoside analogues cross the placenta in primates, ddI and ddC undergo less placental transfer than is noted for ZDV, d4T, and 3TC.[84]

Non-nucleoside Reverse Transcriptase Inhibitors

The safety and pharmacokinetics of nevaripine, a non-nucleoside reverse transcriptase inhibitor (NNRTI), were studied in seven HIV-1 infected pregnant women, who received a single 200-mg oral dose at the onset of labor, and whose newborns received a single dose of 2 mg/kg of body weight at 2 to 3 days of age.[84] The drug was well tolerated by both mothers and infants with prolonged half-life and elimination in both populations. This single dose of nevaripine was sufficient to maintain levels associated with antiviral activity for the first week of life.[84] A phase III perinatal transmission prevention clinical trial using a similar dosing schedule for nevaripine is currently under way.

Delavirdine and efavirenz have not been studied in phase I pharmacokinetic and safety trials in pregnant women. Of seven women who inadvertently became pregnant while on clinical trials of antiviral regimens containing delavirdine, three had ectopic pregnancies, three had three healthy infants, and 1 woman delivered a premature infant with a muscular ventricular septal defect.[84] Delavirdine is known to be teratogenic in rodents when administered in high doses. Studies using efavirenz in pregnant monkeys at doses similar to those being studied in humans showed newborn abnormalities at birth. Three of 13 monkeys were born with birth defects including one with a cleft palate, one with microphthalmia, and another with anencephaly and anophthalmia.[144]

Long-term and transplacental animal carcinogenicity studies are not available for these three non-nucleosides. Until additional data are available, efavirenz and delavirdine should be given to pregnant women only if the benefits outweigh the potential risks. These two FDA-approved NNRTIs are classified as FDA Pregnancy Category C agents.

Protease Inhibitors

No data are available regarding drug dosage, safety, and tolerance of any of the protease inhibitors in pregnant women or in neonates, although phase I studies of several of these agents—indinavir, ritonavir, nelfinavir, and saquinavir in combination with ZDV and 3TC—in HIV-1–infected pregnant women and their infants are currently under way in the United States. Some preliminary data are available on placental passage in animals (see Table 113–3), but long-term animal carcinogenicity studies are not yet completed. Indinavir is associated with infrequent side effects (i.e., hyperbilirubinemia and renal stones) that could be problematic for the newborn if transplacental passage occurs and the drug is administered near the time of delivery.[84] Neonates may have immature hepatic metabolic enzymes, which may result in prolonged drug half-life and possibly exacerbation of the physiologic hyperbilirubinemia observed in newborns. In addition, neonates may be at higher risk of renal stone formation secondary to crystallization of indinavir because of their immature renal function and inability to voluntarily ensure adequate hydration.[84] Ritonavir, nelfinavir, and saquinavir are classified as FDA Pregnancy Category B agents, and indinavir is classified as a Category C drug.

All four of the currently approved protease inhibitors have been associated with onset of diabetes, hyperglycemia, diabetic ketoacidosis, and exacerbation of existing diabetes mellitus.[145–147] Because pregnancy is a risk factor for hyperglycemia, and because it is unknown whether protease inhibitors will exacerbate the risk for pregnancy-associated hyperglycemia, HIV-1–infected pregnant women receiving these agents should be aware of the risk of hyperglycemia and taught to recognize the early manifestations of hyperglycemia to ensure prompt medical care if such signs and symptoms develop.

Management of Pregnant Human Immunodeficiency Virus–Infected Women

An HIV-infected pregnant woman should be managed closely by her obstetrician and the HIV specialist caring for her when she is not pregnant. A thorough history should be taken and physical examination conducted to document baseline findings and to allow for early detection of abnormalities. The history should identify any factors known to be associated with enhanced perinatal transmission including a history of STDs, drug and alcohol use, tobacco use, and high-risk sexual activity including lack of condom use, because altering these practices may reduce perinatal transmission risk nonpharmacologically. A complete physical examination including a pelvic examination can reveal concurrent conditions that may warrant therapy. The woman's HIV-1 disease status should be evaluated at presentation and at least every trimester with lymphocyte marker studies (i.e., $CD4^+/CD8^+$ subsets) and viral load assessment. Ongoing routine obstetric care and decisions about initiating, continuing, or adjusting antiretroviral therapy should be the same as for non–HIV-infected women. Pregnant women should be given an antiretroviral

TABLE 113-3 Preclinical and Clinical Data Relevant to Use of Antiretrovirals in Pregnancy

Antiretroviral Drug	FDA Category*	Placental Passage (newborn : maternal drug ratio)	Long-term Animal Carcinogenicity Studies	Rodent Teratogenicity
Nucleoside Analogue RTIs				
Zidovudine (ZDV, AZT)	C	Yes, in humans [0.85]	Positive (rodent, noninvasive vaginal epithelial/gynecologic tumors)	Positive (near lethal dose)
Zalcitabine (ddC)	C	Yes, in rhesus monkeys [0.30–0.50]	Positive (rodent, thymic lymphomas)	Positive (hydrocephalus at high dose)
Didanosine (ddI)	B	Yes, in humans [0.5]	Negative (no tumors, lifetime rodent study)	Negative
Stavudine (d4T)	C	Yes, in rhesus monkeys [0.76]	Not completed	Negative (decreased sternal bone calcium)
Lamivudine (3TC)	C	Yes, in humans [~1.0]	Negative (no tumors, lifetime rodent study)	Negative
Abacavir	C	Yes, in rats	Not completed	Positive (fetal anasarca at high dose)
Non-nucleoside Analogue RTIs				
Nevirapine	C	Yes, in humans [~1.0]	Not completed	Negative (impaired fertility)
Delavirdine	C	Yes, in rats [late-term fetus, blood 0.15; late-term fetus, liver 0.04]	Not completed	Positive (ventral septal defect)
Efavirenz (DMP-266)	C	Yes, in cynomolgus monkeys [~1.0]	Not completed (but structural abnormalities in 3/20 monkeys including one with anencephaly)	Not completed
Protease Inhibitors				
Saquinavir	B	Unknown	Not completed	Negative
Indinavir	C	Yes, in rats ["significant" in rats, low in rabbits]	Not completed	Negative (extra ribs in rats)
Ritonavir	B	Yes, in rats [mid-term fetus, 1.15; late-term fetus, 0.15–0.64]	Not completed	Negative (cryptorchidism in rats)
Nelfinavir	B	Unknown	Not completed	Negative

*FDA Pregnancy categories are as follows:
A—Adequate and well-controlled studies of pregnant women fail to demonstrate a risk to the fetus during the first trimester of pregnancy (and there is no evidence of risk during later trimesters).
B—Animal reproduction studies fail to demonstrate a risk to the fetus and adequate but well-controlled studies of pregnant women have not been conducted.
C—Safety in human pregnancy has not been determined, animal studies either are positive for fetal risk or have not been conducted, and the drug should not be used unless the potential benefit outweighs the potential risk to the fetus.
D—Positive evidence of human fetal risk exists based on adverse reaction data from investigational or marketing experiences, but the potential benefits from the use of drug in pregnant women may be acceptable despite its potential risks.
X—Studies in animals or reports of adverse reactions have indicated that the risk associated with the use of the drug for pregnant women clearly outweighs any possible benefit.
Abbreviation: RTIs, Reverse transcriptase inhibitors.
Adapted from Centers for Disease Control and Prevention. Public Health Service Task Force recommendations for the use of antiretroviral drugs in pregnant women infected with HIV-1 for maternal health and for reducing perinatal HIV-1 transmission in the United States. MMWR Morb Mortal Wkly Rep. 1998;47(N0.RR-2):5.

regimen that suppresses HIV replication to below detectable levels. Viral load testing should also be repeated approximately 4 weeks after changing antiretroviral medications to provide feedback on the effectiveness of the antiretroviral regimen. The U.S. Public Health Service recommends that infected women in the United States refrain from breast-feeding to avoid postnatal transmission of HIV-1 to their infants through breast milk.[130]

Decisions about antiretroviral medication in pregnancy should be decided by the woman after discussion with her health care provider about the known and unknown benefits and risks of therapy. Because the risk of teratogenicity is greatest during the first trimester, many health care providers advocate waiting until the end of the first trimester before starting new medications. The clinical, immunologic, and virologic status of the mother must be weighed against the potential effect on the fetus. The HIV-infected woman who is already receiving antiretroviral therapy and who discovers she is pregnant may choose either to continue her therapy or temporarily discontinue it until 14 weeks' gestation.[84] If therapy is discontinued, all drugs should be stopped and reintroduced simultaneously to avoid the development of antiretroviral drug resistance. However, discontinuing antiretroviral medications may result in a rebound of viral load, which may have an impact on HIV transmission and the subsequent ability to obtain virologic control.

Because zidovudine is the only antiretroviral agent that has been shown to reduce perinatal transmission, independent of its effect on reducing maternal viral load, the addition of ZDV or substitution of ZDV for another nucleoside analogue antiretroviral is recommended after 14 weeks' gestation.[84] The standard ZDV dosing regimen for adults is 200 mg three times a day or 300 mg twice daily, but because the mechanism by which ZDV reduces perinatal transmission is unknown, the regimen of ZDV taken two or three times daily may not be equivalent to that observed in ACTG 076. However, maternal adherence is expected to be enhanced with this simpler regimen. ZDV administration is recommended for the pregnant woman during labor and for the newborn regardless of the antepartum antiretroviral regimen.[84] Likewise, the 6-week neonatal ZDV component of the ZDV chemoprophylactic regimen should be initiated as soon as possible after delivery, preferably within 12 to 24 hours of birth, even if ZDV was not given during pregnancy or labor. Discussion of treatment options and recommendations should not be coercive, however, and the decision regarding whether to take antiretroviral drugs ultimately resides with the pregnant woman.

Practitioners who provide health care for HIV-1 infected pregnant women and their newborns should report all cases of prenatal exposure to any antiretroviral medication (either alone or in combination) to the Antiretroviral Pregnancy Registry (Post Office Box 13398, Research Triangle Park, NC 22709-3398; telephone 1-919-483-9437 or 1-800-722-9292, ext. 38465; fax 1-919-315-8981).[84]

Treatment and prophylaxis of opportunistic infections during pregnancy should follow guidelines similar to those for nonpregnant women.[148] Pregnant women who develop active opportunistic infections including tuberculosis should receive a drug regimen developed by obstetric and infectious diseases specialists. As with antiretroviral medications, the potential benefits of prophylactic agents must be weighed against their potential risks. Pneumococcal, hepatitis B, and influenza vaccines may be given if indicated during pregnancy. Live vaccines such as rubella, measles, mumps, and varicella are contraindicated during pregnancy and labor and in the early postpartum period.

In summary, guidelines for the prevention of perinatal HIV transmission now include use of optimal combination therapy, as clinically indicated, with inclusion of ZDV in the regimen when possible.[149] Although minimal data are available concerning the pharmacokinetics and safety of antiretrovirals other than ZDV during pregnancy, the overall health of the woman is considered to be of primary importance.[84]

CLINICAL MANIFESTATIONS AND NATURAL HISTORY OF HUMAN IMMUNODEFICIENCY VIRUS INFECTION IN WOMEN

At the beginning of the AIDS epidemic, initial data on the natural history of HIV infection were derived from predominantly male cohorts. The more recently obtained data on the clinical manifestations of HIV infection in women suggest there is little gender difference in nongynecologic opportunistic processes and HIV disease progression. However, it is clear that women can present with gynecologic disease that is influenced by their HIV-induced immune suppression.

Initial Manifestations and Human Immunodeficiency Virus Infection–Related Symptomatology

Historically, it became apparent that recurrent *Candida* vulvovaginitis (defined as the occurrence of at least four discrete episodes over 1 year) was a frequent presenting HIV-related symptom in a study of 117 women from Rhode Island. In this study, recurrent *Candida* vulvovaginitis occurred in 38% of the women and was the most common initial complaint.[150] Other presenting HIV-related signs and symptoms that have been described in women are similar to those that have been noted in men.[150–152] Additional frequent presenting complaints among the Rhode Island cohort included lymphadenopathy (in 15%), constitutional signs and symptoms (unexplained fatigue associated with weight loss or diarrhea or both) (in 7%), and oral candidiasis (in 5%).[150] Clinical manifestations common among immunosuppressed women with a CD4$^+$ cell count of 200/mm^3 in a second study of 224 women from New Orleans[151] were oral candidiasis (reported in 55%), herpes zoster (in 14%), weight loss of 10% (in 34%), and anemia (or hemoglobin less than 11.0 g/dl) (in 48%).

A comparison of the frequencies of HIV-related symptoms in men and women was performed in a third cohort consisting of 2393 men and 582 women evaluated through outpatient clinics in New York City.[152] Although women were more likely to be diagnosed with oral candidiasis (risk ratio of 1.6, 95% confidence interval of 1.2–2.0), none of the other reported symptoms—herpes zoster, oral hairy leukoplakia, lymphadenopathy, weight loss, diarrhea, fever, neuropathy, and seborrheic dermatitis—differed significantly in men and women.

Serious bacterial infections are most apt to occur among HIV-infected women who are moderately immunocompromised[151] and often constitute the initial diagnosis signaling HIV infection and declining immunity. In the Rhode Island study, bacterial pneumonia was the third most common initial clinical manifestation and occurred in 13% of the patients.[150] In the New Orleans study, 9% of the women had at least one serious bacterial infection, and 2% had recurrent infections.[151] In both of these studies, the etiologic agent was often not identified, but *Streptococcus pneumoniae* and *Haemophilus influenzae* were implicated in the majority of the patients for whom culture results were known. Available data conflict regarding whether or not HIV-infected women are actually at higher risk than men for serious bacterial infections,[152, 153] but it is probable that both a history of IDU and the degree of immune compromise are important risk factors.[153]

AIDS-Defining Opportunistic Processes

Overview

In 1993, the most frequent 1987 CDC-reported AIDS-defining opportunistic processes[154] among both men and women were *Pneumocystis carinii* pneumonia (PCP), *Candida* esophagitis, and wasting syndrome. *Candida* esophagitis accounted for a larger proportion of the AIDS-defining events in women (19.6%) than in either heterosexual men (14.6%) or homosexual or bisexual men (12.3%).[155] The increased propensity for *Candida* esophagitis is reflected by findings from the Rhode Island study in which this was the most common diagnosis.[150] Using the 1993 CDC data, multivariate analyses adjusted for race, age, and geographic region showed that female injection drug users were more likely than heterosexual male injection drug users to have had *Candida* esophagitis, cytomegalovirus (CMV) disease, or herpes simplex virus (HSV) disease and less apt to have been diagnosed with either Kaposi's sarcoma (KS) or extrapulmonary tuberculosis.[155]

Kaposi's Sarcoma

Although KS is an infrequent complication, there is evidence that this malignancy may have a different presentation in women than in men. In a review of 15 women with KS, the median CD4$^+$ cell count was only 13/mm^3, and the median crude survival time was only 8.9 months, compared with 23.3 months for men.[156] Women with KS may have a more highly aggressive disease course, or their prognosis may be worse owing in part to delay in diagnosis and treatment. Women with KS have also been noted to have an increased incidence of noncutaneous disease, lymphedema, lymph node disease, and visceral disease.[157] Women may have gynecologic involvement. There is at least one case report of KS presenting as a vulvar mass[158] and two cases of KS diagnosed by cervical biopsy.[159]

Wasting Syndrome

Although HIV-related weight loss does not have a unique presentation in women compared with that in men, the management has differed by gender. Decreased testosterone levels among patients with HIV-related wasting have been demonstrated in both men[160] and women.[161] Although anabolic agents are used increasingly in the management of HIV-related weight loss in men because they cause increases in body cell mass,[162] there is little information on the use of these therapies in women. Currently, studies to evaluate the safety and efficacy of selected anabolic agents that are less virilizing, such as nandrolone and oxandrolone, for treatment of HIV-related weight loss in women are under way.

Breast Cancer

There is little information on breast cancer, a malignancy relatively common among non–HIV-infected women. Even though the incidence of breast cancer has not been noted to be increased among HIV-infected women, data from the Women's Interagency HIV Study (WIHS) for seven women showed unusual pathologic types of breast cancer and a relatively low median age (47 years).[163] At this time, there are no unique recommendations for mammogram screening of HIV-infected women, and guidelines should follow those published for noninfected women.

Gynecologic Manifestations and Sexually Transmitted Diseases

Cervical Disease

The "transformation zone" of the cervix, characterized by transition of the normal cellular lining from a multilayered squamous epithelium to single-layered columnar epithelium, is the most vulnerable to infection by the potentially oncogenic human papillomavirus (HPV) and is therefore the location in which cervical cancer is anticipated to occur. HIV-infected women are two to three times more likely than noninfected women to have detectable levels of HPV DNA in cervicovaginal specimens[63, 164–168] and approximately five times more likely to have squamous intraepithelial lesions (SILs), vulvovaginal condylomata acuminata, or anal intraepithelial neoplasia.[63, 166–171] Not surprisingly, the prevalence of SIL among HIV-infected women is high, with reported rates of approximately 12 to 40%.[150, 151, 172] Adolescent women are particularly susceptible, with prevalence rates for SIL of up to 55%.[173]

Among HIV-infected women, it is clear that HPV disease, as manifested by SIL or cervical intraepithelial neoplasia (CIN) on cervical examination, is influenced by HIV-induced immunosuppression. Both SIL and clinically evident HPV infections have been associated with a declining CD4+ cell count.[151, 174] In addition, women with high plasma HIV RNA levels are at increased risk for both cervical HPV infection with high-risk HPV types and cervical cytologic abnormalities.[175–176] Although the majority of HIV-infected women with SIL present with low-grade lesions,[164, 165, 169] SIL has been reported to be more severe and extensive in HIV-infected women than in noninfected women and can present as multifocal extensive cervical and lower genital tract lesions.[177] The increased incidence of HPV-related disease among HIV-infected women may potentially be due to the demonstrated high rate of persistent HPV infections, particularly among patients with marked immune suppression, with the oncogenic HPV types associated with high-grade lesions and cervical cancer.[178]

Although the risk of cervical disease progression among HIV-infected women with either low-grade SIL or grade 1 CIN is relatively low, or about 14% to 20% annually,[179–181] the risk of recurrent disease after treatment among women with CIN 2 or CIN 3 approaches 40% to 60% annually and is correlated with a low CD4+ cell count.[182, 183] A clinical trial evaluating the efficacy of topical intravaginal 5-fluorouracil treatment for prevention of recurrence following ablative therapy for CIN 2 or CIN 3 in 101 HIV-infected women was completed recently.[183a] Topical 5-fluorouracil treatment was significantly protective, reducing the recurrence rate from 47% on the observation arm to 28% on the 5-fluorouracil arm.[183a].

Cervical carcinoma became an AIDS-defining diagnosis in 1993. Fortunately, the incidence remains low among HIV-infected women even though the prevalence of SIL and CIN is high. However, it is an important AIDS-defining illness and may be the most common AIDS-related malignancy among HIV-infected women in areas with a high prevalence of HPV infection.[184] Compared with noninfected women, HIV-infected women with cervical cancer were more likely to present with advanced clinical disease; to have persistent or recurrent disease at follow-up, a short time to recurrence, and a short survival after diagnosis; and to die of cervical cancer.[185] The median CD4+ cell count is higher (153/mm³ versus 50/mm³) among women with invasive cervical cancer than among women diagnosed with other opportunistic illnesses,[186] but women with low CD4+ cell counts have a particularly poor prognosis.[187]

Because of the increased risk for cervical disease, in 1993 the CDC recommended that HIV-infected women have a Papanicolaou (Pap) smear performed when they are found to be HIV-infected, and if the findings are normal, the smear should be repeated in 6 months. Women who have never had abnormal findings on Pap smear and have had normal findings on at least two smears can undergo Pap screening every 12 months. If inflammation or atypia is present, the Pap smear should be repeated in 3 months. Routine baseline colposcopy screening is not recommended, but women with SIL, HPV disease, and persistent atypia should be referred for colposcopy.[188] Among HIV-infected women, mild cytologic atypia is often associated with CIN.[189]

Pelvic Inflammatory Disease

Several studies performed in the United States or Africa have examined the presentation and course of pelvic inflammatory disease (PID) in HIV-infected and noninfected women. Three of the studies[190–192] found that HIV-infected women had a lower admission white blood cell count on admission to the hospital, and two studies[190, 191] noted that HIV-infected women were more likely to require surgical intervention. Hoegsberg and associates[190] found tubo-ovarian abscesses in 27% (4/15) of HIV-infected women, compared with 14% (13/95) of noninfected women. HIV-infected women were also more likely to have persistent fever refractory to antibiotics in this study. Although Korn and colleagues[191] also reported more frequent surgical intervention, HIV infection did not appear to be associated with the presence of tubo-ovarian abscesses. The third study performed in the United States noted that HIV-infected women were more likely to remain febrile 48 hours after initiation of antimicrobial therapy. However, by the fifth or sixth day of therapy, there was no statistically significant difference in febrile status between HIV-infected and noninfected women.[44] A fourth study performed in Abidjan, Ivory Coast,[193] found that HIV-infected women presented with a significantly higher mean clinical severity score and were more apt to have a temperature of 38°C or higher. The microbiology findings in PID in these studies are similar, although the frequency of *N. gonorrhoeae* and *C. trachomatis* is low compared with that usually reported.[194] Taken together, these studies suggest that HIV infection may influence the morbidity of PID but that HIV-infected women should respond to conventional recommended antibiotic regimens.

Candida *Vulvovaginitis*

Although one study has demonstrated that recurrent vulvovaginitis occurs early in the disease process (median CD4+ cell count of 506/mm³),[195] this finding has not been substantiated in other studies. Some investigators have found that the frequency of *Candida* vulvovaginitis noticeably increases only when the CD4+ cell count falls below 100/mm³.[196] Limited data on the molecular epidemiology of mucosal candidiasis in HIV-infected women reveal that the dominant strains of *Candida* colonizing the oropharynx and the vagina are different, suggesting that the development of disease in these body sites may proceed by differing mechanisms.[197] Although there is concern over the emergence of resistance with chronic triazole use, fluconazole at a dose of 200 mg weekly for the prevention of mucosal candidiasis among HIV-infected women has been shown to be safe and efficacious and does not precipitate clinical resistance.[198]

Idiopathic Genital Ulcers

A rare manifestation described in women with advanced HIV disease is idiopathic vulvar or vaginal ulcers, which can be intractable, progress to fistula formation, and cause severe bleeding.[151, 199–202] In a national retrospective review of 29 women with idiopathic genital ulcers (defined by either negative results on HSV and syphilis testing or nondiagnostic findings on ulcer biopsy), the median CD4+ cell count was only 50/mm³, and 68% of the patients had a prior AIDS-defining event.[201] Thirty-seven percent had coexistent oral ulcers, and in 19%, the genital ulcer progressed to fistula formation. Although the data were limited, there was often a good response to either corticosteroid treatment (topical, intralesional, or systemic) or initiation of antiretroviral treatment in antiretroviral-naive women.[201] A case report has also suggested that genital aphthous ulcers may respond to thalidomide.[203]

Sexually Transmitted Infections

In three retrospective cohort studies performed in Rhode Island, New Orleans, and New York,[153, 156, 170] the proportions of HIV-infected women diagnosed with specific STDs were as follows: syphilis, 3 to 22%; *N. gonorrhoeae* cervicitis, 2 to 7%; *C. trachomatis* cervicitis, 12%; HSV genital ulcers, 4 to 18%; and trichomoniasis, 9 to 27%. In a cohort of 91 adolescent HIV-infected girls, 75% were diagnosed with an STD either at presentation or during follow-up evaluation, and *N. gonorrhoeae* infection, an incidental infection in 42% of the patients, was the most common STD.[173] Factors associated with specific STDs among HIV-infected women included a history of IDU (associated with syphilis and trichomoniasis) and a low CD4+ cell count (associated with active herpes simplex virus [HSV] infection).[151] Incident STDs among HIV-infected women have also been associated with progestin-only contraceptive agents (Depo-Provera and Norplant), possibly owing to different behavioral patterns and inconsistent barrier use.[204] These data support routine surveillance screening for STDs, particularly among populations shown to be at very high risk such as adolescent girls.

Hormonal and Menstrual Function

Little information pertaining to hormonal functioning in HIV-infected women is available. One study has evaluated hormonal levels among 16 HIV-infected women with normal menstrual cycles (in whom the stage of disease was unknown) and found the mean serum progesterone, estradiol, and cortisol levels during each phase of the cycle were similar to values in the literature.[205] Although findings in this study suggest that HIV infection does not influence the endocrine system, at least two studies evaluating menstrual function imply that there is an effect on pituitary-gonadal functioning from the virus or subsequent immune dysfunction. In one study of 248 HIV-infected women and 82 noninfected controls, HIV-infected women were more likely to experience intervals longer than 6 weeks without menstrual bleeding or amenorrhea longer than 3 months and were less likely to have typical premenstrual symptoms, suggesting that anovulatory cycles may be more common in this population.[206] A second study of 797 HIV-infected women and 205 noninfected controls found the prevalence of amenorrhea, defined as no menstrual periods for greater than 90 days, was 7% among HIV-infected women and 5% among noninfected controls. On multivariate analysis, HIV infection, heroin use, low albumin level, and live birth in the past year each were independently associated with amenorrhea.[207] Amenorrhea was also more common among women with low CD4+ cell counts (<50/mm³) and was associated with low or normal levels of follicle-stimulating hormone and low levels of estradiol in approximately 80% of HIV-infected women.[207] In contrast to these studies, two additional studies did not find that HIV infection status or CD4+ cell count was associated with menstrual dysfunction.[208, 209]

There has been at least one case report of an HIV-infected woman diagnosed with high-grade, immunoblastic, non-Hodgkin's lymphoma that originated in the endometrium. The patient presented with intractable menometrorrhagia and subsequently underwent a hysterectomy. This unusual presentation demonstrates the need for a thorough evaluation of dysfunctional uterine bleeding among HIV-infected women.[210]

Human Immunodeficiency Virus Disease Progression

Although initial observations of survival of HIV-infected women and men suggested that women possibly had a worse prognosis than that typical for men,[211, 212] more recent data have not revealed gender differences in the rate of HIV disease progression.[213–215] This observation possibly reflects the fact that in the early years of the epidemic, women often had delayed access to health care, possibly because of delayed recognition of their HIV infection or family and child care obligations.[216] Two recent studies have implied that women may progress at lower HIV-1 plasma RNA levels when compared to men,[216a, b] whereas a third study contradicted these results and found no sex differences in the CD4 to HIV-1 viral load level ratio.[216c]

Studies that evaluated selected demographic, epidemiologic, and clinical and laboratory features for determination of HIV disease progression among cohorts of HIV-infected women have shown that predictive markers are similar to those identified in men. These include high HIV RNA levels, low CD4+ cell counts, rapid declines in CD4+ cell counts, a baseline CDC AIDS-defining opportunistic process, a low body mass index, and pathologic conditions attributable to HIV infection such as chronic diarrhea, herpes zoster, and oral candidiasis.[217–219] Several studies have evaluated the effect of pregnancy on disease progression, with conflicting conclusions.[115–119] However, pregnancy does not appear to be an independent risk factor for disease progression if the analysis takes into account the stage of disease.

MANAGEMENT ISSUES

Several studies have shown that HIV-infected women are less likely than men to receive health care services, including medications.[216, 220] This reflects the fact that delivery of health care to HIV-infected women can be a challenge. Barriers specific for this population have been identified in several studies. These barriers include child care responsibilities and the need for several services, such as gynecologic or obstetric care, that may not be offered on site in the HIV primary care clinic, thus necessitating multiple visits to different locations.[220–222] In addition, IDU has been shown to interfere with access to health care and compliance with treatment,[223] and a substantial proportion (41% in 1994) of women reported to the CDC with a diagnosis of AIDS have had a history of IDU.[224]

Strategies shown to improve accrual and retention of HIV-infected women into health care include combining clinics for mothers and their children, integrating gynecologic or colposcopy services on site into primary care clinics, daily availability of health care provider services, and provision of on-site child care and transportation services.[225]

In young HIV-infected women or infected adolescents, several specific management issues should be addressed. The frequency of STDs has been shown to be disturbingly high among adolescent girls. Seventy-five percent of a New Orleans cohort of HIV-infected females 13 to 18 years of age were diagnosed with an STD at clinic entry or during follow-up evaluation.[173] There is also a high prevalence of psychosocial problems including a history of sexual abuse,[226, 227] substance abuse,[226, 227] and psychiatric diagnoses[226] among HIV-infected adolescents. These findings emphasize the importance of discussing both optimal methods for contraception and STD protection and of incorporating psychosocial management into the comprehensive care for this population.

Older HIV-infected women are unique because they are at risk for various medical conditions because of age and should receive the routine recommended health maintenance screening examinations, such as mammography. Underlying medical conditions, including but not limited to hypertension, diabetes, coronary artery disease, angina, chronic obstructive pulmonary disease, asthma, and arthritis, are common.[228] HIV-infected women at least 40 years of age are also more likely than younger HIV-infected women to be diagnosed with psychiatric illnesses such as substance abuse, anxiety, depression, psychosis, and dementia.[13]

The influence of both menopause and hormone replacement therapy (HRT) on HIV disease progression is unknown. However, one small retrospective study has suggested that in women taking HRT, a trend toward improved survival exists.[13] Although data are limited, HRT should be considered in the management of postmenopausal HIV-infected women, in view of its documented benefit in populations of women not infected with HIV.[229]

Physician experience has been linked to improved outcomes for persons with HIV infection.[230] A recent study found that women with AIDS receiving care in high-experience clinics in New York State survived longer after AIDS diagnosis than those in low-experience clinics.[231] Ideally, HIV-infected women should be cared for by providers with experience in managing patients with HIV infection.

Offering enrollment into clinical trials is an advantageous management option for HIV-infected women. At least one study has shown that women who participate in antiretroviral therapy clinical trials have significantly longer survival.[172] Historically, a relatively low proportion of HIV-infected women has been enrolled into clinical trials. Although efforts to increase women's enrollment became a priority in the early 1990s within the AIDS Clinical Trials Group (ACTG), the percentage of female enrollment increased only from 6.5% to 7.8% between 1990 and 1992.[232] It has therefore been difficult to study the influence of gender on either the toxicity or efficacy of antiretroviral therapies.

One clinical trial statistically powered to evaluate gender differences was the ACTG protocol 175, which compared monotherapy and combination nucleoside analogue therapies in 438 women and 2029 men.[233] Women were significantly more likely than men to discontinue therapy if they were antiretroviral agent–naive or had been randomized to a ddI-containing regimen. Although gender was not associated with either survival or overall response to therapy, among the subgroup of antiretroviral-naive patients randomized to ZVD monotherapy, men were four times more likely ($p < .05$) to experience a 50% decline in CD4$^+$ cells during follow-up evaluation in analyses adjusted for weight, race, and IDU history.[233] These results demonstrate the need to increase enrollment of women into clinical trials, and the influence of gender on efficacy and toxicity should be the subject of selected antiretroviral studies.

REFERENCES

1. UNAIDS/WHO. AIDS Epidemic update: December, 1998. London. http://www.UNAIDS.org/highband/document/epidemio/index.html.
1a. UNAIDS/WHO. Report on Global HIV/AIDS Epidemic. 1997. Geneva, Switzerland. http://www.UNAIDS.org/highband/document/epidemio/index.html.
2. Centers for Disease Control and Prevention. HIV/AIDS Surveillance Report. 1996;8:2–39.
3. Ward JW, Karon J, Fleming P, et al. Trends in AIDS incidence in the United States, 1990–1994. Abstract Mo. C332. Presented at the Eleventh International Conference on AIDS, Vancouver, BC, July 1996.
4. Wortley PM, Fleming PL. AIDS in Women in the United States recent trends. JAMA. 1997;278:911–916.
5. Wold C, Seage GR III, Lenderking WR, et al. Unsafe sex in men who have sex with both men and women. J Acquir Immune Defic Syndr Hum Retrovirol. 1998;17:361–367.
6. Kahn JG, Gurvey J, Pollack LM, et al. How many HIV infections cross the bisexual bridge? An estimate from the United States. AIDS. 1997;11:1031–1037.
7. Wortley PM, Chu SY, Berkelman RL. Epidemiology of HIV/AIDS in women and the impact of the expanded 1993 CDC surveillance definition of AIDS. In: Cotton D, Watts DH, eds. The Medical Management of AIDS in Women. New York: Wiley-Liss; 1997:3–14.
8. Centers for Disease Control and Prevention. Update: Mortality attributable to HIV infection among persons aged 25–44 years—United States, 1994. MMWR Morb Mortal Wkly Rep. 1996;45:121–125.
9. Palella F, Moorman A, Delaney K, et al. Dramatically declining morbidity and mortality in an ambulatory HIV-infected population. Abstract 198. Presented at the Fifth Conference on Retroviruses and Opportunistic Infections, Chicago, Ill, 1998.
10. Palella F, Delaney KM, Moorman AC, et al. Declining morbidity and mortality among patients with advanced human immunodeficiency virus infection. N Engl J Med. 1998;338:853–860.
11. Hogg RS, Heath KV, Yip B, et al. Improved survival among HIV-infected individuals following initiation of antiretroviral therapy. JAMA. 1998;279:450–454.
12. Centers for Disease Control and Prevention. AIDS among persons aged 50 years—United States, 1991–1996. MMWR Morb Mortal Wkly Rep. 1998;47:21–27.
13. Clark RA, Bessinger R. Clinical manifestations and predictors of survival in older women infected with HIV. J Acquir Immune Defic Syndr Hum Retrovirol. 1997;15:341–345.
14. Schable B, Chu SY, Diaz T. Characteristics of women 50 years of age or older with heterosexually acquired AIDS. Am J Public Health. 1996;86:1616–1618.
15. Chaisson RE, Bacchetti P, Osmond D, et al. Cocaine use and HIV infection in intravenous drug users in San Francisco. JAMA. 1989;261:561–565.
16. Edlin BR, Irwin KL, Faruque S, et al. Intersecting epidemics—crack cocaine use and HIV infection among inner-city young adults. Multicenter Crack Cocaine and HIV Infection Study Team. N Engl J Med. 1994;331:1422–1427.
17. Fullilove RE, Fullilove MT, Bowser BP, et al. Risk of sexually transmitted disease among black adolescent crack users in Oakland and San Francisco, Calif. JAMA 1990;263:851–855.
18. Chu SY, Hammett TA, Buehler JW. Update: Epidemiology of reported cases of AIDS in women who report sex only with other women, United States, 1980–1991. AIDS. 1992;518–519.
19. Lemp GF, Jones M, Kellogg TA, et al. HIV seroprevalence and risk behaviors among lesbians and bisexual women in San Francisco and Berkeley, California. Am J Public Health. 1995;85:1549–1552.
20. Centers for Disease Control and Prevention. HIV-1 infection and artificial insemination with processed semen. MMWR Morb Mortal Wkly Rep. 1990;39:249.
21. Stewart GL, Typer JP, Cunningham AL, et al. Transmission of human T-cell lymphotropic virus type III by artificial insemination by donor. Lancet. 1985;2:581–584.
22. Chiasson MA, Stoneburner RL, Joseph SC. Human immunodeficiency virus transmission through artificial insemination. J Acquir Immune Defic Syndr. 1990;3:69–72.
23. Lurie P, Wolfe SM. Unethical trials of interventions to reduce perinatal transmission of the human immunodeficiency virus in developing countries. N Engl J Med. 1997;337:853–856.
24. Cohn SE, Klein JD, Mohr JE, et al. The geography of AIDS: Patterns of urban and rural migration. South Med J. 1994;87:599–606.
25. Fowler MG, Melnick SL, Mathieson BJ. Women and HIV. Epidemiology and global overview. Obstet Gynecol Clin North Am. 1997;24:705–729.
26. Michaels D, Levine C. Estimates of the number of motherless youth orphaned by AIDS in the United States. JAMA. 1992;268:3456–3461.
27. Neal JJ, Fleming PL, Green TA, et al. Trends in heterosexually acquired AIDS in the United States, 1988 through 1995. J Acquir Immune Defic Syndr Hum Retrovirol. 1997;14:465–474.
28. Padian N, Marquis L, Francis DP, et al. Male-to-female transmission of human immunodeficiency virus. JAMA. 1987;258:788–790.
29. Padian NS, Shiboski SC, Jewell NP. Female-to-male transmission of human immunodeficiency virus. JAMA. 1991;266:1664–1667.
30. Fowler MG. Update: Transmission of HIV-1 from mother to child. Curr Opin Obstet Gynecol. 1997;9:343–348.
31. Peterman TA, Stoneburner RL, Allen JR, et al. Risk of human immunodeficiency virus transmission from heterosexual adults with transfusion-associated infections. JAMA. 1988;259:55–58.
32. Padian NS, Shiboski SC, Jewell NP. The effect of number of exposures on the risk of heterosexual HIV transmission. J Infect Dis. 1990;161:883–887.
33. Fowke KR, Nagelkerke NJ, Kimani J, et al. Resistance to HIV-1 infection among persistently seronegative prostitutes in Nairobi, Kenya. Lancet. 1996;348:1347–1351.
34. Lambert, J. AIDS and Women. In: Leppert PC, Howard FM, eds. The Primary Care of Women. Philadelphia: Lippincott-Raven; 1997:560–574.
35. Holmes KK, Johnson DW, Trostle HJ. An estimate of the risk of men acquiring gonorrhea by sexual contact with infected females. Am J Epidemiol. 1970;91:170–174.
36. Platt R, Rice PA, McCormack WM. Risk of acquiring gonorrhea and prevalence of abnormal adnexal findings among women recently exposed to gonorrhea. JAMA. 1983;250:3205–3209.
37. DeGruttola V, Seage GR III, Mayer KH, et al. Infectiousness of HIV between male homosexual partners. J Clin Epidemiol. 1989;42:849–856.
38. Nicolosi A, Correa Leite ML, Musicco M, et al. A The efficiency of male-to-female and female-to-male sexual transmission of the human immunodeficiency virus: A study of 730 stable couples. Italian Study Group on HIV Heterosexual Transmission. Epidemiology. 1994;5:570–575.
39. Skurnick JH, Kennedy CA, Perez G, et al. Behavioral and demographic risk factors for transmission of human immunodeficiency virus type 1 in heterosexual couples: Report from the Heterosexual HIV Transmission Study. Clin Infect Dis. 1998;26:855–864.
40. Guimaraes MD, Vlahov D, Castilho EA. Postcoital vaginal bleeding as a risk factor for transmission of the human immunodeficiency virus in a heterosexual partner study in Brazil. Rio de Janeiro Heterosexual Study Group. Arch Intern Med. 1997;157:1362–1368.
41. Liuzzi G, Chirianni A, Clementi M, et al. Analysis of HIV-1 load in blood, semen and saliva: Evidence for different viral compartments in a cross-sectional and longitudinal study. AIDS. 1996;10:F51–F56.
42. Vernazza PL, Gilliam BL, Flepp M, et al. Effect of antiviral treatment on the shedding of HIV-1 in semen. AIDS. 1997;11:1249–1254.
43. Cu-Uvin SC, Caliendo AM. Cervicovaginal human immunodeficiency virus secretion and plasma viral load in human immunodeficiency virus–seropositive women. Obstet Gynecol. 1997;90:739–743.

44. Gupta P, Mellors J, Kingsley L, et al. High viral load in semen of human immunodeficiency virus type 1–infected men at all stages of disease and its reduction by therapy with protease and nonnucleoside reverse transcriptase inhibitors. J Virol. 1997;71:6271–6275.
45. Levine WC, Pope V, Bhoomkar A, et al. Increase in endocervical CD4+ lymphocytes among women with nonulcerative sexually transmitted diseases. J Infect Dis. 1998;177:167–174.
46. Wasserheit JN. Epidemiological synergy. Interrelationships between human immunodeficiency virus infection and other sexually transmitted diseases. Sex Transm Dis. 1992;19:61–77.
47. Wasserheit JN. STD-HIV interactions: From epidemiological synergy to patient management and public health. Abstract P31. Presented at the Thirty-fifth Annual Meeting of the Infectious Diseases Society of America, Chicago, Ill, September 13–16, 1997.
48. Mayer KH, Anderson DJ. Heterosexual transmission of HIV. In: Minkoff H, DeHovitz JA, Duerr A, eds. HIV Infection in Women. New York: Raven; 1995: 73–85.
49. Laga M, Manoka A, Kivuvu M, et al. Non-ulcerative sexually transmitted diseases as risk factors for HIV-1 transmission in women: Results from a cohort study. AIDS. 1993;7:95–102.
50. de Vincenzi I. A longitudinal study of human immunodeficiency virus transmission by heterosexual partners. European Study Group on Heterosexual Transmission of HIV. N Engl J Med. 1994;331:341–346.
51. Cohen MS, Hoffman IF, Royce RA, et al. Reduction of concentration of HIV-1 in semen after treatment of urethritis: Implications for prevention of sexual transmission of HIV-1. AIDSCAP Malawi Research Group. Lancet. 1997;349:1868–1873.
52. Goulston C, McFarland W, Katzenstein D. Human immunodeficiency virus type 1 RNA shedding in the female genital tract. J Infect Dis. 1998;177:1100–1103.
53. Cu-Uvin S, Caliendo A, Russo R, et al. HIV-1 RNA levels in the genital tract of women on antiretroviral therapy. Abstract 713. Presented at the Fifth Conference on Retroviruses and Opportunistic Infections, Chicago, Ill, February 1–5, 1998.
54. Xu C, Politch JA, Tucker L, et al. Factors associated with increased levels of human immunodeficiency virus type 1 DNA in semen. J Infect Dis. 1997;176:941–947.
55. Rasheed S, Li Z, Xu D, Kovacs A. Presence of cell-free human immunodeficiency virus in cervicovaginal secretions is independent of viral load in the blood of human immunodeficiency virus–infected women. Am J Obstet Gynecol. 1996;175:122–129.
56. Coombs RW, Speck CE, Hughes JP, et al. Association between culturable human immunodeficiency virus type 1 (HIV-1) in semen and HIV-1 RNA levels in semen and blood: Evidence for compartmentalization of HIV-1 between semen and blood. J Infect Dis. 1998;177:320–330.
57. Subbarao S, Wright T, Ellerbrock T, et al. Genotypic evidence of local HIV expression in the female genital tract. Abstract 708. Presented at the Fifth Conference on Retroviruses and Opportunistic Infections, Chicago, Ill, February 1–5, 1998.
58. Shaheen FA, Sison A, Bagasra O, et al. Genotypic and phenotypic characterization of HIV-1 in the blood and genital sectrion of HIV-1 seropositive women. Abstract 710. Presented at the Fifth Conference on Retroviruses and Opportunistic Infections, Chicago, Ill, February 1–5, 1998.
59. Rybo G. Menstrual blood loss in relation to parity and menstrual pattern. Acta Obstet Gynecol Scand. 1966;45:25–45.
60. Tevi-Benissan C, Belec L, Levy M, et al. In vivo semen-associated pH neutralization of cervicovaginal secretions. Clin Diagn Lab Immunol. 1997;4:367–374.
61. Moller BR, Kasperson P. Acidity of the vagina. In: Horowitz BJ, Mardh P-A, eds. Vaginitis and Vaginosis. New York: Wiley-Liss; 1991:63–67.
62. Rosenstein IJ, Stafford MK, Kitchen VS, et al. Effect on normal vaginal flora of three intravaginal microbicidal agents potentially active against human immunodeficiency virus type 1. J Infect Dis. 1998;177:1386–1390.
63. Kreiss JK, Kiviat NB, Plummer FA, et al. Human immunodeficiency virus, human papillomavirus, and cervical intraepithelial neoplasia in Nairobi prostitutes. Sex Transm Dis. 1992;19:54–59.
64. Stafford MK, Ward H, Flanagan A, et al. Safety study of nonoxynol-9 as a vaginal microbicide: Evidence of adverse effects. J Acquir Immune Defic Syndr Hum Retrovirol. 1998;17:327–331.
65. Wainberg MA. The need for vaginal microbicides with antiviral specificity. AIDS. 1998;12:4–6.
66. Biggar RJ, Miotti PG, Taha TE, et al. Perinatal intervention trial in Africa: Effect of a birth canal cleansing intervention to prevent HIV transmission. Lancet. 1996;347:1647–1650.
67. Taha TE, Biggar RJ, Broadhead RL, et al. Effect of cleansing the birth canal with antiseptic solution on maternal and newborn morbidity and mortality in Malawi: Clinical trial. BMJ. 1997;315:216–219.
68. Clemetson DB, Moss GB, Willerford DM, et al. Detection of HIV DNA in cervical and vaginal secretions. Prevalence and correlates among women in Nairobi, Kenya. JAMA. 1993;289:2860–2864.
69. Sha BE, D'Amico RD, Landay AL, et al. Evaluation of immunologic markers in cervicovaginal fluid of HIV-infected and uninfected women: Implications for the immunologic response to HIV in the female genital tract. J Acquir Immune Defic Syndr Hum Retrovirol. 1997;16:161–168.
70. Critchlow CW, Kiviat NB. Detection of human immunodeficiency virus type 1 and type 2 in the female genital tract: Implications for the understanding of virus transmission. Obstet Gynecol Surv. 1997;52:314–324.
71. Ghys PD, Fransen K, Diallo MO, Ettiegne-Traore V, et al. The associations between cervicovaginal HIV shedding, sexually transmitted diseases and immunosuppression in female sex workers in Abidjan, Cote d'Ivoire. AIDS. 1997;11:F85–F93.
72. Grosskurth H, Mosha F, Todd J, et al. Impact of improved treatment of sexually transmitted diseases on HIV infection in rural Tanzania: Randomised controlled trial. Lancet. 1995;346:530–536.
73. European Collaborative Study. Risk factors for mother-to-child transmission of HIV-1. Lancet. 1992;339:1007–1012.
74. Mofenson LM. Mother-child HIV-1 transmission: Timing and determinants. Obstet Gynecol Clin North Am. 1997;24:759–784.
75. Viscarello RR, Cullen MT, DeGennaro NJ, et al. Fetal blood sampling in HIV-seropositive women before elective midtrimester termination of pregnancy. Am J Obstet Gynecol. 1992;167:1075–1079.
76. Lewis SH, Reynolds-Kohler C, Fox HE, et al. HIV-1 in trophoblastic and villous Hofbauer cells, and haematological precursors in eight-week fetuses. Lancet. 1990;335:565–568.
77. Maury W, Potts BJ, Rabson AB. HIV-1 infection of first-trimester and term human placental tissue: A possible mode of maternal-fetal transmission. J Infect Dis. 1989;160:583–588.
78. Jovius E, Koch MA, Schafer A, et al. LAV/HTLV-III in a 20 week fetus. Lancet. 1985;2:1129.
79. Sprecher S, Soumenkoff G, Puissant F, et al. Vertical transmission in a 15 week fetus. Lancet. 1986;2:288.
80. Levine AM. HIV disease in women. Clinical Care Options for HIV. Healthcare Communications Group, L.L.C. 1997;9:3–24.
81. Kalish LA, Pitt J, Lew J, et al. Defining the time of fetal or perinatal acquisition of human immunodeficiency virus type 1 infection on the basis of age at first positive culture. Women and Infants Transmission Study (WITS). J Infect Dis. 1997;175:712–715.
82. Quinn TC, Ruff A, Modlin J. HIV infection and AIDS in children. Annu Rev Public Health. 1992;13:1–30.
83. Blanche S, Tardieu M, Duliege A-M, et al. Longitudinal study of 94 symptomatic infants with perinatally acquired human immunodeficiency virus infection. Evidence for a bimodal expression of clinical and biological symptoms. Am J Dis Child. 1990;144:1210–1215.
84. Centers for Disease Control and Prevention. Public Health Service Task Force recommendations for the use of antiretroviral drugs in pregnant women infected with HIV-1 for maternal health and for reducing perinatal HIV-1 transmission in the United States. MMWR Morb Mortal Wkly Rep. 1998;47:1–30.
85. Ehrnst A, Lindgren S, Dictor M, et al. HIV in pregnant women and their offspring: Evidence for late transmission. Lancet. 1991;338:203–207.
86. Rouzioux C, Costagliola D, Burgard M, et al. Estimating timing of mother-to-child human immunodeficiency virus type-1 (HIV-1) transmission by use of a Markov model: The HIV Infection in Newborns French Collaborative Study Group. Am J Epidemiol. 1995;142:1330–1337.
87. Goedert JJ, Duliege AM, Amos CI, et al. High risk of HIV-1 infection for first-born twins. The International Registry of HIV-Exposed Twins. Lancet. 1991;338:1471–1475.
88. Duliege A-M, Amos CI, Felton S, et al. Birth order, delivery route, and concordance in the transmission of human immunodeficiency virus type-1 from mothers to twins. J Pediatr. 1995;126:625–632.
89. Mayaux MJ, Dussaix E, Isopet J, et al. Maternal virus load during pregnancy and mother-to-child transmission of human immunodeficiency virus type 1: The French perinatal cohort studies. SEROGEST Cohort Group. J Infect Dis. 1997;175:172–175.
90. Coll O, Hernandez M, Boucher CA, et al. Vertical HIV-1 transmission correlates with a high maternal viral load at delivery. J Acquir Immune Defic Syndr Hum Retrovirol. 1997;4:26–30.
91. Pitt J, Brambilla D, Reichelderfer P, et al. Maternal immunologic and virologic risk factors for infant human immunodeficiency virus type 1 infection: Findings from the Women and Infants Transmission Study. J Infect Dis. 1997;175:567–575.
92. St. Louis ME, Kamenga M, Brown C, et al. Risk for perinatal HIV-1 transmission according to maternal immunologic, virologic, and placental factors. JAMA. 1993;269:2853–2859.
93. Report of a Consensus Workshop, Siena, Italy, January 17–18, 1992. Maternal factors involved in mother-to-child transmission of HIV-1. J Acquir Immune Defic Syndr Hum Retrovirol. 1992;5:1019–1029.
94. Thea DM, Steketee RW, Pliner V, et al. The effect of maternal viral load on the risk of perinatal transmission of HIV-1. New York City Perinatal HIV Transmission Collaborative Study Group. AIDS. 1997;11:437–444.
95. Sperling RS, Shapiro DE, Coombs RW, et al. Maternal viral load, zidovudine treatment, and the risk of transmission of human immunodeficiency virus type 1 from mother to infant. Pediatric AIDS Clinical Trials Group Protocol 076 Study Group. N Engl J Med. 1996;335:1621–1629.
96. MacDonald KS, Embree J, Njenga S, et al. Mother-child class I HLA concordance increases perinatal human immunodeficiency virus type 1 transmission. J Infect Dis. 1998;177:551–556.
97. John GC, Nduati RW, Mbori-Ngacha D, et al. Genital shedding of human immunodeficiency virus type 1 DNA during pregnancy: Association with immunosuppression, abnormal cervical or vaginal discharge, and severe vitamin A deficiency. J Infect Dis. 1997;175:57–62.
98. Semba RD, Miotti PG, Chiphangwi JD, et al. Maternal vitamin A deficiency and mother-to-child transmission of HIV-1. Lancet. 1994;343:1593–1597.
99. Mostad SB, Overbaugh J, DeVange DM, et al. Hormonal contraception, vitamin A deficiency, and other risk factors for shedding of HIV-1 infected cells from the cervix and vagina. Lancet. 1997;350:922–927.

100. Rodriguez EM, Mofenson LM, Chang BH, et al. Association of maternal drug use during pregnancy with maternal HIV culture positivity and perinatal HIV transmission. AIDS. 1996;10:273–282.
101. Van't Wout AB, Kootstra NA, Mulder-Kampinga GA, et al. Macrophage-tropic variants initiate human immunodeficiency virus type 1 infection after sexual, parenteral, and vertical transmission. J Clin Invest. 1995;94:2060–2067.
102. Reinhardt PP, Reinhardt B, Lathey JL, et al. Human cord blood mononuclear cells are preferentially infected by non–syncytium inducing macrophage-tropic human immunodeficiency virus type 1 isolates. J Clin Microbiol. 1995;33:292–297.
103. Kunanusont C, Foy HM, Kreiss JK, et al. HIV-1 subtypes and male-to-female transmission in Thailand. Lancet. 1995;345:1078–1083.
104. Bulterys M, Landesman S, Burns DN, et al. Sexual behavior and injection drug use during pregnancy and vertical transmission of HIV-1. J Acquir Immune Defic Syndr. 1997;15:76–82.
105. Matheson PB, Thomas PA, Abrams EJ, et al. Heterosexual behavior during pregnancy and perinatal transmission of HIV-1. New York City Perinatal HIV Transmission Collaborative Study Group. AIDS. 1996;10:1249–1256.
106. Landesman SH, Kalish LA, Burns DN, et al. Obstetrical factors and the transmission of human immunodeficiency virus type 1 from mother to child. N Engl J Med. 1996;334:1617–1623.
107. Zorrilla CD. Obstetric factors and mother-to-infant transmission of HIV-1. Infect Dis Clin North Am. 1997;11:109–118.
108. The International Perinatal HIV Group. The mode of delivery and the risk of vertical transmission of human immunodeficiency virus type 1. A meta-analysis of 15 prospective cohort studies. N Engl J Med. 1999;340:977–987.
109. The European Mode of Delivery Collaboration. Elective caesarean-section versus vaginal delivery in prevention of vertical transmission: A randomized clinical trial. Lancet. 1999;353:1035–1039.
110. Landers DV, Sweet RL. Reducing mother-to-infant transmission of HIV—the door remains open. N Engl J Med. 1996;334:1664–1665.
111. Oxtoby MJ. Human immunodeficiency virus and other viruses in human milk: Placing the issues in broader perspective. Pediatr Infect Dis J. 1988;7:825–835.
112. Van de Perre P, Simonon A, Msellati P, et al. Postnatal transmission of human immunodeficiency virus type 1 from mother to infant. A prospective cohort study in Kigali, Rwanda. N Engl J Med. 1991;325:593–598.
113. Lewis P, Nduati R, Kreiss JK, et al. Cell-free human immunodeficiency virus type 1 in breast milk. J Infect Dis. 1998;177:34–39.
114. Nduati RW, John GC, Richardson BA, et al. Human immunodeficiency virus type 1–infected cells in breast milk: Association with immunosuppression and vitamin A deficiency. J Infect Dis. 1995;172:1461–1468.
115. Dunn DT, Newell ML, Ades AE, et al. Risk of human immunodeficiency virus type 1 transmission through breastfeeding. Lancet. 1992;340:585–588.
116. Berrebia A, Kobuch WE, Puel J, et al. Influence of pregnancy on human immunodeficiency virus disease. Eur J Obstet Gynecol Reprod Biol. 1990;37:211–217.
117. Weisser M, Rudin C, Battegay M, et al. Does pregnancy influence the course of HIV infection? Evidence from two large Swiss cohort studies. J Acquir Immune Defic Syndr Hum Retrovirol. 1998;17:404–410.
118. Minkoff HL, Henderson C, Mendez H, et al. Pregnancy outcomes among mothers infected with HIV and uninfected control subjects. Am J Obstet Gynecol. 1990;163:1598–1604.
119. Bessinger R, Clark R, Kissinger P, et al. Pregnancy is not associated with the progression of HIV disease in women attending an HIV outpatient program. Am J Epidemiol. 1998;147:434–440.
120. Deschamps MM, Papa JW, Desvarieux M, et al. A prospective study of HIV-seropositive asymptomatic women of childbearing age in a developing country. J Acquir Immune Defic Syndr. 1993;6:446–451.
121. Landers DV, Martinez de Tejada B, Coyne BA. Immunology of HIV and pregnancy. The effects of each on the other. Obstet Gynecol Clin North Am. 1997;24:821–831.
122. Marion RW, Wiznia AA, Hutcheon G, Rubinstein A. Human T cell lymphotrophic virus type embryopathy. A new dysmorphia syndrome. Am J Dis Child. 1986;140:638–640.
123. Marion RW, Wiznia AA, Hutcheon RG, Rubinstein A. Fetal AIDS syndrome score. Correlation between severity of dysmorphism and age at diagnosis of immunodeficiency. Am J Dis Child. 1987;141:429–431.
124. Nicholas SW. Is there an HIV associated facial dysmorphism? Pediatr Ann. 1988;17:353.
125. Qazi QH, Sheikh TM, Fikrig S. Lack of evidence for craniofacial dysmorphism in perinatal HIV infection. J Pediatr. 1988;112:7–11.
126. Temmerman M, Chomba EN, Ndinya-Achola J, et al. Maternal human immunodeficiency virus-1 infection and pregnancy outcome. Obstet Gynecol, 1994;83: 495–501.
127. Miotti PG, Dallabetta G, Ndovi E, et al. HIV-1 and pregnant women: Associated factors, prevalence, estimate of incidence and role in fetal wastage in central Africa. AIDS. 1990;4:733–736.
128. Connor EM, Sperling RS, Gelber R, et al. Reduction of maternal-infant transmission of human immunodeficiency virus type 1 with zidovudine treatment. Pediatric AIDS Clinical Trials Group Protocol 076 Study Group. N Engl J Med. 1994;331:1173–1180.
129. Centers for Disease Control and Prevention. Recommendations of the U.S. Public Health Service Task Force on the use of zidovudine to reduce perinatal transmission of human immunodeficiency virus. MMWR Morb Mortal Wkly Rep. 1994;43: 1–20.
130. Centers for Disease Control and Prevention. U.S. Public Health Service recommendations for human immunodeficiency virus counseling and voluntary testing for pregnant women. MMWR Morb Mortal Wkly Rep. 1995;44:1–14.
131. Fiscus SA, Adimora AA, Schoenbach VJ, et al. Perinatal HIV infection and the effect of zidovudine therapy on transmission in rural and urban counties. JAMA. 1996;275:1483–1488.
132. Cooper ER, Nugent RP, Diaz C, et al. After AIDS clinical trial 076: The changing pattern of zidovudine use during pregnancy, and the subsequent reduction in the vertical transmission of human immunodeficiency virus in a cohort of infected women and their infants. Women and Infants Transmission Study Group. J Infect Dis. 1996;174:1207–1211.
133. Forbes J, Burdge D, Money D. Impact of antiretroviral therapy (ART) on the outcome of infants born to HIV seropositive mothers in British Columbia. Abstract 248. Presented at the Fifth Conference on Retroviruses and Opportunistic Infections, Chicago, Ill, February 1–5, 1998.
134. National Institute of Allergy and Infectious Disease–National Institutes of Health. Summary of a meeting of a panel to review studies of transplacental toxicity of AZT. NIAID Fact Sheet. 1997.
135. Khalsa AM, Currier J. Women and HIV. A review of current epidemiology, gynecologic manifestations, and perinatal transmission. Prim Care. 1997;24:617–641.
136. Aleixo LF, Goodenow MM, Sleasman JW. Zidovudine administered to women infected with human immunodeficiency virus type 1 and to their neonates reduces pediatric infection independent of an effect on levels of maternal virus. J Pediatr. 1997;130:906–914.
137. Centers for Disease Control and Prevention. Administration of zidovudine during late pregnancy and delivery to prevent perinatal HIV infection—Thailand, 1996–98. MMWR Morb Mortal Wkly Rep. 1998;4:151–154.
138. Wade NA, Birkhead GS, Warren BL, et al. Abbreviated regimens of zidovudine prophylaxis and perinatal transmission of the human immunodeficiency virus. N Engl J Med. 1998;339:1409–1414.
139. Eastman PS, Shapiro DE, Coombs RW, et al. Maternal viral genotypic zidovudine resistance and infrequent failure of zidovudine therapy to prevent perinatal transmission of human immunodeficiency virus type 1 in pediatric AIDS Clinical Trials Group Protocol 076. J Infect Dis. 1998;177:557–564.
140. Frenkel LM, Wagner LE 2nd, Demeter LM, et al. Effects of zidovudine use during pregnancy on resistance and vertical transmission of human immunodeficiency virus type 1. Clin Infect Dis. 1995;20:1321–1326.
141. Centers for Disease Control and Prevention. Report of the NIH panel to define principles of therapy of HIV infection and guidelines for the use of antiretroviral agents in HIV-infected adults and adolescents. MMWR Morb Mortal Wkly Rep. 1998;47:1–82.
142. Carpenter CC, Fischl MA, Hammer SM, et al. Antiretroviral therapy for HIV infection in 1997. Updated recommendations of the International AIDS Society—USA panel. JAMA. 1997;277:1962–1969.
143. Patil S, Livingston E, McKinney RE, et al. Does pregnancy affect the pharmacokinetics of didanosine (ddI) in HIV-1 infected women? Abstract 225. Presented at the Fifth Conference on Retroviruses and Opportunistic Infections, Chicago, Ill, February 1–5, 1998.
144. National Institute of Allergy and Infectious Disease–National Institutes of Health. Safety information of DMP-266. 1998.
145. FDA Public Health Advisory. Reports of diabetes and hyperglycemia in patients receiving protease inhibitors for the treatment of human immunodeficiency virus (HIV). JAMA. 1997;278:379.
146. Dube M, Johnson D, Currier J, et al. Protease inhibitor–associated hyperglycaemia (Letter). Lancet. 1997;350:713–714.
147. Visnegarwala F, Krause K, Musher D. Severe diabetes associated with protease inhibitor therapy (Letter). Ann Intern Med. 1997;127:947.
148. Centers for Disease Control and Prevention. 1997 USPHS/IDSA guidelines for the prevention of opportunistic infections in persons infected with human immunodeficiency virus. USPHS/IDSA Prevention of Opportunistic Infections Working Group. MMWR Morb Mortal Wkly Rep. 1997;46:1–46.
149. Bryson YJ. Perinatal HIV-1 transmission: Recent advances and therapeutic interventions. AIDS. 1996;3:S33–S42.
150. Carpenter CJC, Mayer KH, Stein MD, et al. Human immunodeficiency virus infection in North American women: Experience with 200 cases and a review of the literature. Medicine. 1991;70:307–325.
151. Clark RA, Brandon W, Dumestre J, Pindaro C. Clinical manifestations of infection with the human immunodeficiency virus in women in Louisiana. Clin Infect Dis. 1993;17:173–177.
152. Greenberg AE, Thomas PA, Landesman SH, et al. The spectrum of HIV-1–related disease among outpatients in New York City. AIDS. 1992;6:849–859.
153. Clark RA, Kissinger P. Is gender associated with serious pyogenic infections diagnosed in HIV infected persons? Am J Epidemiol. 1995;141:176.
154. Centers for Disease Control and Prevention. Revision of the CDC surveillance case definition for acquired immunodeficiency syndrome. MMWR. 1987;36:S3–11S.
155. Fleming PJ, Ciesielski CA, Byers RH, Castro KG, Berkelman RL. Gender differences in reported AIDS-indicative diagnoses. J Infect Dis. 1993;168:61–67.
156. Blair JM, Kovacs A, Beall G, et al. Kaposi's sarcoma in women with AIDS. Abstract 106.4. Presented at the National Conference of Women and HIV, Pasadena, Calif, May 4–7, 1997.
157. Cooley TP, Hirschhorn LR, O'Keane JC. Kaposi's sarcoma in women with AIDS. AIDS. 1996;10:1221–1225.
158. Macasaet MA, Duerr A, Thelmo W, et al. Kaposi's sarcoma presenting as a vulvar mass. Obstet Gynecol. 1995;86:695–697.

159. Darai E, Vlastos G, Madelenat P. Acquired immunodeficiency syndrome–related Kaposi's sarcoma: Two cervical cases. Am J Obstet Gynecol. 1995;173:979.
160. Coodley GO, Loveless MO, Nelson HD, Coodley MK. Endocrine function in the HIV wasting syndrome. J Acquir Immune Defic Syndr. 1994;7:46–51.
161. Grinspoon S, Corcoran C, Miller K, et al. Body composition and endocrine function in women with acquired immunodeficiency syndrome and wasting. J Clin Endocrinol Metab. 1997;82:1332–1337.
162. Engleson RD, Rabkin JG, Rabkin R, Kotler D. Effects of testosterone upon body composition. J Acquir Immune Defic Syndr. 1996;11:510–514.
163. Levine AM, Preston-Martin S, Fruchter R, et al. Unusual cases of breast cancer in HIV-infected women: Data from Women's Interagency HIV Study (WIHS). Abstract 123.1. Presented at the National Conference of Women and HIV, Pasadena, Calif, May 4–7, 1997.
164. Sun XW, Ellerbrock TV, Lungu O, et al. Human papillomavirus infection in human immunodeficiency virus–seropositive women. Obstet Gynecol. 1995;85:680–686.
165. Vermund SH, Kelley KF, Klein RS, et al. High risk of human papillomavirus infection and cervical squamous intrepithelial lesions among women with symptomatic human immunodeficiency virus infection. Am J Obstet Gynecol. 1991;165:392–400.
166. Hillemanns P, Ellerbrock TV, McPhillips S, et al. Prevalence of anal human papillomavirus infection and anal cytologic abnormalities in HIV-seropositive women. AIDS. 1996;10:1641–1647.
167. Laga M, Icenogle JP, Marsella R, et al. Genital papillomavirus infection and cervical dysplasia—opportunistic complications of HIV infection. Int J Cancer. 1992;50:45–48.
168. Chiasson MA, Ellerbrock TV, Bush TJ, et al. Increased prevalence of vulvovaginal condyloma and vulvar intraepithelial neoplasia in women infected with the human immunodeficiency virus. Obstet Gynecol. 1997;89:690–694.
169. Wright TC, Ellerbrock TV, Chiasson MA, et al. Cervical intraepithelial neoplasia in women infected with human immunodeficiency virus; prevalence, risk factors, and validity of Papanicolaou smears; New York Cervical Disease Study. Obstet Gynecol. 1994;84:591–597.
170. Williams AB, Darragh TM, Vranizan K, et al. Anal and cervical human papillomavirus infection and risk of anal and cervical abnormalities in human immunodeficiency virus–infected women. Obstet Gynecol. 1994;83:205–211.
171. Korn A, Landers DV. Gynecological disease in women infected with human immunodeficiency virus type 1. J Acquir Immune Defic Syndr. 1995;9:361–70.
172. Sha BE, Benson CA, Pottage JC, et al. HIV infection in women: An observational study of clinical characteristics, disease progression, and survival for a cohort of women in Chicago. J Acquir Immune Defic Syndr. 1995;8:486–495.
173. Fuller C, Clark RA, Kissinger P, Abdalian SE. Clinical manifestations of infection with human immunodeficiency virus among adolescents in Louisiana. J Adol Health 1996;18:422–428.
174. Maiman M, Tarricone N, Vieira J, et al. Colposcopic evaluation of HIV infected women. Obstet Gynecol 1991;78:84–88.
175. Luque A, Demeter L, Raubertas R, Reichman R. Prediction of cervical human papillomavirus infection and disease by magnitude of HIV-1 in plasma RNA level. Abstract 258. Presented at the Fifth Conference on Retroviruses and Opportunistic Infections, Chicago, Ill, February 1–5, 1998.
176. Assad LS, Riester K, Fruchter RG, et al. HIV RNA level is a risk factor for abnormal cervical cytology. Abstract 716. Presented at the Fifth Conference on Retroviruses and Opportunistic Infections, Chicago, Ill, February 1–5, 1998.
177. Centers for Disease Control and Prevention. Risk for cervical disease in HIV infected women—New York City. MMWR Morb Mortal Wkly Rep. 1990;39:846–849.
178. Sun W, Kuhn L, Ellerbrock TV, et al. Human papillomavirus infection in women infected with human immunodeficiency virus. N Engl J Med. 1997;337:1343–1349.
179. Belafsky P, Clark RA, Kissinger P, Torres J. Natural history of low-grade squamous intraepithelial lesions in women infected with human immunodeficiency virus. J Acquir Immune Defic Syndr. 1996;11:511–512.
180. Biggers SD, LaGuardia KD. The natural history of low grade squamous intraepithelial lesions of the cervix in women with human immunodeficiency virus infection; evidence for an algorithm for management. Abstract Th.B4138. Presented at the Eleventh International Conference on AIDS, Vancouver, BC, July 1996.
181. Olaitan A, Mocroft A, McCarthy K, et al. Cervical abnormality and sexually transmitted disease screening in human immunodeficiency virus–positive women. Obstet Gynecol. 1997;89:71–75.
182. Wright TC, Koulos J, Schnoll F, et al. Cervical intraepithelial neoplasia in women infected with the human immunodeficiency virus: Outcome after loop electrosurgical excision. Gynecol Oncol. 1994;55:253–238.
183. Maiman M, Fruchter RG, Serur E, et al. Recurrent cervical intraepithelial neoplasia in human immunodeficiency virus–seropositive women. Obstet Gynecol. 1993;82:170–174.
183a. Maiman M, Watts DH, Andersen J. A phase three randomized trial of topical vaginal 5-fluorouracil maintenance therapy versus observation after standard treatment for high grade cervical dysplasia in HIV-infected women: ACTG-200. Abstract 466. Presented at the Sixth Conference on Retroviruses and Opportunistic Infections. Chicago, Ill, February 1–5, 1999.
184. Maiman M, Fruchter RG, Clark M, et al. Cervical cancer as an AIDS-defining illness. Obstet Gynecol. 1997;89:76–80.
185. Maiman M, Fruchter RG, Serur E, et al. Human immunodeficiency virus infection and cervical neoplasia. Gynecol Oncol. 1990;38:377–382.
186. Klevens RM, Fleming PL, Mays MA, Frey R. Characteristics of women with AIDS and invasive cervical cancer. Obstet Gynecol. 1996;88:269–273.
187. Maiman M, Fruchter RG, Guy L, et al. Human immunodeficiency virus infection and invasive cervical carcinoma. Cancer. 1993;71:402–406.
188. Centers for Disease Control and Prevention. 1993 sexually transmitted diseases treatment guidelines. MMWR Morb Mortal Wkly Rep. 1993;42(RR14):14.
189. Wright TC, Moscarelli RD, Dole P, et al. Significance of mild cytologic atypia in women infected with human immunodeficiency virus. Obstet Gynecol. 1996;87:515–519.
190. Hoegsberg B, Abulafia O, Sedlis A, et al. Sexually transmitted diseases and human immunoficiency virus infection among women with pelvic inflammatory disease. Am J Obstet Gynecol. 1990;163:1135–1139.
191. Korn AP, Landers DV, Green JR, Sweet RL. Pelvic inflammatory disease in human immunodeficiency virus–infected women. Obstet Gynecol. 1993;82:765–768.
192. Barbosa C, Macasaet M, Brockmann S, et al. Pelvic inflammatory disease and human immunodeficiency virus infection. Obstet Gynecol. 1997;89:65–70.
193. Kamenga M, DeCock KM, St Louis ME, et al. The impact of human immunodeficiency virus infection on pelvic inflammatory disease: A case-control study in Abidjan, Ivory Coast. Am J Obstet Gynecol. 1995;172:919–925.
194. Sweet RL, Landers DV. Pelvic inflammatory disease in HIV-positive women. Lancet 1997;349:1266–1267.
195. Imam N, Carpenter CC, Mayer KH, et al. Hierarchical pattern of mucosal *Candida* infections in HIV-seropositive women. Am J Med. 1990;89:142–146.
196. Duerr A, Sierra M, Clarke L, et al. Vaginal candidiasis among HIV-infected women. Abstract PO-B01-0880. Presented at the Ninth International Conference on AIDS. Berlin, Germany, June 6–11, 1993.
197. Dahl KM, Keath EJ, Powderly WG. Molecular epidemiology of mucosal candidiasis in HIV-positive women. AIDS Res Hum Retroviruses. 1997;13:485–491.
198. Schuman P, Capps L, Peng G, et al. Weekly fluconazole for the prevention of mucosal candidiasis in women with HIV infection. Ann Intern Med. 1997;126:689–696.
199. Schuman P, Christensen C, Sobel J. Aphthous vaginal ulceration in two women with AIDS. Am J Obstet Gynecol. 1990;14:1660–1663.
200. Covino JM, McCormack WM. Vulvar ulcer of unknown etiology in a human immunodeficiency virus-infected woman: Response to treatment with zidovudine. Am J Obstet Gynecol. 1990;153:116–118.
201. Anderson J, Clark RA, Watts H, et al. Idiopathic genital ulcers in women infected with human immunodeficiency virus. J Acquir Immune Defic Syndr. 1996;13:343–347.
202. LaGuardia KD, White M, Saigo PE, et al. Genital ulcer disease in women infected with human immunodeficiency virus infection. Am J Gynecol. 1995;172:553–562.
203. Verberkmoes A, Boer K, Wertheim PM, et al. Thalidomide for genital ulcer in HIV-positive women. Lancet. 1996;347:974.
204. Clark R, Kissinger P, Williams T. Contraception among HIV infected women and adolescents. Int J STD AIDS. 1996;7:439–442.
205. Shelton M, Adams J, Gugino L, et al. Menstrual cycle hormone patterns in HIV-infected women. Presented at the Third Conference on Retroviruses and Opportunistic Infections, Washington, DC, January 28–February 1, 1996.
206. Chirgwin KD, Feldman J, Muneyyirci-Delale O, et al. Menstrual function in human immunodeficiency virus–infected women without acquired immunodeficiency syndrome. J Acquir Immune Defic Syndr. 1996;12:489–494.
207. Cohen M, Greenblatt R, Minkoff H, et al. Menstrual abnormalities in women with HIV infection. Abstract Mo.B540. Presented at the Eleventh International Conference on AIDS, Vancouver, BC, 1996.
208. Ellerbrock TV, Wright TC, Bush T, et al. Characteristics of menstruation in women infected with human immunodeficiency virus. Obstet Gynecol. 1996;87:1030–1034.
209. Shah PN, Smith JR, Wells C, et al. Menstrual symptoms in women infected by the human immunodeficiency virus. Obstet Gynecol. 1994;83:397–400.
210. Gates EJ, Diaz-Arrastia C, DiMaio T, Maiman M. Non-Hodgkin lymphoma of the endometrium in human immunodeficiency virus infection. Obstet Gynecol. 1997;90:697–699.
211. Friedland GH, Saltzman B, Vileno J, et al. Survival differences in patients with AIDS. J Acquir Immune Defic Syndr. 1991;4:144–153.
212. Rothenberg R, Woelfel M, Stoneburner R, et al. Survival with the acquired immunodeficiency syndrome. N Engl J Med. 1987;317:1297–1302.
213. Chaisson RE, Keruly JC, Moore RD. Race, sex, drug use, and progression of HIV disease. N Engl J Med. 1995;333:751–756.
214. Melnick S, Shere R, Louis TA, et al. Survival and disease progression according to gender of patients with HIV infection. JAMA. 1993;272:1915–1921.
215. Flanigan TP, Imam N, Lange N, et al. Decline of $CD4^+$ lymphocyte counts from the time of seroconversion in HIV-positive women. J Women's Health. 1992;1:231–234.
216. Hellinger FJ. The use of health services by women with HIV infection. Health Serv Res. 1993;28:543–561.
216a. Farzadegan H, Hoover DR, Astemborski J, et al. Sex differences in HIV-1 viral load and progression to AIDS. Lancet. 1998;352:1510–1514.
216b. Anastos K, Gange SJ, Lau B, et al. Gender specific differences in quantitative HIV-1 RNA levels. Abstract 274. Presented at the Sixth Conference on Retroviruses and Opportunistic Infections. Chicago, Ill, February 1–5, 1999.
216c. Moore RD, Cheever L, Keruly JC, Chaisson RE. Lack of sex difference in CD4 to HIV-1 RNA viral load ratio. Lancet. 1999;353:463–464.
217. Clark RA, Brandon W, Rice J, Blakley S. Predictors of HIV disease progression in women. J Acquir Immune Defic Syndr. 1995;9:43–50.
218. Lindan CP, Allen S, Serufilira A, et al. Predictors of mortality among HIV infected women in Kigali, Rwanda. Ann Intern Med. 1992;116:320–328.
219. Anastos K, Kovacs A, Kalish L, et al. Quantitative HIV-1 RNA and other factors

associated with survival in the Women's Interagency HIV Study (WIHS). Abstract 207. Presented at the Fifth Conference on Retroviruses and Opportunistic Processes, Chicago, Ill, February 1–5, 1998.
220. Stein MD, Liebman B, Waachtel TJ, et al. HIV-positive women: Reasons they are tested for HIV and their clinical characteristics on entry into health care system. J Gen Intern Med. 1991;6:286–289.
221. Hogan AJ, Soloman DJ, Boukight RR, et al. Under-utilization of medical care services by HIV-infected women? Some preliminary results from Michigan Medicaid Program. AIDS. 1991;5:338–339.
222. Butz AM, Hutton N, Joyner M, et al. HIV-infected women and infants; social and health factors impeding utilization of health care. J Nurse Midwifery. 1993;38:103–109.
223. Lowinson JH, Ruiz P, Millman RB, et al. Substance Abuse. Baltimore: Williams and Wilkins; 1992:734–788.
224. Centers for Disease Control and Prevention. MMWR Morb Mortal Wkly Rep. 1995;44:81–83.
225. Kissinger P, Clark RA, Rice J, Kutzen H, Morse A, Brandon W. Evaluation of a program to remove barriers to public health care for women with HIV infection. South Med J. 1995;88:1121–1125.
226. Kissinger P, Fuller C, Clark RA, Abdalian SE. Psychosocial characteristics of HIV-infected adolescents in New Orleans. J Adol Health. 1997;20:258.
227. Hein K, Dell R, Futterman D, Rotheram-Borus MJ, Shaffer N. Comparison of HIV+ and HIV− adolescents: Risk factors and psychosocial determinants. Pediatrics. 1995;96–104.
228. Schneider DJ, Kloser P. HIV disease in the older inner-city women. [Abstract PoC 4730] Presented at the Eighth International Conference on AIDS, Amsterdam, The Netherlands, July 19–24, 1992.
229. Belchetz PE. Hormonal treatment of postmenopausal women. N Engl J Med. 1994;330:1062–1071.
230. Kitahata MM, Koepsell TD, Deyo RA, Maxwell CL, Dodge WT, Wagner EH. Physicians' experience with the acquired immunodeficiency syndrome as a factor in patients' survival. N Engl J Med. 1996;334(11):701–706.
231. Laine C, Markson LE, McKee LJ, et al. The relationship of clinic experience with advanced HIV and survival of women with AIDS. AIDS. 1998;12:417–424.
232. Cotton DJ, Powderly WG, Feinberg J. Determinants of accrual of women to a large multicenter clinical trials program of HIV infection. J Acquir Immunodefic Syndr. 1993;6:1322–1328.
233. Currier JS, Spino CS, Grimes J, Cotton DH, the ACTG 175 team. Gender differences in toxicity rates and CD4 responses to nucleoside analogue therapy in ACTG 175. (Abstract Th.B.290) Presented at the Eleventh International Conference on AIDS. Vancouver, BC, July 1996.

***Chapter* 114**

Pediatric Human Immunodeficiency Virus Infection

GEOFFREY A. WEINBERG

The epidemic of acquired immunodeficiency syndrome (AIDS) was first recognized in adults in the United States in 1981, although sporadic cases in the United States and Europe had occurred since at least the mid-1970s.[1–5] In retrospect, we know that pediatric cases occurred almost as early as adult cases.[6–9] The infection has reached pandemic proportions in many areas of the world.[10] In the United States, human immunodeficiency virus (HIV) infection and AIDS occur primarily (98%) in adults; globally, pediatric AIDS may represent as much as 25% of the cumulative case number.[10, 11]

Although the pathogenesis of HIV infection and the general virologic and immunologic principles underlying the use of antiretroviral therapy are similar for HIV-infected children and adults, unique considerations are needed for infants, children, and adolescents. These include (1) the acquisition of infection through perinatal exposure for the majority of children (implying a relatively newly acquired infection at birth within the confines of an immature immune system); (2) in utero exposure to antiretroviral medications; (3) differences in immunologic markers, viral load, and serologic diagnostic strategies in young infants; (4) changes in pharmacokinetic parameters with age; (5) considerations related to the formulation and palatability of medications; and (6) issues of adherence in infants and young children dependent on others for medication administration, and in adolescents facing adherence challenges from developmental issues including peer pressure. This chapter addresses the salient pediatric-specific issues in the epidemiology, clinical manifestations, diagnosis, and therapy of pediatric HIV infection.

EPIDEMIOLOGY

Cases of AIDS in children have accounted for only 2% of all reported cases in the United States.[11] The total number of reported cases of AIDS in children and adolescents, however, continues to increase, and the acquisition of HIV infection during adolescence significantly contributes to the large number of cases in young adults. If the average incubation period of adult AIDS is 5 to 10 years, then the roughly 110,000 individuals diagnosed with AIDS at the age of 20 to 29 years (18% of the total U.S. case number) may be assumed to have initially acquired their HIV infection as adolescents. Routes of transmission of HIV in adolescents are similar to those in adults, that is, sexual contact or injecting drug use.

More than 90% of infected children younger than 13 years in the United States acquired their infection from their mother (i.e., vertical transmission).[11] The remainder, including patients with hemophilia or other coagulation disorders, received contaminated blood, its components, or clotting factor concentrates. Transfusion of blood, blood components, or clotting factor concentrates, once a prominent cause of pediatric HIV infection, particularly among boys with hemophilia, is now rarely a mode of HIV transmission. A few cases of HIV infection in children have resulted from sexual abuse by an HIV-seropositive individual. Breast-feeding remains a possible mode of transmission, hence the recommendation contraindicating the use of breast milk from HIV-infected mothers in countries where infant formula is easily available.[12] Less than 3% of cases have been reported to have no identifiable risk factor, and after careful investigation, most are reclassified into one of the established risk factor groups.[11] Transmission of HIV has rarely been demonstrated to occur in families or households, in schools or child care settings, or with routine care in hospitals or clinics.[13, 14]

The risk of infection for an infant born to an HIV-seropositive mother who did not receive antiretroviral therapy during pregnancy is estimated to be between 13 and 39%.[15, 16] The exact timing of transmission from an infected mother to her infant is uncertain, but evidence suggests that transmission may occur in utero, around the time of delivery, or postpartum through breast-feeding.[12, 16, 17] The available evidence suggests that the majority of infections occur close to the time of or during delivery (see Chapter 113).[18] Some studies suggest higher rates of perinatal transmission in women who seroconvert during pregnancy, women with advanced disease, low peripheral CD4$^+$ T-lymphocyte counts, prolonged rupture of membranes, preterm delivery, or high viral loads.[16, 17, 17a] In vaginal deliveries, a firstborn twin is at greater risk of HIV-infection than is a secondborn twin.[19, 20] Prevention of transmission by cesarean section has been suggested by some, but not all, studies.[21–24] However, it is clear that vertical transmission is reduced significantly by the use of zidovudine therapy of pregnant women and their newborn infants (see Chapter 113).[15, 25, 26]

HIV has been detected in both the cellular and the cell-free fractions of human breast milk, and breast-feeding has been implicated in the transmission of HIV infection.[12, 26a] A high maternal plasma viral concentration (load) may also be a factor in the frequency of transmission by breast-feeding.[12]

CLINICAL MANIFESTATIONS

General

HIV-infected infants usually are asymptomatic during the first few months of life. Although the mean age of onset of symptoms is

TABLE 114–1 1993 Revised Case Definition of AIDS-Defining Conditions for Adults and Adolescents 13 Years of Age and Older

Candidiasis of bronchi, trachea, or lungs
Candidiasis, esophageal
Cervical cancer, invasive
Coccidioidomycosis, disseminated or extrapulmonary
Cryptococcosis, extrapulmonary
Cryptosporidiosis, chronic intestinal (>1 mo duration)
Cytomegalovirus disease (other than liver, spleen, or nodes)
Cytomegalovirus retinitis (with loss of vision)
Encephalopathy, HIV-related
Herpes simplex: chronic ulcer(s) (>1 mo duration); or bronchitis, pneumonitis, or esophagitis
Histoplasmosis, disseminated or extrapulmonary
Isosporiasis, chronic intestinal (>1 mo duration)
Kaposi's sarcoma
Lymphoma, Burkitt's (or equivalent term)
Lymphoma, immunoblastic (or equivalent term)
Lymphoma, primary or brain
Mycobacterium avium complex or *M. kansasii*, disseminated or extrapulmonary
Mycobacterium tuberculosis, any site (pulmonary or extrapulmonary)
Mycobacterium, other species or unidentified species, disseminated or extrapulmonary
Pneumocystis carinii pneumonia
Pneumonia, recurrent
Progressive multifocal leukoencephalopathy
Salmonella septicemia, recurrent
Toxoplasmosis of brain
Wasting syndrome due to HIV
CD4$^+$ T-lymphocyte count less than 200 cells/μl or CD4$^+$ percentage <15%

Abbreviations: AIDS, Acquired immundeficiency syndrome; HIV, human immunodeficiency virus.
Modified from Centers for Disease Control and Prevention. 1993 Revised classification system for HIV infection and expanded surveillance definition for AIDS among adolescents and adults. MMWR Morb Mortal Wkly Rep. 1992;41:(RR–17):1–19.

estimated to be about 1 year for perinatally infected infants, increasing numbers of children are remaining asymptomatic for more than 5 years.[27–32] Two categories of infection based on the incubation period and progression of symptoms have been recognized. Approximately 10 to 15% of children die before 4 years of age, most of whom succumb before 18 months of age, whereas the majority of children survive beyond 5 years of age.[27–37]

HIV infection in children causes a varied clinical course. AIDS represents the most severe end of the clinical spectrum, as is the case with adult AIDS infection. The current surveillance definitions of the Centers for Disease Control and Prevention for AIDS in adults and adolescents and the Centers for Disease Control and Prevention pediatric classification system for children younger than 13 years who are born to HIV-infected mothers or who are known to be infected with HIV are given in Tables 114–1 and 114–2, respectively. Although the pediatric classification system was established for surveillance of HIV infection, its clinical categories (Table 114–3) are used to help define progression of the disease.[38]

The manifestations of pediatric HIV infection include generalized lymphadenopathy, hepatomegaly, splenomegaly, failure to thrive, oral candidiasis, recurrent diarrhea, parotitis, cardiomyopathy, hepatitis, nephropathy, central nervous system disease (including developmental delay, which can be progressive), lymphoid interstitial pneumonia, recurrent invasive bacterial infections (*Streptococcus pneumoniae, Haemophilus influenzae,* and *Salmonella* spp.), opportunistic infections, and specified malignancies.[17, 39, 40]

Pneumocystis carinii pneumonia (PCP) is the most common, serious opportunistic infection in children with HIV infection and is associated with a high mortality.[11, 41–44] PCP occurs most frequently in infants between 3 and 6 months of age who acquired the infection before or at birth, but it can occur in younger infants, beginning as early as 4 to 6 weeks.[44] Infants and children characteristically develop a subacute, diffuse pneumonitis with dyspnea at rest, tachypnea, oxygen desaturation, nonproductive cough, and fever.[44] However, the magnitude of these signs may vary. The chest roentgenogram often has bilateral diffuse interstitial disease; rarely, lobar, miliary, and nodular lesions occur as well. Occasionally, the chest roentgenogram at the time of diagnosis appears normal. Mortality in immunocompromised patients is high, ranging from 5 to 40% if treated, and close to 100% if untreated.[39, 40, 44]

Other common opportunistic infections in children include *Candida* esophagitis, disseminated cytomegalovirus infection, and chronic or disseminated herpes simplex and varicella-zoster virus infections. Infections with *Mycobacterium tuberculosis* or *Mycobacterium avium* complex, chronic enteritis caused by *Cryptosporidium* or other agents, and disseminated or central nervous system cryptococcal or *Toxoplasma gondii* infections are distinctly less common in children than in adults (≤14% *M. avium* and ≤1% *Cryptococcus* infections in children compared with 18 to 36% and 5 to 15% in adults, respectively).[17, 40, 45, 45a, 46]

The development of opportunistic infections, particularly PCP, progressive neurologic disease, and severe wasting is associated with a poor prognosis.[17, 27, 29, 39] The prognosis for survival is also poor in children infected perinatally in whom virus is detected early (i.e., by 7 days of life) and in those who become symptomatic in the first year of life.[17a, 27–33, 35–37] With earlier and more effective treatment, survival is likely to improve.

Differences between the Clinical Manifestations of Pediatric and Adult HIV Infection

Although many aspects of adult HIV infection apply to children, a number of presentations of clinical syndromes are unique to children. The overall progression of illness in young children is more rapid than that of adults, perhaps because of the relative immaturity of the child's immune system, and end organs (e.g., undermyelinated central

TABLE 114–2 Pediatric HIV Classification for Children Younger than 13 Years

Immunologic Definitions	Immunologic Categories: Age-Specific, CD4+ T-Lymphocyte Count and Percentage of Total Lymphocytes						Clinical Classifications*			
	<12 mo		*1–5 yr*		*6–12 hr*		*N: No Signs or Symptoms*	*A: Mild Signs or Symptoms*	*B: Moderate Signs or Symptoms†*	*C: Severe Signs or Symptoms†*
	Cells/μl	*%*	*Cells/μl*	*%*	*Cells/μl*	*%*				
1: No evidence of suppression	≥1500	≥25	≥1000	≥25	≥500	≥25	N1	A1	B1	C1
2: Evidence of moderate suppression	750–1499	15–24	500–999	15–24	200–499	15–24	N2	A2	B2	C2
3: Severe suppression	<750	<15	<500	<15	<200	<15	N3	A3	B3	C3

*Children whose HIV infection status is not confirmed are classified by using this grid with a letter E (for perinatally exposed) placed before the appropriate classification code (e.g., EN2).
†Lymphoid interstitial pneumonitis in category B or category C is reportable to state and local health departments as AIDS (see Table 114–3 for further definition of clinical categories).
Abbreviations: AIDS, Acquired immunodeficiency syndrome; HIV, human immunodeficiency virus.
Modified from Centers for Disease Control and Prevention. 1994 revised classification system for HIV infection in children less than 13 years of age; official authorized addenda: Human immunodeficiency virus infection codes and official guidelines for coding and reporting ICD-9-CM. MMWR Morb Mortal Wkly Rep. 1994;43(RR-12), 1–19.

TABLE 114–3 Clinical Categories for Children Younger than 13 Years with HIV Infection

Category N: Not Symptomatic

Children who have no signs or symptoms considered to be the result of human immunodeficiency virus (HIV) infection or have only one of the conditions listed in category A

Category A: Mildly Symptomatic

Children with two or more of the conditions listed below but none of the conditions listed in categories B and C
- Lymphadenopathy (≥0.5 cm at more than two sites; bilateral = one site)
- Hepatomegaly
- Splenomegaly
- Dermatitis
- Parotitis
- Recurrent or persistent upper respiratory tract infection, sinusitis, or otitis media

Category B: Moderately Symptomatic

Children who have symptomatic conditions other than those listed for category A or C that are attributed to HIV infection. Examples of conditions in clinical category B include but are not limited to
- Anemia (<8 g/dl), neutropenia (<1000/mm^3), or thrombocytopenia (<100,000/mm^3) persisting ≥30 d
- Bacterial meningitis, pneumonia, or sepsis (single episode)
- Candidiasis, oropharyngeal (thrush), persisting (>2 mo) in children ≥6 mo of age
- Cardiomyopathy
- Cytomegalovirus infection, with onset before 1 mo of age
- Diarrhea, recurrent or chronic
- Hepatitis
- Herpes simplex virus (HSV) stomatitis, recurrent (more than two episodes within 1 yr)
- HSV bronchitis, pneumonitis, or esophagitis with onset before 1 mo of age
- Herpes zoster (shingles) involving at least two distinct episodes or more than 1 dermatome
- Leiomyosarcoma
- Lymphoid interstitial pneumonia or pulmonary lymphoid hyperplasia complex
- Nephropathy
- Nocardiosis
- Persistent fever (lasting >1 mo)
- Toxoplasmosis, onset before 1 mo of age
- Varicella, disseminated (complicated chickenpox)

Category C: Severely Symptomatic

- Serious bacterial infections, multiple or recurrent (i.e., any combination of at least two culture-confirmed infections within a 2-yr period), of the following types: septicemia, pneumonia, meningitis, bone or joint infection, or abscess of an internal organ or body cavity (excluding otitis media, superficial skin or mucosal abscesses, and indwelling catheter-related infections)
- Candidiasis, esophageal or pulmonary (bronchi, traceha, lungs)
- Coccidioidomycosis, disseminated (at site other than or in addition to lungs or cervical or hilar lymph nodes)
- Cryptococcosis, extrapulmonary
- Cryptosporidiosis or isosporiasis with diarrhea persisting >1 mo
- Cytomegalovirus disease with onset of symptoms at age >1 mo (at a site other than liver, spleen, or lymph nodes)
- Encephalopathy (at least one of the following progressive findings present for at least 2 mo in the absence of a concurrent illness other than HIV infection that could explain the findings): (1) failure to attain or loss of developmental milestones or loss of intellectual ability, verified by standard developmental scale or neuropsychological tests; (2) impaired brain growth or acquired microcephaly demonstrated by head circumference measurements or brain atrophy demonstrated by computed tomography or magnetic resonance imaging (serial imaging is required for children <2 yr of age); (3) acquired symmetric motor deficit manifested by two or more of the following: paresis, pathologic reflexes, ataxia, or gait disturbance
- Herpes simplex viral infection causing a mucocutaneous ulcer that persists for >1 mo; or bronchitis, pneumonitis, or esophagitis for any duration affecting a child >1 mo of age
- Histoplasmosis, disseminated (at a site other than or in addition to lungs or cervical or hilar lymph nodes)
- Kaposi's sarcoma
- Lymphoma, primary, in brain
- Lymphoma, small, noncleaved cell (Burkitt's), or immunoblastic, or large cell lymphoma of B-cell or unknown immunologic phenotype
- *Mycobacterium tuberculosis*, disseminated or extrapulmonary
- *Mycobacterium*, other species or unidentified species, disseminated (at a site other than or in addition to lungs, skin or cervical or hilar lymph nodes)
- *Pneumocystis carinii* pneumonia
- Progressive multifocal leukoencephalopathy
- *Salmonella* (nontyphoid) septicemia, recurrent
- Toxoplasmosis of the brain with onset at >1 mo of age
- Wasting syndrome in the absence of a concurrent illness other than HIV infection that could explain the following findings: (1) persistent weight loss >10% of baseline *or* (2) downward crossing of at least two of the following percentile lines on the weight-for-age chart (e.g., 95th, 75th, 50th, 25th, 5th) in a child ≥1 yr of age *or* (3) <5th percentile on weight-for-height chart on two consecutive measurements, ≥30 d apart *plus* (1) chronic diarrhea (i.e., at least two loose stools per day for ≥30 d) *or* (2) documented fever (for ≥30 d, intermittent or constant)

Modified from Centers for Disease Control and Prevention. 1994 revised classification system for HIV infection in children less than 13 years of age; official authorized addenda: human immunodeficiency virus infection codes and official guidelines for coding and reporting ICD-9-CM. MMWR Morb Mortal Wkly Rep. 1994;43(RR–12):1–19.

nervous system), and the expansion of target cells (e.g., a functioning thymus and greater CD4$^+$ cell counts than in adults).[40]

Recurrent invasive bacterial infections historically are more prominent in pediatric HIV infection than in adult HIV infection, although such infections may decline with the use of antiretrovirals and trimethoprim-sulfamethoxazole for prophylaxis against PCP.[47, 48] Rates of invasive pneumococcal infection among HIV-infected children were three times those of controls in one study[47]; in another study, pneumococcal infection rates among HIV-infected children approached 100 to 300 times those of non–HIV-infected controls.[48]

Pulmonary complications of pediatric HIV infection are notable for the frequency of lymphocytic interstitial pneumonitis, a chronic lymphoproliferative disorder affecting 30 to 40% of children but rarely adults.[49, 50] Lymphocytic interstitial pneumonitis is characterized by diffuse infiltration of the alveoli and small airways by lymphocytes and plasma cells. Clinically, the child may have a nonproductive cough and the insidious onset of hypoxia, bronchiectasis, and pulmonary decompensation during otherwise minor upper or lower respiratory tract infections; some children exhibit clubbing of the digits.[49, 50] Radiographs show interstitial infiltrates and reticulonodular patterns easily confused with tuberculosis or PCP. Lymphocytic interstitial pneumonitis has responded to both antiretroviral therapy and corticosteroids.[49, 50] The cause of lymphocytic interstitial pneumonitis is unclear, although it is speculated that an exaggerated local response to Epstein-Barr virus or HIV, or both, may be causative.[49, 50] Lymphocytic interstitial pneumonitis, although contained within clinical category B, is nevertheless an A105-defining condition (see Tables 114–2 and 114–3).

Central nervous system complications in pediatric HIV infection are frequent, and encephalopathy is an AIDS-defining condition (see Table 114–3). In the early years of the epidemic, 50 to 60% of children with advanced HIV infection exhibited progressive encephalopathy; more recent estimates from cohorts of children including asymptomatic, mildly symptomatic, and symptomatic children range from 20 to 40%. Pediatric HIV encephalopathy is manifested as either a progressive form characterized by impaired brain growth, acquired microcephaly, progressive motor dysfunction, and loss of developmental milestones; or a static form in which children acquire skills and abilities at a continued but subnormal rate, with varied degrees of motor involvement.[51–53] A middle "plateau" form has also been described, with retention of previously acquired developmental milestones but no further development after some point in time.[52] Pure dementia is more commonly seen in adults, not children. A delay in early language development may be seen in the absence of other abnormalities.[54] Neuroimaging findings in pediatric HIV encephalopathy commonly include variable degrees of cerebral atrophy and bilateral symmetric calcification of the basal ganglia and frontal white matter.[52, 55, 56]

Chronic diarrhea, wasting, and gastrointestinal *Candida* infections are common in both adults and children infected with HIV. Failure to thrive is nearly universal in HIV-infected children; severe wasting is an AIDS-defining condition (see Table 114–3). Reductions in both growth and lean body mass appear early, although the pathogenetic basis is not known.[39, 57–60] A reduction in food intake, increased metabolic needs, and impaired nutrient absorption may all play a role.[57–60] Gastrostomy tube supplementation has been shown to be useful in improving weight and fat mass[61]; the role of other therapies such as megestrol, tetrahydrocannabinol, or human growth hormone is uncertain.[39, 62] Esophagitis from *Candida,* cytomegalovirus, or herpes simplex virus occurs in children as in adults, as does bacterial enteritis and to a lesser extent, cryptosporidiosis, aphthous ulcers, and pancreatitis.[57, 63]

Cardiologic manifestations of HIV infection in children have been recognized.[40, 64] Although generally not clinically significant, left ventricular dysfunction and dilated cardiomyopathy are detected frequently by echocardiography and possibly may be related to the occurrence of congestive heart failure and arrhythmias and sudden cardiorespiratory arrests.[65, 66] Cardiomyopathy appears to be associated with HIV encephalopathy.[53, 67] A large ongoing pediatric study has been designed to understand the clinical role of cardiologic manifestations of pediatric HIV infection.[68]

The kidney is also affected by HIV infection, in both adults and children.[69–71] Both glomerulonephropathy and tubular lesions are noted.[69–71]

Hematologic complications such as leukopenia, anemia, and thrombocytopenia occur in both children and adults infected with HIV.[72] Circulating antineutrophil antibodies are common but do not appear to cause neutropenia.[73] Newborns may be more susceptible to bone marrow suppression by antiretroviral agents than adults and older children.[74]

Malignancies in pediatric HIV infection have been relatively uncommon, but leiomyosarcomas and certain lymphomas, including those of the central nervous system and non-Hodgkin's B-cell lymphomas of the Burkitt's type, occur much more frequently in children with HIV infection than in nonimmunocompromised children.[75–78]

A number of complications commonly seen in adult HIV infection occur only rarely in children; these include cerebral toxoplasmosis, cryptococcal meningitis and pneumonia, progressive multifocal leukoencephalopathy, all forms of Kaposi's sarcoma, bacillary angiomatosis, cytomegalovirus retinitis, and hypersensitivity to trimethoprim-sulfamethoxazole.[39, 40, 44, 52] Peripheral neuropathy and myopathy appears to be rarer in children than adults, although symptoms may be missed in preverbal children.[52]

LABORATORY FINDINGS

The most notable finding, particularly as the disease progresses, is an increasing loss of cell-mediated immunity, similar to that in adult HIV infection.[79] The peripheral blood lymphocyte count initially can be normal, but eventually lymphopenia develops because of a decrease in the total number of circulating T lymphocytes. The cells most affected are the $CD4^+$ helper T lymphocytes. The $CD8^+$ suppressor T lymphocytes usually increase in number initially and are not depleted until late in the course of the infection. These changes in cell populations result in a decrease of the normal $CD4^+$/$CD8^+$ cell ratio. The normal values for peripheral $CD4^+$ T-lymphocyte counts and percentages are distinctly different from those of adults and are directly related to age.[38, 80, 81] The lower limits of normal values for children are given in Table 114–2. Responses of T lymphocytes to plant lectin mitogens (phytohemagglutinin, concanavalin A, and particularly pokeweed) are decreased or absent, and HIV-infected children may be anergic to skin test antigens such as mumps, *Candida, Trichophyton,* tetanus, and tuberculin (purified protein derivative), as are HIV-infected adults.[40, 79]

Although B-lymphocyte numbers remain normal or are somewhat increased, humoral immune dysfunction accompanies cellular dysfunction. Serum immunoglobulin concentrations, particularly IgG and IgA, frequently are elevated in HIV-infected children, and have been used as surrogate diagnostic markers for pediatric HIV infection.[82] Some children develop panhypogammaglobulinemia. Specific antibody responses to antigens to which the patient has not previously been exposed can be abnormal.[40, 79]

Circulating concentrations of virus (viral load) in children younger than 12 months are very high (mean of approximately 200,000 RNA copies/ml).[83–85] By 24 months of age, viral concentrations decrease (to a mean of approximately 40,000 RNA copies/ml). Data suggest that plasma viral concentration determinations in conjunction with the $CD4^+$ cell count determinations are more accurate predictors than each marker alone of the prognosis and of survival.[84, 85, 85a] However, there appears to be considerable overlap in RNA levels in infants and children with or without rapid disease progression, making RNA levels less predictive than in adults.[83, 84] In general, high levels of HIV RNA (>300,000 copies/ml in infants younger than 12 months and >100,000 in young children) are associated with higher long-term risk for death, especially if the $CD4^+$ T-lymphocyte percentage is less than 15%.[84] The predictive quartiles of baseline HIV RNA associated with risks for disease progression or death in children are much wider than those reported in adult studies.[85]

The diurnal variation in HIV RNA levels appears to be greater in infants and young children also, such that only fivefold or greater (0.7 $\log_{10}$) changes may be significant in children younger than 2 years (as opposed to a threefold [0.5 $\log_{10}$] or greater changes in older children and adults).[86, 87]

DIAGNOSTIC TESTS

Diagnosis of pediatric HIV infection is usually made by serum antibody tests except in children younger than 18 months, in whom passively acquired maternal antibody may be present.[40] Other than infants born of infected mothers, children infected with HIV usually develop serum antibody to HIV by 6 to 12 weeks after infection, as do adults.

Enzyme immunoassays (EIAs) are used most widely to screen for serum HIV antibody. These tests are highly sensitive and specific, but false-positive results occur in a small percentage of cases. Repeat EIA testing of initially reactive specimens is required to reduce the likelihood of laboratory error; repeatedly reactive tests are highly reliable. Western blot or immunofluorescent antibody tests should be used for confirmation. A positive HIV-antibody test in a child 18 months of age or older usually is indicative of infection.[14, 38] Serum antibodies to HIV are present eventually in virtually all infected children. Occasional children with HIV infection may lack HIV antibody because they have hypogammaglobulinemia or may be unable to produce antibody if they have advanced disease.[82]

Diagnosis in Infants Born to HIV-Seropositive Women

Infants born to HIV-seropositive women (Table 114–4) pose a special diagnostic challenge since they are almost always seropositive at birth, whether or not they are infected, as a result of the transplacental acquisition of maternal antibody, which can be detectable in the infant for as long as 18 months after birth. Thus, IgG antibody tests for HIV are not useful for diagnosis in the child younger than 18 months. The preferred tests are HIV culture and the detection of HIV by using the polymerase chain reaction (PCR), which are the most sensitive and specific tests to detect HIV infection in children born to HIV-infected mothers.[14, 38, 82, 86]

Using these assays (culture or PCR), only approximately 30 to 50% of infected newborns are diagnosed at birth, but nearly 100% of infected infants can be diagnosed by 4 to 6 months of age.[88–91] For an infant born to an HIV-seropositive mother, an initial diagnostic assay of PCR or viral culture should be performed by approximately 1 month of age or as soon as possible thereafter.[14] It is possible that earlier testing (at 48 hours and 14 days of life) may be advantageous for early detection and therapy of infection.[86] If the assay is negative, testing between 4 and 6 months of age should be repeated. A positive HIV culture, PCR, or p24-antigen detection assay constitutes presumptive evidence of HIV infection, and a second diagnostic test should be performed subsequently using either the same assay or one of the other two assays, to confirm the diagnosis. The modified (i.e., after acid dissociation) p24-antigen assay is less sensitive than viral culture or PCR and should be used only if the other tests are not available.[14, 38, 90] If an infant younger than 18 months who has a positive serologic test for HIV develops an AIDS-defining illness (category C; see Table 114–3), the diagnosis of HIV infection is established even if virologic tests are negative.

The child who has two negative virologic tests, both of which are performed at 1 month of age or more and one of which is performed at 4 months of age or more, is considered to have had HIV infection reasonably excluded in the absence of any clinical illness.[14, 41] Follow-up serologic tests should be performed to confirm exclusion of HIV infection and seroreversion. Such tests include either two negative EIA tests performed between 6 and 18 months of age or one negative EIA test at more than 18 months of age.[14, 41] Some experts recommend that the final EIA test be performed at 24 months of age.

TABLE 114–4 Diagnosis of HIV Infection in Children Younger than 13 Years

Diagnosis: HIV Infected
Child <18 mo who
Is known to be HIV-seropositive or born to an HIV-infected mother and has positive results on two separate determinations* (excluding cord blood) from one or more of the following HIV detection tests:
HIV culture
HIV polymerase chain reaction
HIV antigen (p24)
or
Meets criteria for AIDS diagnosis based on 1987 AIDS surveillance case definition†
Child ≥18 mo of age born to an HIV-infected mother or any child infected by blood, blood products, or other known modes of transmission (e.g., sexual contact) who
Is HIV-antibody-positive by repeatedly reactive EIA and confirmatory test (e.g., Western blot or IFA)
or
Meets any of the criteria above
Diagnosis: Perinatally Exposed (Prefix E‡)
Child who does not meet the criteria above who
Is HIV-seropositive by EIA and confirmatory test (e.g., Western blot or IFA) and is <18 mo of age at time of test
or
Has unknown antibody status, but was born to a mother known to be infected with HIV
Diagnosis: Seroreverter
Child who is born to an HIV-infected mother and who
Has been documented as HIV-antibody-negative (i.e., two or more negative EIA tests performed at 6–18 mo of age or one negative EIA test after 18 mo of age)
and
Has had no other laboratory evidence of infection (has not had two positive viral detection tests, if performed)
and
Has not had an AIDS-defining condition

*Both determinations performed at or beyond 1 month of age and at least one determination at or beyond 4 months of age.
†Centers for Disease Control. Revision of the CDC surveillance case definition for acquired immunodeficiency syndrome. MMWR Morb Mortal Wkly Rep. 1987;36 (Supp 11):1S–15S. See Tables 114–2 and 114–3.
‡See Table 114–2.
Abbreviations: AIDS, Acquired immunodeficiency syndrome; EIA, enzyme immunoassay; HIV, human immunodeficiency virus; IFA, immunofluorescence assay.
Modified from Centers for Disease Control and Prevention. 1994 revised classification system for HIV infection in children less than 13 years of age; official authorized addenda: human immunodeficiency virus infection codes and official guidelines for coding and reporting ICD-9-CM. MMWR Morb Mortal Wkly Rep. 1994;43(RR–12):1–19.

Perinatal HIV Serologic Testing

The American Academy of Pediatrics has published recommendations that state that, on the basis of advances in therapy to reduce the rate of perinatal HIV transmission and the continued occurrence of life-threatening illness in young infants with unrecognized HIV infection, documented, routine HIV education and routine testing with consent for all pregnant women in the United States should be carried out.[14] Documented consent for maternal or newborn HIV testing, or both, may be obtained in a variety of ways, including by right of refusal (documented patient education, with testing to take place unless rejected in writing by the patient). In addition, it is recommended that routine education about HIV infection and testing become part of a comprehensive program of health care for women, particularly for women of childbearing age, and that all testing programs for the detection of HIV infection evaluate periodically the proportion of women who refuse HIV testing after HIV education. Those programs in which a proportionately low number of women receive HIV testing should examine the reasons for poor acceptance, with appropriate program modifications made as needed. For women who are seen by a health care professional for the first time in labor and who either have not received prenatal care or have previously tested negative but have not been tested for HIV infection during the current pregnancy, education about HIV infection and maternal HIV testing are recommended during the perinatal period. For newborns whose mothers' HIV serostatus was not determined during the recent pregnancy or the postpartum period, the infant's health care provider should educate the mother concerning the potential benefits of HIV testing for her infant, and the possible risks and benefits to herself of knowing the child's serostatus; and then recommend HIV testing for the newborn. Finally, the health care provider for the infant needs to be informed of the maternal HIV serostatus so that appropriate care and testing of the infant can be accomplished. Similarly, if the infant is found to be seropositive when the maternal serostatus is unknown, the health care provider for the child should ensure that information about the serostatus and its significance be provided to the mother and, with her consent, to her health care provider. The mother should receive appropriate referral to adult HIV-relater services. Some state health departments (e.g., New York) now mandate HIV testing with consent of pregnant women, as well as routine HIV testing of all newborns, as the standard of care.

Informed Consent for HIV Serologic Testing

Testing for HIV infection is unlike most routine blood testing in that substantial psychosocial risks can be incurred.[14] Before testing an infant or child, the parents or other primary caregivers, and the patient, if old enough to comprehend, should be counseled about the possible risks and benefits of testing and the consequences of HIV infection. Oral consent should be obtained from the parent or legal guardian and recorded in the patient's chart. Special written consent procedures for HIV testing should be discouraged as they can inhibit the performance of testing without adding significant benefit. State and local laws and hospital regulations, nevertheless, should be considered in deciding whether written consent is required. The necessity for counseling and consent should not deter efforts to undertake appropriate diagnostic testing for HIV infection. The parents' or patients' refusal to give consent does not relieve physicians of the professional and legal responsibilities to their patients. If the physician believes that testing is essential to the child's health, authorization for testing needs to be obtained by other means (e.g., court order). The results of serologic tests should be discussed in person with the family, primary caregiver, and, if appropriate according to age, the patient; if positive, appropriate counseling and subsequent follow-up care must be provided. Maintaining confidentiality in all cases is essential to preserving the patients' and parents' trust and consent.

TREATMENT

Table 114–5 provides a list of currently available antiretroviral drugs and their recommended dosages for children (updated versions can be obtained via the internet: http://www.hivatis.org).[14, 86] Primary care physicians are encouraged to participate actively in the care of HIV-infected patients in consultation with specialists who have expertise in the treatment of pediatric HIV infection. Expert opinions and knowledge about diagnostic and therapeutic strategies are changing rapidly. In areas of the United States in which enrollment into clinical trials is possible, enrollment of the HIV-infected child into available clinical trials should be encouraged. Information about trials for adolescents and children can be obtained by calling the Pediatric AIDS Clinical Trials Group (PACTG; 800-TRIALS-A).

An increasing number of studies are examining the pharmacokinetics of antiretrovirals in infants, children, and adolescents since drug distribution may differ from that of adults. Many experts feel that dosage for medications for adolescents should be prescribed according to Tanner's staging of puberty besides age.[86] Adolescents in early puberty (i.e., Tanner stages I and II) would be administered doses using the pediatric schedules given in Table 114–5, whereas those in late puberty (Tanner stage V) may require adult dosing schedules.[87] Adolescents in their growth spurt (Tanner stages III and IV) may require dose modification to ensure efficacy and minimize toxicity.[86]

Adherence to complex drug regimens may be especially difficult for children who depend on others for the administration of medication. In addition, not all necessary antiretroviral medications for the prevention of opportunistic infections are available as palatable liquids suitable for administration to infants and children. Other barriers, such as variable absorption of medicines by infants who require frequent feeding, difficulty in providing midday doses if the child is at school, and the reluctance of parents to have antiretroviral medication at home while maintaining secrecy, can all act to reduce compliance. Adolescents may have further challenges because of developmental issues such as not wanting to be different from peers, not understanding why medications are required during asymptomatic

TABLE 114–5 Dosage and Administration of Antiretroviral Drugs for Children

Drug Name [Trade Name]	Available Preparations	Recommended Dosage*
Zidovudine (ZDV, AZT, azidothymidine) [Retrovir]	100-mg capsules 300-mg tablets 10-mg/ml syrup (Combivir = 300 mg ZDV and 150 mg 3TC)	0–6 wk: 2 mg/kg/dose q6h 4 wk–13 yr: 160 mg/m²/dose q8h (range 90–180 mg/m²/dose q6h–q8h) ≥13 yr: 200 mg q8h or 300 mg q12h
Didanosine (ddI, dideoxyinosine) [Videx]	25-, 50-, 100-, 150-mg chewable tablets 100-, 167-, 250-mg buffered powder 10-mg/ml pediatric solution	<13 yr: 90 mg/m²/dose q12h (90–150 mg/m²/dose q12h) ≥13 yr: <60 kg: tablets, 125 mg q12h buffered powder, 167 mg q12h ≥60 kg: tablets, 200 mg q12h buffered powder, 250 mg q12h
Zalcitabine (ddC, dideoxycytidine) [Hivid]	0.375-, 0.75-mg tablets	<13 yr: 0.01 mg/kg/dose q8h ≥13 yr: 0.75 mg q8h
Stavudine (d4T) [Zerit]	15-, 20-, 30-, 40-mg capsules	<13 yr: 1 mg/kg/dose q12h ≥13 yr: 30–40 mg q12h
Lamivudine (3TC) [Epivir]	150-mg tablets 10-mg/ml syrup (Combivir = 300 mg ZDV and 150 mg 3TC)	3 mo–12 yr: 4 mg/kg/dose q12h ≥12 yr: 150 mg q12h
Abacavir (1592U89) [Ziagen]	300–mg tablets 10–mg/ml syrup	<13 yr: 8 mg/kg/dose q12h ≥13 yr: 300 mg q12h
Nevirapine (NVP) [Viramune]	200-mg tablets 10–mg/ml syrup	<13 yr: Unknown; 120–200 mg/m²/dose q12h under study by PACTG ≥13 yr: 200 mg q12h (dose escalation lead-in period reduces complications at all ages)
Delvaridine (DLV) [Rescriptor]	100-mg tablets	<13 yr: Unknown ≥13 yr: 400 mg q8h
Efavirenz (DMP266) [Sustiva]	50-, 100-, 200-mg tablets	<13 yr: 200–400 mg q24h depending on body weight (see package insert) ≥13 yr: 600 mg q24h
Saquinavir (SQV) [Invirase, Fortovase]	Invirase: 200-mg hard gel capsules Fortovase: 200-mg soft gel capsules	<13 yr: Unknown ≥13 yr: 600 mg of Invirase q8h or 1200 mg of Fortovase q8h
Indinavir (IDV) [Crixivan]	200-, 400-mg capsules	<13 yr: Unknown; 350–500 mg/m²/dose q8h under study by PACTG ≥13 yr: 800 mg q8h
Ritonavir (RTV) [Norvir]	100-mg capsules 80-mg/ml elixir	<13 yr: 350–400 mg/m²/dose q12h ≥13 yr: 600 mg q12h (dose escalation lead-in period reduces complications at all ages)
Nelfinavir (NFV) [Viracept]	50-mg/level scoop powder 250-mg tablets	<13 yr: 20–30 mg/kg/dose q8h ≥13 yr: 750 mg q8h

*All dosages listed are by mouth. Dosages listed do not include those for newborns (see guidelines cited).
Abbreviation: PACTG, Pediatric AIDS Clinical Trials Group.
Modified from American Academy of Pediatrics. 1997 Red Book: Report of the Committee on Infectious Diseases. 24th ed. Elk Grove Village, Ill: American Academy of Pediatrics, 1997; and Centers for Disease Control and Prevention. Guidelines for the use of antiretroviral agents in pediatric infection. MMWR Morb Mortal Wkly Rep. 1998;47(RR–4):1–43 http://www.hivatis.org.

periods, and social issues such as a lack of family support, distrust of the medical establishment, and denial and fear of HIV infection. All these issues need to be addressed if medications are to be prescribed for children and adolescents.[86]

Although fewer data are available from pediatric controlled trials, antiretroviral therapy has become the standard of care for HIV-infected children as it is in adults. Substantial improvements in neurodevelopment, growth, immunologic status, and virologic status have been demonstrated in studies of zidovudine (ZDV), didanosine (ddI), lamivudine, and stavudine monotherapy[92–97]; therapy with two nucleoside reverse transcriptase inhibitors (NRTIs)[98, 99]; and combination therapy with one or two NRTIs plus a protease inhibitor or two NRTIs plus the non-nucleoside reverse transcriptase inhibitor nevirapine.[100–105] The results of PACTG study 152 showed that the combination of ZDV and ddI was more effective than ZDV or ddI therapy alone (although ddI alone had some beneficial effects in children older than 3 years).[99] Subsequently, the results from PACTG study 300 showed that combination therapy with ZDV plus lamivudine or ZDV plus ddI, was superior to ddI alone when analyzed by either clinical or virologic end points.[98] Preliminary data from PACTG study 338 has shown that combination therapy including a protease inhibitor is more effective in suppressing viral replication than is dual NRTI therapy.[101] Finally, a preliminary study of aggressive early therapy of HIV-infected infants aged 2 to 3 months administered ZDV, ddI, and an investigational nevirapine syrup reported impressive viral suppression.[102] On the basis of these data and on extrapolations from adult studies (see Chapter 115), the Working Group on Antiretroviral Therapy and Medical Management of HIV-Infected Children has formulated guidelines for the use of antiretroviral agents in pediatric infection[86] as a companion to those recently published for adults and adolescents.[87] A synopsis of these guidelines is in Tables 114–6 through 114–8; the guidelines should be consulted for details of the choice of medication, the dosage for young infants, the timing of the initiation of therapy, and factors indicating a change in therapy.[86, 87, 106] Adverse effects of antiretroviral medications in children are similar to those experienced by adults, in general.[86, 87]

Other new antiretroviral drugs, immunomodulators, and vaccines for therapeutic use are under evaluation. Further information on therapeutic trials in HIV-infected children can be obtained from the PACTG.

The value of intravenous immune globulin (IGIV) in children with HIV infection has been evaluated in several trials. IGIV therapy in combination with antiviral agents may be given for children with humoral immunodeficiency including (1) children with hypogammaglobulinemia (IgG level <250 mg/dl); (2) children with recurrent, serious bacterial infections (defined as two or more serious bacterial infections such as bacteremia, meningitis, or pneumonia in a 1-year period); (3) children who fail to form antibodies to common antigens; and (4) children living in areas where measles is highly prevalent who have not developed an antibody response after two doses (1 month or more apart) of measles-mumps-rubella (MMR) vaccine.[14] The dose of IGIV is 400 mg/kg per dose given every 4 weeks. Intravenous immune globulin may also be useful in the treatment of HIV-associated thrombocytopenia in a dose of 500 to 1000 mg/kg per day for 3 to 5 days.[14] In addition, children with bronchiectasis despite treatment with the standard medical regimen of cyclic antibiotics and aggressive respiratory therapy may benefit from adjunctive IGIV therapy at 600 mg/kg per dose, given monthly.[14]

TABLE 114–6 Indications for Initiation of Antiretroviral Therapy in Children with HIV Infection

Clinical symptoms associated with HIV infection (i.e., clinical categories A, B, or C in Table 114–3)
Evidence of immune suppression, indicated by CD4+ T-lymphocyte absolute number or percentage (i.e., immune category 2 or 3 in Table 114–2)
Age <12 mo—regardless of clinical, immunologic, or virologic status.
For asymptomatic children aged ≥1 yr with normal immune status, two options can be considered:
- Preferred approach
  - Initiate therapy—regardless of age or symptom status
- Alternative approach
  - Defer treatment in situations in which the risk for clinical disease progression is low and other factors (e.g., concern for the durability of response, safety, and adherence) favor postponing treatment. In such cases, the health care provider should regularly monitor virologic, immunologic, and clinical status. Factors to be considered in deciding to initiate therapy include the following:
    - High or increasing HIV RNA copy number
    - Rapidly declining CD4+ T-lymphocyte number or percentage to values approaching those indicative of moderate immune suppression (i.e., immune category 2 in Table 114–2)
    - Development of clinical symptoms

Abbreviation: HIV, Human immunodeficiency virus.
Modified from Centers for Disease Control and Prevention. Guidelines for the use of antiretroviral agents in pediatric infection. MMWR Morb Mortal Wkly Rep. 1998;47(RR–4):1–43.

TABLE 114–7 Recommended Antiretroviral Regimens for Initial Therapy for HIV Infection in Children

Preferred Regimen

Evidence of clinical benefit and sustained suppression of human immunodeficiency virus (HIV) RNA in clinical trials in HIV-infected adults; clinical trials in HIV-infected children are ongoing.
- One highly active protease inhibitor plus two nucleoside analogue reverse transcriptase inhibitors (NRTIs).
  - Preferred protease inhibitor for infants and children who cannot swallow pills or capsules: nelfinavir or ritonavir. Alternative for children who can swallow pills or capsules: indinavir.
  - Recommended dual NRTI combinations: the most data on use in children are available for the combinations of zidovudine (ZDV) and dideoxyinosine (ddI) and for ZDV and lamivudine (3TC). More limited data are available for the combinations of stavudine (d4T) and ddI; d4T and 3TC; and ZDV and zalcitabine (ddC).*
- Alternative for children who can swallow capsules: efavirenz plus 2NRTI; or efavirenz plus nelfinavir and 1NRTI

Alternative Regimen

Less likely to produce sustained HIV RNA suppression in infected adults; the combination of nevirapine, ZDV, and ddI produced substantial and sustained suppression of viral replication in two of six infants first treated at age <4 mo.†
- Nevirapine and two NRTIs

Secondary Alternative Regimen

Clinical benefit demonstrated in clinical trials involving infected adults and/or children, but initial viral suppression may not be sustained.
- Two NRTIs

Not Recommended

Evidence against use because of overlapping toxicity and/or because use may be virologically undesirable.
- Any monotherapy‡
- d4T and ZDV
- ddC and ddI
- ddC and d4T
- ddC and 3TC

*ddC is not available in a liquid preparation commercially, although a liquid formulation is available through a compassionate use program of the manufacturer (Hoffman-LaRoche Inc., Nutley, N.J.). ZDV and ddC is a less preferred choice for use in combination with a protease inhibitor.
†Source: Luzuriaga K, Bryson Y, Krogstad P, et al. Combination treatment with zidovudine, didanosine, and nevirapine in infants with human immunodeficiency virus type 1 infection. N Engl J Med. 1997;336:1343–1349.
‡Except for ZDV chemoprophylaxis administered to HIV-exposed infants during the first 6 weeks of life to prevent preinatal HIV transmission; if an infant is identified as HIV-infected while receiving ZDV prophylaxis, therapy should be changed to a combination antiretroviral drug regimen.
Modified from Centers for Disease Control and Prevention. Guidelines for the use of antiretroviral agents in pediatric infection. MMWR Morb Mortal Wkly Rep. 1998;47(RR–4):1–43.

Prophylaxis of Opportunistic Infections

Early diagnosis and aggressive treatment of opportunistic infections may prolong survival (see Chapter 115).[14, 42, 43] Prophylaxis against a first episode of PCP is indicated for most patients with significant immunocompromise including those with HIV infection and those with primary or acquired immunodeficiency, such as from chemotherapy or other immunosuppressive therapy. Lifelong chemoprophylaxis, regardless of the CD4+ T-lymphocyte count, is strongly recom-

TABLE 114–8 Considerations for Changing Antiretroviral Therapy for HIV-Infected Children

Virologic Considerations*

Less than a minimally acceptable virologic response after 8–12 wk of therapy. For children receiving antiretroviral therapy with two nucleoside analogue reverse transcriptase inhibitors (NRTIs) and a protease inhibitor, such a response is defined as a <10-fold (1.0 $\log_{10}$) decrease from baseline human immunodeficiency virus (HIV) RNA levels. For children who are receiving less potent antiretroviral therapy (i.e., dural NRTI combinations), an insufficient response is defined as a less than fivefold (0.7 $\log_{10}$) decrease in HIV RNA levels from baseline.

HIV RNA not suppressed to undetectable levels after 4–6 mo of antiretroviral therapy.†

Repeated detection of HIV RNA in children who initially responded to antiretroviral therapy with undetectable levels.‡

A reproducible increase in HIV RNA copy number among children who have had a substantial HIV RNA response but still have low levels of detectable HIV RNA. Such an increase would warrant change in therapy if, after initiation of the therapeutic regimen, a greater than threefold (0.5 $\log_{10}$) increase in copy number for children aged ≥2 yr and a greater than fivefold (0.7 $\log_{10}$) increase is observed for children aged <2 yr.

Immunologic Considerations*

Change in immunologic classification (Table 114–2)§

For children with CD4$^+$ T-lymphocyte percentages of <15% (i.e., those in immune category 3), a persistent decline of 5 percentiles or more in CD4$^+$ cell percentage (e.g., from 15 to 10%).

A rapid and substantial decrease in absolute CD4$^+$ T-lymphocyte count (e.g., a >30% decline in <6 mo).

Clinical Considerations

Progressive neurodevelopment deterioration.

Growth failure defined as persistent decline in weight-growth velocity despite adequate nutritional support and without other explanation.

Disease progression defined as advancement from one pediatric clinical category to another (e.g., from clinical category A to clinical category B).‖

*At least two measurements (taken 1 week apart) should be performed before considering a change in therapy.

†The initial HIV RNA level of the child at the start of therapy and the level achieved with therapy should be considered when contemplating potential drug changes. For example, an immediate change in therapy may not be warranted if there is a sustained 1.5 to 2.0 $\log_{10}$ decrease in HIV RNA copy number, even if RNA remains detectable at low levels.

‡More frequent evaluation of HIV RNA levels should be considered if the HIV RNA increase is limited (e.g., if when using an HIV RNA assay with a lower limit of detection of 1000 copies/ml, there is a 0.7 $\log_{10}$ increase from undetectable to approximately 5000 copies/ml in an infant aged <2 yr).

§Minimal changes in CD4$^+$ T-lymphocyte percentile that may result in a change in immunologic category (e.g., from 26 to 24%, or 16 to 14%) may not be as great a concern as a rapid substantial change in CD4$^+$ percentile within the same immunologic category (e.g., a drop from 35 to 25%).

‖In patients with stable immunologic and virologic parameters, progression from one clinical category to another may not represent an indication to change therapy. Thus, in patients whose disease progression is not associated with neurologic deterioration or growth failure, virologic and immunologic considerations are important in deciding whether to change therapy.

Modified from Centers for Disease Control and Prevention. Guidelines for the use of antiretroviral agents in pediatric infection. MMWR Morb Mortal Wkly Rep. 1998;47(RR–4):1–43. http://www.hivatis.org.

mended for any HIV-infected persons, including children of any age, who already have had an episode of PCP.

Because half of all cases of PCP in children with perinatally acquired HIV occur in infants 3 to 6 months of age, early identification of infants who have been perinatally exposed to HIV is essential so that prophylaxis can be initiated before they are at risk. The most effective means to implement this recommendation is by diagnosing maternal HIV infection before or during pregnancy. Prophylaxis for PCP is recommended for all infants born to HIV-infected women beginning at 4 to 6 weeks of age and regardless of the CD4$^+$ T-lymphocyte counts (see Table 114–9). Prophylaxis for PCP should be discontinued for children in whom HIV infection has been excluded. Children whose HIV infection status is not yet determined should continue prophylaxis throughout the first year of life.

Prophylaxis should be continued after 1 year of age for HIV-infected children who have had any CD4$^+$ T-lymphocyte determination in the first 12 months of life indicating severe immunosuppression (i.e., a total count less than 750 cells/μl or a CD4$^+$ percentage of total circulating lymphocytes less than 15%). Prophylaxis may be discontinued at 1 year of age when CD4$^+$ T-lymphocyte monitoring has been appropriate and counts have remained greater than these threshold values that define immunosuppression (see Table 114–9).

For HIV-infected children 1 to 5 years of age, PCP prophylaxis should be administered if (1) any CD4$^+$ T-lymphocyte count is less than 500 cells/μl or the CD4$^+$ percentage is less than 15% (2) a rapidly declining CD4$^+$ T-lymphocyte count occurs; or (3) severely symptomatic HIV disease (category C) is present. Criteria are the same for older children and adolescents except for different age-specific definitions of low absolute CD4$^+$ cell counts. For children 6 years of age or older, any CD4$^+$ count less than 200 cells/μl is an indication for chemoprophylaxis. For adolescents or adults, PCP prophylaxis is indicated if the CD4$^+$ cell count is less than 200/μl, or the patient has unexplained fever for 2 or more weeks or a history of oropharyngeal candidiasis.

HIV-infected children older than 1 year, not previously receiving PCP prophylaxis (e.g., those children not previously identified or whose PCP prophylaxis was discontinued) should begin prophylaxis if at any time their CD4$^+$ cell counts indicate severe immunosuppression (see Table 114–9).

The recommended drug regimen for prophylaxis in all immunocompromised patients (whether from HIV infection, malignancy, or other causes) is trimethroprim-sulfamethoxazole (150 mg trimethroprim/m^2/day with 750 mg sulfamethoxazole/m^2/day) administered orally in divided doses twice a day three times per week on consecutive days (e.g., Monday-Tuesday-Wednesday); alternative dosing schedules include administering the same total dose once daily, 3 days per week, or dividing the dose and giving it every day of the week or on alternate days). For patients who cannot tolerate trimethoprim-sulfamethoxazole, aerosolized pentamidine (300 mg via Respirgard II inhaler monthly) for those 5 years or older is considered to be an alternative; daily oral dapsone (2 mg/kg, not to exceed 100 mg) is another alternate drug for prophylaxis in children, especially those younger than 5 years. Intravenous pentamidine has also been used, but it appears to be less effective and potentially more toxic than other prophylactic regimens.

Other drugs with potential for prophylaxis include pyrimethamine with dapsone, pyrimethamine-sulfadoxine, and oral atovaquone. Experience with these drugs in both adults and children is limited. These agents should be considered only in unusual situations in which the recommended regimens are not tolerated or cannot be used.

Although prophylaxis substantially reduces the risk of PCP, pulmonary and extrapulmonary *P. carinii* infections have occurred in HIV-infected adults and children receiving prophylaxis. The drug of

TABLE 114–9 Recommendations for *Pneumocystis carinii* Pneumonia Prophylaxis for HIV-Exposed Infants and Children, by Age and HIV-Infection Status

Age and HIV-Infection Status	PCP Prophylaxis*
Birth to 4–6 wk, HIV-exposed	No prophylaxis
4–6 wk to 4 mo, HIV-exposed	Prophylaxis
4–12	
HIV-infected or indeterminate	Prophylaxis
HIV-infection excluded†	No prophylaxis
1–5 yr, HIV-infected‡	Prophylaxis if CD4$^+$ T-lymphocyte count is <500 cells/μl or percentage is <15%‡§
≥6 yr, HIV-infected‡	Prophylaxis if CD4$^+$ T-lymphocyte count is <200 cells/μl or percentage is <15%§

*Children who have had PCP should receive lifelong PCP prophylaxis.

†HIV infection can be reasonably excluded among children who have had two or more negative HIV diagnostic tests (i.e., HIV culture or polymerase chain reaction), both of which are performed at ≥1 month of age and one of which is performed at ≥4 months of age, or two or more negative HIV IgG antibody tests performed at ≥6 months of age among children who have no clinical evidence of HIV disease.

‡Children 1 to 2 years of age who were receiving PCP prophylaxis and had a CD4$^+$ count of less than 750 cells/μl or a percentage of less than 15% at less than 12 months of age should continue prophylaxis.

§Prophylaxis should be considered on a case-by-case basis for children who might otherwise be at risk for PCP, such as children with rapidly declining CD4$^+$ counts or percentages or children with category C status of HIV infection.

Abbreviations: HIV, Human immunodeficiency virus; PCP, *Pneumocystis carinii* pneumonia.

Modified from American Academy of Pediatrics. 1997 Red Book: Report of the Committee on Infectious Diseases. 24th ed. Elk Grove Village, Ill: American Academy of Pediatrics, 1997.

choice for therapy of *P. carinii* infections in children is trimethoprim-sulfamethoxazole; parenterally administered pentamidine is an alternative. In children, experience with other agents such as atovaquone, trimetrexate with leucovorin, dapsone with trimethoprim, and clindamycin with primaquine is limited.[44] Corticosteroids may be a useful adjunctive therapy for moderate to severe PCP in children, as has been proved to be the case in adults.[44, 107–111]

Chemoprophylaxis is also suggested to prevent *M. avium* complex infections in children older than 6 years of age with CD4+ cell counts less than 50 cells/μl; weekly azithromycin or daily clarithromycin are the drugs of choice, with daily rifabutin as an alternative.[42, 43] Younger children are given prophylaxis at higher CD4+ cell counts in accordance with age-adjusted normal values.[42, 43] Prophylaxis for other opportunistic infections such as cytomegalovirus infections, fungal disease, and toxoplasmic encephalitis may also warrant chemoprophylaxis in children, but data are lacking to provide clear indications.[42, 43]

Immunization Recommendations

Table 114–10 summarizes recommended immunizations for children with HIV infection.[14] Specific comments are grouped according to whether the child is symptomatic, asymptomatic, or a seronegative contact of a person with HIV infection.[14]

Children with Symptomatic HIV Infection

In general, live-viral (e.g., oral poliovirus, varicella) vaccines and live-bacterial (e.g., Calmette-Guérin bacillus) vaccines should not be given to patients with AIDS or other clinical manifestations of HIV infection indicative of immunosuppression. MMR vaccine in patients who are not severely immunocompromised is an exception. Children receiving IGIV prophylaxis may not respond to MMR vaccine. Other routinely recommended vaccines, that is, diphtheria and tetanus toxoids and acellular pertussis (DTaP) or diphtheria and tetanus toxoids and pertussis (DTP), hepatitis B, *H. influenzae* type B conjugate, and inactivated poliovirus vaccines, should be given according to the usual immunization schedule. Pneumococcal vaccine at 2 years of age and yearly influenza vaccination beginning at the age of 6 months also are recommended.

TABLE 114–10 Recommendations for Routine Immunization of HIV-Infected Children in the United States

Vaccine	Known Asymptomatic HIV Infection	Symptomatic HIV Infection
Hepatitis B	Yes	Yes
DTaP (or DTP)	Yes	Yes
IPV*	Yes	Yes
MMR	Yes	Yes†
Hib	Yes	Yes
Pneumococcal‡	Yes	Yes
Influenza§	Yes	Yes
Varicella‖	No	No

*Only IPV should be used for HIV-infected children, HIV-exposed infants whose status is indeterminate and household contacts of HIV-infected persons.

†Severely immunocompromised HIV-infected children should not receive MMR vaccine (see text).

‡Pneumococcal vaccine should be administered at 2 years of age to all HIV-infected children. Children who are older than 2 years should receive pneumococcal vaccine at the time of diagnosis. Revaccination after 3 to 5 years is recommended.

§Influenza vaccine should be provided seasonally and repeated annually for HIV-exposed infants 6 months of age and older, HIV-infected children, and adolescents, and household contacts of HIV-infected persons.

‖Varicella vaccine is not currently indicated for HIV-exposed or HIV-infected persons, but studies are in progress to determine safety and possible indications.

Abbreviations: DTaP, Diphtheria and tetanus toxoids and acellular pertussis vaccine; DTP, diphtheria and tetanus toxoids and pertussis vaccine; Hib, *Haemophilus influenzae* type B conjugate; HIV, human immunodeficiency virus; IPV, inactivated poliovirus vaccine; MMR, live-virus measles, mumps, and rubella.

From American Academy of Pediatrics. 1997 Red Book: Report of the Committee on Infectious Diseases. 24th ed. Elk Grove Village, Ill: American Academy of Pediatrics; 1997.

Because of the occurrence of severe measles in symptomatic HIV-infected children and the lack of reported serious or unusual reactions to immunization with MMR, measles immunization (given as MMR) of HIV-infected children is recommended unless they are severely immunocompromised. Vaccine should be given at 12 months of age in order to enhance the likelihood of an immune response, that is, before deterioration of the immune system, if possible. The second dose may be administered as soon as 1 month (4 weeks) later in an attempt to induce seroconversion as early as possible. If the risk of exposure to measles is increased, such as during an outbreak, the vaccine should be given at an earlier age, such as at 6 to 9 months.

Based on the case report of an HIV-infected adolescent with severe immunocompromise who developed severe pneumonitis associated with measles vaccine virus, MMR vaccine is contraindicated in severely immunocompromised (as defined in Table 114–2) persons with HIV infection.[112, 113]

In general, children with symptomatic HIV infection have poor immunologic responses to vaccines. Hence, such children, when exposed to a vaccine-preventable disease such as measles or tetanus, should be considered susceptible regardless of the history of vaccination and should receive, if indicated, passive immunoprophylaxis. Immune globulin should also be given to any unimmunized household member who is exposed to measles infection.

Children with Asymptomatic HIV Infection

Children with asymptomatic HIV infection should receive DTaP or DTP, inactivated poliovirus, *H. influenzae* type B conjugate, hepatitis B, and MMR vaccines, according to the usual immunization schedules. Although oral poliovirus vaccine has been given to these patients without adverse effects, inactivated poliovirus vaccine is recommended because both the child and the family members may be immunosuppressed as the result of HIV infection and, therefore, may be at risk for vaccine-associated paralytic poliomyelitis caused by vaccine viral infection.

Varicella vaccine is currently contraindicated in persons with known HIV infection, regardless of the presence or absence of symptoms. The only exception is participants in studies to assess the safety and efficacy of varicella vaccine in HIV-infected persons.

Pneumococcal vaccination is indicated for HIV-infected children 2 years and older as they are at increased risk of invasive pneumococcal infection. Revaccination once after 3 to 5 years is recommended. Yearly influenza vaccination should be considered for HIV-infected children 6 months of age or older.

In the United States and in areas of low prevalence of tuberculosis, Calmette-Guérin bacillus vaccine (BCG) is not recommended. However, in developing countries where the prevalence of tuberculosis is high, the World Health Organization recommends that Calmette-Guérin bacillus vaccine be given to all infants at birth if they are asymptomatic, regardless of maternal HIV infection.

Seronegative Children Residing in the Household of a Patient with Symptomatic HIV Infection

In a household with an adult or child immunocompromised as the result of HIV infection, seronegative as well as seropositive children should receive inactivated poliovirus vaccine because the live polioviruses in oral poliovirus vaccine can be excreted and transmitted to immunosuppressed contacts. MMR may be given because MMR vaccine viruses are not transmitted. To reduce the risk of transmission of influenza to patients with symptomatic HIV infection, yearly influenza vaccination is indicated for their household contacts.

Although person-to-person transmission of the varicella vaccine virus has been reported rarely, varicella vaccination of siblings and susceptible adult caregivers of patients with HIV infection is strongly encouraged to prevent the acquisition of the wild-type varicella-zoster infection, which can cause severe disease in immunocompromised hosts.

Passive Immunization of Children with HIV Infection

Measles. Symptomatic HIV-infected children who are exposed to measles should receive immune globulin prophylaxis (0.5 ml/kg, maximum 15 ml), regardless of vaccination status. Exposed, asymptomatic HIV-infected patients who are susceptible should also receive immune globulin; the recommended dose is 0.25 ml/kg. Children who have received IGIV within 3 weeks of exposure do not require additional passive immunization.

Tetanus. In the management of wounds classified as tetanus prone, children with HIV infection should receive tetanus immune globulin regardless of their vaccination status.

Varicella. Children infected with HIV who are exposed to varicella or herpes zoster and who are susceptible should receive varicella-zoster immune globulin. Children who have received IGIV or varicella-zoster immune globulin within 3 weeks of exposure do not require additional passive immunization.

Treatment of Pregnant Women to Prevent Perinatal Transmission of HIV Infection

Zidovudine therapy of HIV-infected pregnant women and their newborns reduces by approximately two thirds the risk of perinatal transmission of HIV.[15, 25, 26] Supplemental antiretroviral therapy may improve the woman's health and possibly lower the HIV vertical transmission rate even further.[15] Antiretroviral therapy should always be offered during pregnancy (see Chapter 113). When safe and alternative sources of feeding are readily available and affordable (e.g., United States and Europe), HIV-infected women should be counseled not to breast-feed their infants.[12, 14]

HIV INFECTION IN ADOLESCENTS

Adolescents are at special risk for HIV infection; they should be educated about this disease and have access to HIV testing and knowledge of their serostatus.[14] Particular efforts should be targeted at those adolescents with known risk factors for the acquisition of HIV infection. Informed consent for either testing or the release of information regarding serostatus is necessary. Decisions regarding the disclosure of HIV status to a sexual partner without the consent of the patient should be based on several factors, including whether the partner has a reasonable cause to suspect the risk and to take precautions without specific warning, the likelihood that the partner is at risk, relevant law that may prohibit or require such disclosure, and the possible effects of such disclosure on future relationships.[14]

Information regarding HIV infection and AIDS should be regarded as an important component of the anticipatory guidance provided by physicians to their adolescent patients.[14] This guidance should include information about transmission, implications of infection, and strategies for prevention including abstinence from behaviors that place adolescents at risk and safer sex practices for those who decide to be sexually active. Diagnostic testing should be available and offered. Parental involvement in adolescent health care is a desirable goal. The consent of the adolescent alone, however, should be sufficient to provide evaluation and treatment for suspected or confirmed HIV infection.[14]

HIV-infected adolescents may have more specific problems with medication adherence as well.[86, 87] They are frequently inexperienced with medication regimens and health care provision systems, they may fear or deny their HIV infection, and they may distrust any information given to them by the medical establishment.[86] Adolescents may also have complex biopsychosocial issues such as low self-esteem, chaotic and unstructured life styles, peer pressures not to be singled out with illness, and a lack of family support, all of which may reduce adherence. The concrete thought process of adolescents might make it difficult for them to understand why medications are necessary during periods of asymptomatic infection, especially if they have experienced any medication adverse effects. Thus, treatment regimens for adolescents must balance the goal of prescribing a maximally potent antiretroviral regimen with a realistic assessment of existing and potential support systems for the adolescent to adhere to such a regimen.[86, 87]

SCHOOL ATTENDANCE AND EDUCATION OF CHILDREN WITH HIV INFECTION

In the absence of blood exposure, HIV infection is not acquired through the types of contact that usually occur in a school setting, including contact with saliva or tears. Hence, children with HIV infection should not be excluded from school for the protection of other children or personnel.[13, 14] Most school-aged children and adolescents infected with HIV should be allowed to attend school without restrictions, provided the child's physician gives approval.[14] The need for a more restricted school environment for some infected children should be evaluated on a case-by-case basis with consideration of conditions that may pose an increased risk to others, such as aggressive biting behavior or the presence of exudative, weeping skin lesions that cannot be covered. This risk should be assessed regularly by the child's physician. Only the child's parents, other guardians, and physician have an absolute need to know that the child is HIV infected.[13, 14] The number of personnel aware of the child's condition should be kept to the minimum needed to ensure proper care of the child. The family has the right to inform the school, if they so choose. Persons involved in the care and education of an infected student must respect the student's right to privacy. All schools should adopt routine procedures for handling blood or blood-contaminated fluids, including the disposal of sanitary napkins, regardless of whether students with HIV infection are known to be in attendance.[14]

As the life expectancy of HIV-infected children and adolescents increases, the school population of children and adolescents with this disease will also increase. An understanding of the effect of chronic illness and the recognition of neurodevelopmental problems in these children is essential to provide appropriate educational programs.

CHILD CARE AND FOSTER CARE

No reason exists to restrict foster care or adoptive placement of children who have HIV infection to protect the health of other family members.[14] The risk of transmission of HIV infection in family environments is negligible. No need exists to restrict the placement of HIV-infected children in child care settings to protect personnel or other children because the risk of transmission of HIV in these settings is negligible.[14] Child care personnel need not be informed of the HIV status of a child to protect the health of caregivers or other children in the child care environment.[14] In some jurisdictions, the child's diagnosis cannot be divulged without the written consent of the parent or legal guardian. Parents may choose to inform the child care provider of the child's diagnosis in order to support a request that the caregiver observe the child closely for signs of illness that may require medical attention and assist the parents with the child's special emotional and social needs. The recommended standard precautions should be followed in all child care settings when blood or bloody fluids are handled to minimize the possibility of transmission of any blood-borne disease. All preschool child care programs routinely should inform all families whenever a highly contagious illness, such as varicella or measles, occurs in any child in that setting.[14]

ADULTS WITH HIV INFECTION WORKING IN CHILD CARE OR SCHOOLS

Asymptomatic HIV-infected adults may care for children in school or child care settings provided that they do not have exudative skin lesions or other conditions that would allow contact with their body fluids.[14] No data indicate that HIV-infected adults have transmitted HIV in the course of normal child care or school responsibilities.[14]

Adults with symptomatic HIV infection are immunocompromised and at increased risk from infections diseases of young children. They should consult their physicians regarding the safety of continuing work.

MANAGEMENT AND COUNSELING OF FAMILIES

Infection acquired by children before or during birth is a disease of the family.[14] Serologic screening of siblings and parents is recommended. In each case, the physician needs to provide education and ongoing counseling regarding HIV and its transmission and to outline precautions to be taken within the household and the community to prevent spread of this virus.

Infected women need to be made aware of the risk of having an infected child if they become pregnant, and they should be referred for family planning counseling.[14] Infected persons must not donate blood, plasma, sperm, organs, corneas, bone, other tissues, or breast milk.

The infected child should be taught good hygiene and behavior. How much he or she is told about the illness depends on the child's age and maturity.[14] Older children and adolescents should be made aware that the disease can be transmitted sexually and should be provided with appropriate counseling. Most families are not willing to share the diagnosis with others because it can create social isolation. Feelings of guilt are common. Family members, including children, can become clinically depressed and require psychiatric counseling.

SEXUAL ABUSE

After sexual abuse by a person with or at risk for HIV infection, the child should be tested serologically at the time of abuse and at 6 weeks, 3 months, and 6 months after sexual contact.[14] If feasible, serologic evaluation of the abuser for HIV infection should be obtained. Counseling of the child and family needs to be provided.

CHILDREN WITH ACCIDENTAL HIV EXPOSURE

Injuries from hypodermic needles and syringes discarded in public places, usually by injection drug users, are perceived by victims as a significant risk for transmitting HIV infection, although these injuries pose less of a risk than that resulting from needlestick injuries in health care settings.[14] The risk of HIV transmission from a discarded needle in public places appears to be low, and data on the efficacy of postexposure prophylaxis are not available. Consultation with a specialist in HIV infection should be obtained when deciding whether to give a child postexposure chemoprophylaxis (see Chapter 296).[14] The schedule of testing the child for serum HIV antibody is controversial, but some authorities recommend baseline testing along with tests after 6 weeks, 12 weeks, and 6 months.[14] If postexposure chemoprophylaxis is recommended, the adult health care worker guidelines[114] seem reasonable to follow, with the exception that if a decision is made to use a protease inhibitor, nelfinavir (20 to 30 mg/kg/dose given every 8 hours) or ritonavir (350 mg/m^2/dose given every 12 hours) are preferred for younger children because of their availability in powder (nelfinavir) or suspension (ritonavir) formulations.

REFERENCES

1. Centers for Disease Control and Prevention. *Pneumocystis* pneumonia—Los Angeles. MMWR Morb Mortal Wkly Rep. 1981;30:250–252.
2. Centers for Disease Control and Prevention. Kaposi's sarcoma and *Pneumocystis* pneumonia among homosexual men—New York City and California. MMWR Morb Mortal Wkly Rep. 1981;30:305–308.
3. Gottlieb MS, Schroff R, Schanker HM, et al. *Pneumocystis carinii* pneumonia and mucosal candidiasis in previously healthy homosexual men: Evidence of a new acquired cellular immunodeficiency. N Engl J Med. 1981;305:1425–1431.
4. Masur H, Michelis MA, Greene JB, et al. An outbreak of community acquired *Pneumocystis carinii* pneumonia: Initial manifestation of cellular immune dysfunction. N Engl J Med. 1981;305:1431–1438.
5. Huminer D, Rosenfeld JB, Pitlik SD. AIDS in the pre-AIDS era. Rev Infect Dis. 1987;9:1102–1108.
6. Ammann AJ, Cowan MJ, Wara DW, et al: Acquired immunodeficiency in an infant: Possible transmission by means of blood products. Lancet. 1983;1:956–958.
7. Oleske J, Minnefor A, Cooper R Jr, Thomas K, et al. Immune deficiency syndrome in children. JAMA. 1983;249:2345–2349.
8. Rubinstein A, Sicklick M, Gupta A, et al. Acquired immunodeficiency with reversed T4/T8 ratios in infants born to promiscuous and drug-addicted mothers. JAMA. 1983;249:2350–2356.
9. Scott GB, Buck BE, Leterman JG, et al. Acquired immunodeficiency syndrome in infants. N Engl J Med. 1984;310:76–81.
10. Mertens TE, Low-Beer D. HIV and AIDS: Where is the epidemic going? Bull World Health Organ. 1996;74:121–129.
11. Centers for Disease Control and Prevention. HIV/AIDS Surveillance Report. 1997;9(2):1–43.
12. Committee on Pediatric AIDS, American Academy of Pediatrics. Human milk, breastfeeding, and transmission of human immunodeficiency virus in the United States. Pediatrics. 1995;96:977–979.
13. Simonds RJ, Chanock S. Medical issues related to caring for human immunodeficiency virus–infected children in and out of the home. Pediatr Infect Dis J. 1993;12:845–852.
14. American Academy of Pediatrics. HIV infection. In: Peter G, ed. 1997 Red Book: Report of the Committee on Infectious Diseases. 24th ed. Elk Grove Village, Ill: American Academy of Pediatrics; 1997:279–304.
15. Centers for Disease Control and Prevention. Public Health Services Task Force recommendations for the use of antiretroviral drugs in pregnant women infected with HIV-1 for maternal health and for reducing perinatal HIV-1 transmission in the United States. MMWR Morb Mortal Wkly Rep. 1998;47(RR–2):1–30.
16. Tudor-Williams G, Lyall EGH. Perinatal transmission of HIV. Curr Opin Infect Dis. 1997;10:239–245.
17. Scarlatti G. Pediatric HIV infection. Lancet. 1996;348:863–868.
17a. Kuhn L, Steketeern RW, Weedon J, et al: Distinct risk factors for intrauterine and intrapartum human immunodeficiency virus transmission and consequences for disease progression in infected children. J Infect Dis. 1997;179:52–58.
18. Mofenson LM. Mother-child HIV-1 transmission: Timing and determinants. Obstet Gynecol Clin North Am. 1997;24:759–784.
19. Goedert JJ, Duliege AM, Amos CI, et al. High risk of HIV-1 infection for first-born twins. The International Registry of HIV-Exposed Twins. Lancet. 1991;338:1471–1475.
20. Duliege AM, Amos CI, Felton S, et al. Birth order, delivery route, and concordance in the transmission of HIV-1 from mothers to twins. J Pediatr. 1995;126:625–632.
21. European Collaborative Study. Caesarian section and risk of vertical transmission of HIV-1 infection. Lancet. 1994;343:1464–1467.
22. Landesman SH, Kalish CA, Burns DN, et al. Obstetrical factors and the transmission of human immunodeficiency virus type 1 from mother to child. N Engl J Med. 1996;334:1617–1623.
23. Mandelbrot L, Le Chenadec J, Berrebi A, et al. Perinatal HIV-1 transmission. Interaction between zidovudine prophylaxis and mode of delivery in the French Perinatal Cohort. JAMA. 1998;280:55–60.
24. The International Perinatal HIV Group. The mode of delivery and the risk of vertical transmission of human immunodeficiency virus type 1–a meta-analysis of 15 prospective cohort studies. N Eng J Med. 1999, in press.
25. Centers for Disease Control and Prevention. Recommendations of the Public Health Service Task Force on use of zidovudine to reduce perinatal transmission of human immunodeficiency virus. MMWR Morb Mortal Wkly Rep. 1994;43(RR–11):1–21.
26. Connor EM, Sperling RS, Gelber R, et al. Reduction of maternal-infant transmission of human immunodeficiency virus type 1 with zidovudine treatment. N Engl J Med. 1994;331:1173–1180.
26a. Leroy V, Newell M-L, Dabis F, et al. International multicentre pooled analysis of late postnatal mother-to-child transmission of HIV-1 infection. Lancet. 1998;352:597–600
27. Morris CR, Araba-Owoyele L, Spector SA, Maldonado YA. Disease patterns and survival after acquired immunodeficiency syndrome diagnosis in human immunodeficiency virus–infected children. Pediatr Infect Dis J. 1996;15:321–328.
28. Bamji M, Thea DM, Weedon J, et al. Prospective study of human immunodeficiency virus 1–related disease among 512 infants born to infected women in New York City. Pediatr Infect Dis J. 1996;15:891–898.
29. Italian Register for HIV Infection in Children. Features of children perinatally infected with HIV-1 surviving longer than 5 years. Lancet. 1994;343:191–195.
30. Galli L, de Martino M, Pier-Angelo T, et al. Onset of clinical signs in children with HIV-1 perinatal infections. AIDS. 1995;9:455–461.
31. Grubman S, Gross E, Lerner-Weiss N, et al. Older children and adolescents living with perinatally acquired human immunodeficiency virus infection. Pediatrics. 1995;95:657–663.
32. Barnhart HX, Caldwell MB, Thomas P, et al. Natural history of human immunode-

ficiency virus disease in perinatally infected children: An analysis from the Pediatric Spectrum of Disease Project. Pediatrics. 1996;97:710–716.
33. Mayaux M-J, Burgard M, Teglas J-P, et al. Neonatal characteristics in rapidly progressive perinatally acquired HIV-1 disease. JAMA. 1996;275:606–610.
34. Rosenberg PS, Biggar RJ. Trends in HIV incidence among young adults in the United States. JAMA. 1998;279:1894–1899.
35. Scott GB, Hutto C, Makuch RW, et al. Survival in children with perinatally acquired human immunodeficiency virus type 1 infection. N Engl J Med. 1989;321:1791–1796.
36. Turner BJ, Denison M, Eppes SC, et al. Survival experience of 789 children with the acquired immunodeficiency syndrome. Pediatr Infect Dis J. 1993;12:310–20.
37. Abrams EJ, Matheson PB, Thomas PA, et al. Neonatal predictors of infection status and early death among 332 infants at risk of HIV-1 infection monitored prospectively from birth. Pediatrics. 1995;96:451–458.
38. Centers for Disease Control and Prevention. 1994 revised classification system for human immunodeficiency virus infection in children less than 13 years of age; official authorized addenda: Human immunodeficiency virus infection codes and official guidelines for coding and reporting ICD-9-CM. MMWR Morb Mortal Wkly Rep. 1994;43(RR–12):1–19.
39. Domachowske J. Pediatric human immunodeficiency virus infection. Clin Microbiol Rev. 1996;9:448–468.
40. Hanson IC, Shearer WT. AIDS and other acquired immunodeficiency diseases. In: Feigin RD, Cherry JD, eds. Textbook of Pediatric Infectious Diseases. 4th ed. Philadelphia: WB Saunders, 1998:954–979.
41. Centers for Disease Control and Prevention. 1995 revised guidelines for prophylaxis against *Pneumocystis carinii* pneumonia for children infected with or perinatally exposed to human immunodeficiency virus. MMWR Morb Mortal Wkly Rep. 1995;44(RR–4):1–11.
42. Kaplan JE, Masur H, Holmes KK. Prevention of opportunistic infections in persons infected with human immunodeficiency virus. Clin Infect Dis. 1997;25(Suppl 3):S299–S335.
43. Centers for Disease Control and Prevention. 1997 USPHS/IDSA guidelines for the prevention of opportunistic infections in persons infected with human immunodeficiency virus. MMWR Morb Mortal Wkly Rep. 1997;46(RR–12):1–46.
44. Weinberg GA, White AC Jr, Rathore MH. Other infectious agents (*Pneumocystis carinii, Legionella pneumophila,* and protozoan & helminthic pulmonary infections). In: Taussig L, Landau L, LeSouëf PN, et al, eds. Pediatric Respiratory Medicine. St. Louis: Mosby; 1999:762–784.
45. Gonzalez CE, Shetty D, Lewis L, et al. Cryptococcosis in human immunodeficiency virus–infected children. Pediatr Infect Dis J. 1996;15:796–800.
45a. Abadi J, Nachman S, Kressel AB, Pirofski L. Cryptococcosis in children with AIDS. Clin Infect Dis. 1999;28:309–313.
46. Hoyt L, Oleske J, Holland B, Connor E. Nontuberculous mycobacteria in children with acquired immunodeficiency syndrome. Pediatr Infect Dis J. 1992;11:354–360.
47. Andiman WA, Mezger J, Shapiro E. Invasive bacterial infections in children born to women infected with human immunodeficiency virus type 1. J Pediatr. 1994;124:846–852.
48. Mao C, Harper M, McIntosh K, et al. Invasive pneumococcal infections in human immunodeficiency virus–infected children. J Infect Dis. 1996;173:870–876.
49. Connor EM, Andiman WA. Lymphoid interstitial pneumonitis. In: Pizzo PA, Wilfert CM, eds. Pediatric AIDS—The Challenge of HIV Infection in Infants, Children, and Adolescents. 2nd ed. Baltimore: Williams & Wilkins; 1994:467–481.
50. Pitt J. Lymphocytic interstitial pneumonia. Pediatr Clin North Am. 1991;38:89–95.
51. Epstein LG, Sharer LR, Oleske JM, et al. Neurologic manifestations of HIV infection in children. Pediatrics. 1986;78:678–687.
52. Browers P, Belman AL, Epstein L. Central nervous system involvement: Manifestations, evaluation, and pathogenesis. In: Pizzo PA, Wilfert CM, eds. Pediatric AIDS—The Challenge of HIV Infection in Infants, Children, and Adolescents. 2nd ed. Baltimore: Williams & Wilkins; 1994:433–456.
53. Cooper ER, Hanson C, Diaz C, et al. Encephalopathy and progression of human immunodeficiency virus disease in a cohort of children with perinatally acquired human immunodeficiency virus infection. J Pediatr. 1998;132:808–812.
54. Coplan J, Contello KA, Cunningham CK, et al. Early language development in children exposed to or infected with human immunodeficiency virus. Pediatrics. 1998;102:1, electronic pages http://www.pediatrics.org/cgi/content/full/102/1/e8.
55. Belman AL, Diamond G, Dickson D, et al. Pediatric acquired immunodeficiency syndrome. Neurologic syndromes. Am J Dis Child. 1988;142:29–35.
56. Scarmatov V, Frank Y, Rozenstein A. Central brain atrophy in childhood AIDS encephalopathy. AIDS. 1996;10:1227–1231.
57. Winters HS, Miller TL. Gastrointestinal and nutritional problems in pediatric HIV disease. In: Pizzo PA, Wilfert CM, eds. Pediatric AIDS—The Challenge of HIV Infection in Infants, Children, and Adolescents. 2nd ed. Baltimore: Williams & Wilkins; 1994:513–533.
58. Laue L, Cutler GB Jr. Abnormalities in growth and development. In: Pizzo PA, Wilfert CM, eds. Pediatric AIDS—The Challenge of HIV Infection in Infants, Children, and Adolescents. 2nd ed. Baltimore: Williams & Wilkins; 1994:575–589.
59. Saavedra JM, Henderson RA, Permon JA, et al. Longitudinal assessment of growth in children born to mothers with human immunodeficiency virus infection. Arch Pediatr Adolesc Med. 1995;149:497–502.
60. Moye J Jr, Rich KC, Kalish LA, et al. Natural history of somatic growth in infants born to women infected by human immunodeficiency virus. J Pediatr. 1996;128:58–69.
61. Miller TL, Awnetwant EL, Evans S, et al. Gastrostomy tube supplementation for HIV-infected children. Pediatrics. 1995;96:696–702.
62. Jospe N, Powell KR. Growth hormone deficiency in an 8-year-old girl with human immunodeficiency virus infection. Pediatrics. 1990;86:309–312.
63. Miller TL, Winter HS, Luginbuhl LM, et al. Pancreatitis in pediatric human immunodeficiency virus infection. J Pediatr. 1992;120:223–227.
64. Lipshultz SE. Cardiovascular problems. In: Pizzo PA, Wilfert CM, eds. Pediatric AIDS—The Challenge of HIV Infection in Infants, Children, and Adolescents. 2nd ed. Baltimore: Williams & Wilkins; 1994;483–511.
65. Lipshultz SE, Chanock S, Sanders SP, et al. Cardiovascular manifestations of human immunodeficiency virus in infants and children. Am J Cardiol. 1989;63:1489–1497.
66. Luginbuhl LM, Orav EJ, McIntosh K, Lipshultz SE. Cardiac morbidity and related mortality in children with HIV infection. JAMA. 1993;269:2869–2875.
67. Lipshultz SE, Orav EJ, Sanders SP, et al. Cardiac structure and function in children with human immunodeficiency virus infection treated with zidovudine. N Engl J Med. 1992;327:1260–1265.
68. P[2]C[2] HIV Study Group. The pediatric pulmonary and cardiovascular complication of vertically transmitted human immunodeficiency virus (P[2]C[2] HIV) infection study: Design and methods. J Clin Epidemiol. 1996;49:1285–1294.
69. Wigfall DR. Renal problems. In: Pizzo PA, Wilfert CM, eds. Pediatric AIDS—The Challenge of HIV Infection in Infants, Children, and Adolescents. 2nd ed. Baltimore: Williams & Wilkins; 1994:547–557.
70. Strauss J, Zilleruelo G, Abitbol C, et al. Human immunodeficiency virus nephropathy. Pediatr Nephrol. 1993;7:220–225.
71. Strauss J, Abitbol C, Zilleruelo G, et al. Renal disease in children with the acquired immunodeficiency syndrome. N Engl J Med. 1989;321:625–630.
72. Mueller BU. Hematological problems and their management in children with HIV infection. In: Pizzo PA, Wilfert CM, eds. Pediatric AIDS—The Challenge of HIV Infection in Infants, Children, and Adolescents. 2nd ed. Baltimore: Williams & Wilkins; 1994:591–601.
73. Weinberg GA, Gigliotti F, Stroncek DF, et al. Lack of relation of granulocyte antibodies (antineutrophil antibodies) to neutropenia in children with human immunodeficiency virus infection. Pediatr Infect Dis J. 1997;16:881–884.
74. Watson WJ, Stevens TP, Weinberg GA. Profound anemia in a newborn infant of a mother receiving antiretroviral therapy. Pediatr Infect Dis J. 1998;17:435–436.
75. Goedert JJ, Coté TR, Virgo P, et al. Spectrum of AIDS-associated malignant disorders. Lancet. 1998;351:1833–1839.
76. Mueller BU, Pizzo PA. Malignancies in pediatric AIDS. Curr Opin Pediatr. 1996;8:45–49.
77. Chadwick EG, Connor EJ, Hanson ICG, et al. Tumors of smooth-muscle origin in HIV-infected children. JAMA. 1990;263:3182–3184.
78. Mueller BU, Shad AT, Magrath IT, Horowitz ME. Malignancies in children with HIV infection. In: Pizzo PA, Wilfert CM, eds. Pediatric AIDS—The Challenge of HIV Infection in Infants, Children, and Adolescents. 2nd ed. Baltimore: Williams & Wilkins; 1994:603–22.
79. Koup RA, Wilson CB. Clinical immunology of HIV-infected children. In: Pizzo PA, Wilfert CM, eds. Pediatric AIDS—The Challenge of HIV Infection in Infants, Children, and Adolescents. 2nd ed. Baltimore: Williams & Wilkins; 1994:129–157.
80. Comans-Bitter WM, de Groot R, van den Beemd R, et al. Immunophenotyping of blood lymphocytes in childhood: Reference values for lymphocyte subpopulations. J Pediatr. 1997;130:388–393.
81. European Collaborative Study. Age-related standards for T lymphocyte subsets based on uninfected children born to human immunodeficiency virus 1–infected women. Pediatr Infect Dis J. 1992;11:1018–1026.
82. Committee on Pediatric AIDS, American Academy of Pediatrics. Evaluation and medical treatment of the HIV-exposed infant. Pediatrics. 1997;99:909–917.
83. Shearer WT, Quinn TC, LaRussa P, et al. Viral load and disease progression in infants infected with human immunodeficiency virus type 1. N Engl J Med. 1997;336:1337–1342.
84. Mofenson LM, Korelitz J, Meyer WA, et al. The relationship between serum human immunodeficiency virus type 1 (HIV-1) RNA level, CD4 lymphocyte percent, and long-term mortality risk in HIV-1-infected children. J Infect Dis. 1997;175:1029–1038.
85. Palumbo PE, Raskino C, Fiscus S, et al. Predictive value of quantitative plasma HIV RNA and $CD4^+$ lymphocyte count in HIV-infected infants and children. JAMA. 1998;279:756–761.
85a. Palumbo PE, Raskino C, Fiscus S, et al. Virologic and immunologic response to nucleoside reverse transcriptase inhibitor therapy among human immunodeficiency virus—infected infants and children. J Infect Dis. 1999;179:576–583.
86. Centers for Disease Control and Prevention. Guidelines for the use of antiretroviral agents in pediatric infection. MMWR Morb Mortal Wkly Rep. 1998;47(RR–4): 1–43.
87. Centers for Disease Control and Prevention. Report of the NIH Panel to Define Principles of Therapy of HIV Infection and guidelines for the use of antiretroviral agents in HIV-infected adults and adolescents. MMWR Morb Mortal Wkly Rep. 1998;47(RR–5):1–82.
88. Dunn DT, Brandt CD, Kirvine A, et al. The sensitivity of HIV-1 DNA polymerase chain reaction in the neonatal period and the relative contributions of intra-uterine and intrapartum transmission. AIDS. 1995;9:F7–F11.
89. McIntosh K, Pitt J, Brambilla D, et al. Blood culture in the first 6 months of life for diagnosis of vertically transmitted human immunodeficiency virus infection. J Infect Dis. 1994;170:996–1000.
90. Nesheim S, Lee F, Kalish ML, et al. Diagnosis of perinatal human immunodeficiency virus infection by polymerase chain reaction and p24 antigen detection after immune complex dissociation in an urban community hospital. J Infect Dis. 1997;175:1333–1336.

91. Bryson YJ, Luzuriaga K, Sullivan JL, Wara DW. Proposed definitions for in utero versus intrapartum transmission of HIV-1. N Engl J Med. 1993;327:1246–1247.
92. Pizzo PA, Eddy J, Falloon J, et al. Effect of continuous intravenous infusion of zidovudine (AZT) in children with symptomatic HIV infection. N Engl J Med. 1988;319:889–896.
93. McKinney RE, Maha MA, Connor EM, et al. A multicenter trial of oral zidovudine in children with advanced human immunodeficiency virus disease. N Engl J Med. 1991;324:1018–1025.
94. Butler KM, Husson RN, Balis FM, et al. Dideoxyinosine in children with symptomatic human immunodeficiency virus infection. N Engl J Med. 1991;324:137–144.
95. Lewis LL, Venzon D, Church J, et al. Lamivudine in children with human immunodeficiency virus infection: A phase I/II study. J Infect Dis. 1996;174:16–25.
96. Kline MW, Dunkle LM, Church JA, et al. A phase I/II evaluation of stavudine (d4T) in children with human immunodeficiency virus infection. Pediatrics. 1995;96:247–252.
97. Kline MW, Van Dyke RB, Lindsey JC, et al. A randomized comparative trial of stavudine (d4T) versus zidovudine (ZDV, AZT) in children with human immunodeficiency virus infection. Pediatrics. 1998;101:214–220.
98. McKinney RE for the PACTG Protocol 300 Team. Pediatric ACTG 300: Clinical efficacy of ZDV/3TC vs ddI vs ZDV/ddI in symptomatic, HIV-infected children. Abstract 768. In: Programs and Abstracts of the 35th Annual Meeting of the Infectious Diseases Society of America, San Francisco, California, September 13–16, 1997, Alexandria, VA: Infectious Diseases Society of America, 1997.
99. Englund JA, Baker CJ, Raskino C, et al. Zidovudine, didanosine or both as the initial treatment for symptomatic HIV-infected children. N Engl J Med. 1997;336:1704–1712.
100. Krogstad P, Kerr B, Anderson R, et al. Phase I study of the HIV-protease inhibitor nelfinavir mesylate (NFV) in HIV-positive children. Abstract 721. In: Abstracts of the 4th Conference on Retroviruses and Opportunistic Infections, Washington, DC, January 22–26, 1997, Alexandria, VA: Foundation for Retrovirology and Human Health, 1997.
101. Yogev R, Stanley K, Nachman SA, et al. for the PACTG 338 Protocol Team. Virologic efficacy of ZDV + 3TC vs d4T + ritonavir (RTV) vs ZDV + 3TC + RTV in stable antiretroviral experienced HIV-infected children (Pediatric ACTG Trial 338). Abstract LB-6. In: Proceedings of the 37th Interscience Conference on Antimicrobial Agents and Chemotherapy, Toronto, Canada, September 28–October 1, 1997. Washington, DC: American Society for Microbiology; 1997.
102. Luzuriaga K, Bryson Y, Krogstad P, et al. Combination treatment with zidovudine, didanosine and nevirapine in infants with human immunodeficiency virus type 1 infection. N Engl J Med. 1997;336:1343–1349.
103. Mueller BU, Nelson RP Jr, Sleasman J, et al. A phase I/II study of the protease inhibitor ritonavir in children with human immunodeficiency virus infection. Pediatrics. 1998;101:335–343.
104. Mueller BU, Sleasman S, Nelson RP Jr, et al. A phase I/II study of the protease inhibitor indinavir in children with HIV infection. Pediatrics. 1998;102:101–109.
105. Burchett SK, Carey V, Yong F, et al. Virologic activity of didanosine (ddI), zidovudine (ZDV), and nevirapine (NVP) combinations in pediatric subjects with advanced HIV disease (ACTG 245). Abstract 271. In: Abstracts of the 5th Conference on Retroviruses and Opportunistic Infections, Chicago, Ill, February 1–5, 1998, Alexandria, VA: Foundation for Human Retrovirology and Human Health; 1998.
106. Mirochnick M, Capparelli E, Dankner W, et al. Zidovudine pharmacokinetics in premature infants exposed to human immunodeficiency virus. Antimicrob Agents Chemother. 1998;42:808–812.
107. Sleasman JW, Hemenway C, Klein AS, Barrett DJ. Corticosteroids improve survival of children with AIDS and *Pneumocystis carinii* pneumonia. Am J Dis Child. 1993;147:30–34.
108. Bye MR, Cairas-Bazarian C, Ewig JM. Markedly reduced mortality associated with corticosteroid therapy of *Pneumocystis carinii* pneumonia in children with acquired immunodeficiency syndrome. Arch Pediatr Adolesc Med. 1994;148:638–641.
109. Barone SR, Aiuto LT, Krilov LR. Increased survival of young infants with *Pneumocystis carinii* pneumonia and acute respiratory failure with early steroid administration. Clin Infect Dis. 1994;19:212–213.
110. McLaughlin GE, Virdee SS, Schleien CL, et al. Effect of corticosteroid on survival of children with acquired immunodeficiency syndrome and *Pneumocystis carinii*–related respiratory failure. J Pediatr. 1995;126:821–4.
111. National Institutes of Health–University of California Expert Panel for Corticosteroids as Adjunctive Therapy for *Pneumocystis* Pneumonia. Consensus statement on the use of corticosteroids as adjunctive therapy for *Pneumocystis* pneumonia in the acquired immunodeficiency syndrome. N Engl J Med. 1990;323:1500–1504.
112. Centers for Disease Control and Prevention. Measles pneumonitis following measles-mumps-rubella vaccination of a patient with HIV infection, 1993. MMWR Morb Mortal Wkly Rep. 1996;45:603–606.
113. Angel JB, Walpita P, Lerch RA, et al. Vaccine-associated measles pneumonitis in an adult with AIDS. Ann Intern Med. 1998;129:104–106.
114. Centers for Disease Control and Prevention. Public Health Service guidelines for the management of health-care worker exposures to HIV and recommendations for postexposure prophylaxis. MMWR Morb Mortal Wkly Rep. 1998;47:(RR–7)1–34.

Chapter 115

Antiretroviral Therapy of Human Immunodeficiency Virus Infection

GEORGE J. HANNA
MARTIN S. HIRSCH

The treatment of human immunodeficiency virus type 1 (HIV-1) infection has evolved at a rapid pace. In 1987, less than 4 years after HIV-1 was identified as the agent that causes the acquired immunodeficiency syndrome (AIDS), zidovudine was approved for treatment of HIV-1 infection. In the next 8 years, three other nucleoside analogues that also inhibit the HIV-1 enzyme reverse transcriptase (RT) were introduced. From 1995 to 1998, eight new antiretroviral agents were approved, including HIV-1 protease inhibitors and non-nucleoside RT inhibitors, in effect almost tripling the number of antiretroviral drugs available for clinical use. Concurrently, a better understanding of the dynamics of HIV-1 replication and drug resistance mechanisms caused a shift from single- to combination-drug therapy. In addition, technologic advances in quantifying HIV-1 RNA led to a reliance on plasma HIV-1 RNA levels, also known as *viral load*, for monitoring infection. The treatment of HIV-1 infection today requires an understanding of viral replication dynamics, antiviral potency, pharmacokinetics and toxicities of individual drugs, and interactions between drugs used in combination. Moreover, appropriate therapeutic strategies require a knowledge of the limitations imposed by failure of one drug on the future use of the same and related drugs.

ANTIRETROVIRAL AGENTS

HIV-1 is an enveloped virus that contains two copies of genomic RNA.[1] Through its gp120 surface glycoprotein, the virus binds to cellular receptors, most commonly CD4 in association with a chemokine receptor. Once inside the cytoplasm, the viral RT, along with other viral proteins and possibly cellular proteins, converts the viral genomic RNA into a double-stranded DNA molecule by sequential steps, first using the viral RNA as a template to polymerize DNA and form a RNA:DNA hybrid, then degrading the RNA with the RNase H activity associated with the enzyme.[2] The resulting single-stranded DNA is then used as a template to polymerize the second DNA strand. Once double-stranded viral DNA is formed, it is transported to the nucleus, where it is integrated into the cellular genome with the aid of the viral integrase enzyme. Most of the currently available antiretroviral drugs are specific inhibitors of the viral RT.

After integration, HIV-1 DNA is transcribed and translated using predominantly cellular transcription and protein synthesis machinery, although several HIV-1 regulatory genes may influence these processes. Certain viral proteins, including those that form the protein components of the viral core, are synthesized as precursor polyproteins (gag and gag-pol) and require cleavage by a viral protease to yield mature proteins.[1] Immature viral structural proteins, genomic RNA, and replicative enzymes assemble initially as an immature viral core particle in the cytoplasm. This particle associates with envelope glycoproteins at the plasma membrane and buds out as an enveloped viral particle. During the process of budding, the viral protease cleaves the polyproteins in the core, converting the immature viral particle into an infectious virion. Drugs that inhibit the viral protease enzyme prevent cleavage of the polyproteins so that the viral particles remain immature and replication-defective.

Nucleoside Analogue Reverse Transcriptase Inhibitors

Several drugs inhibit viral replication by acting as nucleoside analogues and interfering with the DNA polymerase function of the viral RT (Fig. 115–1, Table 115–1). After uptake by host cells, nucleoside analogues are converted to their triphosphate forms by cellular kinases.[3] Phosphorylation by nucleoside kinases is crucial for rendering the drugs active in suppressing viral replication. Since nucleoside kinase activity may vary in different cell types and in different cell activation states, this may affect the ability of nucleoside analogues to inhibit RT. For instance, the nucleoside kinase activity of macrophages or monocytes at rest may be insufficient to yield adequate intracellular levels of zidovudine triphosphate, whereas the levels of the triphosphate form of didanosine appear to be adequate in resting cells.[4] The triphosphate forms of the drugs have high affinity for the HIV-1 RT and compete with the natural enzyme substrates (deoxynucleoside triphosphates) for binding to the RT. They are incorporated into the growing DNA chain, leading to premature chain termination since they lack a 3′-hydroxyl group to form a phosphodiester bond with the incoming nucleotide. Nucleoside analogue RT inhibitors generally have activity against a broad range of retroviruses, including HIV-1, HIV-2, and human T-lymphotropic virus type 1 (HTLV-1).[3, 5]

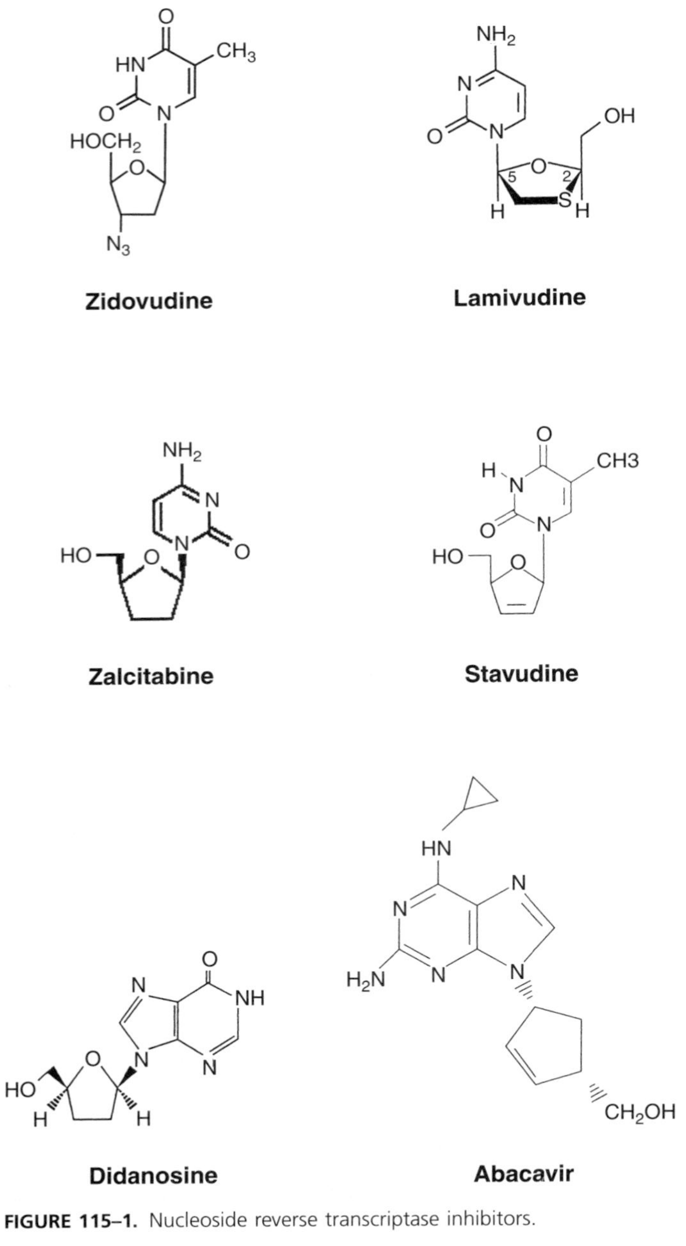

Zidovudine

Lamivudine

Zalcitabine

Stavudine

Didanosine

Abacavir

FIGURE 115–1. Nucleoside reverse transcriptase inhibitors.

Zidovudine

Zidovudine (3′-azido-2′,3′-dideoxythymidine; AZT or ZDV) is an analogue of the nucleoside thymidine. It is available in both oral and parenteral formulations and, in its oral formulation, is well absorbed, with an average bioavailability of 63%.[3, 6] Although its plasma half-life is only 1.1 hours, the half-life of the intracellular biologically active triphosphate form is 3 to 4 hours, allowing dosing intervals of 8 to 12 hours. Zidovudine penetrates the blood-brain barrier well (cerebrospinal fluid [CSF]/plasma concentration ratio of 0.6), and antiviral concentrations in the CSF are easily achieved. Zidovudine is metabolized primarily in the liver by glucuronidation to an inactive compound, and 90% of the absorbed dose is excreted in urine. Current adult dosing for zidovudine is 200 mg orally every 8 hours or 300 mg every 12 hours. In severe renal failure and hemodialysis dependence, dosing should be adjusted to 100 mg orally every 6 to 8 hours. The parenteral formulation of zidovudine is used primarily peripartum to decrease maternal transmission of HIV-1.

The first blinded placebo-controlled trial of zidovudine monotherapy was in adults with AIDS or advanced AIDS-related complex (ARC).[7] The 6-month trial compared zidovudine at 1500 mg/day to placebo and was terminated early when it showed significantly lower rates of opportunistic infections and death in the zidovudine-treated group. Although CD4 T-cell counts initially increased with zidovudine treatment, there was a gradual decline toward baseline values after 3 months. Many of the clinical benefits of zidovudine observed in this study (increases in survival, weight, and Karnofsky score) were more marked among patients with CD4 T-cell counts of 100/mm^3 or lower. Longer follow-up of all patients on open-label zidovudine therapy suggested decreasing clinical benefits of zidovudine within a year of starting therapy.[8] Subsequent studies of zidovudine in adults with mildly symptomatic HIV-1 infection without AIDS and in adults with asymptomatic HIV-1 infection with CD4 T-cell counts less than 500/mm^3 showed a decrease in progression to AIDS or advanced ARC in zidovudine-treated subjects when they were followed up to 18 months.[9, 10] Similarly, in adults with asymptomatic HIV-1 infection and CD4 T-cell counts greater than 400/mm^3, zidovudine treatment was associated with a decrease in overall disease progression over a period of 2 years.[11] However, longer follow-up of subjects with asymptomatic HIV-1 infection and CD4 T-cell counts less than 500/mm^3 suggested that the benefit of zidovudine in delaying progression to AIDS was transient, lasting approximately 2 years.[12] Increases in CD4 T-cell counts were also temporary, and no effect on survival could be demonstrated. Another study of adults with symptomatic HIV-1 infection and CD4 T-cell counts of 200 to 500/mm^3 compared early initiation of zidovudine therapy to withholding zidovudine until progression to AIDS or a CD4 T-cell count drop to less than 200/mm^3.[13] Although the early initiation of zidovudine treatment was associated with a decrease in progression to AIDS, the increase in CD4 T-cell counts was transient, and there was no difference in survival between the two strategies.

Two more recent large trials compared the early initiation of zidovudine therapy to a strategy of withholding therapy until the development of either symptoms or persistently decreased CD4 T-cell counts in subjects with asymptomatic HIV-1 infection. In one study ("Concorde"), a delay in progression to a clinical end point (AIDS, ARC, or death) and a short-term increase in the CD4 T-cell count was seen with early zidovudine use, but these benefits were not maintained after 1 year of therapy.[14] Overall, this trial failed to demonstrate any difference in survival or the rate of progression to a clinical end point over a mean follow-up of 3 years. The other trial examined asymptomatic adults with CD4 T-cell counts of 500/mm^3

TABLE 115-1 Approved Nucleoside Reverse Transcriptase Inhibitors

Agent	Trade Name	Oral Bioavailability (%)	Serum Half-Life (H)	Intracellular Half-Life of Triphosphate (H)	Elimination	Dose*	Availability	Major Adverse Effects‡
Zidovudine	Retrovir	63	1.1	3–4	Hepatic glucuronidation Renal excretion	Adults: 200 mg PO q8h or 300 mg PO q12h Pediatric: 90–180 mg/m² PO q6–12h, up to adult dose	300-mg tablets 100-mg capsules 10-mg/ml syrup 10-mg/ml solution for IV infusion	Headache Insomnia Gastrointestinal intolerance Fatigue Anemia Neutropenia Myositis
Didanosine	Videx	40	1.5	8–24	Cellular metabolism Renal excretion	Adult ≥60 kg: powder 250 mg PO q12h; tablets 200 mg PO q12h Adult <60 kg: powder 167 mg PO q12h; tablets 125 mg PO q12h Pediatric: 90–150 mg/m² PO q12h of solution up to adult dose	25-mg, 50-mg, 100-mg, 150-mg chewable tablets 100-mg, 167-mg, 250-mg powder packets 10-mg/ml solution	Diarrhea Abdominal discomfort Nausea Peripheral neuropathy Pancreatitis
Zalcitabine	Hivid	87	1.2	2.6	Renal excretion	Adult: 0.75 mg PO q8h	0.375-mg, 0.75-mg tablets	Peripheral neuropathy Pancreatitis Oral ulcers
Stavudine	Zerit	86	1.1	3	Renal excretion	Adult ≥60 kg: 40 mg PO q12h Adult <60 kg: 30 mg PO q12h Pediatric: 1 mg/kg q12h, up to adult dose	15-mg, 20-mg, 30-mg, 40-mg capsules 1-mg/ml solution	Peripheral neuropathy
Lamivudine	Epivir	86	2.5	11–14	Renal excretion	Adult: 150 mg PO q12h Pediatric: 4 mg/kg PO q12h, up to adult dose	150-mg tablets 10-mg/ml solution	Headache Fatigue
Abacavir	Ziagen	83	1.5	3.3	Hepatic glucuronidation and carboxylation	Adult: 300 mg PO q12h Pediatric: 8 mg/kg PO q12h, up to adult dose	300-mg tablets 20-mg/ml solution	Hypersensitivity reaction
Zidovudine + Lamivudine	Combivir†					Adult: One tablet PO q12h	300-mg zidovudine/150-mg lamivudine tablet	

*Neonatal dose may differ significantly from pediatric dose described here.
†Pharmacokinetic properties, adverse effects and drug interactions are similar to those of lamivudine and zidovudine used separately.
‡All nucleoside reverse transcriptase inhibitors may also be associated with rare occurrence of potentially fatal lactic acidosis and hepatomegaly with steatosis.

or greater.[15] Although the time interval before CD4 T-cell counts decreased to less than 500/mm³ was 6 months longer in subjects receiving early zidovudine therapy, there was no difference in the rates of progression to AIDS or death during a median follow-up of around 5 years. In summary, therapy with zidovudine as a single-drug regimen confers only transient clinical benefits that are most pronounced in the first few months of therapy but dissipate by 2 years.

Zidovudine has in vitro additive or synergistic antiviral effects with didanosine, zalcitabine, and lamivudine, with several non-nucleoside RT inhibitors (NNRTIs), and with currently available protease inhibitors.[16–19] In contrast, zidovudine and stavudine display antagonistic antiviral effects.[19] These findings have been confirmed in clinical studies where, in contrast to zidovudine monotherapy, several combinations that include zidovudine have produced potent and durable suppression of HIV-1. These are reviewed subsequently.

At the time of its introduction, zidovudine was used at doses of 1000 to 1500 mg/day, which caused significant toxicity. Later studies confirmed that zidovudine at doses of 500 to 600 mg/day has benefits equivalent to those seen at higher doses, but with reduced toxicity.[10, 20] Adverse effects of zidovudine are also seen more commonly in patients with more advanced disease.[21] The most serious toxicity of zidovudine is bone marrow suppression. Although macrocytosis not related to vitamin deficiency is seen in virtually all patients who are on therapeutic doses of zidovudine, severe anemia or neutropenia can also develop, especially in situations where bone marrow reserves are poor secondary to vitamin B_{12} deficiency or opportunistic infections.[21] The incidence of granulocytopenia (neutrophil count <750 cells/mm³) has ranged from 1.8% in asymptomatic individuals receiving 500 mg/day to 47% in persons with AIDS receiving 1500 mg/day.[10, 21] Similarly, severe anemia (hemoglobin levels <8 g/dl) was seen in 1.1% of asymptomatic individuals on 500 mg/day but in at least 29% of persons with AIDS receiving 1500 mg/day.[10, 21] Less commonly, chronic zidovudine use may cause myopathy and myositis that improve after zidovudine discontinuation, unlike primary HIV-1 myopathy.[22] Less serious but more common adverse reactions include headache, insomnia, myalgia, fatigue, nail pigmentation, nausea, bloating, and dyspepsia.[9, 21] Although there is tachyphylaxis to these effects in most patients, some may remain intolerant to zidovudine. Mild elevations in serum hepatic enzyme levels may also be seen, although these occur usually with the concomitant administration of other potential hepatotoxins.[8] Hematologic indices should be monitored while zidovudine is being used, especially if it is taken with other potentially myelosuppressive drugs, such as ganciclovir, or drugs that decrease the clearance of zidovudine, such as methadone or probenecid. If other therapeutic options are not available and if bone marrow toxicity does not improve despite lower doses of zidovudine (300 to 600 mg/day), recombinant erythropoietin can be used to manage anemia and granulocyte-macrophage or granulocyte colony-stimulating factors to control neutropenia.

Didanosine

Didanosine (2′, 3′-dideoxyinosine; ddI) is a purine dideoxynucleoside that is phosphorylated to dideoxyadenosine triphosphate in cells. Since didanosine is inactivated by gastric acid, it must be administered as a buffered solution or buffered tablet.[3, 6] This buffer may in turn interfere with the absorption of several medications, including delavirdine, indinavir, ketoconazole, itraconazole, and fluoroquinolones. These agents should be administered at least 2 hours before didanosine. Didanosine absorption in its current formulations is best when the drug is taken in a fasting state, with an oral bioavailability of 40%. Although didanosine's plasma half-life is approximately 1.5 hours, the relatively long intracellular half-life of its triphosphate form (8 to 24 hours) makes once- or twice-daily dosing possible. Didanosine has limited central nervous system (CNS) penetration with a CSF/plasma concentration ratio of 0.2. The drug is eliminated both by metabolism in cells of diverse tissues with hypoxanthine as an intermediate and by renal excretion. For an adult weighing 60 kg or more, didanosine dosing is 200 mg in tablet form or 250 mg of the powder formulation, orally every 12 hours. For an adult weighing less than 60 kg, the dose should be decreased to 125 mg of the tablet form or 167 mg of the powder formulation orally every 12 hours. Dosing regimens of once-daily administration are currently under study. In severe renal failure and hemodialysis dependence, dosing should be adjusted to one fourth of the total daily dose and given once a day.

Initial studies of didanosine compared its efficacy to that of zidovudine in trials of single-drug therapy. In persons with AIDS or ARC or with a CD4 T-cell count of 200 to 500 cells/mm^3 and previous zidovudine experience, switching to didanosine decreased the rate of new AIDS-defining events or death.[23–25] However, no statistically significant difference in mortality alone could be detected in these studies, and the benefit of didanosine, as measured by increases in CD4 T-cell counts, appeared to be transient. In adults with little or no prior zidovudine experience, the advantages of didanosine over zidovudine were less evident. In one trial of adults with AIDS, ARC, or a CD4 T-cell count of 200 cells/mm^3 or less who were either zidovudine-naive or had very limited zidovudine experience ($\leq$ 16 weeks), no difference in the rate of nonrecurrent AIDS-defining events or death was found when comparing zidovudine to didanosine.[26] However, in another trial involving antiretroviral-naive adults without AIDS and with a CD4 T-cell count of 200 to 500 cells/mm^3, didanosine had more potent activity compared with zidovudine, as measured by a mean decrease in HIV-1 RNA levels at 8 weeks (0.8 $\log_{10}$ for didanosine versus 0.5 $\log_{10}$ for zidovudine), by a mean increase in CD4 T-cell counts, and by rates of progression to clinical end points (AIDS-defining illness, death, or $\geq$ 50% decrease in CD4 T-cell count).[27] This trial found similar benefits of didanosine over zidovudine in zidovudine-experienced patients.

When used as part of a combination regimen, didanosine provides more pronounced and durable clinical benefits than when used as a single-drug regimen. These benefits are most pronounced in antiretroviral-naive individuals. An early trial comparing the combination of didanosine and zidovudine to zidovudine alone in adults with limited zidovudine experience (<4 months) and with a CD4 T-cell count less than 400 cells/mm^3 showed marked increases in CD4 T-cell counts with combination therapy.[28] In antiretroviral-naive adults without AIDS and with a CD4 T-cell count of 200 to 500 cells/mm^3, the combination of zidovudine and didanosine decreased the rate of clinical progression (AIDS-defining illness, death, or $\geq$ 50% decrease in CD4 T-cell count) compared with zidovudine alone.[27] In another trial comparing the combination of didanosine and zidovudine with zidovudine alone in zidovudine-naive adults with more advanced disease (symptomatic HIV disease or asymptomatic disease with a CD4 T-cell count of <350 cells/mm^3), combination therapy decreased both mortality rates and rates of disease progression compared with zidovudine monotherapy.[29]

However, the potency of combination therapy is less if didanosine is added to zidovudine therapy in individuals with a considerable history of prior zidovudine monotherapy. In a study of adults with a CD4 T-cell count of 200 to 500 cells/mm^3 and without AIDS, subjects with a median of 20 months of prior zidovudine use had clinical benefits when switched to zidovudine and didanosine, although the increase in CD4 T-cell counts and the decrease in HIV-1 RNA levels at 8 weeks were blunted compared with those in antiretroviral-naive subjects.[27, 30] In a study on adults with symptomatic HIV disease or with asymptomatic disease and a CD4 T-cell count of less than 350 cells/mm^3, the combination of didanosine and zidovudine was superior to continued zidovudine use in its ability to decrease mortality and clinical progression in zidovudine-experienced individuals (median 17 months of prior use), but these benefits were again less than those in zidovudine-naive patients.[29] In a third study of individuals with more advanced disease (CD4 counts <200 cells/mm^3, median 12 months of prior zidovudine use), the benefit of combining didanosine and zidovudine for delaying death or progression of the disease was noted only in a subset of zidovudine-naive patients.[31]

Hydroxyurea has been proposed for use with didanosine to augment didanosine's antiviral effects.[32] Hydroxyurea inhibits cellular ribonucleotide reductase, thereby decreasing intracellular concentrations of deoxynucleoside triphosphates, particularly deoxyadenosine triphosphate. By itself, hydroxyurea has limited antiretroviral activity. However, because of its ability to decrease levels of intracellular deoxyadenosine triphosphate, with which the active metabolite of didanosine (dideoxyadenosine triphosphate) competes for binding to the viral RT, hydroxyurea displays synergistic antiretroviral activity with didanosine in resting and in active cells. The combination of hydroxyurea and didanosine causes a greater decrease in HIV-1 RNA levels than didanosine alone.[33] Hydroxyurea also improves the antiviral activity of the combination of didanosine and stavudine, although it blunts the CD4 T-cell increase induced by these agents.[34] Clinical studies of combinations including hydroxyurea are ongoing. The most common adverse effect associated with hydroxyurea has been neutropenia, which resolves when the drug is discontinued.

The most serious toxicity associated with didanosine is pancreatitis. Although up to 20% of individuals treated with didanosine may develop increases in serum amylase levels, the rate of clinical pancreatitis may approach 7%.[23, 26] The risk of pancreatitis is higher with more advanced immunosuppression and if didanosine is taken with other agents that increase the risk of pancreatitis (such as ethanol or intravenous pentamidine). Although pancreatitis often resolves after didanosine therapy is discontinued, fatalities have been observed. A peripheral neuropathy, predominantly sensory and characterized by distal numbness, tingling, or pain, has been noted in up to 13% of persons taking didanosine.[23, 26] Neuropathy occurs more commonly in patients with a prior history of neuropathy or previous neurotoxic drug therapy and generally resolves if didanosine is stopped promptly. Asymptomatic hyperuricemia and hypertriglyceridemia have also been noted.[35] Diarrhea, abdominal discomfort, and nausea, though less serious, are common adverse effects and sometimes limit the use of current formulations of didanosine. Newer formulations are under development.

Zalcitabine

Zalcitabine (2′, 3′-dideoxycytidine; ddC) is a cytidine analogue that is well absorbed orally (bioavailability of 87%), but its absorption diminishes significantly when it is administered with food.[3] Its plasma half-life is 1.2 hours, and the intracellular half-life of its triphosphate form is 2.6 hours. Zalcitabine has limited CNS penetration with a CSF/plasma ratio of 0.2. It is excreted largely unchanged in the urine/and dosing may need to be modified in patients with decreased creatinine clearance. The adult dose is 0.75 mg orally every 8 hours.

Initial studies of zalcitabine compared its efficacy to that of zidovudine and didanosine. Two trials comparing zalcitabine to continued zidovudine administration in adults with advanced disease (AIDS or advanced ARC in one study; a CD4 T-cell count of $\leq$ 200 cells/mm^3 or symptomatic HIV-1 disease and a CD4 T-cell count $\leq$ 300 cells/mm^3 in another) who received and tolerated zidovudine for a mean of 18 months failed to show differences in survival or clinical progression between the two regimens.[36, 37] A community-based trial comparing zalcitabine to didanosine in patients who were intolerant to or had clinical progression despite zidovudine therapy did not demonstrate statistically significant differences in the rates of clinical disease progression or death between these two regimens.[38]

Despite its limitations for monotherapy, zalcitabine has shown some efficacy in combination therapy. An early study showed that in antiretroviral-naive individuals with AIDS or ARC, a combination of zidovudine and zalcitabine provided increases in CD4 T-cell counts that were sustained for several months.[39] Clinical benefits in antiretroviral-naive patients were noted in one study of subjects with a CD4 T-cell count of 200 to 500 cells/mm^3 and in another of subjects with symptomatic HIV disease or asymptomatic disease with a CD4 T-cell count of less than 350 cells/mm^3.[27, 29] Benefits were also suggested in a third study of antiretroviral-naive individuals with advanced HIV infection who had either AIDS or a CD4 T-cell count less than 200 cells/mm^3.[31] In contrast, the efficacy of zalcitabine with zidovudine was less in zidovudine-experienced subjects. In persons with CD4 T-cell count of 200 to 500 cells/mm^3 without AIDS who were zidovudine experienced (median 20 months of prior zidovudine), the combination of zidovudine and zalcitabine resulted in fewer clinical end points (AIDS-defining illness, death, or $\geq$50% decrease in CD4 T-cell count) compared with zidovudine alone.[27] In patients with more advanced disease, the combination of zalcitabine and zidovudine decreased the relative risk of disease progression or death compared with zidovudine alone only in individuals with less than a year's experience with zidovudine.[31] Two other studies of adults with advanced disease and considerable zidovudine experience (means of 17 to 18 months of prior zidovudine therapy) failed to show any benefits of the combination over continued zidovudine monotherapy.[29, 37]

A major toxicity of zalcitabine is peripheral neuropathy, which is seen more frequently than with didanosine therapy.[38] The incidence of neuropathy increases with higher doses of the drug, lower creatinine clearance, and lower CD4 T-cell counts and may be up to one third of patients with advanced disease.[36] Neuropathy is generally reversible if the drug is discontinued promptly.[40] Pancreatitis has also been observed in 1 to 2% of all patients taking zalcitabine and is seen more commonly in patients who also have other risks for pancreatitis.[29] Other reactions include oral ulcers, which may be severe in 3% of patients, and fixed drug eruptions.

Stavudine

Stavudine (2,′,3′-didehydro-2′,3′-dideoxythymidine; d4T) is a thymidine nucleoside analogue that is well absorbed after oral administration, with oral bioavailability of 86%. Its plasma half-life is approximately 1.1 hours, and the intracellular half-life of its triphosphate form is approximately 3 hours.[41] Stavudine penetrates the CNS with a CSF/plasma concentration ratio of 0.4.[42] Approximately 40% of an oral dose is eliminated through the kidneys, and the dose should be reduced in patients with renal insufficiency. The metabolic fate of 60% of an oral dose is unknown, but pharmacokinetics of the drug do not appear to be altered in patients with hepatic impairment. The adult dose of stavudine is 40 mg orally twice a day in a person weighing 60 kg or more and 30 mg orally twice a day if the weight is less than 60 kg.

In adults with over 6 months of prior zidovudine use and CD4 T-cell counts of 50 to 500 cells/mm^3, changing therapy to stavudine was beneficial compared with continuing zidovudine.[43] Subjects who received stavudine had higher CD4 T-cell counts and experienced fewer clinical end points (AIDS-defining events or death) compared with those who received zidovudine. However, stavudine monotherapy appears to be inferior to didanosine monotherapy in zidovudine-experienced individuals in its ability to decrease HIV-1 RNA levels and increase CD4 T-cell counts.[44] In vitro, stavudine has shown additive to synergistic antiviral activity against HIV-1 in combination with didanosine, zalcitabine, and lamivudine.[19] Preliminary reports from clinical trials evaluating the combinations of stavudine with didanosine or with lamivudine in treatment of naive patients show potent, durable suppression of HIV-1 RNA with either combination.[45–47] In contrast, stavudine in combination with zidovudine in vitro shows antagonistic activity against HIV-1.[19] In clinical trials, the combination of zidovudine and stavudine failed to demonstrate improved antiviral activity compared with stavudine alone, whether used in zidovudine-experienced or -naive individuals.[44]

Stavudine's major adverse reaction is a sensory peripheral neuropathy, similar to that seen with didanosine and zalcitabine.[48] Neuropathy develops in approximately 13% of stavudine-treated patients.[43] The incidence is increased in patients with advanced disease (up to 25%) and in those with other current or prior risk factors for neuropathy. Neuropathy is generally reversible if the drug is discontinued promptly. If symptoms resolve completely, stavudine may be restarted at half the recommended dose. Although macrocytosis can be seen in many patients, there does not appear to be an increased rate of anemia associated with stavudine in adults.[48]

Lamivudine

Lamivudine ((−)-β-enantiomer of 2′,3′-dideoxy-3′-thiacytidine; 3TC) is a cytidine analogue that is absorbed well orally, with a bioavailability of 86%. Its serum half-life is 2.5 hours, and the intracellular half-life of the biologically active triphosphate form is 11 to 14 hours.[49] Initial studies on adults suggest that lamivudine penetration into the CSF is poor, with a CSF/serum concentration ratio of 0.06.[50] Approximately 70% of a dose is excreted unchanged in urine, and lamivudine dosing should be adjusted in patients with renal impairment. Dosing in adults is 150 mg orally every 12 hours.

When used alone, lamivudine causes a decrease in plasma viral RNA levels and an increase in CD4 T-cell counts, but these effects are largely transient, with a return of both measures toward baseline by 8 weeks of therapy.[51] Lamivudine has shown synergistic activity when combined with either zidovudine or stavudine in vitro.[19] Two clinical trials evaluated the combination of lamivudine and zidovudine in antiretroviral-naive individuals. In adults with 200 to 500 CD4 T cells/mm^3, zidovudine with lamivudine produced a maximal decrease in plasma HIV-1 RNA of 1.6 $\log_{10}$ at week 4 of therapy.[52] Antiviral effects were durable with decreases from baseline HIV-1 RNA levels of 0.9 $\log_{10}$ by week 24 and 0.8 $\log_{10}$ at 1 year, In contrast, zidovudine monotherapy caused a maximal decrease of 0.5 $\log_{10}$, which diminished to 0.2 $\log_{10}$ by 1 year, and lamivudine monotherapy produced a maximal decrease of 1.6 $\log_{10}$, which diminished to 0.4 $\log_{10}$ by 1 year. In the combination arm, increases in CD4 T-cell counts of 61 cells/mm^3 were sustained after a year of therapy compared with a decline of 53 cells/mm^3 in subjects treated with zidovudine alone. Another trial in adults who were largely antiretroviral-naive (5% had previously received less than a month of zidovudine) showed similar sustained benefits in plasma HIV-1 RNA levels and in CD4 T-cell counts.[53]

Two trials examined the combination of zidovudine with lamivudine in zidovudine-experienced subjects and showed antiviral and immunologic benefits that were less than those in antiretroviral-naive subjects. In adults with CD4 T-cell counts of 100 to 400 cells/mm^3 who had a mean previous zidovudine exposure of almost 2 years, the combination of zidovudine and lamivudine produced a decrease in plasma HIV-1 RNA of 0.9 $\log_{10}$ and an increase in CD4 T-cell counts of 40 cells/mm^3 at 24 weeks of therapy, whereas continuation of zidovudine therapy resulted in increased HIV-1 RNA levels and decreased CD4 T-cell counts.[54] A second trial compared the combinations of zidovudine and lamivudine to zidovudine and zalcitabine in adults with CD4 T-cell counts of 100 to 300 cells/mm^3 who had a median previous zidovudine exposure of 20 months.[55] Although both combinations caused HIV-1 RNA decreases of 0.4 to 0.5 $\log_{10}$ at 1 year of therapy, zidovudine with lamivudine increased CD4 T-cell counts by 38 cells/mm^3 at 1 year, whereas zidovudine with zalcitabine produced a decrease of four cells/mm^3. A third trial examined the addition of lamivudine to previous treatment regimens of zidovudine alone or zidovudine with didanosine or zalcitabine in adults with CD4 T-cell counts of 25 to 250 cells/mm^3.[56] Combination therapy that included lamivudine was associated with a 60% decrease in mortality and a 57% decrease in clinical progression to a new AIDS-defining illness or death.

The use of lamivudine in combinations that do not include zidovudine is under investigation. The combination of lamivudine and stavudine can provide potent and durable viral suppression and CD4 T-cell increases in antiretroviral-naive individuals, and similar benefits, though less pronounced, can still be seen in persons with prior experience with zidovudine, didanosine, or zalcitabine.[47] In contrast, the combination of lamivudine with didanosine in antiretroviral-naive individuals may not have significantly increased antiviral potency compared with didanosine alone.[46]

Lamivudine is generally very well tolerated in adults.[52–56] The most frequent adverse events have been headache, dizziness, malaise, or fatigue.

Abacavir

Abacavir is a guanosine analogue that is well absorbed orally. Although the plasma half-life of abacavir is less than 2 hours, the intracellular half-life of its biologically active form, carbovir triphosphate, is 3.3 hours. CSF penetration appears to be limited, with a CSF/serum concentration ratio of 0.18. Abacavir is metabolized primarily by glucuronidation and carboxylation. The adult dose is 300 mg orally every 12 hours. Abacavir produces a median drop of 1.1 log_{10} in HIV-1 RNA levels and a median increase of 92 CD4 T cells/mm^3 at week 4 of therapy when used alone in individuals with CD4 T-cell counts of 200 to 500 cells/mm^3.[57] When combined with zidovudine and lamivudine or with any of the currently available protease inhibitors, it can provide a drop in HIV-1 RNA levels of approximately 2.0 log_{10}, which lasts at least 16 weeks.[58, 59] Abacavir has been generally well tolerated, with the most common adverse effects being nausea, headache, weakness, insomnia, and abdominal pain. Its most serious adverse effect has been a hypersensitivity reaction, which occurs in approximately 3% of treated individuals. Symptoms appear 1 to 4 weeks after starting therapy and include fever and malaise, often with nausea, vomiting, diarrhea, myalgia, arthralgia, and rash, although rash may be absent. Laboratory abnormalities have included acute lymphopenia, elevated liver function tests, and elevated creatine phosphokinase levels. Symptoms resolve within 1 to 2 days of discontinuing abacavir. However rechallenge with the drug, even at decreased dose, may cause the return of symptoms within hours with increased severity and often with life-threatening hypotension and facial or throat swelling. Thus, individuals with hypersensitivity reactions to abacavir should not be rechallenged with the drug.

Mechanisms of Resistance

A major determinant of antiretroviral drug failure is viral genotypic variation conferring drug resistance.[60, 61] HIV-1 infection is a dynamic process with high rates of replication and a great potential for genetic variation.[62–64] Given that HIV-1 RT lacks a proofreading function and is estimated to have an in vivo forward mutation rate of about 10^{-5} mutations/base pair/cycle, a mutation may occur on average at each nucleotide position as often as 10^4 times a day in an untreated individual.[65] HIV-1 genetic variants conferring resistance to single antiretroviral agents may exist in the infected individual before any therapy. When a patient starts a drug regimen, the regimen selects for preexisting mutations as well as additional mutations that appear in different genetic backgrounds. Mutations continue to accumulate unless replication is slowed enough to curtail genetic diversification. Genotypic resistance has been reported for each of the antiretroviral agents in current use.

Viral isolates with reduced sensitivity to zidovudine were documented within 3 years of its introduction.[66] In HIV-1 infected individuals on zidovudine monotherapy, the first mutation to arise in RT is usually a change in codon 70 from Lys to Arg (Lys70→Arg), which is seen transiently and is usually replaced by Thr215→Tyr after a few months of therapy.[67–69] During ongoing therapy, other mutations (including Met41→Leu, Asp67→Asn, Leu210→Trp, Lys219→Glu or Gln, and reappearance of Lys70→Arg,) accumulate and confer augmented resistance to zidovudine.[68–72] Although single-codon mutations confer only minimal resistance to zidovudine, a highly zidovudine-resistant virus with a 100-fold increase in 50% inhibitory concentration (IC_{50}) arises after three or four substitutions.[70, 71, 73, 74] Zidovudine-resistant HIV-1 has shown remarkable fitness, often persisting despite the discontinuation of zidovudine, and its transmissibility does not appear to be impaired.[69, 75–77] In clinical studies, individuals with highly zidovudine-resistant viruses actually do worse than those with zidovudine-susceptible isolates, regardles of whether they continue on zidovudine or switch to didanosine.[78] Although zidovudine-resistant mutants are often susceptible to other RT inhibitors, a large study of viral isolates from individuals on chronic zidovudine monotherapy found that each 10-fold decrease in zidovudine susceptibility was accompanied by a twofold decrease in susceptibility to either didanosine or zalcitabine.[79]

Resistance to didanosine or zalcitabine arises slowly in patients during monotherapy. Mutations in RT associated with decreased susceptibility include Lys65→Arg and Thr69→Asp for zalcitabine and Leu74→Val for didanosine and confer only a fourfold to tenfold increase in IC_{50} relative to wild-type virus.[80–83] Isolates with resistance to didanosine are often also resistant to zalcitabine. In vitro selection with stavudine may produce a virus with the RT Val75→Thr mutation, which confers a sevenfold increase in IC_{50}.[84] This mutation also confers decreased susceptibility to didanosine and zalcitabine. However, prolonged treatment with stavudine (over 1.5 years) is not commonly associated with the emergence of significant genotypic or phenotypic resistance.[85] Resistance to abacavir is also slow to arise and has been associated with RT mutations Lys65→Arg, Leu74→Val, Tyr115→Phe, and Met184→Val, which, in combination, may increase the IC_{50} of the drug by up to 10-fold.[86] However, virus with multiple zidovudine resistance mutations often displays decreased susceptibility to abacavir.[87]

Resistance dynamics for lamivudine are different from those for other nucleoside analogues. In individuals treated with lamivudine alone, high-level resistance (>100-fold increase in IC_{50}) appears within 4 to 8 weeks, conferred by mutations at RT codon 184.[51, 88] Met184→Ile is observed initially followed by Met184→Val. Met184→Val by itself confers low-level cross-resistance (twofold to fivefold increase in IC_{50}) to didanosine, zalcitabine, and abacavir, but no cross-resistance to zidovudine.[88, 89]

Interactions among various drug-selected substitutions may be important in the virologic activity of multidrug combinations.[60] For example, the zidovudine-selected RT mutations Thr215→Tyr and Lys219→Gln may augment didanosine resistance mediated by Leu74→Val.[83] Conversely, the didanosine resistance RT mutation Leu74→Val suppresses the phenotypic increase in IC_{50} seen with some but not all zidovudine resistance mutations.[82, 83] Similarly, the lamivudine resistance mutation RT Met184→Val suppresses the zidovudine resistance conferred by several zidovudine-selected mutations.[90] The clinical relevance of these mutational interactions has not yet been established.

Mutations that individually confer resistance to various drugs in a particular combination play an important role in the development of resistance during therapy with that combination. Sequential use of zidovudine followed by didanosine selects for a virus with zidovudine resistance mutations and the didanosine resistance mutation RT Leu74→Val; this virus is resistant to didanosine but regains sensitivity to zidovudine unless the zidovudine-selected RT Met41→Leu is present.[83] For the combination of zidovudine and lamivudine, the RT Met184→Val mutant virus emerges rapidly whereas zidovudine resistance mutations develop at a slower rate than during zidovudine monotherapy; this virus is resistant to lamivudine but remains sensitive to zidovudine for some time after zidovudine-selected mutations evolve.[90]

However, novel combinations of unexpected mutations conferring multidrug resistance have also been described in patients on multidrug regimens. A virus resistant to both zidovudine and lamivudine emerges after long-term combination therapy. Resistance appears to involve complex selection for newly recognized substitutions in RT (including at codon 333) in addition to persistent zidovudine resistance mutations and the lamivudine resistance mutation at codon 184.[91] This virus maintains the lamivudine resistance phenotype and augments the zidovudine IC_{50}, thus abrogating the Met184→Val suppression of zidovudine phenotypic resistance. A multinucleoside-resistant virus with several novel mutations in RT (Ala62→Val, Val75→Ile, Phe77→Leu, Pro116→Tyr, and Gln151→Met) has also been described in some patients on long-term therapy with zidovudine and didanosine or zidovudine and zalcitabine.[92–94] This virus is resistant to zidovudine, didanosine, zalcitabine, stavudine, abacavir, and to some degree lamivudine. Insertion of two extra amino acids at codon 69 has been seen in several individuals with extensive treatment with nucleoside RT inhibitors.[94a] This insertion, in the context of zidovudine resistance mutations, confers decreased susceptibility to all currently approved nucleoside RT inhibitors.

The determinants of phenotypic resistance to the effects of antiretroviral agents may not reside solely in viral genes. Alterations in cells of individuals exposed to a drug may allow an otherwise susceptible virus to replicate despite the presence of adequate serum levels of the antiretroviral agent. For instance, chronic zidovudine exposure may alter cellular phosphorylation mechanisms, rendering cells inefficient in phosphorylating nucleoside analogue RT inhibitors to their biologically active triphosphate forms.[95] Although this mechanism may be partly responsible for the poorer virologic and clinical response of zidovudine-experienced individuals to other nucleoside RT inhibitors, its role in antiretroviral failure remains to be clarified.[96–98]

Nevirapine

Delavirdine

Efavirenz

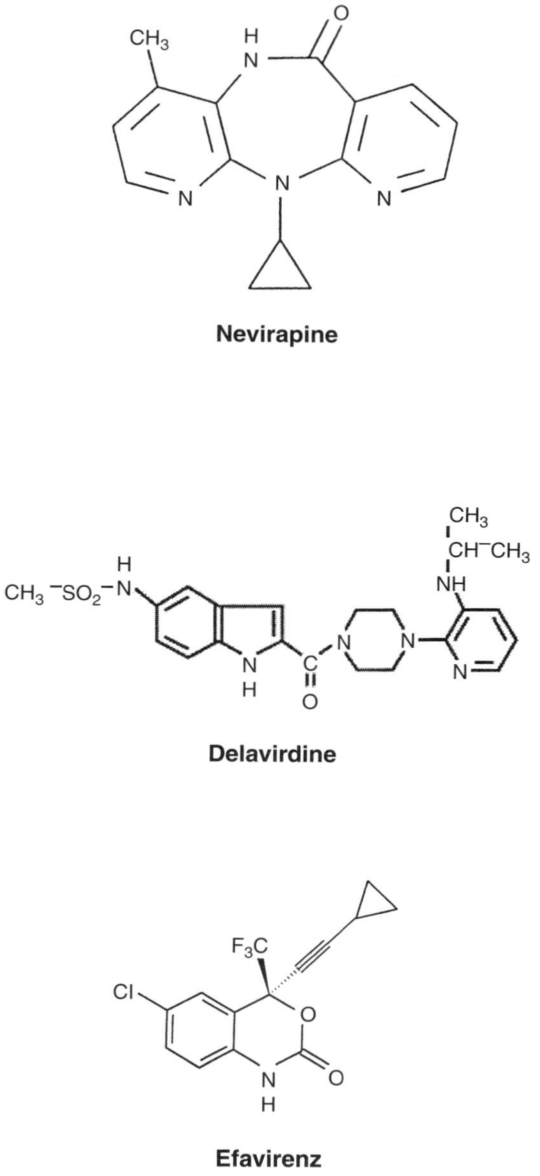

FIGURE 115–2. Non-nucleoside reverse transcriptase inhibitors.

Non-nucleoside Reverse Transcriptase Inhibitors

NNRTIs (Fig. 115–2, Table 115–2) include compounds with widely divergent chemical structures. They do not require phosphorylation or intracellular processing to become activated.[99] They are noncompetitive inhibitors of RT and cause allosteric inhibition of enzyme function by binding at sites distinct from the nucleoside-binding site. Nevirapine and delavirdine cause a disruption of the RT catalytic site and block the DNA polymerase activity of RT. All have excellent activity against HIV-1 but none against HIV-2.

Nevirapine

Nevirapine is well absorbed orally with a bioavailability of greater than 90%, which is not altered by taking the drug with meals or antacid. Its plasma half-life is more than 24 hours.[100] Nevirapine penetrates the CNS well, with a CSF/serum concentration ratio of 0.45. The drug is metabolized extensively in the liver through the cytochrome P-450 enzyme complex. Nevirapine induces its own metabolism and causes a twofold increase in its apparent oral clearance in the first 2 to 4 weeks of therapy. For this reason, and to decrease the incidence of drug-induced rash, the initial adult dose is 200 mg once a day for the first 2 weeks followed by 200 mg twice a day thereafter. Nevirapine also induces the metabolism of other drugs that are metabolized by cytochrome P-450, including oral contraceptive agents, rifampin, rifabutin, and some protease inhibitors (saquinavir and indinavir). The clinical significance of these observations is unclear. Nevirapine does not alter blood levels of ritonavir, nor do saquinavir, ritonavir, or indinavir alter nevirapine levels significantly.

Used alone, nevirapine produces a drop in viral RNA of 1 to 2 $\log_{10}$ by 2 weeks of therapy.[101] However, these values return to baseline by 4 weeks of therapy in conjunction with the emergence of virus resistant to nevirapine.[102, 103] The rapid appearance of resistance has limited the use of nevirapine monotherapy. In vitro, nevirapine has additive to synergistic activity against HIV-1 when used in combination with zidovudine, didanosine, stavudine, lamivudine, and saquinavir. Nevirapine can have potent and durable clinical benefits when used as part of a combination with nucleoside analogue RT inhibitors. In antiretroviral-naive adults with a CD4 T-cell count of 200 to 600 cells/mm^3, the combination of nevirapine with zidovudine and didanosine produced maximal decreases in HIV-1 RNA of 2.2 $\log_{10}$ at week 8 that were sustained through the first year of therapy.[104] After a year of treatment, the mean CD4 T-cell count increased by 139 cells/mm^3 and 45% of subjects had levels of plasma HIV-1 RNA that were undetectable (<20 copies/ml). In contrast, decreases in HIV-1 RNA were transient, and improvements in CD4 T-cell counts were smaller for combinations of zidovudine with didanosine or zidovudine with nevirapine. In antiretroviral-naive adults with more advanced disease (with AIDS or a CD4 T-cell count <200 cells/

TABLE 115-2 Approved Non-nucleoside Reverse Transcriptase Inhibitors

Agent	Trade Name	Oral Bioavail-ability (%)	Serum Half-Life (H)	Elimination	Dose*	Availability	Major Adverse Effects
Nevirapine	Viramune	>90	>24	Hepatic cytochrome P450	Adult: 200 mg PO qd for 14 d, then 200 mg PO q12h if no rash develops Pediatric: 120 mg/m² PO qd for 14 d then increase to 120–200 mg/m² PO q12h if no rash develops, up to adult dose	200-mg tablets	Rash Elevated hepatic transaminases
Delavirdine	Rescriptor	85	5.8	Hepatic cytochrome P450	Adult: 400 mg PO q8h	100-mg tablets	Rash
Efavirenz	Sustiva		>24	Hepatic cytochrome P450	Adult: 600 mg PO qd	50 mg-, 100 mg-, 200 mg- capsules	Dizziness Headache Rash

*Neonatal dose may differ significantly from pediatric dose described here.

mm³), the combination of nevirapine, zidovudine, and didanosine had similarly greater virologic and immunologic benefits compared with the combination of zidovudine and didanosine.[105] However, the efficacy of nevirapine in combination with zidovudine and didanosine may be limited by prior antiretroviral use. In adults with CD4 T-cell counts of less than 350 cells/mm³ and extensive prior use of nucleoside analogue RT inhibitors (nearly all with zidovudine with or without didanosine or zalcitabine for a median of 25 months), the three-drug combination of nevirapine, zidovudine, and didanosine produced a maximal HIV-1 RNA drop of 1.1 $\log_{10}$ at 4 weeks, compared with 0.4 $\log_{10}$ in the two-drug combination of zidovudine and didanosine.[106] By week 48, HIV-1 RNA levels were not different from baseline in the three-drug arm and were slightly above baseline in the two-drug arm. Subjects whose prior treatment consisted of only zidovudine responded better than those who also had experience with didanosine or zalcitabine.

The most frequent adverse effect of nevirapine has been rash, usually presenting as an erythematous maculopapular eruption sparing the palms and soles.[103, 104] It occurs in approximately 22% of patients during the first 1 to 8 weeks of therapy. Generally mild and self-limited, the rash can be monitored on a stable dose of nevirapine, with escalation of the dose after the first 2 weeks of therapy when the rash dissipates. However, in 9% of patients, severe rash can develop, possibly leading to Stevens-Johnson syndrome.[106] If the rash is severe, extensive, or involves the mucous membranes, nevirapine should be discontinued. Elevated hepatic enzyme levels are seen frequently (up to 22% of subjects) although clinical hepatitis has been noted infrequently.[104]

Delavirdine

Delavirdine is well absorbed orally with bioavailability of 85%. It requires an acidic environment for optimal absorption. The use of antacids within 1 hour of delavirdine administration or the use of H_2 blockers may reduce its absorption. The half-life of delavirdine is 5.8 hours. It is highly protein-bound (98%) and has poor CNS penetration.[107] Delavirdine is metabolized primarily by the hepatic cytochrome P-450 enzyme complex. Several drugs may induce hepatic metabolism of delavirdine and thereby decrease its plasma levels. These include nelfinavir, rifabutin, rifampin, and several anticonvulsant agents. Conversely, delavirdine inhibits the hepatic metabolism of several drugs. Significant increases in plasma levels of saquinavir, indinavir, nelfinavir, clarithromycin, and rifabutin have been documented, and potentially serious adverse events have been predicted for dihydropyridine calcium channel blockers (such as nifedipine), cisapride, warfarin, quinidine, ergot derivatives, some nonsedating antihistamines (such as terfenadine and astemizole), and several benzodiazepines. The usual adult does of delavirdine is 400 mg three times a day.

An early study investigated responses in plasma HIV-1 RNA levels and CD4 T-cell counts in nucleoside analogue RT inhibitor–experienced adults receiving delavirdine alone, delavirdine with zidovudine, delavirdine with zidovudine and didanosine, or zidovudine with didanosine.[107] The mean CD4 T-cell counts before therapy were 189 to 222 cells/mm³ in the various arms. Individuals who received delavirdine alone or delavirdine with zidovudine had only small decreases in HIV-1 RNA levels and small increases in CD4 T-cell counts that failed to persist into 1 month of therapy. Changes in these measurements were greatest and most durable in the three-drug arm, with a peak increase in CD4 T-cell counts of 50 cells/mm³ and a maximal decrease in HIV-1 RNA of 0.5 $\log_{10}$. However, by week 24, these values had returned to baseline and were not different from those seen in the zidovudine-with-didanosine arm. Delavirdine appears to have greater efficacy when used in a combination in antiretroviral-naive individuals with less advanced disease. In a group of mostly antiretroviral-naive adults with mean CD4 T-cell counts of approximately 360 cells/mm³, the combination of delavirdine with zidovudine and lamivudine produced a greater decrease in HIV-1 RNA levels (2.25 $\log_{10}$ at 24 weeks of therapy than either zidovudine with lamivudine (1.32 $\log_{10}$) or zidovudine with delavirdine (0.55 $\log_{10}$).[108] Viral RNA levels were undetectable (<400 copies/ml) by week 24 in 71% of individuals on the three-drug regimen, whereas only 23% of those taking zidovudine with lamivudine achieved this level of viral suppression. At the same time, the three-drug combination produced mean increases in CD4 T-cell counts of 105 cells/mm³, whereas zidovudine with lamivudine caused an increase of 75 cells/mm³ and zidovudine with delavirdine showed little change from baseline.

Similarly to nevirapine, rash may occur in approximately 18% of patients receiving delavirdine in the first 1 to 3 weeks of therapy. This is usually an erythematous maculopapular mildly pruritic eruption that is often confluent.[107] In most cases, the rash is transient, peaks over 2 to 3 days, and then resolves gradually. Although the rash is usually mild and does not require discontinuation of delavirdine, it may be severe in 3 to 4% of patients, necessitating discontinuation of therapy. Elevated hepatic transminase levels have also been observed.

Efavirenz

Efavirenz is well absorbed orally and has no significant food effects. Its half-life is over 24 hours, allowing once-daily dosing. Efavirenz is highly protein-bound (99.5%) but appears to have good CNS penetration.[109] It is metabolized primarily by the hepatic cytochrome P-450 enzyme complex. It alters the hepatic metabolism of several drugs, decreasing plasma levels of some (such as clarithromycin, saquinavir, indinavir, and amprenavir). The adult dosage is 600 mg once daily. When combined with indinavir, efavirenz produced a mean decrease in the HIV-1 RNA level of 2.5 $\log_{10}$, which was sustained through 60 weeks of therapy.[110] HIV-1 RNA was undetectable (<400 copies/ml) in 91% of subjects on this regimen, and remained undetectable in 76% with an ultrasensitive text (<20 copies/ml). This combination also produced a mean increase in the CD4 T-cell count of 267 cells/mm^3 at 60 weeks of therapy. The combination of efavirenz with zidovudine and lamivudine in antiretroviral-naive patients provided similarly impressive results when recipients were followed at up to 24 weeks of therapy.[111] One study suggested that, in antiretroviral naïve subjects, virologic response to efavirenz, zidovudine, and lamivudine was at least as effective as that to indinavir, zidovudine, and lamivudine when followed up to 48 weeks.[111a] The most frequent adverse effects have been CNS complaints including lightheadedness, dizziness, a sense of disengagement, or headache. These often diminish with continued therapy, and dosing at bedtime may improve the tolerability of these symptoms. Rash has also been observed, but generally is not severe or does not require drug discontinuation.

Mechanisms of Resistance

Mutations that confer high-level resistance to nevirapine (most commonly Lys103→Asn, Tyr181→Cys, Tyr188→Cys, Gly190→Ala) are selected rapidly during nevirapine monotherapy.[101, 102] These mutants may persist long after withdrawal of nevirapine. A similar pattern has been observed for delavirdine, with resistance mutations that include RT Lys103→Asn, Tyr181→Cys, and Pro236→Leu.[112] In contrast to nevirapine and delavirdine, efavirenz monotherapy may be associated with a slower development of high-level resistance that requires more than one mutation.[113] Efavirenz resistance in treated patients has been most commonly due to RT Lys103→Asn, though other substitutions (including Tyr188→Leu, Gly190→Ser) have also been seen.[114]

Cross-resistance does not occur between nucleoside analogue RT inhibitors and NNRTIs, allowing the potential use of NNRTIs in dividuals in whom a nucleoside analogue–resistant virus is suspected. Mutations conferring resistance to one NNRTI often confer cross-resistance to several other NNRTIs. The considerable overlap in the resistance profile of these drugs makes broad cross-resistance to this class likely.

Nucleotide Analogue Reverse Transcriptase Inhibitors

The expression of the nucleoside kinase responsible for the first phosphorylation step of the nucleoside analogues varies in different tissues and in cells during different states of activation. This may limit the ability of cells to activate nucleoside analogue RT inhibitors. Nucleotide (or nucleoside monophosphate) analogues, in contrast, require only the last two phosphorylation steps. Because enzymes responsible for these steps are ubiquitous, nucleotide RT inhibitors may have antiviral activity in a broader range of tissues and cell types. Once converted intracellularly to its diphosphate form, the nucleotide analogue competes with RT's natural substrates and can function as a chain terminator.

Adefovir (9-(2-phosphonomethoxyethyl)adenine, PMEA) is an analogue of adenine that has activity against a broad array of viruses, including HIV-1, hepatitis B virus, and some herpesviruses. In its native form, adefovir is poorly absorbed orally. However, attaching two pivalic acid moieties to it (forming adefovir dipivoxil) produces a prodrug with an oral bioavailability of 40%. The intracellular half-life of the biologically active diphosphate is 16 to 18 hours allowing for once daily dosing. The drug is excreted renally.

In adults with a mean CD4 T-cell count of 344 cells/mm^3, adefovir monotherapy (125 mg daily) provided a decrease in HIV-1 RNA levels of 0.5 $\log_{10}$ and an increase in mean CD4 T-cell counts of 57 cells/mm^3, both of which were sustained through 12 weeks of therapy.[114a] Although in vitro experiments suggested that the RT mutations Lys65→Arg and Lys70→Glu can confer a 10-fold decrease in susceptibility to adefovir, treatment with adefovir for 1 year did not appear to be associated with emergence of significant genotypic or phenotypic resistance.[114b] The presence of the lamivudine selected RT Met184→Val may increase the susceptibility of HIV-1 to adefovir.[114c]

Long-term use of adefovir may produce serious renal toxicity, including Fanconi syndrome, which may occur in more than 20% of individuals treated at 125 mg daily for longer than 20 weeks. The syndrome rarely appears before 24 weeks and is usually reversible on drug discontinuation. Recent studies suggest that 60 mg of adefovir daily may also show anti-HIV-1 activity, at least over a 4-week period (0.25 log reduction of HIV-1 RNA) with an improved safety profile. In a study comparing nephrotoxicity of adefovir-containing combinations over 42 weeks, adefovir doses of 60 mg daily led to creatinine elevations of 0.5 mg/dl above baseline in 29% of patients, whereas 120 mg daily resulted in creatinine elevations in 42%.[114d] Other common adverse effects of adefovir have included nausea, diarrhea, weakness, and elevations in hepatic enzymes. The pivalic acid derivatives that improve adefovir's bioavailability are associated with reduced carnitine concentrations. Although no clinical sequelae of reduced carnitine were noted in up to 12 weeks of adefovir dipivoxil use without carnitine supplementation, the use of carnitine supplements during long-term therapy would be prudent.

Protease Inhibitors

The HIV protease (or proteinase) enzyme is an aspartyl protease that is essential for post-translational cleavage of gag and gag-pol polyprotein.[1] Several viral proteins, including those that form the protein components of the viral core, as well as protease itself, RT, and integrase, are synthesized as polyproteins that require cleavage by the viral protease to produce mature proteins. Protease inhibitors appear to block the necessary cleavage of these polyproteins in the late stages of the viral replicative cycle, causing the production of immature, defective viral particles.[115, 116] Unlike nucleoside analogue RT inhibitors, protease inhibitors do not need intracellular processing to be activated. Protease inhibitors are active against HIV-1 and HIV-2.

Currently available protease inhibitors (Fig. 115–3, Table 115–3) are extensively metabolized by the hepatic cytochrome P-450 enzyme complex, primarily through the isoenzyme cytochrome P-450_{IIIA4}. Protease inhibitors may interfere, to varied degrees, with the hepatic metabolism of other drugs by acting as cytochrome P-450 inducers or inhibitors.[117, 118] Although these effects are most prominent with ritonavir, the use of any protease inhibitor should prompt a careful review of concurrently used medications to avoid potential adverse effects. For instance, protease inhibitors may increase plasma levels of the antihistamines terfenadine and astemizole, which may decrease the threshold for life-threatening arrythmias. These agents should be avoided when using currently available protease inhibitors. Other drugs may alter blood levels of protease inhibitors by altering their metabolism. Inhibitors of cytochrome P-450 (such as ketoconazole) may increase levels markedly, whereas inducers (such as rifampin and rifabutin) may decrease levels significantly.

Several metabolic adverse effects have been associated with the chronic use of protease inhibitors. Hyperglycemia and new-onset or exacerbation of previous diabetes mellitus have been noted.[119] A lipodystrophy syndrome with symmetric loss of subcutaneous fat from the face and extremities was seen after the initiation of protease inhibitor therapy.[120] Abnormal fat deposits at the posterior base of the neck and in the abdominal viscera, often with elevated serum triglyceride levels, have also been reported.[121, 122] However, it is not clear whether these metabolic alterations are causally related to protease inhibitors as they have also been observed in patients on regimens not containing these drugs.[121, 123]

Saquinavir

Two formulations of oral saquinavir have been developed, a hard capsule and a soft gel capsule. Although the bioavailability of the

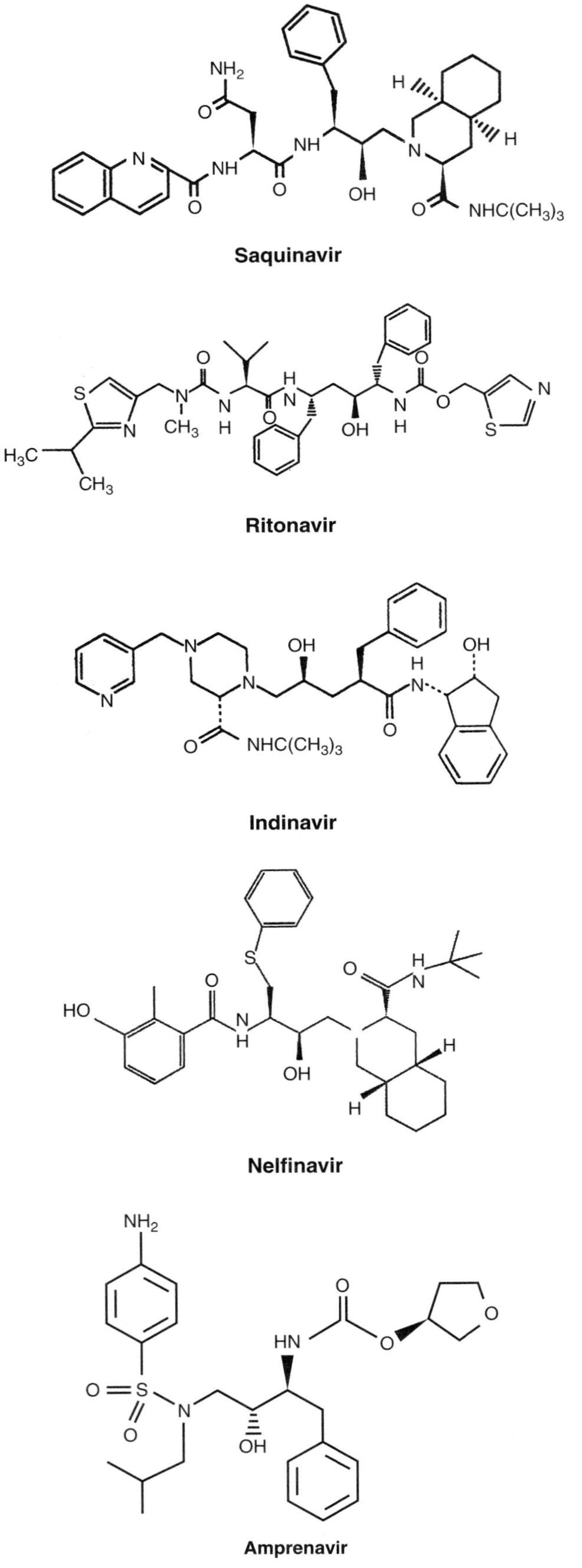

Saquinavir

Ritonavir

Indinavir

Nelfinavir

Amprenavir

FIGURE 115–3. Protease inhibitors.

hard capsule formulation has been low (average of 4%), the newer soft gel capsule has substantially improved bioavailability.[118] Saquinavir should preferably be taken with meals with a high fat content to maximize absorption. It is highly protein-bound (97%). Several drugs, including rifampin, rifabutin, nevirapine, efavirenz, and many anticonvulsants (phenobarbital, phenytoin, carbamazepine) induce metabolism of saquinavir and may decrease its plasma concentration considerably. In contrast, drugs such as ketoconazole, clarithromycin, ritonavir, indinavir, nelfinavir, and delavirdine inhibit the metabolism of saquinavir and may increase its levels markedly. Saquinavir may inhibit the metabolism of cisapride, ergot derivatives, many benzodiazepine sedatives (such as triazolam and midazolam) and several nonsedating antihistamines (such as terfenidine and astemizole), potentially causing dangerously high levels of these drugs. The usual adult dose of the soft gel capsule formulation of saquinavir is 1200 mg orally every 8 hours, but lower doses should be used in combination with some protease inhibitors.

Initial studies of saquinavir in the hard capsule formulation showed that when used alone at a dose of 600 mg three times a day, saquinavir provides a 0.7 $\log_{10}$ decrease in HIV-1 RNA levels and a mean CD4 T-cell count increase of 50 cells/mm^3.[124] However, these benefits dissipate by week 16 of therapy. Subsequent studies using higher doses of the hard capsule formulation demonstrated improved plasma HIV-1 RNA levels and CD4 T-cell count responses (a maximal mean decrease of 1.3 $\log_{10}$ and a mean increase of 121 cells/mm^3 with 2400 mg three times a day).[125] Although these effects diminished with time, they remained better than baseline through week 24 of therapy. Studies of saquinavir in combination with nucleoside analogue RT inhibitors have shown more durable responses than those with saquinavir monotherapy. In adults with CD4 T-cell counts of 50 to 300 cells/mm^3 and with an extensive prior history of zidovudine use (mean of 27 months), the combination of a saquinavir hard capsule at 600 mg three times a day with zidovudine and zalcitabine was superior to zidovudine with zalcitabine or to zidovudine with saquinavir in terms of the maximal decrease in HIV-1 RNA levels (0.8 $\log_{10}$ for the three-drug regimen) and increase in CD4 T-cell counts.[126] These responses were durable in the three-drug arm up to 48 weeks of therapy, although the study was unable to demonstrate differences in clinical outcomes between the various regimens. A more recent trial compared the combination of zalcitabine with saquinavir (hard capsule at 600 mg three times a day) to each of the drugs as monotherapy in zidovudine-experienced adults (mean of 17 months of previous zidovudine) with CD4 T-cell counts of 50 to 300 cells/mm^3.[127] Combination therapy was associated with a decrease in viral RNA levels of 0.6 $\log_{10}$ sustained through 48 weeks of therapy and an increase in CD4 T-cell counts, whereas monotherapy demonstrated more limited virologic and immunologic responses. Despite the low dose of saquinavir used, combination therapy resulted in a 49% reduction in the risk of progression to AIDS and a 68% reduction in mortality by 1 year after the initiation of therapy.

More recent studies have used the soft gel capsule formulation with better results. In adults who were antiretroviral-naive, the saquinavir soft gel capsule administered at 1200 mg three times daily was compared with the hard tablet formulation at 600 mg three times daily, each in combination with two nucleoside analogue RT inhibitors of choice.[128] At 16 weeks of therapy, combinations with the soft gel formulation produced a mean reduction in plasma viral RNA of 2 $\log_{10}$ whereas those with the hard gel formulation resulted in 1.6 $\log_{10}$ reduction. Furthermore, 80% of subjects taking the soft gel form had undetectable HIV-1 RNA levels ($<$ 400 copies/ml), whereas only 43% of those taking the hard tablet achieved similar levels of viral suppression. Taking advantage of ritonavir's marked inhibitory effects on saquinavir metabolism, the combination of saquinavir and ritonavir, which causes at least a 20-fold increase in saquinavir levels compared with that of saquinavir used alone, has been shown to have potent antiretroviral activity.[129, 130] The benefits in viral suppression were more prominent in individuals who were protease inhibi-

TABLE 115–3 Approved Protease Inhibitors

Agent	Trade Name	Oral Bioavailability (%)	Serum Half-Life (H)	Elimination	Dose*	Availability	Major Adverse Effects†
Saquinavir (soft gel capsule)	Fortovase		1–2	Hepatic cytochrome P450	Adult: 1200 mg PO q8h	200-mg soft gel capsules	Nausea Diarrhea Abdominal discomfort
Saquinavir (hard capsule)	Invirase	4	1–2	Hepatic cytochrome P450	Adult: When used in combination with ritonavir, 400–600 mg PO q12h	200-mg hard capsules	Nausea Diarrhea Abdominal discomfort
Ritonavir	Norvir	70	3.2	Hepatic cytochrome P450	Adult: 300 mg PO q12h with escalation over 1–2 wk to 600 mg PO q12h When used in combination with saquinavir, dose often decreased to 400 mg PO q12h Pediatric: 250 mg/m² of solution PO q12h with escalation over 1–2 wk to 400 mg/m² PO q12h, up to adult dose	100-mg capsules 80-mg/ml solution	Nausea, vomiting Diarrhea Abdominal discomfort Circumoral or peripheral paresthesias Fatigue Altered taste Hypercholesterolemia Hypertriglyceridemia Elevated hepatic transaminases
Indinavir	Crixivan	60–65	1.8	Hepatic cytochrome P450	Adults: 800 mg PO q8h	200-mg, 400-mg capsules	Nausea Abdominal discomfort Nephrolithiasis Hyperbilirubinemia
Nelfinavir	Viracept	20–80	3.5–5	Hepatic cytochrome P450	Adult: 750 mg PO q8h Pediatric: 20–30 mg/kg q8h, up to adult dose	250-mg tablets 50-mg/g powder	Diarrhea
Amprenavir	Agenerase		9	Hepatic cytochrome P450	Adult: Capsule 1200 mg PO q12h Pediatric: Capsule 20 mg/kg PO q12h or 15 mg/kg PO q8h, up to adult dose; solution 22.5 mg/kg PO q12h or 17 mg/kg PO q8h, up to 2800	50 mg, 150-mg capsules 15 mg/ml solution	Nausea, vomiting Rash

*Neonatal dose may differ significantly from pediatric dose described here.
†All protease inhibitors may be associated with hyperglycemia and changes in body fat distribution. They may also be associated with rare episodes of hemorrhage in persons with hemophilia.

tor–naive. When used with ritonavir, saquinavir can be given on a twice-daily regimen, although the optimal dose has not been established.

Adverse reactions to saquinavir have included diarrhea, nausea, abdominal discomfort, and dyspepsia. These were infrequent with the hard capsule formulation but appear more frequent and severe with the soft gel capsule.[131] Elevated triglyceride levels and asymptomatic elevations in liver enzyme and creatine phosphokinase levels have also been noted.[125]

Ritonavir

Ritonavir is well absorbed orally with a bioavailability of approximately 70%, is highly protein-bound in plasma (>98%), and has a half-life of 3.2 hours.[118, 132, 133] Other drugs may alter the metabolism of ritonavir, thereby either increasing its serum levels (as observed with clarithromycin, fluconazole, and fluoxetine) or decreasing its levels (as observed with rifampin and some anticonvulsant agents). Conversely, ritonavir itself can cause marked alterations in the metabolism of other drugs. It induces hepatic metabolism of itself as well as of several drugs, thereby decreasing the bioavailability of ethinyl estradiol in oral contraceptive agents, theophylline, and possibly atovaquone and some analgesic agents (including morphine, codeine, naproxen, and ketoprofen). Ritonavir may also inhibit the metabolism of other drugs, potentially causing serious adverse effects when used with rifabutin, several antiarrhythmic agents (amiodarone, quinidine, flecainide, encainide, and quinidine), some nonsedating antihistamines (astemizole and terfenidine), cisapride, meperidine, propoxyphene, ergot derivatives, and several benzodiazepines. It may also cause large increases in plasma levels of saquinavir, indinavir, nelfinavir, erythromycin, clarithromycin, ketoconazole, itraconazole, quinine, carbamazepine, calcium channel blockers, warfarin, analgesic agents (including methadone, fentanyl, and piroxicam), antidepressants (including desipramine, bupropion, sertraline, trazodone, and fluoxetine), some neuroleptics, several hypolipidemic agents, corticosteroids, and others. Since the liquid formulation of ritonavir contains alcohol, patients on metronidazole or disulfiram may have severe reactions if taking liquid ritonavir concomitantly. The usual adult dose of ritonavir is 600 mg orally every 12 hours, though lower doses may be used in combination with some other protease inhibitors. Ritonavir should be stored in a refrigerator and shielded from light.

Used alone, ritonavir produced a maximal decrease in HIV-1 RNA levels of at least 1 $\log_{10}$ at weeks 2 to 4 of therapy.[133, 134] Although HIV-1 RNA levels subsequently rose, they remained significantly lower than baseline by week 32 of therapy. In one study, mean increases in CD4 T-cell counts of up to 230 cells/mm³ above a baseline mean of 130 cells/mm³ were sustained through the 32 weeks of observation.[133] In combination therapy, ritonavir has shown potent and durable clinical benefits. Among adults with advanced HIV disease (CD4 T-cell count of < 100 cells/mm³) whose median length of prior antiretroviral therapy was 3 years (though protease inhibitor–naive), the addition of ritonavir to the nucleoside analogue RT inhibitor regimen resulted in a decreased viral RNA level of 0.6 $\log_{10}$ from baseline and a mean increase in CD4 T-cell counts of more than 50 cells/mm³ after 1 year of therapy.[135] In the ritonavir-treated group, the rate of clinical progression was 42% lower and the death rate was 30% lower during the first year of therapy compared with controls. Ritonavir has also shown potent antiviral activity in combination with other protease inhibitors, including saquinavir, indinavir, and nelfinavir.

Adverse reactions to ritonavir have included gastrointestinal disturbances (nausea, vomiting, or diarrhea in up to 52% and, less frequently, anorexia and abdominal pain), weakness, circumoral or peripheral paresthesias, altered taste, and headache.[133, 135] Adverse effects appear to be more common in patients with more advanced disease. They are also related to plasma levels of ritonavir and are greatest at the time of initiating therapy, before ritonavir induces an increase in its own metabolism. Toxicities often improve with continued therapy and may be less severe if ritonavir is taken with meals.

Also, starting the dosage at 300 mg orally every 12 hours and escalating over 1 to 2 weeks to the full adult dose of 600 mg orally every 12 hours decreases the severity of adverse effects. Most patients experience some elevations in cholesterol levels (30 to 40%) and in triglyceride levels (200 to 300%), and many also develop elevated levels of liver transaminases and creatine phosphokinase.[133, 135]

Indinavir

Indinavir requires an acidic environment for optimal solubility, and food with high protein or fat content interferes with its absorption.[116, 118] Therefore, indinavir should be taken in a fasting state (1 hour before a meal or 2 hours after a meal) or with a light, low-fat snack for optimal bioavailability of 60 to 65%. Indinavir has a half-life of 1.8 hours and exhibits less protein binding (60%) in blood than other protease inhibitors. Certain drugs inhibit indinavir's metabolism, increasing its plasma concentration. These include ritonavir, delavirdine, ketoconazole, and clarithromycin. Other drugs, including nevirapine, efavirenz, rifampin, rifabutin and fluconazole, may increase the metabolism of indinavir, thereby decreasing its plasma concentration. In turn, indinavir inhibits the metabolism of saquinavir, clarithromycin, ketoconazole, and rifabutin and may similarly affect rifampin, some nonsedating antihistamines (terfenidine, astemizole), ergotamines, cisapride, and several benzodiazepines. The usual adult dose of indinavir is 800 mg orally every 8 hours.

Indinavir provides potent and durable benefits, especially when used as part of a combination regimen. In adults with a median CD4 T-cell count of 144 cells/mm^3 who were previously treated with zidovudine for a median of 30 months, treatment with indinavir monotherapy or with zidovudine and lamivudine showed a transient decrease in viral RNA levels that diminished with an increasing time on therapy.[136] However, treatment with zidovudine, lamivudine, and indinavir produced a decrease in HIV-1 RNA levels of 2 $\log_{10}$ that persisted for over 1 year of therapy. At week 24 of therapy, 90% of subjects receiving the three-drug regimen had undetectable HIV-1 RNA levels (<500 copies/ml) whereas only 43% of those on indinavir monotherapy and 30% of those on zidovudine-with-lamivudine therapy had equivalent viral suppression.

A larger study with adults who were zidovudine experienced (median length of prior zidovudine of 21 months) and had more advanced disease (CD4 T-cell counts of 200 cells/mm^3 or less with a mean of 87 cells/mm^3) demonstrated a durable antiviral effect with the combination regimen of zidovudine, lamivudine, and indinavir.[137] The three-drug regimen provided a decrease in viral RNA levels of 2.8 $\log_{10}$ at week 24 with 60% of subjects having undetectable HIV-1 RNA levels (<500 copies/ml). In contrast, the combination of zidovudine and lamivudine without a protease inhibitor produced a decrease in viral RNA levels of 1 $\log_{10}$ at week 24 with only 9% of subjects having undetectable plasma HIV-1 RNA. By week 40, CD4 T-cell counts increased by 121 cells/mm^3 in the three-drug arm and by 40 cells/mm^3 in the two-drug arm. With a median duration of follow-up of only 38 weeks, the study showed a 47% decrease in the rate of clinical progression to a new AIDS-defining diagnosis or death in the protease inhibitor–containing arm.

A third study compared indinavir monotherapy with the combination of zidovudine and lamivudine and to the combination of all three drugs in adults with advanced HIV disease (CD4 T-cell counts ≤50 cells/mm^3) who were zidovudine experienced.[138] After 24 weeks, the median decreases in viral RNA were 2.2 $\log_{10}$ in the three-drug arm but only 0.17 $\log_{10}$ in the indinavir-monotherapy arm and 0.16 $\log_{10}$ in those taking two nucleoside analogue RT inhibitors. The proportion of individuals with undetectable viral RNA levels (< 500 copies/ml) was 65% for the three-drug regimen, 4% for indinavir monotherapy, and 0% for zidovudine combined with lamivudine. Median increases in CD4 T-cell counts were 86 cells/mm^3 in those on the three-drug regimen, 61 cells/mm^3 in those on indinavir monotherapy, and zero cells/mm^3 in the two-drug arm. Long-term follow-up of subjects who initially received the triple-drug regimen showed sustained suppression of plasma viral RNA for up to 84 weeks and persistent CD4 T-cell increases for up to 72 weeks.[139]

The most serious adverse effect of indinavir has been nephrolithiasis, with stones consisting of crystallized indinavir causing symptoms in 4 to 9% of treated individuals.[137, 140, 141] The frequency of nephrolithiasis can be reduced with high oral fluid intake (at least 1.5 liters/day) throughout the day. Indinavir-associated nephrolithiasis is treated supportively with hydration and analgesia, and interruption of indinavir therapy is usually not necessary. Gastrointestinal irritation (abdominal discomfort and nausea) is commonly observed when indinavir is taken in a fasting state. To improve tolerability, the drug may be taken with a small low-fat, low-protein meal without significantly compromising its absorption. Other adverse reactions may include insomnia, dry throat, and dry skin. An indirect hyperbilirubinemia is often observed (at least 10% of individuals) but does not lead to clinically significant liver disease.

Nelfinavir

Nelfinavir has good bioavailability, and its absorption is optimal when administered with food.[116, 118] It is highly protein-bound in plasma (>98%) and has a half-life of 3.5 to 5 hours. Drugs that decrease nelfinavir's metabolism and increase its levels include delavirdine, ritonavir, and ketoconazole. Rifampin and rifabutin increase nelfinavir's metabolism and reduce its plasma levels. Nelfinavir may affect the metabolism of several drugs. It decreases levels of ethinyl estradiol and norethindrone in oral contraceptive agents and may markedly increase levels of delavirdine, saquinavir, rifabutin, cisapride, ergot derivatives, some nonsedating antihistamines (terfenidine, astemizole), and several antiarrhythmics and benzodiazepines. The recommended adult dose of nelfinavir is 750 mg orally every 8 hours, though 1250 mg every 12 hours appears to be equally efficacious.

When nelfinavir was studied as monotherapy and in combination either with stavudine or with zidovudine and lamivudine, the most potent and durable antiviral effects were seen with the three-drug combination.[142] In a population of antiretroviral-naive adults with a mean CD4 T-cell count of 283 cells/mm^3, the combination of zidovudine, lamivudine, and nelfinavir resulted in a mean increase in CD4 T-cell counts of 155 cells/mm^3 and a decrease in plasma HIV-1 RNA of 2 $\log_{10}$ at 6 months of therapy.[143] By 6 months of therapy, 66% of subjects receiving the three-drug regimen had undetectable HIV-1 RNA levels (<50 copies/ml), and this response was maintained through 1 year of therapy.[144] Nelfinavir is being studied in combination therapy with other nucleoside analogue RT inhibitors as well as with other protease inhibitors.

Nelfinavir is generally well tolerated. Gastrointestinal complaints are common and include flatulence and mild to moderate diarrhea that can usually be controlled with antidiarrheal medications such as loperamide.

Amprenavir

Amprenavir is well absorbed orally and has no food effects. It has a half-life of 9 hours. The adult dose is 1200 mg every 12 hours. A study comparing amprenavir alone with the combination of amprenavir with zidovudine and lamivudine found that 63% of subjects taking the combination regimen had undetectable viral RNA levels (<500 copies/ml) at week 24 of therapy.[145] Amprenavir has also shown potency when used with other protease inhibitors. A study of combinations of amprenavir with each of saquinavir, indinavir, and nelfinavir demonstrated median decreases of HIV-1 RNA levels of greater than 2.5 $\log_{10}$ by week 4 that were sustained through week 16 of therapy.[146] In contrast, amprenavir monotherapy produced a peak decrease in viral load of less than 1.5 $\log_{10}$ at week 2 that was not sustained. Amprenavir is usually well tolerated. The most frequent side effects have been headache, gastrointestinal complaints (nausea and diarrhea), and rash.

Mechanisms of Resistance

The initial resistance mutations in HIV protease that arise during selection with protease inhibitors may be unique to the particular inhibitor used. However, other mutations accumulate over time and confer greater resistance to the drug. For saquinavir, one or two mutations in the protease (most commonly Leu90→Met, less often Gly48→Val, or rarely both) are enough to increase IC_{50} significantly and are associated with increased plasma viral RNA levels.[147] One or two mutations selected by ritonavir (first usually being Val82→Ala or Phe) are needed to reduce drug susceptibility, and the accumulation of further mutations (including Lys20→Arg, Leu33→Phe, Met36→Ile or Leu, Met46→Ile or Leu, Ile54→Val, Ala71→Val or Thr, Val82→Thr or Ser, Ile84→Val, and Leu90→Met) confers increasing levels of resistance.[148] Initial viral variants with Val82→Ala or Ile84→Val have a twofold decrease in susceptibility to ritonavir; additions of other mutations (including Met36→Ile, Ile54→Val, and Ala71→Val) can confer a more than 20-fold increase in resistance. For indinavir, a large number of mutations are selected in various combinations and sequential orders in different patients. Most commonly, these include Val82→Ala or Phe or Thr or Met46→Ile or Leu, but other changes include Leu10→Ile or Val or Arg, Lys20→Met or Arg, Leu24→Ile, Ile54→Val or Ala, Leu63→Pro, Ala71→Val or Thr, Ile84→Val, and Leu90→Met.[149, 150] Single or double substitutions do not appear to decrease in vitro susceptibility to indinavir significantly, but an increased number of resistance substitutions are associated with a greater magnitude of phenotypic resistance to the drug. Resistance to nelfinavir often arises first in conjunction with Asp30→Asn.[151] Frequently, this change in the protease is accompanied or followed by other changes, including Glu35→ASP, Met36→Ile, Met46→Ile, Ala71→Val or Thr, Val77→Ile, and Asn88→Asp, or ser. Amprenavir-selected substitutions in the protease have included Leu10→Phe, Met46→Ile, Ile47→Val, and Ile50→Val.[152]

A virus that contains only the initial resistance mutations to a particular protease inhibitor may have little cross-resistance to other protease inhibitors. For example, a nelfinavir-resistant virus with the protease Asp30→Asn substitution often remains susceptible to saquinavir, ritonavir, indinavir, and amprenavir.[151] Similarly, early ritonavir-selected isolates may remain susceptible to saquinavir and amprenavir.[148] However, with longer therapy, a highly resistant virus can evolve that contains many mutations that are common to several protease inhibitors and that confer broad cross-resistance to the entire class. Indinavir-selected resistant viruses are generally also resistant to ritonavir, and a substantial proportion have decreased susceptibility to saquinavir.[150] A study on cross-resistance of viruses obtained from protease inhibitor–treated individuals with resistance to saquinavir, ritonavir, indinavir, or nelfinavir demonstrated broad cross-resistance.[153] Indinavir and ritonavir were most consistently cross-resistant. However, approximately 40% of isolates resistant to saquinavir, ritonavir, or indinavir remained susceptible to nelfinavir.

Although certain protease inhibitor–resistant mutants may have decreased protease enzymatic function and replicative capacity, compensatory mutations in the *gag* region (including protease cleavage sites) may at least partially restore viral replicative fitness.[154] Mutations in protease cleavage sites have been documented for viruses resistant to indinavir and amprenavir.[155, 156]

CLINICAL ISSUES

In untreated HIV-1 infection, ongoing viral replication generally leads to progressive damage to the immune system, ultimately resulting in opportunistic infections or neoplasms and death.[157] Although the rate of disease progression varies widely, exceptions to this principle are rare. Antiretroviral therapy should be considered for all HIV-1–infected individuals with any evidence of ongoing viral replication. The ultimate goals of antiretroviral therapy are to prevent and possibly reverse immunologic deterioration, avert opportunistic infections and other morbidity related to HIV-1 disease, and thereby prolong survival.

Assays for Monitoring Infection

The recent widespread use of plasma HIV-1 RNA levels to monitor HIV-1 infection and antiretroviral therapy has transformed the clinical care of HIV-1–infected individuals. The level of HIV-1 RNA reflects the magnitude of viral replication. It correlates with the rate of CD4 T-cell decline, the relative risk of clinical disease progression, and the time to death.[158–160] On antiretroviral therapy, the magnitude of decrease in HIV-1 RNA levels is related to the relative risk of disease progression and death.[30, 161, 162] Baseline HIV-1 RNA levels should be checked before antiretroviral therapy is initiated to estimate the risk of progression and to guide subsequent therapy.[163] Ideally, this should be done when the patient is clinically stable, as HIV-1 RNA levels may be transiently elevated for several weeks after the initial HIV-1 infection, during an intercurrent illness, or for up to a month after an immunization. Two measurements separated by 1 to 2 weeks minimize the effects of technical and biologic variance that may cause HIV-1 RNA levels to vary by up to threefold (0.5 $\log_{10}$).[161] With potent antiretroviral therapy capable of halting detectable viral replication, the viral load usually decreases by 1 to 2 $\log_{10}$ within 2 weeks of therapy and reaches a nadir by 8 weeks, although up to 16 to 24 weeks may be required to reach a nadir in situations in which initial plasma HIV-1 RNA levels are very high. After therapy is initiated or changed, it is prudent to check HIV-1 RNA levels at least monthly until the nadir is reached and then at least every 3 months. A consistent increase in viral load of more than 0.5 $\log_{10}$ suggests a failing antiretroviral regimen. Even if the patient declines antiretroviral therapy, periodic HIV-1 RNA measurements are useful for monitoring progression of the infection, as increases in HIV-1 RNA levels above baseline may herald a more rapid immunologic or clinical decline. For an individual patient, it is important to follow HIV-1 RNA levels using the same assay since different methods of quantifying viral RNA levels do not always give directly comparable values.

The CD4 T-cell count reflects the extent of immune damage that has already occurred because of HIV-1 infection. CD4 T-cell counts correlate with the risk of developing opportunistic infections or neoplasms and with the time to death. Baseline CD4 T-cell counts should be checked before antiretroviral therapy is initiated to assess the prognosis and to guide the prophylaxis of opportunistic infections. Two measurements separated by 1 to 2 weeks reduce the effects of biologic and technical variance that may alter the cell counts by up to 30%.[164] After therapy is initiated, CD4 T-cell counts should be followed periodically, at least every 3 to 4 months, to monitor immunologic improvement. Although substantial increases in the CD4 T-cell count are common with combination antiretroviral therapy, it is unknown whether the particular CD4 T-cell count increase after therapy reflects the same functional activity as an equivalent CD4 T-cell count obtained before therapy. If the patient declines antiretroviral therapy, CD4 T-cell counts can be useful in monitoring the progression of the disease and in suggesting the need for prophylaxis of opportunistic infections.

Design of Combination Therapy

Several considerations are important in the design of combination regimens. First, the drugs in the combination should offer additive or synergistic intracellular antiviral activity. Such interactions have been documented for several commonly used combinations, including zidovudine with didanosine, zalcitabine, or lamivudine; stavudine with didanosine, zalcitabine, or lamivudine; nucleoside analogue RT inhibitors with NNRTIs and nucleoside analogue RT inhibitors with protease inhibitors.[19, 165] However, some combinations, notably zidovudine and stavudine, can be antagonistic in vitro and may offer relatively poor efficacy when used together clinically.[19, 44]

Second, pharmacokinetic interactions between the drugs in a combination may lead to clinically significant alterations in the absorption or metabolism of the drugs. Didanosine is buffered and cannot be taken simultaneously with antiretrovirals that require an acidic environment for adequate absorption, such as delavirdine and indinavir, making for somewhat unwieldy and complicated regimens with these drugs. Delavirdine and ritonavir increase plasma levels of certain protease inhibitors through the inhibition of hepatic metabolism. In contrast, nevirapine and efavirenz may increase the metabolism of indinavir and decrease its plasma level, necessitating increased dosage of indinavir if used with either of these agents.

Third, different drugs may be able to target cells at different levels of activation or cells in different tissue reservoirs. Because of different phosphorylation dynamics, didanosine, zalcitabine, and lamivudine are active in quiescent cells whereas zidovudine and stavudine are more active in replicating cells.[4] Combinations that include one drug from each category may provide broader antiretroviral coverage, though this has not been demonstrated clinically. The CNS penetration of zidovudine, stavudine, and nevirapine is good whereas it is relatively poor for didanosine, zalcitabine, lamivudine, and delavirdine and remains to be studied carefully for protease inhibitors. However, the relationship between CSF/plasma concentration ratios and antiretroviral activity within the CNS has not been established. The use of a combination regimen capable of suppressing HIV-1 replication in all body compartments may be necessary for long-term efficacy.

Fourth, care must be taken in combining drugs with overlapping toxicities. The use of didanosine and zalcitabine in combination increases the risk of peripheral neuropathy to unacceptable levels. Similarly, the simultaneous use of two bone marrow–suppressive agents, such as zidovudine and hydroxyurea, should be avoided. Whereas combination therapy offers the theoretical advantage that toxicity may be reduced if doses of individual drugs can be decreased, suboptimal dosing may promote the development of drug resistance.

Fifth, the likelihood of adherence to the regimen should be taken into account. A regimen involving multiple pills taken many times in the course of a day around a regimented meal schedule poses major challenges. A regimen involving few pills taken once or twice a day regardless of meals is far more likely to foster adherence. In this regard, a formulation combining zidovudine 300 mg with lamivudine 150 mg in the same tablet simplifies a regimen of two nucleoside RT inhibitors into one pill taken twice a day.

Finally, antiretroviral drugs should be combined with attention to the ability of HIV-1 to develop drug resistance to the individual components. Genotypic resistance may be expected to arise for any new antiretroviral regimen that incompletely inhibits viral replication.[65] Combination regimens that produce more potent inhibition of viral replication may delay or prevent resistance from arising by limiting the opportunity for new mutations to occur or accumulate.[166] Regimens that are not expected to provide complete suppression of HIV-1 RNA should not contain agents for which high-level resistance develops rapidly, such as lamivudine, nevirapine, or delavirdine. In contrast, combinations should be designed to create significant hurdles for the viral evolution of resistance. For instance, a multidrug combination for which significant resistance to all drugs can arise with only one or two mutations may have less durable efficacy compared with an equipotent combination that requires many more mutations in order for the virus to escape from the suppression of replication. The possibility of preexisting virus resistant to one or more drugs must also be kept in mind, especially in patients with a prior history of antiretroviral therapy. A broader antiretroviral coverage, especially with agents that do not share cross-resistance patterns with previously experienced drugs, is more likely to produce lasting benefits. An antiretroviral agent may give rise to a specific resistance mutation that may resensitize a virus that was previously resistant to another drug used in the same combination. An example of this phenomenon is the lamivudine resistance mutation in RT codon 184 that, in a background of some zidovudine resistance mutations, resensitizes the virus to zidovudine.[90] This may explain why the combination of zidovudine and lamivudine confers some long-term benefits as measured by levels of HIV-1 RNA and CD4 T-cell counts in previously heavily zidovudine-treated patients despite the development of the mutation of RT codon 184 in them. Finally, a choice in regimens should be made based in part on preserving future therapeutic options in case the initial combination fails. Once resistant virus arises in an infected individual, it may persist indefinitely, at least as a minority population. Therefore, choices for current and previous therapies significantly influence future therapeutic options.

Clinical Experience with Combination Therapy

The use of two nucleoside RT inhibitors that display synergistic or additive antiviral effects in vitro often results in greater and more durable clinical benefits than the use of one of them alone. These benefits have been most apparent in antiretroviral-naive individuals. For example, the combinations of zidovudine and didanosine or zidovudine and zalcitabine in antiretroviral-naive individuals decrease the rate of disease progression or death compared with zidovudine alone.[27, 29] Similarly, zidovudine with lamivudine provides potent and durable decreases in viral RNA levels and sustained increases in CD4 T-cell counts compared with zidovudine or lamivudine monotherapy in antiretroviral-naive individuals.[52, 53] Potent and durable antiviral benefits have also been noted for stavudine with didanosine and stavudine with lamivudine.[45, 46] However, some combinations have failed to show improved clinical antiviral activity compared with their individual components. Examples include the combination of zidovudine with stavudine compared with stavudine alone[44] and the combination of lamivudine and didanosine compared with didanosine alone.[46] The comparative efficacy of several commonly used combinations (such as zidovudine with lamivudine, stavudine with didanosine, stavudine with lamivudine, and zidovudine with didanosine) is unclear.

Despite the improved efficacy of combinations of two nucleoside RT inhibitors over monotherapy, no two-drug combination of nucleoside analogues has shown potent and durable suppression of viral replication. In contrast, the addition of a protease inhibitor to such a combination has often provided suppression of viral replication that was impressive in its level and duration. In zidovudine-experienced individuals, indinavir combined with zidovudine and lamivudine produced a mean of greater than 2 $\log_{10}$ drop in HIV-1 RNA at 24 weeks of therapy, and more than 50% of subjects had undetectable HIV-1 RNA levels (<500 copies/ml).[136–138] In antiretroviral-naive adults, the use of the soft gel formulation of saquinavir in combination with two nucleoside RT inhibitors or the combination of nelfinavir with zidovudine and lamivudine has provided similarly strong viral suppression.[128, 143] Trials comparing the different protease inhibitors to each other in combination therapies are in progress. Combinations of two nucleoside RT inhibitors with an NNRTI may produce viral suppression and immunologic improvements, which are equivalent to those seen in combinations that include protease inhibitors. Immunologic and virologic benefits of a combination of nevirapine, zidovudine, and didanosine in antiretroviral-naive individuals with 200 to 600 CD4 T-cells/mm^3 did not appear to be substantially inferior to those seen in protease inhibitor–containing regimens.[104] Similar results have been reported for the combination of efavirenz with zidovudine and lamivudine in antiretroviral-naive adults.[111, 111a] Whether there is a difference in relative efficacy between combinations containing a potent protease inhibitor and regimens containing a potent NNRTI remains to be determined.

Although combinations of two nucleoside analogue RT inhibitors with either a protease inhibitor or an NNRTI are commonly used, other combinations have also shown promise in suppressing viral replication and improving immune status. Combinations of two protease inhibitors, with or without nucleoside analogue RT inhibitors, have demonstrated potent and durable viral suppression as demonstrated by saquinavir with ritonavir or by amprenavir with other protease inhibitors.[130, 146] Combinations that include a protease inhibitor and an NNRTI can similarly demonstrate potent viral suppression as demonstrated by efavirenz with indinavir.[110] A combination of three nucleoside analogue RT inhibitors (such as abacavir with zidovudine and lamivudine) has also shown potent viral suppression in preliminary studies.

The background antiretroviral drug experience has a large impact on the likelihood of success of a certain combination regimen. Although the combination of didanosine and zidovudine decreased the rate of disease progression or death compared with zidovudine alone in zidovudine-experienced adults, the clinical benefits were less compared with those in zidovudine-naive subjects.[27, 29] In previously zidovudine-treated adults, zalcitabine with zidovudine has also shown decreased benefits in some studies[27, 31] and no clinical benefits in others.[29, 37] Lamivudine with zidovudine produced sustained decreases in HIV-1 RNA levels and increases in CD4 T-cell counts, but these effects again were less than those in antiretroviral-naive individuals.[54, 55] Nevertheless, these benefits can sometimes translate into decreased disease progression and lower mortality rates.[56] A similar pattern of decreased antiviral efficacy and immunologic improvement was noted for the combination of stavudine with lamivudine in individuals with prior treatment with zidovudine, didanosine, or zalcitabine.[47]

Similar observations can be made for three-drug combinations. Although the addition of ritonavir to a stable regimen of nucleoside analogue RT inhibitors in heavily nucleoside analogue–experienced individuals with advanced HIV disease significantly reduced the rate of clinical progression and death in the first year of therapy, the decrease in viral load at 1 year of therapy was only 0.6 $\log_{10}$, far less than usually observed in antiretroviral-naive individuals receiving combination therapy.[135] In individuals with advanced disease and with considerable prior exposure to nucleoside analogue RT inhibitors, the combination of nevirapine with zidovudine and didanosine, though better than zidovudine with didanosine alone, produced only a transient benefit in viral suppression in contrast to durable benefits obtained in antiretroviral-naive individuals.[106]

Some general principles can be deduced from these trials. First, the long-term efficacy of a regimen is related to the overall potency of the combination. Combinations that produce a greater nadir in viral load are more likely to have durable benefits. Second, the antiviral potency of a combination is not related simply to the type or number of drugs in the combination. Third, the most impressive benefits from a particular combination are usually seen in individuals who are antiretroviral-naive and those who have higher CD4 T-cell counts. This argues for early and aggressive treatment of HIV-1 infection. Fourth, in antiretroviral-experienced individuals, the addition of a single drug to a failing regimen is inferior to changing to a regimen with at least two new drugs to which cross-resistance is unlikely.

Initiating Therapy

The decision to start antiretroviral therapy must be individualized, taking into account the relative risks and benefits of therapy.[167, 168] The CD4 T-cell count and the HIV-1 RNA level can serve as powerful predictors of disease progression and survival in untreated patients. For both measurements, there is a continuum of increasing risk of disease progression and death associated with decreasing CD4 T-cell counts and increasing HIV-1 RNA levels.[158–160] Current understanding of the pathogenesis of AIDS suggests that therapy may be beneficial for patients with any detectable plasma HIV-1 RNA level regardless of the CD4 T-cell count. Antiretroviral therapy should be offered to HIV-1–infected individuals with significantly decreased CD4 T-cell counts or with symptomatic disease, regardless of their plasma HIV-1 RNA levels. In contrast, untreated individuals with normal CD4 T-cell counts and undetectable HIV-1 RNA levels appear to be at extremely low risk for disease progression in the short run. For these individuals, as well as for any persons who choose to defer treatment, CD4 T-cell counts and HIV-1 RNA levels should be monitored regularly.

The potential benefit of antiretroviral therapy must be balanced against possible adverse effects as well as the inconvenience of taking multiple drugs several times a day, often in a strict regimen around meals. Patients must be committed to therapy for an indefinite period of time in order to realize the full benefits of antiretroviral therapy. Given the potential for drug resistance and for extensive cross-resistance within a class of antiretrovirals, the haphazard use of these drugs may render current as well as later antiretroviral therapy ineffective. Thus, deferring antiretroviral therapy to a time when a patient is able to take medications consistently is preferable to using suboptimal therapy. A thorough and informed discussion between the health care provider and the patient is essential for successful long-term therapy.

Several combinations have offered potent and durable benefits in antiretroviral-naive individuals.[167, 168] Combinations of two nucleoside analogue RT inhibitors (such as zidovudine with lamivudine, zidovudine with didanosine, stavudine with didanosine, or stavudine with lamivudine) with a potent protease inhibitor (such as indinavir, ritonavir, nelfinavir, or soft gel capsule formulation of saquinavir) have shown clinical efficacy or virologic activity, or both. Two nucleoside analogue RT inhibitors with a potent NNRTI (such as efavirenz) have shown similar antiretroviral activity and are acceptable alternatives. Other combinations, including two protease inhibitors (such as saquinavir and ritonavir) with one or more nucleoside analogue RT inhibitors, three nucleoside analogue RT inhibitors (e.g., zidovudine, lamivudine, and abacavir), or a combination that includes both a protease inhibitor and an NNRTI, are less well studied but also may prove to be acceptable options. When choosing a regimen, consideration should be given to potential drug toxicity, interactions of antiretrovirals within the combination as well as with other drugs used by the patient, and the patient's ability to adhere to the regimen. These issues are particularly relevant to the patient with opportunistic infections or malignancy who may require several other medications.

Drugs in a combination should be started simultaneously; the sequential addition of drugs over an extended period of time runs an increased risk of having resistance develop. Close attention should be paid to the medication's dosing schedule. Adherence often requires extensive education of the patient and is enhanced by a continuing collaboration between the health care providers and the patient. If it is necessary to stop one drug temporarily, it is generally preferable to stop the entire combination temporarily in order to avoid selecting resistance to the rest of the drugs in the regimen at a time when antiretroviral potency is compromised.

Once a decision to start antiretroviral therapy is made, the aim of treatment should be the suppression of plasma HIV-1 RNA to below detectable limits of the most sensitive available HIV-1 RNA assay. Less profound suppression of viral replication may be associated with the evolution of resistant virus that will result in continuing immune system damage and may compromise current and future antiretroviral therapy options. Predictors of failures include advanced immunodeficiency, prior therapy with a nucleoside analogue RT inhibitor, and nonadherence to a regimen.[136–138, 169] If successful in suppressing viral replication completely, treatment with the full regimen should be continued indefinitely. Two trials examined whether simpler maintenance regimens could be used after induction therapy for 3 to 6 months with zidovudine, lamivudine, and indinavir among adults who achieved undetectable HIV-1 RNA levels ($<$200 to 500 copies/ml).[170, 171] Maintenance regimens of zidovudine with lamivudine, zidovudine with indinavir, or indinavir alone were associated with a higher rate of failure than continuation of the three-drug regimen when assessed several months after changing to maintenance therapy. Replication-competent virus can be isolated from individuals on combination therapy despite having undetectable HIV-1 RNA levels (<50 copies/ml) for up to 2 years.[172, 173]

Changing Therapy

Clinical assessment of the patient along with the HIV-1 RNA levels and the CD4 T-cell counts should be used to assess the need to change therapy. If the patient experiences drug toxicity or intolerance or is unable to adhere to therapy, a change in therapy is required. In these situations, it may be appropriate simply to replace the offending drug by another that is better tolerated and exhibits similar potency in the combination. A change in therapy should also be contemplated if a patient is on suboptimal therapy, such as monotherapy with any antiretroviral agent or a combination of two nucleoside analogue RT inhibitors, as these regimens are associated with a high risk of failure to suppress viral replication. If the patient has undetectable HIV-1 RNA with these regimens, an option is simply to add other drugs to form a regimen that is more likely to produce long-term viral suppression.

The plasma HIV-1 RNA level is the most sensitive indicator of viral replication, and a persistently detectable level while on therapy indicates suboptimal control of viral infection. If viral RNA levels are elevated due to immunization or intercurrent infection, they should return to baseline within 2 to 4 weeks of immunization or recovery from the illness. The HIV-1 RNA level may also be high secondary to incomplete adherence to the drug regimen, decreased absorption of drugs, or altered metabolism. Addressing the cause of the elevation in these cases may return the viral load to undetectable levels without necessarily changing the drug regimen.

Clinical situations that should prompt consideration for changing therapy include (1) a poor early virologic response to therapy, defined as a decrease in viral RNA of less than 1 $\log_{10}$ by 2 months of therapy; (2) failure to suppress plasma HIV-1 RNA to undetectable levels by 4 to 6 months of starting therapy; (3) repeated detection of virus in plasma after initial suppression to undetectable levels, suggesting the development of resistance; (4) a reproducible and significant increase ($\geq$0.5 $\log_{10}$ or threefold) in viral RNA levels from the nadir, not secondary to a self-limiting or correctable cause; (5) a persistent and significant decline in the CD4 T-cell count; (6) clinical deterioration while on a stable regimen.[168] Although it may be ideal to change therapy for any persistently detectable HIV-1 RNA level, this suggestion is tempered by the frequent limitations on remaining treatment options, especially in the heavily pretreated patient. Nevertheless, the consideration for change is more urgent with higher rebound in plasma HIV-1 RNA levels.

When considering changing therapy, an assessment of the likelihood of resistance to each previously used drug should be made since this may limit the use of drugs that share cross-resistance patterns. Assays are available for determining genotypic resistance (by assessing the presence of mutations associated with resistance to specific drugs) or phenotypic susceptibility (by testing the isolate's susceptibility in vitro to different drugs). However, all have significant limitations, and their clinical utility is not yet established.[61]

There are few clinical data to guide changes in therapy in individuals with failing multidrug regimens.[167–168] If the failing regimen consists of monotherapy with a nucleoside analogue RT inhibitor or therapy with two nucleoside analogues, possible alternatives include two new nucleoside analogues (that do not share cross-resistance patterns with the failing nucleoside analogues) with either a protease inhibitor or an NNRTI, or a combination of two protease inhibitors with one or two new nucleoside analogues. A failing regimen of two nucleoside analogues and an NNRTI may be replaced by two new nucleoside analogues and a protease inhibitor, or by a combination of two protease inhibitors with one or two new nucleoside analogues. Alternatives for a failing regimen of two nucleoside analogues and a protease inhibitor depend in part on the particular protease inhibitor in the failing combination and its pattern of cross-resistance. Salvage regimens are often complicated and are evolving at a rapid pace. Consultation with a physician experienced with antiretroviral therapy should be considered.

The aim of treatment after changing therapy should still be to suppress the plasma HIV-1 RNA levels to below detectable limits of the most sensitive available HIV-1 RNA assay. If complete suppression of viral replication cannot be attained with any regimen, the goal should be modified to attain as low a plasma HIV-1 RNA level as possible for as long as possible. Minimizing viral replication is likely to slow further immune deterioration. There is a continuum of increasing clinical benefits (in terms of disease progression and survival) with decreasing HIV-1 RNA levels, and regimens that produced only a 0.6 $\log_{10}$ mean decrease in HIV-1 RNA levels still can result in lower rates of clinical progression and death.[127, 135]

SPECIAL CIRCUMSTANCES

Postexposure Prophylaxis

Certain occupational exposures to HIV-1 may lead to infection. Blood, tissue, semen, vaginal secretions, CSF, serosal fluids, amniotic fluid, any bodily fluids contaminated with visible blood from infected individuals, and concentrated HIV-1 in a laboratory are potential sources of infectious virus, whereas sweat, tears, and nonbloody saliva, urine, and feces are unlikely to cause occupational transmission.[175] The average risk for percutaneous exposure to blood from an infected person is estimated to be 0.2 to 0.5%, whereas mucous membrane exposure carries a risk of approximately 0.1% and exposure through intact skin carries a negligible risk in the majority of situations.[175] However, several factors relating to the viral inoculum alter the actual risk in specific cases.[176] For instance, if the source patient has advanced AIDS and a high level of plasma HIV-1 RNA, the risks are likely to be substantially higher. Similarly, exposure to a large volume of infected fluid can also increase the risk, as noted for deep penetrating injuries, for injuries caused by a sharp device covered with visible blood, or for injuries caused by needles used to enter a blood vessel of the source patient.

A case-control study demonstrated that the administration of zidovudine in the immediate postoccupational exposure period decreased the odds of transmission by approximately 80%.[176] The ability of combination therapy to suppress viral replication better than monotherapy has prompted consideration of its use in postexposure prophylaxis. Furthermore, concern over the presence and transmissibility of virus resistant to zidovudine or other antiretroviral agents argues for both broader coverage and flexibility in designing the prophylaxis regimen. However, data on the efficacy of prophylaxis with a multidrug regimen are lacking. The fact that an average of more than 99.5% of occupational exposures to HIV-1–containing blood will not result in the transmission of the virus suggests the need to use agents with minimal toxicity and high tolerability.

Guidelines on the use of chemoprophylaxis after occupational exposures have been published (see Chapter 296).[177, 178] For each case of exposure, both the source and the patient should be assessed for HIV-1 infection before the incident and the likelihood of a high plasma HIV-1 RNA level and drug resistance in any source known to have HIV-1 infection. The basic prophylaxis regimen is a combination of two nucleoside analogue RT inhibitors with or without a potent protease inhibitor. If drug resistance in the source patient is a concern, alternative antiretroviral regimens should be considered. Chemoprophylaxis should be initiated as soon as possible, preferably within a few hours of the incident, as its efficacy is expected to wane with time. The optimal duration of chemoprophylaxis is unknown, although current guidelines recommend 4 weeks of therapy. Exposed individuals should be followed with antibody testing for HIV-1 infection at baseline, 6 weeks, 12 weeks, and 6 months after exposure.

The evidence that antiretroviral treatment can decrease the rate of HIV-1 transmission in occupational exposure has led to its consideration for individuals with recent sexual exposures to HIV-1.[179] There are no data on the efficacy of this intervention or, if effective, on the optimal drug regimen or timing of therapy. Situations should be assessed individually for the risk of transmission and the potential risks and benefit of prophylaxis with an antiretroviral regimen. Like occupational chemoprophylaxis, prophylaxis with two nucleoside analogue RT inhibitors, with or without a protease inhibitor, for 4 weeks may be considered in specific situations with a significant risk of transmission.

Acute HIV-1 Infection

Although acute infection with HIV-1 mimics several viral syndromes, it can be diagnosed by the detection of an elevated plasma HIV-1 RNA level in the context of a negative or indeterminate HIV-1 antibody test.[180] Several unique considerations favor treatment during this phase of infection. Treatment may limit the extent of viral dissemination throughout the body, possibly into compartments that may be difficult to treat during chronic infection. It may attenuate the progress of HIV-1 disease both acutely and later by producing a lower plasma viral RNA setpoint. Early treatment may also limit the extent of viral genetic variability that accumulates with time and that may allow resistance to drugs to occur readily. It may also allow salvage of a CD4 T-cell–specific immune response that may be important in the immune control of HIV-1 infection.[181]

Principles of therapy in acute infection are the same as for chronic infection. There are limited data on the long-term response to potent therapy, but studies have shown virologic and immunologic responses similar to those expected in chronically infected individuals.[182–185] Treatment should continue indefinitely.

Pregnancy

Pregnancy should not preclude women from receiving optimal antiretroviral therapy.[186] However, several issues that are unique to pregnancy should be considered. These include pharmacokinetic changes produced by pregnancy, potential adverse effects of antiretroviral agents on the fetus, and the efficacy of a regimen in decreasing the rate of perinatal transmission of HIV. Decisions regarding therapy should be made by the woman in consultation with her physician after discussions of known and unknown risks and benefits to her and the fetus (see Chapter 113).

Although there is information on zidovudine use during pregnancy, there is little information on other antiretrovirals.[187] Pharmacokinetics of zidovudine and lamivudine during pregnancy appear to be similar to those observed in the nonpregnant state.[188, 189] Furthermore, both these drugs, as well as nevirapine, cross the placenta well.[190] In contrast, clearance of didanosine is significantly increased during pregnancy, and it may not penetrate the placenta as readily.[191, 192] All appear to be well tolerated during pregnancy with no unexpected adverse effects. Zidovudine does not appear to cause fetal malformation, fetal distress, or premature birth.[193] Although experience with other antiretrovirals during pregnancy is more limited, no pattern of adverse effects on the fetus or newborn has been reported in humans. Efavirenz has shown teratogenicity in nonhuman primates and should be avoided in this setting. There are no data on the pharmacokinetics or potential adverse effects of protease inhibitors in pregnant women.

In a landmark study, zidovudine was shown to decrease the rate of transmission of HIV-1 to the newborn by almost 70%.[194, 195] This double-blind, placebo-controlled trial enrolled HIV-1–infected women with more than 200 CD4 T-cells/mm^3 who were at 14 to 34 weeks of gestation, the large majority of whom were zidovudine-naive. The zidovudine regimen consisted of zidovudine 100 mg orally five times daily continued throughout pregnancy, intravenous zidovudine 2 mg/kg given over 1 hour followed by continuous infusion of 1 mg/kg/hour during labor until delivery, and zidovudine for the newborn at 2 mg/kg orally every 6 hours until 6 weeks of age. Zidovudine decreased perinatal transmission of HIV-1 from 22.6 to 7.6%. Results from another trial using the same zidovudine regimen in women with more advanced disease and with more extensive history of previous zidovudine use showed a transmission rate of approximately 5%.[196] Although combination therapy often produces more profound viral suppression than zidovudine monotherapy, its ability to decrease the rate of perinatal transmission further is still uncertain, particularly since perinatal transmission may occur despite an undetectable HIV-1 RNA level in treated or untreated women, and since the benefits of zidovudine in this setting can not be fully explained by reductions in the maternal viral load.[195, 197]

The evaluation and treatment of HIV-1 infection in a pregnant woman is the same as that in a nonpregnant woman with the added considerations of the impact of pregnancy on the therapy and the impact of therapy of the fetus and risk of perinatal HIV-1 transmission.[187] The first trimester of gestation is a period in which the fetus is most vulnerable to potential teratogenic effects of drugs. If a woman is not yet receiving antiretroviral therapy, she may wish to delay, if feasible, the initiation of antiretroviral therapy until after 10 to 12 weeks of gestation. If a woman is already receiving antiretroviral therapy when pregnancy is diagnosed, she may choose either to continue with antiretroviral therapy or to stop all antiretroviral agents till the end of the first trimester. The goals of therapy during pregnancy are the same as those in other situations: HIV-1 RNA levels should be decreased to levels undetectable by the most sensitive test available. Higher viral loads are associated not only with increased morbidity, mortality, and resistance, but also with increased risk of transmission to the newborn.[195] Given the proven efficacy and safety of zidovudine in decreasing perinatal transmission, the three-part chemoprophylaxis zidovudine regimen described previously (substituting the prenatal part with the more usual dose of 200 mg three times daily or 300 mg twice daily) should be offered as part of or in addition to any regimen used during pregnancy whenever possible. Even if the prenatal use of zidovudine is not possible (due to prior maternal toxicity or choice, or maternal use of stavudine, with which zidovudine displays pharmacologic antagonism), it should be considered for use in the intrapartum period and in the neonate. Infants should be tested with virologic assays at 48 hours, 14 days, 1 to 2 months, and 3 to 6 months of life. If any of these tests show active HIV-1 infection, antiretroviral therapy should be changed to combination therapy recommended for established HIV-1 infection.

Children

Although the pathogenesis of HIV-1 infection in children is similar to that in adults, there are several unique considerations that affect antiretroviral therapy in children (see Chapter 114).[174] Clinical manifestations differ between adults and children, with children often showing deficiencies in growth and in physical and neurologic development during chronic disease. Immunologic differences include markedly higher CD4 T-cell counts at birth that decline slowly to adult levels by the age of 6 years in normal children. Criteria to assess the level of immunodeficiency based on absolute CD4 T-cell counts used in adults are therefore unreliable in young children, and age-specific absolute count criteria or the percentage of CD4 T cells should be used instead. Neonates with HIV-1 infection often have levels of plasma HIV-1 RNA that are very high compared with those of adults, that persist for longer periods, and that may decline slowly over the next few years without therapy.[198] The high level of viremia may cause a slower decline in HIV-1 RNA levels during therapy compared with adults and may produce fewer instances of suppression to undetectable levels with currently available combinations. As observed in adults, lower levels of CD4 T-cell counts and higher levels of plasma HIV-1 RNA are predictive of HIV-1 related morbidity and mortality.[198, 199] Furthermore, each antiretroviral therapy–

associated reduction in HIV-1 RNA of 1 $\log_{10}$ may produce a 49 to 64% reduction in progression of the disease.[199]

Pharmacokinetic properties of antiretroviral agents may differ markedly in various age groups. For instance, the clearance of zidovudine, lamivudine, and nevirapine in neonates is decreased significantly compared with that of older children, necessitating reductions in dosing.[189, 190, 200] The toxicity profile of drugs may also be different in children. For example, lamivudine therapy was associated with several cases of pancreatitis in children, a complication that is uncommon with lamivudine use in adults.[201] Adherence to therapy is a significant problem in children and relates in part to the availability and palatability of pediatric formulations of antiretrovirals. Among the RT inhibitors, liquid formulations are currently available for zidovudine, didanosine, lamivudine, stavudine, and abacavir. Among protease inhibitors, ritonavir is available in liquid formulation and nelfinavir is available as a powder that can be mixed with food or water. In adolescents, pediatric dosing should be used for those in early puberty (Tanner's stage I or II) whereas adult dosing should be used for those in late puberty (Tanner's stage V). Adolescents in their growth spurts should be followed closely for drug efficacy and toxicity using either adult or pediatric dosing with dose changes as necessary.

Monotherapy with several nucleoside analogue RT inhibitors, including zidovudine, didanosine, lamivudine, and stavudine, has been shown to be safe and to have clinical, immunologic, or virologic efficacy in children.[201–204] Combinations of two RT inhibitors are often better than therapy with a single nucleoside analogue RT inhibitor, as demonstrated for zidovudine with didanosine compared with zidovudine monotherapy or zidovudine with lamivudine compared with didanosine alone.[205, 206] The addition of a protease inhibitor to nucleoside analogue RT inhibitors has demonstrated further virologic, immunologic, and clinical benefits.[207–209] Preliminary studies have also shown greater benefits when nevirapine is added to zidovudine and didanosine, especially in antiretroviral-naive children.[210]

FUTURE DIRECTIONS

Several novel nucleoside and nucleotide analogue RT inhibitors, NNRTIs, and protease inhibitors are under development. Viral attachment to and fusion with host cells are potentially accessible targets. One fusion inhibitor, T-20, has shown promise in early clinical pilot studies.[211] Compounds that inhibit the function of coreceptors used by HIV-1 are available, but the ability of HIV-1 to use different coreceptors poses a challenge in formulating therapy based on this concept. Agents that bind to viral envelope proteins (such as gp120 or gp41) may interfere with viral attachment to host cells. The HIV-1 integrase enzyme is crucial for HIV-1 proviral DNA integration into the host genome and for the establishment of infection. Integrase inhibitors are expected to inhibit viral replication, but no potentially useful agents have been described. The viral nucleocapsid protein is important for RNA encapsidation and virus maturation and may also serve as a promising target for therapy. Retroviral nucleocapsid proteins have zinc-finger motifs (specific sequence of amino acids rich in cysteine) that coordinate a zinc ion that is crucial for their function. Compounds that attack the sulfur atoms in cysteine and allow the ejection of zinc inactivate the protein and inhibit viral replication. Although bioavailable compounds with these properties have been described, useful agents for human HIV-1 infection have not yet been reported.

REFERENCES

1. Greene WC. The molecular biology of human immunodeficiency virus type 1 infection. N Engl J Med. 1991;324:308–317.
2. Goff SP. Retroviral reverse transcriptase: Synthesis, structure, and function. J Acquir Immune Defic Syndr. 1990;3:817–831.
3. Yarchoan R, Mitsuya H, Myers CE, Broder S. Clinical pharmacology of 3′-azido-2′,3′-dideoxythymidine (zidovudine) and related dideoxynucleosides [published erratum appears in N Engl J Med. 1990;322:280]. N Engl J Med. 1989;321:726–738.
4. Gao WY, Shirasaka T, Johns DG, et al. Differential phosphorylation of azidothymidine, dideoxycytidine, and dideoxyinosine in resting and activated peripheral blood mononuclear cells. J Clin Invest. 1993;91:2326–2333.
5. Palmer S, Alaeus A, Albert J, Cox S. Drug susceptibility of subtypes A, B, C, D and E human immunodeficiency virus type 1 primary isolates. AIDS Res Hum Retroviruses. 1998;14:157–162.
6. Connolly KJ, Hammer SM. Antiretroviral therapy: Reverse transcriptase inhibition. Antimicrob Agents Chemother. 1992;36:245–254.
7. Fischl MA, Richman DD, Grieco MH, et al. The efficacy of azidothymidine (AZT) in the treatment of patients with AIDS and AIDS-related complex. A double-blind, placebo-controlled trial. N Engl J Med. 1987;317:185–191.
8. Fischl MA, Richman DD, Causey DM, et al. Prolonged zidovudine therapy in patients with AIDS and advanced AIDS-related complex. AZT Collaborative Working Group. JAMA. 1989;262:2405–2410.
9. Fischl MA, Richman DD, Hansen N, et al. The safety and efficacy of zidovudine (AZT) in the treatment of subjects with mildly symptomatic human immunodeficiency virus type 1 (HIV) infection. A double-blind, placebo-controlled trial. The AIDS Clinical Trials Group. Ann Intern Med. 1990;112:727–737.
10. Volberding PA, Lagakos SW, Koch MA, et al. Zidovudine in asymptomatic human immunodeficiency virus infection. A controlled trial in persons with fewer than 500 CD4-positive cells per cubic millimeter. The AIDS Clinical Trials Group of the National Institute of Allergy and Infectious Diseases. N Engl J Med. 1990;322:941–949.
11. Cooper DA, Gatell JM, Kroon S, et al. Zidovudine in persons with asymptomatic HIV infection and CD4+ cell counts greater than 400 per cubic millimeter. The European-Australian Collaborative Group. N Engl J Med. 1993;329:297–303.
12. Volberding PA, Lagakos SW, Grimes JM, et al. The duration of zidovudine benefit in persons with asymptomatic HIV infection. Prolonged evaluation of protocol 019 of the AIDS Clinical Trials Group. JAMA. 1994;272:437–442.
13. Hamilton JD, Hartigan PM, Simberkoff MS, et al. A controlled trial of early versus late treatment with zidovudine in symptomatic human immunodeficiency virus infection. Results of the Veterans Affairs Cooperative Study. N Engl J Med. 1992;326:437–443.
14. Concorde: MRC/ANRS randomised double-blind controlled trial of immediate and deferred zidovudine in symptom-free HIV infection. Concorde Coordinating Committee. Lancet. 1994;343:871–881.
15. Volberding PA, Lagakos SW, Grimes JM, et al. A comparison of immediate with deferred zidovudine therapy for asymptomatic HIV-infected adults with CD4 cell counts of 500 or more per cubic millimeter. AIDS Clinical Trials Group. N Engl J Med. 1995;333:401–407.
16. Johnson VA, Merrill DP, Videler JA, et al. Two-drug combinations of zidovudine, didanosine, and recombinant interferon-alpha A inhibit replication of zidovudine-resistant human immunodeficiency virus type 1 synergistically in vitro. J Infect Dis. 1991;164:646–655.
17. Johnson VA, Merrill DP, Chou TC, Hirsch MS. Human immunodeficiency virus type 1 (HIV-1) inhibitory interactions between protease inhibitor Ro 31-8959 and zidovudine, 2′,3′-dideoxycytidine, or recombinant interferon-alpha A against zidovudine-sensitive or -resistant HIV-1 in vitro. J Infect Dis. 1992;166:1143–1146.
18. Eron JJ Jr, Johnson VA, Merrill DP, et al. Synergistic inhibition of replication of human immunodeficiency virus type 1, including that of a zidovudine-resistant isolate, by zidovudine and 2′,3′-dideoxycytidine in vitro. Antimicrob Agents Chemother. 1992;36:1559–1562.
19. Merrill DP, Moonis M, Chou TC, Hirsch MS. Lamivudine or stavudine in two- and three-drug combinations against human immunodeficiency virus type 1 replication in vitro. J Infect Dis. 1996;173:355–364.
20. Fischl MA, Parker CB, Pettinelli C, et al. A randomized controlled trial of a reduced daily dose of zidovudine in patients with the acquired immunodeficiency syndrome. The AIDS Clinical Trials Group. N Engl J Med. 1990;323:1009–1014.
21. Richman DD, Fischl MA, Grieco MH, et al. The toxicity of azidothymidine (AZT) in the treatment of patients with AIDS and AIDS-related complex. A double-blind, placebo-controlled trial. N Engl J Med. 1987;317:192–197.
22. Dalakas MC, Illa I, Pezeshkpour GH, et al. Mitochondrial myopathy caused by long-term zidovudine therapy. N Engl J Med. 1990;322:1098–1105.
23. Kahn JO, Lagakos SW, Richman DD, et al. A controlled trial comparing continued zidovudine with didanosine in human immunodeficiency virus infection. The NIAID AIDS Clinical Trials Group. N Engl J Med. 1992;327:581–587.
24. Spruance SL, Pavia AT, Peterson D, et al. Didanosine compared with continuation of zidovudine in HIV-infected patients with signs of clinical deterioration while receiving zidovudine. A randomized, double-blind clinical trial. The Bristol-Myers Squibb AI454-010 Study Group. Ann Intern Med. 1994;120:360–368.
25. Montaner JS, Schechter MT, Rachlis A, et al. Didanosine compared with continued zidovudine therapy for HIV-infected patients with 200 to 500 CD4 cells/mm3. A double-blind, randomized, controlled trial. Canadian HIV Trials Network Protocol 002 Study Group. Ann Intern Med. 1995;123:561–571.
26. Dolin R, Amato DA, Fischl MA, et al. Zidovudine compared with didanosine in patients with advanced HIV type 1 infection and little or no previous experience with zidovudine. AIDS Clinical Trials Group [published erratum appears in Arch Intern Med. 1995;155:2255]. Arch Intern Med. 1995;155:961–974.
27. Hammer SM, Katzenstein DA, Hughes MD, et al. A trial comparing nucleoside monotherapy with combination therapy in HIV-infected adults with CD4 cell

counts from 200 to 500 per cubic millimeter. AIDS Clinical Trials Group Study 175 Study Team. N Engl J Med. 1996;335:1081–1090.
28. Collier AC, Coombs RW, Fischl MA, et al. Combination therapy with zidovudine and didanosine compared with zidovudine alone in HIV-1 infection. Ann Intern Med. 1993;119:786–793.
29. Delta: A randomised double-blind controlled trial comparing combinations of zidovudine plus didanosine or zalcitabine with zidovudine alone in HIV-infected individuals. Delta Coordinating Committee [published erratum appears in Lancet. 1996;348:834]. Lancet. 1996;348:283–291.
30. Katzenstein DA, Hammer SM, Hughes MD, et al. The relation of virologic and immunologic markers to clinical outcomes after nucleoside therapy in HIV-infected adults with 200 to 500 CD4 cells per cubic millimeter. AIDS Clinical Trials Group Study 175 Virology Study Team [published erratum appears in N Engl J Med. 1997;337:1097]. N Engl J Med. 1996;335:1091–1098.
31. Saravolatz LD, Winslow DL, Collins G, et al. Zidovudine alone or in combination with didanosine or zalcitabine in HIV-infected patients with the acquired immunodeficiency syndrome or fewer than 200 CD4 cells per cubic millimeter. Investigators for the Terry Beirn Community Programs for Clinical Research on AIDS. N Engl J Med. 1996;335:1099–1106.
32. Lori F, Malykh A, Cara A, et al. Hydroxyurea as an inhibitor of human immunodeficiency virus-type 1 replication. Science. 1994;266:801–805.
33. Montaner JS, Zala C, Conway B, et al. A pilot study of hydroxyurea among patients with advanced human immunodeficiency virus (HIV) disease receiving chronic didanosine therapy: Canadian HIV trials network protocol 080. J Infect Dis. 1997;175:801–806.
34. Rutschmann OT, Opravil M, Iten A, et al. A placebo-controlled trial of didanosine plus stavudine, with and without hydroxyurea, for HIV infection. The Swiss HIV Cohort Study. AIDS. 1998;12:F71–F77.
35. Yarchoan R, Pluda JM, Thomas RV, et al. Long-term toxicity/activity profile of 2′,3′-dideoxyinosine in AIDS or AIDS-related complex. Lancet. 1990;336:526–529.
36. Fischl MA, Olson RM, Follansbee SE, et al. Zalcitabine compared with zidovudine in patients with advanced HIV-1 infection who received previous zidovudine therapy. Ann Intern Med. 1993;118:762–769.
37. Fischl MA, Stanley K, Collier AC, et al. Combination and monotherapy with zidovudine and zalcitabine in patients with advanced HIV disease. The NIAID AIDS Clinical Trials Group. Ann Intern Med. 1995;122:24–32.
38. Abrams DI, Goldman AI, Launer C, et al. A comparative trial of didanosine or zalcitabine after treatment with zidovudine in patients with human immunodeficiency virus infection. The Terry Beirn Community Programs for Clinical Research on AIDS. N Engl J Med. 1994;330:657–662.
39. Meng TC, Fischl MA, Boota AM, et al. Combination therapy with zidovudine and dideoxycytidine in patients with advanced human immunodeficiency virus infection. A phase I/II study. Ann Intern Med. 1992;116:13–20.
40. Skowron G, Bozzette SA, Lim L, et al. Alternating and intermittent regimens of zidovudine and dideoxycytidine in patients with AIDS or AIDS-related complex. Ann Intern Med. 1993;118:321–330.
41. Dudley MN, Graham KK, Kaul S, et al. Pharmacokinetics of stavudine in patients with AIDS or AIDS-related complex. J Infect Dis. 1992;166:480–485.
42. Haworth SJ, Christofalo B, Anderson RD, Dunkle LM. A single-dose study to assess the penetration of stavudine into human cerebrospinal fluid in adults. J Acquir Immune Defic Syndr Hum Retrovirol. 1998;17:235–238.
43. Spruance SL, Pavia AT, Mellors JW, et al. Clinical efficacy of monotherapy with stavudine compared with zidovudine in HIV-infected, zidovudine-experienced patients. A randomized, double-blind, controlled trial. Bristol-Myers Squibb Stavudine/019 Study Group. Ann Intern Med. 1997;126:355–363.
44. Havlir DV, Friedland G, Pollard R, et al. Combination zidovudine (ZDV) and stavudine (d4T) therapy versus other nucleosides: Report of two randomized trials (ACTG 290 and 298). Abstract 2. In: 5th Conference on Retroviruses and Opportunistic Infections. Chicago; 1998:79.
45. Fisher M, Stoehr A, Podzamczer D, et al. A randomized double-blind study of d4T + ddI vs ZDV + ddI as initial treatment in subjects with CD4 count less than or equal to 500 cells/mm.[3] Abstract 661. In: 5th Conference on Retroviruses and Opportunistic Infections. Chicago; 1998:204.
46. Kuritzkes DR, Marschner IC, Johnson VA, et al. A randomized, double-blind, placebo-controlled trial of lamivudine (3TC) in combination with zidovudine (ZDV), stavudine (d4T), or didanosine (ddI) in treatment naive patients. Abstract 1. In: 5th Conference on Retroviruses and Opportunistic Infections. Chicago; 1998:79.
47. Katlama C, Valantin MA, Matheron S, et al. Efficacy and tolerability of stavudine plus lamivudine in treatment-naive and treatment-experienced patients with HIV-1 infection. Ann Intern Med. 1998;129:525–531.
48. Browne MJ, Mayer KH, Chafee SB, et al. 2′,3′-Didehydro-3′-deoxythymidine (d4T) in patients with AIDS or AIDS-related complex: A phase I trial. J Infect Dis. 1993;167:21–29.
49. Van Leeuwen R, Lange JM, Hussey EK, et al. The safety and pharmacokinetics of a reverse transcriptase inhibitor, 3TC, in patients with HIV infection: A phase I study. AIDS. 1992;6:1471–1475.
50. Van Leeuwen R, Katlama C, Kitchen V, et al. Evaluation of safety and efficacy of 3TC (lamivudine) in patients with asymptomatic or mildly symptomatic human immunodeficiency virus infection: A phase I/II study. J Infect Dis. 1995;171:1166–1171.
51. Schuurman R, Nijhuis M, van Leeuwen R, et al. Rapid changes in human immunodeficiency virus type 1 RNA load and appearance of drug-resistant virus populations in persons treated with lamivudine (3TC). J Infect Dis. 1995;171:1411–1419.
52. Eron JJ, Benoit SL, Jemsek J, et al. Treatment with lamivudine, zidovudine, or both in HIV-positive patients with 200 to 500 CD4+ cells per cubic millimeter. North American HIV Working Party. N Engl J Med. 1995;333:1662–1669.
53. Katlama C, Ingrand D, Loveday C, et al. Safety and efficacy of lamivudine-zidovudine combination therapy in antiretroviral-naive patients. A randomized controlled comparison with zidovudine monotherapy. Lamivudine European HIV Working Group. JAMA. 1996;276:118–125.
54. Staszewski S, Loveday C, Picazo JJ, et al. Safety and efficacy of lamivudine-zidovudine combination therapy in zidovudine-experienced patients. A randomized controlled comparison with zidovudine monotherapy. Lamivudine European HIV Working Group. JAMA. 1996;276:111–117.
55. Bartlett JA, Benoit SL, Johnson VA, et al. Lamivudine plus zidovudine compared with zalcitabine plus zidovudine in patients with HIV infection. A randomized, double-blind, placebo-controlled trial. North American HIV Working Party. Ann Intern Med. 1996;125:161–172.
56. Randomised trial of addition of lamivudine or lamivudine plus loviride to zidovudine-containing regimens for patients with HIV-1 infection: The CAESAR trial. Lancet. 1997;349:1413–1421.
57. Saag MS, Sonnerborg A, Torres R, et al. Antiretroviral effect and safety of abacavir alone and in combination with zidovudine in HIV-infected adults. Abacavir Phase 2 Clinical Team. AIDS. 1998;12:F203–F209.
58. Staszewski S, Katlama C, Harrer T, et al. A dose-ranging study to evaluate the safety and efficacy of abacavir alone or in combination with zidovudine and lamivudine in antiretroviral treatment-naive subjects. AIDS. 1998;12:F197–F202.
59. Mellors J, Lederman M, Haas D, et al. Antiretroviral effects of therapy combining abacavir (1592) with HIV protease inhibitors (PIs). Abstract 4. In: 5th Conference on Retroviruses and Opportunistic Infections. Chicago; 1998:79.
60. D'Aquila RT. HIV-1 drug resistance. Molecular pathogenesis and laboratory monitoring. Clin Lab Med. 1994;14:393–422.
61. Hirsch MS, Conway B, D'Aquila RT, et al. Antiretroviral drug resistance testing in adults with HIV infection: implications for clinical management. International AIDS Society—USA Panel. JAMA. 1998;279:1984–1991.
62. Ho DD, Neumann AU, Perelson AS, et al. Rapid turnover of plasma virions and CD4 lymphocytes in HIV-1 infection. Nature. 1995;373:123–126.
63. Wei X, Ghosh SK, Taylor ME, et al. Viral dynamics in human immunodeficiency virus type 1 infection. Nature. 1995;373:117–122.
64. Perelson AS, Neumann AU, Markowitz M, et al. HIV-1 dynamics in vivo: Virion clearance rate, infected cell life-span, and viral generation time. Science. 1996;271:1582–1586.
65. Coffin JM. HIV population dynamics in vivo: Implications for genetic variation, pathogenesis, and therapy. Science. 1995;267:483–489.
66. Larder BA, Darby G, Richman DD. HIV with reduced sensitivity to zidovudine (AZT) isolated during prolonged therapy. Science. 1989;243:1731–1734.
67. Boucher CA, Tersmette M, Lange JM, et al. Zidovudine sensitivity of human immunodeficiency viruses from high-risk, symptom-free individuals during therapy. Lancet. 1990;336:585–590.
68. Boucher CA, O'Sullivan E, Mulder JW, et al. Ordered appearance of zidovudine resistance mutations during treatment of 18 human immunodeficiency virus-positive subjects. J Infect Dis. 1992;165:105–110.
69. Loveday C, Kaye S, Tenant-Flowers M, et al. HIV-1 RNA serum-load and resistant viral genotypes during early zidovudine therapy. Lancet. 1995;345:820–824.
70. Larder BA, Kellam P, Kemp SD. Zidovudine resistance predicted by direct detection of mutations in DNA from HIV-infected lymphocytes. AIDS. 1991;5:137–144.
71. Kellam P, Boucher CA, Larder BA. Fifth mutation in human immunodeficiency virus type 1 reverse transcriptase contributes to the development of high-level resistance to zidovudine. Proc Natl Acad Sci U S A. 1992;89:1934–1938.
72. Hooker DJ, Tachedjian G, Solomon AE, et al. An in vivo mutation from leucine to tryptophan at position 210 in human immunodeficiency virus type 1 reverse transcriptase contributes to high-level resistance to 3′-azido-3′-deoxythymidine. J Virol. 1996;70:8010–8008.
73. Larder BA, Kemp SD. Multiple mutations in HIV-1 reverse transcriptase confer high-level resistance to zidovudine (AZT). Science. 1989;246:1155–1158.
74. Larder BA, Coates KE, Kemp SD. Zidovudine-resistant human immunodeficiency virus selected by passage in cell culture. J Virol. 1991;65:5232–5236.
75. Boucher CA, van Leeuwen R, Kellam P, et al. Effects of discontinuation of zidovudine treatment on zidovudine sensitivity of human immunodeficiency virus type 1 isolates. Antimicrob Agents Chemother. 1993;37:1525–1530.
76. Erice A, Mayers DL, Strike DG, et al. Brief report: Primary infection with zidovudine-resistant human immunodeficiency virus type 1. N Engl J Med. 1993;328:1163–1165.
77. Fitzgibbon JE, Gaur S, Frenkel LD, et al. Transmission from one child to another of human immunodeficiency virus type 1 with a zidovudine-resistance mutation. N Engl J Med. 1993;329:1835–1841.
78. D'Aquila RT, Johnson VA, Welles SL, et al. Zidovudine resistance and HIV-1 disease progression during antiretroviral therapy. AIDS Clinical Trials Group Protocol 116B/117 Team and the Virology Committee Resistance Working Group. Ann Intern Med. 1995;122:401–408.
79. Mayers DL, Japour AJ, Arduino JM, et al. Dideoxynucleoside resistance emerges with prolonged zidovudine monotherapy. The RV43 Study Group. Antimicrob Agents Chemother. 1994;38:307–314.
80. Fitzgibbon JE, Howell RM, Haberzettl CA, et al. Human immunodeficiency virus type 1 pol gene mutations which cause decreased susceptibility to 2′,3′-dideoxycytidine. Antimicrob Agents Chemother. 1992;36:153–157.
81. Zhang D, Caliendo AM, Eron JJ, et al. Resistance to 2′,3′-dideoxycytidine conferred by a mutation in codon 65 of the human immunodeficiency virus type 1 reverse transcriptase. Antimicrob Agents Chemother. 1994;38:282–287.

82. St Clair MH, Martin JL, Tudor-Williams G, et al. Resistance to ddI and sensitivity to AZT induced by a mutation in HIV-1 reverse transcriptase. Science. 1991;253:1557–1559.
83. Eron JJ, Chow YK, Caliendo AM, et al. *pol* mutations conferring zidovudine and didanosine resistance with different effects in vitro yield multiply resistant human immunodeficiency virus type 1 isolates in vivo. Antimicrob Agents Chemother. 1993;37:1480–1487.
84. Lacey SF, Larder BA. Novel mutation (V75T) in human immunodeficiency virus type 1 reverse transcriptase confers resistance to 2′,3′-didehydro-2′,3′-dideoxythymidine in cell culture. Antimicrob Agents Chemother. 1994;38:1428–1432.
85. Lin PF, Samanta H, Rose RE, et al. Genotypic and phenotypic analysis of human immunodeficiency virus type 1 isolates from patients on prolonged stavudine therapy. J Infect Dis. 1994;170:1157–1164.
86. Tisdale M, Alnadaf T, Cousens D. Combination of mutations in human immunodeficiency virus type 1 reverse transcriptase required for resistance to the carbocyclic nucleoside 1592U89. Antimicrob Agents Chemother. 1997;41:1094–1098.
87. Miller V, Sturmer M, Staszewski S, et al. The M184V mutation in HIV-1 reverse transcriptase (RT) conferring lamivudine resistance does not result in broad cross-resistance to nucleoside analogue RT inhibitors. AIDS. 1998;12:705–712.
88. Gao Q, Gu Z, Parniak MA, et al. The same mutation that encodes low-level human immunodeficiency virus type 1 resistance to 2′,3′-dideoxyinosine and 2′,3′-dideoxycytidine confers high-level resistance to the (−) enantiomer of 2′,3′-dideoxy-3′-thiacytidine. Antimicrob Agents Chemother. 1993;37:1390–1392.
89. Gu Z, Gao Q, Li X, et al. Novel mutation in the human immunodeficiency virus type 1 reverse transcriptase gene that encodes cross-resistance to 2′,3′-dideoxyinosine and 2′,3′-dideoxycytidine. J Virol. 1992;66:7128–7135.
90. Larder BA, Kemp SD, Harrigan PR. Potential mechanism for sustained antiretroviral efficacy of AZT-3TC combination therapy. Science. 1995;269:696–699.
91. Kemp SD, Shi C, Bloor S, et al. A novel polymorphism at codon 333 of human immunodeficiency virus type 1 reverse transcriptase can facilitate dual resistance to zidovudine and L-2′,3′-dideoxy-3′-thiacytidine. J Virol. 1998;72:5093–5098.
92. Shirasaka T, Kavlick MF, Ueno T, et al. Emergence of human immunodeficiency virus type 1 variants with resistance to multiple dideoxynucleosides in patients receiving therapy with dideoxynucleosides. Proc Natl Acad Sci U S A. 1995;92:2398–2402.
93. Shafer RW, Kozal MJ, Winters MA, et al. Combination therapy with zidovudine and didanosine selects for drug-resistant human immunodeficiency virus type 1 strains with unique patterns of pol gene mutations. J Infect Dis. 1994;169:722–729.
94. Shafer RW, Iversen AK, Winters MA, et al. Drug resistance and heterogeneous long-term virologic responses of human immunodeficiency virus type 1-infected subjects to zidovudine and didanosine combination therapy. The AIDS Clinical Trials Group 143 Virology Team. J Infect Dis. 1995;172:70–78.
94a. Winters MA, Coolley KL, Girard YA, et al. A 6-basepair insert in the reverse transcriptase gene of human immunodeficiency virus type 1 confers resistance to multiple nucleoside inhibitors. J Clin Invest. 1998;102:1769–1775.
95. Medina DJ, Tung PP, Lerner-Tung MB, et al. Sanctuary growth of human immunodeficiency virus in the presence of 3′-azido-3′-deoxythymidine. J Virol. 1995;69(3):1606-1611.
96. Sommadossi JP, Valantin MA, Zhou XJ, et al. Intracellular phosphorylation of stavudine (d4T) and 3TC correlates with their antiviral activity in naive and zidovudine (ZDV) experienced HIV-infected patients. Abstract 362. In: 5th Conference on Retroviruses and Opportunistic Infections. Chicago; 1998:146.
97. Sommadossi JP, Zhou XJ, Moore J, et al. Impairment of stavudine (d4T) phosphorylation in patients receiving a combination of zidovudine (ZDV) and d4T (ACTG 290). Abstract 3, In: 5th Conference on Retroviruses and Opportunistic Infections. Chicago; 1998:79.
98. Back DJ, Hoggard PG, Gibbons SE, et al. Zidovudine (ZDV) phosphorylation determined at intervals over 12 months in naive and antiretroviral experienced HIV+ patients. Abstract LB10. In: 5th Conference on Retroviruses and Opportunistic Infections. Chicago; 1998:224.
99. De Clercq E. Antiviral therapy for human immunodeficiency virus infections. Clin Microbiol Rev. 1995;8:200–239.
100. Cheeseman SH, Hattox SE, McLaughlin MM, et al. Pharmacokinetics of nevirapine: Initial single-rising-dose study in humans. Antimicrob Agents Chemother. 1993;37:178–182.
101. Havlir DV, Eastman S, Gamst A, Richman DD. Nevirapine-resistant human immunodeficiency virus: Kinetics of replication and estimated prevalence in untreated patients. J Virol. 1996;70:7894–7899.
102. Richman DD, Havlir D, Corbeil J, et al. Nevirapine resistance mutations of human immunodeficiency virus type 1 selected during therapy. J Virol. 1994;68:1660–1666.
103. Havlir D, Cheeseman SH, McLaughlin M, et al. High-dose nevirapine: Safety, pharmacokinetics, and antiviral effect in patients with human immunodeficiency virus infection. J Infect Dis. 1995;171:537–545.
104. Montaner JS, Reiss P, Cooper D, et al. A randomized, double-blind trial comparing combinations of nevirapine, didanosine, and zidovudine for HIV-infected patients: The INCAS Trial. Italy, The Netherlands, Canada and Australia Study. JAMA. 1998;279:930–937.
105. Floridia M, Bucciardini R, Ricciardulli D, et al. A randomized, double-blind trial on the use of a triple combination including nevirapine, a nonnucleoside reverse transcriptase HIV inhibitor, in antiretroviral-naive patients with advanced disease. J Acquir Immune Defic Syndr Hum Retrovirol. 1992;20:11–19.
106. D'Aquila RT, Hughes MD, Johnson VA, et al. Nevirapine, zidovudine, and didanosine compared with zidovudine and didanosine in patients with HIV-1 infection. A randomized, double-blind, placebo-controlled trial. National Institute of Allergy and Infectious Diseases AIDS Clinical Trials Group Protocol 241 Investigators. Ann Intern Med. 1996;124:1019–1030.
107. Davey RT Jr, Chaitt DG, Reed GF, et al. Randomized, controlled phase I/II, trial of combination therapy with delavirdine (U-90152S) and conventional nucleosides in human immunodeficiency virus type 1-infected patients. Antimicrob Agents Chemother. 1996;40:1657–1664.
108. Sargent S, Green S, Para M, et al. Sustained plasma viral burden reductions and CD4 increases in HIV-1 infected patients with rescriptor (DLV) + retrovir (ZDV) + epivir (3TC). Abstract 699. In: 5th Conference on Retroviruses and Opportunistic Infections. Chicago; 1998:209.
109. Fiske WD, Nibbelink DW, Brennan JM, et al. DMP 266 cerebrospinal fluid concentrations (CSF) after oral administration. Abstract A-12. In: 37th Interscience Conference on Antimicrobial Agents and Chemotherapy. Toronto; 1997.
110. Kahn J, Mayers D, Riddler S, et al. Durable clinical anti-HIV-1 activity (60 weeks) and tolerability for efavirenz (DMP 266) in combination with indinavir (IDV) suppression to "less than 1 copy/ml" (OD = background) by Amplicor as a predictor of virologic treatment response [DMP 266-003, cohort IV]. Abstract 692. In: 5th Conference on Retroviruses and Opportunistic Infections. Chicago; 1998:208.
111. Hicks C, Hass D, Seekins D, et al. A phase II, double-blind, placebo-controlled, dose ranging study to assess the antiretroviral activity and safety of DMP 266 (efavirenz, SUSTIVA) in combination with open-label zidovudine (ZDV) with lamivudine (3TC) [DMP 266-005]. Abstract 698. In: 5th Conference on Retroviruses and Opportunistic Infections. Chicago; 1998:209.
111a. Tashima K, Staszewski S, Stryker R, et al. A phase III, multicenter, randomized, open-label study to compare the antiretroviral activity and tolerability of efavirenz (EFV) + indinavir (IDV) versus EFV + zidovudine (ZDV) + lamivudine (3TC) versus IDV + ZDV + 3TC at 48 weeks. Study 006 Investigator Team. Abstract LB16. In: Sixth Conference on Retroviruses and Opportunistic Infections. Chicago; 1999:208.
112. Demeter L, Shafer R, Para M, et al. Delavirdine (DLV) susceptibility of HIV-1 isolates obtained from patients (pts) receiving DLV monotherapy (ACTG 260). In: 3rd Conference on Retroviruses and Opportunistic Infections. Washington, DC; 1996:113.
113. Young SD, Britcher SF, Tran LO, et al. L-743, 726 (DMP-266): A novel, highly potent nonnucleoside inhibitor of the human immunodeficiency virus type 1 reverse transcriptase. Antimicrob Agents Chemother. 1995;39:2602–2605.
114. Bacheler L, George H, Hollis G, Abremski K. Resistance to efavirenz (SUSTIVA) in vivo. Abstract 703. In: 5th Conference on Retroviruses and Opportunistic Infections. Chicago; 1998:210.
114a. Deeks SG, Collier A, Lalezari J, et al. The safety and efficacy of adefovir dipivoxil, a novel anti-human immunodeficiency virus (HIV) therapy, in HIV-infected adults: a randomized, double-blind, placebo-controlled trial. J Infect Dis. 1997;176:1517–1523.
114b. Mulato AS, Lamy PD, Miller MD, et al. Genotypic and phenotypic characterization of human immunodeficiency virus type 1 variants isolated from AIDS patients after prolonged adefovir dipivoxil therapy. Antimicrob Agents Chemother. 1998;42:1620–1628.
114c. Miller MD, Anton KE, Mulato AS, et al. Human immunodeficiency virus type 1 expressing the lamivudine-associated M184V mutation in reverse transcriptase shows increased susceptibility to adefovir and decreased replication capability in vitro. J Infect Dis. 1999;179:92–100.
114d. Gilead Sciences. Press release. March 19, 1999.
115. Deeks SG, Smith M, Holodniy M, Kahn JO. HIV-1 protease inhibitors. A review for clinicians. JAMA. 1997;277:145–153.
116. McDonald CK, Kuritzkes DR. Human immunodeficiency virus type 1 protease inhibitors. Arch Intern Med. 1997;157:951–959.
117. Piscitelli SC, Flexner C, Minor JR, et al. Drug interactions in patients infected with human immunodeficiency virus. Clin Infect Dis. 1996;23:685–693.
118. Flexner C. HIV-protease inhibitors. N Engl J Med. 1998;338:1281–1292.
119. Dube MP, Johnson DL, Currier JS, Leedom JM. Protease inhibitor-associated hyperglycaemia. Lancet. 1997;350:713–714.
120. Viraben R, Aquilina C. Indinavir-associated lipodystrophy. AIDS. 1998;12:F37–F39.
121. Lo JC, Mulligan K, Tai VW, et al."Buffalo hump" in men with HIV-1 infection. Lancet. 1998;351:867–870.
122. Miller KD, Jones E, Yanovski JA, et al. Visceral abdominal-fat accumulation associated with use of indinavir. Lancet. 1998;351:871–875.
123. Hirsch MS, Klibanski A. What price progress? Pseudo-Cushing's syndrome associated with antiretroviral therapy in patients with human immunodeficiency virus infection. Clin Infect Dis. 1998;27:68–72.
124. Kitchen VS, Skinner C, Ariyoshi K, et al. Safety and activity of saquinavir in HIV infection. Lancet. 1995;345:952–955.
125. Schapiro JM, Winters MA, Stewart F, et al. The effect of high-dose saquinavir on viral load and CD4+ T-cell counts in HIV-infected patients. Ann Intern Med. 1996;124:1039–1050.
126. Collier AC, Coombs RW, Schoenfeld DA, et al. Treatment of human immunodeficiency virus infection with saquinavir, zidovudine, and zalcitabine. AIDS Clinical Trials Group. N Engl J Med 1996;334:1011–1017.
127. Haubrich R, Lalezani J, Follansbee SE, et al. Improved survival and reduced clinical progression in HIV-infected patients with advanced disease treated with saquinavir plus zalcitabine. NV14256 Study Team. Antiviral Ther. 1998;3:33–42.
128. Mitsuyasu RT, Skolnik PR, Cohen SR, et al. Activity of the soft gelatin formulation of saquinavir in combination therapy in antiretroviral-naive patients. NV15355 Study Team. AIDS. 1998;12:F103–F109.

129. Merry C, Barry MG, Mulcahy F, et al. Saquinavir pharmacokinetics alone and in combination with ritonavir in HIV-infected patients. AIDS. 1997;11:F29–F33.
130. Rhone SA, Hogg RS, Yip B, et al. The antiviral effect of ritonavir and saquinavir in combination amongst HIV-infected adults: Results from a community-based study. AIDS. 1998;12:619–624.
131. Gill MJ. Safety profile of soft gelatin formulation of saquinavir in combination with nucleosides in a broad patient population. NV15182 Study Team. AIDS. 1998;12:1400–1402.
132. Kempf DJ, Marsh KC, Denissen JF, et al. ABT-538 is a potent inhibitor of human immunodeficiency virus protease and has high oral bioavailability in humans. Proc Natl Acad Sci U S A. 1995;92:2484–2488.
133. Danner SA, Carr A, Leonard JM, et al. A short-term study of the safety, pharmacokinetics, and efficacy of ritonavir, an inhibitor of HIV-1 protease. European-Australian Collaborative Ritonavir Study Group. N Engl J Med. 1995;333:1528–1533.
134. Markowitz M, Saag M, Powderly WG, et al. A preliminary study of ritonavir, an inhibitor of HIV-1 protease, to treat HIV-1 infection. N Engl J Med. 1995;333:1534–1539.
135. Cameron DW, Heath-Chiozzi M, Danner S, et al. Randomised placebo-controlled trial of ritonavir in advanced HIV-1 disease. The Advanced HIV Disease Ritonavir Study Group. Lancet. 1998;351:543–549.
136. Gulick RM, Mellors JW, Havlir D, et al. Treatment with indinavir, zidovudine, and lamivudine in adults with human immunodeficiency virus infection and prior antiretroviral therapy. N Engl J Med. 1997;337:734–739.
137. Hammer SM, Squires KE, Hughes MD, et al. A controlled trial of two nucleoside analogues plus indinavir in persons with human immunodeficiency virus infection and CD4 cell counts of 200 per cubic millimeter or less. AIDS Clinical Trials Group 320 Study Team. N Engl J Med. 1997;337:725–733.
138. Hirsch M, Steigbigel R, Staszewski S, et al. A randomized, controlled trial of indinavir, zidovudine and lamivudine in adults with advanced HIV-infection and prior antiretroviral therapy. J Infect Dis. 1999. In press.
139. Hirsch M, Meibohm A, Rawlins S, Leavitt R. Indinavir (IDV) in combination with ZDV and 3TC in ZDV-experienced patients with CD4 cell count less than or equal to 50 cells/mm^3—-60 week followup. Abstract 383. In: 5th Conference on Retroviruses and Opportunistic Infections. Chicago; 1998:150.
140. Kopp JB, Miller KD, Mican JA, et al. Crystalluria and urinary tract abnormalities associated with indinavir. Ann Intern Med. 1997;127:119–125.
141. Merck Research Laboratories. Letter to investigators. April 8, 1998.
142. Powderly W, Sension M, Conant M, et al. The efficacy of Viracept (nelfinavir mesylate, NFV) in pivotal phase II/III double-blind randomized controlled trials as monotherapy and in combination with d4T or AZT/3TC. Abstract 370. In: 4th Conference on Retroviruses and Opportunistic Infections. Washington, DC; 1997:132.
143. Saag M, Knowles M, Chang Y, et al. Durable effect of VIRACEPT (nelfinavir mesylate, NFV) in triple combination therapy. Abstract I-101. In: 37th Interscience Conference on Antimicrobial Agents and Chemotherapy. Toronto; 1997.
144. Clendeninn N, Quart B, Anderson R, et al. Analysis of long-term virologic data from the VIRACEPT (nelfinavir, NFV) 511 protocol using 3 HIV-RNA assays. Abstract 372. In: 5th Conference on Retroviruses and Opportunistic Infections. Chicago; 1998:148.
145. Murphy RL, Gulick RM, DeGruttola V, et al. Treatment with amprenavir alone or amprenavir with zidovudine and lamivudine in adults with human immunodeficiency virus infection. J Infect Dis. 1999;179:808–816.
146. Eron J, Haubrich R, Richman D, et al. Preliminary assessment of 141W94 in combination with other protease inhibitors. Abstract 6. In: 5th Conference on Retroviruses and Opportunistic Infections. Chicago; 1998:80.
147. Jacobsen H, Hanggi M, Ott M, et al. In vivo resistance to a human immunodeficiency virus type 1 proteinase inhibitor: Mutations, kinetics, and frequencies. J Infect Dis. 1996;173:1379–1387.
148. Molla A, Korneyeva M, Gao Q, et al. Ordered accumulation of mutations in HIV protease confers resistance to ritonavir. Nat Med. 1996;2:760–766.
149. Condra JH, Schleif WA, Blahy OM, et al. In vivo emergence of HIV-1 variants resistant to multiple protease inhibitors. Nature. 1995;374:569–571.
150. Condra JH, Holder DJ, Schleif WA, et al. Genetic correlates of in vivo viral resistance to indinavir, a human immunodeficiency virus type 1 protease inhibitor. J Virol. 1996;70:8270–8276.
151. Patick AK, Duran M, Cao Y, et al. Genotypic and phenotypic characterization of human immunodeficiency virus type 1 variants isolated from patients treated with the protease inhibitor nelfinavir. Antimicrob Agents Chemother. 1998;42:2637–2644.
152. Partaledis JA, Yamaguchi K, Tisdale M, et al. In vitro selection and characterization of human immunodeficiency virus type 1 (HIV-1) isolates with reduced sensitivity to hydroxyethylamino sulfonamide inhibitors of HIV-1 aspartyl protease. J Virol. 1995;69:5228–5235.
153. Hertogs K, Mellors JW, Schel P, et al. Patterns of cross-resistance among protease inhibitors in 483 clinical HIV-1 isolates. Abstract 395. In: Fifth Conference on Retroviruses and Opportunistic Infections. Chicago; 1998:153.
154. Doyon L, Croteau G, Thibeault D, et al. Second locus involved in human immunodeficiency virus type 1 resistance to protease inhibitors. J Virol. 1996;70:3763–3769.
155. Zhang YM, Imamichi H, Imamichi T, et al. Drug resistance during indinavir therapy is caused by mutations in the protease gene and in its Gag substrate cleavage sites. J Virol. 1997;71:6662–6670.
156. De Pasquale MP, Murphy R, Gulick R, et al. Mutations selected in HIV plasma RNA during 141W94 therapy. Abstract 406a. In: 5th Conference on Retroviruses and Opportunistic Infections. Chicago; 1998:155.
157. Report of the NIH Panel to Define Principles of Therapy of HIV Infection. MMWR Morb Mortal Wkly Rep. 1998;47:1–41.
158. Mellors JW, Rinaldo CR Jr, Gupta P, et al. Prognosis in HIV-1 infection predicted by the quantity of virus in plasma [published erratum appears in Science. 1997;275:14]. Science. 1996;272:1167–1170.
159. Mellors JW, Munoz A, Giorgi JV, et al. Plasma viral load and CD4 + lymphocytes as prognostic markers of HIV-1 infection. Ann Intern Med. 1997;126:946–954.
160. Vlahov D, Graham N, Hoover D, et al. Prognostic indicators for AIDS and infectious disease death in HIV-infected injection drug users: Plasma viral load and CD4 + cell count. JAMA. 1998;279:35–40.
161. Hughes MD, Johnson VA, Hirsch MS, et al. Monitoring plasma HIV-1 RNA levels in addition to CD4+ lymphocyte count improves assessment of antiretroviral therapeutic response. ACTG 241 Protocol Virology Substudy Team. Ann Intern Med. 1997;126:929–938.
162. O'Brien WA, Hartigan PM, Daar ES, et al. Changes in plasma HIV RNA levels and CD4+ lymphocyte counts predict both response to antiretroviral therapy and therapeutic failure. VA Cooperative Study Group on AIDS. Ann Intern Med. 1997;126:939–945.
163. Saag MS, Holodniy M, Kuritzkes DR, et al. HIV viral load markers in clinical practice. Nat Med. 1996;2:625–629.
164. Sax PE, Boswell SL, White-Guthro M, Hirsch MS. Potential clinical implications of interlaboratory variability in CD4+ T-lymphocyte counts of patients infected with human immunodeficiency virus. Clin Infect Dis. 1995;21:1121–1125.
165. Caliendo AM, Hirsch MS. Combination therapy for infection due to human immunodeficiency virus type 1 [published erratum appears in Clin Infect Dis. 1994;19:379]. Clin Infect Dis. 1994;18:516–524.
166. Havlir DV, Richman DD. Viral dynamics of HIV: Implications for drug development and therapeutic strategies. Ann Intern Med. 1996;124:984–994.
167. Carpenter CC, Fischl MA, Hammer SM, et al. Antiretroviral therapy for HIV infection in 1998. Updated recommendations of the International AIDS Society-USA panel. JAMA. 1998;280:78–86.
168. Guidelines for the use of antiretroviral agents in HIV-infected adults and adolescents. Department of Health and Human Services and Henry J. Kaiser Family Foundation. MMWR Morb Mortal Wkly Rep. 1998;47:43–82.
169. Vanhove GF, Schapiro JM, Winters MA, et al. Patient compliance and drug failure in protease inhibitor monotherapy. JAMA. 1996;276:1955–1956.
170. Pialoux G, Raffi F, Brun-Vezinet F, et al. A randomized trial of three maintenance regimens given after three months of induction therapy with zidovudine, lamivudine, and indinavir in previously untreated HIV-1-infected patients. Trilege (Agence Nationale de Recherches sur le SIDA 072) Study Team. N Engl J Med. 1998;339:1269–1276.
171. Havlir DV, Marschner IC, Hirsch MS, et al. Maintenance antiretroviral therapies in HIV infected patients with undetectable plasma HIV RNA after triple-drug therapy. AIDS Clinical Trials Group Study 343 Team. N Engl J Med. 1998;339:1261–1268.
172. Finzi D, Hermankova M, Pierson T, et al. Identification of a reservoir for HIV-1 in patients on highly active antiretroviral therapy. Science. 1997;278:1295–1300.
173. Wong JK, Hezareh M, Gunthard HF, et al. Recovery of replication-competent HIV despite prolonged suppression of plasma viremia. Science. 1997;278:1291–1295.
174. Guidelines for the use of antiretroviral agents in pediatric HIV infection. Center for Disease Control and Prevention. MMWR Morb Mortal Wkly Rep. 1998;47:1–43.
175. Gerberding JL. Management of occupational exposures to blood-borne viruses. N Engl J Med. 1995;332:444–451.
176. Cardo DM, Culver DH, Ciesielski CA, et al. A case-control study of HIV seroconversion in health care workers after percutaneous exposure. Centers for Disease Control and Prevention Needlestick Surveillance Group. N Engl J Med. 1997;337:1485–1490.
177. Gerberding JL. Prophylaxis for occupational exposure to HIV. Ann Intern Med. 1996;125:497–501.
178. Public Health Service guidelines for the management of health-care worker exposures to HIV and recommendations for postexposure prophylaxis. MMWR Morb Mortal Wkly Rep. 1998;47:1–34.
179. Katz MH, Gerberding JL. The care of persons with recent sexual exposure to HIV. Ann Intern Med. 1998;128:306–312.
180. Schacker T, Collier AC, Hughes J, et al. Clinical and epidemiologic features of primary HIV infection [published erratum appears in Ann Intern Med. 1997;126:174]. Ann Intern Med. 1996;125:257–264.
181. Rosenberg ES, Billingsley JM, Caliendo AM, et al. Vigorous HIV-1–specific CD4+ T cell responses associated with control of viremia. Science. 1997;278:1447–1450.
182. Kinloch-De Loes S, Hirschel BJ, Hoen B, et al. A controlled trial of zidovudine in primary human immunodeficiency virus infection [published erratum appears in N Engl J Med. 1995;333:1367]. N Engl J Med. 1995;333:408–413.
183. Lafeuillade A, Poggi C, Tamalet C, et al. Effects of a combination of zidovudine, didanosine, and lamivudine on primary human immunodeficiency virus type 1 infection. J Infect Dis. 1997;175:1051–1055.
184. Perrin L, Markowitz M, Calandra G, Chung M. An open treatment study of acute HIV infection with zidovudine, lamivudine and indinavir sulfate. Abstract 238. In: 4th Conference on Retroviruses and Opportunistic Infections. Washington, DC; 1997:108.
185. Hoen B, Harzic M, Dumon B, et al. Efficacy of zidovudine, lamivudine and ritonavir combination in patients with symptomatic primary HIV-1 infection: The

ANRS 053/53b trial. Can eradication be obtained? Abstract 524. In: 5th Conference on Retroviruses and Opportunistic Infections. Chicago; 1998:178.

186. Minkoff H, Augenbraun M. Antiretroviral therapy for pregnant women. Am J Obstet Gynecol. 1997;176:478–489.
187. Public Health Service Task Force recommendations for the use of antiretroviral drugs in pregnant women infected with HIV-1 for maternal health and for reducing perinatal HIV-1 transmission in the United States. Centers for Disease Control and Prevention. MMWR Morb Mortal Wkly Rep. 1998;47: 1–30.
188. O'Sullivan MJ, Boyer PJ, Scott GB, et al. The pharmacokinetics and safety of zidovudine in the third trimester of pregnancy for women infected with human immunodeficiency virus and their infants: Phase I acquired immunodeficiency syndrome clinical trials group study (protocol 082). Zidovudine Collaborative Working Group. Am J Obstet Gynecol. 1993;168: 1510–1516.
189. Moodley J, Moodley D, Pillay K, et al. Pharmacokinetics and antiretroviral activity of lamivudine alone or when coadministered with zidovudine in human immunodeficiency virus type 1-infected pregnant women and their offspring. J Infect Dis. 1998;178:1327–1333.
190. Mirochnick M, Fenton T, Gagnier P, et al. Pharmacokinetics of nevirapine in human immunodeficiency virus type 1-infected pregnant women and their neonates. Pediatric AIDS Clinical Trials Group Protocol 250 Team. J Infect Dis. 1998;178:368–374.
191. Patil SD, Livingston E, McKinney RE, et al. Does pregnancy affect the pharmacokinetics of didanosine (ddI) in HIV-1 infected women? Abstract 225. In: 5th Conference on Retroviruses and Opportunistic Infections. Chicago; 1998:121.
192. Livingston E, Patil S, Unadkat J, et al. Placental transfer of didanosine (ddI) and initial evaluation of didanosine toxicity in HIV-1 infected pregnant women and their offspring. Abstract 226. In: 5th Conference on Retroviruses and Opportunistic Infections. Chicago; 1998:121.
193. Sperling RS, Stratton P, O'Sullivan MJ, et al. A survey of zidovudine use in pregnant women with human immunodeficiency virus infection. N Engl J Med. 1992;326:857–861.
194. Connor EM, Sperling RS, Gelber R, et al. Reduction of maternal-infant transmission of human immunodeficiency virus type 1 with zidovudine treatment. Pediatric AIDS Clinical Trials Group Protocol 076 Study Group. N Engl J Med. 1994;331:1173–1180.
195. Sperling RS, Shapiro DE, Coombs RW, et al. Maternal viral load, zidovudine treatment, and the risk of transmission of human immunodeficiency virus type 1 from mother to infant. Pediatric AIDS Clinical Trials Group Protocol 076 Study Group. N Engl J Med. 1996;335:1621–1629.
196. Stiehm ER, Lambert JS, Mofenson LM, et al. Efficacy of zidovudine and human immunodeficiency virus (HIV) hyperimmune immunoglobulin for reducing perinatal HIV transmission from HIV-infected women with advanced disease: results of Pediatric AIDS Clinical Trials Group protocol 185. J Infect Dis. 1999;179:567–575.
197. Cao Y, Krogstad P, Korber BT, et al. Maternal HIV-1 viral load and vertical transmission of infection: The Ariel Project for the prevention of HIV transmission from mother to infant. Nat Med. 1997;3:549–552.
198. Shearer WT, Quinn TC, LaRussa P, et al. Viral load and disease progression in infants infected with human immunodeficiency virus type 1. Women and Infants Transmission Study Group. N Engl J Med. 1997;336:1337–1342.
199. Palumbo PE, Raskino C, Fiscus S, et al. Predictive value of quantitative plasma HIV RNA and CD4+ lymphocyte count in HIV-infected infants and children. JAMA. 1998;279:756–761.
200. Boucher FD, Modlin JF, Weller S, et al. Phase I evaluation of zidovudine administered to infants exposed at birth to the human immunodeficiency virus. J Pediatr. 1993;122:137–144.
201. Lewis LL, Venzon D, Church J, et al. Lamivudine in children with human immunodeficiency virus infection: A phase I/II study. The National Cancer Institute Pediatric Branch-Human Immunodeficiency Virus Working Group. J Infect Dis. 1996;174:16–25.
202. McKinney RE Jr, Maha MA, Connor EM, et al. A multicenter trial of oral zidovudine in children with advanced human immunodeficiency virus disease. The Protocol 043 Study Group. N Engl J Med. 1991;324:1018–1025.
203. Mueller BU, Butler KM, Stocker VL, et al. Clinical and pharmacokinetic evaluation of long-term therapy with didanosine in children with HIV infection. Pediatrics. 1994;94:724–731.
204. Kline MW, Van Dyke RB, Lindsey JC, et al. A randomized comparative trial of stavudine (d4T) versus zidovudine (ZDV, AZT) in children with human immunodeficiency virus infection. AIDS Clinical Trials Group 240 Team. Pediatrics. 1998;101:214–220.
205. Englund JA, Baker CJ, Raskino C, et al. Zidovudine, didanosine, or both as the initial treatment for symptomatic HIV-infected children. AIDS Clinical Trials Group (ACTG) Study 152 Team. N Engl J Med. 1997;336:1704–1712.
206. McKinney RE, Jr, Johnson GM, Stanley K, et al. A randomized study of combined zidovudine-lamivudine versus didanosine monotherapy in children with symptomatic therapy-naive HIV-1 infection. The Pediatric AIDS Clinical Trials Group Protocol 300 Study Team. J Pediatr. 1998;133:500–508.
207. Melvin AJ, Mohan KM, Arcuino LA, et al. Clinical, virologic and immunologic responses of children with advanced human immunodeficiency virus type 1 disease treated with protease inhibitors. Pediatr Infect Dis J. 1997;16:968–974.
208. Mueller BU, Nelson RP, Jr, Sleasman J, et al. A phase I/II study of the protease inhibitor ritonavir in children with human immunodeficiency virus infection. Pediatrics. 1998;101:335–343.
209. Krogstad P, Wiznia A, Luzuriaga K, et al. Evidence of potent antiviral activity in a phase I/II study of nelfinavir mesylate (Viracept) in HIV infected children. Abstract 270. In: 5th Conference on Retroviruses and Opportunistic Infections. Chicago; 1998:130.
210. Luzuriaga K, Bryson Y, Krogstad P, et al. Combination treatment with zidovudine, didanosine, and nevirapine in infants with human immunodeficiency virus type 1 infection. N Engl J Med. 1997;336:1343–1349.
211. Kilby JM, Hopkins S, Venetta TM, et al. Potent suppression of HIV-1 replication in humans by T-20, a peptide inhibitor of gp41-mediated virus entry. Nat Med. 1998;4:1302–1307.

Chapter 116

Management of Opportunistic Infections Associated with Human Immunodeficiency Virus Infection

HENRY MASUR

The quality and duration of survival for patients with human immunodeficiency virus (HIV) infection has improved remarkably since the acquired immunodeficiency disease (AIDS) was first recognized in the early 1980s.[1–10] Much of the early improvement in prognosis was due to anti-*Pneumocystis* prophylaxis and to nucleoside antiretroviral therapy.[3, 5, 6] Since 1995, an increasing number of patients have received highly active antiretroviral therapy (HAART): for patients who respond in terms of a significantly reduced HIV viral burden and a stable or increased circulating CD4 cell count there has been a dramatic decrease in clinical complications.[1, 2, 2a] This sharp reduction in the number of AIDS-associated opportunistic infections has redirected the focus of management to maximizing the potency, durability, and tolerability of antiretroviral therapy. HIV-infected patients continue to develop opportunistic infections, however, because many patients are unaware of their HIV status until they present with an opportunistic infection and because patients fail HAART owing to drug nonadherence, drug interactions, poor drug absorption, and development of resistant virus.[9, 10]

For patients who do not receive sustained benefit from HAART, health care providers need to be cognizant that a substantial contribution to improved prognosis can be made by more effective management of the opportunistic processes that complicate the immunosuppression caused by HIV.[5–8] Management has become more successful because of advances in several convergent areas: understanding unique features of the natural history of HIV-associated opportunistic infections; recognizing the relationship between the course of immunologic decline and the occurrence of opportunistic processes developing new diagnostic techniques; identifying more effective therapies; designing more effective, more comprehensive preventive strategies; and vastly improving the education of health care workers and patients.

The range and diversity of new approaches to the management of opportunistic infections in patients with HIV infection present problems as well as opportunities. Many patients have difficulty affording the cost of medical care or cannot take time from work or family responsibilities to obtain optimal management. Most patients find it difficult to comply with highly complex schedules of assessments and medications, especially considering the complicated regimens associated with HAART. Moreover, familiar pathogens such as cytomegalovirus (CMV) and *Mycobacterium avium* complex (MAC) may be associated with novel manifestations when patients are receiving HAART.[11–13] Pathogens are increasingly resistant to the most widely used agents. In addition, previously unrecognized or seldom-identified pathogens such as *Nosema, Cyclospora*, human herpesvirus-6, hepatitis C, and *Penicillium* are now producing clinical disease as patients live longer, travel, or reside in diverse geographic areas and receive preventive management for the more frequently recognized pathogens.

Aggressive preventive, diagnostic, and therapeutic management of opportunistic infections in patients with HIV infection are crucial elements of the increasingly successful efforts to improve the prognosis for this patient population. Health care resources expended to manage opportunistic infections are unequivocally well spent if applied with a strategy that emphasizes prevention and that provides aggressive recognition and therapy of acute syndromes.[14]

PROSPECTIVE MONITORING

Prospective clinical and laboratory assessment is vital to the effective management of opportunistic infections in patients with HIV infection, just as it is important for determining prognosis and for deciding the optimal time for antiretroviral intervention.

The CD4+ T-lymphocyte count is a valuable marker to determine when patients are at increased risk for developing a specific opportunistic infection.[10, 15–19] For example, *Pneumocystis carinii* pneumonia (PCP) occurs rarely in patients who have more than 200 to 250 cells/mm^3,[15–17] and disseminated MAC occurs rarely in patients with CD4+ T-lymphocyte counts higher than 50 cells/mm^3.[20, 21] This information is very helpful for focusing a diagnostic evaluation. When a patient with a CD4+ T-lymphocyte count of 700 cells/mm^3 develops cough and fever, for instance, the likelihood that this syndrome is caused by PCP is slim (but not zero). Thus, sputum examination for *Pneumocystis* is generally unnecessary, and most attention, when processing respiratory secretions, should be directed at common bacterial and viral pathogens. In contrast, when the CD4+ T-lymphocyte count is 25 cells/mm^3, a search for *Pneumocystis* in sputum or bronchoalveolar lavage is a very important focus because PCP is so common in this patient population. There is considerable variability, however, in how quickly immune function deteriorates in individual patients, whether or not that patient is being treated with antiretroviral therapy.[19, 22, 23]

Although CD4+ T lymphocyte counts provide a useful estimate of susceptibility to infections, they are not perfect predictive tools. More than 90% of cases of PCP, for example, occur in patients with CD4+ T-lymphocyte counts under 200 cells/mm^3. Some cases, however, occur in patients with measured counts in the 200 to 300 cells/mm^3 range, and a few cases occur in patients with counts greater than 300 cells/mm^3.[15–17] For some of these patients, errors have been due to inaccurate laboratory measurements. Other patients may have rapidly falling CD4+ T-lymphocyte counts such that a value obtained 2 to 4 weeks previously is not a true reflection of the patient's current immunologic status.

A frequent concern is that CD4+ T-lymphocyte counts counts in patients receiving antiretroviral therapy, especially HAART, may not be accurate reflections of clinical susceptibility to opportunistic infections. To date, there are no published studies that have examined large databases, but small series do not provide evidence that opportunistic infections are occurring at "unexpected" CD4+ T-lymphocyte counts regardless of what antiretroviral therapy or immunotherapy patients are receiving and regardless of how low the nadir CD4+ T-lymphocyte counts fell before initiation of HAART.[23a] There is concern that the phenotype or functional capacity of lymphocytes in patients responding to HAART may not be identical to the characteristics of cells in patients with similar CD4+ T-lymphocyte counts who have never received antiretroviral therapy.[24] Although differences in laboratory characteristics have been documented, there is no evidence that these differences in laboratory markers are clinically relevant.

CD4+ T-lymphocyte counts are not the only laboratory predictors of opportunistic infection.[10, 19, 22, 23, 25] HIV viral load in the circulation is an independent predictor: With each log increase in titer, the likelihood of an opportunistic infection occurring increases.[19, 25]

Specific tests for individual pathogens may also be useful predictors of the occurrence (or relapse) of opportunistic infection. Highly sensitive detection systems, such as polymerase chain reaction (PCR) assays of buffy coat or serum for CMV, have the potential to be quite useful.[26]

Clinical findings can be useful predictors of susceptibility to supplement the information derived from CD4+ T-lymphocyte counts and HIV viral loads. For example, the development of otherwise unexplained oropharyngeal candidiasis, persistent fever, previous PCP, wasting, or any type of pneumonia is a good indicator of current susceptibility to PCP and of the need for prophylaxis, independent of the CD4+ T-lymphocyte count and the HIV viral load.[16, 27–29]

MANAGEMENT OF HIGHLY ACTIVE ANTIRETROVIRAL THERAPY FOR PATIENTS WITH ACUTE OPPORTUNISTIC INFECTION

When patients develop acute PCP, severe microsporidial diarrhea, or some other acute or severe opportunistic infection, the question often arises whether to initiate or continue HAART. Unquestionably, the immune augmentation that HAART can produce is likely to be beneficial ultimately in clearing the offending pathogen. However, the potential benefit of HAART must be weighed against two factors: first, the initiation of HAART could produce an enhanced inflammatory response that could be detrimental; HAART-related immune-reactivation retinitis[12] or lymphadenitis[11] has been reported. Second, administration of HAART at a time when adherence may be poor or oral absorption may be unpredictable, or when new drugs could alter pharmacokinetics can result in suboptimal serum drug concentrations. Such suboptimal levels will enhance the likelihood of development of HIV resistance to antiretroviral agents. Thus, in some circumstances, withholding all antiretroviral therapy until an acute opportunistic infection resolves might be the most prudent course. Such a strategy allows the HIV viral load to rise toward its "set point" but does not produce suboptimal antiretroviral pharmacokinetics and thus selective pressure favoring the production of drug-resistant virus.

SPECTRUM OF OPPORTUNISTIC PATHOGENS

Patients with HIV infection are highly susceptible to a unique constellation of pathogens. The opportunistic infections that an individual patient develops are a function of the degree of immunosuppression and of exposure as well as other factors.

Traditionally, most HIV-associated opportunistic infections have been thought to be due to reactivation of latent infection, but this conclusion is based primarily on speculation rather than data. Some episodes of opportunistic infection, such as involvement in outbreaks of multidrug-resistant *Mycobacterium tuberculosis*, clearly represent primary infection. Exogenous reinfection with new strains of tuberculosis, identified by molecular typing systems, for example, has been described.[30, 31] As techniques to identify strain variants are more widely applied, additional information will be forthcoming about how often serial episodes of *Pneumocystis, Candida*, or CMV infection, for example, represent reinfection rather than reactivation.[32, 33] Such information will influence strategies for preventing subsequent episodes of opportunistic processes.

It is apparent that the infectious manifestations of HIV-induced immunosuppression vary geographically because of different exposure patterns. Histoplasmosis, for example, is very common as a cause of pulmonary infiltrates in the Ohio River Valley[34]; *Trypanosoma cruzii* is recognized as a cause of fever and cerebral mass lesions in Brazil[35, 36]; *M. tuberculosis* is very common in certain parts of New York City, Miami, Africa, and Haiti[37, 38]; *Penicillium marneffei* is well recognized in southern China and Thailand[39]; and isosporiasis is common in Haiti.[40] Specific behavior patterns also influence exposure and thus the infectious manifestations of HIV-induced immunosuppression: homosexual men are much more likely to develop Kaposi's sarcoma[41] or ulcerative perirectal herpes simplex than are patients with other behavioral risk factors.

Many of the opportunistic infections characteristic of HIV-induced immunosuppression occur in patients with HIV infection much more frequently than in almost any other patient group. For example, without prophylaxis or effective HAART therapy, PCP will ultimately develop in 60 to 80% of HIV-infected patients in North America.[10, 16] The annual attack rate for patients with CD4+ T-lymphocyte counts below 100 cells/mm^3 is probably twice that for patients with severe combined immunodeficiency syndrome and more than 10 times that for patients with organ transplants, solid tumors, or most hematologic malignant neoplasms.[16, 42] Disseminated MAC was rarely recognized in humans before the advent of HIV infection, yet disseminated MAC occurs in as many as 30 to 40% of patients with advanced HIV infection in the absence of HAART and specific chemoprophylaxis.[20, 21, 43]

Tuberculosis, cerebral toxoplasmosis, persistent cryptosporidiosis, microsporidiosis, and Kaposi's sarcoma are examples of other processes that cause disease so much more commonly in patients with HIV infection than with other immunodeficiencies that their presence should strongly suggest the utility of HIV testing. If a routine HIV test result is negative but the CD4 count is low, consideration should be given to an unusual strain of HIV that might be missed by the assay kit being used (e.g., HIV-1 type O) or an immunoglobulin synthetic defect. In such cases, the utility of an alternative serologic technique or a plasma viral load assay for HIV should be explored (see Chapter 106).

PATHOGENS NOT TRADITIONALLY CONSIDERED OPPORTUNISTIC

Patients with HIV infection develop acute and chronic infections that are due to pathogens that are not classically considered "opportunistic." However, some of those pathogens (e.g., *Streptococcus pneumoniae*) do cause disease with greater frequency or severity in patients with HIV infection than in immunologically normal patients. Others occur because of AIDS-related processes such as lymphedema related to Kaposi's sarcoma (e.g., streptococcal cellulitis) or fungemia related to indwelling intravenous catheters (e.g., candidema). When patients present with infectious syndromes, common community-acquired processes such as influenza, *Escherichia coli*, urinary tract infection, or streptococcal cellulitis must be considered even though these processes may not be more frequent or more severe in this population.

In addition, infectious processes must be considered that reflect patient behavior. Thus, men who have sex with men may develop hepatitis A, rectal gonorrhea, or giardiasis related to their behavior. Intravenous drug abusers may develop staphylococcal sepsis or hepatitis C owing to contaminated needles. Patients with HIV infection may also develop infectious complications caused by procedures or devices: staphylococcal sepsis due to an infected Groshong catheter implanted for ganciclovir administration or cholangitis following an endoscopic retrograph cholangiographic procedure, for example.

DRUG INTERACTIONS

Some drugs used for therapy or prevention of opportunistic infections can interact with each other or with other drugs such as antiretroviral agents. These interactions can alter the efficacy and toxicity of prescribed drugs. This most often occurs with drugs that share the same hepatic cytochrome metabolic pathway. The protease inhibitors, the non-nucleoside reverse transcriptase inhibitors, and rifampin, rifabutin, azoles, or quinolones need special attention. The interaction of rifampin with saquinavir (Fortovase) or ritonavir, for example, can result in very low serum protease inhibitor levels, increasing the likelihood that retroviral resistance will develop. The interaction of fluconazole or a quinolone with rifabutin can augment rifabutin or protease inhibitor levels, increasing the likelihood of rifabutin-related uveitis. Thus, the influence of newly introduced drugs on the pharmacokinetics of concurrent drugs needs to be carefully thought out.[44]

GENERAL PRINCIPLES OF MANAGEMENT

Opportunistic pathogens commonly seen in HIV-infected patients can be categorized into two groups: those that may respond to conventional or investigational drugs but have a high likelihood of recurring when therapy is discontinued and those for which no therapy currently appears to be effective. (Tuberculosis is one of the few opportunistic infections that rarely recurs after one of the recommended courses of therapy.) The successful management of those opportunistic infections that are treatable depends on (1) prompt diagnosis and initiation of therapy before the clinical syndrome is severe, (2) recognition that a poor response to therapy may indicate that a pathogen other than the one initially identified may be present or that the pathogen is resistant to the therapeutic agent employed, and (3) recognition that most therapies must be lifelong to prevent relapses or recurrences.

The management of opportunistic infections in HIV-infected patients differs from management in other patient populations because the natural history of specific processes such as PCP[45] or cryptococcal meningitis[46] is different in patients who do not have AIDS. The tolerance of HIV-infected patients for therapeutic agents such as trimethoprim-sulfamethoxazole or clindamycin may be less than that of other patient groups,[47] and consideration must be given to interactions between the drug directed against opportunistic pathogens and the multiplicity of drugs (prescription and nonprescription) directed against HIV itself and other concomitant processes.[44] The success of long-term management of opportunistic infections, as in many other diseases, is highly dependent on the degree of immunosuppression caused by the underlying disease. In HIV infection, the immunosuppression, as measured by CD4 count and by HIV viral load, must be a major focus of management if the opportunistic infection is to be managed or prevented over the long term with maximum efficacy and success.

An issue that frequently arises is whether to use empirical antimicrobial regimens or to withhold therapy until a specific diagnosis is established.[48–52] For some clinical scenarios such as the presence of a central nervous system mass lesion[50, 51] or the presence of active retinitis,[52] empirical therapy is usually reasonable because clinical features, immune profiles, and certain other noninvasive laboratory tests make correct diagnosis highly likely. In other situations such as meningitis, fever and wasting, or chronic diarrhea, the clinical presentation is so nonspecific that a definitive diagnosis should be sought.

More frequently, cost is an issue that is increasing the attractiveness of empirical diagnosis and therapy in certain situations, especially those involving mild presentations, such as a patient with fever, cough, and pulmonary infiltrates but a Po_2 greater than 95 mmHg on room air.[48, 49] The empirical approach should differ based on the CD4+ T-lymphocyte count and HIV viral load, but a logical management plan employing initial empirical therapy can be designed. Thus, in some settings a clinical rather than a laboratory diagnosis is appropriate.

Patients who respond to HAART, as manifested by sustained increases in CD4+ T-lymphocyte counts, appear to derive substantial protection against opportunistic infection.[10, 53–56b] In 1999, sufficient data recommended that for patients who have raised CD4+ T-lymphocyte counts from below 200 cells/mm^3 to above 200 cells/mm^3, for 3 to 6 months, primary PCP prophylaxis can be discontinued. This prophylaxis should be restarted if the CD4+ T-lymphocyte count subseqently falls below 200 cells/mm^3. It may be reasonable to stop secondary PCP prophylaxis in such patients and to stop prophylaxis for MAC for patients whose CD4+ T-lymphocyte counts rise above 100 cells/mm³, but there are fewer data on which to base a well-founded recommendation. For patients receiving maintenance therapy for CMV retinitis, there are enoungh data to merit recommending that maintenance can be stopped if the CD4+ T-lymphocyte count is above 150 cells/mm³, lesions are inactive, lesions are not sight threatening, and regular ophthalmologic examinations are feasible. There are insufficient data with which to make a well-founded recommendation about stopping long-term maintenance therapy for other opportunistic infections, such as toxoplasmosis, cryptococcosis, and MAC disease for patients who respond to HAART. Until more data are available, such regimens should probably be continued for life regardless of the CD4+ T-lymphocyte count even if patients are receiving HAART.

OPPORTUNISTIC INFECTIONS

Pneumocystis carinii Pneumonia

PCP continues to be a common complication of HIV infection in North America, although in some areas of the world it is much less common (see Chapter 104).[57, 58] Although specific prophylaxis and HAART have reduced the number of cases, many patients do not recognize that they have HIV infection until they present with PCP. Other patients fail to take prophylactic medications; some patients develop PCP despite prophylaxis, especially if the regimen does not include trimethoprim-sulfamethoxazole; and some patients do not have a sustained response to HAART.[27–29, 59] Thus, PCP continues to be a substantial cause of morbidity and mortality.

Pneumocystis disease most often manifests as as pulmonary dysfunction in patients with HIV infection. Patients may have chest tightness or exercise intolerance as very early symptoms, before chest radiograph results are abnormal and before arterial blood gases reveal hypoxemia.[45] If therapy is to have the greatest chance to succeed, patients and clinicians must be trained to initiate diagnostic evaluation at this stage, before pulmonary dysfunction is severe.[60, 61] Even with very mild manifestations of disease, organisms can be recovered readily from sputum or bronchoalveolar lavage, allowing initiation of therapy on an outpatient basis at a stage when prognosis is excellent.[62, 63]

In large series of patients, PCP can be distinguished from bacterial pneumonia or tuberculosis by the duration of symptoms, the character of the sputum, and the radiologic manifestations. However, in individual cases, it is much more difficult to reliably distinguish PCP from a variety of other infectious and noninfectious processes, including tuberculosis, histoplasmosis, and nonspecific interstitial pneumonitis.[34, 64, 65] Thus, it is important to establish a specific diagnosis to ascertain that the correct pathogen is being treated and to avoid the toxicities, cost, and inconvenience of unnecessary drugs. Establishing a specific diagnosis also has epidemiologic implications in terms of ascertaining the isolation precautions or contact tracing that is needed. However, given the cost of a diagnostic evaluation, in some settings it may be necessary to treat mild cases of presumptive PCP empirically.[48, 49] If patients do not improve, the yield of a diagnostic evaluation of *Pneumocystis* infection should not be diminished substantially. Empirical diagnoses by definition preclude the possibility of screening for tuberculosis, which is very important in many communities for early identification of cases and reduction of the transmission of tuberculosis. The availability of induced sputum examination provides a very sensitive, relatively low-cost method for diagnosis of PCP and for detection of tuberculosis.[63, 66] Nucleic acid detection systems utilizing oral washes or gargles offer promise for outpatient assessments, but their utility remains to be established.[67, 68]

The likelihood that an AIDS patient will survive an episode of PCP depends on the severity of pulmonary dysfunction at the time therapy is initiated, the patient's ability to tolerate available regimens, the presence of concomitant pathology, and the severity of the patient's immunologic dysfunction. A poor prognosis correlates best with an alveolar-arterial gradient greater than 30 mmHg, a severely abnormal chest radiograph result, or a large number of organisms detected on lavage or biopsy.[60] Thus, any drug therapy is more likely to be successful if therapy is started at a time when pulmonary dysfunction is mild and if other severe opportunistic infections or neoplasms are absent. Second, third, or subsequent episodes of PCP do not carry a worse prognosis than the first episode.[69]

Oral trimethoprim-sulfamethoxazole is the treatment of choice for acute PCP because of its convenience of administration, high degree of efficacy, and manageability of associated toxicities (Table 116–1).[42, 70, 71] No agent has ever been shown to have a higher efficacy for PCP. There is no clear reason to prefer intravenous over oral trimethoprim-sulfamethoxazole in compliant patients without obvious gastrointestinal dysfunction. Patients usually improve clinically in terms of fever, respiratory rate, arterial-alveolar gradient, and dyspnea within 4 to 8 days, although there may be an initial worsening during the first 48 to 72 hours of therapy.[45, 71, 72]

Survival for mild episodes treated with trimethoprim-sulfamethoxazole has improved steadily over the past decade. For patients with an initial room air partial pressure of oxygen (Po_2) higher than 70 mmHg, survival has improved from 85 to 90% to 95 to 99% in optimal circumstances.[71, 73] (Noncompliant patients and patients with significant concomitant disorders will not have such good results.) This improvement presumably reflects the better understanding that trimethoprim-sulfamethoxazole can be continued despite non–life-threatening toxicities and that the dose may be altered to maximize tolerability yet maintain trimethoprim levels in the 5 to 8 μg/ml range, which appears to be optimal. In addition, better alternative agents are available for patients who are truly failing trimethoprim-sulfamethoxazole or who are unable to tolerate the drug.[42, 70]

Microbiologic resistance of *Pneumocystis* to trimethoprim-sulfamethoxazole has not been proved because the organism isolated from humans cannot be grown in vitro reliably. Recent reports document that some human isolates contain mutations in their dihydropteroate synthase (the target enzyme for sulfonamides), which in other organisms produces microbiologic and clinical resistance.[74, 75] Further information is needed to determine whether these mutations in fact confer sulfonamide resistance to *Pneumocystis* that is clinically significant and whether the frequency of such resistance will become sufficient to warrant new therapeutic and prophylactic strategies.

For trimethoprim-sulfamethoxazole, common adverse reactions include rash, nausea, vomiting, granulocytopenia, transaminase elevations, nephritis, and hyperkalemia.[71, 76–79] These adverse reactions do not invariably require discontinuation of trimethoprim-sulfamethoxazole therapy. The rashes, which commonly occur between the 8th and 12th days of therapy, may be limited in extent and associated with a degree of pruritus that the patient can tolerate for 21 days. They are more frequent in patients with higher CD4+ T-lymphocyte counts.[78] Life-threatening desquamating processes such as Stevens-Johnson syndrome are extraordinarily rare in AIDS patients, although a few fatal cases have been reported. Severe febrile, hypotensive episodes that resemble septic shock in terms of hemodynamics have also been reported. Thus, the development of a rash associated with trimethoprim-sulfamethoxazole therapy is not necessarily an indication to discontinue this drug regimen. Granulocytopenia appears to be a dose-related phenomenon that may resolve partially or completely if the dose of trimethoprim-sulfamethoxazole is reduced by 25%.[70] Granulocytopenia responds to leucovorin administration only rarely. A report that leucovorin administration can diminish the likelihood of therapeutic response to trimethoprim-sulfamethoxazole is intriguing but not conclusive.[80] Nausea and vomiting can be troublesome complications of trimethoprim-sulfamethoxazole therapy. Severe nausea may be due to very high sulfonamide levels and may resolve if the dose is reduced. Transaminase levels may fluctuate until therapy is stopped; they usually return promptly to baseline values.

Overall, adverse reactions in the past have required discontinua-

TABLE 116-1 Therapy for Opportunistic Infections in Patients with HIV Infection

Clinical Disease	Drug	Dose	Route	Interval	Duration
Pneumocystis pneumonia	Trimethoprim with sulfamethoxazole *or*	5 mg/kg with 25 mg/kg	PO, IV	q8h	21 d
	Trimethoprim plus dapsone *or*	300 mg 100 mg	PO PO	q8h qd	21 d
	Pentamidine *or*	3–4 mg/kg	IV (IM)	qd	21 d
	Atovaquone *or*	750 mg	PO	q12h	21 d
	Clindamycin plus primaquine *or*	300–450 mg 15 mg	PO, IV PO	q6h qd	21 d
	Trimetrexate plus leucovorin	45 mg/m² 20 mg/m²	IV PO, IV	q24h q6h	21 d
	Prednisone (adjunctive therapy for severe episode)	40 mg	PO	q12h*	21 d
Pneumocystis pneumonia (maintenance)	Trimethoprim plus sulfamethoxazole *or*	1 single or double-strength tablet	PO	q24h	Lifelong‖
	Dapsone	100 mg	PO	q24h	Lifelong
Toxoplasmosis	Sulfadiazine plus pyrimethamine plus leucovorin *or*	1–2 g 100 mg† 10–25 mg	PO PO PO, IV	q6h qd qd	Lifelong Lifelong Lifelong
	Clindamycin plus pyrimethamine	450–600 mg 50–100 mg†	PO PO	q6h qd	Lifelong Lifelong
Cryptosporidiosis	Paromomycin	1.0 g	PO	bid	Lifelong
Microsporidiosis	Albendazole	400 mg	PO	bid	Lifelong
Isosporiasis	Trimethoprim with sulfamethoxazole *followed by*	160 mg 800 mg	PO, IV	q6h	10 d
	Trimethoprim plus sulfamethaxazole	160 mg 800 mg	PO	bid	14 d
Candidiasis					
Oral	Fluconazole	100–200 mg	PO, IV	q24h	5–10 d
Esophageal	Fluconazole	100–400 mg	PO, IV	q24h	14–21 d
Vaginal	Fluconazole	150 mg	PO	—	one dose
Coccidioidomycosis	Amphotericin B *followed by*	0.5–1.0 mg/kg	IV	q24h	≥56 d
	Itraconazole *followed by*	300 mg 200 mg	PO PO	bid bid	3 d Lifelong
(Pulmonary)	Fluconazole	400–800 mg	PO	q24h	Lifelong
Cryptococcal infection	Amphotericin B with flucytosine *followed by*	0.7 mg/kg with 25 mg/kg	IV PO	q24h q6h	≥14 d ≥14 d
	Fluconazole *followed by*	400 mg	PO	q24h	8 wk
	Fluconazole	200 mg	PO	q24h	Lifelong
Histoplasmosis	Amphotericin B *followed by*	0.5–1.0 mg/kg	IV	q24h	≥28–56 d
	Itraconazole	200 mg	PO	q24h	Lifelong

tion of trimethoprim-sulfamethoxazole therapy in about 25% of cases. Although it has not been proved by a prospective study, adverse reactions can probably be reduced without sacrificing efficacy by lowering the recommended dose of trimethoprim-sulfamethoxazole from trimethoprim, 20 mg/kg/day (with sulfamethoxazole, 100 mg/kg/day) to trimethoprim, 15 mg/kg/day (with sulfamethoxazole, 75 mg/kg/day).[70] About 70 to 80% of sulfonamide-intolerant individuals can tolerate dapsone for significant lengths of time.[81] Gradual dose escalation of trimethoprim-sulfamethoxazole can reduce the impact of adverse effects, but this approach is appropriate for selected patients for prophylaxis, not for therapy for patients with acute illness.[82, 83]

Parenteral pentamidine is effective therapy for PCP.[42, 70] This regimen is inconvenient to administer, however, and the adverse reactions associated with it can be life-threatening. Renal dysfunction, hypoglycemia, hyperglycemia, granulocytopenia, and hypotension are reported in 10 to 50% of patients.[42, 70] For many years pentamidine was administered intramuscularly because early reports described fatal hypotension when the drug was given intravenously.[84, 85] However, intramuscular administration of pentamidine is no longer recommended except in unusual circumstances, because the intramuscular injections are often associated with painful sterile abscesses that can become superinfected. Moreover, the hypotension originally associated with intravenous pentamidine was probably related to the rate of infusion. When pentamidine is administered over at least a 60-minute period in 100 to 150 ml of dextrose in water, clinically important hypotension is unusual.[85] The renal dysfunction associated with pentamidine can be severe. If the serum creatinine level rises by more than 1.0 to 2.0 mg/dl, strong consideration should be given to withholding therapy for a few days or

TABLE 116-1 Therapy for Opportunistic Infections in Patients with HIV Infection *Continued*

Clinical Disease	Drug	Dose	Route	Interval	Duration
Herpes simplex	Acyclovir *or*	200 mg	PO	5/day	10–14 d
	Famciclovir *or*	125–250 mg	PO	q12h	10–14 d
	Valacyclovir	500 mg	PO	q12h	10–14 d
Varicella-zoster virus					
Dermatomal	Acyclovir *or*	800 mg	PO	5/d	7–10 d
	Famciclovr *or*	500 mg	PO	q8h	7–10 d
	Valacyclovir	1000 mg	PO	q8h	7–10 d
Disseminated	Acyclovir	10–12 mg/kg	IV	q8h	7–14 d
Cytomegalovirus	Ganciclovir *followed by*	5 mg/kg	IV	q12h	14–21 d
	Ganciclovir *or*	5 mg/kg	IV	q24h	Lifelong‖
	Foscarnet *followed by*	60 mg/kg	IV	q8h	14–21 d
	Foscarnet *or*	90–120 mg/kg	IV	q24h	Lifelong‖
	Ganciclovir implant *or*	—	—	q6–9m	Lifelong‖
	Cidofovir‡ *followed by*	5 mg/kg 5 mg/kg	IV IV	qwk q2wk	2 wk Lifelong‖
Mycobacterium tuberculosis	Isoniazid§ *and*	300 mg	PO, IM	q24h	At least 6 mo
	Rifampin *and*	600 mg	PO, IV	q24h	At least 6 mo
	Ethambutol *and*	15–25 mg/kg	PO	q24h	Depends on sensitivity
	Pyrazinamide	15–25 mg/kg	PO	q24h	2 mo
Mycobacterium avium complex	Clarithromycin Ethambutol	500 mg 15 mg/kg	PO PO	q12h q24h	Lifelong Lifelong
Bartonella (Rochalimaea) spp.	Erythromycin *or*	500 mg	PO	q6h	≥12 wk
	Doxycycline	100 mg	PO	q12h	≥12 wk

*Prednisone, 40 mg q12h × 5 d, followed by 20 mg bid × 5 d, followed by 20 mg qd × 11 d.
†Following a single loading dose of pyrimethamine, 200 mg.
‡With probenecid as described in package insert.
§With pyridoxine 50 mg PO qd.
‖For patients who have sustained response to HAART (see text for criteria for discontinuation of maintenance therapy).

changing to an alternative agent. Hypoglycemia can be a life-threatening complication of pentamidine therapy and occurs at any juncture during therapy or for many weeks after therapy has been completed.[86] Hypoglycemia occurs more frequently in patients who have pentamidine-induced renal dysfunction. The unpredictability of the hypoglycemia adds an element of risk to the inpatient or outpatient use of this drug. Life-threatening hypoglycemia is sufficiently uncommon, however, that this effective agent is still recommended for patients who cannot tolerate trimethoprim-sulfamethoxazole or trimethoprim-dapsone and who have severe disease. Lowering the dose of parenteral pentamidine from 4 to 3 mg/kg/day has been advocated to reduce toxicity: whether this also reduces efficacy is unknown.[87]

Dapsone (100 mg orally [PO] every day [qd]) plus trimethoprim (5 mg/kg PO every 8 hours or 300 mg PO every 8 hours) appears to be as effective as trimethoprim-sulfamethoxazole but less toxic.[71, 88] Skin rashes are very common among AIDS patients treated with dapsone, but a 21-day course of therapy can usually be completed without interruption. Dapsone alone has some efficacy when 100 mg PO qd is used for 21 days, but there is probably not enough activity to warrant use of this agent as single-drug therapy.[89] Higher doses are not well tolerated.

Atovaquone is a hydroxynaphthoquinone that appears to affect mitochondrial electron transport in microorganisms and thus has a mechanism of action distinct from trimethoprim-sulfamethoxazole or pentamidine.[73] Atovaquone is available as an oral suspension but is not available as a parenteral form. For patients with mild or moderate PCP, it has a high degree of efficacy and is extremely well tolerated. A large, prospective, double-blind study has demonstrated that although atovaquone is very effective, and although it is much better tolerated than trimethoprim-sulfamethoxazole, it is associated with more treatment failures.[73] One possible explanation for a component of the higher rate of treatment failures and the higher death rate in the atovaquone-treated group is that, unlike trimethoprim-sulfamethoxazole, atovaquone has no antibacterial activity, and thus patients in the atovaquone groups were more likely to die of unrecognized, concurrent bacterial processes. Atovaquone is better tolerated than intravenous pentamidine.[90] The absorption of atovaquone suspension can be erratic, especially in patients who cannot consume fatty foods with this medication. It should not be used in patients with significant gastrointestinal dysfunction. Mutations that could confer atovaquone resistance has been identified in human isolates.[91] Their clinical relevance remains to be determined. The primary toxicity due to atovaquone is skin rash. Atovaquone is a reasonable treatment option for patients with mild or moderate PCP who cannot tolerate trimethoprim-sulfamethoxazole and who are good candidates for oral therapy.

Clindamycin plus primaquine is also effective for the therapy of PCP.[71] Despite the fact that primaquine can only be given orally, this regimen has been used successfully in patients with mild, moderate, and severe disease.[71, 92] Clindamycin plus primaquine can be associated with considerable toxicity, including rash, serum transaminase elevation, diarrhea, and hemolysis. It is a reasonable oral regimen for patients who are unable to tolerate other regimens.

Trimetrexate is a potent inhibitor of dihydrofolate reductase that is effective therapy against PCP when used either alone (45 mg/m^2 intravenously [IV] qd) or in combination with a sulfonamide.[93, 94] Because trimetrexate inhibits the dihydrofolate reductase of human cells as well as the enzyme of *Pneumocystis*, it must be given in conjunction with high-dose leucovorin (20 mg/kg IV or PO every 6 hours), which rescues mammalian cells without diminishing the anti-*Pneumocystis* effect of the drug. Trimetrexate is well tolerated when given with leucovorin. Leukopenia is its major adverse effect. Trimetrexate has a high degree of efficacy and has the advantage of being available as a parenteral agent. However, a large, multicenter, double-blind study has demonstrated that trimetrexate therapy is associated with a higher rate of poor response and death than is therapy with trimethoprim-sulfamethoxazole.[94] The relapse rate after trimetrexate therapy is high: 40 to 60% of patients experience relapse within the first 60 days. This relapse rate is probably much lower if a few days of sulfonamide therapy is given concurrently.

Regardless of which specific agent is chosen as the initial therapy for PCP, adjunctive corticosteroid therapy is indicated for any patient whose initial room air Po_2 is lower than 70 mmHg.[95–98] Three prospective trials[95–97] have demonstrated that the frequencies of ventilatory failure and mortality can be reduced substantially by the prompt use of corticosteroids. The precise mechanism by which corticosteroids provide benefit is not well delineated. Physiologically, adjunctive corticosteroids appear to prevent much of the decline in oxygenation that characteristically occurs during the first 3 days of treatment.[72] This decline may be caused by the inflammatory response elicited by dying organisms. Adjunctive corticosteroids may also provide benefit for patients with an initial room air Po_2 higher than 70 mmHg. There is physiologic evidence that shows improved lung function in such patients, but so few patients with mild PCP develop respiratory failure or die that it is difficult to substantiate a survival benefit. The safety of the 21-day regimen is well substantiated: reactivation of tuberculosis, CMV, or Kaposi's sarcoma is unusual[99]; interestingly, the frequency of trimethoprim-sulfamethoxazole–related rash is not diminished by corticosteroids.[100]

When an HIV-infected patient with PCP fails to improve while receiving conventional therapy, there are no controlled data to indicate which modifications in therapy are optimal.[42] The mean time to improvement for HIV-infected patients treated with conventional therapy is 4 to 8 days,[45, 70] so patients should probably not be considered therapeutic failures until they have received 7 to 10 days of therapy. Clinicians often feel compelled to alter therapy earlier, however, especially if the patient is deteriorating rapidly. If a patient has not improved after 5 to 10 days of therapy, a repeat diagnostic procedure should be considered to determine whether another treatable pathogen is present. Bronchoscopy with transbronchial biopsies is the procedure of choice, because lung tissue is usually necessary to assess the presence of CMV and can be very helpful in establishing the presence of fungal or mycobacterial processes, which are the major diagnostic considerations. *Pneumocystis* is often present in lavage or tissue for at least 3 to 4 weeks after initiating therapy even in patients who respond promptly, so its presence after 7 to 10 days of therapy does not necessarily imply that therapy is ineffective.[101] The presence of extensive intra-alveolar exudate or extensive fibrosis after 7 to 10 days of therapy is probably a more ominous sign. Open lung biopsy is rarely necessary to establish a diagnosis of PCP, but this procedure can be useful for identifying other processes. Kaposi's sarcoma of the lung is usually apparent on bronchoscopy because of endobronchial lesions that are obvious to the bronchoscopist. However, if such lesions are not seen on bronchoscopy, Kaposi's sarcoma of the lung is one treatable process that is difficult or impossible to diagnose reliably from cytology or from transbronchial biopsy specimens.[42, 102] Nodular lesions on chest computed tomography (CT) scan, extensive intrabronchial lesions, and the presence of a bloody pleural effusion may be helpful clues.

If *Pneumocystis* infection is the only identifiable cause of the pulmonary dysfunction after 7 to 10 days of therapy and the patient has failed to improve, there are several therapeutic alternatives: (1) switch from trimethoprim-sulfamethoxazole to parenteral pentamidine or vice versa, (2) add corticosteroids to conventional therapy if they have not already been added, (3) switch to intravenous trimetrexate (with or without parenteral sulfonamide in the form of trimethoprim-sulfamethoxazole), (4) switch to intravenous clindamycin with oral primaquine, or (5) use two specific therapies concurrently (e.g., trimethoprim-sulfamethoxazole plus pentamidine). Each of these approaches has been associated with a successful outcome in some cases. A controlled trial is needed to determine the best approach, but such trials are difficult to perform because of the large size, complexity, and cost of a valid study. Whether AIDS patients with PCP should be supported aggressively with intensive care, mechanical ventilation, or other interventions is a controversial issue.[103–105] The most reasonable approach would be to individualize each management plan in terms of the days of therapy that have been received, the therapeutic alternatives that are available, and the concomitant processes that may be present. The patient's wishes and the availability of resources need to be taken into account. Published data indicate that AIDS patients with PCP can survive intubation and mechanical ventilation and lead independent lives for many months after hospital discharge.[60] The best candidates for intensive care and mechanical ventilation are patients who have presented with no other serious opportunistic processes, those who have received fewer than 7 days of therapy, and those who have clearly articulated a desire for aggressive support.

The prevention of PCP is a major priority for the management of patients with HIV infection.[10] Prevention of PCP is logical because episodes are frequent (at least 60 to 80% of patients in North America develop an episode at some point during their HIV infection if they received neither anti-*Pneumocystis* prophylaxis nor antiretroviral therapy), morbidity and mortality due to PCP can be substantial, low-cost drugs are available that are effective, and the period of high susceptibility can be defined.[10, 16, 42] Prospective and retrospective studies have shown that most primary episodes of PCP occur in patients with CD4$^+$ T-lymphocyte counts below 200 cells/mm^3 or in patients, regardless of CD4$^+$ T-lymphocyte count, with otherwise unexplained persistent fever or oropharyngeal candidiasis.[15, 16] Thus, these are the indications for primary prophylaxis. Other documented predictors of the occurrence of PCP, independent of CD4 count, are high HIV viral load,[19, 22, 106] wasting syndrome,[28] previous AIDS-defining event,[27] or prior pneumonia of any type.[27] These parameters should probably be added to the list of indicators for primary prophylaxis. A few cases of PCP will occur in patients with CD4$^+$ T-lymphocyte counts higher than 200 cells/mm^3 who do not have fever or mucocutaneous candidiasis, and thus some clinicians prefer to initiate prophylaxis at somewhat earlier time points. However, such a strategy puts a relatively large patient population on prophylaxis to prevent a relatively small incremental number of treatable cases. Secondary prophylaxis (the prevention of second or subsequent episodes of PCP) is conventionally indicated for everyone who has had a documented PCP episode, because the 1-year recurrence rate is approximately 65% for patients who receive no prophylaxis.[10] As mentioned earlier, there is considerable evidence suggesting that if patients respond to HAART and manifest CD4 counts that are persistently about 200 cells/mm³, it may be reasonable to discontinue prophylaxis, especially if the other listed risk factors are absent and if patients can be trained to seek medical care promptly if symptoms suggestive of PCP develop.

Trimethoprim-sulfamethoxazole is the preferred prophylactic regimen for any HIV-infected patient who can tolerate it (Table 116–2).[10, 107, 108] When administered at a dose of trimethoprim (160 mg) plus sulfamethoxazole (800 mg) (i.e., one double-strength tablet once daily), episodes of PCP are extremely uncommon in patients who adhere to the regimen. Trials have demonstrated that for either primary or secondary prophylaxis, trimethoprim-sulfamethoxazole is much more effective than aerosolized pentamidine or dapsone-containing regimens.[107–116] Trimethoprim-sulfamethoxazole also has the benefit, based on retrospective analyses, of reducing the frequency of toxoplasmosis[117] and may have a beneficial effect on reducing the frequency of pneumococcal and *Haemophilus* infections when daily regimens are used.[107]

Comparative trials have confirmed that trimethoprim-sulfamethoxazole is not nearly as well tolerated as aerosolized pentamidine. About 20 to 40% of patients cannot tolerate trimethoprim-sulfamethoxazole because of the side effects of rash, pruritus, fever, granulocytopenia, thrombocytopenia, anemia, hepatitis, nephritis, nausea, or vomiting. Reducing the dose of trimethoprim-sulfamethoxazole by 50% (i.e., a single-strength tablet daily) or reducing the frequency to two or three times weekly lowers toxicity.[111] In a study comparing trimethoprim-sulfamethoxazole at a dose of one double-strength tablet daily with one double-strength tablet three times weekly, there was no difference in efficacy when the data were evaluated based on an intent-to-treat analysis.[118] However, when occurrences of PCP were analyzed based on the regimen patients were actually taking at the time that PCP was diagnosed, there were more failures on the intermittent regimen. This finding has suggested to some investigators that the intermittent regimen is less effective.

Because trimethoprim-sulfamethoxazole is the preferred regimen, strategies to increase patient tolerance of this regimen are important. Gradual dose escalation of trimethoprim-sulfamethoxazole at the time prophylaxis is initiated has been shown to increase tolerability in two controlled studies.[82, 83]

For patients who cannot tolerate trimethoprim-sulfamethoxazol, there are several alternatives. Daily dapsone or weekly dapsone-pyrimethamine has an efficacy comparable to that of aerosolized pentamidine (i.e., they are not as effective as daily trimethoprim-sulfamethoxazole as prophylaxis for PCP). Dapsone-containing regimens are effective as prophylaxis against toxoplasmosis.[112, 113] Dapsone or dapsone-pyrimethamine, like trimethoprim-sulfamethoxazole, is poorly tolerated by a substantial number of patients: fever, rash, pruritus, and hemolysis occur. About 20% of patients who cannot tolerate trimethoprim-sulfamethoxazole also cannot tolerate dapsone-containing regimens.[81] Aerosolized pentamidine, although not as effective as trimethoprim-sulfamethoxazole, has a definite ability to reduce the frequency of PCP when used for primary or secondary prophylaxis. How aerosolized pentamidine is delivered to the patient is a major determinant of efficacy and safety.[119] Different nebulizers deliver different spectra and different densities of particle sizes and thus deliver different amounts of drug to the lung. Thus, the dosing regimens for the Respirgard II nebulizer and the Fisons nebulizer are quite different. Only the Respirgard II jet nebulizer and the Fisons ultrasonic nebulizer have been studied in large, well-controlled trials with clinical endpoints. Aerosolized pentamidine is well tolerated by most patients. Coughing and wheezing can be ameliorated or prevented by nebulized albuterol. A bitter taste is often reported. Cases of pancreatitis and renal dysfunction have been attributed to aerosolized pentamidine, but it is not certain that aerosolized pentamidine was the cause. A major concern related to the use of aerosolized pentamidine is the environmental contamination with drug and respiratory secretions that is created when patients

TABLE 116–2 Prophylaxis for Human Immunodeficiency Virus–Related Opportunistic Infections

Pathogen	Indication for Prophylaxis	First Choice	Alternatives	Comments
Pneumocystis	CD4⁺ <200/mm³ Persistent unexplained fever Chronic oropharyngeal candidiasis	Trimethoprim-sulfamethoxazole, 1 DS qd or SS	Dapsone, 50 mg qd, + pyrimethamine, 50 mg/wk Dapsone alone (100 mg qd) Aerosolized pentamidine	SS tablets are effective and may be less toxic than DS. Aerosol pentamidine should be delivered by Respirgard nebulizer.
Mycobacterium avium complex	CD4⁺ <100/mm³	Clarithromycin, 500 mg bid	Azithromycin (1200 mg qwk) Rifabutin, 300 mg qd	Rifabutin increases hepatic metabolism of other drugs.
Toxoplasma	No consensus	Trimethoprim-sulfamethoxazole, 1 DS qd	—	Pyrimethamine alone is not effective.
Mycobacterium tuberculosis	PPD >5 mm "High risk"	Sensitive: Isoniazid, 300 mg × 9 mo Resistant: ?	Rifampin* 600 mg, or Rifabutin* 300 mg, and pyrizinamide (15–25 mg/kg qd × 2 mo)	For resistant strains, two-drug regimens using combinations of rifampin, pyrazinamide, or a quinolone can be considered. Include pyridoxine, 500 mg qd for isoniazid-containing regimens. Recommended only if recurrences are severe or frequent.
Candida	Multiple recurrences	Fluconazole, 200 mg daily	Itraconazole, 100 mg qd	
Herpes simplex	Multiple recurrences	Acyclovir, 200 mg qd 3–4 ×/day Famciclovir, 125 mg PO bid Valacyclovir, 500 mg PO bid	—	
Cytomegalovirus	None	—	—	Oral ganciclovir is not recommended currently.
Pneumococcus	All patients	Pneumovax	—	Trimethoprim-sulfamethoxazole, clarithromycin, and azithromycin appear to prevent some disease.
Influenza	All patients	Influenza vaccine	—	—

*For patients receiving HAART, dose adjustments may be necessary.
Abbreviations: DS, Double strength; PPD, purified protein derivative; SS, single strength.

cough or become disconnected from the nebulizer. Health care workers and patients may inhale enough pentamidine to develop detectable urine levels of the drug.[120] The clinical importance of this is unknown. More important, if the patient has pulmonary tuberculosis, the environmental contamination produced by dispersed respiratory particles has considerable potential to spread tuberculosis.[121] Patients need to be carefully screened for pulmonary tuberculosis before aerosolized pentamidine prophylaxis is initiated.

Atovaquone has been assessed as prophylaxis in trials comparing it with either dapsone alone or aerosolized pentamidine.[122, 123] In both trials, atovaquone was equally effective as the alternative, and it was better tolerated than dapsone.

If patients cannot tolerate trimethoprim-sulfamethoxazole and they have an excessive number of breakthroughs while receiving dapsone-containing regimens, aerosolized pentamidine, or atovaquone, there are several poorly studied options. The best option is to try to maximize the patient's ability to tolerate trimethoprim-sulfamethoxazole by using a dose escalation strategy and perhaps an intermittent (three times weekly) regimen. Aerosolized pentamidine can be administered employing doses higher than the approved regimen (300 mg twice monthly or 600 mg once monthly),[124] perhaps with dapsone or azithromycin in addition.[124, 125] Results with clindamycin-primaquine have been disappointing. Whether the need for alternative regimens will grow substantially remains to be seen and depends on the clinical relevance of sulfonamide resistance and the long-term success of HAART therapy.

Patients who "break through" prophylaxis are usually those who are not receiving trimethoprim-sulfamethoxazole, who are not compliant, or who have very low CD4 counts.[126, 127] For such patients, education to reinforce adherence to prophylactic regimens, the use of strategies to enhance tolerability of trimethoprim-sulfamethoxazole, and efforts to augment CD4 counts by HAART are recommended.

Toxoplasma gondii

Toxoplasma gondii (see Chapter 268) causes disease in patients with HIV infection by reactivation rather than by primary infection in most cases.[128] Thus, patients usually have IgG antibodies against *Toxoplasma*, have fairly advanced disease ($CD4^+$ T-lymphocyte counts below 100 cells/mm^3), and have not been receiving trimethoprim-sulfamethoxazole prophylaxis or HAART.[128, 129] Because the seroprevalence of toxoplasmosis is much higher in some areas such as Western Europe and South America than in the United States, those areas have much higher frequencies of AIDS-associated toxoplasmosis.

In patients with HIV infection, toxoplasmosis manifests more often as cerebral disease. Retinochoroiditis, pneumonitis, disseminated disease, and a sepsis-like syndrome have all been reported, but these are not as frequent as focal lesions of the central nervous system. When an HIV-infected patient with a $CD4^+$ T-lymphocyte count below 100 cells/mm^3 presents with a space-occupying cerebral lesion that involves gray matter, the differential diagnosis primarily includes toxoplasmosis and lymphoma. Fungal, mycobacterial, and viral processes manifest as space-occupying lesions infrequently, and progressive multifocal leukoencephalopathy should manifest differently because it affects primarily white matter.

In the era of HAART, central nervous system lymphoma appears to be increasing in frequency compared with central nervous system toxoplasmosis. In large groups of patients, clinical or imaging characteristics distinguish lymphoma from toxoplasmosis.[50, 51, 128] There is some diagnostic utility for immunoglobulin or PCR tests[130] of cerebrospinal fluid, for single photon emission computed tomography (SPECT) or positron emission tomography (PET) scanning,[131] or for magnetic resonance imaging (MRI) scanning.[132] Although a positive cerebrospinal fluid PCR assay for Epstein-Barr virus[133] may prove to be highly specific for primary central nervous system lymphoma, in general this test or these imaging studies are not yet sufficiently specific to justify their sole use for therapeutic decisions. In individual cases, establishing a diagnosis with confidence requires a definitive biopsy or, in the case of toxoplasmosis, a response to empirical therapy. Given the fact that therapy for toxoplasmosis is highly successful and therapy for central nervous system lymphoma remains disappointing, an empirical approach focusing initially on toxoplasmosis is usually considered reasonable.[50] A definitive diagnostic study (i.e., brain biopsy) has some morbidity associated with it, and the diagnostic yield may be only 50% if toxoplasmosis is the etiology.[134] The cysts and tachyzoites of *T. gondii* can be very difficult to recognize in fragments of necrotic brain tissue, and even several small needle biopsy samples may miss the area that has abundant organisms. Because toxoplasmosis is the only common etiology for gray matter lesions that clearly benefits from therapy and because needle biopsy has diagnostic limitations, empirical therapy with pyrimethamine (200 mg orally the first day followed by 50 to 100 mg PO qd) plus sulfadiazine (1 to 2 g PO every 6 hours) is reasonable (see Table 116–1). If a lumbar puncture can be performed safely and if a PCR test for Epstein-Barr virus is available, a positive result would be suggestive of primary central nervous system lymphoma and could prompt either immediate biopsy or therapy directed at the neoplastic process.

Regarding sulfadiazine and pyrimethamine, some clinicians use higher doses of both drugs, but there is no clear evidence that higher doses are more effective, and they almost certainly produce more toxicity. If unequivocal improvement using clinical and radiologic criteria does not occur within 10 to 21 days, a biopsy should be performed to establish whether the etiology is an infectious or a neoplastic process other than toxoplasmosis.[50] Corticosteroids to reduce inflammation may be necessary in patients with substantial or progressive neurologic dysfunction or signs of increased intracranial pressure. The administration of corticosteroids may make evaluation of the clinical and radiologic response to specific therapy difficult because the observed improvement may be solely due to the corticosteroid therapy and unrelated to the anti-*Toxoplasma* regimen employed. Long-term antiseizure medication may be necessary. Although some clinicians institute this prophylactically, it is reasonable to initiate it only if a seizure occurs. For patients who respond, anti-*Toxoplasma* therapy should be continued for life because relapses occur in the same sites as those manifesting initially if therapy is discontinued, even after 8 to 12 months of treatment.[50, 134, 135] Whether the long-term suppressive regimen will be as effective if both pyrimethamine and sulfadiazine are not included at full doses remains to be demonstrated. Even if HAART is initiated and the CD4 cell count rises dramatically, (e.g., to levels higher than 200 cells/mm^3), many clinicians are reluctant to discontinue anti-*Toxoplasma* therapy until more definitive data indicate that this approach is safe, because this is a life-threatening process that causes irreversible brain damage (necrosis).

Treatment failures are unusual for patients with toxoplasmosis who are able to tolerate both pyrimethamine and sulfadiazine. Radiologically proven failures in patients who are taking their drugs should raise the possibility that toxoplasmosis is not the correct or the only diagnosis. Adverse reactions to sulfadiazine (leukopenia, rash, elevated levels of transaminases, nausea, nephritis) and to pyrimethamine (leukopenia, thrombocytopenia) are common.[50, 134, 135] The leukopenia often does not respond to leucovorin therapy, although a short course of leucovorin (10 to 20 mg PO or IV every 6 hours) should be administered.

For patients unable to tolerate sulfadiazine, clindamycin plus pyrimethamine is also quite effective (see Table 116–1).[134, 135] Atovaquone plus pyrimethamine,[136, 137] clarithromycin plus pyrimethamine,[138] doxycycline,[139] or dapsone plus pyrimethamine[140] may also be useful regimens. Pyrimethamine by itself does not appear efficacious,[141] nor is trimetrexate[142] alone effective for long periods of time. Immunotherapy with interferon-γ or interleukin-12 might also be useful.

Trimethoprim-sulfamethoxazole offers considerable protection as primary prophylaxis.[114] Dapsone-pyrimethamine also has substantial efficacy.[112]

Herpes Simplex and Varicella-Zoster Virus Infections

Herpes simplex (see Chapter 125) is a frequent cause of genital and perirectal ulcerations in patients with HIV infection. Oral acyclovir (200 mg every 4 hours) is very effective therapy for herpes simplex virus genital lesions, perirectal lesions, proctitis, oral lesions, digital lesions, and esophagitis.[143–145] Disseminated herpes simplex viral infections and focal visceral manifestations are unusual in HIV-infected patients. Intravenous therapy is rarely necessary unless the patient has a major gastrointestinal disorder that prevents oral absorption. Topical acyclovir has not been demonstrated to be highly effective in patients with HIV infection. The response of acyclovir-sensitive herpes simplex lesions is usually prompt and occurs within 3 to 10 days. Famciclovir or valacyclovir are probably as effective and safe and are more convenient because they can be given twice or three times daily.[146–148] Therapy should continue until the lesions are crusted over or epithelialized. Relapses occur with high frequency. If relapses occur quickly or often, long-term suppression may be necessary. A regimen of oral acyclovir, 400 mg twice daily or 200 mg three or four times per day, is often used, although valacyclovir or famciclovir might be pharmacokinetically more advantageous. Acyclovir-resistant isolates are being recognized.[149, 150] Foscarnet and cidofovir are active against herpes simplex and have been used successfully against acyclovir-resistant strains.[151, 152] Foscarnet-resistant herpes simplex virus has also been reported.[153] Favorable experience has been reported with topical preparations of trifluridine, foscarnet, or cidofovir.[154–156] Clinicians should be cognizant that when lesions recur, the causative virus may be a drug-susceptible strain.

Dermatomal herpes zoster lesions are usually similar in extent and distribution to those seen in immunocompetent patients (see Chapter 126). About 20 to 30% of HIV-infected patients have at least one recurrence. Dissemination of the varicella-zoster virus is an unusual event. When dessimination occurs, lesions may be atypical[157–159]: A high index of suspicion should be maintained that hyperkeratotic, verrucous, or ecthymatous lesions could be due to varicella-zoster virus infection. Even when extensive disseminated cutaneous lesions have been observed, however, clinically apparent visceral disease has rarely been documented. When organ involvement does occur, those of the central nervous system, including the retina, are the most common organs affected. Varicella-zoster virus may produce a characteristic retinal lesion designated as "progressive outer retinal necrosis."

For dermatomal disease, acyclovir therapy probably has a role in hastening the crusting of lesions, in preventing postherpetic neuralgia, and in preventing recurrences in HIV-infected patients (see Table 116–1). Acyclovir appears to be indicated if the initial lesion occurred within 72 hours or new vesicles have recently appeared, or if evidence of dissemination or ophthalmic involvement is apparent. Treatment should probably continue until all lesions are scabbed or crusted, even if this requires more than 7 to 10 days. Patients with zoster ophthalmicus might be logical candidates for high-dose acyclovir (10 mg/kg IV every 8 hours). Corticosteroid therapy to prevent postherpetic neuralgia is not recommended in patients with HIV infection.[160, 161] Acyclovir-resistant isolates do occur.[162, 163] Some have been treated successfully with foscarnet or cidofovir.

About 5% of patients with HIV infection do not have detectable antibodies to varicella-zoster virus. When exposed to this virus, primary varicella can be severe.[164] Acyclovir therapy is probably beneficial for such patients.

Cytomegalovirus

CMV infection, as assessed by serology, is almost universal among HIV-infected patients who have acquired disease by homosexual contact (see Chapter 127). In contrast, only about 75% of patients who are heterosexual will be seropositive for CMV.[165, 166]

Historically, before either specific anti-CMV prophylaxis or HAART was available, 21 to 44% of patients developed CMV-associated disease at some point during their illness.[167] HIV-infected patients with circulating $CD4^+$ T-lymphocyte cell counts lower than 50 cells/mm^3 are often viremic and viruric with CMV.[26, 168] The likelihood of development of CMV-associated disease is related to both the degree of immunosuppression and the quantity of circulating CMV. The latter can be assessed by a variety of quantitative systems that detect antigen or nucleic acid in circulating blood.[26, 169] A strategy to intervene in high-risk patients, that is, those with low CD4 counts and detectable CMV above some defined threshold, is logical because oral agents and long-acting parenteral agents are available, but such an approach has yet to be definitively evaluated.

Retinitis is the most commonly recognized disorder caused by CMV.[170, 171] CMV retinitis has the potential to involve the macula and optic disk rapidly, to cause retinal detachments, and to result in visual impairment and ultimately in blindness. Thus, therapy is urgent when disease is recognized unless lesions are small and very peripheral. CMV retinitis responds to either ganciclovir, administered IV at a dose of 5 mg/kg every 12 hours, or foscarnet, administered IV at 60 mg/kg every 8 hours (see Table 116–1).[52] Empirical therapy without a specific histologic or virologic diagnosis is reasonable because obtaining retinal or vitreous material for examination is risky (detached retinas or secondary infections may result), the appearance of CMV retinitis is quite characteristic to an experienced ophthalmologist, and CMV causes almost all the retinitis that occurs in HIV-infected patients.[172]

Intravenous ganciclovir and intravenous foscarnet are equally effective in terms of inducing remission of retinitis. Intravenous cidofovir is also effective.[173, 174] New lesions or progressive disease may be identified during the first 7 days of therapy, and these do not necessarily imply a poor response. Considerable improvement in inflammation, edema, and hemorrhage will be recognized in responders before the end of 21 days of therapy. For patients treated with a 21-day course of intravenous therapy but no maintenance therapy, relapse at the same site as the initial lesions and at new sites almost invariably occurs within a few weeks or months unless the patients respond to HAART with a substantial rise in $CD4^+$ T-lymphocyte count. Maintenance regimens using intravenous ganciclovir, 5 to 6 mg/kg daily for 5 to 7 days per week, or intravenous foscarnet, 90 mg daily, are often administered, but these regimens only prolong the interval until relapse by several weeks (mean time to progression for patients receiving ganciclovir or foscarnet maintenance regimens is 50 to 59 days).[52]

An oral maintenance regimen is clearly more attractive than a parenteral regimen.[52, 175, 175a] Oral ganciclovir, however, is not as effective as parenteral ganciclovir when used for long-term maintenance.[52, 175] Oral ganciclovir is expensive, requires 12 tablets per day, can be marrow suppressive, and thus has substantial disadvantages. At the time of relapse, patients usually respond to reinstitution of ganciclovir or foscarnet, although resistant CMV isolates do occur.[176] The major toxicity of ganciclovir is bone marrow suppression with neutropenia and thrombocytopenia. Confusion, nausea, vomiting, transaminase elevation, and inhibition of spermatogenesis also occur. When patients with sight-threatening CMV lesions become neutropenic owing to ganciclovir administration, other infectious, neoplastic, immunologic, and drug-related causes of the neutropenia should be sought. Granulocyte colony-stimulating factor may be useful to permit continued ganciclovir therapy. Alternatively, another therapy such as a ganciclovir implant or parenteral foscarnet may be tried. Foscarnet is nephrotoxic and can cause nausea, vomiting, anorexia, seizures, hypocalcemia, and hypomagnesemia.[52, 173] Foscarnet generally must be infused over 60 minutes following a 60-minute infusion of normal saline and thus requires more infusion time than ganciclovir therapy. Foscarnet has in vitro activity against HIV. This feature may be responsible for the apparent survival benefit of foscarnet compared with that of ganciclovir in a large prospective trial of CMV retinitis.[173] Cidofovir has the advantage that it can be given once every 2 weeks after two consecutive weekly doses, thus obviating the need for permanent intravenous access.[177] Cidofovir is nephrotoxic, and each dose should be administered with probenecid following hydration with 1 liter of normal saline.

Local instillation into the globe of an agent active against CMV would be a logical approach to therapy for CMV retinitis. Local instillation of ganciclovir, foscarnet, and antisense nucleic acid has been tried with some success.[177–179] The most widely used approach is surgical implantation of an intraocular device impregnated with ganciclovir. This approach has a very high success rate and enables the patient to avoid regular intravenous or oral maintenance regimens.[175a, 180, 181] Current implants fail after about 6 months owing to depletion of drug and must be replaced. The implantation of these devices can be associated with retinal detachments or endophthalmitis. Obviously, these implants provide local therapy only; thus, their use is associated with a high rate of CMV disease in the contralateral eye and at extraocular loci, unless the patient has had a sustained responses to HAART.

Esophagitis, enteritis, colitis, and pneumonitis are life-threatening syndromes caused by CMV that have been documented to respond to therapy.[182, 183] For these syndromes, a specific diagnosis should be established by histology because the syndromes are indistinguishable from those caused by other pathogens if clinical criteria alone are used. Culture of CMV from tissue, secretions, or excretions is insufficiently specific for CMV-caused disease to be used as a basis for therapy.

For patients with esophagitis, colitis, or rectal ulcers, improvement in clinical symptoms is usually noted during the first week of therapy with ganciclovir or foscarnet.[184, 185] Improved performance status and increased weight are often noted, especially if therapy results in reduced dysphagia or reduced diarrhea. There is considerably less experience with ganciclovir therapy for CMV pneumonia.[183] No consensus exists regarding the specific criteria for establishing the diagnosis, and many patients who failed ganciclovir therapy had very severe and advanced lung damage before ganciclovir treatment was started. Ganciclovir therapy alone has not been reported to be effective in bone marrow transplant recipients unless immune serum globulin or hyperimmune globulin is given concurrently,[183] and thus immune serum globulin is often administered to patients with HIV infection and suspected CMV pneumonia as an adjunct to ganciclovir or foscarnet. How often ganciclovir will be effective in treating CMV pneumonia in AIDS patients either alone or in conjunction with immunoglobulin remains to be determined.

Does maintenance therapy for CMV disease need to be continued for life in patients who manifest a sustained immunologic and virologic response to HAART? Data are accumulating that recurrence of CMV retinitis is extremely unusual if the $CD4^+$ T-lymphocyte count rises above 50 to 100 cells/mm^3 following institution of HAART. It is reasonable to stop maintenance therapy if the $CD4^+$ T-lymphocyte count has been higher than >50 to 100 cells/mm^3, the lesion is inactive, the lesion is not vision threatening, and regular ophthalmologic follow-up is possible. Clinicians need to distinguish between the recurence of CMV retinitis and immune reconstitution vitritis, because management of these syndromes is quite different.[11, 12]

Ganciclovir-resistant and foscarnet-resistant isolates are being recognized with increasing frequency by research laboratories, especially in patients receiving oral ganciclovir.[185–188] Ganciclovir-resistant isolates usually have mutations in the *UL97* gene and maintain susceptibility to foscarnet or cidofovir.[185] Some CMV isolates have mutations in the DNA polymerase gene, however, which can confer resistance to both foscarnet and cidofovir.[188] There is some evidence that ganciclovir in combination with foscarnet may be synergistic.[174]

Because CMV frequently causes specific organ damage in patients with HIV infection and may contribute to the febrile wasting syndromes associated with HIV disease, prevention of CMV disease is a logical goal. Oral ganciclovir has been assessed in prospective studies: Its efficacy is small compared with its toxicities, cost, and the inconvenience of taking 12 tablets daily.[189, 190] Strategies based on intervention with intravenous or oral regimens when CMV is detected by a nucleic acid or antigen assay of serum or peripheral white blood cells are currently being assessed. Patients might also wish to consider methods to reduce infection or reinfection by practicing safe sex, by avoiding infected needles, and by receiving blood products that have been determined to be CMV free or have been filtered.

Epstein-Barr Virus

Epstein-Barr virus (see Chapter 128) can be cultivated from the oropharynx and peripheral mononuclear cells of a substantial number of AIDS patients. This virus has been implicated in the pathogenesis of hairy leukoplakia and primary central nervous system lymphoma and may have a role in the pathogenesis of nonspecific pneumonitis, lymphadenopathy, lymphoma, fever, or wasting. There is insufficient evidence to warrant specific therapy for Epstein-Barr virus at this point, and no drug that would clearly be effective. Detection of EBV by PCR in the cerebrospinal fluid, however, appears to be suggestive of primary central nervous system lymphoma.[133]

Progressive Multifocal Leukoencephalopathy

Progressive multifocal leukoencephalopathy is a unifocal or multifocal demyelinating process caused by the JC virus (see Chapter 134).[191] This disorder produces characteristic white matter lesions. It must be distinguished from AIDS dementia complex and cerebral infarction. Detection of JC virus in the cerebrospinal fluid by nucleic acid amplification is helpful diagnostically.[191, 192] Specific therapy has not been effective. In particular, a recent trial assessing intravenous and intrathecal cytosine arabinoside demonstrated no benefit from either of these interventions.[193] However, several examples of dramatic clinical and radiologic improvement following institution of HAART have been reported.[194–196]

Candida Species

Stomatitis, esophagitis, vaginitis, and proctitis due to *Candida* species infection are common and often respond to topical therapy (nystatin, clotrimazole, or oral amphotericin B), oral therapy (ketoconazole, itraconazole, or fluconazole), or intravenous therapy (fluconazole or one of several amphotericin B preparations).[197–204] Fluconazole (50 to 200 mg PO every 24 hours) is the most convenient regimen and is therefore preferred. For oropharyngeal disease, single-dose therapy with 400 mg may be adequate, but a variety of daily doses (50 to 400 mg) and durations of therapy (1 to 28 days) have been studied, and most have reasonable response rates: 100 mg PO qd for 7 to 14 days is often recommended. If esophagitis is present, a longer course (14 to 21 days) is often employed. Itraconazole is also effective. For vulvovaginal candidiasis, one oral dose of fluconazole (150 mg) is equivalent in efficacy to a 7-day course of topical therapy. Ketoconazole is less expensive than fluconazole or itraconazole but can cause adrenal suppression and is poorly absorbed in the absence of gastric acidity, which is a common occurrence in patients with advanced HIV disease. Fluconazole, itraconazole, and ketoconazole all inhibit certain hepatic enzymes of the cytochrome P-450 class, resulting in elevated levels of drugs such as protease inhibitors and non-nucleoside reverse transcriptase inhibitors.

There is usually no urgency to institute antifungal therapy for any of these candidal mucosal disorders: Esophagitis is rarely associated with bleeding, perforation, fungemia, or disseminated fungal disease. Stomatitis, esophagitis, and proctitis often recur when therapy is discontinued. Fluconazole administration may have to be continued for life if recurrences are frequent or severe. Patients who do not respond to topical or oral azole therapy after 2 weeks usually have CD4 cell counts below 50 cells/mm^3 and extensive prior exposure to fluconazole.[32] The reasons for therapeutic failure need to be assessed, focusing on adherence to dosage regimens and drug interactions, as well as to resistance to fluconazole. If patients fail to respond to a 7-day course of fluconazole (200 mg or more PO qd), higher doses of fluconazole are rarely effective. Other options include itraconazole cyclodextrin solution, oral amphotericin B, or intravenous amphotericin B.[202–205] Patients with refractory candidiasis almost universally require lifelong therapy unless they manifest substantial immunologic and virologic response to HAART. *Candida* species that are clinically and microbiologically resistant to fluconazole are being described with increasing frequency. Amphotericin B resistance has also been reported, although the criteria for defining in vitro resistance to amphotericin B are less well defined.

Disseminated candidiasis is not a common occurrence in HIV-infected patients unless they are receiving drug therapy that makes them neutropenic (especially cytotoxic antineoplastic therapy) or they have a contaminated intravenous catheter. Treatment is similar to that in other patient populations, with particular attention directed at removing contaminated intravenous lines or discontinuing therapies that may be producing neutropenia.

Cryptococcus neoformans, Histoplasma capsulatum, and *Coccidioides immitis*

Most experience with therapy of cryptococcal disease in patients with HIV is derived from patients with meningitis.[206, 207] Patients with factors predicting a poor outcome need more aggressive therapy than patients with mild disease. Baseline factors predicting poor therapeutic response for patients with meningitis include altered mental status (including confusion, lethargy, and obtundation), cerebrospinal fluid antigen titer greater than 1:32 to 1:1024, decreased cerebrospinal fluid leukocyte count (fewer than 20 cells/mm^3), age younger than 35 years, positive blood cultures for *Cryptoccus*, and perhaps hyponatremia and positive central nervous system cultures for *Cryptococcus*. Thus, as for other opportunistic infections, early recognition and institution of therapy are important for maximizing the likelihood of a favorable response. Diagnosis is readily established by culture and cryptococcal antigen testing of blood and cerebrospinal fluid.

The preferred therapy for cryptococcal meningitis is amphotericin B, 0.7 to 1.0 mg/kg/day (with or without flucytosine) IV for at least 2 weeks, followed by fluconazole, 400 mg PO qd for 8 weeks, followed by fluconazole, 200 mg PO qd for life.[208, 209] In early trials, there was a suggestion that amphotericin B was comparable in efficacy to fluconazole, but these trials used low doses of amphotericin B. Subsequent experience with initial fluconazole or itraconazole therapy was less promising. Currently, many clinicians are reluctant to use either drug as initial therapy, although some physicians might use such a regimen for patients with very mild disease. Flucytosine is associated with potential bone marrow suppression, hepatoxicity, and nephrotoxicity, but its addition to amphotericin B probably reduces the relapse rate. For maintenance therapy, prospective data document that fluconazole is more effective than itraconazole when patients are followed for at least 24 weeks.[171] Using the recommended regimen of amphotericin B plus flucytosine followed by fluconazole maintenance therapy, a large prospective trial showed an acute mortality rate of 6%.[208, 209]

There is considerable interest in using alternative drugs to amphotericin B to improve convenience, reduce toxicity, and further improve efficacy. The role for lipid formulations of amphotericin B, for newer triazoles, and for echinocandins is still being investigated.

Patients with cryptococcal disease may deteriorate owing to the consequences of increased intracranial pressure.[210] Clinical signs of increased pressure need to be sought, especially at presentation and during acute induction therapy. The baseline opening pressure should be measured at the time of the initial lumbar puncture. An imaging study of the central nervous system may be useful before the initial lumbar puncture and subsequently if the clinical status deteriorates. If the opening pressure is high (i.e., higher than 25 cm H_2O), consideration should be given to reducing this pressure by repeated lumbar punctures or by insertion of a cerebrospinal fluid drain or shunt.

Patients being treated successfully for cryptococcal meningitis should demonstrate a decline in cerebrospinal fluid cryptococcal antigen titer. There is no well-defined value, however, to follow serum antigen titers serially; such titers do not correlate closely with outcome.[211, 212]

Histoplasmosis is a particularly common, life-threatening, opportunistic infection in patients with HIV infection in certain geographic areas such as Indianapolis, Kansas City, and Puerto Rico.[34] Diagnosis is often established by direct microscopy or culture of bronchoalveolar lavage, bone marrow, or blood. Antigen detection in an appropriate reference laboratory is also highly sensitive for identification of disease. Although a sensitive and specific assay is available only from specialized laboratories, the sensitivity of the test is high in urine (95%), serum (80%), bronchoalveolar lavage (70%), and cerebrospinal fluid (50%).[34, 213] Acute therapy should consist of intravenous amphotericin B, 0.5 to 1.0 mg/kg daily for 3 to 14 days, for most patients. Itraconazole (200 mg PO twice a day [bid]) or fluconazole (800 mg PO qd) is also effective but should probably be reserved as initial therapy for patients with very mild disease. For long-term maintenance therapy, either itraconazole (200 mg PO bid to maintain serum levels higher than 1 μg/ml) or amphotericin B (0.5 to 0.8 mg/kg IV every week) is adequate.[34, 214, 215] Serum and urine *Histoplasma capsulatum* polysaccharide antigens are useful for monitoring both the initial and the long-term phases of treatment; they predict treatment failure or relapse.

Coccidioidomycosis is a common complication of HIV infection in the southwestern United States.[216, 217] Diagnosis can be established by direct microscopy or culture of bronchoalveolar lavage, blood, or cerebrospinal fluid. Serum IgG titers can be helpful; they are usually positive in the presence of active disease. For patients with diffuse pulmonary infiltrates and CD4 counts lower than 50 cells/mm^3, therapy should consist of amphotericin B, 1.0 to 1.5 mg/kg/day. If meningeal involvement is present, either intrathecal amphotericin B (0.3 to 0.5 mg via intrathecal reservoir) twice weekly or fluconazole is a necessary addition to systemic amphotericin B. Focal pneumonia in patients with CD4 counts higher than 50 cells/mm^3 and relatively mild disease can probably be treated adequately with fluconazole alone, 400 mg PO qd. Lifelong maintenance therapy with either fluconazole or itraconazole is recommended. The maintenance dose of azole therapy can be adjusted based on duration of therapy, clinical status, and anti-*Coccidioides* antibody titer.

Aspergillosis is recognized with increasing frequency as a cause of pseudomembranous tracheobronchitis, pneumonia, sinusitis, and disseminated disease.[218, 219] Diagnosis is difficult to confirm without visualization of hyphae in tissue. Therapy is often unsuccessful because of both poor host immune function (patients often have a CD4 count lower than 50 cells/mm^3 and a neutrophil count lower than 500 cells/mm^3) and the presence of extensive disease at the time of diagnosis. Strong consideration should be given to surgical resection of the most obviously affected tissue as an adjunct to medical therapy. Treatment with high-dose amphotericin B (1.0 to 1.5 mg/kg) is the standard approach. Whether lipid formulations of amphotericin B offer any advantage remains to be determined. Itraconazole has activity against *Aspergillus* but is not the preferred choice for single-agent therapy. Whether it is useful in combination with amphotericin B remains to be determined. For patients unable to tolerate high doses of amphotericin B, either itraconazole or liposomal amphotericin B preparations are options.

Streptococcus pneumoniae, Haemophilus influenzae, and Other Bacterial Processes

Patients with HIV infection report a higher incidence of respiratory infections than patients without HIV infection.[220, 221] The frequency of these respiratory infections is inversely related to the CD4+ T-lymphocyte count. These respiratory infections include upper tract diseases (sinusitis, otitis, and bronchitis) and lower tract disease (pneumonia). *S. pneumoniae* and nonencapsulated *Haemophilus influenzae* are common causes. Diagnosis and therapy do not differ from approaches established for patients who are not infected with HIV.

The frequency of bacterial infections can be reduced by prophylactic regimens employing trimethoprim-sulfamethoxazole,[107] clarithromycin,[222] or azithromycin.[223] These drugs are rarely prescribed specifically for their prophylactic antibacterial effect, but they reduce bacterial infections when prescribed to prevent PCP (trimethoprim-sulfamethoxazole) or disseminated MAC. Granulocyte colony-stimulating-factor can reduce the frequency of bacterial infections in severely neutropenic patients. Because pneumococcal disease can be reduced by the administration of pneumococcal vaccine to patients with CD4+ T-lymphocyte counts higher than 200 cells/mm^3, routine immunization should be part of standard care.[10] Immunization should be repeated periodically and should probably be repeated if the initial vaccine was administered when the CD4+ T-lymphocyte count was below 200 cells/mm^3 and the count has subsequently risen above 200 cells/mm^3 owing to HAART.

Other bacterial processes have also been described to occur with increased frequency among patients with HIV infection. Some are due to the use of intravascular devices that, when contaminated, have the potential to cause bacteremias (or fungemias). Some are related to neutropenia, which can complicate advanced HIV disease or which can occur as a complication of the use of certain drugs such as ganciclovir, pentamidine, pyrimethamine, sulfonamides, or antineoplastic agents. Others, such as *Corynebacterium equi*, occur with increased frequency for unclear reasons.

Mycobacterium Species Infection

Mycobacterium tuberculosis

Tuberculosis most often manifests in patients with HIV infection as a pulmonary process. Radiographic appearances are diverse. Extrapulmonary manifestations are more likely to occur in patients infected with HIV than in immunocompetent patients.[224, 225] Diagnosis is established by identification of *M. tuberculosis* in respiratory secretion, tissue, blood, or any other material using culture, nucleic acid probes, or demonstration of suggestive organism by staining. Therapy for tuberculosis is reviewed in Chapter 240. For patients with HIV infection, initial therapy generally consists of daily oral isoniazid (300 mg qd), rifampin (600 mg qd), and pyrazinamide (15 to 25 mg/kg qd) (see Table 116–1).[226] Ethambutol (15 to 25 mg/kg qd) should be added to the initial regimen if there is any reason to suspect drug resistance and should be a routine part of the initial regimen in communities in which drug-resistant strains occur. Thus, in most areas in the United States, a four-drug initial regimen will be appropriate. If the organism is susceptible to all drugs being used, isoniazid and pyrazinamide and rifampin should be continued to complete an initial 2 months of therapy; isoniazid plus rifampin should then be continued for 4 additional months or 6 months after sputum culture conversion, whichever is longer. Because peripheral neuropathy is a major concern in patients with HIV infection, pyridoxine, 50 mg PO qd, should be administered concurrently with isoniazid. The optimal duration of therapy is controversial. Some experts prefer a 9- or 12-month regimen rather than a 6-month regimen (6 months is recommended by the Centers for Disease Control and Prevention for sensitive isolates being treated with daily regimens, starting with isoniazid, rifabutin, ethambutol, and pyrizinamide). A study of HIV-infected patients showed a lower relapse or recurrence rate for patients treated for 12 months (1.9%) compared with that for patients treated for 6 months (9%).[227] It is not certain whether this difference was in fact due to relapses or to reinfections. Whatever regimen is chosen, directly observed therapy should be considered for every patient. If response to therapy is not optimal based on clinical or microbiologic grounds after 8 weeks of therapy, a chest radiograph and drug susceptibility testing should be repeated. Measurement of serum drug levels may also be helpful.

A major problem associated with antituberculosis therapy is management of drug interactions between antituberculous and antiretroviral medications, especially the interaction among rifamycins, protease inhibitors, and non-nucleoside reverse transcriptase inhibitors. The Centers for Disease Control and Prevention has made recommendations for patients receiving HAART that includes protease inhibitors and non-nucleoside reverse transcriptase inhibitors: For regimens that include a rifamycin, rifabutin at 150 mg PO qd rather than rifampin should be used with soft gel saquinavir, nelfinavir mesylate, indinavir, amprenavir, or nevirapine. If efavirenz is used, the dose of rifabutin should be increased to 450 mg daily or twice weekly. Rifamycins should not be used with hard gel saquinavir, ritonavir, or delavirdine; in those cases, therapy for at least 9 months with a regimen that includes streptomycin (or another injectable antituberculous drug) along with isoniazid and pyrazinamide and ethambutol should be considered (see also Chapter 240).[226]

Treatment of drug-resistant tuberculosis is discussed in Chapter 240. Drug-resistant strains have been particular problems in primary tuberculous infections associated with outbreaks at health care facilities and other institutional settings.[31] Therapy is chosen based on prior drug exposure and drug susceptibility patterns.

Chemoprophylaxis should be administered to any HIV-infected patient with a tuberculin skin test induration that is at least 5 mm in diameter if that patient has never received adequate prophylaxis.[228] In addition, HIV-infected patients should receive chemoprophylaxis regardless of tuberculin skin test status if they meet the following criteria: (1) a history of a positive tuberculin skin test result that was not adequately treated, (2) a close contact with a patient with infectious tuberculosis, and (3) a chest radiograph result that is consistent with previous untreated tuberculosis.

Nine months of isoniazid prophylaxis is preferred over a 6-month regimen (see Table 116–2).[226] Isoniazid can be administered either daily or twice weekly at appropriate doses. Alternative regimens not employing isoniazid should be considered in patients with severe liver disease. It is important to recognize that in areas such as Haiti, where tuberculosis is endemic, isoniazid prophylaxis can have a major impact on survival.[37] A combination of pyrazinamide plus rifampin administered for 2 months is also a highly effective regimen for prophylaxis.[229] This regimen has the advantage of a shorter duration than the isoniazid regimen and can be given daily for 2 months, or twice weekly for 2 to 3 months, using recommended dosing guidelines.[190] Protease inhibitors should not be used concurrently with rifampin. If protease inhibitors must be used, rifabutin (150 mg per day) can be substituted for rifampin, and drug toxicity and efficacy should be monitored closely. A third major option for prophylaxis is a 3-month course of isoniazid plus rifampin: As noted previously this regimen is not recommended for patients receiving protease inhibitors unless rifabutin is substituted for rifampin. If rifabutin is used, dose adjustments may be necessary when concurrent HAART is administered.

In addition to considering chemoprophylaxis, patients with HIV infection should reduce the likelihood of exposure to tuberculosis. Thus, employment in homeless shelters, correctional facilities, or respiratory disease health care facilities, for example, should be considered with caution.

Mycobacterium avium Complex

MAC disease has been much less common since the widespread use of HAART.[230] MAC most often manifests as a systemic process characterized by fever, weight loss, elevated serum alkaline phosphatase levels, and substantial anemia. Localized lung disease, diarrhea, or lymphadenopathy can be seen. Immune reactivation lymphadenitis occurs soon after the initiation of HAART. Diagnosis is most readily established by blood culture. Culture of organisms from respiratory secretions, stool, or urine does not unequivocally establish the presence of invasive disease.

Studies to date have demonstrated that several individual drugs or multiple drug regimens can reduce or eliminate mycobacteria over a period of weeks or months.[231–236] Most patients having a favorable microbiologic response experience an improvement in symptoms and signs. Drugs with microbiologic activity and satisfactory toxicity profiles include clarithromycin, azithromycin, rifabutin, ethambutol, amikacin, and several quinolones.

Initial treatment regimens usually include either clarithromycin or azithromycin plus ethambutol (see Table 116–1). There is more experience with clarithromycin than with azithromycin, and thus the former drug is usually preferred. The recommended dose of clarithromycin is 500 mg PO bid; higher doses have been associated with higher mortality.[10] The explanation for this higher mortality is not clear. When clarithromycin or azithromycin is used as monotherapy, relapse occurs in the majority of patients in less than 1 year. If other drugs are added to the macrolide, especially ethambutol, the relapse rate and time to relapse are reduced substantially.

Many clinicians recommend that initial therapy consist of clarithromycin plus ethambutol; additional drugs such as rifabutin or amikacin or ciprofloxacin are added if the disease is severe or extensive. Clofazimine is no longer recommended owing to an association with increased mortality.[10] It is not generally recommended that susceptibility testing of isolates be performed routinely unless the likelihood of drug resistance is high, for example, the patient has developed mycobacteremia while receiving macrolide therapy. Susceptibility testing has been best validated for clarithromycin, azithromycin, and perhaps rifabutin.

Most patients demonstrate defervescence and lower quantities of circulating MAC within 2 to 4 weeks of initiating therapy unless the disease is extensive, drug adherence is poor, or absorption or pharmacokinetic issues result in suboptimal serum tissue concentrations of drug. In such cases, MAC susceptibility testing and serum drug level monitoring are likely to be useful.

When MAC bacteremia relapses after a period of clinical and mycobacterial improvement, organisms are often resistant to the drugs used in the treatment regimen. It is logical to choose a new regimen based on susceptibility results, although, as noted, such testing has not been validated as clinically useful for most drugs. A multidrug regimen employing rifabutin and other agents to which the patient has not been exposed is often recommended. Whether the macrolide should be continued despite clinical or in vitro resistance is controversial.

The optimal duration of therapy for patients demonstrating sustained clinical and microbiologic response is increasingly uncertain. Conventionally, guidelines and recommendations have emphasized the need for lifelong therapy. Evidence suggests that therapy does not need to be lifelong in selected patients who respond to HAART in terms of augmented CD4 T-lymphocyte cell counts. It is reasonable to consider stopping therapy after 1 year for patients who are asymptomatic and who have CD4 counts higher than 100 cells/mm^3, and who have negative cultures of blood and other affected sites. However, the validity of such an approach is unproven.

Chemoprophylaxis for MAC disease is a logical management strategy because this disease is frequent, severe, and difficult to treat long term and because there are parameters for identifying patients who are at highest risk. Patients at risk include those with a CD4 count below 50 cell/mm^3, a previous opportunistic infection (especially CMV disease), and a respiratory or gastrointestinal tract that is colonized with MAC.[43] Clarithromycin, azithromycin, and rifabutin are each effective chemoprophylactic agents in terms of reducing the incidence of disease and in reducing mortality.[237, 238]) Clarithromycin (500 mg PO bid) or azithromycin (1200 mg once per week) is more effective than rifabutin and produces fewer important drug interactions (see Table 116–2). The combination of rifabutin plus azithromycin is more effective than either drug alone, but few clinicians employ this regimen because of the adverse effects and cost associated with this combination regimen. When patients break through clarithromycin prophylaxis, some isolates will be clarithromycin resistant. This is less often the case when breakthroughs occur during rifabutin or azithromycin prophylaxis.

The risk of disseminated *Mycobacterium avium-intracellulare* is markedly reduced in patients with low CD4 counts in whom highly active antiretroviral therapy produces a sustained immunologic and virologic response. Current Guidelines from the U.S. Public Health Service and the Infectious Disease Society of America recommend that prophylaxis can be discontinued if patients have a sustained rise in CD4$^+$ T-lymphocyte count after initiation of HAART.

Enteric Pathogens: *Salmonella* Species, *Shigella* Species, *Campylobacter* Species, *Entamoeba histolytica*, and *Giardia lamblia*

Enteric disease due to *Salmonella, Shigella*, and *Campylobacter* is common. Amoebiasis and giardiasis also occur, but their manifestations are not necessarily different from those in immunocompetent patients.

Initial therapy for *Salmonella, Shigella, Campylobacter, Entamoeba*, and *Giardia* infections follows standard guidelines. Persons with *Salmonella*, and perhaps *Shigella* and *Campylobacter*, infections tend to relapse if long-term suppressive therapy is not administered.

Cryptosporidia, Isospora, Cyclospora, and *Microsporidia*

These four protozoa cause chronic diarrheal syndromes. Each can cause biliary disease as well. Microsporidia (see Chapter 274) can cause systemic disease and can produce keratitis. These pathogens can be identified in stool by appropriate direct microscopic techniques or by tissue biopsy; microsporidia can also be identified by corneal scrapings.

Therapy for cryptosporidiosis (see Chapter 272) has been disappointing. Symptomatic therapy employing antimotility drugs and dietary alterations is often helpful. Octreotide probably offers little benefit beyond that achievable with more readily available agents.[239] Some results with immunoglobulin preparations such as hyperimmune bovine colostrum have been promising.[240, 241] Many clinicians report some transient benefit from paromomycin, but a controlled trial of this agent showed no substantial difference between the effects of this drug and placebo.[242] Several reports suggest that for some patients who respond favorably to HAART, dramatic improvement in cryptosporidial diarrhea and nutritional status can occur for some patients who respond favorably to HAART.[243, 244]

Prevention of cryptosporidiosis should focus on environmental control because no drugs are known to be effective. In some areas where outbreaks have been linked to the local drinking water supply or where contamination is likely, water needs to be boiled for 1 minute or filtered through a device capable of removing particles 1 μm in diameter. Whether all individuals infected with HIV should drink bottled or filtered water exclusively is controversial. Individuals at risk should also avoid contact with farm animals, infected humans, or pets that are at high risk (e.g., dogs and cats younger than 6 months of age, stray animals, or animals with diarrhea).

Isospora and *Cyclospora* (see Chapter 273) can each be treated effectively with trimethoprim-sulfamethoxazole.[245, 246] Patients usually respond symptomatically within 7 to 10 days, but the relapse rate is high unless trimethoprim-sulfamethoxazole is continued over the lifetime for patients whose CD4 counts remain low. If patients respond to HAART with sustained increases in CD4 counts and sustained suppression of HIV viral load, it is logical to presume that long-term maintenance therapy for isosporiasis or cyclosporiasis can be discontinued.

Both albendazole and fumagillin have activity in vitro and in vivo against microsporidia.[247–252] There are numerous reports that albendazole can have a beneficial effect on diarrhea due to *Encephalitozoon intestinalis*, or disseminated disease due to *Encephalitozoon hellem* and *Encephalitozoon cuniculi*, or disease due to *Nosema* or *Tachipleistophora*. Albendazole has not been as effective, unfortunately, treating the major cause of microsporidial diarrhea: *Enterocytozoon bieneusi*.[251] Some patients with *E. bieneusi* diarrhea will experience transient symptomatic improvement after albendazole therapy, but there is little evidence for microbiologic improvement or improvement in D-xylose absorption, and relapse often occurs promptly when drug therapy is discontinued. Oral fumagillin,[253] octreotide,[254] and thalidomide[255] have been reported to decrease diarrhea due to *E. bieneusi* in small series.

Microsporidial keratitis has been treated successfully with lifelong topical fumagillin. Patients with microsporidial keratitis should be assessed for systemic microsporidiosis, and systemic therapy with albendazole should be considered.

Because little is known about the transmission of microsporidia to humans, no specific recommendations for prevention can be made. It is logical to presume that prevention of food and water contamination by animals would decrease transmission of this organism.

Treponema pallidum

Syphilis is often recognized in HIV-infected patients either because of characteristic lesions of primary or secondary disease or because a screening serology for *Treponema pallidum* is positive. It is becoming increasingly apparent that, in patients with primary and secondary syphilis, central nervous system involvement is relatively common (see Chapter 227). If careful diagnostic studies are employed, as many as 40% of patients with primary or secondary syphilis will have serologic or microbiologic evidence of *T. pallidum* in their cerebrospinal fluid regardless of their HIV status. It is also becoming increasingly apparent that, in HIV-infected patients with primary, secondary, or latent syphilis, a single dose of 2.4 mIU benzathine penicillin may be inadequate to cure the central nervous system involvement or to prevent systemic relapses as measured by subsequent rises in serum Venereal Disease Research Laboratory titers. The optimal treatment for HIV-infected patients with early or latent syphilis has not been established: procaine penicillin (1.2 mIU daily for 10 to 14 days) may be preferred over serial doses of benzathine penicillin (2.4 mIU every week for 3 or 4 weeks) in terms of preventing relapses.

Bartonella

Bartonella henselae and *Bartonella quintana* (see Chapter 224) have been described as the causes of a spectrum of clinical syndromes in patients with HIV infection. These syndromes include cutaneous and subcutaneous angiomatous papules that can be confused with Kaposi's sarcoma, and angiomatous masses in the liver (peliosis hepatis), bone, lymph nodes, lungs, and central nervous system, which appear to be mass lesions. Bartonellosis can also manifest as fever and bacteremia. The diagnosis is usually established by Warthin-Starry stain of tissue or by culture of blood or tissue using enriched agar. Most experience with therapy has been with either erythromycin or doxycycline. At least 2 g daily of erythromycin should be given for at least 8 to 12 weeks for patients with cutaneous disease.[256] Doxycycline should be given at a dose of 100 mg every 12 hours. There is no major difference in response rate of bacillary angiomatosis caused by *B. quintana* and *B. henselae*. Clinical response may be seen during the first week. Cutaneous lesions may require 1 to 2 months to resolve; hepatic lesions may require 2 to 3 months. Hepatic and osseous lesions should be treated initially with intravenous erythromycin. Rifampin may be useful as an adjunct to the primary drug. A Jarisch-Herxheimer reaction may be seen in response to the first few drug doses. Treatment failures and relapses occur.

Prevention of bartonellosis should focus on reducing exposure to the vectors, namely, the body louse (for *B. quintana*) and cats and cat fleas (for *B. henselae*).

Kaposi's Sarcoma

The presence of Kaposi's sarcoma does not necessarily mandate institution of specific therapy, especially if lesions are few in number and inconspicuous. Lesions may regress in patients who respond to HAART. Local measures can be useful, including excision, radiation,[257] and intralesional injection with chemotherapy.[258] When lesions in the oropharynx are radiated, mucositis seems to be especially common.

When cutaneous Kaposi's sarcoma is extensive, recombinant interferon-α therapy (10 to 30 million units/m^2 IM, IV, or subcutaneously qd) can be useful, especially for patients with circulating CD4$^+$ T-lymphocyte counts greater than 100 to 200 cells/mm^3.[259] Objective tumor responses can be seen in 4 to 8 weeks, with maximal responses in 12 to 24 weeks. Late initial responses after many months of therapy occasionally occur. Because the tumor response is not rapid, interferon-α therapy is not desirable for urgent, life-threatening situations such as laryngeal or extensive pulmonary involvement. Adverse effects of interferon-α include confusion, fatigue, myalgia, leukopenia, thrombocytopenia, hepatitis, and cardiomyopathy.

Kaposi's sarcoma can cause life-threatening disease by obstructing a vital structure such as the larynx, bronchus, biliary tract, or bowel. Kaposi's sarcoma can occasionally infiltrate a vital organ such as the lung and cause, for instance, fatal hypoxemia. In these life-threatening situations, either radiation therapy or cytotoxic chemotherapy is necessary to produce a rapid and substantial response. The optimal mode of therapy depends on the location and extent of the tumor. A variety of chemotherapeutic regimens have been used with some success, including liposomal vinblastine; etoposide; vincristine; vincristine and vinblastine; vinblastine and bleomycin; and doxorubicin, bleomycin, and vincristine.[28] The optimal drug regimens for specific situations have not been determined. Preliminary evidence suggests that ganciclovir or foscarnet therapy may reduce the risk of Kaposi's sarcoma.

Lymphoma

Lymphomas of the Hodgkin's, non-Hodgkin's, and Burkitt's types are increasingly common as patients with HIV infection survive longer (see Chapter 111). The risk of lymphoma is not confined to specific CD4 count ranges. After a diagnosis is established by tissue biopsy, a staging workup is appropriate. Chemotherapy and radiation therapy each have potential therapeutic value. Long-term remissions are being reported, especially for patients who have none of the following risk factors: CD4 count lower than 100 cells/mm^3, bone marrow involvement, Karnofsky performance status less than 70%, stage IV disease, or prior AIDS-defining illness.[260] The optimal therapeutic approach is controversial: chemotherapy and radiation therapy can each have beneficial roles, and long-term remission should be the goal.[261]

REFERENCES

1. Palella FJ, Delaney KM, Moorman AC, et al. Declining morbidity and mortality among patients with advanced immunodeficiency virus infection. N Engl J Med. 1998;338:853–860.

2. Hogg RS, Heath KV, Yip B, et al. Improved survival among HIV infected individuals following initiation of antiretroviral therapy. JAMA. 1998;279:450–454.

2a. Jones JL, Hanson DL, Dworken MS, et al. Surveillance for AIDS-defining opportunistic illnesses, 1992–1997. MMWR Morb Mortal Wkly Rep. 1999;48(SS-2):1–22.

3. Moore RD, Hidalgo J, Sugland BW, Chaisson RE. Zidovudine and the natural history of the acquired immunodeficiency syndrome. N Engl J Med. 1991;324:1412–1416.

4. Lemp GF, Payne SF, Neal D, et al. Survival trends for patients with AIDS. JAMA. 1990;263:402–406.
5. Chaisson RE, Keruly J, Richman DD, et al. *Pneumocystis* prophylaxis and survival in patients with advanced HIV infection treated with zidovudine. Arch Intern Med. 1992;152:2009–2013.
6. Graham NM, Zeger SL, Park LP, et al. Effect of zidovudine and *Pneumocystis carinii* pneumonia prophylaxis on progression of HIV-1 infection to AIDS. Lancet. 1991;338:265–269.
7. Selik RM, Chu SY, Ward JW. Trends in infectious diseases and cancers among persons dying of HIV infection in the United States from 1987 to 1992. Ann Intern Med. 1995;123:933.
8. Moore RD, Chaisson RE. Natural history of opportunistic disease in an HIV-infected urban clinical cohort. Ann Intern Med. 1996;124:633–642.
9. Centers for Disease Control and Prevention. Report of the NIH panel to define principles of therapy of HIV infection and guidelines for the use of antiretroviral agents in HIV infected adults and adolescents. MMWR Morb Mortal Wkly Rep. 1998;47(RR-5).
10. USPHS/IDSA Prevention of Opportunistic Infections Working Group. USPHS/IDSA guidelines for the prevention of opportunistic infections in persons infected with human immunodeficiency virus. MMWR Morb Mortal Wkly Rep. 1997;46(RR-12):1–48.
11. Race EM, Adelson-Mitty J, Kriegel GR, et al. Focal mycobacterial lymphadenitis following initiation of protease-inhibitor therapy in patients with advanced HIV-1 disease. Lancet. 1998;351:252–255.
12. Zegans ME, Walton RC, Holland GN, et al. Transient vitreous inflammatory reactions associated with combination antiretroviral therapy in patients with AIDS and cytomegalovirus retinitis. Am J Ophthalmol. 1998;125:292–300.
13. Sepkowitz KA. Effect of HAART on natural history of AIDS-related opportunistic disorders. Lancet. 1998;351:228–230.
14. Freedberg KA, Scharfstein JA, Seage GR III, et al. The cost-effectiveness of preventing AIDS-related opportunistic infections. JAMA. 1998;279:130–136.
15. Masur H, Ognibene FP, Yarchoan R, et al. CD4 counts as predictors of opportunistic pneumonias in human immunodeficiency virus (HIV) infection. Ann Intern Med. 1989;111:223–231.
16. Phair J, Munoz A, Detels R, et al. The risk of *Pneumocystis carinii* pneumonia among men infected with human immunodeficiency virus type 1. N Engl J Med. 1990;322:161–165.
17. Chu SY, Hanson DL, Ciesielski C, et al. Prophylaxis against *Pneumocystis carinii* pneumonia at higher CD4+ T-cell counts (Letter). JAMA. 1995;273:848.
18. Yarchoan R, Venzon DJ, Pluda JM, et al. CD4 count and the risk for death in patients infected with HIV receiving antiretroviral therapy. Ann Intern Med. 1991;115:184–189.
19. Mellors JW, Munoz A, Giorgi JV, et al. Plasma viral load and CD4+ lymphocytes as prognostic markers of HIV-1 infection. Ann Intern Med. 1997;126:946–954.
20. Nightingale SD, Cameron DW, Gordin FM, et al. Two controlled trials of rifabutin prophylaxis against *Mycobacterium avium* complex infection in AIDS. N Engl J Med. 1993;329:828–833.
21. Havlik JA Jr, Horsburgh CR Jr, Metchock B, et al. Disseminated *Mycobacterium avium* complex infection: Clinical identification and epidemiologic trends. J Infect Dis. 1992;165:577–580.
22. Marschner IC, Collier AC, Coombs RW, et al. Use of changes in plasma levels of human immunodeficiency virus type 1 RNA to assess clinical benefit of antiretroviral therapy. J Infect Dis. 1998;177:40–47.
23. Katzenstein DA, Hammer SM, Hughes MD, et al. The relation of virologic and immunologic markers to clinical outcomes after nucleoside therapy in HIV-infected adults with 200 to 500 CD4+ cells per cubic millimeter. N Engl J Med. 1996;335:1091–1098.
23a. Miller V, Mocroft A, Reiss P, et al. Relations among CD4 lymphocyte count nadir, antiretroviral therapy, and HIV-1 disease progression: Results from the Eurosida Study. Ann Intern Med 1999;130:570–577.
24. Connors M, Kovacs JA, Krevat S, et al. HIV infection induces changes in CD4+ T-cell phenotype and depletions within the CD4+ T-cell repertoire that are not immediately restored by antiviral or immune-based therapies. Nat Med. 1997;3:533–540.
25. Saag MS, Holodniy M, Kuritzkes DR, et al. HIV viral load markers in clinical practice. Nat Med. 1996;2:625-629.
26. Spector SA, Wong R, Hsia K, et al. Plasma cytomegalovirus (CMV) DNA load predicts CMV disease and survival in AIDS patients. J Clin Invest. 1998;101:497.
27. Kaplan JE, Hanson D, Jones J. Risk factors for primary PCP in HIV-infected adolescents and adults in the U.S. Should history of AIDS-defining illness be included in the criteria for PCP prophylaxis? Abstract 290. In: Abstracts of the Fourth Conference on Retroviruses and Opportunistic Infections, American Society of Microbiology, Washington, DC; January 22–26, 1997.
28. Lundgren JD, Barton SE, Lazzarin A, et al. Factors associated with the development of *Pneumocystis carinii* pneumonia in 5,025 European patients with AIDS. Clin Infect Dis. 1995;21:106–113.
29. Saah AJ, Hoover DR, Peng Y, et al. Predictors for failure of *Pneumocystis carinii* pneumonia prophylaxis. JAMA. 1995;273:1197–1202.
30. Small PM, Shafer RW, Hopewell PC, et al. Exogenous reinfection with multidrug-resistant *Mycobacterium tuberculosis* in patients with advanced HIV infection. N Engl J Med. 1993;328:1137–1144.
31. Daley CL, Small PM, Schecter GF, et al. An outbreak of tuberculosis with accelerated progression among persons infected with human immunodeficiency virus: An analysis using restriction-fragment-length polymorphisms. N Engl J Med. 1992;326:231–235.
32. Maenza JR, Keruly JC, Moore RD, et al. Risk factors for fluconazole-resistant candidiasis in human immunodeficiency virus–infected patients. Clin Infect Dis. 1996;173:219
33. Beard CB, Navin TR. Molecular epidemiology of *Pneumocystis carinii* pneumonia (Commentary). Emerg Infect Dis. 1996;2:147.
34. Wheat LJ, Connolly-Stringfield PA, Baker RL, et al. Disseminated histoplasmosis in the acquired immunodeficiency syndrome: Clinical findings, diagnosis and treatment, and review of the literature. Medicine (Baltimore). 1990;69:361–374.
35. Silva N, O'Bryan L, Medeiros E, et al. *Trypanosoma cruzi* meningoencephalitis in HIV infected patients. J Acquir Immune Defic Synd Human Retrovirol. 1999;20:342–349.
36. Ferreira MS, Nishioka SA, Silvestre MT, et al. Reactivation of Chagas' disease in patients with AIDS: Report of three new cases and review of the literature. Clin Infect Dis. 1997;25:1397–1400.
37. Pape JW, Jean Simone S, Ho JL, et al. Effect of isoniazid prophylaxis on incidence of active tuberculosis and progression in HIV infection. Lancet. 1993;342:268–272.
38. Mukadi Y, Perriens JH, St. Louis ME, et al. Spectrum of immunodeficiency in HIV-1 infected patients with pulmonary tuberculosis in Zaire. Lancet. 1993;342:143–146.
39. Duong TA. Infection due to *Penicillium marneffei*, an emerging pathogen: Review of 155 reported cases. Clin Infect Dis. 1996;23:125–130.
40. Pape JW, Verdier R, Johnson WD, et al. Treatment and prophylaxis of *Isospora belli* infection. N Engl J Med. 1989;320:1044–1047.
41. Kahn JO, Northfelt DW, Miles SA. AIDS associated Kaposi's sarcoma. AIDS Clin Rev. 1992;261–280.
42. Masur H. Prevention and treatment of *Pneumocystis* pneumonia. N Engl J Med. 1992;327:1853–1860.
43. Masur H (Chairman) and the U.S. Public Health Service Task Force on Prophylaxis and Therapy for *Mycobacterium avium* Complex. Recommendations on prophylaxis and therapy for disseminated *Mycobacterium avium* complex disease in patients infected with the human immunodeficiency virus. N Engl J Med. 1993;329:898–904.
44. Piscitelli SC, Flexner C, Minor JR, et al. Drug interactions in patients infected with human immunodeficiency virus. Clin Infect Dis. 1996;23:685.
45. Kovacs JA, Hiemenz JW, Macher AM, et al. *Pneumocystis carinii* pneumonia: A comparison between patients with the acquired immunodeficiency syndrome and patients with other immunodeficiencies. Ann Intern Med. 1984;100:663–671.
46. Kovacs JA, Kovacs AA, Polis M. Cryptococcosis in the acquired immunodeficiency syndrome. Ann Intern Med. 1985;103:533–538.
47. Lee BL, Safrin S. Interactions and toxicities of drugs used in patients with AIDS. Clin Infect Dis 1992;14:773–779.
48. Tu JV, Biem J, Detsky AS. Bronchoscopy versus empirical therapy in HIV-infected patients with presumptive *Pneumocystis carinii* pneumonia. Am Rev Respir Dis. 1993;148:370–377.
49. Masur H, Shelhamer JS. Empiric outpatient management of HIV related pneumonia: Economical or unwise? (Editorial). Ann Intern Med. 1996;124:451–453.
50. Luft BJ, Hafner R, Korzun AH. Toxoplasmic encephalitis in patients with the acquired immunodeficiency syndrome. N Engl J Med. 1993;329:995–1000.
51. Mathews C, Barba D, Fullerton SC. Early biopsy versus empiric treatment with delayed biopsy of non-responders in suspected HIV associated cerebral toxoplasmosis: A decision analysis. AIDS. 1995;9:1243.
52. Jacobson MA. Treatment of cytomegalovirus retinitis in patients with the acquired immunodeficiency syndrome. N Engl J Med.1997;337:105.
53. Macdonald JC, Torriani FJ, Morse LS, et al. Lack of reactivation of cytomegalovirus (CMV) retinitis after stopping CMV maintenance therapy in AIDS patients with sustained elevations in CD4 T cells in response to highly active antiretroviral therapy. J Infect Dis. 1998;177:1182–1187.
54. Tural C, Romeu J, Sirera G, et al. Long-lasting remission of cytomegalovirus retinitis without maintenance therapy in human immunodeficiency virus–infected patients. J Infect Dis. 1998;177:1080–1083.
55. Grube H, Ramratnam B, Ley C, et al. Resolution of AIDS associated cryptosporidiosis after treatment with indinavir. Am J Gastroenterol. 1997;92:726.
56. Carr A, Marriott D, Field A, et al. Treatment of HIV-1-associated microsporidiosis and cryptosporidiosis with combination antiretroviral therapy. Lancet. 1998;351:256–261.
56a. Famer H, Egger M, Opravil M, et al. Discontinuation of primary prophylaxis against *Pneumocystis carinii* pneumonia in HIV-1 infected adults treated with combination antiretroviral therapy. N Engl J Med. 1999;340:1301–1306.
56b. Masur H, Kaplan J. Does *Pneumocystis carinii* prophylaxis still need to be lifelong? N Engl J Med. 1999;340:1356–1357.
57. Abouya YL, Beaumel A, Lucas A, et al. *Pneumocystis* pneumonia—an uncommon cause of death in African patients with acquired immunodeficiency syndrome. Am Rev Respir Dis. 1992;145:617–620.
58. Russian DA, Kovacs J. *Pneumocystis carinii* in Africa: An emerging pathogen? Lancet. 1995;346:1242–1243.
59. Holtzer CD, Jacobson MA, Hadley WK, et al. Decline in the rate of specific opportunistic infections at San Francisco General Hospital, 1994–1997. AIDS. 1998;12:1931–1933.
60. Brenner M, Ognibene FP, Lack EE, et al. Prognostic factors and life expectancy of acquired immunodeficiency syndrome patients with *Pneumocystis carinii* pneumonia. Am Rev Respir Dis.1987;136:1199–1206.
61. el Sadr WM, Simberkoff MS. Survival and prognostic factors in severe *Pneumocystis carinii* pneumonia requiring mechanical ventilation. Am Rev Respir Dis. 1988;137:1264–1267.
62. Ognibene FP, Shelhamer J, Gill V, et al. The diagnosis of *Pneumocystis carinii*

pneumonia in patients with the acquired immunodeficiency syndrome using subsegmental bronchoalveolar lavage. Am Rev Respir Dis.1984;129:933–937.

63. Kovacs JA, Ng VL, Leoung G, et al. Diagnosis of *Pneumocystis* pneumonia: Improved detection in sputum with use of monoclonal antibodies. N Engl J Med. 1988;318:589–593.
64. Barnes PF, Steele MA, Young SMM, Vachon LA. Tuberculosis in patients with human immunodeficiency virus infection—how often does it mimic *Pneumocystis carinii* pneumonia? Chest. 1992;102:428–432.
65. Ognibene FP, Masur H, Rogers P, et al. Nonspecific interstitial pneumonitis without evidence of *Pneumocystis carinii* in asymptomatic patients infected with human immunodeficiency virus (HIV). Ann Intern Med. 1988;109:874–879.
66. Ng VL, Geaghan SM, Leoung G, et al. Lack of effect of prophylactic aerosolized pentamidine on the detection of *Pneumocystis carinii* in induced sputum or bronchoalveolar lavage specimens. Arch Pathol Lab Med. 1993;117:493–496.
67. Wakefield AE, Guiver L, Miller RJ, Hopkin J. DNA amplification in induced sputum samples for diagnosis of *Pneumocystis carinii* pneumonia. Lancet. 1991;337:1378.
68. Helweg-Larson J, Jensen JS, Benfield-Svendsen UG, et al. Diagnostic use of PCR for detection of *Pneumocystis carinii* in oral wash samples. J Clin Microbiol. 36:2068–2072, 1998.
69. Dohn MN, Baughman RP, Vigdorth EM, Frame D. Equal survival rates for first, second and third episodes of *Pneumocystis carinii* pneumonia in patients with AIDS. Arch Intern Med. 1992;152:2465–2470.
70. Sattler FR, Cowan R, Nielsen DM, et al. Trimethoprim-sulfamethoxazole versus pentamidine for therapy of *Pneumocystis* pneumonia: A prospective non-crossover study in patients with AIDS. Ann Intern Med. 1988;109:280–287.
71. Safrin, S, Finkelstein DM, Feinberg J, et al. Comparison of three regimens for treatment of mild to moderate *Pneumocystis carinii* pneumonia in patients with AIDS. A double blind, randomized trial of oral trimethoprim-sulfamethoxazole, dapsone trimethoprim, and clindamycin-primaquine. ACTG 108 Study Group. Ann Intern Med. 1996;124:792–802.
72. Montaner JSG, Lawson LM, Levitt N, et al. Oral corticosteroids prevent early deterioration in patients with moderately severe AIDS-related *Pneumocystis carinii* pneumonia. Ann Intern Med. 1990;113:14–20.
73. Hughes W, Leoung G, Kramer F, et al. Comparision of atovaquone (566C80) with trimethoprim-sulfamethoxazole to treat *Pneumocystis carinii* pneumonia in patients with AIDS. N Engl J Med. 1993;328:1521–1527.
74. Mei Q, Gurunathan S, Masur H, Kovacs J. Failure of co-trimoxazole in *Pneumocystis carinii* infection and the mutations in dihydropteroate synthase gene. Lancet. 1998;351:1631–1632.
75. Kazanjian P, Locke AB, Hossler PA. *Pneumocystis carinii* mutations associated with sulfa and sulfone prophylaxis failures in AIDS patients. AIDS. 1998;12:873–878.
76. Lee BL, Medina I, Benowitz NL, et al. Dapsone, trimethoprim, and sulfamethoxazole plasma levels during treatment of *Pneumocystis* pneumonia in patients with the acquired immunodeficiency syndrome (AIDS): Evidence of drug interactions. Ann Intern Med. 1989;110:606–611.
77. Gordin FM, Simon GL, Wofsy CB, et al. Adverse reactions to trimethoprim-sulfamethoxazole in patients with the acquired immunodeficiency syndrome. Ann Intern Med. 1984;100:495–499.
78. O'Brien JG, Dong BJ, Coleman RL, et al. A 5-year retrospective review of adverse drug reactions and their risk factors in human immunodeficiency virus–infected patients who were receiving intravenous pentamidine therapy for *Pneumocystis carinii* pneumonia. Clin Infect Dis. 1997;24:854–859.
79. Carr A, Swanson C, Penny R, Cooper DA. Clinical and laboratory markers of hypersensitivity to trimethoprim-sulfamethoxazole in patients with *Pneumocystis* pneumonia and AIDS. Clin Infect Dis. 1993;167:180–185.
80. Safrin S, Lee BL, Sande MA. Adjunctive folinic acid with trimethoprim-sulfamethoxazole for *Pneumocystis carinii* pneumonia in AIDS patients is associated with an increased risk of therapeutic failure and death. J Infect Dis. 1994;170:912–917.
81. Holtzer C, Coleman R, Flaherty J. Cross-reactivity and patient outcomes in HIV-infected patients switched from TMP/SMZ to dapsone due to hypersensitivity reactions during PCP prophylaxis. Abstract No. 292. In: Abstracts of the Fourth Conference on Retroviruses and Opportunistic Infections, American Society of Microbiology, Washington, DC; January 22–26, 1997.
82. Para MF, Dohn M, Fram P, et al. ACTG 268 Trial—gradual initiation of trimethoprim/sulfamethoxazole (T/S) as primary prophylaxis for *Pneumocystis carinii* pneumonia (PCP). Abstract No. 2. In: Abstracts of the Fourth Conference on Retroviruses and Opportunistic Infections, American Society of Microbiology, Washington, DC; January 22–26, 1997.
83. Leoung G, Stanford J, Giordano M, et al. A randomized, double-blind trial of TMP/SMX dose escalation vs. direct rechallenge in HIV⁺ persons at risk for PCP and with prior treatment-limiting rash or fever. Abstract No. LB-10. In: Abstracts of the 37th Interscience Conference on Antimicrobial Agents and Chemotherapy, Toronto, Ontario, September 28–October 1, 1997.
84. Navin TR, Fontaine RE. Intravenous versus intramuscular administration of pentamidine. N Engl J Med. 1984;311:1701–1702.
85. Mallory DL, Parrillo JE, Bailey KR, et al. Cardiovascular effects and safety of intravenous and intramuscular pentamidine isethionate. Crit Care Med. 1987;15:503–505.
86. Waskin H, Stehr-Green JK, Helmick CG, et al. Risk factors for hypoglycemia associated with pentamidine therapy for *Pneumocystis* pneumonia. JAMA. 1988;260:345–347.
87. Conte JE, Chernoff D, Feigal DW, et al. Intravenous or inhaled pentamidine for treating *Pneumocystis carinii* pneumonia in AIDS. Ann Intern Med. 1990;113:203–209.
88. Medina I, Mills J, Leoung G, et al. Oral therapy for *Pneumocystis carinii* pneumonia in the acquired immunodeficiency syndrome—a controlled trial of trimethoprim-sulfamethoxazole versus trimethoprim-dapsone. N Engl J Med. 1990;323:776–782.
89. Mills J, Leoung G, Medina J, et al. Dapsone treatment of *Pneumocystis carinii* pneumonia in the acquired immunodeficiency syndrome. Antimicrob Agents Chemother. 1988;32:1057–1060.
90. Dohn MN, Weinberg WG, Torres RA, et al. Oral atovaquone compared with intravenous pentamidine for *Pneumocystis carinii* pneumonia in patients with AIDS. Ann Intern Med. 1994;121:174–180.
91. Walker DJ, Wakefield AE, Dohn MN, et al. Sequence polymorphism in the *Pneumocystis carinii* cytochrome b gene and thus association with atovaquone failure. J Infect Dis. 1998;178:1767–1775.
92. Noskin GA, Murphy RL, Black JR, Phair JP. Salvage therapy with clindamycin/primaquine for *Pneumocystis carinii* pneumonia. Clin Infect Dis. 1992;14:183–188.
93. Allegra CJ, Chabner BA, Tuazon CU, et al. Trimetrexate for the treatment of *Pneumocystis carinii* pneumonia in patients with the acquired immunodeficiency syndrome. N Engl J Med. 1987;317:978–985.
94. Sattler FR, Frame P, Davis R, et al. Trimetrexate with leucovorin versus trimethoprim-sulfamethoxazole for moderate to severe episodes of *Pneumocystis carinii* pneumonia in patients with AIDS: a prospective, controlled multicenter investigation of the AIDS Clinical Trials Group Protocol 029/031. J Infect Dis. 1994;170:165–172.
95. Bozzette SA, Sattler FR, Chiu J, et al. A controlled trial of early adjunctive treatment with corticosteroids for *Pneumocystis carinii* pneumonia in the acquired immunodeficiency syndrome. N Engl J Med. 1990;323:1451–1457.
96. Gagnon S, Boota AM, Fischl MA, et al. Corticosteroids as adjunctive therapy for severe *Pneumocystis carinii* pneumonia in the acquired immunodeficiency syndrome—a double-blind, placebo-controlled trial. N Engl J Med. 1990; 323:1444–1450.
97. Nielsen TL, Eeftinck Schattenkerk JK, Jensen BN, et al. Adjunctive corticosteroid therapy for *Pneumocystis carinii* pneumonia in AIDS: A randomized European multicenter open label study. J Acquir Immune Defic Syndr. 1992;5:726–731.
98. Masur H, et al. Consensus statement on the use of corticosteroids as adjunctive therapy for pneumocystis pneumonia in the acquired immunodeficiency syndrome. N Engl J Med. 1990;323:1500–1504.
99. Jones BD, Taikwel EK, Mercado AL, et al. Tuberculosis in patients with HIV infection who receive corticosteroids for presumed *Pneumocystis carinii* pneumonia. Am J Respir Crit Care Med. 1994;149:1686–1688.
100. Caumes E, Roudier C, Rogeaux O, et al. Effect of corticosteroids on the incidence of adverse cutaneous reactions to trimethoprim-sulfamethoxazole during treatment of AIDS-associated *Pneumocystis carinii* pneumonia. Clin Infect Dis. 1994;18:319–323.
101. Shelhamer JH, Ognibene FP, Macher AM, et al. Persistence of *Pneumocystis carinii* in lung tissue of acquired immunodeficiency syndrome patients treated for *Pneumocystis* pneumonia. Am Rev Respir Dis. 1984;130:1161–1165.
102. Ognibene FP, Steis R, Macher AM, et al. Kaposi's sarcoma–causing infiltrates and respiratory failure in the acquired immunodeficiency syndrome. Ann Intern Med. 1985;102:471–475.
103. Rosen MJ, Clayton K, Schnieder RF, et al. Intensive care of patients with HIV infection: Utilization, critical illnesses, and outcomes. Am J Respir Crit Care Med. 1997;155:67–71.
104. Wachter RM, Luce JM, Hopewell PC. Critical care of patients with AIDS. JAMA. 1992;267:541–547.
105. Randall CL, Horner RD, Bennett CL. Survival from intensive care for patients with HIV-related *Pneumocystis carinii* pneumonia (PCP). Abstract Tu. B. III. In: Abstracts of the XIth International Conference on AIDS, Vancouver, July 7–12, 1996.
106. Swindells S, Currier JS, Williams P. DACS 071: Correlation of viral load and risk for opportunistic infection. Abstract No. 359. In: Abstracts of the Fourth Conference on Retroviruses and Opportunistic Infections, American Society of Microbiology, Washington, DC; January 22–26, 1997.
107. Hardy WD, Feinberg J, Finkelstein DM, et al. A controlled trial of trimethoprim-sulfamethoxazole or aerosolized pentamidine for secondary prophylaxis of *Pneumocystis carinii* pneumonia in patients with the acquired immunodeficiency syndrome: AIDS Clinical Trials Group protocol 021. N Engl J Med. 1992;327:1842–1848.
108. Schneider MME, Hoepelman AIM, Eeftinck Schattenkerk JKM, et al. A controlled trial of aerosolized pentamidine or trimethoprim-sulfamethoxazole as primary prophylaxis against *Pneumocystis carinii* pneumonia in patients with human immunodeficiency virus infection. N Engl J Med. 1992;327:1836–1841.
109. Leoung GS, Feigal DW Jr, Montgomery AB, et al. Aerosolized pentamidine for prophylaxis against *Pneumocystis carinii* pneumonia—the San Francisco Community Prophylaxis Trial. N Engl J Med. 1990;323:769–775.
110. Murphy RL, Lavelle JP, Allan JD, et al. Aerosol pentamidine prophylaxis following *Pneumocystis carinii* pneumonia in AIDS patients: Results of a blinded dose-comparison study using an ultrasonic nebulizer. Am J Med. 1991;90:418–426.
111. Schneider MME, Nielsen TL, Nelsing S, et al. Efficacy and toxicity of two doses of trimethoprim-sulfamethoxazole as primary prophylaxis against *Pneumocystis carinii* pneumonia in patients with human immunodeficiency virus. J Infect Dis. 1995; 171:1632–1636.
112. Girard P-M, Landman R, Gaudebout C, et al. Dapsone-pyrimethamine compared with aerosolized pentamidine as primary prophylaxis against *Pneumocystis carinii*

pneumonia and toxoplasmosis in HIV infection. N Engl J Med. 1993;328:1514–1520.
113. Blum RN, Miller LA, Gaggini LC, Cohn DL. Comparative trial of dapsone vs. trimethoprim-sulfamethoxazole for primary prophylaxis of *Pneumocystis carinii* pneumonia. J Acquir Immune Defic Syndr. 1992;15:341–347.
114. Kemper CA, Tucker RM, Lang DS, et al. Low dose dapsone prophylaxis of *Pneumocystis carinii* pneumonia in AIDS and AIDS-related complex. AIDS. 1990;4:1145–1148.
115. Montaner JSG, Lawson LM, Gervais A, et al. Aerosol pentamidine for secondary prophylaxis of AIDS-related *Pneumocystis carinii* pneumonia: A randomized, placebo-controlled study. Ann Intern Med. 1991;114:948–953.
116. Hirschel B, Lazzarin A, Chopard P, et al. A controlled study of inhaled pentamidine for primary prevention of *Pneumocystis carinii* pneumonia. N Engl J Med. 1991;324:1079–1083.
117. Carr A, Tindall B, Brew BJ, et al. Low-dose trimethoprim-sulfamethoxazole prophylaxis for toxoplasmic encephalitis in patients with AIDS. Ann Intern Med. 1992;117:106–111.
118. El-Sadr W, Luskin-Hawk R, Pulling C, et al. Daily versus thrice weekly trimethoprim-sulfamethoxazole in the prevention of *P. carinii* pneumonia (CPCRA 006). Abstract I-146. In: Abstracts of the 35th Annual Meeting of the Infectious Diseases Society of America, San Francisco, September 13–16, 1997.
119. O'Doherty MJ, Thomas S, Page C, et al. Differences in relative efficacy of nebulizers for pentamidine administration. Lancet. 1988;2:1283–1286.
120. O'Riordan TG, Smaldone GC. Exposure of health care workers to aerosolized pentamidine. Chest. 1992;101:1494–1499.
121. Centers for Disease Control. *Mycobacterium tuberculosis* transmission in a health clinic—Florida, 1988. MMWR Morb Mortal Wkly Rep. 1988;38:256–258, 263–264.
122. El-Sadr W, Murphy R, Luskin-Hawk R, et al. Atovaquone vs. dapsone in the prevention of *P. carinii* pneumonia in patients intolerant to trimethoprim and/or sulfamethoxazole. Abstract No. 769. In: Abstracts of the 35th Annual Meeting of the Infectious Disease Society of America, San Francisco, September 13–16, 1997.
123. Caldwell P, Murphy R, Chan C. Atovaquone suspension for prophylaxis of *Pneumocystis carinii* pneumonia: Effects of baseline prophylaixs on safety and efficacy. Abstract No. 22178. In: Conference Records, 12th World AIDS Conference, Geneva, June 28, 1998.
124. Golden JA, Katz MH, Chernoff DN, et al. A randomized comparison of once monthly or twice monthly high dose aerosolized pentamidine prophylaxis. Chest. 1993;104:743–750.
125. Dunne MW, Bozzette S, McCutchan JA, et al., and the California Collaborative Treatment Group. Prevention of *Pneumocystis carinii* pneumonia with azithromycin. In preparation.
126. Stansell JD, Osmond DH, Charlebois E, et al. Predictors of *Pneumocystis carinii* pneumonia in HIV-infected persons. Am J Respir Crit Care Med. 1997;155:60–66.
127. Moorman A, Von Bargen J, Palella F, et al. Determinants of "breakthrough" *Pneumocystis carinii* pneumonia (PCP) in the HIV outpatient study (HOPS). Abstract No. 294. In: Abstracts of the Fourth Conference on Retroviruses and Opportunistic Infections, American Society of Microbiology, Washington, DC; January 22–26, 1997.
128. Porter SB, Sande MA. Toxoplasmosis of the central nervous system in the acquired immunodeficiency syndrome. N Engl J Med. 1992;327:1643–1648.
129. Israelski DM, Chmiel JS, Poggenser L, et al. Prevalence of *Toxoplasma* infection in a cohort of homosexual men at risk of AIDS and toxoplasmic encephalitis. J Acquir Immune Defic Syndr. 1993;6:414–418.
130. Cingolani A, De Luca A, Ammassari A, et al. PCR detection of *Toxoplasma gondii* DNA in CSF for the differential diagnosis of AIDS-related focal brain lesions. J Med Microbiol. 1996;45:472.
131. Barker DE, Trepashko D, DeMarais P, et al. Utility of thallium brain SPECT in the exclusion of CNS lymphoma in AIDS. Abstract No. 708. In: Abstracts of the Fourth Conference on Retroviruses and Opportunistic Infections, Washington, DC, January 22–26, 1996.
132. Jarvik JG, Hesselink JR, Kennedy C, et al. Acquired immunodeficiency syndrome: Magnetic resonance patterns of brain involvement with pathologic correlation. Arch Neurol. 1998;45:731–736.
133. Antinori A, Ammassari A, DeLuca A, et al. Diagnosis of AIDS- related focal brain lesions: A decision making analysis based on clinical and neurological characteristics combined with polymerase chain reaction assays in CSF. Neurology. 1997;48:687.
134. Dannemann B, McCutchan JA, Israelski D, et al. Treatment of toxoplasmic encephalitis in patients with AIDS: A randomized trial comparing pyrimethamine plus clindamycin to pyrimethamine plus sulfonamides. Ann Intern Med. 1992; 116:33–43.
135. Katlama C, De Wit S, O'Doherty E, et al. Pyrimethamine-clindamycin vs. pyrimethamine-sulfadiazine as acute and long-term therapy for toxoplasmic encephalitis in patients with AIDS. Clin Infect Dis. 1996;22:268.
136. Kovacs JA, O'Neill D, Feuerstein I, et al. Efficacy of atovaquone in treatment of toxoplasmosis in patients with AIDS. Lancet. 1992;340:637–638.
137. Torres RA, Winberg W, Stansell J, et al. Atovaquone for salvage treatment and suppression of toxoplasmic encephalitis in patients with AIDS. Clin Infect Dis. 1997;24:422.
138. Fernandez-Martin J, Leport C, Morlat P, et al. Pyrimethamine-clarithromycin combination for therapy of acute *Toxoplasma encephalitis* in patients with AIDS. Antimicrob Agents Chemother. 1991;35:2049.
139. Morris JT, Kelly JW. Effective treatment of cerebral toxoplasmosis with doxycycline. Am J Med. 1992;93:107.
140. Derouin F, Piketty C, Chastang C, et al. Antitoxoplasma effects of dapsone alone and combined with pyrimethamine. Antimicrob Agents Chemother. 1991;35:252–255.
141. de Gans J, Portegies P, Reiss P, et al. Pyrimethamine as maintenance therapy for central nervous system toxoplasmosis in 38 patients with AIDS. J Acquir Immune Defic Syndr. 1992;5:137–142.
142. Masur H, Polis MA, Tuazon CU, et al. Salvage trial of trimetrexate-leucovorin for the treatment of cerebral toxoplasmosis in patients with AIDS. J Infect Dis. 1993;167:1422–1426.
143. Kalb RE, Grossman ME. Chronic perianal herpes simplex in immunocompromised hosts. Am J Med. 1986;80:486–490.
144. Stewart JA, Reef SE, Pellett PE, et al. Herpes virus infection in persons with HIV. Clin Infect Dis. 1995;21(Suppl):S114.
145. LaGuardia RD, White MH, Saigo PE, et al. Genital ulcer disease in women infected with human immunodeficiency virus. Am J Obstet Gynecol. 1995;172:553.
146. Sacks SL, Aoki FY, Diaz-Mitoma F, et al. Patient initiated, twice-daily oral famciclovir for early recurrent genital herpes: A randomized double blind multicenter trial. JAMA. 1996;276:44.
147. Smiley ML, for the International Valaciclovir HSV Study Group. Valaciclovir and acyclovir for the treatment of recurrent genital herpes simplex virus infections. Abstract No. 1210. In: Abstracts of the 37th Interscience Conference on Antimicrobial Agents and Chemotherapy, Toronto. Washington, DC: American Society for Microbiology; 1997.
148. Mertz GJ, Loveless MO, Levin MJ, et al. Oral famciclovir for suppression of recurrent gential herpes simplex virus infection in women: A multicenter, double blind placebo controlled study. Arch Intern Med. 1997;157:343.
149. Pottage JC Jr, Kessler HA. Herpes simplex virus resistance to acyclovir: Clinical relevance. Infect Agents Dis. 1995;4:115–124.
150. Reyes M, Graber J, Reeves WC. Acyclovir-resistant HSV: Initial results from a National Surveillance System. Abstract No. 55. In: Abstracts of the 35th Annual Meeting of the Infectious Diseases Society of America, San Francisco. Alexandria, Va: Infectious Diseases Society of America; 1997.
151. Chatis PA, Miller CH, Schrager LE, et al. Successful treatment with foscarnet of an acyclovir-resistant mucocutaneous infection with herpes simplex virus in a patient with acquired immunodeficiency syndrome. N Engl J Med. 1989;320:297.
152. Lalezari JP, Drew WL, Glutzer E, et al. Treatment with intravenous (s)-1-(3-hydroxy-2-phosphonylmethoxypropyl) cytosine of acyclovir-resistant mucocutaneous infection with herpes simplex virus in a patient with AIDS. J Infect Dis. 1994;170:550.
153. Safrin S, Kemmerly S, Plotkin B, et al. Foscarnet-resistant herpes simplex virus infection in patients with AIDS. J Infect Dis. 1994;169:193.
154. Birch CJ, Tyssen DP, Tacheddjian G, et al. Clinical effects and in vitro studies of trifluorothymidine combined with interferon-α for treatment of drug resistant and sensitive herpes simplex virus infections. J Infect Dis. 1992;166:108.
155. Kessler HA, Hurwitz C, Farthing C, et al. Pilot study of topical trifluridine for the treatment of acyclovir-resistant mucocutanous herpes simplex disease in patients with AIDS (ACTG 172). J Acquir Immun Defic Syndr. 1996;12:147.
156. Lalezari J, Schacker T, Feinberg J, et al. A randomized, double blind, placebo-controlled study of cidofovir gel for the treatment of acyclovir-unresponsive mucocutanous herpes simplex virus infections in patients with AIDS. J Infect Dis. 1997;17:862.
157. LeBoit PE, Limova M, Yen TSB, et al. Chronic verrucous varicella zoster infection in patients with the acquired immunodeficiency syndrome (AIDS): Histologic and molecular biologic findings. Am J Dermatopathol. 1992;12:1.
158. Hoppenjans WB, Bibler MR, Orme RL, et al. Prolonged cutaneous herpes zoster in acquired immunodeficiency syndrome. Arch Dermatol. 1990;126:1048–1050.
159. Janier M, Hillion B, Baccard M, et al. Chronic varicella zoster infection in acquired immunodeficiency syndrome. J Am Acad Dermatol. 1988;18:584–585.
160. Whitley RJ, Weiss J, Gnann JW, et al. A randomized placebo-controlled trial of acyclovir with and without steroids for the treatment of herpes zoster. Ann Intern Med. 1996;125:376–383.
161. Wood MJ, Johnson RW, McKendrick MW, et al. A randomized trial of acyclovir for 7 days or 21 days with and without prednisone for treatment of acute herpes zoster. N Engl J Med. 1994;330:896–900.
162. Boivin G, Edelman CK, Pedneault L, et al. Phenotypic and genotypic characterization of acyclovir resistant varicella zoster viruses isolated from persons with AIDS. J Infect Dis. 1994;170:68.
163. Lyall EGH, Ogilvie MM, Smith NM, et al. Acyclovir resistant varicella zoster and HIV infection. Arch Dis Child. 1994;70:133.
164. Perronne C, Lazamas M, Leport C, et al. Varicella in patients infected with the human immunodeficiency virus. Arch Dermatol. 1990;126:1033.
165. Collier AC, Meyers JD, Corey L, et al. Cytomegalovirus infection in homosexual men: Relationship to sexual practices, antibody to human immunodeficiency virus, and cell-mediated immunity. Am J Med. 1987;23:593.
166. Drew WL, Miner RC, Ziegler JL, et al. Cytomegalovirus and Kaposi's sarcoma in young homosexual men. Lancet. 1982;1:125.
167. Hoover DR, Saah AJ, Bacellar H, et al. Clinical manifestations of AIDS in the era of *Pneumocystis* prophylaxis. N Engl J Med. 1993;329:1922.
168. Zurlo JJ, O'Neill D, Polis MA, et al. Lack of clinical utility of cytomegalovirus blood and urine cultures in patients with HIV infection. Ann Intern Med. 1993;118:12–17.
169. Wetherill PE, Landry ML, Alcabes P, et al. Use of a quantitative cytomegalovirus (CMV) antigenemia test in evaluation of HIV^+ patients with and without CMV disease. J Acquir Immune Defic Syndr. 1996;12:33.

170. Jacobson MA, Mills J. Serious cytomegalovirus disease in the acquired immunodeficiency syndrome (AIDS). Ann Intern Med. 1988;108:585–594.
171. Drew WL. Cytomegalovirus infection in patients with AIDS. Clin Infect Dis. 1992;14:608–615.
172. Bloom JN, Palestine AG. The diagnosis of cytomegalovirus retinitis. Ann Intern Med. 1988;109:963–969.
173. Studies of the Ocular Complications of AIDS Research Group, AIDS Clinical Trials Group. Mortality in patients with the acquired immunodeficiency syndrome treated with either foscarnet or ganciclovir for cytomegalovirus retinitis. N Engl J Med. 1992;326:213–220.
174. Studies of the Ocular Complications of AIDS Research Group in Collaboration with the AIDS Clinical Trials Group. Combination foscarnet and ganciclovir therapy vs. monotherapy for the treatment of relapsed cytomegalovirus retinitis in patients with AIDS. Arch Ophthalmol. 1996;114:23.
175. Drew WL, Ives D, Lalezari J, et al. Oral ganciclovir as maintenance treatment for cytomegalovirus retinitis in patients with AIDS. N Engl J Med. 1995;333:615.
175a. Martin DF, Kupferman BD, Welitz RA, et al. Oral ganciclovir for patients with cytomegalovirus retinitis treated with a ganciclovir implant. N Engl J Med. 1999;340:1063–1070.
176. Studies of the Ocular Complications of AIDS (SOCA) in collaboration with the AIDS Clinical Trials Group. Cytomegalovirus (CMV) culture results, drug resistance, and clinical outcomes in patients with AIDS and CMV retinitis treated with either foscarnet or ganciclovir. J Infect Dis. 1997;176:50–58.
177. Lalezari FP, Kemper C, Stagg R, et al. A randomized, controlled study of the safety and efficacy of intravenous cidofovir (CDV, HPMPC) for the treatment of relapsing cytomegalovirus retinitis in patients with AIDS. In: Abstracts of the XIth International Conference on AIDS, Vancouver, July 7–12, 1996.
177. Kirsch LS, Arevalo JF, DeClercq E, et al. Phase I/II study of intravitreal cidofovir for the treatment of cytomegalovirus retinitis in patients with the acquired immunodeficiency syndrome. Am J Ophthalmol. 1995;119:466.
178. Rahhal FM, Arevalo JF, Chavez de la Paz E, et al. Treatment of cytomegalovirus retinitis with intravitreous cidofovir in patients with AIDS: A preliminary report. Ann Intern Med. 1996;125:98.
179. Hutcherson SL, Palestine AG, Cantrill HL, et al. Antisense oligonucleotide safety for CMV retinitis in AIDS patients. Abstract No. H136. In: Abstracts of the 35th Interscience Conference on Antimicrobial Agents and Chemotherapy, San Francisco. Washington, DC: American Society of Microbiology; 1995.
180. Musch DC, Martin DF, Gordon JF, et al. Treatment of cytomegalovirus retinitis with a sustained release intraocular ganciclovir implant. N Engl J Med. 1997;337:83.
181. Marx JL, Kapusta MA, Patel SS, et al. Use of the ganciclovir implant in the treatment of recurrent cytomegalovirus retinitis. Arch Ophthalmol. 1996;114:815.
182. Uberti-Foppa C, Lazzerin A, Gianolti N, et al. Cytomegalovirus pneumonia in AIDS patients: Value of cytomegalovirus culture from BAL fluid and correlation with lung disease. Chest. 1998;113:919–923.
183. Emanuel D, Cunningham I, Jules-Elysee K, et al. Cytomegalovirus pneumonia after bone-marrow transplantation successfully treated with the combination of ganciclovir and high-dose intravenous immune globulin. Ann Intern Med. 1988;109:777–782.
184. Parente F, Bianchi-Porro G. Treatment of cytomegalovirus esophagitis in patients with AIDS: A randomized controlled study of foscarnet versus ganciclovir. Am J Gastroenterol. 1998;93:317–322.
185. Erice A, Gil-Roda C, Perez JL, et al. Antiviral susceptibilities and analysis of UP97 and DNA polymerase sequences of clinical cytomegalovirus isolates from immunocompromised patients. J Infect Dis. 1997;175:1087.
186. Drew WL, Miner RC, Crager M, et al. Prevalence of ganciclovir-resistant cytomegalovirus during oral ganciclcovir prophylaxis. Abstract No. LB16. In: Abstracts of the Third Conference on Retroviruses and Opportunistic Infections. Alexandria, Va: Westover Management Group; 1996.
187. Jabs DA, for the CMV Retinitis and Viral Resistance Study Group. Incidence of resistant cytomegalovirus (CMV) in patients being treated for CMV retinitis. Abstract No. 262. In: Abstracts of the Fifth Conference on Retroviruses and Opportunistic Infections, Chicago: Westover Management Group; 1998.
188. Sullivan V, Coen DM. Isolation of foscarnet-resistant human cytomegalovirus patterns of resistance and sensitivity to other antiviral drugs. J Infect Dis. 1991;164:781–784.
189. Spector SA, McKinley GF, Lalezari JP, et al. Oral ganciclovir for the prevention of cytomegalovirus retinitis in persons with AIDS. N Engl J Med. 1996;334:1491.
190. Brosgart CL, Torres RA, Thompson MA, et al. A randomized, placebo controlled trial of the safety and efficacy of oral ganciclovir for prophylaxis of cytomegalovirus disease in HIV infected individuals. AIDS. 1998;12:269–277.
191. Major EO, Amemiya K, Tornatore CS, et al. Pathogenesis and molecular biology of progressive multifocal leukoencephalopathy, the JC virus-induced demyelinating disease of the human brain. Clin Microbiol. Rev. 1992;5:49–73.
192. Matsiota-Bernard P, De Truchis P, Gray F, et al. JC virus detection in the cerebrospinal fluid of AIDS patients with progressive multifocal leucoencephalopathy and monitoring of the antiviral treatment by a PCR method. J Med Microbiol. 1997;46:256.
193. Hall C, Dafni U, Simpson D, et al. Failure of cytosine arabinoside therapy for human immunodeficiency virus-1 associated progressive multifocal leukoencephalopathy. N Engl J Med. 1998;338:1345–1351.
194. Domingo P, Guardiola JM, Iranzo A, et al. Remission of progressive multifocal leucoencephalopathy after antitretroviral therapy (Letter; Comment). Lancet. 1997;349:1554.
195. Baldeweg T, Catalan J. Remission of progressive multifocal leucoencephalopathy after antiretroviral therapy (Letter; Comment). Lancet. 1997;349:1554.
196. Elliot B, Aromin I, Gold R, et al. 2.5 year remission of AIDS-associated progressive multifocal leukoencephalopathy with combined antiretroviral therapy (Letter) (see comments). Lancet. 1997;349:850.
197. De Wit S, Goosens H, Weerts D, et al. Comparison of fluconazole and ketoconazole for oropharyngeal candidiasis in AIDS. Lancet. 1989;1:746.
198. Koletar SL, Russell JA, Fass RJ, et al. Comparison of oral fluconazole and clotrimazole troches as treatment for oral candidiasis in patients infected with human immunodeficiency virus. Antimicrob Agents Chemother. 1990;34:2267.
199. Laine L, Dretler RH, Conteas CN, et al. Fluconazole compared with ketoconazole for the treatment of *Candida* esophagitis in AIDS. Ann Intern Med. 1992;117:655.
200. de Repentigny L, Ratelle J. Comparison of itraconazole and ketoconazole in HIV-positive patients with oropharyngeal or esophageal candidiasis. Chemotherapy. 1996;42:374.
201. Van Huesden AM, Merkus HM, Corbeij RS, et al. Single-dose oral fluconazole versus single-dose topical miconazole for the treatment of acute vulvovaginal candidiosis. Acta Obstet Gynecol Scand. 1990;69:417.
202. Wooley PD, Higgins SP. Comparison of clotrimazole, fluconazole and itraconazole in vaginal candidiasis. Br J Clin Pract. 1995;49:65.
203. Zingman B, Zackin R, Wheat J, et al. Amphotericin B oral suspension for fluconazole-resistant oral candidiasis in HIV-infected patients. Abstract No. 152. In: Abstracts of the 37th Interscience Conference on Antimicrobial Agents and Chemotherapy, Toronto, September 28–October 1, 1997.
204. Sobel JD, Brooker D, Stein GE, et al. Single oral dose fluconazole compared with conventional clotrimazole topical therapy of *Candida* vaginitis. Am J Obstet Gynecol. 1995;172:1263.
205. Moskovitz B, Wu J, Baruch A, et al. Long term safety and efficacy of itraconazole oral solution for the treatment of fluconazole refractory oropharyngeal candidiasis in HIV-positive patients. Abstract No. 325. In: Proceedings of the Fourth Conference on Retroviruses and Opportunistic Infections, Washington, DC, January 22–26, 1997.
206. Zuger A, Louis E, Holzman RS, et al. Cryptococcal disease in patients with the acquired immunodeficiency syndrome: Diagnostic features and outcome of treatment. Ann Intern Med. 1986;104:234–240.
207. Chuck SL, Sande MA. Infections with *Cryptococcus neoformans* in the acquired immunodeficiency syndrome. N Engl J Med. 1989;321:794–799.
208. Van der Horst CM, Saag MS, Cloud GA, et al. Treatment of cryptococcal meningitis associated with the acquired immunodeficiency syndrome. N Engl J Med. 1997;337:15.
209. Saag MS, and the NIAID Mycoses Study Group. Comparison of fluconazole versus itraconazole as maintenance therapy of AIDS-associated cryptococcal meningitis. Clin Infect Dis. 1999;28:291–296.
210. Denning DW, Armstrong RW, Lewis BH, et al. Elevated cerebrospinal fluid pressures in patients with cryptococcal meningitis and acquired immunodeficiency syndrome. Am J Med. 1991;91:267.
211. Powderly WG, Cloud GA, Dismukes WE, et al. Measurement of cryptococcal antigen in serum and cerebrospinal fluid: Value in the management of AIDS-associated cryptococcal meningitis. Clin Infect Dis. 1994;18:789.
212. Powderly WG, Tuazon C, Cloud GA, et al., for the MSG 17/ACTG 159 Team. Serum and CSF cryptococcal antigen in the management of cryptococcal meningitis in AIDS. Abstract No. 6. In: Abstracts of the Fourth National Conference on Human Retroviruses and Related Infections, Washington, DC. Alexandria, Va. Westover Management Group; 1997.
213. Wheat LJ, Connolly-Stringfield P, Blair R, et al. Histoplasmosis relapse in patients with AIDS: Detection using *Histoplasma capsulatum* variety *capsulatum* antigen levels. Ann Intern Med. 1991;115:936–941.
214. Wheat LJ, Hafner R, Wulfsohn M, et al. Prevention of relapse of histoplasmosis with itraconazole in patients with the acquired immunodeficiency syndrome. The National Institute of Allergy and Infectious Diseases Clinical Trials and Mycoses Study Group Collaborators. Ann Intern Med. 1993;118:610–616.
215. Wheat J, Hafner R, Korzun AH, et al. Itraconazole treatment of disseminated histoplasmosis in patients with the acquired immunodeficiency syndrome. Am J Med. 1995;98:336
216. Stevens DA. Coccidioidomycosis. N Engl J Med. 1995;332:1077
217. Singh VR, Smith KD, Lawrence J, et al. Coccidioidomycosis in patients infected with human immunodeficiency virus: Review of 91 cases at a single institution. Clin Infect Dis. 1996;23:563.
218. Mylonakis E, Barlam TF, Flanigan T, et al. Pulmonary aspergillosis and invasive disease in AIDS—Review of 342 cases. Chest. 1998; 114:251–262.
219. Kemper CA, Hostetler JS, Follansbee SE, et al. Ulcerative and plaque-like tracheobronchitis due to infection with *Aspergillus* in patients with AIDS. Clin Infect Dis. 1993;17:344.
220. Wallace JM, Hansen NI, LaVange L, et al. Respiratory disease trends in the Pulmonary Complications of HIV Infection Study cohort. Am J Respir Crit Care Med. 1997;155:72.
221. Hirschtick RE, Glassroth J, Jordan MC, et al. Bacterial pneumonia in persons infected with the human immunodeficiency virus. N Engl J Med. 1995;333:845.
222. Pierce M, Crampton S, Henry D, et al. A randomized trial of clarithromycin as prophylaxis against disseminated *Mycobacterium avium* complex infection in patients with advanced acquired immunodeficiency syndrome. N Engl J Med. 1996;335:392.
223. Currier J, Williams P, Feinberg J, et al. ACTG 815: A prospective study of bacterial infections in advanced HIV disease. Abstract No. 364. In: Abstracts of the Fourth

Conference on Retroviruses and Opportunistic Infections, Washington, DC. Alexandria, Va. Westover Management Group, 1997.
224. Barnes PF, Bloch AB, Davidson PT, Snider DE. Tuberculosis in patients with human immunodeficiency virus infection. N Engl J Med. 1991;324:1644–1650.
225. Barnes PR, Barrows SA. Tuberculosis in the 1990's. Ann Intern Med. 1993; 119:400–410.
226. Centers for Disease Control and Prevention. Prevention and Treatment of Tuberculosis Among Patients Infected with Human Immunodeficiency Virus: Principles of Therapy and Revised Recommendations. MMWR Morb Mortal Wkly Rep. 1998;47(RR-20):1–58.
227. Perriens JH, St. Louis ME, Mukadi YB, et al. Pulmonary tuberculosis in HIV-infected patients in Zaire. N Engl J Med. 1995;332:779.
228. Alwood K, Keruly J, Moore-Rice K, et al. Effectiveness of supervised, intermittent therapy for tuberculosis in HIV-infected patients. AIDS. 1994;8:1103.
229. Chaisson RE, Gordin F, Matts J, et al. A randomized trial of rifampin/pyrizinamide for 2 months vs. INH for 12 months in HIV$^+$tuberculin$^+$adults (CPCRA 004/ ACTG 175 CDC/PAHO). Abstract no.22126. In: Abstracts of the Conference Record, Twelfth World AIDS Conference, June 28, 1998, Geneva, Switzerland.
230. Gordin FM, Cohn DL, Sullam PM, et al. Early manifestations of disseminated *Mycobacterium avium* complex disease: A prospective evaluation. J Infect Dis. 1997;176:126.
231. Chaisson RE, Benson CA, Dube MP, et al. Clarithromycin therapy for bacteremic *Mycobacterium avium* complex disease in patients with AIDS. Ann Intern Med. 1994;121:905.
232. Kemper CA, Meng RC, Nussbaum J, et al. Treatment of *Mycobacterium avium* complex bacteremia in AIDS with a four-drug oral regimen. Ann Intern Med. 1992;116:466.
233. Shafran SD, Singer J, Zarowney DP, et al. A comparison of two regimens for the treatment of *Mycobacterium avium* complex bacteremia in AIDS: Rifabutin, ethambutol, and clarithromycin versus rifampin, ethambutol, clofazimine, and ciprofloxacin. N Engl J Med. 1996;335:377.
234. May T, Brel F, Beuscart C, et al. Comparison of combination therapy regimens for treatment of human immunodeficiency virus–infected patients with disseminated bacteremia due to *Mycobacterium avium*. Clin Infect Dis. 1997;25:621.
235. Gordin F, Sullam P, Shafran S, et al. A placebo controlled trial of rifabutin added to a regimen of clarithromycin and ethambutol in the treatment of *M. avium* complex bacteremia. Abstract No. 22176. In: Abstracts of the Conference Record, Twelfth World AIDS Conference, June 28, 1998, Geneva, Switzerland.
236. Dube MP, Sattler F, Torriani F, et al. A randomized evaluation of ethambutol for prevention of relapse and drug resistance during treatment of *Mycobacterium avium* complex bacteremia with clarithromycin-based combination therapy. J Infect Dis. 1997;176:1225.
237. Benson CA, Cohn DL, Williams P, and the ACTG 196/CPCRA 009 Study Team. A phase III prospective, randomized, double-blind study of the safety and efficacy of clarithromycin (CLA) vs. rifabutin (RBT) vs. CLA + RBT for prevention of *Mycobacterium avium* complex (MAC) disease in HIV$^+$ patients with CD4 counts $<$ 100 cells/uL. Abstract No. 205. In: Abstracts of the Third Conference on Retroviruses and Opportunistic Infections, Washington, DC. Alexandria, Va: Westover Management Group; 1996.
238. Havlir DV, Dube MP, Sattler FR, et al. Prophylaxis against disseminated *Mycobacterium avium* complex with weekly azithromycin, daily rifabutin, or both. N Engl J Med. 1996;335:392.
239. Simon DM, Cello JP, Valenzuela J, et al. Multicenter trial of octreotide in patients with refractory acquired immunodeficiency syndrome–associated diarrhea. Gastroenterology. 1995;108:1753.
240. Ungar BLP, Ward DJ, Fayer R, et al. Cessation of *Cryptosporidium*-associated diarrhea in an acquired immunodeficiency syndrome patient after treatment with hyperimmune bovine colostrum. Gastroenterology. 1990;98:486.
241. Tzipori S, Robertson D, Chapman C. Remission of diarrhea due to cryptosporidiosis in an immunodeficient child treated with hyperimmune bovine colostrum. BMJ. 1986;293:2283.
242. Hewitt RG, Yiannoutsos CT, Higgs ES, et al. for the AIDS Clinical Trials Group. Paromomycin for the treatment of cryptosporidiosis in patients with advanced HIV infection: A randomized, double-blind, placebo-controlled trial. Submitted.
243. Grube H, Ramratnam B, Ley C, et al. Resolution of AIDS associated cryptosporidiosis after treatment with indinavir. Am J Gastroenterol. 1997;92:726.
244. Carr A, Marriott D, Field A, et al. Treatment of HIV-associated microsporidiosis and cryptosporidiosis with combination antiretroviral therapy. Lancet. 1998;351:256.
245. Pape JW, Verdier RI, Johnson WD Jr. Treatment and prophylaxis of *Isospora belli* infection in patients with the acquired immunodeficiency syndrome. N Engl J Med. 1989;320:1044.
246. Pape JW, Verdier RI, Boncy M, et al. Cyclospora infection in adults infected with HIV: Clinical manifestations, treatment, and prophylaxis. Ann Intern Med. 1994;121:654.
247. Dore GJ, Marriott DJ, Hing MC, et al. Disseminated microsporidiosis due to *Septata intestinalis* in nine patients infected with the human immunodeficiency virus: Response to therapy with albendazole. Clin Infect Dis. 1995;21:70.
248. Rosenberger DF, Serdarevic ON, Erlandson RA, et al. Successful treatment of microsporidial keratoconjunctivitis with topical fumagillin in a patient with AIDS. Cornea. 1993;12:261.
249. Diesenhouse MC, Wilson LA, Corrent GF, et al. Treatment of microsporidial keratoconjunctivitis with topical fumagillin. Am J Ophthalmol. 1993;115:293.
250. Lecuit M, Oksenhendler E, Sarfati C. Use of albendazole for disseminated microsporidian infection in a patient with AIDS. Clin Infect Dis. 1994;19:332.
251. Dieterich DT, Lew EA, Kotler DP, et al. Treatment with albendazole for intestinal disease due to *Enterocytozoon bieneusi* in patients with AIDS. J Infect Dis. 1994;169:178.
252. Molina JM, Oksenhendler E, Beauvais B, et al. Disseminated microsporidiosis due to *Septata intestinalis* in patients with AIDS: Clinical features and response to albendazole therapy. J Infect Dis. 1995;171:245.
253. Molina JM, Goguel J, Sarfati C, et al. Drug screening for treatment of *Enterocytozoon bieneusi* infections in patients with HIV infection (ANRS 034). Abstract No. 687. In: Abstracts of the Fourth International Conference on Retroviruses and Opportunistic Infections, Washington, DC, January 22–26, 1996.
254. Cello JP, Grendell JH, Basuk P, et al. Effect of octreotide on refractory AIDS-associated diarrhea. Ann Intern Med. 1991;115:705.
255. Sharpstone D, Rowbotton A, Nelson M, et al. The treatment of microsporidial diarrhea with thalidomide. AIDS. 1995;9:658.
256. Koehler JE. Bartonellosis. In: Dolin R, Masur H, Saag MS. AIDS Therapy. Philadelphia: WB Saunders; 1999:392–399.
257. Berson AM, Quivey JM, Harris JW, et al. Radiation therapy for AIDS-related Kaposi's sarcoma. Int J Radiat Oncol Biol Phys. 1993;27:1057.
258. Boudreaux AA, Smith LL, Cosby CD, et al. Intralesional vinblastine for cutaneous Kaposi's sarcoma associated with acquired immunodeficiency syndrome: A clinical trial to evaluate efficacy and discomfort associated with injection. J Am Acad Dermatol. 1993;28:61.
259. Krown SE, Gold JWM, Niedzwiecki D, et al. Interferon-α with zidovudine: Safety, tolerance, and clinical and virologic effects in patients with Kaposi's sarcoma associated with the acquired immunodeficiency syndrome (AIDS). Ann Intern Med. 1990;112:812.
260. Levine AM, Sullivan-Halley J, Pike MC, et al. HIV-related lymphoma: Prognostic factors predictive of survival. Cancer. 1991;68:2466.
261. Saleh M, Scadden D. Non-Hodgkin's lymphoma. In: Dolin R, Masur H, Saag MS. AIDS Therapy. Philadelphia: WB Saunders; 1999:592–604.

Chapter 117

Vaccines for Human Immunodeficiency Virus-1 Infection

RAPHAEL DOLIN
MICHAEL C. KEEFER

The development of safe and effective vaccines against human immunodeficiency virus-1 (HIV-1) infection or associated disease, or both, is the object of intensive research efforts throughout the world. It is becoming increasingly clear that effective vaccination offers the best hope for containing the epidemic of HIV-1 infection, particularly in areas of the world where extraordinarily rapid spread is being observed (see Chapter 104). The effects of the newly developed highly active antiretroviral therapy remain of uncertain duration, and in any case, because of high cost and limited availability, highly active antiretroviral therapy is beyond the reach of most individuals at risk for HIV infection, except perhaps for segments of the population in developed countries. Attempts to modify high-risk behavior to control the spread of HIV-1 have met with variable success, although in some areas, extensive implementation of such efforts is just now beginning to get under way. Thus, national and international public health agencies have afforded the highest priority to efforts to develop HIV vaccines. The explosive spread of acquired immunodeficiency syndrome in the developing world has imparted a particular sense of urgency to these efforts.

The development of vaccines against HIV-1 presents formidable scientific, logistic, and social challenges, and these have been the subject of several recent reviews.[1–3] Among the most important problems is a current lack of understanding of the critical parameters of immunity that would protect against HIV infection or disease, or both. Additionally, substantial genotypic variation occurs among HIV-1 strains, along with high frequencies of mutation and recombination in the replication of individual isolates. The relationship of these genotypic variations to the expression of antigens that might induce protective immunity remains poorly defined. However, it appears likely that an effective vaccine will have to stimulate broadly directed immune responses, that is, those that are able to inhibit antigenically diverse strains of HIV-1.

Historically, investigation of these types of questions has been greatly facilitated by the use of animal model systems. In this regard, nonhuman primate models of infection with simian immunodeficiency virus (SIV) have provided important information and will likely continue to do so in the future. However, nonhuman primates do not represent a fully satisfactory model for HIV infection in humans at present (see further on). Thus, carefully conducted studies of candidate HIV-1 vaccines in human volunteers have been undertaken and have provided a substantial body of information regarding responses to HIV-1 immunogens. Data from these studies, along with those from studies of immune responses in HIV-1–infected patients, form the basis for the current approaches to the development of HIV-1 vaccines reviewed in this chapter.

IMMUNE RESPONSES TO HUMAN IMMUNODEFICIENCY VIRUS-1 INFECTION

In recent years, the molecular virology and antigenic characteristics of HIV-1 have been elucidated in extraordinary detail (See Chapters 107 and 157). In humans infected with HIV-1, humoral and cell-mediated immune responses directed at a variety of viral antigens have been described. However, as noted earlier, the correlation of specific immune responses with protection from infection or disease, or both, has not yet been accomplished. The implications for vaccine development of HIV-1–specific immune responses in HIV-1–infected patients are reviewed further on.

NEUTRALIZING ANTIBODIES

The level of neutralizing antibodies has been correlated with vaccine efficacy in several viral infections; thus, there has been particular interest in the role that stimulation of such antibodies might play in an efficacious HIV vaccine. Antibodies that neutralize HIV in vitro are directed against a variety of epitopes on HIV-1 proteins, most extensively on the envelope glycoproteins gp120 and gp41.[4–6] These include antibodies directed at a 35–amino acid linear portion of the third variable region of gp120 ("V3 loop")[7] as well as to the CD4 binding domain of the envelope protein.[8] The latter is a discontinuous and highly conformationally dependent site.[9] Neutralizing antibodies directed against the V3 loop are generally more narrow (strain-specific) in their activity than are the more broadly active antibodies directed against the CD4 binding domain.[8, 10] Additional epitopes for neutralization antibodies have been described on the V2 region of gp120[11] and on gp41.[12] Neutralizing antibodies have also been detected against gag, pol, and various regulatory proteins, but they likely play minor roles in neutralizing activity against HIV-1.[13, 14]

For measurement of neutralizing activity, the passage history of isolates of HIV-1 employed in the test is an important variable. T-cell line–adapted (TCLA) viruses are considerably "easier" to neutralize than are non–laboratory-adapted ("primary") isolates.[15] In fact, antibodies generated by vaccine candidates studied in phase I/II trials, thus far, have not been able to neutralize primary isolates, even when high titers of neutralizing activity against laboratory-adapted strains are present. The reasons for this are currently unclear; but this observation suggests that neutralization epitopes may differ between primary and laboratory-adapted isolates, or perhaps are differentially expressed or presented in TCLA viruses and primary isolates. The recent elucidation of the three-dimensional structure of the HIV-1 envelope indicates that it has a highly dynamic configuration, with important differences based on the state of activation and binding to cellular receptors.[16] Factors such as glycosylation, protein folding, and oligomerization may also be important to the antigenic properties of HIV envelope proteins.

Various levels of neutralizing antibodies are present throughout the course of HIV-1 infection. They can be detected within weeks after the onset of symptoms in primary HIV-1 infection and may play a role in the early reduction of plasma viremia, although they are clearly inadequate over time to clear the HIV infection.[17] The reasons for the relative lack of effectiveness of the neutralizing response is not fully understood. In part, it may be related to the generation of "escape mutants" during active virus replication, which leads to viruses that are less susceptible to neutralization by the initial immune responses to infection.[18] Overall, a consistent correlation between levels of neutralizing antibodies and the clinical course of HIV-associated disease has not been found, although some studies indicated that the presence of broadly neutralizing antibodies is a favorable prognostic indicator.[19]

In addition to neutralization activity, antibody-dependent cellular cytotoxicity against HIV-1 can be detected in HIV-infected patients. Antibody-dependent cellular cytotoxicity is directed primarily against sites on the viral envelope, including the V3 loop[20] and the extracellular domain of gp41.[21] The significance of antibody-dependent cellular cytotoxicity as a host defense against HIV-1 infection remains undefined.

CELL-MEDIATED IMMUNE RESPONSES

Cell-mediated responses are considered to be important in the restriction of virus replication and thus in the resolution of a number of viral infections. In particular, T-cell cytotoxic activity, mediated by $CD8^+$ T cells in the context of major histocompatibility (MHC) class I restriction, is an important mechanism for elimination of virus-infected host cells. Cytotoxic T-cell (CTL) activity against HIV antigens, including both $CD4^+$ and $CD8^+$ effector cells, has been detected in HIV-1–seropositive individuals and appears to wane as HIV-1 disease progresses.[22–24] $CD4^+$ and $CD8^+$ CTL activities have also been detected in humans immunized with candidate HIV-1 vaccines (see further on). CTL activity is directed against antigens on a variety of HIV-1 proteins, including envelope glycoproteins, and internal structural proteins (p17, p24, p15), as well as against the products of regulatory genes, including *nef* and *vif,* and *pol* products.[22, 25–29] In recipients of candidate acquired immunodeficiency syndrome vaccines, $CD8^+$ CTL has been detected only after administration of live-virus vector vaccines.[30–33] The administration of subunit vaccines alone has generated only $CD4^+$ CTL to date.[3]

CTLs are capable of lysis of cells infected with primary isolates of HIV-1 and demonstrate broad-based activity against isolates from different clades.[34, 35] CTL activity induced by HIV-2 can also lyse HIV-1–infected cells.[36] Several lines of evidence suggest that $CD8^+$ CTL activity may be important in the control of HIV-1 replication in vivo. As noted earlier, CTL activity decreases as HIV-1–associated disease progresses. In commercial sex workers in the Gambia and Kenya who remain uninfected with HIV-1 despite multiple sexual exposures, HIV-1–specific $CD8^+$ CTL activity has been detected.[37, 38] HIV-1–specific CTLs have also been detected in uninfected infants born to HIV-1–infected mothers.[39] The significance of $CD4^+$ CTL activity directed against HIV-1 in vivo is not known.

Recently, patients with stable, low levels of HIV-1 viremia ("nonprogressors") have been noted to have high levels of HIV-1–specific lymphoproliferative responses,[40] and it has been suggested that this is a marker for the ability of the immune response to control viral replication. The means by which lymphoproliferative responses might exert an inhibitory effect on HIV infection (e.g., by providing helper functions to $CD8^+$ CTLs or through another effector mechanism) is not known.

POTENTIALLY DELETERIOUS IMMUNE RESPONSES

The possibility that HIV-1 infection or immunization may induce immune responses that are deleterious to the host has been an ongoing concern in efforts to develop HIV-1 vaccines. Antibody-dependent enhancement of in vitro infection with HIV-1, either by complement-mediated or Fc-mediated mechanisms, has been reported.[41, 42] This apparently occurs by the interaction of virus-antibody complexes, with or without complement, with cells that bear Fc or complement receptors. This interaction may facilitate (enhance) entry of virus into cells that otherwise might not be infected by the virus. Such enhancing antibodies have been detected in vitro in serum specimens from patients with HIV-1 infection, as well as following immunization with recombinant HIV-1 envelope glycoproteins.[43, 44] Complement-mediated antibody-dependent enhancement of epitopes have been detected on gp41,[45, 46] and an Fc-mediated conformational epitope has been identified on gp120.[47] However, enhancement of infection has not been observed in vivo,[43, 44] and the biologic significance of enhancing antibodies is not known.

As is the case with proteins contained in other viruses, HIV-1 proteins have areas of homology with naturally occurring host regulatory and structural proteins. These include areas of homology between gp120 and interleukin-2,[48] neuroleukin,[49] and β-chains of MHC class II molecules[50]; between gp41 and HLA-DR molecules[51]; and between gag protein and thymosin α1.[52] The significance of these observations is unknown. Although the potential for deleterious immune responses remains a consideration in the development of HIV-1 vaccines, it should be noted that autoimmunity, immunosuppression, enhancement of infection, or other deleterious effects have not been detected in studies of candidate HIV vaccines in humans or in animal models to date (see further on).

TYPES OF CANDIDATE HUMAN IMMUNODEFICIENCY VIRUS-1 VACCINES

Because of the uncertainty regarding the optimal type of immune responses that should be generated by an HIV-1 vaccine, a variety of different approaches to candidate HIV-1 vaccines has been proposed. Some of these are currently at various stages of preclinical development, whereas others have entered or completed phase I and II trials in humans (Table 117–1). One candidate vaccine, a recombinant gp120, is being evaluated in two phase III efficacy trials (see further on). The major types of candidate vaccines under development or consideration are discussed in the following sections.

Whole Virus Vaccines

Traditionally, the initial approach to the development of virus vaccines has been to generate an inactivated or "killed" whole virus preparation. This may be particularly advantageous when the parameters of immunity are not defined and, therefore, when the critical antigenic components of a vaccine are difficult to predict. Compared with a subunit preparation, a whole virus vaccine offers inclusion of a larger number of potentially relevant antigens. In HIV-1 vaccine development, this approach has received relatively little emphasis, primarily because of considerations of safety. The chief concern is related to the potential hazard of retained genetic material in such a vaccine (i.e., the potential risk of transmission of infectious HIV-1). Whole virus vaccines can now be prepared by techniques that render any remaining nucleic acid extremely unlikely to be infectious, and such vaccines can be ascertained to be free of nucleic acids by techniques of extraordinarily high sensitivity. However, the lack of an entirely appropriate animal model in which to demonstrate that a vaccine preparation is free of infectious HIV-1 still poses a significant problem.

Envelope Proteins

Vaccines composed of HIV-1 envelope proteins have undergone the most extensive study. As noted earlier, important neutralizing epitopes, as well as T-cell epitopes, have been identified on HIV-1 envelope proteins. Envelope HIV-1 vaccines studied in humans have been generated through recombinant DNA expression systems, which provide an efficient means to prepare large quantities of purified proteins and also bypass concerns about possible contamination with other HIV-1 components. These recombinant proteins have been generated from laboratory-adapted HIV strains with a number of different vectors and cell systems, including insect,[53] yeast,[54] and mammalian cell cultures.[55–57] Depending on the vector and cell system employed, as well as on the purification procedures, these recombinant proteins may have important differences when compared with their naturally occurring analogues, including differences in tertiary structure, glycosylation, and oligomerization. Envelope protein vaccine candidates that have been evaluated in human trials include an rgp160 generated via a baculovirus vector and produced in insect cells (LAI strain)[44, 44a]; a fully glycosylated rgp160 made via a vaccinia vector in Vero cells (LAI and MN strains)[57]; a nonglycosylated rgp120 made in yeast cells (SF-2 strain)[58]; an rgp120 generated in Chinese hamster ovary cells (SF-2)[59]; and an rgp120 generated in Chinese hamster ovary cells (IIIB and MN strains).[60, 61] The preceding rgp120 vaccines have been derived from TCLA viruses. However, rgp120 subunit candidate vaccines have been generated from primary isolates from clade B (GNE8) and clade E (A244) viruses.

Synthetic Peptides

Another approach to the development of envelope vaccines is the generation of synthetic peptides that include only epitopes of immunologic interest rather than the entire gp160 or gp120 proteins themselves. This affords the opportunity to include only those epitopes that are most important for a protective response in the vaccine and to exclude minor or even potentially deleterious epitopes, such as ones that might be associated with enhancement of infection or immunopathogenesis. Conversely, a potential disadvantage of this approach is that synthetic peptides may not stimulate immune responses to noncontiguous or conformationally dependent epitopes. In addition, synthetic peptides are generally not as immunogenic as whole or native proteins. However, this problem might be overcome by coupling peptides to protein carriers or by addition of more potent adjuvants, or by both. An example of this approach is a vaccine candidate that consists of synthetically produced peptides from the V3 loops of multiple strains of HIV-1, linked to an oligolysine backbone.[62] Another example of this approach is a hybrid linear peptide that consists of multiple epitopes that are recognized by B cells, T-helper cells and CTLs.[63, 64]

Internal or Core Proteins

Vaccine candidates comprised of HIV-1 internal proteins, either entirely or in part, have received relatively less attention. As noted earlier, it is believed that core proteins are particularly important in the generation of cell-mediated immune responses and especially CTLs, although neutralizing antibodies against internal proteins have been reported as well. Examples of vaccine candidates based on internal proteins include a 30–amino acid peptide of p17 of HIV-1 (HGP-30)[65]; a portion of p17/p24 proteins formulated as a virus-like particle by introduction into the yeast retrotransposon Ty (Ty-Gag)[66]; and a p24 protein generated via a baculovirus vector or via Chinese hamster ovary cells.[67]

LIVE VECTORS

Considerable interest exists in the development of a live vector vaccine for HIV-1. Such a vaccine has the potential to present HIV-1 antigens in the context of a replicating microbial system and, in the case of an obligate intracellular organism such as a virus, the antigens are expressed by host cells. Presentation of antigen to the host in this manner may result in a more efficient immune response,

TABLE 117-1 Phase I Studies of Candidate HIV-1 Vaccines in HIV-1 Seronegative Volunteers

Vaccine Type	Cell Type, Production Method	HIV-1 Strain	Sponsor	Reference
Envelope Proteins				
rgp 160	Insect (baculovirus)	LAI	MicroGeneSys	44, 44a, 124
rgp 160	Vero (vaccinia)	LAI, MN	ImmunoAG	93, 93a, 125, 125a
rgp 120 (Env 2-3)	Yeast	SF-2	Chiron/Biocine	58, 91
rgp 120	CHO	LAI/MN	Genentech	60, 61
rgp 120	CHO	SF-2	Chiron/Biocine	59, 92
Peptides				
gp120-V3 loop peptides	Synthetic octameric peptides	MN, 15 strains	United Biomedical Inc.	104, 104a
p14HGP 30	Synthetic linear peptide (p17)	LAI	Viral Technologies Inc.	101–103
Gag lipopeptide P3C541b	Synthetic linear peptide	—	United Biomedical Inc.	AVEG 021*
p14/p24:Ty-VLP	VLP, yeast transposon	LAI	British Biotech PLC	126, AVEG 019*
HIV-1 gp120 C4-V3 peptides	Hybrid synthetic peptides	MN, EV91, RF, CANO	Wyeth-Lederle, Haynes	AVEG 020*
Live Vectors				
HIVAC-1e	Vaccinia construct with gp160	LAI	Bristol-Myers-Squibb (Oncogen)	109, 112
Vaccinia-HIV (TBC-3B)	Vaccinia construct with gp160, gag, pol	IIIB	Therion Biologics	111
Canarypox vCP 125	Canarypox construct with gp160	MN	Pasteur-Merieux-Connaught	114–116
Canarypox vCP 205	Canarypox with gp120, TM gp41, gag, protease	MN/LAI	Pasteur-Merieux-Connaught	116a, 127
Canarypox vCP 300	Canarypox with gp120, TM gp41, gag, protease, CTL epitopes in pol and nef	MN/LAI	Pasteur-Merieux-Connaught	116b
Canarypox vCP 1433	Canarypox with gp120, TM gp41, gag, protease CTL epitopes in pol and nef	MN/LAI	Pasteur-Merieux-Connaught	AVEG 034*
Canarypox vCP 1452	Canarypox as 1433 with two vaccinia virus coding sequences		Pasteur-Merieux-Connaught	AVEG 034*
Salmonella typhi CVD 908 VVG 203	*S. typhi* vector expressing gp120	LAI	Univ. of Maryland Center for Vaccine Development	AVEG 028*
Live Vector + Subunit Boost				
HIVAC-1e + rgp160 (baculovirus)	—†	LAI	Oncogen/MicroGeneSys	30, 113, 117
HIVAC-le + rgp160		LAI + MN	Oncogen/ImmunoAG	128
HIVAC-1e + rgp120 (CHO)	—	LAI + SF-2	Oncogen/Chiron	128
HIVAC-1e + rgp120 (CHO)	—	LAI + LAI or MN	Oncogen/Genentech	128
TBC-3B + rgp120 (CHO)	—	+ MN	Theron/VaxGen	111
vCP125 + rgp120 (CHO)	—	MN + SF-2	PMC+/Chiron	114
vCP205 + rgp120 (CHO)	—	MN + SF-2	PMC/Chiron	116a
vCP300 + rgp120 (CHO)	—	MN + SF-2	PMC/Chiron	116b
DNA Vaccines				
HIV-1 env/rev (APL 400-003)	GeneVax-HIV DNA plasmid backbone	MN	Wyeth-Lederle	—
HIV-1 core (APL 400-047)	GeneVax-HIV DNA plasmid backbone	HXB2 (LAI)	Wyeth-Lederle	78

*AVEG, AIOS Vaccine Evaluation Group protocol number—studies in progress.
†As noted above.

particularly with respect to the generation of MHC class I restricted $CD8^+$ CTLs. The development of an efficiently replicating, genetically stable, live vector also offers important advantages for the large-scale production of vaccines. Some live vectors, such as vaccinia virus, are also resistant to environmental inactivation, which is of practical importance for the use of vaccines in field conditions in developing countries. However, live vectors need to be selected carefully because they can contribute morbidity of their own in certain clinical settings (e.g., administration of a vaccinia vector to individuals with eczema or depressed cell-mediated immune defenses). An additional limitation of live vector vaccines is the development of immunity to the vector after initial immunization so that repeated doses (boosts) with the vector may not be possible, at least over the short term. However, it may be possible to boost with the protein product of the HIV-1 gene inserted in the vector (e.g., with gp160) rather than with the live vector itself, as discussed further on.

The most extensively studied live vectors for HIV-1 vaccine development are the poxvirus vectors vaccinia[68] and canarypox.[69] They are well characterized, contain large DNA genomes into which multiple genes can be inserted, and infect multiple cell types. Stable constructs have been generated that contain various combinations of HIV-1 *env, gag, pol,* and regulatory genes, and these have undergone or are undergoing evaluations in clinical trials (see further on). As noted earlier, vaccinia vectors have the potential risk of causing serious illness in immunosuppressed subjects or those with eczematoid skin disorders, either as a result of vaccination or by spread from vaccines. Further attenuated vaccinia vectors are being developed to address this concern.[70, 71] Canarypox has the advantage of undergoing a single-cycle, nonproductive infection in mammalian cells and therefore does not result in disease or transmission when administered to humans. However, the canarypox vectors appear somewhat less immunogenic overall than vaccinia vectors.

Additional vectors for HIV-1 vaccines that have been proposed and are at various stages of development include adenovirus,[72] poliovirus,[73] salmonella,[74] and bacille Calmette-Guérin.[75] A vector of particular interest is Venezuelan equine encephalitis virus.[76] This virus has a predilection for infection of dendritic cells and can stimulate high levels of both systemic immunity and local IgA production.

Venezuelan equine encephalitis–HIV-1 constructs have been generated that are under evaluation in primate model systems.

Nucleic Acid Vaccination

The observation that segments of nucleic acid genome or plasmids ("naked DNA") could be administered intramuscularly, and subsequently undergo transcription and express proteins, has led to the use of this technique as a means to deliver antigens for immunization. This technique permits the construction of a vaccine that consists only of the component of immunologic interest. The proteins are also presented through the MHC class I–restricted pathway, thus stimulating CTLs. DNA vaccination is being studied for a variety of potential viral vaccines, including phase I studies with HIV-1 vaccines[77, 78] (see Table 117–1).

Live Attenuated Virus Vaccines

The use of live attenuated vaccines has been highly successful in the control of several important viral diseases, such as measles, rubella, and polio. Live attenuated vaccines have the advantage of presenting vaccine antigens in a manner that most closely resembles naturally occurring infection and also stimulates a broad array of humoral and cell-mediated immune responses. With some live attenuated vaccines, immunity may be particularly long-lasting. Depending on the site of immunization, live attenuated viruses (or live vectors) may be highly efficient in stimulation of local (mucosal) immunity, which may be especially important in the prevention of HIV-1 infection transmitted by the sexual route. Boosting by repeated mucosal immunization may also be possible, depending on the intensity and duration of local immune responses stimulated by initial immunization.

Clearly, the major concern in the development of live attenuated HIV-1 vaccine candidates is safety. The problem of devising adequate safety tests, particularly with the lack of an entirely suitable animal model for HIV-1 disease, was noted earlier. The incomplete understanding of the pathogenesis of HIV-1–associated disease, and therefore the associated difficulty of identification of "virulence" factors, has also inhibited attempts to develop live attenuated viruses. HIV-1 is known to have a number of regulatory genes that affect different points of the virus replicative cycle (see Chapter 157). One approach to the development of a live attenuated vaccine has been to delete one or more regulatory genes, which can result in a mutant virus that has lost pathogenicity. Because such a virus has a genetic deletion, it would appear less likely to revert to its pathogenic parent, at least by reconstruction of the deleted gene. The attenuated mutant virus would nonetheless have to replicate sufficiently well to stimulate humoral and cell-mediated immunity. One such live attenuated SIV vaccine, in which the *nef* gene has been deleted,[79] has provided the most impressive protection against virulent SIV challenge among the candidate SIV vaccines tested in macaques thus far (see further on). The precise mechanism of protection for the *nef*-deleted vaccine is unclear but may depend on the continued presence of replicating virus in various cellular compartments. As with other live virus vaccines, attenuation is a relative term and is highly dependent on host factors. *Nef*-deleted SIV viruses that are nonpathogenic in adult monkeys have caused disease when administered to neonatal animals.[80, 80a] Even in adult monkeys, *nef*-deleted mutants have been observed to undergo repair with restoration of virulence, illustrating the risks inherent in such an approach.[81] Nonetheless, the development of a live attenuated vaccine to HIV-1 continues to be an important area for investigation.

ANIMAL MODELS

The availability of an appropriate and practical animal model would be of great importance to studies of the pathogenesis of HIV-1 disease and to the development of vaccines and chemotherapeutic agents. For the development of vaccines, the availability of an animal model is particularly important because it offers the opportunity to conduct experimental virus challenges and thus study the protective effects of candidate vaccines directly. Despite the fact that considerable progress has been made in this area, there is as yet no entirely suitable animal model of HIV-1 infection. Chimpanzees are the only established animal model system in which experimental infection with HIV-1 can be consistently achieved. After infection, chimpanzees mount immune responses to HIV-1, and virus can be isolated from peripheral blood mononuclear cells, although this becomes increasingly difficult as time passes. HIV-1–infected chimpanzees do not show consistent evidence of HIV-related disease, although recently HIV-1 strains have been adapted that have been reported to cause disease in chimpanzees.[82, 83] In addition, chimpanzees are extraordinarily expensive and in short supply so that only small numbers are available for experimental studies of candidate vaccines. The most extensively developed primate model is the macaque, most frequently *Macaca mulatta,* or rhesus macaque, which can be infected with SIV.[84] This model has the advantage that SIV causes disease in macaques, and macaques are much more readily available and less expensive than chimpanzees. After an incubation period that is considerably shorter than that seen in humans infected with HIV, SIV infection results in immunosuppression and in the development of opportunistic infections. Death often results within 3 to 5 months. A particularly virulent strain, $SIV_{pbj,}$ exists that can cause overwhelming disease 1 to 2 weeks after infection.[85] Although differences in the frequency and type of opportunistic processes exist between SIV-induced disease in macaques and HIV-1–induced disease in humans, overall the disease patterns have many features in common. SIV- and HIV-1 are also similar in structure and organization, although some differences exist.[86, 87] The inability to infect macaques with HIV-1 has prevented candidate HIV-1 vaccines from being directly examined in that animal model. Recently, chimeric viruses (SHIV) have been developed that have an envelope derived from HIV-1 and internal proteins from SIV; these viruses can infect macaques.[88] SHIVs offer promise of great utility in studies of candidate HIV-1 vaccines in macaques.

More than 500 studies of the effects of vaccination have been carried out in primate models using a variety of vaccine approaches. As noted earlier, there are SIV strains that have a broad range of virulence, ranging from persistent infection with little or no disease, to rapid, lethal infection. As might be anticipated, candidate vaccines have been generally more effective in inducing protection against less virulent experimental infection, such as $SIVmac_{Bk28}$ or HIV-1 in chimpanzees, than against a more virulent challenge such as $SIVsm_{pbj14}$. In infections with this latter agent, the greatest levels of protection were associated with the use of a live attenuated SIV vaccine.[79] In addition to the virulence of the challenge strain of virus, important variables to be considered in interpretation of primate challenge studies are the dose of challenge virus, the route of administration of virus (intravenous versus intrarectal or intravaginal), the homology between immunizing virus and challenge strain, and the type of end point that was used for evidence of efficacy. The heterogeneity of experimental conditions under which primate challenge studies have been carried out has resulted in apparent inconsistencies of results among some studies and difficulty in generalizing conclusions from others. Overall, a definition of the critical in vitro correlates of protection has not yet emerged from these studies. Nonetheless, as primate models continue to be refined and experimental conditions are further standardized, primate models will undoubtedly play an important role in efforts to develop HIV vaccines. For a detailed description of the results of immunization and virus challenge studies in primate model systems, the reader is referred to excellent recent reviews of the subject.[89–90a]

HUMAN TRIALS

The study of candidate HIV-1 vaccines in humans poses several unique problems above and beyond those encountered in studies of

TABLE 117–2 Phase II Studies of Candidate HIV-1 Vaccines in HIV-1–Seronegative Volunteers

Vaccine	Cell Type, Production Method	HIV-1 Strain	Sponsor	Reference
rgp 120	CHO cells	SF-2 + MN	Chiron/Biocine, Pasteur-Mérieux-Connaught	94
VCP 205 + rgp 120	Canarypox-gp120, TM gp41, gag, protease, CHO cells	MN/LAI, SF-2	Pasteur-Mérieux-Connaught, Chiron/Biocine	AVEG 202*

*AVEG, AIDS Vaccine Evaluation Group protocol number—studies in progress.

other experimental vaccines. Volunteers need to be fully informed of the potential hazards of immunization and of the limitations of our knowledge regarding the pathogenesis of HIV-1–associated disease. Volunteers must be made aware that they may become seropositive for HIV-1 by conventional "screening assays" and of the possible difficulties of employment, eligibility for insurance, and immigration that might result. Volunteers must also be counseled not to abandon behaviors to reduce risk of acquisition of HIV-1 infection because of a hope that the vaccine under study will provide protection against such infection. A detailed description of the procedures employed in the conduct of phase I studies of HIV-1 candidate vaccines in humans, including measures taken to address the preceding issues, has been published.[44]

The purpose of the initial trials (phase I studies) that have been undertaken is to examine the immunogenicity and safety of various vaccine candidates in humans. As noted earlier, studies in primates have not clearly established the superiority of one vaccine approach over another, and therefore several different types of vaccine candidates are being evaluated in humans (see Table 117–1). Studies directed at the development of preventive vaccines have been carried out in healthy, HIV-1 seronegative volunteers. For phase I studies, these individuals have been determined to be at low risk for acquisition of HIV-1 infection to avoid the potentially confounding effects of an intercurrent HIV-1 infection in the study. Phase II studies have been carried out in subjects at higher risk for the acquisition of HIV-1 infection (Table 117–2). Vaccines intended for immunotherapy have been studied in HIV-1–seropositive subjects (see further on) (Table 117–3).

Recombinant Envelope Proteins

Recombinant envelope proteins (rgp160 and rgp 120) have undergone the most extensive study in humans thus far. The viruses from which the envelope proteins were derived were mostly from clade B (LAI, SF-2, and MN strains) and were from TCLA-adapted X4 viruses. Exceptions to this were the recently generated rgp120 from a primary isolate of clade B, and rgp120 from a primary isolate from clade E. Combinations of these latter rgp120s are intended for use in phase III efficacy trials that are currently either under way or planned to get under way shortly (see further on).

The majority of studies with the preceding vaccines were phase I studies of safety and immunogenicity carried out in relatively small numbers of volunteers at "low risk" for acquisition of HIV-1 infection as noted previously.[44, 44a, 58–61, 91–93a] These studies also examined the effects of varying dosages and schedules of immunization. A phase II study compared two rgp120s derived from MN and SF-2 strains in a larger group of 220 subjects who were at high risk for acquisition of HIV-1 infection[94] and who perhaps might be more representative of the ultimate target groups for an HIV-1 vaccine. The recombinant envelope vaccines were administered intramuscularly in multiple-dose schedules, combined with various adjuvants. Overall, the recombinant envelope HIV-1 candidate vaccines were very well tolerated.[94a] Vaccinees experienced mild local reactions comparable in frequency and magnitude to those seen with administration of licensed vaccines. An exception to this was the combination of rgp120 with MTP-PE, a synthetic lipophilic muramyl tripeptide adjuvant, which had a significantly higher rate of local and systemic reactions.[91]

Immunization with at least three doses of these recombinant envelope proteins resulted in high rates (>90%) of binding antibodies to specific HIV-1 proteins as determined by western blot or enzyme-linked immunosorbent assay. High rates of neutralizing antibodies were also induced by the rgp120 immunogens, particularly those generated in Chinese hamster ovary cells.[59–61, 92] In general, rgp120 immunogens induced more neutralizing, but less binding, antibodies than did the rgp160 immunogens.

Neutralizing antibodies were generally restricted to type-specific activity against the homologous isolate. Perhaps most troubling was the unanticipated observation that serum neutralizing activity from the vaccinees was effective only against laboratory-adapted viruses grown in T-cell lines, whereas non-laboratory–adapted HIV-1 viruses ("primary isolates") were not neutralized.[95–97] Subsequent discoveries of HIV coreceptors and structural definition of the HIV envelope have helped to explain why the immune responses to T-cell line–adapted viruses might be different from those to primary isolates. It is now appreciated that the process of attachment of envelope proteins to receptors and coreceptors is extraordinarily complex. This process "triggers" conformational changes in envelope proteins that may result in unmasking or display of epitopes critical for neutralization that may be otherwise hidden.[16] In addition, the highly conformational nature of certain neutralization epitopes may mean that factors such as protein folding, state of oligomerization, patterns of glycosylation and other post-translational changes may be important to the induction of effective neutralizing antibodies to primary isolates.[3]

TABLE 117–3 HIV-1 Vaccines Studied in HIV-1–Infected Patients

Vaccine	Cell Type, Production Method	HIV-1 Strain	Sponsor	Reference
Whole Virus	Inactivated by beta-propiolactone and gamma-irradiation	HZ-321	Immune Research Corp.	118, 118a
Envelope Proteins				
rgp160	Insect (baculovirus)	LAI	MicroGeneSys	119, 119a, 123
rgp160	Vero (vaccinia)	LAI	ImmunoAg	129
rgp120	CHO cells	LAI/MN	Genentech	120–122
rgp120	CHO cells	SF-2	Chiron/Biocine	121, 122
rgp120 (Env 2–3)	Yeast	SF-2	Chiron/Biocine	130
Core Protein				
p211 + rgp 160	Insect (baculovirus)	LAI	MicroGeneSys	67

In addition to circulating antibodies, the recombinant immunogens also readily induced T-cell proliferative responses to HIV-1–specific antigens.[98, 99] However, as might be predicted from the known pathway for processing peptide antigens that results in an association with MHC class II molecules, recombinant protein immunogens did not induce CD8$^+$ CTLs, although some CD4$^+$ CTL activity was detected.[100] The phase II study of rgp120s carried out in subjects with higher risks for HIV-1 infection did not show significantly different safety and immunogenicity profiles from those seen in the phase I studies.[94]

Synthetic Peptides

Synthetic peptides that have undergone phase I studies in humans include peptides from envelope or gag proteins derived from clade B viruses or from multiple other clades (see Table 117–1). Several techniques have been employed for the presentation of immunogens in these vaccine formulations, including conjugation with an oligolysine backbone or with a lipopeptide, encapsulation in polyactide copolymers, or as a fusion protein particle in a self-assembling yeast protein, Ty. In general, these peptide vaccines have been poorly immunogenic, whether administered intramuscularly or by rectal or oral routes.[101–107] Low levels of binding antibodies and little or no neutralizing activity were seen. Studies with more complex peptides containing epitopes of neutralizing antibodies, CTLs, and T-helper activity are currently under way.

Live Virus Vector Vaccines

Vaccinia and canarypox vector constructs with inserts of HIV-1 genes have also undergone extensive phase I studies in humans (see Table 117–1). Vaccinia virus vectors that express gp160 alone or multiple HIV-1 proteins (gp160, gag, and pol) have been administered to normal volunteers in studies similar to those previously carried out with the recombinant envelope immunogens.[108–113] The vaccinia constructs were administered by scarification and resulted in local lesions indistinguishable in character from those seen with the vaccinia parent. The vaccinia vectors induced only low levels of humoral antibody. The neutralizing activity that was seen was also relatively restricted, directed at the homologous virus strain, and active only against TCLA viruses but not against primary isolates. However, induction of CD8$^+$ CTLs directed against HIV-1–infected target cells regularly developed.[30, 32, 108] The presence of preexisting immunity to vaccinia reduced immunogenicity of the vector constructs, and initial immunization with the vaccinia vector provided solid immunity against subsequent infection or "takes" with the vector.[30, 109, 112]

Although the vaccinia constructs were generally well tolerated, the possibility exists of serious problems if vaccinia were inadvertently administered or spread to immunosuppressed patients or to those with eczematoid skin disorders. Because of this, vectors were sought that might have less of a risk in this regard. Canarypox is an avian pox virus that undergoes an abortive replicative cycle in mammalian cells. Administration of canarypox to humans does not result in the production of infectious virus, and therefore it provides a greater margin of safety than does vaccinia. Canarypox constructs have been generated that express gp160, gp120/gp41 (transmembrane protein)/gag/protease, with and without the addition of epitopes in nef/pol. In several phase I studies and one phase II study, intramuscularly administered canarypox was very well tolerated and did not result in detectable lesions.[114–116b] The immune responses to the canarypox vectors were similar to those seen with the vaccinia vector. Relatively weak humoral antibody responses were observed, but HIV-1–specific CD8$^+$ CTL responses were seen in 15 to 30% of subjects at any single point in time, and at least once in 35 to 65% of subjects over the duration of the study.[114–116b] Vectors that express multiple HIV antigens appear to induce CTLs with higher frequency than do those that express only one antigen. The kinetics and duration of the CTL responses are not fully defined, but they appear to last for at least 6 months. CTLs induced by the canarypox vectors killed cells infected with primary isolates as well as cells infected with viruses from clades other than the homologous clade B.[34]

Studies from animal models have suggested that administration of a "boost" with the protein product of the gene inserted in the construct may augment the humoral antibody responses observed after administration of the vector alone. This was seen in trials in humans, in which administration of two booster doses of rgp120 after "priming" with vaccinia vectors resulted in high titers of neutralizing antibodies, similar to those seen after three or four doses of rgp120 alone.[30, 117] However, the neutralizing antibodies induced were still relatively type-specific and neutralized TCLA viruses but not primary isolates of HIV-1.

EFFICACY TRIALS OF CANDIDATE HUMAN IMMUNODEFICIENCY VIRUS-1 VACCINES

Determination of the efficacy of a candidate HIV vaccine requires the conduct of large scale, rigorously controlled clinical trials. Such trials present formidable scientific, logistic, and social challenges, and require extensive resources. The appropriate criteria to determine that a candidate HIV vaccine has sufficient promise to proceed to an efficacy trial remain a matter of substantial controversy. This is particularly so because of the lack of understanding of the critical parameters of immunity noted previously and the limitations of information that can be obtained from the animal model systems. Nonetheless, it is increasingly appreciated that properly conducted efficacy trials themselves may provide important information regarding correlates of protection that may not be obtained otherwise, even if the candidate vaccine is only minimally effective. This information could then be "fed back" to investigators for appropriate modification or revision of vaccine development efforts.

As of this writing, a large scale placebo controlled efficacy trial is under way in the United States of an rgp120 vaccine, AIDSVax B/B, which is a combination of envelope subunits from two clade B strains, MN and a primary isolate, GNE8 (Vaxgen, Inc.). An analogous trial with a clade E–based vaccine (Vaxgen, Inc.) is under way in Thailand. The U.S. trial is studying 5000 subjects for at least a 3-year period, with HIV-1 infection as the primary end point of efficacy. An "intermediate size" efficacy trial has been proposed to study the "prime-boost" approach. This involves vaccination with a canarypox vector that expresses HIV-1 *env, gag, protease, pol,* and *nef* gene sequences, followed by a "boost" with an rgp120 protein. This trial is projected to have 920 to 1750 subjects per arm, to be placebo-controlled, and at the end of 3.5 years to have sufficient power to reject a vaccine with less than 30% efficacy. Detailed laboratory studies to investigate possible correlates of immunity are planned. Potential sites are under discussion for the conduct of such a trial, including multiple sites in the United States and in developing countries.

STUDIES IN HIV-1 SEROPOSITIVE PERSONS (IMMUNOTHERAPY)

The goal of vaccination of HIV-1 seropositive persons (immunotherapy) is to induce an immune response in the host that will retard progression of disease, through either inhibition of virus replication or spread, or by other, as yet undefined mechanisms. Several HIV-1 vaccine candidates have undergone study in HIV-1–seropositive individuals. These include the inactivated virus preparation of Salk,[118, 118a] recombinant gp160 and gp120 proteins,[119, 119a, 120] and p24 preparations.[67] These candidate vaccines have been studied primarily in asymptomatic individuals with CD4 counts of 400 and greater, although some studies in patients with lower CD4 counts have also been carried out. Available results from phase 1 studies indicate that these vaccines are generally well tolerated and that they induce a variety of humoral and cellular immune responses to the immunogen that were either previously undetectable or present at low levels only. These responses have included serum antibody rises to specific epitopes on the immunogen, increased T-cell proliferative responses, and increased CTL activity.

The most extensive controlled trial of this approach was conducted by the AIDS Clinical Trial Group (ACTG 214),[121] which investigated the effect of four rgp120 vaccines: a CHO-derived rgp120 (LAI) in an alum adjuvant, a CHO-derived rgp120 (MN) in alum, a CHO-derived rgp120 (SF-2) in MF59, and a yeast-derived rgp120 from SF-2 (Env 2-3) in MF59. These were studied under a double-blind, placebo (adjuvant only)–controlled experimental design in HIV-1–infected patients with CD4 counts greater than 500/mm^3 who were not receiving antiretroviral therapy. The vaccines were very well tolerated, and the LAI- and MN-derived rgp120s induced HIV-specific lymphoproliferative responses in 29 and 24% of subjects, respectively. The SF-2–derived vaccines were less immunogenic. No effects on CD4 counts were noted among the treatment arms. A companion trial was conducted in subjects who had CD4 counts of less than 500/mm^3 on entry, which showed overall lower rates of induction of HIV-specific lymphocyte responses.[121, 122] No effects on CD4 counts or on disease progression were noted. Other studies using rgp160 or rgp120 vaccines in HIV-1–infected subjects have also failed to demonstrate an effect on decline of T cells or on disease progression.[120, 123]

With the advent of highly active antiretroviral therapy, renewed interest has emerged in the use of HIV vaccines in individuals whose virus replication is effectively suppressed. Some have suggested that for this purpose, vaccine preparations should be derived from the patient's own virus. The hope would be that an augmented immune response, in combination with the effects of highly active antiretroviral therapy, might lead to effective control of viral replication and spread. Studies are planned in children and adults with early HIV infection to evaluate this approach.

SUMMARY

A large body of information has been generated concerning the immune responses to HIV-1 infection and to the administration of candidate HIV-1 vaccines in phase I and II studies in humans. Multiple vaccine approaches have been undertaken, the most extensive of which have been of recombinant envelope proteins (rgp120s) and poxvirus vector constructs. Overall, the vaccines have been well tolerated and without serious toxicities. Rgp120s administered in multiple-dose regimens induce binding and neutralizing antibodies that are type-specific. Neutralizing antibodies are active against laboratory-adapted viruses but not against primary isolates. Lymphocyte proliferative responses are seen, but rgp120s do not induce CD8$^+$ CTLs. Poxvirus constructs are poor inducers of humoral antibodies, but they induce CD8$^+$ CTLs that can kill virus-infected cells from multiple clades. Boosting with rgp120s after immunization with pox vectors significantly raises the titers of neutralizing antibodies, although they are still active only against laboratory-adapted viruses. Phase III efficacy trials of an rgp120 vaccine are under way in the United States and Thailand, and plans are being formulated for an "intermediate-sized efficacy trial" of a canarypox vector followed by an rgp120 boost. Novel vectors, DNA vaccines, and other vaccine approaches are in various stages of development.

REFERENCES

1. Johnston MI. HIV vaccines: problem and prospects. Hosp Pract. 1997;5:125–140.
2. Letvin NL. Progress in the development of an HIV vaccine. Science. 1998;280:1875–1880.
3. Graham B, Karzon DT. AIDS vaccine development. In: Merigan TC, Bartlett JG, Bolognesi D (eds). AIDS Medicine. Baltimore, MD: Williams & Wilkins; 1999:689–724.
4. Palker TJ, Clark ME, Langlois AJ, et al. Type-specific neutralization of the human immunodeficiency virus with antibiotics to env-encoded synthetic peptides. Proc Natl Acad Sci U S A. 1988;85:1932–1936.
5. Javaherian K, Langlois AJ, McDanal C, et al. Principal neutralizing domain of the human immunodeficiency virus type 1 envelope protein. Proc Natl Acad Sci U S A. 1989;86:6768–6772.
6. Ivanoff LA, Looney DJ, McDanal C, et al. Alteration of HIV-1 infectivity and neutralization by a single amino acid replacement in the V3 loop domain. AIDS Res Hum Retroviruses. 1991;7:595–603.
7. Javaherian K, Langlois AJ, LaRosa GJ, et al. Broadly neutralizing antibodies elicited by the hypervariable neutralizing determinant of HIV-1. Science. 1990;250:1590–1593.
8. Ho DD, McKeating JA, Li XL, et al. Conformational epitope on gp120 important in CD4 binding and human immunodeficiency virus type 1 neutralization identified by a human monoclonal antibody. J Virol. 1991;65:489–493.
9. Thali M, Olshevsky U, Furman C, et al. Characterization of a discontinuous human immunodeficiency virus type 1 gp120 epitope recognized by a broadly reactive neutralizing human monoclonal antibody. J Virol. 1991;65:6188–6193.
10. Thali M, Furman C, Ho DD, et al. Discontinuous, conserved neutralization epitopes overlapping the CD4-binding region of human immunodeficiency virus type 1 gp120 envelope glycoprotein. J Virol. 1992;66:5635–5641.
11. McKeating JA, Shotton C, Cordell J, et al. Characterization of neutralizing monoclonal antibodies to linear and conformation-dependent epitopes within the first and second variable domains of human immunodeficiency virus type 1 gp120. J Virol. 1993;67:4932–4944.
12. Muster T, Steindl F, Purtscher M, et al. A conserved neutralizing epitope on gp41 of human immunodeficiency virus type 1. J Virol. 1993;67:6642–6647.
13. Papsidero LD, Sheu M, Ruscetti FW. Human immunodeficiency virus type 1 neutralizing monoclonal antibodies which react with p17 core protein characterization and epitope mapping. J Virol. 1989;63:267–272.
14. Sano K, Lee MH, Morales F, et al. Antibody that inhibits human immunodeficiency virus reverse transcriptase and association with inability to isolate virus. J Clin Microbiol. 1987;25:2415–2417.
15. Moore JP, Cao Y, Qing L, et al. Primary isolates of human immunodeficiency virus type 1 are relatively resistant to neutralization by monoclonal antibodies to gp120, and their neutralization is not predicted by studies with monomeric gp120. J Virol. 1995;69:101–109.
16. Wyatt R, Sodroski J. The HIV-1 envelope glycoproteins: Fusogens, antigens, and immunogens. Science. 1998;280:1884–1888.
17. Clark SJ, Saag MS, Decker WD, et al. High titers of cytopathic virus in plasma of patients with symptomatic primary HIV-1 infection. N Engl J Med. 1991;324:954–960.
18. Arendrup M, Nielsen C, Hansen JE, et al. Autologous HIV-1 neutralizing antibodies: Emergence of neutralization-resistant escape virus and subsequent development of escape virus neutralizing antibodies. J Acquir Immune Defic Syndr. 1992;5:303–307.
19. Montefiori DC, Pantaleo G, Fink LM, et al. Neutralizing and infection-enhancing antibody responses to human immunodeficiency virus type 1 in long term nonprogressors. J Infect Dis. 1996;173:60–67.
20. Baum LL, Cassutt KJ, Knigge K, et al. HIV-1 gp120-specific antibody-dependent cell mediated cytotoxicity correlates with rate of disease progression. J Immunol. 1996;157:2168–2173.
21. Tyler DS, Stanley SD, Zolla-Pazner SB, et al. Identifications of sites within gp41 that serve as targets for antibody-dependent cellular cytotoxicity by using human monoclonal antibodies. J Immunol. 1990;145:3276–3282.
22. Plata F. Implications of HIV-specific cytotoxic T lymphocytes in AIDS. Biotherapy. 1992;5:31–45.
23. Takahashi H, Germain RN, Moses B, et al. An immunodominant class I–restricted cytotoxic T lymphocyte determinant of human immunodeficiency virus type 1 induces CD4 class II–restricted help for itself. J Exp Med. 1990;171:571–576.
24. Rosenberg ZF, Fauci AS. The immunopathogenesis of HIV infection. Adv Immunol. 1989;47:377–431.
25. Langlade-Demoyen P, Michel F, Hoffenbach A, et al. Immune recognition of AIDS virus antigens by human and murine cytotoxic T lymphocytes. J Immunol. 1988;141:1949–1957.
26. Riviere Y, Tanneau-Salvadori F, Regnault A, et al. Human immunodeficiency virus–specific cytotoxic responses of seropositive individuals: Distinct types of effector cells mediate killing of targets expressing gag and env proteins. J Virol. 1989;63:2270–2277.
27. Walker BD, Flexner C, Paradis TJ, et al. HIV-1 reverse transcriptase is a target for cytotoxic T lymphocytes in infected individuals. Science. 1988;240:64–66.
28. Chenciner N, Michel F, Dadaglio G, et al. Multiple subsets of HIV-specific cytotoxic T lymphocytes in humans and mice. Eur J Immunol. 1989;19:1537–1544.
29. Walker BD, Flexner C, Birch-Limberger K, et al. Long-term culture and fine specificity of human cytotoxic T-lymphocyte clones reactive with human immunodeficiency virus type 1. Proc Natl Acad Sci U S A. 1989;86:9514–9518.
30. Cooney EL, McElrath MJ, Corey L, et al. Enhanced immunity to human immunodeficiency virus (HIV) envelope elicited by a combined vaccine regimen consisting of priming with vaccinia recombinant expressing HIV envelope and boosting with gp160 protein. Proc Natl Acad Sci U S A. 1993;90:1882–1886.
31. Hammond SA, Bollinger RC, Stanhope PE, et al. Comparative clonal analysis of human immunodeficiency virus type 1 (HIV-1)–specific CD4$^+$ and CD8$^+$ cytolytic T lymphocytes isolated from seronegative humans immunized with candidate HIV-1 vaccines. J Exp Med. 1992;176:1531–1542.
32. El-Daher N, Keefer MC, Reichman RC, et al. Persisting human immunodeficiency

virus type 1 gp160-specific human T lymphocyte responses including CD8+ cytotoxic activity after receipt of envelope vaccines. J Infect Dis. 1993;168:306–313.
33. Graham BS, Keefer MC, McElrath MJ, et al. Safety and immunogenicity of a candidate HIV-1 vaccine in healthy adults: Recombinant glycoprotein (rgp)120, a randomized, double-blind trial. Ann Intern Med. 1996;125:270–279.
34. Ferrari G, Humphrey W, McElrath MJ, et al. Clade B–based HIV-1 vaccines elicit cross-clade cytotoxic T lymphocyte reactivities in uninfected volunteers. Proc Natl Acad Sci U S A. 1997;94:1396–1401.
35. Cao H, Kanki P, Sankale JL, et al. Cytotoxic T-lymphocyte cross-reactivity among different human immunodeficiency virus type 1 clades: Implications for vaccine development. J Virol 1997;71:8615–8623.
36. Bertoletti A, Cham F, McAdam S, et al. Cytotoxic T cells from human immunodeficiency virus type 2–infected patients frequently crossreact with different human immunodeficiency virus type 1 clades. J Virol. 1998;72:2439–2448.
37. Fowke KR, Nagelkerke NJ, Kimani J, et al. Resistance to HIV-1 infection among persistently seronegative prostitutes in Nairobi, Kenya. Lancet. 1996;348:1347–1351.
38. Rowland-Jones S, Sutton J, Ariyoshi K, et al. HIV-specific cytotoxic T cells in HIV-exposed but uninfected Gambian women. Nature Med. 1995;1:59–64.
39. Rowland-Jones SL, Nixon DF, Aldhous MC, et al. HIV-specific cytotoxic T-cell activity in an HIV-exposed but uninfected infant. Lancet. 1993;341:860–861.
40. Rosenberg ES, Billingsley JM, Caliendo AM, et al. Vigorous HIV-1–specific CD4+ T cell responses associated with control of viremia. Science. 1997;278:1447–1450.
41. Robinson WE Jr, Montefiori DC, Mitchell WM. Antibody-dependent enhancement of human immunodeficiency virus type 1 infection. Lancet. 1988;1:790–794.
42. Takeda A, Tuazon CU, Ennis FA. Antibody-enhanced infection by HIV-1 via Fc receptor–mediated entry. Science. 1988;242:580–583.
43. Montefiori DC, Lefkowitz LB Jr, Keller RE, et al. Absence of a clinical correlation for complement mediated, infection-enhancing antibodies in plasma or sera from HIV-1 infected individuals. AIDS. 1991;5:413–417.
44. Dolin R, Graham B, Greenberg S, et al and the AIDS vaccine Clinical Trials Network. Safety and immunogenicity of an HIV-1 recombinant gp160 candidate vaccine in humans. Ann Intern Med. 1991;114:119–127.
44a. Keefer MC, Graham BS, Belshe RB, et al. Studies of high doses of a human immunodeficiency virus type 1 recombinant glycoprotein 160 candidate vaccine in HIV-1 seronegative humans. AIDS Res Hum Retroviruses. 1994;10:1713–1723.
45. Robinson WE Jr, Gorny MK, Xu JY, et al. Two immunodominant domains of gp41 bind antibodies which enhance human immunodeficiency virus type 1 infection in vitro. J Virol. 1991;65:4169–4176.
46. Jiang SB, Lin K, Neurath AR. Enhancement of human immunodeficiency virus type 1 infection by antisera to peptides from the envelope glycoproteins gp120/gp41. J Exp Med. 1991;174:1557–1563.
47. Takeda A, Robinson JE, Ho DD, et al. Distinction of human immunodeficiency virus type 1 neutralization and infection enhancement by human monoclonal antibodies to glycoprotein 120. J Clin Invest. 1992;89:1952–1957.
48. Reiher WE, Blalock JE, Brunck TK. Sequence homology between acquired immunodeficiency syndrome virus envelope protein and interleukin-2. Proc Natl Acad Sci USA. 1986;83:9188–9192.
49. Lee MR, Ho DD, Gurney ME. Functional interaction and partial homology between human immunodeficiency virus and neuroleukin. Science. 1987;237:1047–1051.
50. Pugliese O, Viora M, Camponeschi B, et al. A gp120 HIV peptide with high similarity to HLA class II beta chains enhances PPD-specific and autoreactive T cell activation. Clin Exp Immunol. 1992;90:170–174.
51. Golding H, Robey FA, Gates FT, et al. Identification of homologous regions in human immunodeficiency virus 1 gp41 and human MHC class II beta I domain. J Exp Med. 1988;167:914–923.
52. Sarin PS, Sun DK, Thornton AH, et al. Neutralization of HTLV-III/LAV replication by antiserum to thymosin α-1. Science. 1986;232:1135–1137.
53. Cochran MA, Ericson BL, Knell JD, et al. Use of baculovirus recombinants as general method for the production of subunit vaccines. In: Ginsberg H, Brown F, Lerner RA, et al, eds. Vaccines 87. Cold Springs Harbor, NY: Cold Springs Harbor Press: 1987:384–388.
54. Steimer KS, van Nest G, Dina D, et al. Genetically engineering human immunodeficiency virus envelope glycoprotein gp 120 produced in yeast is the target of neutralizing antibodies. In: Ginsberg H, Brown F, Lerner RA, et al, eds. Vaccines 87. Cold Springs Harbor, NY: Cold Springs Harbor Press; 1987;236–241.
55. Haigwood NL, Nara PL, Brooks E, et al. Native but not denatured recombinant human immunodeficiency virus type 1 gp120 generates broad-spectrum neutralizing antibodies in baboons. J Virol. 1992;66:172–182.
56. Lasky LA, Groopman JE, Fennie CW, et al. Neutralization of the AIDS retrovirus by antibodies to a recombinant envelope glycoprotein. Science. 1986;233:209–212.
57. Barrett N, Mitterer A, Mundt W, et al. Large scale production and purification of a vaccinia derived HIV-1 gp160 and analysis of its immunogenicity. AIDS Res Hum Retroviruses. 1989;25:159–171.
58. Wintsch J, Chaignat CL, Braun DG, et al. Safety and immunogenicity of a genetically engineered human immunodeficiency virus vaccine. J Infect Dis. 1991;163:219–225.
59. Kahn JO, Sinangil F, Baenziger J, et al. Clinical and immunologic responses to human immunodeficiency virus (HIV) type 1 SF2 gp120 subunit vaccine combined with MF59 adjuvant with or without muramyl tripeptide dipalmitoyl phosphatidylethanolamine in non–HIV-infected human volunteers. J Infect Dis. 1994;170:1288–1291.
60. Schwartz DH, Gorse G, Clements ML, et al. Induction of HIV-1 neutralising and syncytium-inhibiting antibodies in unifected recipients of HIV-IIIB rgp120 subunit vaccine. Lancet. 1993;342:69–73.
61. Belshe RB, Graham BS, Keefer MC, et al. Neutralizing antibodies to HIV-1 in seronegative volunteers immunized with recombinant gp120 from the MN strain of HIV-1. JAMA. 1994;272:475–480.
62. Defoort NP, Nardelli B, Huang W, et al. Macromolecular assemblage in the design of a synthetic AIDS vaccine. Proc Natl Sci U S A. 1992;89:3879–3883.
63. Palker TJ, Matthews TJ, Langlois A, et al. Polyvalent human immunodeficiency virus synthetic immunogen comprised of envelope gp120 T helper cell sites and B cell neutralization epitopes. J Immunol. 1989;142:3612–3619.
64. Ahlers JD, Dunlop N, Pendleton CD, et al. Candidate HIV type 1 multideterminant cluster peptide-P18MN vaccine constructs elicit type 1 helper T cells, cytotoxic T cells, and neutralizing antibody, all using the same adjuvant immunization. AIDS Res Hum Retroviruses 1996;12:259–272.
65. Naylor PH, Sztein MB, Wada S, et al. Preclinical and clinical studies on immunogenicity and safety of the HIV-1 p17 based synthetic peptide AIDS vaccine: HGP-30-KLH. Int J Immunopharmacol. 1991;13(Suppl 1):117–127.
66. Adams SE, Dawson KM, Gull K, et al. The expression of hybrid HIV: Ty virus-like particles in yeast. Nature. 1987;329:68–70.
67. Blick G, Crook S, Buchanan S, et al. A phase I/II study of the toxicity, immunogenicity and efficacy of recombinant gp160 and p24 vaccines (Vax-Syn) in HIV-infected individuals regardless of CD4+ cell count (Abstract TuB0562). Eighth International Conference on AIDS/III STD, World Congress, Amsterdam, July 1992.
68. Hu SL, Kosowski SG, Dalrymple JM. Expression of AIDS virus envelope in recombinant vaccinia viruses. Nature. 1986;320:537–540.
69. Tartaglia J, Cox WI, Taylor J, et al. Highly attenuated poxvirus vectors. AIDS Res Hum Retroviruses. 1992;8:1445–1447.
70. Tartaglia J, Perkus ME, Taylor J, et al. NYVAC: A highly attenuated strain of vaccinia virus. Virology. 1992;188:217–232.
71. Paoletti E. Applications of pox virus vectors to vaccination: An update. Proc Natl Acad Sci U S A. 1996;93:11349–11353.
72. Chanda PK, Natuk RJ, Mason BB, et al. High-level expression of the envelope glycoprotein of the human immunodeficiency virus type 1 in presence of rev gene using helper-independent adenovirus type 7 recombinants. Virology. 1990; 175:535–547.
73. Porter DC, Ansardi DC, Choi WS, et al. Encapsidation of genetically engineered poliovirus minireplicons which express human immunodeficiency virus type 1 gag and pol proteins upon infection. J Virol 1993;67:3712–3719.
74. Cattozzo EM, Stocker BA, Radaelli A, et al. Expression and immunogenicity of V3 loop epitopes of HIV-1, isolates SC and WMJ2, inserted in *Salmonella* flagellin. J Biotechnol. 1997;56:191–203.
75. Aldovini A, Young RA. Humoral and cell-mediated immune responses to live recombinant BCG-HIV vaccines. Nature. 1991;351:479–482.
76. Caley IJ, Betts MR, Irlbeck DM, et al. Humoral, mucosal, and cellular immunity in response to a human immunodeficiency virus type 1 immunogen expressed by a Venezuelan equine encephalitis virus vaccine vector. J Virol. 1997;71:3031–3038.
77. Klinman DM, Takeno M, Icheno M, et al. DNA vaccines: Safety and efficiency issues. Springer Semin Immunopathol. 1997;19:245–256.
78. Mulligan M, Goepfert P, Corey L, et al. AVEG 031: Phase 1 evaluation of a *gag-pol* facilitated DNA vaccine for HIV-1 prevention. Poster presentation 12th World AIDS Conference, Geneva, Switzerland, June 28–July 3, 1998.
79. Daniel MD, Kirchhoff F, Czajak SC, et al. Protective effects of a live attenuated SIV vaccine with a deletion in the *nef* gene. Science. 1992;258:1938–1941.
80. Ruprecht RM, Baba TW, Liska V. Attenuated HIV vaccine: Caveats. Science. 1996;271:1790–1792.
80a. Baba TW, Liska V, Khimani AH, et al. Live attenuated multiply deleted simian immunodeficiency virus causes AIDs in infants and adult macaques. Nat Med. 1999;5:194–203.
81. Whatmore AM, Cook N, Hall GA, et al. Repair and evolution of *nef* in vivo modulates simian immunodeficiency virus virulence. J Virol. 1995;69:5117–5123.
82. Villinger F, Brar SS, Brice GT, et al. Immune and hematopoietic parameters in HIV-1 infected chimpanzees during clinical progression toward AIDS. J Med Primatol. 1997;26:11–18.
83. Novembre FJ, Saucier M, Anderson DC, et al. Development of AIDS in a chimpanzee infected with human immunodeficiency virus type 1. J Virol. 1997;71:4086–4091.
84. Letvin NL, King NW. Immunologic and pathologic manifestations of the infection of rhesus monkeys with simian immunodeficiency virus of macaques. J Acquir Immune Defic Syndr. 1990;3:1023–1040.
85. Fultz PN, McClure HM, Anderson DC, et al. Identification and biologic characterization of an acutely lethal variant of simian immunodeficiency virus from sooty mangabeys (SIV/SMM). AIDS Res Hum Retroviruses 1989;5:397–409.
86. Desrosiers RC. The simian immunodeficiency viruses. Annu Rev Immunol. 1990;8:557–578.
87. Kodama T, Wooley DP, Naidu YM, et al. The significance of premature stop codons in env of SIV. J Virol. 1989;63:4709–4714.
88. Lu YC, Salvato MS, Pauza CD, et al. Utility of SHIV for testing HIV-1 vaccine candidates in macaques. J Acquir Immune Defic Syndr Hum Retrovirol. 1996;12:99–106.
89. Warren JT, Dolatshahi M. Annual updated survey of worldwide HIV, SIV, and SHIV challenge studies in vaccinated nonhuman primates. J Med Primatol. 1994;23:184–225.
90. Warren JT, Levinson MA. Preclinical AIDS vaccine development: Formal survey of global HIV, SIV and SHIV in vivo challenge studies in vaccinated nonhuman primates. J Med Primatol. 1997;26:63–81.

90a. Almond NM, Heeney JL. AIDS vaccine development in primate models. AIDS. 1998;12(Suppl A):S133–S140.
91. Keefer MC, Graham BS, McElrath MJ, NIAID AIDS Vaccine Evaluation Group. Safety and immunogenicity of ENV 2-3, a human immunodeficiency virus type 1 candidate vaccine, in combination with a novel adjuvant, MTP-PE/MF59. AIDS Res Hum Retroviruses. 1996;12:683–693.
92. Graham BS, Keefer MC, McElrath MJ, NIAID AIDS Vaccine Evaluation Group. Safety and immunogenicity of a candidate HIV-1 vaccine in healthy adults: Recombinant glycoprotein (rgp)120. A randomized, double-blind trial. Ann Intern Med. 1996;125:270–279.
93. Gorse GJ, McElrath MJ, Matthews TJ, et al. Modulation of immunologic responses to HIV-1 recombinant gp160 vaccine by dose and schedule of administration. Vaccine. 1998;16:493–506.
93a. Gorse GJ, Corey L, Patel GB, et al. HIV_{MN} recombinant glycoprotein 160 vaccine-induced cellular and humoral immunity boosted by $HIV\text{-}1_{MN}$ recombinant glycoprotein 120 vaccine. AIDS Res and Human Retroviruses. 1999;2:115–132.
94. McElrath MJ, Corey L, Montefiori D, AIDS Vaccine Evaluation Group. A phase II study of two HIV-1 gp120 subunit vaccines comparing their immunogenicity in populations at risk for acquiring HIV-1 infection. Submitted, 1999.
94a Keefer MC, Wolff M, Gorse GJ, et al. Safety profile of phase I and II preventive HIV type 1 envelope vaccination: Experience of the NIAID AIDS Vaccine Evaluation Group. AIDS Res Hum Retroviruses. 1997;14:1163–1197.
95. Mascola JR, Snyder SW, Weislow OS, et al. Immunization with envelope subunit vaccine products elicits neutralizing antibodies against laboratory-adapted but not primary isolates of human immunodeficiency virus type-1. J Infect Dis. 1996;173:340–348.
96. Moore JP, Cao Y, Qing L, et al. Primary isolates of human immunodeficiency virus type 1 are relatively resistant to neutralization by monoclonal antibodies to gp120 and their neutralization is not predicted by studies with monomeric gp120. J Virol. 1995;69:101–109.
97. Burton DR. A vaccine for HIV type-1: The antibody perspective. Proc Natl Acad Sci U S A. 1997;94:10018–10023.
98. Keefer MC, Bonnez W, Roberts NJ Jr, et al. Human immunodeficiency virus (HIV-1) gp160-specific lymphocyte proliferative responses of mononuclear leukocytes from HIV-1 recombinant gp160 vaccine recipients. J Infect Dis. 1991;163:448–453.
99. Gorse GJ, Belshe RB, Newman FK, et al. Lymphocyte proliferative responses following immunization with human immunodeficiency virus recombinant gp160. Vaccine. 1992;10:383–388.
100. Orentas RJ, Hildreth JEK, Obah E, et al. Induction of $CD4^+$ human cytolytic T cells specific for HIV-infected cells by a gp160 subunit vaccine. Science. 1990;248:1234–1237.
101. Sarin PS, Mora CA, Naylor PH, et al. HIV-1 p17 synthetic peptide vaccine HGP-30: Induction of immune response in human subjects and preliminary evidence of protection against HIV challenge in SCID mice. Cell Mol Biol. 1995;41:401–407.
102. Kahn JO, Stites DP, Scillian J, et al. A phase I study of HGP-30, a 30 amino acid subunit of the human immunodeficiency virus (HIV) p17 synthetic peptide analogue subunit vaccine in seronegative subjects. AIDS Res Hum Retroviruses 1992;8:1321–1325.
103. Naylor PH, Sztein MB, Wada S, et al. Preclinical and clinical studies on immunogenicity and safety of the HIV-1 p17 based synthetic peptide AIDS vaccine: HGP-30-KLH. Int J Immunopharmacol. 1991;13(Suppl 1):117–127.
104. Gorse GJ, Keefer MC, Belshe RB, et al. A dose-ranging study of a prototype synthetic HIV-1 V3 branched peptide vaccine. J Infect Dis. 1996;173:330–339.
104a. Keefer ML, Lambert JS, Koff W, et al. A phase I study of a multivalent HIV-1 peptide vaccine in HIV-1 uninfected subjects. Abstract #403. Thirty-third Infectious Disease Society of America Annual Meeting, San Francisco, Calif, September 16–18, 1995.
105. Li D, Forrest BD, Li Z, et al. International clinical trials of HIV vaccines: II. Phase I trial of an HIV-1 synthetic peptide vaccine evaluating an accelerated immunization schedule in Yunnan, China. Asian Pac J Allergy Immunol. 1997;15:105–113.
106. Kelleher AD, Emery S, Cunningham P, et al. Safety and immunogenicity of UBI HIV-1 (MN) octameric V3 peptide vaccine administered by subcutaneous injection. AIDS Res Hum Retroviruses. 1997;13:29–32.
107. Phanuphak P, Teeratakulpixarn S, Sarangbin S, et al. International clinical trials of HIV vaccines. I. Phase I trial of an HIV-1 synthetic peptide vaccine in Bangkok, Thailand. Asian Pac J Allergy Immunol. 1997;15:41–48.
108. Zagury D, Bernard J, Cheynier R, et al. A group specific anamnestic immune reaction against HIV-1 induced by a candidate vaccine against AIDS. Nature. 1988;332:728–731.
109. Cooney EL, Collier AC, Greenberg PD, et al. Safety and immunologic response to a recombinant vaccinia virus vaccine expressing HIV envelope glycoprotein. Lancet. 1991;337:567–572.
110. Stanhope PE, Clements ML, Siliciano RF. Human $CD4^+$ cytolytic T lymphocyte responses to a human immunodeficiency virus type 1 gp160 subunit vaccine. J Infect Dis. 1993;168:92–100.
111. Keefer MC, McElrath MJ, Weinhold K, et al. A phase I trial of vaccinia-env/gag/pol (TBC-3B) given by alternative routes, boosted with rgp120MN [AVEG 014C]. Poster Presentation, Twelfth World AIDS Conference, Geneva, Switzerland, June 28–July 3, 1998.
112. Graham BS, Belshe RB, Clements ML, et al. Vaccination of vaccinia-naïve adults with human immunodeficiency virus type 1 gp160 recombinant vaccinia virus in a blinded, controlled randomized clinical trial. J Infect Dis. 1992;166:244–252.
113. Graham BS, Gorse GJ, Schwartz DH, et al. Determinants of antibody response after recombinant gp160 boosting in vaccinia-naïve volunteers primed with gp160-recombinant vaccinia virus. J Infect Dis. 1994;170:782–786.
114. Clements-Mann ML, Weinthold K, Matthews TJ, et al. Immune responses to human immunodeficiency virus (HIV) type 1 induced by canarypox expressing $HIV\text{-}1_{MN}$ gp120, $HIV\text{-}1_{SF\text{-}2}$ recombinant gp120, or both vaccines in seronegative adults. J Infect Dis. 1998;177:1230–1246.
115. Pialoux G, Excler JL, Riviere Y, et al. A prime-boost approach to HIV preventive vaccine using a recombinant canarypox virus expressing glycoprotein 160 (MN/LAI). AIDS Res Hum Retroviruses. 1995;11:373–381.
116. Fleury B, Janvier G, Pialoux G, et al. Memory cytotoxic T lymphocyte responses in human immunodeficiency virus type I (HIV-1)–negative volunteers immunized with a recombinant canarypox expressing gp160 of HIV-1 and boosted with a recombinant gp160. J Infect Dis. 1996;174:734–738.
116a. Belshe RB, Gorse GJ, Mulligan MJ, et al. Induction of immune responses to HIV-1 by canarypox (ALVAC) HIV-1 and gp120 SF-2 recombinant vaccines in uninfected volunteers. AIDS. 1998;12:2407–2415.
116b. Evans TG, Keefer MC, Wolff M, et al. A canarypox vaccine expressing multiple HIV-1 genes given alone or with vgp120 elicits broad and durable $CD8^+$ CTL in seronegative volunteers. J Infect Dis. 1999. In press.
117. Graham BS, Matthews TJ, Belshe RB, et al. Augmentation of human immunodeficiency virus type 1 neutralizing antibody by priming with gp160 recombinant vaccinia and boosting with rpg160 in vaccinia naïve adults. J Infect Dis. 1993;167:533–537.
118. Salk J. Prospects for the control of AIDS by immunizing seropositive individuals. Nature. 1987;327:473–476.
118a. Levine AM, Groshen S, Allen J, et al. Initial studies on active immunization of HIV-infected subjects using a gp120-depleted HIV-1 immunogen: Long-term follow-up. J Acquir Immune Defic Syndr Hum Retrovirol. 1996;114:351–364.
119. Redfield RR, Birx DL, Ketter N, et al. A phase I evaluation of the safety and immunogenicity of recombinant gp160 in patients with early human immunodeficiency virus infection. N Engl J Med. 1991;324:1677–1684.
119a. Valentine FT, Kundu S, Haslett PAJ, et al. A randomized, placebo-controlled study of the immunogenicity of human immunodeficiency virus (HIV) rgp160 vaccine in HIV-infected subjects with $\geq 400/mm^3$ CD4 T lymphocyte (AIDS Clinical Trial Group Protocol 137). J Infect Dis. 1996;143:1336–1346.
120. Eron JJ, Ashby MA, Giordano MF, et al. Randomised trial of MN rgp120 HIV-1 vaccine in symptomless HIV-1 infection. Lancet. 1996;348:1547–1551.
121. Schooley RT, Spino C, Chiu S, et al. Poor immunogenicity of HIV-1 envelope vaccines with alum or MF59 adjuvant in HIV-1 infected individuals: Results of two randomized trials. Abstract 756. Presented at the Fourth Conference on Retroviruses and Opportunistic Infections. Washington, DC, January 22–26, 1997.
122. Kuritzkes DR, Spino C, Valentine F, et al. Associations of plasma HIV-1 RNA, CD4 count, and immune response in patients with 50-500 CD4 cells/μl. Abstract 757. Presented at Fourth Conference on Retroviruses and Opportunistic Infections. Washington, DC, January 22–26, 1997.
123. Birx DL, Davis C, Ruiz N, et al. Results of a phase II double-blinded multicenter placebo controlled HIV therapeutic vaccine trial. Abstract Tu.A.275. Presented at the Eleventh International Conference on AIDS, Vancouver, 1996.
124. Kovacs JA, Vasudevachari MB, Easter M, et al. Induction of humoral and cell-mediated anti-human immunodeficiency virus (HIV) responses in HIV sero-negative volunteers by immunization with recombinant gp160. J Clin Invest. 1993;92:919–928.
125. Belshe RB, Clements ML, Dolin R, et al. Safety and immunogenicity of a fully glycosylated recombinant gp160 human immunodeficiency virus type 1 vaccine in subjects at low risk of infection. J Infect Dis. 1993;168:1387–1395.
125a. Gorse, GJ, Schwartz DH, Graham BS, et al. HIV-1 recombinant gp160 vaccine given in accelerated dose schedules. Clin Exp Immunol. 1994;98:178–184.
126. Martin S, Weber J, Rott I, et al. Recombinant HIV-1 gag p24-Ty virus-like-particles (VLPs) induce HIV-1 p24 specific T helper cells in seronegative subjects vaccinated with these particles. Abstract POA2194. Presented at the Eight International Conference on AIDS/III STD World Congress, Amsterdam, July 1992.
127. Corey L, Weinhold K, McElrath J, et al. Safety and immunogenicity of live recombinant canarypox vector containing the envelope, gag and protease genes of HIV-1 in seronegative adult volunteers. Oral Abstract. Presented at the Eleventh International Conference on AIDS, Vancouver, Canada, July 7–12, 1996 [Mo.A.282].
128. Corey L, McElrath MJ, Weinhold K, et al. (AIDS Vaccine Evaluation Group). Cytotoxic T cell and neutralizing antibody responses to human immunodeficiency virus type 1 envelope with a combination vaccine regimen. J Infect Dis. 1998;177:301–309.
129. Schwartz D, Clements ML, Belshe R, et al. Interim results of rgp160 vaccine trial in HIV^+ volunteers. Poster presentation. Presented at the Ninth International Conference on AIDS/Fourth Sexually Transmitted Diseases World Congress, Berlin, Germany, June 6–11, 1993 [PO-A28-0668].
130. McElrath MJ, Keefer M, Paxton WB, et al. A phase I randomized, blinded, controlled vaccine trial in asymptomatic HIV-infected individuals using ENV 2-3 in MF-59 with or without MTP-PE. Abstract. Annual Meeting, Infectious Diseases Society of America, New Orleans, La, October 16–18, 1993 [200].

SECTION P
MISCELLANEOUS SYNDROMES

Chapter 118
Chronic Fatigue Syndrome

N. CARY ENGLEBERG

Chronic fatigue syndrome designates an illness that consists of profound, prolonged fatigue associated with other somatic or neuropsychological symptoms. The diagnosis is based on the patient's subjective report of a compatible symptom cluster and the absence of any medical or psychiatric condition that might account for the complaints. Attempts to ascribe this syndrome to a single, coherent cause have been fruitless. To the contrary, the available evidence favors the notion that the syndromal definition identifies a heterogenous population of patients in whom fatigue, pain, cognitive complaints, and "viral"-like symptoms, such as low-grade fever, sore throat, and tender lymph nodes, are the final common pathophysiologic consequences of a variety of different causes.

Other names for this disorder include *myalgic encephalomyelitis* (in Great Britain and Canada) and *chronic fatigue and immune dysfunction syndrome* (in the United States). Most authorities in the United States prefer the name *chronic fatigue syndrome* since there is no convincing evidence that either inflammation of the central nervous system or immune system dysfunction is responsible for the symptoms of the disorder. *Postviral fatigue* and *postinfectious fatigue* are less strictly defined designations for chronic idiopathic fatigue when it is perceived to be induced by an infectious disease and persists through a prolonged convalescence.

HISTORY

Although popular interest in chronic fatigue syndrome has been a relatively recent phenomenon, a historical perspective suggests that the illness is not new.[1] For several centuries, an illness resembling chronic fatigue syndrome has been repeatedly described in the medical literature by different names. The illness has been variously attributed to neurologic, cardiovascular, and endocrine causes, as well as to infectious diseases. The proximate association of infections, especially influenza, with chronic fatigue (i.e., neuraesthenia) was appreciated in the late 19th century.[2] In the 1950s, Spink found that nearly 20% of patients with serologic evidence of brucellosis developed lingering symptoms of fatigue, weakness, myalgic pain, mental confusion, and depression in the absence of evidence for continued, active infection, whether or not they had received treatment.[3] He hypothesized that the development of "chronic brucellosis" involved both an infection and a psychological predisposition. Later studies by Imboden and coworkers confirmed this impression by showing that chronic brucellosis patients scored unfavorably on the Minnesota Multiphasic Personality Inventory relative to patients who had recovered from acute brucellosis.[4] To test the hypothesis that a psychological propensity precedes the chronic fatigue illness, these authors conducted a retrospective cohort analysis of military personnel and dependents in Maryland after an outbreak of Asian influenza during the winter of 1957–1958.[5] All subjects had completed the Minnesota inventory in August 1957, just prior to the epidemic. Prolonged convalescence from influenza was correlated with preexisting, unfavorable scores on certain subscales of this test. Moreover, the typical Minnesota Multiphasic Personality Inventory profile associated with prolonged postinfluenzal symptoms was nearly identical to that observed in patients with chronic brucellosis.[5]

In 1985, two large series of patients with prolonged fatigue and other symptoms were reported to have elevated antibody titers against Epstein-Barr virus (EBV) compared with healthy controls.[6, 7] In the same year, a large outbreak of chronic fatigue with associated symptoms and serologic tests suggesting chronic EBV infection occurred in the area of Lake Tahoe, Nevada.[8] It was proposed that idiopathic chronic fatigue might be due to "chronic mononucleosis." This hypothesis was appealing since it had long been observed that persistent fatigue may follow documented acute mononucleosis in a small proportion of cases.[9–11] However, several subsequent investigations failed to confirm a role for active EBV replication in the persistence of this clinical syndrome.[12–16] Numerous other infectious agents have been proposed as the cause of this syndrome. They include *Candida albicans, Borrelia burgdorferi*, enteroviruses, cytomegalovirus, human herpesvirus 6, spumavirus, retroviruses, and Borna virus (Table 118–1). The evidence that active infection with any of these agents causes a significant proportion of chronic fatigue cases is either inconclusive or refuted by subsequent investigations.

In addition to stimulating a search for alternate causes, the definition of a common clinical syndrome without no apparent cause led to a series of conferences sponsored by the National Institutes of Health and the Centers for Disease Control and Prevention from 1985 to 1994. The purpose of these conferences was to arrive at a consensus definition of the clinical syndrome that could be applied uniformly by investigators studying the epidemiology, clinical features, etiology, and treatment of the disorder.

EPIDEMIOLOGY

Fatigue is one of the most common complaints encountered in general medical practice. In most patients, the complaint is eventually attributed to a diagnosable medical condition or is short-lived. According to the most recent consensus conference definition, severe fatigue that remains unexplained after baseline physical and laboratory examinations and persists for more than 6 months is designated as *idiopathic chronic fatigue*. Patients with idiopathic chronic fatigue who also complain of four or more of the associated symptoms listed in Table 118–2 may be considered to have chronic fatigue syndrome.[17]

Since the case definition requires a medical evaluation, it can only be applied to study the prevalence of chronic fatigue syndrome

TABLE 118–1 Proposed Infectious Causes of Chronic Fatigue Syndrome

Proposed Etiologic Agent	Suggestive Studies	Negative Studies
Epstein-Barr virus	6, 7, 68	12, 14–16
Cytomegalovirus	69, 70	14, 16
Human herpesvirus 6	34, 71, 72	14, 16
Enteroviruses	73–75	14, 16, 76–79
Parvovirus	32	80, 81
Human spumavirus	82	
Human retrovirus	83	84, 85
Borna virus	86	87
Borrelia burgdorferi	88	89, 90
Brucella spp.	91	3
Candida albicans	92, 93	94

TABLE 118–2 CDC/NIH Censensus Conference Definition of Chronic Fatigue Syndrome

Clinically evaluated, unexplained chronic fatigue for more than 6 months' duration, which is not lifelong or the result of ongoing exertion and is not substantially alleviated by rest. The fatigue is associated with a significant reduction in occupational, educational, social, or personal activities.
PLUS
Four or more of the following concurrent symptoms:
- Impaired memory or concentration
- Sore throat
- Tender cervical or axillary lymph nodes
- Muscle pain
- Multijoint pain
- New headaches
- Unrefreshing sleep
- Postexertion malaise

Abbreviations: CDC, Centers for Disease Control and Prevention; NIH, National Institutes of Health. Adapted from Fukuda K, Straus SE, Hickie I, et al. The chronic fatigue syndrome: A comprehensive approach to its definition and study. International Chronic Fatigue Syndrome Study Group. Ann Intern Med. 1994;121:953–959.

in populations who seek medical attention. In a general medical practice in Boston, idiopathic chronic fatigue was reported by 8.5% of patients, but only 0.3% could be diagnosed with chronic fatigue syndrome.[18] The Centers for Disease Control and Prevention attempted to ascertain the national prevalence of chronic fatigue syndrome by conducting case finding through a network of physicians in four cities. The prevalence, age, and sex distribution were remarkably similar in the four cities. The prevalence ranged from 3 to 11 per 100,000 population. Patients were predominantly female (7:1) and clustered in the fourth and fifth decades of life.[19] Similar estimates of prevalence were reported from studies in Australia and the United Kingdom.[20, 21] The repeatedly demonstrated predominance of upper middle class white women in their thirties and forties resulted in the pejorative term *yuppie flu*. However, these and other observations are biased by reliance on clinic-based case ascertainment. When a random telephone survey was conducted in the San Francisco area, a very different epidemiologic pattern emerged.[22] The overall prevalence of subjects reporting a chronic fatigue syndrome–like illness was 0.2% of the population, and the female predominance was less dramatic (2.9:1). The age distribution was the same as that seen in clinic-based studies, but the distribution of cases by income showed higher rates in persons with family incomes less than $40,000, suggesting that the perception of "yuppie flu" is an artifact of health care utilization by the affected populations. Moreover, the rates of chronic fatigue syndrome–like illness were higher in African Americans and Hispanics than in whites and Asian Americans, and there was no preponderance of cases in any individual occupational group.

Outbreaks of idiopathic illness consistent with chronic fatigue syndrome have been reported occasionally during the past 60 years.[23] In many of these outbreaks, the involvement of an infectious agent is unlikely because certain subgroups of the population at risk were affected disproportionately. Large hospital outbreaks in Los Angeles and London, England, affected the professional staff, but not the hospitalized patients or nonprofessional staff.[24, 25] An acute outbreak of neuromyesthenia in New Zealand resulted in chronic fatigue syndrome in many of the affected individuals. A 10-year follow-up of these cases indicated that most patients had recovered partially or completely.[26]

ETIOLOGY AND PATHOGENESIS

Attempts to elucidate the pathophysiology of chronic fatigue syndrome have been hampered by several methodologic problems. Foremost among these is the problem of selecting a homogenous group of subjects for study from among patients identified by the working definition. In a symptom cluster analysis of patients meeting the Centers for Disease Control and Prevention criteria, at least two distinct subgroups emerged, one having numerous syndromal and nonsyndromal symptoms with very high severity scores, and a second, larger group with limited numbers of symptoms and only moderate severity.[27] Similarly, some patients have an acute onset that is sometimes associated with an infectious disease or other definable stressor, whereas others describe an insidious and progressive onset. A majority of patients have past or current psychiatric disorders,[28–30] whereas some have no psychiatric symptomology, past or present. There is no a priori reason to assume that patients with these diverse clinical circumstances have the same disorders simply because they meet the Centers for Disease Control and Prevention criteria at the time of presentation.

A second methodologic problem is that a variety of infectious and noninfectious causes have been proposed (see Table 118–1), but there is no reproducible evidence that any single agent is responsible for a significant proportion of these illnesses. Many of the other proposed chronic infectious causes are also exceedingly common in the healthy human population. Since some cases of chronic fatigue have followed specific infectious diseases, chronic persistent infection has frequently been evoked as one possible pathophysiology. For example, prolonged convalescence from infectious mononucleosis is a well-recognized phenomenon. Although there was never any direct virologic evidence favoring chronic EBV infection as a cause of chronic fatigue syndrome, a significant body of negative research has accumulated to reject this hypothesis. These studies showed no significant differences in serologic titers,[14, 16] shedding of virus in saliva,[13] blood lymphocyte–transforming activity,[13, 15] and EBV-specific cytotoxic lymphocytes[15] between patients and healthy controls. In addition, a large treatment study compared intravenous and oral acyclovir with placebo and failed to show any benefit.[12] Similar negative data have been collected for other specific infectious agents (see Table 118–1).

Chronic fatigue syndrome has been observed to follow several different specific infections (e.g., EBV infection, influenza, brucellosis), including some that are highly localized geographically (e.g., Lyme disease, Q fever, Ross River virus infection).[5, 31–33] Since these illnesses represent a small minority of all idiopathic chronic fatigue cases, these events support the notion that prolonged fatigue is a nonspecific sequel to a variety of illnesses rather than a disease with a specific infectious cause. Controversy persists about whether chronic fatigue can be triggered by any infectious or traumatic event, or whether only a particular type of infection or trauma is necessary.

Pathophysiologic hypotheses focus on various biologic systems as potential targets for these prolonged fatigue disorders (e.g., the immune system, skeletal muscle, heart, central nervous system). Although subtle alterations in some of these systems have been identified in patients, similar changes are also observed in individuals without symptoms, and many of the studies are inconsistent with one another or have not been reproduced. Since chronic idiopathic fatigue usually includes neuropsychological symptoms and minor alterations of hormones regulated at the hypothalamic level (see later), the hypothesis that the central nervous system is the site of these disorders has gained support in recent years. Accumulating data from central nervous system imaging studies supports this notion, but the significance of these findings is still unclear.[34–37]

There may be a genetic predisposition for persistent fatigue after an appropriate stimulus, although large kindred studies have not been done to confirm this hypothesis. Two brief reports have noted that the frequency of a defect in bilirubin glucuronidase (Gilbert's disease) is five times greater in chronic fatigue patients than in the general population.[38, 39] Since Gilbert's disease is generally believed to be a benign defect, one may speculate that the association with chronic fatigue syndrome reflects coinheritance of a genetically linked locus. Similarly, a past history of a depressive disorder is often present in chronic fatigue states and may represent an important predisposing condition[40]; some depressive disorders may have a genetic basis.

CLINICAL MANIFESTATIONS

Chronic fatigue syndrome often begins during the convalescence from an acute flulike illness. On occasion, the syndrome develops in the aftermath of an identifiable infectious disease, such as infectious mononucleosis or influenza. More often, however, the infectious nature of the triggering event is not confirmed. Flulike symptoms may persist or develop de novo after the acute onset. These include sore throat, low-grade fever, tender adenopathy, generalized myalgia, migratory arthralgia, and headache. In contrast, objective physical findings corresponding to these subjective complaints, such as pharyngitis, a temperature greater than 100.5°F, and palpable adenopathy, are rare after the resolution of the initial illness. The presence of significant objective muscle weakness or frank arthritis should suggest an alternative diagnosis.

Persistent, disabling fatigue is the cardinal symptom of the syndrome. Patients often report that they have a limited allotment of energy each day and cannot function once it is depleted. Consequently, exhausting fatigue that lasts from hours to a few days may follow even modest exertion.

Fatigue is often accompanied by neurocognitive difficulties and disturbances of sleep. Patients may describe difficulty with concentration and memory, although actual deficits are not consistently demonstrable using neuropsychological testing. Either insomnia or excessive sleep may be reported. A thorough sleep history helps to determine whether formal polysomnography is indicated to rule out a primary sleep disorder. Sleep disorders are common among patients who present with fatigue, even among those who meet symptomatic criteria for chronic fatigue syndrome.[41] Any or all of the symptoms may occur persistently or occur with striking seasonality. Some cases of chronic fatigue syndrome have seasonal variation comparable to that seen with seasonal affective disorder.[42]

The majority of patients who meet symptom criteria for chronic fatigue syndrome also have a past or current history of a psychiatric disorder (e.g., depression or anxiety disorder).[28–30] The treating physician must determine whether a preexisting psychiatric disorder accounts for all of the patient's complaints. If so, chronic fatigue syndrome should not be diagnosed. Altered mood states that occur in the context of the chronic fatigue syndrome are often transient and reactive to the physical disability and discomfort.

LABORATORY FINDINGS

There are no laboratory tests that are diagnostic for the chronic fatigue syndrome. Therefore, an evaluation for this condition includes laboratory tests only for the purpose of ruling out unrecognized medical conditions that account for the symptoms. The minimal evaluation consists of a complete blood count, serum chemistry profile, urinalysis, and thyroid function testing.[17] Additional tests may be indicated when the history or the quality of the patient's symptoms suggest specific alternate diseases (e.g., chronic infection, collagen vascular disease, neurologic disorder, or neoplasm). A low-titer antinuclear antibody test is found in 15 to 54% of patients with chronic fatigue syndrome.[43, 44] Antibodies against DNA and extractable nuclear antigens are typically absent. Instead, antibodies directed against insoluble nuclear matrix proteins are responsible for the nuclear fluorescence.[44, 45] The significance of these autoantibodies is unknown.

When groups of patients with chronic fatigue syndrome are compared with control groups, significant differences have been found in a number of laboratory or radiologic results (e.g., in hormone levels, central nervous system radiologic tests, measures of cellular immunity, autonomic function). These findings may provide some insight into the pathophysiology of chronic fatigue states, but they have no diagnostic value in individual patients. In all these examples, there is a significant overlap between the fatigued and normal groups so that the tests cannot be used as a reliable marker for the disorder in any individual.

Urinary free cortisol levels have been shown to be lower in patients with chronic fatigue syndrome than in age- and sex-matched healthy controls, although the means of both groups are within the defined normal range.[46, 47] Exaggerated adrenal responsiveness to corticotropin infusions in these patients suggests that a subtle defect in hypothalamic-pituitary-adrenal (HPA)-axis activity may exist at the level of pituitary or above. Similarly reduced HPA-axis activity has also been observed in fibromyalgia and in post-traumatic stress disorder, whereas the opposite is found in major depressive disorder, that is, an increased HPA-axis activity driven from the hypothalamus.[48] These findings suggest the presence of a common pathophysiology in chronic fatigue syndrome and other stress-related disorders that is centered in the central nervous system. However, cortisol levels are not sufficiently discriminatory to be of value in diagnosis. Levels should be obtained only when clinical findings indicate a need to rule out frank adrenal insufficiency.

Small bright objects have been reportedly found more frequently in the brain magnetic resonance imaging studies of chronic fatigue patients than of healthy controls.[34] Similarly, changes in the perfusion of certain areas of the brain are suggested by studies using single photon emission computed tomography scanning.[35–37] The causes of these findings are unknown, and their relationship to symptoms is not clear. Since the findings are not specific for chronic fatigue syndrome, central nervous system imaging should be used only when it is medically indicated to rule out a structural abnormality.

Differences in various measures of immune function (e.g., cytokine levels, in vitro lymphocyte function, flow cytometry) have been observed by comparing chronic fatigue syndrome patients and healthy persons. Many of these reports are inconsistent, but a few of the findings have been demonstrated reproducibly in more than one research laboratory. For example, there appears to be a small but significant increase in the number of lymphocytes bearing the CD45RA phenotype.[49] This phenotype is a marker for activated memory T cells, and the observation of an increase in their number suggests that an ongoing immune response is occurring. Another repeated immunologic finding involves natural killer cells. Both the number of cells bearing the natural killer cell surface marker, CD16, and functional assays of natural killer cell function are reduced in groups of fatigued patients.[50] One concern raised by this latter observation was the possibility that malignancies might occur at an increased rate. Analysis of cancer registries following the large 1985 Lake Tahoe outbreak did not support this notion.[51] The potential consequences of reduced natural killer cell function are unknown; however, this phenomenon is not specific, and experimental data suggest that similar reductions may also follow a variety of other physical and emotional stresses. There is no significant deficiency in any arm of the immune system, and in no instance have any of these laboratory findings been linked to the clinical manifestations of the disorder. Since these tests have no diagnostic or prognostic significance, they are of value only in the context of a research study and should not be ordered as part of the routine evaluation for idiopathic chronic fatigue.

MANAGEMENT

General Principles

Chronic fatigue syndrome is defined as an idiopathic disorder (see Table 118–2). Therefore, specific medical or psychiatric therapy is rational only when an alternate or coexisting diagnosis is present. Antimicrobial therapy is not indicated unless there is clear evidence of a specific, active infection producing disease manifestations. In fact, failed trials of antimicrobial therapy have been cited as evidence that conventional infectious agents are not a perpetuating factor in chronic fatigue syndrome.

Conservative therapy for idiopathic fatigue syndromes is appropriately nonspecific and should be focused on remediation of symptoms and physical rehabilitation instead of specific, presumed causes.[52] Unfortunatley, there is no general consensus about which nonspecific therapies are most appropriate, and controlled studies have given inconsistent results. Since chronic fatigue syndrome is a heterogeneous disorder, the outcomes of treatment studies are heavily influenced by the method of selecting patients. Also, noncontrolled treatment observations are of minimal value in these disorders, because most controlled trials have demonstrated a robust placebo effect.

The treatment of individual patients is empirical. Therefore, it is useful to objectify the symptoms as much as possible so that the response to any intervention can be assessed independently. Medications should be evaluated in an additive or sequential manner so that there can be no confusion about their efficacy or adverse effects. With the large range of symptoms that these patients present, physicians are faced with a variety of treatments from which to choose, and patients may inquire about unconventional or alternative therapies. In the absence of evidence for efficacy, empirical treatment choices should be guided by a concern for safety and cost.

Pharmacologic Therapy

Medications may be useful for the treatment of symptoms: nonnarcotic pain relievers for myalgia, arthralgia, or headache; nonaddictive sleep aids for sleep disruption; psychoactive agents for depression or anxiety. Various vitamins and "nutrisupplements" have no proven benefit and may be quite costly.[53, 54] Costly "immune-enhancing" therapies, such as intravenous immune globulin, immunostimulants, and cytokines, have failed to provide benefit in controlled studies.[55–58]

Carefully controlled treatment trials do not show a consistent benefit from any single pharmacologic agent. It has been useful to extrapolate from more conclusive studies of fibromyalgia patients, since this idiopathic condition has significant overlap with chronic fatigue syndrome. Although the diagnosis of fibromyalgia is based on subjective pain and musculoskeletal tenderness, symptoms of profound fatigue, sleep disruption, and cognitive or emotional difficulties are common accompaniments. In addition, fibromyalgia and chronic fatigue syndrome share certain biologic features (e.g., autonomic and neuroendocrine findings). Tricyclic antidepressants and other drugs with serotonergic activity have benefit in fibromyalgia, and common experience suggests that chronic fatigue patients with pain and sleep disorder may respond in a similar fashion.[59, 60] One large placebo-controlled trial of fluoxetine therapy failed to show benefit; however, this study was criticized because the treatment subjects had already experienced disabling symptoms for many years.[61] Antidepressants are safe and relatively inexpensive, and a large body of evidence suggests that they may have favorable effects on symptoms of depression, pain, and insomnia in other groups of patients.

Researchers at the Johns Hopkins University reported that chronic fatigue patients had abnormal responses to a 45-minute tilt-table test protocol.[62] Virtually all the patients had syncope or reproduction of fatigue symptoms, whereas only about one third of healthy controls had an abnormal response. These investigators proposed that the persistent fatigue may be attributable to neurally mediated hypotension and therefore treatable as such. They used combinations of fludrocortisone, atenolol, and sertraline with increased salt intake and reported a favorable durable response in 39% of their patients. Until these treatments are tested in a placebo-controlled trial, this therapeutic approach remains experimental.

The finding of depressed HPA-axis activity as a feature of chronic fatigue states motivated a study at the National Institutes of Health in which patients received either replacement hydrocortisone or placebo for a 3-month course. This study, and a subsequent trial, suggest that there was minor improvement in the hydrocortisone group during treatment.[63, 63a] However, there was also profound and sustained suppression of the HPA axis that prompted investigators to recommend against the use of steroids for treatment.[63]

Nonpharmacologic Therapy

All patients should be counseled regarding exercise and sleep hygiene. Exercise has traditionally been advocated in the treatment of fibromyalgia. A recent study of chronic fatigue patients confirmed the widely held view that light aerobic exercise is beneficial.[64] In contrast, there is no evidence to support the prescription of bed rest. Moreover, continuous inactivity may both reinforce illness behavior and lead to complicating myofascial pain sydromes. Since physical activity brings on symptoms in many patients, exercise must be introduced gradually.

Many patients have significant disruptions in their sleep patterns that should be gradually corrected. Daytime napping should be limited or avoided altogether, since this behavior may further disrupt nighttime sleep.

Although occasional patients report relief of symptoms with dietary alterations, there is no reliable experimental evidence to inform changes in diet. Highly restrictive diets that may impair general nutrition should be discouraged.

Discussions about the "reality" of chronic fatigue syndrome are decidedly uphelpful, and often insulting, to patients. Similarly, framing the illness in a manner that is inconsistent with the patient's perceptions (e.g., as "depression" in the absence of formal psychiatric criteria) is likely to evoke resistance and noncompliance. The best approach is the one that is most consistent with our current understanding of chronic fatigue syndrome: to recognize and to validate the patient's symptoms as part of an idiopathic syndrome. In doing so, it is essential to educate the patients about the unexplained nature of their fatiguing illness and to correct any misinformation that they may have about its cause or treatment. This approach allows the physician to enlist the patient's support in pursuing the rational management agenda previously described. Along similar lines, several studies have demonstrated the value of formal cognitive-behavioral therapy.[65–67] This approach involves a restructuring of the patient's beliefs concerning the causes of the illness and an objective assessment of the symptoms and disabilities. Classical insight-oriented psychotherapy is rarely indicated but may be helpful in patients who experience significant, ongoing emotional stress at home or work.

SUMMARY

Prolonged idiopathic fatigue states may arise spontaneously or during the convalescence from an infectious disease. When associated with other symptoms, the diagnostic criteria for chronic fatigue syndrome may be met, although the distinction between syndromal and nonsyndromal chronic fatigue may be artificial. There are no laboratory tests that confirm or exclude the diagnosis of chronic fatigue syndrome. Various infections have been proposed as occult causes of the syndrome, but none have been implicated in any significant proportion of the patients who meet the clinical definition. In contrast, most experimental evidence points to a reversible derangement of certain central nervous system functions, and treatment modalities such as exercise, cognitive-behavioral therapy, and medications that act in the central nervous system seem to provide the most benefit.

REFERENCES

1. Straus SE. History of chronic fatigue syndrome. Rev Infect Dis. 1991;13(Suppl 1):S2–S7.
2. Wessely S. The history of chronic fatigue syndrome. In: Straus SE, ed. Chronic Fatigue Syndrome. New York: Marcel Dekker; 1994:3–44.
3. Spink WW. What is chronic brucellosis? Ann Intern Med. 1951;35:358–374.
4. Imboden JB, Canter A, Cluff LE, Trever RN. Brucellosis. III. Psychological aspects of delayed convalescence. Arch Intern Med. 1959;103:406–414.
5. Imboden JB, Canter A, Cluff LE. Convalescence from influenza. A study of the psychological and clinical determinants. Arch Intern Med. 1961;108:393–399.
6. Straus SE, Tosato G, Armstrong G, et al. Persisting illness and fatigue in adults with evidence of Epstein-Barr virus infection. Ann Intern Med. 1985;102:7–16.
7. Jones JF, Ray CG, Minnich LL, et al. Evidence for active Epstein-Barr virus infection in patients with persistent, unexplained illnesses: Elevated anti–early antigen antibodies. Ann Intern Med. 1985;102:1–7.
8. Holmes GP, Kaplan JE, Stewart JA, et al. A cluster of patients with a chronic mononucleosis–like syndrome. JAMA. 1987;257:2297–2302.

9. Issacs R. Chronic infectious mononucleosis. Blood. 1948;3:858–861.
10. Thompson DS, Godleski J, Herman S. Prognosis of post infectious mononucleosis. J Am Coll Health Assoc. 1969;17:453–457.
11. White PD, Grover SA, Kangro HO, et al. The validity and reliability of the fatigue syndrome that follows glandular fever. Psychol Med. 1995;25:917–924.
12. Straus SE, Dale JK, Tobi M, et al. Acyclovir treatment of the chronic fatigue syndrome. N Engl J Med. 1988;319:1692–1698.
13. Sumaya C. Serologic and virologic epidemiology of Epstein-Barr virus. Relevance to chronic fatigue syndrome. Rev Infect Dis. 1991;13 (Suppl 1):S19–S25.
14. Mawle AC, Nisenbaum R, Dobbins JG, et al. Seroepidemiology of chronic fatigue syndrome: A case-control study. Clin Infect Dis. 1995;21:1386–1389.
15. Swanink CM, van der Meer JW, Vercoulen JH, et al. Epstein-Barr virus (EBV) and the chronic fatigue syndrome: Normal virus load in blood and normal immunologic reactivity in the EBV regression assay. Clin Infect Dis. 1995;20:1390–1392.
16. Buchwald D, Ashley RL, Pearlman T, et al. Viral serologies in patients with chronic fatigue and chronic fatigue syndrome. J Med Virol. 1996;50:25–30.
17. Fukuda K, Straus SE, Hickie I, et al. The chronic fatigue syndrome: A comprehensive approach to its definition and study. International Chronic Fatigue Syndrome Study Group. Ann Intern Med 1994;121:953–959.
18. Bates DW, Schmitt W, Buchwald D, et al. Prevalence of fatigue and chronic fatigue syndrome in a primary care practice. Arch Intern Med. 1993;153:2759–2765.
19. Gunn WJ, Connell DB, Randall B. Epidemiology of chronic fatigue syndrome: The Centers for Disease Control Study. Ciba Found Symp. 1993;173:83–93.
20. Lloyd AR, Hickie I, Boughton CR, et al. Prevalence of chronic fatigue syndrome in an Australian population. Med J Austr. 1990;153:522–528.
21. Price RK, North CS, Wessely S, Fraser VJ. Estimating the prevalence of chronic fatigue syndrome and associated symptoms in the community. Public Health Rep. 1992;107:514–522.
22. Steele L, Dobbins JG, Fukuda K, et al. The epidemiology of chronic fatigue in San Francisco. Am J Med. 1998;105(3A):83S–90S.
23. Briggs NC, Levine PH. A comparative review of systemic and neurological symptomatology in 12 outbreaks collectively described as chronic fatigue syndrome, epidemic neuromyasthenia, and myalgic encephalomyelitis. Clin Infect Dis. 1994;18 (Suppl 1):S32–S42.
24. Stevans G. The 1934 epidemic of poliomyelitis in Southern California. Am J Public Health. 1934;12:1213–1214.
25. Crowley N, Nelson M, Stovin S. Epidemiological aspects of an outbreak of encephalomyelitis at the Royal Free Hospital. J Hyg. 1957;55:102–122.
26. Levine PH, Snow PG, Ranum BA, et al. Epidemic neuromyasthenia and chronic fatigue syndrome in west Otago, New Zealand. A 10-year follow-up. Arch Intern Med. 1997;157:750–754.
27. Hickie I, Lloyd A, Hadzi-Pavlovic D, et al. Can the chronic fatigue syndrome be defined by distinct clinical features? Psychol Med. 1995;25:925–935.
28. Kroenke K, Wood DR, Mangelsdorff AD, et al. Chronic fatigue in primary care: Prevalence, patient characteristics and outcome. JAMA. 1988;260:929–934.
29. Pawlikowska T, Chalder T, Hirsch SR, et al. Population based study of fatigue and psychological distress. BMJ. 1994;308:763–766.
30. Manu P, Matthews DA, Lane TJ. The mental health of patients with a chief complaint of chronic fatigue: A prospective evaluation and follow-up. Arch Intern Med. 1988;148:2213–2217.
31. Gaudino EA, Coyle PK, Krupp LB. Post-Lyme syndrome and chronic fatigue syndrome. Neuropsychiatric similarities and differences. Arch Neurol. 1997;54:1372–1376.
32. Jacobson SK, Daly JS, Thorne GM, McIntosh K. Chronic parvovirus B19 infection resulting in chronic fatigue syndrome: Case history and review. Clin Infect Dis. 1997;24:1048–1051.
33. Ayres JG, Smith EG, Flint N. Protracted fatigue and debility after acute Q fever (Letter) Lancet. 1996;347:978–979.
34. Buchwald D, Cheney PR, Peterson DL, et al. A chronic illness characterized by fatigue, neurologic and immunologic disorders, and active human herpesvirus type 6 infection (see Comments). Ann Intern Med. 1992;116:103–113.
35. Schwartz RB, Komaroff AL, Garada BM, et al. SPECT imaging of the brain. Comparison of findings in patients with chronic fatigue syndrome, AIDS dementia complex, and major unipolar depression. Am J Roentgenol. 1994;162:943–951.
36. Costa DC, Tannock C, Brostoff J. Brainstem perfusion is impaired in chronic fatigue syndrome. Q J Med. 1995;88:767–773.
37. Fischler B, D'Haenen H, Cluydts R, et al. Comparison of 99m Tc HMPAO SPECT scan between chronic fatigue syndrome, major depression and healthy controls: An exploratory study of clinical correlates of regional cerebral blood flow. Neuropsychobiology. 1996;34:175–183.
38. Cleary KJ, White PD. Gilbert's and chronic fatigue syndromes in men. Lancet. 1993;341:842.
39. Valesini G, Conti F, Priori R, Balsano F. Gilbert's syndrome and chronic syndrome. Lancet. 1993;341:1162–1163.
40. Wessely S, Chalder T, Hirsch S, et al. Psychological symptoms, somatic symptoms, and psychiatric disorder in chronic fatigue and chronic fatigue syndrome: A prospective study in the primary care setting. Am J Psychiatr. 1996;153:1050–1059.
41. Buchwald D, Pascualy R, Bombardier C, Kith P. Sleep disorders in patients with chronic fatigue. Clin Infect Dis. 1994;18 (Suppl 1):S68–S72.
42. Zubieta JK, Engleberg NC, Yargic LI, et al. Seasonal symptom variation in patients with chronic fatigue: Comparison with major mood disorders. Psychiatr Res. 1994;28:13–22.
43. Bates DW, Buchwald D, Lee J, et al. Clinical laboratory test findings in patients with chronic fatigue syndrome. Arch Intern Med. 1995;155:97–103.
44. Konstantinov K, von Mikecz A, Buchwald D, et al. Autoantibodies to nuclear envelope antigens in chronic fatigue syndrome. J Clin Invest. 1996;98:1888–1896.
45. Von Mikecz A, Konstantinov K, Buchwald DS, et al. High frequency of autoantibodies to insoluble cellular antigens in patients with chronic fatigue syndrome. Arthritis Rheum. 1997;40:295–305.
46. Demitrack MA. Neuroendocrine correlates of chronic fatigue syndrome: A brief review. J Psychiatr Res. 1997;31:69–82.
47. Scott LV, Dinan TG. Urinary free cortisol excretion in chronic fatigue syndrome, major depression and in healthy volunteers. J Affect Disord. 1998;47:49–54.
48. Crofford LJ, Engleberg NC, Demitrack MA. Neurohormonal perturbations in fibromyalgia. In: Chikanza IC, ed. Balliere's Clinical Rheumatology, 10. Philadelphia: Balliere Tindall; 1996:365–378.
49. Straus SE, Fritz S, Dale JK, et al. Lymphocyte phenotype and function in the chronic fatigue syndrome. J Clin Immunol. 1993;13:30–40.
50. Caliguri M, Murray C, Buchwald D, et al. Phenotypic and functional deficency of natural killer cells in patients with chronic fatigue syndrome. J Immunol. 1987;139:3303–3313.
51. Levine PH, Atherton M, Fears T, Hoover R. An approach to studies of cancer subsequent to clusters of chronic fatigue syndrome: Use of data from the Nevada State Cancer Registry. Clin Infect Dis. 1994;18(Suppl 1):S49–S53.
52. Engleberg NC. Medically-oriented therapy for chronic fatigue syndrome and related conditions. In: Demitrack MA, Abbey SE, eds. Chronic Fatigue Syndrome: An Integrative Approach to Evaluation and Treatment. New York: Guilford; 1996:287–309.
53. Kaslow JE, Rucker L, Onishi R. Liver extract–folic acid–cyanocobalamin vs placebo for chronic fatigue syndrome. Arch Intern Med. 1989;149:2501–2503.
54. McCluskey DR. Pharmacological approaches to the therapy of chronic fatigue syndrome. Ciba Found Symp. 1993;173:280–297.
55. Lloyd A, Hickie I, Wakefield D, et al. A double-blind, placebo-controlled trial of intravenous immunoglobulin therapy in patients with chronic fatigue syndrome. Am J Med. 1990;561–568.
56. Peterson PK, Shepard J, Macres M, et al. A controlled trial of intravenous immunoglobulin G in chronic fatigue syndrome. Am J Med. 1990;89:554–560.
57. Straus SE. Intravenous immunoglobulin treatment for the chronic fatigue syndrome. Am J Med. 1990;89:551–553.
58. Lloyd AR, Hickie I, Brockman A, et al. Immunologic and psychologic therapy for patients with chronic fatigue syndrome: A double-blind, placebo controlled trial. Am J Med. 1993;94:197–203.
59. Goldenberg DL. A review of the role of tricyclic medications in the treatment of fibromyalgia syndrome. J Rheumatol. 1989;16(Suppl 19):S137–S139.
60. Gracious B, Wisner KL. Nortriptyline in chronic fatigue syndrome: A double-blind, placebo-controlled single case study. Biol Psychiatry. 1991;30:405–408.
61. Vercoulen JH, Swanink CM, Zitman FG, et al. Randomised, double-blind, placebo-controlled study of fluoxetine in chronic fatigue syndrome. Lancet. 1996;347:858–861.
62. Bou-Holaigah I, Rowe PC, Kan J, Calkins H. The relationship between neurally mediated hypotension and the chronic fatigue syndrome. JAMA. 1995;274:961–967.
63. McKenzie R, O'Fallon A, Dale J, et al. Low-dose hydrocortisone treatment of chronic fatigue syndrome: Results of a placebo controlled study of its efficacy and safety. JAMA. 1998;280:1061–1066.
63a. Cleare AJ, Heap E, Malhi GS, et al. Low-dose hydrocortisone in chronic fatigue syndrome: A randomised crossover trial. Lancet. 1999;353:455–458.
64. Fulcher KY, White PD. Randomised controlled trial of graded exercise in patients with the chronic fatigue syndrome. BMJ. 1997;314:1647–1652.
65. Sharpe M, Hawton K, Simkin S, et al. Cognitive behaviour therapy for the chronic fatigue syndrome: A randomized controlled trial BMJ 1996;312:22–26.
66. Deale A, Chalder T, Marks I, Wessely S. Cognitive behavior therapy for chronic fatigue syndrome: A randomized controlled trial. Am J Psychiatry. 1997;154:408–414.
67. Sharpe MC. Cognitive-behavioral therapy for patients with chronic syndrome: How? In: Demitrack MA, Abbey SE, eds. Chronic Fatigue Syndrome: An Integrative Approach to Evaluation and Treatment. New York: Guilford; 1996:240–262.
68. Natelson BH, Ye N, Moul DE, et al. High titers of anti-Epstein-Barr virus DNA polymerase are found in patients with severe fatiguing illness. J Med Virol. 1994;42:42–46.
69. Lerner MA, Zervos M, Dworkin HJ, et al. A unified theory of the cause of chronic fatigue syndrome. Infect Dis Clin Pract. 1997;6:239–243.
70. Lerner AM, Zervos M, Dworkin HJ, et al. New cardiomyopathy: Pilot study of intravenous ganciclovir in a subset of the chronic fatigue syndrome. Infect Dis Clin Pract. 1997;6:110–117.
71. Patnaik M, Komaroff AL, Conley E, et al. Prevalence of IgM antibodies to human herpesvirus 6 early antigen (p41/38) in patients with chronic fatigue syndrome. J Infect Dis. 1995;172:1364–1367.
72. Di Luca D, Zorzenon M, Mirandola P, et al. Human herpesvirus 6 and human herpesvirus 7 in chronic syndrome. J Clin Microbiol. 1995;33:1660–1661.
73. Yousef GE, Bell EJ, Mann GF, et al. Chronic enterovirus infection in patients with postviral fatigue syndrome. Lancet. 1988;1:146–150.
74. Cunningham L, Bowles NE, Lane RJ, et al. Persistence of enteroviral RNA in chronic fatigue syndrome is associated with the abnormal production of equal amounts of positive and negative strands of enteroviral RNA. J Gen Virol. 1990;71:1399–1402.
75. Gow JW, Behan WM, Clements GB, et al. Enteroviral RNA sequences detected by polymerase chain reaction in muscle of patients with postviral fatigue syndrome. BMJ. 1991;302:692–696.

76. McArdle A, McArdle F, Jackson MJ, et al. Investigation by polymerase chain reaction of enterovioral infection in patients with chronic fatigue syndrome. Clin Sci (Colch). 1996;90:295–300.
77. Gow JW, Behan WM, Simpson K, et al. Studies on enterovirus in patients with chronic fatigue syndrome. Clin Infect Dis. 1994;18(Suppl 1):S126–S129.
78. Lindh G, Samuelson A, Hedlund KO, et al. No findings of enteroviruses in Swedish patients with chronic fatigue syndrome. Scand J Infect Dis. 1996;28:305–307.
79. Nairn C, Galbraith DN, Clements GB. Comparison of coxsackie B neutralisation and enteroviral PCR in chronic fatigue patients. J Med Virol. 1995;46:310–313.
80. Berg AM, Naides SJ, Simms RW. Established fibromyalgia syndrome and parvovirus B19 infection. J Rheumatol. 1993;20:1941–1943.
81. Iaria RL Jr, Komaroff AL, Fagioli LR, et al. Absence of parvovirus B19 infection in chronic fatigue syndrome. Arthritis Rheum. 1995;38:638–641.
82. Martin WJ. Chronic fatigue syndrome (Letter). Science. 1992;255:663.
83. DeFreitas E, Hilliard B, Cheney PR, et al. Retroviral sequences related to human T-lymphotropic virus II in patients with chronic fatigue immune dysfunction syndrome. Proc Natl Acad Sci U S A. 1991;88:2922–2926.
84. Heneine W, Woods TC, Sinha SD, et al. Lack of evidence for infection with known human and animal retroviruses in patients with chronic fatigue syndrome. Clin Infect Dis. 1994;18(Suppl 1):S121–S125.
85. Khan AS, Heneine WM, Chapman LE, et al. Assessment of a retrovirus sequence and other possible risk factors for the chronic fatigue syndrome in adults. Ann Intern Med. 1993;118:241–245.
86. Kitani T, Kuratsune H, Fuke I, et al. Possible correlation between Borna disease virus infection and Japanese patients with chronic fatigue syndrome. Microbiol Immunol. 1996;40:459–462.
87. Bode L, Komaroff AL, Ludwig H. No serologic evidence of Borna disease virus in patients with chronic fatigue syndrome. Clin Infect Dis. 1992;15:1049.
88. Asch ES, Bujak DI, Weiss M, et al. Lyme disease: An infectious and postinfectious syndrome. J Rheumatol. 1994;21:454–461.
89. Dinerman H, Steere AC. Lyme disease associated with fibromyalgia. Ann Intern Med. 1992;117:281 –285.
90. Lightfoot RWJ, Luft BJ, Rahn DW, et al. Empiric parenteral antibiotic treatment of patients with fibromyalgia and fatigue and a positive serologic result for Lyme disease. A cost-effectiveness analysis. Ann Intern Med. 1993;119:503–509.
91. Evans AC. Chronic brucellosis. JAMA. 1934;103:665–667.
92. Crook WG. The Yeast Connection: A Medical Breakthrough. 3rd ed. Jackson, Tenn: Professional Books; 1983.
93. Truss CO. The role of *Candida albicans* in human illness. Orthomol Psychiatry. 1981;10:228–238.
94. Dismukes WE, Wade JS, Lee JY, et al. A randomized, double-blind trial of nystatin therapy for the candidiasis hypersensitivity syndrome. N Engl J Med. 1990;323:1717–1723.

Index

Note: Page numbers in *italics* refer to illustrations; page numbers followed by t refer to tables.

B

C

D

E

F

G

H

I

J

K

L

M

N

O

P

Q

R

S

W

X

Y

ISBN 0-443-07983-8